MEDICINES COMPENDIUM 2006

Published by

DataPharm Communications

Datapharm Communications Ltd
Stocks House
9 North Street
Leatherhead
Surrey
KT22 7AX

Tel: +44 (0)1372 388381
Fax: +44 (0)1372 388384
Email: datapharm@medicines.org.uk

DISCLAIMER

The Summaries of Product Characteristics (SPCs) and Data Sheets contained within this Compendium are prepared independently by each participating pharmaceutical company. The information is only applicable to the United Kingdom. Neither Datapharm Communications Ltd (DCL) nor the Association of the British Pharmaceutical Industry (ABPI) gives any guarantee whatsoever as to the recency or accuracy of the information contained within this publication, including that found in the SPCs or Data Sheets. A doctor or other appropriately qualified healthcare professional should always be consulted before taking or administering any of the products referred to within this book. To the maximum extent permitted by law neither DCL nor the ABPI accept any liability whatsoever in respect of any loss, damage or expense of whatever kind arising from any information contained in this publication or for any error or omission in the Data Sheets or SPCs.

Typeset by AJS Solutions, Huddersfield, West Yorkshire.
Printed in Great Britain by William Clowes Ltd, Beccles, Suffolk.

ISSN 1475-326X
ISBN 0 907102 24 7

ACKNOWLEDGEMENTS

With special thanks to:

- Those members of the pharmaceutical industry who regularly contribute information to the *e*MC (*electronic* Medicines Compendium, http://www.emc.medicines.org.uk)
- The Association of the British Pharmaceutical Industry (ABPI) for their continued support and enthusiasm.
- The Compendium team:

Nicky Helyer	–	Operations Director
Alan Henderson	–	Senior Developer
Millie Martin	–	Information and Quality Control Executive
Joan Terry	–	Customer Support
Julie Woods	–	Projects Co-ordinator

ARE YOU UP TO DATE?

There are over 20,000 changes to medicines information in the UK each year. The electronic Medicines Compendium (eMC) at **http://www.emc.medicines.org.uk** provides daily real time updates directly from the manufacturers. No registration is required and the information is provided free of charge. PILs are also available on the eMC.

CONTENTS

INTRODUCTION

This is the eighth edition of the Compendium in which Summaries of Product Characteristics (SPCs) appear. New requirements came into effect in 1995 replacing Data Sheets with SPCs for new products and those products coming up for licence renewal. Over the last ten years, the majority of Data Sheets have been replaced with SPCs.

This edition is the fifth to be produced directly from the *electronic* Medicines Compendium (*e*MC) which may be found at www.emc.medicines.org.uk.

Where the information comes from

SPCs and Data Sheets are prepared by the individual companies concerned and follow either the requirements laid down by the European Commission's guideline on Summary of Product Characteristics (for SPCs) or the 'The Medicines (Data Sheet) Regulations 1972', as amended (for Data Sheets).

The SPCs and Data Sheets included in this Compendium were the most up-to-date approved versions available as of 30th September 2005 and were sourced from the *e*MC which is updated daily. Due to the constantly evolving nature of the information contained within this book (there are an estimated 20,000 changes a year to UK regulatory medicines information) readers are advised to refer to the *e*MC for the most up-to-date approved versions. Patient Information Leaflets (PILs), where available, can also be found on the *e*MC. Access to the *e*MC is provided free of charge.

SPCs and Data Sheets are intended for members of the medical and pharmacy professions and are written with them in mind. Any member of the public who reads them should bear in mind the need to take professional advice before making any decision affecting his or her own medication based upon their contents.

Revised SPCs/Data Sheets

Individual participating companies may issue loose-leaf SPCs or Data Sheets which supersede those included in the Medicines Compendium. It is advisable to retain any such revised SPCs/Data Sheets which are received and to indicate that fact on the corresponding documents within the Compendium.

Legal category

The following abbreviations may be found under the heading 'Legal Category' in certain documents contained within the Compendium.

GSL A preparation which is included in the General Sale List and can be sold from any retail outlet.

P A Pharmacy sale medicine which can be sold only from a retail pharmacy. A Pharmacist must oversee the dispensing of this medicine although it can be purchased without a prescription.

POM A Prescription-Only Medicine.

CD Controlled Drug: a preparation controlled by the Misuse of Drugs Act 1971 and Regulations. The CD is followed by (Sch 1), (Sch 2), (Sch 3), (Sch 4) or (Sch 5) depending on the schedule to the Misuse of Drugs Regulations 2001, as amended, in which the preparation is included.

Doctors are reminded that certain particulars must be in their own handwriting on prescriptions for certain preparations.

Reporting of adverse reactions

When a new medicine is first licensed there is only limited information on its safety profile from clinical trials data. Further understanding about any medicine is dependent on the availability of information on the safety of the medicine as used in normal clinical practice.

The black triangle symbol (▼) is used to identify newly licensed medicines that are being kept under intensive monitoring by the Medicines and Healthcare products Regulatory Agency (MHRA)/Committee on Safety of Medicines (CSM). This includes medicines that have been licensed for administration via a novel route or drug delivery system, or for a significant new indication which may alter the established risk/benefit profile of that drug. There is no standard time for a product to retain black triangle status. However, an assessment is usually made following two years of post-marketing experience, when all available safety data is reviewed.

In order to recognise possible new hazards rapidly, spontaneous reporting is particularly important. For medicines showing the black triangle symbol the MHRA/CSM asks that all suspected reactions, including those considered to be non serious, are reported via the Yellow Card Scheme. Reporting should be irrespective of uncertainty about the causal relationship, whether the reaction is well recognised or if other drugs have been given concurrently.

A link to the list of the drugs/products currently under intensive surveillance can be found within the CSM area of the MHRA website (http://www.mhra.gov.uk).

Yellow cards can be found at the end of the book. Yellow cards are also available by writing to:

MHRA (medicines)
CSM FREEPOST
London
SW8 5BR

or by e-mailing the Medicines and Healthcare products Regulatory Agency at: info@mhra.gsi.gov.uk or by calling the National Yellow Card Information Service on 0800 731 6789.

Abelcet

(Zeneus Pharma Ltd)

1. NAME OF THE MEDICINAL PRODUCT

Abelcet is the trade name for Amphotericin B Lipid Complex.

2. QUALITATIVE AND QUANTITATIVE COMPOSITION

Abelcet is supplied as a sterile, pyrogen-free suspension in isotonic saline. Each ml of the suspension contains 5.0 mg (5 000 IU) of amphotericin B

3. PHARMACEUTICAL FORM

Abelcet is supplied as a suspension containing 5.0 mg amphotericin B per ml, in vials containing either 10 ml (50 mg, 50,000 IU), or 20 ml (100 mg, 100 000 IU of amphotericin B) which must be diluted before intravenous infusion, according to Section 4.2 (Posology and method of administration).

4. CLINICAL PARTICULARS

4.1 Therapeutic indications

Abelcet is indicated for the treatment of severe invasive candidiasis.

Abelcet is also indicated as second line therapy for the treatment of severe systemic fungal infections in patients who have not responded to conventional amphotericin B or other systemic antifungal agents, in those who have renal impairment or other contra-indications to conventional amphotericin B, or in patients who have developed amphotericin B nephrotoxicity. Abelcet treatment is indicated as second line treatment for invasive aspergillosis, cryptococcal meningitis and disseminated cryptococcosis in HIV patients, fusariosis, coccidiomycosis, zygomycosis and blastomycosis.

4.2 Posology and method of administration

Abelcet is a sterile, pyrogen-free suspension to be diluted for intravenous infusion only.

For severe systemic infections treatment is generally recommended at 5.0 mg/kg for at least 14 days. Abelcet should be administered by intravenous infusion at a rate of 2.5 mg/kg/hr. When commencing treatment with Abelcet for the first time it is recommended to administer a test dose immediately prior to the first infusion. The first infusion should be prepared according to the instructions then, over a period of approximately 15 minutes, 1mg of the infusion should be administered to the patient. After this amount has been administered the infusion should be stopped and the patient observed carefully for 30 minutes. If the patient shows no signs of hypersensitivity the infusion may be continued. As for use with all amphotericin B products, facilities for cardiopulmonary resuscitation should be readily at hand when administering Abelcet for the first time, due to the possible occurrence of anaphylactoid reactions. Abelcet has been administered for as long as 28 months, and cumulative doses have been as high as 73.6g without significant toxicity.

An in-line filter may be used for intravenous infusion of Abelcet. The mean pore diameter of the filter should be no less than 15 microns.

Abelcet may be administered to diabetic patients.

Paediatric use

Systemic fungal infections in children have been treated successfully with Abelcet at doses comparable to the recommended adult dose on a bodyweight basis. Adverse events seen in paediatric patients are similar to those seen in adults.

Use in elderly patients

Systemic fungal infections in elderly patients have been treated successfully with Abelcet at doses comparable to the recommended dose on a bodyweight basis.

Use in neutropenic patients

Abelcet has been used successfully to treat systemic fungal infections in patients who are severely neutropenic as a consequence of haematological malignancy or the use of cytotoxic or immunosuppressive drugs.

Use in patients with renal or liver disease

Systemic fungal infections in patients with renal or liver disease have been treated successfully with Abelcet at doses comparable to the recommended dose on a body weight basis (see special warnings and precautions for further information).

4.3 Contraindications

Abelcet is contraindicated in patients with known hypersensitivity to any of its constituents, unless in the opinion of the physician the advantages of using Abelcet outweigh the risks of hypersensitivity.

4.4 Special warnings and special precautions for use

Systemic Fungal Infections

Abelcet should not be used for treating common or superficial, clinically inapparent fungal infections that are detectable only by positive skin or serologic tests.

Renal Disease

Since Abelcet is a potentially nephrotoxic drug, monitoring of renal function should be performed before initiating treatment in patients with pre-existing renal disease, and at least once weekly during therapy. Abelcet can be administered to patients during renal dialysis or haemofiltration.Serum potassium and magnesium levels should be monitored regularly.

Liver Disease

Patients with concurrent hepatic impairment due to infection, graft-versus-host disease, other liver disease or administration of hepatotoxic drugs have been successfully treated with Abelcet. In cases where serum bilirubin, alkaline phosphatase or serum transaminases increased, factors other than Abelcet were present and possibly accounted for the abnormalities. These factors included infection, hyperalimentation, concomitant hepatotoxic drugs and graft-versus-host disease.

4.5 Interaction with other medicinal products and other forms of Interaction

Nephrotoxic Drugs

Abelcet is a potentially nephrotoxic drug, and particularly close monitoring of renal function is required in patients receiving nephrotoxic drugs concomitantly.

Zidovudine

In dogs, exacerbated myelotoxicity and nephrotoxicity were observed when Abelcet was administered concomitantly with zidovudine. If concomitant treatment with zidovudine is required, renal and haematologic function should be closely monitored.

Cyclosporin

Preliminary data suggest that patients receiving Abelcet concomitantly with high dose cyclosporin experience an increase in serum creatinine. The data also suggest that the increase in serum creatinine is caused by cyclosporin and not Abelcet.

The interaction of Abelcet with other drugs has not been studied to date. Conventional amphotericin B has been reported to interact with antineoplastic agents, corticosteroids and corticotrophin (ACTH), digitalis glycosides and skeletal muscle relaxants.

Leukocyte transfusions

Acute pulmonary toxicity has been reported in patients receiving intravenous amphotericin B and leukocyte transfusions.

4.6 Pregnancy and lactation

Conventional amphotericin B has been used successfully to treat systemic fungal infections in pregnant women with no obvious effects on the foetus, but only a small number of cases have been reported. Reproductive toxicity studies of Abelcet in rats and rabbits showed no evidence of embryotoxicity, foetotoxicity or teratogenicity. However, safety for use in pregnant or lactating women has not been established for Abelcet. Therefore, Abelcet should be administered to pregnant or lactating women only for life-threatening disease when the likely benefit exceeds the risk to the mother and foetus.

4.7 Effects on ability to drive and use machines

Abelcet is unlikely to affect the ability of an individual to drive or use machines, since adverse reactions are usually infusion-related. However, the clinical condition of patients who require Abelcet generally precludes driving or operating machinery.

4.8 Undesirable effects

Adverse reactions that have been reported to occur with conventional amphotericin B may occur with Abelcet. In general, the physician should monitor the patient for any type of adverse event associated with conventional amphotericin B.

Patients in whom significant renal toxicity was observed following conventional amphotericin B frequently did not experience similar effects when Abelcet was substituted. Adverse reactions related to the administration of Abelcet have generally been mild or moderate, and have been most prevalent during the first 2 days of dosing.

Premedication (e.g. paracetamol) may be administered for the prevention of infusion related adverse events. The most common clinical adverse events have been chills, fever, nausea and vomiting, which may occur during the first 2 days of treatment.

Declines in renal function, shown by increased serum creatinine, azotaemia and hypokalaemia, have not typically required discontinuation of treatment.

Abnormal liver function tests have been reported with Abelcet and other amphotericin B products. Although other factors such as infection, hyperalimentation, concomitant hepatotoxic drugs and graft-versus-host disease may be contributory, a causal relationship with Abelcet cannot be excluded. Patients with abnormal liver function tests should be carefully monitored and cessation of treatment considered if liver function deteriorates.

Rarely, encephalopathy and peripheral neuropathy have been reported.

Allergic reactions including anaphylaxis, bronchospasm, dyspnoea and hypotension have also been reported with Abelcet.

4.9 Overdose

No instance of toxicity due to overdose with Abelcet has been reported.One paediatric patient received a single dose of 13.1mg/kg on one occasion, without adverse effects. Should an overdose occur, the patient should be treated as deemed appropriate by the physician.

5. PHARMACOLOGICAL PROPERTIES

Abelcet consists of the antifungal agent, amphotericin B, complexed to two phospholipids. Amphotericin B is a macrocyclic, polyene, broad-spectrum antifungal antibiotic produced by *Streptomyces nodosus*.The lipophilic moiety of amphotericin B allows molecules of the drug to be complexed in a ribbon-like structure with the phospholipids.

5.1 Pharmacodynamic properties

Mechanism of action

Amphotericin B, the active antifungal agent in Abelcet, may be fungistatic or fungicidal, depending on its concentration and on fungal susceptibility. The drug probably acts by binding to ergosterol in the fungal cell membrane causing subsequent membrane damage. As a result, cell contents leak from the fungal cell, and, ultimately, cell death occurs. Binding of the drug to sterols in human cell membranes may result in toxicity, although amphotericin B has greater affinity for fungal ergosterol than for the cholesterol of human cells.

Microbiological activity

Amphotericin B is active against many fungal pathogens *in vitro,* including *Candida* spp., *Cryptococcus neoformans, Aspergillus* spp., *Mucor* spp., *Sporothrix schenckii, Blastomyces dermatitidis, Coccidioides immitis* and *Histoplasma capsulatum.* Most strains are inhibited by amphotericin B concentrations of 0.03-1.0 μg/ml. Amphotericin B has little or no activity against bacteria or viruses. The activity of Abelcet against fungal pathogens *in vitro* is comparable to that of amphotericin B. However, activity of Abelcet *in vitro* may not predict activity in the infected host.

5.2 Pharmacokinetic properties

Amphotericin B is complexed to phospholipids in Abelcet. The pharmacokinetic properties of Abelcet and conventional amphotericin B are different. Pharmacokinetic studies in animals showed that, after administration of Abelcet, amphotericin B levels were highest in the liver, spleen and lung. Amphotericin B in Abelcet was rapidly distributed to tissues. The ratio of drug concentrations in tissues to those in blood increased disproportionately with increasing dose, suggesting that elimination of the drug from the tissues was delayed. Peak blood levels of amphotericin B were lower after administration of Abelcet than after administration of equivalent amounts of conventional drug. Administration of conventional amphotericin B resulted in much lower tissue levels than did dosing with Abelcet. However, in dogs, conventional amphotericin B produced 20-fold higher kidney concentrations than did Abelcet given at comparable doses.

The pharmacokinetics of Abelcet in whole blood were determined in patients with mucocutaneous leishmaniasis. Results for mean pharmacokinetic parameters at 5.0 mg/kg/day were as follows:

	Abelcet
Dose: (mg/kg/day)	5.0
Peak blood level C_{max}: (μg/ml)	1.7
Area under time-concentration curve AUC_{0-24}: (μg.hr/ml)	9.5
Clearance: (ml/hr.kg)	211.0
Volume of distribution Vd: (l/kg)	2286.0
Half-life $T_{½}$: (hr)	173.4

The rapid clearance and large volume of distribution of Abelcet result in a relatively low AUC and are consistent with preclinical data showing high tissue concentrations. The kinetics of Abelcet are linear, the AUC increases proportionately with dose.

Details of the tissue distribution and metabolism of Abelcet in humans, and the mechanisms responsible for reduced toxicity, are not well understood. The following data are available from necropsy in a heart transplant patient who received Abelcet at a dose of 5.3 mg/kg for 3 consecutive days immediately before death:

Organ	Abelcet tissue concentration expressed as amphotericin B content (mg/kg)
Spleen	290.0
Lung	222.0
Liver	196.0

Kidney	6.9
Lymph node	7.6
Heart	5.0
Brain	1.6

5.3 Preclinical safety data

Acute toxicity studies in rodents showed that Abelcet was 10-fold to 20-fold less toxic than conventional amphotericin B. Multiple-dose toxicity studies in dogs lasting 2-4 weeks showed that on a mg/kg basis, Abelcet was 8-fold to 10-fold less nephrotoxic than conventional amphotericin B. This decreased nephrotoxicity was presumably a result of lower drug concentrations in the kidney.

5.4 Carcinogenesis, Mutagenesis and Impairment of Fertility

Since conventional amphotericin B first became available, there have been no reports of drug-related carcinogenicity, mutagenicity, teratogenicity or adverse effect on fertility. Abelcet has been shown not to be mutagenic by the *in vivo* mouse micronucleus assay, *in vitro* bacterial and lymphoma mutation assays, and an *in vivo* cytogenetic assay. It has been shown not to be teratogenic in mice and rabbits.

Phospholipids are essential constituents of human cell membranes. The average diet provides several grams of phospholipids each day. There is no evidence that phospholipids, including DMPC and DMPG, are carcinogenic, mutagenic or teratogenic.

6. PHARMACEUTICAL PARTICULARS

6.1 List of excipients

Each ml of Abelcet contains 3.4 mg L-α-dimyristoylphosphatidylcholine (DMPC), 1.5 mg L-α-dimyristoylphosphatidylglycerol (sodium and ammonium salts) (DMPG), 9.0 mg sodium chloride, and Water for Injection, q.s. ad 1.0 ml.

6.2 Incompatibilities

Abelcet should not be mixed with other drugs or electrolytes.

6.3 Shelf life

Results of stability studies substantiate a shelf-life of 24 months at 5°C.

6.4 Special precautions for storage

Abelcet should be stored under refrigeration at +2 to +8°C. Do not freeze. Protect from light.

6.5 Nature and contents of container

Abelcet is a sterile, pyrogen-free yellow suspension in a single use vial containing 10 or 20 ml (50 mg or 100 mg amphotericin B). The vial is sealed with a rubber stopper and aluminum seal. Vials are packaged in cartons of 10 vials.

6.6 Instructions for use and handling

Abelcet is a sterile, pyrogen-free suspension to be diluted for intravenous infusion only.

Preparation of the suspension for infusion

ASEPTIC TECHNIQUE MUST BE STRICTLY OBSERVED THROUGHOUT HANDLING OF Abelcet, SINCE NO BACTERIOSTATIC AGENT OR PRESERVATIVE IS PRESENT.

Allow the suspension to come to room temperature. Shake gently until there is no evidence of any yellow settlement at the bottom of the vial. Withdraw the appropriate dose of Abelcet from the required number of vials into one or more sterile 20 ml syringes using a 17 to 19 gauge needle. Remove the needle from each syringe filled with Abelcet and replace with the 5 micron high flow filter needle (supplied by B. Braun Medical, Inc.) provided with each vial. Insert the filter needle of the syringe into an IV bag containing 5.0% Dextrose for Injection and empty the contents of the syringe into the bag using either manual pressure or an infusion pump. The final infusion concentration should be 1 mg/ml. For paediatric patients and patients with cardiovascular disease the drug may be diluted with 5.0% Dextrose for Injection to a final infusion concentration of 2 mg/ml. Do not use the agent after dilution with 5.0% Dextrose for Injection if there is any evidence of foreign matter. Vials are single use. Unused material should be discarded. The infusion is best administered by means of an infusion pump.

DO NOT DILUTE WITH SALINE SOLUTIONS OR MIX WITH OTHER DRUGS OR ELECTROLYTES. The compatibility of Abelcet with these materials has not been established. An existing intravenous line should be flushed with 5.0% Dextrose for Injection before infusion of Abelcet or a separate infusion line should be used.

The diluted ready for use suspension may be stored under refrigeration (+2 to +8°C) for up to 24 hours prior to use. Shake vigorously before use. Do not store for later use.

7. MARKETING AUTHORISATION HOLDER

Zeneus Pharma Limited
The Magdalen Centre
Oxford Science Park
Oxford
OX4 4GA
UK

8. MARKETING AUTHORISATION NUMBER(S)

PL: 21799/0001

9. DATE OF FIRST AUTHORISATION/RENEWAL OF THE AUTHORISATION

1 October 2001

10. DATE OF REVISION OF THE TEXT

September 2005

11. LEGAL CATEGORY

POM

Abilify (Otsuka Pharmaceuticals (UK) Ltd)

(Otsuka Pharmaceuticals (UK) Ltd)

1. NAME OF THE MEDICINAL PRODUCT

ABILIFY ▼ 5 mg tablets
ABILIFY ▼ 10 mg tablets
ABILIFY ▼ 15 mg tablets
ABILIFY ▼ 30 mg tablets

2. QUALITATIVE AND QUANTITATIVE COMPOSITION

Each ABILIFY 5 mg tablet contains 5 mg of aripiprazole.

Each ABILIFY 10 mg tablet contains 10 mg of aripiprazole.

Each ABILIFY 15 mg tablet contains 15 mg of aripiprazole.

Each ABILIFY 30 mg tablet contains 30 mg of aripiprazole.

For excipients, see section 6.1.

3. PHARMACEUTICAL FORM

Tablet

ABILIFY 5 mg tablets are rectangular and blue, engraved with A-007 and 5 on one side.

ABILIFY 10 mg tablets are rectangular and pink, engraved with A-008 and 10 on one side.

ABILIFY 15 mg tablets are round and yellow, engraved with A-009 and 15 on one side.

ABILIFY 30 mg tablets are round and pink, engraved with A-011 and 30 on one side.

4. CLINICAL PARTICULARS

4.1 Therapeutic indications

ABILIFY is indicated for the treatment of schizophrenia.

4.2 Posology and method of administration

Oral use.

The recommended starting and maintenance dose for ABILIFY is 15 mg/day administered on a once-a-day schedule without regard to meals.

ABILIFY is effective in a dose range of 15 to 30 mg/day. Enhanced efficacy at doses higher than the recommended daily dose of 15 mg has not been demonstrated although individual patients may benefit from a higher dose. The maximum daily dose should not exceed 30 mg.

Children and adolescents: ABILIFY has not been studied in subjects under 18 years of age.

Patients with hepatic impairment: no dosage adjustment is required for patients with mild to moderate hepatic impairment. In patients with severe hepatic impairment, the data available are insufficient to establish recommendations. In these patients dosing should be managed cautiously. However, the maximum daily dose of 30 mg should be used with caution in patients with severe hepatic impairment (see section 5.2).

Patients with renal impairment: no dosage adjustment is required in patients with renal impairment.

Elderly: the effectiveness of ABILIFY in the treatment of schizophrenia in patients 65 years of age or older has not been established. Owing to the greater sensitivity of this population, a lower starting dose should be considered when clinical factors warrant (see section 4.4).

Gender: no dosage adjustment is required for female patients as compared to male patients (see section 5.2).

Smoking status: according to the metabolic pathway of ABILIFY no dosage adjustment is required for smokers (see section 4.5).

When concomitant administration of potent CYP3A4 or CYP2D6 inhibitors with aripiprazole occurs, the aripiprazole dose should be reduced. When the CYP3A4 or CYP2D6 inhibitor is withdrawn from the combination therapy, aripiprazole dose should then be increased (see section 4.5).

When concomitant administration of potent CYP3A4 inducers with aripiprazole occurs, the aripiprazole dose should be increased. When the CYP3A4 inducer is withdrawn from the combination therapy, the aripiprazole dose should then be reduced to the recommended dose (see section 4.5).

4.3 Contraindications

ABILIFY is contraindicated in patients with hypersensitivity to aripiprazole or to any of the excipients.

4.4 Special warnings and special precautions for use

During antipsychotic treatment, improvement in the patient's clinical condition may take several days to some weeks. Patients should be closely monitored throughout this period.

Tardive Dyskinesia: in premarketing studies of one year or less duration, there were uncommon reports of treatment emergent dyskinesia during treatment with aripiprazole. If signs and symptoms of tardive dyskinesia appear in a patient on ABILIFY, dose reduction or discontinuation should be considered. These symptoms can temporarily deteriorate or can even arise after discontinuation of treatment.

Neuroleptic Malignant Syndrome (NMS): NMS is a potentially fatal symptom complex associated with antipsychotic medicinal products. In premarketing studies, rare cases of NMS were reported during treatment with aripiprazole. Clinical manifestations of NMS are hyperpyrexia, muscle rigidity, altered mental status and evidence of autonomic instability (irregular pulse or blood pressure, tachycardia, diaphoresis and cardiac dysrhythmia). Additional signs may include elevated creatine phosphokinase, myoglobinuria (rhabdomyolysis), and acute renal failure. If a patient develops signs and symptoms indicative of NMS, or presents with unexplained high fever without additional clinical manifestations of NMS, all antipsychotic drugs, including ABILIFY, must be discontinued.

Seizure: in premarketing studies, uncommon cases of seizure were reported during treatment with aripiprazole. Therefore, aripiprazole should be used with caution in patients who have a history of seizure disorder or have conditions associated with seizures.

Cerebrovascular Adverse Events, including stroke, in elderly patients with dementia-related psychosis: in three placebo-controlled trials of aripiprazole in elderly patients with psychosis associated with Alzheimer's disease, cerebrovascular adverse events (e.g. stroke, transient ischaemic attack), including fatalities, were reported in patients (mean age: 84 years; range: 78-88 years). Overall, 1.3% of aripiprazole-treated patients reported cerebrovascular adverse events compared with 0.69% of placebo-treated patients in these trials. This difference was not statistically significant. However, in one of these trials, a fixed-dose trial, there was a significant dose response relationship for cerebrovascular adverse events in patients treated with aripiprazole. Abilify is not approved for the treatment of dementia-related psychosis.

Hyperglycaemia and Diabetes Mellitus: Hyperglycaemia, in some cases extreme and associated with ketoacidosis or hyperosmolar coma or death, has been reported in patients treated with atypical antipsychotic agents. In clinical trials with aripiprazole, there were no significant differences in the incidence rates of hyperglycaemia-related adverse events (including diabetes) or in abnormal glycaemia laboratory values compared to placebo. Precise risk estimates for hyperglycaemia-related adverse events in patients treated with Abilify and with other atypical antipsychotic agents are not available to allow direct comparisons. Patients treated with any antipsychotic agents, including Abilify, should be observed for signs and symptoms of hyperglycaemia (such as polydipsia, polyuria, polyphagia and weakness) and patients with diabetes mellitus or with risk factors for diabetes mellitus should be monitored regularly for worsening of glucose control.

4.5 Interaction with other medicinal products and other forms of Interaction

Due to its α1-adrenergic receptor antagonism, aripiprazole has the potential to enhance the effect of certain antihypertensive agents.

Given the primary CNS effects of aripiprazole, caution should be used when aripiprazole is taken in combination with alcohol or other CNS drugs with overlapping side effects such as sedation (see section 4.8).

Potential for other medicinal products to affect ABILIFY:

A gastric acid blocker, the H2 antagonist famotidine, reduces aripiprazole rate of absorption but this effect is deemed not clinically relevant.

Aripiprazole is metabolised by multiple pathways involving the CYP2D6 and CYP3A4 enzymes but not CYP1A enzymes. Thus, no dosage adjustment is required for smokers.

In a clinical study in healthy subjects, a potent inhibitor of CYP2D6 (quinidine) increased aripiprazole AUC by 107%, while Cmax was unchanged. The AUC and Cmax of dehydro-aripiprazole, the active metabolite, decreased by 32% and 47%. ABILIFY dose should be reduced to approximately one-half of its prescribed dose when concomitant administration of ABILIFY with quinidine occurs. Other potent inhibitors of CYP2D6, such as fluoxetine and paroxetine, may be expected to have similar effects and similar dose reductions should therefore be applied.

In a clinical study in healthy subjects, a potent inhibitor of CYP3A4 (ketoconazole) increased aripiprazole AUC and Cmax by 63% and 37%, respectively. The AUC and Cmax of dehydro-aripiprazole increased by 77% and 43%, respectively. In CYP2D6 poor metabolisers, concomitant use of potent inhibitors of CYP3A4 may result in higher plasma concentrations of aripiprazole compared to that in CYP2D6 extensive metabolisers. When considering concomitant administration of ketoconazole or other potent CYP3A4 inhibitors with ABILIFY, potential benefits should outweigh the potential risks to the patient. When concomitant administration of ketoconazole with ABILIFY occurs, ABILIFY dose should be reduced to approximately one-half of its prescribed dose. Other potent inhibitors of CYP3A4, such as itraconazole and HIV protease inhibitors, may be expected to have similar effects and similar dose reductions should therefore be applied.

Upon discontinuation of the CYP2D6 or 3A4 inhibitor, the dosage of ABILIFY should be increased to the level prior to the initiation of the concomitant therapy.

Following concomitant administration of carbamazepine, a potent inducer of CYP3A4, the geometric means of Cmax and AUC for aripiprazole were 68% and 73% lower, respectively, compared to when aripiprazole (30 mg) was administered alone. Similarly, for dehydro-aripiprazole the geometric means of Cmax and AUC after carbamazepine co-administration were 69% and 71% lower, respectively, than those following treatment with aripiprazole alone.

ABILIFY dose should be doubled when concomitant administration of ABILIFY occurs with carbamazepine. Other potent inducers of CYP3A4 (such as rifampicin, rifabutin, phenytoin, phenobarbital, primidone, efavirenz, nevirapine and St. John's Wort) may be expected to have similar effects and similar dose increases should therefore be applied. Upon discontinuation of potent CYP3A4 inducers, the dosage of ABILIFY should be reduced to the recommended dose.

When either valproate or lithium were administered concomitantly with aripiprazole, there was no clinically significant change in aripiprazole concentrations.

Potential for ABILIFY to affect other medicinal products:

In clinical studies, 10-30 mg/day doses of aripiprazole had no significant effect on the metabolism of substrates of CYP2D6 (dextromethorphan/3-methoxymorphinan ratio), 2C9 (warfarin), 2C19 (omeprazole), and 3A4 (dextromethorphan). Additionally, aripiprazole and dehydroaripiprazole did not show potential for altering CYP1A2-mediated metabolism *in vitro*. Thus, aripiprazole is unlikely to cause clinically important drug interactions mediated by these enzymes.

4.6 Pregnancy and lactation

Pregnancy:

There are no adequate and well-controlled studies of aripiprazole in pregnant women. Animal studies could not exclude potential developmental toxicity (see section 5.3). Patients should be advised to notify their physician if they become pregnant or intend to become pregnant during treatment with aripiprazole. Due to insufficient safety information in humans and concerns raised by animal reproductive studies, this medicinal product should not be used in pregnancy unless the expected benefit clearly justifies the potential risk to the foetus.

Lactation:

Aripiprazole was excreted in the milk of treated rats during lactation. It is not known whether aripiprazole is excreted in human milk. Patients should be advised not to breast feed if they are taking aripiprazole.

4.7 Effects on ability to drive and use machines

As with other antipsychotics, patients should be cautioned about operating hazardous machines, including motor vehicles, until they are reasonably certain that aripiprazole does not affect them adversely.

4.8 Undesirable effects

The following undesirable effects occurred more often (≥ *1/100*) than placebo, or were identified as possibly medically relevant adverse drug reactions (*):

Nervous system disorders
Common (> 1/100m < 1/10): lightheadedness, insomnia, akathisia, somnolence, tremor
Eye disorders
Common (> 1/100, < 1/10): blurred vision
Cardiac disorders
Uncommon (> 1/1,000, < 1/100): tachycardia*
Vascular disorders
Uncommon (> 1/1,000, < 1/100): orthostatic hypotension*
Gastrointestinal disorders
Common (> 1/100, < 1/10): nausea, vomiting, dyspepsia, constipation
General disorders and administration site conditions
Common (> 1/100, < 1/10): headache, asthenia

Extrapyramidal symptoms (EPS): in a long term 52-week controlled study, aripiprazole-treated patients had an overall-lower incidence (27.1%) of EPS including parkinsonism, akathisia, dystonia and dyskinesia compared with those treated with haloperidol (59.2%). In a long term 26-week placebo-controlled study, the incidence of EPS was 20.3% for aripiprazole-treated patients and 13.1% for placebo-treated patients. In another long-term 26-week controlled study, the incidence of EPS was 16.8% for aripiprazole-treated patients and 15.7% for olanzapine-treated patients.

Comparisons between aripiprazole and placebo in the proportions of patients experiencing potentially clinically significant changes in routine laboratory parameters revealed no medically important differences. Elevations of CPK (Creatine Phosphokinase), generally transient and asymptomatic, were observed in 3.9% of aripiprazole treated patients as compared to 3.6% of patients who received placebo.

Other findings:

Undesirable effects known to be associated with antipsychotic therapy and also reported during treatment with aripiprazole include neuroleptic malignant syndrome, tardive dyskinesia, seizure, cerebrovascular adverse events in elderly demented patients, hyper-glycaemia and diabetes mellitus (see section 4.4).

Post-Marketing

The following adverse events have also been reported very rarely during post-marketing surveillance (the calculation for the frequency is based on an estimate of patient exposure):

Immune system disorders:	allergic reaction (e.g. anaphylactic reaction, angioedema, pruritis or urticaria)
Psychiatric disorders:	nervousness, agitation
Nervous system disorders:	speech disorder
Vascular disorders:	syncope
Gastrointestinal disorders:	increased salivation, pancreatitis
Musculoskeletal, connective tissue and bone disorders:	stiffness, myalgia, rhabdomyolysis
General disorders and administration site conditions:	chest pain
Investigations	increased Creatine Phosphokinase, increased Alanine Amino-transferase (ALT), increased Aspartate Aminotransferase (AST)

4.9 Overdose

In clinical studies, accidental or intentional acute overdosage of aripiprazole was identified in patients with estimated doses up to 1080 mg with no fatalities. The reported signs and symptoms observed with aripiprazole overdose included nausea, vomiting, asthenia, diarrhoea and somnolence.

During post-marketing experience, the reported signs and symptoms observed in adult patients who overdosed with aripiprazole alone at doses up to 450 mg included tachycardia and vomiting. In addition, reports of accidental overdose with aripiprazole (up to 195 mg) in children have been received. The potentially medically serious signs and symptoms reported included extrapyramidal symptoms and transient loss of consciousness.

Management of overdose should concentrate on supportive therapy, maintaining an adequate airway, oxygenation and ventilation, and management of symptoms. The possibility of multiple drug involvement should be considered. Therefore cardiovascular monitoring should be started immediately and should include continuous electrocardiographic monitoring to detect possible arrhythmias. Following any confirmed or suspected overdose with aripiprazole, close medical supervision and monitoring should continue until the patient recovers.

Activated charcoal (50 g), administered one hour after aripiprazole, decreased aripiprazole Cmax by about 41% and AUC by about 51%, suggesting that charcoal may be effective in the treatment of overdose.

Although there is no information on the effect of haemodialysis in treating an overdose with aripiprazole, haemodialysis is unlikely to be useful in overdose management since aripiprazole is highly bound to plasma proteins.

5. PHARMACOLOGICAL PROPERTIES

5.1 Pharmacodynamic properties

Pharmacotherapeutic group: antipsychotics, ATC code; N05 AX12

It has been proposed that aripiprazole's efficacy in schizophrenia is mediated through a combination of partial agonism at dopamine D2 and serotonin 5HT1a receptors and antagonism of serotonin 5HT2a receptors. Aripiprazole exhibited antagonist properties in animal models of dopaminergic hyperactivity and agonist properties in animal models of dopaminergic hypoactivity. Aripiprazole exhibited high binding affinity *in vitro* for dopamine D2 and D3, serotonin 5HT1a and 5HT2a receptors and moderate affinity for dopamine D4, serotonin 5HT2c and 5HT7, alpha-1 adrenergic and histamine H1 receptors. Aripiprazole also exhibited moderate binding affinity for the serotonin reuptake site and no appreciable affinity for muscarinic receptors. Interaction with receptors other than dopamine and serotonin subtypes may explain some of the other clinical effects of aripiprazole.

Aripiprazole doses ranging from 0.5 to 30 mg administered once a day to healthy subjects for 2 weeks produced a dose-dependent reduction in the binding of ^{11}C-raclopride, a D2/D3 receptor ligand, to the caudate and putamen detected by positron emission tomography.

Further information on clinical trials:

Schizophrenia: in three short-term (4 to 6 week) placebo-controlled trials involving 1,228 schizophrenic patients, presenting with positive or negative symptoms, aripiprazole was associated with statistically significantly greater improvements in psychotic symptoms compared to placebo.

ABILIFY is effective in maintaining the clinical improvement during continuation therapy in patients who have shown an initial treatment response. In a haloperidol-controlled trial, the proportion of responder patients maintaining response to medication at 52-weeks was similar in both groups (aripiprazole 77% and haloperidol 73%). The overall completion rate was significantly higher for patients on aripiprazole (43%) than for haloperidol (30%). Actual scores in rating scales used as secondary endpoints, including PANSS and the Montgomery-Asberg Depression Rating Scale showed a significant improvement over halperidol.

In a 26-week, placebo-controlled trial in stabilised patients with chronic schizophrenia, aripiprazole had significantly greater reduction in relapse rate, 34% in aripiprazole group and 57% in placebo.

Weight gain: in clinical trials aripiprazole has not been shown to induce clinically relevant weight gain. In a 26-week, olanzapine-controlled, double-blind, multi-national study of schizophrenia which included 314 patients and where the primary end-point was weight gain, significantly fewer patients had at least 7% weight gain over baseline (i.e. a gain of at least 5.6 kg for a mean baseline weight of ~80.5 kg) on aripiprazole (N=18, or 13% of evaluable patients), compared to olanzapine (N=45, or 33% of evaluable patients).

5.2 Pharmacokinetic properties

Absorption:

Aripiprazole is well absorbed, with peak plasma concentrations occurring within 3-5 hours after dosing. Aripiprazole undergoes minimal pre-systemic metabolism. The absolute oral bioavailability of the tablet formulation is 87%. There is no effect of a high fat meal on the pharmacokinetics of aripiprazole.

Distribution:

Aripiprazole is widely distributed throughout the body with an apparent volume of distribution of 4.9 l/kg, indicating extensive extravascular distribution. At therapeutic concentrations, aripiprazole and dehydroaripiprazole are greater than 99% bound to serum proteins, binding primarily to albumin.

Metabolism:

Aripiprazole is extensively metabolised by the liver primarily by three biotransformation pathways: dehydrogenation, hydroxylation and N-dealkylation. Based on *in vitro* studies, CYP3A4 and CYP2D6 enzymes are responsible for dehydrogenation and hydroxylation of aripiprazole, and N-dealkylation is catalysed by CYP3A4. Aripiprazole is the predominant medicinal product moiety in systemic circulation. At steady state, dehydroaripiprazole, the active metabolite, represents about 40% of aripiprazole AUC in plasma.

Elimination:

The mean elimination half-lives for aripiprazole are approximately 75 hours in extensive metabolisers of CYP2D6 and approximately 146 hours in poor metabolisers of CYP2D6.

The total body clearance of aripiprazole is 0.7 ml/min/kg, which is primarily hepatic.

Following a single oral dose of $[^{14}C]$-labelled aripiprazole, approximately 27% of the administered radioactivity was recovered in the urine and approximately 60% in the faeces. Less than 1% of unchanged aripiprazole was excreted in the urine and approximately 18% was recovered unchanged in the faeces.

Pharmacokinetics in special patient groups

Elderly:

There are no differences in the pharmacokinetics of aripiprazole between healthy elderly and younger adult subjects, nor is there any detectable effect of age in a population pharmacokinetic analysis in schizophrenic patients.

Gender:

There are no differences in the pharmacokinetics of aripiprazole between healthy male and female subjects nor is there any detectable effect of gender in a population pharmacokinetic analysis in schizophrenic patients.

Smoking and Race:

Population pharmacokinetic evaluation has revealed no evidence of clinically significant race-related differences or effects from smoking upon the pharmacokinetics of aripiprazole.

Renal Disease:

The pharmacokinetic characteristics of aripiprazole and dehydroaripiprazole were found to be similar in patients with severe renal disease compared to young healthy subjects.

Hepatic Disease:

A single-dose study in subjects with varying degrees of liver cirrhosis (Child-Pugh Classes A, B and C) did not reveal a significant effect of hepatic impairment on the pharmacokinetics of aripiprazole and dehydroaripiprazole, but the study included only 3 patients with Class C liver cirrhosis, which is insufficient to draw conclusions on their metabolic capacity.

5.3 Preclinical safety data

Preclinical safety data revealed no special hazard for humans based on conventional studies of safety pharmacology, repeat-dose toxicity, genotoxicity, carcinogenicity and reproductive toxicity.

Toxicologically significant effects were observed only at doses or exposures that were sufficiently in excess of the maximum human dose or exposure, indicating that these effects were limited or of no relevance to clinical use. These included: dose-dependent adrenocortical toxicity (lipofuscin pigment accumulation and/or parenchymal cell loss) in rats after 104 weeks at 20 to 60 mg/kg/day (3 to 14 times the mean steady-state AUC at the maximum recommended human dose) and increased adrenocortical carcinomas and combined adrenocortical adenomas/carcinomas in female rats at 60 mg/kg/day (14 times the mean steady-state AUC at the maximum recommended human dose).

An additional finding was cholelithiasis as a consequence of precipitation of sulphate conjugates of hydroxy metabolites of aripiprazole in the bile of monkeys after repeated oral dosing at 25 to 125 mg/kg/day (1 to 3 times the mean steady-state AUC at the maximum recommended clinical dose or 16 to 81 times the maximum recommended human dose based on mg/m^2). However, the concentrations of the sulphate conjugates of hydroxyaripiprazole in human bile at the highest dose proposed, 30 mg per day, were no more than 6% of the bile concentrations found in the monkeys in the 39-week study and are well below (6%) their limits of *in vitro* solubility.

Based on results of a full range of standard genotoxicity tests, aripiprazole was considered non-genotoxic. Aripiprazole did not impair fertility in reproductive toxicity studies. Developmental toxicity, including dose-dependent delayed foetal ossification and possible teratogenic effects, were observed in rats at doses resulting in subtherapeutic exposures (based on AUC) and in rabbits at doses resulting in exposures 3 and 11 times the mean steady-state AUC at the maximum recommended clinical dose. Maternal toxicity occurred at doses similar to those eliciting developmental toxicity.

6. PHARMACEUTICAL PARTICULARS

6.1 List of excipients

Lactose monohydrate

Maize starch

Microcrystalline cellulose

Hydroxypropyl cellulose

Magnesium stearate

Red iron oxide E172 (10 mg and 30 mg tablets)

Yellow iron oxide E172 (15 mg tablets)

Indigo carmine E132 aluminium lake (5 mg tablets)

6.2 Incompatibilities

Not applicable.

6.3 Shelf life

3 years

6.4 Special precautions for storage

Store in the original package in order to protect from moisture.

6.5 Nature and contents of container

ABILIFY tablets are available in aluminium perforated unit dose blisters in cartons of 28 × 1 tablets.

6.6 Instructions for use and handling

No special requirements.

7. MARKETING AUTHORISATION HOLDER

Otsuka Pharmaceutical Europe Ltd.

Commonwealth House, 2 Chalkhill Road

Hammersmith - London W6 8DW - United Kingdom

8. MARKETING AUTHORISATION NUMBER(S)

EU/1/04/276/002 Abilify 5mg tablets, 28s

EU/1/04/276/007 Abilify 10mg tablets, 28s

EU/1/04/276/012 Abilify 15mg tablets, 28s

EU/1/04/276/017 Abilify 15mg tablets, 28s

9. DATE OF FIRST AUTHORISATION/RENEWAL OF THE AUTHORISATION

June 2004

10. DATE OF REVISION OF THE TEXT

March 2005

Abilify Tablets 5 mg, 10 mg, 15 mg and 30 mg Tablets (Bristol-Myers Squibb Pharmaceuticals Ltd)

(Bristol-Myers Squibb Pharmaceuticals Ltd)

1. NAME OF THE MEDICINAL PRODUCT

ABILIFY ▼ 5 mg tablets

ABILIFY ▼ 10 mg tablets

ABILIFY ▼ 15 mg tablets

ABILIFY ▼ 30 mg tablets

2. QUALITATIVE AND QUANTITATIVE COMPOSITION

Each ABILIFY 5 mg tablet contains 5 mg of aripiprazole.

Each ABILIFY 10 mg tablet contains 10 mg of aripiprazole.

Each ABILIFY 15 mg tablet contains 15 mg of aripiprazole.

Each ABILIFY 30 mg tablet contains 30 mg of aripiprazole.

For excipients, see section 6.1.

3. PHARMACEUTICAL FORM

Tablet

ABILIFY 5 mg tablets are rectangular and blue, engraved with A-007 and 5 on one side.

ABILIFY 10 mg tablets are rectangular and pink, engraved with A-008 and 10 on one side.

ABILIFY 15 mg tablets are round and yellow, engraved with A-009 and 15 on one side.

ABILIFY 30 mg tablets are round and pink, engraved with A-011 and 30 on one side.

4. CLINICAL PARTICULARS

4.1 Therapeutic indications

ABILIFY is indicated for the treatment of schizophrenia.

4.2 Posology and method of administration

Oral use.

The recommended starting and maintenance dose for ABILIFY is 15 mg/day administered on a once-a-day schedule without regard to meals.

ABILIFY is effective in a dose range of 15 to 30 mg/day. Enhanced efficacy at doses higher than the recommended daily dose of 15 mg has not been demonstrated although individual patients may benefit from a higher dose. The maximum daily dose should not exceed 30 mg.

Children and adolescents: ABILIFY has not been studied in subjects under 18 years of age.

Patients with hepatic impairment: no dosage adjustment is required for patients with mild to moderate hepatic impairment. In patients with severe hepatic impairment, the data available are insufficient to establish recommendations. In these patients dosing should be managed cautiously. However, the maximum daily dose of 30 mg should be used with caution in patients with severe hepatic impairment (see section 5.2).

Patients with renal impairment: no dosage adjustment is required in patients with renal impairment.

Elderly: the effectiveness of ABILIFY in the treatment of schizophrenia in patients 65 years of age or older has not been established. Owing to the greater sensitivity of this population, a lower starting dose should be considered when clinical factors warrant (see section 4.4).

Gender: no dosage adjustment is required for female patients as compared to male patients (see section 5.2).

Smoking status: according to the metabolic pathway of ABILIFY no dosage adjustment is required for smokers (see section 4.5).

When concomitant administration of potent CYP3A4 or CYP2D6 inhibitors with aripiprazole occurs, the aripiprazole dose should be reduced. When the CYP3A4 or CYP2D6 inhibitor is withdrawn from the combination therapy, aripiprazole dose should then be increased (see section 4.5).

When concomitant administration of potent CYP3A4 inducers with aripiprazole occurs, the aripiprazole dose should be increased. When the CYP3A4 inducer is withdrawn from the combination therapy, the aripiprazole dose should then be reduced to the recommended dose (see section 4.5).

4.3 Contraindications

ABILIFY is contraindicated in patients with hypersensitivity to aripiprazole or to any of the excipients.

4.4 Special warnings and special precautions for use

During antipsychotic treatment, improvement in the patient's clinical condition may take several days to some weeks. Patients should be closely monitored throughout this period.

Tardive Dyskinesia: in premarketing studies of one year or less duration, there were uncommon reports of treatment emergent dyskinesia during treatment with aripiprazole. If signs and symptoms of tardive dyskinesia appear in a patient on ABILIFY, dose reduction or discontinuation should be considered. These symptoms can temporarily deteriorate or can even arise after discontinuation of treatment.

Neuroleptic Malignant Syndrome (NMS): NMS is a potentially fatal symptom complex associated with antipsychotic medicinal products. In premarketing studies, rare cases of NMS were reported during treatment with aripiprazole. Clinical manifestations of NMS are hyperpyrexia, muscle rigidity, altered mental status and evidence of autonomic instability (irregular pulse or blood pressure, tachycardia, diaphoresis and cardiac dysrhythmia). Additional signs may include elevated creatine phosphokinase, myoglobinuria (rhabdomyolysis), and acute renal failure. If a patient develops signs and symptoms indicative of NMS, or presents with unexplained high fever without additional clinical manifestations of NMS, all antipsychotic drugs, including ABILIFY, must be discontinued.

Seizure: in premarketing studies, uncommon cases of seizure were reported during treatment with aripiprazole. Therefore, aripiprazole should be used with caution in patients who have a history of seizure disorder or have conditions associated with seizures.

Cerebrovascular Adverse Events, including stroke, in elderly patients with dementia-related psychosis: in three placebo-controlled trials of aripiprazole in elderly patients with psychosis associated with Alzheimer's disease, cerebrovascular adverse events (e.g. stroke, transient ischaemic attack), including fatalities, were reported in patients (mean age: 84 years; range: 78-88 years). Overall, 1.3% of aripiprazole-treated patients reported cerebrovascular adverse events compared with 0.69% of placebo-treated patients in these trials. This difference was not statistically significant. However, in one of these trials, a fixed-dose trial, there was a significant dose response relationship for cerebrovascular adverse events in patients treated with aripiprazole. Abilify is not approved for the treatment of dementia-related psychosis.

Hyperglycaemia and Diabetes Mellitus: Hyperglycaemia, in some cases extreme and associated with ketoacidosis or hyperosmolar coma or death, has been reported in patients treated with atypical antipsychotic agents. In clinical trials with aripiprazole, there were no significant differences in the incidence rates of hyperglycaemia-related adverse events (including diabetes) or in abnormal glycaemia laboratory values compared to placebo. Precise risk estimates for hyperglycaemia-related adverse events in patients treated with Abilify and with other atypical antipsychotic agents are not available to allow direct comparisons. Patients treated with any antipsychotic agents, including Abilify, should be observed for signs and symptoms of hyperglycaemia (such as polydipsia, polyuria, polyphagia and weakness) and patients with diabetes mellitus or with risk factors for diabetes mellitus should be monitored regularly for worsening of glucose control.

4.5 Interaction with other medicinal products and other forms of Interaction

Due to its α1-adrenergic receptor antagonism, aripiprazole has the potential to enhance the effect of certain antihypertensive agents.

Given the primary CNS effects of aripiprazole, caution should be used when aripiprazole is taken in combination with alcohol or other CNS drugs with overlapping side effects such as sedation (see section 4.8).

Potential for other medicinal products to affect ABILIFY:

A gastric acid blocker, the H2 antagonist famotidine, reduces aripiprazole rate of absorption but this effect is deemed not clinically relevant.

Aripiprazole is metabolised by multiple pathways involving the CYP2D6 and CYP3A4 enzymes but not CYP1A enzymes. Thus, no dosage adjustment is required for smokers.

In a clinical study in healthy subjects, a potent inhibitor of CYP2D6 (quinidine) increased aripiprazole AUC by 107%, while Cmax was unchanged. The AUC and Cmax of dehydro-aripiprazole, the active metabolite, decreased by 32% and 47%. ABILIFY dose should be reduced to approximately one-half of its prescribed dose when concomitant administration of ABILIFY with quinidine occurs. Other potent inhibitors of CYP2D6, such as fluoxetine and paroxetine, may be expected to have similar effects and similar dose reductions should therefore be applied.

In a clinical study in healthy subjects, a potent inhibitor of CYP3A4 (ketoconazole) increased aripiprazole AUC and Cmax by 63% and 37%, respectively. The AUC and Cmax of dehydro-aripiprazole increased by 77% and 43%, respectively. In CYP2D6 poor metabolisers, concomitant use of potent inhibitors of CYP3A4 may result in higher plasma concentrations of aripiprazole compared to that in CYP2D6 extensive metabolisers. When considering concomitant administration of ketoconazole or other potent CYP3A4 inhibitors with ABILIFY, potential benefits should outweigh the potential risks to the patient. When concomitant administration of ketoconazole with ABILIFY occurs, ABILIFY dose should be reduced to approximately one-half of its prescribed dose. Other potent inhibitors of CYP3A4, such as itraconazole and HIV protease inhibitors, may be expected to have similar effects and similar dose reductions should therefore be applied.

Upon discontinuation of the CYP2D6 or 3A4 inhibitor, the dosage of ABILIFY should be increased to the level prior to the initiation of the concomitant therapy.

Following concomitant administration of carbamazepine, a potent inducer of CYP3A4, the geometric means of Cmax and AUC for aripiprazole were 68% and 73% lower, respectively, compared to when aripiprazole (30 mg) was administered alone. Similarly, for dehydro-aripiprazole the geometric means of Cmax and AUC after carbamazepine co-administration were 69% and 71% lower, respectively, than those following treatment with aripiprazole alone.

ABILIFY dose should be doubled when concomitant administration of ABILIFY occurs with carbamazepine. Other potent inducers of CYP3A4 (such as rifampicin, rifabutin, phenytoin, phenobarbital, primidone, efavirenz, nevirapine and St. John's Wort) may be expected to have similar effects and similar dose increases should therefore be applied. Upon discontinuation of potent CYP3A4 inducers, the dosage of ABILIFY should be reduced to the recommended dose.

When either valproate or lithium were administered concomitantly with aripiprazole, there was no clinically significant change in aripiprazole concentrations.

Potential for ABILIFY to affect other medicinal products:

In clinical studies, 10-30 mg/day doses of aripiprazole had no significant effect on the metabolism of substrates of CYP2D6 (dextromethorphan/3-methoxymorphinan ratio), 2C9 (warfarin), 2C19 (omeprazole), and 3A4 (dextromethorphan). Additionally, aripiprazole and dehydroaripiprazole did not show potential for altering CYP1A2-mediated metabolism *in vitro*. Thus, aripiprazole is unlikely to cause clinically important drug interactions mediated by these enzymes.

4.6 Pregnancy and lactation

Pregnancy:

There are no adequate and well-controlled studies of aripiprazole in pregnant women. Animal studies could not exclude potential developmental toxicity (see section 5.3). Patients should be advised to notify their physician if they become pregnant or intend to become pregnant during treatment with aripiprazole. Due to insufficient safety information in humans and concerns raised by animal reproductive studies, this medicinal product should not be used in pregnancy unless the expected benefit clearly justifies the potential risk to the foetus.

Lactation:

Aripiprazole was excreted in the milk of treated rats during lactation. It is not known whether aripiprazole is excreted in human milk. Patients should be advised not to breast feed if they are taking aripiprazole.

4.7 Effects on ability to drive and use machines

As with other antipsychotics, patients should be cautioned about operating hazardous machines, including motor vehicles, until they are reasonably certain that aripiprazole does not affect them adversely.

4.8 Undesirable effects

The following undesirable effects occurred more often (≥ *1/100*) than placebo, or were identified as possibly medically relevant adverse drug reactions (*):

Nervous system disorders
Common (> 1/100m < 1/10): lightheadedness, insomnia, akathisia, somnolence, tremor
Eye disorders
Common (> 1/100, < 1/10): blurred vision
Cardiac disorders
Uncommon (> 1/1,000, < 1/100): tachycardia*
Vascular disorders
Uncommon (> 1/1,000, < 1/100): orthostatic hypotension*
Gastrointestinal disorders
Common > 1/100, < 1/10): nausea, vomiting, dyspepsia, constipation
General disorders and administration site conditions
Common > 1/100, < 1/10): headache, asthenia

Extrapyramidal symptoms (EPS): in a long term 52-week controlled study, aripiprazole-treated patients had an overall-lower incidence (27.1%) of EPS including parkinsonism, akathisia, dystonia and dyskinesia compared with those treated with haloperidol (59.2%). In a long term 26-week placebo-controlled study, the incidence of EPS was 20.3% for aripiprazole-treated patients and 13.1% for placebo-treated patients. In another long-term 26-week controlled study, the incidence of EPS was 16.8% for aripiprazole-treated patients and 15.7% for olanzapine-treated patients.

Comparisons between aripiprazole and placebo in the proportions of patients experiencing potentially clinically significant changes in routine laboratory parameters revealed no medically important differences. Elevations of CPK (Creatine Phosphokinase), generally transient and asymptomatic, were observed in 3.9% of aripiprazole treated patients as compared to 3.6% of patients who received placebo.

Other findings:

Undesirable effects known to be associated with antipsychotic therapy and also reported during treatment with aripiprazole include neuroleptic malignant syndrome, tardive dyskinesia, seizure, cerebrovascular adverse events in elderly demented patients, hyper-glycaemia and diabetes mellitus (see section 4.4).

Post-Marketing

The following adverse events have also been reported very rarely during post-marketing surveillance (the calculation for the frequency is based on an estimate of patient exposure):

Immune system disorders:	allergic reaction (e.g. anaphylactic reaction, angioedema, pruritis or urticaria)
Psychiatric disorders:	nervousness, agitation
Nervous system disorders:	speech disorder
Vascular disorders:	syncope
Gastrointestinal disorders:	increased salivation, pancreatitis
Musculoskeletal, connective tissue and bone disorders:	stiffness, myalgia, rhabdomyolysis
General disorders and administration site conditions:	chest pain
Investigations	increased Creatine Phosphokinase, increased Alanine Amino-transferase (ALT), increased Aspartate Aminotransferase (AST)

4.9 Overdose

In clinical studies, accidental or intentional acute overdosage of aripiprazole was identified in patients with estimated doses up to 1080 mg with no fatalities. The reported signs and symptoms observed with aripiprazole overdose included nausea, vomiting, asthenia, diarrhoea and somnolence.

During post-marketing experience, the reported signs and symptoms observed in adult patients who overdosed with aripiprazole alone at doses up to 450 mg included tachycardia and vomiting. In addition, reports of accidental overdose with aripiprazole (up to 195 mg) in children have been received. The potentially medically serious signs and symptoms reported included extrapyramidal symptoms and transient loss of consciousness.

Management of overdose should concentrate on supportive therapy, maintaining an adequate airway, oxygenation and ventilation, and management of symptoms. The possibility of multiple drug involvement should be considered. Therefore cardiovascular monitoring should be started immediately and should include continuous electrocardiographic monitoring to detect possible arrhythmias. Following any confirmed or suspected overdose with aripiprazole, close medical supervision and monitoring should continue until the patient recovers.

Activated charcoal (50 g), administered one hour after aripiprazole, decreased aripiprazole Cmax by about 41% and AUC by about 51%, suggesting that charcoal may be effective in the treatment of overdose.

Although there is no information on the effect of haemodialysis in treating an overdose with aripiprazole, haemodialysis is unlikely to be useful in overdose management since aripiprazole is highly bound to plasma proteins.

5. PHARMACOLOGICAL PROPERTIES

5.1 Pharmacodynamic properties

Pharmacotherapeutic group: antipsychotics, ATC code; N05 AX12

It has been proposed that aripiprazole's efficacy in schizophrenia is mediated through a combination of partial agonism at dopamine D2 and serotonin 5HT1a receptors and antagonism of serotonin 5HT2a receptors. Aripiprazole exhibited antagonist properties in animal models of dopaminergic hyperactivity and agonist properties in animal models of dopaminergic hypoactivity. Aripiprazole exhibited high binding affinity *in vitro* for dopamine D2 and D3, serotonin 5HT1a and 5HT2a receptors and moderate affinity for dopamine D4, serotonin 5HT2c and 5HT7, alpha-1 adrenergic and histamine H1 receptors. Aripiprazole also exhibited moderate binding affinity for the serotonin reuptake site and no appreciable affinity for muscarinic receptors. Interaction with receptors other than dopamine and serotonin subtypes may explain some of the other clinical effects of aripiprazole.

Aripiprazole doses ranging from 0.5 to 30 mg administered once a day to healthy subjects for 2 weeks produced a dose-dependent reduction in the binding of ^{11}C-raclopride, a D2/D3 receptor ligand, to the caudate and putamen detected by positron emission tomography.

Further information on clinical trials:

Schizophrenia: in three short-term (4 to 6 week) placebo-controlled trials involving 1,228 schizophrenic patients, presenting with positive or negative symptoms, aripiprazole was associated with statistically significantly greater improvements in psychotic symptoms compared to placebo.

ABILIFY is effective in maintaining the clinical improvement during continuation therapy in patients who have shown an initial treatment response. In a haloperidol-controlled trial, the proportion of responder patients maintaining response to medication at 52-weeks was similar in both groups (aripiprazole 77% and haloperidol 73%). The overall completion rate was significantly higher for patients on aripiprazole (43%) than for haloperidol (30%). Actual scores in rating scales used as secondary endpoints, including PANSS and the Montgomery-Asberg Depression Rating Scale showed a significant improvement over halperidol.

In a 26-week, placebo-controlled trial in stabilised patients with chronic schizophrenia, aripiprazole had significantly greater reduction in relapse rate, 34% in aripiprazole group and 57% in placebo.

Weight gain: in clinical trials aripiprazole has not been shown to induce clinically relevant weight gain. In a 26-week, olanzapine-controlled, double-blind, multi-national study of schizophrenia which included 314 patients and where the primary end-point was weight gain, significantly fewer patients had at least 7% weight gain over baseline (i.e. a gain of at least 5.6 kg for a mean baseline weight of ~80.5 kg) on aripiprazole (N=18, or 13% of evaluable patients), compared to olanzapine (N=45, or 33% of evaluable patients).

5.2 Pharmacokinetic properties

Absorption:

Aripiprazole is well absorbed, with peak plasma concentrations occurring within 3-5 hours after dosing. Aripiprazole undergoes minimal pre-systemic metabolism. The absolute oral bioavailability of the tablet formulation is 87%. There is no effect of a high fat meal on the pharmacokinetics of aripiprazole.

Distribution:

Aripiprazole is widely distributed throughout the body with an apparent volume of distribution of 4.9 l/kg, indicating extensive extravascular distribution. At therapeutic concentrations, aripiprazole and dehydroaripiprazole are greater than 99% bound to serum proteins, binding primarily to albumin.

Metabolism:

Aripiprazole is extensively metabolised by the liver primarily by three biotransformation pathways: dehydrogenation, hydroxylation and N-dealkylation. Based on *in vitro* studies, CYP3A4 and CYP2D6 enzymes are responsible for dehydrogenation and hydroxylation of aripiprazole, and N-dealkylation is catalysed by CYP3A4. Aripiprazole is the predominant medicinal product moiety in systemic circulation. At steady state, dehydroaripiprazole, the active metabolite, represents about 40% of aripiprazole AUC in plasma.

Elimination:

The mean elimination half-lives for aripiprazole are approximately 75 hours in extensive metabolisers of CYP2D6 and approximately 146 hours in poor metabolisers of CYP2D6.

The total body clearance of aripiprazole is 0.7 ml/min/kg, which is primarily hepatic.

Following a single oral dose of [^{14}C]-labelled aripiprazole, approximately 27% of the administered radioactivity was recovered in the urine and approximately 60% in the faeces. Less than 1% of unchanged aripiprazole was excreted in the urine and approximately 18% was recovered unchanged in the faeces.

Pharmacokinetics in special patient groups

Elderly:

There are no differences in the pharmacokinetics of aripiprazole between healthy elderly and younger adult subjects, nor is there any detectable effect of age in a population pharmacokinetic analysis in schizophrenic patients.

Gender:

There are no differences in the pharmacokinetics of aripiprazole between healthy male and female subjects nor is there any detectable effect of gender in a population pharmacokinetic analysis in schizophrenic patients.

Smoking and Race:

Population pharmacokinetic evaluation has revealed no evidence of clinically significant race-related differences or effects from smoking upon the pharmacokinetics of aripiprazole.

Renal Disease:

The pharmacokinetic characteristics of aripiprazole and dehydroaripiprazole were found to be similar in patients with severe renal disease compared to young healthy subjects.

Hepatic Disease:

A single-dose study in subjects with varying degrees of liver cirrhosis (Child-Pugh Classes A, B and C) did not reveal a significant effect of hepatic impairment on the pharmacokinetics of aripiprazole and dehydroaripiprazole, but the study included only 3 patients with Class C liver cirrhosis, which is insufficient to draw conclusions on their metabolic capacity.

5.3 Preclinical safety data

Preclinical safety data revealed no special hazard for humans based on conventional studies of safety pharmacology, repeat-dose toxicity, genotoxicity, carcinogenicity and reproductive toxicity.

Toxicologically significant effects were observed only at doses or exposures that were sufficiently in excess of the maximum human dose or exposure, indicating that these effects were limited or of no relevance to clinical use. These included: dose-dependent adrenocortical toxicity (lipofuscin pigment accumulation and/or parenchymal cell loss) in rats after 104 weeks at 20 to 60 mg/kg/day (3 to 14 times the mean steady-state AUC at the maximum recommended human dose) and increased adrenocortical carcinomas and combined adrenocortical adenomas/carcinomas in female rats at 60 mg/kg/day (14 times the mean steady-state AUC at the maximum recommended human dose).

An additional finding was cholelithiasis as a consequence of precipitation of sulphate conjugates of hydroxy metabolites of aripiprazole in the bile of monkeys after repeated oral dosing at 25 to 125 mg/kg/day (1 to 3 times the mean steady-state AUC at the maximum recommended clinical dose or 16 to 81 times the maximum recommended human dose based on mg/m^2). However, the concentrations of the sulphate conjugates of hydroxyaripiprazole in human bile at the highest dose proposed, 30 mg per day, were no more than 6% of the bile concentrations found in the monkeys in the 39-week study and are well below (6%) their limits of *in vitro* solubility.

Based on results of a full range of standard genotoxicity tests, aripiprazole was considered non-genotoxic. Aripiprazole did not impair fertility in reproductive toxicity studies. Developmental toxicity, including dose-dependent delayed foetal ossification and possible teratogenic effects, were observed in rats at doses resulting in subtherapeutic exposures (based on AUC) and in rabbits at doses resulting in exposures 3 and 11 times the mean steady-state AUC at the maximum recommended clinical dose. Maternal toxicity occurred at doses similar to those eliciting developmental toxicity.

6. PHARMACEUTICAL PARTICULARS

6.1 List of excipients

Lactose monohydrate

Maize starch

Microcrystalline cellulose

Hydroxypropyl cellulose

Magnesium stearate

Red iron oxide E172 (10 mg and 30 mg tablets)

Yellow iron oxide E172 (15 mg tablets)

Indigo carmine E132 aluminium lake (5 mg tablets)

6.2 Incompatibilities

Not applicable.

6.3 Shelf life

3 years

6.4 Special precautions for storage

Store in the original package in order to protect from moisture.

6.5 Nature and contents of container

ABILIFY tablets are available in aluminium perforated unit dose blisters in cartons of 28 × 1 tablets.

6.6 Instructions for use and handling

No special requirements.

7. MARKETING AUTHORISATION HOLDER

Otsuka Pharmaceutical Europe Ltd.

Commonwealth House, 2 Chalkhill Road

Hammersmith - London W6 8DW - United Kingdom

8. MARKETING AUTHORISATION NUMBER(S)

EU/1/04/276/002 Abilify 5mg tablets, 28s

EU/1/04/276/007 Abilify 10mg tablets, 28s

EU/1/04/276/012 Abilify 15mg tablets, 28s

EU/1/04/276/017 Abilify 30mg tablets, 28s

9. DATE OF FIRST AUTHORISATION/RENEWAL OF THE AUTHORISATION

June 2004

10. DATE OF REVISION OF THE TEXT

March 2005

Accolate

(AstraZeneca UK Limited)

1. NAME OF THE MEDICINAL PRODUCT

ACCOLATE®

2. QUALITATIVE AND QUANTITATIVE COMPOSITION

'Accolate' contains 20 mg zafirlukast in each tablet.

For excipients, see 6.1.

3. PHARMACEUTICAL FORM

Film-coated tablet.

White to off white, round, biconvex film coated tablet.

4. CLINICAL PARTICULARS

4.1 Therapeutic indications

'Accolate' is indicated for the treatment of asthma.

4.2 Posology and method of administration

'Accolate' should be taken continuously.

Adults and children aged 12 years and over:

The dosage is one 20 mg tablet twice daily. This dosage should not be exceeded. Higher doses may be associated with elevations of one or more liver enzymes consistent with hepatotoxicity.

As food may reduce the bioavailability of zafirlukast, 'Accolate' should not be taken with meals.

Elderly:

The clearance of zafirlukast is significantly reduced in elderly patients (over 65 years old), and C_{max} and AUC are approximately double those of younger adults. However, accumulation of zafirlukast is no greater than that seen in multiple-dose trials conducted in adult subjects with asthma, and the consequences of the altered kinetics in the elderly are unknown.

Clinical experience with 'Accolate' in the elderly (over 65 years) is limited and caution is recommended until further information is available.

Children:

There is no clinical experience of the use of 'Accolate' in children under 12 years of age.

Until safety information is available, the use of 'Accolate' in children is contraindicated.

Renal impairment:

No dosage adjustment is necessary in patients with mild renal impairment. However, experience is limited in patients with moderate to severe renal impairment (see section 5.2) so clear dose recommendations cannot be given; 'Accolate' should be used with caution in this patient group.

4.3 Contraindications

'Accolate' should not be given to patients who have previously experienced hypersensitivity to the product or any of its ingredients.

'Accolate' is contraindicated in patients with hepatic impairment or cirrhosis; it has not been studied in patients with hepatitis or in long term studies of patients with cirrhosis.

'Accolate' is contraindicated in children under 12 years of age until safety information is available.

4.4 Special warnings and special precautions for use

'Accolate' should be taken regularly to achieve benefit, even during symptom free periods. 'Accolate' therapy should normally be continued during acute exacerbations of asthma.

'Accolate' does not allow a reduction in existing steroid treatment.

As with inhaled steroids and cromones (disodium cromoglycate, nedocromil sodium), 'Accolate' is not indicated for use in the reversal of bronchospasm in acute asthma attacks.

'Accolate' has not been evaluated in the treatment of labile (brittle) or unstable asthma.

Cases of eosinophilic conditions, including Churg-Strauss Syndrome and eosinophilic pneumonia have been reported in association with Accolate usage. Presentations may involve various body systems including vasculitic rash, worsening pulmonary symptoms, cardiac complications or neuropathy. A causal relationship has neither been confirmed nor refuted. If a patient develops an eosinophilic condition, or a Churg-Strauss Syndrome type illness, Accolate should be stopped. A rechallenge test should not be performed and treatment should not be restarted.

Elevations in serum transaminases can occur during treatment with 'Accolate'. These are usually asymptomatic and transient but could represent early evidence of hepatotoxicity, and have very rarely been associated with more severe hepatocellular injury, fulminant hepatitis and liver failure (see section 4.8). In extremely rare post-marketing cases, no prior clinical symptoms or signs suggestive of liver dysfunction preceded the severe hepatic injury.

If clinical symptoms or signs suggestive of liver dysfunction occur (e.g. anorexia, nausea, vomiting, right upper quadrant pain, fatigue, lethargy, flu-like symptoms, enlarged liver, pruritus and jaundice), Accolate should be discontinued. The serum transaminases, in particular serum ALT, should be measured immediately and the patient managed accordingly.

Physicians may consider the value of routine liver function testing. Periodic serum transaminase testing has not proven to prevent serious injury but is generally believed that early detection of drug-induced hepatic injury along with immediate withdrawal of the suspect drug may enhance the likelihood of recovery. If liver function testing shows evidence of hepatotoxicity 'Accolate' should be discontinued immediately and the patient managed accordingly.

Patients in whom 'Accolate' was withdrawn because of hepatotoxicity should not be re-exposed to 'Accolate'.

4.5 Interaction with other medicinal products and other forms of Interaction

'Accolate' may be administered with other therapies routinely used in the management of asthma and allergy. Inhaled steroids, inhaled and oral bronchodilator therapy, antibiotics and antihistamines are examples of agents which have been co-administered with 'Accolate' without adverse interaction.

'Accolate' may be administered with oral contraceptives without adverse interaction.

Co-administration with warfarin results in an increase in maximum prothrombin time by approximately 35%. It is therefore recommended that if 'Accolate' is co-administered with warfarin, prothrombin time should be closely monitored. The interaction is probably due to an inhibition by zafirlukast of the cytochrome P450 2C9 isoenzyme system.

In clinical trials co-administration with theophylline resulted in decreased plasma levels of zafirlukast, by approximately 30%, but with no effect on plasma theophylline levels. However, during post-marketing surveillance, there have been rare cases of patients experiencing increased theophylline levels when co-administered 'Accolate'.

Co-administration with terfenadine resulted in a 54% decrease in AUC for zafirlukast, but with no effect on plasma terfenadine levels.

Co-administration withacetylsalicylic acid ("aspirin", 650 mg four times a day) may result in increased plasma levels of zafirlukast, by approximately 45%.

Co-administration with erythromycin will result in decreased plasma levels of zafirlukast, by approximately 40%.

The clearance of zafirlukast in smokers may be increased by approximately 20%.

At concentrations of 10 microgram/ml and above, zafirlukast causes increases in the assay value for bilirubin in animal plasma. However, zafirlukast has not been shown to interfere with the 2,5-dichlorophenyl diazonium salt method of bilirubin analysis of human plasma.

4.6 Pregnancy and lactation

The safety of 'Accolate' in human pregnancy has not been established. In animal studies, zafirlukast did not have any apparent effect on fertility and did not appear to have any teratogenic or selective toxic effect on the foetus. The potential risks should be weighed against the benefits of continuing therapy during pregnancy and 'Accolate' should be used during pregnancy only if clearly needed.

Zafirlukast is excreted in human breast milk. 'Accolate' should not be administered to mothers who are breast-feeding.

4.7 Effects on ability to drive and use machines

There is no evidence that 'Accolate' affects the ability to drive and use machinery.

4.8 Undesirable effects

The following have been reported in association with the administration of 'Accolate':

Gastrointestinal: nausea, vomiting, abdominal pain (common)

Hepatobiliary: Symptomatic hepatitis with and without hyperbilirubinaemia (rare), hyperbilirubinaemia, without elevated liver function tests (rare), hepatic failure (very rare), fulminant hepatitis (very rare)

General: malaise (common)

Musculoskeletal: arthralgia (rare), myalgia (rare)

Skin: rash (including blistering), pruritus, hypersensitivity reactions including urticaria and angioedema (rare) and oedema (uncommon)

Neurological: insomnia, headache (common)

Haematologic: bruising (rare), bleeding disorders, including menorrhagia (rare), thrombocytopenia (rare), and agranulocytosis (very rare)

The above events have usually resolved following cessation of therapy. Headache and gastrointestinal disturbance are usually mild and do not necessitate withdrawal from therapy.

In placebo-controlled clinical trials, an increased incidence of infection has been observed in elderly patients given 'Accolate' (7.8% vs 1.4%). Infections were usually mild, predominantly affecting the respiratory tract.

4.9 Overdose

Limited information exists with regard to the effects of overdosage of 'Accolate' in humans.

Management should be supportive. Removal of excess medication by gastric lavage may be helpful.

5. PHARMACOLOGICAL PROPERTIES

5.1 Pharmacodynamic properties

ATC Code: R03D C01.

Pharmacotherapeutic Group: Leukotriene receptor antagonists.

The cysteinyl leukotrienes (LTC_4, LTD_4 and LTE_4) are potent inflammatory eicosanoids released from various cells including mast cells and eosinophils. These important pro-asthmatic mediators bind to cysteinyl leukotriene receptors found in the human airway. Leukotriene production and receptor occupation has been implicated in the pathophysiology of asthma. Effects include smooth muscle contraction, airway oedema and altered cell activity associated with the inflammatory process, including eosinophil influx to the lung.

'Accolate' is a competitive highly selective and potent oral peptide leukotriene antagonist of LTC_4, LTD_4 and LTE_4 components of slow reacting substance of anaphylaxis. In vitro studies have shown that 'Accolate' antagonises the contractile activity of all three peptide leukotrienes (leukotriene C_4, D_4, and E_4) in human conducting airway smooth muscle to the same extent. Animal studies have shown 'Accolate' to be effective in preventing peptide leukotriene-induced increases in vascular permeability, which give rise to oedema in the airways, and to inhibit peptide leukotriene-induced influx of eosinophils into airways.

The specificity of 'Accolate' has been shown by its action on leukotriene receptors and not prostaglandin, thromboxane, cholinergic and histamine receptors.

In a placebo-controlled study where segmental bronchoprovocation with allergen was followed by bronchoalveolar lavage 48 hours later, zafirlukast decreased the rise in basophils, lymphocytes and histamine, and reduced the stimulated production of superoxide by alveolar macrophages.

'Accolate' attenuated the increase in bronchial hyperresponsiveness that follows inhaled allergen challenge. Further, methacholine sensitivity was diminished by long-term dosing with 'Accolate' 20 mg twice daily.

Further, in clinical trials evaluating chronic therapy with 'Accolate', the lung function measured when plasma levels were at trough showed sustained improvements over baseline.

'Accolate' shows a dose dependent inhibition of bronchoconstriction induced by inhaled LTD_4. Asthmatic patients are approximately 10-fold more sensitive to the bronchoconstricting activity of inhaled LTD_4. A single oral dose of 'Accolate' can enable an asthmatic patient to inhale 100 times more LTD_4 and shows significant protection at 12 and 24 hours.

'Accolate' inhibits the bronchoconstriction caused by several kinds of challenge, such as the response to sulphur dioxide, exercise and cold air. 'Accolate' attenuates the early and late phase inflammatory reaction caused by various antigens such as grass, cat dander, ragweed and mixed antigens.

In asthmatic patients not adequately controlled by beta-agonist therapy (given as required) 'Accolate' improves symptoms (reducing daytime and nocturnal asthmatic symptoms), improves lung function, reduces the need for concomitant beta-agonist medication and reduces incidence of exacerbations. Similar benefits have been seen in patients with more severe asthma receiving high dose inhaled steroids.

In clinical studies, there was a significant first-dose effect on baseline bronchomotor tone observed within 2 hours of dosing, when peak plasma concentrations had not yet been achieved. Initial improvements in asthma symptoms occurred within the first week, and often the first few days, of treatment with 'Accolate'.

5.2 Pharmacokinetic properties

Peak plasma concentrations of zafirlukast are achieved approximately 3 hours after oral administration of 'Accolate'.

Administration of 'Accolate' with food increased the variability in the bioavailability of zafirlukast and reduced bioavailability in most (75%) subjects. The net reduction was approximately 40%.

Following twice-daily administration of 'Accolate' (30 to 80 mg bd), accumulation of zafirlukast in plasma was low (not detectable - 2.9 times first dose values; mean 1.45; median 1.27). The terminal half-life of zafirlukast is approximately 10 hours. Steady-state plasma concentrations of zafirlukast were proportional to the dose and predictable from single-dose pharmacokinetic data.

Zafirlukast is extensively metabolised. Following a radiolabelled dose the urinary excretion accounts for approximately 10% dose and faecal excretion for 89%. Zafirlukast is not detected in urine. The metabolites identified in human plasma were found to be at least 90-fold less potent than zafirlukast in a standard in-vitro test of activity.

Zafirlukast is approximately 99% protein bound to human plasma proteins, predominantly albumin, over the concentration range 0.25 to 4.0 microgram/ml.

Pharmacokinetic studies in special populations have been performed in a relatively small number of subjects, and the clinical significance of the following kinetic data is not established.

Pharmacokinetics of zafirlukast in adolescents and adults with asthma were similar to those of healthy adult males. When adjusted for body weight, the pharmacokinetics of zafirlukast are not significantly different between men and women.

Elderly subjects and subjects with stable alcoholic cirrhosis demonstrated an approximately two-fold increase in C_{max} and AUC compared to normal subjects given the same doses of 'Accolate'.

There are no significant differences in the pharmacokinetics of zafirlukast in patients with mild renal impairment and in normal subjects. However, there are no conclusive data available in patients with moderate or severe renal impairment, hence the recommendation for caution is used in this patient population.

5.3 Preclinical safety data

After multiple doses of greater than 40 mg/kg/day for up to 12 months, liver enlargement associated with degenerative/fatty change or glycogen deposition was seen in rats, mice and dogs. Histiocytic aggregates were seen in a number of tissues of dogs.

Male mice given 300 mg/kg zafirlukast daily had an increased incidence of hepatocellular adenomas compared to control animals. Rats given 2000 mg/kg zafirlukast daily had an increased incidence of urinary bladder papilloma compared to control animals. Zafirlukast was not mutagenic in a range of tests. The clinical significance of these findings during the long term use of 'Accolate' in man is uncertain.

There were no other notable findings from the pre-clinical testing.

6. PHARMACEUTICAL PARTICULARS

6.1 List of excipients

Croscarmellose sodium

Hypromellose E464

Lactose Monohydrate

Magnesium Stearate E572

Microcrystalline Cellulose E460

Povidone

Titanium Dioxide E171

6.2 Incompatibilities

None known

6.3 Shelf life

3 years

6.4 Special precautions for storage

Do not store above 30°C.

6.5 Nature and contents of container

Aluminium laminate/foil blister packs containing 56 or 100 tablets.

6.6 Instructions for use and handling

No special precautions.

7. MARKETING AUTHORISATION HOLDER

AstraZeneca UK Limited,

600 Capability Green,

Luton, LU1 3LU, UK.

8. MARKETING AUTHORISATION NUMBER(S)

PL 17901/0001

9. DATE OF FIRST AUTHORISATION/RENEWAL OF THE AUTHORISATION

1 June 2000

10. DATE OF REVISION OF THE TEXT

7th December 2004

Accupro Tablets 10mg

(Pfizer Limited)

1. NAME OF THE MEDICINAL PRODUCT

Accupro® Tablets 10 mg

2. QUALITATIVE AND QUANTITATIVE COMPOSITION

Each 10mg tablet contains quinapril hydrochloride 10.832 mg (equivalent to 10 mg quinapril base)

3. PHARMACEUTICAL FORM

10mg tablet: brown, scored, triangular, film coated tablet imprinted with the dosage strength

4. CLINICAL PARTICULARS

4.1 Therapeutic indications

Hypertension

For the treatment of all grades of essential hypertension. Accupro is effective as monotherapy or concomitantly with diuretics in patients with hypertension.

Congestive Heart Failure

For the treatment of congestive heart failure when given concomitantly with a diuretic and/or cardiac glycoside. Treatment of congestive heart failure with Accupro should always be initiated under close medical supervision.

4.2 Posology and method of administration

For oral use

Adults

Hypertension

Monotherapy: The recommended initial dosage is 10 mg once daily in uncomplicated hypertension. Depending upon clinical response, patient's dosage may be titrated (by doubling the dose allowing adequate time for dosage adjustment) to a maintenance dosage of 20 to 40 mg/day given as a single dose or divided into 2 doses. Long-term control is maintained in most patients with a single daily dosage regimen. Patients have been treated with dosages up to 80 mg/day. Take either with or without food. The dose should always be taken at about the same time of day to help increase compliance.

Concomitant Diuretics: In order to determine if excess hypotension will occur, an initial dosage of 2.5 mg of Accupro is recommended in patients who are being treated with a diuretic. After this the dosage of Accupro should be titrated (as described above) to the optimal response.

Congestive Heart Failure

In order to closely monitor patients for symptomatic hypotension, a single 2.5 mg initial dosage is recommended. After this, patients should be titrated to an effective dose: (up to 40 mg/day) given in 1 or 2 doses with concomitant diuretic and/or cardiac glycoside therapy. Patients are usually maintained effectively on doses of 10-20 mg/day given with concomitant therapy. Take either with or without food. The dose should always be taken at about the same time of day to help increase compliance.

Severe Heart Failure

In the treatment of severe or unstable congestive heart failure, Accupro should always be initiated in hospital under close medical supervision.

Other patients who may also be considered to be at higher risk and should have treatment initiated in hospital include: patients who are on high dose loop diuretics (e.g. > 80 mg frusemide) or on multiple diuretic therapy, have hypovolaemia, hyponatraemia (serum sodium < 130 mgEq/l) or systolic blood pressure < 90 mm Hg, are on high dose vasodilator therapy, have a serum creatinine > 150 μmol/l or are aged 70 years or over.

Elderly/Renal Impairment

In elderly patients and in patients with a creatinine clearance of less than 40 ml/min, an initial dosage in essential hypertension of 2.5 mg is recommended followed by titration to the optimal response.

Children

(6 - 12 years)

Not recommended. Safety and efficacy in children have not been established.

4.3 Contraindications

Accupro is contraindicated in patients with hypersensitivity to any of the ingredients.

Accupro is contraindicated throughout pregnancy (see section 4.6).

Accupro is contraindicated in nursing mothers.

Accupro is contraindicated in patients with a history of angioedema related to previous treatment with ACE inhibitors.

Accupro is contraindicated in patients with hereditary/idiopathic angioneurotic oedema.

4.4 Special warnings and special precautions for use

Accupro should not be used in patients with aortic stenosis or outflow obstruction.

Patients haemodialysed using high-flux polyacrylonitrile ('AN69') membranes are highly likely to experience anaphylactoid reactions if they are treated with ACE inhibitors. This combination should therefore be avoided, either by use of alternative antihypertensive drugs or alternative membranes for haemodialysis. Similar reactions have been observed during low density lipoprotein apheresis with dextran-sulphate. This method should therefore not be used in patients treated with ACE inhibitors.

Anaphylactoid reactions: Patients receiving ACE inhibitors during desensitising treatment with hymenoptera venom have experienced life threatening anaphylactoid reactions. These reactions were avoided by temporarily withholding ACE inhibitor therapy prior to each desensitisation.

In patients with renal insufficiency, monitoring of renal function during therapy should be performed as deemed appropriate, although in the majority renal function will not alter or may improve.

As a consequence of inhibiting the renin-angiotensin-aldosterone system, changes in renal function may be anticipated in susceptible individuals. In patients with severe heart failure whose renal function may depend on the activity of the renin-angiotensin-aldosterone system, treatment with ACE inhibitors including quinapril, may be associated with oliguria and/or progressive azotemia and rarely acute renal failure and/or death.

The half-life of quinaprilat is prolonged as creatinine clearance falls. Patients with a creatinine clearance of <40 ml/min require a lower initial dosage of quinapril. These patients' dosage should be titrated upwards based upon therapeutic response, and renal function should be closely monitored although initial studies do not indicate that quinapril produces further deterioration in renal function.

In clinical studies in hypertensive patients with unilateral or bilateral renal artery stenosis, increases in blood urea nitrogen and serum creatinine have been observed in some patients following ACE inhibitor therapy. These increases were almost always reversible upon discontinuation of the ACE inhibitor and/or diuretic therapy. In such patients, renal function should be monitored during the first few weeks of therapy.

Some patients with hypertension or heart failure with no apparent pre-existing renal vascular disease have developed increases >1.25 times the upper limit of normal) in blood urea and serum creatinine, usually minor and transient, especially when quinapril has been given concomitantly with a diuretic and has been observed in 4% and 3% respectively of patients on monotherapy. This is more likely to occur in patients with pre-existing renal impairment. Dosage reduction and/or discontinuation of a diuretic and/or quinapril may be required.

Angioedema: Angioedema has been reported in patients treated with angiotensin-converting enzyme inhibitors. If laryngeal stridor or angioedema of the face, tongue, or glottis occur, treatment should be discontinued immediately, the patient treated appropriately in accordance with accepted medical care, and carefully observed until the swelling disappears. In instances where swelling is confined to the face and lips, the condition generally resolves without treatment; antihistamines may be useful in relieving symptoms. Angioedema associated with laryngeal involvement may be fatal. Where there is involvement of the tongue, glottis, or larynx likely to cause airway obstruction, appropriate therapy e.g., subcutaneous adrenaline solution 1:1000 (0.3 to 0.5 ml) should be promptly administered.

Black patients receiving ACE inhibitor therapy generally have a higher incidence of angioedema than non-black patients.

Intestinal angioedema: Intestinal angioedema has been reported in patients treated with ACE inhibitors. These patients presented with abdominal pain (with or without nausea or vomiting); in some cases there was no prior history of facial angioedema and C-1 esterase levels were normal. The angioedema was diagnosed by procedures including abdominal CT scan or ultrasound, or at surgery, and symptoms resolved after stopping the ACE inhibitor. Intestinal angioedema should be included in the differential diagnosis of patients on ACE inhibitors presenting with abdominal pain.

Hypotension: Symptomatic hypotension was rarely seen in hypertensive patients treated with Accupro but it is a possible consequence of ACE inhibition therapy particularly in salt/volume depleted patients such as those previously treated with diuretics, who have a dietary salt reduction, or who are on dialysis. If symptomatic hypotension occurs, the patient should be placed in the supine position and, if necessary, receive an intravenous infusion of normal saline. A transient hypotensive response is not a contraindication to further doses; however, lower doses of quinapril or any concomitant diuretic therapy should be considered if this event occurs.

Neutropenia/agranulocytosis: ACE inhibitors have been rarely associated with agranulocytosis and bone marrow depression in patients with uncomplicated hypertension but more frequently in patients with renal impairment, especially if they also have collagen vascular disease. As with other ACE inhibitors, monitoring of white blood cell counts in patients with collagen vascular disease and/or renal diseases should be considered.

4.5 Interaction with other medicinal products and other forms of Interaction

Tetracycline: Because of the presence of magnesium carbonate in the formulation, Accupro has been shown in healthy volunteers to reduce the absorption of tetracycline in concomitant administration by 28-37%. It is recommended that concomitant administration with tetracycline be avoided.

Concomitant diuretic therapy: Patients treated with diuretics may occasionally experience an excessive reduction of blood pressure after initiation of therapy with Accupro. This hypotensive effect may be effectively minimised by either discontinuing the diuretic or increasing the salt intake prior to the initial dose of Accupro. If discontinuation of the diuretic is not possible, medical supervision should be provided for up to two hours following administration of the initial dose.

Agents increasing serum potassium: Concomitant treatments with potassium sparing diuretics, potassium supplements or potassium salts should be used with caution and with appropriate monitoring of serum potassium. As with other ACE inhibitors, patients on quinapril alone may have increased serum potassium levels. When administered concomitantly, quinapril may reduce the hypokalaemia induced by thiazide diuretics.

Surgery/anaesthesia: Although no data are available to indicate there is an interaction between Accupro and anaesthetic agents that produces hypotension, caution should be exercised when patients undergo major surgery or anaesthesia since angiotensin converting enzyme inhibitors have been shown to block angiotensin II formation secondary to compensatory renin release. This may lead to hypotension which can be corrected by volume expansion.

Lithium: Increased serum lithium levels and symptoms of lithium toxicity have been reported in patients receiving concomitant lithium and ACE inhibitor therapy due to the sodium-losing effect of these agents. These drugs should be co-administered with caution and frequent monitoring of serum lithium levels is recommended. If a diuretic is also used, it may increase the risk of lithium toxicity.

Non-steroidal anti-inflammatory drugs: In some patients, the administration of a non-steroidal anti-inflammatory agent may reduce the antihypertensive effect of ACE inhibitors. Furthermore, it has been described that NSAIDs and ACE inhibitors exert an additive effect on the increase in serum potassium, whereas renal function may decrease. These effects are in principle reversible and occur especially in patients with compromised renal function.

Allopurinol, cytostatic and immunosuppressive agents, systemic corticosteroids or procainamide: Concomitant administration with ACE inhibitors may lead to an increased risk for leucopenia.

Alcohol, barbiturates or narcotics: Potentiation of orthostatic hypotension may occur.

Other hypertensive drugs: There may be an additive effect or potentiation.

Antacids: May decrease the bioavailability of Accupro.

Antidiabetic drugs (oral hypoglycaemic agents and insulin): Dosage adjustments of the antidiabetic drug may be required.

4.6 Pregnancy and lactation

Pregnancy: Accupro is contraindicated throughout pregnancy.

Quinapril has been shown to be foetotoxic in rabbits. When ACE inhibitors have been used during the second or third trimesters of pregnancy, there have been reports of hypotension, renal failure, skull hypoplasia, and/or death in the newborn. Oligohydramnios has also been reported, presumably representing decreased renal function in the foetus, limb contractures, craniofacial deformities, hypoplastic lung development and intrauterine growth retardation have been reported in association with oligohydramnios. Should a woman become pregnant while receiving Accupro, the drug should be discontinued as soon as possible. Infants exposed *in utero* to ACE inhibitors should be closely monitored for hypotension, oliguria and hyperkalaemia. If oliguria occurs, attention should be directed towards support of blood pressure and renal perfusion.

Lactation: Accupro should not be used in nursing mothers.

4.7 Effects on ability to drive and use machines

There are no studies on the effect of this medicine on the ability to drive. When driving vehicles or operating machines it should be taken into account that occasionally dizziness or weariness may occur.

4.8 Undesirable effects

The most frequent clinical adverse reactions in hypertension and congestive heart failure are headache, dizziness, rhinitis, coughing, upper respiratory tract infection, fatigue, and nausea and vomiting. Other less frequent side effects are dyspepsia, myalgia, chest pain, abdominal pain, diarrhoea, back pain, sinusitis, insomnia, paraesthesia, nervousness, asthenia, pharyngitis, hypotension, palpitations, flatulence, depression, pruritus, rash, impotence, oedema, arthralgia, amblyopia.

Renal dysfunction, angioedema, hypotension, hyperkalaemia, neutropenia, agranulocytosis - see warnings and precautions.

The following side effects have been observed associated with ACE inhibitor therapy:

Cardiac Disorders: Myocardial infarction, tachycardia

Nervous System Disorders: Cerebral haemorrage, disorders of balance, syncope, taste disturbances, transient ischaemic attacks

Respiratory, Thoracic and Mediastinal Disorders: Bronchitis, bronchospasm, dyspnoea

In individual cases angioneurotic oedema involving the upper airways has caused fatal airway obstruction.

Gastrointestinal Disorders: Constipation, dry mouth, glossitis, ileus, intestinal angioedema. Pancreatitis has been reported rarely in patients treated with ACE inhibitors; in some cases this has proved fatal.

Hepatobiliary Disorders: Cholestatic icterus, hepatitis

Skin and Subcutaneous Tissue Disorders: Alopecia, erythema multiforme, epidermic necrolysis, psoriasis-like efflorescences, Steven Johnson syndrome, urticaria. May be accompanied by fever, eosinophilia and/or increased ANA-titers.

Psychiatric Disorders: Confusion

Eye Disorders: Blurred vision

Ear and Labyrinth Disorders: Tinnitus

Investigations: Increases in blood urea and plasma creatinine may occur. Decreases in haematocrit, platelets and white cell count as well as elevation of liver enzymes and serum bilirubin. In patients with a congential deficiency concerning G-6-PDH individual cases of haemolytic anaemia have been reported.

4.9 Overdose

No data are available with respect to overdosage in humans. The most likely clinical manifestation would be symptoms attributable to severe hypotension, which should normally be treated by intravenous volume expansion.

Haemodialysis and peritoneal dialysis have little effect on the elimination of quinapril and quinaprilat.

Treatment is symptomatic and supportive consistent with established medical care.

5. PHARMACOLOGICAL PROPERTIES

5.1 Pharmacodynamic properties

Quinapril is rapidly de-esterified to quinaprilat (quinapril diacid, the principal metabolite) which is a potent angiotensin-converting enzyme (ACE) inhibitor.

ACE is a peptidyl dipeptidase that catalyses the conversion of angiotensin I to the vasoconstrictor angiotensin II which is involved in vascular control and function through many different mechanisms, including stimulation of aldosterone secretion by the adrenal cortex. The mode of action of quinapril in humans and animals is to inhibit circulating and tissue ACE activity, thereby decreasing vasopressor activity and aldosterone secretion.

In animal studies, the antihypertensive effect of quinapril outlasts its inhibitory effect on circulating ACE, whereas, tissue ACE inhibition more closely correlates with the duration of antihypertensive effects. Administration of 10-40 mg of quinapril to patients with mild to severe hypertension results in a reduction of both sitting and standing blood pressure with minimal effect on heart rate. Antihypertensive activity commences within one hour with peak effects usually achieved by two to four hours after dosing. Achievement of maximum blood pressure lowering effects may require two weeks of therapy in some patients. At the recommended doses, antihypertensive effects are maintained in most patients throughout the 24 hour dosing interval and continue during long term therapy.

5.2 Pharmacokinetic properties

Peak plasma Accupro concentrations are observed within 1 hour of oral administration. The extent of absorption is approximately 60%, and is not influenced by food. Following absorption, Accupro is de-esterified to its major active metabolite, quinaprilat, and to minor inactive metabolites. Accupro has an apparent half-life of approximately one hour. Peak plasma quinaprilat concentrations are observed approximately 2 hours following an oral dose of quinapril. Quinaprilat is eliminated primarily by renal excretion and has an effective accumulation half-life of 3 hours. In patients with renal insufficiency and creatinine clearance of $\leq$40ml/min, peak and trough quinaprilat concentrations increase, time to peak concentration increases, apparent half-life increases, and time to steady state may be delayed. The elimination of quinaprilat is also reduced in elderly patients >65 years) and correlates well with the impaired renal function which frequently occurs in the elderly. Quinaprilat concentrations are reduced in patients with alcoholic cirrhosis due to impaired de-esterification of Accupro. Studies in rats indicate that Accupro and its metabolites do not cross the blood-brain barrier.

5.3 Preclinical safety data

The results of the preclinical tests do not add anything of further significance to the prescriber.

6. PHARMACEUTICAL PARTICULARS

6.1 List of excipients

Magnesium carbonate

Hydrous lactose

Gelatin

Crospovidone

Magnesium stearate

Candelilla wax

Colourings (Opadry Y-5-9020):

Hydroxypropylmethylcellulose

Hydroxypropylcellulose

Macrogol 400

Red iron oxide (E172)

Titanium Dioxide (E171)

6.2 Incompatibilities

None known.

6.3 Shelf life

3 years

6.4 Special precautions for storage

Do not store above 25°C

6.5 Nature and contents of container

Tampertainer with dessicant containing 56 or 100 tablets

Polyamide/aluminium/PVC blister strip. Supplied in packs of 7, 28, 56 or 100 tablets

6.6 Instructions for use and handling

No special instructions needed

7. MARKETING AUTHORISATION HOLDER

Pfizer Limited

Ramsgate Road

Sandwich

Kent

CT13 9NJ

United Kingdom

8. MARKETING AUTHORISATION NUMBER(S)

PL 00057/0515

9. DATE OF FIRST AUTHORISATION/RENEWAL OF THE AUTHORISATION

1 August 2003

10. DATE OF REVISION OF THE TEXT
September 2003
11 LEGAL STATUS
POM
Ref: AC 4_0 UK

Accupro Tablets 20 mg

(Pfizer Limited)

1. NAME OF THE MEDICINAL PRODUCT
Accupro® Tablets 20 mg

2. QUALITATIVE AND QUANTITATIVE COMPOSITION
Each 20mg tablet contains quinapril hydrochloride 21.664 mg (equivalent to 20 mg quinapril base)

3. PHARMACEUTICAL FORM
20mg tablet: brown, scored, round, film coated tablet imprinted with the dosage strength.

4. CLINICAL PARTICULARS

4.1 Therapeutic indications

Hypertension
For the treatment of all grades of essential hypertension. Accupro is effective as monotherapy or concomitantly with diuretics in patients with hypertension.

Congestive Heart Failure
For the treatment of congestive heart failure when given concomitantly with a diuretic and/or cardiac glycoside. Treatment of congestive heart failure with Accupro should always be initiated under close medical supervision.

4.2 Posology and method of administration
For oral use

Adults

Hypertension

Monotherapy: The recommended initial dosage is 10 mg once daily in uncomplicated hypertension. Depending upon clinical response, patient's dosage may be titrated (by doubling the dose allowing adequate time for dosage adjustment) to a maintenance dosage of 20 to 40 mg/day given as a single dose or divided into 2 doses. Long-term control is maintained in most patients with a single daily dosage regimen. Patients have been treated with dosages up to 80 mg/day. Take either with or without food. The dose should always be taken at about the same time of day to help increase compliance.

Concomitant Diuretics: In order to determine if excess hypotension will occur, an initial dosage of 2.5 mg of Accupro is recommended in patients who are being treated with a diuretic. After this the dosage of Accupro should be titrated (as described above) to the optimal response.

Congestive Heart Failure

In order to closely monitor patients for symptomatic hypotension, a single 2.5 mg initial dosage is recommended. After this, patients should be titrated to an effective dose: (up to 40 mg/day) given in 1 or 2 doses with concomitant diuretic and/or cardiac glycoside therapy. Patients are usually maintained effectively on doses of 10-20 mg/day given with concomitant therapy. Take either with or without food. The dose should always be taken at about the same time of day to help increase compliance.

Severe Heart Failure
In the treatment of severe or unstable congestive heart failure, Accupro should always be initiated in hospital under close medical supervision.

Other patients who may also be considered to be at higher risk and should have treatment initiated in hospital include: patients who are on high dose loop diuretics (e.g. > 80 mg frusemide) or on multiple diuretic therapy, have hypovolaemia, hyponatraemia (serum sodium < 130 mgEq/l) or systolic blood pressure < 90 mm Hg, are on high dose vasodilator therapy, have a serum creatinine > 150 μmol/l or are aged 70 years or over.

Elderly/Renal Impairment

In elderly patients and in patients with a creatinine clearance of less than 40 ml/min, an initial dosage in essential hypertension of 2.5 mg is recommended followed by titration to the optimal response.

Children
(6 - 12 years)

Not recommended. Safety and efficacy in children have not been established.

4.3 Contraindications
Accupro is contraindicated in patients with hypersensitivity to any of the ingredients.

Accupro is contraindicated throughout pregnancy (see section 4.6).

Accupro is contraindicated in nursing mothers.

Accupro is contraindicated in patients with a history of angioedema related to previous treatment with ACE inhibitors.

Accupro is contraindicated in patients with hereditary/idiopathic angioneurotic oedema.

4.4 Special warnings and special precautions for use
Accupro should not be used in patients with aortic stenosis or outflow obstruction.

Patients haemodialysed using high-flux polyacrylonitrile ('AN69') membranes are highly likely to experience anaphylactoid reactions if they are treated with ACE inhibitors. This combination should therefore be avoided, either by use of alternative antihypertensive drugs or alternative membranes for haemodialysis. Similar reactions have been observed during low density lipoprotein apheresis with dextran-sulphate. This method should therefore not be used in patients treated with ACE inhibitors.

Anaphylactoid reactions: Patients receiving ACE inhibitors during desensitising treatment with hymenoptera venom have experienced life threatening anaphylactoid reactions. These reactions were avoided by temporarily withholding ACE inhibitor therapy prior to each desensitisation.

In patients with renal insufficiency, monitoring of renal function during therapy should be performed as deemed appropriate, although in the majority renal function will not alter or may improve.

As a consequence of inhibiting the renin-angiotensin-aldosterone system, changes in renal function may be anticipated in susceptible individuals. In patients with severe heart failure whose renal function may depend on the activity of the renin-angiotensin-aldosterone system, treatment with ACE inhibitors including quinapril, may be associated with oliguria and/or progressive azotemia and rarely acute renal failure and/or death.

The half-life of quinaprilat is prolonged as creatinine clearance falls. Patients with a creatinine clearance of <40 ml/min require a lower initial dosage of quinapril. These patients' dosage should be titrated upwards based upon therapeutic response, and renal function should be closely monitored although initial studies do not indicate that quinapril produces further deterioration in renal function.

In clinical studies in hypertensive patients with unilateral or bilateral renal artery stenosis, increases in blood urea nitrogen and serum creatinine have been observed in some patients following ACE inhibitor therapy. These increases were almost always reversible upon discontinuation of the ACE inhibitor and/or diuretic therapy. In such patients, renal function should be monitored during the first few weeks of therapy.

Some patients with hypertension or heart failure with no apparent pre-existing renal vascular disease have developed increases >1.25 times the upper limit of normal) in blood urea and serum creatinine, usually minor and transient, especially when quinapril has been given concomitantly with a diuretic and has been observed in 4% and 3% respectively of patients on monotherapy. This is more likely to occur in patients with pre-existing renal impairment. Dosage reduction and/or discontinuation of a diuretic and/or quinapril may be required.

Angioedema: Angioedema has been reported in patients treated with angiotensin-converting enzyme inhibitors. If laryngeal stridor or angioedema of the face, tongue, or glottis occur, treatment should be discontinued immediately, the patient treated appropriately in accordance with accepted medical care, and carefully observed until the swelling disappears. In instances where swelling is confined to the face and lips, the condition generally resolves without treatment; antihistamines may be useful in relieving symptoms. Angioedema associated with laryngeal involvement may be fatal. Where there is involvement of the tongue, glottis, or larynx likely to cause airway obstruction, appropriate therapy e.g., subcutaneous adrenaline solution 1:1000 (0.3 to 0.5 ml) should be promptly administered.

Black patients receiving ACE inhibitor therapy generally have a higher incidence of angioedema than non-black patients.

Intestinal angioedema: Intestinal angioedema has been reported in patients treated with ACE inhibitors. These patients presented with abdominal pain (with or without nausea or vomiting); in some cases there was no prior history of facial angioedema and C-1 esterase levels were normal. The angioedema was diagnosed by procedures including abdominal CT scan or ultrasound, or at surgery, and symptoms resolved after stopping the ACE inhibitor. Intestinal angioedema should be included in the differential diagnosis of patients on ACE inhibitors presenting with abdominal pain.

Hypotension: Symptomatic hypotension was rarely seen in hypertensive patients treated with Accupro but it is a possible consequence of ACE inhibition therapy particularly in salt/volume depleted patients such as those previously treated with diuretics, who have a dietary salt reduction, or who are on dialysis. If symptomatic hypotension occurs, the patient should be placed in the supine position and, if necessary, receive an intravenous infusion of normal saline. A transient hypotensive response is not a contraindication to further doses; however, lower doses of quinapril or any concomitant diuretic therapy should be considered if this event occurs.

Neutropenia/agranulocytosis: ACE inhibitors have been rarely associated with agranulocytosis and bone marrow depression in patients with uncomplicated hypertension but more frequently in patients with renal impairment, especially if they also have collagen vascular disease. As with other ACE inhibitors, monitoring of white blood cell counts in patients with collagen vascular disease and/or renal diseases should be considered.

4.5 Interaction with other medicinal products and other forms of Interaction
Tetracycline: Because of the presence of magnesium carbonate in the formulation, Accupro has been shown in healthy volunteers to reduce the absorption of tetracycline in concomitant administration by 28-37%. It is recommended that concomitant administration with tetracycline be avoided.

Concomitant diuretic therapy: Patients treated with diuretics may occasionally experience an excessive reduction of blood pressure after initiation of therapy with Accupro. This hypotensive effect may be effectively minimised by either discontinuing the diuretic or increasing the salt intake prior to the initial dose of Accupro. If discontinuation of the diuretic is not possible, medical supervision should be provided for up to two hours following administration of the initial dose.

Agents increasing serum potassium: Concomitant treatments with potassium sparing diuretics, potassium supplements or potassium salts should be used with caution and with appropriate monitoring of serum potassium. As with other ACE inhibitors, patients on quinapril alone may have increased serum potassium levels. When administered concomitantly, quinapril may reduce the hypokalaemia induced by thiazide diuretics.

Surgery/anaesthesia: Although no data are available to indicate there is an interaction between Accupro and anaesthetic agents that produces hypotension, caution should be exercised when patients undergo major surgery or anaesthesia since angiotensin converting enzyme inhibitors have been shown to block angiotensin II formation secondary to compensatory renin release. This may lead to hypotension which can be corrected by volume expansion.

Lithium: Increased serum lithium levels and symptoms of lithium toxicity have been reported in patients receiving concomitant lithium and ACE inhibitor therapy due to the sodium-losing effect of these agents. These drugs should be co-administered with caution and frequent monitoring of serum lithium levels is recommended. If a diuretic is also used, it may increase the risk of lithium toxicity.

Non-steroidal anti-inflammatory drugs: In some patients, the administration of a non-steroidal anti-inflammatory agent may reduce the antihypertensive effect of ACE inhibitors. Furthermore, it has been described that NSAIDs and ACE inhibitors exert an additive effect on the increase in serum potassium, whereas renal function may decrease. These effects are in principle reversible and occur especially in patients with compromised renal function.

Allopurinol, cytostatic and immunosuppressive agents, systemic corticosteroids or procainamide: Concomitant administration with ACE inhibitors may lead to an increased risk for leucopenia.

Alcohol, barbiturates or narcotics: Potentiation of orthostatic hypotension may occur.

Other hypertensive drugs: There may be an additive effect or potentiation.

Antacids: May decrease the bioavailability of Accupro.

Antidiabetic drugs (oral hypoglycaemic agents and insulin): Dosage adjustments of the antidiabetic drug may be required.

4.6 Pregnancy and lactation
Pregnancy: Accupro is contraindicated throughout pregnancy.

Quinapril has been shown to be foetotoxic in rabbits. When ACE inhibitors have been used during the second or third trimesters of pregnancy, there have been reports of hypotension, renal failure, skull hypoplasia, and/or death in the newborn. Oligohydramnios has also been reported, presumably representing decreased renal function in the foetus, limb contractures, craniofacial deformities, hypoplastic lung development and intrauterine growth retardation have been reported in association with oligohydramnios. Should a woman become pregnant while receiving Accupro, the drug should be discontinued as soon as possible. Infants exposed *in utero* to ACE inhibitors should be closely monitored for hypotension, oliguria and hyperkalaemia. If oliguria occurs, attention should be directed towards support of blood pressure and renal perfusion.

Lactation: Accupro should not be used in nursing mothers.

4.7 Effects on ability to drive and use machines
There are no studies on the effect of this medicine on the ability to drive. When driving vehicles or operating machines it should be taken into account that occasionally dizziness or weariness may occur.

4.8 Undesirable effects
The most frequent clinical adverse reactions in hypertension and congestive heart failure are headache, dizziness, rhinitis, coughing, upper respiratory tract infection, fatigue, and nausea and vomiting. Other less frequent side effects are dyspepsia, myalgia, chest pain, abdominal pain, diarrhoea, back pain, sinusitis, insomnia, paraesthesia, nervousness, asthenia, pharyngitis, hypotension, palpitations, flatulence, depression, pruritus, rash, impotence, oedema, arthralgia, amblyopia.

Renal dysfunction, angioedema, hypotension, hyperkalaemia, neutropenia, agranulocytosis - see warnings and precautions.

The following side effects have been observed associated with ACE inhibitor therapy:

Cardiac Disorders: Tachycardia, myocardial infarction

Nervous System Disorders: Cerebral haemorrage, disorders of balance, syncope, taste disturbances, transient ischaemic attacks

Respiratory, Thoracic and Mediastinal Disorders: Bronchitis, bronchospasm, dyspnoea.

In individual cases angioneurotic oedema involving the upper airways has caused fatal airway obstruction.

Gastrointestinal Disorders: Constipation, dry mouth, glossitis, ileus, intestinal angioedema. Pancreatitis has been reported rarely in patients treated with ACE inhibitors; in some cases this has proved fatal.

Hepatobiliary Disorders: Cholestatic icterus, hepatitis

Skin and Subcutaneous Tissue Disorders: Alopecia, erythema multiforme, epidermic necrolysis, psoriasis-like efflorescences, Steven Johnson syndrome, urticaria. May be accompanied by fever, eosinophilia and/or increased ANA-titers.

Psychiatric Disorders: Confusion

Eye Disorders: Blurred vision

Ear and Labyrinth Disorders: Tinnitus

Investigations: Increases in blood urea and plasma creatinine may occur. Decreases in haematocrit, platelets and white cell count as well as elevation of liver enzymes and serum bilirubin. In patients with a congential deficiency concerning G-6-PDH individual cases of haemolytic anaemia have been reported.

4.9 Overdose

No data are available with respect to overdosage in humans. The most likely clinical manifestation would be symptoms attributable to severe hypotension, which should normally be treated by intravenous volume expansion.

Haemodialysis and peritoneal dialysis have little effect on the elimination of quinapril and quinaprilat.

Treatment is symptomatic and supportive consistent with established medical care.

5. PHARMACOLOGICAL PROPERTIES

5.1 Pharmacodynamic properties

Quinapril is rapidly de-esterified to quinaprilat (quinapril diacid, the principal metabolite) which is a potent angiotensin-converting enzyme (ACE) inhibitor.

ACE is a peptidyl dipeptidase that catalyses the conversion of angiotensin I to the vasoconstrictor angiotensin II which is involved in vascular control and function through many different mechanisms, including stimulation of aldosterone secretion by the adrenal cortex. The mode of action of quinapril in humans and animals is to inhibit circulating and tissue ACE activity, thereby decreasing vasopressor activity and aldosterone secretion.

In animal studies, the antihypertensive effect of quinapril outlasts its inhibitory effect on circulating ACE, whereas, tissue ACE inhibition more closely correlates with the duration of antihypertensive effects. Administration of 10-40 mg of quinapril to patients with mild to severe hypertension results in a reduction of both sitting and standing blood pressure with minimal effect on heart rate. Antihypertensive activity commences within one hour with peak effects usually achieved by two to four hours after dosing. Achievement of maximum blood pressure lowering effects may require two weeks of therapy in some patients. At the recommended doses, antihypertensive effects are maintained in most patients throughout the 24 hour dosing interval and continue during long term therapy.

5.2 Pharmacokinetic properties

Peak plasma Accupro concentrations are observed within 1 hour of oral administration. The extent of absorption is approximately 60%, and is not influenced by food. Following absorption, Accupro is de-esterified to its major active metabolite, quinaprilat, and to minor inactive metabolites. Accupro has an apparent half-life of approximately one hour. Peak plasma quinaprilat concentrations are observed approximately 2 hours following an oral dose of quinapril. Quinaprilat is eliminated primarily by renal excretion and has an effective accumulation half-life of 3 hours. In patients with renal insufficiency and creatinine clearance of ≤40ml/min, peak and trough quinaprilat concentrations increase, time to peak concentration increases, apparent half-life increases, and time to steady state may be delayed. The elimination of quinaprilat is also reduced in elderly patients >65 years) and correlates well with the impaired renal function which frequently occurs in the elderly. Quinaprilat concentrations are reduced in patients with alcoholic cirrhosis due to impaired de-esterification of Accupro. Studies in rats indicate that Accupro and its metabolites do not cross the blood-brain barrier.

5.3 Preclinical safety data

The results of the preclinical tests do not add anything of further significance to the prescriber.

6. PHARMACEUTICAL PARTICULARS

6.1 List of excipients

Magnesium carbonate

Hydrous lactose

Gelatin

Crospovidone

Magnesium stearate

Candelilla wax

Colourings (Opadry Y-5-9020):

Hydroxypropylmethylcellulose

Hydroxypropylcellulose

Macrogol 400

Red iron oxide (E172)

Titanium Dioxide (E171)

6.2 Incompatibilities

None known.

6.3 Shelf life

3 years

6.4 Special precautions for storage

Do not store above 25°C

6.5 Nature and contents of container

Tampertainer with dessicant containing 56 or 100 tablets

Polyamide/aluminium/PVC blister strip. Supplied in packs of 7, 28, 56 or 100 tablets

6.6 Instructions for use and handling

No special instructions needed

7. MARKETING AUTHORISATION HOLDER

Pfizer Limited

Ramsgate Road

Sandwich

Kent

CT13 9NJ

United Kingdom

8. MARKETING AUTHORISATION NUMBER(S)

PL 00057/0516

9. DATE OF FIRST AUTHORISATION/RENEWAL OF THE AUTHORISATION

1 August 2003

10. DATE OF REVISION OF THE TEXT

June 2004

11 LEGAL STATUS

POM

Ref: AC 4_0 UK

Accupro Tablets 40mg

(Pfizer Limited)

1. NAME OF THE MEDICINAL PRODUCT

Accupro™ Tablets 40 mg

2. QUALITATIVE AND QUANTITATIVE COMPOSITION

Each 40mg tablet contains quinapril hydrochloride 43.328 mg (equivalent to 40 mg quinapril base)

3. PHARMACEUTICAL FORM

40mg tablet: brown, elliptical, film coated tablet imprinted with the dosage strength.

4. CLINICAL PARTICULARS

4.1 Therapeutic indications

Hypertension

For the treatment of all grades of essential hypertension. Accupro is effective as monotherapy or concomitantly with diuretics in patients with hypertension.

Congestive Heart Failure

For the treatment of congestive heart failure when given concomitantly with a diuretic and/or cardiac glycoside. Treatment of congestive heart failure with Accupro should always be initiated under close medical supervision.

4.2 Posology and method of administration

For oral use

Adults

Hypertension

Monotherapy: The recommended initial dosage is 10 mg once daily in uncomplicated hypertension. Depending upon clinical response, patient's dosage may be titrated (by doubling the dose allowing adequate time for dosage adjustment) to a maintenance dosage of 20 to 40 mg/day given as a single dose or divided into 2 doses. Long-term control is maintained in most patients with a single daily dosage regimen. Patients have been treated with dosages up to 80 mg/day. Take either with or without food. The dose should always be taken at about the same time of day to help increase compliance.

Concomitant Diuretics: In order to determine if excess hypotension will occur, an initial dosage of 2.5 mg of Accupro is recommended in patients who are being treated with a diuretic. After this the dosage of Accupro should be titrated (as described above) to the optimal response.

Congestive Heart Failure

In order to closely monitor patients for symptomatic hypotension, a single 2.5 mg initial dosage is recommended. After this, patients should be titrated to an effective dose: (up to 40 mg/day) given in 1 or 2 doses with concomitant diuretic and/or cardiac glycoside therapy. Patients are usually maintained effectively on doses of 10-20 mg/day given with concomitant therapy. Take either with or without food. The dose should always be taken at about the same time of day to help increase compliance.

Severe Heart Failure

In the treatment of severe or unstable congestive heart failure, Accupro should always be initiated in hospital under close medical supervision.

Other patients who may also be considered to be at higher risk and should have treatment initiated in hospital include: patients who are on high dose loop diuretics (e.g. > 80 mg frusemide) or on multiple diuretic therapy, have hypovolaemia, hyponatraemia (serum sodium < 130 mgEq/l) or systolic blood pressure < 90 mm Hg, are on high dose vasodilator therapy, have a serum creatinine > 150 μmol/l or are aged 70 years or over.

Elderly/Renal Impairment

In elderly patients and in patients with a creatinine clearance of less than 40 ml/min, an initial dosage in essential hypertension of 2.5 mg is recommended followed by titration to the optimal response.

Children

(6 - 12 years)

Not recommended. Safety and efficacy in children have not been established.

4.3 Contraindications

Accupro is contraindicated in patients with hypersensitivity to any of the ingredients.

Accupro is contraindicated throughout pregnancy (see section 4.6).

Accupro is contraindicated in nursing mothers.

Accupro is contraindicated in patients with a history of angioedema related to previous treatment with ACE inhibitors.

Accupro is contraindicated in patients with hereditary/idiopathic angioneurotic oedema.

4.4 Special warnings and special precautions for use

Accupro should not be used in patients with aortic stenosis or outflow obstruction.

Patients haemodialysed using high-flux polyacrylonitrile ('AN69') membranes are highly likely to experience anaphylactoid reactions if they are treated with ACE inhibitors. This combination should therefore be avoided, either by use of alternative antihypertensive drugs or alternative membranes for haemodialysis. Similar reactions have been observed during low density lipoprotein apheresis with dextran-sulphate. This method should therefore not be used in patients treated with ACE inhibitors.

Anaphylactoid reactions: Patients receiving ACE inhibitors during desensitising treatment with hymenoptera venom have experienced life threatening anaphylactoid reactions. These reactions were avoided by temporarily withholding ACE inhibitor therapy prior to each desensitisation.

In patients with renal insufficiency, monitoring of renal function during therapy should be performed as deemed appropriate, although in the majority renal function will not alter or may improve.

As a consequence of inhibiting the renin-angiotensin-aldosterone system, changes in renal function may be anticipated in susceptible individuals. In patients with severe heart failure whose renal function may depend on the activity of the renin-angiotensin-aldosterone system, treatment with ACE inhibitors including quinapril, may be associated with oliguria and/or progressive azotemia and rarely acute renal failure and/or death.

The half-life of quinaprilat is prolonged as creatinine clearance falls. Patients with a creatinine clearance of <40 ml/min require a lower initial dosage of quinapril. These patients' dosage should be titrated upwards based upon therapeutic response, and renal function should be closely monitored although initial studies do not indicate that quinapril produces further deterioration in renal function.

In clinical studies in hypertensive patients with unilateral or bilateral renal artery stenosis, increases in blood urea nitrogen and serum creatinine have been observed in some patients following ACE inhibitor therapy. These increases were almost always reversible upon discontinuation of the ACE inhibitor and/or diuretic therapy. In such patients, renal function should be monitored during the first few weeks of therapy.

Some patients with hypertension or heart failure with no apparent pre-existing renal vascular disease have developed increases >1.25 times the upper limit of normal) in blood urea and serum creatinine, usually minor and transient, especially when quinapril has been given concomitantly with a diuretic and has been observed in 4% and 3% respectively of patients on monotherapy. This is more likely to occur in patients with pre-existing renal impairment. Dosage reduction and/or discontinuation of a diuretic and/or quinapril may be required.

Angioedema: Angioedema has been reported in patients treated with angiotensin-converting enzyme inhibitors. If laryngeal stridor or angioedema of the face, tongue, or glottis occur, treatment should be discontinued immediately, the patient treated appropriately in accordance with accepted medical care, and carefully observed until the swelling disappears. In instances where swelling is confined to the face and lips, the condition generally resolves without treatment; antihistamines may be useful in relieving symptoms. Angioedema associated with laryngeal involvement may be fatal. Where there is involvement of the tongue, glottis, or larynx likely to cause airway obstruction, appropriate therapy e.g., subcutaneous adrenaline solution 1:1000 (0.3 to 0.5 ml) should be promptly administered.

Black patients receiving ACE inhibitor therapy generally have a higher incidence of angioedema than non-black patients.

Intestinal angioedema: Intestinal angioedema has been reported in patients treated with ACE inhibitors. These patients presented with abdominal pain (with or without nausea or vomiting); in some cases there was no prior history of facial angioedema and C-1 esterase levels were normal. The angioedema was diagnosed by procedures including abdominal CT scan or ultrasound, or at surgery, and symptoms resolved after stopping the ACE inhibitor. Intestinal angioedema should be included in the differential diagnosis of patients on ACE inhibitors presenting with abdominal pain.

Hypotension: Symptomatic hypotension was rarely seen in hypertensive patients treated with Accupro but it is a possible consequence of ACE inhibition therapy particularly in salt/volume depleted patients such as those previously treated with diuretics, who have a dietary salt reduction, or who are on dialysis. If symptomatic hypotension occurs, the patient should be placed in the supine position and, if necessary, receive an intravenous infusion of normal saline. A transient hypotensive response is not a contraindication to further doses; however, lower doses of quinapril or any concomitant diuretic therapy should be considered if this event occurs.

Neutropenia/agranulocytosis: ACE inhibitors have been rarely associated with agranulocytosis and bone marrow depression in patients with uncomplicated hypertension but more frequently in patients with renal impairment, especially if they also have collagen vascular disease. As with other ACE inhibitors, monitoring of white blood cell counts in patients with collagen vascular disease and/or renal diseases should be considered.

4.5 Interaction with other medicinal products and other forms of Interaction

Tetracycline: Because of the presence of magnesium carbonate in the formulation, Accupro has been shown in healthy volunteers to reduce the absorption of tetracycline in concomitant administration by 28-37%. It is recommended that concomitant administration with tetracycline be avoided.

Concomitant diuretic therapy: Patients treated with diuretics may occasionally experience an excessive reduction of blood pressure after initiation of therapy with Accupro. This hypotensive effect may be effectively minimised by either discontinuing the diuretic or increasing the salt intake prior to the initial dose of Accupro. If discontinuation of the diuretic is not possible, medical supervision should be provided for up to two hours following administration of the initial dose.

Agents increasing serum potassium: Concomitant treatments with potassium sparing diuretics, potassium supplements or potassium salts should be used with caution and with appropriate monitoring of serum potassium. As with other ACE inhibitors, patients on quinapril alone may have increased serum potassium levels. When administered concomitantly, quinapril may reduce the hypokalaemia induced by thiazide diuretics.

Surgery/anaesthesia: Although no data are available to indicate there is an interaction between Accupro and anaesthetic agents that produces hypotension, caution should be exercised when patients undergo major surgery or anaesthesia since angiotensin converting enzyme inhibitors have been shown to block angiotensin II formation secondary to compensatory renin release. This may lead to hypotension which can be corrected by volume expansion.

Lithium: Increased serum lithium levels and symptoms of lithium toxicity have been reported in patients receiving concomitant lithium and ACE inhibitor therapy due to the sodium-losing effect of these agents. These drugs should be co-administered with caution and frequent monitoring of serum lithium levels is recommended. If a diuretic is also used, it may increase the risk of lithium toxicity.

Non-steroidal anti-inflammatory drugs: In some patients, the administration of a non-steroidal anti-inflammatory agent may reduce the antihypertensive effect of ACE inhibitors. Furthermore, it has been described that NSAIDs and ACE inhibitors exert an additive effect on the increase in serum potassium, whereas renal function may decrease. These effects are in principle reversible and occur especially in patients with compromised renal function.

Allopurinol, cytostatic and immunosuppressive agents, systemic corticosteroids or procainamide: Concomitant administration with ACE inhibitors may lead to an increased risk for leucopenia.

Alcohol, barbiturates or narcotics: Potentiation of orthostatic hypotension may occur.

Other hypertensive drugs: There may be an additive effect or potentiation.

Antacids: May decrease the bioavailability of Accupro.

Antidiabetic drugs (oral hypoglycaemic agents and insulin): Dosage adjustments of the antidiabetic drug may be required.

4.6 Pregnancy and lactation

Pregnancy: Accupro is contraindicated throughout pregnancy.

Quinapril has been shown to be foetotoxic in rabbits. When ACE inhibitors have been used during the second or third trimesters of pregnancy, there have been reports of hypotension, renal failure, skull hypoplasia, and/or death in the newborn. Oligohydramnios has also been reported, presumably representing decreased renal function in the foetus, limb contractures, craniofacial deformities, hypoplastic lung development and intrauterine growth retardation have been reported in association with oligohydramnios. Should a woman become pregnant while receiving Accupro, the drug should be discontinued as soon as possible. Infants exposed *in utero* to ACE inhibitors should be closely monitored for hypotension, oliguria and hyperkalaemia. If oliguria occurs, attention should be directed towards support of blood pressure and renal perfusion.

Lactation: Accupro should not be used in nursing mothers.

4.7 Effects on ability to drive and use machines

There are no studies on the effect of this medicine on the ability to drive. When driving vehicles or operating machines it should be taken into account that occasionally dizziness or weariness may occur.

4.8 Undesirable effects

The most frequent clinical adverse reactions in hypertension and congestive heart failure are headache, dizziness, rhinitis, coughing, upper respiratory tract infection, fatigue, and nausea and vomiting. Other less frequent side effects are dyspepsia, myalgia, chest pain, abdominal pain, diarrhoea, back pain, sinusitis, insomnia, paraesthesia, nervousness, asthenia, pharyngitis, hypotension, palpitations, flatulence, depression, pruritus, rash, impotence, oedema, arthralgia, amblyopia.

Renal dysfunction, angioedema, hypotension, hyperkalaemia, neutropenia, agranulocytosis - see warnings and precautions.

The following side effects have been observed associated with ACE inhibitor therapy:

Cardiac Disorders: Myocardial infarction, tachycardia

Nervous System Disorders: Cerebral haemorrage, disorders of balance, syncope, taste disturbances, transient ischaemic attacks

Respiratory, Thoracic and Mediastinal Disorders: Bronchitis, bronchospasm, dyspnoea

In individual cases angioneurotic oedema involving the upper airways has caused fatal airway obstruction.

Gastrointestinal Disorders: Constipation, dry mouth, glossitis, ileus, intestinal angioedema. Pancreatitis has been reported rarely in patients treated with ACE inhibitors; in some cases this has proved fatal.

Hepatobiliary Disorders: Cholestatic icterus, hepatitis

Skin and Subcutaneous Tissue Disorders: Alopecia, erythema multiforme, epidermic necrolysis, psoriasis-like efflorescences, Steven Johnson syndrome, urticaria. May be accompanied by fever, eosinophilia and/or increased ANA-titers.

Psychiatric Disorders: Confusion

Eye Disorders: Blurred vision

Ear and Labyrinth Disorders: Tinnitus

Investigations: Increases in blood urea and plasma creatinine may occur. Decreases in haematocrit, platelets and white cell count as well as elevation of liver enzymes and serum bilirubin. In patients with a congential deficiency concerning G-6-PDH individual cases of haemolytic anaemia have been reported.

4.9 Overdose

No data are available with respect to overdosage in humans. The most likely clinical manifestation would be symptoms attributable to severe hypotension, which should normally be treated by intravenous volume expansion.

Haemodialysis and peritoneal dialysis have little effect on the elimination of quinapril and quinaprilat.

Treatment is symptomatic and supportive consistent with established medical care.

5. PHARMACOLOGICAL PROPERTIES

5.1 Pharmacodynamic properties

Quinapril is rapidly de-esterified to quinaprilat (quinapril diacid, the principal metabolite) which is a potent angiotensin-converting enzyme (ACE) inhibitor.

ACE is a peptidyl dipeptidase that catalyses the conversion of angiotensin I to the vasoconstrictor angiotensin II which is involved in vascular control and function through many different mechanisms, including stimulation of aldosterone secretion by the adrenal cortex. The mode of action of quinapril in humans and animals is to inhibit circulating and tissue ACE activity, thereby decreasing vasopressor activity and aldosterone secretion.

In animal studies, the antihypertensive effect of quinapril outlasts its inhibitory effect on circulating ACE, whereas, tissue ACE inhibition more closely correlates with the duration of antihypertensive effects. Administration of 10-40 mg of quinapril to patients with mild to severe hypertension results in a reduction of both sitting and standing blood pressure with minimal effect on heart rate. Antihypertensive activity commences within one hour with peak effects usually achieved by two to four hours after dosing. Achievement of maximum blood pressure lowering effects may require two weeks of therapy in some patients. At the recommended doses, antihypertensive effects are maintained in most patients throughout the 24 hour dosing interval and continue during long term therapy.

5.2 Pharmacokinetic properties

Peak plasma Accupro concentrations are observed within 1 hour of oral administration. The extent of absorption is approximately 60%, and is not influenced by food. Following absorption, Accupro is de-esterified to its major active metabolite, quinaprilat, and to minor inactive metabolites. Accupro has an apparent half-life of approximately one hour. Peak plasma quinaprilat concentrations are observed approximately 2 hours following an oral dose of quinapril. Quinaprilat is eliminated primarily by renal excretion and has an effective accumulation half-life of 3 hours. In patients with renal insufficiency and creatinine clearance of ≤40ml/min, peak and trough quinaprilat concentrations increase, time to peak concentration increases, apparent half-life increases, and time to steady state may be delayed. The elimination of quinaprilat is also reduced in elderly patients >65 years) and correlates well with the impaired renal function which frequently occurs in the elderly. Quinaprilat concentrations are reduced in patients with alcoholic cirrhosis due to impaired de-esterification of Accupro. Studies in rats indicate that Accupro and its metabolites do not cross the blood-brain barrier.

5.3 Preclinical safety data

The results of the preclinical tests do not add anything of further significance to the prescriber.

6. PHARMACEUTICAL PARTICULARS

6.1 List of excipients

Magnesium carbonate

Hydrous lactose

Gelatin

Crospovidone

Magnesium stearate

Candelilla wax

Colourings (Opadry Y-5-9020):

Hydroxypropylmethylcellulose

Hydroxypropylcellulose

Macrogol 400

Red iron oxide (E172)

Titanium Dioxide (E171)

6.2 Incompatibilities

None known.

6.3 Shelf life

3 years

6.4 Special precautions for storage

Do not store above 25°C

6.5 Nature and contents of container

Tampertainer with dessicant containing 56 or 100 tablets

Polyamide/aluminium/PVC blister strip. Supplied in packs of 7, 28, 56 or 100 tablets

6.6 Instructions for use and handling

No special instructions needed

7. MARKETING AUTHORISATION HOLDER

Pfizer Limited

Ramsgate Road

Sandwich

Kent

CT13 9NJ

United Kingdom

8. MARKETING AUTHORISATION NUMBER(S)

PL 00057/0517

9. DATE OF FIRST AUTHORISATION/RENEWAL OF THE AUTHORISATION

1 August 2003

10. DATE OF REVISION OF THE TEXT

June 2004

11 LEGAL STATUS

POM

Ref: AC 4_0 UK

Accupro Tablets 5mg

(Pfizer Limited)

1. NAME OF THE MEDICINAL PRODUCT

Accupro® Tablets 5 mg

2. QUALITATIVE AND QUANTITATIVE COMPOSITION

Each 5 mg tablet contains quinapril hydrochloride 5.416 mg (equivalent to 5 mg quinapril base)

3. PHARMACEUTICAL FORM

Brown, scored, elliptical, film coated tablet imprinted with the dosage strength.

4. CLINICAL PARTICULARS

4.1 Therapeutic indications

Hypertension

For the treatment of all grades of essential hypertension. Accupro is effective as monotherapy or concomitantly with diuretics in patients with hypertension.

Congestive Heart Failure

For the treatment of congestive heart failure when given concomitantly with a diuretic and/or cardiac glycoside. Treatment of congestive heart failure with Accupro should always be initiated under close medical supervision.

4.2 Posology and method of administration

For oral use.

Adults

Hypertension

Monotherapy: The recommended initial dosage is 10 mg once daily in uncomplicated hypertension. Depending upon clinical response, patient's dosage may be titrated (by doubling the dose allowing adequate time for dosage adjustment) to a maintenance dosage of 20 to 40 mg/day given as a single dose or divided into 2 doses. Long-term control is maintained in most patients with a single daily dosage regimen. Patients have been treated with dosages up to 80 mg/day.

Take either with or without food. The dose should always be taken at about the same time of day to help increase compliance.

Concomitant Diuretics: In order to determine if excess hypotension will occur, an initial dosage of 2.5 mg of Accupro is recommended in patients who are being treated with a diuretic. After this the dosage of Accupro should be titrated (as described above) to the optimal response.

Congestive Heart Failure

In order to closely monitor patients for symptomatic hypotension, a single 2.5 mg initial dosage is recommended. After this, patients should be titrated to an effective dose: (up to 40 mg/day) given in 1 or 2 doses with concomitant diuretic and/or cardiac glycoside therapy. Patients are usually maintained effectively on doses of 10-20 mg/day given with concomitant therapy. Take either with or without food. The dose should always be taken at about the same time of day to help increase compliance.

Severe Heart Failure

In the treatment of severe or unstable congestive heart failure, Accupro should always be initiated in hospital under close medical supervision.

Other patients who may also be considered to be at higher risk and should have treatment initiated in hospital include: patients who are on high dose loop diuretics (e.g.> 80 mg frusemide) or on multiple diuretic therapy, have hypovolaemia, hyponatraemia (serum sodium < 130 mgEq/l) or systolic blood pressure < 90 mm Hg, are on high dose vasodilator therapy, have a serum creatinine > 150 μmol/l or are aged 70 years or over.

Elderly/Renal Impairment

In elderly patients and in patients with a creatinine clearance of less than 40 ml/min, an initial dosage in essential hypertension of 2.5 mg is recommended followed by titration to the optimal response.

Children

(6 - 12 years)

Not recommended. Safety and efficacy in children have not been established.

4.3 Contraindications

Accupro is contraindicated in patients with hypersensitivity to any of the ingredients.

Accupro is contraindicated throughout pregnancy (see section 4.6).

Accupro is contraindicated in nursing mothers.

Accupro is contraindicated in patients with a history of angioedema related to previous treatment with ACE inhibitors.

Accupro is contraindicated in patients with hereditary/idiopathic angioneurotic oedema.

4.4 Special warnings and special precautions for use

Accupro should not be used in patients with aortic stenosis or outflow obstruction.

Patients haemodialysed using high-flux polyacrylonitrile ('AN69') membranes are highly likely to experience anaphylactoid reactions if they are treated with ACE inhibitors. This combination should therefore be avoided, either by use of alternative antihypertensive drugs or alternative membranes for haemodialysis. Similar reactions have been observed during low density lipoprotein apheresis with dextran-sulphate. This method should therefore not be used in patients treated with ACE inhibitors.

Anaphylactoid reactions: Patients receiving ACE inhibitors during desensitising treatment with hymenoptera venom have experienced life threatening anaphylactoid reactions. These reactions were avoided by temporarily withholding ACE inhibitor therapy prior to each desensitisation.

In patients with renal insufficiency, monitoring of renal function during therapy should be performed as deemed appropriate, although in the majority renal function will not alter or may improve.

As a consequence of inhibiting the renin-angiotensin-aldosterone system, changes in renal function may be anticipated in susceptible individuals. In patients with severe heart failure whose renal function may depend on the activity of the renin-angiotensin-aldosterone system, treatment with ACE inhibitors including quinapril, may be associated with oliguria and/or progressive azotemia and rarely acute renal failure and/or death.

The half-life of quinaprilat is prolonged as creatinine clearance falls. Patients with a creatinine clearance of <40 ml/min require a lower initial dosage of quinapril. These patients' dosage should be titrated upwards based upon therapeutic response, and renal function should be closely monitored although initial studies do not indicate that quinapril produces further deterioration in renal function.

In clinical studies in hypertensive patients with unilateral or bilateral renal artery stenosis, increases in blood urea nitrogen and serum creatinine have been observed in some patients following ACE inhibitor therapy. These increases were almost always reversible upon discontinuation of the ACE inhibitor and/or diuretic therapy. In such patients, renal function should be monitored during the first few weeks of therapy.

Some patients with hypertension or heart failure with no apparent pre-existing renal vascular disease have developed increases >1.25 times the upper limit of normal) in blood urea and serum creatinine, usually minor and transient, especially when quinapril has been given concomitantly with a diuretic and has been observed in 4% and 3% respectively of patients on monotherapy. This is more likely to occur in patients with pre-existing renal impairment. Dosage reduction and/or discontinuation of a diuretic and/or quinapril may be required.

Angioedema: Angioedema has been reported in patients treated with angiotensin-converting enzyme inhibitors. If laryngeal stridor or angioedema of the face, tongue, or glottis occur, treatment should be discontinued immediately, the patient treated appropriately in accordance with accepted medical care, and carefully observed until the swelling disappears. In instances where swelling is confined to the face and lips, the condition generally resolves without treatment; antihistamines may be useful in relieving symptoms. Angioedema associated with laryngeal involvement may be fatal. Where there is involvement of the tongue, glottis, or larynx likely to cause airway obstruction, appropriate therapy e.g., subcutaneous adrenaline solution 1:1000 (0.3 to 0.5 ml) should be promptly administered.

Black patients receiving ACE inhibitor therapy generally have a higher incidence of angioedema than non-black patients.

Intestinal angioedema: Intestinal angioedema has been reported in patients treated with ACE inhibitors. These patients presented with abdominal pain (with or without nausea or vomiting); in some cases there was no prior history of facial angioedema and C-1 esterase levels were normal. The angioedema was diagnosed by procedures including abdominal CT scan or ultrasound, or at surgery, and symptoms resolved after stopping the ACE inhibitor. Intestinal angioedema should be included in the differential diagnosis of patients on ACE inhibitors presenting with abdominal pain.

Hypotension: Symptomatic hypotension was rarely seen in hypertensive patients treated with Accupro but it is a possible consequence of ACE inhibition therapy particularly in salt/volume depleted patients such as those previously treated with diuretics, who have a dietary salt reduction, or who are on dialysis. If symptomatic hypotension occurs, the patient should be placed in the supine position and, if necessary, receive an intravenous infusion of normal saline. A transient hypotensive response is not a contraindication to further doses; however, lower doses of quinapril or any concomitant diuretic therapy should be considered if this event occurs.

Neutropenia/agranulocytosis: ACE inhibitors have been rarely associated with agranulocytosis and bone marrow depression in patients with uncomplicated hypertension but more frequently in patients with renal impairment, especially if they also have collagen vascular disease. As with other ACE inhibitors, monitoring of white blood cell counts in patients with collagen vascular disease and/or renal diseases should be considered.

4.5 Interaction with other medicinal products and other forms of Interaction

Tetracycline: Because of the presence of magnesium carbonate in the formulation, Accupro has been shown in healthy volunteers to reduce the absorption of tetracycline in concomitant administration by 28-37%. It is recommended that concomitant administration with tetracycline be avoided.

Concomitant diuretic therapy: Patients treated with diuretics may occasionally experience an excessive reduction of blood pressure after initiation of therapy with Accupro. This hypotensive effect may be effectively minimised by either discontinuing the diuretic or increasing the salt intake prior to the initial dose of Accupro. If discontinuation of the diuretic is not possible, medical supervision should be provided for up to two hours following administration of the initial dose.

Agents increasing serum potassium: Concomitant treatments with potassium sparing diuretics, potassium supplements or potassium salts should be used with caution and with appropriate monitoring of serum potassium. As with other ACE inhibitors, patients on quinapril alone may have increased serum potassium levels. When administered concomitantly, quinapril may reduce the hypokalaemia induced by thiazide diuretics.

Surgery/anaesthesia: Although no data are available to indicate there is an interaction between Accupro and anaesthetic agents that produces hypotension, caution should be exercised when patients undergo major surgery or anaesthesia since angiotensin converting enzyme inhibitors have been shown to block angiotensin II formation secondary to compensatory renin release. This may lead to hypotension which can be corrected by volume expansion.

Lithium: Increased serum lithium levels and symptoms of lithium toxicity have been reported in patients receiving concomitant lithium and ACE inhibitor therapy due to the sodium-losing effect of these agents. These drugs should be co-administered with caution and frequent monitoring of serum lithium levels is recommended. If a diuretic is also used, it may increase the risk of lithium toxicity.

Non-steroidal anti-inflammatory drugs:

In some patients, the administration of a non-steroidal anti-inflammatory agent may reduce the antihypertensive effect of ACE inhibitors. Furthermore, it has been described that NSAIDs and ACE inhibitors exert an additive effect on the increase in serum potassium, whereas renal function may decrease. These effects are in principle reversible and occur especially in patients with compromised renal function.

Allopurinol, cytostatic and immunosuppressive agents, systemic corticosteroids or procainamide: Concomitant administration with ACE inhibitors may lead to an increased risk for leucopenia.

Alcohol, barbiturates or narcotics: Potentiation of orthostatic hypotension may occur.

Other hypertensive drugs: There may be an additive effect or potentiation.

Antacids: May decrease the bioavailability of Accupro.

Antidiabetic drugs (oral hypoglycaemic agents and insulin): Dosage adjustments of the antidiabetic drug may be required.

4.6 Pregnancy and lactation

Pregnancy: Accupro is contraindicated throughout pregnancy.

Quinapril has been shown to be foetotoxic in rabbits. When ACE inhibitors have been used during the second or third trimesters of pregnancy, there have been reports of hypotension, renal failure, skull hypoplasia, and/or death in the newborn. Oligohydramnios has also been reported, presumably representing decreased renal function in the foetus, limb contractures, craniofacial deformities, hypoplastic lung development and intrauterine growth retardation have been reported in association with oligohydramnios. Should a woman become pregnant while receiving Accupro, the drug should be discontinued as soon as possible. Infants exposed *in utero* to ACE inhibitors should be closely monitored for hypotension, oliguria and hyperkalaemia. If oliguria occurs, attention should be directed towards support of blood pressure and renal perfusion.

Lactation: Accupro should not be used in nursing mothers.

4.7 Effects on ability to drive and use machines

There are no studies on the effect of this medicine on the ability to drive. When driving vehicles or operating machines it should be taken into account that occasionally dizziness or weariness may occur.

4.8 Undesirable effects

The most frequent clinical adverse reactions in hypertension and congestive heart failure are headache, dizziness, rhinitis, coughing, upper respiratory tract infection, fatigue, and nausea and vomiting. Other less frequent side effects are dyspepsia, myalgia, chest pain, abdominal pain, diarrhoea, back pain, sinusitis, insomnia, paraesthesia, nervousness, asthenia, pharyngitis, hypotension, palpitations, flatulence, depression, pruritus, rash, impotence, oedema, arthralgia, amblyopia.

Renal dysfunction, angioedema, hypotension, hyperkalaemia, neutropenia, agranulocytosis -see warnings and precautions.

The following side effects have been observed associated with ACE inhibitor therapy:

Cardiac Disorders: Tachycardia, myocardial infarction

Nervous System Disorders: Cerebral haemorrage, disorders of balance, syncope, taste disturbances, transient ischaemic attacks

Respiratory, Thoracic and Mediastinal Disorders: Bronchitis, bronchospasm, dyspnoea.

In individual cases angioneurotic oedema involving the upper airways has caused fatal airway obstruction.

Gastrointestinal Disorders: Constipation, dry mouth, glossitis, ileus, intestinal angioedema. Pancreatitis has been reported rarely in patients treated with ACE inhibitors; in some cases this has proved fatal.

Hepatobiliary Disorders: Cholestatic icterus, hepatitis

Skin and Subcutaneous Tissue Disorders: Alopecia, erythema multiforme, epidermic necrolysis, psoriasis-like efflorescences, Steven Johnson syndrome, urticaria. May be accompanied by fever, eosinophilia and/or increased ANA-titers.

Psychiatric Disorders: Confusion

Eye Disorders: Blurred vision

Ear and Labyrinth Disorders: Tinnitus

Investigations: Increases in blood urea and plasma creatinine may occur. Decreases in haematocrit, platelets and white cell count as well as elevation of liver enzymes and serum bilirubin. In patients with a congential deficiency concerning G-6-PDH individual cases of haemolytic anaemia have been reported.

4.9 Overdose

No data are available with respect to overdosage in humans. The most likely clinical manifestation would be symptoms attributable to severe hypotension, which should normally be treated by intravenous volume expansion.

Haemodialysis and peritoneal dialysis have little effect on the elimination of quinapril and quinaprilat.

Treatment is symptomatic and supportive consistent with established medical care.

5. PHARMACOLOGICAL PROPERTIES

5.1 Pharmacodynamic properties

Quinapril is rapidly de-esterified to quinaprilat (quinapril diacid, the principal metabolite) which is a potent angiotensin-converting enzyme (ACE) inhibitor.

ACE is a peptidyl dipeptidase that catalyses the conversion of angiotensin I to the vasoconstrictor angiotensin II which is involved in vascular control and function through many different mechanisms, including stimulation of aldosterone secretion by the adrenal cortex. The mode of action of quinapril in humans and animals is to inhibit circulating and tissue ACE activity, thereby decreasing vasopressor activity and aldosterone secretion.

In animal studies, the antihypertensive effect of quinapril outlasts its inhibitory effect on circulating ACE, whereas, tissue ACE inhibition more closely correlates with the duration of antihypertensive effects. Administration of 10-40 mg of quinapril to patients with mild to severe hypertension results in a reduction of both sitting and standing blood pressure with minimal effect on heart rate. Antihypertensive activity commences within one hour with peak effects usually achieved by two to four hours after dosing. Achievement of maximum blood pressure lowering effects may require two weeks of therapy in some patients. At the recommended doses, antihypertensive effects are maintained in most patients throughout the 24 hour dosing interval and continue during long term therapy.

5.2 Pharmacokinetic properties

Peak plasma Accupro concentrations are observed within 1 hour of oral administration. The extent of absorption is approximately 60%, and is not influenced by food. Following absorption, Accupro is de-esterified to its major active metabolite, quinaprilat, and to minor inactive metabolites. Accupro has an apparent half-life of approximately one hour. Peak plasma quinaprilat concentrations are observed approximately 2 hours following an oral dose of quinapril. Quinaprilat is eliminated primarily by renal excretion and has an effective accumulation half-life of 3 hours. In patients with renal insufficiency and creatinine clearance of $\leq$40ml/min, peak and trough quinaprilat concentrations increase, time to peak concentration increases, apparent half-life increases, and time to steady state may be delayed. The elimination of quinaprilat is also reduced in elderly patients >65 years) and correlates well with the impaired renal function which frequently occurs in the elderly. Quinaprilat concentrations are reduced in patients with alcoholic cirrhosis due to impaired de-esterification of Accupro. Studies in rats indicate that Accupro and its metabolites do not cross the blood-brain barrier.

5.3 Preclinical safety data

The results of the preclinical tests do not add anything of further significance to the prescriber.

6. PHARMACEUTICAL PARTICULARS

6.1 List of excipients

Magnesium carbonate

Hydrous lactose

Gelatin

Crospovidone

Magnesium stearate

Candelilla wax

Colourings (Opadry Y-5-9020):

Hydroxypropylmethylcellulose

Hydroxypropylcellulose

Macrogol 400

Red iron oxide (E172)

Titanium Dioxide (E171)

6.2 Incompatibilities

None known

6.3 Shelf life

3 years

6.4 Special precautions for storage

Do not store above 25°C

6.5 Nature and contents of container

Tampertainer with dessicant containing 56 or 100 tablets.

Polyamide/aluminium/PVC blister strip. Supplied in packs of 7, 28, 56 or 100 tablets.

6.6 Instructions for use and handling

No special instructions needed

7. MARKETING AUTHORISATION HOLDER

Pfizer Limited

Ramsgate Road

Sandwich

Kent

CT13 9NJ

United Kingdom

8. MARKETING AUTHORISATION NUMBER(S)

PL 0057/0514

9. DATE OF FIRST AUTHORISATION/RENEWAL OF THE AUTHORISATION

1 August 2003

10. DATE OF REVISION OF THE TEXT

June 2004

11 LEGAL STATUS

POM

Ref: AC4_0 UK

Accuretic 10/12.5mg Tablets

(Pfizer Limited)

1. NAME OF THE MEDICINAL PRODUCT

Accuretic 10/12.5 mg

2. QUALITATIVE AND QUANTITATIVE COMPOSITION

Each tablet contains:

Quinapril hydrochloride 10.85 mg

(Equivalent to 10 mg quinapril base)

and

hydrochlorothiazide PhEur 12.5 mg

3. PHARMACEUTICAL FORM

Film-coated tablet

4. CLINICAL PARTICULARS

4.1 Therapeutic indications

For the treatment of all grades of essential hypertension in patients who have been stabilised on the individual components given in the same proportions.

4.2 Posology and method of administration

For oral use

Adults:

The recommended initial dosage of Accuretic is 10/12.5mg daily. As indicated by blood pressure response, the dosage may be increased to a maximum of 20/25mg daily.

Take either with or without food. The dose should always be taken at about the same time of day to help increase compliance.

In patients with congestive heart failure, with or without associated renal insufficiency, ACE inhibitor therapy for hypertension may cause an excessive drop in blood pressure. Accuretic therapy should be started under close medical supervision. Patients should be followed closely for the first two weeks of treatment and whenever the dosage is increased.

Renal Impairment:

Accuretic is not recommended for use in patients with creatinine clearance of less than 40 ml/min.

Elderly:

The dose should be kept as low as possible commensurate with achievement of adequate blood pressure control.

Children:

Not recommended. Safety and efficacy in children has not been established.

4.3 Contraindications

Accuretic is contra-indicated throughout pregnancy (see section 4.6).

Accuretic is contra-indicated in nursing mothers.

Accuretic is contra-indicated in patients with hypersensitivity to any of the ingredients.

Accuretic is contra-indicated in patients with anuria or hypersensitivity to quinapril, thiazides or any sulphonamide derived drug.

Accuretic is contra-indicated in patients with aortic stenosis or outflow obstruction.

Accuretic is contra-indicated in patients with a history of angioedema related to previous treatment with ACE inhibitors.

Accuretic is contra-indicated in patients with hereditary/idiopathic angioneurotic oedema.

4.4 Special warnings and special precautions for use

Hypotension:

Accuretic can cause symptomatic hypotension, usually not more frequently than either drug as monotherapy. Symptomatic hypotension was rarely seen in uncomplicated hypertensive patients treated with quinapril but is a possible consequence of ACE inhibition therapy in salt/volume depleted patients such as those previously treated with diuretics, who have a dietary salt restriction, or who are on dialysis. The thiazide component of Accuretic may potentiate the action of other antihypertensive drugs. If symptomatic hypotension occurs, the patient should be placed in the supine position and, if necessary, receive an intravenous infusion of normal saline. A transient hypotensive response is not a contraindication to further doses; however, lower doses of the drug should be considered if this event occurs.

Sensitivity reactions may occur in patients with or without a history of allergy or bronchial asthma, e.g. purpura, photosensitivity, urticaria, necrotising angiitis, respiratory distress including pneumonitis and pulmonary oedema, anaphylactic reactions.

Stevens-Johnson syndrome and exacerbations or activation of systemic lupus erythematosus have been reported with thiazides.

Renal Disease:

Accuretic should be used with caution in patients with severe renal disease. Thiazides may precipitate azotemia in such patients, and the effects of repeated dosing may be cumulative.

As a consequence of inhibiting the renin-angiotensin-aldosterone system, changes in renal function may be anticipated in susceptible individuals. In patients with severe heart failure, whose renal function may depend on the activity of the renin- angiotensin-aldosterone system, treatment with ACE inhibitors including quinapril, may be associated with oliguria and/or progressive azotemia and rarely acute renal failure and/or death.

The half-life of quinaprilat is prolonged as creatinine clearance falls. Patients with a creatinine clearance of <40 ml/min require a lower initial dosage of quinapril. These patients' dosage should be titrated upwards based upon therapeutic response, and renal function should be closely monitored although initial studies do not indicate that quinapril produces further deterioration in renal function.

In clinical studies in hypertensive patients with unilateral or bilateral renal artery stenosis, increases in blood urea nitrogen and serum creatinine have been observed in some patients following ACE inhibitor therapy. These increases were almost always reversible upon discontinuation of the ACE inhibitor and/or diuretic therapy. In such patients, renal function should be monitored during the first few weeks of therapy.

Some hypertensive patients with no apparent pre-existing renal vascular disease have developed increases in blood urea and serum creatinine, usually minor and transient, especially when quinapril has been given concomitantly with a diuretic. This is more likely to occur in patients with pre-existing renal impairment. Dosage reduction and/or discontinuation of any diuretic and/or quinapril may be required.

Anaphylactoid reactions:

Desensitisation: Patients receiving ACE inhibitors during desensitising treatment with hymenoptera venom have sustained life-threatening anaphylactoid reactions. In the same patients, these reactions have been avoided when ACE inhibitors were temporarily withheld, but they have reappeared upon inadvertant rechallenge.

LDL apheresis: Patients undergoing low-density lipoprotein apheresis with dextran-sulfate absorption when treated concomitantly with an ACE inhibitor, have reported anaphylactoid reactions.

Patients haemodialysed using high-flux polyacrylonitrile ('AN69') membranes are highly likely to experience anaphylactoid reactions if they are treated with ACE inhibitors. This combination should therefore be avoided, either by use of alternative antihypertensive drugs or alternative membranes for haemodialysis.

Angioedema:

Angioedema has been reported in patients treated with angiotensin-converting enzyme inhibitors. If laryngeal stridor or angioedema of the face, tongue or glottis occurs, treatment with Accuretic should be discontinued immediately; the patient should be treated in accordance with accepted medical care and carefully observed until the swelling disappears. In instances where the swelling is confined to the face and lips, the condition generally resolves without treatment; antihistamines may be useful in relieving symptoms. Angioedema associated with laryngeal involvement may be fatal. Where there is involvement of the tongue, glottis or larynx likely to cause airway obstruction, emergency therapy including, but not limited to, subcutaneous adrenaline solution 1:1000 (0.3 to 0.5 ml) should be promptly administered.

Intestinal angioedema: Intestinal angioedema has been reported in patients treated with ACE inhibitors. These patients presented with abdominal pain (with or without nausea or vomiting); in some cases there was no prior history of facial angioedema and C-1 esterase levels were normal. The angioedema was diagnosed by procedures including abdominal CT scan or ultrasound, or at surgery, and symptoms resolved after stopping the ACE inhibitor. Intestinal angioedema should be included in the differential diagnosis of patients on ACE inhibitors presenting with abdominal pain.

Accuretic should be used cautiously in patients with impaired hepatic function or progressive liver disease because of the known risks associated with alterations in fluid and electrolyte imbalance resulting from thiazide treatment.

Patients receiving Accuretic should be observed for clinical signs of thiazide induced fluid or electrolyte imbalance. In such patients periodic determination of serum electrolytes should be performed. Because quinapril reduces the production of aldosterone, its combination with hydrochlorothiazide may minimise diuretic induced hypokalaemia. However, some patients may still require potassium supplements.

Neutropenia/Agranulocytosis:

ACE inhibitors have been rarely associated with agranulocytosis and bone marrow depression in patients with uncomplicated hypertension but more frequently in patients with renal impairment, especially if they also have a collagen vascular disease. Agranulocytosis has been rarely reported during treatment with quinapril. As with other ACE inhibitors, periodic monitoring of the white blood cell counts in quinapril-treated patients with collagen vascular disease and/or renal disease should be considered.

Black patients receiving ACE inhibitor therapy have been reported to have a higher incidence of angioedema compared to non-black patients.

4.5 Interaction with other medicinal products and other forms of Interaction

Tetracycline:

Because of the presence of magnesium carbonate in the formulation it is recommended that concomitant administration of Accuretic with tetracycline be avoided.

Agents increasing serum potassium:

Accuretic contains a diuretic. The addition of a potassium sparing diuretic or potassium supplement is not recommended since this may cause a significant increase in serum potassium.

Other diuretics:

Accuretic contains a diuretic. Concomitant use of another diuretic may have an additive effect. Also, patients on diuretics, especially those who are volume and/or salt depleted, may experience an excessive reduction of blood pressure on initiation of therapy, or with increased dosage of an ACE inhibitor.

Surgery/anaesthesia:

Although no data are available to indicate that there is an interaction between Accuretic and anaesthetic agents that produce hypotension, caution should be exercised when patients undergo major surgery or anaesthesia since ACE inhibitors have been shown to block angiotensin II formation secondary to compensatory resin release. This may lead to hypotension which can be corrected by volume expansion.

Thiazides may decrease the arterial response to noradrenaline. In emergency surgery pre-anaesthetic and anaesthetic agents should be administered in reduced doses. Thiazides may increase the response to tubocurarine.

Lithium:

Increased serum lithium levels and symptoms of lithium toxicity have been reported in patients receiving concomitant lithium and ACE inhibitor therapy or lithium and thiazide therapy. Lithium should not generally be given with Accuretic since the risk of lithium toxicity may be increased.

Corticosteroids, ACTH:

Intensified electrolyte depletion, particularly hypokalaemia has been observed.

Non-steroidal anti-inflammatory drugs:

In some patients, the administration of a non-steroidal anti-inflammatory agent can reduce the diuretic, natriuretic, and antihypertensive effects of loop, potassium sparing, and thiazide diuretics and may reduce the antihypertensive effect of ACE inhibitors. Therefore, when Accuretic and non-steroidal anti-inflammatory agents are used concomitantly the patients should be observed closely to determine if the desired effect of Accuretic is obtained. Furthermore, it has been described that NSAIDs and ACE inhibitors exert an additive effect on the increase in serum potassium, whereas renal function may decrease. These effects are in principle reversible and occur especially in patients with compromised renal function.

Allopurinol, cytostatic and immunosuppressive agents, systemic corticosteroids or procainamide:

Concomitant administration with ACE inhibitors may lead to an increased risk for leucopenia.

Alcohol, barbiturates or narcotics:

Potentiation of orthostatic hypotension may occur.

Other antihypertensive drugs:

There may be an additive effect or potentiation.

Antacids:

May decrease the bioavailability of Accuretic.

Antidiabetic drugs (oral hypoglycaemic agents and insulin):

Dosage adjustments of the antidiabetic drug may be required.

4.6 Pregnancy and lactation

Pregnancy:

Accuretic is contraindicated throughout pregnancy. Quinapril has been shown to be foetoxic in rabbits. When ACE inhibitors have been used during the second and third trimesters of pregnancy, there have been reports of hypotension, renal failure, skull hypoplasia, and/or death in the newborn. Oligohydramnios has also been reported, presumably resulting from decreased renal function in the foetus; limb contractures, craniofacial deformities, hypoplastic lung development and intrauterine growth retardation have been reported in association with oligohydramnios. Should a woman become pregnant while receiving Accuretic, the drug should be discontinued as soon as possible. Infants exposed *in utero* to ACE inhibitors should be closely observed for hypotension, oliguria and hyperkalemia. If oliguria occurs, attention should be directed toward support of blood pressure and renal perfusion.

Lactation:

ACE inhibitors, including quinapril, are secreted in human milk to a limited extent. Thiazides appear in human milk. Accuretic should therefore not be used in nursing mothers.

4.7 Effects on ability to drive and use machines

There are no studies on the effect of this medicine on the ability to drive. When driving vehicles or operating machines it should be taken into account that occasionally dizziness or weariness may occur.

4.8 Undesirable effects

The most frequent clinical adverse reactions in hypertension are headache, dizziness, rhinitis, coughing and fatigue. Other adverse experiences include myalgia, viral infection, nausea and vomiting, abdominal pains, back pain and upper respiratory infection. Less frequent side-effects are dyspepsia, chest pain, diarrhoea, insomnia, bronchitis, somnolence, asthenia, pharyngitis, vasodilation and vertigo.

Renal dysfunction, angioedema, hypotension, hyperkalemia, neutropenia, agranulocytosis (See 4.4 Special warnings and special precautions for use).

Increases in cholesterol and triglyceride levels may be associated with thiazide diuretic therapy. Increases >1.25 times the upper limit of normal) in serum creatinine and blood urea nitrogen were observed in 3% and 4% respectively of the patients treated with Accuretic. These increases were almost always reversible upon discontinuation of ACE inhibitor therapy. In such patients renal function should be monitored during the first few weeks of therapy.

Hyperuricaemia may occur or frank gout be precipitated by thiazides in certain patients. Insulin requirements in diabetic patients may be altered by thiazides and latent diabetes mellitus may occur.

Adverse events seen only occasionally in clinical trials and post-marketing experience included:

Cardiovascular: Tachycardia, palpitations, syncope

Gastrointestinal: Flatulence, dry mouth or throat, intestinal angioedema

Respiratory: Dyspnea, sinusitis, bronchospasm. In individual cases angioneurotic oedema involving the upper airways has caused fatal airway obstruction.

Skin, vessels: Erythema multiforme, exfoliative dermatitis, alopecia, pemphigus, pruritus, rash, Stevens Johnson syndrome

Nervous/psychiatric: Paresthesia, nervousness

Urogenital: Impotence, urinary tract infection

Other: Arthralgia, peripheral edema, hemolytic anaemia

The following side-effects have been observed associated with ACE Inhibitor therapy:

Cardiovascular: Myocardial infarction, transient ischaemic attacks, cerebral haemorrhage

Gastro-intestinal: Cholestatic icterus, hepatitis, ileus and intestinal angioedema. Pancreatitis has been reported rarely in patients treated with ACE inhibitors; in some cases this has proved fatal.

Skin, vessels: Urticaria, epidermic necrolysis, psoriasis like efflorescences. May be accompanied by fever, eosinophilia and/or increased ANA-titers.

Nervous: Rarely depressions, confusion, tinnitus, blurred vision and taste disturbances.

Drug/Laboratory: Decreases in hematocrit, platelets and white cell count as well as elevation of liver enzymes and serum bilirubin. In patients with a congenital deficiency concerning G-6-PDH, individual cases of hemolytic anaemia have been reported.

4.9 Overdose

No data are available for Accuretic with respect to overdosage in humans. The most likely clinical manifestation would be symptoms attributable to quinapril monotherapy overdosage such as severe hypotension, which would usually be treated by infusion of intravenous normal saline.

The most common signs and symptoms observed for HCTZ monotherapy overdosage are those caused by electrolyte depletion (hypokalemia, hypochloremia, hyponatremia) and dehydration resulting from excessive diuresis. If digitalis has also been administered, hypokalemia may accentuate cardiac arrythmias.

No specific information is available on the treatment of overdosage with quinapril/HCTZ. Haemodialysis and peritoneal dialysis have little effect on the elimination of quinapril and quinaprilat. Treatment is symptomatic and supportive consistent with established medical care.

5. PHARMACOLOGICAL PROPERTIES

5.1 Pharmacodynamic properties

Quinapril is rapidly de-esterified to quinaprilat (quinapril diacid, the principal metabolite), which is a potent angiotensin-converting enzyme (ACE) inhibitor.

Quinapril and hydrochlorothiazide lower blood pressure by different, though complementary mechanisms. With diuretic treatment, blood pressure and blood volume fall, resulting in a rise in angiotensin II levels which tend to blunt the hypotensive effect. Quinapril blocks this rise in angiotensin II. The antihypertensive effects of quinapril and hydrochlorothiazide are additive.

It should be noted that in controlled clinical trials, ACE inhibitors have an effect on blood pressure that is less in black patients than in non-blacks, although this difference is reported to disappear when a diuretic is added.

5.2 Pharmacokinetic properties

Quinapril:

Peak plasma quinapril concentrations are observed within 1 hour of oral administration. The extent of absorption is approximately 60%, and is not influenced by food. Following absorption, quinapril is deesterified to its major active metabolite, quinaprilat, and to minor inactive metabolites. Quinapril has an apparent half-life of approximately one hour. Peak plasma quinaprilat concentrations are observed approximately 2 hours following an oral dose of quinapril. Quinaprilat is eliminated primarily by renal excretion and has an effective accumulation half-life of 7 hours. In patients with renal insufficiency and creatinine clearance of $\leq$40ml/min, peak and trough quinaprilat concentrations increase, time to peak concentration increases, apparent half-life increases, and time to steady state may be delayed. The elimination of quinaprilat is also reduced in elderly patients >65 years) and correlates well with the impaired renal function which frequently occurs in the elderly. Quinaprilat concentrations are reduced in patients with alcoholic cirrhosis due to impaired deesterification of Accuretic. Studies in rats indicate that Accuretic and its metabolites do not cross the blood-brain barrier.

Hydrochlorothiazide:

After oral administration of hydrochlorothiazide, diuresis begins within 2 hours, peaks in about 4 hours, and lasts about 6 to 12 hours. Hydrochlorothiazide is excreted unchanged by the kidney. When plasma levels have been followed for at least 24 hours, the plasma half-life has been observed to vary between 4 to 15 hours. At least 61% of the oral dose is eliminated unchanged within 24 hours. Hydrochlorothiazide crosses the placenta but not the blood-brain barrier.

5.3 Preclinical safety data

The results of the preclinical tests do not add anything of further significance to the prescriber.

6. PHARMACEUTICAL PARTICULARS

6.1 List of excipients

Accuretic tablets contain the following excipients:

Magnesium carbonate, lactose, povidone, crospovidone, magnesium stearate, candelilla wax, colourings: opadry pink OY-S-6937 (contains iron dioxide E172 and titanium dioxide E171 hydroxypropylmethyl cellulose, hydroxypropyl cellulose and polyethylene glycol).

6.2 Incompatibilities

None known.

6.3 Shelf life

3 years.

6.4 Special precautions for storage

Do not store above 25°C.

Store in the original package.

6.5 Nature and contents of container

Double sided aluminium foil blister enclosed in printed carton. Available in pack sizes of 7, 28, 30, 100 and 156.

6.6 Instructions for use and handling
No special instructions needed.

7. MARKETING AUTHORISATION HOLDER
Pfizer Limited
Ramsgate Road
Sandwich
Kent
CT13 9NJ
United Kingdom

8. MARKETING AUTHORISATION NUMBER(S)
PL 00057/0518

9. DATE OF FIRST AUTHORISATION/RENEWAL OF THE AUTHORISATION
1st May 2003.

10. DATE OF REVISION OF THE TEXT
July 2004.

Company Reference: AH 5_0.

Acepril Tablets 12.5 mg, 25 mg and 50 mg

(E. R. Squibb & Sons Limited)

1. NAME OF THE MEDICINAL PRODUCT
Acepril Tablets 12.5mg, 25mg and 50mg

2. QUALITATIVE AND QUANTITATIVE COMPOSITION
Each tablet contains captopril 12.5 mg, 25mg or 50mg.

For excipients, see 6.1

3. PHARMACEUTICAL FORM
Tablets.

4. CLINICAL PARTICULARS
4.1 Therapeutic indications
Hypertension: Acepril is indicated for the treatment of hypertension.

Heart Failure: Acepril is indicated for the treatment of chronic heart failure with reduction of systolic ventricular function, in combination with diuretics and, when appropriate, digitalis and beta-blockers.

Myocardial Infarction:

- *short-term (4 weeks) treatment:* Acepril is indicated in any clinically stable patient within the first 24 hours of an infarction.

- *long-term prevention of symptomatic heart failure:* Acepril is indicated in clinically stable patients with asymptomatic left ventricular dysfunction (ejection fraction (ejection fraction ≤40%).

Type I Diabetic Nephropathy: Acepril is indicated for the treatment of macroproteinuric diabetic nephropathy in patients with type I diabetes.

(See Section 5.1).

4.2 Posology and method of administration
Dose should be individualised according to patient's profile (see 4.4) and blood pressure response. The recommended maximum daily dose is 150 mg.

Acepril may be taken before, during and after meals.

Hypertension: the recommended starting dose is 25-50 mg daily in two divided doses. The dose may be increased incrementally, with intervals of at least 2 weeks, to 100-150 mg/day in two divided doses as needed to reach target blood pressure. Captopril may be used alone or with other antihypertensive agents, especially thiazide diuretics. A once-daily dosing regimen may be appropriate when concomitant antihypertensive medication such as thiazide diuretics is added.

In patients with a strongly active renin-angiotensin-aldosterone system (hypovolaemia, renovascular hypertension, cardiac decompensation) it is preferable to commence with a single dose of 6.25 mg or 12.5 mg. The inauguration of this treatment should preferably take place under close medical supervision. These doses will then be administered at a rate of two per day. The dosage can be gradually increased to 50 mg per day in one or two doses and if necessary to 100 mg per day in one or two doses.

Heart failure: treatment with captopril for heart failure should be initiated under close medical supervision. The usual starting dose is 6.25 mg - 12.5 mg BID or TID. Titration to the maintenance dose (75 - 150 mg per day) should be carried out based on patient's response, clinical status and tolerability, up to a maximum of 150 mg per day in divided doses. The dose should be increased incrementally, with intervals of at least 2 weeks to evaluate patient's response.

Myocardial infarction:

- *short-term treatment:* Acepril treatment should begin in hospital as soon as possible following the appearance of the signs and/or symptoms in patients with stable haemodynamics. A 6.25 mg test dose should be administered, with a 12.5 mg dose being administered 2 hours afterwards and a 25 mg dose 12 hours later. From the following day, captopril should be administered in a 100 mg/day dose, in two daily administrations, for 4 weeks, if warranted by the absence of adverse haemodynamic reactions. At the end of the 4 weeks of treatment, the patient's state should be reassessed before a decision is taken concerning treatment for the post-myocardial infarction stage.

- *chronic treatment:* if captopril treatment has not begun during the first 24 hours of the acute myocardial infarction stage, it is suggested that treatment be instigated between the 3rd and 16th day post-infarction once the necessary treatment conditions have been attained (stable haemodynamics and management of any residual ischaemia). Treatment should be started in hospital under strict surveillance (particularly of blood pressure) until the 75 mg dose is reached. The initial dose must be low (see 4.4), particularly if the patient exhibits normal or low blood pressure at the initiation of therapy. Treatment should be initiated with a dose of 6.25 mg followed by 12.5 mg 3 times daily for 2 days and then 25 mg 3 times daily if warranted by the absence of adverse haemodynamic reactions. The recommended dose for effective cardioprotection during long-term treatment is 75 to 150 mg daily in two or three doses. In cases of symptomatic hypotension, as in heart failure, the dosage of diuretics and/or other concomitant vasodilators may be reduced in order to attain the steady state dose of captopril. Where necessary, the dose of captopril should be adjusted in accordance with the patient's clinical reactions. Captopril may be used in combination with other treatments for myocardial infarction such as thrombolytic agents, beta-blockers and acetylsalicylic acid.

Type I Diabetic nephropathy: in patients with type I diabetic nephropathy, the recommended daily dose of captopril is 75-100 mg in divided doses. If additional lowering of blood pressure is desired, additional antihypertensive medications may be added.

Renal impairment: since captopril is excreted primarily via the kidneys, dosage should be reduced or the dosage interval should be increased in patients with impaired renal function. When concomitant diuretic therapy is required, a loop diuretic (e.g. furosemide), rather than a thiazide diuretic, is preferred in patients with severe renal impairment.

In patients with impaired renal function, the following daily dose may be recommended to avoid accumulation of captopril.

Creatinine clearance (ml/min/1.73 m^2)	Daily starting dose (mg)	Daily maximum dose (mg)
>40	25-50	150
21-40	25	100
10-20	12.5	75
<10	6.25	37.5

Elderly patients: as with other antihypertensive agents, consideration should be given to initiating therapy with a lower starting dose (6.25 mg BID) in elderly patients who may have reduced renal function and other organ dysfunctions (see above and section 4.4).

Dosage should be titrated against the blood pressure response and kept as low as possible to achieve adequate control.

Children and adolescents: the efficacy and safety of captopril have not been fully established. The use of captopril in children and adolescents should be initiated under close medical supervision. The initial dose of captopril is about 0.3 mg/kg body weight. For patients requiring special precautions (children with renal dysfunction, premature infants, new-borns and infants, because their renal function is not the same with older children and adults) the starting dose should be only 0.15 mg captopril/kg weight. Generally, captopril is administered to children 3 times a day, but dose and interval of dose should be adapted individually according to patient's response.

4.3 Contraindications
1. History of hypersensitivity to captopril, to any of the excipients or any other ACE inhibitor.

2. History of angioedema associated with previous ACE inhibitor therapy.

3. Hereditary / idiopathic angioneurotic oedema.

4. Second and third trimester of pregnancy (see 4.6)

5. Lactation (see 4.6).

4.4 Special warnings and special precautions for use
Hypotension: rarely hypotension is observed in uncomplicated hypertensive patients. Symptomatic hypotension is more likely to occur in hypertensive patients who are volume and/or sodium depleted by vigorous diuretic therapy, dietary salt restriction, diarrhoea, vomiting or haemodialysis. Volume and/or sodium depletion should be corrected before the administration of an ACE inhibitor and a lower starting dose should be considered.

Patients with heart failure are at higher risk of hypotension and a lower starting dose is recommended when initiating therapy with an ACE inhibitor. Caution should be used whenever the dose of captopril or diuretic is increased in patients with heart failure.

As with any antihypertensive agent, excessive blood pressure lowering in patients with ischaemic cardiovascular or cerebrovascular disease may increase the risk of myocardial infarction or stroke. If hypotension develops, the patient should be placed in a supine position. Volume repletion with intravenous normal saline may be required.

Renovascular hypertension: there is an increased risk of hypotension and renal insufficiency when patients with bilateral renal artery stenosis or stenosis of the artery to a single functioning kidney are treated with ACE inhibitors. Loss of renal function may occur with only mild changes in serum creatinine. In these patients, therapy should be initiated under close medical supervision with low doses, careful titration and monitoring of renal function.

Renal impairment: in cases of renal impairment (creatinine clearance ≤40 ml/min), the initial dosage of captopril must be adjusted according to the patient's creatinine clearance (se 4.2), and then as a function of the patient's response to treatment. Routine monitoring of potassium and creatinine are part of normal medical practice for these patients.

Angioedema: angioedema of the extremities, face, lips, mucous membranes, tongue, glottis or larynx may occur in patients treated with ACE inhibitors particularly during the first weeks of treatment. However, in rare cases, severe angioedema may develop after long-term treatment with an ACE inhibitor. Treatment should be discontinued promptly. Angioedema involving the tongue, glottis or larynx may be fatal. Emergency therapy should be instituted. The patient should be hospitalised and observed for at least 12 to 24 hours and should not be discharged until complete resolution of symptoms has occurred.

Cough: cough has been reported with the use of ACE inhibitors. Characteristically, the cough is non-productive, persistent and resolves after discontinuation of therapy.

Hepatic failure: rarely, ACE inhibitors have been associated with a syndrome that starts with cholestatic jaundice and progresses to fulminant hepatic necrosis and (sometimes) death. The mechanism of this syndrome is not understood. Patients receiving ACE inhibitors who develop jaundice or marked elevations of hepatic enzymes should discontinue the ACE inhibitor and receive appropriate medical follow-up.

Hyperkalaemia: elevations in serum potassium have been observed in some patients treated with ACE inhibitors, including captopril. Patients at risk for the development of hyperkalaemia include those with renal insufficiency, diabetes mellitus, or those using concomitant potassium-sparing diuretics, potassium supplements or potassium-containing salt substitutes; or those patients taking other drugs associated with increases in serum potassium (e.g. heparin). If concomitant use of the above mentioned agents is deemed appropriate, regular monitoring of serum potassium is recommended.

Lithium: the combination of lithium and captopril is not recommended (see 4.5)

Aortic and mitral valve stenosis/Obstructive hypertropic cardiomyopathy: ACE inhibitors should be used with caution in patients with left ventricular valvular and outflow tract obstruction and avoided in cases of cardiogenic shock and haemodynamically significant obstruction.

Neutropenia/Agranulocytosis: neutropenia/agranulocytosis, thrombocytopenia and anaemia have been reported in patients receiving ACE inhibitors, including captopril. In patients with normal renal function and no other complicating factors, neutropenia occurs rarely. Captopril should be used with extreme caution in patients with collagen vascular disease, immunosuppressant therapy, treatment with allopurinol or procainamide, or a combination of these complicating factors, especially if there is pre-existing impaired renal function. some of these patients developed serious infections which in a few instances did not respond to intensive antibiotic therapy.

If captopril is used in such patients, it is advised that white blood cell count and differential counts should be performed prior to therapy, every 2 weeks during the first 3 months of captopril therapy, and periodically thereafter. During treatment all patients should be instructed to report any sign of infection (e.g. sore throat, fever) when a differential white blood cell count should be performed. Captopril and other concomitant medication (see 4.5) should be withdrawn if neutropenia (neutrophils less than 1000/mm^3) is detected or suspected.

In most patients neutrophil counts rapidly return to normal upon discontinuing captopril.

Proteinuria: proteinuria may occur particularly in patients with existing renal function impairment or on relatively high doses of ACE inhibitors.

Total urinary proteins greater than 1 g per day were seen in about 0.7% of patients receiving captopril. The majority of patients had evidence of prior renal disease or had received relatively high doses of captopril (in excess of 150 mg/day), or both. Nephrotic syndrome occurred in about one-fifth of proteinuric patients. In most cases, proteinuria subsided or cleared within six months whether or not captopril was continued. Parameters of renal function, such as BUN and creatinine, were seldom altered in the patients with proteinuria.

Patients with prior renal disease should have urinary protein estimations (dip-stick on first morning urine) prior to treatment, and periodically thereafter.

Anaphylactoid reactions during desensitisation: sustained life-threatening anaphylactoid reactions have been rarely reported for patients undergoing desensitising treatment with hymenoptera venom while receiving another ACE inhibitor. In the same patients, these reactions were avoided when the ACE inhibitor was temporarily withheld, but they reappeared upon inadvertent rechallenge. Therefore, caution should be used in patients treated with ACE inhibitors undergoing such desensitisation procedures.

Anaphylactoid reactions during high-flux dialysis / lipoprotein apheresis membrane exposure: anaphylactoid reactions have been reported in patients haemodialysed with high-flux dialysis membranes or undergoing low-density lipoprotein apheresis with dextran sulphate absorption. In these patients, consideration should be given to using a different type of dialysis; membrane or a different class of medication.

Surgery/Anaesthesia: hypotension may occur in patients undergoing major surgery or during treatment with anaesthetic agents that are known to lower blood pressure. If hypotension occurs, it may be corrected by volume expansion.

Diabetic patients: the glycaemia levels should be closely monitored in diabetic patients previously treated with oral antidiabetic drugs or insulin, namely during the first month of treatment with an ACE inhibitor.

Lactose: Acepril contains lactose, therefore it should not be used in cases of congenital galactosaemia, glucose and galactose malabsorption or lactase deficiency syndromes (rare metabolic diseases).

Ethnic differences: as with other angiotensin converting enzyme inhibitors, captopril is apparently less effective in lowering blood pressure in black people than in non-blacks, possibly because of a higher prevalence of low-renin states in the black hypertensive population.

4.5 Interaction with other medicinal products and other forms of Interaction

Potassium sparing diuretics or potassium supplements: ACE inhibitors attenuate diuretic induced potassium loss. Potassium sparing diuretics (e.g. spironolactone, triamterene or amiloride), potassium supplements, or potassium-containing salt substitutes may lead to significant increases in serum potassium. If concomitant use is indicated because of demonstrated hypokalaemia they should be used with caution and with frequent monitoring of serum potassium (see 4.4).

Diuretics (thiazide or loop diuretics): prior treatment with high dose diuretics may result in volume depletion and a risk of hypotension when initiating therapy with captopril (see 4.4). The hypotensive effects can be reduced by discontinuation of the diuretic, by increasing volume or salt intake or by initiating therapy with a low dose of captopril. However, no clinically significant drug interactions have been found in specific studies with hydrochlorothiazide or furosemide.

Other antihypertensive agents: captopril has been safely co-administered with other commonly used anti-hypertensive agents (e.g. beta-blockers and long-acting calcium channel blockers). Concomitant use of these agents may increase the hypotensive effects of captopril. Treatment with nitroglycerine and other nitrates, or other vasodilators, should be used with caution.

Treatments of acute myocardial infarction: captopril may be used concomitantly with acetylsalicylic acid (at cardiologic doses), thrombolytics, beta-blockers and/or nitrates in patients with myocardial infarction.

Lithium: reversible increases in serum lithium concentrations and toxicity have been reported during concomitant administration of lithium with ACE inhibitors. Concomitant use of thiazide diuretics may increase the risk of lithium toxicity and enhance the already increased risk of lithium toxicity with ACE inhibitors. Use of captopril with lithium is not recommended, but if the combination proves necessary, careful monitoring of serum lithium levels should be performed (see 4.4)

Tricyclic antidepressants / Antipsychotics: ACE inhibitors may enhance the hypotensive effects of certain tricyclic antidepressants and antipsychotics (see 4.4). Postural hypotension may occur.

Allopurinol, procainamide, cytostatic or immunosuppressive agents: concomitant administration with ACE inhibitors may lead to an increased risk for leucopenia especially when the latter are used at higher than currently recommended doses.

Non-steroidal anti-inflammatory medicinal products: it has been described that non-steroidal anti-inflammatory medicinal products (NSAIDs) and ACE inhibitors exert an additive effect on the increase in serum potassium whereas renal function may decrease. These effects are, in principle, reversible. Rarely, acute renal failure may occur, particularly in patients with compromised renal function such as the elderly or dehydrated. Chronic administration of NSAIDs may reduce the antihypertensive effect of an ACE inhibitor.

Sympathomimetics: may reduce the antihypertensive effects of ACE inhibitors; patients should be carefully monitored.

Antidiabetics: pharmacological studies have shown that ACE inhibitors, including captopril, can potentiate the blood glucose-reducing effects of insulin and oral antidiabetics such as sulphonylurea in diabetics. Should this very rare interaction occur, it may be necessary to reduce the dose of the antidiabetic during simultaneous treatment with ACE inhibitors.

Clinical Chemistry

Captopril may cause a false-positive urine test for acetone.

4.6 Pregnancy and lactation

Pregnancy: Acepril is not recommended during the first trimester of pregnancy. When a pregnancy is planned or confirmed, the switch to an alternative treatment should be initiated as soon as possible. Controlled studies with ACE inhibitors have not been done in humans, but limited number of cases of first trimester exposures have not shown malformations.

Acepril is contraindicated during the second and third trimesters of pregnancy. Prolonged captopril exposure during the second and third trimesters is known to induce toxicity in foetuses (decreased renal function, oligohydramnios, skull ossification retardation) and in neonates (neonatal renal failure, hypotension, hyperkalaemia) (see also 5.3).

Lactation: Acepril is contraindicated in the lactation period.

4.7 Effects on ability to drive and use machines

As with other antihypertensives, the ability to drive and use machines may be reduced, namely at the start of the treatment, or when posology is modified, and also when used in combination with alcohol, but these effects depend on the individual's susceptibility.

4.8 Undesirable effects

Undesirable effects reported for captopril and/or ACE inhibitor therapy include:

Blood and lymphatic disorders:

very rare: neutropenia/agranulocytosis (see 4.4), pancytopenia particularly in patients with renal dysfunction (see 4.4), anaemia (including aplastic and haemolytic), thrombocytopenia, lymphadenopathy, eosinophilia, autoimmune diseases and/or positive ANA-titres.

Metabolism and nutrition disorders:

rare: anorexia

very rare: hyperkalaemia, hypoglycaemia (see 4.4)

Psychiatric disorders:

common: sleep disorders

very rare: confusion, depression.

Nervous system disorders:

common: taste impairment, dizziness

rare: drowsiness, headache and paraesthesia

very rare: cerebrovascular incidents, including stroke, and syncope.

Eye disorders:

very rare: blurred vision

Cardiac disorders:

uncommon: tachycardia or tachyarrhythmia, angina pectoris, palpitations.

very rare: cardiac arrest, cardiogenic shock

Vascular disorders:

uncommon: hypotension (see 4.4), Raynaud syndrome, flush, pallor

Respiratory, thoracic and mediastinal disorders:

common: dry, irritating (non-productive) cough (see 4.4) and dyspnoea

very rare: bronchospasm, rhinitis, allergic alveolitis / eosinophilic pneumonia

Gastrointestinal disorders:

common: nausea, vomiting, gastric irritations, abdominal pain, diarrhoea, constipation, dry mouth.

rare: stomatitis/aphthous ulcerations

very rare: glossitis, peptic ulcer, pancreatitis.

Hepato-biliary disorders:

very rare: impaired hepatic function and cholestasis (including jaundice), hepatitis including necrosis, elevated liver enzymes and bilirubin.

Skin and subcutaneous tissue disorders:

common: pruritus with or without a rash, rash, and alopecia.

uncommon: angioedema (see 4.4)

very rare: urticaria, Stevens Johnson syndrome, erythema multiforme, photosensitivity, erythroderma, pemphigoid reactions and exfoliative dermatitis.

Musculoskeletal, connective tissue and bone disorders:

very rare: myalgia, arthralgia.

Renal and urinary disorders:

rare: renal function disorders including renal failure, polyuria, oliguria, increased urine frequency.

very rare: nephrotic syndrome.

Reproductive system and breast disorders:

very rare: impotence, gynaecomastia.

General disorders:

uncommon: chest pain, fatigue, malaise

very rare: fever

Investigations:

very rare: proteinuria, eosinophilia, increase of serum potassium, decrease of serum sodium, elevation of BUN, serum creatinine and serum bilirubin, decreases in haemoglobin, haematocrit, leucocytes, thrombocytes, positive ANA-titre, elevated ESR.

4.9 Overdose

Symptoms of overdosage are severe hypotension, shock, stupor, bradycardia, electrolyte disturbances and renal failure.

Measures to prevent absorption (e.g. gastric lavage, administration of adsorbents and sodium sulphate within 30 minutes after intake) and hasten elimination should be applied if ingestion is recent. If hypotension occurs, the patient should be placed in the shock position and salt and volume supplementations should be given rapidly. Treatment with angiotensin-II should be considered. Bradycardia or extensive vagal reactions should be treated by administering atropine. The use of a pacemaker may be considered.

Captopril may be removed from circulation by haemodialysis.

5. PHARMACOLOGICAL PROPERTIES

5.1 Pharmacodynamic properties

Pharmacotherapeutic group: ACE inhibitors, plain, ATC code: C09AA01.

Captopril is a highly specific, competitive inhibitor of angiotensin-I converting enzyme (ACE inhibitors).

The beneficial effects of ACE inhibitors appear to result primarily from the suppression of the plasma renin-angiotensin-aldosterone system. Renin is an endogenous enzyme synthesised by the kidneys and released into the circulation where it converts angiotensinogen to angiotensin-I, a relatively inactive decapeptide. Angiotensin-I is then converted by angiotensin converting enzyme, a peptidyldipeptidase, to angiotensin-II. Angiotensin-II is a potent vasoconstrictor responsible for arterial vasoconstriction and increased blood pressure, as well as for stimulation of the adrenal gland to secrete aldosterone. Inhibition of ACE results in decreased plasma angiotensin-II, which leads to decreased vasopressor activity and to reduced aldosterone secretion. Although the latter decrease is small, small increases in serum potassium concentrations may occur, along with sodium and fluid loss. The cessation of the negative feedback of angiotensin-II on the renin secretion results in an increase of the plasma renin activity.

Another function of the converting enzyme is to degrade the potent vasodepressive kinin peptide bradykinin to inactive metabolites. Therefore, inhibition of ACE results in an increased activity of circulating and local kallikrein-kinin-system which contributes to peripheral vasodilation by activating the prostaglandin system; it is possible that this mechanism is involved in the hypotensive effect of ACE inhibitors and is responsible for certain adverse reactions.

Reductions of blood pressure are usually maximal 60 to 90 minutes after oral administration of an individual dose of captopril. The duration of effect is dose related. The reduction in blood pressure may be progressive, so to achieve maximal therapeutic effects, several weeks of therapy may be required. The blood pressure lowering effects of captopril and thiazide-type diuretics are additive.

In patients with hypertension, captopril causes a reduction in supine and erect blood pressure, without inducing any compensatory increase in heart rate, nor water and sodium retention.

In haemodynamic investigations, captopril caused a marked reduction in peripheral arterial resistance. In general there were no clinically relevant changes in renal plasma flow or glomerular filtration rate. In most patients, the antihypertensive effect began about 15 to 30 minutes after oral administration of captopril; the peak effect was achieved after 60 to 90 minutes. The maximum reduction in blood pressure of a defined captopril dose was generally visible after three to four weeks.

In the recommended daily dose, the antihypertensive effect persists even during long-term treatment. Temporary withdrawal of captopril does not cause any rapid, excessive increase in blood pressure (rebound). The treatment of hypertension with captopril leads also to a decrease in left ventricular hypertrophy.

Haemodynamic investigations in patients with heart failure, showed that captopril caused a reduction in peripheral systemic resistance and a rise in venous capacity. This resulted in a reduction in pre-load and after-load of the heart (reduction in ventricular filling pressure). In addition, rises in cardiac output, work index and exercise capacity have been observed during treatment with captopril. In a large, placebo-controlled study in patients with left ventricular dysfunction (LVEF ≤40%) following myocardial infarction, it was shown that captopril (initiated between the 3rd to the 16th day after infarction) prolonged the survival time and reduced cardiovascular mortality. The latter was manifested as a delay in the development of symptomatic heart failure and a reduction in the necessity for hospitalisation due to heart failure compared to placebo. There was also a reduction in re-infarction and in cardiac revascularisation procedures and/or in the need for additional medication with diuretics and/or digitalis or an increase in their dosage compared to placebo.

A retrospective analysis showed that captopril reduced recurrent infarcts and cardiac revascularisation procedures (neither were target criteria of the study).

Another large, placebo-controlled study in patients with myocardial infarction showed that captopril (given within 24 hours of the event and for a duration of one month) significantly reduced overall mortality after 5 weeks compared to placebo. The favourable effect of captopril on total mortality was still detectable even after one year. No indication of a negative effect in relation to early mortality on the first day of treatment was found.

Captopril cardioprotection effects are observed regardless of the patient's age or gender, location of the infarction and concomitant treatments with proven efficacy during the post-infarction period (thrombolytic agents, beta-blockers and acetylsalicylic acid).

Type I diabetic nephropathy

In a placebo-controlled, multicentre double blind clinical trial in insulin-dependent (Type I) diabetes with proteinuria, with or without hypertension (simultaneous administration of other antihypertensives to control blood pressure was allowed), captopril significantly reduced (by 51%) the time to doubling of the baseline creatinine concentration compared to placebo; the incidence of terminal renal failure (dialysis, transplantation) or death was also significantly less common under captopril than under placebo (51%). In patients with diabetes and microalbuminuria, treatment with captopril reduced albumin excretion within two years.

The effects of treatment with captopril on the preservation of renal function are in addition to any benefit that may have been derived from the reduction in blood pressure.

5.2 Pharmacokinetic properties

Captopril is an orally active agent that does not require biotransformation for activity. The average minimal absorption is approximately 75%. Peak plasma concentrations are reached within 60-90 minutes. The presence of food in the gastrointestinal tract reduces absorption by about 30-40%. Approximately 25-30% of the circulating drug is bound to plasma proteins.

The apparent elimination half-life of unchanged captopril in blood is about 2 hours. Greater than 95% of the absorbed dose is eliminated in the urine within 24 hours; 40-50% is unchanged drug and the remainder are inactive disulphide metabolites (captopril disulphide and captopril cysteine disulphide). Impaired renal function could result in drug accumulation. Therefore, in patients with impaired renal function the dose should be reduced and/or dosage interval prolonged (see 4.2).

Studies in animals indicate that captopril does not cross the blood-brain barrier to any significant extent.

5.3 Preclinical safety data

Animal studies performed during organogenesis with captopril have not shown any teratogenic effect but captopril has produced foetal toxicity in several species, including foetal mortality during late pregnancy, growth retardation and postnatal mortality in the rat. Preclinical data reveal no other specific hazard for humans based on conventional studies of safety pharmacology, repeated dose toxicology, genotoxicity and carcinogenicity.

6. PHARMACEUTICAL PARTICULARS

6.1 List of excipients

Lactose, corn starch, microcrystalline cellulose, stearic acid.

6.2 Incompatibilities

None.

6.3 Shelf life

48 Months.

6.4 Special precautions for storage

Store below 30°C.

Protect from moisture.

6.5 Nature and contents of container

The 12.5mg tablets are available in blister packs of 56 tablets. The 25mg & 50mg tablets are available in blister packs of 56 and 84 tablets.

6.6 Instructions for use and handling

No special instructions.

7. MARKETING AUTHORISATION HOLDER

E.R. Squibb & Sons Limited
Uxbridge Business Park
Sanderson Road
Uxbridge
Middlesex UB8 1DH

8. MARKETING AUTHORISATION NUMBER(S)

12.5mg: 0034/0298

25mg: 0034/0299

50mg: 0034/0300

9. DATE OF FIRST AUTHORISATION/RENEWAL OF THE AUTHORISATION

3rd December 1995

10. DATE OF REVISION OF THE TEXT

June 2005

Acezide Tablets

(E. R. Squibb & Sons Limited)

1. NAME OF THE MEDICINAL PRODUCT

Acezide Tablets

2. QUALITATIVE AND QUANTITATIVE COMPOSITION

Each tablet contains 50 mg captopril and 25 mg hydrochlorothiazide.

For excipients, see 6.1.

3. PHARMACEUTICAL FORM

Tablets

4. CLINICAL PARTICULARS

4.1 Therapeutic indications

Treatment of essential hypertension.

This fixed dose combination is indicated in patients whose blood pressure is not adequately controlled by captopril alone or hydrochlorothiazide alone.

4.2 Posology and method of administration

Acezide can be administered in a single or two divided doses/day with or without food in patients whose blood pressure is not adequately controlled by captopril alone or hydrochlorothiazide alone. A maximum daily dose of 100 mg captopril/30 mg hydrochlorothiazide should not be exceeded. If satisfactory reduction of blood pressure has not been achieved, additional antihypertensive medication may be added (see 4.5).

Adults: The administration of the fixed combination of captopril and hydrochlorothiazide is usually recommended after dosage titration with the individual components. The usual maintenance dose is 50/25 mg, once a day, in the morning. When clinically appropriate a direct change from monotherapy to the fixed combination may be considered. The 25/25mg strength may be used once a day for patients whose blood pressure is not adequately controlled by hydrochlorothiazide 25 mg monotherapy and before titration of the captopril component. The 50/25mg and 25/25mg strengths are intended to be used once daily, as two tablets would result in an inappropriately high dose of hydrochlorothiazide (50mg/day). The 50/15 mg strength may be administered to start the fixed combination in patients whose blood pressure is not adequately controlled by 50 mg captopril monotherapy, and/or when a lower dose of hydrochlorothiazide is preferred.

The 25/25mg and 50/15mg tablet strengths are not available in the U.K.

Renal impairment: Creatinine clearance between 30 and 80 ml/min: the initial dose is usually 25/12.5 mg once a day, in the morning.

The combination captopril/hydrochlorothiazide is contraindicated in patients with severe renal impairment (creatinine clearance < 30 ml/min).

Special populations: In salt/volume depleted patients, elderly patients and diabetic patients, the usual starting dose is 25/12.5 mg once a day.

Children: The safety and efficacy of Acezide in children has not been established.

4.3 Contraindications

- History of hypersensitivity to captopril, to any of the excipients or any other ACE inhibitor.
- History of hypersensitivity to hydrochlorothiazide or other sulphonamide-derived drugs.
- History of angioedema associated with previous ACE inhibitor therapy.
- Hereditary/idiopathic angioneurotic oedema
- Severe renal impairment (creatinine clearance < 30 ml/min)
- Severe hepatic impairment.
- Second and third trimester of pregnancy (see 4.6)
- Lactation (see 4.6)

4.4 Special warnings and special precautions for use CAPTOPRIL

Hypotension: Rarely hypotension is observed in uncomplicated hypertensive patients. Symptomatic hypotension is more likely to occur in hypertensive patients who are volume and/or sodium depleted by vigorous diuretic therapy, dietary salt restriction, diarrhoea, vomiting, or haemodialysis. Volume and/or sodium depletion should be corrected before the administration of an ACE inhibitor and a lower starting dose should be considered.

As with any antihypertensive agent, excessive blood pressure lowering in patients with ischaemic cardiovascular or cerebrovascular disease may increase the risk of myocardial infarction or stroke. If hypotension develops, the patient should be placed in a supine position. Volume repletion with intravenous normal saline may be required.

Renovascular hypertension: There is an increased risk of hypotension and renal insufficiency when patients with bilateral renal artery stenosis or stenosis of the artery to a single functioning kidney are treated with ACE inhibitors. Loss of renal function may occur with only mild changes in serum creatinine. In these patients, therapy should be initiated under close medical supervision with low doses, careful titration and monitoring of renal function.

Angioedema: Angioedema of the extremities, face, lips, mucous membranes, tongue, glottis or larynx may occur in patients treated with ACE inhibitors, particularly during the first weeks of treatment. However, in rare cases, severe angioedema may develop after long-term treatment with an ACE inhibitor. Treatment should be discontinued promptly. Angioedema involving the tongue, glottis or larynx may be fatal. Emergency therapy should be instituted. The patient should be hospitalised and observed for at least 12 to 24 hours and should not be discharged until complete resolution of symptoms has occurred.

Cough: Cough has been reported with the use of ACE inhibitors. Characteristically, the cough is non-productive, persistent and resolves after discontinuation of therapy.

Hepatic failure: Rarely, ACE inhibitors have been associated with a syndrome that starts with cholestatic jaundice and progresses to fulminant hepatic necrosis and (sometimes) death. The mechanism of this syndrome is not understood. Patients receiving ACE inhibitors who develop jaundice or marked elevations of hepatic enzymes should discontinue the ACE inhibitors and receive appropriate medical follow-up.

Hyperkalaemia: Elevations in serum potassium have been observed in some patients treated with ACE inhibitors, including captopril. Patients at risk for the development of hyperkalaemia include those with renal insufficiency, diabetes mellitus, or those using concomitant potassium-sparing diuretics, potassium supplements or potassium-containing salt substitutes; or those patients taking other drugs associated with increases in serum potassium (e.g. heparin). If concomitant use of the above mentioned agents is deemed appropriate, regular monitoring of serum potassium is recommended.

Aortic and mitral valve stenosis / Obstructive hypertrophic cardiomyopathy / Cardiogenic shock: ACE inhibitors should be used with caution in patients with left ventricular valvular and outflow tract obstruction and avoided in cases of cardiogenic shock and haemodynamically significant obstruction.

Neutropenia/Agranulocytosis: Neutropenia/agranulocytosis, thrombocytopenia and anaemia have been reported in patients receiving ACE inhibitors, including captopril. In patients with normal renal function and no other complicating factors, neutropenia occurs rarely. Captopril should be used with extreme caution in patients with collagen vascular disease, immunosuppressant therapy, treatment with allopurinol or procainamide, or a combination of these complicating factors, especially if there is pre-existing impaired renal function. Some of these patients developed serious infections which in a few instances did not respond to intensive antibiotic therapy.

If captopril is used in such patients, it is advised that white blood cell count and differential counts should be performed prior to therapy, every 2 weeks during the first 3 months of captopril therapy, and periodically thereafter. During treatment all patients should be instructed to report any sign of infection (e.g. sore throat, fever) when a differential white blood cell count should be performed. Captopril and other concomitant medication (see 4.5) should be withdrawn if neutropenia (neutrophils less than 1000/mm^3) is detected or suspected.

In most patients neutrophil counts rapidly return to normal upon discontinuing captopril.

Proteinurea: proteinuria may occur particularly in patients with existing renal function impairment or on relatively high doses of ACE inhibitors.

Total urinary proteins greater than 1 g per day were seen in about 0.7% of patients receiving captopril. The majority of patients had evidence of prior renal disease or had received relatively high doses of captopril (in excess of 150 mg/day), or both. Nephrotic syndrome occurred in about one-fifth of proteinuric patients. In most cases, proteinuria subsided or cleared within six months whether or not captopril was continued. Parameters of renal function, such as BUN and creatinine, were seldom altered in the patients with proteinuria.

Patients with prior renal disease should have urinary protein estimations (dip-stick on first morning urine) prior to treatment, and periodically thereafter.

Anaphylactoid reactions during desensitisation: sustained life-threatening anaphylactoid reactions have been rarely reported for patients undergoing desensitising treatment with hymenoptera venom while receiving another ACE inhibitor. In the same patients, these reactions were avoided when the ACE inhibitor was temporarily withheld, but they reappeared upon inadvertent rechallenge. Therefore, caution should be used in patients treated with ACE inhibitors undergoing such desensitisation procedures.

Anaphylactoid reactions during high-flux dialysis/ lipoprotein apheresis membrane exposure: Anaphylactoid reactions have been reported in patients haemodialysed with high-flux dialysis membranes or undergoing low-density lipoprotein apheresis with dextran sulphate absorption. In these patients, consideration should be given to using a different type of dialysis membrane or a different class of medication.

Surgery/Anaesthesia: Hypotension may occur in patients undergoing major surgery or during treatment with anaesthetic agents that are known to lower blood pressure. If hypotension occurs, it may be corrected by volume expansion.

Diabetic patients: The glycaemia levels should be closely monitored in diabetic patients previously treated with oral antidiabetic drugs or insulin, namely during the first month of treatment with an ACE inhibitor.

As with other angiotensin converting enzyme inhibitors, Acezide is apparently less effective in lowering blood pressure in black people than in non-blacks, possibly because of higher prevalence of low-renin states in the black hypertensive population.

HYDROCHLOROTHIAZIDE

Renal impairment: In patients with renal disease, thiazides may precipitate azotaemia. Cumulative effects of the drug may develop in patients with impaired renal function. If progressive renal impairment becomes evident, as indicated by a rising non-protein nitrogen, careful reappraisal of therapy is necessary, with consideration given to discontinuing diuretic therapy (see 4.3).

Hepatic impairment: Thiazides should be used with caution in patients with impaired hepatic function or progressive liver disease, since minor alterations of fluid and electrolyte balance may precipitate hepatic coma (see 4.3).

Metabolic and endocrine effects: Thiazide therapy may impair glucose tolerance. In diabetic patients dosage adjustments of insulin or oral hypoglycaemic agents may be required. Latent diabetes mellitus may become manifest during thiazide therapy.

Increases in cholesterol and triglyceride levels have been associated with thiazide diuretic therapy.

Hyperuricaemia may occur or frank gout may be precipitated in certain patients receiving thiazide therapy.

Electrolyte imbalance: As for any patient receiving diuretic therapy, periodic determination of serum electrolytes should be performed at appropriate intervals.

Thiazides, including hydrochlorothiazide, can cause fluid or electrolyte imbalance (hypokalaemia, hyponatraemia and hypochloraemic alkalosis). Warning signs of fluid or electrolyte imbalance are dryness of mouth, thirst, weakness, lethargy, drowsiness, restlessness, muscle pain or cramps, muscular fatigue, hypotension, oliguria, tachycardia and gastrointestinal disturbances such as nausea or vomiting.

Although hypokalaemia may develop with the use of thiazide diuretics, concurrent therapy with captopril may reduce diuretic-induced hypokalaemia. The risk of hypokalaemia is greatest in patients with cirrhosis of the liver, in patients experiencing brisk diuresis, in patients who are receiving inadequate oral intake of electrolytes and in patients receiving concomitant therapy with corticosteroids or ACTH (see 4.5).

Dilutional hyponatraemia may occur in oedematous patients in hot weather. Chloride deficit is generally mild and usually does not require treatment.

Thiazides may decrease urinary calcium excretion and cause an intermittent and slight elevation of serum calcium in the absence of known disorders of calcium metabolism. Marked hypercalcaemia may be evidence of hidden hyperparathyroidism. Thiazides should be discontinued before carrying out tests for parathyroid function.

Thiazides have been shown to increase the urinary excretion of magnesium, which may result in hypomagnesaemia.

Anti-doping test: hydrochlorothiazide contained in this medication could produce a positive analytical result in an anti-doping test.

Other: Sensitivity reactions may occur in patients with or without a history of allergy or bronchial asthma. The possibility of exacerbation or activation of systemic lupus erythematosus has been reported.

CAPTOPRIL/HYDROCHLOROTHIAZIDE COMBINATION

Pregnancy: Acezide is not recommended during the first trimester of pregnancy (see 4.6). If treatment is discontinued due to pregnancy, the prescriber should decide whether treatment of hypertension should be continued.

Risk of hypokalaemia: The combination of an ACE inhibitor with a thiazide diuretic does not rule out the occurrence of hypokalaemia. Regular monitoring of kalaemia should be performed.

Combination with lithium: Acezide is not recommended in association with lithium due to the potentiation of lithium toxicity (see 4.5).

Lactose: Acezide contains lactose. Therefore, it should not be used in cases of congenital galactosaemia, glucose and galactose malabsorption or lactase deficiency syndromes (rare metabolic diseases).

4.5 Interaction with other medicinal products and other forms of Interaction

CAPTOPRIL

Potassium sparing diuretics or potassium supplements: ACE inhibitors attenuate diuretic induced potassium loss. Potassium sparing diuretics (e.g. spironolactone, triamterene or amiloride), potassium supplements, or potassium-containing salt substitutes may lead to significant increases in serum potassium. If concomitant use is indicated because of demonstrated hypokalaemia they should be used with caution and with frequent monitoring of serum potassium (see 4.4).

Diuretics (thiazide or loop diuretics): Prior treatment with high dose diuretics may result in volume depletion and a risk of hypotension when initiating therapy with captopril (see 4.4). The hypotensive effects can be reduced by discontinuation of the diuretic, by increasing volume or salt intake or by initiating therapy with a low dose of captopril. However, no clinically significant drug interactions have been found in specific studies with hydrochlorothiazide or furosemide.

Other antihypertensive agents: captopril has been safely co-administered with other commonly used anti-hypertensive agents (e.g. beta-blockers and long-acting calcium channel blockers). Concomitant use of these agents may increase the hypotensive effects of captopril. Nitroglycerine and other nitrates, or other vasodilators, should be used with caution.

Treatments of acute myocardial infarction: Captopril may be used concomitantly with acetylsalicylic acid (at cardiological doses), thrombolytics, beta-blockers and/or nitrates in patients with myocardial infarction.

Tricyclic antidepressants/Antipsychotics: ACE inhibitors may enhance the hypotensive effects of certain tricyclic antidepressants and antipsychotics (see 4.4). Postural hypotension may occur.

Allopurinol, procainamide, cytostatic or immunosuppressant agents: Concomitant administration with ACE inhibitors may lead to an increased risk of leucopenia, especially when the latter are used at higher than currently recommended doses.

Sympathomimetics: may reduce the antihypertensive effects of ACE inhibitors; patients should be carefully monitored.

Antidiabetics: Pharmacological studies have shown that ACE inhibitors, including captopril, can potentiate the blood glucose-reducing effects of insulin and oral antidiabetics, such as sulphonylurea, in diabetics. Should this very rare interaction occur, it may be necessary to reduce the dose of the antidiabetic during simultaneous treatment with ACE inhibitors.

HYDROCHLOROTHIAZIDE

Amphotericin B (parenteral), carbenoxolone, corticosteroids, corticotropin (ACTH) or stimulant laxatives: hydrochlorothiazide may intensify electrolyte imbalance, particularly hypokalaemia.

Calcium salts: Increased serum calcium levels due to decreased excretion may occur when administered concurrently with thiazide diuretics.

Cardiac glycosides: Enhanced possibility of digitalis toxicity associated with thiazide induced hypokalaemia.

Cholestyramine resin and colestipol: may delay or decrease absorption of hydrochlorothiazide. Sulphonamide diuretics should be taken at least one hour before or four to six hours after these medications.

Nondepolarising muscle relaxants (e.g. tubocurarine chloride): effects of these agents may be potentiated by hydrochlorothiazide.

Drugs associated with torsades de pointes: Because of the risk of hypokalaemia, caution should be used when hydrochlorothiazide is coadministered with drugs associated with torsades de pointes, e.g. some anti-arrhythmics, some antipsychotics and other drugs known to induce torsades de pointes.

CAPTOPRIL/HYDROCHLOROTHIAZIDE COMBINATION

Lithium: Reversible increases in serum lithium concentrations and toxicity have been reported during concomitant administration of lithium with ACE inhibitors. Concomitant use of thiazide diuretics may increase the risk of lithium toxicity and enhance the already increased risk of lithium toxicity with ACE inhibitors. The combination of captopril and hydrochlorothiazide with lithium is therefore not recommended and careful monitoring of serum lithium levels should be performed if the combination proves necessary.

Non-steroidal anti-inflammatory medicinal products: It has been described that non-steroidal anti-inflammatory medicinal products (NSAIDs) and ACE inhibitors exert an additive effect on the increase in serum potassium, whereas renal function may decrease. These effects are, in principle, reversible. Rarely, acute renal failure may occur, particularly in patients with compromised renal function such as the elderly or dehydrated. Chronic administration of NSAIDs may reduce the antihypertensive effect of an ACE inhibitor. The administration of NSAIDs may reduce the diuretic, natriuretic and antihypertensive effects of thiazide diuretics.

Clinical Chemistry

Captopril may cause a false-positive urine test for acetone. Hydrochlorothiazide may cause diagnostic interference of the bentiromide test. Thiazides may decrease serum PBI (Protein Bound Iodine) levels without signs of thyroid disturbance.

4.6 Pregnancy and lactation

Pregnancy: Acezide is not recommended during the first trimester of pregnancy. When a pregnancy is planned or confirmed, an alternative treatment should be initiated as soon as possible. Controlled studies with ACE inhibitors have not been done in humans, but a limited number of cases of first trimester exposures has not shown malformations.

Acezide is contraindicated during the second and third trimesters of pregnancy. Prolonged captopril exposure during the second and third trimesters is known to induce toxicity in foetuses (decreased renal function, oligohydramnios, skull ossification retardation) and in neonates (neonatal renal failure, hypotension, hyperkalaemia) (see also 5.3).

Hydrochlorothiazide, in cases of prolonged exposure during the third trimester of pregnancy, may cause a foetoplacental ischaemia and risk of growth retardation. Moreover, rare cases of hypoglycaemia and thrombocytopenia in neonates have been reported in case of exposure near term.

Hydrochlorothiazide can reduce plasma volume as well as the uteroplacental blood flow.

Should exposure to Acezide have occurred from the second trimester of pregnancy, ultrasound check of renal function and skull is recommended.

Lactation: Acezide is contraindicated in the lactation period.

Both captopril and hydrochlorothiazide are excreted in human milk. Thiazides during breast feeding by lactating mothers have been associated with a decrease or even suppression of lactation. Hypersensitivity to sulphonamide-derived drugs, hypokalaemia and nuclear icterus might occur.

Because of the potential for serious adverse reactions in nursing infants from both drugs, a decision should be made whether to discontinue nursing or to discontinue therapy, taking into account the importance of this therapy to the mother.

4.7 Effects on ability to drive and use machines

As with other antihypertensives, the ability to drive and use machines may be reduced, e.g. at the start of the treatment or when the dose is modified, and also when used in combination with alcohol, but these effects depend on the individual's susceptibility.

4.8 Undesirable effects

CAPTOPRIL

Undesirable effects reported for captopril and/or ACE inhibitor therapy include:

Blood and lymphatic disorders:

very rare: neutropenia/agranulocytosis (see 4.4), pancytopenia, particularly in patients with renal dysfunction (see 4.4), anaemia (including aplastic and haemolytic), thrombocytopenia, lymphadenopathy, eosinophilia, autoimmune diseases and/or positive ANA-titres.

Metabolism and nutrition disorders:

rare: anorexia

very rare: hyperkalaemia, hypoglycaemia (see 4.4)

Psychiatric disorders:

common: sleep disorders

very rare: confusion, depression

Nervous system disorders:

common: taste impairment, dizziness

rare: drowsiness, headache and paraesthesia

very rare: cerebrovascular incidents, including stroke, and syncope

Eye disorders:

very rare: blurred vision.

Cardiac disorders:

uncommon: tachycardia or tachyarrhythmia, angina pectoris, palpitations

very rare: cardiac arrest, cardiogenic shock.

Vascular disorders:

uncommon: hypotension (see 4.4), Raynaud syndrome, flush, pallor

Respiratory, thoracic and mediastinal disorders:

common: dry, irritating (non-productive) cough (see 4.4) and dyspnoea

very rare: bronchospasm, rhinitis, allergic alveolitis/ eosinophilic pneumonia

Gastrointestinal disorders:

common: nausea, vomiting, gastric irritations, abdominal pain, diarrhoea, constipation, dry mouth

rare: stomatitis/aphthous ulcerations

very rare: glossitis, peptic ulcer, pancreatitis

Hepato-biliary disorders:

very rare: impaired hepatic function and cholestasis (including jaundice), hepatitis including necrosis, elevated liver enzymes and bilirubin.

Skin and subcutaneous tissue disorders:

common: pruritus with or without a rash, rash, and alopecia

uncommon: angioedema (see 4.4)

very rare: urticaria, Stevens Johnson syndrome, erythema multiforme, photo-sensitivity, erythroderma, pemphigoid reactions and exfoliative dermatitis.

Musculoskeletal, connective tissue and bone disorders:

very rare: myalgia, arthralgia

Renal and urinary disorders:

rare: renal function disorders, including renal failure, polyuria, oliguria, increased urine frequency

very rare: nephrotic syndrome

Reproductive system and breast disorders:

very rare: impotence, gynaecomastia

General disorders;

uncommon: chest pain, fatigue, malaise

very rare: fever

Investigations:

very rare: proteinuria, eosinophilia, increase of serum potassium, decrease of serum sodium, elevation of BUN, serum creatinine and serum bilirubin, decreases in haemoglobin, haematocrit, leucocytes, thrombocytes, positive ANA-titre, elevated ESR.

HYDROCHLOROTHIAZIDE

Infections and infestations: sialadenitis

Blood and lymphatic system disorders:

leucopenia, neutropenia/agranulocytosis, thrombocytopenia, aplastic anaemia, haemolytic anaemia, bone marrow depression

Metabolism and nutrition disorders:

anorexia, hyperglycaemia, glycosuria, hyperuricaemia, electrolyte imbalance (including hyponatraemia and hypokalaemia), increases in cholesterol and triglycerides.

Psychiatric disorders:

restlessness, depression, sleep disturbances

Nervous system disorders:

loss of appetite, paraesthesia, light-headedness

Eye disorders:

xanthopsia, transient blurred vision

Ear and labyrinth disorders: vertigo

Cardiac disorders:

postural hypotension, cardiac arrhythmias

Vascular disorders:

necrotising angiitis (vasculitis, cutaneous vasculitis)

Respiratory, thoracic and mediastinal disorders:

respiratory distress (including pneumonitis and pulmonary oedema).

Gastrointestinal disorders:

gastric irritation, diarrhoea, constipation, pancreatitis

Hepato-biliary disorders:

jaundice (intrahepatic cholestatic jaundice)

Skin and subcutaneous tissue disorders:

photosensitivity reactions, rash, cutaneous lupus erythematosus-like reactions, reactivation of cutaneous lupus erythematosus, urticaria, anaphylactic reactions, toxic epidermal necrolysis.

Musculoskeletal, connective tissue and bone disorders: muscle spasm

Renal and urinary disorders:

renal dysfunction, interstitial nephritis

General disorders

fever, weakness

4.9 Overdose

Symptoms of overdosage are: increased diuresis, electrolyte imbalance, severe hypotension, depression of consciousness (including coma), convulsions, paresis, cardiac arrhythmias, bradycardia, renal failure.

Measures to prevent absorption (e.g. gastric lavage, administration of absorbing agents and sodium sulphate within 30 minutes of intake) and to hasten elimination should be applied if ingestion is recent. If hypotension occurs, the patient should be placed in the shock position and sodium chloride and volume supplementation should be given rapidly. Treatment with angiotensin-II can be considered. Bradycardia or extensive vagal reactions should be treated by administering atropine. The use of a pacemaker may be considered. Constant monitoring of water, electrolyte and acid base balance, and blood glucose is essential. In the event of hypokalaemia, potassium substitution is necessary.

Captopril may be removed from circulation by haemodialysis. The degree to which hydrochlorothiazide is removed by haemodialysis has not been established.

5. PHARMACOLOGICAL PROPERTIES

5.1 Pharmacodynamic properties

Pharmacotherapeutic group: ACE (Angiotensin-Converting-Enzyme) inhibitors, combinations, ATC code: C09BA01.

Acezide is a combination of an ACE inhibitor, captopril, and an antihypertensive diuretic, hydrochlorothiazide. The combination of these agents has an additive antihypertensive effect, reducing blood pressure to a greater degree than either component alone.

- Captopril is an angiotensin converting enzyme (ACE) inhibitor, i.e. it inhibits ACE, the enzyme involved in the conversion of angiotensin I to angiotensin II - a vasoconstrictor which also stimulates aldosterone secretion by the adrenal cortex.

Such inhibition leads to:

- reduced aldosterone secretion,

- increased plasma renin activity, since aldosterone no longer exerts negative feedback,

- a drop in total peripheral resistance (with a preferential effect on muscles and kidneys) which is not accompanied by water and sodium retention or reflex tachycardia during long-term treatment. Captopril also exerts its antihypertensive effect in subjects with low or normal renin concentrations.

Captopril is effective at all stages of hypertension, i.e. mild, moderate or severe. A reduction in supine and standing systolic and diastolic blood pressures is observed.

After a single dose, the antihypertensive effect is evident fifteen minutes post-dose and reaches a maximum between 1 h and 1.5 h after administration of the drug. Its duration of action is dose-dependent and varies from 6 to 12 hours.

Blood pressure becomes normalised (seated DBP <90mmHg) in patients after two weeks to one month of treatment and the drug retains its effectiveness over the course of time. Patients are also classified as responders if seated DBP decreased by 10% or more from baseline-BP.

Rebound hypertension does not occur when treatment is discontinued.

The treatment of hypertension with captopril leads to an increase in arterial compliance, a rise in renal blood flow without any significant drop in the glomerular filtration rate and a decrease in left ventricular hypertrophy.

- Hydrochlorothiazide is a thiazide diuretic which acts by inhibiting the reabsorption of sodium in the cortical diluting segment of renal tubules. It increases the excretion of sodium and chloride in urine and, to a lesser extent, the excretion of potassium and magnesium thereby increasing urinary output and exerting an antihypertensive effect.

The time to onset of diuretic activity is approximately 2 hours. Diuretic activity reaches a peak after 4 hours and is maintained for 6 to 12 hours. Above a certain dose, thiazide diuretics reach a plateau in terms of therapeutic effect whereas adverse reactions continue to multiply. When treatment is ineffective, increasing the dose beyond recommended doses serves no useful purpose and often gives rise to adverse reactions.

- The concomitant administration of captopril and hydrochlorothiazide in clinical trials led to greater reductions in blood pressure than when either of the products was administered alone.

The administration of captopril inhibits the renin angiotensin aldosterone system and tends to reduce hydrochlorothiazide-induced potassium loss.

Combination of an ACE inhibitor with a thiazide diuretic produces a synergistic effect and also lessens the risk of hypokalaemia provoked by the diuretic alone.

5.2 Pharmacokinetic properties

Captopril is quickly absorbed after oral administration and maximum serum concentrations are obtained around one hour after administration. Minimum mean absorption is approximately 75%. Peak plasma concentrations are reached within 60-90 minutes. The presence of food in the gastrointestinal tract reduces absorption by about 30-40%. Approximately 25-30% of the circulating drug is bound to plasma proteins. The apparent elimination half-life of unchanged captopril in blood is about 2 hours. Greater than 95% of the absorbed dose is eliminated in the urine within 24 hours; 40-50% is unchanged drug and the remainder are inactive disulphide metabolites (captopril disulphide and captopril cysteine disulphide). Impaired renal function could result in drug accumulation. Studies in animals indicate that captopril does not cross the blood-brain barrier to any significant extent.

Oral absorption of hydrochlorothiazide is relatively rapid. The mean plasma half-life in fasted individuals has been reported to be 5 to 15 hours. Hydrochloro-thiazide is eliminated rapidly by the kidney and excreted unchanged >95%) in the urine.

5.3 Preclinical safety data

Animal studies performed during organogenesis with captopril and/or hydrochlorothiazide have not shown any teratogenic effect but captopril has produced foetal toxicity in several species, including foetal mortality during late pregnancy, growth retardation and postnatal mortality in the rat. Preclinical data reveal no other specific hazard for humans based on conventional studies of safety pharmacology, repeated dose toxicology, genotoxicity and carcinogenicity.

6. PHARMACEUTICAL PARTICULARS

6.1 List of excipients

Lactose, magnesium stearate, maize starch, microcrystalline cellulose, stearic acid.

6.2 Incompatibilities

None.

6.3 Shelf life

36 months.

6.4 Special precautions for storage

Store below 30°C. Protect from moisture.

6.5 Nature and contents of container

The tablets are packaged in PVC/PVDC blister / foil strips of 28 tablets per carton.

6.6 Instructions for use and handling

No special instructions.

7. MARKETING AUTHORISATION HOLDER

E.R. Squibb & Sons Limited
Uxbridge Business Park
Sanderson Road
Uxbridge
Middlesex UB8 1DH

8. MARKETING AUTHORISATION NUMBER(S)

PL 0034/0301

9. DATE OF FIRST AUTHORISATION/RENEWAL OF THE AUTHORISATION

28th November 1990 / 8th November 2001

10. DATE OF REVISION OF THE TEXT

June 2005

Distributed in the United Kingdom by: Ashbourne Pharmaceuticals Limited, Victors Farm, Hill Farm, Brixworth, Northampton NN6 9DQ

Achromycin Capsules 250mg

(Wyeth Pharmaceuticals)

1. NAME OF THE MEDICINAL PRODUCT

Achromycin capsules 250mg.

2. QUALITATIVE AND QUANTITATIVE COMPOSITION

Each capsule contains Tetracycline hydrochloride BP 250mg.

3. PHARMACEUTICAL FORM

Orange capsule printed with "Lederle 4874" in black ink.

For oral administration.

4. CLINICAL PARTICULARS

4.1 Therapeutic indications

ACHROMYCIN is a broad-spectrum antibiotic used for the treatment of infections caused by tetracycline-sensitive organisms.

For example, ACHROMYCIN is highly effective in the treatment of infections caused by Borrellia recurrentis (relapsing fever), Calymmatobacterium granulomatis (granuloma inguinale), Chlamydia species (psittacosis, lymphogranuloma venereum, trachoma, inclusion conjunctivitis), Francisella tularensis (tularaemia), Haemophilus ducreyi (chancroid), Leptospira (meningitis, jaundice), Mycoplasma pneumoniae (non-gonococcal urethritis), Pseudomonas mallei and pseudomallei (glanders and melioidosis), Rickettsiae (typhus fever, Q fever, rocky mountain spotted fever), Vibrio species (cholera). It is also highly effective, alone or in combination with streptomycin, in the treatment of infections due to Brucella species (brucellosis) and Yersinia pestis (bubonic plague). Severe acne vulgaris.

Other sensitive organisms include: Actinomyces israelii, Bacillus anthracis (pneumonia), Clostridium species (gas gangrene, tetanus). Entamoeba histolytica (dysentery), Neisseria gonorrhoeae, and anaerobic species, Treponema pallidum and pertenu (syphilis and yaws).

4.2 Posology and method of administration

Adults: One capsule four times a day. This may be increased to six or eight capsules daily in severe infections.

Children: Not recommended for children under 12 years of age. For children above the age of twelve years, the dose is 25-50mg/kg a day divided in 2 or 4 equal doses. The maximum dose should not exceed the recommended adult dosage.

Elderly: ACHROMYCIN should be used with caution in the treatment of elderly patients where accumulation is a possibility.

In patients with renal and/or liver impairment: Tetracyclines should be used cautiously in patients with impaired liver function. Total dosage should be decreased by reduction of recommended individual doses and/or extending the time intervals between doses. See Section 4.4 Special Warnings and Special Precautions for Use

Administration: ACHROMYCIN should be swallowed whole with plenty of fluid while sitting or standing to wash down the drugs and reduce the risk of oesophageal irritation and ulceration. Doses should be taken at least an hour before or two hours after meals. It should be noted that absorption of tetracyclines is impaired by foods and some dairy products, antacids containing aluminium, calcium or magnesium, and by iron-containing preparations. Therapy should be continued for up to three days after characteristic symptoms of the infection have subsided.

4.3 Contraindications
A history of hypersensitvity to tetracyclines or any of the components of the formulation. Overt renal insufficiency. Children under 12 years of age. Use during pregnancy or during lactation in women breast feeding infants is contraindicated (see also Section 4.6 Pregnancy and Lactation).

4.4 Special warnings and special precautions for use
Use in children:

The use of tetracyclines during tooth development in children under the age of 12 years may cause permanent discolouration. Enamel hypoplasia has also been reported.

ACHROMYCIN should be used with caution in patients with renal or hepatic dysfunction or in conjunction with other potentially hepatotoxic or nephrotoxic drugs.

Concurrent use with the anaesthetic methoxyflurane increases the risk of kidney failure and has been reported to result in fatal kidney failure. The anti-anabolic action of the tetracyclines may cause an increase in BUN.

Lower doses are indicated in cases of renal impairment to avoid excessive systemic accumulation, and if therapy is prolonged, serum level determinations are advisable. Patients who have known liver disease should not receive more than 1g daily. In long term therapy, periodic laboratory evaluation of organ systems, including haematopoietic, renal and hepatic studies should be performed.

Photosensitivity manifested by an exaggerated sunburn reaction has been observed in some individuals taking tetracyclines. Patients apt to be exposed to direct sunlight or ultraviolet light should be advised that this reaction can occur with tetracycline drugs, be warned to avoid direct exposure to natural or artificial sunlight and that treatment should be discontinued at the first evidence of skin erythema or skin discomfort.

Cross resistance between tetracyclines may develop in micro-organisms and cross-sensitisation in patients. ACHROMYCIN should be discontinued if there are signs/symptoms of overgrowth of resistant organisms including candida, enteritis, glossitis, stomatitis, vaginitis, pruritis ani or Staphylococcal enterocolitis.

Patients taking oral contraceptives should be warned that if diarrhoea or breakthrough bleeding occur there is a possibility of contraceptive failure.

4.5 Interaction with other medicinal products and other forms of Interaction
ACHROMYCIN should not be used with penicillins. Tetracyclines depress plasma prothrombin activity and reduced doses of concomitant anticoagulants may be required.

Absorption of ACHROMYCIN is impaired by the concomitant administration of iron, calcium, zinc, magnesium and particularly aluminium salts, commonly used in antacids. Absorption of tetracyclines is also impaired by food and some dairy products.

The concomitant use of tetracyclines may reduce the efficacy of oral contraceptives; an increased incidence of breakthrough bleeding may also be experienced.

The concurrent use of tetracycline and methoxyflurane has been reported to result in fatal renal toxicity.

4.6 Pregnancy and lactation
Use in pregnancy:

Contraindicated in pregnancy.

Results of animal studies indicate that tetracyclines cross the placenta, are found in foetal tissues and can have toxic effects on the developing foetus (often related to retardation of skeletal development). Evidence of embryotoxicity has also been noted in animals treated early in pregnancy. ACHROMYCIN therefore, should not be used in pregnancy unless considered essential in which case the maximum daily dose should be 1g. If any tetracycline is used during pregnancy, or if the patient becomes pregnant while taking these drugs, the patient should be informed of the potential hazard to the foetus.

The use of drugs of the tetracycline class during tooth development (last half of pregnancy) may cause permanent discolouration of the teeth (yellow-grey-brown). This adverse reaction is more common during long-term use of the drugs but has been observed after repeated short term courses. Enamel hypoplasia has also been reported.

Use in lactation:

Contraindicated during lactation in women breast feeding infants.

Tetracyclines have been found in the milk of lactating women who are taking a drug in this class. Permanent tooth discolouration may occur in the developing infant and enamel hypoplasia has been reported. Therefore ACHROMYCIN should not be administered to lactating women.

4.7 Effects on ability to drive and use machines
Headache, dizziness, visual disturbances and rarely impaired hearing have been reported with tetracyclines and patients should be warned about the possible hazards of driving or operating machinery during treatment.

4.8 Undesirable effects
Blood and Lymphatic System Disorders:

Haemolytic anaemia, thrombocytopenia, neutropenia, eosinophilia, agranulocytosis, aplastic anaemia

Ear and Labyrinth Disorders:

Tinnitus

Eye Disorders:

Visual disturbances

Gastrointestinal Disorders:

Nausea, vomiting, diarrhoea, glossitis, dysphagia, enterocolitis, pancreatitis, increases in liver enzymes, hepatitis and liver failure. Instances of oesophagitis and oesophageal ulcerations have been reported in patients receiving particularly the capsule and also the tablet forms of tetracyclines. Most of these patients were reported to have taken the medication immediately before going to bed.

Tooth discolouration in paediatric patients less than 12 years of age and also, rarely, in adults.

Immune System Disorders:

Anaphylaxis, anaphylactoid purpura, serum sickness-like reactions

Infections and Infestations:

Candidal overgrowth in the anogenital region.

Metabolism and Nutrition Disorders:

Anorexia

Nervous System Disorders:

Pseudomotor cerebri (benign intracranial hypertension) in adults, bulging fontanels in infants, dizziness, headache

Renal and Urinary Disorders:

Elevations in urea are often dose related. Acute renal failure.

Skin and Subcutaneous Tissue Disorders:

Urticaria, angioneurotic oedema, maculopapular and erythematous rashes, exfoliative dermatitis, fixed drug eruptions including balanitis, erythema multiforme, Stevens-Johnson syndrome, photosensitivity.

4.9 Overdose
No specific antidote. In case of overdosage, discontinue medication, treat symptomatically, and institute supportive measures (gastric lavage plus oral administration of milk or antacids). Tetracyclines are not removed in significant quantities by haemodialysis or peritoneal dialysis.

5. PHARMACOLOGICAL PROPERTIES

5.1 Pharmacodynamic properties
Tetracycline hydrochloride is a broad spectrum antibiotic.

It is active against a large number of Gram-negative and Gram-positive pathogenic bacteria, including some which are resistant to penicillin.

5.2 Pharmacokinetic properties
Tetracyclines are incompletely and irregularly absorbed from the gastro-intestinal tract. Absorption is affected by soluble salts of divalent and trivalent metals, milk and food. Doses of 250 to 500mg orally every six hours usually produce therapeutically effective plasma concentrations ranging from 1 to 3μg per ml and 1.5 to 5μg per ml respectively. 24 to 65% of circulating tetracycline is bound to plasma proteins. They are distributed throughout the body tissues and fluids. Tetracyclines are retained at sites of new bone formation and recent calcification.

The biological half-life of tetracycline is approximately 8.5 hours. The tetracyclines are excreted in the urine and faeces.

5.3 Preclinical safety data
Carcinogenesis, Mutagenesis, Impairment of Fertility

Dietary administration of tetracycline hydrochloride at levels of 0, 12, 500, or 25000 ppm to rats and mice in long-term carcinogenesis studies produced no evidence of carcinogenic activity of tetracycline hydrochloride. However there has been evidence of oncogenic activity in rats in studies with the related antibiotics oxytetracycline (adrenal and pituitary tumours) and minocycline (thyroid tumours).

In two *in vitro* mammalian cell assay systems (i.e., mouse lymphoma and Chinese hamster lung cells), there was evidence of mutagenicity at tetracycline hydrochloride concentrations of 60 and 10 μg/mL, respectively.

Tetracycline hydrochloride had no effect on fertility when administered in the diet to male and female rats at a daily intake of 25 times the human dose.

6. PHARMACEUTICAL PARTICULARS

6.1 List of excipients
Starch modified - dried, Magnesium stearate.

Capsule shell contains: Gelatin, Erythrocine (E127), Quinoline yellow (E104), Titanium dioxide (E171).

Ink used for the capsule marking contains: Shellac, N-Butyl alcohol, Purified water, Soya lecithin MC thin, Simethicone, Industrial methylated spirit 74 OP, Iron oxide black CI 77499 (E172).

6.2 Incompatibilities
None known.

6.3 Shelf life
36 months.

6.4 Special precautions for storage
Store at room temperature in the original container.

6.5 Nature and contents of container
Tamper evident, polypropylene bottles with screw on caps or screw capped glass bottle (pack size: 20, 28).

Polypropylene bottles with screw on caps or blister packs (pack size: 100, 1000).

6.6 Instructions for use and handling
None.

7. MARKETING AUTHORISATION HOLDER
Cyanamid of Great Britain Ltd, Cyanamid House, Fareham Road, GOSPORT, Hampshire, PO13 0AS, UK.

8. MARKETING AUTHORISATION NUMBER(S)
PL 0095/0041.

9. DATE OF FIRST AUTHORISATION/RENEWAL OF THE AUTHORISATION
26 August 1977/25 February 1999

10. DATE OF REVISION OF THE TEXT
25th July 2002.

Aciclovir 200mg Tablets

(Pharmacia Limited)

1. NAME OF THE MEDICINAL PRODUCT
Aciclovir 200mg Tablets

2. QUALITATIVE AND QUANTITATIVE COMPOSITION
Each tablet contains 200mg Aciclovir Ph Eur.

3. PHARMACEUTICAL FORM
Dispersible tablet.

4. CLINICAL PARTICULARS

4.1 Therapeutic indications
Management of herpes simplex, especially herpes genitalis infections of skin and mucous membranes (first as well as recurrent episodes of herpes genitalis).

Prophylactic treatment with Aciclovir 200mg Tablets is indicated in patients with severe recurrent episodes of herpes simplex.

4.2 Posology and method of administration
Dose:
Adults with herpes simplex infections:
200mg of aciclovir every four hours, (five times daily).

In severely immunocompromised patients or in patients where enteral absorption is reduced, aciclovir may be administered by intravenous infusion.

Prevention of severe and recurrent episodes of herpes simplex genitalis infections:
Immunocompetent patients should receive 200mg of aciclovir every six hours (four times daily) or as an alternative, 400mg of aciclovir every twelve hours, (twice daily). In some cases, effective prophylactic treatment with doses of 200mg aciclovir every eight hours, (three times daily) or 200mg of aciclovir every twelve hours, (twice daily) may be sufficient.

In case of relapse despite the daily administration of 800mg aciclovir, 200mg aciclovir every four hours, (five times daily) for five days is recommended (see recommended dosage for herpes simplex infections). Following this a four times daily dose should be administered.

Immunocompromised patients should receive 200mg of aciclovir every six hours, (four times daily) for prophylactic treatment.

Severely immunocompromised patients (e.g. following transplantations) should receive 400mg aciclovir every six hours (four times per day). In patients where enteral absorption is reduced, aciclovir may be administered by intravenous infusion.

Children:
For the treatment of herpes simplex infections, children over the age of two years should receive the dosage recommended for adults. Children under the age of two years should receive half of the adult dosage.

Dosage for patients with Renal Impairment:
(see Table 1 on next page)

Length of treatment:
Therapy with Aciclovir 200mg Tablets should be initiated at the earliest sign or symptom of an infection. In recurrent episodes of herpes simplex infections therapy with Aciclovir 200mg Tablets should be started at the earliest sign of recurrence (e.g. itching, burning, first vesicles).

In herpes simplex infections, treatment should be continued for five days. If the clinical benefit observed is not satisfactory, treatment may be prolonged.

For the prevention of recurrent episodes of herpes simplex in nonimmuno-compromised patients, the length of treatment depends on the severity and frequency of recurrent episodes. Six to twelve months should not be exceeded.

In severely immunocompromised patients, the length of prophylactic treatment depends on the severity of the immunodeficiency and on how long a higher risk of infection persists.

Patients with renal impairment (particularly elderly patients) should drink sufficient quantities of fluid during treatment with Aciclovir 200mg Tablets.

Table 1 Dosage for patients with Renal Impairment

Indication	Creatinine clearance (mg/ml/1.73m²)	Serum creatinine (μmol/l or mg/dl)		Dosage
		Women	Men	
Herpes simplex	< 10	> 550 / > 6.22	> 750 / > 8.48	200mg aciclovir twice daily (every 12 hours)

Method of administration:
Tablets should be taken after meals. They may be dissolved in a quarter of a glass of water with stirring before drinking or swallowed whole with a drink of water.

4.3 Contraindications
Aciclovir 200mg Tablets should not be given to patients with hypersensitivity to aciclovir.

There are no adequate studies concerning the prophylactic use of Aciclovir 200mg Tablets in patients with renal impairment or anuria, Aciclovir 200mg Tablets should not be used in these patients.

4.4 Special warnings and special precautions for use
None.

4.5 Interaction with other medicinal products and other forms of Interaction
Probenecid has been shown to reduce the renal clearance of aciclovir by approximately 30%, resulting in an increase of its mean elimination half-life.

4.6 Pregnancy and lactation
Pregnancy:
There is little experience of the administration of oral aciclovir during pregnancy. The use of Aciclovir 200mg Tablets in women who are, or may become pregnant requires that an expected benefit is weighed against the possible risks, particularly in the first trimester.

Systemic administration (oral and intravenous administration) of aciclovir during the second and third trimester of pregnancy has been described in at least 72 cases without any harm to the foetus.

Lactation:
After oral administration of 200mg aciclovir, five times daily, aciclovir concentrations found in breast milk were 0.6 — 4.1 times the corresponding aciclovir plasma concentrations. The infant would then receive up to 0.3mg/kg/day. Mothers should stop nursing during treatment with Aciclovir 200mg Tablets.

4.7 Effects on ability to drive and use machines
Aciclovir 200mg Tablets are unlikely to impair a patient's ability to drive or to use machines.

4.8 Undesirable effects
The following side effects have been observed after administration of Aciclovir 200mg Tablets:

Cutaneous reactions that usually disappear after cessation of therapy, gastrointestinal disorders such as nausea, vomiting, diarrhoea and abdominal pain.

Occasionally: Neurological reactions such as vertigo, confusion, hallucinations, somnolence. The side effects disappear after cessation of therapy and are usually observed in patients suffering from renal impairment or other diseases favouring the occurrence of these side effects.

Rarely: Increased levels of bilirubin, liver enzymes, serum urea and creatinine; decrease in haematological parameters.

Rare cases of headache, exhaustion, insomnia or fatigue have been observed. In isolated cases, depersonalization occurred which disappeared after treatment was discontinued. Rare cases of respiratory disorders have been reported.

Anaphylaxis, hepatitis, jaundice and acute renal failure have been reported on very rare occasions.

Occasionally, diffuse loss of hair occurred. A causal relationship with aciclovir could not been determined.

Reports on convulsive seizures and psychoses have occurred with aciclovir infusions (i.v.).

4.9 Overdose
Aciclovir is only partly absorbed from the gastrointestinal tract. Given the pharmacokinetic properties of aciclovir, intoxication from overdosage is not expected after oral administration.

Doses of 5g of aciclovir have been administered without signs of intoxication. An unvoluntary intravenous dose of 80mg/kg has been administered without acute side effects.

Treatment for overdose:
Aciclovir may be removed by haemodialysis.

5. PHARMACOLOGICAL PROPERTIES

5.1 Pharmacodynamic properties
Aciclovir is a pharmacologically inactive guanosine analogue that only becomes a virustatic agent after penetrating into a cell infected by herpes simplex virus (HSV) or varicella zoster virus (VZV). The activation of the aciclovir is catalysed by HSV or VZV thymidine kinase, an enzyme that the virus depends on for replication. In simplified terms, the virus synthesizes its own virustatic agent. The process goes as follows:

1. Aciclovir preferentially penetrates into cells infected with the herpes virus.

2. The enzyme thymidine kinase of these cells converts aciclovir to aciclovir monophosphate.

3. Cellular enzymes further convert aciclovir monophosphate to the virustatic agent aciclovir triphosphate.

4. The affinity of aciclovir triphosphate to viral DNA polymerase is 10 to 30 times higher than its affinity to cellular DNA polymerase. It thus selectively inhibits viral enzyme activity.

5. Furthermore, viral DNA polymerase incorporates aciclovir into viral DNA. This causes termination of DNA chain synthesis.

These steps lead to an efficient reduction of virus production.

With the plaque reduction test, an ED_{50} of 0.1μmol aciclovir/l was found in HSV infected Vero cells (green monkey kidney parechyma cells). However, an ED_{50} of 300μmol aciclovir/l was necessary to inhibit growth of uninfected Vero cells. Thus therapeutic indices of up to 3000 were found for cultured cells.

In vitro susceptibility:
Very sensitive: Herpes simplex virus type 1 and 2 (HSV-1, HSV-2),

Varicella zoster virus

Sensitive: Epstein Barr virus

Less sensitive or resistant: Cytomegalovirus

Resistant: RNA viruses, Adenoviruses, Poxviruses

In severely immunocompromised patients, prolonged or repeated treatment may lead to a selection of viral strains with diminished sensitivity, with the consequence that these patients possibly do not respond any more to treatment with aciclovir.

Most of less sensitive HSV clinical isolates have been relatively deficient in the viral thymidine kinase. However, strains with alterations in viral thymidine kinase or viral DNA polymerase have also been reported. Exposure of HSV isolates to aciclovir in vitro may also result in the emergence of less sensitive strains. The relationship between in vitro susceptibility of HSV isolates to aciclovir and the clinical response to therapy has not been established yet.

5.2 Pharmacokinetic properties
Aciclovir is only partly absorbed from the gastrointestinal tract. Mean steady state peak plasma levels following repeated oral administration of 200mg, 400mg and 800mg aciclovir every four hours (five times per day) were 3.02 ± 0.5μmol/l (200mg), 5.21 ± 1.32 μmol/l (400mg) and 8.16 ± 1.98 μmol/l (800mg), respectively.

These concentrations were reached after about 1.5 ± 0.6 hours. The corresponding basic plasma values about four hours after oral administration of aciclovir were 1.61 ± 0.3 μmol/l (200mg), 2.59 ± 0.52 μmol/l (400mg) and 4.0± 0.72 μmol/l (800mg), respectively. 24 hours after aciclovir treatment is discontinued there is no aciclovir detectable in the organism.

In immunocompromised children aged three to eleven years receiving aciclovir orally in doses of 400mg five times per day (corresponding to 300 — 650mg aciclovir/m² body surface), mean peak plasma levels reached 5.7 — 15.1 μmol/l. In infants aged one to six weeks receiving aciclovir orally in doses of 600mg aciclovir/m² body surface every six hours, mean peak plasma levels reached 17.3 and 8.6 μmol/l, respectively.

It can be deduced from the biexponential character of aciclovir kinetics that aciclovir enters tissues and organs in high concentrations and that aciclovir is only slowly eliminated.

The distribution volume in adults (steady state) is 50 ± 8.7 l/1.73m², in new-born and infants up to three months it is 28.8 ± 9.3 l/1.73m².

Protein binding ranged between 9% and 33%.

Distribution in body organs:
Animal studies show that, compared to serum concentrations, higher levels are reached in intestine, kidney, liver and lung, while lower levels are reached in muscle, heart, ovaries and testes.

Post mortem examinations in man have shown that aciclovir reaches high concentrations in the saliva, vaginal secretion, in the liquid found inside the herpes vesicles and in some other body organs. 50% of the respective serum concentrations are reached in liquor.

Metabolism and elimination:
In patients with normal renal function aciclovir is renally eliminated as unchanged drug (62 — 91%) and as 9-carboxymethoxymethyl-guanine (10 — 15%). Plasma half-life ($t_{1/2\beta}$) after intravenous administration of aciclovir is 2.87± 0.76 hours for adults and 4.1 ± 1.2 hours for new-born and infants under the age of three months. There is glomerular filtration as well as tubular secretion of aciclovir. When aciclovir is administered one hour after the administration of 1g of probenecid, plasma half-life ($t_{1/2\beta}$) is prolonged by 18% and the area under the curve for plasma concentrations is enlarged by 40%. Bioavailability is about 20%; 80% of the total aciclovir administered is excreted with faeces.

In patients suffering from chronic renal insufficiency, average plasma half-life is about 19.5 hours. Mean plasma half-life during haemodialysis is 5.7 hours. During haemodialysis a decrease of aciclovir plasma levels of about 60% occurs.

Although the treatment of herpes simplex infections in patients with renal impairment did not produce higher aciclovir concentrations n plasma than those normally found after intravenous administration, the dosage should be reduced if clearance of creatinine is below 10ml/min/1.73m² (see section 4.2 on dosage).

In patients with impaired renal function there is a risk of aciclovir accumulation if clearance of creatinine is < 25ml/min/1.73m² (for a dosage of 800mg five times per day). A dosage reduction is then indicated (see also section 4.2 on dosage).

5.3 Preclinical safety data
Acute toxicity:
The LD_{50} after oral aciclovir in mice and rats could not be determined because doses of 10g/kg in mice and 20g/kg in rats could not be exceeded for physiological reasons. The animals survived administration of these doses.

Subacute toxicity:
Mice were administered aciclovir orally for a period of four weeks in doses up to 450 mg/kg. All animals survived and showed no abnormalities.

Chronic toxicity:
Beagles were administered aciclovir orally for a period of twelve months in doses of up to 60 mg/kg per day. Under this dosage mucoid diarrhoea and vomiting occurred frequently. In some dogs, paw abnormalities and loss of claws were observed. However, these signs were reversible. No other abnormalities were observed.

Rats and mice were administered aciclovir for a period of 775 days in daily doses up to 450 mg/kg without abnormalities.

Mutagenesis:
The following tests showed no mutagenic effects:

Ames test with Salmonella typhimurium, mammalian cells (CHO cells), mouse lymphoma test (6-thioguanine-, AA- and Ouabaine resistance) in vitro, dominant lethal study in vivo in mice (25 and 50 mg/kg i.p.) and lymphocytes of patients having received 5 mg/kg of aciclovir i.v. three times daily for five days or 200mg aciclovir orally five times daily.

In the following tests mutagenicity was observed for high, partly cytotoxic concentrations of aciclovir:

Mouse lymphoma cells at thymidine kinase ($TK^{+/-}$) locus. Since the TK locus is special as far as the activation of aciclovir is concerned, clones may have appeared as a result of chromosomal damage but also as a result of selection.

In cultured human lymphocytes (in vitro) a positive response for chromosomal breaks was only seen at concentrations higher than 550 μmol/l. In vivo, chromosomal breaks were observed in bone marrow cells of female rats at concentrations of 100 mg/kg i.v. There was no chromosomal damage in cells of male rats.

While i.p. administration of 100 mg/kg aciclovir caused no chromosomal damage in Chinese hamsters, treatment with 500 mg/kg, a dose which is generally toxic, did. Doses of 50 mg/kg i.v. administered to rats and Chinese hamsters did not lead to any chromosomal breaks. This corresponds to a no-effect-level of 200 μmol/l.

Determination of gonadal aciclovir levels after intravenous administration of aciclovir to male and female rats revealed concentrations that were 1/3 of the "no-effect-level" in female rats and less than 1/10 of the "no-effect-level" in male rats.

Even if an oral maximum dose of five times 800mg aciclovir is administered, a potential threshold value for a possible mutagenic effect of aciclovir will not be reached. Therefore, a mutagenic risk is not to be expected.

Carcinogenesis:
In in vitro cell transformation assays with mouse fibroblasts, aciclovir caused an altered proliferation behaviour of the monolayer cell cultures (type 111 foci) at a concentration of 220 μmol/l.

Long-term studies (two years) conducted in rats and mice showed no carcinogenicity of aciclovir.

Reproduction toxicology:
Teratogenic effect/embryotoxicity
In rats, no maternal toxic effects or abnormalities/anomalies of foetuses or newborn animals were observed following subcutaneous administration of up to 25mg aciclovir twice daily during organogenesis between day 7 and day 17/day 6 and day 15 of pregnancy.

In studies conducted with rabbits, no maternal toxic effects or negative effects on the development of the foetuses or embryos were observed following intravenous or subcutaneous administration of up to 25mg aciclovir/kg twice daily during organogenesis between day six and day eighteen of pregnancy.

In a further test in rats using subcutaneous administration of 100mg aciclovir/kg three times on day ten of pregnancy (during organogenesis) foetal abnormalities such as anophthalmia and tail abnormalities were observed.

At the same dose, maternal toxic effects (nephrotoxicity) were observed. In addition, maternal aciclovir plasma concentrations were 43-58, 67-90 and 153-167 times higher than those found in man (steady state, mean plasma concentrations) after repeated administration of 800mg, 400mg or 200mg every four hours (five times daily). The clinical relevance of these findings is uncertain.

Fertility

Mostly reversible impairment of spermatogenesis in rats and beagles was observed after administration of aciclovir at very high doses, higher than normal therapeutic doses.

Aciclovir did not impair fertility over two generations of mice who received up to 450 mg/kg/day orally.

There are no adequate studies of orally administered aciclovir and fertility in women. In men, orally administered aciclovir has no effect on the number, morphology and motility of sperms.

6. PHARMACEUTICAL PARTICULARS

6.1 List of excipients

Microcrystalline Cellulose Ph Eur, Sodium Starch Glycollate Ph Eur, Colloidal Anhydrous Silica Ph Eur, Magnesium Stearate Ph Eur.

6.2 Incompatibilities

None.

6.3 Shelf life

The shelf life is three years.

6.4 Special precautions for storage

Store below +25°C.

6.5 Nature and contents of container

Blister strip comprising aluminium foil on one side and PVC on the other and containing 25 tablets per strip. One strip is contained in a carton.

6.6 Instructions for use and handling

None.

7. MARKETING AUTHORISATION HOLDER

TAD Pharma GmbH

Heinz-Lohmann-Strasse 5

27472 Cuxhaven

Germany

Tel: +49 (0) 4721/606-0

Fax: +49 (0) 4721/606-266

8. MARKETING AUTHORISATION NUMBER(S)

United Kingdom: PL 04986/0004

9. DATE OF FIRST AUTHORISATION/RENEWAL OF THE AUTHORISATION

22 November 1996

10. DATE OF REVISION OF THE TEXT

June 2001

LEGAL CATEGORY

POM

Aciclovir 400mg Tablets

(Pharmacia Limited)

1. NAME OF THE MEDICINAL PRODUCT

Aciclovir 400mg Tablets

2. QUALITATIVE AND QUANTITATIVE COMPOSITION

Each tablet contains 400mg Aciclovir Ph Eur.

3. PHARMACEUTICAL FORM

Dispersible tablet

4. CLINICAL PARTICULARS

4.1 Therapeutic indications

Management of herpes zoster (shingles).

Treatment with Aciclovir 400mg Tablets is indicated for the prevention of severe herpes simplex infections in severely immunocompromised adult patients when there is a high risk of infection, e.g. following transplantations.

4.2 Posology and method of administration

Dose:

Adults with herpes zoster (shingles):

Single doses of 800mg of aciclovir (two tablets) every four hours (five times daily).

In severely immunocompromised patients or in patients where enteral absorption is reduced, aciclovir may be administered by intravenous infusion.

Prevention of herpes simplex infections in certain cases:

For prophylaxis in severely immunocompromised patients with a high risk of infection (e.g. following transplantations, a dose of 400mg aciclovir every six hours (four times per day) should be administered. As an alternative in patients where enteral absorption is reduced, aciclovir may be administered by intravenous infusion.

Dosage for patients with Renal Impairment: (see Table 1 above)

Table 1 Dosage for patients with Renal Impairment

Indication	Creatinine clearance (mg/ml/1.73m^2)	Serum creatinine (μmol/l or mg/dl)		Dosage
		Women	Men	
Herpes zoster	25 — 10	280 — 550 / 3.17 — 6.22	370 — 750 / 4.18 — 8.48	800mg aciclovir (2 tablets) 3 times per day (every 8 hours)
	< 10	> 550 / > 6.22	> 750 / > 8.48	800mg aciclovir (2 tablets) twice a day (every 12 hours)

Length of treatment:

Therapy with Aciclovir 400mg Tablets should be initiated at the earliest sign or symptom of an infection.

Clinical studies have shown that patients suffering from herpes zoster benefit from early treatment with 400mg aciclovir.

Patients suffering from renal impairment (particularly elderly patients) should drink sufficient quantities of fluid during treatment with Aciclovir 400mg Tablets.

In severely immunocompromised patients, the length of prophylactic treatment depends on the severity of the immunodeficiency and on how long a higher risk of infection persists.

Method of administration:

Tablets should be taken after meals. They may be dissolved in a quarter of a glass of water with stirring before drinking or swallowed whole with a drink of water.

4.3 Contraindications

Aciclovir 400mg Tablets should not be given to patients with hypersensitivity to aciclovir.

There are no adequate studies concerning the prophylactic use of Aciclovir 400mg Tablets in patients with renal impairment or anuria and aciclovir should not be used in these patients.

4.4 Special warnings and special precautions for use

None.

4.5 Interaction with other medicinal products and other forms of Interaction

Probenecid has been shown to reduce the renal clearance of aciclovir by approximately 30%, resulting in an increase of its mean elimination half-life.

4.6 Pregnancy and lactation

Pregnancy:

There is little experience with oral administration of aciclovir during pregnancy. The use of Aciclovir 400mg Tablets in women who are, or may become pregnant requires that an expected benefit is weighed against the possible risks, particularly in the first trimester.

Systemic administration (oral and intravenous administration) of aciclovir during the second and third trimester of pregnancy has been described in at least 72 cases without any harm to the foetus.

Lactation:

After oral administration of 200mg aciclovir, five times daily, aciclovir concentrations found in breast milk were 0.6 — 4.1 times the corresponding aciclovir plasma concentrations. The infant would then receive up to 0.3mg/kg/day. Mothers should stop nursing during treatment with Aciclovir 400mg Tablets.

4.7 Effects on ability to drive and use machines

Aciclovir 400mg Tablets are unlikely to impair a patient's ability to drive or to use machines.

4.8 Undesirable effects

The following side effects have been observed after administration of Aciclovir 400mg Tablets:

Cutaneous reactions that usually disappear after cessation of therapy, gastrointestinal disorders such as nausea, vomiting, diarrhoea and abdominal pain.

Occasionally: Neurological reactions such as vertigo, confusion, hallucinations, somnolence. The side effects disappear after cessation of therapy and are usually observed in patients suffering from renal impairment or other diseases favouring the occurrence of these side effects.

Rarely: Increased levels of bilirubin, liver enzymes, serum urea and creatinine; decrease in haematological parameters.

Rare cases of headache, exhaustion, insomnia or fatigue have been observed. In isolated cases, depersonalization occurred which disappeared after treatment was discontinued. Rare cases of respiratory disorders have been reported.

Anaphylaxis, hepatitis, jaundice and acute renal failure have been reported on very rare occasions.

Occasionally, diffuse loss of hair occurred. A causal relationship with aciclovir could not been determined.

4.9 Overdose

Aciclovir is only partly absorbed from the gastrointestinal tract. Given the pharmacokinetic properties of aciclovir, intoxication from overdosage is not expected after oral administration.

Doses of 5g of aciclovir have been administered without signs of intoxication. An unvoluntary intravenous dose of 80mg/kg has been administered without acute side effects.

Treatment for overdose:

Aciclovir may be removed by haemodialysis.

5. PHARMACOLOGICAL PROPERTIES

5.1 Pharmacodynamic properties

Aciclovir is a pharmacologically inactive guanosine analogue that only becomes a virustatic agent after penetrating into a cell infected by herpes simplex virus (HSV) or varicella zoster virus (VZV). The activation of the aciclovir is catalysed by HSV or VZV thymidine kinase, an enzyme that the virus depends on for replication. In simplified terms, the virus synthesizes its own virustatic agent. The process goes as follows:

1. Aciclovir preferentially penetrates into cells infected with the herpes virus.

2. The enzyme thymidine kinase of these cells converts aciclovir to aciclovir monophosphate.

3. Cellular enzymes further convert aciclovir monophosphate to the virustatic agent aciclovir triphosphate.

4. The affinity of aciclovir triphosphate to viral DNA polymerase is 10 to 30 times higher than its affinity to cellular DNA polymerase. It thus selectively inhibits viral enzyme activity.

5. Furthermore, viral DNA polymerase incorporates aciclovir into viral DNA. This causes termination of DNA chain synthesis.

These steps lead to an efficient reduction of virus production.

With the plaque reduction test, an ED_{50} of 0.1μmol aciclovir/l was found in HSV infected Vero cells (green monkey kidney parechyma cells). However, an ED_{50} of 300μmol aciclovir/l was necessary to inhibit growth of uninfected Vero cells. Thus therapeutic indices of up to 3000 were found for cultured cells.

In vitro susceptibility:

Very sensitive: Herpes simplex virus type 1 and 2 (HSV-1, HSV-2),

Varicella zoster virus

Sensitive: Epstein Barr virus

Less sensitive or resistant: Cytomegalovirus

Resistant: RNA viruses, Adenoviruses, Poxviruses

In severely immunocompromised patients, prolonged or repeated treatment may lead to a selection of viral strains with diminished sensitivity, with the consequence that these patients possibly do not respond any more to treatment with aciclovir.

Most of less sensitive HSV clinical isolates have been relatively deficient in the viral thymidine kinase. However, strains with alterations in viral thymidine kinase or viral DNA polymerase have also been reported. Exposure of HSV isolates to aciclovir in vitro may also result in the emergence of less sensitive strains. The relationship between in vitro susceptibility of HSV isolates to aciclovir and the clinical response to therapy has not been established yet.

5.2 Pharmacokinetic properties

Aciclovir is only partly absorbed from the gastrointestinal tract. Mean steady state peak plasma levels following repeated oral administration of 200mg, 400mg and 800mg aciclovir every four hours (five times per day) were 3.02 ± 0.5μmol/l (200mg), 5.21 ± 1.32 μmol/l (400mg) and 8.16± 1.98 μmol/l (800mg), respectively.

These concentrations were reached after about 1.5 ± 0.6 hours. The corresponding basic plasma values about four hours after oral administration of aciclovir were 1.61 ± 0.3 μmol/l (200mg), 2.59 ± 0.52 μmol/l (400mg) and 4.0 ± 0.72 μmol/l (800mg), respectively. 24 hours after aciclovir treatment is discontinued there is no aciclovir detectable in the organism.

In immunocompromised children aged three to eleven years receiving aciclovir orally in doses of 400mg five times per day (corresponding to 300 — 650mg aciclovir/m^2 body surface), mean peak plasma levels reached 5.7 — 15.1 μmol/l. In infants aged one to six weeks receiving aciclovir orally in doses of 600mg aciclovir/m^2 body surface every six hours, mean peak plasma levels reached 17.3 and 8.6 μmol/l, respectively.

It can be deduced from the biexponential character of aciclovir kinetics that aciclovir enters tissues and organs in high concentrations and that aciclovir is only slowly eliminated.

The distribution volume in adults (steady state) is 50 ± 8.7 l/ 1.73m^2, in new-born and infants up to three months it is 28.8 ± 9.3 l/1.73m^2.

Protein binding ranged between 9% and 33%.

Distribution in body organs:

Animal studies show that, compared to serum concentrations, higher levels are reached in intestine, kidney, liver and lung, while lower levels are reached in muscle, heart, ovaries and testes.

Post mortem examinations in man have shown that aciclovir reaches high concentrations in the saliva, vaginal secretion, in the liquid found inside the herpes vesicles and in some other body organs. 50% of the respective serum concentrations are reached in liquor.

Metabolism and elimination:

In patients with normal renal function aciclovir is renally eliminated as unchanged drug (62 — 91%) and as 9-carboxymethoxymethyl-guanine (10 — 15%). Plasma half-life ($t_{1/2\beta}$) after intravenous administration of aciclovir is 2.87 ± 0.76 hours for adults and 4.1 ± 1.2 hours for new-born and infants under the age of three months. There is glomerular filtration as well as tubular secretion of aciclovir. When aciclovir is administered one hour after the administration of 1g of probenecid, plasma half-life ($t_{1/2\beta}$) is prolonged by 18% and the area under the curve for plasma concentrations is enlarged by 40%. Bioavailability is about 20%; 80% of the total aciclovir administered is excreted with faeces.

In patients suffering from chronic renal insufficiency, average plasma half-life is about 19.5 hours. Mean plasma half-life during haemodialysis is 5.7 hours. During haemodialysis a decrease of aciclovir plasma levels of about 60% occurs.

Although the treatment of herpes simplex infections in patients with renal impairment did not produce higher aciclovir concentrations n plasma than those normally found after intravenous administration, the dosage should be reduced if clearance of creatinine is below 10ml/min/ 1.73m^2 (see section 4.2 on dosage).

In patients with impaired renal function there is a risk of aciclovir accumulation if clearance of creatinine is < 25ml/ min/1.73m^2 (for a dosage of 800mg five times per day). A dosage reduction is then indicated (see also section 4.2 on dosage).

5.3 Preclinical safety data

Acute toxicity:

The LD_{50} after oral aciclovir in mice and rats could not be determined because doses of 10g/kg in mice and 20g/kg in rats could not be exceeded for physiological reasons. The animals survived administration of these doses.

Subacute toxicity:

Mice were administered aciclovir orally for a period of four weeks in doses up to 450 mg/kg. All animals survived and showed no abnormalities.

Chronic toxicity:

Beagles were administered aciclovir orally for a period of twelve months in doses of up to 60 mg/kg per day. Under this dosage mucoid diarrhoea and vomiting occurred frequently. In some dogs, paw abnormalities and loss of claws were observed. However, these signs were reversible. No other abnormalities were observed.

Rats and mice were administered aciclovir for a period of 775 days in daily doses up to 450 mg/kg without abnormalities.

Mutagenesis:

The following tests showed no mutagenic effects:

Ames test with Salmonella typhimurium, mammalian cells (CHO cells), mouse lymphoma test (6-thioguanine-, AA- and Ouabaine resistance) in vitro, dominant lethal study in vivo in mice (25 and 50 mg/kg i.p.) and lymphocytes of patients having received 5 mg/kg of aciclovir i.v. three times daily for five days or 200mg aciclovir orally five times daily.

In the following tests mutagenicity was observed for high, partly cytotoxic concentrations of aciclovir:

Mouse lymphoma cells at thymidine kinase (TK$^{+/-}$) locus. Since the TK locus is special as far as the activation of aciclovir is concerned, clones may have appeared as a result of chromosomal damage but also as a result of selection.

In cultured human lymphocytes (in vitro) a positive response for chromosomal breaks was only seen at concentrations higher than 550 μmol/l. In vivo, chromosomal breaks were observed in bone marrow cells of female rats at concentrations of 100 mg/kg i.v. There was no chromosomal damage in cells of male rats.

While i.p. administration of 100 mg/kg aciclovir caused no chromosomal damage in Chinese hamsters, treatment with 500 mg/kg, a dose which is generally toxic, did. Doses of 50 mg/kg i.v. administered to rats and Chinese hamsters did not lead to any chromosomal breaks. This corresponds to a no-effect-level of 200 μmol/l.

Determination of gonadal aciclovir levels after intravenous administration of aciclovir to male and female rats revealed concentrations that were 1/3 of the "no-effect-level" in female rats and less than 1/10 of the "no-effect-level" in male rats.

Even if an oral maximum dose of five times 800mg aciclovir is administered, a potential threshold value for a possible mutagenic effect of aciclovir will not be reached. Therefore, a mutagenic risk is not to be expected.

Carcinogenesis:

In in vitro cell transformation assays with mouse fibroblasts, aciclovir caused an altered proliferation behaviour of the monolayer cell cultures (type 111 foci) at a concentration of 220 μmol/l.

Long-term studies (two years) conducted in rats and mice showed no carcinogenicity of aciclovir.

Reproduction toxicology:

Teratogenic effect/embryotoxicity

In rats, no maternal toxic effects or abnormalities/anomalies of foetuses or newborn animals were observed following subcutaneous administration of up to 25mg aciclovir twice daily during organogenesis between day 7 and day 17/day 6 and day 15 of pregnancy.

In studies conducted with rabbits, no maternal toxic effects or negative effects on the development of the foetuses or embryos were observed following intravenous or subcutaneous administration of up to 25mg aciclovir/kg twice daily during organogenesis between day six and day eighteen of pregnancy.

In a further test in rats using subcutaneous administration of 100mg aciclovir/kg three times on day ten of pregnancy (during organogenesis) foetal abnormalities such as anophthalmia and tail abnormalities were observed.

At the same dose, maternal toxic effects (nephrotoxicity) were observed. In addition, maternal aciclovir plasma concentrations were 43-58, 67-90 and 153-167 times higher than those found in man (steady state, mean plasma concentrations) after repeated administration of 800mg, 400mg or 200mg every four hours (five times daily). The clinical relevance of these findings is uncertain.

Fertility

Mostly reversible impairment of spermatogenesis in rats and beagles was observed after administration of aciclovir at very high doses, higher than normal therapeutic doses.

Aciclovir did not impair fertility over two generations of mice who received up to 450 mg/kg/day orally.

There are no adequate studies of orally administered aciclovir and fertility in women. In men, orally administered aciclovir has no effect on the number, morphology and motility of sperms.

6. PHARMACEUTICAL PARTICULARS

6.1 List of excipients

Microcrystalline Cellulose Ph Eur, Sodium Starch Glycollate Ph Eur, Colloidal Anhydrous Silica Ph Eur, Magnesium Stearate Ph Eur.

6.2 Incompatibilities

None.

6.3 Shelf life

The shelf life is three years.

6.4 Special precautions for storage

Store below +25°C.

Keep drugs out of the reach of children.

Unused drugs should be returned to the pharmacy.

6.5 Nature and contents of container

Blister strip comprising aluminium foil on one side and PVC on the other. The strips are packed in cartons to contain 25, 35 or 56 tablets.

6.6 Instructions for use and handling

None.

7. MARKETING AUTHORISATION HOLDER

TAD Pharma GmbH
Heinz-Lohmann-Strasse 5
27472 Cuxhaven
Germany
Tel: +49 (0) 4721/606-0
Fax: +49 (0) 4721/606-266

8. MARKETING AUTHORISATION NUMBER(S)

United Kingdom: PL 04986/0005

9. DATE OF FIRST AUTHORISATION/RENEWAL OF THE AUTHORISATION

22 November 1996

10. DATE OF REVISION OF THE TEXT

June 2001

LEGAL CATEGORY

POM

Aciclovir 800mg Tablets

(Pharmacia Limited)

1. NAME OF THE MEDICINAL PRODUCT

Aciclovir 800mg Tablets

2. QUALITATIVE AND QUANTITATIVE COMPOSITION

Each tablet contains 800mg Aciclovir Ph Eur.

3. PHARMACEUTICAL FORM

Dispersible tablet

4. CLINICAL PARTICULARS

4.1 Therapeutic indications

Management of herpes zoster (shingles).

4.2 Posology and method of administration

Dose:

Adults with herpes zoster (shingles):

800mg of aciclovir (one tablet) every four hours (five times daily).

In severely immunocompromised patients or in patients where enteral absorption is reduced, aciclovir may be administered by intravenous infusion.

Dosage for patients with Renal Impairment:

(see Table 1 below)

Length of treatment:

Therapy with Aciclovir 800mg Tablets should be initiated at the earliest sign or symptom of an infection.

Clinical studies have shown that patients suffering from herpes zoster benefit from early treatment with 800mg aciclovir.

Patients suffering from renal impairment (particularly elderly patients) should drink sufficient quantities of fluid during treatment with Aciclovir 800mg Tablets.

In herpes zoster infections, treatment should be continued for five to seven days.

Method of administration:

Tablets should be taken after meals. They may be dissolved in a quarter of a glass of water with stirring before drinking or swallowed whole with a drink of water.

4.3 Contraindications

Aciclovir 800mg Tablets should not be given to patients with hypersensitivity to aciclovir.

There are no adequate studies concerning the prophylactic use of Aciclovir 800mg Tablets in patients with renal impairment or anuria and aciclovir should not be used in these patients.

4.4 Special warnings and special precautions for use

None.

4.5 Interaction with other medicinal products and other forms of Interaction

Probenecid has been shown to reduce the renal clearance of aciclovir by approximately 30%, resulting in an increase of its mean elimination half-life.

4.6 Pregnancy and lactation

Pregnancy:

There is little experience of oral administration of aciclovir during pregnancy. The use of Aciclovir 800mg Tablets in women who are, or may become pregnant requires that an expected benefit is weighed against the possible risks, particularly in the first trimester.

Systemic administration (oral and intravenous administration) of aciclovir during the second and third trimester of pregnancy has been described in at least 72 cases without any harm to the foetus.

Lactation:

After oral administration of 200mg aciclovir, five times daily, aciclovir concentrations found in breast milk were 0.6 — 4.1 times the corresponding aciclovir plasma concentrations. The infant would then receive up to 0.3mg/kg/ day. Mothers should stop nursing during treatment with Aciclovir 800mg Tablets.

4.7 Effects on ability to drive and use machines

Aciclovir 800mg Tablets are unlikely to impair a patient's ability to drive or to use machines.

4.8 Undesirable effects

The following side effects have been observed after administration of Aciclovir 800mg Tablets:

Cutaneous reactions that usually disappear after cessation of therapy, gastrointestinal disorders such as nausea, vomiting, diarrhoea and abdominal pain.

Table 1 Dosage for patients with Renal Impairment

Indication	Creatinine clearance (mg/ml/1.73m^2)	Serum creatinine (μmol/l or mg/dl)		Dosage
		Women	Men	
Herpes zoster	25 — 10	280 — 550 / 3.17 — 6.22	370 — 750 / 4.18 — 8.48	800mg aciclovir (1 tablet) 3 times per day (every 8 hours)
	< 10	> 550 / > 6.22	> 750 / > 8.48	800mg aciclovir (1 tablet) twice a day (every 12 hours)

Occasionally: Neurological reactions such as vertigo, confusion, hallucinations, somnolence. The side effects disappear after cessation of therapy and are usually observed in patients suffering from renal impairment or other diseases favouring the occurrence of these side effects.

Rarely: Increased levels of bilirubin, liver enzymes, serum urea and creatinine; decrease in haematological parameters.

Rare cases of headache, exhaustion, insomnia or fatigue have been observed. In isolated cases, depersonalization occurred which disappeared after treatment was discontinued. Rare cases of respiratory disorders have been reported.

Anaphylaxis, hepatitis, jaundice and acute renal failure have been reported on very rare occasions.

Occasionally, diffuse loss of hair occurred. A causal relationship with aciclovir could not been determined.

Reports on convulsive seizures and psychoses refer to aciclovir infusions (i.v.) in complicated episodes.

4.9 Overdose

Aciclovir is only partly absorbed from the gastrointestinal tract. Given the pharmacokinetic properties of aciclovir, intoxication from overdosage is not expected after oral administration.

Doses of 5g of aciclovir have been administered without signs of intoxication. An unvoluntary intravenous dose of 80mg/kg has been administered without acute side effects.

Treatment for overdose:

Aciclovir may be removed by haemodialysis.

5. PHARMACOLOGICAL PROPERTIES

5.1 Pharmacodynamic properties

Aciclovir is a pharmacologically inactive guanosine analogue that only becomes a virustatic agent after penetrating into a cell infected by herpes simplex virus (HSV) or varicella zoster virus (VZV). The activation of the aciclovir is catalysed by HSV or VZV thymidine kinase, an enzyme that the virus depends on for replication. In simplified terms, the virus synthesizes its own virustatic agent. The process goes as follows:

1. Aciclovir preferentially penetrates into cells infected with the herpes virus.

2. The enzyme thymidine kinase of these cells converts aciclovir to aciclovir monophosphate.

3. Cellular enzymes further convert aciclovir monophosphate to the virustatic agent aciclovir triphosphate.

4. The affinity of aciclovir triphosphate to viral DNA polymerase is 10 to 30 times higher than its affinity to cellular DNA polymerase. It thus selectively inhibits viral enzyme activity.

5. Furthermore, viral DNA polymerase incorporates aciclovir into viral DNA. This causes termination of DNA chain synthesis.

These steps lead to an efficient reduction of virus production.

With the plaque reduction test, an ED_{50} of 0.1μmol aciclovir/l was found in HSV infected Vero cells (green monkey kidney parechyma cells). However, an ED_{50} of 300μmol aciclovir/l was necessary to inhibit growth of uninfected Vero cells. Thus therapeutic indices of up to 3000 were found for cultured cells.

In vitro susceptibility:

Very sensitive: Herpes simplex virus type 1 and 2 (HSV-1, HSV-2),

Varicella zoster virus

Sensitive: Epstein Barr virus

Less sensitive or resistant: Cytomegalovirus

Resistant: RNA viruses, Adenoviruses, Poxviruses

In severely immunocompromised patients, prolonged or repeated treatment may lead to a selection of viral strains with diminished sensitivity, with the consequence that these patients possibly do not respond any more to treatment with aciclovir.

Most of less sensitive HSV clinical isolates have been relatively deficient in the viral thymidine kinase. However, strains with alterations in viral thymidine kinase or viral DNA polymerase have also been reported. Exposure of HSV isolates to aciclovir in vitro may also result in the emergence of less sensitive strains. The relationship between in vitro susceptibility of HSV isolates to aciclovir and the clinical response to therapy has not been established yet.

5.2 Pharmacokinetic properties

Aciclovir is only partly absorbed from the gastrointestinal tract. Mean steady state peak plasma levels following repeated oral administration of 200mg, 400mg and 800mg aciclovir every four hours (five times per day) were 3.02 ± 0.5μmol/l (200mg), 5.21 ± 1.32 μmol/l (400mg) and 8.16 ± 1.98 μmol/l (800mg), respectively.

These concentrations were reached after about 1.5 ± 0.6 hours. The corresponding basic plasma values about four hours after oral administration of aciclovir were 1.61 ± 0.3 μmol/l (200mg), 2.59 ± 0.52 μmol/l (400mg) and 4.0± 0.72 μmol/l (800mg), respectively. 24 hours after aciclovir treatment is discontinued there is no aciclovir detectable in the organism.

In immunocompromised children aged three to eleven years receiving aciclovir orally in doses of 400mg five times per day (corresponding to 300 — 650mg aciclovir/m^2 body surface), mean peak plasma levels reached 5.7 — 15.1 μmol/l. In infants aged one to six weeks receiving aciclovir orally in doses of 600mg aciclovir/m^2 body surface every six hours, mean peak plasma levels reached 17.3 and 8.6 μmol/l, respectively.

It can be deduced from the biexponential character of aciclovir kinetics that aciclovir enters tissues and organs in high concentrations and that aciclovir is only slowly eliminated.

The distribution volume in adults (steady state) is 50± 8.7 l/ 1.73m^2, in new-born and infants up to three months it is 28.8 ± 9.3 l/1.73m^2.

Protein binding ranged between 9% and 33%.

Distribution in body organs:

Animal studies show that, compared to serum concentrations, higher levels are reached in intestine, kidney, liver and lung, while lower levels are reached in muscle, heart, ovaries and testes.

Post mortem examinations in man have shown that aciclovir reaches high concentrations in the saliva, vaginal secretion, in the liquid found inside the herpes vesicles and in some other body organs. 50% of the respective serum concentrations are reached in liquor.

Metabolism and elimination:

In patients with normal renal function aciclovir is renally eliminated as unchanged drug (62 — 91%) and as 9-carboxymethoxymethyl-guanine (10 — 15%). Plasma half-life ($t_{1/2\beta}$) after intravenous administration of aciclovir is 2.87 ± 0.76 hours for adults and 4.1 ± 1.2 hours for new-born and infants under the age of three months. There is glomerular filtration as well as tubular secretion of aciclovir. When aciclovir is administered one hour after the administration of 1g of probenecid, plasma half-life ($t_{1/2\beta}$) is prolonged by 18% and the area under the curve for plasma concentrations is enlarged by 40%. Bioavailability is about 20%; 80% of the total aciclovir administered is excreted with faeces.

In patients suffering from chronic renal insufficiency, average plasma half-life is about 19.5 hours. Mean plasma half-life during haemodialysis is 5.7 hours. During haemodialysis a decrease of aciclovir plasma levels of about 60% occurs.

Although the treatment of herpes simplex infections in patients with renal impairment did not produce higher aciclovir concentrations n plasma than those normally found after intravenous administration, the dosage should be reduced if clearance of creatinine is below 10ml/min/ 1.73m^2 (see section 4.2 on dosage).

In patients with impaired renal function there is a risk of aciclovir accumulation if clearance of creatinine is < 25ml/ min/1.73m^2 (for a dosage of 800mg five times per day). A dosage reduction is then indicated (see also section 4.2 on dosage).

5.3 Preclinical safety data

Acute toxicity:

The LD_{50} after oral aciclovir in mice and rats could not be determined because doses of 10g/kg in mice and 20g/kg in rats could not be exceeded for physiological reasons. The animals survived administration of these doses.

Subacute toxicity:

Mice were administered aciclovir orally for a period of four weeks in doses up to 450 mg/kg. All animals survived and showed no abnormalities.

Chronic toxicity:

Beagles were administered aciclovir orally for a period of twelve months in doses of up to 60 mg/kg per day. Under this dosage mucoid diarrhoea and vomiting occurred frequently. In some dogs, paw abnormalities and loss of claws were observed. However, these signs were reversible. No other abnormalities were observed.

Rats and mice were administered aciclovir for a period of 775 days in daily doses up to 450 mg/kg without abnormalities.

Mutagenesis:

The following tests showed no mutagenic effects:

Ames test with Salmonella typhimurium, mammalian cells (CHO cells), mouse lymphoma test (6-thioguanine-, AA- and Ouabaine resistance) in vitro, dominant lethal study in vivo in mice (25 and 50 mg/kg i.p.) and lymphocytes of patients having received 5 mg/kg of aciclovir i.v. three times daily for five days or 200mg aciclovir orally five times daily.

In the following tests mutagenicity was observed for high, partly cytotoxic concentrations of aciclovir:

Mouse lymphoma cells at thymidine kinase ($TK^{+/-}$) locus. Since the TK locus is special as far as the activation of aciclovir is concerned, clones may have appeared as a result of chromosomal damage but also as a result of selection.

In cultured human lymphocytes (in vitro) a positive response for chromosomal breaks was only seen at concentrations higher than 550 μmol/l. In vivo, chromosomal breaks were observed in bone marrow cells of female rats at concentrations of 100 mg/kg i.v. There was no chromosomal damage in cells of male rats.

While i.p. administration of 100 mg/kg aciclovir caused no chromosomal damage in Chinese hamsters, treatment with 500 mg/kg, a dose which is generally toxic, did. Doses of 50 mg/kg i.v. administered to rats and Chinese hamsters did not lead to any chromosomal breaks. This corresponds to a no-effect-level of 200 μmol/l.

Determination of gonadal aciclovir levels after intravenous administration of aciclovir to male and female rats revealed concentrations that were 1/3 of the "no-effect-level" in female rats and less than 1/10 of the "no-effect-level" in male rats.

Even if an oral maximum dose of five times 800mg aciclovir is administered, a potential threshold value for a possible mutagenic effect of aciclovir will not be reached. Therefore, a mutagenic risk is not to be expected.

Carcinogenesis:

In in vitro cell transformation assays with mouse fibroblasts, aciclovir caused an altered proliferation behaviour of the monolayer cell cultures (type 111 foci) at a concentration of 220 μmol/l.

Long-term studies (two years) conducted in rats and mice showed no carcinogenicity of aciclovir.

Reproduction toxicology:

Teratogenic effect/embryotoxicity

In rats, no maternal toxic effects or abnormalities/anomalies of foetuses or newborn animals were observed following subcutaneous administration of up to 25mg aciclovir twice daily during organogenesis between day 7 and day 17/day 6 and day 15 of pregnancy.

In studies conducted with rabbits, no maternal toxic effects or negative effects on the development of the foetuses or embryos were observed following intravenous or subcutaneous administration of up to 25mg aciclovir/kg twice daily during organogenesis between day six and day eighteen of pregnancy.

Following subcutaneous administration of 100mg aciclovir/kg three times on day ten of pregnancy (during organogenesis) in a further test in rats, using subcutaneous administration, foetal abnormalities, such as anophthalmia and tail abnormalities, were observed.

At the same dose, maternal toxic effects (nephrotoxicity) were observed. In addition, maternal aciclovir plasma concentrations were 43-58, 67-90 and 153-167 times higher than those found in man (steady state, mean plasma concentrations) after repeated administration of 800mg, 400mg or 200mg every four hours (five times daily). The clinical relevance of these findings is uncertain.

Fertility

Mostly reversible impairment of spermatogenesis in rats and beagles was observed after administration of aciclovir at very high doses, higher than normal therapeutic doses.

Aciclovir did not impair fertility over two generations of mice who received up to 450 mg/kg/day orally.

There are no adequate studies of orally administered aciclovir and fertility in women. In men, orally administered aciclovir has no effect on the number, morphology and motility of sperms.

6. PHARMACEUTICAL PARTICULARS

6.1 List of excipients

Microcrystalline Cellulose Ph Eur, Sodium Starch Glycollate Ph Eur, Colloidal Anhydrous Silica Ph Eur, Magnesium Stearate Ph Eur.

6.2 Incompatibilities

None.

6.3 Shelf life

The shelf life is three years.

6.4 Special precautions for storage

Store below +25°C.

Keep drugs out of the reach of children.

Unused drugs should be returned to the pharmacy.

6.5 Nature and contents of container

Blister strip comprising aluminium foil on one side and PVC on the other and containing five tablets per strip. Seven strips are contained in a carton.

6.6 Instructions for use and handling

None.

7. MARKETING AUTHORISATION HOLDER

TAD Pharma GmbH

Heinz-Lohmann-Strasse 5

27472 Cuxhaven

Germany

Tel: +49 (0) 4721/606-0

Fax: +49 (0) 4721/606-266

8. MARKETING AUTHORISATION NUMBER(S)

United Kingdom: PL 04986/0006

9. DATE OF FIRST AUTHORISATION/RENEWAL OF THE AUTHORISATION

22 November 1996

10. DATE OF REVISION OF THE TEXT

June 2001

LEGAL CATEGORY

POM

Aciclovir Cream 5% w/w

(Pharmacia Limited)

1. NAME OF THE MEDICINAL PRODUCT
Aciclovir Cream 5% w/w

2. QUALITATIVE AND QUANTITATIVE COMPOSITION
5% w/w (50mg per g) Aciclovir Ph Eur.

3. PHARMACEUTICAL FORM
Cream

4. CLINICAL PARTICULARS
4.1 Therapeutic indications
Aciclovir Cream 5% w/w is indicated for the treatment of recurrent herpes labialis and herpes genitalis.

4.2 Posology and method of administration
Dose:
Unless otherwise instructed, apply a thin layer of cream over the site of infection every four hours, five times a day.

Length of treatment:
The cream should be applied to the lesion or developing lesion as soon as possible after the start of the infection. Treatment with Aciclovir Cream 5% w/w is normally continued for five days. If the situation deteriorates or, if after ten days there is no clinical benefit (crusted vesicles, healing of lesions), treatment should be discontinued and patients should consult their physician.

Method of administration:
A cotton bud should be used to apply a sufficient quantity of Aciclovir Cream 5% w/w to cover all lesions. The cream should be applied to visibly infected sites (vesicles, swelling, erythema) and the adjoining areas. If hands are used to apply the cream, they should be thoroughly washed before and after application to prevent further infection of the lesions by bacteria and to prevent autoinoculation of the virus to other mucous membrane and cutaneous sites not yet infected.

4.3 Contraindications
Hypersensitivity to aciclovir, polyoxyethylene fatty acid esters, cetyl alcohol, dimethicone or propylene glycol.

4.4 Special warnings and special precautions for use
Aciclovir Cream 5% w/w should not be used on mucous membranes (e.g. oral cavity, eyes, vagina) since local reactions may occur.

Severely immunocompromised patients should consult their physician before starting treatment with Aciclovir Cream 5% w/w. For these patients, oral administration should be considered.

Because of possible infections of partners, patients with herpes genitalis should be advised to abstain from sexual contact if any lesions are visible.

4.5 Interaction with other medicinal products and other forms of Interaction
No interactions known.

4.6 Pregnancy and lactation
Pregnancy:
Systemic administration of aciclovir in internationally accepted studies did not produce teratogenic effects in mice, rats or rabbits.

In one other study a teratogenic effect was seen, but only at high doses and the clinical relevance of these findings is uncertain.

No evidence of malformations was observed in a group of several hundred patients exposed to aciclovir during the first trimester of pregnancy.

No foetotoxic effect was observed after aciclovir administration during the second and third trimesters of pregnancy.

Only about 0.1% of the aciclovir applied to the skin is detectable in the plasma. Concentrations are minimal so that no systemic effect should occur.

Consequently, topical administration of aciclovir for the specified indications is acceptable.

Lactation:
As there is only minimal systemic absorption of aciclovir, adverse effects on the infant during lactation are unlikely.

4.7 Effects on ability to drive and use machines
Aciclovir Cream 5% w/w is unlikely to impair a patients ability to drive or to use machines.

4.8 Undesirable effects
Transient burning and itching may occur after application of Aciclovir Cream 5% w/w.

Occasionally erythema, dryness, pruritus and desquamation of cutaneous sites have been observed.

Rarely, contact dermatitis has been reported after administration of Aciclovir Cream 5% w/w. Examination showed that in most cases the contact dermatitis was caused by one of the excipients rather than by the active ingredient aciclovir. The contact dermatitis is characterized by the occurrence of the cutaneous reactions as described above, with a widespread distribution.

4.9 Overdose
As only 0.1% of the aciclovir applied to the skin is detectable in the plasma, overdose is unlikely.

5. PHARMACOLOGICAL PROPERTIES
5.1 Pharmacodynamic properties
After penetrating into a cell infected by herpes simplex virus, aciclovir converts to aciclovir triphosphate. Viral replication is selectively inhibited by viral DNA polymerase.

Aciclovir does not eradicate latent virus.

5.2 Pharmacokinetic properties
Concentrations in the plasma are minimal so that there should be no systemic effect.

5.3 Preclinical safety data
Local effects:
Aciclovir cream was applied to guinea pig and rabbit skin (damaged and normal) once a day for 21 days. A mild irritation occurred after repeated application.

Since the amount of active ingredient absorbed from the cream does not lead to significant plasma levels (see paragraph 5.2 on pharmacokinetics) there were no further studies on this form of administration.

6. PHARMACEUTICAL PARTICULARS
6.1 List of excipients
Glycerin monostearate/polyoxyethylen-30-stearate (Arlatone 983S), Dimeticone Ph Eur, Cetyl Alcohol Ph Eur, Liquid Paraffin Ph Eur, White Soft Paraffin USP/DAB10, Propylene Glycol Ph Eur, Purified Water Ph Eur.

6.2 Incompatibilities
None.

6.3 Shelf life
The proposed shelf life is thirty six months.

6.4 Special precautions for storage
Store below 25°C. Do not refrigerate.

6.5 Nature and contents of container
Aluminium tube containing 2*, 5, 10* or 15g of Aciclovir Cream 5% w/w.

One tube is packed in a carton together with a patient information leaflet.

*These tubes only are available in the UK.

6.6 Instructions for use and handling
None.

7. MARKETING AUTHORISATION HOLDER
TAD Pharma GmbH
Heinz-Lohmann-Strasse 5
27472 Cuxhaven
Germany
Tel: +49 (0)4721/606-0
Fax: +49 (0)4721/606-333

8. MARKETING AUTHORISATION NUMBER(S)
United Kingdom: PL 04986/0008

9. DATE OF FIRST AUTHORISATION/RENEWAL OF THE AUTHORISATION
21 November 1996

10. DATE OF REVISION OF THE TEXT
November 1999

LEGAL CATEGORY
POM.

Aci-Jel Therapeutic Vaginal Jelly

(Janssen-Cilag Ltd)

1. NAME OF THE MEDICINAL PRODUCT
Aci-Jel® Therapeutic Vaginal Jelly

2. QUALITATIVE AND QUANTITATIVE COMPOSITION
Glacial acetic acid BP, 0.9386% w/w.

3. PHARMACEUTICAL FORM
Gel.

4. CLINICAL PARTICULARS
4.1 Therapeutic indications
Non-specific chronic vaginitis where the encouragement of vaginal acidity is considered appropriate.

4.2 Posology and method of administration
One applicatorful intravaginally once or twice daily for up to two weeks or as prescribed.

4.3 Contraindications
None known.

4.4 Special warnings and special precautions for use
Compatibility with barrier methods of contraception have not been demonstrated, therefore do not use with condoms and diaphragms.

4.5 Interaction with other medicinal products and other forms of Interaction
None known.

4.6 Pregnancy and lactation
Use with caution.

4.7 Effects on ability to drive and use machines
None known.

4.8 Undesirable effects
Rarely, local irritation and inflammation.

4.9 Overdose
Aci-Jel Therapeutic Vaginal Jelly is intended for intravaginal use. If accidental ingestion occurs, an appropriate method of gastric emptying may be used.

5. PHARMACOLOGICAL PROPERTIES
5.1 Pharmacodynamic properties
Aci-Jel Therapeutic Vaginal Jelly helps restore vaginal pH. Acetic acid is also bactericidal or bacteriostatic to many types of organism.

5.2 Pharmacokinetic properties
There have been no pharmacokinetic studies of absorption of the excipients used in Aci-Jel Jelly. It is unlikely that there is any systemic absorption of any of the ingredients of the product.

5.3 Preclinical safety data
Not applicable.

6. PHARMACEUTICAL PARTICULARS
6.1 List of excipients
Glycerin
Castor oil
Propyl hydroxybenzoate
Tragacanth
Acacia
Egg albumin impalpable powder
Perfume lavender compound 13091
Potassium hydroxide pellets
Potassium bitartrate
Purified water

6.2 Incompatibilities
None known.

6.3 Shelf life
36 months.

6.4 Special precautions for storage
Store at room temperature (at or below 25°C).

6.5 Nature and contents of container
Epoxy resin lined, blind end aluminium tubes with polyethylene caps.

Each tube contains 85 g of jelly.

6.6 Instructions for use and handling
Not applicable.

7. MARKETING AUTHORISATION HOLDER
Janssen-Cilag Ltd
Saunderton
High Wycombe
Buckinghamshire
HP14 4HJ

8. MARKETING AUTHORISATION NUMBER(S)
0242/0205

9. DATE OF FIRST AUTHORISATION/RENEWAL OF THE AUTHORISATION
1 September 1995

10. DATE OF REVISION OF THE TEXT
Not applicable.

Acnecide 5% w/w Gel

(Galderma (U.K.) Ltd)

1. NAME OF THE MEDICINAL PRODUCT
Acnecide 5% w/w Gel

2. QUALITATIVE AND QUANTITATIVE COMPOSITION
Hydrous benzoyl peroxide equivalent to Benzoyl Peroxide 5% w/w

For excipients see 6.1

3. PHARMACEUTICAL FORM
Topical Gel

White, smooth gel

4. CLINICAL PARTICULARS
4.1 Therapeutic indications
Topical therapy for the treatment of acne vulgaris

4.2 Posology and method of administration
For external use only.

Adults and children:

After washing with a mild cleanser, apply once or twice daily or as directed to the affected areas. Initially Acnecide 5 should be used; treatment may be continued with Acnecide 10 provided Acnecide 5 has been well tolerated. The extent of any drying or peeling may be adjusted by modifying the dosage schedule.

4.3 Contraindications
Persons having known sensitivity to benzoyl peroxide.

4.4 Special warnings and special precautions for use
A mild burning sensation will probably be felt on first application and some reddening and peeling of the skin will occur within a few days. During the first weeks of treatment a sudden increase in peeling will occur in most patients. This is not harmful and will normally subside

within a day or two if treatment is temporarily discontinued. If severe irritation occurs, patients should be directed to use the medication less frequently, to temporarily discontinue use or to discontinue use altogether.

Benzoyl peroxide gel should not come into contact with the eyes, mouth, angles of the nose or mucous membranes. If the preparation enters the eye, wash thoroughly with water. Caution should be exercised when applying the drug to the neck and other sensitive areas.

Repeated exposure to sunlight or UV radiation should be avoided.

Contact with any coloured material including hair and dyed fabrics may result in bleaching or discoloration.

Due to the risk of sensitisation, benzoyl peroxide gel should not be applied on damaged skin.

4.5 Interaction with other medicinal products and other forms of Interaction
There are no known interaction with other medications which might be used cutaneously and concurrently with benzoyl peroxide; however, drugs with desquamative, irritant and drying effects should not be used concurrently with benzoyl peroxide gel.

4.6 Pregnancy and lactation
There are no published reports relating to the effects of benzoyl peroxide on reproductive function, fertility, teratogenicity, embryotoxicity, or peri- and post- natal development in animals. In widespread clinical use for the cutaneous treatment of acne vulgaris, at concentrations up to 10% w/w for several decades, benzoyl peroxide has never been associated with effects on these parameters in humans. Caution should be exercised when prescribing to pregnant women.

It is not known whether benzoyl peroxide is excreted in animal or human milk. Because many drugs are excreted in human milk, caution should be exercised when benzoyl peroxide gel is administered to a nursing woman and the preparation should not be applied on the chest to avoid accidental transfer to the infant.

4.7 Effects on ability to drive and use machines
Based on the pharmacodynamic profile and extensive clinical experience, performance related to driving and using machines should not be affected during treatment with Benzoyl peroxide.

4.8 Undesirable effects
The major adverse reaction reported to date with benzoyl peroxide cutaneous therapy is irritation of the skin including erythema, burning, peeling, dryness, itching, stinging, feeling of skin tension locally at the site of application. This is reversible when treatment is reduced in frequency or discontinued. Allergic contact dermatitis, including face oedema, may occur.

4.9 Overdose
Benzoyl peroxide gel is a preparation indicated for topical treatment only. If the medication is applied excessively, no more rapid or better results will be obtained and severe irritation might develop. In this event, treatment must be discontinued and appropriate symptomatic therapy should be instituted.

5. PHARMACOLOGICAL PROPERTIES
5.1 Pharmacodynamic properties
Benzoyl peroxide is an established and effective keratolytic agent with antibacterial properties. It has been shown to be effective in reducing the local population of Propionibacterium acnes leading to a reduction in the production of irritant fatty acids in the sebaceous glands.

5.2 Pharmacokinetic properties
Not applicable. Acnecide is a topical preparation.

5.3 Preclinical safety data
In animal studies by the cutaneous route, benzoyl peroxide is associated with a minimal to moderate skin irritation potential including erythema and oedema. Phototoxic and photoallergic reactions have been reported for benzoyl peroxide therapy.

6. PHARMACEUTICAL PARTICULARS
6.1 List of excipients
Docusate sodium

Disodium edetate

Poloxamer 182

Carbomer 940

Propylene glycol

Acrylates copolymer or glycerol microsponge

Glycerol

Colloidal Anhydrous Silica

Purified water

Sodium hydroxide to adjust the pH.

6.2 Incompatibilities
Not applicable

6.3 Shelf life
3 Years

6.4 Special precautions for storage
Do not store above 25°C.

Do not freeze.

6.5 Nature and contents of container
White low density polyethylene tubes containing 60g gel.

6.6 Instructions for use and handling
No special requirements.

7. MARKETING AUTHORISATION HOLDER
Galderma (UK) Limited,
Galderma House,
Church Lane,
Kings Langley,
Hertfordshire, WD4 8JP,
England.

8. MARKETING AUTHORISATION NUMBER(S)
PL 10590/0006

9. DATE OF FIRST AUTHORISATION/RENEWAL OF THE AUTHORISATION
13th July 1992

10. DATE OF REVISION OF THE TEXT
November 2004.

Acnisal
(Alliance Pharmaceuticals)

1. NAME OF THE MEDICINAL PRODUCT
Acnisal.

2. QUALITATIVE AND QUANTITATIVE COMPOSITION
Salicylic acid 2.0% w/w.

For excipients, see 6.1.

3. PHARMACEUTICAL FORM
Cutaneous solution

An opaque off-white cutaneous emollient solution.

4. CLINICAL PARTICULARS
4.1 Therapeutic indications
Acnisal is for the management of acne. It helps prevent new comedones (blackheads and whiteheads) papules and pustules (acne pimples).

4.2 Posology and method of administration
For topical administration.

Adults:

Acnisal is used to wash the affected area 2 to 3 times daily. Lather with warm water, massage into skin, rinse and dry.

Children:

As for adults.

Elderly:

As for adults.

4.3 Contraindications
Acnisal is contra-indicated in persons with a sensitivity to salicylic acid.

4.4 Special warnings and special precautions for use
For external use only. Avoid contact with the mouth, eyes and other mucous membranes to avoid irritation.

As with other topical preparations containing salicylic acid, excessive prolonged use may result in symptoms of salicylism.

4.5 Interaction with other medicinal products and other forms of Interaction
None known.

4.6 Pregnancy and lactation
No limitations to the use of Acnisal during pregnancy or lactation are known.

4.7 Effects on ability to drive and use machines
None known.

4.8 Undesirable effects
Salicylic acid is a mild irritant and may cause skin irritation. If undue skin irritation develops or increases adjust the usage schedule or consult your physician.

4.9 Overdose
Not applicable.

5. PHARMACOLOGICAL PROPERTIES
5.1 Pharmacodynamic properties
Human comedones, naturally or coal tar induced, are firmly anchored and are dislodged with great difficulty. Most classic "peeling" agents are ineffective: they are merely irritants which cause scaling, creating the illusion of comedolysis. While salicylic acid is an irritant its efficacy is dependent on specific pharmacological effects. It seems to detach horny cells from each other by weakening the intercellular cement. As a result, the comedones tend to undergo disorganisation. The effect is probably a good deal more complex. Salicylic acid penetrates skin readily and increases turnover which also favours exfoliation of the comedo. In concentrations of 0.5 to 2% it significantly reduces the formation of microcomedones, which are the precursors of all other acne lesions.

5.2 Pharmacokinetic properties
There is no evidence of any systemic absorption from the use of Acnisal.

5.3 Preclinical safety data
None presented.

6. PHARMACEUTICAL PARTICULARS
6.1 List of excipients
Purified water

Benzyl alcohol

Sodium chloride

Sodium C14-C16 olefin sulphonate

Lauramide DEA (monoamide 716)

PEG-7 Glyceryl cocoate

Lytron 614 (styrene/acrylate copolymer, octoxynol-9 and sodium dodecylbenzene sulphonate).

6.2 Incompatibilities
Not applicable.

6.3 Shelf life
3 years.

6.4 Special precautions for storage
Store below 25°C.

6.5 Nature and contents of container
Acnisal is supplied in a white HDPE bottle with a white polypropylene screw cap. Each bottle contains either 30ml or 177ml of Acnisal.

6.6 Instructions for use and handling
No special requirements.

Administrative Data
7. MARKETING AUTHORISATION HOLDER
Alliance Pharmaceuticals Ltd
Avonbridge House
Bath Road
Chippenham
Wiltshire
SN15 2BB

8. MARKETING AUTHORISATION NUMBER(S)
PL 16853/0070

9. DATE OF FIRST AUTHORISATION/RENEWAL OF THE AUTHORISATION
11th September 1998.

10. DATE OF REVISION OF THE TEXT
August 2004

Actidose-Aqua Advance
(Cambridge Laboratories)

1. NAME OF THE MEDICINAL PRODUCT
Actidose-Aqua Advance

2. QUALITATIVE AND QUANTITATIVE COMPOSITION
Actidose-Aqua Advance contains 1.04 g of Activated Charcoal/5 ml.

3. PHARMACEUTICAL FORM
Suspension for oral administration.

4. CLINICAL PARTICULARS
4.1 Therapeutic indications
For the emergency treatment of acute poisoning and drug overdosage where substances such as those listed in section 5.1 have been ingested. The list is not exhaustive and Actidose-Aqua Advance may be of benefit following ingestion of many other toxins.

Also indicated for a limited number of systemic poisonings resulting from parenteral overdosage or when the ingested toxin has been totally absorbed. This usually involves repeated doses of Actidose-Aqua Advance to remove compounds which undergo enterohepatic recycling or which can diffuse into the gastrointestinal tract along a concentration gradient. Under these circumstances multiple doses of Actidose-Aqua Advance adsorb the toxin thereby preventing its reabsorption and increasing the concentration gradient in favour of further diffusion of the toxin into the gastrointestinal tract. Compounds most effectively transferred by this mechanism are lipophilic, uncharged and not excessively protein-bound. Examples of compounds which can be eliminated more rapidly by "gastrointestinal dialysis" in this way are phenobarbitone and theophylline.

4.2 Posology and method of administration
The container should be shaken thoroughly prior to administration. If the dose of poison that has been ingested is known, a ratio of 10:1 (activated charcoal:toxin) may be used to determine the optimal dose of activated charcoal, subject to the limits of practicality. In the absence of any information regarding the amount of poison ingested, the following doses are recommended:

Adults (including the elderly) and children over 12 years of age:

For single dose therapy, 50-100 grams of activated charcoal (240-480 ml) taken as soon as possible after ingestion of the poison.

For multiple dose therapy, 25-50 grams of activated charcoal (120-240 ml) every 4-6 hours.

Children aged 1-12 years

For single dose therapy, 25-50 grams of activated charcoal (120-240 ml) taken as soon as possible after ingestion of the poison. For multiple dose therapy, the dose may be repeated every 4-6 hours.

Children under one year of age:

For single dose therapy, 1 g or 5 ml per kg bodyweight taken as soon as possible after ingestion of the poison. For multiple dose therapy, the dose may be repeated every 4-6 hours.

When syrup of ipecac is used to produce emesis, administration of Actidose-Aqua Advance should be delayed until 30-60 minutes after vomiting has ceased. If gastric lavage is being used to facilitate stomach evacuation a single dose of Actidose-Aqua Advance may be administered early in the procedure. This has the advantage of prompt administration of activated charcoal, but the gastric lavage returns will be black which may make it difficult to evaluate what the patient ingested by visual examination.

Actidose-Aqua Advance may be effective even when several hours have elapsed after ingestion of the poison if gastrointestinal motility is reduced by the toxin or if the drug is subject to enterohepatic or enteroenteric recycling.

4.3 Contraindications

Use of Actidose-Aqua Advance is contra-indicated in persons who are not fully conscious.

4.4 Special warnings and special precautions for use

Actidose-Aqua Advance is not recommended for patients who have ingested corrosive agents such as strong acids or alkalis since the activated charcoal may obscure endoscopic visualisation of oesophageal and gastric lesions produced by the toxin. Actidose-Aqua Advance is of little or no value in the treatment of poisoning with cyanides, alcohols, iron salts, malathion and DDT.

Actidose-Aqua Advance is an adjunct in the management of poisoning emergencies. Prior to its use, proper basic life support measures must be implemented where required as well as the appropriate gastric emptying technique if indicated.

Actidose-Aqua Advance should be used with caution in patients who have been exposed to toxins which interfere with gastrointestinal motility (e.g. anticholinergics, opioids). Bowel sounds should be monitored frequently to assess peristaltic action, especially in patients undergoing multiple dose activated charcoal therapy.

4.5 Interaction with other medicinal products and other forms of Interaction

Actidose-Aqua Advance will adsorb most medicaments and many other chemical substances. If a specific antidote is to be administered the likelihood of its adsorption by activated charcoal should be borne in mind, and a parenteral route of administration used if possible. Thus in the case of paracetamol, Actidose-Aqua Advance should not be given as well as oral methionine but may be used alone or in conjunction with intravenous N-acetylcysteine.

Other concurrent medications to counteract shock or associated infection should also be given parenterally since orally administered drugs may be bound to the activated charcoal in the gut.

4.6 Pregnancy and lactation

The safety of this medicinal product for use in human pregnancy has not been established. Experimental animal studies are insufficient to assess the safety with respect to the development of the embryo or foetus, the course of gestation and peri- and postnatal development.

Activated charcoal is however essentially inert pharmacologically and is not absorbed from the gastrointestinal tract. No hazard is therefore anticipated from its use during pregnancy or lactation.

4.7 Effects on ability to drive and use machines

None known

4.8 Undesirable effects

Both the patient and health care professionals should be aware that Actidose-Aqua Advance will produce black stools. A laxative may be given concurrently to accelerate the removal of the activated charcoal-toxin complex, but should be used with caution and only intermittently during multiple dose activated charcoal therapy since profuse and protracted diarrhoea may lead to fluid and electrolyte imbalance.

Aspiration of activated charcoal has been reported to produce airways obstruction and appropriate precautions should be taken. Gastrointestinal obstruction associated with the use of multiple dose activated charcoal therapy has been reported rarely.

4.9 Overdose

Actidose-Aqua Advance is well tolerated and due to its lack of toxicity overdosage requiring treatment is unlikely. A laxative may be administered to enhance elimination of the product.

5. PHARMACOLOGICAL PROPERTIES

5.1 Pharmacodynamic properties

Activated charcoal has a high adsorptive capacity for a wide range of compounds including many of those which are most commonly encountered in deliberate and accidental poisoning. Substances adsorbed include the following:

Aspirin and other salicylates
Barbiturates
Benzodiazepines
Chlormethiazole
Chloroquine
Chlorpromazine and related phenothiazines
Clonidine
Cocaine and other stimulants
Digoxin and digitoxin
Ibuprofen
Mefenamic acid
Mianserin
Nicotine
Paracetamol
Paraquat
Phenelzine and other monoamine oxidase inhibitors
Phenytoin
Propranolol and other beta-blockers
Quinine
Theophylline
Zidovudine

5.2 Pharmacokinetic properties

Activated charcoal is not absorbed from the gastrointestinal tract or subject to any metabolic processes. It is eliminated in the faeces.

5.3 Preclinical safety data

Activated charcoal is essentially inert pharmacologically and it would therefore be expected to be virtually devoid of toxicity, other than any ill effects arising from mechanical obstruction of the gut, or, if inhaled, the lungs.

The excipients in the product are all well known and widely used in medicinal products and should not give rise to any toxicological problems.

6. PHARMACEUTICAL PARTICULARS

6.1 List of excipients

Sucrose
Propylene glycol
Glycerine
Citric Acid
Purified water

6.2 Incompatibilities

None known.

6.3 Shelf life

Two years

6.4 Special precautions for storage

Store at 15 - 30°C. Do not refrigerate.

6.5 Nature and contents of container

(1) Low density polyethylene bottles containing 120 ml.
(2) Low density polyethylene bottles containing 240 ml.
(3) Low density polyethylene tubes containing 120 ml.

6.6 Instructions for use and handling

Shake well before use.

7. MARKETING AUTHORISATION HOLDER

Cambridge Laboratories Limited
Deltic House
Kingfisher Way
Silverlink Business Park
Wallsend
Tyne & Wear NE28 9NX

8. MARKETING AUTHORISATION NUMBER(S)

PL 12070/0011

9. DATE OF FIRST AUTHORISATION/RENEWAL OF THE AUTHORISATION

26 March 1996.

10. DATE OF REVISION OF THE TEXT

February 2000

Actilyse

(Boehringer Ingelheim Limited)

1. NAME OF THE MEDICINAL PRODUCT

Actilyse

2. QUALITATIVE AND QUANTITATIVE COMPOSITION

Active ingredient:

1 vial with 467 mg powder contains: 10 mg alteplase or

1 vial with 933 mg powder contains: 20 mg alteplase or

1 vial with 2333 mg powder contains: 50 mg alteplase

Alteplase is produced by recombinant DNA technique using a Chinese hamster ovary cell-line. The specific activity of alteplase in-house reference material is 580,000 IU/mg. This has been confirmed by comparison with the second international WHO standard for t-PA. The specification for the specific activity of alteplase is 522,000 to 696,000 IU/mg.

For excipients, see 6.1.

3. PHARMACEUTICAL FORM

Powder and solvent for solution for injection and infusion.

4. CLINICAL PARTICULARS

4.1 Therapeutic indications

Thrombolytic treatment in acute myocardial infarction

- 90 minutes (accelerated) dose regimen (see posology and method of administration): for patients in whom treatment can be started within 6 h after symptom onset

- 3 h dose regimen (see posology and method of administration): for patients in whom treatment can be started between 6 - 12 h after symptom onset provided that the diagnosis has been clearly confirmed.

Actilyse has proven to reduce 30-day-mortality in patients with acute myocardial infarction.

Thrombolytic treatment in acute massive pulmonary embolism with haemodynamic instability

The diagnosis should be confirmed whenever possible by objective means such as pulmonary angiography or non-invasive procedures such as lung scanning. There is no evidence for positive effects on mortality and late morbidity related to pulmonary embolism.

Fibrinolytic treatment of acute ischaemic stroke

Treatment must be started within 3 hours of onset of the stroke symptoms and after prior exclusion of intracranial haemorrhage by means of appropriate imaging techniques.

4.2 Posology and method of administration

Actilyse should be given as soon as possible after symptom onset. The following dose guidelines apply.

Under aseptic conditions the content of an injection vial of Actilyse (10 mg or 20 mg or 50 mg) is dissolved with water for injections according to the following table to obtain either a final concentration of 1 mg alteplase/ml or 2 mg alteplase/ml:

The transfer cannulas provided with the packs of Actilyse 20 mg and Actilyse 50 mg are to be used. In the case of Actilyse 10 mg a syringe should be used.

(see Table 1 on next page)

The reconstituted solution should then be administered intravenously. It may be diluted further with sterile physiological saline solution (0.9 %) up to a minimal concentration of 0.2 mg/ml.

Myocardial infarction

a) 90 minutes (accelerated) dose regimen for patients with myocardial infarction, in whom treatment can be started within 6 hours after symptom onset:

	Concentration of alteplase	
	1mg/ml	2mg/ml
	ml	ml
15 mg as an intravenous bolus	15	7.5
50 mg as an infusion over 30 minutes	50	25
followed by an infusion of 35 mg over 60 minutes until the maximal dose of 100 mg	35	17.5

In patients with a body weight below 65 kg the dose should be weight adjusted according to the following table:

	Concentration of alteplase	
	1mg/ml	2mg/ml
	ml	ml
15 mg as an intravenous bolus	15	7.5
	ml/kg bw	ml/kg bw
and 0.75 mg/kg body weight (bw) over 30 minutes (maximum 50 mg)	0.75	0.375
followed by an infusion of 0.5 mg/kg body weight (bw) over 60 minutes (maximum 35 mg)	0.5	0.25

Table 1

Actilyse vial	10mg	20mg	50mg
Volume of Water for Injections to be added to dry powder:			
Final concentration			
(a) 1mg alteplase/ml (ml)	10	20	50
(b) 2mg alteplase/ml (ml)	5	10	25

b) 3 h dose regimen for patients, in whom treatment can be started between 6 and 12 hours after symptom onset:

	Concentration of alteplase	
	1mg/ml	2mg/ml
	ml	ml
10 mg as an intravenous bolus	10	5
50 mg as an infusion over the first hour	50	25
	ml/30 min	ml/ 30 min
followed by infusions of 10 mg over 30 minutes until the maximal dose of 100 mg over 3 hours	10	5

In patients with a body weight below 65 kg the total dose should not exceed 1.5 mg/kg.

The maximum dose of alteplase is 100 mg.

Adjunctive therapy:

Acetylsalicylic acid should be initiated as soon as possible after symptom onset and continued for the first months after myocardial infarction. The recommended dose is 160 - 300 mg/d.

Heparin should be administered concomitantly at least for 24 hours or longer (at least 48 hours with the accelerated dose regimen). It is recommended to start with an initial intravenous bolus of 5,000 IU prior to thrombolytic therapy and to continue with an infusion of 1,000 IU/hour. The dose of heparin should be adjusted according to repeated measurements of aPTT values of 1.5 to 2.5 times the initial value.

Pulmonary embolism

A total dose of 100 mg of alteplase should be administered in 2 hours. Most experience is available with the following dose regimen:

	Concentration of alteplase	
	1mg/ml	2mg/ml
	ml	ml
10 mg as an intravenous bolus over 1 - 2 minutes	10	5
followed by an intravenous infusion of 90 mg over 2 hours	90	45

The total dose should not exceed 1.5 mg/kg in patients with a body weight below 65 kg.

Adjunctive therapy:

After treatment with Actilyse heparin therapy should be initiated (or resumed) when aPTT values are less than twice the upper limit of normal. The infusion should be adjusted according to aPTT values of 1.5 to 2.5 times the initial value.

Acute ischaemic stroke

Treatment must be performed by a physician specialised in neurological care. (See Contra-indications and Special Warnings/Precautions for Use.)

The recommended dose is 0.9 mg alteplase/kg body weight (maximum of 90 mg) infused intravenously over 60 minutes with 10% of the total dose administered as an initial intravenous bolus.

Treatment with Actilyse must be started within 3 hours of the onset of symptoms.

Adjunctive therapy:

The safety and efficacy of this regimen with concomitant administration of heparin and acetylsalicylic acid within the first 24 hours of onset of the symptoms have not been sufficiently investigated. Administration of acetylsalicylic acid or intravenous heparin should be avoided in the first 24 hours after treatment with Actilyse. If heparin is required for other indications (e.g. prevention of deep vein thrombosis) the dose should not exceed 10,000 IU per day, administered subcutaneously.

4.3 Contraindications

Actilyse should not be used in cases where there is a high risk of haemorrhage such as:

- known haemorrhagic diathesis
- patients receiving oral anticoagulants, e.g. warfarin sodium
- manifest or recent severe or dangerous bleeding
- known history of or suspected intracranial haemorrhage
- suspected subarachnoid haemorrhage or condition after subarachnoid haemorrhage from aneurysm
- any history of central nervous system damage (i.e. neoplasm, aneurysm, intracranial or spinal surgery)
- recent (less than 10 days) traumatic external heart massage, obstetrical delivery, recent puncture of a non-compressible blood-vessel (e.g. subclavian or jugular vein puncture)
- severe uncontrolled arterial hypertension
- bacterial endocarditis, pericarditis
- acute pancreatitis
- documented ulcerative gastrointestinal disease during the last 3 months, oesophageal varices, arterial-aneurysm, arterial/venous malformations
- neoplasm with increased bleeding risk
- severe liver disease, including hepatic failure, cirrhosis, portal hypertension (oesophageal varices) and active hepatitis
- major surgery or significant trauma in past 3 months.

Additional contraindications in acute myocardial infarction:

any history of stroke.

Additional contraindications in acute pulmonary embolism:

any history of stroke.

Additional contraindications in acute ischaemic stroke:

- symptoms of ischaemic attack beginning more than 3 hours prior to infusion start or when time of symptom onset is unknown,
- minor neurological deficit or symptoms rapidly improving before start of infusion,
- severe stroke as assessed clinically (e.g. NIHSS>25) and/or by appropriate imaging techniques,
- seizure at onset of stroke,
- evidence of intracranial haemorrhage (ICH) on the CT-scan,
- symptoms suggestive of subarachnoid haemorrhage, even if CT-scan is normal,
- administration of heparin within the previous 48 hours and a thromboplastin time exceeding the upper limit of normal for laboratory,
- patients with any history of prior stroke and concomitant diabetes
- prior stroke within the last 3 months
- platelet count of below 100,000/mm3
- systolic blood pressure > 185 or diastolic BP > 110 mm Hg, or aggressive management (IV medication) necessary to reduce BP to these limits
- blood glucose < 50 or > 400 mg/dl.

Use in children and elderly patients

Actilyse is not indicated for the treatment of acute stroke in children under 18 years or adults over 80 years of age.

4.4 Special warnings and special precautions for use

Thrombolytic/ fibrinolytic treatment requires adequate monitoring. Actilyse should only be used by physicians trained and experienced in the use of thrombolytic treatments and with the facilities to monitor that use. It is recommended that when Actilyse is administered standard resuscitation equipment and medication be available in all circumstances.

The risk of intracranial haemorrhage is increased in elderly patients, therefore in these patients the risk/benefit evaluation should be carried out carefully.

As yet, there is only limited experience with the use of Actilyse in children.

As with all thrombolytic agents, the expected therapeutic benefit should be weighed up particularly carefully against the possible risk, especially in patients with

- small recent traumas, such as biopsies, puncture of major vessels, intramuscular injections, cardiac massage for resuscitation
- conditions with an increased risk of haemorrhage which are not mentioned in chapter 4.3.

The use of rigid catheters should be avoided.

Additional special warnings and precautions in acute myocardial infarction:

A dose exceeding 100 mg of alteplase must not be given because it has been associated with an additional increase in intracranial bleeding.

Therefore special care must be taken to ensure that the dose of alteplase infused is as described in section 4.2 Posology and Method of Administration.

There is limited experience with readministration of Actilyse. Actilyse is not suspected to cause anaphylactic reactions. If an anaphylactoid reaction occurs, the infusion should be discontinued and appropriate treatment initiated.

The expected therapeutic benefit should be weighed up particularly carefully against the possible risk, especially in patients with systolic blood pressure > 160 mm Hg.

Additional special warnings and precautions in acute pulmonary embolism:

same as for acute myocardial infarction (see above)

Additional special warnings and special precautions in acute ischaemic stroke:

- Special precautions for use

Treatment must be performed only by a physician trained and experienced in neurological care.

- Special warnings / conditions with a decreased benefit/ risk ratio

Compared to other indications patients with acute ischaemic stroke treated with Actilyse have a markedly increased risk of intracranial haemorrhage as the bleeding occurs predominantly into the infarcted area. This applies in particular in the following cases:

- all situations listed in Section 4.3. and in general all situations involving a high risk of haemorrhage
- small asymptomatic aneurysms of the cerebral vessels
- patients pre-treated with acetyl salicylic acid (ASA) may have a greater risk of intracerebral haemorrhage, particularly if Actilyse treatment is delayed. Not more than 0.9 mg alteplase/kg bodyweight (max. of 90 mg) should be administered in view of the increased risk of cerebral haemorrhage.

Patients treatment should not be initiated later than 3 hours after the onset of symptoms (see 4.3 Contra-indications) because of an unfavourable benefit/risk ratio mainly based on the following:

- positive treatment effects decrease over time
- mortality rate increases particularly in patients with prior ASA treatment
- risk increases with regard to symptomatic haemorrhages

Blood pressure (BP) monitoring during treatment administration and up to 24 hours seems justified; an i.v. antihypertensive therapy is also recommended if systolic BP > 180 mm Hg or diastolic BP > 105 mm Hg.

The therapeutic benefit is reduced in patients that had a prior stroke or in those with known uncontrolled diabetes, thus the benefit/risk ratio is considered less favourable, but still positive in these patients.

In patients with very mild stroke, the risks outweigh the expected benefit (see 4.3 Contra-indications).

Patients with very severe stroke are at higher risk for intracerebral haemorrhage and death and should not be treated (see 4.3 Contra-indications).

Patients with extensive infarctions are at greater risk of poor outcome including severe haemorrhage and death. In such patients, the benefit/risk ratio should be thoroughly considered.

In stroke patients the likelihood of good outcomes decreases with increasing age, increasing stroke severity and increased levels of blood glucose on admission while the likelihood of severe disability and death or relevant intracranial bleedings increases, independently from treatment. Patients over 80, patients with severe stroke (as assessed clinically and/or by appropriate imaging techniques) and patients with blood glucose levels < 50 mg/dl or >400 mg/dl at baseline should not be treated with Actilyse (see 4.3 Contra-indications).

- Other special warnings

Reperfusion of the ischaemic area may induce cerebral oedama in the infarcted zone. Due to an increased haemorrhagic risk, treatment with platelet aggregation inhibitors should not be initiated within the first 24 hours following thrombolysis with alteplase.

4.5 Interaction with other medicinal products and other forms of Interaction

The risk of haemorrhage is increased if coumarine derivatives, oral anticoagulants, platelet aggregation inhibitors, unfractionated heparin or LMWH or other agents inhibiting coagulation are administered (before, during or within the first 24 hours after treatment with Actilyse) (see 4.3 Contra-indications).

Concomitant treatment with ACE inhibitors may enhance the risk of suffering an anaphylactoid reaction, as in the cases describing such reactions a relatively larger proportion of patients were receiving ACE inhibitors concomitantly.

4.6 Pregnancy and lactation
There is very limited experience with the use of Actilyse during pregnancy and lactation. In cases of an acute life-threatening disease the benefit has to be evaluated against the potential risk.

In pregnant animals no teratogenic effects were observed after iv. infusion of pharmacologically effective doses. In rabbits embryotoxicity (embryolethality, growth retardation) was induced by more than 3 mg/kg/day. No effects on peri-postnatal development or on fertility parameters were observed in rats with doses up to 10 mg/kg/day.

It is not known if alteplase is excreted into breast milk.

4.7 Effects on ability to drive and use machines
Not applicable.

4.8 Undesirable effects
General description

The most frequent adverse reaction associated with Actilyse is bleeding resulting in a fall in haematocrit and/or haemoglobin values. The type of bleeds associated with thrombolytic therapy can be divided into two broad categories:

- superficial bleeding, normally from punctures or damaged blood vessels,
- internal bleedings into the gastro-intestinal or uro-genital tract, retro-peritoneum or CNS or bleeding of parenchymatous organs.

Death and permanent disability are reported in patients who have experienced stroke (including intracranial bleeding) and other serious bleeding episodes.

Table of undesirable effects (according to MedDRA System Organ Class List) based on the reported events which may be causally related to Actilyse treatment

The frequencies given below are based on corresponding occurrences in a clinical trial involving 8,299 patients treated with Actilyse for myocardial infarction.

The classification of cholesterol crystal embolisation, which was not observed in the clinical trial population, was based on spontaneous reporting.

The number of patients treated in clinical trials in the indications pulmonary embolism and stroke (within the 0 - 3 hours time window) is very small in comparison to the number in the trial for myocardial infarction described above. Therefore, small numerical differences observed in comparison with the number in myocardial infarction were presumably attributable to the small sample size.

Except for intracranial haemorrhage as side effect in the indication stroke as well as for reperfusion arrhythmias in the indication myocardial infarction there is no medical reason to assume that the qualitative and quantitative side effect profile of Actilyse in the indications pulmonary embolism and acute ischaemic stroke is different from the profile in the indication myocardial infarction.

[1]very common: > 10 %; [2]common: > 1 % and $\leqslant 10$ %; [3]uncommon: > 0.1 % and $\leqslant 1$ %; [4]rare: > 0.01 % and $\leqslant 0.1$ %

Indication myocardial infarction:

Cardiac disorders:

[1]very common: reperfusion arrhythmias, which can be life threatening and may require the use of conventional anti-arrhythmic therapies

Indications myocardial infarction and pulmonary embolism:

Nervous system disorders

[3]uncommon: intracranial haemorrhage

Indication acute ischaemic stroke:

Nervous system disorders:

[2]common: intracranial haemorrhage. Symptomatic intracerebral haemorrhages represents the major adverse event (up to 10 % of patients). However, this had not shown an increased overall morbidity or mortality.

Indications myocardial infarction, pulmonary embolism and acute ischaemic stroke:

Immune system disorders:

[3]uncommon: anaphylactoid reactions, which are usually mild, but can be life threatening in isolated cases. They may appear as rash, urticaria, bronchospasm, angio-oedema, hypotension, shock or any other symptom associated with allergic reactions. If they occur, conventional anti-allergic therapy should be initiated. In such cases a relatively larger proportion of patients were receiving concomitant Angiotensin Converting Enzymes inhibitors. No definite anaphylactic (IgE mediated) reactions to ACTILYSE® are known. Transient antibody formation to ACTILYSE® has been observed in rare cases and with low titres, but a clinical relevance of this finding could not be established.

Vascular disorders:

[1]very common: bleeding

[2]common: ecchymosis

[3]uncommon: thrombotic embolisation, which may lead to corresponding consequences in the organs concerned

[4]rare: bleeding of parenchymatous organs

[4]rare: cholesterol crystal embolisation, which may lead to corresponding consequences in the organs concerned

[5]very rare: eye haemorrhage

Respiratory, thoracic and mediastinal disorders:

[2]common: epistaxis

Gastrointestinal disorders:

[2]common: bleeding into gastro-intestinal tract, nausea, vomiting. Nausea and vomiting can also occur as symptoms of myocardial infarction.

[3]uncommon: bleeding into retroperitoneum, gingival bleeding

Renal and urinary disorders:

[2]common: bleeding into urogenital tract

General disorders and administration site conditions:

[1]very common: superficial bleeding, normally from punctures or damaged blood vessels

Investigations:

[1]very common: drop in blood pressure

[2]common: increased temperature

Surgical and medical procedures:

[2]common: blood transfusion necessary

Additional information on certain severe or common events

In studies, where patients were treated according to clinical routine, i.e. without acute left-heart catheterisation, a blood transfusion was only occasionally necessary.

If a potentially dangerous haemorrhage occurs in particular cerebral haemorrhage, the fibrinolytic therapy must be discontinued. In general, however, it is not necessary to replace the coagulation factors because of the short half-life and the minimal effect on the systemic coagulation factors. Most patients who have bleeding can be managed by interruption of thrombolytic and anticoagulant therapy, volume replacement, and manual pressure applied to an incompetent vessel. Protamine should be considered if heparin has been administered within 4 hours of the onset of bleeding. In the few patients who fail to respond to these conservative measures, judicious use of transfusion products may be indicated. Transfusion of cryoprecipitate, fresh frozen plasma, and platelets should be considered with clinical and laboratory reassessment after each administration. A target fibrinogen level of 1 g/l is desirable with cryoprecipitate infusion. Antifibrinolytic agents are available as a last alternative. Patients with myocardial infarction or pulmonary embolism may experience disease-related events such as cardiac failure, recurrent ischaemia, angina, cardiac arrest, cardiogenic shock, reinfarction, valve disorders (e.g. aortic valve rupture), and pulmonary embolism. These events have also been reported following thrombolytic therapy and can be life-threatening and may lead to death.

Undesirable effects assigned to the pharmacological substance class

As with other thrombolytic agents, events related to the central nervous system (e.g. convulsions) have been reported in isolated cases, often in association with concurrent ischaemic or haemorrhagic cerebrovascular events.

4.9 Overdose
The relative fibrin specificity notwithstanding, a clinical significant reduction in fibrinogen and other blood coagulation components may occur after overdosage. In most cases, it is sufficient to await the physiological regeneration of these factors after the Actilyse therapy has been terminated. If, however, severe bleeding results, the infusion of fresh frozen plasma or fresh blood is recommended and if necessary, synthetic antifibrinolytics may be administered.

5. PHARMACOLOGICAL PROPERTIES

5.1 Pharmacodynamic properties
Pharmaco-therapeutic group: antithrombotic agent, ATC-code: B 01 A D 02

The active ingredient of Actilyse is alteplase, a recombinant human tissue-type plasminogen activator, a glycoprotein, which activates plasminogen directly to plasmin. When administered intravenously, alteplase remains relatively inactive in the circulatory system. Once bound to fibrin, it is activated, inducing the conversion of plasminogen to plasmin leading to the dissolution of the fibrin clot.

In a study including more than 40,000 patients with an acute myocardial infarction (GUSTO) the administration of 100 mg alteplase over 90 minutes, with concomitant iv. heparin infusion, led to a lower mortality after 30 days (6.3 %) as compared to the administration of streptokinase, 1.5 million U over 60 minutes, with s.c. or iv. heparin (7.3 %). Actilyse-treated patients showed higher infarct related vessel patency rates at 60 and 90 minutes after thrombolysis than the streptokinase-treated patients. No differences in patency rates were noted at 180 minutes or longer.

30-day-mortality is reduced as compared to patients not undergoing thrombolytic therapy.

The release of alpha-hydroxybutyrate-dehydrogenase (HBDH) is reduced. Global ventricular function as well as regional wall motion is less impaired as compared to patients receiving no thrombolytic therapy.

Myocardial infarction

A placebo controlled trial with 100 mg alteplase over 3 hours (LATE) showed a reduction of 30-day-mortality compared to placebo for patients treated within 6-12 hours after symptom onset. In cases, in which clear signs of myocardial infarction are present, treatment initiated up to 24 hours after symptom onset may still be beneficial.

Pulmonary embolism

In patients with acute massive pulmonary embolism with haemodynamic instability thrombolytic treatment with Actilyse leads to a fast reduction of the thrombus size and a reduction of pulmonary artery pressure. Mortality data are not available.

Acute stroke

In two USA studies (NINDS A/B) a significant higher proportion of patients, when compared to placebo, had a favourable outcome (no or minimal disability). These findings were not confirmed in two European studies and an additional USA study. In the latter studies however, the majority of patients were not treated within 3 hours of stroke onset. In a meta-analysis of all patients treated within 3 hours after stroke onset the beneficial effect of alteplase was confirmed. The risk difference versus placebo for a good recovery was 14.9% (CI 95% 8.1% to 21.7%) despite an increased risk of severe and fatal intracranial haemorrhage. The data do not allow a definite conclusion to be drawn on the treatment effect on death. Nevertheless overall, the benefit/risk of alteplase, given within 3 hours of stroke onset and taking into account the precautions stated elsewhere in the SPC, is considered favourable.

Meta-analysis of all clinical data show that the agent is less effective in patients treated after 3 hours of onset (3 to 6 hours) compared with those treated within 3 hours of onset of symptoms, while the risks are higher, which makes the benefit/risk ratio of alteplase unfavourable outside the 0-3 h time frame.

Due to its relative fibrin-specificity alteplase at a dose of 100 mg leads to a modest decrease of the circulating fibrinogen levels to about 60 % at 4 hours, which is generally reverted to more than 80 % after 24 hours. Plasminogen and alpha-2-antiplasmin decrease to about 20 % and 35 % respectively after 4 hours and increase again to more than 80 % at 24 hours. A marked and prolonged decrease of the circulating fibrinogen level is only seen in few patients.

5.2 Pharmacokinetic properties
Alteplase is cleared rapidly from the circulating blood and metabolised mainly by the liver (plasma clearance 550 - 680 ml/min.). The relevant plasma half-life $t_{1/2}$ alpha is 4-5 minutes. This means that after 20 minutes less than 10% of the initial value is present in the plasma. For the residual amount remaining in a deep compartment, a beta-half-life of about 40 minutes was measured.

5.3 Preclinical safety data
In subchronic toxicity studies in rats and marmosets no unexpected side effects were found. No indications of a mutagenic potential were found in mutagenic tests.

6. PHARMACEUTICAL PARTICULARS

6.1 List of excipients
Powder for solution:

L-arginine

Phosphoric acid

Polysorbate 80

Solvent:

Water for injections

The pH of the reconstituted solution is 7.3 +/- 0.5.

6.2 Incompatibilities
The reconstituted solution may be diluted further with sterile physiological saline solution (0.9 %) up to 1:5.

The reconstituted solution must not, however, be diluted further with water for injections or carbohydrate infusion solutions, e.g. glucose.

Actilyse must not be mixed with other medicinal products in the same infusion-vial or via the same catheter (not even with heparin).

6.3 Shelf life
3 years

After reconstitution, an immediate use is recommended. However, the in-use stability has been demonstrated for 24 hours at 2 °C - 8 °C and for 8 hours at 25 °C.

6.4 Special precautions for storage
Do not store above 25°C.

Store in the original package in order to protect from light.

6.5 Nature and contents of container
Powder for solution:

10 ml, 20 ml or 50 ml sterilised glass vials, sealed with sterile siliconised grey butyl-type stoppers with aluminium/plastic flip-off caps.

Solvent:

The water for injections is filled into either 10 ml, 20 ml or 50 ml vials, depending on the size of the rt-PA vials. The water for injections vials are sealed with rubber stoppers and aluminium/plastic flip-off caps.

Transfer cannulas(included with pack-sizes of 20 mg and 50 mg only)

Pack sizes:

10 mg

1 vial with 467 mg powder for solution for infusion

1 vial with 10 ml of water for injections

20 mg

1 vial with 933 mg powder for solution for infusion

1 vial with 20 ml of water for injections

1 transfer cannula

50 mg

1 vial with 2333 mg powder for solution for infusion

1 vial with 50 ml of water for injections

1 transfer cannula

6.6 Instructions for use and handling

None

7. MARKETING AUTHORISATION HOLDER

Boehringer Ingelheim Limited

Ellesfield Avenue

Bracknell

Berkshire

RG12 8YS

8. MARKETING AUTHORISATION NUMBER(S)

PL 00015/0120

9. DATE OF FIRST AUTHORISATION/RENEWAL OF THE AUTHORISATION

12th October 1998 / 26th April 1999

10. DATE OF REVISION OF THE TEXT

December 2003

11. LEGAL CATEGORY

POM

A1/UK/SPC/5

Actiq 200 micrograms, 400 micrograms, 600 micrograms, 800 micrograms, 1200 micrograms, 1600 micrograms compressed lozenge with integral oromucosal applicator.

(Cephalon UK Limited)

1. NAME OF THE MEDICINAL PRODUCT

Actiq® 200 micrograms, 400 micrograms, 600 micrograms, 800 micrograms, 1200 micrograms, 1600 micrograms compressed lozenge with integral oromucosal applicator.

2. QUALITATIVE AND QUANTITATIVE COMPOSITION

One lozenge contains:

200 micrograms fentanyl (equivalent to 314.2 micrograms fentanyl citrate)

400 micrograms fentanyl (equivalent to 628.4 micrograms fentanyl citrate)

600 micrograms fentanyl (equivalent to 942.6 micrograms fentanyl citrate)

800 micrograms fentanyl (equivalent to 1256.8 micrograms fentanyl citrate)

1200 micrograms fentanyl (equivalent to 1885.2 micrograms fentanyl citrate)

1600 micrograms fentanyl (equivalent to 2513.6 micrograms fentanyl citrate)

For excipients, see 6.1.

3. PHARMACEUTICAL FORM

Compressed lozenge with integral oromucosal applicator.

Actiq is formulated as a white to off-white compressed powder drug matrix attached using edible glue to a fracture resistant radio opaque plastic applicator, marked with the dosage strength.

4. CLINICAL PARTICULARS

4.1 Therapeutic indications

Actiq is indicated for the management of breakthrough pain in patients already receiving maintenance opioid therapy for chronic cancer pain. Breakthrough pain is a transitory exacerbation of pain that occurs on a background of otherwise controlled persistent pain.

4.2 Posology and method of administration

In order to minimise the risks of opioid-related side-effects and to identify the "successful" dose, it is imperative that patients be monitored closely by health professionals during the titration process. Any unused Actiq units that the patient no longer requires must be disposed of properly. Patients must be reminded of the requirements to keep Actiq stored in a location away from children.

Method of administration

Actiq is intended for oromucosal administration, and therefore should be placed in the mouth against the cheek and should be moved around the mouth using the applicator, with the aim of maximising the amount of mucosal exposure to the product. The Actiq unit should be sucked, not chewed, as absorption of fentanyl via the buccal mucosa is rapid in comparison with systemic absorption via the gastrointestinal tract. Water may be used to moisten the buccal mucosa in patients with a dry mouth.

The Actiq unit should be consumed over a 15 minute period. If signs of excessive opioid effects appear before the Actiq unit is fully consumed it should be immediately removed, and consideration given to decreasing future dosages.

Dose titration and maintenance therapy

Actiq should be individually titrated to a "successful" dose that provides adequate analgesia and minimises side effects. In clinical trials the successful dose of Actiq for breakthrough pain was not predicted from the daily maintenance dose of opioid.

a) Titration

Before patients are titrated with Actiq, it is expected that their background persistent pain will be controlled by use of opioid therapy and that they are typically experiencing no more than 4 episodes of breakthrough pain per day.

The initial dose of Actiq used should be 200 micrograms, titrating upwards as necessary through the range of available dosage strengths (200, 400, 600, 800, 1200 and 1600 micrograms). Patients should be carefully monitored until a dose is reached that provides adequate analgesia with acceptable side effects using a single dosage unit per episode of breakthrough pain. This is defined as the successful dose.

During titration, if adequate analgesia is not obtained within 15 minutes after the patient completes consumption of a single Actiq unit, a second Actiq unit of the same strength may be consumed. No more than two Actiq units should be used to treat any individual pain episode. At 1600 micrograms, a second dose is only likely to be required by a minority of patients.

If treatment of consecutive breakthrough pain episodes requires more than one dosage unit per episode, an increase in dose to the next higher available strength should be considered.

Actiq® Titration Process

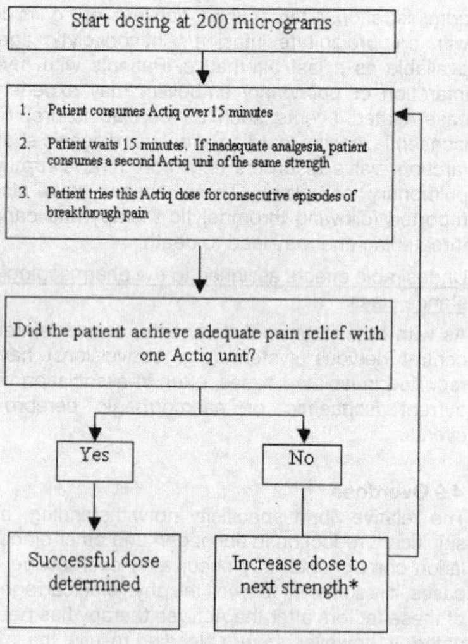
Start dosing at 200 micrograms
1. Patient consumes Actiq over 15 minutes
2. Patient waits 15 minutes. If inadequate analgesia, patient consumes a second Actiq unit of the same strength
3. Patient tries this Actiq dose for consecutive episodes of breakthough pain
Did the patient achieve adequate pain relief with one Actiq unit?
Yes
No
Successful dose determined
Increase dose to next strength*

*Available dosage strengths include: 200, 400, 600, 800, 1200 and 1600 micrograms

b) Maintenance

Once a successful dose has been established (i.e., on average, an episode is effectively treated with a single unit), patients should be maintained on this dose and should limit consumption to a maximum of four Actiq units per day.

Patients should be monitored by a health professional to ensure that the maximum consumption of four units of Actiq per day is not exceeded.

c) Dose re-adjustment

If more than four episodes of breakthrough pain are experienced per day, over a period of more than four consecutive days the dose of the long acting opioid used for persistent pain should be re-evaluated. If the dose of the long acting opioid is increased, the dose of Actiq to treat breakthrough pain may need to be reviewed.

It is imperative that any dose re-titration of any analgesic is monitored by a health professional.

d) Discontinuation of therapy

Actiq therapy may usually be immediately discontinued if no longer required for breakthrough pain only, in patients who continue to take their chronic opioid therapy for persistent pain.

For patients requiring discontinuation of all opioid therapy, account should be taken of the Actiq dose in consideration of a gradual downward opioid titration to avoid the possibility of abrupt withdrawal effects.

Use in Children

The appropriate posology and safety of Actiq have not been established in children and adolescents.

Use in the elderly

Elderly patients have been shown to be more sensitive to the effects of fentanyl when administered intravenously. Therefore dose titration needs to be approached with particular care. In the elderly, elimination of fentanyl is slower and the terminal elimination half-life is longer, which may result in accumulation of the active substance and to a greater risk of undesirable effects.

Formal clinical trials with Actiq have not been conducted in the elderly. It has been observed, however, in clinical trials that patients over 65 years of age required lower doses of Actiq for successful relief of breakthrough pain.

Use in special patient populations

Special care should be taken during the titration process in patients with kidney or liver dysfunction.

4.3 Contraindications

Hypersensitivity to fentanyl or to any of the excipients.

Simultaneous use of monoamine-oxidase (MAO) inhibitors, or within 2 weeks after the cessation of the use of MAO inhibitors.

Severe respiratory depression or severe obstructive lung conditions.

4.4 Special warnings and special precautions for use

It is important that the long acting opioid treatment used to treat the patient's persistent pain has been stabilised before Actiq therapy begins.

Tolerance and physical and/or psychological dependence may develop upon repeated administration of opioids such as fentanyl. However, iatrogenic addiction following therapeutic use of opioids is rare.

As with all opioids, there is a risk of clinically significant respiratory depression associated with the use of Actiq. Particular caution should be used when titrating Actiq in patients with non-severe chronic obstructive pulmonary disease or other medical conditions predisposing them to respiratory depression, as even normally therapeutic doses of Actiq may further decrease respiratory drive to the point of respiratory failure.

The product should not be given to opioid-naïve patients as there is an increased risk of respiratory depression and the appropriate dose in this patient population has not yet been determined.

Actiq should only be administered with extreme caution in patients who may be particularly susceptible to the intracranial effects of CO_2 retention, such as those with evidence of increased intracranial pressure, or impaired consciousness. Opioids may obscure the clinical course of a patient with a head injury and should be used only if clinically warranted.

Intravenous fentanyl may produce bradycardia. Therefore, Actiq should be used with caution in patients with bradyarrhythmias.

In addition, Actiq should be administered with caution to patients with liver or kidney dysfunction. The influence of liver and renal impairment on the pharmacokinetics of the medicinal product has not been evaluated, however, when administered intravenously the clearance of fentanyl has been shown to be altered in hepatic and renal disease due to alterations in metabolic clearance and plasma proteins. After administration of Actiq, impaired liver and renal function may both increase the bioavailability of swallowed fentanyl and decrease its systemic clearance, which could lead to increased and prolonged opioid effects. Therefore, special care should be taken during the titration process in patients with moderate or severe hepatic or renal disease.

Careful consideration should be given to patients with hypovolaemia and hypotension.

Diabetic patients should be advised that the medicine product contains dextrates (dextrates are composed of 93% dextrose monohydrate and 7% maltodextrin. The total glucose load per dosage unit is approximately 1.89 grams per dose).

Normal oral hygiene is recommended to avoid any potential harm to the teeth.

An evaluation of each out-patient concerning possible accidental child exposures should be undertaken.

Lozenges must be kept out of reach and sight of children and non-patients at all times before and after use. For instructions on handling and disposal, see Section 6.6.

4.5 Interaction with other medicinal products and other forms of Interaction

Fentanyl is metabolised by the CYP3A4 isoenzyme in the liver and intestinal mucosa. Potent inhibitors of CYP3A4 such as macrolide antibiotics, e.g. erythromycin, ketoconazole and certain protease inhibitors, e.g. ritonavir, may increase the bioavailability of swallowed fentanyl and may also decrease its systemic clearance which may result in increased or prolonged opioid effects. Similar effects could be seen after concurrent ingestion of grapefruit juice, which is known to inhibit CYP3A4. Hence caution is advised if fentanyl is given concomitantly with CYP3A4 inhibitors.

The concomitant use of other CNS depressants, including other opioids, sedatives or hypnotics, general anaesthetics, phenothiazines, tranquillisers, skeletal muscle relaxants, sedating antihistamines and alcohol may produce additive depressant effects.

Withdrawal symptoms may be precipitated through the administration of drugs with opioid antagonist activity, e.g., naloxone, or mixed agonist/antagonist analgesics (e.g., pentazocine, butorphanol, buprenorphine, nalbuphine).

4.6 Pregnancy and lactation
There are no adequate data from the use of fentanyl in pregnant women. Studies in animals have shown reproductive toxicity (see Section 5.3). Opioid analgesic agents can cause neonatal respiratory depression. With long-term use during pregnancy, there is a risk of neonatal withdrawal symptoms. Actiq should not be used in pregnancy unless clearly necessary.

It is advised not to use fentanyl during delivery because fentanyl passes through the placenta and may cause respiratory depression in the fœtus. The placental transfer ratio is 0.44 (foetal:maternal ratio 1.00:2.27). Fentanyl passes into breast milk, therefore women should not breast-feed while taking Actiq because of the possibility of sedation and/or respiratory depression in their infants. Breast feeding should not be restarted until at least 24 hours after the last administration of fentanyl.

4.7 Effects on ability to drive and use machines
No studies of the effects on the ability to drive and use machines have been performed. However, opioid analgesics may impair the mental and/or physical ability required for the performance of potentially dangerous tasks (e.g., driving a car or operating machinery). Patients should be advised not to drive or operate machinery if they experience somnolence or dizziness while taking Actiq.

4.8 Undesirable effects
The adverse events seen with Actiq are typical opioid side effects. Frequently, these opioid side effects will cease or decrease in intensity with continued use of Actiq, as the patient is titrated to the proper dose. Opioid side effects should be expected and managed accordingly.

Because the clinical trials of Actiq were designed to evaluate safety and efficacy in treating breakthrough pain, all patients were also taking concomitant opioids, such as sustained-release morphine or transdermal fentanyl, for their persistent pain. Thus it is not possible to definitively separate the effects of Actiq alone.

The adverse events considered to be at least possibly-related to treatment, from clinical trials involving 659 patients taking Actiq were as follows (very common >10%, common >1 - 10%, uncommon >0.1 - 1%):

Body as a whole	
Common:	asthenia, headache
Uncommon:	abdomen enlarged, abdominal pain, accidental injury, hangover effect, malaise
Cardiovascular system	
Uncommon:	*hypotension, tachycardia, vasodilatation
Digestive system	
Very common:	nausea/vomiting
Common:	constipation, dyspepsia
Uncommon:	anorexia, cheilitis, dysphagia, eructation, flatulence, gingivitis, gum haemorrhage, increased salivation, intestinal obstruction, jaundice, mouth ulcers, stomatitis, tongue disorder
Metabolic and nutritional disorders	
Uncommon:	thirst
Nervous system	
Common:	anxiety, confusion, dizziness, dry mouth, insomnia, somnolence
Uncommon:	abnormal co-ordination, abnormal dreams, abnormal thinking, agitation, amnesia, ataxia, circumoral paraesthesia, decreased reflexes, delusions, depersonalisation, depression, emotional lability, euphoria, hallucinations, hyperaesthesia, hypokinesia, myoclonus, stupor
Respiratory system	
Common:	dyspnoea
Uncommon:	asthma, *hypoventilation, pharyngitis, *respiratory failure
Skin and appendages	
Common:	pruritis, sweating
Uncommon:	rash, urticaria
Special senses	
Common:	abnormal vision
Uncommon:	taste perversion
Urogenital system	
Uncommon:	urinary retention

* The most serious adverse events associated with all opioids are respiratory depression (potentially leading to apnoea or respiratory arrest), circulatory depression, hypotension and shock. All patients should be followed for symptoms of respiratory depression.

4.9 Overdose
The symptoms of fentanyl overdosage are expected to be similar in nature to those of intravenous fentanyl and other opioids, and are an extension of its pharmacological actions, with the most serious significant effect being respiratory depression.

Immediate management of opioid overdose includes removal of the Actiq unit via the applicator, if still in the mouth, ensuring a patent airway, physical and verbal stimulation of the patient, assessment of the level of consciousness, ventilatory and circulatory status, and assisted ventilation (ventilatory support) if necessary.

For treatment of overdosage (accidental ingestion) in the opioid naïve person, intravenous access should be obtained, and naloxone or other opioid antagonists should be employed as clinically indicated. The duration of respiratory depression following overdose may be longer than the effects of the opioid antagonist's action (e.g., the half-life of naloxone ranges from 30 to 81 minutes) and repeated administration may be necessary. Consult the Summary of Product Characteristics of the individual opioid antagonist for details about such use.

For treatment of overdose in opioid-maintained patients, intravenous access should be obtained. The judicious use of naloxone or another opioid antagonist may be warranted in some instances, but it is associated with the risk of precipitating an acute withdrawal syndrome.

Although muscle rigidity interfering with respiration has not been seen following the use of Actiq, this is possible with fentanyl and other opioids. If it occurs, it should be managed by the use of assisted ventilation, by an opioid antagonist, and as a final alternative, by a neuromuscular blocking agent.

5. PHARMACOLOGICAL PROPERTIES

5.1 Pharmacodynamic properties
Pharmacotherapeutic group: Opioid analgesic, phenylpiperidone derivative ATC code N02A BO3.

Fentanyl, a pure opioid agonist, acts primarily through interaction with mu-opioid receptors located in the brain, spinal cord and smooth muscle. The primary site of therapeutic action is the central nervous system (CNS). The most clinically useful pharmacological effect of the interaction of fentanyl with mu-opioid receptors is analgesia. The analgesic effects of fentanyl are related to the blood level of the active substance, if proper allowance is made for the delay into and out of the CNS (a process with a 3-5 minute half-life). In opioid-naïve individuals, analgesia occurs at blood levels of 1 to 2 ng/ml, while blood levels of 10-20 ng/ml would produce surgical anaesthesia and profound respiratory depression.

In patients with chronic cancer pain on stable doses of regularly scheduled opioids to control their persistent pain, Actiq produced significantly more breakthrough pain relief compared with placebo at 15, 30, 45, and 60 minutes following administration.

Secondary actions include increase in the tone and decrease in the contractions of the gastrointestinal smooth muscle, which results in prolongation of gastrointestinal transit time and may be responsible for the constipatory effect of opioids.

While opioids generally increase the tone of urinary tract smooth muscle, the overall effect tends to vary, in some cases producing urinary urgency, in others difficulty in urination.

All opioid mu-receptor agonists, including fentanyl, produce dose dependent respiratory depression. The risk of respiratory depression is less in patients with pain and those receiving chronic opioid therapy who develop tolerance to respiratory depression and other opioid effects. In non-tolerant subjects, typically peak respiratory effects are seen 15 to 30 minutes following the administration of Actiq, and may persist for several hours.

5.2 Pharmacokinetic properties
General introduction
Fentanyl is highly lipophilic and can be absorbed very rapidly through the oral mucosa and more slowly by the conventional gastrointestinal route. It is subject to first-pass hepatic and intestinal metabolism and the metabolites do not contribute to fentanyl's therapeutic effects.

Absorption
The absorption pharmacokinetics of fentanyl from Actiq are a combination of rapid oromucosal absorption and slower gastrointestinal absorption of swallowed fentanyl. Approximately 25% of the total dose of Actiq is rapidly absorbed from the buccal mucosa. The remaining 75% of the dose is swallowed and slowly absorbed from the gastrointestinal tract. About 1/3 of this amount (25% of the total dose) escapes hepatic and intestinal first-pass elimination and becomes systemically available. Absolute bioavailability is about 50% compared to intravenous fentanyl, divided equally between rapid oromucosal and slower gastrointestinal absorption. C_{max} ranges from 0.39 to 2.51 ng/ml after consumption of Actiq (200 micrograms to 1600 micrograms). T_{max} is around 20 to 40 minutes after consumption of an Actiq unit (range 20 – 480 minutes).

Distribution
Animal data show that fentanyl is rapidly distributed to the brain, heart, lungs, kidneys and spleen followed by a slower redistribution to muscles and fat. The plasma protein binding of fentanyl is 80-85%. The main binding protein is alpha-1-acid glycoprotein, but both albumin and lipoproteins contribute to some extent. The free fraction of fentanyl increases with acidosis. The mean volume of distribution at steady state (V_{ss}) is 4 l/kg.

Biotransformation
Fentanyl is metabolised in the liver and in the intestinal mucosa to norfentanyl by CYP3A4 isoform.

Norfentanyl is not pharmacologically active in animal studies. More than 90% of the administered dose of fentanyl is eliminated by biotransformation to N-dealkylated and hydroxylated inactive metabolites.

Elimination
Less than 7% of the dose is excreted unchanged in the urine, and only about 1% is excreted unchanged in the faeces. The metabolites are mainly excreted in the urine, while faecal excretion is less important. The total plasma clearance of fentanyl is 0.5 l/hr/kg (range 0.3-0.7 l/hr/kg). The terminal elimination half-life after Actiq administration is about 7 hours.

Linearity/non-linearity
Dose proportionality across the available range of dosages (200 micrograms to 1600 micrograms) of Actiq has been demonstrated.

5.3 Preclinical safety data
Preclinical data from general toxicity studies and *in vivo* and *in vitro* genotoxicity studies reveal no special hazard for humans, beyond the information included in other sections of the SPC.

In reproductive toxicity studies reduced fertility and increased embryonic death, but no teratogenicity was observed in rats.

6. PHARMACEUTICAL PARTICULARS

6.1 List of excipients
Lozenge:
Dextrates (93% dextrose monohydrate, as D-glucose, and 7% maltodextrin)
Citric acid
Dibasic sodium phosphate
Artificial berry flavour (maltodextrin, propylene glycol, artificial flavours and triethylcitrate)
Magnesium stearate

Edible glue used to attach the lozenge to the handle:
Purity gum BE (E1450, a modified maize based food starch)
Confectioner's sugar (sucrose and corn starch)
Distilled water

Imprinting ink:
Ethanol
De-ionised water
De-waxed white shellac
Propylene glycol
FD & C Blue No. 1 (E133)

6.2 Incompatibilities
Not applicable.

6.3 Shelf life
3 years

6.4 Special precautions for storage
Do not store above 30°C.

Keep Actiq stored in a location away from children, at all times.

6.5 Nature and contents of container
Each Actiq dosage unit is contained in a heat sealed blister package consisting of a paper/foil laminated lid, and a PVC/Aclar thermoformed blister, supplied in cartons of 3, 6, 15 or 30 individual units.

Not all pack sizes may be marketed.

6.6 Instructions for use and handling
Patients and their carers must be instructed that Actiq contains an active substance in an amount that can be

fatal to a child. Patients and their carers must be instructed to keep all units out of the reach of children and to discard open units appropriately.

Lozenges with residual active substance should at no time be discarded or misplaced. Any used product or waste material should be disposed of in accordance with local requirements.

7. MARKETING AUTHORISATION HOLDER

Cephalon UK Limited
11/13 Frederick Sanger Road
Surrey Research Park
Guildford
Surrey
GU2 7YD

8. MARKETING AUTHORISATION NUMBER(S)

Actiq 200 microgram compressed lozenge with integral oromucosal applicator

PL 16260/0003

Actiq 400 microgram compressed lozenge with integral oromucosal applicator

PL 16260/0004

Actiq 600 microgram compressed lozenge with integral oromucosal applicator

PL 16260/0005

Actiq 800 microgram compressed lozenge with integral oromucosal applicator

PL 16260/0006

Actiq 1200 microgram compressed lozenge with integral oromucosal applicator

PL 16260/0007

Actiq 1600 microgram compressed lozenge with integral oromucosal applicator

PL 16260/0008

9. DATE OF FIRST AUTHORISATION/RENEWAL OF THE AUTHORISATION

10th August 2002

10. DATE OF REVISION OF THE TEXT

August 2002

Legal Category

CD (Sch2), POM

Actonel 30mg Film Coated Tablets

(Procter & Gamble Pharmaceuticals UK Limited)

1. NAME OF THE MEDICINAL PRODUCT

Actonel 30 mg film-coated tablets.

2. QUALITATIVE AND QUANTITATIVE COMPOSITION

Each film-coated tablet contains 30 mg risedronate sodium (equivalent to 27.8 mg risedronic acid).

For excipients, see section 6.1.

3. PHARMACEUTICAL FORM

Film-coated tablets.

Oval white film-coated tablet with RSN on one side and 30 mg on the other.

4. CLINICAL PARTICULARS

4.1 Therapeutic indications

Treatment of Paget's disease of the bone.

4.2 Posology and method of administration

The recommended daily dose in adults is one 30 mg tablet orally for 2 months. If re-treatment is considered necessary (at least two months post-treatment), a new treatment with the same dose and duration of therapy could be given. The absorption of Actonel is affected by food, thus to ensure adequate absorption patients should take Actonel:

• Before breakfast: At least 30 minutes before the first food, other medicinal product or drink (other than plain water) of the day.

In the particular instance that before breakfast dosing is not practical, Actonel can be taken between meals or in the evening at the same time everyday, with strict adherence to the following instructions, to ensure Actonel is taken on an empty stomach:

• Between meals: Actonel should be taken at least 2 hours before and at least 2 hours after any food, medicinal product or drink (other than plain water).

• In the evening: Actonel should be taken at least 2 hours after the last food, medicinal product or drink (other than plain water) of the day. Actonel should be taken at least 30 minutes before going to bed.

If an occasional dose is missed, Actonel can be taken before breakfast, between meals, or in the evening according to the instructions above.

The tablet must be swallowed whole and not sucked or chewed. To aid delivery of the tablet to the stomach Actonel is to be taken while in an upright position with a glass of plain water (≥120 ml). Patients should not lie down for 30 minutes after taking the tablet (see section 4.4).

Physicians should consider the administration of supplemental calcium and vitamin D if dietary intake is inadequate, especially as bone turnover is significantly elevated in Paget's disease.

Elderly: No dosage adjustment is necessary since bioavailability, distribution and elimination were similar in elderly >60 years of age) compared to younger subjects.

Children: Safety and efficacy of Actonel have not been established in children and adolescents.

4.3 Contraindications

Known hypersensitivity to risedronate sodium or to any of its excipients.

Hypocalcaemia (see section 4.4).

Pregnancy and lactation.

Severe renal impairment (creatinine clearance <30ml/min).

4.4 Special warnings and special precautions for use

Foods, drinks (other than plain water) and medicinal products containing polyvalent cations (such as calcium, magnesium, iron and aluminium) may interfere with the absorption of bisphosphonates and should not be taken at the same time as Actonel (see section 4.5). In order to achieve the intended efficacy, strict adherence to the dosing recommendations is necessary (see section 4.2).

Some bisphosphonates have been associated with oesophagitis and oesophageal ulcerations. Therefore patients should pay attention to the dosing instructions (see section 4.2). In patients who have a history of oesophageal disorders which delay oesophageal transit or emptying e.g. stricture or achalasia, or who are unable to stay in the upright position for at least 30 minutes after taking the tablet, risedronate sodium should be used with special caution because of limited clinical experience in these patients. Prescribers should emphasise the importance of the dosing instructions to these patients.

Hypocalcaemia should be treated before starting Actonel therapy. Other disturbances of bone and mineral metabolism (e.g. parathyroid dysfunction, hypovitaminosis D) should be treated at the time of starting Actonel therapy.

This medicine contains lactose. Patients with rare hereditary problems of galactose intolerance, the Lapp lactase deficiency or glucose-galactose malabsorption should not take this medicine.

4.5 Interaction with other medicinal products and other forms of Interaction

No formal interaction studies have been performed, however no clinically relevant interactions with other medicinal products were found during clinical trials.

Concomitant ingestion of medications containing polyvalent cations (e.g. calcium, magnesium, iron and aluminium) will interfere with the absorption of Actonel (see section 4.4).

Actonel is not systemically metabolised, does not induce cytochrome P450 enzymes, and has low protein binding.

4.6 Pregnancy and lactation

There are no adequate data from the use of risedronate sodium in pregnant women. Studies in animals have shown reproductive toxicity (see section 5.3). The potential risk for humans is unknown.

Actonel must not be used during pregnancy or by breast-feeding women.

4.7 Effects on ability to drive and use machines

No effects on ability to drive and use machines have been observed.

4.8 Undesirable effects

Risedronate has been studied in phase III clinical trials involving more than 15,000 patients.The majority of undesirable effects observed in clinical trials were mild to moderate in severity and usually did not require cessation of therapy.

Adverse experiences reported in phase III clinical trials in postmenopausal women with osteoporosis treated for up to 36 months with risedronate 5mg/day (n=5020) or placebo (n=5048) and considered possibly or probably related to risedronate are listed below using the following convention (incidences versus placebo are shown in brackets): very common (≥1/10); common (≥1/100; <1/10); uncommon (≥1/1,000; <1/100); rare (≥1/10,000; <1/1,000); very rare (<1/10,000).

Nervous system disorders:

Common: headache (1.8% vs. 1.4%)

Eye disorders:

Uncommon: iritis*

Gastrointestinal disorders:

Common: constipation (5.0% vs. 4.8%), dyspepsia (4.5% vs. 4.1%), nausea (4.3% vs. 4.0%), abdominal pain (3.5% vs. 3.3%), diarrhoea (3.0% vs. 2.7%)

Uncommon: gastritis (0.9% vs. 0.7%), oesophagitis (0.9% vs. 0.9%), dysphagia (0.4% vs. 0.2%), duodenitis (0.2% vs. 0.1), oesophageal ulcer (0.2% vs. 0.2%)

Rare: glossitis (<0.1% vs. 0.1%), oesophageal stricture (<0.1% vs. 0.0%),

Musculoskeletal and connective tissues disorders:

Common: musculoskeletal pain (2.1% vs. 1.9%)

Investigations (hepatobiliary):

Rare: abnormal liver function tests*

In a phase III Paget's Disease clinical trial comparing risedronate vs. etidronate (61 patients in each group), the following additional adverse experiences considered possibly or probably drug related by investigators have been reported (incidence greater in risedronate than in etidronate): arthralgia (9.8% vs. 8.2%); amblyopia, apnoea, bronchitis, colitis, corneal lesion, cramps leg, dizziness, dry eye, flu syndrome, hypocalcaemia, myasthenia, neoplasm, nocturia, oedema peripheral, pain bone, pain chest, rash, sinusitis, tinnitus, and weight decrease (all at 1.6% vs. 0.0%).

Laboratory findings: Early, transient, asymptomatic and mild decreases in serum calcium and phosphate levels have been observed in some patients.

The following additional adverse reactions have been reported during post-marketing use:

Skin and subcutaneous tissue disorders:

Very rare (<1/10,000): hypersensitivity and skin reactions, including angioedema, generalised rash, and bullous skin reactions, some severe.

* No relevant incidences from Phase III osteoporosis studies; frequency based on adverse event/laboratory/rechallenge findings in earlier clinical trials.

4.9 Overdose

No specific information is available on the treatment of overdose with risedronate sodium.

Decreases in serum calcium following substantial overdose may be expected. Signs and symptoms of hypocalcaemia may also occur in some of these patients.

Milk or antacids containing magnesium, calcium or aluminium should be given to bind risedronate and reduce absorption of the drug. In cases of substantial overdose, gastric lavage may be considered to remove unabsorbed drug.

5. PHARMACOLOGICAL PROPERTIES

5.1 Pharmacodynamic properties

Pharmaco-therapeutic group: Bisphosphonates

ATC Code: M05 BA07

Risedronate sodium is a pyridinyl bisphosphonate that binds to bone hydroxyapatite and inhibits osteoclast-mediated bone resorption. The bone turnover is reduced while the osteoblast activity and bone mineralisation is preserved.

Paget's disease of the bone: In the clinical programme Actonel was studied in patients with Paget's disease. After treatment with Actonel 30 mg/day for 2 months the following was seen:

• serum alkaline phosphatase normalised in 77% of patients compared to 11% in the control group (etidronate 400 mg/day for 6 months). Significant reductions were observed in urinary hydroxyproline/creatinine and urinary deoxypyridinoline/creatinine,

• radiographs taken at baseline and after 6 months demonstrated a decrease in the extent of osteolytic lesions in both the appendicular and axial skeleton. No new fractures were observed.

The observed response was similar in pagetic patients regardless of whether they had previously received other treatments for Paget's disease, or the severity of the disease.

53% of patients followed for 18 months after initiation of a single 2 month course of Actonel remained in biochemical remission.

In a trial comparing before-breakfast dosing and dosing at other times of the day in women with postmenopausal osteoporosis, lumbar spine BMD gains were statistically higher with before-breakfast dosing.

5.2 Pharmacokinetic properties

Absorption: Absorption after an oral dose is relatively rapid (t_{max} ~1 hour) and is independent of dose over the range studied (2.5 to 30 mg). Mean oral bioavailability of the tablet is 0.63% and is decreased when risedronate sodium is administered with food. Bioavailability was similar in men and women.

Distribution: The mean steady state volume of distribution is 6.3 l/kg in humans. Plasma protein binding is about 24%.

Metabolism: There is no evidence of systemic metabolism of risedronate sodium.

Elimination: Approximately half of the absorbed dose is excreted in urine within 24 hours, and 85% of an intravenous dose is recovered in the urine after 28 days. Mean renal clearance is 105 ml/min and mean total clearance is 122 ml/min, with the difference probably attributed to clearance due to adsorption to bone. The renal clearance is not concentration dependent, and there is a linear relationship between renal clearance and creatinine clearance. Unabsorbed risedronate sodium is eliminated unchanged in faeces. After oral administration the concentration-time profile shows three elimination phases with a terminal half-life of 480 hours.

Special populations:

Elderly: no dosage adjustment is necessary.

5.3 Preclinical safety data
In toxicological studies in rat and dog dose dependent liver toxic effects of risedronate sodium were seen, primarily as enzyme increases with histological changes in rat. The clinical relevance of these observations is unknown. Testicular toxicity occurred in rat and dog at exposures considered in excess of the human therapeutic exposure. Dose related incidences of upper airway irritation were frequently noted in rodents. Similar effects have been seen with other bisphosphonates. Lower respiratory tract effects were also seen in longer term studies in rodents, although the clinical significance of these findings is unclear. In reproduction toxicity studies at exposures close to clinical exposure ossification changes were seen in sternum and/or skull of foetuses from treated rats and hypocalcemia and mortality in pregnant females allowed to deliver. There was no evidence of teratogenesis at 3.2mg/kg/day in rat and 10mg/kg/day in rabbit, although data are only available on a small number of rabbits. Maternal toxicity prevented testing of higher doses. Studies on genotoxicity and carcinogenesis did not show any particular risks for humans.

6. PHARMACEUTICAL PARTICULARS
6.1 List of excipients
Tablet core: lactose monohydrate, microcrystalline cellulose, crospovidone, magnesium stearate.

Film coating: hypromellose, macrogol 400, hyprolose, macrogol 8000, silicon dioxide, titanium dioxide E171.

6.2 Incompatibilities
Not applicable.

6.3 Shelf life
5 years.

6.4 Special precautions for storage
No special storage conditions.

6.5 Nature and contents of container
Opaque PVC/aluminium foil blister cards of 14 tablets in cardboard carton, tablet count 28 (2 × 14) and tablet count 14 (1 × 14).

Sample pack – Opaque PVC/aluminium foil blister cards of 3 tablets in cardboard carton, tablet count 3 (1 × 3).

Not all pack sizes may be marketed.

6.6 Instructions for use and handling
No special requirements.

7. MARKETING AUTHORISATION HOLDER
Procter & Gamble Pharmaceuticals UK Ltd
Rusham Park, Whitehall Lane
Egham, Surrey, TW20 9NW, UK

8. MARKETING AUTHORISATION NUMBER(S)
PL 00364/0071
PA 170/20/2

9. DATE OF FIRST AUTHORISATION/RENEWAL OF THE AUTHORISATION
1999-10-07/2004-10-07

10. DATE OF REVISION OF THE TEXT
2005-01-28

Actonel 5mg Film Coated Tablets

(Procter & Gamble Pharmaceuticals UK Limited)

1. NAME OF THE MEDICINAL PRODUCT
Actonel 5 mg film-coated tablets.

2. QUALITATIVE AND QUANTITATIVE COMPOSITION
Each film-coated tablet contains 5 mg risedronate sodium (equivalent to 4.64 mg risedronic acid).

For excipients, see section 6.1.

3. PHARMACEUTICAL FORM
Film-coated tablets.

Oval yellow film-coated tablet with RSN on one side and 5 mg on the other.

4. CLINICAL PARTICULARS
4.1 Therapeutic indications
Treatment of postmenopausal osteoporosis, to reduce the risk of vertebral fractures. Treatment of established postmenopausal osteoporosis, to reduce the risk of hip fractures. Prevention of osteoporosis in postmenopausal women with increased risk of osteoporosis (see section 5.1).

To maintain or increase bone mass in postmenopausal women undergoing long-term (more than 3 months), systemic corticosteroid treatment at doses ≥ 7.5mg/day prednisone or equivalent.

4.2 Posology and method of administration
The recommended daily dose in adults is one 5 mg tablet orally. The absorption of Actonel is affected by food, thus to ensure adequate absorption patients should take Actonel:

• Before breakfast: At least 30 minutes before the first food, other medicinal product or drink (other than plain water) of the day.

In the particular instance that before breakfast dosing is not practical, Actonel can be taken between meals or in the evening at the same time everyday, with strict adherence to the following instructions, to ensure Actonel is taken on an empty stomach:

• Between meals: Actonel should be taken at least 2 hours before and at least 2 hours after any food, medicinal product or drink (other than plain water).

• In the evening: Actonel should be taken at least 2 hours after the last food, medicinal product or drink (other than plain water) of the day. Actonel should be taken at least 30 minutes before going to bed.

If an occasional dose is missed, Actonel can be taken before breakfast, between meals, or in the evening according to the instructions above.

The tablets must be swallowed whole and not sucked or chewed. To aid delivery of the tablet to the stomach Actonel is to be taken while in an upright position with a glass of plain water (≥120 ml). Patients should not lie down for 30 minutes after taking the tablet (see section 4.4).

Supplemental calcium and vitamin D should be considered if the dietary intake is inadequate.

Elderly: No dosage adjustment is necessary since bioavailability, distribution and elimination were similar in elderly >60 years of age) compared to younger subjects.

Children: Safety and efficacy of Actonel have not been established in children and adolescents.

4.3 Contraindications
Known hypersensitivity to risedronate sodium or to any of its excipients.

Hypocalcaemia (see section 4.4).

Pregnancy and lactation.

Severe renal impairment (creatinine clearance <30ml/min).

4.4 Special warnings and special precautions for use
Foods, drinks (other than plain water) and medicinal products containing polyvalent cations (such as calcium, magnesium, iron and aluminium) interfere with the absorption of bisphosphonates and should not be taken at the same time as Actonel (see section 4.5). In order to achieve the intended efficacy, strict adherence to dosing recommendations is necessary (see section 4.2)

Efficacy of bisphosphonates in the treatment of postmenopausal osteoporosis is related to the presence of low bone mineral density (BMD T-score at hip or lumbar spine ≤-2.5 SD) and/or prevalent fracture.

High age or clinical risk factors for fracture alone are not reasons to initiate treatment of osteoporosis with a bisphosphonate.

The evidence to support efficacy of bisphosphonates including Actonel in very elderly women >80 years) is limited (see section 5.1).

Some bisphosphonates have been associated with oesophagitis and oesophageal ulcerations. Therefore patients should pay attention to the dosing instructions (see section 4.2). In patients who have a history of oesophageal disorders which delay oesophageal transit or emptying e.g. stricture or achalasia, or who are unable to stay in the upright position for at least 30 minutes after taking the tablet, risedronate sodium should be used with special caution because of limited clinical experience in these patients. Prescribers should emphasise the importance of the dosing instructions to these patients.

Hypocalcaemia should be treated before starting Actonel therapy. Other disturbances of bone and mineral metabolism (e.g. parathyroid dysfunction, hypovitaminosis D) should be treated at the time of starting Actonel therapy.

This medicine contains lactose. Patients with rare hereditary problems of galactose intolerance, the Lapp lactase deficiency or glucose-galactose malabsorption should not take this medicine.

4.5 Interaction with other medicinal products and other forms of Interaction
No formal interaction studies have been performed, however no clinically relevant interactions with other medicinal products were found during clinical trials. In the Actonel Phase III osteoporosis studies, acetyl salicylic acid or NSAID use was reported by 33% and 45% of patients respectively.

If considered appropriate Actonel may be used concomitantly with oestrogen supplementation.

Concomitant ingestion of medications containing polyvalent cations (e.g. calcium, magnesium, iron and aluminium) will interfere with the absorption of Actonel (see section 4.4).

Actonel is not systemically metabolised, does not induce cytochrome P450 enzymes, and has low protein binding.

4.6 Pregnancy and lactation
There are no adequate data from the use of risedronate sodium in pregnant women. Studies in animals have shown reproductive toxicity (see section 5.3). The potential risk for humans is unknown. Actonel must not be used during pregnancy or by breast-feeding women.

4.7 Effects on ability to drive and use machines
No effects on ability to drive and use machines have been observed.

4.8 Undesirable effects
Risedronate has been studied in phase III clinical trials involving more than 15,000 patients. The majority of undesirable effects observed in clinical trials were mild to moderate in severity and usually did not require cessation of therapy.

Adverse experiences reported in phase III clinical trials in postmenopausal women with osteoporosis treated for up to 36 months with risedronate 5mg/day (n=5020) or placebo (n=5048) and considered possibly or probably related to risedronate are listed below using the following convention (incidences versus placebo are shown in brackets): very common (≥1/10); common (≥1/100; <1/10); uncommon (≥1/1,000; <1/100); rare (≥1/10,000; <1/1,000); very rare (<1/10,000).

Nervous system disorders:

Common: headache (1.8% vs. 1.4%)

Eye disorders:

Uncommon: iritis*

Gastrointestinal disorders:

Common: constipation (5.0% vs. 4.8%), dyspepsia (4.5% vs. 4.1%), nausea (4.3% vs. 4.0%), abdominal pain (3.5% vs. 3.3%), diarrhoea (3.0% vs. 2.7%)

Uncommon: gastritis (0.9% vs. 0.7%), oesophagitis (0.9% vs. 0.9%), dysphagia (0.4% vs. 0.2%), duodenitis (0.2% vs. 0.1), oesophageal ulcer (0.2% vs. 0.2%)

Rare: glossitis (<0.1% vs. 0.1%), oesophageal stricture (<0.1% vs. 0.0%),

Musculoskeletal and connective tissues disorders:

Common: musculoskeletal pain (2.1% vs. 1.9%)

Investigations (hepatobiliary):

Rare: abnormal liver function tests*

Laboratory findings: Early, transient, asymptomatic and mild decreases in serum calcium and phosphate levels have been observed in some patients.

The following additional adverse reactions have been reported during post-marketing use:

Skin and subcutaneous tissue disorders:

Very rare (<1/10,000): hypersensitivity and skin reactions, including angioedema, generalised rash, and bullous skin reactions, some severe.

* No relevant incidences from Phase III osteoporosis studies; frequency based on adverse event/laboratory/rechallenge findings in earlier clinical trials.

4.9 Overdose
No specific information is available on the treatment of overdose with risedronate sodium.

Decreases in serum calcium following substantial overdose may be expected. Signs and symptoms of hypocalcaemia may also occur in some of these patients.

Milk or antacids containing magnesium, calcium or aluminium should be given to bind risedronate and reduce absorption of the risedronate sodium. In cases of substantial overdose, gastric lavage may be considered to remove unabsorbed risedronate sodium.

5. PHARMACOLOGICAL PROPERTIES
5.1 Pharmacodynamic properties
Pharmaco-therapeutic group: Bisphosphonates
ATC Code: M05 BA07

Risedronate sodium is a pyridinyl bisphosphonate that binds to bone hydroxyapatite and inhibits osteoclast-mediated bone resorption. The bone turnover is reduced while the osteoblast activity and bone mineralisation is preserved. In preclinical studies risedronate sodium demonstrated potent anti-osteoclast and antiresorptive activity, and dose dependently increased bone mass and biomechanical skeletal strength. The activity of risedronate sodium was confirmed by measuring biochemical markers for bone turnover during pharmacodynamic and clinical studies. Decreases in biochemical markers of bone turnover were observed within 1 month and reached a maximum in 3-6 months.

Treatment and Prevention of Postmenopausal Osteoporosis:

A number of risk factors are associated with postmenopausal osteoporosis including low bone mass, low bone mineral density, early menopause, a history of smoking and a family history of osteoporosis. The clinical consequence of osteoporosis is fractures. The risk of fractures is increased with the number of risk factors.

The clinical programme studied the effect of risedronate sodium on the risk of hip and vertebral fractures and contained early and late postmenopausal women with and without fracture. Daily doses of 2.5 mg and 5 mg were studied and all groups, including the control groups, received calcium and vitamin D (if baseline levels were low). The absolute and relative risk of new vertebral and hip fractures were estimated by use of a time-to-first event analysis.

• Two placebo-controlled trials (n=3,661) enrolled postmenopausal women under 85 years with vertebral fractures at baseline. Risedronate sodium 5 mg daily given for 3 years reduced the risk of new vertebral fractures relative to the control group. In women with respectively at least 2 or at least 1 vertebral fractures, the relative risk reduction was 49% and 41% respectively (incidence of new vertebral fractures with risedronate sodium 18.1% and 11.3%, with placebo 29.0% and 16.3%, respectively). The effect of treatment was seen as early as the end of the first year of treatment. Benefits were also demonstrated in women with multiple fractures at baseline. Risedronate sodium 5 mg daily also reduced the yearly height loss compared to the control group.

• Two further placebo controlled trials enrolled postmenopausal women above 70 years with or without vertebral fractures at baseline. Women 70-79 years were enrolled with femoral neck BMD T-score <-3 SD (manufacturer's range, i.e. -2.5 SD using NHANES III) and at least one additional risk factor. Women ≥80 years could be enrolled on the basis of at least one non-skeletal risk factor for hip fracture or low bone mineral density at the femoral neck. Statistical significance of the efficacy of risedronate sodium versus placebo is only reached when the two treatment groups 2.5 mg and 5 mg are pooled. The following results are only based on *a-posteriori* analysis of subgroups defined by clinical practise and current definitions of osteoporosis:

- In the subgroup of patients with femoral neck BMD T-score ≤-2.5SD (NHANES III) and at least one vertebral fracture at baseline, risedronate sodium given for 3 years reduced the risk of hip fractures by 46% relative to the control group (incidence of hip fractures in combined risedronate sodium 2.5 and 5 mg groups 3.8%, placebo 7.4%);

- Data suggest that a more limited protection than this may be observed in the very elderly (≥80 years). This may be due to the increasing importance of non-skeletal factors for hip fracture with increasing age.

- In these trials, data analysed as a secondary endpoint indicated a decrease in the risk of new vertebral fractures in patients with low femoral neck BMD without vertebral fracture and in patients with low femoral neck BMD with or without vertebral fracture. Risedronate sodium 5 mg daily given for 3 years increased bone mineral density (BMD) relative to control at the lumbar spine, femoral neck, trochanter and wrist and prevented bone loss at the mid-shaft radius.

• In a one-year follow-up off therapy after three years treatment with risedronate sodium 5 mg daily there was rapid reversibility of the suppressing effect of risedronate sodium on bone turnover rate.

• In postmenopausal women taking oestrogen, risedronate sodium 5 mg daily increased bone mineral density (BMD) at the femoral neck and mid-shaft radius only, compared to oestrogen alone.

• Bone biopsy samples from postmenopausal women treated with risedronate sodium 5 mg daily for 2 to 3 years, showed an expected moderate decrease in bone turnover. Bone formed during risedronate sodium treatment was of normal lamellar structure and bone mineralisation. These data together with the decreased incidence of osteoporosis related fractures at vertebral sites in women with osteoporosis appear to indicate no detrimental effect on bone quality.

• Endoscopic findings from a number of patients with a number of moderate to severe gastrointestinal complaints in both risedronate sodium and control patients indicated no evidence of treatment related gastric, duodenal or oesophageal ulcers in either group, although duodenitis was uncommonly observed in the risedronate sodium group.

• In a trial comparing before-breakfast dosing and dosing at other times of the day in women with postmenopausal osteoporosis, lumbar spine BMD gains were statistically higher with before-breakfast dosing.

Corticosteroid Induced Osteoporosis:

The clinical programme included patients initiating corticosteroid therapy (≥ 7.5 mg/day prednisone or equivalent) within the previous 3 months or patients who had been taking corticosteroids for more than 6 months. Results of these studies demonstrate that:

• Risedronate sodium 5 mg daily given for one year maintains or increases bone mineral density (BMD) relative to control at the lumbar spine, femoral neck, and trochanter.

• Risedronate sodium 5 mg daily reduced the incidence of vertebral fractures, monitored for safety, relative to control at 1 year in pooled studies.

• histological examination of bone biopsies from patients taking corticosteroids and risedronate sodium 5 mg daily did not show signs of disturbed mineralisation process.

5.2 Pharmacokinetic properties

Absorption: Absorption after an oral dose is relatively rapid (t_{max} ~1 hour) and is independent of dose over the range studied (2.5 to 30 mg). Mean oral bioavailability of the tablet is 0.63% and is decreased when risedronate sodium is administered with food. Bioavailability was similar in men and women.

Distribution: The mean steady state volume of distribution is 6.3 l/kg in humans. Plasma protein binding is about 24%.

Metabolism: There is no evidence of systemic metabolism of risedronate sodium.

Elimination: Approximately half of the absorbed dose is excreted in urine within 24 hours, and 85% of an intravenous dose is recovered in the urine after 28 days. Mean renal clearance is 105 ml/min and mean total clearance is 122 ml/min, with the difference probably attributed to clearance due to adsorption to bone. The renal clearance is not concentration dependent, and there is a linear relationship between renal clearance and creatinine clearance. Unabsorbed risedronate sodium is eliminated unchanged in faeces. After oral administration the concentration-time profile shows three elimination phases with a terminal half-life of 480 hours.

Special populations:

Elderly: no dosage adjustment is necessary.

Acetyl salicylic acid/NSAID users: Among regular acetyl salicylic acid or NSAID users (3 or more days per week) the incidence of upper gastrointestinal adverse events in Actonel treated patients was similar to that in control patients.

5.3 Preclinical safety data

In toxicological studies in rat and dog dose dependent liver toxic effects of risedronate sodium were seen, primarily as enzyme increases with histological changes in rat. The clinical relevance of these observations is unknown. Testicular toxicity occurred in rat and dog at exposures considered in excess of the human therapeutic exposure. Dose related incidences of upper airway irritation were frequently noted in rodents. Similar effects have been seen with other bisphosphonates. Lower respiratory tract effects were also seen in longer term studies in rodents, although the clinical significance of these findings is unclear. In reproduction toxicity studies at exposures close to clinical exposure ossification changes were seen in sternum and/or skull of foetuses from treated rats and hypocalcemia and mortality in pregnant females allowed to deliver. There was no evidence of teratogenesis at 3.2mg/kg/day in rat and 10mg/kg/day in rabbit, although data are only available on a small number of rabbits. Maternal toxicity prevented testing of higher doses. Studies on genotoxicity and carcinogenesis did not show any particular risks for humans.

6. PHARMACEUTICAL PARTICULARS

6.1 List of excipients

Tablet core: lactose monohydrate, microcrystalline cellulose, crospovidone, magnesium stearate.

Film coating: ferric oxide yellow E172, hypromellose, macrogol 400, hyprolose, macrogol 8000, silicon dioxide, titanium dioxide E171.

6.2 Incompatibilities

Not applicable.

6.3 Shelf life

5 years.

6.4 Special precautions for storage

No special storage conditions.

6.5 Nature and contents of container

Opaque PVC/aluminium foil blister cards of 14 tablets in a cardboard carton, tablet count 14, 28 (2 × 14), 84 (6 × 14), 98 (7 × 14) or 10 × 14 (hospital bundle).

2 × 10 count perforated blister strip (hospital unit dose)

Not all pack sizes may be marketed.

6.6 Instructions for use and handling

No special requirements.

7. MARKETING AUTHORISATION HOLDER

Procter & Gamble Pharmaceuticals UK Ltd

Rusham Park, Whitehall Lane

Egham, Surrey, TW20 9NW, UK

8. MARKETING AUTHORISATION NUMBER(S)

PL 00364/0070

PA 170/20/1

9. DATE OF FIRST AUTHORISATION/RENEWAL OF THE AUTHORISATION

1999-10-07/2004-10-07

10. DATE OF REVISION OF THE TEXT

2005-01-28

Actonel Once a Week 35mg film coated tablets.

(Procter & Gamble Pharmaceuticals UK Limited)

1. NAME OF THE MEDICINAL PRODUCT

Actonel Once a Week 35mg film coated tablets.

2. QUALITATIVE AND QUANTITATIVE COMPOSITION

One film-coated tablet contains 35 mg risedronate sodium, which is equivalent to 32.5 mg risedronic acid.

For excipients, see section 6.1.

3. PHARMACEUTICAL FORM

Film-coated tablet.

Oval light-orange film-coated tablet with RSN on one side and 35 mg on the other.

4. CLINICAL PARTICULARS

4.1 Therapeutic indications

Treatment of postmenopausal osteoporosis, to reduce the risk of vertebral fractures. Treatment of established postmenopausal osteoporosis, to reduce the risk of hip fractures.

4.2 Posology and method of administration

The recommended dose in adults is one 35 mg tablet orally once a week. The tablet should be taken on the same day each week.

The absorption of risedronate is affected by food, thus to ensure adequate absorption patients should take Actonel Once a Week 35 mg at least 30 minutes before the first food, other medicinal product or drink (other than water) of the day.

Patients should be instructed that if a dose is missed, one Actonel Once a Week 35 mg tablet should be taken on the day that the tablet is remembered. Patients should then return to taking one tablet once a week on the day the tablet is normally taken. Two tablets should not be taken on the same day.

The tablet must be swallowed whole and not sucked or chewed. To aid delivery of the tablet to the stomach Actonel Once a Week 35 mg is to be taken while in an upright position with a glass of plain water (≥120 ml). Patients should not lie down for 30 minutes after taking the tablet (see section 4.4).

Supplemental calcium and vitamin D should be considered if the dietary intake is inadequate.

Elderly: Since the target population is postmenopausal women, a specific dosage instruction for the elderly is not warranted. This has also been shown in the very elderly, 75 years old and above.

Renal Impairment: No dosage adjustment is required for those patients with mild to moderate renal impairment. The use of risedronate is contraindicated in patients with severe renal impairment (creatinine clearance lower than 30ml/min) (see sections 4.3 and 5.2).

4.3 Contraindications

Known hypersensitivity to risedronate or to any of its excipients.

Hypocalcaemia (see section 4.4).

Pregnancy and lactation.

Severe renal impairment (creatinine clearance <30ml/min).

4.4 Special warnings and special precautions for use

Efficacy of bisphosphonates in the treatment of postmenopausal osteoporosis is related to the presence of low bone mineral density (BMD T-score at hip or lumbar spine ≤-2.5 SD) and/or prevalent fracture.

High age or clinical risk factors for fracture alone are not sufficient reasons to initiate treatment of osteoporosis with a bisphosphonate.

The evidence to support efficacy of bisphosphonates including risedronate in very elderly women >80 years) is limited (see section 5.1).

Some bisphosphonates have been associated with oesophagitis and oesophageal ulcerations. Therefore patients should pay attention to the dosing instructions (see section 4.2). In patients who have a history of oesophageal disorders which delay oesophageal transit or emptying e.g. stricture or achalasia, or who are unable to stay in the upright position for at least 30 minutes after taking the tablet, risedronate should be used with special caution because of limited clinical experience in these patients. Prescribers should emphasise the importance of the dosing instructions to these patients.

Hypocalcaemia should be treated before starting Actonel Once a Week 35 mg therapy. Other disturbances of bone and mineral metabolism (i.e. parathyroid dysfunction, hypovitaminosis D) should be treated at the time of starting Actonel Once a Week 35 mg therapy.

4.5 Interaction with other medicinal products and other forms of Interaction

No formal interaction studies have been performed, however no clinically relevant interactions with other medicinal products were found during clinical trials. In the risedronate Phase III osteoporosis studies with daily dosing, acetyl salicylic acid or NSAID use was reported by 33% and 45% of patients respectively. In the Phase III once a week study, acetyl salicylic acid or NSAID use was reported by 57% and 40% of patients respectively. Among regular acetyl salicylic acid or NSAID users (3 or more days per week) the incidence of upper gastrointestinal adverse events in risedronate treated patients was similar to that in control patients.

If considered appropriate risedronate may be used concomitantly with oestrogen supplementation.

Foods, drinks (other than plain water) and medicinal products containing polyvalent cations (such as calcium, magnesium, iron and aluminium) may interfere with the absorption of risedronate and should not be taken at the same time. Therefore Actonel Once a Week 35 mg should be taken at least 30 minutes before the first food, other medicinal product or drink of the day.

Risedronate is not systemically metabolised, does not induce cytochrome P450 enzymes, and has low protein binding.

4.6 Pregnancy and lactation

There are no adequate data from use of risedronate in pregnant women. Studies in animals have shown

Table 1 Common Adverse Events (>1/100, <1/10) Considered Possibly or Probably Medicinal Product Related[a,b] in Phase III Osteoporosis Trials of up to 3 Years Duration

Body System	One-Year Study: Actonel Once a Week 35mg % (N = 485)	One-Year Study: Actonel 5mg/day % (N = 480)	Up to Three-Year Studies: Actonel 5mg/day % (N = 5020)	Up to Three-Year Studies: Placebo % (N = 5048)
Body as a Whole				
Pain	1.2	0.8	0.6	0.5
Digestive System				
Dyspepsia	3.5	4.2	4.5	4.1
Nausea	2.9	4.2	4.3	4.0
Abdominal pain	2.5	3.5	3.5	3.3
Constipation	1.9	2.1	5.0	4.8
Diarrhoea	1.6	1.9	3.0	2.7
GI disorder	1.6	1.0	0.9	0.8
Musculoskeletal System				
Musculoskeletal pain	3.7	3.1	2.1	1.9
Nervous System				
Headache	1.0	1.3	1.8	1.4

[a] Investigator assessment

[b] Adverse events are presented if they occurred in >1/100 and <1/10 in either treatment group in the one-year study, or in >1/100 and <1/10 of patients treated with Actonel 5 mg daily and at a greater incidence than in patients given placebo in the up to three-year studies.

reproductive toxicity (see section 5.3). The potential risk to humans is unknown. Risedronate must not be used during pregnancy or by breast-feeding women.

4.7 Effects on ability to drive and use machines

No effects on ability to drive and use machines have been observed.

4.8 Undesirable effects

In a one-year, double-blind, multicentre study comparing Actonel 5 mg daily and Actonel Once a Week 35 mg in postmenopausal women with osteoporosis, the overall safety and tolerability profiles were similar. In nine Phase III osteoporosis studies of up to 3 years duration, the overall safety and tolerability profiles of Actonel 5 mg daily and placebo were similar. The majority of undesirable effects observed in clinical trials were mild to moderate in severity and usually did not require cessation of therapy.

(see Table 1 above)

(see Table 2 below)

Additionally, the following has been reported during clinical trials:

Eye disorders:

Uncommon (>1/1000, <1/100): Iritis

Investigations (hepatobiliary):

Rare (>1/10,000, <1/1000): Abnormal liver function tests

Laboratory findings: Early, transient, asymptomatic and mild decreases in serum calcium and phosphate levels have been observed in some patients.

The following additional adverse reactions have been reported during post-marketing use:

Skin and subcutaneous tissue disorders:

Very rare (<1/10,000): hypersensitivity and skin reactions, including angioedema, generalised rash, and bullous skin reactions, some severe.

4.9 Overdose

No specific information is available on the treatment of acute overdose with risedronate.

Decreases in serum calcium following substantial overdose may be expected. Signs and symptoms of hypocalcaemia may also occur in some of these patients.

Milk or antacids containing magnesium, calcium or aluminium should be given to bind risedronate and reduce absorption of risedronate. In cases of substantial overdose, gastric lavage may be considered to remove unabsorbed risedronate.

5. PHARMACOLOGICAL PROPERTIES

5.1 Pharmacodynamic properties

Pharmaco-therapeutic group: Bisphosphonates

ATC Code: M05BA07.

Risedronate is a pyridinyl bisphosphonate that binds to bone hydroxyapatite and inhibits osteoclast-mediated bone resorption. The bone turnover is reduced while the osteoblast activity and bone mineralisation is preserved. In preclinical studies risedronate demonstrated potent antiosteoclast and antiresorptive activity, and dose dependently increased bone mass and biomechanical skeletal

Table 2 Uncommon Adverse Events (≥1/1000, <1/100) Considered Possibly or Probably Medicinal Product Related[a] in Phase III Osteoporosis Trials of up to 3 Years Duration and Associated with Bisphosphonates

Body System	One-Year Study: Actonel Once a Week 35mg % (N = 485)	One-Year Study: Actonel 5mg/day % (N = 480)	Up to Three-Year Studies: Actonel 5mg/day % (N = 5020)	Up to Three-Year Studies: Placebo % (N=5048)
Digestive System				
Oesophagitis	0.6	0.6	0.9	0.9
Oesophageal ulcer	0.2	0.0	0.2	0.2
Gastritis	0.0	1.0	0.9	0.7
Dysphagia	0.0	0.4	0.4	0.2
Duodenitis	0.0	0.4	0.2	0.1
Glossitis	0.0	0.2	<0.1	0.1
Oesophageal stricture	0.0	0.2	<0.1	0.0

[a] Investigator assessment.

strength. The activity of risedronate was confirmed by measuring biochemical markers for bone turnover during pharmacodynamic and clinical studies. Decreases in biochemical markers of bone turnover were observed within 1 month and reached a maximum in 3-6 months. Decreases in biochemical markers of bone turnover were similar with Actonel Once a Week 35 mg and Actonel 5 mg daily at 12 months.

Treatment of Postmenopausal Osteoporosis:

A number of risk factors are associated with postmenopausal osteoporosis including low bone mass, low bone mineral density, early menopause, a history of smoking and a family history of osteoporosis. The clinical consequence of osteoporosis is fractures. The risk of fractures is increased with the number of risk factors.

Based on effects on mean change in lumbar spine BMD, Actonel Once a Week 35 mg (n=485) was shown to be equivalent to Actonel 5 mg daily (n=480) in a one-year, double-blind, multicentre study of postmenopausal women with osteoporosis

The clinical programme for risedronate administered once daily studied the effect of risedronate on the risk of hip and vertebral fractures and contained early and late postmenopausal women with and without fracture. Daily doses of 2.5 mg and 5 mg were studied and all groups, including the control groups, received calcium and vitamin D (if baseline levels were low). The absolute and relative risk of new vertebral and hip fractures were estimated by use of a time-to-first event analysis.

• Two placebo-controlled trials (n=3661) enrolled postmenopausal women under 85 years with vertebral fractures at baseline. Risedronate 5 mg daily given for 3 years reduced the risk of new vertebral fractures relative to the control group. In women with respectively at least 2 or at least 1 vertebral fractures, the relative risk reduction was 49% and 41% respectively (incidence of new vertebral fractures with risedronate 18.1% and 11.3%, with placebo 29.0% and 16.3%, respectively). The effect of treatment was seen as early as the end of the first year of treatment. Benefits were also demonstrated in women with multiple fractures at baseline. Risedronate 5 mg daily also reduced the yearly height loss compared to the control group.

• Two further placebo controlled trials enrolled postmenopausal women above 70 years with or without vertebral fractures at baseline. Women 70-79 years were enrolled with femoral neck BMD T-score <-3 SD (manufacturer's range, i.e. -2.5 SD using NHANES III) and at least one additional risk factor. Women ≥80 years could be enrolled on the basis of at least one non-skeletal risk factor for hip fracture or low bone mineral density at the femoral neck. Statistical significance of the efficacy of risedronate versus placebo is only reached when the two treatment groups 2.5 mg and 5 mg are pooled. The following results are only based on *a-posteriori* analysis of subgroups defined by clinical practise and current definitions of osteoporosis:

In the subgroup of patients with femoral neck BMD T-score ≤-2.5SD (NHANES III) and at least one vertebral fracture at baseline, risedronate given for 3 years reduced the risk of hip fractures by 46% relative to the control group (incidence of hip fractures in combined risedronate 2.5 and 5 mg groups 3.8%, placebo 7.4%);

Data suggest that a more limited protection than this may be observed in the very elderly (≥80 years). This may be due to the increasing importance of non-skeletal factors for hip fracture with increasing age.

In these trials, data analysed as a secondary endpoint indicated a decrease in the risk of new vertebral fractures in patients with low femoral neck BMD without vertebral fracture and in patients with low femoral neck BMD with or without vertebral fracture.

• Risedronate 5 mg daily given for 3 years increased bone mineral density (BMD) relative to control at the lumbar spine, femoral neck, trochanter and wrist and maintained bone density at the mid-shaft radius.

• In a one-year follow-up off therapy after three years treatment with risedronate 5 mg daily there was rapid reversibility of the suppressing effect of risedronate on bone turnover rate.

• Bone biopsy samples from postmenopausal women treated with risedronate 5 mg daily for 2 to 3 years, showed an expected moderate decrease in bone turnover. Bone formed during risedronate treatment was of normal lamellar structure and bone mineralisation. These data together with the decreased incidence of osteoporosis related fractures at vertebral sites in women with osteoporosis appear to indicate no detrimental effect on bone quality.

• Endoscopic findings from a number of patients with a number of moderate to severe gastrointestinal complaints in both risedronate and control patients indicated no evidence of treatment related gastric, duodenal or oesophageal ulcers in either group, although duodenitis was uncommonly observed in the risedronate group.

5.2 Pharmacokinetic properties

Absorption: Absorption after an oral dose is relatively rapid (t_{max} ~1 hour) and is independent of dose over the range studied (single dose study, 2.5 to 30 mg; multiple dose studies, 2.5 to 5 mg daily and up to 50 mg dosed weekly). Mean oral bioavailability of the tablet is 0.63% and is decreased when risedronate is administered with food. Bioavailability was similar in men and women.

Distribution: The mean steady state volume of distribution is 6.3 l/kg in humans. Plasma protein binding is about 24%.

Metabolism: There is no evidence of systemic metabolism of risedronate.

Elimination: Approximately half of the absorbed dose is excreted in urine within 24 hours, and 85% of an intravenous dose is recovered in the urine after 28 days. Mean renal clearance is 105 ml/min and mean total clearance is 122 ml/min, with the difference probably attributed to clearance due to adsorption to bone. The renal clearance is not concentration dependent, and there is a linear relationship between renal clearance and creatinine clearance. Unabsorbed risedronate is eliminated unchanged in faeces. After oral administration the concentration-time profile shows three elimination phases with a terminal half-life of 480 hours.

5.3 Preclinical safety data

In toxicological studies in rat and dog dose dependent liver toxic effects of risedronate were seen, primarily as enzyme increases with histological changes in rat. The clinical relevance of these observations is unknown. Testicular toxicity occurred in rat and dog at oral doses of 20mg/kg/day and 8mg/kg/day respectively. Dose related incidences of upper airway irritation were frequently noted in rodents. Similar effects have been seen with other bisphosphonates. Lower respiratory tract effects were also seen in longer term studies in rodents, although the clinical significance of these findings is unclear. In reproduction toxicity studies at exposures close to clinical exposure ossification changes were seen in sternum and/or skull of foetuses from treated rats and hypocalcaemia and mortality in pregnant females allowed to deliver. There was no evidence of teratogenesis at 3.2mg/kg/day in rat and 10mg/kg/day in rabbit, although data are only available on a small number of rabbits. Maternal toxicity prevented testing of higher doses. Preclinical data reveal no special hazard for humans based on conventional studies of genotoxicity and carcinogenesis.

6. PHARMACEUTICAL PARTICULARS

6.1 List of excipients

Tablet core: lactose monohydrate, microcrystalline cellulose, crospovidone, magnesium stearate.

Film coating: Dri-Klear (hypromellose, macrogol 400, hydroxypropyl cellulose, macrogol 8000, and silicon dioxide), Chroma-Tone White DDB-7536W (titanium dioxide (E171), hypromellose), ferric oxide yellow (E172), ferric oxide red (E172).

6.2 Incompatibilities

Not applicable.

6.3 Shelf life

3 years.

6.4 Special precautions for storage

No special precautions for storage.

6.5 Nature and contents of container

Clear PVC/aluminium foil blisters in a cardboard carton.

Blisters in packs containing 1, 2, 4, 10, 12 (3x4), or 16 (4x4) tablets.

Not all pack sizes may be marketed.

6.6 Instructions for use and handling

No special requirements.

7. MARKETING AUTHORISATION HOLDER

Procter & Gamble Pharmaceuticals UK Ltd.
Rusham Park, Whitehall Lane,
Egham,
Surrey TW20 9NW
UK

8. MARKETING AUTHORISATION NUMBER(S)

PL 00364/0080

PA 170/20/3

9. DATE OF FIRST AUTHORISATION/RENEWAL OF THE AUTHORISATION

13 January 2003

10. DATE OF REVISION OF THE TEXT

October 2004

Actos Tablets

(Takeda UK Ltd)

1. NAME OF THE MEDICINAL PRODUCT

Actos tablets.

2. QUALITATIVE AND QUANTITATIVE COMPOSITION

Each tablet contains 15mg or 30mg or 45mg of pioglitazone as hydrochloride.

For excipients, see 6.1.

3. PHARMACEUTICAL FORM

Tablet.

The 15mg tablets are white to off-white, round, convex and marked '15' on one face.

The 30mg tablets are white to off-white, round, flat and marked '30' on one face.

The 45mg tablets are white to off-white, round, flat and marked '45' on one face.

4. CLINICAL PARTICULARS

4.1 Therapeutic indications

Pioglitazone is indicated as oral monotherapy in type 2 diabetes mellitus patients, particularly overweight patients, inadequately controlled by diet and exercise for whom metformin is inappropriate because of contraindications or intolerance.

Pioglitazone is also indicated for oral combination treatment in type 2 diabetes mellitus patients with insufficient glycaemic control despite maximal tolerated dose of oral monotherapy with either metformin or sulphonylurea:

- in combination with metformin particularly in overweight patients

- in combination with a sulphonylurea only in patients who show intolerance to metformin or for whom metformin is contraindicated

4.2 Posology and method of administration

The long-term benefits of therapy with pioglitazone have not been demonstrated (see section 5.1).

Pioglitazone tablets are taken orally once daily with or without food.

Dosage in adults:

Pioglitazone may be initiated at 15mg or 30mg once daily. The dose may be increased in increments up to 45mg once daily.

In combination with metformin, the current metformin dose can be continued upon initiation of pioglitazone therapy.

In combination with sulphonylurea, the current sulphonylurea dose can be continued upon initiation of pioglitazone therapy. If patients report hypoglycaemia, the dose of sulphonylurea should be decreased.

Elderly:

No dosage adjustment is necessary for elderly patients (see section 5.2).

Patients with renal impairment:

No dosage adjustment is necessary in patients with impaired renal function (creatinine clearance > 4 ml/min) (see section 5.2). No information is available from dialysed patients therefore pioglitazone should not be used in such patients.

Patients with hepatic impairment:

Pioglitazone should not be used in patients with hepatic impairment (see section 4.4).

Children and adolescents:

There are no data available on the use of pioglitazone in patients under 18 years of age, and therefore its use is not recommended in this age group.

4.3 Contraindications

Pioglitazone is contraindicated in patients with:

- known hypersensitivity to pioglitazone or to any of the excipients of the tablet

- cardiac failure or history of cardiac failure (NYHA stages I to IV)

- hepatic impairment.

Pioglitazone is also contraindicated for use in combination with insulin.

4.4 Special warnings and special precautions for use

There is no clinical experience with pioglitazone in triple combination with other oral antidiabetics.

Fluid retention and cardiac failure:

Pioglitazone can cause fluid retention, which may exacerbate or precipitate heart failure. Patients should be observed for signs and symptoms of heart failure, particularly those with reduced cardiac reserve. Pioglitazone should be discontinued if any deterioration in cardiac status occurs. There have been cases of cardiac failure reported from the market when pioglitazone was used in combination with insulin. Therefore pioglitazone is contraindicated in combination with insulin. There also have been cases of cardiac failure reported from the market when pioglitazone was used in patients with a history of cardiac failure. Since NSAIDs and pioglitazone are associated with fluid retention, concomitant administration may increase the risk of oedema.

Monitoring of liver function:

There have been rare reports of hepatocellular dysfunction during post-marketing experience (see section 4.8). It is recommended, therefore, that patients treated with pioglitazone undergo periodic monitoring of liver enzymes. Liver enzymes should be checked prior to the initiation of therapy with pioglitazone in all patients. Therapy with pioglitazone should not be initiated in patients with increased baseline liver enzyme levels (ALT> 2.5 X upper limit of normal) or with any other evidence of liver disease.

Following initiation of therapy with pioglitazone, it is recommended that liver enzymes be monitored periodically based on clinical judgement. If ALT levels are increased to 3 X upper limit of normal during pioglitazone therapy, liver enzyme levels should be reassessed as soon as possible. If ALT levels remain > 3 X the upper limit of normal, therapy should be discontinued. If any patient develops symptoms suggesting hepatic dysfunction, which may include unexplained nausea, vomiting, abdominal pain, fatigue, anorexia and/or dark urine, liver enzymes should be checked. The decision whether to continue the patient on therapy with pioglitazone should be guided by clinical judgement pending laboratory evaluations. If jaundice is observed, drug therapy should be discontinued.

Weight gain:

In clinical trials with pioglitazone there was evidence of weight gain, therefore weight should be closely monitored. Part of the treatment of diabetes is dietary control. Patients should be advised to adhere strictly to a calorie-controlled diet.

Haematology:

There was a small reduction in mean haemoglobin (4 % relative reduction) and haematocrit (4.1 % relative reduction) during therapy with pioglitazone, consistent with haemodilution. Similar changes were seen in metformin (haemoglobin 3 - 4 % and haematocrit 3.6 – 4.1 % relative reductions) and to a lesser extent sulphonylurea (haemoglobin 1 – 2 % and haematocrit 1 – 3.2 % relative reductions) treated patients in comparative controlled trials with pioglitazone.

Others:

As a consequence of enhancing insulin action, pioglitazone treatment in patients with polycystic ovarian syndrome may result in resumption of ovulation. These patients may be at risk of pregnancy. Patients should be aware of the risk of pregnancy and if a patient wishes to become pregnant or if pregnancy occurs, the treatment should be discontinued (see section 4.6).

4.5 Interaction with other medicinal products and other forms of Interaction

Interaction studies have shown that pioglitazone has no relevant effect on either the pharmacokinetics or pharmacodynamics of digoxin, warfarin, phenprocoumon and metformin. Co-administration of pioglitazone with sulphonylureas does not appear to affect the pharmacokinetics of the sulphonylurea. Studies in man suggest no induction of the main inducible cytochrome P450, 1A, 2C8/9 and 3A4. *In vitro* studies have shown no inhibition of any subtype of cytochrome P450. Interactions with substances metabolised by these enzymes, e.g. oral contraceptives, cyclosporin, calcium channel blockers, and HMGCoA reductase inhibitors are not to be expected.

4.6 Pregnancy and lactation

Use in pregnancy:

There are no adequate human data to determine the safety of pioglitazone during pregnancy. Foetal growth restriction was apparent in animal studies with pioglitazone. This was attributable to the action of pioglitazone in diminishing the maternal hyperinsulinaemia and increased insulin resistance that occurs during pregnancy thereby reducing the availability of metabolic substrates for foetal growth. The relevance of such a mechanism in humans is unclear and pioglitazone should not be used in pregnancy.

Use in breast-feeding:

Pioglitazone has been shown to be present in the milk of lactating rats. It is not known whether pioglitazone is secreted in human milk. Therefore, pioglitazone should not be administered to breast-feeding women.

4.7 Effects on ability to drive and use machines

No effects on ability to drive and use machines have been observed.

4.8 Undesirable effects

Adverse reactions reported in excess > 0.5 %) of placebo and as more than an isolated case in patients receiving pioglitazone in double-blind studies are listed below as MedDRA preferred term by system organ class and absolute frequency. Frequencies are defined as: common > 1/100, < 1/10; uncommon > 1/1000, < 1/100; rare > 1/10000, < 1/1000; very rare < 1/10000.

MONOTHERAPY

Eye disorders

Common: visual disturbance

Infection and infestations

Common: upper respiratory tract infection

Uncommon: sinusitis

Investigations

Common: weight increased

Nervous system disorders

Common: hypoaesthesia

Uncommon: insomnia

PIOGLITAZONE IN COMBINATION WITH METFORMIN

Blood and lymphatic system disorders

Common: anaemia

Eye disorders

Common: visual disturbance

Gastrointestinal disorders

Uncommon: flatulence

Investigations

Common: weight increased

Musculoskeletal system and connective tissue disorders

Common: arthralgia

Nervous system disorders

Common: headache

Renal and urinary disorders

Common: haematuria

Reproductive system and breast disorders

Common: erectile dysfunction

PIOGLITAZONE IN COMBINATION WITH SULPHONYLUREA

Ear and labyrinth disorders

Uncommon: vertigo

Eye disorders

Uncommon: visual disturbance

Gastrointestinal disorders

Common: flatulence

General disorders and administration site conditions

Uncommon: fatigue

Investigations

Common: weight increased

Uncommon: increased lactic dehydrogenase

Metabolism and nutritional disorders

Uncommon: appetite increased, hypoglycaemia

Nervous system disorders

Common: dizziness

Uncommon: headache

Renal and urinary disorders

Uncommon: glycosuria, proteinuria

Skin and subcutaneous tissue disorders

Uncommon: sweating

Oedema was reported in 6 – 9 % of patients treated with pioglitazone over one year in controlled clinical trials. The oedema rates for comparator groups (sulphonylurea, metformin) were 2 – 5 %. The reports of oedema were generally mild to moderate and usually did not require discontinuation of treatment.

In active comparator controlled trials mean weight increase with pioglitazone given as monotherapy was 2 – 3 kg over one year. This is similar to that seen in a sulphonylurea active comparator group. In combination trials pioglitazone added to metformin resulted in mean weight increase over one year of 1.5 kg and added to a sulphonylurea of 2.8 kg. In comparator groups addition of sulphonylurea to metformin resulted in a mean weight gain of 1.3 kg and addition of metformin to a sulphonylurea a mean weight loss of 1.0 kg.

Visual disturbance has been reported mainly early in treatment and is related to changes in blood glucose due to temporary alteration in the turgidity and refractive index of the lens as seen with other hypoglycaemic agents.

In clinical trials with pioglitazone the incidence of elevations of ALT greater than three times the upper limit of normal was equal to placebo but less than that seen in metformin or sulphonylurea comparator groups. Mean levels of liver enzymes decreased with treatment with pioglitazone. Rare cases of elevated liver enzymes and hepatocellular dysfunction have occurred in post-marketing experience. Although in very rare cases fatal outcome has been reported, causal relationship has not been established.

In controlled clinical trials the incidence of reports of heart failure with pioglitazone treatment was the same as in placebo, metformin and sulphonylurea treatment groups. Heart failure has been reported rarely with marketing use of pioglitazone.

4.9 Overdose

Patients have taken pioglitazone at higher than the recommended highest dose of 45 mg daily. The maximum reported dose of 120 mg/day for four days, then 180 mg/day for seven days was not associated with any symptoms.

Hypoglycaemia may occur in combination with sulphonylureas or insulin. Symptomatic and general supportive measures should be taken in case of overdose.

5. PHARMACOLOGICAL PROPERTIES

5.1 Pharmacodynamic properties

Pharmacotherapeutic group: oral blood glucose lowering drugs; Thiazolidinediones; ATC code: A10 BG 03.

Pioglitazone effects may be mediated by a reduction of insulin resistance. Pioglitazone appears to act via activation of specific nuclear receptors (peroxisome proliferator activated receptor gamma) leading to increased insulin sensitivity of liver, fat and skeletal muscle cells in animals. Treatment with pioglitazone has been shown to reduce hepatic glucose output and to increase peripheral glucose disposal in the case of insulin resistance.

Fasting and postprandial glycaemic control is improved in patients with type 2 diabetes mellitus. The improved glycaemic control is associated with a reduction in both fasting and postprandial plasma insulin concentrations. A clinical trial of pioglitazone vs. gliclazide as monotherapy was extended to two years in order to assess time to treatment failure (defined as appearance of HbA_{1c} $\geqslant$ 8.0 % after the first six months of therapy). Kaplan-Meier analysis showed shorter time to treatment failure in patients treated with gliclazide, compared with pioglitazone. At two years, glycaemic control (defined as HbA_{1c} $<$ 8.0 %) was sustained in 69 % of patients treated with pioglitazone, compared with 50 % of patients on gliclazide. In a two-year study of combination therapy comparing pioglitazone with gliclazide when added to metformin, glycaemic control measured as mean change from baseline in HbA_{1c} was similar between treatment groups after one year. The rate of deterioration of HbA_{1c} during the second year was less with pioglitazone than with gliclazide.

HOMA analysis shows that pioglitazone improves beta cell function as well as increasing insulin sensitivity. Two-year clinical studies have shown maintenance of this effect.

In one year clinical trials, pioglitazone consistently gave a statistically significant reduction in the albumin/creatinine ratio compared to baseline.

The effect of pioglitazone (45 mg monotherapy *vs.* placebo) was studied in a small 18-week trial in type 2 diabetics. Pioglitazone was associated with significant weight gain. Visceral fat was significantly decreased, while there was an increase in extra-abdominal fat mass. Similar changes in body fat distribution on pioglitazone have been accompanied by an improvement in insulin sensitivity. In most clinical trials, reduced total plasma triglycerides and free fatty acids, and increased HDL-cholesterol levels were observed as compared to placebo, with no statistically significant increases in LDL-cholesterol levels. In clinical trials of up to two years duration, pioglitazone reduced total plasma triglycerides and free fatty acids, and increased HDL cholesterol levels, compared with placebo, metformin or gliclazide. Pioglitazone did not cause statistically significant increases in LDL cholesterol levels compared with placebo, whilst reductions were observed with metformin and gliclazide. In a 20-week study, as well as reducing fasting triglycerides, pioglitazone reduced post prandial hypertriglyceridaemia through an effect on both absorbed and hepatically synthesised triglycerides. These effects were independent of pioglitazone's effects on glycaemia and were statistically significant different to glibenclamide.

An outcome study is underway with pioglitazone, and until this is completed the long-term benefits associated with improved metabolic control have not been demonstrated.

5.2 Pharmacokinetic properties

Absorption:

Following oral administration, pioglitazone is rapidly absorbed, and peak plasma concentrations of unchanged pioglitazone are usually achieved 2 hours after administration. Proportional increases of the plasma concentration were observed for doses from 2 – 60 mg. Steady state is achieved after 4–7 days of dosing. Repeated dosing does not result in accumulation of the compound or metabolites. Absorption is not influenced by food intake. Absolute bioavailability is greater than 80 %.

Distribution:

The estimated volume of distribution in humans is 0.25 l/kg.

Pioglitazone and all active metabolites are extensively bound to plasma protein $>$ 99 %).

Metabolism:

Pioglitazone undergoes extensive hepatic metabolism by hydroxylation of aliphatic methylene groups. This is predominantly via cytochrome P450 3A4 and 2C9 although multiple other isoforms are involved to a lesser degree. Three of the six identified metabolites are active (M-II, M-III, and M-IV). When activity, concentrations and protein binding are taken into account, pioglitazone and metabolite M-III contribute equally to efficacy. On this basis M-IV contribution to efficacy is approximately three-fold that of pioglitazone, whilst the relative efficacy of M-II is minimal.

In vitro studies have shown no evidence that pioglitazone inhibits any subtype of cytochrome P450. There is no induction of the main inducible P450 isoenzymes 1A, 2C8/9, and 3A4 in man.

Interaction studies have shown that pioglitazone has no relevant effect on either the pharmacokinetics or pharmacodynamics of digoxin, warfarin, phenprocoumon and metformin. It is therefore not expected that inducers or inhibitors of P450 isoenzymes will alter pioglitazone or active metabolites in a significant way.

Elimination:

Following oral administration of radiolabelled pioglitazone to man, recovered label was mainly in faeces (55%) and a lesser amount in urine (45 %). In animals, only a small amount of unchanged pioglitazone can be detected in either urine or faeces. The mean plasma elimination half-life of unchanged pioglitazone in man is 5 to 6 hours and for its total active metabolites 16 to 23 hours.

Elderly:

Steady state pharmacokinetics are similar in patients age 65 and over and young subjects.

Patients with renal impairment:

In patients with renal impairment, plasma concentrations of pioglitazone and its metabolites are lower than those seen in subjects with normal renal function, but oral clearance of parent substance is similar. Thus free (unbound) pioglitazone concentration is unchanged.

Patients with hepatic impairment:

Total plasma concentration of pioglitazone is unchanged, but with an increased volume of distribution. Intrinsic clearance is therefore reduced, coupled with a higher unbound fraction of pioglitazone.

5.3 Preclinical safety data

In toxicology studies, plasma volume expansion with haemodilution, anaemia, and reversible eccentric cardiac hypertrophy was consistently apparent after repeated dosing of mice, rats, dogs, and monkeys. In addition, increased fatty deposition and infiltration were observed. These findings were observed across species at plasma concentrations $\leqslant$ 4 times the clinical exposure. Foetal growth restriction was apparent in animal studies with pioglitazone. This was attributable to the action of pioglitazone in diminishing the maternal hyperinsulinaemia and increased insulin resistance that occurs during pregnancy thereby reducing the availability of metabolic substrates for foetal growth.

Pioglitazone was devoid of genotoxic potential in a comprehensive battery of *in vivo* and *in vitro* genotoxicity assays. An increased incidence of hyperplasia (males and females) and tumours (males) of the urinary bladder epithelium was apparent in rats treated with pioglitazone for up to 2 years. The relevance of this finding is unknown. There was no tumorigenic response in mice of either sex. Hyperplasia of the urinary bladder was not seen in dogs or monkeys treated for up to 12 months.

In an animal model of familial adenomatous polyposis (FAP), treatment with two other thiazolidinediones increased tumour multiplicity in the colon. The relevance of this finding is unknown.

6. PHARMACEUTICAL PARTICULARS

6.1 List of excipients

Carmellose calcium, hydroxypropylcellulose, lactose monohydrate and magnesium stearate.

6.2 Incompatibilities

Not applicable.

6.3 Shelf life

3 years.

6.4 Special precautions for storage

No special precautions for storage.

6.5 Nature and contents of container

Aluminium/aluminium blisters, packs of 28 tablets.

6.6 Instructions for use and handling

No special requirements.

7. MARKETING AUTHORISATION HOLDER

Takeda Europe R & D Centre Limited

Savannah House

11-12 Charles II Street

London

SW1Y 4QU

United Kingdom

8. MARKETING AUTHORISATION NUMBER(S)

EU/1/00/150/001 - Actos 15mg × 28

EU/1/00/150/004 - Actos 30mg × 28

EU/1/00/150/012 - Actos 45mg × 28

9. DATE OF FIRST AUTHORISATION/RENEWAL OF THE AUTHORISATION

13-10-2000

10. DATE OF REVISION OF THE TEXT

February 2005

Actrapid 100 IU/ml, Actrapid Penfill 100 IU/ml, Actrapid NovoLet 100 IU/ml

(Novo Nordisk Limited)

1. NAME OF THE MEDICINAL PRODUCT

Actrapid 100 IU/ml

Solution for injection in a vial

Actrapid Penfill 100 IU/ml

Solution for injection in a cartridge

Actrapid NovoLet 100 IU/ml

Solution for injection in a pre-filled pen

2. QUALITATIVE AND QUANTITATIVE COMPOSITION

Insulin human, rDNA (produced by recombinant DNA technology in *Saccharomyces cerevisiae*).

1 ml contains 100 IU of insulin human

1 vial contains 10 ml equivalent to 1000 IU

1 cartridge contains 3 ml equivalent to 300 IU

1 pre-filled pen contains 3 ml equivalent to 300 IU

One IU (International Unit) corresponds to 0.035 mg of anhydrous human insulin.

For excipients, see Section 6.1. List of excipients.

3. PHARMACEUTICAL FORM

Solution for injection in a vial.

Solution for injection in cartridge.

Solution for injection in a pre-filled pen.

Actrapid is a clear, colourless, aqueous solution.

4. CLINICAL PARTICULARS

4.1 Therapeutic indications

Treatment of diabetes mellitus.

4.2 Posology and method of administration

Actrapid is a fast-acting insulin and may be used in combination with long-acting insulins.

Dosage

Dosage is individual and determined in accordance with the needs of the patient. The individual insulin requirement is usually between 0.3 and 1.0 IU/kg/day. The daily insulin requirement may be higher in patients with insulin resistance (e.g. during puberty or due to obesity) and lower in patients with residual, endogenous insulin production.

In patients with diabetes mellitus optimised glycaemic control delays the onset of late diabetic complications. Close blood glucose monitoring is recommended.

An injection should be followed within 30 minutes by a meal or snack containing carbohydrates.

Dosage adjustment

Concomitant illness, especially infections and feverish conditions, usually increases the patient's insulin requirement.

Renal or hepatic impairment may reduce insulin requirement.

Adjustment of dosage may also be necessary if patients change physical activity or their usual diet.

Dosage adjustment may be necessary when transferring patients from one insulin preparation to another (see section 4.4 Special warnings and special precautions for use).

Administration

For subcutaneous and intravenous (vial) use.

Actrapid is usually administered subcutaneously in the abdominal wall. The thigh, the gluteal region or the deltoid region may also be used.

Subcutaneous injection into the abdominal wall ensures a faster absorption than from other injection sites.

Injection into a lifted skin fold minimises the risk of unintended intramuscular injection.

Keep the needle under the skin for at least 6 seconds to make sure the entire dose is injected.

Injection sites should be rotated within an anatomic region in order to avoid lipodystrophy.

Actrapid may also be administered intravenously, which should only be carried out by health care professionals. The intravenous use of Actrapid from any pen or cartridge should be an exemption in situations where vials are not available. In this case Actrapid should be drawn into an insulin syringe, provided air is avoided, or infused with an infusion system.

Actrapid is accompanied by a package leaflet with detailed instruction for use to be followed.

The vials are for use with insulin syringes with a corresponding unit scale. When two types of insulin are mixed, draw the amount of fast-acting insulin first, followed by the amount of long-acting insulin.

The cartridges are designed to be used with Novo Nordisk delivery systems (durable devices for repeated use) and NovoFine needles. Detailed instruction accompanying the delivery system must be followed.

Actrapid NovoLet is designed to be used with NovoFine needles.

NovoLet delivers 2-78 units in increments of 2 units.

The pens should be primed before injection so that the dose selector returns to zero and a drop of insulin appears at the needle tip.

The dose is set by turning the selector, which returns to zero during the injection.

4.3 Contraindications

Hypoglycaemia

Hypersensitivity to human insulin or to any of the excipients (see section 6.1 List of excipients).

4.4 Special warnings and special precautions for use

Inadequate dosage or discontinuation of treatment, especially in type 1 diabetes, may lead to **hyperglycaemia**.

Usually the first symptoms of hyperglycaemia set in gradually, over a period of hours or days. They include thirst, increased frequency of urination, nausea, vomiting, drowsiness, flushed dry skin, dry mouth, loss of appetite as well as acetone odour of breath.

In type 1 diabetes, untreated hyperglycaemic events eventually lead to diabetic ketoacidosis, which is potentially lethal.

Hypoglycaemia may occur if the insulin dose is too high in relation to the insulin requirement (see section 4.8 and 4.9).

Omission of a meal or unplanned, strenuous physical exercise may lead to hypoglycaemia.

Patients whose blood glucose control is greatly improved e.g. by intensified insulin therapy, may experience a change in their usual warning symptoms of hypoglycaemia and should be advised accordingly. Usual warning symptoms may disappear in patients with long-standing diabetes.

Transferring a patient to another type or brand of insulin should be done under strict medical supervision. Changes in strength, brand (manufacturer), type (fast-, dual-, long-acting insulin etc.), origin (animal, human or analogue insulin) and/or method of manufacture (recombinant DNA versus animal source insulin) may result in a need for a change in dosage. If an adjustment is needed when switching the patients to Actrapid, it may occur with the first dose or during the first several weeks or months.

A few patients who have experienced hypoglycaemic reactions after transfer from animal source insulin have reported that early warning symptoms of hypoglycaemia were less pronounced or different from those experienced with their previous insulin.

Before travelling between different time zones, the patient should be advised to consult the doctor, since this may mean that the patient has to take insulin and meals at different times.

Due to the risk of precipitation in pump catheters, Actrapid should not be used in insulin pumps for continuous subcutaneous insulin infusion.

Actrapid contains metacresol, which may cause allergic reactions.

4.5 Interaction with other medicinal products and other forms of Interaction

A number of medicinal products are known to interact with glucose metabolism. The physician must therefore take possible interactions into account and should always ask their patients about any medicinal products they take.

The following substances may reduce insulin requirement:

Oral hypoglycaemic agents (OHA), monoamine oxidase inhibitors (MAOI), non-selective beta-blocking agents, angiotensin converting enzyme (ACE) inhibitors, salicylates and alcohol.

The following substances may increase insulin requirement:

Thiazides, glucocorticoids, thyroid hormones and beta-sympathomimetics, growth hormone and danazol.

Beta-blocking agents may mask the symptoms of hypoglycaemia and delay recovery from hypoglycaemia.

Octreotide/lanreotide may both decrease and increase insulin requirement.

Alcohol may intensify and prolong the hypoglycaemic effect of insulin.

4.6 Pregnancy and lactation

There are no restrictions on treatment of diabetes with insulin during pregnancy, as insulin does not pass the placental barrier.

Both hypoglycaemia and hyperglycaemia, which can occur in inadequately controlled diabetes therapy, increase the risk of malformations and death *in utero*. Intensified control in the treatment of pregnant women with diabetes is therefore recommended throughout pregnancy and when contemplating pregnancy.

Insulin requirements usually fall in the first trimester and increase subsequently during the second and third trimesters.

After delivery, insulin requirements return rapidly to pre-pregnancy values.

Insulin treatment of the nursing mother presents no risk to the baby. However, the Actrapid dosage may need to be adjusted.

4.7 Effects on ability to drive and use machines

The patient's ability to concentrate and react may be impaired as a result of hypoglycaemia. This may constitute a risk in situations where these abilities are of special importance (e.g. driving a car or operating machinery).

Patients should be advised to take precautions to avoid hypoglycaemia whilst driving. This is particularly important in those who have reduced or absent awareness of the warning signs of hypoglycaemia or have frequent episodes of hypoglycaemia. The advisability of driving should be considered in these circumstances.

4.8 Undesirable effects

As for other insulin products, hypoglycaemia, in general is the most frequently occurring undesirable effect. It may occur if the insulin dose is too high in relation to the insulin requirement. In clinical trials and during marketed use the frequency varies with patient population and dose regimens. Therefore, no specific frequency can be presented. Severe hypoglycaemia may lead to unconsciousness and/ or convulsions and may result in temporary or permanent impairment of brain function or even death.

Frequencies of adverse drug reactions from clinical trials, that are considered related to fast-acting insulin human, Actrapid, are listed below. The frequencies are defined as: Uncommon $>1/1000$, $<1/100$). Isolated spontaneous cases are presented as very rare defined as $<1/10{,}000$.

Immune system disorders

Uncommon – Urticaria, rash

Very rare – Anaphylactic reactions

Symptoms of generalized hypersensitivity may include generalized skin rash, itching, sweating, gastrointestinal upset, angioneurotic oedema, difficulties in breathing, palpitation, reduction in blood pressure and fainting/loss of consciousness. Generalised hypersensitivity reactions are potentially life threatening.

Nervous system disorders

Uncommon – Peripheral neuropathy

Fast improvement in blood glucose control may be associated with a condition termed "acute painful neuropathy", which is usually reversible.

Eye disorders

Uncommon – Refraction disorders

Refraction anomalies may occur upon initiation of insulin therapy. These symptoms are usually of transitory nature.

Very rare – Diabetic retinopathy

Long-term improved glycaemic control decreases the risk of progression of diabetic retinopathy. However, intensification of insulin therapy with abrupt improvement in glycaemic control may be associated with temporary worsening of diabetic retinopathy.

Skin and subcutaneous tissue disorders

Uncommon – Lipodystrophy

Lipodystrophy may occur at the injection site as a consequence of failure to rotate injection sites within an area.

General disorders and administration site conditions

Uncommon – Injection site reactions

Injection site reactions (redness, swelling, itching, pain and haematoma at the injection site) may occur during treatment with insulin. Most reactions are transitory and disappear during continued treatment.

Very rare – Oedema

Oedema may occur upon initiation of insulin therapy. These symptoms are usually of transitory nature.

4.9 Overdose

A specific overdose of insulin cannot be defined. However, hypoglycaemia may develop over sequential stages:

- Mild hypoglycaemic episodes can be treated by oral administration of glucose or sugary products. It is therefore recommended that the diabetic patient carry some sugar lumps, sweets, biscuits or sugary fruit juice.
- Severe hypoglycaemic episodes, where the patient has become unconscious, can be treated by glucagon (0.5 to 1 mg) given intramuscularly or subcutaneously by a person who has received appropriate instruction, or by glucose given intravenously by a medical professional. Glucose must also be given intravenously, if the patient does not respond to glucagon within 10 to 15 minutes.

Upon regaining consciousness, administration of oral carbohydrate is recommended for the patient in order to prevent relapse.

5. PHARMACOLOGICAL PROPERTIES

5.1 Pharmacodynamic properties

Pharmacotherapeutic group: insulins and analogues, fast-acting, insulin (human). ATC code: A10A B01.

The blood glucose lowering effect of insulin is due to the facilitated uptake of glucose following binding of insulin to receptors on muscle and fat cells and to the simultaneous inhibition of glucose output from the liver.

A clinical trial in a single intensive care unit treating hyperglycaemia (blood glucose above 10 mmol/L) in 204 diabetic and 1344 non-diabetic patients undergoing major surgery showed that normoglycaemia (blood glucose 4.4 – 6.1 mmol/L) induced by intravenous Actrapid reduced mortality by 42% (8% versus 4.6%).

Actrapid is a fast-acting insulin.

Onset of action is within ½ hour, reaches a maximum effect within 1.5-3.5 hours and the entire time of duration is approximately 7-8 hours.

5.2 Pharmacokinetic properties

Insulin in the blood stream has a half-life of a few minutes. Consequently, the time-action profile of an insulin preparation is determined solely by its absorption characteristics.

This process is influenced by several factors (e.g. insulin dosage, injection route and site, thickness of subcutaneous fat, type of diabetes). The pharmacokinetics of insulins is therefore affected by significant intra- and inter-individual variation.

Absorption

The maximum plasma concentration is reached within 1.5-2.5 hours after subcutaneous administration.

Distribution

No profound binding to plasma proteins, except circulating insulin antibodies (if present) has been observed.

Metabolism

Human insulin is reported to be degraded by insulin protease or insulin-degrading enzymes and possibly protein disulfide isomerase. A number of cleavage (hydrolysis) sites on the human insulin molecule have been proposed; none of the metabolites formed following the cleavage are active.

Elimination

The terminal half-life is determined by the rate of absorption from the subcutaneous tissue. The terminal half-life ($t_{½}$) is therefore a measure of the absorption rather than of the elimination *per se* of insulin from plasma (insulin in the blood stream has a $t_{½}$ of a few minutes). Trials have indicated a $t_{½}$ of about 2-5 hours.

The pharmacokinetic profile of Actrapid has been studied in a small number (n=18) of diabetic children (aged 6-12 years) and adolescents (aged 13-17 years). The data are limited but suggest that the pharmacokinetic profile in children and adolescents may be similar to that in adults. However, there were differences between age groups in C_{max}, stressing the importance of individual titration of human insulin.

5.3 Preclinical safety data
Preclinical data reveal no special hazard for humans based on conventional studies of safety pharmacology, repeated dose toxicity, genotoxicity, carcinogenic potential, toxicity to reproduction.

6. PHARMACEUTICAL PARTICULARS

6.1 List of excipients
Zinc chloride

Glycerol

Metacresol

Sodium hydroxide or/and hydrochloric acid (for pH adjustment)

Water for injections

6.2 Incompatibilities
Medicinal products added to the insulin solution may cause degradation of the insulin, e.g. if the medicinal products contain thiols or sulphites. Upon mixing Actrapid with infusion fluids an unpredictable amount of insulin will be adsorbed to the infusion material. Monitoring of the patient's blood glucose during infusion is therefore recommended.

6.3 Shelf life
30 months.

After first opening: 6 weeks.

6.4 Special precautions for storage
Store in a refrigerator (2°C - 8°C).

Do not freeze.

Actrapid:

Keep the vial in the outer carton in order to protect from light.

During use: do not refrigerate. Do not store above 25°C.

Actrapid Penfill:

Keep the cartridge in the outer carton in order to protect from light.

During use: do not refrigerate. Do not store above 30°C.

Actrapid NovoLet:

During use: do not refrigerate. Do not store above 30°C.

Keep the pen cap on in order to protect the insulin from light.

Protect from excessive heat and sunlight.

6.5 Nature and contents of container
Glass vial (type 1) closed with a bromobutyl/polyisoprene rubber stopper and a protective tamper-proof plastic cap.

Pack size: 1 × 10 ml.

Glass cartridge (type 1) with a bromobutyl rubber plunger and a bromobutyl/polyisoprene rubber stopper.

Pack size: 5 cartridges × 3 ml.

Pre-filled pen (multidose disposable pen) comprising a pen injector with a cartridge (3 ml). The cartridge is made of glass (type 1), containing a bromobutyl rubber plunger and a bromobutyl/polyisoprene rubber stopper. The pen injector is made of plastic.

Pack size: 5 pre-filled pens × 3 ml.

6.6 Instructions for use and handling
Cartridges and pens should only be used in combination with products that are compatible with them and allow the cartridge and pen to function safely and effectively.

Actrapid Penfill and Actrapid NovoLet are for single person use only. The container must not be refilled

Insulin preparations, which have been frozen, must not be used.

Insulin solutions should not be used if they do not appear water clear and colourless.

Actrapid should not be used in insulin pumps for continuous subcutaneous insulin infusion.

7. MARKETING AUTHORISATION HOLDER
Novo Nordisk A/S

Novo Allé

DK-2880 Bagsværd

Denmark

8. MARKETING AUTHORISATION NUMBER(S)
Actrapid 100 IU/ml EU/1/02/230/003

Actrapid Penfill 100 IU/ml EU/1/02/230/006

Actrapid NovoLet 100 IU/ml EU/1/02/230/008

9. DATE OF FIRST AUTHORISATION/RENEWAL OF THE AUTHORISATION
October 2002

10. DATE OF REVISION OF THE TEXT
2 August 2004

Legal Status
POM

Acular

(Allergan Ltd)

1. NAME OF THE MEDICINAL PRODUCT
ACULAR®

2. QUALITATIVE AND QUANTITATIVE COMPOSITION
Ketorolac trometamol 0.5% w/v.

3. PHARMACEUTICAL FORM
Eye drops.

4. CLINICAL PARTICULARS

4.1 Therapeutic indications
ACULAR® is indicated for the prophylaxis and reduction of inflammation and associated symptoms following ocular surgery.

4.2 Posology and method of administration
Route of administration: Ocular.

One drop instilled into the eye three times daily starting 24 hours pre-operatively and continuing for up to three weeks post-operatively.

No special dosage for the elderly.

4.3 Contraindications
ACULAR® is contra-indicated in individuals hypersensitive to any component of the medication.

The potential exists for cross-sensitivity to acetylsalicylic acid and other non-steroidal anti-inflammatory drugs. ACULAR® is contra-indicated in individuals who have previously exhibited sensitivities to these drugs.

ACULAR® is contra-indicated in children, and during pregnancy or lactation.

4.4 Special warnings and special precautions for use
It is recommended that ACULAR® be used with caution in patients with known bleeding tendencies or who are receiving other medications which may prolong bleeding time, or patients with a known history of peptic ulceration.

In common with other anti-inflammatory drugs, ACULAR® may mask the usual signs of infection.

ACULAR® contains benzalkonium chloride as a preservative and should not be used in patients continuing to wear soft (hydrophilic) contact lenses.

4.5 Interaction with other medicinal products and other forms of Interaction
ACULAR® has been safely administered with systemic and ophthalmic medications such as antibiotics, sedatives, beta blockers, carbonic anhydrase inhibitors, miotics, mydriatics, cycloplegics and corticosteroids.

4.6 Pregnancy and lactation
There was no evidence of teratogenicity in rats or rabbits studied at maternally-toxic doses of ketorolac. Prolongation of the gestation period and/or delayed parturition were seen in the rat. Ketorolac and its metabolites have been shown to pass into the foetus and milk of animals. Ketorolac has been detected in human milk at low levels. Safety in human pregnancy has not been established. Ketorolac is therefore contra-indicated during pregnancy, labour or delivery, or in mothers who are breast feeding.

4.7 Effects on ability to drive and use machines
Transient blurring of vision may occur on instillation of eye drops. Do not drive or use hazardous machinery unless vision is clear.

4.8 Undesirable effects
The most frequent adverse events reported with the use of ACULAR® are transient stinging and burning on instillation and other minor symptoms of ocular irritation.

Blurring and/or diminished vision have been reported with the use of ACULAR® and other non-steroidal anti-inflammatory drugs.

None of the typical adverse reactions reported with the use of systemic non-steroidal anti-inflammatory agents (including ketorolac trometamol) have been observed at the doses used in topical ophthalmic therapy.

4.9 Overdose
There is no experience of overdose by the ophthalmic route. Overdose is unlikely to occur via the recommended method of administration.

5. PHARMACOLOGICAL PROPERTIES

5.1 Pharmacodynamic properties
Pharmacotherapeutic classification (ATC): S01B C

ACULAR® (ketorolac trometamol) is a non-steroidal anti-inflammatory agent demonstrating analgesic and anti-inflammatory activity. Ketorolac trometamol inhibits the cyclo-oxygenase enzyme essential for biosynthesis of prostaglandins. ACULAR® has been shown to reduce prostaglandin levels in the aqueous humour after topical ophthalmic administration.

Ketorolac trometamol given systemically does not cause pupil constriction. Results from clinical studies indicate that ACULAR® has no significant effect on intra-ocular pressure.

5.2 Pharmacokinetic properties
a) General characteristics

Absorption

Rabbit aqueous humor bioavailability:

Mean concentration of total radioactivity 0.856 g-equiv./ml @ 0.5 hr

1.607 g-equiv./ml @ 2 hr

Tmax 3.38 hr

Cmax 1.905 g-equiv./ml

AUC (0-8 hr) 9.39 g-equiv. hr/ml

Total AUC 13.53 g-equiv. hr/ml

Half-life 3.77 hr

Absolute ocular bioavailability 3.7%

After topical ocular doses in the rabbit the half life of total radioactivity in aqueous humor was longer than after intracameral injection. This suggests that topical dosing may lead to a "reservoir" effect in the corneal epithelium and continued flux of drug from the reservoir into the aqueous humor.

Distribution
After ophthalmic doses were administered to rabbits, peak concentrations of radioactivity were achieved within 1 hour in the ocular tissues and were highest in the cornea (6.06 mcg-eq/ml). At 1 hour, the majority of the radioactivity (0.9% of administered dose) was recovered from the sclera (0.58%) and cornea (0.24%), and smaller amounts were recovered from the aqueous humor (0.026%), vitreous humor (0.023%), retina-choroid (0.018%), iris-ciliary body (0.007%) and lens (0.002%).

Relative to plasma AUC values, the AUC's in rabbits were higher for cornea (104 fold), sclera (27 fold), iris-ciliary body (5.8 fold), retina-choroid (5.6 fold) aqueous humor (3.3 fold) and approximately one-half in the vitreous humor and lens. After ophthalmic administration, concentrations of drug-related radioactivity were higher in the ocular tissues and lower in plasma compared with those after IV dosing.

Systemic Absorption

After ophthalmic doses in the rabbit, ketorolac was absorbed rapidly into the systemic circulation (Tmax, 15 min). Plasma half-lives after ophthalmic doses (6.6 - 6.9 hr) were longer than those after IV administration (1.1 hr), suggesting that removal of drug from eye into the venous circulation may be rate-limiting. By comparison of drug levels in aqueous humor after intracameral injection vs. plasma levels after IV administration, ketorolac was shown to clear more rapidly from plasma (6 ml/min) than from the anterior chamber (11 mcl/min).

In the cynomolgus monkey, peak plasma levels of ketorolac occurred at 1.1 hr after the ophthalmic dose. The plasma half-life of ketorolac was similar after ophthalmic (1.8 hr) and IV doses (1.6 hr).

The majority of the ophthalmic dose was excreted in urine (66% in rabbit and 75% in monkey) and a small amount in feces (11% in rabbit and 2% in monkey). The extent of systemic absorption after ophthalmic dosing averaged 73% in the rabbit and 76% in the cynomolgus monkey.

Metabolism

After ophthalmic administration in rabbits, ketorolac represented the major component (more than 90%) of radioactivity in aqueous humor and plasma and the p-hydroxy metabolite accounted for 5% of radioactivity in plasma. Ketorolac was also the major component (96%) of plasma radioactivity after ophthalmic dosing in monkeys.

After ophthalmic dosing in the rabbit, 72%, 17% and 6% of the total radioactivity in urine was comprised of intact ketorolac, p-hydroxy ketorolac and other polar metabolites, respectively. After IV dosing, the relative proportions of total radioactivity in urine averaged 6% as intact ketorolac, 68% as p-hydroxy ketorolac and 22% as polar metabolites.

In the monkey, intact ketorolac and its polar metabolite accounted for 32% and 65% of the total radioactivity in urine, respectively, after ophthalmic dosing, and 50% and 49% of the radioactivity in urine, respectively, after IV dosing. Thus, the metabolism of ketorolac was qualitatively similar after ophthalmic and IV administration in the monkey and rabbit.

b) Characteristics in patients

Ketorolac tromethamine solutions (0.1% or 0.5%) or vehicle were instilled into the eyes of patients approximately 12 hours and 1 hour prior to surgery. Concentrations of ketorolac in aqueous humor sampled at the time of surgery were at the lower limit of detection (40 ng/ml) in 1 patient and below the quantitation limit in 7 patients dosed with 0.1% ketorolac tromethamine. The average aqueous humor level of ketorolac in patients treated with 0.5% ketorolac tromethamine was 95 ng/ml. Concentrations of PGE2 in aqueous humor were 80 pg/ml, 40 pg/ml and 28 pg/ml in patients treated with vehicle, 0.1% ketorolac tromethamine and 0.5% ketorolac tromethamine, respectively.

In the 21-day multiple dose (TID) tolerance study in healthy subjects, only 1 of 13 subjects had a detectable plasma level pre-dose (0.021 g/ml). In another group of 13 subjects, only 4 subjects showed very low plasma levels of ketorolac (0.011 to 0.023 g/ml) 15 minutes after the ocular dose.

Thus, higher levels of ketorolac in the aqueous humor and very low or no detectable plasma levels after ophthalmic doses, suggest that the use of ketorolac tromethamine by the ophthalmic route in treatment of ocular disorders results in quite low systemic absorption in patients.

5.3 Preclinical safety data
Acute, sub-acute and chronic studies of ACULAR® in experimental animals have established the safety of the drug. In addition, octoxynol 40 was separately evaluated for its ocular safety. ACULAR® was found to be non-irritating, it did not demonstrate a local anaesthetic effect, it did not influence the healing of experimental corneal wounds in rabbits, it did not enhance the spread of experimental ocular infections of Candida albicans, Herpes simplex virus type one, or Pseudomonas aeruginosa in rabbits, and it did not increase the ocular pressure of normal rabbit eyes.

6. PHARMACEUTICAL PARTICULARS

6.1 List of excipients
Sodium chloride Ph Eur

Benzalkonium chloride Ph Eur

Edetate disodium Ph Eur

Octoxynol 40

1N Sodium hydroxide Ph Eur or 1N Hydrochloric acid Ph Eur, to adjust pH

Purified water Ph Eur

6.2 Incompatibilities
None known.

6.3 Shelf life
24 months, unopened.

Discard any unused contents 28 days after opening the bottle.

6.4 Special precautions for storage
None.

6.5 Nature and contents of container
Bottle with dropper applicator, containing clear, colourless to slightly yellow, sterile ophthalmic solution. Pack size: 5 ml.

6.6 Instructions for use and handling
None.

7. MARKETING AUTHORISATION HOLDER
Allergan Ltd.

Coronation Road

High Wycombe

Bucks HP12 3SH

8. MARKETING AUTHORISATION NUMBER(S)
PL 00426/0082

9. DATE OF FIRST AUTHORISATION/RENEWAL OF THE AUTHORISATION
16 April 1996

10. DATE OF REVISION OF THE TEXT
None

Acupan Tablets

(3M Health Care Limited)

1. NAME OF THE MEDICINAL PRODUCT
Acupan Tablets

2. QUALITATIVE AND QUANTITATIVE COMPOSITION
Nefopam Hydrochloride 30 mg.

3. PHARMACEUTICAL FORM
Tablet

4. CLINICAL PARTICULARS

4.1 Therapeutic indications
Acupan is indicated for the relief of acute and chronic pain, including post-operative pain, dental pain, musculo-skeletal pain, acute traumatic pain and cancer pain.

4.2 Posology and method of administration
ADULTS: Dosage may range from 1 to 3 tablets three times daily depending on response. The recommended starting dosage is 2 tablets three times daily.

ELDERLY: Elderly patients may require reduced dosage due to slower metabolism. It is strongly recommended that the starting dose does not exceed one tablet three times daily as the elderly appear more susceptible to, in particular, the CNS side effects of Acupan and some cases of hallucinations and confusion have been reported in this age group.

CHILDREN: Since Acupan has not been evaluated in children, no dosage recommendation can be given for patients under 12 years.

4.3 Contraindications
Acupan is contra-indicated in patients with a history of convulsive disorders and should not be given to patients taking mono-amine-oxidase (MAO) inhibitors.

4.4 Special warnings and special precautions for use
The side effects of Acupan may be additive to those of other agents with anticholinergic or sympathomimetic activity. It should not be used in the treatment of myocardial infarction since there is no clinical experience in this indication. Hepatic and renal insufficiency may interfere with the metabolism and excretion of nefopam. Acupan should be used with caution in patients with, or at risk of, urinary retention. Rarely a temporary, harmless pink discoloration of the urine has occurred.

4.5 Interaction with other medicinal products and other forms of Interaction
Caution should be exercised when nefopam is administered concurrently with tricyclic antidepressants.

4.6 Pregnancy and lactation
There is no evidence as to the drug safety in human pregnancy, nor is there evidence from animal work that it is free from hazard. Avoid in pregnancy unless there is no safer treatment.

4.7 Effects on ability to drive and use machines
Not applicable.

4.8 Undesirable effects
Nausea, nervousness, dry mouth, light-headedness urinary retention, hypotension, syncope, palpitations, gastro-intestinal disturbances (including abdominal pain and diarrhoea), dizziness, paraesthesia, convulsions, tremor, confusion, hallucination, angioedema, and allergic reactions may occur. Less frequently, vomiting, blurred vision, drowsiness, sweating, insomnia, headache and tachycardia have been reported.

4.9 Overdose
The clinical pattern of nefopam toxicity in overdose is on the neurological (convulsions, hallucinations and agitation) and cardiovascular systems (tachycardia with a hyperdynamic circulation). Routine supportive measures should be taken and prompt removal of ingested drug by gastric lavage or induced vomiting with Syrup of Ipecacuanha should be carried out. Oral administration of activated charcoal may help prevent absorption.

Convulsions and hallucinations should be controlled (e.g. with intravenously or rectally administered diazepam). Beta-adrenergic blockers may help control the cardiovascular complications.

5. PHARMACOLOGICAL PROPERTIES

5.1 Pharmacodynamic properties
Acupan is a potent and rapidly-acting analgesic. It is totally distinct from other centrally-acting analgesics such as morphine, codeine, pentazocine and propoxyphene.

Unlike the narcotic agents, Acupan has been shown not to cause respiratory depression. There is no evidence from pre-clinical research of habituation occurring with Acupan.

5.2 Pharmacokinetic properties
Nefopam is absorbed from the gastro-intestinal tract. Peak plasma concentrations occur about 1-3 hours after oral administration. About 73% is bound to plasma proteins. It has an elimination half-life of about 4 hours. It is extensively metabolised and excreted mainly in urine. Less than 5% of a dose is excreted unchanged in the urine. About 8% of a dose is excreted via the faeces.

5.3 Preclinical safety data
Not applicable

6. PHARMACEUTICAL PARTICULARS

6.1 List of excipients
Dibasic calcium phosphate dihydrate

Microcrystalline cellulose

Pregelatinised maize starch

Magnesium stearate

Hydrogenated vegetable oil

Colloidal silicon dioxide

These tablets are film coated using an aqueous solution containing: hydroxypropyl methylcellulose 2910, titanium dioxide.

6.2 Incompatibilities
None known

6.3 Shelf life
5 years

6.4 Special precautions for storage
Store below 30°C.

6.5 Nature and contents of container
20 micron aluminium foil and 250 micron UPVC

Blister pack of 90 tablets

6.6 Instructions for use and handling
None.

7. MARKETING AUTHORISATION HOLDER
3M Health Care Limited

3M House

Morley Street

Loughborough

Leics

LE11 1EP

8. MARKETING AUTHORISATION NUMBER(S)
00068/0061

9. DATE OF FIRST AUTHORISATION/RENEWAL OF THE AUTHORISATION
2nd March 1978 / 11th January 1995

10. DATE OF REVISION OF THE TEXT
November 2000

ACWY Vax Vaccine

(GlaxoSmithKline UK)

1. NAME OF THE MEDICINAL PRODUCT
ACWY Vax Meningococcal Polysaccharide vaccine PhEur (groups A, C, W_{135} and Y polysaccharides)

2. QUALITATIVE AND QUANTITATIVE COMPOSITION
Each 0.5 ml dose contains at least 50 micrograms each of meningococcal polysaccharides serogroups A, C, W_{135} and Y.

3. PHARMACEUTICAL FORM
Powder and solvent for solution for injection

4. CLINICAL PARTICULARS

4.1 Therapeutic indications
Active immunisation against meningococcal meningitis caused by group A, C, W_{135} and Y meningococci.

The vaccine is particularly recommended for subjects at risk, for example those living in areas or travelling to countries where the disease is epidemic or highly endemic. It is also recommended in epidemic situations and for close contacts of patients with this disease. It may also be used in individuals with terminal complement component deficiency, properdin deficiency and functional or actual splenectomy.

4.2 Posology and method of administration
Adults and children aged two years and over

0.5 ml of reconstituted vaccine (single dose)

Persons who have previously been immunised with a meningococcal serogroup C conjugate vaccine may receive ACWY Vax in order to confer protection against disease caused by A, W_{135}, Y.

ACWY Vax does not elicit a protective immune response to the meningococcal serogroup C antigen in infants, and does not reliably elicit a protective immune response against this serogroup in children of less than two years (see section 4.4).

Immune responses to the serogroup A, W_{135} and Y antigens may be achieved in children of less than two years, but are likely to be short-lived. (See section 5.1). This vaccine is not to be used in infants of less than two months.

Method of administration

Deep subcutaneous injection.

4.3 Contraindications
Do not use in subjects hypersensitive to any component of the vaccine or in subjects having shown signs of hypersensitivity after previous administration of ACWY Vax or in those with febrile conditions.

4.4 Special warnings and special precautions for use
ACWY Vax vaccine gives no protection against meningococcal meningitis caused by meningococci belonging to groups other than group A, C, W_{135} and Y.

This vaccine is not suitable for immunisation of children of less than two years against infections due to Neisseria meningitidis serogroup C disease. Children in this age group should receive a meningococcal serogroup C conjugate vaccine in accordance with current guidance.

This vaccine should not be used in infants of less than two months. ACWY Vax does not provide reliable or long-lived protection against meningococcal disease due to serogroups A, W_{135}, Y in children of less than two years.

Administration of the vaccine to subjects with impaired immune responses may not induce an effective response.

As with all vaccinations, a solution of 1:1000 adrenaline should be available for injection should an anaphylactic reaction occur.

ACWY Vax vaccine should not under any circumstances be injected by the intravenous route.

4.5 Interaction with other medicinal products and other forms of Interaction
Not applicable.

4.6 Pregnancy and lactation
Adequate human data on use during pregnancy or lactation, and adequate animal reproduction studies are not available. ACWY Vax vaccine is not recommended in pregnancy unless there is a definite risk of group A,C, W_{135} or Y meningococcal disease.

4.7 Effects on ability to drive and use machines
The vaccine is unlikely to produce an effect on the ability to drive and use machines.

4.8 Undesirable effects
ACWY Vax may cause erythema, induration and tenderness or pain at the site of injection. Very rarely headache, fatigue, fever, somnolence and allergic reactions, including anaphylactic reactions have been reported. Miscellaneous neurological reactions have been reported very rarely although a causal relationship to ACWY Vax vaccine has not been established.

4.9 Overdose
Not applicable.

5. PHARMACOLOGICAL PROPERTIES

5.1 Pharmacodynamic properties

Active immunisation group A, C, W_{135} and Y meningococcal meningitis.

In adults and children over five years of age immunity will persist for up to 5 years. Children who were aged under 5 years when first vaccinated should be considered for revaccination after 2-3 years if they remain at high risk.

One dose of ACWY Vax will elicit a protective response in over 90% of older children and adults within 2 to 3 weeks. In children below the age of two years protection rates against serogroups C, W_{135} and Y are lower than against serogroup A and antibodies decline more rapidly than in older children and adults (at 15 days seroconversion rates range between 90-96% against serogroup A; 40-90% against serogroup C; 50-85% against serogroup W_{135}, 45-79% against serogroup Y in children aged 6-23 months).

5.2 Pharmacokinetic properties

Not applicable.

5.3 Preclinical safety data

Not applicable.

6. PHARMACEUTICAL PARTICULARS

6.1 List of excipients

Lactose

6.2 Incompatibilities

Not applicable.

6.3 Shelf life

When stored under the prescribed conditions, storage at 2°C - 8°C, shelf-life is two years.

6.4 Special precautions for storage

Store at 2°C - 8°C.

6.5 Nature and contents of container

Powder for reconstitution

ACWY is supplied in a pellet in 3 ml vials (Type I glass) with stoppers (bromobutyl rubber) and overcaps with flip-off tops (aluminium), containing one dose.

Solvent for reconstitution

Sterile saline solution (0.9%) – PL 00002/0236. The solvent is supplied in a pre-filled syringe (Type I glass) containing 0.5 ml, with a plunger stopper (rubber butyl). A 38mm (1.5 inch), 21 gauge needle is supplied for reconstitution of the ACWY vaccine. A 25mm (1 inch), 23 gauge needle is supplied for administration of ACWY. However, a 16mm (5/8 inch), 25 gauge needle may also be used to administer the vaccine.

6.6 Instructions for use and handling

The vaccine should be inspected visually for any foreign particulate matter and/or other colouration prior to administration. In the event of either being observed, discard the vaccine.

ACWY Vax must be reconstituted by adding the entire contents of the supplied diluent to the vial containing the vaccine pellet. After the addition of the diluent to the vaccine pellet, the mixture should be well shaken until the pellet is completely dissolved in the diluent.

The reconstituted vaccine should be used immediately, and certainly within one hour.

Administrative Data

7. MARKETING AUTHORISATION HOLDER

SmithKline Beecham PLC
Great West Road
Brentford
Middlesex TW8 9GS
Trading as:
GlaxoSmithKline UK
Stockley Park West
Uxbridge
Middlesex UB11 1BT

8. MARKETING AUTHORISATION NUMBER(S)

PL 10592/0014

9. DATE OF FIRST AUTHORISATION/RENEWAL OF THE AUTHORISATION

21.12.98

10. DATE OF REVISION OF THE TEXT

10.07.2003

11. Legal Status

POM

Adalat & Adalat 5

(Bayer plc)

1. NAME OF THE MEDICINAL PRODUCT

Adalat
Adalat 5

2. QUALITATIVE AND QUANTITATIVE COMPOSITION

Adalat: One capsule contains 10 mg nifedipine

Adalat 5: One capsule contains 5 mg nifedipine

For excipients see Section 6.1.

3. PHARMACEUTICAL FORM

Capsule, soft.

Orange, gelatin ovoid capsules containing a yellow viscous fluid and overprinted with either 'ADALAT' or 'ADALAT 5' and the Bayer cross.

4. CLINICAL PARTICULARS

4.1 Therapeutic indications

For the prophylaxis of chronic stable angina pectoris, the treatment of Raynaud's phenomenon and hypertension.

4.2 Posology and method of administration

The capsules should be taken orally with a little water. The recommended starting dose is 5 mg every eight hours with subsequent titration of dose according to response. The dose can be increased to a maximum of 20 mg every eight hours.

The pharmacokinetics of nifedipine are altered in the elderly so that lower maintenance doses of nifedipine may be required compared to younger patients.

Nifedipine is metabolised primarily by the liver and therefore patients with liver dysfunction should be carefully monitored, and in severe cases, a dose reduction may be necessary.

Patients with renal impairment should not require adjustment of dosage.

Treatment may be continued indefinitely.

Nifedipine is not recommended for use in children.

Adalat/Adalat 5 should not be taken with grapefruit juice (see Section 4.5).

4.3 Contraindications

Adalat/Adalat 5 should not be administered to patients with known hypersensitivity to nifedipine or other dihydropyridines because of the theoretical risk of cross-reactivity.

Adalat/Adalat 5 should not be administered to women capable of child-bearing or to nursing mothers.

Adalat/Adalat 5 should not be used in cardiogenic shock, clinically significant aortic stenosis, unstable angina pectoris, or during or within one month of a myocardial infarction.

Adalat/Adalat 5 should not be used for the treatment of acute attacks of angina.

The safety of Adalat/Adalat 5 in malignant hypertension has not been established.

Adalat/Adalat 5 should not be used for secondary prevention of myocardial infarction.

Adalat/Adalat 5 should not be administered concomitantly with rifampicin since effective plasma levels of nifedipine may not be achieved owing to enzyme induction (see Section 4.5).

4.4 Special warnings and special precautions for use

Adalat/Adalat 5 is a not beta-blocker and therefore gives no protection against the dangers of abrupt beta-blocker withdrawal; any such withdrawal should be gradual reduction of the dose of beta-blocker, preferably over 8-10 days.

Adalat/Adalat 5 may be used in combination with beta-blocking drugs and other antihypertensive agents but the possibility of an additive effect resulting in postural hypotension should be borne in mind. Adalat will not prevent possible rebound effects after cessation of other antihypertensive therapy.

Adalat/Adalat 5 should be used with caution in patients whose cardiac reserve is poor. Deterioration of heart failure has occasionally been observed with nifedipine.

At doses higher than those recommended, there is some concern about increased mortality and morbidity in the treatment of ischaemic heart disease, in particular after myocardial infarction.

Treatment with short-acting nifedipine may induce an exaggerated fall in blood pressure and reflex tachycardia which can cause cardiovascular complications such as myocardial and cerebrovascular ischaemia.

Caution should be exercised in patients with severe hypotension.

Ischaemic pain has been reported in a small proportion of patients within 30 to 60 minutes of the introduction of Adalat therapy. Although a "steal" effect has not been demonstrated, patients experiencing this effect should discontinue Adalat.

The use of Adalat/Adalat 5 in diabetic patients may require adjustment of their control.

In dialysis patients with malignant hypertension and hypovolaemia, a marked decrease in blood pressure can occur.

Whilst nifedipine is contra-indicated in pregnancy, particular care must be exercised when administering nifedipine in combination with i.v. magnesium sulphate to pregnant women.

4.5 Interaction with other medicinal products and other forms of Interaction

Known Interactions

As with other dihydropyridines, nifedipine should not be taken with grapefruit juice as elevated plasma concentrations occur, due to a decreased first pass metabolism. As a consequence, the blood pressure lowering effect of nifedipine may be increased. After regular intake of grapefruit juice, this effect may last for at least three days after the last ingestion of grapefruit juice.

The antihypertensive effect of Adalat/Adalat 5 may be potentiated by simultaneous administration of cimetidine.

When used in combination with nifedipine, serum quinidine levels have been shown to be suppressed regardless of dosage of quinidine. Therefore, monitoring of quinidine plasma levels and if necessary adjustment of the quinidine dosage are recommended. The pharmacokinetics of nifedipine may also be altered when used in combination with quinidine. It is therefore recommended to monitor blood pressure and if necessary reduce the nifedipine dosage.

The simultaneous administration of nifedipine and digoxin may lead to reduced digoxin clearance and hence an increase in the plasma digoxin level. Plasma digoxin levels should be monitored and, if necessary, the digoxin dose reduced.

Phenytoin induces the cytochrome P450 3A4 system. Upon co-administration with phenytoin, the bioavailability of nifedipine is reduced and thus its efficacy weakened. When both drugs are concomitantly administered, the clinical response to nifedipine should be monitored and, if necessary, an increase of the nifedipine dose considered. If the dose of nifedipine is increased during co-administration of both drugs, a reduction of the nifedipine dose should be considered when the treatment with phenytoin is discontinued.

Diltiazem decreases the clearance of nifedipine and hence increases plasma nifedipine levels. Therefore, caution should be taken when both drugs are used in combination and a reduction of the nifedipine dose may be necessary.

Nifedipine may increase the spectrophotometric values of urinary vanillylmandelic acid falsely. However, HPLC measurements are unaffected.

Adalat/Adalat 5 should not be administered concomitantly with rifampicin since effective plasma levels of nifedipine may not be achieved owing to enzyme induction (see Section 4.3).

Simultaneous administration of cisapride and nifedipine or quinupristin/dalfopristin and nifedipine may lead to increased plasma concentrations of nifedipine. Consequently, the blood pressure should be monitored and, if necessary, the nifedipine dose reduced.

Theoretical Interactions

Nifedipine is metabolised via the cytochrome P450 3A4 system and, therefore, there are theoretical interactions for drugs which are known to inhibit this enzyme system (e.g. erythromycin, ketoconazole, itraconazole, fluconazole, fluoxetine, indinavir, nelfinavir, ritonavir, amprenavir and saquinavir). Although no formal *in vivo* interaction studies have been performed with these drugs, co-administration can be expected to lead to an increase in plasma concentrations of nifedipine. Blood pressure should therefore be monitored and, if necessary, a reduction in the nifedipine dose considered.

A clinical study investigating the potential of a drug interaction between nifedipine and nefazodone has not yet been performed. Nefazodone is known to inhibit the cytochrome P450 3A4 mediated metabolism of other drugs. Therefore an increase in nifedipine plasma concentrations upon co-administration of both drugs cannot be excluded. When nefazodone is given together with nifedipine, the blood pressure should be monitored and, if necessary, a reduction in the nifedipine dose considered.

Tacrolimus has been shown to be metabolised via the cytochrome P450 3A4 system. Upon co-administration of both drugs, the tacrolimus plasma concentrations should be monitored and, if necessary, a reduction in the tacrolimus dose considered.

Although no formal interaction studies have been performed between nifedipine and carbamazipine, phenobarbitone or valproic acid, these drugs have been shown to alter the plasma concentrations of a structurally similar calcium channel blocker. A decrease (carbamazipine, phenobarbitone) or an increase (valproic acid) in nifedipine plasma concentrations and hence an alteration in efficacy cannot be excluded.

Drugs shown not to interact with nifedipine

The following drugs have been shown to have no effect on the pharmacokinetics of nifedipine when administered concomitantly: ajmaline, aspirin, benazepril, candesartan cilexetil, debrisoquine, doxazosin, irbesartan, omeprazole, orlistat, pantoprazole, ranitidine, rosiglitazone, talinolol and triamterene hydrochlorothiazide.

4.6 Pregnancy and lactation

Adalat is contra-indicated in women capable of child-bearing.

The safety of Adalat for use in human pregnancy has not been established. Evaluation of experimental animal studies has shown reproductive toxicity consisting of embryotoxicity and teratogenic effects at maternally toxic doses.

Adalat is contra-indicated in nursing mothers as nifedipine may be present in breast milk.

In single cases of *in vitro* fertilisation calcium antagonists like nifedipine have been associated with reversible biochemical changes in the spermatozoa's head section that may result in impaired sperm function. In those men who are repeatedly unsuccessful in fathering a child by *in vitro* fertilisation, and where no other explanation can be found, calcium antagonists like nifedipine should be considered as possible causes.

4.7 Effects on ability to drive and use machines

Reactions to the drug, which vary in intensity from individual to individual, may impair the ability to drive or to operate machinery. This applies particularly at the start of treatment, on changing the medication and in combination with alcohol.

4.8 Undesirable effects

Most undesirable effects are consequences of the vasodilatory effects of nifedipine and usually regress upon withdrawal of therapy.

In all clinical studies (nifedipine, n = 3223), the following undesirable effects were commonly reported > 1% < 10% incidence): headache and vasodilatation which occur most frequently in the early stages of treatment, nausea, dizziness and peripheral oedema not associated with heart failure or weight gain.

Additionally, uncommon and rare undesirable effects were also reported:

Uncommon > 0.1% < 1%)

Body as a whole:	abdominal pain; lethargy; asthenia; chest pain; oedema; malaise
Cardiovascular:	hypotension; palpitations; postural hypotension; tachycardia
Digestive:	constipation; diarrhoea; dry mouth; dyspepsia; gastrointestinal disorder
Nervous:	agitation; nervousness; sleep disorder; tremor; vertigo
Respiratory:	dyspnoea
Skin:	pruritus; rash; sweating
Special senses:	abnormal vision

As with the use of other short-acting dihydropyridines in patients with ischaemic heart disease, exacerbation of angina pectoris may occur at the start of treatment with nifedipine capsules. The occurrence of myocardial infarction has been described although it is not possible to distinguish such an event from the natural course of ischaemic heart disease.

Rare > 0.01% < 0.1%)

Body as a whole:	enlarged abdomen; allergic reaction; pain; hypersensitivity-type jaundice
Cardiovascular:	syncope
Digestive:	anorexia; flatulence; vomiting
Metabolic:	hyperglycaemia
Musculo-skeletal:	myalgia
Nervous:	hyperaesthesia; insomnia; mood changes; paraesthesia; somnolence
Skin:	skin disorder
Urogenital:	polyuria; impotence

For spontaneous reports the following undesirable effects were reported very rarely worldwide (<0.01%): hypotension which may lead to prolonged QT interval and ventricular fibrillation, liver function test abnormalities, agranulocytosis, purpura, hyperglycaemia, exfoliative dermatitis, photosensitive dermatitis and urticaria. There have also been reports of gingival hyperplasia and, in older men on long-term therapy, gynaecomastia, but these usually regress upon withdrawal of therapy.

4.9 Overdose

Clinical effects

Reports of nifedipine overdosage are limited and symptoms are not necessarily dose-related. Severe hypotension due to vasodilatation, and tachycardia or bradycardia are the most likely manifestations of overdose.

Metabolic disturbances include hyperglycaemia, metabolic acidosis and hypo- or hyperkalaemia.

Cardiac effects may include heart block, AV dissociation and asystole, and cardiogenic shock with pulmonary oedema.

Other toxic effects include nausea, vomiting, drowsiness, dizziness, confusion, lethargy, flushing, hypoxia and unconsciousness to the point of coma.

Treatment

As far as treatment is concerned, elimination of nifedipine and the restoration of stable cardiovascular conditions have priority.

After oral ingestion, gastric lavage is indicated, if necessary in combination with irrigation of the small intestine. Ipecacuanha should be given to children.

Activated charcoal should be given, 50 g for adults, 10-15 g for children.

Blood pressure, ECG, central arterial pressure, pulmonary wedge pressure, urea and electrolytes should be monitored.

Hypotension as a result of cardiogenic shock and arterial vasodilatation should be treated with elevation of the feet and plasma expanders. If these measures are ineffective, hypotension may be treated with 10% calcium gluconate 10-20 ml intravenously over 5-10 minutes. If the effects are inadequate, the treatment can be continued, with ECG monitoring. In addition, beta-sympathomimetics may be given, e.g. isoprenaline 0.2 mg slowly i.v. or as a continuous infusion of 5 μg/min. If an insufficient increase in blood pressure is achieved with calcium and isoprenaline, vasoconstricting sympathomimetics such as dopamine or noradrenaline should be administered. The dosage of these drugs should be determined by the patient's response.

Bradycardia may be treated with atropine, beta-sympathomimetics or a temporary cardiac pacemaker, as required.

Additional fluids should be administered with caution to avoid cardiac overload.

5. PHARMACOLOGICAL PROPERTIES

5.1 Pharmacodynamic properties

ATC code: C08C A 05

Selective Calcium channel blocker (Dihydropyridine derivative) with mainly vascular effects.

As a specific and potent calcium antagonist, the main action of Adalat is to relax arterial smooth muscle both in the coronary and peripheral circulation.

In angina pectoris, Adalat capsules relax peripheral arteries so reducing the load on the left ventricle. Additionally, Adalat dilates submaximally both clear and pre-stenotic, stenotic and post-stenotic coronary arteries, thus protecting the heart against coronary artery spasm and improving perfusion to the ischaemic myocardium.

Adalat capsules reduce the frequency of painful attacks and ischaemic ECG changes, irrespective of the relative contribution from coronary artery spasm or atherosclerosis.

Adalat causes a reduction in blood pressure such that the percentage lowering is directly related to its initial level. In normotensive individuals, Adalat has little or no effect on blood pressure.

5.2 Pharmacokinetic properties

Greater than 90% of a single oral or sub-lingual dose of nifedipine is absorbed. Radioactivity is detected in the serum 20 minutes after an oral dose and 10 minutes after a sub-lingual dose. Maximal equivalent serum concentrations are achieved 1 - 2 hours after enteral administration and these correspond to the equivalent concentrations over the same time period after intravenous administration (the drug is almost completely absorbed).

After enteral or intravenous doses, 70 - 80% of activity is eliminated (primarily as metabolites) via the urine. Remaining excretion is via the faeces.

After 24 hours, 90% of the administered dose is eliminated.

Protein binding of nifedipine exceeds 90% in human serum.

5.3 Preclinical safety data

There are no preclinical safety data of relevance to the prescriber which are additional to those already included in other sections of the Summary of Product Characteristics.

6. PHARMACEUTICAL PARTICULARS

6.1 List of excipients

Adalat capsules contain the following excipients:

Glycerol, purified water, saccharin sodium, peppermint oil and macrogol 400.

The capsule shell contains:

Gelatin, glycerol 85%, titanium dioxide (E171) and yellow orange S (E110).

6.2 Incompatibilities

Not applicable.

6.3 Shelf life

PP blister packs: 36 months

6.4 Special precautions for storage

Store in the original container. The capsules should be protected from strong light. Do not store above 25°C.

6.5 Nature and contents of container

Blister strips composed of PP foil backed with aluminium foil: 90 capsules.

6.6 Instructions for use and handling

No additional information.

7. MARKETING AUTHORISATION HOLDER

Bayer plc
Bayer House
Strawberry Hill
Newbury
Berkshire RG14 1JA
United Kingdom

Trading as: Bayer plc, Pharmaceutical Division, or Baypharm or Baymet.

8. MARKETING AUTHORISATION NUMBER(S)

Adalat: PL 00010/0021
Adalat 5: PL 00010/0079

9. DATE OF FIRST AUTHORISATION/RENEWAL OF THE AUTHORISATION

Adalat: Date of first authorisation: 15 July 1977

Date of last renewal: 14 April 1999

Adalat 5: Date of first authorisation: 27 March 1981

Date of last renewal: 25 January 1999

10. DATE OF REVISION OF THE TEXT

March 2005

LEGAL CATEGORY

POM

Adalat LA 20, 30 AND 60

(Bayer plc)

1. NAME OF THE MEDICINAL PRODUCT

Adalat LA 20

Adalat LA 30

Adalat LA 60

2. QUALITATIVE AND QUANTITATIVE COMPOSITION

Adalat LA 20: one tablet contains 20 mg nifedipine.

Adalat LA 30: one tablet contains 30 mg nifedipine.

Adalat LA 60: one tablet contains 60 mg nifedipine.

Each tablet contains a 10% overage of nifedipine to deliver the label claim.

For excipients see Section 6.1.

3. PHARMACEUTICAL FORM

Prolonged release film-coated tablet.

Pink, circular convex tablets with Adalat 20, 30 or 60 marked on one side.

4. CLINICAL PARTICULARS

4.1 Therapeutic indications

Adalat LA 20: For the treatment of mild to moderate hypertension.

Adalat LA 30 and Adalat LA 60: For the treatment of all grades of hypertension.

For the prophylaxis of chronic stable angina pectoris either as monotherapy or in combination with a beta-blocker.

4.2 Posology and method of administration

For oral administration, the tablets should be swallowed whole with a glass of water. The tablets should be taken at approximately 24-hour intervals, i.e. at the same time each day, preferably during the morning. Adalat LA tablets must be swallowed whole; under no circumstances should they be bitten, chewed or broken up.

In mild to moderate hypertension, the recommended initial dose is one 20 mg tablet once-daily. In severe hypertension, the recommended initial dose is one 30 mg tablet once-daily. If necessary, the dosage can be increased according to individual requirements up to a maximum of 90 mg once-daily.

For the prophylaxis of angina pectoris, the recommended initial dose is one 30 mg tablet once-daily. The dosage can be increased according to individual requirements up to a maximum of 90 mg once-daily.

Patients in whom hypertension or anginal symptoms are controlled on Adalat capsules or Adalat retard may be safely switched to Adalat LA. Prophylactic anti-anginal efficacy is maintained when patients are switched from other calcium antagonists such as diltiazem or verapamil to Adalat LA. Patients switched from other calcium antagonists should initiate therapy at the recommended initial dose of 30 mg Adalat LA once-daily. Subsequent titration to a higher dose may be initiated as warranted clinically.

The pharmacokinetics of nifedipine are altered in the elderly so that lower maintenance doses of nifedipine may be required compared to younger patients.

Patients with renal impairment should not require adjustment of dosage.

Treatment may be continued indefinitely.

Nifedipine is not recommended for use in children.

Adalat LA should not be taken with grapefruit juice (see Section 4.5).

4.3 Contraindications

Adalat LA should not be administered to patients with known hypersensitivity to nifedipine or other dihydropyridines because of the theoretical risk of cross-reactivity.

Adalat LA should not be administered to women capable of child-bearing or to nursing mothers.

Adalat LA should not be used in cardiogenic shock, clinically significant aortic stenosis, unstable angina, or during or within one month of a myocardial infarction.

Adalat LA should not be used for the treatment of acute attacks of angina.

The safety of Adalat LA in malignant hypertension has not been established.

Adalat LA should not be used for secondary prevention of myocardial infarction.

Owing to the duration of action of the formulation, Adalat LA should not be administered to patients with hepatic impairment.

Adalat LA should not be administered to patients with a history of gastro-intestinal obstruction, oesophageal obstruction, or any degree of decreased lumen diameter of the gastro-intestinal tract.

Adalat LA is contra-indicated in patients with inflammatory bowel disease or Crohn's disease.

Adalat LA should not be administered concomitantly with rifampicin since effective plasma levels of nifedipine may not be achieved owing to enzyme induction (see Section 4.5).

4.4 Special warnings and special precautions for use

Adalat LA tablets must be swallowed whole; under no circumstances should they be bitten, chewed or broken up.

The outer membrane of the Adalat LA tablet is not digested and, therefore, what appears to be the complete tablet may be seen in the toilet or associated with the patient's stools.

Caution should be exercised in patients with hypotension as there is a risk of further reduction in blood pressure.

Adalat LA may be used in combination with beta-blocking drugs and other antihypertensive agents but the possibility of an additive effect resulting in postural hypotension should be borne in mind. Adalat LA will not prevent possible rebound effects after cessation of other antihypertensive therapy.

Adalat LA should be used with caution in patients whose cardiac reserve is poor. Deterioration of heart failure has occasionally been observed with nifedipine.

Ischaemic pain has been reported in a small proportion of patients following the introduction of nifedipine therapy. Although a 'steal' effect has not been demonstrated, patients experiencing this effect should discontinue nifedipine therapy.

Diabetic patients taking Adalat LA may require adjustment of their control.

In dialysis patients with malignant hypertension and hypovolaemia, a marked decrease in blood pressure can occur.

Whilst nifedipine is contra-indicated in pregnancy, particular care must be exercised when administering nifedipine in combination with i.v. magnesium sulphate to pregnant women.

As the outer membrane of the Adalat LA tablet is not digested, care should be exercised as obstructive symptoms may occur, particularly in patients with pre-existing severe gastrointestinal narrowing. Bezoars can occur in very rare cases and may require surgical intervention.

Adalat LA must not be administered to patients with Kock pouch (ileostomy after proctocolectomy).

A false positive effect may be experienced when performing a barium contrast x-ray.

4.5 Interaction with other medicinal products and other forms of Interaction

Known Interactions

As with other dihydropyridines, nifedipine should not be taken with grapefruit juice as elevated plasma concentrations occur, due to a decreased first pass metabolism. As a consequence, the blood pressure lowering effect of nifedipine may be increased. After regular intake of grapefruit juice, this effect may last for at least three days after the last ingestion of grapefruit juice.

The antihypertensive effect of Adalat LA may be potentiated by simultaneous administration of cimetidine.

When used in combination with nifedipine, serum quinidine levels have been shown to be suppressed regardless of dosage of quinidine. Therefore, monitoring of quinidine plasma levels and if necessary adjustment of the quinidine dosage are recommended. The pharmacokinetics of nifedipine may also be altered when used in combination with quinidine. It is therefore recommended to monitor blood pressure, and if necessary reduce the nifedipine dosage.

The simultaneous administration of nifedipine and digoxin may lead to reduced digoxin clearance and, hence, an increase in the plasma digoxin level. Plasma digoxin levels should be monitored and, if necessary, the digoxin dose reduced.

Phenytoin induces the cytochrome P450 3A4 system. Upon co-administration with phenytoin, the bioavailability of nifedipine is reduced and thus its efficacy weakened. When both drugs are concomitantly administered, the clinical response to nifedipine should be monitored and, if necessary, an increase of the nifedipine dose considered. If the dose of nifedipine is increased during co-administration of both drugs, a reduction of the nifedipine dose should be considered when the treatment with phenytoin is discontinued.

Diltiazem decreases the clearance of nifedipine and, hence, increases plasma nifedipine levels. Therefore, caution should be taken when both drugs are used in combination and a reduction of the nifedipine dose may be necessary.

Nifedipine may increase the spectrophotometric values of urinary vanillylmandelic acid falsely. However, HPLC measurements are unaffected.

Adalat LA should not be administered concomitantly with rifampicin since effective plasma levels of nifedipine may not be achieved owing to enzyme induction (see Section 4.3).

Simultaneous administration of cisapride and nifedipine or quinupristin/dalfopristin and nifedipine may lead to increased plasma concentrations of nifedipine. Consequently, the blood pressure should be monitored and, if necessary, the nifedipine dose reduced.

Theoretical Interactions

Nifedipine is metabolised via the cytochrome P450 3A4 system and, therefore, there are theoretical interactions for drugs which are known to inhibit this enzyme system (e.g. erythromycin, ketoconazole, itraconazole, fluconazole, fluoxetine, indinavir, nelfinavir, ritonavir, amprenavir and saquinavir). Although no formal *in vivo* interaction studies have been performed with these drugs, co-administration can be expected to lead to an increase in plasma concentrations of nifedipine. Blood pressure should therefore be monitored and, if necessary, a reduction in the nifedipine dose considered.

A clinical study investigating the potential of a drug interaction between nifedipine and nefazodone has not yet been performed. Nefazodone is known to inhibit the cytochrome P450 3A4 mediated metabolism of other drugs. Therefore an increase in nifedipine plasma concentrations upon co-administration of both drugs cannot be excluded. When nefazodone is given together with nifedipine, the blood pressure should be monitored and, if necessary, a reduction in the nifedipine dose considered.

Tacrolimus has been shown to be metabolised via the cytochrome P450 3A4 system. Upon co-administration of both drugs, the tacrolimus plasma concentrations should be monitored and, if necessary, a reduction in the tacrolimus dose considered.

Although no formal interaction studies have been performed between nifedipine and carbamazipine, phenobarbitone or valproic acid, these drugs have been shown to alter the plasma concentrations of a structurally similar calcium channel blocker. A decrease (carbamazipine, phenobarbitone) or an increase (valproic acid) in nifedipine plasma concentrations and hence an alteration in efficacy cannot be excluded.

Drugs shown not to interact with nifedipine

The following drugs have been shown to have no effect on the pharmacokinetics of nifedipine when administered concomitantly: ajmaline, aspirin, benazepril, candesartan cilexetil, debrisoquine, doxazosin, irbesartan, omeprazole, orlistat, pantoprazole, ranitidine, rosiglitazone, talinolol and triamterene hydrochlorothiazide.

4.6 Pregnancy and lactation

Adalat LA is contra-indicated in women capable of child bearing.

The safety of Adalat LA for use in human pregnancy has not been established. Evaluation of experimental animal studies has shown reproductive toxicity consisting of embryotoxicity and teratogenic effects at maternally toxic doses.

Adalat LA is contra-indicated in nursing mothers as nifedipine may be present in breast milk.

In single cases of *in vitro* fertilisation calcium antagonists like nifedipine have been associated with reversible biochemical changes in the spermatozoa's head section that may result in impaired sperm function. In those men who are repeatedly unsuccessful in fathering a child by *in vitro* fertilisation, and where no other explanation can be found, calcium antagonists like nifedipine should be considered as possible causes.

4.7 Effects on ability to drive and use machines

Reactions to the drug, which vary in intensity from individual to individual, may impair the ability to drive or to operate machinery. This applies particularly at the start of treatment, on changing the medication and in combination with alcohol.

4.8 Undesirable effects

Most undesirable effects are consequences of the vasodilatory effects of nifedipine and usually regress upon withdrawal of therapy.

In all clinical studies (nifedipine, n = 9566), the following undesirable effects were commonly reported > 1% < 10% incidence): headache, palpitations and vasodilatation which occur most frequently in the early stages of treatment, lethargy, asthenia, constipation, dizziness and oedema particularly peripheral oedema not associated with heart failure or weight gain.

Additionally, uncommon and rare undesirable effects were also reported:

Uncommon > 0.1% < 1%)

Body as a whole:	abdominal pain; chest pain; leg pain; pain; malaise
Cardiovascular:	hypotension; postural hypotension; syncope; tachycardia
Digestive:	diarrhoea; dry mouth; dyspepsia; flatulence; nausea
Musculo-skeletal:	leg cramps
Nervous:	insomnia; nervousness; paraesthesia; somnolence; vertigo
Respiratory:	dyspnoea
Skin:	pruritus; rash
Urogenital:	nocturia; polyuria

Rare > 0.01% < 0.1%)

Body as a whole:	allergic reaction; chest pain substernal; chills; facial oedema; fever; hypersensitivity-type jaundice
Cardiovascular:	cardiovascular disorder
Digestive:	anorexia; eructation; gastrointestinal disorder; gingivitis; gingival hyperplasia; GGT increased; liver function test abnormalities; vomiting
Musculo-skeletal:	arthralgia; joint disorder; myalgia
Nervous:	hyperaesthesia; sleep disorder; tremor; mood changes
Respiratory:	epistaxis
Skin:	angioedema; maculopapular, pustular and vesiculobullous rash; sweating; urticaria
Special senses:	abnormal vision; eye disorder; eye pain
Urogenital:	dysuria; impotence

As with other sustained release dihydropyridines, exacerbation of angina pectoris may occur rarely at the start of treatment with sustained release formulations of nifedipine. The occurrence of myocardial infarction has been described although it is not possible to distinguish such an event from the natural course of ischaemic heart disease.

For spontaneous reports the following undesirable effects were reported very rarely worldwide (<0.01%): anaphylactic reaction, bezoar, dysphagia, oesophagitis, gum disorder, intestinal obstruction, intestinal ulcer, jaundice, increase in ALT, leucopenia, purpura, hyperglycaemia, weight loss, muscle cramps, exfoliative dermatitis, photosensitive dermatitis and blurred vision. There have also been reports of gynaecomastia in older men on long-term therapy, but this usually regresses upon withdrawal of therapy.

4.9 Overdose

There are no reports of overdosage with Adalat LA.

Clinical effects

Reports of nifedipine overdosage are limited and symptoms are not necessarily dose-related. Severe hypotension due to vasodilatation, and tachycardia or bradycardia are the most likely manifestations of overdose.

Metabolic disturbances include hyperglycaemia, metabolic acidosis and hypo- or hyperkalaemia.

Cardiac effects may include heart block, AV dissociation and asystole, and cardiogenic shock with pulmonary oedema.

Other toxic effects include nausea, vomiting, drowsiness, dizziness, confusion, lethargy, flushing, hypoxia and unconsciousness to the point of coma.

Treatment

As far as treatment is concerned, elimination of nifedipine and the restoration of stable cardiovascular conditions have priority.

After oral ingestion, gastric lavage is indicated, if necessary in combination with irrigation of the small intestine. Ipecacuanha should be given to children.

Elimination must be as complete as possible, including the small intestine, to prevent the otherwise inevitable subsequent absorption of the active substance.

Activated charcoal should be given in 4-hourly doses of 25 g for adults, 10 g for children.

Blood pressure, ECG, central arterial pressure, pulmonary wedge pressure, urea and electrolytes should be monitored.

Hypotension as a result of cardiogenic shock and arterial vasodilatation should be treated with elevation of the feet and plasma expanders. If these measures are ineffective, hypotension may be treated with 10% calcium gluconate 10-20 ml intravenously over 5-10 minutes. If the effects are inadequate, the treatment can be continued, with ECG monitoring. In addition, beta-sympathomimetics may be given, e.g. isoprenaline 0.2 mg slowly i.v. or as a continuous infusion of 5 μg/min. If an insufficient increase in blood pressure is achieved with calcium and isoprenaline, vasoconstricting sympathomimetics such as dopamine or noradrenaline should be administered. The dosage of these drugs should be determined by the patient's response.

Bradycardia may be treated with atropine, beta-sympathomimetics or a temporary cardiac pacemaker, as required.

Additional fluids should be administered with caution to avoid cardiac overload.

5. PHARMACOLOGICAL PROPERTIES

5.1 Pharmacodynamic properties

ATC code: C08C A 05

Selective Calcium channel blocker (Dihydropyridine derivative) with mainly vascular effects.

As a specific and potent calcium antagonist, the main action of nifedipine is to relax arterial smooth muscle, both in the coronary and peripheral circulation. The Adalat LA tablet is formulated to achieve controlled delivery of nifedipine in a release profile sufficient to enable once-daily administration to be effective in clinical use.

In hypertension, the main action of nifedipine is to cause peripheral vasodilatation and thus reduce peripheral resistance. Nifedipine administered once-daily provides 24-hour control of raised blood pressure. Nifedipine causes reduction in blood pressure such that the percentage lowering is proportional to its initial level. In normotensive individuals, nifedipine has little or no effect on blood pressure.

In angina, Adalat LA reduces peripheral and coronary vascular resistance, leading to an increase in coronary blood flow, cardiac output and stroke volume, whilst decreasing after-load. Additionally, nifedipine dilates submaximally both clear and atherosclerotic coronary arteries, thus protecting the heart against coronary artery spasm and improving perfusion to the ischaemic myocardium. Nifedipine reduces the frequency of painful attacks and the ischaemic ECG changes irrespective of the relative contribution from coronary artery spasm or atherosclerosis.

In a multi-national, randomised, double-blind, prospective study involving 6321 hypertensive patients with at least one additional risk factor followed over 3 to 4.8 years, Adalat LA 30 and 60 (nifedipine GITS) were shown to reduce blood pressure to a comparable degree as a standard diuretic combination.

5.2 Pharmacokinetic properties

General characteristics:

Orally administered nifedipine is almost completely absorbed in the gastro-intestinal tract. Nifedipine undergoes first-pass metabolism in the liver, giving a systemic availability of 45-68% following oral administration. At steady-state, the bioavailability of Adalat LA tablets ranges from 68-86% relative to Adalat capsules. Administration in the presence of food slightly alters the early rate of absorption but does not influence the extent of drug availability.

Nifedipine is almost completely metabolised in the liver. Nifedipine is eliminated in the form of its metabolites, predominantly via the kidneys, with approximately 5-15% being excreted via the bile in the faeces. Non-metabolised nifedipine can be detected only in traces (below 1.0%) in the urine. Nifedipine is approximately 95% bound to plasma protein.

The Adalat LA tablet is formulated to release nifedipine in a controlled way to enable once-daily administration.

The pharmacokinetic profile of this formulation is characterised by low peak-trough fluctuation. 0-24 hour plasma concentration versus time profiles at steady-state are plateau-like, rendering the Adalat LA tablet appropriate for once-a-day administration.

Characteristics in patients:

There are no significant differences in the pharmacokinetics of nifedipine between healthy subjects and subjects with renal impairment. Therefore, dosage adjustment is not needed in these patients.

In patients with hepatic impairment, the elimination half-life is distinctly prolonged and the total clearance is reduced. Owing to the duration of action of the formulation, Adalat LA should not be administered in these patients.

5.3 Preclinical safety data

Following acute oral and intravenous administration of nifedipine in various animal species, the following LD_{50} (mg/kg) values were obtained:

Mouse: Oral: 454 (401-572)*; i.v.: 4.2 (3.8-4.6)*.

Rat: Oral: 1022 (950-1087)*; i.v.: 15.5 (13.7-17.5)*.

Rabbit: Oral: 250-500; i.v.: 2-3.

Cat: Oral: ~ 100; i.v.: 0.5-8.

Dog: Oral: > 250; i.v.: 2-3.

* 95% confidence interval.

In subacute and subchronic toxicity studies in rats and dogs, nifedipine was tolerated without damage at doses of up to 50 mg/kg (rats) and 100 mg/kg (dogs) p.o. over periods of thirteen and four weeks, respectively. Following intravenous administration, dogs tolerated up to 0.1 mg/kg nifedipine for six days without damage. Rats tolerated daily intravenous administration of 2.5 mg/kg nifedipine over a period of three weeks without damage.

In chronic toxicity studies in dogs with treatment lasting up to one year, nifedipine was tolerated without damage at doses up to and including 100 mg/kg p.o. In rats, toxic effects occurred at concentrations above 100 ppm in the feed (approximately 5-7 mg/kg bodyweight).

In a carcinogenicity study in rats (two years), there was no evidence of a carcinogenic effect of nifedipine.

In studies in mice, rats and rabbits, a dose which was maternally toxic induced teratogenic effects in some cases and embryotoxicity.

In *in vitro* and *in vivo* tests, nifedipine has not been associated with mutagenic properties.

6. PHARMACEUTICAL PARTICULARS

6.1 List of excipients

Polyethylene oxide, hypromellose, magnesium stearate, sodium chloride, iron oxide (E172), cellulose acetate, macrogol 3350, organic coating which contains hydroxypropylcellulose, hypromellose, propylene glycol, titanium dioxide (E171) and iron oxide red (E172), and printing ink (shellac, iron oxide black (E172)).

6.2 Incompatibilities

Not applicable.

6.3 Shelf life

Adalat LA 20:

PP blister packs: 48 months

Adalat LA 30 and LA 60:

PVC/Aclar blister packs: 48 months

PP blister packs: 48 months

6.4 Special precautions for storage

Store in the original container. The tablets should be protected from strong light.

Adalat LA 30 and LA 60 should not be stored above 30 °C.

6.5 Nature and contents of container

Blister packs composed of PP or PVC/Aclar (Adalat LA 30 and LA 60 only) backed with aluminium foil, each containing 28 tablets.

6.6 Instructions for use and handling

No additional information.

7. MARKETING AUTHORISATION HOLDER

Bayer plc

Bayer House

Strawberry Hill

Newbury

Berkshire RG14 1JA

United Kingdom

Trading as Bayer plc, Pharmaceutical Division or Baypharm or Baymet.

8. MARKETING AUTHORISATION NUMBER(S)

Adalat LA 20: PL 0010/0222

Adalat LA 30: PL 0010/0174

Adalat LA 60: PL 0010/0175

9. DATE OF FIRST AUTHORISATION/RENEWAL OF THE AUTHORISATION

Date of first authorisation: Adalat LA 20: 22 December 1998

Adalat LA 30 and Adalat LA 60: 16 March 1992

Date of last renewal: Adalat LA 20, 30 and 60: 21 April 2002

10. DATE OF REVISION OF THE TEXT

June 2005

LEGAL CATEGORY

POM

Adalat retard

(Bayer plc)

1. NAME OF THE MEDICINAL PRODUCT

Adalat retard

2. QUALITATIVE AND QUANTITATIVE COMPOSITION

One film-coated tablet contains 20 mg nifedipine.

For excipients see Section 6.1.

3. PHARMACEUTICAL FORM

Film-coated tablets.

Grey-pink, circular tablets marked with 1U on one side and a Bayer cross on the reverse.

4. CLINICAL PARTICULARS

4.1 Therapeutic indications

For the prophylaxis of chronic stable angina pectoris and the treatment of hypertension.

4.2 Posology and method of administration

The recommended starting dose of Adalat retard is 10 mg every 12 hours swallowed with water with subsequent titration of dosage according to response. The dose may be adjusted to 40 mg every 12 hours.

Adalat retard 10 permits titration of initial dosage. The recommended dose is one Adalat retard 10 tablet (10 mg) every 12 hours.

Nifedipine is metabolised primarily by the liver and therefore patients with liver dysfunction should be carefully monitored, and in severe cases, a dose reduction may be necessary.

Patients with renal impairment should not require adjustment of dosage.

Treatment may be continued indefinitely.

The pharmacokinetics of nifedipine are altered in the elderly so that lower maintenance doses of nifedipine may be required compared to younger patients.

Nifedipine is not recommended for use in children.

Adalat retard should not be taken with grapefruit juice (see Section 4.5).

4.3 Contraindications

Adalat retard should not be administered to patients with known hypersensitivity to nifedipine or other dihydropyridines because of the theoretical risk of cross-reactivity.

Adalat retard should not be administered to women capable of child-bearing or to nursing mothers.

Adalat retard should not be used in cardiogenic shock, clinically significant aortic stenosis, unstable angina, or during or within one month of a myocardial infarction.

Adalat retard should not be used for the treatment of acute attacks of angina.

The safety of Adalat retard in malignant hypertension has not been established.

Adalat retard should not be used for secondary prevention of myocardial infarction.

Adalat retard should not be administered concomitantly with rifampicin since effective plasma levels of nifedipine may not be achieved owing to enzyme induction (see Section 4.5).

4.4 Special warnings and special precautions for use

Adalat retard is not a beta-blocker and therefore gives no protection against the dangers of abrupt beta-blocker withdrawal; any such withdrawal should be a gradual reduction of the dose of beta-blocker preferably over 8 - 10 days.

Adalat retard may be used in combination with beta-blocking drugs and other antihypertensive agents but the possibility of an additive effect resulting in postural hypotension should be borne in mind. Adalat retard will not prevent possible rebound effects after cessation of other antihypertensive therapy.

Adalat retard should be used with caution in patients whose cardiac reserve is poor. Deterioration of heart failure has occasionally been observed with nifedipine.

Caution should be exercised in patients with severe hypotension.

Ischaemic pain has been reported in a small proportion of patients within one to four hours of the introduction of Adalat retard therapy. Although a "steal" effect has not been demonstrated, patients experiencing this effect should discontinue Adalat retard.

The use of Adalat retard in diabetic patients may require adjustment of their control.

In dialysis patients with malignant hypertension and hypovolaemia, a marked decrease in blood pressure can occur.

Whilst nifedipine is contra-indicated in pregnancy, particular care must be exercised when administering nifedipine in combination with i.v. magnesium sulphate to pregnant women.

4.5 Interaction with other medicinal products and other forms of Interaction

Known Interactions

As with other dihydropyridines, nifedipine should not be taken with grapefruit juice as elevated plasma concentrations occur, due to a decreased first pass metabolism. As a consequence, the blood pressure lowering effect of nifedipine may be increased. After regular intake of grapefruit juice, this effect may last for at least three days after the last ingestion of grapefruit juice.

The antihypertensive effect of Adalat retard may be potentiated by simultaneous administration of cimetidine.

When used in combination with nifedipine, serum quinidine levels have been shown to be suppressed regardless of dosage of quinidine. Therefore, monitoring of quinidine plasma levels and if necessary adjustment of the quinidine dosage are recommended. The pharmacokinetics of nifedipine may also be altered when used in combination with quinidine. It is therefore recommended to monitor blood pressure, and if necessary reduce the nifedipine dosage.

The simultaneous administration of nifedipine and digoxin may lead to reduced digoxin clearance and hence an increase in the plasma digoxin level. Plasma digoxin levels should be monitored and, if necessary, the digoxin dose reduced.

Phenytoin induces the cytochrome P450 3A4 system. Upon co-administration with phenytoin, the bioavailability of nifedipine is reduced and thus its efficacy weakened. When both drugs are concomitantly administered, the clinical response to nifedipine should be monitored and, if necessary, an increase of the nifedipine dose considered. If the dose of nifedipine is increased during co-administration of both drugs, a reduction of the nifedipine dose should be considered when the treatment with phenytoin is discontinued.

Diltiazem decreases the clearance of nifedipine and hence increases plasma nifedipine levels. Therefore, caution should be taken when both drugs are used in combination and a reduction of the nifedipine dose may be necessary.

Nifedipine may increase the spectrophotometric values of urinary vanillylmandelic acid falsely. However, HPLC measurements are unaffected.

Adalat retard should not be administered concomitantly with rifampicin since effective plasma levels of nifedipine may not be achieved owing to enzyme induction (see Section 4.3).

Simultaneous administration of cisapride and nifedipine or quinupristin/dalfopristin and nifedipine may lead to increased plasma concentrations of nifedipine. Consequently, the blood pressure should be monitored and, if necessary, the nifedipine dose reduced.

Theoretical Interactions

Nifedipine is metabolised via the cytochrome P450 3A4 system and, therefore, there are theoretical interactions for drugs which are known to inhibit this enzyme system (e.g. erythromycin, ketoconazole, itraconazole, fluconazole, fluoxetine, indinavir, nelfinavir, ritonavir, amprenavir and saquinavir). Although no formal *in vivo* interaction studies have been performed with these drugs, co-administration can be expected to lead to an increase in plasma concentrations of nifedipine. Blood pressure should therefore be monitored and, if necessary, a reduction in the nifedipine dose considered.

A clinical study investigating the potential of a drug interaction between nifedipine and nefazodone has not yet been performed. Nefazodone is known to inhibit the cytochrome P450 3A4 mediated metabolism of other drugs. Therefore an increase in nifedipine plasma concentrations upon co-administration of both drugs cannot be excluded. When nefazodone is given together with nifedipine, the blood pressure should be monitored and, if necessary, a reduction in the nifedipine dose considered.

Tacrolimus has been shown to be metabolised via the cytochrome P450 3A4 system. Upon co-administration of both drugs, the tacrolimus plasma concentrations should be monitored and, if necessary, a reduction in the tacrolimus dose considered.

Although no formal interaction studies have been performed between nifedipine and carbamazipine, phenobarbitone or valproic acid, these drugs have been shown to alter the plasma concentrations of a structurally similar calcium channel blocker. A decrease (carbamazipine, phenobarbitone) or an increase (valproic acid) in nifedipine plasma concentrations and hence an alteration in efficacy cannot be excluded.

Drugs shown not to interact with nifedipine

The following drugs have been shown to have no effect on the pharmacokinetics of nifedipine when administered concomitantly: ajmaline, aspirin, benazepril, candesartan cilexetil, debrisoquine, doxazosin, irbesartan, omeprazole, orlistat, pantoprazole, ranitidine, rosiglitazone, talinolol and triamterene hydrochlorothiazide.

4.6 Pregnancy and lactation

Adalat retard is contra-indicated in women capable of child-bearing.

The safety of Adalat retard for use in human pregnancy has not been established. Evaluation of experimental animal studies has shown reproductive toxicity consisting of embryotoxicity and teratogenic effects at maternally toxic doses.

Adalat retard is contra-indicated in nursing mothers, as nifedipine may be present in breast milk.

In single cases of *in vitro* fertilisation calcium antagonists like nifedipine have been associated with reversible biochemical changes in the spermatozoa's head section that may result in impaired sperm function. In those men who are repeatedly unsuccessful in fathering a child by *in vitro* fertilisation, and where no other explanation can be found, calcium antagonists like nifedipine should be considered as possible causes.

4.7 Effects on ability to drive and use machines

Reactions to the drug, which vary in intensity from individual to individual, may impair the ability to drive or to operate machinery. This applies particularly at the start of treatment, on changing the medication and in combination with alcohol.

4.8 Undesirable effects

Most undesirable effects are consequences of the vasodilatory effects of nifedipine and usually regress upon withdrawal of therapy.

In all clinical studies (n = 7243), the following undesirable effects were commonly reported > 1% < 10% incidence): headache, vasodilatation and palpitations which occur most frequently in the early stages of treatment, nausea, dizziness, lethargy, asthenia, oedema and peripheral oedema not associated with heart failure or weight gain.

Additionally, uncommon and rare undesirable effects were also reported:

Uncommon > 0.1% < 1%)

Body as a whole:	abdominal pain; chest pain; malaise; pain
Cardiovascular:	postural hypotension; syncope; tachycardia
Digestive:	constipation; diarrhoea; dry mouth; dyspepsia; vomiting
Musculo-skeletal	arthralgia; myalgia
Nervous:	insomnia; nervousness; paraesthesia; somnolence; tremor; vertigo
Respiratory:	dyspnoea
Skin:	pruritus; rash; skin disorder; sweating
Urogenital system	nocturia; polyuria

As with other sustained release dihydropyridines, exacerbation of angina pectoris may occur at the start of treatment with sustained release formulations of nifedipine. The occurrence of myocardial infarction has been described although it is not possible to distinguish such an event from the natural course of ischaemic heart disease.

Rare > 0.01% < 0.1%)

Body as a whole:	enlarged abdomen; allergic reaction; photosensitivity reactions; hypersensitivity-type jaundice
Cardiovascular:	hypotension
Digestive:	flatulence; gastrointestinal disorder; GGTP increase; liver function test abnormalities
Haemic and lymphatic system:	purpura
Nervous:	hyperaesthesia; mood changes
Skin:	urticaria
Special senses:	abnormal vision; ambylopia
Urogenital:	impotence

For spontaneous reports the following undesirable effects were reported very rarely worldwide (<0.01%): gingival hyperplasia, agranulocytosis, erythromelalgia, exfoliative dermatitis and anaphylactic reaction. There have also been reports of gynaecomastia in older men on long-term therapy, but this usually regresses upon withdrawal of therapy.

4.9 Overdose

Clinical effects

Reports of nifedipine overdosage are limited and symptoms are not necessarily dose-related. Severe hypotension due to vasodilatation, and tachycardia or bradycardia are the most likely manifestations of overdose.

Metabolic disturbances include hyperglycaemia, metabolic acidosis and hypo- or hyperkalaemia.

Cardiac effects may include heart block, AV dissociation and asystole, and cardiogenic shock with pulmonary oedema.

Other toxic effects include nausea, vomiting, drowsiness, dizziness, confusion, lethargy, flushing, hypoxia and unconsciousness to the point of coma.

Treatment

As far as treatment is concerned, elimination of nifedipine and the restoration of stable cardiovascular conditions have priority.

After oral ingestion, gastric lavage is indicated, if necessary in combination with irrigation of the small intestine. Ipecacuanha should be given to children.

Elimination must be as complete as possible, including the small intestine, to prevent the otherwise inevitable subsequent absorption of the active substance.

Activated charcoal should be given in 4-hourly doses of 25 g for adults, 10 g for children.

Blood pressure, ECG, central arterial pressure, pulmonary wedge pressure, urea and electrolytes should be monitored.

Hypotension as a result of cardiogenic shock and arterial vasodilatation should be treated with elevation of the feet and plasma expanders. If these measures are ineffective, hypotension may be treated with 10% calcium gluconate 10-20 ml intravenously over 5-10 minutes. If the effects are inadequate, the treatment can be continued, with ECG monitoring. In addition, beta-sympathomimetics may be given, e.g. isoprenaline 0.2 mg slowly i.v., or as a continuous infusion of 5 μg/min. If an insufficient increase in blood pressure is achieved with calcium and isoprenaline, vasoconstricting sympathomimetics such as dopamine or noradrenaline should be administered. The dosage of these drugs should be determined by the patient's response.

Bradycardia may be treated with atropine, beta-sympathomimetics or a temporary cardiac pacemaker, as required.

Additional fluids should be administered with caution to avoid cardiac overload.

5. PHARMACOLOGICAL PROPERTIES

5.1 Pharmacodynamic properties

ATC code: C08C A 05

Selective Calcium channel blocker (Dihydropyridine derivative) with mainly vascular effects.

Nifedipine is a specific and potent calcium antagonist. In hypertension, the main action of Adalat retard is to cause peripheral vasodilatation and thus reduce peripheral resistance.

In angina, Adalat retard reduces peripheral and coronary vascular resistance, leading to an increase in coronary blood flow, cardiac output and stroke volume, whilst decreasing after-load.

Additionally, nifedipine dilates submaximally both clear and atherosclerotic coronary arteries, thus protecting the heart against coronary artery spasm and improving perfusion to the ischaemic myocardium.

Nifedipine reduces the frequency of painful attacks and the ischaemic ECG changes irrespective of the relative contribution from coronary artery spasm or atherosclerosis.

Adalat retard administered twice-daily provides 24-hour control of raised blood pressure. Adalat retard causes reduction in blood pressure such that the percentage lowering is directly related to its initial level. In normotensive individuals, Adalat retard has little or no effect on blood pressure.

5.2 Pharmacokinetic properties

Nifedipine is absorbed almost completely from the gastrointestinal tract regardless of the oral formulation used and undergoes extensive metabolism in the liver to inactive metabolites, with less than 1% of the parent drug appearing unchanged in the urine. The rate of absorption determines the drug's apparent elimination. The apparent elimination phase half-life for Adalat retard 20 mg tablets has been estimated as 2.2 - 2.4 ± 0.8 hours.

After enteral or intravenous doses, 70 - 80% of activity is eliminated (primarily as metabolites) via the urine. Remaining excretion is via the faeces.

After 24 hours, 90% of the administered dose is eliminated.

Protein binding of nifedipine exceeds 90% in human serum.

5.3 Preclinical safety data

There are no preclinical data of relevance to the prescriber, which are additional to those already included in other sections of the Summary of Product Characteristics.

6. PHARMACEUTICAL PARTICULARS

6.1 List of excipients

Microcrystalline cellulose, maize starch, lactose, polysorbate 80, magnesium stearate, hypromellose, macrogol 4000, red iron oxide (E172) and titanium dioxide (E171).

6.2 Incompatibilities

Not applicable.

6.3 Shelf life

PVC blister packs: 48 months

PP blister packs: 30 months

6.4 Special precautions for storage

Store in the original container. The tablets should be protected from strong light.

6.5 Nature and contents of container

Blister strips of 14 tablets in a cardboard outer container, in packs of 56.

Blister strips are composed of red polypropylene (PP) foil 0.3 mm or red polyvinylchloride (PVC) foil 0.25 mm, backed with aluminium foil.

6.6 Instructions for use and handling

No additional information

7. MARKETING AUTHORISATION HOLDER

Bayer plc

Bayer House

Strawberry Hill

Newbury

Berkshire RG14 1JA

United Kingdom

Trading as Bayer plc, Pharmaceutical Division or Baypharm or Baymet.

8. MARKETING AUTHORISATION NUMBER(S)

PL 0010/0078

9. DATE OF FIRST AUTHORISATION/RENEWAL OF THE AUTHORISATION

Date of first authorisation: 12 February 1982

Date of last renewal: 19 May 2002

10. DATE OF REVISION OF THE TEXT

April 2005

Legal category

POM

Adalat retard 10

(Bayer plc)

1. NAME OF THE MEDICINAL PRODUCT

Adalat retard 10

2. QUALITATIVE AND QUANTITATIVE COMPOSITION

One film-coated tablet contains 10 mg nifedipine.

For excipients see Section 6.1.

3. PHARMACEUTICAL FORM

Film-coated tablets.

Grey-pink, circular tablets marked with A10 on one side and a Bayer cross on the reverse.

4. CLINICAL PARTICULARS

4.1 Therapeutic indications

For the prophylaxis of chronic stable angina pectoris and the treatment of hypertension.

4.2 Posology and method of administration

The recommended starting dose of Adalat retard is 10 mg every 12 hours swallowed with water with subsequent titration of dosage according to response. The dose may be adjusted to 40 mg every 12 hours.

Adalat retard 10 permits titration of initial dosage. The recommended dose is one Adalat retard 10 tablet (10 mg) every 12 hours.

Nifedipine is metabolised primarily by the liver and therefore patients with liver dysfunction should be carefully monitored and in severe cases, a dose reduction may be necessary.

Patients with renal impairment should not require adjustment of dosage.

Treatment may be continued indefinitely.

The pharmacokinetics of nifedipine are altered in the elderly so that lower maintenance doses of nifedipine may be required compared to younger patients.

Nifedipine is not recommended for use in children.

Adalat retard 10 should not be taken with grapefruit juice (see Section 4.5).

4.3 Contraindications

Adalat retard 10 should not be administered to patients with known hypersensitivity to nifedipine or other dihydropyridines because of the theoretical risk of cross-reactivity.

Adalat retard 10 should not be administered to women capable of child-bearing or to nursing mothers.

Adalat retard 10 should not be used in cardiogenic shock, clinically significant aortic stenosis, unstable angina, or during or within one month of a myocardial infarction.

Adalat retard 10 should not be used for the treatment of acute attacks of angina.

The safety of Adalat retard 10 in malignant hypertension has not been established.

Adalat retard 10 should not be used for secondary prevention of myocardial infarction.

Adalat retard 10 should not be administered concomitantly with rifampicin since effective plasma levels of nifedipine may not be achieved owing to enzyme induction (see section 4.5).

4.4 Special warnings and special precautions for use

Adalat retard 10 is not a beta-blocker and therefore gives no protection against the dangers of abrupt beta-blocker withdrawal; any such withdrawal should be gradual reduction of the dose of beta-blocker preferably over 8 - 10 days.

Adalat retard 10 may be used in combination with beta-blocking drugs and other antihypertensive agents but the possibility of an additive effect resulting in postural hypotension should be borne in mind. Adalat retard 10 will not prevent possible rebound effects after cessation of other antihypertensive therapy.

Adalat retard 10 should be used with caution in patients whose cardiac reserve is poor. Deterioration of heart failure has occasionally been observed with nifedipine.

Caution should be exercised in patients with severe hypotension.

Ischaemic pain has been reported in a small proportion of patients within one to four hours of the introduction of Adalat retard therapy. Although a "steal" effect has not been demonstrated, patients experiencing this effect should discontinue Adalat retard.

The use of Adalat retard 10 in diabetic patients may require adjustment of their control.

In dialysis patients with malignant hypertension and hypovolaemia, a marked decrease in blood pressure can occur.

Whilst nifedipine is contra-indicated in pregnancy, particular care must be exercised when administering nifedipine in combination with i.v. magnesium sulphate to pregnant women.

4.5 Interaction with other medicinal products and other forms of Interaction

Known Interactions

As with other dihydropyridines, nifedipine should not be taken with grapefruit juice as elevated plasma concentrations occur, due to a decreased first pass metabolism. As a consequence, the blood pressure lowering effect of nifedipine may be increased. After regular intake of grapefruit juice, this effect may last for at least three days after the last ingestion of grapefruit juice.

The antihypertensive effect of Adalat retard 10 may be potentiated by simultaneous administration of cimetidine.

When used in combination with nifedipine, serum quinidine levels have been shown to be suppressed regardless of dosage of quinidine. Therefore, monitoring of quinidine plasma levels and if necessary adjustment of the quinidine dosage are recommended. The pharmacokinetics of nifedipine may also be altered when used in combination with quinidine. It is therefore recommended to monitor blood pressure, and if necessary reduce the nifedipine dosage.

The simultaneous administration of nifedipine and digoxin may lead to reduced digoxin clearance and hence an increase in the plasma digoxin level. Plasma digoxin levels should be monitored and, if necessary, the digoxin dose reduced.

Phenytoin induces the cytochrome P450 3A4 system. Upon co-administration with phenytoin, the bioavailability of nifedipine is reduced and thus its efficacy weakened. When both drugs are concomitantly administered, the clinical response to nifedipine should be monitored and, if necessary, an increase of the nifedipine dose considered. If the dose of nifedipine is increased during co-administration of both drugs, a reduction of the nifedipine dose should be considered when the treatment with phenytoin is discontinued.

Diltiazem decreases the clearance of nifedipine and hence increases plasma nifedipine levels. Therefore, caution should be taken when both drugs are used in combination and a reduction of the nifedipine dose may be necessary.

Nifedipine may increase the spectrophotometric values of urinary vanillylmandelic acid falsely. However, HPLC measurements are unaffected.

Adalat retard 10 should not be administered concomitantly with rifampicin since effective plasma levels of nifedipine may not be achieved owing to enzyme induction (see Section 4.3).

Simultaneous administration of cisapride and nifedipine or quinupristin/dalfopristin and nifedipine may lead to increased plasma concentrations of nifedipine. Consequently, the blood pressure should be monitored and, if necessary, the nifedipine dose reduced.

Theoretical Interactions

Nifedipine is metabolised via the cytochrome P450 3A4 system and, therefore, there are theoretical interactions for drugs which are known to inhibit this enzyme system (e.g. erythromycin, ketoconazole, itraconazole, fluconazole, fluoxetine, indinavir, nelfinavir, ritonavir, amprenavir and saquinavir). Although no formal *in vivo* interaction studies have been performed with these drugs, co-administration can be expected to lead to an increase in plasma concentrations of nifedipine. Blood pressure should therefore be monitored and, if necessary, a reduction in the nifedipine dose considered.

A clinical study investigating the potential of a drug interaction between nifedipine and nefazodone has not yet been performed. Nefazodone is known to inhibit the cytochrome P450 3A4 mediated metabolism of other drugs. Therefore an increase in nifedipine plasma concentrations upon co-administration of both drugs cannot be excluded. When nefazodone is given together with nifedipine, the blood pressure should be monitored and, if necessary, a reduction in the nifedipine dose considered.

Tacrolimus has been shown to be metabolised via the cytochrome P450 3A4 system. Upon co-administration of both drugs, the tacrolimus plasma concentrations should be monitored and, if necessary, a reduction in the tacrolimus dose considered.

Although no formal interaction studies have been performed between nifedipine and carbamazipine, phenobarbitone or valproic acid, these drugs have been shown to alter the plasma concentrations of a structurally similar calcium channel blocker. A decrease (carbamazipine, phenobarbitone) or an increase (valproic acid) in nifedipine plasma concentrations and hence an alteration in efficacy cannot be excluded.

Drugs shown not to interact with nifedipine

The following drugs have been shown to have no effect on the pharmacokinetics of nifedipine when administered concomitantly: ajmaline, aspirin, benazepril, candesartan cilexetil, debrisoquine, doxazosin, irbesartan, omeprazole, orlistat, pantoprazole, ranitidine, rosiglitazone, talinolol and triamterene hydrochlorothiazide.

4.6 Pregnancy and lactation

Adalat retard 10 is contra-indicated in women capable of child-bearing.

The safety of Adalat retard 10 for use in human pregnancy has not been established. Evaluation of experimental animal studies has shown reproductive toxicity consisting of embryotoxicity and teratogenic effects at maternally toxic doses.

Adalat retard 10 is contra-indicated in nursing mothers, as nifedipine may be present in breast milk.

In single cases of *in vitro* fertilisation calcium antagonists like nifedipine have been associated with reversible biochemical changes in the spermatozoa's head section that may result in impaired sperm function. In those men who are repeatedly unsuccessful in fathering a child by *in vitro* fertilisation, and where no other explanation can be found, calcium antagonists like nifedipine should be considered as possible causes.

4.7 Effects on ability to drive and use machines

Reactions to the drug, which vary in intensity from individual to individual, may impair the ability to drive or to operate machinery. This applies particularly at the start of treatment, on changing the medication and in combination with alcohol.

4.8 Undesirable effects

Most undesirable effects are consequences of the vasodilatory effects of nifedipine and usually regress upon withdrawal of therapy.

In all clinical studies (n = 7243), the following undesirable effects were commonly reported > 1% < 10% incidence): headache, vasodilatation and palpitations which occur most frequently in the early stages of treatment, nausea, dizziness, lethargy, asthenia, oedema and peripheral oedema not associated with heart failure or weight gain.

Additionally, uncommon and rare undesirable effects were also reported:

Uncommon > 0.1% < 1%)

Body as a whole:	abdominal pain; chest pain; malaise; pain
Cardiovascular:	postural hypotension; syncope; tachycardia
Digestive:	constipation; diarrhoea; dry mouth; dyspepsia; vomiting
Musculo-skeletal	arthralgia; myalgia
Nervous:	insomnia; nervousness; paraesthesia; somnolence; tremor; vertigo
Respiratory:	dyspnoea
Skin:	pruritus; rash; skin disorder; sweating
Urogenital system	nocturia; polyuria

As with other sustained release dihydropyridines, exacerbation of angina pectoris may occur at the start of treatment with sustained release formulations of nifedipine. The occurrence of myocardial infarction has been described although it is not possible to distinguish such an event from the natural course of ischaemic heart disease.

Rare > 0.01% < 0.1%)

Body as a whole:	enlarged abdomen; allergic reaction; photosensitivity reactions; hypersensitivity-type jaundice
Cardiovascular:	hypotension
Digestive:	flatulence; gastrointestinal disorder; GGTP increase; liver function test abnormalities
Haemic and lymphatic system:	purpura
Nervous:	hyperaesthesia; mood changes
Skin:	urticaria
Special senses:	abnormal vision; ambylopia
Urogenital:	impotence

For spontaneous reports the following undesirable effects were reported very rarely worldwide (<0.01%): gingival hyperplasia, agranulocytosis, erythromelalgia, exfoliative dermatitis and anaphylactic reaction. There have also been reports of gynaecomastia in older men on long-term therapy, but this usually regresses upon withdrawal of therapy.

4.9 Overdose

Clinical effects

Reports of nifedipine overdosage are limited and symptoms are not necessarily dose-related. Severe hypotension due to vasodilatation, and tachycardia or bradycardia are the most likely manifestations of overdose.

Metabolic disturbances include hyperglycaemia, metabolic acidosis and hypo- or hyperkalaemia.

Cardiac effects may include heart block, AV dissociation and asystole, and cardiogenic shock with pulmonary oedema.

Other toxic effects include nausea, vomiting, drowsiness, dizziness, confusion, lethargy, flushing, hypoxia and unconsciousness to the point of coma.

Treatment

As far as treatment is concerned, elimination of nifedipine and the restoration of stable cardiovascular conditions have priority.

After oral ingestion, gastric lavage is indicated, if necessary in combination with irrigation of the small intestine. Ipecacuanha should be given to children.

Elimination must be as complete as possible, including the small intestine, to prevent the otherwise inevitable subsequent absorption of the active substance.

Activated charcoal should be given in 4-hourly doses of 25 g for adults, 10 g for children.

Blood pressure, ECG, central arterial pressure, pulmonary wedge pressure, urea and electrolytes should be monitored.

Hypotension as a result of cardiogenic shock and arterial vasodilatation should be treated with elevation of the feet and plasma expanders. If these measures are ineffective, hypotension may be treated with 10% calcium gluconate 10-20 ml intravenously over 5-10 minutes. If the effects are inadequate, the treatment can be continued, with ECG monitoring. In addition, beta-sympathomimetics may be given, e.g. isoprenaline 0.2 mg slowly i.v., or as a continuous infusion of 5 μg/min. If an insufficient increase in blood pressure is achieved with calcium and isoprenaline, vasoconstricting sympathomimetics such as dopamine or noradrenaline should be administered. The dosage of these drugs should be determined by the patient's response.

Bradycardia may be treated with atropine, beta-sympathomimetics or a temporary cardiac pacemaker, as required.

Additional fluids should be administered with caution to avoid cardiac overload.

5. PHARMACOLOGICAL PROPERTIES

5.1 Pharmacodynamic properties

ATC code: C08C A 05

Selective Calcium channel blocker (Dihydropyridine derivative) with mainly vascular effects.

Nifedipine is a specific and potent calcium antagonist. In hypertension, the main action of Adalat retard is to cause peripheral vasodilatation and thus reduce peripheral resistance.

In angina, Adalat retard 10 reduces peripheral and coronary vascular resistance, leading to an increase in coronary blood flow, cardiac output and stroke volume, whilst decreasing after-load.

Additionally, nifedipine dilates submaximally both clear and atherosclerotic coronary arteries, thus protecting the heart against coronary artery spasm and improving perfusion to the ischaemic myocardium.

Nifedipine reduces the frequency of painful attacks and the ischaemic ECG changes irrespective of the relative contribution from coronary artery spasm or atherosclerosis.

Adalat retard administered twice-daily provides 24-hour control of raised blood pressure. Adalat retard causes reduction in blood pressure such that the percentage lowering is directly related to its initial level. In normotensive individuals, Adalat retard has little or no effect on blood pressure.

5.2 Pharmacokinetic properties

Nifedipine is absorbed almost completely from the gastro-intestinal tract regardless of the oral formulation used and undergoes extensive metabolism in the liver to inactive metabolites, with less than 1% of the parent drug appearing unchanged in the urine. The rate of absorption determines the drug's apparent elimination. The apparent elimination phase half-life for the 10 mg capsule and 20 mg retard tablet has been estimated as 2.2 - 2.4 ± 0.8 hours.

After enteral or intravenous doses, 70 - 80% of activity is eliminated (primarily as metabolites) via the urine. Remaining excretion is via the faeces.

After 24 hours, 90% of the administered dose is eliminated.

Protein binding of nifedipine exceeds 90% in human serum.

5.3 Preclinical safety data

There are no preclinical data of relevance to the prescriber which are additional to those already included in other sections of the Summary of Product Characteristics.

6. PHARMACEUTICAL PARTICULARS

6.1 List of excipients

Microcrystalline cellulose, maize starch, lactose, polysorbate 80, magnesium stearate, hypromellose, macrogol 4000, red iron oxide (E172) and titanium dioxide (E171).

6.2 Incompatibilities

Not applicable.

6.3 Shelf life

PVC blister packs: 48 months

PP blister packs: 30 months

6.4 Special precautions for storage

Store in the original container. The tablets should be protected from strong light.

6.5 Nature and contents of container

Blister strips of 14 tablets in a cardboard outer container, in packs of 56 tablets.

Blister strips are composed of red polypropylene foil 0.3 mm or red polyvinylchloride foil 0.25 mm, backed with aluminium foil.

6.6 Instructions for use and handling

No additional information

7. MARKETING AUTHORISATION HOLDER

Bayer plc

Bayer House

Strawberry Hill

Newbury

Berkshire RG14 1JA

United Kingdom

Trading as Bayer plc, Pharmaceutical Division, Baypharm or Baymet.

8. MARKETING AUTHORISATION NUMBER(S)

PL 0010/0151

9. DATE OF FIRST AUTHORISATION/RENEWAL OF THE AUTHORISATION

Date of first authorisation: 7 May 1987

Date of last renewal: 19 May 2002

10. DATE OF REVISION OF THE TEXT

May 2003

Legal category

POM

Adcal 600mg chewable tablets

(Strakan Pharmaceuticals Ltd)

1. NAME OF THE MEDICINAL PRODUCT

Adcal 600mg chewable tablets

2. QUALITATIVE AND QUANTITATIVE COMPOSITION

Per tablet:

Calcium carbonate 1500mg

equivalent to 600mg of elemental calcium

3. PHARMACEUTICAL FORM

Chewable Tablet

4. CLINICAL PARTICULARS

4.1 Therapeutic indications

Adcal is a chewable tablet recommended as a supplementary source of calcium when normal requirements are high and in the correction of calcium deficiency in the diet. They can be used in osteoporosis therapy as an adjunct to more specific conventional treatments. Adcal chewable tablets can be used as a phosphate binding agent in the management of renal failure.

4.2 Posology and method of administration

Oral.

Adults, elderly and children

Dietary deficiency and as an adjunct in osteoporosis therapy; 2 chewable tablets per day, preferably one tablet each morning and evening.

For use in binding phosphate in the management of renal failure in patients on renal dialysis, the dose should be adjusted for the individual patient and is dependent on the serum phosphate level.

The tablets should be chewed, not swallowed whole and taken just prior to, during or immediately following a meal.

4.3 Contraindications

Absolute contra-indications are hypercalcaemia resulting for example from myeloma, bone metastases or other malignant bone disease, sarcoidosis; primary hyperparathyroidism and vitamin D overdosage. Severe renal failure untreated by renal dialysis. Hypersensitivity to any of the tablet ingredients.

Relative contra-indications are osteoporosis due to prolonged immobilisation, renal stones, severe hypercalciuria.

4.4 Special warnings and special precautions for use

Patients with mild to moderate renal failure or mild hypercalciuria should be supervised carefully. Periodic checks of plasma calcium levels and urinary calcium excretion should be made in patients with mild to moderate renal failure or mild hypercalciuria.

Urinary calcium excretion should also be measured. In patients with a history of renal stones urinary calcium excretion should be measured to exclude hypercalciuria.

With long-term treatment it is advisable to monitor serum and urinary calcium levels and kidney function, and reduce or stop treatment temporarily if urinary calcium exceeds 7.5mmol/24 hours.

Allowances should be made for calcium and vitamin D supplements from other sources.

4.5 Interaction with other medicinal products and other forms of Interaction

The risk of hypercalcaemia should be considered in patients taking thiazide diuretics since these drugs can reduce urinary calcium excretion. Hypercalcaemia must be avoided in digitalised patients.

Certain foods (e.g. those containing oxalic acid, phosphate or phytinic acid) may reduce the absorption of calcium.

The effects of digitalis and other cardiac glycosides may be accentuated with the oral administration of calcium combined with Vitamin D. Strict medical supervision is needed and, if necessary monitoring of ECG and calcium.

Calcium salts may reduce the absorption of thyroxine, bisphosphonates, sodium fluoride, quinolone and tetracycline antibiotics or iron. It is advisable to allow a minimum period of four hours before taking the calcium.

4.6 Pregnancy and lactation

During pregnancy and lactation treatment with Adcal should be under the direction of a physician. During pregnancy and lactation, requirements for calcium are increased but in deciding on the required supplementation allowances should be made for availability of these agents from other sources. If Adcal and iron supplements are both required to be administered to the patient, they should be taken at different times (see Section 4.5).

4.7 Effects on ability to drive and use machines

None known

4.8 Undesirable effects

The use of calcium supplements has, rarely, given rise to mild gastro-intestinal disturbances, such as constipation, flatulence, nausea, gastric pain, diarrhoea.

4.9 Overdose

Overdosage with calcium carbonate has not been reported. Alkalosis is a potential but rare risk. Overdosage may cause gastro-intestinal disturbances but would not be expected to cause hypercalcaemia except in patients treated with excessive doses of vitamin D. Treatment should be aimed at lowering serum calcium levels comprising a high fluid intake and low calcium diet and in severe cases treatment with corticosteroid and other specialist treatment may be necessary

5. PHARMACOLOGICAL PROPERTIES

5.1 Pharmacodynamic properties

Calcium carbonate is a well established medicinal material and is used extensively for supplementation in deficiency states. Calcium carbonate is also widely used as an antacid.

5.2 Pharmacokinetic properties

The pharmacokinetic profiles of calcium and its salts are well known. Calcium carbonate is converted to calcium chloride by gastric acid. Calcium is absorbed to the extent of about 15-25% from the gastro-intestinal tract while the remainder reverts to insoluble calcium carbonate and calcium stearate, and is excreted in the faeces.

5.3 Preclinical safety data

Calcium carbonate is a well known and widely used material and has been used in clinical practice for many years. As such toxicity is only likely to occur in chronic overdosage where hypercalcaemia could result.

6. PHARMACEUTICAL PARTICULARS

6.1 List of excipients

Xylitol, polydextrose, pre-gelatinised starch, sodium saccharin, magnesium stearate, fruit flavour (contains propylene glycol).

6.2 Incompatibilities

Not applicable, oral preparation.

6.3 Shelf life

24 months

6.4 Special precautions for storage

Do not store above 25°C.

Store in the original package. Keep container in the outer carton.

6.5 Nature and contents of container

PVC/PVdC aluminium foil blister packs of 10 (Physicians sample), or 100 tablets in a cardboard carton.

6.6 Instructions for use and handling

No special conditions

Administrative Data

7. MARKETING AUTHORISATION HOLDER

Strakan Ltd.

Buckholm Mill

Buckholm Mill Brae

Galashiels

Scotland, TD1 2HB

8. MARKETING AUTHORISATION NUMBER(S)

PL16508/0005

9. DATE OF FIRST AUTHORISATION/RENEWAL OF THE AUTHORISATION

30 May 2000

10. DATE OF REVISION OF THE TEXT

July 2001

Adcal D3 chewable tablets

(Strakan Pharmaceuticals Ltd)

1. NAME OF THE MEDICINAL PRODUCT

Adcal-D_3 Chewable tablets

2. QUALITATIVE AND QUANTITATIVE COMPOSITION

Per tablet:

Calcium carbonate 1500mg equivalent to 600mg of elemental calcium.

Colecalciferol 400iu equivalent to 10μg vitamin D_3.

For excipients see 6.1

3. PHARMACEUTICAL FORM

Chewable Tablet

4. CLINICAL PARTICULARS

4.1 Therapeutic indications

As an adjunct to specific therapy for osteoporosis and in situations requiring therapeutic supplementation of malnutrition e.g. in pregnancy and established vitamin D dependent osteomalacia.

The prevention and treatment of calcium deficiency/vitamin D deficiency especially in the housebound and institutionalised elderly subjects. Deficiency of the active moieties is indicated by raised levels of PTH, lowered 25-hydroxy vitamin D and raised alkaline phosphatase levels which are associated with increased bone loss.

4.2 Posology and method of administration

Oral.

Adults and Elderly and children above 12 years of age:

2 chewable tablets per day, preferably one tablet each morning and evening.

Children:

Not recommended for children under 12 years.

4.3 Contraindications
Absolute contra-indications are hypercalcaemia resulting for example from myeloma, bone metastases or other malignant bone disease, sarcoidosis; primary hyperparathyroidism and vitamin D overdosage. Severe renal failure. Hypersensitivity to any of the tablet ingredients.

Relative contra-indications are osteoporosis due to prolonged immobilisation, renal stones, severe hypercalciuria.

4.4 Special warnings and special precautions for use
Patients with mild to moderate renal failure or mild hypercalciuria should be supervised carefully. Periodic checks of plasma calcium levels and urinary calcium excretion should be made in patients with mild to moderate renal failure or mild hypercalciuria.

Urinary calcium excretion should also be measured. In patients with a history of renal stones urinary calcium excretion should be measured to exclude hypercalciuria.

With long-term treatment it is advisable to monitor serum and urinary calcium levels and kidney function, and reduce or stop treatment temporarily if urinary calcium exceeds 7.5mmol/24 hours.

Allowances should be made for calcium and vitamin D supplements from other sources.

4.5 Interaction with other medicinal products and other forms of Interaction
The risk of hypercalcaemia should be considered in patients taking thiazide diuretics since these drugs can reduce urinary calcium excretion. Hypercalcaemia must be avoided in digitalised patients.

Certain foods (e.g. those containing oxalic acid, phosphate or phytinic acid) may reduce the absorption of calcium.

Concomitant treatment with phenytoin or barbiturates can decrease the effect of vitamin D because of metabolic activation. Concomitant use of glucocorticoids can decrease the effect of vitamin D.

The effects of digitalis and other cardiac glycosides may be accentuated with the oral administration of calcium combined with Vitamin D. Strict medical supervision is needed and, if necessary monitoring of ECG and calcium.

Calcium salts may reduce the absorption of thyroxine, bisphosphonates, sodium fluoride, quinolone or tetracycline antibiotics or iron. It is advisable to allow a minimum period of four hours before taking the calcium.

4.6 Pregnancy and lactation
During pregnancy and lactation treatment with Adcal-D_3 should always be under the direction of a physician. During pregnancy and lactation, requirements for calcium and vitamin D are increased but in deciding on the required supplementation allowances should be made for availability of these agents from other sources. If Adcal-D_3 and iron supplements are both required to be administered to the patient, they should be taken at different times (see Section 4.5).

Overdoses of vitamin D have shown teratogenic effects in pregnant animals. In humans, long term hypercalcaemia can lead to physical and mental retardation, aortic stenosis and retinopathy in a new born child. Vitamin D and its metabolites pass into the breast milk.

4.7 Effects on ability to drive and use machines
None known.

4.8 Undesirable effects
The use of calcium supplements has, rarely, given rise to mild gastro-intestinal disturbances, such as constipation, flatulence, nausea, gastric pain, diarrhoea. Following administration of vitamin D supplements occasional skin rash has been reported. Hypercalciuria, and in rare cases hypercalcaemia have been seen with long term treatment at high dosages.

4.9 Overdose
The most serious consequence of acute or chronic overdose is hypercalcaemia due to vitamin D toxicity. Symptoms include nausea, vomiting, polyuria, and constipation. Chronic overdoses can lead to vascular and organ calcification as a result of hypercalcaemia. Treatment should consist of stopping all intake of calcium and vitamin D and rehydration.

5. PHARMACOLOGICAL PROPERTIES
5.1 Pharmacodynamic properties
Strong evidence that supplemental calcium and vitamin D_3 can reduce the incidence of hip and other non-vertebral fractures derives from an 18 month randomised placebo controlled study in 3270 healthy elderly women living in nursing homes or apartments for elderly people. A positive effect on bone mineral density was also observed.

In patients treated with 1200mg elemental calcium and 800IU vitamin D_3 daily, i.e. the same dose delivered by two tablets of Adcal-D_3, the number of hip fractures was 43% lower (p=0.043) and the total number of non vertebral fractures was 32% lower than among those who received placebo. Proximal femur bone mineral density after 18 months of treatment increased 2.7% in the calcium/vitamin D_3 group and decreased 4.6% in the placebo group ($p < 0.001$). In the calcium/vitamin D_3 group, the mean serum PTH concentration decreased by 44% from baseline at 18 months and serum 25-hydroxy-vitamin D concentration had increased by 162% over baseline.

Analysis of the intention-to-treat results showed a decreased probability of both hip fractures ($p = 0.004$) and other fractures ($p < 0.001$) in the calcium/vitamin D_3 treatment group. Analysis of the other two populations (active treatment and those treated and followed for 18 months) revealed comparable results to the intention-to-treat analysis. The odds ratio for hip fractures among women in the placebo group compared with those in the calcium/vitamin D_3 group was 1.7 (95% CI 1.0 to 2.8) and that for other nonvertebral fractures was 1.4 (95% CI 1.4 to 2.1). In the placebo group, there was a marked increase in the incidence of hip fractures over time whereas the incidence in the calcium/vitamin D_3 group was stable. Thus treatment reduced the age-related risk of fracture at 18 months ($p = 0.007$ for hip fractures and $p = 0.009$ for all non-vertebral fractures). At 3 years follow-up, the decrease in fracture risk was maintained in the calcium/vitamin D_3 group.

5.2 Pharmacokinetic properties
The pharmacokinetic profiles of calcium and its salts are well known. Calcium carbonate is converted to calcium chloride by gastric acid. Calcium is absorbed to the extent of about 15-25% from the gastro-intestinal tract while the remainder reverts to insoluble calcium carbonate and calcium stearate, and is excreted in the faeces.

The pharmacokinetics of vitamin D is also well known. Vitamin D is well absorbed from the gastro-intestinal tract in the presence of bile. It is hydroxylated in the liver to form 25-hydroxycholecalciferol and then undergoes further hydroxylation in the kidney to form the active metabolite 1, 25 dihydroxycholecalciferol (calcitriol). The metabolites circulate in the blood bound to a specific α - globin, Vitamin D and its metabolites are excreted mainly in the bile and faeces.

5.3 Preclinical safety data
Calcium carbonate and vitamin D are well known and widely used materials and have been used in clinical practice for many years. As such toxicity is only likely to occur in chronic overdosage where hypercalcaemia could result.

6. PHARMACEUTICAL PARTICULARS
6.1 List of excipients
Xylitol, modified maize starch, sodium saccharin, magnesium stearate, DL-α-tocopherol, edible fats, gelatin, soya oil, sucrose and corn starch. 'Tutti-Frutti' flavour (contains propylene glycol).

6.2 Incompatibilities
Not applicable, oral preparation.

6.3 Shelf life
18 months

6.4 Special precautions for storage
Do not store above 25°C.

6.5 Nature and contents of container
Blister packs of 10 (physicians sample), 30, 60, 90 and 100 tablets in a cardboard carton.

6.6 Instructions for use and handling
No special conditions.

Administrative Data
7. MARKETING AUTHORISATION HOLDER
Strakan Ltd.

Buckholm Mill

Buckholm Mill Brae

Galashiels

Scotland

TD1 2HB

8. MARKETING AUTHORISATION NUMBER(S)
PL 16508/0001

9. DATE OF FIRST AUTHORISATION/RENEWAL OF THE AUTHORISATION
1 December 1998

10. DATE OF REVISION OF THE TEXT
June 2004

Adcortyl in Orabase 0.1%

(E. R. Squibb & Sons Limited)

1. NAME OF THE MEDICINAL PRODUCT
Adcortyl® in Orabase® 0.1%

2. QUALITATIVE AND QUANTITATIVE COMPOSITION
Triamcinolone Acetonide Ph.Eur. 0.1% w/w.

3. PHARMACEUTICAL FORM
Oromucosal paste.

4. CLINICAL PARTICULARS
4.1 Therapeutic indications
Adcortyl in Orabase is indicated for aphthous ulcers, ulcerative stomatitis, denture stomatitis, desquamative gingivitis, erosive lichen planus and lesions of the oral mucosa of traumatic origin.

4.2 Posology and method of administration
Adults and Children:
To be applied to the lesion at bedtime and two to four times daily, preferably after meals. Apply to the affected area; do not rub in.

Elderly:
Corticosteroids should be used sparingly and for short periods of time.

4.3 Contraindications
In patients with a history of hypersensitivity to the product components.

In tuberculous and most viral lesions of the skin, particularly herpes simplex and varicella. Should not be used in fungal or bacterial infections without suitable concomitant anti-infective therapy.

4.4 Special warnings and special precautions for use
Adrenal suppression can occur with prolonged use of topical corticosteroids or with occlusion. These effects are more likely to occur in infants and children and courses of treatment in childhood should be limited to 5 days. Dentures may act in the same way as an occlusive dressing.

4.5 Interaction with other medicinal products and other forms of Interaction
None known.

4.6 Pregnancy and lactation
Pregnancy: There is inadequate evidence of safety in human pregnancy. Topical administration of corticosteroids to pregnant animals can cause abnormalities of foetal development including cleft palate and intra-uterine growth retardation. There may, therefore, be a very small risk of such effects in the human foetus.

4.7 Effects on ability to drive and use machines
Not applicable.

4.8 Undesirable effects
Triamcinolone acetonide is well tolerated. Where adverse reactions occur they are usually reversible on cessation of therapy.

The possibility of the systemic effects which are associated with all steroid therapy should be considered.

4.9 Overdose
Topically applied corticosteroids can be absorbed in sufficient amounts to produce systemic effects.

In the event of accidental ingestion, the patient should be observed and treated symptomatically.

5. PHARMACOLOGICAL PROPERTIES
5.1 Pharmacodynamic properties
Triamcinolone acetonide is a potent fluorinated corticosteroid with anti-inflammatory, antipruritic and anti-allergic actions.

5.2 Pharmacokinetic properties
In common with other corticosteroids, triamcinolone is absorbed from sites of local application. When administered under occlusive dressings, or when the skin is broken, sufficient may be absorbed to produce systemic effects.

5.3 Preclinical safety data
See 4.6 "Pregnancy and lactation".

6. PHARMACEUTICAL PARTICULARS
6.1 List of excipients
Gelatin, pectin, sodium carboxymethylcellulose, polyethylene resin and liquid paraffin.

6.2 Incompatibilities
None.

6.3 Shelf life
5 years.

6.4 Special precautions for storage
Do not store above 25°C.

6.5 Nature and contents of container
Aluminium tubes containing 10g paste.

6.6 Instructions for use and handling
Not applicable.

7. MARKETING AUTHORISATION HOLDER
E.R. Squibb & Sons Ltd

Uxbridge Business Park

Sanderson Road

Uxbridge

Middlesex UB8 1DH.

8. MARKETING AUTHORISATION NUMBER(S)
PL 0034/5006R

9. DATE OF FIRST AUTHORISATION/RENEWAL OF THE AUTHORISATION
28 September 1988 / 04 February 2004

10. DATE OF REVISION OF THE TEXT
June 2005

Adcortyl in Orabase for Mouth Ulcers

(E. R. Squibb & Sons Limited)

1. NAME OF THE MEDICINAL PRODUCT
Adcortyl® in Orabase® for Mouth Ulcers
(triamcinolone acetonide in oromucosal paste)

2. QUALITATIVE AND QUANTITATIVE COMPOSITION
Triamcinolone Acetonide 0.1% w/w.

3. PHARMACEUTICAL FORM
Oromucosal paste.

4. CLINICAL PARTICULARS

4.1 Therapeutic indications
For the treatment of common mouth ulcers.

4.2 Posology and method of administration
Adults, Children and the Elderly: Using a clean, dry finger, apply a thin layer to the oral lesion at bedtime and if required two to three times a day. Do not apply more than four times in 24 hours. Do not rub in.

4.3 Contraindications
Contra-indicated in patients with a history of hypersensitivity to the product components.

In tuberculous and most viral lesions, particularly herpes simplex, vaccinia and varicella. The products should not be used in fungal or bacterial infections without suitable concomitant anti-infective therapy.

4.4 Special warnings and special precautions for use
Adrenal suppression can occur with topical corticosteroid therapy and dentures may increase absorption.

If symptoms persist, consult your doctor or dentist. Courses should be limited to 5 days.

Caution in patients with active/history of peptic ulcer and/or diabetes.

4.5 Interaction with other medicinal products and other forms of Interaction
None.

4.6 Pregnancy and lactation
There is inadequate evidence of safety in human pregnancy. Topical administration of corticosteroids to pregnant animals can cause abnormalities of foetal development including cleft palate and intra-uterine growth retardation. There may, therefore, be a very small risk of such effects in the human foetus.

4.7 Effects on ability to drive and use machines
None.

4.8 Undesirable effects
Triamcinolone acetonide is well tolerated. Where adverse reactions occur they are usually reversible on cessation of therapy.

Signs of systemic toxicity such as oedema and electrolyte imbalance have not been observed even when high topical dosage has been used. The possibility of the systemic effects which are associated with all steroid therapy should be considered.

4.9 Overdose
Topically applied corticosteroids can be absorbed in sufficient amounts to produce systemic effects (see undesirable effects).

In the event of accidental ingestion, the patient should be observed and treated symptomatically.

5. PHARMACOLOGICAL PROPERTIES

5.1 Pharmacodynamic properties
Triamcinolone acetonide is a potent fluorinated corticosteroid with rapid anti-inflammatory, antipruritic and anti-allergic actions.

5.2 Pharmacokinetic properties
The plasma half-life of triamcinolone acetonide is 1-2 hours. Triamcinolone is bound to plasma proteins to a relatively small degree, much less than hydrocortisone for example. Triamcinolone acetonide is metabolised largely hepatically but also by the kidney and is excreted in urine. The main metabolic route is 6-beta hydroxylation. No significant hydrolytic cleavage of the acetonide occurs.

5.3 Preclinical safety data
See 4.6 "Pregnancy and lactation".

6. PHARMACEUTICAL PARTICULARS

6.1 List of excipients
Gelatin, pectin, sodium carboxymethylcellulose, polyethylene resin and liquid paraffin.

6.2 Incompatibilities
None.

6.3 Shelf life
5 years.

6.4 Special precautions for storage
Store below 30°C.

6.5 Nature and contents of container
Aluminium tubes containing 5g paste.

6.6 Instructions for use and handling
Not applicable.

7. MARKETING AUTHORISATION HOLDER
E.R. Squibb & Sons Ltd
Uxbridge Business Park
Sanderson Road
Uxbridge
Middlesex UB8 1DH.

8. MARKETING AUTHORISATION NUMBER(S)
PL 0034/0321

9. DATE OF FIRST AUTHORISATION/RENEWAL OF THE AUTHORISATION
3rd January 1995

10. DATE OF REVISION OF THE TEXT
June 2005

Adcortyl Intra-Articular/Intradermal Injection 10mg/ml

(E. R. Squibb & Sons Limited)

1. NAME OF THE MEDICINAL PRODUCT
Adcortyl® Intra-articular/Intradermal Injection 10mg/ml

2. QUALITATIVE AND QUANTITATIVE COMPOSITION
Adcortyl® Intra-articular/Intradermal Injection contains triamcinolone acetonide 10mg per ml of sterile suspension.

3. PHARMACEUTICAL FORM
Sterile aqueous suspension for injection.

4. CLINICAL PARTICULARS

4.1 Therapeutic indications
Intra-articular use: for alleviating the joint pain, swelling and stiffness associated with rheumatoid arthritis and osteoarthrosis, with an inflammatory component; also for bursitis, epicondylitis, and tenosynovitis.

Intradermal use: for lichen simplex chronicus (neuro-dermatitis), granuloma annulare, lichen planus, keloids, alopecia areata and hypertrophic scars.

4.2 Posology and method of administration
Adcortyl is for intra-articular or intra-dermal injection. The safety and efficacy of administration by other routes has yet to be established. Strict aseptic precautions should be observed. Since the duration of effect is variable, subsequent doses should be given when symptoms recur and not at set intervals.

Adults: The dose of Adcortyl injection for intra-articular administration, and injection into tendon sheaths and bursae, is dependent on the size of the joint to be treated and on the severity of the condition. Doses of 2.5-5mg (0.25-0.5ml) for smaller joints and 5-15mg (0.5-1.5ml) for larger joints usually alleviate the symptoms. Triamcinolone acetonide 40mg/ml (Kenalog) is available to facilitate administration of larger doses. (See Precautions re Achilles tendon).

Intradermal dosage is usually 2-3mg (0.2-0.3ml), depending on the size of the lesion. No more than 5mg (0.5ml) should be injected at any one site. If several sites are injected the total dosage administered should not exceed 30mg (3ml). The injection may be repeated if necessary, at one or two week intervals.

Elderly: Treatment of elderly patients, particularly if long term, should be planned bearing in mind the more serious consequences of the common side effects of corticosteroids in old age, especially osteoporosis, diabetes, hypertension, hypokalaemia, susceptibility to infection and thinning of the skin. Close supervision is required to avoid life-threatening reactions.

Children: Adcortyl is not recommended in children under 6 years. Adcortyl intra-articular/intradermal may be used in older children in suitably adjusted dosages. Growth and development of children on prolonged corticosteroid therapy should be carefully observed. Caution should be used in the event of exposure to chickenpox, measles or other communicable diseases. (See 4.4 Special Warnings and Special Precautions for Use.)

4.3 Contraindications
Hypersensitivity to any of the ingredients.

Systemic infections unless specific anti-infective therapy is employed.

Administration by intravenous or intrathecal injection.

4.4 Special warnings and special precautions for use
Warnings (Intra-Articular Injection):

Corticosteroids should not be injected into unstable joints.

Patients should be specifically warned to avoid over-use of joints in which symptomatic benefit has been obtained. Severe joint destruction with necrosis of bone may occur if repeated intra-articular injections are given over a long period of time. Care should be taken if injections are given into tendon sheaths to avoid injection into the tendon itself. Repeated injection into inflamed tendons should be avoided as it has been shown to cause tendon rupture.

Due to the absence of a true tendon sheath, the Achilles tendon should not be injected with depot corticosteroids.

Precautions:

Intra-articular injection should not be carried out in the presence of active infection in or near joints. The preparation should not be used to alleviate joint pain arising from infectious states such as gonococcal or tubercular arthritis.

Undesirable effects may be minimised using the lowest effective dose for the minimum period, and by administering the daily requirement, whenever possible, as a single morning dose on alternate days. Frequent patient review is required to titrate the dose appropriately against disease activity (See dosage section).

Adrenal cortical atrophy develops during prolonged therapy and may persist for years after stopping treatment. Withdrawal of corticosteroids after prolonged therapy must, therefore, always be gradual to avoid acute adrenal insufficiency and should be tapered off over weeks or months according to the dose and duration of treatment. During prolonged therapy any intercurrent illness, trauma or surgical procedure will require a temporary increase in dosage. If corticosteroids have been stopped following prolonged therapy they may need to be reintroduced temporarily. Patients should carry steroid treatment cards which give clear guidance on the precautions to be taken to minimise risk and which provide details of prescriber, drug, dosage and the duration of treatment.

Suppression of the inflammatory response and immune function increases the susceptibility to infections and their severity. The clinical presentation may often be atypical and serious infections such as septicaemia and tuberculosis may be masked and may reach an advanced stage before being recognised.

Chickenpox and measles are of particular concern since these normally minor illnesses may be fatal in immunosuppressed patients.

Unless they have had chickenpox, patients receiving parenteral corticosteroids for purposes other than replacement should be regarded as being *at risk of severe chickenpox*. Manifestations of fulminant illness include pneumonia, hepatitis and disseminated intravascular coagulation; rash is not necessarily a prominent feature.

Passive immunisation with varicella-zoster immunoglobulin is needed for exposed non-immune patients receiving systemic corticosteroids or for those who have used them within the previous 3 months; varicella-zoster immunoglobulin should preferably be given within 3 days of exposure and not later than 10 days. Confirmed chickenpox warrants specialist care and urgent treatment. Corticosteroids should not be stopped and dosage may need to be increased.

Patients should be advised to avoid exposure to measles and to seek medical advice without delay if exposure occurs. Prophylaxis with normal immunoglobulin may be needed.

During corticosteroid therapy antibody response will be reduced and therefore affect the patient's response to vaccines. Live vaccines should not be administered.

Special Precautions:

Particular care is required when considering use of systemic corticosteroids in patients with the following conditions and frequent patient monitoring is necessary.

Recent intestinal anastomoses, diverticulitis, thrombophlebitis, existing or previous history of severe affective disorders (especially previous steroid psychosis), exanthematous disease, chronic nephritis, or renal insufficiency, metastatic carcinoma, osteoporosis (post-menopausal females are particularly at risk); in patients with an active peptic ulcer (or a history of peptic ulcer). Myasthenia gravis. Latent or healed tuberculosis; in the presence of local or systemic viral infection, systemic fungal infections or in active infections not controlled by antibiotics. In acute psychoses; in acute glomerulonephritis. Hypertension; congestive heart failure; glaucoma (or a family history of glaucoma), previous steroid myopathy or epilepsy. Liver failure.

Corticosteroid effects may be enhanced in patients with hypothyroidism or cirrhosis and decreased in hyperthyroid patients.

Diabetes may be aggravated, necessitating a higher insulin dosage. Latent diabetes mellitus may be precipitated.

Menstrual irregularities may occur, and this possibility should be mentioned to female patients.

Rare instances of anaphylactoid reactions have occurred in patients receiving corticosteroids, especially when a patient has a history of drug allergies.

All corticosteroids increase calcium excretion.

Aspirin should be used cautiously in conjunction with corticosteroids in patients with hypoprothrombinaemia.

4.5 Interaction with other medicinal products and other forms of Interaction
Amphotericin B injection and potassium-depleting agents: Patients should be observed for hypokalaemia.

Anticholinesterases: Effects of anticholinesterase agent may be antagonised.

Anticoagulants, oral: Corticosteroids may potentiate or decrease anticoagulant action. Patients receiving oral anticoagulants and corticosteroids should therefore be closely monitored.

Antidiabetics: Corticosteroids may increase blood glucose; diabetic control should be monitored, especially when corticosteroids are initiated, discontinued, or changed in dosage.

Antihypertensives, including diuretics: corticosteroids antagonise the effects of antihypertensives and diuretics. The hypokalaemic effect of diuretics, including acetazolamide, is enhanced.

Anti-tubercular drugs: Isoniazid serum concentrations may be decreased.

Cyclosporin: Monitor for evidence of increased toxicity of cyclosporin when the two are used concurrently.

Digitalis glycosides: Co-administration may enhance the possibility of digitalis toxicity.

Oestrogens, including oral contraceptives: Corticosteroid half-life and concentration may be increased and clearance decreased.

Hepatic Enzyme Inducers (e.g. barbiturates, phenytoin, carbamazepine, rifampicin, primidone, aminoglutethimide): There may be increased metabolic clearance of Adcortyl. Patients should be carefully observed for possible diminished effect of steroid, and the dosage should be adjusted accordingly.

Human growth hormone: The growth-promoting effect may be inhibited.

Ketoconazole: Corticosteroid clearance may be decreased, resulting in increased effects.

Nondepolarising muscle relaxants: Corticosteroids may decrease or enhance the neuromuscular blocking action.

Nonsteroidal anti-inflammatory agents (NSAIDS): Corticosteroids may increase the incidence and/or severity of GI bleeding and ulceration associated with NSAIDS. Also, corticosteroids can reduce serum salicylate levels and therefore decrease their effectiveness. Conversely, discontinuing corticosteroids during high-dose salicylate therapy may result in salicylate toxicity. Aspirin should be used cautiously in conjunction with corticosteroids in patients with hypoprothrombinaemia.

Thyroid drugs: Metabolic clearance of adrenocorticoids is decreased in hypothyroid patients and increased in hyperthyroid patients. Changes in thyroid status of the patient may necessitate adjustment in adrenocorticoid dosage.

Vaccines: Neurological complications and lack of antibody response may occur when patients taking corticosteroids are vaccinated. (See 4.4 Special Warnings and Special Precautions for Use.)

4.6 Pregnancy and lactation

The ability of corticosteroids to cross the placenta varies between individual drugs, however triamcinolone does cross the placenta.

Administration of corticosteroids to pregnant animals can cause abnormalities of foetal development, including cleft palate, intra-uterine growth retardation and effects on brain growth and development. There is no evidence that corticosteroids result in an increased incidence of congenital abnormalities, such as cleft palate / lip in man. However, when administered for prolonged periods or repeatedly during pregnancy, corticosteroids may increase the risk of intra-uterine growth retardation. Hypoadrenalism may, in theory, occur in the neonate following prenatal exposure to corticosteroids but usually resolves spontaneously following birth and is rarely clinically important.

As with all drugs, corticosteroids should only be prescribed when the benefits to the mother and child outweigh the risks. When corticosteroids are essential, however, patients with normal pregnancies may be treated as though they were in the non-gravid state.

Lactation:

Corticosteroids may pass into breast milk, although no data are available for triamcinolone. Infants of mothers taking high doses of systemic corticosteroids for prolonged periods may have a degree of adrenal suppression.

4.7 Effects on ability to drive and use machines

None known.

4.8 Undesirable effects

Where adverse reactions occur they are usually reversible on cessation of therapy. The incidence of predictable side-effects, including hypothalamic-pituitary-adrenal suppression correlate with the relative potency of the drug, dosage, timing of administration and duration of treatment (See Warnings and Precautions).

Absorption of triamcinolone following Adcortyl injection, especially when given by the intra-articular route, is rare. However, patients should be watched closely for the following adverse reactions which may be associated with any corticosteroid therapy:

Anti-inflammatory and immunosuppressive effects: Increased susceptibility and severity of infections with suppression of clinical symptoms and signs, opportunistic infections, recurrence of dormant tuberculosis (See Warnings and Precautions).

Fluid and electrolyte disturbances: sodium retention, fluid retention, congestive heart failure in susceptible patients, potassium loss, cardiac arrhythmias or ECG changes due to potassium deficiency, hypokalaemic alkalosis, increased calcium excretion and hypertension.

Musculoskeletal: muscle weakness, fatigue, steroid myopathy, loss of muscle mass, osteoporosis, avascular osteonecrosis, vertebral compression fractures, delayed healing of fractures, aseptic necrosis of femoral and humeral heads, pathological fractures of long bones and spontaneous fractures, tendon rupture.

Hypersensitivity: Anaphylatic reactions, angiodema, rash, pruritus and urticaria, particularly where there is a history of drug allergies.

Dermatological: impaired wound healing, thin fragile skin, petechiae and ecchymoses, facial erythema, increased sweating, purpura, striae, hirsutism, acneiform eruptions, lupus erythematous-like lesions and suppressed reactions to skin tests.

Gastrointestinal: dyspepsia, peptic ulcer with possible subsequent perforation and haemorrhage, pancreatitis, abdominal distension and ulcerative oesophagitis, candidiasis.

Neurological: euphoria, psychological dependence, depression, insomnia, convulsions, increased intracranial pressure with papilloedema (pseudo-tumour cerebri) usually after treatment, vertigo, headache, neuritis or paraesthesias and aggravation of pre-existing psychiatric conditions and epilepsy.

Endocrine: menstrual irregularities and amenorrhoea; development of the Cushingoid state; suppression of growth in childhood and adolescence; secondary adrenocortical and pituitary unresponsiveness, particularly in times of stress (eg. trauma, surgery or illness); decreased carbohydrate tolerance; manifestations of latent diabetes mellitus and increased requirements for insulin or oral hypoglycaemic agents in diabetes, weight gain. Negative protein and calcium balance. Increased appetite.

Ophthalmic: posterior supcapsular cataracts, increased intraocular pressure, glaucoma, exophthalmos, papilloedema, corneal or scleral thinning, exacerbation of ophthalmic viral or fungal diseases.

Others: necrotising angiitis, thrombophlebitis, thromboembolism, leucocytosis, insomnia and syncopal episodes.

Withdrawal Symptoms and Signs:

On withdrawal, fever, myalgia, arthralgia, rhinitis, conjunctivitis, painful itchy skin nodules and weight loss may occur. Too rapid a reduction in dose following prolonged treatment can lead to acute adrenal insufficiency, hypotension and death (See Warnings and Precautions).

Intra-Articular Injection:

Reactions following intra-articular administration have been rare. In a few instances, transient flushing and dizziness have occurred. Local symptoms such as post-injection flare, transient pain, irritation, sterile abscesses, hyper- or hypo-pigmentation, Charcot-like arthropathy and occasional increase in joint discomfort may occur. Local fat atrophy may occur if the injection is not given into the joint space, but is temporary and disappears within a few weeks to months.

Intradermal Injection:

Local discomfort, sterile abscesses, hyper- and hypo-pigmentation and subcutaneous and cutaneous atrophy (which usually disappears unless the basic disease process is itself atrophic) have occurred. Very rare instances of blindness associated with intralesional therapy around the face and head have been reported.

4.9 Overdose

Not applicable.

5. PHARMACOLOGICAL PROPERTIES

5.1 Pharmacodynamic properties

Triamcinolone acetonide is a synthetic glucocorticoid with marked anti-inflammatory and anti-allergic actions. Following local injection, relief of pain and swelling and greater freedom of movement are usually obtained within a few hours; such administration avoids the more severe systemic side-effects which may accompany parenteral or oral corticosteroid administration.

5.2 Pharmacokinetic properties

Triamcinolone acetonide may be absorbed into the systemic circulation from synovial spaces. However clinically significant systemic levels after intra-articular injection are unlikely to occur except perhaps following treatment of large joints with high doses. Systemic effects do not ordinarily occur with intra-articular injections when the proper techniques of administration and the recommended dosage regimens are observed.

The systemic effects of intradermally administered triamcinolone acetonide have not been extensively studied. The risk of systemic absorption, though minimal, should be taken into consideration especially when repeated intralesional administrations may be necessary.

In common with other corticosteroids, triamcinolone is metabolised largely hepatically but also by the kidney and is excreted in urine. The main metabolic route is 6-beta-hydroxylation; no significant hydrolytic cleavage of the acetonide occurs. In view of the hepatic metabolism and renal excretion of triamcinolone acetonide, functional impairments of the liver or kidney may affect the pharmacokinetics of the drug. This may become clinically significant if large or frequent doses of intradermal or intra-articular triamcinolone acetonide are given.

5.3 Preclinical safety data

See 4.6 Pregnancy and Lactation.

6. PHARMACEUTICAL PARTICULARS

6.1 List of excipients

Benzyl alcohol, polysorbate 80, sodium carboxymethylcellulose, sodium chloride, water.

6.2 Incompatibilities

The injection should not be physically mixed with other medicinal products.

6.3 Shelf life

36 months

6.4 Special precautions for storage

In an upright position. Do not store above 25°C. Avoid freezing.

6.5 Nature and contents of container

Carton containing glass ampoules 5 × 1ml or individually cartoned multidose vials of 5ml.

6.6 Instructions for use and handling

No special handling instructions.

7. MARKETING AUTHORISATION HOLDER

E.R. Squibb & Sons Ltd.
Uxbridge Business Park
Sanderson Road
Uxbridge
Middlesex
UB8 1DH

8. MARKETING AUTHORISATION NUMBER(S)

PL 0034/5002R

9. DATE OF FIRST AUTHORISATION/RENEWAL OF THE AUTHORISATION

25 July 1986 / 8 November 2002

10. DATE OF REVISION OF THE TEXT

June 2005

Adenocor

(sanofi-aventis)

1. NAME OF THE MEDICINAL PRODUCT

Adenocor

2. QUALITATIVE AND QUANTITATIVE COMPOSITION

Each vial contains 6mg of adenosine per 2ml (3mg/ml).

For excipients, see 6.1

3. PHARMACEUTICAL FORM

Solution for injection

Clear, colourless solution

4. CLINICAL PARTICULARS

4.1 Therapeutic indications

Rapid conversion to a normal sinus rhythm of paroxysmal supraventricular tachycardias, including those associated with accessory by-pass tracts (Wolff-Parkinson-White Syndrome).

Diagnostic Indications

Aid to diagnosis of broad or narrow complex supraventricular tachycardias. Although Adenocor will not convert atrial flutter, atrial fibrillation or ventricular tachycardia to sinus rhythm, the slowing of AV condition helps diagnosis of atrial activity.

Sensitisation of intra-cavitary electrophysiological investigations.

4.2 Posology and method of administration

Adenocor is intended for hospital use only with monitoring and cardiorespiratory resuscitation equipment available for immediate use. It should be administered by rapid IV bolus injection according to the ascending dosage schedule below. To be certain the solution reaches the systemic circulation administer either directly into a vein or into an IV line. If given into an IV line it should be injected as proximally as possible, and followed by a rapid saline flush.

Adenocor should only be used when facilities exist for cardiac monitoring. Patients who develop high-level AV block at a particular dose should not be given further dosage increments.

Therapeutic dose

Adult:

Initial dose: 3mg given as a rapid intravenous bolus (over 2 seconds).

Second dose: If the first dose does not result in elimination of the supraventricular tachycardia within 1 to 2 minutes, 6mg should be given also as a rapid intravenous bolus.

Third dose: If the second dose does not result in elimination of the supraventricular tachycardia within 1 to 2 minutes. 12mg should be given also as a rapid intravenous bolus.

Additional or higher doses are not recommended.

Children

No controlled paediatric study has been undertaken. Published uncontrolled studies show similar effects of adenosine in adults and children: effective doses for children were between 0.0375 and 0.25mg/kg.

Elderly

See dosage recommendations for adults.

Diagnostic dose

The above ascending dosage schedule should be employed until sufficient diagnostic information has been obtained.

Method of administration: Rapid intravenous injection only.

4.3 Contraindications

Adenocor is contraindicated for patients suffering from:

- Second or third degree AV block (except in patients with a functioning artificial pacemaker).

- Sick sinus syndrome (except in patients with a functional artificial pacemaker).

- Asthma

- Hypersensitivity to adenosine.

4.4 Special warnings and special precautions for use

Special warnings: Due to the possibility of transient cardiac arrhythmias arising during conversion of the supraventricular tachycardia to normal sinus rhythm, administration should be carried out in hospital with electrocardiographic monitoring.

Since neither the kidney nor the liver are involved in the degradation of exogenous adenosine, Adenocor's efficacy should be unaffected by hepatic or renal insufficiency.

As dipyridamole is a known inhibitor of adenosine uptake, it may potentiate the action of Adenocor. It is therefore suggested that Adenocor should not be administered to patients receiving dipyridamole; if use of Adenocor is essential, its dosage should be reduced (*see Section 4.5 Interactions with other Medicaments and other forms of Interaction*).

Precautions: Patients with atrial fibrillation/flutter and an accessory by-pass tract may develop increased conduction down the anomalous pathway.

Because of the possible risk of torsades de pointes, Adenocor should be used with caution in patients with a prolonged QT interval, whether this is congenital, drug induced or of metabolic origin.

In patients with chronic obstructive pulmonary disease, adenosine may precipitate or aggravate bronchospasm.

4.5 Interaction with other medicinal products and other forms of Interaction

As dipyridamole is a known inhibitor of adenosine uptake, it may potentiate the action of Adenocor; in one study dipyridamole was shown to produce a 4 fold increase in adenosine actions. Asystole has been reported following concomitant administration. It is therefore suggested that Adenocor should not be administered to patients receiving dipyridamole; if use of Adenocor is essential, its dosage should be reduced. *See Section 4.4 Special Warnings and Precautions for Use.*

Theophylline and other xanthines such as caffeine are known strong inhibitors of adenosine.

Adenocor may interact with drugs tending to impair cardiac conduction.

4.6 Pregnancy and lactation

Pregnancy: In the absence of evidence that adenosine does not cause foetal harm, Adenocor should only be used during pregnancy where absolutely necessary.

Lactation: In the absence of clinical experience use of Adenocor during lactation should be considered only if essential.

4.7 Effects on ability to drive and use machines

Not applicable.

4.8 Undesirable effects

Adverse reactions have been ranked under heading of system-organ class and frequency using the following convention: very commonly >= 1/10); commonly >= 1/100, <1/10); uncommonly >= 1/,000, <1/100); rarely >= 1/10,000, <1/1,000); very rarely (<1/10,000).

These side effects are generally mild, of short duration (usually less than 1 minute) and well tolerated by the patient. However severe reactions can occur.

• **Nervous system disorders**

Commonly:

- headache,

- dizziness / lightheadedness

Very rarely: transient, and spontaneously and rapidly reversible worsening of intracranial hypertension

• **Psychiatric disorders**

Commonly: apprehension

• **Special senses disorders**

Uncommonly:

- blurred vision,

- metallic taste

• **Gastro-intestinal system disorders**

Commonly: nausea

• **Cardiovascular disorders:**

Very commonly:

- facial flush

- bradycardia

- asystole

- sinus pause

- atrioventricular block

- atrial extrasystoles

- skipped beats

- ventricular excitability disorders such as ventricular extrasystoles, non-sustained ventricular tachycardia

Uncommonly:

- sinus tachycardia

- palpitations

Very rarely:

- severe bradycardia which is not corrected by atropine and may require temporary pacing

- atrial fibrillation

- torsade de pointes

- ventricular fibrillation

Adenosine induced bradycardia predisposes to ventricular excitability disorders, including ventricular fibrillation and torsade de pointes, which justify the recommendations made in Section 4.2. "*Posology and Method of Administration*". The above mentioned cardiac arrhythmias occur at the time of conversion to normal sinus rhythm.

• **Respiratory system disorders:**

Very commonly: dyspnoea

Uncommonly: hyperventilation

Very rarely: bronchospasm, apnoea (usually in patients with evidence of pre-existing asthma/COPD)

• **General disorders**

Commonly:

- Feeling of thoracic constriction / chest pain / chest pressure,

- burning sensation

Uncommonly:

- head pressure

- heaviness in arms

- arm, neck and back pain

- sweating

Very rarely: feeling of discomfort

• **Application site disorders**

Very rarely: injection site reactions

4.9 Overdose

No cases of overdosage have been reported. As the half life of adenosine in blood is very short, the duration of any effects is expected to be limited. Pharmacokinetic evaluation indicates that methyl xanthines are competitive antagonists to adenosine, and that therapeutic concentrations of theophylline block its exogenous effects.

5. PHARMACOLOGICAL PROPERTIES

5.1 Pharmacodynamic properties

Antiarrhythmic drug.

Adenosine is a purine nucleoside which is present in all cells of the body. Animal pharmacology studies have in several species shown that Adenosine has a negative dromotropic effect on the atrioventricular (AV) node.

In man Adenocor (Adenosine) administered by rapid intravenous injection slows conduction through the AV node. This action can interrupt re-entry circuits involving the AV node and restore normal sinus rhythm in patients with paroxysmal supraventricular tachycardias. Once the circuit has been interrupted, the tachycardia stops and normal sinus rhythm is re-established.

One acute interruption of the circuit is usually sufficient to arrest the tachycardia.

Since atrial fibrillation and atrial flutter do not involve the AV node as part of a re-entry circuit, Adenosine will not terminate these arrhythmias.

By transiently slowing AV conduction, atrial activity is easier to evaluate from ECG recordings and therefore the use of Adenosine can aid the diagnosis of broad or narrow complex tachycardias.

Adenosine may be useful during electrophysiological studies to determine the site of AV block or to determine in some cases of pre-excitation, whether conduction is occurring by an accessory pathway or via the AV node.

5.2 Pharmacokinetic properties

Adenosine is impossible to study via classical ADME protocols. It is present in various forms in all cells of the body where it plays an important role in energy production and utilisation systems. An efficient salvage and recycling system exists in the body, primarily in the erythrocytes and blood vessel endothelial cells. The half life in vitro is estimated to be <10 seconds. The in vivo half life may be even shorter.

5.3 Preclinical safety data

There are no pre-clinical data of relevance to the prescriber which are additional to that already included in other sections of the SPC.

6. PHARMACEUTICAL PARTICULARS

6.1 List of excipients

Sodium Chloride

Water for Injections

6.2 Incompatibilities

Compatibility with other medicines is not known.

6.3 Shelf life

36 months.

Any portion of the vial not used at once should be discarded.

6.4 Special precautions for storage

Do not refrigerate.

6.5 Nature and contents of container

Clear, type I glass vials with chlorobutyl rubber closures secured with aluminium caps. Packs of 6 vials in plastic trays in cardboard cartons.

6.6 Instructions for use and handling

None.

7. MARKETING AUTHORISATION HOLDER

Sanofi-Synthelabo Limited

One Onslow Street

Guildford

Surrey

GU1 4YS

8. MARKETING AUTHORISATION NUMBER(S)

PL 11723/0005

9. DATE OF FIRST AUTHORISATION/RENEWAL OF THE AUTHORISATION

12th March 2002

10. DATE OF REVISION OF THE TEXT

January 2005

Legal category: POM

Adenoscan

(sanofi-aventis)

1. NAME OF THE MEDICINAL PRODUCT

ADENOSCAN® 30 mg/10 ml, solution for intravenous infusion

2. QUALITATIVE AND QUANTITATIVE COMPOSITION

Adenoscan® is a sterile solution for intravenous infusion provided in 10 ml clear glass vials containing 30 mg of adenosine.

For excipients, see section 6.1.

3. PHARMACEUTICAL FORM

Solution for infusion.

4. CLINICAL PARTICULARS

4.1 Therapeutic indications

Intravenous Adenoscan® is a coronary vasodilator for use in conjunction with radionuclide myocardial perfusion imaging in patients who cannot exercise adequately or for whom exercise is inappropriate.

4.2 Posology and method of administration

Adenoscan® is intended for use in hospitals.It should be administered following the same procedure as for exercise testing where facilities for cardiac monitoring and cardio-respiratory resuscitation are available. During administration of Adenoscan® continuous ECG control is necessary as life-threatening arrhythmia might occur. Heart rate and blood pressure should be monitored every minute.

Adults:

1. Adenoscan® should be administered undiluted as a continuous peripheral intravenous infusion at a dose of 140 μg/kg/min for six minutes using an infusion pump. Separate venous sites for Adenoscan® and radionuclide administration are recommended to avoid an adenosine bolus effect.

2. After three minutes of Adenoscan® infusion, the radionuclide is injected to ensure sufficient time for peak coronary blood flow to occur. The optimal vasodilator protocol is achieved with six minutes of Adenoscan® infusion.

3. To avoid an adenosine bolus effect, blood pressure should be measured in the arm opposite to the Adenoscan® infusion.

The table below is given as a guide for adjustment of the infusion rate of undiluted Adenoscan®, in line with body-weight (total dose 0.84 mg/kg).

Patient Weight (kg)	Infusion Rate (ml/min)
45-49	2.1
50-54	2.3
55-59	2.6
60-64	2.8
65-59	3.0

70-74	3.3
75-79	3.5
80-84	3.8
85-89	4.0
90-94	4.2
95-99	4.4
100-104	4.7

Children:

In the absence of data, the use of Adenoscan® in children cannot be recommended.

Elderly:

See dosage recommendations for adults.

4.3 Contraindications

Adenoscan® is contra-indicated in patients suffering from:

- Known hypersensitivity to adenosine
- Second or third degree AV block, sick sinus syndrome except in patients with a functioning artificial pacemaker
- Long QT syndrome
- Severe hypotension
- Unstable angina not successfully stabilised with medical therapy
- Decompensated states of heart failure
- Chronic obstructive lung disease with evidence of bronchospasm (e.g. asthma bronchiale)
- Concomitant use of dipyridamole.

4.4 Special warnings and special precautions for use

Because it has the potential to cause significant hypotension, Adenoscan® should be used with caution in patients with left main coronary stenosis, uncorrected hypovolemia, stenotic valvular heart disease, left to right shunt, pericarditis or pericardial effusion, autonomic dysfunction or stenotic carotid artery disease with cerebrovascular insufficiency. Adenoscan® infusion should be discontinued in any patient who develops persistent or symptomatic hypotension. Adenoscan® should be used with caution in patients with recent myocardial infarction or severe heart failure. Adenoscan® should be used with caution in patients with minor conduction defects (first degree AV block, bundle branch block) that could be transiently aggravated during infusion.

Adenoscan® should be used with caution in patients with atrial fibrillation or flutter and especially in those with an accessory by-pass tract since particularly the latter may develop increased conduction down the anomalous pathway.

Rare cases of severe bradycardia have been reported. Some occurred in early post-transplant patients; in the other cases occult sino-atrial disease was present. The occurrence of severe bradycardia should be taken as a warning of underlying disease and should lead to treatment discontinuation. Severe bradycardia would favour the occurrence of torsades de pointes, especially in patients with prolonged QT intervals. But to date, no case of torsades de pointes has been reported when adenosine is continuously infused.

The occurrence of respiratory failure, asystole, angina or severe hypotension should also lead to treatment discontinuation.

In patients with recent heart transplantation (less than 1 year) an increased sensitivity of the heart to adenosine has been observed.

Safety and effectiveness in paediatric patients have not been established. Therefore Adenoscan® is not recommended for use in children until further data become available.

4.5 Interaction with other medicinal products and other forms of Interaction

Dipyridamole inhibits adenosine cellular uptake and metabolism, and potentiates the action of Adenoscan®. In one study dipyridamole was shown to produce a 4 fold increase in adenosine actions. It is therefore suggested that Adenoscan® should not be administered to patients receiving dipyridamole; if use of Adenoscan® is essential, dipyridamole should be stopped 24 hours before hand, or the dose of Adenoscan® should be greatly reduced.

Aminophylline, theophylline and other xanthines are competitive adenosine antagonists and should be avoided for 24 hours prior to use of Adenoscan®.

Food and drinks containing xanthines (tea, coffee, chocolate and cola) should be avoided for at least 12 hours prior to use of Adenoscan®.

Adenosine can safely be co-administered with other cardioactive or vasoactive drugs (*see 5.1 Pharmacodynamic Properties*).

4.6 Pregnancy and lactation

It is not known whether Adenoscan® can cause harm when administered to pregnant or lactating women. Therefore the use during pregnancy is contraindicated unless the physician considers the benefits outweigh the risk. Adenoscan® should not be used during lactation period.

4.7 Effects on ability to drive and use machines

None known.

4.8 Undesirable effects

Effects related to the known pharmacology of adenosine are frequent, but usually self-limiting and of short duration. Discontinuation of infusion may be necessary if the effect is intolerable.

Methylxanthines, such as IV aminophylline or theophylline have been used to terminate persistent side effects (50-125 mg by slow intravenous injection).

• Cardiovascular system:

- very commonly: flushing
- commonly: hypotension, AV block, ST segment depression, arrhythmia (sustained or non-sustained ventricular tachycardia).

If sustained second or third degree AV block develops the infusion should be discontinued. If first degree AV block occurs, the patient should be observed carefully as a quarter of patients will progress to a higher degree of block.

- rarely: bradycardia
- very rarely: asystole (*see 4.4 Special warnings and special precautions for use*)

• Respiratory system:

- very commonly: dyspnoea (or the urge to breathe deeply)
- rarely: bronchospasm, nasal congestion
- very rarely: respiratory failure (*see 4.4 Special warnings and special precautions for use*)

• Central nervous system:

- very commonly: headache
- commonly: dizziness or feeling light-headed
- uncommonly: paraesthesia,
- rarely: tremors

• Psychiatric disorders:

- uncommonly: nervousness
- rarely: drowsiness,

• Special senses:

- uncommonly: dry mouth, metallic taste
- rarely: tinnitus, blurred vision

• Genital / urinary system:

- rarely: urinary urgency, nipple discomfort

• Body as a whole:

- very commonly: chest pain or pressure
- commonly: abdominal, throat, neck and jaw discomfort
- uncommonly: sweating, discomfort in the leg, arm or back, weakness.

• Application site disorders

- very rarely: injection site reactions

4.9 Overdose

No cases of overdosage have been reported. Overdosage would cause severe hypotension, bradycardia or asystole. The half life of adenosine in blood is very short, and side effects of Adenoscan® (when they occur) would quickly resolve when the infusion is discontinued. Administration of IV aminophylline or theophylline may be needed.

5. PHARMACOLOGICAL PROPERTIES

5.1 Pharmacodynamic properties

ATC Code: Other Cardiac Preparations C01EB 10

Adenosine is a potent vasodilator in most vascular beds, except in renal afferent arterioles and hepatic veins where it produces vasoconstriction. Adenosine exerts its pharmacological effects through activation of purine receptors (cell-surface A_1 and A_2 adenosine receptors). Although the exact mechanism by which adenosine receptor activation relaxes vascular smooth muscle is not known, there is evidence to support both inhibition of the slow inward calcium current reducing calcium uptake, and activation of adenylate cyclase through A_2 receptors in smooth muscle cells. Adenosine may reduce vascular tone by modulating sympathetic neurotransmission. The intracellular uptake of adenosine is mediated by a specific transmembrane nucleoside transport system. Once inside the cell, adenosine is rapidly phosphorylated by adenosine kinase to adenosine monophosphate, or deaminated by adenosine deaminase to inosine. These intracellular metabolites of adenosine are not vasoactive.

Intracoronary Doppler flow catheter studies have demonstrated that intravenous Adenoscan® at 140 μg/kg/min produces maximum coronary hyperaemia (relative to intracoronary papaverine) in approximately 90% of cases within 2-3 minutes of the onset of the infusion. Coronary blood flow velocity returns to basal levels within 1-2 minutes of discontinuing the Adenoscan® infusion.

The increase in blood flow caused by Adenoscan® in normal coronary arteries is significantly more than that in stenotic arteries. Adenoscan® redirects coronary blood flow from the endocardium to the epicardium and may reduce collateral coronary blood flow thereby inducing regional ischaemia.

Continuous infusion of adenosine in man has been shown to produce a mild dose-dependent fall in mean arterial pressure and a dose-related positive chronotropic effect, most likely caused by sympathetic stimulation. The onset of this reflex increase in heart rate occurs later than the negative chronotropic/dromotropic effect. This differential effect is mostly observed after bolus injection thus explaining the potential use of adenosine as a treatment for supraventricular arrhythmias when administered as a bolus or as a coronary vasodilator when administered as an infusion.

Although Adenoscan® affects cardiac conduction, it has been safely and effectively administered in the presence of other cardioactive or vasoactive drugs such as beta adrenergic blocking agents, calcium channel antagonists, nitrates, ACE inhibitors, diuretics, digitalis or anti-arrhythmics.

5.2 Pharmacokinetic properties

It is impossible to study adenosine in classical pharmacokinetic studies. It is present in various forms in all the cells of the body where it plays an important role in energy production and utilisation systems. An efficient salvage and recycling system exists in the body, primarily in erythrocytes and blood vessel endothelial cells. The half-life *in vitro* is estimated to be less than 10 seconds. The *in vivo* half-life may be even shorter.

Since neither the kidney nor the liver are involved in the degradation of exogenous adenosine, the efficacy of Adenoscan® should be unaffected by hepatic or renal insufficiency.

5.3 Preclinical safety data

Because adenosine is naturally present in all living cells, studies in animals to evaluate the carcinogenic potential of Adenoscan® (adenosine) have not been performed.

6. PHARMACEUTICAL PARTICULARS

6.1 List of excipients

Sodium Chloride

Water for Injection

6.2 Incompatibilities

Compatibility with other medicines is not known.

6.3 Shelf life

3 years

6.4 Special precautions for storage

Do not refrigerate. Any portion of the vial not used at once should be discarded.

6.5 Nature and contents of container

Type I glass vials with chlorobutyl rubber stoppers, packs with 6 vials containing 10 ml of solution at 3 mg/ml, i.e. 30 mg of adenosine per vial.

6.6 Instructions for use and handling

See section 4.2. Posology and Method of Administration.

The product should be inspected visually for particulate matter and colouration prior to administration.

7. MARKETING AUTHORISATION HOLDER

Sanofi-Synthelabo

PO Box 597

Guildford

Surrey

8. MARKETING AUTHORISATION NUMBER(S)

11723/0086

9. DATE OF FIRST AUTHORISATION/RENEWAL OF THE AUTHORISATION

2nd May 2000

10. DATE OF REVISION OF THE TEXT

February 2003

Legal Category POM

Adizem-SR capsules

(Napp Pharmaceuticals Limited)

1. NAME OF THE MEDICINAL PRODUCT

ADIZEM®-SR capsules 90 mg, 120 mg, 180 mg

2. QUALITATIVE AND QUANTITATIVE COMPOSITION

Diltiazem hydrochloride 90 mg, 120 mg, 180 mg

For excipients, see section 6.1

3. PHARMACEUTICAL FORM

Prolonged release capsules

ADIZEM-SR capsules 90 mg are white capsules marked "90 mg"

ADIZEM-SR capsules 120 mg are white/brown capsules marked "120 mg"

ADIZEM-SR capsules 180 mg are white/pale brown capsules marked "180 mg"

The capsules contain prolonged release microgranules.

4. CLINICAL PARTICULARS

4.1 Therapeutic indications

For the management of angina pectoris.

For the treatment of mild to moderate hypertension.

4.2 Posology and method of administration

Route of administration

Oral.

Dosage may be taken with or without food, and should be swallowed whole and not chewed.

Angina

Adults: The usual initial dose is 90 mg twice daily. Dosage may be increased gradually to 120 mg twice daily, or 180 mg twice daily if required. Patients' responses may vary and dosage requirements can differ significantly between individual patients.

Elderly and patients with impaired renal or hepatic function:

In the elderly, dosage should commence at 60 mg diltiazem hydrochloride twice daily and the dose carefully titrated as required.

Hypertension:

Adults: the usual dose is one ADIZEM-SR 120 mg tablet or capsule twice daily. Patients may benefit by titrating from a lower total daily dose.

Elderly and patients with impaired renal or hepatic function:

The starting dose should be 60 mg diltiazem hydrochloride twice daily, increasing to one ADIZEM-SR 90 mg capsule twice daily and then to one ADIZEM-SR 120 mg tablet or capsule twice daily if clinically indicated.

Children:

The ADIZEM preparations are not recommended for children. Safety and efficacy in children has not been established.

In order to avoid confusion, it is suggested that patients once titrated to an effective dose using either ADIZEM-SR tablets or capsules should remain on this treatment and should not be changed between different presentations.

4.3 Contraindications

Pregnancy and in women of child bearing capacity. Patients with bradycardia (less than 50 bpm), second or third degree heart block, sick sinus syndrome, decompensated cardiac failure, patients with left ventricular dysfunction following myocardial infarction. Concurrent use with dantrolene infusion because of the risk of ventricular fibrillation.

4.4 Special warnings and special precautions for use

The product should be used with caution in patients with reduced left ventricular function. Patients with mild bradycardia, first degree AV block or prolonged PR interval should be observed closely. Diltiazem is considered unsafe in patients with acute porphyria.

4.5 Interaction with other medicinal products and other forms of Interaction

Due consideration should be given to the possibility of an additive effect when diltiazem is prescribed with drugs which may induce bradycardia or other anti-arrhythmic drugs.

Diltiazem hydrochloride has been used safely in combination with beta-blockers, diuretics, ACE-inhibitors and other anti-hypertensive agents. It is recommended that patients receiving these combinations should be regularly monitored. Concomitant use with alpha-blockers such as prazosin should be strictly monitored because of the possible synergistic hypotensive effect of this combination. Patients with pre-existing conduction defects should not receive the combination of diltiazem and beta-blockers.

Case reports have suggested that blood levels of carbamazepine, cyclosporin and theophylline may be increased when given concurrently with diltiazem hydrochloride. Care should be exercised in patients taking these drugs. In common with other calcium antagonists diltiazem hydrochloride may cause small increases in plasma levels of digoxin.

Concurrent use with H_2 antagonists may increase serum levels of diltiazem.

Treatment with diltiazem has been continued without problem during anaesthesia, but the anaesthetist should be made aware of the treatment regimen.

4.6 Pregnancy and lactation

Diltiazem hydrochloride is contraindicated in pregnant women or women of child bearing potential, and is not recommended in nursing mothers.

4.7 Effects on ability to drive and use machines

None known.

4.8 Undesirable effects

Diltiazem is generally well tolerated. Occasional undesirable effects are nausea, headache, oedema of the legs, flushing, hypotension, fatigue, gastrointestinal disturbance and gingival hyperplasia which disappear on cessation of treatment. Serious skin reactions such as exfoliative dermatitis and allergic skin reactions such as angioneurotic oedema, erythema multiforme and vasculitis have been reported. Diltiazem may cause depression of atrioventricular nodal conduction and bradycardia. Isolated cases of moderate and transient increased liver transaminases have been observed at the start of treatment. Isolated cases of clinical hepatitis have been reported, which resolved when diltiazem was withdrawn.

4.9 Overdose

The clinical symptoms of acute intoxication may include pronounced hypotension or even collapse and sinus bradycardia with or without atrioventricular conduction defects.

The patient should be closely monitored in hospital to exclude arrhythmias or atrioventricular conduction defects. Gastric lavage and osmotic diuresis should be undertaken when considered appropriate. Symptomatic bradycardia and high grade atrioventricular block may respond to atropine, isoprenaline or occasionally temporary cardiac pacing.

Hypotension may require correction with plasma volume expanders, intravenous calcium gluconate and positive inotropic agents. The formulation employs a prolonged release system which will continue to release diltiazem for some hours.

5. PHARMACOLOGICAL PROPERTIES

5.1 Pharmacodynamic properties

Pharmacotherapeutic group: Selective calcium channel blocker with direct cardiac effects

ATC Code: C08D B01

Diltiazem is an antianginal agent and calcium antagonist. Diltiazem inhibits transmembrane calcium entry in myocardial muscle fibres and in vascular smooth muscle fibres, thereby decreasing the quantity of intracellular calcium available to the contractile proteins.

5.2 Pharmacokinetic properties

ADIZEM-SR capsules is a form characterised by prolonged release of diltiazem hydrochloride in the digestive tract. Diltiazem is 80% bound to human plasma proteins (albumin, acid glucoproteins).

The biotransformation routes are:

- Deacetylation
- Oxidative o- and n-demethylation
- Conjugation of the phenolic metabolites.

The primary metabolites, n-demethyldiltiazem and desacetyldiltiazem exert less pharmacological activity than diltiazem. The other metabolites are pharmacologically inactive.

After administration of 180 to 300 mg of ADIZEM-SR capsules, a peak plasma concentration of 80 to 220 ng/ml, respectively, is obtained after about 5.5 hours.

The elimination half-life varies from 6 to 8 hours, depending on the strength.

5.3 Preclinical safety data

There are no pre-clinical data of relevance to the prescriber which are additional to that already included in other sections of the SPC.

6. PHARMACEUTICAL PARTICULARS

6.1 List of excipients

Capsule contents

Sucrose and maize starch SP microgranules

Povidone

Sucrose

Ethylcellulose

Talc

Aquacoat ECD 30

Dibutyl sebacate

Capsule shells

Titanium dioxide (E171)

Gelatin

Iron oxide (E172) – 120 mg and 180 mg capsules only.

Indigotine (E132) - 120 mg capsules only.

6.2 Incompatibilities

None known.

6.3 Shelf life

Three years.

6.4 Special precautions for storage

Do not store above 25°C.

6.5 Nature and contents of container

Blister packs (aluminium/PVC) boxed in cardboard cartons.

Pack sizes: 56 capsules

6.6 Instructions for use and handling

Not applicable

7. MARKETING AUTHORISATION HOLDER

Napp Pharmaceuticals Ltd

Cambridge Science Park

Milton Road

Cambridge CB4 0GW

8. MARKETING AUTHORISATION NUMBER(S)

PL 16950/0006-0008

9. DATE OF FIRST AUTHORISATION/RENEWAL OF THE AUTHORISATION

2 October 1992/23 September 2003

10. DATE OF REVISION OF THE TEXT

June 2003

11. Legal Category

POM

® The Napp device and ADIZEM are Registered Trade Marks

Adizem-SR tablets

(Napp Pharmaceuticals Limited)

1. NAME OF THE MEDICINAL PRODUCT

ADIZEM®-SR tablets 120 mg

2. QUALITATIVE AND QUANTITATIVE COMPOSITION

Diltiazem Hydrochloride 120 mg

For excipients see section 6.1

3. PHARMACEUTICAL FORM

White film-coated capsule-shaped, prolonged release tablets. The tablets are marked 120/DL on one side and with a scoreline on the other.

4. CLINICAL PARTICULARS

4.1 Therapeutic indications

For the management of angina pectoris. For the treatment of mild to moderate hypertension.

4.2 Posology and method of administration

Route of administration

Oral.

Dosage may be taken with or without food, and should be swallowed whole and not chewed.

Angina

Adults:

The usual initial dose is 90 mg twice-daily. Dosage may be increased gradually to 120 mg twice-daily, or 180 mg twice-daily if required. Patients' responses may vary and dosage requirements can differ significantly between individual patients.

Elderly and patients with impaired renal or hepatic function:

In the elderly, dosage should commence at 60 mg diltiazem hydrochloride twice-daily and the dose carefully titrated as required.

Hypertension

Adults:

The usual dose is one ADIZEM-SR 120 mg tablet or capsule twice-daily. Patients may benefit by titrating from a lower total daily dose.

Elderly and patients with impaired renal or hepatic function:

The starting dose should be 60 mg diltiazem hydrochloride twice-daily, increasing to one ADIZEM-SR 90 mg capsule twice-daily and then to one ADIZEM-SR 120 mg tablet or capsule twice-daily if clinically indicated.

Children:

The ADIZEM preparations are not recommended for children. Safety and efficacy in children has not been established.

In order to avoid confusion, it is suggested that patients, once titrated to an effective dose using either ADIZEM tablets or capsules, should remain on this treatment and should not be changed between different presentations.

4.3 Contraindications

Pregnancy and in women of child-bearing capacity. Patients with bradycardia (less than 50 bpm), second or third degree heart block, sick sinus syndrome, decompensated cardiac failure, patients with left ventricular dysfunction following myocardial infarction. Concurrent use with dantrolene infusion because of the risk of ventricular fibrillation.

4.4 Special warnings and special precautions for use

The product should be used with caution in patients with reduced left ventricular function. Patients with mild bradycardia, first degree AV block or prolonged PR interval should be observed closely. Diltiazem is considered unsafe in patients with acute porphyria.

4.5 Interaction with other medicinal products and other forms of Interaction

Due consideration should be given to the possibility of an additive effect when diltiazem is prescribed with drugs which may induce bradycardia or other anti-arrhythmic drugs.

Diltiazem hydrochloride has been used safely in combination with beta-blockers, diuretics, ACE-inhibitors and other anti-hypertensive agents. It is recommended that patients receiving these combinations should be regularly monitored. Concomitant use with alpha-blockers such as prazosin should be strictly monitored because of the possible synergistic hypotensive effect of this combination. Patients with pre-existing conduction defects should not receive the combination of diltiazem and beta-blockers.

Case reports have suggested that blood levels of carbamazepine, cyclosporin and theophylline may be increased when given concurrently with diltiazem hydrochloride. Care should be exercised in patients taking these drugs. In common with other calcium antagonists, diltiazem hydrochloride may cause small increases in plasma levels of digoxin.

Concurrent use with H_2-antagonists may increase serum levels of diltiazem.

Treatment with diltiazem has been continued without problem during anaesthesia, but the anaesthetist should be aware of the treatment regimen.

4.6 Pregnancy and lactation

Diltiazem hydrochloride is contra-indicated in pregnant women or women of child-bearing potential, and is not recommended in nursing mothers.

4.7 Effects on ability to drive and use machines

None known.

4.8 Undesirable effects

Diltiazem is generally well tolerated. Occasional undesirable effects are nausea, headache, oedema of the legs, flushing, hypotension and fatigue, gastrointestinal disturbance and gingival hyperplasia which disappear on cessation of treatment. Serious skin reactions such as exfoliative dermatitis and allergic skin reactions such as angioneurotic oedema, erythema multiforme and vasculitis have been reported. Diltiazem may cause depression of atrioventricular nodal conduction and bradycardia. Isolated cases of moderate and transient increased liver transaminases have been observed at the start of treatment. Isolated cases of clinical hepatitis have been reported, which resolved when diltiazem was withdrawn.

4.9 Overdose

The clinical symptoms of acute intoxication may include pronounced hypotension or even collapse and sinus bradycardia with or without atrioventricular conduction defects.

The patient should be closely monitored in hospital to exclude arrhythmias or atrioventricular conduction defects. Gastric lavage and osmotic diuresis should be undertaken when considered appropriate. Symptomatic bradycardia and high grade atrioventricular block may respond to atropine, isoprenaline or occasionally temporary cardiac pacing.

Hypotension may require correction with plasma volume expanders, intravenous calcium gluconate and positive inotropic agents. The formulation employs a prolonged release system which will continue to release diltiazem for some hours.

5. PHARMACOLOGICAL PROPERTIES

Pharmacotherapeutic group: Selective calcium channel blocker with direct cardiac effects

ATC Code: C08D B01

5.1 Pharmacodynamic properties

Diltiazem is a calcium antagonist which restricts the slow channel entry of calcium ions into the cell and so reduces the liberation of calcium from stores in the endoplasmic reticulum. This results in a reduction in the amount of available intra-cellular calcium and consequently:

1) Reduction of myocardial oxygen consumption.

2) Dilation of small and large coronary arteries.

3) Mild peripheral vasodilation.

4) A negative dromotropic effect.

5) The reflex positive chronotropic and inotropic effects due to reflex sympathetic activity are partially inhibited. This results in a slight reduction or no change in heart rate.

The antianginal effect is due to a reduction in cardiac oxygen demand with maintenance of coronary blood flow. Cardiac contractility and ventricular ejection fraction are unchanged. Treatment with diltiazem increases exercise capacity, improves the indices of myocardial ischaemia in the angina patient and relieves the spasm of vasospastic (Prinzmetal's) angina.

5.2 Pharmacokinetic properties

An oral dose of diltiazem is almost completely absorbed. Despite this, diltiazem has a low bioavailability owing to hepatic first pass metabolism. Diltiazem is metabolised extensively and only 1.0 to 3.0% of the dose is excreted in the urine as unchanged diltiazem. The release of the drug has been prolonged in the 120 mg tablet by special pharmaceutical technology. The high peak concentrations of the absorption phase have been eliminated. This allows the tablet to be administered twice-daily.

5.3 Preclinical safety data

There are no pre-clinical data of relevance to the prescriber which are additional to that already included in other sections of the SPC.

6. PHARMACEUTICAL PARTICULARS

6.1 List of excipients

Lactose

Hydrogenated castor oil

Colloidal aluminium hydroxide

Acrylic resin

Talc

Magnesium stearate

Hypromellose

Sucrose

Glycerol 85%

Titanium dioxide (E171)

Polysorbate 80

6.2 Incompatibilities

None known.

6.3 Shelf life

36 months.

6.4 Special precautions for storage

Do not store above 30°C.

Store in the original package.

6.5 Nature and contents of container

Aluminium foil backed PVdC/PVC blister packs containing 56 tablets.

6.6 Instructions for use and handling

None.

7. MARKETING AUTHORISATION HOLDER

Napp Pharmaceuticals Ltd

Cambridge Science Park

Milton Road

Cambridge

CB4 0GW

8. MARKETING AUTHORISATION NUMBER(S)

PL 16950/0009

9. DATE OF FIRST AUTHORISATION/RENEWAL OF THE AUTHORISATION

21 December 1989/23 September 2003

10. DATE OF REVISION OF THE TEXT

June 2003

11. Legal Category

POM

® ADIZEM and the Napp device are Registered Trade Marks.

Adizem-XL capsules

(Napp Pharmaceuticals Limited)

1. NAME OF THE MEDICINAL PRODUCT

ADIZEM®-XL capsules 120, 180, 200, 240, 300 mg

2. QUALITATIVE AND QUANTITATIVE COMPOSITION

Diltiazem Hydrochloride 120, 180, 200, 240, 300 mg

For excipients, see section 6.1.

3. PHARMACEUTICAL FORM

Prolonged release capsules.

ADIZEM-XL capsules 120 mg have a pale pink body and a navy blue cap, marked DCR 120.

ADIZEM-XL capsules 180 mg have a dark pink body and a royal blue cap marked DCR 180.

ADIZEM-XL capsules 200 mg have a brown body and a brown cap marked DCR 200.

ADIZEM-XL capsules 240 mg have a dark red body and a blue cap marked DCR 240.

ADIZEM-XL capsules 300 mg have a dark maroon body and a pale blue cap marked DCR 300.

4. CLINICAL PARTICULARS

4.1 Therapeutic indications

Management of angina pectoris.

Treatment of mild to moderate hypertension.

4.2 Posology and method of administration

Route of administration

Oral

Posology

Dosage requirements may differ between patients with angina and patients with hypertension. In addition, individual patients' responses may vary necessitating careful titration. This range of capsule strengths facilitates titration to the optimal dose.

The capsules should be swallowed whole and not chewed.

Adults:

For patients new to diltiazem therapy the usual starting dose is one 240 mg capsule daily.

Patients currently receiving a total daily dose of 180 mg diltiazem (as 90 mg b.d. or 60 mg t.i.d.) and transferring to ADIZEM-XL capsules should be given the 240 mg capsule (o.d.). A patient receiving 240 mg/day of diltiazem (as 120 mg b.d.) should commence treatment on the 240 mg capsule (o.d.), titrating to the 300 mg capsule (o.d.) if required.

Elderly and patients with impaired hepatic and renal function:

For patients new to diltiazem therapy, the usual starting dose is one 120 mg capsule daily. If necessary the dose may be gradually increased but careful monitoring of this group of patients is advised.

Elderly patients transferring to ADIZEM-XL capsules should receive the same total daily dose of diltiazem, titrating upwards as required.

Children:

ADIZEM-XL capsules are not recommended for children. Safety and efficacy in children have not been established.

In order to avoid confusion, it is suggested that patients, once titrated to an effective dose using ADIZEM-XL capsules, should remain on this treatment and should not be changed between different presentations.

4.3 Contraindications

Pregnancy and in women of child bearing capacity. Patients with bradycardia (less than 50 bpm), second or third degree heart block, sick sinus syndrome, decompensated cardiac failure, patients with left ventricular dysfunction following myocardial infarction. Concurrent use with dantrolene infusion because of the risk of ventricular fibrillation.

4.4 Special warnings and special precautions for use

The product should be used with caution in patients with reduced left ventricular function. Patients with mild bradycardia, first degree AV block or prolonged PR interval should be observed closely. Diltiazem is considered unsafe in patients with acute porphyria.

4.5 Interaction with other medicinal products and other forms of Interaction

Due consideration should be given to the possibility of an additive effect when diltiazem is prescribed with drugs which may induce bradycardia or other anti-arrhythmic drugs.

Diltiazem hydrochloride has been used safely in combination with beta-blockers, diuretics, ACE-inhibitors and other anti-hypertensive agents. It is recommended that patients receiving these combinations should be regularly monitored. Concomitant use with alpha-blockers such as prazosin should be strictly monitored because of the possible synergistic hypotensive effect of this combination. Patients with pre-existing conduction defects should not receive the combination of diltiazem and beta-blockers.

Case reports have suggested that blood levels of carbamazepine, cyclosporin and theophylline may be increased when given concurrently with diltiazem hydrochloride. Care should be exercised in patients taking these drugs. In common with other calcium antagonists diltiazem hydrochloride may cause small increases in plasma levels of digoxin.

Concurrent use with H_2 -antagonists may increase serum levels of diltiazem.

Treatment with diltiazem has been continued without problem during anaesthesia, but the anaesthetist should be made aware of the treatment regimen.

4.6 Pregnancy and lactation

Diltiazem hydrochloride is contraindicated in pregnant women or women of child bearing potential, and is not recommended in nursing mothers.

4.7 Effects on ability to drive and use machines

None known.

4.8 Undesirable effects

Diltiazem is generally well tolerated. Occasional undesirable effects are nausea, headache, oedema of the legs, flushing, hypotension, fatigue, gastrointestinal disturbance and gingival hyperplasia which disappear on cessation of treatment. Serious skin reactions such as exfoliative dermatitis and allergic skin reactions, such as angioneurotic oedema, erythema multiforme and vasculitis have been reported. Diltiazem may cause depression of atrioventricular nodal conduction and bradycardia. Isolated cases of moderate and transient increased liver transaminases have been observed at the start of treatment. Isolated cases of clinical hepatitis have been reported, which resolved when diltiazem was withdrawn.

4.9 Overdose

The clinical symptoms of acute intoxication may include pronounced hypotension or even collapse and sinus bradycardia with or without atrioventricular conduction defects.

The patient should be closely monitored in hospital to exclude arrhythmias or atrioventricular conduction defects. Gastric lavage and osmotic diuresis should be undertaken when considered appropriate. Symptomatic bradycardia and high grade atrioventricular block may respond to atropine, isoprenaline or occasionally temporary cardiac pacing.

Hypotension may require correction with plasma volume expanders, intravenous calcium gluconate and positive inotropic agents. The formulation employs a prolonged release system which will continue to release diltiazem for some hours.

5. PHARMACOLOGICAL PROPERTIES

Pharmacotherapeutic group: Selective calcium channel blocker with direct cardiac effects

ATC Code: C08D B01

5.1 Pharmacodynamic properties

Diltiazem is a calcium antagonist. It restricts the slow channel entry of calcium ions into the cell and so reduces the liberation of calcium from stores in the sarcoplasmic reticulum. This results in a reduction in the amount of available intra-cellular calcium and consequently a (1) reduction of myocardial oxygen consumption, (2) dilation of small and large coronary arteries, (3) mild peripheral vasodilation, (4) negative dromotropic effects, (5) reflex positive chronotropic and inotropic effects due to reflex sympathetic activity are partially inhibited and result in a slight reduction or no change in heart rate.

The antihypertensive effect is due to the reduction in peripheral vascular resistance.

The antianginal effect is due to a reduction in the peripheral resistance, thereby decreasing the after-load, whilst a reduction in the vasomotor tone of the coronary circulation maintains the coronary blood flow. Cardiac contractility and ventricular ejection fraction are unchanged. Diltiazem increases exercise capacity and improves indices of myocardial ischaemia in the angina patient. Diltiazem relieves the spasm of vasospastic (Prinzmetal) angina.

5.2 Pharmacokinetic properties
An oral dose of diltiazem is almost completely absorbed. Despite this, diltiazem has a low bioavailability owing to extensive first pass metabolism. This process is saturable at higher doses of the drug resulting in a non-linear accumulation and higher blood concentrations at steady state than would be anticipated from those following a single dose.

ADIZEM-XL capsules reduce the degree of saturation by presenting diltiazem in a retarded fashion therefore eliminating the high peak concentrations of the absorption phase. This allows the capsule to be administered once daily.

In pharmacokinetic studies in healthy volunteers, diltiazem was well absorbed. The controlled release capsules provided prolonged absorption of the drug, producing peak steady state plasma concentrations between 4 and 14 hours post-dose. The availability of diltiazem from ADIZEM-XL capsules 120 mg (o.d.) relative to a prolonged release 60 mg diltiazem preparation (b.d.) was approximately 79% at steady state. Similarly, the availability of diltiazem from the 240 mg capsule (o.d.) relative to ADIZEM-SR tablets 120 mg (b.d.) was approximately 78%. The extent of absorption of diltiazem was not affected when ADIZEM-XL capsules were co-administered with a high-fat meal.

5.3 Preclinical safety data
There are no pre-clinical data of relevance to the prescriber which are additional to that already included in other sections of the SPC.

6. PHARMACEUTICAL PARTICULARS

6.1 List of excipients
Capsule Contents
Microcrystalline Cellulose
Ethylcellulose N10
Colloidal Anhydrous Silica
Polysorbate 80
Dibutyl Sebacate
Magnesium Stearate
Capsule shells
Iron oxide (E172)
Titanium dioxide (E171)
Sodium dodecylsulphate
Gelatin
Erythrosine (E127) (not present in the 200 mg capsule)
Indigo carmine (E132) (not present in the 200 mg capsule)
Patent blue V (E131) (300 mg capsule only)
Printing ink
Shellac
Soya lecithin
2-ethoxyethanol
Demeticone
Titanium dioxide (E171)

6.2 Incompatibilities
None known

6.3 Shelf life
2 years

6.4 Special precautions for storage
Do not store above 25°C

6.5 Nature and contents of container
PVC/PVdC blister packs with aluminium foil (containing 28 capsules).

6.6 Instructions for use and handling
None.

Administrative Data

7. MARKETING AUTHORISATION HOLDER
Napp Pharmaceuticals Ltd
Cambridge Science Park
Milton Road
Cambridge CB4 0GW

8. MARKETING AUTHORISATION NUMBER(S)
PL 16950/0010-0013, 0121

9. DATE OF FIRST AUTHORISATION/RENEWAL OF THE AUTHORISATION
ADIZEM-XL capsules 120 mg, 180 mg, 240 mg, 300 mg:
11 August 1993 / 23 September 2003
ADIZEM-XL capsules 200 mg:
10 September 2001/23 September 2003

10. DATE OF REVISION OF THE TEXT
April 2004

11. Legal Category
POM

ADIZEM-XL capsules are the subject of UK Patent GB 2 258 613.

® The Napp device and ADIZEM are Registered Trade Marks.

Adult Meltus Chesty Coughs with Congestion

(SSL International plc)

1. NAME OF THE MEDICINAL PRODUCT
Adult Meltus Chesty Coughs with Congestion.

2. QUALITATIVE AND QUANTITATIVE COMPOSITION
Guaifenesin BP 100mg/5ml; Pseudoephedrine Hydrochloride BP 30mg/5ml.

3. PHARMACEUTICAL FORM
Oral solution.

4. CLINICAL PARTICULARS

4.1 Therapeutic indications
Symptomatic relief of upper respiratory tract disorders accompanied by productive cough which benefit from a combination of a nasal decongestant and an expectorant.

4.2 Posology and method of administration
Oral. Adults and children aged 12 years and over: Two 5ml spoonfuls three times a day. Elderly: No specific studies have been carried out on the elderly, but similar products have been widely used in older people. However, it may be advisable to monitor renal and hepatic function and, if there is serious impairment, caution should be exercised.

4.3 Contraindications
The product is contraindicated in patients who have previously shown intolerance to pseudoephedrine or guaifenesin. It is also contraindicated in persons currently being treated with monoamine oxidase inhibitors, and also within two weeks of stopping treatment. It is also contraindicated in persons with severe hypertension or severe coronary artery disease.

4.4 Special warnings and special precautions for use
Although pseudoephedrine has virtually no presser effect in patients with normal blood pressure, Adult Meltus Chesty Coughs with Congestion should be used with caution in patients taking antihypertensive agents, tricyclic antidepressants, other sympathomimetic agents such as decongestants, appetite suppressants and amphetamine-like psychostimulants. The effects of a single dose of linctus on the blood pressure of these patients should be observed before recommending repeated or unsupervised treatment. As with other sympathomimetic agents, caution should be exercised in patients with uncontrolled diabetes, hyperthyroidism, elevated intraocular pressure and prostatic enlargement.

4.5 Interaction with other medicinal products and other forms of Interaction
The effect of antihypertensive agents which act by modifying sympathetic activity may be partially reversed by Adult Meltus Chesty Coughs with Congestion. Concomitant use of this product with other sympathomimetic agents such as decongestants, tricyclic antidepressants, appetite suppressants and amphetamine-like psychostimulants, or with monoamine oxidase inhibitors which interfere with the catabolism of sympathomimetic amines, may occasionally cause a rise in blood pressure. The antibacterial agent furazolidine is known to cause a dose related inhibition of monoamine oxidase, and although there are reports of hypertensive crises having occurred, it should not be administered concurrently with this product.

4.6 Pregnancy and lactation
Although pseudoephedrine and guaifenesin have been in widespread use for many years without apparent ill consequence, there are no specific data on their use during pregnancy. Caution should therefore be exercised by balancing the potential benefit of treatment against any possible hazards. Systemic administration of pseudoephedrine, up to 50 times the human dose in rats and up to 35 times the human dose in rabbits, did not produce teratogenic effects. It has been estimated that approximately 0.5% - 0.7% of a single dose of pseudoephedrine ingested by a mother will be excreted in the breast milk over 24 hours, but the effects of this on breast-fed infants is not known.

4.7 Effects on ability to drive and use machines
None stated.

4.8 Undesirable effects
Side effects are uncommon. In some patients pseudoephedrine may occasionally cause insomnia. Rarely, sleep disturbances and hallucinations have been reported. A fixed drug eruption to pseudoephedrine, taking the form of erythematous nummular patches, has been reported, but is a rare occurrence. Urinary retention has been reported in male patients in whom prostatic enlargement could have been an important predisposing factor.

4.9 Overdose
As with other sympathomimetic agents, symptoms of overdose include irritability, restlessness, tremor, convulsions, palpitations, hypertension, and difficulty in micturition. Gastric lavage and supportive measures for respiration and circulation should be performed if indicated. Convulsions should be controlled with an anticonvulsant. Catheterisation of the bladder may be necessary.

If desired, the elimination of pseudoephedrine can be accelerated by acid diuresis or by dialysis.

5. PHARMACOLOGICAL PROPERTIES

5.1 Pharmacodynamic properties
Pseudoephedrine has direct and indirect sympathomimetic activity and is an orally effective upper respiratory tract decongestant. Pseudoephedrine is substantially less potent than ephedrine in producing both tachycardia and elevation in systolic blood pressure, and considerably less potent in causing stimulation of the central nervous system. On the basis of widespread and long established clinical use, guaifenesin is recognised as an expectorant in bronchitis.

5.2 Pharmacokinetic properties
Pseudoephedrine is readily and completely absorbed from the gastrointestinal tract following oral administration, with no presystemic metabolism. It achieves peak plasma concentrations between 1 and 3 hours after oral dosing. It is eliminated largely unchanged in urine (55 -90%) in 24 hours, although there is some metabolism in the liver (<1%) by N-demethylation. It has a plasma half-life of 5-8 hours after oral dosing, but its urinary elimination and hence half-life, is pH dependant, such that elimination will be increased in subjects with acidic urine and decreased in subjects with alkaline urine. It is excreted in breast milk at concentrations consistently higher than those in maternal plasma, and is likely to cross the placenta. The elimination is reduced in renal impairment and with deteriorating renal function in the elderly. Guaifenesin is absorbed from the gastrointestinal tract. It is metabolised and excreted in the urine.

5.3 Preclinical safety data
None stated.

6. PHARMACEUTICAL PARTICULARS

6.1 List of excipients
Purified Honey BP; Sucrose (Granular) BP; Glycerin BP; Alcohol (96%) BP; Aniseed Oil BP; Menthol Crystals BP; Caramel (E150) USP; Glucose Liquid (HSE); Purified Water BP.

6.2 Incompatibilities
None stated.

6.3 Shelf life
24 months unopened.

6.4 Special precautions for storage
Store at or below 25°C.

6.5 Nature and contents of container
Amber glass sirop bottles filled with tamper evident cap with fitted polycone liner in printed cartons containing 100ml of product, including a 5ml CE marked polystyrene measuring spoon.

6.6 Instructions for use and handling
Not applicable.

7. MARKETING AUTHORISATION HOLDER
Cupal Limited
Tubiton House
Oldham
OL1 3HS

8. MARKETING AUTHORISATION NUMBER(S)
PL 0338/0088.

9. DATE OF FIRST AUTHORISATION/RENEWAL OF THE AUTHORISATION
23rd September 1996 / 1st November 2002.

10. DATE OF REVISION OF THE TEXT
May 2003.

Adult Meltus Dry Coughs with Congestion

(SSL International plc)

1. NAME OF THE MEDICINAL PRODUCT
Adult Meltus Dry Coughs with Congestion.

2. QUALITATIVE AND QUANTITATIVE COMPOSITION
Dextromethorphan Hydrobromide BP 10mg/5ml; Pseudoephedrine Hydrochloride BP 10mg/5ml.

3. PHARMACEUTICAL FORM
Oral liquid.

4. CLINICAL PARTICULARS
4.1 Therapeutic indications
Symptomatic relief of dry painful tickly coughs and catarrh.

4.2 Posology and method of administration
Oral. Adults, the elderly and children over 12 years of age: One or two 5ml spoonfuls to be taken four times a day. Not to be given to children under 12 years of age.

4.3 Contraindications
Patients with cardiovascular disease, hypertension, hyperthyroidism, hyperexcitability, phaechromocytoma, closed angle glaucoma. Use with caution in patients with liver disease and asthma. May increase the difficulty of micturition in patients with prostatic enlargements. Hypersensitivity to any of the ingredients or if also taking monoamine oxidase inhibitors.

4.4 Special warnings and special precautions for use
Do not exceed the stated dose. If symptoms persist of worsen, seek medical advice. Keep out of reach of children. If pregnant or taking regular medication, consult your doctor before taking this product.

4.5 Interaction with other medicinal products and other forms of Interaction
Monoamine oxidase inhibitors. The activity of the pseudoephedrine content is diminished by guanethidine, reserpine and methyldopa and may be diminished or enhanced by tricyclic antidepressants. The pseudoephedrine may diminish the effects of guanethidine and may increase the possibility of arrhythmias in digitalised patients. Use with caution in patients with diabetes.

4.6 Pregnancy and lactation
Not to be used by pregnant or lactating women.

4.7 Effects on ability to drive and use machines
None stated.

4.8 Undesirable effects
Large doses may cause giddiness, headache, nausea, vomiting, sweating, thirst, tachycardia, precordial pain, palpitations, difficulty in micturition, muscular weakness, tremors, anxiety, restlessness and insomnia.

4.9 Overdose
Management of overdose generally involves supportive and symptomatic therapy, and in cases of severe overdose, aspiration followed by gastric lavage may be used to empty the stomach. Treatment of dextromethorphan hydrobromide overdose is by the specific antidote, naloxone.

5. PHARMACOLOGICAL PROPERTIES
5.1 Pharmacodynamic properties
Adult Meltus Dry Coughs with Congestion contains dextromethorphan hydrobromide and pseudoephedrine hydrochloride to provide cough suppression and bronchodilation in cases of dry irritating coughs.

5.2 Pharmacokinetic properties
Pseudoephedrine is readily and completely absorbed from the gastrointestinal tract following oral administration with no presystemic metabolism, achieving peak plasma concentrations between one and three hours after oral dosing. It has a plasma half-life of 5 to 8 hours following oral dosing but its urinary elimination and hence half-life is pH dependent such that elimination will be increased in patients with acidic urine and decreased in subjects with alkaline urine. Dextromethorphan is well absorbed following oral administration but is subject to extensive presystemic metabolism in the liver. The main metabolite is dextrorphan. Dextromethorphan is extensively biotransformed in the liver with about 50% of the dose excreted in the urine over 24 hours. Less than 1% of a dose is excreted in the faeces. About 8% of the dose is excreted as the unchanged drug in the urine within 6 hours.

5.3 Preclinical safety data
There are no preclinical data of relevance to the prescriber which are additional to that already included in other sections of the SPC.

6. PHARMACEUTICAL PARTICULARS
6.1 List of excipients
Menthol BP; Alcohol (96%) BP; Glycerin BP; Sorbitol Solution BP; Chloroform BP; Sodium Cyclamate BP; Loganberry Flavour 500 195E; Sodium Saccharin BP; Sodium Carboxymethylcellulose BP; Methyl Hydroxybenzoate BP; Propyl Hydroxybenzoate BP; Water.

6.2 Incompatibilities
Monoamine oxidase inhibitors (MAOIs). Antihypertensive therapy. Chloroform, cyclopropane, halothane and other halogenated anaesthetics.

6.3 Shelf life
36 months unopened.

6.4 Special precautions for storage
Store below 25°C.

6.5 Nature and contents of container
100ml: Amber glass bottles with tamper evident cap with fitted polycone liner packed into a carton enclosing a 5ml CE marked polystyrene measuring spoon.

6.6 Instructions for use and handling
Not applicable.

7. MARKETING AUTHORISATION HOLDER
Cupal Limited
Tubiton House
Oldham
OL1 3HS

8. MARKETING AUTHORISATION NUMBER(S)
PL 0338/5029R.

9. DATE OF FIRST AUTHORISATION/RENEWAL OF THE AUTHORISATION
31st January 1990 / 18th May 2001.

10. DATE OF REVISION OF THE TEXT
May 2003.

Aerobec 100 Autohaler

(3M Health Care Limited)

1. NAME OF THE MEDICINAL PRODUCT
AeroBec 100 Autohaler.

2. QUALITATIVE AND QUANTITATIVE COMPOSITION
Each actuation delivers beclometasone dipropionate 100μg (as propellant solvate) into the mouthpiece of the adapter.

3. PHARMACEUTICAL FORM
Pressurised aerosol for inhalation therapy.

4. CLINICAL PARTICULARS
4.1 Therapeutic indications
AeroBec 100 Autohaler is indicated for the prophylactic treatment of chronic reversible obstructive airways disease.

4.2 Posology and method of administration
The dose should be titrated to the lowest dose at which effective control of asthma is maintained.

ADULTS: for maintenance: 1 inhalation (100 μg), three or four times daily or 2 inhalations (200 μg), twice daily. In more severe cases a dose of 600-800 μg (6-8 inhalations) daily is recommended, with subsequent reductions. The maximum recommended daily dose of this preparation is 1 mg. In patients receiving doses of 1500 μg or more daily, adrenal suppression may occur.

CHILDREN: 1 inhalation (100 μg), two to four times daily.

ELDERLY: No special dosage recommendations are made for elderly patients.

4.3 Contraindications
Hypersensitivity to beclometasone is a contra-indication. Caution should be observed in patients with pulmonary tuberculosis.

4.4 Special warnings and special precautions for use
Patients should be instructed on the proper use of the inhaler. They should be made aware of the prophylactic nature of AeroBec Autohaler therapy and that it should be used regularly at the intervals recommended and not when immediate relief is required.

In patients who have been transferred to inhalation therapy, systemic steroid therapy may need to be re-instated rapidly during periods of stress or where airways obstruction or mucus prevents absorption from the inhalation.

Systemic effects of inhaled corticosteroids may occur, particularly at high doses prescribed for prolonged periods. These effects are much less likely to occur than with oral corticosteroids. Possible systemic effects include adrenal suppression, growth retardation in children and adolescents, decrease in bone mineral density, cataract and glaucoma. It is important therefore that the dose of inhaled steroid is titrated to the lowest dose at which effective control of asthma is maintained.

It is recommended that the height of children receiving prolonged treatment with inhaled corticosteroids is regularly monitored. If growth is slowed, therapy should be reviewed with the aim of reducing the dose of inhaled corticosteroid, if possible, to the lowest dose at which effective control of asthma is maintained. In addition, consideration should be given to referring the patient to a paediatric respiratory specialist.

Prolonged treatment with high doses of inhaled corticosteroids, particularly higher than the recommended doses, may result in clinically significant adrenal suppression. Additional systemic corticosteroid cover should be considered during periods of stress or elective surgery.

Patients who have received systemic steroids for long periods of time or at high doses, or both, need special care and subsequent management when transferred to beclometasone therapy. Recovery from impaired adrenocortical function, caused by prolonged systemic steroid therapy, is slow. The patient should be in a reasonably stable state before being given AeroBec Autohaler in addition to his usual maintenance dose of systemic steroid. Withdrawal of the systemic steroid should be gradual, starting after about seven days by reducing the daily oral dose by 1 mg prednisolone, or equivalent, at intervals not less than one week. Adrenocortical function should be monitored regularly.

Most patients can be successfully transferred to AeroBec Autohaler with maintenance of good respiratory function, but special care is necessary for the first months after the transfer until the hypothalamic-pituitary-adrenal (HPA) system has sufficiently recovered to enable the patient to cope with emergencies such as trauma, surgery or infections.

Patients who have been transferred to inhalation therapy should carry a warning card indicating that systemic steroid therapy may need to be re-instated without delay during periods of stress. It may be advisable to provide such patients with a supply of oral steroid to use in emergency, for example when the asthma worsens as a result of a chest infection. The dose of AeroBec Autohaler should be increased at this time and then gradually reduced to the maintenance level after the systemic steroid has been discontinued.

Discontinuation of systemic steroids may cause exacerbation of allergic diseases such as atopic eczema and rhinitis. These should be treated as required with antihistamine and topical therapy.

4.5 Interaction with other medicinal products and other forms of Interaction
None known

4.6 Pregnancy and lactation
There is inadequate evidence of safety in human pregnancy. In animals, systemic administration of relatively high doses can cause abnormalities of foetal development including growth retardation and cleft palate. There may therefore be a very small risk of such effects in the human foetus. However, inhalation of beclometasone dipropionate into the lungs avoids the high level of exposure that occurs with administration by systemic routes.

The use of beclometasone in pregnancy requires that the possible benefits of the drug be weighed against the possible hazards. The drug has been in widespread use for many years without apparent ill consequence.

It is probable that beclometasone is excreted in milk. However, given the relatively low doses used by the inhalation route, the levels are likely to be low. In mothers breast feeding their baby the therapeutic benefits of the drug should be weighed against the potential hazards to mother and baby.

4.7 Effects on ability to drive and use machines
None

4.8 Undesirable effects
Candidiasis of the throat and mouth may develop in some patients, but this can be treated without discontinuation of beclometasone therapy. Hoarseness may also occur.

As with other inhaled therapy, paradoxical bronchospasm with wheezing may occur immediately after dosing. Immediate treatment with an inhaled short-acting bronchodilator is required. Aerobec Autohaler should be discontinued immediately and alternative prophylactic therapy introduced.

Systemic effects of inhaled corticosteroids may occur particularly at high doses prescribed for prolonged periods. These may include adrenal suppression, growth retardation in children and adolescents, decrease in bone mineral density, cataract and glaucoma.

Hypersensitivity reactions including rashes, urticaria, pruritus and erythema and oedema of the eye, face, lips and throat (angioedema) have been reported.

4.9 Overdose
Acute overdosage is unlikely to cause problems. The only harmful effect that follows inhalation of large amounts of the drug over a short time period is suppression of HPA function. Specific emergency action need not be taken. Treatment with AeroBec Autohaler should be continued at the recommended dose to control the asthma; HPA function recovers in a day or two.

If grossly excessive doses of beclometasone dipropionate were taken over a prolonged period a degree of atrophy of the adrenal cortex could occur in addition to HPA suppression. In this event the patient should be treated as steroid-dependent and transferred to a suitable maintenance dose of a systemic steroid such as prednisolone. Once the condition is stabilised the patient should be returned to AeroBec Autohaler by the method recommended above.

5. PHARMACOLOGICAL PROPERTIES
5.1 Pharmacodynamic properties
Inhaled beclometasone dipropionate is now well established in the management of asthma. It is a synthetic glucocorticoid and exerts a topical, anti-inflammatory effect on the lungs, without significant systemic activity.

5.2 Pharmacokinetic properties
The beclometasone dipropionate absorbed directly from the lungs is converted to less active metabolites during its passage through the liver. Peak plasma concentrations are reached 3-5 hours following ingestion. Excretion is via the urine.

5.3 Preclinical safety data
Not applicable.

6. PHARMACEUTICAL PARTICULARS

6.1 List of excipients
Sorbitan trioleate Ph Eur
Trichlorofluoromethane (Propellant 11) BP (1988)
Dichlorodifluoromethane (Propellant 12) BP (1988)
Dichlorotetrafluoroethane (Propellant 114) BP (1988)

6.2 Incompatibilities
None known

6.3 Shelf life
3 years

6.4 Special precautions for storage
Do not store above 30°C. Avoid storage in direct sunlight or heat. Protect from frost.

6.5 Nature and contents of container
10ml aluminium vial closed with a 50μl metering valve containing 200 doses.

6.6 Instructions for use and handling
Pressurised vial. Do not puncture. Do not burn, even when empty.

Administrative Data

7. MARKETING AUTHORISATION HOLDER
3M Health Care Limited
3M House
Morley Street
Loughborough
Leicestershire
LE11 1EP

8. MARKETING AUTHORISATION NUMBER(S)
0068/0145

9. DATE OF FIRST AUTHORISATION/RENEWAL OF THE AUTHORISATION
January 1992

10. DATE OF REVISION OF THE TEXT
November 2004.

Aerobec 50 Autohaler

(3M Health Care Limited)

1. NAME OF THE MEDICINAL PRODUCT
AeroBec 50 Autohaler.

2. QUALITATIVE AND QUANTITATIVE COMPOSITION
Each actuation delivers beclometasone dipropionate 50μg (as propellant solvate) into the mouthpiece of the adapter.

3. PHARMACEUTICAL FORM
Pressurised aerosol for inhalation therapy.

4. CLINICAL PARTICULARS

4.1 Therapeutic indications
AeroBec 50 Autohaler is indicated for the prophylactic treatment of chronic reversible obstructive airways disease.

4.2 Posology and method of administration
The dose should be titrated to the lowest dose at which effective control of asthma is maintained.

ADULTS: for maintenance: 4 inhalations (200 μg), twice daily or 2 inhalations (100 μg), three or four times daily. In more severe cases a dose of 600-800 μg (12 - 16 inhalations) daily is recommended, with subsequent reductions. The maximum recommended daily dose of this preparation is 1 mg. In patients receiving doses of 1500 μg or more daily, adrenal suppression may occur.

CHILDREN: 1 or 2 inhalations (50-100 μg), two to four times daily.

ELDERLY: No special dosage recommendations are made for elderly patients.

4.3 Contraindications
Hypersensitivity to beclometasone is a contra-indication. Caution should be observed in patients with pulmonary tuberculosis.

4.4 Special warnings and special precautions for use
Patients should be instructed on the proper use of the inhaler. They should be made aware of the prophylactic nature of Aerobec Autohaler therapy and that it should be used regularly at the intervals recommended and not when immediate relief is required.

In patients who have been transferred to inhalation therapy, systemic steroid therapy may need to be re-instated rapidly during periods of stress or where airways obstruction or mucus prevents absorption from the inhalation.

Systemic effects of inhaled corticosteroids may occur, particularly at high doses prescribed for prolonged periods. These effects are much less likely to occur than with oral corticosteroids. Possible systemic effects include adrenal suppression, growth retardation in children and adolescents, decrease in bone mineral density, cataract and glaucoma. It is important therefore that the dose of inhaled steroid is titrated to the lowest dose at which effective control of asthma is maintained.

It is recommended that the height of children receiving prolonged treatment with inhaled corticosteroids is regularly monitored. If growth is slowed, therapy should be reviewed with the aim of reducing the dose of inhaled corticosteroid, if possible, to the lowest dose at which effective control of asthma is maintained. In addition, consideration should be given to referring the patient to a paediatric respiratory specialist.

Prolonged treatment with high doses of inhaled corticosteroids, particularly higher than the recommended doses, may result in clinically significant adrenal suppression. Additional systemic corticosteroid cover should be considered during periods of stress or elective surgery.

Patients who have received systemic steroids for long periods of time or at high doses, or both, need special care and subsequent management when transferred to beclometasone therapy. Recovery from impaired adrenocortical function, caused by prolonged systemic steroid therapy, is slow. The patient should be in a reasonably stable state before being given AeroBec Autohaler in addition to his usual maintenance dose of systemic steroid. Withdrawal of the systemic steroid should be gradual, starting after about seven days by reducing the daily oral dose by 1 mg prednisolone, or equivalent, at intervals not less than one week. Adrenocortical function should be monitored regularly.

Most patients can be successfully transferred to AeroBec Autohaler with maintenance of good respiratory function, but special care is necessary for the first months after the transfer until the hypothalamic-pituitary-adrenal (HPA) system has sufficiently recovered to enable the patient to cope with emergencies such as trauma, surgery or infections.

Patients who have been transferred to inhalation therapy should carry a warning card indicating that systemic steroid therapy may need to be re-instated without delay during periods of stress. It may be advisable to provide such patients with a supply of oral steroid to use in emergency, for example when the asthma worsens as a result of a chest infection. The dose of AeroBec Autohaler should be increased at this time and then gradually reduced to the maintenance level after the systemic steroid has been discontinued.

Discontinuation of systemic steroids may cause exacerbation of allergic diseases such as atopic eczema and rhinitis. These should be treated as required with antihistamine and topical therapy.

4.5 Interaction with other medicinal products and other forms of Interaction
None known

4.6 Pregnancy and lactation
There is inadequate evidence of safety in human pregnancy. In animals, systemic administration of relatively high doses can cause abnormalities of foetal development including growth retardation and cleft palate. There may therefore be a very small risk of such effects in the human foetus. However, inhalation of beclometasone dipropionate into the lungs avoids the high level of exposure that occurs with administration by systemic routes.

The use of beclometasone in pregnancy requires that the possible benefits of the drug be weighed against the possible hazards. The drug has been in widespread use for many years without apparent ill consequence.

It is probable that beclometasone is excreted in milk. However, given the relatively low doses used by the inhalation route, the levels are likely to be low. In mothers breast feeding their baby the therapeutic benefits of the drug should be weighed against the potential hazards to mother and baby.

4.7 Effects on ability to drive and use machines
None

4.8 Undesirable effects
Candidiasis of the throat and mouth may develop in some patients, but this can be treated without discontinuation of beclometasone therapy. Hoarseness may also occur.

As with other inhaled therapy, paradoxical bronchospasm with wheezing may occur immediately after dosing. Immediate treatment with an inhaled short-acting bronchodilator is required. Aerobec Autohaler should be discontinued immediately and alternative prophylactic therapy introduced.

Systemic effects of inhaled corticosteroids may occur particularly at high doses prescribed for prolonged periods. These may include adrenal suppression, growth retardation in children and adolescents, decrease in bone mineral density, cataract and glaucoma.

Hypersensitivity reactions including rashes, urticaria, pruritus and erythema and oedema of the eye, face, lips and throat (angioedema) have been reported.

4.9 Overdose
Acute overdosage is unlikely to cause problems. The only harmful effect that follows inhalation of large amounts of the drug over a short time period is suppression of HPA function. Specific emergency action need not be taken. Treatment with AeroBec Autohaler should be continued at the recommended dose to control the asthma; HPA function recovers in a day or two.

If grossly excessive doses of beclometasone dipropionate were taken over a prolonged period a degree of atrophy of the adrenal cortex could occur in addition to HPA suppression. In this event the patient should be treated as steroid-dependent and transferred to a suitable maintenance dose of a systemic steroid such as prednisolone. Once the condition is stabilised the patient should be returned to AeroBec Autohaler by the method recommended above.

5. PHARMACOLOGICAL PROPERTIES

5.1 Pharmacodynamic properties
Inhaled beclometasone dipropionate is now well established in the management of asthma. It is a synthetic glucocorticoid and exerts a topical, anti-inflammatory effect on the lungs, without significant systemic activity.

5.2 Pharmacokinetic properties
The beclometasone dipropionate absorbed directly from the lungs is converted to less active metabolites during its passage through the liver. Peak plasma concentrations are reached 3-5 hours following ingestion. Excretion is via the urine.

5.3 Preclinical safety data
Not applicable.

6. PHARMACEUTICAL PARTICULARS

6.1 List of excipients
Sorbitan trioleate Ph Eur
Trichlorofluoromethane (Propellant 11) BP (1988)
Dichlorodifluoromethane (Propellant 12) BP (1988)
Dichlorotetrafluoroethane (Propellant 114) BP (1988)

6.2 Incompatibilities
None known

6.3 Shelf life
3 years

6.4 Special precautions for storage
Do not store above 30°C. Avoid storage in direct sunlight or heat. Protect from frost.

6.5 Nature and contents of container
10ml Aluminium vial closed with a 50μL metering valve containing 200 doses.

6.6 Instructions for use and handling
Pressurised vial. Do not puncture. Do not burn, even when empty.

Administrative Data

7. MARKETING AUTHORISATION HOLDER
3M Health Care Limited
3M House
Morley Street
Loughborough
Leicestershire
LE11 1EP

8. MARKETING AUTHORISATION NUMBER(S)
0068/0143

9. DATE OF FIRST AUTHORISATION/RENEWAL OF THE AUTHORISATION
October 1991

10. DATE OF REVISION OF THE TEXT
November 2004.

Aerobec Forte Autohaler

(3M Health Care Limited)

1. NAME OF THE MEDICINAL PRODUCT
AeroBec Forte Autohaler.

2. QUALITATIVE AND QUANTITATIVE COMPOSITION
Each actuation delivers beclometasone dipropionate 250μg (as propellant solvate) into the mouthpiece of the adapter.

3. PHARMACEUTICAL FORM
Pressurised aerosol for inhalation therapy.

4. CLINICAL PARTICULARS

4.1 Therapeutic indications
AeroBec Forte Autohaler is indicated for the prophylactic treatment of chronic reversible obstructive airways disease in those patients who require high doses of beclometasone to control their symptoms.

4.2 Posology and method of administration
The dose should be titrated to the lowest dose at which effective control of asthma is maintained.

ADULTS: for maintenance: 2 inhalations (500 μg), twice daily or 1 inhalations (250 μg), four times daily, may be increased to 2 inhalations four times daily if necessary.

In patients receiving doses of 1500 μg or more daily, adrenal suppression may occur. The degree of suppression may not always be clinically significant but it is advisable to provide such patients with a supply of oral steroid to use in stressful situations. The risk of adrenal suppression occurring should be balanced against the therapeutic advantages.

CHILDREN: AeroBec Forte Autohaler is not recommended for use in children.

ELDERLY: No special dosage recommendations are made for elderly patients.

4.3 Contraindications

Hypersensitivity to beclometasone is a contra-indication. Caution should be observed in patients with pulmonary tuberculosis.

4.4 Special warnings and special precautions for use

Patients should be instructed on the proper use of the inhaler. They should be made aware of the prophylactic nature of Aerobec Autohaler therapy and that it should be used regularly at the intervals recommended and not when immediate relief is required.

In patients who have been transferred to inhalation therapy, systemic steroid therapy may need to be re-instated rapidly during periods of stress or where airways obstruction or mucus prevents absorption from the inhalation.

Systemic effects of inhaled corticosteroids may occur, particularly at high doses prescribed for prolonged periods. These effects are much less likely to occur than with oral corticosteroids. Possible systemic effects include adrenal suppression, growth retardation in adolescents, decrease in bone mineral density, cataract and glaucoma. It is important therefore that the dose of inhaled steroid is titrated to the lowest dose at which effective control of asthma is maintained.

It is recommended that the height of adolescents receiving prolonged treatment with inhaled corticosteroids is regularly monitored. If growth is slowed, therapy should be reviewed with the aim of reducing the dose of inhaled corticosteroid, if possible, to the lowest dose at which effective control of asthma is maintained.

Prolonged treatment with high doses of inhaled corticosteroids, particularly higher than the recommended doses, may result in clinically significant adrenal suppression. Additional systemic corticosteroid cover should be considered during periods of stress or elective surgery.

Patients who have received systemic steroids for long periods of time or at high doses, or both, need special care and subsequent management when transferred to beclometasone therapy. Recovery from impaired adrenocortical function, caused by prolonged systemic steroid therapy, is slow. The patient should be in a reasonably stable state before being given AeroBec Autohaler in addition to his usual maintenance dose of systemic steroid. Withdrawal of the systemic steroid should be gradual, starting after about seven days by reducing the daily oral dose by 1 mg prednisolone, or equivalent, at intervals not less than one week. Adrenocortical function should be monitored regularly.

Most patients can be successfully transferred to AeroBec Autohaler with maintenance of good respiratory function, but special care is necessary for the first months after the transfer until the hypothalamic-pituitary-adrenal (HPA) system has sufficiently recovered to enable the patient to cope with emergencies such as trauma, surgery or infections.

Patients who have been transferred to inhalation therapy should carry a warning card indicating that systemic steroid therapy may need to be re-instated without delay during periods of stress. It may be advisable to provide such patients with a supply of oral steroid to use in emergency, for example when the asthma worsens as a result of a chest infection. The dose of AeroBec Autohaler should be increased at this time and then gradually reduced to the maintenance level after the systemic steroid has been discontinued.

Discontinuation of systemic steroids may cause exacerbation of allergic diseases such as atopic eczema and rhinitis. These should be treated as required with antihistamine and topical therapy.

4.5 Interaction with other medicinal products and other forms of Interaction

None known

4.6 Pregnancy and lactation

There is inadequate evidence of safety in human pregnancy. In animals, systemic administration of relatively high doses can cause abnormalities of foetal development including growth retardation and cleft palate. There may therefore be a very small risk of such effects in the human foetus. However, inhalation of beclometasone dipropionate into the lungs avoids the high level of exposure that occurs with administration by systemic routes.

The use of beclometasone in pregnancy requires that the possible benefits of the drug be weighed against the possible hazards. The drug has been in widespread use for many years without apparent ill consequence.

It is probable that beclometasone is excreted in milk. However, given the relatively low doses used by the inhalation route, the levels are likely to be low. In mothers breast feeding their baby the therapeutic benefits of the drug should be weighed against the potential hazards to mother and baby.

4.7 Effects on ability to drive and use machines

None

4.8 Undesirable effects

Candidiasis of the throat and mouth may develop in some patients, but this can be treated without discontinuation of beclometasone therapy. Hoarseness may also occur.

As with other inhaled therapy, paradoxical bronchospasm with wheezing may occur immediately after dosing. Immediate treatment with an inhaled short-acting bronchodilator is required. Aerobec Forte Autohaler should be discontinued immediately and alternative prophylactic therapy introduced.

Systemic effects of inhaled corticosteroids may occur particularly at high doses prescribed for prolonged periods. These may include adrenal suppression, growth retardation in adolescents, decrease in bone mineral density, cataract and glaucoma.

Hypersensitivity reactions including rashes, urticaria, pruritus and erythema and oedema of the eye, face, lips and throat (angioedema) have been reported.

4.9 Overdose

If grossly excessive doses of beclometasone dipropionate were taken over a prolonged period a degree of atrophy of the adrenal cortex could occur in addition to HPA suppression. In this event the patient should be treated as steroid-dependent and transferred to a suitable maintenance dose of a systemic steroid such as prednisolone. Once the condition is stabilised the patient should be returned to AeroBec Forte Autohaler by the method recommended above. To guard against unexpected occurrence of adrenal suppression regular tests of adrenal function are advised.

5. PHARMACOLOGICAL PROPERTIES

5.1 Pharmacodynamic properties

Inhaled beclometasone dipropionate is now well established in the management of asthma. It is a synthetic glucocorticoid and exerts a topical, anti-inflammatory effect on the lungs, without significant systemic activity.

5.2 Pharmacokinetic properties

The beclometasone dipropionate absorbed directly from the lungs is converted to less active metabolites during its passage through the liver. Peak plasma concentrations are reached 3-5 hours following ingestion. Excretion is via the urine.

5.3 Preclinical safety data

Not applicable.

6. PHARMACEUTICAL PARTICULARS

6.1 List of excipients

Sorbitan trioleate Ph Eur

Trichlorofluoromethane (Propellant 11) BP (1988)

Dichlorodifluoromethane (Propellant 12) BP (1988)

Dichlorotetrafluoroethane (Propellant 114) BP (1988)

6.2 Incompatibilities

None known

6.3 Shelf life

3 years

6.4 Special precautions for storage

Do not store above 30°C. Avoid storage in direct sunlight or heat. Protect from frost.

6.5 Nature and contents of container

10ml Aluminium vial closed with a 50μl metering valve containing 200 doses.

6.6 Instructions for use and handling

Pressurised vial. Do not puncture. Do not burn, even when empty.

Administrative Data

7. MARKETING AUTHORISATION HOLDER

3M Health Care Limited

3M House

Morley Street

Loughborough

Leicestershire

LE11 1EP

8. MARKETING AUTHORISATION NUMBER(S)

0068/0140

9. DATE OF FIRST AUTHORISATION/RENEWAL OF THE AUTHORISATION

October 1991

10. DATE OF REVISION OF THE TEXT

November 2004.

Aerodiol

(Servier Laboratories Limited)

1. NAME OF THE MEDICINAL PRODUCT

AERODIOL

2. QUALITATIVE AND QUANTITATIVE COMPOSITION

Each spray delivers 0.07 ml of solution which contains estradiol equivalent to 150 micrograms of estradiol hemihydrate.

For excipients, see 6.1

3. PHARMACEUTICAL FORM

Nasal spray, solution.

4. CLINICAL PARTICULARS

4.1 Therapeutic indications

Hormone replacement therapy (HRT) for oestrogen deficiency symptoms in post menopausal women.

The experience of treating women older than 65 years is limited.

4.2 Posology and method of administration

NASAL ROUTE.

The recommended dose for initiation of treatment is 150 μg (1 spray) in a nostril.

After 2 or 3 cycles the dosage may be adjusted in response to clinical symptoms:

The usual maintenance dose is 300 μg (2 sprays) per 24 hours, i.e. 1 spray in each nostril once daily.

• If symptoms of oestrogen deficiency persist, the number of sprays may be increased up to 3 or 4 per day (450 μg or 600 μg), in divided doses, morning and evening.

• In the event of signs of hyperoestrogenism such as breast tenderness, abdominal bloating, anxiety, nervousness or aggressiveness, the dosage should be reduced to 1 spray (150μg)daily.

For initiation and continuation of treatment of postmenopausal symptoms, the lowest effective dose for the shortest duration (see also section 4.4 "Special warnings and special precautions for use") should be used.

AERODIOL may be administered as cyclical or continuous treatment:

Cyclical treatment: AERODIOL is used cyclically for a duration of 21 to 28 days, followed by a 2- to 7-day treatment-free period.

Continuous treatment: AERODIOL is administered daily without a break in treatment. Continuous (non-cyclical) treatment may be indicated in hysterectomised women and in cases where oestrogen deficiency symptoms occur during the treatment-free period.

For non-hysterectomised women, AERODIOL is recommended to be combined with progestogen treatment for at least 12 days per cycle to avoid oestrogen-induced endometrial hyperplasia. (see section 4.4 "Special warnings and special precautions for use").

Sequential progestogen treatment should be administered as follows:

• if AERODIOL is administered cyclically, a progestogen will be added to estradiol for at least the last 12 days of treatment.

Thus, no hormones will be administered during the treatment-free period of the cycle.

• if AERODIOL is administered continuously, it is recommended to take a progestogen for at least 12 days each month.

In either case, withdrawal bleeding will usually occur when the progestogen is discontinued.

Unless there is a previous diagnosis of endometriosis, it is not recommended to add a progestogen in hysterectomised women.

Patients changing from another cyclic or continuous sequential preparation should complete the cycle and may then change to AERODIOL without a break in therapy. Patients changing from a continuous combined preparation may start therapy at any time.

Priming: before it is first used, the bottle must be primed by firmly activating the pump 3 times.

The bottle should be held vertically during administration. The head is bent slightly forward and the nozzle introduced into each nostril in turn. Pressure is then exerted on the pump. The patient must not breathe in during spraying nor blow the nose immediately afterwards.

In the event of a severely blocked nose, AERODIOL may be administered temporarily via the oromucosal route by administration via the upper gingival sulcus. In such circumstances, the usual dosage should be doubled.

Patients with a runny nose should blow their nose before administration of AERODIOL.

Dosing should preferably take place at the same time every day.

If a dose is forgotten, it can be given at any time up to the next scheduled dose but it should not be doubled. Forgetting a dose may increase the likelihood of breakthrough bleeding and spotting.

The risk/benefit ratio should be re-evaluated regularly to adjust the treatment if needed:

• for the duration of treatment with AERODIOL

• when changing from another hormonal treatment to AERODIOL.

4.3 Contraindications

• Known, past or suspected breast cancer;

- Known or suspected oestrogen-dependent malignant tumours (*e.g.* endometrial cancer);
- Undiagnosed genital bleeding;
- Untreated endometrial hyperplasia;
- Previous idiopathic or current venous thromboembolism (deep venous thrombosis, pulmonary embolism);
- Active or recent arterial thromboembolic disease (*e.g.* angina, myocardial infarction);
- Acute liver disease, or a history of liver disease as long as liver function tests have failed to return to normal;
- Known hypersensitivity to estradiol hemihydrate or to any of the excipients;
- Porphyria.

4.4 Special warnings and special precautions for use

For the treatment of postmenopausal symptoms, HRT should only be initiated for symptoms that adversely affect quality of life. In all cases, a careful appraisal of the risks and benefits should be undertaken at least annually and HRT should only be continued as long as the benefit outweighs the risk.

Medical examination/follow up

Before initiating or reinstituting HRT, a complete personal and family medical history should be taken. Physical (including pelvic and breast) examination should be guided by this and by the contraindications and warnings for use. During treatment, periodic check-ups are recommended of a frequency and nature adapted to the individual woman. Women should be advised what changes in their breasts should be reported to their doctor or nurse. Investigations, including mammography, should be carried out in accordance with currently accepted screening practices, modified to the clinical needs of the individual.

Conditions which need supervision

If any of the following conditions are present, have occurred previously, and/or have been aggravated during pregnancy or previous hormone treatment, the patient should be closely supervised. It should be taken into account that these conditions may recur or be aggravated during treatment with AERODIOL, in particular:

- Leiomyoma (uterine fibroids) or endometriosis
- A history of, or risk factors for, thromboembolic disorders (see below)
- Risk factors for oestrogen-dependent tumours, e.g. first degree heredity for breast cancer
- Hypertension
- Liver disorders (e.g. liver adenoma)
- Diabetes mellitus with or without vascular involvement
- Cholelithiasis
- Migraine or (severe) headache
- Systemic lupus erythematosus
- A history of endometrial hyperplasia (see below)
- Epilepsy
- Asthma
- Otosclerosis
- Recurrent epistaxis

Reasons for immediate withdrawal of therapy:

Therapy should be discontinued if a contraindication is discovered and in the following situations:

- Jaundice or deterioration in liver function
- Significant increase in blood pressure
- New onset of migraine-type headache
- Pregnancy.

Endometrial hyperplasia

The risk of endometrial hyperplasia and carcinoma is increased when oestrogens are administered alone for prolonged periods (see section 4.8). The addition of a progestogen for at least 12 days per cycle in non-hysterectomised women greatly reduces this risk.

For doses of 450 μg/d and 600 μg/d, the endometrial safety of added gestagens has not been studied.

Break-through bleeding and spotting may occur during the first months of treatment. If break-through bleeding or spotting appears after some time on therapy, or continues after treatment has been discontinued, the reason should be investigated. Such investigations may include endometrial biopsy to exclude endometrial malignancy.

Unopposed oestrogen stimulation may lead to premalignant or malignant transformation in the residual foci of endometriosis. Therefore, the addition of progestogens to oestrogen replacement therapy should be considered in women who have undergone hysterectomy because of endometriosis, especially if they are known to have residual endometriosis.

Breast Cancer

A randomised placebo-controlled trial, the Women's Health Initiative study (WHI), and epidemiological studies, including the Million Women Study (MWS), have reported an increased risk of breast cancer in women taking oestrogens or oestrogen-progestogen combinations or tibolone for HRT for several years (see section 4.8 "Undesirable effects").

For all HRT, an excess risk becomes apparent within a few years of use and increases with duration of intake but returns to baseline within a few (at most five) years after stopping treatment.

In the MWS, the relative risk of breast cancer with conjugated equine oestrogens (CEE) or estradiol (E2) was greater when a progestogen was added, either sequentially or continuously, and regardless of type of progestogen. There was no evidence of a difference in risk between the different routes of administration.

In the WHI study, the continuous combined conjugated equine oestrogen and medroxyprogesterone acetate (CEE + MPA) product used was associated with breast cancers that were slightly larger in size and more frequently had local lymph node metastases compared to placebo.

HRT, especially oestrogen-progestogen combined treatment, increases the density of mammographic images which may adversely affect the radiological detection of breast cancer.

Venous Thromboembolism

HRT is associated with a higher relative risk of developing venous thromboembolism (VTE) *i.e.* deep vein thrombosis or pulmonary embolism. One randomised controlled trial and epidemiological studies found a two to threefold higher risk for users compared with non-users. For non-users it is estimated that the number of cases of VTE that will occur over a 5-year period is about 3 per 1,000 women aged 50-59 years and 8 per 1,000 women aged between 60-69 years. It is estimated that in healthy women who use HRT for 5 years, the number of additional cases of VTE over a 5-year period will be between 2 and 6 (best estimate =4) per 1000 women aged 50-59 years and between 5 and 15 (best estimate = 9) per 1000 women aged 60-69 years. The occurrence of such an event is more likely in the first year of HRT than later.

Generally recognised risk factors for VTE include a personal history or family history, severe obesity (Body Mass Index > 30kg/m^2) and systemic lupus erythematosus (SLE). There is no consensus about the role of varicose veins in VTE.

Patients with a history of VTE or known thrombophilic states have an increased risk of VTE. HRT may add to this risk. Personal or strong family history of thromboembolism or recurrent spontaneous abortion should be investigated in order to exclude a thrombophilic predisposition. Until a thorough evaluation of thrombophilic factors has been made or anticoagulant treatment initiated, use of HRT in such patients should be viewed as contraindicated. Those women already on anticoagulant treatment require careful consideration of the benefit-risk of HRT.

The risk of VTE may be temporarily increased with prolonged immobilisation, major trauma or major surgery. As in all post-operative patients, scrupulous attention should be given to prophylactic measures to prevent VTE following surgery. Where prolonged immobilisation is liable to follow elective surgery, particularly abdominal or orthopaedic surgery to the lower limbs, consideration should be given to temporarily stopping HRT four to six weeks earlier, if possible. Treatment should not be restarted until the woman is completely mobilised.

If VTE develops after initiating therapy, the drug should be discontinued. Patients should be told to contact their doctors immediately if they are aware of a potential thromboembolic symptom (*e.g.* painful swelling of a leg, sudden pain in the chest, dyspnoea).

Coronary Artery Disease (CAD)

There is no evidence from randomised controlled trials of cardiovascular benefit with continuous combined conjugated oestrogens and medroxyprogesterone acetate (MPA). Two large clinical trials (WHI and HERS i.e. Heart and Estrogen/progestin Replacement Study) showed a possible increased risk of cardiovascular morbidity in the first year of use and no overall benefit. For other HRT products there are only limited data from randomised controlled trials examining effects in cardiovascular morbidity or mortality. Therefore, it is uncertain whether these findings also extend to other HRT products.

Stroke

One large randomised clinical trial (WHI-trial) found, as a secondary outcome, an increased risk of ischaemic stroke in healthy women during treatment with continuous combined conjugated oestrogens and MPA. For women who do not use HRT, it is estimated that the number of cases of stroke that will occur over a 5 year period is about 3 per 1000 women aged 50-59 years and 11 per 1000 women aged 60-69 years. It is estimated that for women who use conjugated oestrogens and MPA for 5 years, the number of additional cases will be between 0 and 3 (best estimate =1) per 1000 users aged 50-59 years and between 1 and 9 (best estimate =4) per 1000 users aged 60-69 years. It is unknown whether the increased risk also extends to other HRT products.

Ovarian Cancer

Long-term (at least 5-10 years) use of oestrogen-only HRT products in hysterectomised women has been associated with an increased risk of ovarian cancer in some epidemiological studies. It is uncertain whether long-term use of combined HRT confers a different risk than oestrogen-only products.

Other Conditions

Oestrogens may cause fluid retention, and therefore patients with cardiac or renal dysfunction should be carefully observed. Patients with terminal renal insufficiency should be closely observed, since it is expected that the levels of circulating oestrogens from AERODIOL is increased.

Women with pre-existing hypertriglyceridemia should be followed closely during oestrogen replacement or hormone replacement therapy, since rare cases of large increases of plasma triglycerides leading to pancreatitis have been reported with oestrogen therapy in this condition.

Estrogens increase thyroid binding globulin (TBG), leading to increased circulating total thyroid hormone, as measured by protein-bound iodine (PBI), T4 levels (by column or by radio-immunoassay) or T3 levels (by radio-immunoassay). T3 resin uptake is decreased, reflecting the elevated TBG. Free T4 and free T3 concentrations are unaltered. Other binding proteins may be elevated in serum, i.e. corticoid binding globulin (CBG), sex-hormone-binding globulin (SHBG) leading to increased circulating corticosteroids and sex steroids, respectively. Free or biological active hormone concentrations are unchanged. Other plasma proteins may be increased (angiotensinogen/ renin substrate, alpha-I-antitrypsin, ceruloplasmin).

There is no conclusive evidence for improvement of cognitive function. There is some evidence from the WHI trial of increased risk of probable dementia in women who start using continuous combined CEE and MPA after the age of 65. It is unknown whether the findings apply to younger post-menopausal women or other HRT products.

4.5 Interaction with other medicinal products and other forms of Interaction

Combinations requiring precautions for use:

Enzyme Inducers:

The metabolism of oestrogens may be increased by concomitant use of substances known to induce drug-metabolising enzymes, specifically cytochrome P450 enzymes, such as anticonvulsants (*e.g.* phenobarbital, phenytoin, carbamazepine), and anti-infectives (*e.g.* rifampicin, rifabutin, nevirapine, efavirenz).

After nasal administration, the first-pass effect in the liver is avoided and, therefore, nasally administered oestrogens such as AERODIOL might be less affected by enzyme inducers than orally administered hormones.

Antiretroviral agents:

Ritonavir and nelfinavir, although known as strong enzyme inhibitors, by contrast exhibit enzyme inducing properties when used concomitantly with steroid hormones.

Herbal preparations containing St John's Wort (Hypericum perforatum) may induce the metabolism of oestrogens.

Clinically, an increased metabolism of oestrogens and progestogens may lead to a decreased effect and changes in the uterine bleeding profile.

Nasal corticosteroids and nasally administered vasoconstricting agents:

The effect of concomitant administration of nasal corticosteroids or nasal vasoconstricting agents has not been studied.

AERODIOL should not be administered immediately after nasal corticosteroids or nasal vasoconstricting agents.

4.6 Pregnancy and lactation

Pregnancy:

AERODIOL is not indicated during pregnancy. If pregnancy occurs during medication with AERODIOL treatment should be withdrawn immediately.

The results to date of most epidemiological studies relevant to inadvertent foetal exposure to oestrogens indicate no teratogenic or foetotoxic effects.

Lactation:

AERODIOL is not indicated during lactation.

4.7 Effects on ability to drive and use machines

No effects on ability to drive or use machines have been observed.

4.8 Undesirable effects

The most frequently reported undesirable effects >10%) during treatment with AERODIOL are symptoms at the application site: prickling-tingling sensation, sneezing and rhinorrhoea.

Other undesirable effects reported in users of AERODIOL or other non-oral estradiol preparations are listed in the table

(see Table 1 on next page)

Breast cancer

According to evidence from a large number of epidemiological studies and one randomised placebo-controlled trial, the Women's Health Initiative (WHI), the overall risk of breast cancer increases with increasing duration of HRT use in current or recent HRT users.

For oestrogen-only HRT, estimates of relative risk (RR) from a reanalysis of original data from 51 epidemiological studies (in which >80% of HRT use was oestrogen-only HRT) and from the epidemiological Million Women Study

Table 1

Organ system	Common ADRs >1/100, <1/10	Uncommon ADRs >1/1000, <1/100	Rare ADRs >1/10.000, <1/1000
Body as a whole	Headache	Fluid retention/oedema, weight increase/loss, dizziness, fatigue, leg cramps, migraine	
Gastrointestinal	Nausea	Bloating, abdominal cramps	Cholelithiasis, cholestatic jaundice
Reproductive	Breakthrough bleeding, spotting, mastodynia	Dysmenorrhoea, endometrial hyperplasia, benign breast tumours	Increase in size of uterine fibroids
Respiratory tract	Epistaxis		
Skin and appendages		Acne, pruritus	Urticaria
Cardiovascular		Hypertension	
Psychiatric	Increase/decrease in libido		Depression

(MWS) are similar at 1.35 (95%CI 1.21 – 1.49) and 1.30 (95%CI 1.21 – 1.40), respectively.

For oestrogen plus progestogen combined HRT, several epidemiological studies have reported an overall higher risk for breast cancer than with oestrogens alone.

The MWS reported that, compared to never users, the use of various types of oestrogen-progestogen combined HRT was associated with a higher risk of breast cancer (RR = 2.00, 95%CI: 1.88 – 2.12) than use of oestrogens alone (RR = 1.30, 95%CI: 1.21 – 1.40) or use of tibolone (RR=1.45; 95%CI 1.25-1.68).

The WHI trial reported a risk estimate of 1.24 (95%CI 1.01 – 1.54) after 5.6 years of use of oestrogen-progestogen combined HRT (CEE + MPA) in all users compared with placebo.

The absolute risks calculated from the MWS and the WHI trial are presented below:

The MWS has estimated, from the known average incidence of breast cancer in developed countries, that:

- For women not using HRT, about 32 in every 1000 are expected to have breast cancer diagnosed between the ages of 50 and 64 years.
- For 1000 current or recent users of HRT, the number of *additional* cases during the corresponding period will be:

For users of *oestrogen-only* replacement therapy

- between 0 and 3 (best estimate = 1.5) for 5 years' use
- between 3 and 7 (best estimate = 5) for 10 years' use.

For users of *oestrogen plus progestogen* combined HRT

- between 5 and 7 (best estimate = 6) for 5 years' use
- between 18 and 20 (best estimate = 19) for 10 years' use.

The WHI trial estimated that after 5.6 years of follow-up of women between the ages of 50 and 79 years, an additional 8 cases of invasive breast cancer would be due to oestrogen-progestogen combined HRT (CEE + MPA) per 10,000 women years.

According to calculations from the trial data, it is estimated that:

For 1000 women in the placebo group

- about 16 cases of invasive breast cancer would be diagnosed in 5 years.

For 1000 women who used oestrogen + progestogen combined HRT (CEE + MPA)

- the number of additional cases would be between 0 and 9 (best estimate = 4) for 5 years' use.

The number of additional cases of breast cancer in women who use HRT is broadly similar for women who start HRT irrespective of age at start of use (between the ages of 45-65) (see section 4.4 "Special warnings and special precautions for use").

Endometrial Cancer

In women with an intact uterus, the risk of endometrial hyperplasia and endometrial cancer increases with increasing duration of use of unopposed oestrogens. According to data from epidemiological studies, the best estimate of the risk is that for women not using HRT, about 5 in every 1000 are expected to have endometrial cancer diagnosed between the ages of 50 and 65. Depending on the duration of treatment and oestrogen dose, the reported increase in endometrial cancer risk among unopposed oestrogen users varies from 2-to 12-fold greater compared with non-users. Adding a progestogen to oestrogen-only therapy greatly reduces this increased risk.

Other adverse reactions have been reported in association with oestrogen treatment:

- Oestrogen-dependent neoplasms benign and malignant, *e.g.* endometrial cancer;
- Venous thromboembolism, *i.e.* deep leg or pelvic venous thrombosis and pulmonary embolism, is more frequent among HRT users than among non-users. For further information, see sections 4.3 "Contraindications" and 4.4 "Special warnings and special precautions for use";
- Myocardial infarction and stroke;
- Gall bladder disease;
- Skin and subcutaneous disorders: chloasma, erythema multiforme, erythema nodosum, vascular purpura;
- Probable dementia (see section 4.4 "Special warnings and special precautions for use").

4.9 Overdose

The route of administration makes significant acute overdose unlikely. The effects of overdose are generally breast tenderness, abdominal/pelvic bloating, nausea and aggressiveness.

5. PHARMACOLOGICAL PROPERTIES

5.1 Pharmacodynamic properties

ATC Classification: G03CA03

OESTROGENS (Genitourinary system and sex hormones)

The active ingredient, synthetic 17β-estradiol, is chemically and biologically identical to endogenous human estradiol. It substitutes for the loss of oestrogen production in menopausal women, and alleviates menopausal symptoms. AERODIOL constitutes pulsed oestrogen therapy that provides a hormone exposure similar to that found during the early to mid follicular phases of the menstrual cycle.

During treatment, due to the mechanism of action, the minimum FSH values are observed 6 to 8 hours post-dosing and a decrease is still present immediately before the next dose.

Relief of menopausal symptoms was achieved during the first few weeks of treatment with AERODIOL.

5.2 Pharmacokinetic properties

When administered at a dose of 300 μg AERODIOL achieves peak serum estradiol levels around 1000 pg/mL, 10 to 30 minutes post-dosing. 17β-estradiol (E_2) is rapidly distributed. Return to values close to baseline occurs within 12 hours of dosing.

The absolute bioavailability of estradiol when administered by the nasal route is around 25% and is higher than that following oral administration because AERODIOL avoids intestinal and liver first pass effects in contrast to orally administered oestrogens.

Hormone exposure, as expressed by the area under the curve of plasma estradiol concentration against time (AUC_{24h}) is proportional to the dose. Following nasal administration of 300 μg, the AUC_{24h} is similar to that obtained using other administration routes (patch delivering 50 μg/d, 2-mg tablet) but with a different kinetic profile (pulse).

In clinical trials, no case of non-absorption was observed.

E_1 (Estrone)/E_2 ratios are around 1. A 20% decrease in bioavailability of estradiol has been observed in heavy smokers (1 pack/day).

A 20% decrease in bioavailability of estradiol has been observed in heavy smokers (1 pack/day).

Cigarette smoking immediately before AERODIOL administration does not modify the nasal absorption of estradiol.

5.3 Preclinical safety data

Local tolerability studies in animals have shown that nasal administration of estradiol does not damage the nasal mucosa.

6. PHARMACEUTICAL PARTICULARS

6.1 List of excipients

Methyl β-cyclodextrin (RAMEB), sodium chloride, sodium hydroxide or hydrochloric acid, purified water.

6.2 Incompatibilities

Not applicable.

6.3 Shelf life

3 years.

6.4 Special precautions for storage

No special precautions for storage.

6.5 Nature and contents of container

4.2 ml (60 sprays) in a bottle (Type-1 glass) with a metering pump (polypropylene) and a nasal applicator (polypropylene); packs of 1 and 3 bottles.

6.6 Instructions for use and handling

No special requirements.

7. MARKETING AUTHORISATION HOLDER

LES LABORATOIRES SERVIER

22, rue Garnier

92200 Neuilly-sur-Seine

France

8. MARKETING AUTHORISATION NUMBER(S)

PL 05815/0021

9. DATE OF FIRST AUTHORISATION/RENEWAL OF THE AUTHORISATION

25 January 2001

10. DATE OF REVISION OF THE TEXT

May 2004

Agenerase 150mg Soft Capsules

(GlaxoSmithKline UK)

1. NAME OF THE MEDICINAL PRODUCT

Agenerase 150 mg soft capsules

2. QUALITATIVE AND QUANTITATIVE COMPOSITION

Each capsule contains 150 mg amprenavir.

For excipients, see section 6.1.

3. PHARMACEUTICAL FORM

Soft capsule.

The soft capsules are oblong, opaque, off-white to cream coloured, printed with 'GX CC2'.

4. CLINICAL PARTICULARS

4.1 Therapeutic indications

Agenerase, in combination with other antiretroviral agents, is indicated for the treatment of protease inhibitor (PI) experienced HIV-1 infected adults and children above the age of 4 years. Agenerase capsules should normally be administered with low dose ritonavir as a pharmacokinetic enhancer of amprenavir (see sections 4.2 and 4.5). The choice of amprenavir should be based on individual viral resistance testing and treatment history of patients (see section 5.1).

The benefit of Agenerase boosted with ritonavir has not been demonstrated in PI naïve patients (see section 5.1)

4.2 Posology and method of administration

Therapy should be initiated by a physician experienced in the management of HIV infection.

The importance of complying with the full recommended dosing regimen should be stressed to all patients.

Agenerase is administered orally and can be taken with or without food.

Agenerase is also available as an oral solution for use in children or adults unable to swallow capsules. Amprenavir is 14 % less bioavailable from the oral solution than from the capsules; therefore, Agenerase capsules and Agenerase oral solution are not interchangeable on a milligram per milligram basis (see section 5.2).

Adults and adolescents of 12 years of age and older (greater than 50 kg body weight): the recommended dose of Agenerase capsules is 600 mg twice daily with ritonavir, 100 mg twice daily, in combination with other antiretroviral agents.

If Agenerase capsules are used without the boosting effect of ritonavir higher doses of Agenerase (1200 mg twice daily) should be used.

Children (4 to 12 years) and patients less than 50 kg body weight: the recommended dose of Agenerase capsules is 20 mg/kg body weight twice a day, in combination with other antiretroviral agents, without exceeding a total daily dose of 2400 mg.

The pharmacokinetics, efficacy and safety of Agenerase in combination with low doses of ritonavir or other protease inhibitors have not yet been evaluated in children. Therefore, such combinations should be avoided in children.

Children less than 4 years of age: Agenerase is not recommended in children less than 4 years of age (see section 5.3).

Elderly: the pharmacokinetics, efficacy and safety of amprenavir have not been studied in patients over 65 years of age (see section 5.2).

Renal impairment: no dose adjustment is considered necessary in patients with renal impairment (see section 5.2).

Hepatic impairment: the principal route of metabolism of amprenavir is via the liver. Agenerase capsules should be used with caution in patients with hepatic impairment. Clinical efficacy and safety have not been determined in this patient group. For subjects with hepatic impairment, pharmacokinetic data are available for the use of Agenerase capsules without the boosting effect of ritonavir. Based on pharmacokinetic data, the dose of Agenerase capsules should be reduced to 450 mg twice a day for adult patients with moderate hepatic impairment and to 300 mg twice a day for adult patients with severe hepatic impairment. No dose recommendation can be made in children with hepatic impairment (see section 5.2).

The use of amprenavir in combination with ritonavir has not been studied in patients with hepatic impairment. No dose recommendations can be made regarding this combination. Concomitant administration should be used with caution in patients with mild and moderate hepatic impairment and is contraindicated in patients with severe hepatic impairment (see section 4.3).

4.3 Contraindications

Known hypersensitivity to amprenavir or any ingredient of Agenerase capsules.

Agenerase must not be administered concurrently with medicinal products with narrow therapeutic windows that are substrates of cytochrome P450 3A4 (CYP3A4). Co-administration may result in competitive inhibition of the metabolism of these medicinal products and create the potential for serious and/or life-threatening adverse events such as cardiac arrhythmia (e.g. terfenadine, astemizole, cisapride, pimozide), prolonged sedation or respiratory depression (e.g. triazolam, diazepam, flurazepam, midazolam), or peripheral vasospasm or ischaemia and ischaemia of other tissues, including cerebral or myocardial ischaemia (e.g. ergot derivatives).

Agenerase in combination with ritonavir is contraindicated in patients with severe hepatic impairment.

Agenerase must not be given with rifampicin because rifampicin reduces trough plasma concentrations of amprenavir by approximately 92 % (see section 4.5).

Herbal preparations containing St John's wort (*Hypericum perforatum*) must not be used while taking amprenavir due to the risk of decreased plasma concentrations and reduced clinical effects of amprenavir (see section 4.5).

4.4 Special warnings and special precautions for use

Patients should be advised that Agenerase, or any other current antiretroviral therapy does not cure HIV and that they may still develop opportunistic infections and other complications of HIV infection. Current antiretroviral therapies, including Agenerase, have not been proven to prevent the risk of transmission of HIV to others through sexual contact or blood contamination. Appropriate precautions should continue to be taken.

On the basis of current pharmacodynamic data, amprenavir should be used in combination with at least two other antiretrovirals. When amprenavir is administered as monotherapy, resistant viruses rapidly emerge (see section 5.1). Agenerase capsules should normally be given in combination with low dose ritonavir and in combination with other antiretroviral agents (see section 4.2).

Liver Disease: The safety and efficacy of amprenavir has not been established in patients with significant underlying liver disorders. Agenerase capsules are contraindicated in patients with severe hepatic impairment when used in combination with ritonavir (see section4.3). Patients with chronic hepatitis B or C and treated with combination antiretroviral therapy are at an increased risk of severe and potentially fatal hepatic adverse events. In case of concomitant antiviral therapy for hepatitis B or C, please refer also to the relevant product information for these medicinal products.

Patients with pre-existing liver dysfunction, including chronic active hepatitis, have an increased frequency of liver function abnormalities during combination antiretroviral therapy and should be monitored according to standard practice. If there is evidence of worsening liver disease in such patients, interruption or discontinuation of treatment must be considered.

Medicinal products – interactions

Amprenavir, like other HIV protease inhibitors, is an inhibitor of the cytochrome CYP3A4 enzyme. Agenerase should not be administered concurrently with medications with narrow therapeutic windows which are substrates of CYP3A4 (see section 4.3). Combination with other agents may result in serious and/or life-threatening interactions, therefore caution is advised whenever Agenerase is co-administered with medicinal products that are inducers, inhibitors or substrates of CYP3A4 (see section 4.5).

Caution should be exercised when prescribing Agenerase and ritonavir concomitantly with CYP2D6 substrates with a narrow therapeutic index, i.e. flecainide, propafenone and metoprolol (when used in cardiac insufficiency).

The HMG-CoA reductase inhibitors lovastatin and simvastatin are highly dependent on CYP3A4 for metabolism, thus concomitant use of Agenerase with simvastatin or lovastatin is not recommended due to an increased risk of myopathy, including rhabdomyolysis. Caution must also be exercised if Agenerase is used concurrently with atorvastatin, which is metabolized to a lesser extent by CYP3A4. In this situation, a reduced dose of atorvastatin should be considered. If treatment with a HMG-CoA reductase inhibitor is indicated, pravastatin or fluvastatin are recommended (see section 4.5).

For some medicinal products that can cause serious or life-threatening undesirable effects, such as amiodarone, phenobarbital, phenytoin, lidocaine (systemic), tricyclic antidepressants, quinidine and warfarin (monitor International Normalised Ratio), concentration monitoring is available; this should minimise the risk of potential safety problems with concomitant use.

Because of the potential for metabolic interactions with amprenavir, the efficacy of hormonal contraceptives may be modified, but there is insufficient information to predict the nature of the interactions. Therefore, alternative reliable methods of contraception are recommended for women of childbearing potential (see section 4.5).

Co-administration of amprenavir with methadone leads to a decrease of methadone concentrations. Therefore, when methadone is co-administered with amprenavir, patients should be monitored for opiate abstinence syndrome, in particular if low-dose ritonavir is also given. No recommendations can currently be made regarding adjustment of amprenavir dose when amprenavir is co-administered with methadone.

Agenerase capsules contain vitamin E (109 IU/150 mg capsule), therefore additional vitamin E supplementation is not recommended.

Due to the potential risk of toxicity from the high propylene glycol content of Agenerase oral solution, this formulation is contraindicated in children below the age of four years and should be used with caution in certain other patient populations. The Summary of Product Characteristics of Agenerase oral solution should be consulted for full prescribing information.

Rash / cutaneous reactions

Rashes/cutaneous reactions: most patients with mild or moderate rash can continue Agenerase. Appropriate antihistamines (e.g. cetirizine dihydrochloride) may reduce pruritus and hasten the resolution of rash. Agenerase should be permanently discontinued when rash is accompanied with systemic symptoms or allergic symptoms or mucosal involvement (see section 4.8).

Hyperglycaemia

New onset of diabetes mellitus, hyperglycaemia or exacerbations of existing diabetes mellitus have been reported in patients receiving antiretroviral therapy, including protease inhibitors. In some of these, the hyperglycaemia was severe and in some cases also associated with ketoacidosis. Many of the patients had confounding medical conditions, some of which required therapy with agents that have been associated with the development of diabetes mellitus or hyperglycaemia.

Lipodystrophy

Combination antiretroviral therapy has been associated with the redistribution of body fat (lipodystrophy) in HIV patients. The long-term consequences of these events are currently unknown. Knowledge about the mechanism is incomplete. A connection between visceral lipomatosis and protease inhibitors and lipoatrophy and nucleoside reverse transcriptase inhibitors has been hypothesised. A higher risk of lipodystrophy has been associated with individual factors such as older age, and with drug related factors such as longer duration of antiretroviral treatment and associated metabolic disturbances. Clinical examination should include evaluation for physical signs of fat redistribution. Consideration should be given to the measurement of fasting serum lipids and blood glucose. Lipid disorders should be managed as clinically appropriate (see section 4.8).

Haemophiliac patients

There have been reports of increased bleeding, including spontaneous skin haematomas and haemarthroses, in haemophiliac patients type A and B treated with protease inhibitors. In some patients, additional factor VIII was given. In more than half of the reported cases, treatment with protease inhibitors was continued, or reintroduced if treatment had been discontinued. A causal relationship has been evoked, although the mechanism of action has not been elucidated. Haemophiliac patients should therefore be made aware of the possibility of increased bleeding.

Immune Reactivation Syndrome

In HIV-infected patients with severe immune deficiency at the time of institution of combination antiretroviral therapy (CART), an inflammatory reaction to asymptomatic or residual opportunistic pathogens may arise and cause serious clinical conditions, or aggravation of symptoms. Typically, such reactions have been observed within the first few weeks or months of initiation of CART. Relevant examples are cytomegalovirus retinitis, generalised and/or focal mycobacterium infections, and *Pneumocystis carinii* pneumonia. Any inflammatory symptoms should be evaluated and treatment instituted when necessary.

4.5 Interaction with other medicinal products and other forms of Interaction

Interaction studies have been performed with amprenavir as the sole protease inhibitor. When amprenavir and ritonavir are co-administered, the ritonavir metabolic drug interaction profile may predominate because ritonavir is a more potent CYP3A4 inhibitor. Ritonavir also inhibits CYP2D6 and induces CYP3A4, CYP1A2, CYP2C9 and glucuronosyl transferase. The full prescribing information for ritonavir must therefore be consulted prior to initiation of therapy with Agenerase and ritonavir.

Amprenavir and ritonavir are primarily metabolised in the liver by CYP3A4. Therefore, medicinal products that either share this metabolic pathway or modify CYP3A4 activity may modify the pharmacokinetics of amprenavir. Similarly, amprenavir and ritonavir might also modify the pharmacokinetics of other medicinal products that share this metabolic pathway.

Terfenadine, cisapride, pimozide, triazolam, diazepam, midazolam, flurazepam ergotamine, dihydroergotamine and astemizole are contraindicated in patients receiving Agenerase. Concurrent administration can lead to competitive inhibition of the metabolism of these products and thus result in serious, life-threatening events (see section 4.3).

Of note, the following interaction data was obtained in adults.

Antiretroviral agents

• ***Protease inhibitors (PIs):***

Indinavir: the AUC, C_{min} and C_{max} of indinavir were decreased by 38 %, 27 %, and 22 %, respectively, when given with amprenavir. The clinical relevance of these changes is unknown. The AUC, C_{min} and C_{max} of amprenavir were increased by 33 %, 25 %, and 18 %, respectively. No dose adjustment is necessary for either medicinal product when indinavir is administered in combination with amprenavir.

Saquinavir: the AUC, C_{min} and C_{max} of saquinavir were decreased by 19 % and 48 % and increased by 21 %, respectively, when given with amprenavir. The clinical relevance of these changes is unknown. The AUC, C_{min} and C_{max} of amprenavir were decreased by 32 %, 14 %, and 37 %, respectively. No dose adjustment is necessary for either medicinal product when saquinavir is administered in combination with amprenavir.

Nelfinavir: the AUC, C_{min} and C_{max} of nelfinavir were increased by 15 %, 14 %, and 12 %, respectively, when given with amprenavir. The C_{max} of amprenavir was decreased by 14 % whilst the AUC and C_{min} were increased by 9 % and 189 %, respectively. No dose adjustment is necessary for either medicinal product when nelfinavir is administered in combination with amprenavir (see also efavirenz below).

Ritonavir: the AUC and C_{min} of amprenavir were increased by 64% and 508% respectively and the C_{max} decreased by 30% when ritonavir (100 mg twice daily) was coadministered with amprenavir capsules (600 mg twice daily) compared to values achieved after 1200 mg twice daily doses of amprenavir capsules. In clinical trials, doses of amprenavir 600 mg twice daily and ritonavir 100 mg twice daily have been used; confirming the safety and efficacy of this regimen.

Lopinavir / ritonavir (Kaletra): in an open-label, non-fasting pharmacokinetic study, the AUC, C_{max} and C_{min} of lopinavir were decreased by 38%, 28% and 52% respectively when amprenavir (750 mg twice daily) was given in combination with Kaletra (400 mg lopinavir + 100 mg ritonavir twice daily). In the same study, the AUC, C_{max}, and C_{min} of amprenavir were increased 72%, 12%, and 483%, respectively, when compared to values after standard doses of amprenavir (1200 mg twice daily).

The amprenavir plasma C_{min} values achieved with the combination of amprenavir (600 mg twice daily) in combination with Kaletra (400 mg lopinavir + 100 mg ritonavir twice daily) are approximately 40-50% lower than when amprenavir (600 mg twice daily) is given in combination with ritonavir 100 mg twice daily. Adding additional ritonavir to an amprenavir plus Kaletra regimen increase lopinavir C_{min} values, but not amprenavir C_{min} values. No dose recommendation can be given for the co-administration of amprenavir and Kaletra, but close monitoring is advised because the safety and efficacy of this combination is unknown.

• ***Nucleoside analogue reverse transcriptase inhibitors (NRTIs):***

Zidovudine: the AUC and C_{max} of zidovudine were increased by 31 % and 40 %, respectively, when given with amprenavir. The AUC and the C_{max} of amprenavir were unaltered. No dose adjustment for either medicinal product is necessary when zidovudine is administered in combination with amprenavir.

Lamivudine: the AUC and C_{max} of lamivudine and amprenavir, respectively, were both unaltered when these two medicinal products were given concomitantly. No dose adjustment is necessary for either medicinal product when lamivudine is administered in combination with amprenavir.

Abacavir: the AUC, C_{min}, and C_{max} of abacavir were unaltered when given with amprenavir. The AUC, C_{min}, and C_{max} of amprenavir were increased by 29 %, 27 %, and 47 %, respectively. No dose adjustment is necessary for either medicinal product when abacavir is administered in combination with amprenavir.

Didanosine: no pharmacokinetic study has been performed with Agenerase in combination with didanosine, however, due to its antacid component, it is recommended that didanosine and Agenerase should be administered at least one hour apart (see Antacids below).

• *Non-nucleoside reverse transcriptase inhibitors (NNRTIs):*

Efavirenz: efavirenz has been seen to decrease the C_{max}, AUC, and $C_{min,ss}$ of amprenavir by approximately 40 % in adults. When amprenavir is combined with ritonavir, the effect of efavirenz is compensated by the pharmacokinetic booster effect of ritonavir. Therefore, if efavirenz is given in combination with amprenavir (600 mg twice daily) and ritonavir (100 mg twice daily), no dose adjustment is necessary.

Further, if efavirenz is given in combination with amprenavir and nelfinavir, no dosage adjustment is necessary for any of the medicinal products.

Treatment with efavirenz in combination with amprenavir and saquinavir is not recommended as the exposure to both protease inhibitors would be decreased.

No dose recommendation can be given for co-administration of amprenavir with another protease inhibitor and efavirenz in children. Such combinations should be avoided in patients with hepatic impairment.

Nevirapine : The effect of nevirapine on other protease inhibitors and the limited evidence available suggest that nevirapine may decrease the serum concentrations of amprenavir.

Delavirdine: the AUC, C_{max} and C_{min} of delavirdine were decreased by 61%, 47% and 88% respectively when given with amprenavir. The AUC, C_{max} and C_{min} of amprenavir were increased by 130%, 40% and 125% respectively.

No dose recommendations can be given for the co-administration of amprenavir and delavirdine. If these medicinal products are used concomitantly care is advised, as delavirdine may be less effective due to decreased and potentially sub-therapeutic plasma concentrations.

No dose recommendations can be given for the co-administration of amprenavir and low dose ritonavir with delavirdine. If these medicinal products are used concomitantly care is advised, and close clinical and virological monitoring should be performed since it is difficult to predict the effect of the combination of amprenavir and ritonavir on delavirdine.

Antibiotics/antifungals

Rifampicin: rifampicin is a potent inducer of CYP3A4. Concomitant administration with amprenavir resulted in a reduction of amprenavir C_{min} and AUC by 92 % and 82 %, respectively. Rifampicin must not be used concomitantly with amprenavir (see section 4.3).

Rifabutin: co-administration of amprenavir with rifabutin resulted in a 193 % increase in rifabutin AUC and an increase of rifabutin-related adverse events. The increase in rifabutin plasma concentration is likely to result from inhibition of rifabutin CYP3A4 mediated metabolism by amprenavir. When it is clinically necessary to co-administer rifabutin with Agenerase, a dosage reduction of at least half the recommended dose of rifabutin is advised, although no clinical data are available. When ritonavir is co-administered a larger increase in rifabutin concentration may occur.

Clarithromycin: the AUC and C_{min} of clarithromycin were unaltered and the C_{max} decreased by 10 % when given with amprenavir. The AUC, C_{min} and C_{max} of amprenavir were increased by 18 %, 39 %, and 15 % respectively. No dose adjustment is necessary for either medicinal product when clarithromycin is administered in combination with amprenavir. When ritonavir is co-administered an increase in clarithromycin concentrations may occur.

Erythromycin: no pharmacokinetic study has been performed with Agenerase in combination with erythromycin, however, plasma levels of both medicinal products may be increased when co-administered.

Ketoconazole: the AUC and C_{max} of ketoconazole were increased by 44 % and 19 % respectively when given with amprenavir. The AUC and C_{max} of amprenavir were increased by 31 % and decreased by 16 %, respectively. No dose adjustment for either medicinal product is necessary when ketoconazole is administered in combination with amprenavir. When ritonavir is co-administered a larger increase in ketoconazole concentrations may occur.

Other possible interactions

Other medicinal products, listed below, including examples of substrates, inhibitors or inducers of CYP3A4, may lead to interactions when administered with Agenerase. The clinical significance of these possible interactions is not known and has not been investigated. Patients should therefore be monitored for toxic reactions associated with these medicinal products when these are administered in combination with Agenerase.

Antacids: on the basis of the data for other protease inhibitors, it is advisable not to take antacids at the same time as Agenerase, since its absorption may be impaired. It is recommended that antacids and Agenerase should be administered at least one hour apart.

Benzodiazepines: the serum concentrations of alprazolam, triazolam, midazolam, clonazepam, diazepam and flurazepam may be increased by amprenavir resulting in enhanced sedation (see section 4.3).

Calcium-channel blockers: amprenavir may lead to increased serum concentrations of diltiazem, nicardipine, nifedipine or nimodipine, possibly resulting in enhanced activity and toxicity of these medicinal products.

Erectile dysfunction agents: based on data for other protease inhibitors caution should be used when prescribing sildenafil to patients receiving Agenerase. Co-administration of Agenerase with sildenafil may substantially increase sildenafil plasma concentrations and may result in sildenafil-associated adverse events.

HMG-CoA reductase inhibitors: HMG-CoA reductase inhibitors which are highly dependent on CYP3A4 for metabolism, such as lovastatin and simvastatin, are expected to have markedly increased plasma concentrations when co-administered with Agenerase. Since increased concentrations of HMG-CoA reductase inhibitors may cause myopathy, including rhabdomyolysis, the combination of these medicinal products with Agenerase is not recommended. Atorvastatin is less dependent on CYP3A4 for metabolism. When used with Agenerase, the lowest possible dose of atorvastatin should be administered. The metabolism of pravastatin and fluvastatin is not dependent on CYP3A4, and interactions are not expected with protease inhibitors. If treatment with a HMG-CoA reductase inhibitor is indicated, pravastatin or fluvastatin is recommended.

Methadone and opiate derivatives: co-administration of methadone with amprenavir resulted in a decrease in the C_{max} and AUC of the active methadone enantiomer (R-enantiomer) of 25% and 13% respectively, whilst the C_{max}, AUC and C_{min} of the inactive methadone enantiomer (S-enantiomer) were decreased by 48%, 40% and 23% respectively. When methadone is co-administered with amprenavir, patients should be monitored for opiate abstinence syndrome, in particular if low-dose ritonavir is also given.

As compared to a non-matched historical control group, co-administration of methadone and amprenavir resulted in a 30%, 27% and 25% decrease in serum amprenavir AUC, C_{max} and C_{min} respectively. No recommendations can currently be made regarding adjustment of amprenavir dose when amprenavir is co-administered with methadone due to the inherent low reliability of non-matched historical controls.

Steroids: oestrogens, progestogens and some glucocorticoids may interact with amprenavir. However, the information currently available is not sufficient for determining the nature of the interaction. Co-administration of Ortho-Novum 1/35 (0.035 mg ethinyl estradiol plus 1.0 mg norethindrone) resulted in a decrease of the amprenavir AUC and C_{min} of 22% and 20% respectively, C_{max} being unchanged. The C_{min} of ethinyl estradiol was increased by 32%, whilst the AUC and C_{min} of norethindrone were increased by 18% and 45% respectively. Alternative methods of contraception are recommended for women of childbearing potential. When ritonavir is co-administered, the effect on hormonal contraceptive concentrations cannot be predicted, therefore, alternative methods of contraception are also recommended.

St John's wort: serum levels of amprenavir can be reduced by concomitant use of the herbal preparation St John's wort (*Hypericum perforatum*). This is due to induction of drug metabolising enzymes by St John's wort. Herbal preparations containing St John's wort should therefore not be combined with Agenerase. If a patient is already taking St John's wort, check amprenavir and if possible viral levels and stop St John's wort. Amprenavir levels may increase on stopping St John's wort. The dose of amprenavir may need adjusting. The inducing effect may persist for at least 2 weeks after cessation of treatment with St John's wort (see section 4.3).

Other substances: plasma concentrations of other substances may be increased by amprenavir. These include substances such as: clozapine, carbamazepine, cimetidine, dapsone, itraconazole and loratadine.

4.6 Pregnancy and lactation

Pregnancy: the safe use of amprenavir in human pregnancy has not been established. Placental transfer of amprenavir and/or its related metabolites has been shown to occur in animals (see section 5.3).

This medicinal product should be used during pregnancy only after careful weighing of the potential benefits compared to the potential risk to the foetus.

Lactation: amprenavir-related material was found in rat milk, but it is not known whether amprenavir is excreted in human milk. A reproduction study in pregnant rats dosed from the time of uterine implantation through lactation showed reduced body weight gains in the offspring during the nursing period. The systemic exposure to the dams associated with this finding was similar to exposure in humans, following administration of the recommended dose. The subsequent development of the offspring, including fertility and reproductive performance, was not affected by the maternal administration of amprenavir.

It is therefore recommended that mothers being treated with Agenerase do not breast-feed their infants. Additionally, it is recommended that HIV infected women do not breast-feed their infants in order to avoid transmission of HIV.

4.7 Effects on ability to drive and use machines

No studies on the effects on ability to drive and use machines have been performed.

4.8 Undesirable effects

The safety of Agenerase has been studied in adults and children of at least 4 years of age, in controlled clinical trials, in combination with various other antiretroviral agents. Adverse events considered associated with the use of Agenerase are gastro-intestinal symptoms, rash and oral/peri-oral paraesthesia. Most undesirable effects associated with Agenerase therapy were mild to moderate in severity, early in onset, and rarely treatment-limiting. For many of these events, it is unclear whether they are related to Agenerase, to concomitant treatment used in the management of HIV disease or to the disease process.

In children, the nature of the safety profile is similar to that seen in adults.

Adverse reactions are listed below by MedDRA body system organ class and by frequency. The frequency categories used are:

Very common ⩾ 1 in 10

Common ⩾ 1 in 100 and < 1 in 10

Uncommon ⩾ 1 in 1,000 and < 1 in 100

Rare ⩾1 in 10,000 and < 1 in 1,000

Frequency categories for the events below have been based on clinical trials and postmarketing data.

Most of the adverse events below come from two clinical trials (PROAB3001, PROAB3006) involving PI naïve subjects receiving Agenerase 1200mg twice daily. Events (grade 2-4) reported by study investigators as attributable to study medication and occurring in >1% of patients, are included as well as grade 3-4 treatment emergent laboratory abnormalities. Note that the background rates in comparator groups were not taken into account.

Metabolism and nutrition disorders

Common: Elevated triglycerides, elevated amylase, abnormal fat redistribution, anorexia

Uncommon: Hyperglycaemia, hypercholesterolaemia

Elevated triglycerides, elevated amylase and hyperglycaemia (grade 3-4) were reported primarily in patients with abnormal values at baseline.

Elevations in cholesterol were of grade 3-4 intensity.

Combination antiretroviral therapy has been associated with redistribution of body fat (lipodystrophy) in HIV patients including the loss of peripheral and facial subcutaneous fat, increased intra-abdominal and visceral fat, breast hypertrophy and dorsocervical fat accumulation (buffalo hump).

Symptoms of abnormal fat redistribution were infrequent in PROAB3001 with amprenavir. Only one case (a buffalo hump) was reported in 113 (< 1 %) antiretroviral naive subjects treated with amprenavir in combination with lamivudine/zidovudine for a median duration of 36 weeks. In study PROAB3006, seven cases (3 %) were reported in 245 NRTI-experienced subjects treated with amprenavir and in 27 (11 %) of 241 subjects treated with indinavir, in combination with various NRTIs for a median duration of 56 weeks ($p < 0.001$).

Combination antiretroviral therapy has been associated with metabolic abnormalities such as hypertriglyceridaemia, hypercholesterolaemia, insulin resistance, hyperglycaemia and hyperlactataemia (see section 4.4).

Psychiatric disorders

Common: Mood disorders, depressive disorders

Nervous system disorders

Very Common: Headache

Common: Oral/perioral paraesthesia, tremors, sleep disorders

Gastrointestinal disorders

Very Common: Diarrhoea, nausea, flatulence, vomiting

Common: Abdominal pain, abdominal discomfort, dyspeptic symptoms, loose stools

Hepatobiliary disorders

Common: Elevated transaminases

Uncommon: Hyperbilirubinaemia

Elevated transaminases and hyperbilirubinaemia (grade 3-4) were reported primarily in patients with abnormal values at baseline. Almost all subjects with abnormal liver function tests were co-infected with Hepatitis B or C virus.

Skin and subcutaneous tissue disorders

Very Common: Rash

Rare: Stevens Johnson syndrome

Rashes were usually mild to moderate, erythematous or maculopapular cutaneous eruptions, with or without pruritus, occurring during the second week of therapy and resolving spontaneously within two weeks, without discontinuation of treatment with amprenavir. A higher incidence of rash was reported in patients treated with amprenavir in combination with efavirenz. Severe or life-threatening skin reactions have also occurred in patients treated with amprenavir (see section 4.4).

Musculoskeletal and connective tissue disorders

Increased CPK, myalgia, myositis, and rarely rhabdomyolysis have been reported with protease inhibitors, particularly in combination with nucleoside analogues.

General disorders and administration site conditions

Very Common: Fatigue

In HIV-infected patients with severe immune deficiency at the time of initiation of combination antiretroviral therapy (CART), an inflammatory reaction to asymptomatic or residual opportunistic infections may arise (see section 4.4).

In PI experienced patients receiving Agenerase capsules 600 mg twice daily and low dose ritonavir, 100 mg twice daily, the nature and frequency of adverse events (grade 2-4) and Grade 3/4 laboratory abnormalities were similar to those observed with Agenerase alone, with the exception of elevated triglyceride levels, and elevated CPK levels which were very common in patients receiving Agenerase and low dose ritonavir.

4.9 Overdose

There are limited reports of overdose with Agenerase. If overdose occurs, the patient should be monitored for evidence of toxicity (see section 4.8), and standard supportive treatment provided as necessary. Since amprenavir is highly protein bound, dialysis is unlikely to be helpful in reducing blood levels of amprenavir.

5. PHARMACOLOGICAL PROPERTIES

5.1 Pharmacodynamic properties

Pharmacotherapeutic group; protease inhibitor; ATC Code: JO5A E05

Amprenavir is a competitive inhibitor of the HIV protease. It blocks the ability of the viral protease to cleave the precursor polyproteins necessary for viral replication.

Amprenavir is a potent and selective inhibitor of HIV-1 and HIV-2 replication *in vitro*. In isolated experimental settings, synergy was shown *in vitro* in combination with nucleoside analogues including didanosine, zidovudine, abacavir and the protease inhibitor, saquinavir. It has been shown to have an additive effect in combination with indinavir, ritonavir and nelfinavir.

Serial passage experiments have demonstrated the protease mutation I50V to be key to the development of amprenavir resistance *in vitro*, with the triple variant, I50V+M46I/L+I47V, resulting in a greater than 10-fold increase in IC_{50} to amprenavir. This triple mutation resistance profile has not been observed with other protease inhibitors either from *in vitro* studies or in clinical settings. *In vitro* variants resistant to amprenavir remained sensitive to saquinavir, indinavir and nelfinavir, but showed three to five-fold reduced susceptibility to ritonavir. The triple mutant, I50V+M46I/L+I47V, was unstable during *in vitro* passage in the presence of saquinavir, with loss of the I47V mutation, and the development of resistance to saquinavir resulted in resensitisation to amprenavir. Passage of the triple mutant in either indinavir, nelfinavir or ritonavir resulted in additional protease mutations being selected, leading to dual resistance. Mutation I84V, observed transiently *in vitro* has rarely been selected during amprenavir therapy.

The resistance profile seen with amprenavir in clinical practice is different from that observed with other protease inhibitors. Consistent with *in vitro* experiments, the development of amprenavir resistance during therapy, is in the majority cases, associated with the mutation I50V. However, three alternative mechanisms have also been observed to result in the development of amprenavir resistance in the clinic, and involve either mutations I54L/M or V32I+I47V or, rarely, I84V. Each of the four genetic patterns produces viruses with reduced susceptibility to amprenavir, some cross-resistance to ritonavir, but susceptibility to indinavir, nelfinavir and saquinavir is retained.

The following table summarises the mutations associated with the development of reduced phenotypic susceptibility to amprenavir in subjects treated with amprenavir.

Protease mutations acquired on amprenavir-containing therapy which have been demonstrated to result in reduced phenotypic susceptibility to amprenavir:
I50V or I54L/M or I84V or V32I with I47V

The pre-existence of resistance to other components of a first-line PI-containing regimen is significantly associated with subsequent development of protease mutations, highlighting the importance of considering all components of a treatment regimen when change is indicated.

Many *in vitro* PI-resistant variants, and 322 of 433 (74 %) clinical PI-resistant variants with multiple protease inhibitor resistance mutations were susceptible to amprenavir. The principal protease mutation associated with cross-resistance to amprenavir following treatment failure with other protease inhibitors was I84V, particularly when mutations L10I/V/F were also present.

In multiple PI-experienced subjects, the likelihood of a successful virological response is increased with an increasing number of active drugs (ie. agents to which the virus is susceptible) in the rescue regimen. The presence at the time of therapy change in PI-experienced subjects of multiple key mutations associated with PI-resistance, or the development of such mutations during PI therapy, is significantly associated with treatment outcome. The total number of all types of protease mutations present at the time of therapy change was also correlated with outcome in PI-experienced populations. The presence of 3 or more mutations from M46I/L, I54L/M/V, V82A/F/I/T, I84V and L90M in a population of multiple PI-experienced subjects was significantly related to amprenavir treatment failure.

The following table summarises the mutations, identified in clinical isolates from highly PI- experienced patients, associated with an increased risk of treatment failure of amprenavir-containing regimens.

Protease mutations in virus from PI-experienced patients associated with reduced virological response to subsequent amprenavir containing regimens:
COMBINATION OF AT LEAST THREE OF: M46I/L or I54L/M/V or V82A/F/I/T or I84V or L90M.

The number of key PI-resistance mutations increases markedly the longer a failing PI-containing regimen is continued. Early discontinuation of failing therapies is recommended in order to limit the accumulation of multiple mutations, which may be detrimental to a subsequent rescue regimen.

Amprenavir is not recommended for use as monotherapy, due to the rapid emergence of resistant virus.

Cross resistance between amprenavir and reverse transcriptase inhibitors, is unlikely to occur because the enzyme targets are different.

Clinical experience:

Agenerase in combination with low dose ritonavir and nucleoside analogues (NRTI) has been shown to be effective in the treatment of PI-experienced HIV–1 infected adults.

In a randomised, open-label study in PI-experienced adults experiencing virological failure (viral load $\geqslant$1000 copies/ml), Agenerase (600 mg twice daily) / ritonavir (100 mg twice daily) was compared to other PIs. The study comprised two separate components. Analyses described are intent to treat (Exposed).

Sub-study A (n=163) compared Agenerase / ritonavir to other, predominantly ritonavir boosted PIs, in a standard of care regimen, in patients with virus sensitive to Agenerase, at least one other PI, and at least one NRTI. After 16 weeks, the antiviral response to Agenerase/ritonavir, as measured by time-averaged change from baseline in plasma HIV-1 RNA (AAUCMB), was shown to be non-inferior to that in the patients in the other PI treatment group [mean plasma HIV-1 RNA AAUCMB 1.315 $\log_{10}$ copies/ml and 1.343 $\log_{10}$ copies/ml respectively, mean stratified difference 0.043 $\log_{10}$ copies/ml (95% CI: –0.25, 0.335), ITT(E) population, Observed analysis]. The proportion of subjects with plasma HIV-1 RNA $<$400 copies/ml was similar across the treatment groups (66% and 70% respectively).

Sub-study B (n=43) compared Agenerase / ritonavir to continued current PI therapy in patients with virus resistant to indinavir, ritonavir, nelfinavir and saquinavir. Agenerase/ritonavir demonstrated superior efficacy as measured by AAUCMB after four weeks [mean strata adjusted treatment difference –0.669 $\log_{10}$ copies/ml (95% CI -0.946, -0.391), p=0.00002, ITT(E) population, Observed analysis]. Additionally, the proportion of subjects with plasma HIV-1 RNA below 400 copies/ml was higher in the Agenerase/ritonavir group (48%) than in the group maintained on the PI regimen current at study start (0%), p=0.00048.

Agenerase without low dose ritonavir in combination with other antiretroviral agents including nucleoside analogues, non-nucleoside analogues and protease inhibitors, has been shown to be effective in antiretroviral naïve and NRTI-experienced PI-naïve HIV-1 infected adults and heavily pre-treated children aged 4 years or more.

In a double-blind study in antiretroviral naive HIV-infected adults (n = 232), amprenavir (1200 mg twice daily) in combination with zidovudine and lamivudine was significantly superior to zidovudine and lamivudine. In an intent-to-treat analysis (any missing value or premature discontinuation considered as failure i.e. $\geqslant$ 400 copies/ml), the proportion of subjects with plasma HIV-1 RNA $<$ 400 copies/ml through week 48 was 41 % in the amprenavir/lamivudine/zidovudine group and 3 % in the lamivudine/zidovudine group ($p < 0.001$).

In an open-label randomised study in NRTI experienced PI naive adults (n = 504), in combination with various NRTIs amprenavir (1200 mg twice daily) was found to be less effective than indinavir: the proportion of subjects with plasma HIV-1 RNA $<$ 400 copies/ml at week 48 was 30 % in the amprenavir arm and 46 % in the indinavir arm in the intent-to-treat analysis (any missing value or premature discontinuation considered as failure, i.e. $\geqslant$ 400 copies/ml).

Results from two paediatric studies with amprenavir oral solution and/or capsules in 268 heavily pre-treated children aged 2 to 18 years indicate that amprenavir is an effective antiretroviral agent in children. Decreases in median HIV-1 RNA greater than 1 $\log_{10}$ copies/ml were observed in protease inhibitor naive subjects and improvements in immune category (CD4 %) were reported.

The use of Agenerase, without the boosting effect of low dose ritonavir, has not been sufficiently studied in heavily pretreated protease inhibitor experienced patients.

5.2 Pharmacokinetic properties

Absorption: after oral administration, amprenavir is rapidly and well absorbed. The absolute bioavailability is unknown due to the lack of an acceptable intravenous formulation for use in man. Approximately 90 % of an orally administered radiolabelled amprenavir dose was recovered in the urine and the faeces, primarily as amprenavir metabolites. Following oral administration, the mean time (t_{max}) to maximal serum concentrations of amprenavir is between 1-2 hours for the capsule and 0.5 to 1 hour for the oral solution. A second peak is observed after 10 to 12 hours and may represent either delayed absorption or enterohepatic recirculation.

At therapeutic dosages (1200 mg twice daily), the mean maximum steady state concentration ($C_{max,ss}$) of amprenavir capsules is 5.36 μg/ml (0.92-9.81) and the minimum steady state concentration ($C_{min,ss}$) is 0.28 μg/ml (0.12-0.51). The mean AUC over a dosing interval of 12 hours is 18.46 μg.h/ml (3.02-32.95). The 50 mg and 150 mg capsules have been shown to be bioequivalent. The bioavailability of the oral solution at equivalent doses is lower than that of the capsules, with an AUC and C_{max} approximately 14 % and 19 % lower, respectively (see section 4.2).

The AUC and C_{min} of amprenavir were increased by 64% and 508% respectively and the C_{max} decreased by 30% when ritonavir (100 mg twice daily) was coadministered with amprenavir (600 mg twice daily) compared to values achieved after 1200 mg twice daily doses of amprenavir.

While administration of amprenavir with food results in a 25 % reduction in AUC, it had no effect on the concentration of amprenavir 12 hours after dosing (C_{12}). Therefore, although food affects the extent and rate of absorption, the steady-state trough concentration ($C_{min,ss}$) was not affected by food intake.

Distribution: the apparent volume of distribution is approximately 430 litres (6 l/kg assuming a 70 kg body weight), suggesting a large volume of distribution, with penetration of amprenavir freely into tissues beyond the systemic circulation. The concentration of amprenavir in the cerebrospinal fluid is less than 1 % of plasma concentration.

In *in vitro* studies, the protein binding of amprenavir is approximately 90 %. Amprenavir is primarily bound to the alpha–1-acid glycoprotein (AAG), but also to albumin. Concentrations of AAG have been shown to decrease during the course of antiretroviral therapy. This change will decrease the total active substance concentration in the plasma, however the amount of unbound amprenavir, which is the active moiety, is likely to be unchanged. While absolute free active substance concentrations remain constant, the percent of free active substance will fluctuate directly with total active substance concentrations at steady-state go from $C_{max,ss}$ to $C_{min,ss}$ over the course of the dosing interval. This will result in a fluctuation in the apparent volume of distribution of total active substance but the volume of distribution of free active substance does not change.

Clinically significant binding displacement interactions involving medicinal products primarily bound to AAG are generally not observed. Therefore, interactions with amprenavir due to protein binding displacement are highly unlikely.

Metabolism: amprenavir is primarily metabolised by the liver with less than 3 % excreted unchanged in the urine. The primary route of metabolism is via the cytochrome P450 CYP3A4 enzyme. Amprenavir is a substrate of and inhibits CYP3A4. Therefore medicinal products that are inducers, inhibitors or substrates of CYP3A4 must be used with caution when administered concurrently with Agenerase (see sections 4.3, 4.4 and 4.5).

Elimination: the plasma elimination half-life of amprenavir ranges from 7.1 to 10.6 hours. The plasma amprenavir half-life is increased when Agenerase capsules are co-administered with ritonavir. Following multiple oral doses of amprenavir (1200 mg twice a day), there is no significant active substance accumulation. The primary route of elimination of amprenavir is via hepatic metabolism with less than 3 % excreted unchanged in the urine. The metabolites and unchanged amprenavir account for approximately 14 % of the administered amprenavir dose in the urine, and approximately 75 % in the faeces.

Special populations:

Paediatrics: the pharmacokinetics of amprenavir in children (4 years of age and above) are similar to those in adults. Dosages of 20 mg/kg twice a day and 15 mg/kg three times a day with Agenerase capsules provided similar daily amprenavir exposure to 1200 mg twice a day in adults. Amprenavir is 14 % less bioavailable from the oral solution than from the capsules; therefore, Agenerase capsules and Agenerase oral solution are not interchangeable on a milligram per milligram basis.

Elderly: the pharmacokinetics of amprenavir have not been studied in patients over 65 years of age.

Renal impairment: patients with renal impairment have not been specifically studied. Less than 3 % of the therapeutic dose of amprenavir is excreted unchanged in the urine. The impact of renal impairment on amprenavir elimination should be minimal, therefore, no initial dose adjustment is considered necessary. Renal clearance of ritonavir is also negligible; therefore the impact of renal impairment on amprenavir and ritonavir elimination should be minimal.

Hepatic impairment: the pharmacokinetics of amprenavir are significantly altered in patients with moderate to severe hepatic impairment. The AUC increased nearly three fold in patients with moderate impairment and four fold in patients with severe hepatic impairment. Clearance also decreased in a corresponding manner to the AUC. The dosage should therefore be reduced in these patients (see section 4.2). These dosing regimens will provide plasma amprenavir levels comparable to those achieved in healthy subjects given a 1200 mg dose twice daily without concomitant administration of ritonavir.

5.3 Preclinical safety data

In long-term carcinogenicity studies with amprenavir in mice and rats, there were benign hepatocellular adenomas in males at exposure levels equivalent to 2.0-fold (mice) or 3.8-fold (rats) those in humans given 1200 mg twice daily of amprenavir alone. In male mice altered hepatocellular foci were seen at doses that were at least 2.0 times human therapeutic exposure.

A higher incidence of hepatocellular carcinoma was seen in all amprenavir male mouse treatment groups. However, this increase was not statistically significantly different from male control mice by appropriate tests. The mechanism for the hepatocellular adenomas and carcinomas found in these studies has not been elucidated and the significance of the observed effects for humans is uncertain. However, there is little evidence from the exposure data in humans, both in clinical trials and from marketed use, to suggest that these findings are of clinical significance.

Amprenavir was not mutagenic or genotoxic in a battery of *in vivo* and *in vitro* genetic toxicity assays, including bacterial reverse mutation (Ames Test), mouse lymphoma, rat micronucleus, and chromosome aberration in human peripheral lymphocytes.

In toxicological studies with mature animals, the clinically relevant findings were mostly confined to the liver and gastrointestinal disturbances. Liver toxicity consisted of increases in liver enzymes, liver weights and microscopic findings including hepatocyte necrosis. This liver toxicity can be monitored for and detected in clinical use, with measurements of AST, ALT and alkaline phosphatase activity. However, significant liver toxicity has not been observed in patients treated in clinical studies, either during administration of Agenerase or after discontinuation.

Amprenavir did not affect fertility. Local toxicity and sensitising potential was absent in animal studies, but slight irritating properties to the rabbit eye were identified.

Toxicity studies in young animals, treated from four days of age, resulted in high mortality in both the control animals and those receiving amprenavir. These results imply that young animals lack fully developed metabolic pathways enabling them to excrete amprenavir or some critical components of the formulation (e.g. propylene glycol, PEG400). However, the possibility of anaphylactic reaction related to PEG400 cannot be excluded. In clinical studies, the safety and efficacy of amprenavir have not yet been established in children below four years of age.

In pregnant mice, rabbits and rats there were no major effects on embryo-foetal development. However, at systemic plasma exposures significantly below (rabbits) or not significantly higher (rat) than the expected human exposures during therapeutic dosing, a number of minor changes, including thymic elongation and minor skeletal variations were seen, indicating developmental delay. A dose-dependent increase in placental weight was found in the rabbit and rat which may indicate effects on placental function. It is therefore recommended that women of childbearing potential taking Agenerase should practice effective contraception (e.g. barrier methods).

6. PHARMACEUTICAL PARTICULARS

6.1 List of excipients

Capsule shell: gelatin, glycerol, d-sorbitol and sorbitans solution, titanium dioxide, red printing ink.

Capsule contents: d-alpha tocopheryl polyethylene glycol 1000 succinate (TPGS), macrogol 400 (PEG 400), propylene glycol.

6.2 Incompatibilities

Not applicable.

6.3 Shelf life

3 years.

6.4 Special precautions for storage

Do not store above 30°C.

Keep the container tightly closed.

6.5 Nature and contents of container

One or two white High Density Polyethylene (HDPE) bottles, each containing 240 capsules.

6.6 Instructions for use and handling

No special requirements.

Administrative Data

7. MARKETING AUTHORISATION HOLDER

Glaxo Group Ltd

Greenford Road

Greenford

Middlesex UB6 0NN

United Kingdom

8. MARKETING AUTHORISATION NUMBER(S)

EU/1/00/148/002

EU/1/00/148/003

9. DATE OF FIRST AUTHORISATION/RENEWAL OF THE AUTHORISATION

20th October 2000

10. DATE OF REVISION OF THE TEXT

17 December 2004

Agenerase 15mg/ml Oral Solution

(GlaxoSmithKline UK)

1. NAME OF THE MEDICINAL PRODUCT

Agenerase 15 mg/ml oral solution

2. QUALITATIVE AND QUANTITATIVE COMPOSITION

Agenerase oral solution contains 15 mg/ml of amprenavir.

For excipients, see section 6.1.

3. PHARMACEUTICAL FORM

Oral solution.

The oral solution is clear, pale yellow to yellow with grape, bubblegum and peppermint flavouring.

4. CLINICAL PARTICULARS

4.1 Therapeutic indications

Agenerase oral solution, in combination with other antiretroviral agents, is indicated for the treatment of protease inhibitor (PI) experienced HIV-1 infected adults and children above the age of 4 years. The choice of amprenavir should be based on individual viral resistance testing and treatment history of patients (see section 5.1).

In protease inhibitor naive patients, Agenerase is less effective than indinavir.

4.2 Posology and method of administration

Therapy should be initiated by a physician experienced in the management of HIV infection.

The importance of complying with the full recommended dosing regimen should be stressed to all patients.

Agenerase oral solution is administered orally and can be taken with or without food.

Agenerase is also available as capsules. Amprenavir is 14 % less bioavailable from the Agenerase oral solution than from the capsules; therefore, Agenerase capsules and Agenerase oral solution are not interchangeable on a milligram per milligram basis (see section 5.2).

Patients should discontinue Agenerase oral solution as soon as they are able to swallow the capsule formulation (see section 4.4).

Patients of 4 years and older unable to swallow Agenerase capsules: the recommended dose of Agenerase oral solution is 17 mg (1.1 ml)/kg three times a day, in combination with other antiretroviral agents, without exceeding a total daily dose of 2800 mg.

The pharmacokinetic interactions between amprenavir and low doses of ritonavir or other protease inhibitors have not yet been evaluated in children. Additionally, as no dosing recommendations can be made regarding the concomitant use of Agenerase oral solution and low dose ritonavir, the use of this combination must be avoided in these patient populations.

Children less than 4 years of age: Agenerase oral solution is contraindicated in children less than 4 years of age. (see sections 4.3and 5.3).

Elderly: the pharmacokinetics, efficacy and safety of amprenavir have not been studied in patients over 65 years of age. (see section 5.2).

Renal impairment: although no dose adjustment is considered necessary for amprenavir, Agenerase oral solution is contraindicated in patients with renal failure (see section 4.3).

Hepatic impairment: Agenerase oral solution is contraindicated in patients with hepatic impairment or failure (see section 4.3) (see Summary of Product Characteristics of Agenerase Capsules for prescribing information)

4.3 Contraindications

Known hypersensitivity to amprenavir or any ingredient of Agenerase oral solution.

Because of the potential risk of toxicity from the large amount of the excipient propylene glycol, Agenerase oral solution is contraindicated in infants and children below the age of 4 years, pregnant women, patients with hepatic impairment or failure and patients with renal failure. Agenerase oral solution is also contraindicated in patients treated with disulfiram or other medicinal products that reduce alcohol metabolism (e.g. metronidazole) and preparations that contain alcohol (e.g. ritonavir oral solution) or additional propylene glycol (see section 4.4and 5.1).

Agenerase must not be administered concurrently with medicinal products with narrow therapeutic windows that are substrates of cytochrome P450 3A4 (CYP3A4). Co-administration may result in competitive inhibition of the metabolism of these medicinal products and create the potential for serious and/or life-threatening adverse events such as cardiac arrhythmia (e.g. terfenadine, astemizole, cisapride, pimozide), prolonged sedation or respiratory depression (e.g. triazolam, diazepam, flurazepam, midazolam), or peripheral vasospasm or ischaemia and ischaemia of other tissues, including cerebral or myocardial ischaemia (e.g. ergot derivatives).

Agenerase must not be given with rifampicin because rifampicin reduces trough plasma concentrations of amprenavir by approximately 92 % (see section 4.5).

Herbal preparations containing St John's wort (*Hypericum perforatum*) must not be used while taking amprenavir due to the risk of decreased plasma concentrations and reduced clinical effects of amprenavir (see section 4.5).

4.4 Special warnings and special precautions for use

Patients should be advised that Agenerase, or any other current antiretroviral therapy does not cure HIV and that they may still develop opportunistic infections and other complications of HIV infection. Current antiretroviral therapies, including Agenerase, have not been proven to prevent the risk of transmission of HIV to others through sexual contact or blood contamination. Appropriate precautions should continue to be taken.

On the basis of current pharmacodynamic data amprenavir should be used in combination with at least two other antiretrovirals. When amprenavir is administered as monotherapy, resistant viruses rapidly emerge (see section 5.1).

Liver Disease: The principal route of metabolism of amprenavir and the propylene glycol excipient is via the liver, Agenerase oral solution is contraindicated in patients with hepatic impairment or failure (see section 4.3).

Patients taking the oral solution of Agenerase, particularly those with renal impairment or those with decreased ability to metabolise propylene glycol (e.g. those of Asian origin), should be monitored for adverse reactions potentially related to the high propylene glycol content (550 mg/ml), such as seizures, stupor, tachycardia, hyperosmolarity, lactic acidosis, renal toxicity, haemolysis. For patients with renal failure, hepatic impairment or failure, children and pregnant women, see section 4.3. The concomitant administration of Agenerase oral solution with disulfiram or other medicinal products that reduce alcohol metabolism (e.g. metronidazole), or preparations that contain alcohol (e.g. ritonavir oral solution) or additional propylene glycol is contraindicated (see sections 4.3and 4.5).

Medicinal products – interactions

Amprenavir, like other HIV protease inhibitors, is an inhibitor of the cytochrome CYP3A4 enzyme. Agenerase should not be administered concurrently with medications with narrow therapeutic windows which are substrates of CYP3A4 (see section 4.3). Combination with other agents may result in serious and/or life-threatening interactions, therefore caution is advised whenever Agenerase is co-administered with medicinal products that are inducers, inhibitors or substrates of CYP3A4 (see section 4.5).

The HMG-CoA reductase inhibitors lovastatin and simvastatin are highly dependent on CYP3A4 for metabolism, thus concomitant use of Agenerase with simvastatin or lovastatin is not recommended due to an increased risk of myopathy, including rhabdomyolysis. Caution must also be exercised if Agenerase is used concurrently with atorvastatin, which is metabolized to a lesser extent by CYP3A4. In this situation, a reduced dose of atorvastatin should be considered. If treatment with a HMG-CoA reductase inhibitor is indicated, pravastatin or fluvastatin are recommended (see section 4.5).

For some medicinal products that can cause serious or life-threatening undesirable effects, such as amiodarone, phenobarbital, phenytoin, lidocaine (systemic), tricyclic antidepressants, quinidine and warfarin (monitor International Normalised Ratio), concentration monitoring is available; this should minimise the risk of potential safety problems with concomitant use.

Because of the potential for metabolic interactions with amprenavir, the efficacy of hormonal contraceptives may be modified, but there is insufficient information to predict the nature of the interactions. Therefore, alternative reliable methods of contraception are recommended for women of childbearing potential (see section 4.5).

Co-administration of amprenavir with methadone leads to a decrease of methadone concentrations. Therefore, when methadone is co-administered with amprenavir, patients should be monitored for opiate abstinence syndrome, in particular if low-dose ritonavir is also given. No recommendations can currently be made regarding adjustment of amprenavir dose when amprenavir is co-administered with methadone.

Agenerase oral solution contains vitamin E (46 IU/ml), therefore additional vitamin E supplementation is not recommended.

Rash / cutaneous reactions

Rashes/cutaneous reactions: most patients with mild or moderate rash can continue Agenerase. Appropriate antihistamines (e.g. cetirizine dihydrochloride) may reduce pruritus and hasten the resolution of rash. Agenerase should be permanently discontinued when rash is accompanied with systemic symptoms or allergic symptoms or mucosal involvement (see section 4.8).

Hyperglycaemia

New onset of diabetes mellitus, hyperglycaemia or exacerbations of existing diabetes mellitus have been reported in patients receiving antiretroviral therapy, including protease inhibitors. In some of these, the hyperglycaemia was severe and in some cases also associated with ketoacidosis. Many of the patients had confounding medical conditions, some of which required therapy with agents that have been associated with the development of diabetes mellitus or hyperglycaemia.

Lipodystrophy

Combination antiretroviral therapy has been associated with the redistribution of body fat (lipodystrophy) in HIV patients. The long-term consequences of these events are currently unknown. Knowledge about the mechanism is incomplete. A connection between visceral lipomatosis and protease inhibitors and lipoatrophy and nucleoside reverse transcriptase inhibitors has been hypothesised. A higher risk of lipodystrophy has been associated with individual factors such as older age, and with drug related factors such as longer duration of antiretroviral treatment and associated metabolic disturbances. Clinical examination should include evaluation for physical signs of fat redistribution. Consideration should be given to the measurement of fasting serum lipids and blood glucose. Lipid disorders should be managed as clinically appropriate (see section 4.8).

Haemophiliac patients

There have been reports of increased bleeding, including spontaneous skin haematomas and haemarthroses in haemophiliac patients type A and B treated with protease inhibitors. In some patients, additional factor VIII was given. In more than half of the reported cases, treatment with protease inhibitors was continued, or reintroduced if treatment had been discontinued. A causal relationship has been evoked, although the mechanism of action has not been elucidated. Haemophiliac patients should therefore be made aware of the possibility of increased bleeding.

Immune Reactivation Syndrome

In HIV-infected patients with severe immune deficiency at the time of institution of combination antiretroviral therapy (CART), an inflammatory reaction to asymptomatic or residual opportunistic pathogens may arise and cause serious clinical conditions, or aggravation of symptoms. Typically, such reactions have been observed within the first few weeks or months of initiation of CART. Relevant examples are cytomegalovirus retinitis, generalised and/or focal mycobacterium infections, and *Pneumocystis carinii* pneumonia. Any inflammatory symptoms should be evaluated and treatment instituted when necessary.

4.5 Interaction with other medicinal products and other forms of Interaction

Amprenavir is primarily metabolised in the liver by CYP3A4. Therefore, medicinal products that either share this metabolic pathway or modify CYP3A4 activity may modify the pharmacokinetics of amprenavir. Similarly, amprenavir might also modify the pharmacokinetics of other medicinal products that share this metabolic pathway.

Terfenadine, cisapride, pimozide, triazolam, diazepam, midazolam, flurazepam, ergotamine, dihydroergotamine and astemizole are contraindicated in patients receiving Agenerase. Concurrent administration can lead to competitive inhibition of the metabolism of these products and thus result in serious, life-threatening events (see section 4.3).

Of note, the following interaction data was obtained in adults.

Antiretroviral agents

• ***Protease inhibitors (PIs)***

Indinavir: the AUC, C_{min} and C_{max} of indinavir were decreased by 38 %, 27 %, and 22 %, respectively, when given with amprenavir. The clinical relevance of these changes is unknown. The AUC, C_{min} and C_{max} of amprenavir were increased by 33 %, 25 %, and 18 %, respectively. No dose adjustment is necessary for either medicinal product when indinavir is administered in combination with amprenavir.

Saquinavir: the AUC, C_{min} and C_{max} of saquinavir were decreased by 19 % and 48 % and increased by 21 %, respectively, when given with amprenavir. The clinical relevance of these changes is unknown. The AUC, C_{min} and C_{max} of amprenavir were decreased by 32 %, 14 % and 37 %, respectively. No dose adjustment is necessary for either medicinal product when saquinavir is administered in combination with amprenavir.

Nelfinavir: the AUC, C_{min} and C_{max} of nelfinavir were increased by 15 %, 14 %, and 12 % respectively when given with amprenavir. The C_{max} of amprenavir was decreased by 14 % whilst the AUC and C_{min} were increased by 9 % and 189 %, respectively. No dose adjustment is necessary for either medicinal product when nelfinavir is administered in combination with amprenavir (see also efavirenz below).

Ritonavir: the AUC and C_{min} of amprenavir were increased by 64% and 508% respectively and the C_{max} decreased by 30% when ritonavir (100 mg twice daily) was co-administered with amprenavir capsules (600 mg twice daily) compared to values achieved after 1200 mg twice daily doses of amprenavir capsules. In clinical trials, doses of amprenavir 600 mg twice daily and ritonavir 100 mg twice daily have been used; confirming the safety and efficacy of this regimen.

Agenerase oral solution and ritonavir oral solution should not be co-administered (see section 4.3).

Lopinavir / ritonavir (Kaletra): in an open-label, non-fasting pharmacokinetic study, the AUC, C_{max} and C_{min} of lopinavir were decreased by 38%, 28% and 52% respectively when amprenavir (750 mg twice daily) was given in combination with Kaletra (400 mg lopinavir + 100 mg ritonavir twice daily). In the same study, the AUC, C_{max}, and C_{min} of amprenavir were increased 72%, 12%, and 483%, respectively, when compared to values after standard doses of amprenavir (1200 mg twice daily).

The amprenavir plasma C_{min} values achieved with the combination of amprenavir (600 mg twice daily) in combination with Kaletra (400 mg lopinavir + 100 mg ritonavir twice daily) are approximately 40-50% lower than when amprenavir (600 mg twice daily) is given in combination with ritonavir 100 mg twice daily. Adding additional ritonavir to an amprenavir plus Kaletra regimen increase lopinavir C_{min} values, but not amprenavir C_{min} values. No dose recommendation can be given for the co-administration of amprenavir and Kaletra, but close monitoring is advised because the safety and efficacy of this combination is unknown.

• **Nucleoside analogue reverse transcriptase inhibitors (NRTIs):**

Zidovudine: the AUC and C_{max} of zidovudine were increased by 31 % and 40 %, respectively, when given with amprenavir. The AUC and the C_{max} of amprenavir were unaltered. No dose adjustment for either medicinal product is necessary when zidovudine is administered in combination with amprenavir.

Lamivudine: the AUC and C_{max} of lamivudine and amprenavir, respectively, were both unaltered when these two medicinal products were given concomitantly. No dose adjustment is necessary for either medicinal product when lamivudine is administered in combination with amprenavir.

Abacavir: the AUC, C_{min} and C_{max} of abacavir were unaltered when given with amprenavir. The AUC, C_{min}, and C_{max} of amprenavir were increased by 29 %, 27 %, and 47 % respectively. No dose adjustment is necessary for either medicinal product when abacavir is administered in combination with amprenavir.

Didanosine: no pharmacokinetic study has been performed with Agenerase in combination with didanosine, however, due to its antacid component, it is recommended that didanosine and Agenerase should be administered at least one hour apart (see Antacids below).

• *Non-nucleoside reverse transcriptase inhibitors (NNRTIs):*

Efavirenz: efavirenz has been seen to decrease the C_{max}, AUC, and $C_{min,ss}$ of amprenavir by approximately 40 % in adults. When amprenavir is combined with ritonavir, the effect of efavirenz is compensated by the pharmacokinetic booster effect of ritonavir. Therefore, if efavirenz is given in combination with amprenavir (600 mg twice daily) and ritonavir (100 mg twice daily), no dose adjustment is necessary.

Further, if efavirenz is given in combination with amprenavir and nelfinavir, no dosage adjustment is necessary for any of the medicinal products.

Treatment with efavirenz in combination with amprenavir and saquinavir is not recommended, as the exposure to both protease inhibitors would be decreased.

No dose recommendation can be given for the co-administration of amprenavir with another protease inhibitor and efavirenz in children.

Nevirapine: The effect of nevirapine on other protease inhibitors and the limited evidence available suggest that nevirapine may decrease the serum concentrations of amprenavir.

Delavirdine: the AUC, C_{max} and C_{min} of delavirdine were decreased by 61%, 47% and 88% respectively when given with amprenavir. The AUC, C_{max} and C_{min} of amprenavir were increased by 130%, 40% and 125% respectively.

No dose recommendations can be given for the co-administration of amprenavir and delavirdine. If these medicinal products are used concomitantly care is advised, as delavirdine may be less effective due to decreased and potentially sub-therapeutic plasma concentrations.

Antibiotics/antifungals

Rifampicin: rifampicin is a potent inducer of CYP3A4. Concomitant administration with amprenavir resulted in a reduction of amprenavir C_{min} and AUC by 92 % and 82 % respectively. Rifampicin must not be used concomitantly with amprenavir (see section 4.3).

Rifabutin: co-administration of amprenavir with rifabutin resulted in a 193 % increase in rifabutin AUC and an increase of rifabutin-related adverse events. The increase in rifabutin plasma concentration is likely to result from inhibition of rifabutin CYP3A4 mediated metabolism by amprenavir. When it is clinically necessary to co-administer rifabutin with Agenerase, a dosage reduction of at least half the recommended dose of rifabutin is advised, although no clinical data are available.

Clarithromycin: the AUC and C_{min} of clarithromycin were unaltered and the C_{max} decreased by 10 % when given with amprenavir. The AUC, C_{min} and C_{max} of amprenavir were increased by 18 %, 39 %, and 15 % respectively. No dose adjustment is necessary for either medicinal product when clarithromycin is administered in combination with amprenavir.

Erythromycin: no pharmacokinetic study has been performed with Agenerase in combination with erythromycin, however, plasma levels of both medicinal products may be increased when co-administered.

Ketoconazole: the AUC and C_{max} of ketoconazole were increased by 44 % and 19 % respectively when given with amprenavir. The AUC and C_{max} of amprenavir were increased by 31 % and decreased by 16 % respectively. No dose adjustment for either medicinal product is necessary when ketoconazole is administered in combination with amprenavir.

Metronidazole: Agenerase oral solution is contraindicated in patients treated with metronidazole (see section 4.3).

Other possible interactions

Other medicinal products, listed below, including examples of substrates, inhibitors or inducers of CYP3A4, may lead to interactions when administered with Agenerase. The clinical significance of these possible interactions is not known and has not been investigated. Patients should therefore be monitored for toxic reactions associated with these medicinal products when these are administered in combination with Agenerase.

Alcohol and inhibitors of alcohol metabolism: Agenerase oral solution contains propylene glycol (550 mg/ml), which is primarily metabolised via alcohol dehydrogenase. Therefore, concomitant administration with disulfiram or other medicinal products that reduce alcohol metabolism (e.g. metronidazole) or preparations that contain alcohol (e.g. ritonavir oral solution) or propylene glycol is contraindicated (see sections 4.3 and 4.4).

Antacids: on the basis of the data for other protease inhibitors, it is advisable not to take antacids at the same time as Agenerase, since its absorption may be impaired. It is recommended that antacids and Agenerase should be administered at least one hour apart.

Benzodiazepines: the serum concentrations of alprazolam, triazolam, midazolam, clonazepam, diazepam and flurazepam may be increased by amprenavir resulting in enhanced sedation (see section 4.3).

Calcium-channel blockers: amprenavir may lead to increased serum concentrations of diltiazem, nicardipine, nifedipine or nimodipine, possibly resulting in enhanced activity and toxicity of these medicinal products.

Erectile dysfunction agents: based on data for other protease inhibitors caution should be used when prescribing sildenafil to patients receiving Agenerase. Co-administration of Agenerase with sildenafil may substantially increase sildenafil plasma concentrations and may result in sildenafil-associated adverse events.

HMG-CoA reductase inhibitors: HMG-CoA reductase inhibitors which are highly dependent on CYP3A4 for metabolism, such as lovastatin and simvastatin, are expected to have markedly increased plasma concentrations when co-administered with Agenerase. Since increased concentrations of HMG-CoA reductase inhibitors may cause myopathy, including rhabdomyolysis, the combination of these medicinal products with Agenerase is not recommended. Atorvastatin is less dependent on CYP3A4 for metabolism. When used with Agenerase, the lowest possible dose of atorvastatin should be administered. The metabolism of pravastatin and fluvastatin is not dependent on CYP3A4, and interactions are not expected with protease inhibitors. If treatment with a HMG-CoA reductase inhibitor is indicated, pravastatin or fluvastatin is recommended.

Methadone and opiate derivatives: co-administration of methadone with amprenavir resulted in a decrease in the C_{mxc} and AUC of the active methadone enantiomer (R-enantiomer) of 25% and 13% respectively, whilst the C_{max}, AUC and C_{min} of the inactive methadone enantiomer (S-enantiomer) were decreased by 48%, 40% and 23% respectively. When methadone is co-administered with amprenavir, patients should be monitored for opiate abstinence syndrome, in particular if low-dose ritonavir is also given.

As compared to a non-matched historical control group, co-administration of methadone and amprenavir resulted in a 30%, 27% and 25% decrease in serum amprenavir AUC, C_{max} and C_{min} respectively. No recommendations can currently be made regarding adjustment of amprenavir dose when amprenavir is co-administered with methadone due to the inherent low reliability of non-matched historical controls.

Steroids: oestrogens, progestogens and some glucocorticoids may interact with amprenavir. However, the information currently available is not sufficient for determining the nature of the interaction. Co-administration of Ortho-Novum 1/35 (0.035 mg ethinyl estradiol plus 1.0 mg norethindrone) resulted in a decrease of the amprenavir AUC and C_{min} of 22% and 20% respectively, C_{max} being unchanged. The C_{min} of ethinyl estradiol was increased by 32%, whilst the AUC and C_{min} of norethindrone were increased by 18% and 45% respectively. Alternative methods of contraception are recommended for women of childbearing potential.

St John's wort: serum levels of amprenavir can be reduced by concomitant use of the herbal preparation St John's wort (*Hypericum perforatum*). This is due to induction of drug metabolising enzymes by St John's wort. Herbal preparations containing St John's wort should therefore not be combined with Agenerase. If a patient is already taking St John's wort, check amprenavir and if possible viral levels and stop St John's wort. Amprenavir levels may increase on stopping St John's wort. The dose of amprenavir may need adjusting. The inducing effect may persist for at least 2 weeks after cessation of treatment with St John's wort (see section 4.3).

Other substances: plasma concentrations of other substances may be increased by amprenavir. These include substances such as: clozapine, carbamazepine, cimetidine, dapsone, itraconazole and loratadine.

4.6 Pregnancy and lactation

Pregnancy: the safe use of amprenavir in human pregnancy has not been established. Agenerase oral solution should not be used during pregnancy due to the potential risk of toxicity to the foetus from the propylene glycol content (see section 4.3).

Lactation: amprenavir-related material was found in rat milk, but it is not known whether amprenavir is excreted in human milk. A reproduction study in pregnant rats dosed from the time of uterine implantation through lactation showed reduced body weight gains in the offspring during the nursing period. The systemic exposure to the dams associated with this finding was similar to exposure in humans, following administration of the recommended dose. The subsequent development of the offspring, including fertility and reproductive performance, was not affected by the maternal administration of amprenavir.

It is therefore recommended that mothers being treated with Agenerase do not breast-feed their infants. Additionally, it is recommended that HIV infected women do not breast-feed their infants in order to avoid transmission of HIV.

4.7 Effects on ability to drive and use machines

No studies on the effects on ability to drive and use machines have been performed.

4.8 Undesirable effects

The safety of Agenerase has been studied in adults and children of at least 4 years of age in controlled clinical trials, in combination with various other antiretroviral agents. Adverse events considered associated with the use of Agenerase are gastro-intestinal symptoms, rash and oral/peri-oral paraesthesia. Most undesirable effects associated with Agenerase therapy were mild to moderate in severity, early in onset, and rarely treatment limiting. For many of these events it is unclear whether they are related to Agenerase, to concomitant treatment used in the management of HIV disease or to the disease process.

In children, the nature of the safety profile is similar to that seen in adults.

Adverse reactions are listed below by MedDRA body system organ class and by frequency. The frequency categories used are:

Very common $\geqslant$ 1 in 10

Common $\geqslant$ 1 in 100 and $<$ 1 in 10

Uncommon $\geqslant$ 1 in 1,000 and $<$ 1 in 100

Rare $\geqslant$1 in 10,000 and $<$ 1 in 1,000

Frequency categories for the events below have been based on clinical trials and postmarketing data.

Most of the adverse events below come from two clinical trials (PROAB3001, PROAB3006) involving PI naïve subjects receiving Agenerase 1200mg twice daily. Events (grade 2-4) reported by study investigators as attributable to study medication and occurring in $>$1% of patients, are included as well as grade 3-4 treatment emergent laboratory abnormalities. Note that the background rates in comparator groups were not taken into account.

Metabolism and nutrition disorders

Common: Elevated triglycerides, elevated amylase, abnormal fat redistribution, anorexia

Uncommon: Hyperglycaemia, hypercholesterolaemia

Elevated triglycerides, elevated amylase and hyperglycaemia (grade 3-4) were reported primarily in patients with abnormal values at baseline.

Elevations in cholesterol were of grade 3-4 intensity.

Combination antiretroviral therapy has been associated with redistribution of body fat (lipodystrophy) in HIV patients including the loss of peripheral and facial subcutaneous fat, increased intra-abdominal and visceral fat, breast hypertrophy and dorsocervical fat accumulation (buffalo hump).

Symptoms of abnormal fat redistribution were infrequent in PROAB3001 with amprenavir. Only one case (a buffalo hump) was reported in 113 ($<$ 1 %) antiretroviral naive subjects treated with amprenavir in combination with lamivudine/zidovudine for a median duration of 36 weeks. In study PROAB3006, seven cases (3 %) were reported in 245 NRTI-experienced subjects treated with amprenavir and in 27 (11 %) of 241 subjects treated with indinavir, in combination with various NRTIs for a median duration of 56 weeks ($p < 0.001$).

Combination antiretroviral therapy has been associated with metabolic abnormalities such as hypertriglyceridaemia, hypercholesterolaemia, insulin resistance, hyperglycaemia and hyperlactataemia (see section 4.4).

Psychiatric disorders

Common: Mood disorders, depressive disorders

Nervous system disorders

Very Common: Headache

Common: Oral/perioral paraesthesia, tremors, sleep disorders

Gastrointestinal disorders

Very Common: Diarrhoea, nausea, flatulence, vomiting

Common: Abdominal pain, abdominal discomfort, dyspeptic symptoms, loose stools

Hepatobiliary disorders

Common: Elevated transaminases

Uncommon: Hyperbilirubinaemia

Elevated transaminases and hyperbilirubinaemia (grade 3-4) were reported primarily in patients with abnormal values at baseline. Almost all subjects with abnormal liver function tests were co-infected with Hepatitis B or C virus.

Skin and subcutaneous tissue disorders

Very Common: Rash

Rare: Stevens Johnson syndrome

Rashes were usually mild to moderate, erythematous or maculopapular cutaneous eruptions, with or without pruritus, occurring during the second week of therapy and resolving spontaneously within two weeks, without discontinuation of treatment with amprenavir. A higher incidence of rash was reported in patients treated with amprenavir in combination with efavirenz. Severe or life-threatening skin reactions have also occurred in patients treated with amprenavir (see section 4.4).

Musculoskeletal and connective tissue disorders

Increased CPK, myalgia, myositis, and rarely rhabdomyolysis have been reported with protease inhibitors, particularly in combination with nucleoside analogues.

General disorders and administration site conditions

Very Common: Fatigue

In HIV-infected patients with severe immune deficiency at the time of initiation of combination antiretroviral therapy (CART), an inflammatory reaction to asymptomatic or residual opportunistic infections may arise (see section 4.4).

Limited experience with Agenerase oral solution indicate a similar safety profile as for the capsules. In PI experienced patients receiving Agenerase capsules 600 mg twice daily and low dose ritonavir, 100 mg twice daily, the nature and frequency of adverse events (grade 2-4) and Grade 3/4 laboratory abnormalities were similar to those observed with Agenerase alone, with the exception of elevated triglyceride levels, and elevated CPK levels which were very common in patients receiving Agenerase and low dose ritonavir.

4.9 Overdose

There are limited reports of overdose with Agenerase. If overdose occurs, the patient should be monitored for evidence of toxicity (see section 4.8), and standard supportive treatment provided as necessary. Agenerase oral solution contains a large amount of propylene glycol (see section 4.4). In the event of overdosage, monitoring and management of acid-base abnormalities are recommended. Propylene glycol can be removed by hemodialysis. However, since amprenavir is highly protein bound, dialysis is unlikely to be helpful in reducing blood levels of amprenavir.

5. PHARMACOLOGICAL PROPERTIES

5.1 Pharmacodynamic properties

Pharmacotherapeutic group: protease inhibitor; ATC Code: JO5A E05

Amprenavir is a competitive inhibitor of the HIV protease. It blocks the ability of the viral protease to cleave the precursor polyproteins necessary for viral replication.

Amprenavir is a potent and selective inhibitor of HIV-1 and HIV-2 replication *in vitro*. In isolated experimental settings, synergy was shown *in vitro* in combination with nucleoside analogues including didanosine, zidovudine, abacavir and the protease inhibitor, saquinavir. It has been shown to have an additive effect in combination with indinavir, ritonavir and nelfinavir.

Serial passage experiments have demonstrated the protease mutation I50V to be key to the development of amprenavir resistance *in vitro*, with the triple variant, I50V+M46I/L+I47V, resulting in a greater than 10-fold increase in IC_{50} to amprenavir. This triple mutation resistance profile has not been observed with other protease inhibitors either from *in vitro* studies or in clinical settings. *In vitro* variants resistant to amprenavir remained sensitive to saquinavir, indinavir and nelfinavir, but showed three to five-fold reduced susceptibility to ritonavir. The triple mutant, I50V+M46I/L+I47V, was unstable during *in vitro* passage in the presence of saquinavir, with loss of the I47V mutation, and the development of resistance to saquinavir resulted in resensitisation to amprenavir. Passage of the triple mutant in either indinavir, nelfinavir or ritonavir resulted in additional protease mutations being selected, leading to dual resistance. Mutation I84V, observed transiently *in vitro* has rarely been selected during amprenavir therapy.

The resistance profile seen with amprenavir in clinical practice is different from that observed with other protease inhibitors. Consistent with *in vitro* experiments, the development of amprenavir resistance during therapy, is in the majority cases, associated with the mutation I50V. However, three alternative mechanisms have also been observed to result in the development of amprenavir resistance in the clinic, and involve either mutations I54L/M or V32I+I47V or, rarely, I84V. Each of the four genetic patterns produces viruses with reduced susceptibility to amprenavir, some cross-resistance to ritonavir, but susceptibility to indinavir, nelfinavir and saquinavir is retained.

The following table summarises the mutations associated with the development of reduced phenotypic susceptibility to amprenavir in subjects treated with amprenavir.

Protease mutations acquired on amprenavir-containing therapy which have been demonstrated to result in reduced phenotypic susceptibility to amprenavir:
I50V or I54L/M or I84V or V32I with I47V

The pre-existence of resistance to other components of a first-line PI-containing regimen is significantly associated with subsequent development of protease mutations, highlighting the importance of considering all components of a treatment regimen when change is indicated.

Many *in vitro* PI-resistant variants, and 322 of 433 (74%) clinical PI-resistant variants with multiple protease inhibitor resistance mutations were susceptible to amprenavir. The principal protease mutation associated with cross-resistance to amprenavir following treatment failure with other protease inhibitors was I84V, particularly when mutations L10I/V/F were also present.

In multiple protease inhibitor-experienced subjects, the likelihood of a successful virological response is increased with an increasing number of active drugs (ie. agents to which the virus is susceptible) in the rescue regimen. The presence at the time of therapy change in PI-experienced subjects of multiple key mutations associated with PI-resistance, or the development of such mutations during PI therapy, is significantly associated with treatment outcome. The total number of all types of protease mutations present at the time of therapy change was also correlated with outcome in PI-experienced populations. The presence of 3 or more mutations from M46I/L, I54L/M/V, V82A/F/I/T, I84V and L90M in a population of multiple PI-experienced subjects was significantly related to amprenavir treatment failure.

The following table summarises the mutations, identified in clinical isolates from highly PI- experienced patients, associated with an increased risk of treatment failure of amprenavir-containing regimens.

Protease mutations in virus from PI-experienced patients associated with reduced virological response to subsequent amprenavir containing regimens:
COMBINATION OF AT LEAST THREE OF: M46I/L or I54L/M/V or V82A/F/I/T or I84V or L90M.

The number of key PI-resistance mutations increases markedly the longer a failing PI-containing regimen is continued. Early discontinuation of failing therapies is recommended in order to limit the accumulation of multiple mutations, which may be detrimental to a subsequent rescue regimen.

Amprenavir is not recommended for use as monotherapy, due to the rapid emergence of resistant virus.

Cross resistance between amprenavir and reverse transcriptase inhibitors, is unlikely to occur because the enzyme targets are different.

Clinical experience:

Agenerase in combination with low dose ritonavir and nucleoside analogues (NRTI) has been shown to be effective in the treatment of PI-experienced HIV–1 infected adults.

In a randomised, open-label study in PI-experienced adults experiencing virological failure (viral load $\geqslant$1000 copies/ml), Agenerase (600 mg twice daily) / ritonavir (100 mg twice daily) was compared to other PIs. The study comprised two separate components. Analyses described are intent to treat (Exposed).

Sub-study A (n=163) compared Agenerase / ritonavir to other, predominantly ritonavir boosted PIs, in a standard of care regimen, in patients with virus sensitive to Agenerase, at least one other PI, and at least one NRTI. After 16 weeks, the antiviral response to Agenerase/ritonavir, as measured by time-averaged change from baseline in plasma HIV-1 RNA (AAUCMB), was shown to be non-inferior to that in the patients in the other PI treatment group [mean plasma HIV-1 RNA AAUCMB 1.315 $\log_{10}$ copies/ml and 1.343 $\log_{10}$ copies/ml respectively, mean stratified difference 0.043 $\log_{10}$ copies/ml (95% CI: –0.25, 0.335), ITT(E) population, Observed analysis]. The proportion of subjects with plasma HIV-1 RNA $<$400 copies/ml was similar across the treatment groups (66% and 70% respectively).

Sub-study B (n=43) compared Agenerase / ritonavir to continued current PI therapy in patients with virus resistant to indinavir, ritonavir, nelfinavir and saquinavir. Agenerase/ritonavir demonstrated superior efficacy as measured by AAUCMB after four weeks [mean strata adjusted treatment difference –0.669 $\log_{10}$ copies/ml (95% CI -0.946, -0.391), p=0.00002, ITT(E) population, Observed analysis]. Additionally, the proportion of subjects with plasma HIV-1 RNA below 400 copies/ml was higher in the Agenerase/ritonavir group (48%) than in the group maintained on the PI regimen current at study start (0%), p=0.00048.

Agenerase without low dose ritonavir in combination with other antiretroviral agents including nucleoside analogues, non-nucleoside analogues and protease inhibitors, has been shown to be effective in antiretroviral naïve and NRTI-experienced PI-naïve HIV-1 infected adults and heavily pre-treated children aged 4 years or more.

In a double-blind study in antiretroviral naive HIV-infected adults (n = 232), amprenavir (1200 mg twice daily) in combination with zidovudine and lamivudine was significantly superior to zidovudine and lamivudine. In an intent-to-treat analysis (any missing value or premature discontinuation considered as failure i.e. $\geqslant$ 400 copies/ml), the proportion of subjects with plasma HIV-1 RNA $<$ 400 copies/ml through week 48 was 41 % in the amprenavir/lamivudine/zidovudine group and 3 % in the lamivudine/zidovudine group ($p < 0.001$).

In an open-label randomised study in NRTI-experienced PI-naive adults (n = 504), in combination with various NRTIs amprenavir (1200 mg twice daily) was found to be less effective than indinavir: the proportion of subjects with plasma HIV-1 RNA $<$ 400 copies/ml at week 48 was 30 % in the amprenavir arm and 46 % in the indinavir arm in the intent-to-treat analysis (any missing value or premature discontinuation considered as failure, i.e. $\geqslant$ 400 copies/ml).

Results from two paediatric studies with amprenavir oral solution and/or capsules in 268 heavily pre-treated children aged 2 to 18 years indicate that amprenavir is an effective antiretroviral agent in children. Decreases in median HIV-1 RNA greater than 1 $\log_{10}$ copies/ml were observed in protease inhibitor naive subjects and improvements in immune category (CD4 %) were reported.

The use of Agenerase, without the boosting effect of low dose ritonavir, has not been sufficiently studied in heavily pretreated protease inhibitor experienced patients.

5.2 Pharmacokinetic properties

Absorption: after oral administration, amprenavir is rapidly and well absorbed. The absolute bioavailability is unknown due to the lack of an acceptable intravenous formulation for use in man. Approximately 90 % of an orally administered radiolabelled amprenavir dose was recovered in the urine and the faeces, primarily as amprenavir metabolites. Following oral administration, the mean time (t_{max}) to maximal serum concentrations of amprenavir is between 1-2 hours for the capsule and 0.5 to 1 hour for the oral solution. A second peak is observed after 10 to 12 hours and may represent either delayed absorption or enterohepatic recirculation.

At therapeutic dosages (1200 mg twice daily), the mean maximum steady state concentration ($C_{max,ss}$) of amprenavir capsules is 5.36 μg/ml (0.92-9.81) and the minimum steady state concentration ($C_{min,ss}$) is 0.28 μg/ml (0.12-0.51). The mean AUC over a dosing interval of 12 hours is 18.46 μg.h/ml (3.02-32.95). The 50 mg and 150 mg capsules have been shown to be bioequivalent. The bioavailability of the oral solution at equivalent doses is lower than that of the capsules, with an AUC and C_{max} approximately 14 % and 19 % lower, respectively (see section 4.2).

While administration of amprenavir with food results in a 25 % reduction in AUC, it had no effect on the concentration of amprenavir 12 hours after dosing (C_{12}). Therefore, although food affects the extent and rate of absorption, the steady-state trough concentration ($C_{min,ss}$) was not affected by food intake.

Distribution: the apparent volume of distribution is approximately 430 litres (6 l/kg assuming a 70 kg body weight), suggesting a large volume of distribution, with penetration of amprenavir freely into tissues beyond the systemic circulation. The concentration of amprenavir in the cerebrospinal fluid is less than 1 % of plasma concentration.

In *in vitro* studies, the protein binding of amprenavir is approximately 90 %. Amprenavir is primarily bound to the alpha–1-acid glycoprotein (AAG), but also to albumin. Concentrations of AAG have been shown to decrease during the course of antiretroviral therapy. This change will decrease the total active substance concentration in the plasma, however the amount of unbound amprenavir, which is the active moiety, is likely to be unchanged. While absolute free active substance concentrations remain constant, the percent of free active substance will fluctuate directly with total active substance concentrations at steady-state go from $C_{max,ss}$ to $C_{min,ss}$ over the course of the dosing interval. This will result in a fluctuation in the apparent volume of distribution of total active substance, but the volume of distribution of free active substance does not change.

Clinically significant binding displacement interactions involving medicinal products primarily bound to AAG are generally not observed. Therefore, interactions with amprenavir due to protein binding displacement are highly unlikely.

Metabolism: amprenavir is primarily metabolised by the liver with less than 3 % excreted unchanged in the urine. The primary route of metabolism is via the cytochrome P450 CYP3A4 enzyme. Amprenavir is a substrate of and inhibits CYP3A4. Therefore medicinal products that are inducers, inhibitors or substrates of CYP3A4 must be used with caution when administered concurrently with Agenerase (see sections 4.3, 4.4 and 4.5).

Elimination: the plasma elimination half-life of amprenavir ranges from 7.1 to 10.6 hours. Following multiple oral doses of amprenavir (1200 mg twice a day), there is no significant active substance accumulation. The primary route of elimination of amprenavir is via hepatic metabolism with less than 3 % excreted unchanged in the urine. The metabolites and unchanged amprenavir account for approximately 14 % of the administered amprenavir dose in the urine, and approximately 75 % in the faeces.

Special populations:

Paediatrics: the pharmacokinetics of amprenavir in children (4 years of age and above) are similar to those in adults. Dosages of 20 mg/kg twice a day and 15 mg/kg three times a day with Agenerase capsules provided similar daily amprenavir exposure to 1200 mg twice a day in adults. Amprenavir is 14 % less bioavailable from the oral solution than from the capsules; therefore, Agenerase capsules and Agenerase oral solution are not interchangeable on a milligram per milligram basis.

Elderly: the pharmacokinetics of amprenavir have not been studied in patients over 65 years of age.

Renal impairment: patients with renal impairment have not been specifically studied. Less than 3 % of the therapeutic dose of amprenavir is excreted unchanged in the urine. The impact of renal impairment on amprenavir elimination should be minimal, therefore, no initial dose adjustment is considered necessary.

Hepatic impairment: the pharmacokinetics of amprenavir are significantly altered in patients with moderate to severe hepatic impairment. The AUC increased nearly three fold in patients with moderate impairment and four fold in patients with severe hepatic impairment. Clearance also decreased in a corresponding manner to the AUC. Agenerase oral solution should not be used in patients with hepatic impairment or failure (see section 4.3).

5.3 Preclinical safety data

In long-term carcinogenicity studies with amprenavir in mice and rats, there were benign hepatocellular adenomas in males at exposure levels equivalent to 2.0-fold (mice) or 3.8-fold (rats) those in humans given 1200 mg twice daily of amprenavir alone. In male mice altered hepatocellular foci were seen at doses that were at least 2.0 times human therapeutic exposure.

A higher incidence of hepatocellular carcinoma was seen in all amprenavir male mouse treatment groups. However, this increase was not statistically significantly different from male control mice by appropriate tests. The mechanism for the hepatocellular adenomas and carcinomas found in these studies has not been elucidated and the significance of the observed effects for humans is uncertain. However, there is little evidence from the exposure data in humans, both in clinical trials and from marketed use, to suggest that these findings are of clinical significance.

Amprenavir was not mutagenic or genotoxic in a battery of *in vivo* and *in vitro* genetic toxicity assays, including bacterial reverse mutation (Ames Test), mouse lymphoma, rat micronucleus, and chromosome aberration in human peripheral lymphocytes.

In toxicological studies with mature animals, the clinically relevant findings were mostly confined to the liver and gastrointestinal disturbances. Liver toxicity consisted of increases in liver enzymes, liver weights and microscopic findings including hepatocyte necrosis. This liver toxicity can be monitored for and detected in clinical use, with measurements of AST, ALT and alkaline phosphatase activity. However, significant liver toxicity has not been observed in patients treated in clinical studies, either during administration of Agenerase or after discontinuation.

Amprenavir did not affect fertility. Local toxicity and sensitising potential was absent in animal studies, but slight irritating properties to the rabbit eye were identified.

Toxicity studies in young animals, treated from four days of age, resulted in high mortality in both the control animals and those receiving amprenavir. These results imply that young animals lack fully developed metabolic pathways enabling them to excrete amprenavir or some critical components of the formulation (e.g. propylene glycol, PEG 400). However, the possibility of anaphylactic reaction related to PEG 400 cannot be excluded. In clinical studies, the safety and efficacy of amprenavir have not yet been established in children below four years of age.

In pregnant mice, rabbits and rats there were no major effects on embryo-foetal development. However, at systemic plasma exposures significantly below (rabbits) or not significantly higher (rat) than the expected human exposures during therapeutic dosing, a number of minor changes, including thymic elongation and minor skeletal variations were seen, indicating developmental delay. A dose-dependent increase in placental weight was found in the rabbit and rat which may indicate effects on placental function. It is therefore recommended that women of childbearing potential taking Agenerase should practice effective contraception (e.g. barrier methods).

6. PHARMACEUTICAL PARTICULARS

6.1 List of excipients

Propylene glycol, macrogol 400 (PEG 400), d-alpha tocopheryl polyethylene glycol 1000 succinate, acesulfame potassium, saccharin sodium, sodium chloride, artificial grape bubblegum flavour, natural peppermint flavour, menthol, citric acid, anhydrous, sodium citrate dihydrate, purified water.

6.2 Incompatibilities

Not applicable.

6.3 Shelf life

3 years.

6.4 Special precautions for storage

Do not store above 25°C.

Discard the oral solution 15 days after first opening the bottle.

6.5 Nature and contents of container

White High Density Polyethylene (HDPE) bottles containing 240 ml of oral solution. A 20 ml measuring cup is provided in the pack.

6.6 Instructions for use and handling

No special requirements.

Administrative Data

7. MARKETING AUTHORISATION HOLDER

Glaxo Group Ltd

Greenford Road

Greenford

Middlesex UB6 0NN

United Kingdom

8. MARKETING AUTHORISATION NUMBER(S)

EU/1/00/148/004

9. DATE OF FIRST AUTHORISATION/RENEWAL OF THE AUTHORISATION

20th October 2000

10. DATE OF REVISION OF THE TEXT

17 December 2004

Agenerase 50mg Soft Capsules

(GlaxoSmithKline UK)

1. NAME OF THE MEDICINAL PRODUCT

Agenerase 50 mg soft capsules

2. QUALITATIVE AND QUANTITATIVE COMPOSITION

Each capsule contains 50 mg of amprenavir.

For excipients, see section 6.1.

3. PHARMACEUTICAL FORM

Soft capsule.

The soft capsules are oblong, opaque, off-white to cream coloured, printed with 'GX CC1'.

4. CLINICAL PARTICULARS

4.1 Therapeutic indications

Agenerase, in combination with other antiretroviral agents, is indicated for the treatment of protease inhibitor (PI) experienced HIV-1 infected adults and children above the age of 4 years. Agenerase capsules should normally be administered with low dose ritonavir as a pharmacokinetic enhancer of amprenavir (see sections 4.2 and 4.5). The choice of amprenavir should be based on individual viral resistance testing and treatment history of patients (see section 5.1).

The benefit of Agenerase boosted with ritonavir has not been demonstrated in PI naïve patients (see section 5.1)

4.2 Posology and method of administration

Therapy should be initiated by a physician experienced in the management of HIV infection.

The importance of complying with the full recommended dosing regimen should be stressed to all patients.

Agenerase is administered orally and can be taken with or without food.

Agenerase is also available as an oral solution for use in children or adults unable to swallow capsules. Amprenavir is 14 % less bioavailable from the oral solution than from the capsules; therefore, Agenerase capsules and Agenerase oral solution are not interchangeable on a milligram per milligram basis (see section 5.2).

Adults and adolescents of 12 years of age and older (greater than 50 kg body weight): the recommended dose of Agenerase capsules is 600 mg twice daily with ritonavir, 100 mg twice daily, in combination with other antiretroviral agents.

If Agenerase capsules are used without the boosting effect of ritonavir higher doses of Agenerase (1200 mg twice daily) should be used.

Children (4 to 12 years) and patients less than 50 kg body weight: the recommended dose of Agenerase capsules is 20 mg/kg body weight twice a day, in combination with other antiretroviral agents, without exceeding a total daily dose of 2400 mg.

The pharmacokinetics, efficacy and safety of Agenerase in combination with low doses of ritonavir or other protease inhibitors have not yet been evaluated in children. Therefore, such combinations should be avoided in children.

Children less than 4 years of age: Agenerase is not recommended in children less than 4 years of age (see section 5.3).

Elderly: the pharmacokinetics, efficacy and safety of amprenavir have not been studied in patients over 65 years of age (see section 5.2).

Renal impairment: no dose adjustment is considered necessary in patients with renal impairment (see section 5.2).

Hepatic impairment: the principal route of metabolism of amprenavir is via the liver. Agenerase capsules should be used with caution in patients with hepatic impairment. Clinical efficacy and safety have not been determined in this patient group. For subjects with hepatic impairment, pharmacokinetic data are available for the use of Agenerase capsules without the boosting effect of ritonavir. Based on pharmacokinetic data, the dose of Agenerase capsules should be reduced to 450 mg twice a day for adult patients with moderate hepatic impairment and to 300 mg twice a day for adult patients with severe hepatic impairment. No dose recommendation can be made in children with hepatic impairment (see section 5.2).

The use of amprenavir in combination with ritonavir has not been studied in patients with hepatic impairment. No dose recommendations can be made regarding this combination. Concomitant administration should be used with caution in patients with mild and moderate hepatic impairment and is contraindicated in patients with severe hepatic impairment (see section 4.3).

4.3 Contraindications

Known hypersensitivity to amprenavir or any ingredient of Agenerase capsules.

Agenerase must not be administered concurrently with medicinal products with narrow therapeutic windows that are substrates of cytochrome P450 3A4 (CYP3A4). Co-administration may result in competitive inhibition of the metabolism of these medicinal products and create the potential for serious and/or life-threatening adverse events such as cardiac arrhythmia (e.g. terfenadine, astemizole, cisapride, pimozide), prolonged sedation or respiratory depression (e.g. triazolam, diazepam, flurazepam, midazolam), or peripheral vasospasm or ischaemia and ischaemia of other tissues, including cerebral or myocardial ischaemia (e.g. ergot derivatives).

Agenerase in combination with ritonavir is contraindicated in patients with severe hepatic impairment.

Agenerase must not be given with rifampicin because rifampicin reduces trough plasma concentrations of amprenavir by approximately 92 % (see section 4.5).

Herbal preparations containing St John's wort (*Hypericum perforatum*) must not be used while taking amprenavir due to the risk of decreased plasma concentrations and reduced clinical effects of amprenavir (see section 4.5).

4.4 Special warnings and special precautions for use

Patients should be advised that Agenerase, or any other current antiretroviral therapy does not cure HIV and that they may still develop opportunistic infections and other complications of HIV infection. Current antiretroviral therapies, including Agenerase, have not been proven to prevent the risk of transmission of HIV to others through sexual contact or blood contamination. Appropriate precautions should continue to be taken.

On the basis of current pharmacodynamic data, amprenavir should be used in combination with at least two other antiretrovirals. When amprenavir is administered as monotherapy, resistant viruses rapidly emerge (see section 5.1). Agenerase capsules should normally be given in combination with low dose ritonavir and in combination with other antiretroviral agents (see section 4.2).

Liver Disease: The safety and efficacy of amprenavir has not been established in patients with significant underlying liver disorders. Agenerase capsules are contraindicated in patients with severe hepatic impairment when used in combination with ritonavir (see section 4.3). Patients with chronic hepatitis B or C and treated with combination antiretroviral therapy are at an increased risk of severe and potentially fatal hepatic adverse events. In case of concomitant antiviral therapy for hepatitis B or C, please refer also to the relevant product information for these medicinal products.

Patients with pre-existing liver dysfunction, including chronic active hepatitis, have an increased frequency of liver function abnormalities during combination antiretroviral therapy and should be monitored according to standard practice. If there is evidence of worsening liver disease in such patients, interruption or discontinuation of treatment must be considered.

Medicinal products – interactions

Amprenavir, like other HIV protease inhibitors, is an inhibitor of the cytochrome CYP3A4 enzyme. Agenerase should not be administered concurrently with medications with narrow therapeutic windows which are substrates of CYP3A4 (see section 4.3). Combination with other agents may result in serious and/or life-threatening interactions, therefore caution is advised whenever Agenerase is co-administered with medicinal products that are inducers, inhibitors or substrates of CYP3A4 (see section 4.5).

Caution should be exercised when prescribing Agenerase and ritonavir concomitantly with CYP2D6 substrates with a narrow therapeutic index, i.e. flecainide, propafenone and metoprolol (when used in cardiac insufficiency).

The HMG-CoA reductase inhibitors lovastatin and simvastatin are highly dependent on CYP3A4 for metabolism, thus concomitant use of Agenerase with simvastatin or lovastatin is not recommended due to an increased risk of myopathy, including rhabdomyolysis. Caution must also be exercised if Agenerase is used concurrently with atorvastatin, which is metabolized to a lesser extent by CYP3A4. In this situation, a reduced dose of atorvastatin should be considered. If treatment with a HMG-CoA reductase inhibitor is indicated, pravastatin or fluvastatin are recommended (see section 4.5).

For some medicinal products that can cause serious or life-threatening undesirable effects, such as amiodarone, phenobarbital, phenytoin, lidocaine (systemic), tricyclic antidepressants, quinidine and warfarin (monitor International Normalised Ratio), concentration monitoring is available; this should minimise the risk of potential safety problems with concomitant use.

Because of the potential for metabolic interactions with amprenavir, the efficacy of hormonal contraceptives may be modified, but there is insufficient information to predict the nature of the interactions. Therefore, alternative reliable methods of contraception are recommended for women of childbearing potential (see section 4.5).

Co-administration of amprenavir with methadone leads to a decrease of methadone concentrations. Therefore, when methadone is co-administered with amprenavir, patients should be monitored for opiate abstinence syndrome, in particular if low-dose ritonavir is also given. No recommendations can currently be made regarding adjustment of amprenavir dose when amprenavir is co-administered with methadone.

Agenerase capsules contain vitamin E (36 IU/50 mg capsule), therefore additional vitamin E supplementation is not recommended.

Due to the potential risk of toxicity from the high propylene glycol content of Agenerase oral solution, this formulation is contraindicated in children below the age of four years and should be used with caution in certain other patient populations. The Summary of Product Characteristics of Agenerase oral solution should be consulted for full prescribing information.

Rash / cutaneous reactions

Rashes/cutaneous reactions: most patients with mild or moderate rash can continue Agenerase. Appropriate antihistamines (e.g. cetirizine dihydrochloride) may reduce pruritus and hasten the resolution of rash. Agenerase should be permanently discontinued when rash is accompanied with systemic symptoms or allergic symptoms or mucosal involvement (see section 4.8).

Hyperglycaemia

New onset of diabetes mellitus, hyperglycaemia or exacerbations of existing diabetes mellitus have been reported in patients receiving antiretroviral therapy, including protease inhibitors. In some of these, the hyperglycaemia was severe and in some cases also associated with ketoacidosis. Many of the patients had confounding medical conditions, some of which required therapy with agents that have been associated with the development of diabetes mellitus or hyperglycaemia.

Lipodystrophy

Combination antiretroviral therapy has been associated with the redistribution of body fat (lipodystrophy) in HIV patients. The long-term consequences of these events are currently unknown. Knowledge about the mechanism is incomplete. A connection between visceral lipomatosis and protease inhibitors and lipoatrophy and nucleoside reverse transcriptase inhibitors has been hypothesised. A higher risk of lipodystrophy has been associated with individual factors such as older age, and with drug related factors such as longer duration of antiretroviral treatment and associated metabolic disturbances. Clinical examination should include evaluation for physical signs of fat redistribution. Consideration should be given to the measurement of fasting serum lipids and blood glucose. Lipid disorders should be managed as clinically appropriate (see section 4.8).

Haemophiliac patients

There have been reports of increased bleeding, including spontaneous skin haematomas and haemarthroses, in haemophiliac patients type A and B treated with protease inhibitors. In some patients, additional factor VIII was given. In more than half of the reported cases, treatment with protease inhibitors was continued, or reintroduced if treatment had been discontinued. A causal relationship has been evoked, although the mechanism of action has not been elucidated. Haemophiliac patients should therefore be made aware of the possibility of increased bleeding.

Immune Reactivation Syndrome

In HIV-infected patients with severe immune deficiency at the time of institution of combination antiretroviral therapy (CART), an inflammatory reaction to asymptomatic or residual opportunistic pathogens may arise and cause serious clinical conditions, or aggravation of symptoms. Typically, such reactions have been observed within the first few weeks or months of initiation of CART. Relevant examples are cytomegalovirus retinitis, generalised and/or focal mycobacterium infections, and *Pneumocystis carinii* pneumonia. Any inflammatory symptoms should be evaluated and treatment instituted when necessary.

4.5 Interaction with other medicinal products and other forms of Interaction

Interaction studies have been performed with amprenavir as the sole protease inhibitor. When amprenavir and ritonavir are co-administered, the ritonavir metabolic drug interaction profile may predominate because ritonavir is a more potent CYP3A4 inhibitor. Ritonavir also inhibits CYP2D6 and induces CYP3A4, CYP1A2, CYP2C9 and glucuronosyl transferase. The full prescribing information for ritonavir must therefore be consulted prior to initiation of therapy with Agenerase and ritonavir.

Amprenavir and ritonavir are primarily metabolised in the liver by CYP3A4. Therefore, medicinal products that either share this metabolic pathway or modify CYP3A4 activity may modify the pharmacokinetics of amprenavir. Similarly, amprenavir and ritonavir might also modify the pharmacokinetics of other medicinal products that share this metabolic pathway.

Terfenadine, cisapride, pimozide, triazolam, diazepam, midazolam, flurazepam, ergotamine, dihydroergotamine and astemizole are contraindicated in patients receiving Agenerase. Concurrent administration can lead to competitive inhibition of the metabolism of these products and thus result in serious, life-threatening events (see section 4.3).

Of note, the following interaction data was obtained in adults.

Antiretroviral agents

• ***Protease inhibitors (PIs):***

Indinavir: the AUC, C_{min} and C_{max} of indinavir were decreased by 38 %, 27 %, and 22 %, respectively, when given with amprenavir. The clinical relevance of these changes is unknown. The AUC, C_{min} and C_{max} of amprenavir were increased by 33 %, 25 %, and 18 %, respectively. No dose adjustment is necessary for either medicinal product when indinavir is administered in combination with amprenavir.

Saquinavir: the AUC, C_{min} and C_{max} of saquinavir were decreased by 19 % and 48 % and increased by 21 %, respectively, when given with amprenavir. The clinical relevance of these changes is unknown. The AUC, C_{min} and C_{max} of amprenavir were decreased by 32 %, 14 %, and 37 %, respectively. No dose adjustment is necessary for either medicinal product when saquinavir is administered in combination with amprenavir.

Nelfinavir: the AUC, C_{min} and C_{max} of nelfinavir were increased by 15 %, 14 %, and 12 %, respectively, when given with amprenavir. The C_{max} of amprenavir was decreased by 14 % whilst the AUC and C_{min} were increased by 9 % and 189 %, respectively. No dose adjustment is necessary for either medicinal product when nelfinavir is administered in combination with amprenavir (see also efavirenz below).

Ritonavir: the AUC and C_{min} of amprenavir were increased by 64% and 508% respectively and the C_{max} decreased by 30% when ritonavir (100 mg twice daily) was co-administered with amprenavir capsule (600 mg twice daily) compared to values achieved after 1200 mg twice daily doses of amprenavir capsules. In clinical trials, doses of amprenavir 600 mg twice daily and ritonavir 100 mg twice daily have been used; confirming the safety and efficacy of this regimen.

Lopinavir / ritonavir (Kaletra): in an open-label, non-fasting pharmacokinetic study, the AUC, C_{max} and C_{min} of lopinavir were decreased by 38%, 28% and 52% respectively when amprenavir (750 mg twice daily) was given in combination with Kaletra (400 mg lopinavir + 100 mg ritonavir twice daily). In the same study, the AUC, C_{max}, and C_{min} of amprenavir were increased 72%, 12%, and 483%, respectively, when compared to values after standard doses of amprenavir (1200 mg twice daily).

The amprenavir plasma C_{min} values achieved with the combination of amprenavir (600 mg twice daily) in combination with Kaletra (400 mg lopinavir + 100 mg ritonavir twice daily) are approximately 40-50% lower than when amprenavir (600 mg twice daily) is given in combination with ritonavir 100 mg twice daily. Adding additional ritonavir to an amprenavir plus Kaletra regimen increase lopinavir C_{min} values, but not amprenavir C_{min} values. No dose recommendation can be given for the co-administration of amprenavir and Kaletra, but close monitoring is advised because the safety and efficacy of this combination is unknown.

• ***Nucleoside analogue reverse transcriptase inhibitors (NRTIs):***

Zidovudine: the AUC and C_{max} of zidovudine were increased by 31 % and 40 %, respectively, when given with amprenavir. The AUC and the C_{max} of amprenavir were unaltered. No dose adjustment for either medicinal product is necessary when zidovudine is administered in combination with amprenavir.

Lamivudine: the AUC and C_{max} of lamivudine and amprenavir, respectively, were both unaltered when these two medicinal products were given concomitantly. No dose adjustment is necessary for either medicinal product when lamivudine is administered in combination with amprenavir.

Abacavir: the AUC, C_{min} and C_{max} of abacavir were unaltered when given with amprenavir. The AUC, C_{min} and C_{max} of amprenavir were increased by 29 %, 27 %, and 47 %, respectively. No dose adjustment is necessary for either medicinal product when abacavir is administered in combination with amprenavir.

Didanosine: no pharmacokinetic study has been performed with Agenerase in combination with didanosine, however, due to its antacid component, it is recommended that didanosine and Agenerase should be administered at least one hour apart (see Antacids below).

• *Non-nucleoside reverse transcriptase inhibitors (NNRTIs):*

Efavirenz: efavirenz has been seen to decrease the C_{max}, AUC and $C_{min,ss}$ of amprenavir by approximately 40 % in adults. When amprenavir is combined with ritonavir, the effect of efavirenz is compensated by the pharmacokinetic booster effect of ritonavir. Therefore, if efavirenz is given in combination with amprenavir (600 mg twice daily) and ritonavir (100 mg twice daily), no dose adjustment is necessary.

Further, if efavirenz is given in combination with amprenavir and nelfinavir, no dosage adjustment is necessary for any of the medicinal products.

Treatment with efavirenz in combination with amprenavir and saquinavir is not recommended, as the exposure to both protease inhibitors would be decreased.

No dose recommendation can be given for the co-administration of amprenavir with another protease inhibitor and efavirenz in children. Such combinations should be avoided in patients with hepatic impairment.

Nevirapine: The effect of nevirapine on other protease inhibitors and the limited evidence available suggest that nevirapine may decrease the serum concentrations of amprenavir.

Delavirdine: the AUC, C_{max} and C_{min} of delavirdine were decreased by 61%, 47% and 88% respectively when given with amprenavir. The AUC, C_{max} and C_{min} of amprenavir were increased by 130%, 40% and 125% respectively.

No dose recommendations can be given for the co-administration of amprenavir and delavirdine. If these medicinal products are used concomitantly care is advised, as delavirdine may be less effective due to decreased and potentially sub-therapeutic plasma concentrations.

No dose recommendations can be given for the co-administration of amprenavir and low dose ritonavir with delavirdine. If these medicinal products are used concomitantly care is advised, and close clinical and virological monitoring should be performed since it is difficult to predict the effect of the combination of amprenavir and ritonavir on delavirdine.

Antibiotics/antifungals

Rifampicin: rifampicin is a potent inducer of CYP3A4. Concomitant administration with amprenavir resulted in a reduction of amprenavir C_{min} and AUC by 92 % and 82 %, respectively. Rifampicin must not be used concomitantly with amprenavir (see section 4.3).

Rifabutin: co-administration of amprenavir with rifabutin resulted in a 193 % increase in rifabutin AUC and an increase of rifabutin-related adverse events. The increase in rifabutin plasma concentration is likely to result from inhibition of rifabutin CYP3A4 mediated metabolism by amprenavir. When it is clinically necessary to co-administer rifabutin with Agenerase, a dosage reduction of at least half the recommended dose of rifabutin is advised, although no clinical data are available. When ritonavir is co-administered a larger increase in rifabutin concentration may occur.

Clarithromycin: the AUC and C_{min} of clarithromycin were unaltered and the C_{max} decreased by 10 % when given with amprenavir. The AUC, C_{min} and C_{max} of amprenavir were increased by 18 %, 39 % and 15 %, respectively. No dose adjustment is necessary for either medicinal product when clarithromycin is administered in combination with amprenavir. When ritonavir is co-administered an increase in clarithromycin concentrations may occur.

Erythromycin: no pharmacokinetic study has been performed with Agenerase in combination with erythromycin, however, plasma levels of both medicinal products may be increased when co-administered.

Ketoconazole: the AUC and C_{max} of ketoconazole were increased by 44 % and 19 %, respectively when given with amprenavir. The AUC and C_{max} of amprenavir were increased by 31 % and decreased by 16 %, respectively. No dose adjustment for either medicinal product is necessary when ketoconazole is administered in combination with amprenavir. When ritonavir is co-administered a larger increase in ketoconazole concentrations may occur.

Other possible interactions

Other medicinal products, listed below, including examples of substrates, inhibitors or inducers of CYP3A4, may lead to interactions when administered with Agenerase. The clinical significance of these possible interactions is not known and has not been investigated. Patients should therefore be monitored for toxic reactions associated with these medicinal products when these are administered in combination with Agenerase.

Antacids: on the basis of the data for other protease inhibitors, it is advisable not to take antacids at the same time as Agenerase, since its absorption may be impaired. It is recommended that antacids and Agenerase should be administered at least one hour apart.

Benzodiazepines: the serum concentrations of alprazolam, triazolam, midazolam, clonazepam, diazepam and flurazepam may be increased by amprenavir resulting in enhanced sedation (see section 4.3).

Calcium-channel blockers: amprenavir may lead to increased serum concentrations of diltiazem, nicardipine, nifedipine or nimodipine, possibly resulting in enhanced activity and toxicity of these medicinal products.

Erectile dysfunction agents: based on data for other protease inhibitors caution should be used when prescribing sildenafil to patients receiving Agenerase. Co-administration of Agenerase with sildenafil may substantially increase sildenafil plasma concentrations and may result in sildenafil-associated adverse events.

HMG-CoA reductase inhibitors: HMG-CoA reductase inhibitors which are highly dependent on CYP3A4 for metabolism, such as lovastatin and simvastatin, are expected to have markedly increased plasma concentrations when co-administered with Agenerase. Since increased concentrations of HMG-CoA reductase inhibitors may cause myopathy, including rhabdomyolysis, the combination of these medicinal products with Agenerase is not recommended. Atorvastatin is less dependent on CYP3A4 for metabolism. When used with Agenerase, the lowest possible dose of atorvastatin should be administered. The metabolism of pravastatin and fluvastatin is not dependent on CYP3A4, and interactions are not expected with protease inhibitors. If treatment with a HMG-CoA reductase inhibitor is indicated, pravastatin or fluvastatin is recommended.

Methadone and opiate derivatives: co-administration of methadone with amprenavir resulted in a decrease in the C_{max} and AUC of the active methadone enantiomer (R-enantiomer) of 25% and 13% respectively, whilst the C_{max}, AUC and C_{min} of the inactive methadone enantiomer (S-enantiomer) were decreased by 48%, 40% and 23% respectively. When methadone is co-administered with amprenavir, patients should be monitored for opiate abstinence syndrome, in particular if low-dose ritonavir is also given.

As compared to a non-matched historical control group, co-administration of methadone and amprenavir resulted in a 30%, 27% and 25% decrease in serum amprenavir AUC, C_{max} and C_{min} respectively. No recommendations can currently be made regarding adjustment of amprenavir dose when amprenavir is co-administered with methadone due to the inherent low reliability of non-matched historical controls.

Steroids: oestrogens, progestogens and some glucocorticoids may interact with amprenavir. However, the information currently available is not sufficient for determining the nature of the interaction. Co-administration of Ortho-Novum 1/35 (0.035 mg ethinyl estradiol plus 1.0 mg norethindrone) resulted in a decrease of the amprenavir AUC and C_{min} of 22% and 20% respectively, C_{max} being unchanged. The C_{min} of ethinyl estradiol was increased by 32%, whilst the AUC and C_{min} of norethindrone were increased by 18% and 45% respectively. Alternative methods of contraception are recommended for women of childbearing potential. When ritonavir is co-administered, the effect on hormonal contraceptive concentrations cannot be predicted, therefore, alternative methods of contraception are also recommended.

St John's wort: serum levels of amprenavir can be reduced by concomitant use of the herbal preparation St John's wort (*Hypericum perforatum*). This is due to induction of drug metabolising enzymes by St John's wort. Herbal preparations containing St John's wort should therefore not be combined with Agenerase. If a patient is already taking St John's wort, check amprenavir and if possible viral levels and stop St John's wort. Amprenavir levels may increase on stopping St John's wort. The dose of amprenavir may need adjusting. The inducing effect may persist for at least 2 weeks after cessation of treatment with St John's wort (see section 4.3).

Other substances: plasma concentrations of other substances may be increased by amprenavir. These include substances such as: clozapine, carbamazepine, cimetidine, dapsone, itraconazole and loratadine.

4.6 Pregnancy and lactation

Pregnancy: the safe use of amprenavir in human pregnancy has not been established. Placental transfer of amprenavir and/or its related metabolites has been shown to occur in animals (see section 5.3).

This medicinal product should be used during pregnancy only after careful weighing of the potential benefits compared to the potential risk to the foetus.

Lactation: amprenavir-related material was found in rat milk, but it is not known whether amprenavir is excreted in human milk. A reproduction study in pregnant rats dosed from the time of uterine implantation through lactation showed reduced body weight gains in the offspring during the nursing period. The systemic exposure to the dams associated with this finding was similar to exposure in humans, following administration of the recommended dose. The subsequent development of the offspring, including fertility and reproductive performance, was not affected by the maternal administration of amprenavir.

It is therefore recommended that mothers being treated with Agenerase do not breast-feed their infants. Additionally, it is recommended that HIV infected women do not breast feed their infants in order to avoid transmission of HIV.

4.7 Effects on ability to drive and use machines

No studies on the effects on ability to drive and use machines have been performed.

4.8 Undesirable effects

The safety of Agenerase has been studied in adults and children at least 4 years of age, in controlled clinical trials, in combination with various other antiretroviral agents. Adverse events considered associated with the use of Agenerase are gastro-intestinal symptoms, rash and oral/peri-oral paraesthesia. Most undesirable effects associated with Agenerase therapy were mild to moderate in severity, early in onset, and rarely treatment limiting. For many of these events, it is unclear whether they are related to Agenerase, to concomitant treatment used in the management of HIV disease or to the disease process.

In children, the nature of the safety profile is similar to that seen in adults.

Adverse reactions are listed below by MedDRA body system organ class and by frequency. The frequency categories used are:

Very common $\geqslant$ 1 in 10

Common $\geqslant$ 1 in 100 and $<$ 1 in 10

Uncommon $\geqslant$ 1 in 1,000 and $<$ 1 in 100

Rare $\geqslant$1 in 10,000 and $<$ 1 in 1,000

Frequency categories for the events below have been based on clinical trials and postmarketing data.

Most of the adverse events below come from two clinical trials (PROAB3001, PROAB3006) involving PI naïve subjects receiving Agenerase 1200mg twice daily. Events (grade 2-4) reported by study investigators as attributable to study medication and occurring in $>$1% of patients, are included as well as grade 3-4 treatment emergent laboratory abnormalities. Note that the background rates in comparator groups were not taken into account.

Metabolism and nutrition disorders

Common: Elevated triglycerides, elevated amylase, abnormal fat redistribution, anorexia

Uncommon: Hyperglycaemia, hypercholesterolaemia

Elevated triglycerides, elevated amylase and hyperglycaemia (grade 3-4) were reported primarily in patients with abnormal values at baseline.

Elevations in cholesterol were of grade 3-4 intensity.

Combination antiretroviral therapy has been associated with redistribution of body fat (lipodystrophy) in HIV patients including the loss of peripheral and facial subcutaneous fat, increased intra-abdominal and visceral fat, breast hypertrophy and dorsocervical fat accumulation (buffalo hump).

Symptoms of abnormal fat redistribution were infrequent in PROAB3001 with amprenavir. Only one case (a buffalo hump) was reported in 113 ($<$ 1 %) antiretroviral naive subjects treated with amprenavir in combination with lamivudine/zidovudine for a median duration of 36 weeks. In study PROAB3006, seven cases (3 %) were reported in 245 NRTI-experienced subjects treated with amprenavir and in 27 (11 %) of 241 subjects treated with indinavir, in combination with various NRTIs for a median duration of 56 weeks ($p < 0.001$).

Combination antiretroviral therapy has been associated with metabolic abnormalities such as hypertriglyceridaemia, hypercholesterolaemia, insulin resistance, hyperglycaemia and hyperlactataemia (see section 4.4).

Psychiatric disorders

Common: Mood disorders, depressive disorders

Nervous system disorders

Very Common: Headache

Common: Oral/perioral paraesthesia, tremors, sleep disorders

Gastrointestinal disorders

Very Common: Diarrhoea, nausea, flatulence, vomiting

Common: Abdominal pain, abdominal discomfort, dyspeptic symptoms, loose stools

Hepatobiliary disorders

Common: Elevated transaminases

Uncommon: Hyperbilirubinaemia

Elevated transaminases and hyperbilirubinaemia (grade 3-4) were reported primarily in patients with abnormal values at baseline. Almost all subjects with abnormal liver function tests were co-infected with Hepatitis B or C virus.

Skin and subcutaneous tissue disorders

Very Common: Rash

Rare: Stevens Johnson syndrome

Rashes were usually mild to moderate, erythematous or maculopapular cutaneous eruptions, with or without pruritus, occurring during the second week of therapy and resolving spontaneously within two weeks, without discontinuation of treatment with amprenavir. A higher incidence of rash was reported in patients treated with amprenavir in combination with efavirenz. Severe or life-threatening skin reactions have also occurred in patients treated with amprenavir (see section 4.4).

Musculoskeletal and connective tissue disorders

Increased CPK, myalgia, myositis, and rarely rhabdomyolysis have been reported with protease inhibitors, particularly in combination with nucleoside analogues.

General disorders and administration site conditions

Very Common: Fatigue

In HIV-infected patients with severe immune deficiency at the time of initiation of combination antiretroviral therapy (CART), an inflammatory reaction to asymptomatic or residual opportunistic infections may arise (see section 4.4).

In PI experienced patients receiving Agenerase capsules 600 mg twice daily and low dose ritonavir, 100 mg twice daily, the nature and frequency of adverse events (grade 2-4) and Grade 3/4 laboratory abnormalities were similar to those observed with Agenerase alone, with the exception of elevated triglyceride levels, and elevated CPK levels which were very common in patients receiving Agenerase and low dose ritonavir.

4.9 Overdose

There are limited reports of overdose with Agenerase. If overdose occurs, the patient should be monitored for evidence of toxicity (see section 4.8) and standard supportive treatment provided as necessary. Since amprenavir is highly protein bound, dialysis is unlikely to be helpful in reducing blood levels of amprenavir.

5. PHARMACOLOGICAL PROPERTIES

5.1 Pharmacodynamic properties

Pharmacotherapeutic group; protease inhibitor; ATC Code: JO5A E05

Amprenavir is a competitive inhibitor of the HIV protease. It blocks the ability of the viral protease to cleave the precursor polyproteins necessary for viral replication.

Amprenavir is a potent and selective inhibitor of HIV-1 and HIV-2 replication *in vitro*. In isolated experimental settings, synergy was shown *in vitro* in combination with nucleoside analogues including didanosine, zidovudine, abacavir and the protease inhibitor, saquinavir. It has been shown to have an additive effect in combination with indinavir, ritonavir and nelfinavir.

Serial passage experiments have demonstrated the protease mutation I50V to be key to the development of amprenavir resistance *in vitro*, with the triple variant, I50V+M46I/L+I47V, resulting in a greater than 10-fold increase in IC_{50} to amprenavir. This triple mutation resistance profile has not been observed with other protease inhibitors either from in *vitro* studies or in clinical settings. *In vitro* variants resistant to amprenavir remained sensitive to saquinavir, indinavir and nelfinavir, but showed three to five-fold reduced susceptibility to ritonavir. The triple mutant, I50V+M46I/L+I47V, was unstable during *in vitro* passage in the presence of saquinavir, with loss of the I47V mutation, and the development of resistance to saquinavir resulted in resensitisation to amprenavir. Passage of the triple mutant in either indinavir, nelfinavir or ritonavir resulted in additional protease mutations being selected, leading to dual resistance. Mutation I84V, observed transiently *in vitro* has rarely been selected during amprenavir therapy.

The resistance profile seen with amprenavir in clinical practice is different from that observed with other protease inhibitors. Consistent with *in vitro* experiments, the development of amprenavir resistance during therapy, is in the majority cases, associated with the mutation I50V. However, three alternative mechanisms have also been observed to result in the development of amprenavir resistance in the clinic, and involve either mutations I54L/M or V32I+I47V or, rarely, I84V. Each of the four genetic patterns produces viruses with reduced susceptibility to amprenavir, some cross-resistance to ritonavir, but susceptibility to indinavir, nelfinavir and saquinavir is retained.

The following table summarises the mutations associated with the development of reduced phenotypic susceptibility to amprenavir in subjects treated with amprenavir.

Protease mutations acquired on amprenavir-containing therapy which have been demonstrated to result in reduced phenotypic susceptibility to amprenavir:
I50V or I54L/M or I84V or V32I with I47V

The pre-existence of resistance to other components of a first-line PI-containing regimen is significantly associated with subsequent development of protease mutations, highlighting the importance of considering all components of a treatment regimen when change is indicated.

Many *in vitro* PI-resistant variants, and 322 of 433 (74 %) clinical PI-resistant variants with multiple protease inhibitor resistance mutations were susceptible to amprenavir. The principal protease mutation associated with cross-resistance to amprenavir following treatment failure with other protease inhibitors was I84V, particularly when mutations L10I/V/F were also present.

In multiple protease inhibitor-experienced subjects, the likelihood of a successful virological response is increased with an increasing number of active drugs (i.e. agents to which the virus is susceptible) in the rescue regimen. The presence at the time of therapy change in PI-experienced subjects of multiple key mutations associated with PI-resistance, or the development of such mutations during PI therapy, is significantly associated with treatment outcome. The total number of all types of protease mutations present at the time of therapy change was also correlated with outcome in PI-experienced populations. The presence of 3 or more mutations from M46I/L, I54L/M/V, V82A/F/I/T, I84V and L90M in a population of multiple PI-experienced subjects was significantly related to amprenavir treatment failure.

The following table summarises the mutations, identified in clinical isolates from highly PI- experienced patients, associated with an increased risk of treatment failure of amprenavir-containing regimens.

Protease mutations in virus from PI-experienced patients associated with reduced virological response to subsequent amprenavir containing regimens:
COMBINATION OF AT LEAST THREE OF: M46I/L or I54L/M/V or V82A/F/I/T or I84V or L90M.

The number of key PI-resistance mutations increases markedly the longer a failing PI-containing regimen is continued. Early discontinuation of failing therapies is recommended in order to limit the accumulation of multiple mutations, which may be detrimental to a subsequent rescue regimen.

Amprenavir is not recommended for use as monotherapy, due to the rapid emergence of resistant virus.

Cross resistance between amprenavir and reverse transcriptase inhibitors is unlikely to occur because the enzyme targets are different.

Clinical experience:

Agenerase in combination with low dose ritonavir and nucleoside analogues (NRTI) has been shown to be effective in the treatment of PI-experienced HIV–1 infected adults.

In a randomised, open-label study in PI-experienced adults experiencing virological failure (viral load ⩾1000 copies/ml), Agenerase (600 mg twice daily) / ritonavir (100 mg twice daily) was compared to other PIs. The study comprised two separate components. Analyses described are intent to treat (Exposed).

Sub-study A (n=163) compared Agenerase / ritonavir to other, predominantly ritonavir boosted PIs, in a standard of care regimen, in patients with virus sensitive to Agenerase, at least one other PI, and at least one NRTI. After 16 weeks, the antiviral response to Agenerase/ritonavir, as measured by time-averaged change from baseline in plasma HIV-1 RNA (AAUCMB), was shown to be non-inferior to that in the patients in the other PI treatment group [mean plasma HIV-1 RNA AAUCMB 1.315 $\log_{10}$ copies/ml and 1.343 $\log_{10}$ copies/ml respectively, mean stratified difference 0.043 $\log_{10}$ copies/ml (95% CI: –0.25, 0.335), ITT(E) population, Observed analysis]. The proportion of subjects with plasma HIV-1 RNA <400 copies/ml was similar across the treatment groups (66% and 70% respectively).

Sub-study B (n=43) compared Agenerase / ritonavir to continued current PI therapy in patients with virus resistant to indinavir, ritonavir, nelfinavir and saquinavir. Agenerase/ritonavir demonstrated superior efficacy as measured by AAUCMB after four weeks [mean strata adjusted treatment difference –0.669 $\log_{10}$ copies/ml (95% CI -0.946, -0.391), p=0.00002, ITT(E) population, Observed analysis]. Additionally, the proportion of subjects with plasma HIV-1 RNA below 400 copies/ml was higher in the Agenerase/ritonavir group (48%) than in the group maintained on the PI regimen current at study start (0%), p=0.00048.

Agenerase without low dose ritonavir, in combination with other antiretroviral agents including nucleoside analogues, non-nucleoside analogues and protease inhibitors, has been shown to be effective in antiretroviral naïve and NRTI-experienced HIV-1 infected adults and heavily pretreated children aged 4 years or more.

In a double-blind study in antiretroviral naive HIV-infected adults (n = 232), amprenavir (1200 mg twice daily) in combination with zidovudine and lamivudine was significantly superior to zidovudine and lamivudine. In an intent-to-treat analysis (any missing value or premature discontinuation considered as failure i.e. ⩾ 400 copies/ml), the proportion of subjects with plasma HIV-1 RNA < 400 copies/ml through week 48 was 41 % in the amprenavir/lamivudine/zidovudine group and 3 % in the lamivudine/zidovudine group (p < 0.001).

In an open-label randomised study in NRTI-experienced PI-naive adults (n = 504), in combination with various NRTIs amprenavir (1200 mg twice daily) was found to be less effective than indinavir: the proportion of subjects with plasma HIV-1 RNA < 400 copies/ml at week 48 was 30 % in the amprenavir arm and 46 % in the indinavir arm in the intent-to-treat analysis (any missing value or premature discontinuation considered as failure, i.e. ⩾ 400 copies/ml).

Results from two paediatric studies with amprenavir oral solution and/or capsules in 268 heavily pre-treated children aged 2 to 18 years indicate that amprenavir is an effective antiretroviral agent in children. Decreases in median HIV-1 RNA greater than 1 $\log_{10}$ copies/ml were observed in protease inhibitor naive subjects and improvements in immune category (CD4 %) were reported.

The use of Agenerase, without the boosting effect of low dose ritonavir, has not been sufficiently studied in heavily pretreated protease inhibitor experienced patients.

5.2 Pharmacokinetic properties

Absorption: after oral administration, amprenavir is rapidly and well absorbed. The absolute bioavailability is unknown due to the lack of an acceptable intravenous formulation for use in man. Approximately 90 % of an orally administered radiolabelled amprenavir dose was recovered in the urine and the faeces, primarily as amprenavir metabolites. Following oral administration, the mean time (t_{max}) to maximal serum concentrations of amprenavir is between 1-2 hours for the capsule and 0.5 to 1 hour for the oral solution. A second peak is observed after 10 to 12 hours and may represent either delayed absorption or enterohepatic recirculation.

At therapeutic dosages (1200 mg twice daily), the mean maximum steady state concentration ($C_{max,ss}$) of amprenavir capsules is 5.36 μg/ml (0.92-9.81) and the minimum steady state concentration ($C_{min,ss}$) is 0.28 μg/ml (0.12-0.51). The mean AUC over a dosing interval of 12 hours is 18.46 μg.h/ml (3.02-32.95). The 50 mg and 150 mg capsules have been shown to be bioequivalent. The bioavailability of the oral solution at equivalent doses is lower than that of the capsules, with an AUC and C_{max} approximately 14 % and 19 % lower, respectively (see section 4.2).

The AUC and C_{min} of amprenavir were increased by 64% and 508% respectively and the C_{max} decreased by 30% when ritonavir (100 mg twice daily) was coadministered with amprenavir (600 mg twice daily) compared to values achieved after 1200 mg twice daily doses of amprenavir.

While administration of amprenavir with food results in a 25 % reduction in AUC, it had no effect on the concentration of amprenavir 12 hours after dosing (C_{12}). Therefore, although food affects the extent and rate of absorption, the steady-state trough concentration ($C_{min,ss}$) was not affected by food intake.

Distribution: the apparent volume of distribution is approximately 430 litres (6 l/kg assuming a 70 kg body weight), suggesting a large volume of distribution, with penetration of amprenavir freely into tissues beyond the systemic circulation. The concentration of amprenavir in the cerebrospinal fluid is less than 1 % of plasma concentration.

In *in vitro* studies, the protein binding of amprenavir is approximately 90 %. Amprenavir is primarily bound to the alpha-1-acid glycoprotein (AAG), but also to albumin. Concentrations of AAG have been shown to decrease during the course of antiretroviral therapy. This change will decrease the total active substance concentration in the plasma, however the amount of unbound amprenavir, which is the active moiety, is likely to be unchanged. While absolute free active substance concentrations remain constant, the percent of free active substance will fluctuate directly with total active substance concentrations at steady-state go from $C_{max,ss}$ to $C_{min,ss}$ over the course of the dosing interval. This will result in a fluctuation in the apparent volume of distribution of total active substance, but the volume of distribution of free active substance does not change.

Clinically significant binding displacement interactions involving medicinal products primarily bound to AAG are generally not observed. Therefore, interactions with amprenavir due to protein binding displacement are highly unlikely.

Metabolism: amprenavir is primarily metabolised by the liver with less than 3 % excreted unchanged in the urine. The primary route of metabolism is via the cytochrome P450 CYP3A4 enzyme. Amprenavir is a substrate of and inhibits CYP3A4. Therefore, medicinal products that are inducers, inhibitors or substrates of CYP3A4 must be used with caution when administered concurrently with Agenerase (see sections 4.3, 4.4 and 4.5).

Elimination: the plasma elimination half-life of amprenavir ranges from 7.1 to 10.6 hours. The plasma amprenavir half-life is increased when Agenerase capsules are co-administered with ritonavir. Following multiple oral doses of amprenavir (1200 mg twice a day), there is no significant active substance accumulation. The primary route of elimination of amprenavir is via hepatic metabolism with less than 3 % excreted unchanged in the urine. The metabolites and unchanged amprenavir account for approximately 14 % of the administered amprenavir dose in the urine, and approximately 75 % in the faeces.

Special populations:

Paediatrics: the pharmacokinetics of amprenavir in children (4 years of age and above) are similar to those in adults. Dosages of 20 mg/kg twice a day and 15 mg/kg three times a day with Agenerase capsules provided similar daily amprenavir exposure to 1200 mg twice a day in adults. Amprenavir is 14 % less bioavailable from the oral solution than from the capsules; therefore, Agenerase capsules and Agenerase oral solution are not interchangeable on a milligram per milligram basis.

Elderly: the pharmacokinetics of amprenavir have not been studied in patients over 65 years of age.

Renal impairment: patients with renal impairment have not been specifically studied. Less than 3 % of the therapeutic dose of amprenavir is excreted unchanged in the urine. The impact of renal impairment on amprenavir elimination should be minimal, therefore, no initial dose adjustment is considered necessary. Renal clearance of ritonavir is also negligible; therefore the impact of renal impairment on amprenavir and ritonavir elimination should be minimal.

Hepatic impairment: the pharmacokinetics of amprenavir are significantly altered in patients with moderate to severe hepatic impairment. The AUC increased nearly three-fold in patients with moderate impairment and four fold in patients with severe hepatic impairment. Clearance also decreased in a corresponding manner to the AUC. The dosage should therefore be reduced in these patients (see section 4.2). These dosing regimens will provide plasma amprenavir levels comparable to those achieved in healthy subjects given a 1200 mg dose twice daily without concomitant administration of ritonavir.

5.3 Preclinical safety data

In long-term carcinogenicity studies with amprenavir in mice and rats, there were benign hepatocellular adenomas in males at exposure levels equivalent to 2.0-fold (mice) or 3.8-fold (rats) those in humans given 1200 mg twice daily of amprenavir alone. In male mice altered hepatocellular foci were seen at doses that were at least 2.0 times human therapeutic exposure.

A higher incidence of hepatocellular carcinoma was seen in all amprenavir male mouse treatment groups. However, this increase was not statistically significantly different from male control mice by appropriate tests. The mechanism for the hepatocellular adenomas and carcinomas found in these studies has not been elucidated and the significance of the observed effects for humans is uncertain. However, there is little evidence from the exposure data in humans, both in clinical trials and from marketed use, to suggest that these findings are of clinical significance.

Amprenavir was not mutagenic or genotoxic in a battery of *in vivo* and *in vitro* genetic toxicity assays, including bacterial reverse mutation (Ames Test), mouse lymphoma, rat micronucleus, and chromosome aberration in human peripheral lymphocytes.

In toxicological studies with mature animals, the clinically relevant findings were mostly confined to the liver and gastrointestinal disturbances. Liver toxicity consisted of increases in liver enzymes, liver weights and microscopic findings including hepatocyte necrosis. This liver toxicity can be monitored for and detected in clinical use, with measurements of AST, ALT and alkaline phosphatase activity. However, significant liver toxicity has not been observed in patients treated in clinical studies, either during administration of Agenerase or after discontinuation.

Amprenavir did not affect fertility.

Local toxicity and sensitising potential was absent in animal studies, but slight irritating properties to the rabbit eye were identified.

Toxicity studies in young animals, treated from four days of age, resulted in high mortality in both the control animals and those receiving amprenavir. These results imply that young animals lack fully developed metabolic pathways enabling them to excrete amprenavir or some critical components of the formulation (e.g. propylene glycol, PEG 400). However, the possibility of anaphylactic reaction related to PEG 400 cannot be excluded. In clinical studies, the safety and efficacy of amprenavir have not yet been established in children below four years of age.

In pregnant mice, rabbits and rats there were no major effects on embryo-foetal development. However, at systemic plasma exposures significantly below (rabbits) or not significantly higher (rat) than the expected human exposures during therapeutic dosing, a number of minor changes, including thymic elongation and minor skeletal variations were seen, indicating developmental delay. A dose-dependent increase in placental weight was found in the rabbit and rat which may indicate effects on placental function. It is therefore recommended that women of childbearing potential taking Agenerase should practice effective contraception (e.g. barrier methods).

6. PHARMACEUTICAL PARTICULARS

6.1 List of excipients

Capsule shell: gelatin, glycerol, d-sorbitol and sorbitans solution, titanium dioxide, red printing ink.

Capsule contents: d-alpha tocopheryl polyethylene glycol 1000 succinate (TPGS), macrogol 400 (PEG 400), propylene glycol.

6.2 Incompatibilities

Not applicable.

6.3 Shelf life

3 years.

6.4 Special precautions for storage

Do not store above 30°C.

Keep the container tightly closed.

6.5 Nature and contents of container

White High Density Polyethylene (HDPE) bottles containing 480 capsules.

6.6 Instructions for use and handling

No special requirements.

7. MARKETING AUTHORISATION HOLDER

Glaxo Group Ltd

Greenford Road

Greenford

Middlesex UB6 0NN

United Kingdom

8. MARKETING AUTHORISATION NUMBER(S)

EU/1/00/148/001

9. DATE OF FIRST AUTHORISATION/RENEWAL OF THE AUTHORISATION

20th October 2000

10. DATE OF REVISION OF THE TEXT

17 December 2004

AGGRASTAT solution for infusion and concentrate for solution for infusion

(Merck Sharp & Dohme Limited)

1. NAME OF THE MEDICINAL PRODUCT

AGGRASTAT® * (50 MICROGRAMS/ML) SOLUTION FOR INFUSION

AGGRASTAT® * (250 MICROGRAMS/ML) CONCENTRATE FOR SOLUTION FOR INFUSION

* in the following document the abbreviated terms detailed below are used.

• 'Aggrastat' means 'Aggrastat' Solution for Infusion or 'Aggrastat' Concentrate for Solution for Infusion.

• 'Aggrastat' Solution will be used when referring to 'Aggrastat' Solution for Infusion i.e. the 250 ml bag.

• 'Aggrastat' Concentrate will be used when referring to 'Aggrastat' Concentrate for Solution for Infusion i.e. the 50 ml vial.

2. QUALITATIVE AND QUANTITATIVE COMPOSITION

'Aggrastat' Solution:

1 ml of solution for infusion contains 56 micrograms of tirofiban hydrochloride monohydrate which is equivalent to 50 micrograms tirofiban.

'Aggrastat' Concentrate:

1 ml of concentrate for solution for infusion contains 281 micrograms of tirofiban hydrochloride monohydrate which is equivalent to 250 micrograms tirofiban.

For excipients, see section 6.1.

3. PHARMACEUTICAL FORM

'Aggrastat' Solution: Solution for Infusion

(250 ml bag)

A clear, colourless concentrated solution.

'Aggrastat' Concentrate: Concentrate for solution for infusion.

A clear, colourless concentrated solution.

4. CLINICAL PARTICULARS

4.1 Therapeutic indications

'Aggrastat' is indicated for the prevention of early myocardial infarction in patients presenting with unstable angina or non-Q-wave myocardial infarction with the last episode of chest pain occurring within 12 hours and with ECG changes and/or elevated cardiac enzymes.

Patients most likely to benefit from 'Aggrastat' treatment are those at high risk of developing myocardial infarction within the first 3-4 days after onset of acute angina symptoms including for instance those that are likely to undergo an early PTCA (see also 4.2 'Posology and method of administration' and 5.1 'Pharmacodynamic properties').

'Aggrastat' is intended for use with acetylsalicylic acid and unfractionated heparin.

4.2 Posology and method of administration

This product is for hospital use only, by specialist physicians experienced in the management of acute coronary syndromes.

'Aggrastat' concentrate for solution for infusion must be diluted before use.

'Aggrastat' is given intravenously at an initial infusion rate of 0.4 microgram/kg/min for 30 minutes. At the end of the initial infusion, 'Aggrastat' should be continued at a maintenance infusion rate of 0.1 microgram/kg/min. 'Aggrastat' should be given with unfractionated heparin (usually an intravenous bolus of 5,000 units [U] simultaneously with the start of 'Aggrastat' therapy, then approximately 1,000 U per hour, titrated on the basis of the activated thromboplastin time [APTT], which should be about twice the normal value) and ASA (see 5.1 'Pharmacodynamic properties', *PRISM-PLUS study*), unless contra-indicated.

No dosage adjustment is necessary for the elderly (see also 4.4 'Special warnings and precautions for use').

Patients with severe kidney failure

In severe kidney failure (creatinine clearance <30 ml/min) the dosage of 'Aggrastat' should be reduced by 50% (see also 4.4 'Special warnings and precautions for use' and 5.2 'Pharmacokinetic properties').

The following table is provided as a guide to dosage adjustment by weight.

'Aggrastat' Concentrate for Solution for Infusion must be diluted to the same strength as 'Aggrastat' Injection Premixed, as noted under *Instructions for Use.*

(see Table 1 on next page)

Start and duration of therapy with 'Aggrastat'

'Aggrastat' optimally should be initiated within 12 hours after the last anginal episode. The recommended duration should be at least 48 hours. Infusion of 'Aggrastat' and unfractionated heparin may be continued during coronary angiography and should be maintained for at least 12 hours and not more than 24 hours after angioplasty/atherectomy. Once a patient is clinically stable and no coronary intervention procedure is planned by the treating physician, the infusion should be discontinued. The entire duration of treatment should not exceed 108 hours.

Concurrent therapy (unfractionated heparin, ASA)

Treatment with unfractionated heparin is initiated with an i.v. bolus of 5,000 U and then continued with a maintenance infusion of 1,000 U per hour. The heparin dosage is titrated to maintain an APTT of approximately twice the normal value.

Unless contra-indicated, all patients should receive ASA orally before the start of 'Aggrastat' (see 5.1 'Pharmacodynamic properties', *PRISM-PLUS study*). This medication should be continued at least for the duration of the infusion of 'Aggrastat'.

If angioplasty (PTCA) is required, heparin should be stopped after PTCA, and the sheaths should be withdrawn once coagulation has returned to normal, e.g. when the activated clotting time (ACT) is less than 180 seconds (usually 2-6 hours after discontinuation of heparin).

AGGRASTAT SOLUTION

Instructions for use

Do not withdraw solution directly from the container with a syringe.

Directions for use of IntraVia ™† containers

To open: Tear foil overpouch or plastic dust cover down side at slit and remove IntraVia™ container. Some opacity of the plastic due to moisture absorption during the sterilisation process may be observed. This is normal and does not affect the solution quality or safety. The opacity will diminish gradually. Check for minute leaks by squeezing inner bag firmly. If leaks are found, discard solution as sterility may be impaired.

†IntraVia is the tradename for the infusion bag used for 'Aggrastat' Solution.

Do not use unless solution is clear and seal is intact.

Do not add supplementary medication or withdraw solution directly from the bag with a syringe.

CAUTION: Do not use plastic containers in series connections. Such use could result in air embolism due to residual air being drawn from the primary container before administration of the fluid from the secondary container is completed.

Preparation for administration

1. Suspend container from eyelet support.

2. Remove plastic protector from outlet port at bottom of container.

3. Attach administration set. Refer to complete directions accompanying set.

Use according to the dosage table above.

Where the solution and container permit, parenteral drugs should be inspected for visible particles or discoloration before use.

'Aggrastat' should only be given intravenously and may be administered with unfractionated heparin through the same infusion tube.

It is recommended that 'Aggrastat' be administered with a calibrated infusion set using sterile equipment.

Care should be taken to ensure that no prolongation of the infusion of the initial dose occurs and that miscalculation of the infusion rates for the maintenance dose on the basis of the patient's weight is avoided.

Table 1 'Aggrastat' Concentrate for Solution for Infusion must be diluted to the same strength as 'Aggrastat' Injection Premixed, as noted under *Instructions for Use*.

	Most Patients		Severe Kidney Failure	
Patient Weight (kg)	30 min Loading Infusion Rate (ml/hr)	Maintenance Infusion Rate (ml/hr)	30 min Loading Infusion Rate (ml/hr)	Maintenance Infusion Rate (ml/hr)
30-37	16	4	8	2
38-45	20	5	10	3
46-54	24	6	12	3
55-62	28	7	14	4
63-70	32	8	16	4
71-79	36	9	18	5
80-87	40	10	20	5
88-95	44	11	22	6
96-104	48	12	24	6
105-112	52	13	26	7
113-120	56	14	28	7
121-128	60	15	30	8
129-137	64	16	32	8
138-145	68	17	34	9
146-153	72	18	36	9

AGGRASTAT CONCENTRATE

Instructions for use

'Aggrastat' Concentrate must be diluted before use:

1. Draw 50 ml from a 250 ml container of sterile 0.9% saline or 5% glucose in water and replace with 50 ml 'Aggrastat' (from one 50 ml puncture vial) to make up a concentration of 50 microgram/ml. Mix well before use.

2. Use according to the dosage table above.

FOR BOTH FORMULATIONS

Where the solution and container permit, parenteral drugs should be inspected for visible particles or discoloration before use.

'Aggrastat' should only be given intravenously and may be administered with unfractionated heparin through the same infusion tube.

It is recommended that 'Aggrastat' be administered with a calibrated infusion set using sterile equipment.

Care should be taken to ensure that no prolongation of the infusion of the initial dose occurs and that miscalculation of the infusion rates for the maintenance dose on the basis of the patient's weight is avoided.

4.3 Contraindications

'Aggrastat' is contra-indicated in patients who are hypersensitive to the active substance or to any of the excipients of the preparation or who developed thrombocytopenia during earlier use of a GP IIb/IIIa receptor antagonist.

Since inhibition of platelet aggregation increases the bleeding risk, 'Aggrastat' is contra-indicated in patients with:

• History of stroke within 30 days or any history of haemorrhagic stroke.

• Known history of intracranial disease (e.g. neoplasm, arteriovenous malformation, aneurysm).

• Active or recent (within the previous 30 days of treatment) clinically relevant bleeding (e.g. gastro-intestinal bleeding).

• Malignant hypertension.

• Relevant trauma or major surgical intervention within the past six weeks.

• Thrombocytopenia (platelet count $<100{,}000/mm^3$), disorders of platelet function.

• Clotting disturbances (e.g. prothrombin time >1.3 times normal or INR [International Normalised Ratio] >1.5).

• Severe liver failure.

4.4 Special warnings and special precautions for use

The administration of 'Aggrastat' alone without unfractionated heparin is not recommended.

There is limited experience with concomitant administration of 'Aggrastat' with enoxaparin (see also 5.1 'Pharmacodynamic properties' and 5.2 'Pharmacokinetic properties'). The concomitant administration of 'Aggrastat' with enoxaparin is associated with a higher frequency of cutaneous and oral bleeding events, but not in TIMI bleeds**, when compared with the concomitant administration of 'Aggrastat' and unfractionated heparin. An increased risk of serious bleeding events associated with the concomitant administration of 'Aggrastat' and enoxaparin cannot be excluded, particularly in patients given additional unfractionated heparin in conjunction with angiography and/or PCI. The efficacy of 'Aggrastat' in combination with enoxaparin has not been established. The safety and efficacy of 'Aggrastat' with other low molecular weight heparins has not been investigated.

There is insufficient experience with the use of tirofiban hydrochloride in the following diseases and conditions, however, an increased risk of bleeding is suspected. Therefore, tirofiban hydrochloride is not recommended in:

• Traumatic or protracted cardiopulmonary resuscitation, organ biopsy or lithotripsy within the past two weeks

• Severe trauma or major surgery >6 weeks but <3 months previously

• Active peptic ulcer within the past three months

• Uncontrolled hypertension $>180/110$ mm Hg)

• Acute pericarditis

• Active or a known history of vasculitis

• Suspected aortic dissection

• Haemorrhagic retinopathy

• Occult blood in the stool or haematuria

• Thrombolytic therapy (see 4.5 'Interaction with other medicinal products and other forms of interaction').

• Concurrent use of drugs that increase the risk of bleeding to a relevant degree (see 4.5 'Interaction with other medicinal products and other forms of interaction').

**TIMI major bleeds are defined as a haemoglobin drop of >50 g/l with or without an identified site, intracranial haemorrhage, or cardiac tamponade. TIMI minor bleeds are defined as a haemoglobin drop of >30 g/l by $\leqslant 50$ g/l with bleeding from a known site or spontaneous gross haematuria, haematemesis, or haemoptysis. TIMI "loss no site" is defined as a haemoglobin drop >40 g/l but <50 g/l without an identified bleeding site.

There is no therapeutic experience with tirofiban hydrochloride in patients for whom thrombolytic therapy is indicated (e.g. acute transmural myocardial infarction with new pathological Q-waves or elevated ST-segments or left bundle-branch block in the ECG). Consequently, the use of tirofiban hydrochloride is not recommended in these circumstances.

'Aggrastat' infusion should be stopped immediately if circumstances arise that necessitate thrombolytic therapy (including acute occlusion during PTCA) or if the patient must undergo an emergency coronary artery bypass graft (CABG) operation or requires an intra-aortic balloon pump.

There are limited efficacy data in patients immediately undergoing PTCA.

There is no therapeutic experience with 'Aggrastat' in children, thus, the use of 'Aggrastat' is not recommended in these patients.

Other precautionary notes and measures

There are insufficient data regarding the re-administration of 'Aggrastat'.

Patients should be carefully monitored for bleeding during treatment with 'Aggrastat'. If treatment of haemorrhage is necessary, discontinuation of 'Aggrastat' should be considered (see also 4.9 'Overdose'). In cases of major or uncontrollable bleeding, tirofiban hydrochloride should be discontinued immediately.

'Aggrastat' should be used with special caution in the following conditions and patient groups:

• Recent clinically relevant bleeding (less than one year)

• Puncture of a non-compressible vessel within 24 hours before administration of 'Aggrastat'

• Recent epidural procedure (including lumbar puncture and spinal anaesthesia)

• Severe acute or chronic heart failure

• Cardiogenic shock

• Mild to moderate liver insufficiency

• Platelet count $<150{,}000/mm^3$, known history of coagulopathy or platelet function disturbance or thrombocytopenia

• Haemoglobin concentration less than 11 g/dl or haematocrit $<34\%$.

Special caution should be used during concurrent administration of, ticlopidine, clopidogrel, adenosine, dipyridamole, sulfinpyrazone, and prostacyclin.

Elderly patients, female patients, and patients with low body weight

Elderly and/or female patients had a higher incidence of bleeding complications than younger or male patients, respectively. Patients with a low body weight had a higher incidence of bleeding than patients with a higher body weight. For these reasons 'Aggrastat' should be used with caution in these patients and the heparin effect should be carefully monitored.

Impaired renal function

There is evidence from clinical studies that the risk of bleeding increases with decreasing creatinine clearance and hence also reduced plasma clearance of tirofiban. Patients with decreased renal function (creatinine clearance <60ml/min) should therefore be carefully monitored for bleeding during treatment with 'Aggrastat' and the heparin effect should be carefully monitored. In severe kidney failure the 'Aggrastat' dosage should be reduced (see also 4.2 'Posology and method of administration').

Femoral artery line

During treatment with 'Aggrastat' there is a significant increase in bleeding rates, especially in the femoral artery area, where the catheter sheath is introduced. Care should be taken to ensure that only the anterior wall of the femoral artery is punctured. Arterial sheaths may be removed when coagulation has returned to normal, e.g. when activated clotting time (ACT) is less than 180 seconds, (usually 2–6 hours after discontinuation of heparin).

After removal of the introducer sheath, careful haemostasis should be ensured under close observation.

General nursing care

The number of vascular punctures, and intramuscular injections should be minimised during the treatment with 'Aggrastat'. I.V. access should only be obtained at compressible sites of the body. All vascular puncture sites should be documented and closely monitored. The use of urinary catheters, nasotracheal intubation and nasogastric tubes should be critically considered.

Monitoring of laboratory values

Platelet count, haemoglobin and haematocrit levels should be determined before treatment with 'Aggrastat' as well as within 2-6 hours after start of therapy with 'Aggrastat' and at least once daily thereafter while on therapy (or more often if there is evidence of a marked decrease). In patients who have previously received GPIIb/IIIa receptor antagonists (cross reactivity can occur), the platelet count should be monitored immediately e.g. within the first hour of administration after re-exposure (see also 4.8 Undesirable effects). If the platelet count falls below $90{,}000/mm^3$, further platelet counts should be carried out in order to rule out pseudothrombocytopenia. If thrombocytopenia is confirmed, 'Aggrastat' and heparin should be discontinued. Patients should be monitored for bleeding and treated if necessary (see also 4.9 'Overdose').

In addition, activated thromboplastin time (APTT) should be determined before treatment and the anticoagulant effects of heparin should be carefully monitored by repeated determinations of APTT and the dose should be adjusted accordingly (see also 4.2 'Posology and method of administration'). Potentially life-threatening bleeding may occur especially when heparin is administered with other products affecting haemostasis, such as GPIIb/IIIa receptor antagonists.

4.5 Interaction with other medicinal products and other forms of Interaction

The use of several platelet aggregation inhibitors increases the risk of bleeding, likewise their combination with heparin, warfarin and thrombolytics. Clinical and biological parameters of haemostasis should be regularly monitored.

The concomitant administration of 'Aggrastat' and ASA (acetylsalicyclic acid or aspirin) increases the inhibition of platelet aggregation to a greater extent than aspirin alone, as measured by *ex vivo* APD-induced platelet aggregation test. The concomitant administration of 'Aggrastat' and unfractionated heparin increases the prolongation of the bleeding time to a greater extent as compared to unfractionated heparin alone.

With the concurrent use of 'Aggrastat' and unfractionated heparin and ASA there was a higher incidence of bleeding than when only unfractionated heparin and ASA were used together (see also 4.4 'Special warnings and special precautions for use' and 4.8 'Undesirable effects').

'Aggrastat' prolonged bleeding time; however, the combined administration of 'Aggrastat' and ticlopidine did not additionally affect bleeding time.

Concomitant use of warfarin with 'Aggrastat' plus heparin was associated with an increased risk of bleeding.

'Aggrastat' is not recommended in thrombolytic therapy - concurrent or less than 48 hours before administration of tirofiban hydrochloride or concurrent use of drugs that increase the risk of bleeding to a relevant degree (e.g. oral anticoagulants, other parenteral GP IIb/IIIa inhibitors, dextran solutions). There is insufficient experience with the use of tirofiban hydrochloride in these conditions; however, an increased risk of bleeding is suspected.

4.6 Pregnancy and lactation

Pregnancy

For tirofiban hydrochloride, no clinical data on exposed pregnancies are available. Animal studies provide limited information with respect to effects on pregnancy, embryonal/foetal development, parturition, and postnatal development. 'Aggrastat' should not be used during pregnancy unless clearly necessary.

Lactation

It is not known whether 'Aggrastat' is excreted in human milk but it is known to be excreted in rat milk. Because of the potential for adverse effects on the nursing infant, a decision should be made whether to discontinue nursing or discontinue the drug, taking into account the importance of the drug to the mother.

4.7 Effects on ability to drive and use machines

No data are available on whether 'Aggrastat' impairs the ability to drive or operate machinery.

4.8 Undesirable effects

Bleeding

The adverse event causally related to 'Aggrastat' therapy (used concurrently with unfractionated heparin and ASA) most commonly reported was bleeding, which was usually of a milder nature.

In the PRISM-PLUS study, the overall incidence of major bleeding using the TIMI criteria (defined as a haemoglobin drop of >50 g/l with or without an identified site, intracranial haemorrhage, or cardiac tamponade) in patients treated with 'Aggrastat' in combination with heparin was not significantly higher than in the control group. The incidence of major bleeding using the TIMI criteria was 1.4% for 'Aggrastat' in combination with heparin and 0.8% for the control group (which received heparin). The incidence of minor bleeding using the TIMI criteria (defined as a haemoglobin drop of >30 g/l with bleeding from a known site, spontaneous gross haematuria, haematemesis or haemoptysis) was 10.5% for 'Aggrastat' in combination with heparin and 8.0% for the control group. There were no reports of intracranial bleeding for 'Aggrastat' in combination with heparin or in the control group. The incidence of retroperitoneal bleeding reported for 'Aggrastat' in combination with heparin was 0.0% and 0.1% for the control group. The percentage of patients who received a transfusion (including packed red blood cells, fresh frozen plasma, whole blood cryoprecipitates and platelets) was 4.0% for 'Aggrastat' and 2.8% for the control group.

'Aggrastat' given with unfractionated heparin and ASA was associated with gastro-intestinal, haemorrhoidal and postoperative bleeding, epistaxis, gum bleeds and surface dermatorrhagia as well as oozing haemorrhage (haematoma) in the area of intravascular puncture sites (e.g. in cardiac catheter examinations) significantly more often than was unfractionated heparin and ASA alone.

Non-bleeding-associated adverse reactions

The most common adverse drug reactions (incidence over 1%) associated with 'Aggrastat' given concurrently with heparin, apart from bleeding, were nausea (1.7%), fever (1.5%) and headache (1.1%); nausea, fever and headache occurred with incidences of 1.4%, 1.1% and 1.2%, respectively, in the control group.

The incidence of adverse non-bleeding-related events was higher in women (compared to men) and older patients (compared to younger patients). However, the incidences of non-bleeding-related adverse events in these patients were comparable for the 'Aggrastat' with heparin' group and the 'heparin alone' group.

[*Common*: >1/100, <1/10)]

Nervous system and psychiatric disorders:

Common: headache

Gastro-intestinal disorders:

Common: nausea

General disorders and administration site conditions:

Common: fever

Investigations

The most common changes of laboratory parameters associated with 'Aggrastat' related to bleeding: reduction of haemoglobin and haematocrit levels and an increased occurrence of occult blood in urine and faeces.

Occasionally during 'Aggrastat' therapy an acute fall in the platelet count or thrombocytopenia occurred. The percentage of patients in whom the platelet count fell to below 90,000/mm^3 was 1.5%. The percentage of patients in whom the platelet count fell to less than 50,000/mm^3 was 0.3%. These decreases were reversible upon discontinuation of 'Aggrastat'. Acute and severe platelet decreases have been observed in patients with no prior history of thrombocytopenia upon re-administration of GPIIb/IIIa receptor antagonists.

The following additional adverse reactions have been reported infrequently in post-marketing experience; they are derived from spontaneous reports for which precise incidences cannot be determined:

Blood and lymphatic system disorders:

Intracranial bleeding, retroperitoneal bleding, haemopericardium, pulmonary (alveolar) haemorrhage, and epidural haematoma in the spinal region. Fatal bleedings have been reported rarely.

Acute and/or severe (<20,000/mm^3) decreases in platelet counts which may be associated with chills, low-grade fever or bleeding complications (see 'Investigations' above)

Immune system disorders:

Severe allergic reactions (e.g., bronchospasm, urticaria) including anaphylactic reactions. The reported cases have occurred during initial treatment (also on the first day) and during readministration of tirofiban. Some cases have been associated with severe thrombocytopenia (platelet counts <10,000/mm^3).

4.9 Overdose

Inadvertent overdosage with tirofiban hydrochloride occurred in the clinical studies, up to 50 microgram/kg as a three minute bolus or 1.2 microgram/kg/min as an initial infusion. Overdosage with up to 1.47 microgram/kg/min as a maintenance infusion rate has also occurred.

a) Symptoms of overdosage

The symptom of overdosage most commonly reported was bleeding, usually mucosal bleeding and localised bleeding at the arterial puncture site for cardiac catheterisation but also single cases of intracranial haemorrhages and retroperitoneal bleedings (see also 4.4 'Special warnings and precautions for use' and 5.1 'Pharmacodynamic properties', *PRISM-PLUS study*).

b) Measures

Overdosage with tirofiban hydrochloride should be treated in accordance with the patient's condition and the attending physician's assessment. If treatment of haemorrhage is necessary, the 'Aggrastat' infusion should be discontinued. Transfusions of blood and/or thrombocytes should also be considered. 'Aggrastat' can be removed by haemodialysis.

5. PHARMACOLOGICAL PROPERTIES

5.1 Pharmacodynamic properties

ATC-Code: B01A C17

Tirofiban hydrochloride is a non-peptidal antagonist of the GP IIb/IIIa receptor, an important platelet surface receptor involved in platelet aggregation. Tirofiban hydrochloride prevents fibrinogen from binding to the GP IIb/IIIa receptor, thus blocking platelet aggregation.

Tirofiban hydrochloride leads to inhibition of platelet function, evidenced by its ability to inhibit *ex vivo* ADP-induced platelet aggregation and to prolong bleeding time (BT). Platelet function returns to baseline within eight hours after discontinuation.

The extent of this inhibition runs parallel to the tirofiban hydrochloride plasma concentration.

In the target population the recommended dosage of 'Aggrastat', in the presence of unfractionated heparin and ASA, produced a more than 70% (median 89%) inhibition of *ex vivo* ADP-induced platelet aggregation in 93% of the patients, and a prolongation of the bleeding time by a factor of 2.9 during infusion. Inhibition was achieved rapidly with the 30-minute loading infusion and was maintained over the duration of the infusion.

PRISM-PLUS study

The double-blind, multicentre, controlled PRISM-PLUS study compared the efficacy of tirofiban and unfractionated heparin (n=773) versus unfractionated heparin (n=797) in patients with unstable angina or acute non-Q-wave myocardial infarction (NQWMI).

Patients had to have prolonged, repetitive anginal pain, or post-infarction angina within 12 hours prior to randomisation, accompanied by new transient or persistent ST-T wave changes (ST depression or elevation ⩾0.1 mV; T-wave inversions ⩾0.3 mV) or elevated cardiac enzymes (total CPK ⩾ 2 times upper limit of normal, or CK-MB fraction elevated at the time of enrollment >5 % or greater than upper limit of normal]).

In this study, patients were randomised to either

– 'Aggrastat' (30 minute loading infusion of 0.4 microgram/kg/min followed by a maintenance infusion of 0.10 microgram/kg/min) and heparin (bolus of 5,000 units (U) followed by an infusion of 1,000 U/hr titrated to maintain an activated partial thromboplastin time (APTT) of approximately two times control),

– or heparin alone (bolus of 5,000 U followed by an infusion of 1,000 U/hr titrated to maintain an APTT of approximately two times control).

All patients received ASA unless contra-indicated; 300-325 mg orally per day were recommended for the first 48 hours and thereafter 80-325 mg orally per day (as determined by the physician). Study drug was initiated within 12 hours after the last anginal episode. Patients were treated for 48 hours, after which they underwent angiography and possibly angioplasty/atherectomy, if indicated, while tirofiban hydrochloride was continued. Tirofiban hydrochloride was infused for a mean period of 71.3 hours.

The combined primary study end-point was the occurrence of refractory ischaemia, myocardial infarction or death at seven days after the start of tirofiban hydrochloride.

The mean age of the population was 63 years; 32% of patients were female. At baseline approximately 58% of patients had ST segment depression; 53% had T-wave inversions; 46% of patients presented with elevated cardiac enzymes. During the study approximately 90% of patients underwent coronary angiography; 30% underwent early angioplasty and 23% underwent early coronary artery bypass surgery.

At the primary end-point, there was a 32% risk reduction (RR) (12.9% vs. 17.9%) in the tirofiban hydrochloride group for the combined end-point (p=0.004): this represents approximately 50 events avoided for 1,000 patients treated. Results of the primary end-point were principally attributed to the occurrence of myocardial infarction and refractory ischaemic conditions.

After 30 days the RR for the combined end-point (death/myocardial infarction/refractory ischaemic conditions/readmissions for unstable angina) was 22% (18.5% vs. 22.3%; p=0.029).

After six months the risk of the combined end-point (death/myocardial infarction/refractory ischaemic conditions/readmissions for unstable angina) was reduced by 19% (27.7% vs. 32.1%; p=0.024).

Regarding the most commonly used double combined end-point, death or myocardial infarction, the results at seven days, 30 days and six months were as follows: at seven days for the tirofiban group there was a 43% RR (4.9% vs. 8.3%; p=0.006); at 30 days the RR was 30% (8.7% vs. 11.9%; p=0.027) and at 6 months the RR was 23% (12.3% vs. 15.3%; p=0.063).

The reduction in the incidence of myocardial infarctions in patients receiving 'Aggrastat' appeared early during treatment (within the first 48 hours) and this reduction was maintained through six months, without significant effect on mortality.

In the 30% of patients who underwent angioplasty/atherectomy during initial hospitalisation, there was a 46% RR (8.8% vs. 15.2%) for the primary combined end-point at 30 days as well as a 43% RR (5.9% vs. 10.2%) for 'myocardial infarction or death'.

Based on a safety study, the concomitant administration of 'Aggrastat' with enoxaparin (n=315) was compared to the concomitant administration of 'Aggrastat' with unfractionated heparin (n=210) in patients presenting with unstable angina and non-Q-wave myocardial infarction. A 30 minute loading dose of tirofiban (0.4 microgram/kg/min) was followed by a maintenance infusion of 0.1 microgram/kg/min for up to 108 hours. Patients randomised to the enoxaparin group received a 1.0 mg/kg subcutaneous injection of enoxaparin every 12 hours for a period of at least 24 hours and a maximum duration of 96 hours. Patients randomised to the unfractionated heparin group received a 5000-unit intravenous bolus of unfractionated heparin followed by a maintenance infusion of 1000 units per hour for at least 24 hours and a maximum duration of 108 hours. The total TIMI bleed rate was 3.5% for the tirofiban/enoxaparin group and 4.8% for the tirofiban/unfractionated heparin group. Cutaneous bleeds and oral bleeds occurred more frequently in patients randomised to the enoxaparin group versus the unfractionated heparin group. Catheter site bleeds were more common in the enoxaparin group as compared to the unfractionated heparin group. Patients randomised to the enoxaparin group who subsequently required PCI were switched to unfractionated heparin peri-procedurally with the dose titrated to maintain an ACT of 250 seconds or higher. Although there was a signifcant difference in the rates of cutaneous bleeds between the two groups (29.2% in the enoxaparin converted to unfractionated heparin group and 15.2% in the unfractionated heparin group), there were no TIMI major bleeds (see also 4.4 'Special warnings and precautions for use') in either group. The efficacy of 'Aggrastat' in combination with enoxaparin has not been established.

Patients most likely to benefit from 'Aggrastat' treatment are those at high risk of developing myocardial infarction within the 3-4 days after onset of acute angina symptoms. According to epidemiological findings, a higher incidence of cardiovascular events has been associated with certain indicators, for instance: age, elevated heart rate or blood pressure, persistent or recurrent ischaemic cardiac pain, marked ECG changes (in particular ST-segment abnormalities), raised cardiac enzymes or markers (e.g. CK-MB, troponins) and heart failure.

5.2 Pharmacokinetic properties

Distribution

Tirofiban is not strongly bound to plasma protein, and protein binding is concentration-independent in the range of 0.01–25 microgram/ml. The unbound fraction in human plasma is 35%.

The distribution volume of tirofiban in the steady state is about 30 litres.

Biotransformation

Experiments with ^{14}C-labelled tirofiban showed the radioactivity in urine and faeces to be emitted chiefly by unchanged tirofiban. The radioactivity in circulating plasma originates mainly from unchanged tirofiban (up to 10 hours after administration). These data suggested limited metabolisation of tirofiban.

Elimination

After intravenous administration of ^{14}C-labelled tirofiban to healthy subjects, 66% of the radioactivity was recovered in the urine, 23% in the faeces. The total recovery of radioactivity was 91%. Renal and biliary excretion contribute significantly to the elimination of tirofiban.

In healthy subjects the plasma clearance of tirofiban is about 250 ml/min. Renal clearance is 39–69% of plasma clearance. The half-life is about 1.5 hours.

Gender

The plasma clearance of tirofiban in patients with coronary heart disease is similar in men and women.

Elderly patients

The plasma clearance of tirofiban is about 25% less in elderly >65 years) patients with coronary heart disease in comparison to younger (≤65 years) patients.

Ethnic groups

No difference was found in the plasma clearance between patients of different ethnic groups.

Coronary Artery Disease

In patients with unstable angina pectoris or NQWMI the plasma clearance was about 200 ml/min, the renal clearance 39% of the plasma clearance. The half-life is about two hours.

Impaired renal function

In clinical studies, patients with decreased renal function showed a reduced plasma clearance of tirofiban depending on the degree of impairment of creatinine clearance. In patients with a creatinine clearance of less than 30 ml/min, including haemodialysis patients, the plasma clearance of tirofiban is reduced to a clinically relevant extent (over 50%) (see also 4.2 'Posology and method of administration'). Tirofiban is removed by haemodialysis.

Liver failure

There is no evidence of a clinically significant reduction of the plasma clearance of tirofiban in patients with mild to moderate liver failure. No data are available on patients with severe liver failure.

Effects of other drugs

The plasma clearance of tirofiban in patients receiving one of the following drugs was compared to that in patients not receiving that drug in a sub-set of patients (n=762) in the PRISM study. There were no substantial >15%) effects of these drugs on the plasma clearance of tirofiban: acebutolol, alprazolam, amlodipine, aspirin preparations, atenolol, bromazepam, captopril, diazepam, digoxin, diltiazem, docusate sodium, enalapril, furosemide, glibenclamide, unfractionated heparin, insulin, isosorbide, lorazepam, lovastatin, metoclopramide, metoprolol, morphine, nifedipine, nitrate preparations, oxazepam, paracetamol, potassium chloride, propranolol, ranitidine, simvastatin, sucralfate and temazepam.

The pharmacokinetics and pharmacodynamics of 'Aggrastat' were investigated when concomitantly administered with enoxaparin (1mg/kg subcutaneously every 12 hours) and compared with the combination of 'Aggrastat' and unfractionated heparin. There was no difference in the clearance of 'Aggrastat' between the two groups.

5.3 Preclinical safety data

Preclinical data reveal no special hazard for humans based on conventional studies of safety pharmacology, repeated dose toxicity and genotoxicity.

Tirofiban crosses the placenta in rats and rabbits.

6. PHARMACEUTICAL PARTICULARS

6.1 List of excipients

Sodium chloride, sodium citrate dihydrate, citric acid anhydrous, water for injections, hydrochloric acid and/or sodium hydroxide (for pH adjustment).

6.2 Incompatibilities

Incompatibility has been found with diazepam. Therefore, 'Aggrastat' and diazepam should not be administered in the same intravenous line.

6.3 Shelf life

'Aggrastat' Solution: 2 years

'Aggrastat Concentrate: 3 years.

From a microbiological point of view the diluted solution for infusion should be used immediately. If not used immediately, in use storage conditions are the responsibility of the user and would normally not be longer than 24 hours at 2-8°C, unless reconstitution has taken place in controlled and validated aseptic conditions.

6.4 Special precautions for storage

'Aggrastat' Solution:

Do not freeze. Keep container in either foil overpouch (250 ml solution for infusion) or outer carton (500 ml solution for infusion), to protect from light.

'Aggrastat' Concentrate:

Do not freeze. Keep container in outer carton to protect from light.

6.5 Nature and contents of container

'Aggrastat' Solution:

250 ml IntraVia™ container (PL 2408 plastic), colourless, 3-layer polyolefine film with outlet port and PVC tube with blue top. It is packed in a preprinted foil overpouch.

500 ml IntraVia™ container (PL 2408 plastic), colourless, 3-layer polyolefine film with outlet port and PVC tube with blue top. It is packed in a dust cover made from polyolefine transparent without print.

Pack sizes: 1 or 3 containers with 250 ml solution for infusion. 1 container with 500 ml solution for infusion. Not all pack sizes may be marketed.

'Aggrastat' Concentrate:

50 ml Type I glass vial.

6.6 Instructions for use and handling

No incompatibilities have been found with 'Aggrastat' and the following intravenous formulations: atropine sulfate, dobutamine, dopamine, epinephrine HCl, furosemide, heparin, lidocaine, midazolam HCl, morphine sulfate, nitroglycerin, potassium chloride, propanolol HCl and famotidine injection.

'Aggrastat' Solution:

Some opacity of the plastic due to moisture absorption during the sterilisation process may be observed. This is normal and does not affect the solution quality or safety. The opacity will diminish gradually. Check for minute leaks by squeezing inner bag firmly. If leaks are found, discard solution as sterility may be impaired.

'Aggrastat' Concentrate:

'Aggrastat' concentrate for solution for infusion must be diluted before use.

See 4.2 'Posology and method of administration'.

Any unused solution should be discarded.

7. MARKETING AUTHORISATION HOLDER

Merck Sharp & Dohme Limited

Hertford Road, Hoddesdon, Hertfordshire EN11 9BU, UK

8. MARKETING AUTHORISATION NUMBER(S)

'Aggrastat' Solution: PL0025/0375

'Aggrastat' Concentrate: PL0025/0376

9. DATE OF FIRST AUTHORISATION/RENEWAL OF THE AUTHORISATION

First authorisation: 15 July 1999.

First renewal: 14 May 2003

10. DATE OF REVISION OF THE TEXT

April 2005.

® denotes registered trademark of Merck & Co., Inc., Whitehouse Station, NJ, USA.

SPC.ARSC.03.UK.0877 (JOINT)

Agrippal

(Wyeth Pharmaceuticals)

1. NAME OF THE MEDICINAL PRODUCT

AGRIPPAL®

Suspension for injection in pre-filled syringe

Influenza vaccine (surface antigen, inactivated)

(2005/2006 season)

2. QUALITATIVE AND QUANTITATIVE COMPOSITION

Influenza virus surface antigens (haemagglutinin and neuraminidase)*, of strains:

A/New Caledonia/20/99 (H1N1) - like strain (A/New Caledonia/20/99 IVR-116)

15 micrograms **

A/California/7/2004 (H3N2) – like strain (A/New York/55/2004 NYMC X-157)

15 micrograms**

B/Shanghai/361/2002 - like strain (B/Jiangsu/10/2003)

15 micrograms **

For one dose of 0.5 ml.

*propagated in eggs, inactivated by formaldehyde

**haemagglutinin

This vaccine complies with the WHO recommendations (northern hemisphere) and EU decision for the 2005/2006 season.

For excipients see 6.1

3. PHARMACEUTICAL FORM

Suspension for injection in pre-filled syringe.

4. CLINICAL PARTICULARS

4.1 Therapeutic indications

Prophylaxis of influenza, especially in those who run an increased risk of associated complications.

4.2 Posology and method of administration

- Adults and children from 36 months: 0.5 ml

- Children from 6 months to 35 months: Clinical data are limited. Dosages of 0.25 ml or 0.5 ml have been used.

For children who have not previously been vaccinated, a second dose should be given after an interval of at least 4 weeks.

Immunisation should be carried out by intramuscular or deep subcutaneous injection.

4.3 Contraindications

Hypersensitivity to the active substances, to any of the excipients and to eggs, chicken proteins, kanamycin and neomycin sulphate, formaldehyde, cetyltrimethylammonium bromide (CTAB) and polysorbate 80.

Immunisation shall be postponed in patients with febrile illness or acute infection.

4.4 Special warnings and special precautions for use

As with all injectable vaccines, appropriate medical treatment and supervision should always be readily available in case of a rare anaphylactic event following the administration of the vaccine.

The vaccine (AGRIPPAL) should under no circumstances be administered intravascularly.

Antibody response in patients with endogenous or iatrogenic immunosuppression may be insufficient.

4.5 Interaction with other medicinal products and other forms of Interaction

The vaccine (AGRIPPAL) may be given at the same time as other vaccines. Immunisation should be carried out on separate limbs. It should be noted that the adverse reactions may be intensified.

The immunological response may be diminished if the patient is undergoing immunosuppressant treatment.

Following influenza vaccination, false positive results in serology tests using the ELISA method to detect antibodies against HIV1, Hepatitis C and especially HTLV1 have been observed. The Western Blot technique disproves the results. The transient false positive reactions could be due to the IgM response to the vaccine.

4.6 Pregnancy and lactation

Limited data from vaccinations in pregnant women do not indicate that adverse foetal and maternal outcomes were attributable to the vaccine. The use of this vaccine may be considered from the second trimester of pregnancy. For pregnant women with medical conditions that increase their risk of complications from influenza, administration of the vaccine is recommended, irrespective of their stage of pregnancy.

The vaccine (AGRIPPAL) may be used during lactation.

4.7 Effects on ability to drive and use machines

The vaccine is unlikely to produce an effect on the ability to drive and use machines.

4.8 Undesirable effects

Adverse reactions from clinical trials

The safety of trivalent inactivated influenza vaccines is assessed in open label, uncontrolled clinical trials performed as annual update requirement, including at least 50 adults aged 18 – 60 years of age and at least 50 elderly aged 60 years or older. Safety evaluation is performed during the first 3 days following vaccination.

Undesirable effects reported are listed according to the following frequency.

Adverse events from clinical trials:

Common (>1/100, <1/10):

Local reactions: redness, swelling, pain, ecchymosis, induration.

Systemic reactions: fever, malaise, shivering, fatigue, headache, sweating, myalgia, arthralgia.

These reactions usually disappear within 1-2 days without treatment.

From Post-marketing surveillance additionally, the following adverse events have been reported:

Uncommon (>1/1,000, <1/100):

Generalised skin reactions including pruritus, urticaria or non-specific rash.

Rare (>1/10,000, <1/1,000): neuralgia, paraesthesia, convulsions, transient thrombocytopenia.

Allergic reactions, in rare cases leading to shock, have been reported.

Very rare (<1/10,000):

Vasculitis with transient renal involvement.

Neurological disorders, such as encephalomyelitis, neuritis and Guillain Barré syndrome.

4.9 Overdose

Overdosage is unlikely to have any untoward effect.

5. PHARMACOLOGICAL PROPERTIES

5.1 Pharmacodynamic properties

Seroprotection is generally obtained within 2 to 3 weeks. The duration of postvaccinal immunity to homologous strains or to strains closely related to the vaccine strains varies but is usually 6-12 months.

ATC code J07BB02.

5.2 Pharmacokinetic properties

Not applicable

5.3 Preclinical safety data

Not applicable

6. PHARMACEUTICAL PARTICULARS

6.1 List of excipients

Sodium chloride, Potassium chloride, Potassium dihydrogen phosphate, Disodium phosphate dihydrate, Magnesium chloride, Calcium chloride, and Water for Injections.

6.2 Incompatibilities

In the absence of compatibility studies, this medicinal product must not be mixed with other medicinal products.

6.3 Shelf life

1 year.

6.4 Special precautions for storage

This product should be stored at +2°C to +8°C (in a refrigerator).

Do not freeze. Protect from light.

6.5 Nature and contents of container

0.5 ml of suspension for injection in a pre-filled syringe (type I glass) equipped with a rubber plunger stopper, presented with or without a needle.

Pack of 1, with needle (23 G, 1" or 25 G, 1" or 25 G, 5/8") or without needle.

Pack of 10x, with needle (23 G, 1" or 25 G 1" or 25 G, 5/8") or without needle.

6.6 Instructions for use and handling

The vaccine should be allowed to reach room temperature before use.

Shake before use.

If half a dose (0.25 ml) is to be administered, discard half the contained volume

(up to the mark indicated on the syringe barrel), before injection.

7. MARKETING AUTHORISATION HOLDER

Chiron S.r.l., Via Fiorentina 1, SIENA, Italy

8. MARKETING AUTHORISATION NUMBER(S)

PL 13767/0004

9. DATE OF FIRST AUTHORISATION/RENEWAL OF THE AUTHORISATION

8 March 1999

10. DATE OF REVISION OF THE TEXT

June 2005

Further information may be obtained from:

For the UK:

Wyeth Vaccines, Huntercombe Lane South,

Taplow, Maidenhead, Berkshire, SL6 OPH

Telephone: 01628 415330

® Registered trade mark of Chiron S.r.l., Italy

Aldactide 25mg and 50mg Tablets

(Pharmacia Limited)

1. NAME OF THE MEDICINAL PRODUCT

Aldactide 25.

Aldactide 50.

2. QUALITATIVE AND QUANTITATIVE COMPOSITION

Each tablet contains 25mg spironolactone BP and 25mg hydroflumethiazide BP

Each tablet contains 50mg spironolactone BP and 50mg hydroflumethiazide BP

3. PHARMACEUTICAL FORM

Buff, film coated tablets engraved "SEARLE 101" on one side.

Buff, film coated tablets engraved "SEARLE 180" on one side.

4. CLINICAL PARTICULARS

4.1 Therapeutic indications

Congestive cardiac failure.

4.2 Posology and method of administration

Administration of Aldactide once daily with a meal is recommended.

Adults

Most patients will require an initial dosage of 100mg spironolactone daily. The dosage should be adjusted as necessary and may range from 25mg to 200mg spironolactone daily.

Elderly

It is recommended that treatment is started with the lowest dose and titrated upwards as required to achieve maximum benefit. Care should be taken with severe hepatic and renal impairment which may alter drug metabolism and excretion.

Children

Although clinical trials using Aldactide have not been carried out in children, as a guide, a daily dosage providing 1.5 to 3mg of spironolactone per kilogram body weight given in divided doses, may be employed.

4.3 Contraindications

Aldactide is contraindicated in patients with anuria, acute renal insufficiency, rapidly deteriorating or severe impairment of renal function, hyperkalaemia, significant hypercalcaemia, Addison's disease and in patients who are hypersensitive to spironolactone, thiazide diuretics or to other sulphonamide derived drugs.

Aldactide should not be administered with other potassium conserving diuretics and potassium supplements should not be given routinely with Aldactide as hyperkalemia may be induced.

4.4 Special warnings and special precautions for use

Warnings

Sulphonamide derivatives including thiazides have been reported to exacerbate or activate systemic lupus erythematosus.

Precautions

Fluid and electrolyte balance: Fluid and electrolyte status should be regularly monitored particularly in the elderly, in those with significant renal and hepatic impairment, and in patients receiving digoxin and drugs with pro-arrhythmic effects.

Hyperkalaemia may occur in patients with impaired renal function or excessive potassium intake and can cause cardiac irregularities which may be fatal. Should hyperkalaemia develop Aldactide should be discontinued, and if necessary, active measures taken to reduce the serum potassium to normal. *(See 4.3 Contraindications)*

Hypokalaemia may develop as a result of profound diuresis, particularly when Aldactide is used concomitantly with loop diuretics, glucocorticoids or ACTH.

Hyponatraemia may be induced especially when Aldactide is administered in combination with other diuretics.

Hepatic impairment: Caution should be observed in patients with acute or severe liver impairment as vigorous diuretic therapy may precipitate encephalopathy in susceptible patients. Regular estimation of serum electrolytes is essential in such patients.

Reversible hyperchloraemic metabolic acidosis usually in association with hyperkalaemia has been reported to occur in some patients with decompensated hepatic cirrhosis, even in the presence of normal renal function.

Urea and uric acid: Reversible increases in blood urea have been reported, particularly accompanying vigorous diuresis or in the presence of impaired renal function.

Thiazides may cause hyperuricaemia and precipitate attacks of gout in some patients.

Diabetes mellitus: Thiazides may aggravate existing diabetes and the insulin requirements may alter. Diabetes mellitus which has been latent may become manifest during thiazide administration.

Hyperlipidaemia: Caution should be observed as thiazides may raise serum lipids.

4.5 Interaction with other medicinal products and other forms of Interaction

Spironolactone has been reported to increase serum digoxin concentration and to interfere with certain serum digoxin assays. In patients receiving digoxin and spironolactone the digoxin response should be monitored by means other than serum digoxin concentrations, unless the digoxin assay used has been proven not to be affected by spironolactone therapy. If it proves necessary to adjust the dose of digoxin, patients should be carefully monitored for evidence of enhanced or reduced digoxin effect. Potentiation of the effect of antihypertensive drugs occurs and their dosage may need to be reduced when Aldactide is added to the treatment regime and then adjusted as necessary. Since ACE inhibitors decrease aldosterone production they should not routinely be used with Aldactide, particularly in patients with marked renal impairment.

As carbenoxolone may cause sodium retention and thus decrease the effectiveness of Aldactide, concurrent use should be avoided.

Non-steroidal anti-inflammatory drugs may attenuate the natriuretic efficacy of diuretics due to inhibition of intrarenal synthesis of prostaglandins.

Concurrent use of lithium and thiazides may reduce lithium clearance leading to intoxication.

Spironolactone and thiazides may reduce vascular responsiveness to noradrenaline. Caution should be exercised in the management of patients subjected to regional or general anaesthesia while they are being treated with Aldactide.

Concomitant use of aldactide with other potassium-sparing diuretics, ACE inhibitors, angiotensin II antagonists, aldosterone blockers, potassium supplements, a diet rich in potassium, or salt substitutes containing potassium, may lead to severe hyperkalaemia.

In fluorimetric assays, spironolactone may interfere with the estimation of compounds with similar flourescence characteristics.

Spironolactone has been shown to increase the half-life of digoxin.

Aspirin, indomethacin, and mefanamic acid have been shown to attenuate the diuretic effect of spironolactone.

Spironolactone enhances the metabolism of antipyrine.

Spironolactone can interfere with assays for plasma digoxin concentrations

The absorption of a number of drugs including thiazides is decreased when co-administered with cholestyramine and colestipol.

Thiazide co-administered with calcium and/or vitamin D may increase the risk of hypercalcaemia. Thiazides may delay the elimination of quinidine.

4.6 Pregnancy and lactation

Pregnancy

Spironolactone or its metabolites may, and hydroflumethiazide does, cross the placental barrier. With spironolactone, feminisation has been observed in male rat foetuses, thiazides may decrease placental perfusion, increase uterine inertia and inhibit labour. In the foetus or neonate thiazides may cause jaundice, thrombocytopenia, hypoglycaemia, electrolyte imbalance and death from maternal complications. The use of Aldactide in pregnant women requires that the anticipated benefit be weighed against the possible hazards to the mother and foetus.

Lactation

Metabolites of spironolactone and hydroflumethiazide, have been detected in breast milk. If use of Aldactide is considered essential, an alternative method of infant feeding should be instituted.

4.7 Effects on ability to drive and use machines

Somnolence and dizziness have been reported to occur in some patients. Caution is advised when driving or operating machinery until the response to initial treatment has been determined.

4.8 Undesirable effects

Gynaecomastia may develop in association with the use of spironolactone. Development appears to be related to both dosage level and duration of therapy and is normally reversible when the drug is discontinued. In rare instances some breast enlargement may persist.

The following adverse events have been reported in association with spironolactone therapy:

Body as a Whole: malaise

Endocrine Disorders: benign breast neoplasm, breast pain

Gastrointestinal Disorders: gastrointestinal disturbances, nausea

Hematologic Disorders: leukopenia (including agranulocytosis), thrombocytopenia

Liver Disorders: hepatic function abnormal

Metabolic and Nutritional Disorders: electrolyte disturbances, hyperkalemia

Musculoskeletal Disorders: leg cramps

Nervous System Disorders: dizziness

Psychiatric Disorders: changes in libido, confusion

Reproductive Disorders: menstrual disorders

Skin and Appendages: alopecia, hypertrichosis, pruritus, rash, urticaria,

Urinary System Disorders: acute renal failure

The following isolated adverse event has been reported in association with spironolactone therapy:

Skin and Appendages: Stevens Johnson Syndrome

Adverse reactions reported in association with thiazides include: gastrointestinal upsets, skin rashes, photosensitivity, blood dyscrasias, raised serum lipids, aplastic anaemia, purpura muscle cramps, weakness, restlessness, headache, dizziness, vertigo, jaundice, orthostatic hypotension, impotence, paraesthesia, and rarely pancreatitis, necrotising vasculitis and xanthopsia. Rarely hypercalcaemia has been reported in association with thiazides, usually in patients with pre-existing metabolic bone disease or parathyroid dysfunction.

4.9 Overdose

Acute overdosage may be manifested by drowsiness, mental confusion, nausea, vomiting, dizziness or diarrhoea. Hyponatraemia, Hypokalaemia or hyperkalaemia may be induced or hepatic coma may be precipitated in patients with severe liver disease, but these effects are unlikely to be associated with acute overdosage. Symptoms of hyperkalaemia may manifest as paraesthesia, weakness, flaccid paralysis or muscle spasm and may be difficult to distinguish clinically from hypokalaemia. Electro-cardiographic changes are the earliest specific signs of potassium disturbances. No specific antidote has been identified. Improvement may be expected after withdrawal of the drug. General supportive measures including replacement of fluids and electrolytes may be indicated. For hyperkalaemia, reduce potassium intake, administer potassium-excreting diuretics, intravenous glucose with regular insulin or oral ion-exchange resins.

5. PHARMACOLOGICAL PROPERTIES

5.1 Pharmacodynamic properties

Spironolactone, as a competitive aldosterone antagonist, increases sodium excretion whilst reducing potassium loss at the distal renal tubule. It has a gradual and prolonged action.

Hydroflumethiazide is a thiazide diuretic. Diuresis is initiated usually within 2 hours and lasts for about 12-18 hours.

5.2 Pharmacokinetic properties

Spironolactone is well absorbed orally and is principally metabolised to active metabolites: sulphur containing metabolites (80%) and partly canrenone (20%). Although the plasma half life of spironolactone itself is short (1.3 hours) the half lives of the active metabolites are longer (ranging from 2.8 to 11.2 hours). Elimination of metabolites occurs primarily in the urine and secondarily through biliary excretion in the faeces.

Following the administration of 100 mg of spironolactone daily for 15 days in non-fasted healthy volunteers, time to peak plasma concentration (t_{max}), peak plasma concentration (C_{max}), and elimination half-life ($t_{1/2}$) for spironolactone is 2.6 hr., 80 ng/ml, and approximately 1.4 hr., respectively. For the 7-alpha-(thiomethyl) spironolactone and canrenone metabolites, t_{max} was 3.2 hr. and 4.3 hr., C_{max} was 391 ng/ml and 181 ng/ml, and $t_{1/2}$ was 13.8 hr. and 16.5 hr., respectively.

The renal action of a single dose of spironolactone reaches its peak after 7 hours, and activity persists for at least 24 hours

Hydroflumethiazide is incompletely but fairly rapidly absorbed from the gastro-intestinal tract. It appears to have a biphasic biological half-life with an estimated alpha-phase of about 2 hours and an estimated beta-phase of about 17 hours; it has a metabolite with a longer half-life, which is extensively bound to the red blood cells. Hydroflumethiazide is excreted in the urine; its metabolite has also been detected in the urine.

5.3 Preclinical safety data

Carcinogenicity: Spironolactone has been shown to produce tumours in rats when administered at high doses over a long period of time. The significance of these findings with respect to clinical use is not certain. However, the long term use of spironolactone in young patients requires careful consideration of the benefits and the potential hazard involved. Spironolactone or its metabolites may cross the placental barrier. With spironolactone, feminisation has been observed in male rat foetuses. The use of Aldactone in pregnant women requires that the anticipated benefit be weighed against the possible hazards to the mother and foetus.

6. PHARMACEUTICAL PARTICULARS

6.1 List of excipients

Aldactide 25 and 50 contains: Calcium sulphate dihydrate, corn starch, polyvinyl pyrrolidone, magnesium stearate, felocofix peppermint, hydroxypropyl methylcellulose, polyethylene glycol and opaspray yellow (contains E172 and E171).

6.2 Incompatibilities

None stated.

6.3 Shelf life

The shelf life of Aldactide tablets is 5 years.

6.4 Special precautions for storage

Store in a dry place below 30°C.

6.5 Nature and contents of container

Aldactide 25mg and 50mg tablets may be packaged in the following containers: Amber glass bottles, HDPE containers or PVC/foil blister packs containing 100 and 500 tablets.

6.6 Instructions for use and handling

There are no special instructions for handling.

7. MARKETING AUTHORISATION HOLDER

Pharmacia Limited

Davy Avenue

Knowlhill

Milton Keynes

MK5 8PH

United Kingdom

8. MARKETING AUTHORISATION NUMBER(S)

Aldactide 25 - PL 00032/0391

Aldactide 50 - PL 00032/0392

9. DATE OF FIRST AUTHORISATION/RENEWAL OF THE AUTHORISATION

Aldactide 25 - 6 July 2002

Aldactide 50 – 23 May 2002

10. DATE OF REVISION OF THE TEXT

July 2004

11. LEGAL CATEGORY

POM

Aldactone 25mg, 50mg and 100mg Tablets

(Pharmacia Limited)

1. NAME OF THE MEDICINAL PRODUCT

Aldactone 25mg

Aldactone 50mg

Aldactone 100 mg

2. QUALITATIVE AND QUANTITATIVE COMPOSITION

Each tablet contains 25mg spironolactone BP

Each tablet contains 50mg spironolactone BP

Each tablet contains 100 mg spironolactone BP

3. PHARMACEUTICAL FORM

Buff, film coated tablets engraved "SEARLE 39" on one side.

White, film coated tablets engraved "SEARLE 916" on one side.

Buff, film coated tablets engraved "SEARLE 134" on one side.

4. CLINICAL PARTICULARS

4.1 Therapeutic indications

Congestive cardiac failure.

Hepatic cirrhosis with ascites and oedema.

Malignant ascites

Nephrotic syndrome.

Diagnosis and treatment of primary aldosteronism.

4.2 Posology and method of administration

Administration of Aldactone once daily with a meal is recommended.

Adults

Congestive cardiac failure

Usual dose- 100mg/day. In difficult or severe cases the dosage may be gradually increased up to 400mg/day. When oedema is controlled, the usual maintenance level is 25mg-200mg/day.

Hepatic cirrhosis with ascites and oedema.

If urinary Na+/K+ ratio is greater than 1.0, 100mg/day. If the ratio is less than 1.0, 200-400mg/day. Maintenance dosage should be individually determined.

Malignant ascites

Initial dose usually 100-200mg/day. In severe cases the dosage may be gradually increased up to 400mg/day. When oedema is controlled, maintenance dosage should be individually determined.

Nephrotic syndrome

Usual dose 100-200mg/day. Spironolactone has not been shown to be anti-inflammatory, nor to affect the basic pathological process. Its use is only advised if glucocorticoids by themselves are insufficiently effective.

Diagnosis and treatment of primary aldosteronism.

Aldactone may be employed as an initial diagnostic measure to provide presumptive evidence of primary hyperaldosteronism while patients are on normal diets.

Long test: Aldactone is administered at a daily dosage of 400mg for three to four weeks. Correction of hypokalaemia and of hypertension provides presumptive evidence for the diagnosis of primary hyperaldosteronism.

Short test: Aldactone is administered at a daily dosage of 400mg for four days. If serum potassium increases during Aldactone administration but drops when Aldactone is discontinued, a presumptive diagnosis of primary hyperaldosteronism should be considered.

After the diagnosis of hyperaldosteronism has been established by more definitive testing procedures, Aldactone may be administered at doses of 100mg-400mg daily in preparation for surgery. For patients who are considered unsuitable for surgery, Aldactone may be employed for long-term maintenance therapy at the lowest effective dosage determined for the individual patient.

Elderly

It is recommended that treatment is started with the lowest dose and titrated upwards as required to achieve maximum benefit. Care should be taken with severe hepatic and renal impairment which may alter drug metabolism and excretion.

Children

Initial daily dosage should provide 3mg of spironolactone per kilogram body weight given in divided doses. Dosage should be adjusted on the basis of response and tolerance. If necessary a suspension may be prepared by crushing Aldactone tablets.

4.3 Contraindications

Aldactone is contraindicated in patients with anuria, acute renal insufficiency, rapidly deteriorating or severe impairment of renal function, hyperkalaemia, Addison's disease and in patients who are hypersensitive to spironolactone.

Aldactone should not be administered concurrently with other potassium conserving diuretics and potassium supplements should not be given routinely with Aldactone as hyperkalemia may be induced.

4.4 Special warnings and special precautions for use

Fluid and electrolyte balance: Fluid and electrolyte status should be regularly monitored particularly in the elderly, in those with significant renal and hepatic impairment

Hyperkalaemia may occur in patients with impaired renal function or excessive potassium intake and can cause cardiac irregularities which may be fatal. Should hyperkalaemia develop Aldactone should be discontinued, and if necessary, active measures taken to reduce the serum potassium to normal.(*See 4.3 Contraindications*)

Hyponatremia may be induced, especially when Aldactone is administered in combination with other diuretics.

Reversible hyperchloraemic metabolic acidosis, usually in association with hyperkalaemia has been reported to occur in some patients with decompensated hepatic cirrhosis, even in the presence of normal renal function.

Urea: Reversible increases in blood urea have been reported in association with Aldactone therapy, particularly in the presence of impaired renal function.

4.5 Interaction with other medicinal products and other forms of Interaction

Spironolactone has been reported to increase serum digoxin concentration and to interfere with certain serum digoxin assays. In patients receiving digoxin and spironolactone the digoxin response should be monitored by means other than serum digoxin concentrations, unless the digoxin assay used has been proven not to be affected by spironolactone therapy. If it proves necessary to adjust the dose of digoxin patients should be carefully monitored for evidence of enhanced or reduced digoxin effect.

Potentiation of the effect of antihypertensive drugs occurs and their dosage may need to be reduced when Aldactone is added to the treatment regime and then adjusted as necessary. Since ACE inhibitors decrease aldosterone production they should not routinely be used with Aldactone, particularly in patients with marked renal impairment.

As carbenoxolone may cause sodium retention and thus decrease the effectiveness of Aldactone concurrent use should be avoided.

Non-steroidal anti-inflammatory drugs may attenuate the natriuretic efficacy of diuretics due to inhibition of intrarenal synthesis of prostaglandins.

Spironolactone reduces vascular responsiveness to noradrenaline. Caution should be exercised in the management of patients subjected to regional or general anaesthesia while they are being treated with Aldactone.

Concomitant use of aldactone with other potassium-sparing diuretics, ACE inhibitors, angiotensin II antagonists, aldosterone blockers, potassium supplements, a diet rich in potassium, or salt substitutes containing potassium, may lead to severe hyperkalaemia.

In fluorimetric assays, spironolactone may interfere with the estimation of compounds with similar fluorescence characteristics.

Spironolactone has been shown to increase the half-life of digoxin.

Aspirin, indomethacin, and mefanamic acid have been shown to attenuate the diuretic effect of spironolactone.

Spironolactone enhances the metabolism of antipyrine.

Spironolactone can interfere with assays for plasma digoxin concentrations

4.6 Pregnancy and lactation

Pregnancy

Spironolactone or its metabolites may cross the placental barrier. With spironolactone, feminisation has been observed in male rat foetuses. The use of Aldactone in pregnant women requires that the anticipated benefit be weighed against the possible hazards to the mother and foetus.

Lactation

Metabolites of spironolactone have been detected in breast milk. If use of Aldactone is considered essential, an alternative method of infant feeding should be instituted.

4.7 Effects on ability to drive and use machines

Somnolence and dizziness have been reported to occur in some patients. Caution is advised when driving or operating machinery until the response to initial treatment has been determined.

4.8 Undesirable effects

Gynaecomastia may develop in association with the use of spironolactone. Development appears to be related to both dosage level and duration of therapy and is normally reversible when the drug is discontinued. In rare instances some breast enlargement may persist.

The following adverse events have been reported in association with spironolactone therapy:

Body as a Whole: malaise

Endocrine Disorders: benign breast neoplasm, breast pain

Gastrointestinal Disorders: gastrointestinal disturbances, nausea

Hematologic Disorders: leukopenia (including agranulocytosis), thrombocytopenia

Liver Disorders: hepatic function abnormal

Metabolic and Nutritional Disorders: electrolyte disturbances, hyperkalemia

Musculoskeletal Disorders: leg cramps

Nervous System Disorders: dizziness

Psychiatric Disorders: changes in libido, confusion

Reproductive Disorders: menstrual disorders

Skin and Appendages: alopecia, hypertrichosis, pruritus, rash, urticaria,

Urinary System Disorders: acute renal failure

The following isolated adverse event has been reported in association with spironolactone therapy:

Skin & Appendages: Stevens Johnson Syndrome

4.9 Overdose

Acute overdosage may be manifested by drowsiness, mental confusion, nausea, vomiting, dizziness or diarrhoea. Hyponatraemia, or hyperkalaemia may be induced, but these effects are unlikely to be associated with acute overdosage. Symptoms of hyperkalaemia may manifest as paraesthesia, weakness, flaccid paralysis or muscle spasm and may be difficult to distinguish clinically from hypokalaemia. Electrocardiographic changes are the earliest specific signs of potassium disturbances. No specific antidote has been identified. Improvement may be expected after withdrawal of the drug. General supportive measures including replacement of fluids and electrolytes may be indicated. For hyperkalaemia, reduce potassium intake, administer potassium-excreting diuretics, intravenous glucose with regular insulin or oral ion-exchange resins.

5. PHARMACOLOGICAL PROPERTIES

5.1 Pharmacodynamic properties

Spironolactone, as a competitive aldosterone antagonist, increases sodium excretion whilst reducing potassium loss at the distal renal tubule. It has a gradual and prolonged action.

5.2 Pharmacokinetic properties

Spironolactone is well absorbed orally and is principally metabolised to active metabolites: sulphur containing metabolites (80%) and partly canrenone (20%). Although the plasma half life of spironolactone itself is short (1.3 hours) the half lives of the active metabolites are longer (ranging from 2.8 to 11.2 hours). Elimination of metabolites occurs primarily in the urine and secondarily through biliary excretion in the faeces.

Following the administration of 100 mg of spironolactone daily for 15 days in non-fasted healthy volunteers, time to peak plasma concentration (t_{max}), peak plasma concentration (C_{max}), and elimination half-life ($t_{1/2}$) for spironolactone is 2.6 hr., 80 ng/ml, and approximately 1.4 hr., respectively. For the 7-alpha-(thiomethyl) spironolactone and canrenone metabolites, t_{max} was 3.2 hr. and 4.3 hr., C_{max} was 391 ng/ml and 181 ng/ml, and $t_{1/2}$ was 13.8 hr. and 16.5 hr., respectively.

The renal action of a single dose of spironolactone reaches its peak after 7 hours, and activity persists for at least 24 hours

5.3 Preclinical safety data

Carcinogenicity: Spironolactone has been shown to produce tumours in rats when administered at high doses over a long period of time. The significance of these findings with respect to clinical use is not certain. However the long term use of spironolactone in young patients requires careful consideration of the benefits and the potential hazard involved. Spironolactone or its metabolites may cross the placental barrier. With spironolactone, feminisation has been observed in male rat foetuses. The use of Aldactone in pregnant women requires that the anticipated benefit be weighed against the possible hazards to the mother and foetus.

6. PHARMACEUTICAL PARTICULARS

6.1 List of excipients

Aldactone 25mg, 50mg & 100mg contain: Calcium sulphate dihydrate, corn starch, polyvinyl pyrrolidone, magnesium stearate, felocofix peppermint, hydroxypropyl methylcellulose, polyethylene glycol and opaspray yellow (contains E171 and E172).

6.2 Incompatibilities

None stated.

6.3 Shelf life

The shelf life of Aldactone tablets is 5 years.

6.4 Special precautions for storage

Store in a dry place below 30°C.

6.5 Nature and contents of container

Aldactone 25mg, 50mg & 100mg tablets may be packaged in the following containers:

Amber glass or plastic bottles containing 100 or 500 tablets.

HDPE containers of 50 or 1,000 tablets.

PVC/foil blister packs containing 100 or 500 tablets and PVC/foil blister calender pack of 28 tablets.

6.6 Instructions for use and handling

None

7. MARKETING AUTHORISATION HOLDER

Pharmacia Limited
Davy Avenue
Knowlhill
Milton Keynes
MK5 8PH
United Kingdom

8. MARKETING AUTHORISATION NUMBER(S)

Aldactone 25mg - PL 00032/0394

Aldactone 50mg - PL 00032/0395

Aldactone 100mg - PL 00032/0393

9. DATE OF FIRST AUTHORISATION/RENEWAL OF THE AUTHORISATION

Aldactone 25mg - 10 February 2002

Aldactone 50mg - 14 February 2002

Aldactone 100mg - 7 February 2002

10. DATE OF REVISION OF THE TEXT

March 2004

11. LEGAL CATEGORY

POM.

Ref: AN1_1

Aldara 5% Cream

(3M Health Care Limited)

1. NAME OF THE MEDICINAL PRODUCT

ALDARA 5% cream

2. QUALITATIVE AND QUANTITATIVE COMPOSITION

Each sachet contains 12.5 mg of imiquimod in 250 mg cream (5 %).

For excipients, see 6.1.

3. PHARMACEUTICAL FORM

Cream

White to slightly yellow cream.

4. CLINICAL PARTICULARS

4.1 Therapeutic indications

Imiquimod cream is indicated for the topical treatment of external genital and perianal warts (condylomata acuminata) and small superficial basal cell carcinomas (sBCCs) in adult patients.

4.2 Posology and method of administration

Posology

The application frequency and duration of treatment with imiquimod cream is different for each indication

External genital warts in adults:

Imiquimod cream should be applied 3 times per week (example: Monday, Wednesday, and Friday; or Tuesday, Thursday, and Saturday) prior to normal sleeping hours, and should remain on the skin for 6 to 10 hours. Imiquimod cream treatment should continue until the clearance of visible genital orperianal warts or for a maximum of 16 weeks per episode of warts.

Superficial basal cell carcinoma in adults:

Apply imiquimod cream for 6 weeks, 5 times per week (example: Monday to Friday) prior to normal sleeping hours, and leave on the skin for approximately 8 hours.

Method of administration

External genital warts:

Imiquimod cream should be applied in a thin layer and rubbed on the clean wart area until the cream vanishes. Only apply to affected areas and avoid any application on internal surfaces. Imiquimod cream should be applied prior to normal sleeping hours. During the 6 to 10 hour treatment period, showering or bathing should be avoided. After this period it is essential that imiquimod cream is removed with mild soap and water. Application of an excess of cream or prolonged contact with the skin may result in a severe application site reaction (see sections 4.4, 4.8 and 4.9). A single-use sachet is sufficient to cover a wart area of 20 cm^2 (approx. 3 $inches^2$). Sachets should not be re-used once opened. Hands should be washed carefully before and after application of cream.

Uncircumcised males treating warts under the foreskin should retract the foreskin and wash the area daily (see section 4.4).

Superficial basal cell carcinoma:

Before applying imiquimod cream, patients should wash the treatment area with mild soap and water and dry thoroughly. Sufficient cream should be applied to cover the treatment area, including one centimetre of skin surrounding the tumour. The cream should be rubbed into the treatment area until the cream vanishes. The cream should be applied prior to normal sleeping hours and remain on the skin for approximately 8 hours. During this period, showering and bathing should be avoided. After this period it is essential that imiquimod cream is removed with mild soap and water.

Sachets should not be re-used once opened. Hands should be washed carefully before and after application of cream.

Response of the treated tumour to imiquimod cream should be assessed 12 weeks after the end of treatment. If the treated tumour shows an incomplete response, a different therapy should be used (see section 4.4).

A rest period of several days may be taken (see section 4.4) if the local skin reaction to imiquimod cream causes excessive discomfort to the patient, or if infection is observed at the treatment site. In this latter case, appropriate other measures should be taken.

4.3 Contraindications

Imiquimod cream is contraindicated in patients with known hypersensitivity to imiquimod or any of the excipients of the cream.

4.4 Special warnings and special precautions for use

External genital warts and superficial basal cell carcinoma:

Avoid contact with the eyes.

Imiquimod has the potential to exacerbate inflammatory conditions of the skin.

Imiquimod cream therapy is not recommended until the skin has healed after any previous drug or surgical treatment.

The use of an occlusive dressing is not recommended with imiquimod cream therapy.

The excipients methylhydroxybenzoate, propylhydroxybenzoate, cetyl alcohol and stearyl alcohol may cause allergic reactions.

External genital warts:

There is limited experience in the use of imiquimod cream in the treatment of men with foreskin-associated warts. The safety database in uncircumcised men treated with imiquimod cream three times weekly and carrying out a daily foreskin hygiene routine is less than 100 patients. In other studies, in which a daily foreskin hygiene routine was not followed, there were two cases of severe phimosis and one case of stricture leading to circumcision. Treatment in this patient population is therefore recommended only in men who are able or willing to follow the daily foreskin hygiene routine. Early signs of stricture may include local skin reactions (e.g. erosion, ulceration, edema, induration), or increasing difficulty in retracting the foreskin. If these symptoms occur, the treatment should be stopped immediately. Based on current knowledge, treating urethral, intra-vaginal, cervical, rectal or intra-anal warts is not recommended. Imiquimod cream therapy should not be initiated in tissues where open sores or wounds exist until after the area has healed.

Local skin reactions such as erythema, erosion, excoriation, flaking and oedema are common. Other local reactions such as induration, ulceration, scabbing, and vesicles have also been reported. Should an intolerable skin reaction occur, the cream should be removed by washing the area with mild soap and water. Treatment with imiquimod cream can be resumed after the skin reaction has moderated.

The risk of severe local skin reactions may be increased when imiquimod is used at higher than recommended doses (see section 4.2). However, in rare cases severe local reactions that have required treatment and/or caused temporary incapacitation have been observed in patients who have used imiquimod according to the instructions. Where such reactions have occurred at the urethral meatus, some women have experienced difficulty in urinating, sometimes requiring emergency catheterisation and treatment of the affected area.

No clinical experience exists with imiquimod cream immediately following treatment with other cutaneously applied drugs for treatment of external genital or perianal warts. Imiquimod cream should be washed from the skin before sexual activity. Imiquimod creammay weaken condoms and diaphragms, therefore concurrent use with imiquimod creamis not recommended. Alternative forms of contraception should be considered.

The safety data with imiquimod cream in patients older than 65 years are limited to four patients.

In immunocompromised patients, repeat treatment with imiquimod cream is not recommended.

While limited data have shown an increased rate of wart reduction in HIV positive patients, imiquimod cream has not been shown to be as effective in terms of wart clearance in this patient group.

Superficial basal cell carcinoma:

Imiquimod has not been evaluated for the treatment of basal cell carcinoma within 1 cm of the eyelids, nose, lips or hairline.

During therapy and until healed, affected skin is likely to appear noticeably different from normal skin. Local skin reactions are common but these reactions generally decrease in intensity during therapy or resolve after cessation of imiquimod cream therapy. There is an association between the complete clearance rate and the intensity of local skin reactions (e.g. erythema). These local skin reactions may be related to the stimulation of local immune response. If required by the patient's discomfort or the severity of the local skin reaction, a rest period of several days may be taken. Treatment with imiquimod cream can be resumed after the skin reaction has moderated.

The clinical outcome of therapy can be determined after regeneration of the treated skin, approximately 12 weeks after the end of treatment.

As data on long-term clearance rates beyond 12 months post-treatment are not currently available, other appropriate therapeutic modalities should be considered for sBCC.

No clinical experience exists with the use of imiquimod cream in immunocompromised patients.

No clinical experience exists in patients with recurrent and previously treated BCCs, therefore use for previously treated tumours is not recommended.

Data from an open label clinical trial suggest that large tumours >7.25 cm^2) are less likely to respond to imiquimod therapy.

The skin surface area treated should be protected from solar exposure.

4.5 Interaction with other medicinal products and other forms of Interaction

Interactions with other medicinal products, including immunosuppressive drugs, have not been studied; such interactions with systemic drugs would be limited by the minimal percutaneous absorption of imiquimod cream.

4.6 Pregnancy and lactation

In animal teratology (rat and rabbit) and reproductive studies (rat), no teratogenic nor embryo-fetotoxic effects were observed (see 5.3). In the absence of such effects in animals, malformative effects in man are generally considered unlikely to occur. Historically, drugs responsible for malformations in man were teratogenic in well-conducted studies using two animal species. Data on a limited number of pregnancies are available but no general conclusion can be drawn from these.

Caution should be exercised when prescribing to pregnant women.

As no quantifiable levels >5 ng/ml) of imiquimod are detected in the serum after single and multiple topical doses, no specific advice can be given on whether to use or not in lactating mothers.

4.7 Effects on ability to drive and use machines

No studies on the effects on the ability to drive and use machines have been performed. From the undesirable effects noted in section 4.8, it is unlikely that treatment will have any effect on the ability to drive and use machines.

4.8 Undesirable effects

a) General Description:

External genital warts:

In the pivotal trials with 3 times a week dosing, the most frequently reported adverse drug reactions judged to be probably or possibly related to imiquimod cream treatment were application site reactions at the wart treatment site (33.7% of imiquimod treated patients). Some systemic adverse reactions, including headache (3.7%), influenza-like symptoms (1.1%), and myalgia (1.5%) were also reported.

Patient reported adverse reactions from 2292 patients treated with imiquimod cream in placebo controlled and open clinical studies are presented below. These adverse events are considered at least possibly causally related to treatment with imiquimod.

Superficial basal cell carcinoma:

In trials with 5x per week dosing 58% of patients experienced at least one adverse event. The most frequently reported adverse events from the trials judged probably or possibly related to imiquimod cream are application site disorders, with a frequency of 28.1%. Some systemic adverse reactions, including back pain (1.1%) and influenza-like symptoms (0.5%) were reported by imiquimod cream patients.

Patient reported adverse reactions from 185 patients treated with imiquimod cream in placebo controlled phase III clinical studies for superficial basal cell carcinoma are presented below. These adverse events are considered at least possibly causally related to treatment with imiquimod.

b) Tabular Listing of adverse events:

Frequencies are defined as Very common (greater than 10%), Common (1% - 10%), Uncommon (0.1% - 1%). Lower frequencies from clinical trials are not reported here.

	External genital warts (3x wk/16wks) N = 2292	**Superficial basal cell carcinoma (5x/wk, 6 wks) N = 185**
Infections and infestations:		
Infection	Common	Common
Herpes simplex	Uncommon	
Genital candidiasis	Uncommon	
Vaginitis	Uncommon	
Bacterial infection	Uncommon	
Fungal infection	Uncommon	
Upper respiratory tract infection	Uncommon	
Vulvitis	Uncommon	
Pustules		Common
Blood and lymphatic system disorders:		
Lymphadenopathy	Uncommon	Common
Metabolism and nutrition disorders:		
Anorexia	Uncommon	
Psychiatric disorders:		
Insomnia	Uncommon	
Depression	Uncommon	
Irritability		Uncommon
Nervous system disorders:		
Headache	Common	
Paraesthesia	Uncommon	
Dizziness	Uncommon	
Migraine	Uncommon	
Somnolence	Uncommon	
Ear and labyrinth disorders:		
Tinnitus	Uncommon	
Vascular disorders:		
Flushing	Uncommon	
Respiratory, thoracic and mediastinal disorders:		
Pharyngitis	Uncommon	
Rhinitis	Uncommon	
Gastrointestinal disorders:		
Nausea	Common	Uncommon
Abdominal pain	Uncommon	
Diarrhoea	Uncommon	
Vomiting	Uncommon	
Rectal disorder	Uncommon	
Rectal tenesmus	Uncommon	
Dry mouth		Uncommon
Skin and subcutaneous tissue disorders:		
Pruritus	Uncommon	
Dermatitis	Uncommon	Uncommon
Folliculitis	Uncommon	
Rash erythematous	Uncommon	
Eczema	Uncommon	
Rash	Uncommon	
Sweating increased	Uncommon	
Urticaria	Uncommon	
Musculoskeletal and connective tissue disorders:		
Myalgia	Common	
Arthralgia	Uncommon	
Back pain	Uncommon	Common
Renal and urinary disorders:		
Dysuria	Uncommon	
Reproductive system and breast disorders:		
Genital pain male	Uncommon	
Penile disorder	Uncommon	
Dyspareunia	Uncommon	
Erectile dysfunction	Uncommon	
Uterovaginal prolapse	Uncommon	
Vaginal pain	Uncommon	
Vaginitis atrophic	Uncommon	
Vulval disorder	Uncommon	
General disorders and administration site conditions:		
Application site pruritus	Very common	Very common
Application site pain	Very common	Common
Application site burning	Common	Common
Application site irritation	Common	Common
Fatigue	Common	
Pyrexia	Uncommon	
Influenza-like illness	Uncommon	Uncommon
Pain	Uncommon	
Asthenia	Uncommon	
Malaise	Uncommon	
Rigors	Uncommon	
Application site bleeding		Common
Application site discharge		Uncommon
Application site erythema		Common
Application site inflammation		Uncommon
Application site oedema		Uncommon
Application site papules		Common
Application site paraesthesia		Common
Application site rash		Common
Application site scabbing		Uncommon
Application site skin breakdown		Uncommon
Application site vesicles		Uncommon
Application site swelling		Uncommon
Lethargy		Uncommon

c) Frequently occurring adverse events:

External genital warts:

Investigators of placebo controlled trials were required to evaluate protocol mandated clinical signs (skin reactions). These protocol mandated clinical sign assessments indicate that local skin reactions including erythema (61%), erosion (30%), excoriation/flaking/scaling (23%) and oedema (14%) were common in these placebo controlled clinical trials with imiquimod cream applied three times weekly (see section 4.4 for further details). Local skin reactions, such as erythema, are probably an extension of the pharmacologic effects of imiquimod cream.

Remote site skin reactions, mainly erythema (44%), were also reported in the placebo controlled trials. These reactions were at non-wart sites which may have been in contact with imiquimod cream. Most skin reactions were mild to moderate in severity and resolved within 2 weeks of treatment discontinuation. However, in some cases these reactions have been severe, requiring treatment and/or causing incapacitation. In very rare cases, severe reactions at the urethral meatus have resulted in dysuria in women (see section 4.4).

Superficial basal cell carcinoma:

Investigators of the placebo controlled clinical trials were required to evaluate protocol mandated clinical signs (skin reactions). These protocol mandated clinical sign assessments indicate that severe erythema (31%) severe erosions (13%) and severe scabbing and crusting (19%) were very common in these trials with imiquimod cream applied 5x weekly. Local skin reactions, such as erythema, are probably an extension of the pharmacologic effect of imiquimod cream.

Skin infections during treatment with imiquimod have been observed. While serious sequelae have not resulted, the possibility of infection in broken skin should always be considered.

d) Adverse events applicable to all indications:

Reports have been received of localised hypopigmentation and hyperpigmentation following imiquimod cream use. Follow-up information suggests that these skin colour changes may be permanent in some patients.

Reductions in haemoglobin, white blood cell count, absolute neutrophils and platelets have been observed in clinical trials. These reductions are not considered to be clinically significant in patients with normal haematologic reserve. Patients with reduced haematologic reserve have not been studied in clinical trials.

4.9 Overdose

When applied topically, systemic overdosage with imiquimod cream is unlikely due to minimal percutaneous absorption. Studies in rabbits reveal a dermal lethal dose of greater than 5g/kg. Persistent dermal overdosing of imiquimod cream could result in severe local skin reactions.

Following accidental ingestion, nausea, emesis, headache, myalgia and fever could occur after a single dose of 200 mg imiquimod which corresponds to the content of approximately 16 sachets. The most clinically serious adverse event reported following multiple oral doses of $\geqslant$ 200 mg was hypotension which resolved following oral or intravenous fluid administration.

5. PHARMACOLOGICAL PROPERTIES

5.1 Pharmacodynamic properties

External genital warts and superficial basal cell carcinoma:

Pharmacotherapeutic group: Chemotherapeutics for topical use, antivirals: ATC Code: D06BB10.

Imiquimod is an immune response modifier. Saturable binding studies suggest a membrane receptor for imiquimod exists on responding immune cells. Imiquimod has no direct antiviral activity. In animal models imiquimod is effective against viral infections and acts as an antitumour agent principally by induction of alpha interferon and other cytokines. The induction of alpha interferon and other cytokines following imiquimod cream application to genital wart tissue has also been demonstrated in clinical studies.

Increases in systemic levels of alpha interferon and other cytokines following topical application of imiquimod were demonstrated in a pharmacokinetic study.

External genital warts:

Clinical Efficacy

The results of 3 phase III pivotal efficacy studies showed that treatment with imiquimod for sixteen weeks was significantly more effective than treatment with vehicle as measured by total clearance of treated warts.

In 119 imiquimod-treated female patients, the combined total clearance rate was 60% as compared to 20% in 105 vehicle-treated patients (95%CI for rate difference: 20% to 61%, $p < 0.001$). In those imiquimod patients who achieved total clearance of their warts, the median time to clearance was 8 weeks.

In 157 imiquimod-treated male patients, the combined total clearance rate was 23% as compared to 5% in 161 vehicle-treated patients (95%CI for rate difference: 3% to 36%, $p < 0.001$). In those imiquimod patients who achieved total clearance of their warts, the median time to clearance was 12 weeks.

Superficial basal cell carcinoma:

Clinical efficacy:

The efficacy of imiquimod 5 times per week for 6 weeks was studied in two double-blind vehicle controlled clinical trials. Target tumours were histologically confirmed single primary superficial basal cell carcinomas with a minimum size of 0.5 cm^2 and a maximum diameter of 2 cm. Tumours located within 1 cm of the eyes, nose, mouth, ears or hairline were excluded. In a pooled analysis of these two studies, histological clearance was noted in 82% (152/185) of patients. When clinical assessment was also included, clearance judged by this composite endpoint was noted in 75% (139/185) of patients. These results were statistically significant ($p < 0.001$) by comparison with the vehicle group, 3% (6/179) and 2% (3/179) respectively. There was a significant association between the intensity of local skin reactions (e.g. erythema) seen during the treatment period and complete clearance of the basal cell carcinoma.

Interim results from a long-term open-label uncontrolled study indicate an estimated sustained clearance of 92%. Data on recurrence rates beyond 12 months are not yet available.

5.2 Pharmacokinetic properties

External genital warts and superficial basal cell carcinoma:

Less than 0.9% of a topically applied single dose of radiolabeled imiquimod was absorbed through the skin of human subjects. The small amount of drug which was absorbed into the systemic circulation was promptly excreted by both urinary and faecal routes at a mean ratio of approximately 3 to 1. No quantifiable levels > 5 ng/ml) of drug were detected in serum after single or multiple topical doses.

Systemic exposure (percutaneous penetration) was calculated from recovery of carbon-14 from [14C] imiquimod in urine and faeces.

Minimal systemic absorption of imiquimod 5% cream across the skin of 58 patients with actinic keratosis was observed with 3 times per week dosing for 16 weeks. The extent of percutaneous absorption did not change significantly between the first and last doses of this study. Peak serum drug concentrations at the end of week 16 were observed between 9 and 12 hours and were 0.1, 0.2, and 1.6 ng/mL for the applications to face (12.5 mg, 1 single-use sachet), scalp (25 mg, 2 sachets) and hands/arms (75 mg, 6 sachets), respectively. The application surface area was not controlled in the scalp and hands/ arms groups. Dose proportionality was not observed. An apparent half-life was calculated that was approximately 10 times greater than the 2 hour half-life seen following subcutaneous dosing in a previous study, suggesting prolonged retention of drug in the skin. Urinary recovery was less than 0.6% of the applied dose at week 16 in these patients.

5.3 Preclinical safety data

Preclinical data revealed no special hazard for humans based on conventional studies of safety pharmacology, mutagenicity and teratogenicity.

In a four-month rat dermal toxicity study, significantly decreased body weight and increased spleen weight were observed at 0.5 and 2.5 mg/kg; similar effects were not seen in a four month mouse dermal study. Local dermal irritation, especially at higher doses, was observed in both species.

A two-year mouse carcinogenicity study by dermal administration on three days a week did not induce tumours at the application site. However, the incidences of hepatocellular tumours among treated animals were greater than those for controls. The mechanism for this is not known, but as imiquimod has low systemic absorption from human skin, and is not mutagenic, any risk to humans from systemic exposure is likely to be low. Furthermore, tumours were not seen at any site in a 2-year oral carcinogenicity study in rats.

Imiquimod cream was evaluated in a photocarcinogenicity bioassay in albino hairless mice exposed to simulated solar ultraviolet radiation (UVR). Animals were administered imiquimod cream three times per week and were irradiated 5 days per week for 40 weeks. Mice were maintained for an additional 12 weeks for a total of 52 weeks. Tumours occurred earlier and in greater number in the group of mice administered the vehicle cream in comparison with the low UVR control group. The significance for man is unknown. Topical administration of imiquimod cream resulted in no tumour enhancement at any dose, in comparison with the vehicle cream group.

6. PHARMACEUTICAL PARTICULARS

6.1 List of excipients

isostearic acid

benzyl alcohol

cetyl alcohol

stearyl alcohol

white soft paraffin

polysorbate 60

sorbitan stearate

glycerol

methyl hydroxybenzoate

propyl hydroxybenzoate

xanthan gum

purified water.

6.2 Incompatibilities

Not applicable.

6.3 Shelf life

2 years.

6.4 Special precautions for storage

Do not store above 25°C.

Sachets should not be re-used once opened.

6.5 Nature and contents of container

Boxes of 12 single-use polyester/aluminium foil sachets, containing 250 mg of cream.

6.6 Instructions for use and handling

No special requirements.

7. MARKETING AUTHORISATION HOLDER

Laboratoires 3M Santé

Boulevard de l'Oise

F-95029 Cergy Pontoise Cedex

France

8. MARKETING AUTHORISATION NUMBER(S)

EU/1/98/080/001

9. DATE OF FIRST AUTHORISATION/RENEWAL OF THE AUTHORISATION

18/09/2003

10. DATE OF REVISION OF THE TEXT

July 2004

Aldomet 250 and 500 mg Tablets

(Merck Sharp & Dohme Limited)

1. NAME OF THE MEDICINAL PRODUCT

ALDOMET® Tablets 250 mg

ALDOMET® Tablets 500 mg

2. QUALITATIVE AND QUANTITATIVE COMPOSITION

'Aldomet' Tablets 250 mg, contain methyldopa equivalent to 250 mg anhydrous methyldopa.

'Aldomet' Tablets 500 mg, contain methyldopa equivalent to 500 mg anhydrous methyldopa.

3. PHARMACEUTICAL FORM

Yellow, film-coated tablets.

'Aldomet' Tablets 250 mg are marked 'ALDOMET MSD 401'.

'Aldomet' Tablets 500 mg are marked 'ALDOMET MSD 516'.

4. CLINICAL PARTICULARS

4.1 Therapeutic indications

In the treatment of hypertension.

4.2 Posology and method of administration

General considerations: Methyldopa is largely excreted by the kidney, and patients with impaired renal function may respond to smaller doses.

Withdrawal of 'Aldomet' is followed by return of hypertension, usually within 48 hours. This is not complicated generally by an overshoot of blood pressure.

Therapy with 'Aldomet' may be initiated in most patients already on treatment with other antihypertensive agents by terminating these antihypertensive medications gradually, as required. Following such previous antihypertensive therapy, 'Aldomet' should be limited to an initial dose of not more than 500 mg daily and increased as required at intervals of not less than two days.

When methyldopa is given to patients on other antihypertensives the dose of these agents may need to be adjusted to effect a smooth transition.

When 500 mg of 'Aldomet' is added to 50 mg of hydrochlorothiazide, the two agents may be given together once daily.

Many patients experience sedation for two or three days when therapy with 'Aldomet' is started or when the dose is increased. When increasing the dosage, therefore, it may be desirable to increase the evening dose first.

Oral therapy - Adults: Initial dosage: Usually 250 mg two or three times a day, for two days.

Adjustment: Usually adjusted at intervals of not less than two days, until an adequate response is obtained. The maximum recommended daily dosage is 3 g.

Oral therapy - Children: initial dosage is based on 10 mg/kg of bodyweight daily in 2-4 oral doses. The daily dosage is then increased or decreased until an adequate response is achieved. The maximum dosage is 65 mg/kg or 3.0 g daily, whichever is less.

Use in the elderly: The initial dose in elderly patients should be kept as low as possible, not exceeding 250 mg daily; an appropriate starting dose in the elderly would be 125 mg b.d. increasing slowly as required, but not to exceed a maximum daily dosage of 2 g. Syncope in older patients may be related to an increased sensitivity and advanced arteriosclerotic vascular disease. This may be avoided by lower doses.

4.3 Contraindications

'Aldomet' is contra-indicated in patients with:

- active hepatic disease, such as acute hepatitis and active cirrhosis

- hypersensitivity (including hepatic disorders associated with previous methyldopa therapy) to any component of these products
- depression
- on therapy with monoamine oxidase inhibitors (MAOIs).

'Aldomet' is not recommended for the treatment of phaeochromocytoma (see 4.4 'Special warnings and precautions for use').

4.4 Special warnings and special precautions for use

Acquired haemolytic anaemia has occurred rarely; should symptoms suggest anaemia, haemoglobin and/or haematocrit determinations should be made. If anaemia is confirmed, tests should be done for haemolysis. If haemolytic anaemia is present, 'Aldomet' should be discontinued. Stopping therapy, with or without giving a corticosteroid, has usually brought prompt remission. Rarely, however, deaths have occurred.

Some patients on continued therapy with methyldopa develop a positive Coombs test. From the reports of different investigators, the incidence averages between 10% and 20%. A positive Coombs test rarely develops in the first six months of therapy, and if it has not developed within 12 months, it is unlikely to do so later on continuing therapy. Development is also dose-related, the lowest incidence occurring in patients receiving 1 g or less of methyldopa per day. The test becomes negative usually within weeks or months of stopping methyldopa.

Prior knowledge of a positive Coombs reaction will aid in evaluating a cross-match for transfusion. If a patient with a positive Coombs reaction shows an incompatible minor cross-match, an indirect Coombs test should be performed. If this is negative, transfusion with blood compatible in the major cross-match may be carried out. If positive, the advisability of transfusion should be determined by a haematologist.

Reversible leucopenia, with primary effect on granulocytes has been reported rarely. The granulocyte count returned to normal on discontinuing therapy. Reversible thrombocytopenia has occurred rarely.

Occasionally, fever has occurred within the first three weeks of therapy, sometimes associated with eosinophilia or abnormalities in liver-function tests. Jaundice, with or without fever, also may occur. Its onset is usually within the first two or three months of therapy. In some patients the findings are consistent with those of cholestasis. Rare cases of fatal hepatic necrosis have been reported. Liver biopsy, performed in several patients with liver dysfunction, showed a microscopic focal necrosis compatible with drug hypersensitivity. Liver-function tests and a total and differential white blood-cell count are advisable before therapy and at intervals during the first six weeks to twelve weeks of therapy, or whenever an unexplained fever occurs.

Should fever, abnormality in liver function, or jaundice occur, therapy should be withdrawn. If related to methyldopa, the temperature and abnormalities in liver function will then return to normal. Methyldopa should not be used again in these patients. Methyldopa should be used with caution in patients with a history of previous liver disease or dysfunction.

Patients may require reduced doses of anaesthetics when on methyldopa. If hypotension does occur during anaesthesia, it can usually be controlled by vasopressors. The adrenergic receptors remain sensitive during treatment with methyldopa.

Dialysis removes methyldopa; therefore, hypertension may recur after this procedure.

Rarely, involuntary choreoathetotic movements have been observed during therapy with methyldopa in patients with severe bilateral cerebrovascular disease. Should these movements occur, therapy should be discontinued.

'Aldomet' should be used with extreme caution in patients, or in near relatives of patients, with hepatic porphyria.

Interference with laboratory tests:

Methyldopa may interfere with the measurement of urinary uric acid by the phosphotungstate method, serum creatinine by the alkaline picrate method, and AST (SGOT) by colorimetric method. Interference with spectrophotometric methods for AST (SGOT) analysis has not been reported.

As methyldopa fluoresces at the same wavelengths as catecholamines, spuriously high amounts of urinary catecholamines may be reported interfering with a diagnosis of phaeochromocytoma.

It is important to recognise this phenomenon before a patient with a possible phaeochromocytoma is subjected to surgery. Methyldopa does not interfere with measurements of VMA (vanillylmandelic acid) by those methods which convert VMA to vanillin.

Rarely, when urine is exposed to air after voiding, it may darken because of breakdown of methyldopa or its metabolites.

4.5 Interaction with other medicinal products and other forms of Interaction

Lithium:

When methyldopa and lithium are given concomitantly the patient should be monitored carefully for symptoms of lithium toxicity.

Other antihypertensive drugs:

When methyldopa is used with other antihypertensive drugs, potentiation of antihypertensive action may occur. The progress of patients should be carefully followed to detect side reactions or manifestations of drug idiosyncrasy.

Other classes of drug:

The antihypertensive effect of 'Aldomet' may be diminished by sympathomimetics, phenothiazines, tricyclic antidepressants and MAOIs (see 4.3 'Contra-indications'). In addition, phenothiazines may have additive hypotensive effects.

Iron:

Several studies demonstrate a decrease in the bioavailability of methyldopa when it is ingested with ferrous sulphate or ferrous gluconate. This may adversely affect blood pressure control in patients treated with methyldopa.

4.6 Pregnancy and lactation

'Aldomet' has been used under close medical supervision for the treatment of hypertension during pregnancy. There was no clinical evidence that 'Aldomet' caused foetal abnormalities or affected the neonate.

Published reports of the use of methyldopa during all trimesters indicate that if this drug is used during pregnancy the possibility of foetal harm appears remote.

Methyldopa crosses the placental barrier and appears in cord blood and breast milk.

Although no obvious teratogenic effects have been reported, the possibility of foetal injury cannot be excluded and the use of the drug in women who are, or may become, pregnant or who are breast-feeding their newborn infant requires that anticipated benefits be weighed against possible risks.

4.7 Effects on ability to drive and use machines

'Aldomet' may cause sedation, usually transient, during the initial period of therapy or whenever the dose is increased. If affected, patients should not carry out activities where alertness is necessary, such as driving a car or operating machinery.

4.8 Undesirable effects

Sedation, usually transient, may occur during the initial period of therapy or whenever the dose is increased. If affected, patients should not attempt to drive, or operate machinery. Headache, asthenia or weakness may be noted as early and transient symptoms.

The following reactions have been reported:

Central nervous system: Sedation (usually transient), headache, asthenia or weakness, paraesthesiae, Parkinsonism, Bell's palsy, involuntary choreoathetotic movements. Psychic disturbances including nightmares, impaired mental acuity and reversible mild psychoses or depression. Dizziness, light-headedness, and symptoms of cerebrovascular insufficiency (may be due to lowering of blood pressure).

Cardiovascular: Bradycardia, prolonged carotid sinus hypersensitivity, aggravation of angina pectoris. Orthostatic hypotension (decrease daily dosage). Oedema (and weight gain) usually relieved by use of a diuretic. (Discontinue methyldopa if oedema progresses or signs of heart failure appear.)

Gastro-intestinal: Nausea, vomiting, distension, constipation, flatus, diarrhoea, colitis, mild dryness of mouth, sore or 'black' tongue, pancreatitis, sialadenitis.

Hepatic: Liver disorders including hepatitis, jaundice, abnormal liver-function tests.

Haematological: Positive Coombs test, haemolytic anaemia, bone-marrow depression, leucopenia, granulocytopenia, thrombocytopenia, eosinophilia. Positive tests for antinuclear antibody. LE cells, and rheumatoid factor.

Allergic: Drug-related fever and lupus-like syndrome, myocarditis, pericarditis.

Dermatological: Rash as in eczema or lichenoid eruption, toxic epidermal necrolysis.

Other: Nasal stuffiness, rise in blood urea, breast enlargement, gynaecomastia, hyperprolactinaemia, amenorrhoea, lactation, impotence, decreased libido, failure of ejaculation, mild arthralgia with or without joint swelling, myalgia.

4.9 Overdose

Acute overdosage may produce acute hypotension with other responses attributable to brain and gastro-intestinal malfunction (excessive sedation, weakness, bradycardia, dizziness, light-headedness, constipation, distension, flatus, diarrhoea, nausea, and vomiting).

If ingestion is recent, emesis may be induced or gastric lavage performed. There is no specific antidote. Methyldopa is dialysable. Treatment is symptomatic. Infusions may be helpful to promote urinary excretion. Special attention should be directed towards cardiac rate and output, blood volume, electrolyte balance, paralytic ileus, urinary function and cerebral activity. Administration of sympathomimetic agents may be indicated. When chronic overdosage is suspected, 'Aldomet' should be discontinued.

5. PHARMACOLOGICAL PROPERTIES

5.1 Pharmacodynamic properties

It appears that several mechanisms of action account for the clinically useful effects of methyldopa and the current generally accepted view is that its principal action is on the central nervous system.

The antihypertensive effect of methyldopa is probably due to its metabolism to alpha-methylnoradrenaline, which lowers arterial pressure by stimulation of central inhibitory alpha-adrenergic receptors, false neurotransmission, and/or reduction of plasma renin activity. Methyldopa has been shown to cause a net reduction in the tissue concentration of serotonin, dopamine, epinephrine (adrenaline) and norepinephrine (noradrenaline).

5.2 Pharmacokinetic properties

Absorption of oral methyldopa is variable and incomplete. Bioavailability after oral administration averages 25%. Peak concentrations in plasma occur at two to three hours, and elimination of the drug is biphasic regardless of the route of administration. Plasma half-life is 1.8 ± 0.2 hours. Renal excretion accounts for about two thirds of drug clearance from plasma.

5.3 Preclinical safety data

No relevant information.

6. PHARMACEUTICAL PARTICULARS

6.1 List of excipients

Tablet-core: cellulose powder, anhydrous citric acid; colloidal silicon dioxide; ethylcellulose; guar gum; magnesium stearate; sodium calcium edetate;

Tablet-coating: propylene glycol; anhydrous citric acid; hypromellose; quinoline yellow aluminium lake E104; red iron oxide E172; talc; titanium dioxide, carnauba wax.

6.2 Incompatibilities

None known.

6.3 Shelf life

36 months.

6.4 Special precautions for storage

Keep containers well closed and store below 25°C, protected from light.

6.5 Nature and contents of container

'Aldomet' 250 mg: White polyethylene bottle of 100 and 500 tablets with turquoise polyethylene closure, or PVC aluminium blister packs of 60 and 90 tablets.

'Aldomet' 500 mg: White polyethylene bottle of 100 and 500 tablets with turquoise polyethylene closure, or PVC aluminium blister packs of 30 tablets.

6.6 Instructions for use and handling

None.

7. MARKETING AUTHORISATION HOLDER

Merck Sharp & Dohme Limited

Hertford Road, Hoddesdon, Hertfordshire EN11 9BU, UK

8. MARKETING AUTHORISATION NUMBER(S)

Tablets 250 mg: PL0025/0099

Tablets 500 mg: PL0025/0100

9. DATE OF FIRST AUTHORISATION/RENEWAL OF THE AUTHORISATION

Licence first granted: 21 February 1974

Licence last renewed: 5 September 2001

10. DATE OF REVISION OF THE TEXT

August 2001

LEGAL CATEGORY

POM

SPC.ADMT.01.UK.0625

Alimta 500mg powder for concentrate for solution for infusion

(Eli Lilly and Company Limited)

1. NAME OF THE MEDICINAL PRODUCT

Alimta*▼ 500mg powder for concentrate for solution for infusion.

2. QUALITATIVE AND QUANTITATIVE COMPOSITION

Each vial contains 500mg of pemetrexed (as pemetrexed disodium).

Each vial must be reconstituted with 20ml of sodium chloride 9mg/ml (0.9%) solution for injection resulting in 25mg/ml of solution. The appropriate volume of required dose is removed from the vial and further diluted to 100ml with sodium chloride 9mg/ml (0.9%) solution for injection (see section 6.6.).

For excipients, see section 6.1.

3. PHARMACEUTICAL FORM

Powder for concentrate for solution for infusion.

A white to either light yellow or green-yellow lyophilised powder.

4. CLINICAL PARTICULARS

4.1 Therapeutic indications

Alimta in combination with cisplatin is indicated for the treatment of chemotherapy naive patients with unresectable malignant pleural mesothelioma.

Alimta is indicated as monotherapy for the treatment of patients with locally advanced or metastatic non-small cell lung cancer after prior chemotherapy.

4.2 Posology and method of administration

Alimta must only be administered under the supervision of a physician qualified in the use of anti-cancer chemotherapy.

The Alimta solution must be prepared according to the instructions provided in section 6.6.

Malignant Pleural Mesothelioma

In patients treated for malignant pleural mesothelioma, the recommended dose of Alimta is 500mg/m^2 of body surface area (BSA) administered as an intravenous infusion over 10 minutes on the first day of each 21-day cycle. The recommended dose of cisplatin is 75mg/m^2 BSA infused over two hours approximately 30 minutes after completion of the pemetrexed infusion on the first day of each 21-day cycle. Patients must receive adequate anti-emetic treatment and appropriate hydration prior to and/or after receiving cisplatin (see also cisplatin Summary of Product Characteristics for specific dosing advice).

Non-Small Cell Lung Cancer

In patients treated for non-small cell lung cancer, the recommended dose of Alimta is 500mg/m^2 BSA administered as an intravenous infusion over 10 minutes on the first day of each 21-day cycle.

Pre-Medication Regimen

To reduce the incidence and severity of skin reactions, a corticosteroid should be given the day prior to, on the day of, and the day after pemetrexed administration. The corticosteroid should be equivalent to 4mg of dexamethasone administered orally twice a day (see section 4.4).

To reduce toxicity, patients treated with pemetrexed must also receive vitamin supplementation (see section 4.4). Patients must take oral folic acid or a multivitamin containing folic acid (350 to 1,000 micrograms) on a daily basis. At least five doses of folic acid must be taken during the seven days preceding the first dose of pemetrexed, and dosing must continue during the full course of therapy and for 21 days after the last dose of pemetrexed. Patients must also receive an intramuscular injection of vitamin B_{12} (1000 micrograms) in the week preceding the first dose of pemetrexed and once every three cycles thereafter. Subsequent vitamin B_{12} injections may be given on the same day as pemetrexed.

Monitoring

Patients receiving pemetrexed should be monitored before each dose with a complete blood count, including a differential white cell count (WCC) and platelet count. Prior to each chemotherapy administration, blood chemistry tests should be collected to evaluate renal and hepatic function. Before the start of any cycle of chemotherapy, patients are required to have the following: absolute neutrophil count (ANC) should be ⩾1,500 cells/mm^3 and platelets should be ⩾100,000 cells/mm^3.

Creatinine clearance should be ⩾45ml/min.

The total bilirubin should be ⩽1.5-times upper limit of normal. Alkaline phosphatase (AP), aspartate transaminase (AST or SGOT), and alanine transaminase (ALT or SGPT) should be ⩽3-times upper limit of normal. Alkaline phosphatase, AST, and ALT ⩽5-times upper limit of normal is acceptable if liver has tumour involvement.

Dose Adjustments

Dose adjustments at the start of a subsequent cycle should be based on nadir haematologic counts or maximum non-haematologic toxicity from the preceding cycle of therapy. Treatment may be delayed to allow sufficient time for recovery. Upon recovery, patients should be retreated using the guidelines in *Tables 1, 2, and 3*, which are applicable for Alimta used as a single-agent or in combination with cisplatin.

Table 1. **Dose Modification Table for Alimta (as Single-Agent or in Combination) and Cisplatin - Haematologic Toxicities**

Nadir ANC <500/mm^3 and nadir platelets ⩾50,000/mm^3	75% of previous dose (both Alimta and cisplatin)
Nadir platelets ⩽50,000/mm^3 regardless of nadir ANC	50% of previous dose (both Alimta and cisplatin)

If patients develop non-haematologic toxicities ⩾Grade 3 (excluding neurotoxicity), Alimta should be withheld until resolution to less than or equal to the patient's pre-therapy value. Treatment should be resumed according to the guidelines in *Table 2*.

Table 2. **Dose Modification Table for Alimta (as Single-Agent or in Combination) and Cisplatin - Non-Haematologic Toxicities**[a, b]

	Dose of Alimta (mg/m^2)	Dose for Cisplatin (mg/m^2)
Any Grade 3 or 4 toxicities except mucositis	75% of previous dose	75% of previous dose
Any diarrhoea requiring hospitalisation (irrespective of grade) or Grade 3 or 4 diarrhoea	75% of previous dose	75% of previous dose
Grade 3 or 4 mucositis	50% of previous dose	100% of previous dose

[a]National Cancer Institute Common Toxicity Criteria (CTC).

[b]Excluding neurotoxicity.In the event of neurotoxicity, the recommended dose adjustment for Alimta and cisplatin is documented in *Table 3*. Patients should discontinue therapy if Grade 3 or 4 neurotoxicity is observed.

Table 3. **Dose Modification Table for Alimta (as Single-Agent or in Combination) and Cisplatin - Neurotoxicity**

CTC* Grade	Dose of Alimta (mg/m^2)	Dose for Cisplatin (mg/m^2
0-1	100% of previous dose	100% of previous dose
2	100% of previous dose	50% of previous dose

*Common Toxicity Criteria (CTC).

Treatment with Alimta should be discontinued if a patient experiences any haematologic or non-haematologic Grade 3 or 4 toxicity after 2 dose reductions or immediately if Grade 3 or 4 neurotoxicity is observed.

Elderly: In clinical studies, there has been no indication that patients 65 years of age or older are at increased risk of adverse events compared to patients younger than 65 years old. No dose reductions other than those recommended for all patients are necessary.

Children and adolescents: Alimta is not recommended for use in patients under 18 years of age, as safety and efficacy have not been established in this group of patients.

Patients with renal impairment (standard Cockcroft and Gault formula or glomerular filtration rate measured Tc99m-DPTA serum clearance method): Pemetrexed is primarily eliminated unchanged by renal excretion. In clinical studies, patients with creatinine clearance of ⩾45ml/min required no dose adjustments other than those recommended for all patients. There are insufficient data on the use of pemetrexed in patients with creatinine clearance below 45ml/min; therefore, the use of pemetrexed is not recommended (see section 4.4).

Patients with hepatic impairment: No relationships between AST (SGOT), ALT (SGPT), or total bilirubin and pemetrexed pharmacokinetics were identified. However, patients with hepatic impairment, such as bilirubin >1.5-times the upper limit of normal and/or transaminase >3.0-times the upper limit of normal (hepatic metastases absent) or >5.0-times the upper limit of normal (hepatic metastases present), have not been specifically studied.

4.3 Contraindications

Hypersensitivity to pemetrexed or to any of the excipients.

Breast-feeding must be discontinued during pemetrexed therapy (see section 4.6).

Concomitant yellow fever vaccine (see section 4.5).

4.4 Special warnings and special precautions for use

Pemetrexed can suppress bone marrow function as manifested by neutropenia, thrombocytopenia, and anaemia (see section 4.8). Myelosuppression is usually the dose-limiting toxicity. Patients should be monitored for myelosuppression during therapy and pemetrexed should not be given to patients until absolute neutrophil count (ANC) returns to ⩾1500 cells/mm^3 and platelet count returns to ⩾100,000 cells/mm^3. Dose reductions for subsequent cycles are based on nadir ANC, platelet count, and maximum non-haematologic toxicity seen from the previous cycle (see section 4.2).

In the Phase 3 mesothelioma trial, overall less toxicity and reduction in Grade 3/4 haematologic and non-haematologic toxicities, such as neutropenia, febrile neutropenia, and infection with Grade 3/4 neutropenia, were reported when pre-treatment with folic acid and vitamin B_{12} was administered. Therefore patients treated with pemetrexed must be instructed to take folic acid and vitamin B_{12} as a prophylactic measure to reduce treatment-related toxicity (see section 4.2).

Skin reactions have been reported in patients not pre-treated with a corticosteroid. Pre-treatment with dexamethasone (or equivalent) can reduce the incidence and severity of skin reactions (see section 4.2).

An insufficient number of patients has been studied with creatinine clearance of below 45ml/min. Therefore, the use of pemetrexed in patients with creatinine clearance of <45ml/min is not recommended (see section 4.2).

Patients with mild to moderate renal insufficiency (creatinine clearance from 45 to 79ml/min) should avoid taking non-steroidal anti-inflammatory drugs (NSAIDs), such as ibuprofen, and aspirin (>1.3g daily), for 2 days before, on the day of, and 2 days following pemetrexed administration (see section 4.5).

All patients eligible for pemetrexed therapy should avoid taking NSAIDs with long elimination half-lives for at least 5 days prior to, on the day, and at least 2 days following pemetrexed administration (see section 4.5).

The effect of third space fluid, such as pleural effusion or ascites, on pemetrexed is unknown. In patients with clinically significant third space fluid, consideration should be given to draining the effusion prior to pemetrexed administration.

Due to the gastro-intestinal toxicity of pemetrexed given in combination with cisplatin, severe dehydration has been observed. Therefore, patients should receive adequate anti-emetic treatment and appropriate hydration prior to and/or after receiving treatment.

Serious cardiovascular events, including myocardial infarction and cerebrovascular events, have been uncommonly reported during clinical studies with pemetrexed, usually when given in combination with another cytotoxic agent. Most of the patients in whom these events have been observed had pre-existing cardiovascular risk factors (see section 4.8).

Immunodepressed status is common in cancer patients. As a result, concomitant use of live attenuated vaccines (except yellow fever) is not recommended (see section 4.5).

Pemetrexed can have genetically damaging effects. Sexually mature males are advised not to father a child during the treatment and up to 6 months thereafter. Contraceptive measures or abstinence are recommended. Owing to the possibility of pemetrexed treatment causing irreversible infertility, men are advised to seek counselling on sperm storage before starting treatment.

Women of childbearing potential must use effective contraception during treatment with pemetrexed (see section 4.6).

4.5 Interaction with other medicinal products and other forms of Interaction

Pemetrexed is mainly eliminated unchanged renally by tubular secretion and to a lesser extent by glomerular filtration. Concomitant administration of nephrotoxic drugs (eg, aminoglycoside, loop diuretics, platinum compounds, cyclosporin) could potentially result in delayed clearance of pemetrexed. This combination should be used with caution. If necessary, creatinine clearance should be closely monitored.

Concomitant administration of substances that are also tubularly secreted (eg, probenecid, penicillin) could potentially result in delayed clearance of pemetrexed. Caution should be made when these drugs are combined with pemetrexed. If necessary, creatinine clearance should be closely monitored.

In patients with normal renal function (creatinine clearance ⩾80ml/min), high doses of non-steroidal anti-inflammatory drugs (NSAIDs, such as ibuprofen >1600mg/day) and aspirin at higher dosage (⩾1.3g daily) may decrease pemetrexed elimination and, consequently, increase the occurrence of pemetrexed adverse events. Therefore, caution should be made when administering higher doses of NSAIDs or aspirin at higher dosage, concurrently with pemetrexed to patients with normal function (creatinine clearance ⩾80ml/min).

In patients with mild to moderate renal insufficiency (creatinine clearance from 45 to 79ml/min), the concomitant administration of pemetrexed with NSAIDs (eg, ibuprofen) or aspirin at higher dosage should be avoided for 2 days before, on the day of, and 2 days following pemetrexed administration (see section 4.4).

In the absence of data regarding potential interaction with NSAIDs having longer half-lives, such as piroxicam or rofecoxib, the concomitant administration with pemetrexed should be avoided for at least 5 days prior to, on the day, and at least 2 days following pemetrexed administration (see section 4.4).

Pemetrexed undergoes limited hepatic metabolism. Results from *in vitro* studies with human liver microsomes indicated that pemetrexed would not be predicted to cause clinically significant inhibition of the metabolic clearance of drugs metabolised by CYP3A, CYP2D6, CYP2C9, and CYP1A2.

Interactions Common to all Cytotoxics

Due to the increased thrombotic risk in patients with cancer, the use of anticoagulation treatment is frequent. The high intra-individual variability of the coagulation status during diseases and the possibility of interaction between oral anticoagulants and anti-cancer chemotherapy require increased frequency of INR (International Normalised Ratio) monitoring, if it is decided to treat the patient with oral anticoagulants.

Concomitant Use Contra-Indicated

Yellow fever vaccine: Risk of fatal generalised vaccinale disease (see section 4.3).

Concomitant Use Not Recommended

Live attenuated vaccines (except yellow fever): Risk of systemic, possibly fatal, disease. The risk is increased in subjects who are already immunosuppressed by their underlying disease. Use an inactivated vaccine where it exists (poliomyelitis) (see section 4.4).

4.6 Pregnancy and lactation

There are no data from the use of pemetrexed in pregnant women but pemetrexed, like other anti-metabolites, is suspected to cause serious birth defects when administered during pregnancy. Animal studies have shown reproductive toxicity (see section 5.3). Pemetrexed should not be used during pregnancy unless clearly necessary, after a careful consideration of the needs of the mother and the risk for the foetus (see section 4.4).

Women of childbearing potential must use effective contraception during treatment with pemetrexed.

Pemetrexed can have genetically damaging effects. Sexually mature males are advised not to father a child during the treatment and up to 6 months thereafter. Contraceptive measures or abstinence are recommended. Owing to the possibility of pemetrexed treatment causing irreversible infertility, men are advised to seek counselling on sperm storage before starting treatment.

It is not known whether pemetrexed is excreted in human milk and adverse effects on the suckling child cannot be excluded. Breast-feeding must be discontinued during pemetrexed therapy (see section 4.3).

4.7 Effects on ability to drive and use machines

No studies on the effects on the ability to drive and use machines have been performed. However, it has been reported that pemetrexed may cause fatigue. Therefore, patients should be cautioned against driving or operating machines if this event occurs.

4.8 Undesirable effects

The table below provides the frequency and severity of undesirable effects that have been reported in >5% of 168 patients with mesothelioma who were randomised to receive cisplatin and pemetrexed and 163 patients with mesothelioma randomised to receive single-agent cisplatin. In both treatment arms, these chemonaive patients were fully supplemented with folic acid and vitamin B_{12}.

(see Table 4)

Table 4

System Organ Class	Frequency	Event*	Pemetrexed/Cisplatin (n = 168)		Cisplatin (n = 163)	
			All Grades Toxicity (%)	Grade 3-4 Toxicity (%)	All Grades Toxicity (%)	Grade 3-4 Toxicity (%)
Blood and lymphatic system disorders	Very common	Neutrophils/ granulocytes decreased	56.0	23.2	13.5	3.1
		Leucocytes decreased	53.0	14.9	16.6	0.6
		Haemoglobin decreased	26.2	4.2	10.4	0.0
		Platelets decreased	23.2	5.4	8.6	0.0
Eye disorders	Common	Conjunctivitis	5.4	0.0	0.6	0.0
Gastro-intestinal disorders	Very common	Nausea	82.1	11.9	76.7	5.5
		Vomiting	56.5	10.7	49.7	4.3
		Stomatitis/ pharyngitis	23.2	3.0	6.1	0.0
		Anorexia	20.2	1.2	14.1	0.6
		Diarrhoea	16.7	3.6	8.0	0.0
		Constipation	11.9	0.6	7.4	0.6
	Common	Dyspepsia	5.4	0.6	0.6	0.0
General disorders	Very common	Fatigue	47.6	10.1	42.3	9.2
Metabolism and nutrition disorders	Common	Dehydration	6.5	4.2	0.6	0.6
Nervous system disorders	Very common	Neuropathy-sensory	10.1	0.0	9.8	0.6
	Common	Dysgeusia	7.7	0.0	6.1	0.0
Renal and urinary disorders	Very common	Creatinine elevation	10.7	0.6	9.8	1.2
		Creatinine clearance decreased**	16.1	0.6	17.8	1.8
Skin and subcutaneous tissue disorders	Very common	Rash	16.1	0.6	4.9	0.0
		Alopecia	11.3	0.0	5.5	0.0

*Refer to National Cancer Institute CTC version 2 for each grade of toxicity, except the term "creatinine clearance decreased"** which is derived from the term "renal/genitourinary other".
Very common - ⩾ 10%; common is normally defined as >1% and <10%. For the purpose of this table, a cut-off of 5% was used for inclusion of all events where the reporter considered a possible relationship to pemetrexed and cisplatin

Clinically relevant CTC toxicities that were reported in >1% and ⩽5% (common) of the patients that were randomly assigned to receive cisplatin and pemetrexed include increased AST, ALT, and GGT, infection, pyrexia, febrile neutropenia, renal failure, chest pain, and urticaria.

Clinically relevant CTC toxicities that were reported in ⩽1% of the patients that were randomly assigned to receive cisplatin and pemetrexed include arrhythmia and motor neuropathy.

The table below provides the frequency and severity of undesirable effects that have been reported in >5% of 265 patients randomly assigned to receive single-agent pemetrexed with folic acid and vitamin B_{12} supplementation and 276 patients randomly assigned to receive single-agent docetaxel. All patients were diagnosed with locally advanced or metastatic non-small cell lung cancer and received prior chemotherapy.

(see Table 5 on next page)

Clinically relevant CTC toxicities that were reported in >1% and ⩽5% (common) of the patients that were randomly assigned to pemetrexed include sensory neuropathy, motor neuropathy, abdominal pain, increased creatinine, febrile neutropenia, infection without neutropenia, allergic reaction/hypersensitivity and erythema multiforme.

Clinically relevant CTC toxicities that were reported in ⩽1% of the patients that were randomly assigned to pemetrexed include supraventricular arrhythmias.

Clinically relevant Grade 3 and Grade 4 laboratory toxicities were similar between integrated Phase 2 results from three single-agent pemetrexed studies (n = 164) and the Phase 3 single-agent pemetrexed study described above, with the exception of neutropenia (12.8% versus 5.3%, respectively) and alanine transaminase elevation (15.2% versus 1.9%, respectively). These differences were likely due to differences in the patient population, since the Phase 2 studies included both chemonaive and heavily pre-treated breast cancer patients with pre-existing liver metastases and/or abnormal baseline liver function tests.

Serious cardiovascular and cerebrovascular events, including myocardial infarction, angina pectoris, cerebrovascular accident, and transient ischaemic attack, have been uncommonly reported during clinical studies with pemetrexed, usually when given in combination with another cytotoxic agent. Most of the patients in whom these events have been observed had pre-existing cardiovascular risk factors.

Rare cases of hepatitis, potentially serious, have been reported during clinical studies with pemetrexed.

4.9 Overdose

Reported symptoms of overdose include neutropenia, anaemia, thrombocytopenia, mucositis, and rash. Anticipated complications of overdose include bone marrow suppression as manifested by neutropenia, thrombocytopenia, and anaemia. In addition, infection with or without fever, diarrhoea, and/or mucositis may be seen. In the event of suspected overdose, patients should be monitored with blood counts and should receive supportive therapy as necessary. The use of calcium folinate/folinic acid in the management of pemetrexed overdose should be considered.

5. PHARMACOLOGICAL PROPERTIES

5.1 Pharmacodynamic properties

Pharmacotherapeutic group: Folic acid analogues. *ATC code:* L01BA04.

Alimta is a multi-targeted anti-cancer antifolate agent that exerts its action by disrupting crucial folate-dependent metabolic processes essential for cell replication.

In vitro studies have shown that pemetrexed behaves as a multi-targeted antifolate by inhibiting thymidylate synthase (TS), dihydrofolate reductase (DHFR), and glycinamide ribonucleotide formyltransferase (GARFT), which are key folate-dependent enzymes for the *de novo* biosynthesis of thymidine and purine nucleotides. Pemetrexed is transported into cells by both the reduced folate carrier and membrane folate binding protein transport systems. Once in the cell, pemetrexed is rapidly and efficiently converted to polyglutamate forms by the enzyme folylpolyglutamate synthetase. The polyglutamate forms are retained in cells and are even more potent inhibitors of TS and GARFT. Polyglutamation is a time- and concentration-dependent process that occurs in tumour cells and, to a lesser extent, in normal tissues. Polyglutamated metabolites have an increased intracellular half-life resulting in prolonged drug action in malignant cells.

Clinical Efficacy

EMPHACIS, a multi-centre, randomised, single-blind Phase 3 study of Alimta plus cisplatin versus cisplatin in chemonaive patients with malignant pleural mesothelioma, has shown that patients treated with Alimta and cisplatin had a clinically meaningful 2.8-month median survival advantage over patients receiving cisplatin alone.

During the study, low-dose folic acid and vitamin B_{12} supplementation was introduced to patients' therapy to reduce toxicity. The primary analysis of this study was performed on the population of all patients randomly assigned to a treatment arm who received study drug (randomised and treated). A subgroup analysis was performed on patients who received folic acid and vitamin B_{12} supplementation during the entire course of study therapy (fully supplemented). The results of these analyses of efficacy are summarised in the table below.

Efficacy of Alimta Plus Cisplatin vs Cisplatin in Malignant Pleural Mesothelioma

(see Table 6 on next page)

A statistically significant improvement of the clinically relevant symptoms (pain and dyspnoea) associated with malignant pleural mesothelioma in the Alimta/cisplatin arm (212 patients) versus the cisplatin arm alone (218 patients) was demonstrated using the Lung Cancer Symptom Scale. Statistically significant differences in pulmonary function tests were also observed. The separation between the treatment arms was achieved by improvement in lung function in the Alimta/cisplatin arm and deterioration of lung function over time in the control arm.

There are limited data in patients with malignant pleural mesothelioma treated with Alimta alone. Alimta at a dose of 500mg/m^2 was studied as a single-agent in 64 chemonaive patients with malignant pleural mesothelioma. The overall response rate was 14.1%.

Table 5

System Organ Class	Frequency	Event*	Pemetrexed n = 265		Docetaxel n = 276	
			All Grades Toxicity (%)	Grade 3-4 Toxicity (%)	All Grades Toxicity (%)	Grade 3-4 Toxicity (%)
Blood and lymphatic system disorders	Very common	Haemoglobin decreased	19.2	4.2	22.1	4.3
		Leucocytes decreased	12.1	4.2	34.1	27.2
		Neutrophils/ granulocytes decreased	10.9	5.3	45.3	40.2
	Common	Platelets decreased	8.3	1.9	1.1	0.4
Gastro-intestinal disorders	Very common	Nausea	30.9	2.6	16.7	1.8
		Anorexia	21.9	1.9	23.9	2.5
		Vomiting	16.2	1.5	12.0	1.1
		Stomatitis/ pharyngitis	14.7	1.1	17.4	1.1
		Diarrhoea	12.8	0.4	24.3	2.5
	Common	Constipation	5.7	0.0	4.0	0.0
General disorders	Very common	Fatigue	34.0	5.3	35.9	5.4
	Common	Fever	8.3	0.0	7.6	0.0
Hepatobiliary disorders	Common	SGPT (ALT) elevation	7.9	1.9	1.4	0.0
		SGOT (AST) elevation	6.8	1.1	0.7	0.0
Skin and subcutaneous tissue disorders	Very common	Rash/ desquamation	14.0	0.0	6.2	0.0
	Common	Pruritus	6.8	0.4	1.8	0.0
		Alopecia	6.4	0.4	37.7	2.2

*Refer to National Cancer Institute CTC version 2 for each grade of toxicity.
Very common - ≥10%; common is normally defined as >1% and <10%. For the purpose of this table, a cut-off of 5% was used for inclusion of all events where the reporter considered a possible relationship to pemetrexed.

Table 6 Efficacy of Alimta Plus Cisplatin vs Cisplatin in Malignant Pleural Mesothelioma

Efficacy Parameter	Randomised and Treated Patients		Fully Supplemented Patients	
	Alimta/Cisplatin	Cisplatin	Alimta/Cisplatin	Cisplatin
	(n = 226)	(n = 222)	(n = 168)	(n = 163)
Median overall survival (months)	12.1	9.3	13.3	10.0
(95% CI)	(10.0-14.4)	(7.8-10.7)	(11.4-14.9)	(8.4-11.9)
Log rank *P*-value*	0.020		0.051	
Median time to tumour progression (months)	5.7	3.9	6.1	3.9
(95% CI)	(4.9-6.5)	(2.8-4.4)	(5.3-7.0)	(2.8-4.5)
Log rank *P*-value*	0.001		0.008	
Time to treatment failure (months)	4.5	2.7	4.7	2.7
(95% CI)	(3.9-4.9)	(2.1-2.9)	(4.3-5.6)	(2.2-3.1)
Log rank *P*-value*	0.001		0.001	
Overall response rate**	41.3%	16.7%	45.5%	19.6%
(95% CI)	(34.8-48.1)	(12.0-22.2)	(37.8-53.4)	(13.8-26.6)
Fisher's exact *P*-value*	<0.001		<0.001	

Abbreviation: CI = confidence interval.
**P*-value refers to comparison between arms.
**In the Alimta/cisplatin arm, randomised and treated (n = 225) and fully supplemented (n = 167).

A multi-centre, randomised, open-label Phase 3 study of Alimta versus docetaxel in patients with locally advanced or metastatic NSCLC after prior chemotherapy has shown median survival times of 8.3 months for patients treated with Alimta (intent to treat population n = 283) and 7.9 months for patients treated with docetaxel (ITT n = 288).

Efficacy of Alimta vs Docetaxel in NSCLC - ITT Population

	Alimta	Docetaxel
Survival time (months)	(n = 283)	(n = 288)
Median (m)	8.3	7.9
95% CI for median	(7.0-9.4)	(6.3-9.2)
HR	0.99	
95% CI for HR	(.82-1.20)	
Non-inferiority *P*-value (HR)	.226	
Progression free survival (months)	(n = 283)	(n = 288)
Median	2.9	2.9
HR (95% CI)	0.97 (.82-1.16)	
Time to treatment failure (TTTF - months)	(n =283)	(n =288)
Median	2.3	2.1
HR (95% CI)	0.84 (.71-.997)	
Response (n: qualified for response)	(n = 264)	(n = 274)
Response rate (%) (95% CI)	9.1 (5.9-13.2)	8.8 (5.7-12.8)
Stable disease (%)	45.8	46.4

Abbreviations: CI = confidence interval; HR = hazard ratio; ITT = intent to treat; n = total population size.

5.2 Pharmacokinetic properties

The pharmacokinetic properties of pemetrexed following single-agent administration have been evaluated in 426 cancer patients with a variety of solid tumours at doses ranging from 0.2 to 838mg/m^2 infused over a 10-minute period. Pemetrexed has a steady-state volume of distribution of 9 l/m^2. *In vitro* studies indicate that pemetrexed is approximately 81% bound to plasma proteins. Binding was not notably affected by varying degrees of renal impairment. Pemetrexed undergoes limited hepatic metabolism. Pemetrexed is primarily eliminated in the urine, with 70% to 90% of the administered dose being recovered unchanged in urine within the first 24 hours following administration. Pemetrexed total systemic clearance is 91.8ml/min and the elimination half-life from plasma is 3.5 hours in patients with normal renal function (creatinine clearance of 90ml/min). Between patient variability in clearance is moderate at 19.3%. Pemetrexed total systemic exposure (AUC) and maximum plasma concentration increase proportionally with dose. The pharmacokinetics of pemetrexed are consistent over multiple treatment cycles.

The pharmacokinetic properties of pemetrexed are not influenced by concurrently administered cisplatin. Oral folic acid and intramuscular vitamin B_{12} supplementation do not affect the pharmacokinetics of pemetrexed.

5.3 Preclinical safety data

Administration of pemetrexed to pregnant mice resulted in decreased foetal viability, decreased foetal weight, incomplete ossification of some skeletal structures, and cleft palate.

Administration of pemetrexed to male mice resulted in reproductive toxicity characterised by reduced fertility rates and testicular atrophy. This suggests that pemetrexed may impair male fertility. Female fertility was not investigated.

Pemetrexed was not mutagenic in either the *in vitro* chromosome aberration test in Chinese hamster ovary cells, or the Ames test. Pemetrexed has been shown to be clastogenic in the *in vivo* micronucleus test in the mouse.

Studies to assess the carcinogenic potential of pemetrexed have not been conducted.

6. PHARMACEUTICAL PARTICULARS

6.1 List of excipients

Mannitol

Hydrochloric acid

Sodium hydroxide

6.2 Incompatibilities

Pemetrexed is physically incompatible with diluents containing calcium, including lactated Ringer's injection and Ringer's injection. In the absence of compatibility studies (with other drugs and diluents), this medicinal product must not be mixed with other medicinal products.

6.3 Shelf life
Two years.

6.4 Special precautions for storage
Unopened vial: This medicinal product does not require any special storage conditions.

Reconstituted and infusion solutions: When prepared as directed, reconstitution and infusion solutions of Alimta contain no antimicrobial preservatives. Chemical and physical in-use stability of reconstituted and infusion solutions of pemetrexed were demonstrated for 24 hours at refrigerated temperature or 25°C. From a microbiological point of view, the product should be used immediately. If not used immediately, in-use storage times and conditions prior to use are the responsibility of the user and would normally not be longer than 24 hours at 2 to 8°C, unless reconstitution/dilution has taken place in controlled and validated aseptic conditions.

6.5 Nature and contents of container
Powder in Type I glass vial. Rubber stopper.

Pack of 1 vial.

6.6 Instructions for use and handling
1. Use aseptic technique during the reconstitution and further dilution of pemetrexed for intravenous infusion administration.

2. Calculate the dose and the number of Alimta vials needed. Each vial contains an excess of pemetrexed to facilitate delivery of label amount.

3. Reconstitute 500mg vials with 20ml of sodium chloride 9mg/ml (0.9%) solution for injection, without preservative, resulting in a solution containing 25mg/ml pemetrexed. Gently swirl each vial until the powder is completely dissolved. The resulting solution is clear and ranges in colour from colourless to yellow or green-yellow without adversely affecting product quality. The pH of the reconstituted solution is between 6.6 and 7.8. **Further dilution is required.**

4. The appropriate volume of reconstituted pemetrexed solution should be further diluted to 100ml with sodium chloride 9mg/ml (0.9%) solution for injection, without preservative, and administered as an intravenous infusion over 10 minutes.

5. Pemetrexed infusion solutions prepared as directed above are compatible with polyvinyl chloride and polyolefin lined administration sets and infusion bags.

6. Parenteral medicinal products should be inspected visually for particulate matter and discolouration prior to administration. If particulate matter is observed, do not administer.

7. Pemetrexed solutions are for single use only. Any unused product or waste material should be disposed of in accordance with local requirements.

Preparation and administration precautions: As with other potentially toxic anti-cancer agents, care should be exercised in the handling and preparation of pemetrexed infusion solutions. The use of gloves is recommended. If a pemetrexed solution contacts the skin, wash the skin immediately and thoroughly with soap and water. If pemetrexed solutions contact the mucous membranes, flush thoroughly with water. Pemetrexed is not a vesicant. There is not a specific antidote for extravasation of pemetrexed. There have been few reported cases of pemetrexed extravasation, which were not assessed as serious by the investigator. Extravasation should be managed by local standard practice as with other non-vesicants.

7. MARKETING AUTHORISATION HOLDER
Eli Lilly Nederland BV, Grootslag 1-5, NL-3991 RA Houten, The Netherlands.

8. MARKETING AUTHORISATION NUMBER(S)
EU/1/04/290/001

9. DATE OF FIRST AUTHORISATION/RENEWAL OF THE AUTHORISATION
Date of first authorisation: 20 September 2004

Date of renewal of authorisation: -

10. DATE OF REVISION OF THE TEXT
-

LEGAL CATEGORY
POM

*ALIMTA (pemetrexed) is a trademark of Eli Lilly and Company.

AT1M

Alka-Seltzer Original

(Bayer plc)

1. NAME OF THE MEDICINAL PRODUCT
Alka-Seltzer Original

2. QUALITATIVE AND QUANTITATIVE COMPOSITION
One tablet contains 324mg acetylsalicylic acid (aspirin) Ph.Eur, 965mg citric acid Ph.Eur and 1625mg sodium hydrogen carbonate Ph.Eur. The active ingredients in water become sodium citrate 1296mg, sodium acetylsalicylate 364mg and sodium hydrogen carbonate 209mg.

3. PHARMACEUTICAL FORM
Effervescent tablets for oral administration.

4. CLINICAL PARTICULARS

4.1 Therapeutic indications
For fast and effective symptomatic relief of headache with upset stomach, particularly when due to too much to eat or drink. Alka-Seltzer Original is especially effective when taken before bed and again in the morning.

Symptomatic relief of sprains, strains, rheumatic pain, sciatica, lumbago, fibrositis, muscular aches and pains, joint swelling and stiffness.

For mild to moderate pain including headache, migraine, neuralgia, toothache, sore throat, period pains, aches and pains.

Symptomatic relief of influenza, feverishness, feverish colds.

4.2 Posology and method of administration
Alka-Seltzer Original tablets must always be dissolved in a glass of water prior to oral administration. The tablets dissolve more quickly in warm water.

The dose in adults, elderly and children aged 16 years and over, is two tablets in water. The dose may be repeated every four hours, as required, with a maximum of four dosages in 24 hours. These dosages should not be continued for more than three days without consulting a physician. The stated dose must not be exceeded.

Do not give to children under 16 years, unless specifically indicated (e.g. for Kawasaki's disease).

4.3 Contraindications
Alka-Seltzer Original should not be administered to patients:

• with known hypersensitivity reactions (e.g. bronchospasm, rhinitis, urticaria) in response to acetylsalicylic acid, other salicylates or substances with similar actions e.g non-steroidal anti-inflammatory drug.

• with known hypersensitivity to any of the other ingredients, refer to section 6.1.

• with active peptic ulceration or a history of peptic ulceration.

• with haemorrhagic diseases such as haemophilia.

• in the last trimester of pregnancy (see sections 4.4 and 4.6).

• receiving doses of methotrexate at 15mg/week or greater (see section 4.5).

4.4 Special warnings and special precautions for use
Acetylsalicylic acid may precipitate bronchospasm and induce asthma attacks or other hypersensitivity reactions in susceptible individuals.

Caution should be exercised in patients:

• whose renal or hepatic function is impaired

• with a history of gastrointestinal disorders

• in the first or second trimester of pregnancy or who are breast-feeding (see sections 4.3 and 4.6)

• taking anticoagulants (e.g. coumarin derivatives or heparin)

Aspirin can cause gout in patients with low uric acid excretion.

There is a possible association between aspirin and Reye's syndrome when given to children. Reye's syndrome is a very rare disease, which affects the brain, and liver, and can be fatal. For this reason aspirin should not be given to children aged under 16 unless specifically indicated (e.g. Kawasaki's disease).

Home medications should be considered only for minor or temporary ailments and should be used as directed. If symptoms persist or recur frequently, a physician should be consulted.

Due to its inhibitory effect on platelet aggregation aspirin may cause increased bleeding during and after surgery.

4.5 Interaction with other medicinal products and other forms of Interaction
Alka-Seltzer Original may:

• Enhance the activity of anticoagulants, insulin and sulphonylurea hypoglycaemic agents.

• Enhance the activity of methotrexate and increase its toxicity (see section 4.3).

• Diminish the effects of uricosuric agents.

• Diminish the effects of diuretics.

• Potentiate the risk of gastro-intestinal bleeding during concomitant therapy with corticosteroids.

• Potentiate the effects and side-effects of other non-steroidal anti-inflammatory drugs.

• Enhance the plasma concentrations of digoxin.

• Enhance the effects of some anti-epileptics, such as sodium valproate and phenytoin.

• Interact with antihypertensive medicines.

• Increase the risk of bleeding with thrombolytics and other anti-platelet agents e.g. ticlopidine.

Decreased blood salicylate levels may occur when aspirin is taken concomitantly with glucocorticoids. There is a risk of salicylate overdose when glucocorticoids treatment is stopped.

At doses of 3g/day or more, aspirin may:

• Increase risk of ulcers and gastro-intestinal bleeding when taken with other NSAIDs.

• Decrease glomerular filtration when taken with diuretics.

• Decrease glomerular filtration and anti-hypertensive effect when taken with ACE inhibitors.

4.6 Pregnancy and lactation
(see sections 4.3 and 4.4)

Although clinical and epidemiological evidence suggests the safety of acetylsalicylic acid for use in pregnancy, caution should be exercised when administered to pregnant patients.

Acetylsalicylic acid has the ability to alter platelet function and, therefore, there may be a risk of haemorrhage in infants whose mothers have consumed acetylsalicylic acid during pregnancy. The onset of labour may be delayed and the duration increased, with an increase in maternal blood loss. Therefore, analgesic doses should be avoided during the last trimester.

High doses of acetylsalicylic acid may result in closure of foetal ductus arteriosus *in utero* and possibly persistent pulmonary hypertension in the new born. Kernicterus may be a consequence of jaundice in neonates.

Administration of aspirin at doses greater than 300mg/day, shortly before birth can lead to intra-cranial haemorrhages, particularly in premature babies.

The intake of acetylsalicylic acid by breast-feeding patients should be avoided as there is a risk of Reye's syndrome. Regular use of high doses could impair platelet function and produce hypoprothrombinaemia in the infant if neonatal vitamin K stores are low.

When aspirin has been taken regularly or high doses have been taken then breast-feeding should be discontinued early.

4.7 Effects on ability to drive and use machines
None known.

4.8 Undesirable effects
Gastro-intestinal disorders have been reported for acetylsalicylic acid containing products e.g. nausea, diarrhoea, vomiting and gastro-intestinal bleeding which can lead to anaemia in some cases. Gastro-intestinal ulcers may develop, which may lead to haemorrhaging and perforation.

Rare cases of bronchospasm, asthmatic or hypersensitivity reactions have been reported for acetylsalicylic acid containing products.

Isolated cases of liver function disturbances and severe skin reactions have also been reported.

Due to the effect on platelet aggregation aspirin may be associated with an increased risk of bleeding.

Dizziness and tinnitus have also been reported but these side effects are more commonly indicative of an overdose.

4.9 Overdose
Salicylates / Aspirin
Salicylate poisoning is usually associated with plasma concentrations >350 mg/L (2.5 mmol/L). Most adult deaths occur in patients whose concentrations exceed 700 mg/L (5.1 mmol/L). Single doses less than 100 mg/kg are unlikely to cause serious poisoning.

Symptoms

Common features include vomiting, dehydration, tinnitus, vertigo, deafness, sweating, warm extremities with bounding pulses, increased respiratory rate and hyperventilation. Some degree of acid-base disturbance is present in most cases.

A mixed respiratory alkalosis and metabolic acidosis with normal or high arterial pH (normal or reduced hydrogen ion concentration) is usual in adults and children over the age of four years. In children aged four years or less, a dominant metabolic acidosis with low arterial pH (raised hydrogen ion concentration) is common. Acidosis may increase salicylate transfer across the blood brain barrier.

Uncommon features include haematemesis, hyperpyrexia, hypoglycaemia, hypokalaemia, thrombocytopaenia, increased INR/PTR, intravascular coagulation, renal failure and non-cardiac pulmonary oedema.

Central nervous system features including confusion, disorientation, coma and convulsions are less common in adults than in children.

Management

Give activated charcoal if an adult presents within one hour of ingestion of more than 250 mg/kg. The plasma salicylate concentration should be measured, although the severity of poisoning cannot be determined from this alone and the clinical and biochemical features must be taken into account. Elimination is increased by urinary alkalinisation, which is achieved by the administration of 1.26% sodium hydrogen carbonate. The urine pH should be monitored. Correct metabolic acidosis with intravenous 8.4% sodium hydrogen carbonate (first check serum potassium). Forced diuresis should not be used since it does not enhance salicylate excretion and may cause pulmonary oedema.

Haemodialysis is the treatment of choice for severe poisoning and should be considered in patients with plasma salicylate concentrations >700 mg/L (5.1 mmol/L), or lower concentrations associated with severe clinical or metabolic features. Patients under ten years or over 70 have increased risk of salicylate toxicity and may require dialysis at an earlier stage.

5. PHARMACOLOGICAL PROPERTIES

5.1 Pharmacodynamic properties
The therapeutic uses of Alka-Seltzer Original are based on the following pharmacological properties of the active ingredients. Acetylsalicylate has analgesic, anti-pyretic and anti-inflammatory properties. The buffer converts acetylsalicylic acid to sodium acetylsalicylate and promotes gastric emptying.

5.2 Pharmacokinetic properties
Acetylsalicylate is rapidly absorbed from the small intestine after oral ingestion of Alka-Seltzer Original and rapidly distributed to all body tissues. Peak plasma levels occur at approximately 20 minutes. Excretion is mainly renal.

5.3 Preclinical safety data
None relevant.

6. PHARMACEUTICAL PARTICULARS

6.1 List of excipients
Alka-Seltzer Original tablets contain no additional excipients.

6.2 Incompatibilities
None known.

6.3 Shelf life
Shelf-life of the product as packaged for sale: 36 months.

6.4 Special precautions for storage
Do not store above 25°C. Store in the original package.

6.5 Nature and contents of container
Primary packaging consists of laminated paper/polyethylene/aluminium foil with surlyn heat foil or a direct printed lamination of aluminium and surlyn heat seal.

Aluminium foil pouches, each containing two tablets. Available in pack sizes of 2, 8, 10, 12, 20 or 30 tablets.

6.6 Instructions for use and handling
The tablets should not be removed from the foil pouches until immediately before use.

If only one tablet from the foil pouch is used, the remaining one should be disposed of.

If a foil pouch is damaged and/or the tablets are powdery or discoloured, they should not be used. However, in the event that tablets are used, they are not harmful.

Alka-Seltzer Original must not be used after the expiry date.

Keep out of the reach of children.

7. MARKETING AUTHORISATION HOLDER
Bayer Diagnostics Manufacturing Limited

Bayer House

Strawberry Hill

Newbury, Berkshire

RG14 1JA

8. MARKETING AUTHORISATION NUMBER(S)
PL 0055/0115

9. DATE OF FIRST AUTHORISATION/RENEWAL OF THE AUTHORISATION
Date of first authorisation: 10 June 1988

Date of last renewal: 10 June 1993

10. DATE OF REVISION OF THE TEXT
July 2004

Legal Category
GSL

Alka-Seltzer XS

(Bayer plc)

1. NAME OF THE MEDICINAL PRODUCT
Alka-Seltzer XS

2. QUALITATIVE AND QUANTITATIVE COMPOSITION
Each tablet contains acetylsalicylic acid (aspirin) Ph.Eur 267mg, paracetamol Ph.Eur 133mg, caffeine Ph.Eur 40mg, sodium hydrogen carbonate Ph.Eur 1.606g and citric acid Ph.Eur 954mg.

3. PHARMACEUTICAL FORM
Effervescent tablets.

4. CLINICAL PARTICULARS

4.1 Therapeutic indications
For rapid relief of pain including migraine, headache, period pains, neuralgia, toothache, sore throat.

Headache with upset stomach.

Symptomatic relief of rheumatic pain, sciatica, lumbago, fibrositis, muscular aches and pains.

Symptomatic relief of influenza, feverishness, feverish colds.

4.2 Posology and method of administration
Alka-Seltzer XS is for oral ingestion after dissolution in water. It dissolves more quickly in warm water.

Adults: Two tablets in water. This dose may be repeated every four hours up to four doses in 24 hours but the dosage should not be continued for more than three days without consulting a doctor. Do not exceed the stated dose.

Do not give to children under 16 years, unless specifically indicated (e.g. for Kawasaki's disease).

4.3 Contraindications
Alka-Seltzer XS should not be administered to patients:

• with known hypersensitivity reactions (e.g. bronchospasm, rhinitis, urticaria) in response to acetylsalicylic acid, other salicylates, or substances with similar actions e.g. non-steroidal anti-inflammatory drugs.

• with known hypersensitivity to paracetamol or any of the other ingredients, refer to section 2.

• with active peptic ulceration or a history of peptic ulceration.

• with haemorrhagic diseases such as haemophilia.

• in the last trimester of pregnancy (see sections 4.4 and 4.6).

• receiving doses of methotrexate at 15mg/week or greater (see section 4.5).

4.4 Special warnings and special precautions for use
Acetylsalicylic acid may precipitate bronchospasm and induce asthma attacks or other hypersensitivity reactions in susceptible individuals.

Caution should be exercised in patients:

• with a history of gastrointestinal disorders

• in the first or second trimester of pregnancy or who are breast-feeding (see sections 4.3 and 4.6)

• taking anticoagulants (e.g. coumarin derivatives or heparin)

• whose renal or hepatic function is impaired. The hazards of overdose are greater in those with non-cirrhotic alcoholic liver disease.

Aspirin can cause gout in patients with low uric acid excretion.

Alka-Seltzer XS contains paracetamol and so other paracetamol-containing preparations should be avoided. The maximum dose of paracetamol for adults is 4g daily.

Do not exceed the recommended dose. If symptoms persist consult your doctor. Keep out of the reach of children.

There is a possible association between aspirin and Reye's syndrome when given to children.Reye's syndrome is a very rare disease, which affects the brain and liver, and can be fatal. For this reason aspirin should not be given to children aged under 16 years unless specifically indicated (e.g. Kawasaki's disease).

Due to its inhibitory effect on platelet aggregation aspirin may cause increased bleeding during and after surgery.

Leaflet warning: Immediate medical advice should be sought in the event of an overdose, even if you feel well, because of the risk of delayed, serious liver damage.

Label warning: Immediate medical advice should be sought in the event of an overdose, even if you feel well. Do not take with any other paracetamol-containing products.

4.5 Interaction with other medicinal products and other forms of Interaction
Alka-Seltzer XS may:

• Enhance the activity of anticoagulants such as warfarin and other coumarins.

• Enhance the activity of insulin and sulphonylurea hypoglycaemic agents.

• Enhance the activity of methotrexate and increase its toxicity (see section 4.3).

• Diminish the effects of uricosuric agents.

• Diminish the effects of diuretics.

• Potentiate the risk of gastro-intestinal bleeding during concomitant therapy with corticosteroids.

• Potentiate the effects and side-effects of other non-steroidal anti-inflammatory drugs.

• Enhance the plasma concentrations of digoxin.

• Enhance the effects of some anti-epileptics, such as sodium valproate and phenytoin.

• Interact with antihyperstensive medicines.

• Increase risk of bleeding with thrombolytics and other anti-platelet agents e.g. ticlopidine.

The speed of absorption of paracetamol may be increased by metoclopramide or domperidone and absorption reduced by cholestyramine.

Decreased blood salicylate levels may occur when aspirin is taken concomitantly with glucocorticoids. There is a risk of salicylate overdose when glucocorticoids treatment is stopped.

At doses of 3g/day or more, aspirin may:

• Increase risk of ulcers and gastro-intestinal bleeding when taken with other NSAIDs.

• Decrease glomerular filtration when taken with diuretics.

• Decrease glomerular filtration and anti-hypertensive effect when taken with ACE inhibitors.

When taken with alcohol, the effects of acetylsalicylic acid on the gastro-intestinal tract may increase.

4.6 Pregnancy and lactation
(see sections 4.3 and 4.4)

Alka-Seltzer XS should not be taken by pregnant or nursing women unless directed by a doctor.

Pregnancy

Acetylsalicylic acid:

Although clinical and epidemiological evidence suggests the safety of acetylsalicylic acid for use in pregnancy, caution should be exercised when administered to pregnant patients.

Acetylsalicylic acid has the ability to alter platelet function and, therefore, there may be a risk of haemorrhage in infants whose mothers have consumed acetylsalicylic acid during pregnancy. The onset of labour may be delayed and the duration increased, with an increase in maternal blood loss. Therefore, analgesic doses should be avoided during the last trimester of pregnancy.

High doses of acetylsalicylic acid may result in closure of foetal ductus arteriosus *in utero* and possibly persistent pulmonary hypertension in the new born. Kernicterus may be a consequence of jaundice in neonates.

Administration of aspirin at doses greater than 300mg/day, shortly before birth can lead to intra-cranial haemorrhages, particularly in premature babies.

Paracetamol:

Epidemiological studies in human pregnancy have shown no ill effects due to paracetamol used in the recommended dosage, but patients should follow the advice of their doctor regarding its use.

Lactation

Acetylsalicylic acid:

The intake of acetylsalicylic acid by breast-feeding patients should be avoided as there is a risk of Reye's syndrome. Regular use of high doses could impair platelet function and produce hypoprothrombinaemia in the infant if neonatal vitamin K stores are low.

When aspirin has been taken regularly or high doses have been taken then breast-feeding should be discontinued early.

Paracetamol:

Paracetamol is excreted in breast milk but not in a clinically significant amount. Available published data on paracetamol does not contraindicate it for breast feeding.

4.7 Effects on ability to drive and use machines
None.

4.8 Undesirable effects

Acetylsalicylic acid:

Gastrointestinal disorders have been reported for acetylsalicylic acid containing products e.g. nausea, diarrhoea, vomiting and gastro-intestinal bleeding which can lead to anaemia in some cases. Gastrointestinal ulcers may develop, which may lead to haemorraging and perforation.

Rare cases of bronchospasm, asthmatic or hypersensitivity reactions have been reported for acetylsalicylic acid containing products.

Isolated cases of liver function disturbances and severe skin reactions have also been reported.

Due to the effect on platelet aggregation, acetylsalicylic acid may be associated with an increased risk of bleeding.

Dizziness and tinnitus have also been reported for acetylsalicylic acid but these side effects are more commonly indicative of an overdose.

Paracetamol:

Adverse effects of paracetamol are rare but hypersensitivity including skin rash may occur. There have been reports of blood dyscrasias including thrombocytopenia and agranulocytosis, but these were not necessarily causality related to paracetmaol.

There have been reports of blood dyscrasis including thrombocytopenia and agranulocytosis, but these were not necessarily causally related to paracetamol.

4.9 Overdose

Paracetamol

Liver damage is possible in adults who have taken 10g or more of paracetamol.

Symptoms

Symptoms of paracetamol overdosage in the first 24 hours are pallor, nausea, vomiting, anorexia and abdominal pain. Liver damage may become apparent 12 to 48 hours after ingestion. Abnormalities of glucose metabolism and metabolic acidosis may occur. In severe poisoning, hepatic failure may progress to encephalopathy, coma and death. Acute renal failure with acute tubular necrosis may develop even in the absence of severe liver damage. Cardiac arrhythmias and pancreatitis have been reported.

Management

Immediate treatment is essential in the management of paracetamol overdose. Despite a lack of significant early symptoms, patients should be referred to hospital urgently for immediate medical attention and any patient who had ingested around 7.5g or more of paracetamol in the preceding 4 hours should undergo gastric lavage. Administration of oral methionine or intravenous N-acetylcysteine which may have a beneficial effect up to at least 48 hours after the overdose, may be required. General supportive measures must be available.

Acetysalicyclic acid

Salicylate poisoning is usually associated with plasma concentrations >350 mg/L (2.5 mmol/L). Most adult deaths occur in patients whose concentrations exceed 700 mg/L (5.1 mmol/L). Single doses less than 100 mg/kg are unlikely to cause serious poisoning.

Symptoms

Common features include vomiting, dehydration, tinnitus, vertigo, deafness, sweating, warm extremities with bounding pulses, increased respiratory rate and hyperventilation. Some degree of acid-base disturbance is present in most cases.

A mixed respiratory alkalosis and metabolic acidosis with normal or high arterial pH (normal or reduced hydrogen ion concentration) is usual in adults and children over the age of four years. In children aged four years or less, a dominant metabolic acidosis with low arterial pH (raised hydrogen ion concentration) is common. Acidosis may increase salicylate transfer across the blood brain barrier.

Uncommon features include haematemesis, hyperpyrexia, hypoglycaemia, hypokalaemia, thrombocytopaenia, increased INR/PTR, intravascular coagulation, renal failure and non-cardiac pulmonary oedema.

Central nervous system features including confusion, disorientation, coma and convulsions are less common in adults than in children.

Management

Give activated charcoal if an adult presents within one hour of ingestion of more than 250 mg/kg. The plasma salicylate concentration should be measured, although the severity of poisoning cannot be determined from this alone and the clinical and biochemical features must be taken into account. Elimination is increased by urinary alkalinisation, which is achieved by the administration of 1.26% sodium bicarbonate. The urine pH should be monitored. Correct metabolic acidosis with intravenous 8.4% sodium bicarbonate (first check serum potassium). Forced diuresis should not be used since it does not enhance salicylate excretion and may cause pulmonary oedema.

Haemodialysis is the treatment of choice for severe poisoning and should be considered in patients with plasma salicylate concentrations >700 mg/L (5.1 mmol/L), or lower concentrations associated with severe clinical or metabolic features. Patients under ten years or over 70 have increased risk of salicylate toxicity and may require dialysis at an earlier stage.

5. PHARMACOLOGICAL PROPERTIES

5.1 Pharmacodynamic properties

The therapeutic uses of Alka-Seltzer XS are based on the following pharmacological properties of the active ingredients:

Acetylsalicylate - analgesic, antipyretic and anti-inflammatory.

Paracetamol - analgesic, antipyretic.

Caffeine - central nervous system stimulant.

The buffer converts acetylsalicylic acid to sodium acetylsalicylate and promotes gastric emptying.

5.2 Pharmacokinetic properties

Acetylsalicylate is rapidly absorbed from the small intestine after oral ingestion of Alka-Seltzer XS and rapidly distributed to all body tissues.

Acetylsalicylate is hydrolysed to its active primary metabolite salicylic acid and completely excreted in the urine, principally as glucoronic acid and glycine conjugates of salicylic acid, but also as salicylic acid itself. Salicylates are extensively bound to plasma proteins. Peak plasma levels occur at approximately 20 minutes. Following administration of acetylsalicylic acid, salicylic acid can be detected in breast milk, cerebral spinal fluid and synovial fluid. The substance crosses the placenta.

Paracetamol is rapidly absorbed from the upper gastrointestinal tract after oral administration of Alka-Seltzer XS, with the small intestine being an important site of absorption. Peak plasma concentration occurs about 30 minutes to 2 hours after ingestion. It is rapidly distributed throughout the body and is primarily metabolised in the liver with excretion via the kidney. Elimination half-life varies from about 1 to 4 hours. Paracetamol crosses the placental barrier and is present in breast milk.

Caffeine is readily absorbed after oral administration and passes readily into the central nervous system. Excretion is renal.

5.3 Preclinical safety data

There are no preclinical data of relevance to the prescriber which are additional to the information included in other sections of the Summary of Product Characteristics.

6. PHARMACEUTICAL PARTICULARS

6.1 List of excipients

Not applicable.

6.2 Incompatibilities

None known.

6.3 Shelf life

36 months.

6.4 Special precautions for storage

Laminated paper/polyethylene/aluminium surlyn heat sealed foil:

Do not store above 25°C. Store in the original package.

Laminated aluminium/polyethylene surlyn heat sealed foil:

Do not store above 25°C. Store in the original package.

6.5 Nature and contents of container

Laminated paper/polyethylene/aluminium surlyn heat sealed foil, or laminated aluminium/polyethylene surlyn heat sealed foil.

Pack sizes available are 2, 10, 12, 20, and 30 tablets.

6.6 Instructions for use and handling

None applicable.

7. MARKETING AUTHORISATION HOLDER

Bayer Diagnostics Manufacturing Limited
T/A Bayer Bridgend
Bayer House
Strawberry Hill
Newbury, Berkshire
RG14 1JA

8. MARKETING AUTHORISATION NUMBER(S)

PL 0055/5017R

9. DATE OF FIRST AUTHORISATION/RENEWAL OF THE AUTHORISATION

Date of first authorisation: 23 April 1982

Date of last renewal: 10 August 2004

10. DATE OF REVISION OF THE TEXT

October 2004

LEGAL STATUS

GSL

Alkeran Injection 50 mg

(GlaxoSmithKline UK)

1. NAME OF THE MEDICINAL PRODUCT

Alkeran Injection 50 mg

2. QUALITATIVE AND QUANTITATIVE COMPOSITION

Melphalan Hydrochloride BP equivalent to 50 mg mephalan per vial.

3. PHARMACEUTICAL FORM

Freeze-dried powder for injection.

4. CLINICAL PARTICULARS

4.1 Therapeutic indications

Alkeran Injection, at conventional intravenous dosage, is indicated in the treatment of multiple myeloma and ovarian cancer.

Alkeran Injection, at high intravenous dosage, is indicated, with or without haematopoietic stem cell transplantation, for the treatment of multiple myeloma and childhood neuroblastoma.

Alkeran Injection, administered by regional arterial perfusion, is indicated in the treatment of localised malignant melanoma of the extremities and localised soft tissue sarcoma of the extremities.

In the above indications, Alkeran may be used alone or in combination with other cytotoxic drugs.

4.2 Posology and method of administration

Parenteral administration:

Alkeran Injection is for intravenous use and regional arterial perfusion only. Alkeran Injection should not be given without haematopoietic stem cell rescue at doses of above 140 mg/m^2.

For intravenous administration, it is recommended that Alkeran Injection solution is injected slowly into a fast-running infusion solution via a swabbed injection port.

If direct injection into a fast-running infusion is not appropriate, Alkeran Injection solution may be administered diluted in an infusion bag.

Alkeran is not compatible with infusion solutions containing dextrose and it is recommended that only sodium chloride intravenous infusion 0.9% w/v is used.

When further diluted in an infusion solution, Alkeran has reduced stability and the rate of degradation increases rapidly with rise in temperature. If Alkeran is infused at a room temperature of approximately 25°C, the total time from preparation of the injection solution to the completion of infusion should not exceed 1.5 hours.

Should any visible turbidity or crystallisation appear in the reconstituted or diluted solutions, the preparation must be discarded.

Care should be taken to avoid possible extravasation of Alkeran and in cases of poor peripheral venous access, consideration should be given to use of a central venous line.

If high dose Alkeran Injection is administered with or without autologous bone marrow transplantation, administration via a central venous line is recommended.

For regional arterial perfusion, the literature should be consulted for detailed methodology.

Multiple myeloma: Alkeran Injection is administered on an intermittent basis alone, or in combination with other cytotoxic drugs. Administration of prednisone has also been included in a number of regimens.

When used as a single agent, a typical intravenous Alkeran dosage schedule is 0.4 mg/kg body weight (16 mg/m^2 body surface area) repeated at appropriate intervals (e.g. once every 4 weeks), provided there has been recovery of the peripheral blood count during this period.

High-dose regimens generally employ single intravenous doses of between 100 and 200 mg/m^2 body surface area (approximately 2.5 to 5.0 mg/kg body weight), but haematopoietic stem cell rescue becomes essential following doses in excess of 140 mg/m^2 body surface area. Hydration and forced diuresis are also recommended.

Ovarian adenocarcinoma: When used intravenously as a single agent, a dose of 1 mg/kg body weight (approximately 40 mg/m^2 body surface area) given at intervals of 4 weeks has often been used.

When combined with other cytotoxic drugs, intravenous doses of between 0.3 and 0.4 mg/kg body weight (12 to 16 mg/m^2 body surface area) have been used at intervals of 4 to 6 weeks.

Advanced neuroblastoma: Doses of between 100 and 240 mg/m^2 body surface area (sometimes divided equally over 3 consecutive days) together with haematopoietic stem cell rescue, have been used either alone or in combination with radiotherapy and/or other cytotoxic drugs.

Malignant melanoma: Hyperthermic regional perfusion with Alkeran has been used as an adjuvant to surgery for early malignant melanoma and as palliative treatment for advanced but localised disease. The scientific literature should be consulted for details of perfusion technique and dosage used. A typical dose range for upper extremity perfusions is 0.6-1.0 mg/kg bodyweight and for lower extremity perfusions is 0.8-1.5 mg/kg body weight.

Soft tissue sarcoma: Hyperthermic regional perfusion with Alkeran has been used in the management of all stages of localised soft tissue sarcoma, usually in combination with surgery. A typical dose range for upper extremity perfusions is 0.6-1.0 mg/kg body weight and for lower extremity perfusions is 1-1.4 mg/kg body weight.

Use in Children

Alkeran, at conventional dosage, is only rarely indicated in children and dosage guidelines cannot be stated.

High dose Alkeran Injection, in association with haematopoietic stem cell rescue, has been used in childhood neuroblastoma and dosage guidelines based on body surface area, as for adults, may be used.

Use in the elderly

Although Alkeran is frequently used at conventional dosage in the elderly, there is no specific information available relating to its administration to this patient subgroup.

Experience in the use of high dose Alkeran in elderly patients is limited. Consideration should therefore be given to ensure adequate performance status and organ function, before using high dose Alkeran Injection in elderly patients.

Dosage in renal impairment

Alkeran clearance, though variable, may be decreased in renal impairment.

Currently available pharmacokinetic data do not justify an absolute recommendation on dosage reduction when administering Alkeran Tablets to patients with renal impairment, but it may be prudent to use a reduced dosage initially until tolerance is established.

When Alkeran Injection is used at conventional intravenous dosage (16-40 mg/m^2 body surface area), it is recommended that the initial dose should be reduced by 50% and subsequent dosage determined according to the degree of haematological suppression.

For high intravenous doses of Alkeran (100 to 240 mg/m^2 body surface area), the need for dose reduction depends upon the degree of renal impairment, whether haematopoietic stem cells are re-infused, and therapeutic need. Alkeran Injection should not be given without haematopoietic stem cell rescue at doses of above 140 mg/m^2.

As a guide, for high dose Alkeran treatment without haematopoietic stem cell rescue in patients with moderate renal impairment (creatinine clearance 30 to 50 ml/min) a dose reduction of 50% is usual. High dose Alkeran (above 140 mg/m^2) without haematopoietic stem cell rescue should not be used in patients with more severe renal impairment.

High dose Alkeran with haematopoietic stem cell rescue has been used successfully even in dialysis dependent patients with end-stage renal failure. The relevant literature should be consulted for details.

4.3 Contraindications

Alkeran should not be given to patients who have suffered a previous hypersensitivity reaction to melphalan.

4.4 Special warnings and special precautions for use

Alkeran is a cytotoxic drug, which falls into the general class of alkylating agents. It should be prescribed only by physicians experienced in the management of malignant disease with such agents. As with all high dose chemotherapy, precautions should be taken to prevent tumour lysis syndrome.

Immunisation using a live organism vaccine has the potential to cause infection in immunocompromised hosts. Therefore, immunisations with live organism vaccines are not recommended.

Since Alkeran is myelosuppressive, frequent blood counts are essential during therapy and the dosage should be delayed or adjusted if necessary.

Alkeran Injection solution can cause local tissue damage, should extravasation occur and consequently, it should not be administered by direct injection into a peripheral vein. It is recommended that Alkeran Injection solution is administered by injecting slowly into a fast-running intravenous infusion via a swabbed injection port, or via a central venous line.

In view of the hazards involved and the level of supportive care required, the administration of high dose Alkeran Injection should be confined to specialist centres, with the appropriate facilities and only be conducted by experienced clinicians.

In patients receiving high dose Alkeran Injection, consideration should be given to the prophylactic administration of anti-infective agents and the administration of blood products as required.

Consideration should be given to ensure adequate performance status and organ function before using high dose Alkeran Injection. Alkeran Injection should not be given without haematopoietic stem cell rescue at doses of above 140 mg/m^2.

As with all cytotoxic chemotherapy, adequate contraceptive precautions should be practised when either partner is receiving Alkeran.

Safe handling of Alkeran

The handling of Alkeran formulations should follow guidelines for the handling of cytotoxic drugs according to the Royal Pharmaceutical Society of Great Britain Working Party on the handling of cytotoxic drugs.

Monitoring

Since Alkeran is a potent myelosuppressive agent, it is essential that careful attention should be paid to the monitoring of blood counts, to avoid the possibility of excessive myelosuppression and the risk of irreversible bone marrow aplasia. Blood counts may continue to fall after treatment is stopped, so at the first sign of an abnormally large fall in leukocyte or platelet counts, treatment should be temporarily interrupted. Alkeran should be used with caution in patients who have undergone recent radiotherapy or chemotherapy in view of increased bone marrow toxicity.

Renal Impairment

Alkeran clearance may be reduced in patients with renal impairment who may also have uraemic marrow suppression. Dose reduction may therefore be necessary (see Posology and Method of Administration). See Undesirable Effects for elevation of blood urea.

Mutagenicity

Melphalan is mutagenic in animals and chromosome aberrations have been observed in patients being treated with the drug.

Carcinogenicity

Melphalan, in common with other alkylating agents, may be leukaemogenic in man. There have been reports of acute leukaemia occurring after prolonged melphalan treatment for diseases such as amyloid, malignant melanoma, multiple myeloma, macroglobulinaemia, cold agglutinin syndrome and ovarian cancer.

A comparison of patients with ovarian cancer who received alkylating agents with those who did not, showed that the use of alkylating agents, including melphalan, significantly increased the incidence of acute leukaemia.

The leukaemogenic risk must be balanced against the potential therapeutic benefit when considering the use of melphalan.

Effects on Fertility

Alkeran causes suppression of ovarian function in premenopausal women resulting in amenorrhoea in a significant number of patients.

There is evidence from some animal studies that Alkeran can have an adverse effect on spermatogenesis. Therefore, it is possible that Alkeran may cause temporary or permanent sterility in male patients.

The label for the product will contain the following statements:

Keep out of the reach of children.

Store below 30° C

Do not refrigerate.

Protect from light

4.5 Interaction with other medicinal products and other forms of Interaction

Vaccinations with live organism vaccines are not recommended in immunocompromised individuals (see Warnings and Precautions).

Nalidixic acid together with high-dose intravenous melphalan has caused deaths in children due to haemorrhagic enterocolitis.

Impaired renal function has been described in bone marrow transplant patients who received high dose intravenous melphalan and who subsequently received ciclosporin to prevent graft-versus-host disease.

4.6 Pregnancy and lactation

The teratogenic potential of Alkeran has not been studied. In view of its mutagenic properties and structural similarity to known teratogenic compounds, it is possible that melphalan could cause congenital defects in the offspring of patients treated with the drug.

The use of melphalan should be avoided whenever possible during pregnancy, particularly during the first trimester. In any individual case, the potential hazard to the foetus must be balanced against the expected benefit to the mother.

Mothers receiving Alkeran should not breastfeed.

4.7 Effects on ability to drive and use machines

None known.

4.8 Undesirable effects

The most common side-effect is bone marrow depression, leading to leucopenia and thrombocytopenia.

Gastro-intestinal effects such as nausea and vomiting have been reported in up to 30% of patients receiving conventional oral doses of Alkeran.

Stomatitis occurs rarely following conventional doses of Alkeran.

The incidence of diarrhoea, vomiting and stomatitis becomes the dose limiting toxicity in patients given high intravenous doses of Alkeran in association with haematopoietic stem cell transplantation.

Allergic reactions to Alkeran such as urticaria, oedema, skin rashes and anaphylactic shock have been reported uncommonly following initial or subsequent dosing, particularly after intravenous administration. Cardiac arrest has also been reported rarely in association with such events.

Maculopapular rashes and pruritus have occasionally been noted.

Hepatic disorders ranging from abnormal liver function tests to clinical manifestations such as hepatitis and jaundice have been reported. Veno-occlusive disease has been reported in association with these cases.

There have been case reports of interstitial pneumonitis and pulmonary fibrosis; fatal reports of pulmonary fibrosis have been received.

There have also been case reports of haemolytic anaemia occurring after melphalan treatment.

Temporary significant elevation of the blood urea has been seen in the early stages of melphalan therapy in myeloma patients with renal damage.

Alopecia has been reported but is uncommon at conventional doses.

A subjective and transient sensation of warmth and/or tingling was described in approximately two thirds of patients with haematological malignancies who were given high dose Alkeran Injection via a central line.

4.9 Overdose

Gastro-intestinal effects, including nausea, vomiting and diarrhoea are the most likely signs of acute oral overdosage. The immediate effects of acute intravenous overdosage are nausea and vomiting. Damage to the gastrointestinal mucosa may also ensue and diarrhoea, sometimes haemorrhagic, has been reported after overdosage. The principal toxic effect is bone marrow suppression, leading to leucopenia, thrombocytopenia and anaemia.

General supportive measures, together with appropriate blood and platelet transfusions, should be instituted if necessary and consideration given to hospitalisation, antibiotic cover, the use of haematological growth factors.

There is no specific antidote. The blood picture should be closely monitored for at least four weeks following overdosage until there is evidence of recovery.

5. PHARMACOLOGICAL PROPERTIES

5.1 Pharmacodynamic properties

Melphalan is a bifunctional alkylating agent. Formation of carbonium intermediates from each of the two bis-2-chloroethyl groups enables alkylation through covalent binding with the 7-nitrogen of guanine on DNA, cross-linking the two DNA strands and thereby preventing cell replication.

5.2 Pharmacokinetic properties

The absorption of melphalan was found to be highly variable in 13 patients given 0.6 mg/kg orally, with respect to both the time to first appearance of the drug in plasma (range 0 to 336 minutes) and peak plasma concentration (range 70 to 630 ng/ml). In 5 of the patients who were given an equivalent intravenous dose, the mean bioavailability of melphalan was found to be 56 ± 7%. The terminal plasma half-life was 90 ± 57 minutes with 11% of the drug being recovered in the urine over 24 hours.

The administration of Alkeran Tablets immediately after food delayed the time to achieving peak plasma concentrations and reduced the area under the plasma concentration-time curves by between 39 and 45%.

The pharmacokinetics of intravenous Alkeran given at both conventional and high doses are best described by a bi-exponential, 2-compartment model. In 8 patients given a single bolus dose of 0.5 to 0.6 mg/kg, the composite initial and terminal half-lives were reported to be 7.7 ± 3.3 minutes and 108 ± 20.8 minutes, respectively. Following injection of melphalan, monohydroxymelphalan and dihydroxymelphalan were detected in the patients' plasma, reaching peak levels at approximately 60 minutes and 105 minutes, respectively. A similar half life of 126 ± 6 minutes was seen when melphalan was added to the patients' serum *in vitro* (37°C) suggesting that spontaneous degradation rather than enzymic metabolism may be the major determinant of the drug's half life in man.

Following administration of a 2 minute infusion of doses ranging from 5 to 23 mg/m^2 (approximately 0.1 to 0.6 mg/kg) to 10 patients with ovarian cancer or multiple myeloma, the pooled initial and terminal half-lives were, respectively, 8.1 ± 6.6 minutes and 76.9 ± 40.7 minutes. In this study, the mean volumes of distribution at steady state and central compartment were 29.1 ± 13.6 litres and 12.2 ± 6.5 litres, respectively and a mean clearance of 342.7 ± 96.8 ml/minute was recorded.

In 15 children and 11 adults given high-dose intravenous Alkeran (140 mg/m^2) with forced diuresis, the mean initial and terminal half-lives were found to be 6.5 ± 3.6 minutes and 41.4 ± 16.5 minutes, respectively. Mean initial and terminal half-lives of 8.8 ± 6.6 minutes and 73.1 ± 45.9 minutes, respectively, were recorded in 28 patients with various malignancies who were given doses of between 70 and 200 mg/m^2 as a 2 to 20 minute infusion. The mean volumes of distribution at steady state and central compartment were respectively, 40.2 ± 18.3 litres and 18.2 ± 11.7 litres and the mean clearance was 564.6 ± 159.1 ml/minute.

Following hyperthermic (39°C) perfusion of the lower limb with 1.75 mg/kg body weight, mean initial and terminal half-lives of 3.6 ± 1.5 minutes and 46.5 ± 17.2 minutes respectively, were recorded in 11 patients with advanced malignant melanoma. Mean volumes of distribution at steady state and central compartment were, respectively, 2.87 ± 0.8 litres and 1.01 ± 0.28 litres and a mean clearance of 55.0 ± 9.4 ml/minute was recorded.

5.3 Preclinical safety data

There are no pre-clinical data of relevance to the prescriber which are additional to that already included in other sections of the SmPC.

6. PHARMACEUTICAL PARTICULARS

6.1 List of excipients

Hydrochloric Acid Ph.Eur.

Povidone K12 Ph.Eur.

Water for Injections BP

6.2 Incompatibilities

None known.

6.3 Shelf life

36 months.

6.4 Special precautions for storage

Store below 30° C

Protect from light

Do not refrigerate.

6.5 Nature and contents of container

Clear, neutral glass vial and bromobutyl rubber stopper with an aluminium collar.

Pack size: 50 mg

6.6 Instructions for use and handling

Preparation of Alkeran Injection Solution: Alkeran Injection should be prepared at room temperature, by reconstituting the freeze-dried powder with the solvent-diluent provided. 10 ml of this vehicle should be added, as a single quantity, and the vial immediately shaken vigorously until solution is complete. The resulting solution contains the equivalent of 5 mg per ml anhydrous melphalan and has a pH of approximately 6.5.

Alkeran Injection solution has limited stability and should be prepared immediately before use. Any unused solution should be discarded according to standard guidelines for handling and disposal of cytotoxic drugs.

The reconstituted solution should not be refrigerated as this will cause precipitation.

Administrative Data

7. MARKETING AUTHORISATION HOLDER

The Wellcome Foundation Limited

Greenford

Middlesex

UB6 0NN

trading as:

GlaxoSmithKline UK

Stockley Park West

Uxbridge

Middlesex

UB11 1BT

8. MARKETING AUTHORISATION NUMBER(S)
PL 00003/0323.

9. DATE OF FIRST AUTHORISATION/RENEWAL OF THE AUTHORISATION
19 January 1999

10. DATE OF REVISION OF THE TEXT
25 February 2005

11. Legal Status
POM

Alkeran Injection Diluent

(GlaxoSmithKline UK)

1. NAME OF THE MEDICINAL PRODUCT
SOLVENT-DILUENT (for Alkeran Injection)

2. QUALITATIVE AND QUANTITATIVE COMPOSITION
No active ingredient present

3. PHARMACEUTICAL FORM
Liquid for reconstitution of Alkeran

4. CLINICAL PARTICULARS

4.1 Therapeutic indications
The Solvent-Diluent is used to reconstitute Alkeran Injection.

4.2 Posology and method of administration
The reconstituted injection is administered by infusion.

4.3 Contraindications
Not Applicable.

4.4 Special warnings and special precautions for use
Not Applicable.

The label for this product will contain the following statements:

Keep out of the reach of children.

Store below 30° C

Do not refrigerate.

Protect from light

4.5 Interaction with other medicinal products and other forms of Interaction
Not Applicable.

4.6 Pregnancy and lactation
Not Applicable.

4.7 Effects on ability to drive and use machines
Not Applicable.

4.8 Undesirable effects
Not Applicable.

4.9 Overdose
Not Applicable.

5. PHARMACOLOGICAL PROPERTIES

5.1 Pharmacodynamic properties
Not Applicable.

5.2 Pharmacokinetic properties
Not Applicable.

5.3 Preclinical safety data
Not Applicable.

6. PHARMACEUTICAL PARTICULARS

6.1 List of excipients

Excipient	Specification
Sodium citrate	Ph.Eur
Propylene glycol	Ph.Eur
Ethanol (96%)	BP
Water for injections	Ph.Eur

6.2 Incompatibilities
Not Applicable.

6.3 Shelf life
36 months

6.4 Special precautions for storage
Store below 30° C, protect from light, do not refrigerate.

6.5 Nature and contents of container
Clear neutral glass vial and chlorobutyl rubber stopper or fluoro-resin butyl rubber stopper with aluminium collar.

Pack size: 10 ml

6.6 Instructions for use and handling
Not Applicable.

Administrative Data

7. MARKETING AUTHORISATION HOLDER
The Wellcome Foundation Ltd

Greenford

Middlesex UB6 0NN

trading as:

GlaxoSmithKline UK

Stockley Park West

Uxbridge

Middlesex UB11 1BT

8. MARKETING AUTHORISATION NUMBER(S)
PL 00003/0324

9. DATE OF FIRST AUTHORISATION/RENEWAL OF THE AUTHORISATION
19 January 2005

10. DATE OF REVISION OF THE TEXT
08 July 2003

11. Legal Status
POM

Alkeran Tablets 2mg

(GlaxoSmithKline UK)

1. NAME OF THE MEDICINAL PRODUCT
Alkeran Tablets 2 mg

2. QUALITATIVE AND QUANTITATIVE COMPOSITION
Each tablet contains 2 mg melphalan.

3. PHARMACEUTICAL FORM
Film-coated tablets

ALKERAN are white to off-white film-coated, round, biconvex tablets engraved "GX EH3" on one side and "A" on the other.

4. CLINICAL PARTICULARS

4.1 Therapeutic indications
Alkeran Tablets are indicated in the treatment of multiple myeloma and advanced ovarian adenocarcinoma.

Alkeran either alone or in combination with other drugs has a significant therapeutic effect in a proportion of patients suffering from advanced breast carcinoma.

Alkeran is effective in the treatment of a proportion of patients suffering from polycythaemia vera.

Alkeran has also been used as an adjuvant to surgery in the management of breast carcinoma.

4.2 Posology and method of administration
GENERAL:

Since Alkeran is myelosuppressive, frequent blood counts are essential during therapy and the dosage should be delayed or adjusted if necessary (see *Special Warnings and Precautions for Use*).

Oral administration in Adults: The absorption of Alkeran after oral administration is variable. Dosage may need to be cautiously increased until myelosuppresion is seen, in order to ensure that potentially therapeutic levels have been reached.

Multiple Myleloma:

Numerous regimes have been used and the scientific literature should be consulted for details. The administration of Alkeran and prednisone is more effective than Alkeran alone. The combination is usually given on an intermittent basis, although the superiority of this technique over continuous therapy is not established. A typical oral dosage schedule is 0.15 mg/kg bodyweight/day in divided doses for 4 days repeated at intervals of six weeks. Prolonging treatment beyond one year in responders does not appear to improve results.

Ovarian adenocarcinoma:

A typical regimen is 0.2 mg/kg bodyweight/day orally for 5 days. This is repeated every 4-8 weeks, or as soon as the bone marrow has recovered. Alkeran has also been used intravenously in the treatment of ovarian carcinoma.

Advanced carcinoma of the breast:

Alkeran has been given orally at a dose of 0.15 mg/kg bodyweight or 6 mg/m^2 body surface area/day for 5 days and repeated every 6 weeks. The dose was decreased if bone marrow toxicity was observed.

Polycythaemia vera:

For remission induction the usual dose is 6-10 mg daily for 5-7 days, after which 2-4 mg daily is given until satisfactory disease control is achieved. Therapy is maintained with a dose of 2-6 mg per week. During maintenance therapy, careful haematological control is essential with dosage adjustment according to the results of frequent blood counts.

Children:

Alkeran is very rarely indicated in children and dosage guidelines cannot be stated.

Use in the elderly:

There is no specific information available on the use of Alkeran in elderly patients.

Dosage in renal impairment:

In patients with moderate to severe renal impairment currently available pharmacokinetic data do not justify an absolute recommendation on dosage reduction when administering the oral preparation to these patients, but it may be prudent to use a reduced dose initially.

4.3 Contraindications
Alkeran should not be given to patients who have suffered a previous hypersensitivity reaction to melphalan.

4.4 Special warnings and special precautions for use
Alkeran is an active cytotoxic agent for use only under the direction of physicians experienced in the administration of such agents.

Immunisation using a live organism vaccine has the potential to cause infection in immunocompromised hosts. Therefore, immunisations with live organism vaccines are not recommended.

Safe Handling of ALKERAN tablets:

See 6.6 Instructions for Use/Handling

Monitoring:

Since Alkeran is a potent myelosuppresive agent, it is essential that careful attention should be paid to the monitoring of blood counts to avoid the possibility of excessive myelosuppression and the risk of irreversible bone marrow aplasia. Blood counts may continue to fall after treatment is stopped, so at the first sign of an abnormally large fall in leucocyte or platelet counts, treatment should be temporarily interrupted. Alkeran should be used with caution in patients who have undergone recent radiotherapy or chemotherapy in view of increased bone marrow toxicity.

Renal impairment:

Patients with renal impairment should be closely observed as they may have uraemic marrow suppression. (See undesirable effects for elevation of blood urea Section 4.8)

Mutagenicity:

Alkeran is mutagenic in animals and chromosome aberrations have been observed in patients being treated with the drug.

Carcinogenicity:

The evidence is growing that melphalan in common with other alkylating agents may be leukaemogenic in man. There have been reports of acute leukaemia occurring after prolonged melphalan treatment for diseases such as amyloid, malignant melanoma, macroglobulinaemia, cold agglutinin syndrome and ovarian cancer.

A comparison of patients with ovarian cancer who received alkylating agents with those who did not, showed that the use of alkylating agents, including melphalan, significantly increased the incidence of acute leukaemia. The leukaemogenic risk must be balanced against the potential therapeutic benefit when considering the use of melphalan.

Alkeran causes suppression of ovarian function in premenopausal women resulting in amenorrhoea in a significant number of patients.

4.5 Interaction with other medicinal products and other forms of Interaction
Vaccinations with live organism vaccines are not recommended in immunocompromised individuals (see Warnings and Precautions).

Nalidixic acid together with high-dose intravenous melphalan has caused deaths in children due to haemorrhagic enterocolitis.

Impaired renal function has been described in bone marrow transplant patients who were pre-conditioned with high dose intravenous melphalan and who subsequently received ciclosporin to prevent graft-versus-host disease.

4.6 Pregnancy and lactation
As with all cytotoxic chemotherapy, adequate contraceptive precautions should be advised when either partner is receiving Alkeran.

Teratogenicity:

The teratogenic potential of Alkeran has not been studied. In view of its mutagenic properties and structural similarity to known teratogenic compounds, it is possible that melphalan could cause congenital defects in the offspring of patients treated with the drug.

Pregnancy:

The use of melphalan should be avoided whenever possible during pregnancy, particularly during the first trimester. In any individual case the potential hazard to the foetus must be balanced against the expected benefit to the mother.

Lactation:

Mother receiving Alkeran should not breast-feed.

4.7 Effects on ability to drive and use machines
Not known.

4.8 Undesirable effects
The most common side-effect is bone marrow depression, leading to leucopenia and thrombocytopenia.

Gastro-intestinal effects such as nausea and vomiting occur in up to 30 per cent of patients receiving conventional dose of Alkeran.

Stomatitis occurs rarely following conventional doses of Alkeran. The incidence of diarrhoea, vomiting and stomatitis is likely to increase in patients given high intravenous doses of Alkeran. Cyclophosphamide pre-treatment has been shown to reduce the severity of Alkeran-induced gastro-intestinal damage.

Rare cases of allergic reactions to Alkeran such as urticaria, oedema, skin rashes and anaphylaxis have been reported in patients who were treated over several months. Two incidences of cardiac arrest were also recorded among these patients although a relationship to Alkeran administration was not demonstrated.

Maculopapular rashes and pruritus have occasionally been noted

There have also been case reports of haemolytic anaemia occurring after melphalan treatment.

Alopecia has been reported but is uncommon.

Hepatic Disorders ranging from Abnormal liver function tests to clinical manifestations such as hepatitis and jaundice have been reported.

There have been case reports of interstitial pneumonitis and pulmonary fibrosis: fatal reports of pulmonary fibrosis have been received.

Temporary significant elevation of blood urea has been seen in the early stages of melphalan therapy in myeloma patients with renal damage

4.9 Overdose

Symptoms and signs:

Gastro-intestinal effects, including nausea, vomiting and diarrhoea are the most likely signs of acute oral overdosage. Diarrhoea, sometimes haemorrhagic, has been reported after intravenous overdosage. The principal toxic effect is bone marrow aplasia, leading to neutropenia and thrombocytopenia.

Treatment:

There is no specific antidote. The blood picture should be closely monitored for at least four weeks following overdosage until there is evidence of recovery.

General supportive measures, together with appropriate blood transfusion, should be instituted if necessary.

5. PHARMACOLOGICAL PROPERTIES

5.1 Pharmacodynamic properties

Melphalan is a bifunctional alkylating agent. Formation of carbonium intermediates from each of the two bis-2-chlorethyl groups enables alkylation through covalent binding with the 7-nitrogen of guanine on DNA, cross-linking two DNA strands and thereby preventing cell replication.

5.2 Pharmacokinetic properties

The absorption of melphalan was found to be highly variable in 13 patients given 0.6mg/kg orally, with respect to both the time to first appearance of the drug in plasma (range 0 to 336 minutes) and peak plasma concentration (range 70 to 630 ng/ml). In 5 of the patients who were given an equivalent intravenous dose, the mean absolute bioavailability of melphalan was found to be 56 $\pm$ 27%. The plasma mean terminal elimination half-life was 90 $\pm$ 57 minutes with 11% of the drug being recovered in the urine over 24 hours.

In a study of 18 patients administered melphalan 0.2 to 0.25 mg/kg bodyweight orally, a maximum plasma concentration (range 87 to 350 ng/ml) was reached within 0.5 to 2.0 hours. The mean elimination half-life was 1.12 $\pm$ 0.15 hours.

The administration of Alkeran tablets immediately after food delayed the time to achieving peak plasma concentrations and reduced the area under the plasma concentration-time curves by between 39 and 45%.

5.3 Preclinical safety data

There are no preclinical data of relevance to the prescriber, which are additional to that in other sections of the SmPC.

6. PHARMACEUTICAL PARTICULARS

6.1 List of excipients

Tablet Core:

Microcrystalline cellulose

Crospovidone

Colloidal anhydrous silica

Magnesium stearate

Tablet Film Coating:

Hypromellose

Titanium dioxide

Macrogol

6.2 Incompatibilities

None known

6.3 Shelf life

24 months

6.4 Special precautions for storage

Store at 2°C to 8°C.

6.5 Nature and contents of container

Supplied in amber glass bottles with a child resistant closure containing 25 or 50 tablets.

6.6 Instructions for use and handling

Safe handling of ALKERAN tablets:

The handling of Alkeran tablets should follow guidelines for the handling of cytotoxic drugs according to prevailing local recommendations and/or regulations (for example Royal Pharmaceutical Society of Great Britain Working Party on the Handling of Cytotoxic Drugs).

Provided the outer coating of the tablet is intact, there is no risk in handling Alkeran tablets.

Alkeran tablets should not be divided.

Disposal:

Alkeran tablets should be destroyed in accordance with relevant local regulatory requirements concerning the disposal of cytotoxic drugs.

Administrative Data

7. MARKETING AUTHORISATION HOLDER

The Wellcome Foundation Limited

Glaxo Wellcome House

Berkeley Avenue

Greenford

Middlesex, UB6 ONN

Trading as

GlaxoSmithKline UK

Stockley Park West

Uxbridge

Middlesex, UB11 1BT

8. MARKETING AUTHORISATION NUMBER(S)

PL 00003/5008R

9. DATE OF FIRST AUTHORISATION/RENEWAL OF THE AUTHORISATION

11 November 2002

10. DATE OF REVISION OF THE TEXT

25 February 2005

11. Legal Status

POM

ALLEGRON

(King Pharmaceuticals Ltd)

1. NAME OF THE MEDICINAL PRODUCT

ALLEGRON TABLETS

2. QUALITATIVE AND QUANTITATIVE COMPOSITION

Tablets containing Nortriptyline Hydrochloride EP equivalent to 10mg nortriptyline base tablets are white, unscored and have a diameter of 5.5mm. Marked 'KING'.

Tablets containing Nortriptyline Hydrochloride EP equivalent to 25mg nortriptyline base tablets are orange, scored and have a diameter of 8mm. Marked 'KING'.

3. PHARMACEUTICAL FORM

Tablet

4. CLINICAL PARTICULARS

4.1 Therapeutic indications

Allegron is indicated for the relief of symptoms of depression. It may also be used for the treatment of some cases of nocturnal enuresis.

4.2 Posology and method of administration

For oral administration.

Adults: The usual adult dose is 25mg three or four times daily. Dosage should begin at a low level and be increased as required. Alternatively, the total daily dose may be given once a day. When doses above 100mg daily are administered, plasma levels of nortriptyline should be monitored and maintained in the optimum range of 50 to 150ng/ml. Doses above 150mg per day are not recommended.

Lower than usual dosages are recommended for elderly patients and adolescents. Lower dosages are also recommended for outpatients than for hospitalised patients who will be under close supervision. The physician should initiate dosage at a low level and increase it gradually, noting carefully the clinical response and any evidence of intolerance. Following remission, maintenance medication may be required for a longer period of time at the lowest dose that will maintain remission.

If a patient develops minor side-effects, the dosage should be reduced. The drug should be discontinued promptly if adverse effects of a serious nature or allergic manifestations occur.

The elderly: 30 to 50mg/day in divided doses.

Adolescent patients: 30 to 50mg/day in divided doses.

Plasma levels: Optimal responses to nortriptyline have been associated with plasma concentrations of 50 to 150ng/ml. Higher concentrations may be associated with more adverse experiences. Plasma concentrations are difficult to measure, and physicians should consult the laboratory professional staff.

Many antidepressants (tricyclic antidepressants, including nortriptyline, selective serotonin re-uptake inhibitors and others) are metabolised by the hepatic cytochrome P450 isoenzyme P450IID6. Three to ten per cent of the population have reduced isoenzyme activity ('poor metabolisers') and may have higher than expected plasma concentrations at usual doses. The percentage of 'poor metabolisers' in a population is also affected by its ethnic origin.

Older patients have been reported to have higher plasma concentrations of the active nortriptyline metabolite 10-hydroxynortriptyline. In one case, this was associated with apparent cardiotoxicity, despite the fact that nortriptyline concentrations were within the 'therapeutic range'. Clinical findings should predominate over plasma concentrations as primary determinants of dosage changes.

Children: (for nocturnal enuresis only).

Age (years)	Weight kg	lb	Dose (mg)
6-7	20-25	44-55	10
8-11	25-35	55-77	10-20
>11	35-54	77-119	25-35

The dose should be administered thirty minutes before bedtime.

The maximum period of treatment should not exceed three months. A further course of treatment should not be started until a full physical examination, including an ECG, has been made.

4.3 Contraindications

Hypersensitivity to nortriptyline.

Recent myocardial infarction, any degree of heart block or other cardiac arrhythmias.

Severe liver disease.

Mania.

Nortriptyline is contra-indicated for the nursing mother and for children under the age of six years.

Please also refer to 'Drug interactions' section.

4.4 Special warnings and special precautions for use

Warnings: As improvement may not occur during the initial weeks of therapy, patients, especially those posing a high suicidal risk, should be closely monitored during this period.

Withdrawal symptoms, including insomnia, irritability and excessive perspiration, may occur on abrupt cessation of therapy.

The use of nortriptyline in schizophrenic patients may result in an exacerbation of the psychosis or may activate latent schizophrenic symptoms. If administered to overactive or agitated patients, increased anxiety and agitation may occur. In manic-depressive patients, nortriptyline may cause symptoms of the manic phase to emerge.

Cross sensitivity between nortriptyline and other tricyclic antidepressants is a possibility.

Patients with cardiovascular disease should be given nortriptyline only under close supervision because of the tendency of the drug to produce sinus tachycardia and to prolong the conduction time. Myocardial infarction, arrhythmia and strokes have occurred. Great care is necessary if nortriptyline is administered to hyperthyroid patients or to those receiving thyroid medication, since cardiac arrhythmias may develop.

The use of nortriptyline should be avoided, if possible, in patients with a history of epilepsy. If it is used, however, the patients should be observed carefully at the beginning of treatment, for nortriptyline is known to lower the convulsive threshold.

The elderly are particularly liable to experience adverse reactions, especially agitation, confusion and postural hypotension.

Troublesome hostility in a patient may be aroused by the use of nortriptyline.

Behavioural changes may occur in children receiving therapy for nocturnal enuresis.

If possible, the use of nortriptyline should be avoided in patients with narrow angle glaucoma or symptoms suggestive of prostatic hypertrophy.

The possibility of a suicide attempt by a depressed patient remains after the initiation of treatment. This possibility should be considered in relation to the quantity of drug dispensed at any one time.

When it is essential, nortriptyline may be administered with electroconvulsive therapy, although the hazards may be increased.

Both elevation and lowering of blood sugar levels have been reported. Significant hypoglycaemia was reported in a Type II diabetic patient maintained on chlorpropamide (250mg/day), after the addition of nortriptyline (125mg/day).

4.5 Interaction with other medicinal products and other forms of Interaction

Drug interactions: Under no circumstances should nortriptyline be given concurrently with, or within two weeks of cessation of, therapy with monoamine oxidase inhibitors. Hyperpyretic crises, severe convulsions and fatalities have occurred when similar tricyclic antidepressants were used in such combinations.

Nortriptyline should not be given with sympathomimetic agents such as adrenaline, ephedrine, isoprenaline, noradrenaline, phenylephrine and phenylpropanolamine.

Nortriptyline may decrease the antihypertensive effect of guanethidine, debrisoquine, bethanidine and possibly clonidine. Concurrent administration of reserpine has been shown to produce a 'stimulating' effect in some depressed patients. It would be advisable to review all antihypertensive therapy during treatment with tricyclic antidepressants.

Barbiturates may increase the rate of metabolism of nortriptyline.

Anaesthetics given during tricyclic antidepressant therapy may increase the risk of arrhythmias and hypotension. If surgery is necessary, the drug should be discontinued, if possible, for several days prior to the procedure, or the anaesthetist should be informed if the patient is still receiving therapy.

Tricyclic antidepressants may potentiate the CNS depressant effect of alcohol.

The potentiating effect of excessive consumption of alcohol may lead to increased suicidal attempts or overdosage, especially in patients with histories of emotional disturbances or suicidal ideation.

Steady-state serum concentrations of the tricyclic antidepressants are reported to fluctuate significantly as cimetidine is either added to or deleted from the drug regimen. Higher than expected steady-state serum concentrations of the tricyclic antidepressant have been observed when therapy is initiated in patients already taking cimetidine. A decrease may occur when cimetidine therapy is discontinued.

Because nortriptyline's metabolism (like other tricyclic and SSRI antidepressants) involves the hepatic cytochrome P450IID6 isoenzyme system, concomitant therapy with drugs also metabolised by this system may lead to drug interactions. Lower doses than are usually prescribed for either the tricyclic antidepressant or the other drug may therefore be required.

Greater than two-fold increases in previously stable plasma levels of nortriptyline have occurred when fluoxetine was administered concomitantly. Fluoxetine and its active metabolite, norfluoxetine, have long half-lives (4-16 days for norfluoxetine).

Concomitant therapy with other drugs that are metabolised by this isoenzyme, including other antidepressants, phenothiazines, carbamazepine, propafenone, flecainide and encainide, or that inhibit this enzyme (eg, quinidine), should be approached with caution.

Supervision and adjustment of dosage may be required when nortriptyline is used with other anticholinergic drugs.

4.6 Pregnancy and lactation

Usage in pregnancy: The safety of nortriptyline for use during pregnancy has not been established, nor is there evidence from animal studies that it is free from hazard; therefore the drug should not be administered to pregnant patients or women of childbearing age unless the potential benefits clearly outweigh any potential risk.

Usage in nursing mothers: See 'Contra-indications'.

4.7 Effects on ability to drive and use machines

Nortriptyline may impair the mental and/or physical abilities required for the performance of hazardous tasks, such as operating machinery or driving a car; therefore the patient should be warned accordingly.

4.8 Undesirable effects

Included in the following list are a few adverse reactions that have not been reported with this specific drug. However, the pharmacological similarities among the tricyclic antidepressant drugs require that each of the reactions be considered when nortriptyline is administered.

Cardiovascular: Hypotension, hypertension, tachycardia, palpitation, myocardial infarction, arrhythmias, heart block, stroke.

Psychiatric: Confusional states (especially in the elderly) with hallucinations, disorientation, delusions; anxiety, restlessness, agitation; insomnia, panic, nightmares; hypomania; exacerbation of psychosis.

Neurological: Numbness, tingling, paraesthesia of extremities; inco-ordination, ataxia, tremors; peripheral neuropathy; extrapyramidal symptoms; seizures, alteration of EEG patterns; tinnitus.

Anticholinergic: Dry mouth and, rarely, associated sublingual adenitis or gingivitis; blurred vision, disturbance of accommodation, mydriasis; constipation, paralytic ileus; urinary retention, delayed micturition, dilation of the urinary tract.

Allergic: Rash, petechiae, urticaria, itching, photosensitisation (avoid excessive exposure to sunlight); oedema (general or of face and tongue), drug fever, cross-sensitivity with other tricyclic drugs.

Haematological: Bone-marrow depression, including agranulocytosis; aplastic anaemia; eosinophilia; purpura; thrombocytopenia.

Gastro-intestinal: Nausea and vomiting, anorexia, epigastric distress, diarrhoea; peculiar taste, stomatitis, abdominal cramps, black tongue, constipation, paralytic ileus.

Endocrine: Gynaecomastia in the male; breast enlargement and galactorrhoea in the female; increased or decreased libido, impotence; testicular swelling; elevation or depression of blood sugar levels; syndrome of inappropriate secretion of antidiuretic hormone.

Other: Jaundice (simulating obstructive); altered liver function, hepatitis and liver necrosis; weight gain or loss; sweating; flushing; urinary frequency, nocturia; drowsiness, dizziness, weakness, fatigue; headache; parotid swelling; alopecia.

Withdrawal symptoms: Though these are not indicative of addiction, abrupt cessation of treatment after prolonged therapy may produce nausea, headache and malaise.

4.9 Overdose

Signs and symptoms: 50mg of a tricyclic antidepressant can be an overdose in a child. Of patients who are alive at presentation, mortality of 0-15% has been reported. Symptoms may begin within several hours and may include blurred vision, confusion, restlessness, dizziness, hypothermia, hyperthermia, agitation, vomiting, hyperactive reflexes, dilated pupils, fever, rapid heart rate, decreased bowel sounds, dry mouth, inability to void, myoclonic jerks, seizures, respiratory depression, myoglobinuric renal failure, nystagmus, ataxia, dysarthria, choreoathetosis, coma, hypotension and cardiac arrhythmias. Cardiac conduction may be slowed, with prolongation of QRS complex and QT intervals, right bundle branch and AV block, ventricular tachyarrhythmias (including Torsade de pointes and fibrillation) and death. Prolongation of QRS duration to more than 100msec is predictive of more severe toxicity. The absence of sinus tachycardia does not ensure a benign course. Hypotension may be caused by vasodilatation, central and peripheral alpha-adrenergic blockade and cardiac depression. In a healthy young person, prolonged resuscitation may be effective; one patient survived 5 hours of cardiac massage.

Treatment: Symptomatic and supportive therapy is recommended. Activated charcoal may be more effective than emesis or lavage to reduce absorption.

Ventricular arrhythmias, especially when accompanied by lengthened QRS intervals, may respond to alkalinisation by hyperventilation or administration of sodium bicarbonate. Serum electrolytes should be monitored and managed. Refractory arrhythmias may respond to propranolol, bretylium or lignocaine. Quinidine and procainamide usually should not be used because they may exacerbate arrhythmias and conduction already slowed by the overdose.

Seizures may respond to diazepam. Phenytoin may treat seizures and cardiac rhythm disturbances. Physostigmine may antagonise atrial tachycardia, gut immotility, myoclonic jerks and somnolence. The effects of physostigmine may be short-lived.

Diuresis and dialysis have little effect. Haemoperfusion is unproven. Monitoring should continue, at least until the QRS duration is normal.

5. PHARMACOLOGICAL PROPERTIES

5.1 Pharmacodynamic properties

Nortriptyline is a tricyclic antidepressant with actions and uses similar to these of Amitriplyline. It is the principal active metabolite of Amitriplyline.

In the treatment of depression Nortriptyline is given by mouth as the hydrochloride in doses equivalent to Nortriptyline 10mg 3 or 4 times daily initially, gradually increased to 25mg 4 times daily as necessary. A suggested initial dose for adolescents and the elderly is 10mg thrice daily. Inappropriately high plasma concentrations of Nortriptyline have been associated with deterioration in antidepressant response. Since Nortriptyline has prolonged half-life, once daily dosage regimens are also suitable, usually given at night.

5.2 Pharmacokinetic properties

Parts of metabolism of Nortriptyline include hydroxylation (possibly to active metabolites). N-oxidation and conjugation with glucuronic acid. Nortriptyline is widely distributed throughout the body and is extensively bound to plasma and tissue protein. Plasma concentrations of Nortriptyline vary very widely between individuals and no simple correlation with therapeutic response has been established.

5.3 Preclinical safety data

There are no preclinical data of relevance to the prescriber

6. PHARMACEUTICAL PARTICULARS

6.1 List of excipients

10 mg Tablets:

Maize Starch, Magnesium Stearate, Lactose Monohydrate, Calcium Phosphate, Purified Water. **Coat**: Glycerol, Methylhydroxpropyl Cellulose

25 mg Tablets:

Maize Starch, Magnesium Stearate, Lactose Monohydrate, Calcium Phosphate, Sunset Yellow, Purified Water. **Coat**: Glycerol, Methylhydroxpropyl Cellulose, Ethylcellulose, Methyl Alcohol, Isopropyl Alcohol, Methylene Chloride.

6.2 Incompatibilities

None Stated

6.3 Shelf life

36 months

6.4 Special precautions for storage

No special requirements

6.5 Nature and contents of container

High density polyethylene bottles containing 100 and 500 tablets

UPVC blister strips with aluminium foil backing containing 25 tablets

6.6 Instructions for use and handling

Not applicable

7. MARKETING AUTHORISATION HOLDER

King Pharmaceuticals Ltd

Donegal Street

Ballybofey

County Donegal

8. MARKETING AUTHORISATION NUMBER(S)

10mg 14385/0001; 25mg 14385/0002

9. DATE OF FIRST AUTHORISATION/RENEWAL OF THE AUTHORISATION

30th March 1998

10. DATE OF REVISION OF THE TEXT

March 2003

11. Legal Classification

POM

Almogran 12.5mg Tablets

(Organon Laboratories Limited)

1. NAME OF THE MEDICINAL PRODUCT

Almogran 12.5 mg Filmcoated tablet

2. QUALITATIVE AND QUANTITATIVE COMPOSITION

Each tablet contains almotriptan 12.5 mg as almotriptan D,L-hydrogen malate.

For excipients, see 6.1.

3. PHARMACEUTICAL FORM

Film-coated tablet.

White, circular, biconvex film-coated tablet with a blue A printed on one side.

4. CLINICAL PARTICULARS

4.1 Therapeutic indications

Acute treatment of the headache phase of migraine attacks with or without aura.

4.2 Posology and method of administration

Almogran should be taken with liquids after the onset of migraine-associated headache.

Almotriptan should not be used for migraine prophylaxis.

The tablets can be taken with or without food.

Adults (18-65 years of age)

The recommended dose is one tablet containing 12.5 mg of almotriptan. A second dose may be taken if the symptoms reappear within 24 hours. This second dose may be taken provided that there is a minimum interval of two hours between the two doses.

The efficacy of a second dose for the treatment of the same attack when an initial dose is ineffective has not been examined in controlled trials. Therefore if a patient does not respond to the first dose, a second dose should not be taken for the same attack.

The maximum recommended dose is two doses in 24 hours.

Children and adolescents (under 18 years of age)

There are no data concerning the use of almotriptan in children and adolescents, therefore its use in this age group is not recommended.

Elderly (over 65 years of age)

No dosage adjustment is required in the elderly. The safety and effectiveness of almotriptan in patients older than 65 years has not been systematically evaluated.

Renal Impairment

Dosage adjustment is not required in patients with mildor moderate renal impairment. Patients with severe renal impairment should take no more than one 12.5 mg tablet in a 24 hour period.

Hepatic Impairment

There are no data concerning the use of almotriptan in patients with hepatic impairment (see Section 4.3 Contra-indications and 4.4 Special warning and precautions for use).

4.3 Contraindications

Hypersensitivity to the active substance or to any of the excipients.

As with other 5-$HT_{1B/1D}$ receptor agonists, almotriptan should not be used in patients with a history, symptoms or signs of ischaemic heart disease (myocardial infarction, angina pectoris, documented silent ischaemia, Prinzmetal's angina) or severe hypertension and uncontrolled mild or moderate hypertension.

Patients with a previous cerebrovascular accident (CVA) or transient ischaemic attack (TIA). Peripheral vascular disease.

Concomitant administration with ergotamine, ergotamine derivatives (including methysergide) and other 5-$HT_{1B/1D}$ agonists is contraindicated.

Patients with severe hepatic impairment (see Section 4.2. Posology and method of administration).

4.4 Special warnings and special precautions for use

Almotriptan should only be used where there is a clear diagnosis of migraine. It should not be used to treat basilar, hemiplegic or ophthalmoplegic migraine.

As with other acute migraine therapies, before treating headaches in patients not previously diagnosed as migraine sufferers and in migraine sufferers who present atypical symptoms, care should be taken to exclude other potentially serious neurological conditions.

In very rare cases, as with other 5-$HT_{1B/1D}$ receptor agonists, coronary vasospasm and myocardial infarction have been reported. Therefore almotriptan should not be administered to patients who could have an undiagnosed coronary condition without prior evaluation of potential underlying cardiovascular disease. Such patients include postmenopausal women, males over 40 and patients with other risk factors for coronary disease such as uncontrolled hypertension, hypercholesterolaemia, obesity, diabetes, smoking or a clear family history of cardiovascular disease. These evaluations however, may not identify every patient who has cardiac disease and in very rare case, serious cardiac events have occurred in patients without underlying cardiovascular disease when 5-HT_1 agonists have been administered.

Following administration, almotriptan can be associated with transient symptoms including chest pain and tightness which may be intense and involve the throat (see Section 4.8 Undesirable effects). Where such symptoms are thought to indicate ischaemic heart disease, no further dose should be taken and appropriate evaluation should be carried out.

Caution should be exercised when prescribing almotriptan to patients with known hypersensitivity to sulphonamides.

It is advised to wait at least 6 hours following use of almotriptan before administering ergotamine. At least 24 hours should elapse after the administration of an ergotamine-containing preparation before almotriptan is given. Although additive vasospastic effects were not observed in a clinical trial in which 12 healthy subjects received oral almotriptan and ergotamine, such additive effects are theoretically possible (see Section 4.3 Contraindications).

Patients with severe renal impairment should not take more than one 12.5 mg tablet in a 24 hour period.

Caution is recommended in patients with mild to moderate hepatic disease and treatment is contraindicated in patients with severe hepatic disease (see section 5.2 Pharmacokinetic properties)

Undesirable effects may be more common during concomitant use of triptans and herbal preparations containing St John's Wort (Hypericum perforatum).

As with other 5-$HT_{1B/1D}$ receptor agonists, almotriptan may cause mild, transient increases in blood pressure, which may be more pronounced in the elderly.

Excessive use of an anti-migraine medicinal product can lead to daily chronic headache requiring a dosage adjustment.

The maximum recommended dose of almotriptan should not be exceeded.

4.5 Interaction with other medicinal products and other forms of Interaction

Interaction studies were performed with monoamine oxidase A inhibitors, beta-blockers, selective serotonin reuptake inhibitors, ergot derivatives, calcium channel blockers or inhibitors of Cytochrome P450 isoenzymes 3A4 and 2D6. The results of these studies are detailed below in this section. There are no in vivo interaction studies assessing the effect of almotriptan on other drugs.

Concomitant use of almotriptan and ergotamine did not cause pharmacokinetic differences in the rate and extent of absorption of almotriptan. Only a small decrease of C_{max} and non-relevant delay of T_{max} by one hour were observed (see Section 4.3 Contraindications and 4.4 Special warning and precautions for use).

Multiple dosing with moclobemide, a reversible MAO-A inhibitor, resulted in a 37% increase in AUC of almotriptan, without any clinically relevant changes in C_{max} or half-life. The increase in AUC is not considered clinically relevant. No clinically significant interactions were observed.

Multiple dosing with the selective serotonin re-uptake inhibitor fluoxetine, an inhibitor of CYP2D6 and CYP3A4, resulted in a small increase in AUC (<10%) and a 20% increase in C_{max} of almotriptan. These changes are without clinical relevance. No clinically significant interactions were observed.

Multiple dosing with the calcium channel blocker verapamil, a substrate of CYP3A4, resulted in a 20% increase in C_{max} and AUC of almotriptan. The increase is not considered clinically relevant. No clinically significant interactions were observed.

Multiple dosing with propranolol did not alter the pharmacokinetics of almotriptan. No clinically significant interactions were observed.

In vitro studies performed to evaluate the ability of almotriptan to inhibit the major CYP enzymes in human liver microsomes and human monoamine oxidase (MAO) showed that almotriptan would not be expected to alter the metabolism of drugs metabolised by CYP or MAO-A and MAO-B enzymes.

4.6 Pregnancy and lactation

Pregnancy

The safety of almotriptan for use in human pregnancy has not been established.

Studies in animals have shown that almotriptan has no harmful effects on gestation, parturition or postnatal development, and no birth defects associated with the drug have been observed in rats or rabbits.

Because animal reproduction studies are not always predictive of human response, administration of almotriptan should only be considered if the expected benefit to the mother outweighs any possible risk to the foetus.

Lactation

There are no data regarding excretion of almotriptan in human milk. Studies in rats have shown that almotriptan and/or its metabolites are excreted in milk.

Caution should therefore be exercised when prescribing during lactation. Infant exposure may be minimised by avoiding breast feeding for 24 hours after treatment.

4.7 Effects on ability to drive and use machines

There are no studies on the effect of almotriptan on the ability to drive or operate machinery. However, since somnolence may occur during a migraine attack and has been reported as a side effect of treatment with almotriptan, caution is recommended in patients performing skilled tasks.

4.8 Undesirable effects

Almogran was evaluated in over 2700 patients for up to one year in clinical trials. The most common adverse reactions at the therapeutic dose were dizziness, somnolence, nausea, vomiting and fatigue. None of the adverse reactions had an incidence superior to 1.5%.

In the following classification additional adverse reactions in patients taking one or two doses of Almogran 12.5 mg within 24 hours during acute or long term clinical trials (irrespective of the incidence for placebo) are listed by System Organ Class (SOC) and in descending order of frequency:

Nervous system disorders:	Common (>1/100, <1/10):	dizziness, somnolence.
	Uncommon (>1/1,000, <1/100):	paraesthesia, headache.
Ear and labyrinth disorders:	Uncommon (>1/1,000, <1/100):	tinnitus.
Cardiac disorders:	Uncommon (>1/1,000, <1/100):	palpitations.
	Very rare (<1/10,000):	coronary vasospasm, myocardial infarction, and tachycardia.
Respiratory, thoracic and mediastinal disorders:	Uncommon (>1/1,000, <1/100):	throat tightness.
Gastrointestinal Disorders:	Common (>1/100, <1/10):	nausea, vomiting.
	Uncommon (>1/1,000, <1/100):	diarrhoea, dyspepsia, dry mouth.
Musculoskeletal, connective tissue and bone disorders:	Uncommon (>1/1,000, <1/100):	myalgia, bone pain.
General Disorders:	Common (>1/100, <1/10):	fatigue.
	Uncommon (>1/1,000, <1/100):	chest pain, asthenia.

4.9 Overdose

There are no reports of overdose.

The most frequently reported adverse event in patients receiving 150 mg (the highest dose administered to patients) was somnolence.

Overdose should be treated symptomatically and vital functions should be maintained. Since the elimination half-life is around 3.5 hours monitoring should continue for at least 12 hours or while symptoms or signs persist.

5. PHARMACOLOGICAL PROPERTIES

5.1 Pharmacodynamic properties

Pharmacotherapeutic group: Antimigraine. Selective 5-HT_1 receptor agonist.

ATC code: N02C C.

Mechanism of action

Almotriptan is a selective 5-HT_{1B} and 5-HT_{1D} receptor agonist. These receptors mediate vasoconstriction of certain cranial vessels, as demonstrated in studies using isolated human tissue preparations. Almotriptan also interacts with the trigeminovascular system, inhibiting extravasation of plasma proteins from dural vessels following trigeminal ganglionic stimulation, which is a feature of neuronic inflammation thatseems to be involved in the physiopathology of migraine. Almotriptan has no significant activity on other 5-HT receptor subtypes and no significant affinity for adrenergic, adenosine, angiotensin, dopamine, endothelin or tachykinin binding sites.

Pharmacodynamic effects

The efficacy of almotriptan in the acute treatment of migraine attacks was established in four multicentre, placebo-controlled clinical trials including more than 700 patients who were administered 12.5 mg. The decrease in pain began 30 minutes after administration, and the percentage of response (reduction of headache from moderate-severe to mild or absent) after 2 hours was 57-70% with almotriptan and 32-42% after placebo. In addition, almotriptan relieved nausea, photophobia and phonophobia associated with migraine attacks.

5.2 Pharmacokinetic properties

Almotriptan is well absorbed, with an oral bioavailability of about 70%. Maximum plasma concentrations (C_{max}) occur approximately between 1.5 and 3.0 hours after administration. The rate and extent of absorption is unaffected by concomitant ingestion of food. In healthy subjects administered single oral doses ranging from 5 mg to 200 mg, C_{max} and AUC were proportional to dose, indicating linear pharmacokinetic behaviour. The elimination half-life ($t_{1/2}$) is about 3.5 h in healthy subjects. There is no evidence of any gender-related effect on the pharmacokinetics of almotriptan.

More than 75% of the dose administered is eliminated in urine, and the remainder in faeces. Approximately, the 50% of the urinary and faecal excretion is unchanged almotriptan. The major biotransformation route is via monoamine oxidase (MAO-A) mediated oxidative deamination to the indole acetic metabolite. Cytochrome P450 (3A4 and 2D6 isozymes) and flavin mono-oxygenase are other enzymes involved in the metabolism of almotriptan. None of the metabolites is significantly active pharmacologically.

After an intravenous dose of almotriptan administered to healthy volunteers the average values for the distribution volume, total clearance and elimination half-life were 195 L, 40 L/h and 3.4 h respectively. Renal clearance (CL_R) accounted for about two-thirds of total clearance and renal tubular secretion is probably also involved. The CL_R correlates well with renal function in patients with mild (creatinine clearance: 60-90 ml/min), moderate (creatinine clearance: 30-59 ml/min) and severe (creatinine clearance: < 30 ml/min) renal impairment. The increase of the mean $t_{1/2}$ (up to 7 hours) is statistically and clinically significant in the case of patients with severe renal impairment only. Compared with healthy subjects, the increase in the maximum plasma concentration (C_{max}) of almotriptan was 9%, 84% and 72% respectively for patients with slight, moderate and severe renal impairment, whereas the increase in exposure (AUC) was 23%, 80% and 195% respectively. According to these results, the reduction of the total clearance of almotriptan was -20%, -40% and -65% respectively for patients with slight, moderate and severe renal impairment.As expected, total (CL) and renal (CL_R) clearances were reduced but without clinical relevance in healthy elderly volunteers compared with a young control group.

Based on the mechanisms of almotriptan clearance in man, approximately 45% of almotriptan elimination appears to be due to hepatic metabolism. Therefore, even if these clearance mechanisms were totally blocked or impaired, plasma almotriptan levels would be increased a maximum of two-fold over the control state, assuming that renal function (and almotriptan renal clearance) are not altered by hepatic impairment. In patients with severe renal impairment, C_{max} is increased twofold, and AUC is increased approximately threefold relative to healthy volunteers. Maximal changes in pharmacokinetic parameters in patients with significant hepatic impairment would not exceed these ranges. For this reason, no study of the pharmacokinetics of almotriptan in patients with hepatic impairment was performed.

5.3 Preclinical safety data

In safety pharmacology, repeated dose toxicity and reproduction toxicity studies, adverse effects were observed only at exposures well above the maximum human exposure.

Almotriptan did not show any mutagenic activity in a standard battery of *in vitro* and *in vivo* genotoxicity studies, and no carcinogenic potential was revealed in studies conducted in mice and rats.

As occurs with other 5-$HT_{1B/1D}$ receptor agonists, almotriptan binds to melanin. However, no ocular adverse effects associated with the drug have been observed in dogs after treatment for up to one year.

6. PHARMACEUTICAL PARTICULARS

6.1 List of excipients

Tablet core:	**Coating material:**	**Printing ink:**
Mannitol	Hypromellose	Hypromellose
Microcrystalline cellulose	Titanium dioxide (E-171)	Propylene glycol
Povidone	Macrogol 400	Indigo carmine (E-132)
Sodium starch glycolate	Carnauba wax	
Sodium stearyl fumarate		

6.2 Incompatibilities
Not applicable.

6.3 Shelf life
3 years

6.4 Special precautions for storage
This medicinal product does not require any special storage conditions.

6.5 Nature and contents of container
Boxes containing aluminium foil blisters with 2, 3, 4, 6, 7, 9, 12, 14 or 18 tablets.

Not all pack sizes may be marketed.

6.6 Instructions for use and handling
No special requirements.

Administrative Data

7. MARKETING AUTHORISATION HOLDER
ALMIRALL PRODESFARMA, S.A.

General Mitre 151,

08022 BARCELONA- Spain.

8. MARKETING AUTHORISATION NUMBER(S)
PL 16973/0005

9. DATE OF FIRST AUTHORISATION/RENEWAL OF THE AUTHORISATION
Date of first authorisation: 26 October 2000

Date of last renewal: December 2004

10. DATE OF REVISION OF THE TEXT
March 2005

11. Legal category
POM

Distributed in the UK by:

Organon Laboratories Ltd,
Science Park, Cambridge CB4 0FL Tel: 01223 432700

Aloxi 250micrograms solution for injection

(Cambridge Laboratories)

1. NAME OF THE MEDICINAL PRODUCT
Aloxi▼ 250 micrograms solution for injection.

2. QUALITATIVE AND QUANTITATIVE COMPOSITION
One ml of solution contains 50 micrograms palonosetron (as hydrochloride).

Each vial of 5 ml of solution contains 250 micrograms palonosetron (as hydrochloride).

For excipients, see section 6.1.

3. PHARMACEUTICAL FORM
Solution for injection.

Clear, colourless solution.

4. CLINICAL PARTICULARS

4.1 Therapeutic indications
Aloxi is indicated for: the prevention of acute nausea and vomiting associated with highly emetogenic cancer chemotherapy and the prevention of nausea and vomiting associated with moderately emetogenic cancer chemotherapy

4.2 Posology and method of administration
For intravenous use.

Adults:

250 micrograms palonosetron administered as a single intravenous bolus approximately 30 minutes before the start of chemotherapy. Aloxi should be injected over 30 seconds.

Repeated dosing of Aloxi within a seven day interval is not recommended.

The efficacy of Aloxi in the prevention of nausea and vomiting induced by highly emetogenic chemotherapy may be enhanced by the addition of a corticosteroid administered prior to chemotherapy.

Elderly:

No dosage adjustment is necessary for the elderly.

Children and adolescents:

Use in patients under 18 years of age is not recommended until further data becomes available.

Hepatic impaired patients

No dose adjustment is necessary for patients with impaired hepatic function.

Renal impaired patients

No dose adjustment is necessary for patients with impaired renal function.

No data are available for patients with end stage renal disease undergoing haemodialysis.

4.3 Contraindications
Hypersensitivity to the active substance or to any of the excipients.

4.4 Special warnings and special precautions for use
As palonosetron may increase large bowel transit time, patients with a history of constipation or signs of subacute intestinal obstruction should be monitored following administration. Two cases of constipation with faecal impaction requiring hospitalisation have been reported in association with palonosetron 750 micrograms.

At all dose levels tested, palonosetron did not induce clinically relevant prolongation of the QT interval. However, as for other 5-HT3 antagonists, caution should be exercised in the concomitant use of palonosetron with medicinal products that increase the QT interval or in patients who have or are likely to develop prolongation of the QT interval.

4.5 Interaction with other medicinal products and other forms of Interaction
Palonosetron is mainly metabolised by CYP2D6, with minor contribution by CYP3A4 and CYP1A2 isoenzymes. Based on in vitro studies, palonosetron does not inhibit or induce cytochrome P450 isoenzyme at clinically relevant concentrations.

Chemotherapeutic agents:

In preclinical studies, palonosetron did not inhibit the antitumour activity of the five chemotherapeutic agents tested (cisplatin, cyclophosphamide, cytarabine, doxorubicin and mitomycin C).

Metoclopramide:

In a clinical study, no significant pharmacokinetic interaction was shown between a single intravenous dose of palonosetron and steady state concentration of oral metoclopramide, which is a CYP2D6 inhibitor.

CYP2D6 inducers and inhibitors:

In a population pharmacokinetic analysis, it has been shown that there was no significant effect on palonosetron clearance when co-administered with CYP2D6 inducers (dexamethasone and rifampicin) and inhibitors (including amiodarone, celecoxib, chlorpromazine, cimetidine, doxorubicin, fluoxetine, haloperidol, paroxetine, quinidine, ranitidine, ritonavir, sertraline or terbinafine).

Corticosteroids:

Palonosetron has been administered safely with corticosteroids.

Other medicinal products:

Palonosetron has been administered safely with analgesics, antiemetic/antinauseants, antispasmodics and anticholinergic medicinal products.

4.6 Pregnancy and lactation
Animal studies do not indicate direct or indirect harmful effects with respect to pregnancy, embryonal/foetal development, parturition or postnatal development. Only limited data from animal studies are available regarding the placental transfer (see section 5.3).

There is no experience of palonosetron in human pregnancy so palonosetron should not be used in pregnant women unless it is considered essential by the physician. As there are no data concerning palonosetron excretion in breast milk, breast-feeding should be discontinued during therapy.

4.7 Effects on ability to drive and use machines
No studies on the effects on the ability to drive and use machines have been performed.

Since palonosetron may induce dizziness, somnolence or fatigue, patients should be cautioned when driving or operating machines.

4.8 Undesirable effects
In clinical studies at a dose of 250 micrograms (total 633 patients) the most frequently observed adverse reactions, at least possibly related to Aloxi, were headache (9%) and constipation (5%).

In the clinical studies the following adverse reactions (ARs) were observed as possibly or probably related to Aloxi. These were classified as common (between 1% and 10%) or uncommon (between 0.1% and 1%).

(see table 1 below)

Very rare cases (<1/10,000) of hypersensitivity reactions and injection site reactions (burning, induration, discomfort and pain) were reported from post-marketing experience.

4.9 Overdose
No case of overdose has been reported.

Doses of up to 6 mg have been used in clinical trials. The highest dose group showed a similar incidence of adverse events compared to the other dose groups and no dose response effects were observed. In the unlikely event of overdose with Aloxi, this should be managed with supportive care. Dialysis studies have not been performed, however, due to the large volume of distribution, dialysis is unlikely to be an effective treatment for Aloxi overdose.

5. PHARMACOLOGICAL PROPERTIES

5.1 Pharmacodynamic properties
Pharmacotherapeutic group: Antiemetics and antinauseants, serotonin (5HT3) antagonists. ATC code: [proposed: under application]

Palonosetron is a selective high-affinity receptor antagonist of the 5HT3 receptor.

In two randomised, double-blind studies with a total of 1,132 patients receiving moderately emetogenic chemotherapy that included cisplatin ≤ 50 mg/m^2,

Table 1

System Organ Class	Common ARs (>1/100 to <1/10)	Uncommon ARs (>1/1,000 to <1/100)
Metabolism and nutrition disorders		Hyperkalaemia, metabolic disorders, hypocalcaemia, anorexia, hyperglycaemia, appetite decreased
Psychiatric disorders		Anxiety, euphoric mood
Nervous system disorders	Headache Dizziness	Somnolence, insomnia, paraesthesia, hypersomnia, peripheral sensory neuropathy
Eye disorders		Eye irritation, amblyopia
Ear and labyrinth disorders		Motion sickness, tinnitus
Cardiac disorders		Tachycardia, bradycardia, extrasystoles, myocardial ischaemia, sinus tachycardia, sinus arrhythmia, supraventricular extrasystoles
Vascular disorders		Hypotension, hypertension, vein discolouration, vein distended
Respiratory, thoracic and mediastinal disorders		Hiccups
Gastrointestinal disorders	Constipation Diarrhoea	Dyspepsia, abdominal pain, abdominal pain upper, dry mouth, flatulence
Hepato-biliary disorders		Hyperbilirubinaemia
Skin and subcutaneous tissue disorders		Dermatitis allergic, pruritic rash
Musculoskeletal and connective tissue disorders		Arthralgia
Renal and urinary disorders		Urinary retention, glycosuria
General disorders and administration site conditions		Asthenia, pyrexia, fatigue, feeling hot, influenza like illness
Investigations		Elevated transaminases, hypokalaemia, electrocardiogram QT prolonged

carboplatin, cyclophosphamide $\leqslant$ 1,500 mg/m^2 and doxorubicin > 25 mg/m^2, palonosetron 250 micrograms and 750 micrograms were compared with ondansetron 32 mg (half-life 4 hours) or dolasetron 100 mg (half-life 7.3 hours) administered intravenously on Day 1, without dexamethasone.

In a randomised, double-blind study with a total of 667 patients receiving highly emetogenic chemotherapy that included cisplatin $\geqslant$60 mg/m^2, cyclophosphamide > 1,500 mg/m^2 and dacarbazine, palonosetron 250 micrograms and 750 micrograms were compared with ondansetron 32 mg administered intravenously on Day 1. Dexamethasone was administered prophylactically before chemotherapy in 67% of patients.

The pivotal studies were not designed to assess efficacy of palonosetron in delayed onset nausea and vomiting. The antiemetic activity was observed during 0-24 hours, 24-120 hours and 0-120 hours. Results for the studies on moderately emetogenic chemotherapy and for the study on highly emetogenic chemotherapy are summarised in the following tables.

Palonosetron was non-inferior versus the comparators in the acute phase of emesis both in moderately and highly emetogenic setting.

Although comparative efficacy of palonosetron in multiple cycles has not been demonstrated in controlled clinical trials, 875 patients enrolled in the three phase 3 trials continued in an open label safety study and were treated with palonosetron 750 micrograms for up to 9 additional cycles of chemotherapy. The overall safety was maintained during all cycles.

TABLE 2: PERCENTAGE OF PATIENTS[a] RESPONDING BY TREATMENT GROUP AND PHASE IN THE MODERATELY EMETOGENIC CHEMOTHERAPY STUDY VERSUS ONDANSETRON

(see Table 2)

TABLE 3: PERCENTAGE OF PATIENTS[a] RESPONDING BY TREATMENT GROUP AND PHASE IN THE MODERATELY EMETOGENIC CHEMOTHERAPY STUDY VERSUS DOLASETRON

(see Table 3)

TABLE 4: PERCENTAGE OF PATIENTS[a] RESPONDING BY TREATMENT GROUP AND PHASE IN THE HIGHLY EMETOGENIC CHEMOTHERAPY STUDY VERSUS ONDANSETRON

(see Table 4 on next page)

Table 2 PERCENTAGE OF PATIENTS[a] RESPONDING BY TREATMENT GROUP AND PHASE IN THE MODERATELY EMETOGENIC CHEMOTHERAPY STUDY VERSUS ONDANSETRON

	Aloxi 250 micrograms (n= 189)	Ondansetron 32 milligrams (n= 185)	Delta	
	%	%	%	
Complete Response (No Emesis and No Rescue Medication)				97.5% CI [b]
0 – 24 hours	81.0	68.6	12.4	[1.8%, 22.8%]
24 – 120 hours	74.1	55.1	19.0	[7.5%, 30.3%]
0 – 120 hours	69.3	50.3	19.0	[7.4%, 30.7%]
Complete Control (Complete Response and No More Than Mild Nausea)				p-value [c]
0 – 24 hours	76.2	65.4	10.8	NS
24 – 120 hours	66.7	50.3	16.4	0.001
0 – 120 hours	63.0	44.9	18.1	0.001
No Nausea (Likert Scale)				p-value [c]
0 – 24 hours	60.3	56.8	3.5	NS
24 – 120 hours	51.9	39.5	12.4	NS
0 – 120 hours	45.0	36.2	8.8	NS

a Intent-to-treat cohort.

b The study was designed to show non-inferiority. A lower bound greater than –15% demonstrates non-inferiority between Aloxi and comparator.

c Chi-square test. Significance level at α=0.05.

Table 3 PERCENTAGE OF PATIENTS[a] RESPONDING BY TREATMENT GROUP AND PHASE IN THE MODERATELY EMETOGENIC CHEMOTHERAPY STUDY VERSUS DOLASETRON

	Aloxi 250 micrograms (n= 185)	Dolasetron 100 milligrams (n= 191)	Delta	
	%	%	%	
Complete Response (No Emesis and No Rescue Medication)				97.5% CI [b]
0 – 24 hours	63.0	52.9	10.1	[-1.7%, 21.9%]
24 – 120 hours	54.0	38.7	15.3	[3.4%, 27.1%]
0 – 120 hours	46.0	34.0	12.0	[0.3%, 23.7%]
Complete Control (Complete Response and No More Than Mild Nausea)				p-value [c]
0 – 24 hours	57.1	47.6	9.5	NS
24 – 120 hours	48.1	36.1	12.0	0.018
0 – 120 hours	41.8	30.9	10.9	0.027
No Nausea (Likert Scale)				p-value [c]
0 – 24 hours	48.7	41.4	7.3	NS
24 – 120 hours	41.8	26.2	15.6	0.001
0 – 120 hours	33.9	22.5	11.4	0.014

a Intent-to-treat cohort.

b The study was designed to show non-inferiority. A lower bound greater than –15% demonstrates non-inferiority between Aloxi and comparator.

c Chi-square test. Significance level at α=0.05.

5.2 Pharmacokinetic properties

Absorption

Following intravenous administration, an initial decline in plasma concentrations is followed by slow elimination from the body with a mean terminal elimination half-life of approximately 40 hours. Mean maximum plasma concentration (Cmax) and area under the concentration-time curve (AUC0-∞) are generally dose-proportional over the dose range of 0.3–90 μg/kg in healthy subjects and in cancer patients.

Distribution

Palonosetron at the recommended dose is widely distributed in the body with a volume of distribution of approximately 6.9 to 7.9 l/kg. Approximately 62% of palonosetron is bound to plasma proteins.

Metabolism

Palonosetron is eliminated by dual route, about 40 % eliminated through the kidney and with approximately 50% metabolised to form two primary metabolites, which have less than 1% of the 5HT3 receptor antagonist activity of palonosetron. In vitro metabolism studies have shown that CYP2D6 and to a lesser extent, CYP3A4 and CYP1A2 isoenzymes are involved in the metabolism of palonosetron. However, clinical pharmacokinetic parameters are not significantly different between poor and extensive metabolisers of CYP2D6 substrates. Palonosetron does not inhibit or induce cytochrome P450 isoenzymes at clinically relevant concentrations.

Elimination

After a single intravenous dose of 10 micrograms/kg [^{14}C]-palonosetron, approximately 80% of the dose was recovered within 144 hours in the urine with palonosetron representing approximately 40% of the administered dose, as unchanged active substance. After a single intravenous bolus administration in healthy subjects the total body clearance of palonosetron was 173 ± 73 ml/min and renal clearance was 53 ± 29 ml/min. The low total body clearance and large volume of distribution resulted in a terminal elimination half-life in plasma of approximately 40 hours. Ten percent of patients have a mean terminal elimination half-life greater than 100 hours.

Pharmacokinetics in special populations

Elderly:

Age does not affect the pharmacokinetics of palonosetron. No dosage adjustment is necessary in elderly patients.

Gender:

Gender does not affect the pharmacokinetics of palonosetron. No dosage adjustment is necessary based on gender.

Paediatric patients:

No pharmacokinetic data are available in patients below 18 years of age.

Renal impairment:

Mild to moderate renal impairment does not significantly affect palonosetron pharmacokinetic parameters. Severe renal impairment reduces renal clearance, however total body clearance in these patients is similar to healthy subjects. No dosage adjustment is necessary in patients with renal insufficiency. No pharmacokinetic data in haemodialysis patients are available.

Hepatic impairment:

Hepatic impairment does not significantly affect total body clearance of palonosetron compared to the healthy subjects. While the terminal elimination half-life and mean systemic exposure of palonosetron is increased in the subjects with severe hepatic impairment, this does not warrant dose reduction.

5.3 Preclinical safety data

Preclinical effects were observed only at exposures considered sufficiently in excess of the maximum human exposure indicating little relevance to clinical use.

Nonclinical studies indicate that palonosetron, only at very high concentrations, may block ion channels involved in ventricular de- and re-polarisation and prolong action potential duration.

Animal studies do not indicate direct or indirect harmful effects with respect to pregnancy, embryonal/foetal development, parturition or postnatal development. Only limited data from animal studies are available regarding the placental transfer (see section 4.6).

Palonosetron is not mutagenic. High doses of palonosetron (each dose causing at least 30 times the human therapeutic exposure) applied daily for two years caused an increased rate of liver tumours, endocrine neoplasms (in thyroid, pituitary, pancreas, adrenal medulla) and skin tumours in rats but not in mice. The underlying mechanisms are not fully understood, but because of the high doses employed and since Aloxi is intended for single application in humans, these findings are not considered relevant for clinical use.

Table 4 PERCENTAGE OF PATIENTS[a] RESPONDING BY TREATMENT GROUP AND PHASE IN THE HIGHLY EMETOGENIC CHEMOTHERAPY STUDY VERSUS ONDANSETRON

	Aloxi 250 micrograms (n= 223)	Ondansetron 32 milligrams (n= 221)	Delta	
	%	%	%	
Complete Response (No Emesis and No Rescue Medication)				97.5% CI [b]
0 – 24 hours	59.2	57.0	2.2	[-8.8%, 13.1%]
24 – 120 hours	45.3	38.9	6.4	[-4.6%, 17.3%]
0 – 120 hours	40.8	33.0	7.8	[-2.9%, 18.5%]
Complete Control (Complete Response and No More Than Mild Nausea)				p-value [c]
0 – 24 hours	56.5	51.6	4.9	NS
24 – 120 hours	40.8	35.3	5.5	NS
0 – 120 hours	37.7	29.0	8.7	NS
No Nausea (Likert Scale)				p-value [c]
0 – 24 hours	53.8	49.3	4.5	NS
24 – 120 hours	35.4	32.1	3.3	NS
0 – 120 hours	33.6	32.1	1.5	NS

a Intent-to-treat cohort.

b The study was designed to show non-inferiority. A lower bound greater than –15% demonstrates non-inferiority between Aloxi and comparator.

c Chi-square test. Significance level at α=0.05.

6. PHARMACEUTICAL PARTICULARS

6.1 List of excipients

Mannitol

Disodium edetate

Sodium citrate

Citric acid monohydrate

Water for injections

Sodium hydroxide solution

Hydrochloric acid solution

6.2 Incompatibilities

This medicinal product must not be mixed with other medicinal products.

6.3 Shelf life

3 years.

Upon opening of the vial, any unused solution should be discarded.

6.4 Special precautions for storage

This medicinal product does not require any special storage conditions

6.5 Nature and contents of container

Type I glass vial with chlorobutyl siliconised rubber stopper and aluminium cap. Available in packs of 1 vial containing 5 ml of solution.

6.6 Instructions for use and handling

Single use only, any unused solution should be discarded.

7. MARKETING AUTHORISATION HOLDER

Helsinn Birex Pharmaceuticals Ltd.

Damastown

Mulhuddart

Dublin 15

Republic of Ireland

8. MARKETING AUTHORISATION NUMBER(S)

EU/1/04/306/001

9. DATE OF FIRST AUTHORISATION/RENEWAL OF THE AUTHORISATION

22 March 2005

10. DATE OF REVISION OF THE TEXT

22 March 2005

Alpha Keri Bath Oil

(Bristol-Myers Pharmaceuticals)

1. NAME OF THE MEDICINAL PRODUCT

Alpha Keri Bath Oil.

2. QUALITATIVE AND QUANTITATIVE COMPOSITION

Bath oil containing Mineral oil 91.7% w/w and Lanolin oil 3% w/w.

3. PHARMACEUTICAL FORM

Bath oil for topical use.

4. CLINICAL PARTICULARS

4.1 Therapeutic indications

Alpha Keri Bath Oil effectively deposits a thin uniform emulisified film of oil over the skin, and this retards evaporation of moisture, helps to relieve itching, lubricates and softens the skin.

Alpha Keri Bath Oil is valuable as an aid in the management of dry pruritic skin, especially in senile pruritus, ichthyosis and other dermotases where dermal hydration is an important part of the therapy (as in the prevention of decubitus ulcer).

Alpha Keri Bath Oil is particularly suitable for infant bathing. The preparation also overcomes the problem of cleansing the skin in conditions where the use of soaps, soap substitutes and colloid or oat-meal baths prove irritating.

4.2 Posology and method of administration

Adults and Children

Alpha Keri Bath Oil should always be either added to water or rubbed onto wet skin.

Because of its inherent cleansing properties soap should not be used with Alpha Keri.

Bath:

Add 10-20 ml to the bath water. Soak for 10-20 minutes.

Sponge Bath

Add 10-20 ml to basin of warm water. Apply over the entire body with a sponge or flannel.

Skin Cleansing

Rub a small amount onto wet skin, rinse and pat dry.

Infant Bath

Add 5ml to bath water.

Shower

Pour a small amount onto a wet sponge or flannel and rub onto wet skin, rinse and pat dry.

Elderly

No dosage adjustment is necessary.

4.3 Contraindications

Alpha Keri Bath Oil contains lanolin oil and is therefore contra-indicated in those patients allergic to lanolin.

4.4 Special warnings and special precautions for use

None known.

4.5 Interaction with other medicinal products and other forms of Interaction

None known.

4.6 Pregnancy and lactation

No special precautions.

4.7 Effects on ability to drive and use machines

None known.

4.8 Undesirable effects

Alpha Keri Bath Oil deposits a film of oil over the skin, special care should be taken to guard against slipping, especially in the bath or shower.

4.9 Overdose

Not applicable.

5. PHARMACOLOGICAL PROPERTIES

5.1 Pharmacodynamic properties

Mineral and lanolin oils have emollient properties. The product deposits a thin uniform emulsified film of oil over the skin and thus retards the evaporation of moisture, helping to relieve itching, lubricates and softens the skin.

5.2 Pharmacokinetic properties

Not applicable for this type of product.

5.3 Preclinical safety data

No further relevant information.

6. PHARMACEUTICAL PARTICULARS

6.1 List of excipients

Oxybenzone, perfume, PEG-4-dilaurate (polyethylene dilaurate).

6.2 Incompatibilities

None known.

6.3 Shelf life

36 months.

6.4 Special precautions for storage

Store Alpha Keri Bath Oil at room temperature (below 25°C).

6.5 Nature and contents of container

Clear PVC bottles, closures are polypropylene with pulp/SA-66 liners or linerless polypropylene dispenser closure with hinge (flip-top closure) in pack sizes of 240 or 480 ml.

6.6 Instructions for use and handling

None known.

7. MARKETING AUTHORISATION HOLDER

Bristol-Myers Squibb Holdings Ltd.,

t/a Bristol-Myers Pharmaceuticals or

Westwood Pharmaceuticals,

Uxbridge Business Park,

Sanderson Road,

Uxbridge,

Middlesex

UB8 1DH

8. MARKETING AUTHORISATION NUMBER(S)

PL 0125/0141

9. DATE OF FIRST AUTHORISATION/RENEWAL OF THE AUTHORISATION

23rd June 1992

10. DATE OF REVISION OF THE TEXT

22 July 2005

Alphaderm Cream 30g & 100g

(Alliance Pharmaceuticals)

1. NAME OF THE MEDICINAL PRODUCT

Alphaderm Cream

2. QUALITATIVE AND QUANTITATIVE COMPOSITION

Alphaderm cream contains the active ingredients Hydrocortisone, PhEur 1% w/w and Urea, BP 10% w/w.

3. PHARMACEUTICAL FORM

Translucent white cream.

4. CLINICAL PARTICULARS

4.1 Therapeutic indications

For the treatment of all dry ichthyotic, eczematous conditions of the skin, including atopic, infantile, chronic allergic and irritant eczema, asteatotic, hyperkeratotic and lichenified eczema, neurodermatitis and prurigo.

4.2 Posology and method of administration

Adults, children and the elderly. A small amount should be applied topically to the preferably dry affected areas twice daily. In resistant lesions occlusive dressings may be used but this is usually unnecessary because of the self occlusive nature of the special base.

4.3 Contraindications

Primary bacterial, viral and fungal diseases of the skin and secondarily infected eczemas or intertrigo acne, perioral dermatitis, rosacea and, in general, should not be used on weeping surfaces.

Known hypersensitivity to the active ingredients or any of its excipients.

4.4 Special warnings and special precautions for use

Caution should be exercised when using in children. In infants and children, long term continuous therapy should be avoided, as adrenal suppression can occur even without occlusion. Excessive absorption may occur when applied under napkins. Where possible treatment in infants should be limited to 5-7 days.

Application to moist or fissured skin may cause temporary irritation.

As with corticosteroids in general, prolonged application to the face and eyelids is undesirable and the cream should be kept away from the eyes.

4.5 Interaction with other medicinal products and other forms of Interaction
None known.

4.6 Pregnancy and lactation
There is inadequate evidence for safety in human pregnancy. Topical administration of corticosteroids to pregnant animals can cause abnormalities of foetal development including cleft palate and intra-uterine growth retardation. There may, therefore, be a very small risk of such effects in the human foetus.

4.7 Effects on ability to drive and use machines
Alphaderm does not interfere with the ability to drive or use machines.

4.8 Undesirable effects
If used correctly Alphaderm is unlikely to cause side effects. However, the following events have been observed with topical steroids, and although are rare with hydrocortisone, may occur, especially with long-term use; spread and worsening of untreated infection; thinning of the skin; irreversible striae atrophicae and telangiectasia; contact dermatitis, perioral dermatitis; acne; mild depigmentation which may be reversible. Atrophic changes may occur in intertriginous areas or nappy areas in young children.

4.9 Overdose
Chronically, grossly excessive over-use on large areas of skin in, for example, children could result in adrenal suppression of the hypothalamic-pituitary axis (HPA) as well as topical and systemic signs and symptoms of high corticosteroid dosage. In such cases, treatment should not stop abruptly. Adrenal insufficiency may require treatment with systemic hydrocortisone. Ingestion of a large amount of Alphaderm would be expected to result in gastrointestinal irritation, nausea, and possibly vomiting. Symptomatic and supportive care should be given. Liberal oral administration of milk or water may be helpful.

5. PHARMACOLOGICAL PROPERTIES

5.1 Pharmacodynamic properties
Hydrocortisone is a naturally occurring glucocorticoid with proven anti-inflammatory and vasoconstrictive properties. Urea has been demonstrated to have hydrating, keratolytic and anti-pruritic properties. As such, urea has additional therapeutic effect in dry hyperkeratotic skin conditions. Alphaderm cream contains hydrocortisone and urea in a specially formulated base which assists the percutaneous transportation of the active ingredients to the site of action. Due to this formulation, Alphaderm acts as a moderately potent topical corticosteroid. The base is self-occlusive and fulfils the functions of both an ointment and a cream.

5.2 Pharmacokinetic properties
Therapeutic activity of hydrocortisone depends upon the adequate penetration through the horny layer of the skin. The urea in the formulation solubilises part of the hydrocortisone and has a keratolytic effect. Both these factors increase penetration of the hydrocortisone

5.3 Preclinical safety data
None stated

6. PHARMACEUTICAL PARTICULARS

6.1 List of excipients
White soft paraffin, maize starch, isopropyl myristate, sycrowax HR-C, palmitic acid, sorbitan laurate and Arlatone G.

6.2 Incompatibilities
None known.

6.3 Shelf life
Two years

6.4 Special precautions for storage
Do not store above 25°C.

6.5 Nature and contents of container
Supplied in tubes of 30g and 100g.

6.6 Instructions for use and handling
A patient leaflet is provided with details of use and handling of the product.

7. MARKETING AUTHORISATION HOLDER
Alliance Pharmaceuticals Ltd

Avonbridge House

Bath Road

Chippenham

Wiltshire

SN15 2BB

8. MARKETING AUTHORISATION NUMBER(S)
PL 16853/0060.

9. DATE OF FIRST AUTHORISATION/RENEWAL OF THE AUTHORISATION
13 February 1990

10. DATE OF REVISION OF THE TEXT
November 2004

11. LEGAL STATUS
POM

Alphagan

(Allergan Ltd)

1. NAME OF THE MEDICINAL PRODUCT
Alphagan® 0.2% (2 mg/ml) eye drops, solution.

2. QUALITATIVE AND QUANTITATIVE COMPOSITION
Brimonidine [(R,R)-tartrate] 0.2% (2.0 mg/ml)

(equivalent to brimonidine base 0.13%, 1.3 mg/ml)

1 drop of Alphagan® = approximately 35 μl = 70 μg brimonidine tartrate

For excipients, see 6.1.

3. PHARMACEUTICAL FORM
Eye drops, solution.

Clear, greenish-yellow to light greenish-yellow solution.

4. CLINICAL PARTICULARS

4.1 Therapeutic indications
Reduction of elevated intraocular pressure (IOP) in patients with open angle glaucoma or ocular hypertension.

- As monotherapy in patients in whom topical beta-blocker therapy is contraindicated.
- As adjunctive therapy to other intraocular pressure lowering medications when the target IOP is not achieved with a single agent (see Section 5.1).

4.2 Posology and method of administration
The recommended dose is one drop of Alphagan® in the affected eye(s) twice daily, approximately 12 hours apart. No dosage adjustment is required for the use in elderly patients.

As with any eye drops, to reduce possible systemic absorption, it is recommended that the lachrymal sac be compressed at the medial canthus (punctal occlusion) for one minute. This should be performed immediately following the instillation of each drop.

If more than one topical ophthalmic drug is to be used, the different drugs should be instilled 5-15 minutes apart.

Alphagan® has not been studied in patients with hepatic or renal impairment - see section 4.4.

Alphagan® should not be used in neonates and is not recommended for use in children (see Section 4.3 Contra-indications; Section 4.4 Special warning and precautions for use and Section 4.9 Overdose). It is known that severe adverse reactions can occur in neonates. The safety and efficacy of Alphagan® have not been established in children.

4.3 Contraindications
Alphagan® is contraindicated for use in neonates and in patients with hypersensitivity to brimonidine tartrate or any component of this medication. Alphagan®is also contraindicated in patients receiving monoamine oxidase (MAO) inhibitor therapy and patients on antidepressants which affect noradrenergic transmission (e.g. tricyclic antidepressants and mianserin).

4.4 Special warnings and special precautions for use
Symptoms of brimonidine overdose have been reported in a few neonates receiving Alphagan® as part of medical treatment of congenital glaucoma.

Caution should be exercised in treating patients with severe or unstable and uncontrolled cardiovascular disease.

Some (12.7%)patients in clinical trials experienced an ocularallergic type reaction with Alphagan® (see section 4.8 for details). If allergic reactions are observed, treatment with Alphagan® should be discontinued.

Alphagan® should be used with caution in patients with depression, cerebral or coronary insufficiency, Raynaud's phenomenon, orthostatic hypotension or thromboangiitis obliterans.

Alphagan® has not been studied in patients with hepatic or renal impairment; caution should be used in treating such patients.

The preservative in Alphagan®, benzalkonium chloride, may cause eye irritation. Remove contact lenses prior to application and wait at least 15 minutes before reinsertion. Known to discolour soft contact lenses.

4.5 Interaction with other medicinal products and other forms of Interaction
Although specific drug interactions studies have not been conducted with Alphagan®, the possibility of an additive or potentiating effect with CNS depressants (alcohol, barbiturates, opiates, sedatives, or anaesthetics) should be considered.

No data on the level of circulating catecholamines after Alphagan® administration are available. Caution, however, is advised in patients taking medications which can affect the metabolism and uptake of circulating amines e.g. chlorpromazine, methylphenidate, reserpine.

After the application of Alphagan®, clinically insignificant decreases in blood pressure were noted in some patients. Caution is advised when using drugs such as antihypertensives and/or cardiac glycosides concomitantly with Alphagan®.

Caution is advised when initiating (or changing the dose of) a concomitant systemic agent (irrespective of pharmaceutical form) which may interact with α-adrenergic agonists or interfere with their activity i.e. agonists or antagonists of the adrenergic receptor e.g. (isoprenaline, prazosin).

4.6 Pregnancy and lactation
The safety of use during human pregnancy has not been established. In animal studies, brimonidine tartrate did not cause any teratogenic effects. In rabbits, brimonidine tartrate, at plasma levels higher than are achieved during therapy in humans, has been shown to cause increased preimplantation loss and postnatal growth reduction. Alphagan® should be used during pregnancy only if the potential benefit to the mother outweighs the potential risk to the foetus.

It is not known if brimonidineis excreted in human milk. The compound is excreted in the milk of the lactating rat. Alphagan® should not be used by women nursing infants.

4.7 Effects on ability to drive and use machines
Alphagan® may cause fatigue and/or drowsiness, which may impair the ability to drive or operate machinery. Alphagan® may cause blurred and/or abnormal vision, which may impair the ability to drive or to use machinery, especially at night or in reduced lighting.

4.8 Undesirable effects
a) The most commonly reported ADRs are oral dryness, ocular hyperaemia and burning/stinging, all occurring in 22 to 25% of patients. They are usually transient and not commonly of a severity requiring discontinuation of treatment.

Symptoms of ocular allergic reactions occurred in 12.7% of subjects (causing withdrawal in 11.5% of subjects) in clinical trials with the onset between 3 and 9 months in the majority of patients.

(see Table 1 on next page)

4.9 Overdose
Ophthalmic overdose:

There is no experience in adults with the unlikely case of an overdosage via the ophthalmic route. However, symptoms of brimonidine overdose such as hypotension, bradycardia, hypothermia and apnea have been reported in a few neonates receiving Alphagan® as part of medical treatment of congenital glaucoma.

Systemic overdose resulting from accidental ingestion:

One report of accidental human adult ingestion of Alphagan® has been received. The patient ingested about 10 drops of Alphagan®. He experienced a hypotensive episode a few hours after the ingestion and then a rebound hypertension approximately 8 hours after ingestion.

Oral overdoses of other alpha-2-agonists have been reported to cause symptoms such as hypotension, asthenia, vomiting, lethargy, sedation, bradycardia, arrhythmias, miosis, apnea, hypotonia, hypothermia, respiratory depression and seizure.

5. PHARMACOLOGICAL PROPERTIES

5.1 Pharmacodynamic properties
ATC code = *S01E A* 05.

Brimonidine is an alpha-2 adrenergic receptor agonist that is 1000-fold more selective for the alpha-2 adrenoceptor than the alpha-1 adrenoreceptor.

This selectivity results in no mydriasis and the absence of vasoconstriction in microvessels associated with human retinal xenografts.

Topical administration of brimonidine tartrate decreases intraocular pressure (IOP) in humans with minimal effect on cardiovascular or pulmonary parameters.

Limited data are available for patients with bronchial asthma showing no adverse effects.

Alphagan® has a rapid onset of action, with peak ocular hypotensive effect seen at two hours post-dosing. In two 1 year studies, Alphagan® lowered IOP by mean values of approximately 4-6 mmHg.

Fluorophotometric studies in animals and humans suggest that brimonidine tartrate has a dual mechanism of action. It is thought that Alphagan® may lower IOP by reducing aqueous humour formation and enhancing uveoscleral outflow.

Clinical trials show that Alphagan is effective in combination with topical beta-blockers. Shorter term studies also suggest that Alphagan has a clinically relevant additive effect in combination with travoprost (6 weeks) and latanoprost (3 months).

5.2 Pharmacokinetic properties
a) General characteristics

After ocular administration of a 0.2% solution twice daily for 10 days, plasma concentrations were low (mean Cmax was 0.06 ng/ml). There was a slight accumulation in the blood after multiple (2 times daily for 10 days) instillations. The area under the plasma concentration-time curve over 12 hours at steady state ($AUC_{0\text{-}12h}$) was 0.31 ng·hr/ml, as compared to 0.23 ng·hr/ml after the first dose. The mean apparent half-life in the systemic circulation was approximately 3 hours in humans after topical dosing.

Table 1

b)	Ocular effects	Very Common: (>1 in 10)	- ocular irritation including allergic reactions (hyperaemia, burning and stinging, pruritis, foreign body sensation, conjunctival follicles). - blurred vision.
		Common: (>1 in 100 and <1 in 10)	- local irritation (eyelid hyperaemia and oedema, blepharitis, conjunctival oedema and discharge, ocular pain and tearing). - photophobia - corneal erosion and staining - ocular dryness - conjunctival blanching - abnormal vision - conjunctivitis.
		Very Rare: (<1 in 10,000)	Iritis (anterior uveitis) Miosis
	Systemic effects	Very Common: (>1 in 10)	Headache Oral dryness Fatigue/drowsiness
		Common: (>1 in 100 and <1 in 10)	Upper respiratory symptoms Dizziness Gastrointestinal symptoms Asthenia Abnormal taste
		Uncommon: (>1 in 1,000 and <1 in 100)	Palpitations/arrythmias (including bradycardia and tachycardia) Systemic allergic reactions Depression Nasal dryness
		Rare: (>1 in 10,000 and <1 in 1,000)	Dyspnoea
		Very Rare: (<1 in 10,000)	Syncope Hypertension Hypotension Insomnia
c)	Symptoms of brimonidine overdose such as hypotension, bradycardia, hypothermia and apnea have been reported in a few neonates receiving Alphagan® as part of medical treatment of congenital glaucoma.		

The plasma protein binding of brimonidine after topical dosing in humans is approximately 29%.

Brimonidine binds reversibly to melanin in ocular tissues, in vitro and in vivo. Following 2 weeks of ocular instillation, the concentrations of brimonidine in iris, ciliary body and choroid-retina were 3- to 17-fold higher than those after a single dose. Accumulation does not occur in the absence of melanin.

The significance of melanin binding in humans is unclear. However, no significant ocular adverse reaction was found during biomicroscopic examination of eyes in patients treated with Alphagan® for up to one year, nor was significant ocular toxicity found during a one year ocular safety study in monkeys given approximately four times the recommended dose of brimonidine tartrate.

Following oral administration to man, brimonidine is well absorbed and rapidly eliminated. The major part of the dose (around 75% of the dose) was excreted as metabolites in urine within five days; no unchanged drug was detected in urine. In vitro studies, using animal and human liver, indicate that the metabolism is mediated largely by aldehyde oxidase and cytochrome P450. Hence, the systemic elimination seems to be primarily hepatic metabolism.

Kinetics profile:

No great deviation from dose proportionality for plasma Cmax and AUC was observed following a single topical dose of 0.08%, 0.2% and 0.5%.

b) Characteristics in patients

Characteristics in elderly patients:

The C_{max}, AUC, and apparent half-life of brimonidine are similar in the elderly (subjects 65 years or older)after a single dose compared with young adults, indicating that its systemic absorption and elimination are not affected by age.

Based on data from a 3 month clinical study, which included elderly patients, systemic exposure to brimonidine was very low.

5.3 Preclinical safety data

The available mutagenicity and carcinogenicity data indicate that Alphagan® will exert neither mutagenic nor carcinogenic activities under the conditions of clinical use.

6. PHARMACEUTICAL PARTICULARS

6.1 List of excipients

Benzalkonium Chloride

Polyvinyl alcohol

Sodium chloride

Sodium citrate, dihydrate

Citric acid, monohydrate

Purified water

Hydrochloric acid or

Sodium hydroxide to adjust pH

6.2 Incompatibilities

Not applicable.

6.3 Shelf life

Before first opening:	2 years for the 2.5ml container.
	3 years for the 5ml and 10ml containers.
After first opening:	Use within 28 days.

6.4 Special precautions for storage

Do not store above 25°C.

6.5 Nature and contents of container

White low density polyethylene dropper bottles with a 35 microlitre tip. The cap is either a conventional white or purple screw cap or a Compliance Cap (C-Cap).

2.5 ml, 5 ml and 10 ml bottles in packs of 1, 3 or 6.

Not all pack sizes may be marketed.

6.6 Instructions for use and handling

No special requirements.

7. MARKETING AUTHORISATION HOLDER

Allergan Limited

Coronation Road

High Wycombe

Buckinghamshire

HP12 3SH

UK

8. MARKETING AUTHORISATION NUMBER(S)

PL 00426/0088

9. DATE OF FIRST AUTHORISATION/RENEWAL OF THE AUTHORISATION

18th March 2002

10. DATE OF REVISION OF THE TEXT

3rd February 2005

Alu-Cap Capsules

(3M Health Care Limited)

1. NAME OF THE MEDICINAL PRODUCT

Alu-Cap Capsules

2. QUALITATIVE AND QUANTITATIVE COMPOSITION

Each capsule contains 475 mg Dried Aluminium Hydroxide Gel Ph Eur as a white powder.

3. PHARMACEUTICAL FORM

Hard gelatin capsules

4. CLINICAL PARTICULARS

4.1 Therapeutic indications

Alu-Cap is recommended for use as a phosphate binding agent in the management of renal failure. It may also be used as an antacid.

4.2 Posology and method of administration

FOR PHOSPHATE BINDING

ADULTS AND CHILDREN: The dosage must be selected in accordance with individual patient requirements, and may range from 4 to 20 capsules of Alu-Cap daily (approximately 2 to 10 g dried aluminium hydroxide gel), taken with meals.

AS AN ANTACID

ADULTS: One Alu-Cap four times daily and on retiring.

CHILDREN: Alu-Cap is not suitable for antacid therapy in children.

ELDERLY: No special dosage recommendations are made for elderly patients.

Route of Administration: Oral

4.3 Contraindications

Alu-Cap is contra-indicated in patients with hypophosphataemia and acute porphyria.

4.4 Special warnings and special precautions for use

Serum phosphate levels should be monitored in all patients receiving phosphate binders, to prevent the development of a phosphate depletion syndrome.

4.5 Interaction with other medicinal products and other forms of Interaction

Aluminium hydroxide may form complexes with certain antibiotics (eg tetracyclines); concomitant administration may result in reduced absorption of the antibiotic.

4.6 Pregnancy and lactation

There is no evidence of safety of the drug in human pregnancy but it has been in wide use for many years without apparent ill consequence, animal studies having shown no hazard.

4.7 Effects on ability to drive and use machines

None

4.8 Undesirable effects

Aluminium hydroxide is astringent and may cause constipation.

4.9 Overdose

SYMPTOMS AND TREATMENT: A single massive dose of aluminium hydroxide is unlikely to have harmful sequelae, as aluminium is not absorbed systemically to any great extent. Gastric lavage should be administered, followed by a mild aperient if required.

5. PHARMACOLOGICAL PROPERTIES

5.1 Pharmacodynamic properties

In the gut, aluminium hydroxide absorbs phosphate ions. This reduces absorption of phosphate into the body, and thereby reduces serum phosphate levels.

Aluminium hydroxide gel is a slow-acting antacid. It is used to provide symptomatic relief in gastric hyperacidity. In addition, the antipeptic and demulcent activity of aluminium hydroxide helps to protect inflamed gastric mucosa against further irritation by gastric secretions.

5.2 Pharmacokinetic properties

Aluminium hydroxide is slowly but perhaps incompletely converted to aluminium chloride in the stomach. Some absorption of soluble aluminium salts occurs from the gastro-intestinal tract with some excretion in the urine. Some unabsorbed aluminium hydroxide combines with phosphates and some form carbonates and salts of fatty acids, all these salts are excreted in the faeces.

5.3 Preclinical safety data
Not applicable.

6. PHARMACEUTICAL PARTICULARS
6.1 List of excipients
Polyethylene Glycol 6000

Purified Talc

'Solka Floc' BW 100, Special

Capsule shell: E104, E110, E127, E131

6.2 Incompatibilities
None known.

6.3 Shelf life
5 years

6.4 Special precautions for storage
Store below 30°C.

6.5 Nature and contents of container
Amber glass bottles with screw cap containing 120 capsules.

6.6 Instructions for use and handling
None

7. MARKETING AUTHORISATION HOLDER
3M Health Care Limited

3M House

Morley Street

Loughborough

Leics

LE11 1EP

8. MARKETING AUTHORISATION NUMBER(S)
PL 00068/0052

9. DATE OF FIRST AUTHORISATION/RENEWAL OF THE AUTHORISATION
6 June 1974/27 September 1994

10. DATE OF REVISION OF THE TEXT
June 1999.

Alupent Syrup

(Boehringer Ingelheim Limited)

1. NAME OF THE MEDICINAL PRODUCT
ALUPENT® Syrup

2. QUALITATIVE AND QUANTITATIVE COMPOSITION
Each 5 ml contains orciprenaline sulphate 10 mg.

3. PHARMACEUTICAL FORM
Syrup.

4. CLINICAL PARTICULARS
4.1 Therapeutic indications
ALUPENT is indicated for the relief of reversible airways obstruction.

ALUPENT Syrup is suggested for maintenance therapy.

4.2 Posology and method of administration
Adults: The usual dose is 2 × 5 ml four times daily. The maximum recommended daily dosage is 8 × 5 ml spoonfuls.

Children 3-12 years: The usual starting dose is 1 × 5 ml four times daily. This may be increased to 2 × 5 ml three times daily as necessary. The maximum recommended daily dosage is 6 × 5 ml spoonfuls.

Children 1-3 years: The usual starting dose is ½ × 5 ml four times daily. This may be increased to 1 × 5 ml four times daily as necessary. The maximum recommended daily dosage is 4 × 5 ml spoonfuls.

Children 0-1 year: The usual starting dose is ½ × 5 ml three times daily. This may be increased to 1 × 5 ml three times daily as necessary. The maximum recommended daily dosage is 3 × 5 ml spoonfuls.

Diluents: ALUPENT Syrup may be diluted with either Syrup BP or Sorbitol Solution BP.

No specific information on the use of this product in the elderly is available.

Clinical trials have included patients over 65 years and no adverse reactions specific to this age group have been reported.

4.3 Contraindications
Hypertrophic obstructive cardiomyopathy, tachyarrhythmia. Hypersensitivity to any of the ingredients in ALUPENT Syrup.

4.4 Special warnings and special precautions for use
A chronic requirement for treatment would suggest the need for clinical review of the management of the patient's asthma. The patient's need for anti-inflammatory therapy (e.g. corticosteroids), or the adequacy of such therapy in patients already receiving it should be assessed.

Patients must be warned not to exceed the prescribed dose. In the case of acute rapidly worsening dyspnoea a doctor should be consulted immediately.

Sympathomimetic agents can cause unwanted effects. The concomitant use of other sympathomimetic drugs should be avoided or only used under strict medical supervision. ALUPENT and anticholinergic bronchodilators have been administered concurrently in reversible airways obstruction. In some situations, co-administered sympathomimetic agents and anticholinergics have been shown to produce greater bronchodilatation than the use of either agent alone (but see Interactions).

In the following conditions ALUPENT should only be used after careful risk/benefit assessment, especially when doses higher than those recommended are used:

Insufficiently controlled diabetes mellitus, recent myocardial infarction, severe organic heart or vascular disorders, phaeochromocytoma, hyperthyroidism.

Potentially serious hypokalaemia may result from excessive beta-agonist therapy. This effect may be potentiated by concomitant treatment with xanthine derivatives, glucocorticosteroids and diuretics.

Additionally, hypoxia may aggravate the effects of hypokalaemia on cardiac rhythm. It is recommended that serum potassium levels are monitored in such situations.

4.5 Interaction with other medicinal products and other forms of Interaction
In view of the possible interaction between beta-adrenergics and monoamine oxidase inhibitors or tricyclic antidepressants, care should be exercised if it is proposed to administer these compounds concurrently with ALUPENT.

Beta-adrenergics, anticholinergics and xanthine derivatives (such as theophylline) may enhance the bronchodilator effect of orciprenaline.

The concurrent administration of the other beta-adrenergics, systemically absorbed anticholinergics and xanthine derivatives (e.g. theophylline) may increase the frequency and severity of unwanted effects.

Beta$_2$-receptor blockers counteract the action of ALUPENT.

Potentially serious bronchospasm may occur during concurrent administration of beta-blockers to patients with reversible airways obstruction.

Inhalation of halogenated hydrocarbon anaesthetics such as halothane, trichloroethylene and enflurane may increase the susceptibility to the cardiovascular effects of beta-agonists.

4.6 Pregnancy and lactation
Although orciprenaline sulphate has been in general use for several years, there is no definite evidence of ill-consequence following administration of the drug during human pregnancy. Only in doses far in excess of the equivalent maximum human dose were effects on foetal development seen in animals.

ALUPENT should only be used during pregnancy, especially the first trimester, if the potential benefit outweighs the potential risk to the foetus.

The inhibitory effect of orciprenaline sulphate on uterine contraction should be taken into account.

Safety in breast-fed infants has not been established.

4.7 Effects on ability to drive and use machines
None stated.

4.8 Undesirable effects
The most frequently reported undesirable effects observed with ALUPENT are tremor and nervousness, headache, dizziness, tachycardia, palpitations, gastro-intestinal discomfort, nausea and vomiting. Some patients have experienced a feeling of tightness of the chest.

Potentially serious hypokalaemia may result from beta$_2$-agonist therapy.

As with other beta-mimetics, sweating, weakness and myalgia/muscle cramps may occur. In rare cases decrease in diastolic blood pressure, increase in systolic blood pressure, arrhythmias, particularly after higher doses may occur.

In rare cases, local irritation, skin reactions or allergic reactions have been reported. There have been isolated cases of anaphylactic or anaphylactoid reactions.

In individual cases psychological alterations have been reported under inhalational therapy with beta-mimetics.

4.9 Overdose
Symptoms
The expected symptoms of overdosage with ALUPENT are those of excessive beta-stimulation such as flushing, tremor, nausea, restlessness, tachycardia, palpitation, dizziness, headache, hypotension, hypertension, a feeling of pressure in the chest, excitation, angina, increased pulse pressure and arrhythmia. Hypokalaemia may occur following overdose with orciprenaline. Serum potassium levels should be monitored.

Therapy
Treatment of overdosage should primarily be supportive and symptom-oriented.

If specific therapy is considered necessary, cardioselective beta-blockers are to be preferred. These should be administered with extreme caution to patients with asthma because of the risk of precipitating severe bronchospasm.

5. PHARMACOLOGICAL PROPERTIES
5.1 Pharmacodynamic properties
ALUPENT is a sympathomimetic amine with bronchodilator properties.

Following oral administration, the effect is usually noted within 30 minutes. The peak effect of bronchodilator activity following orciprenaline sulphate generally occurs within 60-90 minutes, and lasts for 1 to 5 hours.

5.2 Pharmacokinetic properties
Following oral administration orciprenaline is absorbed from the GI tract and undergoes extensive first-pass metabolism; about 40% of an oral dose is reported to reach the circulation unchanged. It is excreted in the urine primarily as glucuronide conjugates.

5.3 Preclinical safety data
There is no additional information available other than that already provided.

6. PHARMACEUTICAL PARTICULARS
6.1 List of excipients
Sodium metabisulphite

Disodium edetate dihydrate

Methyl parahydroxybenzoate

Propyl parahydroxybenzoate

Hydroxyethylcellulose

Saccharin

Sorbitol solution

Woodruff aroma

Sodium hydroxide

Purified water

6.2 Incompatibilities
None stated.

6.3 Shelf life
5 years

6.4 Special precautions for storage
Do not store above 25°C. Keep container in the outer carton.

6.5 Nature and contents of container
ALUPENT Syrup is available in pack sizes of 50ml, 250ml, 300ml and 2L in amber type III glass bottles with tamper-evident, child resistant polypropylene caps with expanded polyethylene liners. Not all pack sizes may be marketed.

6.6 Instructions for use and handling
None stated.

7. MARKETING AUTHORISATION HOLDER
Boehringer Ingelheim Limited

Ellesfield Avenue

Bracknell

Berkshire

RG12 8YS

United Kingdom

8. MARKETING AUTHORISATION NUMBER(S)
00015/0001R

9. DATE OF FIRST AUTHORISATION/RENEWAL OF THE AUTHORISATION
21/2/96

10. DATE OF REVISION OF THE TEXT
February 2003

11. Legal category
Prescription Only Medicine

A5b/UK/SPC/8

Alvedon Suppositories 60, 125, 250 mg

(AstraZeneca UK Limited)

1. NAME OF THE MEDICINAL PRODUCT
Alvedon Suppositories 60, 125, 250 mg.

2. QUALITATIVE AND QUANTITATIVE COMPOSITION
Each suppository contains Paracetamol 60, 125 or 250 mg.

For excipients see 6.1.

3. PHARMACEUTICAL FORM
Suppositories.

4. CLINICAL PARTICULARS
4.1 Therapeutic indications
For the treatment of mild to moderate pain and pyrexia in children:

up to the age of 1 year - 60 mg suppositories

aged 1-5 years - 125 mg suppositories

aged 6-12 years - 250 mg suppositories

Alvedon suppositories may be especially useful in patients unable to take oral forms of paracetamol, e.g. post-operatively or with nausea and vomiting.

4.2 Posology and method of administration
60 mg suppositories
Children 3 months to 1 year, 1-2 suppositories:

The dosage should be based on age and weight i.e.

3 months (5 kg) - 60mg (1 suppository)

1 year (10 kg) - 120mg (2 suppositories)

Infants under 3 months:

One suppository (60 mg) is suitable for babies who develop a fever following immunisation at 2 months. Otherwise only use in babies aged less than 3 months on a doctor's advice.

125 mg suppositories

Children 1-5 years, 1-2 suppositories.

The dosage should be based on age and weight i.e.

1 year (10 Kg) - 125mg (1 suppository)

5 years (20 Kg) -250mg (2 suppositories)

250 mg suppositories

Children 6 to 12 years 1-2 suppositories:

The dosage should be based on age and weight i.e.

6 years (20 Kg) - 250mg (1 suppository)

12 years (40 Kg) - 500mg (2 suppositories)

These doses may be repeated up to a maximum of 4 times in 24 hours. The dose should not be repeated more frequently than every 4 hours. The recommended dose should not be exceeded. Higher doses do not produce any increase in analgesic effect. Only whole suppositories should be administered – do not break suppository before administration.

4.3 Contraindications

Hypersensitivity to paracetamol or hard fat

4.4 Special warnings and special precautions for use

Alvedon Suppositories should not be combined with other analgesic medications that contain paracetamol. Paracetamol should be given with care to patients with impaired kidney or liver function.

Label and Leaflet will state the following warnings:

Label:

"Immediate medical advice should be sought in the event of an overdose, even if the child seems well".

"Do not give with any other Paracetamol-containing products."

Leaflet:

"Immediate medical advice should be sought in the event of an overdose, even if the child seems well, because of the risk of delayed, serious liver damage."

4.5 Interaction with other medicinal products and other forms of Interaction

Drugs which induce hepatic microsomal enzymes such as alcohol, barbiturates and other anticonvulsants, may increase the hepatotoxicity of paracetamol, particularly after overdosage.

The anti-coagulant effect of warfarin and other coumarins may be enhanced by prolonged regular use of paracetamol with increased risk of bleeding. The effect appears to increase as the dose of paracetamol is increased, but can occur with doses as low as 1.5 – 2 g paracetamol per day for at least 5 – 7 days. Occasional doses have no significant effect.

Enzyme-inducing medicines, such as some antiepileptic drugs (phenytoin, phenobarbital, carbamazepine) have been shown in pharmacokinetic studies to reduce the plasma AUC of paracetamol to approx. 60 %. Other substances with enzyme-inducing properties, e.g. rifampicin and St. John's wort (hypericum) are also suspected of causing lowered concentrations of paracetamol. In addition, the risk of liver damage during treatment with maximum recommended doses of paracetamol will be higher in patients being treated with enzyme-inducing agents.

4.6 Pregnancy and lactation

Not applicable.

4.7 Effects on ability to drive and use machines

None known.

4.8 Undesirable effects

Side-effects at therapeutic doses are rare.

Common >1/100	*Miscellaneous:*	Redness of the rectal mucous membranes
Rare <1/1000	*General:*	Allergic reactions
	Skin:	Exanthema, urticaria
	Liver:	Liver damage
	Genitourinary:	Increase in creatinine (mostly secondary to hepatorenal syndrome)

There have been reports of blood dyscrasias including thrombocytopenia and agranulocytosis, but these were not necessarily causally related to paracetamol.

Hepatic necrosis may occur after overdosage (see below).

4.9 Overdose

Immediate treatment is essential in the management of paracetamol overdose. Despite a lack of significant early symptoms, patients should be referred to a hospital urgently for immediate medical attention. Administration of oral methionine or intravenous N-acetylcysteine which may have a beneficial effect up to at least 48 hours after the overdose, may be required. General supportive measures must be available.

Symptoms of paracetamol overdose in the first 24 hours are pallor, nausea, vomiting, anorexia and abdominal pain. Liver damage may become apparent 12 to 48 hours after ingestion ingestion and clinical symptoms generally culminate after 4-6 days.

Abnormalities of glucose metabolism and metabolic acidosis may occur. In severe poisoning, hepatic failure may progress to encephalopathy, coma and death. Acute renal failure with acute tubular necrosis may develop even in the absence of severe liver damage. Cardiac arrhythmias and pancreatitis have been reported.

Toxicity: 5 g during 24 hours in a child aged 3 ½ years, 15-20 g in adults, caused fatal intoxication. The toxic dose for children and adults is generally >140 mg/kg. Malnutrition, dehydration, medication with enzyme-inducing drugs such as some antiepileptic drugs (phenytoin, phenobarbital, carbamazepine), rifampicin and St. John's wort (hypericum) are risk factors, and even slight overdosage can then cause marked liver damage. Even subacute "therapeutic" overdose has resulted in severe intoxication with doses varying from 6 g/24 hours for a week, 20 g for 2-3 days, etc.

5. PHARMACOLOGICAL PROPERTIES

5.1 Pharmacodynamic properties

ATC code: N02BE01

Paracetamol is an aniline derivative with analgesic and antipyretic actions similar to those of aspirin but with no demonstrable anti-inflammatory activity. Paracetamol is less irritant to the stomach than aspirin. It does not affect thrombocyte aggregation or bleeding time. Paracetamol is generally well tolerated by patients hypersensitive to acetylsalicylic acid.

5.2 Pharmacokinetic properties

Paracetamol is well absorbed by both oral and rectal routes. Peak plasma concentrations occur about 2 to 3 hours after rectal administration. The plasma half life is about 2 hours.

Paracetamol is primarily metabolised in the liver by conjugation to glucuronide and sulphate. A small amount (about 3-10% of a therapeutic dose) is metabolised by oxidation and the reactive intermediate metabolite thus formed is bound preferentially to the liver glutathione and excreted as cystein and mercapturic acid conjugates. Excretion occurs via the kidneys. 2-3% of a therapeutic dose is excreted unchanged; 80-90% as glucuronide and sulphate and a smaller amount as cystein and mercapturic acid derivatives.

5.3 Preclinical safety data

Not applicable

6. PHARMACEUTICAL PARTICULARS

6.1 List of excipients

Hard fat (Witepsol H12)

6.2 Incompatibilities

None known.

6.3 Shelf life

3 years.

6.4 Special precautions for storage

Do not store above 25°C.

6.5 Nature and contents of container

PVC/polyethylene blister strips each containing 5 suppositories. Packs of 5 or 10 suppositories.

PCV/polyethylene blister strips each containing 1 suppository. Packs of 10 suppositories.

Not all pack sizes may be marketed.

6.6 Instructions for use and handling

Peel the wrapper apart to remove the suppository, gently push into the rectum pointed end first.

7. MARKETING AUTHORISATION HOLDER

AstraZeneca UK Ltd.,

600 Capability Green,

Luton,

LU1 3LU,

UK

8. MARKETING AUTHORISATION NUMBER(S)

PL 17901/0096, 0097, 0098

9. DATE OF FIRST AUTHORISATION/RENEWAL OF THE AUTHORISATION

16th June 2002

10. DATE OF REVISION OF THE TEXT

23 June 2003

Alvesco 160 Inhaler

(ALTANA Pharma Limited)

1. NAME OF THE MEDICINAL PRODUCT

Alvesco® ▼160 Inhaler

2. QUALITATIVE AND QUANTITATIVE COMPOSITION

1 actuation (delivered dose from the mouthpiece) contains 160 micrograms of ciclesonide.

For excipients, see section 6.1.

3. PHARMACEUTICAL FORM

Pressurised inhalation, solution

Clear and colourless

4. CLINICAL PARTICULARS

4.1 Therapeutic indications

Treatment to control persistent asthma in adults (18 years and older).

4.2 Posology and method of administration

The medicinal product is for inhalation use only.

The recommended starting dose of Alvesco® is 160 micrograms once daily which is usually also the maximum dose. Dose reduction to 80 micrograms once daily may be an effective maintenance dose for some patients.

Alvesco® should preferably be administered in the evening although morning dosing of Alvesco® has also been shown to be effective. The final decision on evening or morning dosing should be left to the discretion of the physician.

Symptoms start to improve with Alvesco® within 24 hours of treatment. Once control is achieved, the dose of Alvesco® should be individualised and titrated to the minimum dose needed to maintain good asthma control.

Patients with severe asthma are at risk of acute attacks and should have regular assessments of their asthma control including pulmonary function tests. Increasing use of short-acting bronchodilators to relieve asthma symptoms indicates deterioration of asthma control. If patients find that short-acting relief bronchodilator treatment becomes less effective, or they need more inhalations than usual, medical attention must be sought. In this situation, patients should be reassessed and consideration given to the need for increased anti-inflammatory treatment therapy (e.g. higher doses of Alvesco® or a course of oral corticosteroids). Severe asthma exacerbations should be managed the usual way.

To address specific patient needs, such as finding it difficult to press the inhaler and breathe in at the same time, Alvesco® can be used with the AeroChamber Plus(TM) spacer device.

Specific patient groups:

There is no need to adjust the dose in elderly patients or those with hepatic or renal impairment.

To date, there are insufficient data available in the treatment of adolescents and children 17 years and younger with Alvesco®.

Instructions for use / handling:

The patient needs to be instructed how to use the inhaler correctly.

If the inhaler is new or has not been used for one week or more, three puffs should be released into the air. No shaking is necessary as this is a solution aerosol.

During inhalation, the patient should preferably sit or stand, and the inhaler should be held upright with the thumb on the base, below the mouthpiece.

Instruct the patient to remove the mouthpiece cover, place the inhaler into their mouth, close their lips around the mouthpiece, and breathe in slowly and deeply. While breathing in through the mouth, the top of the inhaler should be pressed down. Then, patients should remove the inhaler from their mouth, and hold their breath for about 10 seconds, or as long as is comfortable. The patient is not to breathe out into the inhaler. Finally, patients should breathe out slowly and replace the mouthpiece cover.

The mouthpiece should be cleaned with a dry tissue or cloth weekly. The inhaler should not be washed or put in water.

For detailed instructions see Patient Information Leaflet.

4.3 Contraindications

Hypersensitivity to ciclesonide or any of the excipients.

4.4 Special warnings and special precautions for use

As with all inhaled corticosteroids, Alvesco® should be administered with caution in patients with active or quiescent pulmonary tuberculosis, fungal, viral or bacterial infections, and only if these patients are adequately treated.

As with all inhaled corticosteroids, Alvesco® is not indicated in the treatment of status asthmaticus or other acute episodes of asthma where intensive measures are required.

As with all inhaled corticosteroids, Alvesco® is not designed to relieve acute asthma symptoms for which an inhaled short-acting bronchodilator is required. Patients should be advised to have such rescue medication available.

Systemic effects of inhaled corticosteroids may occur, particularly at high doses prescribed for prolonged periods. These effects are much less likely to occur than with oral corticosteroids. Possible systemic effects include adrenal suppression, growth retardation in children and adolescents, decrease in bone mineral density, cataract and glaucoma. It is therefore important that the dose of inhaled corticosteroid is titrated to the lowest dose at which effective control of asthma is maintained.

There is no data available in patients with severe hepatic impairment. An increased exposure in patients with severe hepatic impairment is expected and these patients should therefore be monitored for potential systemic effects.

The benefits of inhaled ciclesonide should minimise the need for oral steroids. However, patients transferred from oral steroids remain at risk of impaired adrenal reserve for a considerable time after transferring to inhaled ciclesonide. The possibility of respective symptoms may persist for some time.

These patients may require specialised advice to determine the extent of adrenal impairment before elective procedures. The possibility of residual impaired adrenal response should always be considered in an emergency (medical or surgical) and elective situations likely to produce stress, and appropriate corticosteroid treatment considered.

Lack of response or severe exacerbations of asthma should be treated by increasing the dose of inhaled ciclesonide and, if necessary, by giving a systemic steroid and/or an antibiotic if there is an infection.

For the transfer of patients being treated with oral corticosteroids:

The transfer of oral steroid-dependent patients to inhaled ciclesonide, and their subsequent management, needs special care as recovery from impaired adrenocortical function, caused by prolonged systemic steroid therapy, may take a considerable time.

Patients who have been treated with systemic steroids for long periods of time, or at a high dose, may have adrenocortical suppression. With these patients adrenocortical function should be monitored regularly and their dose of systemic steroid reduced cautiously.

After approximately a week, gradual withdrawal of the systemic steroid is started by reducing the dose by 1 mg prednisolone per week, or its equivalent. For maintenance doses of prednisolone in excess of 10 mg daily, it may be appropriate to cautiously use larger reductions in dose at weekly intervals.

Some patients feel unwell in a non-specific way during the withdrawal phase despite maintenance or even improvement of respiratory function. They should be encouraged to persevere with inhaled ciclesonide and to continue withdrawal of systemic steroid, unless there are objective signs of adrenal insufficiency.

Patients transferred from oral steroids whose adrenocortical function is still impaired should carry a steroid warning card indicating that they need supplementary systemic steroid during periods of stress, e.g. worsening asthma attacks, chest infections, major intercurrent illness, surgery, trauma, etc.

Replacement of systemic steroid treatment with inhaled therapy sometimes unmasks allergies such as allergic rhinitis or eczema previously controlled by systemic drug.

Paradoxical bronchospasm with an immediate increase of wheezing or other symptoms of bronchoconstriction after dosing should be treated with an inhaled short-acting bronchodilator, which usually results in quick relief. The patient should be assessed and therapy with Alvesco® should only be continued, if after careful consideration the expected benefit is greater than the possible risk. Correlation between severity of asthma and general susceptibility for acute bronchial reactions should be kept in mind (see section 4.8).

Patients' inhaler technique should be checked regularly to make sure that inhaler actuation is synchronised with inhaling to ensure optimum delivery to the lungs.

4.5 Interaction with other medicinal products and other forms of Interaction

In vitro data indicate that CYP3A4 is the major enzyme involved in the metabolism of the active metabolite of ciclesonide M1 in man.

The serum levels of ciclesonide and its metabolite M1 are low. However, co-administration with a potent inhibitor of the cytochrome P 450 3A4 system (e.g. ketoconazole, itraconazole and ritonavir or nelfinavir) should be considered with caution because there might be an increase in ciclesonide / metabolite serum levels. The risk of clinical adverse effect (e.g. cushingoid syndrome) cannot be excluded.

4.6 Pregnancy and lactation

There are no adequate and well-controlled studies in pregnant women.

In animal studies glucocorticoids have been shown to induce malformations (see section 5.3). This is not likely to be relevant for humans given recommended inhalation doses.

As with other glucocorticoids, ciclesonide shouldonly be usedduring pregnancy if the potential benefit to the mother justifies the potential riskto the foetus. The lowest effective dose of ciclesonide needed to maintain adequate asthma control should be used.

Infants born of mothers who received corticosteroids during pregnancy are to be observed carefully for hypoadrenalism.

It is unknown whether inhaled ciclesonide is excreted in human breast milk. Administration of ciclesonide to women who are breastfeeding should only be considered if the expected benefit to the mother is greater than any possible risk to the child.

4.7 Effects on ability to drive and use machines

Inhaled ciclesonide has no or negligibleinfluence on the ability to drive and use machines.

4.8 Undesirable effects

Approximately 4% of patients experienced adverse reactions in clinical trials with Alvesco® given in the dose range 80 to 1280 micrograms per day. In the majority of cases, these were mild and did not require discontinuation of treatment with Alvesco®.

Frequency / Organ System	Common [> 1/100, < 1/10]	Uncommon [> 1/1,000, < 1/100]
Gastrointestinal Disorders		Bad taste
General disorders and administration site conditions		Application site reactions such as burning, inflammation, and irritation; Application site dryness
Respiratory, thoracic and mediastinal disorders	Paradoxical bronchospasm	Hoarseness of voice Cough after inhalation
Skin and subcutaneous tissue disorders		Rash and eczema

Paradoxical bronchospasm may occur immediately after dosing and is an unspecific acute reaction to all inhaled medicinal products, which may be related to the active substance, the excipient, or evaporation cooling in the case of metered dose inhalers. In severe cases, withdrawal of Alvesco® should be considered.

Systemic effects of inhaled corticosteroids may occur, particularly at high doses prescribed for prolonged periods (see also section 4.4).

4.9 Overdose

Acute:

Inhalation by healthy volunteers of a single dose of 2880 micrograms of ciclesonide was well tolerated.

The potential for acute toxic effects following overdose of inhaled ciclesonide is low. After acute overdosage no specific treatment is necessary.

Chronic:

After prolonged administration of 1280 micrograms of ciclesonide, no clinical signs of adrenal suppression were observed. However, if higher than recommended dosage is continued over prolonged periods, some degree of adrenal suppression cannot be excluded. Monitoring of adrenal reserve may be necessary.

5. PHARMACOLOGICAL PROPERTIES

5.1 Pharmacodynamic properties

Pharmacotherapeutic group: Other drugs for obstructive airway diseases, Inhalants, Glucocorticoids, ATC Code: R03B A08

Ciclesonide exhibits low binding affinity to the glucocorticoid-receptor. Once orally inhaled, ciclesonide is enzymatically converted in the lungs to the principal metabolite (C21-des-methylpropionyl-ciclesonide) which has a pronounced anti-inflammatory activity and is thus considered as the active metabolite.

In three clinical trials, ciclesonide has been shown to reduce airway reactivity to adenosine monophosphate in hyperreactive patients. In another trial, pre-treatment with ciclesonide for seven days significantly attenuated the early and late phase reactions following inhaled allergen challenge. Inhaled ciclesonide treatment was also shown to attenuate the increase in inflammatory cells (total eosinophils) and inflammatory mediators in induced sputum.

A controlled study compared 24-hour plasma cortisol AUC in 26 adult asthmatic patients following 7 days of treatment. Compared to placebo, treatment with ciclesonide 320, 640, and 1280 micrograms/day did not statistically significantly lower the 24-hour time averages of plasma cortisol ($AUC_{(0-24)}$/24 hours) nor was a dose-dependent effect seen.

In a clinical trial involving 164 adult male and female asthmatic patients, ciclesonide was given at doses of 320 micrograms or 640 micrograms/day over 12 weeks. After stimulation with 1 and 250 micrograms cosyntropin, no significant changes in plasma cortisol levels were observed versus placebo.

Double-blind placebo-controlled trials of 12-weeks duration have shown that treatment with ciclesonide resulted in improved lung function as measured by FEV_1 and peak expiratory flow, improved asthma symptom control, and decreased need for inhaled beta-2 agonist.

5.2 Pharmacokinetic properties

Ciclesonide is presented in HFA-134a propellant and ethanol as a solution aerosol, which demonstrates a linear relationship between different doses, puff strengths and systemic exposure.

ABSORPTION:

Studies with oral and intravenous dosing of radiolabeled ciclesonide have shown an incomplete extent of oral absorption (24.5%). The oral bioavailability of both ciclesonide and the active metabolite is negligible (<0.5% for ciclesonide, <1% for the metabolite). Based on a γ-scintigraphy experiment, lung deposition in healthy subjects is 52%. In line with this figure, the systemic bioavailability for the active metabolite is >50% by using the ciclesonide metered dose inhaler. As the oral bioavailability for the active metabolite is <1%, the swallowed portion of the inhaled ciclesonide does not contribute to systemic absorption.

DISTRIBUTION:

Following intravenous administration to healthy subjects, the initial distribution phase for ciclesonide was rapid and consistent with its high lipophilicity. The volume of distribution averaged 2.9 l/kg. The total serum clearance of ciclesonide is high (average 2.0 l/h/kg) indicating a high hepatic extraction. The percentage of ciclesonide bound to human plasma proteins averaged 99%, and that of the active metabolite 98-99%, indicating an almost complete binding of circulating ciclesonide/active metabolite to plasma proteins.

METABOLISM:

Ciclesonide is primarily hydrolysed to its biologically active metabolite by esterase enzymes in the lung. Investigation of the enzymology of further metabolism by human liver microsomes showed that this compound is mainly metabolised to hydroxylated inactive metabolites by CYP3A4 catalysis. Furthermore, reversible lipophilic fatty acid ester conjugates of the active metabolite were detected in the lung.

EXCRETION:

Ciclesonide is predominantly excreted via the faeces (67%), after oral and intravenous administration, indicating that excretion via the bile is the major route of elimination.

Pharmacokinetic characteristics in patients:

ASTHMATIC PATIENTS

Ciclesonide shows no pharmacokinetic changes in mild asthmatic patients compared to healthy subjects.

RENAL OR HEPATIC INSUFFICIENCY, ELDERLY

According to population pharmacokinetics, age has no impact on the systemic exposure of the active metabolite.

Reduced liver function may affect the elimination of corticosteroids. In a study including patients with hepatic impairment suffering from liver cirrhosis, a higher systemic exposure to the active metabolite was observed.

Due to the lack of renal excretion of the active metabolite, studies on renal impaired patients have not been performed.

5.3 Preclinical safety data

Preclinical data with ciclesonide reveal no special hazard for humans based on conventional studies of safety pharmacology, repeated dose toxicity, genotoxicity, or carcinogenic potential.

In animal studies on reproductive toxicity, glucocorticosteroids have been shown to induce malformations (cleft palate, skeletal malformations). However, these animal results do not seem to be relevant for humans given recommended doses.

Animal studies with other glucocorticoids indicate that administration of pharmacological doses of glucocorticoids during pregnancy may increase the risk for intrauterine growth retardation, adult cardiovascular and/or metabolic disease and/or permanent changes in glucocorticoid receptor density, neurotransmitter turnover and behaviour. The relevance of these data to humans administered ciclesonide by inhalation is unknown.

6. PHARMACEUTICAL PARTICULARS

6.1 List of excipients

Norflurane (HFA-134a)

Ethanol, anhydrous

6.2 Incompatibilities

Not applicable.

6.3 Shelf life

2 years.

6.4 Special precautions for storage

This medicinal product does not require any special storage conditions.

The container contains a pressurised liquid. Do not expose to temperatures higher than 50°C.

The container should not be punctured, broken or burnt even when apparently empty.

6.5 Nature and contents of container

The inhaler comprises a pressurised container made from aluminium and is sealed with a metering valve, mouthpiece, and cap.

60 metered actuations

120 metered actuations

Hospital packs:

10 × 60 metered actuations

10 × 120 metered actuations

[Not all pack sizes may be marketed]

6.6 Instructions for use and handling

Patients should be carefully instructed in the proper use of their inhaler (see Patient Information Leaflet).

As with most inhaled medicinal products in pressurised containers, the therapeutic effect of this medicinal product may decrease when the container is cold. However, Alvesco® delivers a consistent dose from –10°C to 40°C.

7. MARKETING AUTHORISATION HOLDER

ALTANA Pharma AG

Byk-Gulden-Str. 2

D-78467 Konstanz

Germany

8. MARKETING AUTHORISATION NUMBER(S)

PL 20141/0006

9. DATE OF FIRST AUTHORISATION/RENEWAL OF THE AUTHORISATION

16 April 2004

10. DATE OF REVISION OF THE TEXT

22 February 2005

11. LEGAL CLASSIFICATION

POM

Alvesco 80 Inhaler

(ALTANA Pharma Limited)

1. NAME OF THE MEDICINAL PRODUCT

Alvesco® ▼ 80 Inhaler

2. QUALITATIVE AND QUANTITATIVE COMPOSITION

1 actuation (delivered dose from the mouthpiece) contains 80 micrograms of ciclesonide.

For excipients, see section 6.1.

3. PHARMACEUTICAL FORM

Pressurised inhalation, solution

Clear and colourless

4. CLINICAL PARTICULARS

4.1 Therapeutic indications

Treatment to control persistent asthma in adults (18 years and older).

4.2 Posology and method of administration

The medicinal product is for inhalation use only.

The recommended starting dose of Alvesco® is 160 micrograms once daily which is usually also the maximum dose. Dose reduction to 80 micrograms once daily may be an effective maintenance dose for some patients.

Alvesco® should preferably be administered in the evening although morning dosing of Alvesco® has also been shown to be effective. The final decision on evening or morning dosing should be left to the discretion of the physician.

Symptoms start to improve with Alvesco® within 24 hours of treatment. Once control is achieved, the dose of Alvesco® should be individualised and titrated to the minimum dose needed to maintain good asthma control.

Patients with severe asthma are at risk of acute attacks and should have regular assessments of their asthma control including pulmonary function tests. Increasing use of short-acting bronchodilators to relieve asthma symptoms indicates deterioration of asthma control. If patients find that short-acting relief bronchodilator treatment becomes less effective, or they need more inhalations than usual, medical attention must be sought. In this situation, patients should be reassessed and consideration given to the need for increased anti-inflammatory treatment therapy (e.g. higher doses of Alvesco® or a course of oral corticosteroids). Severe asthma exacerbations should be managed the usual way.

To address specific patient needs, such as finding it difficult to press the inhaler and breathe in at the same time, Alvesco® can be used with the AeroChamber Plus™ spacer device.

Specific patient groups:

There is no need to adjust the dose in elderly patients or those with hepatic or renal impairment.

To date, there are insufficient data available in the treatment of adolescents and children 17 years and younger with Alvesco®.

Instructions for use / handling:

The patient needs to be instructed how to use the inhaler correctly.

If the inhaler is new or has not been used for one week or more, three puffs should be released into the air. No shaking is necessary as this is a solution aerosol.

During inhalation, the patient should preferably sit or stand, and the inhaler should be held upright with the thumb on the base, below the mouthpiece.

Instruct the patient to remove the mouthpiece cover, place the inhaler into their mouth, close their lips around the mouthpiece, and breathe in slowly and deeply. While breathing in through the mouth, the top of the inhaler should be pressed down. Then, patients should remove the inhaler from their mouth, and hold their breath for about 10 seconds, or as long as is comfortable. The patient is not to breathe out into the inhaler. Finally, patients should breathe out slowly and replace the mouthpiece cover.

The mouthpiece should be cleaned with a dry tissue or cloth weekly. The inhaler should not be washed or put in water.

For detailed instructions see Patient Information Leaflet.

4.3 Contraindications

Hypersensitivity to ciclesonide or any of the excipients.

4.4 Special warnings and special precautions for use

As with all inhaled corticosteroids, Alvesco® should be administered with caution in patients with active or quiescent pulmonary tuberculosis, fungal, viral or bacterial infections, and only if these patients are adequately treated.

As with all inhaled corticosteroids, Alvesco® is not indicated in the treatment of status asthmaticus or other acute episodes of asthma where intensive measures are required.

As with all inhaled corticosteroids, Alvesco® is not designed to relieve acute asthma symptoms for which an inhaled short-acting bronchodilator is required. Patients should be advised to have such rescue medication available.

Systemic effects of inhaled corticosteroids may occur, particularly at high doses prescribed for prolonged periods. These effects are much less likely to occur than with oral corticosteroids. Possible systemic effects include adrenal suppression, growth retardation in children and adolescents, decrease in bone mineral density, cataract and glaucoma. It is therefore important that the dose of inhaled corticosteroid is titrated to the lowest dose at which effective control of asthma is maintained.

There is no data available in patients with severe hepatic impairment. An increased exposure in patients with severe hepatic impairment is expected and these patients should therefore be monitored for potential systemic effects.

The benefits of inhaled ciclesonide should minimise the need for oral steroids. However, patients transferred from oral steroids remain at risk of impaired adrenal reserve for a considerable time after transferring to inhaled ciclesonide. The possibility of respective symptoms may persist for some time.

These patients may require specialised advice to determine the extent of adrenal impairment before elective procedures. The possibility of residual impaired adrenal response should always be considered in an emergency (medical or surgical) and elective situations likely to produce stress, and appropriate corticosteroid treatment considered.

Lack of response or severe exacerbations of asthma should be treated by increasing the dose of inhaled ciclesonide and, if necessary, by giving a systemic steroid and/or an antibiotic if there is an infection.

For the transfer of patients being treated with oral corticosteroids:

The transfer of oral steroid-dependent patients to inhaled ciclesonide, and their subsequent management, needs special care as recovery from impaired adrenocortical function, caused by prolonged systemic steroid therapy, may take a considerable time.

Patients who have been treated with systemic steroids for long periods of time, or at a high dose, may have adrenocortical suppression. With these patients adrenocortical function should be monitored regularly and their dose of systemic steroid reduced cautiously.

After approximately a week, gradual withdrawal of the systemic steroid is started by reducing the dose by 1 mg prednisolone per week, or its equivalent. For maintenance doses of prednisolone in excess of 10 mg daily, it may be appropriate to cautiously use larger reductions in dose at weekly intervals.

Some patients feel unwell in a non-specific way during the withdrawal phase despite maintenance or even improvement of respiratory function. They should be encouraged to persevere with inhaled ciclesonide and to continue withdrawal of systemic steroid, unless there are objective signs of adrenal insufficiency.

Patients transferred from oral steroids whose adrenocortical function is still impaired should carry a steroid warning card indicating that they need supplementary systemic steroid during periods of stress, e.g. worsening asthma attacks, chest infections, major intercurrent illness, surgery, trauma, etc.

Replacement of systemic steroid treatment with inhaled therapy sometimes unmasks allergies such as allergic rhinitis or eczema previously controlled by systemic drug.

Paradoxical bronchospasm with an immediate increase of wheezing or other symptoms of bronchoconstriction after dosing should be treated with an inhaled short-acting bronchodilator, which usually results in quick relief. The patient should be assessed and therapy with Alvesco® should only be continued, if after careful consideration the expected benefit is greater than the possible risk. Correlation between severity of asthma and general susceptibility for acute bronchial reactions should be kept in mind (see section 4.8).

Patients' inhaler technique should be checked regularly to make sure that inhaler actuation is synchronised with inhaling to ensure optimum delivery to the lungs.

4.5 Interaction with other medicinal products and other forms of Interaction

In vitro data indicate that CYP3A4 is the major enzyme involved in the metabolism of the active metabolite of ciclesonide M1 in man.

The serum levels of ciclesonide and its metabolite M1 are low. However, co-administration with a potent inhibitor of the cytochrome P 450 3A4 system (e.g. ketoconazole, itraconazole and ritonavir or nelfinavir) should be considered with caution because there might be an increase in ciclesonide / metabolite serum levels. The risk of clinical adverse effect (e.g. cushingoid syndrome) cannot be excluded.

4.6 Pregnancy and lactation

There are no adequate and well-controlled studies in pregnant women.

In animal studies glucocorticoids have been shown to induce malformations (see section 5.3). This is not likely to be relevant for humans given recommended inhalation doses.

As with other glucocorticoids, ciclesonide shouldonly be usedduring pregnancy if the potential benefit to the mother justifies the potential riskto the foetus. The lowest effective dose of ciclesonide needed to maintain adequate asthma control should be used.

Infants born of mothers who received corticosteroids during pregnancy are to be observed carefully for hypoadrenalism.

It is unknown whether inhaled ciclesonide is excreted in human breast milk. Administration of ciclesonide to women who are breastfeeding should only be considered if the expected benefit to the mother is greater than any possible risk to the child.

4.7 Effects on ability to drive and use machines

Inhaled ciclesonide has no or negligibleinfluence on the ability to drive and use machines.

4.8 Undesirable effects

Approximately 4% of patients experienced adverse reactions in clinical trials with Alvesco® given in the dose range 80 to 1280 micrograms per day. In the majority of cases, these were mild and did not require discontinuation of treatment with Alvesco®.

Frequency Organ System	Common [> 1/100, < 1/10]	Uncommon [> 1/1,000, < 1/100]
Gastrointestinal Disorders		Bad taste
General disorders and administration site conditions		Application site reactions such as burning, inflammation, and irritation; Application site dryness
Respiratory, thoracic and mediastinal disorders	Paradoxical bronchospasm	Hoarseness of voice Cough after inhalation
Skin and subcutaneous tissue disorders		Rash and eczema

Paradoxical bronchospasm may occur immediately after dosing and is an unspecific acute reaction to all inhaled medicinal products, which may be related to the active substance, the excipient, or evaporation cooling in the case of metered dose inhalers. In severe cases, withdrawal of Alvesco® should be considered.

Systemic effects of inhaled corticosteroids may occur, particularly at high doses prescribed for prolonged periods (see also section 4.4).

4.9 Overdose

Acute:

Inhalation by healthy volunteers of a single dose of 2880 micrograms of ciclesonide was well tolerated.

The potential for acute toxic effects following overdose of inhaled ciclesonide is low. After acute overdosage no specific treatment is necessary.

Chronic:

After prolonged administration of 1280 micrograms of ciclesonide, no clinical signs of adrenal suppression were observed. However, if higher than recommended dosage is continued over prolonged periods, some degree of adrenal suppression cannot be excluded. Monitoring of adrenal reserve may be necessary.

5. PHARMACOLOGICAL PROPERTIES

5.1 Pharmacodynamic properties

Pharmacotherapeutic group: Other drugs for obstructive airway diseases, Inhalants, Glucocorticoids, ATC Code: R03B A08

Ciclesonide exhibits low binding affinity to the glucocorticoid-receptor. Once orally inhaled, ciclesonide is enzymatically converted in the lungs to the principal metabolite (C21-des-methylpropionyl-ciclesonide) which has a pronounced anti-inflammatory activity and is thus considered as the active metabolite.

In three clinical trials, ciclesonide has been shown to reduce airway reactivity to adenosine monophosphate in hyperreactive patients. In another trial, pre-treatment with ciclesonide for seven days significantly attenuated the early and late phase reactions following inhaled allergen challenge. Inhaled ciclesonide treatment was also shown to attenuate the increase in inflammatory cells (total eosinophils) and inflammatory mediators in induced sputum.

A controlled study compared 24-hour plasma cortisol AUC in 26 adult asthmatic patients following 7 days of treatment. Compared to placebo, treatment with ciclesonide 320, 640, and 1280 micrograms/day did not statistically significantly lower the 24-hour time averages of plasma cortisol ($AUC_{(0-24)}$/24 hours) nor was a dose-dependent effect seen.

In a clinical trial involving 164 adult male and female asthmatic patients, ciclesonide was given at doses of 320 micrograms or 640 micrograms/day over 12 weeks. After stimulation with 1 and 250 micrograms cosyntropin, no significant changes in plasma cortisol levels were observed versus placebo.

Double-blind placebo-controlled trials of 12-weeks duration have shown that treatment with ciclesonide resulted in improved lung function as measured by FEV_1 and peak expiratory flow, improved asthma symptom control, and decreased need for inhaled beta-2 agonist.

5.2 Pharmacokinetic properties

Ciclesonide is presented in HFA-134a propellant and ethanol as a solution aerosol, which demonstrates a linear relationship between different doses, puff strengths and systemic exposure.

ABSORPTION:

Studies with oral and intravenous dosing of radiolabeled ciclesonide have shown an incomplete extent of oral absorption (24.5%). The oral bioavailability of both ciclesonide and the active metabolite is negligible (<0.5% for ciclesonide, <1% for the metabolite). Based on a γ-scintigraphy experiment, lung deposition in healthy subjects is 52%. In line with this figure, the systemic bioavailability for the active metabolite is >50% by using the ciclesonide metered dose inhaler. As the oral bioavailability for the active metabolite is <1%, the swallowed portion of the inhaled ciclesonide does not contribute to systemic absorption.

DISTRIBUTION:

Following intravenous administration to healthy subjects, the initial distribution phase for ciclesonide was rapid and consistent with its high lipophilicity. The volume of distribution averaged 2.9 l/kg. The total serum clearance of ciclesonide is high (average 2.0 l/h/kg) indicating a high hepatic extraction. The percentage of ciclesonide bound to human plasma proteins averaged 99%, and that of the active metabolite 98-99%, indicating an almost complete binding of circulating ciclesonide/active metabolite to plasma proteins.

METABOLISM:

Ciclesonide is primarily hydrolysed to its biologically active metabolite by esterase enzymes in the lung. Investigation of the enzymology of further metabolism by human liver microsomes showed that this compound is mainly metabolised to hydroxylated inactive metabolites by CYP3A4 catalysis. Furthermore, reversible lipophilic fatty acid ester conjugates of the active metabolite were detected in the lung.

EXCRETION:

Ciclesonide is predominantly excreted via the faeces (67%), after oral and intravenous administration, indicating that excretion via the bile is the major route of elimination.

Pharmacokinetic characteristics in patients:

ASTHMATIC PATIENTS

Ciclesonide shows no pharmacokinetic changes in mild asthmatic patients compared to healthy subjects.

RENAL OR HEPATIC INSUFFICIENCY, ELDERLY

According to population pharmacokinetics, age has no impact on the systemic exposure of the active metabolite.

Reduced liver function may affect the elimination of corticosteroids. In a study including patients with hepatic impairment suffering from liver cirrhosis, a higher systemic exposure to the active metabolite was observed.

Due to the lack of renal excretion of the active metabolite, studies on renal impaired patients have not been performed.

5.3 Preclinical safety data

Preclinical data with ciclesonide reveal no special hazard for humans based on conventional studies of safety pharmacology, repeated dose toxicity, genotoxicity, or carcinogenic potential.

In animal studies on reproductive toxicity, glucocorticosteroids have been shown to induce malformations (cleft palate, skeletal malformations). However, these animal results do not seem to be relevant for humans given recommended doses.

Animal studies with other glucocorticoids indicate that administration of pharmacological doses of glucocorticoids during pregnancy may increase the risk for intrauterine growth retardation, adult cardiovascular and/or metabolic disease and/or permanent changes in glucocorticoid receptor density, neurotransmitter turnover and behaviour. The relevance of these data to humans administered ciclesonide by inhalation is unknown.

6. PHARMACEUTICAL PARTICULARS

6.1 List of excipients

Norflurane (HFA-134a)

Ethanol, anhydrous

6.2 Incompatibilities

Not applicable.

6.3 Shelf life

2 years.

6.4 Special precautions for storage

This medicinal product does not require any special storage conditions.

The container contains a pressurised liquid. Do not expose to temperatures higher than 50°C.

The container should not be punctured, broken or burnt even when apparently empty.

6.5 Nature and contents of container

The inhaler comprises a pressurised container made from aluminium and is sealed with a metering valve, mouthpiece, and cap.

60 metered actuations

120 metered actuations

[Not all pack sizes may be marketed]

6.6 Instructions for use and handling

Patients should be carefully instructed in the proper use of their inhaler (see Patient Information Leaflet).

As with most inhaled medicinal products in pressurised containers, the therapeutic effect of this medicinal product may decrease when the container is cold. However, Alvesco® delivers a consistent dose from −10°C to 40°C.

7. MARKETING AUTHORISATION HOLDER

ALTANA Pharma AG

Byk-Gulden-Str. 2

D-78467 Konstanz

Germany

8. MARKETING AUTHORISATION NUMBER(S)

PL 20141/0005

9. DATE OF FIRST AUTHORISATION/RENEWAL OF THE AUTHORISATION

16 April 2004

10. DATE OF REVISION OF THE TEXT

22 February 2005

11. LEGAL CLASSIFICATION

POM

Amaryl

(sanofi-aventis)

1. NAME OF THE MEDICINAL PRODUCT

Amaryl 1mg, tablet

Amaryl 2mg, tablet

Amaryl 3mg, tablet

Amaryl 4mg, tablet

2. QUALITATIVE AND QUANTITATIVE COMPOSITION

Each tablet contains 1 or 2 or 3 or 4mg glimepiride.

For excipients see 6.1.

3. PHARMACEUTICAL FORM

Tablet.

The tablets are oblong and scored on both sides. Amaryl 1mg is pink, Amaryl 2mg is green, Amaryl 3mg is pale yellow and Amaryl 4mg is light blue.

4. CLINICAL PARTICULARS

4.1 Therapeutic indications

Amaryl is indicated for the treatment of type 2 diabetes mellitus, when diet, physical exercise and weight reduction alone are not adequate.

4.2 Posology and method of administration

The basis for successful treatment of diabetes is a good diet, regular physical activity, as well as routine checks of blood and urine. Tablets or insulin cannot compensate if the patient does not keep to the recommended diet.

Dosage is determined by the results of blood and urinary glucose determinations.

The starting dose is 1 mg glimepiride per day. If good control is achieved this dosage should be used for maintenance therapy.

If control is unsatisfactory the dosage should be increased, based on the glycaemic control, in a stepwise manner with an interval of about 1 to 2 weeks between each step, to 2, 3 or 4 mg glimepiride per day.

A dosage of more than 4 mg glimepiride per day gives better results only in exceptional cases. The maximum recommended dose is 6 mg glimepiride per day.

In patients not adequately controlled with the maximum daily dose of metformin, concomitant glimepiride therapy can be initiated. While maintaining the metformin dose, glimepiride therapy is started with a low dose, and is then titrated up depending on the desired level of metabolic control up to the maximum daily dose. The combination therapy should be initiated under close medical supervision.

In patients not adequately controlled with the maximum daily dose of Amaryl, concomitant insulin therapy can be initiated if necessary. While maintaining the glimepiride dose, insulin treatment is started at low dose and titrated up depending on the desired level of metabolic control. The combination therapy should be initiated under close medical supervision.

Normally a single daily dose of glimepiride is sufficient. It is recommended that this dose be taken shortly before or during a substantial breakfast or - if none is taken - shortly before or during the first main meal.

If a dose is forgotten, this should not be corrected by increasing the next dose.

Tablets should be swallowed whole with some liquid.

If a patient has a hypoglycaemic reaction on 1 mg glimepiride daily, this indicates that they can be controlled by diet alone.

In the course of treatment, as an improvement in control of diabetes is associated with higher insulin sensitivity, glimepiride requirements may fall. To avoid hypoglycaemia timely dose reduction or cessation of therapy must therefore be considered. Change in dosage may also be necessary, if there are changes in weight or life style of the patient, or other factors that increase the risk of hypo- or hyperglycaemia.

Switch over from other oral hypoglycaemic agents to Amaryl:

A switch over from other oral hypoglycaemic agents to Amaryl can generally be done. For the switch over to Amaryl the strength and the half life of the previous medication has to be taken into account. In some cases, especially in antidiabetics with a long half life (e.g. chlorpropamide), a wash out period of a few days is advisable in order to minimise the risk of hypoglycaemic reactions due to the additive effect. The recommended starting dose is 1 mg glimepiride per day. Based on the response the glimepiride dosage may be increased stepwise, as indicated earlier.

Switch over from Insulin to Amaryl:

In exceptional cases, where type 2 diabetic patients are regulated on insulin, a changeover to Amaryl may be indicated. The changeover should be undertaken under close medical supervision.

Use in renal or hepatic impairment:

See section 4.3 Contraindications.

4.3 Contraindications

Amaryl should not be used in the following cases: insulin dependent diabetes, diabetic coma, ketoacidosis, severe renal or hepatic function disorders, hypersensitivity to glimepiride, other sulphonylureas or sulphonamides or excipients in the tablet.

In case of severe renal or hepatic function disorders, a change over to insulin is required.

Amaryl is contra-indicated in pregnancy and lactation.

4.4 Special warnings and special precautions for use

Amaryl must be taken shortly before or during a meal.

When meals are taken at irregular hours or skipped altogether, treatment with Amaryl may lead to hypoglycaemia. Possible symptoms of hypoglycaemia include: headache, ravenous hunger, nausea, vomiting, lassitude, sleepiness, disordered sleep, restlessness, aggressiveness, impaired concentration, alertness and reaction time, depression, confusion, speech and visual disorders, aphasia, tremor, paresis, sensory disturbances, dizziness, helplessness, loss of self-control, delirium, cerebral convulsions, somnolence and loss of consciousness up to and including coma, shallow respiration and bradycardia.

In addition, signs of adrenergic counter-regulation may be present such as sweating, clammy skin, anxiety, tachycardia, hypertension, palpitations, angina pectoris and cardiac arrhythmias.

The clinical picture of a severe hypoglycaemic attack may resemble that of a stroke. Symptoms can almost always be promptly controlled by immediate intake of carbohydrates (sugar). Artificial sweeteners have no effect.

It is known from other sulphonylureas that, despite initially successful countermeasures, hypoglycaemia may recur.

Severe hypoglycaemia or prolonged hypoglycaemia, only temporarily controlled by the usual amounts of sugar, require immediate medical treatment and occasionally hospitalisation.

Factors favouring hypoglycaemia include:

- unwillingness or (more commonly in older patients) incapacity of the patient to cooperate,
- under nutrition, irregular mealtimes or missed meals or periods of fasting,
- alterations in diet,
- imbalance between physical exertion and carbohydrate intake,
- consumption of alcohol, especially in combination with skipped meals,
- impaired renal function,
- serious liver dysfunction,
- over dosage with Amaryl,
- certain uncompensated disorders of the endocrine system affecting carbohydrate metabolism or counter regulation of hypoglycaemia (as for example in certain disorders of thyroid function and in anterior pituitary or adrenocortical insufficiency),
- concurrent administration of certain other medicines (see "Interactions").

Treatment with Amaryl requires regular monitoring of glucose levels in blood and urine. In addition determination of the proportion of glycosylated haemoglobin is recommended.

Regular hepatic and haematological monitoring (especially leucocytes and thrombocytes) are required during treatment with Amaryl.

In stress-situations (e.g. accidents, acute operations, infections with fever, etc.) a temporary switch to insulin may be indicated.

No experience has been gained concerning the use of Amaryl in patients with severe impairment of liver function or dialysis patients. In patients with severe impairment of renal or liver function change over to insulin is indicated.

4.5 Interaction with other medicinal products and other forms of Interaction

If Amaryl is taken simultaneously with certain other medicines, both undesired increases and decreases in the hypoglycaemic action of glimepiride can occur. For this reason, other medicines should only be taken with the knowledge (or at the prescription) of the doctor.

Glimepiride is metabolised by cytochrome P450 2CY (CYP2C9). Its metabolism is known to be influenced by concomitant administration of CYP2C9 inducers (e.g. rifampicin) or inhibitors (e.g. fluconazole).

Results from an *in-vivo* interaction study reported in literature show that Glimepiride AUC is increased approximately 2-fold by fluconazole, one of the most potent CYP2C9 inhibitors.

Based on the experience with Amaryl and with other sulphonylureas the following interactions have to be mentioned.

Potentiation of the blood-glucose-lowering effect and, thus, in some instances hypoglycaemia may occur when one of the following drugs is taken, for example:

phenylbutazone, azapropazon and oxyfenbutazone	sulphinpyrazone
insulin and oral antidiabetic products	certain long acting sulphonamides
metformin	tetracyclines
salicylates and p-amino-salicylic acid	MAO-inhibitors
anabolic steroids and male sex hormones	quinolone antibiotics
chloramphenicol	probenecid
coumarin anticoagulants	miconazol
fenfluramine	pentoxifylline (high dose parenteral)
fibrates	tritoqualine
ACE inhibitors	fluconazole
fluoxetine	
allopurinol	
sympatholytics	
cyclo-, tro- and iphosphamides	

Weakening of the blood-glucose-lowering effect and, thus raised blood glucose levels may occur when one of the following drugs is taken, for example:

- oestrogens and progestagens,
- saluretics, thiazide diuretics,
- thyroid stimulating agents, glucocorticoids,
- phenothiazine derivatives, chlorpromazine,
- adrenaline and sympathicomimetics,
- nicotinic acid (high dosages) and nicotinic acid derivatives,
- laxatives (long term use),
- phenytoin, diazoxide,
- glucagon, barbiturates and rifampicin,
- acetozolamide.

H_2 antagonists, beta blockers, clonidine and reserpine may lead to either potentiation or weakening of the blood glucose lowering effect.

Under the influence of sympatholytic drugs such as beta-blockers, clonidine, guanethidine and reserpine, the signs of adrenergic counter regulation to hypoglycaemia may be reduced or absent.

Alcohol intake may potentiate or weaken the hypoglycaemic action of glimepiride in an unpredictable fashion.

Glimepiride may either potentiate or weaken the effects of coumarin derivatives.

4.6 Pregnancy and lactation

Pregnancy

Amaryl is contra-indicated during pregnancy. The use of insulin is required under such circumstances. Patients who consider pregnancy should inform their physician.

Lactation

Because sulphonylurea derivatives like glimepiride pass into the breast milk, Amaryl must not be taken by breast-feeding women.

4.7 Effects on ability to drive and use machines

The patient's ability to concentrate and react may be impaired as a result of hypoglycaemia or hyperglycaemia or, for example, as a result of visual impairment. This may constitute a risk in situations where these abilities are of special importance (e.g. driving a car or operating machinery).

Patients should be advised to take precautions to avoid hypoglycaemia whilst driving. This is particularly important in those who have reduced or absent awareness of the warning symptoms of hypoglycaemia or have frequent episodes of hypoglycaemia. It should be considered whether it is advisable to drive or operate machinery in these circumstances.

4.8 Undesirable effects

Based on experience with Amaryl and with other sulphonylureas the following side effects have to be mentioned.

Immune system disorders

In very rare cases mild hypersensitivity reactions may develop into serious reactions with dyspnoea, fall in blood pressure and sometimes shock. Allergic vasculitis is possible in very rare cases.

Cross allergenicity with sulphonylureas, sulphonamides or related substances is possible.

Blood and lymphatic system disorders

Changes in haematology are rare during Amaryl treatment. Moderate to severe thrombocytopenia, leucopenia, erythrocytopenia, granulocytopenia, agranulocytosis, haemolytic anaemia and pancytopenia may occur.

These are in general reversible upon discontinuation of medication.

Metabolism and nutrition disorders

In rare cases hypoglycaemic reactions have been observed after administration of Amaryl. These reactions mostly occur immediately, may be severe and are not always easy to correct. The occurrence of such reactions depends, as with other hypoglycaemic therapies, on individual factors such as dietary habits and the dosage (see further under "Special warnings and special precautions for use").

Eye disorders

Transient visual disturbances may occur especially on initiation of treatment, due to changes in blood glucose levels.

Gastrointestinal disorders

Gastrointestinal complaints like nausea, vomiting and diarrhoea, pressure or a feeling of fullness in the stomach and abdominal pain are very rare and seldom lead to discontinuation of therapy.

Hepato-biliary disorders

Elevation of liver enzymes may occur. In very rare cases, impairment of liver function (e.g. with cholestasis and jaundice) may develop, as well as hepatitis which may progress to liver failure.

Skin and subcutaneous tissue disorders

Hypersensitivity reactions of the skin may occur as itching, rash and urticaria.

In very rare cases hypersensitivity to light may occur.

Investigations

In very rare cases, a decrease in the sodium serum concentrations may occur.

4.9 Overdose

After ingestion of an overdosage hypoglycaemia may occur, lasting from 12 to 72 hours, and may recur after an initial recovery. Symptoms may not be present for up to 24 hours after ingestion. In general observation in hospital is recommended. Nausea, vomiting and epigastric pain may occur. The hypoglycaemia may in general be accompanied by neurological symptoms like restlessness, tremor, visual disturbances, co-ordination problems, sleepiness, coma and convulsions.

Treatment primarily consists of preventing absorption by inducing vomiting and then drinking water or lemonade with activated charcoal (adsorbent) and sodium-sulphate (laxative). If large quantities have been ingested, gastric lavage is indicated, followed by activated charcoal and sodium-sulphate. In case of (severe) overdosage hospitalisation in an intensive care department is indicated. Start the administration of glucose as soon as possible, if necessary by a bolus intravenous injection of 50 ml of a 50% solution, followed by an infusion of a 10% solution with strict monitoring of blood glucose. Further treatment should be symptomatic.

In particular when treating hypoglycaemia due to accidental intake of Amaryl in infants and young children, the dose of glucose given must be carefully controlled to avoid the possibility of producing dangerous hyperglycaemia. Blood glucose should be closely monitored.

5. PHARMACOLOGICAL PROPERTIES

5.1 Pharmacodynamic properties

Pharmacotherapeutic group: Oral blood glucose lowering drugs: Sulfonamides, urea derivatives. ATC Code: A10B B12.

Glimepiride is an orally active hypoglycaemic substance belonging to the sulphonylurea group. It may be used in non-insulin dependent diabetes mellitus.

Glimepiride acts mainly by stimulating insulin release from pancreatic beta cells.

As with other sulphonylureas this effect is based on an increase of responsiveness of the pancreatic beta cells to the physiological glucose stimulus. In addition, glimepiride seems to have pronounced extrapancreatic effects also postulated for other sulphonylureas.

<u>**Insulin release:**</u>

Sulphonylureas regulate insulin secretion by closing the ATP-sensitive potassium channel in the beta cell membrane. Closing the potassium channel induces depolarisation of the beta cell and results - by opening of calcium channels - in an increased influx of calcium into the cell.

This leads to insulin release through exocytosis.

Glimepiride binds with a high exchange rate to a beta cell membrane protein which is associated with the ATP-sensitive potassium channel but which is different from the usual sulphonylurea binding site.

<u>**Extrapancreatic activity:**</u>

The extrapancreatic effects are for example an improvement of the sensitivity of the peripheral tissue for insulin and a decrease of the insulin uptake by the liver.

The uptake of glucose from blood into peripheral muscle and fat tissues occurs via special transport proteins, located in the cells membrane. The transport of glucose in these tissues is the rate limiting step in the use of glucose. Glimepiride increases very rapidly the number of active glucose transport molecules in the plasma membranes of muscle and fat cells, resulting in stimulated glucose uptake.

Glimepiride increases the activity of the glycosyl-phosphatidylinositol-specific phospholipase C which may be correlated with the drug-induced lipogenesis and glycogenesis in isolated fat and muscle cells.

Glimepiride inhibits the glucose production in the liver by increasing the intracellular concentration of fructose-2,6-bisphosphate, which in its turn inhibits the gluconeogenesis.

General

In healthy persons, the minimum effective oral dose is approximately 0.6 mg. The effect of glimepiride is dose-dependent and reproducible. The physiological response to acute physical exercise, reduction of insulin secretion, is still present under glimepiride.

There was no significant difference in effect regardless of whether the drug was given 30 minutes or immediately before a meal. In diabetic patients, good metabolic control over 24 hours can be achieved with a single daily dose.

Although the hydroxy metabolite of glimepiride caused a small but significant decrease in serum glucose in healthy persons, it accounts for only a minor part of the total drug effect.

Combination therapy with metformin

Improved metabolic control for concomitant glimepiride therapy compared to metformin alone in patients not adequately controlled with the maximum daily dosage of metformin has been shown in one study.

Combination therapy with insulin

Data for combination therapy with insulin are limited. In patients not adequately controlled with the maximum dosage of glimepiride, concomitant insulin therapy can be initiated. In two studies, the combination achieved the same improvement in metabolic control as insulin alone; however, a lower average dose of insulin was required in combination therapy.

5.2 Pharmacokinetic properties

Absorption: The bioavailability of glimepiride after oral administration is complete. Food intake has no relevant influence on absorption, only absorption rate is slightly diminished. Maximum serum concentrations (C_{max}) are reached approx. 2.5 hours after oral intake (mean 0.3 μg/ml during multiple dosing of 4 mg daily) and there is a linear relationship between dose and both C_{max} and AUC (area under the time/concentration curve).

Distribution: Glimepiride has a very low distribution volume (approx. 8.8 litres) which is roughly equal to the albumin distribution space, high protein binding (>99%), and a low clearance (approx. 48 ml/min).

In animals, glimepiride is excreted in milk. Glimepiride is transferred to the placenta. Passage of the blood brain barrier is low.

Biotransformation and elimination: Mean dominant serum half-life, which is of relevance for the serum concentrations under multiple-dose conditions, is about 5 to 8 hours. After high doses, slightly longer half-lives were noted.

After a single dose of radiolabelled glimepiride, 58% of the radioactivity was recovered in the urine, and 35% in the faeces. No unchanged substance was detected in the urine. Two metabolites - most probably resulting from hepatic metabolism (major enzyme is CYP2C9) - were identified both in urine and faeces: the hydroxy derivative and the carboxy derivative. After oral administration of glimepiride, the terminal half-lives of these metabolites were 3 to 6 and 5 to 6 hours respectively.

Comparison of single and multiple once-daily dosing revealed no significant differences in pharmacokinetics, and the intra individual variability was very low. There was no relevant accumulation.

Pharmacokinetics were similar in males and females, as well as in young and elderly (above 65 years) patients. In patients with low creatinine clearance, there was a tendency for glimepiride clearance to increase and for average serum concentrations to decrease, most probably resulting from a more rapid elimination because of lower protein binding. Renal elimination of the two metabolites was impaired. Overall no additional risk of accumulation is to be assumed in such patients.

Pharmacokinetics in five non-diabetic patients after bile duct surgery were similar to those in healthy persons.

5.3 Preclinical safety data

Preclinical effects observed occurred at exposures sufficiently in excess of the maximum human exposure as to indicate little relevance to clinical use, or were due to the pharmacodynamic action (hypoglycaemia) of the compound. This finding is based on conventional safety pharmacology, repeated dose toxicity, genotoxicity, carcinogenicity, and reproduction toxicity studies. In the latter (covering embryotoxicity, teratogenicity and developmental toxicity), adverse effects observed were considered to be secondary to the hypoglycaemic effects induced by the compound in dams and in offspring.

6. PHARMACEUTICAL PARTICULARS

6.1 List of excipients

Lactose

sodium starch glycollate

magnesium stearate

microcrystallinecellulose

povidone 25000

Further as colouring agents:

Amaryl 1 mg: red iron oxide (E172)

Amaryl 2 mg: yellow iron oxide (E172), indigo-carmine aluminium lake (E132)

Amaryl 3 mg: yellow iron oxide (E172)

Amaryl 4 mg: indigo-carmine aluminium lake (E132)

6.2 Incompatibilities

Not applicable.

6.3 Shelf life

1, 2, 3, and 4 mg: 3 years.

6.4 Special precautions for storage

Do not store above 25°C.

In order to protect from moisture store in the original package.

6.5 Nature and contents of container

PVC/Aluminium blisters

30 tablets Amaryl (in blister packs of 10 tablets each).

6.6 Instructions for use and handling

No special information.

7. MARKETING AUTHORISATION HOLDER

Hoechst Marion Roussel Limited

Broadwater Park

Denham

Uxbridge

Middlesex UB9 5HP

8. MARKETING AUTHORISATION NUMBER(S)

Amaryl Tablets, 1mg: PL 13402/0006

Amaryl Tablets, 2mg: PL 13402/0007

Amaryl Tablets, 3mg: PL 13402/0008

Amaryl Tablets, 4mg: PL 13402/0009

9. DATE OF FIRST AUTHORISATION/RENEWAL OF THE AUTHORISATION

8 November 1996

10. DATE OF REVISION OF THE TEXT

July 2004

11. Legal Category

POM

Ambisome

(Gilead Sciences International Limited)

1. NAME OF THE MEDICINAL PRODUCT

AmBisome Injection (liposomal amphotericin).

2. QUALITATIVE AND QUANTITATIVE COMPOSITION

AmBisome is a sterile lyophilized product for intravenous infusion. Each vial contains 50 mg of amphotericin (50,000 units) encapsulated in liposomes. For excipients, see Section 6.1.

Amphotericin B has a molecular weight of 924.10 and is represented by the formula and structure shown below:

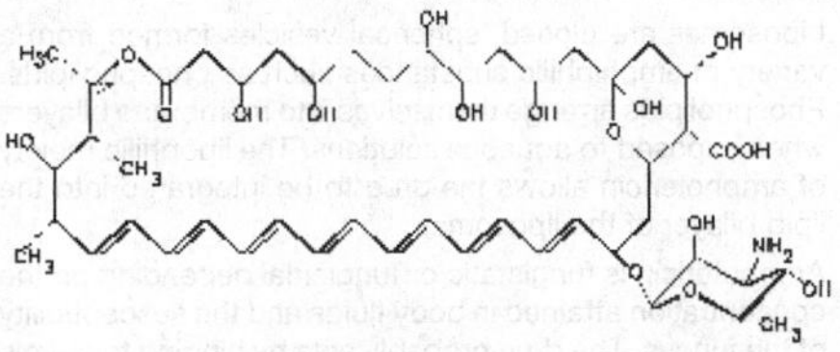

$C_{47}H_{73}NO_{17}$

3. PHARMACEUTICAL FORM

AmBisome is a sterile, lyophilized product for intravenous infusion. After reconstitution, the product is an injectable intended to be administered by intravenous infusion.

4. CLINICAL PARTICULARS

4.1 Therapeutic indications

AmBisome is indicated in:

the treatment of severe systemic and/or deep mycoses where toxicity (particularly nephrotoxicity) precludes the use of conventional systemic amphotericin B in effective dosages.

the treatment of visceral leishmaniasis in immunocompetent patients including both adults and children.

the empirical treatment of presumed fungal infections in febrile neutropenic patients, where the fever has failed to respond to broad spectrum antibiotics and appropriate investigations have failed to define a bacterial or viral cause.

Infections successfully treated with AmBisome include: disseminated candidiasis, aspergillosis, mucormycosis, chronic mycetoma, cryptococcal meningitis and visceral leishmaniasis.

This drug should not be used to treat the common clinically in apparent forms of fungal disease which show only positive skin or serologic tests.

4.2 Posology and method of administration

AmBisome should be administered by intravenous infusion over a 30 - 60 minute period. The recommended concentration for intravenous infusion is 0.20 mg/ml to 2.00 mg/ml amphotericin as AmBisome. AmBisome therapy has been administered for as long as three months, with a cumulative dose of 16.8 g of amphotericin as AmBisome without significant toxicity.

Treatment of mycoses:

Therapy is usually instituted at a daily dose of 1.0 mg/kg of body weight, and increased stepwise to 3.0 mg/kg, as required. Data are presently insufficient to define total dosage requirements and duration of treatment necessary for resolution of mycoses. However, a cumulative dose of 1.0 - 3.0 g of amphotericin as AmBisome over 3 - 4 weeks has been typical. Dosage of amphotericin as AmBisome must be adjusted to the specific requirements of each patient.

Treatment of visceral leishmaniasis:

A total dose of 21.0 - 30.0 mg/kg of body weight given over 10 -21 days may be used in the treatment of visceral leishmaniasis. Particulars as to the optimal dosage and the eventual development of resistance are as yet incomplete. The product should be administered under strict medical supervision.

Empirical treatment of febrile neutropenia:

The recommended daily dose is 3 mg/kg body weight per day. Treatment should be continued until the recorded temperature is normalised for 3 consecutive days. In any event, treatment should be discontinued after a maximum of 42 days.

Paediatric Patients: Both systemic fungal infections in children and presumed fungal infections in children with febrile neutropenia have been successfully treated with

AmBisome, without reports of unusual adverse events. Paediatric patients have received

AmBisome at doses comparable to those used in adults on a per kilogram body weight basis.

Elderly Patients: No specific dosage recommendations or precautions.

Renal Impairment: AmBisome has been successfully administered to a large number of patients with pre-existing renal impairment at starting doses ranging from 1-3 mg/kg/day in clinical trials, and no adjustment in dose or frequency of administration was required.

4.3 Contraindications

AmBisome is contraindicated in those patients who have shown hypersensitivity to any of its constituents unless, in the opinion of the physician, the condition requiring treatment is life-threatening and amenable only to AmBisome therapy.

4.4 Special warnings and special precautions for use

Anaphylaxis has been reported rarely in association with AmBisome infusion. Allergic type reactions, including severe infusion-related reactions can occur during administration of amphotericin -containing products, including AmBisome. Therefore, administration of a test dose is still advisable before a new course of treatment. For this purpose a small amount of an AmBisome infusion (e.g. 1 mg) can be administered for about 10 minutes, the infusion stopped and the patient observed carefully for the next 30 minutes. If there have been no severe allergic or anaphylactic reactions the infusion of AmBisome dose can be continued. If a severe allergic or anaphylactic reaction occurs, the patient should not receive further infusions of AmBisome.

Although infusion-related reactions are not usually serious, consideration of precautionary measures for the prevention or treatment of these reactions should be given to patients who receive AmBisome therapy. Slower infusion rates or routine doses of diphenhydramine, paracetamol, pethidine, and/or hydrocortisone have been reported as successful in their prevention or treatment.

AmBisome has been shown to be substantially less toxic than conventional amphotericin; however, adverse events may still occur. In particular, caution should be exercised when prolonged therapy is required. Laboratory evaluation of renal, hepatic and haematopoietic function should be performed regularly, and at least once weekly. Levels of serum electrolytes, particularly serum potassium and magnesium, should be monitored regularly. Particular attention should be paid to patients receiving concomitant therapy with nephrotoxic drugs. Renal function should be closely monitored in these patients. If clinically significant reduction in renal function or worsening of other parameters occurs, subsequent dosages should be reduced or interrupted on the basis of laboratory measures.

AmBisome may be nephrotoxic despite being tolerated significantly better than other amphotericin products. If the renal function deteriorates significantly during AmBisome therapy, consideration should be given to dose reduction or discontinuation until renal function improves, however, this decision should take into account any concomitant therapy with known nephrotoxic drugs.

In the Treatment of Diabetic Patients: It should be noted that AmBisome contains approximately 900 mg of sucrose in each vial.

4.5 Interaction with other medicinal products and other forms of Interaction

No specific pharmacokinetic interaction studies have been performed with AmBisome. Although no clinically significant interactions of AmBisome with other drugs have been reported in clinical trials, patients requiring concomitant drug therapy should be monitored closely. Conventional amphotericin has been reported to interact with the following drugs:

antineoplastic agents, corticosteroids and corticotrophin (ACTH), digitalis glycosides and skeletal muscle relaxants. Loop diuretics or thiazides and related diuretics increase the risk of hypokalaemia when given with amphotericin.

No evidence of benefit from the use of flucytosine with AmBisome has been observed. Whilst synergy between amphotericin and flucytosine has been reported, amphotericin may enhance the toxicity of flucytosine by increasing its cellular uptake and impeding its renal excretion.

Concurrent administration of AmBisome with other nephrotoxic agents, for example cyclosporine and aminoglycosides, polymixins and tacrolimus may increase the risk of nephrotoxicity in some patients. However, in patients receiving concomitant cyclosporin and/or aminoglycosides, AmBisome was associated with significantly less nephrotoxicity as compared to amphotericin.

4.6 Pregnancy and lactation

Teratogenicity studies in both rats and rabbits have concluded that AmBisome has no teratogenic potential in these species (See also section 5.3).

No reproductive toxicity studies have been conducted with AmBisome in pregnant women. Systemic fungal infections have been successfully treated in pregnant women with conventional amphotericin without obvious effect on the foetus, but the number of cases reported has been small. Safety for use in pregnant women has not been established with AmBisome.

It is not known if AmBisome is excreted in human milk

AmBisome should only be used during pregnancy or breast-feeding if the possible benefits to be derived outweigh the potential risks involved

4.7 Effects on ability to drive and use machines

The effects of AmBisome on the ability to drive and /or use machines have not been investigated. Some of the undesirable effects of AmBisome presented below may impact the ability to drive and use machines, however, the clinical condition of most patients treated with AmBisome precludes driving vehicles or operating machinery.

4.8 Undesirable effects

Fever and chills/rigors are the most frequent infusion-related reactions expected to occur during the first AmBisome dose administration when no premedication to prevent these reactions is provided. In two double-blind, comparative studies, AmBisome treated patients experienced a significantly lower incidence of infusion-related reactions, as compared to patients treated with conventional amphotericin B or amphotericin B lipid complex. Less frequent infusion-related reactions may consist of one or more of the following symptoms including back pain and/or chest tightness or pain, dyspnoea, bronchospasm, flushing, tachycardia, and hypotension, and these resolved rapidly when the infusion was stopped. These reactions may not occur with every subsequent dose or when slower infusion rates (over 2 hours) are used (see Special Warnings and Precautions for Use on prevention or treatment of these reactions).

In pooled study data from randomised, controlled clinical trials comparing AmBisome with conventional amphotericin B therapy in greater than 1,000 patients, reported adverse reactions were considerably less severe and less frequent in AmBisome treated patients as compared with conventional amphotericin B treated patients.

Nephrotoxicity occurs to some degree with conventional amphotericin B, in most patients receiving the drug intravenously. In a double-blind study involving 687 patients, the incidence of nephrotoxicity with AmBisome (as measured by serum creatinine increase greater than 2.0 times baseline measurement), was approximately half that for conventional amphotericin B. In another double-blind study involving 244 patients, the incidence of nephrotoxicity with AmBisome (as measured by serum creatinine increase greater than 2.0 times baseline measurement) was approximately half that for Amphotericin B lipid complex.

The following adverse reactions have been attributed to AmBisome. The incidence is based on analysis from pooled clinical trials of 688 AmBisome treated patients. The adverse reactions are listed below by body system organ class using MedDRA and are sorted by absolute frequency.

Frequencies are defined as:

Very common	$\geqslant$ 10%
Common	$\geqslant$ 1% and < 10%
Uncommon	$\geqslant$ 0.1 % and < 1%
Rare	> 0.01% and <0.1%
Very rare	< 0.01%

Blood and Lymphatic System Disorders

Uncommon: thrombocytopenia

Immune System Disorders

Uncommon: anaphylactoid reaction

Metabolism and Nutrition disorders

Very common: hypokalemia

Common: hypomagnaesemia, hypocalcaemia, hyperglycaemia, hyponatraemia

Nervous System Disorders

Common: headache

Uncommon: convulsion

Cardiac Disorders

Common: tachycardia

Vascular disorders

Common: vasodilatation, flushing, hypotension

Respiratory, thoracic and mediastinal disorders

Common: dyspnoea

Uncommon: bronchospasm

Gastrointestinal Disorders

Very common: nausea, vomiting

Common: diarrhoea, abdominal pain

Hepatobiliary disorders

Common: hyperbilirubinemia

Skin and Subcutaneous Disorders

Common: rash

Musculoskeletal and Connective Tissue Disorders

Common: back pain

General Disorders and Administration Site Conditions

Very Common: pyrexia, rigors

Common: chest pain

Investigations

Common: increased creatinine, blood urea increased, alkaline phosphatase increased, liver function tests abnormal

In addition to adverse reaction reports from clinical trials, the following possible adverse reactions have also been identified during post-marketing use of AmBisome.

Immune System Disorders

Very Rare: anaphylactic reactions, hypersensitivity

Skin and Subcutaneous Disorders

Very rare: angioneurotic oedema

Renal and Urinary Disorders

Very rare: renal failure, renal insufficiency.

4.9 Overdose

The toxicity of AmBisome due to overdose has not been defined. Repeated daily doses up to 10 mg/kg in paediatric patients and 15 mg/kg in adult patients have been administered in clinical trials with no reported dose dependent toxicity. If overdose should occur, cease administration immediately. Carefully monitor clinical status including renal and hepatic function, serum electrolytes and haematological status. Haemodialysis or peritoneal dialysis does not appear to affect the elimination of AmBisome.

5. PHARMACOLOGICAL PROPERTIES

5.1 Pharmacodynamic properties

Amphotericin is a macrocyclic, polyene antifungal antibiotic produced by *Streptomyces nodosus.*

Liposomes are closed, spherical vesicles formed from a variety of amphiphilic substances such as phospholipids. Phospholipids arrange themselves into membrane bilayers when exposed to aqueous solutions. The lipophilic moiety of amphotericin allows the drug to be integrated into the lipid bilayer of the liposomes.

Amphotericin is fungistatic or fungicidal depending on the concentration attained in body fluids and the susceptibility of the fungus. The drug probably acts by binding to sterols in the fungal cell membrane, with a resultant change in membrane permeability, allowing leakage of a variety of small molecules. Mammalian cell membranes also contain sterols, and it has been suggested that the damage to human cells and fungal cells caused by amphotericin B may share common mechanisms.

Microbiology: Amphotericin, the antifungal component of AmBisome, shows a high order of in vitro activity against many species of fungi. Most strains of *Histoplasma capsulatum, Coccidioides immitis, Candida spp., Blastomyces dermatitidis, Rhodotorula, Cryptococcus neoformans, Sporothrix schenkii, Mucor mucedo* and *Aspergillus fumigatus,* are inhibited by concentrations of amphotericin ranging from 0.03 to 1.0 mcg/ml in vitro. Amphotericin has minimal or no effect on bacteria and viruses.

5.2 Pharmacokinetic properties

The pharmacokinetic profile of AmBisome, based upon total plasma concentrations of amphotericin B, was determined in cancer patients with febrile neutropenia and bone marrow transplant patients who received 1 hour infusions of 1.0 to 7.5mg/kg/day AmBisome for 3 to 20 days. AmBisome has a significantly different pharmacokinetic profile from that reported in the literature for conventional presentations of amphotericin B, with higher amphotericin B plasma concentrations (Cmax) and increased exposure (AUC_{0-24}) following administration of AmBisome as compared to conventional amphotericin B. After the first dose and last dose, the pharmacokinetic parameters of AmBisome (mean ± standard deviation) ranged from:

C max	7.3 μg/ml (± 3.8) to 83.7 μg/ml (± 43.0)
$T_{1/2}$	6.3 hr (± 2.0) to 10.7 hr (± 6.4)
AUC_{0-24}	27 μg.hr/ml (±14) to 555 μg.hr/ml (± 311)
Clearance (Cl)	11 ml/hr/kg (± 6) to 51 ml/hr/kg (± 44)
Volume of distribution (Vss)	0.10 L/kg (± 0.07) to 0.44 L/kg (±0.27)

Minimum and maximum pharmacokinetic values do not necessarily come from the lowest and highest doses, respectively. Following administration of AmBisome steady state was reached quickly (generally within 4 days of dosing). AmBisome pharmacokinetics following the first dose appear non-linear such that serum AmBisome concentrations are greater than proportional with increasing dose. This non-proportional dose response is believed to be due to saturation of reticuloendothelial AmBisome clearance. There was no significant drug accumulation in the plasma following repeated administration of 1 to 7.5mg/kg/day. Volume of distribution on day 1 and at steady state suggests that there is extensive tissue distribution of AmBisome. After repeated administration of AmBisome, the terminal elimination half-life ($t_{1/2\beta}$) for AmBisome was approximately 7 hours. The excretion of AmBisome has not been studied. The metabolic pathways of amphotericin B and AmBisome are not known. Due to the size of the liposomes, there is no glomerular filtration and renal elimination of AmBisome, thus avoiding interaction of amphotericin B with the cells of the distal tubuli and reducing the potential for nephrotoxicity seen with conventional amphotericin B presentations.

Renal Impairment

The effect of renal impairment on the pharmacokinetics of AmBisome has not been formally studied. Data suggest that no dose adjustment is required in patients undergoing haemodialysis or filtration procedures, however, AmBisome administration should be avoided during the procedure.

5.3 Preclinical safety data

In subchronic toxicity studies in dogs (1 month), rabbits (1 month) and rats (3 months) at systemic exposure levels similar to or less than the exposure seen in man at therapeutic doses, the target organs for AmBisome toxicity were the liver and kidneys with thrombocytopenia also observed. All are known targets for amphotericin B toxicity.

Neither amphotericin B nor AmBisome was mutagenic in *in vitro* systems, and AmBisome gave a negative result in a mouse micronucleus test

Carcinogenicity studies have not been conducted with AmBisome.

No adverse effects on male or female reproductive function were noted in rats and no foetal developmental toxicity was noted in teratogenicity studies in rats and rabbits.

6. PHARMACEUTICAL PARTICULARS

6.1 List of excipients

Hydrogenated soy phosphatidylcholine, cholesterol, distearoylphosphatidylglycerol, alpha tocopherol, sucrose, disodium succinate hexahydrate, sodium hydroxide and hydrochloric acid.

6.2 Incompatibilities

AmBisome is incompatible with saline solutions and may not be mixed with other drugs or electrolytes.

6.3 Shelf life

36 months.

Shelf -life of AmBisome after first opening

As AmBisome does not contain any bacteriostatic agent, from a microbiological point of view, the reconstituted or diluted product should be used immediately.

In-use storage times and conditions prior to administration are the responsibility of the user and would normally not be longer than 24 hours at 2-8°C, unless reconstitution has taken place in controlled and validated aseptic conditions.

However, the following chemical and physical in-use stability data for AmBisome has been demonstrated:

- **Shelf-life after reconstitution:**

Glass vials for 24 hours at 25±2°C exposed to ambient light

Glass vials and polypropylene syringes up to 7 days at 2-8°C

- **Shelf-life after dilution with Dextrose:**

PVC or Polyolefin infusion bags: see table below for recommendations

(see Table 1 on next page)

6.4 Special precautions for storage

AmBisome: Unopened vials; Do not store above 25°C. Do not freeze. Keep container in the outer carton.

Reconstituted Concentrate:

Glass vials at 25±2°C exposed to ambient light

Glass vials and polypropylene syringes: 2-8°C. Do not freeze

DO NOT STORE partially used vials for future patient use

Diluted with Dextrose:

PVC or Polyolefin infusion bags: 25±2°C exposed to ambient light or at 2-8°C. Do not freeze.

6.5 Nature and contents of container

AmBisome is presented in 15 ml or 30ml sterile, Type I glass vials. The currently marketed presentation is the 15ml vial. The closure consists of a grey butyl rubber stopper and aluminium ring seal fitted with a removable plastic cap. Single-dose vials are packed ten per carton with 10 filters.

6.6 Instructions for use and handling

READ THIS ENTIRE SECTION CAREFULLY BEFORE BEGINNING RECONSTITUTION

Table 1

Diluent	Dilution	Concentration of Amphotericin B mg/mL	Maximum duration of storage at 2-8°C	Maximum duration of storage at 25±2°C
5% Dextrose	1:2	2.0	7 days	48 hours
	1:8	0.5	7 days	48 hours
	1:20	0.2	4 days	24 hours
10% Dextrose	1:2	2.0	48 hours	72 hours
20% Dextrose	1:2	2.0	48 hours	72 hours

AmBisome Must Be Reconstituted By Suitably Trained Staff

AmBisome must be reconstituted using Sterile Water for Injection **(without a bacteriostatic agent).**

Vials of AmBisome Containing 50 mg of Amphotericin are Prepared as Follows:

1. Add 12 ml of Sterile Water for Injection to each AmBisome vial, to yield a preparation containing 4 mg/ml amphotericin.
2. IMMEDIATELY after the addition of water, SHAKE THE VIAL VIGOROUSLY for 30 seconds to completely disperse the AmBisome. Visually inspect the vial for particulate matter and continue shaking until complete dispersion is obtained.
3. Calculate the amount of reconstituted (4 mg/ml) AmBisome to be further diluted.
4. The infusion solution is obtained by dilution of the reconstituted AmBisome with between one (1) and nineteen (19) parts Dextrose Injection by volume, to give a final concentration in the recommended range of 2.00 mg/ml to 0.20 mg/ml amphotericin as AmBisome.
5. Withdraw the calculated volume of reconstituted AmBisome into a sterile syringe. Using the 5 micron filter provided, instill the AmBisome preparation into a sterile container with the correct amount of Dextrose Injection.

Do not reconstitute the lyophilized powder/cake with saline or add saline to the reconstituted concentrate, or mix with other drugs.

Use only Water for Injection to reconstitute the powder/cake. Use only 5% Dextrose Injection to dilute the reconstituted product to the appropriate concentration for infusion.

Aseptic technique must be strictly observed in all handling, since no preservative or bacteriostatic agent is present in AmBisome, or in the materials specified for reconstitution and dilution. The use of any solution other than those recommended, or the presence of a bacteriostatic agent (e.g. benzyl alcohol) in the solution, may cause precipitation of AmBisome. Do not use material if there is any evidence of precipitation of foreign matter.

An in-line membrane filter may be used for intravenous infusion of AmBisome. However, **the mean pore diameter of the filter should not be less than 1.0 micron.**

Note: AmBisome is not physically compatible with saline solutions and should not be mixed with other drugs or electrolytes. An existing intravenous line must be flushed with 5% Dextrose Injection prior to infusion of AmBisome. If this is not feasible, AmBisome should be administered through a separate line.

7. MARKETING AUTHORISATION HOLDER

Gilead Sciences International Limited,
Granta Park,
Abington,
Cambridge,
CB1 6GT.

8. MARKETING AUTHORISATION NUMBER(S)

PL: 16807/0001.

9. DATE OF FIRST AUTHORISATION/RENEWAL OF THE AUTHORISATION

11 September 1998/24 September 2004.

10. DATE OF REVISION OF THE TEXT

29 April 2005.

Amias Tablets

(Takeda UK Ltd)

1. NAME OF THE MEDICINAL PRODUCT

Amias 2 mg Tablets.
Amias 4 mg Tablets.
Amias 8 mg Tablets.
Amias 16 mg Tablets.
Amias 32 mg Tablets.

2. QUALITATIVE AND QUANTITATIVE COMPOSITION

Each tablet contains 2 mg candesartan cilexetil.
Each tablet contains 4 mg candesartan cilexetil.
Each tablet contains 8 mg candesartan cilexetil.
Each tablet contains 16 mg candesartan cilexetil.
Each tablet contains 32 mg candesartan cilexetil.
For excipients, see 6.1.

3. PHARMACEUTICAL FORM

Tablet.

Amias 2 mg Tablets are round white tablets.

Amias 4 mg Tablets are round white tablets with a single score line on both sides.

Amias 8 mg Tablets are round pale pink tablets with a single score line on both sides.

Amias 16 mg Tablets are round light pink tablets with one convex side and one scored flat side, embossing 16 on scored convex side.

Amias 32 mg Tablets are round light pink tablets with convex faces, debossed 32 on one face.

4. CLINICAL PARTICULARS

4.1 Therapeutic indications

Essential hypertension.

Treatment of patients with heart failure and impaired left ventricle systolic function (left ventricular ejection fraction ⩽ 40%) as add-on therapy to ACE-inhibitors or when ACE-inhibitors are not tolerated (see section 5.1 Pharmacodynamic properties).

4.2 Posology and method of administration

Dosage in Hypertension

The recommended initial dose and usual maintenance dose is 8 mg once daily. The dose may be increased to 16 mg once daily. If blood pressure is not sufficiently controlled after 4 weeks of treatment with 16 mg once daily, the dose may be further increased to a maximum of 32 mg once daily (see section 5.1 Pharmacodynamic properties). If blood pressure control is not achieved with this dose, alternative strategies should be considered.

Therapy should be adjusted according to blood pressure response. Most of the antihypertensive effect is attained within 4 weeks of initiation of treatment.

Use in the elderly

No initial dosage adjustment is necessary in elderly patients.

Use in patients with intravascular volume depletion

An initial dose of 4 mg may be considered in patients at risk for hypotension, such as patients with possible volume depletion (see also 4.4 Special warnings and special precautions for use).

Use in impaired renal function

The starting dose is 4 mg in patients with renal impairment, including patients on haemodialysis. The dose should be titrated according to response. There is limited experience in patients with very severe or end-stage renal impairment ($Cl_{creatinine}$ < 15 ml/min). See section 4.4 special warnings and special precautions for use.

Use in impaired hepatic function

An initial dose of 2 mg once daily is recommended in patients with mild to moderate hepatic impairment. The dose may be adjusted according to response. There is no experience in patients with severe hepatic impairment.

Concomitant therapy

Addition of a thiazide-type diuretic such as hydrochlorothiazide has been shown to have an additive antihypertensive effect with Amias.

Dosage in Heart Failure

The usual recommended initial dose of Amias is 4 mg once daily. Up-titration to the target dose of 32 mg once daily or the highest tolerated dose is done by doubling the dose at intervals of at least 2 weeks (see section 4.4 Special warnings and special precautions for use).

Special patient populations

No initial dose adjustment is necessary for elderly patients or in patients with intravascular volume depletion, renal impairment or mild to moderate hepatic impairment.

Concomitant therapy

Amias can be administered with other heart failure treatment, including ACE inhibitors, beta-blockers, diuretics and digitalis or a combination of these medicinal products (see also section 4.4 Special warnings and special precautions for use and 5.1 Pharmacodynamic properties).

Administration

Amias should be taken once daily with or without food.

Use in black patients

The antihypertensive effect of candesartan is less in black than non-black patients. Consequently, uptitration of Amias and concomitant therapy may be more frequently needed for blood pressure control in black than non-black patients (see section 5.1 Pharmacodynamic properties).

Use in children and adolescents

The safety and efficacy of Amias have not been established in children and adolescents (under 18 years).

4.3 Contraindications

Hypersensitivity to candesartan cilexetil or to any of the excipients.

Pregnancy and lactation (see section 4.6 Pregnancy and lactation).

Severe hepatic impairment and/or cholestasis.

4.4 Special warnings and special precautions for use

Renal impairment

As with other agents inhibiting the renin-angiotensin-aldosterone system, changes in renal function may be anticipated in susceptible patients treated with Amias.

When Amias is used in hypertensive patients with renal impairment, periodic monitoring of serum potassium and creatinine levels is recommended. There is limited experience in patients with very severe or end-stage renal impairment ($Cl_{creatinine}$ < 15 ml/min). In these patients Amias should be carefully titrated with thorough monitoring of blood pressure.

Evaluation of patients with heart failure should include periodic assessments of renal function, especially in elderly patients 75 years or older, and patients with impaired renal function. During dose titration of Amias, monitoring of serum creatinine and potassium is recommended. Clinical trials in heart failure did not include patients with serum creatinine >265 μmol/L >3 mg/dL).

Concomitant therapy with an ACE inhibitor in heart failure

The risk of adverse events, especially renal function impairment and hyperkalaemia, may increase when candesartan is used in combination with an ACE inhibitor (see section 4.8 Undesirable effects). Patients with such treatment should be monitored regularly and carefully.

Haemodialysis

During dialysis the blood pressure may be particularly sensitive to AT_1-receptor blockade as a result of reduced plasma volume and activation of the renin-angiotensin-aldosterone system. Therefore Amias should be carefully titrated with thorough monitoring of blood pressure in patients on haemodialysis.

Renal artery stenosis

Other medicinal products that affect the renin-angiotensin-aldosterone system, i.e. angiotensin converting enzyme (ACE) inhibitors, may increase blood urea and serum creatinine in patients with bilateral renal artery stenosis or stenosis of the artery to a solitary kidney. A similar effect may be anticipated with angiotensin II receptor antagonists.

Kidney transplantation

There is no experience regarding the administration of Amias in patients with a recent kidney transplantation.

Hypotension

Hypotension may occur during treatment with Amias in heart failure patients. As described for other agents acting on the renin-angiotensin-aldosterone system, it may also occur in hypertensive patients with intravascular volume depletion such as those receiving high dose diuretics. Caution should be observed when initiating therapy and correction of hypovolemia should be attempted.

Anaesthesia and surgery

Hypotension may occur during anaesthesia and surgery in patients treated with angiotensin II antagonists due to blockade of the renin-angiotensin system. Very rarely, hypotension may be severe such that it may warrant the use of intravenous fluids and/or vasopressors.

Aortic and mitral valve stenosis (obstructive hypertrophic cardiomyopathy)

As with other vasodilators, special caution is indicated in patients suffering from haemodynamically relevant aortic or mitral valve stenosis, or obstructive hypertrophic cardiomyopathy.

Primary hyperaldosteronism

Patients with primary hyperaldosteronism will not generally respond to antihypertensive medicinal products acting through inhibition of the renin-angiotensin-aldosterone system. Therefore, the use of Amias is not recommended.

Hyperkalaemia

Based on experience with the use of other medicinal products that affect the renin-angiotensin-aldosterone system, concomitant use of Amias with potassium-sparing diuretics, potassium supplements, salt substitutes containing potassium, or other medicinal products that may increase potassium levels (e.g. heparin) may lead to increases in serum potassium in hypertensive patients.

In heart failure patients treated with Amias, hyperkalaemia may occur. During treatment with Amias in patients with heart failure, periodic monitoring of serum potassium is recommended, especially when taken concomitantly with ACE inhibitors and potassium-sparing diuretics such as spironolactone.

General

In patients whose vascular tone and renal function depend predominantly on the activity of the renin-angiotensin-aldosterone system (e.g. patients with severe congestive heart failure or underlying renal disease, including renal artery stenosis), treatment with other medicinal products that affect this system has been associated with acute hypotension, azotaemia, oliguria or, rarely, acute renal failure. The possibility of similar effects cannot be excluded with angiotensin II receptor antagonists. As with any antihypertensive agent, excessive blood pressure decrease in patients with ischaemic cardiopathy or ischaemic cerebrovascular disease could result in a myocardial infarction or stroke.

Patients with rare hereditary problems of galactose intolerance, the Lapp lactase deficiency or glucose-galactose malabsorption should not take this medicinal product.

4.5 Interaction with other medicinal products and other forms of Interaction

No drug interactions of clinical significance have been identified.

Compounds which have been investigated in clinical pharmacokinetic studies include hydrochlorothiazide, warfarin, digoxin, oral contraceptives (i.e. ethinylestradiol/ levonorgestrel), glibenclamide, nifedipine and enalapril.

Candesartan is eliminated only to a minor extent by hepatic metabolism (CYP2C9). Available interaction studies indicate no effect on CYP2C9 and CYP3A4 but the effect on other cytochrome P450 isoenzymes is presently unknown.

The antihypertensive effect of candesartan may be enhanced by other medicinal products with blood pressure lowering properties, whether prescribed as an antihypertensive or prescribed for other indications.

Based on experience with the use of other medicinal products that affect the renin-angiotensin-aldosterone system concomitant use of potassium-sparing diuretics, potassium supplements, salt substitutes containing potassium, or other medicinal products that may increase potassium levels (e.g. heparin) may lead to increases in serum potassium.

Reversible increases in serum lithium concentrations and toxicity have been reported during concomitant administration of lithium with ACE inhibitors. A similar effect may occur with angiotensin II receptor antagonists and careful monitoring of serum lithium levels is recommended during concomitant use.

As with other antihypertensive agents, the antihypertensive effect of candesartan may be attenuated by non-steroidal anti-inflammatory drugs such as indomethacin.

The bioavailability of candesartan is not affected by food.

4.6 Pregnancy and lactation

Use in pregnancy

There are very limited data from the use of Amias in pregnant women. These data are insufficient to allow conclusions about potential risk for the foetus when used during the first trimester. In humans, foetal renal perfusion, which is dependent upon the development of the renin-angiotensin-aldosterone system, begins in the second trimester. Thus, risk to the foetus increases if Amias is administered during the second or third trimesters of pregnancy. When used in pregnancy during the second and third trimesters, medicinal products that act directly on the renin-angiotensin system can cause foetal and neonatal injury (hypotension, renal dysfunction, oliguria and/or anuria, oligohydramnios, skull hypoplasia, intrauterine growth retardation) and death. Cases of lung hypoplasia, facial abnormalities and limb contractures have also been described.

Animal studies with candesartan cilexetil have demonstrated late foetal and neonatal injury in the kidney. The mechanism is believed to be pharmacologically mediated through effects on the renin-angiotensin-aldosterone system.

Based on the above information, Amias should not be used in pregnancy. If pregnancy is detected during treatment, Amias should be discontinued (see section 4.3 Contraindications).

Use in lactation

It is not known whether candesartan is excreted in human milk. However, candesartan is excreted in the milk of lactating rats. Because of the potential for adverse effects on the nursing infant Amias should not be given during breast-feeding (see section 4.3 Contraindications).

4.7 Effects on ability to drive and use machines

The effect of candesartan on the ability to drive and use machines has not been studied but based on its pharmacodynamic properties candesartan is unlikely to affect this ability. When driving vehicles or operating machines it should be taken into account that dizziness or weariness may occur during treatment.

4.8 Undesirable effects

Treatment of Hypertension

In controlled clinical studies adverse events were mild and transient and comparable to placebo. The overall incidence of adverse events showed no association with dose or age. Withdrawals from treatment due to adverse events were similar with candesartan cilexetil (3.1%) and placebo (3.2%).

In a pooled analysis of clinical trial data, the following common >1/100) adverse reactions with candesartan cilexetil were reported based on an incidence of adverse events with candesartan cilexetil at least 1% higher than the incidence seen with placebo:

Nervous system disorders:

Dizziness/vertigo, headache.

Infections and infestations:

Respiratory infection.

Laboratory findings

In general, there were no clinically important influences of Amias on routine laboratory variables. As for other inhibitors of the renin-angiotensin-aldosterone system, small decreases in haemoglobin have been seen. Increases in creatinine, urea or potassium and decrease in sodium have been observed. Increases in S-ALAT (S-GPT) were reported as adverse events slightly more often with Amias than with placebo (1.3% vs 0.5%). No routine monitoring of laboratory variables is usually necessary for patients receiving Amias. However, in patients with renal impairment, periodic monitoring of serum potassium and creatinine levels is recommended.

Treatment of Heart Failure

The adverse experience profile of Amias in heart failure patients was consistent with the pharmacology of the drug and the health status of the patients. In the CHARM clinical programme, comparing Amias in doses up to 32 mg (n=3,803) to placebo (n=3,796), 21.0% of the candesartan cilexetil group and 16.1% of the placebo group discontinued treatment because of adverse events. Adverse reactions commonly (≥1/100, <1/10) seen were:

Vascular disorders:

Hypotension

Metabolism and nutrition disorders:

Hyperkalaemia

Renal and urinary disorders:

Renal impairment

Laboratory findings:

Increases in creatinine, urea and potassium. Periodic monitoring of serum creatinine and potassium is recommended (see section 4.4 Special warnings and special precautions for use).

Post Marketing

The following adverse reactions have been reported very rarely (<1/10.000) in post marketing experience:

Blood and lymphatic system disorders:

Leukopenia, neutropenia and agranulocytosis.

Metabolism and nutrition disorders:

Hyperkalaemia, hyponatraemia.

Nervous system disorders:

Dizziness, headache.

Gastrointestinal disorders:

Nausea.

Hepato-biliary disorders:

Increased liver enzymes, abnormal hepatic function or hepatitis.

Skin and subcutaneous tissue disorders:

Angioedema, rash, urticaria, pruritus.

Musculoskeletal, connective tissue and bone disorders:

Back pain, arthralgia, myalgia.

Renal and urinary disorders:

Renal impairment, including renal failure in susceptible patients.

(see section 4.4 Special warnings and special precautions for use).

4.9 Overdose

Symptoms

Based on pharmacological considerations, the main manifestation of an overdose is likely to be symptomatic hypotension and dizziness. In individual case reports of overdose (of up to 672 mg candesartan cilexetil), patient recovery was uneventful.

Management

If symptomatic hypotension should occur, symptomatic treatment should be instituted and vital signs monitored. The patient should be placed supine with the legs elevated. If this is not sufficient, plasma volume should be increased by infusion of, for example, isotonic saline solution. Sympathomimetic medicinal products may be administered if the above-mentioned measures are not sufficient.

Candesartan is not removed by haemodialysis.

5. PHARMACOLOGICAL PROPERTIES

5.1 Pharmacodynamic properties

Pharmacotherapeutic group: Angiotensin II antagonists (candesartan), ATC code C09C A06.

Angiotensin II is the primary vasoactive hormone of the renin-angiotensin-aldosterone system and plays a role in the pathophysiology of hypertension, heart failure and other cardiovascular disorders. It also has a role in the pathogenesis of end organ hypertrophy and damage. The major physiological effects of angiotensin II, such as vasoconstriction, aldosterone stimulation, regulation of salt and water homeostasis and stimulation of cell growth, are mediated via the type 1 (AT_1) receptor.

Candesartan cilexetil is a prodrug suitable for oral use. It is rapidly converted to the active substance, candesartan, by ester hydrolysis during absorption from the gastrointestinal tract. Candesartan is an angiotensin II receptor antagonist, selective for AT_1 receptors, with tight binding to and slow dissociation from the receptor. It has no agonist activity.

Candesartan does not inhibit ACE, which converts angiotensin I to angiotensin II and degrades bradykinin. There is no effect on ACE and no potentiation of bradykinin or substance P. In controlled clinical trials comparing candesartan with ACE inhibitors, the incidence of cough was lower in patients receiving candesartan cilexetil. Candesartan does not bind to or block other hormone receptors or ion channels known to be important in cardiovascular regulation. The antagonism of the angiotensin II (AT_1) receptors results in dose related increases in plasma renin levels, angiotensin I and angiotensin II levels, and a decrease in plasma aldosterone concentration.

Hypertension

In hypertension, candesartan causes a dose-dependent, long-lasting reduction in arterial blood pressure. The antihypertensive action is due to decreased systemic peripheral resistance, without reflex increase in heart rate. There is no indication of serious or exaggerated first dose hypotension or rebound effect after cessation of treatment.

After administration of a single dose of candesartan cilexetil, onset of antihypertensive effect generally occurs within 2 hours. With continuous treatment, most of the reduction in blood pressure with any dose is generally attained within four weeks and is sustained during long-term treatment. According to a meta-analysis, the average additional effect of a dose increase from 16 mg to 32 mg once daily was small. Taking into account the inter-individual variability, a more than average effect can be expected in some patients. Candesartan cilexetil once daily provides effective and smooth blood pressure reduction over 24 hours with little difference between maximum and trough effects during the dosing interval. The antihypertensive effect and tolerability of candesartan and losartan were compared in two randomised, double-blind studies in a total of 1,268 patients with mild to moderate hypertension. The trough blood pressure reduction (systolic/diastolic) was 13.1/10.5 mmHg with candesartan cilexetil 32 mg once daily and 10.0/8.7 mmHg with losartan potassium 100 mg once daily (difference in blood pressure reduction 3.1/1.8 mmHg, $p < 0.0001/p < 0.0001$). The most common adverse events were respiratory infection (candesartan 6.6%, losartan 8.9%), headache (candesartan 5.8%, losartan 5.6%) and dizziness (candesartan 4.4%, losartan 1.9%).

When candesartan cilexetil is used together with hydrochlorothiazide, the reduction in blood pressure is additive. Concomitant administration of candesartan cilexetil with hydrochlorothiazide or amlodipine is well tolerated.

Candesartan is similarly effective in patients irrespective of age and gender. Medicinal products that block the renin-angiotensin-aldosterone system have less pronounced antihypertensive effect in black patients (usually a low-renin population) than in non-black patients. This is also the case for candesartan. In an open-label clinical experience trial in 5,156 patients with diastolic hypertension, the blood pressure reduction during candesartan treatment was significantly less in black than non-black patients (14.4/10.3 mmHg vs 19.0/12.7 mmHg, $p < 0.0001/p < 0.0001$).

Candesartan increases renal blood flow and either has no effect on, or increases glomerular filtration rate while renal vascular resistance and filtration fraction are reduced. In a 3-month clinical study in hypertensive patients with type 2 diabetes mellitus and microalbuminuria, antihypertensive treatment with candesartan cilexetil reduced urinary albumin excretion (albumin/creatinine ratio, mean 30%, 95% confidence level interval 15-42%). There are currently no data on the effect of candesartan on the progression to diabetic nephropathy. In hypertensive patients with type II diabetes mellitus, 12 weeks treatment with candesartan cilexetil 8 mg to 16 mg had no adverse effects on blood glucose or lipid profile.

The effects of candesartan cilexetil 8-16 mg (mean dose 12 mg) once daily, on cardiovascular morbidity and mortality were evaluated in a randomised clinical trial with 4,937 elderly patients (aged 70-89 years; 21% aged 80 or above) with mild to moderate hypertension followed for a mean of 3.7 years (Study on COgnition and Prognosis in the Elderly). Patients received candesartan cilexetil or placebo with other antihypertensive treatment added as needed. The blood pressure was reduced from 166/90 to 145/80 mmHg in the candesartan group, and from 167/90 to 149/82mmHg in the control group. There was no statistically significant difference in the primary endpoint, major cardiovascular events (cardiovascular mortality, non-fatal stroke and non-fatal myocardial infarction). There were 26.7 events per 1000 patient-years in the candesartan group versus 30.0 events per 1000 patient-years in the control group (relative risk 0.89, 95% CI 0.75 to 1.06, p=0.19).

Heart Failure

Treatment with candesartan cilexetil reduces mortality, reduces hospitalisation due to heart failure and improves symptoms in patients with left ventricular systolic dysfunction as shown in the Candesartan in Heart failure – Assessment of Reduction in Mortality and morbidity (CHARM) programme.

This multinational, placebo controlled, double-blind study programme in chronic heart failure (CHF) patients with NYHA functional class II to IV consisted of three separate studies: CHARM-Alternative (n=2,028) in patients with LVEF $\leqslant$40% not treated with an ACE inhibitor because of intolerance (mainly due to cough, 72%), CHARM-Added (n=2,548) in patients with LVEF $\leqslant$40% and treated with an ACE inhibitor, and CHARM-Preserved (n=3,023) in patients with LVEF>40%. Patients on optimal CHF therapy at baseline were randomised to placebo or candesartan cilexetil (titrated from 4 mg or 8 mg once daily to 32 mg once daily or the highest tolerated dose, mean dose 24 mg) and followed for a median of 37.7 months. After 6 months of treatment 63% of the patients still taking candesartan cilexetil (89%) were at the target dose of 32 mg.

In CHARM-Alternative, the composite endpoint of cardiovascular mortality or first CHF hospitalisation was significantly reduced with candesartan in comparison with placebo (hazard ratio (HR) 0.77, 95% CI 0.67-0.89, p <0.001). This corresponds to a relative risk reduction of 23%. Fourteen patients needed to be treated for the duration of the study to prevent one patient from dying of a cardiovascular event or being hospitalised for treatment of heart failure. The composite endpoint of all-cause mortality or first CHF hospitalisation was also significantly reduced with candesartan (HR 0.80, 95% CI 0.70-0.92, p=0.001). Both the mortality and morbidity (CHF hospitalisation) components of these composite endpoints contributed to the favourable effects of candesartan. Treatment with candesartan cilexetil resulted in improved NYHA functional class (p=0.008).

In CHARM-Added, the composite endpoint of cardiovascular mortality or first CHF hospitalisation was significantly reduced with candesartan in comparison with placebo (HR 0.85, 95% CI 0.75-0.96, p=0.011). This corresponds to a relative risk reduction of 15%. Twenty-three patients needed to be treated for the duration of the study to prevent one patient from dying of a cardiovascular event or being hospitalised for treatment of heart failure. The composite endpoint of all-cause mortality or first CHF hospitalisation was also significantly reduced with candesartan (HR 0.87, 95% CI 0.78-0.98, p=0.021). Both the mortality and morbidity components of these composite endpoints contributed to the favourable effects of candesartan. Treatment with candesartan cilexetil resulted in improved NYHA functional class (p=0.020).

In CHARM-Preserved, no statistically significant reduction was achieved in the composite endpoint of cardiovascular mortality or first CHF hospitalisation (HR 0.89, 95% CI 0.77-1.03, p=0.118). The numerical reduction was attributable to reduced CHF hospitalisation. There was no evidence of effect on mortality in this study.

All-cause mortality was not statistically significant when examined separately in each of the three CHARM studies. However, all-cause mortality was also assessed in pooled populations, CHARM-Alternative and CHARM-Added (HR 0.88, 95% CI 0.79-0.98, p=0.018) and all three studies (HR 0.91, 95% CI 0.83-1.00, p=0.055).

The beneficial effects of candesartan on cardiovascular mortality and CHF hospitalisation were consistent irrespective of age, gender and concomitant medication. Candesartan was effective also in patients taking both beta-blockers and ACE inhibitors at the same time, and the benefit was obtained whether or not patients were taking ACE inhibitors at the target dose recommended by treatment guidelines.

In patients with CHF and depressed left ventricular systolic function (left ventricular ejection fraction, LVEF $\leqslant$40%), candesartan decreases systemic vascular resistance and pulmonary capillary wedge pressure, increases plasma renin activity and angiotensin II concentration, and decreases aldosterone levels.

5.2 Pharmacokinetic properties

Absorption and distribution

Following oral administration, candesartan cilexetil is converted to the active substance candesartan. The absolute bioavailability of candesartan is approximately 40% after an oral solution of candesartan cilexetil. The relative bioavailability of the tablet formulation compared with the same oral solution is approximately 34% with very little variability. The estimated absolute bioavailability of the tablet is therefore 14%. The mean peak serum concentration (C_{max}) is reached 3-4 hours following tablet intake. The candesartan serum concentrations increase linearly with increasing doses in the therapeutic dose range. No gender related differences in the pharmacokinetics of candesartan have been observed. The area under the serum concentration *versus* time curve (AUC) of candesartan is not significantly affected by food.

Candesartan is highly bound to plasma protein (more than 99%). The apparent volume of distribution of candesartan is 0.1 l/kg.

Metabolism and elimination

Candesartan is mainly eliminated unchanged via urine and bile and only to a minor extent eliminated by hepatic metabolism. The terminal half-life of candesartan is approximately 9 hours. There is no accumulation following multiple doses.

Total plasma clearance of candesartan is about 0.37 ml/min/kg, with a renal clearance of about 0.19 ml/min/kg. The renal elimination of candesartan is both by glomerular filtration and active tubular secretion. Following an oral dose of ^{14}C-labelled candesartan cilexetil, approximately 26% of the dose is excreted in the urine as candesartan and 7% as an inactive metabolite while approximately 56% of the dose is recovered in the faeces as candesartan and 10% as the inactive metabolite.

Pharmacokinetics in special populations

In the elderly (over 65 years) C_{max} and AUC of candesartan are increased by approximately 50% and 80%, respectively in comparison to young subjects. However, the blood pressure response and the incidence of adverse events are similar after a given dose of Amias in young and elderly patients (see section 4.2 Posology and method of administration).

In patients with mild to moderate renal impairment C_{max} and AUC of candesartan increased during repeated dosing by approximately 50% and 70%, respectively, but $t_{1/2}$ was not altered, compared to patients with normal renal function. The corresponding changes in patients with severe renal impairment were approximately 50% and 110%, respectively. The terminal $t_{1/2}$ of candesartan was approximately doubled in patients with severe renal impairment. The AUC of candesartan in patients undergoing haemodialysis was similar to that in patients with severe renal impairment.

In patients with mild to moderate hepatic impairment, there was a 23% increase in the AUC of candesartan (see section 4.2 Posology and method of administration).

5.3 Preclinical safety data

There was no evidence of abnormal systemic or target organ toxicity at clinically relevant doses. In preclinical safety studies candesartan had effects on the kidneys and on red cell parameters at high doses in mice, rats, dogs and monkeys. Candesartan caused a reduction of red blood cell parameters (erythrocytes, haemoglobin, haematocrit). Effects on the kidneys (such as interstitial nephritis, tubular distension, basophilic tubules; increased plasma concentrations of urea and creatinine) were induced by candesartan which could be secondary to the hypotensive effect leading to alterations of renal perfusion. Furthermore, candesartan induced hyperplasia/hypertrophy of the juxtaglomerular cells. These changes were considered to be caused by the pharmacological action of candesartan. For therapeutic doses of candesartan in humans, the hyperplasia/hypertrophy of the renal juxtaglomerular cells does not seem to have any relevance.

Foetotoxicity has been observed in late pregnancy (see section 4.6 Pregnancy and lactation).

Data from *in vitro* and *in vivo* mutagenicity testing indicate that candesartan will not exert mutagenic or clastogenic activities under conditions of clinical use. There was no evidence of carcinogenicity.

6. PHARMACEUTICAL PARTICULARS

6.1 List of excipients

Carmellose calcium

Hydroxypropyl cellulose

Iron oxide red (E172) (8, 16 and 32 mg tablets only)

Lactose monohydrate

Magnesium stearate

Maize starch

Macrogol

6.2 Incompatibilities

Not applicable.

6.3 Shelf life

3 years.

6.4 Special precautions for storage

Do not store above 30°C.

6.5 Nature and contents of container

Polypropylene blister.

2mg Tablets: Blister packs of 7 and 14 tablets.

4mg, 8mg,16mg and 32 mg tablets: Blister packs of 7, 14, 20, 28, 50, 56, 98, 98x1 (single dose unit), 100 or 300 tablets.

Not all pack sizes may be marketed.

6.6 Instructions for use and handling

No special requirements.

7. MARKETING AUTHORISATION HOLDER

Takeda UK Limited

Takeda House

Mercury Park, Wycombe Lane

Wooburn Green, High Wycombe

Buckinghamshire HP10 0HH

8. MARKETING AUTHORISATION NUMBER(S)

PL 16189/0001

PL 16189/0002

PL 16189/0003

PL 16189/0004

PL 16189/0007

9. DATE OF FIRST AUTHORISATION/RENEWAL OF THE AUTHORISATION

15 December 1998/29 April 2002

10. DATE OF REVISION OF THE TEXT

December 2004

Amikin Injection 100 mg/2 ml and 500 mg/2 ml

(Bristol-Myers Pharmaceuticals)

1. NAME OF THE MEDICINAL PRODUCT

AMIKIN INJECTION 100MG / 2ML and 500MG / 2ML

2. QUALITATIVE AND QUANTITATIVE COMPOSITION

Each vial contains in 2 ml amikacin sulphate equivalent to amikacin activity 100mg (100,000 international units).

Each vial contains in 2 ml amikacin sulphate equivalent to amikacin activity 500mg (500,000 international units).

3. PHARMACEUTICAL FORM

Solution for administration to human beings by injection.

4. CLINICAL PARTICULARS

4.1 Therapeutic indications

Amikacin sulphate is an aminoglycoside antibiotic which is active against a broad spectrum of Gram-negative organisms, including *Pseudomonas* spp., *Escherichia coli*, indole-positive and indole-negative *Proteus* spp. *Klebsiella-Enterobacter-Serratia* spp, *Salmonella*, *Shigella*, *Minea-Herellae*, *Citrobacter freundii* and *Providencia* spp.

Many strains of these gram-negative organisms resistant to gentamicin and tobramycin may show sensitivity to amikacin *in vitro*. The principal Gram-positive organism sensitive to amikacin is *Staphylococcus aureus*, including methicillin-resistant strains. Amikacin has some activity against other Gram-positive organisms including certain strains of *Streptococcus pyogenes*, Enterococci and *Diplococcus pneumoniae*.

Amikin is indicated in the short-term treatment of serious infections due to susceptible strains of Gram-negative bacteria. It may also be indicated for the treatment of known or suspected staphylococcal disease.

4.2 Posology and method of administration

For most infections the intramuscular route is preferred, but in life-threatening infections, or in patients in whom intramuscular injection is not feasible the intravenous route, either slow bolus (2 to 3 minutes) or infusion (0.25% over 30 minutes) may be used.

Intramuscular and intravenous administration

At the recommended dosage level, uncomplicated infections due to sensitive organisms should respond to therapy within 24 to 48 hours.

If clinical response does not occur within three to five days consideration should be given to alternative therapy.

Adults and children

15mg/kg/day in two equally divided doses (equivalent to 500mg b.i.d. in adults): use of the 100mg/2ml strength is recommended for children for the accurate measurement of the appropriate dose.

Neonates and premature infants

An initial loading dose of 10mg/kg followed by 15mg/kg/day in two equally divided doses.

Elderly

Amikacin is excreted by the renal route. Renal function should be assessed whenever possible and dosage adjusted as described under impaired renal function.

Life-threatening infections and/or those caused by Pseudomonas

The adult dose may be increased to 500mg every eight hours but should neither exceed 1.5g/day nor be administered for a period longer than 10 days. A maximum total adult dose of 15g should not be exceeded.

Urinary tract infections: (other than pseudomonal infections)

7.5mg/kg/day in two equally divided doses (equivalent to 250mg b.i.d. in adults). As the activity of amikacin is enhanced by increasing the pH, a urinary alkalising agent may be administered concurrently.

Impaired renal function

In patients with impaired renal function, the daily dose should be reduced and/or the intervals between doses increased to avoid accumulation of the drug. A suggested method for estimating dosage in patients with known or suspected diminished renal function is to multiply the serum creatinine concentration (in mg/100ml) by 9 and use the resulting figure as the interval in hours between doses.

Serum Creatinine Concentration (mg/100ml)		Interval between AMIKACIN doses of 7.5mg/kg/IM (hours)
1.5		13.5
2.0		18
2.5		22.5
3.0	X 9 =	27
3.5		31.5
4.0		36
4.5		40.5
5.0		45
5.5		49.5
6.0		54

As renal function may alter appreciably during therapy, the serum creatinine should be checked frequently and the dosage regimen modified as necessary.

Intraperitoneal use

Following exploration for established peritonitis, or after peritoneal contamination due to faecal spill during surgery, Amikin may be used as an irrigant after recovery from anaesthesia in concentrations of 0.25% (2.5mg/ml). If instillation is desired in adults, a single dose of 500mg is diluted in 20ml of sterile distilled water and may be instilled through a polyethylene catheter sutured into the wound at closure. If possible, instillation should be postponed until the patient has fully recovered from the effects of anaesthesia and muscle-relaxing drugs.

Other routes of administration

Amikin in concentrations of 0.25% may be used satisfactorily as an irrigating solution in abscess cavities, the pleural space, the peritoneum and the cerebral ventricles.

4.3 Contraindications

Hypersensitivity to any of the components of the product.

Myasthenia gravis.

4.4 Special warnings and special precautions for use

Patients should be well hydrated during amikacin therapy.

In patients with impaired renal function or diminished glomerular filtration, amikacin should be used cautiously. In such patients, renal function should be assessed by the usual methods prior to therapy and periodically during therapy. Daily doses should be reduced and/or the interval between doses lengthened in accordance with serum creatinine concentrations to avoid accumulation of abnormally high blood levels and to minimise the risk of ototoxicity.

As with other aminoglycosides, ototoxicity and/or nephrotoxicity can result from the use of amikacin; precautions on dosage and adequate hydration should be observed.

If signs of renal irritation appear (such as albumin, casts, red or white blood cells), hydration should be increased and a reduction in dosage may be desirable. These findings usually disappear when treatment is completed. However, if azotaemia or a progressive decrease in urine output occurs, treatment should be stopped.

The use of amikacin in patients with a history of allergy to aminoglycosides or in patients who may have subclinical renal or eighth nerve damage induced by prior administration of nephrotoxic and/or ototoxic agents such as streptomycin, dihydrostreptomycin, gentamicin, tobramycin, kanamycin, bekanamycin, neomycin, polymyxin B, colistin, cephaloridine, or viomycin should be considered with caution, as toxicity may be additive.

In these patients amikacin should be used only if, in the opinion of the physician, therapeutic advantages outweigh the potential risks.

Aminoglycosides may impair neuromuscular transmission and should be used with caution in patients with muscular disorders such as parkinsonism. Large doses given during surgery have been responsible for a transient myasthenic syndrome.

The intraperitoneal use of amikacin is not recommended in young children.

4.5 Interaction with other medicinal products and other forms of Interaction

Concurrent use with other potentially nephrotoxic or ototoxic drug substances should be avoided. Where this is not possible, monitor carefully.The risk of ototoxicity is increased when amikacin is used in conjunction with rapidly acting diuretic drugs, particularly when the diuretic is administered intravenously. Such agents include frusemide and ethacrynic acid which is itself an ototoxic agent. Irreversible deafness may result.

The intraperitoneal use of amikacin is not recommended in patients under the influence of anaesthetics or muscle-relaxing drugs (including ether, halothane, d-tubocurarine, succinylcholine and decamethonium) as neuromuscular blockade and consequent respiratory depression may occur.

Indomethacin may increase the plasma concentration of amikacin in neonates.

In patients with severely impaired renal function, a reduction in activity of aminoglycosides may occur with concomitant use of penicillin-type drugs.

4.6 Pregnancy and lactation

Amikacin rapidly crosses the placenta into the foetal circulation and amniotic fluid and there is a potential risk of ototoxicity in the foetus.

4.7 Effects on ability to drive and use machines

None stated.

4.8 Undesirable effects

When the recommended precautions and dosages are followed the incidence of toxic reactions, such as tinnitus, vertigo, partial reversible or irreversible deafness, skin rash, drug fever, headache, paraesthesia, nausea and vomiting is low. Urinary signs of renal irritation (albumin, casts and red or white blood cells), azotaemia and oliguria have been reported. There have been reports of retinal toxicity following intravitreal injection of amikacin.

4.9 Overdose

In the event of overdosage or toxic reaction, peritoneal dialysis or haemodialysis will aid in the removal of amikacin from the blood.

5. PHARMACOLOGICAL PROPERTIES

5.1 Pharmacodynamic properties

Amikacin sulphate is an aminoglycoside antibiotic which is active against a broad spectrum of Gram-negative organisms, including *Pseudomonas* spp, *Escherichia coli*, indole-positive and indole-negative *Proteus* spp. *Klebsiella-Enterobacter-Serratia* spp, *Salmonella, Shigella, Minea-Herellae*, *Citrobacter Freundii* and *Providencia* spp.

Many strains of these Gram-negative organisms resistant to gentamicin and tobramycin may show sensitivity to amikacin *in vitro*. The principal Gram-positive organism sensitive to amikacin is *Staphylococcus aureus*, including methicillin-resistant strains. Amikacin has some activity against other Gram-positive organisms including certain strains of *Streptococcus pyogenes*, Enterococci and *Diplococcus pneumoniae*.

5.2 Pharmacokinetic properties

Amikin is rapidly absorbed after intramuscular injection. Peak serum levels of approximately 11mg/l and 23mg/l are reached one hour after i.m. doses of 250mg and 500mg respectively. Levels 10 hours after injection are of the order of 0.3mg/l and 2.1mg/l respectively.

Twenty per cent or less is bound to serum protein and serum concentrations remain in the bactericidal range for sensitive organisms for 10 to 12 hours.

Amikin diffuses readily through extracellular fluids and is excreted in the urine unchanged, primarily by glomerular filtration. Half-life in individuals with normal renal functions is two to three hours.

Following intramuscular administration of a 250mg dose, about 65% is excreted in six hours and 91% within 24 hours. The urinary concentrations average 563 mg/l in the first 6 hours and 163 mg/l over 6 to 12 hours. Mean urine concentrations after a 500mg i.m. dose average 832 mg/l in the first six hours.

Single doses of 500mg administered to normal adults as an intravenous infusion over a period of 30 minutes produce a mean peak serum concentration of 38mg/l at the end of the infusion. Repeated infusions do not produce drug accumulation.

Amikin has been found in cerebrospinal fluid, pleural fluid, amniotic fluid and in the peritoneal cavity following parenteral administration.

5.3 Preclinical safety data

No further relevant information.

6. PHARMACEUTICAL PARTICULARS

6.1 List of excipients

Sodium bisulphite, sodium citrate, sulphuric acid, water for injection.

6.2 Incompatibilities

None.

6.3 Shelf life

36 months.

6.4 Special precautions for storage

Store below 25°C.

6.5 Nature and contents of container

Five 2 ml flint glass Type 1 vial with butyl rubber stopper and aluminium seal in a cardboard carton.

6.6 Instructions for use and handling

None stated.

7. MARKETING AUTHORISATION HOLDER

Bristol-Myers Squibb Holdings Ltd

Uxbridge Business Park

Sanderson Road

Uxbridge

Middlesex UB8 1DH

8. MARKETING AUTHORISATION NUMBER(S)

Amikin 100mg/2ml: 0125/0090R

Amikin 500mg/2ml: 0125/0092R

9. DATE OF FIRST AUTHORISATION/RENEWAL OF THE AUTHORISATION

30th January 1991

10. DATE OF REVISION OF THE TEXT

July 2005

Amilamont

(Rosemont Pharmaceuticals Limited)

1. NAME OF THE MEDICINAL PRODUCT

Amilamont

2. QUALITATIVE AND QUANTITATIVE COMPOSITION

Amiloride Hydrochloride BP 5.675mg

equivalent to

anhydrous Amiloride Hydrochloride 5mg

3. PHARMACEUTICAL FORM

Solution for oral administration

4. CLINICAL PARTICULARS

4.1 Therapeutic indications

Potassium - conserving agent; diuretic.

Although Amiloride Hydrochloride may be used alone, its principal indication is as concurrent therapy with thiazides or more potent diuretics to conserve potassium during periods of vigorous diuresis and during long term maintenance therapy.

In hypertension, it is used as an adjunct to prolonged therapy with thiazides and similar agents to prevent potassium depletion.

In congestive heart failure, Amiloride Hydrochloride may be effective alone, but its principal indication is for concomitant use in patients receiving thiazides or more potent diuretic agents.

In hepatic cirrhosis with ascites, Amiloride Hydrochloride usually provides adequate diuresis, with diminished potassium loss and less risk of metabolic alkalosis, when used alone. It may be used with more potent diuretics when a greater diuresis is required while maintaining a more balanced serum electrolyte pattern.

4.2 Posology and method of administration

Adults:

Amiloride Hydrochloride alone. The usual initial dosage is 10mg (as a single dose or 5mg twice a day). The total daily dose should not exceed 20mg (20ml) a day. After diuresis has been achieved, the dosage may be reduced by 5mg (5ml) increments to the least amount required.

Amiloride Hydrochloride with other diuretic therapy

When Amiloride is used with a diuretic which is given on an intermittent basis, it should be given at the same time as the diuretic.

Hypertension

Usually 2.5mg (2.5ml) given once a day together with the usual antihypertensive dosage of the thiazide concurrently employed. If necessary, increase to 5mg (5ml) given once a day or in divided doses.

Congestive heart failure

Initially 2.5mg (2.5ml) a day together with the usual dose of the diuretic concurrently employed, subsequently adjusted if required, but not exceeding 10mg (10ml) a day. Optimal dosage is determined by the diuretic response and the plasma potassium level. Once an initial diuresis has been achieved, reduction in dosage may be attempted for maintenance therapy. Maintenance therapy may be on an intermittent basis.

Hepatic Cirrhosis with ascites

Initiate therapy with a low dose. A single daily dose of 5mg (5ml) plus a low dosage of the other diuretic agent may be increased gradually until there is an effective diuresis. The dosage of Amiloride Hydrochloride should not exceed 10mg (10ml) a day. Maintenance dosages may be lower than those required to initiate diuresis; dosage reduction should therefore be attempted when the patient's weight is stabilised. A gradual weight reduction is especially desirable in cirrhotic patients to reduce the likelihood of untoward reactions associated with diuretic therapy.

Children

The use of Amiloride Hydrochloride in children under 18 years of age is not recommended as safety and efficacy have not been established.

Elderly

The elderly are more susceptible to electrolyte imbalance, and are more likely to experience hyperkalaemia since renal reserve may be reduced. The dosage should be carefully adjusted according to renal function, blood electrolytes and diuretic response.

4.3 Contraindications

Hyperkalaemia (plasma potassium over 5.5mmol/l) other potassium-conserving agents or potassium supplements (see Precautions); anuria; acute renal failure, severe progressive renal disease, diabetic nephropathy (see Precautions); prior sensitivity to this product. Safety for use in children is not established. See also 'Use in Pregnancy' and 'Use in the Breast Feeding mother'.

4.4 Special warnings and special precautions for use

Diabetes Mellitus

To minimise the risk of hyperkalaemia in known or suspected diabetic patients, the status of renal function should be determined before initiating therapy. Amiloride Hydrochloride should be discontinued for at least three days before a glucose-tolerance test.

Metabolic or Respiratory Acidosis

Potassium-conserving therapy should be initiated only with caution in severely ill patients in whom metabolic or respiratory acidosis may occur e.g. patients with cardiopulmonary disease or decompensated diabetes. Shifts in acid-base balance alter the balance of extracellular-intracellular potassium, and the development of acidosis may be associated with rapid increases in plasma potassium.

Hyperkalaemia

This has been observed in patients receiving Amiloride Hydrochloride, alone or with other diuretics. These patients should be observed carefully for clinical, laboratory or ECG evidence of hyperkalaemia.

Some deaths have been reported in this group of patients. Hyperkalaemia has been noted particularly in the elderly and in hospital patients with hepatic cirrhosis or cardiac oedema who have known renal involvement, who were seriously ill, or were undergoing vigorous diuretic therapy.

Neither potassium-conserving agents nor a diet rich in potassium should be used with Amiloride Hydrochloride except in severe and/or refractory cases of hypokalaemia. If the combination is used, plasma potassium levels must be continuously monitored.

Impaired Renal Function

Patients with increases in blood urea over 10mmol/l, serum creatinine over 130μmol/l, or with diabetes mellitus, should not receive Amiloride Hydrochloride without careful, frequent monitoring of serum electrolytes and blood urea levels. In renal impairment, use of a potassium conserving agent may result in rapid development of hyperkalaemia.

Treatment of Hyperkalemia

If hyperkalaemia occurs, Amiloride Hydrochloride should be discontinued immediately and, if necessary, active measures taken to reduce the plasma potassium level.

Electrolyte Imbalance and Reversible Blood Urea Increases.

Hyponatraemia and hypochloraemia may occur when Amiloride Hydrochloride is used with other diuretics. Reversible increases in blood urea levels have been reported accompanying vigorous diuresis, especially when diuretics were used in seriously ill patients, such as those with hepatic cirrhosis with ascites and metabolic alkalosis, or those with resistant oedema. Careful monitoring of serum electrolytes and blood urea levels should therefore be carried out when Amiloride Hydrochloride is given with other diuretics to such patients.

Cirrhotic patients

Oral diuretic therapy is more frequently accompanied by side effects in patients with hepatic cirrhosis with or without ascites, because these patients are intolerant of acute shifts in electrolyte balance, and because they often already have hypokalaemia as a result of associated aldosteronism.

In patients with pre-existing severe liver disease, hepatic encephalopathy manifested by tremors, confusion and coma, and increased jaundice has been reported in association with diuretics, including Amiloride Hydrochloride.

4.5 Interaction with other medicinal products and other forms of Interaction

Lithium should not be given with diuretics because they reduce its renal clearance and add a high risk of lithium toxicity.

When combined with thiazide diuretics, Amiloride can act synergistically with chlorthiazide to increase the risk of hyponatraemia.

When Amiloride Hydrochloride is administered concomitantly with an angiotensin-converting enzyme inhibitor, the risk of hyperkalaemia may be increased. Therefore, if concomitant use of these agents is indicated because of demonstrated hypokalaemia, they should be used with caution and with frequent monitoring of serum potassium.

The concomitant administration of Amiloride and NSAIDs may lead to an increased risk of nephrotoxicity, an antagonism of the diuretic effect and possibly an increased risk of hyperkalaemia.

4.6 Pregnancy and lactation

Because clinical experience is limited, Amiloride Hydrochloride is not recommended for use during pregnancy. The routine use of diuretics in otherwise healthy pregnant women with or without mild oedema is not indicated because they may be associated with hypovolaemia, increased blood viscosity and decreased placental perfusion.

Foetal and neonatal jaundice, foetal bone marrow depression and thrombocytopenia have also been described. The potential benefits of the drug must be weighed against the possible hazards to the foetus if it is administered to a woman of child bearing age.

It is not known whether Amiloride Hydrochloride is excreted in human milk. Because many drugs are excreted by this route, and because there is a risk that it might take this route of excretion and that it might then cause serious side effects in the breast feeding infant, the mother should either stop breast feeding or stop taking the drug. The decision depends on the importance of the drug to the mother.

4.7 Effects on ability to drive and use machines

None known

4.8 Undesirable effects

Amiloride Hydrochloride is normally well tolerated, although minor side effects are reported relatively frequently. Except for hyperkalaemia, significant side effects are infrequent. Nausea, anorexia, abdominal pain, flatulence and mild skin rash are probably due to Amiloride; but other side effects are generally associated with diuresis or with the underlying condition being treated.

Body as a whole

Headache, weakness, fatigue, back pain, chest pain, neck/shoulder ache, pain in the extremities.

Cardiovascular

Angina pectoris, orthostatic hypotension, arrhythmias, palpitation, one patient with partial heart block developed complete heartblock.

Digestive

Anorexia, nausea, vomiting, diarrhoea, constipation, abdominal pain, GI bleeding, jaundice, thirst, dyspepsia, flatulence.

Metabolic

Elevated plasma potassium levels above 5.5mmol/l, hyponatraemia

Integumentary

Pruritus, rash, dryness of mouth, alopecia

Musculoskeletal

Muscle cramps, joint pain

Nervous

Dizziness, vertigo, paraesthesiae, tremors, encephalopathy.

Psychiatric

Nervousness, mental confusion, insomnia, decreased libido, depression, somnolence.

Respiratory

Cough, dyspnoea

Special Senses

Nasal congestion, visual disturbances, increased intraocular pressure, tinnitus.

Urogenital

Impotence, polyuria, dysuria, bladder spasm, frequency of micturition.

Reactions in which no causal relationship could be established were activation of probable pre-existing peptic ulcer, aplastic anaemia, neutropenia and abnormal liver function tests. In a few cirrhotic patients, jaundice associated with the underlying disease had deepened but the drug relationship is uncertain.

4.9 Overdose

No data are available; and it is not known whether the drug is dialysable.

The most likely signs and symptoms are dehydration and electrolyte imbalance which should be treated by established methods. Therapy should be discontinued and the patient observed closely. No specific antidote is available. If ingestion is recent, emesis should be induced or gastric lavage performed. Treatment is symptomatic and supportive. If hyperkalaemia occurs, active measures should be taken to reduce plasma potassium levels.

The plasma half life of amiloride is about six hours.

5. PHARMACOLOGICAL PROPERTIES

5.1 Pharmacodynamic properties

Amiloride has mild diuretic and anti-hypertensive activity. It acts primarily in the distal tubule and does not require aldosterone for its action. Amiloride is a mild natriuretic which does not initiate a concomitant decrease in potassium levels. The mechanism of action includes inhibition of the electrogenic entry of sodium thus causing a fall in the electrical potential across the tubular epithelium. Since this potential is one of the main causes of the secretion of potassium, this mechanism is likely to be the basis of the potassium sparing effect. By blocking the sodium channels, Amiloride may also reduce exchange of Na+ ions and H+ ions. A combination of the Amiloride with a benzothiadazine diuretic will cause less magnesium excretion than the diuretic alone.

5.2 Pharmacokinetic properties

Amiloride is incompletely absorbed from the gastro-intestinal tract, only about 50% is recovered unchanged in the urine following an oral dose. The drug is not metabolised and can, therefore, be useful in patients with liver disease. Peak plasma concentrations are reached about 3 - 4 hours after oral administration and the plasma half-life is in the range of 6 - 9 hours.

In a 70Kg man, the distribution volume is about 5L/Kg, suggesting that the drug is widely distributed in the tissues. Amiloride appears to be weakly bound to plasma proteins as determined by electrophoretic and gel filtration studies. It is not known whether the drug is excreted in breast milk, although studies have shown the presence of Amiloride in the breast milk of rats.

Amiloride is excreted unchanged in the urine. In two studies in which single doses of 14C-Amiloride were used, approximately 50% was recovered in urine and 40% in the faeces within 72 hours. In radioactive studies, peak plasma levels of 38 - 40μg/L were seen three to four hours after a single 20mg oral dose. These low plasma levels are thought to be due to extravascular distribution as evidenced by the large volume of distribution.

In man, the calculate renal clearance of Amiloride exceed in the glomerular filtration, suggesting that there is a tubular secretory pathway. Renal clearance of the drug does not appear to be affected by probenecid, pH of the urine or urinary flow rate.

5.3 Preclinical safety data

None stated

6. PHARMACEUTICAL PARTICULARS

6.1 List of excipients

Citric Acid Monohydrate BP, Methyl Hydroxybenzoate BP, Propyl Hydroxybenzoate BP, Propylene Glycol BP, Vanillin BP, Compound Orange Spirit BP, Liquid Maltitol Ph Eur, Purified Water BP.

6.2 Incompatibilities

None known

6.3 Shelf life

Shelf life in marketed pack 24 months

6.4 Special precautions for storage

Store at or below 25°C, out of reach of children

6.5 Nature and contents of container

Glass (Type III) amber bottle, with capacities of 125ml, 150ml, 200ml, 300ml

Closures: a)aluminium, EPE wadded ROPP caps

b) HDPE, EPE wadded, tamper evident

c) HDPE EPE wadded, tamper evident, child resistant

6.6 Instructions for use and handling

None stated

7. MARKETING AUTHORISATION HOLDER

Rosemont Pharmaceuticals Ltd

Rosemont House

Yorkdale Industrial Park

Braithwaite Street

Leeds

LS11 9XE

8. MARKETING AUTHORISATION NUMBER(S)

PL 00427/0091

9. DATE OF FIRST AUTHORISATION/RENEWAL OF THE AUTHORISATION

21 November 1995

10. DATE OF REVISION OF THE TEXT

22.12.00

Aminophylline Injection BP Minijet

(International Medication Systems (UK) Ltd)

1. NAME OF THE MEDICINAL PRODUCT

Aminophylline Injection BP Minijet

2. QUALITATIVE AND QUANTITATIVE COMPOSITION

Theophylline anhydrous BP 20.995 mg/ml

Ethylenediamine BP 6.058 mg/ml

(equivalent to aminophylline 25 mg/ml).

3. PHARMACEUTICAL FORM

Sterile aqueous solution for intravenous administration.

4. CLINICAL PARTICULARS

4.1 Therapeutic indications

For the treatment of acute asthma and acute exacerbation of chronic obstructive lung disease.

4.2 Posology and method of administration

Aminophylline should only be given by **SLOW** intravenous injection or infusion at about 1 ml per minute. Plasma theophylline levels should be maintained between 10 and 20 mg/l. Levels should be monitored pre and post dosing.

Loading dose:

5mg/kg over 20-30 minutes.

If patient already has plasma level of theophylline, (e.g. from previous tablets or capsules), reduce loading dose accordingly. Assume each mg/kg aminophylline will increase plasma concentration by 2mg/l.

Maintenance dose (by slow iv infusion):

Age group	*Dose*
6 months - 9 years	1mg/kg/hr
10-16 years	0.8mg/kg/hr.
Adults	0.5mg/kg/hr
Elderly or patients with cor pulmonale	0.3mg/kg/hr
Congestive heart failure or liver failure	0.1-0.2mg/kg/hr

4.3 Contraindications
Hypersensitivity to ethylene diamine, theophylline or other xanthines. Also contraindicated in patients with acute porphyria.

4.4 Special warnings and special precautions for use
Theophylline clearance is reduced in patients with severe congestive heart failure, pulmonary oedema, cor pulmonale, hepatic dysfunction, and hypoxaemic states. The dose may need to be lowered in these patients to reduce toxicity. Use with caution in patients with peptic ulceration, hyperthyroidism, hypertension, cardiac arrhythmias or other cardiovascular disease, acute febrile illness, epilepsy, glaucoma and diabetes mellitus.

Patients on oral theophylline preparations must have their plasma level measured prior to administration of i.v. aminophylline. The margin between therapeutic and toxic plasma levels is narrow so adverse events may easily occur; plasma levels should be monitored, the concentration for optimum response is 10-20 mg/l.

4.5 Interaction with other medicinal products and other forms of Interaction
Plasma theophylline levels may be increased by macrolide antibiotics (eg erythromycin), calcium channel blockers (verapamil and diltiazem), propranolol, some quinolone antibiotics, allopurinol (600 mg daily), cimetidine, oralcontraceptives, fluvoxamine and viloxazine and by influenza vaccines. The concomitant use of fluvoxamine and aminophylline should usually be avoided. Where this is not possible, patients should have their aminophylline dose halved and plasma aminophylline/theophylline should be monitored closely.

Plasma theophylline levels are reduced by rifampicin, lithium, sulphinpyrazone and anticonvulsants such as phenobarbitone, phenytoin, carbamazepine and primidone. Clearance is increased by 40-60% in people who smoke.

The risk of cardiac arrhythmias is increased with the concomitant use of pancuronium bromide, halothane or sympathomimetic drugs.

The direct stimulating effect of theophylline on the myocardium may enhance sensitivity to cardiac glycosides.

Caution is required in severe asthma, as the hypokalaemic effect of beta2-adrenoceptor stimulants may be potentiated by concomitant treatment with aminophylline. Plasma potassium levels should be monitored in severe asthma.

Plasma concentration of theophylline can be reduced by concomitant use of the herbal remedy St John's wort (Hypericum perforatum).

4.6 Pregnancy and lactation
Pregnancy

Theophylline crosses the placenta. Its safety in pregnancy has not been established.

Neonates of mothers taking theophylline during pregnancy should be monitored for signs of theophylline toxicity. In some neonates, tachycardia, jitteriness, irritability, gagging and vomiting have been reported.

Lactation

Theophylline is excreted in breast milk. Based on relative weight, a nursing infant receives as much as 10 to 15% of the mother's dose. Use of aminophylline by nursing mothers may cause irritability or other signs of toxicity in nursing infants.

4.7 Effects on ability to drive and use machines
Not applicable; this preparation is intended for use only in emergencies.

4.8 Undesirable effects
Adverse events are usually associated with the cardiovascular system, central nervous system or gastrointestinal tract. The frequency and severity of side effects increases as the plasma theophylline concentration increases. Excessive doses of theophylline may cause cardiac or neurotoxicity, resulting in life-threatening cardiac arrhythmias, death or convulsions. Serious adverse effects may occur before any other signs of toxicity, so it is important to monitor plasma theophylline levels.

The most common adverse events are nausea, anorexia and tremor. At higher doses or in more sensitive patients tachycardia, palpitations and arrhythmias may occur. Rapid administration may be associated with a lowering of blood pressure. Headache, anxiety, insomnia and convulsions may occur, especially if the injection is administered too fast.

On rare occasions, hypersensitivity reactions have been reported.

4.9 Overdose
Symptoms: nausea, vomiting and haematemesis, agitation, restlessness, dilated pupils and convulsions, hypotension and life-threatening cardiac arrhythmias. Profound hypokalaemia and a metabolic acidosis may develop.

Treatment: repeated oral doses of activated charcoal enhance the clearance of theophylline. Haemoperfusion through a charcoal cartridge or haemodialysis are two other methods of treatment. Hypokalaemia can be corrected by IV infusion of potassium chloride and convulsions can be controlled by IV diazepam and/or phenobarbital.

Other measures should be supportive, to maintain cardiac and respiratory function. Plasma theophylline concentration should be measured at least every 4 hours.

5. PHARMACOLOGICAL PROPERTIES

5.1 Pharmacodynamic properties
Aminophylline is a methylxanthine; its effects may be mediated by inhibition of cyclic nucleotide phosphodiesterase which results in increased concentrations of intracellular cAMP. The actions of theophylline on the myocardium and on neuromuscular transmission may result from intracellular translocation of ionised calcium.

Theophylline relaxes the smooth muscle of the respiratory tract producing bronchodilatation, increasing flow rate and vital capacity; the effect is concentration-dependent. Theophylline stimulates all levels of the central nervous system. It increases blood pressure, heart rate and force of contraction; increases gastric acid output; causes a transient diuresis and increases plasma free fatty acid concentration and catecholamine release from the adrenal medulla.

5.2 Pharmacokinetic properties
Aminophylline releases free theophylline in vivo. Theophylline is rapidly distributed to all body tissues; it crosses the placenta and is present in breast milk. It is about 60% bound to plasma protein. For bronchodilatation, serum levels should be between 10 and 20 mg/l.

Elimination half life depends on the patients age and condition, it is reduced in smokers and heavy drinkers:

premature neonates	- 30 hours (12-57)
1 to 6 months	- 12 hours (5.7-29)
6 months to 1 year	- 5.3 hours (2.2-10)
1 to 4 years	- 3.4 hours (1.9-5.5)
6 to 17 years	- 3.7 hours (1.4-7.9)
healthy adults	- 8.2 hours (3.6-12.8)

There is a wide interindividual variability in plasma theophylline clearance at all ages Decreased theophylline clearance is associated with liver cirrhosis, severe congestive heart failure and cor pulmonale, and some drugs (see 4.5).

Excretion is primarily by hepatic biotransformation with about 10% excreted unchanged in the urine; in premature infants urinary excretion ranges from 90 to 50% depending on age. The metabolic pathways are capacity-limited.

5.3 Preclinical safety data
Teratogenesis has been reported in mice given caffeine at doses 30 times the usual human adult dose but this has not been seen in rats or confirmed by human epidemiological studies. An association between caffeine ingestion and pancreatic cancer has been reported and a similar excess risk of pancreatic cancer was reported in US male veteran asthmatics treated with various bronchodilators including theophylline. The significance of these studies is not clear.

6. PHARMACEUTICAL PARTICULARS

6.1 List of excipients
Water for Injection USP

6.2 Incompatibilities
None known.

6.3 Shelf life
18 months.

6.4 Special precautions for storage
Store below 25°C. Protect from light.

6.5 Nature and contents of container
The solution is contained in a USP type I glass vial with an elastomeric closure which meets all the relevant USP specifications. The product is available as 10 ml and 20ml.

6.6 Instructions for use and handling
The container is specially designed for use with the IMS Minijet injector. Do not use the injection if crystals have separated.

Administrative Data

7. MARKETING AUTHORISATION HOLDER
International Medication Systems (UK) Ltd
208 Bath Road
Slough
Berkshire
SL1 3WE
UK

8. MARKETING AUTHORISATION NUMBER(S)
PL 03265/0012R

9. DATE OF FIRST AUTHORISATION/RENEWAL OF THE AUTHORISATION
Date first granted: 27 March 1991

Date renewed: 22 April 1997

10. DATE OF REVISION OF THE TEXT
April 2001
POM

Amiodarone Injection Minijet 30mg/ml

(International Medication Systems (UK) Ltd)

1. NAME OF THE MEDICINAL PRODUCT
Amiodarone Injection Minijet 30mg/ml. Solution for injection.

2. QUALITATIVE AND QUANTITATIVE COMPOSITION
Amiodarone Hydrochloride 30mg/ml
(Each 10ml vial contains 300mg)
For excipients, see section 6.1.

3. PHARMACEUTICAL FORM
Solution for injection.

4. CLINICAL PARTICULARS
Treatment should be initiated and normally monitored only under hospital or specialist supervision. Amiodarone injection is indicated only for the treatment of severe rhythm disorders not responding to other therapies or when other treatments cannot be used.

4.1 Therapeutic indications
Tachyarrhythmias associated with Wolff-Parkinson-White Syndrome.

All types of tachyarrhythmias including: supraventricular, nodal and ventricular tachycardias; atrial flutter and fibrillation; ventricular fibrillation; when other drugs cannot be used. The injection is to be used where a rapid response is required.

4.2 Posology and method of administration
Amiodarone injection should only be used when facilities exist for cardiac monitoring, defibrillation and cardiac pacing.

In children, amiodarone injection normally should be given under the supervision of a paediatric cardiologist.

IV infusion is preferred to bolus due to the haemodynamic effects sometimes associated with rapid injection.

Amiodarone injection may be used prior to DC conversion.

Repeated or continuous infusion via peripheral veins may lead to local discomfort and inflammation. When repeated or continuous infusion is anticipated, administration by a central venous catheter is recommended.

The standard recommended dose is 5mg/kg bodyweight given by intravenous infusion over a period of 20 minutes to 2 hours. This should be administered as a dilute solution in 250ml 5% dextrose. This may be followed by repeat infusion up to 1,200mg (approximately 15mg/kg bodyweight) in up to 500ml 5% dextrose per 24 hours, the rate of infusion being adjusted on the basis of clinical response.

In extreme clinical emergency the drug may, at the discretion of the clinician, be given as a slow injection of 150-300mg in 10-20ml 5% dextrose over a minimum of 3 minutes. This should not be repeated for at least 15 minutes.

Patients treated with amiodarone injection must be continuously monitored e.g. in an intensive care unit.

When given by infusion amiodarone injection may reduce the drop size and, if appropriate, adjustments should be made to the rate of infusion.

Changeover from intravenous to oral therapy: as soon as an adequate response has been obtained, oral therapy should be initiated concomitantly at the usual loading dose (200mg three times a day). Amiodarone injection should then be phased out gradually.

Elderly: as with all patients it is important that the minimum effective dose is used. Whilst there is no evidence that dosage requirements are different for this group of patients they may be more susceptible to bradycardia and conduction effects if too high a dose is employed. Particular attentions should be paid to monitoring thyroid function. See Contraindications, Section 4.3 and Precautions, Section 4.4.

4.3 Contraindications
Sinus bradycardia and sino-atrial heart block. In patients with severe conduction disturbances (high grade AV block, bifascicular or trifascicular block) or sinus node disease, amiodarone injection should only be used in conjunction with a pacemaker.

Evidence or history of thyroid dysfunction. Thyroid function tests should be performed prior to therapy in all patients.

Severe respiratory failure, cardiovascular collapse, or severe arterial hypotension; congestive heart failure and cardiomyopathy are also contraindications when using amiodarone injection as a bolus injection.

Known hypersensitivity to iodine or to amiodarone (one ampoule contains approximately 112mg iodine).

The combination of amiodarone injection with drugs which may induce torsades de pointes is contraindicated (see Interactions, Section 4.5).

Lactation (see section 4.6 Lactation)

Amiodarone Injection Minijet contains benzyl alcohol. There have been reports of fatal "gasping syndrome" in neonates (hypotension, bradycardia and cardiovascular collapse) following the administration of intravenous solution containing this preservative. Amiodarone Injection Minijet is therefore contraindicated in infants or young children up to 3 years old.

4.4 Special warnings and special precautions for use
Amiodarone Injection Minijet should only be used in a special care unit under continuous monitoring (ECG and blood pressure).

Too high a dose may lead to severe bradycardia and to conduction disturbances with the appearance of an idioventricular rhythm, particularly in elderly patients or during digitalis therapy. In these circumstances, amiodarone treatment should be withdrawn. If necessary beta-adrenostimulants or glucagon may be given.

Caution should be exercised in patients with hypotension and decompensated cardiomyopathy.

Amiodarone induces ECG changes; QT interval lengthening corresponding to prolonged repolarisation with the possible development of U and deformed T waves; these changes are evidence of its pharmacological action and do not reflect toxicity.

Although there have been no literature reports on the potentiation of hepatic adverse effects of alcohol, patients should be advised to moderate their alcohol intake while being treated with amiodarone.

Anaesthesia:

Before surgery, the anaesthetist should be informed that the patient is being treated with amiodarone (see section 4.5 Interactions with other Medicinal Products and other Forms of Interaction).

Increased plasma levels of flecainide have been reported with co-administration of amiodarone. The flecainide dose should be reduced accordingly and the patient closely monitored (see section 4.5 Interactions with other Medicinal Products and other Forms of Interaction).

4.5 Interaction with other medicinal products and other forms of Interaction
Some of the more important drugs that interact with amiodarone include warfarin, digoxin, phenytoin and any drug which prolongs QT interval.

Amiodarone raises the plasma concentrations of highly protein bound drugs, for example oral anticoagulants and phenytoin. The dose of warfarin should be reduced accordingly. More frequent monitoring of prothrombin time both during and after amiodarone treatment is recommended. Phenytoin dosage should be reduced if signs of overdosage appear and plasma levels may be measured.

Administration of amiodarone injection to a patient already receiving digoxin will bring about an increase in the plasma digoxin concentration and thus precipitate symptoms and signs associated with high digoxin levels. Monitoring is recommended and digoxin dosage usually has to be reduced. A synergistic effect on heart rate and atrioventricular conduction is also possible.

Combined therapy with the following drugs which prolong the QT interval is contraindicated (see Contraindications, Section 4.3) due to the increased risk of torsades de pointes: for example:

- Class Ia anti-arrhythmic drugs e.g. quinidine, procainamide, disopyramide
- Class III anti-arrhythmic drugs e.g. sotalol, bretylium
- Intravenous erythromycin, co-trimoxazole or pentamidine injection
- Anti-psychotics e.g. chlorpromazine, thioridazine, pimozide, haloperidol
- Lithium and tricyclic anti-depressants e.g. doxepin, maprotiline, amitriptyline
- Certain antihistamines e.g. terfenadine, astemizole
- Anti-malarials e.g. quinine, mefloquine, chloroquine, halofantrine

Combined therapy with the following drugs is not recommended; beta blockers and certain calcium channel blockers (diltiazem, verapamil); potentiation of negative chronotropic properties and conduction slowing effects may occur.

Stimulant laxatives may cause hypokalaemia thus increasing the risk of torsades de pointes; other types of laxatives should be used.

Caution should be exercised over combined therapy with the following drugs which may cause hypokalaemia and/or hypomagnesaemia: diuretics, systemic corticosteroids, tetracosactrin, intravenous amphotericin.

In case of hypokalaemia, corrective action should be taken and QT interval monitored. In case of torsades de pointes antiarrhythmic agents should not be given; pacing may be instituted and IV magnesium may be used.

Caution is advised in patients undergoing general anaesthesia, or receiving high dose oxygen therapy.

Potentially severe complications have been reported in patients taking amiodarone undergoing general anaesthesia: bradycardia unresponsive to atropine, hypotension, disturbances of conduction, decreased cardiac output.

A few cases of adult respiratory distress syndrome, most often in the period immediately after surgery, have been observed. A possible interaction with high oxygen concentration may be implicated. The anaesthetist should be informed that the patient is taking amiodarone.

Amiodarone may increase the plasma levels of ciclosporin when used in combination, due to a decrease in the clearance of this drug.

Amiodarone can increase serum levels of dextromethorphan.

Probable increase in flecainide plasma levels; it is advised to reduce the flecainide dose by 50% and to monitor the patient closely for adverse effects. Monitoring of flecainide plasma levels is strongly recommended in such circumstances.

4.6 Pregnancy and lactation
Pregnancy: Although no teratogenic effects have been observed in animals, there are insufficient data on the use of amiodarone during pregnancy in humans to judge any possible toxicity. However, in view of the pharmacological properties of the drug on the foetus and its effects on the foetal thyroid gland, amiodarone is contraindicated during pregnancy, except in exceptional circumstances.

Lactation: Amiodarone is excreted into the breast milk in significant quantities and breast-feeding is contraindicated.

4.7 Effects on ability to drive and use machines
No studies on the effects on the ability to drive and use machines have been performed.

4.8 Undesirable effects
Following intravenous infusion, inflammation of veins is possible. This may be avoided by the use of a central venous catheter.

Rapid administration of amiodarone injection has been associated with hot flushes, sweating and nausea. A moderate and transient reduction in blood pressure may occur. Circulatory collapse may be precipitated by too rapid administration or overdosage (atropine has been used successfully in such patients presenting with bradycardia). In case of respiratory failure, notably in asthmatics, bronchospasm and/or apnoea may also occur. Isolated cases of anaphylactic shock have been reported.

Amiodarone can cause serious adverse reactions affecting the eyes, heart, lung, liver, thyroid gland, skin and peripheral nervous system (see below). Because these reactions can be delayed, patients on long term treatment should be carefully supervised.

Ophthalmological: Patients on continuous therapy almost always develop microdeposits in the cornea. The deposits are usually only discernable by slit-lamp examinations and may rarely cause subjective symptoms such as visual haloes and blurring of vision. The deposits are considered essentially benign, do not require discontinuation of amiodarone and regress following termination of treatment. Rare cases of impaired visual acuity due to optic neuritis have been reported, although at present, the relationship with amiodarone has not been established. Unless blurred or decreased vision occurs, opthalmological examination is recommended annually.

Cardiac: Bradycardia, which is generally moderate and dose dependent, has been reported. In some cases (sinus node disease, elderly patients) marked bradycardia or more exceptionally sinus arrest has occurred. There have been rare instances of conduction disturbances (sino-atrial block, various degrees of AV-block). Because of the long half life of amiodarone, if bradycardia is severe and symptomatic the insertion of a pacemaker should be considered. Amiodarone has a low proarrhythmic effect. However arrhythmia (new occurrence or aggravation) followed in some cases by cardiac arrest has been reported; with current knowledge it is not possible to differentiate a drug effect from the underlying cardiac condition or lack of therapeutic efficacy. This has usually occurred in combination with other precipitating factors particularly other antiarrhythmic agents, hypokalaemia and digoxin.

Pulmonary: Amiodarone can cause pulmonary toxicity (hypersensitivity pneumonitis, alveolar/interstitial pneumonia or fibrosis, pleuritis, bronchiolitis obliterans organising pneumonia). Sometimes this toxicity can be fatal.

Presenting features can include dyspnoea (which may be severe and unexplained by the current cardiac status), non-productive cough and deterioration in general health (fatigue, weight loss and fever). The onset is usually slow but may be rapidly progressive. Whilst the majority of cases have been reported with long-term therapy, a few have occurred soon after starting treatment.

Patients should be carefully evaluated clinically and consideration given to chest X-ray before starting therapy. During treatment, if pulmonary toxicity is suspected, this should be repeated and associated with lung function testing including where possible measurement of transfer factor. Initial radiological changes may be difficult to distinguish from pulmonary venous congestion. Pulmonary toxicity has usually been reversible following early withdrawal of amiodarone therapy, with or without corticosteroid therapy. Clinical symptoms often resolve within a few weeks followed by slower radiological and lung function improvement. Some patients can deteriorate despite discontinuing amiodarone. A few cases of adult respiratory distress syndrome, most often in the period after surgery, have been observed, resulting sometimes in fatalities (see Interactions, Section 4.5).

A few cases of bronchospasm have been reported in patients with severe respiratory failure and especially in asthmatic patients.

Hepatic: Amiodarone may be associated with a variety of hepatic effects, including cirrhosis, hepatitis and jaundice. Some fatalities have been reported, mainly following long-term therapy, although rarely they have occurred soon after starting treatment. It is advisable to monitor hepatic functions particularly transaminases before treatment and six monthly thereafter.

At the beginning of therapy, elevation of serum transaminases which can be in isolation (1.5 to 3 times normal) may occur. These may return to normal with dose reduction, or sometimes spontaneously.

Isolated cases of acute liver disorders with elevated serum transaminases and/or jaundice may occur; in such cases treatment should be discontinued.

There have been reports of chronic liver disease. Alteration of of laboratory tests which may be minimal (transaminases elevated 1.5 to 5 times normal) or clinical signs (possible hepatomegaly) during treatment for longer than 6 months should suggest this diagnosis. Routine monitoring of liver function tests is therefore advised. Abnormal clinical and laboratory test results usually regress upon cessation of treatment. Histological findings may resemble pseudo-alcoholic hepatitis, but they can be variable and include chirrosis.

Thyroid: Both thyrotoxicosis and hypothyroidism have occurred during or soon after amiodarone treatment. Simple monitoring of the usual biochemical tests is confusing because some tests such as free T4 and free T3 may be altered where the patient is euthyroid. Clinical monitoring is therefore recommended before start of treatment, then six monthly and should be continued for some months after discontinuation of treatment. This is particularly important in the elderly. In patients whose history indicates an increased risk of thyroid dysfunction, regular assessment is recommended.

Hyperthyroidism: Clinical features such as weight loss, asthenia, restlessness, increase in heart rate, recurrence of the cardiac dysrhythmia, angina, or congestive heart failure, should alert the clinician. The diagnosis may be supported by an elevated serum T3, a low level of thyroid stimulating hormone (TSH) as measured by high sensitivity methods and a reduced TSH response to TRH. Elevation of reverse T3 (r T3) may also be found. In the case of hyperthyroidism, therapy should be withdrawn. Clinical recovery usually occurs within a few weeks, although severe cases, sometimes resulting in fatalities, have been reported.

Courses of anti-thyroid drugs have been used for the treatment of severe thyroid hyperactivity; large doses may be required initially. These may not always be effective and concomitant high dose corticosteroid therapy (eg 1mg/kg prednisolone) may be required for several weeks.

Hypothyroidism: Clinical features such as weight gain, reduced activity or excessive bradycardia should suggest the diagnosis. This may be supported by an elevated serum TSH level and an exaggerated TSH response to TRH. T_4 and T_3 levels may be low. Thyroid hypofunction usually resolves within 3 months of cessation of therapy; it may be treated cautiously with L-thyroxine. Concomitant use of amiodarone should be continued only in life threatening situations, when TSH levels may provide a guide to L-thyroxin dosage.

Dermatological: Patients taking amiodarone can become unduly sensitive to sunlight and should be warned of this possibility. In most cases, symptoms are limited to tingling, burning and erythema of sun exposed skin but severe phototoxic reactions with blistering may be seen. Photosensitivity may persist for several months after discontinuation of amiodarone. Photosensitivity may be minimised by limiting exposure to UV light, wearing suitable protective hats and clothing and by using a broad spectrum sun screening preparation. Rarely, a slate grey or bluish discolouration of light exposed skin, particularly on the face may occur. Resolution of this pigmentation may be very slow once the drug is discontinued. Other types of skin rashes including rash maculo-papular and isolated cases of exfoliative dermatitis have been reported. Cases of erythema have been reported during radiotherapy.

Neurological: Peripheral neuropathy can be caused by amiodarone. Myopathy has occasionally been reported. Both these conditions may be severe although they are usually reversible on drug withdrawal. Nightmares, vertigo, headaches, sleeplessness and paraesthesia may also occur. Tremor and ataxia have also infrequently been reported usually with complete regression after reduction of dose or withdrawal of the drug. Benign intracranial hypertension (pseudo-tumour cerebri) has been reported.

Other: Other unwanted effects occasionally reported include nausea, vomiting, metallic taste (which usually occur with loading dosage which regress on dose reduction), fatigue, impotence, epididymo-orchitis, and alopecia. Isolated cases suggesting a hypersensitivity reaction involving vasculitis, renal involvement with moderate elevation of creatinine levels or thrombocytopenia have been observed. Haemolytic or aplastic anaemia have rarely been reported. Isolated cases of anapylatic shock have been reported.

4.9 Overdose

Little information is available regarding acute overdosage with amiodarone. Few cases of sinus bradycardia, heart block, attacks of ventricular tachycardia, torsades de pointes, circulatory failure and hepatic injury have been reported.

In the event of overdose, treatment should be symptomatic in addition to general supportive measures. The patient should be monitored and if bradycardia occurs beta-adrenostimulants or glucagon may be given. Spontaneously resolving attacks of ventricular tachycardia may also occur. Due to the pharmacokinetics of amiodarone, adequate and prolonged surveillance of the patient, particularly cardiac status, is recommended. Neither amiodarone nor its metabolites are dialysable.

5. PHARMACOLOGICAL PROPERTIES

5.1 Pharmacodynamic properties

Pharmacotherapeutic group: antiarrhythmic, Class III; ATC code: C01BD 01.

Amiodarone is a product for the treatment of tachyarrythmias and has complex pharmacological actions. Its effects are anti-adrenergic (partial alpha and beta blockers). It has haemodynamic effects (increased blood flow and systematic/coronary vasodilatation). The drug reduces myocardial oxygen consumption and has been shown to have a sparing effect of rat myocardial ATP utilisation, with decreased oxidative processes. Amiodarone inhibits the metallic and biochemical effects of catecholamines on the heart and inhibits Na+ and K+ activated ATP-ase.

5.2 Pharmacokinetic properties

Pharmacokinetics of amiodarone are unusual and complex, and have not been completely elucidated. Absorption following oral administration is variable and may be prolonged, with enterohepatic cycling. The major metabolite is desethylamiodarone. Amiodarone is highly protein bound (> 95%). Renal excretion is minimal and faecal excretion is the major route. A study in both healthy volunteers and patients after intravenous administration of amiodarone reported that the calculated volumes of distribution and total blood clearance using a two-compartment open model were similar for both groups. Elimination of amiodarone after intravenous injection appeared to be biexponential with a distribution phase lasting about 4 hours. The very high volume of distribution combined with a relatively low apparent volume for the central compartment suggests extensive tissue distribution. A bolus IV injection of 400mg gave a terminal T½ of approximately 11 hours.

5.3 Preclinical safety data

There are no pre-clinical data of relevance to the prescriber which are additional to that already included in other sections of the SmPC.

6. PHARMACEUTICAL PARTICULARS

6.1 List of excipients

Benzyl alcohol

Polysorbate 80

Water for injections

6.2 Incompatibilities

Amiodarone Injection is incompatible with saline and when diluted should be administered solely in 5% dextrose solution. Solutions containing less than 300mg amiodarone hydrochloride in 500ml dextrose 5% are unstable and should not be used.

The use of administration equipment or devices containing plasticizers such as DEHP (di-2-ethylhexyphthalate) in the presence of amiodarone may result in leaching out of DEHP. In order to minimise patient exposure to DEHP, the final amiodarone dilution for infusion should preferably be administered through non DEHP-containing sets.

6.3 Shelf life

36 months.

6.4 Special precautions for storage

Do not store above 25°C. Keep vial in the outer carton.

6.5 Nature and contents of container

The solution is contained in a type I glass vial with an elastomeric closure and a plastic vial cap.

An IMS Minijet® injector is supplied in the carton.

The product is available as 10ml.

6.6 Instructions for use and handling

The container is specially designed for use with the IMS Minijet® injector. The instructions for the use of the injector can be found on the side of the outer carton and are as follows;

- Remove the protective caps
- Carefully thread glass vial into injector 3 half turns or until the needle penetrates the stopper
- Remove the needle cap, point needle upwards and expel air.

All infusions longer than 2 hours should be made in glass containers.

7. MARKETING AUTHORISATION HOLDER

International Medication Systems (UK) Ltd

208 Bath Road

Slough

Berkshire

SL1 3WE

UK

8. MARKETING AUTHORISATION NUMBER(S)

PL 03265/0076

9. DATE OF FIRST AUTHORISATION/RENEWAL OF THE AUTHORISATION

28 January 2004

10. DATE OF REVISION OF THE TEXT

March 2005.

Amoxicillin Sodium for Injection

(Wockhardt UK Ltd)

1. NAME OF THE MEDICINAL PRODUCT

Amoxicillin Sodium for Injection BP 250mg

Amoxicillin Sodium for Injection BP 500mg

Amoxicillin Sodium for Injection BP 1g

2. QUALITATIVE AND QUANTITATIVE COMPOSITION

Sodium Amoxicillin equivalent to Amoxicillin Ph Eur 250mg

Sodium Amoxicillin equivalent to Amoxicillin Ph Eur 500mg

Sodium Amoxicillin equivalent to Amoxicillin Ph Eur 1g

3. PHARMACEUTICAL FORM

Powder for solution for injection.

4. CLINICAL PARTICULARS

4.1 Therapeutic indications

Amoxicillin is a broad-spectrum aminopenicillin and is indicated in the treatment of bacterial infections such as actinomycosis, biliary-tract infections, bone and joint infections, acute exacerbations of chronic bronchitis, gastroenteritis, (including *Escherichia coli* enteritis and *Salmonella* enteritis, but not shigellosis), gonorrhoea, mouth infections, sinusitis, otitis media, pneumonia (except where *Mycoplasma* suspected), typhoid and paratyphoid fever, urinary-tract infections, bacterial meningitis and the prophylaxis of endocarditis.

It is also used in the treatment of Lyme disease.

4.2 Posology and method of administration

Treatment of Infections in Adults and the Elderly

By intramuscular injection:	500mg every eight hours.
By intravenous injection or infusion:	500mg every eight hours (or in severe infection 1g every six hours) may be given by slow iv injection over three to four minutes or by infusion over 30 to 60 minutes.

Treatment of Infection in Children up to 10 years

By intramuscular or intravenous injection or infusion:	50-100mg per kg bodyweight daily in divided doses.

Renal impairment

It may be necessary to reduce the total daily dosage depending on the degree of renal impairment.

As amoxicillin is removed by haemodialysis, patients receiving haemodialysis may require another dose of amoxicillin at the end of their dialysis.

Endocarditis prophylaxis

Dental procedures under general anaesthesia Upper respiratory tract procedures under general anaesthesia:	No special risk (ie, no prosthetic heart valves, no history of endocarditis, not more than a single dose of a penicillin in the previous month)	**Adults and the elderly:** 1g amoxicillin iv at induction, followed by 500mg oral, iv or im amoxicillin six hours later **Children under 5 years:** Quarter adult dose **Children 5-10 years:** Half adult dose
	Special risk (with prosthetic heart valves, history of endocarditis, or receipt of more than a single dose of a penicillin in the previous month)	**Adults and the elderly:** 1g amoxicillin iv with im or iv gentamicin at induction, followed by 500mg oral, iv or im amoxicillin six hours later **Children under 5 years:** Quarter adult dose plus gentamicin **Children 5-10 years:** Half adult dose plus gentamicin *NB Amoxicillin and gentamicin should not be mixed in the same syringe*
Genito-urinary procedures under general anaesthesia in patients with no urinary tract infection: Gastrointestinal, obstetric and gynaecological procedures under general anaesthesia for patients with prosthetic heart valves or history of endocarditis:		**Adults and the elderly:** 1g amoxicillin iv with im or iv gentamicin at induction, followed by 500mg oral, iv or im amoxicillin six hours later **Children under 5 years:** Quarter adult dose plus gentamicin **Children 5-10 years:** Half adult dose plus gentamicin *NB Amoxicillin and gentamicin should not be mixed in the same syringe*

Method of Administration

Intravenous Injection:	Dissolve 250mg in 5mL Water forInjections Ph Eur (final volume 5.2mL). Dissolve 500mg in 10mL Water for Injections Ph Eur (final volume 10.4mL). Dissolve 1g in 20mL Water for Injections Ph Eur (final volume 20.8mL).

Amoxicillin Sodium for Injection BP, when diluted may be injected slowly into a vein or infusion line over three to four minutes.

Intravenous Infusion:

Prepare as above and add to an iv solution in a minibag or in-line burette. Administer over 30 to 60 minutes. Alternatively the appropriate volume of iv fluid may be transferred from the infusion bag into the vial, using a suitable reconstitution device, and drawn back into the bag after dissolution.

Intramuscular Injection: Add 1.5mL Water for Injections Ph Eur to 250mg and shake vigorously (final volume 1.7mL).

Add 2.5mL Water for Injections Ph Eur to 500mg and shake vigorously (final volume 2.9mL).

4.3 Contraindications

Penicillin hypersensitivity.

Glandular fever and lymphatic lymphoma.

Bacterial resistance to amoxicillin or ampicillin.

4.4 Special warnings and special precautions for use

Amoxicillin should be given with caution to patients with a history of allergy, especially to drugs. Desensitisation may be necessary if treatment is essential.

Amoxicillin should not be used in patients with underlying defects of the urinary tract or for long-term treatment of recurrent urinary tract infection, as resistance may develop in the enteric flora.

Care is necessary if very high doses of amoxicillin are given, especially if renal function is poor, because of the risk of nephrotoxicity. The intrathecal route should be avoided. Care is also necessary if large doses of sodium (as amoxicillin sodium) are given to patients with impaired renal function or heart failure. Renal and haematological status should be monitored during prolonged and high-dose therapy.

Care is required when treating some patients with syphilis because of the Jarisch- Herxheimer reaction.

Contact with amoxicillin should be avoided since skin sensitisation may occur.

Amoxicillin should preferably not be given to patients with undiagnosed pharyngitis (who may have mononucleosis) or patients with lymphatic leukaemia or possibly HIV infection who may also be at increased risk of developing skin rashes with amoxicillin.

4.5 Interaction with other medicinal products and other forms of Interaction

Amoxicillin may decrease the efficacy of oestrogen-containing oral contraceptives. Plasma concentrations of amoxicillin are enhanced if probenecid is given concurrently. There is reduced excretion of methotrexate (increased risk of toxicity).

There may be antagonism between amoxicillin and bacteriostatic agents such as chloramphenicol. An increased frequency of skin rashes has been reported in patients receiving amoxicillin together with allopurinol, compared to those receiving amoxicillin alone.

4.6 Pregnancy and lactation

There has been no evidence of a teratogenic effect in animals or untoward effect in humans. When antibiotic therapy is required during pregnancy, Amoxicillin may be considered appropriate.

Trace quantities of amoxicillin can be detected in breast milk.

4.7 Effects on ability to drive and use machines

None.

4.8 Undesirable effects

The most common adverse effects are sensitivity reactions including urticaria, maculo- papular rashes (often appearing more than seven days after commencing treatment), fever, joint pains and angioedema. Anaphylaxis occasionally occurs and has sometimes been fatal. Late sensitivity reactions may include serum sickness-like reactions, haemolytic anaemia and acute interstitial nephritis.

Other adverse effects are generally associated with large intravenous doses of amoxicillin or impaired renal function. These include transient leucopenia and thrombocytopenia, haemolytic anaemia and neutropenia (which might have some immunological basis); prolongation of bleeding time and defective platelet function; convulsions and other signs of central nervous system toxicity (encephalopathy has been reported following intrathecal administration and can be fatal); electrolyte disturbances due to administration of large amounts of sodium.

Most patients with infectious mononucleosis develop a maculopapular rash when treated with amoxicillin, and patients with other lymphoid disorders such as lymphatic leukaemia also appear to be at higher risk.

Some patients with syphilis may experience a Jarisch-Herxheimer reaction shortly after treatment is started. Symptoms include fever, chills, headache and reaction at the site of lesions. The reaction can be dangerous in cardiovascular syphilis or where there is a serious risk of increased local damage such as with optic atrophy.

Gastrointestinal effects (diarrhoea and nausea) reported with amoxicillin commonly occur after oral administration, not parenteral administration. Pseudomembranous colitis has been reported with most antibiotics.

Erythema multiforme (including Stevens-Johnson syndrome, toxic epidermal necrolysis, exfoliative dermatitis, hepatitis and cholestatic jaundice have been reported with combined amoxicillin and clavulanic acid therapy.

4.9 Overdose

Symptoms: gross overdosage will produce very high urinary concentrations, particularly after parenteral administration. Problems are unlikely if adequate fluid intake and urinary output are maintained but crystalluria is a possibility.

Treatment: is symptomatic. More specific measures may be necessary in patients with impaired renal function. Amoxicillin is removed by haemodialysis.

5. PHARMACOLOGICAL PROPERTIES

5.1 Pharmacodynamic properties

Amoxicillin is a member of the penicillin family. The penicillin nucleus consists of a thiazolidine ring connected to a β-lactam ring to which is attached a side-chain. The side-chain determines most of the pharmacological and antibacterial properties of the penicillin in question. In the case of amoxicillin the benzyl ring in the side chain extends the range of antimicrobial activity into the Gram-negative bacteria. Amoxicillin kills bacteria by interfering with the synthesis of the bacterial cell wall. As a result the bacterial cell wall is weakened, the cell swells and then ruptures. Amoxicillin is readily hydrolysed by the staphylococcal penicillinase. Its spectrum of activity is extended by administration with the β-lactamase inhibitor clavulanic acid.

5.2 Pharmacokinetic properties

After the equivalent of 500mg intramuscular amoxicillin, given as amoxicillin sodium, the serum level peaks at one hour at approximately 14mg L^{-1}

Amoxicillin is rapidly distributed throughout the body but penetrates the uninflamed meninges poorly. Its distribution into the cerebrospinal fluid is known to be less efficient than that of ampicillin. Amoxicillin concentrations in interstitial fluid peak around one hour after the serum peak, according to skin window tests. Concentrations in umbilical cord blood have been found to be a fraction of those in maternal blood. Concentrations in amniotic fluid are variable but less than 50% of maternal blood levels. The volume of blood distribution is 0.3 Lkg^{-1} bodyweight. Plasma protein binding is around 20%. Only small amounts of the drug are excreted in breast-milk.

Elimination of amoxicillin occurs via the kidneys by glomerular filtration and tubular secretion. After parenteral administration, 75% of the dose is excreted via the kidneys within the following six hours. High concentrations have been recorded in the bile, but in the presence of biliary tract obstruction amoxicillin may be undetectable.

A small amount (10-20%) of the drug is metabolised by hydrolysis of the β-lactam ring to penicilloic acid, which is excreted in the urine. There is limited enterohepatic circulation of the antibiotic.

5.3 Preclinical safety data

There are no pre-clinical data of relevance to the prescriber which are additional to those included in other sections.

6. PHARMACEUTICAL PARTICULARS

6.1 List of excipients

None

6.2 Incompatibilities

If amoxicillin is prescribed concurrently with an aminoglycoside, the antibiotics should not be mixed in the syringe, intravenous fluid container or giving set because under these conditions, loss of activity of the aminoglycoside can occur.

Amoxicillin should not be mixed with blood products or other proteinaceous fluids (eg protein hydrolysates) or with intravenous lipid emulsions.

6.3 Shelf life

36 months.

6.4 Special precautions for storage

Store below 25°C

Reconstituted solutions should be administered immediately after preparation.

6.5 Nature and contents of container

Vials containing 250mg or 500mg of amoxicillin sodium for injection in packs of 10 vials. Vials containing 1g of amoxicillin sodium for injection in single packs.

6.6 Instructions for use and handling

The vials are not suitable for multidose use.

Administrative Data

7. MARKETING AUTHORISATION HOLDER

CP Pharmaceuticals Ltd,
Ash Road North,
Wrexham
LL13 9UF

8. MARKETING AUTHORISATION NUMBER(S)

Amoxicillin Sodium for Injection BP 250mg - PL 4543/0398.

Amoxicillin Sodium for Injection BP 500mg - PL 4543/0399.

Amoxicillin Sodium for Injection BP 1g - PL 4543/0400.

9. DATE OF FIRST AUTHORISATION/RENEWAL OF THE AUTHORISATION

N/A

10. DATE OF REVISION OF THE TEXT

September 1998

Amoxil 3g Sachet

(GlaxoSmithKline UK)

1. NAME OF THE MEDICINAL PRODUCT

Amoxil® Sachets 3 G Sucrose-Free

2. QUALITATIVE AND QUANTITATIVE COMPOSITION

Amoxil Sachets 3 G Sucrose-Free contain 3 G amoxicillin per sachet

The amoxicillin is present as the trihydrate.

3. PHARMACEUTICAL FORM

Amoxil Sachets SF: sucrose-free sachets in a sorbitol base, for reconstitution in water.

Each sachet carries instructions for preparation.

4. CLINICAL PARTICULARS

4.1 Therapeutic indications

Treatment of Infection: Amoxil is a broad spectrum antibiotic indicated for the treatment of commonly occurring bacterial infections such as:

Upper respiratory tract infections

Otitis media

Acute and chronic bronchitis

Chronic bronchial sepsis

Lobar and bronchopneumonia

Cystitis, urethritis, pyelonephritis

Bacteriuria in pregnancy

Gynaecological infections including puerperal sepsis and septic abortion

Gonorrhoea

Peritonitis

Intra-abdominal sepsis

Septicaemia

Bacterial endocarditis

Typhoid and paratyphoid fever

Skin and soft tissue infections

Osteomyelitis

Dental abscess (as an adjunct to surgical management)

In children with urinary tract infection the need for investigation should be considered.

Prophylaxis of endocarditis: Amoxil may be used for the prevention of bacteraemia, associated with procedures such as dental extraction, in patients at risk of developing bacterial endocarditis.

The wide range of organisms sensitive to the bactericidal action of Amoxil include:

Gram-positive	Gram-negative
Streptococcus faecalis	*Haemophilus influenzae*
Streptococcus pneumoniae	*Escherichia coli*
Streptococcus pyogenes	*Proteus mirabilis*
Streptococcus viridans	*Salmonella* species
Staphylococcus aureus	*Shigella* species
(penicillin-sensitive)	*Bordetella pertussis*
Clostridium species	*Brucella* species
Corynebacterium species	*Neisseria gonorrhoeae*
Bacillus anthracis	*Neisseria meningitidis*
Listeria monocytogenes	*Vibrio cholerae*
	Pasteurella septica

4.2 Posology and method of administration

Administration:

Oral:

Treatment of Infection:

Adult dosage (including elderly patients):

Standard adult dosage: 250 mg three times daily, increasing to 500 mg three times daily for more severe infections.

High dosage therapy (maximum recommended oral dosage 6 g daily in divided doses): A dosage of 3 g twice daily is recommended in appropriate cases for the treatment of severe or recurrent purulent infection of the respiratory tract.

Short course therapy: Simple acute urinary tract infection: two 3 g doses with 10-12 hours between the doses. Dental abscess: two 3 g doses with 8 hours between the doses. Gonorrhoea: single 3 g dose.

Children's dosage (up to 10 years of age):

Standard children's dosage: 125 mg three times daily, increasing to 250 mg three times daily for more severe infections.

Amoxil Paediatric Suspension is recommended for children under six months of age.

In severe or recurrent acute otitis media, especially where compliance may be a problem, 750 mg twice a day for two days may be used as an alternative course of treatment in children aged 3 to 10 years.

Prophylaxis of endocarditis:

(see Table 1 on next page)

In renal impairment the excretion of the antibiotic will be delayed and, depending on the degree of impairment, it may be necessary to reduce the total daily dosage.

Prophylaxis of endocarditis: see table on previous page.

4.3 Contraindications

Amoxil is a penicillin and should not be given to penicillin-hypersensitive patients. Attention should be paid to possible cross-sensitivity with other beta-lactam antibiotics eg. cephalosporins.

4.4 Special warnings and special precautions for use

Serious and occasionally fatal hypersensitivity (anaphylactoid) reactions have been reported in patients on penicillin

Table 1 Prophylaxis of endocarditis

CONDITION		ADULTS' DOSAGE (INCLUDING ELDERLY)	CHILDREN'S DOSAGE	NOTES
Dental procedures: prophylaxis for patients undergoing extraction, scaling or surgery involving gingival tissues and who have not received a penicillin in the previous month. (N.B. Patients with prosthetic heart valves should be referred to hospital - see below).	Patient not having general anaesthetic.	3 g 'Amoxil' orally, 1 hour before procedure. A second dose may be given 6 hours later, if considered necessary.	Under 10: half adult dose. Under 5: quarter adult dose.	Note 1. If prophylaxis with 'Amoxil' is given twice within one month, emergence of resistant streptococci is unlikely to be a problem. Alternative antibiotics are recommended if more frequent prophylaxis is required, or if the patient has received a course of treatment with a penicillin during the previous month. Note 2 To minimise pain on injection, 'Amoxil' may be given as two injections of 500 mg dissolved in sterile 1% lignocaine solution (see *Administration*).
	Patient having general anaesthetic: if oral antibiotics considered to be appropriate.	Initially 3 g 'Amoxil' orally 4 hours prior to anaesthesia, followed by 3 g orally (or 1 g IV or IM if oral dose not tolerated) as soon as possible after the operation.		
	Patient having general anaesthetic: if oral antibiotics not appropriate.	1 g 'Amoxil' IV or IM immediately before induction; with 500 mg orally, 6 hours later.		
Dental procedures: patients for whom referral to hospital is recommended: a) Patients to be given a general anaesthetic who have been given a penicillin in the previous month. b) Patients to be given a general anaesthetic who have a prosthetic heart valve. c) Patients who have had one or more attacks of endocarditis.		Initially: 1 g 'Amoxil' IV or IM with 120 mg gentamicin IV or IM immediately prior to anaesthesia (if given) or 15 minutes prior to dental procedure. Followed by (6 hours later): 500 mg 'Amoxil' orally.	Under 10: the doses of 'Amoxil' should be half the adult dose; the dose of gentamicin should be 2 mg/kg. Under 5: the doses of 'Amoxil' should be quarter the adult dose; the dose of gentamicin should be 2 mg/kg.	See Note 2. Note 3. 'Amoxil' and gentamicin should not be mixed in the same syringe. Note 4. Please consult the appropriate data sheet for full prescribing information on gentamicin.
Genitourinary Surgery or Instrumentation: prophylaxis for patients who have no urinary tract infection and who are to have genito-urinary surgery or instrumentation under general anaesthesia. In the case of *Obstetric and Gynaecological Procedures* and *Gastrointestinal Procedures* – routine prophylaxis is recommended only for patients with prosthetic heart valves.		Initially: 1 g 'Amoxil' IV or IM with 120 mg gentamicin IV or IM, immediately before induction. Followed by (6 hours later): 500 mg 'Amoxil' orally or IV or IM according to clinical condition.		See Notes 2, 3 and 4 above.
Surgery or Instrumentation of the Upper Respiratory Tract	Patients other than those with prosthetic heart valves.	1 g 'Amoxil' IV or IM immediately before induction; 500 mg 'Amoxil' IV or IM 6 hours later.	Under 10: half adult dose. Under 5: quarter adult dose.	See Note 2 above. Note 5. The second dose of 'Amoxil' may be administered orally as 'Amoxil' Syrup SF/DF.
	Patients with prosthetic heart valves.	Initially: 1 g 'Amoxil' IV or IM with 120 mg gentamicin IV or IM, immediately before induction; followed by (6 hours later) 500 mg 'Amoxil' IV or IM.	Under 10: the dose of 'Amoxil' should be half the adult dose; the gentamicin dose should be 2 mg/kg. Under 5: the dose of 'Amoxil' should be quarter the adult dose; the dose of gentamicin should be 2 mg/kg.	See Notes 2, 3, 4 and 5 above.

therapy. These reactions are more likely to occur in individuals with a history of hypersensitivity to beta-lactam antibiotics (see 4.3).

Erythematous (morbilliform) rashes have been associated with glandular fever in patients receiving amoxicillin.

Prolonged use may also occasionally result in overgrowth of non-susceptible organisms.

In patients with reduced urine output, crystalluria has been observed very rarely, predominantly with parenteral therapy. During the administration of high doses of amoxicillin, it is advisable to maintain adequate fluid intake and urinary output in order to reduce the possibility of amoxicillin crystalluria (see Section 4.9 Overdose).

Dosage should be adjusted in patients with renal impairment (see 4.2).

4.5 Interaction with other medicinal products and other forms of Interaction

In common with other broad spectrum antibiotics, amoxicillin may reduce the efficacy of oral contraceptives and patients should be warned accordingly.

Concurrent administration of allopurinol during treatment with amoxicillin can increase the likelihood of allergic skin reactions.

Prolongation of prothrombin time has been reported rarely in patients receiving amoxicillin. Appropriate monitoring should be undertaken when anticoagulants are prescribed concurrently.

It is recommended that when testing for the presence of glucose in urine during amoxicillin treatment, enzymatic glucose oxidase methods should be used. Due to the high urinary concentrations of amoxicillin, false positive readings are common with chemical methods.

4.6 Pregnancy and lactation

Use in pregnancy:

Animal studies with Amoxil have shown no teratogenic effects. The product has been in extensive clinical use since 1972 and its suitability in human pregnancy has been well documented in clinical studies. When antibiotic therapy is required during pregnancy, Amoxil may be considered appropriate when the potential benefits outweigh the potential risks associated with treatment.

Use in lactation:

Amoxicillin may be given during lactation. With the exception of the risk of sensitisation associated with the excretion of trace quantities of amoxicillin in breast milk, there are no known detrimental effects for the breast-fed infant.

4.7 Effects on ability to drive and use machines

Adverse effects on the ability to drive or operate machinery have not been observed.

4.8 Undesirable effects

The following convention has been utilised for the classification of undesirable effects:-

Very common $>1/10$), common $>1/100$, $<1/10$), uncommon $>1/1000$, $<1/100$), rare $>1/10,000$, $<1/1000$), very rare ($<1/10,000$)

The majority of side effects listed below are not unique to amoxicillin and may occur when using other penicillins.

Unless otherwise stated, the frequency of adverse events has been derived from more than 30 years of post-marketing reports.

Blood and lymphatic system disorders

Very rare: Reversible leucopenia (including severe neutropenia or agranulocytosis), reversible thrombocytopenia and haemolytic anaemia.

Prolongation of bleeding time and prothrombin (see Section 4.5 - Interaction with other Medicaments and other Forms of Interaction)

Immune system disorders

Very rare: As with other antibiotics, severe allergic reactions, including angioneurotic oedema, anaphylaxis (see Section 4.4 - Special Warnings and Precautions for Use), serum sickness and hypersensitivity vasculitis.

If a hypersensitivity reaction is reported, the treatment must be discontinued. (See also Skin and subcutaneous tissue disorders).

Nervous system disorders

Very rare: Hyperkinesia, dizziness and convulsions. Convulsions may occur in patients with impaired renal function or in those receiving high doses.

Gastrointestinal disorders

Clinical Trial Data

***Common:** Diarrhoea and nausea.

***Uncommon:** Vomiting.

Post-marketing Data

Very rare: Mucocutaneous candidiasis and antibiotic associated colitis (including pseudomembraneous colitis and haemorrhagic colitis).

Superficial tooth discolouration has been reported in children. Good oral hygiene may help to prevent tooth discolouration as it can usually be removed by brushing.

Hepato-biliary disorders

Very rare: Hepatitis and cholestatic jaundice. A moderate rise in AST and/or ALT.

The significance of a rise in AST and/or ALT is unclear.

Skin and subcutaneous tissue disorders

Clinical Trial Data

***Common:** Skin rash

***Uncommon:** Urticaria and pruritus

Post-marketing Data

Very rare: Skin reactions such as erythema multiforme, Stevens-Johnson syndrome, toxic epidermal necrolysis, bullous and exfoliative dermatitis and acute generalised exanthematous pustulosis (AGEP)

(See also Immune system disorders).

Renal and urinary tract disorders

Very rare: Interstitial nephritis.

Very rare: Crystalluria (see Section 4.9 Overdose)

*The incidence of these AEs was derived from clinical studies involving a total of approximately 6,000 adult and paediatric patients taking amoxicillin.

4.9 Overdose

Gastrointestinal effects such as nausea, vomiting and diarrhoea may be evident and should be treated symptomatically with attention to the water/electrolyte balance. Amoxicillin crystalluria, in some cases leading to renal failure, has been observed (see Section 4.4 Special warnings and special precautions for use).

Amoxicillin may be removed from the circulation by haemodialysis.

5. PHARMACOLOGICAL PROPERTIES

5.1 Pharmacodynamic properties

Amoxil is a broad spectrum antibiotic.

It is rapidly bactericidal and possesses the safety profile of a penicillin.

5.2 Pharmacokinetic properties

Amoxil is well absorbed by the oral and parenteral routes. Oral administration, usually at convenient t.d.s. dosage, produces high serum levels independent of the time at which food is taken. Amoxil gives good penetration into bronchial secretions and high urinary concentrations of unchanged antibiotic.

5.3 Preclinical safety data

Not applicable.

6. PHARMACEUTICAL PARTICULARS

6.1 List of excipients

Amoxil Sachet SF

Each sachet contains quinoline yellow (E104), saccharin sodium, xanthan gum (E415), peach, strawberry and lemon dry flavours and sorbitol (E420).

6.2 Incompatibilities

None stated.

6.3 Shelf life

Sachet SF: 36 Months

6.4 Special precautions for storage

Amoxil Sachets SF should be stored in a dry place below 25°C.

6.5 Nature and contents of container

Amoxil Sachet 3 G Sucrose Free: Original packs of 2 and 14. Each sachet carries instructions for preparation and each pack contains a Patient Information Leaflet.

6.6 Instructions for use and handling

To be taken immediately following reconstitution.

Administrative Data

7. MARKETING AUTHORISATION HOLDER

Beecham Group plc
980 Great West Road
Brentford
Middlesex TW8 9GS
Trading as:
GlaxoSmithKline UK
Stockley Park West
Uxbridge
Middlesex UB11 1BT

8. MARKETING AUTHORISATION NUMBER(S)

Amoxil 3 G Sachet Sucrose-Free PL 00038/0334

9. DATE OF FIRST AUTHORISATION/RENEWAL OF THE AUTHORISATION

Amoxil 3 G Sachet Sucrose-Free 03 December 2002

10. DATE OF REVISION OF THE TEXT

01 February 2005

11. Legal Status

POM

Amoxil Capsules 250mg

(GlaxoSmithKline UK)

1. NAME OF THE MEDICINAL PRODUCT

Amoxil® Capsules 250 mg

2. QUALITATIVE AND QUANTITATIVE COMPOSITION

Amoxil Capsules 250 mg contain 250 mg amoxicillin per capsule

The amoxicillin is present as the trihydrate.

3. PHARMACEUTICAL FORM

Amoxil Capsules: maroon and gold capsules overprinted 'Amoxil 250'.

4. CLINICAL PARTICULARS

4.1 Therapeutic indications

Treatment of Infection: Amoxil is a broad spectrum antibiotic indicated for the treatment of commonly occurring bacterial infections such as:

Upper respiratory tract infections
Otitis media
Acute and chronic bronchitis
Chronic bronchial sepsis
Lobar and bronchopneumonia
Cystitis, urethritis, pyelonephritis
Bacteriuria in pregnancy
Gynaecological infections including puerperal sepsis and septic abortion
Gonorrhoea
Peritonitis
Intra-abdominal sepsis
Septicaemia
Bacterial endocarditis
Typhoid and paratyphoid fever
Skin and soft tissue infections
Dental abscess (as an adjunct to surgical management)
Helicobacter pylori eradication in peptic (duodenal and gastric) ulcer disease.

In children with urinary tract infection the need for investigation should be considered.

Prophylaxis of endocarditis: Amoxil may be used for the prevention of bacteraemia, associated with procedures such as dental extraction, in patients at risk of developing bacterial endocarditis.

Consideration should be given to official local guidance (e.g. national requirements) on the appropriate use of antibacterial agents. "Susceptibility of the causative organisms to the treatment should be tested (if possible), although the therapy may be initiated before the results are available.

4.2 Posology and method of administration

Treatment of Infection:

Adult dosage (including elderly patients):

Standard adult dosage: 250 mg three times daily, increasing to 500 mg three times daily for more severe infections.

High dosage therapy (maximum recommended oral dosage 6 g daily in divided doses): A dosage of 3 g twice daily is recommended in appropriate cases for the treatment of severe or recurrent purulent infection of the respiratory tract.

Short course therapy: Simple acute urinary tract infection: two 3 g doses with 10-12 hours between the doses. Dental abscess: two 3 g doses with 8 hours between the doses. Gonorrhoea: single 3 g dose.

Renal impairement:

Glomerular filtration rat >30ml/min No adjustment necessary.

Glomerular filtration rate 10-30ml/min: Amoxicillin. max. 500mg b.d

Glomerular filtration rate <10ml/min: Amoxicillin. Max. 500mg/day

Helicobacter eradication in peptic (duodenal and gastric) ulcer disease:

Amoxil is recommended at a dose of twice daily in association with a proton pump inhibitor and antimicrobial agents as detailed below:

Omeprazole 40 mg daily, Amoxicillin 1G BID, Clarithromycin 500mg

BID × 7days

or

Omeprazole 40mg daily, Amoxicillin750mg-1G BID, Metronidazole 400mg

TID × 7 days

Children's dosage (up to 10 years of age):

Standard children's dosage: 125 mg three times daily, increasing to 250 mg three times daily for more severe infections.

Renal impairement in children under 40 kg:

Creatnine clearance >30mL/min: No adjustment necessary.

Creatinine clearance 10-30mL/min: 15 mg/kg given b.i.d

Creatinine clearance <10mL/min: 15 mg/kg given as a single daily dose

Amoxil Paediatric Suspension is recommended for children under six months of age.

In severe or recurrent acute otitis media, especially where compliance may be a problem, 750 mg twice a day for two days may be used as an alternative course of treatment in children aged 3 to 10 years.

In renal impairment the excretion of the antibiotic will be delayed and, depending on the degree of impairment, it may be necessary to reduce the total daily dosage.

Prophylaxis of endocarditis: see table on next page.

Administration: Oral:

Treatment should be continued for 2 to 3 days following the disappearance of symptoms. It is recommended that at least 10 days treatment be given for any infection caused by beta-haemolytic streptococci in order to achieve eradication of the organism.

4.3 Contraindications

Amoxil is a penicillin and should not be given to penicillin-hypersensitive patients. Attention should be paid to possible cross-sensitivity with other beta-lactam antibiotics eg. cephalosporins.

4.4 Special warnings and special precautions for use

Before initiating therapy with amoxicillin, careful enquiry should be made concerning previous hypersensitivity reactions to penicillins, cephalosporins.

Serious and occasionally fatal hypersensitivity (anaphylactoid) reactions have been reported in patients on penicillin therapy. These reactions are more likely to occur in individuals with a history of hypersensitivity to beta-lactam antibiotics (see 4.3).

Erythematous (morbilliform) rashes have been associated with glandular fever in patients receiving amoxicillin.

Prolonged use may also occasionally result in overgrowth of non-susceptible organisms.

In patients with reduced urine output, crystalluria has been observed very rarely, predominantly with parenteral therapy. During the administration of high doses of amoxicillin, it is advisable to maintain adequate fluid intake and urinary output in order to reduce the possibility of amoxicillin crystalluria (see Section 4.9 Overdose).

In patients with renal impairment, the rate of excretion of amoxicillin will be reduced depending on the degree of impairment and it may be necessary to reduce the total daily unit amoxicillin dosage accordingly (see section 4.2).

4.5 Interaction with other medicinal products and other forms of Interaction

In common with other broad spectrum antibiotics, amoxicillin may reduce the efficacy of oral contraceptives and patients should be warned accordingly.

Concurrent administration of allopurinol during treatment with amoxicillincan increase the likelihood of allergic skin reactions.

Prolongation of prothrombin time has been reported rarely in patients receiving amoxicillin. Appropriate monitoring should be undertaken when anticoagulants are prescribed concurrently.

It is recommended that when testing for the presence of glucose in urine during amoxicillin treatment, enzymatic glucose oxidase methods should be used. Due to the high urinary concentrations of amoxicillin, false positive readings are common with chemical methods.

Probenecid decreases the renal tubular secretion of amoxicillin. Concurrent use with amoxicillin may result in increased and prolonged blood levels of amoxicillin.

Prophylaxis of endocarditis:

(see Table 1 on next page)

4.6 Pregnancy and lactation

Use in pregnancy:

Animal studies with Amoxil have shown no teratogenic effects. The product has been in extensive clinical use since 1972 and its suitability in human pregnancy has been well documented in clinical studies. When antibiotic therapy is required during pregnancy, Amoxil may be considered appropriate when the potential benefits outweigh the potential risks associated with treatment.

Use in lactation:

Amoxicillin may be given during lactation. With the exception of the risk of sensitisation associated with the excretion of trace quantities of amoxicillinin breast milk, there are no known detrimental effects for the breast-fed infant.

4.7 Effects on ability to drive and use machines

Adverse effects on the ability to drive or operate machinery have not been observed.

4.8 Undesirable effects

The following convention has been utilised for the classification of undesirable effects:-

Very common (>1/10), common (>1/100, <1/10), uncommon (>1/1000,<1/100), rare (>1/10,000, <1/1000), very rare (<1/10,000)

The majority of side effects listed below are not unique to amoxicillin and may occur when using other pencillins.

Unless otherwise stated, the frequency of adverse events has been derived from more than 30 years of post-marketing reports.

Blood and lymphatic system disorders

Very rare: Reversible leucopenia (including severe neutropenia or agranulocytosis), reversible thrombocytopenia and haemolytic anaemia.

Prolongation of bleeding time and prothrombin (see Section 4.5 - Interaction with other Medicaments and other Forms of Interaction)

Immune system disorders

Very rare: As with other antibiotics, severe allergic reactions, including angioneurotic oedema, anaphylaxis (see Section 4.4 - Special Warnings and Precautions for Use), serum sickness and hypersensitivity vasculitis.

If a hypersensitivity reaction is reported, the treatment must be discontinued. (See also Skin and subcutaneous tissue disorders).

Nervous system disorders

Very rare: Hyperkinesia, dizziness and convulsions. Convulsions may occur in patients with impaired renal function or in those receiving high doses.

Gastrointestinal disorders

Clinical Trial Data

***Common**: Diarrhoea and nausea.

***Uncommon**: Vomiting.

Post-marketing Data

Very rare: Mucocutaneous candidiasis and antibiotic associated colitis (including pseudomembraneous colitis and haemorrhagic colitis).

Table 1 Prophylaxis of endocarditis

CONDITION		ADULTS' DOSAGE (INCLUDING ELDERLY)	CHILDREN'S DOSAGE	NOTES
Dental procedures: prophylaxis for patients undergoing extraction, scaling or surgery involving gingival tissues and who have not received a penicillin in the previous month. (N.B. Patients with prosthetic heart valves should be referred to hospital - see below).	Patient not having general anaesthetic.	3 g 'Amoxil' orally, 1 hour before procedure. A second dose may be given 6 hours later, if considered necessary.	Under 10: half adult dose. Under 5: quarter adult dose.	Note 1. If prophylaxis with 'Amoxil' is given twice within one month, emergence of resistant streptococci is unlikely to be a problem. Alternative antibiotics are recommended if more frequent prophylaxis is required, or if the patient has received a course of treatment with a penicillin during the previous month. Note 2 To minimise pain on injection, 'Amoxil' may be given as two injections of 500 mg dissolved in sterile 1% lignocaine solution (see *Administration*).
	Patient having general anaesthetic: if oral antibiotics considered to be appropriate.	Initially 3 g 'Amoxil' orally 4 hours prior to anaesthesia, followed by 3 g orally (or 1 g IV or IM if oral dose not tolerated) as soon as possible after the operation.		
	Patient having general anaesthetic: if oral antibiotics not appropriate.	1 g 'Amoxil' IV or IM immediately before induction; with 500 mg orally, 6 hours later.		
Dental procedures: patients for whom referral to hospital is recommended: a) Patients to be given a general anaesthetic who have been given a penicillin in the previous month. b) Patients to be given a general anaesthetic who have a prosthetic heart valve. c) Patients who have had one or more attacks of endocarditis.		Initially: 1 g 'Amoxil' IV or IM with 120 mg gentamicin IV or IM immediately prior to anaesthesia (if given) or 15 minutes prior to dental procedure. Followed by (6 hours later): 500 mg 'Amoxil' orally.	Under 10: the doses of 'Amoxil' should be half the adult dose; the dose of gentamicin should be 2 mg/kg. Under 5: the doses of 'Amoxil' should be quarter the adult dose; the dose of gentamicin should be 2 mg/kg.	See Note 2. Note 3. 'Amoxil' and gentamicin should not be mixed in the same syringe. Note 4. Please consult the appropriate data sheet for full prescribing information on gentamicin.
Genitourinary Surgery or Instrumentation: prophylaxis for patients who have no urinary tract infection and who are to have genito-urinary surgery or instrumentation under general anaesthesia. In the case of *Obstetric and Gynaecological Procedures* and *Gastrointestinal Procedures* – routine prophylaxis is recommended only for patients with prosthetic heart valves.		Initially: 1 g 'Amoxil' IV or IM with 120 mg gentamicin IV or IM, immediately before induction. Followed by (6 hours later): 500 mg 'Amoxil' orally or IV or IM according to clinical condition.		See Notes 2, 3 and 4 above.
Surgery or Instrumentation of the Upper Respiratory Tract	Patients other than those with prosthetic heart valves.	1 g 'Amoxil' IV or IM immediately before induction; 500 mg 'Amoxil' IV or IM 6 hours later.	Under 10: half adult dose. Under 5: quarter adult dose.	See Note 2 above. Note 5. The second dose of 'Amoxil' may be administered orally as 'Amoxil' Syrup SF/DF.
	Patients with prosthetic heart valves.	Initially: 1 g 'Amoxil' IV or IM with 120 mg gentamicin IV or IM, immediately before induction; followed by (6 hours later) 500 mg 'Amoxil' IV or IM.	Under 10: the dose of 'Amoxil' should be half the adult dose; the gentamicin dose should be 2 mg/kg. Under 5: the dose of 'Amoxil' should be quarter the adult dose; the dose of gentamicin should be 2 mg/kg.	See Notes 2, 3, 4 and 5 above.

Superficial tooth discolouration has been reported in children. Good oral hygiene may help to prevent tooth discolouration as it can usually be removed by brushing.

Hepato-biliary disorders

Very rare: Hepatitis and cholestatic jaundice. A moderate rise in AST and/or ALT.

The significance of a rise in AST and/or ALT is unclear.

Skin and subcutaneous tissue disorders

Clinical Trial Data

*Common: Skin rash

*Uncommon: Urticaria and pruritus

Post-marketing Data

Very rare: Skin reactions such as erythema multiforme, Stevens-Johnson syndrome, toxic epidermal necrolysis, bullous and exfoliative dermatitis and acute generalised exanthematous pustulosis (AGEP)

(See also Immune system disorders).

Renal and urinary tract disorders

Very rare: Interstitial nephritis.

Very rare: Crystalluria (see Section 4.9 Overdose)

*The incidence of these AEs was derived from clinical studies involving a total of approximately 6,000 adult and paediatric patients taking amoxicillin.

4.9 Overdose

Gastrointestinal effects such as nausea, vomiting and diarrhoea may be evident and should be treated symptomatically with attention to the water/electrolyte balance. Amoxicillin crystalluria, in some cases leading to renal failure, has been observed (see Section 4.4 Special warnings and special precautions for use).

Amoxicillin may be removed from the circulation by haemodialysis.

5. PHARMACOLOGICAL PROPERTIES

5.1 Pharmacodynamic properties

Amoxil is a broad spectrum antibiotic.

It is rapidly bactericidal and possesses the safety profile of a penicillin.

The wide range of organisms sensitive to the bactericidal action of Amoxil include:

Aerobes:

Gram-positive	Gram-negative
Streptococcus faecalis	*Haemophilus influenzae*
Streptococcus pneumoniae	*Escherichia coli*
Streptococcus pyogenes	*Proteus mirabilis*
Streptococcus viridans	*Salmonella* species
Staphylococcus aureus (penicillin-sensitive strains only)	*Shigella* species
	Bordetella pertussis
	Brucella species
Corynebacterium species	*Neisseria gonorrhoeae*
Bacillus anthracis	*Neisseria meningitidis*
Listeria monocytogenes	*Vibrio cholerae*
	Pasteurella septica

Anaerobes:

Clostridium species

5.2 Pharmacokinetic properties

Amoxil is well absorbed by the oral and parenteral routes. Oral administration, usually at convenient t.d.s. dosage, produces high serum levels independent of the time at which food is taken. Amoxil gives good penetration into bronchial secretions and high urinary concentrations of unchanged antibiotic.

5.3 Preclinical safety data

Not applicable.

6. PHARMACEUTICAL PARTICULARS

6.1 List of excipients

Amoxil Capsules 250 Mg

Each capsule contains magnesium stearate (E572) and erythrosine (E127), indigo carmine (E132), titanium dioxide (E171), yellow iron oxide (E172) and gelatin.

6.2 Incompatibilities

None known.

6.3 Shelf life

Capsules 60M

6.4 Special precautions for storage

Amoxil Capsules should be stored in a dry place.

6.5 Nature and contents of container

Amoxil Capsules: 250 mg Original Pack of 21 with Patient Information Leaflet; also container of 500. Also packs of 3, 6, 12, 50, 100 and 50,000.

6.6 Instructions for use and handling

Not applicable.

Administrative Data

7. MARKETING AUTHORISATION HOLDER

Beecham Group plc

Great West Road, Brentford, Middlesex TW8 9GS

Trading as GlaxoSmithKline UK, Stockley Park West, Uxbridge, Middlesex UB11 1BT

And/or

Bencard or SmithKline Beecham Pharmaceuticals, Mundells, Welwyn Garden City, Hertfordshire, AL7 1EY.

8. MARKETING AUTHORISATION NUMBER(S)

Amoxil Capsules 250 mg 0038/0103

9. DATE OF FIRST AUTHORISATION/RENEWAL OF THE AUTHORISATION

19 April 1972 / 13 January 1998

10. DATE OF REVISION OF THE TEXT

01 February 2005

11. Legal Category

POM

Amoxil Capsules 500mg

(GlaxoSmithKline UK)

1. NAME OF THE MEDICINAL PRODUCT

Amoxil® Capsules 500 mg

2. QUALITATIVE AND QUANTITATIVE COMPOSITION

Amoxil Capsules 500 mg contain 500 mg amoxicillin per capsule

The amoxicillin is present as the trihydrate.

3. PHARMACEUTICAL FORM

Amoxil Capsules: maroon and gold capsules overprinted 'Amoxil 500'.

4. CLINICAL PARTICULARS

4.1 Therapeutic indications

Treatment of Infection: Amoxil is a broad spectrum antibiotic indicated for the treatment of commonly occurring bacterial infections such as:

Upper respiratory tract infections

Otitis media

Acute and chronic bronchitis

Chronic bronchial sepsis

Lobar and bronchopneumonia

Cystitis, urethritis, pyelonephritis

Bacteriuria in pregnancy

Gynaecological infections including puerperal sepsis and septic abortion

Gonorrhoea

Peritonitis

Intra-abdominal sepsis

Septicaemia

Bacterial endocarditis

Typhoid and paratyphoid fever

Skin and soft tissue infections

Dental abscess (as an adjunct to surgical management)

Helicobacter pylori eradication in peptic (duodenal and gastric) ulcer disease.

In children with urinary tract infection the need for investigation should be considered.

Prophylaxis of endocarditis: Amoxil may be used for the prevention of bacteraemia, associated with procedures such as dental extraction, in patients at risk of developing bacterial endocarditis.

Consideration should be given to official local guidance (e.g. national requirements) on the appropriate use of antibacterial agents.''Susceptibility of the causative organism to the treatment should be tested (if possible), although the therapy may be initiated before the results are available.

4.2 Posology and method of administration

Treatment of Infection:

Adult dosage (including elderly patients):

Standard adult dosage: 250 mg three times daily, increasing to 500 mg three times daily for more severe infections.

High dosage therapy (maximum recommended oral dosage 6 g daily in divided doses): A dosage of 3 g twice daily is recommended in appropriate cases for the treatment of severe or recurrent purulent infection of the respiratory tract.

Short course therapy: Simple acute urinary tract infection: two 3 g doses with 10-12 hours between the doses. Dental abscess: two 3 g doses with 8 hours between the doses. Gonorrhoea: single 3 g dose.

Helicobacter eradication in peptic (duodenal and gastric) ulcer disease:

Amoxil is recommended at a dose of twice daily in association with a proton pump inhibitor and antimicrobial agents as detailed below:

Omeprazole 40 mg daily, Amoxicillin 1G BID, Clarithromycin 500mg

BID × 7days

or

Omeprazole 40mg daily, Amoxicillin 750mg-1G BID, Metronidazole 400mg

TID × 7 days

Renal impairment:

Glomerular filtration rate >30ml/min No adjustment necessary.

Glomerular filtration rate 10-30ml/min: Amoxicillin. max. 500mg b.d

Glomerular filtration rate <10ml/min: Amoxicillin. max. 500mg/day

Children's dosage (up to 10 years of age):

Standard children's dosage: 125 mg three times daily, increasing to 250 mg three times daily for more severe infections.

Renal impairment in children under 40 kg:

Creatinine clearance >30mL/min: No adjustment necessary.

Creatinine clearance 10-30mL/min: 15 mg/kg given b.i.d

Creatinine clearance <10mL/min: 15 mg/kg given as a single daily dose

Amoxil Paediatric Suspension is recommended for children under six months of age.

In severe or recurrent acute otitis media, especially where compliance may be a problem, 750 mg twice a day for two days may be used as an alternative course of treatment in children aged 3 to 10 years.

In renal impairment the excretion of the antibiotic will be delayed and, depending on the degree of impairment, it may be necessary to reduce the total daily dosage.

Prophylaxis of endocarditis: see table on next page.

Administration: Oral:

Treatment should be continued for 2 to 3 days following the disappearance of symptoms. It is recommended that at least 10 days treatment be given for any infection caused by beta-haemolytic streptococci in order to achieve eradictaion of the organism.

4.3 Contraindications

Amoxil is a penicillin and should not be given to penicillin-hypersensitive patients. Attention should be paid to possible cross-sensitivity with other beta-lactam antibiotics eg. cephalosporins.

4.4 Special warnings and special precautions for use

Before initiating therapy with amoxicillin, careful enquiry should be made concerning previous hypersensitivity reactions to penicillins, cephalosporins.

Serious and occasionally fatal hypersensitivity (anaphylactoid) reactions have been reported in patients on penicillin therapy. These reactions are more likely to occur in individuals with a history of hypersensitivity to beta-lactam antibiotics (see 4.3).

Erythematous (morbilliform) rashes have been associated with glandular fever in patients receiving amoxicillin.

Prolonged use may also occasionally result in overgrowth of non-susceptible organisms.

In patients with reduced urine output, crystalluria has been observed very rarely, predominantly with parenteral therapy. During the administration of high doses of amoxicillin, it is advisable to maintain adequate fluid intake and urinary output in order to reduce the possibility of amoxicillin crystalluria (see Section 4.9 Overdose).

In patients with renal impairment, the rate of excretion of amoxicillin will be reduced depending on the degree of impairment and it may be necessary to reduce the total daily unit amoxicillin dosage accordingly (see section 4.2).

4.5 Interaction with other medicinal products and other forms of Interaction

In common with other broad spectrum antibiotics, amoxicillin may reduce the efficacy of oral contraceptives and patients should be warned accordingly.

Concurrent administration of allopurinol during treatment with amoxicillin can increase the likelihood of allergic skin reactions.

Prolongation of prothrombin time has been reported rarely in patients receiving amoxicillin. Appropriate monitoring should be undertaken when anticoagulants are prescribed concurrently.

It is recommended that when testing for the presence of glucose in urine during amoxicillin treatment, enzymatic glucose oxidase methods should be used. Due to the high urinary concentrations of amoxicillin, false positive readings are common with chemical methods.

Table 1 Prophylaxis of endocarditis

CONDITION		ADULTS' DOSAGE (INCLUDING ELDERLY)	CHILDREN'S DOSAGE	NOTES
Dental procedures: prophylaxis for patients undergoing extraction, scaling or surgery involving gingival tissues and who have not received a penicillin in the previous month. (N.B. Patients with prosthetic heart valves should be referred to hospital - see below).	Patient not having general anaesthetic.	3 g 'Amoxil' orally, 1 hour before procedure. A second dose may be given 6 hours later, if considered necessary.	Under 10: half adult dose. Under 5: quarter adult dose.	Note 1. If prophylaxis with 'Amoxil' is given twice within one month, emergence of resistant streptococci is unlikely to be a problem. Alternative antibiotics are recommended if more frequent prophylaxis is required, or if the patient has received a course of treatment with a penicillin during the previous month. Note 2 To minimise pain on injection, 'Amoxil' may be given as two injections of 500 mg dissolved in sterile 1% lignocaine solution (see *Administration*).
	Patient having general anaesthetic: if oral antibiotics considered to be appropriate.	Initially 3 g 'Amoxil' orally 4 hours prior to anaesthesia, followed by 3 g orally (or 1 g IV or IM if oral dose not tolerated) as soon as possible after the operation.		
	Patient having general anaesthetic: if oral antibiotics not appropriate.	1 g 'Amoxil' IV or IM immediately before induction; with 500 mg orally, 6 hours later.		
Dental procedures: patients for whom referral to hospital is recommended: a) Patients to be given a general anaesthetic who have been given a penicillin in the previous month. b) Patients to be given a general anaesthetic who have a prosthetic heart valve. c) Patients who have had one or more attacks of endocarditis.		Initially: 1 g 'Amoxil' IV or IM with 120 mg gentamicin IV or IM immediately prior to anaesthesia (if given) or 15 minutes prior to dental procedure. Followed by (6 hours later): 500 mg 'Amoxil' orally.	Under 10: the doses of 'Amoxil' should be half the adult dose; the dose of gentamicin should be 2 mg/kg. Under 5: the doses of 'Amoxil' should be quarter the adult dose; the dose of gentamicin should be 2 mg/kg.	See Note 2. Note 3. 'Amoxil' and gentamicin should not be mixed in the same syringe. Note 4. Please consult the appropriate data sheet for full prescribing information on gentamicin.
Genitourinary Surgery or Instrumentation: prophylaxis for patients who have no urinary tract infection and who are to have genito-urinary surgery or instrumentation under general anaesthesia. In the case of *Obstetric and Gynaecological Procedures* and *Gastrointestinal Procedures* – routine prophylaxis is recommended only for patients with prosthetic heart valves.		Initially: 1 g 'Amoxil' IV or IM with 120 mg gentamicin IV or IM, immediately before induction. Followed by (6 hours later): 500 mg 'Amoxil' orally or IV or IM according to clinical condition.		See Notes 2, 3 and 4 above.
Surgery or Instrumentation of the Upper Respiratory Tract	Patients other than those with prosthetic heart valves.	1 g 'Amoxil' IV or IM immediately before induction; 500 mg 'Amoxil' IV or IM 6 hours later.	Under 10: half adult dose. Under 5: quarter adult dose.	See Note 2 above. Note 5. The second dose of 'Amoxil' may be administered orally as 'Amoxil' Syrup SF/DF.
	Patients with prosthetic heart valves.	Initially: 1 g 'Amoxil' IV or IM with 120 mg gentamicin IV or IM, immediately before induction; followed by (6 hours later) 500 mg 'Amoxil' IV or IM.	Under 10: the dose of 'Amoxil' should be half the adult dose; the gentamicin dose should be 2 mg/kg. Under 5: the dose of 'Amoxil' should be quarter the adult dose; the dose of gentamicin should be 2 mg/kg.	See Notes 2, 3, 4 and 5 above.

Probenecid decreases the renal tubular secretion of amoxicillin. Concurrent use with amoxicillin may result in increased and prolonged blood levels of amoxicillin.

Prophylaxis of endocarditis:

(see Table 1 on previous page)

4.6 Pregnancy and lactation

Use in pregnancy:

Animal studies with Amoxil have shown no teratogenic effects. The product has been in extensive clinical use since 1972 and its suitability in human pregnancy has been well documented in clinical studies. When antibiotic therapy is required during pregnancy, Amoxil may be considered appropriate when the potential benefits outweigh the potential risks associated with treatment.

Use in lactation:

Amoxicillin may be given during lactation. With the exception of the risk of sensitisation associated with the excretion of trace quantities of amoxicillin in breast milk, there are no known detrimental effects for the breast-fed infant.

4.7 Effects on ability to drive and use machines

Adverse effects on the ability to drive or operate machinery have not been observed.

4.8 Undesirable effects

The following convention has been utilised for the classification of undesirable effects:-

Very common (>1/10), common (>1/100, <1/10), uncommon (>1/1000,<1/100), rare (>1/10,000, <1/1000), very rare (<1/10,000)

The majority of side effects listed below are not unique to amoxicillin and may occur when using other penicillins.

Unless otherwise stated, the frequency of adverse events has been derived from more than 30 years of post-marketing reports.

Blood and lymphatic system disorders

Very rare: Reversible leucopenia (including severe neutropenia or agranulocytosis), reversible thrombocytopenia and haemolytic anaemia.

Prolongation of bleeding time and prothrombin (see Section 4.5 - Interaction with other Medicaments and other Forms of Interaction)

Immune system disorders

Very rare: As with other antibiotics, severe allergic reactions, including angioneurotic oedema, anaphylaxis (see Section 4.4 - Special Warnings and Precautions for Use), serum sickness and hypersensitivity vasculitis.

If a hypersensitivity reaction is reported, the treatment must be discontinued. (See also Skin and subcutaneous tissue disorders).

Nervous system disorders

Very rare: Hyperkinesia, dizziness and convulsions. Convulsions may occur in patients with impaired renal function or in those receiving high doses.

Gastrointestinal disorders

Clinical Trial Data

*__Common__: Diarrhoea and nausea.

*__Uncommon__: Vomiting.

Post-marketing Data

Very rare: Mucocutaneous candidiasis and antibiotic associated colitis (including pseudomembraneous colitis and haemorrhagic colitis).

Superficial tooth discolouration has been reported in children. Good oral hygiene may help to prevent tooth discolouration as it can usually be removed by brushing.

Hepato-biliary disorders

Very rare: Hepatitis and cholestatic jaundice. A moderate rise in AST and/or ALT.

The significance of a rise in AST and/or ALT is unclear.

Skin and subcutaneous tissue disorders

Clinical Trial Data

*__Common__: Skin rash

*__Uncommon__: Urticaria and pruritus

Post-marketing Data

Very rare: Skin reactions such as erythema multiforme, Stevens-Johnson syndrome, toxic epidermal necrolysis, bullous and exfoliative dermatitis and acute generalised exanthematous pustulosis (AGEP)

(See also Immune system disorders).

Renal and urinary tract disorders

Very rare: Interstitial nephritis.

Very rare: Crystalluria (see Section 4.9 Overdose)

*The incidence of these AEs was derived from clinical studies involving a total of approximately 6,000 adult and paediatric patients taking amoxicillin.

4.9 Overdose

Gastrointestinal effects such as nausea, vomiting and diarrhoea may be evident and should be treated symptomatically with attention to the water/electrolyte balance. Amoxicillin crystalluria, in some cases leading to renal failure, has been observed (see Section 4.4 Special warnings and special precautions for use).

Amoxicillin may be removed from the circulation by haemodialysis.

5. PHARMACOLOGICAL PROPERTIES

5.1 Pharmacodynamic properties

Amoxil is a broad spectrum antibiotic.

It is rapidly bactericidal and possesses the safety profile of a penicillin.

The wide range of organisms sensitive to the bactericidal action of Amoxil include:

Aerobes:

Gram-positive Gram-negative

Streptococcus faecalis Haemophilus influenzae

Streptococcus pneumoniae Escherichia coli

Streptococcus pyogenes Proteus mirabilis

Streptococcus viridans Salmonella species

Staphylococcus aureus Shigella species

(penicillin-sensitive strains only) *Bordetella pertussis*

Brucella species

Corynebacterium species *Neisseria gonorrhoeae*

Bacillus anthracis Neisseria meningitidis

Listeria monocytogenesVibrio cholerae

Pasteurella septica

Anaerobes:

Clostridium species

5.2 Pharmacokinetic properties

Amoxil is well absorbed by the oral and parenteral routes. Oral administration, usually at convenient t.d.s. dosage, produces high serum levels independent of the time at which food is taken. Amoxil gives good penetration into bronchial secretions and high urinary concentrations of unchanged antibiotic.

5.3 Preclinical safety data

Not applicable.

6. PHARMACEUTICAL PARTICULARS

6.1 List of excipients

Amoxil Capsules 500 Mg

Each capsule contains magnesium stearate (E572) and erythrosine (E127), indigo carmine (E132), titanium dioxide (E171), yellow iron oxide (E172) and gelatin.

6.2 Incompatibilities

None known.

6.3 Shelf life

Capsules 60M

6.4 Special precautions for storage

Amoxil Capsules should be stored in a dry place.

6.5 Nature and contents of container

Amoxil Capsules: 500 mg Original Pack of 21 with Patient Information Leaflet; also container of 100. Also packs of 3, 6, 12, 50 and 500.

6.6 Instructions for use and handling

Not applicable.

Administrative Data

7. MARKETING AUTHORISATION HOLDER

Beecham Group plc

Great West Road, Brentford, Middlesex TW8 9GS

Trading as GlaxoSmithKline UK, Stockley Park West, Uxbridge, Middlesex UB11 1BT

And/or

Bencard or SmithKline Beecham Pharmaceuticals, Mundells, Welwyn Garden City, Hertfordshire AL7 1EY.

8. MARKETING AUTHORISATION NUMBER(S)

Amoxil Capsules 500 mg 0038/0105

9. DATE OF FIRST AUTHORISATION/RENEWAL OF THE AUTHORISATION

19 April 1972 / 13 January 1998

10. DATE OF REVISION OF THE TEXT

01 February 2005

11. Legal Status

POM

Amoxil Paediatric Suspension

(GlaxoSmithKline UK)

1. NAME OF THE MEDICINAL PRODUCT

Amoxil® Paediatric Suspension

2. QUALITATIVE AND QUANTITATIVE COMPOSITION

Amoxil Paediatric Suspension contains 125 mg amoxicillin per 1.25 ml dose

The amoxicillin is present as the trihydrate.

3. PHARMACEUTICAL FORM

Amoxil Paediatric Suspension: citrus flavoured suspension. Presented as powder in bottles for preparing 20 ml.

4. CLINICAL PARTICULARS

4.1 Therapeutic indications

Treatment of Infection: Amoxil is a broad spectrum antibiotic indicated for the treatment of commonly occurring bacterial infections such as:

Upper respiratory tract infections

Otitis media

Acute and chronic bronchitis

Chronic bronchial sepsis

Lobar and bronchopneumonia

Cystitis, urethritis, pyelonephritis

Bacteriuria in pregnancy

Gynaecological infections including puerperal sepsis and septic abortion

Gonorrhoea

Peritonitis

Intra-abdominal sepsis

Septicaemia

Bacterial endocarditis

Typhoid and paratyphoid fever

Skin and soft tissue infections

Osteomyelitis

Dental abscess (as an adjunct to surgical management)

In children with urinary tract infection the need for investigation should be considered.

Prophylaxis of endocarditis: Amoxil may be used for the prevention of bacteraemia, associated with procedures such as dental extraction, in patients at risk of developing bacterial endocarditis.

Consideration should be given to official local guidance (e.g. national requirements) on the appropriate use of antibacterial agents.''Susceptibility of the causative organism to the treatment should be tested (if possible), although the therapy may be initiated before the results are available.

4.2 Posology and method of administration

Treatment of Infection:

Adult dosage (including elderly patients):

Oral:

Standard adult dosage: 250 mg three times daily, increasing to 500 mg three times daily for more severe infections.

High dosage therapy (maximum recommended oral dosage 6 g daily in divided doses): A dosage of 3 g twice daily is recommended in appropriate cases for the treatment of severe or recurrent purulent infection of the respiratory tract.

Short course therapy: Simple acute urinary tract infection: two 3 g doses with 10-12 hours between the doses. Dental abscess: two 3 g doses with 8 hours between the doses. Gonorrhoea: single 3 g dose.

Renal impairment:

Glomerular filtration rate >30ml/min No adjustment necessary.

Glomerular filtration rate 10-30ml/min: Amoxicillin. max. 500mg b.d

Glomerular filtration rate <10ml/min: Amoxicillin. max. 500mg/day

Children's dosage (up to 10 years of age):

Oral:

Standard children's dosage: 125 mg three times daily, increasing to 250 mg three times daily for more severe infections.

Renal impairment in children under 40 kg:

Creatinine clearance >30mL/min: No adjustment necessary.

Creatinine clearance 10-30mL/min: 15 mg/kg given b.i.d

Creatinine clearance <10mL/min: 15 mg/kg given as a single daily dose

Amoxil Paediatric Suspension is recommended for children under six months of age.

In severe or recurrent acute otitis media, especially where compliance may be a problem, 750 mg twice a day for two days may be used as an alternative course of treatment in children aged 3 to 10 years.

Prophylaxis of endocarditis:

(see Table 1 on next page)

In renal impairment the excretion of the antibiotic will be delayed and, depending on the degree of impairment, it may be necessary to reduce the total daily dosage.

Prophylaxis of endocarditis: see table on previous page.

Administration:

Oral.

Treatment should be continued for 2 to 3 days following the disappearance of symptoms. It is recommended that at least 10 days treatment be given for any infection caused by beta-haemolytic streptococci in order to achieve eradictaion of the organism.

4.3 Contraindications

Amoxil is a penicillin and should not be given to penicillin-hypersensitive patients. Attention should be paid to

Table 1 Prophylaxis of endocarditis

CONDITION		ADULTS' DOSAGE (INCLUDING ELDERLY)	CHILDREN'S DOSAGE	NOTES
Dental procedures: prophylaxis for patients undergoing extraction, scaling or surgery involving gingival tissues and who have not received a penicillin in the previous month. (N.B. Patients with prosthetic heart valves should be referred to hospital - see below).	Patient not having general anaesthetic.	3 g 'Amoxil' orally, 1 hour before procedure. A second dose may be given 6 hours later, if considered necessary.	Under 10: half adult dose. Under 5: quarter adult dose.	Note 1. If prophylaxis with 'Amoxil' is given twice within one month, emergence of resistant streptococci is unlikely to be a problem. Alternative antibiotics are recommended if more frequent prophylaxis is required, or if the patient has received a course of treatment with a penicillin during the previous month. Note 2 To minimise pain on injection, 'Amoxil' may be given as two injections of 500 mg dissolved in sterile 1% lignocaine solution (see *Administration*).
	Patient having general anaesthetic: if oral antibiotics considered to be appropriate.	Initially 3 g 'Amoxil' orally 4 hours prior to anaesthesia, followed by 3 g orally (or 1 g IV or IM if oral dose not tolerated) as soon as possible after the operation.		
	Patient having general anaesthetic: if oral antibiotics not appropriate.	1 g 'Amoxil' IV or IM immediately before induction; with 500 mg orally, 6 hours later.		
Dental procedures: patients for whom referral to hospital is recommended: a) Patients to be given a general anaesthetic who have been given a penicillin in the previous month. b) Patients to be given a general anaesthetic who have a prosthetic heart valve. c) Patients who have had one or more attacks of endocarditis.		Initially: 1 g 'Amoxil' IV or IM with 120 mg gentamicin IV or IM immediately prior to anaesthesia (if given) or 15 minutes prior to dental procedure. Followed by (6 hours later): 500 mg 'Amoxil' orally.	Under 10: the doses of 'Amoxil' should be half the adult dose; the dose of gentamicin should be 2 mg/kg. Under 5: the doses of 'Amoxil' should be quarter the adult dose; the dose of gentamicin should be 2 mg/kg.	See Note 2. Note 3. 'Amoxil' and gentamicin should not be mixed in the same syringe. Note 4. Please consult the appropriate data sheet for full prescribing information on gentamicin.
Genitourinary Surgery or Instrumentation: prophylaxis for patients who have no urinary tract infection and who are to have genito-urinary surgery or instrumentation under general anaesthesia. In the case of *Obstetric and Gynaecological Procedures* and *Gastrointestinal Procedures* – routine prophylaxis is recommended only for patients with prosthetic heart valves.		Initially: 1 g 'Amoxil' IV or IM with 120 mg gentamicin IV or IM, immediately before induction. Followed by (6 hours later): 500 mg 'Amoxil' orally or IV or IM according to clinical condition.		See Notes 2, 3 and 4 above.
Surgery or Instrumentation of the Upper Respiratory Tract	Patients other than those with prosthetic heart valves.	1 g 'Amoxil' IV or IM immediately before induction; 500 mg 'Amoxil' IV or IM 6 hours later.	Under 10: half adult dose. Under 5: quarter adult dose.	See Note 2 above. Note 5. The second dose of 'Amoxil' may be administered orally as 'Amoxil' Syrup SF/DF.
	Patients with prosthetic heart valves.	Initially: 1 g 'Amoxil' IV or IM with 120 mg gentamicin IV or IM, immediately before induction; followed by (6 hours later) 500 mg 'Amoxil' IV or IM.	Under 10: the dose of 'Amoxil' should be half the adult dose; the gentamicin dose should be 2 mg/kg. Under 5: the dose of 'Amoxil' should be quarter the adult dose; the dose of gentamicin should be 2 mg/kg.	See Notes 2, 3, 4 and 5 above.

possible cross-sensitivity with other beta-lactam antibiotics eg. cephalosporins.

4.4 Special warnings and special precautions for use

Before initiating therapy with amoxicillin, careful enquiry should be made concerning previous hypersensitivity reactions to penicillins, cephalosporins.

Serious and occasionally fatal hypersensitivity (anaphylactoid) reactions have been reported in patients on penicillin therapy. These reactions are more likely to occur in individuals with a history of hypersensitivity to beta-lactam antibiotics (see 4.3).

Erythematous (morbilliform) rashes have been associated with glandular fever in patients receiving amoxicillin.

Prolonged use may also occasionally result in overgrowth of non-susceptible organisms.

In patients with reduced urine output, crystalluria has been observed very rarely, predominantly with parenteral therapy. During the administration of high doses of amoxicillin, it is advisable to maintain adequate fluid intake and urinary output in order to reduce the possibility of amoxicillin crystalluria (see Section 4.9 Overdose).

In patients with renal impairment, the rate of excretion of amoxicillin will be reduced depending on the degree of impairment and it may be necessary to reduce the total daily unit amoxicillin dosage accordingly (see section 4.2).

4.5 Interaction with other medicinal products and other forms of Interaction

In common with other broad spectrum antibiotics, amoxicillin may reduce the efficacy of oral contraceptives and patients should be warned accordingly.

Concurrent administration of allopurinol during treatment with amoxicillin can increase the likelihood of allergic skin reactions.

Prolongation of prothrombin time has been reported rarely in patients receiving amoxicillin. Appropriate monitoring should be undertaken when anticoagulants are prescribed concurrently.

It is recommended that when testing for the presence of glucose in urine during amoxicillin treatment, enzymatic glucose oxidase methods should be used. Due to the high urinary concentrations of amoxicillin, false positive readings are common with chemical methods.

Probenecid decreases the renal tubular secretion of amoxicillin. Concurrent use with amoxicillin may result in increased and prolonged blood levels of amoxicillin.

4.6 Pregnancy and lactation

Use in pregnancy:

Animal studies with Amoxil have shown no teratogenic effects. The product has been in extensive clinical use since 1972 and its suitability in human pregnancy has been well documented in clinical studies. When antibiotic therapy is required during pregnancy, Amoxil may be considered appropriate when the potential benefits outweigh the potential risks associated with treatment.

Use in lactation:

Amoxicillin may be given during lactation. With the exception of the risk of sensitisation associated with the excretion of trace quantities of amoxicillin in breast milk, there are no known detrimental effects for the breast-fed infant.

4.7 Effects on ability to drive and use machines

Adverse effects on the ability to drive or operate machinery have not been observed.

4.8 Undesirable effects

The following convention has been utilised for the classification of undesirable effects:-

Very common (>1/10), common (>1/100, <1/10), uncommon (>1/1000,<1/100), rare (>1/10,000, <1/1000), very rare (<1/10,000)

The majority of side effects listed below are not unique to amoxicillin and may occur when using other penicillins.

Unless otherwise stated, the frequency of adverse events has been derived from more than 30 years of post-marketing reports.

Blood and lymphatic system disorders

Very rare: Reversible leucopenia (including severe neutropenia or agranulocytosis), reversible thrombocytopenia and haemolytic anaemia.

Prolongation of bleeding time and prothrombin (see Section 4.5 - Interaction with other Medicaments and other Forms of Interaction)

Immune system disorders

Very rare: As with other antibiotics, severe allergic reactions, including angioneurotic oedema, anaphylaxis (see Section 4.4 - Special Warnings and Precautions for Use), serum sickness and hypersensitivity vasculitis.

If a hypersensitivity reaction is reported, the treatment must be discontinued. (See also Skin and subcutaneous tissue disorders).

Nervous system disorders

Very rare: Hyperkinesia, dizziness and convulsions. Convulsions may occur in patients with impaired renal function or in those receiving high doses.

Gastrointestinal disorders

Clinical Trial Data

*__Common__: Diarrhoea and nausea.

*__Uncommon__: Vomiting.

Post-marketing Data

Very rare: Mucocutaneous candidiasis and antibiotic associated colitis (including pseudomembraneous colitis and haemorrhagic colitis).

Superficial tooth discolouration has been reported in children. Good oral hygiene may help to prevent tooth discolouration as it can usually be removed by brushing.

Hepato-biliary disorders

Very rare: Hepatitis and cholestatic jaundice. A moderate rise in AST and/or ALT.

The significance of a rise in AST and/or ALT is unclear.

Skin and subcutaneous tissue disorders

Clinical Trial Data

*__Common__: Skin rash

*__Uncommon__: Urticaria and pruritus

Post-marketing Data

Very rare: Skin reactions such as erythema multiforme, Stevens-Johnson syndrome, toxic epidermal necrolysis, bullous and exfoliative dermatitis and acute generalised exanthematous pustulosis (AGEP)

(See also Immune system disorders).

Renal and urinary tract disorders

Very rare: Interstitial nephritis.

Very rare: Crystalluria (see Section 4.9 Overdose).

*The incidence of these AEs was derived from clinical studies involving a total of approximately 6,000 adult and paediatric patients taking amoxicillin.

4.9 Overdose

Gastrointestinal effects such as nausea, vomiting and diarrhoea may be evident and should be treated symptomatically with attention to the water/electrolyte balance. Amoxicillin crystalluria, in some cases leading to renal failure, has been observed (see Section 4.4 Special warnings and special precautions for use).

Amoxicillin may be removed from the circulation by haemodialysis.

5. PHARMACOLOGICAL PROPERTIES

5.1 Pharmacodynamic properties

Amoxil is a broad spectrum antibiotic.

It is rapidly bactericidal and possesses the safety profile of a penicillin.

The wide range of organisms sensitive to the bactericidal action of Amoxil include:

Aerobes:

Gram-positive Gram-negative

Streptococcus faecalis Haemophilus influenzae

Streptococcus pneumoniae Escherichia coli

Streptococcus pyogenes Proteus mirabilis

Streptococcus viridans Salmonella species

Staphylococcus aureus Shigella species

(penicillin-sensitive strains only) *Bordetella pertussis*

Brucella species

Corynebacterium species *Neisseria gonorrhoeae*

Bacillus anthracis Neisseria meningitidis

Listeria monocytogenesVibrio cholerae

Pasteurella septica

Anaerobes:

Clostridium species

5.2 Pharmacokinetic properties

Amoxil is well absorbed by the oral and parenteral routes. Oral administration, usually at convenient t.d.s. dosage, produces high serum levels independent of the time at which food is taken. Amoxil gives good penetration into bronchial secretions and high urinary concentrations of unchanged antibiotic.

5.3 Preclinical safety data

Not applicable.

6. PHARMACEUTICAL PARTICULARS

6.1 List of excipients

Amoxil Paediatric Suspension

The powder contains sodium benzoate (E211), sodium carboxymethylcellulose (E466), quinoline yellow (E104), peach, strawberry and lemon dry flavours and sucrose (0.6 g per 1.25 ml dose).

6.2 Incompatibilities

None known.

6.3 Shelf life

Paediatric Suspension 36M (once reconstituted: 14 days)

6.4 Special precautions for storage

Prior to use, Amoxil Paediatric Suspension should be stored in a dry place.

Once dispensed, Amoxil Paediatric Suspension should be stored at 25°C or below and used within 14 days. Amoxil Paediatric Suspension may be diluted with water or Syrup BP.

6.5 Nature and contents of container

Amoxil Paediatric Suspension: 125 mg per 1.25 ml: Original Pack of 20 ml with pipette and Patient Information Leaflet.

6.6 Instructions for use and handling

None.

Administrative Data

7. MARKETING AUTHORISATION HOLDER

Beecham Group plc

Great West Road, Brentford, Middlesex TW8 9GS

Trading as GlaxoSmithKline UK Stockley Park West, Uxbridge, Middlesex UB11 1BT

And/or

Bencard or SmithKline Beecham Pharmaceuticals, Mundells, Welwyn Garden City, Hertfordshire AL7 1EY

8. MARKETING AUTHORISATION NUMBER(S)

Amoxil Paediatric Suspension

125 mg per 1.25 ml 0038/0107

9. DATE OF FIRST AUTHORISATION/RENEWAL OF THE AUTHORISATION

07 March 1972 / 13 January 1998

10. DATE OF REVISION OF THE TEXT

01 February 2005

11. Legal Status

POM

Amoxil Syrup Sucrose-Free/Dye-Free 125mg/5ml

(GlaxoSmithKline UK)

1. NAME OF THE MEDICINAL PRODUCT

Amoxil® Syrup Sucrose-Free/Dye-Free 125 mg/5 ml

2. QUALITATIVE AND QUANTITATIVE COMPOSITION

Amoxil Syrup SF/DF 125 mg contains 125 mg amoxicillin per 5 ml dose.

The amoxicillin is present as the trihydrate.

3. PHARMACEUTICAL FORM

Amoxil Syrup SF/DF 125 mg/5 ml: citrus-flavoured sucrose-free/dye-free suspension in a sorbitol base. Presented as powder in bottles for preparing 100 ml.

4. CLINICAL PARTICULARS

4.1 Therapeutic indications

Treatment of Infection: Amoxil is a broad spectrum antibiotic indicated for the treatment of commonly occurring bacterial infections such as:

Upper respiratory tract infections

Otitis media

Acute and chronic bronchitis

Chronic bronchial sepsis

Lobar and bronchopneumonia

Cystitis, urethritis, pyelonephritis

Bacteriuria in pregnancy

Gynaecological infections including puerperal sepsis and septic abortion

Gonorrhoea

Peritonitis

Intra-abdominal sepsis

Septicaemia

Bacterial endocarditis

Typhoid and paratyphoid fever

Skin and soft tissue infections

Osteomyelitis

Dental abscess (as an adjunct to surgical management)

In children with urinary tract infection the need for investigation should be considered.

Prophylaxis of endocarditis: Amoxil may be used for the prevention of bacteraemia, associated with procedures such as dental extraction, in patients at risk of developing bacterial endocarditis.

The wide range of organisms sensitive to the bactericidal action of Amoxil include:

Gram-positive Gram-negative

Streptococcus faecalis Haemophilus influenzae

Streptococcus pneumoniae Escherichia coli

Streptococcus pyogenes Proteus mirabilis

Streptococcus viridans Salmonella species

Staphylococcus aureus Shigella species

(penicillin-sensitive) *Bordetella pertussis*

Clostridium species *Brucella* species

Corynebacterium species *Neisseria gonorrhoeae*

Bacillus anthracis Neisseria meningitidis

Listeria monocytogenesVibrio cholerae

Pasteurella septica

4.2 Posology and method of administration

Treatment of Infection:

Adult dosage (including elderly patients):

Oral:

Standard adult dosage: 250 mg three times daily, increasing to 500 mg three times daily for more severe infections.

High dosage therapy (maximum recommended oral dosage 6 g daily in divided doses): A dosage of 3 g twice daily is recommended in appropriate cases for the treatment of severe or recurrent purulent infection of the respiratory tract.

Short course therapy: Simple acute urinary tract infection: two 3 g doses with 10-12 hours between the doses. Dental abscess: two 3 g doses with 8 hours between the doses. Gonorrhoea: single 3 g dose.

Injectable:

500 mg IM eight hourly (or more frequently if necessary) in moderate infections. (This dose may be given by slow IV injection if more convenient.)

1 g IV six hourly in severe infections.

Children's dosage (up to 10 years of age):

Oral:

Standard children's dosage: 125 mg three times daily, increasing to 250 mg three times daily for more severe infections.

Amoxil Paediatric Suspension is recommended for children under six months of age.

Prophylaxis of endocarditis:

(see Table 1 on next page)

In severe or recurrent acute otitis media, especially where compliance may be a problem, 750 mg twice a day for two days may be used as an alternative course of treatment in children aged 3 to 10 years.

Injectable:

50-100 mg/kg body weight a day, in divided doses.

Parenteral therapy is indicated if the oral route is considered impracticable or unsuitable, and particularly for the urgent treatment of severe infection.

In renal impairment the excretion of the antibiotic will be delayed and, depending on the degree of impairment, it may be necessary to reduce the total daily dosage.

Prophylaxis of endocarditis: see table on previous page.

Administration:

Oral

4.3 Contraindications

Amoxil is a penicillin and should not be given to penicillin-hypersensitive patients. Attention should be paid to possible cross-sensitivity with other beta-lactam antibiotics eg. cephalosporins.

4.4 Special warnings and special precautions for use

Serious and occasionally fatal hypersensitivity (anaphylactoid) reactions have been reported in patients on penicillin therapy. These reactions are more likely to occur in individuals with a history of hypersensitivity to beta-lactam antibiotics (see 4.3).

Erythematous (morbilliform) rashes have been associated with glandular fever in patients receiving amoxicillin.

Prolonged use may also occasionally result in overgrowth of non-susceptible organisms.

In patients with reduced urine output, crystalluria has been observed very rarely, predominantly with parenteral therapy. During the administration of high doses of amoxicillin, it is advisable to maintain adequate fluid intake and urinary output in order to reduce the possibility of amoxicillin crystalluria (see Section 4.9 Overdose).

Dosage should be adjusted in patients with renal impairment (see 4.2).

4.5 Interaction with other medicinal products and other forms of Interaction

In common with other broad spectrum antibiotics, amoxicillin may reduce the efficacy of oral contraceptives and patients should be warned accordingly.

Concurrent administration of allopurinol during treatment with amoxicillin can increase the likelihood of allergic skin reactions.

Prolongation of prothrombin time has been reported rarely in patients receiving amoxicillin. Appropriate monitoring should be undertaken when anticoagulants are prescribed concurrently.

It is recommended that when testing for the presence of glucose in urine during amoxicillin treatment, enzymatic glucose oxidase methods should be used. Due to the high urinary concentrations of amoxicillin, false positive readings are common with chemical methods.

4.6 Pregnancy and lactation

Use in pregnancy:

Animal studies with Amoxil have shown no teratogenic effects. The product has been in extensive clinical use since 1972 and its suitability in human pregnancy has been well documented in clinical studies. When antibiotic therapy is required during pregnancy, Amoxil may be considered appropriate when the potential benefits outweigh the potential risks associated with treatment.

Use in lactation:

Amoxicillin may be given during lactation. With the exception of the risk of sensitisation associated with the excretion of trace quantities of amoxicillin in breast milk, there are no known detrimental effects for the breast-fed infant.

4.7 Effects on ability to drive and use machines

Adverse effects on the ability to drive or operate machinery have not been observed.

4.8 Undesirable effects

The following convention has been utilised for the classification of undesirable effects:-

Very common (>1/10), common (>1/100, <1/10), uncommon (>1/1000,<1/100), rare (>1/10,000, <1/1000), very rare (<1/10,000)

The majority of side effects listed below are not unique to amoxicillin and may occur when using other pencillins.

Unless otherwise stated, the frequency of adverse events has been derived from more than 30 years of post-marketing reports.

Blood and lymphatic system disorders

Very rare: Reversible leucopenia (including severe neutropenia or agranulocytosis), reversible thrombocytopenia and haemolytic anaemia.

Prolongation of bleeding time and prothrombin (see Section 4.5 - Interaction with other Medicaments and other Forms of Interaction)

Immune system disorders

Very rare: As with other antibiotics, severe allergic reactions, including angioneurotic oedema, anaphylaxis (see Section 4.4 - Special Warnings and Precautions for Use), serum sickness and hypersensitivity vasculitis.

If a hypersensitivity reaction is reported, the treatment must be discontinued. (See also Skin and subcutaneous tissue disorders).

Table 1 Prophylaxis of endocarditis

CONDITION		ADULTS' DOSAGE (INCLUDING ELDERLY)	CHILDREN'S DOSAGE	NOTES
Dental procedures: prophylaxis for patients undergoing extraction, scaling or surgery involving gingival tissues and who have not received a penicillin in the previous month. (N.B. Patients with prosthetic heart valves should be referred to hospital - see below).	Patient not having general anaesthetic.	3 g 'Amoxil' orally, 1 hour before procedure. A second dose may be given 6 hours later, if considered necessary.	Under 10: half adult dose. Under 5: quarter adult dose.	Note 1. If prophylaxis with 'Amoxil' is given twice within one month, emergence of resistant streptococci is unlikely to be a problem. Alternative antibiotics are recommended if more frequent prophylaxis is required, or if the patient has received a course of treatment with a penicillin during the previous month. Note 2 To minimise pain on injection, 'Amoxil' may be given as two injections of 500 mg dissolved in sterile 1% lignocaine solution (see *Administration*).
	Patient having general anaesthetic: if oral antibiotics considered to be appropriate.	Initially 3 g 'Amoxil' orally 4 hours prior to anaesthesia, followed by 3 g orally (or 1 g IV or IM if oral dose not tolerated) as soon as possible after the operation.		
	Patient having general anaesthetic: if oral antibiotics not appropriate.	1 g 'Amoxil' IV or IM immediately before induction; with 500 mg orally, 6 hours later.		
Dental procedures: patients for whom referral to hospital is recommended: a) Patients to be given a general anaesthetic who have been given a penicillin in the previous month. b) Patients to be given a general anaesthetic who have a prosthetic heart valve. c) Patients who have had one or more attacks of endocarditis.		Initially: 1 g 'Amoxil' IV or IM with 120 mg gentamicin IV or IM immediately prior to anaesthesia (if given) or 15 minutes prior to dental procedure. Followed by (6 hours later): 500 mg 'Amoxil' orally.	Under 10: the doses of 'Amoxil' should be half the adult dose; the dose of gentamicin should be 2 mg/kg. Under 5: the doses of 'Amoxil' should be quarter the adult dose; the dose of gentamicin should be 2 mg/kg.	See Note 2. Note 3. 'Amoxil' and gentamicin should not be mixed in the same syringe. Note 4. Please consult the appropriate data sheet for full prescribing information on gentamicin.
Genitourinary Surgery or Instrumentation: prophylaxis for patients who have no urinary tract infection and who are to have genito-urinary surgery or instrumentation under general anaesthesia. In the case of *Obstetric and Gynaecological Procedures* and *Gastrointestinal Procedures* – routine prophylaxis is recommended only for patients with prosthetic heart valves.		Initially: 1 g 'Amoxil' IV or IM with 120 mg gentamicin IV or IM, immediately before induction. Followed by (6 hours later): 500 mg 'Amoxil' orally or IV or IM according to clinical condition.		See Notes 2, 3 and 4 above.
Surgery or Instrumentation of the Upper Respiratory Tract	Patients other than those with prosthetic heart valves.	1 g 'Amoxil' IV or IM immediately before induction; 500 mg 'Amoxil' IV or IM 6 hours later.	Under 10: half adult dose. Under 5: quarter adult dose.	See Note 2 above. Note 5. The second dose of 'Amoxil' may be administered orally as 'Amoxil' Syrup SF/DF.
	Patients with prosthetic heart valves.	Initially: 1 g 'Amoxil' IV or IM with 120 mg gentamicin IV or IM, immediately before induction; followed by (6 hours later) 500 mg 'Amoxil' IV or IM.	Under 10: the dose of 'Amoxil' should be half the adult dose; the gentamicin dose should be 2 mg/kg. Under 5: the dose of 'Amoxil' should be quarter the adult dose; the dose of gentamicin should be 2 mg/kg.	See Notes 2, 3, 4 and 5 above.

Nervous system disorders

Very rare: Hyperkinesia, dizziness and convulsions. Convulsions may occur in patients with impaired renal function or in those receiving high doses.

Gastrointestinal disorders

Clinical Trial Data

*__Common__: Diarrhoea and nausea.

*__Uncommon__: Vomiting.

Post-marketing Data

Very rare: Mucocutaneous candidiasis and antibiotic associated colitis (including pseudomembraneous colitis and haemorrhagic colitis).

Superficial tooth discolouration has been reported in children. Good oral hygiene may help to prevent tooth discolouration as it can usually be removed by brushing.

Hepato-biliary disorders

Very rare: Hepatitis and cholestatic jaundice. A moderate rise in AST and/or ALT.

The significance of a rise in AST and/or ALT is unclear.

Skin and subcutaneous tissue disorders

Clinical Trial Data

*__Common__: Skin rash

*__Uncommon__: Urticaria and pruritus

Post-marketing Data

Very rare: Skin reactions such as erythema multiforme, Stevens-Johnson syndrome, toxic epidermal necrolysis, bullous and exfoliative dermatitis and acute generalised exanthematous pustulosis (AGEP)

(See also Immune system disorders).

Renal and urinary tract disorders

Very rare: Interstitial nephritis.

Very rare: Crystalluria (see Section 4.9 Overdose).

*The incidence of these AE's was derived from clinical studies involving a total of approximately 6,000 adult and paediatric patients taking amoxicillin.

4.9 Overdose

Gastrointestinal effects such as nausea, vomiting and diarrhoea may be evident and should be treated symptomatically with attention to the water/electrolyte balance. Amoxicillin crystalluria, in some cases leading to renal failure, has been observed (see Section 4.4 Special warnings and special precautions for use).

Amoxicillin may be removed from the circulation by haemodialysis.

5. PHARMACOLOGICAL PROPERTIES

5.1 Pharmacodynamic properties

Amoxil is a broad spectrum antibiotic.

It is rapidly bactericidal and possesses the safety profile of a penicillin.

5.2 Pharmacokinetic properties

Amoxil is well absorbed by the oral and parenteral routes. Oral administration, usually at convenient t.d.s. dosage, produces high serum levels independent of the time at which food is taken. Amoxil gives good penetration into bronchial secretions and high urinary concentrations of unchanged antibiotic.

5.3 Preclinical safety data

Not applicable.

6. PHARMACEUTICAL PARTICULARS

6.1 List of excipients

Amoxil Syrup SF/DF 125 mg/5ml

The powder contains disodium edetate, sodium benzoate (E211), saccharin sodium, silica (E551), xanthan gum (E415), peach, strawberry and lemon dry flavours and sorbitol (E420).

6.2 Incompatibilities

None.

6.3 Shelf life

Amoxil Syrup SF/DF 125 mg /5 ml — 60M (once reconstituted: 14 days)

6.4 Special precautions for storage

Store powder in a dry place. Once dispensed, Amoxil Syrup SF/DF should be used within 14 days. If dilution of the reconstituted SF/DF product is required, water should be used.

6.5 Nature and contents of container

Amoxil Syrup SF/DF 125 mg/5 ml: Original Pack of 100 ml with Patient InformationLeaflet.

6.6 Instructions for use and handling

None

Administrative Data

7. MARKETING AUTHORISATION HOLDER

Beecham Group plc

Great West Road

Brentford

Middlesex TW8 9GS

Trading as:

GlaxoSmithKline UK, Stockley Park West, Uxbridge, Middlesex UB11 1BT

And/or

Bencard or SmithKline Beecham Pharmaceuticals all at Mundells Welwyn Garden City, Hertfordshire AL7 1EY

8. MARKETING AUTHORISATION NUMBER(S)

Amoxil Syrup SF/DF 125 mg/5 ml — 0038/0326

9. DATE OF FIRST AUTHORISATION/RENEWAL OF THE AUTHORISATION

14 May 1985 / 16 January 1998

10. DATE OF REVISION OF THE TEXT

5th July 2005

11. Legal Status

POM

Amoxil Syrup Sucrose-Free/Dye-Free 250mg/5ml

(GlaxoSmithKline UK)

1. NAME OF THE MEDICINAL PRODUCT

Amoxil® Syrup Sucrose-Free/Dye-Free 250 mg/5 ml

2. QUALITATIVE AND QUANTITATIVE COMPOSITION

Amoxil Syrup SF/DF 250 mg contains 250 mg amoxicillin per 5 ml dose.

The amoxicillin is present as the trihydrate.

3. PHARMACEUTICAL FORM

Amoxil Syrup SF/DF 250 mg/5 ml: citrus-flavoured sucrose-free/Dye Freesuspension in a sorbitol base. Presented as powder in bottles for preparing 100 ml.

4. CLINICAL PARTICULARS

4.1 Therapeutic indications

Treatment of Infection: Amoxil is a broad spectrum antibiotic indicated for the treatment of commonly occurring bacterial infections such as:

Upper respiratory tract infections

Otitis media

Acute and chronic bronchitis
Chronic bronchial sepsis
Lobar and bronchopneumonia
Cystitis, urethritis, pyelonephritis
Bacteriuria in pregnancy
Gynaecological infections including puerperal sepsis and septic abortion
Gonorrhoea
Peritonitis
Intra-abdominal sepsis
Septicaemia
Bacterial endocarditis
Typhoid and paratyphoid fever
Skin and soft tissue infections
Osteomyelitis
Dental abscess (as an adjunct to surgical management)

In children with urinary tract infection the need for investigation should be considered.

Prophylaxis of endocarditis: Amoxil may be used for the prevention of bacteraemia, associated with procedures such as dental extraction, in patients at risk of developing bacterial endocarditis.

The wide range of organisms sensitive to the bactericidal action of Amoxil include:

Gram-positive	Gram-negative
Streptococcus faecalis	*Haemophilus influenzae*
Streptococcus pneumoniae	*Escherichia coli*
Streptococcus pyogenes	*Proteus mirabilis*
Streptococcus viridans	*Salmonella* species
Staphylococcus aureus (penicillin-sensitive)	*Shigella* species
	Bordetella pertussis
Clostridium species	*Brucella* species
Corynebacterium species	*Neisseria gonorrhoeae*
Bacillus anthracis	*Neisseria meningitidis*
Listeria monocytogenes	*Vibrio cholerae*
	Pasteurella septica

4.2 Posology and method of administration

Treatment of Infection:

Adult dosage (including elderly patients):

Oral:

Standard adult dosage: 250 mg three times daily, increasing to 500 mg three times daily for more severe infections.

High dosage therapy (maximum recommended oral dosage 6 g daily in divided doses): A dosage of 3 g twice daily is recommended in appropriate cases for the treatment of severe or recurrent purulent infection of the respiratory tract.

Short course therapy: Simple acute urinary tract infection: two 3 g doses with 10-12 hours between the doses. Dental abscess: two 3 g doses with 8 hours between the doses. Gonorrhoea: single 3 g dose.

Injectable:

500 mg IM eight hourly (or more frequently if necessary) in moderate infections. (This dose may be given by slow IV injection if more convenient.)

1 g IV six hourly in severe infections.

Children's dosage (up to 10 years of age):

Oral:

Standard children's dosage: 125 mg three times daily, increasing to 250 mg three times daily for more severe infections.

Amoxil Paediatric Suspension is recommended for children under six months of age.

Prophylaxis of endocarditis:

(see Table 1)

In severe or recurrent acute otitis media, especially where compliance may be a problem, 750 mg twice a day for two days may be used as an alternative course of treatment in children aged 3 to 10 years.

Injectable:

50-100 mg/kg body weight a day, in divided doses.

Parenteral therapy is indicated if the oral route is considered impracticable or unsuitable, and particularly for the urgent treatment of severe infection.

In renal impairment the excretion of the antibiotic will be delayed and, depending on the degree of impairment, it may be necessary to reduce the total daily dosage.

Prophylaxis of endocarditis: see table on previous page.

Administration:

Oral

Table 1 Prophylaxis of endocarditis

CONDITION		ADULTS' DOSAGE (INCLUDING ELDERLY)	CHILDREN'S DOSAGE	NOTES
Dental procedures: prophylaxis for patients undergoing extraction, scaling or surgery involving gingival tissues and who have not received a penicillin in the previous month. (N.B. Patients with prosthetic heart valves should be referred to hospital - see below).	Patient not having general anaesthetic.	3 g 'Amoxil' orally, 1 hour before procedure. A second dose may be given 6 hours later, if considered necessary.	Under 10: half adult dose. Under 5: quarter adult dose.	Note 1. If prophylaxis with 'Amoxil' is given twice within one month, emergence of resistant streptococci is unlikely to be a problem. Alternative antibiotics are recommended if more frequent prophylaxis is required, or if the patient has received a course of treatment with a penicillin during the previous month. Note 2 To minimise pain on injection, 'Amoxil' may be given as two injections of 500 mg dissolved in sterile 1% lignocaine solution (see *Administration*).
	Patient having general anaesthetic: if oral antibiotics considered to be appropriate.	Initially 3 g 'Amoxil' orally 4 hours prior to anaesthesia, followed by 3 g orally (or 1 g IV or IM if oral dose not tolerated) as soon as possible after the operation.		
	Patient having general anaesthetic: if oral antibiotics not appropriate.	1 g 'Amoxil' IV or IM immediately before induction; with 500 mg orally, 6 hours later.		
Dental procedures: patients for whom referral to hospital is recommended: a) Patients to be given a general anaesthetic who have been given a penicillin in the previous month. b) Patients to be given a general anaesthetic who have a prosthetic heart valve. c) Patients who have had one or more attacks of endocarditis.		Initially: 1 g 'Amoxil' IV or IM with 120 mg gentamicin IV or IM immediately prior to anaesthesia (if given) or 15 minutes prior to dental procedure. Followed by (6 hours later): 500 mg 'Amoxil' orally.	Under 10: the doses of 'Amoxil' should be half the adult dose; the dose of gentamicin should be 2 mg/kg. Under 5: the doses of 'Amoxil' should be quarter the adult dose; the dose of gentamicin should be 2 mg/kg.	See Note 2. Note 3. 'Amoxil' and gentamicin should not be mixed in the same syringe. Note 4. Please consult the appropriate data sheet for full prescribing information on gentamicin.
Genitourinary Surgery or Instrumentation: prophylaxis for patients who have no urinary tract infection and who are to have genito-urinary surgery or instrumentation under general anaesthesia. In the case of *Obstetric and Gynaecological Procedures* and *Gastrointestinal Procedures* – routine prophylaxis is recommended only for patients with prosthetic heart valves.		Initially: 1 g 'Amoxil' IV or IM with 120 mg gentamicin IV or IM, immediately before induction. Followed by (6 hours later): 500 mg 'Amoxil' orally or IV or IM according to clinical condition.		See Notes 2, 3 and 4 above.
Surgery or Instrumentation of the Upper Respiratory Tract	Patients other than those with prosthetic heart valves.	1 g 'Amoxil' IV or IM immediately before induction; 500 mg 'Amoxil' IV or IM 6 hours later.	Under 10: half adult dose. Under 5: quarter adult dose.	See Note 2 above. Note 5. The second dose of 'Amoxil' may be administered orally as 'Amoxil' Syrup SF/DF.
	Patients with prosthetic heart valves.	Initially: 1 g 'Amoxil' IV or IM with 120 mg gentamicin IV or IM, immediately before induction; followed by (6 hours later) 500 mg 'Amoxil' IV or IM.	Under 10: the dose of 'Amoxil' should be half the adult dose; the gentamicin dose should be 2 mg/kg. Under 5: the dose of 'Amoxil' should be quarter the adult dose; the dose of gentamicin should be 2 mg/kg.	See Notes 2, 3, 4 and 5 above.

4.3 Contraindications

Amoxil is a penicillin and should not be given to penicillin-hypersensitive patients. Attention should be paid to possible cross-sensitivity with other beta-lactam antibiotics eg. cephalosporins.

4.4 Special warnings and special precautions for use

Serious and occasionally fatal hypersensitivity (anaphylactoid) reactions have been reported in patients on penicillin therapy. These reactions are more likely to occur in individuals with a history of hypersensitivity to beta-lactam antibiotics (see 4.3).

Erythematous (morbilliform) rashes have been associated with glandular fever in patients receiving amoxicillin.

Prolonged use may also occasionally result in overgrowth of non-susceptible organisms.

In patients with reduced urine output, crystalluria has been observed very rarely, predominantly with parenteral therapy. During the administration of high doses of amoxicillin, it is advisable to maintain adequate fluid intake and urinary output in order to reduce the possibility of amoxicillin crystalluria (see Section 4.9 Overdose).

Dosage should be adjusted in patients with renal impairment (see 4.2).

4.5 Interaction with other medicinal products and other forms of Interaction

In common with other broad spectrum antibiotics, amoxicillin may reduce the efficacy of oral contraceptives and patients should be warned accordingly.

Concurrent administration of allopurinol during treatment with amoxicillin can increase the likelihood of allergic skin reactions.

Prolongation of prothrombin time has been reported rarely in patients receiving amoxicillin. Appropriate monitoring should be undertaken when anticoagulants are prescribed concurrently.

It is recommended that when testing for the presence of glucose in urine during amoxicillin treatment, enzymatic glucose oxidase methods should be used. Due to the high urinary concentrations of amoxicillin, false positive readings are common with chemical methods.

4.6 Pregnancy and lactation

Use in pregnancy:

Animal studies with Amoxil have shown no teratogenic effects. The product has been in extensive clinical use since 1972 and its suitability in human pregnancy has been well documented in clinical studies. When antibiotic therapy is required during pregnancy, Amoxil may be considered appropriate when the potential benefits outweigh the potential risks associated with treatment.

Use in lactation:

Amoxicillin may be given during lactation. With the exception of the risk of sensitisation associated with the excretion of trace quantities of amoxicillin in breast milk, there are no known detrimental effects for the breast-fed infant.

4.7 Effects on ability to drive and use machines
Adverse effects on the ability to drive or operate machinery have not been observed.

4.8 Undesirable effects
The following convention has been utilised for the classification of undesirable effects:-

Very common (>1/10), common (>1/100, <1/10), uncommon (>1/1000,<1/100), rare (>1/10,000, <1/1000), very rare (<1/10,000)

The majority of side effects listed below are not unique to amoxycillin and may occur when using other pencillins.

Unless otherwise stated, the frequency of adverse events has been derived from more than 30 years of post-marketing reports.

Blood and lymphatic system disorders

Very rare: Reversible leucopenia (including severe neutropenia or agranulocytosis), reversible thrombocytopenia and haemolytic anaemia.

Prolongation of bleeding time and prothrombin (see Section 4.5 - Interaction with other Medicaments and other Forms of Interaction)

Immune system disorders

Very rare: As with other antibiotics, severe allergic reactions, including angioneurotic oedema, anaphylaxis (see Section 4.4 - Special Warnings and Precautions for Use), serum sickness and hypersensitivity vasculitis.

If a hypersensitivity reaction is reported, the treatment must be discontinued. (See also Skin and subcutaneous tissue disorders).

Nervous system disorders

Very rare: Hyperkinesia, dizziness and convulsions. Convulsions may occur in patients with impaired renal function or in those receiving high doses.

Gastrointestinal disorders

Clinical Trial Data

***Common**: Diarrhoea and nausea.

***Uncommon**: Vomiting.

Post-marketing Data

Very rare: Mucocutaneous candidiasis and antibiotic associated colitis (including pseudomembraneous colitis and haemorrhagic colitis).

Superficial tooth discolouration has been reported in children. Good oral hygiene may help to prevent tooth discolouration as it can usually be removed by brushing.

Hepato-biliary disorders

Very rare: Hepatitis and cholestatic jaundice. A moderate rise in AST and/or ALT.

The significance of a rise in AST and/or ALT is unclear.

Skin and subcutaneous tissue disorders

Clinical Trial Data

***Common**: Skin rash

***Uncommon**: Urticaria and pruritus

Post-marketing Data

Very rare: Skin reactions such as erythema multiforme, Stevens-Johnson syndrome, toxic epidermal necrolysis, bullous and exfoliative dermatitis and acute generalised exanthematous pustulosis (AGEP)

(See also Immune system disorders).

Renal and urinary tract disorders

Very rare: Interstitial nephritis.

Very rare: Crystalluria (see Section 4.9 Overdose).

*The incidence of these AEs was derived from clinical studies involving a total of approximately 6,000 adult and paediatric patients taking amoxicillin.

4.9 Overdose
Gastrointestinal effects such as nausea, vomiting and diarrhoea may be evident and should be treated symptomatically with attention to the water/electrolyte balance. Amoxicillin crystalluria, in some cases leading to renal failure, has been observed (see Section 4.4 Special warnings and special precautions for use).

Amoxicillin may be removed from the circulation by haemodialysis.

5. PHARMACOLOGICAL PROPERTIES
5.1 Pharmacodynamic properties
Amoxil is a broad spectrum antibiotic.

It is rapidly bactericidal and possesses the safety profile of a penicillin.

5.2 Pharmacokinetic properties
Amoxil is well absorbed by the oral and parenteral routes. Oral administration, usually at convenient t.d.s. dosage, produces high serum levels independent of the time at which food is taken. Amoxil gives good penetration into bronchial secretions and high urinary concentrations of unchanged antibiotic.

5.3 Preclinical safety data
Not applicable.

6. PHARMACEUTICAL PARTICULARS
6.1 List of excipients
Amoxil Syrup SF/DF 250 mg / 5ml

The powder contains disodium edetate, sodium benzoate (E211), saccharin sodium, silica (E551), xanthan gum (E415), peach, strawberry and lemon dry flavours and sorbitol (E420).

6.2 Incompatibilities
None.

6.3 Shelf life

Amoxil Syrup SF/DF 250 mg / 5 ml	60M (once reconstituted: 14 days)

6.4 Special precautions for storage
Store powder in a dry place. Once dispensed, Amoxil Syrup SF/DF should be used within 14 days. If dilution of the reconstituted SF/DF product is required, water should be used.

6.5 Nature and contents of container
Amoxil Syrup SF/DF 250 mg/5 ml: Original Pack of 100 ml with Patient InformationLeaflet.

6.6 Instructions for use and handling
None

Administrative Data
7. MARKETING AUTHORISATION HOLDER
Beecham Group plc

Great West Road, Brentford

Middlesex TW8 9GS

Trading as:

GlaxoSmithKline UK, Stockley Park West, Uxbridge, Middlesex UB11 1BT

And/or

Bencard or SmithKline Beecham Pharmaceuticals all at Mundells Welwyn Garden City, Hertfordshire AL7 1EY

8. MARKETING AUTHORISATION NUMBER(S)
Amoxil Syrup SF/DF 250 mg/5 ml 0038/0327

9. DATE OF FIRST AUTHORISATION/RENEWAL OF THE AUTHORISATION
14 May 1985 / 16 January 1998

10. DATE OF REVISION OF THE TEXT
5th July 2005

11. Legal Status
POM

Amoxil Vials for Injection 1g

(GlaxoSmithKline UK)

1. NAME OF THE MEDICINAL PRODUCT
Amoxil® Vials For Injection 1 G

2. QUALITATIVE AND QUANTITATIVE COMPOSITION
Amoxil Vials for Injection 1 g contain 1 g amoxicillin

The amoxicillin is present as the sodium salt in Amoxil injections (each 1 g vial contains approximately 3.3 mmol of sodium).

3. PHARMACEUTICAL FORM
Amoxil Vials: vials containing sterile powder for reconstitution.

4. CLINICAL PARTICULARS
4.1 Therapeutic indications
Treatment of Infection: Amoxil is a broad spectrum antibiotic indicated for the treatment of commonly occurring bacterial infections such as:

Upper respiratory tract infections

Otitis media

Acute and chronic bronchitis

Chronic bronchial sepsis

Lobar and bronchopneumonia

Cystitis, urethritis, pyelonephritis

Bacteriuria in pregnancy

Gynaecological infections including puerperal sepsis and septic abortion

Gonorrhoea

Peritonitis

Intra-abdominal sepsis

Septicaemia

Bacterial endocarditis

Typhoid and paratyphoid fever

Skin and soft tissue infections

In children with urinary tract infection the need for investigation should be considered.

Prophylaxis of endocarditis: Amoxil may be used for the prevention of bacteraemia, associated with procedures such as dental extraction, in patients at risk of developing bacterial endocarditis.

The wide range of organisms sensitive to the bactericidal action of Amoxil include:

Gram-positive	Gram-negative
Streptococcus faecalis	*Haemophilus influenzae*
Streptococcus pneumoniae	*Escherichia coli*
Streptococcus pyogenes	*Proteus mirabilis*
Streptococcus viridans	*Salmonella* species
Staphylococcus aureus (penicillin-sensitive)	*Shigella* species
	Bordetella pertussis
Clostridium species	*Brucella* species
Corynebacterium species	*Neisseria gonorrhoeae*
Bacillus anthracis	*Neisseria meningitidis*
Listeria monocytogenes	*Vibrio cholerae*
	Pasteurella septica

4.2 Posology and method of administration
Treatment of infection:

Adult dosage (including elderly patients):

Injectable:

500 mg IM eight hourly (or more frequently if necessary) in moderate infections. (This dose may be given by slow IV injection if more convenient.)

1 g IV six hourly in severe infections.

Children's dosage (*up to 10 years of age*):

Injectable:

50-100 mg/kg body weight a day, in divided doses.

Parenteral therapy is indicated if the oral route is considered impracticable or unsuitable, and particularly for the urgent treatment of severe infection.

In renal impairment the excretion of the antibiotic will be delayed and, depending on the degree of impairment, it may be necessary to reduce the total daily dosage.

Prophylaxis of endocarditis: see table on next page.

Prophylaxis of endocarditis:

(see Table 1 on next page)

Administration:

Intravenous Injection, Intravenous Infusion, Intramuscular: Using vials for injection (See Section 6.6)

4.3 Contraindications
Amoxil is a penicillin and should not be given to penicillin-hypersensitive patients. Attention should be paid to possible cross-sensitivity with other beta-lactam antibiotics, e.g. cephalosporins.

4.4 Special warnings and special precautions for use
Serious and occasionally fatal hypersensitivity (anaphylactoid) reactions have been reported in patients on penicillin therapy. These reactions are more likely to occur in individuals with a history of hypersensitivity to beta-lactam antibiotics (see Section 4.3).

Erythematous (morbilliform) rashes have been associated with glandular fever in patients receiving amoxicillin.

Prolonged use may also occasionally result in overgrowth of non-susceptible organisms.

In patients with reduced urine output, crystalluria has been observed very rarely, predominantly with parenteral therapy. During the administration of high doses of amoxicillin, it is advisable to maintain adequate fluid intake and urinary output in order to reduce the possibility of amoxicillin crystalluria (See Section 4.9 Overdose). Amoxicillin has been reported to precipitate in bladder catheters after intravenous administration of large doses. A regular check of patency should be maintained.

Dosage should be adjusted in patients with renal impairment (see Section 4.2).

When prepared for intramuscular or direct intravenous injection, Amoxil should be administered immediately after reconstitution. The stability of Amoxil in various infusion fluids is given in the Package Enclosure Leaflet.

4.5 Interaction with other medicinal products and other forms of Interaction
In common with other broad spectrum antibiotics, amoxicillin may reduce the efficacy of oral contraceptives and patients should be warned accordingly.

Concurrent administration of allopurinol during treatment with amoxicillin can increase the likelihood of allergic skin reactions.

Prolongation of prothrombin time has been reported rarely in patients receiving amoxicillin. Appropriate monitoring should be undertaken when anticoagulants are prescribed concurrently.

It is recommended that when testing for the presence of glucose in urine during amoxicillin treatment, enzymatic glucose oxidase methods should be used. Due to the high urinary concentrations of amoxicillin, false positive readings are common with chemical methods.

4.6 Pregnancy and lactation
Use in pregnancy:

Animal studies with Amoxil have shown no teratogenic effects. The product has been in extensive clinical use since 1972 and its suitability in human pregnancy has been

Table 1 Prophylaxis of endocarditis

CONDITION		ADULTS' DOSAGE (INCLUDING ELDERLY)	CHILDREN'S DOSAGE	NOTES
Dental procedures: prophylaxis for patients undergoing extraction, scaling or surgery involving gingival tissues and who have not received a penicillin in the previous month. (N.B. Patients with prosthetic heart valves should be referred to hospital - see below).	Patient not having general anaesthetic.	3 g 'Amoxil' orally, 1 hour before procedure. A second dose may be given 6 hours later, if considered necessary.	Under 10: half adult dose. Under 5: quarter adult dose.	Note 1. If prophylaxis with 'Amoxil' is given twice within one month, emergence of resistant streptococci is unlikely to be a problem. Alternative antibiotics are recommended if more frequent prophylaxis is required, or if the patient has received a course of treatment with a penicillin during the previous month. Note 2 To minimise pain on injection, 'Amoxil' may be given as two injections of 500 mg dissolved in sterile 1% lignocaine solution (see *Administration*).
	Patient having general anaesthetic: if oral antibiotics considered to be appropriate.	Initially 3 g 'Amoxil' orally 4 hours prior to anaesthesia, followed by 3 g orally (or 1 g IV or IM if oral dose not tolerated) as soon as possible after the operation.		
	Patient having general anaesthetic: if oral antibiotics not appropriate.	1 g 'Amoxil' IV or IM immediately before induction; with 500 mg orally, 6 hours later.		
Dental procedures: patients for whom referral to hospital is recommended: a) Patients to be given a general anaesthetic who have been given a penicillin in the previous month. b) Patients to be given a general anaesthetic who have a prosthetic heart valve. c) Patients who have had one or more attacks of endocarditis.		Initially: 1 g 'Amoxil' IV or IM with 120 mg gentamicin IV or IM immediately prior to anaesthesia (if given) or 15 minutes prior to dental procedure. Followed by (6 hours later): 500 mg 'Amoxil' orally.	Under 10: the doses of 'Amoxil' should be half the adult dose; the dose of gentamicin should be 2 mg/kg. Under 5: the doses of 'Amoxil' should be quarter the adult dose; the dose of gentamicin should be 2 mg/kg.	See Note 2. Note 3. 'Amoxil' and gentamicin should not be mixed in the same syringe. Note 4. Please consult the appropriate data sheet for full prescribing information on gentamicin.
Genitourinary Surgery or Instrumentation: prophylaxis for patients who have no urinary tract infection and who are to have genito-urinary surgery or instrumentation under general anaesthesia. In the case of *Obstetric and Gynaecological Procedures* and *Gastrointestinal Procedures* – routine prophylaxis is recommended only for patients with prosthetic heart valves.		Initially: 1 g 'Amoxil' IV or IM with 120 mg gentamicin IV or IM, immediately before induction. Followed by (6 hours later): 500 mg 'Amoxil' orally or IV or IM according to clinical condition.		See Notes 2, 3 and 4 above.
Surgery or Instrumentation of the Upper Respiratory Tract	Patients other than those with prosthetic heart valves.	1 g 'Amoxil' IV or IM immediately before induction; 500 mg 'Amoxil' IV or IM 6 hours later.	Under 10: half adult dose. Under 5: quarter adult dose.	See Note 2 above. Note 5. The second dose of 'Amoxil' may be administered orally as 'Amoxil' Syrup SF/DF.
	Patients with prosthetic heart valves.	Initially: 1 g 'Amoxil' IV or IM with 120 mg gentamicin IV or IM, immediately before induction; followed by (6 hours later) 500 mg 'Amoxil' IV or IM.	Under 10: the dose of 'Amoxil' should be half the adult dose; the gentamicin dose should be 2 mg/kg. Under 5: the dose of 'Amoxil' should be quarter the adult dose; the dose of gentamicin should be 2 mg/kg.	See Notes 2, 3, 4 and 5 above.

well documented in clinical studies. When antibiotic therapy is required during pregnancy, Amoxil may be considered appropriate when the potential benefits outweigh the potential risks associated with treatment.

Use in lactation:

Amoxicillin may be given during lactation. With the exception of the risk of sensitisation associated with the excretion of trace quantities of amoxicillin in breast milk, there are no known detrimental effects for the breast-fed infant.

4.7 Effects on ability to drive and use machines

Adverse effects on the ability to drive or operate machinery have not been observed.

4.8 Undesirable effects

The following convention has been utilised for the classification of undesirable effects:-

Very common (>1/10), common (>1/100, <1/10), uncommon (>1/1000,<1/100), rare (>1/10,000, <1/1000), very rare (<1/10,000)

The majority of side effects listed below are not unique to amoxycillin and may occur when using other penicillins.

Unless otherwise stated, the frequency of adverse events has been derived from more than 30 years of post-marketing reports.

Blood and lymphatic system disorders

Very rare: Reversible leucopenia (including severe neutropenia or agranulocytosis), reversible thrombocytopenia and haemolytic anaemia.

Prolongation of bleeding time and prothrombin (see Section 4.5 - Interaction with other Medicaments and other Forms of Interaction)

Immune system disorders

Very rare: As with other antibiotics, severe allergic reactions, including angioneurotic oedema, anaphylaxis (see Section 4.4 - Special Warnings and Precautions for Use), serum sickness and hypersensitivity vasculitis.

If a hypersensitivity reaction is reported, the treatment must be discontinued. (See also Skin and subcutaneous tissue disorders).

Nervous system disorders

Very rare: Hyperkinesia, dizziness and convulsions. Convulsions may occur in patients with impaired renal function or in those receiving high doses.

Gastrointestinal disorders

Clinical Trial Data

Common: Diarrhoea and nausea.

Uncommon: Vomiting.

Post-marketing Data

Very rare: Mucocutaneous candidiasis and antibiotic associated colitis (including pseudomembraneous colitis and haemorrhagic colitis).

Hepato-biliary disorders

Very rare: Hepatitis and cholestatic jaundice. A moderate rise in AST and/or ALT.

The significance of a rise in AST and/or ALT is unclear.

Skin and subcutaneous tissue disorders

Clinical Trial Data

Common: Skin rash

Uncommon: Urticaria and pruritus

Post-marketing Data

Very rare: Skin reactions such as erythema multiforme, Stevens-Johnson syndrome, toxic epidermal necrolysis, bullous and exfoliative dermatitis and acute generalised exanthematous pustulosis (AGEP)

(See also Immune system disorders).

Renal and urinary tract disorders

Very rare: Interstitial nephritis, crystalluria (See Section 4.9 Overdose).

The incidence of these AEs was derived from clinical studies involving a total of approximately 6,000 adult and paediatric patients taking amoxycillin.

4.9 Overdose

Gastrointestinal effects such as nausea, vomiting and diarrhoea may be evident and should be treated symptomatically with attention to the water/electrolyte balance. Amoxicillin crystalluria, in some cases leading to renal failure, has been observed (see Section 4.4 Special warnings and special precautions for use).

Amoxicillin may be removed from the circulation by haemodialysis.

5. PHARMACOLOGICAL PROPERTIES

5.1 Pharmacodynamic properties

Amoxil is a broad spectrum antibiotic.

It is rapidly bactericidal and possesses the safety profile of a penicillin.

5.2 Pharmacokinetic properties

Amoxil is well absorbed by the oral and parenteral routes. Amoxil gives good penetration into bronchial secretions and high urinary concentrations of unchanged antibiotic.

5.3 Preclinical safety data

Not applicable.

6. PHARMACEUTICAL PARTICULARS

6.1 List of excipients

Amoxil Injection

None

6.2 Incompatibilities

Amoxil should not be mixed with blood products, other proteinaceous fluids such as protein hydrolysates, or with intravenous lipid emulsions.

If Amoxil is prescribed concurrently with an aminoglycoside, the antibiotics should not be mixed in the syringe, intravenous fluid container or giving set because loss of activity of the aminoglycoside can occur under these conditions.

6.3 Shelf life

Injection Vials 18 months

6.4 Special precautions for storage

Amoxil Vials for Injection should be stored in a cool, dry place.

When prepared for intramuscular or direct intravenous injection, Amoxil should be administered immediately after reconstitution. The stability of Amoxil in various infusion fluids is dependent upon the concentration and temperature: stability times are given in the Package Enclosure Leaflet.

6.5 Nature and contents of container

Amoxil Vials for Injection: Clear Type I glass vials fitted with a butyl rubber closure and an aluminium seal. 1 g: packs of 5 or 10. Each pack carries instructions for use.

6.6 Instructions for use and handling

Intravenous Injection:

Dissolve 1 g in 20 ml Water for Injections BP (Final volume=20.8 ml).

Amoxil injection, suitably diluted, may be injected directly into a vein or the infusion line over a period of three to four minutes.

Intravenous Infusion:

Solutions may be prepared as described for intravenous injections and then added to an intravenous solution in a minibag or in-line burette and administered over a period of half to one hour. Alternatively, using a suitable reconstitution device, the appropriate volume of intravenous fluid may be transferred from the infusion bag into the vial and then drawn back into the bag after dissolution.

Intramuscular:

1 g: Add 2.5 ml Water for Injections BP ‡ and shake vigorously (Final volume=3.3 ml).

‡ The 1 g vial will not dissolve in sterile 1% solution of lignocaine hydrochloride at the required concentration. To minimise pain on injection, 1 g of Amoxil may be given as two separate injections of 500 mg dissolved in a sterile solution of 1% lignocaine hydrochloride.

A transient pink colouration or slight opalescence may appear during reconstitution. Reconstituted solutions are normally a pale straw colour.

Administrative Data

7. MARKETING AUTHORISATION HOLDER

Beecham Group plc

Great West Road, Brentford, Middlesex TW8 9GS

Trading as GlaxoSmithKline UK, Stockley Park West, Uxbridge, Middlesex UB11 1BT

And/or

Bencard or SmithKline Beecham Pharmaceuticals at Mundells Welwyn Garden City, Hertfordshire AL7 1 EY

8. MARKETING AUTHORISATION NUMBER(S)

Amoxil Vials for Injection 1 g 0038/0225

9. DATE OF FIRST AUTHORISATION/RENEWAL OF THE AUTHORISATION

Amoxil Vials for Injection 1 g 13.10.98

10. DATE OF REVISION OF THE TEXT

01 February 2005

11. Legal Status

POM

Amoxil Vials for Injection 500mg

(GlaxoSmithKline UK)

1. NAME OF THE MEDICINAL PRODUCT

Amoxil® Vials for Injection 500 Mg

2. QUALITATIVE AND QUANTITATIVE COMPOSITION

Amoxil Vials for Injection 500 mg contain 500 mg amoxicillin

The amoxicillin is present as the sodium salt in Amoxil injections (each 1 g vial contains approximately 3.3 mmol of sodium).

3. PHARMACEUTICAL FORM

Amoxil Vials: vials containing sterile powder for reconstitution.

4. CLINICAL PARTICULARS

4.1 Therapeutic indications

Treatment of Infection: Amoxil is a broad spectrum antibiotic indicated for the treatment of commonly occurring bacterial infections such as:

Upper respiratory tract infections

Otitis media

Acute and chronic bronchitis

Chronic bronchial sepsis

Lobar and bronchopneumonia

Cystitis, urethritis, pyelonephritis

Bacteriuria in pregnancy

Gynaecological infections including puerperal sepsis and septic abortion

Gonorrhoea

Peritonitis

Intra-abdominal sepsis

Septicaemia

Bacterial endocarditis

Typhoid and paratyphoid fever

Skin and soft tissue infections

In children with urinary tract infection the need for investigation should be considered.

Prophylaxis of endocarditis: Amoxil may be used for the prevention of bacteraemia, associated with procedures such as dental extraction, in patients at risk of developing bacterial endocarditis.

The wide range of organisms sensitive to the bactericidal action of Amoxil include:

Gram-positive Gram-negative

Streptococcus faecalis *Haemophilus influenzae*

Streptococcus pneumoniae *Escherichia coli*

Streptococcus pyogenes *Proteus mirabilis*

Streptococcus viridans *Salmonella* species

Staphylococcus aureus *Shigella* species

(penicillin-sensitive) *Bordetella pertussis*

Clostridium species *Brucella* species

Corynebacterium species *Neisseria gonorrhoeae*

Bacillus anthracis *Neisseria meningitidis*

*Listeria monocytogenes**Vibrio cholerae*

Pasteurella septica

4.2 Posology and method of administration

Treatment of infection:

Adult dosage (including elderly patients):

Injectable:

500 mg IM eight hourly (or more frequently if necessary) in moderate infections. (This dose may be given by slow IV injection if more convenient.)

1 g IV six hourly in severe infections.

Children's dosage (up to 10 years of age):

Injectable:

50-100 mg/kg body weight a day, in divided doses.

Parenteral therapy is indicated if the oral route is considered impracticable or unsuitable, and particularly for the urgent treatment of severe infection.

In renal impairment the excretion of the antibiotic will be delayed and, depending on the degree of impairment, it may be necessary to reduce the total daily dosage.

Prophylaxis of endocarditis: see table on next page.

Prophylaxis of endocarditis:

(see Table 1 on next page)

Administration:

Intravenous Injection, Intravenous Infusion, Intramuscular:

Using vials for injection (See Section 6.6)

4.3 Contraindications

Amoxil is a penicillin and should not be given to penicillin-hypersensitive patients. Attention should be paid to possible cross-sensitivity with other beta-lactam antibiotics, e.g. cephalosporins.

4.4 Special warnings and special precautions for use

Serious and occasionally fatal hypersensitivity (anaphylactoid) reactions have been reported in patients on penicillin therapy. These reactions are more likely to occur in individuals with a history of hypersensitivity to beta-lactam antibiotics (see Section 4.3).

Erythematous (morbilliform) rashes have been associated with glandular fever in patients receiving amoxicillin.

Prolonged use may also occasionally result in overgrowth of non-susceptible organisms.

In patients with reduced urine output, crystalluria has been observed very rarely, predominantly with parenteral therapy. During the administration of high doses of amoxicillin, it is advisable to maintain adequate fluid intake and urinary output in order to reduce the possibility of amoxicillin crystalluria (see Section 4.9 Overdose). Amoxicillin has been reported to precipitate in bladder catheters after intravenous administration of large doses. A regular check of patency should be maintained.

Dosage should be adjusted in patients with renal impairment (see Section 4.2).

When prepared for intramuscular or direct intravenous injection, Amoxil should be administered immediately after reconstitution. The stability of Amoxil in various infusion fluids is given in the Package Enclosure Leaflet.

4.5 Interaction with other medicinal products and other forms of Interaction

In common with other broad spectrum antibiotics, amoxicillin may reduce the efficacy of oral contraceptives and patients should be warned accordingly.

Concurrent administration of allopurinol during treatment with amoxicillin can increase the likelihood of allergic skin reactions.

Prolongation of prothrombin time has been reported rarely in patients receiving amoxicillin. Appropriate monitoring should be undertaken when anticoagulants are prescribed concurrently.

It is recommended that when testing for the presence of glucose in urine during amoxicillin treatment, enzymatic glucose oxidase methods should be used. Due to the high urinary concentrations of amoxicillin, false positive readings are common with chemical methods.

4.6 Pregnancy and lactation

Use in pregnancy

Animal studies with Amoxil have shown no teratogenic effects. The product has been in extensive clinical use since 1972 and its suitability in human pregnancy has been well documented in clinical studies. When antibiotic therapy is required during pregnancy, Amoxil may be considered appropriate when the potential benefits outweigh the potential risks associated with treatment.

Use in lactation:

Amoxicillin may be given during lactation. With the exception of the risk of sensitisation associated with the excretion of trace quantities of amoxicillin in breast milk, there are no known detrimental effects for the breast-fed infant.

4.7 Effects on ability to drive and use machines

Adverse effects on the ability to drive or operate machinery have not been observed.

4.8 Undesirable effects

The following convention has been utilised for the classification of undesirable effects:-

Very common ($>1/10$), common ($>1/100$, $<1/10$), uncommon ($>1/1000$, $<1/100$), rare ($>1/10{,}000$, $<1/1000$), very rare ($<1/10{,}000$)

The majority of side effects listed below are not unique to amoxycillin and may occur when using other penicillins.

Unless otherwise stated, the frequency of adverse events has been derived from more than 30 years of post-marketing reports.

Blood and lymphatic system disorders

Very rare: Reversible leucopenia (including severe neutropenia or agranulocytosis), reversible thrombocytopenia and haemolytic anaemia.

Prolongation of bleeding time and prothrombin (see Section 4.5 - Interaction with other Medicaments and other Forms of Interaction)

Immune system disorders

Very rare: As with other antibiotics, severe allergic reactions, including angioneurotic oedema, anaphylaxis (see Section 4.4 - Special Warnings and Precautions for Use), serum sickness and hypersensitivity vasculitis.

If a hypersensitivity reaction is reported, the treatment must be discontinued. (See also Skin and subcutaneous tissue disorders).

Nervous system disorders

Very rare: Hyperkinesia, dizziness and convulsions. Convulsions may occur in patients with impaired renal function or in those receiving high doses.

Gastrointestinal disorders

Clinical Trial Data

Common: Diarrhoea and nausea.

Uncommon: Vomiting.

Post-marketing Data

Very rare: Mucocutaneous candidiasis and antibiotic associated colitis (including pseudomembraneous colitis and haemorrhagic colitis).

Hepato-biliary disorders

Very rare: Hepatitis and cholestatic jaundice. A moderate rise in AST and/or ALT.

The significance of a rise in AST and/or ALT is unclear.

Skin and subcutaneous tissue disorders

Clinical Trial Data

Common: Skin rash

Uncommon: Urticaria and pruritus

Post-marketing Data

Very rare: Skin reactions such as erythema multiforme, Stevens-Johnson syndrome, toxic epidermal necrolysis, bullous and exfoliative dermatitis and acute generalised exanthematous pustulosis (AGEP)

(See also Immune system disorders).

Renal and urinary tract disorders

Very rare: Interstitial nephritis, crystalluria (See Section 4.9 Overdose).

The incidence of these AEs was derived from clinical studies involving a total of approximately 6,000 adult and paediatric patients taking amoxycillin.

4.9 Overdose

Gastrointestinal effects such as nausea, vomiting and diarrhoea may be evident and should be treated symptomatically with attention to the water/electrolyte balance. Amoxicillin crystalluria, in some cases leading to renal failure, has been observed (see Section 4.4 Special warnings and special precautions for use).

Amoxicillin may be removed from the circulation by haemodialysis.

5. PHARMACOLOGICAL PROPERTIES

5.1 Pharmacodynamic properties

Amoxil is a broad spectrum antibiotic.

It is rapidly bactericidal and possesses the safety profile of a penicillin.

5.2 Pharmacokinetic properties

Amoxil is well absorbed by the oral and parenteral routes. Amoxil gives good penetration into bronchial secretions and high urinary concentrations of unchanged antibiotic.

5.3 Preclinical safety data

Not applicable.

6. PHARMACEUTICAL PARTICULARS

6.1 List of excipients

Amoxil Injection: None

6.2 Incompatibilities

Amoxil should not be mixed with blood products, other proteinaceous fluids such as protein hydrolysates, or with intravenous lipid emulsions.

If Amoxil is prescribed concurrently with an aminoglycoside, the antibiotics should not be mixed in the syringe, intravenous fluid container or giving set because loss of activity of the aminoglycoside can occur under these conditions.

Table 1 Prophylaxis of endocarditis

CONDITION		ADULTS' DOSAGE (INCLUDING ELDERLY)	CHILDREN'S DOSAGE	NOTES
Dental procedures: prophylaxis for patients undergoing extraction, scaling or surgery involving gingival tissues and who have not received a penicillin in the previous month. (N.B. Patients with prosthetic heart valves should be referred to hospital - see below).	Patient not having general anaesthetic.	3 g 'Amoxil' orally, 1 hour before procedure. A second dose may be given 6 hours later, if considered necessary.	Under 10: half adult dose. Under 5: quarter adult dose.	Note 1. If prophylaxis with 'Amoxil' is given twice within one month, emergence of resistant streptococci is unlikely to be a problem. Alternative antibiotics are recommended if more frequent prophylaxis is required, or if the patient has received a course of treatment with a penicillin during the previous month. Note 2 To minimise pain on injection, 'Amoxil' may be given as two injections of 500 mg dissolved in sterile 1% lignocaine solution (see *Administration*).
	Patient having general anaesthetic: if oral antibiotics considered to be appropriate.	Initially 3 g 'Amoxil' orally 4 hours prior to anaesthesia, followed by 3 g orally (or 1 g IV or IM if oral dose not tolerated) as soon as possible after the operation.		
	Patient having general anaesthetic: if oral antibiotics not appropriate.	1 g 'Amoxil' IV or IM immediately before induction; with 500 mg orally, 6 hours later.		
Dental procedures: patients for whom referral to hospital is recommended: a) Patients to be given a general anaesthetic who have been given a penicillin in the previous month. b) Patients to be given a general anaesthetic who have a prosthetic heart valve. c) Patients who have had one or more attacks of endocarditis.		Initially: 1 g 'Amoxil' IV or IM with 120 mg gentamicin IV or IM immediately prior to anaesthesia (if given) or 15 minutes prior to dental procedure. Followed by (6 hours later): 500 mg 'Amoxil' orally.	Under 10: the doses of 'Amoxil' should be half the adult dose; the dose of gentamicin should be 2 mg/kg. Under 5: the doses of 'Amoxil' should be quarter the adult dose; the dose of gentamicin should be 2 mg/kg.	See Note 2. Note 3. 'Amoxil' and gentamicin should not be mixed in the same syringe. Note 4. Please consult the appropriate data sheet for full prescribing information on gentamicin.
Genitourinary Surgery or Instrumentation: prophylaxis for patients who have no urinary tract infection and who are to have genito-urinary surgery or instrumentation under general anaesthesia. In the case of *Obstetric and Gynaecological Procedures* and *Gastrointestinal Procedures* – routine prophylaxis is recommended only for patients with prosthetic heart valves.		Initially: 1 g 'Amoxil' IV or IM with 120 mg gentamicin IV or IM, immediately before induction. Followed by (6 hours later): 500 mg 'Amoxil' orally or IV or IM according to clinical condition.		See Notes 2, 3 and 4 above.
Surgery or Instrumentation of the Upper Respiratory Tract	Patients other than those with prosthetic heart valves.	1 g 'Amoxil' IV or IM immediately before induction; 500 mg 'Amoxil' IV or IM 6 hours later.	Under 10: half adult dose. Under 5: quarter adult dose.	See Note 2 above. Note 5. The second dose of 'Amoxil' may be administered orally as 'Amoxil' Syrup SF/DF.
	Patients with prosthetic heart valves.	Initially: 1 g 'Amoxil' IV or IM with 120 mg gentamicin IV or IM, immediately before induction; followed by (6 hours later) 500 mg 'Amoxil' IV or IM.	Under 10: the dose of 'Amoxil' should be half the adult dose; the gentamicin dose should be 2 mg/kg. Under 5: the dose of 'Amoxil' should be quarter the adult dose; the dose of gentamicin should be 2 mg/kg.	See Notes 2, 3, 4 and 5 above.

6.3 Shelf life

Injection Vials 18 months

6.4 Special precautions for storage

Amoxil Vials for Injection should be stored in a cool, dry place.

When prepared for intramuscular or direct intravenous injection, Amoxil should be administered immediately after reconstitution. The stability of Amoxil in various infusion fluids is dependent upon the concentration and temperature: stability times are given in the Package Enclosure Leaflet.

6.5 Nature and contents of container

Amoxil Vials for Injection: Clear Type I glass vials fitted with a butyl rubber closure and an aluminium seal. 500 mg: packs of 5 or 10. Each pack carries instructions for use.

6.6 Instructions for use and handling

Intravenous Injection:

Dissolve 500 mg in 10 ml Water for Injections BP (Final volume=10.4 ml).

Amoxil injection, suitably diluted, may be injected directly into a vein or the infusion line over a period of three to four minutes.

Intravenous Infusion:

Solutions may be prepared as described for intravenous injections and then added to an intravenous solution in a minibag or in-line burette and administered over a period of half to one hour. Alternatively, using a suitable reconstitution device, the appropriate volume of intravenous fluid may be transferred from the infusion bag into the vial and then drawn back into the bag after dissolution.

Intramuscular:

500 mg: Add 2.5 ml Water for Injections BP † and shake vigorously (Final volume=2.9 ml).

If pain is experienced on intramuscular injection, a sterile 1% solution of lignocaine hydrochloride or 0.5% solution of procaine hydrochloride may be used in place of Water for Injections.

A transient pink colouration or slight opalescence may appear during reconstitution. Reconstituted solutions are normally a pale straw colour.

Administrative Data

7. MARKETING AUTHORISATION HOLDER

Beecham Group plc

Great West Road, Brentford, Middlesex TW8 9GS

Trading as GlaxoSmithKline UK Stockley Park West, Uxbridge, Middlesex UB11 1BT

And/or

Bencard or SmithKline Beecham Pharmaceuticals at Mundells Welwyn Garden City, Hertfordshire AL7 1 EY

8. MARKETING AUTHORISATION NUMBER(S)

Amoxil Vials for Injection 500 mg 0038/0222

9. DATE OF FIRST AUTHORISATION/RENEWAL OF THE AUTHORISATION

Amoxil Vials for Injection 500 mg 13.10.98

10. DATE OF REVISION OF THE TEXT

1st February 2005

11. Legal Status

POM

Amphocil

(Cambridge Laboratories)

1. NAME OF THE MEDICINAL PRODUCT

AMPHOCIL™.

2. QUALITATIVE AND QUANTITATIVE COMPOSITION

Ingredient	Specification Reference	Quantity (W/W)
Amphotericin B	USP	5.060
Sodium cholesteryl sulphate	House	2.672
Tromethamine	USP	0.571
Disodium edetate	Ph Eur	0.034
Lactose monohydrate	Ph Eur	91.311
Hydrocholoric acid	Ph Eur	0.353[a]
Water for injection	Ph Eur	b
Nitrogen	NF	c

[a]HCl qs to a target pH of 7.0 ± 0.5.

[b]Mean NMT 2.0% residual moisture and no individual vial greater than 2.5%.

[c]Used to fill vial headspace.

3. PHARMACEUTICAL FORM

Amphotericin B USP, 5% (W/W), lyophilisate for reconstitution. Each vial contains either 50 mg (50,000 IU) or 100 mg (100,000 IU) of amphotericin B USP as a complex with sodium cholesteryl sulphate.

4. CLINICAL PARTICULARS

4.1 Therapeutic indications

AMPHOCIL is indicated for the treatment of severe systemic and/or deep mycoses in cases where toxicity or renal failure precludes the use of conventional amphotericin B in effective doses, and in cases where prior systemic antifungal therapy has failed. Fungal infections successfully treated with AMPHOCIL include disseminated candidiasis and aspergillosis. AMPHOCIL has been used successfully in severely neutropenic patients.

AMPHOCIL is not intended for use in common, clinically inapparent fungal diseases diagnosed only by skin tests or serological determinations.

4.2 Posology and method of administration

Dosage: Therapy may begin at a daily dose of 1.0 mg/kg of body weight, increasing to the recommended dose of 3.0-4.0 mg/kg as required. Doses as high as 6 mg/kg have been used in patients. Dosage should be adjusted to the individual requirements of each patient. The median cumulative dose in clinical studies was 3.5 g and the median treatment duration was 16 days. Ten percent (10%) of patients received 13 g or more of AMPHOCIL over a period of 27 to 409 days.

Administration: AMPHOCIL is administered by intravenous infusion at a rate of 1 to 2 mg/kg/hour. If the patient experiences acute reactions or cannot tolerate the infusion volume, the infusion time may be extended. Pre-medication (e.g. paracetamol, antihistamines, antiemetics) may be administered to patients who have previously suffered infusion-related adverse reactions.

Paediatric patients: A limited number of paediatric patients have been treated with AMPHOCIL at daily doses (mg/kg) similar to those in adults. No unusual adverse events were reported.

Elderly patients: A limited number of elderly patients have been treated with AMPHOCIL; available data do not indicate the need for specific dose recommendations or precautions in elderly patients.

4.3 Contraindications
AMPHOCIL should not be administered to patients who have documented hypersensitivity to any of its components, unless, in the opinion of the physician, the advantages of using AMPHOCIL outweigh the risks of hypersensitivity.

4.4 Special warnings and special precautions for use
A test dose which is advisable when commencing all new courses of treatment should immediately precede the first dose; a small amount of drug (e.g. 20 ml of a solution containing 0.1 g per litre) should be infused over 10 minutes and the patient carefully observed for the next 30 minutes.

In the treatment of diabetic patients: It should be noted that each vial of AMPHOCIL contains lactose monohydrate.

In the treatment of renal dialysis patients: AMPHOCIL should be administered only at the end of each dialysis period. Serum electrolytes, particularly potassium and magnesium, should be regularly monitored.

4.5 Interaction with other medicinal products and other forms of Interaction
There have been no reported interactions between AMPHOCIL and other drugs including cyclosporine. However, caution should be used in patients receiving concomitant therapy with drugs known to interact with conventional amphotericin B such as nephrotoxic drugs (aminoglycosides, cisplatin and pentamidine), corticosteroids and corticotropin (ACTH) that may potentiate hypokalaemia and digitalis glycosides, muscle relaxants and antiarrhythmic agents whose effects may be potentiated in the presence of hypokalaemia.

The use of flucytosine with AMPHOCIL has not been studied. While the synergy between amphotericin B and flucytosine has been reported, amphotericin B may enhance the toxicity of flucytosine by increasing its cellular uptake and impeding its renal excretion.

4.6 Pregnancy and lactation
Pregnancy: Animal reproductive toxicology studies with AMPHOCIL have shown no evidence of harm to the foetus. Although the active ingredient, amphotericin B, has been in wide use for many years without apparent ill consequence, there is inadequate evidence of safety of AMPHOCIL in human pregnancy. Therefore, it is recommended that administration of AMPHOCIL is avoided in pregnancy unless the anticipated benefit to the patient outweighs the potential risk to the foetus.

Nursing mothers: It is not known whether amphotericin B is excreted in human milk. Consideration should be given to discontinuation of nursing during treatment with AMPHOCIL.

4.7 Effects on ability to drive and use machines
Not applicable to current indication or expected use.

4.8 Undesirable effects
In general, the physician should monitor the patient for any type of adverse event associated with conventional amphotericin B. The appearance of adverse reactions does not generally prevent the patient completing the course of treatment. Caution should be exercised when high doses or prolonged therapy is indicated.

Acute reactions including fever, chills and rigours may occur. Anaphylactoid reactions including hypotension, tachycardia, bronchospasm, dyspnoea, hypoxia and hyperventilation have also been reported. Most acute reactions are successfully treated by reducing the rate of infusion and prompt administration of anti-histamines and adrenal corticosteroids. Serious anaphylactoid effects may necessitate discontinuation of AMPHOCIL and treatment with additional supportive therapy (e.g. adrenaline).

Clinical studies conducted so far have shown AMPHOCIL to be less nephrotoxic than conventional amphotericin B. Serum creatinine levels tend to remain consistent throughout the course of therapy even in patients with renal insufficiency. Patients who developed renal insufficiency during treatment with conventional amphotericin B, were stabilised or improved when AMPHOCIL was substituted. Decreases in renal function attributable to AMPHOCIL treatment were rare. However, as with conventional amphotericin B, renal function should be monitored with particular attention to those patients receiving concomitant therapy with nephrotoxic drugs.

There have been no reports of unequivocal hepatic toxicity of AMPHOCIL. Changes in alkaline phosphatase and bilirubin levels were infrequent.

Changes in coagulation, thrombocytopenia and hypomagnesemia were sometimes observed on AMPHOCIL. Anaemia, which is a very common adverse event during treatment with conventional amphotericin B, developed in only 2.5% of the patients treated with AMPHOCIL.

Other reported events include nausea, vomiting, hypertension, headache, backache, diarrhoea and abdominal pain.

4.9 Overdose
In case of overdose, stop administration immediately and carefully monitor the patient's clinical status (renal, liver and cardiac function, haematological status, serum electrolytes) and institute symptomatic treatment.

5. PHARMACOLOGICAL PROPERTIES

5.1 Pharmacodynamic properties
Amphotericin B is a macrocyclic polyene antibiotic isolated from *Streptomyces nodosus*. Amphotericin B has a high affinity for ergosterol, the primary sterol in fungal cell membranes, and a lesser affinity for cholesterol, the predominant sterol of mammalian cell membranes. Binding of amphotericin B to ergosterol results in damage to the fungal cell membrane, enhanced membrane permeability and eventual cell death. Mammalian cell membranes also contain sterols, and it has been suggested that the damage caused by amphotericin B to human cells follows a similar mode of action to that of fungal cells. AMPHOCIL is considered to have the same mode of action as conventional amphotericin B, but with reduced toxicity.

AMPHOCIL is a novel formulation of amphotericin B based on its unique affinity for sterols. AMPHOCIL is a stable complex of amphotericin B and sodium cholesteryl sulphate, a naturally occurring cholesterol metabolite. Amphotericin B and sodium cholesteryl sulphate are complexed in a near equimolar ratio to form uniform disc-shaped microparticles. AMPHOCIL is not a liposomal formulation but a colloidal dispersion of amphotericin B and sodium cholesteryl sulphate.

Pharmacological studies indicated that overall, AMPHOCIL is essentially equivalent, *in vitro*, to conventional amphotericin B against a variety of fungal pathogens. Higher doses of AMPHOCIL are tolerated, thus it is generally more effective in eradicating fungal infections than conventional amphotericin B in several *in vivo* models.

5.2 Pharmacokinetic properties
Pharmacokinetic studies in animals demonstrate that the distribution of AMPHOCIL and conventional amphotericin B are notably different. Lower peak plasma levels of amphotericin B and greater total area under the curve values after AMPHOCIL treatment, compared to comparable doses of conventional amphotericin B have been observed. Higher concentrations of amphotericin B measured in the liver, spleen and bone marrow after AMPHOCIL administration were not accompanied by evidence of increased toxicity in these organ systems. Levels in the kidney, a primary site of toxicity of conventional amphotericin B, were 4- to 5-fold lower after treatment with AMPHOCIL and correlated with reduced nephrotoxicity compared to conventional amphotericin B. Maximum plasma concentrations of amphotericin B were lower in AMPHOCIL treated animals. The terminal half-life was longer in the AMPHOCIL treated animals owing to the accumulation of amphotericin B in the liver and its subsequent slow release.

In bone marrow transplant patients administered AMPHOCIL at doses of 0.5 to 8.0 mg/kg/day, there was an increase in both the volume of distribution (V_{ss}) and the total plasma clearance (Cl_t) as the dose escalated. The mean values for V_{ss}, Cl_t and terminal half-life for doses $\leqslant$ 2.0 mg/kg were 2.25 l/kg, 0.0855 l/h/kg and 22.1 hours, respectively. The mean values for doses $>$ 2.0 mg/kg were 3.61 l/kg, 0.116 l/h/kg and 27.2 hours respectively. The maximum steady-state concentrations achievable after multiple dosing ranged from 658 to 6212 μg/l for doses of 0.5 to 8.0 mg/kg/day respectively. There was no evidence of continued accumulation of AMPHOCIL at doses of 8.0 mg/kg/day. There was no net change in renal function over the duration of AMPHOCIL treatment (range from 1 to 108 days, median 28 days).

5.3 Preclinical safety data
AMPHOCIL was found to be generally less toxic than conventional amphotericin B in a series of acute and repeat dose studies, with a 4- to 5-fold increased margin of safety. There were no unique toxicities observed following treatment with AMPHOCIL relative to conventional amphotericin B. Nephrotoxicity was diminished during AMPHOCIL treatment even at dose levels 4- to 5-fold higher than toxic doses of conventional amphotericin B. Accumulation of amphotericin B in the liver following AMPHOCIL administration was observed; however, there were no associated signs of increased hepatotoxicity relative to conventional amphotericin B. In-vitro and in-vivo tests on induction of gene and chromosome mutations were negative for amphotericin B. Carcinogenicity studies have not been conducted with amphotericin B or AMPHOCIL. To date there have been no clinical reports of carcinogenicity associated with the use of amphotericin B.

Embryo-feotal studies in rats and rabbits, at doses of 2.5 mg/kg/day or greater showed maternal toxicity i.e. reduced weight gain and loss of appetite. There were no adverse effects on embryo-foetal development up to 10 mg/kg/day. There are no specific data for the effect of AMPHOCIL on human fertility, but in multiple dose toxicity studies of up to 13 weeks (in rats and dogs) there was no effect on ovarian or testicular histology. Although, amphotericin B has not been associated with peri- or post-natal effects no studies with AMPHOCIL are available.

6. PHARMACEUTICAL PARTICULARS

6.1 List of excipients
The following excipients are contained in each vial of lyophilised product:

Sodium cholesteryl sulphate

Tromethamine, USP

Disodium edetate, Ph Eur

Hydrocholoric acid, Ph Eur

Water for injection, Ph Eur

Lactose monohydrate, Ph Eur

6.2 Incompatibilities
Do not reconstitute lyophilised powder/cake with saline or dextrose solutions. Do not add saline or electrolytes to the reconstituted concentrate, or mix with other drugs.

If administered through an existing intravenous line, flush with 5% Dextrose for Injection prior to infusion of AMPHOCIL, otherwise administer via a separate line.

The use of any solution other than those recommended, or the presence of a bacteriostatic agent (e.g., benzyl alcohol) in the solution may cause precipitation of AMPHOCIL.

Do not use material that shows evidence of precipitation or any other particulate matter. Strict aseptic technique should always be followed during reconstitution and dilution since no preservatives are present in the lyophilised drug or in the solutions used for reconstitution and dilution.

6.3 Shelf life
Unopened vials of lyophilised material have a shelf-life of 36months and should be stored below 30°C (86°F). After reconstitution, the drug should be refrigerated at 2-8°C (36-46°F) and used within 24 hours. Do not freeze. After further dilution with 5% Dextrose for Injection, the infusion should be stored in a refrigerator (2-8°C) and used within 24 hours. Partially used vials should be discarded.

6.4 Special precautions for storage
Store below 30°C (86°F).

6.5 Nature and contents of container
The container is a Type I moulded glass vial, the stopper is a grey butyl lyophilisation type stopper, and the cap is an aluminium ring with either a green or yellow polypropylene flip-off top.

6.6 Instructions for use and handling
Directions for reconstitution and dilution: AMPHOCIL must be reconstituted by addition of sterile Water for Injection, Ph Eur, using a sterile syringe and a 20-gauge needle.

Rapidly inject into the vial:

50 mg/vial • 10 ml sterile Water for Injection

100 mg/vial • 20 ml sterile Water for Injection

Shake gently by hand, rotating the vial, until the yellow fluid becomes clear. Note that the fluid may be opalescent. The liquid in each reconstituted vial will contain 5 mg of amphotericin B per ml. For infusion, further dilute to a final concentration of 0.625mg/ml by diluting 1 volume of the reconstituted AMPHOCIL with 7 volumes of 5% Dextrose for Injection.

7. MARKETING AUTHORISATION HOLDER
SEQUSS Pharmaceuticals, Incorporated
1050 Hamilton Court
Menlo Park, CA 94025, USA

8. MARKETING AUTHORISATION NUMBER(S)
PLs 11866/0002-3

9. DATE OF FIRST AUTHORISATION/RENEWAL OF THE AUTHORISATION
August 1993

10. DATE OF REVISION OF THE TEXT
December 21, 1995

Amytal
(Flynn Pharma Ltd)

1. NAME OF THE MEDICINAL PRODUCT
AMYTAL

2. QUALITATIVE AND QUANTITATIVE COMPOSITION
Each tablet contains 50mg Amylobarbitone BP

3. PHARMACEUTICAL FORM
Tablet (white, coded T37)

4. CLINICAL PARTICULARS

4.1 Therapeutic indications
For the short-term treatment of severe, intractable insomnia in patients already taking barbiturates. New patients should not be started on this preparation. Attempts should be made to wean patients off this preparation by gradual reduction of the dose over a period of days or weeks (*see drug abuse and dependence*). Abrupt discontinuation should be avoided as this may precipitate withdrawal effects (*see warnings*).

4.2 Posology and method of administration
For oral administration to adults only. Normal dosage is 100-200mg at bedtime.

THE ELDERLY

Amytal is not recommended for use in elderly or debilitated patients.

CHILDREN

Amytal should not be administered to children or young adults

Amylobarbitone is expected to lose most its effectiveness for both inducing and maintaining sleep after about two weeks of continued drug administration, even with the use of multiple doses.

4.3 Contraindications

Hypersensitivity to barbiturates, a history of manifest or latent porphyria, marked impairment of liver function or respiratory disease in which dyspnoea or obstruction is evident.

Barbiturates should not be administered to children, young adults, patients with a history of drug or alcohol addiction or abuse, the elderly and the debilitated.

4.4 Special warnings and special precautions for use

Addiction potential: Barbiturates have a high addiction potential. Long-term use, or use of high dosage for short periods, may lead to tolerance and subsequently to physical and psychological dependence. Patients who have psychological dependence on barbiturates may increase the dosage or decrease the dosage interval without consulting a doctor, and subsequently may develop a physical dependence on barbiturates.

To minimise the possibility of overdosage or development of dependence, the amount prescribed should be limited to that required for the interval until the next appointment.

Withdrawal symptoms occur after long-term normal use (and particularly after abuse) on rapid cessation of barbiturate treatment. Symptoms include nightmares, irritability and insomnia, and in severe cases, tremors, delirium, convulsions and death.

Barbiturates should be withdrawn gradually from any patient known to be taking excessive doses over long periods.

Caution should be exercised when oral barbiturates are administered in the presence of acute or chronic pain, because paradoxical excitement may be induced or important symptoms may be masked.

Information for patients: The following information should be given to patients receiving amylobarbitone:

1. The use of amylobarbitone carries with it an associated risk of psychological and/or physical dependence. The patient should be warned against increasing the dose of the drug without consulting a doctor.

2. Amylobarbitone may impair the mental and/or physical abilities required for the performance of potentially hazardous tasks, such as driving a car or operating machinery. The patient should be cautioned accordingly.

3. Alcohol should not be consumed while taking amylobarbitone. The concurrent use of amylobarbitone with other CNS depressants (eg, alcohol, narcotics, tranquillisers and antihistamines) may result in additional CNS depressant effects.

Drug abuse and dependence: Barbiturates may be habit forming; tolerance, psychological and physical dependence may occur especially following prolonged use of high doses. Daily administration in excess of 400 mg secobarbitone, for approximately 90 days, is likely to produce some degree of physical dependence.

A dosage of 600 - 800 mg, for at least 35 days, is sufficient to produce withdrawal seizures. The average daily dose for the barbiturate addict is usually about 1.5g.

As tolerance to barbiturates develops, the amount needed to maintain the same level of intoxication increases; tolerance to a fatal dosage, however, does not increase more than twofold. As this occurs, the margin between intoxicating dosage and fatal dosage becomes smaller. The lethal dose of a barbiturate is far less if alcohol is also ingested.

Symptoms of acute intoxication include unsteady gait, slurred speech and sustained nystagmus. Mental signs of chronic intoxication include confusion, poor judgement, irritability, insomnia and somatic complaints.

The symptoms of barbiturate withdrawal can be severe and may cause death. Minor withdrawal symptoms may appear 8 to 12 hours after the last dose of a barbiturate. These symptoms usually appear in the following order: anxiety, muscle twitching, tremor of hands and fingers, progressive weakness, dizziness, distortion in visual perception, nausea, vomiting, insomnia and orthostatic hypotension. Major withdrawal symptoms (convulsions and delirium) may occur within 16 hours and last up to five days after abrupt cessation of barbiturates. Intensity of withdrawal symptoms gradually declines over a period of approximately 15 days. Individuals susceptible to barbiturate abuse and dependence include alcoholics and opiate abusers, as well as other sedative-hypnotic and amphetamine abusers.

Dependence on barbiturates arises from repeated administration on a continuous basis, generally in amounts exceeding therapeutic dose levels. Treatment of dependence consists of cautious and gradual withdrawal of the drug. Barbiturate-dependent patients can be withdrawn by using a number of withdrawal regimens. In all cases, withdrawal takes an extended period. One method involves substituting a 30 mg dose of phenobarbitone for each 100 - 200 mg dose of barbiturate that the patient has been taking. The total daily amount of phenobarbitone is then administered in three or four divided doses, not to exceed 600 mg daily. Should signs of withdrawal occur on the first day of treatment, a loading dose of 100 to 200 mg of phenobarbitone may be administered intramuscularly in addition to the oral dose. After stabilisation on phenobarbitone, the total daily dose is decreased by 30 mg a day as long as withdrawal is proceeding smoothly. A modification of this regimen involves initiating treatment at the patient's regular dosage level and decreasing the daily dosage by 10% as tolerated by the patient.

Infants that are physically dependent on barbiturates may be given phenobarbitone, 3 to 10 mg/kg/day. After withdrawal symptoms (hyperactivity, disturbed sleep, tremors and hyperreflexia) are relieved, the dosage of phenobarbitone should be gradually decreased and completely withdrawn over a two week period.

Carcinogenesis: Animal data show that phenobarbitone can be carcinogenic after lifetime administration.

Human data: In a 29 year epidemiological study of 9136 patients who were treated on an anticonvulsant protocol that included phenobarbitone, results indicated a higher than normal incidence of hepatic carcinoma. Previously some of these patients had been treated with thorotrast, a drug that is known to produce hepatic carcinomas. Thus, this study did not provide sufficient evidence that phenobarbitone is carcinogenic in humans.

A retrospective study of 84 children with brain tumours, matched to 73 normal controls and 78 cancer controls (malignant disease other than brain tumours), suggested an association between exposure to barbiturates prenatally and an increased incidence of brain tumours.

Barbiturates should be administered with caution, if at all, to patients who are mentally depressed or have suicidal tendencies. They should also be used with great caution and at reduced dosage in those with hepatic disease, marked renal dysfunction, shock or respiratory depression.

Elderly or debilitated patients may react to barbiturates with marked excitement, depression or confusion (see 'Contra-indications'). In some persons, barbiturates repeatedly produce excitement rather than depression.

Barbiturates should not be administered to patients showing the premonitory signs of hepatic coma(see 'Contra-indications').

A cumulative effect may occur with the barbiturates leading to features of chronic poisoning including headache, depression and slurred speech.

Automatism may follow the use of a hypnotic dose of barbiturate

The systemic effects of exogenous and endogenous corticosteroids may be diminished by amylobarbitone. This product should therefore be administered with caution to patients with borderline hypoadrenal function, regardless of whether it is of pituitary or of primary adrenal origin.

Laboratory tests: Prolonged therapy with barbiturates should be accompanied by periodic evaluation of, for example, the haematopoietic, renal and hepatic systems (but see 'Uses).

4.5 Interaction with other medicinal products and other forms of Interaction

Toxic effects and fatalities have occurred following overdoses of amylobarbitone alone and in combination with other CNS depressants. Caution should be exercised in prescribing unnecessarily large amounts of amylobarbitone for patients who have a history of emotional disturbances or suicidal ideation or who have misused alcohol or other CNS drugs.

Anticoagulants: Barbiturates cause induction of the liver microsomal enzymes responsible for metabolising many other drugs. In particular they may result in increased metabolism and decreased anticoagulant response of oral anticoagulants (eg warfarin). Patients stabilised on anticoagulant therapy may require dosage adjustments if barbiturates are added to or withdrawn from their regimen.

Corticosteroids: Barbiturates appear to enhance the metabolism of exogenous corticosteroids and steroid dosage may also need adjustment.

Griseofulvin: Barbiturates may interfere with the absorption of oral griseofulvin, thus decreasing its blood level. Concomitant administration should be avoided if possible.

Doxycycline: Barbiturates may shorten the half-life of doxycycline for as long as two weeks after the barbiturate is discontinued. If administered concomitantly the clinical response to doxycycline should be monitored closely.

Phenytoin, Sodium Valproate, Valproic Acid: The effect of barbiturates on phenytoin metabolism is variable. Phenytoin and barbiturate blood levels should be monitored more frequently if administered concomitantly. Sodium valproate and valproic acid increase amylobarbitone serum levels. Therefore these levels should be monitored and dosage adjustments made as clinically indicated.

CNS Depressants: Concomitant use of other CNS depressants, including other sedatives or hypnotics, antihistamines, tranquillisers or alcohol, may produce additive depressant effects.

Monoamine Oxidase Inhibitors (MAOIS): Prolong the effects of barbiturates.

Oestradiol, oestrone, progesterone and other steroidal hormones: There have been reports of patients treated with antiepileptic drugs (eg phenobarbitone) who became pregnant while taking oral contraceptives. Barbiturates may decrease the effect of oestradiol. An alternative contraceptive method might be suggested to women taking barbiturates.

4.6 Pregnancy and lactation

Usage in Pregnancy: Barbiturates are contraindicated during pregnancy since they can cause foetal harm. A higher than expected incidence of foetal abnormalities may be connected with maternal consumption of barbiturates. Barbiturates readily cross the placental barrier and are distributed throughout foetal tissues with highest concentrations in placenta, foetal liver and brain. Withdrawal symptoms occur in infants born to women who receive barbiturates during the last trimester of pregnancy. If a patient becomes pregnant whilst taking this drug, she should be told of the potential hazard to the foetus.

Reports of infants suffering from long term barbiturate exposure *in utero* included the acute withdrawal syndrome of seizures and hyper-irritability from birth to a delayed onset of up to 14 days.

Labour and Delivery: Respiratory depression has been noted in infants born following the use of barbiturates during labour. Premature infants are particularly susceptible. Resuscitation equipment should be available.

Nursing Mothers: Small amounts of barbiturates are excreted in the milk and they are therefore contraindicated for the nursing mother.

4.7 Effects on ability to drive and use machines

Amylobaritone may impair the mental and/or physical abilities required for the performance of potentially hazardous tasks such as driving a car or operating machinery. The patient should be cautioned accordingly

4.8 Undesirable effects

The following adverse reactions and their incidences were compiled from surveillance of thousands of hospitalised patients who received barbiturates. As such patients may be less aware of certain of the milder adverse effects of barbiturates, the incidence of these reactions may be somewhat higher in fully ambulatory patients.

More than 1 in 100 patients: The most common adverse reaction, estimated to occur at a rate of 1 to 3 patients per 100, is the following:

NERVOUS SYSTEM: Somnolence

LESS THAN 1 IN 100 PATIENTS: Adverse reactions estimated to occur at a rate of less than 1 in 100 patients are listed below grouped by organ system and by decreasing frequency:

NEUROLOGICAL: Agitation, confusion, hyperkinesia, ataxia, CNS depression, nightmares, nervousness, psychiatric disturbance, hallucinations, insomnia, anxiety, dizziness, abnormal thinking.

RESPIRATORY: Hypoventilation, apnoea.

CARDIOVASCULAR: Bradycardia, hypotension, syncope.

DIGESTIVE: Nausea, vomiting, constipation

OTHER: Headache, hypersensitivity reactions (angioneurotic oedema, rashes, exfoliative dermatitis), fever, liver damage. Hypersensitivity is more likely to occur in patients with asthma, urticaria or angioneurotic oedema. Megaloblastic anaemia has followed chronic phenobarbitone use.

4.9 Overdose

The toxic dose of barbiturates varies considerably. In general, an oral dose of 1g of most barbiturates produces serious poisoning in an adult. Death commonly occurs after 2 to 10g of ingested barbiturate. The sedative, therapeutic blood levels of amylobarbitone ranges between 2 and 10 mg/1; the usual lethal blood level ranges from 40 to 80 mg/l. Barbiturate intoxication may be confused with alcoholism, bromide intoxication, and various neurological disorders. Potential tolerance must be considered when evaluating significance of dose and plasma concentration.

Signs and Symptoms: Symptoms of oral overdose may occur within 15 minutes and begin with CNS depression, absent or sluggish reflexes, underventilation, hypotension and hypothermia, which may progress to pulmonary oedema and death. Haemorrhagic blisters may develop, especially at pressure points.

In extreme overdose, all electrical activity in the brain may cease, in which case a 'flat' EEG normally equated with clinical death cannot be accepted. This effect is fully reversible unless hypoxic damage occurs. Consideration should be given to the possibility of barbiturate intoxication even in situations that appear to involve trauma.

Complications such as pneumonia, pulmonary oedema, cardiac arrhythmias, congestive heart failure and renal failure may occur. Uraemia may increase CNS sensitivity to barbiturates if renal function is impaired. Differential diagnosis should include hypoglycaemia, head trauma, cerebrovascular accidents, convulsive states and diabetic coma.

Treatment: General management should consist of symptomatic and supportive therapy. Activated charcoal may be more effective than emesis or lavage. Diuresis and peritoneal dialysis are of little value. Haemodialysis and haemoperfusion enhance drug clearance and should be considered in serious poisoning. If the patient has chronically abused sedatives, withdrawal reactions may be manifest following acute overdose.

5. PHARMACOLOGICAL PROPERTIES

5.1 Pharmacodynamic properties

Amytal (amylobarbitone), a barbiturate with a moderate duration of action, is a CNS depressant. In ordinary doses the drug acts as a sedative and hypnotic.

Barbiturates are capable of producing all levels of CNS mood alteration, from excitation to mild sedation, hypnosis and deep coma. Overdosage can product death. Barbiturates depress the sensory cortex, decrease motor activity, alter cerebellar function and produce drowsiness, sedation and hypnosis.

Barbiturate-induced sleep differs from physiologic sleep. Sleep laboratory studies have demonstrated that barbiturates reduce the amount of time spent in the rapid eye movement (REM) phase of sleep, or dreaming stage. Also stages III and IV sleep are decreased. Following abrupt cessation of barbiturates used regularly, patients may experience markedly increased dreaming, nightmares and/or insomnia. Therefore, withdrawal of a single therapeutic dose over five or six days has been recommended to lessen the REM rebound and disturbed sleep which contribute to drug withdrawal syndrome (for example, decrease the dose from 3 to 2 doses a day for 1 week).

5.2 Pharmacokinetic properties

Barbiturates are weak acids that are absorbed and rapidly distributed to all tissues and fluids, with high concentrations in the brain, liver and kidneys. Lipid solubility of the barbiturates is the dominant factor in their distribution within the body. Barbiturates are bound to plasma and tissue proteins; the degree of binding increases as a function of lipid solubility.

Amylobarbitone is readily absorbed from the gastro-intestinal tract (the onset of action being from 45 to 60 minutes and the duration ranging from 6 to 8 hours) and following absorption some 60% is bound to plasma proteins. It has a half-life of about 20 to 25 hours, which is considerably extended in neonates. It is metabolised in the liver; up to about 50% is excreted in the urine as 3- hydroxyamylobarbitone and up to about 30% as *N*-hydroxyamylobarbitone. Less than 1% appears unchanged in urine and up to about 5% in faeces.

5.3 Preclinical safety data

Carcinogenesis: Animal data show that phenobarbitone can be carcinogenic after lifetime administration.

6. PHARMACEUTICAL PARTICULARS

6.1 List of excipients

Starch, Gelatin, Magnesium Stearate

6.2 Incompatibilities

Not applicable

6.3 Shelf life

60 months

6.4 Special precautions for storage

Store below 25°C. Keep lid tightly closed.

6.5 Nature and contents of container

High density polyethylene bottles with screw caps containing 500 tablets.

6.6 Instructions for use and handling

Not applicable

7. MARKETING AUTHORISATION HOLDER

Flynn Pharma Ltd.

Alton House

4 Herbert Street

Dublin 2

Republic of Ireland

8. MARKETING AUTHORISATION NUMBER(S)

PL 13621/0001

9. DATE OF FIRST AUTHORISATION/RENEWAL OF THE AUTHORISATION

1995

10. DATE OF REVISION OF THE TEXT

December 1995

11. LEGAL CATEGORY

CD (Sch 3), POM

Anadin Extra Soluble Tablets

(Wyeth Consumer Healthcare)

1. NAME OF THE MEDICINAL PRODUCT

Anadin Extra Soluble Tablets

2. QUALITATIVE AND QUANTITATIVE COMPOSITION

Active Ingredients

Aspirin BP 300 mg/tablet

Paracetamol Ph Eur 200 mg/tablet

Caffeine Citrate 90 mg/tablet

Equivalent to Caffeine Ph Eur 45 mg/tablet

3. PHARMACEUTICAL FORM

Soluble tablet for oral administration.

4. CLINICAL PARTICULARS

4.1 Therapeutic indications

For the treatment of mild to moderate pain including headache, migraine, neuralgia, toothache, sore throat, period pains, symptomatic relief of sprains, strains, rheumatic pain, sciatica, lumbago, fibrositis, muscular aches and pains, joint swelling and stiffness, influenza, feverishness and feverish colds.

4.2 Posology and method of administration

Dissolve 2 tablets in water

Adults, the elderly and young persons aged 16 and over:

2 tablets every 4 hours to a maximum of 8 tablets in 24 hours.

Do not give to children aged under 16 years, unless on the advice of a doctor.

4.3 Contraindications

Hypersensitivity to the active ingredients or any of the other constituents. Peptic ulceration and those with a history of peptic ulceration; haemophilia, concurrent anti-coagulant therapy; children under 16 years and when breast feeding because of possible risk of Reye's Syndrome.

4.4 Special warnings and special precautions for use

Caution should be exercised in patients with asthma, allergic disease, impairment of hepatic or renal function (avoid if severe) and dehydration.

Do not take if you have a stomach ulcer.

Do not exceed the stated dose.

Do not take other paracetamol-containing products.

If symptoms persist for more than 3 days consult your doctor.

Keep out of the reach of children.

Immediate medical advice should be sought in the case of an overdose, even if you feel well.

There is a possible association between aspirin and Reye's syndrome when given to children. Reye's syndrome is a very rare disease which affects the brain and liver, and can be fatal. For this reason aspirin should not be given to children under 16 years.

The leaflet will state:

There is a possible association between aspirin and Reye's syndrome when given to children. Reye's syndrome is a very rare disease which can be fatal. For this reason aspirin should not be given to children under 16 years unless on the advice of a doctor.

4.5 Interaction with other medicinal products and other forms of Interaction

Aspirin

Other NSAIDS and corticosteroids: Concurrent use of other NSAIDs or corticosteroids may increase the likelihood of GI side effects.

Diuretics: Antagonism of the diuretic effect.

Anticoagulants: Increased risk of bleeding due to antiplatelet effect.

Metoclopramide: Metoclopramide increases the rate of absorption of aspirin. However, concurrent use need not be avoided.

Phenytoin: The effect of phenytoin may be enhanced by aspirin. However, no special precautions are needed.

Valproate: The effect of valproate may be enhanced by aspirin.

Methotrexate: Delayed excretion and increased toxicity of methotrexate.

Paracetamol

Cholestyramine: The absorption of paracetamol is reduced by cholestyramine. Therefore the cholestyramine should not be taken within one hour if maximal analgesia is required.

Metoclopramide and Domperidone: The absorption of paracetamol is increased by metoclopramide and domperidone. However, concurrent use need not be avoided.

Warfarin: Potentiation of warfarin with continual high dosage of paracetamol with increased risk of bleeding; occasional doses have no significant effect.

Chloramphenicol: Increased plasma concentration of chloramphenicol.

4.6 Pregnancy and lactation

There is clinical and epidemiological evidence of safety of aspirin in pregnancy, but it may prolong labour and contribute to maternal and neonatal bleeding, and so should not be used in late pregnancy.

Aspirin appears in breast milk, and regular high doses may affect neonatal clotting. Not recommended while breast feeding due to possible risk of Reye's Syndrome as well as neonatal bleeding due to hypoprothrombinaemia.

There is epidemiological evidence of safety of paracetamol in human pregnancy. Paracetamol is excreted in breast milk but not in a clinically significant amount. Available published data do not contraindicate breast feeding.

Caffeine appears in breast milk. Irritability and poor sleeping pattern in the infant have been reported.

4.7 Effects on ability to drive and use machines

None known

4.8 Undesirable effects

Side effects are mild and infrequent, but there is a high incidence of gastro-intestinal irritation with slight asymptomatic blood loss. Increased bleeding time. Aspirin may precipitate bronchospasm and induce asthma attacks or other hypersensitivity reactions in susceptible individuals. Aspirin may induce gastro-intestinal haemorrhage, occasionally major. It may precipitate gout in susceptible individuals. Possible risk of Reye's Syndrome in children under 16 years.

Adverse effects of paracetamol are rare but hypersensitivity including skin rash may occur. There have been reports of blood dyscrasias including thrombocytopenia and agranulocytosis, but these were not necessarily causality related to paracetamol.

High doses of caffeine can cause tremor and palpitations.

4.9 Overdose

Aspirin

Severe intoxication from heavy overdosage is shown by hyperventilation, fever, restlessness, ketosis, respiratory alkalosis, metabolic acidosis and convulsions.

Paracetamol

Symptoms of paracetamol overdosage in the first 24 hours are pallor, nausea, vomiting, anorexia and abdominal pain. Liver damage may become apparent 12 to 48 hours after ingestion. Abnormalities of glucose metabolism and metabolic acidosis may occur.

In severe poisoning, hepatic failure may progress to encephalopathy, coma and death. Acute renal failure with acute tubular necrosis may develop even in the absence of severe liver damage. Cardiac arrhythmias and pancreatitis have been reported.

Liver damage is likely in adults who have taken 10g or more of paracetamol. It is considered that excess quantities of toxic metabolite (usually adequately detoxified by glutathione when normal doses of paracetamol are ingested), become irreversibly bound to liver tissue.

Treatment

Aspirin

A worthwhile recovery of salicylates can be achieved up to 24 hours after ingestion. Treatment must be in hospital where plasma salicylate pH and electrolytes can be measured. Fluid losses are replaced and forced alkaline diuresis is considered when the plasma salicylate concentration is greater than 500mg/litre (3.6 mmol/litre) in adults or 300mg/litre (2.2 mmol/litre) in children.

Paracetamol

Immediate treatment is essential in the management of paracetamol overdose. Despite a lack of significant early symptoms, patients should be referred to hospital urgently for immediate medical attention and any patient who has ingested around 7.5 g or more of paracetamol in the preceding 4 hours should undergo gastric lavage administration of oral methionine or intravenous n-acetylcysteine, which may have a beneficial effect up to at least 48 hours after the overdose, may be required. General supportive measures must be available.

5. PHARMACOLOGICAL PROPERTIES

5.1 Pharmacodynamic properties

ASPIRIN

Mechanisms of action/effect

Salicylates inhibit the activity of the enzyme cyclo-oxygenase to decrease the formation of precursors of prostaglandins and thromboxanes from arachidonic acid. Although many of the therapeutic effects may result from inhibition of prostaglandin synthesis (and consequent reduction of prostaglandin activity) in various tissues, other actions may also contribute significantly to the therapeutic effects.

Analgesic

Produces analgesia through a peripheral action by blocking pain impulse generation and via a central action, possibly in the hypothalamus.

Anti-inflammatory (Nonsteroidal)

Exact mechanisms have not been determined. Salicylates may act peripherally in inflamed tissue probably by inhibiting the synthesis of prostaglandins and possibly by inhibiting the synthesis and/or actions of other mediators of the inflammatory response.

Antipyretic

May produce antipyresis by acting centrally on the hypothalamic heat regulating centre to produce peripheral vasodilation resulting in increased cutaneous blood flow, sweating and heat loss.

PARACETAMOL

Mechanism of action/effect

Analgesic - the mechanism of analgesic action has not been fully determined. Paracetamol may act predominantly by inhibiting prostaglandin synthesis in the central nervous system (CNS) and, to a lesser extent, through a peripheral action by blocking pain-impulse generation.

The peripheral action may also be due to inhibition of prostaglandin synthesis or to inhibition of the synthesis or actions of other substances that sensitise pain receptors to mechanical or chemical stimulation.

Antipyretic - paracetamol probably produces antipyresis by acting centrally on the hypothalamic heat-regulation centre to produce peripheral vasodilation resulting in increased blood flow through the skin, sweating, and heat loss. The central action probably involves inhibition of prostaglandin synthesis in the hypothalamus.

CAFFEINE

Mechanisms of action/effect

Central nervous system stimulant - caffeine stimulates all levels of the CNS, although its cortical effects are milder and of shorter duration than those of amphetamines.

Analgesia adjunct

Caffeine constricts cerebral vasculature with an accompanying decrease in the cerebral blood flow and in the oxygen tension of the brain. It is believed that caffeine helps to relieve headache by providing more rapid onset on action and/or enhanced pain relief with lower doses of analgesic. Recent studies with ergotamine indicate that the enhancement of effect by the addition of caffeine may also be due to improved gastrointestinal absorption of ergotamine when administered with caffeine.

5.2 Pharmacokinetic properties

ASPIRIN

Absorption and fate

Absorption is generally rapid and complete following oral administration. It is largely hydrolysed in the gastrointestinal tract, liver and blood to salicylate which is further metabolised primarily in the liver.

PARACETAMOL

Absorption and Fate

Paracetamol is readily absorbed from the gastro-intestinal tract with peak plasma concentrations occurring about 30 minutes to 2 hours after ingestion. It is metabolised in the liver and excreted in the urine mainly as the glucuronide and sulphate conjugates. Less than 5% is excreted as unchanged paracetamol. The elimination half-life varies from about 1 to 4 hours. Plasma-protein binding is negligible at usual therapeutic concentrations but increases with increasing concentrations.

A minor hydroxylated metabolite which is usually produced in very small amounts by mixed-function oxidases in the liver and which is usually detoxified by conjugation with liver glutathione may accumulate following paracetamol overdosage and cause liver damage.

CAFFEINE

Absorption and fate

Caffeine is completely and rapidly absorbed after oral administration with peak concentrations occurring between 5 and 90 minutes after dose in fasted subjects. There is no evidence of presystemic metabolism. Elimination is almost entirely by hepatic metabolism in adults.

In adults, marked individual variability in the rate of elimination occurs. The mean plasma elimination half life is 4.9 hours with a range of 1.9 -12.2 hours. Caffeine distributes into all body fluids. The mean plasma protein binding of caffeine is 35%.

Caffeine is metabolised almost completely via oxidation, demethylation, and acetylation, and is excreted in the urine. The major metabolites are 1-methylxanthine, 7-methylxanthine, 1,7-dimethylxanthine (paraxanthine). Minor metabolites include 1-methyluric acid and 5-acetylamino-6 formylamino-3-methyluracil (AMFU).

5.3 Preclinical safety data

The active ingredients in Anadin Extra Soluble Tablets have a well established safety record. This combination of ingredients has been marketed for a number of years.

6. PHARMACEUTICAL PARTICULARS

6.1 List of excipients

Citric Acid Anhydrous Ph Eur

Calcium Carbonate Ph Eur

Lactose Ph Eur

Microcrystalline Cellulose Ph Eur

Maize Starch Ph Eur

Hydrogenated Vegetable Oil BP

Lemon Flavour 6334

Saccharin Sodium BP

Aspartame NF

Dioctyl Sodium Sulphosuccinate BP

Water Ph Eur

Pregelatinised Starch

Polyvinylpyrollidone

Potato Starch

Colloidal Silicon Dioxide

6.2 Incompatibilities

None stated

6.3 Shelf life

36 months.

6.4 Special precautions for storage

Do not store above 25°C

6.5 Nature and contents of container

PET/AL/PE blisters of 4 tablets in packs of 8, 16, 20, 24 or 32 tablets within a cardboard carton.

6.6 Instructions for use and handling

Tablets should be dissolved in water.

7. MARKETING AUTHORISATION HOLDER

Whitehall Laboratories Ltd

trading as Wyeth Consumer Healthcare

Huntercombe Lane South

Taplow

Maidenhead

Berkshire SL6 OPH

8. MARKETING AUTHORISATION NUMBER(S)

PL 0165/0075

9. DATE OF FIRST AUTHORISATION/RENEWAL OF THE AUTHORISATION

31 December 1991

10. DATE OF REVISION OF THE TEXT

March 2005

Anadin Extra Tablets

(Wyeth Consumer Healthcare)

1. NAME OF THE MEDICINAL PRODUCT

Anadin Extra Tablets/Powerin Tablets

2. QUALITATIVE AND QUANTITATIVE COMPOSITION

Aspirin BP 300 mg/tablet

Paracetamol Ph Eur 200 mg/tablet

Caffeine Ph Eur 45 mg/tablet

3. PHARMACEUTICAL FORM

Tablet for oral administration.

4. CLINICAL PARTICULARS

4.1 Therapeutic indications

For the treatment of mild to moderate pain including headache, migraine, neuralgia, toothache, sore throat, period pains, symptomatic relief of sprains, strains, rheumatic pain, sciatica, lumbago, fibrositis, muscular aches and pains, joint swelling and stiffness, influenza, feverishness and feverish colds.

4.2 Posology and method of administration

Adults, the elderly and young persons aged 16 and over:

2 tablets every 4 hours to a maximum of 8 tablets in 24 hours.

Do not give to children aged under 16 years, unless on the advice of a doctor.

4.3 Contraindications

Hypersensitivity to the active ingredients or any of the other constituents. Peptic ulceration and those with a history of peptic ulceration; haemophilia, concurrent anti-coagulant therapy; children under 16 years and when breast feeding because of possible risk of Reyes Syndrome.

4.4 Special warnings and special precautions for use

Caution should be exercised in patients with asthma, allergic disease, impairment of hepatic or renal function (avoid if severe) and dehydration.

Do not take if you have a stomach ulcer.

Do not exceed the stated dose.

Do not take other paracetamol containing products.

Taking too many tablets may be harmful and you should get medical advice straight away even if you do not feel ill.

If symptoms continue for more than 3 days consult your doctor.

Keep out of reach of children.

There is a possible association between aspirin and Reye's syndrome when given to children. Reye's syndrome is a very rare disease which affects the brain and liver, and can be fatal. For this reason aspirin should not be given to children under 16 years.

4.5 Interaction with other medicinal products and other forms of Interaction

Aspirin:

Other NSAIDS and corticosteroids: Concurrent use of other NSAIDS or corticosteroids may increase the likelihood of GI side effects.

Diuretics: Antagonism of the diuretic effect.

Anticoagulants: Increased risk of bleeding due to antiplatelet effect.

Metoclopramide: Metoclopramide increases the rate of absorption of aspirin. However, concurrent use need not be avoided.

Phenytoin: The effect of phenytoin may be enhanced by aspirin. However, no special precautions are needed.

Valproate: The effect of valproate may be enhanced by aspirin.

Methotrexate: Delayed excretion and increased toxicity of methotrexate.

Paracetamol:

Cholestyramine: The absorption of paracetamol is reduced by cholestyramine. Therefore, the cholestyramine should not be taken within one hour if maximal analgesia is required.

Metoclopramide and Domperidone: The absorption of paracetamol is increased by metoclopramide and domperidone. However, concurrent use need not be avoided.

Warfarin: Potentiation of warfarin with continual high dosage of paracetamol.

Chloramphenicol: Increased plasma concentration of chloramphenicol.

4.6 Pregnancy and lactation

There is clinical and epidemiological evidence of safety of aspirin in pregnancy, but it may prolong labour and contribute to material and neonatal bleeding, and so should not be used in late pregnancy.

Aspirin appears in breast milk, and regular high doses may affect neonatal clotting. Not recommended while breast feeding due to possible risk of Reye's Syndrome as well as neonatal bleeding due to hypoprothrombinaemia.

There is epidemiological evidence of safety of paracetamol in human pregnancy.

Caffeine appears in breast milk. Irritability and poor sleeping pattern in the infant have been reported.

4.7 Effects on ability to drive and use machines

None stated.

4.8 Undesirable effects

Side effects are mild and infrequent, but there is a high incidence of gastro-intestinal irritation with slight asymptomatic blood loss. Increased bleeding time. Bronchospasm and skin reactions in hypersensitive patients. Aspirin may induce gastro-intestinal haemorrhage, occasionally major. It may precipitate gout in susceptible individuals. Possible risk of Reye's Syndrome in children under 16 years. Isolated reports of thrombocytopenia purpura, methaemoglobinaemia and agranulocytosis.

High doses of caffeine can cause tremor and palpitations.

4.9 Overdose

Aspirin:

Severe intoxication from heavy overdosage is shown by hyperventilation, fever, restlessness, ketosis, respiratory alkalosis, metabolic acidosis and convulsions.

Paracetamol:

Symptoms of paracetamol overdosage in the first 24 hours are pallor, nausea, vomiting, anorexia and abdominal pain. Liver damage may become apparent 12 to 48 hours after ingestion. Abnormalities of glucose metabolism and metabolic acidosis may occur. In severe poisoning, hepatic failure may progress to encephalopathy, coma and death. Acute renal failure with acute tubular necrosis may develop even in the absence of severe liver damage. Cardiac arrhythmias and pancreatitis have been reported.

Liver damage is likely in adults who have taken 10g or more of paracetamol. It is considered that excess quantities of toxic metabolite (usually adequately detoxified by glutathione when normal doses of paracetamol are ingested), become irreversibly bound to liver tissue.

Treatment

Aspirin:

A worthwhile recovery of salicylates can be achieved up to 24 hours after ingestion. Treatment must be in hospital where plasma salicylate, pH and electrolytes can be measured. Fluid losses are replaced and forced alkaline diuresis is considered when plasma salicylate concentration is greater than 500 mg/litre (3.6 mmol/litre) in adults or 300 mg/litre (2.2 mmol/litre) in children.

Paracetamol:

Immediate treatment is essential in the management of paracetamol overdosage. Despite a lack of significant early symptoms, patients should be referred to hospital urgently for medical attention and any patient who has ingested around 7.5 g or more of paracetamol in the preceding 4 hours should undergo gastric lavage, administration of oral methionine or intravenous n-acetylcysteine, which may have a beneficial effect up to at least 48 hours after the overdose, may be required. General supportive measures must be available.

5. PHARMACOLOGICAL PROPERTIES

5.1 Pharmacodynamic properties

Aspirin

Mechanisms of action/effect

Salicylates inhibit the activity of the enzyme cyclo-oxygenase to decrease the formation of precursors of prostaglandins and thromboxanes from arachidonic acid. Although many of the therapeutic effects may result from inhibition of prostaglandin synthesis (and consequent reduction of prostaglandin activity) in various tissues, other actions may also contribute significantly to the therapeutic effects.

Analgesic

Produces analgesia through a peripheral action by blocking pain impulse generation and via a central action, possibly in the hypothalamus.

Anti-inflammatory (Nonsteroidal)

Exact mechanisms have not been determined. Salicylates may act peripherally in inflamed tissue probably by inhibiting the synthesis of prostaglandins and possibly by inhibiting the synthesis and/or actions of other mediators of the inflammatory response.

Antipyretic

May produce antipyresis by acting centrally on the hypothalamic heat-regulating centre to produce peripheral vasodilation resulting in increased cutaneous blood flow, sweating and heat loss.

Paracetamol

Mechanism of action/effect

Analgesic - the mechanism of analgesic action has not been fully determined. Paracetamol may act predominantly by inhibiting prostaglandin synthesis in the central nervous system (CNS) and, to a lesser extent, through a peripheral action by blocking pain-impulse generation.

The peripheral action may also be due to inhibition of prostaglandin synthesis or to inhibition of the synthesis or actions of other substances that sensitise pain receptors to mechanical or chemical stimulation.

Antipyretic - paracetamol probably produces antipyresis by acting centrally on the hypothalamic heat-regulation centre to produce peripheral vasodilation resulting in increased blood flow through the skin, sweating, and heat loss. The central action probably involves inhibition of prostaglandin synthesis in the hypothalamus.

Caffeine

Mechanisms of action/effect

Central nervous system stimulant - caffeine stimulates all levels of the CNS, although its cortical effects are milder and of shorter duration than those of amphetamines.

Analgesia adjunct

Caffeine constricts cerebral vasculature with an accompanying decrease in the cerebral blood flow and in the oxygen tension of the brain. It is believed that caffeine helps to relieve headache by providing more rapid onset on action and/or enhanced pain relief with lower doses of analgesic. Recent studies with ergotamine indicate that the enhancement of effect by the addition of caffeine may also be due to improved gastrointestinal absorption of ergotamine when administered with caffeine.

5.2 Pharmacokinetic properties

Aspirin

Absorption and fate

Absorption is generally rapid and complete following oral administration. It is largely hydrolysed in the gastrointestinal tract, liver and blood to salicylate which is further metabolised primarily in the liver.

Paracetamol

Absorption and fate

Paracetamol is readily absorbed from the gastro-intestinal tract with peak plasma concentrations occurring about 30 minutes to 2 hours after ingestion. It is metabolised in the liver and excreted in the urine mainly as the glucuronide and sulphate conjugates. Less than 5% is excreted as unchanged paracetamol. The elimination half-life varies from about 1 to 4 hours. Plasma-protein binding is negligible at usual therapeutic concentrations but increases with increasing concentrations.

A minor hydroxylated metabolite which is usually produced in very small amounts by mixed-function oxidases in the liver and which is usually detoxified by conjugation with liver glutathione may accumulate following paracetamol overdosage and cause liver damage.

Caffeine

Absorption and fate

Caffeine is completely and rapidly absorbed after oral administration with peak concentrations occurring between 5 an 90 minutes after dose in fasted subjects. There is no evidence of presystemic metabolism. Elimination is almost entirely by hepatic metabolism in adults.

In adults, marked individual variability in the rate of elimination occurs. The mean plasma elimination half life is 4.9 hours with a range of 1.9 - 12.2 hours. Caffeine distributes into all body fluids. The mean plasma protein binding of caffeine is 35%.

Caffeine is metabolised almost completely via oxidation, demethylation, and acetylation, and is excreted in the urine as 1-methyluric acid, 1-methylxanthine, 7-methylxanthine, 1,7-dimethylixanthine (paraxanthine) and 5-acethylamine-6-formylamine-3-methyluracil (AFMU).

5.3 Preclinical safety data

The active ingredients in Anadin Extra tablets have a well established safety record. This combination of ingredients has been marketed for a number of years.

6. PHARMACEUTICAL PARTICULARS

6.1 List of excipients

Maize Starch

Microcrystalline Cellulose

Hydrogenated vegetable oil

Hydroxypropyl Methylcellulose

Carbowax

Pregelatinised Starch

Polyvinylpyrollidone

6.2 Incompatibilities

None stated

6.3 Shelf life

24 months

6.4 Special precautions for storage

"Do not store above 25°C"

6.5 Nature and contents of container

Cartons containing blister (UPVC/hard tempered Aluminium foil) strips.

Polypropylene pack with a polypropylene label attached to it containing blister (UPVC/hard tempered Aluminium foil) strips.

8, 12, 16, 24, 32 tablets.

6.6 Instructions for use and handling

Not applicable

7. MARKETING AUTHORISATION HOLDER

Whitehall Laboratories Ltd

trading as Wyeth Consumer Healthcare

Huntercombe Lane South

Taplow

Maidenhead

Berkshire

SL6 0PH

8. MARKETING AUTHORISATION NUMBER(S)

PL 0165/5013R

9. DATE OF FIRST AUTHORISATION/RENEWAL OF THE AUTHORISATION

20 July 1990

10. DATE OF REVISION OF THE TEXT

September 2004

Anadin Ibuprofen 200mg Tablets

(Wyeth Consumer Healthcare)

1. NAME OF THE MEDICINAL PRODUCT

Anadin Ibuprofen Tablets

2. QUALITATIVE AND QUANTITATIVE COMPOSITION

Each tablet contains Ibuprofen 200mg.

For excipients see 6.1.

3. PHARMACEUTICAL FORM

Coated tablet.

White, sugar coated tablets smooth in texture with a polished surface. Black Anadin I printed on one side.

4. CLINICAL PARTICULARS

4.1 Therapeutic indications

For the relief of mild to moderate pain including rheumatic and muscular pain, backache, headache, dental pain, migraine, neuralgia, dysmenorrhoea and feverishness. For relief of the symptoms of cold and influenza.

4.2 Posology and method of administration

For oral administration and short-term use only.

Adults, the elderly and children over the age of 12:

The minimum effective dose should be used for the shortest time necessary to relieve symptoms. If the product is required for more than 10 days, the patient should consult a doctor.

1 or 2 tablets to be taken with a drink of water up to three times a day, as required.

Not to be given to children under 12 years of age.

The dose should not be repeated more frequently than every four hours and not more than 6 tablets should be taken in any 24 hour period.

4.3 Contraindications

Hypersensitivity to any of the constituents.

Ibuprofen is contra-indicated in patients who have previously shown hypersensitivity reactions (e.g. asthma, rhinitis, or urticaria) in response to aspirin or other non-steroidal anti-inflammatory drugs.

Active or previous peptic ulcer.

History of upper gastrointestinal bleeding or perforation, related to previous NSAID therapy.

Use with concomitant NSAIDs including cyclo-oxygenase-2 specific inhibitors.

4.4 Special warnings and special precautions for use

Bronchospasm may be precipitated in patients suffering from or with previous history of bronchial asthma or allergic disease.

Caution is required in patients with renal, cardiac or hepatic impairment since renal function may deteriorate.

Undesirable effects may be minimised by using the minimum effective dose for the shortest possible duration.

The elderly are at increased risk of the serious consequences of adverse reactions.

There is some evidence that drugs, which inhibit cyclo-oxygenase/prostaglandin synthesis, may cause impairment of female fertility by an effect on ovulation. This is reversible on withdrawal of treatment.

Gastro-intestinal bleeding, ulceration, or perforation, which can be fatal, has been reported with all NSAIDs at anytime during treatment, with or without warning symptoms or a previous history of serious GI effects.

Patients with a history of GI toxicity, particularly when elderly, should report any unusual abdominal symptoms (especially GI bleeding) particularly in the initial stages of treatment.

Caution should be advised in patients receiving concomitant medications which could increase the risk of gastro-toxicity or bleeding, such as corticosteroids, or anticoagulants such as warfarin or anti-platelet agents such as aspirin (see section 4.5).

Where GI bleeding or ulceration occurs in patients receiving ibuprofen, the treatment should be withdrawn.

The label will state:

Do not use if you have or have ever had a stomach ulcer or are allergic to ibuprofen or aspirin. Do not use if you have ever had stomach bleeding or perforation after taking a non-steroidal anti-inflammatory medicine. If you are allergic to or are taking any other painkiller, are pregnant, or suffer from asthma, speak to your doctor before taking ibuprofen. Do not exceed the stated dose. Keep out of the sight and reach of children. If symptoms persist, consult your doctor.

4.5 Interaction with other medicinal products and other forms of Interaction

NSAIDs may enhance the effects of anti-coagulants, such as warfarin, and diminish the effect of anti-hypertensives or diuretics.

Concurrent aspirin or other NSAIDs may result in an increased incidence of adverse reactions.

Corticosteroids: may increase the risk of adverse reaction in the gastrointestinal tract.

4.6 Pregnancy and lactation

While no teratogenic effects have been demonstrated in animal experiments, use of Ibuprofen during pregnancy should be avoided. The onset of labour may be delayed and duration of labour increased.

Ibuprofen does appear in the breast milk in very low concentrations and is unlikely to affect the breast fed infant adversely.

4.7 Effects on ability to drive and use machines

None.

4.8 Undesirable effects

Gastro-intestinal and skin disorders are most frequently reported. Adverse effects include the following:

Gastro-intestinal: abdominal pain, nausea and dyspepsia. Occasionally peptic ulcer, perforation or gastrointestinal haemorrhage, sometimes fatal, particularly in the elderly, may occur (see section 4.4).

Hypersensitivity reactions have been reported following treatment with NSAIDs. These may consist of

a) Non specific allergic reactions and anaphylaxis,

b) b) respiratory tract reactivity comprising asthma, aggravated asthma, bronchospasm or dyspnoea or

c) c) assorted skin disorders, including rashes of various types, pruritus, urticaria, purpura, angioedema, and more rarely bullous dermatoses (including epidermal necrolysis, exfoliative dermatitis and erythema multiforme).

Haematological: Thrombocytopenia.

Renal: Papillary necrosis which can lead to renal failure.

Other: Rarely hepatic dysfunction, headache, hearing disturbances, exacerbation of colitis, aseptic meningitis and dizziness.

4.9 Overdose

Symptoms include headache, vomiting, drowsiness and hypotension. Gastric lavage and correction of severe electrolyte abnormalities should be considered.

5. PHARMACOLOGICAL PROPERTIES

5.1 Pharmacodynamic properties

Ibuprofen has analgesic, antipyretic and anti-inflammatory properties.

Ibuprofen inhibits prostaglandin synthesis.

5.2 Pharmacokinetic properties

Ibuprofen is rapidly absorbed following administration and is rapidly distributed throughout the whole body. The excretion is rapid and complete via the kidneys.

Maximum plasma concentrations are reached 45 minutes after ingestion if taken on an empty stomach. When taken with food, peak levels are observed after 1 to 2 hours. These times may vary with different dosage forms.

The half life of ibuprofen is about 2 hours.

In limited studies, ibuprofen appears in the breast milk in very low concentrations.

5.3 Preclinical safety data
Not applicable.

6. PHARMACEUTICAL PARTICULARS
6.1 List of excipients
Maize starch
Pregelatinised starch
Colloidal Anhydrous Silica
Stearic acid
Sucrose
Macrogol
Perfectamyl Gel
Povidone
Carnauba wax
Polysorbate
Titanium dioxide
Talc
Calcium Carbonate
Opacode S-1-8152 HV Black *.

*The colouring agents contain Iron oxide(E172), Shellac, Butyl alcohol, Soya lecithin(E322), Antifoam.

6.2 Incompatibilities
None stated

6.3 Shelf life
3 years

6.4 Special precautions for storage
Do not store above 25C. Store in the original packaging.

6.5 Nature and contents of container
PVC/PE/PVDC and paper/aluminium blister pack

or

250micron UPVC/20micron aluminium blister pack.

Packaged in a carton containing 16 tablets.

6.6 Instructions for use and handling
Not applicable.

7. MARKETING AUTHORISATION HOLDER
Whitehall Laboratories Limited trading as
Wyeth Consumer Healthcare
Huntercombe Lane South
Taplow
Maidenhead
Berkshire SL6 0PH

8. MARKETING AUTHORISATION NUMBER(S)
PL 0165/0136

9. DATE OF FIRST AUTHORISATION/RENEWAL OF THE AUTHORISATION
06 January 2004

10. DATE OF REVISION OF THE TEXT
6th January 2004

Anadin Original

(Wyeth Consumer Healthcare)

1. NAME OF THE MEDICINAL PRODUCT
Anadin Original

2. QUALITATIVE AND QUANTITATIVE COMPOSITION
Active Ingredients:

Aspirin BP	325mg/tablet
Caffeine PhEur	15mg/tablet

3. PHARMACEUTICAL FORM
Tablet for oral administration.

4. CLINICAL PARTICULARS
4.1 Therapeutic indications
For the treatment of mild to moderate pain including headache, migraine, neuralgia, toothache, sore throat, period pains and aches and pains.

For the symptomatic treatment of sprains, strains, rheumatic pain, sciatica, lumbago, fibrositis, muscular aches and pains, joint swelling and stiffness, influenza, feverishness and feverish colds.

4.2 Posology and method of administration
Adults, the elderly and young persons aged 16 and over:

2 tablets every 4 hours.

Do not exceed 12 tablets in 24 hours.

Do not give to children aged under 16, unless on the advice of a doctor.

4.3 Contraindications
Hypersensitivity to the active ingredient or any of the other constituents. Peptic ulceration and those with a history of peptic ulceration, haemophilia, concurrent anti-coagulant therapy, children under 16 years and when breast feeding because of possible risk of Reyes.

4.4 Special warnings and special precautions for use
- Caution should be exercised in patients with asthma, allergic disease, impairment of hepatic or renal function (avoid if severe) and dehydration.
- Do not take if you have a stomach ulcer.
- Do not exceed the stated dose.
- If symptoms persist for more than 3 days consult your doctor.
- Do not exceed 12 tablets in 24 hours.
- Keep all medicines out of the reach of children.

There is a possible association between aspirin and Reye's syndrome when given to children. Reye's syndrome is a very rare disease which affects the brain and liver, and can be fatal. For this reason aspirin should not be given to children under 16 years.

4.5 Interaction with other medicinal products and other forms of Interaction
Aspirin
- Other NSAIDS and corticosteroids: Concurrent use of other NSAIDS or corticosteroids may increase the likelihood of GI side effects.
- Diuretics: Antagonism of the diuretic effect.
- Anticoagulants: Increased risk of bleeding due to antiplatelet effect.
- Metoclopramide: Metoclopramide increases the rate of absorption of aspirin. However, concurrent use need not be avoided.
- Phenytoin: The effect of phenytoin may be enhanced by aspirin. However, no special precautions are needed.
- Valproate: The effect of valproate may be enhanced by aspirin.
- Methotrexate: Delayed excretion and increased toxicity of methotrexate.

4.6 Pregnancy and lactation
There is clinical and epidemiological evidence of safety of aspirin in pregnancy, but it may prolong labour and contribute to maternal and neonatal bleeding, and so should not be used in late pregnancy.

Aspirin appears in breast milk, and regular high doses may affect neonatal clotting. Not recommended while breast feeding due to possible risk of Reye's Syndrome as well as neonatal bleeding due to hypoprothrombinaemia.

Caffeine appears in breast milk. Irritability and poor sleeping pattern in the infant have been reported.

4.7 Effects on ability to drive and use machines
None known.

4.8 Undesirable effects
Side effects are mild and infrequent, but there is a high incidence of gastro-intestinal irritation with slight asymptomatic blood loss. Increased bleeding time. Aspirin may precipitate bronchospasm and induce asthma attacks or other hypersensitivity reactions in susceptible individuals. Aspirin may induce gastro-intestinal haemorrhage, occasionally major. It may precipitate gout in susceptible individuals. Possible risk of Reye's Syndrome in children under 16 years.

High doses of caffeine can cause tremor and palpitations.

4.9 Overdose
Severe intoxication from heavy overdosage is shown by hyperventilation, fever, restlessness, ketosis, respiratory alkalosis, metabolic acidosis and convulsions.

Treatment

A worthwhile recovery of salicylates can be achieved up to 24 hours after ingestion. Treatment must be in hospital where plasma salicylate pH and electrolytes can be measured. Fluid losses are replaced and forced alkaline diuresis is considered when the plasma salicylate concentration is greater than 500mg/litre (3.6 mmol/litre) in adults or 300mg/litre (2.2 mmol/litre) in children.

5. PHARMACOLOGICAL PROPERTIES
5.1 Pharmacodynamic properties
ASPIRIN
Mechanisms of action/effect

Salicylates inhibit the activity of the enzyme cyclo-oxygenase to decrease the formation of precursors of prostaglandins and thromboxanes from arachidonic acid. Although many of the therapeutic effects may result from inhibition of prostaglandin synthesis (and consequent reduction of prostaglandin activity) in various tissues, other actions may also contribute significantly to the therapeutic effects.

Analgesic

Produces analgesia through a peripheral action by blocking pain impulse generation and via a central action, possibly in the hypothalamus.

Anti-inflammatory (Nonsteroidal)

Exact mechanisms have not been determined. Salicylates may act peripherally in inflamed tissue probably by inhibiting the synthesis of prostaglandins and possibly by inhibiting the synthesis and/or actions of other mediators of the inflammatory response.

Antipyretic

May produce antipyresis by acting centrally on the hypothalamic heat regulating centre to produce peripheral vasodilation resulting in increased cutaneous blood flow, sweating and heat loss.

Caffeine
Mechanisms of action/effect

Central nervous system stimulant – caffeine stimulates all levels of the CNS, although its cortical effects are milder and of shorter duration than those of amphetamines.

Analgesia adjunct

Caffeine constricts cerebral vasculature with an accompanying decrease in the cerebral blood flow and in the oxygen tension of the brain. It is believed that caffeine helps to relieve headache by providing more rapid onset on action and/or enhanced pain relief with lower doses of analgesic. Recent studies with ergotamine indicate that the enhancement of effect by the addition of caffeine may also be due to improved gastrointestinal absorption of ergotamine when administered with caffeine.

5.2 Pharmacokinetic properties
Aspirin
Absorption and fate

Absorption is generally rapid and complete following oral administration. It is largely hydrolysed in the gastrointestinal tract, liver and blood to salicylate which is further metabolised primarily in the liver.

Caffeine
Absorption and fate

Caffeine is completely and rapidly absorbed after oral administration with peak concentration occurring between 5 and 90 minutes after dose in fasted subjects. There is no evidence of presystemic metabolism. Elimination is almost entirely by hepatic metabolism in adults.

In adults, marked individual variability in the rate of elimination occurs. The mean plasma elimination half life is 4.9 hours with a range of 1.9 –12.2 hours. Caffeine distributes into all body fluids. The mean plasma protein binding of caffeine is 35%.

Caffeine is metabolised almost completely via oxidation, demethylation, and acetylation, and is excreted in the urine. The major metabolites are 1-methylxanthine, 7-methylxanthine, 1,7-dimethylxanthine (paraxanthine). Minor metabolites include 1-methyluric acid and 5-acetylamino-6 formylamino-3-methyluracil (AMFU).

5.3 Preclinical safety data
None stated.

6. PHARMACEUTICAL PARTICULARS
6.1 List of excipients
Quinine Sulphate Ph Eur
Maize Starch PhEur
Microcrystalline Cellulose Ph Eur
Hydroxypropyl Methylcellulose (Methocel E5) Ph Eur
Hydroxypropyl Methylcellulose (Methocel E15) Ph Eur
Polyethylene Glycol (Carbowax 3350) USNF
Calcium Stearate USNF

6.2 Incompatibilities
None known.

6.3 Shelf life
24 months

6.4 Special precautions for storage
Do not store above 25°C.

6.5 Nature and contents of container
Paper/Polyethylene strip 4, 8

Cartons containing PVC/PVdC hard tempered aluminium foil with glassine paper blister strip 4, 6, 8, 12, 16, 24, 32

Polypropylene drum with CRC cap 24, 32

Aluminium containers with approved polyethylene CRC Cap 16, 32

Paper/Polyethylene laminated strip packs 4, 8

6.6 Instructions for use and handling
Not applicable.

7. MARKETING AUTHORISATION HOLDER
Whitehall Laboratories Limited
trading as Wyeth Consumer Healthcare
Huntercombe Lane South
Taplow
Maidenhead
Berkshire
SL6 OPH

8. MARKETING AUTHORISATION NUMBER(S)
PL 0165/0060

9. DATE OF FIRST AUTHORISATION/RENEWAL OF THE AUTHORISATION
31 August 1993

10. DATE OF REVISION OF THE TEXT
January 2005

Anadin Paracetamol Tablets

(Wyeth Consumer Healthcare)

1. NAME OF THE MEDICINAL PRODUCT
Anadin Paracetamol Tablets

2. QUALITATIVE AND QUANTITATIVE COMPOSITION
Active Ingredients mg/tablet

Paracetamol Ph Eur 500.00

3. PHARMACEUTICAL FORM
Tablet for oral administration.

4. CLINICAL PARTICULARS

4.1 Therapeutic indications
For the treatment of mild to moderate pain including headache, migraine, neuralgia, toothache, sore throat, period pains, aches and pains, symptomatic relief of rheumatic aches and pains and of influenza, feverishness and feverish colds.

4.2 Posology and method of administration
Adults, the elderly and young persons over 12 years:

2 tablets every 4 hours to a maximum of 8 tablets in 24 hours.

Children 6 – 12 years:

½ to 1 tablet every 4 hours to a maximum of 4 tablets in 24 hours.

Children under 6 years:

Not recommended.

4.3 Contraindications
Hypersensitivity to paracetamol or any of the constituents.

4.4 Special warnings and special precautions for use
Care is advised in the administration of paracetamol to patients with severe renal or severe hepatic impairment. The hazards of overdose are greater in those with non-cirrhotic alcoholic liver disease.

The label will state:

Do not exceed the stated dose.

Keep out of the reach of children.

Contains Paracetamol.

Do not take with any other paracetamol-containing products.

If symptoms persist for more than 3 days consult your doctor.

Immediate medical advice should be sought in the event of an overdose, even if you feel well.

4.5 Interaction with other medicinal products and other forms of Interaction
Cholestyramine: The absorption of paracetamol is reduced by cholestyramine. Therefore, the cholestyramine should not be taken within one hour if maximal analgesia is required.

Metoclopramide and Domperidone: The absorption of paracetamol is increased by metoclopramide and domperidone. However, concurrent use need not be avoided.

Warfarin: Potentiation of warfarin with continual high dosage of paracetamol.

Chloramphenicol: Increased plasma concentration of chloramphenicol.

4.6 Pregnancy and lactation
There is clinical and epidemiological evidence of safety of paracetamol in pregnancy. Paracetamol is excreted in breast milk but not in a clinically significant amount. Available published data do not contraindicate breast feeding.

4.7 Effects on ability to drive and use machines
None known.

4.8 Undesirable effects
Side effects are rare but hypersensitivity, including skin rash may occur.

Isolated reports of thrombocytopenia purpura, methaemoglobinaemia and agranulocytosis.

4.9 Overdose
Liver damage is possible in adults who have taken 10g or more of paracetamol. Ingestion of 5g or more of paracetamol may lead to liver damage if the patient has risk factors (see below).

Risk Factors:

If the patient;

a. Is on long term treatment with carbamazepine, phenobarbitone, phenytoin, primidone, rifampicin, St John's Wort or other drugs that induce liver enzymes.

Or

b, Regularly consumes ethanol in excess of recommended amounts.

Or

c, Is likely to be glutathione deplete e.g. eating disorders, cystic fibrosis, HIV infection, starvation, cachexia.

Symptoms
Symptoms of paracetamol overdosage in the first 24 hours are pallor, nausea, vomiting, anorexia and abdominal pain. Liver damage may become apparent 12 to 48 hours after ingestion. Abnormalities of glucose metabolism and metabolic acidosis may occur. In severe poisoning, hepatic failure may progress to encephalopathy, haemorrhage, hypoglycaemia, cerebral oedema, and death. Acute renal failure with acute tubular necrosis, strongly suggested by loin pain, haematuria and proteinuria, may develop even in the absence of severe liver damage. Cardiac arrhythmias and pancreatitis have been reported.

Management
Immediate treatment is essential in the management of paracetamol overdose. Despite a lack of significant early symptoms, patients should be referred to hospital urgently for immediate medical attention. Symptoms may be limited to nausea or vomiting and may not reflect the severity of overdose or the risk of organ damage. Management should be in accordance with established treatment guidelines, see BNF overdose section.

Treatment with activated charcoal should be considered if the overdose has been taken within 1 hour. Plasma paracetamol concentration should be measured at 4 hours or later after ingestion (earlier concentrations are unreliable) but results should not delay initiation of treatment beyond 8 hours after ingestion, as the effectiveness of the antidote declines sharply after this time. If required the patient should be given intravenous-N-acetylcysteine, in line with the established dosage schedule. If vomiting is not a problem, oral methionine may be a suitable alternative for remote areas, outside hospital.

5. PHARMACOLOGICAL PROPERTIES

5.1 Pharmacodynamic properties
Mechanisms of Action/Effect

Analgesic – the mechanism of analgesic action has not been fully determined. Paracetamol may act predominantly by inhibiting prostaglandin synthesis in the central nervous system (CNS) and to a lesser extent, through a peripheral action by blocking pain-impulse generation.

The peripheral action may also be due to inhibition of prostaglandin synthesis or to inhibition of the synthesis or actions of other substances that sensitise pain receptors to mechanical or chemical stimulation.

Antipyretic – paracetamol probably produces antipyresis by acting centrally on the hypothalamic heat-regulation centre to produce peripheral vasodilation resulting in increased blood flow through the skin, sweating and heat loss. The central action probably involves inhibition of prostaglandin synthesis in the hypothalamus.

5.2 Pharmacokinetic properties
Absorption and Fate

Paracetamol is readily absorbed from the gastro-intestinal tract with peak plasma concentrations occurring about 30 minutes to 2 hours after ingestion. It is metabolised in the liver and excreted in the urine mainly as the glucuronide and sulphate conjugates. Less than 5% is excreted as unchanged paracetamol. The elimination half-life varies from about 1 to 4 hours. Plasma-protein binding is negligible at usual therapeutic concentrations but increases with increasing concentrations.

A minor hydroxylated metabolite which is usually produced in very small amounts by mixed-function oxidases in the liver and which is usually detoxified by conjugation with liver glutathione may accumulate following paracetamol overdosage and cause liver damage.

5.3 Preclinical safety data
None stated

6. PHARMACEUTICAL PARTICULARS

6.1 List of excipients
Croscarmellose Sodium

Povidone

Pregelatinised Maize Starch

Hydroxypropyl Methylcellulose

Polyethylene Glycol

6.2 Incompatibilities
None known.

6.3 Shelf life
5 years

6.4 Special precautions for storage
Do not store above 25°C.

6.5 Nature and contents of container
PVC/PVdC hard tempered aluminium foil with glassine paper blister packs 8, 16, 32 tablets.

6.6 Instructions for use and handling
Not applicable.

7. MARKETING AUTHORISATION HOLDER
Whitehall Laboratories Ltd

trading as Wyeth Consumer Healthcare

Huntercombe Lane South

Taplow

Maidenhead

Berkshire

SL6 OPH

8. MARKETING AUTHORISATION NUMBER(S)
PL 0165/0056

9. DATE OF FIRST AUTHORISATION/RENEWAL OF THE AUTHORISATION
30 July 1987/11 February 1997

10. DATE OF REVISION OF THE TEXT
January 2005

Anadin Ultra

(Wyeth Consumer Healthcare)

1. NAME OF THE MEDICINAL PRODUCT
Anadin Ultra

2. QUALITATIVE AND QUANTITATIVE COMPOSITION
Each capsule contains 200mg Ibuprofen

3. PHARMACEUTICAL FORM
Capsule, soft
For oral administration

4. CLINICAL PARTICULARS

4.1 Therapeutic indications
Pharmacy only:

For the relief of mild to moderate pain including rheumatic and muscular pain, backache, headache, dental pain, migraine, neuralgia, dysmenorrhoea, feverishness and for the relief of symptoms of cold and influenza. Also, for the symptomatic relief of the pain of non-serious arthritic conditions.

GSL only:

For the relief of mild to moderate pain including rheumatic and muscular pain, backache, headache, dental pain, migraine, neuralgia, dysmenorrhoea, feverishness and for the relief of symptoms of cold and influenza.

4.2 Posology and method of administration
For all indications:

Adults, the elderly and children over 12 years of age:

1 or 2 capsules every 4 to 6 hours as required.

The capsules should be taken with water.

Do not exceed 6 capsules (1200mg) in 24 hours.

Not to be used for children under 12 years of age.

4.3 Contraindications
Use in patients hypersensitive to any of the ingredients. Use in patients hypersensitive to aspirin or with bronchospasm, asthma, rhinitis or urticaria associated with non-steroidal anti-inflammatory drugs. Ibuprofen should not be given to patients with current or previous peptic ulceration.

4.4 Special warnings and special precautions for use
Bronchospasm may be precipitated in patients suffering from or with a previous history of bronchial asthma or allergic disease.

Caution is required in patients with renal, cardiac or hepatic impairment since renal function may deteriorate. The dose should be as low as possible and renal function should be monitored.

Undesirable effects may be minimised by using the minimum effective dose for the shortest possible duration. The elderly are at increased risk of the serious consequences of adverse reactions.

The label will state:

Do not exceed the stated dose

If symptoms persist, consult your doctor

Keep out of the reach of children

Do not use if you have ever had a stomach ulcer

Do not use if you are allergic to Ibuprofen, aspirin or any of the other ingredients

Do not take with any other painkillers

If you are allergic to or taking any other painkiller, are pregnant, or suffer from asthma, consult your doctor

4.5 Interaction with other medicinal products and other forms of Interaction
NSAIDs may enhance the effects of anti-coagulants and diminish the effect of anti-hypertensives or thiazide diuretics.

Concurrent aspirin or other NSAIDs may result in an increased incidence of adverse reactions.

Increases in serum lithium concentrations following administration of ibuprofen may be clinically significant.

Concomitant administration of ibuprofen with moderate and high doses of methotrexate may lead to serious and fatal methotrexate toxicity. Patients with reduced renal function may be at additional risk of toxicity from the combination even when low doses of methotrexate ($\leq$20mg/week) are used.

4.6 Pregnancy and lactation
While no teratogenic effect has been demonstrated in animal experiments, use of Ibuprofen during pregnancy should, if possible, be avoided. The onset of labour may be delayed and duration of labour increased.

Ibuprofen does appear in breast milk in very low concentrations, and is unlikely to affect the breast fed infant adversely.

4.7 Effects on ability to drive and use machines
None known.

4.8 Undesirable effects
Gastro-intestinal and skin disorders are most frequently reported. Adverse effects include the following:

Gastro-intestinal: Abdominal pain, nausea and dyspepsia, constipation, diarrhoea and occasionally peptic ulcer and gastro-intestinal haemorrhage.

Hypersensitivity reactions which may consist of non-specific allergic reactions and anaphylaxis. These may be experienced as:

a) respiratory tract reactivity comprising of asthma, aggravated asthma, bronchospasm or dyspnoea.

b) assorted skin disorders, including rashes of various types, pruritis, urticaria, purpura, angioedema, and more rarely bullous dermatoses (including epidermal necrolysis and erythema multiforme).

Haematological: Most frequent thrombocytopenia, but occasionally agranulocytosis and aplastic anaemia.

Renal: Haematuria, interstitial nephritis, renal papillary necrosis and renal failure have occasionally been reported.

Other: Rarely hepatic dysfunction, headache, hearing disturbances and dizziness.

4.9 Overdose
In cases of overdosage, headache, vomiting, drowsiness and hypotension have been reported. Hyperkalaemia may develop. Treatment is supportive with gastric lavage and correction of severe electrolyte imbalance if required.

5. PHARMACOLOGICAL PROPERTIES

5.1 Pharmacodynamic properties
Ibuprofen is a phenylpropionic acid derivative which has analgesic, anti-inflammatory and anti-pyretic actions.

5.2 Pharmacokinetic properties

Absorption:

After oral administration, solubilised ibuprofen (Anadin Ultra) is quickly absorbed when administered under fasting conditions. Cmax is achieved within 0.6 hours compared with conventional tablets (0.75 – 1.5 hours). When taken with food, peak levels are observed after 1 to 2 hours. It is over 90% plasma protein bound in the circulation and has a short elimination half life of 0.9 – 2.5 hours.

Distribution:

The short plasma half life does not lead to accumulation phenomena. In the synovial fluid, ibuprofen is found with stable concentrations between the 2nd and 8th hour after ingestion, the synovial Cmax being approximately equal to one third of the plasma Cmax. Following ingestion of 400mg of ibuprofen every 6 hours by nursing women, the quantity of ibuprofen found in their milk is less than 1mg in 24 hours.

Metabolism:

Ibuprofen does not have any enzyme-inducing effect. If is 90% metabolised in the liver to 2 hydroxyibuprofen and 2-carboxyibuprofen.

Excretion:

The metabolites are excreted in the urine along with approximately 9% of unchanged drug.

5.3 Preclinical safety data
No relevant information additional to that already contained is elsewhere in the SPC.

6. PHARMACEUTICAL PARTICULARS

6.1 List of excipients
Polyethylene Glycol, Potassium Hydroxide, Anidrisorb 85/70 (mixture of Sorbitans and Sorbitols, Mannitol), Gelatin, E104, E131, Purified water, Opacode White Ink (E171, Propylene Glycol, Polyvinyl acetate phthalate, Polyethylene Glycol).

6.2 Incompatibilities
None known.

6.3 Shelf life
24 months

6.4 Special precautions for storage
Do not store above 25°C.

6.5 Nature and contents of container
Anadin Ultra is packed into blister strips of 4, 6, 8, 10, 12, 16, 20, 24, 30, 32, 36, 40, 48, 50, 60, 70, 72, 80, 90, 96 and 100 capsules in a cardboard box.

Pack A: PVdC (60gsm)/white opaque PVC (200μm)/heat sealed to the foil.

Foil: Hard temper aluminium foil (20 um)/Heatseal lacquer (7 gsm).

Pack B: Blister: White opaque thermoformed unplasticised PVC (250 um)/

PVdC coating (60 gsm) heat sealed to the foil.

Foil: Glassine (35 gsm)/Lamination adhesive/Aluminium foil (9 um)/Heatseal lacquer (7 gsm).

6.6 Instructions for use and handling
No special instructions.

7. MARKETING AUTHORISATION HOLDER
Whitehall Laboratories Ltd
trading as Wyeth Consumer Healthcare
Huntercombe Lane South
Taplow
Maidenhead
Berkshire
SL6 0PH
United Kingdom

8. MARKETING AUTHORISATION NUMBER(S)
PL 00165/0142

9. DATE OF FIRST AUTHORISATION/RENEWAL OF THE AUTHORISATION
22 September 1999

10. DATE OF REVISION OF THE TEXT
July 2002

Anafranil 75mg SR Tablets

(Cephalon UK Limited)

1. NAME OF THE MEDICINAL PRODUCT
Anafranil® 75mg SR Tablets.

2. QUALITATIVE AND QUANTITATIVE COMPOSITION
Chemical name: 3-Chloro-5-[3-(dimethylamino)-propyl] 10,11-dihydro-5H-dibenz[b,f] azepine hydrochloride (= clomipramine hydrochloric).

Each tablet contains 75mg Clomipramine hydrochloride B.P.

3. PHARMACEUTICAL FORM
Slow release, film coated tablets.

4. CLINICAL PARTICULARS

4.1 Therapeutic indications
Antidepressant: Symptoms of depressive illness especially where sedation is required. Obsessional and phobic states. Adjunctive treatment of cataplexy associated with narcolepsy.

4.2 Posology and method of administration
Before initiating treatment with Anafranil, hypokalemia should be treated (see 4.4. Special warnings and precautions for use).

As a precaution against possible serotonergic toxicity, adherence to the recommended doses of Anafranil is advised and any increase in dose should be made with caution if other serotonergic agents are co-administered (see 4.4 Special warnings and precautions for use).

Adults:

Oral - 10mg/day initially, increasing gradually to 30-150mg/day, if required, in divided doses throughout the day or as a single dose at bedtime. Many patients will be adequately maintained on 30-50mg/day. Higher doses may be needed in some patients, particularly those suffering from obsessional or phobic disorders. In severe cases this dosage can be increased up to a maximum of 250mg per day. Once a distinct improvement has set in, the daily dosage may be adjusted to a maintenance level averaging either 2-4 capsules of 25mg or 1 tablet of 75mg.

Elderly:

The initial dose should be 10mg/day, which may be increased with caution under close supervision to an optimum level of 30-75mg daily which should be reached after about 10 days and then maintained until the end of treatment.

Children:

Not recommended.

Obsessional/phobic states:

The maintenance dosage of Anafranil is generally higher than that used in depression. It is recommended that the dose be built up to 100-150mg Anafranil daily, according to the severity of the condition. This should be attained gradually over a period of 2 weeks starting with 1 × 25mg Anafranil daily. In elderly patients and those sensitive to tricyclic antidepressants a starting dose of 1 × 10mg Anafranil daily is recommended. Again where a higher dosage is required the SR 75mg formulation may be preferable.

Adjunctive treatment of cataplexy associated with narcolepsy:

(Oral treatment): 10-75mg daily. It is suggested that treatment is commenced with 10mg Anafranil daily and gradually increased until a satisfactory response occurs. Control of cataplexy should be achieved within 24 hours of reaching the optimal dose. Where necessary, therapy may be combined with capsules and syrup up to the maximum dose of 75mg per day.

Route of Administration

Oral

4.3 Contraindications
Known hypersensitivity to clomipramine or any of the excipients, or cross-sensitivity to tricyclic antidepressants of the dibenzazepine group. Recent myocardial infarction. Any degree of heart block or other cardiac arrhythmias. Mania, severe liver disease, narrow angle glaucoma. Retention of urine. Anafranil should not be given in combination with or within 3 weeks before or after treatment with an MAO inhibitor (see Interactions).

The concomitant treatment with selective, reversible MAO-A inhibitors such as moclobamide, is also contraindicated.

4.4 Special warnings and special precautions for use
As improvement in depression may not occur for the first two to four weeks treatment, patients should be closely monitored during this period.

Tricyclic antidepressants are known to lower the convulsion threshold and Anafranil should therefore be used with extreme caution in patients with epilepsy and other predisposing factors, e.g. brain damage of varying aetiology, concomitant use of neuroleptics, withdrawal from alcohol or drugs with anticonvulsive properties (e.g. benzodiazepines). It appears that the occurrence of seizures is dose dependent, therefore the recommended total daily dose of Anafranil should not be exceeded.

Caution is called for when giving tricyclic antidepressants to patients with tumours of the adrenal medulla (e.g. phaeochromocytoma, neuroblastoma), in whom they may provoke hypertensive crises.

Concomitant treatment of Anafranil and electroconvulsive therapy should only be resorted to under careful supervision.

Elderly patients are particularly liable to experience adverse effects, especially agitation, confusion, and postural hypotension.

Many patients with panic disorders experience intensified anxiety symptoms at the start of the treatment with antidepressants. This paradoxical initial increase in anxiety is most pronounced during the first few days of treatment and generally subsides within two weeks.

Precautions:

Before initiating treatment it is advisable to check the patient's blood pressure, because individuals with hypotension or a labile circulation may react to the drug with a fall in blood pressure.

Although changes in the white blood cell count have been reported with Anafranil only in isolated cases, periodic blood cell counts and monitoring for symptoms such as fever and sore throat are called for, particularly during the first few months of therapy. They are also recommended during prolonged therapy.

It is advisable to monitor cardiac and hepatic function during long-term therapy with Anafranil. In patients with liver disease, periodic monitoring of hepatic enzyme levels is recommended.

There may be a risk of QTc prolongation and Torsade de Pointes, particularly at supra-therapeutic doses or supra-therapeutic plasma concentrations of clomipramine, as occur in the case of co-medication with selective serotonin reuptake inhibitors (SSRIs). Therefore, concomitant administration of drugs that can cause accumulation of clomipramine should be avoided. Equally, concomitant administration of drugs that can prolong the QTc interval should be avoided. (see 4.5 Interactions with other medicinal products and other forms of interaction). It is established that hypokalemia is a risk-factor of QTc prolongation and Torsade de Pointes. Therefore, hypokalemia should be treated before initiating treatment with Anafranil and Anafranil should be used with caution when combined with SSRIs or diuretics (see 4.5. Interactions with other medicinal products and other forms of interaction.)Caution is indicated in patients with hyperthyroidism or during concomitant treatment with thyroid preparations since aggravation of unwanted cardiac effects may occur.

Because of its anticholinergic properties, Anafranil should be used with caution in patients with a history of increased intra-ocular pressure, narrow angle glaucoma or urinary retention (e.g. diseases of the prostate).

An increase in dental caries has been reported during long-term treatment with tricyclic antidepressants. Regular dental check-ups are therefore advisable during long-term treatment.

Caution is called for in patients with chronic constipation. Tricyclic antidepressants may cause paralytic ileus, particularly in the elderly and in bedridden patients.

Decreased lacrimation and accumulation of mucoid secretions due to the anticholinergic properties of tricyclic antidepressants may cause damage to the corneal epithelium in patients with contact lenses.

Risk of suicide is inherent to severe depression and may persist until significant remission occurs. Patients posing a high suicide risk require close initial supervision.

Activation of psychosis has occasionally been observed in schizophrenic patients receiving tricyclic antidepressants. Hypomanic or manic episodes have also been reported during a depressive phase in patients with cyclic affective disorders receiving treatment with a tricyclic antidepressant. In such cases it may be necessary to reduce the dosage of Anafranil or to withdraw it and administer an antipsychotic agent. After such episodes have subsided, low dose therapy with Anafranil may be resumed if required.

Anafranil may cause anxiety, feelings of unrest, and hyperexcitation in agitated patients and patients with accompanying schizophrenic symptoms.

In predisposed and elderly patients, Anafranil may, particularly at night, provoke pharmacogenic (delirious) psychoses, which disappear without treatment within a few days of withdrawing the drug.

Before general or local anaesthesia, the anaesthetist should be aware that the patient has been receiving Anafranil and of the possible interactions (see 4.5 Interactions with other medicinal products and other forms of interaction).

As a precaution against possible serotonergic toxicity, adherence to the recommended doses of Anafranil is advised and any increase in dose should be made with caution if other serotonergic agents are co-administered.

Abrupt withdrawal should be avoided because of possible adverse reactions (see 4.8 Undesirable Effects).

4.5 Interaction with other medicinal products and other forms of Interaction

MAO inhibitors:

Do not give Anafranil for at least 3 weeks after discontinuation of treatment with MAO inhibitors (there is a risk of severe symptoms consistent with Serotonin Syndrome such as hypertensive crisis, hyperpyrexia, myoclonus, agitation, seizures, delirium and coma). The same applies when giving a MAO inhibitor after previous treatment with Anafranil. In both instances the treatment should initially be given in small gradually increasing doses and its effects monitored. There is evidence to suggest that Anafranil may be given as little as 24 hours after a reversible MAO-A inhibitor such as moclobemide, but the 3 week wash-out period must be observed if the MAO-A inhibitor is used after Anafranil.

Serotonergic Agents:

Serotonin Syndrome can possibly occur when Anafranil is administered with other serotonergic co-medications such as selective serotonin reuptake inhibitors, tricyclic antidepressants and lithium. For fluoxetine a washout period of two to three weeks is advised before and after treatment with fluoxetine.

CNS depressants:

Tricyclic antidepressants may potentiate the effects of alcohol and other central depressant substances (e.g. barbiturates, benzodiazepines, or general anaesthetics).

Neuroleptics:

Comedication may result in increased plasma levels of tricyclic antidepressants, a lowered convulsion threshold, and seizures. Combination with thioridazine may produce severe cardiac arrhythmias.

Anticoagulants:

Tricyclic antidepressants may potentiate the anticoagulant effect of coumarin drugs by inhibiting their metabolism by the liver. Careful monitoring of plasma prothrombin is therefore advised.

Anticholinergic agents:

Tricyclic antidepressants may potentiate the effects of these drugs (e.g. phenothiazine, antiparkinsonian agents, antihistamines, atropine, biperiden) on the eye, central nervous system, bowel and bladder).

Adrenergic neurone blockers:

Anafranil may diminish or abolish the antihypertensive effects of guanethidine, betanidine, reserpine, clonidine and alpha-methyldopa. Patients requiring comedication for hypertension should therefore be given antihypertensives of a different type (e.g. vasodilators, or beta-blockers).

Sympathomimetic drugs:

Anafranil may potentiate the cardiovascular effects of adrenaline, ephedrine, isoprenaline, noradrenaline, phenylephrine, and phenylpropanolamine (e.g. as contained in local and general anaesthetic preparations and nasal decongestants).

Quinidine:

Tricyclic antidepressants should not be employed in combination with antiarrhythmic agents of the quinidine type.

Liver-enzyme inducers:

Drugs which activate the hepatic mono-oxygenase enzyme system (e.g. barbiturates, carbamazepine, phenytoin, nicotine and oral contraceptives) may accelerate the metabolism and lower the plasma concentrations of clomipramine, resulting in decreased efficacy. Plasma levels of phenytoin and carbamazepine may increase, with corresponding adverse effects. It may be necessary to adjust the dosage of these drugs.

Diuretics:

Diuretics may lead to hypokalemia, which increases the risk of QTc prolongation and Torsade de Pointes, Hypokalaemia should therefore be treated prior to administration of Anafranil. (see 4.2 Posology and 4.4 Special warnings and precautions).

Drugs that can cause increase plasma clomipramine levels or which in themselves prolong the QTc interval:

The risk of QTc prolongation and Torsade de Pointes is likely to be increased if Anafranil is co-administered with other drugs that can cause QTc prolongation. Therefore concomitant use of such agents with Anafranil is not recommended. (see 4.4 Special warnings and precautions). Examples include certain anti-arrhythmics, such as those of Class 1A (such as quinidine, disopyramide and procainamide) and Class III (such as amiodarone and sotalol), tricyclic antidepressants (such as amitriptyline); certain tetracyclic antidepressants (such as maprotiline); certain antipsychotic medications (such as phenothiazines and pimozide); certain antihistamines (such as terfenadine); lithium, quinine and pentamidine. This list is not exhaustive. The risk of QTc prolongation and Torsade de Pointes is likely to be increased if Anafranil is co-administered with drugs that can cause increased plasma clomipramine levels. Anafranil is metabolised by cytochrome P450 2D6 and the plasma concentration of Anafranil may therefore be increased by drugs that are either substrates and/or inhibitors of this P450 isoform. Therefore, concurrent use of these drugs with Anafranil is not recommended (section section 4.4 Special warnings). Examples of drugs which are substrates or inhibitors of cytochrome P450 2D6 include anti-arrhythmics, certain antidepressants including SSRIs, tricyclic antidepressants and moclobemide; certain antipsychotics; β-blockers; protease inhibitors, opiates, ecstasy (MDMA) and cimetidine. This list is not exhaustive.

Methylphenidate and Oestrogens:

these drugs may also increase plasma concentrations of tricyclic antidepressants, whose dosage should therefore be reduced.

4.6 Pregnancy and lactation

There is inadequate evidence of safety of Anafranil in human pregnancy. Do not use, especially during the first and last trimesters unless there are compelling reasons. Animal work has not shown clomipramine to be free from hazard.

Neonates whose mothers had taken tricyclic antidepressants up till delivery have developed dyspnoea, lethargy, colic, irritability, hypotension or hypertension, tremor or spasms, during the first few hours or days. Anafranil should - if this is at all justifiable - be withdrawn at least 7 weeks before the calculated date of confinement.

The active substance of Anafranil passes into the breast milk in small quantities. Therefore nursing mothers should be advised to withdraw the medication or cease breastfeeding.

4.7 Effects on ability to drive and use machines

Patients receiving Anafranil should be warned that blurred vision, drowsiness and other CNS symptoms (see Undesirable Effects) may occur, in which case they should not drive, operate machinery or do anything else which may require alertness or quick actions. Patients should also be warned that alcohol or other drugs may potentiate these effects (see Interactions).

4.8 Undesirable effects

Unwanted effects are usually mild and transient, disappearing under continued treatment or with a reduction in the dosage. They do not always correlate with plasma drug levels or dose. It is often difficult to distinguish certain undesirable effects from symptoms of depression such as fatigue, sleep disturbances, agitation, anxiety, constipation, and dry mouth.

If severe neurological or psychiatric reactions occur, Anafranil should be withdrawn.

Elderly patients are particularly sensitive to anticholinergic, neurological, psychiatric, or cardiovascular effects. Their ability to metabolise and eliminate drugs may be reduced, leading to a risk of elevated plasma concentrations at therapeutic doses.

The following side-effects, although not necessarily observed with Anafranil, have occurred with tricyclic antidepressants.

Frequency estimates: Very common $\geqslant$ 10%, Common $\geqslant$ 1% to $<$ 10%, Uncommon $\geqslant$ 0.1 to $<$ 1%, Rare $<$ 0.01% to $<$ 0.1%, Very rare $<$ 0.01%.

Anticholinergic effects:

Very common: dryness of the mouth, sweating, constipation, disorders of visual accommodation and blurred vision, disturbances of micturition.

Common: hot flushes, mydriasis.

Very rare: glaucoma.

Central nervous system

Psychiatric effects:

Very common: drowsiness, transient fatigue, feelings of unrest, increased appetite.

Common: confusion accompanied by disorientation and hallucinations (particularly in geriatric patients and patients suffering from Parkinson's disease), anxiety states, agitation, sleep disturbances, mania, hypomania, aggressiveness, impaired memory, yawning, depersonalisation, insomnia, nightmares, aggravated depression, impaired concentration.

Uncommon: activation of psychotic symptoms.

Neurological effects:

Very common: dizziness, tremor, headache, myoclonus.

Common: delirium, speech disorders, paraesthesia, muscle weakness, muscle hypertonia.

Uncommon: convulsions, ataxia.

Very rare: EEG changes, hyperpyrexia.

Cardiovascular system:

Common: postural hypotension, sinus tachycardia, and clinically irrelevant ECG changes in patients of normal cardiac status (e.g. T and ST changes), palpitations.

Uncommon: arrhythmias, increased blood pressure.

Very rare: conduction disorders (e.g. widening of QRS complex, prolonged QTc interval, PQ changes, bundle-branch block), Torsade de Pointes, particularly in patients with hypokalemia).

Gastro-intestinal tract:

Very common: nausea.

Common: vomiting, abdominal disorders, diarrhoea, anorexia.

Hepatic effects:

Common: elevated transaminases.

Very rare: hepatitis with or without jaundice.

Skin:

Common: allergic skin reactions (skin rash, urticaria), photosensitivity, pruritus.

Very rare: local reactions after intravenous injections (thrombophlebitis, lymphangitis, burning sensation, and allergic skin reactions), oedema (local or generalised), hair loss.

Endocrine system and metabolism:

Very common: weight gain, disturbances of libido and potency.

Common: galactorrhoea, breast enlargement.

Very rare: SIADH (inappropriate antidiuretic hormone secretion syndrome).

Hypersensitivity:

Very rare: allergic alveolitis (pneumonitis) with or without eosinophilia, systemic anaphylactic/anaphylactoid reactions including hypotension.

Blood:

Very rare: leucopenia, agranulocytosis, thrombocytopenia, eosinophilia, and purpura.

Sense organs:

Common: taste disturbances, tinnitus.

Others:

The following symptoms commonly occur after abrupt withdrawal or reduction of the dose: nausea, vomiting, abdominal pain, diarrhoea, insomnia, headache, nervousness and anxiety.

4.9 Overdose

The signs and symptoms of overdose with Anafranil are similar to those reported with other tricyclic antidepressants. Cardiac abnormalities and neurological disturbances are the main complications. In children accidental ingestion of any amount should be regarded as serious and potentially fatal.

Signs and symptoms:

Symptoms generally appear within 4 hours of ingestion and reach maximum severity after 24 hours. Owing to delayed absorption (anticholinergic effect), long half-life, and enterohepatic recycling of the drug, the patient may be at risk for up to 4-6 days.

The following signs and symptoms may be seen:

Central nervous system:

Drowsiness, stupor, coma, ataxia, restlessness, agitation, enhanced reflexes, muscular rigidity, choreoathetoid movements, convulsions, Serotonin Syndrome (e.g. hypertensive crisis, hyperpyrexia, myoclonus, delirium and coma) may be observed.

Cardiovascular system:

Hypotension, tachycardia,, QTc prolongation and arrhythmia including Torsade de Pointes, conduction disorders, shock, heart failure; in very rare cases cardiac arrest.

Respiratory depression, cyanosis, vomiting, fever, mydriasis, sweating and oliguria or anuria may also occur.

Treatment

There is no specific antidote, and treatment is essentially symptomatic and supportive.

Anyone suspected of receiving an overdose of Anafranil, particularly children, should be hospitalised and kept under close surveillance for at least 72 hours.

Perform gastric lavage or induce vomiting as soon as possible if the patient is alert. If the patient has impaired consciousness, secure the airway with a cuffed endotracheal tube before beginning lavage, and do not induce vomiting. These measures are recommended for up to 12 hours or even longer after the overdose, since the anticholinergic effect of the drug may delay gastric emptying. Administration of activated charcoal may help to reduce drug absorption.

Treatment of symptoms is based on modern methods of intensive care, with continuous monitoring of cardiac function, blood gases, and electrolytes and, if necessary, emergency measures such as:

- anticonvulsive therapy
- artificial respiration,

- insertion of a temporary cardiac pacemaker,
- plasma expander, dopamine or dobutamine administered by intravenous drip,
- resuscitation.

Treatment of Torsade de Pointes:

If Torsade de Pointes should occur during treatment with Anafranil, the drug should be discontinued and hypoxia, electrolyte abnormalities and acid base disturbances should be corrected. Persistent Torsade de Pointes may be treated with magnesium sulphate 2g (20ml of 10% solution) intravenously over 30-120 seconds, repeated twice at intervals of 5-15 minutes if necessary. Alternatively, if these measures fail, the arrhythmia may be abolished by increasing the underlying heart rate. This can be achieved by atrial and ventricular pacing or by isoprenaline (isproterenol) infusion to achieve a heart rate of 90-110 beats/minute. Torsade de Pointes is usually not helped by antiarrhythmic drugs and those which prolong the QTc interval (e.g. amiodarone, quinidine) may make it worse.

Since it has been reported that physostigmine may cause severe bradycardia, asystole and seizures, its use is not recommended in cases of overdosage with Anafranil. Haemodialysis or peritoneal dialysis are ineffective because of the low plasma concentrations of clomipramine.

5. PHARMACOLOGICAL PROPERTIES

5.1 Pharmacodynamic properties

Clomipramine is a tricyclic antidepressant and its pharmacological action includes alpha-adrenolytic, anticholinergic, anti-histaminic, and 5-HT receptor blocking properties. The therapeutic activity of Anafranil is thought to be based on its ability to inhibit the neuronal re-uptake of noradrenaline and 5-HT. Inhibition of the latter is the dominant component.

5.2 Pharmacokinetic properties

Absorption:

The active substance is completely absorbed following oral administration and intramuscular injection.

The systemic bioavailability of unchanged clomipramine is reduced by 50% by "first-pass" metabolism to desmethylclomipramine (an active metabolite). The bioavailability of clomipramine is not markedly affected by the ingestion of food but the onset of absorption and therefore the time to peak may be delayed. Coated tablets and sustained release tablets are bioequivalent with respect to amount absorbed.

During oral administration of constant daily doses of Anafranil the steady state plasma concentration of clomipramine and desmethylclomipramine (active metabolite) and the ratio between these concentrations show a high variability between patients e.g. 75mg Anafranil daily produced steady state concentrations of clomipramine ranging from about 20 to 175ng/ml. Levels of desmethylclomipramine follow a similar pattern but are 40-85% higher.

Distribution:

Clomipramine is 97.6% bound to plasma proteins. The apparent volume of distribution is about 12-17 L/kg of bodyweight. Concentrations in cerebrospinal fluid are about 2% of the plasma concentration.

Biotransformation:

The major route of transformation of clomipramine is demethylation to the desmethylclomipramine. In addition, clomipramine and desmethylclomipramine are hydroxylated to 8-hydroxy-clomipramine and 8-hydroxy-desmethylclomipramine but little is known about their activity *in vivo*. The hydroxylation of clomipramine and desmethylclomipramine is under genetic control similar to that of debrisoquine. In poor metabolisers of debrisoquine this may lead to high concentrations of desmethylclomipramine, concentrations of clomipramine are less significantly influenced.

Elimination:

Clomipramine is eliminated from the blood with a mean half-life of 21 hours (range 12-36h), and desmethylclomipramine with a half-life of 36 hours.

About two thirds of a single dose of clomipramine is excreted in the form of water-soluble conjugates in the urine, and approximately one third in the faeces. The quantity of unchanged clomipramine and desmethylclomipramine excreted in the urine amounts to about 2% and 0.5% of the administered dose respectively.

Characteristics in patients:

In elderly patients, plasma clomipramine concentrations may be higher for a given dose than would be expected in younger patients because of reduced metabolic clearance.

The effects of hepatic and renal impairment on the pharmacokinetics of clomipramine have not been determined.

5.3 Preclinical safety data

None stated.

6. PHARMACEUTICAL PARTICULARS

6.1 List of excipients

Colloidal silicon dioxide (Aerosil 200), calcium hydrogen phosphate, Eudrogit E 30D (dry substance), calcium stearate. The coating constituents are hydroxypropylmethylcellulose 3CPS (2910), red iron oxide (E172), polyethoxylated castor oil (cremophor RH40), purified talc special, titanium dioxide (E171) and purified water.

6.2 Incompatibilities

None.

6.3 Shelf life

60 months.

6.4 Special precautions for storage

Protect from moisture.

6.5 Nature and contents of container

The tablets are dull greyish-red film coated, round, slightly convex with bevelled edges, imprinted "Geigy" on one face and GD on the other, and come in PVC blister packs of 28 tablets.

6.6 Instructions for use and handling

None.

7. MARKETING AUTHORISATION HOLDER

Novartis Pharmaceuticals UK Limited
trading as Geigy Pharmaceuticals
Frimley Business Park
Frimley
Camberley
Surrey
GU16 7SR

8. MARKETING AUTHORISATION NUMBER(S)

PL 00101/0436

9. DATE OF FIRST AUTHORISATION/RENEWAL OF THE AUTHORISATION

04 July 1997 / 28 October 1999

10. DATE OF REVISION OF THE TEXT

19 July 2004

Legal Category: POM

Anafranil Capsules

(Cephalon UK Limited)

1. NAME OF THE MEDICINAL PRODUCT

Anafranil® Capsules 10mg, 25mg and 50mg.

2. QUALITATIVE AND QUANTITATIVE COMPOSITION

Chemical name: 3-chloro-5-[3-(dimethylamino)-propyl] 10, 11- dihydro-5H-dibenz [b,f] azepine hydrochloride (= clomipramine hydrochloric).

Each capsule contains 10mg, 25mg or 50mg clomipramine hydrochloride B.P.

3. PHARMACEUTICAL FORM

Capsule

4. CLINICAL PARTICULARS

4.1 Therapeutic indications

Symptoms of depressive illness especially where sedation is required. Obsessional and phobic states. Adjunctive treatment of cataplexy associated with narcolepsy.

4.2 Posology and method of administration

Before initiating treatment with Anafranil, hypokalemia should be treated (see 4.4. Special warnings and precautions for use).

As a precaution against possible serotonergic toxicity, adherence to the recommended doses of Anafranil is advised and any increase in dose should be made with caution if other serotonergic agents are co-administered (see 4.4 Special warnings and precautions for use).

Adults:

Oral - 10mg/day initially, increasing gradually to 30-150mg/day, if required, in divided doses throughout the day or as a single dose at bedtime. Many patients will be adequately maintained on 30-50mg/day. Higher doses may be needed in some patients, particularly those suffering from obsessional or phobic disorders. In severe cases this dosage can be increased up to a maximum of 250mg per day. Once a distinct improvement has set in, the daily dosage may be adjusted to a maintenance level averaging either 2-4 capsules of 25mg or 1 tablet of 75mg.

Elderly:

The initial dose should be 10mg/day, which may be increased with caution under close supervision to an optimum level of 30-75mg daily which should be reached after about 10 days and then maintained until the end of treatment.

Children:

Not recommended.

Obsessional/phobic states:

The maintenance dosage of Anafranil is generally higher than that used in depression. It is recommended that the dose be built up to 100-150mg Anafranil daily, according to the severity of the condition. This should be attained gradually over a period of 2 weeks starting with 1 × 25mg Anafranil daily. In elderly patients and those sensitive to tricyclic antidepressants a starting dose of 1 × 10mg Anafranil daily is recommended. Again where a higher dosage is required the SR 75mg formulation may be preferable.

Adjunctive treatment of cataplexy associated with narcolepsy:

(Oral treatment): 10-75mg daily. It is suggested that treatment is commenced with 10mg Anafranil daily and gradually increased until a satisfactory response occurs. Control of cataplexy should be achieved within 24 hours of reaching the optimal dose. Where necessary, therapy may be combined with capsules and syrup up to the maximum dose of 75mg per day.

Route of Administration:

Oral

4.3 Contraindications

Known hypersensitivity to clomipramine, or any of the excipients or cross-sensitivity to tricyclic antidepressants of the dibenzazepine group. Recent myocardial infarction. Any degree of heart block or other cardiac arrhythmias. Mania, severe liver disease, narrow angle glaucoma. Retention of urine. Anafranil should not be given in combination or within 3 weeks before or after treatment with a MAO inhibitor (see Drug Interactions). The concomitant treatment with selective, reversible MAO-A inhibitors, such as moclobamide, is also contra-indicated.

4.4 Special warnings and special precautions for use

As improvement in depression may not occur for the first two to four weeks treatment, patients should be closely monitored during this period.

Tricyclic antidepressants are known to lower the convulsion threshold and Anafranil should therefore be used with extreme caution in patients with epilepsy and other predisposing factors, e.g. brain damage of varying aetiology, concomitant use of neuroleptics, withdrawal from alcohol or drugs with anticonvulsive properties (e.g. benzodiazepines). It appears that the occurrence of seizures is dose dependent, therefore the recommended total daily dose of Anafranil should not be exceeded.

Caution is called for when giving tricyclic antidepressants to patients with tumours of the adrenal medulla (e.g. phaeochromocytoma, neuroblastoma), in whom they may provoke hypertensive crises.

Concomitant treatment of Anafranil and electroconvulsive therapy should only be resorted to under careful supervision.

Elderly patients are particularly liable to experience adverse effects, especially agitation, confusion, and postural hypotension.

Many patients with panic disorders experience intensified anxiety symptoms at the start of the treatment with antidepressants. This paradoxical initial increase in anxiety is most pronounced during the first few days of treatment and generally subsides within two weeks.

Precautions:

Before initiating treatment it is advisable to check the patient's blood pressure, because individuals with hypotension or a labile circulation may react to the drug with a fall in blood pressure.

Although changes in the white blood cell count have been reported with Anafranil only in isolated cases, periodic blood cell counts and monitoring for symptoms such as fever and sore throat are called for, particularly during the first few months of therapy. They are also recommended during prolonged therapy.

It is advisable to monitor cardiac and hepatic function during long-term therapy with Anafranil. In patients with liver disease, periodic monitoring of hepatic enzyme levels is recommended.

There may be a risk of QTc prolongation and Torsade de Pointes, particularly at supra-therapeutic doses or supra-therapeutic plasma concentrations of clomipramine, as occur in the case of co-medication with selective serotonin reuptake inhibitors (SSRIs). Therefore, concomitant administration of drugs that can cause accumulation of clomipramine should be avoided. Equally, concomitant administration of drugs that can prolong the QTc interval should be avoided. (see 4.5 Interactions with other medicinal products and other forms of interaction). It is established that hypokalemia is a risk-factor of QTc prolongation and Torsade de Pointes. Therefore, hypokalemia should be treated before initiating treatment with Anafranil and Anafranil should be used with caution when combined with SSRIs or diuretics (see 4.5. Interactions with other medicinal products and other forms of interaction.)Caution is indicated in patients with hyperthyroidism or during concomitant treatment with thyroid preparations since aggravation of unwanted cardiac effects may occur.

Because of its anticholinergic properties, Anafranil should be used with caution in patients with a history of increased intra-ocular pressure, narrow angle glaucoma or urinary retention (e.g. diseases of the prostate).

An increase in dental caries has been reported during long-term treatment with tricyclic antidepressants. Regular dental check-ups are therefore advisable during long-term treatment.

Caution is called for in patients with chronic constipation. Tricyclic antidepressants may cause paralytic ileus, particularly in the elderly and in bedridden patients.

Decreased lacrimation and accumulation of mucoid secretions due to the anticholinergic properties of tricyclic antidepressants may cause damage to the corneal epithelium in patients with contact lenses.

Risk of suicide is inherent to severe depression and may persist until significant remission occurs. Patients posing a high suicide risk require close initial supervision.

Activation of psychosis has occasionally been observed in schizophrenic patients receiving tricyclic antidepressants. Hypomanic or manic episodes have also been reported during a depressive phase in patients with cyclic affective disorders receiving treatment with a tricyclic antidepressant. In such cases it may be necessary to reduce the dosage of Anafranil or to withdraw it and administer an antipsychotic agent. After such episodes have subsided, low dose therapy with Anafranil may be resumed if required.

Anafranil may cause anxiety, feelings of unrest, and hyperexcitation in agitated patients and patients with accompanying schizophrenic symptoms.

In predisposed and elderly patients, Anafranil may, particularly at night, provoke pharmacogenic (delirious) psychoses, which disappear without treatment within a few days of withdrawing the drug.

Before general or local anaesthesia, the anaesthetist should be aware that the patient has been receiving Anafranil and of the possible interactions (see 4.5 Interactions with other medicinal products and other forms of interaction).

As a precaution against possible serotonergic toxicity, adherence to the recommended doses of Anafranil is advised and any increase in dose should be made with caution if other serotonergic agents are co-administered.

Abrupt withdrawal should be avoided because of possible adverse reactions (see 4.8 Undesirable Effects).

4.5 Interaction with other medicinal products and other forms of Interaction

MAO inhibitors:

Do not give Anafranil for at least 3 weeks after discontinuation of treatment with MAO inhibitors (there is a risk of severe symptoms consistent with Serotonin Syndrome such as hypertensive crisis, hyperpyrexia, myoclonus, agitation, seizures, delirium and coma). The same applies when giving a MAO inhibitor after previous treatment with Anafranil. In both instances the treatment should initially be given in small gradually increasing doses and its effects monitored. There is evidence to suggest that Anafranil may be given as little as 24 hours after a reversible MAO-A inhibitor such as moclobemide, but the 3 week wash-out period must be observed if the MAO-A inhibitor is used after Anafranil.

Serotonergic Agents:

Serotonin Syndrome can possibly occur when Anafranil is administered with other serotonergic co-medications such as selective serotonin reuptake inhibitors, tricyclic antidepressants and lithium. For fluoxetine a washout period of two to three weeks is advised before and after treatment with fluoxetine.

CNS depressants:

Tricyclic antidepressants may potentiate the effects of alcohol and other central depressant substances (e.g. barbiturates, benzodiazepines, or general anaesthetics).

Neuroleptics:

Comedication may result in increased plasma levels of tricyclic antidepressants, a lowered convulsion threshold, and seizures. Combination with thioridazine may produce severe cardiac arrhythmias.

Anticoagulants:

Tricyclic antidepressants may potentiate the anticoagulant effect of coumarin drugs by inhibiting their metabolism by the liver. Careful monitoring of plasma prothrombin is therefore advised.

Anticholinergic agents:

Tricyclic antidepressants may potentiate the effects of these drugs(e.g. phenothiazine, antiparkinsonian agents, antihistamines, atropine, biperiden) on the eye, central nervous system, bowel and bladder.

Adrenergic neurone blockers:

Anafranil may diminish or abolish the antihypertensive effects of guanethidine, betanidine, reserpine, clonidine and alpha-methyldopa. Patients requiring comedication for hypertension should therefore be given antihypertensives of a different type (e.g. vasodilators, or beta-blockers).

Sympathomimetic drugs:

Anafranil may potentiate the cardiovascular effects of adrenaline, ephedrine, isoprenaline, noradrenaline, phenylephrine, and phenylpropanolamine (e.g. as contained in local and general anaesthetic preparations and nasal decongestants).

Quinidine:

Tricyclic antidepressants should not be employed in combination with antiarrhythmic agents of the quinidine type.

Liver-enzyme inducers:

Drugs which activate the hepatic mono-oxygenase enzyme system (e.g. barbiturates, carbamazepine, phenytoin, nicotine and oral contraceptives) may accelerate the metabolism and lower the plasma concentrations of clomipramine, resulting in decreased efficacy. Plasma levels of phenytoin and carbamazepine may increase, with corresponding adverse effects. It may be necessary to adjust the dosage of these drugs.

Diuretics:

Diuretics may lead to hypokalemia, which increases the risk of QTc prolongation and Torsade de Pointes. Hypokalaemia should therefore be treated prior to administration of Anafranil. (see 4.2 Posology and 4.4 Special warnings and precautions).

Drugs that can cause increase plasma clomipramine levels or which in themselves prolong the QTc interval:

The risk of QTc prolongation and Torsade de Pointes is likely to be increased if Anafranil is co-administered with other drugs that can cause QTc prolongation. Therefore concomitant use of such agents with Anafranil is not recommended. (see 4.4 Special warnings and precautions). Examples include certain anti-arrhythmics, such as those of Class 1A (such as quinidine, disopyramide and procainamide) and Class III (such as amiodarone and sotalol), tricyclic antidepressants (such as amitriptyline); certain tetracyclic antidepressants (such as maprotiline); certain antipsychotic medications (such as phenothiazines and pimozide); certain antihistamines (such as terfenadine); lithium, quinine and pentamidine. This list is not exhaustive. The risk of QTc prolongation and Torsade de Pointes is likely to be increased if Anafranil is co-administered with drugs that can cause increased plasma clomipramine levels. Anafranil is metabolised by cytochrome P450 2D6 and the plasma concentration of Anafranil may therefore be increased by drugs that are either substrates and/or inhibitors of this P450 isoform. Therefore, concurrent use of these drugs with Anafranil is not recommended (section section 4.4 Special warnings). Examples of drugs which are substrates or inhibitors of cytochrome P450 2D6 include anti-arrhythmics, certain antidepressants including SSRIs, tricyclic antidepressants and moclobemide; certain antipsychotics; β-blockers; protease inhibitors, opiates, ecstasy (MDMA) and cimetidine. This list is not exhaustive.

Methylphenidate and Oestrogens:

These drugs may also increase plasma concentrations of tricyclic antidepressants, whose dosage should therefore be reduced.

4.6 Pregnancy and lactation

There is inadequate evidence of safety of Anafranil in human pregnancy. Do not use unless there are compelling reasons, especially during the first and last trimesters. Animal work has not shown clomipramine to be free from hazard.

Neonates whose mothers had taken tricyclic antidepressants up until delivery have developed dyspnoea, lethargy, colic, irritability, hypotension or hypertension, tremor or spasms, during the first few hours or days. Anafranil should - if this is at all justifiable - be withdrawn at least 7 weeks before the calculated date of confinement.

The active substance of Anafranil passes into the breast milk in small quantities. Therefore nursing mothers should be advised to withdraw the medication or cease breast-feeding.

4.7 Effects on ability to drive and use machines

Patients receiving Anafranil should be warned that blurred vision, drowsiness and other CNS symptoms (see Undesirable Effects) may occur in which case they should not drive, operate machinery or do anything else which may require alertness or quick actions. Patients should also be warned that consumption of alcohol or other drugs may potentiate these effects (see Drug Interactions).

4.8 Undesirable effects

Unwanted effects are usually mild and transient, disappearing under continued treatment or with a reduction in the dosage. They do not always correlate with plasma drug levels or dose. It is often difficult to distinguish certain undesirable effects from symptoms of depression such as fatigue, sleep disturbances, agitation, anxiety, constipation, and dry mouth.

If severe neurological or psychiatric reactions occur, Anafranil should be withdrawn.

Elderly patients are particularly sensitive to anticholinergic, neurological, psychiatric, or cardiovascular effects. Their ability to metabolise and eliminate drugs may be reduced, leading to a risk of elevated plasma concentrations at therapeutic doses.

The following side-effects, although not necessarily observed with Anafranil, have occurred with tricyclic antidepressants.

Frequency estimates: Very common $\geqslant$ 10%, Common $\geqslant$ 1% to $<$ 10%, Uncommon $\geqslant$ 0.1 to $<$ 1%, Rare $<$ 0.01% to $<$ 0.1%, Very rare $<$ 0.01%.

Anticholinergic effects

Very common: dryness of the mouth, sweating, constipation, disorders of visual accommodation and blurred vision, disturbances of micturition.

Common: hot flushes, mydriasis.

Very rare: glaucoma.

Central nervous system

Psychiatric effects:

Very common: drowsiness, transient fatigue, feelings of unrest, increased appetite.

Common: confusion accompanied by disorientation and hallucinations (particularly in geriatric patients and patients suffering from Parkinson's disease), anxiety states, agitation, sleep disturbances, mania, hypomania, aggressiveness, impaired memory, yawning, depersonalisation, insomnia, nightmares, aggravated depression, impaired concentration.

Uncommon: activation of psychotic symptoms.

Neurological effects

Very common: dizziness, tremor, headache, myoclonus.

Common: delirium, speech disorders, paraesthesia, muscle weakness, muscle hypertonia.

Uncommon: convulsions, ataxia.

Very rare: EEG changes, hyperpyrexia.

Cardiovascular system

Common: postural hypotension, sinus tachycardia, and clinically irrelevant ECG changes in patients of normal cardiac status (e.g. T and ST changes), palpitations.

Uncommon: arrhythmias, increased blood pressure.

Very rare: conduction disorders (e.g. widening of QRS complex, prolonged QTc interval, PQ changes, bundle-branch block), Torsade de Pointes, particularly in patients with hypokalemia).

Gastro-intestinal tract

Very common: nausea.

Common: vomiting, abdominal disorders, diarrhoea, anorexia.

Hepatic effects

Common: elevated transaminases.

Very rare: hepatitis with or without jaundice.

Skin

Common: allergic skin reactions (skin rash, urticaria), photosensitivity, pruritus.

Very rare: local reactions after intravenous injections (thrombophlebitis, lymphangitis, burning sensation, and allergic skin reactions), oedema (local or generalised), hair loss.

Endocrine system and metabolism

Very common: weight gain, disturbances of libido and potency.

Common: galactorrhoea, breast enlargement.

Very rare: SIADH (inappropriate antidiuretic hormone secretion syndrome).

Hypersensitivity

Very rare: allergic alveolitis (pneumonitis) with or without eosinophilia, systemic anaphylactic/anaphylactoid reactions including hypotension.

Blood:

Very rare: leucopenia, agranulocytosis, thrombocytopenia, eosinophilia, and purpura.

Sense organs

Common: taste disturbances, tinnitus.

Others

The following symptoms commonly occur after abrupt withdrawal or reduction of the dose: nausea, vomiting, abdominal pain, diarrhoea, insomnia, headache, nervousness and anxiety.

4.9 Overdose

The signs and symptoms of overdose with Anafranil are similar to those reported with other tricyclic antidepressants. Cardiac abnormalities and neurological disturbances are the main complications. In children accidental ingestion of any amount should be regarded as serious and potentially fatal.

Signs and symptoms

Symptoms generally appear within 4 hours of ingestion and reach maximum severity after 24 hours. Owing to delayed absorption (anticholinergic effect), long half-life, and enterohepatic recycling of the drug, the patient may be at risk for up to 4-6 days.

The following signs and symptoms may be seen:

Central nervous system:

Drowsiness, stupor, coma, ataxia, restlessness, agitation, enhanced reflexes, muscular rigidity, choreoathetoid movements, convulsions, Serotonin Syndrome (e.g. hypertensive crisis, hyperpyrexia, myoclonus, delirium and coma) may be observed.

Cardiovascular system:

Hypotension, tachycardia,, QTc prolongation and arrhythmia including Torsade de Pointes, conduction disorders, shock, heart failure; in very rare cases cardiac arrest.

Respiratory depression, cyanosis, vomiting, fever, mydriasis, sweating and oliguria or anuria may also occur.

Treatment

There is no specific antidote, and treatment is essentially symptomatic and supportive.

Anyone suspected of receiving an overdose of Anafranil, particularly children, should be hospitalised and kept under close surveillance for at least 72 hours.

Perform gastric lavage or induce vomiting as soon as possible if the patient is alert. If the patient has impaired consciousness, secure the airway with a cuffed endotracheal tube before beginning lavage, and do not induce vomiting. These measures are recommended for up to 12 hours or even longer after the overdose, since the anticholinergic effect of the drug may delay gastric emptying. Administration of activated charcoal may help to reduce drug absorption.

Treatment of symptoms is based on modern methods of intensive care, with continuous monitoring of cardiac function, blood gases, and electrolytes and, if necessary, emergency measures such as:

- anticonvulsive therapy
- artificial respiration,
- insertion of a temporary cardiac pacemaker,
- plasma expander, dopamine or dobutamine administered by intravenous drip,
- resuscitation.

Treatment of Torsade de Pointes:

If Torsade de Pointes should occur during treatment with Anafranil, the drug should be discontinued and hypoxia, electrolyte abnormalities and acid base disturbances should be corrected. Persistent Torsade de Pointes may be treated with magnesium sulphate 2g (20ml of 10% solution) intravenvenously over 30-120 seconds, repeated twice at intervals of 5-15 minutes if necessary. Alternatively, if these measures fail, the arrhythmia may be abolished by increasing the underlying heart rate. This can be achieved by atrial and ventricular pacing or by isoprenaline (isproterenol) infusion to achieve a heart rate of 90-110 beats/minute. Torsade de Pointes is usually not helped by antiarrhythmic drugs and those which prolong the QTc interval (e.g. amiodarone, quinidine) may make it worse.

Since it has been reported that physostigmine may cause severe bradycardia, asystole and seizures, its use is not recommended in cases of overdosage with Anafranil. Haemodialysis or peritoneal dialysis are ineffective because of the low plasma concentrations of clomipramine.

5. PHARMACOLOGICAL PROPERTIES

5.1 Pharmacodynamic properties

Clomipramine is a tricyclic antidepressant and its pharmacological action includes alpha-adrenolytic, anticholinergic, anti-histaminic and 5-HT receptor blocking properties. The therapeutic activity of Anafranil is thought to be based on its ability to inhibit the neuronal re-uptake of noradrenaline and 5-HT. Inhibition of the latter is the dominant component.

5.2 Pharmacokinetic properties

Absorption:

The active substance is completely absorbed following oral administration and intramuscular injection.

The systemic bioavailability of unchanged clomipramine is reduced by 50% by "first-pass" metabolism to desmethylclomipramine (an active metabolite). The bioavailability of clomipramine is not markedly affected by the ingestion of food but the onset of absorption and therefore the time to peak may be delayed. Coated tablets and sustained release tablets are bioequivalent with respect to amount absorbed.

During oral administration of constant daily doses of Anafranil the steady state plasma concentrations of clomipramine and desmethylclomipramine (active metabolite) and the ratio between these concentrations show a high variability between patients, e.g. 75mg Anafranil daily produces steady state concentrations of clomipramine ranging from about 20 to 175ng/ml. Levels of desmethylclomipramine follow a similar pattern but are 40-85% higher.

Distribution:

Clomipramine is 97.6% bound to plasma proteins. The apparent volume of distribution is about 12-17 L/kg bodyweight. Concentrations in cerebrospinal fluid are about 2% of the plasma concentration.

Biotransformation:

The major route of transformation of clomipramine is demethylation to desmethylclomipramine. In addition, clomipramine and desmethylclomipramine are hydroxylated to 8-hydroxy-clomipramine and 8-hydroxy-desmethylclomipramine but little is known about their activity *in vivo*. The hydroxylation of clomipramine and desmethylclomipramine is under genetic control similar to that of debrisoquine. In poor metabolisers of debrisoquine this may lead to high concentrations of desmethylclomipramine; concentrations of clomipramine are less significantly influenced.

Elimination:

Oral clomipramine is eliminated from the blood with a mean half-life of 21 hours (range 12-36 h), and desmethylclomipramine with a half-life of 36 hours.

About two-thirds of a single dose of clomipramine is excreted in the form of water-soluble conjugates in the urine, and approximately one-third in the faeces. The quantity of unchanged clomipramine and desmethylclomipramine excreted in the urine amounts to about 2% and 0.5% of the administered dose respectively.

Characteristics in patients:

In elderly patients, plasma clomipramine concentrations may be higher for a given dose than would be expected in younger patients because of reduced metabolic clearance.

The effects of hepatic and renal impairment on the pharmacokinetics of clomipramine have not been determined.

5.3 Preclinical safety data

None stated

6. PHARMACEUTICAL PARTICULARS

6.1 List of excipients

Lactose, gelatin and magnesium stearate, yellow iron oxide (E172), black iron oxide (E172), red iron oxide (E172), titanium dioxide and brown printing ink.

6.2 Incompatibilities

None.

6.3 Shelf life

60 months

6.4 Special precautions for storage

Protect from moisture. Store below 30°C.

6.5 Nature and contents of container

The 10mg capsules are two tone brownish-caramel cap/greyish yellow body, hard gelatin size 4, imprinted 'Geigy' and come in PVC/aluminium blister packs in pack sizes of 84.

The 25mg capsules are two tone brownish-orange/caramel-coloured, hard gelatin size 4, imprinted 'Geigy' and come in PVC/aluminium blister packs in pack sizes of 84.

The 50mg capsules are two tone light grey/caramel-coloured, hard gelatin size 4, imprinted 'Geigy' and come in PVC/aluminium blister packs in pack sizes of 56.

6.6 Instructions for use and handling

None.

7. MARKETING AUTHORISATION HOLDER

Novartis Pharmaceuticals UK Limited

Trading as Geigy Pharmaceuticals

Frimley Business Park

Frimley

Camberley

Surrey

GU16 7SR

8. MARKETING AUTHORISATION NUMBER(S)

10mg: PL 00101/0438

25mg: PL 00101/0439

50mg: PL 00101/0440

9. DATE OF FIRST AUTHORISATION/RENEWAL OF THE AUTHORISATION

04 July 1997 / 28 October 1999

10. DATE OF REVISION OF THE TEXT

19 July 2004

Legal Category

POM

Anapen

(Celltech Pharmaceuticals Limited)

1. NAME OF THE MEDICINAL PRODUCT

Anapen 300 micrograms in 0.3ml solution for injection in a pre-filled syringe

2. QUALITATIVE AND QUANTITATIVE COMPOSITION

Each millilitre contains 1mg of adrenaline

One dose of 0.3ml contains 300 micrograms of adrenaline

3. PHARMACEUTICAL FORM

Solution for injection. Clear colourless solution practically free from particles.

4. CLINICAL PARTICULARS

4.1 Therapeutic indications

Emergency treatment for acute allergic reactions (anaphylaxis) caused by peanuts or other foods, drugs, insect bites or stings, and other allergens as well as exercise-induced or idiopathic anaphylaxis.

4.2 Posology and method of administration

Use only by the intramuscular route.

Anapen consists of a pre-filled syringe of adrenaline contained in an auto-injection device. The whole is referred to as an auto-injector.

One Anapen injection should be administered intramuscularly immediately on the appearance of the signs and symptoms of anaphylactic shock. These may occur within minutes of exposure to the allergen and are most commonly manifested by urticaria, flushing or angioedema; more severe reactions involve the circulatory and respiratory systems. Inject Anapen only into the anterolateral aspect of the thigh, not the buttock. The injected area may be lightly massaged for 10 seconds following injection.

The effective dose is typically in the range 0.005-0.01mg/kg but higher doses may be necessary in some cases.

Use in adults: The usual dose is 300 micrograms. Larger adults may require more than one injection to reverse the effect of an allergic reaction. In some circumstances a single dose of adrenaline may not completely reverse the effects of an acute allergic reaction and for such patients a repeat injection may be given after 10-15 minutes.

Use in children: The appropriate dose may be 150 micrograms (Anapen Junior) or 300 micrograms (Anapen) of adrenaline, depending on the body weight of the child and the discretion of the doctor. The auto-injector of Anapen Junior is designed to deliver a single dose of 150 micrograms epinephrine. A dosage below 150 micrograms cannot be administered in sufficient accuracy in children weighing less than 15 kg and use is therefore not recommended unless in a life-threatening situation and under medical advice.

A double syringe pack is available in certain markets.

Anapen auto-injector is intended for immediate self-administration by a person with a history of anaphylaxis and is designed to deliver a single dose of 300 micrograms (0.3ml) adrenaline. For stability reasons 0.75ml is left in the syringe after use but the unit cannot be used again and should be safely discarded.

4.3 Contraindications

Hypersensitivity to adrenaline or to any of the excipients

4.4 Special warnings and special precautions for use

All patients who are prescribed Anapen should be thoroughly instructed to understand the indications for use and the correct method of administration. Anapen is indicated as emergency supportive therapy only and patients should be advised to seek immediate medical attention following administration.

Use with caution in patients with heart disease e.g coronary heart and cardiac muscle diseases (angina may be induced), cor pulmonale, cardiac arrythmias or tachycardia. There is a risk of adverse reactions following adrenaline administration in patients with hyperthyroidism, cardiovascular disease (severe angina pectoris, obstructive cardiomyopathy and ventricular arrhythmia and hypertension), phaeochromocytoma, high intraocular pressure, severe renal impairment, prostatic adenoma leading to residual urine, hypercalcemia, hypokalemia, diabetes, or in elderly or pregnant patients. Also, Anapen contains sodium metabisulphite, which can cause allergic-type reactions including anaphylactic symptoms and bronchospasm in susceptible people, especially those with a history of asthma. Patients with these conditions must be carefully instructed in regard to the circumstances under which Anapen should be used.

Repeated local injection can result in necrosis at sites of injection from vascular constriction. Accidental intravascular injection may result in cerebral haemorrhage due to a sudden rise in blood pressure. Accidental injection into hands or feet may cause loss of blood flow to adjacent areas due to vasoconstriction.

4.5 Interaction with other medicinal products and other forms of Interaction

The effects of adrenaline may be potentiated by tricyclic antidepressants mixed noradrenargic-serotoninergic antidepressants like venlafaxine, sibutramine or milnacipran and monoamine oxidase inhibitors (sudden blood pressure increase and possible cardiac arrhythmia), COMT blocking agent, thyroid hormones, theophylline, oxytocin, parasympatholytics, certain antihistamines (diphenhydramine, chlorpheniramine), levodopa and alcohol.

Severe hypertension and bradykardia may occur when adrenaline is administered with non-selective beta-blocking medicinal products.

Concurrent therapy with sympathomimetics may potentiate the effects of adrenaline.

Use Anapen with caution in patients receiving medicinal products which may sensitise the heart to arrhythmias, e.g. digitalis, quinidine, halogenated anaesthetics.

The pressor effects of adrenaline may be counteracted by administration of rapidly acting vasodilators or alpha adrenergic blocking medicinal products. Anaphylactic effects can be antagonised by beta-blocking agents, especially non-selective beta-blockers.

Adrenaline inhibits insulin secretion and diabetic patients may require upward adjustment of their insulin or other hypoglycaemic therapy.

4.6 Pregnancy and lactation

There are no adequate or well-controlled studies of adrenaline in pregnant women. Adrenaline should only be used in pregnancy if the potential benefit justifies the potential risk to the foetus. Adrenaline may dramatically reduce placental blood flow, although anaphylactic shock will do this too. Adrenaline is not orally bioavailable; any adrenaline excreted in breast milk would not be expected to have any effect on the nursing infant.

4.7 Effects on ability to drive and use machines

It is not recommended that patients should drive or use machines following administration of adrenaline, since patients will be affected by symptoms of the anaphylactic shock.

4.8 Undesirable effects

The occurrence of undesirable effects depends on the sensitivity of the individual patient and the dose applied.

Common adverse reactions even at low doses due to adrenaline include palpitations, tachycardia, sweating, nausea, vomiting, respiratory difficulty, pallor, dizziness, weakness, tremor, headache, apprehension, nervousness, anxiety and coldness of extremities.

Less frequently reported effects include hallucinations, syncopes,, hyperglycaemia, hypokalaemia, metabolic acidosis, mydriasis, difficulty in micturition with urinary retention, muscle tremor.

Adverse reactions which occur at higher doses or in susceptible individuals are cardiac arrhythmias (ventricular fibrillation /cardiac arrest), sudden rise of blood pressure (sometimes leading to cerebral haemorrhage), as well as vasoconstriction (e.g. in the skin, mucous tissues and kidneys).

Anapen contains a sulphite that may cause allergic-type reactions including anaphylactic reactions or life- threatening or less severe asthmatic episodes in certain susceptible patients.

4.9 Overdose

Overdose or accidental intravascular injection of adrenaline may cause cerebral haemorrhage from a sudden rise of blood pressure. Death may result from acute pulmonary oedema arising from peripheral vascular constriction and cardiac stimulation.

The pressor effects of adrenaline may be counteracted by rapidly acting vasodilators or alpha-adrenergic blocking medicinal products. Should prolonged hypotension follow such measures, it may be necessary to administer another pressor medicinal product, such as noradrenaline.

Acute pulmonary oedema with respiratory embarrassment following adrenaline overdose should be managed by administration of a rapidly acting alpha-adrenergic blocking medicinal product such as phentolamine and/or with intermittent positive pressure respiration.

Adrenaline overdose may also result in transient bradycardia followed by tachycardia; these can be followed by potentially fatal cardiac arrhythmias, which may be treated by beta-adrenergic blocking medicinal products. These must be preceded or accompanied by an alpha-adrenergic blocker to control the alpha-mediated effects on the peripheral circulation.

5. PHARMACOLOGICAL PROPERTIES

5.1 Pharmacodynamic properties

Pharmacotherapeutic group: adrenergic and dopaminergic agents, adrenaline

ATC code: C01 CA 24.

Adrenaline is a naturally occurring catecholamine secreted by the adrenal medulla in response to exertion or stress. It is a sympathomimetic amine which is a potent stimulant of both alpha and beta adrenergic receptors and its effects on target organs are, therefore, complex. It is the medicinal product of choice to provide rapid relief of hypersensitivity reactions to allergies or to idiopathic or exercise induced anaphylaxis.

Adrenaline has a strong vasoconstrictor action through alpha adrenergic stimulation. This activity counteracts the vasodilatation and increased vascular permeability leading to loss of intravascular fluid and subsequent hypotension, which are the major pharmacotoxicological features in anaphylactic shock. Through its stimulation of bronchial beta adrenergic receptors, adrenaline has a powerful bronchodilator action which alleviates wheezing and dyspnoea. Adrenaline also alleviates pruritus, urticaria and angioedema associated with anaphylaxis.

5.2 Pharmacokinetic properties

Adrenaline is rapidly inactivated in the body, mostly in the liver by the enzymes COMT and MAO. Much of a dose of adrenaline is excreted as metabolites in urine. The plasma half-life is about 2-3 minutes. However, when given by subcutaneous or intramuscular injection, local vasoconstriction may delay absorption so that the effects may last longer than the half life suggests.

5.3 Preclinical safety data

Adrenaline has been widely used in the clinical management of allergic emergencies for many years. There are no pre-clinical data of relevance to the prescriber which are additional to that already included in other sections of the SPC.

6. PHARMACEUTICAL PARTICULARS

6.1 List of excipients

Sodium chloride,

Sodium metabisulphite (E223),

Hydrochloric acid

Water for injections.

6.2 Incompatibilities

Not applicable.

6.3 Shelf life

24 months.

6.4 Special precautions for storage

Do not store above 25°C. Store in the original package.

6.5 Nature and contents of container

Anapen consists of a pre-filled syringe contained in a single use auto-injection device.

The syringe contains adrenaline solution. The auto-injection device delivers 0.3ml of this solution.

The immediate container is a glass syringe sealed by a rubber plunger at one end, and at the other end by a rubber needle shield.

Syringe

BD (Becton Dickinson) borosilicate glass type 1, 27G 1/2"

Plunger

BD (Becton Dickinson) black chlorobutyl rubber PH 701/50

6.6 Instructions for use and handling

For single use only. Discard safely immediately after use.

Full graphics are shown on label and in patient leaflet.

Remove the black needle cap, which pulls the rubber protective shield off the needle. Remove the black safety cap from the red firing button. Hold the needle end of the device against the outer thigh and press the firing button. The injection may be made, if necessary, through light clothing. Hold in position for 10 seconds and then remove. Replace the black needle cap after use.

A needle-free trainer auto injector device is available

7. MARKETING AUTHORISATION HOLDER

Lincoln Medical Ltd

13 Boathouse Meadow Business Park

Cherry Orchard Lane

Salisbury SP2 7LD

United Kingdom

8. MARKETING AUTHORISATION NUMBER(S)

PL 18813/0001

9. DATE OF FIRST AUTHORISATION/RENEWAL OF THE AUTHORISATION

11 July 2001

10. DATE OF REVISION OF THE TEXT

14/10/02 and 20/11/03

Anapen Junior 150 micrograms/0.3ml solution for injection in a pre-filled syringe.

(Celltech Pharmaceuticals Limited)

1. NAME OF THE MEDICINAL PRODUCT

Anapen Junior 150 micrograms/0.3ml solution for injection in a pre-filled syringe.

2. QUALITATIVE AND QUANTITATIVE COMPOSITION

Each millilitre contains 0.5mg of adrenaline.

One dose of 0.3ml contains 150 micrograms of adrenaline.

3. PHARMACEUTICAL FORM

Solution for injection. Clear colourless solution practically free from particles.

4. CLINICAL PARTICULARS

4.1 Therapeutic indications

Emergency treatment for acute allergic reactions (anaphylaxis) caused by peanuts or other foods, drugs, insect bites or stings, and other allergens as well as exercise-induced or idiopathic anaphylaxis.

4.2 Posology and method of administration

Use only by the intramuscular route.

Anapen Junior consists of a pre-filled syringe of adrenaline contained in an auto-injection device. The whole is referred to as an auto-injector.

One Anapen Junior injection should be administered intramuscularly immediately on the appearance of the signs and symptoms of anaphylactic shock. These may occur within minutes of exposure to the allergen and are most commonly manifested by urticaria, flushing or angioedema; more severe reactions involve the circulatory and respiratory systems. Inject Anapen Junior only into the anterolateral aspect of the thigh, not the buttock. The injected area may be lightly massaged for 10 seconds following injection.

The effective dose is typically in the range 0.005-0.01mg/kg but higher doses may be necessary in some cases.

Use in children: The appropriate dose may be 150 micrograms (Anapen Jnr) or 300 micrograms (Anapen) of epinephrine (adrenaline), depending on the body weight of the child and the discretion of the doctor. Larger children may require more than one injection to reverse the effect of an allergic reaction. In some circumstances a single dose of adrenaline may not completely reverse the effects of an acute allergic reaction and for such patients a repeat injection with a second syringe) may be given after 10-15 minutes.

The auto-injector of Anapen Junior is designed to deliver a single dose of 150 micrograms epinephrine. A dosage below 150 micrograms cannot be administered in sufficient accuracy in children weighing less than 15 kg and use is therefore not recommended unless in a life threatening situation and under medical advice.

A double syringe pack is available in certain markets.

Anapen Junior auto-injector is intended for immediate self-administration by a person with a history of anaphylaxis and is designed to deliver a single dose of 150 micrograms (0.3ml) adrenaline. For stability reasons 0.75ml is left in the syringe after use but the unit cannot be used again and should be safely discarded.

4.3 Contraindications

Hypersensitivity to epinephrine or to any of the excipients.

4.4 Special warnings and special precautions for use

All patients who are prescribed Anapen Junior should be thoroughly instructed to understand the indications for use and the correct method of administration. Anapen Junior is indicated as emergency supportive therapy only and patients should be advised to seek immediate medical attention following administration.

Use with caution in patients with heart disease e.g coronary heart and cardiac muscle diseases (angina may be induced), cor pulmonale, cardiac arrythmias or tachycardia. There is a risk of adverse reactions following adrenaline administration in patients with hyperthyroidism, cardiovascular disease (severe angina pectoris, obstructive cardiomyopathy and ventricular arrhythmia and hypertension), phaeochromocytoma, high intraocular pressure, severe renal impairment, prostatic adenoma leading to residual urine, hypercalcemia, hypokalemia, diabetes, or in elderly or pregnant patients. Also, Anapen Junior contains sodium metabisulphite which can cause allergic-type reactions including anaphylactic symptoms and bronchospasm in susceptible people, especially those with a history of asthma.

Patients with these conditions must be carefully instructed in regard to the circumstances under which Anapen Junior should be used.

Repeated local injection can result in necrosis at sites of injection from vascular constriction. Accidental intravascular injection may result in cerebral haemorrhage due to a sudden rise in blood pressure. Accidental injection into hands or feet may cause loss of blood flow to adjacent areas due to vasoconstriction.

4.5 Interaction with other medicinal products and other forms of Interaction

The effects of adrenaline may be potentiated by tricyclic antidepressants mixed noradrenargic-serotoninergic antidepressants like venlafaxine, sibutramine or milnacipran and monoamine oxidase inhibitors (sudden blood pressure increase and possible cardiac arrhythmia), COMT blocking agent, thyroid hormones, theophylline, oxytocin, parasympatholytics, certain antihistamines (diphenhydramine, chlorpheniramine), levodopa and alcohol.

Severe hypertension and bradykardia may occur when adrenaline is administered with non-selective beta-blocking medicinal products.

Concurrent therapy with sympathomimetics may potentiate the effects of adrenaline.

Use Anapen Junior with caution in patients receiving medicinal products which may sensitise the heart to arrhythmias, e.g. digitalis, quinidine halogenated anaesthetics.

The pressor effects of adrenaline may be counteracted by administration of rapidly acting vasodilators or alpha adrenergic blocking medicinal products. Anaphylactic effects can be antagonised by beta-blocking agents, especially non-selective beta-blockers.

Adrenaline inhibits insulin secretion and diabetic patients may require upward adjustment of their insulin or other hypoglycaemic therapy.

4.6 Pregnancy and lactation

There are no adequate or well-controlled studies of adrenaline in pregnant women. Adrenaline should only be used in pregnancy if the potential benefit justifies the potential risk to the foetus. Adrenaline may dramatically reduce placental blood flow, although anaphylactic shock will do this too. Adrenalineis not orally bioavailable; any adrenaline excreted in breast milk would not be expected to have any effect on the nursing infant.

4.7 Effects on ability to drive and use machines

It is not recommended that patients should drive or use machines following administration of adrenaline, since patients will be affected by symptoms of the anaphylactic shock.

4.8 Undesirable effects

The occurrence of undesirable effects depends on the sensitivity of the individual patient and the dose applied.

Common adverse reactions even at low doses due to adrenaline include palpitations, tachycardia, sweating, nausea, vomiting, respiratory difficulty, pallor, dizziness, weakness, tremor, headache, apprehension, nervousness, anxiety coldness of extremities. Less frequently reported effects include hallucinations, syncopes,, hyperglycaemia, hypokalaemia, metabolic acidosis, mydriasis, difficulty in micturition with urinary retention, muscle tremor.

Adverse reactions which occur at higher doses or in susceptible individuals are cardiac arrhythmias (ventricular fibrillation /cardiac arrest), sudden rise of blood pressure (sometimes leading to cerebral haemorrhage), as well as vasoconstriction (e.g. in the skin, mucous tissues and kidneys).

Anapen contains a sulphite that may cause allergic-type reactions including anaphylactic reactions or life-threatening or less severe asthmatic episodes in certain susceptible patients.

4.9 Overdose

Overdose or accidental intravascular injection of adrenaline may cause cerebral haemorrhage from a sudden rise of blood pressure. Death may result from acute pulmonary oedema arising from peripheral vascular constriction and cardiac stimulation.

The pressor effects of adrenaline may be counteracted by rapidly acting vasodilators or alpha-adrenergic blocking medicinal products. Should prolonged hypotension follow such measures, it may be necessary to administer another pressor medicinal product, such as noradrenaline.

Acute pulmonary oedema with respiratory embarrassment following adrenaline overdose should be managed by administration of a rapidly acting alpha-adrenergic blocking medicinal product such as phentolamine and/or with intermittent positive pressure respiration.

Adrenaline overdose may also result in transient bradycardia followed by tachycardia; these can be followed by potentially fatal cardiac arrhythmias, which may be treated by beta-adrenergic blocking medicinal products. These must be preceded or accompanied by an alpha-adrenergic blocker to control the alpha-mediated effects on the peripheral circulation.

5. PHARMACOLOGICAL PROPERTIES

5.1 Pharmacodynamic properties

Pharmacotherapeutic group: adrenergic and dopaminergic agents, adrenaline

ATC code: C01 CA 24

Adrenaline is a naturally occurring catecholamine secreted by the adrenal medulla in response to exertion or stress. It is a sympathomimetic amine which is a potent stimulant of both alpha and beta adrenergic receptors and its effects on target organs are, therefore, complex. It is the medicinal product of choice to provide rapid relief of hypersensitivity reactions to allergies or to idiopathic or exercise induced anaphylaxis.

Adrenaline has a strong vasoconstrictor action through alpha-adrenergic stimulation. This activity counteracts the vasodilatation and increased vascular permeability leading to loss of intravascular fluid and subsequent hypotension, which are the major pharmacotoxicological features in anaphylactic shock. Through its stimulation of bronchial beta adrenergic receptors, adrenaline has a powerful bronchodilator action which alleviates wheezing and dyspnoea. Adrenaline also alleviates pruritus, urticaria and angioedema associated with anaphylaxis.

5.2 Pharmacokinetic properties

Adrenaline is rapidly inactivated in the body, mostly in the liver by the enzymes COMT and MAO. Much of a dose of adrenaline is excreted as metabolites in urine. The plasma half-life is about 2-3 minutes. However, when given by subcutaneous or intramuscular injection, local vasoconstriction may delay absorption so that the effects may last longer than the half-life suggests.

5.3 Preclinical safety data

Adrenaline has been widely used in the clinical management of allergic emergencies for many years. There are no pre-clinical data of relevance to the prescriber which are additional to that already included in other sections of the SPC.

6. PHARMACEUTICAL PARTICULARS

6.1 List of excipients

Sodium chloride,

Sodium metabisulphite (E223)

Hydrochloric acid

Water for injections

6.2 Incompatibilities

Not applicable.

6.3 Shelf life

21 months.

6.4 Special precautions for storage

Do not store above 25°C. Store in the original package.

6.5 Nature and contents of container

Anapen Junior consists of a pre-filled syringe contained in a single use auto-injection device.

The syringe contains adrenaline solution. The auto-injection device delivers 0.3ml of this solution.

The immediate container is a glass syringe sealed by a rubber plunger at one end, and at the other end by a rubber needle shield.

Syringe

BD (Becton Dickinson) borosilicate glass type 1, 27G 1/2"

Plunger

BD (Becton Dickinson) black chlorobutyl rubber PH 701/50

6.6 Instructions for use and handling

For single use only. Discard safely immediately after use.

Full graphics are shown on label and in patient leaflet.

Remove the black needle cap, which pulls the rubber protective shield off the needle. Remove the black safety cap from the red firing button. Hold the needle end of the device against the outer thigh and press the firing button. The injection may be made, if necessary, through light clothing. Hold in position for 10 seconds and then remove. Replace the black needle cap after use.

A needle-free trainer auto injector device is available.

7. MARKETING AUTHORISATION HOLDER

Lincoln Medical Ltd

13 Boathouse Meadow Business Park

Cherry Orchard Lane

Salisbury SP2 7LD

United Kingdom

8. MARKETING AUTHORISATION NUMBER(S)

PL 18813/0002

9. DATE OF FIRST AUTHORISATION/RENEWAL OF THE AUTHORISATION

11 July 2001

10. DATE OF REVISION OF THE TEXT

February 2004

Anbesol Liquid

(SSL International plc)

1. NAME OF THE MEDICINAL PRODUCT

Anbesol Liquid.

2. QUALITATIVE AND QUANTITATIVE COMPOSITION

Lidocaine Hydrochloride Ph Eur 0.9% w/w; Chlorocresol Ph Eur 0.1% w/w; and Cetylpyridinium Chloride Ph Eur 0.02% w/w.

3. PHARMACEUTICAL FORM

Liquid for oral administration.

4. CLINICAL PARTICULARS

4.1 Therapeutic indications

For the temporary relief of pain caused by recurrent mouth ulcers, denture irritation and teething.

4.2 Posology and method of administration

Adults, children and the elderly: apply undiluted to the affected area with the fingertip. Two applications immediately will normally be sufficient to obtain pain relief. Use up to eight times a day. Babies teething: One application only. Do not repeat for at least half an hour. Use up to eight times a day.

4.3 Contraindications

Patients with a known history of hypersensitivity or allergic type reactions to any of the constituents of the product.

4.4 Special warnings and special precautions for use

If symptoms persist for more than 7 days, consult your doctor or dentist. For babies teething, do not repeat for at least half an hour. Keep all medicines out of the reach of children. Do not exceed the stated dose.

4.5 Interaction with other medicinal products and other forms of Interaction

None known.

4.6 Pregnancy and lactation

No special precautions required.

4.7 Effects on ability to drive and use machines

None known.

4.8 Undesirable effects

There have been reports of non-specific ulceration following oral cetylpyridinium chloride therapy.

4.9 Overdose

Ingestion of the complete contents of the marketed pack would not be expected to cause any adverse effects.

5. PHARMACOLOGICAL PROPERTIES

5.1 Pharmacodynamic properties

Lidocaine hydrochloride: White crystalline powder soluble in water and alcohol. Mechanism of action/effect: Lidocaine is a local anaesthetic of the amide type, which acts by reversible inhibition of nerve impulse generation and transmission. Chlorocresol: Colourless crystals or a white crystalline powder slightly soluble in water and alcohol. Chlorocresol has a disinfectant action. Cetylpyridinium chloride: A white unctuous powder soluble in water and alcohol. Mechanism of action/effect: cetylpyridinium chloride has a disinfectant action.

5.2 Pharmacokinetic properties

Lidocaine hydrochloride: Absorption and fate: Lidocaine is readily absorbed from mucous membranes and through damaged skin. Lidocaine undergoes first-pass metabolism in the liver and about 90% is dealkylated to form monoethylglycinexylidide and glycinexylidide. Further metabolism occurs and the metabolites are excreted in the urine with less than 10% as unchanged lidocaine. Chlorocresol: Absorption: there is no significant absorption of chlorocresol through the skin or mucous. Cetylpyridinium chloride: Absorption: there is no significant absorption of cetylpyridinium chloride through the skin or mucous membranes.

5.3 Preclinical safety data

None stated.

6. PHARMACEUTICAL PARTICULARS

6.1 List of excipients

Alcohol 96% BP, Menthol BP, Glycerin Ph Eur, Caramel Colour (containing colourants E110, E104, E123, E142), Purified Water Ph Eur.

6.2 Incompatibilities

None known.

6.3 Shelf life

36 months.

6.4 Special precautions for storage

Store at a temperature not exceeding 25°C.

6.5 Nature and contents of container

6.5ml, 15 ml: glass bottles

6.6 Instructions for use and handling

Not applicable.

7. MARKETING AUTHORISATION HOLDER

Seton Products Limited, Tubiton House, Oldham, OL1 3HS.

8. MARKETING AUTHORISATION NUMBER(S)

PL 11314/0117.

9. DATE OF FIRST AUTHORISATION/RENEWAL OF THE AUTHORISATION

11th July 1998/ 24th May 2001.

10. DATE OF REVISION OF THE TEXT

May 2001.

Anbesol Teething Gel

(SSL International plc)

1. NAME OF THE MEDICINAL PRODUCT

Anbesol Teething Gel.

2. QUALITATIVE AND QUANTITATIVE COMPOSITION

Lidocaine Hydrochloride Ph Eur 1.0% w/w; Chlorocresol Ph Eur 0.1% w/w; and Cetylpyridinium Chloride Ph Eur 0.02% w/w.

3. PHARMACEUTICAL FORM

Gel for oral administration.

4. CLINICAL PARTICULARS

4.1 Therapeutic indications

For the temporary relief of pain caused by recurrent mouth ulcers, denture irritation and teething.

4.2 Posology and method of administration

Adults, children and the elderly: apply a small amount to the affected area with a clean fingertip. Two applications immediately will normally be sufficient to obtain pain relief. Use up to four times a day. Babies teething: apply a small amount to the affected area with a clean fingertip. Use up to four times a day.

4.3 Contraindications

Patients with a known history of hypersensitivity or allergic type reactions to any of the constituents of the product.

4.4 Special warnings and special precautions for use

The following statements appear on the packaging: (i) if symptoms persist for more than 7 days, consult your doctor or pharmacist; (ii) keep all medicines out of the reach of children.

4.5 Interaction with other medicinal products and other forms of Interaction

None known.

4.6 Pregnancy and lactation

No special precautions required.

4.7 Effects on ability to drive and use machines

None known.

4.8 Undesirable effects

There have been reports of non-specific ulceration following oral cetylpyridinium chloride therapy.

4.9 Overdose

Overdose is extremely unlikely considering the small size of the tube used for sale.

5. PHARMACOLOGICAL PROPERTIES

5.1 Pharmacodynamic properties

Lidocaine: Lidocaine is a local anaesthetic of the amide type which acts by reversible inhibition of nerve impulse generation and transmission. Chlorocresol: Chlorocresol has a disinfectant action. Cetylpyridinium chloride: Cetylpyridinium chloride has a disinfectant action.

5.2 Pharmacokinetic properties

Lidocaine hydrochloride: Absorption and Fate: Lidocaine is readily absorbed from mucous membranes and through damaged skin. Lidocaine undergoes first-pass metabolism in the liver and about 90% is dealkylated to form monoethylglycinexylidide and glycinexylidide. Further metabolism occurs and the metabolites are excreted in the urine with less than 10% as unchanged lidocaine. Chlorocresol: There is no significant absorption of chlorocresol through the skin or mucous membranes. Cetylpyridinium chloride: Absorption: There is no significant absorption of cetylpyridinium chloride through the skin or mucous membranes.

5.3 Preclinical safety data
The active ingredients in Anbesol Teething Gel have a well established safety record.

6. PHARMACEUTICAL PARTICULARS

6.1 List of excipients
Alcohol 96% BP; Glycerin Ph Eur; Clove Oil BP; Sodium Saccharin BP; Hydroxypropyl Cellulose Ph Eur; Ponceau 4R (E124); Purified Water Ph Eur.

6.2 Incompatibilities
None known.

6.3 Shelf life
36 months.

6.4 Special precautions for storage
Store at a temperature not exceeding 25°C.

6.5 Nature and contents of container
Membrane sealed lacquered aluminium tubes fitted with plastic caps containing 10g gel.

6.6 Instructions for use and handling
None.

7. MARKETING AUTHORISATION HOLDER
Seton Products Limited, Tubiton House, Oldham, OL1 3HS.

8. MARKETING AUTHORISATION NUMBER(S)
PL 11314/0115.

9. DATE OF FIRST AUTHORISATION/RENEWAL OF THE AUTHORISATION
11th December 1998 / 11th October 2003.

10. DATE OF REVISION OF THE TEXT
October 2003.

Ancotil 2.5g/250 ml Solution for Infusion

(Valeant Pharmaceuticals Ltd)

1. NAME OF THE MEDICINAL PRODUCT
Ancotil 2.5g/250 ml Solution for Infusion.

2. QUALITATIVE AND QUANTITATIVE COMPOSITION
Flucytosine Ph. Eur. 2.5g in 250 mL.

3. PHARMACEUTICAL FORM
Infusion bottles containing 2.5g flucytosine Ph. Eur. in 250 mL isotonic sodium chloride solution.

4. CLINICAL PARTICULARS

4.1 Therapeutic indications
Ancotil is indicated for the treatment of systemic yeast and fungal infections due to sensitive organisms: such infections include cryptococcosis, candidiasis, chromomycosis and infections due to *torulopsis glabrata* and *hansenula*.

In the treatment of cryptococcal meningitis and severe systemic candidiasis it is recommended that Ancotil should be given in combination with amphotericin-B. Amphotericin-B may also be given in combination with Ancotil in severe or long-standing infections due to other organisms. In cases of cryptococcal meningitis, where toxicity of amphotericin B, or a combination of flucytosine with amphotericin B is dose limiting, a combination of flucytosine with fluconazole has demonstrated successful cure, but at a lower rate than in combination with amphotericin B.

4.2 Posology and method of administration
Adults and Children
Ancotil for Infusion should be administered using a giving set. It may be administered directly into a vein, through a central venous catheter, or by intra-peritoneal infusion. The recommended daily dosage in adults and children is 200 mg/kg body-weight divided into four doses over the 24 hours. In patients harboring extremely sensitive organisms a total daily dose of 100 to 150 mg/kg body-weight may be sufficient. Adequate effects can, however, often be obtained with a lower dose.

It is suggested that the duration of the infusion should be of the order of 20 to 40 minutes provided this is balanced with the fluid requirements of the patient. As a rule, treatment with Ancotil for Infusion should rarely be required for periods of more than one week.

Since Ancotil is excreted primarily by the kidneys, patients with renal impairment should be given smaller doses. The following is suggested as a guide for dosage in patients with severe infection associated with renal impairment:

In patients with:

Creatinine clearance <40 to >20 mL/min: 50 mg/kg every 12 hours.

Creatinine clearance <20 to >10 mL/min: 50 mg/kg every 24 hours.

Creatinine clearance <10 mL/min: an initial single dose of 50 mg/kg; subsequent doses should be calculated according to the results of regular monitoring of the serum concentration of the drug, which should not be allowed to exceed 80 micrograms/mL. Blood levels of <25 to 50 micrograms/mL are normally effective.

The duration of treatment should be determined on an individual basis.

The outcome of therapy will be affected by variations in the sensitivity of the infection organism, its accessibility and its susceptibility to Ancotil, as well as by differences in the response of individual patients. In cases of cryptococcal meningitis, treatment should last for at least four months.

Neonates
The dose in neonates should be calculated in the same way as for adults and children, but the high possibility of renal impairment should be considered in this group either as intrinsic to their age or as a result of other nephrotoxic therapies. It is advised to closely monitor the serum levels of flucytosine in this group and adjust the dose according to levels. In cases where renal impairment is present the dose interval should be extended (as with adults and children). Where renal impairment is not a feature but serum levels are above those recommended, the does should be reduced but the dosing interval should remain the same.

Elderly
Although no specific studies have been performed to establish the use of Ancotil in the elderly, documented use indicated that the dosage requirements and side effects profile are similar to those of younger patients. Particular attention should be paid to renal function in this group.

Ancotil for Infusion may be given concurrently with other infusions of normal saline, glucose or glucose/saline. No other agent should be added to or mixed with Ancotil for Infusion.

4.3 Contraindications
Ancotil is contra-indicated in patients who have shown hypersensitivity to flucytosine or any of the excipients.

4.4 Special warnings and special precautions for use
The product should be used with great caution in patients with depression of bone marrow function or blood dyscrasias. Blood counts and tests of renal and hepatic function should be performed before and during treatment. This should occur at least weekly in patients with renal insufficiency or blood dyscrasias.

Ancotil should not be used in patients with impaired renal function in the absence of facilities for monitoring blood levels of the drug.

When measuring drug serum levels, it should be noted that levels of the drug in blood samples, taken during or immediately after administration of Ancotil for Infusion, are not a reliable guide to subsequent levels; it is advisable to remove blood for monitoring of blood levels of Ancotil shortly before starting the next infusion.

In calculating the fluid and electrolyte intake of patients with impaired renal function, cardiac failure or electrolyte imbalance, due allowance should be made for the volume and sodium content (138 millimole/litre) of Ancotil for Infusion.

Sensitivity testing:
It is recommended that cultures for sensitivity testing be taken before treatment and repeated at regular intervals during therapy. However, it is not necessary to delay treatment until results of these tests are known.

To determine sensitivities, the methods of Shadomy (Appl. Microbiol., 1969, 17, 871) and Scholer (Mykosen, 1970, 13, 179) are recommended.

For sensitivity testing it is essential that culture media are free of antagonists to flucytosine.

Creatinine Measurement:
Flucytosine may interfere with the dual-slide enzymatic measurement of creatinine used with the manual desk top Vitros DT 60 analyser, giving the false impression of azetomia. Other suitable methods should be used for creatinine assessment. The current creatinine method used with automated Vitros analysers is not affected by flucytosine.

4.5 Interaction with other medicinal products and other forms of Interaction
There is contradictory evidence concerning a drug interaction between Ancotil and cytarabine. Strict monitoring of blood levels is required if the two medicines are given concurrently.

4.6 Pregnancy and lactation
Teratogenic effects have been seen in rats, in which species flucytosine is metabolised to fluorouracil. The metabolism may differ in man: nevertheless, the use of Ancotil in pregnancy and in women of childbearing age requires that the potential benefits of therapy be weighed against its possible hazards. The drug should not be given to women breast feeding infants.

4.7 Effects on ability to drive and use machines
Not applicable.

4.8 Undesirable effects
Nausea, vomiting, diarrhoea and skin rashes may occur but are usually of a transient nature.

Less frequently observed side effects include allergic reactions, Lyell's Syndrome, myocardial toxicity and ventricular dysfunction, confusion, hallucinations, convulsions, headache, sedation and vertigo. Alterations in tests of liver function are generally dose related and reversible but hepatitis and hepatic necrosis have been reported. Acute liver injury with possible fatal outcome in debilitated patients may occur in isolated cases.

Heamatological changes, mainly leucopenia, thrombocytopenia, agranulocytosis or aplastic anaemia have been reported. This is more common when serum levels of flucytosine are high in patients with renal impairment and when amphotericin-B has been co. prescribed. In isolated cases, bone marrow toxicity may be irreversible and could lead to death in patients with pre-existing immunosuppression, Local irritation or phlebitis does not appear to be a problem with Ancotil for Infusion.

4.9 Overdose
Haemodialysis produces a rapid fall in the serum concentration of Ancotil.

5. PHARMACOLOGICAL PROPERTIES

5.1 Pharmacodynamic properties
Ancotil is a fluorinated pyrimidine effective in the treatment of certain systemic fungal infections. In fungi sensitive to the preparation, it acts as a competitive inhibitor of uracil metabolism.

5.2 Pharmacokinetic properties
Ancotil is widely distributed in body tissues and fluids (including cerebrospinal fluid). Binding to plasma proteins is minimal. Half-life of elimination is 3-6 hours in patients with normal renal function but this value increases in renal failure. About 90% of the dose administered is excreted unchanged in the urine. Flucytosine is metabolised to 5-flurouracil. The area under the curves (AUC) ratio of 5-flurouracil to flucytosine is 4%. Flucytosine can be removed by haemodialysis.

5.3 Preclinical safety data
Not relevant.

6. PHARMACEUTICAL PARTICULARS

6.1 List of excipients
Sodium chloride Ph. Eur., tromethamine USP, hydrochloric acid 25% and water for injections Ph. Eur.

6.2 Incompatibilities
Ancotil for Infusion may be given concurrently with other infusions of Sodium Chloride Intravenous infusion (0.9% w/v) BP, Glucose Intravenous Infusion (5% w/v) BP, or Sodium Chloride (0.18% w/v) and Glucose (4% w/v) Intravenous infusion BP. No other agent should be added to or mixed with Ancotil for Infusion.

6.3 Shelf life
2 years.

6.4 Special precautions for storage
Ancotil for Infusion should be stored between 18°C and 25°C. If stored below 18°C, precipitation of Ancotil substance may occur, which should be redissolved by heating to 80°C for not more than 30 minutes.

Prolonged storage above 25°C could lead to the decomposition of Ancotil resulting in the formation of 5-fluorouracil.

6.5 Nature and contents of container
250 mL neutral glass bottle (DIN 58363) with a teflon coated butyl rubber stopper. Bottles are in packs of 5.

6.6 Instructions for use and handling
Ancotil for Infusion is available to hospitals only.

7. MARKETING AUTHORISATION HOLDER
Valeant Pharmaceuticals Limited
Cedarwood
Chineham Business Park
Crockford Lane
Basingstoke
Hampshire RG24 8WD

8. MARKETING AUTHORISATION NUMBER(S)
PL 15142/0002
PA 513/3/1

9. DATE OF FIRST AUTHORISATION/RENEWAL OF THE AUTHORISATION
8th November 1994
8th June 1991

10. DATE OF REVISION OF THE TEXT
November 2004

Androcur

(Schering Health Care Limited)

1. NAME OF THE MEDICINAL PRODUCT
Androcur® 50mg tablets

2. QUALITATIVE AND QUANTITATIVE COMPOSITION
Each tablet contains 50 mg cyproterone acetate.

For excipients, see 6.1

3. PHARMACEUTICAL FORM
Tablet.

White, round tablet, scored on one side and embossed with the letters "BV" in a regular hexagon on the other side.

4. CLINICAL PARTICULARS

4.1 Therapeutic indications

Control of libido in severe hypersexuality and/or sexual deviation in the adult male.

4.2 Posology and method of administration

Adults including the elderly:

One tablet twice daily, after the morning and evening meals.

Children:

Androcur should not be given to youths under 18.

For oral administration.

4.3 Contraindications

Liver diseases, malignant tumours (except for carcinoma of the prostate) and wasting diseases (because of transient catabolic action). A history of or existing thrombosis or embolism. Severe diabetes with vascular changes. Sickle cell anaemia. Severe chronic depression.

Androcur should not be given to youths under 18 or to those whose bone maturation and testicular development are incomplete.

Hypersensitivity to any of the components of Androcur.

4.4 Special warnings and special precautions for use

Liver: Direct hepatic toxicity, including jaundice, hepatitis and hepatic failure, which has been fatal in some cases, has been reported in patients treated with 200-300 mg cyproterone acetate. Most reported cases are in men with prostatic cancer. Toxicity is dose-related and develops, usually, several months after treatment has begun. Liver function tests should be performed pre-treatment, regularly during treatment and whenever any symptoms or signs suggestive of hepatotoxicity occur. If hepatotoxicity is confirmed, cyproterone acetate should normally be withdrawn, unless the hepatotoxicity can be explained by another cause, e.g. metastatic disease, in which case cyproterone acetate should be continued only if the perceived benefit outweighs the risk.

As with other sex steroids, benign and malignant liver changes have been reported in isolated cases.

In very rare cases, liver tumours may lead to life-threatening intra-abdominal haemorrhage. If severe upper abdominal complaints, liver enlargement or signs of intra-abdominal haemorrhage occur, a liver tumour should be considered in the differential diagnosis.

Thromboembolism: In extremely rare cases, the occurrence of thromboembolic events has been reported in temporal association with the use of Androcur. however, a causal relationship seems to be questionable. (See section 4.3)

Breathlessness: Shortness of breath may occur. This may be due to the stimulatory effect of progesterone and synthetic progestogens on breathing, which is accompanied by hypocapnia and compensatory alkalosis, and which is not considered to require treatment.

Adrenocortical function: During treatment adrenocortical function should be checked regularly, since suppression has been observed.

Diabetes: Androcur can influence carbohydrate metabolism. Parameters of carbohydrate metabolism should be examined carefully in all diabetics before and regularly during treatment. See also section 4.5.

Haemoglobin: Hypochromic anaemia has been found rarely during long-term treatment, and blood-counts before and at regular intervals during treatment are advisable.

Spermatogenesis: A spermatogram should be recorded before starting treatment in patients of procreative age, as a guard against attribution of pre-existing infertility to Androcur at a later stage. It should be noted that the decline in spermatogenesis is slow, and Androcur should, therefore, not be regarded as a male contraceptive.

Medico-legal considerations: Doctors are advised to ensure that the fully informed consent of the patient to Androcur treatment is witnessed and can be verified.

4.5 Interaction with other medicinal products and other forms of Interaction

Diabetes: The requirement for oral antidiabetics or insulin can change. See also section 4.4.

Chronic alcoholism: Alcohol appears to reduce the effect of Androcur which is of no value in chronic alcoholics.

4.6 Pregnancy and lactation

Not applicable

4.7 Effects on ability to drive and use machines

Fatigue and lassitude are common - patients should be warned about this and if affected should not drive or operate machinery.

4.8 Undesirable effects

Thromboembolism: See section 4.4.

Inhibition of spermatogenesis: The sperm count and the volume of ejaculate are reduced, infertility is usual, and there may be azoospermia after 8 weeks. There is usually slight atrophy of the seminiferous tubules. Follow-up examinations have shown these changes to be reversible, spermatogenesis usually reverting to its previous state about 3-5 months after stopping Androcur, or in some users, up to 20 months. That spermatogenesis can recover even after very long treatment is not yet known. There is evidence that abnormal sperms which might give rise to malformed embryos are produced during treatment with Androcur.

Tiredness: Fatigue and lassitude are common.

Gynaecomastia: About one patient in five develops transient or perhaps in some cases permanent enlargement of the mammary glands. In rare cases galactorrhoea and tender benign nodules have been reported. Symptoms mostly subside after discontinuation of treatment or reduction of dosage.

Bodyweight: During long-term treatment, changes in bodyweight have been reported, chiefly weight gains.

Osteoporosis: Rarely cases of osteoporosis have also been reported.

Other changes that have been reported include:

- reduction of sebum production leading to dryness of the skin and improvement of existing acne vulgaris;
- transient patchy loss and reduced growth of body hair, increased growth of scalp hair, lightening of hair colour and female type of pubic hair growth;
- occasionally depressive moods can occur;
- breathlessness can occur (see section 4.4);
- in rare cases, hypersensitivity reactions and rashes may occur.

4.9 Overdose

There have been no reports of ill-effects from overdosage, which it is, therefore, generally unnecessary to treat. There are no specific antidotes and if treatment is required it should be symptomatic.

5. PHARMACOLOGICAL PROPERTIES

5.1 Pharmacodynamic properties

Cyproterone acetate acts as an antiandrogen by blocking androgen receptors. It also has progestogenic activity, which exerts a negative feedback effect on hypothalamic receptors, so leading to a reduction in gonadotrophin release, and hence to diminished production of testicular androgens. Sexual drive and potency are reduced and gonadal function is inhibited.

An occasional tendency for the prolactin levels to increase slightly has been observed under higher doses of cyproterone acetate.

5.2 Pharmacokinetic properties

Following oral administration, cyproterone acetate is completely absorbed over a wide dose range. The ingestion of two cyproterone acetate 50 mg tablets gives maximum serum levels of about 285 ng/ml at about 3 hours. Thereafter, drug serum levels declined during a time interval of typically 24 to 120 h, with a terminal half-life of 43.9 ± 12.8 h. The total clearance of cyproterone acetate from serum is 3.5 ± 1.5 ml/min/kg. Cyproterone acetate is metabolised by various pathways, including hydroxylations and conjugations. The main metabolite in human plasma is the 15β-hydroxy derivative.

Some drug is excreted unchanged with bile fluid. Most of the dose is excreted in the form of metabolites at a urinary to biliary ratio of 3:7. The renal and biliary excretion proceeds with a half-life of 1.9 days. Metabolites from plasma are eliminated at a similar rate (half-life of 1.7 days).

Cyproterone acetate is almost ex-clusively bound to plasma albumin. About 3.5 - 4 % of total drug levels are present unbound. Because protein binding is non-specific, changes in SHBG (sex hormone binding globulin) levels do not affect the pharmacokinetics of cyproterone acetate.

The absolute bioavailability of cyproterone acetate is almost complete (88 % of dose).

5.3 Preclinical safety data

Recognised first-line tests of genotoxicity gave negative results when conducted with cyproterone acetate. However, further tests showed that cyproterone acetate was capable of producing adducts with DNA (and an increase in DNA repair activity) in liver cells from rats and monkeys and also in freshly isolated human hepatocytes. This DNA-adduct formation occurred at exposures that might be expected to occur in the recommended dose regimens for cyproterone acetate. *In vivo* consequences of cyproterone acetate treatment were the increased incidence of focal, possibly preneoplastic, liver lesions in which cellular enzymes were altered in female rats, and an increase of mutation frequency in transgenic rats carrying a bacterial gene as target for mutation. The clinical relevance of these findings is presently uncertain. Clinical experience to date would not support an increased incidence of hepatic tumours in man. However, it must be borne in mind that sex steroids can promote the growth of certain hormone dependent tissues and tumours.

6. PHARMACEUTICAL PARTICULARS

6.1 List of excipients

Lactose

Maize starch

Povidone 25 000

Silicon dioxide (aerosil) (E551)

Magnesium stearate (E572)

6.2 Incompatibilities

None known

6.3 Shelf life

5 years

6.4 Special precautions for storage

No special precautions for storage

6.5 Nature and contents of container

PVC/Aluminium bister pack.

Pack size: 56 tablets

6.6 Instructions for use and handling

Keep out of the reach of children.

7. MARKETING AUTHORISATION HOLDER

Schering Health Care Limited

The Brow

Burgess Hill

West Sussex RH15 9NE

8. MARKETING AUTHORISATION NUMBER(S)

PL 0053/0023

9. DATE OF FIRST AUTHORISATION/RENEWAL OF THE AUTHORISATION

26th April 2002

10. DATE OF REVISION OF THE TEXT

2nd April 2004

LEGAL CATEGORY

POM

Andropatch 2.5mg

(GlaxoSmithKline UK)

1. NAME OF THE MEDICINAL PRODUCT

Andropatch 2.5 mg

2. QUALITATIVE AND QUANTITATIVE COMPOSITION

Each Andropatch 2.5 mg System contains 12.2 mg testosterone BP.

3. PHARMACEUTICAL FORM

Andropatch 2.5 mg is a transdermal drug delivery system consisting of a self-adhesive patch surrounding a central drug reservoir of testosterone dissolved in an alcohol-based gel.

Each Andropatch 2.5 mg System delivers *in vivo* approximately 2.5 mg of testosterone over 24 hours across skin of average permeability. (Active surface area 7.5 cm^2).

4. CLINICAL PARTICULARS

4.1 Therapeutic indications

Andropatch 2.5 mg is indicated for testosterone replacement therapy in conditions with a deficiency or an absence of endogenous testosterone associated with primary or secondary hypogonadism.

4.2 Posology and method of administration

Adults and Elderly

The usual dose is two Andropatch 2.5 mg Systems applied nightly (approximately 10 pm) and worn for 24 hours, providing approximately 5 mg testosterone per day. The dose can be adjusted up to the equivalent of 7.5 mg nightly or down to 2.5 mg nightly depending on the serum testosterone measured in the morning after application. Measurement of serum testosterone should be repeated taking care to ensure proper system adhesion and correct time of application before the dose is adjusted. Three systems per day may be required for men with a higher body weight >130 kg). Treatment in non-virilised patients may be initiated with one system applied nightly. The dose should be adjusted as appropriate.

The duration of treatment and frequency of testosterone measurements is determined by the physician.

The adhesive side of the Andropatch 2.5 mg System should be applied to a clean, dry area of the skin on the back, abdomen, upper arms, or thighs. Bony prominences, such as the shoulder and hip areas, and areas that may be subjected to prolonged pressure during sleeping or sitting should be avoided. Application to these sites has been associated with burn-like blister reactions (see Section 4.8). Do not apply to broken or damaged skin. Do not apply to the scrotum. The sites of application should be rotated, with an interval of seven days between applications to the same site. The area selected should not be oily, damaged or irritated.

The system should be applied immediately after opening the pouch and removing the protective release liner. The system should be pressed firmly in place, making sure there is good contact with the skin, especially around the edges.

Children

Andropatch 2.5 mg is not indicated for use in children as there has been no clinical experience of its use below the age of 15.

4.3 Contraindications

Androgens are contra-indicated in men with carcinoma of the breast or known or suspected carcinoma of the prostate, nephrotic syndrome, hypercalcaemia and known hypersensitivity to testosterone.

Andropatch 2.5 mg is contra-indicated in men with known hypersensitivity to other constituents of the patch.

Andropatch 2.5 mg has not been evaluated in women and must not be used in women. Testosterone may be harmful to the foetus.

4.4 Special warnings and special precautions for use
Elderly men treated with androgens may be at an increased risk for the development of prostatic hyperplasia.

Elderly men and others with an increased risk of developing prostatic cancer, should be assessed before starting testosterone replacement therapy because testosterone may promote the growth of subclinical prostate cancer.

As in men without testosterone deficiency, patients on testosterone replacement therapy should be periodically evaluated for prostate cancer.

Care should be taken in patients with skeletal metastases due to the risk of hypercalcaemia/hypercalcuria developing from androgen therapy.

If the patient develops an application site reaction, treatment should be reviewed and discontinued if necessary.

Testosterone may cause a rise in blood pressure and Andropatch 2.5 mg should be used with caution in patients with hypertension.

Oedema, with or without congestive heart failure, may result from androgen treatment in patients with pre-existing cardiac, renal, or hepatic disease. In addition to discontinuation of the drug, diuretic therapy may be required.

Andropatch 2.5 mg should be used with caution in patients with ischaemic heart disease, epilepsy and migraine as these conditions may be aggravated.

4.5 Interaction with other medicinal products and other forms of Interaction
When given simultaneously with anticoagulants the anticoagulant effect can increase. Patients receiving oral anticoagulants require close monitoring especially when androgens are started or stopped.

Concurrent administration of oxyphenbutazone and androgens may result in elevated serum levels of oxyphenbutazone.

In diabetic patients, the metabolic effects of androgens may alter blood glucose and, therefore, insulin requirements.

4.6 Pregnancy and lactation
Andropatch 2.5 mg therapy has not been evaluated in and must not be used in women under any circumstances. Testosterone may be harmful to the foetus.

4.7 Effects on ability to drive and use machines
There is no evidence that Andropatch 2.5 mg will affect the ability of a patient to drive or to use machines.

4.8 Undesirable effects
In the majority of cases, transient mild to moderate skin reactions have been observed at the site of application at some time during treatment. These include pruritus; irritation with erythema, induration or burning, rash and allergic contact dermatitis. Burn-like lesions characterised by blisters, skin necrosis, and ulceration that healed over several weeks with scarring in some cases have also been observed.

The burn-like lesions occurred sporadically, usually only at one site, (most commonly over bony prominences or areas that may have been subjected to prolonged pressure during sleeping or sitting). Such lesions should be treated as burns.

As seen with other testosterone treatments, prostate abnormalities, prostate cancer, headache, depression and gastrointestinal bleeding were also observed.

Other known undesirable effects associated with testosterone treatments include hirsuitism, male pattern baldness, seborrhoea, acne, excessive frequency and duration of penile erections, nausea, cholestatic jaundice, increased or decreased libido, anxiety, generalised paraesthaesia. Oligospermia may occur at high doses. Prolonged testosterone administration may cause electrolyte disturbances, e.g. retention of sodium, chloride, potassium, calcium, inorganic phosphates and water.

4.9 Overdose
This is not likely due to the mode of administration. Serum testosterone has a half-life of 70 minutes and therefore falls rapidly once the Andropatch 2.5 mg Systems are removed.

5. PHARMACOLOGICAL PROPERTIES

5.1 Pharmacodynamic properties
Andropatch 2.5 mg delivers physiologic amounts of testosterone producing circulating testosterone concentrations that mimic the normal circadian rhythm of healthy young men.

Testosterone, the primary androgenic hormone is responsible for the normal growth and development of the male sex organs and for maintenance of secondary sex characteristics.

Male hypogonadism results from insufficient secretion of testosterone and is characterised by low serum testosterone concentrations. Symptoms associated with male hypogonadism include the following: impotence and decreased sexual desire; fatigue and loss of energy; mood depression; regression of secondary sexual characteristics.

Androgens promote retention of nitrogen, sodium, potassium and phosphorus, decreases urinary excretion of calcium, increase protein anabolism, decrease protein catabolism, are also responsible for the growth spurt of adolescence and for the eventual termination of linear growth and stimulate the production of red blood cells by enhancing erythropoietin production.

Exogenous administration of androgens inhibits endogenous testosterone release. With large doses of exogenous androgens, spermatogenesis may be suppressed.

5.2 Pharmacokinetic properties
Following Andropatch 2.5 mg application to non-scrotal skin, testosterone is continuously absorbed during the 24-hour dosing period. Daily application of two Andropatch 2.5 mg patches at approximately 10 pm results in a serum testosterone concentration profile which mimics the normal circadian variation observed in healthy young men. Maximum concentrations occur in the early morning hours with minimum concentrations in the evening.

In hypogonadal men, application of two Andropatch 2.5 mg Systems to the back, abdomen, thighs or upper arms resulted in average testosterone absorption of 4 to 5 mg over 24 hours. Applications to the chest and shins resulted in greater inter individual variability and average 24-hour absorption of 3 to 4 mg. The serum testosterone concentration profiles during application were similar for all sites.

Normal range morning serum testosterone concentrations are reached during the first day of dosing. There is no accumulation of testosterone during continuous treatment.

Upon removal of the Andropatch 2.5 mg Systems, serum testosterone concentrations decrease with an apparent half-life of approximately 70 minutes. Hypogonadal concentrations are reached within 24 hours following system removal.

5.3 Preclinical safety data
None therapeutically relevant.

6. PHARMACEUTICAL PARTICULARS

6.1 List of excipients
Ethanol, Purified Water, Glycerol, glycerol mono-oleate, methyl laurate, Carbomer 1342, Sodium Hydroxide.

6.2 Incompatibilities
No specific incompatabilities.

6.3 Shelf life
24 months.

6.4 Special precautions for storage
Do not store above 25°C. Apply to skin immediately upon removal from the protective pouch. Do not store outside the pouch provided.

6.5 Nature and contents of container
Each Andropatch 2.5 mg System contains 12.2 mg testosterone BP for delivery of 2.5 mg testosterone per day. Each Andropatch 2.5 mg System is individually pouched and supplied in cartons of 10, 30 and 60 pouches. The pouch is made from paper, low density polyethylene and aluminium foil.

6.6 Instructions for use and handling
Andropatch 2.5 mg may be discarded with household waste in a manner that avoids accidental contact by others.

Damaged systems should not be used.

The drug reservoir may be burst by excessive heat or pressure.

Administrative Data

7. MARKETING AUTHORISATION HOLDER
SmithKline Beecham plc
980 Great West Road
Brentford
Middlesex TW8 9GS
Trading as:
GlaxoSmithKline UK
Stockley Park West
Uxbridge
Middlesex UB11 1BT

8. MARKETING AUTHORISATION NUMBER(S)
PL 10592/0069

9. DATE OF FIRST AUTHORISATION/RENEWAL OF THE AUTHORISATION
02 January 2002

10. DATE OF REVISION OF THE TEXT
29 August 2002

11. Legal Status
POM

Andropatch 5mg

(GlaxoSmithKline UK)

1. NAME OF THE MEDICINAL PRODUCT
Andropatch 5 mg

2. QUALITATIVE AND QUANTITATIVE COMPOSITION
Each Andropatch System contains 24.3 mg testosterone BP.

3. PHARMACEUTICAL FORM
Andropatch is a transdermal drug delivery system consisting of a self-adhesive patch surrounding a central drug reservoir of testosterone dissolved in an alcohol-based gel.

Each Andropatch System delivers *in vivo* approximately 5 mg of testosterone over 24 hours across skin of average permeability. (Active surface area $15cm^2$)

4. CLINICAL PARTICULARS

4.1 Therapeutic indications
Andropatch is indicated for testosterone replacement therapy in conditions with a deficiency or an absence of endogenous testosterone associated with primary or secondary hypogonadism.

4.2 Posology and method of administration
Adults and Elderly
The usual dose is one Andropatch System applied nightly (approximately 10 pm) and worn for 24 hours, providing approximately 5 mg testosterone per day. The dose can be adjusted up to the equivalent of 7.5 mg nightly or down to 2.5 mg patch nightly depending on the serum testosterone measured in the morning after application. Measurement of serum testosterone should be repeated taking care to ensure proper system adhesion and correct time of application before the dose is adjusted. The equivalent of 7.5 mg per day may be required for men with a higher body weight >130 kg). Treatment in non-virilised patients may be initiated with one 2.5 mg system applied nightly. The dose should be adjusted as appropriate.

The duration of treatment and frequency of testosterone measurements is determined by the physician.

The adhesive side of the Andropatch System should be applied to a clean, dry area of the skin on the back, abdomen, upper arms, or thighs. Bony prominences, such as the shoulder and hip areas, and areas that may be subjected to prolonged pressure during sleeping or sitting should be avoided. Application to these sites has been associated with burn-like blister reactions (see Section 4.8). Do not apply to broken or damaged skin.Do not apply to the scrotum. The sites of application should be rotated, with an interval of seven days between applications to the same site. The area selected should not be oily, damaged or irritated.

The system should be applied immediately after opening the pouch and removing the protective release liner. The system should be pressed firmly in place, making sure there is good contact with the skin, especially around the edges.

Children
Andropatch is not indicated for use in children as there has been no clinical experience of its use below the age of 15.

4.3 Contraindications
Androgens are contra-indicated in men with carcinoma of the breast or known or suspected carcinoma of the prostate, nephrotic syndrome, hypercalcaemia and known hypersensitivity to testosterone.

Andropatch is contra-indicated in men with known hypersensitivity to other constituents of the patch.

Andropatch has not been evaluated in women and must not be used in women. Testosterone may be harmful to the foetus.

4.4 Special warnings and special precautions for use
Elderly men treated with androgens may be at an increased risk for the development of prostatic hyperplasia.

Elderly men and others with an increased risk of developing prostatic cancer, should be assessed before starting testosterone replacement therapy because testosterone may promote the growth of subclinical prostate cancer.

As in men without testosterone deficiency, patients on testosterone replacement therapy should be periodically evaluated for prostate cancer.

Care should be taken in patients with skeletal metastases due to the risk of hypercalcaemia/hypercalcuria developing from androgen therapy.

If the patient develops an application site reaction, treatment should be reviewed and discontinued if necessary.

Testosterone may cause a rise in blood pressure and Andropatch should be used with caution in patients with hypertension.

Oedema, with or without congestive heart failure, may result from androgen treatment in patients with pre-existing cardiac, renal, or hepatic disease. In addition to discontinuation of the drug, diuretic therapy may be required.

Andropatch should be used with caution in patients with ischaemic heart disease, epilepsy and migraine as these conditions may be aggravated.

4.5 Interaction with other medicinal products and other forms of Interaction
When given simultaneously with anticoagulants the anticoagulant effect can increase. Patients receiving oral anticoagulants require close monitoring especially when androgens are started or stopped.

Concurrent administration of oxyphenbutazone and androgens may result in elevated serum levels of oxyphenbutazone.

In diabetic patients, the metabolic effects of androgens may alter blood glucose and, therefore, insulin requirements.

4.6 Pregnancy and lactation
Andropatch therapy has not been evaluated in and must not be used in women under any circumstances. Testosterone may be harmful to the foetus.

4.7 Effects on ability to drive and use machines
There is no evidence that Andropatch will affect the ability of a patient to drive or to use machines.

4.8 Undesirable effects
In the majority of cases, transient mild to moderate skin reactions have been observed at the site of application at some time during treatment. These include pruritus; irritation with erythema, induration or burning, rash and allergic contact dermatitis. Burn-like lesions characterised by blisters, skin necrosis, and ulceration that healed over several weeks with scarring in some cases have also been observed.

The burn-like lesions occurred sporadically, usually only at one site, (most commonly over bony prominences or areas that may have been subjected to prolonged pressure during sleeping or sitting). Such lesions should be treated as burns.

As seen with other testosterone treatments, prostate abnormalities, prostate cancer, headache, depression and gastrointestinal bleeding were also observed.

Other known undesirable effects associated with testosterone treatments include hirsuitism, male pattern baldness, seborrhoea, acne, excessive frequency and duration of penile erections, nausea, cholestatic jaundice, increased or decreased libido, anxiety, generalised paraesthaesia. Oligospermia may occur at high doses. Prolonged testosterone administration may cause electrolyte disturbances, e.g. retention of sodium, chloride, potassium, calcium, inorganic phosphates and water.

4.9 Overdose
This is not likely due to the mode of administration. Serum testosterone has a half-life of 70 minutes and therefore falls rapidly once the Andropatch Systems are removed.

5. PHARMACOLOGICAL PROPERTIES
5.1 Pharmacodynamic properties
Andropatch delivers physiologic amounts of testosterone producing circulating testosterone concentrations that mimic the normal circadian rhythm of healthy young men.

Testosterone, the primary androgenic hormone is responsible for the normal growth and development of the male sex organs and for maintenance of secondary sex characteristics.

Male hypogonadism results from insufficient secretion of testosterone and is characterised by low serum testosterone concentrations. Symptoms associated with male hypogonadism include the following: impotence and decreased sexual desire; fatigue and loss of energy; mood depression; regression of secondary sexual characteristics.

Androgens promote retention of nitrogen, sodium, potassium and phosphorus, decreases urinary excretion of calcium, increase protein anabolism, decrease protein catabolism, are also responsible for the growth spurt of adolescence and for the eventual termination of linear growth and stimulate the production of red blood cells by enhancing erythropoietin production.

Exogenous administration of androgens inhibits endogenous testosterone release. With large doses of exogenous androgens, spermatogenesis may be suppressed.

5.2 Pharmacokinetic properties
Following Andropatch application to non-scrotal skin, testosterone is continuously absorbed during the 24-hour dosing period. Daily application of two 2.5 mg or one 5 mg Andropatch patches at approximately 10 pm results in a serum testosterone concentration profile which mimics the normal circadian variation observed in healthy young men. Maximum concentrations occur in the early morning hours with minimum concentrations in the evening.

In hypogonadal men, application of two 2.5 mg or one 5 mg Andropatch Systems to the back, abdomen, thighs or upper arms resulted in average testosterone absorption of 4 to 5 mg over 24 hours. Applications to the chest and shins resulted in greater inter individual variability and average 24-hour absorption of 3 to 4 mg. The serum testosterone concentration profiles during application were similar for all sites.

Normal range morning serum testosterone concentrations are reached during the first day of dosing. There is no accumulation of testosterone during continuous treatment.

Upon removal of the Andropatch Systems, serum testosterone concentrations decrease with an apparent half-life of approximately 70 minutes. Hypogonadal concentrations are reached within 24 hours following system removal.

5.3 Preclinical safety data
None therapeutically relevant.

6. PHARMACEUTICAL PARTICULARS
6.1 List of excipients
Ethanol, Purified Water, Glycerol, glycerol mono-oleate, methyl laurate, Carbomer 1342, Sodium Hydroxide.

6.2 Incompatibilities
No specific incompatabilities.

6.3 Shelf life
24 months.

6.4 Special precautions for storage
Do not store above 25°C. Apply to skin immediately upon removal from the protective pouch. Do not store outside the pouch provided.

6.5 Nature and contents of container
Each Andropatch System contains 24.3mg testosterone BP for delivery of 5mg testosterone per day. Each Andropatch System is individually pouched and supplied in cartons of 5, 15 and30 pouches. The pouch is made from paper, low density polyethylene and aluminium foil.

6.6 Instructions for use and handling
Andropatch may be discarded with household waste in a manner that avoids accidental contact by others.

Damaged systems should not be used.

The drug reservoir may be burst by excessive heat or pressure.

Administrative Data
7. MARKETING AUTHORISATION HOLDER
SmithKline Beecham plc
980 Great West Road
Brentford
Middlesex TW8 9GS
Trading as:
GlaxoSmithKline UK
Stockley Park West
Uxbridge
Middlesex UB11 1BT

8. MARKETING AUTHORISATION NUMBER(S)
PL 10592/0106

9. DATE OF FIRST AUTHORISATION/RENEWAL OF THE AUTHORISATION
26 August 2002

10. DATE OF REVISION OF THE TEXT
29 August 2002

11. Legal Status
POM

Anectine Injection

(GlaxoSmithKline UK)

1. NAME OF THE MEDICINAL PRODUCT
Anectine Injection.

2. QUALITATIVE AND QUANTITATIVE COMPOSITION
Suxamethonium Chloride Injection BP 100mg in 2ml.

3. PHARMACEUTICAL FORM
Injection.

4. CLINICAL PARTICULARS
4.1 Therapeutic indications
Used in anaesthesia as a muscle relaxant to facilitate endotracheal intubation, mechanical ventilation and a wide range of surgical and obstetric procedures.

It is also used to reduce the intensity of muscular contractions associated with pharmacologically or electrically-induced convulsions.

4.2 Posology and method of administration
Usually by bolus intravenous injection.

Adults: The dose is dependent on body weight, the degree of muscular relaxation required, the route of administration, and the response of individual patients.

To achieve endotracheal intubation Anectine is usually administered intravenously in a dose of 1 mg/kg. This dose will usually produce muscular relaxation in about 30 to 60 seconds and has a duration of action of about 2 to 6 minutes. Larger doses will produce more prolonged muscular relaxation, but doubling the dose does not necessarily double the duration of relaxation. Supplementary doses of Anectine of 50% to 100% of the initial dose administered at 5 to 10 minute intervals will maintain muscle relaxation during short surgical procedures performed under general anaesthesia.

For prolonged surgical procedures Anectine may be given by intravenous infusion as a 0.1% to 0.2% solution, diluted in 5% glucose solution or sterile isotonic saline solution, at a rate of 2.5 to 4 mg per minute. The infusion rate should be adjusted according to the response of individual patients.

The total dose of Anectine given by repeated intravenous injection or continuous infusion should not exceed 500 mg per hour.

Children: Infants and young children are more resistant to Anectine compared with adults.

The recommended intravenous dose of Anectine for neonates and infants is 2 mg/kg. A dose of 1 mg/kg in older children is recommended.

When Anectine is given as intravenous infusion in children, the dosage is as for adults with a proportionately lower initial infusion rate based on body weight.

Anectine may be given intramuscularly to infants at doses up to 4 to 5mg/kg and in older children up to 4 mg/kg. These doses produce muscular relaxation within about 3 minutes. A total dose of 150 mg should not be exceeded.

Use in the elderly: Dosage requirements of Anectine in the elderly are comparable to those for younger adults.

The elderly may be more susceptible to cardiac arrhythmias, especially if digitalis-like drugs are also being taken. See also '*Special warnings and precautions for use*'.

Instructions to open the ampoule

Ampoules are equipped with the OPC (One Point Cut) opening system and must be opened using the following instructions:

hold with the hand the bottom part of the ampoule as indicated in picture 1

put the other hand on the top of the ampoule positioning the thumb above the coloured point and press as indicated in picture 2

Picture 1

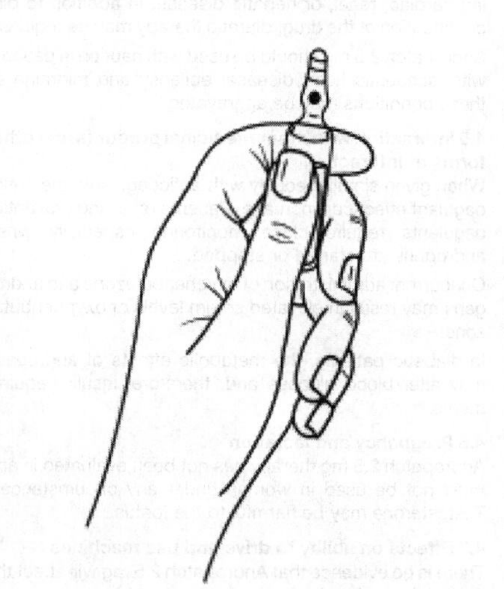

Picture 2

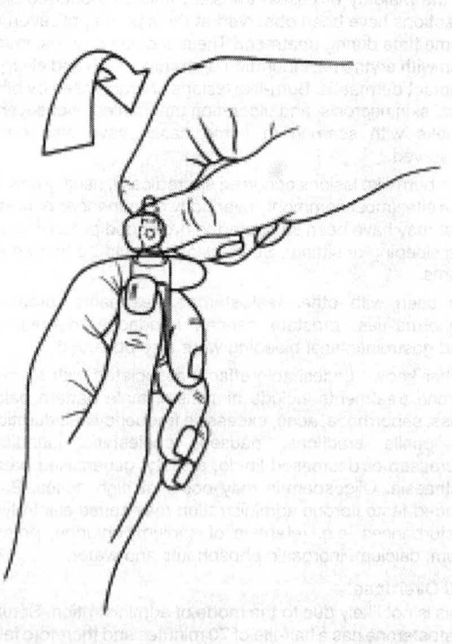

4.3 Contraindications
Anectine has no effect on the level of consciousness and should not be administered to a patient who is not fully anaesthetised.

Hypersensitivity to suxamethonium may exist in rare instances, and Anectine should not be administered to patients known to be hypersensitive to the drug.

As suxamethonium can act as a trigger of sustained myofibrillar contraction in susceptible individuals, Anectine is contra-indicated in patients with a personal or family history of malignant hyperthermia. If this condition occurs unexpectedly, all anaesthetic agents known to be associated with its development (including Anectine) must be immediately discontinued, and full supportive measures must be immediately instituted. Intravenous dantrolene sodium is the primary specific therapeutic drug and is recommended as soon as possible after the diagnosis is made.

Anectine is contra-indicated in patients known to have an inherited atypical plasma cholinesterase activity.

An acute transient rise in serum potassium often occurs following the administration of Anectine in normal individuals; the magnitude of this rise is of the order of 0.5 mmol/litre. In certain pathological states or conditions this increase in serum potassium following Anectine administration may be excessive and cause serious cardiac arrhythmias and cardiac arrest. For this reason the use of Anectine is contra-indicated in:

In patients recovering from major trauma or severe burns; the period of greatest risk of hyperkalaemia is from about 5 to 70 days after the injury and may be further prolonged if there is delayed healing due to persistent infection.

Patients with neurological deficits involving acute major muscle wasting (upper and/or lower motor neurone lesions); the potential for potassium release occurs within the first 6 months after the acute onset of the neurological deficit and correlates with the degree and extent of muscle paralysis. Patients who have been immobilised for prolonged periods of time may be at similar risk.

Patients with pre-existing hyperkalaemia. In the absence of hyperkalaemia and neuropathy, renal failure is not a contra-indication to the administration of a normal single dose of Anectine Injection, but multiple or large doses may cause clinically significant rises in serum potassium and should not be used.

Suxamethonium causes a significant transient rise in intra-ocular pressure, and should therefore not be used in the presence of open eye injuries or where an increase in intra-ocular pressure is undesirable unless the potential benefit of its use outweighs the potential risk to the eye.

Anectine should be avoided in patients with a personal or family history of congenital myotonic diseases such as myotonia congenita and dystrophia myotonica since its administration may on occasion be associated with severe myotonic spasms and rigidity.

Anectine should be avoided in patients with Duchenne muscular dystrophy since its administration may be associated with rigidity, hyperthermia, hyperkalaemia, myoglobinaemia, cardiac arrest, and post-operative respiratory depression.

4.4 Special warnings and special precautions for use

Anectine should be administered only by or under close supervision of an anaesthetist familiar with its action, characteristics and hazards, who is skilled in the management of artificial respiration and only where there are adequate facilities for immediate endotracheal intubation with administration of oxygen by intermittent positive pressure ventilation.

Anectine should not be mixed in the same syringe with any other agent, especially thiopentone.

During prolonged administration of Anectine, it is recommended that the patient is fully monitored with a peripheral nerve stimulator in order to avoid overdosage.

Anectine is rapidly hydrolysed by plasma cholinesterase which thereby limits the intensity and duration of the neuromuscular blockade.

Prolonged and intensified neuromuscular blockade following Anectine Injection may occur secondary to reduced plasma cholinesterase activity in the following states or pathological conditions: physiological variation as in pregnancy and the puerperium; genetically determined abnormal plasma cholinesterase; severe generalised tetanus, tuberculosis, other severe or chronic infections; following severe burns; chronic debilitating disease, malignancy, chronic anaemia and malnutrition; end-stage hepatic failure, acute or chronic renal failure; auto-immune diseases: myxoedema, collagen diseases; iatrogenic: following plasma exchange, plasmapheresis, cardiopulmonary bypass, and as a result of concomitant drug therapy (see *Interactions*).

If Anectine is given over a prolonged period, the characteristic depolarising neuromuscular (or Phase I) block may change to one with characteristics of a non-depolarising (or Phase II) block. Although the characteristics of a developing Phase II block resemble those of a true non-depolarising block, the former cannot always be fully or permanently reversed by anticholinesterase agents. When a Phase II block is fully established, its effects will then usually be fully reversible with standard doses of neostigmine accompanied by an anticholinergic agent.

Tachyphylaxis occurs after repeated administration of Anectine.

Caution should be exercised when using suxamethonium in children, since paediatric patients are more likely to have an undiagnosed myopathy or an unknown predisposition to malignant hyperthermia, which places them at increased risk of serious adverse events following suxamethonium.

In patients with severe sepsis, the potential for hyperkalaemia seems to be related to the severity and duration of infection.

It is inadvisable to administer Anectine to patients with advanced myasthenia gravis. Although these patients are resistant to suxamethonium they develop a state of Phase II block which can result in delayed recovery. Patients with myasthenic Eaton-Lambert syndrome are more sensitive than normal to Anectine, necessitating dosage reduction.

In healthy adults, Anectine occasionally causes a mild transient slowing of the heart rate on initial administration. Bradycardias are more commonly observed in children and on repeated administration of suxamethonium in both children and adults. Pre-treatment with intravenous atropine or glycopyrrolate significantly reduces the incidence and severity of suxamethonium-related bradycardia.

In the absence of pre-existing or evoked hyperkalaemia, ventricular arrhythmias are rarely seen following suxamethonium administration. Patients taking digitalis-like drugs are however more susceptible to such arrhythmias. The action of suxamethonium on the heart may cause changes in cardiac rhythm including cardiac arrest.

4.5 Interaction with other medicinal products and other forms of Interaction

Certain drugs or chemicals are known to reduce normal plasma cholinesterase activity and may therefore prolong the neuromuscular blocking effects of Anectine. These include: organophosphorous insecticides and metriphonate; ecothiopate eye drops; trimetaphan; specific anticholinesterase agents: neostigmine, pyridostigmine, physostigmine, edrophonium; tacrine hydrochloride; cytotoxic compounds: cyclophosphamide, mechlorethamine, triethylene-melamine, and thiotepa; psychiatric drugs: phenelzine, promazine and chlorpromazine; anaesthetic agents and drugs: ketamine, morphine and morphine antagonists, pethidine, pancuronium, propanidid.

Other drugs with potentially deleterious effects on plasma cholinesterase activity include aprotinin, diphenhydramine, promethazine, oestrogens, oxytocin, high-dose steroids, and oral contraceptives, terbutaline and metoclopramide.

Certain drugs or substances may enhance or prolong the neuromuscular effects of Anectine by mechanisms unrelated to plasma cholinesterase activity. These include: magnesium salts; lithium carbonate; azathioprine; quinine and chloroquinine; antibiotics such as the aminoglycosides, clindamycin and polymyxins; antiarrhythmic drugs: quinidine, procainamide, verapamil, beta-blockers, lignocaine and procaine; volatile inhalational anaesthetic agents: halothane, enflurane, desflurane, isoflurane, diethylether and methoxyflurane have little effect on the Phase I block of Anectine injection but will accelerate the onset and enhance the intensity of a Phase II suxamethonium-induced block.

Patients receiving digitalis-like drugs are more susceptible to the effects of suxamethonium-exacerbated hyperkalaemia.

4.6 Pregnancy and lactation

No studies of the effect of suxamethonium on female fertility or pregnancy have been performed.

Suxamethonium has no direct action on the uterus or other smooth muscle structures. In normal therapeutic doses it does not cross the placental barrier in sufficient amounts to affect the respiration of the infant.

The benefits of the use of suxamethonium as part of a rapid sequence induction for general anaesthesia normally outweigh the possible risk to the foetus.

Plasma cholinesterase levels fall during the first trimester of pregnancy to about 70 to 80% of their pre-pregnancy values; a further fall to about 60 to 70% of the pre-pregnancy levels occurs within 2 to 4 days after delivery. Plasma cholinesterase levels then increase to reach normal over the next 6 weeks. Consequently, a high proportion of pregnant and puerperal patients may exhibit mildly prolonged neuromuscular blockade following Anectine injection.

It is not known whether suxamethonium or its metabolites are excreted in human milk.

4.7 Effects on ability to drive and use machines

Not applicable.

4.8 Undesirable effects

Muscle pains are frequently experienced after administration of suxamethonium and most commonly occur in ambulatory patients undergoing short surgical procedures under general anaesthesia. There appears to be no direct connection between the degree of visible muscle fasciculation after Anectine administration and the incidence or severity of pain. The use of small doses of non-depolarising muscle relaxants given minutes before suxamethonium administration has been advocated for the reduction of incidence and severity of suxamethonium-associated muscle pains. This technique may require the use of doses of suxamethonium in excess of 1mg/kg to achieve satisfactory conditions for endotracheal intubation.

The following adverse reactions have been reported after administration of Anectine:

Cardiovascular: bradycardia, tachycardia, hypertension, hypotension, arrhythmias; (including ventricular arrhythmias) and cardiac arrest.

Respiratory: bronchospasm, prolonged respiratory depression and apnoea;

Musculoskeletal: muscle fasciculation, post-operative muscle pains, myoglobinaemia, myoglobinuria;

Other: anaphylactic reactions, hyperthermia, increased intra-ocular pressure, increased intragastric pressure, rash, skin flushing, excessive salivation.

There are case reports of hyperkalaemia-related cardiac arrests following the administration of suxamethonium to patients with congenital cerebral palsy, tetanus, Duchenne muscular dystrophy, and closed head injury.

4.9 Overdose

Apnoea and prolonged muscle paralysis are the main serious effects of overdosage. It is essential, therefore, to maintain the airway and adequate ventilation until spontaneous respiration occurs.

The decision to use neostigmine to reverse a Phase II suxamethonium-induced block depends on the judgement of the clinician in the individual case. Valuable information in regard to this decision will be gained by monitoring neuromuscular function. If neostigmine is used its administration should be accompanied by appropriate doses of an anticholinergic agent such as atropine.

5. PHARMACOLOGICAL PROPERTIES

5.1 Pharmacodynamic properties

Short-acting depolarising neuromuscular blocking agent.

5.2 Pharmacokinetic properties

None stated.

5.3 Preclinical safety data

Genotoxicity:-

No bacterial mutation assays have been conducted.

There are some data to suggest a weak clastogenic effect in mice, but not in patients who had received suxamethonium chloride.

Carcinogenicity:-

Carcinogenicity studies have not been performed.

Embryo-foetal Development:-

Animal reproduction studies have not been conducted with suxamethonium. It is also not known whether suxamethonium can affect reproductive capacity or cause foetal harm when administered to a pregnant woman.

6. PHARMACEUTICAL PARTICULARS

6.1 List of excipients

Water for Injections EP.

6.2 Incompatibilities

None known.

6.3 Shelf life

18 months.

6.4 Special precautions for storage

Store between 2 – 8 °C. Do not freeze. Keep in the outer carton.

6.5 Nature and contents of container

Neutral glass. 2ml ampoules.

6.6 Instructions for use and handling

For intravenous injection under medical direction.

Administrative Data

7. MARKETING AUTHORISATION HOLDER

The Wellcome Foundation Limited

Glaxo Wellcome House

Berkeley Avenue

Greenford UB6 ONN

trading as

GlaxoSmithKline UK

Stockley Park West

Uxbridge

Middlesex UB11 1BT

8. MARKETING AUTHORISATION NUMBER(S)

PL 00003/5203R

9. DATE OF FIRST AUTHORISATION/RENEWAL OF THE AUTHORISATION

25 July 1996

10. DATE OF REVISION OF THE TEXT

2 April 2003

11. Legal Status

POM

Anexate 500 micrograms/5ml Ampoule

(Roche Products Limited)

1. NAME OF THE MEDICINAL PRODUCT

Anexate 500 micrograms/5ml Ampoule

2. QUALITATIVE AND QUANTITATIVE COMPOSITION

Each 5ml ampoule contains 500 micrograms of flumazenil (100 micrograms per ml).

For excipients, *see 6.1.*

3. PHARMACEUTICAL FORM

Solution for Injection or infusion.

A clear, almost colourless, sterile aqueous solution.

4. CLINICAL PARTICULARS

4.1 Therapeutic indications

Anexate is indicated for the complete or partial reversal of the central sedative effects of benzodiazepines. It may therefore be used in anaesthesia and intensive care in the following situations:

Termination of general anaesthesia induced and/or maintained with benzodiazepines.

Reversal of benzodiazepine sedation in short diagnostic and therapeutic procedures.

For the specific reversal of the central effects of benzodiazepines, to allow return to spontaneous respiration and consciousness, in patients in intensive care.

4.2 Posology and method of administration

Anexate is for slow intravenous injection or infusion. It should only be administered under the supervision of an experienced physician.

Anexate may be used concurrently with other resuscitative procedures.

Adults

The recommended initial dose is 200 micrograms administered intravenously over 15 seconds. If the desired level of consciousness is not obtained within 60 seconds a further dose of 100 micrograms can be injected and repeated at 60-second intervals where necessary, up to a maximum total dose of 1mg or in intensive care situations, 2mg. The usual dose required is 300 - 600 micrograms.

If drowsiness recurs, an intravenous infusion of 100 - 400 micrograms per hour may be employed. The rate of infusion should be individually adjusted to achieve the desired level of arousal.

The individually titrated, slow injections or infusions of Anexate should not produce withdrawal symptoms, even in patients exposed to high doses of benzodiazepines and/or for long periods of time. If, however, unexpected signs of overstimulation occur, an individually titrated dose of diazepam (Valium) or midazolam (Hypnovel) should be given by slow intravenous injection.

If a significant improvement in consciousness or respiratory function is not obtained after repeated doses of Anexate, a non-benzodiazepine aetiology must be assumed.

Elderly

No specific data are available on the use of Anexate in the elderly, but it should be remembered that this population is more sensitive to the effects of benzodiazepines and should be treated with due caution.

Children

There are insufficient data to make dosage recommendations for Anexate in children. It should, therefore, be administered only if the potential benefits to the patient outweigh the possible risks.

Use in renal and hepatic insufficiency

No dosage adjustments are necessary in patients with renal impairment. However, since flumazenil is primarily metabolised in the liver, careful titration of dosage is recommended in patients with impaired hepatic function.

4.3 Contraindications

Anexate is contraindicated in patients with known hypersensitivity to flumazenil, benzodiazepines or any of the excipients.

Anexate is contraindicated in patients who have been given a benzodiazepine for control of a potentially life-threatening condition (e.g. control of intracranial pressure or status epilepticus).

In mixed intoxications with benzodiazepines and tricyclic and/or tetracyclic antidepressants, the toxicity of the antidepressants can be masked by protective benzodiazepine effects. In the presence of autonomic (anticholinergic), neurological (motor abnormalities) or cardiovascular symptoms of severe intoxication with tricyclics/tetracyclics, Anexate should not be used to reverse benzodiazepine effects.

4.4 Special warnings and special precautions for use

In view of the short duration of action of Anexate and the possible need for repeat doses, the patient should remain under close observation until all possible central benzodiazepine effects have subsided.

The use of Anexate is not recommended in epileptic patients who have been receiving benzodiazepine treatment for a prolonged period. Although Anexate exerts a slight intrinsic anticonvulsant effect, its abrupt suppression of the protective effect of a benzodiazepine agonist can give rise to convulsions in epileptic patients.

Anexate should be used with caution in patients with head injury as it may be capable of precipitating convulsions or altering cerebral blood flow in patients receiving benzodiazepines.

Benzodiazepines have a dependence potential when used chronically. Symptoms such as depression, nervousness, rebound insomnia, irritability, sweating and diarrhoea may arise following abrupt cessation of benzodiazepines in patients treated with high doses and/or for prolonged periods of time. Rapid injection of Anexate in such patients may trigger these withdrawal symptoms, even in patients who stopped taking the benzodiazepine in the weeks preceding Anexate administration (depending on the half-life of the benzodiazepine used) and should therefore be avoided. There is also a possibility of mild and transient withdrawal reactions occurring even after a short period of administration of benzodiazepines.

When Anexate is used with neuromuscular blocking agents, it should not be injected until the effects of neuromuscular blockade have been fully reversed.

In high-risk patients, the advantages of counteracting the central nervous system depression associated with benzodiazepines should be weighed against the drawbacks of rapid awakening.

The dosage of Anexate should be adjusted individually to the needs of patients suffering from pre-operative anxiety or having a history of chronic or episodic anxiety. In anxious patients, particularly those with coronary heart disease, it is preferable to maintain a degree of sedation throughout the early post-operative period rather than bring about complete arousal.

The pain felt by patients in the post-operative period must be taken into account. Following a major intervention, it is preferable to maintain a moderate degree of sedation.

Anexate is not recommended either as a treatment for benzodiazepine dependence or for the management of protracted benzodiazepine abstinence syndromes.

4.5 Interaction with other medicinal products and other forms of Interaction

Anexate blocks the central effects of benzodiazepines by competitive interaction at the receptor level; the effects of non-benzodiazepines acting via the benzodiazepine receptor, such as zopiclone, are also blocked by Anexate. However, Anexate is ineffective when unconsciousness is due to other substances.

Interaction with other central nervous system depressants has not been observed. However, particular caution is necessary when using Anexate in cases of intentional overdosage since the toxic effects of other psychotropic drugs (especially tricyclic antidepressants) taken concurrently may increase with the subsidence of the benzodiazepine effect.

The pharmacokinetics of benzodiazepines are unaltered in the presence of Anexate and vice versa.

4.6 Pregnancy and lactation

Like other benzodiazepine compounds, Anexate is expected to cross the placenta and to enter into breast milk, although the total quantities involved would be small. There has been little human usage but animal studies have shown no teratogenic potential. The established medical principle of only administering drugs in early pregnancy when considered absolutely necessary should therefore be observed.

Emergency use of Anexate during lactation is not contraindicated.

4.7 Effects on ability to drive and use machines

Patients who have received Anexate to reverse the effects of benzodiazepine sedation should be warned not to drive, to operate machinery or to engage in any other physically or mentally demanding activity for at least 24 hours, since the effect of the benzodiazepine may return.

4.8 Undesirable effects

Anexate is generally well tolerated. In post-operative use, nausea and/or vomiting are occasionally observed, particularly if opiates have also been employed. Flushing has also been noted. If patients are awakened too rapidly, they may become agitated, anxious or fearful. Very rarely, seizures have been reported, particularly in patients known to suffer from epilepsy or severe hepatic impairment, particularly after long-term treatment with benzodiazepines or in cases of mixed drug overdose. Transient increases in blood pressure and heart rate may occur on awakening in intensive care patients.

Any side-effects associated with Anexate usually subside rapidly without the need for special treatment.

Excessive and/or rapidly injected doses of Anexate may induce benzodiazepine withdrawal symptoms such as anxiety attacks, tachycardia, dizziness and sweating in patients on long-term and/or high dose benzodiazepine treatment ending at any time within the weeks preceding Anexate administration (depending on the half-life of the benzodiazepine used). Such symptoms may be treated by slow intravenous injection of diazepam or midazolam (see section *4.2 Posology and method of administration*). There is also a possibility of mild and transient withdrawal reactions occurring even after a short period of administration of benzodiazepines.

Anexate has been reported to provoke panic attacks in patients with a history of panic disorders.

Hypersensitivity reactions (including anaphylaxis) have occurred very rarely.

4.9 Overdose

Even when given intravenously at doses of 100mg, no symptoms of overdosage attributable to Anexate have been observed.

5. PHARMACOLOGICAL PROPERTIES

5.1 Pharmacodynamic properties

Anexate, an imidazobenzodiazepine, is a specific competitive inhibitor of substances which act via the benzodiazepine receptors, specifically blocking their central effects. The hypnotic-sedative effects of the agonist are rapidly reversed by Anexate and may then reappear gradually within a few hours, depending on the half-life and dose ratio of the agonist and antagonist.

5.2 Pharmacokinetic properties

The pharmacokinetics of flumazenil are dose-proportional within and above the therapeutic range (up to 100mg).

Distribution

Flumazenil, a weak lipophilic base, is about 50% bound to plasma proteins. Albumin accounts for two thirds of plasma protein binding. Flumazenil is extensively distributed in the extravascular space. Plasma concentrations of flumazenil decrease with a half-life of 4 - 11 minutes during the distribution phase. The volume of distribution at steady state is 0.9 – 1.1 l/kg.

Metabolism

Flumazenil is extensively metabolised in the liver. The carboxylic acid metabolite is the main metabolite in plasma (free form) and urine (free form and its glucuronide). This main metabolite showed no benzodiazepine agonist or antagonist activity in pharmacological tests.

Elimination

Flumazenil is almost completely (99%) eliminated by non-renal routes. Practically no unchanged flumazenil is excreted in the urine, suggesting complete metabolic degradation of the drug. Elimination of radiolabelled drug is essentially complete within 72 hours, with 90 - 95% of the radioactivity appearing in urine and 5 - 10% in the faeces. Elimination is rapid, as shown by a short elimination half-life of 40 - 80 minutes. The total plasma clearance of flumazenil is 0.8 – 1.0 l/hr/kg and can be attributed almost entirely to hepatic clearance.

Ingestion of food during an intravenous infusion of flumazenil results in a 50% increase in clearance, most likely due to the increased hepatic blood flow that accompanies a meal.

Pharmacokinetics in special populations

In patients with impaired liver function, the elimination half-life of flumazenil is longer and the total body clearance lower than in healthy subjects. The pharmacokinetics of flumazenil are not significantly affected in the elderly, by gender, haemodialysis or renal failure.

5.3 Preclinical safety data

There are no preclinical data of relevance to the prescriber which are additional to that already included in other sections of the SPC.

6. PHARMACEUTICAL PARTICULARS

6.1 List of excipients

Disodium Edetate

Glacial Acetic Acid

Sodium Chloride

Sodium Hydroxide

Water for Injections

6.2 Incompatibilities

None stated.

6.3 Shelf life

Unopened: 5 years.

The product should be used immediately after opening.

6.4 Special precautions for storage

Do not store above 30°C.

6.5 Nature and contents of container

Clear glass 5ml ampoules. Cartons of 5 or 25.

6.6 Instructions for use and handling

Anexate ampoule solution may be diluted with Sodium Chloride Intravenous Infusion BP or Dextrose 5% Intravenous Infusion BP. Chemical and physical stability has been demonstrated for 24 hours at room temperature.

Anexate infusion should be administered within 3 hours of preparation.

No preparations other than those recommended should be added to the Anexate ampoule or mixed with the Anexate infusion solution.

For single use only. Discard any unused contents.

7. MARKETING AUTHORISATION HOLDER

Roche Products Limited, 40 Broadwater Road, Welwyn Garden City, Hertfordshire, AL7 3AY.

8. MARKETING AUTHORISATION NUMBER(S)

PL 0031/0228

9. DATE OF FIRST AUTHORISATION/RENEWAL OF THE AUTHORISATION

19 July 1999

10. DATE OF REVISION OF THE TEXT

July 2005

Anexate, Hypnovel and Valium are registered trade marks

Angeliq film-coated tablets

(Schering Health Care Limited)

1. NAME OF THE MEDICINAL PRODUCT

▼Angeliq film-coated tablets

2. QUALITATIVE AND QUANTITATIVE COMPOSITION

Each film-coated tablet contains: 1 mg estradiol (as estradiol hemihydrate) and 2mg drospirenone

For excipients, see 6.1

3. PHARMACEUTICAL FORM

Film-coated tablet

Medium red, round tablet with convex faces, one side embossed with the letters DL in a regular hexagon.

4. CLINICAL PARTICULARS

4.1 Therapeutic indications

Hormone replacement therapy for oestrogen deficiency symptoms in postmenopausal women more than 1 year post menopause.

Prevention of osteoporosis in postmenopausal women at high risk of future fractures who are intolerant of, or contra-indicated for, other medicinal products approved for the prevention of osteoporosis.

(See also Section 4.4)

The experience treating women older than 65 years is limited.

4.2 Posology and method of administration

Women who do not take hormone replacement therapy (HRT) or women who change from another continuous combined product may start treatment at any time. Women changing from a cyclic, sequential combined HRT regimen, treatment should begin the day following completion of the prior regimen.

• Dosage

One tablet is taken daily. Each blister pack is for 28 days of treatment.

• Administration

The tablets are to be swallowed whole with some liquid irrespective of food intake. Treatment is continuous, which means that the next pack follows immediately without a break. The tablets should preferably be taken at the same time every day. If a tablet is forgotten it should be taken as soon as possible. If more than 24 hours have elapsed no extra tablet needs to be taken. If several tablets are forgotten, bleeding may occur.

For treatment of postmenopausal symptoms, the lowest effective dose should be used.

For initiation and continuation of treatment of postmenopausal symptoms, the lowest effective dose for the shortest duration (see also Section 4.4) should be used.

4.3 Contraindications

• Undiagnosed genital bleeding

• Known past or suspected cancer of the breast

• Known or suspected oestrogen-dependent malignant tumours (e.g. endometrial cancer)

• Untreated endometrial hyperplasia

• Previous idiopathic or current venous thromboembolism (deep venous thrombosis, pulmonary embolism)

• Active or recent arterial thromboembolic disease (e.g. angina, myocardial infarction)

• Acute liver disease, or a history of liver disease as long as liver function tests have failed to return to normal

• Porphyria

• Severe renal insufficiency or acute renal failure

• Known hypersensitivity to the active substances or to any of the excipients

4.4 Special warnings and special precautions for use

For the treatment of postmenopausal symptoms, HRT should only be initiated for symptoms that adversely affect quality of life. In all cases, a careful appraisal of the risks and benefits should be undertaken at least annually and HRT should only be continued as long as the benefit outweighs the risk.

Medical examination/follow-up

Before initiating or reinstituting HRT, a complete personal and family medical history should be taken. Physical (including pelvic and breast) examination should be guided by this and by the contraindications and warnings for use. During treatment, periodic check-ups are recommended of a frequency and nature adapted to the individual woman. Women should be advised what changes in their breasts should be reported to their doctor or nurse. Investigations, including mammography, should be carried out in accordance with currently accepted screening practices, modified to the clinical needs of the individual.

Conditions which need supervision

If any of the following conditions are present, have occurred previously, and/or have been aggravated during pregnancy or previous hormone treatment, the patient should be closely supervised. It should be taken into account that these conditions may recur or be aggravated during treatment with Angeliq, in particular:

- Leiomyoma (uterine fibroids) or endometriosis
- A history of, or risk factors for, thromboembolic disorders (see below)
- Risk factors for oestrogen dependent tumours, e.g. 1st degree heredity for breast cancer
- Hypertension
- Liver disorders (e.g. liver adenoma)
- Diabetes mellitus with or without vascular involvement
- Cholelithiasis
- Migraine or (severe) headache
- Systemic lupus erythematosus.
- A history of endometrial hyperplasia (see below)
- Epilepsy
- Asthma
- Otosclerosis

Reasons for immediate withdrawal of therapy:

-Therapy should be discontinued in case a contraindication is discovered and in the following situations:

- Jaundice or deterioration in liver function
- Significant increase in blood pressure
- New onset of migraine-type headache
- Pregnancy

Endometrial hyperplasia

• The risk of endometrial hyperplasia and carcinoma is increased when oestrogens are administered alone for prolonged periods (see section 4.8). The addition of a progestogen for at least 12 days per cycle in non-hysterectomised women greatly reduces this risk.

• Break-through bleeding and spotting may occur during the first months of treatment. If break-through bleeding or spotting appears after some time on therapy, or continues after treatment has been discontinued, the reason should be investigated, which may include endometrial biopsy to exclude endometrial malignancy

Breast cancer

• A randomised placebo-controlled trial, the Women's Health Initiative study (WHI), and epidemiological studies, including the Million Women Study (MWS), have reported an increased risk of breast cancer in women taking oestrogens, oestrogen-progestogen combinations or tibolone for HRT for several years (see Section 4.8). For all HRT, an excess risk becomes apparent within a few years of use and increases with duration of intake but returns to baseline within a few (at most five) years after stopping treatment.

• In the MWS, the relative risk of breast cancer with conjugated equine oestrogens (CEE) or estradiol (E2) was greater when a progestogen was added, either sequentially or continuously, and regardless of type of progestogen. There was no evidence of a difference in risk between the different routes of administration.

• In the WHI study, the continuous combined conjugated equine oestrogen and medroxyprogesterone acetate (CEE + MPA) product used was associated with breast cancers that were slightly larger in size and more frequently had local lymph node metastases compared to placebo.

• HRT, especially oestrogen-progestogen combined treatment, increases the density of mammographic images which may adversely affect the radiological detection of breast cancer.

Venous thromboembolism

• HRT is associated with a higher relative risk of developing venous thromboembolism (VTE), i.e. deep vein thrombosis or pulmonary embolism. One randomised controlled trial and epidemiological studies found a two - to threefold higher risk for users compared with non-users. For non-users it is estimated that the number of cases of VTE that will occur over a 5 year period is about 3 per 1000 women aged 50-59 years and 8 per 1000 women aged between 60-69 years. It is estimated that in healthy women who use HRT for 5 years, the number of additional cases of VTE over a 5 year period will be between 2 and 6 (best estimate=4) per 1000 women aged 50-59 years and between 5 and 15 (best estimate=9) per 1000 women aged 60-69 years. The occurrence of such an event is more likely in the first year of HRT than later.

• Generally recognised risk factors for VTE include a personal history or family history, severe obesity (BMI > 30 kg/m ^{2}) and systemic lupus erythematosus (SLE). There is no consensus about the possible role of varicose veins in VTE.

• Patients with a history of VTE or known thrombophilic states have an increased risk of VTE. HRT may add to this risk. Personal or strong family history of thromboembolism or recurrent spontaneous abortion should be investigated in order to exclude a thrombophilic predisposition. Until a thorough evaluation of thrombophilic factors has been made or anticoagulant treatment initiated, use of HRT in such patients should be viewed as contraindicated. Those women already on anticoagulant treatment require careful consideration of the benefit-risk of use of HRT.

• The risk of VTE may be temporarily increased with prolonged immobilisation, major trauma or major surgery. As in all postoperative patients, scrupulous attention should be given to prophylactic measures to prevent VTE following surgery. Where prolonged immobilisation is liable to follow elective surgery, particularly abdominal or orthopaedic surgery to the lower limbs, consideration should be given to temporarily stopping HRT 4 to 6 weeks earlier, if possible. Treatment should not be restarted until the woman is completely mobilised.

• If VTE develops after initiating therapy, the drug should be discontinued. Patients should be told to contact their doctors immediately when they are aware of a potential thromboembolic symptom (e.g., painful swelling of a leg, sudden pain in the chest, dyspnoea).

Coronary artery disease (CAD)

• There is no evidence from randomised controlled trials of cardiovascular benefit with continuous combined conjugated oestrogens and medroxyprogesterone acetate (MPA). Two large clinical trials (WHI and HERS i.e. Heart and Estrogen/progestin Replacement Study) showed a possible increased risk of cardiovascular morbidity in the first year of use and no overall benefit. For other HRT products there are only limited data from randomised controlled trials examining effects in cardiovascular morbidity or mortality. Therefore, it is uncertain whether these findings also extend to other HRT products.

Stroke

• One large randomised clinical trial (WHI-trial) found, as a secondary outcome, an increased risk of ischaemic stroke in healthy women during treatment with continuous combined conjugated oestrogens and MPA. For women who do not use HRT, it is estimated that the number of cases of stroke that will occur over a 5 year period is about 3 per 1000 women aged 50-59 years and 11 per 1000 women aged 60-69 years. It is estimated that for women who use conjugated oestrogens and MPA for 5 years, the number of additional cases will be between 0 and 3 (best estimate=1) per 1000 users aged 50-59 years and between 1 and 9 (best estimate=4) per 1000 users aged 60-69 years. It is unknown whether the increased risk also extends to other HRT products.

Ovarian cancer

• Long-term (at least 5-10 years) use of oestrogen-only HRT products in hysterectomised women has been associated with an increased risk of ovarian cancer in some epidemiological studies. It is uncertain whether long-term use of combined HRT confers a different risk than oestrogen-only products.

Other conditions

• Oestrogens may cause fluid retention, and therefore patients with cardiac or renal dysfunction should be carefully observed.

• Women with pre-existing hypertriglyceridaemia should be followed closely during oestrogen replacement or hormone replacement therapy, since rare cases of large increases of plasma triglycerides leading to pancreatitis have been reported with oestrogen therapy in this condition.

• Oestrogens increase thyroid binding globulin (TBG), leading to increased circulating total thyroid hormone, as measured by protein-bound iodine (PBI), T4 levels (by column or by radioimmunoassay) or T3 levels (by radioimmunoassay). T3 resin uptake is decreased, reflecting the elevated TBG. Free T4 and free T3 concentrations are unaltered. Other binding proteins may be elevated in serum, ie. corticoid binding globulin (CBG), sex-hormone-binding globulin (SHBG) leading to increased circulating corticosteroids and sex steroids, respectively. Free or biological active hormone concentrations are unchanged. Other plasma proteins may be increased (angiotensinogen/renin substrate, alpha-I-antitrypsin, ceruloplasmin).

• There is no conclusive evidence for improvement of cognitive function. There is some evidence from the WHI trial of increased risk of probable dementia in women who start using continuous combined CEE and MPA after the age of 65. It is unknown whether the findings apply to younger post-menopausal women or other HRT products.

• The progestin component in Angeliq is an aldosterone antagonist with potassium sparing properties. In most cases, no increase of potassium levels is to be expected. In a clinical study, however in some patients with mild or moderate renal impairment and concomitant use of potassium-sparing medicinal products serum potassium levels slightly, but not significantly, increased during drospirenone intake. Potassium excretion may be decreased in patients presenting with renal insufficiency and a pretreatment serum potassium in the upper reference range, particularly during concomitant use of potassium sparing medicinal products. Further checks of serum potassium during the first treatment cycle are recommended in these patients. See also section 4.5.

• Chloasma may occasionally occur, especially in women with a history of chloasma gravidarum. Women with a tendency to chloasma should avoid exposure to the sun or ultraviolet radiation whilst taking HRT.

4.5 Interaction with other medicinal products and other forms of Interaction

• Effects of other medicinal products on Angeliq

The metabolism of oestrogens [and progestogens] may be increased by concomitant use of substances known to induce drug-metabolising enzymes, specifically cytochrome P450 enzymes, such as anticonvulsants (e.g. phenobarbital, phenytoin, carbamazepine) and anti-infectives (e.g. rifampicin, rifabutin, nevirapine, efavirenz).

Ritonavir and nelfinavir, although known as strong inhibitors, by contrast exhibit inducing properties when used concomitantly with steroid hormones. Herbal preparations containing St. John's wort (Hypericum perforatum) may induce the metabolism of oestrogens [and progestogens].

Clinically, an increased metabolism of oestrogens and progestogens may lead to decreased effect and changes in the uterine bleeding profile.

The main metabolites of drospirenone are generated without involvement of the cytochrome P450 system. Inhibitors of this enzyme system are therefore unlikely to influence the metabolism of drospirenone.

• Interaction of Angeliq with other medicinal products

Based on *in vitro* enzymatic inhibition studies and on an *in vivo* drug-drug interaction study in female volunteers using omeprazole as marker substrate, drospirenone shows no potential to increase plasma levels of concomitantly administered drugs.

• In patients without renal insufficiency, the concomitant use of drospirenone and ACE-inhibitors or NSAIDs did not show a significant effect on serum potassium. Nevertheless, concomitant use of Angeliq with aldosterone antagonists or potassium-sparing diuretics has not been studied. In this case, serum potassium should be tested during the first treatment cycle. See also section 4.4.

4.6 Pregnancy and lactation

• Pregnancy

Angeliq is not indicated during pregnancy. If pregnancy occurs during medication with Angeliq, treatment should be discontinued promptly. No clinical data on exposed pregnancies are available for drospirenone. Animal studies have shown reproductive toxicity (see Section 5.3). The potential risk for humans is unknown. The results of most epidemiological studies to date relevant to inadvertent foetal exposure to combinations of oestrogens with other progestogens have not indicated a teratogenic or foetotoxic effect.

• Lactation

Angeliq is not indicated during lactation.

4.7 Effects on ability to drive and use machines

No effects on the ability to drive and use machines have been observed.

4.8 Undesirable effects

The table below (HARTS Body System and Dictionary Term) attributes frequencies to the undesirable effects of Angeliq. These frequencies are based on the frequencies of adverse events, which were recorded in 4 phase III clinical studies (n = 1532 women at risk) and considered at least possibly related to treatment with 1 mg E2 in combination with 1, 2, or 3 mg DRSP.

During treatment, breakthrough bleeding and spotting is very common. The frequency of bleeding decreases during the first few months of treatment. For further information on bleeding pattern see section 5.1. Breast pain was a very common symptom, reported in approximately one out of five women.

(see Table 1)

According to evidence from a large number of epidemiological studies and one randomised placebo-controlled trial, the Women's Health Initiative (WHI), the overall risk of breast cancer increases with increasing duration of HRT use in current or recent HRT users.

For *oestrogen-only* HRT, estimates of relative risk (RR) from a reanalysis of original data from 51 epidemiological studies (in which >80% of HRT use was oestrogen-only HRT) and from the epidemiological Million Women Study (MWS) are similar at 1.35 (95% CI 1.21 – 1.49) and 1.30 (95% CI 1.21 – 1.40), respectively.

For *oestrogen plus progestogen* combined HRT, several epidemiological studies have reported an overall higher risk for breast cancer than with oestrogens alone.

The MWS reported that, compared to never users, the use of various types of oestrogen-progestogen combined HRT was associated with a higher risk of breast cancer (RR = 2.00, 95% CI: 1.88 – 2.12) than use of oestrogens alone (RR = 1.30, 95% CI: 1.21 – 1.40) or use of tibolone (RR = 1.45, 95% CI: 1.25 – 1.68).

The WHI trial reported a risk estimate of 1.24 (95% CI: 1.01 – 1.54) after 5.6 years of use of oestrogen-progestogen combined HRT (CEE + MPA) in all users compared with placebo.

The absolute risks calculated from the MWS and the WHI trial are presented below:

The MWS has estimated, from the known average incidence of breast cancer in developed countries, that:

• For women not using HRT, about 32 in every 1000 are expected to have breast cancer diagnosed between the ages of 50 and 64 years.

• For 1000 current or recent users of HRT, the number of additional cases during the corresponding period will be . . .

• *For users of oestrogen-only replacement therapy:*

• Between 0 and 3 (best estimate = 1.5) for 5 years use

• Between 3 and 7 (best estimate = 5) for 10 years use

• *For users of oestrogen plus progestogen combined HRT:*

• Between 5 and 7 (best estimate = 6) for 5 years use

• Between 18 and 20 (best estimate = 19) for 10 years use

The WHI trial estimated that after 5.6 years of follow-up of women between the ages of 50 and 79 years, an *additional* 8 cases of invasive breast cancer would be due to *oestrogen-progestogen combined* HRT (CEE + MPA) per 10,000 women years.

According to calculations from the trial data, it is estimated that:

• *For 1000 women in the placebo group,*

• About 16 cases of invasive breast cancer would be diagnosed in 5 years.

• *For 1000 women who used oestrogen + progestogen combined HRT (CEE + MPA),* the number of additional cases would be,

• Between 0 and 9 (best estimate = 4) for 5 years use.

The number of additional cases of breast cancer in women who use HRT is broadly similar for women who start HRT irrespective of age at start of use (between the ages of 45-65) (see section 4.4).

Endometrial cancer

In women with an intact uterus, the risk of endometrial hyperplasia and endometrial cancer increases with increasing duration of use of unopposed oestrogens.

According to data from epidemiological studies, the best estimate of the risk is that for women not using HRT, about 5 in every 1000 are expected to have endometrial cancer diagnosed between the ages of 50 and 65. Depending on the duration of treatment and oestrogen dose, the reported increase in endometrial cancer risk among unopposed oestrogen users varies from 2-to 12-fold greater compared with non-users. Adding a progestogen to oestrogen-only therapy greatly reduces this increased risk.

Other adverse reactions have been reported in association with oestrogen/progestogen treatment:

- Oestrogen-dependent neoplasms benign and malignant, e.g. endometrial cancer.
- Venous thromboembolism, i.e. deep leg or pelvic venous thrombosis and pulmonary embolism, is more frequent among hormone replacement therapy users than among non-users. For further information, see section 4.3 Contra-indications and 4.4 Special warning and precautions for use.
- Myocardial infarction and stroke
- Gall bladder disease.
- Skin and subcutaneous disorders: chloasma, erythema multiforme, erythema nodosum, vascular purpura.
- Probable dementia (see section 4.4)

4.9 Overdose

In clinical studies in male volunteers doses up to 100 mg of drospirenone were well tolerated. Based on general experience with combined oral contraceptives, symptoms that may possibly occur are nausea and vomiting and – in young girls and some women – vaginal bleeding. There are no specific antidotes, and, therefore, treatment should be symptomatic.

5. PHARMACOLOGICAL PROPERTIES

5.1 Pharmacodynamic properties

Pharmacotherapeutic group: Progestogens and oestrogens, fixed combination; ATC code G 03F A

Estradiol

Angeliq contains synthetic 17β-estradiol, which is chemically and biologically identical to endogenous human estradiol. It substitutes for the loss of oestrogen production in menopausal women, and alleviates menopausal symptoms. Oestrogens prevent bone loss following menopause or ovariectomy.

Drospirenone

Drospirenone is a synthetic progestogen.

As oestrogens promote the growth of the endometrium, unopposed oestrogens increase the risk of endometrial hyperplasia and cancer. The addition of a progestogen reduces, but does not eliminate the oestrogen-induced risk of endometrial hyperplasia in non-hysterectomised women.

Drospirenone displays aldosterone antagonistic activity. Therefore, increases in sodium and water excretion and decreases in potassium excretion may be observed.

In animal studies, drospirenone has no oestrogenic, glucocorticoid or antiglucocorticoid activity.

Clinical trial information

• **Relief of oestrogen-deficiency symptoms and bleeding patterns**

Relief of menopausal symptoms was achieved during the first few weeks of treatment.

Amenorrhea was seen in 73 % of the women during months 10-12 of treatment. Break through bleeding and / or spotting appeared in 59 % of the women during the first three months of treatment and in 27% during months 10-12 of treatment.

• **Prevention of osteoporosis**

Oestrogen deficiency at menopause is associated with an increasing bone turnover and decline in bone mass. The effect of oestrogen on the bone mineral density is dose-dependent. Protection appears to be effective as long as treatment is continued. After discontinuation of HRT, bone mass is lost at a rate similar to that in untreated women.

Evidence from WHI trial and meta-analysed trials shows that current use of HRT, alone or in combination with a progestogen – given to predominantly healthy women – reduces the risk of hip, vertebral, and other osteoporotic fractures. HRT may also prevent fractures in women with low bone density and/or established osteoporosis, but the evidence for that is limited.

After 2 years of treatment with Angeliq, the increase in hip bone mineral density (BMD) was 3.96 +/- 3.15% (mean +/- SD) in osteopenic patients and 2.78 +/- 1.89 % (mean +/- SD) in non-osteopenic patients. The percentage of women who maintained or gained BMD in hip zone during treatment was 94.4 % in osteopenic patients and 96.4 % in non-osteopenic patients.

Angeliq also had an effect on lumbar spine BMD. The increase after 2 years was 5.61 +/- 3.34 % (mean +/- SD) in osteopenic women and 4.92+/- 3.02 % (mean +/- SD) in non-osteopenic women. The percentage of osteopenic women who maintained or gained BMD in lumbar zone during treatment was 100%, whereas this percentage was 96.4 % in non-osteopenic women.

Table 1

Organ system	Common (≥ 1/100, < 1/10)	Uncommon (≥ 1/1000, < 1/100)
BODY AS A WHOLE	Abdominal pain or bloating, asthenia, pain in extremity.	Pain in back or pelvis, chills, malaise
CARDIOVASCULAR SYSTEM	-	Migraine, hypertension, chest pain, palpitations, varicose veins, venous thrombosis, superficial thrombophlebitis, vasodilatation.
DIGESTIVE	Nausea	Gastrointestinal disorder, increased appetite, abnormal liver function tests.
METABOLIC AND NUTRITIONAL	-	Generalised or localised oedema, weight gain, hyperlipaemia.
MUSCULOSKELETAL SYSTEM	-	Muscle cramps, arthralgia.
NERVOUS SYSTEM	Headache, mood swings, hot flushes, nervousness.	Insomnia, dizziness, decreased libido, impaired concentration, paraesthesia, increased sweating, anxiety, dry mouth, vertigo.
RESPIRATORY SYSTEM	-	Dyspnoea
SKIN and APPENDAGES	-	Alopecia, skin or hair disorder, hirsutism
SPECIAL SENSES	-	Taste disturbance
UROGENITAL AND BREAST	Uterine fibroids enlarged, cervix neoplasm, leukorrhea, breakthrough bleeding, benign breast neoplasms, breast enlargement.	Vulvovaginitis, endometrial or cervical disorder, dysmenorrhoea, ovarian cyst, urinary tract infections or incontinence, breast engorgement.

5.2 Pharmacokinetic properties
DROSPIRENONE

• Absorption

After oral administration drospirenone is rapidly and completely absorbed. With a single administration, peak serum levels of approx. 21.9 ng/ml are reached about 1 hour after ingestion. After repeated administration, a maximum steady-state concentration of 35.9 ng/ml is reached after about 10 days. The absolute bioavailability is between 76 and 85%. Concomitant ingestion of food had no influence on the bioavailability.

• Distribution

After oral administration, serum drospirenone levels decrease in two phases which are characterised by a mean terminal half-life of about 35 – 39 h. Drospirenone is bound to serum albumin and does not bind to sex hormone binding globulin (SHBG) or corticoid binding globulin (CBG). Only 3 - 5 % of the total serum drug concentrations are present as free steroid. The mean apparent volume of distribution of drospirenone is 3.7 - 4.2 l/kg.

• Metabolism

Drospirenone is extensively metabolised after oral administration. The major metabolites in the plasma are the acid form of drospirenone, generated by opening of the lactone ring, and the 4,5-dihydro-drospirenone-3-sulphate, both of which are formed without involvement of the P450 system. Both major metabolites are pharmacologically inactive. Drospirenone is metabolised to a minor extent by cytochrome P450 3A4 based on *in vitro* data. In vitro and clinical studies do not indicate an inhibitory effect of DRSP on CYP enzymes after administration of Angeliq.

• Elimination

The metabolic clearance rate of drospirenone in serum is 1.2 - 1.5 ml/min/kg showing an intersubject variability of about 25 %. Drospirenone is excreted only in trace amounts in unchanged form. The metabolites of drospirenone are excreted with the faeces and urine at an excretion ratio of about 1.2 to 1.4. The half-life of metabolite excretion with the urine and faeces is about 40 h.

• Steady-state conditions and linearity

Following daily oral administration of Angeliq, drospirenone concentrations reached a steady-state after about 10 days. Serum drospirenone levels accumulated by a factor of about 2 to 3 as a consequence of the ratio of terminal half-life and dosing interval. At steady-state, mean serum levels of drospirenone fluctuate in the range of 14 – 36 ng/ml after administration of Angeliq. Pharmacokinetics of drospirenone are dose-proportional within the dose range of 1 to 4 mg.

ESTRADIOL

• Absorption

Following oral administration, estradiol is rapidly and completely absorbed. During the absorption and the first liver passage, estradiol undergoes extensive metabolism, thus reducing the absolute bioavailability of oestrogen after oral administration to about 5% of the dose. Maximum concentrations of about 22 pg/ml were reached 6-8 h after single oral administration of Angeliq. The intake of food had no influence on the bioavailability of estradiol as compared to drug intake on an empty stomach.

• Distribution

Following oral administration of Angeliq only gradually changing serum levels of estradiol are observed within an administration interval of 24 hours. Because of the large circulating pool of oestrogen sulphates and glucuronides on the one hand and the enterohepatic recirculation on the other hand, the terminal half-life of estradiol represents a composite parameter that is dependent on all of these processes and is in the range of about 13-20 h after oral administration.

Estradiol is bound non-specifically to serum albumin and specifically to SHBG. Only about 1-2 % of the circulating estradiol is present as free steroid, 40-45 % is bound to SHBG. The apparent volume of distribution of estradiol after single intravenous administration is about 1 l/kg.

• Metabolism

Estradiol is rapidly metabolised, and besides estrone and estrone sulphate, a large number of other metabolites and conjugates are formed. Estrone and estriol are known as pharmacologically active metabolites of estradiol; only estrone occurs in relevant concentrations in plasma. Estrone reaches about 6-fold higher serum levels than estradiol. The serum levels of the estrone conjugates are about 26 times higher than the corresponding concentrations of free estrone.

• Elimination

The metabolic clearance has been found to be about 30 ml/min/kg. The metabolites of estradiol are excreted via urine and bile with a half-life of about 1 day.

• Steady-state conditions

Following daily oral administration of Angeliq, estradiol concentrations reached a steady-state after about five days. Serum estradiol levels accumulate approx. 2-fold. Orally administered estradiol induces the formation of SHBG which influences the distribution with respect to the serum proteins, causing an increase of the SHBG-bound fraction and a decrease in the albumin-bound and unbound fraction indicating non-linearity of the pharmacokinetics of estradiol after ingestion of Angeliq. With a dosing interval of 24 hours, mean steady-state serum levels of estradiol fluctuate in the range of 20-43 pg/ml following administration of Angeliq. Pharmacokinetics of estradiol are dose-proportional at doses of 1 and 2 mg.

Special Populations

Hepatic Dysfunction

The pharmacokinetics of a single oral dose of 3 mg DRSP in combination with 1 mg estradiol (E2) was evaluated in 10 female patients with moderate hepatic impairment (Child Pugh B) and 10 healthy female subjects matched for age, weight, and smoking history. Mean serum DRSP concentration-time profiles were comparable in both groups of women during the absorption/distribution phases with similar Cmax and tmax values, suggesting that the rate of absorption was not affected by the hepatic impairment. The mean terminal half-life was about 1.8 times greater and an about 50% decrease in apparent oral clearance (CL/f) was seen in volunteers with moderate hepatic impairment as compared to those with normal liver function.

Renal Insufficiency

The effect of renal insufficiency on the pharmacokinetics of DRSP (3 mg daily for 14 days) were investigated in female subjects with normal renal function and mild and moderate renal impairment. At steady-state of DRSP treatment, serum DRSP levels in the group with mild renal impairment (creatinine clearance CLcr, 50-80 ml/min) were comparable to those in the group with normal renal function (CLcr, >80 ml/min). The serum DRSP levels were on average 37% higher in the group with moderate renal impairment (CLcr, 30-50 ml/min) compared to those in the group with normal renal function. Linear regression analysis of the DRSP AUC(0-24h) values in relation to the creatinine clearance revealed a 3.5% increase with a 10 ml/min reduction of creatinine clearance. This slight increase is not expected to be of clinical relevance.

5.3 Preclinical safety data

Animal studies with estradiol and drospirenone have shown expected oestrogenic and gestagenic effects. There are no preclinical data of relevance to the prescriber that are additional to those already included in other sections of the SPC.

6. PHARMACEUTICAL PARTICULARS

6.1 List of excipients

Tablet Core:

Lactose monohydrate

Maize starch

Maize starch, pregelatinised

Povidone

Magnesium stearate

Film coating material:

Hypromellose

Macrogol 6000

Talc

Titanium dioxide (E171)

Ferric oxide, red (E172)

6.2 Incompatibilities

Not applicable

6.3 Shelf life

Three years

6.4 Special precautions for storage

No special precautions for storage

6.5 Nature and contents of container

Transparent polyvinyl film (250 μm) / aluminium foil (20 μm) blister strips of 28 tablets with imprinted days of the week

The pack size is 3 × 28 tablets

6.6 Instructions for use and handling

No special requirements.

7. MARKETING AUTHORISATION HOLDER

Schering Health Care Limited

The Brow

Burgess Hill

West Sussex

RH15 9NE

8. MARKETING AUTHORISATION NUMBER(S)

PL 00053/0341

9. DATE OF FIRST AUTHORISATION/RENEWAL OF THE AUTHORISATION

10 March 2004

10. DATE OF REVISION OF THE TEXT

9 March 2004

LEGAL CATEGORY

POM

Angettes 75

(Bristol-Myers Pharmaceuticals)

1. NAME OF THE MEDICINAL PRODUCT

Angettes 75

2. QUALITATIVE AND QUANTITATIVE COMPOSITION

Each tablet contains: Aspirin BP 75 mg

3. PHARMACEUTICAL FORM

Tablet.

4. CLINICAL PARTICULARS

4.1 Therapeutic indications

For the secondary prevention of thrombotic cerebrovascular or cardiovascular disease and following by-pass surgery. The advice of a doctor should be sought before commencing therapy for the first time.

4.2 Posology and method of administration

Adults

The usual dosage, for long-term use, is 75mg - 150mg once daily. In some circumstances a higher dose may be appropriate, especially in short-term, and up to 300mg a day may be used on the advice of a doctor.

Elderly

The risk/benefit ratios in the elderly have not been fully established.

Children

Do not give to children aged under 16 years, unless specifically indicated (e.g. for Kawasaki's disease).

4.3 Contraindications

Active or history of peptic ulceration, haemophilia and other bleeding disorders, hypersensitivity to aspirin.

4.4 Special warnings and special precautions for use

Aspirin may induce gastro-intestinal haemorrhage, occasionally major. Patients with hypertension should be carefully monitored.

There is a possible association between aspirin and Reye's syndrome when given to children. Reye's syndrome is a very rare disease, which affects the brain and liver, and can be fatal. For this reason aspirin should not be given to children aged under 16 years unless specifically indicated (e.g. for Kawasaki's disease).

4.5 Interaction with other medicinal products and other forms of Interaction

Aspirin may enhance the effects of anticoagulants and may inhibit the action of uricosurics.

4.6 Pregnancy and lactation

There is clinical and epidemiological evidence of safety in human pregnancy. Aspirin may prolong labour and contribute to maternal and neonatal bleeding, and should be avoided at term.

4.7 Effects on ability to drive and use machines

None known.

4.8 Undesirable effects

Aspirin may enhance the effects of anticoagulants and may inhibit the action of uricosurics. Aspirin may precipitate bronchospasm and may induce attacks of asthma in susceptible subjects. Hypersensitivity reactions have been reported in susceptible individuals.

4.9 Overdose

Overdosage is unlikely due to the low level of aspirin in Angettes. If necessary gastric lavage, forced alkaline diuresis and supportive therapy may be employed. Restoration of acid/base balance may be required.

5. PHARMACOLOGICAL PROPERTIES

5.1 Pharmacodynamic properties

Aspirin has antiplatelet, analgesic, antipyretic and anti-inflammatory properties.

5.2 Pharmacokinetic properties

After a single oral dose of a salicylate, the plasma concentration becomes appreciable within 30 minutes, reaches a peak in about 2 hours and then slowly declines.

The highest concentrations occur in plasma, kidney, liver, heart and lung.

From 50-80% of salicylic acid in plasma is bound to plasma proteins, mainly albumin.

Salicylate is metabolised chiefly in the smooth endoplasmic reticulum of liver cells.

5.3 Preclinical safety data

There are no preclinical safety data of relevance to the prescriber which are additional to that already included in other sections of the SPC.

6. PHARMACEUTICAL PARTICULARS

6.1 List of excipients

Lactose, maize starch, sodium saccharin.

6.2 Incompatibilities

None.

6.3 Shelf life

36 months.

6.4 Special precautions for storage

Do not store above 30°C.

6.5 Nature and contents of container

28 tablets as 2 blister strips of PVC/PVDC with 20 micron lacquered aluminium/PVC film (20micron/15micron), each containing 2 × 7 tablets.

6.6 Instructions for use and handling

None.

7. MARKETING AUTHORISATION HOLDER
Bristol-Myers Squibb Holdings Ltd
Uxbridge Business Park
Sanderson Road
Uxbridge, Middlesex UB8 1DH

8. MARKETING AUTHORISATION NUMBER(S)
0125/5020R

9. DATE OF FIRST AUTHORISATION/RENEWAL OF THE AUTHORISATION
6th June 1990

10. DATE OF REVISION OF THE TEXT
July 2005

Anhydrol Forte

(Dermal Laboratories Limited)

1. NAME OF THE MEDICINAL PRODUCT
ANHYDROL® FORTE

2. QUALITATIVE AND QUANTITATIVE COMPOSITION
Aluminium Chloride Hexahydrate 20.0% w/v.

3. PHARMACEUTICAL FORM
Clear, colourless evaporative topical solution.

4. CLINICAL PARTICULARS

4.1 Therapeutic indications
For the topical treatment of hyperhidrosis specifically involving axillae, hands or feet.

4.2 Posology and method of administration
For adults, children and the elderly: Apply to the affected sites at night, as required, and allow to dry. Wash off in the morning.

4.3 Contraindications
Not to be used in cases of sensitivity to any of the ingredients.

4.4 Special warnings and special precautions for use
Care should be taken to restrict the application to the affected sites only. Keep away from the eyes and mucous membranes. Care should be taken to avoid Anhydrol Forte coming into direct contact with clothing, polished surfaces, jewellery or metal. Replace cap tightly after use. For external use only.

4.5 Interaction with other medicinal products and other forms of Interaction
Do not bathe immediately before use and, if the axillae are treated, do not shave or use depilatories on this area within 12 hours before or after use.

4.6 Pregnancy and lactation
No special precautions.

4.7 Effects on ability to drive and use machines
None known.

4.8 Undesirable effects
If applied too frequently, Anhydrol Forte may cause irritation which should be treated with a mild topical hydrocortisone cream.

4.9 Overdose
See section above (undesirable effects).

5. PHARMACOLOGICAL PROPERTIES

5.1 Pharmacodynamic properties
Aluminium chloride is believed to denature the protein content of sweat issuing from eccrine glands, and to combine with the intraductal keratin fibrils, producing a functional closure. The antibacterial action of the aluminium ion also precludes the development of miliaria. Accordingly, there is no secondary inflammation. The intraluminal pressure rises to the point where it acts as a feedback system, shutting off acinar secretion.

The formulation of Anhydrol Forte has been tested in widespread clinical practice, and has been shown to be effective when used in accordance with the recommended instructions.

5.2 Pharmacokinetic properties
As the active ingredient is applied in an alcoholic solution of low surface tension, it therefore penetrates into the terminal pores of the sweat ducts, when applied, as recommended, to dry skin. The alcohol then evaporates off, leaving the salt deposited in close contact with the lining of the duct. The use of the preparation is restricted to small areas of skin, namely the axillae, hands or feet, to ensure that there are no detrimental effects from widespread obstruction of sweating.

5.3 Preclinical safety data
No special information.

6. PHARMACEUTICAL PARTICULARS

6.1 List of excipients
IMS.

6.2 Incompatibilities
None known.

6.3 Shelf life
36 months.

6.4 Special precautions for storage
Highly flammable. Do not store above 25°C. Store upright and away from flames.

6.5 Nature and contents of container
60 ml plastic bottle with roll-on applicator and screwcap. This is supplied as an original pack (OP).

6.6 Instructions for use and handling
Not applicable.

7. MARKETING AUTHORISATION HOLDER
Dermal Laboratories
Tatmore Place, Gosmore
Hitchin, Herts SG4 7QR, UK.

8. MARKETING AUTHORISATION NUMBER(S)
0173/0030.

9. DATE OF FIRST AUTHORISATION/RENEWAL OF THE AUTHORISATION
16 December 2001.

10. DATE OF REVISION OF THE TEXT
December 2001.

Antabuse Tablets 200mg

(Alpharma Limited)

1. NAME OF THE MEDICINAL PRODUCT
Antabuse® tablets 200 mg.
Disulfiram tablets 200 mg.

2. QUALITATIVE AND QUANTITATIVE COMPOSITION
Each tablet contains 200 mg disulfiram.

3. PHARMACEUTICAL FORM
Tablets.

4. CLINICAL PARTICULARS

4.1 Therapeutic indications
Alcohol deterrent compound. Disulfiram may be indicated as an adjuvant in the treatment of carefully selected and co-operative patients with drinking problems. Its use must be accompanied by appropriate supportive treatment.

4.2 Posology and method of administration
Adults and elderly patients only:
It is recommended that treatment with Disulfiram should be initiated only in a hospital or specialised clinic and by physicians experienced in its use. The patient should have adequate social and family support to avoid ingestion of alcohol. Suitable patients should not have ingested alcohol for at least 24 hours and must be warned that a Disulfiram-alcohol reaction is potentially dangerous.

On the first day of treatment, the patient should be given no more than 4 tablets of Disulfiram in one dose (800 mg). The next day the patient should take 3 tablets followed on the third day by 2 tablets and on the fourth and fifth days by 1 tablet. Subsequently, daily dosing should continue at 1 or half a tablet daily for as long as advised by the physician but no longer than six months without review.

In the routine management of the alcoholic it is not recommended to carry out an alcohol challenge test. If the clinician feels an alcohol challenge test is essential for the success of the therapy, full information of the procedure and risks of this test can be obtained from the company. As severe reactions can occur any alcohol challenge should be carried out in specialised units by physicians acquainted with the procedure. Full resuscitation facilities must be immediately available.

Children:
Not applicable.

4.3 Contraindications
Presence of cardiac failure, coronary artery disease, previous history of CVA, hypertension, severe personality disorder, suicidal risk or psychosis.

4.4 Special warnings and special precautions for use
Caution should be exercised in the presence of renal failure, hepatic or respiratory disease, diabetes mellitus and epilepsy.

Before initiating treatment it is advised that appropriate examinations should be carried out to establish the suitability of the patient for treatment. Patients must not ingest alcohol during or for 1 week after ceasing Disulfiram therapy. Patients must be warned of the unpredictable and potentially severe nature of a Disulfiram-alcohol reaction as, in rare cases deaths have been reported following the drinking of alcohol by patients receiving Disulfiram. Certain foods, liquid medicines, remedies, tonics, toiletries, perfumes and aerosol sprays may contain sufficient alcohol to elicit a Disulfiram-alcohol reaction and patients should be made aware of this. Caution should also be exercised with low alcohol and "non-alcohol" or "alcohol-free" beers and wines, which may provoke a reaction when consumed in sufficient quantities. All personnel involved in the administration of Disulfiram to the patient know that Disulfiram should not be given during a drinking episode.

4.5 Interaction with other medicinal products and other forms of Interaction
Disulfiram blocks the metabolism of alcohol and leads to an accumulation of acetaldehyde in the blood stream. The Disulfiram-alcohol reaction can occur within 10 minutes of ingestion of alcohol and may last several hours. It is characterised by intense flushing, dyspnoea, headache, palpitations, tachycardia, hypotension, nausea and vomiting.

Supportive therapy should be available and measures may be necessary to counteract hypotension. Severe vomiting might occur requiring administration of intravenous fluids.

Disulfiram may potentiate the toxic effects of warfarin, antipyrine, phenytoin, chlordiazepoxide and diazepam by inhibiting their metabolism. Animal studies have indicated similar inhibition of metabolism of pethidine, morphine and amphetamines. A few case reports of increase in confusion and changes in affective behaviour have been noted with the concurrent administration of metronidazole, isoniazid or paraldehyde. Potentiation of organic brain syndrome and choreoatphetosis following pimozide have occurred very rarely. The intensity of the Disulfiram-alcohol reaction may be increased by amitriptyline and decreased by diazepam. Chlorpromazine while decreasing certain components of the reaction may increase the overall intensity of the reaction. Disulfiram inhibits the oxidation and renal excretion of rifampicin.

4.6 Pregnancy and lactation
Pregnancy: The use of Disulfiram in the first trimester of pregnancy is not advised. The risk/benefit ratio in assessing adverse effects of alcoholism in pregnancy should be taken into account when considering the use of Disulfiram in pregnant patients.

There have been rare reports of congenital abnormalities in infants whose mothers have received Disulfiram in conjunction with other medicines.

Lactation: Should not be used. No information is available on whether Disulfiram is excreted in breast milk. Its use during breast feeding is not advised especially where there is a possibility of interaction with medicines that the baby may be taking.

4.7 Effects on ability to drive and use machines
Presumed to be safe or unlikely to produce an effect.

4.8 Undesirable effects
During initial treatment, drowsiness and fatigue may occur, nausea, vomiting, halitosis and reduction in libido have been reported. If side effects are marked the dosage may be reduced. Psychotic reactions, including depression, paranoia, schizophrenia and mania occur rarely in patients receiving Disulfiram. Allergic dermatitis, peripheral neuritis and hepatic cell damage have also been reported.

4.9 Overdose
Disulfiram alone has low toxicity. Reports of the ingestion of quantities of up to 25 g refer to central and peripheral neurological symptoms which have resolved without sequel. Treatment should be symptomatic, gastric lavage and observation are recommended.

Disulfiram blocks the metabolism of alcohol and leads to an accumulation of acetaldehyde in the blood stream. The Disulfiram-alcohol reaction can occur within 10 minutes of ingestion of alcohol and may last several hours. It is characterised by intense flushing, dyspnoea and vomiting.

Supportive therapy should be available and measures may be necessary to counteract hypotension. Severe vomiting might occur requiring administration of intravenous fluids.

Symptoms: Vomiting, headache, drowsiness, fatigue, apathy, ataxia.

Treatment: Gastric lavage. Observation. Disulfiram by itself has low toxicity.

5. PHARMACOLOGICAL PROPERTIES

5.1 Pharmacodynamic properties
The effect of Disulfiram is primarily due to irreversible inactivation of liver ALDH. In the absence of this enzyme, the metabolism of ethanol is blocked and the intracellular acetaldehyde concentration rises. The symptoms of the Disulfiram-alcohol reaction (DAR) are due partly to the high levels of acetaldehyde. The conversion of dopamine to noradrenaline is also inhibited and the depletion of noradrenaline in the heart and blood vessels allows acetaldehyde to act directly on these tissues to cause flushing, tachycardia and hypotension.

In addition to its affect on acetaldehyde dehydrogenase, disulfiram inhibits other enzyme systems including dopamine-beta-hydroxylase (which converts dopamine and noradrenaline) and hepatic microsomal mixed function oxidases (which are responsible for the metabolism of many drugs). Disulfiram may thus potentiate the action of drugs which are metabolised by these enzymes.

5.2 Pharmacokinetic properties
Following oral administration, absorption is variable, distribution is primarily to the kidney, pancreas, liver, intestines and fat. Disulfiram is rapidly metabolised to diethyldithiocarbamic acid (DDC), is conjugated with glucuronic acid, oxidised to sulphate, methylated and decomposed to diethylamine and carbon disulphide. Excretion is primarily through the kidneys.

5.3 Preclinical safety data
None.

6. PHARMACEUTICAL PARTICULARS

6.1 List of excipients
Lactose, potato starch, povidone, microcrystalline cellulose, polysorbate 20, tartaric acid, colloidal anhydrous silica, sodium bicarbonate, maize starch, magnesium stearate.

6.2 Incompatibilities
None.

6.3 Shelf life
3 years.

6.4 Special precautions for storage
Store below 25°C in a dry place and keep tightly closed. Protect from light.

6.5 Nature and contents of container
Polyethylene container with a polyethylene screw cap tamper evident closure, pack size of 50 tablets.

6.6 Instructions for use and handling
Not applicable.

Administration Details

7. MARKETING AUTHORISATION HOLDER
Dumex-Alpharma A/S
Dalslandsgade 11
DK-2300 Copenhagen S.

8. MARKETING AUTHORISATION NUMBER(S)
PL 04938/0011

9. DATE OF FIRST AUTHORISATION/RENEWAL OF THE AUTHORISATION
16 August 1994

10. DATE OF REVISION OF THE TEXT
19 August 1999

Antepsin Suspension

(Chugai Pharma UK Limited)

1. NAME OF THE MEDICINAL PRODUCT
Antepsin Suspension.

2. QUALITATIVE AND QUANTITATIVE COMPOSITION
Antepsin Suspension: each 5 mL dose contains 1 gram sucralfate.

3. PHARMACEUTICAL FORM
Antepsin Suspension is a white to off-white viscous suspension with an odour of aniseed/caramel.

4. CLINICAL PARTICULARS

4.1 Therapeutic indications
Antepsin Suspension: Treatment of duodenal ulcer, gastric ulcer, chronic gastritis, and the prophylaxis of gastrointestinal haemorrhage from stress ulceration in seriously ill patients.

4.2 Posology and method of administration
For oral administration.

Duodenal ulcer, gastric ulcer, chronic gastritis:

Adults: The usual dose is 2 grams twice daily to be taken on rising and at bedtime, or 1 gram 4 times a day to be taken 1 hour before meals and at bedtime. Maximum daily dose: 8 grams. For ease of administration Antepsin Tablets may be dispersed in 10-15 mL of water.

Four to six weeks' treatment is usually needed for ulcer healing, but up to twelve weeks may be necessary in resistant cases.

Antacids may be used as required for relief of pain, but should not be taken half an hour before or after Antepsin.

Children and Elderly: see below

Prophylaxis of gastrointestinal haemorrhage from stress ulceration:

Adults: The usual dose is 1 gram six times a day. A maximum dose of 8 grams daily should not be exceeded. Antacids may be used as required for relief of pain, but should not be taken half an hour before or after Antepsin.

Elderly: There are no special dosage requirements for elderly patients but as with all medicines, the lowest effective dose should be used.

Children: Safety and effectiveness in children has not been established.

4.3 Contraindications
Contraindicated in individuals who are hypersensitive to any of the ingredients of Antepsin.

4.4 Special warnings and special precautions for use
The product should only be used with caution in patients with renal dysfunction, due to the possibility of increased aluminium absorption.

In patients with severe renal impairment or on dialysis, Antepsin should be used with extreme caution and only for short-term treatment. The concomitant use of other aluminium containing medications is not recommended in view of the enhanced potential for aluminium absorption and toxicity.

Bezoars (an insoluble mass formed with the gastric lumen) have been reported occasionally in patients taking Antepsin Suspension. The majority of these patients had underlying conditions that may predispose to bezoar formation such as delayed gastric emptying, or were receiving concomitant enteral feeding (see under Interactions). Bezoars have been reported after administration of Antepsin Suspension to severely ill patients in ITU, especially in premature infants in whom the use of sucralfate is not recommended.

4.5 Interaction with other medicinal products and other forms of Interaction
Concomitant administration of Antepsin may reduce the bioavailability of certain drugs including tetracycline, ciprofloxacin, norfloxacin, ketoconazole, digoxin, warfarin, phenytoin, and H2 antagonists. The bioavailability of these agents may be restored by separating the administration of these agents from Antepsin by two hours. This interaction appears to be non systemic in origin presumably resulting from these agents being bound by Antepsin in the gastrointestinal tract. Because of the potential of Antepsin to alter the absorption of some drugs from the gastrointestinal tract, the separate administration of Antepsin from that of other agents should be considered when alterations in bioavailability are felt to be critical for concomitantly administered drugs.

The administration of Antepsin Suspension and enteral feeds by nasogastric tube should be separated by one hour in patients receiving Antepsin Suspension for the prophylaxis of stress ulceration. In rare cases bezoar formation has been reported when Antepsin and enteral feeds have been given too closely together.

4.6 Pregnancy and lactation
Teratogenicity studies in mice, rats and rabbits at doses up to 50 times the human dose have revealed no evidence of harm to the foetus. Safety in pregnant women has not been established and Antepsin should be used during pregnancy only if clearly needed.

It is not known whether this drug is excreted in human milk. Caution should be exercised when Antepsin is administered to nursing women.

4.7 Effects on ability to drive and use machines
None stated (presumed to be safe or unlikely to produce any effect).

4.8 Undesirable effects
Adverse reactions to Antepsin in clinical trials were minor and only rarely led to discontinuation of the drug. Adverse events seen during use of Antepsin have included constipation, diarrhoea, nausea, vomiting, gastric discomfort, indigestion, flatulence, dry mouth, rash, back pain, dizziness, headache, vertigo, drowsiness and hypersensitivity reactions including pruritus, oedema and urticaria.

4.9 Overdose
There is no experience in humans with overdosage. Acute oral toxicity studies in animals, however, using doses to 12 g/kg body weight, could not find a lethal dose. Risks associated with overdosage, should, therefore, be minimal.

5. PHARMACOLOGICAL PROPERTIES

5.1 Pharmacodynamic properties
The action of Antepsin is non-systemic as the drug is only minimally absorbed from the gastro-intestinal tract. The small amounts that are absorbed are excreted primarily in the urine. Antepsin exerts a generalised cytoprotective effect by preventing gastro-intestinal mucosal injury.

Studies in humans and animal models show that Antepsin forms an ulcer adherent complex with the proteinaceous exudate of the ulcer site. This property enables Antepsin to form a protective barrier over the ulcer lesion giving sustained protection against the penetration and action of gastric acid, pepsin and bile. Studies both in humans and animals demonstrate that Antepsin protects the gastric mucosa against various irritants such as alcohol, acetylsalicylic acid and sodium taurocholate.

Antepsin also directly inhibits pepsin activity and absorbs bile salts. It has only weak antacid activity. It does not alter gastric emptying time, nor normal digestive function. Antepsin has no demonstrated pharmacological effect on the cardiovascular or central nervous systems.

5.2 Pharmacokinetic properties
Sucralfate is only minimally absorbed from the gastro-intestinal tract. The small amounts that are absorbed are excreted primarily in the urine. Absorption of aluminium from sucralfate may be increased in patients on dialysis or with renal dysfunction (see also "other special warnings and precautions").

5.3 Preclinical safety data
There was no evidence of carcinogenesis in mice and rats receiving oral sucralfate in dosages of up to 1 gm/kg daily (12 times the usual human dosage) for 2 years. In animal studies there was no effect evidence of impaired fertility. The effect of sucralfate on human fertility is not known.

6. PHARMACEUTICAL PARTICULARS

6.1 List of excipients
Sodium saccharin, sodium dihydrogen phosphate, glycerol, E217, E219, xantham gum, aniseed flavour and caramel flavour.

6.2 Incompatibilities
None known.

6.3 Shelf life
36 months.

6.4 Special precautions for storage
Store below 25°C.

6.5 Nature and contents of container
Glass bottle (pack size 250 mL)

6.6 Instructions for use and handling
None stated.

7. MARKETING AUTHORISATION HOLDER
Chugai Pharma UK Ltd.
Mulliner House
Flanders Road
Turnham Green
London
W4 1NN

8. MARKETING AUTHORISATION NUMBER(S)
PL 12185/0010

9. DATE OF FIRST AUTHORISATION/RENEWAL OF THE AUTHORISATION
1 December 1998

10. DATE OF REVISION OF THE TEXT
April 2003

Antepsin Tablets 1g

(Chugai Pharma UK Limited)

1. NAME OF THE MEDICINAL PRODUCT
Antepsin Tablets 1 g.

2. QUALITATIVE AND QUANTITATIVE COMPOSITION
Each Antepsin (1 g) tablet contains 1 gram of the active ingredient sucralfate.

3. PHARMACEUTICAL FORM
Antepsin Tablets 1 gram are biconvex, oblong white tablets with a dividing score on one side.

4. CLINICAL PARTICULARS

4.1 Therapeutic indications
Treatment of duodenal ulcer, gastric ulcer, chronic gastritis.

4.2 Posology and method of administration
For oral administration.

Duodenal ulcer, gastric ulcer, chronic gastritis:

Adults: The usual dose is 2 grams twice daily to be taken on rising and at bedtime, or 1 gram 4 times a day to be taken 1 hour before meals and at bedtime. For ease of administration, Antepsin Tablets may be dispersed in 10-15 mL of water. Four to six weeks' treatment is usually needed for ulcer healing, but up to twelve weeks may be necessary in resistant cases.

Antacids may be used as required for relief of pain, but should not be taken half an hour before or after Antepsin.

Children and Elderly: see below

Prophylaxis of gastrointestinal haemorrhage from stress ulceration:

Adults: The usual dose is 1 gram six times a day. A maximum dose of 8 grams daily should not be exceeded. Antacids may be used as required for relief of pain, but should not be taken half an hour before or after Antepsin.

Elderly: There are no special dosage requirements for elderly patients but, as with all medicines, the lowest effective dose should be used.

Children: Safety and effectiveness in children has not been established.

4.3 Contraindications
Contraindicated in individuals who are hypersensitive to any of the ingredients of Antepsin.

4.4 Special warnings and special precautions for use
The product should only be used with caution in patients with renal dysfunction, due to the possibility of increased aluminium absorption. In patients with severe renal impairment or on dialysis, Antepsin should be used with extreme caution and only for short-term treatment. The concomitant use of other aluminium containing medications is not recommended in view of the enhanced potential for aluminium absorption and toxicity.

4.5 Interaction with other medicinal products and other forms of Interaction
Concomitant administration of Antepsin may reduce the bioavailability of certain drugs including tetracycline, ciprofloxacin, norfloxacin, ketoconazole, digoxin, warfarin, phenytoin, and H2 antagonists. The bioavailability of these agents may be restored by separating the administration of these agents from Antepsin by two hours. This interaction appears to be non systemic in origin presumably resulting from these agents being bound by Antepsin in the gastrointestinal tract. Because of the potential of Antepsin to alter the absorption of some drugs from the gastrointestinal tract, the separate administration of Antepsin from that of other agents should be considered when

alterations in bioavailability are felt to be critical for concomitantly administered drugs.

4.6 Pregnancy and lactation

Teratogenicity studies in mice, rats and rabbits at doses up to 50 times the human dose have revealed no evidence of harm to the foetus. Safety in pregnant women has not been established and Antepsin should be used during pregnancy only if clearly needed.

It is not known whether this drug is excreted in human milk. Caution should be exercised when Antepsin is administered to nursing women.

4.7 Effects on ability to drive and use machines

None stated (presumed to be safe or unlikely to produce any effect).

4.8 Undesirable effects

Adverse reactions to Antepsin in clinical trials were minor and only rarely led to discontinuation of the drug. Adverse events seen during use of Antepsin have included constipation, diarrhoea, nausea, vomiting, gastric discomfort, indigestion, flatulence, dry mouth, rash, back pain, dizziness, headache, vertigo, drowsiness and hypersensitivity reactions including pruritus, oedema and urticaria.

4.9 Overdose

There is no experience in humans with overdosage. Acute oral toxicity studies in animals, however, using doses to 12g/kg body weight, could not find a lethal dose. Risks associated with overdosage, should, therefore, be minimal.

5. PHARMACOLOGICAL PROPERTIES

5.1 Pharmacodynamic properties

The action of Antepsin is non-systemic as the drug is only minimally absorbed from the gastro-intestinal tract. The small amounts that are absorbed are excreted primarily in the urine. Antepsin exerts a generalised cytoprotective effect by preventing gastro-intestinal mucosal injury. Studies in humans and animal models show that Antepsin forms an ulcer adherent complex with the proteinaceous exudate of the ulcer site. This property enables Antepsin to form a protective barrier over the ulcer lesion giving sustained protection against the penetration and action of gastric acid, pepsin and bile. Studies both in humans and animals demonstrate that Antepsin protects the gastric mucosa against various irritants such as alcohol, acetylsalicylic acid and sodium taurocholate.

Antepsin also directly inhibits pepsin activity and absorbs bile salts. It has only weak antacid activity. It does not alter gastric emptying time, nor normal digestive function. Antepsin has no demonstrated pharmacological effect on the cardiovascular or central nervous systems.

5.2 Pharmacokinetic properties

Sucralfate is only minimally absorbed from the gastro-intestinal tract. The small amounts that are absorbed are excreted primarily in the urine. Absorption of aluminium from sucralfate may be increased in patients on dialysis or with renal dysfunction (see also "other special warnings and precautions").

5.3 Preclinical safety data

There was no evidence of carcinogenesis in mice and rats receiving oral sucralfate in dosages of up to 1 gm/kg daily (12 times the usual human dosage) for 2 years. In animal studies there was no effect evidence of impaired fertility. The effect of sucralfate on human fertility is not known.

6. PHARMACEUTICAL PARTICULARS

6.1 List of excipients

Polyethylene glycol 6000, microcrystalline cellulose, calcium carboxymethyl cellulose, magnesium stearate.

6.2 Incompatibilities

None known.

6.3 Shelf life

36 months.

6.4 Special precautions for storage

Store below 25°C.

6.5 Nature and contents of container

Blister packs (pack size 50 tablets).

6.6 Instructions for use and handling

None stated.

7. MARKETING AUTHORISATION HOLDER

Chugai Pharma UK Ltd.

Mulliner House

Flanders Road

Turnham Green

London

W4 1NN

8. MARKETING AUTHORISATION NUMBER(S)

PL 12185/0008

9. DATE OF FIRST AUTHORISATION/RENEWAL OF THE AUTHORISATION

1 December 1998

10. DATE OF REVISION OF THE TEXT

January 2004

Anturan Tablets 100 mg and 200 mg

(Amdipharm)

1. NAME OF THE MEDICINAL PRODUCT

ANTURAN® Tablets 100mg

ANTURAN® Tablets 200mg

2. QUALITATIVE AND QUANTITATIVE COMPOSITION

The active ingredient is 1,2-Diphenyl-3,5-dioxo-4-(2-phenylsulphinylethyl)-

pyrazolidine (= sulfinpyrazone B.P.)

Each coated tablet contains 100 mg or 200 mg sulfinpyrazone.

3. PHARMACEUTICAL FORM

Coated tablets.

4. CLINICAL PARTICULARS

4.1 Therapeutic indications

Chronic, including tophaceous gout; recurrent gouty arthritis; hyperuricaemia.

4.2 Posology and method of administration

Anturan is administered orally in tablet form with meals or milk.

Adults: 100-200mg daily increasing gradually (over the first two or three weeks) to 600mg daily (rarely 800mg), and maintained until the serum urate level has fallen within the normal range. Subsequent dosage should be reduced, to the lowest level which maintains serum urate within the normal range. Maintenance dose may be as low as 200mg daily. Reduced dose required in renal impairment. Not to be used in severe renal impairment.

Children: Paediatric usage not established.

4.3 Contraindications

Acute attacks of gout. Treatment with Anturan should not be initiated during an acute attack of gout.

Gastric and duodenal ulcer (overt or case-history).

Known hypersensitivity to sulfinpyrazone and other pyrazolone derivatives. Sulfinpyrazone is contra-indicated in patients in whom attacks of asthma, urticaria, or acute rhinitis are precipitated by acetylsalicylic acid or by other drugs with prostaglandin-synthetase inhibiting activity.

Severe parenchymal lesions of the liver or kidneys (also in the case history). Porphyria. Blood dyscrasias (also in the case history). Haemorrhagic diatheses (e.g. blood coagulation disorders).

In the treatment of chronic gout salicylates antagonise the action of Anturan and should not be given concurrently.

4.4 Special warnings and special precautions for use

During the early stages of treatment in patients with hyperuricaemia or gout, acute attacks of gout may be precipitated. To help prevent episodes of urolithiasis or renal colic, ensure adequate fluid intake and alkalinisation of the urine during initial stages of therapy.

Since Anturan may cause salt and water retention, caution is called for in patients with overt or latent heart failure.

For the early detection of a haematological abnormality, careful clinical supervision and full blood count should be done before and at regular intervals during treatment.

Use with caution in patients with impaired renal function.

In patients with an elevated plasma uric acid level and/or with a history of nephrolithiasis or renal colic, and also when resuming treatment after interruption of the medication, a cautious incremental dosage schedule should be adopted. As with any form of long-term uricosuric medication, renal function tests should be performed regularly, particularly in cases where there is pre-existing evidence of renal failure.

4.5 Interaction with other medicinal products and other forms of Interaction

Since Anturan may potentiate the action of coumarin-type anticoagulants, frequent estimation of prothrombin time should be undertaken when these drugs are given concurrently, and the dosage of anticoagulant adjusted accordingly.

Anturan may also potentiate the action of other plasma protein binding drugs such as hypoglycaemic agents and sulphonamides, which may necessitate a modification in dosage.

Penicillins (e.g. penicillin G): Inhibition of tubular secretion may raise the plasma concentrations of penicillins.

Theophylline: Activation of microsomal liver enzymes and resultant acceleration of metabolism lowers the plasma concentration of theophylline.

Phenytoin: Displacement of phenytoin from its plasma protein-binding sites as well as inhibition of microsomal liver enzymes delays the metabolism of phenytoin, thus prolonging its half-life and raising its plasma concentration.

Substances affecting haemostasis: Such substances, e.g. non-steroidal antirheumatic drugs, may exert a synergistic effect on the blood coagulation system and thus increase the risk of haemorrhage.

4.6 Pregnancy and lactation

Anturan should be used with caution in pregnant women, weighing the potential risk against the possible benefits.

It is not known whether the active substance of Anturan and/or its metabolite(s) pass into breast milk. For safety reasons mothers should refrain from taking the drug.

4.7 Effects on ability to drive and use machines

None known.

4.8 Undesirable effects

Gastro-intestinal tract:

Frequent: mild transient gastro-intestinal upsets, such as nausea, vomiting, diarrhoea.

In isolated cases: gastro-intestinal bleeding and ulcers.

Urogenital system:

Rare: acute renal failure (mostly reversible), especially with high initial dosages.

In isolated cases: salt and water retention.

Skin:

Rare: allergic skin reactions (e.g. drug rash, urticaria).

Blood:

In isolated cases: leucopenia, thrombocytopenia, agranulocytosis, aplastic anaemia.

Liver:

In isolated cases: hepatic dysfunction (increase in transaminases and alkaline phosphatase), jaundice, and hepatitis.

4.9 Overdose

Signs and symptoms: Nausea, vomiting, abdominal pains, diarrhoea, hypotension, cardiac arrhythmias, hyperventilation, respiratory disorders, impairment of consciousness, coma, epileptic seizures, oliguria or anuria, acute renal failure, renal colic.

Treatment: Immediate treatment consists of forced emesis to recover undigested tablets. This is followed by gastric lavage preferably with mild alkaline solution such as sodium bicarbonate solution and supportive therapy as indicated.

Note that forced diuresis is of no value.

5. PHARMACOLOGICAL PROPERTIES

5.1 Pharmacodynamic properties

Anturan lowers serum urate levels by blocking tubular reabsorption, thereby increasing renal excretion of uric acid. As a result of increased excretion, serum urate deposits are mobilised and tophi are no longer formed.

5.2 Pharmacokinetic properties

After oral administration the active substance is absorbed rapidly and almost completely ($> 85\%$).

Following a single oral dose of 100mg or 200mg sulfinpyrazone, peak plasma concentrations of 5-6μg/ml or 13-22μg/ml, respectively, are attained after 1-2 hours. Sulfinpyrazone has a half-life of 2-4 hours.

Following repeated administration of sulfinpyrazone in a dosage of 400mg b.i.d. for 23 days, a significant decrease in the AUC values and an increase in the drug's clearance was observed as compared with the values recorded after a single dose. After multiple dosing with 400mg b.i.d., the mean steady-state concentration of sulfinpyrazone amounts to 5.1μg/ml, which corresponds to only half of the calculated value after a single dose (9.6μg/ml). The reason for this is an increase in total clearance brought about by the fact that the drug induces its own metabolism.

Sulfinpyrazone is metabolised by reduction to the sulphide and by oxidation to the sulphone and to hydroxy-compounds. The sulphide metabolite inhibits platelet aggregation in vitro about 12 times more strongly than sulfinpyrazone itself. In comparison with sulfinpyrazone the plasma concentrations of the sulphide metabolite are low. Peak sulphide concentrations are reached approx. 19 hours after administration of a single dose.

5.3 Preclinical safety data

Animal experimental findings indicate that Anturan is neither mutagenic nor carcinogenic or teratogenic.

6. PHARMACEUTICAL PARTICULARS

6.1 List of excipients

Lactose, maize starch, aerosil 200, magnesium stearate, gelatin, sodium starch glycollate, sucrose, talc, povidone, titanium dioxide (E 171), polyethylene glycol, avicel, yellow iron oxide (E 172) and printing ink brown.

6.2 Incompatibilities

None known.

6.3 Shelf life

60 months.

6.4 Special precautions for storage

Protect from moisture and store below 25°C.

6.5 Nature and contents of container

Anturan Tablets 100 mg:

Containers and blister packs of 84 tablets.

Anturan Tablets 200 mg:

Securitainers (polypropylene body with polyethylene cap) and child resistant/tamper evident loose fill packs of 84, blister packs of 84 and 112 and amber glass bottles of 100 tablets.

6.6 Instructions for use and handling

None.

7. MARKETING AUTHORISATION HOLDER
Amdipharm plc
Regency House
Miles Gray Road
Basildon
Essex
SS14 3AF

8. MARKETING AUTHORISATION NUMBER(S)
Anturan Tablets 100 mg: PL 20072/0024
Anturan Tablets 200 mg: PL 20072/0025

9. DATE OF FIRST AUTHORISATION/RENEWAL OF THE AUTHORISATION
1 January 2005

10. DATE OF REVISION OF THE TEXT
February 2005

Anugesic HC Cream

(Pfizer Limited)

1. NAME OF THE MEDICINAL PRODUCT
ANUGESIC HC CREAM

2. QUALITATIVE AND QUANTITATIVE COMPOSITION
Each 100g of cream contains zinc oxide EP 12.35g, balsam peru EP 1.85g, benzyl benzoate EP 1.2g, pramoxine hydrochloride USP 1g, bismuth oxide 0.875g, hydrocortisone acetate EP 0.5g.

3. PHARMACEUTICAL FORM
A smooth, homogeneous, buff coloured cream with the characteristic odour of balsam peru.

4. CLINICAL PARTICULARS
4.1 Therapeutic indications
Anugesic HC cream provides antiseptic, astringent, emollient and decongestant properties. In addition hydrocortisone exerts an anti-inflammatory effect. Pramoxine is a rapidly acting local anaesthetic. The cream may be used to provide lubrication for suppositories.

Anugesic HC cream is indicated for the comprehensive symptomatic treatment of severe and acute discomfort or pain associated with internal and external haemorrhoids and pruritus ani.

4.2 Posology and method of administration
For topical use.

Adults:
Apply cream to the affected area at night, in the morning and after each evacuation. Thoroughly cleanse the affected area, dry and apply cream by gently smoothing onto the affected area. For internal conditions use rectal nozzle provided and clean it after each use.

Not to be taken orally.

Elderly (over 65 years):
As for adults.

Children:
Not recommended.

4.3 Contraindications
Tubercular, fungal and most viral lesions including herpes simplex, vaccinia and varicella. History of sensitivity to any of the constituents.

4.4 Special warnings and special precautions for use
As with all products containing topical steroids the possibility of systemic absorption should be borne in mind.

Prolonged or excessive use may produce systemic corticosteroid effects and use for periods longer than seven days is not recommended.

Following symptomatic relief definite diagnosis should be established.

4.5 Interaction with other medicinal products and other forms of Interaction
None known.

4.6 Pregnancy and lactation
There is inadequate evidence of safety in human pregnancy and there may be a very small risk of cleft palate and intrauterine growth retardation as well as suppression of the neonatal HPA axis. There is evidence of harmful effects in animals. Use in pregnancy only when there is no safer alternative and when the disease itself carries risks for the mother or child.

4.7 Effects on ability to drive and use machines
None known.

4.8 Undesirable effects
Rarely, sensitivity reactions. Patients may occasionally experience transient burning on application, especially if the anoderm is not intact.

4.9 Overdose
If swallowed, fever, nausea, vomiting, stomach cramps and diarrhoea may develop 3-12 hours after ingestion.

Pramoxine is relatively non-toxic and less sensitising than other local anaesthetics. Hydrocortisone does not normally produce toxic effects in an acute single overdose.

Treatment of a large acute overdosage should include gastric lavage, purgation with magnesium sulphate and complete bed rest. If necessary, give oxygen and general supportive measures. Methaemoglobinaemia should be treated by intravenous methylene blue.

5. PHARMACOLOGICAL PROPERTIES
5.1 Pharmacodynamic properties
Pramoxine hydrochloride is a surface anaesthetic used on the skin and mucous membranes to relieve surface pain and pruritis.

Hydrocortisone acetate has the general properties of hydrocortisone and the anti-inflammatory action is of primary interest in this product.

Benzyl benzoate is used as a solubilizing agent and has mild antiseptic and preservative properties.

Bismuth oxide exerts a protective action on mucous membranes and raw surfaces. It is weakly astringent and is reported to have antiseptic properties.

Balsam peru has protective properties and a very mild antiseptic action by virtue of its content of cinnamic and benzoic acids. It is believed to promote the growth of epithelial cells.

Zinc oxide acts as an astringent and mild antiseptic.

5.2 Pharmacokinetic properties
It is well known that topically applied corticosteroids can be absorbed percutaneously. This appears to be more likely upon repeated or prolonged use.

The remaining active ingredients in Anugesic HC Cream exert their therapeutic effect without being absorbed into the systemic circulation. These observations are supported by evidence from various studies and reviews.

5.3 Preclinical safety data
The results of the preclinical tests do not add anything of further significance to the prescriber.

6. PHARMACEUTICAL PARTICULARS
6.1 List of excipients
Liquid paraffin, glyceryl monostearate, propylene glycol, polysorbate 60, sorbitan monostearate, titanium dioxide E171, methyl hydroxybenzoate, propyl hydroxybenzoate and purified water.

6.2 Incompatibilities
None known

6.3 Shelf life
2 years

6.4 Special precautions for storage
Do not store above 25°C.

6.5 Nature and contents of container
Aluminium tube externally printed and internally lacquered with plastic cap. Supplied in packs of 15, 25 and 30 g.

6.6 Instructions for use and handling
No special instructions needed.

7. MARKETING AUTHORISATION HOLDER
Pfizer Limited
Sandwich
Kent CT13 9NJ
United Kingdom

8. MARKETING AUTHORISATION NUMBER(S)
PL 00057/0520

9. DATE OF FIRST AUTHORISATION/RENEWAL OF THE AUTHORISATION
27th June 2003

10. DATE OF REVISION OF THE TEXT

Anugesic HC Suppositories

(Pfizer Limited)

1. NAME OF THE MEDICINAL PRODUCT
Anugesic HC Suppositories.

2. QUALITATIVE AND QUANTITATIVE COMPOSITION
Each 2.8g suppository contains pramoxine hydrochloride USP 27mg, hydrocortisone acetate EP 5mg, benzyl benzoate EP 33mg, bismuth oxide 24mg, bismuth subgallate BP 59mg, balsam peru EP 49mg, zinc oxide EP 296mg.

3. PHARMACEUTICAL FORM
Buff coloured suppositories having the characteristic odour of balsam peru.

4. CLINICAL PARTICULARS
4.1 Therapeutic indications
Anugesic HC Suppositories provide antiseptic, astringent, emollient and decongestant properties. In addition hydrocortisone exerts an anti-inflammatory effect. Pramoxine is a rapidly acting local anaesthetic.

Anugesic HC Suppositories are indicated for the comprehensive symptomatic treatment of severe and acute discomfort or pain associated with internal and external haemorrhoids and pruritus ani.

4.2 Posology and method of administration
For rectal use. Not to be taken orally.

Adults:
Remove plastic cover and insert one suppository into the anus at night, in the morning and after each evacuation.

Elderly (over 65 years):
As for adults.

Children:
Not recommended.

4.3 Contraindications
Tubercular, fungal and most viral lesions including herpes simplex, vaccinia and varicella. History of sensitivity to any of the constituents.

4.4 Special warnings and special precautions for use
Following symptomatic relief definitive diagnosis should be established.

4.5 Interaction with other medicinal products and other forms of Interaction
None known.

4.6 Pregnancy and lactation
There is inadequate evidence of safety in human pregnancy and there may be a very small risk of cleft palate and intrauterine growth retardation as well as suppression of the neonatal HPA axis. There is evidence of harmful effects in animals. Use in pregnancy only when there is no safer alternative and when the disease itself carries risks for the mother or child.

4.7 Effects on ability to drive and use machines
None known.

4.8 Undesirable effects
As with all products containing topical steroids the possibility of systemic absorption should be borne in mind.

Prolonged or excessive use may produce systemic corticosteroid effects and use for periods longer than seven days is not recommended.

Rarely, sensitivity reactions.

Patients may occasionally experience transient burning on application, especially if the anoderm is not intact.

4.9 Overdose
If swallowed, fever, nausea, vomiting, stomach cramps and diarrhoea may develop 3-12 hours after ingestion.

Pramoxine is relatively non-toxic and less sensitising than other local anaesthetics. Hydrocortisone does not normally produce toxic effects in an acute single overdose.

Treatment of a large acute overdosage should include gastric lavage, purgation with magnesium sulphate and complete bed rest. If necessary, give oxygen and general supportive measures. Methaemoglobinaemia should be treated by intravenous methylene blue.

5. PHARMACOLOGICAL PROPERTIES
5.1 Pharmacodynamic properties
Pramoxine hydrochloride is a surface anaesthetic used on the skin and mucous membranes to relieve surface pain and pruritis.

Hydrocortisone acetate has the general properties of hydrocortisone and the anti-inflammatory action is of primary interest in this product.

Benzyl benzoate is used as a solubilizing agent and has mild antiseptic and preservative properties.

Bismuth oxide, zinc oxide and bismuth subgallate exert a protective action on mucous membranes and raw surfaces. They are mildly astringent and are reported to have antiseptic properties.

Balsam peru has protective properties and a very mild antiseptic action by virtue of its content of cinnamic and benzoic acids. It is believed to promote the growth of epithelial cells.

5.2 Pharmacokinetic properties
It is well known that topically applied corticosteroids can be absorbed percutaneously. This appears to be more likely upon repeated or prolonged use.

The remaining active ingredients in Anugesic HC Suppositories exert their therapeutic effect without being absorbed into the systemic circulation. These observations are supported by evidence from various studies and reviews.

5.3 Preclinical safety data
The results of the preclinical tests do not add anything of further significance to the prescriber.

6. PHARMACEUTICAL PARTICULARS
6.1 List of excipients
Calcium hydrogen phosphate, hard fat "A", hard fat "B" and cocoa butter.

6.2 Incompatibilities
None known

6.3 Shelf life
3 years.

6.4 Special precautions for storage
Store below 25°C.

6.5 Nature and contents of container
Printed strip pack consisting of white opaque PVC/polyethylene laminated film. Supplied in packs of 12 and 24 suppositories.

6.6 Instructions for use and handling
No special instructions needed.

7. MARKETING AUTHORISATION HOLDER
Pfizer Limited

Sandwich

Kent CT13 9NJ

United Kingdom

8. MARKETING AUTHORISATION NUMBER(S)
PL 00057/0521

9. DATE OF FIRST AUTHORISATION/RENEWAL OF THE AUTHORISATION
1st July 2003

10. DATE OF REVISION OF THE TEXT

Anusol Cream

(Pfizer Consumer Healthcare)

1. NAME OF THE MEDICINAL PRODUCT
ANUSOL cream

2. QUALITATIVE AND QUANTITATIVE COMPOSITION
ANUSOL cream contains -

Zinc oxide Ph Eur	10.75 g
Bismith oxide	2.14 g
Balsam Peru Ph Eur	1.8 g

3. PHARMACEUTICAL FORM
A buff coloured cream

4. CLINICAL PARTICULARS
4.1 Therapeutic indications
ANUSOL cream provides antiseptic, astringent and emollient properties which help to relieve discomfort associated with minor ano-rectal conditions.

ANUSOL cream also provides lubricating properties for use with suppositories.

Indicated for the symptomatic relief of uncomplicated internal and external haemorrhoids, pruritus ani, proctitis and fissures. Also indicated post-operatively in ano-rectal surgical procedures and after incision of thrombosed or sclerosed ano-rectal veins.

4.2 Posology and method of administration
Topical

Adults and elderly (over 65 years): apply to the affected area at night, in the morning and after each evacuation until the condition is controlled. Thoroughly cleanse the affected area, dry and apply cream. ANUSOL cream is prepared in a vanishing cream base and may be gently smoothed on to the affected area without the need to apply a gauze dressing. For internal conditions, use rectal nozzle provided. Remove the nozzle cap. Clean the nozzle after each use.

Not to be taken orally.

Children: Not Recommended.

4.3 Contraindications
Known hypersensitivity to any of the constituents.

4.4 Special warnings and special precautions for use
None known.

4.5 Interaction with other medicinal products and other forms of Interaction
None known.

4.6 Pregnancy and lactation
Whilst formal studies on the effect of this product during human pregnancy have not been conducted, there is no epidemiological evidence of adverse effect, either to the pregnant mother or foetus.

4.7 Effects on ability to drive and use machines
None known.

4.8 Undesirable effects
Rarely, sensitivity reactions. Patients may occasionally experience transient burning on application, especially if the anoderm is not intact.

4.9 Overdose
Treatment of a large acute overdose should include gastric lavage, purgation with magnesium sulphate and complete bed rest. If necessary, apply oxygen and give general supportive measures.

5. PHARMACOLOGICAL PROPERTIES
5.1 Pharmacodynamic properties
ANUSOL cream provides antiseptic, astringent and emollient properties which help to relieve discomfort associated with minor ano-rectal conditions. It also provides lubricating properties for use with suppositories.

Bismuth oxide is weakly astringent with supposed antiseptic properties and has a protective action on mucous membranes and raw surfaces. Zinc oxide is an astringent and mild antiseptic and probably owes its actions to the ability of the zinc ion to precipitate protein, but other mechanisms may be involved. Zinc oxide is also used to absorb skin moisture and decrease friction and discourage growth of certain bacteria. Balsam Peru has a very mild antiseptic action by virtue of its content of cinnamic and benzoic acids. It is believed to promote the growth of epithelial cells.

5.2 Pharmacokinetic properties
The active ingredients exert their therapeutic effect without being absorbed into the systemic circulation. These observations are supported by evidence from various studies and reviews.

5.3 Preclinical safety data
The active ingredients of ANUSOL are well known constituents of medicinal products and their safety profiles are well documented.

6. PHARMACEUTICAL PARTICULARS
6.1 List of excipients
Glycerol monostearate Ph Eur

Liquid paraffin Ph Eur

Propylene glycol Ph Eur

Polysorbate 60 Ph Eur

Sorbitan stearate BP

Titanium dioxide Ph Eur

Methyl p-hydroxybenzoate Ph Eur

Propyl p-hydroxybenzoate Ph Eur

Purified water Ph Eur

6.2 Incompatibilities
None known.

6.3 Shelf life
3 years when stored in the original packaging.

6.4 Special precautions for storage
Store at a temperature not exceeding 25°C.

6.5 Nature and contents of container
Pack size 23g, 30g or 43g, externally printed and internally lacquered aluminium tube with plastic cap. A plastic nozzle with cap is also provided for internal application.

6.6 Instructions for use and handling
No special requirements.

7. MARKETING AUTHORISATION HOLDER
Pfizer Consumer Healthcare

Alternative Trading Style

Warner Lambert Consumer Healthcare

Walton Oaks

Dorking Road

Walton-on-the-Hill

Surrey KT20 7NS

United Kingdom

8. MARKETING AUTHORISATION NUMBER(S)
PL 15513/0041

9. DATE OF FIRST AUTHORISATION/RENEWAL OF THE AUTHORISATION
15 September 1997

10. DATE OF REVISION OF THE TEXT
January 2005

Anusol Ointment

(Pfizer Consumer Healthcare)

1. NAME OF THE MEDICINAL PRODUCT
Anusol Ointment

2. QUALITATIVE AND QUANTITATIVE COMPOSITION
Each 100g ointment contains:

Zinc Oxide 10.75 g

Bismuth Subgallate 2.25 g

Balsam Peru 1.875 g

Bismuth Oxide 0.875 g

3. PHARMACEUTICAL FORM
A light buff coloured ointment.

4. CLINICAL PARTICULARS
4.1 Therapeutic indications
Symptomatic relief of uncomplicated internal and external haemorrhoids, pruritus ani, proctitis and fissures. Also indicated post operatively in ano-rectal surgical procedures and after incision of thrombosed or sclerosed anorectal veins.

Anusol Ointment provides antiseptic, astringent and emollient properties which help to relieve discomfort associated with minor ano-rectal conditions.

4.2 Posology and method of administration
Topical.

Adults and Elderly (over 65 years): Apply to the affected area at night, in the morning and after each evacuation until the condition is controlled. Thoroughly cleanse the affected area, dry and apply ointment. Anusol Ointment should be applied on a gauze dressing. For internal conditions use rectal nozzle provided. Remove the nozzle cap. Clean the nozzle after each use. Not to be taken orally.

Children: Not recommended

4.3 Contraindications
Known hypersensitivity to any of the constituents.

4.4 Special warnings and special precautions for use
None known.

4.5 Interaction with other medicinal products and other forms of Interaction
None known.

4.6 Pregnancy and lactation
Whilst formal studies on the effect of this product during pregnancy have not been conducted, there is no epidemiological evidence of adverse effects either to the pregnant mother or foetus.

4.7 Effects on ability to drive and use machines
None known.

4.8 Undesirable effects
Rarely, sensitivity reactions. Patients may occasionally experience transient burning on application, especially if the anoderm is not intact.

4.9 Overdose
Treatment of a large acute overdose should include gastric lavage, purgation with magnesium sulphate and complete bed rest. If necessary, apply oxygen and give general supportive measures.

5. PHARMACOLOGICAL PROPERTIES
5.1 Pharmacodynamic properties
Anusol Ointment provides antiseptic, astringent and emollient properties which help to relieve discomfort associated with minor ano-rectal conditions.

Bismuth Oxide is weakly astringent with supposed antiseptic properties and has a protective action on mucous membranes and raw surfaces.

Zinc Oxide is an astringent and mild antiseptic and probably owes its actions to the ability of the zinc ion to precipitate protein but other mechanisms may be involved. Zinc Oxide is also used to absorb skin moisture and decrease friction and discourage growth of certain bacteria.

Balsam Peru has a very mild antiseptic action by virtue of its content of cinnamic and benzoic acids. It is believed to promote the growth of epithelial cells.

5.2 Pharmacokinetic properties
The active ingredients exert their therapeutic effect without being absorbed into the systemic circulation. These observations are supported by evidence from various studies and reviews.

5.3 Preclinical safety data
The active ingredients of Anusol are well known constituents of medicinal products and their safety profile is well documented.

6. PHARMACEUTICAL PARTICULARS
6.1 List of excipients
Anusol Ointment contains the following excipients:-

Magnesium stearate

Cocoa butter

Lanolin anhydrous

Castor oil

Kaolin light

Petroleum Jelly White

6.2 Incompatibilities
None known.

6.3 Shelf life
Not less than 3 years when stored in the original packing.

6.4 Special precautions for storage
Do not store above 25° C.

6.5 Nature and contents of container
Externally printed and internally lacquered 25 g aluminium tube with plastic cap. A plastic nozzle with cap is also provided for internal application.

6.6 Instructions for use and handling
No special requirements.

7. MARKETING AUTHORISATION HOLDER
Pfizer Consumer Healthcare

Alternative Trading Style

Warner Lambert Consumer Healthcare

Walton Oaks

Dorking Road

Walton-on-the-Hill

Surrey KT20 7NS

United Kingdom

8. MARKETING AUTHORISATION NUMBER(S)
15513/0042

9. DATE OF FIRST AUTHORISATION/RENEWAL OF THE AUTHORISATION
14 March 1997

10. DATE OF REVISION OF THE TEXT
January 2005

Anusol Plus HC Ointment

(Pfizer Consumer Healthcare)

1. NAME OF THE MEDICINAL PRODUCT
ANUSOL PLUS HC OINTMENT

2. QUALITATIVE AND QUANTITATIVE COMPOSITION
Each 100 g of ointment contains the following active ingredients:-

Hydrocortisone acetate Ph Eur 0.25 g

Benzyl benzoate Ph Eur 1.25 g

Bismuth subgallate FP 2.25 g

Bismuth oxide 0.875 g

Balsam peru Ph Eur 1.875 g

Zinc oxide Ph Eur 10.75 g

3. PHARMACEUTICAL FORM
Ointment.

4. CLINICAL PARTICULARS
4.1 Therapeutic indications
Symptomatic treatment of internal and external haemorrhoids and pruritus ani.

4.2 Posology and method of administration
Topical administration.

ADULTS (over 18 years)

To be applied sparingly to the affected area at night, in the morning and after each evacuation up to a maximum of 4 applications a day. Thoroughly cleanse the affected area, dry and apply ointment on a gauze dressing. For internal conditions use rectal nozzle provided. Remove the nozzle cap. Clean the nozzle after each use. Use for a maximum period of one week.

ELDERLY (over 65 years)

As for adults

CHILDREN (under 18 years)

Not recommended.

4.3 Contraindications
Tubercular, fungal and most viral lesions including herpes simplex, vaccinia and varicella. History of sensitivity to any of the constituents.

4.4 Special warnings and special precautions for use
As with all products containing topical steroids, the possibility of systemic absorption should be borne in mind.

Prolonged or excessive use may produce systemic corticosteroid effects, and use for periods longer than seven days is not recommended.

The product should be discontinued and the patient advised to consult a medical practitioner if symptoms do not improve or worsen or if rectal bleeding occurs.

4.5 Interaction with other medicinal products and other forms of Interaction
Concurrent use with other corticosteroid preparations, either topically or orally may increase the likelihood of systemic effects.

4.6 Pregnancy and lactation
There is inadequate evidence of safety in human pregnancy and there may be a very small risk of cleft palate and intrauterine growth retardation as well as suppression of the neonatal hypothalamic-pituitary-adrenal axis. There is evidence of harmful effects in animals. To be used in pregnancy only when there is no safer alternative and when the disease itself carries risks for the mother or child.

No special precautions required for use during lactation.

4.7 Effects on ability to drive and use machines
No effects have been reported on ability to drive or use machinery.

4.8 Undesirable effects
Rarely, sensitivity reactions may occur. Patients may occasionally experience transient burning on application, especially if the anoderm is not intact.

4.9 Overdose
If swallowed, fever, nausea, vomiting, stomach cramps and diarrhoea may develop 3-12 hours after ingestion.

Hydrocortisone normally does not produce toxic effects in an acute single overdose.

Treatment of a large acute overdose should include gastric lavage, purgation with magnesium sulphate and complete bed rest. If necessary oxygen and general supportive measures should be given. Methaemoglobinaemia should be treated by intravenous methylthioninium chloride.

5. PHARMACOLOGICAL PROPERTIES
5.1 Pharmacodynamic properties
ANUSOL PLUS HC provides antiseptic, astringent, emollient and decongestant properties. In addition hydrocortisone exerts anti-inflammatory actions.

Bismuth oxide, zinc oxide, and bismuth subgallate exert a protective action on mucous membranes and raw surfaces. They are mildly astringent and are reported to have antiseptic properties.

Balsam Peru has protective properties and a very mild antiseptic action by virtue of its contents of cinnamic and benzoic acids. It is believed to promote the growth of epithelial cells.

Benzyl benzoate is used as a solubilizing agent and has mild antiseptic and preservative properties.

Hydrocortisone acetate has the general properties of hydrocortisone and this anti-inflammatory action is of primary interest of this product.

5.2 Pharmacokinetic properties
Systemic absorption of hydrocortisone acetate from the rectum may occur but estimates of the extent of absorption have been variable and have always been less than 30%. Following absorption it is metabolised in the liver and most body tissues before being excreted in the urine. Biological half life is approximately 100 minutes and it is 90% bound to plasma protein.

The other active ingredients in Anusol Plus HC Ointment exert their therapeutic effect without being absorbed into the systemic circulation. These are supported by evidence from various studies and reviews.

5.3 Preclinical safety data
The active ingredients of Anusol are well known constituents of medicinal products and their safety profile is well documented.

6. PHARMACEUTICAL PARTICULARS
6.1 List of excipients
Kaolin light

Magnesium stearate

Castor oil

Cocoa butter

Lanolin anhydrous

Petroleum jelly white

Calcium hydrogen phosphate

6.2 Incompatibilities
No incompatibilities have been reported.

6.3 Shelf life
3 years.

6.4 Special precautions for storage
Do not store above 25°C

6.5 Nature and contents of container
Externally printed aluminium tube with wadded plastic cap, containing 15 g of ointment. A plastic nozzle with cap is also provided for internal application.

6.6 Instructions for use and handling
No Special Requirements.

7. MARKETING AUTHORISATION HOLDER
Pfizer Consumer Healthcare

Alternative Trading Style

Warner Lambert Consumer Healthcare

Walton Oaks

Dorking Road

Walton-on-the-Hill

Surrey KT20 7NS

United Kingdom

8. MARKETING AUTHORISATION NUMBER(S)
PL 15513/0039

9. DATE OF FIRST AUTHORISATION/RENEWAL OF THE AUTHORISATION
02 January 2000 / 26 January 2001

10. DATE OF REVISION OF THE TEXT
January 2005

Anusol Plus HC Suppositories

(Pfizer Consumer Healthcare)

1. NAME OF THE MEDICINAL PRODUCT
Anusol Plus HC Suppositories

2. QUALITATIVE AND QUANTITATIVE COMPOSITION
Anusol Plus HC Suppositories contain:

Hydrocortisone acetate 10 mg

Benzyl benzoate 33 mg

Bismuth subgallate 59 mg

Bismuth oxide 24 mg

Balsam peru 49 mg

Zinc oxide 296 mg

3. PHARMACEUTICAL FORM
Suppository

4. CLINICAL PARTICULARS
4.1 Therapeutic indications
Symptomatic treatment of internal haemorrhoids and pruritus ani.

4.2 Posology and method of administration
Anal insertion

Adults (over 18 years)

Remove wrapper and insert one suppository into the anus at night, in the morning and after each evacuation up to a maximum of three per day for a maximum period of one week.

Elderly (over 65 years)

As for adults

Children (under 18 years)

Not recommended.

4.3 Contraindications
Tubercular, fungal and most viral lesions including herpes simplex, vaccinia and varicella. History of sensitivity to any of the constituents.

4.4 Special warnings and special precautions for use
As with all products containing topical steroids, the possibility of systemic absorption should be borne in mind.

Prolonged or excessive use may produce systemic corticosteroid effects, and use for periods longer than seven days is not recommended.

The product should be discontinued and the patient advised to consult a medical practitioner if symptoms do not improve or worsen or if rectal bleeding occurs.

4.5 Interaction with other medicinal products and other forms of Interaction
Concurrent use with other corticosteroid preparations, either topically or orally, may increase the likelihood of systemic effects.

4.6 Pregnancy and lactation
There is inadequate evidence of safety in human pregnancy and there may be a very small risk of cleft palate and intrauterine growth retardation as well as suppression of the neonatal hypothalamic-pituitary-adrenal axis. There is evidence of harmful effects in animals. To be used in pregnancy only when there is no safer alternative and when the disease itself carries risks for the mother or child.

No special precautions required for use during lactation.

4.7 Effects on ability to drive and use machines
No effects have been reported on ability to drive or use machinery.

4.8 Undesirable effects
Rarely, sensitivity reactions may occur. Patients may occasionally experience transient burning on application, especially if the anoderm is not intact.

4.9 Overdose
If swallowed, fever, nausea, vomiting, stomach cramps and diarrhoea may develop 3-12 hours after ingestion.

Hydrocortisone normally does not produce toxic effects in an acute single overdose.

Treatment of a large acute overdose should include gastric lavage, purgation with magnesium sulphate and complete bed rest. If necessary give oxygen and general supportive measures. Methaemoglobinaemia should be treated by intravenous methylene blue.

5. PHARMACOLOGICAL PROPERTIES
5.1 Pharmacodynamic properties
Anusol Plus HC provides antiseptic, astringent, emollient and decongestant properties. In addition, hydrocortisone exerts an anti-inflammatory action.

Bismuth oxide, zinc oxide and bismuth subgallate exert a protective action on mucous membranes and raw surfaces. They are mildly astringent and are reported to have antiseptic properties

Balsam Peru has protective properties and very mild antiseptic action by virtue of its content of cinnamic and benzoic acids. It is believed to promote the growth of epithelial cells.

Benzyl benzoate is used as a solubilizing agent and has mild antiseptic and preservative properties.

Hydrocortisone acetate has the general properties of hydrocortisone and the anti-inflammatory action is of primary interest in the product.

5.2 Pharmacokinetic properties
Systemic absorption of hydrocortisone acetate from the rectum may occur but estimates of the extent of absorption have been variable and have always been less than 30%. Following absorption it is metabolised in the liver and most body tissues before being excreted in the urine. Biological half-life is approximately 100 minutes and it is 90% bound to plasma protein.

The other active ingredients in Anusol HC Plus Suppositories exert their therapeutic effect without being absorbed into the systemic circulation. These observations are supported by evidence from various studies and reviews.

5.3 Preclinical safety data
The active ingredients of Anusol are well known constituents of medicinal products and their safety profile is well documented.

6. PHARMACEUTICAL PARTICULARS
6.1 List of excipients
Kaolin light

Hard Fat (Suppocire BS2)

6.2 Incompatibilities
No incompatibilities have been reported.

6.3 Shelf life
3 years.

6.4 Special precautions for storage
Do not store above 25°C.

6.5 Nature and contents of container
Printed strip pack consisting of white opaque PVC/polyethylene laminated film. Each pack contains 12 suppositories.

6.6 Instructions for use and handling
No special requirements.

Administrative Data

7. MARKETING AUTHORISATION HOLDER
Pfizer Consumer Healthcare

Alternative Trading Style

Warner Lambert Consumer Healthcare

Walton Oaks

Dorking Road

Walton-on-the-Hill

Surrey KT20 7NS

United Kingdom

8. MARKETING AUTHORISATION NUMBER(S)
PL 15513/0040

9. DATE OF FIRST AUTHORISATION/RENEWAL OF THE AUTHORISATION
31st October 1997 / 26th January 2001

10. DATE OF REVISION OF THE TEXT
February 2004

Anusol Suppositories

(Pfizer Consumer Healthcare)

1. NAME OF THE MEDICINAL PRODUCT
Anusol Suppositories

2. QUALITATIVE AND QUANTITATIVE COMPOSITION
Each suppository contains:

Zinc oxide 296 mg

Bismuth subgallate 59 mg

Balsam peru 49 mg

Bismuth oxide 24 mg

3. PHARMACEUTICAL FORM
Suppository

4. CLINICAL PARTICULARS

4.1 Therapeutic indications
For the relief of internal haemorrhoids and other related ano-rectal conditions.

4.2 Posology and method of administration
Anal insertion

Adults
Remove wrapper and insert one suppository into the anus at night, in the morning and after each evacuation. Not to be taken orally.

Elderly (over 65 years)

As for adults

Children

Not recommended.

4.3 Contraindications
History of sensitivity to any of the constituents.

4.4 Special warnings and special precautions for use
None known.

4.5 Interaction with other medicinal products and other forms of Interaction
None known.

4.6 Pregnancy and lactation
Whilst formal studies on the effect of this product during human pregnancy have not been conducted, there is no epidemiological evidence of adverse effect, either to the pregnant mother or foetus.

4.7 Effects on ability to drive and use machines
None known.

4.8 Undesirable effects
Rarely, sensitivity reactions. Patients may occasionally experience transient burning on application, especially if the anoderm is not intact.

4.9 Overdose
Treatment of a large acute overdose should include gastric lavage, purgation with magnesium sulphate and complete bed rest. If necessary, give oxygen and general supportive measures.

5. PHARMACOLOGICAL PROPERTIES

5.1 Pharmacodynamic properties
Anusol Suppositories provide antiseptic, astringent and emollient properties which help to relieve discomfort associated with minor ano-rectal conditions.

Bismuth Oxide, Zinc Oxide and Bismuth Subgallate exert a protective action on mucous membranes and raw surfaces. They are mildly astringent and are reported to have antiseptic properties.

Balsam Peru has protective properties and a very mild antiseptic action by virtue of its content of Cinnamic and Benzoic Acids. It is believed to promote the growth of epithelial cells.

5.2 Pharmacokinetic properties
The active ingredients in Anusol Suppositories exert their therapeutic effect without being absorbed into the systemic circulation. These observations are supported by evidence from various studies and reviews.

5.3 Preclinical safety data
The active ingredients of Anusol are well known constituents of medicinal products and their safety profile is well documented.

6. PHARMACEUTICAL PARTICULARS

6.1 List of excipients
Hard Fat (Suppocire BS2)

Kaolin light

Titanium Dioxide

Miglyol 812

6.2 Incompatibilities
None known.

6.3 Shelf life
3 years.

6.4 Special precautions for storage
Store at a temperature not exceeding 25°C.

6.5 Nature and contents of container
12 and 24 pack printed strip pack consisting of white opaque PVC/polyethylene laminated film.

6.6 Instructions for use and handling
No special requirements.

Administrative Data

7. MARKETING AUTHORISATION HOLDER
Pfizer Consumer Healthcare

Alternative Trading Style

Warner Lambert Consumer Healthcare

Walton Oaks

Dorking Road

Walton-on-the-Hill

Surrey KT20 7NS

United Kingdom

8. MARKETING AUTHORISATION NUMBER(S)
PL 15513/0043

9. DATE OF FIRST AUTHORISATION/RENEWAL OF THE AUTHORISATION
15th September 1997 / 19th July 2001

10. DATE OF REVISION OF THE TEXT
February 2004

Anzemet IV

(Amdipharm)

1. NAME OF THE MEDICINAL PRODUCT
Anzemet IV 20 mg/ml Solution for injection ▼

2. QUALITATIVE AND QUANTITATIVE COMPOSITION
Dolasetron mesilate 20 mg/ml

Ampoules each contain:

9.3 mg Dolasetron (as 12.5 mg mesilate salt) in 0.625 ml solution for injection

74 mg Dolasetron (as 100 mg mesilate salt) in 5 ml solution for injection

For excipients, see 6.1.

3. PHARMACEUTICAL FORM
Solution for injection.

Clear, colourless solution, free from visible particles.

4. CLINICAL PARTICULARS

4.1 Therapeutic indications
- Management of nausea and vomiting in patients receiving initial and repeat courses of cancer chemotherapy (including high dose cisplatin).

- Treatment of post operative nausea and vomiting.

- Prevention of post operative nausea and vomiting in patients at high risk, such as intra-abdominal gynaecological surgery or with a known history of post operative nausea and vomiting.

4.2 Posology and method of administration
Anzemet IV can be injected over 30 seconds or diluted to 50 ml in normal saline, 5% dextrose or other compatible intravenous fluids (see Section 6.2 Incompatibilities) and infused over a period of 30 seconds to 15 minutes. More rapid iv administration should be avoided. See 4.8 Undesirable Effects.

CANCER THERAPY INDUCED NAUSEA AND VOMITING

Adults

For prevention of nausea and vomiting in patients receiving emetogenic chemotherapy, a 100 mg single dose of Anzemet IV is recommended approximately 30 minutes prior to each chemotherapy treatment. To protect against delayed nausea and vomiting after the cessation of a chemotherapy cycle, a 200 mg single daily dose of Anzemet tablets is recommended. Anzemet IV or tablets may be administered for up to a maximum of 4 consecutive days in relation to any one chemotherapy cycle.

The efficacy of Anzemet IV in controlling nausea and vomiting can be improved by coadministration of corticosteroids.

Children

Anzemet IV is not recommended for use in children.

Elderly

Patient and volunteer data indicate that the pharmacokinetics of Dolasetron and the active metabolite are unaltered in patients 65 years of age or older and thus no dosage adjustment is required.

Patients with renal impairment

Plasma levels of the active metabolite are increased after oral or intravenous administration of Anzemet IV in patients with severe renal failure (creatinine clearance < 10 ml/min). No dosage adjustment is required.

A small percentage of renally impaired patients may be poor metabolisers and therefore plasma levels in these patients may be higher.

Patients with hepatic impairment

Plasma levels of the active metabolite are increased after oral and unchanged after intravenous administration of Anzemet IV in patients with severe hepatic failure (Child-Pugh Class B or C). No dosage adjustment is required.

POST-OPERATIVE NAUSEA AND VOMITING

Adults

For treatment a single dose should be administered as soon as nausea or emesis presents. The recommended dose for treatment is 12.5 mg.

For prevention of post-operative nausea and vomiting a single dose of Anzemet IV is recommended at cessation of anaesthesia. The recommended dose for prevention is 12.5 mg.

Children

Anzemet IV is not recommended for use in children.

Elderly

Patient and volunteer data indicate that the pharmacokinetics of Dolasetron and the active metabolite are unaltered in patients 65 years of age or older and thus no dosage adjustment is required.

Patients with renal impairment

Plasma levels of the active metabolite are increased after oral or intravenous administration of Anzemet IV in patients with severe renal failure (creatinine clearance < 10 ml/min). No dosage adjustment is required.

A small percentage of renally impaired patients may be poor metabolisers and therefore plasma levels in these patients may be higher.

Patients with hepatic impairment

Plasma levels of the active metabolite are increased after oral and unchanged after intravenous administration of Anzemet IV in patients with severe hepatic failure (Child-Pugh Class B or C). No dosage adjustment is required.

4.3 Contraindications
Patients with a markedly prolonged QTc interval (for example, in association with congenital QT interval prolongation), patients with AV block II-III, and patients receiving concomitant Class I and III antiarrhythmics should not receive Anzemet IV.

There is insufficient information in such patients on the effects of Anzemet IV on the electrocardiogram to conclude that the drug may be safely administered in these circumstances.

Hypersensitivity to the active substance or to any of the excipients.

4.4 Special warnings and special precautions for use
5-HT_3 receptor antagonists, including Anzemet IV, have been shown to cause ECG interval prolongations, including QTc.

Use of 5-HT_3 receptor antagonists and other drugs which prolong ECG intervals requires that caution be exercised in patients who have existing prolongation of cardiac conduction intervals, particularly QTc, patients with significant electrolyte disturbances, bundle branch block or underlying cardiac diseases such as congestive heart failure. See Sections 4.3 Contraindications and 4.8 Undesirable Effects.

Anzemet IV should not be administered by intramuscular injection.

Cross-hypersensitivity reactions have been reported in patients who received other selective 5-HT_3 receptor antagonists. Although these type of reactions have not, as yet, been reported with Dolasetron mesilate, patients who have experienced hypersensitivity reactions with other 5-HT_3 receptor antagonists should be closely monitored following the administration of Anzemet IV.

4.5 Interaction with other medicinal products and other forms of Interaction

The potential for clinically significant drug-drug interactions posed by Dolasetron mesilate and its active metabolite appears to be low for drugs commonly used in chemotherapy or surgery, because the active metabolite is eliminated by multiple routes. Inhibition or induction of cytochrome P450 does not cause large changes in clearance of Dolasetron as demonstrated by concomitant administration of cimetidine for 7 days (peak plasma concentrations and systemic exposure of the active metabolite increased by 15% and 24%, respectively) and concomitant administration of rifampicin for 7 days (peak plasma concentrations and systemic exposure of the metabolite decreased by 17% and 28%, respectively).

The efficacy of Anzemet IV may be enhanced by the coadministration of dexamethasone.

4.6 Pregnancy and lactation

There is no experience in humans. Anzemet IV should not be used during pregnancy unless the expected benefit to the patient is thought to outweigh any possible risk to the foetus.

Dolasetron mesilate is not teratogenic when administered to animals and did not affect male or female fertility, nor perinatal or postnatal development.

It is not known if Dolasetron or its metabolites are excreted in human milk. Therefore, it is recommended that mothers receiving Anzemet IV should not breast feed their babies.

4.7 Effects on ability to drive and use machines

No known effects.

4.8 Undesirable effects

The most frequently reported undesirable effects in cancer patients receiving Anzemet IV in single dose studies were headache 21.9%, diarrhoea 9.9%, tachycardia 3.3%, fever 3.2% and fatigue 3.2%; these events occurred with similar frequency with the comparator 5-HT_3 receptor antagonists.

In a study where Anzemet IV was administered to cancer patients for seven consecutive days, the most frequently reported undesirable effects were headache 43.7%, constipation 32.1%, fatigue 24.2%, sleep disorder 16.9%, dyspepsia 16.3%, diarrhoea 16.3%, abdominal pain 15.7%, dizziness 14.0%, drowsiness 12.0%, flushing 11.4%, pain 11.4%, anorexia 10.8%, taste perversion 8.7%, chills/shivering 7.9% and flatulence 6.1%; these events occurred with similar frequency with the comparator 5-HT_3 receptor antagonist.

The most frequently reported undesirable effects in surgical patients receiving Anzemet IV in single dose studies were bradycardia 10.0%, headache 8.3%, T wave change 4.6% and dizziness 4.0%; these events occurred with similar frequency with placebo.

Over all clinical trials, hypotension occurred in 1.9% of Dolasetron patients; this event occurred at a similar frequency with placebo or active comparator. Similarly, occasional transient asymptomatic increases in serum transaminases have been reported. There have been rare ($<0.1\%$) reports of intestinal obstruction, pancreatitis, jaundice, seizure, cardiac arrhythmia, bronchospasm, severe bradycardia and oedema. The relationship of these events to Anzemet IV has not been established.

Reversible ECG interval changes (PR and QT_c prolongation, QRS widening) may occur and are related in magnitude and frequency to blood levels of the active metabolite. These changes are self limiting with declining blood levels. Some patients have interval prolongations for 24 hours or longer. Interval prolongation could lead to cardiovascular consequences, including heart block or cardiac arrhythmias. These have been rarely reported.

In very rare cases, severe hypotension, bradycardia and possibly loss of consciousness may occur immediately or closely following iv bolus administration of dolasetron mesilate.

There are very rare reports of wide complex tachycardia or ventricular tachycardia and of ventricular fibrillation/cardiac arrest following intravenous administration.

Local pain or burning may be experienced on intravenous administration.

As with other 5-HT_3 receptor antagonists, there have been reports of hyper-sensitivity reactions such as rash, pruritus, urticaria, bronchospasm and very rare reports of angio-oedema and anaphylaxis. See 4.4 Special warnings and precautions for use.

4.9 Overdose

There is no specific antidote for Dolasetron mesilate. Following a suspected overdose, patients should be managed with symptomatic and supportive therapy as part of expectant management. If clinically indicated, the patient should have cardiac monitoring.

Severe hypotension and dizziness were reported soon after intravenous infusion of 13 mg/kg: normal sinus rhythm with prolongation of the PR, QRS and QTc intervals was recorded on ECG at 2 hours after the infusion. See 4.8 Undesirable Effects for information on asymptomatic ECG interval prolongations. In a child who received 6 mg/kg orally, no clinical symptoms occurred and no treatment was given.

5. PHARMACOLOGICAL PROPERTIES

5.1 Pharmacodynamic properties

Pharmacotherapeutic group: Serotonin (5-HT_3) antagonists,

ATC code: A04A A04

Dolasetron mesilate and its major metabolite are selective serotonin 5-HT_3 antagonists. The precise mode of action as an antiemetic is not known. The serotonin 5-HT_3 receptors are located on the nerve terminals of the vagus in the periphery and are centrally located in the chemoreceptor trigger zone of the area postrema. It is thought that chemotherapeutic agents produce nausea and vomiting by releasing serotonin from the enterochromaffin cells of the small intestine and that the released serotonin can then activate 5-HT_3 receptors located on vagal efferents to initiate the vomiting reflex. The effect of Anzemet IV in the management of cancer therapy induced nausea and vomiting is due to antagonism of 5-HT_3 receptors on neurons either peripherally and/or centrally located.

The mechanisms of action in post-operative nausea and vomiting are not known but there may be pathways common to chemotherapy induced nausea and vomiting.

5.2 Pharmacokinetic properties

a) General characteristics of the active substance

Dolasetron mesilate is rapidly ($t_{½} < 10$ minutes) and completely metabolised to the active reduced metabolite, which is widely distributed in the body with mean apparent volume of distribution of 5.0-7.9 l/kg. The plasma protein binding of the active metabolite is approximately 69-77%.

The absolute bioavailability of an oral solution is approximately 75%.

The active metabolite is eliminated by renal excretion (approximately 30%) and metabolism, mainly glucuronidation and hydroxylation.

In man, the $t_{½}$ of the active metabolite is 7-9 hours. The pharmacokinetics of the active metabolite are linear over the therapeutic dose range.

b) Characteristics in patients

The pharmacokinetics of the active metabolite are similar in cancer patients, elderly subjects and healthy young male and female subjects.

Although Anzemet IV is not recommended in children, the following data are available. In paediatric cancer patients, clearance of active metabolite increased 1.3 to 2-fold (12-17 years) and 2 to 3-fold (3-11 years) compared to adult cancer patients or healthy volunteers. In paediatric surgery patients, clearance of active metabolite increased approximately 1.4-fold (2-12 years) compared to adult healthy volunteers. These changes resulted in significantly lower plasma levels and systemic exposures compared to adults administered the same doses.

In patients with severe renal impairment (creatinine clearance <10 ml/min), maximum plasma levels of metabolite are increased 17% or 34%, respectively, after intravenous or oral administration of Dolasetron mesilate, and systemic exposure is increased approximately 2-fold.

In patients with severe hepatic impairment (Child-Pugh Class B or C), maximum plasma levels of metabolite are increased 18% and systemic exposure increases 66% after oral administration of Dolasetron mesilate. Systemic exposure is not altered after intravenous administration of Dolasetron mesilate to this patient population.

In poor metabolisers of sparteine/debrisoquine, maximum plasma levels of metabolite are unchanged whilst systemic exposure is increased up to 2-fold.

5.3 Preclinical safety data

Repeated daily intravenous administration of Dolasetron mesilate to rats and dogs produced CNS effects at plasma concentrations in the same range as the maximum plasma concentration in humans given the highest recommended intravenous dose (100 mg). Similar effects have not been reported in humans at a frequency greater than active comparator or placebo.

Seizures were observed following repeat intravenous dosing in rats (60 mg/kg/day) which resulted in plasma concentrations equal to or greater than 7 times the maximum plasma concentrations in humans given the highest recommended intravenous dose (100 mg). Seizures were also observed following single intravenous doses of 140 and 126 mg/kg in mice and rats, respectively.

Dolasetron mesilate was not mutagenic in a variety of *in vitro* and *in vivo* mutagenicity tests, including the mouse micronucleus assay. Tumour findings in the high dose group of the mouse oral carcinogenicity study were not considered relevant for the clinical short-term use.

In μmolar concentrations, Dolasetron and its metabolite MDL 74,156, as with other 5-HT_3 antagonists, blocked cloned human cardiac Na^+ and HERG K^+ ion channels.

6. PHARMACEUTICAL PARTICULARS

6.1 List of excipients

Mannitol for Injection.

Sodium acetate trihydrate.

Glacial acetic acid.

Water for Injections.

6.2 Incompatibilities

In general, Anzemet IV should not be mixed in solution with other drugs. It is important that when any drugs are administered at the same time as Anzemet IV that the tubing and Y-site are thoroughly and completely flushed with a compatible infusion fluid between administration of the two drug solutions.

6.3 Shelf life

Undiluted product: 3 years

Diluted product: 24 hours

6.4 Special precautions for storage

Undiluted product: Keep the container in the outer carton in order to protect from light.

Diluted product: Dilutions of intravenous fluids should be used immediately after preparation. If storage cannot be avoided, the maximum storage time of dilutions is 24 hours at 2 – 8°C.

6.5 Nature and contents of container

The ampoules are either a 1 ml (12.5 mg) or 5 ml (100 mg) clear glass type I ampoule, packed in a cardboard carton. Cartons are bundled by transparent foil.

Package quantities: 12.5 mg - ten ampoules

100 mg - one ampoule

100 mg - five ampoules

6.6 Instructions for use and handling

The container and solution should be visually inspected before use. Use only clear particle-free, colourless solution. Do not use if the container is damaged.

Compatibility with infusion fluids: Anzemet IV should only be admixed with those infusion fluids which are recommended. Anzemet IV is physically and chemically stable at concentrations up to 2 mg/ml in the following infusion fluids:

5% Glucose

0.9% Sodium chloride

10% Mannitol

Compound sodium lactate

0.18% Sodium chloride/4% Glucose

Anzemet IV is compatible with polypropylene syringes.

7. MARKETING AUTHORISATION HOLDER

Amdipharm plc
Regency House
Miles Gray Road
Basildon
Essex SS14 3AF
United Kingdom

8. MARKETING AUTHORISATION NUMBER(S)

PL 20072/0001

9. DATE OF FIRST AUTHORISATION/RENEWAL OF THE AUTHORISATION

22 December 2003

10. DATE OF REVISION OF THE TEXT

Anzemet IV and tablets

(Amdipharm)

1. NAME OF THE MEDICINAL PRODUCT

ANZEMET IV 20 mg/ml Solution for injection ▼

ANZEMET 50 mg tablets ▼

ANZEMET 200 mg tablets ▼

2. QUALITATIVE AND QUANTITATIVE COMPOSITION

Anzemet IV solution for injection:

Each ampoule contains Dolasetron Mesilate 20 mg/ml:

9.3 mg dolasetron (as **12.5 mg** mesilate salt) in 0.625 ml solution for injection

74 mg dolasetron (as **100 mg** mesilate salt) in 5 ml solution for injection

Anzemet Tablets:

37 mg dolasetron (as **50 mg** mesilate salt).

148 mg dolasetron (as **200 mg** mesilate salt).

For excipients, see 6.1.

3. PHARMACEUTICAL FORM

Anzemet IV solution for injection:

Clear, colourless solution, free from visible particles.

Anzemet film-coated tablets:

The 50mg tablets are round and pale pink, the 200mg tablets are oval and dark pink. Both strengths of tablets are imprinted with the product logo on one side.

4. CLINICAL PARTICULARS

4.1 Therapeutic indications

- Anzemet IV and Anzemet Tablets:

- Management of nausea and vomiting in patients receiving initial and repeat courses of cancer chemotherapy (including high dose cisplatin).

- Prevention of post operative nausea and vomiting in patients at high risk, such as intra-abdominal gynaecological surgery or with a known history of post operative nausea and vomiting.

- Additionally for Anzemet IV:

- Treatment of post operative nausea and vomiting.

4.2 Posology and method of administration

Anzemet IV can be injected over 30 seconds or diluted to 50 ml in normal saline, 5% dextrose or other compatible intravenous fluids (see Section 6.2 Incompatibilities) and infused over a period of 30 seconds to 15 minutes. More rapid i.v. administration should be avoided. See 4.8 Undesirable Effects.

CANCER THERAPY INDUCED NAUSEA AND VOMITING

Adults

For prevention of nausea and vomiting in patients receiving emetogenic chemotherapy, a 100 mg single dose of Anzemet IV approximately 30 minutes prior to each chemotherapy treatment or a 200 mg single dose of Anzemet tablets approximately one hour prior to each chemotherapy treatment, is recommended. To protect against delayed nausea and vomiting after the cessation of a chemotherapy cycle, a 200 mg single daily dose of Anzemet tablets is recommended. Anzemet IV or tablets may be administered for up to a maximum of 4 consecutive days in relation to any one chemotherapy cycle.

The efficacy of Anzemet in controlling nausea and vomiting can be improved by co-administration of corticosteroids.

Children

Anzemet IV and Anzemet tablets are not recommended for use in children.

Elderly

Patient and volunteer data indicate that the pharmacokinetics of Dolasetron and the active metabolite are unaltered in patients 65 years of age or older and thus no dosage adjustment is required.

Patients with renal impairment

Plasma levels of the active metabolite are increased after oral or intravenous administration of Dolasetron mesilate in patients with severe renal failure (creatinine clearance < 10 ml/min). No dosage adjustment is required.

A small percentage of renally impaired patients may be poor metabolisers and therefore plasma levels in these patients may be higher.

Patients with hepatic impairment

Plasma levels of the active metabolite are increased after oral and unchanged after intravenous administration of Dolasetron mesilate in patients with severe hepatic failure (Child-Pugh Class B or C). No dosage adjustment is required.

POST-OPERATIVE NAUSEA AND VOMITING

TREATMENT

Adults

For treatment a single dose of Anzemet IV should be administered as soon as nausea or emesis presents. The recommended dose for treatment is 12.5 mg IV.

PREVENTION

Adults

For prevention of post-operative nausea and vomiting a single 12.5 mg dose of Anzemet IV at cessation of anaesthesia or a single 50 mg dose of Anzemet tablets prior to the induction of anaesthesia, is recommended.

Children

Anzemet IV and tablets are not recommended for use in children.

Elderly

Patient and volunteer data indicate that the pharmacokinetics of Dolasetron and the active metabolite are unaltered in patients 65 years of age or older and thus no dosage adjustment is required.

Patients with renal impairment

Plasma levels of the active metabolite are increased after oral or intravenous administration of Anzemet in patients with severe renal failure (creatinine clearance < 10 ml/min). No dosage adjustment is required.

A small percentage of renally impaired patients may be poor metabolisers and therefore plasma levels in these patients may be higher.

Patients with hepatic impairment

Plasma levels of the active metabolite are increased after oral and unchanged after intravenous administration of Dolasetron mesilate in patients with severe hepatic failure (Child-Pugh Class B or C). No dosage adjustment is required.

4.3 Contraindications

Patients with a markedly prolonged QTc interval (for example, in association with congenital QT interval prolongation), patients with AV block II-III, and patients receiving concomitant Class I and III antiarrhythmics should not receive Anzemet.

There is insufficient information in such patients on the effects of Anzemet on the electrocardiogram to conclude that the drug may be safely administered in these circumstances.

Hypersensitivity to the active substance or to any of the excipients.

4.4 Special warnings and special precautions for use

5-HT_3 receptor antagonists, including Anzemet, have been shown to cause ECG interval prolongations, including QTc.

Use of 5-HT_3 receptor antagonists and other drugs which prolong ECG intervals requires that caution be exercised in patients who have existing prolongation of cardiac conduction intervals, particularly QTc, patients with significant electrolyte disturbances, bundle branch block or underlying cardiac diseases such as congestive heart failure. See Sections 4.3 Contraindications and 4.8 Undesirable Effects.

Anzemet IV should not be administered by intramuscular injection.

Cross-hypersensitivity reactions have been reported in patients who received other selective 5-HT_3 receptor antagonists. Although these type of reactions have not, as yet, been reported with dolasetron mesilate, patients who have experienced hypersensitivity reactions with other 5-HT_3 receptor antagonists should be closely monitored following the administration of Anzemet.

4.5 Interaction with other medicinal products and other forms of Interaction

The potential for clinically significant drug-drug interactions posed by Anzemet and its active metabolite appears to be low for drugs commonly used in chemotherapy or surgery, because the active metabolite is eliminated by multiple routes. Inhibition or induction of cytochrome P450 does not cause large changes in clearance of Dolasetron as demonstrated by concomitant administration of cimetidine for 7 days (peak plasma concentrations and systemic exposure of the active metabolite increased by 15% and 24%, respectively) and concomitant administration of rifampicin for 7 days (peak plasma concentrations and systemic exposure of the metabolite decreased by 17% and 28%, respectively).

The efficacy of Anzemet may be enhanced by the co-administration of dexamethasone.

4.6 Pregnancy and lactation

There is no experience in humans. Anzemet should not be used during pregnancy unless the expected benefit to the patient is thought to outweigh any possible risk to the foetus.

Dolasetron mesilate is not teratogenic when administered to animals and did not affect male or female fertility, nor perinatal or postnatal development.

It is not known if Dolasetron or its metabolites are excreted in human milk. Therefore, it is recommended that mothers receiving Anzemet should not breast feed their babies.

4.7 Effects on ability to drive and use machines

No known effects.

4.8 Undesirable effects

The most frequently reported undesirable effects in cancer patients receiving Anzemet in single dose studies were headache 21.9%, diarrhoea 9.9%, tachycardia 3.3%, fever 3.2% and fatigue 3.2%; these events occurred with similar frequency with the comparator 5-HT_3 receptor antagonists.

In a study where Anzemet was administered to cancer patients for seven consecutive days, the most frequently reported undesirable effects were headache 43.7%, constipation 32.1%, fatigue 24.2%, sleep disorder 16.9%, dyspepsia 16.3%, diarrhoea 16.3%, abdominal pain 15.7%, dizziness 14.0%, drowsiness 12.0%, flushing 11.4%, pain 11.4%, anorexia 10.8%, taste perversion 8.7%, chills/shivering 7.9% and flatulence 6.1%; these events occurred with similar frequency with the comparator 5-HT_3 receptor antagonist.

The most frequently reported undesirable effects in surgical patients receiving Anzemet in single dose studies were bradycardia 10.0%, headache 8.3%, T wave change 4.6% and dizziness 4.0%; these events occurred with similar frequency with placebo.

Over all clinical trials, hypotension occurred in 1.9% of Dolasetron patients; this event occurred at a similar frequency with placebo or active comparator. Similarly, occasional transient asymptomatic increases in serum transaminases have been reported. There have been rare (<0.1%) reports of intestinal obstruction, pancreatitis, jaundice, seizure, cardiac arrhythmia, bronchospasm, severe bradycardia and oedema. The relationship of these events to Anzemet has not been established.

Reversible ECG interval changes (PR and QT_c prolongation, QRS widening) may occur and are related in magnitude and frequency to blood levels of the active metabolite. These changes are self limiting with declining blood levels. Some patients have interval prolongations for 24 hours or longer. Interval prolongation could lead to cardiovascular consequences, including heart block or cardiac arrhythmias. These have been rarely reported.

In very rare cases, severe hypotension, bradycardia and possibly loss of consciousness may occur immediately or closely following i.v. bolus administration of dolasetron mesilate.

In patients given the intravenous form, very rare reports of wide complex tachycardia or ventricular tachycardia and of ventricular fibrillation/cardiac arrest have been reported.

Local pain or burning may be experienced on intravenous administration.

As with other 5-HT_3 receptor antagonists, there have been reports of hyper-sensitivity reactions such as rash, pruritus, urticaria, bronchospasm and very rare reports of angio-oedema and anaphylaxis. See 4.4 Special warnings and precautions for use.

4.9 Overdose

There is no specific antidote for Dolasetron mesilate. Following a suspected overdose, patients should be managed with symptomatic and supportive therapy as part of expectant management. If clinically indicated, the patient should have cardiac monitoring.

Severe hypotension and dizziness were reported soon after intravenous infusion of 13 mg/kg: normal sinus rhythm with prolongation of the PR, QRS and QTc intervals was recorded on ECG at 2 hours after the infusion. See 4.8 Undesirable Effects for information on asymptomatic ECG interval prolongations. In a child who received 6 mg/kg orally, no clinical symptoms occurred and no treatment was given.

5. PHARMACOLOGICAL PROPERTIES

5.1 Pharmacodynamic properties

Pharmacotherapeutic group: Serotonin (5-HT_3) antagonists, ATC code: A04A A04

Dolasetron mesilate and its major metabolite are selective serotonin 5-HT_3 antagonists. The precise mode of action as an antiemetic is not known. The serotonin 5-HT_3 receptors are located on the nerve terminals of the vagus in the periphery and are centrally located in the chemoreceptor trigger zone of the area postrema. It is thought that chemotherapeutic agents produce nausea and vomiting by releasing serotonin from the enterochromaffin cells of the small intestine and that the released serotonin can then activate 5-HT_3 receptors located on vagal efferents to initiate the vomiting reflex. The effect of Anzemet in the management of cancer therapy induced nausea and vomiting is due to antagonism of 5-HT_3 receptors on neurons either peripherally and/or centrally located.

The mechanisms of action in post-operative nausea and vomiting are not known but there may be pathways common to chemotherapy induced nausea and vomiting.

5.2 Pharmacokinetic properties

a) **General characteristics of the active substance**

Dolasetron mesilate is rapidly ($t_{½}$ <10 minutes) and completely metabolised to the active reduced metabolite, which is widely distributed in the body with mean apparent volume of distribution of 5.0-7.9 l/kg. The plasma protein binding of the active metabolite is approximately 69-77%.

The absolute bioavailability of an oral solution is approximately 75%.

The active metabolite is eliminated by renal excretion (approximately 30%) and metabolism, mainly glucuronidation and hydroxylation.

In man, the $t_{½}$ of the active metabolite is 7-9 hours. The pharmacokinetics of the active metabolite are linear over the therapeutic dose range.

b) **Characteristics in patients**

The pharmacokinetics of the active metabolite are similar in cancer patients, elderly subjects and healthy young male and female subjects.

Although Anzemet is not recommended in children, the following data are available. In paediatric cancer patients, clearance of active metabolite increased 1.3 to 2-fold (12-17 years) and 2 to 3-fold (3-11 years) compared to adult cancer patients or healthy volunteers. In paediatric surgery patients, clearance of active metabolite increased approximately 1.4-fold (2-12 years) compared to adult healthy volunteers. These changes resulted in significantly lower plasma levels and systemic exposures compared to adults administered the same doses.

In patients with severe renal impairment (creatinine clearance <10 ml/min), maximum plasma levels of metabolite are increased 17% or 34%, respectively, after intravenous or oral administration of Dolasetron mesilate, and systemic exposure is increased approximately 2-fold.

In patients with severe hepatic impairment (Child-Pugh Class B or C), maximum plasma levels of metabolite are increased 18% and systemic exposure increases 66% after oral administration of Dolasetron mesilate. Systemic exposure is not altered after intravenous administration of Dolasetron mesilate to this patient population.

In poor metabolisers of sparteine/debrisoquine, maximum plasma levels of metabolite are unchanged whilst systemic exposure is increased up to 2-fold.

5.3 Preclinical safety data

Repeated daily oral or intravenous administration of Dolasetron mesilate to rats and dogs produced CNS effects at plasma concentrations in the same range as the maximum plasma concentration in humans given the highest recommended intravenous (100 mg) or oral (200 mg) dose. Similar effects have not been reported in humans at a frequency greater than active comparator or placebo.

Seizures were observed following repeat intravenous or oral dosing in rats (60 mg/kg/day and 75 mg/kg/day respectively) and repeat oral dosing in dogs (10 mg/kg BD), which resulted in plasma concentrations equal to or greater than 7 (rats, intravenous or oral) and 1.2 (dogs) times the maximum plasma concentrations in humans given the highest recommended intravenous (100 mg) or oral (200 mg) dose. Seizures were also observed following single intravenous doses of 140 and 126 mg/kg in mice and rats, respectively, and single oral doses of 525 and 700 mg/kg in mice and rats, respectively.

Dolasetron mesilate was not mutagenic in a variety of in vitro and in vivo mutagenicity tests, including the mouse micronucleus assay. Tumour findings in the high dose group of the mouse oral carcinogenicity study were not considered relevant for the clinical short-term use.

In μmolar concentrations, dolasetron and its metabolite MDL 74,156, as with other 5-HT_3 antagonists, blocked cloned human cardiac Na^+ and HERG K^+ ion channels.

6. PHARMACEUTICAL PARTICULARS

6.1 List of excipients

Anzemet IV Solution for injection:

Mannitol for Injection, Sodium Acetate Trihydrate, Glacial Acetic Acid, Water for Injections.

Anzemet Tablets:

Tablet core: Lactose, Pregelatinised Starch, Croscarmellose Sodium, Magnesium Stearate.

Tablet coat: Opadry pink film contains: Hydroxypropylmethylcellulose, Polyethylene Glycol, Polysorbate 80, Titanium Dioxide (E171), Red Iron Oxide (E172).

Polish: Carnauba Wax, White Beeswax.

Printing ink: Ammonium Hydroxide, Ethylene Monoethyl Ether, Lecithin, Propylene Glycol, Pharmaceutical Glaze, Synthetic Black Iron Oxide.

6.2 Incompatibilities

In general, Anzemet IV should not be mixed in solution with other drugs. It is important that when any drugs are administered at the same time as Anzemet IV that the tubing and Y-site are thoroughly and completely flushed with a compatible infusion fluid between administration of the two drug solutions.

Not applicable for tablets.

6.3 Shelf life

3 years for undiluted solution for injection.

24 hours for diluted solution for injection.

3 years for tablets.

6.4 Special precautions for storage

Anzemet IV:

Undiluted product: Keep the container in the outer carton in order to protect from light.

Diluted product: Dilutions of intravenous fluids should be used immediately after preparation. If storage cannot be avoided, the maximum storage time of dilutions is 24 hours at 2 - 8 °C.

Anzemet Tablets:

No special precautions for storage of tablets

6.5 Nature and contents of container

Anzemet IV:

The ampoules are either a 1 ml (12.5 mg) or 5 ml (100 mg) clear glass type I ampoule, packed in a cardboard carton. Cartons are bundled by transparent foil.

Package quantities:

12.5 mg - ten ampoules

100 mg - one ampoule

100 mg - five ampoules

Anzemet Tablets:

Tablets are packaged in PVC/PVDC and aluminium foil blister pack contained in a cardboard carton.

Package quantities:

50 mg and 200 mg tablets:

3 tablets

200 mg tablets only:

6 tablets

6.6 Instructions for use and handling

Anzemet IV:

The container and solution should be visually inspected before use. Use only clear particle-free, colourless solution. Do not use if the container is damaged.

Compatibility with infusion fluids: Anzemet IV should only be admixed with those infusion fluids which are recommended. Anzemet IV is physically and chemically stable at concentrations up to 2 mg/ml in the following infusion fluids:

5% Glucose

0.9% Sodium Chloride

10% Mannitol

Compound Sodium Lactate

0.18% Sodium Chloride/4% Glucose

Anzemet IV is compatible with polypropylene syringes.

Anzemet Tablets:

No special requirements.

7. MARKETING AUTHORISATION HOLDER

Amdipharm plc

Regency House

Miles Gray Road

Basildon

Essex SS14 3AF

United Kingdom

8. MARKETING AUTHORISATION NUMBER(S)

Anzemet IV Solution for Injection: PL 20072/0001

Anzemet 50 mg Tablets: PL 20072/0002

Anzemet 200 mg Tablets: PL 20072/0003

9. DATE OF FIRST AUTHORISATION/RENEWAL OF THE AUTHORISATION

22nd December 2003

10. DATE OF REVISION OF THE TEXT

Anzemet tablets

(Amdipharm)

1. NAME OF THE MEDICINAL PRODUCT

Anzemet 50 mg Tablets ▼

Anzemet 200 mg Tablets ▼

2. QUALITATIVE AND QUANTITATIVE COMPOSITION

37 mg Dolasetron (as 50 mg mesilate salt).

148 mg Dolasetron (as 200 mg mesilate salt).

For excipients, see 6.1

3. PHARMACEUTICAL FORM

Film-coated tablets.

50 mg tablets are round and pale pink.

200 mg tablets are oval and dark pink.

Both strengths are imprinted with the product logo on one side.

4. CLINICAL PARTICULARS

4.1 Therapeutic indications

- Management of nausea and vomiting in patients receiving initial and repeat courses of cancer chemotherapy (including high dose cisplatin).

- Prevention of post operative nausea and vomiting in patients at high risk, such as intra-abdominal gynaecological surgery or with a known history of post operative nausea and vomiting.

4.2 Posology and method of administration

CANCER THERAPY INDUCED NAUSEA AND VOMITING

Adults

For prevention of nausea and vomiting in patients receiving emetogenic chemotherapy, a 200 mg single dose of Anzemet tablets is recommended approximately one hour prior to each chemotherapy treatment. To protect against delayed nausea and vomiting after the cessation of a chemotherapy cycle, a 200 mg single daily dose of Anzemet tablets is recommended. Anzemet IV or tablets may be administered for up to a maximum of 4 consecutive days in relation to any one chemotherapy cycle.

The efficacy of Anzemet tablets in controlling nausea and vomiting can be improved by coadministration of corticosteroids.

Children

Anzemet is not recommended for use in children.

Elderly

Patient and volunteer data indicate that the pharmacokinetics of Dolasetron and the active metabolite are unaltered in patients 65 years of age or older and thus no dosage adjustment is required.

Patients with renal impairment

Plasma levels of the active metabolite are increased after oral or intravenous administration of Dolasetron mesilate in patients with severe renal failure (creatinine clearance < 10 ml/min). No dosage adjustment is required.

A small percentage of renally impaired patients may be poor metabolisers and therefore plasma levels in these patients may be higher.

Patients with hepatic impairment

Plasma levels of the active metabolite are increased after oral and unchanged after intravenous administration of Dolasetron mesilate in patients with severe hepatic failure (Child-Pugh Class B or C). No dosage adjustment is required.

POST-OPERATIVE NAUSEA AND VOMITING

Adults

For prevention of post-operative nausea and vomiting a single 50 mg dose of Anzemet tablets is recommended prior to the induction of anaesthesia.

Children

Anzemet is not recommended for use in children.

Elderly

Patient and volunteer data indicate that the pharmacokinetics of Dolasetron and the active metabolite are unaltered in patients 65 years of age or older and thus no dosage adjustment is required.

Patients with renal impairment

Plasma levels of the active metabolite are increased after oral or intravenous administration of Dolasetron mesilate in patients with severe renal failure (creatinine clearance < 10 ml/min). No dosage adjustment is required.

A small percentage of renally impaired patients may be poor metabolisers and therefore plasma levels in these patients may be higher.

Patients with hepatic impairment

Plasma levels of the active metabolite are increased after oral and unchanged after intravenous administration of Dolasetron mesilate in patients with severe hepatic failure (Child-Pugh Class B or C). No dosage adjustment is required.

4.3 Contraindications

Patients with a markedly prolonged QTc interval (for example, in association with congenital QT interval prolongation), patients with AV block II-III, and patients receiving concomitant Class I and III antiarrhythmics should not receive Anzemet.

There is insufficient information in such patients on the effects of Anzemet on the electrocardiogram to conclude that the drug may be safely administered in these circumstances.

Hypersensitivity to the active substance or to any of the excipients.

4.4 Special warnings and special precautions for use

5-HT_3 receptor antagonists, including Anzemet, have been shown to cause ECG interval prolongations, including QTc.

Use of 5-HT_3 receptor antagonists and other drugs which prolong ECG intervals requires that caution be exercised in patients who have existing prolongation of cardiac conduction intervals, particularly QTc, patients with significant electrolyte disturbances, bundle branch block or underlying cardiac diseases such as congestive heart failure. See Sections 4.3 Contraindications and 4.8 Undesirable Effects.

Cross-hypersensitivity reactions have been reported in patients who received other selective 5-HT_3 receptor antagonists. Although these type of reactions have not, as yet, been reported with Dolasetron mesilate, patients who have experienced hypersensitivity reactions with other 5-HT_3 receptor antagonists should be closely monitored following the administration of Anzemet.

4.5 Interaction with other medicinal products and other forms of Interaction

The potential for clinically significant drug-drug interactions posed by Dolasetron mesilate and its active metabolite appears to be low for drugs commonly used in chemotherapy or surgery, because the active metabolite is eliminated by multiple routes. Inhibition or induction of cytochrome P450 does not cause large changes in clearance of Dolasetron as demonstrated by concomitant administration of cimetidine for 7 days (peak plasma concentrations and systemic exposure of the active metabolite increased by 15% and 24%, respectively) and concomitant administration of rifampicin for 7 days (peak plasma concentrations and systemic exposure of the metabolite decreased by 17% and 28%, respectively).

The efficacy of Anzemet may be enhanced by the coadministration of dexamethasone.

4.6 Pregnancy and lactation

There is no experience in humans. Anzemet tablets should not be used during pregnancy unless the expected benefit to the patient is thought to outweigh any possible risk to the foetus.

Dolasetron mesilate is not teratogenic when administered to animals and did not affect male or female fertility, nor perinatal or postnatal development.

It is not known if Dolasetron or its metabolites are excreted in human milk. Therefore, it is recommended that mothers receiving Anzemet tablets should not breast feed their babies.

4.7 Effects on ability to drive and use machines

No known effects.

4.8 Undesirable effects

The most frequently reported undesirable effects in cancer patients receiving Anzemet in single dose studies were headache 21.9%, diarrhoea 9.9%, tachycardia 3.3%, fever 3.2% and fatigue 3.2%; these events occurred with similar frequency with the comparator 5-HT_3 receptor antagonists.

In a study where Anzemet was administered to cancer patients for seven consecutive days, the most frequently reported undesirable effects were headache 43.7%, constipation 32.1%, fatigue 24.2%, sleep disorder 16.9%, dyspepsia 16.3%, diarrhoea 16.3%, abdominal pain 15.7%, dizziness 14.0%, drowsiness 12.0%, flushing 11.4%, pain 11.4%, anorexia 10.8%, taste perversion 8.7%, chills/shivering 7.9% and flatulence 6.1%; these events occurred with similar frequency with the comparator 5-HT_3 receptor antagonist.

The most frequently reported undesirable effects in surgical patients receiving Anzemet in single dose studies were bradycardia 10.0%, headache 8.3%, T wave change 4.6%

and dizziness 4.0%; these events occurred with similar frequency with placebo.

Over all clinical trials, hypotension occurred in 1.9% of Dolasetron patients; this event occurred at a similar frequency with placebo or active comparator.

Similarly, occasional transient asymptomatic increases in serum transaminases have been reported. There have been rare (<0.1%) reports of intestinal obstruction, pancreatitis, jaundice, seizure, cardiac arrhythmia, bronchospasm, severe bradycardia and oedema. The relationship of these events to Anzemet has not been established.

Reversible ECG interval changes (PR and QT_c prolongation, QRS widening) may occur and are related in magnitude and frequency to blood levels of the active metabolite. These changes are self limiting with declining blood levels. Some patients have interval prolongations for 24 hours or longer. Interval prolongation could lead to cardiovascular consequences, including heart block or cardiac arrhythmias. These have been rarely reported.

In patients given the intravenous form, very rare reports of wide complex tachycardia or ventricular tachycardia and of ventricular fibrillation/cardiac arrest have been reported.

As with other 5-HT_3 receptor antagonists, there have been reports of hyper- sensitivity reactions such as rash, pruritus, urticaria, bronchospasm and very rare reports of angio-oedema and anaphylaxis. See 4.4 Special warnings and special precautions for use.

4.9 Overdose

There is no specific antidote for Dolasetron mesilate. Following a suspected overdose, patients should be managed with symptomatic and supportive therapy as part of expectant management. If clinically indicated, the patient should have cardiac monitoring.

Severe hypotension and dizziness were reported soon after intravenous infusion of 13 mg/kg: normal sinus rhythm with prolongation of the PR, QRS and QTc intervals was recorded on ECG at 2 hours after the infusion. See 4.8 Undesirable Effects for information on asymptomatic ECG interval prolongations. In a child who received 6 mg/kg orally, no clinical symptoms occurred and no treatment was given.

5. PHARMACOLOGICAL PROPERTIES

5.1 Pharmacodynamic properties

Pharmacotherapeutic group: Serotonin (5-HT_3) antagonists,

ATC code: A04A A04

Dolasetron mesilate and its major metabolite are selective serotonin 5-HT_3 antagonists. The precise mode of action as an antiemetic is not known. The serotonin 5-HT_3 receptors are located on the nerve terminals of the vagus in the periphery and are centrally located in the chemoreceptor trigger zone of the area postrema. It is thought that chemotherapeutic agents produce nausea and vomiting by releasing serotonin from the enterochromaffin cells of the small intestine and that the released serotonin can then activate 5-HT_3 receptors located on vagal efferents to initiate the vomiting reflex. The effect of Anzemet in the management of cancer therapy induced nausea and vomiting is due to antagonism of 5-HT_3 receptors on neurons either peripherally and/or centrally located.

The mechanisms of action in post-operative nausea and vomiting are not known but there may be pathways common to chemotherapy induced nausea and vomiting.

5.2 Pharmacokinetic properties

a) General characteristics of the active substance

Dolasetron mesilate is rapidly ($t_{½}$ <10 minutes) and completely metabolised to the active reduced metabolite, which is widely distributed in the body with mean apparent volume of distribution of 5.0-7.9 l/kg. The plasma protein binding of the active metabolite is approximately 69-77%.

The absolute bioavailability of an oral solution is approximately 75%.

The active metabolite is eliminated by renal excretion (approximately 30%) and metabolism, mainly glucuronidation and hydroxylation.

In man, the $t_{½}$ of the active metabolite is 7-9 hours. The pharmacokinetics of the active metabolite are linear over the therapeutic dose range.

b) Characteristics in patients

The pharmacokinetics of the active metabolite are similar in cancer patients, elderly subjects and healthy young male and female subjects.

Although Anzemet is not recommended in children, the following data are available. In paediatric cancer patients, clearance of active metabolite increased 1.3 to 2-fold (12-17 years) and 2 to 3-fold (3-11 years) compared to adult cancer patients or healthy volunteers. In paediatric surgery patients, clearance of active metabolite increased approximately 1.4-fold (2-12 years) compared to adult healthy volunteers. These changes resulted in significantly lower plasma levels and systemic exposures compared to adults administered the same doses.

In patients with severe renal impairment (creatinine clearance <10 ml/min), maximum plasma levels of metabolite are increased 17% or 34%, respectively, after intravenous or oral administration of Dolasetron mesilate, and systemic exposure is increased approximately 2-fold.

In patients with severe hepatic impairment (Child-Pugh Class B or C), maximum plasma levels of metabolite are increased 18% and systemic exposure increases 66% after oral administration of Dolasetron mesilate. Systemic exposure is not altered after intravenous administration of Dolasetron mesilate to this patient population.

In poor metabolisers of sparteine/debrisoquine, maximum plasma levels of metabolite are unchanged whilst systemic exposure is increased up to 2-fold.

5.3 Preclinical safety data

Repeated daily oral administration of Dolasetron mesilate to rats and dogs produced CNS effects at plasma concentrations in the same range as the maximum plasma concentration in humans given the highest recommended oral dose (200 mg). Similar effects have not been reported in humans at a frequency greater than active comparator or placebo.

Seizures were observed following repeat oral dosing in rats (75 mg/kg/day) and in dogs (10 mg/kg BID) which resulted in plasma concentrations equal to or greater than 7 and 1.2, respectively, times the maximum plasma concentrations in humans given the highest recommended oral dose (200 mg). Seizures were also observed following single oral doses of 525 and 700 mg/kg in mice and rats, respectively.

Dolasetron mesilate was not mutagenic in a variety of *in vitro* and *in vivo* mutagenicity tests, including the mouse micronucleus assay. Tumour findings in the high dose group of the mouse oral carcinogenicity study were not considered relevant for the clinical short-term use.

In μmolar concentrations, Dolasetron and its metabolite MDL 74,156, as with other 5-HT_3 antagonists, blocked cloned human cardiac Na^+ and HERG K^+ ion channels.

6. PHARMACEUTICAL PARTICULARS

6.1 List of excipients

Tablet core:

Lactose

Pregelatinised starch

Croscarmellose sodium

Magnesium stearate

Tablet coat:

Opadry pink film contains:

Hydroxypropylmethylcellulose

Polyethylene glycol

Polysorbate 80

Titanium dioxide (E171)

Red iron oxide (E172)

Polish:

Carnauba wax

White beeswax

Printing ink:

Ammonium hydroxide, ethylene monoethyl ether, lecithin, propylene glycol, pharmaceutical glaze, synthetic black iron oxide.

6.2 Incompatibilities

Not applicable.

6.3 Shelf life

3 years.

6.4 Special precautions for storage

No special precautions for storage.

6.5 Nature and contents of container

Tablets are packaged in PVC/PVDC and aluminium foil blister pack contained in a cardboard carton.

Package quantities:

50 mg and 200 mg tablets:

3 tablets

200 mg tablets only:

6 tablets

6.6 Instructions for use and handling

No special requirements.

7. MARKETING AUTHORISATION HOLDER

Amdipharm plc

Regency House

Miles Gray Road

Basildon

Essex, SS14 3AF

United Kingdom

8. MARKETING AUTHORISATION NUMBER(S)

PL 20072/0002

PL 20072/0003

9. DATE OF FIRST AUTHORISATION/RENEWAL OF THE AUTHORISATION

22 December 2003

10. DATE OF REVISION OF THE TEXT

Apidra 100 U/ml, solution for injection

(sanofi-aventis)

1. NAME OF THE MEDICINAL PRODUCT

Apidra ▼ 100 U/ml, solution for injection in vial

Apidra ▼100 U/ml, solution for injection in cartridge.

2. QUALITATIVE AND QUANTITATIVE COMPOSITION

Each ml contains 100 U insulin glulisine (equivalent to 3.49 mg).

Each vial contains 10 ml of solution for injection, equivalent to 1000 U.

Each cartridge contains 3 ml of solution for injection, equivalent to 300 U.

Insulin glulisine is produced by recombinant DNA technology in *Escherichia coli*.

For excipients, see section 6.1.

3. PHARMACEUTICAL FORM

Solution for injection in vial.

Solution for injection in cartridge.

Clear, colourless, aqueous solution.

4. CLINICAL PARTICULARS

4.1 Therapeutic indications

Treatment of adult patients with diabetes mellitus.

4.2 Posology and method of administration

Apidra should be given shortly (0-15 min) before or soon after meals.

Apidra should be used in regimens that include an intermediate or long acting insulin or basal insulin analogue and can be used with oral hypoglycaemic agents.

The dosage of Apidra should be individually adjusted.

Administration

Apidra should be given by subcutaneous injection or by continuous subcutaneous pump infusion.

Apidra should be administered subcutaneously in the abdominal wall, thigh or deltoid or by continuous infusion in the abdominal wall. Injection sites and infusion sites within an-injection area (abdomen, thigh or deltoid) should be rotated from one injection to the next. The rate of absorption, and consequently the onset and duration of action, may be affected by the injection site, exercise and other variables. Subcutaneous injection in the abdominal wall ensures a slightly faster absorption than other injection sites (see section 5.2).

Care should be taken to ensure that a blood vessel has not been entered. After injection, the site of injection should not be massaged. Patients must be educated to use proper injection techniques.

Mixing with insulins

Apidra must not be mixed with any preparations other than NPH (Neutral Protamine Hagedorn) human insulin.

Continuous subcutaneous infusion pump

When used with an insulin infusion pump, Apidra must not be mixed with diluents or any other insulin.

For further details on handling, see section 6.6

Special populations

Renal impairment

The pharmacokinetic properties of insulin glulisine are generally maintained in patients with renal impairment. However, insulin requirements may be reduced in the presence of renal impairment (see section 5.2).

Hepatic impairment

The pharmacokinetic properties of insulin glulisine have not been investigated in patients with decreased liver function. In patients with hepatic impairment, insulin requirements may be diminished due to reduced capacity for gluconeogenesis and reduced insulin metabolism.

Elderly

Limited pharmacokinetic data are available in elderly patients with diabetes mellitus. Deterioration of renal function may lead to a decrease in insulin requirements.

Children and adolescents

There is no adequate clinical information on the use of Apidra in children and adolescents.

4.3 Contraindications

Hypersensitivity to insulin glulisine or to any of the excipients.

Hypoglycaemia.

4.4 Special warnings and special precautions for use

Transferring a patient to a new type or brand of insulin should be done under strict medical supervision. Changes in strength, brand (manufacturer), type (regular, NPH, lente, etc.), species (animal) and/or method of manufacturing may result in a change in dosage. Concomitant oral antidiabetic treatment may need to be adjusted.

The use of inadequate dosages or discontinuation of treatment, especially in insulin-dependent diabetic, may lead to hyperglycaemia and diabetic ketoacidosis; conditions which are potentially lethal.

Hypoglycaemia

The time of occurrence of hypoglycaemia depends on the action profile of the insulins used and may, therefore, change when the treatment regimen is changed.

Conditions which may make the early warning symptoms of hypoglycaemia different or less pronounced include long duration of diabetes, intensified insulin therapy, diabetic nerve disease, medicinal products such as beta blockers or after transfer from animal-source insulin to human insulin.

Adjustment of dosage may be also necessary if patients undertake increased physical activity or change their usual meal plan. Exercise taken immediately after a meal may increase the risk of hypoglycaemia.

When compared with soluble human insulin, if hypoglycaemia occurs after an injection with rapid acting analogues, it may occur earlier.

Uncorrected hypoglycaemic or hyperglycaemic reactions can cause loss of consciousness, coma, or death.

Insulin requirements may be altered during illness or emotional disturbances.

4.5 Interaction with other medicinal products and other forms of Interaction

Studies on pharmacokinetic interactions have not been performed. Based on empirical knowledge from similar medicinal products, clinically relevant pharmacokinetic interactions are unlikely to occur.

A number of substances affect glucose metabolism and may require dose adjustment of insulin glulisine and particularly close monitoring.

Substances that may enhance the blood-glucose-lowering activity and increase susceptibility to hypoglycaemia include oral antidiabetic agents, angiotensin converting enzyme (ACE) inhibitors, disopyramide, fibrates, fluoxetine, monoamide oxidase inhibitors (MAOIs), pentoxifylline, propoxyphene, salicylates and sulfonamide antibiotics.

Substances that may reduce the blood-glucose-lowering activity include corticosteroids, danazol, diazoxide, diuretics, glucagon, isoniazid, phenothiazine derivatives, somatropin, sympathomimetic agents (e.g. epinephrine [adrenaline], salbutamol, terbutaline), thyroid hormones, estrogens, progestins (e.g. in oral contraceptives), protease inhibitors and atypical antipsychotic medicinal products (e.g. olanzapine and clozapine).

Beta-blockers, clonidine, lithium salts or alcohol may either potentiate or weaken the blood-glucose-lowering activity of insulin. Pentamidine may cause hypoglycaemia, which may sometimes be followed by hyperglycaemia.

In addition, under the influence of sympatholytic medicinal products such as beta-blockers, clonidine, guanethidine and reserpine, the signs of adrenergic counter-regulation may be reduced or absent.

4.6 Pregnancy and lactation

Pregnancy

There are no adequate data on the use of insulin glulisine in pregnant women.

Animal reproduction studies have not revealed any differences between insulin glulisine and human insulin regarding pregnancy, embryonal/foetal development, parturition or postnatal development (see section 5.3).

Caution should be exercised when prescribing to pregnant women. Careful monitoring of glucose control is essential.

It is essential for patients with pre-existing or gestational diabetes to maintain good metabolic control throughout pregnancy. Insulin requirements may decrease during the first trimester and generally increase during the second and third trimesters. Immediately after delivery, insulin requirements decline rapidly.

Lactation

It is unknown whether insulin glulisineis excreted in human milk, but in general insulin does not pass into breast milk and is not absorbed after oral administration.

Breast-feeding mothers may require adjustments in insulin dose and diet.

4.7 Effects on ability to drive and use machines

The patient's ability to concentrate and react may be impaired as a result of hypoglycaemia or hyperglycaemia or, for example, as a result of visual impairment. This may constitute a risk in situations where these abilities are of special importance (e.g. driving a car or operating machinery).

Patients should be advised to take precautions to avoid hypoglycaemia whilst driving. This is particularly important in those who have reduced or absent awareness of the warning symptoms of hypoglycaemia or have frequent episodes of hypoglycaemia. The advisability of driving should be considered in these circumstances.

4.8 Undesirable effects

Hypoglycaemia, the most frequent undesirable effect of insulin therapy, may occur if the insulin dose is too high in relation to the insulin requirement.

The following related adverse reactions from clinical investigations were listed below by system organ class and in order of decreasing incidence (very common: > 1/10; common: > 1/100, < 1/10; uncommon: > 1/1,000, < 1/100; rare: > 1/10,000, < 1/1,000; very rare: < 1/10,000).

Figure 1

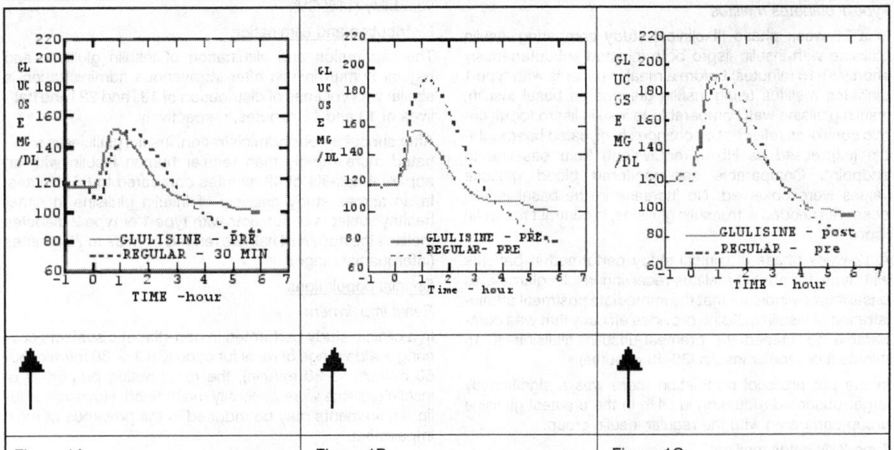

Figure 1A | Figure 1B | Figure 1C

Figure 1: Average glucose-lowering effect over 6 hours in 20 patients with type 1 diabetes mellitus. Insulin glulisine given 2 minutes (GLULISINE pre) before the start of a meal compared to regular human insulin given 30 minutes (REGULAR 30 min) before the start of the meal (figure 1A) and compared to regular human insulin given 2 minutes (REGULAR pre) before a meal (figure 1B). Insulin glulisine given 15 minutes (GLULISINE post) after start of a meal compared to regular human insulin given 2 minutes (REGULAR pre) before start of the meal (figure 1C). On the x-axis, zero (arrow) is the start of a 15-minute meal.

Metabolism and nutrition disorders

Very common: Hypoglycaemia

Symptoms of hypoglycaemia usually occur suddenly. They may include cold sweats, cool pale skin, fatigue, nervousness or tremor, anxiousness, unusual tiredness or weakness, confusion, difficulty in concentration, drowsiness, excessive hunger, vision changes, headache, nausea and palpitation. Hypoglycaemia can become severe and may lead to unconsciousness and/or convulsions and may result in temporary or permanent impairment of brain function or even death.

Skin and subcutaneous tissue disorders

Common: injection site reactions and local hypersensitivity reactions.

Local hypersensitivity reactions (redness, swelling and itching at the injection site) may occur during treatment with insulin. These reactions are usually transitory and normally they disappear during continued treatment.

Rare: Lipodystrophy

Lipodystrophy may occur at the injection site as a consequence of failure to rotate injection sites within an area.

General disorders

Uncommon: Systemic hypersensitivity reactions

Systemic hypersensitivity reactions may include urticaria, chest tightness, dyspnea, allergic dermatitis and pruritus. Severe cases of generalized allergy, including anaphylactic reaction, may be life-threatening.

4.9 Overdose

Hypoglycaemia may occur as a result of an excess of insulin activity relative to food intake and energy expenditure.

There are no specific data available concerning overdose with insulin glulisine. However, hypoglycaemia may develop over sequential stages:

Mild hypoglycaemic episodes can be treated by oral administration of glucose or sugary products. It is therefore recommended that the diabetic patient constantly carries some sugar lumps, sweets, biscuits or sugary fruit juice.

Severe hypoglycaemic episodes, where the patient has become unconscious, can be treated by glucagon (0.5 to 1 mg) given intramuscularly or subcutaneously by a person who has received appropriate instruction, or by glucose given intravenously by a medical professional. Glucose must also be given intravenously, if the patient does not respond to glucagon within 10 to 15 minutes.

Upon regaining consciousness, administration of oral carbohydrate is recommended for the patient in order to prevent relapse.

After an injection of glucagon, the patient should be monitored in a hospital in order to find the reason for this severe hypoglycaemia and prevent other similar episodes.

5. PHARMACOLOGICAL PROPERTIES

5.1 Pharmacodynamic properties

Pharmacotherapeutic group: insulin and analogues, fast-acting. ATC code: A10AB06

Insulin glulisine is a recombinant human insulin analogue that is equipotent to regular human insulin. Insulin glulisine has a more rapid onset of action and a shorter duration of action than regular human insulin.

The primary activity of insulins and insulin analogues, including insulin glulisine, is regulation of glucose metabolism. Insulins lower blood glucose levels by stimulating peripheral glucose uptake, especially by skeletal muscle and fat, and by inhibiting hepatic glucose production. Insulin inhibits lipolysis in the adipocyte, inhibits proteolysis and enhances protein synthesis.

Studies in healthy volunteers and patients with diabetes demonstrated that insulin glulisine is more rapid in onset of action and of shorter duration of action than regular human insulin when given subcutaneously. When insulin glulisine is injected subcutaneously, the glucose lowering activity will begin within 10 – 20 minutes. The glucose-lowering activities of insulin glulisine and regular human insulin are equipotent when administered by intravenous route. One unit of insulin glulisine has the same glucose-lowering activity as one unit of regular human insulin.

A phase I study in patients with type 1 diabetes mellitus assessed the glucose lowering profiles of insulin glulisine and regular human insulin administered subcutaneously at a dose of 0.15 U/kg, at different times in relation to a 15-minute standard meal. Data indicated that insulin glulisine administered 2 minutes before the meal gives similar postprandial glycemic control compared to regular human insulin given 30 minutes before the meal. When given 2 minutes prior to meal, insulin glulisine provided better postprandial control than regular human insulin given 2 minutes before the meal. Insulin glulisine administered 15 minutes after starting the meal gives similar glycemic control as regular human insulin given 2 minutes before the meal (see figure 1).

(See Figure 1 above)

Obesity

A phase I study carried out with insulin glulisine, lispro and regular human insulin in an obese population has demonstrated that insulin glulisine maintains its rapid-acting properties. In this study, the time to 20% of total AUC and the AUC (0-2h) representing the early glucose lowering activity were respectively of 114 minutes and 427mg.kg^{-1} for insulin glulisine, 121 minutes and 354mg.kg^{-1} for lispro, 150 minutes and 197mg.kg^{-1} for regular human insulin (see figure 2).

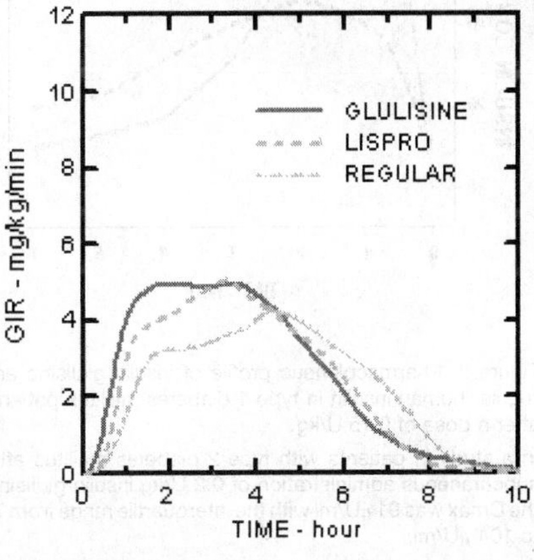

Figure 2: Glucose infusion rates after subcutaneous injection of 0.3 U/kg of insulin glulisine (GLULISINE) or insulin lispro (LISPRO) or regular human insulin (REGULAR) in an obese population.

Clinical studies

Type 1 diabetes mellitus

In a 26-week phase III clinical study comparing insulin glulisine with insulin lispro both injected subcutaneously shortly (0-15 minutes) before a meal in patients with type 1 diabetes mellitus using insulin glargine as basal insulin, insulin glulisine was comparable to insulin lispro for glycemic control as reflected by changes in glycated haemoglobin (expressed as HbA_{1c} equivalent) from baseline to endpoint. Comparable self-monitored blood glucose values were observed. No increase in the basal insulin dose was needed with insulin glulisine, in contrast to insulin lispro.

A 12-week phase III clinical study performed in patients with type 1 diabetes mellitus receiving insulin glargine as basal therapy indicate that the immediate postmeal administration of insulin glulisine provides efficacy that was comparable to immediate premeal insulin glulisine (0-15 minutes) or regular insulin (30-45 minutes).

In the per protocol population there was a significantly larger observed reduction in GHb in the premeal glulisine group compared with the regular insulin group.

Type 2 diabetes mellitus

A 26-week phase III clinical study followed by a 26-week extension safety study was conducted to compare insulin glulisine (0-15 minutes before a meal) with regular human insulin (30-45 minutes before a meal) injected subcutaneously in patients with type 2 diabetes mellitus also using NPH insulin as basal insulin. The average body mass index (BMI) of patients was 34.55 kg/m^2. Insulin glulisine was shown to be comparable to regular human insulin with regard to glycated haemoglobin (expressed as HbA_{1c} equivalent) changes from baseline to the 6-month endpoint (-0.46% for insulin glulisine and -0.30% for regular human insulin, p=0.0029) and from baseline to the 12-month endpoint (-0.23% for insulin glulisine and -0.13% for regular human insulin, difference not significant). In this study, the majority of patients (79%) mixed their short acting insulin with NPH insulin immediately prior to injection and 58 % of subjects used oral hypoglycemic agents at randomization and were instructed to continue to use them at the same dose.

Race and Gender

In controlled clinical trials in adults, insulin glulisine did not show differences in safety and efficacy in subgroup analyses based on race and gender.

5.2 Pharmacokinetic properties

In insulin glulisine the replacement of the human insulin amino acid asparagine in position B3 by lysine and the lysine in position B29 by glutamic acid favors more rapid absorption.

Absorption and bioavailability

Pharmacokinetic profiles in healthy volunteers and diabetes patients (type 1 or 2) demonstrated that absorption of insulin glulisine was about twice as fast with a peak concentration approximately twice as high as compared to regular human insulin.

In a study in patients with type 1 diabetes mellitus after subcutaneous administration of 0.15 U/kg, for insulin glulisine the T_{max} was 55 minutes and C_{max} was 82 ± 1.3 μU/ml compared to a T_{max} of 82 minutes and a C_{max} of 46 ± 1.3 μU/ml for regular human insulin. The mean residence time of insulin glulisine was shorter (98 min) than for regular human insulin (161 min) (see figure3).

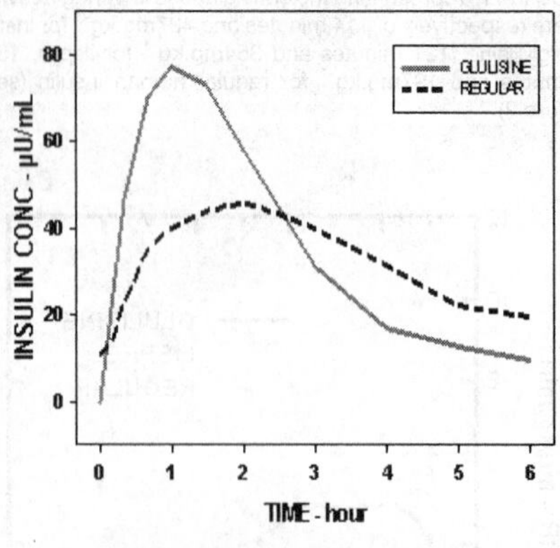

Figure 3: Pharmacokinetic profile of insulin glulisine and regular human insulin in type 1 diabetes mellitus patients after a dose of 0.15 U/kg.

In a study in patients with type 2 diabetes mellitus after subcutaneous administration of 0.2 U/kg insulin glulisine, the Cmax was 91 μU/ml with the interquartile range from 78 to 104 μU/ml.

When insulin glulisine was injected subcutaneously into abdomen, deltoid and thigh, the concentration-time profiles were similar with a slightly faster absorption when administered in the abdomen compared to the thigh. Absorption from deltoid sites was in-between (see section 4.2). The absolute bioavailability (70%) of insulin glulisine was similar between injection sites and of low intra-subject variability (11%CV).

Distribution and elimination

The distribution and elimination of insulin glulisine and regular human insulin after intravenous administration is similar with volumes of distribution of 13 l and 22 l and half-lives of 13 and 18 minutes, respectively.

After subcutaneous administration, insulin glulisine is eliminated more rapidly than regular human insulin with an apparent half-life of 42 minutes compared to 86 minutes. In an across study analysis of insulin glulisine in either healthy subjects or subjects with type 1 or type 2 diabetes mellitus the apparent half-life ranged from 37 to 75 minutes (interquartile range).

Special populations

Renal impairment

In a clinical study performed in non-diabetic subjects covering a wide range of renal function (CrCl > 80 ml/min, 30-50 ml/min, < 30 ml/min), the rapid-acting properties of insulin glulisine were generally maintained. However, insulin requirements may be reduced in the presence of renal impairment.

Hepatic impairment

The pharmacokinetic properties have not been investigated in patients with impaired liver function.

Elderly

Very limited pharmacokinetic data are available for elderly patients with diabetes mellitus.

Children and adolescents

The pharmacokinetic and pharmacodynamic properties of insulin glulisine were investigated in children (7-11 years) and adolescents (12-16 years) with type 1 diabetes mellitus. Insulin glulisine was rapidly absorbed in both age groups, with similar T_{max} and C_{max} as in adults (see section 4.2). Administered immediately before a test meal, insulin glulisine provided better postprandial control than regular human insulin, as in adults (see section 5.1). The glucose excursion (AUC_{0-6h}) was 641 mg.h.dl^{-1} for insulin glulisine and 801mg.h.dl^{-1} for regular human insulin.

5.3 Preclinical safety data

Preclinical data did not reveal toxicity findings others than those linked to the blood glucose lowering pharmacodynamic activity (hypoglycemia), different from regular human insulin or of clinical relevance for humans.

6. PHARMACEUTICAL PARTICULARS

6.1 List of excipients

Metacresol

Sodium chloride

Trometamol

Polysorbate 20

Hydrochloric acid, concentrated

Sodium hydroxide

Water for injections

6.2 Incompatibilities

In the absence of compatibility studies insulin glulisine must not be mixed with any preparations other than NPH human insulin.

When used with an insulin infusion pump, Apidra must not be mixed with other medicinal products.

6.3 Shelf life

2 years.

Shelf life after first use:

4 weeks.

6.4 Special precautions for storage

Unopened

Store in a refrigerator (2°C - 8°C)

Keep the vial and cartridge in the outer carton in order to protect from light.

Do not freeze.

Ensure that the container is not directly touching the freezer compartment or freezer packs.

In use conditions:

Do not store above 25°C.

Keep the vial in the outer carton in order to protect from light.

6.5 Nature and contents of container

Vial:

Colourless glass vial (type I) with flanged aluminium overseal, elastomeric rubber stopper and tear-off lid. Each vial contains 10 ml solution. Packs of 1 vial are available.

Cartridge:

Colourless glass cartridge (type I) with elastomeric rubber plunger and flanged aluminium overseal with elastomeric rubber stopper. Each cartridge contains 3 ml. Packs of 5 cartridges are available.

6.6 Instructions for use and handling

Apidra vials are for use with insulin syringes with the corresponding unit scale and for use with an insulin pump system (see section 4.2).

Inspect the vial before use. It must only be used if the solution is clear, colourless, with no solid particles visible. Since Apidra is a solution, it does not require resuspension before use.

The cartridges are to be used in conjunction with an insulin pen such as OptiPen and as recommended in the information provided by the device manufacturer.

The manufacturer's instructions for using the pen must be followed carefully for loading the cartridge, attaching the needle, and administering the insulin injection. Inspect the cartridge before use. It must only be used if the solution is clear, colourless, with no solid particles visible. Before insertion of the cartridge into the reusable pen, the cartridge must be stored at room temperature for 1 to 2 hours. Air bubbles must be removed from the cartridge before injection (see instruction for using pen). Empty cartridges must not be refilled.

If OptiPen is damaged, it should not be used.

If the pen malfunctions, the solution may be drawn from the cartridge into a syringe (suitable for an insulin with 100 U/ml) and injected.

To prevent any kind of contamination, the re-usable pen should be used by a single patient only.

Mixing with insulins

When mixed with NPH human insulin, Apidra should be drawn into the syringe first. Injection should be given immediately after mixing as no data are available regarding the mixtures made up a significant time before injection.

Continuous subcutaneous infusion pump

Apidra may be used for Continuous Subcutaneous Insulin Infusion (CSII) in pump systems suitable for insulin infusion with the appropriate catheters and reservoirs.

Patients using CSII should be comprehensively instructed on the use of the pump system. The infusion set and reservoir should be changed every 48 hours using aseptic technique.

Patients administering Apidra by CSII must have alternative insulin available in case of pump system failure.

7. MARKETING AUTHORISATION HOLDER

Aventis Pharma Deutschland GmbH, Brueningstrasse 50, D-65926 Frankfurt am Main, Germany.

8. MARKETING AUTHORISATION NUMBER(S)

Vial: EU/1/04/285/001

Cartridge: EU/1/04/285/008

9. DATE OF FIRST AUTHORISATION/RENEWAL OF THE AUTHORISATION

27 September 2004

10. DATE OF REVISION OF THE TEXT

July 2005

Legal category:

POM

APO-go ampoules 10mg/ml

(Britannia Pharmaceuticals Limited)

1. NAME OF THE MEDICINAL PRODUCT

APO-go AMPOULES 10 mg/ml Solution for Injection

or

APO-go AMPUL 10 mg/ml Solution for Injection (Denmark)

or

APO-go 10 mg/ml Solution for Injection (Sweden)

or

APOgo 10 mg/ml Solution for Injection (France)

2. QUALITATIVE AND QUANTITATIVE COMPOSITION

1ml contains 10mg apomorphine hydrochloride 0.5 H_2O

2ml contains 20mg apomorphine hydrochloride 0.5 H_2O

5ml contains 50mg apomorphine hydrochloride 0.5 H_2O

For excipients, see section 6.1

3. PHARMACEUTICAL FORM

Solution for Injection

Solution is clear and colourless.

4. CLINICAL PARTICULARS

4.1 Therapeutic indications

The treatment of disabling motor fluctuations ("on-off" phenomena) in patients with Parkinson's disease which persist despite individually titrated treatment with levodopa (with a peripheral decarboxylase inhibitor) and/or other dopamine agonists.

4.2 Posology and method of administration

APO-go Ampoules 10 mg/ml Solution for Injection is for subcutaneous use by intermittent bolus injection. APO-go ampoules 10 mg/ml Solution for Injection may also be administered as a continuous subcutaneous infusion by minipump and or syringe-driver (see section 6.6, instructions for use and handling).

Apomorphine must not be used via the intravenous route.

Dosage

Adults

Administration

Selection of Patients Suitable for APO-go injections:

Patients selected for treatment with APO-go should be able to recognise the onset of their 'off' symptoms and be capable of injecting themselves or else have a responsible carer able to inject for them when required.

It is essential that the patient is established on domperidone, usually 20 mg three times daily for at least two days prior to initiation of therapy.

Apomorphine should be initiated in the controlled environment of a specialist clinic. The patient should be supervised by a physician experienced in the treatment of Parkinson's disease (e.g. neurologist). The patient's treatment with levodopa, with or without dopamine agonists, should be optimised before starting APO-go treatment.

Determination of the threshold dose.

The appropriate dose for each patient is established by incremental dosing schedules. The following schedule is suggested:-

1mg of apomorphine HCl (0.1ml), that is approximately 15-20 micrograms/kg, may be injected subcutaneously during a hypokinetic, or 'off' period and the patient is observed over 30 minutes for a motor response.

If no response, or an inadequate response, is obtained a second dose of 2 mg of apomorphine HCl (0.2ml) is injected subcutaneously and the patient observed for an adequate response for a further 30 minutes.

The dosage may be increased by incremental injections with at least a forty minute interval between succeeding injections, until a satisfactory motor response is obtained.

Establishment of treatment.

Once the appropriate dose is determined a single subcutaneous injection may be given into the lower abdomen or outer thigh at the first signs of an 'off' episode. It cannot be excluded that absorption may differ with different injection sites within a single individual. Accordingly, the patient should then be observed for the next hour to assess the quality of their response to treatment. Alterations in dosage may be made according to the patient's response.

The optimal dosage of apomorphine hydrochloride varies between individuals but, once established, remains relatively constant for each patient.

Precautions on continuing treatment.

The daily dose of APO-go varies widely between patients, typically within the range of 3-30 mg, given as 1-10 injections and sometimes as many as 12 separate injections per day.

It is recommended that the total daily dose of apomorphine HCl should not exceed 100 mg and that individual bolus injections should not exceed 10 mg.

In clinical studies it has usually been possible to make some reduction in the dose of levodopa; this effect varies considerably between patients and needs to be carefully managed by an experienced physician.

Once treatment has been established domperidone therapy may be gradually reduced in some patients but successfully eliminated only in a few, without any vomiting or hypotension.

Continuous Infusion

Patients who have shown a good 'on' period response during the initiation stage, but whose overall control remains unsatisfactory using intermittent injections, or who require many and frequent injections (more than 10 per day), may be commenced on or transferred to continuous subcutaneous infusion by minipump and or syringe-driver (see section 6.6, instructions for use and handling) as follows:-

Continuous infusion is started at a rate of 1 mg apomorphine HCl (0.1 ml) per hour then increased according to the individual response. Increases in the infusion rate should not exceed 0.5 mg per hour at intervals of not less than 4 hours. Hourly infusion rates may range between 1 mg and 4 mg (0.1 ml and 0.4 ml), equivalent to 0.015 - 0.06 mg/kg/hour. Infusions should run for waking hours only. Unless the patient is experiencing severe night-time problems, 24 hour infusions are not advised. Tolerance to the therapy does not seem to occur as long as there is an overnight period without treatment of at least 4 hours. In any event, the infusion site should be changed every 12 hours.

Patients may need to supplement their continuous infusion with intermittent bolus boosts via the pump system as necessary, and as directed by their physician.

A reduction in dosage of other dopamine agonists may be considered during continuous infusion.

Children and adolescents:

APO-go Ampoules 10 mg/ml Solution for Injection is contraindicated for children and adolescents under 18 years of age (see section 4.3, contraindications).

Elderly:

The elderly are well represented in the population of patients with Parkinson's disease and constitute a high proportion of those studied in clinical trials of APO-go. The management of elderly patients treated with APO-go has not differed from that of younger patients.

Renal impairment:

A dose schedule similar to that recommended for adults, and the elderly, can be followed for patients with renal impairment (see section 4.4, special warning and precautions for use).

4.3 Contraindications

In patients with respiratory depression, dementia, psychotic diseases or hepatic insufficiency.

Intermittent apomorphine HCl treatment is not suitable for patients who have an 'on' response to levodopa which is marred by severe dyskinesia or dystonia.

APO-go should not be administered to patients who have a known hypersensitivity to apomorphine or any excipients of the medicinal product.

APO-go is contraindicated for children and adolescents under 18 years of age.

Pregnancy and lactation (see section 4.6, pregnancy and lactation)

4.4 Special warnings and special precautions for use

Apomorphine HCl should be given with caution to patients with renal, pulmonary or cardiovascular disease and persons prone to nausea and vomiting.

Extra caution is recommended during initiation of therapy in elderly and/or debilitated patients.

Since apomorphine may produce hypotension, even when given with domperidone pretreatment, care should be exercised in patients with pre-existing cardiac disease or in patients taking vasoactive medicinal products such as antihypertensives, and especially in patients with pre-existing postural hypotension.

APO-go Ampoules 10mg/ml Solution for Injection contains sodium metabisulphite which may rarely cause severe allergic reactions and bronchospasm.

Coombs' positive haemolytic anaemia has been reported rarely in patients treated with levodopa and the incidence in patients taking levodopa and apomorphine is unaltered. Coombs' positive anaemia has not been reported in patients taking apomorphine in association with other therapy. Haematology tests should be undertaken at regular intervals as with levodopa when given concomitantly with apomorphine.

Caution is advised when combining apomorphine with other medicinal products, especially those with a narrow therapeutic range (see section 4.5, interaction with other medicinal products and other forms of interaction)

Neuropsychiatric problems co-exist in many patients with advanced Parkinson's disease. There is evidence that for some patients neuropsychiatric disturbances may be exacerbated by apomorphine.

Special care should be exercised when apomorphine is used in these patients.

Apomorphine has been associated with somnolence, and other dopamine agonists can be associated with sudden sleep onset episodes, particularly in patients with Parkinson's disease. Patients must be informed of this and advised to exercise caution while driving or operating machines during treatment with apomorphine. Patients who have experienced somnolence must refrain from driving or operating machines. Furthermore a reduction of dosage or termination of therapy may be considered.

4.5 Interaction with other medicinal products and other forms of Interaction

Patients selected for treatment with apomorphine HCl are almost certain to be taking concomitant medications for their Parkinson's disease. In the initial stages of apomorphine HCl therapy the patient should be monitored for unusual side-effects or signs of potentiation of effect.

Neuroleptic medicinal products may have an antagonistic effect if used with apomorphine. There is a potential interaction between clozapine and apomorphine, however clozapine may also be used to reduce the symptoms of neuropsychiatric complications.

If neuroleptic medicinal products have to be used in patients with Parkinson's disease treated by dopamine agonists, a gradual reduction in apomorphine dose may be considered when administration is by minipump and or syringe-driver (symptoms suggestive of neuroleptic malignant syndrome have been reported rarely with abrupt withdrawal of dopaminergic therapy).

The possible effects of apomorphine on the plasma concentrations of other medicinal products have not been studied. Therefore caution is advised when combining apomorphine with other medicinal products, especially those with a narrow therapeutic range.

Antihypertensive and Cardiac Active Medicinal Products

Even when co-administered with domperidone, apomorphine may potentiate the antihypertensive effects of these medicinal products. See section 4.4 special warnings and precautions for use above.

4.6 Pregnancy and lactation

Animal reproduction studies have not been conducted with apomorphine HCl. Neither is there any experience of apomorphine in pregnant women. Therefore, apomorphine HCl should not be used in women of child bearing potential.

It is anticipated that apomorphine is excreted in breast milk. Breast-feeding should be avoided during apomorphine HCl therapy.

4.7 Effects on ability to drive and use machines

Patients being treated with apomorphine and presenting with somnolence and/or sudden sleep episodes must be informed to refrain from driving or engaging in activities (e.g. operating machines) where impaired alertness may put themselves or others at risk of serious injury or death until such recurrent episodes and somnolence have resolved (see also section 4.4, special warning and precautions for use).

4.8 Undesirable effects

very common (>10%):

Local induration and nodules (usually asymptomatic) often develop at subcutaneous sites of injection in most patients, particularly with continuous use. In patients on high doses of apomorphine HCl these may persist and give rise to areas of erythema, tenderness and induration. Panniculitis has been reported from these patients where a skin biopsy has been undertaken. Care should be taken to ensure that areas of ulceration do not become infected. Pruritus may occur at the site of injection.

These local subcutaneous effects can sometimes be reduced by rotation of injection sites or possibly by the use of ultrasound (if available) to areas of nodularity and induration.

Common (1-10%):

Nausea and vomiting, particularly when apomorphine treatment is first initiated, usually as a result of the omission of domperidone (See section 4.2, posology and method of administration)

Transient sedation with each dose of apomorphine HCl at the start of therapy may occur; this usually resolves over the first few weeks.

Apomorphine is associated with somnolence.

Neuropsychiatric disturbances are common in parkinsonian patients. Apo-go should be used with special caution in these patients. Transient mild confusion and visual hallucinations have occurred during apomorphine HCl therapy.

Uncommon (0.1-1%):

Postural hypotension is seen infrequently and is usually transient. (See section 4.4, special warnings and precautions for use).

Apomorphine may induce dyskinesias during 'on' periods which can be severe in some cases, and in a few patients may result in cessation of therapy.

Coombs' positive haemolytic anaemia has rarely been reported in patients treated with levodopa and apomorphine.

Rare (0.01%-0.1%):

Eosinophilia has rarely occurred during treatment with apomorphine HCl.

Due to the presence of sodium metabisulphite, allergic reactions (including anaphylaxis and bronchospasm may occur.

4.9 Overdose

There is little clinical experience of overdose with apomorphine by this route of administration. Symptoms of overdose may be treated empirically as suggested below:-

Excessive emesis may be treated with domperidone.

Respiratory depression may be treated with naloxone.

Hypotension: appropriate measures should be taken, e.g. raising the foot of the bed.

Bradycardia may be treated with atropine.

5. PHARMACOLOGICAL PROPERTIES

5.1 Pharmacodynamic properties

Pharmacotherapeutic group: Dopamine agonists

ATC Classification: N04B C07

Apomorphine is a direct stimulant of dopamine receptors and while possessing both D1 and D2 receptor agonist properties does not share transport or metabolic pathways with levodopa.

Although in intact experimental animals, administration of apomorphine suppresses the rate of firing of nigro-striatal cells and in low dose has been found to produce a reduction in locomotor activity (thought to represent pre-synaptic inhibition of endogenous dopamine release) its actions on parkinsonian motor disability are likely to be mediated at post-synaptic receptor sites. This biphasic effect is also seen in humans.

5.2 Pharmacokinetic properties

After subcutaneous injection of apomorphine its fate can be described by a two-compartment model, with a distribution half-life of 5 (±1.1) minutes and an elimination half-life of 33 (±3.9) minutes. Clinical response correlates well with levels of apomorphine in the cerebrospinal fluid; the active substance distribution being best described by a two-compartment model. Apomorphine is rapidly and completely absorbed from subcutaneous tissue, correlating with the rapid onset of clinical effects (4-12 minutes), and that the brief duration of clinical action of the active substance (about 1 hour) is explained by its rapid clearance. The metabolism of apomorphine is by glucuronidation and sulphonation to at least ten per cent of the total; other pathways have not been described.

5.3 Preclinical safety data
Repeat dose subcutaneous toxicity studies reveal no special hazard for humans, beyond the information included in other sections of the SmPC.

In vitro genotoxicity studies demonstrated mutagenic and clastogenic effects, most likely due to products formed by oxidation of apomorphine. However, apomorphine was not genotoxic in the *in vivo* studies performed.

There are no data on fertility and embryo-foetal toxicity. No carcinogenicity studies have been performed.

6. PHARMACEUTICAL PARTICULARS

6.1 List of excipients
Sodium metabisulphite (E223)

Hydrochloric acid (37%), (to adjust pH to 3.0-4.0)

Sodium hydroxide (99%), (to adjust pH to 3.0-4.0)

Water for Injections

6.2 Incompatibilities
In the absence of compatibility studies, this medicinal product must not be mixed with other medicinal products.

6.3 Shelf life
2 years

6.4 Special precautions for storage
Keep the container in the outer carton.

Do not store above 25°C.

6.5 Nature and contents of container
Type I glass ampoules containing 2ml solution for injection, in packs of 5 ampoules.

Type I glass ampoules containing 5ml solution for injection, in packs of 5 ampoules.

6.6 Instructions for use and handling
Do not use if the solution has turned green.

The solution should be inspected visually prior to use. Only clear and colourless solutions should be used.

For single use only. Any unused solution should be discarded.

Continuous infusion and the use of a minipump and or syringe-driver.

The choice of which minipump and or syringe-driver to use, and the dosage settings required, will be determined by the physician in accordance with the particular needs of the patient.

7. MARKETING AUTHORISATION HOLDER
Forum Products Limited

41 - 51 Brighton Road

Redhill

Surrey

RH1 6YS

8. MARKETING AUTHORISATION NUMBER(S)
PL 05928/0020

9. DATE OF FIRST AUTHORISATION/RENEWAL OF THE AUTHORISATION
January 2002

10. DATE OF REVISION OF THE TEXT
June 2002

APO-go Pen 10mg/ml

(Britannia Pharmaceuticals Limited)

1. NAME OF THE MEDICINAL PRODUCT
APO-go PEN 10 mg/ml Solution for Injection

2. QUALITATIVE AND QUANTITATIVE COMPOSITION
1ml contains 10mg apomorphine hydrochloride

For excipients see 6.1

3. PHARMACEUTICAL FORM
Solution for injection.

Solution is clear and colourless.

4. CLINICAL PARTICULARS

4.1 Therapeutic indications
The treatment of disabling motor fluctuations ("on-off" phenomena) in patients with Parkinson's disease which persist despite individually titrated treatment with levodopa (with a peripheral decarboxylase inhibitor) and/or other dopamine agonists.

4.2 Posology and method of administration
APO-go Pen 10 mg/ml Solution for Injection is for subcutaneous use by intermittent bolus injection.

(See section 4.4. Special warnings and precautions for use).

Dosage

Adults

Administration

Selection of patients suitable for APO-go injections:

Patients selected for treatment with APO-go should be able to recognise the onset of their 'off' symptoms and be capable of injecting themselves or else have a responsible carer able to inject for them when required.

It is essential that the patient is established on domperidone, usually 20mg three times daily for at least two days prior to initiation of therapy.

Apomorphine should be initiated in the controlled environment of a specialist clinic. The treatment should be supervised by a physician experienced in the treatment of Parkinson's disease (e.g. Neurologist). The patient's treatment with levodopa, with or without dopamine agonists, should be optimised before starting APO-go treatment.

Determination of the threshold dose.

The appropriate dose for each patient is established by incremental dosing schedules. The following schedule is suggested:-

1mg of apomorphine HCl (0.1ml), that is approximately 15-20 micrograms/kg, may be injected subcutaneously during a hypokinetic, or 'off' period and the patient is observed over 30 minutes for a motor response.

If no response, or an inadequate response, is obtained a second dose of 2 mg of apomorphine HCl (0.2ml) is injected subcutaneously and the patient observed for an adequate response for a further 30 minutes.

The dosage may be increased by incremental injections with at least a forty minute interval between succeeding injections, until a satisfactory motor response is obtained.

Establishment of treatment.

Once the appropriate dose is determined a single subcutaneous injection may be given into the lower abdomen or outer thigh at the first signs of an "off" episode. It cannot be excluded that absorption may differ with different injection sites within a single individual. Accordingly, the patient should then be observed for the next hour to assess the quality of their response to treatment. Alterations in dosage may be made according to the patient's response.

The optimal dosage of apomorphine hydrochloride varies between individuals but, once established, remains relatively constant for each patient.

Precautions on continuing treatment.

The daily dose of APO-go varies widely between patients, typically within the range of 3-30 mg, given as 1-10 injections and sometimes as many as 12 separate injections per day.

It is recommended that the total daily dose of apomorphine HCl should not exceed 100 mg and that individual bolus injections should not exceed 10 mg.

In clinical studies it has usually been possible to make some reduction in the dose of levodopa; this effect varies considerably between patients and needs to be carefully managed by an experienced physician.

Once treatment has been established domperidone therapy may be gradually reduced in some patients but successfully eliminated only in a few, without any vomiting or hypotension.

Children and adolescents.

APO-go Pen 10 mg/ml Solution for Injection is contra-indicated for children and adolescents under 18 years of age (see section 4.3 Contra-indications).

Elderly

The elderly are well represented in the population of patients with Parkinson's disease and constitute a high proportion of those studied in clinical trials of APO-go. The management of elderly patients treated with APO-go has not differed from that of younger patients.

Renal impairment

A dose schedule similar to that recommended for adults, and the elderly, can be followed for patients with renal impairment (see section 4.4, precautions for use).

4.3 Contraindications
In patients with respiratory depression, dementia, psychotic diseases or hepatic insufficiency.

Intermittent apomorphine HCl treatment is not suitable for patients who have an 'on' response to levodopa, which is marred by severe dyskinesia or dystonia.

APO-go is contra-indicated for children and adolescents under 18 years of age.

APO-go should not be administered to patients who have a known hypersensitivity to apomorphine or any of the excipients of the medicinal product.

Pregnancy and lactation (see section 4.6)

4.4 Special warnings and special precautions for use
Apomorphine HCl should be given with caution to patients with renal, pulmonary or cardiovascular disease and persons prone to nausea and vomiting.

Extra caution is recommended during initiation of therapy in elderly and/or debilitated patients.

Since apomorphine may produce hypotension, even when given with domperidone pretreatment, care should be exercised in patients with pre-existing cardiac disease or in patients taking vasoactive medicinal productssuch as antihypertensives, especially in patients with pre-existing postural hypotension.

APO-go Pen 10mg/ml Solution for Injectioncontains sodium bisulphite which may rarely cause severe allergic reactions and bronchospasm.

Coombs' positive haemolytic anaemia has been reported rarely in patients treated with levodopa and the incidence in patients taking levodopa and apomorphine is unaltered. Coombs' positive anaemia has not been reported in patients taking apomorphine in association with other therapy. Haematology tests should be undertaken at regular intervals, as with levodopa, when given concomitantly with apomorphine.

Caution is advised when combining apomorphine with other drugs, especially those with a narrow therapeutic range (see section 4.5).

Neuropsychiatric problems co-exist in many patients with advanced Parkinson's disease. There is evidence that for some patients neuropsychiatric disturbances may be exacerbated by apomorphine.

Special care should be exercised when apomorphine is used in these patients.

Apomorphine has been associated with somnolence, and other dopamine agonists can be associated with sudden sleep onset episodes, particularly in patients with Parkinson's disease. Patients must be informed of this and advised to exercise caution while driving or operating machines during treatment with apomorphine. Patients who have experienced somnolence must refrain from driving or operating machines. Furthermore a reduction of dosage or termination of therapy may be considered.

4.5 Interaction with other medicinal products and other forms of Interaction
Patients selected for treatment with apomorphine HCl are almost certain to be taking concomitant medications for their Parkinson's disease. In the initial stages of apomorphine HCl therapy the patient should be monitored for unusual side-effects or signs of potentiation of effect.

Neuroleptic medicinal products may have an antagonistic effect if used with apomorphine. There is a potential interaction between clozapine and apomorphine, however clozapine may also be used to reduce the symptoms of neuropsychiatric complications.

The possible effects of apomorphine on the plasma concentrations of other drugs have not been studied. Therefore caution is advised when combining apomorphine with other drugs, especially those with a narrow therapeutic range.

Antihypertensive and Cardiac Active Medicinal Drugs

Even when co-administered with domperidone, apomorphine may potentiate the antihypertensive effects of these drugs. See *Special warnings and precautions for use* above.

4.6 Pregnancy and lactation
Animal reproduction studies have not been conducted with apomorphine HCl. Neither is there any experience of the use of apomorphine in pregnant women. Therefore, apomorphine HCl should not be used in women of child bearing potential.

It is anticipated thatapomorphine is excreted in breast milk. Breast-feeding should be avoided during apomorphine HCl therapy.

4.7 Effects on ability to drive and use machines
Apomorphine may have a sedative effect and patients affected should not drive or operate machinery.

Patients being treated with apomorphine and presenting with somnolence must be informed to refrain from driving or engaging in activities (e.g. operating machines) where impaired alertness may put themselves or others at risk of serious injury or death unless patients have overcome such experiences of somnolence (see also Section 4.4).

4.8 Undesirable effects
Very common (> 10%):

Local induration and nodules (usually asymptomatic) often develop at subcutaneous sites of injection in most patients. In patients on high doses of apomorphine HCl these may persist and give rise to areas of erythema, tenderness and induration. Panniculitus has been reported from these patients where a skin biopsy has been undertaken. Care should be taken to ensure that areas of ulceration do not become infected.

Pruritus may occur at the site of injection.

These local subcutaneous effects can sometimes be reduced by rotation of injection sites or possibly by the use of ultrasound (if available) to areas of nodularity and induration.

Common (1 - 10%):

Nausea and vomiting, particularly when apomorphine treatment is first initiated, usually as a result of the omission of domperidone (See section 4.2 Posology and Method of Administration)

Transient sedation with each dose of apomorphine HCl at the start of therapy may occur; this usually resolves over the first few weeks.

Apomorphine is associated with somnolence.

Neuropsychiatric disturbances are common in parkinsonian patients. Apo-go should be used with special caution in these patients. Transient mild confusion and visual hallucinations have occurred during apomorphine HCl therapy.

Uncommon (0.1 - 1%):

Postural hypotension is seen infrequently and is usually transient

(See section 4.4 Special Warnings and Precautions for Use).

Apomorphine may induce dyskinesias during 'on' periods which can be severe in some cases, and in a few patients may result in cessation of therapy.

Coombs' positive haemolytic anaemia has rarely been reported in patients treated with levodopa and apomorphine.

Breathing difficulties have been reported.

Rare (0.01% - 0.1%):

Eosinophilia has rarely occurred during treatment with apomorphine HCl.

Due to the presence of sodium bisulphite, allergic reactions (including anaphylaxis and bronchospasm may occur).

4.9 Overdose

There is little clinical experience of overdosewith apomorphine by this route of administration. Symptoms of overdose may be treated empirically as suggested below:-

Excessive emesis may be treated with domperidone.

Respiratory depression may be treated with naloxone.

Hypotension: appropriate measures should be taken, e.g. raising the foot of the bed.

Bradycardia may be treated with atropine.

5. PHARMACOLOGICAL PROPERTIES

5.1 Pharmacodynamic properties

Pharmatherapeutic group: Dopamine agonists ATC Classification: N04B C07

Apomorphine is a direct stimulant of dopamine receptors and while possessing both D1 and D2 receptor agonist properties does not share transport or metabolic pathways with levodopa.

Although in intact experimental animals, administration of apomorphine suppresses the rate of firing of nigro-striatal cells and in low dose has been found to produce a reduction in locomotor activity (thought to represent pre-synaptic inhibition of endogenous dopamine release) its actions on parkinsonian motor disability are likely to be mediated at post-synaptic receptor sites. This biphasic effect is also seen in humans.

5.2 Pharmacokinetic properties

After subcutaneous injection of apomorphineits fate can be described by a two-compartment model, with a distribution half-life of 5 (± 1.1) minutes and an elimination half-life of 33 (± 3.9) minutes. Clinical response correlates well with levels of apomorphine in the cerebrospinal fluid; the drug distribution being best described by a two- compartment model. Apomorphine is rapidly and completely absorbed from subcutaneous tissue, correlating with the rapid onset of clinical effects (4-12 minutes), and that the brief duration of clinical action of the drug (about 1 hour) is explained by its rapid clearance. The metabolism of apomorphine is by glucuronidation and sulphonation to at least ten per cent of the total; other pathways have not been described.

5.3 Preclinical safety data

Repeat dose subcutaneous toxicity studies reveal no special hazard for humans, beyond the information included in other sections of the SmPC.

In vitro genotoxicity studies demonstrated mutagenic and clastogenic effects, most likely due to products formed by oxidation of apomorphine. However, apomorphine was not genotoxic in the in vivo studies performed.

There are no data on fertility and embryo-foetal toxicity. No carcinogenicity studies have been performed.

6. PHARMACEUTICAL PARTICULARS

6.1 List of excipients

Sodium bisulphite (E222)

Hydrochloric Acid (37%), concentrated (to adjust pH to 3.0 –4.0)

Water for Injection

6.2 Incompatibilities

In the absence of incompatability studies, this medicinal product must not be mixed with other medicinal products.

6.3 Shelf life

2 years

48 hours after first opening

6.4 Special precautions for storage

Do not store above 25°C.

Store in the original container.

6.5 Nature and contents of container

Cartridge.

APO-go Pen 10 mg/ml is a disposable multiple dose pen injector system incorporating a clear glass (type I) cartridge containing a clear solution for injection. The glass cartridge is sealed at one end with a bromobutyl rubber piston, and at the other end with a bromobutylrubber/aluminium membrane.

Each pen contains 3ml of solution for injection.

Packs containing 1, 5, or 10 × 3ml pens in a moulded plastic tray in an outer cardboard carton.

6.6 Instructions for use and handling

APO-go PEN

Do not use if solution has turned green.

Discard each pen no later than 48 hours from first use.

(see attached diagram)

1. Dosage dial
2. Arrow showing the dosage selected
3. Numbers indicating the dose per injection (1-10 mg)
4. Graduations *(in mg)* on cartridge showing total amount of apomorphine in the pen
5. Membrane
6. Needle
7. Needle protector
8. Outer sleeve of pen
9. Protective cone
10. Needle in sealed unit

* The pack does NOT contain needles for use with your Pen. Use pen needles for use with your Pen. Use pen needles not less than 12mm (½") in length and not finer than 0.33mm (29G).

Pen needles recommended for use with insulin pens are compatible with APO-go Pen

HOW TO USE YOUR APO-go PEN

Read these instructions carefully

DO NOT PULL THE RED DIAL BEFORE YOU HAVE SET THE DOSAGE (See f)

(see attached diagram)

ATTACHING THE NEEDLE

(a) Before using your pen system you will need a surgical wipe and one needle in its protective cone (see 9). Take the pen out of its box and remove the outer sleeve (see 8).

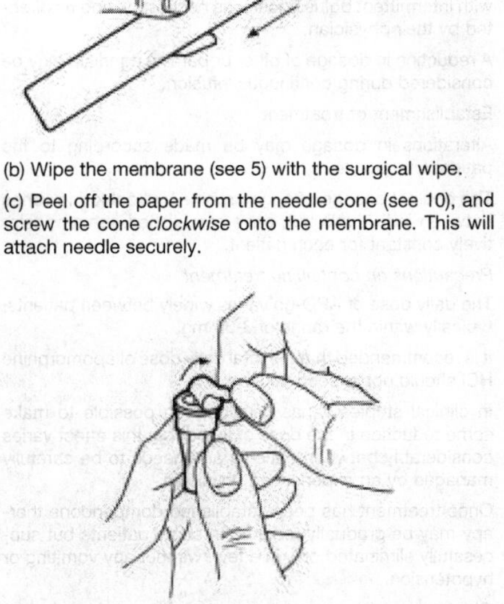

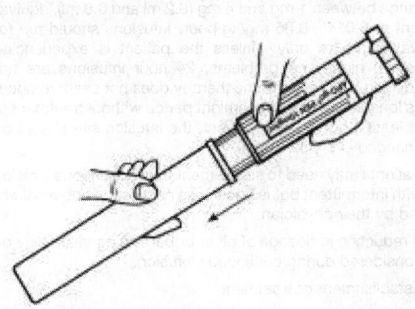

(b) Wipe the membrane (see 5) with the surgical wipe.

(c) Peel off the paper from the needle cone (see 10), and screw the cone *clockwise* onto the membrane. This will attach needle securely.

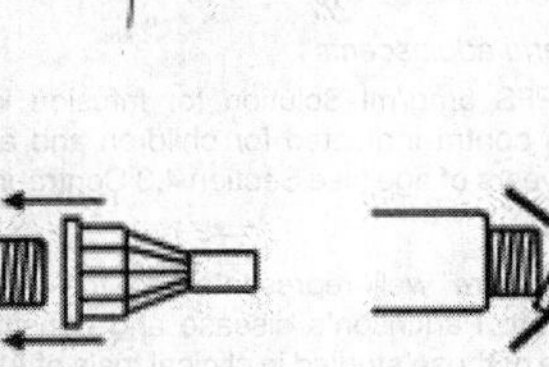

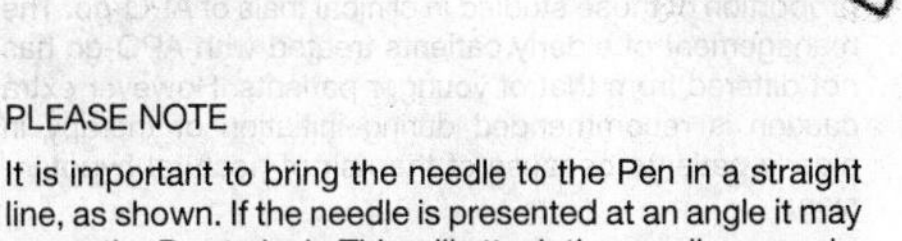

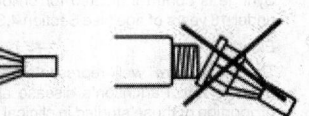

PLEASE NOTE

It is important to bring the needle to the Pen in a straight line, as shown. If the needle is presented at an angle it may cause the Pen to leak. This will attach the needle securely.

(d) Remove the protective cone, *but do not throw it away*. Do not remove the needle protector at this stage (see 7).

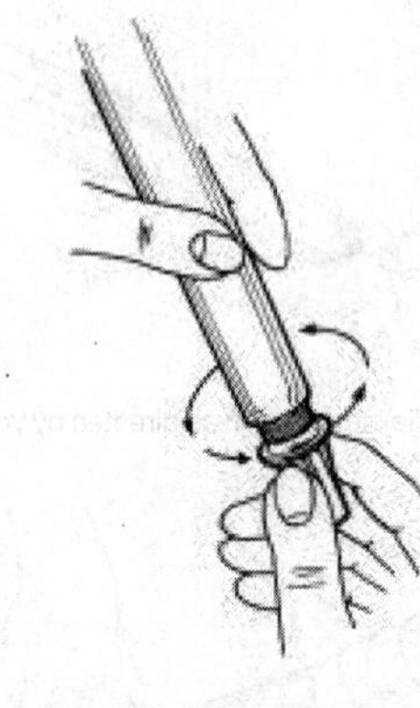

(e) Replace the pen's outer sleeve.

HOW TO SELECT YOUR CORRECT DOSAGE

(see attached diagram)

(f) Press the red dosage dial (see 1) and turn the dial clockwise until the arrow points to your prescribed dosage (see 2,3). Then release downward pressure on the red dial. The dose is now set, and you do not need to redial for subsequent injections.

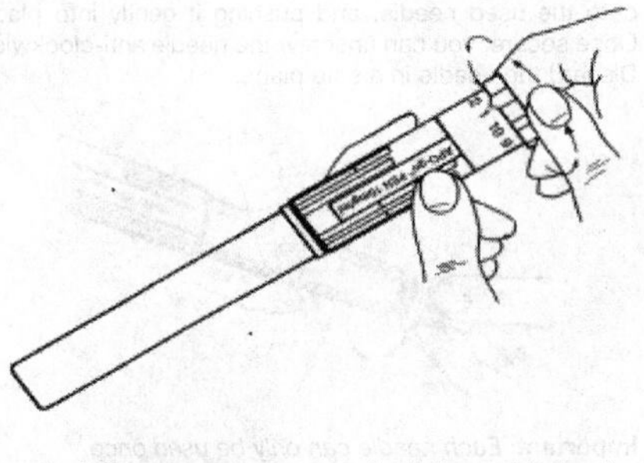

Important; If you pass your prescribed dose while turning the dial, just continue pressing and turning in the same direction until you arrive at it again. *Never pull and turn the red dosage dial at the same time.*

If your prescribed dose is 2mg or less, it is necessary to "prime" the pen before injecting the first dose. Do this by emptying the first 2mg dose onto a paper tissue and discard. Then, set the dose you require for injection and inject in the usual way (see below under "INJECTING"). If the first dose required is more than 2mg, then it is not necessary to "prime" the pen.

INJECTING

(see attached diagram)

(g) Pull out the red dosage dial as far as it will go. Check the white scale on the plunger and inject only if the highest number visible corresponds to the intended dose.

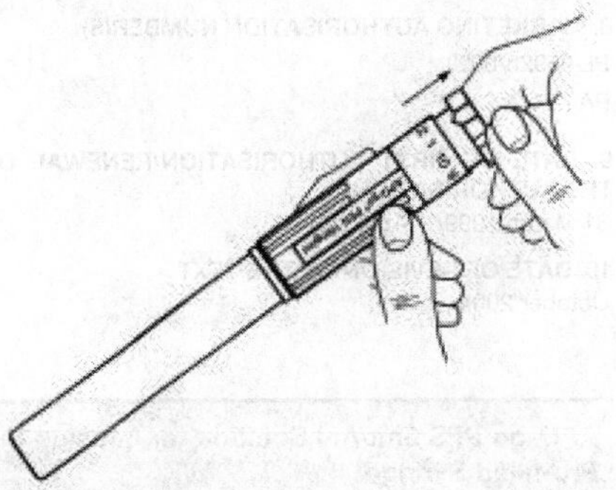

(h) Using a surgical wipe, clean the area of skin around the proposed site of injection.

Remove the pen's outer sleeve.

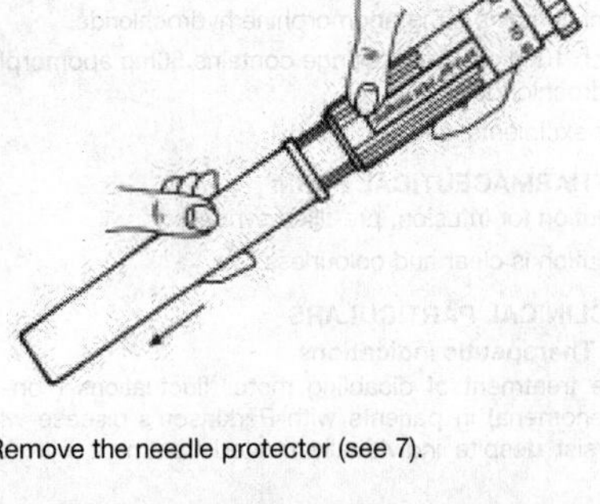

(i) Remove the needle protector (see 7).

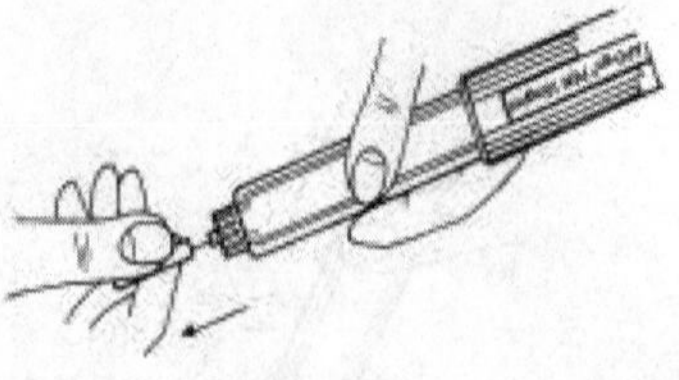

(j) Insert the needle into the skin as directed by your doctor.

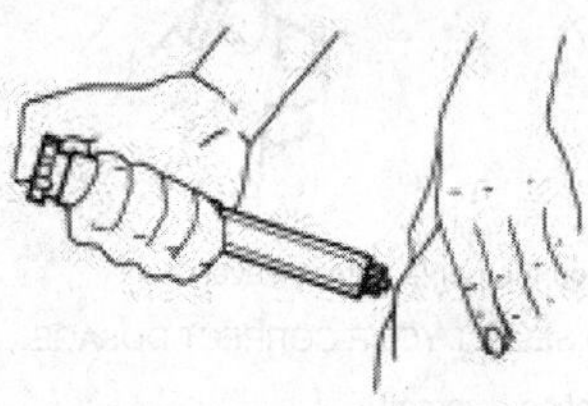

To inject, press the red dosage dial down as far as it will go, using your thumb if possible. Once the red dosage dial is fully depressed, count to three before withdrawing the needle.

(k) Remove and discard the needle, using the protective cone (see 9). This is done by replacing the protective cone onto the used needle, and pushing it gently into place. Once secure, you can unscrew the needle anti-clockwise. Discard the needle in a safe place.

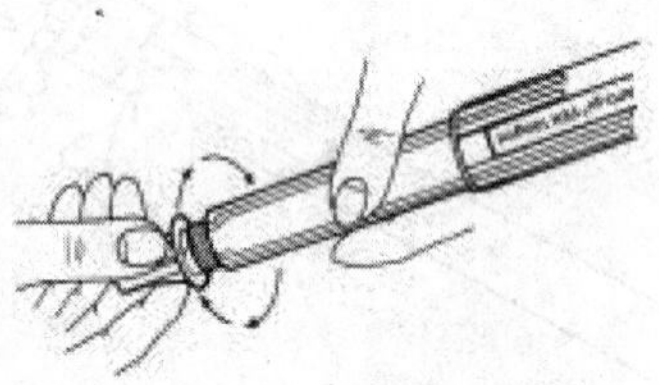

Important: *Each needle can only be used once.*

PREPARING FOR THE NEXT INJECTION:

Check that there is enough apomorphine left in the cartridge for the next injection (see 4). If there is, put a new needle in place, following the same procedure as before. (*Remember not to throw away the protective cone*).

If there is not enough apomorphine left for another injection, prepare another pen.

Finally, replace the outer sleeve of the pen.

7. MARKETING AUTHORISATION HOLDER

Forum Products Limited

41 - 51 Brighton Road

Redhill

Surrey

RH1 6YS

United Kingdom

8. MARKETING AUTHORISATION NUMBER(S)

PL 05928/0021

PA 454/2/1

9. DATE OF FIRST AUTHORISATION/RENEWAL OF THE AUTHORISATION

31 March 1999/ 1 April 2004

10. DATE OF REVISION OF THE TEXT

October 2004

APO-go PFS 5mg/ml Solution for Infusion in Pre-filled Syringe

(Britannia Pharmaceuticals Limited)

1. NAME OF THE MEDICINAL PRODUCT

APO-go PFS 5mg/ml Solution for Infusion in Pre-filled Syringe

2. QUALITATIVE AND QUANTITATIVE COMPOSITION

1 ml contains 5 mg apomorphine hydrochloride.

Each 10ml pre-filled syringe contains 50mg apomorphine hydrochloride.

For excipients, see Section 6.1

3. PHARMACEUTICAL FORM

Solution for Infusion, pre-filled syringe

Solution is clear and colourless

4. CLINICAL PARTICULARS

4.1 Therapeutic indications

The treatment of disabling motor fluctuations ("on-off" phenomena) in patients with Parkinson's disease which persist despite individually titrated treatment with levodopa (with a peripheral decarboxylase inhibitor) and/or other dopamine agonists.

4.2 Posology and method of administration

APO-go PFS 5mg/ml Solution for Infusion in Pre-filled Syringe is a pre-diluted pre-filled syringe intended for use as a continuous subcutaneous infusion by minipump and / or syringe-driver (see Section 6.6 Instruction for Use/ Handling that provides information on how to use the APO-go PFS 5mg/ml Solution for Infusion in Pre-filled Syringe with different types of minipumps and/or syringe driver).

Apomorphine must not be used via the intravenous route.

Dosage

Adults

Administration

Selection of Patients Suitable for APO-go:

> Patients selected for treatment with APO-go should be able to recognise the onset of their 'off' symptoms and be capable of injecting themselves or else have a responsible carer able to inject for them when required. It is essential that the patient is established on domperidone, usually 20 mg three times daily for at least two days prior to initiation of therapy.
> Apomorphine should be initiated in the controlled environment of a specialist clinic. The patient should be supervised by a physician experienced in the treatment of Parkinson's disease (e.g. neurologist). The patient's treatment with levodopa, with or without dopamine agonists, should be optimised before starting APO-go treatment.

Continuous Infusion

Patients who have shown a good 'on' period response during the initiation stage of apomorphine therapy, but whose overall control remains unsatisfactory using intermittent injections, or who require many and frequent injections (more than 10 per day), may be commenced on or transferred to continuous subcutaneous infusion by minipump and / or syringe driver (see Section 6.6 Instruction for Use/Handling) as follows:-

The threshold dose for continuous infusion should be determined as follows: Continuous infusion is started at a rate of 1 mg apomorphine HCl (0.2 ml) per hour then increased according to the individual response each day. Increases in the infusion rate should not exceed 0.5 mg at intervals of not less than 4 hours. Hourly infusion rates may range between 1 mg and 4 mg (0.2 ml and 0.8 ml), equivalent to 0.014 - 0.06 mg/kg/hour. Infusions should run for waking hours only. Unless the patient is experiencing severe night-time problems, 24 hour infusions are not advised. Tolerance to the therapy does not seem to occur as long as there is an overnight period without treatment of at least 4 hours. In any event, the infusion site should be changed every 12 hours.

Patients may need to supplement their continuous infusion with intermittent bolus boosts, as necessary, and as directed by their physician.

A reduction in dosage of other dopamine agonists may be considered during continuous infusion.

Establishment of treatment

Alterations in dosage may be made according to the patient's response.

The optimal dosage of apomorphine hydrochloride varies between individuals but, once established, remains relatively constant for each patient.

Precautions on continuing treatment

The daily dose of APO-go varies widely between patients, typically within the range of 3-30 mg.

It is recommended that the total daily dose of apomorphine HCl should not exceed 100 mg.

In clinical studies it has usually been possible to make some reduction in the dose of levodopa; this effect varies considerably between patients and needs to be carefully managed by an experienced physician.

Once treatment has been established domperidone therapy may be gradually reduced in some patients but successfully eliminated only in a few, without any vomiting or hypotension.

Children and adolescents

APO-go PFS 5mg/ml Solution for Infusion in Pre-filled Syringe is contra-indicated for children and adolescents under 18 years of age (see Section 4.3 Contra-indications).

Elderly

The elderly are well represented in the population of patients with Parkinson's disease and constitute a high proportion of those studied in clinical trials of APO-go. The management of elderly patients treated with APO-go has not differed from that of younger patients. However extra caution is recommended during initiation of therapy in elderly patients because of the risk of postural hypotension.

Renal impairment

A dose schedule similar to that recommended for adults, and the elderly, can be followed for patients with renal impairment (see Section 4.4 Special Warnings and Precautions for Use).

4.3 Contraindications

In patients with respiratory depression, dementia, psychotic diseases or hepatic insufficiency.

Apomorphine HCl treatment is not suitable for patients who have an 'on' response to levodopa which is marred by severe dyskinesia or dystonia.

APO-go should not be administered to patients who have a known hypersensitivity to apomorphine or any excipients of the medicinal product.

APO-go is contra-indicated for children and adolescents under 18 years of age.

Pregnancy and lactation (see Section 4.6 Pregnancy and Lactation)

4.4 Special warnings and special precautions for use

Apomorphine HCl should be given with caution to patients with renal, pulmonary or cardiovascular disease and persons prone to nausea and vomiting.

Extra caution is recommended during initiation of therapy in elderly and/or debilitated patients.

Since apomorphine may produce hypotension, even when given with domperidone pretreatment, care should be exercised in patients with pre-existing cardiac disease or in patients taking vasoactive medicinal products such as antihypertensives, and especially in patients with pre-existing postural hypotension.

APO-go PFS 5mg/ml Solution for Infusion in Pre-filled Syringe contains sodium metabisulphite which may rarely cause severe allergic reactions and bronchospasm.

Coombs' positive haemolytic anaemia has been reported rarely in patients treated with levodopa and the incidence in patients taking levodopa and apomorphine is unaltered. Coombs' positive haemolytic anaemia has not been reported in patients taking apomorphine in association with other therapy. Haematology tests should be undertaken at regular intervals as with levodopa when given concomitantly with apomorphine.

Caution is advised when combining apomorphine with other medicinal products, especially those with a narrow therapeutic range (see Section 4.5 Interactions with other Medicinal Products and Other Forms of Interaction)

Neuropsychiatric problems co-exist in many patients with advanced Parkinson's disease. There is evidence that for some patients neuropsychiatric disturbances may be exacerbated by apomorphine. Special care should be exercised when apomorphine is used in these patients.

Apomorphine has been associated with somnolence, and other dopamine agonists can be associated with sudden sleep onset episodes, particularly in patients with Parkinson's disease. Patients must be informed of this and advised to exercise caution while driving or operating machines during treatment with apomorphine. Patients who have experienced somnolence must refrain from driving or operating machines. Furthermore a reduction of dosage or termination of therapy may be considered.

This medicinal product contains 33.89 mg sodium per 10ml dose. This should be taken into consideration by patients on a controlled sodium diet.

4.5 Interaction with other medicinal products and other forms of Interaction

Patients selected for treatment with apomorphine HCl are almost certain to be taking concomitant medications for their Parkinson's disease. In the initial stages of apomorphine HCl therapy the patient should be monitored for unusual side-effects or signs of potentiation of effect.

Neuroleptic medicinal products may have an antagonistic effect if used with apomorphine. There is a potential interaction between clozapine and apomorphine, however clozapine may also be used to reduce the symptoms of neuropsychiatric complications.

If neuroleptic medicinal products have to be used in patients with Parkinson's disease treated by dopamine agonists, a gradual reduction in apomorphine dose may be considered when administration is by minipump and / or syringe- driver (symptoms suggestive of neuroleptic malignant syndrome have been reported rarely with abrupt withdrawal of dopaminergic therapy).

The possible effects of apomorphine on the plasma concentrations of other medicinal products have not been studied. Therefore caution is advised when combining apomorphine with other medicinal products, especially those with a narrow therapeutic range.

Antihypertensive and Cardiac Active Medicinal Products

Even when co-administered with domperidone, apomorphine may potentiate the antihypertensive effects of these medicinal products (see Section 4.4 Special Warnings and Precautions for Use).

4.6 Pregnancy and lactation

Animal reproduction studies have not been conducted with apomorphine HCl.

Neither is there any experience of apomorphine usage in pregnant women. Therefore, apomorphine HCl should not be used in women of child-bearing potential.

It is anticipated that apomorphine is excreted in breast milk. Breast-feeding should be avoided during apomorphine HCl therapy.

4.7 Effects on ability to drive and use machines
Patients being treated with apomorphine and presenting with somnolence and/or sudden sleep episodes must be informed to refrain from driving or engaging in activities (e.g. operating machines) where impaired alertness may put themselves or others at risk of serious injury or death until such recurrent episodes and somnolence have resolved (see also Section 4.4 Special Warnings and Precautions for Use).

4.8 Undesirable effects
Very common (>10%):

Local induration and nodules (usually asymptomatic) often develop at subcutaneous sites of injection in most patients, particularly with continuous use. In patients on high doses of apomorphine HCl these may persist and give rise to areas of erythema, tenderness and induration. Panniculitus has been reported from these patients where a skin biopsy has been undertaken. Care should be taken to ensure that areas of ulceration do not become infected. Pruritus may occur at the site of injection.

These local subcutaneous effects can sometimes be reduced by rotation of injection sites or possibly by the use of ultrasound (if available) to areas of nodularity and induration.

Common (1-10%):

Nausea and vomiting, particularly when apomorphine treatment is first initiated, usually as a result of the omission of domperidone (See Section 4.2 Posology and Method of Administration)

Transient sedation with each dose of apomorphine HCl at the start of therapy may occur; this usually resolves over the first few weeks.

Apomorphine is associated with somnolence.

Neuropsychiatric disturbances are common in parkinsonian patients. APO-go should be used with special caution in these patients. Transient mild confusion and visual hallucinations have occurred during apomorphine HCl therapy.

Uncommon (0.1-1%):

Postural hypotension is seen infrequently and is usually transient (See Section 4.4 Special Warnings and Precautions for Use).

Apomorphine may induce dyskinesias during 'on' periods, which can be severe in some cases, and in a few patients may result in cessation of therapy.

Coombs' positive haemolytic anaemia has rarely been reported in patients treated with levodopa and apomorphine.

Rare (0.01%-0.1%):

Eosinophilia has rarely occurred during treatment with apomorphine HCl.

Due to the presence of sodium metabisulphite, allergic reactions (including anaphylaxis and bronchospasm) may occur.

4.9 Overdose
There is little clinical experience of overdose with apomorphine by this route of administration. Symptoms of overdose may be treated empirically as suggested below:-

Excessive emesis may be treated with domperidone.

Respiratory depression may be treated with naloxone.

Hypotension: appropriate measures should be taken, e.g. raising the foot of the bed.

Bradycardia may be treated with atropine.

5. PHARMACOLOGICAL PROPERTIES

5.1 Pharmacodynamic properties
Pharmatherapeutic group: Dopamine agonists

ATC Classification: N04B C07

Apomorphine is a direct stimulant of dopamine receptors and while possessing both D1 and D2 receptor agonist properties does not share transport or metabolic pathways with levodopa.

Although in intact experimental animals, administration of apomorphine suppresses the rate of firing of nigro-striatal cells and in low dose has been found to produce a reduction in locomotor activity (thought to represent pre-synaptic inhibition of endogenous dopamine release) its actions on parkinsonian motor disability are likely to be mediated at post-synaptic receptor sites. This biphasic effect is also seen in humans.

5.2 Pharmacokinetic properties
After subcutaneous injection of apomorphine its fate can be described by a two-compartment model, with a distribution half-life of 5 (±1.1) minutes and an elimination half-life of 33 (±3.9) minutes. Clinical response correlates well with levels of apomorphine in the cerebrospinal fluid; the active substance distribution being best described by a two-compartment model. Apomorphine is rapidly and completely absorbed from subcutaneous tissue, correlating with the rapid onset of clinical effects (4-12 minutes), and the brief duration of clinical action of the active substance (about 1 hour) is explained by its rapid clearance.

The metabolism of apomorphine is by glucuronidation and sulphonation to at least ten per cent of the total; other pathways have not been described.

5.3 Preclinical safety data
Repeat dose subcutaneous toxicity studies reveal no special hazard for humans, beyond the information included in other sections of the SmPC.

In vitro genotoxicity studies demonstrated mutagenic and clastogenic effects, most likely due to products formed by oxidation of apomorphine. However, apomorphine was not genotoxic in the in vivo studies performed.

There are no data on fertility and embryo-foetal toxicity. No carcinogenicity studies have been performed.

6. PHARMACEUTICAL PARTICULARS

6.1 List of excipients
Sodium chloride

Sodium metabisulphite (E223)

Hydrochloric acid (37%), to adjust pH to 3.0-4.0

Water for Injections

6.2 Incompatibilities
In the absence of compatibility studies, this medicinal product must not be mixed with other medicinal products.

6.3 Shelf life
Unopened 2 years

Once opened the pre-filled syringe should be used immediately.

6.4 Special precautions for storage
Keep the container in the outer carton.

Do not store above 25°C.

6.5 Nature and contents of container
Clear glass (Type I) pre-filled syringe with a chlorobutyl rubber stopper and tip.

Packs contain 5 × 10ml Pre-filled Syringes in a cardboard tray in an outer cardboard carton.

6.6 Instructions for use and handling
There is no need to dilute APO-go PFS 5mg/ml Solution for Infusion in Pre-filled Syringe prior to use.

Do not use if the solution has turned green. The solution should be inspected visually prior to use. Only clear, colourless and particle free solution should be used.

APO-go PFS 5mg/ml Solution for Infusion in Pre-filled Syringe is for single use only. Any unused solution should be discarded.

Continuous infusion and the use of a minipump and / or syringe-driver

The choice, of which minipump and / or syringe-driver to use, and the dosage settings required, will be determined by the physician in accordance with the particular needs of the patient.

After single use, adaptors and plastic syringes should be discarded and disposed of in a Sharps bin.

APO-go PFS 5mg/ml Solution for Infusion in Pre-filled Syringe has been designed for continuous infusion of apomorphine therapy via a syringe driver. It is not intended to be used for intermittent injection.

APO-go PFS 5mg/ml Solution for Infusion in Pre-filled Syringe can be used with suitable pumps/syringe drivers, e.g. APO-go pump or Graseby syringe driver. Detailed explanations will be provided by the Distributor.

7. MARKETING AUTHORISATION HOLDER
Forum Products Limited

41 - 51 Brighton Road

Redhill

Surrey

RH1 6YS

United Kingdom

8. MARKETING AUTHORISATION NUMBER(S)
PL 05928/0025

9. DATE OF FIRST AUTHORISATION/RENEWAL OF THE AUTHORISATION
September 2004

10. DATE OF REVISION OF THE TEXT
April 2005

Apresoline Ampoules 20 mg

(Sovereign Medical)

1. NAME OF THE MEDICINAL PRODUCT
Apresoline Ampoules 20 mg

2. QUALITATIVE AND QUANTITATIVE COMPOSITION
The active ingredient is 1-hydralainophthalazine hydrochloride (hydralazine hydrochloride). Each 2 ml ampoule contains 20mg hydralazine hydrochloride.

3. PHARMACEUTICAL FORM
Ampoules

4. CLINICAL PARTICULARS

4.1 Therapeutic indications

1. Treatment of hypertensive emergencies, particularly those associated with pre-eclampsia and toxaemia of pregnancy.
2. Treatment of hypertension with renal complications.

4.2 Posology and method of administration
Adults:

Initially 5 to 10 mg by slow intravenous injection, to avoid precipitous decreases in arterial pressure with a critical reduction in cerebral or utero-placental perfusion. If necessary a repeat injection can be given after an interval of 20-30 minutes, throughout which blood pressure and heart rate should be monitored. A satisfactory response can be defined as a decrease in diastyloic blood pressure to 90/100 mmHg. The contents of the vial should be reconstituted by dissolving in 1 ml of water for injection BP. This should then be further diluted with 10 ml of Sodium Chloride injection BP 0.9% and be administered by slow intravenous injection. The injection must be given immediately and any remainder discarded. Apresoline may also be given by continuous intravenous infusion, beginning with a flow rate of 200-300μg/min. Maintenance flow rates must be determined individually and are usually within the range 50-150μg/min. The product reconstituted as for direct iv injection may be added via the infusion container to 500 ml of Sodium Chloride Injection BP 0.9% and given by continuous infusion. The addition should be made immediately before administration and the mixture should not be stored. Apresoline for infusion can also be used with 5% sorbitol solution or isotonic inorganic infusion solutions such as Ringers solution.

Children:

Not recommended

Elderly:

Clinical evidence would indicate that no special dosage regime is necessary. Advancing age does not affect either blood concentration or systemic clearance. Renal elimination may however be affected in so far as kidney function diminishes with age.

4.3 Contraindications
Known hypersensitivity to hydralazine of dihydralazine.

Idiopathic systemic lupus erythematosus (SLE) and related diseases.

Severe tachycardia and heart failure with a high cardiac output (e.g. in thyrotoxicosis).

Myocardial insufficiency due to mechanical obstruction (e.g. in the presence of aortic or mitral stenosis or constructive pericarditis).

Isolated right ventricular failure due to pulmonary hypertension (cor pulmonale).

Dissecting aortic aneurysm.

4.4 Special warnings and special precautions for use
Warnings
The overall 'hyperdynamic' state of the circulation induced by hydralazine may accentuate certain clinical conditions. Myocardial stimulation may provoke or aggravate angina pectoris. Patients with suspected or confirmed coronary artery disease should therefore be given Apresoline only under cover beta-blocker or in combination with other suitable sympatholytic agents. It is important that the beta-blocker medication should be commenced a few days before the start of treatment with Apresoline.

Patients who have survived a myocardial infarction should not receive Apresoline until a post-infarction stabilisation phase has been achieved.

Prolonged treatment with hydralazine (i.e. usually for more than 6 months) may provoke a lupus erythematosus (LE) like syndrome, especially where doses exceed 100 mg daily. First symptoms are likely to be arthralgia, sometimes associated with fever and rash and are reversible after withdrawal of the drug. In its more severe form it resembles acute SLE, and in rare cases renal and ocular involvement have been reported. Long-term treatment with corticosteroids may be required to reverse these changes. Since such reactions tend to occur more frequently the higher the dose and the longer its duration, and since they are more common in slow acetylators, it is recommended that for maintenance therapy the lowest effective dose should be used. If 100 mg daily fails to elicit an adequate clinical effect, the patient's acetylator status should be evaluated. Slow acetylators and women run greater risk of developing the LE like syndrome and every effort should therefore be made to keep the dosage below 100 mg daily and a careful watch kept for signs and symptoms suggestive of this syndrome. If such symptoms do develop the drug should be gradually withdrawn. Rapid acetylators often respond inadequately even to doses of 100 mg daily and therefore the dose can be raised with only a slightly increased risk of an LE-like syndrome.

During long term treatment with Apresoline it is advisable to determine the antinuclear factors and conduct urine analysis at intervals of approximately 6 months. Microhaematuria and / or proteinuria, in particular together with positive titres of ANF, may be initial signs of immune-complex glomerulonephritis associated with the SLE like syndrome. If overt clinical signs or symptoms develop, the drug should be withdrawn immediately.

Skin rash, febrile reactions and change in blood count occur rarely and drug should be withdrawn. Peripheral neuritis in the form of paraesthesia has been reported, and may respond to pyridoxine administration or drug withdrawal.

In high (cyto-) toxic concentrations, hydralazine induces gene mutations in single cell organisms and in mammalian cells in vitro. No unequivocally mutagenic effects have been detected *in vivo* in a great number of test systems.

Hydralazine in lifetime carcinogenicity studies, caused, towards the end of the experiments, small but statistically significant increases in lung tumours in mice and in hepatic and testicular tumours in rats. These tumours also occur spontaneously with fairly high frequency in aged rodents.

With due consideration of these animals and in-vitro toxicological findings, hydralazine in therapeutic doses does not appear to bear risk that would necessitate a limitation of its administration. Many years of clinical experience have not suggested that human cancer is associated with hydralazine use.

Precautions

In patients with renal impairment (creatine clearance < 30 ml/min or serum creatinine concentrations > 2.5 mg / 100 ml or 221 μmol / l) and in patients with hepatic dysfunction the dose or interval between doses should be adjusted according to clinical response, in order to avoid accumulation of the 'apparent' active substance.

Apresoline should be used with caution in patients with coronary artery disease (since it may increase angina) or cerebrovascular disease.

When undergoing surgery, patients treated with Apresoline may show a fall in blood pressure, in which case one should not use adrenaline to correct the hypotension, since it enhances the cardiac-accelerating effects of hydralazine.

4.5 Interaction with other medicinal products and other forms of Interaction

Potentiation of effects: Concurrent therapy with other anti-hypertensives (vasodilators, calcium antagonists, ACE inhibitors, diuretics), anaesthetics tricyclic antidepressants, major tranquillisers or drugs exerting central depressant actions (including alcohol).

Administration of Apresoline shortly before of after diazoxide may give rise to marked hypotension.

MAO inhibitors should be used with caution in patients receiving Apresoline.

Concurrent administration of Apresoline with beta-blockers subject to a strong first pass effect (e.g. propranolol) may increase their bioavailability. Download adjustment of these drugs may be required when they are given concomitantly with Apresoline.

4.6 Pregnancy and lactation

Use of Apresoline in pregnancy, before the third trimester should be avoided but the drug maybe employed in later pregnancy if there is no safer alternative or when the disease itself carries serious risks for the mother or child e.g. pre-eclampsia and /or eclampsia.

No serious adverse effects in human pregnancy have been reported to date with Apresoline, although experience in the third trimester is extensive.

Hydralazine passes into breast milk but reports available so far have not shown adverse effects on the infant. Mothers in whom use of Apresoline proves unavoidable may breast feed their infant provided that the infant is observed for possible adverse effects.

4.7 Effects on ability to drive and use machines

Apresoline may impair the patient's reactions especially at the start of the treatment. The patient should be warned of the hazard when driving or operating machinery.

4.8 Undesirable effects

Some of the adverse effects listed below e.g. tachycardia, palpitation, angina symptoms, flushing, headache, dizziness, nasal congestion and gastro-intestinal disturbances are commonly seen at the start of treatment, especially if the dose is raised quickly. However such effects generally subside in the further course of treatment.

(The following frequency estimates are used: frequent > 10 %, occasional 1-10% rare 0.001-1% isolated cases < 0.001%)

Cardiovascular system:

Frequently: tachycardia, palpitation.

Occasionally: flushing, hypotension, anginal symptoms.

Rarely: oedema, heart failure.

Isolated cases: paradoxical pressor responses.

Central and peripheral nervous system:

Frequently: headache.

Rarely: dizziness.

Isolated cases: peripheral neuritis, polyneuritis, paraesthesiae (these unwanted effects may be reversed by administering pyridoxine).

Musculo-skeletal system:

Occasionally:arthralgia, joint swelling, myalgia.

Skin and appendages:

Rarely: rash.

Urogenital system:

Rarely: proteinuria, increased plasma creatinine, haematuria sometimes in association with glomerulonephritis.

Isolated cases: acute renal failure, urinary retention.

Gastro-intestinal tract:

Occasionally: gastro-intestinal disturbances, diarrhoea, nausea, vomiting. Rarely: jaundice, liver enlargement, abnormal liver function sometimes in association with hepatitis.

Isolated cases: paralytic ileus.

Blood:

Rarely: anaemia, leucopenia, neutropenia, thrombocytopenia with or without purpura.

Isolated cases: haemolytic anaemia, leucocytosis, lymphadenopathy, pancytopenia, splenomegaly, agranulocytosis.

Psyche:

Rarely: agitation, anorexia, anxiety.

Isolated cases: depression, hallucinations.

Sense organs:

Rarely: increased lacrimination, conjunctivitis, nasal congestion.

Hypersensitivity reactions:

Occasionally: SLE-like syndrome (see under 'Warnings')

Rarely: hypersensitivity reactions such as pruritus, urticaria, vasculitis, eosinophilia, hepatitis.

Respiratory tract:

Rarely: dyspnoea, pleural pain.

Miscellaneous:

Rarely: fever, weight decrease, malaise.

Isolated cases: exophthalmos.

4.9 Overdose

Signs and symptoms

Symptoms include hypotension, tachycardia, myocardial ischaemia dysrhythmias and coma.

Treatment

Supportive measures including intravenous fluids are also indicated. If hypotension is present, an attempt should be made to raise the blood pressure without increasing the tachycardia. Adrenaline should therefore be avoided.

5. PHARMACOLOGICAL PROPERTIES

5.1 Pharmacodynamic properties

Pharmacotherapeutic group

Hydralazine is a peripheral vasodilator.

Mechanism of action

Hydralazine is a direct acting vasodilator which exerts its effects principally on the arterioles. Its precise mode of action is not known. Administration of hydralazine produces a fall in peripheral resistance and a decrease in arterial blood pressure, effects which induce reflux sympathetic cardiovascular responses. The concomitant use of a beta-blocker will reduce these reflex effects and enhance the anti-hypertensive effect. The use of hydralazine can result in sodium and fluid retention, producing oedema and reduced urinary volume. These effects can be prevented by concomitant administration of a diuretic.

5.2 Pharmacokinetic properties

Absorption

None stated

Distribution

Apresoline is rapidly distributed in the body and displays a particular affinity for the blood-vessel walls. Plasma protein binding is of the order of 90%.

Biotransformation

None stated

Elimination

Plasma half-life averages 2-3 hours but is prolonged up to 16 hours in severe renal failure (creatinine clearance less than 20 ml / min) and shortened to approximately 45 minutes in rapid acetylators.

Characteristics in patients

None stated

5.3 Preclinical safety data

Hydralazine has been found to be teratogenic in mice producing a small incidence of cleft palate and certain other bony malformations, in oral doses ranging from 20-120 mg / kg i.e. 20-30 times the maximum human daily dose. It was not teratogenic in rats or rabbits.

6. PHARMACEUTICAL PARTICULARS

6.1 List of excipients

Hydrochloric acid

6.2 Incompatibilities

Dextrose infusion solutions are not compatible because contact between hydralazine and glucose causes hydralazine to be rapidly broken down.

6.3 Shelf life

5 years

6.4 Special precautions for storage

The ampoules should be protected from light and stored below 30°C. Single use only. Use immediately after reconstitution.

Medicines should be kept out of reach of children.

6.5 Nature and contents of container

Colourless Type I glass 2 ml ampoule. Five ampoules are packed in a cupboard printed carton.

6.6 Instructions for use and handling

None

Administrative Data

7. MARKETING AUTHORISATION HOLDER

Waymade Plc

Trading as Sovereign Medical
Sovereign House,
Miles Gray Road
Basildon,
Essex, SS14 3FR.
United Kingdom

8. MARKETING AUTHORISATION NUMBER(S)

PL 06464/1239

9. DATE OF FIRST AUTHORISATION/RENEWAL OF THE AUTHORISATION

15 November 2001

10. DATE OF REVISION OF THE TEXT

Apresoline Tablets 25 mg

(Amdipharm)

1. NAME OF THE MEDICINAL PRODUCT

Apresoline Tablets 25 mg

2. QUALITATIVE AND QUANTITATIVE COMPOSITION

The active ingredient is 1-hydrazinophthalazine hydrochloride (hydralazine hydrochloride).

One coated tablet contains 25 mg hydralazine hydrochloride B.P.

3. PHARMACEUTICAL FORM

Sugar-coated tablets.

4. CLINICAL PARTICULARS

4.1 Therapeutic indications

For the treatment of moderate to severe hypertension as an adjunct to other anti-hypertensive agents.

For use in combination with long-acting nitrates in moderate to severe chronic congestive cardiac failure in patients in whom optimal doses of diuretics and cardiac glycosides have proved insufficient.

4.2 Posology and method of administration

See "Precautions" before use.

Adults:

Hypertension: the dose should be adjusted to the individual requirements of the patient. Treatment should begin with low doses of Apresoline which, depending on the patient's response should be increased stepwise to achieve optimal therapeutic effect whilst keeping unwanted effects to a minimum.

Initially 25 mg bid. This can be increased gradually to a dose not exceeding 200 mg daily. The dose should not be increased beyond 100 mg daily without first checking the patient's acetylator status.

Chronic congestive heart failure: Treatment with Apresoline Tablets should always be initiated in hospital, where the patient's individual haemodynamic values can be reliably determined with the help of invasive monitoring. It should then be continued in hospital until the patient has become stabilised on the requisite maintenance dose. Doses vary greatly between individual patients and are generally higher than those used for treating hypertension. After progressive titration (initially 25 mg tid or qid increasing every second day) the maintenance dosage averages 50-75 mg qid.

Children:

Not recommended

Elderly:

Clinical evidence would indicate that no special dosage regime is necessary. Advancing age does not affect either blood concentration or systemic clearance. Renal elimination may however be affected in so far as kidney function diminishes with age.

4.3 Contraindications

Known hypersensitivity to hydralazine or dihydralazine.

Idiopathic systemic lupus erythematosus (SLE) and related diseases.

Severe tachycardia and heart failure with a high cardiac output (e.g. in thyrotoxicosis).

Myocardial insufficiency due to mechanical obstruction (e.g. in the presence of aortic or mitral stenosis or constrictive pericarditis).

Isolated right ventricular failure due to pulmonary hypertension.

4.4 Special warnings and special precautions for use

Warnings

The overall 'hyperdynamic' state of the circulation induced by hydralazine may accentuate certain clinical conditions. Myocardial stimulation may provoke or aggravate angina pectoris. Patients with suspected or confirmed coronary artery disease should therefore be given Apresoline Tablets only under cover of beta-blocker or in combination with other suitable sympatholytic agents. It is important that the beta-blocker medication should be commenced a few days before the start of treatment with Apresoline Tablets.

Patients who have survived a myocardial infarction should not receive Apresoline Tablets until a post-infarction stabilisation *state* has been achieved.

Prolonged treatment with hydralazine (i.e. usually for more than 6 months) may provoke a lupus erythematosus (LE) like syndrome, especially where doses exceed 100 mg daily. First symptoms are likely to be arthralgia, sometimes associated with fever and rash and are reversible after withdrawal of the drug. In its more severe form it resembles acute SLE, and in rare cases renal and ocular involvement have been reported. Long term treatment with corticosteroids may be required to reverse these changes. Since such reactions tend to occur more frequently the higher the dose and the longer its duration, and since they are also more common in slow acetylators, it is recommended that for maintenance therapy the lowest effective dose should be used. If 100 mg daily fails to elicit an adequate clinical effect, the patient's acetylator status should be evaluated. Slow acetylators and women run greater risk of developing the LE like syndrome and every effort should therefore be made to keep the dosage below 100 mg daily and a careful watch kept for signs and symptoms suggestive of this syndrome. If such symptoms do develop the drug should be gradually withdrawn.

Rapid acetylators often respond inadequately even to doses of 100 mg daily and therefore the dose can be raised with only a slightly increased risk of an LE like syndrome.

During long term treatment with Apresoline Tablets it is advisable to determine the antinuclear factors and conduct urine analysis at intervals of approximately 6 months. Microhaematuria and / or proteinuria, in particular together with positive titres of ANF, may be initial signs of immune-complex glomerulonephritis associated with the SLE like syndrome. If overt clinical signs or symptoms develop, the drug should be withdrawn immediately.

Skin rash, febrile reactions and change in blood count occur rarely and drug should be withdrawn. Peripheral neuritis in the form of paraesthesia has been reported, and may respond to pyridoxine administration or drug withdrawal.

Precautions

In patients with renal impairment (creatinine clearance < 30 ml/min or serum creatinine concentrations > 2.5 mg / 100 ml or 221 μmol/l) and in patients with hepatic dysfunction the dose or interval between doses should be adjusted according to clinical response, in order to avoid accumulation of the 'apparent' active substance.

Apresoline Tablets should be used with caution in patients with coronary artery disease (since it may increase angina) or cerebrovascular disease.

When undergoing surgery, patients treated with Apresoline Tablets may show a fall in blood pressure, in which case one should not use adrenaline to correct the hypotension, since it enhances the cardiac-accelerating effects of hydralazine.

When initiating therapy in heart failure, particular caution should be exercised and the patient kept under surveillance and/or haemodynamic monitoring for early detection of postural hypotension or tachycardia. Where discontinuation of therapy in heart failure is indicated, Apresoline Tablets should be withdrawn gradually (except in serious situations, such as SLE-like syndrome or blood dyscrasias) in order to avoid precipitation and/or exacerbation of heart failure.

4.5 Interaction with other medicinal products and other forms of Interaction

Potentiation of effects: Concurrent therapy with other antihypertensives (vasodilators, calcium antagonists, ACE inhibitors, diuretics), anaesthetics, tricyclic antidepressants, major tranquillisers or drugs exerting central depressant actions (including alcohol).

Administration of Apresoline Tablets shortly before or after diazoxide may give rise to marked hypotension.

MAO inhibitors should be used with caution in patients receiving Apresoline Tablets.

Concurrent administration of Apresoline Tablets with beta-blockers subject to a strong first pass effect (e.g. propranolol) may increase their bioavailability. Downward adjustment of these drugs may be required when they are given concomitantly with Apresoline Tablets.

4.6 Pregnancy and lactation

Use of Apresoline Tablets in pregnancy, before the third trimester should be avoided but the drug may be employed in later pregnancy if there is no safer alternative or when the disease itself carries serious risks for the mother or child e.g. pre-eclampsia and /or eclampsia.

No serious adverse effects in human pregnancy have been reported to date with Apresoline, although experience in the third trimester is extensive.

Hydralazine passes into breast milk but reports available so far have not shown adverse effects on the infant. Mothers in whom use of Apresoline Tablets is unavoidable may breast feed their infant provided that the infant is observed for possible adverse effects.

4.7 Effects on ability to drive and use machines

Apresoline may impair the patient's reactions especially at the start of the treatment. The patient should be warned of the hazard when driving or operating machinery.

4.8 Undesirable effects

Some of the adverse effects listed below e.g. tachycardia, palpitation, angina symptoms, flushing, headache, dizziness, nasal congestion and gastro-intestinal disturbances are commonly seen at the start of treatment, especially if the dose is raised quickly. However such effects generally subside in the further course of treatment.

(The following frequency estimates are used: frequent > 10 %, occasional 1-10%, rare 0.001-1%, isolated cases < 0.001%)

Cardiovascular system:

Frequently: tachycardia, palpitation.

Occasionally: flushing, hypotension, anginal symptoms.

Rarely: oedema, heart failure.

Isolated cases: paradoxical pressor responses.

Central and peripheral nervous system:

Frequently: headache.

Rarely: dizziness.

Isolated cases: peripheral neuritis, polyneuritis, paraesthesiae (these unwanted effects may be reversed by administering pyridoxine).

Musculo-skeletal system:

Occasionally: arthralgia, joint swelling, myalgia.

Skin and appendages:

Rarely: rash.

Urogenital system:

Rarely: proteinuria, increased plasma creatinine, haematuria sometimes in association with glomerulonephritis.

Isolated cases: acute renal failure, urinary retention.

Gastro-intestinal tract:

Occasionally: gastro-intestinal disturbances, diarrhoea, nausea, vomiting.

Rarely: jaundice, liver enlargement, abnormal liver function sometimes in association with hepatitis.

Isolated cases: paralytic ileus.

Blood:

Rarely: anaemia, leucopenia, neutropenia, thrombocytopenia with or without purpura.

Isolated cases: haemolytic anaemia, leucocytosis, lymphadenopathy, pancytopenia, splenomegaly, agranulocytosis.

Psyche:

Rarely: agitation, anorexia, anxiety.

Isolated cases: depression, hallucinations.

Sense organs:

Rarely: increased lacrimation, conjunctivitis, nasal congestion.

Hypersensitivity reactions:

Occasionally: SLE-like syndrome (see under 'Warnings').

Rarely: hypersensitivity reactions such as pruritus, urticaria, vasculitis, eosinophilia, hepatitis.

Respiratory tract:

Rarely: dyspnoea, pleural pain.

Miscellaneous:

Rarely: fever, weight decrease, malaise.

Isolated cases: exophthalmos.

4.9 Overdose

Signs and symptoms

Symptoms include hypotension, tachycardia, myocardial ischaemia dysrhythmias and coma.

Treatment

Gastric lavage should be instituted as soon as possible. Supportive measures including intravenous fluids are also indicated. If hypotension is present, an attempt should be made to raise the blood pressure without increasing the tachycardia.

5. PHARMACOLOGICAL PROPERTIES

5.1 Pharmacodynamic properties

Pharmacotherapeutic group

Hydralazine is a peripheral vasodilator.

Mechanism of action

Hydralazine is a direct acting vasodilator which exerts its effects principally on the arterioles. Its precise mode of action is not known. Administration of hydralazine produces a fall in peripheral resistance and a decrease in arterial blood pressure, effects which induce reflex sympathetic cardiovascular responses. The concomitant use of a beta-blocker will reduce these reflex effects and enhance the anti-hypertensive effect. The use of hydralazine can result in sodium and fluid retention, producing oedema and reduced urinary volume. These effects can be prevented by concomitant administration of a diuretic.

5.2 Pharmacokinetic properties

Absorption

Orally administered hydralazine is rapidly and completely absorbed but is subject to a dose dependent first pass effect (systemic bioavailability: 26-55%) which is dependent upon the individual's acetylator status. Peak plasma concentrations are attained after 0.5 to 1.5 hours.

Distribution

Hydralazine is rapidly distributed in the body and displays a particular affinity for the blood vessel walls. Plasma protein binding is of the order of 90%. Within 24 hours after an oral dose, the quantity recovered in the urine averages 80% of the dose.

Biotransformation

Nil.

Elimination

Hydralazine appears in the plasma chiefly in the form of a readily hydrolysable conjugate with pyruvic acid. Plasma half-life averages 2-3 hours but is prolonged up to 16 hours in severe renal failure (creatinine clearance less than 20 ml/min) and shortened to approximately 45 minutes in rapid acetylators.

The bulk of the dose is excreted as acetylated and hydroxylated metabolites, some of which are conjugated with glucuronic acid.

Characteristics in patients

None relevant.

5.3 Preclinical safety data

Hydralazine has been found to be teratogenic in mice producing a small incidence of cleft palate and certain other bony malformations, in oral doses ranging from 20-120 mg / kg i.e. 20-30 times the maximum human daily dose. It was not teratogenic in rats or rabbits.

In high (cyto-) toxic concentrations, hydralazine induces gene mutations in single cell organisms and in mammalian cells in vitro. No unequivocally mutagenic effects have been detected in vivo in a great number of test systems.

Hydralazine in lifetime carcinogenicity studies, caused, towards the end of the experiments, small but statistically significant increases in lung tumours in mice and in hepatic and testicular tumours in rats. These tumours also occur spontaneously with fairly high frequency in aged rodents.

With due consideration of these animals and in-vitro toxicological findings, hydralazine in therapeutic doses does not appear to bear risk that would necessitate a limitation of its administration. Many years of clinical experience have not suggested that human cancer is associated with hydralazine use.

6. PHARMACEUTICAL PARTICULARS

6.1 List of excipients

Sugar-coated tablets of 25 mg contain silicon dioxide, microcrystalline cellulose, magnesium stearate, polyvinylpyrrolidone, wheat starch, hydroxypropylmethylcellulose, povidone, talc, titanium dioxide, polyethylene glycol, sucrose, yellow iron oxide and water.

6.2 Incompatibilities

None.

6.3 Shelf life

4 years.

6.4 Special precautions for storage

Protect from moisture and heat. Store below 30°C.

6.5 Nature and contents of container

Securitainers of 84.

6.6 Instructions for use and handling

None.

7. MARKETING AUTHORISATION HOLDER

Amdipharm plc
Regency House
Miles Gray Road
Basildon
Essex
SS14 3AF
U.K.

8. MARKETING AUTHORISATION NUMBER(S)

PL 20072/0026

9. DATE OF FIRST AUTHORISATION/RENEWAL OF THE AUTHORISATION

30 March 2005

10. DATE OF REVISION OF THE TEXT
March 2005

Aprinox 2.5 and 5mg Tablets
(Sovereign Medical)

1. NAME OF THE MEDICINAL PRODUCT
Aprinox Tablets 2.5 mg

Aprinox Tablets 5 mg

2. QUALITATIVE AND QUANTITATIVE COMPOSITION
Each Aprinox Tablet 2.5 mg contains bendroflumethiazide 2.5 mg

Each Aprinox Tablet 5 mg contains bendroflumethiazide 5 mg

For excipients, see section 6.1

3. PHARMACEUTICAL FORM
White tablets

4. CLINICAL PARTICULARS
4.1 Therapeutic indications
For the treatment of oedema and hypertension. Aprinox may also be used to suppress lactation.

4.2 Posology and method of administration
For oral administration.

Adults:
Oedema
Initially, 5-10 mg in the morning, daily or on alternate days; maintenance dose 5-10 mg one to three times weekly.

Hypertension
The usual dose is 2.5 mg taken in the morning. Higher doses are rarely necessary.

Suppression of lactation
5 mg in the morning and 5 mg at midday for about five days.

Children: Dosage in children may be up to 400 mcg/kg bodyweight initially, reducing to 50-100 mcg/kg bodyweight daily for maintenance.

Elderly: The dosage of thiazide diuretics may need to be reduced in the elderly, particularly when renal function is impaired, because of the possibility of electrolyte imbalance.

4.3 Contraindications
Aprinox is contra-indicated in patients with known hypersensitivity to thiazides; refractory hypokalaemia, hyponatraemia, hypercalcaemia; severe renal and hepatic impairment; symptomatic hyperuricaemia and Addison's disease.

4.4 Special warnings and special precautions for use
Bendroflumethiazide should be used with caution in patients with mild to moderate hepatic or renal impairment (avoid if severe). Renal function should be continuously monitored during thiazide therapy. Thiazide diuretics may exacerbate or activate systemic lupus erythematosus in susceptible patients.

All thiazide diuretics can produce a degree of electrolyte imbalance, especially in patients with renal or hepatic impairment or when dosage is high or prolonged. Serum electrolytes should be checked for abnormalities, particularly hypokalaemia, and the latter corrected by the addition of a potassium supplement to the regimen. Aggravates diabetes and gout; increased risk of hypomagnesaemia in alcoholic cirrhosis.

4.5 Interaction with other medicinal products and other forms of Interaction
Sensitivity to digitalis glycosides may be increased by the hypokalaemic effect of concurrent bendroflumethiazide. Patients should be observed for signs of digitalis intoxication, in particular arrhythmias, and if these appear, the dosage of the digitalis glycoside should be temporarily reduced and a potassium supplement given to restore stability.

Serum lithium concentrations may be increased by concurrent use of thiazide diuretics.

Non-steroidal anti-inflammatory agents may blunt the diuretic and antihypertensive effects of thiazide diuretics. Diuretics may increase the risk of nephrotoxicity of NSAIDs

ACTH, corticosteroids, acetazolamide and carbenoxolone may exacerbate the hypokalaemia associated with thiazide use. Thiazide diuretics may enhance the neuromuscular blocking effects of the non-depolarising muscle relaxants, e.g. tubocurarine.

Thiazides may enhance the effects of antihypertensive agents, while postural hypotension associated with therapy may be enhanced by concomitant ingestion of alcohol, barbiturates or opioids.

Concomitant use of carbamazepine may increase the risk of hyponatraemia.

There is an increased risk of hyponatraemia if thiazides are given with amphotericin.

The risk of hypercalcaemia is increased by the concomitant intake of calcium salts or vitamin D preparations.

Concomitant use with cisplatin can lead to an increased risk of nephrotoxicity and ototoxicity.

The cardiac toxicity of disopyramide, amiodarone, flecainide and quinidine is increased if hypokalaemia occurs. The action of lidocaine and mexiletine is antagonised by hypokalaemia.

There is an increased risk of hyponatraemia when thiazides are used concomitantly with aminoglutethimide. Thiazides can cause an increased risk of hypercalcaemia with toremifene.

Colestipol and colestyramine may reduce the absorption of thiazide diuretics and should therefore be given 2 hours prior to, or after the ingestion of bendroflumethiazide.

Calcium-channel blockers and moxisylyte can cause an enhanced hypotensive effect.

There is an increased risk of postural hypotension with tricyclic antidepressants. There may also be an increased risk of hypokalaemia if thiazides are given with reboxetine. Concomitant use with monoamine oxidase inhibitors (MAOIs), baclofen or tizanidine may also give an increased hypotensive effect.

Oestrogens and combined oral contraceptives may antagonise the diuretic effect of thiazides.

There is an increased risk of first-dose hypotensive effect of post-synaptic alpha-blockers such as prazosin.

Hypokalaemia increases the risk of ventricular arrhythmias with pimozide or thioridazine, therefore, concomitant use should be avoided. Hypokalaemia or other electrolyte imbalance also increases the risk of ventricular arrhythmias with terfenadine.

Bendroflumethiazide may interfere with a number of laboratory tests, including estimation of serum protein-bound iodine and tests of parathyroid function.

4.6 Pregnancy and lactation
Diuretics are best avoided for the management of oedema of pregnancy or hypertension in pregnancy as their use may be associated with hypokalaemia, increased blood viscosity and reduced placental perfusion.

There is inadequate evidence of safety in human pregnancy and foetal bone marrow depression and thrombocytopenia have been described. Foetal and neonatal jaundice have also been described.

As diuretics pass into breast milk and bendroflumethiazide can suppress lactation, its use should be avoided in mothers who wish to breast feed.

4.7 Effects on ability to drive and use machines
No adverse effects known.

4.8 Undesirable effects
All thiazide diuretics can produce a degree of electrolyte imbalance, e.g. hypokalaemia.

Thiazide diuretics may raise the serum uric acid levels with subsequent exacerbation of gout in susceptible subjects.

Thiazide diuretics sometimes lower carbohydrate tolerance and the insulin dosage of the diabetic patient may require adjustment. Care is necessary when bendroflumethiazide is administered to those with a known predisposition to diabetes.

Postural hypotension and mild gastro-intestinal effects; hypokalaemia, hypomagnesaemia, hyponatraemia, hypercalcaemia, hypochloraemic alkalosis, hyperuricaemia, gout, hyperglycaemia, and altered plasma lipid concentration.

Less commonly, rashes, photosensitivity; blood disorders (including neutropenia and thrombocytopenia – when given in late pregnancy neonatal thrombocytopenia has been reported); pancreatitis, intrahepatic cholestasis, and hypersensitivity reactions (including pneumonitis, pulmonary oedema, severe skin reactions) also reported.

Rarely, blood dyscrasias, including agranulocytosis, aplastic anaemia, thrombocytopenia and leucopenia, and pancreatitis have been reported with long term therapy. Skin rashes and impotence (reversible on withdrawal of treatment) have occasionally been reported.

4.9 Overdose
Symptoms of overdosage include anorexia, nausea, vomiting, diarrhoea, diuresis, dehydration, hypotension, dizziness, weakness, muscle cramps, paraesthesia, tetany, gastrointestinal bleeding, hyponatraemia, hypo- or hyperglycaemia, hypokalaemia and metabolic alkalosis. Initial treatment consists of either emesis or gastric lavage, if appropriate. Otherwise treatment should be symptomatic and supportive including the correction of fluid and electrolyte imbalance.

Blood pressure should also be monitored.

There is no specific antidote.

5. PHARMACOLOGICAL PROPERTIES
5.1 Pharmacodynamic properties
Bendroflumethiazide is a thiazide diuretic which reduces the absorption of electrolytes from the renal tubules, thereby increasing the excretion of sodium and chloride ions, and consequently of water. The excretion of other electrolytes, notably potassium and magnesium, is also increased. The excretion of calcium is reduced. Thiazides also reduce carbonic anhydrase activity so that bicarbonate excretion is increased, but this effect is generally small and does not appreciably alter the acid base balance or the pH of the urine. Thiazides also have a hypotensive effect, due to a reduction in peripheral resistance and enhance the effects of other antihypertensive agents.

5.2 Pharmacokinetic properties
Bendroflumethiazide is completely absorbed from the gastrointestinal tract and it is fairly extensively metabolised. About 30% is excreted unchanged in the urine. The onset of diuretic action of the thiazides following oral administration occurs within two hours and the peak effect between three and six hours after administration. The duration of the diuretic action of bendroflumethiazide is between 18 and 24 hours. The onset of the hypotensive action is generally three or four days.

5.3 Preclinical safety data
Not applicable

6. PHARMACEUTICAL PARTICULARS
6.1 List of excipients
Lactose

Maize Starch

Stearic acid

French chalk for tablets.

6.2 Incompatibilities
Not applicable.

6.3 Shelf life
36 months

6.4 Special precautions for storage
None

6.5 Nature and contents of container
Amber glass bottle having a tin-plate cap with a waxed aluminium-faced pulpboard liner.

Pack size: 100 and 500 tablets.

PVC/Al blister pack

Pack size: 28 Tablets

6.6 Instructions for use and handling
None

7. MARKETING AUTHORISATION HOLDER
Waymade PLC Trading as Sovereign Medical

Sovereign House

Miles Gray Road

Basildon, Essex SS14 3FR

8. MARKETING AUTHORISATION NUMBER(S)
Aprinox Tablets 2.5 mg: PL 06464/0706

Aprinox Tablets 5 mg: PL 06464/0707

9. DATE OF FIRST AUTHORISATION/RENEWAL OF THE AUTHORISATION
11 January 1999

10. DATE OF REVISION OF THE TEXT
November 2004

Aprovel 75 mg, 150 mg and 300 mg Film-Coated Tablet (Bristol-Myers Squibb Pharmaceuticals Ltd)
(Bristol-Myers Squibb Pharmaceuticals Ltd)

1. NAME OF THE MEDICINAL PRODUCT
Aprovel 75 mg film-coated tablets.

Aprovel 150 mg film-coated tablets.

Aprovel 300 mg film-coated tablets.

2. QUALITATIVE AND QUANTITATIVE COMPOSITION
Each film-coated tablet contains 75 mg, 150 mg or 300 mg irbesartan.

For excipients, see 6.1.

3. PHARMACEUTICAL FORM
Film-coated tablet.

White to off-white, biconvex, and oval-shaped with a heart debossed on one side. The other side is engraved with the number 2871 on the 75 mg tablet, 2872 on the 150 mg tablet and 2873 on the 300 mg tablet.

4. CLINICAL PARTICULARS
4.1 Therapeutic indications
Treatment of essential hypertension.

Treatment of renal disease in patients with hypertension and type 2 diabetes mellitus as part of an antihypertensive drug regimen (see 5.1).

4.2 Posology and method of administration
The usual recommended initial and maintenance dose is 150 mg once daily, with or without food. Aprovel at a dose of 150 mg once daily generally provides a better 24 hour blood pressure control than 75 mg. However, initiation of therapy with 75 mg could be considered, particularly in haemodialysed patients and in the elderly over 75 years.

In patients insufficiently controlled with 150 mg once daily, the dose of Aprovel can be increased to 300 mg, or other anti-hypertensive agents can be added. In particular, the addition of a diuretic such as hydrochlorothiazide has been shown to have an additive effect with Aprovel (see 4.5).

In hypertensive type 2 diabetic patients, therapy should be initiated at 150 mg irbesartan once daily and titrated up to 300 mg once daily as the preferred maintenance dose for treatment of renal disease. The demonstration of renal benefit of Aprovel in hypertensive type 2 diabetic patients is based on studies where irbesartan was used in addition to other antihypertensive agents, as needed, to reach target blood pressure (see 5.1).

Renal impairment: No dosage adjustment is necessary in patients with impaired renal function. A lower starting dose (75 mg) should be considered for patients undergoing haemodialysis.

Intravascular volume depletion: Volume and/or sodium depletion should be corrected prior to administration of Aprovel.

Hepatic impairment: No dosage adjustment is necessary in patients with mild to moderate hepatic impairment. There is no clinical experience in patients with severe hepatic impairment.

Elderly patients: Although consideration should be given to initiating therapy with 75 mg in patients over 75 years of age, dosage adjustment is not usually necessary for the elderly.

Children: Safety and efficacy of Aprovel have not been established in children.

4.3 Contraindications

Hypersensitivity to any component of the product (see 6.1).

Second and third trimester of pregnancy (see 4.6).

Lactation (see 4.6).

4.4 Special warnings and special precautions for use

Intravascular volume depletion: Symptomatic hypotension, especially after the first dose, may occur in patients who are volume and/or sodium depleted by vigorous diuretic therapy, dietary salt restriction, diarrhoea or vomiting. Such conditions should be corrected before the administration of Aprovel.

Renovascular hypertension: There is an increased risk of severe hypotension and renal insufficiency when patients with bilateral renal artery stenosis or stenosis of the artery to a single functioning kidney are treated with drugs that affect the renin-angiotensin-aldosterone system. While this is not documented with Aprovel, a similar effect should be anticipated with angiotensin-II receptor antagonists.

Renal impairment and kidney transplantation: When Aprovel is used in patients with impaired renal function, a periodic monitoring of potassium and creatinine serum levels is recommended. There is no experience regarding the administration of Aprovel in patients with a recent kidney transplantation.

Hypertensive patients with type 2 diabetes and renal disease: The effects of irbesartan both on renal and cardiovascular events were not uniform across all subgroups, in an analysis carried out in the study with patients with advanced renal disease. In particular, they appeared less favourable in women and non-white subjects (see 5.1).

Hyperkalaemia: As with other drugs that affect the renin-angiotensin-aldosterone system, hyperkalaemia may occur during the treatment with Aprovel, especially in the presence of renal impairment, overt proteinuria due to diabetic renal disease and/or heart failure. Close monitoring of serum potassium in patients at risk is recommended (see 4.5).

Lithium The combination of lithium and Aprovel is not recommended (see 4. 5).

Aortic and mitral valve stenosis, obstructive hypertrophic cardiomyopathy: As with other vasodilators, special caution is indicated in patients suffering from aortic or mitral stenosis, or obstructive hypertrophic cardiomyopathy.

Primary aldosteronism: Patients with primary aldosteronism generally will not respond to anti-hypertensive drugs acting through inhibition of the renin-angiotensin system. Therefore, the use of Aprovel is not recommended.

General: In patients whose vascular tone and renal function depend predominantly on the activity of the renin-angiotensin-aldosterone system (e.g. patients with severe congestive heart failure or underlying renal disease, including renal artery stenosis), treatment with angiotensin converting enzyme inhibitors or angiotensin-II receptor antagonists that affect this system has been associated with acute hypotension, azotaemia, oliguria, or rarely, acute renal failure. As with any anti-hypertensive agent, excessive blood pressure decrease in patients with ischaemic cardiopathy or ischaemic cardiovascular disease could result in a myocardial infarction or stroke.

As observed for angiotensin converting enzyme inhibitors, irbesartan and the other angiotensin antagonists are apparently less effective in lowering blood pressure in black people than in non-blacks, possibly because of higher prevalence of low-renin states in the black hypertensive population (see 5.1).

4.5 Interaction with other medicinal products and other forms of Interaction

Diuretics and other antihypertensive agents: Other antihypertensive agents may increase the hypotensive effects of irbesartan; however Aprovel has been safely administered with other antihypertensive agents, such as beta-blockers, long-acting calcium channel blockers, and thiazide diuretics. Prior treatment with high dose diuretics may result in volume depletion and a risk of hypotension when initiating therapy with Aprovel (see 4.4).

Potassium supplements and potassium-sparing diuretics: Based on experience with the use of other drugs that affect the renin-angiotensin system, concomitant use of potassium-sparing diuretics, potassium supplements, salt substitutes containing potassium or other drugs that may increase serum potassium levels (e.g. heparin) may lead to increases in serum potassium and is, therefore, not recommended (see 4.4).

Lithium: Reversible increases in serum lithium concentrations and toxicity have been reported during concomitant administration of lithium with angiotensin converting enzyme inhibitors. Similar effects have been very rarely reported with irbesartan. Therefore, this combination is not recommended (see 4.4). If the combination proves necessary, careful monitoring of serum lithium levels is recommended.

Non-steroidal anti-inflammatory drugs: When angiotensin II antagonists are administered simultaneously with non-steroidal anti-inflammatory drugs (i.e. selective COX-2 inhibitors, acetylsalicylic acid >3 g/day) and non-selective NSAIDs), attenuation of the antihypertensive effect may occur.

As with ACE inhibitors, concomitant use of angiotensin II antagonists and NSAIDs may lead to an increased risk of worsening of renal function, including possible acute renal failure, and an increase in serum potassium, especially in patients with poor pre-existing renal function. The combination should be administered with caution, especially in the elderly. Patients should be adequately hydrated and consideration should be given to monitoring renal function after initiation of concomitant therapy, and periodically thereafter.

Additional information on irbesartan interactions: In clinical studies, the pharmacokinetics of irbesartan are not affected by hydrochlorothiazide. Irbesartan is mainly metabolised by CYP2C9 and to a lesser extent by glucuronidation. No significant pharmacokinetic or pharmacodynamic interactions were observed when irbesartan was co-administered with warfarin, a drug metabolised by CYP2C9. The effects of CYP2C9 inducers such as rifampicin on the pharmacokinetics of irbesartan have not been evaluated. The pharmacokinetics of digoxin were not altered by coadministration of irbesartan.

4.6 Pregnancy and lactation

Pregnancy: see 4.3.

As a precautionary measure, irbesartan should preferably not be used during the first trimester of pregnancy. A switch to a suitable alternative treatment should be carried out in advance of a planned pregnancy. In the second and third trimesters, substances that act directly on the renin-angiotensin-system can cause foetal or neonatal renal failure, foetal skull hypoplasia and even foetal death. Therefore, irbesartan is contraindicated in the second and third trimesters of pregnancy. If pregnancy is diagnosed, irbesartan should be discontinued as soon as possible. Skull and renal function should be checked with echography if, inadvertently, the treatment was taken for a long period.

Lactation: Aprovel is contraindicated during lactation. It is not known whether irbesartan is excreted in human milk. Irbesartan is excreted in the milk of lactating rats (see 4.3).

4.7 Effects on ability to drive and use machines

The effect of irbesartan on ability to drive and use machines has not been studied, but, based on its pharmacodynamic properties, irbesartan is unlikely to affect this ability. When driving vehicles or operating machines, it should be taken into account that occasionally dizziness or weariness may occur during treatment.

4.8 Undesirable effects

The frequency of adverse reactions listed below is defined using the following convention: very common (≥1/10); common (≥1/100, <1/10); uncommon (≥1/1,000, <1/100); rare (≥1/10,000, <1/1,000); very rare (<1/10,000).

Hypertension: In placebo-controlled trials in patients with hypertension, the overall incidence of adverse events did not differ between the irbesartan (56.2%) and the placebo groups (56.5%). Discontinuation due to any clinical or laboratory adverse event was less frequent for irbesartan-treated patients (3.3%) than for placebo-treated patients (4.5%). The incidence of adverse events was not related to dose (in the recommended dose range), gender, age, race, or duration of treatment.

In placebo-controlled trials in which 1965 patients received irbesartan, the following adverse drug reactions were reported:

Nervous system disorders:

Common: dizziness

Cardiac disorders:

Uncommon: tachycardia

Vascular disorders:

Uncommon: flushing

Respiratory, thoracic and mediastinal disorders:

Uncommon: cough

Gastrointestinal disorders:

Common: nausea/vomiting

Uncommon: diarrhoea, dyspepsia/heartburn

Reproductive system and breast disorders:

Uncommon: sexual dysfunction

General disorders and administration site conditions:

Common: fatigue

Uncommon: chest pain

Investigations:

Common: significant increases in plasma creatinine kinase were commonly observed (1.7%) in irbesartan treated subjects. None of these increases was associated with identifiable clinical musculoskeletal events.

Hypertension and type 2 diabetes with renal disease: In addition to the adverse drug reactions mentioned under hypertension, in diabetic hypertensive patients with microalbuminuria and normal renal function, orthostatic dizziness and orthostatic hypotension were reported in 0.5% of the patients (i.e., uncommon) but in excess of placebo.

In diabetic hypertensive patients with chronic renal insufficiency and overt proteinuria, the following additional adverse reactions were reported in >2% of patients and in excess of placebo:

Nervous system disorders:

Common: Orthostatic dizziness

Vascular disorders:

Common: Orthostatic hypotension

Musculoskeletal, connective tissue and bone disorders:

Common: Musculoskeletal pain

Investigations:

Hyperkalaemia occurred more often in diabetic patients treated with irbesartan than with placebo. In diabetic hypertensive patients with microalbuminuria and normal renal function, hyperkalaemia (≥5.5 mEq/l) occurred in 29.4% (i.e. very common) of the patients in the irbesartan 300 mg group and 22% of the patients in the placebo group. In diabetic hypertensive patients with chronic renal insufficiency and overt proteinuria, hyperkalaemia (≥5.5 mEq/l) occurred in 46.3% (i.e. very common) of the patients in the irbesartan group and 26.3% of the patients in the placebo group. A decrease in haemoglobin, which was not clinically significant, has been observed in 1.7% (i.e. common) of hypertensive patients with advanced diabetic renal disease treated with irbesartan.

In addition, since introduction of irbesartan in the market, the following adverse drug reactions have also been reported:

Immune system disorders:

Rare: as with other angiotensin-II receptor antagonists, rare cases of hypersensitivity reactions such as rash, urticaria, angioedema have been reported

Metabolism and nutrition disorders:

Very rare: hyperkalaemia

Nervous system disorders:

Very rare: headache

Ear and labyrinth disorders:

Very rare: tinnitus

Gastrointestinal disorders:

Very rare: dysgeusia

Hepato-biliary disorders:

Very rare: abnormal liver function, hepatitis

Musculoskeletal, connective tissue and bone disorders:

Very rare: myalgia, arthralgia

Renal and urinary disorders:

Very rare: impaired renal function including isolated cases of renal failure in patients at risk (see 4.4)

4.9 Overdose

Experience in adults exposed to doses of up to 900 mg/day for 8 weeks revealed no toxicity. The most likely manifestations of overdosage are expected to be hypotension and tachycardia; bradycardia might also occur from overdose. No specific information is available on the treatment of overdosage with Aprovel. The patient should be closely monitored, and the treatment should be symptomatic and supportive. Suggested measures include induction of emesis and/or gastric lavage. Activated charcoal may be useful in the treatment of overdosage. Irbesartan is not removed by haemodialysis.

5. PHARMACOLOGICAL PROPERTIES

5.1 Pharmacodynamic properties

Pharmacotherapeutic group: Angiotensin-II antagonists, ATC code C09C A04.

Irbesartan is a potent, orally active, selective angiotensin-II receptor (type AT_1) antagonist.

Mechanism of Action: It is expected to block all actions of angiotensin-II mediated by the AT_1 receptor, regardless of the source or route of synthesis of angiotensin-II. The selective antagonism of the angiotensin-II (AT_1) receptors results in increases in plasma renin levels and angiotensin-II levels, and a decrease in plasma aldosterone concentration. Serum potassium levels are not significantly affected by irbesartan alone at the recommended doses. Irbesartan does not inhibit ACE (kininase-II), an enzyme which generates angiotensin-II and also degrades bradykinin into inactive metabolites. Irbesartan does not require metabolic activation for its activity.

Clinical efficacy:

Hypertension

Irbesartan lowers blood pressure with minimal change in heart rate. The decrease in blood pressure is dose-related for once a day doses with a tendency towards plateau at doses above 300 mg. Doses of 150-300 mg once daily lower supine or seated blood pressures at trough (i.e. 24 hours after dosing) by an average of 8-13/5-8 mm Hg (systolic/diastolic) greater than those associated with placebo.

Peak reduction of blood pressure is achieved within 3-6 hours after administration and the blood pressure lowering effect is maintained for at least 24 hours. At 24 hours the reduction of blood pressure was 60-70% of the corresponding peak diastolic and systolic responses at the recommended doses. Once daily dosing with 150 mg produced trough and mean 24 hour responses similar to twice daily dosing on the same total dose.

The blood pressure lowering effect of Aprovel is evident within 1-2 weeks, with the maximal effect occurring by 4-6 weeks after start of therapy. The antihypertensive effects are maintained during long term therapy. After withdrawal of therapy, blood pressure gradually returns toward baseline. Rebound hypertension has not been observed.

The blood pressure lowering effects of irbesartan and thiazide-type diuretics are additive. In patients not adequately controlled by irbesartan alone, the addition of a low dose of hydrochlorothiazide (12.5 mg) to irbesartan once daily results in a further placebo-adjusted blood pressure reduction at trough of 7-10/3-6 mm Hg (systolic/diastolic).

The efficacy of Aprovel is not influenced by age or gender. As is the case with other drugs that affect the renin-angiotensin system, black hypertensive patients have notably less response to irbesartan monotherapy. When irbesartan is administered concomitantly with a low dose of hydrochlorothiazide (e.g. 12.5 mg daily), the antihypertensive response in black patients approaches that of white patients.

There is no clinically important effect on serum uric acid or urinary uric acid secretion.

Hypertension and type 2 diabetes with renal disease

The "Irbesartan Diabetic Nephropathy Trial (IDNT)" shows that irbesartan decreases the progression of renal disease in patients with chronic renal insufficiency and overt proteinuria. IDNT was a double blind, controlled, morbidity and mortality trial comparing Aprovel, amlodipine and placebo. In 1715 hypertensive patients with type 2 diabetes, proteinuria ≥900 mg/day and serum creatinine ranging from 1.0-3.0 mg/dl, the long-term effects (mean 2.6 years) of Aprovel on the progression of renal disease and all-cause mortality were examined. Patients were titrated from 75 mg to a maintenance dose of 300 mg Aprovel, from 2.5 mg to 10 mg amlodipine, or placebo as tolerated. Patients in all treatment groups typically received between 2 and 4 antihypertensive agents (e.g. diuretics, beta blockers, alpha blockers) to reach a predefined blood pressure goal of ≤135/85 mmHg or a 10 mmHg reduction in systolic pressure if baseline was > 160 mmHg. Sixty per cent (60%) of patients in the placebo group reached this target blood pressure whereas this figure was 76% and 78% in the irbesartan and amlodipine groups, respectively. Irbesartan significantly reduced the relative risk in the primary combined endpoint of doubling serum creatinine, end-stage renal disease (ESRD) or all-cause mortality. Approximately 33% of patients in the irbesartan group reached the primary renal composite endpoint, compared to 39% and 41% in the placebo and amlodipine groups [20% relative risk reduction versus placebo ($p = 0.024$) and 23% relative risk reduction compared to amlodipine ($p = 0.006$)]. When the individual components of the primary endpoint were analysed, no effect in all cause mortality was observed, while a positive trend in the reduction in ESRD and a significant reduction in doubling of serum creatinine were observed.

Subgroups consisting of gender, race, age, duration of diabetes, baseline blood pressure, serum creatinine and albumin excretion rate were assessed for treatment effect. In the female and black subgroups which represented 32% and 26% of the overall study population, respectively, a renal benefit was not evident, although the confidence intervals do not exclude it. As for the secondary endpoint of fatal and non-fatal cardiovascular events, there was no difference among the three groups in the overall population, although an increased incidence of non-fatal MI was seen for women and a decreased incidence of non-fatal MI was seen in males in the irbesartan group versus the placebo-based regimen. An increased incidence of non-fatal MI and stroke was seen in females in the irbesartan-based regimen versus the amlodipine-based regimen, while hospitalisation due to heart failure was reduced in the overall population. However, no proper explanation for these findings in women has been identified.

The study of the "Effects of Irbesartan on Microalbuminuria in Hypertensive Patients with type 2 Diabetes Mellitus (IRMA 2)" shows that irbesartan 300 mg delays progression to overt proteinuria in patients with microalbuminuria. IRMA 2 was a placebo-controlled double blind morbidity study in 590 patients with type 2 diabetes, microalbuminuria (30-300 mg/day) and normal renal function (serum creatinine ≤1.5 mg/dl in males and < 1.1 mg/dl in females). The study examined the long-term effects (2 years) of Aprovel on the progression to clinical (overt) proteinuria (urinary albumin excretion rate (UAER) > 300 mg/day, and an increase in UAER of at least 30% from baseline). The predefined blood pressure goal was ≤135/85 mmHg. Additional antihypertensive agents (excluding ACE inhibitors, angiotensin-II receptor antagonists and dihydropyridine calcium blockers) were added as needed to help achieve the blood pressure goal. While similar blood pressure was achieved in all treatment groups, fewer subjects in the irbesartan 300 mg group (5.2%) than in the placebo (14.9%) or in the irbesartan 150 mg group (9.7%) reached the endpoint of overt proteinuria, demonstrating a 70% relative risk reduction versus placebo ($p = 0.0004$) for the higher dose. An accompanying improvement in the glomerular filtration rate (GFR) was not observed during the first three months of treatment. The slowing in the progression to clinical proteinuria was evident as early as three months and continued over the 2 year period. Regression to normoalbuminuria (< 30 mg/day) was more frequent in the Aprovel 300 mg group (34%) than in the placebo group (21%).

5.2 Pharmacokinetic properties

After oral administration, irbesartan is well absorbed: studies of absolute bioavailability gave values of approximately 60-80%. Concomitant food intake does not significantly influence the bioavailability of irbesartan.

Plasma protein binding is approximately 96%, with negligible binding to cellular blood components. The volume of distribution is 53-93 litres.

Following oral or intravenous administration of ^{14}C irbesartan, 80-85% of the circulating plasma radioactivity is attributable to unchanged irbesartan. Irbesartan is metabolised by the liver via glucuronide conjugation and oxidation. The major circulating metabolite is irbesartan glucuronide (approximately 6%). *In vitro* studies indicate that irbesartan is primarily oxidised by the cytochrome P450 enzyme *CYP2C9*; isoenzyme *CYP3A4* has negligible effect.

Irbesartan exhibits linear and dose proportional pharmacokinetics over the dose range of 10 to 600 mg. A less than proportional increase in oral absorption at doses beyond 600 mg (twice the maximal recommended dose) was observed; the mechanism for this is unknown. Peak plasma concentrations are attained at 1.5-2 hours after oral administration. The total body and renal clearance are 157-176 and 3-3.5 ml/min, respectively. The terminal elimination half-life of irbesartan is 11-15 hours. Steady-state plasma concentrations are attained within 3 days after initiation of a once-daily dosing regimen. Limited accumulation of irbesartan (< 20%) is observed in plasma upon repeated once-daily dosing. In a study, somewhat higher plasma concentrations of irbesartan were observed in female hypertensive patients. However, there was no difference in the half-life and accumulation of irbesartan. No dosage adjustment is necessary in female patients. Irbesartan AUC and C_{max} values were also somewhat greater in elderly subjects (≥ 65 years) than those of young subjects (18-40 years). However the terminal half-life was not significantly altered. No dosage adjustment is necessary in elderly patients.

Irbesartan and its metabolites are eliminated by both biliary and renal pathways. After either oral or IV administration of ^{14}C irbesartan, about 20% of the radioactivity is recovered in the urine, and the remainder in the faeces. Less than 2% of the dose is excreted in the urine as unchanged irbesartan.

Renal impairment: In patients with renal impairment or those undergoing haemodialysis, the pharmacokinetic parameters of irbesartan are not significantly altered. Irbesartan is not removed by haemodialysis.

Hepatic impairment: In patients with mild to moderate cirrhosis, the pharmacokinetic parameters of irbesartan are not significantly altered.

Studies have not been performed in patients with severe hepatic impairment.

5.3 Preclinical safety data

There was no evidence of abnormal systemic or target organ toxicity at clinically relevant doses. In preclinical safety studies, high doses of irbesartan (≥ 250 mg/kg/day in rats and ≥ 100 mg/kg/day in macaques) caused a reduction of red blood cell parameters (erythrocytes, haemoglobin, haematocrit). At very high doses (≥ 500 mg/kg/day) degenerative changes in the kidney (such as interstitial nephritis, tubular distension, basophilic tubules, increased plasma concentrations of urea and creatinine) were induced by irbesartan in the rat and the macaque and are considered secondary to the hypotensive effects of the drug which led to decreased renal perfusion. Furthermore, irbesartan induced hyperplasia/hypertrophy of the juxtaglomerular cells (in rats at ≥ 90 mg/kg/day, in macaques at ≥ 10 mg/kg/day). All of these changes were considered to be caused by the pharmacological action of irbesartan. For therapeutic doses of irbesartan in humans, the hyperplasia / hypertrophy of the renal juxtaglomerular cells does not appear to have any relevance.

There was no evidence of mutagenicity, clastogenicity or carcinogenicity.

Animal studies with irbesartan showed transient toxic effects (increased renal pelvic cavitation, hydroureter or subcutaneous oedema) in rat foetuses, which were resolved after birth. In rabbits, abortion or early resorption were noted at doses causing significant maternal toxicity, including mortality. No teratogenic effects were observed in the rat or rabbit.

6. PHARMACEUTICAL PARTICULARS

6.1 List of excipients

Tablet core: lactose monohydrate, microcrystalline cellulose, croscarmellose sodium, hypromellose, silicon dioxide, magnesium stearate.

Film-coating: lactose monohydrate, hypromellose, titanium dioxide (E171), macrogol, carnauba wax.

6.2 Incompatibilities

Not applicable.

6.3 Shelf life

3 years.

6.4 Special precautions for storage

Do not store above 30°C. Store in the original package.

6.5 Nature and contents of container

Aprovel film-coated tablets are packaged in blister packs containing 28 tablets in PVC/PVDC/Aluminium strips.

6.6 Instructions for use and handling

No special requirements.

7. MARKETING AUTHORISATION HOLDER

SANOFI PHARMA BRISTOL-MYERS SQUIBB SNC

174 avenue de France

F-75013 Paris - France

8. MARKETING AUTHORISATION NUMBER(S)

Aprovel 75 mg film-coated tablets: EU/1/97/046/17

Aprovel 150 mg film-coated tablets: EU/1/97/046/22

Aprovel 300 mg film-coated tablets: EU/1/97/046/27

9. DATE OF FIRST AUTHORISATION/RENEWAL OF THE AUTHORISATION

02 March 2004

10. DATE OF REVISION OF THE TEXT

02 August 2004

Aprovel Film-Coated Tablets

(sanofi-aventis)

1. NAME OF THE MEDICINAL PRODUCT

Aprovel 75 mg film-coated tablets.

Aprovel 150 mg film-coated tablets.

Aprovel 300 mg film-coated tablets.

2. QUALITATIVE AND QUANTITATIVE COMPOSITION

Each film-coated tablet contains 75 mg, 150 mg or 300 mg irbesartan.

For excipients, see 6.1.

3. PHARMACEUTICAL FORM

Film-coated tablet.

White to off-white, biconvex, and oval-shaped with a heart debossed on one side. The other side is engraved with the number 2871 on the 75 mg tablet, 2872 on the 150 mg tablet and 2873 on the 300 mg tablet.

4. CLINICAL PARTICULARS

4.1 Therapeutic indications

Treatment of essential hypertension.

Treatment of renal disease in patients with hypertension and type 2 diabetes mellitus as part of an antihypertensive drug regimen (see 5.1).

4.2 Posology and method of administration

The usual recommended initial and maintenance dose is 150 mg once daily, with or without food. Aprovel at a dose of 150 mg once daily generally provides a better 24 hour blood pressure control than 75 mg. However, initiation of therapy with 75 mg could be considered, particularly in haemodialysed patients and in the elderly over 75 years.

In patients insufficiently controlled with 150 mg once daily, the dose of Aprovel can be increased to 300 mg, or other anti-hypertensive agents can be added. In particular, the addition of a diuretic such as hydrochlorothiazide has been shown to have an additive effect with Aprovel (see 4.5).

In hypertensive type 2 diabetic patients, therapy should be initiated at 150 mg irbesartan once daily and titrated up to

300 mg once daily as the preferred maintenance dose for treatment of renal disease. The demonstration of renal benefit of Aprovel in hypertensive type 2 diabetic patients is based on studies where irbesartan was used in addition to other antihypertensive agents, as needed, to reach target blood pressure (see 5.1).

Renal impairment: No dosage adjustment is necessary in patients with impaired renal function. A lower starting dose (75 mg) should be considered for patients undergoing haemodialysis.

Intravascular volume depletion: Volume and/or sodium depletion should be corrected prior to administration of Aprovel.

Hepatic impairment: No dosage adjustment is necessary in patients with mild to moderate hepatic impairment. There is no clinical experience in patients with severe hepatic impairment.

Elderly patients: Although consideration should be given to initiating therapy with 75 mg in patients over 75 years of age, dosage adjustment is not usually necessary for the elderly.

Children: Safety and efficacy of Aprovel have not been established in children.

4.3 Contraindications

Hypersensitivity to any component of the product (see 6.1).

Second and third trimester of pregnancy (see 4.6).

Lactation (see 4.6).

4.4 Special warnings and special precautions for use

Intravascular volume depletion: Symptomatic hypotension, especially after the first dose, may occur in patients who are volume and/or sodium depleted by vigorous diuretic therapy, dietary salt restriction, diarrhoea or vomiting. Such conditions should be corrected before the administration of Aprovel.

Renovascular hypertension: There is an increased risk of severe hypotension and renal insufficiency when patients with bilateral renal artery stenosis or stenosis of the artery to a single functioning kidney are treated with drugs that affect the renin-angiotensin-aldosterone system. While this is not documented with Aprovel, a similar effect should be anticipated with angiotensin-II receptor antagonists.

Renal impairment and kidney transplantation: When Aprovel is used in patients with impaired renal function, a periodic monitoring of potassium and creatinine serum levels is recommended. There is no experience regarding the administration of Aprovel in patients with a recent kidney transplantation.

Hypertensive patients with type 2 diabetes and renal disease: The effects of irbesartan both on renal and cardiovascular events were not uniform across all subgroups, in an analysis carried out in the study with patients with advanced renal disease. In particular, they appeared less favourable in women and non-white subjects (see 5.1).

Hyperkalaemia: As with other drugs that affect the renin-angiotensin-aldosterone system, hyperkalaemia may occur during the treatment with Aprovel, especially in the presence of renal impairment, overt proteinuria due to diabetic renal disease and/or heart failure. Close monitoring of serum potassium in patients at risk is recommended (see 4.5).

Lithium The combination of lithium and Aprovel is not recommended (see 4. 5).

Aortic and mitral valve stenosis, obstructive hypertrophic cardiomyopathy: As with other vasodilators, special caution is indicated in patients suffering from aortic or mitral stenosis, or obstructive hypertrophic cardiomyopathy.

Primary aldosteronism: Patients with primary aldosteronism generally will not respond to anti-hypertensive drugs acting through inhibition of the renin-angiotensin system. Therefore, the use of Aprovel is not recommended.

General: In patients whose vascular tone and renal function depend predominantly on the activity of the renin-angiotensin-aldosterone system (e.g. patients with severe congestive heart failure or underlying renal disease, including renal artery stenosis), treatment with angiotensin converting enzyme inhibitors or angiotensin-II receptor antagonists that affect this system has been associated with acute hypotension, azotaemia, oliguria, or rarely, acute renal failure. As with any anti-hypertensive agent, excessive blood pressure decrease in patients with ischaemic cardiopathy or ischaemic cardiovascular disease could result in a myocardial infarction or stroke.

As observed for angiotensin converting enzyme inhibitors, irbesartan and the other angiotensin antagonists are apparently less effective in lowering blood pressure in black people than in non-blacks, possibly because of higher prevalence of low-renin states in the black hypertensive population (see 5.1).

4.5 Interaction with other medicinal products and other forms of Interaction

Diuretics and other antihypertensive agents: Other antihypertensive agents may increase the hypotensive effects of irbesartan; however Aprovel has been safely administered with other antihypertensive agents, such as beta-blockers, long-acting calcium channel blockers, and thiazide diuretics. Prior treatment with high dose diuretics may result in volume depletion and a risk of hypotension when initiating therapy with Aprovel (see 4.4).

Potassium supplements and potassium-sparing diuretics: Based on experience with the use of other drugs that affect the renin-angiotensin system, concomitant use of potassium-sparing diuretics, potassium supplements, salt substitutes containing potassium or other drugs that may increase serum potassium levels (e.g. heparin) may lead to increases in serum potassium and is, therefore, not recommended (see 4.4).

Lithium: Reversible increases in serum lithium concentrations and toxicity have been reported during concomitant administration of lithium with angiotensin converting enzyme inhibitors. Similar effects have been very rarely reported with irbesartan. Therefore, this combination is not recommended (see 4.4). If the combination proves necessary, careful monitoring of serum lithium levels is recommended.

Non-steroidal anti-inflammatory drugs: When angiotensin II antagonists are administered simultaneously with non-steroidal anti-inflammatory drugs (i.e. selective COX-2 inhibitors, acetylsalicylic acid >3 g/day) and non-selective NSAIDs), attenuation of the antihypertensive effect may occur.

As with ACE inhibitors, concomitant use of angiotensin II antagonists and NSAIDs may lead to an increased risk of worsening of renal function, including possible acute renal failure, and an increase in serum potassium, especially in patients with poor pre-existing renal function. The combination should be administered with caution, especially in the elderly. Patients should be adequately hydrated and consideration should be given to monitoring renal function after initiation of concomitant therapy, and periodically thereafter.

Additional information on irbesartan interactions: In clinical studies, the pharmacokinetics of irbesartan are not affected by hydrochlorothiazide. Irbesartan is mainly metabolised by CYP2C9 and to a lesser extent by glucuronidation. No significant pharmacokinetic or pharmacodynamic interactions were observed when irbesartan was co-administered with warfarin, a drug metabolised by CYP2C9. The effects of CYP2C9 inducers such as rifampicin on the pharmacokinetics of irbesartan have not been evaluated. The pharmacokinetics of digoxin were not altered by coadministration of irbesartan.

4.6 Pregnancy and lactation

Pregnancy: see 4.3.

As a precautionary measure, irbesartan should preferably not be used during the first trimester of pregnancy. A switch to a suitable alternative treatment should be carried out in advance of a planned pregnancy. In the second and third trimesters, substances that act directly on the renin-angiotensin-system can cause foetal or neonatal renal failure, foetal skull hypoplasia and even foetal death. Therefore, irbesartan is contraindicated in the second and third trimesters of pregnancy. If pregnancy is diagnosed, irbesartan should be discontinued as soon as possible. Skull and renal function should be checked with echography if, inadvertently, the treatment was taken for a long period.

Lactation: Aprovel is contraindicated during lactation. It is not known whether irbesartan is excreted in human milk. Irbesartan is excreted in the milk of lactating rats (see 4.3).

4.7 Effects on ability to drive and use machines

The effect of irbesartan on ability to drive and use machines has not been studied, but, based on its pharmacodynamic properties, irbesartan is unlikely to affect this ability. When driving vehicles or operating machines, it should be taken into account that occasionally dizziness or weariness may occur during treatment.

4.8 Undesirable effects

The frequency of adverse reactions listed below is defined using the following convention: very common ($\geqslant$1/10); common ($\geqslant$1/100, <1/10); uncommon ($\geqslant$1/1,000, <1/100); rare ($\geqslant$1/10,000, <1/1,000); very rare (<1/10,000).

Hypertension: In placebo-controlled trials in patients with hypertension, the overall incidence of adverse events did not differ between the irbesartan (56.2%) and the placebo groups (56.5%). Discontinuation due to any clinical or laboratory adverse event was less frequent for irbesartan-treated patients (3.3%) than for placebo-treated patients (4.5%). The incidence of adverse events was not related to dose (in the recommended dose range), gender, age, race, or duration of treatment.

In placebo-controlled trials in which 1965 patients received irbesartan, the following adverse drug reactions were reported:

Nervous system disorders:

Common: dizziness

Cardiac disorders:

Uncommon: tachycardia

Vascular disorders:

Uncommon: flushing

Respiratory, thoracic and mediastinal disorders:

Uncommon: cough

Gastrointestinal disorders:

Common: nausea/vomiting

Uncommon: diarrhoea, dyspepsia/heartburn

Reproductive system and breast disorders:

Uncommon: sexual dysfunction

General disorders and administration site conditions:

Common: fatigue

Uncommon: chest pain

Investigations:

Common: significant increases in plasma creatinine kinase were commonly observed (1.7%) in irbesartan treated subjects. None of these increases was associated with identifiable clinical musculoskeletal events.

Hypertension and type 2 diabetes with renal disease: In addition to the adverse drug reactions mentioned under hypertension, in diabetic hypertensive patients with microalbuminuria and normal renal function, orthostatic dizziness and orthostatic hypotension were reported in 0.5% of the patients (i.e., uncommon) but in excess of placebo.

In diabetic hypertensive patients with chronic renal insufficiency and overt proteinuria, the following additional adverse reactions were reported in >2% of patients and in excess of placebo:

Nervous system disorders:

Common: Orthostatic dizziness

Vascular disorders:

Common: Orthostatic hypotension

Musculoskeletal, connective tissue and bone disorders:

Common: Musculoskeletal pain

Investigations:

Hyperkalaemia occurred more often in diabetic patients treated with irbesartan than with placebo. In diabetic hypertensive patients with microalbuminuria and normal renal function, hyperkalaemia ($\geqslant$5.5 mEq/l) occurred in 29.4% (i.e. very common) of the patients in the irbesartan 300 mg group and 22% of the patients in the placebo group. In diabetic hypertensive patients with chronic renal insufficiency and overt proteinuria, hyperkalaemia ($\geqslant$5.5 mEq/l) occurred in 46.3% (i.e. very common) of the patients in the irbesartan group and 26.3% of the patients in the placebo group. A decrease in haemoglobin, which was not clinically significant, has been observed in 1.7% (i.e. common) of hypertensive patients with advanced diabetic renal disease treated with irbesartan.

In addition, since introduction of irbesartan in the market, the following adverse drug reactions have also been reported:

Immune system disorders:

Rare: as with other angiotensin-II receptor antagonists, rare cases of hypersensitivity reactions such as rash, urticaria, angioedema have been reported

Metabolism and nutrition disorders:

Very rare: hyperkalaemia

Nervous system disorders:

Very rare: headache

Ear and labyrinth disorders:

Very rare: tinnitus

Gastrointestinal disorders:

Very rare: dysgeusia

Hepato-biliary disorders:

Very rare: abnormal liver function, hepatitis

Musculoskeletal, connective tissue and bone disorders:

Very rare: myalgia, arthralgia

Renal and urinary disorders:

Very rare: impaired renal function including isolated cases of renal failure in patients at risk (see 4.4)

4.9 Overdose

Experience in adults exposed to doses of up to 900 mg/day for 8 weeks revealed no toxicity. The most likely manifestations of overdosage are expected to be hypotension and tachycardia; bradycardia might also occur from overdose. No specific information is available on the treatment of overdosage with Aprovel. The patient should be closely monitored, and the treatment should be symptomatic and supportive. Suggested measures include induction of emesis and/or gastric lavage. Activated charcoal may be useful in the treatment of overdosage. Irbesartan is not removed by haemodialysis.

5. PHARMACOLOGICAL PROPERTIES

5.1 Pharmacodynamic properties

Pharmacotherapeutic group: Angiotensin-II antagonists, ATC code C09C A04.

Irbesartan is a potent, orally active, selective angiotensin-II receptor (type AT_1) antagonist.

Mechanism of Action: It is expected to block all actions of angiotensin-II mediated by the AT_1 receptor, regardless of the source or route of synthesis of angiotensin-II. The selective antagonism of the angiotensin-II (AT_1) receptors results in increases in plasma renin levels and angiotensin-II levels, and a decrease in plasma aldosterone concentration. Serum potassium levels are not significantly affected by irbesartan alone at the recommended doses. Irbesartan does not inhibit ACE (kininase-II), an enzyme which generates angiotensin-II and also degrades bradykinin into inactive metabolites. Irbesartan does not require metabolic activation for its activity.

Clinical efficacy:

Hypertension

Irbesartan lowers blood pressure with minimal change in heart rate. The decrease in blood pressure is dose-related for once a day doses with a tendency towards plateau at doses above 300 mg. Doses of 150-300 mg once daily lower supine or seated blood pressures at trough (i.e. 24 hours after dosing) by an average of 8-13/5-8 mm Hg (systolic/diastolic) greater than those associated with placebo.

Peak reduction of blood pressure is achieved within 3-6 hours after administration and the blood pressure lowering effect is maintained for at least 24 hours. At 24 hours the reduction of blood pressure was 60-70% of the corresponding peak diastolic and systolic responses at the recommended doses. Once daily dosing with 150 mg produced trough and mean 24 hour responses similar to twice daily dosing on the same total dose.

The blood pressure lowering effect of Aprovel is evident within 1-2 weeks, with the maximal effect occurring by 4-6 weeks after start of therapy. The antihypertensive effects are maintained during long term therapy. After withdrawal of therapy, blood pressure gradually returns toward baseline. Rebound hypertension has not been observed.

The blood pressure lowering effects of irbesartan and thiazide-type diuretics are additive. In patients not adequately controlled by irbesartan alone, the addition of a low dose of hydrochlorothiazide (12.5 mg) to irbesartan once daily results in a further placebo-adjusted blood pressure reduction at trough of 7-10/3-6 mm Hg (systolic/diastolic).

The efficacy of Aprovel is not influenced by age or gender. As is the case with other drugs that affect the renin-angiotensin system, black hypertensive patients have notably less response to irbesartan monotherapy. When irbesartan is administered concomitantly with a low dose of hydrochlorothiazide (e.g. 12.5 mg daily), the antihypertensive response in black patients approaches that of white patients.

There is no clinically important effect on serum uric acid or urinary uric acid secretion.

Hypertension and type 2 diabetes with renal disease

The "Irbesartan Diabetic Nephropathy Trial (IDNT)" shows that irbesartan decreases the progression of renal disease in patients with chronic renal insufficiency and overt proteinuria. IDNT was a double blind, controlled, morbidity and mortality trial comparing Aprovel, amlodipine and placebo. In 1715 hypertensive patients with type 2 diabetes, proteinuria ⩾900 mg/day and serum creatinine ranging from 1.0-3.0 mg/dl, the long-term effects (mean 2.6 years) of Aprovel on the progression of renal disease and all-cause mortality were examined. Patients were titrated from 75 mg to a maintenance dose of 300 mg Aprovel, from 2.5 mg to 10 mg amlodipine, or placebo as tolerated. Patients in all treatment groups typically received between 2 and 4 antihypertensive agents (e.g. diuretics, beta blockers, alpha blockers) to reach a predefined blood pressure goal of ⩽135/85 mmHg or a 10 mmHg reduction in systolic pressure if baseline was > 160 mmHg. Sixty per cent (60%) of patients in the placebo group reached this target blood pressure whereas this figure was 76% and 78% in the irbesartan and amlodipine groups, respectively. Irbesartan significantly reduced the relative risk in the primary combined endpoint of doubling serum creatinine, end-stage renal disease (ESRD) or all-cause mortality. Approximately 33% of patients in the irbesartan group reached the primary renal composite endpoint, compared to 39% and 41% in the placebo and amlodipine groups [20% relative risk reduction versus placebo (p = 0.024) and 23% relative risk reduction compared to amlodipine (p = 0.006)]. When the individual components of the primary endpoint were analysed, no effect in all cause mortality was observed, while a positive trend in the reduction in ESRD and a significant reduction in doubling of serum creatinine were observed.

Subgroups consisting of gender, race, age, duration of diabetes, baseline blood pressure, serum creatinine and albumin excretion rate were assessed for treatment effect. In the female and black subgroups which represented 32% and 26% of the overall study population, respectively, a renal benefit was not evident, although the confidence intervals do not exclude it. As for the secondary endpoint of fatal and non-fatal cardiovascular events, there was no difference among the three groups in the overall population, although an increased incidence of non-fatal MI was seen for women and a decreased incidence of non-fatal MI was seen in males in the irbesartan group versus the placebo-based regimen. An increased incidence of non-fatal MI and stroke was seen in females in the irbesartan-based regimen versus the amlodipine-based regimen, while hospitalisation due to heart failure was reduced in the overall population. However, no proper explanation for these findings in women has been identified.

The study of the "Effects of Irbesartan on Microalbuminuria in Hypertensive Patients with type 2 Diabetes Mellitus (IRMA 2)" shows that irbesartan 300 mg delays progression to overt proteinuria in patients with microalbuminuria. IRMA 2 was a placebo-controlled double blind morbidity study in 590 patients with type 2 diabetes, microalbuminuria (30-300 mg/day) and normal renal function (serum creatinine ⩽1.5 mg/dl in males and < 1.1 mg/dl in females). The study examined the long-term effects (2 years) of Aprovel on the progression to clinical (overt) proteinuria (urinary albumin excretion rate (UAER) > 300 mg/day, and an increase in UAER of at least 30% from baseline). The predefined blood pressure goal was ⩽135/85 mmHg. Additional antihypertensive agents (excluding ACE inhibitors, angiotensin-II receptor antagonists and dihydropyridine calcium blockers) were added as needed to help achieve the blood pressure goal. While similar blood pressure was achieved in all treatment groups, fewer subjects in the irbesartan 300 mg group (5.2%) than in the placebo (14.9%) or in the irbesartan 150 mg group (9.7%) reached the endpoint of overt proteinuria, demonstrating a 70% relative risk reduction versus placebo (p = 0.0004) for the higher dose. An accompanying improvement in the glomerular filtration rate (GFR) was not observed during the first three months of treatment. The slowing in the progression to clinical proteinuria was evident as early as three months and continued over the 2 year period. Regression to normoalbuminuria (< 30 mg/day) was more frequent in the Aprovel 300 mg group (34%) than in the placebo group (21%).

5.2 Pharmacokinetic properties

After oral administration, irbesartan is well absorbed: studies of absolute bioavailability gave values of approximately 60-80%. Concomitant food intake does not significantly influence the bioavailability of irbesartan.

Plasma protein binding is approximately 96%, with negligible binding to cellular blood components. The volume of distribution is 53-93 litres.

Following oral or intravenous administration of ^{14}C irbesartan, 80-85% of the circulating plasma radioactivity is attributable to unchanged irbesartan. Irbesartan is metabolised by the liver via glucuronide conjugation and oxidation. The major circulating metabolite is irbesartan glucuronide (approximately 6%). *In vitro* studies indicate that irbesartan is primarily oxidised by the cytochrome P450 enzyme *CYP2C9*; isoenzyme *CYP3A4* has negligible effect.

Irbesartan exhibits linear and dose proportional pharmacokinetics over the dose range of 10 to 600 mg. A less than proportional increase in oral absorption at doses beyond 600 mg (twice the maximal recommended dose) was observed; the mechanism for this is unknown. Peak plasma concentrations are attained at 1.5-2 hours after oral administration. The total body and renal clearance are 157-176 and 3-3.5 ml/min, respectively. The terminal elimination half-life of irbesartan is 11-15 hours. Steady-state plasma concentrations are attained within 3 days after initiation of a once-daily dosing regimen. Limited accumulation of irbesartan (< 20%) is observed in plasma upon repeated once-daily dosing. In a study, somewhat higher plasma concentrations of irbesartan were observed in female hypertensive patients. However, there was no difference in the half-life and accumulation of irbesartan. No dosage adjustment is necessary in female patients. Irbesartan AUC and C_{max} values were also somewhat greater in elderly subjects (⩾ 65 years) than those of young subjects (18-40 years). However the terminal half-life was not significantly altered. No dosage adjustment is necessary in elderly patients.

Irbesartan and its metabolites are eliminated by both biliary and renal pathways. After either oral or IV administration of ^{14}C irbesartan, about 20% of the radioactivity is recovered in the urine, and the remainder in the faeces. Less than 2% of the dose is excreted in the urine as unchanged irbesartan.

Renal impairment: In patients with renal impairment or those undergoing haemodialysis, the pharmacokinetic parameters of irbesartan are not significantly altered. Irbesartan is not removed by haemodialysis.

Hepatic impairment: In patients with mild to moderate cirrhosis, the pharmacokinetic parameters of irbesartan are not significantly altered.

Studies have not been performed in patients with severe hepatic impairment.

5.3 Preclinical safety data

There was no evidence of abnormal systemic or target organ toxicity at clinically relevant doses. In preclinical safety studies, high doses of irbesartan (⩾ 250 mg/kg/day in rats and ⩾ 100 mg/kg/day in macaques) caused a reduction of red blood cell parameters (erythrocytes, haemoglobin, haematocrit). At very high doses (⩾ 500 mg/kg/day) degenerative changes in the kidney (such as interstitial nephritis, tubular distension, basophilic tubules, increased plasma concentrations of urea and creatinine) were induced by irbesartan in the rat and the macaque and are considered secondary to the hypotensive effects of the drug which led to decreased renal perfusion. Furthermore, irbesartan induced hyperplasia/hypertrophy of the juxtaglomerular cells (in rats at ⩾ 90 mg/kg/day, in macaques at ⩾ 10 mg/kg/day). All of these changes were considered to be caused by the pharmacological action of irbesartan. For therapeutic doses of irbesartan in humans, the hyperplasia / hypertrophy of the renal juxtaglomerular cells does not appear to have any relevance.

There was no evidence of mutagenicity, clastogenicity or carcinogenicity.

Animal studies with irbesartan showed transient toxic effects (increased renal pelvic cavitation, hydroureter or subcutaneous oedema) in rat foetuses, which were resolved after birth. In rabbits, abortion or early resorption were noted at doses causing significant maternal toxicity, including mortality. No teratogenic effects were observed in the rat or rabbit.

6. PHARMACEUTICAL PARTICULARS

6.1 List of excipients

Tablet core: lactose monohydrate, microcrystalline cellulose, croscarmellose sodium, hypromellose, silicon dioxide, magnesium stearate.

Film-coating: lactose monohydrate, hypromellose, titanium dioxide (E171), macrogol, carnauba wax.

6.2 Incompatibilities

Not applicable.

6.3 Shelf life

3 years.

6.4 Special precautions for storage

Do not store above 30°C. Store in the original package.

6.5 Nature and contents of container

Aprovel film-coated tablets are packaged in blister packs containing 28 tablets in PVC/PVDC/Aluminium strips.

6.6 Instructions for use and handling

No special requirements.

7. MARKETING AUTHORISATION HOLDER

SANOFI PHARMA BRISTOL-MYERS SQUIBB SNC

174 avenue de France

F-75013 Paris - France

8. MARKETING AUTHORISATION NUMBER(S)

Aprovel 75 mg film-coated tablets: EU/1/97/046/17

Aprovel 150 mg film-coated tablets: EU/1/97/046/22

Aprovel 300 mg film-coated tablets: EU/1/97/046/27

9. DATE OF FIRST AUTHORISATION/RENEWAL OF THE AUTHORISATION

02 March 2004

10. DATE OF REVISION OF THE TEXT

02 August 2004

Legal category: POM

Aprovel Film-Coated Tablets (Sanofi Pharma Bristol-Myers Squibb SNC)

(Sanofi Pharma Bristol-Myers Squibb SNC)

1. NAME OF THE MEDICINAL PRODUCT

Aprovel 75 mg film-coated tablets.

Aprovel 150 mg film-coated tablets.

Aprovel 300 mg film-coated tablets.

2. QUALITATIVE AND QUANTITATIVE COMPOSITION

Each film-coated tablet contains 75 mg, 150 mg or 300 mg irbesartan.

For excipients, see 6.1.

3. PHARMACEUTICAL FORM

Film-coated tablet.

White to off-white, biconvex, and oval-shaped with a heart debossed on one side. The other side is engraved with the number 2871 on the 75 mg tablet, 2872 on the 150 mg tablet and 2873 on the 300 mg tablet.

4. CLINICAL PARTICULARS

4.1 Therapeutic indications

Treatment of essential hypertension.

Treatment of renal disease in patients with hypertension and type 2 diabetes mellitus as part of an antihypertensive drug regimen (see 5.1).

4.2 Posology and method of administration

The usual recommended initial and maintenance dose is 150 mg once daily, with or without food. Aprovel at a dose of 150 mg once daily generally provides a better 24 hour blood pressure control than 75 mg. However, initiation of therapy with 75 mg could be considered, particularly in haemodialysed patients and in the elderly over 75 years.

In patients insufficiently controlled with 150 mg once daily, the dose of Aprovel can be increased to 300 mg, or other anti-hypertensive agents can be added. In particular, the addition of a diuretic such as hydrochlorothiazide has been shown to have an additive effect with Aprovel (see 4.5).

In hypertensive type 2 diabetic patients, therapy should be initiated at 150 mg irbesartan once daily and titrated up to 300 mg once daily as the preferred maintenance dose for treatment of renal disease. The demonstration of renal benefit of Aprovel in hypertensive type 2 diabetic patients is based on studies where irbesartan was used in addition to other antihypertensive agents, as needed, to reach target blood pressure (see 5.1).

Renal impairment: No dosage adjustment is necessary in patients with impaired renal function. A lower starting dose (75 mg) should be considered for patients undergoing haemodialysis.

Intravascular volume depletion: Volume and/or sodium depletion should be corrected prior to administration of Aprovel.

Hepatic impairment: No dosage adjustment is necessary in patients with mild to moderate hepatic impairment. There is no clinical experience in patients with severe hepatic impairment.

Elderly patients: Although consideration should be given to initiating therapy with 75 mg in patients over 75 years of age, dosage adjustment is not usually necessary for the elderly.

Children: Safety and efficacy of Aprovel have not been established in children.

4.3 Contraindications

Hypersensitivity to any component of the product (see 6.1).

Second and third trimester of pregnancy (see 4.6).

Lactation (see 4.6).

4.4 Special warnings and special precautions for use

Intravascular volume depletion: Symptomatic hypotension, especially after the first dose, may occur in patients who are volume and/or sodium depleted by vigorous diuretic therapy, dietary salt restriction, diarrhoea or vomiting. Such conditions should be corrected before the administration of Aprovel.

Renovascular hypertension: There is an increased risk of severe hypotension and renal insufficiency when patients with bilateral renal artery stenosis or stenosis of the artery to a single functioning kidney are treated with drugs that affect the renin-angiotensin-aldosterone system. While this is not documented with Aprovel, a similar effect should be anticipated with angiotensin-II receptor antagonists.

Renal impairment and kidney transplantation: When Aprovel is used in patients with impaired renal function, a periodic monitoring of potassium and creatinine serum levels is recommended. There is no experience regarding the administration of Aprovel in patients with a recent kidney transplantation.

Hypertensive patients with type 2 diabetes and renal disease: The effects of irbesartan both on renal and cardiovascular events were not uniform across all subgroups, in an analysis carried out in the study with patients with advanced renal disease. In particular, they appeared less favourable in women and non-white subjects (see 5.1).

Hyperkalaemia: As with other drugs that affect the renin-angiotensin-aldosterone system, hyperkalaemia may occur during the treatment with Aprovel, especially in the presence of renal impairment, overt proteinuria due to diabetic renal disease and/or heart failure. Close monitoring of serum potassium in patients at risk is recommended (see 4.5).

Lithium The combination of lithium and Aprovel is not recommended (see 4. 5).

Aortic and mitral valve stenosis, obstructive hypertrophic cardiomyopathy: As with other vasodilators, special caution is indicated in patients suffering from aortic or mitral stenosis, or obstructive hypertrophic cardiomyopathy.

Primary aldosteronism: Patients with primary aldosteronism generally will not respond to anti-hypertensive drugs acting through inhibition of the renin-angiotensin system. Therefore, the use of Aprovel is not recommended.

General: In patients whose vascular tone and renal function depend predominantly on the activity of the renin-angiotensin-aldosterone system (e.g. patients with severe congestive heart failure or underlying renal disease, including renal artery stenosis), treatment with angiotensin converting enzyme inhibitors or angiotensin-II receptor antagonists that affect this system has been associated with acute hypotension, azotaemia, oliguria, or rarely, acute renal failure. As with any anti-hypertensive agent, excessive blood pressure decrease in patients with ischaemic cardiopathy or ischaemic cardiovascular disease could result in a myocardial infarction or stroke.

As observed for angiotensin converting enzyme inhibitors, irbesartan and the other angiotensin antagonists are apparently less effective in lowering blood pressure in black people than in non-blacks, possibly because of higher prevalence of low-renin states in the black hypertensive population (see 5.1).

4.5 Interaction with other medicinal products and other forms of Interaction

Diuretics and other antihypertensive agents: Other antihypertensive agents may increase the hypotensive effects of irbesartan; however Aprovel has been safely administered with other antihypertensive agents, such as beta-blockers, long-acting calcium channel blockers, and thiazide diuretics. Prior treatment with high dose diuretics may result in volume depletion and a risk of hypotension when initiating therapy with Aprovel (see 4.4).

Potassium supplements and potassium-sparing diuretics: Based on experience with the use of other drugs that affect the renin-angiotensin system, concomitant use of potassium-sparing diuretics, potassium supplements, salt substitutes containing potassium or other drugs that may increase serum potassium levels (e.g. heparin) may lead to increases in serum potassium and is, therefore, not recommended (see 4.4).

Lithium: Reversible increases in serum lithium concentrations and toxicity have been reported during concomitant administration of lithium with angiotensin converting enzyme inhibitors. Similar effects have been very rarely reported with irbesartan. Therefore, this combination is not recommended (see 4.4). If the combination proves necessary, careful monitoring of serum lithium levels is recommended.

Non-steroidal anti-inflammatory drugs: When angiotensin II antagonists are administered simultaneously with non-steroidal anti-inflammatory drugs (i.e. selective COX-2 inhibitors, acetylsalicylic acid >3 g/day) and non-selective NSAIDs), attenuation of the antihypertensive effect may occur.

As with ACE inhibitors, concomitant use of angiotensin II antagonists and NSAIDs may lead to an increased risk of worsening of renal function, including possible acute renal failure, and an increase in serum potassium, especially in patients with poor pre-existing renal function. The combination should be administered with caution, especially in the elderly. Patients should be adequately hydrated and consideration should be given to monitoring renal function after initiation of concomitant therapy, and periodically thereafter.

Additional information on irbesartan interactions: In clinical studies, the pharmacokinetics of irbesartan are not affected by hydrochlorothiazide. Irbesartan is mainly metabolised by CYP2C9 and to a lesser extent by glucuronidation. No significant pharmacokinetic or pharmacodynamic interactions were observed when irbesartan was co-administered with warfarin, a drug metabolised by CYP2C9. The effects of CYP2C9 inducers such as rifampicin on the pharmacokinetics of irbesartan have not been evaluated. The pharmacokinetics of digoxin were not altered by coadministration of irbesartan.

4.6 Pregnancy and lactation

Pregnancy: see 4.3.

As a precautionary measure, irbesartan should preferably not be used during the first trimester of pregnancy. A switch to a suitable alternative treatment should be carried out in advance of a planned pregnancy. In the second and third trimesters, substances that act directly on the renin-angiotensin-system can cause foetal or neonatal renal failure, foetal skull hypoplasia and even foetal death. Therefore, irbesartan is contraindicated in the second and third trimesters of pregnancy. If pregnancy is diagnosed, irbesartan should be discontinued as soon as possible. Skull and renal function should be checked with echography if, inadvertently, the treatment was taken for a long period.

Lactation: Aprovel is contraindicated during lactation. It is not known whether irbesartan is excreted in human milk. Irbesartan is excreted in the milk of lactating rats (see 4.3).

4.7 Effects on ability to drive and use machines

The effect of irbesartan on ability to drive and use machines has not been studied, but, based on its pharmacodynamic properties, irbesartan is unlikely to affect this ability. When driving vehicles or operating machines, it should be taken into account that occasionally dizziness or weariness may occur during treatment.

4.8 Undesirable effects

The frequency of adverse reactions listed below is defined using the following convention: very common (≥1/10); common (≥1/100, <1/10); uncommon (≥1/1,000, <1/100); rare (≥1/10,000, <1/1,000); very rare (<1/10,000).

Hypertension: In placebo-controlled trials in patients with hypertension, the overall incidence of adverse events did not differ between the irbesartan (56.2%) and the placebo groups (56.5%). Discontinuation due to any clinical or laboratory adverse event was less frequent for irbesartan-treated patients (3.3%) than for placebo-treated patients (4.5%). The incidence of adverse events was not related to dose (in the recommended dose range), gender, age, race, or duration of treatment.

In placebo-controlled trials in which 1965 patients received irbesartan, the following adverse drug reactions were reported:

<u>Nervous system disorders</u>:

Common: dizziness

<u>Cardiac disorders</u>:

Uncommon: tachycardia

<u>Vascular disorders</u>:

Uncommon: flushing

<u>Respiratory, thoracic and mediastinal disorders</u>:

Uncommon: cough

<u>Gastrointestinal disorders</u>:

Common: nausea/vomiting

Uncommon: diarrhoea, dyspepsia/heartburn

<u>Reproductive system and breast disorders</u>:

Uncommon: sexual dysfunction

<u>General disorders and administration site conditions</u>:

Common: fatigue

Uncommon: chest pain

<u>Investigations</u>:

Common: significant increases in plasma creatinine kinase were commonly observed (1.7%) in irbesartan treated subjects. None of these increases was associated with identifiable clinical musculoskeletal events.

Hypertension and type 2 diabetes with renal disease: In addition to the adverse drug reactions mentioned under hypertension, in diabetic hypertensive patients with microalbuminuria and normal renal function, orthostatic dizziness and orthostatic hypotension were reported in 0.5% of the patients (i.e., uncommon) but in excess of placebo.

In diabetic hypertensive patients with chronic renal insufficiency and overt proteinuria, the following additional adverse reactions were reported in >2% of patients and in excess of placebo:

<u>Nervous system disorders</u>:

Common: Orthostatic dizziness

<u>Vascular disorders</u>:

Common: Orthostatic hypotension

<u>Musculoskeletal, connective tissue and bone disorders</u>:

Common: Musculoskeletal pain

<u>Investigations</u>:

Hyperkalaemia occurred more often in diabetic patients treated with irbesartan than with placebo. In diabetic hypertensive patients with microalbuminuria and normal renal function, hyperkalaemia (≥5.5 mEq/l) occurred in 29.4% (i.e. very common) of the patients in the irbesartan 300 mg group and 22% of the patients in the placebo group. In diabetic hypertensive patients with chronic renal insufficiency and overt proteinuria, hyperkalaemia (≥5.5 mEq/l) occurred in 46.3% (i.e. very common) of the patients in the irbesartan group and 26.3% of the patients in the placebo group. A decrease in haemoglobin, which was not clinically significant, has been observed in 1.7% (i.e. common) of hypertensive patients with advanced diabetic renal disease treated with irbesartan.

In addition, since introduction of irbesartan in the market, the following adverse drug reactions have also been reported:

<u>Immune system disorders</u>:

Rare: as with other angiotensin-II receptor antagonists, rare cases of hypersensitivity reactions such as rash, urticaria, angioedema have been reported

<u>Metabolism and nutrition disorders</u>:

Very rare: hyperkalaemia

<u>Nervous system disorders</u>:

Very rare: headache

<u>Ear and labyrinth disorders</u>:

Very rare: tinnitus

<u>Gastrointestinal disorders</u>:

Very rare: dysgeusia

<u>Hepato-biliary disorders</u>:

Very rare: abnormal liver function, hepatitis

<u>Musculoskeletal, connective tissue and bone disorders</u>:

Very rare: myalgia, arthralgia

<u>Renal and urinary disorders</u>:

Very rare: impaired renal function including isolated cases of renal failure in patients at risk (see 4.4)

4.9 Overdose

Experience in adults exposed to doses of up to 900 mg/day for 8 weeks revealed no toxicity. The most likely manifestations of overdosage are expected to be hypotension and tachycardia; bradycardia might also occur from overdose. No specific information is available on the treatment of overdosage with Aprovel. The patient should be closely monitored, and the treatment should be symptomatic and supportive. Suggested measures include induction of emesis and/or gastric lavage. Activated charcoal may be useful in the treatment of overdosage. Irbesartan is not removed by haemodialysis.

5. PHARMACOLOGICAL PROPERTIES

5.1 Pharmacodynamic properties

Pharmacotherapeutic group: Angiotensin-II antagonists, ATC code C09C A04.

Irbesartan is a potent, orally active, selective angiotensin-II receptor (type AT_1) antagonist.

Mechanism of Action: It is expected to block all actions of angiotensin-II mediated by the AT_1 receptor, regardless of the source or route of synthesis of angiotensin-II. The selective antagonism of the angiotensin-II (AT_1) receptors results in increases in plasma renin levels and angiotensin-II levels, and a decrease in plasma aldosterone concentration. Serum potassium levels are not significantly affected by irbesartan alone at the recommended doses. Irbesartan does not inhibit ACE (kininase-II), an enzyme which generates angiotensin-II and also degrades bradykinin into inactive metabolites. Irbesartan does not require metabolic activation for its activity.

Clinical efficacy:

Hypertension

Irbesartan lowers blood pressure with minimal change in heart rate. The decrease in blood pressure is dose-related for once a day doses with a tendency towards plateau at doses above 300 mg. Doses of 150-300 mg once daily lower supine or seated blood pressures at trough (i.e. 24 hours after dosing) by an average of 8-13/5-8 mm Hg (systolic/diastolic) greater than those associated with placebo.

Peak reduction of blood pressure is achieved within 3-6 hours after administration and the blood pressure lowering effect is maintained for at least 24 hours. At 24 hours the reduction of blood pressure was 60-70% of the corresponding peak diastolic and systolic responses at the recommended doses. Once daily dosing with 150 mg produced trough and mean 24 hour responses similar to twice daily dosing on the same total dose.

The blood pressure lowering effect of Aprovel is evident within 1-2 weeks, with the maximal effect occurring by 4-6 weeks after start of therapy. The antihypertensive effects are maintained during long term therapy. After withdrawal of therapy, blood pressure gradually returns toward baseline. Rebound hypertension has not been observed.

The blood pressure lowering effects of irbesartan and thiazide-type diuretics are additive. In patients not adequately controlled by irbesartan alone, the addition of a low dose of hydrochlorothiazide (12.5 mg) to irbesartan once daily results in a further placebo-adjusted blood pressure reduction at trough of 7-10/3-6 mm Hg (systolic/diastolic).

The efficacy of Aprovel is not influenced by age or gender. As is the case with other drugs that affect the renin-angiotensin system, black hypertensive patients have notably less response to irbesartan monotherapy. When irbesartan is administered concomitantly with a low dose of hydrochlorothiazide (e.g. 12.5 mg daily), the antihypertensive response in black patients approaches that of white patients.

There is no clinically important effect on serum uric acid or urinary uric acid secretion.

Hypertension and type 2 diabetes with renal disease

The "Irbesartan Diabetic Nephropathy Trial (IDNT)" shows that irbesartan decreases the progression of renal disease in patients with chronic renal insufficiency and overt proteinuria. IDNT was a double blind, controlled, morbidity and mortality trial comparing Aprovel, amlodipine and placebo. In 1715 hypertensive patients with type 2 diabetes, proteinuria ⩾900 mg/day and serum creatinine ranging from 1.0-3.0 mg/dl, the long-term effects (mean 2.6 years) of Aprovel on the progression of renal disease and all-cause mortality were examined. Patients were titrated from 75 mg to a maintenance dose of 300 mg Aprovel, from 2.5 mg to 10 mg amlodipine, or placebo as tolerated. Patients in all treatment groups typically received between 2 and 4 antihypertensive agents (e.g. diuretics, beta blockers, alpha blockers) to reach a predefined blood pressure goal of ⩽135/85 mmHg or a 10 mmHg reduction in systolic pressure if baseline was > 160 mmHg. Sixty per cent (60%) of patients in the placebo group reached this target blood pressure whereas this figure was 76% and 78% in the irbesartan and amlodipine groups, respectively. Irbesartan significantly reduced the relative risk in the primary combined endpoint of doubling serum creatinine, end-stage renal disease (ESRD) or all-cause mortality. Approximately 33% of patients in the irbesartan group reached the primary renal composite endpoint, compared to 39% and 41% in the placebo and amlodipine groups [20% relative risk reduction versus placebo (p = 0.024) and 23% relative risk reduction compared to amlodipine (p = 0.006)]. When the individual components of the primary endpoint were analysed, no effect in all cause mortality was observed, while a positive trend in the reduction in ESRD and a significant reduction in doubling of serum creatinine were observed.

Subgroups consisting of gender, race, age, duration of diabetes, baseline blood pressure, serum creatinine and albumin excretion rate were assessed for treatment effect. In the female and black subgroups which represented 32% and 26% of the overall study population, respectively, a renal benefit was not evident, although the confidence intervals do not exclude it. As for the secondary endpoint of fatal and non-fatal cardiovascular events, there was no difference among the three groups in the overall population, although an increased incidence of non-fatal MI was seen for women and a decreased incidence of non-fatal MI was seen in males in the irbesartan group versus the placebo-based regimen. An increased incidence of non-fatal MI and stroke was seen in females in the irbesartan-based regimen versus the amlodipine-based regimen, while hospitalisation due to heart failure was reduced in the overall population. However, no proper explanation for these findings in women has been identified.

The study of the "Effects of Irbesartan on Microalbuminuria in Hypertensive Patients with type 2 Diabetes Mellitus (IRMA 2)" shows that irbesartan 300 mg delays progression to overt proteinuria in patients with microalbuminuria. IRMA 2 was a placebo-controlled double blind morbidity study in 590 patients with type 2 diabetes, microalbuminuria (30-300 mg/day) and normal renal function (serum creatinine ⩽1.5 mg/dl in males and < 1.1 mg/dl in females). The study examined the long-term effects (2 years) of Aprovel on the progression to clinical (overt) proteinuria (urinary albumin excretion rate (UAER) > 300 mg/day, and an increase in UAER of at least 30% from baseline). The predefined blood pressure goal was ⩽135/85 mmHg. Additional antihypertensive agents (excluding ACE inhibitors, angiotensin-II receptor antagonists and dihydropyridine calcium blockers) were added as needed to help achieve the blood pressure goal. While similar blood pressure was achieved in all treatment groups, fewer subjects in the irbesartan 300 mg group (5.2%) than in the placebo (14.9%) or in the irbesartan 150 mg group (9.7%) reached the endpoint of overt proteinuria, demonstrating a 70% relative risk reduction versus placebo (p = 0.0004) for the higher dose. An accompanying improvement in the glomerular filtration rate (GFR) was not observed during the first three months of treatment. The slowing in the progression to clinical proteinuria was evident as early as three months and continued over the 2 year period. Regression to normoalbuminuria (< 30 mg/day) was more frequent in the Aprovel 300 mg group (34%) than in the placebo group (21%).

5.2 Pharmacokinetic properties

After oral administration, irbesartan is well absorbed: studies of absolute bioavailability gave values of approximately 60-80%. Concomitant food intake does not significantly influence the bioavailability of irbesartan.

Plasma protein binding is approximately 96%, with negligible binding to cellular blood components. The volume of distribution is 53-93 litres.

Following oral or intravenous administration of ^{14}C irbesartan, 80-85% of the circulating plasma radioactivity is attributable to unchanged irbesartan. Irbesartan is metabolised by the liver via glucuronide conjugation and oxidation. The major circulating metabolite is irbesartan glucuronide (approximately 6%). *In vitro* studies indicate that irbesartan is primarily oxidised by the cytochrome P450 enzyme *CYP2C9*; isoenzyme *CYP3A4* has negligible effect.

Irbesartan exhibits linear and dose proportional pharmacokinetics over the dose range of 10 to 600 mg. A less than proportional increase in oral absorption at doses beyond 600 mg (twice the maximal recommended dose) was observed; the mechanism for this is unknown. Peak plasma concentrations are attained at 1.5-2 hours after oral administration. The total body and renal clearance are 157-176 and 3-3.5 ml/min, respectively. The terminal elimination half-life of irbesartan is 11-15 hours. Steady-state plasma concentrations are attained within 3 days after initiation of a once-daily dosing regimen. Limited accumulation of irbesartan (< 20%) is observed in plasma upon repeated once-daily dosing. In a study, somewhat higher plasma concentrations of irbesartan were observed in female hypertensive patients. However, there was no difference in the half-life and accumulation of irbesartan. No dosage adjustment is necessary in female patients. Irbesartan AUC and C_{max} values were also somewhat greater in elderly subjects (⩾ 65 years) than those of young subjects (18-40 years). However the terminal half-life was not significantly altered. No dosage adjustment is necessary in elderly patients.

Irbesartan and its metabolites are eliminated by both biliary and renal pathways. After either oral or IV administration of ^{14}C irbesartan, about 20% of the radioactivity is recovered in the urine, and the remainder in the faeces. Less than 2% of the dose is excreted in the urine as unchanged irbesartan.

Renal impairment: In patients with renal impairment or those undergoing haemodialysis, the pharmacokinetic parameters of irbesartan are not significantly altered. Irbesartan is not removed by haemodialysis.

Hepatic impairment: In patients with mild to moderate cirrhosis, the pharmacokinetic parameters of irbesartan are not significantly altered.

Studies have not been performed in patients with severe hepatic impairment.

5.3 Preclinical safety data

There was no evidence of abnormal systemic or target organ toxicity at clinically relevant doses. In preclinical safety studies, high doses of irbesartan (⩾ 250 mg/kg/day in rats and ⩾ 100 mg/kg/day in macaques) caused a reduction of red blood cell parameters (erythrocytes, haemoglobin, haematocrit). At very high doses (⩾ 500 mg/kg/day) degenerative changes in the kidney (such as interstitial nephritis, tubular distension, basophilic tubules, increased plasma concentrations of urea and creatinine) were induced by irbesartan in the rat and the macaque and are considered secondary to the hypotensive effects of the drug which led to decreased renal perfusion. Furthermore, irbesartan induced hyperplasia/hypertrophy of the juxtaglomerular cells (in rats at ⩾ 90 mg/kg/day, in macaques at ⩾ 10 mg/kg/day). All of these changes were considered to be caused by the pharmacological action of irbesartan. For therapeutic doses of irbesartan in humans, the hyperplasia / hypertrophy of the renal juxtaglomerular cells does not appear to have any relevance.

There was no evidence of mutagenicity, clastogenicity or carcinogenicity.

Animal studies with irbesartan showed transient toxic effects (increased renal pelvic cavitation, hydroureter or subcutaneous oedema) in rat foetuses, which were resolved after birth. In rabbits, abortion or early resorption were noted at doses causing significant maternal toxicity, including mortality. No teratogenic effects were observed in the rat or rabbit.

6. PHARMACEUTICAL PARTICULARS

6.1 List of excipients

Tablet core: lactose monohydrate, microcrystalline cellulose, croscarmellose sodium, hypromellose, silicon dioxide, magnesium stearate.

Film-coating: lactose monohydrate, hypromellose, titanium dioxide (E171), macrogol, carnauba wax.

6.2 Incompatibilities

Not applicable.

6.3 Shelf life

3 years.

6.4 Special precautions for storage

Do not store above 30°C. Store in the original package.

6.5 Nature and contents of container

Aprovel film-coated tablets are packaged in blister packs containing 28 tablets in PVC/PVDC/Aluminium strips.

6.6 Instructions for use and handling

No special requirements.

7. MARKETING AUTHORISATION HOLDER

SANOFI PHARMA BRISTOL-MYERS SQUIBB SNC
174 avenue de France
F-75013 Paris - France

8. MARKETING AUTHORISATION NUMBER(S)

Aprovel 75 mg film-coated tablets: EU/1/97/046/17

Aprovel 150 mg film-coated tablets: EU/1/97/046/22

Aprovel 300 mg film-coated tablets: EU/1/97/046/27

9. DATE OF FIRST AUTHORISATION/RENEWAL OF THE AUTHORISATION

02 March 2004

10. DATE OF REVISION OF THE TEXT

02 August 2004

Legal category: POM

Aquadrate Cream 30g & 100g

(Alliance Pharmaceuticals)

1. NAME OF THE MEDICINAL PRODUCT

Aquadrate Cream

2. QUALITATIVE AND QUANTITATIVE COMPOSITION

Aquadrate cream contains urea Ph Eur 10% w/w.

3. PHARMACEUTICAL FORM

A smooth, unperfumed, non greasy, off white cream for topical administration.

4. CLINICAL PARTICULARS

4.1 Therapeutic indications

For the treatment of ichthyosis and hyperkeratotic skin conditions associated with atopic eczema, xeroderma, iasteatosis and other chronic dry skin conditions.

4.2 Posology and method of administration

Aquadrate is applied topically. Wash affected areas well, rinse off all traces of soap, dry, and apply sparingly twice daily. Occlusive dressings may be used but are usually unnecessary because of the self-occlusive nature of the cream.

4.3 Contraindications

Known hypersensitivity to the product.

4.4 Special warnings and special precautions for use

Avoid application to moist or broken skin.

4.5 Interaction with other medicinal products and other forms of Interaction

Aquadrate may increase the penetration through the skin barrier of other topically applied medicaments.

4.6 Pregnancy and lactation

Animal reproduction studies have not been conducted with Aquadrate. Aquadrate should only be used if the anticipated benefits outweigh the risks.

4.7 Effects on ability to drive and use machines

Aquadrate does not interfere with the ability to drive or use machines.

4.8 Undesirable effects

May produce stinging if applied to sensitive, moist or fissured skin.

4.9 Overdose

Topical applications of excessive amounts of Aquadrate might cause skin irritation but no other effects would be expected. Ingestion of a large amount of Aquadrate would be expected to result in gastrointestinal irritation (nausea and vomiting). Symptomatic and supportive care should be given. Liberal oral administration of milk or water may be helpful.

5. PHARMACOLOGICAL PROPERTIES

5.1 Pharmacodynamic properties

Urea has a therapeutic effect in chronic dry skin conditions through its hydrating, keratolytic and anti-pruritic properties.

5.2 Pharmacokinetic properties

There is no information available on the pharmacokinetics of urea.

6. PHARMACEUTICAL PARTICULARS

6.1 List of excipients

The cream also contains white soft paraffin, maize starch, isopropyl myristate, syncrowax HR-C, palmitic acid, sorbitan laurate and arlatone G.

6.2 Incompatibilities

None known.

6.3 Shelf life

Two years.

6.4 Special precautions for storage

Store below 30°C.

6.5 Nature and contents of container

Aquadrate is available in tubes of 30g and 100g.

6.6 Instructions for use and handling

A patient leaflet is provided with details of use and handling of the product.

7. MARKETING AUTHORISATION HOLDER

Alliance Pharmaceuticals Ltd
Avonbridge House
Bath Road
Chippenham
Wiltshire
SN15 2BB

8. MARKETING AUTHORISATION NUMBER(S)

PL 16853/0061

9. DATE OF FIRST AUTHORISATION/RENEWAL OF THE AUTHORISATION

10 September 1991

10. DATE OF REVISION OF THE TEXT

November 2004

11. LEGAL STATUS

P

Aquasept Skin Cleanser

(Medlock Medical Ltd)

1. NAME OF THE MEDICINAL PRODUCT

Aquasept Skin Cleanser.

2. QUALITATIVE AND QUANTITATIVE COMPOSITION

Triclosan 2.0% w/v.

3. PHARMACEUTICAL FORM

Clear blue solution.

4. CLINICAL PARTICULARS

4.1 Therapeutic indications

This product has an antibacterial effect and is intended for the following uses: prevention of cross infection; prevention of self infection; preoperative hand disinfection; antiseptic skin cleansing; whole body bathing prior to elective surgery; whole body bathing to help eliminate the carriage of pathogens.

4.2 Posology and method of administration

For preoperative hand disinfection (250 ml and 500 ml): wet area to be cleaned. Apply about 5 ml of Aquasept and wash for one minute, paying particular attention to the area around the fingernails and cuticles and between the fingers. Rinse and repeat for two minutes. Rinse thoroughly and dry hands with a sterile towel. For antiseptic skin cleansing (250 ml and 500 ml): wet area to be cleaned and use Aquasept as a liquid soap, washing thoroughly for one minute. Rinse and dry thoroughly. For whole body bathing (28.5 ml, 250 ml and 500 ml): in shower or bath, use Aquasept as a liquid soap, paying particular attention to the hair, perineum, groin, axillae and nares. Take two baths or showers on the two days prior to surgery. Approximately 28.5 ml of Aquasept will suffice for one shower or bath.

4.3 Contraindications

None.

4.4 Special warnings and special precautions for use

For external use only. Avoid contact with eyes. Keep out of reach of children. Some product excipients may give rise to allergic reactions in some people. In this instance, discontinue use and seek medical advice.

4.5 Interaction with other medicinal products and other forms of Interaction

None stated.

4.6 Pregnancy and lactation

None stated.

4.7 Effects on ability to drive and use machines

None stated.

4.8 Undesirable effects

None stated.

4.9 Overdose

Ingestion: Gastric lavage and symptomatic treatment.

5. PHARMACOLOGICAL PROPERTIES

5.1 Pharmacodynamic properties

Triclosan is a bactericide.

5.2 Pharmacokinetic properties

None stated.

5.3 Preclinical safety data

None stated.

6. PHARMACEUTICAL PARTICULARS

6.1 List of excipients

Purified water; MEA lauryl sulphate; cocamide DEA; cocamidopropyl betaine; isopropyl alcohol; propylene glycol; tetrasodium edetate; triethanolamine; chlorocresol; Sea Fresh Perfume; Patent Blue V (E131).

6.2 Incompatibilities

None stated.

6.3 Shelf life

36 months unopened.

6.4 Special precautions for storage

None stated.

6.5 Nature and contents of container

HDPE or HDPP container. Polypropylene wadless screw-caps or compression-moulded screw caps with steran faced pulpboard liners. Sizes: 28.5 ml, 250 ml and 500 ml.

6.6 Instructions for use and handling

Not applicable.

7. MARKETING AUTHORISATION HOLDER

Medlock Medical Limited, Tubiton House, Medlock Street, Oldham, OL1 3HS.

8. MARKETING AUTHORISATION NUMBER(S)

PL 21248/0001.

9. DATE OF FIRST AUTHORISATION/RENEWAL OF THE AUTHORISATION

3rd July 2005.

10. DATE OF REVISION OF THE TEXT

July 2005.

Arava 10, 20 and 100mg Tablets

(sanofi-aventis)

1. NAME OF THE MEDICINAL PRODUCT

Arava™ 10 mg film-coated tablets ▼
Arava™ 20 mg film-coated tablets ▼
Arava™ 100 mg film-coated tablets ▼

2. QUALITATIVE AND QUANTITATIVE COMPOSITION

Arava 10 mg film-coated tablets contain 10 mg of the active ingredient leflunomide.

Arava 20 mg film-coated tablets contain 20 mg of the active ingredient leflunomide.

Arava 100 mg film-coated tablets contain 100 mg of the active ingredient leflunomide.

For excipients, see section 6.1.

3. PHARMACEUTICAL FORM

Film-coated tablet.

Arava 10 mg film-coated tablets are white to almost white, round film-coated tablets with a diameter of about 7 mm, imprinted with ZBN on one side.

Arava 20 mg film-coated tablets are yellowish to ochre and triangular film-coated tablets, imprinted with ZBO on one side.

Arava 100 mg film-coated tablets are white to almost white, round film-coated tablets with a diameter of about 1 cm, imprinted with ZBP on one side.

4. CLINICAL PARTICULARS

4.1 Therapeutic indications

Leflunomide is indicated for the treatment of adult patients with:

- active rheumatoid arthritis as a "disease-modifying anti-rheumatic drug" (DMARD),
- active psoriatic arthritis.

Recent or concurrent treatment with hepatotoxic or haematotoxic DMARDs (e.g. methotrexate) may result in an increased risk of serious adverse reactions; therefore, the initiation of leflunomide treatment has to be carefully considered regarding these benefit/risk aspects.

Moreover, switching from leflunomide to another DMARD without following the washout procedure (see section 4.4) may also increase the risk of serious adverse reactions even for a long time after the switching.

4.2 Posology and method of administration

ALT (SGPT) and a complete blood cell count, including differential white blood cell count and a platelet count, must be checked simultaneously and with the same frequency:

- Before initiation of leflunomide
- every two weeks during the first six months of treatment, and
- every eight weeks thereafter (see also section 4.4).

Leflunomide therapy is started with a loading dose of 100 mg once daily for 3 days.

- The recommended maintenance dose for rheumatoid arthritis is leflunomide 10 mg to 20 mg once daily. Patients may be started on leflunomide 10 mg or 20 mg depending on the severity (activity) of the disease.
- The recommended maintenance dose is 20 mg once daily for patients with psoriatic arthritis (see section 5.1).

The therapeutic effect usually starts after 4 to 6 weeks and may further improve up to 4 to 6 months.

There is no dose adjustment recommended in patients with mild renal insufficiency.

No dosage adjustment is required in patients above 65 years of age.

Arava is not recommended for use in patients under 18 years as its safety and efficacy have not been studied in this age group.

The treatment should be initiated and supervised by specialists experienced in the treatment of rheumatoid arthritis and psoriatic arthritis.

Administration

Arava tablets should be swallowed whole with sufficient amounts of liquid. The extent of leflunomide absorption is not affected if it is taken with food.

4.3 Contraindications

Arava must not be used in patients with hypersensitivity to leflunomide (especially previous Stevens-Johnson syndrome, toxic epidermal necrolysis, erythema multiforme) or to any of the excipients in the tablets.

Leflunomide is contraindicated in:

- patients with impairment of liver function,
- patients with severe immunodeficiency states, e.g. AIDS,
- patients with significantly impaired bone marrow function or significant anaemia, leucopenia, neutropenia or thrombocytopenia due to causes other than rheumatoid or psoriatic arthritis,
- patients with serious infections, (see section 4.4)
- patients with moderate to severe renal insufficiency, because insufficient clinical experience is available in this patient group,
- patients with severe hypoproteinaemia, e.g. in nephrotic syndrome,
- pregnant women, or women of childbearing potential who are not using reliable contraception during treatment with leflunomide and thereafter as long as the plasma levels of the active metabolite are above 0.02 mg/l (see also section 4.6). Pregnancy must be excluded before start of treatment with leflunomide.
- Women must not use leflunomide while breast-feeding. (See also section 4.6)

4.4 Special warnings and special precautions for use

Arava should be administered to patients only under careful medical supervision.

Concomitant administration of hepatotoxic or haematotoxic DMARDs (e.g. methotrexate) is not advisable.

The active metabolite of leflunomide, A771726, has a long half-life, usually 1 to 4 weeks. Serious undesirable effects might occur (e.g. hepatotoxicity, haematotoxicity or allergic reactions, see below), even if the treatment with leflunomide has been stopped. Therefore, when such toxicities occur or when switching to another DMARD (e.g. methotrexate) after treatment with leflunomide a washout procedure should be performed (see below).

For washout procedures and other recommended actions in case of desired or unintended pregnancy see section 4.6.

Liver reactions

Rare cases of severe liver injury, including cases with fatal outcome, have been reported during the treatment with leflunomide. Most of the cases occurred within the first 6 months of treatment.

Co-medication with other hepatotoxic medicinal products was frequently present. It is considered essential that monitoring recommendations are strictly adhered to.

ALT (SGPT) must be checked before initiation of leflunomide and at the same frequency as the complete blood cell count (every two weeks) during the first six months of treatment and every 8 weeks thereafter.

For ALT (SGPT) elevations between 2- and 3-fold the upper limit of normal, dose reduction from 20 mg to 10 mg may be considered and monitoring must be performed weekly. If

ALT (SGPT) elevations of more than 2-fold the upper limit of normal persist or if ALT elevations of more than 3-fold the upper limit of normal are present, leflunomide must be discontinued and wash-out procedures initiated. It is recommended that monitoring of liver enzymes be maintained after discontinuation of leflunomide treatment, until liver enzyme levels have normalised.

Due to a potential for additive hepatotoxic effects, it is recommended that alcohol consumption be avoided during treatment with leflunomide.

Since the active metabolite of leflunomide, A771726, is highly protein bound and cleared via hepatic metabolism and biliary secretion, plasma levels of A771726 are expected to be increased in patients with hypoproteinaemia. Arava is contraindicated in patients with severe hypoproteinaemia or impairment of liver function (see section 4.3).

Haematological reactions

Together with ALT, a complete blood cell count, including differential white blood cell count and platelets, must be performed before start of leflunomide treatment as well as every 2 weeks for the first 6 months of treatment and every 8 weeks thereafter.

In patients with pre-existing anaemia, leucopenia, and/or thrombocytopenia as well as in patients with impaired bone marrow function or those at risk of bone marrow suppression, the risk of haematological disorders is increased. If such effects occur, a washout (see below) to reduce plasma levels of A771726 should be considered.

In case of severe haematological reactions, including pancytopenia, Arava and any concomitant myelosuppressive medication must be discontinued and a leflunomide washout procedure initiated.

Combinations with other treatments

The use of leflunomide with antimalarials used in rheumatic diseases (e.g. chloroquine and hydroxychloroquine), intramuscular or oral gold, D-penicillamine, azathioprine and other immunosuppressive agents (with the exception of methotrexate, see section 4.5) has not been studied up to now.

The risk associated with combination therapy, in particular in long-term treatment, is unknown. Since such therapy can lead to additive or even synergistic toxicity (e.g. hepato- or haematotoxicity), combination with another DMARD (e.g. methotrexate) is not advisable.

Caution is advised when leflunomide is given together with drugs, other than NSAIDs, metabolised by CYP2C9 such as phenytoin, warfarin, phenprocoumon and tolbutamide.

Switching to other treatments

As leflunomide has a long persistence in the body, a switching to another DMARD (e.g. methotrexate) without performing the washout procedure (see below) may raise the possibility of additive risks even for a long time after the switching (i.e. kinetic interaction, organ toxicity).

Similarly, recent treatment with hepatotoxic or haematotoxic drugs (e.g. methotrexate) may result in increased side-effects; therefore, the initiation of leflunomide treatment has to carefully be considered regarding these benefit/risk aspects and closer monitoring is recommended in the initial phase after switching.

Skin reactions

In case of ulcerative stomatitis, leflunomide administration should be discontinued.

Very rare cases of Stevens-Johnson syndrome or toxic epidermal necrolysis have been reported in patients treated with leflunomide. As soon as skin and/or mucosal reactions are observed which raise the suspicion of such severe reactions, Arava and any other possibly associated medication must be discontinued, and a leflunomide washout procedure initiated immediately. A complete washout is essential in such cases. In such cases re-exposure to leflunomide is contra-indicated (see section 4.3).

Infections

It is known that medications with immunosuppressive properties - like leflunomide – may cause patients to be more susceptible to infections, including opportunistic infections. Infections may be more severe in nature and may, therefore, require early and vigorous treatment. In the event that severe, uncontrolled infections occur, it may be necessary to interrupt leflunomide treatment and administer a washout procedure as described below.

Patients with tuberculin reactivity must be carefully monitored because of the risk of tuberculosis reactivation.

Respiratory reactions

Interstitial Lung disease has been reported during treatment with leflunomide (see section 4.8).

Interstitial Lung disease is a potentially fatal disorder, which may occur acutely during therapy. Pulmonary symptoms, such as cough and dyspnoea, may be a reason for discontinuation of the therapy and for further investigation, as appropriate.

Blood Pressure

Blood pressure must be checked before the start of leflunomide treatment and periodically thereafter.

Procreation (recommendations for men)

Male patients should be aware of the possible male-mediated foetal toxicity. Reliable contraception during treatment with leflunomide should also be guaranteed.

There are no specific data on the risk of male-mediated foetal toxicity. However, animal studies to evaluate this specific risk have not been conducted. To minimise any possible risk, men wishing to father a child should consider discontinuing use of leflunomide and taking cholestyramine 8 g 3 times daily for 11 days or 50 g of activated powdered charcoal 4 times daily for 11 days.

In either case the A771726 plasma concentration is then measured for the first time. Thereafter, the A771726 plasma concentration must be determined again after an interval of at least 14 days. If both plasma concentrations are below 0.02 mg/l, and after a waiting period of at least 3 months, the risk of foetal toxicity is very low.

Washout procedure

Cholestyramine 8 g is administered 3 times daily. Alternatively, 50 g of activated powdered charcoal is administered 4 times daily. Duration of a complete washout is usually 11 days. The duration may be modified depending on clinical or laboratory variables.

Lactose

Patients with rare hereditary problems of galactose intolerance, the Lapp lactase deficiency or glucose-galactose malabsorption should not take this medicine.

4.5 Interaction with other medicinal products and other forms of Interaction

Increased side-effects may occur in case of recent or concomitant use of hepatotoxic or haematotoxic drugs or when leflunomide treatment is followed by such drugs without a washout period (see also guidance concerning combination with other treatments, section 4.4). Therefore, closer monitoring of liver and haematological parameters is recommended in the initial phase after switching.

In a small (n=30) study with co-administration of leflunomide (10 to 20 mg per day) with methotrexate (10 to 25 mg per week) a 2-to 3-fold elevation in liver enzymes was seen on 5 of 30 patients. All elevations resolved, 2 with continuation of both drugs and 3 after discontinuation of leflunomide. A more than 3-fold increase was seen in another 5 patients. All of these also resolved, 2 with continuation of both drugs and 3 after discontinuation of leflunomide.

In patients with rheumatoid arthritis, no pharmacokinetic interaction between the leflunomide (10 to 20 mg per day) and methotrexate (10 to 25 mg per week) was demonstrated.

It is recommended that patients receiving leflunomide are not treated with cholestyramine or activated powdered charcoal because this leads to a rapid and significant decrease in plasma A771726 (the active metabolite of leflunomide; see also section 5) concentration. The mechanism is thought to be by interruption of enterohepatic recycling and/or gastrointestinal dialysis of A771726.

If the patient is already receiving nonsteroidal anti-inflammatory drugs (NSAIDs) and/or corticosteroids, these may be continued after starting leflunomide.

The enzymes involved in the metabolism of leflunomide and its metabolites are not exactly known. An *in vivo* interaction study with cimetidine (non-specific cytochrome P450 inhibitor) has demonstrated a lack of a significant interaction. Following concomitant administration of a single dose of leflunomide to subjects receiving multiple doses of rifampicin (non-specific cytochrome P450 inducer) A771726 peak levels were increased by approximately 40%, whereas the AUC was not significantly changed. The mechanism of this effect is unclear.

In vitro studies indicate that A771726 inhibits cytochrome P4502C9 (CYP2C9) activity. In clinical trials no safety problems were observed when leflunomide and NSAIDs metabolised by CYP2C9 were co-administered. Caution is advised when leflunomide is given together with drugs, other than NSAIDs, metabolised by CYP2C9 such as phenytoin, warfarin, phenprocoumon and tolbutamide.

In a study in which leflunomide was given concomitantly with a triphasic oral contraceptive pill containing 30 μg ethinyloestradiol to healthy female volunteers, there was no reduction in contraceptive activity of the pill, and A771726 pharmacokinetics were within predicted ranges.

Vaccinations

No clinical data are available on the efficacy and safety of vaccinations under leflunomide treatment. Vaccination with live attenuated vaccines is, however, not recommended. The long half-life of leflunomide should be considered when contemplating administration of a live attenuated vaccine after stopping Arava.

4.6 Pregnancy and lactation

Pregnancy

The active metabolite of leflunomide, A771726, is suspected to cause serious birth defects when administered during pregnancy.

Arava is contraindicated (see 4.3) in pregnancy.

Women of childbearing potential have to use effective contraception during and up to 2 years after treatment (see "waiting period" below) or up to 11 days after treatment (see abbreviated "washout period" below).

The patient must be advised that if there is any delay in onset of menses or any other reason to suspect pregnancy, they must notify the physician immediately for pregnancy testing, and if positive, the physician and patient must discuss the risk to the pregnancy. It is possible that rapidly lowering the blood level of the active metabolite, by instituting the drug elimination procedure described below, at the first delay of menses may decrease the risk to the foetus from leflunomide.

For women receiving leflunomide treatment and who wish to become pregnant, one of the following procedures is recommended in order to ascertain that the foetus is not exposed to toxic concentrations of A771726 (target concentration below 0.02 mg/l):

Waiting period:

A771726 plasma levels can be expected to be above 0.02 mg/l for a prolonged period. The concentration may be expected to decrease below 0.02 mg/l about 2 years after stopping the treatment with leflunomide.

After a 2-year waiting period, the A771726 plasma concentration is measured for the first time. Thereafter, the A771726 plasma concentration must be determined again after an interval of at least 14 days. If both plasma concentrations are below 0.02 mg/l no teratogenic risk is to be expected.

For further information on the sample testing please contact the Marketing Authorisation Holder or its local representative (see section 7).

Washout procedure:

After stopping treatment with leflunomide:

• cholestyramine 8 g is administered 3 times daily for a period of 11 days.

• alternatively, 50 g of activated powdered charcoal is administered 4 times daily for a period of 11 days.

However, also following either of the washout procedures, verification by 2 separate tests at an interval of at least 14 days and a waiting period of one-and-a-half months between the first occurrence of a plasma concentration below 0.02 mg/l and fertilisation is required.

Women of childbearing potential should be told that a waiting period of 2 years after treatment discontinuation is required before they may become pregnant. If a waiting period of up to approximately 2 years under reliable contraception is considered unpractical, prophylactic institution of a washout procedure may be advisable.

Both cholestyramine and activated powdered charcoal may influence the absorption of oestrogens and progestogens such that reliable contraception with oral contraceptives may not be guaranteed during the washout procedure with cholestyramine or activated powdered charcoal. Use of alternative contraceptive methods is recommended.

Lactation

Animal studies indicate that leflunomide or its metabolites pass into breast milk. Breast-feeding women must, therefore, not receive leflunomide.

4.7 Effects on ability to drive and use machines

In the case of side-effects such as dizziness the patient's ability to concentrate and to react properly may be impaired. In such cases patients should refrain from driving cars and using machines.

4.8 Undesirable effects

Classification of expected frequencies:

Common $>1/100$, $<1/10$; uncommon $>1/1000$, $<1/100$; rare $>1/10,000$, $<1/1000$; very rare $<1/10,000$.

Infections and infestations

Very rare: severe infections, including sepsis which may be fatal.

Like other agents with immunosuppressive potential, leflunomide may increase susceptibility to infections, including opportunistic infections (see also section 4.4). Thus, the overall incidence of infections can increase (in particular of rhinitis, bronchitis and pneumonia).

Blood and lymphatic system disorders

Common: leucopenia (leucocytes >2 G/l)

Uncommon: anaemia, mild thrombocytopenia (platelets <100 G/l)

Rare: eosinophilia, leucopenia (leucocytes <2 G/l), pancytopenia (probably by antiproliferative mechanism)

Very rare: agranulocytosis

Recent, concomitant or consecutive use of potentially myelotoxic agents may be associated with a higher risk of haematological effects.

The risk of malignancy, particularly lymphoproliferative disorders, is increased with use of some immunosuppressive agents.

Immune system disorders

Common: mild allergic reactions

Very rare: severe anaphylactic/anaphylactoid reactions, vasculitis

Metabolism and nutrition disorders

Common: anorexia, weight loss (usually insignificant)

Uncommon: hypokalaemia

Psychiatric disorders

Uncommon: anxiety

Nervous system disorders

Common: headache, dizziness, paraesthesia

Very rare: peripheral neuropathy

Cardiac disorders

Common: mild increase in blood pressure

Rare: severe increase in blood pressure

Respiratory, thoracic and mediastinal disorders

Rare: interstitial lung disease (including interstitial pneumonitis) which may be fatal.

Gastrointestinal disorders

Common: diarrhoea, nausea, vomiting, oral mucosal disorders (e.g., aphthous stomatitis, mouth ulceration), abdominal pain,

Uncommon: taste disturbances

Very rare: pancreatitis

Hepato-biliary disorders

Common: elevation of liver parameters (transaminases [especially ALT], less often gamma-GT, alkaline phosphatase, bilirubin)

Rare: hepatitis, jaundice/cholestasis and very rarely, severe liver injury such as hepatic failure and acute hepatic necrosis that may be fatal

Skin and subcutaneous tissue disorders

Common: increased hair loss, eczema, dry skin, rash (including maculopapular rash), pruritus

Uncommon: urticaria

Very rare: Stevens-Johnson syndrome, toxic epidermal necrolysis, erythema multiforme

Musculoskeletal and connective tissue disorders

Common: tenosynovitis

Uncommon: tendon rupture

General disorders and administration site conditions

Common: asthenia

Mild hyperlipidaemia may occur. Uric acid levels usually decrease.

Laboratory findings for which a clinical relevance could not be established include small increases in LDH and CK. Mild hypophosphataemia is uncommon.

Marginal (reversible) decreases in sperm concentration, total sperm count and rapid progressive motility cannot be excluded.

The active metabolite of leflunomide, A771726, has a long half-life, usually 1 to 4 weeks. If a severe undesirable effect of leflunomide occurs, or if for any other reason A771726 needs to be cleared rapidly from the body, the washout procedure described in section 4.4 has to be followed. The procedure may be repeated as clinically necessary. For suspected severe immunological/allergic reactions such as Stevens-Johnson syndrome or toxic epidermal necrolysis, a complete washout is essential.

4.9 Overdose

Symptoms

There have been reports of chronic overdose in patients taking Arava at daily doses up to five times the recommended daily dose, and reports of acute overdose in adults and children.

There were no adverse events reported in the majority of case reports of overdose. Adverse events consistent with the safety profile for leflunomide were: abdominal pain, nausea, diarrhoea, elevated liver enzymes, anaemia, leucopenia, pruritus and rash.

Management

In the event of an overdose or toxicity, cholestyramine or charcoal is recommended to accelerate elimination. Cholestyramine given orally at a dose of 8 g three times a day for 24 hours to three healthy volunteers decreased plasma levels of A771726 by approximately 40% in 24 hours and by 49% to 65% in 48 hours.

Administration of activated charcoal (powder made into a suspension) orally or via nasogastric tube (50 g every 6 hours for 24 hours) has been shown to reduce plasma concentrations of the active metabolite A771726 by 37% in 24 hours and by 48% in 48 hours.

These washout procedures may be repeated if clinically necessary.

Studies with both hemodialysis and CAPD (chronic ambulatory peritoneal dialysis) indicate that A771726, the primary metabolite of leflunomide, is not dialysable.

5. PHARMACOLOGICAL PROPERTIES

5.1 Pharmacodynamic properties

Pharmacotherapeutic group: selective immunosuppressive agents, ATC Code: L04AA13

Human pharmacology

Leflunomide is a disease-modifying anti-rheumatic agent with antiproliferative properties.

Animal pharmacology

Leflunomide is effective in animal models of arthritis and of other autoimmune diseases and transplantation, mainly if administered during the sensitisation phase. It has immunomodulating/ immunosuppressive characteristics, acts as an antiproliferative agent, and displays anti-inflammatory properties. Leflunomide exhibits the best protective effects on animal models of autoimmune diseases when administered in the early phase of the disease progression.

In vivo, it is rapidly and almost completely metabolised to A771726 which is active *in vitro*, and is presumed to be responsible for the therapeutic effect.

Mode of action

A771726, the active metabolite of leflunomide, inhibits the human enzyme dihydroorotate dehydrogenase (DHODH) and exhibits antiproliferative activity.

Rheumatoid Arthritis

The efficacy of Arava in the treatment of rheumatoid arthritis was demonstrated in 4 controlled trials (1 in phase II and 3 in phase III). The phase II trial, study YU203, randomised 402 subjects with active rheumatoid arthritis to placebo (n=102), leflunomide 5 mg (n=95), 10 mg (n=101) or 25 mg/day (n=104). The treatment duration was 6 months.

All leflunomide patients in the phase III trials used an initial dose of 100 mg for 3 days.

Study MN301 randomised 358 subjects with active rheumatoid arthritis to leflunomide 20 mg/day (n=133), sulphasalazine 2 g/day (n=133), or placebo (n=92). Treatment duration was 6 months.

Study MN303 was an optional 6-month blinded continuation of MN301 without the placebo arm, resulting in a 12-month comparison of leflunomide and sulphasalazine.

Study MN302 randomised 999 subjects with active rheumatoid arthritis to leflunomide 20 mg/day (n=501) or methotrexate at 7.5 mg/week increasing to 15 mg/week (n=498). Folate supplementation was optional and only used in 10% of patients. Treatment duration was 12 months.

Study US301 randomised 482 subjects with active rheumatoid arthritis to leflunomide 20 mg/day (n=182), methotrexate 7.5 mg/week increasing to 15 mg/week (n=182), or placebo (n=118). All patients received folate 1 mg bid. Treatment duration was 12 months.

Leflunomide at a daily dose of at least 10 mg (10 to 25 mg in study YU203, 20 mg in studies MN301 and US301) was statistically significantly superior to placebo in reducing the signs and symptoms of rheumatoid arthritis in all 3 placebo-controlled trials. The ACR (American College of Rheumatology) response rates in study YU203 were 27.7% for placebo, 31.9% for 5 mg, 50.5% for 10 mg and 54.5% for 25 mg/day. In the phase III trials, the ACR response rates for leflunomide 20 mg/day vs. placebo were 54.6% vs. 28.6% (study MN301), and 49.4% vs. 26.3% (study US301). After 12 months with active treatment, the ACR response rates in leflunomide patients were 52.3% (studies MN301/303), 50.5% (study MN302) and 49.4% (study US301), compared to 53.8% (studies MN301/303) in sulphasalazine patients, 64.8% (study MN302), and 43.9% (study US301) in methotrexate patients. In study MN302 leflunomide was significantly less effective than methotrexate. However, in study US301 no significant differences were observed between leflunomide and methotrexate in the primary efficacy parameters. No difference was observed between leflunomide and sulphasalazine (study MN301). The leflunomide treatment effect was evident by 1 month, stabilised by 3 to 6 months and continued throughout the course of treatment.

A randomised, double-blind, parallel group non-inferiority study compared the relative efficacy of two different daily maintenance doses of leflunomide, 10 mg and 20 mg. From the results it can be concluded that efficacy results of the 20 mg maintenance dose were more favourable, on the other hand, the safety results favoured the 10 mg daily maintenance dose.

Psoriatic Arthritis

The efficacy of Arava was demonstrated in one controlled, randomised double blind study 3L01 in 188 patients with psoriatic arthritis, treated at 20 mg/day. Treatment duration was 6 months.

Leflunomide 20 mg/day was significantly superior to placebo in reducing the symptoms of arthritis in patients with psoriatic arthritis: the PsARC (Psoriatic Arthritis treatment Response Criteria) responders were 59% in the leflunomide group and 29.7% in the placebo group by 6 months ($p < 0.0001$). The effect of leflunomide on improvement of function and on reduction of skin lesions was modest.

5.2 Pharmacokinetic properties

Leflunomide is rapidly converted to the active metabolite, A771726, by first-pass metabolism (ring opening) in gut wall and liver. In a study with radiolabelled ^{14}C-leflunomide in three healthy volunteers, no unchanged leflunomide was detected in plasma, urine or faeces. In other studies, unchanged leflunomide levels in plasma have rarely been detected, however, at ng/ml plasma levels. The only plasma radiolabelled metabolite detected was A771726. This metabolite is responsible for essentially all the *in vivo* activity of Arava.

Absorption

Excretion data from the ^{14}C study indicated that at least about 82 to 95% of the dose is absorbed. The time to peak plasma concentrations of A771726 is very variable; peak plasma levels can occur between 1 hour and 24 hours after single administration. Leflunomide can be administered with food, since the extent of absorption is comparable in the fed and fasting state. Due to the very long half-life of A771726 (approximately 2 weeks), a loading dose of 100 mg for 3 days was used in clinical studies to facilitate the rapid attainment of steady-state levels of A771726. Without a loading dose, it is estimated that attainment of steady-state plasma concentrations would require nearly two months of dosing. In multiple dose studies in patients with rheumatoid arthritis, the pharmacokinetic parameters of A771726 were linear over the dose range of 5 to 25 mg. In these studies, the clinical effect was closely related to the plasma concentration of A771726 and to the daily dose of leflunomide. At a dose level of 20 mg/day, average plasma concentration of A771726 at steady state is approximately 35 μg/ml. At steady state plasma levels accumulate about 33-to 35-fold compared with single dose.

Distribution

In human plasma, A771726 is extensively bound to protein (albumin). The unbound fraction of A771726 is about 0.62%. Binding of A771726 is linear in the therapeutic concentration range. Binding of A771726 appeared slightly reduced and more variable in plasma from patients with rheumatoid arthritis or chronic renal insufficiency. The extensive protein binding of A771726 could lead to displacement of other highly-bound drugs. *In vitro* plasma protein binding interaction studies with warfarin at clinically relevant concentrations, however, showed no interaction. Similar studies showed that ibuprofen and diclofenac did not displace A771726, whereas the unbound fraction of A771726 is increased 2- to 3- fold in the presence of tolbutamide. A771726 displaced ibuprofen, diclofenac and tolbutamide but the unbound fraction of these drugs is only increased by 10% to 50%. There is no indication that these effects are of clinical relevance. Consistent with extensive protein binding A771726 has a low apparent volume of distribution (approximately 11 litres). There is no preferential uptake in erythrocytes.

Metabolism

Leflunomide is metabolised to one primary (A771726) and many minor metabolites including TFMA (4-trifluoromethylaniline). The metabolic biotransformation of leflunomide to A771726 and subsequent metabolism of A771726 is not controlled by a single enzyme and has been shown to occur in microsomal and cytosolic cellular fractions. Interaction studies with cimetidine (non-specific cytochrome P450 inhibitor) and rifampicin (non-specific cytochrome P450 inducer), indicate that *in vivo* CYP enzymes are involved in the metabolism of leflunomide only to a small extent.

Elimination

Elimination of A771726 is slow and characterised by an apparent clearance of about 31 ml/hr. The elimination half-life in patients is approximately 2 weeks. After administration of a radiolabelled dose of leflunomide, radioactivity was equally excreted in faeces, probably by biliary elimination, and in urine. A771726 was still detectable in urine and faeces 36 days after a single administration.The principal urinary metabolites were glucuronide products derived from leflunomide (mainly in 0 to 24 hour samples) and an oxanilic acid derivative of A771726. The principal faecal component was A771726.

It has been shown in man that administration of an oral suspension of activated powdered charcoal or cholestyramine leads to a rapid and significant increase in A771726 elimination rate and decline in plasma concentrations (see section 4.9). This is thought to be achieved by a gastrointestinal dialysis mechanism and/or by interrupting enterohepatic recycling.

Pharmacokinetics in renal failure

Leflunomide was administered as a single oral 100 mg dose to 3 haemodialysis patients and 3 patients on continuous peritoneal dialysis (CAPD). The pharmacokinetics of A771726 in CAPD patients appeared to be similar to healthy volunteers. A more rapid elimination of A771726 was observed in haemodialysis subjects which was not due to extraction of drug in the dialysate.

Pharmacokinetics in liver failure

No data are available regarding treatment of patients with hepatic impairment. The active metabolite A771726 is extensively protein bound and cleared via hepatic metabolism and biliary secretion. These processes may be affected by hepatic dysfunction.

Influence of age

Pharmacokinetics in subjects under 18 years have not been studied. Pharmacokinetic data in elderly (> 65 years) are limited but consistent with pharmacokinetics in younger adults.

5.3 Preclinical safety data

Leflunomide, administered orally and intraperitoneally, has been studied in acute toxicity studies in mice and rats. Repeated oral administration of leflunomide to mice for up to 3 months, to rats and dogs for up to 6 months and to monkeys for up to 1 month's duration revealed that the major target organs for toxicity were bone marrow, blood, gastrointestinal tract, skin, spleen, thymus and lymph nodes. The main effects were anaemia, leucopenia, decreased platelet counts and panmyelopathy and reflect the basic mode of action of the compound (inhibition of

DNA synthesis). In rats and dogs, Heinz bodies and/or Howell-Jolly bodies were found. Other effects found on heart, liver, cornea and respiratory tract could be explained as infections due to immunosuppression. Toxicity in animals was found at doses equivalent to human therapeutic doses.

Leflunomide was not mutagenic. However, the minor metabolite TFMA (4-trifluoromethylaniline) caused clastogenicity and point mutations *in vitro*, whilst insufficient information was available on its potential to exert this effect *in vivo*.

In a carcinogenicity study in rats, leflunomide did not show carcinogenic potential. In a carcinogenicity study in mice an increased incidence of malignant lymphoma occurred in males of the highest dose group, considered to be due to the immunosuppressive activity of leflunomide. In female mice an increased incidence, dose-dependent, of bronchiolo-alveolar adenomas and carcinomas of the lung was noted. The relevance of the findings in mice relative to the clinical use of leflunomide is uncertain.

Leflunomide was not antigenic in animal models.

Leflunomide was embryotoxic and teratogenic in rats and rabbits at doses in the human therapeutic range and exerted adverse effects on male reproductive organs in repeated dose toxicity studies. Fertility was not reduced.

6. PHARMACEUTICAL PARTICULARS

6.1 List of excipients

Tablet core:

Arava 10 mg film-coated tablets: Maize starch, povidone (E1201), crospovidone (E1202), silica colloidal anhydrous, magnesium stearate (E470b), lactose monohydrate.

Arava 20 mg film-coated tablets: Maize starch, povidone (E1201), crospovidone (E1202), silica colloidal anhydrous, magnesium stearate (E470b), lactose monohydrate.

Arava 100 mg film-coated tablets: Maize starch, povidone (E1201), crospovidone (E1202), talc (E553b), silica colloidal anhydrous, magnesium stearate (E470b), lactose monohydrate.

Film-Coating:

Arava 10 mg film-coated tablets: Talc (E553b), hypromellose (E464), titanium dioxide (E171), macrogol 8000.

Arava 20 mg film-coated tablets: Talc (E553b), hypromellose (E464), titanium dioxide (E171), macrogol 8000, and yellow ferric oxide (E172).

Arava 100 mg film-coated tablets: Talc (E553b), hypromellose (E464), titanium dioxide (E171), macrogol 8000.

6.2 Incompatibilities

Not applicable.

6.3 Shelf life

3 years.

6.4 Special precautions for storage

Blister: Store in the original package.

Bottle: Keep the container tightly closed.

6.5 Nature and contents of container

Arava 10 mg and Arava 20 mg film-coated tablets:

Bottle: HDPE wide-necked bottle, 100 ml with screw cap with integrated desiccant container. Pack size: 30 film-coated tablets.

Arava 100 mg film-coated tablets:

Aluminium / Aluminium blister. Pack size: 3 film-coated tablets.

6.6 Instructions for use and handling

No special requirements.

7. MARKETING AUTHORISATION HOLDER

Aventis Pharma Deutschland GmbH

D-69526 Frankfurt am Main

Germany

8. MARKETING AUTHORISATION NUMBER(S)

Arava 10 mg film-coated tablets: EU/1/99/118/003

Arava 20 mg film-coated tablets: EU/1/99/118/007

Arava 100 mg film-coated tablets: EU/1/99/118/009

9. DATE OF FIRST AUTHORISATION/RENEWAL OF THE AUTHORISATION

Date of first authorisation: 02 September 1999

Date of last renewal: 13 October 2004

10. DATE OF REVISION OF THE TEXT

December 2004

11. Legal Category

POM

Arcoxia 60 mg, 90 mg & 120 mg Tablets

(Merck Sharp & Dohme Limited)

1. NAME OF THE MEDICINAL PRODUCT

ARCOXIA® 60 mg Film-coated Tablets ▼

ARCOXIA® 90 mg Film-coated Tablets ▼

ARCOXIA® 120 mg Film Coated Tablets ▼

2. QUALITATIVE AND QUANTITATIVE COMPOSITION

Each film-coated tablet contains 60, 90 or 120 mg of etoricoxib.

For excipients, see 6.1.

3. PHARMACEUTICAL FORM

Film-coated tablet.

60 mg Tablets: Green, apple-shaped, biconvex tablets debossed '447' on one side and 'MSD' on the other side.

90 mg Tablets: White, apple-shaped, biconvex tablets debossed '454' on one side and 'MSD' on the other side.

120 mg Tablets: Pale-green, apple-shaped, biconvex tablets debossed '541' on one side and 'MSD' on the other side.

4. CLINICAL PARTICULARS

4.1 Therapeutic indications

For the symptomatic relief of osteoarthritis (OA), rheumatoid arthritis (RA) and the pain and signs of inflammation associated with acute gouty arthritis.

The decision to prescribe a selective COX-2 inhibitor should be based on an assessment of the individual patient's overall risks (see 4.3, 4.4).

4.2 Posology and method of administration

ARCOXIA is administered orally and may be taken with or without food. The onset of drug effect may be faster when ARCOXIA is administered without food. This should be considered when rapid symptomatic relief is needed.

Osteoarthritis

The recommended dose is 60 mg once daily.

Rheumatoid arthritis

The recommended dose is 90 mg once daily.

Acute gouty arthritis

The recommended dose is 120 mg once daily. Etoricoxib 120 mg should be used only for the acute symptomatic period. In clinical trials for acute gouty arthritis, etoricoxib was given for 8 days.

Doses greater than those recommended for each indication have either not demonstrated additional efficacy or have not been studied. Therefore, the dose for each indication is the maximum recommended dose.

The dose for OA should not exceed 60 mg daily.

The dose for RA should not exceed 90 mg daily.

The dose for acute gout should not exceed 120 mg daily, limited to a maximum of 8 days treatment.

As the cardiovascular risks of etoricoxib may increase with dose and duration of exposure, the shortest duration possible and the lowest effective daily dose should be used. The patient's need for symptomatic relief and response to therapy should be re-evaluated periodically, especially in patients with osteoarthritis (see 4.3, 4.4, 4.8 and 5.1).

Elderly: No dosage adjustment is necessary for elderly patients.

Hepatic insufficiency: In patients with mild hepatic dysfunction (Child-Pugh score 5-6) a dose of 60 mg once daily should not be exceeded. In patients with moderate hepatic dysfunction (Child-Pugh score 7-9) the recommended dose of 60 mg ***every other day*** should not be exceeded.

Clinical experience is limited, particularly in patients with moderate hepatic dysfunction and caution is advised. There is no clinical experience in patients with severe hepatic dysfunction (Child-Pugh score ⩾10); therefore, its use is contraindicated in these patients (see 4.3, 4.4 and 5.2).

Renal insufficiency: No dosage adjustment is necessary for patients with creatinine clearance ⩾30 ml/min (see 5.2). The use of etoricoxib in patients with creatinine clearance <30 ml/min is contraindicated (see 4.3 and 4.4).

Paediatric use: Etoricoxib is contraindicated in children and adolescents under 16 years of age.

4.3 Contraindications

History of hypersensitivity to the active substance or to any of the excipients (see 6.1).

Active peptic ulceration or active gastro-intestinal (GI) bleeding.

Patients who have experienced bronchospasm, acute rhinitis, nasal polyps, angioneurotic oedema, urticaria, or allergic-type reactions after taking acetylsalicylic acid or NSAIDs including COX-2 (cyclo-oxygenase-2) inhibitors.

Pregnancy and lactation (see 4.6 and 5.3).

Severe hepatic dysfunction (serum albumin <25 g/l or Child-Pugh score ⩾10).

Estimated renal creatinine clearance <30 ml/min.

Children and adolescents under 16 years of age.

Inflammatory bowel disease.

Congestive heart failure (NYHA II-IV).

Patients with hypertension whose blood pressure has not been adequately controlled.

Established ischaemic heart disease and/or cerebrovascular disease.

4.4 Special warnings and special precautions for use

Gastro-intestinal effects

Upper gastro-intestinal complications [perforations, ulcers or bleedings (PUBs)], some of them resulting in fatal outcome, have occurred in patients treated with etoricoxib.

Caution is advised with treatment of patients most at risk of developing a gastro-intestinal complication with NSAIDs: the elderly, patients using any other NSAID or acetylsalicylic acid concomitantly, or patients with a prior history of gastro-intestinal disease, such as ulceration and GI bleeding.

There is a further increase in the risk of gastro-intestinal adverse effects (gastro-intestinal ulceration or other gastro-intestinal complications) when etoricoxib is taken concomitantly with acetylsalicylic acid (even at low doses). A significant difference in GI safety between selective COX-2 inhibitors + acetylsalicylic acid *vs.* NSAIDs + acetylsalicylic acid has not been demonstrated in long-term clinical trials (see 5.1).

Cardiovascular effects

Clinical trials suggest that the selective COX-2 inhibitor class of drugs may be associated with a risk of thrombotic events (especially MI and stroke), relative to placebo and some NSAIDs. As the cardiovascular risks of etoricoxib may increase with dose and duration of exposure, the shortest duration possible and the lowest effective daily dose should be used. The patient's need for symptomatic relief and response to therapy should be re-evaluated periodically, especially in patients with osteoarthritis (see 4.2, 4.3, 4.8 and 5.1).

Patients with significant risk factors for cardiovascular events (e.g. hypertension, hyperlipidaemia, diabetes mellitus, smoking) or peripheral arterial disease should only be treated with etoricoxib after careful consideration (see 5.1).

COX-2 selective inhibitors are not a substitute for acetylsalicylic acid for prophylaxis of cardiovascular thromboembolic diseases because of their lack of antiplatelet effect. Therefore antiplatelet therapies should not be discontinued (see 4.5 and 5.1).

Renal effects

Renal prostaglandins may play a compensatory role in the maintenance of renal perfusion. Therefore, under conditions of compromised renal perfusion, administration of etoricoxib may cause a reduction in prostaglandin formation and, secondarily, in renal blood flow, and thereby impair renal function. Patients at greatest risk of this response are those with pre-existing significantly impaired renal function, uncompensated heart failure, or cirrhosis. Monitoring of renal function in such patients should be considered.

Fluid retention, oedema and hypertension

As with other drugs known to inhibit prostaglandin synthesis, fluid retention, oedema and hypertension have been observed in patients taking etoricoxib. Caution should be exercised in patients with a history of cardiac failure, left ventricular dysfunction, or hypertension and in patients with pre-existing oedema from any other reason. If there is clinical evidence of deterioration in the condition of these patients, appropriate measures including discontinuation of etoricoxib should be taken.

Etoricoxib may be associated with more frequent and severe hypertension than some other NSAIDs and selective COX-2 inhibitors, particularly at high doses. Therefore, special attention should be paid to blood pressure monitoring during treatment with etoricoxib. If blood pressure rises significantly, alternative treatment should be considered.

Hepatic effects

Elevations of alanine aminotransferase (ALT) and/or aspartate aminotransferase (AST) (approximately three or more times the upper limit of normal) have been reported in approximately 1% of patients in clinical trials treated for up to one year with etoricoxib 60 and 90 mg daily.

Any patients with symptoms and/or signs suggesting liver dysfunction, or in whom an abnormal liver function test has occurred, should be monitored. If signs of hepatic insufficiency occur, or if persistently abnormal liver function tests (three times the upper limit of normal) are detected, etoricoxib should be discontinued.

General

If during treatment, patients deteriorate in any of the organ system functions described above, appropriate measures should be taken and discontinuation of etoricoxib therapy should be considered. Medically appropriate supervision should be maintained when using etoricoxib in the elderly and in patients with renal, hepatic, or cardiac dysfunction.

Caution should be used when initiating treatment with etoricoxib in patients with dehydration. It is advisable to rehydrate patients prior to starting therapy with etoricoxib.

Serious skin reactions, including exfoliative dermatitis, Stevens-Johnson syndrome, and toxic epidermal necrolysis, have been reported in association with the use of NSAIDs including other COX-2 (cyclo-oxygenase-2) inhibitors and cannot be ruled out for etoricoxib (see 4.8). Hypersensitivity reactions (anaphylaxis, angioedema) have been reported in patients receiving etoricoxib (see 4.8). Etoricoxib should be discontinued at the first sign of hypersensitivity.

Etoricoxib may mask fever and other signs of inflammation.

Caution should be exercised when co-administering etoricoxib with warfarin or other oral anticoagulants (see 4.5).

The use of etoricoxib, as with any medicinal product known to inhibit cyclo-oxygenase/prostaglandin synthesis, is not recommended in women attempting to conceive (see 4.6, 5.1 and 5.3).

ARCOXIA tablets contain lactose. Patients with rare hereditary problems of galactose intolerance, the Lapp lactase deficiency or glucose-galactose malabsorption should not take this medicine.

4.5 Interaction with other medicinal products and other forms of Interaction

Pharmacodynamic interactions

Oral anticoagulants: In subjects stabilised on chronic warfarin therapy, the administration of etoricoxib 120 mg daily was associated with an approximate 13% increase in prothrombin time International Normalised Ratio (INR). Therefore, patients receiving oral anticoagulants should be closely monitored for their prothrombin time INR, particularly in the first few days when therapy with etoricoxib is initiated or the dose of etoricoxib is changed (see 4.4).

Diuretics, ACE inhibitors and Angiotensin II Antagonists: NSAIDs may reduce the effect of diuretics and other antihypertensive drugs. In some patients with compromised renal function (e.g. dehydrated patients or elderly patients with compromised renal function) the co-administration of an ACE inhibitor or angiotensin II antagonist and agents that inhibit cyclo-oxygenase may result in further deterioration of renal function, including possible acute renal failure, which is usually reversible. These interactions should be considered in patients taking etoricoxib concomitantly with ACE inhibitors or angiotensin II antagonists. Therefore the combination should be administered with caution, especially in the elderly. Patients should be adequately hydrated and consideration should be given to monitoring of renal function after initiation of concomitant therapy, and periodically thereafter.

Acetylsalicylic Acid: In a study in healthy subjects, at steady state, etoricoxib 120 mg once daily had no effect on the anti-platelet activity of acetylsalicylic acid (81 mg once daily). Etoricoxib can be used concomitantly with acetylsalicylic acid at doses used for cardiovascular prophylaxis (low-dose acetylsalicylic acid). However, concomitant administration of low-dose acetylsalicylic acid with etoricoxib may result in an increased rate of GI ulceration or other complications compared to use of etoricoxib alone. Concomitant administration of etoricoxib with doses of acetylsalicylic acid *above* those for cardiovascular prophylaxis or with other NSAIDs is not recommended. (See 5.1 and 4.4.)

Ciclosporin and tacrolimus: Although this interaction has not been studied with etoricoxib, co-administration of ciclosporin or tacrolimus with any NSAID may increase the nephrotoxic effect of ciclosporin or tacrolimus. Renal function should be monitored when etoricoxib and either of these drugs is used in combination.

Pharmacokinetic interactions

The effect of etoricoxib on the pharmacokinetics of other drugs

Lithium: NSAIDs decrease lithium renal excretion and therefore increase lithium plasma levels. If necessary, monitor blood lithium closely and adjust the lithium dosage while the combination is being taken and when the NSAID is withdrawn.

Methotrexate: Two studies investigated the effects of etoricoxib 60, 90 or 120 mg administered once daily for seven days in patients receiving once-weekly methotrexate doses of 7.5 to 20 mg for rheumatoid arthritis. Etoricoxib at 60 and 90 mg had no effect on methotrexate plasma concentrations or renal clearance. In one study, etoricoxib 120 mg had no effect, but in the other study, etoricoxib 120 mg increased methotrexate plasma concentrations by 28% and reduced renal clearance of methotrexate by 13%. Adequate monitoring for methotrexate-related toxicity is recommended when etoricoxib and methotrexate are administered concomitantly.

Oral contraceptives: Etoricoxib 60 mg given concomitantly with an oral contraceptive containing 35 mcg ethinyl estradiol (EE) and 0.5 to 1 mg norethindrone for 21 days increased the steady state $AUC_{0\text{-}24hr}$ of EE by 37%. Etoricoxib 120 mg given with the same oral contraceptive concomitantly or separated by 12 hours, increased the steady state $AUC_{0\text{-}24hr}$ of EE by 50 to 60%. This increase in EE concentration should be considered when selecting an oral contraceptive for use with etoricoxib. An increase in EE exposure can increase the incidence of adverse events associated with oral contraceptives (e.g. venous thrombo-embolic events in women at risk).

Hormone Replacement Therapy: Administration of etoricoxib 120 mg with hormone replacement therapy consisting of conjugated estrogens (0.625 mg Premarin® Wyeth) for 28 days, increased the mean steady state $AUC_{0\text{-}24hr}$ of unconjugated estrone (41%), equilin (76%) and 17-β-estradiol (22%). The effect of the recommended chronic doses of etoricoxib (60 and 90 mg) has not been studied. The effects of etoricoxib 120 mg on the exposure ($AUC_{0\text{-}24hr}$) to these estrogenic components of Premarin were less than half of those observed when Premarin was administered alone and the dose was increased from 0.625 to 1.25 mg. The clinical significance of these increases is unknown, and higher doses of Premarin were not studied in combination with etoricoxib. These increases in estrogenic concentration should be taken into consideration when selecting post-menopausal hormone therapy for use with etoricoxib because the increase in estrogen exposure might increase the risk of adverse events associated with HRT.

Prednisone/prednisolone: In drug-interaction studies, etoricoxib did not have clinically important effects on the pharmacokinetics of prednisone/prednisolone.

Digoxin: Etoricoxib 120 mg administered once daily for 10 days to healthy volunteers did not alter the steady-state plasma $AUC_{0\text{-}24hr}$ or renal elimination of digoxin. There was an increase in digoxin C_{max} (approximately 33%). This increase is not generally important for most patients. However, patients at high risk of digoxin toxicity should be monitored for this when etoricoxib and digoxin are administered concomitantly.

Effect of etoricoxib on drugs metabolised by sulfotransferases

Etoricoxib is an inhibitor of human sulfotransferase activity, particularly SULT1E1, and has been shown to increase the serum concentrations of ethinyl estradiol. While knowledge about effects of multiple sulfotransferases is presently limited and the clinical consequences for many drugs are still being examined, it may be prudent to exercise care when administering etoricoxib concurrently with other drugs primarily metabolised by human sulfotransferases (e.g. oral salbutamol and minoxidil).

Effect of etoricoxib on drugs metabolised by CYP isoenzymes

Based on *in vitro* studies, etoricoxib is not expected to inhibit cytochromes P450 (CYP) 1A2, 2C9, 2C19, 2D6, 2E1 or 3A4. In a study in healthy subjects, daily administration of etoricoxib 120 mg did not alter hepatic CYP3A4 activity as assessed by the erythromycin breath test.

Effects of other drugs on the pharmacokinetics of etoricoxib

The main pathway of etoricoxib metabolism is dependent on CYP enzymes. CYP3A4 appears to contribute to the metabolism of etoricoxib *in vivo. In vitro* studies indicate that CYP2D6, CYP2C9, CYP1A2 and CYP2C19 also can catalyse the main metabolic pathway, but their quantitative roles have not been studied *in vivo*.

Ketoconazole: Ketoconazole, a potent inhibitor of CYP3A4, dosed at 400 mg once a day for 11 days to healthy volunteers, did not have any clinically important effect on the single-dose pharmacokinetics of 60 mg etoricoxib (43% increase in AUC).

Rifampicin: Co-administration of etoricoxib with rifampicin, a potent inducer of CYP enzymes, produced a 65% decrease in etoricoxib plasma concentrations. This interaction may result in recurrence of symptoms when etoricoxib is co-administered with rifampicin. While this information may suggest an increase in dose, doses of etoricoxib greater than those listed for each indication have not been studied in combination with rifampicin and are therefore not recommended (see 4.2).

Antacids: Antacids do not affect the pharmacokinetics of etoricoxib to a clinically relevant extent.

4.6 Pregnancy and lactation

Pregnancy

The use of etoricoxib, as with any drug substance known to inhibit COX-2, is not recommended in women attempting to conceive.

No clinical data on exposed pregnancies are available for etoricoxib. Studies in animals have shown reproductive toxicity (see 5.3). The potential for human risk in pregnancy is unknown. Etoricoxib, as with other medicinal products inhibiting prostaglandin synthesis, may cause uterine inertia and premature closure of the ductus arteriosus during the last trimester. Etoricoxib is contraindicated in pregnancy (see 4.3). If a woman becomes pregnant during treatment, etoricoxib should be discontinued.

Lactation

It is not known whether etoricoxib is excreted in human milk. Etoricoxib is excreted in the milk of lactating rats. Women who use etoricoxib should not breast feed. (See 4.3 and 5.3.)

4.7 Effects on ability to drive and use machines

No studies on the effect of etoricoxib on the ability to drive or use machines have been performed. However, patients who experience dizziness, vertigo or somnolence while taking etoricoxib should refrain from driving or operating machinery.

4.8 Undesirable effects

In clinical trials, etoricoxib was evaluated for safety in approximately 4,800 individuals, including approximately 3,400 patients with OA, RA or chronic low back pain (approximately 600 patients with OA or RA were treated for one year or longer).

In clinical studies, the undesirable effects profile was similar in patients with OA or RA treated with etoricoxib for one year or longer.

In a clinical study for acute gouty arthritis, patients were treated with etoricoxib 120 mg once daily for eight days. The adverse experience profile in this study was generally similar to that reported in the combined OA, RA, and chronic low back pain studies.

The following undesirable effects were reported at an incidence greater than placebo in clinical trials in patients with OA, RA or chronic low back pain treated with etoricoxib 60 mg or 90 mg for up to 12 weeks or in post-marketing experience:

[Very Common (>1/10) Common (>1/100, <1/10) Uncommon (>1/1000, <1/100) Rare (>1/10,000, <1/1,000) Very rare (<1/10,000) including isolated cases]

Infections and infestations:

Uncommon: gastro-enteritis, upper respiratory infection, urinary tract infection.

Immune system disorder:

Very rare: hypersensitivity reactions, including angioedema, anaphylactic/ anaphylactoid reactions.

Metabolism and nutrition disorders:

Common: oedema/fluid retention.

Uncommon: appetite increase or decrease, weight gain.

Psychiatric disorders:

Uncommon: anxiety, depression, mental acuity decreased.

Nervous system disorder:

Common: dizziness, headache.

Uncommon: dysgeusia, insomnia, paraesthesia/ hypaesthesia, somnolence.

Eye disorders:

Uncommon: blurred vision.

Ear and labyrinth disorders:

Uncommon: tinnitus.

Cardiac disorders:

Uncommon: congestive heart failure, non-specific ECG changes.

Very rare: myocardial infarction.

Vascular disorders:

Common: hypertension.

Uncommon: flushing.

Very rare: cerebrovascular accident.

Respiratory, thoracic and mediastinal disorders:

Uncommon: cough, dyspnoea, epistaxis.

Gastro-intestinal disorders:

Common: gastro-intestinal disorders (e.g. abdominal pain, flatulence, heartburn), diarrhoea, dyspepsia, epigastric discomfort, nausea.

Uncommon: abdominal distention, acid reflux, bowel movement pattern change, constipation, dry mouth, gastroduodenal ulcer, irritable bowel syndrome, oesophagitis, oral ulcer, vomiting.

Very rare: peptic ulcers including gastro-intestinal perforation and bleeding (mainly in the elderly).

Skin and subcutaneous tissue disorders:

Uncommon: ecchymosis, facial oedema, pruritus, rash.

Very rare: urticaria.

Musculoskeletal, connective tissue and bone disorders:

Uncommon: muscular cramp/spasm, musculoskeletal pain/stiffness.

Renal and urinary disorders:

Uncommon: proteinuria.

Very rare: renal insufficiency, including renal failure, usually reversible upon discontinuation of treatment (see 4.4).

General disorders and administration site conditions:

Common: asthenia/fatigue, flu-like disease.

Uncommon: chest pain.

Investigations:

Common: ALT increased, AST increased.

Uncommon: blood urea nitrogen increased, creatine phosphokinase increased, haematocrit decreased, haemoglobin decreased, hyperkalaemia, leukocytes decreased, platelets decreased, serum creatinine increased, uric acid increased.

The following serious undesirable effects have been reported in association with the use of NSAIDs and cannot be ruled out for etoricoxib: nephrotoxicity including interstitial nephritis and nephrotic syndrome; hepatotoxicity including hepatic failure and jaundice; cutaneo-mucosal adverse effects and severe skin reactions (see 4.4).

4.9 Overdose

No overdoses of etoricoxib were reported during clinical trials.

In clinical studies, administration of single doses of etoricoxib up to 500 mg and multiple doses up to 150 mg/day for 21 days did not result in significant toxicity.

In the event of overdose, it is reasonable to employ the usual supportive measures, e.g. remove unabsorbed material from the GI tract, employ clinical monitoring, and institute supportive therapy, if required.

Etoricoxib is not dialysable by haemodialysis; it is not known whether etoricoxib is dialysable by peritoneal dialysis.

5. PHARMACOLOGICAL PROPERTIES

5.1 Pharmacodynamic properties

Pharmacotherapeutic group: Anti-inflammatory and antirheumatic products, non-steroids, coxibs

ATC Code: MO1 AH05

Etoricoxib is an oral, selective cyclo-oxygenase-2 (COX-2) inhibitor within the clinical dose range.

Across clinical pharmacology studies, ARCOXIA produced dose-dependent inhibition of COX-2 without inhibition of COX-1 at doses up to 150 mg daily. Etoricoxib did not inhibit gastric prostaglandin synthesis and had no effect on platelet function.

Cyclo-oxygenase is responsible for generation of prostaglandins. Two isoforms, COX-1 and COX-2, have been identified. COX-2 is the isoform of the enzyme that has been shown to be induced by pro-inflammatory stimuli and has been postulated to be primarily responsible for the synthesis of prostanoid mediators of pain, inflammation, and fever. COX-2 is also involved in ovulation, implantation and closure of the ductus arteriosus, regulation of renal function, and central nervous system functions (fever induction, pain perception and cognitive function). It may also play a role in ulcer healing. COX-2 has been identified in tissue around gastric ulcers in man but its relevance to ulcer healing has not been established.

Approximately 3,100 patients were treated with etoricoxib ⩾60 mg daily for 12 weeks or longer. There was no discernible difference in the rate of serious thrombotic cardiovascular events between patients receiving etoricoxib ⩾60 mg, placebo, or non-naproxen NSAIDs. However, the rate of these events was higher in patients receiving etoricoxib compared with those receiving naproxen 500 mg twice daily. The difference in antiplatelet activity between some COX-1 inhibiting NSAIDs and COX-2 selective inhibitors may be of clinical significance in patients at risk of thrombo-embolic events. COX-2 inhibitors reduce the formation of systemic (and therefore possibly endothelial) prostacyclin without affecting platelet thromboxane. The clinical relevance of these observations has not been established.

A study of approximately 7,100 osteoarthritis patients compared the gastrointestinal tolerability of etoricoxib 90 mg (1.5 times the recommended OA dose) with diclofenac 150 mg. Patients were treated for a median duration of 11 months. Use of gastroprotective agents and low dose aspirin were permitted in the study. The gastrointestinal and cardiovascular safety data are summarised below.

Gastrointestinal tolerability and safety results: Etoricoxib was associated with a statistically significantly lower incidence of patient withdrawals due to a predefined composite endpoint of clinical gastrointestinal adverse events and laboratory adverse events related to elevated liver function tests compared to diclofenac. The incidence of clinical gastrointestinal events leading to withdrawal was statistically significantly lower for etoricoxib versus diclofenac (7.1% versus 9.1% respectively). The rates for confirmed upper gastrointestinal perforations, ulcerations and bleeds were the same for etoricoxib and diclofenac (1.11 events per 100 patient years).

The following additional safety results were observed in the study:

Cardiovascular data:The event rates for serious thrombotic events were: Etoricoxib 1.25 events per 100 patient years versus 1.15 events per 100 patient years for diclofenac (relative risk 1.07, 95% CI: 0.65%, 1.74%). The rates of myocardial infarction were 0.68 versus 0.42 events per 100 patient years on etoricoxib and diclofenac respectively. The rates of ischaemic stroke were 0.14 versus 0.23 per 100 patient years on etoricoxib versus diclofenac respectively.

Cardiorenal events: Statistically significantly more patients treated with etoricoxib than diclofenac experienced adverse effects associated with hypertension (11.7% versus 5.9%) and oedema (7.5% versus 5.9%). A higher rate of discontinuation due to hypertension was seen (2.3% versus 0.7%) and this was statistically significant. The incidence of patient discontinuations due to oedema was 0.9% for etoricoxib versus 0.7% for diclofenac The incidence of congestive heart failure was 0.4% for etoricoxib versus 0.2% for diclofenac.

Hepatic adverse events: Etoricoxib was associated with a statistically significantly lower rate of withdrawals than diclofenac (0.3% versus 5.2%), due largely to elevations in liver function tests. The majority of elevations in liver function tests on diclofenac that resulted in discontinuation were greater than 3 times the upper limit of normal.

In patients with osteoarthritis (OA), etoricoxib 60 mg once daily provided significant improvements in pain and patient assessments of disease status. These beneficial effects were observed as early as the second day of therapy and maintained for up to 52 weeks.

In patients with rheumatoid arthritis (RA), etoricoxib 90 mg once daily provided significant improvements in pain, inflammation, and mobility. These beneficial effects were maintained over the 12-week treatment periods.

In patients experiencing attacks of acute gouty arthritis, etoricoxib 120 mg once daily over an eight-day treatment period, relieved moderate to extreme joint pain and inflammation comparable to indomethacin 50 mg three times daily. Pain relief was observed as early as four hours after initiation of treatment.

In studies specifically designed to measure the onset of action of etoricoxib, the onset of action occurred as early as 24 minutes after dosing.

In two 12-week double-blind endoscopy studies, the cumulative incidence of gastroduodenal ulceration was significantly lower in patients treated with etoricoxib 120 mg once daily than in patients treated with either naproxen 500 mg twice daily or ibuprofen 800 mg three times daily. Etoricoxib had a higher incidence of ulceration as compared to placebo.

A prespecified, combined analysis of eight clinical trials of approximately 4,000 patients with OA, RA, or chronic low back pain assessed the incidence rate for the following end-points: 1) discontinuation for upper GI symptoms; 2) discontinuation for any GI adverse experiences; 3) new use of gastroprotective medications and 4) new use of any GI medications. There was an approximate 50% risk reduction for these end-points in patients treated with etoricoxib (60, 90 or 120 mg daily) as compared to patients treated with naproxen 500 mg twice daily or diclofenac 50 mg three times daily. There were no statistically significant differences between etoricoxib and placebo.

A randomised, double-blind, placebo-controlled, parallel-group study evaluated the effects of 15 days of treatment of etoricoxib (90 mg), celecoxib (200 mg bid), naproxen (500 mg bid) and placebo on urinary sodium excretion, blood pressure, and other renal function parameters in subjects 60 to 85 years of age on a 200-mEq /day sodium diet. Etoricoxib, celecoxib, and naproxen had similar effects on urinary sodium excretion over the 2 weeks of treatment. All active comparators showed an increase relative to placebo with respect to systolic blood pressures; however, etoricoxib was associated with a statistically significant increase at Day 14 when compared to celecoxib and naproxen (mean change from baseline for systolic blood pressure: etoricoxib 7.7 mmHg, celecoxib 2.4 mmHg, naproxen 3.6 mmHg).

5.2 Pharmacokinetic properties

Absorption

Orally administered etoricoxib is well absorbed. The absolute bioavailability is approximately 100%. Following 120 mg once-daily dosing to steady state, the peak plasma concentration (geometric mean C_{max} = 3.6 μg/ml) was observed at approximately 1 hour (T_{max}) after administration to fasted adults. The geometric mean area under the curve (AUC_{0-24hr}) was 37.8 μg•hr/ml. The pharmacokinetics of etoricoxib are linear across the clinical dose range.

Dosing with food (a high-fat meal) had no effect on the extent of absorption of etoricoxib after administration of a 120 mg dose. The rate of absorption was affected, resulting in a 36% decrease in C_{max} and an increase in T_{max} by 2 hours. These data are not considered clinically significant. In clinical trials, etoricoxib was administered without regard to food intake.

Distribution

Etoricoxib is approximately 92% bound to human plasma protein over the range of concentrations of 0.05 to 5 μg/ml. The volume of distribution at steady state (V_{dss}) was approximately 120 l in humans.

Etoricoxib crosses the placenta in rats and rabbits, and the blood-brain barrier in rats.

Metabolism

Etoricoxib is extensively metabolised with <1% of a dose recovered in urine as the parent drug. The major route of metabolism to form the 6'-hydroxymethyl derivative is catalysed by CYP enzymes. CYP3A4 appears to contribute to the metabolism of etoricoxib *in vivo. In vitro* studies indicate that CYP2D6, CYP2C9, CYP1A2 and CYP2C19 also can catalyse the main metabolic pathway, but their quantitative roles *in vivo* have not been studied.

Five metabolites have been identified in man. The principal metabolite is the 6'-carboxylic acid derivative of etoricoxib formed by further oxidation of the 6'-hydroxymethyl derivative. These principal metabolites either demonstrate no measurable activity or are only weakly active as COX-2 inhibitors. None of these metabolites inhibit COX-1.

Elimination

Following administration of a single 25-mg radiolabeled intravenous dose of etoricoxib to healthy subjects, 70% of radioactivity was recovered in urine and 20% in faeces, mostly as metabolites. Less than 2% was recovered as unchanged drug.

Elimination of etoricoxib occurs almost exclusively through metabolism followed by renal excretion. Steady state concentrations of etoricoxib are reached within seven days of once daily administration of 120 mg, with an accumulation ratio of approximately 2, corresponding to a half-life of approximately 22 hours. The plasma clearance after a 25-mg intravenous dose is estimated to be approximately 50 ml/min.

Characteristics in patients

Elderly: Pharmacokinetics in the elderly (65 years of age and older) are similar to those in the young.

Gender: The pharmacokinetics of etoricoxib are similar between men and women.

Hepatic insufficiency: Patients with mild hepatic dysfunction (Child-Pugh score 5-6) administered etoricoxib 60 mg once daily had an approximately 16% higher mean AUC as compared to healthy subjects given the same regimen. Patients with moderate hepatic dysfunction (Child-Pugh score 7-9) administered etoricoxib 60 mg ***every other day*** had similar mean AUC to the healthy subjects given etoricoxib 60 mg once daily. There are no clinical or pharmacokinetic data in patients with severe hepatic dysfunction (Child-Pugh score ⩾10). (See 4.2 and 4.3.)

Renal insufficiency: The pharmacokinetics of a single dose of etoricoxib 120 mg in patients with moderate to severe renal insufficiency and patients with end-stage renal disease on haemodialysis were not significantly different from those in healthy subjects. Haemodialysis contributed negligibly to elimination (dialysis clearance approximately 50 ml/min). (See 4.3 and 4.4.)

Paediatric patients: The pharmacokinetics of etoricoxib in paediatric patients (<12 years old) have not been studied.

In a pharmacokinetic study (n=16) conducted in adolescents (aged 12 to 17) the pharmacokinetics in adolescents weighing 40 to 60 kg given etoricoxib 60 mg once daily and adolescents >60 kg given etoricoxib 90 mg once daily were similar to the pharmacokinetics in adults given etoricoxib 90 mg once daily. Safety and effectiveness of etoricoxib in paediatric patients have not been established. (See 4.2 *'Paediatric use'*.)

5.3 Preclinical safety data

In preclinical studies, etoricoxib has been demonstrated not to be genotoxic. Etoricoxib was not carcinogenic in mice. Rats developed hepatocellular and thyroid follicular cell adenomas at >2-times the daily human dose [90 mg] based on systemic exposure when dosed daily for approximately two years. Hepatocellular and thyroid follicular cell adenomas observed in rats are considered to be a consequence of rat-specific mechanism related to hepatic CYP enzyme induction. Etoricoxib has not been shown to cause hepatic CYP3A enzyme induction in humans.

In the rat, gastro-intestinal toxicity of etoricoxib increased with dose and exposure time. In the 14-week toxicity study, etoricoxib caused gastro-intestinal ulcers at exposures greater than those seen in man at the therapeutic dose. In the 53- and 106-week toxicity study, gastro-intestinal ulcers were also seen at exposures comparable to those seen in man at the therapeutic dose. In dogs, renal and gastro-intestinal abnormalities were seen at high exposures.

Etoricoxib was not teratogenic in reproductive toxicity studies conducted in rats at 15 mg/kg/day (this represents approximately 1.5 times the daily human dose [90 mg] based on systemic exposure). In rabbits, no treatment-related external or skeletal foetal malformations were seen. A non-dose-related low incidence of cardiovascular malformations was observed in etoricoxib-treated rabbits. The relationship to treatment is not established. In rats and rabbits, no embryo/foetal effects were seen at systemic exposures equal to or less than those at the daily human dose [90 mg]. However, there was a decrease in embryo/foetal survival at exposures greater than or equal to 1.5 times the human exposure. (See 4.3 and 4.6.)

Etoricoxib is excreted in the milk of lactating rats at concentrations approximately two-fold those in plasma. There was a decrease in pup body weight following exposure of pups to milk from dams administered etoricoxib during lactation.

6. PHARMACEUTICAL PARTICULARS

6.1 List of excipients

Core: Calcium hydrogen phosphate (anhydrous), croscarmellose sodium, magnesium stearate, microcrystalline cellulose.

Tablet coating: Carnauba wax, lactose monohydrate, hypromellose, titanium dioxide (E171), glycerol triacetate. The 60- and 120-mg tablets also contain indigo carmine lake (E132) and yellow ferric oxide (E172).

6.2 Incompatibilities

Not applicable.

6.3 Shelf life

2 years.

6.4 Special precautions for storage

Bottles: Keep the container tightly closed.

Blisters: Store in the original package.

6.5 Nature and contents of container

Aluminum/aluminium blisters in packs containing 2, 5, 7, 10, 14, 20, 28, 30, 50, 84, 98 or 100 tablets.

Aluminum/aluminium blisters (unit doses) in packs of 50 or 100 tablets.

White, round, HDPE bottles with a white, polypropylene closure containing 30 or 90 tablets.

Not all pack sizes may be marketed.

6.6 Instructions for use and handling
No special requirements.

7. MARKETING AUTHORISATION HOLDER
Merck Sharp & Dohme Limited
Hertford Road, Hoddesdon, Hertfordshire EN11 9BU, UK

8. MARKETING AUTHORISATION NUMBER(S)
60 mg Tablets PL 0025/0422
90 mg Tablets PL 0025/0423
120 mg Tablets PL 0025/0424

9. DATE OF FIRST AUTHORISATION/RENEWAL OF THE AUTHORISATION
60 mg Tablets 13 February 2002
90 mg Tablets 13 February 2002
120 mg Tablets 13 February 2002

10. DATE OF REVISION OF THE TEXT
May 2005

LEGAL CATEGORY
POM

® denotes registered trademark of Merck & Co., Inc., Whitehouse Station, NJ, USA.

SPC.ACX.05.UK-IRL.2183 II-011/007

AREDIA Dry Powder 15mg, 30mg and 90mg

(Novartis Pharmaceuticals UK Ltd)

1. NAME OF THE MEDICINAL PRODUCT
Aredia® Dry Powder 15mg
Aredia® Dry Powder 30mg
Aredia® Dry Powder 90mg

2. QUALITATIVE AND QUANTITATIVE COMPOSITION
The active ingredient is disodium 3-amino-1-hydroxypropylidene-1,1-bisphosphonate pentahydrate (pamidronate disodium).

One vial contains 15mg, 30mg or 90mg of sterile, lyophilised pamidronate disodium. An ampoule containing 5mL sterile water for injections is supplied with each 15mg vial, and a 10mL ampoule with each 30mg or 90mg vial.

3. PHARMACEUTICAL FORM
Powder and solvent for solution for infusion.

4. CLINICAL PARTICULARS
4.1 Therapeutic indications
Treatment of conditions associated with increased osteoclast activity:

Tumour-induced hypercalcaemia

Osteolytic lesions and bone pain in patients with bone metastases associated with breast cancer or multiple myeloma

Paget's disease of bone.

4.2 Posology and method of administration
Aredia must never be given as a bolus injection (see Section 4.4 Special warnings and special precautions for use). The reconstituted solution of Aredia from powder in vials should be diluted in a calcium-free infusion solution (0.9 % w/v sodium chloride solution or 5% w/v glucose solution) and infused slowly.

The infusion rate should never exceed 60mg/hour (1mg/min), and the concentration of Aredia in the infusion solution should not exceed 60mg/250ml. In patients with established or suspected renal impairment (e.g. those with tumour-induced hypercalcaemia or multiple myeloma) it is recommended that the infusion rate does not exceed 20mg/h (see also Section 4.2 Posology and method of administration "Renal impairment"). In order to minimise local reactions at the infusion site, the cannula should be inserted carefully into a relatively large vein.

Tumour-induced hypercalcaemia

It is recommended that patients be rehydrated with 0.9% w/v sodium chloride solution before or during treatment.

The total dose of Aredia to be used for a treatment course depends on the patient's initial serum calcium levels. The following guidelines are derived from clinical data on uncorrected calcium values. However, doses within the ranges given are also applicable for calcium values corrected for serum protein or albumin in rehydrated patients.

Initial serum calcium		Recommended total
(mmol/L)	(mg %)	dose (mg)
up to 3.0	up to 12.0	15 - 30
3.0 - 3.5	12.0 - 14.0	30 - 60
3.5 - 4.0	14.0 - 16.0	60 - 90
> 4.0	> 16.0	90

The total dose of Aredia may be administered either in a single infusion or in multiple infusions over 2-4 consecutive days. The maximum dose per treatment course is 90 mg for both initial and repeated courses.

A significant decrease in serum calcium is generally observed 24-48 hours after administration of Aredia, and normalisation is usually achieved within 3 to 7 days. If normocalcaemia is not achieved within this time, a further dose may be given. The duration of the response may vary from patient to patient, and treatment can be repeated whenever hypercalcaemia recurs. Clinical experience to date suggests that Aredia may become less effective as the number of treatments increases.

Osteolytic lesions and bone pain in multiple myeloma

The recommended dose is 90mg every 4 weeks.

Osteolytic lesions and bone pain in bone metastases associated with breast cancer

The recommended dose is 90mg every 4 weeks. This dose may also be administered at 3 weekly intervals to coincide with chemotherapy if desired.

Paget's disease of Bone

The recommended treatment course consists of a total dose of 180mg administered in unit doses of either 30mg once a week for 6 consecutive weeks, or 60mg every other week over 6 weeks. Experience to date suggests that any mild and transient unwanted effects (see Section 4.8 Undesirable effects) tend to occur after the first dose. For this reason if unit doses of 60mg are used it is recommended that treatment be started with an initial dose of 30mg followed by 60mg every other week (i.e. total dose 210mg). Each dose of 30 or 60mg should be diluted in 125 or 250 ml 0.9% w/v sodium chloride solution respectively, and the infusion rate should not exceed 60mg/hour (1mg/min). This regimen or increased dose levels according to disease severity, up to a maximum total dose of 360mg (in divided doses of 60mg) can be repeated every 6 months until remission of disease is achieved, and if relapse occurs.

Renal Impairment

Aredia should not be administered to patients with severe renal impairment (creatinine clearance < 30 mL/min) unless in cases of life-threatening tumour-induced hypercalcaemia where the benefit outweighs the potential risk. Because there is only limited clinical experience in patients with severe renal impairment no dose recommendations for this patient population can be made (see Section 4.4 "Special warnings and special precautions for use" and Section 5.2 "Pharmacokinetic properties").

As with other i.v. bisphosphonates, renal monitoring is recommended, for instance, measurement of serum creatinine prior to each dose of Aredia. In patients receiving Aredia for bone metastases who show evidence of deterioration in renal function, Aredia treatment should be withheld until renal function returns to within 10% of the baseline value. This recommendation is based on a clinical study, in which renal deterioration was defined as follows:

- For patients with normal baseline creatinine, increase of 0.5mg/dL.
- For patients with abnormal baseline creatinine, increase of 1.0mg/dL.

A pharmacokinetic study conducted in patients with cancer and normal or impaired renal function indicates that the dose adjustment is not necessary in mild (creatinine clearance 61-90 mL/min) to moderate renal impairment (creatinine clearance 30-60 mL/min). In such patients, the infusion rate should not exceed 90 mg/4h (approximately 20-22 mg/h).

Hepatic impairment

Although patients with hepatic impairment exhibited higher mean AUC and Cmax values compared to patients with normal hepatic function, this is not perceived being clinically relevant. As pamidronate is still rapidly cleared from the plasma almost entirely into the bone and as is administered on a monthly basis for chronic treatment, drug accumulation is not expected. Therefore no dose adjustment is necessary in patients with mild to moderate abnormal hepatic function (see Section 5.2 Pharmacokinetic properties "Hepatic impairment"). Clinical data in patients with severe hepatic impairment is not available. Pamidronate should be administered to this patient population with caution.

Children

There is no clinical experience with Aredia in children. Therefore until further experience is gained, Aredia is only recommended for use in adult patients.

4.3 Contraindications
Known hypersensitivity to pamidronate or to other bisphosphonates, or any of the other ingredients of Aredia.

4.4 Special warnings and special precautions for use
Warnings

Aredia should not be given as a bolus injection, but should always be diluted and given as a slow intravenous infusion (see Section 4.2 Posology and method of administration).

Bisphosphonates, including Aredia, have been associated with renal toxicity manifested as deterioration of renal function and potential renal failure. Due to the risk of clinically significant deterioration in renal function which may progress to renal failure, single doses of Aredia should not exceed 90mg, and the recommended infusion time should be observed (See Section 4.2. Posology and method of administration).

As with other i.v. bisphosphonates renal monitoring is recommended, for instance, measurement of serum creatinine prior to each dose of Aredia. Patients treated with Aredia for bone metastases should have the dose withheld if renal function has deteriorated (see Section 4.2. Posology and method of administration).

Aredia should not be administered to patients with severe renal impairment (creatinine clearance < 30 mL/min) unless in cases of life-threatening tumour-induced hypercalcaemia where the benefit outweighs the potential risk. (See section 4.2 Posology and method of administration "Renal impairment"). Because there is only limited pharmacokinetic data with severe renal impairment no dose recommendations for this patient population can be made (See Section 4.2 "Posology and method of administration" and Section 5.2 "Pharmacokinetic properties").Aredia should not be given with other bisphosphonates because their combined effects have not been investigated.

Convulsions have been precipitated in some patients with tumour-induced hypercalcaemia due to the electrolyte changes associated with this condition and its effective treatment.

Precautions

Standard hypercalcaemia-related metabolic parameters including serum, calcium and phosphate should be monitored following initiation of therapy with Aredia. Patients who have undergone thyroid surgery may be particularly susceptible to developing hypocalcaemia due to relative hypoparathyroidism.

Aredia is excreted intact primarily via the kidney (see Section 5.2 Pharmacokinetic properties), thus the risk of renal adverse reactions may be greater in patients with impaired renal function.

Deterioration of renal function (including renal failure) has been reported following long-term treatment with Aredia in patients with multiple myeloma.

As there are no clinical data available in patients with severe hepatic insufficiency, no specific recommendations can be given for this patient population.

There is very little experience of the use of Aredia in patients receiving haemodialysis.

In patients with cardiac disease, especially in the elderly, additional saline overload may precipitate cardiac failure (left ventricular failure or congestive heart failure). Fever (influenza-like symptoms) may also contribute to this deterioration.

Patients with Paget's disease of the bone who are at risk of calcium or Vitamin D deficiency (e.g. through malabsorption or lack of exposure to sunlight) should take oral supplements of both during Aredia therapy to minimise the potential risk of hypocalcaemia.

Osteonecrosis of the jaw has been reported in patients with cancer receiving treatment regimens including bisphosphonates. Many of these patients were also receiving chemotherapy and corticosteroids. The majority of reported cases have been associated with dental procedures such as tooth extraction. Many had signs of local infection including osteomyelitis.

A dental examination with appropriate preventive dentistry should be considered prior to treatment with bisphosphonates in patients with concomitant risk factors (e.g. cancer, chemotherapy, corticosteroids, poor oral hygiene).

While on treatment, these patients should avoid invasive dental procedures if possible. For patients who develop osteonecrosis of the jaw while on bisphosphonate therapy, dental surgery may exacerbate the condition. For patients requiring dental procedures, there are no data available to suggest whether discontinuation of bisphosphonate treatment reduces the risk of osteonecrosis of the jaw. Clinical judgement of the treating physician should guide the management plan of each patient based on individual benefit/risk assessment.

4.5 Interaction with other medicinal products and other forms of Interaction
Aredia has been administered concomitantly with commonly used anticancer agents without interactions occurring.

Aredia has been used in combination with calcitonin in patients with severe hypercalcaemia, resulting in a synergistic effect producing a more rapid fall in serum calcium.

Caution is warranted when Aredia is used with other potentially nephrotoxic drugs.

In multiple myeloma patients, the risk of renal dysfunction may be increased when Aredia is used in combination with thalidomide.

Since pamidronate binds to bone, it could in theory interfere with bone scintigraphy examinations.

4.6 Pregnancy and lactation
In animal experiments, pamidronate showed no teratogenic potential and did not affect general reproductive performance or fertility. In rats, prolonged parturition and reduced survival rate of pups were probably caused by a decrease in maternal serum calcium levels. In pregnant rats, pamidronate has been shown to cross the placental barrier and accumulate in fetal bone in a manner similar to that observed in adult animals.

There is insufficient clinical experience to support the use of Aredia in pregnant women. Therefore, Aredia should not be administered during pregnancy except in cases of life-threatening hypercalcaemia.

A study in lactating rats has shown that pamidronate will pass into the milk. Mothers treated with Aredia should therefore not breast-feed their infants.

4.7 Effects on ability to drive and use machines

Patients should be warned that in rare cases somnolence and/or dizziness may occur following Aredia infusion, in which case they should not drive, operate potentially dangerous machinery, or engage in other activities that may be hazardous because of decreased alertness.

4.8 Undesirable effects

Adverse reactions to Aredia are usually mild and transient. The most common adverse reactions are asymptomatic hypocalcaemia and fever (an increase in body temperature of 1-2°C), typically occurring within the first 48 hours of infusion. Fever usually resolves spontaneously and does not require treatment.

Frequency estimate: very common (≥1/10), common (≥1/100, <1/10), uncommon (≥1/1,000, <1/100), rare (≥1,10,000, <1/1,000), very rare (<1/10,000) including isolated reports.

General disorders and administration site conditions

Very common: fever and influenza-like symptoms sometimes accompanied by malaise, rigor, fatigue and flushes

Common: reactions at the infusion site: pain, redness, swelling, induration, phlebitis, thrombophlebitis

Musculoskeletal system

Common: transient bone pain, arthralgia, myalgia, generalised pain.

Uncommon: muscle cramps.

Gastrointestinal tract

Common: nausea, vomiting, anorexia, abdominal pain, diarrhoea, constipation, gastritis.

Uncommon: dyspepsia.

Central nervous system

Common: symptomatic hypocalcaemia (paresthesia, tetany), headache, insomnia, somnolence.

Uncommon: seizures, agitation, dizziness, lethargy.

Very rare: confusion, visual hallucinations.

Blood

Common: anaemia, thrombocytopenia, lymphocytopenia.

Very rare: leukopenia.

Cardiovascular system

Common: hypertension.

Uncommon: hypotension.

Very rare: left ventricular failure (dyspnoea, pulmonary oedema), congestive heart failure (oedema) due to fluid overload.

Renal system

Uncommon: acute renal failure.

Rare: focal segmental glomerulosclerosis including the collapsing variant, nephrotic syndrome.

Very rare: deterioration of pre-existing renal disease, haematuria.

Skin

Common: rash

Uncommon: pruritus.

Special senses

Common: conjunctivitis.

Uncommon: uveitis (iritis, iridocyclitis).

Very rare: scleritis, episcleritis, xanthopsia.

Infection

Very rare: reactivation of Herpes simplex, reactivation of Herpes zoster.

Immune system

Uncommon: allergic reactions including anaphylactoid reactions, bronchospasm/dyspnoea, Quincke's (angioneurotic) oedema.

Very rare: anaphylactic shock

Biochemical changes

Very common: hypocalcaemia, hypophosphataemia.

Common: hypokalaemia, hypomagnesaemia, increase in serum creatinine.

Uncommon: abnormal liver function tests, increase in serum urea.

Very rare: hyperkalaemia, hypernatraemia.

Postmarketing: Very rare cases of osteonecrosis (primarily of the jaw) have been reported in patients treated with bisphosphonates. Many had signs of local infection including osteomyelitis. The majority of the reports refer to cancer patients following tooth extractions or other dental surgeries. Osteonecrosis of the jaw has multiple well documented risk factors including a diagnosis of cancer, concomitant therapies (e.g. chemotherapy, radiotherapy, corticosteroids) and co-morbid conditions (e.g. anaemia, coagulopathies, infection, pre-existing oral disease). Although causality cannot be determined, it is prudent to avoid dental surgery as recovery may be prolonged (see section 4.4 Special warnings and special precautions for use).

4.9 Overdose

Patients who have received doses higher than those recommended should be carefully monitored. In the event of clinically significant hypocalcaemia with paraesthesia, tetany and hypotension, reversal may be achieved with an infusion of calcium gluconate.

5. PHARMACOLOGICAL PROPERTIES

5.1 Pharmacodynamic properties

Pharmacotherapeutic group: Inhibitor of bone resorption (ATC code MO5B A 03).

Pamidronate disodium, the active substance of Aredia, is a potent inhibitor of osteoclastic bone resorption. It binds strongly to hydroxyapatite crystals and inhibits the formation and dissolution of these crystals *in vitro*. Inhibition of osteoclastic bone resorption *in vivo* may be at least partly due to binding of the drug to the bone mineral.

Pamidronate suppresses the accession of osteoclast precursors onto the bone. However, the local and direct antiresorptive effect of bone-bound bisphosphonate appears to be the predominant mode of action *in vitro* and *in vivo*.

Experimental studies have demonstrated that pamidronate inhibits tumour-induced osteolysis when given prior to or at the time of inoculation or transplantation with tumour cells. Biochemical changes reflecting the inhibitory effect of Aredia on tumour-induced hypercalcaemia, are characterised by a decrease in serum calcium and phosphate and secondarily by decreases in urinary excretion of calcium, phosphate, and hydroxyproline.

Hypercalcaemia can lead to a depletion in the volume of extracellular fluid and a reduction in the glomerular filtration rate (GFR). By controlling hypercalcaemia, Aredia improves GFR and lowers elevated serum creatinine levels in most patients.

Clinical trials in patients with breast cancer and predominantly lytic bone metastases or with multiple myeloma showed that Aredia prevented or delayed skeletal-related events (hypercalcaemia, fractures, radiation therapy, surgery to bone, spinal cord compression) and decreased bone pain

Paget's disease of bone, which is characterised by local areas of increased bone resorption and formation with qualitative changes in bone remodelling, responds well to treatment with Aredia. Clinical and biochemical remission of the disease has been demonstrated by bone scintigraphy, decreases in urinary hydroxyproline and serum alkaline phosphatase, and by symptomatic improvement.

5.2 Pharmacokinetic properties

General characteristics

Pamidronate has a strong affinity for calcified tissues, and total elimination of pamidronate from the body is not observed within the time-frame of experimental studies. Calcified tissues are therefore regarded as site of "apparent elimination".

Absorption

Pamidronate disodium is given by intravenous infusion. By definition, absorption is complete at the end of the infusion.

Distribution

Plasma concentrations of pamidronate rise rapidly after the start of an infusion and fall rapidly when the infusion is stopped. The apparent half-life in plasma is about 0.8 hours. Apparent steady-state concentrations are therefore achieved with infusions of more than about 2-3 hours' duration. Peak plasma pamidronate concentrations of about 10 nmol/mL are achieved after an intravenous infusion of 60 mg given over 1 hour.

In animals and in man, a similar percentage of the dose is retained in the body after each dose of pamidronate disodium. Thus the accumulation of pamidronate in bone is not capacity-limited, and is dependent solely on the total cumulative dose administered.

The percentage of circulating pamidronate bound to plasma proteins is relatively low (about 54 %), and increases when calcium concentrations are pathologically elevated.

Elimination

Pamidronate does not appear to be eliminated by biotransformation and it is almost exclusively eliminated by renal excretion. After an intravenous infusion, about 20-55 % of the dose is recovered in the urine within 72 hours as unchanged pamidronate. Within the time-frame of experimental studies the remaining fraction of the dose is retained in the body. The percentage of the dose retained in the body is independent of both the dose (range 15-180 mg) and the infusion rate (range 1.25-60 mg/h). From the urinary elimination of pamidronate, two decay phases, with apparent half-lives of about 1.6 and 27 hours, can be observed. The apparent total plasma clearance is about 180mL/min and the apparent renal clearance is about 54 mL/min. There is a tendency for the renal clearance to correlate with creatinine clearance.

Characteristics in patients

Hepatic and metabolic clearance of pamidronate are insignificant. Aredia thus displays little potential for drug-drug interactions both at the metabolic level and at the level of protein binding (see above).

Hepatic impairment

The pharmacokinetics of pamidronate were studied in male cancer patients at risk for bone metastases with normal hepatic function (n=6) and mild to moderate hepatic dysfunction (n=9). Each patient received a single 90mg dose of Aredia infused over 4 hours. There was a statistically significant difference in the pharmacokinetics between patients with normal and impaired hepatic function. Patients with hepatic impairment exhibited higher mean AUC (39.7%) and Cmax (28.6%) values. The difference was not considered clinically relevant. The mean ratio based on log transformed parameters of impaired versus normal patients was 1.38 (90% C.I. 1.12 – 1.70, P=0.02) for AUC and 1.23 (90% C.I. 0.89 – 1.70, P=0.27) for Cmax. Nevertheless, pamidronate was still rapidly cleared from the plasma. Drug levels were not detectable in patients by 12-36 hours after drug infusion. Because Aredia is administered on a monthly basis, drug accumulation is not expected. No changes in Aredia dosing regimen are recommended for patients with mild to moderate abnormal hepatic function (see Section 4.2 Posology and method of administration).

Renal impairment

A pharmacokinetic study conducted in patients with cancer showed no differences in plasma AUC of pamidronate between patients with normal renal function and patients with mild to moderate renal impairment. In patients with severe renal impairment (creatinine clearance <30mL/min), the AUC of pamidronate was approximately 3 times higher than in patients with normal renal function (creatinine clearance >90mL/min). Because there is only limited pharmacokinetic data with severe renal impairment no dose recommendations for this patient population can be made (See Section 4.2 "Posology and method of administration" and Section 4.4 "Special warnings and special precautions for use").

5.3 Preclinical safety data

The toxicity of pamidronate is characterised by direct (cytotoxic) effects on organs with a copious blood supply, particularly the kidneys following i.v. exposure. The compound is not mutagenic and does not appear to have carcinogenic potential.

6. PHARMACEUTICAL PARTICULARS

6.1 List of excipients

Vials: Mannitol, phosphoric acid.

Solvent Ampoules: water for injections.

6.2 Incompatibilities

Studies with glass bottles, as well as infusion bags made from polyvinylchloride and polyethylene (prefilled with 0.9% w/v sodium chloride solution or 5% w/v glucose solution) showed no incompatibility with Aredia.

To avoid potential incompatibilities, Aredia reconstituted solution is to be diluted with 0.9% w/v sodium chloride solution or 5% w/v glucose solution.

Aredia reconstituted solution must not be mixed with calcium-containing solution such as Ringer's solution.

6.3 Shelf life

3 years

6.4 Special precautions for storage

Protect vials from heat (store below 30°C). The reconstituted solution is chemically and physically stable for 24 hours at room temperature. However, from a microbiological point of view, it is preferable to use the product immediately after aseptic reconstitution and dilution.

If not used immediately, the duration and conditions of storage prior to use are the care provider's responsibility. The total time between reconstitution, dilution and storage in a refrigerator at 2 to 8°C and end of administration must not exceed 24 hours.

6.5 Nature and contents of container

Colourless glass vials of 10 mL, with closures made from a butyl rubber derivative.

The solvent is packaged in sealed glass ampoules.

6.6 Instructions for use and handling

Powder in vials should be first dissolved in sterile water for injection, i.e. 15mg in 5 mL. The sterile water for injection is available in ampoules which are supplied together with vials. The pH of the reconstituted solution is 6.0-7.0. The reconstituted solution should be further diluted with a calcium-free infusion solution (0.9% w/v sodium chloride or 5% w/v glucose solution) before administration. It is important that the powder be completely dissolved before the reconstituted solution is withdrawn for dilution.

7. MARKETING AUTHORISATION HOLDER

Novartis Pharmaceuticals UK Limited,
trading as Ciba Laboratories.
Frimley Business Park
Frimley,
Camberley,
Surrey,
GU16 7SR

8. MARKETING AUTHORISATION NUMBER(S)

Aredia Dry Powder 15mg: PL 00101/0518

Aredia Dry Powder 30mg: PL 00101/0519

Aredia Dry Powder 90mg: PL 00101/0521

Water for Injections Ph.Eur. PL 00101/0479

9. DATE OF FIRST AUTHORISATION/RENEWAL OF THE AUTHORISATION

Aredia Dry Powder 15mg: 21 October 2002

Aredia Dry Powder 30mg: 21 October 2002

Aredia Dry Powder 90mg: 1 October 2003

Water for Injections Ph.Eur. 21 April 2003

10. DATE OF REVISION OF THE TEXT

4 January 2005

LEGAL CATEGORY

POM

Aricept

(Eisai Ltd)

1. NAME OF THE MEDICINAL PRODUCT

ARICEPT® 5 mg film coated tablets

ARICEPT® 10 mg film coated tablets

2. QUALITATIVE AND QUANTITATIVE COMPOSITION

5 mg donepezil hydrochloride tablets each containing 4.56 mg donepezil free base.

10 mg donepezil hydrochloride tablets each containing 9.12 mg donepezil free base.

For excipients, see 6.1

3. PHARMACEUTICAL FORM

Film-Coated tablets

5 mg donepezil as white, round, biconvex tablets embossed 'ARICEPT' on one side and '5' on the other side.

10 mg donepezil as yellow, round, biconvex tablets embossed 'ARICEPT' on one side and '10' on the other side

4. CLINICAL PARTICULARS

4.1 Therapeutic indications

ARICEPT tablets are indicated for the symptomatic treatment of mild to moderately severe Alzheimer's dementia.

4.2 Posology and method of administration

Adults/Elderly:

Treatment is initiated at 5 mg/day (once-a-day dosing). ARICEPT should be taken orally, in the evening, just prior to retiring. The 5 mg/day dose should be maintained for at least one month in order to allow the earliest clinical responses to treatment to be assessed and to allow steady-state concentrations of donepezil hydrochloride to be achieved. Following a one-month clinical assessment of treatment at 5 mg/day, the dose of ARICEPT can be increased to 10 mg/day (once-a-day dosing). The maximum recommended daily dose is 10 mg. Doses greater than 10 mg/day have not been studied in clinical trials.

Upon discontinuation of treatment, a gradual abatement of the beneficial effects of ARICEPT is seen. There is no evidence of a rebound effect after abrupt discontinuation of therapy.

Renal and hepatic impairment:

A similar dose schedule can be followed for patients with renal impairment, as clearance of donepezil hydrochloride is not affected by this condition.

Due to possible increased exposure in mild to moderate hepatic impairment (see section 5.2), dose escalation should be performed according to individual tolerability. There are no data for patients with severe hepatic impairment.

Children:

ARICEPT is not recommended for use in children.

4.3 Contraindications

ARICEPT is contraindicated in patients with a known hypersensitivity to donepezil hydrochloride, piperidine derivatives, or to any excipients used in the formulation. ARICEPT is contraindicated in pregnancy.

4.4 Special warnings and special precautions for use

Treatment should be initiated and supervised by a physician experienced in the diagnosis and treatment of Alzheimer's dementia. Diagnosis should be made according to accepted guidelines (e.g. DSM IV, ICD 10). Therapy with donepezil should only be started if a caregiver is available who will regularly monitor drug intake for the patient. Maintenance treatment can be continued for as long as a therapeutic benefit for the patient exists. Therefore, the clinical benefit of donepezil should be reassessed on a regular basis. Discontinuation should be considered when evidence of a therapeutic effect is no longer present. Individual response to donepezil cannot be predicted. The use of ARICEPT in patients with severe Alzheimer's dementia, other types of dementia or other types of memory impairment (e.g., age-related cognitive decline), has not been investigated.

Anaesthesia: ARICEPT, as a cholinesterase inhibitor, is likely to exaggerate succinylcholine-type muscle relaxation during anaesthesia.

Cardiovascular Conditions: Because of their pharmacological action, cholinesterase inhibitors may have vagotonic effects on heart rate (e.g., bradycardia). The potential for this action may be particularly important to patients with "sick sinus syndrome" or other supraventricular cardiac conduction conditions, such as sinoatrial or atrioventricular block.

There have been reports of syncope and seizures. In investigating such patients the possibility of heart block or long sinusal pauses should be considered.

Gastrointestinal Conditions: Patients at increased risk for developing ulcers, e.g., those with a history of ulcer disease or those receiving concurrent nonsteroidal anti-inflammatory drugs (NSAIDs), should be monitored for symptoms. However, the clinical studies with ARICEPT showed no increase, relative to placebo, in the incidence of either peptic ulcer disease or gastrointestinal bleeding.

Genitourinary: Although not observed in clinical trials of ARICEPT, cholinomimetics may cause bladder outflow obstruction.

Neurological Conditions: Seizures: Cholinomimetics are believed to have some potential to cause generalised convulsions. However, seizure activity may also be a manifestation of Alzheimer's Disease.

Cholinomimetics may have the potential to exacerbate or induce extrapyramidal symptoms

Pulmonary Conditions: Because of their cholinomimetic actions, cholinesterase inhibitors should be prescribed with care to patients with a history of asthma or obstructive pulmonary disease.

The administeration of ARICEPT concomitantly with other inhibitors of acetylcholinesterase, agonists or antagonists of the cholinergic system should be avoided.

Severe Hepatic Impairment: There are no data for patients with severe hepatic impairment.

4.5 Interaction with other medicinal products and other forms of Interaction

Donepezil hydrochloride and/or any of its metabolites does not inhibit the metabolism of theophylline, warfarin, cimetidine or digoxin in humans. The metabolism of donepezil hydrochloride is not affected by concurrent administration of digoxin or cimetidine. In vitro studies have shown that the cytochrome P450 isoenzymes 3A4 and to a minor extent 2D6 are involved in the metabolism of donepezil. Drug interaction studies performed in vitro show that ketoconazole and quinidine, inhibitors of CYP3A4 and 2D6 respectively, inhibit donepezil metabolism. Therefore these and other CYP3A4 inhibitors, such as itraconazole and erythromycin, and CYP2D6 inhibitors, such as fluoxetine could inhibit the metabolism of donepezil. In a study in healthy volunteers, ketoconazole increased mean donepezil concentrations by about 30%. Enzyme inducers, such as rifampicin, phenytoin, carbamazepine and alcohol may reduce the levels of donepezil. Since the magnitude of an inhibiting or inducing effect is unknown, such drug combinations should be used with care. Donepezil hydrochloride has the potential to interfere with medications having anticholinergic activity. There is also the potential for synergistic activity with concomitant treatment involving medications such as succinylcholine, other neuromuscular blocking agents or cholinergic agonists or beta blocking agents which have effects on cardiac conduction.

4.6 Pregnancy and lactation

Pregnancy:

Teratology studies conducted in pregnant rats at doses up to approximately 80 times the human dose and in pregnant rabbits at doses up to approximately 50 times the human dose did not disclose any evidence for a teratogenic potential. However, in a study in which pregnant rats were given approximately 50 times the human dose from day 17 of gestation through day 20 postpartum, there was a slight increase in stillbirths and a slight decrease in pup survival through day 4 postpartum. No effect was observed at the next lower dose tested, approximately 15 times the human dose. ARICEPT should not be used during pregnancy. For donepezil no clinical data on exposed pregnancies are available.

Lactation:

It is not known whether donepezil hydrochloride is excreted in human breast milk and there are no studies in lactating women. Therefore, women on donepezil should not breast feed.

4.7 Effects on ability to drive and use machines

Alzheimer's Dementia may cause impairment of driving performance or compromise the ability to use machinery. Furthermore, donepezil can induce fatigue, dizziness and muscle cramps, mainly when initiating or increasing the dose. The ability of Alzheimer patients on donepezil to

Table 1

System Organ Class	Common	Uncommon	Rare
Infections and infestations	Common cold		
Metabolism and nutrition disorders	Anorexia		
Psychiatric disorders	Hallucinations** Agitation** Aggressive behaviour**		
Nervous system disorders	Syncope* Dizziness Insomnia	Seizure*	Extrapyramidal symptoms
Cardiac disorders		Bradycardia	Sino-atrial block Atrioventricular block
Gastrointestinal disorders	Diarrhoea Vomiting Nausea Abdominal disturbance	Gastrointestinal haemorrhage Gastric and duodenal ulcers	
Hepato-biliary disorders			Liver dysfunction including hepatitis***
Skin and subcutaneous tissue disorders	Rash Pruritis		
Musculoskeletal, connective tissue and bone disorders	Muscle cramps		
Renal and urinary disorders	Urinary incontinence		
General disorders and administration site conditions	Headache Fatigue Pain		
Investigations		Minor increase in serum concentration of muscle creatine kinase	
Injury and poisoning	Accident		

*In investigating patients for syncope or seizure the possibility of heart block or long sinusal pauses should be considered (see section 4.4)

**Reports of hallucinations, agitation and aggressive behaviour have resolved on dose-reduction or discontinuation of treatment.

***In cases of unexplained liver dysfunction, withdrawal of ARICEPT should be considered.

continue driving or operating complex machines should be routinely evaluated by the treating physician.

4.8 Undesirable effects

The most common adverse events are diarrhoea, muscle cramps, fatigue, nausea, vomiting and insomnia.

Adverse reactions reported as more than an isolated case are listed below, by system organ class and by frequency. Frequencies are defined as: common (> 1/100, < 1/10), uncommon (> 1/1,000, < 1/100) and rare > 1/10,000, < 1/1,000).

(see Table 1 on previos page)

4.9 Overdose

The estimated median lethal dose of donepezil hydrochloride following administration of a single oral dose in mice and rats is 45 and 32 mg/kg, respectively, or approximately 225 and 160 times the maximum recommended human dose of 10 mg per day. Dose-related signs of cholinergic stimulation were observed in animals and included reduced spontaneous movement, prone position, staggering gait, lacrimation, clonic convulsions, depressed respiration, salivation, miosis, fasciculation and lower body surface temperature.

Overdosage with cholinesterase inhibitors can result in cholinergic crisis characterized by severe nausea, vomiting, salivation, sweating, bradycardia, hypotension, respiratory depression, collapse and convulsions. Increasing muscle weakness is a possibility and may result in death if respiratory muscles are involved.

As in any case of overdose, general supportive measures should be utilised. Tertiary anticholinergics such as atropine may be used as an antidote for ARICEPT overdosage. Intravenous atropine sulphate titrated to effect is recommended: an initial dose of 1.0 to 2.0 mg IV with subsequent doses based upon clinical response. Atypical responses in blood pressure and heart rate have been reported with other cholinomimetics when co-administered with quaternary anticholinergics such as glycopyrrolate. It is not known whether donepezil hydrochloride and/or its metabolites can be removed by dialysis (hemodialysis, peritoneal dialysis, or hemofiltration).

5. PHARMACOLOGICAL PROPERTIES

5.1 Pharmacodynamic properties

The pharmacotherapeutic group: drugs for dementia; ATC-code N06DA02.

Donepezil hydrochloride is a specific and reversible inhibitor of acetylcholinesterase, the predominant cholinesterase in the brain. Donepezil hydrochloride is in vitro over 1000 times more potent an inhibitor of this enzyme than of butyrylcholinesterase, an enzyme which is present mainly outside the central nervous system.

In patients with Alzheimer's Dementia participating in clinical trials, administration of single daily doses of 5 mg or 10 mg of ARICEPT produced steady-state inhibition of acetylcholinesterase activity (measured in erythrocyte membranes) of 63.6% and 77.3%, respectively when measured post dose. The inhibition of acetylcholinesterase (AChE) in red blood cells by donepezil hydrochloride has been shown to correlate to changes in ADAS-cog, a sensitive scale which examines selected aspects of cognition. The potential for donepezil hydrochloride to alter the course of the underlying neuropathology has not been studied. Thus Aricept cannot be considered to have any effect on the progress of the disease.

Efficacy of treatment with Aricept has been investigated in four placebo-controlled trials, 2 trials of 6-month duration and 2 trials of 1-year duration.

In the 6 months clinical trial, an analysis was done at the conclusion of donepezil treatment using a combination of three efficacy criteria: the ADAS-Cog (a measure of cognitive performance), the Clinician Interview Based Impression of Change with Caregiver Input (a measure of global function) and the Activities of Daily Living Subscale of the Clinical Dementia Rating Scale (a measure of capabilities in community affairs, home and hobbies and personal care).

Patients who fulfilled the criteria listed below were considered treatment responders.

Response = Improvement of ADAS-Cog of at least 4 points

No deterioration of CIBIC

No Deterioration of Activities of Daily Living Subscale of the Clinical Dementia Rating Scale

	% Response	
	Intent to Treat Population n=365	Evaluable Population n=352
Placebo Group	10%	10%
Aricept 5-mg Group	18%*	18%*
Aricept 10-mg Group	21%*	22%**

* $p < 0.05$

** $p < 0.01$

Aricept produced a dose-dependent statistically significant increase in the percentage of patients who were judged treatment responders.

5.2 Pharmacokinetic properties

General characteristics

Absorption: Maximum plasma levels are reached approximately 3 to 4 hours after oral administration. Plasma concentrations and area under the curve rise in proportion to the dose. The terminal disposition half-life is approximately 70 hours, thus, administration of multiple single-daily doses results in gradual approach to steady-state. Approximate steady-state is achieved within 3 weeks after initiation of therapy. Once at steady-state, plasma donepezil hydrochloride concentrations and the related pharmacodynamic activity show little variability over the course of the day.

Food did not affect the absorption of donepezil hydrochloride.

Distribution: Donepezil hydrochloride is approximately 95% bound to human plasma proteins. The plasma protein binding of the active metabolite 6-O-desmethyldonepezil in not known. The distribution of donepezil hydrochloride in various body tissues has not been definitively studied. However, in a mass balance study conducted in healthy male volunteers, 240 hours after the administration of a single 5 mg dose of ^{14}C-labelled donepezil hydrochloride, approximately 28% of the label remained unrecovered. This suggests that donepezil hydrochloride and/or its metabolites may persist in the body for more than 10 days.

Metabolism/Excretion: Donepezil hydrochloride is both excreted in the urine intact and metabolised by the cytochrome P450 system to multiple metabolites, not all of which have been identified. Following administration of a single 5 mg dose of ^{14}C-labeled donepezil hydrochloride, plasma radioactivity, expressed as a percent of the administered dose, was present primarily as intact donepezil hydrochloride (30%), 6-O-desmethyl donepezil (11% - only metabolite that exhibits activity similar to donepezil hydrochloride), donepezil-cis-N-oxide (9%), 5-O-desmethyl donepezil (7%) and the glucuronide conjugate of 5-O-desmethyl donepezil (3%). Approximately 57% of the total administered radioactivity was recovered from the urine (17% as unchanged donepezil), and 14.5% was recovered from the faeces, suggesting biotransformation and urinary excretion as the primary routes of elimination. There is no evidence to suggest enterohepatic recirculation of donepezil hydrochloride and/or any of its metabolites.

Plasma donepezil concentrations decline with a half-life of approximately 70 hours.

Sex, race and smoking history have no clinically significant influence on plasma concentrations of donepezil hydrochloride. The pharmacokinetics of donepezil has not been formally studied in healthy elderly subjects or in Alzheimer's patients. However mean plasma levels in patients closely agreed with those of young healthy volunteers.

Patients with mild to moderate hepatic impairment had increased donepezil steady state concentrations; mean AUC by 48% and mean C_{max} by 39% (see section 4.2).

5.3 Preclinical safety data

Extensive testing in experimental animals has demonstrated that this compound causes few effects other than the intended pharmacological effects consistent with its action as a cholinergic stimulator (see Section 4.9 above). Donepezil is not mutagenic in bacterial and mammalian cell mutation assays. Some clastogenic effects were observed in vitro at concentrations overtly toxic to the cells and more than 3000 times the steady -state plasma concentrations. No clastogenic or other genotoxic effects were observed in the mouse micronucleus model in vivo. There was no evidence of oncogenic potential in long term carcinogenicity studies in either rats or mice.

Donepezil hydrochloride had no effect on fertility in rats, and was not teratogenic in rats or rabbits, but had a slight effect on still births and early pup survival when administered to pregnant rats at 50 times the human dose (see Section 4.6 above).

6. PHARMACEUTICAL PARTICULARS

6.1 List of excipients

Lactose monohydrate, maize starch, microcrystalline cellulose, hydroxypropyl cellulose and magnesium stearate.

The film coating contains talc, macrogol, hypromellose and titanium dioxide. Additionally the 10mg tablet contains yellow iron oxide.

6.2 Incompatibilities

Not applicable

6.3 Shelf life

3 years

6.4 Special precautions for storage

Do not store above 30°C.

6.5 Nature and contents of container

5 mg and 10mg tablets:

Bottles (HDPE) of 28, 30 and 100

Unit Dose blister strips (PVC/Aluminium)

Pack sizes: 28, 30, 56, 60, 98 or 120 tablets

Not all pack sizes may be marketed.

6.6 Instructions for use and handling

No special requirements

7. MARKETING AUTHORISATION HOLDER

Eisai Ltd., Hammersmith International Centre, 3 Shortlands, London W6 8EE

8. MARKETING AUTHORISATION NUMBER(S)

PL 10555/0006 (5 mg)

PL 10555/0007 (10 mg)

9. DATE OF FIRST AUTHORISATION/RENEWAL OF THE AUTHORISATION

14 February 1997

10. DATE OF REVISION OF THE TEXT

08 January 2002

Arimidex 1mg Film-Coated Tablet

(AstraZeneca UK Limited)

1. NAME OF THE MEDICINAL PRODUCT

Arimidex® 1mg Film-coated Tablets

2. QUALITATIVE AND QUANTITATIVE COMPOSITION

Each tablet contains 1mg anastrozole

For excipients, see 6.1.

3. PHARMACEUTICAL FORM

Film-coated tablet

4. CLINICAL PARTICULARS

4.1 Therapeutic indications

Treatment of advanced breast cancer in postmenopausal women. Efficacy has not been demonstrated in oestrogen receptor negative patients unless they had a previous positive clinical response to tamoxifen.

Adjuvant treatment of postmenopausal women with hormone receptor positive early invasive breast cancer.

4.2 Posology and method of administration

Adults including the elderly: One 1mg tablet to be taken orally once a day

Children: Not recommended for use in children

Renal Impairment: No dose change is recommended in patients with mild or moderate renal impairment

Hepatic Impairment: No dose change is recommended in patients with mild hepatic disease.

For early disease, the recommended duration of treatment should be 5 years.

4.3 Contraindications

Arimidex is contra-indicated in:

- pre-menopausal women.
- pregnant or lactating women.
- patients with severe renal impairment (creatinine clearance less than 20ml/min).
- patients with moderate or severe hepatic disease.
- patients with known hypersensitivity to anastrozole or to any of the excipients as referenced in Section 6.1.

Oestrogen-containing therapies should not be co-administered with Arimidex as they would negate its pharmacological action.

Concurrent tamoxifen therapy (see Section 4.5).

4.4 Special warnings and special precautions for use

Arimidex is not recommended for use in children as safety and efficacy have not been established in this group of patients.

The menopause should be defined biochemically in any patient where there is doubt about hormonal status.

There are no data to support the safe use of Arimidex in patients with moderate or severe hepatic impairment, or patients with severe impairment of renal function (creatinine clearance less than 20ml/min).

Women with osteoporosis or at risk of osteoporosis should have their bone mineral density formally assessed by bone densitometry e.g. DEXA scanning at the commencement of treatment and at regular intervals thereafter. Treatment or prophylaxis for osteoporosis should be initiated as appropriate and carefully monitored.

There are no data available for the use of anastrozole with LHRH analogues. This combination should not be used outside clinical trials.

As Arimidex lowers circulating oestrogen levels it may cause a reduction in bone mineral density. Adequate data to show the effect of bisphosphonates on bone mineral density loss caused by anastrozole, or their utility when used prophylactically, are not currently available.

4.5 Interaction with other medicinal products and other forms of Interaction

Antipyrine and cimetidine clinical interaction studies indicate that the co-administration of Arimidex with other drugs is unlikely to result in clinically significant drug interactions mediated by cytochrome P450.

A review of the clinical trial safety database did not reveal evidence of clinically significant interaction in patients treated with Arimidex who also received other commonly prescribed drugs.

Table 1

Very common (≥ 10%)	*Vascular:*	• Hot flushes, mainly mild or moderate in nature.
Common (≥ 1% and < 10%)	*General:*	• Asthenia, mainly mild or moderate in nature.
	Musculoskeletal, connective tissue and bone:	• Joint pain/stiffness, mainly mild or moderate in nature.
	Reproductive system and breast:	• Vaginal dryness, mainly mild or moderate in nature.
	Skin and subcutaneous tissue:	• Hair thinning, mainly mild or moderate in nature. • Rash, mainly mild or moderate in nature.
	Gastrointestinal:	• Nausea, mainly mild or moderate in nature. • Diarrhoea, mainly mild or moderate in nature.
	Nervous system:	• Headache, mainly mild or moderate in nature.
Uncommon (≥ 0.1% and <1%)	*Reproductive system and breast:*	• Vaginal bleeding, mainly mild or moderate in nature*.
	Metabolism and nutrition:	• Anorexia, mainly mild in nature. • Hypercholesterolaemia, mainly mild or moderate in nature.
	Gastrointestinal:	• Vomiting, mainly mild or moderate in nature.
	Nervous system:	• Somnolence, mainly mild or moderate in nature.
Very rare (<0.01%)	*Skin and subcutaneous tissue:*	• Erythema multiforme • Stevens-Johnson syndrome • Allergic reactions including angioedema, urticaria and anaphylaxis

*Vaginal bleeding has been reported uncommonly, mainly in patients with advanced breast cancer during the first few weeks after changing from existing hormonal therapy to treatment with Arimidex. If bleeding persists, further evaluation should be considered.

Oestrogen-containing therapies should not be co-administered with Arimidex as they would negate its pharmacological action.

Tamoxifen should not be co-administered with Arimidex, as this may diminish its pharmacological action. (See Section 4.3).

4.6 Pregnancy and lactation

Arimidex is contra-indicated in pregnant or lactating women.

4.7 Effects on ability to drive and use machines

Arimidex is unlikely to impair the ability of patients to drive and operate machinery. However, asthenia and somnolence have been reported with the use of Arimidex and caution should be observed when driving or operating machinery while such symptoms persist.

4.8 Undesirable effects

(see Table 1 above)

As Arimidex lowers circulating oestrogen levels, it may cause a reduction in bone mineral density placing some patients at a higher risk of fracture (see Section 4.4).

Elevated gamma-GT and alkaline phosphatase have been reported uncommonly (≥0.1% and <1%). A causal relationship for these changes has not been established.

The table below presents the frequency of pre-specified adverse events in the ATAC study, irrespective of causality, reported in patients receiving trial therapy and up to 14 days after cessation of trial therapy.

Adverse effects	Arimidex (N=3092)	Tamoxifen (N=3094)
Hot flushes	1104 (35.7%)	1264 (40.9%)
Joint pain/stiffness	1100 (35.6%)	911 (29.4%)
Mood disturbances	597 (19.3%)	554 (17.9%)
Fatigue/asthenia	575 (18.6%)	544 (17.6%)
Nausea and vomiting	393 (12.7%)	384 (12.4%)
Fractures	315 (10.2%)	209 (6.8%)
Fractures of the spine, hip, or wrist/Colles	133 (4.3%)	91 (2.9%)
Wrist/Colles fractures	67 (2.2%)	50 (1.6%)
Spine fractures	43 (1.4%)	22 (0.7%)
Hip fractures	28 (0.9%)	26 (0.8%)
Cataracts	182 (5.9%)	213 (6.9%)
Vaginal bleeding	167 (5.4%)	317 (10.2%)
Ischaemic cardiovascular disease	127 (4.1%)	104 (3.4%)
Angina pectoris	71 (2.3%)	51 (1.6%)
Myocardial infarct	37 (1.2%)	34 (1.1%)
Coronary artery disorder	25 (0.8%)	23 (0.7%)
Myocardial ischaemia	22 (0.7%)	14 (0.5%)
Vaginal discharge	109 (3.5%)	408 (13.2%)
Any venous thromboembolic event	87 (2.8%)	140 (4.5%)
Deep venous thromboembolic events including PE	48 (1.6%)	74 (2.4%)
Ischaemic cerebrovascular events	62 (2.0%)	88 (2.8%)
Endometrial cancer	4 (0.2%)	13 (0.6%)

Fracture rates of 22 per 1000 patient-years and 15 per 1000 patient-years were observed for the Arimidex and tamoxifen groups, respectively, after a median follow up of 68 months. The observed fracture rate for Arimidex is similar to the range reported in age-matched postmenopausal populations. It has not been determined whether the rates of fracture and osteoporosis seen in ATAC in patients on anastrozole treatment reflect a protective effect of tamoxifen, a specific effect of anastrozole, or both.

The incidence of osteoporosis was 10.5% in patients treated with Arimidex and 7.3% in patients treated with tamoxifen.

4.9 Overdose

There is limited clinical experience of accidental overdosage. In animal studies, anastrozole demonstrated low acute toxicity. Clinical trials have been conducted with various dosages of Arimidex, up to 60mg in a single dose given to healthy male volunteers and up to 10mg daily given to post-menopausal women with advanced breast cancer; these dosages were well tolerated. A single dose of Arimidex that results in life-threatening symptoms has not been established. There is no specific antidote to overdosage and treatment must be symptomatic.

In the management of an overdose, consideration should be given to the possibility that multiple agents may have been taken. Vomiting may be induced if the patient is alert. Dialysis may be helpful because Arimidex is not highly protein bound. General supportive care, including frequent monitoring of vital signs and close observation of the patient, is indicated.

5. PHARMACOLOGICAL PROPERTIES

5.1 Pharmacodynamic properties

ATC Code: L02B G03 (Enzyme inhibitors)

Arimidex is a potent and highly selective non-steroidal aromatase inhibitor. In post-menopausal women, oestradiol is produced primarily from the conversion of androstenedione to oestrone through the aromatase enzyme complex in peripheral tissues. Oestrone is subsequently converted to oestradiol. Reducing circulating oestradiol levels has been shown to produce a beneficial effect in women with breast cancer. In post-menopausal women, Arimidex at a daily dose of 1mg produced oestradiol suppression of greater than 80% using a highly sensitive assay.

Arimidex does not possess any progestogenic, androgenic or oestrogenic activity.

Daily doses of Arimidex up to 10mg do not have any effect on cortisol or aldosterone secretion, measured before or after standard ACTH challenge testing. Corticoid supplements are therefore not needed.

In a large phase III study conducted in 9366 postmenopausal women with operable breast cancer treated for 5 years, Arimidex was shown to be statistically superior to tamoxifen in disease free survival. A greater magnitude of benefit was observed for disease free survival in favour of Arimidex versus tamoxifen for the prospectively defined hormone receptor positive population. Arimidex was statistically superior to tamoxifen in time to recurrence. The difference was of even greater magnitude than in disease free survival for both the Intention To Treat (ITT) population and hormone receptor positive population. Arimidex was statistically superior to tamoxifen in terms of time to distant recurrence. The incidence of contralateral breast cancer was statistically reduced for Arimidex compared to tamoxifen. Following 5 years of therapy, anastrozole is at least as effective as tamoxifen in terms of overall survival. However, due to low death rates, additional follow-up is required to determine more precisely the long-term survival for anastrozole relative to tamoxifen. With 68 months median follow-up, patients in the ATAC study have not been followed up for sufficient time after 5 years of treatment, to enable a comparison of long-term post treatment effects of Arimidex relative to tamoxifen.

(see Table 2 on next page)

As with all treatment decisions, women with breast cancer and their physician should assess the relative benefits and risks of the treatment.

When Arimidex and tamoxifen were co-administered, the efficacy and safety were similar to tamoxifen when given alone, irrespective of hormone receptor status. The exact mechanism of this is not yet clear. It is not believed to be due to a reduction in the degree of oestradiol suppression produced by Arimidex.

5.2 Pharmacokinetic properties

Absorption of anastrozole is rapid and maximum plasma concentrations typically occur within two hours of dosing (under fasted conditions). Anastrozole is eliminated slowly with a plasma elimination half-life of 40 to 50 hours. Food slightly decreases the rate but not the extent of absorption. The small change in the rate of absorption is not expected to result in a clinically significant effect on steady-state plasma concentrations during once daily dosing of Arimidex tablets. Approximately 90 to 95% of plasma anastrozole steady-state concentrations are attained after 7 daily doses. There is no evidence of time or dose-dependency of anastrozole pharmacokinetic parameters.

Anastrozole pharmacokinetics are independent of age in post-menopausal women.

Pharmacokinetics have not been studied in children.

Anastrozole is only 40% bound to plasma proteins.

Anastrozole is extensively metabolised by post-menopausal women with less than 10% of the dose excreted in the urine unchanged within 72 hours of dosing. Metabolism of anastrozole occurs by N-dealkylation, hydroxylation and glucuronidation. The metabolites are excreted primarily via the urine. Triazole, the major metabolite in plasma, does not inhibit aromatase.

The apparent oral clearance of anastrozole in volunteers with stable hepatic cirrhosis or renal impairment was in the range observed in healthy volunteers.

5.3 Preclinical safety data

Acute toxicity

In acute toxicity studies in rodents the median lethal dose of anastrozole was greater than 100mg/kg/day by the oral route and greater than 50mg/kg/day by the intraperitoneal route. In an oral acute toxicity study in the dog the median lethal dose was greater than 45mg/kg/day.

Table 2

ATAC endpoint summary: 5-year treatment completion analysis

Efficacy endpoints	Number of events (frequency)			
	Intention-to-treat population		Hormone-receptor-positive tumour status	
	Arimidex (N=3125)	Tamoxifen (N=3116)	Arimidex (N=2618)	Tamoxifen (N=2598)
Disease-free survival [a]	575 (18.4)	651 (20.9)	424 (16.2)	497 (19.1)
Hazard ratio	0.87		0.83	
2-sided 95% CI	0.78 to 0.97		0.73 to 0.94	
p-value	0.0127		0.0049	
Distant disease-free survival [b]	500 (16.0)	530 (17.0)	370 (14.1)	394 (15.2)
Hazard ratio	0.94		0.93	
2-sided 95% CI	0.83 to 1.06		0.80 to 1.07	
p-value	0.2850		0.2838	
Time to recurrence [c]	402 (12.9)	498 (16.0)	282 (10.8)	370 (14.2)
Hazard ratio	0.79		0.74	
2-sided 95% CI	0.70 to 0.90		0.64 to 0.87	
p-value	0.0005		0.0002	
Time to distant recurrence [d]	324 (10.4)	375 (12.0)	226 (8.6)	265 (10.2)
Hazard ratio	0.86		0.84	
2-sided 95% CI	0.74 to 0.99		0.70 to 1.00	
p-value	0.0427		0.0559	
Contralateral breast primary	35 (1.1)	59 (1.9)	26 (1.0)	54 (2.1)
Odds ratio	0.59		0.47	
2-sided 95% CI	0.39 to 0.89		0.30 to 0.76	
p-value	0.0131		0.0018	
Overall survival [e]	411 (13.2)	420 (13.5)	296 (11.3)	301 (11.6)
Hazard ratio	0.97		0.97	
2-sided 95% CI	0.85 to 1.12		0.83 to 1.14	
p-value	0.7142		0.7339	

a Disease-free survival includes all recurrence events and is defined as the first occurrence of loco-regional recurrence, contralateral new breast cancer, distant recurrence or death (for any reason).

b Distant disease-free survival is defined as the first occurrence of distant recurrence or death (for any reason).

c Time to recurrence is defined as the first occurrence of loco-regional recurrence, contralateral new breast cancer, distant recurrence or death due to breast cancer.

d Time to distant recurrence is defined as the first occurrence of distant recurrence or death due to breast cancer.

e Number (%) of patients who had died.

Chronic toxicity

Multiple dose toxicity studies utilized rats and dogs. No no-effect levels were established for anastrozole in the toxicity studies, but those effects that were observed at the low doses (1mg/kg/day) and mid doses (dog 3mg/kg/day; rat 5mg/kg/day) were related to either the pharmacological or enzyme inducing properties of anastrozole and were unaccompanied by significant toxic or degenerative changes.

Mutagenicity

Genetic toxicology studies with anastrozole show that it is not a mutagen or a clastogen.

Reproductive toxicology

Oral administration of anastrozole to pregnant rats and rabbits caused no teratogenic effects at doses up to 1.0 and 0.2mg/kg/day respectively. Those effects that were seen (placental enlargement in rats and pregnancy failure in rabbits) were related to the pharmacology of the compound.

The survival of litters born to rats given anastrozole at 0.02mg/kg/day and above (from day 17 of pregnancy to day 22 post-partum) was compromised. These effects were related to the pharmacological effects of the compound on parturition. There were no adverse effects on behaviour or reproductive performance of the first generation offspring attributable to maternal treatment with anastrozole.

Carcinogenicity

A two year rat oncogenicity study resulted in an increase in incidence of hepatic neoplasms and uterine stromal polyps in females and thyroid adenomas in males at the high dose (25mg/kg/day) only. These changes occurred at a dose which represents 100-fold greater exposure than occurs at human therapeutic doses, and are considered not to be clinically relevant to the treatment of patients with anastrozole.

A two year mouse oncogenicity study resulted in the induction of benign ovarian tumours and a disturbance in the incidence of lymphoreticular neoplasms (fewer histiocytic sarcomas in females and more deaths as a result of lymphomas). These changes are considered to be mouse-specific effects of aromatase inhibition and not clinically relevant to the treatment of patients with anastrozole.

6. PHARMACEUTICAL PARTICULARS

6.1 List of excipients

Lactose Monohydrate Ph. Eur.

Povidone Ph. Eur.

Sodium Starch Glycollate B.P.

Magnesium Stearate Ph. Eur.

Hypromellose Ph. Eur.

Macrogol 300 Ph. Eur.

Titanium Dioxide Ph. Eur.

6.2 Incompatibilities

Nil

6.3 Shelf life

The shelf life of Arimidex is 5 years.

6.4 Special precautions for storage

Do not store above 30°C.

6.5 Nature and contents of container

PVC blister/aluminium foil packs of 20, 28, 30, 84, 98, 100 and 300 tablets contained in a carton.

6.6 Instructions for use and handling

Not applicable

Administrative Data

7. MARKETING AUTHORISATION HOLDER

AstraZeneca UK Limited

600 Capability Green

Luton

LU1 3LU

UK

8. MARKETING AUTHORISATION NUMBER(S)

PL 17901/0002

9. DATE OF FIRST AUTHORISATION/RENEWAL OF THE AUTHORISATION

18th June 2000/11th August 2000

10. DATE OF REVISION OF THE TEXT

15th June 2005

Arixtra 2.5mg/0.5ml solution for injection, pre-filled syringe.

(GlaxoSmithKline UK)

1. NAME OF THE MEDICINAL PRODUCT

Arixtra ▼ 2.5 mg/0.5 ml solution for injection, pre-filled syringe.

2. QUALITATIVE AND QUANTITATIVE COMPOSITION

Each pre-filled syringe (0.5 ml) contains 2.5 mg of fondaparinux sodium.

For excipients, see 6.1.

3. PHARMACEUTICAL FORM

Solution for injection, pre-filled syringes.

The solution is a clear and colourless liquid.

4. CLINICAL PARTICULARS

4.1 Therapeutic indications

Prevention of Venous Thromboembolic Events (VTE) in patients undergoing major orthopaedic surgery of the lower limbs such as hip fracture, major knee surgery or hip replacement surgery.

Prevention of Venous Thromboembolic Events (VTE) in patients undergoing abdominal surgery who are judged to be at high risk of thromboembolic complications, such as patients undergoing abdominal cancer surgery (see section 5.1).

Prevention of Venous Thromboembolic Events (VTE) in medical patients who are judged to be at high risk for VTE and who are immobilised due to acute illness such as cardiac insufficiency and/or acute respiratory disorders, and/or acute infectious or inflammatory disease.

4.2 Posology and method of administration

Patients undergoing major orthopaedic or abdominal surgery

The recommended dose of Arixtra is 2.5 mg once daily administered post-operatively by subcutaneous injection.

The initial dose should be given 6 hours following surgical closure provided that haemostasis has been established.

Treatment should be continued until the risk of venous thrombo-embolism has diminished, usually until the patient is ambulant, at least 5 to 9 days after surgery. Experience shows that in patients undergoing hip fracture surgery, the risk of VTE continues beyond 9 days after surgery. In these patients the use of prolonged prophylaxis with Arixtra should be considered for up to an additional 24 days (see section 5.1).

Medical patients who are at high risk for thromboembolic complications based on an individual risk assessment

The recommended dose of Arixtra is 2.5 mg once daily administered by subcutaneous injection. A treatment duration of 6-14 days has been clinically studied in medical patients (see section 5.1).

Special populations

In patients undergoing major orthopaedic surgery, timing of the first Arixtra injection requires strict adherence in patients ≥75 years, and/or with body weight <50 kg and/or with renal impairment with creatinine clearance ranging between 20 to 50 ml/min.

The first Arixtra administration should be given not earlier than 6 hours following surgical closure. The injection should not be given unless haemostasis has been established. (See section 4.4).

Renal impairment: Arixtra should not be used in patients with creatinine clearance < 20ml/min. In patients with creatinine clearance in the range of 20 to 30 ml/min, the use of the Arixtra 1.5 mg dose is recommended.

In patients with creatinine clearance in the range of 30 to 50 ml/min, the use of the Arixtra 1.5 mg dose may be considered for short- term prophylaxis based on pharmacokinetic modelling results. For long term prophylaxis, the 1.5 mg dose should be considered as an alternative to the 2.5 mg dose. (See section 4.4).

Hepatic impairment: no dosing adjustment is necessary. In patients with severe hepatic impairment, Arixtra should be used with care. (See section 4.4).

Paediatric population: the safety and efficacy of Arixtra in patients under the age of 17 has not been studied.

Method of administration

Arixtra is administered by deep subcutaneous injection while the patient is lying down. Sites of administration should alternate between the left and the right anterolateral and left and right posterolateral abdominal wall. To avoid the loss of medicinal product when using the pre-filled syringe do not expel the air bubble from the syringe before the injection. The whole length of the needle should be inserted perpendicularly into a skin fold held between the thumb and the forefinger; the skin fold should be held throughout the injection.

See section 6.6 Instructions for use and handling and disposal.

4.3 Contraindications

known hypersensitivity to fondaparinux or to any of the excipients

active clinically significant bleeding

acute bacterial endocarditis

- severe renal impairment defined by creatinine clearance < 20 ml/min.

4.4 Special warnings and special precautions for use

Arixtra is intended for subcutaneous use only. Do not administer intramuscularly.

Haemorrhage

Arixtra should be used with caution in patients who have an increased risk of haemorrhage, such as those with congenital or acquired bleeding disorders (eg. platelet count <50,000/mm^3), active ulcerative gastrointestinal disease and recent intracranial haemorrhage or shortly after brain, spinal or ophthalmic surgery and in special patient groups as outlined below.

Agents that may enhance the risk of haemorrhage should not be administered concomitantly with fondaparinux. These agents include desirudin, fibrinolytic agents, GP IIb/IIIa receptor antagonists, heparin, heparinoids, or Low Molecular Weight Heparin (LMWH). When required, concomitant therapy with vitamin K antagonist should be administered in accordance with the information of Section 4.5. Other antiplatelet drugs (acetylsalicylic acid, dipyridamole, sulfinpyrazone, ticlopidine or clopidogrel), and NSAIDs should be used with caution. If co-administration is essential, close monitoring is necessary.

Spinal / Epidural anaesthesia

In patients undergoing major orthopaedic surgery, epidural or spinal haematomas that may result in long-term or permanent paralysis cannot be excluded with the concurrent use of Arixtra and spinal/epidural anaesthesia or spinal puncture. The risk of these rare events may be higher with post-operative use of indwelling epidural catheters or the concomitant use of other medicinal products affecting haemostasis.

Elderly patients: the elderly population is at increased risk of bleeding. As renal function is generally decreasing with age, elderly patients may show reduced elimination and increased exposure of fondaparinux. (See section 5.2). Arixtra should be used with caution in elderly patients. (See section 4.2).

Low body weight: patients with body weight <50 kg are at increased risk of bleeding. Elimination of fondaparinux decreases with weight. Arixtra should be used with caution in these patients. (See section 4.2).

Renal impairment: Fondaparinux is known to be mainly excreted by the kidney. Patients with creatinine clearance <50 ml/min are at increased risk of bleeding and should be treated with caution. (See section 4.2 and section 4.3).

Severe hepatic impairment: dosing adjustment of Arixtra is not necessary. However, the use of Arixtra should be considered with caution because of an increased risk of bleeding due to a deficiency of coagulation factors in patients with severe hepatic impairment. (See section 4.2).

Patients with Heparin Induced Thrombocytopenia

Fondaparinux does not bind to platelet factor 4 and does not cross-react with sera from patients with Heparin Induced Thrombocytopenia (HIT) type II. The efficacy and safety of fondaparinux have not been formally studied in patients with HIT type II.

4.5 Interaction with other medicinal products and other forms of Interaction

Bleeding risk is increased with concomitant administration of Arixtra and agents that may enhance the risk of haemorrhage (See section 4.4).

Oral anticoagulants (warfarin), platelet inhibitors (acetylsalicylic acid), NSAIDs (piroxicam) and digoxin did not interact with the pharmacokinetics of Arixtra. The Arixtra dose (10 mg) in the interaction studies was higher than the dose recommended for the present indications. Arixtra neither influenced the INR activity of warfarin, nor the bleeding time under acetylsalicylic acid or piroxicam treatment, nor the pharmacokinetics of digoxin at steady state.

Follow-up therapy with another anticoagulant medicinal product

If follow-up treatment is to be initiated with heparin or LMWH, the first injection should, as a general rule, be given one day after the last Arixtra injection.

If follow up treatment with a Vitamin K antagonist is required, treatment with fondaparinux should be continued until the target INR value has been reached.

4.6 Pregnancy and lactation

There are no adequate data from the use of Arixtra in pregnant women. Animal studies are insufficient with respect to effects on pregnancy, embryo/foetal development, parturition and postnatal development because of limited exposure. Arixtra should not be prescribed to pregnant women unless clearly necessary.

Fondaparinux is excreted in rat milk but it is not known whether fondaparinux is excreted in human milk. Breastfeeding is not recommended during treatment with fondaparinux. Oral absorption by the child is however unlikely.

4.7 Effects on ability to drive and use machines

No studies on the effect on the ability to drive and to use machines have been performed.

4.8 Undesirable effects

The safety of Arixtra 2.5 mg has been evaluated in 3,595 patients undergoing major orthopaedic surgery of the lower limbs treated up to 9 days, in 327 patients undergoing hip fracture surgery treated for 3 weeks following an initial prophylaxis of 1 week, 1407 patients undergoing abdominal surgery treated up to 9 days, and in 425 medical patients who are at risk for thromboembolic complications treated up to 14 days.

The undesirable effects reported by the investigator as at least possibly related to Arixtra are presented within each frequency grouping (common: ⩾ 1 % < 10 %; uncommon: ⩾ 0.1 % < 1 %; rare: ⩾ 0.01 % < 0.1 %) and system organ class by decreasing order of seriousness; these undesirable effects should be interpreted within the surgical and medical context.

(see Table 1 below)

In other studies or in post-marketing experience, rare cases of intracranial / intracerebral and retroperitoneal bleedings have been reported.

4.9 Overdose

Arixtra doses above the recommended regimen may lead to an increased risk of bleeding.

Overdose associated with bleeding complications should lead to treatment discontinuation and search for the primary cause. Initiation of appropriate therapy such as surgical haemostasis, blood replacements, fresh plasma transfusion, plasmapheresis should be considered.

5. PHARMACOLOGICAL PROPERTIES

5.1 Pharmacodynamic properties

Pharmacotherapeutic group: antithrombotic agents.

ATC code: B01AX05

Pharmacodynamic effects

Fondaparinux is a synthetic and selective inhibitor of activated Factor X (Xa). The antithrombotic activity of fondaparinux is the result of antithrombin III (ATIII) mediated selective inhibition of Factor Xa. By binding selectively to ATIII, fondaparinux potentiates (about 300 times) the innate neutralization of Factor Xa by ATIII. Neutralisation of Factor Xa interrupts the blood coagulation cascade and inhibits both thrombin formation and thrombus development. Fondaparinux does not inactivate thrombin (activated Factor II) and has no effects on platelets.

At the 2.5 mg dose, Arixtra does not affect routine coagulation tests such as activated partial thromboplastin time (aPTT), activated clotting time (ACT) or prothrombin time (PT)/International Normalised Ratio (INR) tests in plasma nor bleeding time or fibrinolytic activity.

Fondaparinux does not cross-react with sera from patients with heparin-induced thrombocytopaenia.

Clinical studies

Prevention of Venous Thromboembolic Events (VTE) in patients undergoing major orthopaedic surgery of the lower limbs treated up to 9 days: the Arixtra clinical program was designed to demonstrate the efficacy of Arixtra for the prevention of venous thromboembolic events (VTE), i.e. proximal and distal deep vein thrombosis (DVT) and pulmonary embolism (PE) in patients undergoing major orthopaedic surgery of the lower limbs such as hip fracture, major knee surgery or hip replacement surgery. Over 8,000 patients (hip fracture – 1,711, hip replacement – 5,829, major knee surgery – 1,367) were studied in controlled Phase II and III clinical studies. Arixtra 2.5 mg once daily started 6-8 hours postoperatively was compared with enoxaparin 40 mg once daily started 12 hours before surgery, or 30 mg twice daily started 12-24 hours after surgery.

In a pooled analysis of these studies, the recommended dose regimen of Arixtra versus enoxaparin was associated with a significant decrease (54% - 95% CI, 44 %; 63%) in the rate of VTE evaluated up to day 11 after surgery, irrespective of the type of surgery performed. The majority of endpoint events were diagnosed by a prescheduled venography and consisted mainly of distal DVT, but the incidence of proximal DVT was also significantly reduced. The incidence of symptomatic VTE, including PE was not significantly different between treatment groups.

In studies versus enoxaparin 40 mg once daily started 12 hours before surgery, major bleeding was observed in 2.8% of fondaparinux patients treated with the recommended dose, compared to 2.6% with enoxaparin.

Prevention of Venous Thromboembolic Events (VTE) in patients undergoing hip fracture surgery treated for up to 24 days following an initial prophylaxis of 1 week: In a randomised double-blind clinical trial, 737 patients were treated with Arixtra 2.5 mg once daily for 7 +/- 1 days following hip fracture surgery. At the end of this period, 656 patients were randomised to receive Arixtra 2.5 mg once daily or placebo for an additional 21 +/- 2 days. Fondaparinux provided a significant reduction in the overall rate of VTE compared with placebo [3 patients (1.4%) vs 77 patients (35%), respectively]. The majority (70/80) of the recorded VTE events were venographically detected non-symptomatic cases of DVT. Fondaparinux also provided a significant reduction in the rate of symptomatic VTE (DVT, and / or PE) [1 (0.3%) vs 9 (2.7%) patients, respectively] including two fatal PE reported in the placebo group. Major bleedings, all at surgical site and none fatal, were observed in 8 patients (2.4%) treated with Arixtra 2.5 mg compared to 2 (0.6%) with placebo.

Prevention of Venous Thromboembolic Events (VTE) in patients undergoing abdominal surgery who are judged to be at high risk of thromboembolic complications, such as patients undergoing abdominal cancer surgery: In a double-blind clinical study, 2927 patients were randomized to receive Arixtra 2.5mg once daily or dalteparin 5000 IU once daily, with one 2500 IU preoperative injection

Table 1

System organ class MedDRA	Undesirable effects in patients undergoing major orthopaedic surgery of lower limbs and/or abdominal surgery	Undesirable effects in medical patients
Infections and infestations	*Rare:* post-operative wound infection	
Blood and lymphatic system disorders	*Common:* post-operative haemorrhage, anaemia *Uncommon:* bleeding (epistaxis, gastrointestinal, haemoptysis, hematuria, haematoma) thrombocytopenia, purpura, thrombocythaemia, platelet abnormal, coagulation disorder	*Common:* bleeding (haematoma, haematuria, haemoptysis, gingival bleeding) *Uncommon:* anaemia
Immune system disorders	*Rare:* allergic reaction	
Metabolism and nutrition disorders	*Rare:* hypokalaemia	
Nervous system disorders	*Rare:* anxiety, somnolence, vertigo, dizziness, headache, confusion	
Vascular disorders	*Rare:* hypotension	
Respiratory, thoracic and mediastinal disorders	*Rare:* dyspnoea, coughing	*Uncommon:* dyspnoea
Gastrointestinal disorders	*Uncommon:* nausea, vomiting *Rare:* abdominal pain, dyspepsia, gastritis, constipation, diarrhoea	
Hepatobiliary disorders	*Uncommon:* hepatic enzymes increased, hepatic function abnormal *Rare:* bilirubinaemia	
Skin and subcutaneous tissue disorders	*Uncommon:* rash, pruritus	*Uncommon:* rash, pruritus
General disorders and administration site conditions	*Uncommon:* oedema, oedema peripheral, fever, wound secretion *Rare:* chest pain, fatigue, hot flushes, leg pain, oedema genital, flushing, syncope	*Uncommon:* chest pain

and a first 2500 IU post-operative injection, for 7±2 days. The main sites of surgery were colonic/rectal, gastric, hepatic, cholecystectomy or other biliary. Sixty-nine percent of the patients underwent surgery for cancer. Patients under-going urological (other than kidney) or gynaecological surgery, laparoscopic surgery or vascular surgery were not included in the study.

In this study, the incidence of total VTE was 4.6% (47/1027) with fondaparinux, versus 6.1%: (62/1021) with dalteparin: odds ratio reduction [95%CI] = -25.8% [-49.7%, 9.5%]. The difference in total VTE rates between the treatment groups, which was not statistically significant, was mainly due to a reduction of asymptomatic distal DVT. The incidence of symptomatic DVT was similar between treatment groups: 6 patients (0.4%) in the fondaparinux group vs 5 patients (0.3%) in the dalteparin group. In the large subgroup of patients undergoing cancer surgery (69% of the patient population), the VTE rate was 4.7% in the fondaparinux group, versus 7.7% in the dalteparin group.

Major bleeding was observed in 3.4% of the patients in the fondaparinux group and in 2.4% of the dalteparin group.

Prevention of Venous Thromboembolic Events (VTE) in medical patients who are at high risk for thromboembolic complications due to restricted mobility during acute illness: In a randomised double-blind clinical trial, 839 patients were treated with Arixtra 2.5 mg once daily or placebo for 6 to 14 days. This study included acutely ill medical patients, aged ⩾ 60 years, expected to require bed rest for at least four days, and hospitalized for congestive heart failure NYHA class III/IV and/or acute respiratory illness and/or acute infectious or inflammatory disease. Arixtra significantly reduced the overall rate of VTE compared to placebo [18 patients (5.6%) vs 34 patients (10.5%), respectively]. The majority of events were asymptomatic distal DVT. Arixtra also significantly reduced the rate of adjudicated fatal PE [0 patients (0.0%) vs 5 patients (1.2%), respectively]. Major bleedings were observed in 1 patient (0.2%) of each group.

5.2 Pharmacokinetic properties

Absorption: after subcutaneous dosing, fondaparinux is completely and rapidly absorbed (absolute bioavailability 100%). Following a single subcutaneous injection of Arixtra 2.5 mg to young healthy subjects, peak plasma concentration (mean C_{max} = 0.34 mg/l) is obtained 2 hours post-dosing. Plasma concentrations of half the mean C_{max} values are reached 25 minutes post-dosing.

In elderly healthy subjects, pharmacokinetics of fondaparinux are linear in the range of 2 to 8 mg by subcutaneous route. Following once daily dosing, steady state of plasma levels is obtained after 3 to 4 days with a 1.3-fold increase in C_{max} and AUC.

Mean (CV%) steady state pharmacokinetic parameters estimates of fondaparinux in patients undergoing hip replacement surgery receiving Arixtra 2.5 mg once daily are: C_{max} (mg/l) - 0.39 (31%), T_{max} (h) - 2.8 (18%) and C_{min} (mg/l) -0.14 (56%). In hip fracture patients, associated with their increased age, fondaparinux steady state plasma concentrations are: C_{max} (mg/l) - 0.50 (32%), C_{min} (mg/l) - 0.19 (58%).

Distribution: the distribution volume of fondaparinux is limited (7-11 litres). *In vitro*, fondaparinux is highly and specifically bound to antithrombin protein with a dose-dependant plasma concentration binding (98.6% to 97.0% in the concentration range from 0.5 to 2 mg/l). Fondaparinux does not bind significantly to other plasma proteins, including platelet factor 4 (PF4).

Since fondaparinux does not bind significantly to plasma proteins other than ATIII, no interaction with other medicinal products by protein binding displacement are expected.

Metabolism: although not fully evaluated, there is no evidence of fondaparinux metabolism and in particular no evidence for the formation of active metabolites.

Fondaparinux does not inhibit CYP450s (CYP1A2, CYP2A6, CYP2C9, CYP2C19, CYP2D6, CYP2E1 or CYP3A4) *in vitro*. Thus, Arixtra is not expected to interact with other medicinal products *in vivo* by inhibition of CYP-mediated metabolism.

Excretion/Elimination: the elimination half-life ($t_{½}$) is about 17 hours in healthy young subjects and about 21 hours in healthy elderly subjects. Fondaparinux is excreted to 64 – 77 % by the kidney as unchanged compound.

Special populations:

Paediatric patients: fondaparinux has not been investigated in this population.

Elderly patients: renal function may decrease with age and thus, the elimination capacity for fondaparinux may be reduced in elderly. In patients >75 years undergoing orthopaedic surgery, the estimated plasma clearance was 1.2 to 1.4 times lower than in patients <65 years.

Renal impairment: compared with patients with normal renal function (creatinine clearance > 80 ml/min), plasma clearance is 1.2 to 1.4 times lower in patients with mild renal impairment (creatinine clearance 50 to 80 ml/min) and on average 2 times lower in patients with moderate renal impairment (creatinine clearance 30 to 50 ml/min). In severe renal impairment (creatinine clearance < 30 ml/min), plasma clearance is approximately 5 times lower than in normal renal function. Associated terminal half-life values were 29 h in moderate and 72 h in patients with severe renal impairment.

Gender: no gender differences were observed after adjustment for body weight.

Race: pharmacokinetic differences due to race have not been studied prospectively. However, studies performed in Asian (Japanese) healthy subjects did not reveal a different pharmacokinetic profile compared to Caucasian healthy subjects. Similarly, no plasma clearance differences were observed between black and Caucasian patients undergoing orthopaedic surgery.

Body weight: plasma clearance of fondaparinux increases with body weight (9% increase per 10 kg).

Hepatic impairment: fondaparinux pharmacokinetics has not been evaluated in hepatic impairment.

5.3 Preclinical safety data

Preclinical data reveal no special risk for humans based on conventional studies of safety pharmacology, repeated dose toxicity, and genotoxicity. Animal studies are insufficient with respect to effects on toxicity to reproduction because of limited exposure.

6. PHARMACEUTICAL PARTICULARS

6.1 List of excipients

Sodium chloride

Water for injections

Hydrochloric acid

Sodium hydroxide

6.2 Incompatibilities

In the absence of compatibility studies, Arixtra must not be mixed with other medicinal products.

6.3 Shelf life

3 years.

6.4 Special precautions for storage

Do not freeze.

6.5 Nature and contents of container

Arixtra pre-filled single-use syringes are made of Type I glass barrel (1 ml) affixed with a 27 gauge × 12.7 mm needle and stoppered with a bromobutyl or chlorobutyl elastomer plunger stopper.

Arixtra is available in pack sizes of 2, 7, 10 and 20 pre-filled syringes with a blue automatic safety system. Not all pack sizes may be marketed.

6.6 Instructions for use and handling

The subcutaneous injection is administered in the same way as with a classical syringe.

Parenteral solutions should be inspected visually for particulate matter and discoloration prior to administration.

Instruction for self-administration is mentioned in the Package Leaflet.

The needle protection system of the Arixtra pre-filled syringe has been designed with an automatic safety system to protect from needle stick injuries following injection.

Any unused product or waste material should be disposed of in accordance with local requirements.

Administrative Data

7. MARKETING AUTHORISATION HOLDER

Glaxo Group Ltd

Greenford

Middlesex

UB6 0NN

United Kingdom

8. MARKETING AUTHORISATION NUMBER(S)

EU/1/02/206/001-004

9. DATE OF FIRST AUTHORISATION/RENEWAL OF THE AUTHORISATION

21 March 2002

10. DATE OF REVISION OF THE TEXT

7th July 2005

Arixtra 5mg, 7.5mg, 10mg solution for injection, pre-filled syringe

(GlaxoSmithKline UK)

1. NAME OF THE MEDICINAL PRODUCT

Arixtra ▼ 5 mg/0.4 ml solution for injection, pre-filled syringe.

Arixtra ▼ 7.5 mg/0.6 ml solution for injection, pre-filled syringe.

Arixtra ▼ 10 mg/0.8 ml solution for injection, pre-filled syringe.

2. QUALITATIVE AND QUANTITATIVE COMPOSITION

Each pre-filled syringe (0.4 ml, 0.6 ml or 0.8 ml) contains 5 mg, 7.5 mg or 10 mg of fondaparinux sodium.

For excipients, see 6.1.

3. PHARMACEUTICAL FORM

Solution for injection, pre-filled syringes.

The solution is a clear and colourless to slightly yellow liquid.

4. CLINICAL PARTICULARS

4.1 Therapeutic indications

Treatment of acute Deep Vein Thrombosis (DVT) and treatment of acute Pulmonary Embolism (PE), except in haemodynamically unstable patients or patients who require thrombolysis or pulmonary embolectomy.

4.2 Posology and method of administration

The recommended dose of Arixtra is 7.5 mg (patients with body weight ⩾ 50, ⩽ 100kg) once daily administered by subcutaneous injection. For patients with body weight < 50 kg, the recommended dose is 5 mg. For patients with body weight > 100 kg, the recommended dose is 10 mg.

Treatment should be continued for at least 5 days and until adequate oral anticoagulation is established (International Normalised Ratio 2 to 3). Concomitant oral anticoagulation treatment should be initiated as soon as possible and usually within 72 hours. The average duration of administration in clinical trials was 7 days and the clinical experience from treatment beyond 10 days is limited.

Special populations

Elderly patients: No dosing adjustment is necessary. In patients ⩾75 years, Arixtra should be used with care, as renal function decreases with age. (See section 4.4).

Renal impairment: Arixtra should be used with caution in patients with moderate renal impairment (See section 4.4).

There is no experience in the subgroup of patients with *both* high body weight >100 kg) and moderate renal impairment (creatinine clearance 30-50 ml/min). In this subgroup, after an initial 10 mg daily dose, a reduction of the daily dose to 7.5 mg may be considered, based on pharmacokinetic modelling (see section 4.4).

Arixtra should not be used in patients with severe renal impairment (creatinine clearance < 30 ml/min) (See section 4.3).

Hepatic impairment: No dosing adjustment is necessary. In patients with severe hepatic impairment, Arixtra should be used with care. (See section 4.4).

Paediatric population: The safety and efficacy of Arixtra in patients under the age of 17 has not been studied.

Method of administration

Arixtra is administered by deep subcutaneous injection while the patient is lying down. Sites of administration should alternate between the left and the right anterolateral and left and right posterolateral abdominal wall. To avoid the loss of medicinal product when using the pre-filled syringe do not expel the air bubble from the syringe before the injection. The whole length of the needle should be inserted perpendicularly into a skin fold held between the thumb and the forefinger; the skin fold should be held throughout the injection.

See section 6.6 Instructions for use and handling and disposal.

4.3 Contraindications

- known hypersensitivity to fondaparinux or to any of the excipients;

- active clinically significant bleeding;

- acute bacterial endocarditis;

- severe renal impairment (creatinine clearance < 30 ml/min).

4.4 Special warnings and special precautions for use

Arixtra is intended for subcutaneous use only. Do not administer intramuscularly.

There is limited experience from treatment with Arixtra in haemodynamically unstable patients and no experience in patients requiring thrombolysis, embolectomy or insertion of a vena cava filter.

Haemorrhage

Arixtra should be used with caution in patients who have an increased risk of haemorrhage, such as those with congenital or acquired bleeding disorders (eg. platelet count <50,000/mm^3), active ulcerative gastrointestinal disease and recent intracranial haemorrhage or shortly after brain, spinal or ophthalmic surgery and in special patient groups as outlined below.

As for other anticoagulants, Arixtra should be used with caution in patients who have undergone recent surgery (<3 days) and only once surgical haemostasis has been established.

Agents that may enhance the risk of haemorrhage should not be administered concomitantly with fondaparinux. These agents include desirudin, fibrinolytic agents, GP IIb/IIIa receptor antagonists, heparin, heparinoids, or Low Molecular Weight Heparin (LMWH). During treatment of VTE, concomitant therapy with vitamin K antagonist should be administered in accordance with the information of Section 4.5. Other antiplatelet drugs (acetylsalicylic acid, dipyridamole, sulfinpyrazone, ticlopidine or clopidogrel), and NSAIDs should be used with caution. If co-administration is essential, close monitoring is necessary.

Spinal / Epidural anaesthesia:

In patients receiving Arixtra for treatment of VTE rather than prophylaxis, spinal/epidural anaesthesia in case of surgical procedures should not be used.

Elderly patients: The elderly population is at increased risk of bleeding. As renal function generally decreases with age, elderly patients may show reduced elimination and increased exposure of fondaparinux(see section 5.2). Incidences of bleeding events in patients receiving the recommended regimen in the treatment of DVT or PE and aged <65 years, 65-75 and >75 years were 3.0 %, 4.5 % and 6.5 %, respectively. The corresponding incidences in patients receiving the recommended regimen of enoxaparin in the treatment of DVT were 2.5%, 3.6% and 8.3% respectively, while the incidences in patients receiving the recommended regimen of UFH in the treatment of PE were 5.5%, 6.6% and 7.4%, respectively. Arixtra should be used with caution in elderly patients (see section 4.2).

Low body weight: Clinical experience is limited in patients with body weight <50 kg. Arixtra should be used with caution at a daily dose of 5 mg in this population (see sections 4.2 and 5.2).

Renal impairment: The risk of bleeding increases with increasing renal impairment. Fondaparinux is known to be excreted mainly by the kidney. Incidences of bleeding events in patients receiving the recommended regimen in the treatment of DVT or PE with normal renal function, mild renal impairment, moderate renal impairment and severe renal impairment were 3.0 % (34/1132), 4.4 % (32/733), 6.6% (21/318), and 14.5 % (8/55) respectively. The corresponding incidences in patients receiving the recommended regimen of enoxaparin in the treatment of DVT were 2.3% (13/559), 4.6% (17/368), 9.7% (14/145) and 11.1% (2/18) respectively, and in patients receiving the recommended regimen of unfractionated heparin in the treatment of PE were 6.9% (36/523), 3.1% (11/352), 11.1% (18/162) and 10.7% (3/28), respectively. Arixtra is contra-indicated in severe renal impairment (creatinine clearance <30 ml/min) and should be used with caution in patients with moderate renal impairment (creatinine clearance 30-50 ml/min). The duration of treatment should not exceed that evaluated during clinical trial (mean 7 days) (See sections 4.2, 4.3 and 5.2).

There is no experience in the subgroup of patients with both high body weight >100 kg) and moderate renal impairment (creatinine clearance 30-50 ml/min). Arixtra should be used with care in these patients. After an initial 10 mg daily dose, a reduction of the daily dose to 7.5 mg may be considered, based on pharmacokinetic modelling (see section 4.2).

Severe hepatic impairment: The use of Arixtra should be considered with caution because of an increased risk of bleeding due to a deficiency of coagulation factors in patients with severe hepatic impairment (see section 4.2).

Patients with Heparin Induced Thrombocytopenia: Fondaparinux does not bind to platelet factor 4 and does not cross-react with sera from patients with Heparin Induced Thrombocytopenia (HIT) type II. The efficacy and safety of fondaparinux have not been formally studied in patients with HIT type II.

4.5 Interaction with other medicinal products and other forms of Interaction

Bleeding risk is increased with concomitant administration of Arixtra and agents that may enhance the risk of hemorrhage (See section 4.4).

In clinical studies performed with Arixtra, oral anticoagulants (warfarin) did not interact with the pharmacokinetics of Arixtra; at the 10 mg dose used in the interaction studies, Arixtra did not influence the anticoagulation monitoring (INR) activity of warfarin.

Platelet inhibitors (acetylsalicylic acid), NSAIDs (piroxicam) and digoxin did not interact with the pharmacokinetics of Arixtra. At the 10 mg dose used in the interaction studies, Arixtra did not influence the bleeding time under acetylsalicylic acid or piroxicam treatment, nor the pharmacokinetics of digoxin at steady state.

4.6 Pregnancy and lactation

No clinical data on exposed pregnancies are available. Animal studies are insufficient with respect to effects on pregnancy, embryo/foetal development, parturition and postnatal development because of limited exposure. Arixtra should not be prescribed to pregnant women unless clearly necessary.

Fondaparinux is excreted in rat milk but it is not known whether fondaparinux is excreted in human milk. Breast-feeding is not recommended during treatment with fondaparinux. Oral absorption by the child is however unlikely.

4.7 Effects on ability to drive and use machines

No studies on the effect on the ability to drive and to use machines have been performed.

4.8 Undesirable effects

The safety of Arixtra has been evaluated in 2,517 patients treated for Venous Thrombo-Embolism and treated with fondaparinux for an average of 7 days. The most common adverse reactions were bleeding complications (See section 4.4).

The undesirable effects reported by the investigator as at least possibly related to Arixtra are presented within each frequency grouping (common: ⩾ 1 % < 10 %; uncommon: ⩾ 0.1 % < 1 %; rare: ⩾ 0.01 % < 0.1 %) and system organ class by decreasing order of seriousness.

System organ class	Undesirable effects (1)
Red blood cells disorders	Uncommon: anemia
Platelet, bleeding and clotting disorders	Common: bleeding (gastrointestinal, hematuria, hematoma, epistaxis, haemoptysis, utero-vaginal haemorrhage, haemarthrosis, ocular, purpura, bruise) Uncommon: thrombocytopaenia Rare: other bleeding (hepatic, retroperitoneal, intracranial/ intracerebral), thrombocythaemia
Central and peripheral nervous system disorders	Uncommon: headache Rare: dizziness
Gastro-intestinal system disorders	Uncommon: nausea, vomiting
Liver and biliary disorders	Uncommon: abnormal liver function
Skin and appendage disorders	Rare: rash erythematous, reaction at injection site
Body as a whole-general disorders	Uncommon: pain, oedema Rare: allergic reaction
Metabolic and nutritional disorders	Rare: non-protein-nitrogen (Npn) (2) increased

(1) isolated AEs have not been considered except if they were medically relevant.

(2) Npn stands for non-protein-nitrogen such as urea, uric acid, amino acid, etc..

4.9 Overdose

Arixtra doses above the recommended regimen may lead to an increased risk of bleeding.

There is no known antidote to fondaparinux.

Overdose associated with bleeding complications should lead to treatment discontinuation and search for the primary cause. Initiation of appropriate therapy such as surgical hemostasis, blood replacements, fresh plasma transfusion, plasmapheresis should be considered.

5. PHARMACOLOGICAL PROPERTIES

5.1 Pharmacodynamic properties

Pharmacotherapeutic group: antithrombotic agents.

Proposed ATC code: B01AX05

<u>*Pharmacodynamic effects*</u>

Fondaparinux is a synthetic and selective inhibitor of activated Factor X (Xa). The antithrombotic activity of fondaparinux is the result of antithrombin III (antithrombin) mediated selective inhibition of Factor Xa. By binding selectively to antithrombin, fondaparinux potentiates (about 300 times) the innate neutralization of Factor Xa by antithrombin. Neutralisation of Factor Xa interrupts the blood coagulation cascade and inhibits both thrombin formation and thrombus development. Fondaparinux does not inactivate thrombin (activated Factor II) and has no effects on platelets.

At the doses used for treatment, Arixtra does not, to a clinically relevant extent, affect routine coagulation tests such as activated partial thromboplastin time (aPTT), activated clotting time (ACT) or prothrombin time (PT)/International Normalised Ratio (INR) tests in plasma nor bleeding time or fibrinolytic activity. At higher doses, moderate changes in aPTT can occur. At the 10 mg dose used in interaction studies, Arixtra did not significantly influence the anticoagulation activity (INR) of warfarin.

Fondaparinux does not cross-react with sera from patients with heparin-induced thrombocytopaenia.

<u>*Clinical studies*</u>

The Arixtra clinical program in treatment of Venous Thromboembolism was designed to demonstrate the efficacy of Arixtra for the treatment of deep vein thrombosis (DVT) and pulmonary embolism (PE). Over 4874 patients were studied in controlled Phase II and III clinical studies.

Treatment of Deep Venous Thrombosis

In a randomised, double-blind, clinical trial in patients with a confirmed diagnosis of acute symptomatic DVT, Arixtra 5 mg (body weight < 50 kg), 7.5 mg (body weight ⩾ 50 kg, ⩽ 100 kg) or 10 mg (body weight > 100 kg) SC once daily was compared to enoxaparin sodium 1 mg/kg SC twice daily. A total of 2192 patients were treated; for both groups, patients were treated for at least 5 days and up to 26 days (mean 7 days). Both treatment groups received Vitamin K antagonist therapy usually initiated within 72 hours after the first study drug administration and continued for 90 ± 7 days, with regular dose adjustments to achieve an INR of 2-3. The primary efficacy endpoint was the composite of confirmed symptomatic recurrent non-fatal VTE and fatal VTE reported up to Day 97. Treatment with Arixtra was demonstrated to be non-inferior to enoxaparin (VTE rates 3.9% and 4.1%, respectively).

Major bleeding during the initial treatment period was observed in 1.1% of fondaparinux patients, compared to 1.2% with enoxaparin.

Treatment of Pulmonary Embolism

A randomised, open-label, clinical trial was conducted in patients with acute symptomatic PE. The diagnosis was confirmed by objective testing (lung scan, pulmonary angiography or spiral CT scan). Patients who required thrombolysis or embolectomy or vena cava filter were excluded. Randomised patients could have been pre-treated with UFH during the screening phase but patients treated for more than 24 hours with therapeutic dose of anticoagulant or with uncontrolled hypertension were excluded. Arixtra 5 mg (body weight < 50 kg), 7.5 mg (body weight ⩾ 50kg, ⩽ 100 kg) or 10 mg (body weight >100 kg) SC once daily was compared to unfractionated heparin IV bolus (5000 IU) followed by a continuous IV infusion adjusted to maintain 1.5–2.5 times aPTT control value. A total of 2184 patients were treated; for both groups, patients were treated for at least 5 days and up to 22 days (mean 7 days). Both treatment groups received Vitamin K antagonist therapy usually initiated within 72 hours after the first study drug administration and continued for 90 ± 7 days, with regular dose adjustments to achieve an INR of 2-3. The primary efficacy endpoint was the composite of confirmed symptomatic recurrent non-fatal VTE and fatal VTE reported up to Day 97. Treatment with Arixtra was demonstrated to be non-inferior to unfractionated heparin (VTE rates 3.8% and 5.0%, respectively).

Major bleeding during the initial treatment period was observed in 1.3% of fondaparinux patients, compared to 1.1% with unfractionated heparin.

5.2 Pharmacokinetic properties

The pharmacokinetics of fondaparinux sodium are derived from fondaparinux plasma concentrations quantified via anti factor Xa activity. Only fondaparinux can be used to calibrate the anti-Xa assay (the international standards of heparin or LMWH are not appropriate for this use). As a result, the concentration of fondaparinux is expressed as milligrams (mg).

Absorption: after subcutaneous dosing, fondaparinux is completely and rapidly absorbed (absolute bioavailability 100%). Following a single subcutaneous injection of Arixtra 2.5 mg to young healthy subjects, peak plasma concentration (mean C_{max} = 0.34 mg/l) is obtained 2 hours post-dosing. Plasma concentrations of half the mean C_{max} values are reached 25 minutes post-dosing.

In elderly healthy subjects, pharmacokinetics of fondaparinux is linear in the range of 2 to 8 mg by subcutaneous route. Following once daily dosing, steady state of plasma levels is obtained after 3 to 4 days with a 1.3-fold increase in C_{max} and AUC.

Mean (CV%) steady state pharmacokinetic parameters estimates of fondaparinux in patients undergoing hip replacement surgery receiving Arixtra 2.5 mg once daily are: C_{max} (mg/l) - 0.39 (31%), T_{max} (h) - 2.8 (18%) and C_{min} (mg/l) -0.14 (56%). In hip fracture patients, associated with their increased age, fondaparinux steady state plasma concentrations are: C_{max} (mg/l) - 0.50 (32%), C_{min} (mg/l) - 0.19 (58%).

In DVT and PE treatment, patients receiving Arixtra 5 mg (body weight <50 kg), 7.5 mg (body weight 50-100 kg inclusive) and 10 mg (body weight >100 kg) once daily, the body weight-adjusted doses provide similar exposure across all body weight categories. The mean (CV%) steady state pharmacokinetic parameters estimates of fondaparinux in patients with VTE receiving the fondaparinux proposed dose regimen once daily are: C_{max} (mg/l) - 1.41 (23 %), T_{max} (h) – 2.4 (8%) and C_{min} (mg/l) -0.52 (45 %). The associated 5th and 95th percentiles are, respectively, 0.97 and 1.92 for C_{max} (mg/l), and 0.24 and 0.95 for C_{min} (mg/l).

Distribution: the distribution volume of fondaparinux is limited (7-11 litres). *In vitro*, fondaparinux is highly and specifically bound to antithrombin protein with a dose-dependant plasma concentration binding (98.6% to 97.0% in the concentration range from 0.5 to 2 mg/l). Fondaparinux does not bind significantly to other plasma proteins, including platelet factor 4 (PF4).

Since fondaparinux does not bind significantly to plasma proteins other than antithrombin, no interaction with other medicinal products by protein binding displacement are expected.

Metabolism: although not fully evaluated, there is no evidence of fondaparinux metabolism and in particular no evidence for the formation of active metabolites.

Fondaparinux does not inhibit CYP450s (CYP1A2, CYP2A6, CYP2C9, CYP2C19, CYP2D6, CYP2E1 or CYP3A4) *in vitro*. Thus, Arixtra is not expected to interact with other medicinal products *in vivo* by inhibition of CYP-mediated metabolism.

Excretion/Elimination: the elimination half-life ($t_{1/2}$) is about 17 hours in healthy young subjects and about 21 hours in healthy elderly subjects. Fondaparinux is excreted to 64 – 77 % by the kidney as unchanged compound.

Special populations:

Paediatric patients: fondaparinux has not been investigated in this population.

Elderly patients: renal function may decrease with age and thus, the elimination capacity for fondaparinux may be reduced in elderly. In patients >75 years undergoing orthopaedic surgery and receiving Arixtra 2.5 mg once daily, the estimated plasma clearance was 1.2 to 1.4 times lower than in patients <65 years. A similar pattern is observed in DVT and PE treatment patients.

Renal impairment: compared with patients with normal renal function (creatinine clearance > 80 ml/min) undergoing orthopaedic surgery and receiving Arixtra 2.5 mg once daily, plasma clearance is 1.2 to 1.4 times lower in patients with mild renal impairment (creatinine clearance 50 to 80 ml/min) and on average 2 times lower in patients with moderate renal impairment (creatinine clearance 30 to 50 ml/min). In severe renal impairment (creatinine clearance <30 ml/min), plasma clearance is approximately 5 times lower than in normal renal function. Associated terminal half-life values were 29 h in moderate and 72 h in patients with severe renal impairment. A similar pattern is observed in DVT and PE treatment patients.

Body weight: plasma clearance of fondaparinux increases with body weight (9% increase per 10 kg).

Gender: no gender differences were observed after adjustment for body weight.

Race: pharmacokinetic differences due to race have not been studied prospectively. However, studies performed in Asian (Japanese) healthy subjects did not reveal a different pharmacokinetic profile compared to Caucasian healthy subjects. Similarly, no plasma clearance differences were observed between black and Caucasian patients undergoing orthopaedic surgery.

Hepatic impairment: fondaparinux pharmacokinetics has not been evaluated in hepatic impairment.

5.3 Preclinical safety data

Preclinical data reveal no special risk for humans based on conventional studies of safety pharmacology and genotoxicity. The repeated dose and reproduction toxicity studies did not reveal any special risk but did not provide adequate documentation of safety margins due to limited exposure in the animal species.

6. PHARMACEUTICAL PARTICULARS

6.1 List of excipients

Sodium chloride

Water for injections

Hydrochloric acid

Sodium hydroxide

6.2 Incompatibilities

In the absence of compatibility studies, this medicinal product must not be mixed with other medicinal products.

6.3 Shelf life

3 years

6.4 Special precautions for storage

Do not freeze.

6.5 Nature and contents of container

Arixtra pre-filled single-use syringes are made of Type I glass barrel (1 ml) affixed with a 27 gauge × 12.7 mm needle and stoppered with a chlorobutyl elastomer plunger stopper.

Arixtra 5 mg/0.4 ml is available in pack sizes of 2, 7 and 10 pre-filled syringes with an orange automatic safety system. Not all pack sizes may be marketed.

Arixtra 7.5 mg/0.6 ml is available in pack sizes of 2, 7 and 10 pre-filled syringes with a magenta automatic safety system. Not all pack sizes may be marketed.

Arixtra 10 mg/0.8 ml is available in pack sizes of 2, 7 and 10 pre-filled syringes with a violet automatic safety system. Not all pack sizes may be marketed

6.6 Instructions for use and handling

The subcutaneous injection is administered in the same way as with a classical syringe.

Parenteral solutions should be inspected visually for particulate matter and discoloration prior to administration.

Instruction for self-administration is mentioned in the Package Leaflet.

The Arixtra pre-filled syringe has been designed with an automatic needle protection system to prevent needle stick injuries following injection.

Any unused product or waste material should be disposed of in accordance with local requirements.

This medicinal product is for single use only.

Administrative Data

7. MARKETING AUTHORISATION HOLDER

Glaxo Group Ltd
Greenford
Middlesex
UB6 0NN
United Kingdom

8. MARKETING AUTHORISATION NUMBER(S)

Arixtra 2.5 mg/0.4 ml EU/1/02/206/009-011

Arixtra 7.5 mg/0.6 ml EU/1/02/206/012-014

Arixtra 10 mg/0.8 ml EU/1/02/206/015-017

9. DATE OF FIRST AUTHORISATION/RENEWAL OF THE AUTHORISATION

21 March 2002

10. DATE OF REVISION OF THE TEXT

12 January 2005

11. Legal Status

POM

Aromasin

(Pharmacia Limited)

1. NAME OF THE MEDICINAL PRODUCT

Aromasin® 25 mg coated tablets.

2. QUALITATIVE AND QUANTITATIVE COMPOSITION

Each coated tablet contains 25 mg exemestane.

For Excipients, see 6.1

3. PHARMACEUTICAL FORM

Coated tablet

Round, biconvex, off-white coated tablet marked 7663 on one side.

4. CLINICAL PARTICULARS

4.1 Therapeutic indications

Aromasin® is indicated for the adjuvant treatment of postmenopausal women with oestrogen receptor positive invasive early breast cancer, following 2 -3 years of initial adjuvant tamoxifen therapy.

Aromasin® is indicated for the treatment of advanced breast cancer in women with natural or induced postmenopausal status whose disease has progressed following anti-oestrogen therapy. Efficacy has not been demonstrated in patients with oestrogen receptor negative status.

4.2 Posology and method of administration

Adult and elderly patients

The recommended dose of Aromasin® is one 25 mg tablet to be taken once daily, preferably after a meal.

In patients with early breast cancer, treatment with Aromasin® should continue until completion of five years of combined sequential adjuvant hormonal therapy (tamoxifen followed by Aromasin®), or earlier if tumour relapse occurs.

In patients with advanced breast cancer, treatment with Aromasin® should continue until tumour progression is evident.

No dose adjustments are required for patients with hepatic or renal insufficiency (see 5.2).

Children

Not recommended for use in children

4.3 Contraindications

Aromasin® tablets are contra-indicated in patients with a known hypersensitivity to the active substance or to any of the excipients, in pre-menopausal women and in pregnant or lactating women.

4.4 Special warnings and special precautions for use

Aromasin® should not be administered to women with pre-menopausal endocrine status. Therefore, whenever clinically appropriate, the post-menopausal status should be ascertained by assessment of LH, FSH and oestradiol levels.

Aromasin® should be used with caution in patients with hepatic or renal impairment.

Aromasin® tablets contain sucrose and should not be administered to patients with rare hereditary problems of fructose intolerance, glucose-galactose malabsorption or sucrase-isomaltase insufficiency.

Aromasin® tablets contain methyl-p-hydroxybenzoate which may cause allergic reactions (possibly delayed).

As Aromasin® is a potent oestrogen lowering agent, reductions in bone mineral density can be anticipated. The impact of Aromasin® on long-term fracture risk remains undetermined. During adjuvant treatment with Aromasin®, women with osteoporosis or at risk of osteoporosis should have their bone mineral density formally assessed by bone densitometry at the commencement of treatment. Although adequate data to show the effects of therapy in the treatment of the bone mineral density loss caused by Aromasin® are not available, treatment for osteoporosis should be initiated as appropriate. Patients treated with Aromasin® should be carefully monitored.

4.5 Interaction with other medicinal products and other forms of Interaction

In vitro evidence showed that the drug is metabolised through cytochrome P450 (CYP) 3A4 and aldoketoreductases (see 5.2) and does not inhibit any of the major CYP isoenzymes. In a clinical pharmacokinetic study, the specific inhibition of CYP 3A4 by ketoconazole showed no significant effects on the pharmacokinetics of exemestane.

In an interaction study with rifampicin, a potent CYP450 inducer, at a dose of 600 mg daily and a single dose of exemestane 25 mg, the AUC of exemestane was reduced by 54% and Cmax by 41%. Since the clinical relevance of this interaction has not been evaluated, the co-administration of drugs, such as rifampicin, anticonvulsants (e.g. phenytoin and carbamazepine) and herbal preparations containing *hypericum perforatum* (St John's Wort) known to induce CYP3A4 may reduce the efficacy of Aromasin®.

Aromasin® should be used cautiously with drugs that are metabolised via CYP3A4 and have a narrow therapeutic window. There is no clinical experience of the concomitant use of Aromasin® with other anticancer drugs.

Aromasin® should not be coadministered with oestrogen-containing medicines as these would negate its pharmacological action.

4.6 Pregnancy and lactation

No clinical data on exposed pregnancies are available with Aromasin®. Studies on animals have shown reproductive toxicity (See section 5.3). Aromasin® is therefore contra-indicated in pregnant women. It is not known whether exemestane is excreted into human milk. Aromasin® should not be administered to lactating woman.

4.7 Effects on ability to drive and use machines

Drowsiness, somnolence, asthenia and dizziness have been reported with the use of the drug. Patients should be advised that, if these events occur, their physical and/or mental abilities required for operating machinery or driving a car may be impaired.

4.8 Undesirable effects

Aromasin® was generally well tolerated across all studies and in the clinical studies, conducted with Aromasin®, undesirable effects were usually mild to moderate. The withdrawal rate due to adverse events in studies was 6.3% in patients with early breast cancer receiving adjuvant treatment with Aromasin® following initial adjuvant tamoxifen therapy and 2.8% in the overall patient population with advanced breast cancer receiving the standard dose of 25 mg. In patients with early breast cancer the most commonly reported adverse reactions were hot flushes (22%), arthralgia (17%) and fatigue (17%). In patients with advanced breast cancer the most commonly reported adverse reactions were hot flushes (14%) and nausea (12%).

Most adverse reactions can be attributed to the normal pharmacological consequences of oestrogen deprivation (e.g. hot flushes).

The reported adverse reactions are listed below by system organ class and by frequency.

Frequencies are defined as: very common (> 10%), common (> 1%, ≤ 10%), uncommon (> 0.1%, ≤ 1%), rare (> 0.01%, ≤ 0.1%).

Metabolism and nutrition disorders:	
Common	Anorexia
Psychiatric disorders:	
Very common	Insomnia
Common	Depression
Nervous system disorders:	
Very common	Headache
Common	Dizziness, carpal tunnel syndrome
Uncommon	Somnolence
Vascular disorders:	
Very common	Hot flushes
Gastrointestinal disorders:	
Very common	Nausea
Common	Abdominal pain, vomiting, constipation, dyspepsia, diarrhoea
Skin and subcutaneous tissue disorders:	
Very common	Increased sweating
Common	Rash, alopecia
Musculoskeletal and bone disorders:	
Very common	Joint and musculoskeletal pain (*)
General disorders and administration site conditions:	
Very common	Fatigue

Common	Pain, peripheral oedema
Uncommon	Asthenia

(*) Includes: arthralgia, and less frequently pain in limb, osteoarthritis, back pain, arthritis, myalgia and joint stiffness

Blood and lymphatic system disorders

In patients with Advanced Breast Cancer thrombocytopenia and leucopenia have been rarely reported. An occasional decrease in lymphocytes has been observed in approximately 20% of patients receiving Aromasin®, particularly in patients with pre-existing lymphopenia; however, mean lymphocyte values in these patients did not change significantly over time and no corresponding increase in viral infections was observed. These effects have not been observed in patients treated in Early Breast Cancer studies.

Hepatobiliary disorders

A mild elevation of alkaline phosphatase was very commonly observed possibly related to the increased bone turnover. Mild elevation of bilirubin was commonly observed, although usually not associated with elevation of liver enzymes.

The table below presents the frequency of pre-specified adverse events and illnesses in the Early Breast Cancer study (IES), irrespective of causality, reported in patients receiving trial therapy and up to 30 days after cessation of trial therapy.

Adverse events and illnesses	Exemestane (N = 2252)	Tamoxifen (N = 2279)
Hot flushes	488 (21.7%)	456 (20.0%)
Fatigue	372 (16.5%)	345 (15.1%)
Headache	303 (13.5%)	255 (11.2%)
Insomnia	279 (12.4%)	199 (8.7%)
Sweating increased	270 (12.0%)	242 (10.6%)
Dizziness	225 (10.0%)	197 (8.6%)
Nausea	199 (8.8%)	205 (9.0%)
Osteoporosis	116 (5.2%)	65 (2.9%)
Vaginal haemorrhage	87 (3.9%)	109 (4.8%)
Gynaecological	81 (3.6%)	154 (6.8%)
Other primary cancer	56 (2.5%)	84 (3.7%)
Vomiting	51 (2.3%)	52 (2.3%)
Visual disturbance	44 (2.0%)	48 (2.1%)
Cardiovascular disorder	21 (0.9%)	39 (1.7%)
Osteoporotic fracture	17 (0.8%)	13 (0.6%)
Thromboembolism	15 (0.7%)	40 (1.8%)
Myocardial infarction	14 (0.6%)	4 (0.2%)

4.9 Overdose

Clinical trials have been conducted with Aromasin® given up to 800 mg in a single dose to healthy female volunteers and up to 600 mg daily to postmenopausal women with advanced breast cancer; these dosages were well tolerated. The single dose of Aromasin® that could result in life-threatening symptoms is not known. In rats and dogs, lethality was observed after single oral doses equivalent respectively to 2000 and 4000 times the recommended human dose on a mg/m^2 basis. There is no specific antidote to overdosage and treatment must be symptomatic. General supportive care, including frequent monitoring of vital signs and close observation of the patient, is indicated.

5. PHARMACOLOGICAL PROPERTIES

5.1 Pharmacodynamic properties

Pharmacotherapeutic group: steroidal aromatase inhibitor; anti-neoplastic agent

ATC: L02BG06

Exemestane is an irreversible, steroidal aromatase inhibitor, structurally related to the natural substrate androstenedione. In post-menopausal women, oestrogens are produced primarily from the conversion of androgens into oestrogens through the aromatase enzyme in peripheral tissues. Oestrogen deprivation through aromatase inhibition is an effective and selective treatment for hormone dependent breast cancer in postmenopausal women. In postmenopausal women, Aromasin® p.o. significantly lowered serum oestrogen concentrations starting from a 5 mg dose, reaching maximal suppression (>90%) with a dose of 10-25 mg. In postmenopausal breast cancer patients treated with the 25 mg daily dose, whole body aromatization was reduced by 98%.

Table 1

Endpoint Population	Exemestane Events /N (%)	Tamoxifen Events /N (%)	Hazard Ratio (95% CI)	p-value*
Disease-free survival [a]				
All patients	**213**/2352 (9.1%)	**306**/2372 (12.9%)	0.69 (0.58-0.82)	0.00003
ER+ patients	**164**/2008 (8.2%)	**248**/2011 (12.3%)	0.65 (0.53-0.79)	0.00001
Contralateral breast cancer				
All patients	**8**/2352 (0.3%)	**25**/2372 (1.1%)	0.32 (0.15-0.72)	0.00340
ER+ patients	**5**/2008 (0.3%)	**23**/2011 (1.1%)	0.22 (0.08-0.57)	0.00069
Breast cancer free survival [b]				
All patients	**171**/2352 (7.3%)	**262**/2372 (11.0%)	0.65 (0.54-0.79)	<0.00001
ER+ patients	**128**/2008 (6.4%)	**215**/2011 (10.7%)	0.58 (0.47-0.73)	<0.00001
Distant recurrence free survival [c]				
All patients	**142**/2352 (6.0%)	**204**/2372 (8.6%)	0.70 (0.56-0.86)	0.00083
ER+ patients	**107**/2008 (5.3%)	**163**/2011 (8.1%)	0.65 (0.51-0.83)	0.00048
Overall survival *d*				
All patients	**116**/2352 (4.9%)	**137**/2372 (5.8%)	0.86 (0.67-1.10)	0.22962
ER+ patients	**90**/2008 (4.5%)	**104**/2011 (5.2%)	0.87 (0.66-1.16)	0.33671

* Log-rank test ER+ patients = oestrogen receptor positive patients;

[a] Disease-free survival is defined as the first occurrence of local or distant recurrence, contralateral breast cancer, or death from any cause;

[b] Breast cancer free survival is defined as the first occurrence of local or distant recurrence, contralateral breast cancer or breast cancer death;

[c] Distant recurrence free survival is defined as the first occurrence of distant recurrence or breast cancer death;

[d] Overall survival is defined as occurrence of death from any cause.

Exemestane does not possess any progestogenic or oestrogenic activity. A slight androgenic activity, probably due to the 17-hydro derivative, has been observed mainly at high doses. In multiple daily doses trials, Aromasin® had no detectable effects on adrenal biosynthesis of cortisol or aldosterone, measured before or after ACTH challenge, thus demonstrating its selectivity with regard to the other enzymes involved in the steroidogenic pathway.

Glucocorticoid or mineralocorticoid replacements are therefore not needed. A non dose-dependent slight increase in serum LH and FSH levels has been observed even at low doses: this effect is, however, expected for the pharmacological class and is probably the result of feedback at the pituitary level due to the reduction in oestrogen levels that stimulate the pituitary secretion of gonadotropins also in postmenopausal women.

Adjuvant Treatment of Early Breast Cancer

In a multicentre, randomised, double-blind study, conducted in 4724 postmenopausal patients with oestrogen-receptor-positive or unknown primary breast cancer, patients who had remained disease-free after receiving adjuvant tamoxifen therapy for 2 to 3 years, were randomised to receive 3 to 2 years of Aromasin® (25 mg/day) or tamoxifen (20 or 30 mg/day) to complete a total of 5 years of hormonal therapy.

After a median duration of therapy of about 27 months and a median follow-up of about 35 months, results showed that sequential treatment with Aromasin® after 2 to 3 years of adjuvant tamoxifen therapy was associated with a clinically and statistically significant improvement in disease-free survival (DFS) compared with continuation of tamoxifen therapy. Analysis showed that in the observed study period Aromasin® reduced the risk of breast cancer recurrence by 31% compared with tamoxifen (hazard ratio 0.69; p=0.00003). The beneficial effect of exemestane over tamoxifen with respect to DFS was apparent regardless of nodal status or prior chemotherapy.

Aromasin® also significantly reduced the risk of contralateral breast cancer (hazard ratio 0.32, p=0.0034).

At the time of analysis, overall survival was not significantly different in the two groups with 116 deaths occurring in the Aromasin® group and 137 in the tamoxifen group (hazard ratio 0.86, p=0.23).

Main efficacy results are summarised in the table below:

(see Table 1 above)

It is not possible to state whether the differences in disease-free survival will translate into an overall survival advantage for exemestane.

Preliminary results from a bone substudy demonstrated that women treated for 1 year with Aromasin® following 2 to 3 years of tamoxifen treatment experienced moderate reduction in bone mineral density. In the overall study, at 30 months of treatment, the fracture incidence was not statistically different in patients treated with Aromasin® and tamoxifen (3.8% and 2.7% correspondingly).

Preliminary results from an endometrial substudy indicate that after 2 years of treatment there was a median decrease in endometrial thickness of 28.6% (n=52) in the Aromasin®-treated patients compared to an increase of 5.3% (n=51) in the tamoxifen-treated patients. Endometrial thickening, reported at the start of study treatment, was reversed to normal (< 5 mm) for 50% of patients treated with Aromasin®.

Treatment of Advanced Breast Cancer

In a randomised peer reviewed controlled clinical trial, Aromasin® at the daily dose of 25 mg has demonstrated statistically significant prolongation of survival, Time to Progression (TTP), Time to Treatment Failure (TTF) as compared to a standard hormonal treatment with megestrol acetate in postmenopausal patients with advanced breast cancer that had progressed following, or during, treatment with tamoxifen either as adjuvant therapy or as first-line treatment for advanced disease.

5.2 Pharmacokinetic properties

Absorption:

After oral administration of Aromasin® tablets, exemestane is absorbed rapidly. The fraction of the dose absorbed from the gastrointestinal tract is high. The absolute bioavailability in humans is unknown, although it is anticipated to be limited by an extensive first pass effect. A similar effect resulted in an absolute bioavailability in rats and dogs of 5%. After a single dose of 25 mg, maximum plasma levels of 18 ng/ml are reached after 2 hours. Concomitant intake with food increases the bioavailability by 40%.

Distribution:

The volume of distribution of exemestane, not corrected for the oral bioavailability, is ca 20.000l. The kinetics is linear and the terminal elimination half-life is 24 h. Binding to plasma proteins is 90% and is concentration independent. Exemestane and its metabolites do not bind to red blood cells.

Exemestane does not accumulate in an unexpected way after repeated dosing.

Metabolism and excretion:

Exemestane is metabolised by oxidation of the methylene moiety on the 6 position by CYP 3A4 isoenzyme and/or reduction of the 17-keto group by aldoketoreductase followed by conjugation. The clearance of exemestane is ca 500 l/h, not corrected for the oral bioavailability.

The metabolites are inactive or the inhibition of aromatase is less than the parent compound.

The amount excreted unchanged in urine is 1% of the dose. In urine and faeces equal amounts (40%) of ^{14}C-labelled exemestane were eliminated within a week.

Special populations

Age: No significant correlation between the systemic exposure of Aromasin® and the age of subjects has been observed.

Renal insufficiency:

In patients with severe renal impairment (CL_{cr} < 30 ml/min) the systemic exposure to exemestane was 2-times higher compared with healthy volunteers.

Given the safety profile of exemestane, no dose adjustment is considered to be necessary.

Hepatic insufficiency:

In patients with moderate or severe hepatic impairment the exposure of exemestane is 2-3 fold higher compared with healthy volunteers. Given the safety profile of exemestane, no dose adjustment is considered to be necessary.

5.3 Preclinical safety data

Toxicological studies: Findings in the repeat dose toxicology studies in rat and dog were generally attributable to the pharmacological activity of exemestane, such as effects on reproductive and accessory organs. Other toxicological effects (on liver, kidney or central nervous system) were observed only at exposures considered sufficiently in excess of the maximum human exposure indicating little relevance to clinical use.

Mutagenicity: Exemestane was not genotoxic in bacteria (Ames test), in V79 Chinese hamster cells, in rat hepatocytes or in the mouse micronucleus assay. Although exemestane was clastogenic in lymphocytes *in vitro*, it was not clastogenic in two *in vivo* studies.

Reproductive toxicology: Aromasin was embryotoxic in rats and rabbits at systemic exposure levels similar to those obtained in humans at 25 mg/day. There was no evidence of teratogenicity.

Carcinogenicity: In a two-year carcinogenicity study in female rats, no treatment-related tumors were observed. In male rats the study was terminated on week 92, because of early death by chronic nephropathy. In a two-year carcinogenicity study in mice, an increase in the incidence of hepatic neoplasms in both genders was observed at the intermediate and high doses (150 and 450 mg/kg/day). This finding is considered to be related to the induction of hepatic microsomal enzymes, an effect observed in mice but not in clinical studies. An increase in the incidence of renal tubular adenomas was also noted in male mice at the high dose (450 mg/kg/day). This change is considered to be species- and gender-specific and occurred at a dose which represents 63-fold greater exposure than occurs at the human therapeutic dose. None of these observed effects is considered to be clinically relevant to the treatment of patients with exemestane.

6. PHARMACEUTICAL PARTICULARS

6.1 List of excipients

Tablet core: Silica, colloidal hydrated; crospovidone; hypromellose; magnesium stearate; mannitol; microcrystalline cellulose; sodium starch glycollate (A); polysorbate 80

Sugar-coating: hypromellose; polyvinylalcohol; simethicone; macrogol 6000; sucrose; magnesium carbonate, light; titanium dioxide; methyl-p-hydroxybenzoate (E218); cetyl esters wax; talc; carnauba wax.

Printing ink: ethyl alcohol; shellac; iron oxides black (E172) and titanium oxides (E171)

6.2 Incompatibilities

Not applicable.

6.3 Shelf life

3 years.

6.4 Special precautions for storage

No special precautions for storage.

6.5 Nature and contents of container

30 and 90 tablets in blister packs (Aluminium-PVDC/PVC-PVDC)

6.6 Instructions for use and handling

No special requirements.

7. MARKETING AUTHORISATION HOLDER

Pharmacia Ltd

Ramsgate Road

Sandwich

CT13 9NJ

UK

8. MARKETING AUTHORISATION NUMBER(S)

PL 0032/0236

9. DATE OF FIRST AUTHORISATION/RENEWAL OF THE AUTHORISATION

16th December 1998 / 16th December 2003

10. DATE OF REVISION OF THE TEXT

23 August 2005

Legal category: POM

Company reference AM5_2

Arthrotec 50 Tablets

(Pharmacia Limited)

1. NAME OF THE MEDICINAL PRODUCT

Arthrotec® 50.

2. QUALITATIVE AND QUANTITATIVE COMPOSITION

Each tablet consists of a gastro-resistant core containing 50mg diclofenac sodium surrounded by an outer mantle containing 200mcg misoprostol.

3. PHARMACEUTICAL FORM

White, round, biconvex tablets marked on one side and 'Searle 1411' on the other side.

4. CLINICAL PARTICULARS

4.1 Therapeutic indications

Arthrotec 50 is indicated for patients who require the non-steroidal anti-inflammatory drug diclofenac together with misoprostol.

The diclofenac component of Arthrotec 50 is indicated for the symptomatic treatment of osteoarthritis and rheumatoid arthritis. The misoprostol component of Arthrotec 50 is indicated for patients with a special need for the prophylaxis of NSAID-induced gastric and duodenal ulceration

4.2 Posology and method of administration

Adults

One tablet to be taken with food, two or three times daily. Tablets should be swallowed whole, not chewed.

Elderly/Renal Impairment/Hepatic Impairment

No adjustment of dosage is necessary in the elderly or in patients with hepatic impairment or mild to moderate renal impairment as pharmacokinetics are not altered to any clinically relevant extent. Nevertheless patients with renal or hepatic impairment should be closely monitored (see also Section 4.8 - Undesirable Effects).

Children

The safety and efficacy of Arthrotec 50 in children has not been established.

4.3 Contraindications

Arthrotec 50 is contraindicated in:

- Patients with active gastric or duodenal ulceration or who have active GI bleeding or other active bleedings e.g. cerebrovascular bleedings.

- Pregnant women and in women planning a pregnancy.

- Patients who are lactating or who are breast feeding.

- Patients with a known hypersensitivity to diclofenac, aspirin, other NSAIDs, misoprostol, other prostaglandins, or any other ingredient of the product.

- Patients in whom attacks of asthma, urticaria or acute rhinitis are precipitated by aspirin or other non-steroidal anti-inflammatory agents.

4.4 Special warnings and special precautions for use

Warnings

Use in pre-menopausal women (see also Contraindications)

Arthrotec 50 should not be used in pre-menopausal women unless they use effective contraception and have been advised of the risks of taking the product if pregnant (see section 4.6). The label will state: Not for use by pre-menopausal women unless using effective contraception.

Precautions

Arthrotec 50, in common with other NSAIDs, may decrease platelet aggregation and prolong bleeding time. Extra supervision is recommended in haematopoietic disorders or in conditions with defective coagulation or in patients with a history of cerebrovascular bleeding.

Fluid retention and oedema have been observed in patients taking NSAIDs, including Arthrotec 50. Therefore, Arthrotec 50 should be used with caution in patients with compromised cardiac function and other conditions predisposing to fluid retention.

In patients with renal, cardiac or hepatic impairment caution is required since the use of NSAIDs may result in deterioration of renal function. In the following conditions Arthrotec 50 should be used only in exceptional circumstances and with close clinical monitoring: advanced cardiac failure, advanced kidney failure, advanced liver disease.

Similarly caution is also required in patients with diuretic treatment or otherwise at risk of hypovolaemia.The dose should be kept as low as possible and renal function should be monitored.

Caution is required in patients suffering from ulcerative colitis or Crohn's Disease.

NSAIDs, including Arthrotec, should be used with caution in patients with a history of, or active, GI disease, such as ulceration, bleeding or inflammatory conditions.

NSAIDs may precipitate bronchospasm in patients suffering from, or with a history of, bronchial asthma or allergic disease.

By reducing inflammation, diclofenac may diminish diagnostic signs of infection, such as fever.

All patients who are receiving long-term treatment with NSAIDs should be monitored as a precautionary measure (eg. renal, hepatic function, blood counts and haemoccult testing).

4.5 Interaction with other medicinal products and other forms of Interaction

NSAIDs may attenuate the natriuretic efficacy of diuretics due to inhibition of intrarenal synthesis of prostaglandins. Concomitant treatment with potassium-sparing diuretics may be associated with increased serum potassium levels, hence serum potassium should be monitored.

Because of their effect on renal prostaglandins, cyclo-oxygenase inhibitors such as diclofenac can increase the nephrotoxicity of cyclosporin.

Steady state plasma lithium and digoxin levels may be increased and ketoconazole levels may be decreased.

Pharmacodynamic studies with diclofenac have shown no potentiation of oral hypoglycaemic and anticoagulant drugs. However as interactions have been reported with other NSAIDs, caution and adequate monitoring are, nevertheless advised (see statement on platelet aggregation in Precautions).

Because of decreased platelet aggregation caution is also advised when using Arthrotec 50 with anti-coagulants.

Caution is advised when methotrexate is administered concurrently with NSAIDs because of possible enhancement of its toxicity by the NSAID as a result of increase in methotrexate plasma levels.

Concomitant use with other NSAIDs or with corticosteroids may increase the frequency of side effects generally.

NSAIDs may reduce the effect of anti-hypertensives, including ACE inhibitors. Co-administration of Arthrotec and ACE inhibitors may lead to impaired renal function.

Animal data indicate that NSAIDs can increase the risk of convulsions associated with quinolone antibiotics. Patients taking NSAIDs and quinolones may have an increased risk of developing convulsions.

NSAIDs should not be used for 8-12 days after mifepristone administration as NSAIDs can reduce the effect of mifepristone.

4.6 Pregnancy and lactation

Pregnancy

Arthrotec 50 is contraindicated in pregnant women and in women planning a pregnancy as misoprostol may increase uterine tone and contractions in pregnancy which could produce miscarriage. Use of misoprostol during pregnancy has been associated with birth defects. Also diclofenac may cause premature closure of the ductus arteriosus.

Lactation

Arthrotec 50 should not be administered during breast feeding as there are no data on the excretion into breast milk for either misoprostol or diclofenac. Theoretically, any misoprostol excreted in the breast milk could cause diarrhoea in the nursing infant.

4.7 Effects on ability to drive and use machines

Patients who experience dizziness or other central nervous system disturbances while taking NSAIDs should refrain from driving or operating machinery.

4.8 Undesirable effects

Common:

General: Headache, dizziness.

Gastrointestinal: Abdominal pain, diarrhoea, nausea, dyspepsia, flatulence, vomiting, gastritis and eructation.

Diarrhoea is usually mild to moderate and transient and can be minimised by taking Arthrotec 50 with food and by avoiding the use of predominantly magnesium-containing antacids.

Skin: Skin rashes.

Infrequent:

General: Tiredness, peripheral oedema.

Gastrointestinal: Peptic ulcer, stomatitis, decrease in haemoglobin associated with GI blood loss, oesophageal lesions.

Liver: Elevations of SGPT, SGOT, alkaline phosphatase or bilirubin.

Female reproductive system: Menorrhagia, intermenstrual bleeding and vaginal bleeding have been reported in pre-menopausal women and vaginal bleeding in post-menopausal women.

Rarely or very rarely:

Blood system: Thrombocytopenia, leucopenia, agranulocytosis, haemolytic anaemia, aplastic anaemia.

Gastrointestinal: Anorexia, dry mouth, bleeding (haematemesis, melaena), perforated ulcer, glossitis, other GI complaints (ulcerative colitis, Crohn's disease), constipation.

Liver: Hepatitis with or without jaundice.

Skin/hypersensitivity: Urticaria, erythema multiforme, photosensitivity reactions, Steven-Johnson's syndrome, Lyell's syndrome (acute toxic epidermal necrolysis), hypersensitivity including bronchospasm and angioedema, purpura including allergic purpura and hair loss.

CNS: Drowsiness, paraesthesia, memory disorders, disorientation, visual disturbances, tinnitus, insomnia, irritability, convulsions, depression, anxiety, nightmares, tremors, psychotic reactions, taste disturbance.

Renal: As a class NSAIDs have been associated with renal pathology including papillary necrosis, interstitial nephritis, nephrotic syndrome and renal failure.

Other: In isolated cases worsening of inflammation associated with infections have been reported in association with NSAID treatment.

A number of side effects have been reported in clinical studies or in the literature following use of misoprostol for non-approved indications. These include abnormal uterine contractions, uterine haemorrhage, retained placenta, amniotic fluid embolism, incomplete abortion and premature birth.

4.9 Overdose
The toxic dose of Arthrotec 50 has not been determined and there is no experience of overdosage. Intensification of the pharmacological effects may occur with overdosage. Management of acute poisoning with NSAIDs essentially consists of supportive and symptomatic measures. It is reasonable to take measures to reduce absorption of any recently consumed drug by forced emesis, gastric lavage or activated charcoal.

5. PHARMACOLOGICAL PROPERTIES
5.1 Pharmacodynamic properties
Arthrotec 50 is a non-steroidal, anti-inflammatory drug which is effective in treating the signs and symptoms of arthritic conditions.

This activity is due to the presence of diclofenac which has been shown to have anti-inflammatory and analgesic properties.

Arthrotec 50 also contains the gastroduodenal mucosal protective component misoprostol which is a synthetic prostaglandin E_1 analogue that enhances several of the factors that maintain gastroduodenal mucosal integrity.

5.2 Pharmacokinetic properties
The pharmacokinetic profiles of diclofenac and misoprostol administered as Arthrotec 50 are similar to the profiles when the two drugs are administered as separate tablets and there are no pharmacokinetic interactions between the two components.

5.3 Preclinical safety data
In co-administration studies in animals, the addition of misoprostol did not enhance the toxic effects of diclofenac. The combination was also shown not to be teratogenic or mutagenic. The individual components show no evidence of carcinogenic potential.

Misoprostol in multiples of the recommended therapeutic dose in animals has produced gastric mucosal hyperplasia. This characteristic response to E-series prostaglandins reverts to normal on discontinuation of the compound.

6. PHARMACEUTICAL PARTICULARS
6.1 List of excipients
Arthrotec 50 tablets contain:

Lactose, microcrystalline cellulose, maize starch, povidone K-30, cellulose acetate phthalate, diethyl phthalate, methylhydroxpropylcellulose, crospovidone, magnesium stearate, hydrogenated castor oil, colloidal anhydrous silica.

6.2 Incompatibilities
None known.

6.3 Shelf life
Arthrotec 50 has a shelf-life of 3 years when stored in cold-formed blisters.

6.4 Special precautions for storage
Store in a dry place at or below 25°C.

6.5 Nature and contents of container
Arthrotec 50 is presented in cold formed aluminium blisters in pack sizes of 6, 7, 56, 60, 84, 100, 120 and 140 tablets.

6.6 Instructions for use and handling
None.

7. MARKETING AUTHORISATION HOLDER
Pharmacia Limited
Davy Avenue
Milton Keynes
Buckinghamshire
MK5 8PH
United Kingdom

8. MARKETING AUTHORISATION NUMBER(S)
PL 00032/0396

9. DATE OF FIRST AUTHORISATION/RENEWAL OF THE AUTHORISATION
Date of first authorisation: 15 April 2002

10. DATE OF REVISION OF THE TEXT
March 2003

Legal Category
POM

Arthrotec 75

(Pharmacia Limited)

1. NAME OF THE MEDICINAL PRODUCT
Arthrotec 75 tablets

2. QUALITATIVE AND QUANTITATIVE COMPOSITION
Each tablet consists of a gastro-resistant core containing 75 mg diclofenac sodium surrounded by an outer mantle containing 200 micrograms misoprostol.

For excipients, see section 6.1.

3. PHARMACEUTICAL FORM
Tablet.

White, round, biconvex tablets marked "A" and "75" on one side and 'Searle 1421' on the other side.

4. CLINICAL PARTICULARS
4.1 Therapeutic indications
Arthrotec 75 is indicated for patients who require the non-steroidal anti-inflammatory drug diclofenac together with misoprostol.

The diclofenac component of Arthrotec 75 is indicated for the symptomatic treatment of osteoarthritis and rheumatoid arthritis. The misoprostol component of Arthrotec 75 is indicated for patients with a special need for the prophylaxis of NSAID-induced gastric and duodenal ulceration

4.2 Posology and method of administration
Adults
One tablet to be taken with food, two times daily. Tablets should be swallowed whole, not chewed.

Elderly/Renal Impairment/Hepatic Impairment
No adjustment of dosage is necessary in the elderly or in patients with hepatic impairment or mild to moderate renal impairment as pharmacokinetics are not altered to any clinically relevant extent. Nevertheless, elderly patients and patients with renal or hepatic impairment should be closely monitored (see also Section 4.8 - Undesirable effects).

Children (under 18 years)
The safety and efficacy of Arthrotec 75 in children has not been established.

4.3 Contraindications
Arthrotec 75 is contraindicated in:

- Patients with active gastric or duodenal ulceration or who have active GI bleeding or other active bleedings e.g. cerebrovascular bleedings.
- Pregnant women and in women planning a pregnancy.
- Patients who are lactating or who are breast-feeding.
- Patients with a known hypersensitivity to diclofenac, aspirin, other NSAIDs, misoprostol, other prostaglandins, or any other ingredient of the product.
- Patients in whom, attacks of asthma, urticaria or acute rhinitis are precipitated by aspirin or other non-steroidal anti-inflammatory agents.

4.4 Special warnings and special precautions for use
Warnings
Use in pre-menopausal women (see also section 4.3 - Contraindications)
Arthrotec 75 should not be used in pre-menopausal women unless they use effective contraception and have been advised of the risks of taking the product if pregnant (see section 4.6 – Pregnancy and lactation).

The label will state: 'Not for use in pre-menopausal women unless using effective contraception'.

Precautions
• Renal/Cardiac/Hepatic
In patients with renal, cardiac or hepatic impairment and in the elderly, caution is required since the use of NSAIDs may result in deterioration of renal function. In the following conditions Arthrotec 75 should be used only in exceptional circumstances and with close clinical monitoring: advanced cardiac failure, advanced kidney failure, advanced liver disease. Co-administration with cyclosporin may cause an increased risk of nephrotoxicity (See section 4.5 – Interaction with other medicinal products and other forms of Interaction).

Similarly caution is also required in patients with diuretic treatment or otherwise at risk of hypovolaemia.The dose should be kept as low as possible and renal function should be monitored (See section 4.5 – Interaction with other medicinal products and other forms of Interaction).

Co-administration with ACE inhibitors may cause an impairment of renal function (See section 4.5 – Interaction with other medicinal products and other forms of Interaction).

Fluid retention and oedema have been observed in patients taking NSAIDs, including Arthrotec 75. Therefore, Arthrotec 75 should be used with caution in patients with compromised cardiac function and other conditions predisposing to fluid retention.

• Blood system/Gastrointestinal
Arthrotec 75 in common with other NSAIDs, may decrease platelet aggregation and prolong bleeding time. Extra supervision is recommended in haematopoietic disorders or in conditions with defective coagulation or in patients with a history of cerebrovascular bleeding.

Caution is required in patients suffering from ulcerative colitis or Crohn's Disease.

Care should be taken in elderly patients and in patients treated with corticosteroids, other NSAIDs, or anti-coagulants (See section 4.5 – Interaction with other medicinal products and other forms of Interaction).

• Hypersensitivity
NSAID's may precipitate bronchospasm in patients suffering from, or with a history of bronchial asthma or allergic disease.

• Long-term treatment
All patients who are receiving long-term treatment with NSAIDs should be monitored as a precautionary measure (e.g. renal, hepatic function and blood counts). During long-term, high dose treatment with analgesic/anti-inflammatory drugs, headaches can occur which must not be treated with higher doses of the medicinal product.

• Arthrotec may mask fever and thus an underlying infection.

4.5 Interaction with other medicinal products and other forms of Interaction
NSAIDs may attenuate the natriuretic efficacy of diuretics due to inhibition of intrarenal synthesis of prostaglandins. Concomitant treatment with potassium-sparing diuretics may be associated with increased serum potassium levels; hence serum potassium should be monitored.

Because of their effect on renal prostaglandins, cyclo-oxygenase inhibitors such as diclofenac can increase the nephrotoxicity of cyclosporin (See section 4.4 – Special warnings and precautions for use).

Steady state plasma lithium and digoxin levels may be increased and ketoconazole levels may be decreased.

Pharmacodynamic studies with diclofenac have shown no potentiation of oral hypoglycaemic and anticoagulant drugs. However as interactions have been reported with other NSAIDs, caution and adequate monitoring are, nevertheless advised (see statement on platelet aggregation in Precautions).

Because of decreased platelet aggregation caution is also advised when using Arthrotec 75 with anti-coagulants.

Cases of hypo and hyperglycaemia have been reported when diclofenac was associated with antidiabetic agents.

Caution is advised when methotrexate is administered concurrently with NSAIDs because of possible enhancement of its toxicity by the NSAID as a result of increase in methotrexate plasma levels.

Concomitant use with other NSAIDs or with corticosteroids may increase the frequency of side effects generally.

NSAIDs may reduce the effects of antihypertensives including ACE inhibitors.

Co-administration of NSAIDs and ACE inhibitors may cause an impairment of renal function.

Antacids may delay the absorption of diclofenac. Magnesium-containing antacids have been shown to exacerbate misoprostol-associated diarrhoea.

Animal data indicate that NSAIDs can increase the risk of convulsions associated with quinolone antibiotics. Patients taking NSAIDs and quinolones may have an increased risk of developing convulsions.

NSAIDs should not be used for 8-12 days after mifepristone administration as NSAIDs can reduce the effect of mifepristone.

4.6 Pregnancy and lactation
Pregnancy
Arthrotec 75 is contraindicated in pregnant women and in women planning a pregnancy as misoprostol may increase uterine tone and contractions in pregnancy, which could produce miscarriage. Also diclofenac may cause premature closure of the ductus arteriosus.

Lactation
Arthrotec 75 should not be administered during breast-feeding as there are no data on the excretion into breast milk for either misoprostol or diclofenac.

4.7 Effects on ability to drive and use machines
Patients who experience dizziness or other central nervous system disturbances while taking NSAIDs should refrain from driving or operating machinery.

4.8 Undesirable effects
Gastrointestinal: Abdominal pain, diarrhoea, nausea, dyspepsia, flatulence, vomiting, gastritis and eructation.

Diarrhoea is usually mild to moderate and transient and can be minimised by taking Arthrotec 75 with food and by avoiding the use of predominantly magnesium-containing antacids.

Peptic ulcer, stomatitis, decrease in haemoglobin associated with GI blood loss, oesophageal lesions.

Anorexia, dry mouth, bleeding (haematemesis, melaena), perforated ulcer, glossitis, other GI complaints (exacerbation of ulcerative colitis or Crohn's disease), constipation.

Gastrointestinal ulcers, possibly with haemorrhage and intestinal perforation.

Skin/Hypersensitivity: Rashes (urticaria, erthyema multiforme), photosensitivity reactions, Stevens-Johnson syndrome, Lyell's syndrome (acute toxic epidermal necrolysis), hypersensitivity including, asthma and angioedema, purpura including allergic purpura and hair loss, vasculitis and pneumonitis.

Hypersensitivity reactions such as pruritus. Cutaneous eruptions with vesiculation and erythroderma.

Anaphylactic/anaphylactoid systemic reactions; oedema of the face and tongue, hypotension and shock.

Liver: Elevations of SGPT, SGOT, alkaline phosphotase or bilirubin.

Hepatitis, with or without jaundice.In isolated cases, severe fulminant hepatitis may occur, possibly without prodromal symptoms.

Female reproductive system: Menorrhagia, intermenstrual bleeding and vaginal bleeding have been reported in pre-menopausal women and vaginal bleeding in post-menopausal women.

Blood system: Thrombocytopenia, leucopenia, agranulocytosis, haemolytic anaemia, aplastic anaemia.

CNS: Drowsiness, paraesthesia, memory disorders, disorientation, visual disturbances, tinnitus, insomnia, irritability, convulsions, depression, anxiety, nightmares, tremors, psychotic reactions, taste disturbance, headache, dizziness and tiredness. Symptoms of aseptic meningitis (stiff neck, headache, nausea, vomiting, fever or impaired consciousness have been reported during treatment with NSAIDs. Patients suffering from autimmune disease (e.g. lupus erythematosus, mixed connective tissue disorders) seem to be more susceptible.

Renal: Oedema. As a class NSAIDs have been associated with renal pathology including papillary necrosis, interstitial nephritis, nephrotic syndrome, proteinuria, haematuria, acute renal insufficiency and renal failure.

Cardiovascular System: Hypotension, hypertension, oedema palpitations, chest pain and cardiac failure.

Other: Oedemas (e.g. peripheral oedema), especially in patients with hypertension or impaired renal function.

In isolated cases worsening of inflammation associated with infections have been reported in association with NSAID treatment.

4.9 Overdose

The toxic dose of Arthrotec 75 has not been determined and there is no experience of overdosage. Intensification of the pharmacological effects may occur with overdosage. Management of acute poisoning with NSAIDs essentially consists of supportive and symptomatic measures. It is reasonable to take measures to reduce absorption of any recently consumed drug by forced emesis, gastric lavage or activated charcoal.

5. PHARMACOLOGICAL PROPERTIES

5.1 Pharmacodynamic properties

Pharmacotherapeutic group (ATC code): M01BX

Arthrotec 75 is a non-steroidal, anti-inflammatory drug, which is effective in treating the signs and symptoms of arthritic conditions.

This activity is due to the presence of diclofenac, which has been shown to have anti-inflammatory and analgesic properties.

Arthrotec 75 also contains the gastroduodenal mucosal protective component misoprostol, which is a synthetic prostaglandin E_1 analogue that enhances several of the factors that maintain gastroduodenal mucosal integrity

Arthrotec 75 administered bd provides 200 micrograms less misoprostol than Arthrotec tds, whilst providing the same daily dose (150 mg) of diclofenac and may offer a better therapeutic ratio for certain patients.

5.2 Pharmacokinetic properties

The pharmacokinetic profiles of diclofenac and misoprostol administered as Arthrotec 75 are similar to the profiles when the two drugs are administered as separate tablets and there are no pharmacokinetic interactions between the two components.

Diclofenac sodium is completely absorbed from the gastrointestinal (GI) tract after fasting oral administration. Only 50 % of the absorbed dose is systemically available due to first pass metabolism. Peak plasma levels are achieved in 2 hours (range 1-4 hours), and the area-under-the plasma-concentration curve (AUC) is dose proportional within the range of 25 mg to 150 mg. The extent of diclofenac sodium absorption is not significantly affected by food intake.

The terminal half-life is approximately 2 hours. Clearance and volume of distribution are about 350 ml/min and 550 ml/kg, respectively. More than 99 % of diclofenac sodium is reversibly bound to human plasma albumin, and this has been shown not to be age dependent.

Diclofenac sodium is eliminated through metabolism and subsequent urinary and biliary excretion of the glucuronide and the sulfate conjugates of the metabolites. Approximately 65 % of the dose is excreted in the urine and 35 % in the bile. Less than 1 % of the parent drug is excreted unchanged.

Misoprostol is rapidly and extensively absorbed, and it undergoes rapid metabolism to its active metabolite, misoprostol acid, which is eliminated with an elimination $t_{½}$ of about 30 minutes. No accumulation of misoprostol acid was found in multiple-dose studies, and plasma steady state was achieved within 2 days. The serum protein binding of misoprostol acid is less than 90 %. Approximately 70 % of the administered dose is excreted in the urine, mainly as biologically inactive metabolites.

Single and multiple dose studies have been conducted comparing the pharmacokinetics of Arthrotec 75 with the diclofenac 75 mg and misoprostol 200 micrograms components administered separately. Bioequivalence between the two methods of providing diclofenac were demonstrable for AUC and absorption rate (C_{max}/AUC). In the steady state comparisons under fasted conditions bioequivalence was demonstrable in terms of AUC. Food reduced the rate and extent of absorption of diclofenac for both Arthrotec 75 and co-administered diclofenac. Despite the virtually identical mean AUCs in the fed, steady state, statistical bioequivalence was not established. This however is due to the broad co-efficients of variation in these studies due to the wide inter-individual variability in time to absorption and the extensive first-pass metabolism that occurs with diclofenac.

Bioequivalence in terms of AUC (0-24 h) was demonstrable when comparing steady state pharmacokinetics of Arthrotec 75 given bd with diclofenac 50 mg/misoprostol 200 micrograms given tds, both regimens providing a total daily dose of 150 mg diclofenac.

With respect to administration of misoprostol, bioequivalence was demonstrated after a single dose of Arthrotec 75 or misoprostol administered alone. Under steady state conditions food decreases the misoprostol C_{max} after Arthrotec 75 administration and slightly delays absorption, but the AUC is equivalent.

5.3 Preclinical safety data

In co-administration studies in animals, the addition of misoprostol did not enhance the toxic effects of diclofenac. The combination was also shown not to be teratogenic or mutagenic. The individual components show no evidence of carcinogenic potential.

Misoprostol in multiples of the recommended therapeutic dose in animals has produced gastric mucosal hyperplasia. This characteristic response to E-series prostaglandins reverts to normal on discontinuation of the compound.

6. PHARMACEUTICAL PARTICULARS

6.1 List of excipients

Arthrotec 75 tablets contain:

Lactose, microcrystalline cellulose, maize starch, povidone K-30, methylacrylic acid copolymer type C, sodium hydroxide, talc, triethylcitrate, hypromellose, crospovidone, magnesium stearate, hydrogenated castor oil, colloidal anhydrous silica

6.2 Incompatibilities

Not applicable.

6.3 Shelf life

3 years.

6.4 Special precautions for storage

Do not store above 25 °C. Store in the original package.

6.5 Nature and contents of container

Arthrotec 75 is presented in cold-formed aluminium blisters in pack sizes of 10, 20, 30, 60, 90, 100 and 140 tablets.

Not all pack sizes may be marketed.

6.6 Instructions for use and handling

No special requirements.

7. MARKETING AUTHORISATION HOLDER

Pharmacia Limited
Ramsgate Road
Sandwich
Kent
CT13 9NJ
United Kingdom

8. MARKETING AUTHORISATION NUMBER(S)

PL 00032/0397

9. DATE OF FIRST AUTHORISATION/RENEWAL OF THE AUTHORISATION

Renewed 16th April 2003

10. DATE OF REVISION OF THE TEXT

27 August 2004

Arythmol

(Abbott Laboratories Limited)

1. NAME OF THE MEDICINAL PRODUCT

Arythmol

2. QUALITATIVE AND QUANTITATIVE COMPOSITION

Each tablet contains 150 mg or 300 mg propafenone HCl.

3. PHARMACEUTICAL FORM

Tablets.

4. CLINICAL PARTICULARS

4.1 Therapeutic indications

Arythmol is indicated for the prophylaxis and treatment of ventricular arrhythmias.

Arythmol is also indicated for the prophylaxis and treatment of paroxysmal supraventricular tachyarrhythmias which include paroxysmal atrial flutter/fibrillation and paroxysmal re-entrant tachycardias involving the AV node or accessory bypass tracts, when standard therapy has failed or is contra-indicated.

4.2 Posology and method of administration

It is recommended that Arythmol therapy should be initiated under hospital conditions, by a physician experienced in the treatment of arrhythmias. The individual maintenance dose should be determined under cardiological surveillance including ECG monitoring and blood pressure control. If the QRS interval is prolonged by more than 20%, the dose should be reduced or discontinued until the ECG returns to normal limits.

Adults: Initially, 150 mg three times daily increasing at a minimum of three-day intervals to 300 mg twice daily and if necessary, to a maximum of 300 mg three times daily.

The tablets should be swallowed whole and taken with a drink after food. A reduction in the total daily dose is recommended for patients below 70 kg bodyweight.

Elderly: Higher plasma concentrations of propafenone have been noted during treatment. Elderly patients may therefore respond to a lower dose.

Children: A suitable dosage form of Arythmol for children is not available.

Dosage in impaired liver function: Arythmol is extensively metabolised via a saturable hepatic oxidase pathway. In view of the increased bioavailability and elimination half-life of propafenone, a reduction in the recommended dose may be necessary.

Dosage in impaired renal function: Although the elimination of propafenone and its major metabolite is not affected by renal impairment, Arythmol should be administered cautiously.

4.3 Contraindications

Arythmol is contra-indicated in patients with uncontrolled congestive heart failure, cardiogenic shock (unless arrhythmia-induced), severe bradycardia, uncontrolled electrolyte disturbances, severe obstructive pulmonary disease or marked hypotension.

Arythmol may worsen myasthenia gravis.

Unless patients are adequately paced (see section 4.4, Special Warnings and Precautions for Use), Arythmol should not be used in the presence of sinus node dysfunction, atrial conduction defects, second degree or greater AV block, bundle branch block or distal block.

Minor prolongation of the PR interval and intra-ventricular conduction defects (QRS duration of less than 20%) are to be expected during treatment with Arythmol and do not warrant dose reduction or drug withdrawal.

4.4 Special warnings and special precautions for use

The weak negative inotropic effect of Arythmol may assume importance in patients predisposed to cardiac failure. In common with other anti-arrhythmic drugs, Arythmol has been shown to alter sensitivity and pacing threshold. In patients with pacemakers, appropriate adjustments may be required. Because of the beta-blocking effect, care should be exercised in the treatment of patients with obstructive airways disease or asthma. Patients with structural heart disease may be predisposed to serious adverse effects.

4.5 Interaction with other medicinal products and other forms of Interaction

The effects of Arythmol may be potentiated if it is given in combination with other local anaesthetic type agents or agents which depress myocardial activity.

Arythmol has been shown to increase the plasma levels of digoxin and caution should be exercised with regard to digitalis toxicity.

Arythmol has been shown to increase the plasma levels of warfarin, with an accompanying increase in prothrombin time, which may require a reduction in the dose of warfarin.

Plasma levels of propafenone may be increased by concomitant administration of cimetidine.

Increased propranolol and metoprolol plasma levels have been observed when these beta-blockers were used concurrently with Arythmol. Thus, dose reduction of these beta-blockers may be required. Details of interactions with other beta-blockers are not known.

Concomitant administration of propafenone and quinidine may result in decreased oral clearance with an increase in steady state plasma concentrations of propafenone.

There has been a report of the lowering of propafenone levels by rifampicin, via the hepatic mixed oxidase system. This reduction may lead to breakthrough arrhythmias.

Cases of possible interactions with cyclosporin (levels increased with deterioration in renal function), theophylline (levels increased), desipramine (levels increased) have also been reported.

Due to the arrhythmogenic effects of tricyclic and related antidepressants and/or neuroleptics, these drugs may interact adversely when used concomitantly with anti-arrhythmic drugs including propafenone.

4.6 Pregnancy and lactation
Animal studies have not shown any teratogenic effects but as there is no experience of the use of the drug in human pregnancy, Arythmol should not be used during pregnancy and lactation.

4.7 Effects on ability to drive and use machines
Blurred vision, dizziness, fatigue and postural hypotension may affect the patient's speed of reaction and impair the individual's ability to operate machinery or motor vehicles.

4.8 Undesirable effects
Arythmol may produce minor nervous system and cardiovascular side effects but is generally well tolerated. Occasionally and particularly with higher doses, gastrointestinal disorders (i.e. anorexia, bloating), dizziness, nausea and vomiting, fatigue, bitter taste, constipation, diarrhoea, headache, blurred vision, dry mouth, vertigo and retching have been reported. Very rarely, restlessness, nightmares, sleep disorders, psychological disorders (such as states of anxiety and confusion) and extrapyramidal symptoms may occur.

Allergic skin reactions such as reddening, pruritus, exanthema or urticaria may occur infrequently. Postural hypotension is occasionally seen, particularly in the elderly. These effects disappear after reduction of the dose or discontinuation of the drug.

Bradycardia, sinoatrial, atrioventricular or intraventricular blocks may occur (see section 4.9, Overdose). In common with other anti-arrhythmic drugs, there is a small risk of pro-arrhythmic effects. Convulsions have been observed extremely rarely in cases of overdosage. Rare cases of individual hypersensitivity reactions (manifested by cholestasis, blood dyscrasias, lupus syndrome) and seizures have been reported. All were reversible on discontinuation of treatment. In some cases, a diminution of potency and a drop in sperm count have been observed after high doses of Arythmol. This phenomenon is reversible when treatment is discontinued. However, since treatment with Arythmol may be vital, the drug must not be discontinued without consulting the attending physician. Very rarely, a fully reversible decrease of white cell, granulocyte and platelet counts has been observed. Isolated cases of agranulocytosis have been reported.

4.9 Overdose
Experience with overdosage is limited. No specific antidote is known. Procedures to enhance drug elimination from the body by haemodialysis or haemoperfusion are unlikely to succeed because of the large volume of drug distribution. The usual emergency measures for acute cardiovascular collapse should be applied. In severe conduction disturbance associated with compromised cardiac function, atropine, isoprenaline or pacemaker therapy may be required. If electrical stimulation is not possible, an attempt should be made to shorten the QRS duration and increase the heart rate with high doses of isoprenaline. Bundle branch block by itself is not an indication for isoprenaline. Hypotension may require inotropic support. Convulsions should be treated with i.v. diazepam.

5. PHARMACOLOGICAL PROPERTIES

5.1 Pharmacodynamic properties
Propafenone is a class IC anti-arrhythmic agent.

It has a stabilising action on myocardial membranes, reduces the fast inward current carried by sodium ions with a reduction in depolarisation rate and prolongs the impulse conduction time in the atrium, AV node and primarily, in the His-Purkinje system.

Impulse conduction through accessory pathways, as in WPW syndrome, is either inhibited, by prolongation of the refractory period or blockade of the conduction pathway, both in anterograde but mostly retrograde direction.

At the same time, spontaneous excitability is reduced by an increase of the myocardial stimulus threshold while electrical excitability of the myocardium is decreased by an increase of the ventricular fibrillation threshold.

Anti-arrhythmic effects: Slowing of upstroke velocity of the action potential, decrease of excitability, homogenisation of conduction rates, suppression of ectopic automaticity, lowered myocardial disposition to fibrillation.

Propafenone has moderate beta-sympatholytic activity without clinical relevance. However, the possibility exists that high daily doses (900 - 1200 mg) may trigger a sympatholytic (anti-adrenergic) effect.

In the ECG, propafenone causes a slight prolongation of P, PR and QRS intervals while the QTC interval remains unaffected as a rule.

In digitalised patients with an ejection fraction of 35-50%, contractility of the left ventricle is slightly decreased. In patients with acute transmural infarction and heart failure, the intravenous administration of propafenone may markedly reduce the left ventricular ejection fraction but to an essentially lesser extent in patients in the acute stages of infarction without heart failure. In both cases, pulmonary arterial pressure is minimally raised. Peripheral arterial pressure does not show any significant changes. This demonstrates that propafenone does not exert an unfavourable effect on left ventricular function which would be of clinical relevance. A clinically-relevant reduction of left ventricular function is to be expected only in patients with pre-existing poor ventricular function.

Untreated heart failure might then deteriorate possibly resulting in decompensation.

5.2 Pharmacokinetic properties
Following oral administration, propafenone is nearly completely absorbed from the gastrointestinal tract in a dose-dependent manner and distributed rapidly in the body.

After a single dose of one tablet, bioavailability is about 50%. With repeated doses, plasma concentration and bioavailability rise disproportionately due to saturation of the first pass metabolism in the liver. Steady state is reached after 3 or 4 days, when bioavailability increases to about 100%. Therapeutic plasma levels are in the range of 150 ng/ml to 1500 ng/ml. In the therapeutic concentration range, more than 95% of propafenone is bound to plasma proteins. Comparing cumulative urinary excretion over 24 hours allowed for the calculation that 1.3% of intravenous (70 mg) and 0.65% of oral (600 mg) propafenone is excreted unchanged in the urine, i.e. propafenone is almost exclusively metabolised in the liver. Even in the presence of impaired renal function, reduced elimination of propafenone is not likely, which is confirmed by case reports and single kinetic studies in patients on chronic haemodialysis. Clinical chemistry values did not differ from those of patients with uncompromised kidneys.

Terminal elimination half-life in patients is 5-7 hours (12 hours in single cases) following repeated doses. A close positive correlation between plasma level and AV conduction time was seen in the majority of both healthy volunteers and patients.

After a plasma level of 500 ng/ml, the PR interval is statistically significantly prolonged as compared to baseline values which allows for dose titration and monitoring of the patients with the help of ECG readings. The frequency of ventricular extrasystoles decreases as plasma concentrations increase. Adequate anti-arrhythmic activity has, in single cases, been observed at plasma levels as low as <500 ng/ml.

5.3 Preclinical safety data
None.

6. PHARMACEUTICAL PARTICULARS

6.1 List of excipients
Microcrystalline cellulose, maize starch, hydroxypropylmethylcellulose, croscarmellose sodium, purified water, polyethylene glycol 6000, titanium dioxide, polyethylene glycol 400 and magnesium stearate.

6.2 Incompatibilities
None.

6.3 Shelf life
5 years.

6.4 Special precautions for storage
Do not store above 30°C.

6.5 Nature and contents of container
Arythmol Tablets 150 mg: PVC/aluminium blister strips containing 90 tablets.

Arythmol Tablets 300 mg: PVC/aluminium blister strips containing 60 tablets.

6.6 Instructions for use and handling
None.

7. MARKETING AUTHORISATION HOLDER
Abbott Laboratories Limited

Queenborough

Kent

ME11 5EL

United Kingdom

8. MARKETING AUTHORISATION NUMBER(S)
Arythmol 150 mg Tablets PL 00037/0331

Arythmol 300mg Tablets PL 00037/0332

9. DATE OF FIRST AUTHORISATION/RENEWAL OF THE AUTHORISATION
5 December 2001

10. DATE OF REVISION OF THE TEXT

Asacol 400mg MR Tablets
(Procter & Gamble Pharmaceuticals UK Limited)

1. NAME OF THE MEDICINAL PRODUCT
Asacol® 400mg MR Tablets

2. QUALITATIVE AND QUANTITATIVE COMPOSITION
400 mg mesalazine (5-aminosalicylic acid) per tablet.

3. PHARMACEUTICAL FORM
Red-brown, oblong, modified release tablets.

4. CLINICAL PARTICULARS

4.1 Therapeutic indications
Ulcerative Colitis:

For the treatment of mild to moderate acute exacerbations. For the maintenance of remission.

Crohn's ileo-colitis

For the maintenance of remission.

4.2 Posology and method of administration
ADULTS:

Oral:

Acute disease: Six tablets a day in divided doses, with concomitant corticosteroid therapy where clinically indicated.

Maintenance therapy: Three to six tablets a day in divided doses.

ELDERLY: The normal adult dosage may be used unless renal function is impaired (see section 4.4).

CHILDREN: There is no dosage recommendation.

4.3 Contraindications
A history of sensitivity to salicylates or renal sensitivity to sulphasalazine. Confirmed severe renal impairment (GFR less than 20 ml/min). Children under 2 years of age.

4.4 Special warnings and special precautions for use
Use in the elderly should be cautious and subject to patients having normal renal function.

Renal disorder: Mesalazine is excreted rapidly by the kidney, mainly as its metabolite, N-acetyl-5-aminosalicylic acid. In rats, large doses of mesalazine injected intravenously produce tubular and glomerular toxicity. Asacol should be used with extreme caution in patients with confirmed mild to moderate renal impairment (see section 4.3). Patients on mesalazine should have renal function monitored, (with serum creatinine levels measured) prior to treatment start. Renal function should then be monitored periodically during treatment, for example every 3 months for the first year, then 6 monthly for the next 4 years and annually thereafter, based on individual patient history. Physicians should take into account risk factors such as prior and concomitant medications, duration and severity of disease and concurrent illnesses. Treatment with mesalazine should be discontinued if renal function deteriorates. If dehydration develops, normal electrolyte and fluid balance should be restored as soon as possible.

Serious blood dyscrasias have been reported very rarely with mesalazine. Haematological investigations should be performed if the patient develops unexplained bleeding, bruising, purpura, anaemia, fever or sore throat. Treatment should be stopped if there is suspicion or evidence of blood dyscrasia.

4.5 Interaction with other medicinal products and other forms of Interaction
'Asacol' Tablets should not be given with lactulose or similar preparations, which lower stool pH and may prevent release of mesalazine.

Concurrent use of other known nephrotoxic agents, such as NSAIDs and azathioprine, may increase the risk of renal reactions (see section 4.4).

4.6 Pregnancy and lactation
No information is available with regard to teratogenicity; however, negligible quantities of mesalazine are transferred across the placenta and are excreted in breast milk following sulphasalazine therapy. Use of 'Asacol' during pregnancy should be with caution, and only if the potential benefits are greater than the possible hazards. 'Asacol' should, unless essential, be avoided by nursing mothers.

4.7 Effects on ability to drive and use machines
Not applicable.

4.8 Undesirable effects
The side effects are predominantly gastrointestinal, including nausea, diarrhoea and abdominal pain. Headache has also been reported.

There have been rare reports of leucopenia, neutropenia, agranulocytosis, aplastic anaemia and thrombocytopenia, alopecia, peripheral neuropathy, pancreatitis, abnormalities of hepatic function and hepatitis, myocarditis and pericarditis, allergic and fibrotic lung reactions, lupus erythematosus-like reactions and rash (including urticaria), interstitial nephritis and nephrotic syndrome with oral mesalazine treatment, usually reversible on withdrawal. Renal failure has been reported. Mesalazine-induced nephrotoxicity should be suspected in patients developing renal dysfunction during treatment.

Mesalazine may very rarely be associated with an exacerbation of the symptoms of colitis, Stevens Johnson syndrome and erythema multiforme.

Other side effects observed with sulphasalazine such as depression of sperm count and function, have not been reported with 'Asacol'.

4.9 Overdose
Following tablet ingestion, gastric lavage and intravenous transfusion of electrolytes to promote diuresis. There is no specific antidote.

5. PHARMACOLOGICAL PROPERTIES

5.1 Pharmacodynamic properties
Mesalazine is one of the two components of sulphasalazine, the other being sulphapyridine. It is the latter which is responsible for the majority of the side effects associated with sulphasalazine therapy whilst mesalazine is known to be the active moiety in the treatment of ulcerative colitis.

5.2 Pharmacokinetic properties
'Asacol' Tablets contain 400 mg of available mesalazine. This is released in the terminal ileum and large bowel by the effect of pH. Above pH 7 the Eudragit S coat disintegrates and releases the active constituent. 'Asacol' Tablets contain, in a single tablet, an equivalent quantity of mesalazine to that theoretically available from the complete azo-reduction of 1g of sulphasalazine.

5.3 Preclinical safety data
There are no preclinical data of relevance to the prescriber which are additional to that already included in other sections of the SPC.

6. PHARMACEUTICAL PARTICULARS

6.1 List of excipients
Core: lactose, sodium starch glycollate, magnesium stearate, talc, polyvinylpyrrolidone.

Coating: Eudragit S, dibutylphthalate, iron oxides (E172) and polyethylene glycol.

6.2 Incompatibilities
Not applicable.

6.3 Shelf life
2 years.

6.4 Special precautions for storage
Store tablets in a dry place at a temperature not exceeding 25°C and protect from direct sunlight.

6.5 Nature and contents of container
Tablets in cartons (OP) of 120, each containing 12 opaque PVC blister packs of 10 tablets or cartons (OP) of 90, each containing six opaque PVC blister packs of 15 tablets.

6.6 Instructions for use and handling
Do not chew or crush tablets before swallowing.

Administrative Data

7. MARKETING AUTHORISATION HOLDER
Procter & Gamble Pharmaceuticals UK Ltd.

Rusham Park

Whitehall Lane

Egham

Surrey

TW20 9NW

8. MARKETING AUTHORISATION NUMBER(S)
PL00364/0073

9. DATE OF FIRST AUTHORISATION/RENEWAL OF THE AUTHORISATION
1.2.88 / 21.05.2002

10. DATE OF REVISION OF THE TEXT
April 2003

Asacol Foam Enema

(Procter & Gamble Pharmaceuticals UK Limited)

1. NAME OF THE MEDICINAL PRODUCT
Asacol® Foam Enema.

2. QUALITATIVE AND QUANTITATIVE COMPOSITION
Mesalazine (5-aminosalicylic acid), 1g per metered dose.

3. PHARMACEUTICAL FORM
White, aerosol foam enema.

4. CLINICAL PARTICULARS

4.1 Therapeutic indications
For the treatment of mild to moderate acute exacerbations of ulcerative colitis affecting the distal colon.

4.2 Posology and method of administration
Route of administration: Rectal.

Adults: For disease affecting the rectosigmoid region, one metered dose 1g a day for 4 - 6 weeks; for disease involving the descending colon, two metered doses 2g once a day for 4 - 6 weeks.

Elderly: The normal adult dosage may be used unless renal function is impaired (see Section 4.4).

Children: There is no dosage recommendation.

4.3 Contraindications
A history of sensitivity to salicylates or renal sensitivity to sulphasalazine. Confirmed severe renal impairment (GFR less than 20 ml/min). Children under 2 years of age.

4.4 Special warnings and special precautions for use
Use in the elderly should be cautious and subject to patients having a normal renal function.

Renal disorder: Mesalazine is excreted rapidly by the kidney, mainly as its metabolite, N-acetyl-5-aminosalicylic acid. In rats, large doses of mesalazine injected intravenously produce tubular and glomerular toxicity. Asacol should be used with extreme caution in patients with confirmed mild to moderate renal impairment (see section 4.3). Treatment with mesalazine should be discontinued if renal function deteriorates. If dehydration develops, normal electrolyte and fluid balance should be restored as soon as possible.

Serious blood dyscrasias have been reported very rarely with mesalazine. Haematological investigations should be performed if the patient develops unexplained bleeding, bruising, purpura, anaemia, fever or sore throat. Treatment should be stopped if there is suspicion or evidence of blood dyscrasia.

4.5 Interaction with other medicinal products and other forms of Interaction
Concurrent use of other known nephrotoxic agents, such as NSAIDs and azathioprine, may increase the risk of renal reactions (see section 4.4).

4.6 Pregnancy and lactation
No information is available with regard to teratogenicity; however, negligible quantities of mesalazine are transferred across the placenta and are excreted in breast milk following sulphasalazine therapy. Use of 'Asacol' during pregnancy should be with caution, and only if the potential benefits are greater than the possible hazards. 'Asacol' should, unless essential, be avoided by nursing mothers.

4.7 Effects on ability to drive and use machines
Not applicable.

4.8 Undesirable effects
The side effects are predominantly gastrointestinal, including nausea, diarrhoea and abdominal pain. Headache has also been reported.

There have been rare reports of leucopenia, neutropenia, agranulocytosis, aplastic anaemia and thrombocytopenia, alopecia, peripheral neuropathy, pancreatitis, abnormalities of hepatic function and hepatitis, myocarditis and pericarditis, allergic and fibrotic lung reactions, lupus erythematosus-like reactions and rash (including urticaria), interstitial nephritis and nephrotic syndrome with oral mesalazine treatment, usually reversible on withdrawal. Renal failure has been reported. Mesalazine-induced nephrotoxicity should be suspected in patients developing renal dysfunction during treatment.

Mesalazine may very rarely be associated with an exacerbation of the symptoms of colitis, Stevens Johnson syndrome and erythema multiforme.

Other side effects observed with sulphasalazine such as depression of sperm count and function, have not been reported with 'Asacol'.

Rarely, local irritation may occur after administration of rectal dosage forms containing mesalazine.

4.9 Overdose
Not applicable.

5. PHARMACOLOGICAL PROPERTIES

5.1 Pharmacodynamic properties
Mesalazine is one of the two components of sulphasalazine, the other being sulphapyridine. It is the latter which is responsible for the majority of the side effects associated with sulphasalazine therapy whilst mesalazine is known to be the active moiety in the treatment of ulcerative colitis.

5.2 Pharmacokinetic properties
The foam enema is intended to deliver mesalazine directly to the proposed site of action in the colon and rectum.

5.3 Preclinical safety data
There are no preclinical data of relevance to the prescriber which are additonal to those already included in other sections of the SPC.

6. PHARMACEUTICAL PARTICULARS

6.1 List of excipients
Sorbitan mono-oleate, polysorbate 20, emulsifying wax, colloidal anhydrous silica, sodium metabisulphite, disodium edetate, methylhydroxybenzoate, propylhydroxybenzoate, sodium phosphate dodecahydrate or heptahydrate, sodium acid phosphate, glycerol, Macrogol 300, purified water, propane, iso-butane, n-butane.

6.2 Incompatibilities
Not applicable.

6.3 Shelf life
Three years.

6.4 Special precautions for storage
Store the foam enema below 30°C. This is a pressurised canister, containing a flammable propellant. It should be kept away from any flames or sparks, including cigarettes. It should be protected from direct sunlight and must not be pierced or burned even when empty.

6.5 Nature and contents of container
Cartoned aerosol cans, each carton consisting of one aerosol can containing 14 metered doses, plus 14 disposable applicators and 14 disposable plastic bags.

6.6 Instructions for use and handling
Read the instructions carefully before using 'Asacol' Foam Enema for the first time.

Mix contents by shaking the can vigorously for about five seconds.

Before using the enema for the first time, remove the safety tag from under the dome.

Push the plastic applicator firmly on to the spout of the can and align the notch beneath the dome with the spout.

Hold the can in the palm of one hand with the dome pointing downwards. This product must only be dispensed when the can is upside down, with the dome nearest to the ground. (If the can is not upside down the foam will not come out properly.)

You may find that the easiest way to use the enema is to raise one foot on to a firm surface, such as a stool or chair, and insert the applicator into the rectum as far as is comfortable. You can apply a lubricating jelly to the tip of the applicator for comfort if you wish.

To administer a dose, fully depress the dome once and release it. The foam will not come out of the can until you release the dome. To administer a second dose, press and release the dome again. Wait for 15 seconds before withdrawing the applicator.

Note: the can will only work when held with the dome pointing down.

Remove the applicator and dispose of it in one of the plastic bags provided. Do not flush it down the toilet.

7. MARKETING AUTHORISATION HOLDER
Procter & Gamble Pharmaceuticals UK Ltd.

Rusham Park

Whitehall Lane

Egham

Surrey

TW20 9NW

United Kingdom

8. MARKETING AUTHORISATION NUMBER(S)
PL 00364/0077

9. DATE OF FIRST AUTHORISATION/RENEWAL OF THE AUTHORISATION
3.6.94/21.05.2002

10. DATE OF REVISION OF THE TEXT
October 2002

11. Legal Status
POM

Asacol Suppositories 250 mg & 500 mg

(Procter & Gamble Pharmaceuticals UK Limited)

1. NAME OF THE MEDICINAL PRODUCT
Asacol® Suppositories 250 mg & 500 mg

2. QUALITATIVE AND QUANTITATIVE COMPOSITION
Asacol Suppositories contain 250 or 500 mg mesalazine per suppository.

3. PHARMACEUTICAL FORM
Opaque, beige suppositories, containing 250 mg or 500 mg mesalazine.

4. CLINICAL PARTICULARS

4.1 Therapeutic indications
For the treatment of mild to moderate acute exacerbations of ulcerative colitis.

The suppositories are particularly appropriate in patients with distal disease.

For the maintenance of remission of ulcerative colitis.

4.2 Posology and method of administration
ADULTS:

Suppositories 250 mg: Three to six suppositories a day in divided doses, with the last dose at bedtime.

Suppositories 500 mg: A maximum of three suppositories a day in divided doses, with the last dose at bedtime.

ELDERLY: The normal adult dosage may be used unless renal function is impaired (see section 4.4).

CHILDREN: There is no dosage recommendation.

4.3 Contraindications
A history of sensitivity to salicylates or renal sensitivity to sulphasalazine. Confirmed severe renal impairment (GFR <20 ml/min). Children under 2 years of age.

4.4 Special warnings and special precautions for use
Use in the elderly should be cautious and subject to patients having normal renal function.

Renal disorder: Mesalazine is excreted rapidly by the kidney, mainly as its metabolite, N-acetyl-5-aminosalicylic acid. In rats, large doses of mesalazine injected intravenously produce tubular and glomerular toxicity. Asacol should be used with extreme caution in patients with confirmed mild to moderate renal impairment (see section 4.3). Treatment with mesalazine should be discontinued if renal function deteriorates. If dehydration develops, normal electrolyte and fluid balance should be restored as soon as possible.

Serious blood dyscrasias have been reported very rarely with mesalazine. Haematological investigations should be performed if the patient develops unexplained bleeding, bruising, purpura, anaemia, fever or sore throat. Treatment should be stopped if there is suspicion or evidence of blood dyscrasia.

4.5 Interaction with other medicinal products and other forms of Interaction
Concurrent use of other known nephrotoxic agents, such as NSAIDs and azathioprine, may increase the risk of renal reactions (see section 4.4)

4.6 Pregnancy and lactation
No information is available with regard to teratogenicity; however, negligible quantities of mesalazine are transferred across the placenta and are excreted in breast milk following sulphasalazine therapy. Use of Asacol during pregnancy should be with caution, and only if the potential benefits are greater than the possible hazards. Asacol should, unless essential, be avoided by nursing mothers.

4.7 Effects on ability to drive and use machines
Not applicable.

4.8 Undesirable effects
The side effects are predominantly gastrointestinal, including nausea, diarrhoea and abdominal pain. Headache has also been reported.

There have been rare reports of leucopenia, neutropenia, agranulocytosis, aplastic anaemia and thrombocytopenia, alopecia, peripheral neuropathy, pancreatitis, abnormalities of hepatic function and hepatitis, myocarditis and pericarditis, allergic and fibrotic lung reactions, lupus erythematosus-like reactions and rash (including urticaria), interstitial nephritis and nephrotic syndrome with oral mesalazine treatment, usually reversible on withdrawal. Renal failure has been reported. Mesalazine-induced nephrotoxicity should be suspected in patients developing renal dysfunction during treatment.

Mesalazine may very rarely be associated with an exacerbation of the symptoms of colitis, Stevens Johnson syndrome and erythema multiforme.

Other side effects observed with sulphasalazine such as depression of sperm count and function, have not been reported with Asacol.

Rarely, local irritation may occur after administration of rectal dosage forms containing mesalazine.

4.9 Overdose
There is no specific antidote.

5. PHARMACOLOGICAL PROPERTIES
5.1 Pharmacodynamic properties
Mesalazine is one of the two components of sulphasalazine, the other being sulphapyridine. It is the latter which is responsible for the majority of the side effects associated with sulphasalazine therapy whilst mesalazine is known to be the active moiety in the treatment of ulcerative colitis. Asacol consists only of this active component which is delivered directly by the suppositories.

5.2 Pharmacokinetic properties
The suppository is designed to deliver mesalazine directly to the proposed site of action in the distal bowel.

5.3 Preclinical safety data
There are no preclinical data of relevance to the prescriber which are additional to that already included in other sections of the SPC.

6. PHARMACEUTICAL PARTICULARS
6.1 List of excipients
Witepsol W45 (Hard Fat).

6.2 Incompatibilities
Not applicable.

6.3 Shelf life
Suppositories 250 mg: 4 years.
Suppositories 500 mg: 3 years.

6.4 Special precautions for storage
Store below 25°C. Protect from light.

6.5 Nature and contents of container
Cartoned plastic moulds (OP), each containing 20 suppositories (250 mg) or 10 suppositories (500 mg).

6.6 Instructions for use and handling
For rectal administration.

7. MARKETING AUTHORISATION HOLDER
Procter & Gamble Pharmaceuticals UK Ltd.
Rusham Park
Whitehall Lane
Egham
Surrey
TW20 9NW
United Kingdom

8. MARKETING AUTHORISATION NUMBER(S)
Asacol Suppositories 250 mg 00364/0075
Asacol Suppositories 500 mg 00364/0076

9. DATE OF FIRST AUTHORISATION/RENEWAL OF THE AUTHORISATION
Asacol Suppositories 250 mg 20.4.88/21.05.2002
Asacol Suppositories 500 mg 22.3.90/21.05.2002

10. DATE OF REVISION OF THE TEXT
October 2002

11. Legal Status
POM.

Asasantin Retard
(Boehringer Ingelheim Limited)

1. NAME OF THE MEDICINAL PRODUCT
ASASANTIN Retard

2. QUALITATIVE AND QUANTITATIVE COMPOSITION
Each capsule contains dipyridamole 200 mg and aspirin 25 mg.

3. PHARMACEUTICAL FORM
Capsule containing aspirin in standard release form and dipyridamole in modified release form.

Capsules consisting of a red cap and an ivory body imprinted with the company logo and the figures "01A".

4. CLINICAL PARTICULARS
4.1 Therapeutic indications
Secondary prevention of ischaemic stroke and transient ischaemic attacks.

4.2 Posology and method of administration
For oral administration.

Adults, including the elderly

The recommended dose is one capsule twice daily, usually one in the morning and one in the evening preferably with meals.

The capsules should be swallowed whole without chewing.

Children

ASASANTIN Retard is not indicated for use in children and young people. Do not give to children aged under 16 years, unless specifically indicated (e.g. for Kawasaki's disease).

4.3 Contraindications
Hypersensitivity to any component of the product or salicylates.

Patients with active gastric or duodenal ulcers or with bleeding disorders.

Patients in the last trimester of pregnancy.

4.4 Special warnings and special precautions for use
Among other properties dipyridamole acts as a vasodilator. It should be used with caution in patients with severe coronary artery disease, including unstable angina and/or recent myocardial infarction, left ventricular outflow obstruction, or haemodynamic instability (e.g. decompensated heart failure).

Patients being treated with regular oral doses of ASASANTIN Retard should not receive additional intravenous dipyridamole. Clinical experience suggests that patients being treated with oral dipyridamole who also require pharmacological stress testing with intravenous dipyridamole, should discontinue drugs twenty-four hours prior to stress testing.

ASASANTIN Retard should be used in caution in patients with coagulation disorders.

In patients with myasthenia gravis readjustment of therapy may be necessary after changes in dipyridamole dosage (see Interactions).

Due to the aspirin component, ASASANTIN Retard should be used in caution in patients with asthma, allergic rhinitis, nasal polyps, chronic or recurring gastric or duodenal complaints, impaired renal (avoid if severe) or hepatic function or glucose-6-phosphate dehydrogenase deficiency.

In addition, caution is advised in patients hypersensitive to other non-steroidal anti-inflammatory drugs.

ASASANTIN Retard is not indicated for use in children and young people. There is a possible association between aspirin and Reye's syndrome when given to children. Reye's syndrome is a very rare disease, which affects the brain and liver, and can be fatal. For this reason aspirin should not be given to children aged under 16 years unless specifically indicated (e.g. for Kawasaki's disease).

The dose of aspirin in ASASANTIN Retard has not been studied in secondary prevention of myocardial infarction.

4.5 Interaction with other medicinal products and other forms of Interaction
When dipyridamole is used in combination with aspirin or with warfarin, the statements regarding precautions, warnings and tolerance for these preparations must be observed.

Aspirin may enhance the effect of anticoagulants (e.g. coumarin derivatives and heparin) and increase the risk of gastrointestinal side effects when administered simultaneously with NSAIDs or corticosteroids. Addition of dipyridamole to aspirin does not increase the incidence of bleeding events. When dipyridamole was administered concomitantly with warfarin, bleeding was no greater in frequency or severity than that observed when warfarin was administered alone.

Dipyridamole increases the plasma levels and cardiovascular effects of adenosine. Adjustment of adenosine dosage should therefore be considered if use with dipyridamole is unavoidable.

Dipyridamole may increase the hypotensive effect of blood pressure lowering drugs and may counteract the anticholinesterase effect of cholinesterase inhibitors thereby potentially aggravating myasthenia gravis.

The effect of hypoglycaemic agents and the toxicity of methotrexate may be increased by the concomitant administration of aspirin.

Aspirin may decrease the natriuretic effect of spironolactone and inhibit the effect of uricosuric agents (e.g. probenecid, sulphinpyrazone).

There is some experimental evidence that ibuprofen interferes with aspirin induced inhibition of platelet cyclo-oxygenase. This interaction could reduce the beneficial cardiovascular effects of aspirin, however the evidence for this is not conclusive. Further, in view of the known increased risk of gastrointestinal toxicity associated with NSAID and aspirin co-medication, this combination should be avoided wherever possible. When such a combination is necessary the balance of gastrointestinal and cardiovascular risks should be considered.

4.6 Pregnancy and lactation
There is inadequate evidence of safety of ASASANTIN Retard in human pregnancy.

Animal studies performed with the drug combination revealed no increased teratogenic risk over the individual components alone. Fertility studies and studies covering the peri-postnatal period have not been performed with the combination.

ASASANTIN Retard should be used with caution in the first and second trimester, and, since aspirin is associated with delayed and prolonged labour and an increased risk of bleeding, its use is contraindicated in the third trimester.

Dipyridamole and salicylates are excreted in breast milk. Therefore ASASANTIN Retard should only be administered to nursing mothers if clearly needed.

4.7 Effects on ability to drive and use machines
None stated.

4.8 Undesirable effects
Adverse reactions at therapeutic doses are usually mild. Vomiting, diarrhoea and symptoms such as dizziness, nausea, dyspepsia, headache and myalgia have been observed following treatment with dipyridamole. These tend to occur early after initiating treatment and may disappear with continued treatment.

As a result of its vasodilating properties, dipyridamole may cause hypotension, hot flushes and tachycardia. In rare cases, worsening of the symptoms of coronary heart disease has been observed.

Aspirin produces a prolongation of the bleeding time and in very rare cases increased bleeding during or after surgery has been observed following administration of dipyridamole.

Aspirin may produce epigastric distress, nausea and vomiting, gastro or duodenal ulcers and erosive gastritis which may lead to serious gastrointestinal bleeding. These side effects are more likely to occur when higher doses are administered although they may also occur when low doses are used.

Iron deficiency anaemia may develop as a result of occult gastrointestinal bleeding when aspirin is used for long periods of time.

Hypersensitivity reactions including rash, urticaria, severe bronchospasm and angio-oedema have been reported for both dipyridamole and for aspirin. In addition rhinitis, and severe cutaneous skin eruptions have been observed with aspirin. Very rarely, a reduction in platelet count (thrombocytopenia) may occur following administration of aspirin and isolated cases have been reported in conjunction with treatment with dipyridamole. Dizziness and tinnitus can, particularly in elderly patients, be symptoms of aspirin overdosage.

Dipyridamole has been shown to be incorporated into gallstones.

4.9 Overdose
Because of the dose ratio of dipyridamole to aspirin, overdosage is likely to be dominated by signs and symptoms of dipyridamole overdose.

Due to the low number of observations, experience with dipyridamole overdose is limited.

Symptoms such as a warm feeling, flushes, sweating, accelerated pulse, restlessness, feeling of weakness, dizziness, drop in blood pressure and anginal complaints can be expected.

The signs and symptoms of mild acute aspirin overdose are hyperventilation, tinnitus, nausea, vomiting, impairment of vision and hearing, dizziness and confusional states. In severe poisoning, delirium, tremor, dyspnoea, sweating, bleedings, dehydration, disturbances of the acid base balance and electrolyte composition of the plasma, hypothermia and coma may be seen.

Administration of xanthine derivatives (e.g. aminophylline) may reverse the haemodynamic effects of dipyridamole overdose. Due to its wide distribution to tissues and its predominantly hepatic elimination, dipyridamole is not likely to be accessible to enhanced removal procedures.

Apart from general measures (e.g. gastric lavage), treatment of aspirin overdosage consists chiefly of measures to accelerate the excretion of aspirin (forced alkaline diuresis) and to restore the acid-base and electrolyte balance. Infusions of sodium bicarbonate and potassium chloride solutions may be given. In severe cases haemodialysis may be necessary.

5. PHARMACOLOGICAL PROPERTIES

5.1 Pharmacodynamic properties

The anti-thrombotic action of dipyridamole is based on its ability to modify various aspects of platelet function such as inhibition of platelet adhesion and aggregation, which have been shown to be factors associated with the initiation of thrombus formation, as well as lengthening shortened platelet survival time.

Aspirin inhibits platelet aggregation by its inhibitory effect on cyclo-oxygenase in thrombocytes. Dipyridamole does not affect cyclo-oxygenase activity in human platelets and when given simultaneously with aspirin, does not reduce the inhibitory effect on cyclo-oxygenase activity which is obtained with aspirin alone.

The anti-thrombotic effects of dipyridamole and aspirin are additive.

5.2 Pharmacokinetic properties

Peak plasma concentrations of dipyridamole are reached 2 - 3 hours after administration. Steady state conditions are reached within 3 days.

Metabolism of dipyridamole occurs in the liver predominantly by conjugation with glucuronic acid to form a monoglucuronide. In plasma about 70 - 80% of the total amount is present as parent compound and 20 - 30% as the monoglucuronide.

Renal excretion is very low (1 - 5%).

Aspirin is well absorbed from the upper gastro-intestinal tract after oral administration and is rapidly distributed throughout the whole body.

Salicylates are mainly eliminated by hepatic metabolism although unchanged salicylate is also excreted in the urine.

In ASASANTIN Retard the pharmacokinetics of the individual components remain unchanged.

5.3 Preclinical safety data

Dipyridamole and aspirin separately have been extensively investigated in animal models and no clinically significant findings have been observed at doses equivalent to therapeutic doses in humans. Toxicokinetic evaluations were not included in these studies.

Studies with the drug combination dipyridamole/aspirin in a ratio of 1:4 revealed additive, but no potentiating toxic effects. A single dose study in rats using dipyridamole/aspirin in a ratio of 1:0.125 gave comparable results to studies with the 1:4 combination.

6. PHARMACEUTICAL PARTICULARS

6.1 List of excipients

Tartaric acid
Povidone
Eudragit S 100
Talc
Acacia
Hypromellose phthalate
Hypromellose
Triacetin
Dimethicone 350
Stearic acid
Lactose
Aluminium stearate
Colloidal silica
Maize starch
Microcrystalline cellulose
Sucrose
Titanium dioxide; E171

Capsule Shells:
Gelatin
Titanium dioxide; E171
Red and yellow iron oxides; E172

Printing Ink:
Shellac
Ethyl alcohol
Isopropyl alcohol
Propylene glycol
N-butyl alcohol
Ammonium hydroxide
Potassium hydroxide
Purified water
Red iron oxide; E172

6.2 Incompatibilities

None stated.

6.3 Shelf life

30 months

6.4 Special precautions for storage

Store below 25°C

Discard any capsules remaining 6 weeks after first opening.

6.5 Nature and contents of container

White polypropylene tubes with low-density polyethylene Air-sec stoppers filled with desiccating agent (90% white silicon gel/10% molecular sieves).Packs contain 60 capsules.

6.6 Instructions for use and handling

None stated.

7. MARKETING AUTHORISATION HOLDER

Boehringer Ingelheim limited
Ellesfield Avenue
Bracknell
Berkshire
RG12 8YS
England

8. MARKETING AUTHORISATION NUMBER(S)

PL 00015/0224

9. DATE OF FIRST AUTHORISATION/RENEWAL OF THE AUTHORISATION

12 May 1998

10. DATE OF REVISION OF THE TEXT

May 2004

11. Legal category

Prescription only medicine

A8/UK/SPC 9

Ascabiol Emulsion 25% W/V

(sanofi-aventis)

1. NAME OF THE MEDICINAL PRODUCT

Ascabiol Emulsion 25% w/v.

2. QUALITATIVE AND QUANTITATIVE COMPOSITION

Benzyl benzoate BP 25% w/v.

3. PHARMACEUTICAL FORM

Cutaneous Emulsion

4. CLINICAL PARTICULARS

4.1 Therapeutic indications

Ascabiol is an efficient acaricide and is indicated for the treatment of scabies and pediculosis.

4.2 Posology and method of administration

Route of administration: Topical.

Adults

Scabies: After a hot bath and drying, Ascabiol is applied to the whole body except the head and face. If the application is thorough, one treatment should suffice, but the possibility of failure is lessened if a second application is made within five days of the first.

Alternatively Ascabiol can be applied to the whole body, except the head and face, on three occasions at 12-hourly intervals. The patient has a hot bath 12 hours after the last application and changes to clean clothes and sheets.

Pediculosis: The affected region is coated with Ascabiol followed by a wash 24 hours later with soap and water. In severe cases this procedure may need to be repeated two or three times. An examination should always be made a week after the last treatment to confirm disinfestation.

Elderly patients

No specific recommendations.

Children

Ascabiol can be diluted with an equal quantity of water for older children and with three parts of water for babies.

4.3 Contraindications

None.

4.4 Special warnings and special precautions for use

The emulsion may damage plastic or acrylic bathroom furniture. Care should be taken not to splash the emulsion on such surfaces.

4.5 Interaction with other medicinal products and other forms of Interaction

Not applicable.

4.6 Pregnancy and lactation

There is inadequate evidence of the safety of Ascabiol in human pregnancy, but it has been in widespread use for many years without apparent ill consequence. Nevertheless Ascabiol should not be used during pregnancy unless considered essential.

Breast feeding should be suspended during treatment with Ascabiol. Feeding may be restarted after the emulsion has been washed off the body.

4.7 Effects on ability to drive and use machines

Not applicable.

4.8 Undesirable effects

Ascabiol causes little skin irritation, but may cause a transient burning sensation. This is usually mild but can occasionally be severe in sensitive individuals. In the event of a severe skin reaction the preparation should be washed off using soap and warm water. Ascabiol is also irritating to the eyes therefore these should be protected if it is applied to the scalp.

4.9 Overdose

If Ascabiol is accidentally taken by mouth treatment should consist of gastric lavage or the administration of an emetic. An anticonvulsant should be given if necessary, otherwise treatment is symptomatic.

Urinary retention in adults and convulsions in infants have been reported following excessive use of topical benzyl benzoate. The body should be washed to remove excess benzyl benzoate. Otherwise treatment is symptomatic.

5. PHARMACOLOGICAL PROPERTIES

5.1 Pharmacodynamic properties

Benzyl benzoate is lethal to *Sarcoptes scabei* and to the larval and adult forms of head lice.

5.2 Pharmacokinetic properties

No data available by the topical route.

5.3 Preclinical safety data

There are no preclinical data of relevance to the prescriber which are additional to that already included in other sections of the SPC.

6. PHARMACEUTICAL PARTICULARS

6.1 List of excipients

Stearic acid powder, Trolamine, Terpineol, Oil cinnamon leaf Ceylon, Silicone MS antifoam A, Purified Water.

6.2 Incompatibilities

Not applicable.

6.3 Shelf life

36 months.

6.4 Special precautions for storage

Do not store above 25°C.

6.5 Nature and contents of container

Amber glass bottles with a screw cap in 100ml size.

6.6 Instructions for use and handling

The emulsion may damage plastic or acrylic bathroom furniture. Care should be taken not to splash the emulsion on such surfaces.

7. MARKETING AUTHORISATION HOLDER

Aventis Pharma Ltd
50 Kings Hill Avenue
Kings Hill
West Malling
Kent ME19 4AH
UK

8. MARKETING AUTHORISATION NUMBER(S)

PL 04425/0339

9. DATE OF FIRST AUTHORISATION/RENEWAL OF THE AUTHORISATION

6 June 2005

10. DATE OF REVISION OF THE TEXT

June 2005

Legal category: POM

Ascorbic Acid Injection BPC 500mg/5ml

(UCB Pharma Limited)

1. NAME OF THE MEDICINAL PRODUCT

Ascorbic Acid Injection BPC 500 mg/5 ml

2. QUALITATIVE AND QUANTITATIVE COMPOSITION

Ascorbic Acid 10.0% w/v

For excipients see 6.1

3. PHARMACEUTICAL FORM

Solution for injection

4. CLINICAL PARTICULARS

4.1 Therapeutic indications

The prevention and treatment of scurvy, or other conditions requiring vitamin C supplementation, where the deficiency is acute or oral administration is difficult.

4.2 Posology and method of administration

Route of Administration: Parenteral

Adults

0.5 to 1g daily for scurvy, 200 to 500mg daily for preventative therapy.

Children

100 to 300mg daily for curative purposes, or 30mg daily for protective treatment.

Elderly

No special dosage requirements have been suggested.

4.3 Contraindications

Hyperoxaluria

4.4 Special warnings and special precautions for use

Ascorbic acid should be given with care to patients with hyperoxaluria. Tolerance may be induced in patients taking high doses.

Large doses of Ascorbic Acid have resulted in haemolysis in patients with glucose-6-phosphate dehydrogenase (G6PD) deficiency.

4.5 Interaction with other medicinal products and other forms of Interaction

Drugs which induce tissue desaturation of ascorbic acid include aspirin, nicotine from cigarettes, alcohol, several appetite suppressants, iron, phenytoin, some anti-convulsant drugs, the oestrogen component of oral contraceptives and tetracycline. Large doses of ascorbic acid may cause the urine to become acidic causing unexpected renal tubular reabsorption of acidic drugs, thus producing an exaggerated response. Conversely basic drugs may exhibit decreased reabsorption resulting in a decreased therapeutic effect. Large doses may reduce the response to oral anticoagulants.

It has been reported that concurrent administration of ascorbic acid and fluphenazine has resulted in decreased fluphenazine plasma concentrations.

Ascorbic acid is a strong reducing agent and interferes with numerous laboratory tests based on oxidation - reduction reactions. Specialised references should be consulted for specific information on laboratory test interferences caused by ascorbic acid.

Ascorbic acid given in addition to desferrioxamine in patients with iron overload to achieve better iron excretion may worsen iron toxicity, particularly to the heart, early on in the treatment when there is excessive tissue iron. Therefore it is recommended that in patients with normal cardiac function ascorbic acid should not be given for the first month after starting desferrioxamine. Ascorbic acid should not be given in conjunction with desferrioxamine in patients with cardiac dysfunction.

Aspirin can reduce the absorption of ascorbic acid by approximately a third and decreases urinary excretion by about half. The clinical importance of this is uncertain.

Patients with kidney failure given aluminium antacids and oral citrate can develop a potentially fatal encephalopathy due to marked rise in blood aluminium levels. There is evidence that vitamin C may interact similarly.

Oral contraceptives lower serum levels of ascorbic acid.

4.6 Pregnancy and lactation

Ascorbic acid in doses greater than 1g daily should not be taken during pregnancy since the effect of large doses on the foetus is unknown. Ascorbic acid is excreted in breast milk, but there is no evidence of any hazard.

4.7 Effects on ability to drive and use machines

Ascorbic acid injection is unlikely to affect the patients ability to drive or use machinery.

4.8 Undesirable effects

Large doses may cause gastrointestinal disorders including diarrhoea. Large doses may also result in hyperoxaluria and renal oxalate calculi may form if the urine becomes acidic. Doses of 600mg or more daily have a diuretic action. Induced tolerance with prolonged use of large doses can result in symptoms of deficiency when intake is reduced to normal.

4.9 Overdose

Large doses may cause gastrointestinal disorders including diarrhoea. Large doses may also result in hyperoxaluria and renal oxalate calculi may form if urine is acidic. Doses of 600mg or more daily have a diuretic action. Stop treatment and treat symptomatically.

5. PHARMACOLOGICAL PROPERTIES

5.1 Pharmacodynamic properties

ATC Code: A11G A01

Ascorbic acid, a water-soluble vitamin, is essential for formation of collagen and intercellular material, and therefore necessary for the development of cartilage, bone, teeth and for the healing of wounds. It is also essential for the conversion from folic acid to folinic acid, facilitates iron absorption from the gastro-intestinal tract and influences haemoglobin formation and erythrocyte maturation.

5.2 Pharmacokinetic properties

Distribution - widely distributed in body tissues with about 25% bound to plasma proteins. Large amounts are present in leucocytes and platelets. Ascorbic acid crosses the placenta.

Metabolism - readily oxidised to dehydroascorbic acid where some is metabolised to oxalic acid and the inactive ascorbate - 2 - sulphate. Metabolic turnover appears to be greater in females than males.

Excretion - large doses are rapidly excreted in the urine when in excess of the requirements of the body and after an intravenous dose, about 40% is excreted in 8 hours, which is increased to about 70% after tissue saturation. The amount of unchanged drug is dose dependent; in women the excretion of ascorbic acid appears to vary with the stage of the menstrual cycle and it is decreased when taking oral contraceptives.

Ascorbic acid is excreted in breast milk.

Oxalic acid and ascorbate - 2 - sulphate are excreted in the urine.

5.3 Preclinical safety data

None stated.

6. PHARMACEUTICAL PARTICULARS

6.1 List of excipients

Sodium Bicarbonate

Sodium Metabisulphite

Hydrochloric acid

Water for injections

6.2 Incompatibilities

Incompatible with ferric salts, oxidising agents, and salts of heavy metals, particularly copper.

Injections of ascorbic acid have been reported to be incompatible with aminophylline, bleomycin sulphate, erythromycin lactobionate, nafcillin sodium, nitrofurantoin sodium, conjugated oestrogens, sodium bicarbonate and sulphafurazole diethanolamine. Occasional incompatibility, depending on pH or concentration, has occurred with chloramphenicol sodium succinate.

6.3 Shelf life

12 months

6.4 Special precautions for storage

Do not store above 25°C

6.5 Nature and contents of container

5 ml neutral glass (Type 1) ampoules. Pack size - 10.

6.6 Instructions for use and handling

None stated

7. MARKETING AUTHORISATION HOLDER

UCB Pharma Limited

208 Bath Road

Slough

Berkshire

SL1 3WE

UK

8. MARKETING AUTHORISATION NUMBER(S)

PL 00039/5649R

9. DATE OF FIRST AUTHORISATION/RENEWAL OF THE AUTHORISATION

14th November 1986/2nd June 1994/2 June 1999

10. DATE OF REVISION OF THE TEXT

June 2005

POM

Asendis

(Wyeth Pharmaceuticals)

1. NAME OF THE MEDICINAL PRODUCT

ASENDIS* Tablets 50mg

ASENDIS* Tablets 100mg

2. QUALITATIVE AND QUANTITATIVE COMPOSITION

Asendis Tablets 50mg are orange, flat, heptagonal-shaped tablets, scored on one side and engraved with "LL50" on the other, each containing 50mg of amoxapine.

Asendis Tablets 100 mg are mottled blue, flat, heptagonal-shaped tablets, scored on one side and engraved with "LL100" on the other, each containing 100mg of amoxapine.

3. PHARMACEUTICAL FORM

Tablets.

4. CLINICAL PARTICULARS

4.1 Therapeutic indications

ASENDIS* is an anti-depressant indicated for the symptomatic treatment of depressive illness.

4.2 Posology and method of administration

Adults: Initially 100-150mg daily, increasing slowly according to clinical response up to 300mg daily, in divided doses or one dose which may be given at night.

Usual Maintenance dose: 150-250mg daily.

Elderly patients: An initial dose of 25mg twice a day is recommended. If necessary, the dosage may be increased under close supervision after five to seven days to a maximum of 50mg three times daily. Less than the normal dose may be sufficient to produce a satisfactory clinical response.

Children (under 16 years): Not recommended.

Studies have demonstrated that the initial clinical effect of ASENDIS* can occur within four to seven days. Treatment should be maintained for a minimum period of one month, and current psychiatric practice suggests that several months treatment may be necessary after initial clinical improvement.

4.3 Contraindications

- Recent myocardial infarction or coronary artery insufficiency.
- Heart block or other cardiac arrhythmias.
- Mania.
- Severe liver disease.
- Use in patients hypersensitive to dibenzoxazepines, or in patients who are currently receiving, or have received, monoamine oxidase inhibitors in the preceding two weeks.

4.4 Special warnings and special precautions for use

Tardive dyskinesia, consisting of potentially irreversible, dyskinetic movements, may develop in patients treated with amoxapine. Withdrawal-emergent dyskinesia has been observed with a decrease and/or discontinuation of amoxapine.

A potentially fatal symptom complex sometimes referred to as Neuroleptic Malignant Syndrome (NMS) has been reported in association with amoxapine alone or in combination with antipsychotic drugs. Clinical manifestations of NMS are hyperpyrexia, muscle rigidity, altered mental status and evidence of autonomic instability (irregular pulse or blood pressure, tachycardia, diaphoresis, and cardiac dysrhythmias).

The diagnostic evaluation of patients with this syndrome is complicated. In arriving at a diagnosis, it is important to identify cases where the clinical presentation includes both serious medical illness (eg pneumonia, systemic infection, etc) and untreated or inadequately treated extrapyramidal signs and symptoms (EPS). Other important considerations in the differential diagnosis include central anticholinergic toxicity, heat stroke, drug fever and primary central nervous system (CNS) pathology.

The management of NMS should include 1) immediate discontinuation of antipsychotic drugs, if any, and other drugs not essential to concurrent therapy, 2) intensive symptomatic treatment and medical monitoring, and 3) treatment of any concomitant serious medical problems for which specific treatments are available. There is no general agreement about specific pharmacological treatment regimens for uncomplicated NMS.

In common with other drugs of this class, caution should be exercised when using in patients with any of the following conditions: urinary retention, narrow angle glaucoma, hyperthyroidism, cardiovascular disorders, blood dyscrasias and hepatic or renal impairment. ASENDIS* should be used with particular caution in patients with a history of epilepsy or recent convulsions.

Psychotic manifestations may be exacerbated during treatment with tri/tetracyclic anti-depressants.

A minority of patients may not improve during the first 2 - 4 weeks of treatment. Patients should be closely monitored during this period, especially those posing a high suicidal risk.

Concurrent administration with electroconvulsive therapy may increase the hazards associated with such therapy.

Although not indicative of addiction, withdrawal symptoms may occur on abrupt cessation of therapy (see 4.8 Undesirable effects).

In common with other anti-depressants, the elderly are more prone to experiencing adverse reactions, especially agitation and confusion, hence the importance of initiating treatment at a lower dose (See 4.2. Posology and method of administration).

4.5 Interaction with other medicinal products and other forms of Interaction

The drug interactions experienced with ASENDIS* are those that could be expected from a drug of this class and include the following:

ASENDIS* may decrease the anti-hypertensive effect of guanethidine, debrisoquine, bethanidine and possibly clonidine. It would be advisable to review all anti-hypertensive therapy during treatment.

ASENDIS* should not be given with sympathomimetic agents such as adrenaline, ephedrine, isoprenaline, noradrenaline, phenylephrine, and phenylpropanolamine.

ASENDIS* may potentiate the effects of drugs having an anticholinergic action, ethchlorvynol, thyroid hormone therapy, and the central nervous depressant action of alcohol.

Barbiturates may increase the metabolism of tri/tetracyclic antidepressants.

Anaesthetics given during tri/tetracyclic anti-depressant therapy may increase the risk of arrhythmias and hypotension. If surgery is necessary, the anaesthetist should be informed that a patient is being so treated.

Caution should be exercised if ASENDIS* is given concomitantly with Lithium.

Serum levels of several tricyclic anti-depressants have been reported to be significantly increased when cimetidine is administered concurrently; although such an interaction has not been reported to date with ASENDIS*.

4.6 Pregnancy and lactation

There are no adequately well controlled studies in pregnant women. ASENDIS* should therefore be used during pregnancy only if the potential benefit justifies the potential risk to the foetus. ASENDIS* like many other systemic drugs is excreted in human milk. The effects of the drug on infants are unknown, and hence the administration to nursing mothers cannot be recommended.

4.7 Effects on ability to drive and use machines

As with many other antidepressants, ASENDIS* may initially impair alertness. Patients should be warned of the possible hazard when driving or operating machinery.

4.8 Undesirable effects

In common with certain other drugs of this class, the following adverse effects have been reported with

ASENDIS*. These have been categorised according to incidence.

Incidence greater than 1%

The most frequent types of adverse reactions occurring in clinical trials were sedative and anti-cholinergic. These included; drowsiness (14%), dry mouth (14%), constipation (12%), and blurred vision (7%).

Less frequently reported adverse reactions

CNS and Neuromuscular: anxiety, insomnia, restlessness, nervousness, palpitations, tremors, confusion, excitement, nightmares, ataxia, alterations in EEG patterns.

Allergic: oedema, skin rash.

Endocrine: elevation of prolactin levels.

Gastrointestinal: nausea.

Other: dizziness, headache, fatigue, weakness, excessive appetite, increased perspiration.

Incidence less than 1%

Anticholinergic: disturbances of accommodation, mydriasis, urinary hesitancy and retention, nasal stuffiness.

Cardiovascular: hypotension, hypertension, syncope, tachycardia.

Allergic: drug fever, urticaria, photosensitisation, pruritis, vasculitis, hepatitis.

CNS and Neuromuscular: tingling, paraesthesia of the extremities, tinnitus, disorientation, seizures, hypomania, numbness, inco-ordination, disturbed concentration, hyperthermia, extrapyramidal symptoms including tardive dyskinesia. Neuroleptic malignant syndrome (see Section 4.4 Special warnings and precautions for use). Withdrawal symptoms reported in association with amoxapine discontinuation or dose reduction include tardive dyskinesia, anxiety, irritability, chills, confusion, headache, insomnia, malaise, nausea and sweating.

Haematologic: leukopenia, agranulocytosis.

Gastrointestinal: epigastric distress, vomiting, flatulence, abdominal pain, peculiar taste, diarrhoea.

Endocrine: increased or decreased libido, impotence, menstrual irregularity, breast enlargement and galactorrhoea in the female, syndrome of inappropriate antidiuretic hormone secretion.

Hepatobiliary disorders: hepatitis, abnormal liver function.

Skin and subcutaneous tissue disorders: Erythema multiforme, Stevens-Johnson syndrome, toxic epidermal necrolysis.

Other: lacrimation, weight loss or gain, altered liver function, painful ejaculation.

4.9 Overdose

Toxic manifestations of ASENDIS* overdose differ significantly from those of other tricyclic anti-depressants. Serious cardiovascular effects are rare and tend to be limited to sinus tachycardia. QT prolongation has been observed with overdose. Convulsions may occur frequently (40-50%) in those taking substantial overdoses and status epilepticus is not uncommon. Coma has also been observed with overdose. Respiratory and/or metabolic acidosis may develop, usually in association with repeated seizures. Acute renal failure, usually in association with overdose–associated rhabdomyolysis, may develop 2-5 days after substantial overdose of ASENDIS*. There is a rare potential for permanent neurological damage. Fatal overdoses with amoxapine have occurred.

There is no specific antidote for ASENDIS*; treatment should be symptomatic and supportive with special attention to prevention or control of seizures. If the patient is conscious, emesis should be induced as soon as possible, followed by gastric lavage. Administration of activated charcoal after gastric lavage may reduce absorption and facilitate drug elimination. An adequate airway should be established in unconscious patients, who may also need full support of vital functions and cardiac monitoring. Convulsions, when they occur, typically begin within 12 hours of ingestion and may respond to standard anti-convulsant therapy such as intravenous diazepam and/or phenytoin. More rigorous treatment is required should status epilepticus develop. Drugs which are known to potentiate respiratory depression should be avoided. Treatment for renal impairment, should it occur, is the same as for non-drug-induced renal dysfunction.

5. PHARMACOLOGICAL PROPERTIES

5.1 Pharmacodynamic properties

Amoxapine is a tricyclic antidepressant. It has marked anticholinergic and sedative properties, and prevents re-uptake (and hence inactivation) of noradrenaline and serotonin at nerve terminals. Its mode of action in depression is not fully understood.

5.2 Pharmacokinetic properties

Amoxapine is readily absorbed from the gastro-intestinal tract. Since amoxapine slows gastro-intestinal transit time, absorption can, however, be delayed, particularly in overdosage.

Amoxapine is metabolised by hydroxylation and excreted in the urine mainly as its metabolites in the conjugated form.

Amoxapine has been reported to have a half life of 8 hours and its major metabolite, 8-hydroxy-amoxapine, a half life of 30 hours. Amoxapine is extensively bound to plasma proteins.

5.3 Preclinical safety data

There are no pre-clinical data of relevance to the prescriber which are additional to that already included in other sections of the Summary of Product Characteristics.

6. PHARMACEUTICAL PARTICULARS

6.1 List of excipients

Dibasic calcium phosphate

Maize starch (pregelatinised)

Corn starch

Magnesium stearate

Stearic acid

50mg Tablets: Colourings – E104 and E127

100mg Tablets: Colouring – E132.

6.2 Incompatibilities

None

6.3 Shelf life

36 months

6.4 Special precautions for storage

Store below 25°C.

6.5 Nature and contents of container

White polypropylene bottles with white urea screw on caps of 56, 84, 100 or 500 tablets.

6.6 Instructions for use and handling

None

7. MARKETING AUTHORISATION HOLDER

Cyanamid of Great Britain Limited

Fareham Road

Gosport

Hants

PO13 0AS

8. MARKETING AUTHORISATION NUMBER(S)

ASENDIS* Tablets 50mg: PL 00095/0057

ASENDIS* Tablets 100mg: PL 00095/0058

9. DATE OF FIRST AUTHORISATION/RENEWAL OF THE AUTHORISATION

First Authorisation: 24 April 1981

Last Renewal: 07 January 2004

10. DATE OF REVISION OF THE TEXT

07 January 2004

*Trade Mark.

Asmabec Clickhaler 50, 100, 250

(UCB Pharma Limited)

1. NAME OF THE MEDICINAL PRODUCT

Asmabec Clickhaler 50μg

Asmabec Clickhaler 100μg

Asmabec Clickhaler 250μg.

Inhalation powder.

2. QUALITATIVE AND QUANTITATIVE COMPOSITION

Each metered actuation of 1.3mg contains 50 micrograms of beclometasone dipropionate and delivers 45 micrograms of beclometasone dipropionate.

Each metered actuation of 2.6mg contains 100 micrograms of beclometasone dipropionate and delivers 90 micrograms of beclometasone dipropionate.

Each metered actuation of 6.6mg contains 250 micrograms of beclometasone dipropionate and delivers 225 micrograms of beclometasone dipropionate.

For excipients see 6.1.

3. PHARMACEUTICAL FORM

Inhalation powder

White free-flowing powder.

4. CLINICAL PARTICULARS

4.1 Therapeutic indications

Beclometasone Dipropionate is indicated for the control of persistent asthma.

4.2 Posology and method of administration

The product is intended for oral inhalation only. For optimum results Asmabec Clickhaler should be used regularly.

The initial dose should be appropriate to the severity of the disease and the maintenance dose titrated to the lowest dose at which effective control of asthma is achieved.

Adults:

The initial dose for patients with mild asthma is 200 to 400 micrograms per day; this may be increased to 800 micrograms per day if required.

For patients with moderate asthma and severe asthma the initial dose can be 800 to 1600 micrograms per day, increased to 2000 micrograms in severe cases. The normal maximum daily for adults is 2000 micrograms.

The maintenance dose is normally 200 to 400 micrograms twice daily. If necessary the dose may be increased to 1600 to 2000 micrograms per day divided into two to four doses and be reduced later when asthma is stabilised.

Children aged 6 - 12 years:

Up to 100 micrograms 2 to 4 times daily according to the clinical response.

Normally the maximum daily dose in children is 400μg. However some cases of severe asthma may not be controlled and higher doses may be required in line with international guidelines. Once the asthma is controlled, the dose of Asmabec Clickhaler should be reduced to the minimum to maintain control.

When transferring a patient to Asmabec Clickhaler from other devices, treatment should be individualised taking into consideration the active ingredient and method of administration.

4.3 Contraindications

Asmabec Clickhaler is contra-indicated in patients with hypersensitivity (allergy) to beclometasone dipropionate or to the excipient (see 6.1 List of Excipients).

4.4 Special warnings and special precautions for use

Patients should be instructed in the proper use of the inhaler. They should also be made aware of the prophylactic nature of therapy with Asmabec Clickhaler and that they should use it regularly, every day, even when they are asymptomatic. Beclometasone dipropionate is not suitable for the treatment of an acute asthma attack.

Increasing use of bronchodilators, in particular short-acting inhaled β_2-agonists, to relieve symptoms indicates deterioration of asthma control. If patients find that short-acting relief bronchodilator treatment becomes less effective, or they need more inhalations than usual, medical attention must be sought. In this situation patients should be reassessed and consideration given to the need for increased anti-inflammatory therapy (e.g. higher doses of inhaled corticosteroids or a course of oral corticosteroids). Severe exacerbations of asthma must be treated in the normal way.

Systemic effects of inhaled corticosteroids may occur, particularly at high doses prescribed for prolonged periods. Possible systemic effects include adrenal suppression, growth retardation in children and adolescents, decrease in bone mineral density, cataract and glaucoma. It is important therefore that the dose of inhaled steroids is titrated to the lowest dose at which effective control of symptoms is achieved.

It is recommended that the height of children receiving prolonged treatment with inhaled steroids is regularly monitored. If growth is slowed, therapy should be reviewed with the aim of reducing the dose of inhaled corticosteroid if possible, to the lowest dose at which effective control of symptoms is achieved.

Doses in excess of 1500 micrograms per day may induce adrenal suppression. In such patients the risks of developing adrenal suppression should be balanced against the therapeutic advantages, and precautions should be taken to provide systemic steroid cover in situations of stress or elective surgery.

The transfer to inhaled beclometasone dipropionate of patients who have been treated with systemic steroids for long periods of time, or at high dose, needs special care and subsequent management as recovery from impaired adrenocortical function is slow. With these patients adrenocortical function should be monitored regularly and their dose of systemic steroid reduced cautiously. Gradual withdrawal of the systemic steroid should commence after about one week. Reductions in dosage, appropriate to the level of maintenance systemic steroid, should be introduced at not less than weekly intervals.

Some patients may feel unwell in a non-specific way during withdrawal of the systemic steroid. They should be encouraged to persevere with the inhaled beclometasone dipropionate, unless there are objective signs of adrenal insufficiency.

Patients who have been transferred from oral steroids whose adrenocortical function is impaired should carry a steroid warning card indicating that they may need supplementary systemic steroids during periods of stress, eg. worsening asthma attacks, chest infections, major intercurrent illness, surgery, trauma etc.

Replacement of systemic steroid treatment with inhaled therapy sometimes unmasks allergies such as allergic rhinitis or eczema previously controlled by the systemic drug.

In the case of massive mucus secretion in the respiratory tract, de-obstruction and a short course of oral steroids may be necessary to ensure efficacy of the inhaled beclometasone.

Special care is necessary in patients with active or quiescent pulmonary tuberculosis and in patients with viral, bacterial and fungal infections of the eye, mouth or respiratory tract. In the case of bacterial infection of the respiratory tract adequate antibiotic co-medication may be required.

Treatment with Asmabec Clickhaler especially at high dosesshould not be stopped abruptly.

4.5 Interaction with other medicinal products and other forms of Interaction

Due to the very low plasma concentration achieved after inhaled dosing, clinically significant drug interactions are in general unlikely. Care should be taken when co-administering known strong CYP 3A4 inhibitors (e.g. ketoconazole, itraconazole, nelfinavir, ritonavir) as there is a potential for increased systemic exposure to beclometasone.

4.6 Pregnancy and lactation

Pregnancy: There are insufficient data regarding the safety of beclometasone dipropionate during human pregnancy.- Systemic administration of relatively high doses of corticosteroids to pregnant animals can cause abnormalities of foetal development including cleft palate and intra-uterine growth retardation. There may therefore be a very small risk of such effects in the human foetus. Because beclometasone dipropionate is delivered directly to the lungs by the inhaled route it avoids the high level of exposure that occurs when corticosteroids are given by systemic routes.

The use of beclometasone dipropionate in pregnancy requires that the possible benefits of the drug be weighed against the possible hazards. It should be noted that the drug has been in widespread use for many years without apparent ill consequence.

Lactation It is reasonable to assume that beclometasone dipropionate is secreted in milk, but at the dosages used for direct inhalation there is low potential for significant levels in breast milk.

The use of beclometasone dipropionate in mothers breast feeding their babies requires that the therapeutic benefits of the drug be weighed against the potential hazards to the mother and baby.

4.7 Effects on ability to drive and use machines

None known

4.8 Undesirable effects

Candidiasis of the mouth and throat (thrush) may occur in some patients, which can be treated whilst still continuing with Asmabec Clickhaler. Hoarseness may also occur. It may be helpful to rinse out the mouth thoroughly with water immediately after inhalation.

As with other inhalation therapy, the potential for paradoxical bronchospasm should be kept in mind. If it occurs, the preparation should be discontinued immediately and, if necessary, alternative therapy instituted.

Systemic effects of inhaled corticosteroids may occur, particularly at high doses prescribed for prolonged periods. These may include adrenal suppression, growth retardation in children and adolescents, decrease in bone mineral density, cataract and glaucoma and easy bruising of the skin. Very rarely hypersensitivity, including rash and angioedema may occur.

4.9 Overdose

Acute Inhalation of a large amount of the drug over a short period may lead to temporary suppression of adrenal function. No emergency action is required. Treatment with beclometasone dipropionate by inhalation should be continued at a dose sufficient to control asthma; adrenal function recovers in a few days and can be verified by measuring plasma cortisol.

Chronic Use of excessive doses of inhaled beclometasone dipropionate over a prolonged period may cause adrenal suppression and a degree of atrophy of the adrenal cortex. Transfer to a maintenance dose of a systemic steroid may be required until the condition is stabilised. Treatment with inhaled beclometasone dipropionate should then be continued at a dose sufficient to control asthma.

If higher than approved doses are continued over prolonged periods, significant adrenal suppression and adrenal crisis are possible. Presenting symptoms of adrenal crisis may initially be non-specific and include anorexia, abdominal pain, weight loss, tiredness, headache, nausea, vomiting. Hypoglycaemia with decreased consciousness and/or convulsions is a typical symptom. Situations which could potentially trigger acute adrenal crisis include exposure to trauma, surgery, infection or any rapid reduction in dosage.

5. PHARMACOLOGICAL PROPERTIES

5.1 Pharmacodynamic properties

ATC code: R03B A01. Other anti-asthmatics, inhalants, glucocorticoids.

Beclometasone dipropionate given by inhalation has a glucocorticoid anti-inflammatory action within the lungs.

The exact mechanism responsible for this anti-inflammatory effect is unknown.

5.2 Pharmacokinetic properties

Absorption from the gastrointestinal tract is slow and bioavailability is low, suggesting that most of the absorbed drug is metabolised during its first passage through the liver. Since the dose of oral beclometasone dipropionate needed to suppress plasma cortisol is greater than that required by inhalation, this suggests that the portion absorbed from the lungs is mainly responsible for any systemic effects.

5.3 Preclinical safety data

Studies in a number of animal species, including rats, rabbits and dogs, have shown no unusual toxicity during acute experiments. The effects of beclometasone dipropionate in producing signs of glucocorticoid excess during chronic administration by various routes are dose related. Teratogenicity testing has shown cleft palate in mice, as with other glucocorticoids.Beclometasone dipropionateis non-genotoxic and demonstrates no oncogenic potential in lifetime studies with rats.

6. PHARMACEUTICAL PARTICULARS

6.1 List of excipients

Lactose monohydrate (which contains milk proteins)

6.2 Incompatibilities

Not applicable

6.3 Shelf life

2 years.

6 months when removed from the foil pouch.

6.4 Special precautions for storage

Do not store above 30°C. Store in a dry place.

6.5 Nature and contents of container

A plastic inhaler device incorporating a metering pump and a mouthpiece enclosed within a polyester/ aluminium / polyethylene heat-sealed sachet.

Each 50 microgram inhaler contains 200 actuations.

Each 100 microgram inhaler contains 200 actuations.

Each 250 microgram inhaler contains 100 actuations.

6.6 Instructions for use and handling

1. Remove mouthpiece cover from the inhaler
2. Shake the inhaler well
3. Hold the inhaler upright with thumb on the base and finger on the push button.

Press the dosing button down firmly - once only.

4. Breathe out as far as is comfortable.

Note: do not blow into the device at any time.

5. Place mouthpiece in your mouth. Close lips firmly around it (do not bite it).
6. Breathe in through your mouth steadily and deeply, to draw the medicine into your lungs.
7. Hold your breath, take the inhaler from your mouth and continue holding your breath for about 5 seconds.
8. For the second puff, keep the inhaler upright and repeat steps 2-7.
9. Replace the mouthpiece cover.

7. MARKETING AUTHORISATION HOLDER

UCB Pharma Limited
208 Bath Road
Slough
Berkshire
SL1 3WE
UK

8. MARKETING AUTHORISATION NUMBER(S)

PL 00039/0501 Asmabec Clickhaler 50μg

PL 00039/0502 Asmabec Clickhaler 100μg

PL 00039/0503 Asmabec Clickhaler 250μg

9. DATE OF FIRST AUTHORISATION/RENEWAL OF THE AUTHORISATION

30 October 1998

10. DATE OF REVISION OF THE TEXT

15 Jul 2005

POM

Asmanex Twisthaler 200 and 400 microgrames Inhalation Powder

(Schering-Plough Ltd)

1. NAME OF THE MEDICINAL PRODUCT

Asmanex Twisthaler▼ 200 and 400 micrograms Inhalation Powder

2. QUALITATIVE AND QUANTITATIVE COMPOSITION

Each delivered dose contains 200 or 400 micrograms mometasone furoate.

For excipients, see 6.1.

3. PHARMACEUTICAL FORM

Inhalation powder.

White to off-white powder agglomerates.

4. CLINICAL PARTICULARS

4.1 Therapeutic indications

Regular treatment to control persistent asthma.

4.2 Posology and method of administration

This product is for inhalation use only.

For use in adult and adolescent patients 12 years of age and older.

Dosage recommendations are based on severity of asthma (see criteria below).

Patients with persistent mild to moderate asthma: The recommended starting dose for most of these patients is 400 micrograms once daily. Data suggest that better asthma control is achieved if once daily dosing is administered in the evening. Some patients may be more adequately controlled on 400 micrograms daily, given in two divided doses (200 micrograms twice daily).

The dose of Asmanex Twisthaler 200 or 400 micrograms Inhalation Powder should be individualised and titrated to the lowest dose at which effective control of asthma is maintained. Dose reduction to 200 micrograms once daily given in the evening may be an effective maintenance dose for some patients.

Patients with severe asthma: The recommended starting dose is 400 micrograms twice daily, which is the maximum recommended dose. When symptoms are controlled, titrate Asmanex Twisthaler 200 or 400 micrograms Inhalation Powder to the lowest effective dose.

In patients with severe asthma and previously receiving oral corticosteroids, Asmanex Twisthaler 200 or 400 micrograms Inhalation Powder will be initiated concurrently with the patient's usual maintenance dose of systemic corticosteroid. After approximately one week, gradual withdrawal of the systemic corticosteroid can be initiated by reducing the daily or alternate daily dose. The next reduction is made after an interval of one to two weeks, depending on the response of the patient. Generally, these decrements are not to exceed 2.5 mg of prednisone daily, or its equivalent.

A slow rate of withdrawal is strongly recommended. During withdrawal of oral corticosteroids, patients must be carefully monitored for signs of unstable asthma, including objective measures of airway function, and for adrenal insufficiency (see 4.4).

The patient should be instructed that Asmanex Twisthaler 200 or 400 micrograms Inhalation Powder is not intended to be used "on demand" as a reliever medication to treat acute symptoms and that this product must be taken regularly to maintain therapeutic benefit even when he or she is asymptomatic.

Criteria:

***Mild asthma**: symptoms > 1 time a week but < 1 time per day; exacerbations may affect activity and sleep; night-time asthma symptoms > 2 times a month; PEF or FEV_1 > 80 % predicted, variability 20 – 30 %*

***Moderate asthma**: symptoms daily; exacerbations affect activity and sleep; night-time asthma symptoms > 1 time a week; daily use of short-acting $beta_2$–agonist; PEF or FEV_1 > 60- < 80 % predicted, variability > 30 %*

***Severe asthma**: continuous symptoms; frequent exacerbations; frequent night-time asthma symptoms; physical activities limited by asthma symptoms; PEF or FEV_1 ≤ 60% predicted, variability > 30%*

Special populations

Children less than 12 years of age: Clinical data are not available to recommend use in this age group.

Elderly patients older than 65 years of age: No dosage adjustment is necessary.

The patient needs to be instructed how to use the inhaler correctly (see below).

Method of administration

Prior to removing the cap, be sure the counter and the pointer on the cap are aligned. The inhaler can be opened by removing the white cap while holding unit upright (the pink-coloured base down for 200 micrograms, the maroon-coloured base down for 400 micrograms), gripping the base, and twisting the cap counterclockwise. The counter will register the number down by one count. Instruct the patient to place the inhaler in the mouth, closing the lips around the mouthpiece, and to breathe in rapidly and deeply. Then, the inhaler is removed from the mouth, and the breath held for about 10 seconds, or as long as is comfortable. The patient is not to breathe out through the inhaler. To close, while holding the unit in an upright position, replace the cap immediately after each inhalation, loading for the next dose by rotating the cap clockwise while gently pressing down until a click sound is heard and the cap is fully closed. The arrow on the cap will be fully aligned with the counter window. After inhalation, patients are advised to rinse the mouth and spit out the water. This helps to reduce the risk of candidiasis.

The digital display will indicate when the last dose has been delivered; after dose 01, the counter will read 00 and the cap will lock, at which time the unit must be discarded. The inhaler is to be kept clean and dry at all times. The outside of the mouthpiece can be cleaned with a dry cloth or tissue; do not wash the inhaler; avoid contact with water.

For detailed instructions see Patient Leaflet.

4.3 Contraindications

Hypersensitivity (allergy) to the active substance or to the excipient (see 6.1 List of excipients).

4.4 Special warnings and special precautions for use

During clinical trials, oral candidiasis, which is associated with the use of this class of medicinal product, occurred in some patients. This infection may require treatment with appropriate antifungal therapy and in some patients discontinuance of Asmanex Twisthaler 200 or 400 micrograms Inhalation Powder may be necessary (see 4.8).

Systemic effects of inhaled corticosteroids may occur, particularly at high doses prescribed for prolonged periods. These effects are much less likely to occur than with oral corticosteroids. Possible systemic effects include adrenal suppression, growth retardation in children and adolescents, decrease in bone mineral density, cataracts and glaucoma. Therefore, it is important that the dose of inhaled corticosteroid is titrated to the lowest dose at which effective control of asthma is maintained.

Particular care is needed for patients who are transferred from systemically active corticosteroids to inhaled mometasone furoate, because deaths due to adrenal insufficiency have occurred in asthmatic patients during and after transfer from systemic corticosteroids to less systemically available inhaled corticosteroids. After withdrawal from systemic corticosteroids, a number of months are required for recovery of hypothalamic-pituitary-adrenal (HPA) axis function.

During dose reduction some patients may experience symptoms of systemic corticosteroid withdrawal, e.g. joint and/or muscular pain, lassitude and depression, despite maintenance or even improvement in pulmonary function. Such patients are to be encouraged to continue with both Asmanex Twisthaler 200 or 400 micrograms Inhalation Powder treatment and withdrawal of the systemic corticosteroids, unless objective signs of adrenal insufficiency are present. If evidence of adrenal insufficiency occurs, increase the systemic corticosteroid doses temporarily and thereafter continue withdrawal more slowly.

During periods of stress, including trauma, surgery, or infection, or a severe asthma attack, patients transferred from systemic corticosteroids will require supplementary treatment with a short course of systemic corticosteroids, which is gradually tapered as symptoms subside.

It is recommended that such patients carry a supply of oral corticosteroids and a warning card indicating their need and recommended dosage of systemic corticosteroids during stressful periods. Periodic testing of adrenocortical function, particularly measurement of early morning plasma cortisol levels, is recommended.

Transfer of patients from systemic corticosteroid therapy to Asmanex Twisthaler 200 or 400 micrograms Inhalation Powder may unmask pre-existing allergic conditions previously suppressed by systemic corticosteroid therapy. If this occurs, symptomatic treatment is recommended.

Mometasone furoate is not to be regarded as a bronchodilator and is not indicated for rapid relief of bronchospasm or asthma attacks; thus, patients should be instructed to keep an appropriate short-acting bronchodilator inhaler on hand for use when needed.

Instruct patients to contact their physician immediately when asthmatic episodes are not responsive to bronchodilators during treatment with this product or if peak-flow falls. This may indicate worsening asthma. During such episodes, patients may require systemic corticosteroid therapy. In these patients, dose titration to the maximum recommended maintenance dose of inhaled mometasone furoate may be considered.

Use of Asmanex Twisthaler 200 or 400 micrograms Inhalation Powder will often permit control of asthma symptoms with less suppression of HPA axis function than therapeutically equivalent oral doses of prednisone. Although mometasone furoate has demonstrated low systemic bioavailability at the recommended dosage, it is absorbed into the circulation and can be systemically active at higher doses. Thus, to maintain its profile of limited potential for HPA axis suppression, recommended doses of this product must not be exceeded, and must be titrated to the lowest effective dose for each individual patient.

There is no evidence that the administration of this product in amounts greater than recommended doses increases efficacy.

Use Asmanex Twisthaler 200 or 400 micrograms Inhalation Powder with caution, if at all, in patients with untreated active or quiescent tuberculous infections of the respiratory tract, or in untreated fungal, bacterial, systemic viral infections or ocular herpes simplex.

Advise patients who are receiving corticosteroids or other immunosuppressant medicines of the risk of exposure to certain infections (e.g., chickenpox, measles) and of the importance of obtaining medical advice if such exposure occurs. This is of particular importance in children.

A reduction of growth velocity in children or adolescents may occur as a result of inadequate control of chronic diseases such as asthma or from use of corticosteroids for treatment. Physicians are advised to closely follow the growth of adolescents taking corticosteroids by any route and weigh the benefits of corticosteroid therapy and asthma control against the possibility of growth suppression if an adolescent's growth appears slowed.

It is recommended that the height of children or adolescents receiving prolonged treatment with inhaled corticosteroids is regularly monitored. If growth is slowed, review therapy with the aim of reducing the dose of inhaled corticosteroids if possible, to the lowest dose at which effective control of symptoms is achieved. In addition, consideration should be given to referring the patient to a paediatric respiratory specialist.

When using inhaled corticosteroids, the possibility for clinically significant adrenal suppression may occur, especially after prolonged treatment with high doses and particularly with higher than recommended doses. This is to be considered during periods of stress or elective surgery, when additional systemic corticosteroids may be needed. However, during clinical trials there was no evidence of HPA axis suppression after prolonged treatment with inhaled mometasone furoate at doses $\leq$ 800 micrograms per day.

Lack of response or severe exacerbations of asthma should be treated by increasing the maintenance dose of inhaled mometasone furoate, and if necessary, by giving a systemic corticosteroid and/or an antibiotic if infection is suspected, and by use of beta-agonist therapy.

The patient should be advised against abrupt discontinuation of therapy with Asmanex Twisthaler 200 or 400 micrograms Inhalation Powder.

Patients with lactose intolerance: The maximum recommended daily dose contains lactose 4.64 mg per day. Patients with rare hereditary problems of galactose intolerance, the Lapp lactase deficiency or glucose-galactose malabsorption should not take this medicine.

4.5 Interaction with other medicinal products and other forms of Interaction

Co-administration of inhaled mometasone furoate with the potent CYP3A4 enzyme inhibitor ketoconazole causes small but marginally significant (p= 0.09) decreases in serum cortisol $AUC_{(0-24)}$ and resulted in approximately a 2-fold increase in plasma concentration of mometasone.

4.6 Pregnancy and lactation

There are no adequate studies in pregnant women. Studies in animals with mometasone furoate, like other glucocorticoids, have shown reproductive toxicity (see 5.3); however, the potential risk for humans is unknown.

As with other inhaled corticosteroid preparations, mometasone furoate is not to be used during pregnancy unless the potential benefit to the mother justifies the potential risk to the mother, fetus or infant. Infants born of mothers who received corticosteroids during pregnancy are to be observed carefully for hypoadrenalism.

It is known that mometasone furoate is excreted in low doses in the milk of suckling rats. It is not known if mometasone furoate is excreted in human milk, thus, caution should be used when Asmanex Twisthaler 200 or 400 micrograms Inhalation Powder is administered to breast-feeding women.

4.7 Effects on ability to drive and use machines

Inhaled mometasone furoate has no or negligible influence on the ability to drive and use machines.

4.8 Undesirable effects

In placebo-controlled clinical trials, oral candidiasis was very common > 10%) in the 400 micrograms twice daily treatment group; other common (1-10%), treatment-related undesirable effects were pharyngitis, headache and dysphonia (Table 1).

(see Table 1 below)

With twice daily dosing, oral candidiasis was reported in 6 % and 15 % of patients on the 200 microgram and 400 microgram dose regimens, respectively, and in 2%, on both of the once-daily regimens.

With the twice daily regimen, treatment-related pharyngitis was reported in 4 % (200 micrograms) and 8 % (400 micrograms) of patients. On the once-daily regimen, the incidence was 4% (200 micrograms) and 2% (400 micrograms).

In patients dependent on oral corticosteroids, who were treated with Asmanex Twisthaler 400 micrograms twice daily for 12 weeks, oral candidiasis occurred in 20 %, and dysphonia in 7 %. These effects were considered treatment-related.

Uncommonly reported adverse events were dry mouth and throat, dyspepsia, weight increase and palpitations.

There was no suggestion of an increased risk of undesirable effects in adolescents or patients 65 years of age or older.

As with other inhaled asthma medications, bronchospasm may occur with an immediate increase in wheezing after dosing. If bronchospasm occurs following dosing with the Asmanex Twisthaler 200 or 400 micrograms Inhalation Powder, immediate treatment with a fast-acting inhaled bronchodilator is recommended; thus, the patient should be told to keep an appropriate bronchodilator inhaler on hand at all times. In such cases, treatment with Asmanex Twisthaler 200 or 400 micrograms Inhalation Powder is then discontinued immediately and alternative therapy instituted.

Systemic effects of inhaled corticosteroids may occur, particularly when prescribed at high doses for prolonged periods. These may include adrenal suppression, growth retardation in children and adolescents, decrease in bone mineral density, cataract and glaucoma.

Rare cases of glaucoma, increased intraocular pressure and/or cataracts have been reported with the use of inhaled corticosteroids.

As with other glucocorticoid products, the potential for hypersensitivity reactions including rashes, urticaria, pruritus and erythema and oedema of the eyes, face, lips and throat should be considered.

4.9 Overdose

Because of the low systemic bioavailability of this product, overdose is unlikely to require any therapy other than observation, followed by initiation of the appropriate prescribed dosage. Inhalation or oral administration of excessive doses of corticosteroids may lead to suppression of HPA axis function.

Management of the inhalation of mometasone furoate in doses in excess of the recommended dose regimens should include monitoring of adrenal function. Mometasone furoate therapy in a dose sufficient to control asthma can be continued.

5. PHARMACOLOGICAL PROPERTIES

5.1 Pharmacodynamic properties

Pharmacotherapeutic group: Other Antiasthmatics, Inhalants, - Glucocorticoids, ATC code R03B A07

Mometasone furoate is a topical glucocorticoid with local anti-inflammatory properties.

It is likely that much of the mechanism for the effects of mometasone furoate lies in its ability to inhibit the release of mediators of the inflammatory cascade. *In vitro*, mometasone furoate inhibits the release of leukotrienes from leukocytes of allergic patients. In cell culture, mometasone furoate demonstrated high potency in inhibition of synthesis and release of IL-1, IL-5, IL-6, and TNF-alpha; it is also a potent inhibitor of LT production and in addition it is an extremely potent inhibitor of the production of the Th_2 cytokines, IL-4 and IL-5, from human CD4+ T-cells.

Mometasone furoate has been shown *in vitro* to exhibit a binding affinity for the human glucocorticoid receptor which is approximately 12 times that of dexamethasone, 7 times that of triamcinolone acetonide, 5 times that of budesonide, and 1.5 times that of fluticasone.

In a clinical trial, inhaled mometasone furoate has been shown to reduce airway reactivity to adenosine monophosphate in hyperreactive patients. In another trial, pretreatment using the Asmanex Twisthaler for five days significantly attenuated the early and late phase reactions following inhaled allergen challenge and also reduced allergen-induced hyperresponsiveness to methacholine.

Inhaled mometasone furoate treatment was also shown to attenuate the increase in inflammatory cells (total and activated eosinophils) in induced sputum following allergen and methacholine challenge. The clinical significance of these findings is not known.

Table 1 Frequency*(F) of undesirable effects with Asmanex Twisthaler Inhalation Powder in excess of placebo (P), by treatment regimen

Category	QD (Once Daily Dosing)		BID (Twice Daily Dosing)	
	200 mcg (F)	400 mcg (F)	200 mcg (F)	400 mcg (F)
Infection and infestation Candidiasis	1 % (U)	1 %(U)	5 % (C)	14 % (VC)
Ear & labyrinth disorders Dysphonia	<P (U)	Equal	1 % (C)	2 % (C)
Respiratory disorders Pharyngitis	2 % (C)	Equal	2 % (C)	6 % (C)
General disorders Headache	1 % (C)	1 % (C)	Equal	1 % (C)

***Frequency** (CIOMS): Uncommon (U)= <1%, Common (C)=>1%-10%, Very Common (VC)>10%

In asthmatic patients, repeated administration of inhaled mometasone furoate for 4 weeks at doses of 200 micrograms twice daily to 1200 micrograms once daily showed no evidence of clinically relevant HPA-axis suppression at any dose level and was associated with detectable systemic activity only at a dose of 1600 micrograms per day.

In long-term clinical trials using doses up to 800 micrograms per day, there was no evidence of HPA axis suppression, as assessed by reductions in morning plasma cortisol levels or abnormal responses to cosyntropin.

In a 28 day clinical trial involving 60 asthmatic patients, administration of Asmanex Twisthaler at doses of 400 micrograms, 800 micrograms or 1200 micrograms once daily, or 200 micrograms twice daily, did not result in a statistically significant decrease in 24-hour plasma cortisol AUC.

The potential systemic effect of twice daily dosing of mometasone furoate was evaluated in an active and placebo controlled trial that compared 24-hour plasma cortisol AUC in 64 adult asthmatic patients treated for 28 days with mometasone furoate 400 micrograms twice daily, 800 micrograms twice daily, or prednisone 10 mg once daily. Mometasone furoate 400 micrograms twice daily treatment reduced plasma cortisol $AUC_{(0-24)}$ values from placebo values by 10 - 25 %. Mometasone furoate 800 micrograms twice daily reduced plasma cortisol $AUC_{(0-24)}$ from placebo values by 21 - 40 %. Reduction in cortisol was significantly greater after prednisone 10 mg once daily than with placebo or either of the mometasone treatment groups.

Double-blind placebo-controlled trials of 12-weeks duration have shown that treatment with Asmanex Twisthaler at delivered doses within the range of 200 micrograms (once-daily in the evening) - 800 micrograms per day resulted in improved lung function as measured by FEV_1 and peak expiratory flow, improved asthma symptom control, and decreased need for inhaled $beta_2$-agonist. Improved lung function was observed within 24 hours of the start of treatment in some patients, although maximum benefit was not achieved before 1 to 2 weeks or longer. Improved lung function was maintained for the duration of treatment.

5.2 Pharmacokinetic properties

Absorption: The systemic bioavailability of mometasone furoate following oral inhalation in healthy volunteers is low, due to poor absorption from the lungs and the gut and extensive pre-systemic metabolism. Plasma concentrations of mometasone following inhalation at the recommended doses of 200 micrograms to 400 micrograms per day were generally near or below the limit of quantification (50 pg/ml) of the analytical assay and were highly variable.

Distribution: After intravenous bolus administration, the V_d is 332 l. The *in vitro* protein binding for mometasone furoate is high, 98 % to 99 % in concentration range of 5 to 500 ng/ml.

Metabolism: The portion of an inhaled mometasone furoate dose that is swallowed and absorbed in the gastrointestinal tract undergoes extensive metabolism to multiple metabolites. There are no major metabolites detectable in plasma. In human liver microsomes, mometasone is metabolised by cytochrome P450 3A4 (CYP3A4).

Elimination: After intravenous bolus administration, mometasone furoate has a terminal elimination $T_{1/2}$ of approximately 4.5 hours. A radiolabelled, orally inhaled dose is excreted mainly in the feces (74 %) and to a lesser extent in the urine (8 %).

5.3 Preclinical safety data

All toxicological effects observed are typical of this class of compounds and are related to exaggerated pharmacological effects of glucocorticoids.

Like other glucocorticoids, mometasone furoate is a teratogen in rodents and rabbits.Effects noted were umbilical hernia in rats, cleft palate in mice, and gall bladder agenesis, umbilical hernia, and flexed front paws in rabbits.There were also reductions in maternal body weight gains, effects on fetal growth (lower fetal body weight and/or delayed ossification) in rats, rabbits and mice, and reduced offspring survival in mice.

In long-term carcinogenicity studies in mice and rats, inhaled mometasone furoate demonstrated no statistically significant increase in the incidence of tumours.

Mometasone furoate showed no genotoxic activity in a standard battery of *in vitro* and *in vivo* tests.

6. PHARMACEUTICAL PARTICULARS

6.1 List of excipients

Lactose anhydrous (which contains milk proteins)

6.2 Incompatibilities

Not applicable.

6.3 Shelf life

2 years

3 months after opening.

6.4 Special precautions for storage

Store in original package until opened.

Do not refrigerate or freeze.

Do not store above 30°C.

6.5 Nature and contents of container

Multi-dose powder inhaler.

A counter on the device indicates the number of doses remaining.

The powder inhaler is coloured white with a pink (200 micrograms) or maroon (400 micrograms) base, and is a multi-component device composed of polypropylene copolymer, polybutylene terephthalate, polyester, acrylonitrile-butadiene-styrene, bromo-butyl rubber and stainless steel. It contains a silica gel desiccant cartridge in the white polypropylene cap. The inhaler device is enclosed in an aluminium foil laminate pouch.

Individual units of 14 (400 micrograms only), 30 and 60 metered actuations. Not all pack sizes may be marketed.

6.6 Instructions for use and handling

No special requirements.

7. MARKETING AUTHORISATION HOLDER

Schering-Plough Ltd

Shire Park

Welwyn Garden City

Hertfordshire

AL7 1TW

UK

8. MARKETING AUTHORISATION NUMBER(S)

Asmanex Twisthaler 200 micrograms Inhalation Powder: PL 00201/0254

Asmanex Twisthaler 400 micrograms Inhalation Powder: PL 00201/0255

9. DATE OF FIRST AUTHORISATION/RENEWAL OF THE AUTHORISATION

30 April 2001

10. DATE OF REVISION OF THE TEXT

February 2004

Legal Category

Prescription Only Medicine

Asmanex/07-04/4

Asmasal Clickhaler

(UCB Pharma Limited)

1. NAME OF THE MEDICINAL PRODUCT

Asmasal Clickhaler inhalation powder

2. QUALITATIVE AND QUANTITATIVE COMPOSITION

Each metered actuation of 3 mg of inhalation powder contains 114 micrograms of salbutamol sulphate (95 micrograms salbutamol base) and delivers 110 micrograms of salbutamol sulphate (90 micrograms of salbutamol base).

For excipients see section 6.1.

3. PHARMACEUTICAL FORM

Inhalation powder

4. CLINICAL PARTICULARS

4.1 Therapeutic indications

Asmasal Clickhaler is indicated for the symptomatic treatment of bronchospasm in bronchial asthma and other conditions with associated reversible airways obstruction. Appropriate anti-inflammatory therapy should be considered in line with current practice.

Asmasal Clickhaler may be used when necessary to relieve attacks of acute dyspnoea due to bronchoconstriction.

Asmasal Clickhaler may also be used before exertion to prevent exercise-induced bronchospasm or before exposure to a known unavoidable allergen challenge.

4.2 Posology and method of administration

Adults: For the relief of acute bronchospasm and for managing intermittent episodes of asthma, one inhalation may be administered as a single dose; this may be increased to two inhalations if necessary. If the response is inadequate, higher doses than two inhalations can be used. The maximum recommended dose is two inhalations three or four times a day.

To prevent exercise-induced bronchospasm one or two inhalations should be taken 15 minutes before exertion.

One or two inhalations may also be taken before foreseeable contact with allergens.

Elderly: as for adults

Children: One inhalation is the recommended dose for the relief of acute bronchospasm, in the management of episodic asthma or before exercise. If the response is inadequate, higher doses than one inhalation can be used.

On demand use should not exceed four times daily. The bronchodilator effect of each administration of inhaled salbutamol lasts for at least four hours except in patients whose asthma is becoming worse. Such patients should be warned not to increase their usage of the inhaler, but should seek medical advice since treatment with, or an increased dose of an inhaled and/or systemic glucocorticosteroid is indicated.

As there may be adverse effects associated with excessive dosing, the dosage or frequency of administration should only be increased on medical advice.

The following instructions for use are included in the Patient Information Leaflet:

1. Remove mouthpiece cover from the inhaler
2. Shake the inhaler well
3. Hold the inhaler upright with thumb on the base and finger on the push button. Press the dosing button down firmly - once only
4. Breathe out as far as is comfortable.

Note: do not blow into the device at any time.

5. Place mouthpiece in your mouth. Close lips firmly around it (do not bite it)
6. Breathe in through your mouth steadily and deeply, to draw the medicine into your lungs.
7. Hold your breath, take the inhaler from your mouth and continue holding your breath for about 5 seconds.
8. For the second puff, keep the inhaler upright and repeat steps 2-7.
9. Replace the mouthpiece cover.

4.3 Contraindications

Asmasal Clickhaler is contra-indicated in patients with intolerance or hypersensitivity to the active ingredient or the excipient.

4.4 Special warnings and special precautions for use

Bronchodilators should not be the only or main treatment in patients with moderate to severe or unstable asthma. Severe asthma requires regular medical assessment including lung function testing as patients are at risk of severe attacks and even death. Physicians should consider using the maximum recommended dose of inhaled corticosteroid and/or oral corticosteroid therapy in these patients. Increasing use of bronchodilators, in particular short-acting inhaled beta-2-agonists to relieve symptoms, indicates deterioration of asthma control. If patients find that short-acting bronchodilator treatment becomes less effective or they need more inhalations than usual, they should be warned by the prescriber of the need for consulting immediately. In this situation, patients should be reassessed and consideration given to the need for increased anti-inflammatory therapy (eg. higher doses of inhaled corticosteroids or a course of oral corticosteroids).

Salbutamol should be administered cautiously, especially with systemic therapy, to patients suffering from thyrotoxicosis, myocardial insufficiency, hypertension, known aneurysms, decreased glucose tolerance, manifest diabetes, phaeochromocytoma and concomitant use of cardiac glycosides. Caution should also be applied in patients with myocardial ischemia, tachyarrythmias and hypertrophic obstructive cardiomyopathy.

Salbutamol and non-selective beta-blocking drugs, such as propranolol, should not usually be prescribed together.

Potentially serious hypokalaemia has resulted from systemic b2-agonist therapy. Particular caution is advised in acute severe asthma as this effect may be potentiated by concomitant treatment with xanthine derivatives, steroids, diuretics and by hypoxia. It is recommended that serum potassium levels are monitored in such situations.

4.5 Interaction with other medicinal products and other forms of Interaction

Salbutamol and non-selective beta-blocking drugs, such as propranolol, should not usually be prescribed together. Caution is also advised in patients using cardiac glycosides.

Potentially serious hypokalaemia has resulted from systemic b2-agonist therapy. Particular caution is advised in acute severe asthma as this effect may be potentiated by concomitant treatment with xanthine derivatives, steroids, diuretics and by hypoxia.

Patients should be instructed to discontinue salbutamol at least 6 hours before intended anaesthesia with halogenated anaesthetics, wherever possible.

4.6 Pregnancy and lactation

Pregnancy: Administration of salbutamol during pregnancy should only be considered if the expected benefit to the mother is greater than any possible risk to the fetus. As with the majority of drugs there is little published evidence of its safety in the early stages of pregnancy, but in animal studies, there was evidence of some harmful effects in the fetus at very high dose levels.

Lactation: Salbutamol may be secreted in breast milk. It is not known whether salbutamol has a harmful effect on the neonate and so its use should be restricted to situations where it is felt that the expected benefit to the mother is likely to outweigh any potential risk to the neonate.

4.7 Effects on ability to drive and use machines

Individual reactions, especially at higher doses, may be such that patients' ability to drive or use machines may be affected, particularly so at the beginning of treatment and in conjunction with alcohol.

The possible side effects of salbutamol such as transient muscle cramps and tremor may necessitate caution when using machines.

4.8 Undesirable effects

The side effects are dose dependent and due to the direct mechanism of β_2-agonists.

Hypersensitivity reactions include angioedema and urticaria, bronchospasm, hypotension and collapse and have been reported very rarely.

Blood and the lymphatic system disorders: potentially serious hypokalaemia may result from systemic β_2-agonist therapy. Special precautions should be taken in patients using β_2-agonists with hypokalaemia because of the increased risk of tachycardia and arrhythmias. Hypokalaemia may be potentiated by concomitant therapy with corticosteroids, diuretics and xanthines.

Psychiatric disorders: nervousness, feeling of tenseness. As with other b2 agonists, hyperactivity in children has been reported rarely.

Nervous system disorders: mild tremor, headache, dizziness.

Cardiac disorders: tachycardia, angioedema, hypotension, cardiac arrhythmias (including atrial fibrillation, supraventricular tachycardia and extrasystoles) have been reported in association with b2 agonists, usually in susceptible patients.

Respiratory, thoracic and mediastinal disorders: as with other inhalation therapy, the potential for paradoxical bronchospasm should be kept in mind. If it occurs, the preparation should be discontinued immediately and alternative therapy instituted.

Gastrointestinal disorders: nausea

Skin and subcutaneous tissue disorders: urticaria.

Musculoskeletal, connective tissue and bone disorders: there have been rare reports of transient muscle cramps

General disorders and administration site conditions: oral and pharyngeal irritation can occur.

4.9 Overdose

An overdose should be treated symptomatically.

The preferred antidote for overdosage with salbutamol is a cardioselective beta-blocking agent but beta-blocking drugs should be used with caution in patients with a history of bronchospasm.

If hypokalaemia occurs potassium replacement via the oral route should be given. In patients with severe hypokalaemia intravenous replacement may be necessary.

5. PHARMACOLOGICAL PROPERTIES

5.1 Pharmacodynamic properties

ATC Code: R03A C02

Salbutamol is a beta-adrenergic stimulant which has a selective action on bronchial b2-adrenoceptors at therapeutic doses. Following inhalation, salbutamol exerts a stimulating action on b2 receptors on bronchial smooth muscles, and thus ensures rapid bronchodilation which becomes significant within a few minutes and persists for 4 to 6 hours.

The drug also causes vasodilation leading to a reflex chronotropic effect and widespread metabolic effects, including hypokalaemia.

5.2 Pharmacokinetic properties

Following treatment with salbutamol by inhalation, only approximately 10% or less of the drug is deposited in the airways and the remainder is swallowed. Pre-systemic metabolism of salbutamol is considerable and occurs primarily in the gastrointestinal tract and by conjugation to form an inactive sulphate ester. The systemic clearance for salbutamol is 30 l/hr. Salbutamol is eliminated both through excretion of unchanged drug in urine and through metabolism mainly via sulphate conjugation. The elimination half-life varies between 3 and 7 hours. Salbutamol is well absorbed from the gastrointestinal tract.

5.3 Preclinical safety data

Preclinical data reveal no special hazard for humans based on conventional studies of safety pharmacology, repeated dose toxicity and genotoxicity. Findings concerning teratogenicity in rabbits at high systemic exposure and the induction of benign mesovarian leiomyomas in rats are not considered of clinical concern.

6. PHARMACEUTICAL PARTICULARS

6.1 List of excipients

Lactose monohydrate

6.2 Incompatibilities

Not applicable

6.3 Shelf life

2 years in unopened foil pouch. 6 months when removed from foil pouch.

6.4 Special precautions for storage

Do not store above 30°C. Store in a dry place.

6.5 Nature and contents of container

A plastic inhaler device incorporating an actuating and metering mechanism enclosed within an aluminium foil heat sealed bag. Each device contains 750mg of powder - sufficient for 200 actuations.

6.6 Instructions for use and handling

Instructions for use are included in the patient information leaflet. These are also included in Section 4.2.

7. MARKETING AUTHORISATION HOLDER

UCB Pharma Limited

208 Bath Road

Slough, Berkshire

SL1 3WE

UK

8. MARKETING AUTHORISATION NUMBER(S)

PA 365/78/1

9. DATE OF FIRST AUTHORISATION/RENEWAL OF THE AUTHORISATION

17th April 1998 / 9th May 2002

10. DATE OF REVISION OF THE TEXT

June 2005

POM

Aspav

(Alpharma Limited)

1. NAME OF THE MEDICINAL PRODUCT

ASPAV

2. QUALITATIVE AND QUANTITATIVE COMPOSITION

Each tablet contains 500mg Aspirin PhEur, 7.71mg Papaveretum BP (equivalent to 5mg anhydrous morphine).

3. PHARMACEUTICAL FORM

White uncoated tablets.

4. CLINICAL PARTICULARS

4.1 Therapeutic indications

1) For the relief of moderate to severe pain in post-operative states and in the relief of chronic pain associated with inoperable carcinoma.

4.2 Posology and method of administration

Posology

Adults: One or two tablets to be dispersed in water every 4-6 hours. Not more than eight tablets in any 24 hours.

Children: Do not give to children aged under 16 years, unless specifically indicated (e.g. for Kawasaki's disease).

Method of Administration

To be dispersed in water for oral administration.

4.3 Contraindications

Aspav should not be taken by patients with the following conditions:

- Known hypersensitivity to aspirin, papaveretum, other ingredients in the product, other opioids, other salicylates or non-steroidal anti-inflammatory drugs (a patient may have developed anaphylaxis, angioedema, asthma, rhinitis or urticaria induced by aspirin or other NSAIDs).
- Nasal polyps associated with asthma (high risk of severe sensitivity reactions).
- Active peptic ulceration or a past history of ulceration or dyspepsia.
- Haemophilia or other haemorrhagic disorder (including thrombocytopenia) as there is an increased risk of bleeding.
- Concurrent anticoagulant therapy should be avoided.
- Diarrhoea caused by poisoning until the toxic material has been eliminated, or diarrhoea associated with pseudomembraneous colitis
- respiratory depression
- obstructive airways disease

4.4 Special warnings and special precautions for use

There is a possible association between aspirin and Reye's Syndrome when given to children. Reye's syndrome is a very rare disease which affects the brain and the liver, and can be fatal. For this reason aspirin should not be given to children aged under 16 years unless specifically indicated (e.g. for Kawasaki's disease).

Aspav should be used with caution in patients with:

- allergic disease
- anaemia (may be exacerbated by GI blood loss)
- asthma (increased risk of bronchospastic sensitivity reactions)
- cardiac failure (conditions which predispose to fluid retention)
- dehydration
- glucose-6-phosphate dehydrogenase deficiency (aspirin rarely causes haemolytic anaemia)
- gout (serum urate may be increased)
- hepatic function impairment (avoid if severe)
- renal function impairment
- surgery. Aspirin should be discontinued several days before scheduled surgery (including dental extractions)
- systemic lupus erythematosus and other connective tissue disorders (hepatic and renal function may be impaired in these conditions)
- thyrotoxicosis (may be exacerbated by large doses of salicylates)
- hypothyroidism (risk of depression and prolonged CNS depression is increased)
- inflammatory bowel disease - risk of toxic megacolon
- Opioids should not be administered during an asthma attack
- convulsions - may be induced or exacerbated
- drug abuse, dependence (including alcoholism), enhanced instability, suicidal ideation or attempts - predisposed to drug abuse
- head injuries or conditions where intracranial pressure is raised
- gall bladder disease or gall stones - opioids may cause biliary contraction
- gastro-intestinal surgery - use with caution after recent GI surgery as opioids may alter GI motility
- prostatic hypertrophy or recent urinary tract surgery
- adrenocortical insufficiency, eg Addison's Disease
- hypotension and shock
- myasthenia gravis
- phaeochromocytoma - opioids may stimulate catecholamine release by inducing the release of endogenous histamine

4.5 Interaction with other medicinal products and other forms of Interaction

The following drug interactions should be considered when prescribing aspav:

- Alcohol - may enhance gastro-intestinal side effect of aspirin.
- Analgesics - avoid concomitant administration of other salicylates or other NSAIDs (including topical formulations) as increased risk of side effects.
- Alkalizers of urine (*eg* carbonic anhydrase inhibitors, antacids, citrates) - increased excretion of aspirin.
- Anticoagulants or platelet aggregation inhibitors - increased risk of bleeding.
- Antiepileptic drugs (*eg* phenytoin, sodium valproate) - increased effect.
- Corticosteroids - increased risk of gastro-intestinal bleeding or ulceration.
- Dipyridamole - increase in peak concentration.
- Diuretics - frusemide and acetazolamide (risk of toxic effects), spironolactone (antagonized diuretic action).
- Hypoglycaemics - enhanced activity.
- Methotrexate - increased toxicity.
- Metoclopramide and domperidone - increased rate of absorption of aspirin.
- Mifepristone - avoid aspirin until 8-12 days after mifepristone.
- Ototoxic medicine (*eg* vancomycin) - potential for ototoxicity increased. Hearing loss may occur and may progress to deafness even after discontinuation of the medication. Effects may be reversible but are usually permanent.
- Uricosurics (*eg* probenecid, sulphinpyrazone) - effects of uricosurics reduced.
- Laboratory investigations - aspirin may interfere with some laboratory tests such as urine 5-hydroxyindoleacetic acid determinations and copper sulphate urine sugar tests.
- CNS depressants - enhanced sedative and/or hypotensive effect with alcohol, anaesthetics, hypnotics, anxiolytics, antipsychotics, hydroxyzine, tricyclic antidepressants
- Antibacterials, *eg* ciprofloxacin, - avoid premedication with opioids as reduced plasma ciprofloxacin concentration
- MAOIs - use only with extreme caution
- Cyclizine
- Mexiletine - delayed absorption
- Metoclopramide and domperidone - antagonise GI effects
- Cisapride - possible antagonism of GI effects
- Dopaminergics (*eg* selegiline) - possible risk of hyperpyrexia and CNS toxicity. This risk is greater with pethidine but with other opioids the risk is uncertain
- Ulcer healing drugs - cimetidine inhibits the metabolism of opioid analgesics.
- Anticholinergics (*eg* atropine) - risk of severe constipation which may lead to paralytic illness, and /or urinary retention
- Antidiarrhoeal drugs (*eg* loperamide, kaolin) - increased risk of severe constipation
- Antihypertensive drugs (*eg* guanethidine, diuretics) - enhanced hypotensive effect
- Opioid antagonists (*eg* buprenorphine, naltrexone, naloxone)
- Neuromuscular blocking agents - additive respiratory depressant effects

4.6 Pregnancy and lactation

Controlled trials in humans using aspirin have not shown evidence of teratogenic effects. However, studies in animals have shown that salicylates can cause birth defects including fissure of the spine and skull, facial clefts and malformations of the CNS, viscera and skeleton. Ingestion of aspirin during the last two weeks of pregnancy may increase the risk of fetal or neonatal haemorrhage. Regular or high dose use of salicylates late in pregnancy may result in constriction or premature closing of the fetal ductus arteriosus, increased risk of still birth or neonatal death, decreased birth weight, prolonged labour, complicated deliveries and increased risk of maternal or fetal haemorrhage and possibly persistent pulmonary hypertension of newborn or kernicterus in jaundiced neonates. Pregnant women should be advised not to take aspirin in the last three months of pregnancy unless under medical supervision.

Risk benefit must be considered because opioid analgesics cross the placenta. Studies in animals have shown opioids to cause delayed ossification in mice and increased resorption in rats.

Regular use during pregnancy may cause physical dependence in the fetus, leading to withdrawal symptoms in the neonate. During labour opioids enter the fetal circulation and may cause respiratory depression in the neonate. Administration should be avoided during the late stages of labour and during the delivery of a premature infant.

Aspirin is distributed in breastmilk. Aspirin should be avoided while breastfeeding.

Papaveretum is distributed in breast milk in small amounts. It is advisable to avoid administration opioids in a breastfeeding woman.

4.7 Effects on ability to drive and use machines
Opioid analgesics can impair mental function and can cause blurred vision and dizziness. Patients should make sure they are not affected before driving or operating machinery.

4.8 Undesirable effects
Adverse effects of aspirin treatment which have been reported include:

- Allergic reactions - rhinitis, urticaria, angioneurotic oedema and worsening of asthma and problems with breathing
- Effects on GI system - gastrointestinal bleeding or ulceration which can occasionally be major (may develop bloody or black tarry stools, severe stomach pain and vomiting blood), gastrointestinal irritation (mild stomach pain, heartburn and nausea) and hepatitis (particularly in patients with SLE or connective tissue disease)
- Effects on blood - anaemia, haemolytic anaemia, hypoprothrombinaemia, thrombocytopenia, aplastic anaemia, pancytopenia
- Effects on sensory system - tinnitus
- Salicylism - mild chronic salicylate intoxication may occur after repeated administration of large doses, symptoms include dizziness, tinnitus, deafness, sweating, nausea, vomiting, headache and mental confusion, and may be controlled by reducing the dose
- Effects in children - aspirin may be associated with the development of Reye's Syndrome (encephalopathy and hepatic failure) in children presenting with an acute febrile illness

Adverse effects of opioid treatment which have been reported include:

- Allergic reactions (may be caused by histamine release) - including rash, urticaria, difficulty breathing, increased sweating, redness or flushed face
- effects on CNS - confusion, drowsiness, vertigo, dizziness, changes in mood, hallucinations, CNS excitation (restlessness/excitement), convulsions, mental depression, headache, trouble sleeping, or nightmares, raised intracranial pressure, tolerance or dependence
- effects on GI system - constipation, GI irritation, biliary spasm, nausea, vomiting, loss of appetite, dry mouth, paralytic ileus or toxic megacolon
- effects on CVS - bradycardia, palpitations, hypotension
- effects on sensory system -blurred or double vision
- effects on GU system - ureteral spasm, antidiuretic effect
- other effects - trembling, unusual tiredness or weakness, malaise, miosis, hypothermia
- effects of withdrawal - abrupt withdrawal precipitates a withdrawal syndrome. Symptoms may include tremor, insomnia, nausea, vomiting, sweating and increase in heart rate, respiratory rate and blood pressure. NOTE - tolerance diminishes rapidly after withdrawal so a previously tolerated dose may prove fatal.

4.9 Overdose
Salicylates:

Symptoms of overdose depend upon plasma salicylate concentration.

Concentration greater than 300mgl^{-1} - tinnitus and vertigo

Concentration approx 400mgl^{-1} - hyperventilation

Concentration above 600mgl^{-1} - metabolic acidosis

Concentration range 700-900mgl^{-1} - coma, fever, hypothrombinaemia, cardiovascular collapse, renal failure.

Treatment - Aspirin may remain in the stomach for many hours after ingestion and should be removed by gastric lavage.

Plasma salicylate, pH and electrolytes should be measured. Fluid losses replaced and forced alkaline diuresis (eg with sodium bicarbonate) should be considered when the plasma salicylate concentration is greater than 500mgl^{-1} (3.6 mmol l^{-1}) in adults or 300mgl^{-1} (2.2 mmol l^{-1}) in children. In very severe cases of poisoning haemodialysis may be needed.

Opioids:

Symptoms: cold clammy skin, confusion, convulsions, severe drowsiness, tiredness, low blood pressure, pinpoint pupils of eyes, slow heart beat and respiratory rate coma.

Treatment: Treat respiratory depression or other life-threatening adverse effects first. Empty the stomach via gastric lavage or induction of emesis.

The opioid antagonist naloxone (0.4-2mg subcutaneous) can be given and repeated at 2-3 minute intervals to a maximum of 10mg. Naloxone may also be given by intramuscular injection or intravenous infusion. The patient should be monitored as the duration of opioid analgesic may exceed that of the antagonist.

5. PHARMACOLOGICAL PROPERTIES
5.1 Pharmacodynamic properties
Aspirin has analgesic, anti-inflammatory and antipyretic properties.

Papaveretum has the analgesic and narcotic properties of morphine.

5.2 Pharmacokinetic properties
Absorption of non-ionised aspirin occurs in the stomach. Acetylsalicylates and salicylates are also readily absorbed from the intestine. Hydrolysis to salicylic acid occurs rapidly in the intestine and in the circulation. Salicylates are extensively bound to plasma proteins; aspirin to a lesser degree. Aspirin and the salicylates are rapidly distributed to all body tissues; they appear in milk and cross the placenta. The rate of excretion of aspirin varies with urinary pH, increasing as pH rises and being greatest at pH 7.5 and above. Aspirin is excreted as salicylic acid and as glucuronide conjugates and as salicyluric and gentisic acids.

5.3 Preclinical safety data
Not applicable.

6. PHARMACEUTICAL PARTICULARS
6.1 List of excipients
Also contains: calcium carbonate, citric acid, lactose, maize starch, saccharin.

6.2 Incompatibilities
None known.

6.3 Shelf life
Shelf-life

18 months from the date of manufacture.

Shelf-life after dilution/reconstitution

Not applicable.

Shelf-life after first opening

Not applicable.

6.4 Special precautions for storage
Keep tightly closed and store below 25°C in a dry place.

Protect from light.

6.5 Nature and contents of container
The product containers are rigid injection moulded polypropylene or injection blow-moulded polyethylene containers with polyfoam wad or polypropylene ullage filler and snap-on polyethylene lids; in case any supply difficulties should arise the alternative is amber glass containers with screw caps and steran faced liner with polyfoam wad or cotton wool. An alternative closure for polyethylene containers is a polypropylene, twist on, push down and twist off child-resistant, tamper-evident lid.

Also included in each pack is a 2g silica gel capsule.

Pack sizes: 7s, 10s, 14s, 21s, 25s, 28s, 30s, 50s, 56s, 60s, 84s, 100s, 112s, 250s, 500s, 1000s, 5000s

6.6 Instructions for use and handling
To be dispersed in water for oral administration.

Administrative Data
7. MARKETING AUTHORISATION HOLDER
Name or style and permanent address of registered place of business of the holder of the Marketing Authorisation:

Alpharma Limited (Trading style: Alpharma, Cox Pharmaceuticals)

Whiddon Valley

BARNSTAPLE

N Devon EX32 8NS

8. MARKETING AUTHORISATION NUMBER(S)
PL 0142/5597 R

9. DATE OF FIRST AUTHORISATION/RENEWAL OF THE AUTHORISATION
21 January 1982 / 21 January 1992

10. DATE OF REVISION OF THE TEXT
January 2003

AT10

(Intrapharm Laboratories Ltd)

1. NAME OF THE MEDICINAL PRODUCT
AT10

2. QUALITATIVE AND QUANTITATIVE COMPOSITION
Dihydrotachysterol BP 0.025% w/v

3. PHARMACEUTICAL FORM
Oily solution

4. CLINICAL PARTICULARS
4.1 Therapeutic indications
AT10 is recommended for use in acute, chronic and latent forms of hypocalcaemic tetany due to hypoparathyroidism where its action is to increase the rate of absorption and utilisation of calcium.

4.2 Posology and method of administration
Adults (and the elderly):

In acute cases 3-5ml may be given on each of the first three days of treatment, followed two to three days later by blood and urinary calcium estimations. The maintenance dose of AT10 is usually within the range of 1-7ml each week, but the precise amount depends on the results of serum and urinary calcium determinations. In chronic cases an initial dose of 2ml of AT10 daily, or on alternate days, may be sufficient to maintain normocalcaemia in moderate cases. The dose of AT10 usually has to be increased during menstruation and periods of unusual activity.

Children
No specific dosage recommendations.

Route of Administration
Oral.

4.3 Contraindications
Hypersensitivity to dihydrotachysterol.

Hypercalcaemia.

Hypervitaminosis D.

Allergy to nuts (including peanuts).

4.4 Special warnings and special precautions for use
AT10 contains Arachis oil (peanut oil) and should not be taken by patients known to be allergic to peanut. As there is a possible relationship between allergy to peanut and allergy to Soya, patients with Soya allergy should also avoid AT10.

As with calciferol, uncontrolled prolonged administration of AT10 can result in hypercalcaemia which may lead to nephrocalcinosis. Therefore accurate blood calcium determinations must be made at the beginning of treatment and then periodically until the required maintenance dose has been established. The serum calcium level should subsequently be kept between 2.25-2.5mmol/litre. Serum phosphate, magnesium, and alkaline phosphatase should also be measured periodically to monitor progress.

If nausea and vomiting are present, serum calcium level should be checked.

Monitoring of calciuria is a convenient supplement to blood calcium determinations, but it should not be regarded as a substitute because in hypoparathyroid patients treated with AT10 hypercalciuria can occur in the presence of hypocalcaemia.

Certain individuals, particularly those suffering from sarcoidosis, are very sensitive to the effect of Vitamin D and it is advisable to consult a physician in cases of doubt.

4.5 Interaction with other medicinal products and other forms of Interaction
Several classes of medicine interact with Vitamin D analogues calling for adjustment in the dosage of AT10. Thyroid replacement therapy may increase clearance of dihydrotachysterol; cholestyramine may impair its absorption; thiazide diuretics may enhance the calcaemic response leading to hypercalcaemia; barbiturates, anticonvulsants, rifampicin and isoniazid may reduce the effectiveness of AT10. Hypercalcaemia induced by excessive dosaging of AT10 may enhance the toxic effects of cardiac glycosides.

4.6 Pregnancy and lactation
The safety of dihydrotachysterol in pregnancy is not established. Since there is some evidence that use during pregnancy could lead to foetal damage and hypercalcaemia in the newborn, treatment with AT10 is only justified if potential benefits outweigh possible risks. Dihydrotachysterol is excreted in breast milk and may cause hypercalcaemia in the suckling infant. AT10 is contraindicated in breast feeding mothers.

4.7 Effects on ability to drive and use machines
None stated.

4.8 Undesirable effects
Side effects are most likely to be due to hypercalcaemia, the first signs of which are loss of appetite, listlessness and nausea.

More severe manifestations include vomiting, urgency of micturition, polyuria, dehydration, thirst, vertigo, stupor, headache, abdominal cramps and paralysis.

The calcium and phosphorus concentrations of serum and urine are increased.

With chronic overdosage, calcium may be deposited in many tissues, including arteries and the kidneys, leading to hypertension and renal failure. Plasma cholesterol may also be increased.

4.9 Overdose
Treatment

The symptoms of hypercalcaemia in chronic overdosage will usually respond to withdrawal of medication, bed rest, liberal fluid intake and the use of laxatives.

In acute overdosage, consideration should be given to recovery of AT10 by emesis or gastric lavage if ingestion is recent. Serum calcium estimations should be helpful in determining management.

In massive overdosage of Vitamin D, corticosteroids have been found useful and also neutral phosphate in resistant cases. Several months management may be needed in such cases.

5. PHARMACOLOGICAL PROPERTIES
5.1 Pharmacodynamic properties
Dihydrotachysterol is a synthetic analogue of Vitamin D and is used in the treatment of hypoparathyroidism. However, it is not useful in the treatment of rickets since its antirachitic activity is considerably weaker than that of Vitamin D.

The actions of dihydrotachysterol resemble those of calciferol and Vitamin D_3. It promotes the absorption of calcium from the intestine and the mobilisation of calcium from bone as effectively as calciferol. Dihydrotachysterol acts more rapidly and is more rapidly eliminated than calciferol and its action is therefore more readily controlled; in practice, calciferol is generally used for the treatment of Vitamin D deficiency and dihydrotachysterol for other conditions.

5.2 Pharmacokinetic properties
Vitamin D substances are well absorbed from the gastro-intestinal tract. The presence of bile is essential for adequate intestinal absorption; absorption may be decreased in patients with decreased fat absorption.

Vitamin D compounds and their metabolites are excreted mainly in the bile and faeces with only small amounts appearing in urine.

5.3 Preclinical safety data
There are no preclinical data of relevance to the prescriber which are additional to that already included in other sections of the SPC.

6. PHARMACEUTICAL PARTICULARS
6.1 List of excipients
Arachis oil, Sodium sulphate anhydrous.

6.2 Incompatibilities
None.

6.3 Shelf life
48 months.

6.4 Special precautions for storage
Store in well-closed containers protected from heat and light.

6.5 Nature and contents of container
15ml bottles with a 1ml dropper.

Pack size: 15ml.

6.6 Instructions for use and handling
None.

Administrative Data
7. MARKETING AUTHORISATION HOLDER
Intrapharm Laboratories Limited
Maidstone
Kent
ME15 9QS

8. MARKETING AUTHORISATION NUMBER(S)
PL 17509/0004

9. DATE OF FIRST AUTHORISATION/RENEWAL OF THE AUTHORISATION
30 April 1999

10. DATE OF REVISION OF THE TEXT
May 2003

11. Legal category
P

Atarax Tablets

(Pfizer Limited)

1. NAME OF THE MEDICINAL PRODUCT
ATARAX®

2. QUALITATIVE AND QUANTITATIVE COMPOSITION
Hydroxyzine hydrochloride 10mg
Hydroxyzine hydrochloride 25mg

3. PHARMACEUTICAL FORM
10mg sugar coated tablets, coloured orange and coded on one side with 'Pfizer'

25mg sugar coated tablets, coloured green and coded on one side with 'Pfizer'

4. CLINICAL PARTICULARS
4.1 Therapeutic indications
Atarax is indicated to assist in the management of anxiety in adults.

Atarax is indicated for the management of pruritus associated with acute and chronic urticaria, including cholinergic and physical types, and atopic and contact dermatitis in adults and children.

4.2 Posology and method of administration
Method of administration: oral.

Dosage:

Anxiety
Adults 50-100mg four times daily.

Pruritus
Adults Starting dose of 25mg at night increasing as necessary to 25mg three or four times daily.

Use in the elderly Atarax may be used in elderly patients with no special precautions other than the care always necessary in this age group. The lowest effective maintenance dose and careful observation for side-effects are important.

Use in children From 6 months to 6 years 5-15mg rising to 50mg daily in divided doses and for children over 6 years, 15-25mg rising to 50-100mg daily in divided doses.

As with all medications, the dosage should be adjusted according to the patient's response to therapy.

Renal impairment The total daily dosage should be reduced by half (see 'Special Warnings and Precautions for Use').

4.3 Contraindications
Atarax is contra-indicated in patients who have shown previous hypersensitivity to it.

4.4 Special warnings and special precautions for use
Atarax should be used with caution in patients with impaired renal function (see 'Posology and Method of Administration'). It is uncertain whether the drug may accumulate or have other adverse effects in such patients. Atarax is completely metabolised and one of the metabolites is the active metabolite cetirizine. Cetirizine is renally excreted and clearance is reduced in patients with moderate renal impairment and on dialysis compared to normal volunteers.

4.5 Interaction with other medicinal products and other forms of Interaction
Patients should be warned that Atarax may enhance their response to alcohol, barbiturates and other CNS depressants.

4.6 Pregnancy and lactation
Atarax is contra-indicated in early pregnancy. Hydroxyzine, when administered to the pregnant mouse, rat and rabbit, induced foetal abnormalities at doses substantially above the human therapeutic range. Clinical data in humans are inadequate to establish safety in early pregnancy. There is inadequate evidence of safety in the later stages of pregnancy. Use in pregnancy only when there is no safe alternative or when the disease itself carries risks for the mother or child.

Use in nursing mothers It is not known whether Atarax is excreted in human milk. Since many drugs are so excreted, Atarax should not be given to nursing mothers.

4.7 Effects on ability to drive and use machines
Patients should be warned that Atarax may impair their ability to perform activities requiring mental alertness or physical co-ordination such as operating machinery or driving a vehicle.

4.8 Undesirable effects
Therapeutic doses of Atarax seldom produce marked impairment of mental alertness. Drowsiness may occur; if so, it is usually transitory and may disappear after a few days of continued therapy or upon reduction of the dose. Dryness of the mouth may be encountered at higher doses. Dizziness, weakness, headache and confusion have been reported.

Extensive clinical use has substantiated the absence of toxic effects on the liver or bone marrow when administered for over four years of uninterrupted therapy. The absence of side-effects has been further demonstrated in experimental studies in which excessively high doses were administered.

Involuntary motor activity, including rare instances of tremor and convulsions, have been reported, usually with doses considerably higher than those recommended. Continuous therapy with over 1g/day has been employed in some patients without these effects having been encountered.

4.9 Overdose
The most common manifestation of Atarax overdosage is hypersedation. As in the management of overdosage with any drug, it should be borne in mind that multiple agents may have been taken. If vomiting has not occurred spontaneously in conscious patients it should be induced. Immediate gastric lavage is also recommended. General supportive care, including frequent monitoring of the vital signs and close observation of the patient is indicated. Hypotension, though unlikely, may be controlled with intravenous fluids and noradrenaline, or metaraminol. Adrenaline should not be used in this situation as Atarax counteracts its pressor action.

There is no specific antidote. It is doubtful whether haemodialysis has any value in the treatment of overdosage with Atarax. However, if other agents such as barbiturates have been ingested concomitantly, haemodialysis may be indicated.

5. PHARMACOLOGICAL PROPERTIES
5.1 Pharmacodynamic properties
Atarax is unrelated chemically to phenothiazine, reserpine and meprobamate.

Atarax has been shown clinically to be a rapid-acting anxiolytic with a wide margin of safety. It induces a calming effect in anxious tense adults. It is not a cortical depressant, but its action may be due to a suppression of activity in certain key regions of the subcortical area of the central nervous system.

Antihistamine effects have been demonstrated experimentally and confirmed clinically; it is highly effective in alleviating pruritus.

5.2 Pharmacokinetic properties
Atarax is rapidly absorbed from the gastro-intestinal tract and effects are usually noted within 15 to 30 minutes after oral administration.

5.3 Preclinical safety data
None stated.

6. PHARMACEUTICAL PARTICULARS
6.1 List of excipients
Tablet core: Lactose anhydrous, Calcium Phosphate Dibasic Anhydrous, Pregelatinised Starch, Magnesium Stearate, Sodium Lauryl Sulphate

Tablet coating: Sucrose, Gum Acacia, Calcium Sulphate Dihydrate, Talc, Butyl Parahydroxybenzoate, Beeswax, Carnauba Wax., Dewaxed Orange Shellac, Opalux AS.3563 Dye (10mg only) and Opalux AS.21094 Dye (25mg only)

6.2 Incompatibilities
None stated.

6.3 Shelf life
24 months.

6.4 Special precautions for storage
Do not store above 25°C

6.5 Nature and contents of container
White opaque 250 micron PVC/Aclar - 20 micron aluminium foil blister strips containing 84 × 10mg tablets, (6 blister strips per carton) or 28 × 25mg tablets (2 blister strips per carton).

6.6 Instructions for use and handling
No special requirements.

7. MARKETING AUTHORISATION HOLDER
Pfizer Limited
Ramsgate Road
Sandwich
Kent CT13 9NJ
United Kingdom

8. MARKETING AUTHORISATION NUMBER(S)
Atarax 10mg Tablets PL0057/5003R

Atarax 25mg Tablets PL0057/5004R

9. DATE OF FIRST AUTHORISATION/RENEWAL OF THE AUTHORISATION
Atarax 10mg Tablets 27 April 1987/30 July 1997

Atarax 25mg Tablets 24 July 1985/24 July 1997

10. DATE OF REVISION OF THE TEXT
March 2003

LEGAL CATEGORY
POM

Ref. AT3_0

Atenolol 100mg Tablets BP

(Wockhardt UK Ltd)

1. NAME OF THE MEDICINAL PRODUCT
Atenolol Tablets BP 100mg or Totamol Tablets 100mg

2. QUALITATIVE AND QUANTITATIVE COMPOSITION
Atenolol 100mg

3. PHARMACEUTICAL FORM
Tablet for oral use

4. CLINICAL PARTICULARS
4.1 Therapeutic indications
Atenolol is recommended for the treatment of hypertension, angina pectoris, cardiac dysrhythmia, and for early intervention in the acute phase of myocardial infarction.

4.2 Posology and method of administration

Dosage

Adults:

Hypertension: Usually 50mg daily.

Angina: Usually 100mg daily or 50mg twice daily.

Dysrhythmias: Following control with intravenous atenolol, a suitable oral maintenance dosage is 50-100mg daily, given as a single dose.

Myocardial Infarction: Following treatment with intravenous atenolol, oral atenolol 50mg may be given approximately 15 minutes later, provided no untoward effects occur from the intravenous dose. This should be followed by a further 50mg orally 12 hours after the intravenous dose and subsequent dosage maintained, after a further 12 hours, with 100mg daily. If bradycardia and/or hypotension requiring treatment, or any other untoward effects occur, atenolol should be discontinued.

Renal impairment: The dose may need to be reduced.

Hepatic dysfunction: The dose may need to be reduced.

Elderly Patients:

Dosage requirements may be reduced, especially in patients with impaired renal function.

Children under 12 years of age:

There are inadequate clinical data available on the use of atenolol in children and for this reason it is not recommended.

4.3 Contraindications

Atenolol is contra-indicated in patients with a known hypersensitivity to atenolol, severe bradycardia, second degree or third degree heart block, uncontrolled heart failure, hypotension, severe peripheral vascular disease (includingintermittent claudication), sick sinus syndrome, cardiogenic shock, phaeocromocytoma (without a concomitant alpha-blocker), metabolic acidosis.

Although cardioselective beta-blockers may have less effect on lung function than non-selective beta-blockers, as with all beta-blockers these should be avoided in patients with asthma or a history of reversible obstructive airways disease or bronchospasm (see 4.4 Special Warnings and Precautions for Use), unless there are compelling clinical reasons for their use.

4.4 Special warnings and special precautions for use

Care should be taken when using beta-blockers in patients with poor cardiac reserve. Myocardial contractility must be maintained and signs of failure controlled with digitalis and diuretics.

Therapy should not be withdrawn abruptly, especially in patients with ischaemic heart disease, and replacement therapy should be considered to prevent exacerbation of angina pectoris, rebound hypertension, myocardial infarction, ventricular arrhythmias and sudden cardiac death (see 4.8, Undesirable Effects. Treatment should not be discontinued abruptly in patients on long-term therapy, but should be discontinued over one to two weeks.

If a beta-blocker is withdrawn prior to surgery it should be discontinued for at least 24 hours, if the patient is being anaesthetised. If beta-blockers are not discontinued before anaesthesia, the anaesthetist should be made aware of the beta-blocker therapy. A drug such as atropine may be given to counter increases in vagal tone. Anaesthetics causing myocardial depression such as ether, halothane and enflurane should be avoided (see 4.5, Interactions).

Beta-blockers may increase both the sensitivity towards allergens and seriousness of anaphylactic reactions and may also reduce the response to adrenaline. They may unmask myasthenia gravis or potentiate a myasthenic condition.

Patients with psoriasis should only be given beta-blockers after careful consideration, as psoriasis may be aggravated.

Atenolol should be used with caution in diabetics subject to frequent episodes of hypoglycaemia. Symptoms of hypoglycaemia and of hyperthyroidism may be masked (see 4.5, Interactions).

The product label will carry the warning " Do not take this medicine if there is a history of wheezing or asthma."

If the use of atenolol in patients with asthma or a history of obstructive airways disease is unavoidable, the risk of inducing bronchospasm should be appreciated and appropriate precautions taken. If bronchospasm occurs, this will usually be reversed by commonly used bronchodilators such as salbutamol or isoprenaline.

In patients with renal impairment or hepatic dysfunction, atenolol should be used with caution and reduction of dosage should be considered (see 4.2, Posology and Method of Administration).

4.5 Interaction with other medicinal products and other forms of Interaction

Alcohol: Enhanced hypotensive effect

Aldesleukin: Enhanced hypotensive effect.

Alprostadil: Enhanced hypotensive effect.

Amphetamines: Avoid concomitant use.

Ampicillin: Reduces atenolol serum levels.

Anaethetics: Enhanced hypotensive effect. Avoid anaesthetics which cause myocardial depression, e.g. ether, halothane and enflurane (see 4.4 Special Warnings and Precautions for Use).

Analgesics: Antihypertensive effects of beta-blockers may be impaired by non-steroidal anti-inflammatory drugs (NSAIDs), particularly indomethacin – avoid concomitant use.

Antacids: Reduced absorption may occur if calcium or aluminium hydroxide is administered concurrently.

Antiarrhythmics and other drugs affecting cardiac conduction: (eg, disopyramide, amiodarone, quinidine) additive negative inotropic effects on the heart, with increased risk of bradycardia, hypotension, ventricular fibrillation, heart block or asystole - avoid concomitant use.

Anticholinesterase agents: Increased risk of bradycardia

Antidepressants and antipsychotics: Phenothiazines and tricyclic antidepressants and tropisetron may increase the risk of ventricular arrhythmias Enhanced hypotensive effect with monoamine oxidase inhibitors (MAOIs).

Antidiabetics: Dosage of hypoglycaemic agents requirements may need to be increased (see 4.4 Special Warnings and Precautions for Use). There may be an enhanced hypoglycaemic effect and masking of warning signs with concurrent administration of insulin and oral antidiabetic drugs. Hypoglycaemia is more likely in Type I than in Type II diabetics and may be associated with delayed recovery or hypertension.

Antihypertensives, including angiotensin-converting enzyme (ACE) inhibitors and angiotensin-II antagonists; enhanced hypotension; alpha-blockers; enhanced risk of first dose hypotension - avoid concomitant use. Cardiodepressant calcium channel blocking agents such as diltiazem, nifedipine and verapamil may induce negative inotropic effects such as severe hypotension, bradycardia, asystole and heart failure avoid concomitant use.

Antimalarials: Risk of bradycardia increased with mefloquine.

Anxiolytics and hypnotics: Enhanced hypotensive effect with benzodiazepines.

Cardiac glycosides: Risk of marked bradycardia and AV block.

Clonidine: Increased risk of hypertension on withdrawal – avoid concomitant use

Ergot alkaloids: Increased peripheral vasoconstriction - avoid concomitant use.

Moxisylyte: Increased risk of severe postural hypotension.

Oestrogens and Progesterones: Ooestrogens and combined oral contraceptives may antagonise the antihypertensive effect.

Parasympathomimetics: Increasedrisk of bradycardia

Sympathomimetics: Risk of severe hypertension and bradycardia with such agents as adrenaline, noradrenaline and ephedrine - avoid concomitant use. Beta-blockers may also reduce the response to adrenaline in the management of anaphylaxis (see 4.4 Special Warnings and Precautions for Use).

Theophylline: Atenolol antagonises bronchodilator effect: avoid concomitant use

Ulcer healing drugs:Carbenoxolone may antagonise the hypotensive effect.

4.6 Pregnancy and lactation

Atenolol crosses the placenta. The safety of atenolol if given in early pregnancy has not been established and its use should therefore be avoided. Beta-blockers reduce placental perfusion, which may result in intrauterine foetal death, immature and premature deliveries. In addition, adverse effects (especially hypoglycaemia and bradycardia) may occur in foetus and neonate in the postnatal period.

Administration of atenolol in pregnancy may be associated with reduced foetal growth, which is greatest when started in early pregnancy, such as in the second trimester and is related to the duration of treatment. The risk of adverse effects to the foetus or neonate is greater in severely hypertensive pregnancies.

However, atenolol has been used effectively under close supervision for the treatment of hypertension in the third trimester.

Atenolol is excreted in breast milk. Breast-feeding can be undertaken but infants should be monitored for bradycardia, respiratory depression, hypotension and hypoglycaemia.

4.7 Effects on ability to drive and use machines

Occasionally dizziness or fatigue may occur when taking atenolol tablets. If affected, patients should not drive or operate machinery

4.8 Undesirable effects

Cardiovascular: heart failure, heart block, bradycardia, hypotension, dizziness, peripheral vasoconstriction withcoldness of the extremities (including exacerbation of intermittent claudication and Raynaud's phenomenon). (see 4.4, Special Warnings and Precautions for Use).

Eye: visual disturbances including blurred vision, sore eyes, dry eyes (reversible on withdrawal; discontinuance of the drug should be considered if any such reaction is not otherwise explicable), conjunctivitis.

Gastrointestinal: nausea, vomiting, diarrhoea, constipation and abdominal cramps, sclerosing peritonitisand retroperitoneal fibrosis.

General: fatigue, headache, dry mouth, sleep disturbances of the type noted with other beta-blockers have been reported rarely. An increase in (A)nti (N)uclear (A)ntibodies has been seen: its clinical relevance is not clear.

Haemopoietic: thrombocytopenia, eosinophilia and leucopenia including agranulocytosis.

Hepatic: Elevated liver enzymes and/or bilirubin

Metabolic: Lupus-like syndrome.Hyperglycaemia or hypoglycaemia. Non-diabetic patients susceptible to hypoglycaemia include those on regular dialysis, and long term patients who are nutritionally compromised or have liver disease. Atenolol may increase serum triglyceride levels.

Musculoskeletal, connective tissue and bone disorders: Myopathies including muscle cramps, arthralgia.

Nervous system: Paraesthesia, peripheral neuritis.

Psychiatric: Depression, psychosis, hallucinations, confusion, anxiety and nervousness.

Respiratory: Bronchospasm, pneumonitis, pulmonary fibrosis and pleurisy.

Reproductive: Impotence, Peyronie's disease;

Skin: Purpura, pruritus, reversible alopecia, skin rashes (reversible on withdrawal; discontinuance of the drug should be considered if any such reaction is not otherwise explicable), psoriasiform rash or exacerbation of psoriasis

Withdrawal: Sudden cessation of therapy with a betablockercan cause angina, myocardial infarction, ventricular arrhythmias and sudden cardiac death. (see 4.4 Special Warnings and Precautions for Use).

4.9 Overdose

Symptoms: Many cases of beta-blocker overdosage are uneventful, but some patients develop severe and occasionally fatal cardiovascular depression. Effects can includebradycardia, cardiac conduction block, hypotension, heart failure, and cardiogenic shock. Convulsions, coma, bronchospasm, respiratory depression, and bronchoconstriction can also occur, although infrequently.

Treatment:Absorption of any drug material still present in the gastrointestinal tract can be prevented by gastric lavage and administration of activated charcoal.

Excessive (therapeutic) bradycardia can be countered by atropine sulphate 0.6 to 2.4mg in divided doses of 600 micrograms.

Acute massive overdosage requires hospital management and expert advice should be obtained. Maintenance of a clear airway and adequate ventilation is mandatory. Excessive bradycardia and hypotension may be countered by atropine, (3 mg adult, 40 micrograms/kg child) intravenously. Cardiogenic shock unresponsive to atropine may be treated with an intravenous injection of glucagon (50-50 micrograms/kg in 5% glucose, with precautions to protect the airway in case of vomiting). A further dose of glucagon (or an intravenous infusion) may be required if the response is not maintained. If glucagon is not available intravenous isoprenaline is an alternative.

Administration of calcium ions, or the use of a cardiac pacemaker may also be considered. In patients intoxicated with hydrophilic beta-blocking agents, which include atenolol, haemodialysis or haemoperfusion may be considered.

5. PHARMACOLOGICAL PROPERTIES

5.1 Pharmacodynamic properties

Atenolol is a beta-adrenoceptor blocking agent for use in the management of hypertension and angina pectoris. It is a cardioselective beta-blocker selective for cardiac $beta_1$ receptors and has no partial agonist or membrane stabilising activity.

The mode of action of atenolol and other beta-blockers in the moderation of hypertension is still not fully understood although its effects on plasma renin and cardiac output are probably of primary importance. Atenolol reduces cardiac output, alters baroreceptor reflex sensitivity and blocks peripheral adrenoceptors. Atenolol has been found to reduce systolic and diastolic blood pressures by about 15% in patients with mild to moderate hypertension. Its beta-adrenoceptor antagonist properties reduce cardiac work. This property improves exercise tolerance in anginal patients.

5.2 Pharmacokinetic properties

Atenolol is not completely absorbed from the gastrointestinal tract, its oral bioavailability being of the order 50-60%. It is approximately 5% bound to plasma proteins. The plasma half-life of atenolol is about 6 hours. However, the duration of therapeutic effect is much longer than this, allowing once daily dosing. Atenolol is excreted largely unchanged in the urine and its dosage should be adjusted in renal failure.

5.3 Preclinical safety data

There are no pre-clinical data of relevance to the prescriber which are additional to those already included in other sections

6. PHARMACEUTICAL PARTICULARS

6.1 List of excipients

Maize Starch

Heavy Magnesium Carbonate

Povidone K30

Sodium Starch Glycollate

Magnesium Stearate

Purified Water

Opadry Orange OY-3455

6.2 Incompatibilities

None known

6.3 Shelf life

Three years

6.4 Special precautions for storage

Do not store above 25°C

Store in the original container

6.5 Nature and contents of container

Strip packs consisting of opaque white or clear UPVC coated with UPVDC, and aluminium foil with heat seal coating on bright side and colourless key coating on dull side. Strip packs contain 28 or 504 tablets.

Polypropylene or polyethylene tablet container of 500 tablets.

6.6 Instructions for use and handling

None

Administrative Data

7. MARKETING AUTHORISATION HOLDER

CP Pharmaceuticals Ltd

Ash Road North

Wrexham

LL13 9UF

8. MARKETING AUTHORISATION NUMBER(S)

PL 4543/0265

9. DATE OF FIRST AUTHORISATION/RENEWAL OF THE AUTHORISATION

Date of first authorisation 07/07/88

Date of last renewal 21/05/02

10. DATE OF REVISION OF THE TEXT

May 2003.

Atenolol 25mg Tablets BP

(Wockhardt UK Ltd)

1. NAME OF THE MEDICINAL PRODUCT

Atenolol Tablets BP 25mg or Totamol Tablets 25mg or Kentol Tablets 25mg

2. QUALITATIVE AND QUANTITATIVE COMPOSITION

Atenolol 25mg

For excipients, see 6.1.

3. PHARMACEUTICAL FORM

Tablet for oral use

4. CLINICAL PARTICULARS

4.1 Therapeutic indications

Atenolol is recommended for the treatment of hypertension, angina pectoris, cardiac dysrhythmia, and for early intervention in the acute phase of myocardial infarction.

4.2 Posology and method of administration

Dosage

Adults:

Hypertension: Usually 50mg daily.

Angina: Usually 100mg daily or 50mg twice daily.

Dysrhythmias: Following control with intravenous atenolol, a suitable oral maintenance dosage is 50-100mg daily, given as a single dose.

Myocardial Infarction: Following treatment with intravenous atenolol, oral atenolol 50mg may be given approximately 15 minutes later, provided no untoward effects occur from the intravenous dose. This should be followed by a further 50mg orally 12 hours after the intravenous dose and subsequent dosage maintained, after a further 12 hours, with 100mg daily. If bradycardia and/or hypotension requiring treatment, or any other untoward effects occur, atenolol should be discontinued.

Renal impairment: The dose may need to be reduced.

Hepatic dysfunction: The dose may need to be reduced.

Elderly Patients:

Dosage requirements may be reduced, especially in patients with impaired renal function.

Children under 12 years of age:

There are inadequate clinical data available on the use of atenolol in children and for this reason it is not recommended.

4.3 Contraindications

Atenolol is contra-indicated in patients with a known hypersensitivity to atenolol, severe bradycardia, second degree or third degree heart block, uncontrolled heart failure, hypotension, severe peripheral vascular disease (includingintermittent claudication), sick sinus syndrome, cardiogenic shock, phaeocromocytoma (without a concomitant alpha-blocker), metabolic acidosis.

Although cardioselective beta-blockers may have less effect on lung function than non-selective beta-blockers, as with all beta-blockers these should be avoided in patients with asthma or a history of reversible obstructive airways disease or bronchospasm (see 4.4 Special Warnings and Precautions for Use), unless there are compelling clinical reasons for their use.

4.4 Special warnings and special precautions for use

Care should be taken when using beta-blockers in patients with poor cardiac reserve. Myocardial contractility must be maintained and signs of failure controlled with digitalis and diuretics.

Therapy should not be withdrawn abruptly, especially in patients with ischaemic heart disease, and replacement therapy should be considered to prevent exacerbation of angina pectoris, rebound hypertension, myocardial infarction, ventricular arrhythmias and sudden cardiac death (see 4.8, Undesirable Effects). Treatment should not be discontinued abruptly in patients on long-term therapy, but should be discontinued over one to two weeks.

If a beta-blocker is withdrawn prior to surgery it should be discontinued for at least 24 hours, if the patient is being anaesthetised. If beta blockers are not discontinued before anaesthesia, the anaesthetist should be made aware of the beta-blocker therapy. A drug such as atropine may be given to counter increases in vagal tone. Anaesthetics causing myocardial depression such as ether, halothane and enflurane should be avoided (see 4.5, Interactions).

Atenolol reduces heart rate. In instances when symptoms may be attributable to the slow heart rate, the dose should be reduced. Beta-blockers should be used with caution in first degree AV block.

Beta-blockers may increase both the sensitivity towards allergens and seriousness of anaphylactic reactions and may also reduce the response to adrenaline. They may unmask myasthenia gravis or potentiate a myasthenic condition.

Patients with psoriasis should only be given beta-blockers after careful consideration, as psoriasis may be aggravated.

Atenolol should be used with caution in diabetics subject to frequent episodes of hypoglycaemia. Symptoms of hypoglycaemia and of hyperthyroidism may be masked (see 4.5 Interactions).

The product label will carry the warning " Do not take this medicine if there is a history of wheezing or asthma."

If the use of atenolol in patients with asthma or a history of obstructive airways disease is unavoidable, the risk of inducing bronchospasm should be appreciated and appropriate precautions taken. If bronchospasm occurs, this will usually be reversed by commonly used bronchodilators such as salbutamol or isoprenaline.

In patients with renal impairment or hepatic dysfunction, atenolol should be used with caution and reduction of dosage should be considered (see 4.2, Posology and Method of Administration).

4.5 Interaction with other medicinal products and other forms of Interaction

Alcohol: Enhanced hypotensive effect

A ldesleukin: Enhanced hypotensive effect.

Alprostadil: Enhanced hypotensive effect.

Amphetamines: Avoid concomitant use.

Ampicillin: Reduces atenolol serum levels.

Anaethetics: Enhanced hypotensive effect. Avoid anaesthetics which cause myocardial depression, e.g. ether, halothane and enflurane (see 4.4 Special Warnings and Precautions for Use).

Analgesics: Antihypertensive effects of beta-blockers may be impaired by non-steroidal anti-inflammatory drugs (NSAIDs), particularly indomethacin – avoid concomitant use.

Antacids: Reduced absorption may occur if calcium or aluminium hydroxide is administered concurrently.

Antiarrhythmics and other drugs affecting cardiac conduction: (eg, disopyramide, amiodarone, quinidine)additive negative inotropic effects on the heart, with increased risk of bradycardia, hypotension, ventricular fibrillation, heart block or asystole - avoid concomitant use.

Anticholinesterase agents: Increasedrisk of bradycardia

Antidepressants and antipsychotics: Phenothiazines and tricyclic antidepressants and tropisetron may increase the risk of ventricular arrhythmias.Enhanced hypotensive effect with monoamine oxidase inhibitors (MAOIs).

Antidiabetics: Dosage of hypoglycaemic agents requirements may need to be increased (see 4.4 Special Warnings and Precautions for Use). There may be an enhanced hypoglycaemic effect and masking of warning signs with concurrent administration of insulin and oral antidiabetic drugs. Hypoglycaemia is more likely in Type I than in Type II diabetics and may be associated with delayed recovery or hypertension.

Antihypertensives, including angiotensin-converting enzyme (ACE) inhibitors and angiotensin-II antagonists; enhanced hypotension; alpha-blockers; enhanced risk of first dose hypotension - avoid concomitant use. Cardiodepressant calcium channel blocking agents such as diltiazem, nifedipine and verapamil may induce negative inotropic effects such as severe hypotension, bradycardia, asystole and heart failure avoid concomitant use.

Antimalarials: Risk of bradycardia increased with mefloquine.

Anxiolytics and hypnotics: Enhanced hypotensive effect with benzodiazepines.

Cardiac glycosides: Risk of marked bradycardia and AV block.

Clonidine: Increased risk of hypertension on withdrawal – avoid concomitant use

Ergot alkaloids: Increased peripheral vasoconstriction - avoid concomitant use.

Moxisylyte: Increased risk of severe postural hypotension.

Oestrogens and Progesterones: Oestrogens and combined oral contraceptives may antagonise the antihypertensive effect.

P arasympathomimetics: Increased risk of bradycardia

Sympathomimetics: Risk of severe hypertension and bradycardia with such agents as adrenaline, noradrenaline and ephedrine - avoid concomitant use. Beta-blockers may also reduce the response to adrenaline in the management of anaphylaxis (see 4.4 Special Warnings and Precautions for Use).

Theophylline: Atenolol antagonises bronchodilator effect: avoid concomitant use

Ulcer healing drugs: Carbenoxolone may antagonise the hypotensive effect.

4.6 Pregnancy and lactation

Atenolol crosses the placenta.The safety of atenolol if given in early pregnancy has not been established and its use should therefore be avoided. Beta-blockers reduce placental perfusion, which may result in intrauterine foetal death, immature and premature deliveries. In addition, adverse effects (especially hypoglycaemia and bradycardia) may occur in foetus and neonate in the postnatal period.

Administration of atenolol in pregnancy may be associated with reduced foetal growth, which is greatest when started in early pregnancy, such as in the second trimester and is related to the duration of treatment. The risk of adverse effects to the foetus or neonate is greater in severely hypotensive pregnancies.

However, atenolol has been used effectively under close supervision for the treatment of hypertension in the third trimester.

Atenolol is excreted in breast milk. Breast-feeding can be undertaken but infants should be monitored for bradycardia, respiratory depression, hypotension and hypoglycaemia.

4.7 Effects on ability to drive and use machines

Occasionally dizziness or fatigue may occur when taking atenolol tablets. If affected, patients should not drive or operate machinery

4.8 Undesirable effects

Cardiovascular: heart failure, heart block, bradycardia, hypotension, dizziness, peripheral vasoconstriction withcoldness of the extremities (including exacerbation of intermittent claudication and Raynaud's phenomenon). (see 4.4, Special Warnings and Precautions for Use).

Eye: visual disturbances including blurred vision, sore eyes, dry eyes (reversible on withdrawal; discontinuance of the drug should be considered if any such reaction is not otherwise explicable), conjunctivitis.

Gastrointestinal:nausea, vomiting, diarrhoea, constipation and abdominal cramps, sclerosing peritonitisand retroperitoneal fibrosis.

General: fatigue, headache, dry mouth, sleep disturbances of the type noted with other beta-blockers have been reported rarely. An increase in (A)nti (N)uclear (A)ntibodies has been seen: its clinical relevance is not clear.

Haemopoietic: thrombocytopenia, eosinophilia and leucopenia includingagranulocytosis.

Hepatic: elevated liver enzymes and/or bilirubin

Metabolic: Lupus-like syndrome.Hyperglycaemia or hypoglycaemia. Non-diabetic patients susceptible to hypoglycaemia include those on regular dialysis, and long term patients who are nutritionally compromised or have liver disease. Atenolol may increase serum triglyceride levels.

Musculoskeletal, connective tissue and bone disorders: Myopathies including muscle cramps, arthralgia.

Nervous system: paraesthesia, peripheral neuritis.

Psychiatric: depression, psychosis, hallucinations, confusion, anxiety and nervousness.

Respiratory: bronchospasm, pneumonitis, pulmonary fibrosis and pleurisy.

Reproductive: impotence, Peyronie's disease;

Skin: Purpura, pruritus, reversible alopecia, skin rashes (reversible on withdrawal; discontinuance of the drug should be considered if any such reaction is not otherwise explicable), psoriasiform rash or exacerbation of psoriasis

Withdrawal: Sudden cessation of therapy with a beta-blockercan cause angina, myocardial infarction, ventricular arrhythmias and sudden cardiac death. (see 4.4 Special Warnings and Precautions for Use).

4.9 Overdose

Symptoms: Many cases of beta-blocker overdosage are uneventful, but some patients develop severe and occasionally fatal cardiovascular depression. Effects can include Bbradycardia, cardiac conduction block, hypotension, heart failure, acute cardiac insufficiency and cardiogenic shock. Convulsions, coma, bronchospasm, respiratory depression, and bronchoconstriction can also occur, although infrequently.

Treatment:Absorption of any drug material still present in the gastrointestinal tract can be prevented by gastric lavage and administration of activated charcoal and a laxative.

Excessive (therapeutic) bradycardia can be countered by atropine sulphate 0.6 to 2.4 mg in divided doses of 600 micrograms.

Acute massive overdosage requires hospital management and expert advice should be obtained. Maintenance of a clear airway and adequate ventilation is mandatory. Excessive bradycardia and hypotension may be countered by atropine, (3 mg adult, 40 micrograms/kg child) intravenously. Cardiogenic shock unresponsive to atropine may be treated with an intravenous injection of glucagon (50-50 micrograms/kg in 5% glucose, with precautions to protect the airway in case of vomiting). A further dose of glucagon (or an intravenous infusion) may be required if the response is not maintained. If glucagon is not available intravenous isoprenaline is an alternative.

Administration of calcium ions, or the use of a cardiac pacemaker may also be considered. In patients intoxicated with hydrophilic beta-blocking agents, which include atenolol, haemodialysis or haemoperfusion may be considered.

5. PHARMACOLOGICAL PROPERTIES

5.1 Pharmacodynamic properties

Atenolol is a beta-adrenoceptor blocking agent for use in the management of hypertension and angina pectoris. It is a cardioselective beta-blocker selective for cardiac $beta_1$ receptors and has no partial agonist or membrane stabilising activity.

The mode of action of atenolol and other beta-blockers in the moderation of hypertension is still not fully understood although its effects on plasma renin and cardiac output are probably of primary importance. Atenolol reduces cardiac output, alters baroreceptor reflex sensitivity and blocks peripheral adrenoceptors. Atenolol has been found to reduce systolic and diastolic blood pressures by about 15% in patients with mild to moderate hypertension. Its beta-adrenoceptor antagonist properties reduce cardiac work. This property improves exercise tolerance in anginal patients.

5.2 Pharmacokinetic properties

Atenolol is not completely absorbed from the gastrointestinal tract, its oral bioavailability being of the order 50-60%. It is approximately 5% bound to plasma proteins. The plasma half-life of atenolol is about 6 hours. However, the duration of therapeutic effect is much longer than this, allowing once daily dosing. Atenolol is excreted largely unchanged in the urine and its dosage should be adjusted in renal failure.

5.3 Preclinical safety data

There are no pre-clinical data of relevance to the prescriber which are additional to those already included in other sections

6. PHARMACEUTICAL PARTICULARS

6.1 List of excipients

Maize Starch

Heavy Magnesium Carbonate

Povidone K30

Sodium Starch Glycollate

Magnesium Stearate

Purified Water

6.2 Incompatibilities

None known

6.3 Shelf life

Three years

6.4 Special precautions for storage

Do not store above 25°C

Store in the original container

6.5 Nature and contents of container

Strip packs consisting of opaque white or clear UPVC coated with UPVDC, and aluminium foil with heat seal coating on bright side and colourless key coating on dull side. Strip packs contain 28 or 504 tablets.

Polypropylene or polyethylene tablet container of 500 tablets.

6.6 Instructions for use and handling

None

Administrative Data

7. MARKETING AUTHORISATION HOLDER

CP Pharmaceuticals Ltd

Ash Road North

Wrexham

LL13 9UF

8. MARKETING AUTHORISATION NUMBER(S)

PL 4543/0325

9. DATE OF FIRST AUTHORISATION/RENEWAL OF THE AUTHORISATION

Date of first authorisation 29/11/91

Renewal of authorisation 21/05/02

10. DATE OF REVISION OF THE TEXT

May 2003.

Atenolol 50mg Tablets BP

(Wockhardt UK Ltd)

1. NAME OF THE MEDICINAL PRODUCT

Atenolol Tablets BP 50mg or Totamol Tablets 50mg

2. QUALITATIVE AND QUANTITATIVE COMPOSITION

Atenolol 50mg

For excipients, see 6.1

3. PHARMACEUTICAL FORM

Tablet for oral use

4. CLINICAL PARTICULARS

4.1 Therapeutic indications

Atenolol is recommended for the treatment of hypertension, angina pectoris, cardiac dysrhythmia, and for early intervention in the acute phase of myocardial infarction.

4.2 Posology and method of administration

Dosage

Adults:

Hypertension: Usually 50mg daily.

Angina: Usually 100mg daily or 50mg twice daily.

Dysrhythmias: Following control with intravenous atenolol, a suitable oral maintenance dosage is 50-100mg daily, given as a single dose.

Myocardial Infarction: Following treatment with intravenous atenolol, oral atenolol 50mg may be given approximately 15 minutes later, provided no untoward effects occur from the intravenous dose. This should be followed by a further 50mg orally 12 hours after the intravenous dose and subsequent dosage maintained, after a further 12 hours, with 100mg daily. If bradycardia and/or hypotension requiring treatment, or any other untoward effects occur, atenolol should be discontinued.

Renal impairment: The dose may need to be reduced.

Hepatic dysfunction: The dose may need to be reduced.

Elderly Patients:

Dosage requirements may be reduced, especially in patients with impaired renal function.

Children under 12 years of age:

There are inadequate clinical data available on the use of atenolol in children and for this reason it is not recommended.

4.3 Contraindications

Atenolol is contra-indicated in patients with a known hypersensitivity to atenolol, severe bradycardia, second degree or third degree heart block, uncontrolled heart failure, hypotension, severe peripheral vascular disease (includingintermittent claudication), sick sinus syndrome, cardiogenic shock, phaeocromocytoma (without a concomitant alpha-blocker), metabolic acidosis.

Although cardioselective beta-blockers may have less effect on lung function than non-selective beta-blockers, as with all beta-blockers these should be avoided in patients with asthma or a history of reversible obstructive airways disease or bronchospasm (see 4.4 Special Warnings and Precautions for Use), unless there are compelling clinical reasons for their use.

4.4 Special warnings and special precautions for use

Care should be taken when using beta-blockers in patients with poor cardiac reserve. Myocardial contractility must be maintained and signs of failure controlled with digitalis and diuretics.

Therapy should not be withdrawn abruptly, especially in patients with ischaemic heart disease, and replacement therapy should be considered to prevent exacerbation of angina pectoris, rebound hypertension, myocardial infarction, ventricular arrhythmias and sudden cardiac death (see 4.8, Undesirable Effects. Treatment should not be discontinued abruptly in patients on long-term therapy, but should be discontinued over one to two weeks.

If a beta-blocker is withdrawn prior to surgery it should be discontinued for at least 24 hours, if the patient is being anaesthetised. If beta blockers are not discontinued before anaesthesia, the anaesthetist should be made aware of the beta-blocker therapy. A drug such as atropine may be given to counter increases in vagal tone. Anaesthetics causing myocardial depression such as ether, halothane and enflurane should be avoided (see 4.5, Interactions).

Atenolol reduces heart rate. In instances when symptoms may be attributable to the slow heart rate, the dose should be reduced. Beta-blockers should be used with caution in first degree AV block.

Beta-blockers may increase both the sensitivity towards allergens and seriousness of anaphylactic reactions and may also reduce the response to adrenaline. They may unmask myasthenia gravis or potentiate a myasthenic condition.

Patients with psoriasis should only be given beta-blockers after careful consideration, as psoriasis may be aggravated.

Atenolol should be used with caution in diabetics subject to frequent episodes of hypoglycaemia. Symptoms of hypoglycaemia and of hyperthyroidism may be masked (see 4.5, Interactions).

The product label will carry the warning " Do not take this medicine if there is a history of wheezing or asthma."

If the use of atenolol in patients with asthma or a history of obstructive airways disease is unavoidable, the risk of inducing bronchospasm should be appreciated and appropriate precautions taken. If bronchospasm occurs, this will usually be reversed by commonly used bronchodilators such as salbutamol or isoprenaline.

In patients with renal impairment or hepatic dysfunction, atenolol should be used with caution and reduction of dosage should be considered (see 4.2, Posology and Method of Administration).

4.5 Interaction with other medicinal products and other forms of Interaction

Alcohol: Enhanced hypotensive effect

Aldesleukin: Enhanced hypotensive effect.

Alprostadil: Enhanced hypotensive effect.

Amphetamines: Avoid concomitant use.

Ampicillin: Reduces atenolol serum levels.

Anaethetics: Enhanced hypotensive effect. Avoid anaesthetics which cause myocardial depression, e.g. ether, halothane and enflurane (see 4.4 Special Warnings and Precautions for Use).

Analgesics: Antihypertensive effects of beta-blockers may be impaired by non-steroidal anti-inflammatory drugs (NSAIDs), particularly indomethacin – avoid concomitant use.

Antacids : Reduced absorption may occur if calcium or aluminium hydroxide is administered concurrently.

Antiarrhythmics and other drugs affecting cardiac conduction: (eg, disopyramide, amiodarone, quinidine) additive negative inotropic effects on the heart, with increased risk of bradycardia, hypotension, ventricular fibrillation, heart block or asystole - avoid concomitant use.

Anticholinesterase agents: Increased risk of bradycardia

Antidepressants and antipsychotics: Phenothiazines and tricyclic antidepressants and tropisetron may increase the risk of ventricular arrhythmias*Enhanced hypotensive effect with monoamine oxidase inhibitors (MAOIs).*

Antidiabetics: Dosage of hypoglycaemic agents requirements may need to be increased (see 4.4 Special Warnings and Precautions for Use). There may be an enhanced hypoglycaemic effect and masking of warning signs with concurrent administration of insulin and oral antidiabetic drugs. Hypoglycaemia is more likely in Type I than in Type II diabetics and may be associated with delayed recovery or hypertension.

Antihypertensives, including angiotensin-converting enzyme (ACE) inhibitors and angiotensin-II antagonists; enhanced hypotension; alpha-blockers; enhanced risk of first dose hypotension - avoid concomitant use. Cardiodepressant calcium channel blocking agents such as diltiazem, nifedipine and verapamil may induce negative inotropic effects such as severe hypotension, bradycardia, asystole and heart failure avoid concomitant use.

Antimalarials: Risk of bradycardia increased with mefloquine.

Anxiolytics and hypnotics : Enhanced hypotensive effect with benzodiazepines.

Cardiac glycosides: Risk of marked bradycardia and AV block.

Clonidine: Increased risk of hypertension on withdrawal – avoid concomitant use

Ergot alkaloids: Increased peripheral vasoconstriction - avoid concomitant use.

Moxisylyte: Increased risk of severe postural hypotension.

Oestrogens and Progesterones:Oestrogens and combined oral contraceptives may antagonise the antihypertensive effect.

Parasympathomimetics: Increased risk of bradycardia

Sympathomimetics: Risk of severe hypertension and bradycardia with such agents as adrenaline, noradrenaline and ephedrine - avoid concomitant use. Beta-blockers may also reduce the response to adrenaline in the management of anaphylaxis (see 4.4 Special Warnings and Precautions for Use).

Theophylline: Atenolol antagonises bronchodilator effect: avoid concomitant use

Ulcer healing drugs: Carbenoxolone may antagonise the hypotensive effect.

4.6 Pregnancy and lactation

Atenolol crosses the placenta.The safety of atenolol if given in early pregnancy has not been established and its use should therefore be avoided. Beta-blockers reduce placental perfusion, which may result in intrauterine foetal death, immature and premature deliveries. In addition, adverse effects (especially hypoglycaemia and bradycardia) may occur in foetus and neonate in the postnatal period.

Administration of atenolol in pregnancy may be associated with reduced foetal growth, which is greatest when started in early pregnancy, such as in the second trimester and is related to the duration of treatment. The risk of adverse effects to the foetus or neonate is greater in severely hypertensive pregnancies.

However, atenolol has been used effectively under close supervision for the treatment of hypertension in the third trimester.

Atenolol is excreted in breast milk. Breast-feeding can be undertaken but infants should be monitored for bradycardia, respiratory depression, hypotension and hypoglycaemia.

4.7 Effects on ability to drive and use machines

Occasionally dizziness or fatigue may occur when taking atenolol tablets. If affected, patients should not drive or operate machinery

4.8 Undesirable effects

Cardiovascular: Heart failure, heart block, bradycardia, hypotension, dizziness, peripheral vasoconstriction withcoldness of the extremities (including exacerbation of intermittent claudication and Raynaud's phenomenon). (see 4.4, Special Warnings and Precautions for Use).

Eye: Visual disturbances including blurred vision, sore eyes, dry eyes (reversible on withdrawal; discontinuance of the drug should be considered if any such reaction is not otherwise explicable), conjunctivitis.

Gastrointestinal: Nausea, vomiting, diarrhoea, constipation and abdominal cramps, sclerosing peritonitisand retroperitoneal fibrosis.

General: Fatigue, headache, dry mouth, sleep disturbances of the type noted with other beta-blockers have been reported rarely. An increase in (A)nti (N)uclear (A)ntibodies has been seen: its clinical relevance is not clear.

Haemopoietic: Thrombocytopenia, eosinophilia and leucopenia including agranulocytosis.

Hepatic: Elevated liver enzymes and/or bilirubin

Metabolic: Lupus-like syndrome.Hyperglycaemia or hypoglycaemia. Non-diabetic patients susceptible to hypoglycaemia include those on regular dialysis, and long term patients who are nutritionally compromised or have liver disease. Atenolol may increase serum triglyceride levels.

Musculoskeletal, connective tissue and bone disorders: Myopathies including muscle cramps, arthralgia.

Nervous system: Paraesthesia, peripheral neuritis.

Psychiatric: Depression, psychosis, hallucinations, confusion, anxiety and nervousness.

Respiratory: Bronchospasm, pneumonitis, pulmonary fibrosis and pleurisy.

Reproductive: Impotence, Peyronie's disease;

Skin: Purpura, pruritus, reversible alopecia, skin rashes (reversible on withdrawal; discontinuance of the drug should be considered if any such reaction is not otherwise explicable), psoriasiform rash or exacerbation of psoriasis

Withdrawal: Sudden cessation of therapy with a beta-blockercan cause angina, myocardial infarction, ventricular arrhythmias and sudden cardiac death. (see 4.4 Special Warnings and Precautions for Use).

4.9 Overdose

Symptoms: Many cases of beta-blocker overdosage are uneventful, but some patients develop severe and occasionally fatal cardiovascular depression. Effects can include Bradycardia, cardiac conduction block, hypotension, heart failure, and cardiogenic shock. Convulsions, coma, bronchospasm, respiratory depression, and bronchoconstriction can also occur, although infrequently

Treatment:Absorption of any drug material still present in the gastrointestinal tract can be prevented by gastric lavage andadministration of activated charcoal.

Excessive (therapeutic) bradycardia can be countered by atropine sulphate 0.6 to 2.4 mg in divided doses of 600 micrograms.

Acute massive overdosage requires hospital management and expert advice should be obtained. Maintenance of a clear airway and adequate ventilation is mandatory. Excessive bradycardia and hypotension may be countered by atropine, (3 mg adult, 40 micrograms/kg child) intravenously. Cardiogenic shock unresponsive to atropine may be treated with an intravenous injection of glucagon (50-50 micrograms/kg in 5% glucose, with precautions to protect the airway in case of vomiting). A further dose of glucagon (or an intravenous infusion) may be required if the response is not maintained. If glucagon is not available intravenous isoprenaline is an alternative.

Administration of calcium ions, or the use of a cardiac pacemaker may also be considered. In patients intoxicated with hydrophilic beta-blocking agents, whichinclude atenolol, haemodialysis or haemoperfusion may be considered.

5. PHARMACOLOGICAL PROPERTIES

5.1 Pharmacodynamic properties

Atenolol is a beta-adrenoceptor blocking agent for use in the management of hypertension and angina pectoris. It is a cardioselective beta-blocker selective for cardiac $beta_1$ receptors and has no partial agonist or membrane stabilising activity.

The mode of action of atenolol and other beta-blockers in the moderation of hypertension is still not fully understood although its effects on plasma renin and cardiac output are probably of primary importance. Atenolol reduces cardiac output, alters baroreceptor reflex sensitivity and blocks peripheral adrenoceptors. Atenolol has been found to reduce systolic and diastolic blood pressures by about 15% in patients with mild to moderate hypertension. Its beta-adrenoceptor antagonist properties reduce cardiac work. This property improves exercise tolerance in anginal patients.

5.2 Pharmacokinetic properties

Atenolol is not completely absorbed from the gastrointestinal tract, its oral bioavailability being of the order 50-60%. It is approximately 5% bound to plasma proteins. The plasma half-life of atenolol is about 6 hours. However, the duration of therapeutic effect is much longer than this, allowing once daily dosing. Atenolol is excreted largely unchanged in the urine and its dosage should be adjusted in renal failure.

5.3 Preclinical safety data

There are no pre-clinical data of relevance to the prescriber which are additional to those already included in other sections

6. PHARMACEUTICAL PARTICULARS

6.1 List of excipients

Maize Starch

Heavy Magnesium Carbonate

Povidone K30

Sodium Starch Glycollate

Magnesium Stearate

Purified Water

Opadry Orange OY-3455

6.2 Incompatibilities

None known

6.3 Shelf life

Three years

6.4 Special precautions for storage

Do not store above 25°C

Store in the original container

6.5 Nature and contents of container

Strip packs consisting of opaque white or clear UPVC coated with UPVDC, and aluminium foil with heat seal coating on bright side and colourless key coating on dull side. Strip packs contain 28 or 504 tablets.

Polypropylene or polyethylene tablet container of 500 tablets.

6.6 Instructions for use and handling

None

Administrative Data

7. MARKETING AUTHORISATION HOLDER

CP Pharmaceuticals Ltd

Ash Road North

Wrexham

LL13 9UF

8. MARKETING AUTHORISATION NUMBER(S)

PL 4543/0264

9. DATE OF FIRST AUTHORISATION/RENEWAL OF THE AUTHORISATION

Date of first authorisation 07/07/88

Date of renewal of authorisation 21/05/02

10. DATE OF REVISION OF THE TEXT

May 2003

Ativan Injection

(Wyeth Pharmaceuticals)

1. NAME OF THE MEDICINAL PRODUCT

Ativan* Injection

2. QUALITATIVE AND QUANTITATIVE COMPOSITION

Ativan Injection contains the active ingredient lorazepam BP at a concentration of 4mg/ml.

Lorazepam (INN, BAN) is chemically defined as 7-chloro-5-(o-chlorphenyl)-1,3-dihydro-3-hydroxy-2H-1,4-benzodiazepin-2-one.

3. PHARMACEUTICAL FORM

Ativan Injection is a clear, colourless solution supplied in clear glass ampoules containing 4mg lorazepam in 1ml of solution.

4. CLINICAL PARTICULARS

4.1 Therapeutic indications

Pre-operative medication or premedication for uncomfortable or prolonged investigations, e.g. bronchoscopy, arteriography, endoscopy.

The treatment of acute anxiety states, acute excitement or acute mania.

The control of status epilepticus.

4.2 Posology and method of administration

Dosage and duration of therapy should be individualised. The lowest effective dose should be prescribed for the shortest time possible.

Treatment in all patients should be withdrawn gradually to minimise possible withdrawal symptoms (See Special Warnings and Special Precautions for Use).

Route of administration

Ativan Injection can be given intravenously or intramuscularly. However, the intravenous route is to be preferred. Care should be taken to avoid injection into small veins and intra-arterial injection.

Absorption from the injection site is considerably slower if the intramuscular route is used and as rapid an effect may be obtained by oral administration of Ativan tablets.

Ativan should not be used for long-term chronic treatment.

Preparation of the injection

Ativan Injection is slightly viscid when cool. To facilitate injection it may be diluted 1:1 with normal Saline or Water for Injection BP immediately before administration. If given intramuscularly it should always be diluted.

Ativan Injection is presented as a 1ml solution in a 2ml ampoule to facilitate dilution.

Ativan Injection should not be mixed with other drugs in the same syringe.

Dosage:

1. Premedication:

Adults: 0.05mg/kg (3.5mg for an average 70kg man). By the intravenous route the injection should be given 30-45 minutes before surgery when sedation will be evident after 5-10 minutes and maximal loss of recall will occur after 30-45 minutes.

By the intramuscular route the injection should be given 1-1 $^1/_2$ hours before surgery when sedation will be evident after 30-45 minutes and maximal loss of recall will occur after 60-90 minutes.

Children: Ativan Injection is not recommended in children under 12.

2. Acute Anxiety

Adults: 0.025-0.03mg/kg (1.75-2.1mg for an average 70kg man). Repeat 6 hourly.

Children: Ativan Injection is not recommended in children under 12.

3. Status epilepticus

Adults: 4mg intravenously

Children: 2mg intravenously

Elderly: The elderly may respond to lower doses and half the normal adult dose may be sufficient.

Patients with Renal or Hepatic impairment:

Lower doses may be sufficient in these patients (*See Special Warnings and Precautions for Use*). Use in patients with severe hepatic insufficiency is contraindicated.

4.3 Contraindications

- Acute pulmonary insufficiency.
- Hypersensitivity to benzodiazepines, including Ativan Injection or any of the vehicle constituents (polyethylene glycol, propylene glycol, benzyl alcohol).
- Sleep apnoea syndrome
- Myasthenia gravis
- Severe hepatic insufficiency
- Ativan Injection contains benzyl alcohol and is contraindicated in infants or young children, up to 3 years old.

Ativan Injection is not recommended for out-patient use unless the patient is accompanied.

4.4 Special warnings and special precautions for use

Prior to use, Ativan Injection may be diluted with equal amounts of compatible diluent *(see Posology and Method of Administration)*. Intravenous injection should be made slowly except in the control of status epilepticus where rapid injection is required.

The possibility that respiratory arrest may occur or that the patient may have partial airway obstruction should be considered. Therefore, equipment necessary to maintain a patent airway and to support respiration/ventilation should be available and used where necessary.

It is recommended that patients receiving Ativan Injection should remain under observation for at least eight hours and preferably overnight. When Ativan Injection is used for short procedures on an outpatient basis, the patient should be accompanied when discharged.

Patients should be advised that their tolerance for alcohol and other CNS depressants will be diminished in the presence of Ativan Injection. Alcoholic beverages should not be consumed for at least 24 to 48 hours after receiving Ativan Injection.

Extreme care must be taken in administering Ativan Injection to elderly or very ill patients and to those with limited pulmonary reserve, because of the possibility that apnoea and/or cardiac arrest may occur. Care should also be exercised when administering Ativan Injection to a patient with status epilepticus, especially when the patient has received other central nervous system depressants.

There is no evidence to support the use of Ativan Injection in coma or shock.

Ativan is not intended for the primary treatment of psychotic illness or depressive disorders, and should not be used alone to treat depressed patients. The use of benzodiazepines may have a disinhibiting effect and may release suicidal tendencies in depressed patients.

Pre-existing depression may emerge during benzodiazepine use.

There are no clinical data available for Ativan Injection with regard to abuse or dependence. However, based upon experience with oral benzodiazepines, doctors should be aware that repeated doses of Ativan Injection over a prolonged period of time may lead to physical and psychological dependence. The risk of dependence on Ativan is low when used at the recommended dose and duration, but increases with higher doses and longer term use.The risk of dependence is further increased in patients with a history of alcoholism or drug abuse, or in patients with significant personality disorders. Therefore, use in individuals with a history of alcoholism or drug abuse should be avoided.

Dependence may lead to withdrawal symptoms, especially if treatment is discontinued abruptly. Therefore, **the drug should always be discontinued gradually** - using the oral preparation if necessary.

Symptoms reported following discontinuation of oral benzodiazepines include headaches, muscle pain, anxiety, tension, depression, insomnia, restlessness, confusion, irritability, sweating, and the occurrence of "rebound" phenomena whereby the symptoms that led to treatment with benzodiazepines recur in an enhanced form. These symptoms may be difficult to distinguish from the original symptoms for which the drug was prescribed.

In severe cases the following symptoms may occur: derealisation; depersonalisation; hyperacusis; tinnitus; numbness and tingling of the extremities; hypersensitivity to light, noise, and physical contact; involuntary movements; vomiting; hallucinations; convulsions. Convulsions may be more common in patients with pre-existing seizure disorders or who are taking other drugs that lower the convulsive threshold, such as antidepressants.

It may be useful to inform the patient that treatment will be of limited duration and that it will be discontinued gradually. The patient should also be made aware of the possibility of "rebound" phenomena to minimise anxiety should they occur.

There are indications that, in the case of benzodiazepines with a short duration of action, withdrawal phenomena can become manifest within the dosage interval, especially when the dosage is high.

When benzodiazepines with a long duration of action are being used, it is important to warn against changing to a benzodiazepine with a short duration of action, as withdrawal symptoms may develop.

Abuse of benzodiazepines has been reported.

Anxiety or insomnia may be a symptom of several other disorders. The possibility should be considered that the complaint may be related to an underlying physical or psychiatric disorder for which there is more specific treatment.

Caution should be used in the treatment of patients with acute narrow-angle glaucoma.

Patients with impaired renal or hepatic function should be monitored frequently and have their dosage adjusted carefully according to patient response. Lower doses may be sufficient in these patients. The same precautions apply to elderly or debilitated patients and patients with chronic respiratory insufficiency.

As with all CNS-depressants, the use of benzodiazepines may precipitate encephalopathy in patients with severe hepatic insufficiency. Therefore, use in these patients is contraindicated.

Some patients taking benzodiazepines have developed a blood dyscrasia, and some have had elevations in liver enzymes. Periodic haematologic and liver-function assessments are recommended where repeated courses of treatment are considered clinically necessary.

Transient anterograde amnesia or memory impairment has been reported in association with the use of benzodiazepines. This effect may be advantageous when Ativan is used as a premedicant.

Paradoxical reactions have been occasionally reported during benzodiazepine use (see Undesirable effects). Such reactions may be more likely to occur in children and the elderly. Should these occur, use of the drug should be discontinued.

Although hypotension has occurred only rarely, benzodiazepines should be administered with caution to patients in whom a drop in blood pressure might lead to cardiovascular or cerebrovascular complications. This is particularly important in elderly patients.

Ativan Injection contains the excipients polyethylene glycol and propylene glycol. There have been rare reports of propylene glycol toxicity (e.g. lactic acidosis, hyperosmolality, hypotension) and polyethylene glycol toxicity (e.g. acute tubular necrosis) during administration of Ativan Injection at higher than recommended doses. Central nervous system toxicity, including seizures, as well as unresponsiveness, tachypnoea, tachycardia and diaphoresis have also been associated with propylene glycol toxicity. Symptoms may be more likely to develop in patients with renal or hepatic impairment and in paediatric patients.

4.5 Interaction with other medicinal products and other forms of Interaction

Not recommended: Concommitant intake with alcohol

The sedative effects may be enhanced when the product is used in combination with alcohol. This affects the ability to drive or use machines.

The benzodiazepines, including Ativan Injection, produce additive CNS depressant effects when co-administered with other medications which themselves produce CNS depression, e.g. barbiturates, antipsychotics, sedatives/hypnotics, anxiolytics, antidepressants, narcotic analgesics, sedative antihistamines, anticonvulsants and anaesthetics.

An enhancement of the euphoria induced by narcotic analgesics may occur with benzodiazepine use, leading to an increase in psychic dependence.

Compounds which inhibit certain hepatic enzymes (particularly cytochrome P450) may enhance the activity of benzodiazepines. To a lesser degree this also applies to benzodiazepines which are metabolised only by conjugation.

The addition of scopolamine to Ativan Injection is not recommended, since their combination has been observed to cause an increased incidence of sedation, hallucination and irrational behaviour.

4.6 Pregnancy and lactation

Ativan Injection should not be used during pregnancy, especially during the first and last trimesters, unless in the judgement of the physician such administration is clinically justifiable. Benzodiazepines may cause foetal damage when administered to pregnant women.

If the drug is prescribed to a woman of childbearing potential, she should be warned to contact her physician about stopping the drug if she intends to become, or suspects that she is, pregnant.

Use of Ativan Injection during the late phase of pregnancy may require ventilation of the infant at birth.

If, for compelling medical reasons, the product is administered during the late phase of pregnancy, or during labour at high doses, effects on the neonate, such as hypothermia, hypotonia and moderate respiratory depression, can be expected, due to the pharmacological action of the compound.

Infants of mothers who ingested benzodiazepines for several weeks or more preceding delivery have been reported to have withdrawal symptoms during the postnatal period.

Symptoms such as hypotonia, hypothermia, respiratory depression, apnoea, feeding problems, and impaired metabolic response to cold stress have been reported in neonates born of mothers who have received benzodiazepines during the late phase of pregnancy or at delivery.

There are insufficient data regarding obstetrical safety of parenteral Ativan, including use in cesarean section. Such use, therefore, is not recommended.

Since benzodiazepines are found in breast milk, Ativan Injection should not be given to breast feeding mothers.

4.7 Effects on ability to drive and use machines

Sedation, amnesia, impaired concentration and impaired muscular function may adversely affect the ability to drive or use machines. Therefore, patients should not drive or operate machinery within 24-48 hours of administration of Ativan Injection and should be advised not to take alcohol *(see also Interactions)*.

4.8 Undesirable effects

Lorazepam is well tolerated and imbalance or ataxia are signs of excessive dosage. Drowsiness may occur. Occasional confusion, hangover, headache on waking, dizziness, blurred vision, nausea, vomiting, restlessness, depression, crying, sobbing, hallucinations, diplopia have been reported. In addition, blood dyscrasias and increased liver enzymes have occasionally been reported. On rare occasions visual disturbances, hypotension, hypertension, gastrointestinal disturbances and mild transient skin rashes have been reported. Convulsion/seizure has been reported during or following treatment with lorazepam but causality has not been established.

Tolerance at the injection site is generally good although, rarely, pain and redness have been reported after Ativan Injection.

Transient anterograde amnesia or memory impairment may occur using therapeutic doses, the risk increasing at higher doses *(see Special Warnings and Special Precautions for Use)*.

Paradoxical reactions, such as restlessness, agitation, irritability, aggressiveness, delusion, rage, nightmares, hallucinations, psychoses and inappropriate behaviour, have been occasionally reported during benzodiazepine use. Such reactions may be more likely to occur in children and the elderly *(see Special Warnings and Special Precautions for Use)*.

4.9 Overdose

In the management of overdosage with any drug, it should be borne in mind that multiple agents may have been taken.

Overdosage of benzodiazepines is usually manifested by degrees of central nervous system depression ranging from drowsiness to coma. In mild cases, symptoms include drowsiness, mental confusion and lethargy. In more serious cases, and especially when other CNS-depressant drugs or alcohol are ingested, symptoms may include ataxia, hypotension, hypotonia, respiratory depression, coma and, very rarely, death.

Rarely, propylene glycol toxicity and polyethylene glycol toxicity have been reported following higher than recommended doses of Ativan Injection *(See Section 4.4)*.

Treatment of overdosage is mainly supportive including monitoring of vital signs and close observation of the patient. An adequate airway should be maintained and assisted respiration used as needed. Hypotension, though unlikely, may be controlled with noradrenaline. Lorazepam is poorly dialysable.

The benzodiazepine antagonist, flumazenil, may be useful in hospitalised patients for the management of benzodiazepine overdosage. Flumazenil product information should be consulted prior to use.

5. PHARMACOLOGICAL PROPERTIES

5.1 Pharmacodynamic properties

Ativan is a benzodiazepine with anxiolytic, sedative, hypnotic, anticonvulsant and muscle relaxant properties.

5.2 Pharmacokinetic properties

Ativan Injection is readily absorbed when given intramuscularly. Peak plasma concentrations occur approximately 60-90 minutes following intramuscular administration.

Ativan is metabolised by a simple one-step process to a pharmacologically inactive glucuronide. There is minimal risk of accumulation after repeated doses, giving a wide margin of safety.

There are no major active metabolites. The elimination half-life is about 12-16 hours when given intramuscularly or intravenously.

5.3 Preclinical safety data

Nothing of relevance to the prescriber.

6. PHARMACEUTICAL PARTICULARS

6.1 List of excipients

Polyethylene glycol 400, benzyl alcohol, propylene glycol.

6.2 Incompatibilities

None known

6.3 Shelf life

18 months

6.4 Special precautions for storage

Store and transport refrigerated (2°C to 8°C).

Keep ampoule in the outer carton.

6.5 Nature and contents of container

10 × 1ml solution (in 2ml ampoules) per pack.

6.6 Instructions for use and handling

None.

7. MARKETING AUTHORISATION HOLDER

John Wyeth and Brother Limited

trading as: Wyeth Laboratories

Huntercombe Lane South

Taplow

Maidenhead

Berkshire SL6 0PH

8. MARKETING AUTHORISATION NUMBER(S)

Ativan Injection: PL 0011/0051

9. DATE OF FIRST AUTHORISATION/RENEWAL OF THE AUTHORISATION

First Authorisation: 25 March 1988

Last Renewal: 9 February 1999

10. DATE OF REVISION OF THE TEXT

28 February 2005

Atropine Injection BP Minijet

(International Medication Systems (UK) Ltd)

1. NAME OF THE MEDICINAL PRODUCT
Atropine Injection BP Minijet

2. QUALITATIVE AND QUANTITATIVE COMPOSITION
Atropine Sulphate 0.1 mg/ml

3. PHARMACEUTICAL FORM
Sterile aqueous solution for parenteral administration to humans.

4. CLINICAL PARTICULARS

4.1 Therapeutic indications
Acute myocardial infarction with AV conduction block due to excess vagal tone (Wenkebach Type I, second-degree AV block) and sinus bradycardia, with associated hypotension and increased ventricular irritability.

Atropine can also be used in cardiopulmonary resuscitation for the treatment of sinus bradycardia accompanied by hypotension, hypoperfusion or ectopic arrhythmias.

Parenteral atropine is indicated as an antisialogogue in anaesthetic premedication to prevent or reduce secretions of the respiratory tract.

During anaesthesia, atropine may be used to prevent reflex bradycardia and restore cardiac rate and arterial pressure resulting from increased vagal activity associated with laryngoscopy, tracheal intubation and intra-abdominal manipulation. It may also be administered to block muscarinic effects when neostigmine is used to counteract muscle relaxants such as tubocurarine.

Parenteral atropine is an antidote for cardiovascular collapse following overdose of anticholinesterases; in the treatment of poisoning from organophosphorous insecticides or from chemical warfare 'nerve' gases and in the treatment of mushroom poisoning.

4.2 Posology and method of administration

Adults, children over 12 and the elderly:

Bradyarrhythmias: intramuscular or intravenous, 300 to 600 mcg (0.3 to 0.6 mg) every four to six hours to a total dose of 2 mg.

In cardiac resuscitation, intravenous 500 mcg (0.5 mg) repeated at 5 minute intervals until the desired heart rate is achieved. In asystole, 3 mg may be given intravenously as a once only single dose. If atropine cannot be administered intravenously during resuscitation, 2-3 times the intravenous dose may be administered via an endotracheal tube.

Premedication before anaesthesia: intramuscular or subcutaneous, 300 to 600 mcg (0.3 to 0.6 mg) 30-60 minutes before surgery or the same dose intravenously immediately before surgery.

To control muscarinic side effects of neostigmine: intravenous, 600 to 1200 mcg (0.6 - 1.2 mg).

Anticholinesterase poisoning: intramuscular or intravenous, 1 to 2 mg repeated every 5 to 60 minutes until signs and symptoms disappear, up to a maximum of 100 mg in the first 24 hours.

Children:

The usual intramuscular, intravenous or subcutaneous dose in children is 10 mcg/kg (0.01 mg/kg), but generally not exceeding 400 mcg (0.4 mg). If necessary, these doses may be repeated every 4-6 hours.

Cardiac: for advanced cardiac life support: intravenous, 20mcg/kg (0.02 mg/kg) with a minimum dose of 10 mcg (0.01 mg) repeated at 5 minute intervals, to a maximum dose of 100 mcg (0.1 mg).

Premedication before anaesthesia: intramuscular or subcutaneous; 30-60 minutes before surgery.

Up to 3 kg - 100 mcg (0.1 mg)

7 - 9 kg - 200 mcg (0.2 mg)

12 - 16 kg - 300 mcg (0.3 mg)

Over 20 kg - as for adults.

To control the muscarinic side effects of neostigmine: neonates and infants - 20 mcg/kg (0.02 mg/kg).

Anticholinesterase poisoning: intramuscular or intravenous, 50 mcg/kg (0.05 mg/kg) every 10-30 minutes until muscarinic signs and symptoms disappear.

4.3 Contraindications
Contra-indications are not applicable to the use of atropine in life-threatening emergencies (eg. asystole).

Atropine is contraindicated in patients with known hypersensitivity to the drug, obstruction of the bladder neck eg due to prostatic hypertrophy, reflux oesophagitis, closed angle glaucoma, myasthenia gravis (unless used to treat the adverse effects of an anticholinesterase agent), paralytic ileus, severe ulcerative colitis and obstructive disease of the gastrointestinal tract.

4.4 Special warnings and special precautions for use
Antimuscarinic agents should be used with caution in the elderly and children since these patients may be more susceptible to adverse effects. Atropine should also be used with caution in patients with hyperthyroidism, hepatic or renal disease or hypertension. Use with caution in febrile patients or when ambient temperature is high since antimuscarinics may cause an increase in temperature. Antimuscarinics block vagal inhibition of the SA nodal pacemaker and should thus be used with caution in patients with tachyarrhythmias, congestive heart failure or coronary heart disease. Parenterally administered atropine should be used cautiously in patients with chronic pulmonary disease since a reduction in bronchial secretions may lead to formation of bronchial plugs. Antimuscarinics should be used with extreme caution in patients with autonomic neuropathy.

Antimuscarinics decrease gastric motility, relax the lower oesophageal sphincter and may delay gastric emptying; they should therefore be used with caution in patients with gastric ulcer, oesophageal reflux or hiatus hernia associated with reflux oesophagitis, diarrhoea or GI infection.

4.5 Interaction with other medicinal products and other forms of Interaction
The effects of atropine may be enhanced by the concomitant administration of other drugs with anticholinergic activity eg. tricyclic antidepressants, antispasmodics, anti-parkinsonian drugs, some antihistamines, phenothiazines, disopyramide and quinidine. By delaying gastric emptying, atropine may alter the absorption of other drugs.

4.6 Pregnancy and lactation
Atropine crosses the placenta. Studies in humans have not been done and only limited information is available from animal studies. Intravenous administration of atropine during pregnancy or at term may cause tachycardia in the foetus. Atropine should only be administered to pregnant women if the benefits outweigh the risks to the foetus. Trace amounts of atropine appear in the breast milk and may cause antimuscarinic effects in the infant; lactation may be inhibited.

4.7 Effects on ability to drive and use machines
Not applicable; this preparation is intended for use only in emergencies.

4.8 Undesirable effects
Adverse effects are dose-related and usually reversible when therapy is discontinued. In relatively small doses, atropine reduces salivary, bronchial and sweat secretions; dry mouth and anhidrosis may develop, these effects being intensified as the dosage is increased. Reduced bronchial secretion may cause dehydration of residual secretion and consequent formation of thick bronchial plugs that are difficult to eject from the respiratory tract.

Larger doses dilate the pupil and inhibit accommodation of the eye, and block vagal impulses with consequent increase in heart rate with possible atrial arrhythmias, A-V dissociation and multiple ventricular ectopics; parasympathetic control of the urinary bladder and gastrointestinal tract is inhibited, causing urinary retention and constipation. Further increase in dosage inhibits gastric secretion. Anaphylaxis, urticaria and rash occasionally progressing to exfoliation may develop in some patients. Other effects include hallucinations, increased ocular tension, loss of taste, headache, nervousness, drowsiness, weakness, dizziness, flushing, insomnia, nausea, vomiting and bloated feeling. Mental confusion and/or excitement may occur especially in the elderly.

4.9 Overdose
Symptoms: marked dryness of the mouth accompanied by a burning sensation, difficulty in swallowing, pronounced photophobia, flushing and dryness of the skin, raised body temperature, rash, nausea, vomiting, tachycardia and hypertension. Restlessness, tremor, confusion, excitement, hallucinations and delirium may result from CNS stimulation; this is followed by increasing drowsiness, stupor and general central depression terminating in death from circulatory and respiratory failure.

Treatment: In severe cases, physostigmine, 1 to 4 mg, should be administered intravenously, intramuscularly or subcutaneously, the dose may be repeated if necessary since it is rapidly eliminated from the body. Diazepam may be administered for sedation of the delirious patient but the risk of central depression occurring late in the course of atropine poisoning contraindicates large doses of sedative. An adequate airway should be maintained and respiratory failure may be treated with oxygen and carbon dioxide inhalation. Fever is reduced by the application of cold packs or sponging with tepid water. Adequate fluid intake is important. Urethral catheterisation may be necessary. If photophobia is present or likely, the patient should be nursed in a darkened room.

5. PHARMACOLOGICAL PROPERTIES

5.1 Pharmacodynamic properties
Atropine is an antimuscarinic agent which competitively antagonizes acetylcholine at postganglionic nerve endings, thus affecting receptors of the exocrine glands, smooth muscle, cardiac muscle and the central nervous system.

Peripheral effects include tachycardia, decreased production of saliva, sweat, bronchial, nasal, lachrymal and gastric secretions, decreased intestinal motility and inhibition of micturition.

Atropine increases sinus rate and sinoatrial and AV conduction. Usually heart rate is increased but there may be an initial bradycardia.

Atropine inhibits secretions throughout the respiratory tract and relaxes bronchial smooth muscle producing bronchodilatation.

5.2 Pharmacokinetic properties
Following intravenous administration, the peak increase in heart rate occurs within 2 to 4 minutes. Peak plasma concentrations of atropine after intramuscular administration are reached within 30 minutes, although peak effects on the heart, sweating and salivation may occur nearer one hour after intramuscular administration.

Plasma levels after intramuscular and intravenous injection are comparable at one hour. Atropine is distributed widely throughout the body and crosses the blood brain barrier. The elimination half life is about 2 to 5 hours. Up to 50% of the dose is protein bound. It disappears rapidly from the circulation.

Atropine is metabolised in the liver by oxidation and conjugation to give inactive metabolites.

About 50% of the dose is excreted within 4 hours and 90% in 24 hours in the urine, about 30 to 50% as unchanged drug.

5.3 Preclinical safety data
Not applicable since atropine has been used in clinical practice for many years and its effects in man are well known.

6. PHARMACEUTICAL PARTICULARS

6.1 List of excipients
Sodium Citrate Dihydrate USP

Citric Acid Monohydrate USP

Sodium Chloride USP

Water for Injection USP

6.2 Incompatibilities
None known.

6.3 Shelf life
36 months

6.4 Special precautions for storage
Store below 25°C. Protect from light.

6.5 Nature and contents of container
The solution is contained in a USP type I glass vial with an elastomeric closure which meets all the relevant USP specifications. The product is available either as 5, 10 or 30ml.

6.6 Instructions for use and handling
The container is specially designed for use with the IMS Minijet injector.

7. MARKETING AUTHORISATION HOLDER
International Medication Systems (UK) Ltd

208 Bath Road

Slough

Berkshire

SL1 3WE

UK

8. MARKETING AUTHORISATION NUMBER(S)
PL 03265/0013R

9. DATE OF FIRST AUTHORISATION/RENEWAL OF THE AUTHORISATION
Date first granted: 20.03.91

Date renewed: 17 March 1997

10. DATE OF REVISION OF THE TEXT
November 2001

POM

Atrovent Aerocaps

(Boehringer Ingelheim Limited)

1. NAME OF THE MEDICINAL PRODUCT
Atrovent® Aerocaps®

2. QUALITATIVE AND QUANTITATIVE COMPOSITION
Each capsule contains 40 micrograms of ipratropium bromide.

3. PHARMACEUTICAL FORM
Inhalation powder, hard capsule.

Dark olive/light olive opaque size 3 hard gelatin capsules.

4. CLINICAL PARTICULARS

4.1 Therapeutic indications
ATROVENT AEROCAPS are indicated for the regular treatment of reversible bronchospasm associated with chronic obstructive pulmonary disease (COPD) and chronic asthma.

4.2 Posology and method of administration
Adults (including the elderly):

1 capsule three or four times daily. This dose may be doubled safely in patients who are less responsive.

A total daily dose of 8 capsules should not be exceeded.

Children (under 12 years):

There is limited experience of the use of ATROVENT AEROCAPS in children, therefore the product is not recommended for use in children.

If therapy does not produce a significant improvement or if the patient's condition gets worse, medical advice must be sought. In the case of acute or rapidly worsening dyspnoea (difficulty in breathing) a doctor should be consulted immediately.

One ATROVENT AEROCAP is equivalent to two puffs of ATROVENT Inhaler or one puff of ATROVENT Forte.

Administration

The capsules are only intended for use in the AEROHALER and should not be swallowed. The AEROHALER pierces the AEROCAP so that you can breathe the powder it contains into your lungs. The instructions for use of the AEROHALER should be read carefully to ensure correct administration.

The magazine allows you to load up to six capsules at a time. When using the AEROHALER you will be breathing the medicine (powder) in from one capsule at a time. This means that you will be breathing in an exact dose each time.

1. Remove the inhaler from the protective pouch provided.
2. Opening the inhaler. Open the mouthpiece (white part).
3. Magazine. Load the magazine according to the manufacturer's instructions as detailed on the Patient Information Leaflet. It is important to only load the number of capsules you will need for that day. Close the inhaler by pushing down the mouthpiece until it clicks.
4. Preparing for inhalation. Hold the mouthpiece upwards. Push the white button until it clicks and release it immediately. This pierces the capsule, making the medicine available for inhalation.
5. Inhalation. Breathe out fully, then raise the AEROHALER to your mouth and close your lips around the mouthpiece. Next breathe in slowly but deeply through the AEROHALER. While holding your breath for as long as is comfortable, remove the mouthpiece from your mouth. Finally, breathe out slowly, preferably through your nose, not your mouth. It is important not to breathe out through the AEROHALER.
6. Preparing for the next dose. Follow the manufacturer's instructions as detailed on the Patient Information Leaflet.
7. Removing the capsules. When you have used the last capsule, open up the mouthpiece. Turn the AEROHALER upside down and shake out all the used capsules. Then close, or refill, the inhaler.
8. The AEROHALER should be cleaned from time-to-time following the manufacturer's instructions as detailed on the Patient Information Leaflet.

4.3 Contraindications

Known hypersensitivity to atropine or its derivatives, or to any other component of the product.

4.4 Special warnings and special precautions for use

Caution is advocated in the use of anticholinergic agents in patients with narrow-angle glaucoma, or with prostatic hyperplasia or bladder-outflow obstruction.

As patients with cystic fibrosis may be prone to gastro-intestinal motility disturbances, ATROVENT, as with other anticholinergics, should be used with caution in these patients.

Immediate hypersensitivity reactions following the use of ATROVENT have been demonstrated by rare cases of urticaria, angioedema, rash, bronchospasm, oropharyngeal oedema and anaphylaxis.

There have been isolated reports of ocular complications (i.e. mydriasis, increased intraocular pressure, narrow-angle glaucoma, eye pain) when aerosolised ipratropium bromide, either alone or in combination with an adrenergic beta$_2$-agonist, has come into contact with the eyes.

Patients must be instructed in the correct administration of ATROVENT AEROCAPS and care must be taken not to allow the powder to enter into the eyes. However, since the inhaler device used to aerosolise the powder is breath-actuated, there should be little risk of the powder entering the eyes.

Eye pain or discomfort, blurred vision, visual halos or coloured images in association with red eyes from conjuctival congestion and corneal oedema may be signs of acute narrow-angle glaucoma. Should any of these symptoms develop, treatment with miotic drops should be initiated and specialist advice sought immediately.

4.5 Interaction with other medicinal products and other forms of Interaction

There is evidence that the administration of ATROVENT with beta-adrenergic drugs and xanthine preparations may produce an additive bronchodilatory effect.

4.6 Pregnancy and lactation

The safety of ATROVENT during human pregnancy has not been established. The benefits of using ATROVENT during a confirmed or suspected pregnancy must be weighed against the possible hazards to the unborn child. Preclinical studies have shown no embryotoxic or teratogenic effects following inhalation or intranasal application at doses considerably higher than those recommended in man.

It is not known whether ipratropium bromide is excreted into breast milk. It is unlikely that ipratropium bromide would reach the infant to an important extent, however caution should be exercised when ATROVENT is administered to nursing mothers.

4.7 Effects on ability to drive and use machines

None stated.

4.8 Undesirable effects

The most frequent non-respiratory adverse reactions reported in clinical trials with ATROVENT were headache, nausea (with or without vomiting) and dryness of the mouth.

The following side effects have been observed with ATROVENT: tachycardia, palpitations, supraventricular tachycardia and atrial fibrillation, visual accommodation disturbances, gastro-intestinal motility disturbances and urinary retention. These side effects have been rare and reversible. The risk of urinary retention may be increased in patients with pre-existing urinary outflow tract obstruction.

Ocular side effects have been reported (see: Special Warnings and Special Precautions for Use).

As with other inhaled bronchodilator therapy, cough, local irritation and inhalation induced bronchoconstriction may occur.

Allergic-type reactions such as skin rash, angioedema of the tongue, lips and face, urticaria, laryngospasm and anaphylactic reactions may occur.

4.9 Overdose

No symptoms specific to overdosage have been encountered. In view of the wide therapeutic window and topical administration of ATROVENT, no serious anticholinergic symptoms are to be expected. As with other anticholinergics, dry mouth, visual accommodation disturbances and tachycardia would be the expected symptoms and signs of overdose.

5. PHARMACOLOGICAL PROPERTIES

5.1 Pharmacodynamic properties

ATROVENT is a quaternary ammonium compound with anticholinergic (parasympatholytic) properties. In preclinical studies, it appears to inhibit vagally mediated reflexes by antagonising the action of acetylcholine, the transmitter agent released from the vagus nerve. Anticholinergics prevent the increase in intracellular concentration of cyclic guanosine monophosphate (cyclic GMP) caused by interaction of acetylcholine with the muscarinic receptor on bronchial smooth muscle.

The bronchodilation following inhalation of ATROVENT is induced by local drug concentrations sufficient for anticholinergic efficacy at the bronchial smooth muscle and not by systemic drug concentrations.

In clinical trials using metered dose inhalers in patients with reversible bronchospasm associated with asthma or chronic obstructive pulmonary disease significant improvements in pulmonary function (FEV_1 increases of 15% or more) occurred within 15 minutes, reached a peak in 1-2 hours, and persisted for approximately 4 hours.

Preclinical and clinical evidence suggest no deleterious effect of ATROVENT on airway mucous secretion, mucociliary clearance or gas exchange.

5.2 Pharmacokinetic properties

The therapeutic effect of ATROVENT is produced by a local action in the airways. Therefore time courses of bronchodilation and systemic pharmacokinetics do not run in parallel.

Following inhalation, dose portions from 10 to 30%, depending on the formulation, device and inhalation technique, are generally deposited in the lungs. The major part of the dose is swallowed and passes through the gastro-intestinal tract.

Due to the negligible gastro-intestinal absorption of ipratropium bromide the bioavailability of the swallowed dose portion is only approximately 2%. This fraction of the dose does not make a relevant contribution to the plasma concentrations of the active ingredient. The portion of the dose deposited in the lungs reaches the circulation rapidly (within minutes).

Limited data on total systemic bioavailability (pulmonary and gastro-intestinal portions), based on renal excretion (0 – 24 hours) of ipratropium bromide, suggest a range of 7 to 28% when delivery is via a nebuliser or a MDI product. It is assumed that this is also a valid range for the inhalation from the powder preparation.

Kinetic parameters describing the distribution of ipratropium bromide were calculated from plasma concentrations after i.v. administration.

A rapid biphasic decline in plasma concentrations is observed. The volume of distribution (V_β) is 338 L (≙ 4.6 L/kg). The drug is minimally (less then 20%) bound to plasma proteins. The ipratropium ion does not cross the blood-brain barrier, consistent with the ammonium structure of the molecule.

The half-life of the terminal elimination phase is about 1.6 hours.

The mean total clearance of the drug is determined to be 2.3 L/min. The major portion of approximately 60% of the systemic available dose is eliminated by metabolic degradation, probably in the liver. The main urinary metabolites bind poorly to the muscarinic receptor and have to be regarded as ineffective.

A portion of approximately 40% of the systemic available dose is cleared via urinary excretion corresponding to an experimental renal clearance of 0.9 L/min. A study with radiolabelled material showed that approximately 10% of orally administered ipratropium bromide was absorbed from the gastro-intestinal tract and metabolised. Less than 1% of an oral dose is renally excreted as parent compound.

In excretion balance studies after intravenous administration of a radioactive dose, less than 10% of the drug-related radioactivity (including parent compound and all metabolites) is excreted via the biliary-faecal route. The dominant excretion of drug-related radioactivity occurs via the kidneys.

5.3 Preclinical safety data

There are no pre-clinical data of relevance to the prescriber which are additional to that already included in other sections of the SPC.

6. PHARMACEUTICAL PARTICULARS

6.1 List of excipients

Glucose (ground anhydrous)

Capsule shell: Titanium dioxide (E171), Indigo Carmine (E132), Iron Oxide Yellow (E172), ron Oxide Black (E172), Gelatin.

6.2 Incompatibilities

Not applicable.

6.3 Shelf life

24 months.

6.4 Special precautions for storage

Do not store above 25°C.

Store in the original container.

6.5 Nature and contents of container

PVC/Aluminium blister packs containing 30, 50, 60, 90, 100, 120, 180, 240, 300 or 360 AEROCAPS (currently only the 100 pack size is marketed: Pack containing 100 AEROCAPS and 1 CE marked AEROHALER device and refill pack containing 100 AEROCAPS).

6.6 Instructions for use and handling

None stated.

7. MARKETING AUTHORISATION HOLDER

Boehringer Ingelheim Limited

Ellesfield Avenue

Bracknell

Berkshire

RG12 8YS

United Kingdom

8. MARKETING AUTHORISATION NUMBER(S)

PL 00015/0156

9. DATE OF FIRST AUTHORISATION/RENEWAL OF THE AUTHORISATION

27 February 1992

10. DATE OF REVISION OF THE TEXT

June 2003

11. Legal Category

POM

A9a/UK/SPC/8

Atrovent Inhaler CFC-Free

(Boehringer Ingelheim Limited)

1. NAME OF THE MEDICINAL PRODUCT

▼ATROVENT Inhaler CFC-Free 20 micrograms/actuation pressurised inhalation solution.

2. QUALITATIVE AND QUANTITATIVE COMPOSITION

One metered dose (ex-valve) contains 20 micrograms ipratropium bromide (as the monohydrate).

For excipients, see 6.1.

3. PHARMACEUTICAL FORM

Pressurised inhalation, solution.

Each container is filled with 10 ml of a clear, colourless liquid, free from suspended particles.

ATROVENT Inhaler CFC-Free contains a new propellant, HFA-134a, and does not contain any chlorofluorocarbons (CFCs).

4. CLINICAL PARTICULARS

4.1 Therapeutic indications

ATROVENT Inhaler CFC-Free is indicated for the regular treatment of reversible bronchospasm associated with chronic obstructive pulmonary disease (COPD) and chronic asthma.

4.2 Posology and method of administration

For inhalation use.

Adults (including the elderly):

Usually 1 or 2 puffs three or four times daily, although some patients may need up to 4 puffs at a time to obtain maximum benefit during early treatment.

Children:

6-12 years: Usually 1 or 2 puffs three times daily.

Under 6 years: Usually 1 puff three times daily.

In order to ensure that the inhaler is used correctly, administration should be supervised by an adult.

The recommended dose should not be exceeded.

If therapy does not produce a significant improvement, if the patient's condition gets worse or if a reduced response to treatment becomes apparent, medical advice must be sought. In the case of acute or rapidly worsening dyspnoea (difficulty in breathing) a doctor should be consulted immediately.

Administration

The correct administration of ipratropium bromide from the inhaler is essential for successful therapy. For detailed information on instructions for use please refer to the Patient Information Leaflet.

The canister should be pressed twice to release two metered doses into the air before the inhaler is used for the first time, or when the inhaler has not been used for 3 days or more, to ensure that the inhaler is working properly and that it is ready for use.

Before each occasion on which the inhaler is used the following should be observed:

1. Remove protective cap.
2. Hold the inhaler upright (the arrow on the base of the container should be pointing upwards), breathe out gently and then close the lips over the mouthpiece
3. Breathe in slowly and deeply, pressing the base of the canister firmly at the same time; this releases one metered dose. Hold the breath for 10 seconds or as long as is comfortable, then remove the mouthpiece from the mouth and breathe out slowly.
4. If a second inhalation is required you should wait at least one minute and then repeat Points 2 and 3 above.
5. Replace the protective cap after use.

The inhaler can be used with the Aerochamber Plus™ spacer device. This may be useful for patients, e.g. children, who find it difficult to synchronise breathing in and inhaler actuation.

The canister is not transparent. It is therefore not possible to see when it is empty. The inhaler will deliver 200 actuations. When these have all been used (usually after 3 – 4 weeks of regular use) the inhaler may still appear to contain a small amount of fluid. However the inhaler should be replaced in order to ensure that each metered dose contains the correct amount of medicine.

WARNING:

The plastic mouthpiece has been specially designed for use with ATROVENT Inhaler CFC-Free to ensure that each metered dose contains the correct amount of medicine. The mouthpiece must never be used with any other metered dose inhaler nor must ATROVENT Inhaler CFC-Free be used with any mouthpiece other than the one supplied with the product.

The mouthpiece should always be kept clean. To clean the mouthpiece, the canister and dustcap must be removed. The mouthpiece should then be washed in warm soapy water, rinsed and dried. Care should be taken to ensure that the small hole in the mouthpiece is flushed through thoroughly. The canister and dustcap should be replaced once the mouthpiece is dry.

4.3 Contraindications

ATROVENT Inhaler CFC-Free should not be taken by patients with known hypersensitivity to atropine or its derivatives, or to ipratropium bromide or to any other component of the product.

4.4 Special warnings and special precautions for use

When using ATROVENT Inhaler CFC-Free for the first time, some patients may notice that the taste is slightly different from that of the CFC-containing formulation. Patients should be made aware of this when changing from one formulation to the other. They should also be told that the formulations have been shown to be interchangeable for all practical purposes and that the difference in taste has no consequences in terms of the safety or the efficacy of the new formulation.

Caution is advocated in the use of anticholinergic agents in patients with narrow-angle glaucoma, or with prostatic hyperplasia or bladder-outflow obstruction. As patients with cystic fibrosis may be prone to gastrointestinal motility disturbances, ipratropium bromide, as with other anticholinergics, should be used with caution in these patients.

Hypersensitivity reactions following the use of ipratropium bromide have been seen and have presented as urticaria, angioedema, rash, bronchospasm, oropharyngeal oedema and anaphylaxis.

There have been isolated reports of ocular complications (i.e. mydriasis, increased intraocular pressure, narrow-angle glaucoma, eye pain) when aerosolised ipratropium bromide, either alone or in combination with an adrenergic beta$_2$-agonist, has come into contact with the eyes. Thus patients must be instructed in the correct administration of ATROVENT Inhaler CFC-Free and warned against the accidental release of the contents into the eye. Antiglaucoma therapy is effective in the prevention of acute narrow-angle glaucoma in susceptible individuals and patients who may be susceptible to glaucoma should be warned specifically on the need for ocular protection.

Eye pain or discomfort, blurred vision, visual halos or coloured images in association with red eyes from conjunctival congestion and corneal oedema may be signs of acute narrow-angle glaucoma. Should any combination of these symptoms develop, treatment with miotic drops should be initiated and specialist advice sought immediately.

Patients should be informed when starting treatment that the onset of action of ipratropium bromide is slower than that of inhaled sympathomimetic bronchodilators.

4.5 Interaction with other medicinal products and other forms of Interaction

There is evidence that the administration of ipratropium bromide with beta-adrenergic drugs and xanthine preparations may produce an additive bronchodilatory effect.

4.6 Pregnancy and lactation

There is no experience of the use of this product in pregnancy and lactation in humans. It should not be used in pregnancy or lactation unless the expected benefits to the mother are thought to outweigh any potential risks to the fetus or neonate.

The safety of ipratropium bromide during human pregnancy has not been established. The benefits of using ipratropium bromide during a confirmed or suspected pregnancy must be weighed against the possible hazards to the unborn child. Preclinical studies have shown no embryotoxic or teratogenic effects following inhalation or intranasal application at doses considerably higher than those recommended in man.

It is not known whether ipratropium bromide is excreted into breast milk. It is unlikely that ipratropium bromide would reach the infant to an important extent, however caution should be exercised when ipratropium bromide is administered to nursing mothers.

Studies of HFA-134a administered to pregnant and lactating rats and rabbits have not revealed any special hazard.

4.7 Effects on ability to drive and use machines

On the basis of the pharmacodynamic profile and reported adverse drug reactions it is not likely that ipratropium bromide has an effect on ability to drive and use machines.

4.8 Undesirable effects

The most frequent non-respiratory adverse events reported in clinical trials were headache, nausea (with or without vomiting) and dryness of the mouth.

The following side effects have been observed with ATROVENT: tachycardia, palpitations, supraventricular tachycardia and atrial fibrillation, visual accommodation disturbances, gastrointestinal motility disturbances and urinary retention. These side effects have been rare and reversible. The risk of urinary retention may be increased in patients with pre-existing urinary outflow tract obstruction.

Ocular side effects have been reported (see Section 4.4 - Special Warning and Precautions for Use).

As with other inhalation therapy, cough and local irritation may occur. In addition, as with other inhalation therapy, inhalation induced bronchoconstriction may occur with an immediate increase in wheezing after dosing. This should be treated straight away with a fast acting inhaled bronchodilator. ATROVENT Inhaler CFC-Free should be discontinued immediately, the patient assessed and, if necessary, alternative treatment instituted.

Allergic-type reactions such as skin rash, angioedema of the tongue, lips and face, urticaria (including giant urticaria), laryngospasm and anaphylactic reactions may occur.

When using ATROVENT Inhaler CFC-Free for the first time some patients may notice that the taste is slightly different from that of the CFC-containing formulation. Some patients have described the taste as unpleasant.

4.9 Overdose

No symptoms specific to overdosage have been encountered. In view of the wide therapeutic window and topical administration of ipratropium bromide, no serious anticholinergic symptoms are to be expected. As with other anticholinergics, dry mouth, visual accommodation disturbances and tachycardia would be the expected symptoms and signs of overdose.

5. PHARMACOLOGICAL PROPERTIES

5.1 Pharmacodynamic properties

ATC Code: R03B B01

Trials with a treatment duration of up to three months involving adult asthmatics and COPD patients, and asthmatic children, in which the HFA formulation and the CFC formulation have been compared have shown the two formulations to be therapeutically equivalent.

Ipratropium bromide is a quaternary ammonium compound with anticholinergic (parasympatholytic) properties. In preclinical studies, it appears to inhibit vagally mediated reflexes by antagonising the action of acetylcholine, the transmitter agent released from the vagus nerve. Anticholinergics prevent the increase in intracellular concentration of cyclic guanosine monophosphate (cyclic GMP) caused by interaction of acetylcholine with the muscarinic receptor on bronchial smooth muscle.

The bronchodilation following inhalation of ipratropium bromide is induced by local drug concentrations sufficient for anticholinergic efficacy at the bronchial smooth muscle and not by systemic drug concentrations.

In clinical trials using metered dose inhalers in patients with reversible bronchospasm associated with asthma or chronic obstructive pulmonary disease significant improvements in pulmonary function (FEV_1 increases of 15% or more) occurred within 15 minutes, reached a peak in 1-2 hours, and persisted for approximately 4 hours.

Preclinical and clinical evidence suggest no deleterious effect of ipratropium bromide on airway mucous secretion, mucociliary clearance or gas exchange.

5.2 Pharmacokinetic properties

The therapeutic effect of ipratropium bromide is produced by a local action in the airways. Therefore time courses of bronchodilation and systemic pharmacokinetics do not run in parallel.

Following inhalation, dose portions from 10 to 30%, depending on the formulation, device and inhalation technique, are generally deposited in the lungs. The major part of the dose is swallowed and passes through the gastro-intestinal tract.

Due to the negligible gastrointestinal absorption of ipratropium bromide the bioavailability of the swallowed dose portion is only approximately 2%. This fraction of the dose does not make a relevant contribution to the plasma concentrations of the active ingredient. The portion of the dose deposited in the lungs reaches the circulation rapidly (within minutes).

Limited data on total systemic bioavailability (pulmonary and gastrointestinal portions), based on renal excretion (0 – 24 hours) of ipratropium bromide, suggests a range of 7 to 28% when delivery is via a nebuliser or a MDI product. It is assumed that this is also a valid range for inhalation from the powder preparation. This is also a valid range for inhalation from the metered aerosol with HFA 134a propellant because the kinetic results (renal excretion, AUC and Cmax) from the HFA formulation and the conventional CFC formulation are closely comparable.

Kinetic parameters describing the distribution of ipratropium bromide were calculated from plasma concentrations after i.v. administration.

A rapid biphasic decline in plasma concentrations is observed. The volume of distribution (V_β) is 338 L ($\triangleq$ 4.6 L/kg). The drug is minimally (less then 20%) bound to plasma proteins. The ipratropium ion does not cross the blood-brain barrier, consistent with the ammonium structure of the molecule.

The half-life of the terminal elimination phase is about 1.6 hours.

The mean total clearance of the drug is determined to be 2.3 L/min. The major portion of approximately 60% of the systemic available dose is eliminated by metabolic degradation, probably in the liver. The main urinary metabolites bind poorly to the muscarinic receptor and have to be regarded as ineffective.

A portion of approximately 40% of the systemic available dose is cleared via urinary excretion corresponding to an experimental renal clearance of 0.9 L/min. A study with radiolabelled material showed that approximately 10% of orally administered ipratropium bromide was absorbed from the gastrointestinal tract and metabolised. Less than 1% of an oral dose is renally excreted as parent compound.

In excretion balance studies after intravenous administration of a radioactive dose, less than 10% of the drug-related radioactivity (including parent compound and all metabolites) is excreted via the biliary-faecal route. The dominant excretion of drug-related radioactivity occurs via the kidneys.

5.3 Preclinical safety data

Preclinical data reveal no special hazard for humans based on conventional studies of safety pharmacology, repeated dose toxicity, genotoxicity, carcinogenic potential and toxicity to reproduction.

6. PHARMACEUTICAL PARTICULARS

6.1 List of excipients

1,1,1,2 – Tetrafluoroethane (HFA-134a)

Ethanol anhydrous

Purified water

Citric acid anhydrous.

6.2 Incompatibilities

Not applicable.

6.3 Shelf life

36 months.

6.4 Special precautions for storage

Do not store above 25°C. Protect from direct sunlight, heat and frost.

The canister contains a pressurised liquid. Do not expose to temperatures higher than 50°C. Do not pierce the canister.

6.5 Nature and contents of container

17 ml stainless steel pressurised container with a 50 μl metering valve and oral adaptor. Each canister contains 200 actuations.

6.6 Instructions for use and handling

None.

7. MARKETING AUTHORISATION HOLDER

Boehringer Ingelheim Limited
Ellesfield Avenue
Bracknell
Berkshire
RG12 8YS
United Kingdom

8. MARKETING AUTHORISATION NUMBER(S)

PL 00015/0266

9. DATE OF FIRST AUTHORISATION/RENEWAL OF THE AUTHORISATION

1 March 2004

10. DATE OF REVISION OF THE TEXT

May 2004

11. LEGAL CATEGORY

POM

A9e-UK-SPC-3

Atrovent UDVs

(Boehringer Ingelheim Limited)

1. NAME OF THE MEDICINAL PRODUCT

Atrovent 250 UDVs, 1 ml

Atrovent UDVs, 2 ml

2. QUALITATIVE AND QUANTITATIVE COMPOSITION

Each single dose unit contains 0.025 % w/v ipratropium bromide i.e. 250 micrograms in 1 ml and 500 micrograms in 2 ml.

3. PHARMACEUTICAL FORM

Nebuliser solution.

4. CLINICAL PARTICULARS

4.1 Therapeutic indications

ATROVENT UDVs are indicated for treatment of reversible bronchospasm associated with chronic obstructive pulmonary disease (COPD).

ATROVENT UDVs are indicated, when used concomitantly with inhaled beta$_2$-agonists, for treatment of reversible airways obstruction as in acute and chronic asthma.

4.2 Posology and method of administration

The dosage should be adapted to the individual needs of the patient. In children aged 12 years and under, only ATROVENT 250 UDVs, 1 ml should be used. The following doses are recommended:

Adults (including the elderly) and children over 12 years of age:

250 - 500 micrograms (i.e. one vial of 250 micrograms in 1 ml or 1 vial of 500 micrograms in 2 ml) 3 to 4 times daily.

For treatment of acute bronchospasm, 500 micrograms.

Repeated doses can be administered until the patient is stable. The time interval between the doses may be determined by the physician.

It is advisable not to exceed the recommended daily dose during either acute or maintenance treatment. Daily doses exceeding 2 mg in adults and children over 12 years of age should only be given under medical supervision.

Children 6 - 12 years of age:

250 micrograms (i.e. one vial of 250 micrograms in 1ml) up to a total daily dose of 1mg (4 vials).

The time interval between doses may be determined by the physician.

Children 0 – 5 years of age (for treatment of acute asthma only):

125 – 250 micrograms (i.e. half to one vial of 250 micrograms in 1 ml) up to a total daily dose of 1 mg (4 vials).

Ipratropium bromide should be administered no more frequently than 6 hourly in children under 5 years of age.

For acute bronchospasm, repeated doses may be administered until the patient is stable.

If therapy does not produce a significant improvement or if the patient's condition gets worse, medical advice must be sought. In the case of acute or rapidly worsening dyspnoea (difficulty in breathing) a doctor should be consulted immediately.

ATROVENT UDVs may be combined with a short-acting beta$_2$-agonist in the same nebuliser chamber, for simultaneous administration where co-administration is required. The solution should be used as soon as possible after mixing and any unused solution should be discarded.

ATROVENT UDVs can be administered using a range of commercially available nebulising devices. The dose of nebuliser solution may need to be diluted in order to obtain a final volume suitable for the particular nebuliser being used (usually 2 – 4 ml); if dilution is necessary use only sterile sodium chloride 0.9% solution.

ATROVENT UDVs and disodium cromoglycate inhalation solutions that contain the preservative benzalkonium chloride should not be administered simultaneously in the same nebuliser as precipitation may occur.

Administration

The unit dose vials are intended only for inhalation with suitable nebulising devices and should not be taken orally or administered parenterally.

1. Get your nebuliser ready by following the manufacturer's instructions and the advice of your doctor.

2. Carefully separate a new dose unit from the strip. NEVER use one which has been opened already.

3. Open by simply twisting off the top, always taking care to hold it in an upright position.

4. Unless otherwise instructed by your doctor, squeeze all the contents into the nebuliser chamber. If you have also been prescribed a short-acting beta$_2$-agonist nebuliser solution, the solutions can be combined in the same nebuliser chamber. If dilution is necessary this should be carried out using ONLY sterile sodium chloride 0.9% solution and as instructed by your doctor.

5. Use your nebuliser as directed by your doctor.

6. After you have finished, throw away any leftover solution or partially used vials. Follow the manufacturer's instructions for cleaning your nebuliser. It is important that your nebuliser is kept clean.

4.3 Contraindications

Known hypersensitivity to atropine or its derivatives, or to any other component of the product.

4.4 Special warnings and special precautions for use

Use of the nebuliser solution should be subject to close medical supervision during initial dosing.

Caution is advocated in the use of anticholinergic agents in patients with narrow-angle glaucoma, or with prostatic hyperplasia or bladder-outflow obstruction.

As patients with cystic fibrosis may be prone to gastro-intestinal motility disturbances, ATROVENT, as with other anticholinergics, should be used with caution in these patients.

Immediate hypersensitivity reactions following the use of ATROVENT have been demonstrated by rare cases of urticaria, angioedema, rash, bronchospasm, oropharyngeal oedema and anaphylaxis.

There have been isolated reports of ocular complications (i.e. mydriasis, increased intra-ocular pressure, narrow-angle glaucoma, eye pain) when aerosolised ipratropium bromide, either alone or in combination with an adrenergic beta$_2$-agonist, has come into contact with the eyes during nebuliser therapy.

Eye pain or discomfort, blurred vision, visual halos or coloured images in association with red eyes from conjunctival congestion and corneal oedema may be signs of acute narrow-angle glaucoma. Should any combination of these symptoms develop, treatment with miotic drops should be initiated and specialist advice sought immediately.

Patients must be instructed in the correct administration of ATROVENT UDVs. Care must be taken not to allow the solution or mist to enter the eyes. It is recommended that the nebulised solution is administered via a mouthpiece. If this is not available and a nebuliser mask is used, it must fit properly. Patients who may be predisposed to glaucoma should be warned specifically to protect their eyes.

4.5 Interaction with other medicinal products and other forms of Interaction

There is evidence that the administration of ATROVENT with beta-adrenergic drugs and xanthine preparations may produce an additive bronchodilatory effect.

The risk of acute glaucoma in patients with a history of narrow-angle glaucoma (see Special Warnings and Precautions for Use) may be increased when nebulised ipratropium bromide and beta$_2$-agonists are administered simultaneously.

4.6 Pregnancy and lactation

The safety of ATROVENT during human pregnancy has not been established. The benefits of using ATROVENT during a confirmed or suspected pregnancy must be weighed against the possible hazards to the unborn child. Preclinical studies have shown no embryotoxic or teratogenic effects following inhalation or intranasal application at doses considerably higher than those recommended in man.

It is not known whether ipratropium bromide is excreted into breast milk. It is unlikely that ipratropium bromide would reach the infant to an important extent, however caution should be exercised when ATROVENT is administered to nursing mothers.

4.7 Effects on ability to drive and use machines

None stated.

4.8 Undesirable effects

The most frequent non-respiratory adverse reactions reported in clinical trials with ATROVENT were headache, nausea (with or without vomiting) and dryness of the mouth.

The following side effects have been observed with ATROVENT: tachycardia, palpitations, supraventricular tachycardia and atrial fibrillation, visual accommodation disturbances, gastro-intestinal motility disturbances and urinary retention. These side effects have been rare and reversible. The risk of urinary retention may be increased in patients with pre-existing urinary outflow tract obstruction.

Ocular side effects have been reported (see: Special Warnings and Precautions for Use).

As with other inhaled bronchodilator therapy, cough, local irritation and inhalation induced bronchoconstriction may occur.

Allergic-type reactions such as skin rash, angioedema of the tongue, lips and face, urticaria, laryngospasm and anaphylactic reactions have been reported.

4.9 Overdose

No symptoms specific to overdosage have been encountered. In view of the wide therapeutic window and topical administration of ATROVENT, no serious anticholinergic symptoms are to be expected. As with other anticholinergics, dry mouth, visual accommodation disturbances and tachycardia would be the expected symptoms and signs of overdose.

5. PHARMACOLOGICAL PROPERTIES

5.1 Pharmacodynamic properties

ATROVENT is a quaternary ammonium compound with anticholinergic (parasympatholytic) properties. In preclinical studies, it appears to inhibit vagally mediated reflexes by antagonising the action of acetylcholine, the transmitter agent released from the vagus nerve. Anticholinergics prevent the increase in intracellular concentration of cyclic guanosine monophosphate (cyclic GMP) caused by interaction of acetylcholine with the muscarinic receptor on bronchial smooth muscle.

The bronchodilation following inhalation of ATROVENT is induced by local drug concentrations sufficient for anticholinergic efficacy at the bronchial smooth muscle and not by systemic drug concentrations.

In clinical trials using metered dose inhalers in patients with reversible bronchospasm associated with chronic obstructive pulmonary disease significant improvements in pulmonary function (FEV_1 increases of 15% or more) occurred within 15 minutes, reached a peak in 1-2 hours, and persisted for approximately 4 hours.

Preclinical and clinical evidence suggest no deleterious effect of ATROVENT on airway mucous secretion, mucociliary clearance or gas exchange.

The bronchodilator effect of ATROVENT in the treatment of acute bronchospasm associated with asthma has been shown in studies in adults and children over 6 years of age. In most of these studies ATROVENT was administered in combination with an inhaled beta$_2$-agonist.

5.2 Pharmacokinetic properties

The therapeutic effect of ATROVENT is produced by a local action in the airways. Therefore time courses of bronchodilation and systemic pharmacokinetics do not run in parallel.

Following inhalation, dose portions from 10 to 30%, depending on the formulation, device and inhalation technique, are generally deposited in the lungs. The major part of the dose is swallowed and passes through the gastro-intestinal tract.

Due to the negligible gastro-intestinal absorption of ipratropium bromide the bioavailability of the swallowed dose portion is only approximately 2%. This fraction of the dose does not make a relevant contribution to the plasma concentrations of the active ingredient. The portion of the dose deposited in the lungs reaches the circulation rapidly (within minutes).

Limited data on total systemic bioavailability (pulmonary and gastro-intestinal portions), based on renal excretion (0 – 24 hours) of ipratropium bromide, suggests a range of 7 – 28% when delivery is via a nebuliser or a MDI product. It is assumed that this is also a valid range for inhalation from the powder preparation.

Kinetic parameters describing the distribution of ipratropium bromide were calculated from plasma concentrations after i.v. administration.

A rapid biphasic decline in plasma concentrations is observed. The volume of distribution (V_β) is 338 L (≡ 4.6 L/kg). The drug is minimally (less then 20%) bound to plasma proteins. The ipratropium ion does not cross the blood-brain barrier, consistent with the ammonium structure of the molecule.

The half-life of the terminal elimination phase is about 1.6 hours.

The mean total clearance of the drug is determined to be 2.3 L/min. The major portion of approximately 60% of the systemic available dose is eliminated by metabolic degradation, probably in the liver. The main urinary metabolites bind poorly to the muscarinic receptor and have to be regarded as ineffective.

A portion of approximately 40% of the systemic available dose is cleared via urinary excretion corresponding to an experimental renal clearance of 0.9 L/min. A study with radiolabelled material showed that approximately 10% of orally administered ipratropium bromide was absorbed from the gastro-intestinal tract and metabolised. Less than

1% of an oral dose is renally excreted as parent compound.

In excretion balance studies after intravenous administration of a radioactive dose, less than 10% of the drug-related radioactivity (including parent compound and all metabolites) is excreted via the biliary-faecal route. The dominant excretion of drug-related radioactivity occurs via the kidneys.

5.3 Preclinical safety data
There are no pre-clinical data of relevance to the prescriber which are additional to that already included in other sections of the SPC.

6. PHARMACEUTICAL PARTICULARS

6.1 List of excipients
Sodium Chloride

1N Hydrochloric Acid

Purified Water

6.2 Incompatibilities
None stated.

6.3 Shelf life
36 months (unopened).

As the product contains no preservative, a fresh vial should be used for each dose and the vial should be opened immediately before administration. Any solution left in the vial should be discarded.

6.4 Special precautions for storage
Do not store above 25°C. Protect from direct light.

6.5 Nature and contents of container
Polyethylene unit dose vials packed in cartons. Each single dose unit contains either 1 ml or 2 ml of solution in pack sizes of 10, 20, 30, 50, 60, 80, 100, 120, 150, 200, 300, 500 and 1000.

Pack sizes of 20 and 60 are currently marketed.

6.6 Instructions for use and handling
None.

7. MARKETING AUTHORISATION HOLDER
Boehringer Ingelheim Limited

Ellesfield Avenue

Bracknell

Berkshire

RG12 8YS

8. MARKETING AUTHORISATION NUMBER(S)
PL 0015/0108

9. DATE OF FIRST AUTHORISATION/RENEWAL OF THE AUTHORISATION
27 August 1986/17 January 1997

10. DATE OF REVISION OF THE TEXT
June 2003

11. Legal Category
Prescription Only Medicine

A9d/UK/SPC/13

Audax Ear Drops

(SSL International plc)

1. NAME OF THE MEDICINAL PRODUCT
Audax Ear Drops.

2. QUALITATIVE AND QUANTITATIVE COMPOSITION
Choline Salicylate Solution BP 43.22% w/v; Glycerol BP 12.62% w/v.

3. PHARMACEUTICAL FORM
Solution for topical administration to the ear.

4. CLINICAL PARTICULARS

4.1 Therapeutic indications
For the symptomatic relief of ear pain in acute and chronic otitis media and externa. Patients with ear pain should always seek medical advice. Softening of ear wax as an aid to ear wax removal.

4.2 Posology and method of administration
Adults, the elderly and children: *For pain relief:* With the head tilted to one side, the external ear canal is filled completely with Audax Ear Drops using the dropper provided. The ear should be plugged with cotton wool soaked with the ear drops. A wick may be inserted, if preferred, using the ear drops to keep it moist. Audax Ear Drops should be instilled every three to four hours.

For softening of ear wax: Apply as described above, twice daily, for four days.

4.3 Contraindications
Not to be used in children under one year of age without medical advice being sought. Salicylate sensitivity; perforated ear drum. Hypersensitivity to any of the ingredients in the medicine.

4.4 Special warnings and special precautions for use
None stated.

4.5 Interaction with other medicinal products and other forms of Interaction
None stated.

4.6 Pregnancy and lactation
There is no known hazard with the use of this product during pregnancy and lactation.

4.7 Effects on ability to drive and use machines
None stated.

4.8 Undesirable effects
None stated.

4.9 Overdose
Each bottle of Audax Ear Drops contains 1.6g of choline salicylate, equivalent to 1.2g of aspirin. Accidental or deliberate ingestion of the contents of a bottle of Audax Ear Drops is therefore only of concern in small infants. In such cases, signs of intoxication may include dizziness, tinnitus, sweating, vomiting, confusion and hyperventilation. Gross overdosage may lead to central nervous system depression. Management should include, as appropriate, induced vomiting, correction of fluid and electrolyte balance and measurement of plasma salicylate levels. At concentrations in excess of 300mg/litre measures such as forced alkaline diuresis and haemodialysis to enhance clearance may be appropriate.

5. PHARMACOLOGICAL PROPERTIES

5.1 Pharmacodynamic properties
Choline salicylate has actions similar to those of aspirin, that is, analgesic, anti-inflammatory and antipyretic actions considered to be due to inhibition of the biosynthesis of prostaglandins. Glycerol softens ear wax due to its water-retaining and emollient properties.

5.2 Pharmacokinetic properties
Not applicable as Audax Ear Drops are applied topically.

5.3 Preclinical safety data
None stated.

6. PHARMACEUTICAL PARTICULARS

6.1 List of excipients
Ethylene Oxide Polyoxypropylene Glycol; Chlorbutol (Hemihydrate) BP; Hydrochloric Acid; Propylene Glycol BP.

6.2 Incompatibilities
None stated.

6.3 Shelf life
36 months unopened.

6.4 Special precautions for storage
Store at or below 20°C.

6.5 Nature and contents of container
Cartoned amber glass bottle with screw cap and integral dropper containing 10ml of product.

6.6 Instructions for use and handling
None stated.

7. MARKETING AUTHORISATION HOLDER
Seton Products Limited, Tubiton House, Oldham, OL1 3HS.

8. MARKETING AUTHORISATION NUMBER(S)
PL 11314/0039.

9. DATE OF FIRST AUTHORISATION/RENEWAL OF THE AUTHORISATION
25th July 1995 / 26th March 2001.

10. DATE OF REVISION OF THE TEXT
March 2001.

Augmentin Intravenous

(GlaxoSmithKline UK)

1. NAME OF THE MEDICINAL PRODUCT
Augmentin® Intravenous

2. QUALITATIVE AND QUANTITATIVE COMPOSITION
Vials of sterile powder providing co-amoxiclav 500/100 (600 mg Augmentin) or co-amoxiclav 1000/200 (1.2 g Augmentin). For reconstitution as an intravenous injection or infusion.

The amoxicillin is present as amoxicillin sodium and the clavulanic acid is present as potassium clavulanate.

3. PHARMACEUTICAL FORM
Powder for solution for injection or infusion.

4. CLINICAL PARTICULARS

4.1 Therapeutic indications
Augmentin is an antibiotic agent with a notably broad spectrum of activity against the commonly occurring bacterial pathogens in general practice and hospital. The β-lactamase inhibitory action of clavulanate extends the spectrum of amoxicillin to embrace a wider range of organisms, including many resistant to other β-lactam antibiotics.

Augmentin Intravenous is indicated for short-term treatment of bacterial infections at the following sites when amoxicillin-resistant β-lactamase-producing strains are suspected as the cause. In other situations, amoxicillin alone should be considered.

- *Upper Respiratory Tract Infections (including ENT)* in particular sinusitis, otitis media, recurrent tonsillitis. These infections are often caused by *Streptococcus pneumoniae, Haemophilus influenzae**, *Moraxella catarrhalis** and *Streptococcus pyogenes.*

- *Lower Respiratory Tract Infections* in particular acute exacerbations of chronic bronchitis (especially if considered severe), bronchopneumonia. These infections are often caused by *Streptococcus pneumoniae, Haemophilus influenzae** and *Moraxella catarrhalis**.

- *Genito-urinary Tract and Abdominal Infections* in particular cystitis (especially when recurrent or complicated - excluding prostatitis), septic abortion, pelvic or puerperal sepsis and intra-abdominal sepsis. These infections are often caused by *Enterobacteriaceae** (mainly *Escherichia coli**), *Staphylococcus saprophyticus, Enterococcus* species.*

- *Skin and Soft Tissue Infections* in particular cellulitis, animal bites and severe dental abscess with spreading cellulitis. These infections are often caused by *Staphylococcus aureus**, *Streptococcus pyogenes* and *Bacteroides* species*.

- *Prophylaxis of wound infection associated with surgical procedures* in particular gastrointestinal, pelvic, major head and neck surgery and after limb amputation for infection.

- A comprehensive list of sensitive organisms is provided in Section 5.

* Some members of these species of bacteria produce β-lactamase, rendering them insensitive to amoxicillin alone.

Mixed infections caused by amoxicillin-susceptible organisms in conjunction with Augmentin-susceptible β-lactamase-producing organisms may be treated withAugmentin. These infections should not require the addition of another antibiotic resistant to β-lactamases.

4.2 Posology and method of administration
Dosages for the treatment of infection

Adults and children over 12 years: Usually 1.2 g eight hourly. In more serious infections, increase frequency to six-hourly intervals.

Children 3 months-12 years: Usually 30 mg/kg * Augmentin eight hourly. In more serious infections, increase frequency to six-hourly intervals.

Children 0-3 months: 30 mg/kg* Augmentin every 12 hours in premature infants and in full-term infants during the perinatal period, increasing to eight hours thereafter.

*Each 30 mg Augmentin provides co-amoxiclav 25/5.

Adult dosage for surgical prophylaxis

The usual dose is 1.2 g Augmentin Intravenous given at the induction of anaesthesia. Operations where there is a high risk of infection, e.g. colorectal surgery, may require three, and up to four, doses of 1.2 g Augmentin Intravenous in a 24-hour period. These doses are usually given at 0, 8, 16 (and 24) hours. This regimen can be continued for several days if the procedure has a significantly increased risk of infection.

Clear clinical signs of infection at operation will require a normal course of intravenous or oral Augmentin therapy post-operatively.

Dosage in renal impairment

Adults

Mild impairment (creatinine clearance >30 ml/min)	Moderate impairment (creatinine clearance 10-30 ml/min)	Severe impairment (creatinine clearance <10 ml/min)
No change in dosage.	1.2 g IV stat., followed by 600 mg IV 12 hourly.	1.2 g IV stat., followed by 600 mg IV 24 hourly. Dialysis decreases serum concentrations of Augmentin and an additional 600 mg IV dose may need to be given during dialysis and at the end of dialysis.

Children

Similar reductions in dosage should be made for children.

Dosage in hepatic impairment

Dose with caution; monitor hepatic function at regular intervals.

There are, as yet, insufficient data on which to base a dosage recommendation.

Each 1.2 g vial of Augmentin contains 1.0 mmol of potassium and 2.7 mmol of sodium (approx).

Administration

Augmentin Intravenous may be administered either by intravenous injection or by intermittent infusion (see Section 6.6). It is not suitable for intramuscular administration.

Duration of therapy should be appropriate to the indication and should not exceed 14 days without review.

4.3 Contraindications

Penicillin hypersensitivity. Attention should be paid to possible cross-sensitivity with other β-lactam antibiotics, e.g. cephalosporins.

A previous history of Augmentin- or penicillin-associated jaundice/hepatic dysfunction.

4.4 Special warnings and special precautions for use

Changes in liver function tests have been observed in some patients receiving Augmentin. The clinical significance of these changes is uncertain but Augmentin should be used with caution in patients with evidence of hepatic dysfunction.

Cholestatic jaundice, which may be severe, but is usually reversible, has been reported rarely. Signs and symptoms may not become apparent for several weeks after treatment has ceased.

In patients with renal impairment, dosage should be adjusted according to the degree of impairment (see Section 4.2).

If the parenteral administration of high doses is necessary, the sodium content must be taken into account in patients on a sodium restricted diet.

In patients with reduced urine output crystalluria has been observed very rarely, predominantly with parenteral therapy. During administration of high doses of amoxicillin it is advisable to maintain adequate fluid intake and urinary output in order to reduce the possibility of amoxicillin crystalluria (see Section 4.9 Overdose). Amoxicillin has been reported to precipitate in bladder catheters after intravenous administration of large doses. A regular check of patency should be maintained.

Serious and occasionally fatal hypersensitivity (anaphylactoid) reactions have been reported in patients on penicillin therapy. These reactions are more likely to occur in individuals with a history of penicillin hypersensitivity (see Section 4.3).

Erythematous rashes have been associated with glandular fever in patients receiving amoxicillin.

Prolonged use may also occasionally result in overgrowth of non-susceptible organisms.

4.5 Interaction with other medicinal products and other forms of Interaction

Prolongation of bleeding time and prothrombin time have been reported in some patients receiving Augmentin. Augmentin should be used with care in patients on anti-coagulation therapy.

In common with other broad-spectrum antibiotics, Augmentin may reduce the efficacy of oral contraceptives and patients should be warned accordingly.

Concomitant use of allopurinol during treatment with amoxicillin can increase the likelihood of allergic skin reactions. There are no data on the concomitant use of Augmentin and allopurinol.

4.6 Pregnancy and lactation

Reproduction studies in animals (mice and rats) with orally and parenterally administered Augmentin have shown no teratogenic effects. In a single study in women with preterm, premature rupture of the foetal membrane (pPROM), it was reported that prophylactic treatment with Augmentin may be associated with an increased risk of necrotising enterocolitis in neonates. As with all medicines, use should be avoided in pregnancy, especially during the first trimester, unless considered essential by the physician.

Augmentin may be administered during the period of lactation. With the exception of the risk of sensitisation, associated with the excretion of trace quantities in breast milk, there are no known detrimental effects for the breast-fed infant.

4.7 Effects on ability to drive and use machines

None known.

4.8 Undesirable effects

Side effects are uncommon and mainly of a mild and transitory nature.

Gastrointestinal reactions:

Diarrhoea, indigestion, nausea, vomiting, and mucocutaneous candidiasis have been reported. Antibiotic-associated colitis (including pseudomembranous colitis and haemorrhagic colitis) has been reported rarely. Nausea, although uncommon, is more often associated with higher oral dosages. If gastrointestinal side effects occur with oral therapy they may be reduced by taking Augmentin at the start of meals.

Superficial tooth discolouration has been reported rarely, mostly with the suspension. It can usually be removed by brushing.

Renal and urinary tract disorders:

Crystalluria has been reported very rarely (See Section 4.9 Overdose).

Genito-urinary effects:

Vaginal itching, soreness and discharge may occur.

Hepatic effects:

Moderate and asymptomatic rises in AST and/or ALT and alkaline phosphatases have been reported occasionally. Hepatitis and cholestatic jaundice have been reported rarely. These hepatic reactions have been reported more commonly with Augmentin than with other penicillins.

After Augmentin hepatic reactions have been reported more frequently in males and elderly patients, particularly those over 65 years. The risk increases with duration of treatment longer than 14 days. These reactions have been very rarely reported in children.

Signs and symptoms usually occur during or shortly after treatment but in some cases may not occur until several weeks after treatment has ended. Hepatic reactions are usually reversible but they may be severe and, very rarely, deaths have been reported.

Hypersensitivity reactions:

Urticarial and erythematous skin rashes sometimes occur. Rarely erythema multiforme, Stevens-Johnson syndrome, toxic epidermal necrolysis, bullous exfoliative dermatitis, acute generalised exanthematous pustulosis (AGEP), serum sickness-like syndrome and hypersensitivity vasculitis have been reported. Treatment should be discontinued if one of these disorders occurs. In common with other β-lactam antibiotics angioedema and anaphylaxis have been reported. Interstitial nephritis can occur rarely.

Haematological effects:

As with other β-lactams transient leucopenia (including neutropenia and agranulocytosis), thrombocytopenia and haemolytic anaemia have been reported rarely. Prolongation of bleeding time and prothrombin time has also been reported rarely (see Section 4.5).

CNS effects:

CNS effects have been seen very rarely. These include reversible hyperactivity, dizziness, headache and convulsions. Convulsions may occur with impaired renal function or in those receiving high doses.

Local:

Thrombophlebitis at the site of injection has been reported occasionally.

4.9 Overdose

Gastrointestinal symptoms and disturbance of the fluid and electrolyte balances may be evident. They may be treated symptomatically with attention to the water electrolyte balance. Augmentin may be removed from the circulation by haemodialysis.

Amoxicillin crystalluria, in some cases leading to renal failure, has been observed (see Section 4.4 Special Warnings and Special Precautions for Use)

5. PHARMACOLOGICAL PROPERTIES

5.1 Pharmacodynamic properties

Resistance to many antibiotics is caused by bacterial enzymes which destroy the antibiotic before it can act on the pathogen. The clavulanate in Augmentin anticipates this defence mechanism by blocking the β-lactamase enzymes, thus rendering the organisms sensitive to amoxicillin's rapid bactericidal effect at concentrations readily attainable in the body.

Clavulanate by itself has little antibacterial activity; however, in association with amoxicillin as Augmentin, it produces an antibiotic agent of broad spectrum with wide application in hospital and general practice.

Augmentin is bactericidal to a wide range of organisms including:

Gram-positive

Aerobes: *Enterococcus faecalis**, *Enterococcus faecium**, *Streptococcus pneumoniae, Streptococcus pyogenes, Streptococcus viridans, Staphylococcus aureus**, Coagulase negative *staphylococci** (including *Staphylococcus epidermidis**), *Corynebacterium* species, *Bacillus anthracis**, *Listeria monocytogenes*.

Anaerobes: *Clostridium* species, *Peptococcus* species, *Peptostreptococcus*.

Gram-negative

Aerobes: *Haemophilus influenzae**, *Moraxella catarrhalis** *(Branhamella catarrhalis), Escherichia coli**, *Proteus mirabilis**, *Proteus vulgaris**, *Klebsiella* species*, *Salmonella* species*, *Shigella* species*, *Bordetella pertussis, Brucella* species, *Neisseria gonorrhoeae**, *Neisseria meningitidis**, *Vibrio cholerae, Pasteurella multocida*.

Anaerobes: *Bacteroides* species* including *B. fragilis*.

* Some members of these species of bacteria produce β-lactamase, rendering them insensitive to amoxicillin alone.

5.2 Pharmacokinetic properties

The pharmacokinetics of the two components of Augmentin are closely matched. Both clavulanate and amoxicillin have low levels of serum binding; about 70% remains free in the serum.

Doubling the dosage of Augmentin approximately doubles the serum levels achieved.

5.3 Preclinical safety data

Not relevant

6. PHARMACEUTICAL PARTICULARS

6.1 List of excipients

None

6.2 Incompatibilities

Augmentin Intravenous should not be mixed with blood products, other proteinaceous fluids such as protein hydrolysates or with intravenous lipid emulsions.

If Augmentin is prescribed concurrently with an aminoglycoside, the antibiotics should not be mixed in the syringe, intravenous fluid container or giving set because loss of activity of the aminoglycoside can occur under these conditions.

6.3 Shelf life

Two years

6.4 Special precautions for storage

Augmentin vials should be stored in a dry place. Do not store above 25°C.

6.5 Nature and contents of container

For 1.2g and 600mg:

Clear glass vials (Ph.Eur. Type I) fitted with butyl rubber bungs and aluminium overseals.

or (for 1.2g only):

Clear glass vials (Ph. Eur. Type III, moulded) with butyl rubber bungs and aluminium flip-top lids.

6.6 Instructions for use and handling

600 mg vial: To reconstitute dissolve in 10 ml Water for Injections BP.

(Final volume 10.5 ml.)

1.2 g vial: To reconstitute dissolve in 20 ml Water for Injections BP.

(Final volume 20.9 ml.)

Augmentin Intravenous should be given by slow intravenous injection over a period of three to four minutes and used within 20 minutes of reconstitution. It may be injected directly into a vein or via a drip tube.

Alternatively, Augmentin Intravenous may be infused in Water for Injections BP or Sodium Chloride Intravenous Injection BP (0.9% w/v). Add, without delay, 600 mg reconstituted solution to 50 ml infusion fluid or 1.2 g reconstituted solution to 100 ml infusion fluid (e.g. using a minibag or in-line burette). Infuse over 30-40 minutes and complete within four hours of reconstitution. For other appropriate infusion fluids, see Package Enclosure Leaflet.

Any residual antibiotic solutions should be discarded.

Augmentin Intravenous is less stable in infusions containing glucose, dextran or bicarbonate. Reconstituted solution should, therefore, not be added to such infusions but may be injected into the drip tubing over a period of three to four minutes.

Administrative Data

7. MARKETING AUTHORISATION HOLDER

Beecham Group plc
980 Great West Road
Brentford
Middlesex TW8 9GS

Trading as:

GlaxoSmithKline UK
Stockley Park West
Uxbridge
Middlesex UB11 1BT

8. MARKETING AUTHORISATION NUMBER(S)

PL 00038/0320

9. DATE OF FIRST AUTHORISATION/RENEWAL OF THE AUTHORISATION

2 August 2002

10. DATE OF REVISION OF THE TEXT

11 January 2005

11. Legal Status

POM

Augmentin Tablets 375mg/625mg, Dispersible Tablets 375 mg, 250/62 SF Suspension, 125/31 SF Suspension

(GlaxoSmithKline UK)

1. NAME OF THE MEDICINAL PRODUCT

Augmentin® 375 mg Tablets
Augmentin® 625 mg Tablets
Augmentin® Dispersible Tablets 375 mg
Augmentin® 250/62 SF Suspension
Augmentin® 125/31 SF Suspension

2. QUALITATIVE AND QUANTITATIVE COMPOSITION

Augmentin 375 mg Tablets: Each tablet contains co-amoxiclav 250/125.

Augmentin 625 mg Tablets: Each tablet contains co-amoxiclav 500/125.

Augmentin Dispersible Tablets 375 mg: Each tablet contains co-amoxiclav 250/125.

Augmentin 250/62 SF Suspension: When reconstituted each 5 ml contains co-amoxiclav 250/62.

Augmentin 125/31 SF Suspension: When reconstituted each 5 ml contains co-amoxiclav 125/31.

In all the above presentations the amoxicillin is present as amoxicillin trihydrate and the clavulanic acid is present as potassium clavulanate.

3. PHARMACEUTICAL FORM

Augmentin 375 mg Tablets: White, oval, film-coated tablets engraved Augmentin on one side.

Augmentin 625 mg Tablets: White, oval, film-coated tablets engraved Augmentin

Augmentin Dispersible Tablets: White round tablets engraved Augmentin.

Augmentin 250/62 SF and 125/31 SF Suspension: Dry powder for reconstitution in water, at time of dispensing, to form an oral sugar-free suspension.

4. CLINICAL PARTICULARS

4.1 Therapeutic indications

Augmentin is an antibiotic agent with a notably broad spectrum of activity against the commonly occurring bacterial pathogens in general practice and hospital. The β-lactamase inhibitory action of clavulanate extends the spectrum of amoxicillin to embrace a wider range of organisms, including many resistant to other β-lactam antibiotics.

Augmentin oral preparations are indicated for short-term treatment of bacterial infections at the following sites when amoxicillin resistant β-lactamase-producing strains are suspected as the cause. In other situations, amoxicillin alone should be considered.

- *Upper Respiratory Tract Infections (including ENT)* in particular sinusitis, otitis media, recurrent tonsillitis. These infections are often caused by *Streptococcus pneumoniae, Haemophilus influenzae*, Moraxella catarrhalis** and *Streptococcus pyogenes*.

- *Lower Respiratory Tract Infections* in particular acute exacerbations of chronic bronchitis (especially if considered severe), bronchopneumonia. These infections are often caused by *Streptococcus pneumoniae, Haemophilus influenzae** and *Moraxella catarrhalis**.

- *Genito-urinary Tract and Abdominal Infections* in particular cystitis (especially when recurrent or complicated - excluding prostatitis), septic abortion, pelvic or puerperal sepsis and intra-abdominal sepsis. These infections are often caused by *Enterobacteriaceae** (mainly *Escherichia coli*), Staphylococcus saprophyticus, Enterococcus species.**

- *Skin and Soft Tissue Infections* in particular cellulitis, animal bites and severe dental abscess with spreading cellulitis. These infections are often caused by *Staphylococcus aureus*, Streptococcus pyogenes* and *Bacteroides species**.

- A comprehensive list of sensitive organisms is provided in Section 5.

* Some members of these species of bacteria produce β-lactamase, rendering them insensitive to amoxicillin alone.

Mixed infections caused by amoxicillin-susceptible organisms in conjunction with Augmentin-susceptible β-lactamase-producing organisms may be treated with Augmentin. These infections should not require the addition of another antibiotic resistant to β-lactamases.

4.2 Posology and method of administration

Usual dosages for the treatment of infection

Adults and children over 12 years	One Augmentin 375 mg Tablet or Dispersible Tablet three times a day. In severe infections one Augmentin 625 mg Tablet three times a day. Therapy can be started parenterally and continued with an oral preparation.
Children	The usual recommended daily dosage is 25 mg/kg/day* in divided doses every eight hours. The table below presents guidance for children.

Augmentin Suspension

Under 1 year	25 mg/kg/day*, for example a 7.5 kg child would require 2 ml Augmentin 125/31 SF Suspension t.d.s.
1-6 years (10-18 kg)	5ml Augmentin 125/31 SF Suspension t.d.s.
Over 6 years (18-40 kg)	5ml Augmentin 250/62 SF Suspension t.d.s.

In more serious infections the dosage may be increased up to 50 mg/kg/day in divided doses every eight hours.

* Each 25 mg Augmentin provides co-amoxiclav 20/5.

Augmentin 375 mg and 625 mg Tablets are not recommended in children of 12 years and under.

Dosage in dental infections (e.g. dentoalveolar abscess)

Adults and children over 12 years: one Augmentin Tablet 375 mg three times a day for five days.

Dosage in renal impairment

Adults:

Mild impairment	Moderate impairment	Severe impairment
(Creatinine clear-ance >30 ml/min)	(Creatinine clearance 10-30 ml/min)	(Creatinine clearance <10 ml/min)
No change in dosage.	One 375 mg tablet or one 625 mg tablet 12 hourly.	Not more than one 375 mg tablet 12 hourly; 625 mg tablets are not recommended.

Children:

Similar reductions in dosage should be made for children.

Dosage in hepatic impairment

Dose with caution; monitor hepatic function at regular intervals.

There are, as yet, insufficient data on which to base a dosage recommendation.

Each 375 mg tablet of Augmentin contains 0.63 mmol (25 mg) of potassium.

Administration

Oral: Tablets, dispersible tablets or suspensions. To minimise potential gastrointestinal intolerance, administer at the start of a meal. The absorption of Augmentin is optimised when taken at the start of a meal. Dispersible tablets should be stirred into a little water before taking.

Duration of therapy should be appropriate to the indication and should not exceed 14 days without review.

4.3 Contraindications

Penicillin hypersensitivity. Attention should be paid to possible cross-sensitivity with other β-lactam antibiotics, e.g. cephalosporins.

A previous history of Augmentin- or penicillin-associated jaundice/hepatic dysfunction.

4.4 Special warnings and special precautions for use

Changes in liver function tests have been observed in some patients receiving Augmentin. The clinical significance of these changes is uncertain but Augmentin should be used with caution in patients with evidence of hepatic dysfunction.

Cholestatic jaundice, which may be severe, but is usually reversible, has been reported rarely. Signs and symptoms may not become apparent for several weeks after treatment has ceased.

In patients with renal impairment, dosage should be adjusted according to the degree of impairment (see Section 4.2).

In patients with reduced urine output, crystalluria has been observed very rarely, predominately with parenteral therapy. During the administration of high doses of amoxicillin, it is advisable to maintain adequate fluid intake and urinary output in order to reduce the possibility of amoxicillin crystalluria.

Serious and occasionally fatal hypersensitivity (anaphylactoid) reactions have been reported in patients on penicillin therapy. These reactions are more likely to occur in individuals with a history of penicillin hypersensitivity (see Section 4.3).

Erythematous rashes have been associated with glandular fever in patients receiving amoxicillin.

Prolonged use may also occasionally result in overgrowth of non-susceptible organisms.

Augmentin Suspensions contain 12.5 mg aspartame per 5 ml dose and therefore care should be taken in phenylketonuria.

4.5 Interaction with other medicinal products and other forms of Interaction

Prolongation of bleeding time and prothrombin time have been reported in some patients receiving Augmentin. Augmentin should be used with care in patients on anti-coagulation therapy.

In common with other broad-spectrum antibiotics, Augmentin may reduce the efficacy of oral contraceptives and patients should be warned accordingly.

Concomitant use of allopurinol during treatment with amoxicillin can increase the likelihood of allergic skin reactions. There are no data on the concomitant use of Augmentin and allopurinol.

4.6 Pregnancy and lactation

Reproduction studies in animals (mice and rats) with orally and parenterally administered Augmentin have shown no teratogenic effects. In a single study in women with preterm, premature rupture of the foetal membrane (pPROM), it was reported that prophylactic treatment with Augmentin may be associated with an increased risk of necrotising enterocolitis in neonates. As with all medicines, use should be avoided in pregnancy, especially during the first trimester, unless considered essential by the physician.

Augmentin may be administered during the period of lactation. With the exception of the risk of sensitisation, associated with the excretion of trace quantities in breast milk, there are no known detrimental effects for the breast-fed infant.

4.7 Effects on ability to drive and use machines

None known.

4.8 Undesirable effects

Side effects are uncommon and mainly of a mild and transitory nature.

Gastrointestinal reactions:

Diarrhoea, indigestion, nausea, vomiting, and mucocutaneous candidiasis have been reported. Antibiotic-associated colitis (including pseudomembranous colitis and haemorrhagic colitis) has been reported rarely. Nausea, although uncommon, is more often associated with higher oral dosages. If gastrointestinal side effects occur with oral therapy they may be reduced by taking Augmentin at the start of meals.

As with other antibiotics the incidence of gastrointestinal side effects may be raised in children under two years. In clinical trials, however, only 4% of children under two years were withdrawn from treatment.

Superficial tooth discolouration has been reported rarely, mostly with the suspension. It can usually be removed by brushing.

Renal and urinary tract disorders:

Crystalluria has been reported very rarely.

Genito-urinary effects:

Vaginal itching, soreness and discharge may occur.

Hepatic effects:

Moderate and asymptomatic rises in AST and/or ALT and alkaline phosphatases have been reported occasionally. Hepatitis and cholestatic jaundice have been reported rarely. These hepatic reactions have been reported more commonly with Augmentin than with other penicillins.

After Augmentin hepatic reactions have been reported more frequently in males and elderly patients, particularly those over 65 years. The risk increases with duration of treatment longer than 14 days. These reactions have been very rarely reported in children.

Signs and symptoms usually occur during or shortly after treatment but in some cases may not occur until several weeks after treatment has ended. Hepatic reactions are usually reversible but they may be severe and, very rarely, deaths have been reported.

Hypersensitivity reactions:

Urticarial and erythematous skin rashes sometimes occur. Rarely erythema multiforme, Stevens-Johnson syndrome, toxic epidermal necrolysis, bullous exfoliative dermatitis, acute generalised exanthematous pustulosis (AGEP), serum sickness-like syndrome and hypersensitivity vasculitis have been reported. Treatment should be discontinued if one of these disorders occurs. In common with other β-lactam antibiotics angioedema and anaphylaxis have been reported. Interstitial nephritis can occur rarely.

Haematological effects:

As with other β-lactams transient leucopenia (including neutropenia and agranulocytosis), thrombocytopenia and haemolytic anaemia have been reported rarely. Prolongation of bleeding time and prothrombin time has also been reported rarely (see Section 4.5).

CNS effects:

CNS effects have been seen very rarely. These include reversible hyperactivity, dizziness, headache and convulsions. Convulsions may occur with impaired renal function or in those receiving high doses.

4.9 Overdose

Gastrointestinal symptoms and disturbance of the fluid and electrolyte balances may be evident. They may be treated symptomatically with attention to the water electrolyte balance. Augmentin may be removed from the circulation by haemodialysis.

Amoxicillin crystalluria has been observed (see Section 4.4).

5. PHARMACOLOGICAL PROPERTIES

5.1 Pharmacodynamic properties

Resistance to many antibiotics is caused by bacterial enzymes which destroy the antibiotic before it can act on the pathogen. The clavulanate in Augmentin anticipates this defence mechanism by blocking the β-lactamase enzymes, thus rendering the organisms sensitive to amoxicillin's rapid bactericidal effect at concentrations readily attainable in the body.

Clavulanate by itself has little antibacterial activity; however, in association with amoxicillin as Augmentin, it produces an antibiotic agent of broad spectrum with wide application in hospital and general practice.

Augmentin is bactericidal to a wide range of organisms including:

Gram-positive

Aerobes: *Enterococcus faecalis**, *Enterococcus faecium**, *Streptococcus pneumoniae, Streptococcus pyogenes, Streptococcus viridans, Staphylococcus aureus**, Coagulase negative *staphylococci** (including *Staphylococcus epidermidis**), *Corynebacterium* species, *Bacillus anthracis**, *Listeria monocytogenes.*

Anaerobes: *Clostridium* species, *Peptococcus* species, *Peptostreptococcus.*

Gram-negative

Aerobes: *Haemophilus influenzae**, *Moraxella catarrhalis** (*Branhamella catarrhalis*), *Escherichia coli**, *Proteus mirabilis**, *Proteus vulgaris**, *Klebsiella* species*, *Salmonella* species*, *Shigella* species*, *Bordetella pertussis, Brucella* species, *Neisseria gonorrhoeae**, *Neisseria meningitidis**, *Vibrio cholerae, Pasteurella multocida.*

Anaerobes: *Bacteroides* species* including *B. fragilis*.

* Some members of these species of bacteria produce beta-lactamase, rendering them insensitive to amoxicillin alone.

5.2 Pharmacokinetic properties

The pharmacokinetics of the two components of Augmentin are closely matched. Peak serum levels of both occur about one hour after oral administration. Absorption of Augmentin is optimised at the start of a meal. Both clavulanate and amoxicillin have low levels of serum binding; about 70% remains free in the serum.

Doubling the dosage of Augmentin approximately doubles the serum levels achieved.

5.3 Preclinical safety data

Not relevant

6. PHARMACEUTICAL PARTICULARS

6.1 List of excipients

Augmentin 375 mg and 625 mg tablets:

Each tablet contains magnesium stearate, sodium starch glycollate, colloidal silica, microcrystalline cellulose, titanium dioxide (E171), hydroxypropyl methylcellulose, polyethylene glycol and silicone oil.

Augmentin Dispersible Tablets 375 Mg

Each tablet contains polyvinylpyrrolidone (cross-linked), silica gel, saccharin sodium, pineapple, strawberry and blood orange dry flavours, magnesium stearate and microcrystalline cellulose.

Augmentin 250/62 And 125/31 Sf Suspensions

The powder contains xanthan gum, hydroxypropyl methylcellulose, aspartame, silicon dioxide, colloidal silica, succinic acid, raspberry, orange and golden syrup dry flavours.

6.2 Incompatibilities

None

6.3 Shelf life

Augmentin 375 mg Tablets	Blister enclosed in pouch 24M, Glass bottles 24M
Augmentin 625 mg Tablets	Blister enclosed in pouch 24M, Glass bottles 36M
Augmentin Dispersible Tablets 375 mg	24M
Augmentin 250/62 SF and 125/31 SF Suspension	Dry powder 18M Reconstituted suspensions seven days

6.4 Special precautions for storage

Augmentin 375 mg and 625 mg Tablets should be stored in a dry place at 25°C or below.

Augmentin Dispersible Tablets 375 mg should be stored in a dry place.

Augmentin 250/62 SF and 125/31 SF Suspensions: the dry powder should be stored in a dry place. Reconstituted suspensions should be kept in a refrigerator (but not frozen) for up to seven days.

6.5 Nature and contents of container

Augmentin 375 mg Tablets: Aluminium PVC/PVdC blister enlcosed within an aluminium laminate pouch containing a desiccant sachet. Each pouch contains a plaque of 7 tablets. 3 pouches are enclosed within a carton to provide a pack of 21 tablets. Also amber glass bottles of 100.

Augmentin 625 mg Tablets: Aluminium PVC/PVdC blister enlcosed within an aluminium laminate pouch containing a desiccant sachet. Each pouch contains a plaque of 7 tablets. 3 pouches are enclosed within a carton to provide a pack of 21 tablets.

Augmentin Dispersible Tablets 375 mg: Blister packs of 21 in a carton.

Augmentin 250/62 SF and 125/31 SF Suspensions: Clear glass bottles containing powder for reconstitution to 100 ml.

6.6 Instructions for use and handling

Augmentin 375 mg and 625 mg Tablets: None

Augmentin Dispersible Tablets 375 mg: The dispersible tablets should be stirred with a little water before taking.

Augmentin 250/62 SF and 125/31 SF Suspensions: At time of dispensing, the dry powder should be reconstituted to form an oral suspension as detailed below:

Strength	Volume of water to be added to reconstitute	Nominal bottle size	Final volume of reconstituted oral suspension
125/31	92 ml	150 ml	100 ml
250/62	90 ml	150 ml	100 ml

Administrative Data

7. MARKETING AUTHORISATION HOLDER

Beecham Group plc
980 Great West Road
Brentford
Middlesex TW8 9GS

Trading as:

GlaxoSmithKline UK
Stockley Park West
Uxbridge
Middlesex UB11 1BT

8. MARKETING AUTHORISATION NUMBER(S)

Augmentin 375 mg Tablets	PL 00038/0270
Augmentin 625 mg Tablets	PL 00038/0362
Augmentin Dispersible Tablets 375 mg	PL 00038/0272
Augmentin 250/62 SF Suspension	PL 00038/0337
Augmentin 125/31 SF Suspension	PL 00038/0298

9. DATE OF FIRST AUTHORISATION/RENEWAL OF THE AUTHORISATION

Augmentin 375 mg Tablets	27 July 2002
Augmentin 625 mg Tablets	27 March 2000
Augmentin Dispersible Tablets 375 mg	27 July 2002
Augmentin 250/62 SF Suspension	18 February 2000
Augmentin 125/31 SF Suspension	08 December 1998

10. DATE OF REVISION OF THE TEXT

11 January 2005

11. Legal Status

POM

Augmentin-Duo 400/57

(GlaxoSmithKline UK)

1. NAME OF THE MEDICINAL PRODUCT

Augmentin®-Duo 400/57.

2. QUALITATIVE AND QUANTITATIVE COMPOSITION

Augmentin-Duo 400/57 contains 400 mg amoxicillin and 57 mg clavulanic acid per 5ml (co-amoxiclav 400/57).

The amoxicillin is present as amoxicillin trihydrate and the clavulanic acid is present as potassium clavulanate.

3. PHARMACEUTICAL FORM

Dry powder for reconstitution in water, at time of dispensing, to form an oral sugar-free suspension.

4. CLINICAL PARTICULARS

4.1 Therapeutic indications

Augmentin-Duo 400/57 is an antibiotic agent with a notably broad spectrum of activity against the commonly occurring bacterial pathogens in general practice and hospital. The β-lactamase inhibitory action of clavulanate extends the spectrum of amoxicillin to embrace a wider range of organisms, including many resistant to other β-lactam antibiotics.

Augmentin-Duo 400/57, for twice-daily (b.i.d) oral dosing, is indicated for short-term treatment of bacterial infections at the following sites when amoxicillin resistant β-lactamase-producing strains are suspected as the cause. In other situations, amoxicillin alone should be considered.

- *Upper Respiratory Tract Infections (including ENT)* in particular sinusitis, otitis media, recurrent tonsillitis. These infections are often caused by *Streptococcus pneumoniae, Haemophilus influenzae**, *Moraxella catarrhalis** and *Streptococcus pyogenes.*

- *Lower Respiratory Tract Infections* in particular acute exacerbations of chronic bronchitis (especially if considered severe), bronchopneumonia. These infections are often caused by *Streptococcus pneumoniae, Haemophilus influenzae** and *Moraxella catarrhalis**.

- *Urinary Tract Infections* in particular cystitis (especially when recurrent or complicated - excluding prostatitis). These infections are often caused by *Enterobacteriaceae** (mainly *Escherichia coli**), *Staphylococcus saprophyticus, Enterococcus* species.*

- *Skin and Soft Tissue Infections* in particular cellulitis, animal bites and severe dental abscess with spreading cellulitis. These infections are often caused by *Staphylococcus aureus**, *Streptococcus pyogenes* and *Bacteroides* species*.

- A comprehensive list of sensitive organisms is provided in Section 5.

* Some members of these species of bacteria produce β-lactamase, rendering them insensitive to amoxicillin alone.

Mixed infections caused by amoxicillin-susceptible organisms in conjunction with Augmentin-Duo 400/57-susceptible β-lactamase-producing organisms may be treated with Augmentin-Duo 400/57. These infections should not require the addition of another antibiotic resistant to β-lactamases.

4.2 Posology and method of administration

The usual recommended daily dosage is:

25/3.6 mg/kg/day in mild to moderate infections (upper respiratory tract infections, e.g. recurrent tonsillitis, lower respiratory infections and skin and soft tissue infections)

45/6.4 mg/kg/day for the treatment of more serious infections (upper respiratory tract infections, e.g. otitis media and sinusitis, lower respiratory tract infections, e.g. bronchopneumonia and urinary tract infections)

The tables below give guidance for children.

Children over 2 years

25/3.6 mg/kg/ day	2 - 6 years (13 - 21 kg)	2.5 ml Augmentin-Duo 400/ 57 Suspension b.i.d.
	7 - 12 years (22 - 40 kg)	5.0 ml Augmentin-Duo 400/ 57 Suspension b.i.d.
45/6.4 mg/kg/ day	2 - 6 years (13 - 21 kg)	5.0 ml Augmentin-Duo 400/ 57 Suspension b.i.d.
	7 - 12 years (22 - 40 kg)	10.0 ml Augmentin-Duo 400/57 Suspension b.i.d.

Children aged 2 months to 2 years

Children under 2 years should be dosed according to body weight

Weight (kg)	25/3.6 mg/kg/day) (ml/b.i.d.*)	45/6.4 mg/kg/day (ml/b.i.d.*)
2	0.3	0.6
3	0.5	0.8
4	0.6	1.1
5	0.8	1.4
6	0.9	1.7
7	1.1	2.0
8	1.3	2.3
9	1.4	2.5
10	1.6	2.8
11	1.7	3.1
12	1.9	3.4
13	2.0	3.7
14	2.2	3.9
15	2.3	4.2

* The 35 ml presentation is supplied with a syringe dosing device - See Sections 6.5 and 6.6

There is insufficient experience with Augmentin-Duo' to make dosage recommendations for children under 2 months old.

Infants with immature kidney function

For children with immature renal function Augmentin-Duo 400/57 is not recommended.

Renal impairment

For children with a GFR of >30 ml/min no adjustment in dosage is required. For children with a GFR of <30 ml/min Augmentin-Duo 400/57 is not recommended.

Hepatic impairment

Dose with caution; monitor hepatic function at regular intervals. There is, as yet, insufficient evidence on which to base a dosage recommendation.

Method of administration

To minimise potential gastrointestinal intolerance, administer at the start of a meal. The absorption of co-amoxiclav is optimised when taken at the start of a meal. Duration of therapy should be appropriate to the indication and should not exceed 14 days without review. Therapy can be started parenterally and continued with an oral preparation.

4.3 Contraindications

Penicillin hypersensitivity.

Attention should be paid to possible cross-sensitivity with other β-lactam antibiotics, e.g. cephalosporins.

A previous history of co-amoxiclav- or penicillin-associated jaundice/hepatic dysfunction.

4.4 Special warnings and special precautions for use

Changes in liver function tests have been observed in some patients receiving co-amoxiclav. The clinical significance of these changes is uncertain but co-amoxiclav should be used with caution in patients with evidence of hepatic dysfunction.

Cholestatic jaundice, which may be severe, but is usually reversible, has been reported rarely. Signs and symptoms may not become apparent for several weeks after treatment has ceased.

In patients with renal impairment, dosage should be adjusted according to the degree of impairment (see Section 4.2).In patients with moderate or severe renal impairment Augmentin-Duo 400/57 is not recommended.

In patients with reduced urine output, crystalluria has been observed very rarely, predominantly with parenteral therapy. During the administration of high doses of amoxicillin, it is advisable to maintain adequate fluid intake and urinary output in order to reduce the possibility of amoxicillin crystalluria (see Section 4.9 Overdose).

Serious and occasionally fatal hypersensitivity (anaphylactoid) reactions have been reported in patients on penicillin therapy. These reactions are more likely to occur in individuals with a history of penicillin hypersensitivity (see Section 4.3).

Erythematous rashes have been associated with glandular fever in patients receiving amoxicillin.

Prolonged use may also occasionally result in overgrowth of non-susceptible organisms.

Augmentin-Duo 400/57 contains 16.64 mg aspartame per 5 ml dose and therefore care should be taken in phenylketonuria.

4.5 Interaction with other medicinal products and other forms of Interaction

Prolongation of bleeding time and prothrombin time have been reported in some patients receiving co-amoxiclav. Co-amoxiclav should be used with care in patients on anticoagulation therapy. In common with other broad-spectrum antibiotics, co-amoxiclav may reduce the efficacy of oral contraceptives and patients should be warned accordingly.

Concomitant use of allopurinol during treatment with amoxicillin can increase the likelihood of allergic skin reactions. There are no data on the concomitant use of co-amoxiclav and allopurinol.

4.6 Pregnancy and lactation

Use in pregnancy

Reproduction studies in animals (mice and rats) with orally and parenterally administered co-amoxiclav have shown no teratogenic effects In a single study in women with preterm, premature rupture of the foetal membrane (pPROM), it was reported that prophylactic treatment with Augmentin may be associated with an increased risk of necrotising enterocolitis in neonates. As with all medicines, use should be avoided in pregnancy, especially during the first trimester, unless considered essential by the physician.

Use in lactation

Co-amoxiclav may be administered during the period of lactation. With the exception of the risk of sensitisation, associated with the excretion of trace quantities in breast milk, there are no known detrimental effects for the breast-fed infant.

4.7 Effects on ability to drive and use machines

Adverse effects on the ability to drive or operate machinery have not been observed.

4.8 Undesirable effects

Side effects are uncommon and mainly of a mild and transitory nature.

Gastrointestinal reactions:

Diarrhoea, indigestion, nausea, vomiting, and mucocutaneous candidiasis have been reported. Antibiotic-associated colitis (including pseudomembranous colitis and haemorrhagic colitis) has been reported rarely. Nausea, although uncommon, is more often associated with higher oral dosages. If gastrointestinal side effects occur with oral therapy they may be reduced by taking co-amoxiclav at the start of meals.

Superficial tooth discolouration has been reported rarely, mostly with the suspension. It can usually be removed by brushing.

Renal and urinary tract disorders:

Crystalluria has been reported very rarely (see Section 4.9 Overdose).

Genito-urinary effects:

Vaginal itching, soreness and discharge may occur.

Hepatic effects:

Moderate and asymptomatic rises in AST and/or ALT and alkaline phosphatases have been reported occasionally. Hepatitis and cholestatic jaundice have been reported rarely. These hepatic reactions have been reported more commonly with co-amoxiclav than with other penicillins.

After co-amoxiclav hepatic reactions have been reported more frequently in males and elderly patients, particularly those over 65 years. The risk increases with duration of treatment longer than 14 days. These reactions have been very rarely reported in children.

Signs and symptoms usually occur during or shortly after treatment but in some cases may not occur until several weeks after treatment has ended. Hepatic reactions are usually reversible but they may be severe and, very rarely, deaths have been reported.

Hypersensitivity reactions:

Urticarial and erythematous skin rashes sometimes occur. Rarely erythema multiforme, Stevens- Johnson syndrome, toxic epidermal necrolysis, bullous exfoliative dermatitis, acute generalised exanthematous pustulosis (AGEP), serum sickness-like syndrome and hypersensitivity vasculitis have been reported. Treatment should be discontinued if one of these disorders occurs. In common with other β-lactam antibiotics angioedema and anaphylaxis have been reported. Interstitial nephritis can occur rarely.

Haematological effects:

As with other β-lactams transient leucopenia (including neutropenia and agranulocytosis), thrombocytopenia and haemolytic anaemia have been reported rarely. Prolongation of bleeding time and prothrombin time has also been reported rarely (see Section 4.5).

CNS effects:

CNS effects have been seen very rarely. These include reversible hyperactivity, dizziness, headache and convulsions. Convulsions may occur with impaired renal function or in those receiving high doses.

4.9 Overdose

Overdosage

Gastrointestinal symptoms and disturbance of the fluid and electrolyte balances may be evident. They may be treated symptomatically, with attention to the water/electrolyte balance. Co-amoxiclav may be removed from the circulation by haemodialysis.

Amoxicillin crystalluria, in some cases leading to renal failure, has been observed (see Section 4.4 Special warnings and special precautions for use)

Drug abuse and dependence

Drug dependency, addiction and recreational abuse have not been reported as a problem with this compound.

5. PHARMACOLOGICAL PROPERTIES

Augmentin-Duo400/57 contains a combination of amoxicillin and clavulanic acid, co-amoxiclav 400/57.

5.1 Pharmacodynamic properties

Microbiology

Amoxicillin is a semi-synthetic antibiotic with a broad spectrum of antibacterial activity against many Gram-positive and Gram-negative micro-organisms. Amoxicillin is, however, susceptible to degradation by β-lactamases and therefore the spectrum of activity of amoxicillin alone does not include organisms which produce these enzymes.

Clavulanic acid is a β-lactam, structurally related to the penicillins, which possesses the ability to inactivate a wide range of β-lactamase enzymes commonly found in microorganisms resistant to penicillins and cephalosporins. In particular, it has good activity against the clinically important plasmid mediated beta-lactamases frequently responsible for transferred drug resistance. It is generally less effective against chromosomally-mediated type 1 β-lactamases.

The presence of clavulanic acid in Augmentin-Duo 400/57 protects amoxicillin from degradation by β-lactamase enzymes and effectively extends the antibacterial spectrum of amoxicillin to include many bacteria normally resistant to amoxicillin and other penicillins and cephalosporins. Thus Augmentin-Duo 400/57 possesses the distinctive properties of a broad spectrum antibiotic and a β-lactamase inhibitor. Augmentin-Duo 400/57 is bactericidal to a wide range of organisms including:

Gram-positive

Aerobes: *Enterococcus faecalis**, *Enterococcus faecium**, *Streptococcus pneumoniae, Streptococcus pyogenes, Streptococcus viridans, Staphylococcus aureus**, Coagulase negative *staphylococci** (including *Staphylococcus epidermidis**), *Corynebacterium* species, *Bacillus anthracis**, *Listeria monocytogenes.*

Anaerobes: *Clostridium* species, *Peptococcus* species, *Peptostreptococcus.*

Gram-negative

Aerobes: *Haemophilus influenzae**, *Moraxella catarrhalis** *(Branhamella catarrhalis), Escherichia coli**, *Proteus mirabilis**, *Proteus vulgaris**, *Klebsiella* species*, *Salmonella* species*, *Shigella* species*, *Bordetella pertussis, Brucella* species, *Neisseria gonorrhoeae**, *Neisseria meningitidis**, *Vibrio cholerae, Pasteurella multocida.*

Anaerobes: *Bacteroides* species* including *B. fragilis*.

* Some members of these species of bacteria produce β-lactamase, rendering them insensitive to amoxicillin alone.

5.2 Pharmacokinetic properties

a. Absorption:

The two components of Augmentin-Duo 400/57, amoxicillin and clavulanic acid, are each fully dissociated in aqueous solution at physiological pH. Both components are rapidly and well absorbed by the oral route of administration. Absorption of co-amoxiclav is optimised when taken at the start of a meal.

b. Pharmacokinetics

Pharmacokinetic studies have been performed in children, including one study [25000/382] which has compared co-amoxiclav t.i.d and b.i.d. All of these data indicate that the elimination pharmacokinetics seen in adults also apply to children with mature kidney function.

The mean AUC values for amoxicillin are essentially the same following twice-a-day dosing with the 875/125 mg tablet or three-times-a-day dosing with the 500/125 mg tablet, in adults. No differences between the 875 mg bid and 500mg t.i.d dosing regimes are seen when comparing the amoxicillin $T_{½}$, or C_{max} after normalisation for the different doses of amoxicillin administered. Similarly, no differences are seen for the clavulanate $T_{½}$, C_{max} or AUC values after appropriate dose normalisation [Study 360].

The time of dosing of co-amoxiclav relative to the start of a meal has no marked effects on the pharmacokinetics of amoxicillin in adults. In a study of the 875/125 mg tablet [Study 362], the time of dosing relative to ingestion of a meal had a marked effect on the pharmacokinetics of clavulanate. For clavulanate AUC and C_{max}, the highest mean values and smallest inter-subject variabilities were achieved by administering co-amoxiclav at the start of a meal, compared to the fasting state or 30 or 150 minutes after the start of a meal.

The mean C_{max}, T_{max}, $T_{½}$ and AUC values for amoxicillin and clavulanic acid are given below for an 875 mg/125 mg dose of co-amoxiclav administered at the start of a meal [Study 362].

Mean Pharmacokinetic Parameters

(see Table 1)

Amoxicillin serum concentrations achieved with co-amoxiclav are similar to those produced by the oral administration of equivalent doses of amoxicillin alone.

c. Distribution:

Following intravenous administration therapeutic concentrations of both amoxicillin and clavulanic acid may be detected in the tissues and interstitial fluid. Therapeutic concentrations of both drugs have been found in gall bladder, abdominal tissue, skin, fat, and muscle tissues; fluids found to have therapeutic levels include synovial and peritoneal fluids, bile and pus.

Neither amoxicillin nor clavulanic acid is highly protein bound, studies show that about 25% for clavulanic acid and 18% for amoxicillin of total plasma drug content is bound to protein. From animal studies there is no evidence to suggest that either component accumulates in any organ.

Amoxicillin, like most penicillins, can be detected in breast milk. There are no data available on the passage of clavulanic acid into breast milk.

Reproduction studies in animals have shown that both amoxicillin and clavulanic acid penetrate the placental barrier. However, no evidence of impaired fertility or harm to the foetus was detected.

d. Elimination:

As with other penicillins, the major route of elimination for amoxicillin is via the kidney, whereas for clavulanate elimination is by both non-renal and renal mechanisms. Approximately 60-70% of the amoxicillin and approximately 40-65% of the clavulanic acid are excreted unchanged in urine during the first 6 hours after administration of a single 375 or 625 mg tablet.

Table 1 Mean Pharmacokinetic Parameters

Drug Administration	Dose (mg)	C_{max} (mg/L)	T_{max}* (hours)	AUC (mg.h/L)	$T_{½}$ (hours)
AUGMENTIN 1 g					
Amoxicillin	875 mg	12.4	1.5	29.9	1.36
Clavulanic acid	125 mg	3.3	1.3	6.88	0.92

* Median values

Table 2

Fill Weight	Volume of water to be added to reconstitute	Nominal bottle size	Final volume of reconstituted oral suspension
6.3 g	32 ml	107 ml	35 ml
12.6 g	64 ml	147 ml	70 ml
25.2 g	127 ml	200 ml	140 ml

Amoxicillin is also partly excreted in the urine as the inactive penicilloic acid in quantities equivalent to 10-25% of the initial dose. Clavulanic acid is extensively metabolised in man to 2,5-dihydro-4-(2- hydroxyethyl)-5-oxo-1H-pyrrole-3-carboxylic acid and 1-amino-4-hydroxy- butan-2-one and eliminated in urine and faeces and as carbon dioxide in expired air.

5.3 Preclinical safety data
No further information of relevance.

6. PHARMACEUTICAL PARTICULARS

6.1 List of excipients
Xantham gum, aspartame, colloidal silica, silicon dioxide, crospovidone, carmellose sodium, magnesium stearate, sodium benzoate, strawberry flavour.

6.2 Incompatibilities
None known.

6.3 Shelf life
Glass Bottles

Dry powder: 18 months when stored at temperatures at or below 25°C.

Reconstituted suspensions: seven days when stored in a refrigerator (2-8°C).

Sachets

18 months when stored at temperatures at or below 25°C.

6.4 Special precautions for storage
The dry powder should be stored in well-sealed containers in a dry place.

6.5 Nature and contents of container
Clear, glass bottles containing an off-white dry powder. The 35 ml presentation is supplied in a carton with a polystyrene syringe dosing device.

or

Single-dose sachets. Four sachets are supplied in a carton.

When reconstituted, an off-white suspension is formed

6.6 Instructions for use and handling
Glass bottles:

At time of dispensing, the dry powder should be reconstituted to form an oral suspension, as detailed above:

(see Table 2 above)

The 35 ml presentation is provided with a syringe dosing device which should be used in place of the cap following reconstitution. This device is used to dose patients under 2 years according to the schedule in Section 4.2.

Sachets:

Single-dose sachets contain powder for a 2.5 ml dose.

Directions for use: Check that the sachet is intact before use

1. Cut sachet along dotted line
2. Empty contents into a glass
3. Half fill sachet with water
4. Pour into the glass, stir well and drink immediately

If two or four sachets have to be taken at once then they can be mixed in the same glass.

Administrative Data

7. MARKETING AUTHORISATION HOLDER
SmithKline Beecham plc

980 Great West Road

Brentford

Middlesex TW8 9GS

Trading as:

GlaxoSmithKline UK

Stockley Park West

Uxbridge

Middlesex, UB11 1BT

8. MARKETING AUTHORISATION NUMBER(S)
PL 10592/0070

9. DATE OF FIRST AUTHORISATION/RENEWAL OF THE AUTHORISATION
2 January 2002

10. DATE OF REVISION OF THE TEXT
8th February 2005

11. Legal Status
POM

Aureocort Ointment

(Wyeth Pharmaceuticals)

1. NAME OF THE MEDICINAL PRODUCT
Aureocort Ointment

2. QUALITATIVE AND QUANTITATIVE COMPOSITION
Aureocort Ointment is a topical preparation containing the active ingredients chlortetracycline hydrochloride 3.09 w/w and triamcinolone acetonide 0.1 w/w.

3. PHARMACEUTICAL FORM
Ointment for topical administration.

4. CLINICAL PARTICULARS

4.1 Therapeutic indications
Aureocort combines the anti-inflammatory action of triamcinolone acetonide with the anti-infective properties of chlortetracycline.

It is indicated in the treatment of secondarily infected atopic dermatitis, contact dermatitis, eczema, neurodermatitis, otitis externa, seborrhoeic dermatitis, varicose eczema, vesiculo-pustular dermatitis. It may also be used in the treatment of infected insect bites.

4.2 Posology and method of administration
Recommended doses and dosage schedules:

Adults, children over 8 years and the elderly

Aureocort Ointment should be applied sparingly to the affected area, either directly or on sterile gauze, two or three times daily.

Aureocort treatment should be limited to seven days (see section 4.4)

Avoid contact with eyes (see section 4.4)

In general, dose selection for an elderly patient should be cautious, taking into account physiological changes in ageing skin (see section 4.4)

4.3 Contraindications
The use of Aureocort is contra-indicated in tuberculous, fungal or viral lesions of the skin (herpes simplex, vaccinia and varicella), and primary bacterial infections, e.g. impetigo, pyoderma and furunculosis.

Aureocort Topical preparations are also contra-indicated in patients with a history of hypersensitivity to tetracyclines, corticosteroids, or any other ingredient in the preparations.

4.4 Special warnings and special precautions for use
Corticosteroids, such as triamcinolone, may be absorbed in sufficient amounts to cause systemic corticosteroid effects, if applied to large areas, to broken skin or under occlusive dressings. Systemic absorption of topical corticosteroids has produced reversible hypothalamic-pituitary-adrenal (HPA) axis suppression, manifestations of Cushing's syndrome, hyperglycemia, and glucosuria in some patients.

Minor degrees of adrenal suppression may occur when Aureocort Ointment is applied over relatively small areas under an occlusive dressing. Occlusion should not be used when treating conditions of the face.

Chlortetracycline, like other tetracycline-class antibiotics, may cause foetal harm when administered to a pregnant woman (see section 4.6)

The use of corticosteroids on infected areas should be continuously and carefully observed, bearing in mind the potential spreading of infections (caused by organisms not sensitive to chlortetracycline) by anti-inflammatory corticosteroids. It may be advisable to discontinue corticosteroid therapy and/or initiate alternative antibacterial measures in these circumstances. Generalised dermatological conditions may require systemic corticosteroid therapy.

Steroid-antibiotic combinations should not be continued for more than 7 days in the absence of any clinical improvement, since in this situation occult extension of infection may occur due to the masking effect of the steroid. Extended or recurrent application may increase the risk of contact sensitisation and should be avoided.

Hypersensitivity reactions to the anti-infective component may be masked by the presence of the corticosteroid.

Phototoxic reactions can occur in individuals using chlortetracycline, and are characterized by severe burns of exposed surfaces resulting from direct exposure of patients to sunlight during therapy with chlortetracycline. Patients exposed to direct sunlight or ultraviolet light (artificial sunlight) should be advised that this reaction can occur, and treatment should be discontinued at the first evidence of erythema of the skin.

Caution should also be applied when using this preparation on the periorbital area of the face, as it can induce ocular complications that include cataract, glaucoma, retarded healing or corneal abrasion, extension of herpetic infection, and increased susceptibility of bacterial and fungal infection.

Paediatric Use

Paediatric patients may demonstrate a greater susceptibility to topical corticosteroid induced hypothalmic-pituitary-adrenal (HPA) axis suppression and Cushing's syndrome than mature patients because of a larger skin surface area to body weight ratio and are also therefore more susceptible to systemic toxicity.

HPA axis suppression (and Addisonian crisis upon withdrawal), Cushing's syndrome, and intracranial hypertension have been reported in children receiving topical corticosteroids. Administration of topical corticosteroids to children should be limited to the least amount compatible with an effective therapeutic regimen. Chronic corticosteroid therapy may interfere with growth and development of children.

The use of drugs of the tetracycline class during tooth development may result in permanent discolouration of the teeth (see section 4.6).

This adverse reaction is more common during long-term use of the drug, but has been observed following repeated short-term courses. Enamel hypoplasia has also been reported. Tetracycline drugs, therefore, should not be used during tooth development unless other drugs are not likely to be effective or are contraindicated.

To reduce the theoretical risk of damage to permanent dentition by tetracyclines, Aureocort ointment should not be used in children under 8 years of age, unless other drugs are unlikely to be effective or are contra-indicated.

Geriatric Use

Clinical studies of topical triamcinolone acetonide-chlortetracycline hydrochloride did not include sufficient numbers of subjects aged 65 and over to determine whether they respond differently from younger subjects. Other reported clinical experience has not identified differences in responses between the elderly and younger patients. In general, dose selection for an elderly patient should be cautious, taking into account physiological changes in ageing skin.

Use in cases where the approved indication/s co-exist with psoriasis

Aureocort ointment should be used with caution in patients with psoriasis as it may result in rebound relapses following the development of tolerance, including generalized pustular psoriasis. It may also result in local and systemic toxicity due to impaired barrier function of the skin. Absorption is more likely after repeated applications, possibly by greater skin permeability in psoriatic areas than normal skin.

4.5 Interaction with other medicinal products and other forms of Interaction
Not applicable.

4.6 Pregnancy and lactation

Pregnancy

Topical administration of corticosteroids to pregnant rabbits has been reported to cause abnormalities of foetal development, including cleft palate and intrauterine growth retardation at relatively low doses. There are no adequate and well-controlled studies in pregnant women on teratogenic effects from topically applied triamcinolone acetonide-chlortetracycline hydrochloride preparations. Chlortetracycline, like other tetracycline-class antibiotics, may cause foetal harm when administered to a pregnant woman. As this agent is absorbed percutaneously, teratogenicity following topical application cannot be excluded. If any tetracycline is used during pregnancy or if the patient becomes pregnant while using this drug, the patient should be informed of the potential hazard to the foetus.

The use of corticosteroid/antibiotic preparations, containing drugs of the tetracycline class, during tooth development (last half of pregnancy, infancy and childhood to the age of 8 years) may cause permanent discolouration of the teeth (yellow-grey-brown). This adverse reaction, related only to tetracyclines, is more common during long-term use of the drug, but has been observed following repeated short-term courses. Enamel hypoplasia has also been reported. Tetracycline drugs, therefore, should not be used during tooth development unless other drugs are not likely to be effective or are contraindicated.

Triamcinolone acetonide-chlortetracycline hydrochloride topical preparations should be used during pregnancy only if the potential benefit justifies the potential risk to the foetus.

Lactation

It is not known whether topical administration of corticosteroid-chlortetracycline antibiotic preparations result in systemic absorption to produce quantities in human milk, and it is therefore advised that this preparation is not used during lactation.

4.7 Effects on ability to drive and use machines
Not applicable.

4.8 Undesirable effects
Information on side effects according to the body system are as follows:

System Organ Class	Adverse Reaction
Immune system disorders:	Hypersensitivity
Skin and subcutaneous tissue disorders:	Application site reactions, including contact dermatitis, skin atrophy, steroid purpura, striae, skin fragility, exfoliative dermatitis, burning sensation, acneiform eruption, folliculitis, rosacea, periocular and perioral dermatitis, delayed wound healing, granulomas, telangiectases, erythema, hypopigmentation, hypertrichosis, masking or aggravation of dermatophyte infection and secondary infection or aggravation of existing infection, photosensitivity, rash, urticaria, pruritus

A few patients may be allergic to any of the components. If an adverse reaction occurs, medication should be discontinued.

Systemic absorption of corticosteroids may occur if they are used over extensive body areas, with or without occlusive non-permeable dressings. When occlusive non-permeable dressings are used, miliaria, folliculitis and pyoderma may sometimes develop beneath the occlusive material.

Localised atrophy and striae have been reported with the use of corticosteroids by the occlusive technique.

Use of topical corticosteroids, such as triamcinolone, in the periorbital region may result in ocular complications (see section 4.4).

Under certain circumstances sufficient amounts of topical corticosteroids, such as triamcinolone, can be absorbed to cause systemic corticosteroid effects including adrenal suppression and Cushing's syndrome. Cessation of topical steroid therapy after an extended treatment period can result in Addisonian crisis.

Chlortetracycline, like other tetracycline-class antibiotics, may cause foetal harm when administered to a pregnant woman, and may cause permanent discolouration of the teeth during development in children up to the age of 8 years (see section 4.6).

4.9 Overdose

Under certain circumstances topically applied corticosteroids can be absorbed in sufficient amounts to produce systemic effects including Cushing's syndrome. Cessation of topical steroid therapy after an extended treatment period can result in an Addisonian crisis.

5. PHARMACOLOGICAL PROPERTIES

5.1 Pharmacodynamic properties

Aureocort Ointment contains two active ingredients:

(i) Chlortetracycline hydrochloride is a broad spectrum antibiotic. It is active against a large number of gram-positive and gram-negative bacteria, including some which are resistant to penicillin.

(ii) Triamcinolone Acetonide is a corticosteroid with anti-inflammatory, anti-pruritus and anti-allergic effects.

5.2 Pharmacokinetic properties

Topically applied tetracycline preparations are not absorbed into the general circulation to any significant degree.

Absorption of triamcinolone acetonide from topically applied preparations is usually minimal. However, corticosteroids may be absorbed in sufficient amounts to cause systemic effects if applied to large areas, when the skin is broken, or under occlusive dressings.

5.3 Preclinical safety data

Nothing of any relevance to the prescriber.

6. PHARMACEUTICAL PARTICULARS

6.1 List of excipients

Paraffin white soft, wool fat

6.2 Incompatibilities

None known.

6.3 Shelf life

3 years.

6.4 Special precautions for storage

Do not store above 25°C.

Store in the original pack.

6.5 Nature and contents of container

Collapsible aluminium tubes with white, high density polyethylene caps.

6.6 Instructions for use and handling

Not applicable.

7. MARKETING AUTHORISATION HOLDER

Cyanamid of Great Britain Limited
Fareham Road
Gosport
Hants
PO13 0AS

8. MARKETING AUTHORISATION NUMBER(S)

PL 00095/5076R

9. DATE OF FIRST AUTHORISATION/RENEWAL OF THE AUTHORISATION

First Authorisation: 27 December 1990 (Review).

10. DATE OF REVISION OF THE TEXT

09 September 2004

Avandamet 2mg and 4mg film-coated Tablets

(GlaxoSmithKline UK)

1. NAME OF THE MEDICINAL PRODUCT

Avandamet 2 mg/500 mg film-coated tablets ▼.
Avandamet 2 mg/1000 mg film-coated tablets ▼.
Avandamet 4 mg/1000 mg film-coated tablets ▼.

2. QUALITATIVE AND QUANTITATIVE COMPOSITION

Each tablet contains rosiglitazone maleate corresponding to 2 or 4 mg rosiglitazone in combination with metformin hydrochloride 500 mg or 1000 mg (corresponding to metformin free base 390 mg or 780 mg respectively).

For excipients, see section 6.1.

3. PHARMACEUTICAL FORM

Film-coated tablets.

Avandamet 2 mg/500 mg - Pale pink film-coated tablets marked "gsk" on one side and "2/500" on the other.

Avandamet 2 mg/1000 mg - Yellow film-coated tablets marked "gsk" on one side and "2/1000" on the other.

Avandamet 4 mg/1000 mg - Pink film-coated tablets marked "gsk" on one side and "4/1000" on the other.

4. CLINICAL PARTICULARS

4.1 Therapeutic indications

Avandamet is indicated in the treatment of type 2 diabetes mellitus patients, particularly overweight patients, who are unable to achieve sufficient glycaemic control at their maximally tolerated dose of oral metformin alone.

4.2 Posology and method of administration

For the different dosage regimens, Avandamet is available in appropriate strengths.

The usual starting dose of Avandamet is 4 mg/day rosiglitazone plus 2000 mg/day metformin hydrochloride (this dosage is achievable with one tablet of Avandamet 2 mg/1000 mg, taken twice a day).

Rosiglitazone can be increased to 8 mg/day after 8 weeks if greater glycaemic control is required. The maximum recommended daily dose of Avandamet is 8 mg rosiglitazone plus 2000 mg metformin hydrochloride (this dosage is achievable with two tablets of Avandamet 2 mg/500 mg taken twice a day, or one tablet of Avandamet 4 mg/1000 mg taken twice a day).

Dose titration with rosiglitazone (added to the optimal dose of metformin) may be considered before the patient is switched to Avandamet.

When clinically appropriate, direct change from metformin monotherapy to Avandamet may be considered.

Taking Avandamet with or just after food may reduce gastrointestinal symptoms associated with metformin.

Elderly

As metformin is excreted via the kidney, and elderly patients have a tendency to decreased renal function, elderly patients taking Avandamet should have their renal function monitored regularly (see sections 4.3 and 4.4).

Patients with renal impairment

Avandamet should not be used in patients with renal failure or renal dysfunction e.g. serum creatinine levels > 135 μmol/l in males and > 110 μmol/l in females and/or creatinine clearance < 70 ml/min (see sections 4.3 and 4.4).

Children and adolescents

There are no data available on the use of rosiglitazone in patients under 18 years of age, and therefore use of Avandamet in this age group is not recommended.

4.3 Contraindications

Avandamet is contraindicated in patients with:

- hypersensitivity to rosiglitazone, metformin hydrochloride or to any of the excipients
- cardiac failure or history of cardiac failure (NYHA stages I to IV)
- acute or chronic disease which may cause tissue hypoxia such as:
- cardiac or respiratory failure
- recent myocardial infarction
- shock
- hepatic impairment
- acute alcohol intoxication, alcoholism (see section 4.4)
- diabetic ketoacidosis or diabetic pre-coma
- renal failure or renal dysfunction e.g. serum creatinine levels > 135 μmol/l in males and > 110 μmol/l in females and/or creatinine clearance < 70 ml/min (see section 4.4)
- acute conditions with the potential to alter renal function such as:
- dehydration
- severe infection
- shock
- intravascular administration of iodinated contrast agents (see section 4.4)
- lactation.

Avandamet is also contraindicated for use in combination with insulin (see section 4.4).

4.4 Special warnings and special precautions for use

There is no clinical experience of other oral antihyperglycaemic agents added to treatment with either Avandamet or concomitantly administered metformin and rosiglitazone.

Lactic acidosis

Lactic acidosis is a very rare, but serious, metabolic complication that can occur due to metformin accumulation. Reported cases of lactic acidosis in patients on metformin have occurred primarily in diabetic patients with significant renal failure. The incidence of lactic acidosis can and should be reduced by also assessing other associated risk factors such as poorly controlled diabetes, ketosis, prolonged fasting, excessive alcohol intake, hepatic insufficiency and any conditions associated with hypoxia.

Diagnosis:

Lactic acidosis is characterised by acidotic dyspnoea, abdominal pain and hypothermia followed by coma. Diagnostic laboratory findings are decreased blood pH, plasma lactate levels above 5 mmol/l and an increased anion gap and lactate/pyruvate ratio. If metabolic acidosis is suspected, treatment with the medicinal product should be discontinued and the patient hospitalised immediately (see section 4.9).

Renal function

As metformin is excreted by the kidney, serum creatinine concentrations should be determined regularly:

- at least once a year in patients with normal renal function
- at least two to four times a year in patients with serum creatinine levels at the upper limit of normal and in elderly patients.

Decreased renal function in elderly patients is frequent and asymptomatic. Special caution should be exercised in situations where renal function may become impaired, for example when initiating antihypertensive or diuretic therapy or when starting treatment with an NSAID.

Fluid retention and cardiac failure

Rosiglitazone can cause fluid retention, which may exacerbate or precipitate heart failure. Signs and symptoms of fluid retention, including weight gain, should be monitored. The possible contribution of fluid retention to weight gain should be individually assessed. Rapid and excessive weight gain has been reported very rarely as a sign of fluid retention. Patients should be observed for signs and symptoms of heart failure, particularly those with reduced cardiac reserve. Avandamet must be discontinued if any deterioration in cardiac status occurs. An increased incidence of cardiac failure has been observed in clinical trials when rosiglitazone is used in combination with insulin. Therefore Avandamet is contraindicated in combination with insulin. Heart failure was also reported more frequently in patients with a history of heart failure, in elderly patients and in patients with mild or moderate renal failure. Since NSAIDs and rosiglitazone are associated with fluid retention, concomitant administration may increase the risk of oedema.

Monitoring of liver function

There have been rare reports of hepatocellular dysfunction during post-marketing experience with rosiglitazone (see section 4.8). There is limited experience with rosiglitazone in patients with elevated liver enzymes (ALT > 2.5 times the upper limit of normal). Therefore, liver enzymes should be checked prior to the initiation of therapy with Avandamet in all patients and periodically thereafter based on clinical judgement. Therapy with Avandamet should not be initiated in patients with increased baseline liver enzyme levels (ALT > 2.5 times the upper limit of normal) or with any other evidence of liver disease. If ALT levels are increased to > 3 times the upper limit of normal during Avandamet therapy, liver enzyme levels should be reassessed as soon as possible. If ALT levels remain > 3 times the upper limit of normal, therapy should be discontinued. If any patient develops symptoms suggesting hepatic dysfunction, which may include unexplained nausea, vomiting, abdominal pain, fatigue, anorexia and/or dark urine, liver enzymes should be checked. The decision whether to continue the patient on therapy with Avandamet should be guided by clinical judgement pending laboratory evaluations. If jaundice is observed, therapy should be discontinued.

Weight gain

In clinical trials with rosiglitazone there was evidence of weight gain, therefore weight should be closely monitored.

Anaemia

Rosiglitazone treatment is associated with a reduction of haemoglobin levels. In patients with low haemoglobin levels before initiating therapy, there is an increased risk of anaemia during treatment with Avandamet.

Surgery

As Avandamet contains metformin hydrochloride, the treatment should be discontinued 48 hours before elective surgery with general anaesthesia and should not usually be resumed earlier than 48 hours afterwards.

Administration of iodinated contrast agent

The intravascular administration of iodinated contrast agents in radiological studies can lead to renal failure. Therefore, due to the metformin active substance, Avandamet should be discontinued prior to, or at the time of the test and not reinstituted until 48 hours afterwards, and only after renal function has been re-evaluated and found to be normal (see section 4.5).

Other precautions

Premenopausal women have received rosiglitazone during clinical studies. Although hormonal imbalance has been seen in preclinical studies (see section 5.3), no significant undesirable effects associated with menstrual disorders have been observed. As a consequence of improving insulin sensitivity, resumption of ovulation may occur in patients who are anovulatory due to insulin resistance. Patients should be aware of the risk of pregnancy (see section 4.6).

Rosiglitazone should be used with caution during concomitant administration of CYP2C8 inhibitors (e.g. gemfibrozil) or inducers (e.g. rifampicin). Glycaemic control should be monitored closely. Rosiglitazone dose adjustment within the recommended posology or changes in diabetic treatment should be considered (see section 4.5).

All patients should continue their diet with regular distribution of carbohydrate intake during the day.

Overweight patients should continue their energy-restricted diet.

The usual laboratory tests for diabetes monitoring should be performed regularly.

Avandamet tablets contain lactose and therefore should not be administered to patients with rare hereditary problems of galactose intolerance, the Lapp lactase deficiency or glucose-galactose malabsorption.

4.5 Interaction with other medicinal products and other forms of Interaction

There have been no formal interaction studies for Avandamet, however the concomitant use of the active substances in patients in clinical studies and in widespread clinical use has not resulted in any unexpected interactions. The following statements reflect the information available on the individual active substances (rosiglitazone and metformin).

There is increased risk of lactic acidosis in acute alcohol intoxication (particularly in the case of fasting, malnutrition or hepatic insufficiency) due to the metformin active substance of Avandamet (see section 4.4). Avoid consumption of alcohol and medicinal products containing alcohol.

In vitro studies demonstrate that rosiglitazone is predominantly metabolised by CYP2C8, with CYP2C9 as only a minor pathway.

Co-administration of rosiglitazone with gemfibrozil (an inhibitor of CYP2C8) resulted in a twofold increase in rosiglitazone plasma concentrations. Since there is a potential for an increase in the risk of dose-related adverse reactions, a decrease in rosiglitazone dose may be needed. Close monitoring of glycaemic control should be considered (see section 4.4).

Co-administration of rosiglitazone with rifampicin (an inducer of CYP2C8) resulted in a 66% decrease in rosiglitazone plasma concentrations. It cannot be excluded that other inducers (e.g. phenytoin, carbamazepine, phenobarbital, St John's wort) may also affect rosiglitazone exposure. The rosiglitazone dose may need to be increased. Close monitoring of glycaemic control should be considered (see section 4.4).

Clinically significant interactions with CYP2C9 substrates or inhibitors are not anticipated.

Concomitant administration of rosiglitazone with the oral antihyperglycaemic agents glibenclamide and acarbose did not result in any clinically relevant pharmacokinetic interactions.

No clinically relevant interactions with digoxin, the CYP2C9 substrate warfarin, the CYP3A4 substrates nifedipine, ethinylestradiol or norethindrone were observed after co-administration with rosiglitazone.

Intravascular administration of iodinated contrast agents may lead to renal failure, resulting in metformin accumulation and a risk of lactic acidosis. Metformin should be discontinued prior to, or at the time of the test and not reinstituted until 48 hours afterwards and only after renal function has been re-evaluated and found to be normal.

Combination requiring precautions for use

Glucocorticoids (given by systemic and local routes) beta-2-agonists, and diuretics have intrinsic hyperglycaemic activity. The patient should be informed and more frequent blood glucose monitoring performed, especially at the beginning of treatment. If necessary, the dosage of the antihyperglycaemic medicinal product should be adjusted during therapy with the other medicinal product and on its discontinuation.

ACE-inhibitors may decrease the blood glucose levels. If necessary, the dosage of the antihyperglycaemic medicinal product should be adjusted during therapy with the other medicinal product and on its discontinuation.

4.6 Pregnancy and lactation

For Avandamet no preclinical or clinical data on exposed pregnancies or lactation are available.

There are no adequate data for the use of rosiglitazone in pregnant women. Studies in animals have shown reproductive toxicity (see section 5.3). The potential risk for humans is unknown.

Therefore, Avandamet should not be used during pregnancy. If a patient wishes to become pregnant or if pregnancy occurs, treatment with AVANDAMET should be discontinued unless the expected benefit to the mother outweighs the potential risk to the foetus.

Both rosiglitazone and metformin have been detected in the milk of experimental animals. It is not known whether breast-feeding will lead to exposure of the infant to the medicinal product. Avandamet must therefore not be used in women who are breast-feeding (see section 4.3).

4.7 Effects on ability to drive and use machines

Avandamet has no or negligible influence on the ability to drive or use machines.

4.8 Undesirable effects

There have been no therapeutic clinical trials conducted with Avandamet tablets however bioequivalence of Avandamet with co-administered rosiglitazone and metformin has been demonstrated (see section 5.2). The data presented here relate to the co-administration of rosiglitazone and metformin, where rosiglitazone has been added to metformin. There have been no studies of metformin added to rosiglitazone.

Frequencies for adverse reactions are listed below by system organ class and are defined as: very common ($\geqslant$ 1/10), common ($\geqslant$ 1/100, < 1/10), uncommon ($\geqslant$ 1/1,000, < 1/100), rare ($\geqslant$ 1/10,000, < 1/1,000) and very rare (< 1/10,000).

Rosiglitazone and metformin

Adverse reactions (with suspected/probable relationship to treatment reported as more than an isolated case) in patients receiving concomitantly administered rosiglitazone and metformin in excess of metformin alone in double-blind studies are listed below.

Blood and the lymphatic system disorders

Common: anaemia.

Metabolism and nutrition disorders

Common: hypoglycaemia.

Uncommon: hyperlipaemia, diabetes mellitus aggravated, hypercholesterolaemia, weight increase, anorexia.

Gastrointestinal disorders

Common: flatulence, nausea, gastritis, vomiting.

Uncommon: constipation.

General disorders and administration site conditions

Uncommon: oedema dependent.

In double-blind studies, oedema occurred in 5.2% of patients and hypercholesterolaemia in 2.1% of patients treated with rosiglitazone and metformin. The incidence of anaemia was higher when rosiglitazone was used in combination with metformin. The elevated total cholesterol levels were associated with an increase in both LDLc and HDLc, but the ratio of total cholesterol:HDLc was unchanged or improved in long term studies. Overall, these increases were generally mild to moderate and usually did not require discontinuation of treatment.

In double-blind studies, the incidence of all adverse events relating to liver and biliary systems was 1.1% for rosiglitazone and metformin compared to an incidence of 1.1% for metformin alone.

Heart failure occurred uncommonly during double-blind clinical studies of rosiglitazone in combination with metformin (0.2%) but was reported with a higher incidence during studies of rosiglitazone in combination with insulin (2.5%).

In 24 month studies, rosiglitazone treatment in combination with metformin was associated with a mean increase of 4.5% in weight.

Additional information on the individual active substances of the fixed dose combination

Rosiglitazone

In double-blind clinical trials with rosiglitazone the incidence of elevations of ALT greater than three times the upper limit of normal was equal to placebo (0.2%).

Rare cases of elevated liver enzymes and hepatocellular dysfunction have been reported in post-marketing experience. Although in very rare cases, a fatal outcome has been reported, causal relationship has not been established.

Rare cases of congestive heart failure and pulmonary oedema have been reported in post-marketing experience.

Very rare cases of angioedema and urticaria have been reported in post-marketing experience.

Very rare cases of rapid and excessive weight gain have been reported in post-marketing experience.

Metformin

Gastrointestinal symptoms such as nausea, vomiting, diarrhoea, abdominal pain and loss of appetite are very common. These occur most frequently during initiation of therapy and resolve spontaneously in most cases.

Metallic taste is common.

Mild erythema has been reported very rarely in some hypersensitive individuals.

A decrease of vitamin B12 absorption with decrease of serum levels has been very rarely observed in patients treated long-term with metformin and appears generally to be without clinical significance).

Lactic acidosis (0.03 cases/1,000 patient-years) is very rare (see section 4.4).

4.9 Overdose

No data are available with regard to overdose of Avandamet.

Limited data are available with regard to overdose of rosiglitazone in humans. In clinical studies in volunteers rosiglitazone has been administered at single oral doses of up to 20 mg and was well tolerated.

A large overdose of metformin (or coexisting risks of lactic acidosis) may lead to lactic acidosis, which is a medical emergency and must be treated in hospital.

In the event of an overdose, it is recommended that appropriate supportive treatment is initiated as dictated by the patient's clinical status. The most effective method to remove lactate and metformin is haemodialysis, however rosiglitazone is highly protein bound and is not cleared by haemodialysis.

5. PHARMACOLOGICAL PROPERTIES

5.1 Pharmacodynamic properties

Pharmacotherapeutic group: Combinations of oral blood glucose lowering drugs. ATC code: A10B D03.

Avandamet combines two antihyperglycaemic agents with complimentary mechanisms of action to improve glycaemic control in patients with type 2 diabetes: rosiglitazone maleate, a member of the thiazolidinedione class and metformin hydrochloride, a member of the biguanide class. Thiazolidinediones act primarily by reducing insulin resistance and biguanides act primarily by decreasing endogenous hepatic glucose production.

Rosiglitazone

Rosiglitazone is a selective agonist at the PPARγ (peroxisome proliferator activated receptor gamma) nuclear receptor and is a member of the thiazolidinedione class of antihyperglycaemic agents. It reduces glycaemia by reducing insulin resistance at adipose tissue, skeletal muscle and liver.

The antihyperglycaemic activity of rosiglitazone has been demonstrated in a number of animal models of type 2 diabetes. In addition, rosiglitazone preserved β-cell function as shown by increased pancreatic islet mass and insulin content and prevented the development of overt hyperglycaemia in animal models of type 2 diabetes. Rosiglitazone did not stimulate pancreatic insulin secretion or induce hypoglycaemia in rats and mice. The major metabolite (a para-hydroxy-sulphate) with high affinity to the soluble human PPARγ, exhibited relatively high potency in a glucose tolerance assay in obese mice. The clinical relevance of this observation has not been fully elucidated.

In clinical trials, the glucose lowering effects observed with rosiglitazone are gradual in onset with near maximal reductions in fasting plasma glucose (FPG) evident following approximately 8 weeks of therapy. The improved glycaemic control is associated with reductions in both fasting and post-prandial glucose.

Rosiglitazone was associated with increases in weight. In mechanistic studies, the weight increase was predominantly shown to be due to increased subcutaneous fat with decreased visceral and intra-hepatic fat.

Consistent with the mechanism of action, rosiglitazone in combination with metformin reduced insulin resistance and improved pancreatic β-cell function. Improved glycaemic control was also associated with significant decreases in free fatty acids. As a consequence of different but complementary mechanisms of action, combination therapy of rosiglitazone with metformin resulted in additive effects on glycaemic control in type 2 diabetic patients.

In studies with a maximal duration of three years, rosiglitazone given once or twice daily in combination with metformin produced a sustained improvement in glycaemic control (FPG and HbA1c). A more pronounced glucose-lowering effect was observed in obese patients. An outcome study has not been completed with rosiglitazone, therefore the long-term benefits associated with improved glycaemic control of rosiglitazone have not been demonstrated.

There are no studies completed assessing long-term cardiovascular outcome in patients receiving rosiglitazone in combination with metformin.

Metformin

Metformin is a biguanide with antihyperglycaemic effects, lowering both basal and postprandial plasma glucose. It does not stimulate insulin secretion and therefore does not produce hypoglycaemia.

Metformin may act via three mechanisms:

- by reduction of hepatic glucose production by inhibiting gluconeogenesis and glycogenolysis
- in muscle, by modestly increasing insulin sensitivity, improving peripheral glucose uptake and utilisation
- by delaying intestinal glucose absorption.

Metformin stimulates intracellular glycogen synthesis by acting on glycogen synthase. Metformin increases the transport capacity of specific types of membrane glucose transporters (GLUT-1 and GLUT-4).

In humans, independently of its action on glycaemia, metformin has favourable effects on lipid metabolism. This has been shown at therapeutic doses in controlled, medium-term or long-term clinical studies: metformin reduces total cholesterol, LDLc and triglyceride levels.

The prospective randomised (UKPDS) study has established the long-term benefit of intensive blood glucose control in type 2 diabetes. Analysis of the results for overweight patients treated with metformin after failure of diet alone showed:

- a significant reduction of the absolute risk of any diabetes-related complication in the metformin group (29.8 events/1,000 patient-years) versus diet alone (43.3 events/1,000 patient-years), p=0.0023, and versus the combined sulphonylurea and insulin monotherapy groups (40.1 events/1,000 patient-years), p=0.0034
- a significant reduction of the absolute risk of diabetes-related mortality: metformin 7.5 events/1,000 patient-years, diet alone 12.7 events/1,000 patient-years, p=0.017
- a significant reduction of the absolute risk of overall mortality: metformin 13.5 events/1,000 patient-years versus diet alone 20.6 events/1,000 patient-years (p=0.011), and versus the combined sulphonylurea and insulin monotherapy groups 18.9 events/1,000 patient-years (p=0.021)
- a significant reduction in the absolute risk of myocardial infarction: metformin 11 events/1,000 patient-years, diet alone 18 events/1,000 patient-years (p=0.01).

5.2 Pharmacokinetic properties

Avandamet

Absorption:

No statistically significant difference was observed between the absorption characteristics of rosiglitazone and metformin from the Avandamet tablet and those obtained from rosiglitazone maleate and metformin hydrochloride tablets, respectively.

Food had no effect on the AUC of rosiglitazone or metformin when Avandamet was administered to healthy volunteers. In the fed state, C_{max} was lower (22% rosiglitazone and 15% metformin) and t_{max} delayed (by approx. 1.5 h rosiglitazone and 0.5 h metformin). This food-effect is not considered clinically significant.

The following statements reflect the pharmacokinetic properties of the individual active substances of Avandamet.

Rosiglitazone

Absorption:

Absolute bioavailability of rosiglitazone following both a 4 and an 8 mg oral dose is approximately 99%. Rosiglitazone plasma concentrations peak at around 1 h after dosing. Plasma concentrations are approximately dose proportional over the therapeutic dose range.

Administration of rosiglitazone with food resulted in no change in overall exposure (AUC), although a small decrease in C_{max} (approx. 20-28%) and a delay in t_{max} (approx. 1.75 h) were observed compared to dosing in the fasting state. These small changes are not clinically significant and, therefore, it is not necessary to administer rosiglitazone at any particular time in relation to meals. The absorption of rosiglitazone is not affected by increases in gastric pH.

Distribution:

The volume of distribution of rosiglitazone is approximately 14 l in healthy volunteers. Plasma protein binding of rosiglitazone is high (approximately 99.8%) and is not influenced by concentration or age. The protein binding of the major metabolite (a para-hydroxy-sulphate) is very high > 99.99%).

Metabolism:

Metabolism of rosiglitazone is extensive with no parent compound being excreted unchanged. The major routes of metabolism are N-demethylation and hydroxylation, followed by conjugation with sulphate and glucuronic acid. The contribution of the major metabolite (a para-hydroxy-sulphate) to the overall antihyperglycaemic activity of rosiglitazone has not been fully elucidated in man and it cannot be ruled out that the metabolite may contribute to the activity. However, this raises no safety concern regarding target or special populations as hepatic impairment is contraindicated and the phase III clinical studies included a considerable number of elderly patients and patients with mild to moderate renal impairment.

In vitro studies demonstrate that rosiglitazone is predominantly metabolised by CYP2C8, with a minor contribution by CYP2C9.

Since there is no significant *in vitro* inhibition of CYP1A2, 2A6, 2C19, 2D6, 2E1, 3A or 4A with rosiglitazone, there is a low probability of significant metabolism-based interactions with substances metabolised by these P450 enzymes. Rosiglitazone showed moderate inhibition of CYP2C8 (IC_{50} 18 μM) and low inhibition of CYP2C9 (IC_{50} 50 μM) *in vitro* (see section 4.5). An *in vivo* interaction study with warfarin indicated that rosiglitazone does not interact with CYP2C9 substrates *in vivo*.

Elimination:

Total plasma clearance of rosiglitazone is around 3 l/h and the terminal elimination half-life of rosiglitazone is approximately 3-4 h. There is no evidence for unexpected accumulation of rosiglitazone after once or twice daily dosing. The major route of excretion is the urine with approximately two-thirds of the dose being eliminated by this route, whereas faecal elimination accounts for approximately 25% of dose. No intact active substance is excreted in urine or faeces. The terminal half-life for radioactivity was about 130 h indicating that elimination of metabolites is very slow. Accumulation of the metabolites in plasma is expected upon repeated dosing, especially that of the major metabolite (a para-hydroxy-sulphate) for which an 8-fold accumulation is anticipated.

Special populations:

Gender: In the pooled population pharmacokinetic analysis, there were no marked differences in the pharmacokinetics of rosiglitazone between males and females.

Elderly: In the pooled population pharmacokinetic analysis, age was not found to influence the pharmacokinetics of rosiglitazone to any significant extent.

Hepatic impairment: In cirrhotic patients with moderate (Child-Pugh B) hepatic impairment, unbound C_{max} and AUC were 2- and 3-fold higher than in normal subjects. The inter-subject variability was large, with a 7-fold difference in unbound AUC between patients.

Renal insufficiency: There are no clinically significant differences in the pharmacokinetics of rosiglitazone in patients with renal impairment or end stage renal disease on chronic dialysis.

Metformin

Absorption:

After an oral dose of metformin, t_{max} is reached in 2.5 h. Absolute bioavailability of a 500 mg metformin tablet is approximately 50-60% in healthy subjects. After an oral dose, the non-absorbed fraction recovered in faeces was 20-30%.

After oral administration, metformin absorption is saturable and incomplete. It is assumed that the pharmacokinetics of metformin absorption is non-linear. At the usual metformin doses and dosing schedules, steady state plasma concentrations are reached within 24-48 h and are generally less than 1 μg/ml. In controlled clinical trials, maximum metformin plasma levels (C_{max}) did not exceed 4 μg/ml, even at maximum doses.

Food decreases the extent and slightly delays the absorption of metformin. Following administration of a dose of 850 mg, a 40% lower plasma peak concentration, a 25% decrease in AUC and a 35 min prolongation of time to peak plasma concentration was observed. The clinical relevance of this decrease is unknown.

Distribution:

Plasma protein binding is negligible. Metformin partitions into erythrocytes. The blood peak is lower than the plasma peak and appears at approximately the same time. The red blood cells most likely represent a secondary compartment of distribution. The mean V_d ranged between 63 - 276 l.

Metabolism:

Metformin is excreted unchanged in the urine. No metabolites have been identified in humans.

Elimination:

Renal clearance of metformin is > 400 ml/min, indicating that metformin is eliminated by glomerular filtration and tubular secretion. Following an oral dose, the apparent terminal elimination half-life is approximately 6.5 h. When renal function is impaired, renal clearance is decreased in proportion to that of creatinine and thus the elimination half-life is prolonged, leading to increased levels of metformin in plasma.

5.3 Preclinical safety data

No animal studies have been conducted with the combined products in Avandamet. The following data are findings in studies performed with rosiglitazone or metformin individually.

Rosiglitazone

Undesirable effects observed in animal studies with possible relevance to clinical use were as follows: An increase in plasma volume accompanied by decrease in red cell parameters and increase in heart weight. Increases in liver weight, plasma ALT (dog only) and fat tissue were also observed. Similar effects have been seen with other thiazolidinediones.

In reproductive toxicity studies, administration of rosiglitazone to rats during mid-late gestation was associated with foetal death and retarded foetal development. In addition, rosiglitazone inhibited ovarian oestradiol and progesterone synthesis and lowered plasma levels of these hormones resulting in effects on oestrus/menstrual cycles and fertility (see section 4.4).

In an animal model for familial adenomatous polyposis (FAP), treatment with rosiglitazone at 200 times the pharmacologically active dose increased tumour multiplicity in the colon. The relevance of this finding is unknown. However, rosiglitazone promoted differentiation and reversal of mutagenic changes in human colon cancer cells *in vitro*. In addition, rosiglitazone was not genotoxic in a battery of *in vivo* and *in vitro* genotoxicity studies and there was no evidence of colon tumours in lifetime studies of rosiglitazone in two rodent species.

Metformin

Preclinical data for metformin reveal no special hazard for humans based on conventional studies of safety pharmacology, repeated dose toxicity, genotoxicity, carcinogenic potential, toxicity to reproduction.

6. PHARMACEUTICAL PARTICULARS

6.1 List of excipients

Tablet-core:

Sodium starch glycollate, hypromellose (E464), microcrystalline cellulose (E460), lactose monohydrate, povidone (E1201), magnesium stearate.

Avandamet 2 mg/1000 mg film-coating:

Hypromellose (E464), titanium dioxide (E171), macrogol, iron oxide yellow (E172).

Avandamet 2 mg/500 mg and Avandamet 4 mg/1000 mg film-coating:

Hypromellose (E464), titanium dioxide (E171), macrogol, iron oxide red (E172).

6.2 Incompatibilities

Not applicable.

6.3 Shelf life

2 years.

6.4 Special precautions for storage

This medicinal product does not require any special storage conditions.

6.5 Nature and contents of container

Avandamet 2 mg/500 mg tablets: Opaque blisters (PVC/PVdC/aluminium). Packs of 112 tablets.

Avandamet 2 mg/1000 mg and 4 mg/1000 mg tablets:

Opaque blisters (PVC/PVdC/aluminium). Packs of 56 tablets.

6.6 Instructions for use and handling

No special requirements.

Administrative Data

7. MARKETING AUTHORISATION HOLDER

SmithKline Beecham plc

980 Great West Road

Brentford, Middlesex

TW8 9GS

United Kingdom

8. MARKETING AUTHORISATION NUMBER(S)

EU/1/03/258/006 – Avandamet 2 mg/500 mg – 112 film-coated tablets.

EU/1/03/258/009 – Avandamet 2 mg/1000 mg – 56 film coated tablets

EU/1/03/258/012 – Avandamet 4 mg/1000 mg – 56 film-coated tablets

9. DATE OF FIRST AUTHORISATION/RENEWAL OF THE AUTHORISATION

20 October 2003 - Avandamet 2 mg/500 mg

02 September 2004 – Avandamet 2 mg/1000 mg

02 September 2004 – Avandamet 4 mg/1000 mg

10. DATE OF REVISION OF THE TEXT

20 January 2005

Avandia 4mg & 8mg Tablets

(GlaxoSmithKline UK)

1. NAME OF THE MEDICINAL PRODUCT

AVANDIA* 4 mg film-coated tablets

AVANDIA* 8 mg film-coated tablets

2. QUALITATIVE AND QUANTITATIVE COMPOSITION

Each tablet contains rosiglitazone maleate corresponding to 4 or 8 mg rosiglitazone.

For excipients see section 6.1.

3. PHARMACEUTICAL FORM

Film-coated tablets

4 mg - Orange film-coated tablets debossed with "GSK" on one side and "4" on the other side.

8 mg - Red-brown film-coated tablets debossed with "GSK" on one side and "8" on the other side.

4. CLINICAL PARTICULARS

4.1 Therapeutic indications

Rosiglitazone is indicated in the treatment of type 2 diabetes mellitus:

as **monotherapy**

– in patients (particularly overweight patients) inadequately controlled by diet and exercise for whom metformin is inappropriate because of contraindications or intolerance

as **dual oral therapy** in combination with

– metformin, in patients (particularly overweight patients) with insufficient glycaemic control despite maximal tolerated dose of monotherapy with metformin

– a sulphonylurea, only in patients who show intolerance to metformin or for whom metformin is contraindicated, with insufficient glycaemic control despite monotherapy with a sulphonylurea

as **triple oral therapy** in combination with

– metformin and a sulphonylurea, in patients (particularly overweight patients) with insufficient glycaemic control despite dual oral therapy (see section 4.4).

4.2 Posology and method of administration

Experience from clinical trials with rosiglitazone is currently limited to three years. The long-term benefits of therapy with rosiglitazone have not been demonstrated (see section 5.1).

Rosiglitazone therapy is usually initiated at 4 mg/day. This dose can be increased to 8 mg/day after eight weeks if greater glycaemic control is required.

Rosiglitazone may be given once or twice a day.

Rosiglitazone may be taken with or without food.

Elderly

No dose adjustment is required in the elderly.

Patients with renal impairment

No dose adjustment is required in patients with mild and moderate renal insufficiency. Limited data are available in patients with severe renal insufficiency (creatinine clearance < 30ml/min) and therefore rosiglitazone should be used with caution in these patients.

Patients with hepatic impairment

Rosiglitazone should not be used in patients with hepatic impairment.

Children and adolescents

There are no data available on the use of rosiglitazone in patients under 10 years of age. For children aged 10 to 17 years, there are limited data on rosiglitazone as monotherapy (see sections 5.1 and 5.2). The available data do not support efficacy in the paediatric population and therefore such use is not recommended.

4.3 Contraindications

Use of rosiglitazone is contraindicated in patients with:

known hypersensitivity to rosiglitazone or to any of the excipients of the tablet, or cardiac failure or history of cardiac failure (NYHA class I to IV), or hepatic impairment.

Rosiglitazone is also contraindicated for use in combination with insulin.

4.4 Special warnings and special precautions for use

Fluid retention and cardiac failure

Rosiglitazone can cause dose dependent fluid retention which may exacerbate or precipitate heart failure. Signs and symptoms of fluid retention, including weight gain, should be monitored. The possible contribution of fluid retention to weight gain should be individually assessed. Rapid and excessive weight gain has been reported very rarely as a sign of fluid retention. Patients should be observed for signs and symptoms of heart failure, particularly those with reduced cardiac reserve. Rosiglitazone should be discontinued if any deterioration in cardiac status occurs. An increased incidence of cardiac failure has been observed in clinical trials when rosiglitazone is used in combination with insulin. Therefore rosiglitazone is contraindicated in combination with insulin. Heart failure was also reported more frequently in patients with a history of heart failure, in elderly patients and in patients with mild or moderate renal failure. Since NSAIDs and rosiglitazone are associated with fluid retention, concomitant administration may increase the risk of oedema.

Monitoring of liver function

There have been rare reports of hepatocellular dysfunction during postmarketing experience (see section 4.8). There is limited experience with rosiglitazone in patients with elevated liver enzymes (ALT > 2.5X upper limit of normal). Therefore, liver enzymes should be checked prior to the initiation of therapy with rosiglitazone in all patients and periodically thereafter based on clinical judgement. Therapy with rosiglitazone should not be initiated in patients with increased baseline liver enzyme levels (ALT > 2.5X upper limit of normal) or with any other evidence of liver disease. If ALT levels are increased to > 3X upper limit of normal during rosiglitazone therapy, liver enzyme levels should be reassessed as soon as possible. If ALT levels remain > 3X the upper limit of normal, therapy should be discontinued. If any patient develops symptoms suggesting hepatic dysfunction, which may include unexplained nausea, vomiting, abdominal pain, fatigue, anorexia and/or dark urine, liver enzymes should be checked. The decision whether to continue the patient on therapy with rosiglitazone should be guided by clinical judgement pending laboratory evaluations. If jaundice is observed, drug therapy should be discontinued.

Weight gain

In clinical trials with rosiglitazone there was evidence of dose-related weight gain, therefore weight should be closely monitored.

Anaemia

Rosiglitazone treatment is associated with a dose-related reduction of haemoglobin levels. In patients with low haemoglobin levels before initiating therapy, there is an increased risk of anaemia during treatment with rosiglitazone.

Hypoglycaemia

Patients receiving rosiglitazone in dual or triple oral therapy with a sulphonylurea may be at risk for dose-related hypoglycaemia, and a reduction in the dose of the sulphonylurea may be necessary.

Triple oral therapy

The use of rosiglitazone in triple oral therapy, in combination with metformin and a sulphonylurea, may be associated with increased risks for fluid retention and heart failure, as well as hypoglycaemia (see section 4.8). Increased monitoring of the patient is recommended and adjustment of the dose of sulphonylurea may be necessary. The decision to initiate triple oral therapy should include consideration of the alternative to switch the patient to insulin.

Others

Premenopausal women have received rosiglitazone during clinical studies. Although hormonal imbalance has been seen in preclinical studies (see section 5.3), no significant undesirable effects associated with menstrual disorders have been observed. As a consequence of improving insulin sensitivity, resumption of ovulation may occur in patients who are anovulatory due to insulin resistance. Patients should be aware of the risk of pregnancy and if a patient wishes to become pregnant or if pregnancy occurs the treatment should be discontinued (see section 4.6).

Rosiglitazone should be used with caution in patients with severe renal insufficiency (creatinine clearance < 30ml/min).

Rosiglitazone should be used with caution during concomitant administration of CYP2C8 inhibitors (e.g. gemfibrozil) or inducers (e.g. rifampicin). Glycaemic control should be monitored closely. Rosiglitazone dose adjustment within the recommended posology or changes in diabetic treatment should be considered (see section 4.5).

Avandia tablets contain lactose and therefore should not be administered to patients with rare hereditary problems of galactose intolerance, the Lapp lactase deficiency or glucose-galactose malabsorption.

4.5 Interaction with other medicinal products and other forms of Interaction

In vitro studies demonstrate that rosiglitazone is predominantly metabolised by CYP2C8, with CYP2C9 as only a minor pathway.

Co-administration of rosiglitazone with gemfibrozil (an inhibitor of CYP2C8) resulted in a twofold increase in rosiglitazone plasma concentrations. Since there is a potential for an increase in the risk of dose-related adverse reactions, a decrease in rosiglitazone dose may be needed. Close monitoring of glycaemic control should be considered (see section 4.4).

Co-administration of rosiglitazone with rifampicin (an inducer of CYP2C8) resulted in a 66% decrease in rosiglitazone plasma concentrations. It cannot be excluded that other inducers (e.g. phenytoin, carbamazepine, phenobarbital, St John's wort) may also affect rosiglitazone exposure. The rosiglitazone dose may need to be increased. Close monitoring of glycaemic control should be considered (see section 4.4).

Clinically significant interactions with CYP2C9 substrates or inhibitors are not anticipated.

Concomitant administration with the oral anti-diabetic agents metformin, glibenclamide and acarbose did not result in any clinically relevant pharmacokinetic interactions with rosiglitazone. Moderate ingestion of alcohol with rosiglitazone has no effect on glycaemic control.

No clinically relevant interactions with digoxin, the CYP2C9 substrate warfarin, the CYP3A4 substrates nifedipine, ethinylestradiol or norethindrone were observed after co-administration with rosiglitazone.

4.6 Pregnancy and lactation

There are no adequate data from the use of rosiglitazone in pregnant women. Studies in animals have shown reproductive toxicity (see section 5.3). The potential risk for humans is unknown. Rosiglitazone should not be used during pregnancy.

Rosiglitazone has been detected in the milk of experimental animals. It is not known whether breast-feeding will lead to exposure of the infant to drug. Rosiglitazone should therefore not be used in women who are breast-feeding.

4.7 Effects on ability to drive and use machines

No effects on the ability to drive or operate machinery have been observed.

4.8 Undesirable effects

Adverse reactions* reported in excess > 0.2% of placebo (monotherapy) or comparator (combination therapy), and as more than an isolated case, in patients receiving rosiglitazone in double-blind studies are listed below, by system organ class and absolute frequency. Frequencies are defined as: very common ⩾ 1/10, common ⩾ 1/100, < 1/10; uncommon ⩾ 1/1000, < 1/100.

* defined as events with suspected/probable relationship to treatment as reported by the investigator.

ROSIGLITAZONE MONOTHERAPY

Blood and the lymphatic system disorders

Common: anaemia

Metabolism and nutrition disorders

Common: hypercholesterolaemia

Uncommon: hyperlipaemia, hypertriglyceridaemia, weight increase, appetite increase

Nervous system disorders

Uncommon: paraesthesia

Gastrointestinal disorders

Uncommon: flatulence

Renal and urinary disorders

Uncommon: glycosuria

ROSIGLITAZONE IN DUAL ORAL THERAPY WITH METFORMIN

Blood and the lymphatic system disorders

Common: anaemia

Metabolism and nutrition disorders

Common: hypoglycaemia

Uncommon: hyperlipaemia, diabetes mellitus aggravated, hypercholesterolaemia, weight increase, anorexia

Gastrointestinal disorders

Common: flatulence, nausea, vomiting, gastritis

Uncommon: constipation

General disorders and administration site conditions

Common: oedema dependent

ROSIGLITAZONE IN DUAL ORAL THERAPY WITH SULPHONYLUREA

Blood and the lymphatic system disorders

Common: thrombocytopenia, anaemia

Uncommon: leukopenia

Metabolism and nutrition disorders

Common: hypoglycaemia, weight increase, hyperlipaemia

Uncommon: hypercholesterolaemia, hypertriglyceridaemia, appetite increased

Nervous system disorders

Common: dizziness

Respiratory, thoracic and mediastinal disorders

Uncommon: dyspnoea

Gastrointestinal disorders

Uncommon: flatulence

Hepatobiliary disorders

Uncommon: hepatic function abnormal

Skin and subcutaneous tissue disorders

Common: face oedema

General disorders and administration site conditions

Common: oedema

Uncommon: fatigue

ROSIGLITAZONE IN TRIPLE ORAL THERAPY WITH METFORMIN AND SULPHONYLUREA

Blood and the lymphatic system disorders

Common: anaemia

Uncommon: granulocytopenia

Metabolism and nutrition disorders

Very Common: hypoglycaemia

Common: hypercholesterolaemia, weight increase, hyperlipaemia

Uncommon: anorexia

Nervous system disorders

Uncommon: headache, dizziness

Cardiac disorders

Uncommon: cardiac failure

Gastrointestinal disorders

Common: nausea

Uncommon: dyspepsia

Musculoskeletal and connective tissue disorders

Uncommon: myalgia

General disorders and administration site conditions

Common: oedema

The occurrence of the following events are reported as incidence figures (%).

In double blind studies, oedema (which was generally dose-related) occurred in patients treated with rosiglitazone as monotherapy (5.4%), dual oral therapy with metformin (5.2%), dual oral therapy with sulphonylurea (10.4%) and triple oral therapy (12.1%).

Heart failure occurred uncommonly during double-blind clinical studies of rosiglitazone in monotherapy (0.2%) and in dual oral therapy with sulphonylurea (0.5%) or metformin (0.2%) but was reported with a five-fold higher incidence during studies of rosiglitazone in combination with insulin (2.5%). The incidence of heart failure on triple oral therapy was 1.4% in the main double blind study.

In a placebo-controlled one-year trial in patients with congestive heart failure NYHA class I-II, worsening or possible worsening of heart failure occurred in 6.4% of patients treated with rosiglitazone, compared with 3.5% on placebo.

Rare cases (frequency ⩾ 1/10000, < 1/1000) of congestive heart failure and pulmonary oedema have been reported in post-marketing experience for rosiglitazone as monotherapy and in combination with other oral antidiabetic agents.

In double-blind studies, dose-related hypoglycaemia occurred when rosiglitazone was used in combination with sulphonylurea in dual and triple oral therapy (9.7% and 30.7%, respectively).

Anaemia was generally dose-related and the incidence was highest when rosiglitazone was used in combination with metformin. Adverse experiences of hypercholesterolaemia were reported in up to 5.3% of patients treated with rosiglitazone (monotherapy, dual or triple oral therapy). The elevated total cholesterol levels were associated with increase in both LDLc and HDLc, but the ratio of total cholesterol:HDLc was unchanged or improved in long term studies. Overall, these increases were generally mild to moderate and usually did not require discontinuation of treatment.

In double-blind clinical trials with rosiglitazone the incidence of elevations of ALT greater than three times the upper limit of normal was equal to placebo (0.2%) and less than that of the active comparators (0.5% metformin/sulphonylureas). The incidence of all adverse events relating to liver and biliary systems was < 1.5% in any treatment group and similar to placebo. Rare cases (frequency ⩾1/10000, <1/1000) of elevated liver enzymes and hepatocellular dysfunction have been reported in post-marketing experience. Although in very rare cases fatal outcome has been reported, causal relationship has not been established.

Very rarely cases (frequency < 1/10000) of angioedema and urticaria have been reported in post-marketing experience.

Weight gain was generally dose-related. In 24 month studies, rosiglitazone treatment was associated with a mean increase of 4.5% (4.1 kg) in weight in dual oral therapy with metformin and a mean increase of 4.9% (4.3 kg) in dual oral therapy with sulphonylurea. As monotherapy, rosiglitazone was associated with a mean increase of 3.9% (3.7 kg) in weight at 18 months. As triple oral therapy, rosiglitazone was associated with a mean increase of 4.3% (4.0 kg) at 44 weeks.

Very rarely cases (frequency < 1/10000) of rapid and excessive weight gain have been reported in post-marketing experience.

4.9 Overdose

Limited data are available with regard to overdose in humans. In clinical studies in volunteers rosiglitazone has been administered at single oral doses of up to 20 mg and was well tolerated.

In the event of an overdose, it is recommended that appropriate supportive treatment should be initiated, as dictated by the patient's clinical status. Rosiglitazone is highly protein bound and is not cleared by haemodialysis.

5. PHARMACOLOGICAL PROPERTIES

5.1 Pharmacodynamic properties

Pharmacotherapeutic group: oral blood glucose lowering drugs; thiazolidinediones; ATC code: A10 BG 02

Rosiglitazone is a selective agonist at the PPARγ (peroxisomal proliferator activated receptor gamma) nuclear receptor and is a member of the thiazolidinedione class of anti-diabetic agents. It reduces glycaemia by reducing insulin resistance at adipose tissue, skeletal muscle and liver.

Pre-clinical data

The antihyperglycaemic activity of rosiglitazone has been demonstrated in a number of animal models of type 2 diabetes. In addition, rosiglitazone preserved β-cell function as shown by increased pancreatic islet mass and insulin content and prevented the development of overt hyperglycaemia in animal models of type 2 diabetes. Rosiglitazone did not stimulate pancreatic insulin secretion or induce hypoglycaemia in rats and mice. The major metabolite (para-hydroxy-sulphate) with high affinity to the soluble human PPARγ, exhibited relatively high potency in a glucose tolerance assay in obese mouse. The clinical relevance of this observation has not been fully elucidated.

Clinical trials data

The glucose lowering effects observed with rosiglitazone are gradual in onset with near maximal reductions in fasting plasma glucose (FPG) evident following approximately 8 weeks of therapy. The improved glycaemic control is associated with reductions in both fasting and post-prandial glucose.

Rosiglitazone was associated with increases in weight. In mechanistic studies, the weight increase was predominantly shown to be due to increased subcutaneous fat with decreased visceral and intra-hepatic fat.

Consistent with the mechanism of action, rosiglitazone reduced insulin resistance and improved pancreatic β-cell function. Improved glycaemic control was also associated with significant decreases in free fatty acids. As a consequence of different but complementary mechanisms of action, dual oral therapy of rosiglitazone with a sulphonylurea or metformin resulted in additive effects on glycaemic control in type 2 diabetic patients.

In studies with a maximal duration of three years, rosiglitazone given once or twice daily in combination with a sulphonylurea or metformin produced a sustained improvement in glycaemic control (FPG and HbA1c). A more pronounced glucose-lowering effect was observed in obese patients. An outcome study has not been conducted with rosiglitazone, therefore the long-term benefits associated with improved glycaemic control have not been demonstrated.

At 18 months, in an ongoing long term comparator study, rosiglitazone in dual oral therapy with metformin or a sulphonylurea was non-inferior to the combination of sulphonylurea plus metformin for lowering HbA1c.

An active controlled clinical trial (rosiglitazone up to 8 mg daily or metformin up to 2,000 mg daily) of 24 weeks duration was performed in 197 children (10-17 years of age) with type 2 diabetes. Improvement in HbA1c from baseline achieved statistical significance only in the metformin group. Rosiglitazone failed to demonstrate non-inferiority to metformin. Following rosiglitazone treatment, there were no new safety concerns noted in children compared to adult patients with type 2 diabetes mellitus. No long-term efficacy and safety data are available in paediatric patients.

There are no studies assessing long-term cardiovascular outcome in patients receiving rosiglitazone.

5.2 Pharmacokinetic properties

Absorption:

Absolute bioavailability of rosiglitazone following both a 4 and an 8 mg oral dose is approximately 99%. Rosiglitazone plasma concentrations peak at around 1 hour after dosing. Plasma concentrations are approximately dose proportional over the therapeutic dose range.

Administration of rosiglitazone with food resulted in no change in overall exposure (AUC), although a small decrease in C_{max} (approximately 20 to 28%) and a delay in t_{max} (ca.1.75 h) were observed compared to dosing in the fasting state. These small changes are not clinically significant and, therefore, it is not necessary to administer rosiglitazone at any particular time in relation to meals. The absorption of rosiglitazone is not affected by increases in gastric pH.

Distribution:

The volume of distribution of rosiglitazone is approximately 14 litres in healthy volunteers. Plasma protein binding of rosiglitazone is high (approximately 99.8%) and is not influenced by concentration or age. The protein binding of the major metabolite (para-hydroxy-sulphate) is very high >99.99%).

Metabolism:

Metabolism of rosiglitazone is extensive with no parent compound being excreted unchanged. The major routes of metabolism are N-demethylation and hydroxylation, followed by conjugation with sulphate and glucuronic acid. The contribution of the major metabolite (para-hydroxy-sulphate) to the overall anti-diabetic activity of rosiglitazone has not been fully elucidated in man and it cannot be ruled out that the metabolite may contribute to the activity. However, this raises no safety concern regarding target or special populations as hepatic impairment is contraindicated and the phase III clinical studies included a considerable number of elderly patients and patients with mild to moderate renal impairment.

In vitro studies demonstrate that rosiglitazone is predominantly metabolised by CYP2C8, with a minor contribution by CYP2C9.

Since there is no significant *in vitro* inhibition of CYP1A2, 2A6, 2C19, 2D6, 2E1, 3A or 4A with rosiglitazone, there is a low probability of significant metabolism-based interactions with substances metabolised by these P450 enzymes. Rosiglitazone showed moderate inhibition of CYP2C8 (IC_{50} 18 μM) and low inhibition of CYP2C9 (IC_{50} 50 μM) *in vitro* (see section 4.5). An *in vivo* interaction study with warfarin indicated that rosiglitazone does not interact with CYP2C9 substrates *in vivo*.

Elimination:

Total plasma clearance of rosiglitazone is around 3 l/h and the terminal elimination half-life of rosiglitazone is approximately 3 to 4 hours. There is no evidence for unexpected accumulation of rosiglitazone after once or twice daily dosing. The major route of excretion is the urine with approximately two-thirds of the dose being eliminated by this route, whereas faecal elimination accounts for approximately 25% of dose. No intact drug is excreted in urine or faeces. The terminal half-life for radioactivity was about 130 hours indicating that elimination of metabolites is very slow. Accumulation of the metabolites in plasma is expected upon repeated dosing, especially that of the major metabolite (para-hydroxy-sulphate) for which an 8-fold accumulation is anticipated.

Special populations:

Gender: In the pooled population pharmacokinetic analysis, there were no marked differences in the pharmacokinetics of rosiglitazone between males and females.

Elderly: In the pooled population pharmacokinetic analysis, age was not found to influence the pharmacokinetics of rosiglitazone to any significant extent.

Children and adolescents: Population pharmacokinetic analysis including 96 paediatric patients aged 10 to 18 years and weighing 35 to 178 kg suggested similar mean CL/F in children and adults. Individual CL/F in the paediatric population was in the same range as individual adult data. CL/F seemed to be independent of age, but increased with weight in the paediatric population.

Hepatic impairment: In cirrhotic patients with moderate (Child-Pugh B) hepatic impairment, unbound C_{max} and AUC were 2- and 3-fold higher than in normal subjects. The inter-subject variability was large, with a 7-fold difference in unbound AUC between patients.

Renal insufficiency: There are no clinically significant differences in the pharmacokinetics of rosiglitazone in patients with renal impairment or end stage renal disease on chronic dialysis.

5.3 Preclinical safety data

Adverse effects observed in animal studies with possible relevance to clinical use were as follows: An increase in plasma volume accompanied by decrease in red cell parameters and increase in heart weight. Increases in liver weight, plasma ALT (dog only) and fat tissue were also observed. Similar effects have been seen with other thiazolidinediones.

In reproductive toxicity studies, administration of rosiglitazone to rats during mid-late gestation was associated with foetal death and retarded foetal development. In addition, rosiglitazone inhibited ovarian oestradiol and progesterone synthesis and lowered plasma levels of these hormones resulting in effects on oestrus/menstrual cycles and fertility (see section 4.4).

In an animal model for familial adenomatous polyposis (FAP), treatment with rosiglitazone at 200 times the pharmacologically active dose increased tumour multiplicity in the colon. The relevance of this finding is unknown. However, rosiglitazone promoted differentiation and reversal of mutagenic changes in human colon cancer cells *in vitro*. In addition, rosiglitazone was not genotoxic in a battery of *in vivo* and *in vitro* genotoxicity studies and there was no evidence of colon tumours in lifetime studies of rosiglitazone in two rodent species.

6. PHARMACEUTICAL PARTICULARS

6.1 List of excipients

4 and 8 mg Tablet core:

Sodium starch glycollate (Type A), hypromellose, microcrystalline cellulose, lactose monohydrate, magnesium stearate.

4 mg Film coating:

Opadry orange OY-L-23028 (hypromellose 6cP, titanium dioxide E171, macrogol 3000, purified talc, lactose monohydrate, glycerol triacetate, iron oxide red E172, iron oxide yellow E172).

8 mg Film coating:

Opadry pink OY-L-24803 (hypromellose 6cP, titanium dioxide E171, macrogol 3000, lactose monohydrate, glycerol triacetate, iron oxide red E172).

6.2 Incompatibilities

Not applicable.

6.3 Shelf life

2 years.

6.4 Special precautions for storage

This medicinal product does not require any special storage conditions.

6.5 Nature and contents of container

Opaque blister packs (PVC/ aluminium).

4 mg - 28 and 56 film-coated tablets.

8 mg - 28 film-coated tablets

6.6 Instructions for use and handling

No special requirements.

Administrative Data

7. MARKETING AUTHORISATION HOLDER

SmithKline Beecham plc, 980 Great West Road, Brentford, Middlesex, TW8 9GS, United Kingdom.

8. MARKETING AUTHORISATION NUMBER(S)

EU/1/00/137/006 - Avandia 4 mg - 28 Film-coated tablets

EU/1/00/137/007 - Avandia 4 mg - 56 Film-coated tablets

EU/1/00/137/011 - Avandia 8 mg - 28 Film-coated tablets

9. DATE OF FIRST AUTHORISATION/RENEWAL OF THE AUTHORISATION

Date of first authorisation: 11 July 2000

Date of renewal: 18 July 2005

10. DATE OF REVISION OF THE TEXT

09 August 2005

11. Legal Status

POM

*Avandia is a registered trademark of SmithKline Beecham

Avastin 25mg/ml concentrate for solution for infusion

(Roche Products Limited)

1. NAME OF THE MEDICINAL PRODUCT

Avastin®▼ 25 mg/ml concentrate for solution for infusion.

2. QUALITATIVE AND QUANTITATIVE COMPOSITION

Bevacizumab 25 mg per ml. Each vial contains 100 mg of bevacizumab in 4 ml and 400 mg in 16 ml respectively.

Bevacizumab is a recombinant humanised monoclonal antibody produced by DNA technology in Chinese Hamster ovary cells.

For excipients, see section 6.1.

3. PHARMACEUTICAL FORM

Concentrate for solution for infusion.

Clear to slightly opalescent, colourless to pale brown liquid.

4. CLINICAL PARTICULARS

4.1 Therapeutic indications

Avastin (bevacizumab) in combination with intravenous 5-fluorouracil/folinic acid or intravenous 5-fluorouracil/folinic acid/irinotecan is indicated for first-line treatment of patients with metastatic carcinoma of the colon or rectum.

4.2 Posology and method of administration

Avastin must be administered under the supervision of a physician experienced in the use of antineoplastic medicinal products.

It is recommended that treatment be continued until progression of the underlying disease.

The recommended dose of Avastin is 5 mg/kg of body weight given once every 14 days as an intravenous infusion. Dose reduction for adverse events is not recommended. If indicated, therapy should either be discontinued or temporarily suspended as described in section 4.4.

The initial dose should be delivered over 90 minutes as an intravenous infusion. If the first infusion is well tolerated, the second infusion may be administered over 60 minutes. If the 60-minute infusion is well tolerated, all subsequent infusions may be administered over 30-minutes.

The initial dose should be administered following chemotherapy, all subsequent doses can be given before or after chemotherapy.

Do not administer as an intravenous push or bolus.

Avastin infusions should not be administered or mixed with glucose solutions (see section 6.2).

Special populations

Children and Adolescents: The safety and efficacy in children and adolescents have not been studied. Avastin should not be used in the paediatric group until further data become available (see section 5.3).

Elderly: No dose adjustment is required in the elderly.

Renal impairment: The safety and efficacy have not been studied in patients with renal impairment.

Hepatic impairment: The safety and efficacy have not been studied in patients with hepatic impairment.

4.3 Contraindications

- Hypersensitivity to the active substance or to any of the excipients.
- Hypersensitivity to Chinese hamster ovary (CHO) cell products or other recombinant human or humanised antibodies.
- Pregnancy (see section 4.6).
- Avastin is contraindicated in patients with untreated CNS metastases (see sections 4.4 and 4.8).

4.4 Special warnings and special precautions for use

Gastrointestinal perforations (see section 4.8)

Patients with metastatic carcinoma of the colon or rectum and an intra-abdominal inflammatory process may be at increased risk for the development of gastrointestinal perforation when treated with Avastin and chemotherapy. Therefore, caution should be exercised when treating these patients. Therapy should be permanently discontinued in patients who develop gastrointestinal perforation.

Wound Healing Complications (see section 4.8)

Avastin may adversely affect the wound healing process. Therapy should not be initiated for at least 28 days following major surgery or until the surgical wound is fully healed. In patients who experienced wound healing complications during therapy, treatment should be withheld until the wound is fully healed. Therapy should be withheld for elective surgery.

Hypertension (see section 4.8)

An increased incidence of hypertension was observed in Avastin-treated patients. Clinical safety data suggest that the incidence of hypertension is likely to be dose-dependent. There is no information on the effect of Avastin in patients with uncontrolled hypertension at the time of initiating therapy. Therefore, caution should be exercised before initiating therapy in these patients. Monitoring of blood pressure is generally recommended during therapy.

In patients with severe hypertension requiring medical therapy, temporary interruption of Avastin is recommended until adequate control is achieved. If hypertension cannot be controlled with medical therapy, treatment should be permanently discontinued. Therapy should be permanently discontinued in patients who develop hypertensive crisis.

Proteinuria (see section 4.8)

Patients with a history of hypertension may be at increased risk for the development of proteinuria when treated with Avastin. There is evidence suggesting that Grade 1 [US National Cancer Institute-Common Toxicity Criteria (NCI-CTC) version 2.0] proteinuria may be related to the dose. Monitoring of proteinuria by dipstick urinalysis is recommended prior to starting and during therapy. Therapy should be discontinued in patients who develop Grade 4 proteinuria (nephrotic syndrome).

Arterial Thromboembolism (see section 4.8)

In five randomised clinical trials, the incidence of arterial thromboembolic events including cerebrovascular accidents (CVAs), transient ischaemic attacks (TIAs) and myocardial infarctions (MIs) was higher in patients receiving Avastin in combination with chemotherapy compared to those who received chemotherapy alone.

A history of arterial thromboembolic events or age over 65 years was associated with an increased risk of developing arterial thromboembolic events during therapy. Caution should be taken when treating these patients with Avastin.

Therapy should be permanently discontinued in patients who develop arterial thromboembolic events.

Haemorrhage

The risk of CNS haemorrhage in patients with CNS metastases receiving Avastin could not be fully evaluated, as these patients were excluded from clinical trials. Thus, Avastin should not be used in these patients (see sections 4.3 and 4.8).

Patients with metastatic cancer of the colon or rectum might have an increased risk of developing tumour-associated haemorrhage. Avastin should be discontinued permanently in patients who experience Grade 3 or 4 bleeding during Avastin therapy (see section 4.8).

There is no information on the safety profile of Avastin in patients with congenital bleeding diathesis, acquired coagulopathy or in patients receiving full dose of anticoagulants for the treatment of thromboembolism prior to starting Avastin treatment, as such patients were excluded from clinical trials. Therefore, caution should be exercised before initiating therapy in these patients. However, patients who developed venous thrombosis while receiving therapy did not appear to have an increased rate of serious bleeding when treated with a full dose of warfarin and Avastin concomitantly.

Congestive Heart Failure (CHF)/Cardiomyopathy (see section 4.8)

Prior anthracycline exposure and/or prior radiation to the chest wall may be possible risk factors for the development of CHF. Caution should be exercised before initiating Avastin therapy in patients with these risk factors.

4.5 Interaction with other medicinal products and other forms of Interaction

No formal drug interaction studies with other antineoplastic agents have been conducted. However, the existing data suggest that bevacizumab does not affect the pharmacokinetics of 5-fluorouracil (5-FU), carboplatin, paclitaxel, and doxorubicin to a clinically relevant extent.

In one study, irinotecan concentrations were similar in patients receiving Irinotecan/5-FU/folinic acid (IFL) alone and in combination with bevacizumab. Concentrations of SN38, the active metabolite of irinotecan, were analysed in a subset of patients (approximately 30 per treatment arm). Concentrations of SN38 were on average 33% higher in patients receiving IFL in combination with bevacizumab compared with IFL alone. Due to high inter-patient variability and limited sampling, it is uncertain if the increase in SN38 levels observed was due to bevacizumab. There was a small increase in diarrhoea and leukopenia adverse events (known adverse drug reactions of irinotecan), and also more dose reductions of irinotecan were reported in the IFL + bevacizumab-treated patients.

Patients who develop severe diarrhoea, leukopenia or neutropenia with bevacizumab and irinotecan combination should have irinotecan dose modifications as specified in the Summary of Product Characteristics for the medicinal product containing irinotecan.

4.6 Pregnancy and lactation

Pregnancy

There are no data on the use of Avastin in pregnant women. Studies in animals have shown reproductive toxicity including malformations (see section 5.3). IgGs are known to cross the placenta, and Avastin is anticipated to inhibit angiogenesis in the foetus. Avastin must not be used during pregnancy. In women of childbearing potential, appropriate contraceptive measures must be used during therapy, and for at least 6 months following the last dose of Avastin.

Lactation

It is not known whether bevacizumab is excreted in human milk. As maternal IgG is excreted in milk and bevacizumab could harm infant growth and development (see section 5.3), women must discontinue breast-feeding during therapy and not breast feed for at least six months following the last dose of Avastin.

4.7 Effects on ability to drive and use machines

No studies on the effects on the ability to drive and use machines have been performed. However, there is no evidence that Avastin treatment results in an increase in adverse events that might lead to impairment of the ability to drive or operate machinery or impairment of mental ability.

4.8 Undesirable effects

The overall safety profile of Avastin is based on 1132 patients with metastatic carcinoma of the colon or rectum, locally advanced or metastatic non-small cell lung, metastatic breast and hormone-resistant prostate cancer, who received Avastin either as a single agent or in combination with chemotherapy in clinical trials.

The most serious adverse events were:

- Gastrointestinal perforations (see section 4.4).
- Haemorrhage (see section 4.4).
- Arterial thromboembolism (see section 4.4).

The most frequently observed adverse events across all clinical trials in patients receiving Avastin with or without chemotherapy were asthenia, diarrhoea, nausea and pain NOS (Not Otherwise Specified).

Analyses of the clinical safety data suggest that the occurrence of hypertension and proteinuria with Avastin therapy are likely to be dose-dependent.

In a phase III, randomised, double-blind, active-controlled study in metastatic carcinoma of the colon or rectum (Study AVF2107g), 396 patients were treated with IFL+ placebo (Arm 1), 392 patients were treated with IFL + Avastin (Arm 2), and 109 patients were treated with 5-fluorouracil/folinic acid (5-FU/FA) + Avastin (Arm 3). In a phase II, randomised, double-blind, active-controlled study (Study AVF2192g), the safety of Avastin was investigated in 204 patients with metastatic carcinoma of the colon or rectum who were not optimal candidates for first-line irinotecan. Of these patients, 104 were treated with 5-FU/FA + placebo (Arm 1) and 100 patients were treated with 5-FU/FA + Avastin (Arm 2). The safety overview of these two studies is displayed in Table 1 below:

Table 1: Safety overview of study AVF2107g and AVF2192g

(see Table 1)

In the phase III and II studies in metastatic carcinoma of the colon or rectum (AVF2107g, AVF2192g), Grade 3 and 4

Table 1 Safety overview of study AVF2107g and AVF2192g

	AVF2107g		AVF2192g	
	IFL + placebo N=396	IFL + Avastin N=392	5-FU/FA + placebo N=104	5-FU/FA + Avastin N=100
Death within 60 days of randomisation	4.9%	3.0%	13.5%	5.0%
Median duration of safety observation (weeks)	28	40	23	31
SAEs leading to death	2.8%	2.6%	6.7%	4.0%
AEs leading to study drug discontinuation	7.1%	8.4%	11.5%	10.0%

Data are unadjusted for the differential time on treatment.

adverse events (irrespective of causal relationship) observed in ⩾ 10% and ⩾ 1% - < 10% of Avastin-treated patients as compared to the control groups were as shown in Table 2:

Table 2: Grade 3 and 4 adverse events (irrespective of causal relationship and occurring with ⩾ 2% higher incidence in Avastin-treated arm compared with the control group) observed in ⩾ 10%, and ⩾ 1% - < 10% of Avastin-treated patients: studies AVF2107g and AVF2192g

Frequency of adverse events System organ class	AVF2107g IFL + Avastin	AVF2192g 5-FU/FA + Avastin
⩾ 10%		
Cardiac disorders		Hypertension
⩾ 1% and <10%		
Cardiac disorders	Hypertension	
Blood & lymphatic system disorders	Leukopenia	
General disorders & administration site conditions	Pain	Asthenia Pain
Gastrointestinal disorders	Diarrhoea Abdominal pain	
Infections & infestations disorders		Sepsis Abscess
Nervous system disorders		Cerebral ischaemia Syncope
Vascular disorders	Deep vein thrombosis Thromboembolism (Arterial)*	Thromboembolism (Arterial)*

* *Pooled arterial thromboembolic events including cerebrovascular accident, myocardial infarction, transient ischaemic attack and other arterial thromboembolic events.*

Data are unadjusted for the differential time on treatment.

In the phase III and II studies in metastatic carcinoma of the colon or rectum (AVF2107g, AVF2192g), adverse events of all grades (irrespective of causal relationship) which occurred in ⩾ 10%, and ⩾ 1% - < 10% of Avastin-treated patients as compared to the control groups were as presented in Table 3:

Table 3: Adverse events of all grades (irrespective of causal relationship and occurring with ⩾ 10% higher incidence in Avastin-treated arm compared with the control group) observed in ⩾ 10%, and ⩾ 1%- < 10% of Avastin-treated patients as compared to the control groups: studies AVF2107g and AVF2192g

Frequency of adverse events system organ class	AVF2107g IFL + Avastin	AVF2192g 5-FU/FA + Avastin
⩾ 10%		
Cardiac disorders	Hypertension	Hypertension
Gastrointestinal disorders	Rectal haemorrhage Stomatitis Constipation	Stomatitis
General disorders & administration site conditions	Pain	Asthenia Pain Pyrexia
Metabolism & nutrition disorders	Anorexia	
⩾ 1% and < 10%		
Eye disorders	Eye disorders	
Nervous system disorders	Dysgeusia	
Respiratory, thoracic & mediastinal disorders	Epistaxis Dyspnoea Rhinitis	
Skin & subcutaneous tissue disorders	Dermatitis exfoliative Skin discoloration Dry skin	

Data are unadjusted for the differential time on treatment.

The following adverse events have been observed in Avastin-treated patients, and may be potentially related to Avastin therapy:

Gastrointestinal perforations (see section 4.4):

Avastin has been associated with serious cases of gastrointestinal perforation in patients with metastatic carcinoma of the colon or rectum.

In clinical trials in metastatic carcinoma of the colon or rectum, gastrointestinal perforation was observed in 1.4% - 2.0% of the Avastin-treated patients. Of these, 0.4% - 1% had fatal outcome. The presentation of these events varied in type and severity, ranging from free air seen on the plain abdominal X-ray, which resolved without treatment, to a colonic perforation with abdominal abscess and fatal outcome. The common feature among these cases was intra-abdominal inflammation, either from gastric ulcer disease, tumour necrosis, diverticulitis, or chemotherapy-associated colitis.

Wound healing (see section 4.4):

As Avastin may adversely impact wound healing, patients who had major surgery within the last 28 days were excluded from participation in clinical trials for metastatic cancer of the colon or rectum.

In clinical trials of metastatic carcinoma of the colon or rectum, patients who underwent cancer-related surgery between 28 and 60 days prior to starting therapy did not have increased risk of post-operative bleeding or wound healing complications during treatment compared to the controlled groups. Adverse events consistent with post-operative bleeding or wound healing complication were observed in 10% - 20% of Avastin-treated patients who underwent major surgery while receiving treatment.

Hypertension (see section 4.4):

An increased incidence of hypertension has been observed in Avastin-treated patients. Hypertension was generally treated with oral anti-hypertensives such as angiotensin-converting enzyme inhibitors, diuretics and calcium-channel blockers. It rarely resulted in discontinuation (0.7% of all Avastin-treated patients) or hospitalisation, and resulted in hypertensive encephalopathy in one case (0.1%). The risk of Avastin-associated hypertension did not correlate with the patients' baseline characteristics, underlying disease or concomitant therapy.

In clinical trials of metastatic carcinoma of the colon or rectum, hypertension of any grade occurred in 22.4% - 32.0% of Avastin-treated patients. Grade 3 hypertension (requiring oral anti-hypertensive medication) was reported in 11.0% - 16.0% of Avastin-treated patients. No hypertensive crisis (Grade 4) was reported. At week 24 of treatment, the mean change of blood pressure (BP) from baseline was diastolic BP +4.1 to +5.4 mmHg and systolic BP +5.5 to +8.4 mmHg in the treated patients.

Proteinuria (see section 4.4):

Proteinuria, reported as adverse event, was observed in 23.3% of all Avastin-treated patients. It ranged in severity from clinically asymptomatic, transient, trace proteinuria to nephrotic syndrome, with the great majority as Grade 1 proteinuria. The proteinuria seen in clinical trials was not associated with renal dysfunction and rarely required permanent discontinuation of therapy.

In clinical trials of metastatic carcinoma of the colon or rectum, proteinuria was reported as an adverse event in 21.7% - 38.0% of Avastin-treated patients. No Grade 4 proteinuria was reported.

Haemorrhage (see section 4.4):

Overall, 4.0% of NCI-CTC Grade 3 and 4 bleeding events were observed in all Avastin treated patients. In clinical trials of metastatic carcinoma of the colon or rectum, there was no significant difference in the incidence of grade 3 and 4 bleeding events observed between Avastin-treated patients (3.1% - 5.1%) compared to that observed in the controls (2.5% - 2.9%).

The haemorrhagic events that have been observed in clinical studies were predominantly tumour-associated haemorrhage (see below) and minor mucocutaneous haemorrhage.

Tumour-associated haemorrhage was observed in phase I and phase II studies. In patients with non-small cell lung cancer receiving Avastin, serious haemorrhage was observed in 9% (6% fatal) of treated patients. These events occurred suddenly and presented as major or massive haemoptysis in patients with either squamous cell histology and/or tumours located in the centre of the chest in close proximity to major blood vessels. In some cases, these haemorrhages were preceded by cavitation and/or necrosis of the tumour.

Tumour-associated haemorrhage was also seen rarely in other tumour types and locations, including central nervous system (CNS) bleeding in a patient with hepatoma with occult CNS metastases (see section 4.3) and continuous oozing of blood from a thigh sarcoma with necrosis.

In clinical trials of metastatic carcinoma of the colon or rectum, tumour-associated haemorrhagic events were observed in 1% - 3% of the Avastin-treated patients. The addition of Avastin did not result in significant increase in the incidence or severity of Grade 3 or 4 haemorrhagic events.

Across all clinical trials, ***mucocutaneous haemorrhage*** has been seen in 20% - 40% of Avastin-treated patients. These were most commonly NCI-CTC Grade 1 epistaxis that lasted less than 5 minutes, resolved without medical intervention and did not require any changes in treatment regimen. In clinical trials of metastatic carcinoma of the colon or rectum, epistaxis was reported in 22.0% - 34.3% of Avastin-treated patients.

There have also been less common events of minor mucocutaneous haemorrhage in other locations, such as gingival bleeding and vaginal bleeding.

Thromboembolism (see section 4.4):

In clinical trials of metastatic carcinoma of the colon or rectum, the overall incidence of thromboembolic events was similar between Avastin-treated patients (18.0% - 19.4%) and the controls (16.2% - 18.3%).

Arterial thromboembolism:

In clinical trials of metastatic carcinoma of the colon or rectum, the incidence of arterial thromboembolic events including CVAs, MIs, TIAs, and other arterial thromboembolic events was higher in Avastin-treated patients (3.3% - 10.0%) compared to the controls (1.3% - 4.8%).

In five randomised trials including metastatic carcinoma of the colon or rectum trials (N=1745), arterial thromboembolic events including CVAs, MIs, TIAs, and other thromboembolic events occurred in 4.5% (45/1004) of patients treated with Avastin in combination with chemotherapy compared to 2.0% (15/741) of patients treated with chemotherapy alone. In patients treated with Avastin plus chemotherapy, arterial thromboembolic events led to a fatal outcome in 0.8% (8/1004). In patients treated with chemotherapy alone, a fatal outcome from arterial thromboembolic events was reported in 0.4% (3/741). CVAs (including TIAs) occurred in 2.2% of patients treated with Avastin in combination with chemotherapy and 0.5% of patients treated with chemotherapy alone. MI occurred in 1.9% of patients treated with Avastin in combination with chemotherapy compared to 1.1% of patients treated with chemotherapy alone.

Venous thromboembolism:

In clinical trials of metastatic carcinoma of the colon or rectum, venous thromboembolic events, including deep venous thrombosis, pulmonary embolism and thrombophlebitis occurred in 9.0% - 16.6% of Avastin-treated patients compared to that of 13.5% - 15.2% in the controls. It could not be determined if these events were due to the patients' underlying cancer, their cytotoxic chemotherapy, Avastin or other risk factors.

Congestive Heart Failure (CHF)/Cardiomyopathy

In the phase III controlled clinical trial of metastatic breast cancer, CHF/cardiomyopathy was reported in 3% of the Avastin-treated patients compared with 1% in the controlled group. These events varied in severity from asymptomatic declines in left ventricular ejection fraction to symptomatic CHF requiring hospitalisation and treatment. All the Avastin-treated patients were previously treated with anthracyclines (doxorubicin cumulative dose range 240–360 mg/m^2). Many of these patients also had prior radiotherapy to the left chest wall. Most of these patients showed improved symptoms and/or left ventricular function following appropriate medical therapy.

There was no information on patients with pre-existing CHF (NYHA II-IV) at the time of initiating the therapy, as these patients were excluded from studies. In patients with metastatic cancer of the colon or rectum, there was no increased incidence of CHF in Avastin-treated patients.

Elderly Patients

Data from 5 randomised clinical trials showed that age > 65 years was associated with an increased risk of developing arterial thromboembolic events including cerebrovascular accidents (CVAs), transient ischaemic attacks (TIAs) and myocardial infarctions (MIs) when treated with Avastin (see sections 4.4 and 4.8 under *Thromboembolism*). No increased incidence of Avastin-related events including gastrointestinal perforation, wound healing complications, hypertension, proteinuria, haemorrhage and congestive heart failure/cardiomyopathy was observed in elderly patients (> 65 years) with metastatic cancer of the colon or rectum receiving Avastin compared to those aged ⩽ 65 years treated with Avastin.

In the phase III study in metastatic carcinoma of colon or rectum trial (AVF2107g), 114 out of the 392 patients who received Avastin were older than 65 years. Only Grade 3/4 leukopenia occurred at an incidence of ⩾ 5% in the elderly patients (> 65 years) compared to those patients aged ⩽ 65 years.

In the phase II study in metastatic carcinoma of colon or rectum trial (AVF2192g), the majority of the Avastin-treated patients was older than 65 years (83%). The overall safety profile of Avastin from this study was comparable to the overall safety profile observed in Study AVF2107g.

Laboratory Abnormalities:

Decreased neutrophil count, decreased white blood cell count and presence of urine protein may be associated with Avastin.

Decreased neutrophil count and decreased white blood cell count were the most commonly observed Grade 3 and 4 laboratory abnormalities in Avastin-treated patients across all clinical trials. Grade 3 and 4 laboratory

Table 4 Treatment regimens in study AVF2107g

	Treatment	Starting Dose	Schedule
Arm 1	Irinotecan	125 mg/m^2 IV	Given once weekly for 4 weeks every 6 weeks
	5-Fluorouracil	500 mg/m^2 IV	
	Folinic acid	20 mg/m^2 IV	
	Placebo	IV	Every 2 weeks
Arm 2	Irinotecan	125 mg/m^2 IV	Given once weekly for 4 weeks every 6 weeks
	5-Fluorouracil	500 mg/m^2 IV	
	Folinic acid	20 mg/m^2 IV	
	Avastin	5 mg/kg IV	Every 2 weeks
Arm 3	5-Fluorouracil	500 mg/m^2 IV	Given once weekly for 6 weeks every 8 weeks
	Folinic acid	500 mg/m^2 IV	
	Avastin	5 mg/kg IV	Every 2 weeks

5-Fluorouracil: IV bolus injection immediately after folinic acid.
folinic acid: IV bolus injection (over 1–2 minutes) immediately after each irinotecan dose.

abnormalities occurring in ⩾ 5% of Avastin-treated patients with or without chemotherapy in any trials included decreased neutrophil count, decreased white blood cell count, protein urine present, decreased blood potassium, decreased blood phosphorus, increased blood glucose and increased blood alkaline phosphatase.

The higher incidences of decreased neutrophil count and decreased white blood cell count observed in the IFL + Avastin arm possibly correlated to the increased concentrations of SN38, the active metabolite of irinotecan (see section 4.5).

4.9 Overdose

The highest dose tested in humans (20 mg/kg of body weight, intravenous) was associated with severe migraine in several patients.

5. PHARMACOLOGICAL PROPERTIES

5.1 Pharmacodynamic properties

Pharmacotherapeutic group: Antineoplastic agents, monoclonal antibody, ATC code: L01X C07

Mechanism of action

Bevacizumab binds to vascular endothelial growth factor (VEGF) and thereby inhibits the binding of VEGF to its receptors, Flt-1 (VEGFR-1) and KDR (VEGFR-2), on the surface of endothelial cells. Neutralising the biological activity of VEGF reduces the vascularisation of tumours, thereby inhibiting tumour growth.

Pharmacodynamic effects

Administration of bevacizumab or its parental murine antibody to xenotransplant models of cancer in nude mice resulted in extensive anti-tumour activity in human cancers, including colon, breast, pancreas and prostate. Metastatic disease progression was inhibited and microvascular permeability was reduced.

Clinical efficacy

The safety and efficacy of the recommended dose (5 mg/kg of body weight every two weeks) in metastatic carcinoma of the colon or rectum were studied in three randomised, active-controlled clinical trials in combination with fluoropyrimidine-based first-line chemotherapy. Avastin was combined with two chemotherapy regimens:

- **AVF2107g**: A weekly schedule of irinotecan/bolus 5-fluorouracil/folinic acid (IFL) for a total of 4 weeks of each 6 week-cycle (Saltz regimen).
- **AVF0780g**: In combination with bolus 5-fluorouracil/folinic acid (5-FU/FA) for a total of 6 weeks of each 8 week-cycle (Roswell Park regimen).
- **AVF2192g**: In combination with bolus 5-FU/FA for a total of 6 weeks of each 8 week-cycle (Roswell Park regimen) in patients who were not optimal candidates for first-line irinotecan treatment.

All three trials evaluated Avastin at a dose of 5 mg/kg of body weight every two weeks and enrolled patients with previously untreated metastatic carcinoma of the colon or rectum.

Avastin in Combination with IFL Chemotherapy for First-Line Treatment of Metastatic Carcinoma of the Colon or Rectum (AVF2107g): This was a phase III randomised, double-blind, active-controlled clinical trial evaluating Avastin in combination with IFL as first-line treatment for metastatic carcinoma of the colon or rectum. Eight hundred and thirteen patients were randomised to receive IFL + placebo (Arm 1) or IFL + Avastin (5 mg/kg every 2 weeks, Arm 2) (see Table 4). A third group of 110 patients received bolus 5-FU/FA+Avastin (Arm3). Enrollment in Arm 3 was discontinued, as pre-specified, once safety of Avastin with the IFL regimen was established and considered acceptable. All treatments were continued until disease progression. The overall mean age was 59.4 years; 56.6% of patients had an ECOG performance status of 0, 43% had a value of 1 and 0.4% had a value of 2. 15.5 % had received prior radiotherapy and 28.4 % prior chemotherapy.

Table 4 Treatment regimens in study AVF2107g

(see Table 4 above)

The primary efficacy variable of the trial was duration of survival. The addition of Avastin to IFL resulted in a statistically significant increase in overall survival (see Table 5). The clinical benefit, as measured by overall survival, was seen in all pre-specified patient subgroups, including those defined by age, sex, performance status, location of primary tumour, number of organs involved and duration of metastatic disease.

The efficacy results of Avastin in combination with IFL-chemotherapy are displayed in Table 5.

Table 5 Efficacy results for study AVF2107g

	AVF2107g	
	Arm 1 IFL + Placebo	**Arm 2 IFL + Avastin[a]**
Number of Patients	411	402
Overall survival		
Median time (months)	15.6	20.3
95% Confidence Interval	14.29 – 16.99	18.46 – 24.18
Hazard ratio[b]		0.660
p-value		0.00004
Progression-free survival		
Median time (months)	6.2	10.6
Hazard ratio		0.54
p-value		< 0.0001
Overall response rate		
Rate (%)	34.8	44.8
95% CI	30.2–39.6	39.9–49.8
p-value		0.0036
Duration of response		
Median time (months)	7.1	10.4
25–75 percentile (months)	4.7–11.8	6.7–15.0

[a]5 mg/kg every 2 weeks.
[b]Relative to control arm.

Among the 110 patients randomised to Arm 3 (5-FU/FA + Avastin), the median overall survival was 18.3 months, median progression free survival was 8.8 months, overall response rate was 39% and median duration of response was 8.5 months.

Avastin in Combination with 5-FU/FA Chemotherapy for the First-Line Treatment of Metastatic Carcinoma of the Colon or Rectum in patients who were not optimal candidates for first-line irinotecan treatment (AVF2192g): This was a phase II randomised, double-blind, active-controlled clinical trial evaluating the efficacy and safety of Avastin in combination with 5-FU/FA as first-line treatment for metastatic colorectal cancer in patients who were not optimal candidates for first-line irinotecan treatment. Patients had to be either more susceptible to irinotecan toxicity (⩾ 65 years, prior radiotherapy to pelvis or abdomen) or less likely to benefit from irinotecan treatment (PS ⩾ 1, baseline albumin < 3.5 g/dl) in order to be eligible for enrolment. One hundred and five patients were randomised to 5-FU/FA + placebo arm and 104 patients to 5-FU/FA + Avastin (5 mg/kg every 2 weeks) arm. All treatments were continued until disease progression. The overall mean age was 71 years; 28.2% of patients had a ECOG performance status of 0, 65.1% had a value of 1 and 6.7% had a value of 2. The addition of Avastin 5 mg/kg every two weeks to 5-FU/FA resulted in higher objective response rates, significantly longer progression-free survival, and a trend in longer survival, compared to 5-FU/FA chemotherapy alone (see Table 6). These efficacy data were consistent with the results observed in studies AVF2107g and AVF0780g.

Avastin in Combination with 5-FU/FA Chemotherapy for the First-Line Treatment of Metastatic Carcinoma of the Colon or Rectum (AVF0780g): This was a phase II randomised, active-controlled, open-labelled clinical trial investigating Avastin in combination with 5-FU/FA as first-line treatment of metastatic colorectal cancer. The median age was 64 years. 19 % of the patients had received prior chemotherapy and 14 % prior radiotherapy. Seventy-one patients were randomised to receive bolus 5-FU/FA or 5-FU/FA + Avastin (5 mg/kg every 2 weeks). A third group of 33 patients received bolus 5-FU/FA + Avastin (10 mg/kg every 2 weeks). Patients were treated until disease progression. The primary endpoints of the trial were objective response rate and progression-free survival. The addition of Avastin 5 mg/kg every two weeks to 5-FU/FA resulted in higher objective response rates, longer progression-free survival, and a trend in longer survival, compared with 5-FU/FA chemotherapy alone (see Table 6). These efficacy data are consistent with the results from study AVF2107g.

The efficacy data from studies AVF0780g and AVF2192g investigating Avastin in combination with 5-FU/FA-chemotherapy are summarised in Table 6.

Table 6: Efficacy results for studies AVF0780g and AVF2192g

(see Table 6 on next page)

5.2 Pharmacokinetic properties

The pharmacokinetic data for bevacizumab are available from eight clinical trials in patients with solid tumours. In all clinical trials, bevacizumab was administered as an IV infusion. The rate of infusion was based on tolerability, with an initial infusion duration of 90 minutes. The pharmacokinetics of bevacizumab was linear at doses ranging from 1 to 10 mg/kg.

Absorption

Not applicable.

Distribution

Based on a population pharmacokinetic analysis of 491 subjects receiving Avastin weekly, every 2 weeks, or every 3 weeks, in doses ranging from 1 to 20 mg/kg, the volume of the central compartment (V_c) was 2.92 l. Results also indicated that, after correcting for body weight, male subjects had a larger V_c (+ 22%) than females.

Metabolism

Assessment of bevacizumab metabolism in rabbits following a single IV dose of ^{125}I-bevacizumab indicated that its metabolic profile was similar to that expected for a native IgG molecule which does not bind VEGF.

Elimination

Bevacizumab clearance was 0.231 l/day. The volume of the central compartment (V_c) and clearance correspond to an initial half-life of 1.4 days and a terminal half-life of about 20 days. This half-life is consistent with the terminal elimination half-life for human endogenous IgG, which is 18 to 23 days. In patients with low albumin (⩽ 29g/l) and high alkaline phosphatase (⩾ 484U/l) (both markers of disease severity), clearance was approximately 20% higher than in patients with median laboratory values.

Table 6 Efficacy results for studies AVF0780g and AVF2192g

	AVF0780g			AVF2192g	
	5-FU/FA	5-FU/FA + Avastin[a]	5-FU/FA + Avastin[b]	5-FU/FA + placebo	5-FU/FA + Avastin
Number of Patients	36	35	33	105	104
Overall survival					
Median time (months)	13.6	17.7	15.2	12.9	16.6
95% Confidence Interval				10.35 - 16.95	13.63 – 19.32
Hazard ratio[c]	-	0.52	1.01		0.79
p-value		0.073	0.978		0.16
Progression-free survival					
Median time (months)	5.2	9.0	7.2	5.5	9.2
Hazard ratio		0.44	0.69		0.5
p-value		0.0049	0.217		0.0002
Overall response rate					
Rate (percent)	16.7	40.0	24.2	15.2	26
95% CI	7.0 –33.5	24.4 –57.8	11.7 – 42.6	9.2 - 23.9	18.1 - 35.6
p-value		0.029	0.43	-	0.055
Duration of response					
Median time (months)	NR	9.3	5.0	6.8	9.2
25–75 percentile (months)	5.5 –NR	6.1 –NR	3.8 – 7.8	5.59 - 9.17	5.88 - 13.01

[a]5 mg/kg every 2 weeks.
[b]10 mg/kg every 2 weeks.
[c]Relative to control arm.
NR = Not reached.

Pharmacokinetics in Special Populations

The population pharmacokinetics were analysed to evaluate the effects of demographic characteristics. The results showed no significant difference in the pharmacokinetics of bevacizumab in relation to age.

Children and adolescents: No studies have been conducted to investigate the pharmacokinetics of bevacizumab in paediatric patients.

Renal impairment: No studies have been conducted to investigate the pharmacokinetics of bevacizumab in renally impaired patients.

Hepatic impairment: No studies have been conducted to investigate the pharmacokinetics of bevacizumab in patients with hepatic impairment.

5.3 Preclinical safety data

In studies of up to 26 weeks duration in cynomolgus monkeys, physeal dysplasia was observed in young animals with open growth plates, at bevacizumab average serum concentrations below the expected human therapeutic average serum concentrations. In rabbits, bevacizumab was shown to inhibit wound healing at doses below the proposed clinical dose. Effects on wound healing were shown to be fully reversible.

Studies to evaluate the mutagenic and carcinogenic potential of bevacizumab have not been performed.

No specific studies in animals have been conducted to evaluate the effect on fertility. An adverse effect on female fertility can however be expected as repeat dose toxicity studies in animals have shown inhibition of the maturation of ovarian follicles and a decrease/absence of corpora lutea and associated decrease in ovarian and uterus weight as well as a decrease in the number of menstrual cycles.

Bevacizumab has been shown to be embryotoxic and teratogenic when administered to rabbits. Observed effects included decreases in maternal and foetal body weights, an increased number of foetal resorptions and an increased incidence of specific gross and skeletal foetal malformations. Adverse foetal outcomes were observed at all tested doses, of which the lowest dose resulted in average serum concentrations approximately 3 times larger than in humans receiving 5 mg/kg every 2 weeks.

6. PHARMACEUTICAL PARTICULARS

6.1 List of excipients

Trehalose dihydrate

Sodium phosphate

Polysorbate 20

Water for injections

6.2 Incompatibilities

A concentration dependent degradation profile of bevacizumab was observed when diluted with glucose solutions (5%).

6.3 Shelf life

2 years.

Chemical and physical in-use stability has been demonstrated for 48 hours at 2°C to 30°C in sodium chloride 9 mg/ml (0.9%) solution for injection. From a microbiological point of view, the product should be used immediately. If not used immediately, in-use storage times and conditions are the responsibility of the user and would normally not be longer than 24 hours at 2°C to 8°C, unless dilution has taken place in controlled and validated aseptic conditions.

6.4 Special precautions for storage

Store in a refrigerator (2°C-8°C).

Do not freeze.

Keep the vial in the outer carton in order to protect from light.

6.5 Nature and contents of container

Single-use vial (Type I glass) with a butyl rubber stopper containing 100 mg of bevacizumab in 4 ml of concentrate for solution for infusion.

Single-use vial (Type I glass) with a butyl rubber stopper containing 400 mg of bevacizumab in 16 ml of concentrate for solution for infusion.

Pack of 1 vial containing 4 ml.

Pack of 1 vial containing 16 ml.

6.6 Instructions for use and handling

Avastin does not contain any antimicrobial preservative; therefore, care must be taken to ensure the sterility of the prepared solution.

Avastin should be prepared by a healthcare professional using aseptic technique. Withdraw the necessary amount of bevacizumab for a dose of 5 mg/kg of body weight and dilute with sodium chloride 9 mg/ml (0.9%) solution for injection up to a total volume of 100 ml. Discard any unused portion left in a vial, as the product contains no preservatives. Parenteral medicinal products should be inspected visually for particulate matter and discoloration prior to administration.

No incompatibilities between Avastin and polyvinyl chloride or polyolefine bags or infusion sets have been observed.

7. MARKETING AUTHORISATION HOLDER

Roche Registration Limited
40 Broadwater Road
Welwyn Garden City
Hertfordshire, AL7 3AY
United Kingdom

8. MARKETING AUTHORISATION NUMBER(S)

EU/1/04/300/001 - 100mg/4ml vial

EU/1/04/300/002 - 400mg/16ml vial

9. DATE OF FIRST AUTHORISATION/RENEWAL OF THE AUTHORISATION

12 January 2005

10. DATE OF REVISION OF THE TEXT

Not applicable.

AVAXIM

(Sanofi Pasteur MSD)

1. NAME OF THE MEDICINAL PRODUCT

AVAXIM®, suspension for injection in a pre-filled syringe.

Hepatitis A vaccine (inactivated, adsorbed).

2. QUALITATIVE AND QUANTITATIVE COMPOSITION

One 0.5 mL dose contains:

Hepatitis A virus, GBM strain (inactivated)[1,2] .... 160 U[3]

1 produced in human diploid (MRC-5) cells

2 adsorbed on aluminium hydroxide, hydrated (0.3 milligrams Al)

3 In the absence of an international standardised reference, the antigen content is expressed using an in-house reference

For excipients, see 6.1.

3. PHARMACEUTICAL FORM

Suspension for injection in a pre-filled syringe.

Hepatitis A vaccine (inactivated, adsorbed) is a cloudy and white suspension.

4. CLINICAL PARTICULARS

4.1 Therapeutic indications

AVAXIM® is indicated for active immunisation against infection caused by hepatitis A virus in susceptible adults and adolescents (of 16 years and over).

Individuals having grown up in areas of high endemicity and/or with a history of jaundice may be immune to hepatitis A, in which case the vaccine is unnecessary. Testing for antibodies to hepatitis A prior to a decision on immunisation should be considered in such situations. If not, seropositivity against hepatitis A is not a contraindication. AVAXIM® is as well tolerated in seropositive as in seronegative subjects (see Section 4.8).

4.2 Posology and method of administration

The recommended dosage for subjects of at least 16 years of age is 0.5 millilitre for each injection. As AVAXIM® has not been extensively studied in subjects less than or equal to 15 years of age, it is not indicated in this age group.

Initial protection is achieved with one single dose of vaccine. Protective levels of antibody may not be reached until 14 days after administration of the vaccine. There are serological data to show that there should be continuing protection against hepatitis A for up to 36 months after a first dose in subjects who responded to the initial vaccination.

In order to provide long-term protection, a second dose (booster) of an inactivated hepatitis A vaccine should be given. The second dose is preferably given between 6 and 12 months after the primary immunisation but may be administered up to 36 months after the primary immunisation.

It is predicted that HAV antibodies persist for many years (at least 10 years) after the booster vaccination.

The vaccine may be used as a booster in subjects who received another inactivated hepatitis A vaccine (monovalent or with purified Vi polysaccharide typhoid) 6 months to up to 36 months previously.

Method of administration

AVAXIM® should be administered by intramuscular injection in the deltoid region.

AVAXIM® must not be administered intradermally or intravascularly.

In exceptional circumstances (e.g. in patients with thrombocytopenia or in patients at risk of haemorrhage), the vaccine may be injected by the subcutaneous route.

4.3 Contraindications

Hypersensitivity to any AVAXIM® component or hypersensitivity following a previous injection of this vaccine.

Systemic hypersensitivity to neomycin, which may be present in the vaccine in trace amounts.

Vaccination should be delayed in subjects with an acute severe febrile illness.

4.4 Special warnings and special precautions for use

As with all vaccines, appropriate medical treatment and supervision should be readily available for immediate use in case of rare anaphylactic reaction following vaccination.

AVAXIM® should only be given by a physician or health care worker trained in the administration of vaccines.

Individuals who develop symptoms suggestive of hypersensitivity after an injection of AVAXIM® should not receive further injections of the vaccine (see contraindications).

The vaccine should not be administered into the buttocks, due to the varying amount of fatty tissue in this region, contributing to variability in effectiveness of the vaccine.

Following vaccination with AVAXIM® protection develops against infection caused by hepatitis A virus. This protection does not occur immediately but over 90% of individuals will have protective levels of antibodies after 2 weeks.

In the event that the booster vaccination has been delayed, there may be a decreased anti-hepatitis A antibody response. If long-term protection is required, the serum anti-hepatitis A antibody titre may be determined after AVAXIM® administration.

As with any vaccine, vaccination may not result in a protective response in all susceptible vaccinees.

Because of the incubation period of hepatitis A, infection may be present but not clinically apparent at the time of vaccination. The effect of AVAXIM® on individuals late in the incubation period of hepatitis A has not been documented.

AVAXIM® does not provide protection against infection caused by hepatitis B virus, hepatitis C virus, hepatitis E virus or by other liver pathogens.

AVAXIM® has not been studied in patients with impaired immunity. The immune response to AVAXIM® could be impaired by immunosuppressive treatment or in immunodeficiency states. In such cases, it is recommended to measure the antibody response to be sure of protection and, if possible, to wait for the end of any suppressive treatment before vaccination. Nevertheless, vaccination of subjects with chronic immunodeficiency such as HIV infection is recommended although the antibody response may be limited.

As no studies have been performed with AVAXIM® in subjects with liver disease, the use of this vaccine in such subjects should be considered with care.

4.5 Interaction with other medicinal products and other forms of Interaction

As AVAXIM® is inactivated, concomitant administration with other inactivated vaccine(s) given at another injection site is unlikely to interfere with immune responses. When concurrent administration is considered necessary, AVAXIM® must not be mixed with other vaccines in the same syringe, and other vaccines should be administered at different sites with different syringes and needles.

Seroconversion rates were not modified when AVAXIM® was given at the same time as but at a different injection site to a Vi polysaccharide typhoid vaccine or a yellow fever vaccine reconstituted with a Vi polysaccharide typhoid vaccine. Studies on the concomitant administration of AVAXIM® and recombinant hepatitis B virus vaccine have not been performed.

Concomitant administration of immunoglobulin and AVAXIM® at two separate sites may be performed. Seroconversion rates are not modified, but antibody titres could be lower than after vaccination with AVAXIM® alone. Therefore, consideration should be given to whether or not the subject is likely to be at long-term risk of exposure.

No interaction with other medicinal products is currently known.

4.6 Pregnancy and lactation

The effect of AVAXIM® on embryo foetal development has not been assessed. AVAXIM® is not recommended in pregnancy unless there is a high risk of hepatitis A infection. The vaccine should be given to a pregnant woman only if clearly needed.

There are no data on the effect of administration of AVAXIM® during lactation. AVAXIM® is therefore not recommended during lactation.

4.7 Effects on ability to drive and use machines

None known.

4.8 Undesirable effects

In clinical trials, adverse reactions were usually mild and confined to the first few days after vaccination with spontaneous recovery.

The most common reactions with an incidence of 1% to 10% were mild local pain (10% of injections), asthenia (10%), myalgia/arthralgia (7.9%), headache (7.2%), gastro-intestinal tract disorders (nausea, vomiting, decreased appetite, diarrhoea, abdominal pain) (4.3%) and mild fever (3.7%).

Those with an incidence less than 1% included redness at the injection site (0.5%). On rare occasions a nodule was observed at the injection site (less than 0.1%).

Mild reversible elevation of serum transaminases has been observed on rare occasions.

Reactions were less frequently reported after the booster dose than after the first dose. In subjects seropositive against hepatitis A virus, AVAXIM® was as well tolerated as in seronegative subjects.

In post marketing surveillance, skin reactions such as urticaria, rashes associated or not with pruritus were very rarely observed.

4.9 Overdose

Not applicable.

5. PHARMACOLOGICAL PROPERTIES

5.1 Pharmacodynamic properties

AVAXIM® confers immunity against hepatitis A virus by inducing antibody titres greater than those obtained after passive immunisation with immunoglobulin. Antibody appears shortly after the first injection and 14 days after vaccination more than 90% of immunocompetent subjects are seroprotected (titre above 20 mIU/millilitre).

One month after the first injection, almost 100% of subjects have antibody titres above 20mIU/millilitre. In a study of 103 healthy adults who were followed serologically for three years after the first injection of AVAXIM®, 99% still had at least 20 mIU/ml anti-HAV antibody at month 36.

The long-term persistence of protective antibody levels to hepatitis A virus after a booster dose of AVAXIM® is under evaluation. Antibody titres obtained two years after the first booster are consistent with a projected protection of at least 10 years.

5.2 Pharmacokinetic properties

Not relevant.

5.3 Preclinical safety data

Preclinical safety data reveal no special hazard to humans based on conventional studies of acute toxicity, repeated dose toxicity, local tolerance and hypersensitivity.

6. PHARMACEUTICAL PARTICULARS

6.1 List of excipients

The formulation contains:

2-phenoxyethanol

Formaldehyde

Medium 199 Hanks (complex blend of amino acids, mineral salts, vitamins and other ingredients)

Water for injections

Hydrochloric acid and sodium hydroxide for pH adjustment

6.2 Incompatibilities

This medicinal product must not be mixed with other medicinal products.

6.3 Shelf life

3 years.

6.4 Special precautions for storage

Store between +2°C and +8°C (in a refrigerator).

The vaccine must not be frozen. If frozen, the vaccine should be discarded.

6.5 Nature and contents of container

0.5 ml of suspension in pre-filled syringe (type I glass) with a plunger-stopper (chlorobromobutyl) and attached needle and needle-shield (natural rubber or polyisoprene).

0.5 ml of suspension in pre-filled syringe (type I glass) with a plunger-stopper (chlorobromobutyl) and tip-cap (chlorobromobutyl), without needle.

Packs of 1, 5, 10 and 20 syringes.

0.5 ml of suspension in pre-filled syringe (type I glass) with a plunger-stopper (chlorobromobutyl) and tip-cap (chlorobromobutyl), with 1 or 2 separate needles (for each syringe).

Packs of 1 and 10 syringes.

Not all pack sizes and presentations may be marketed.

6.6 Instructions for use and handling

For needle free syringes, the needle should be pushed firmly on to the end of the pre-filled syringe and rotated through 90 degrees.

Shake before injection to obtain a homogeneous suspension.

7. MARKETING AUTHORISATION HOLDER

Sanofi Pasteur MSD Limited
Mallards Reach
Bridge Avenue
Maidenhead
Berkshire
SL6 1QP

8. MARKETING AUTHORISATION NUMBER(S)

UK: PL 6745/0070

9. DATE OF FIRST AUTHORISATION/RENEWAL OF THE AUTHORISATION

30th April 2001

10. DATE OF REVISION OF THE TEXT

May 2005

Avelox 400 mg Tablets

(Bayer plc)

1. NAME OF THE MEDICINAL PRODUCT

Avelox 400mg film-coated tablets ▼

2. QUALITATIVE AND QUANTITATIVE COMPOSITION

One film-coated tablet contains 436.8mg moxifloxacin hydrochloride equivalent to 400mg moxifloxacin.

For excipients, see 6.1.

3. PHARMACEUTICAL FORM

Film-coated tablets.

Dull red tablets marked with "M400" on one side and "BAYER" on the reverse.

4. CLINICAL PARTICULARS

4.1 Therapeutic indications

Avelox 400 mg film-coated tablets are indicated for the treatment of the following bacterial infections:

- Acute exacerbation of chronic bronchitis
- Community acquired pneumonia, except severe cases
- Acute bacterial sinusitis (adequately diagnosed)

Avelox 400 mg film-coated tablets are indicated for the treatment of the above infections if they are caused by bacteria susceptible to moxifloxacin.

Consideration should be given to official guidance on the appropriate use of antibacterial agents.

4.2 Posology and method of administration

Dosage (adults)

One 400 mg film-coated tablet once daily.

No adjustment of dosage is required in the elderly, in patients with low bodyweight, in patients with mild to severely impaired renal function or in patients on chronic dialysis i.e. hemodialysis and continuous ambulatory peritoneal dialysis (see Section 5.2 for more details).

There is insufficient data in patients with impaired liver function (see Section 4.3).

Method of administration

The film-coated tablet should be swallowed whole with sufficient liquid and may be taken independent of meals.

Duration of administration

Avelox 400 mg tablets should be used for the following treatment durations:

- Acute exacerbation of chronic bronchitis, 5-10 days
- Community acquired pneumonia, 10 days
- Acute sinusitis, 7 days

Avelox 400 mg film-coated tablets have been studied in clinical trials for up to 14 days treatment.

The recommended dose (400 mg once-daily), and duration of therapy for the indication being treated should not be exceeded.

4.3 Contraindications

– Known hypersensitivity to moxifloxacin, other quinolones or any of the excipients.

– Pregnancy and lactation (see Section 4.6).

– Children and growing adolescents.

– Patients with a history of tendon disease/disorder related to quinolone treatment.

Both in preclinical investigations and in humans, changes in cardiac electrophysiology have been observed following exposure to moxifloxacin, in the form of QT prolongation. For reasons of drug safety, Avelox is therefore contra-indicated in patients with:

– Congenital or documented acquired QT prolongation

– Electrolyte disturbances, particularly in uncorrected hypokalaemia

– Clinically relevant bradycardia

– Clinically relevant heart failure with reduced left-ventricular ejection fraction

– Previous history of symptomatic arrhythmias

Avelox should not be used concurrentlywith other drugs that prolong the QT interval (see also Section 4.5).

Due to a lack of data, Avelox is also contra-indicated in patients with impaired liver function (Child Pugh C) and in patients with transaminases increase > 5 fold ULN.

4.4 Special warnings and special precautions for use

- Quinolones are known to trigger seizures. Use should be with caution in patients with CNS disorders which may predispose to seizures or lower the seizure threshold.
- If vision becomes impaired or any effects on the eyes are experienced, an eye specialist should be consulted immediately.
- Tendon inflammation and rupture may occur with quinolone therapy including moxifloxacin, particularly in elderly patients and in those treated concurrently with corticosteroids. At the first sign of pain or inflammation, patients should discontinue treatment with Avelox and rest the affected limb(s).
- Moxifloxacin has been shown to prolong the QTc interval on the electrocardiogram in some patients. In the analysis of ECGs obtained in the clinical trial program, QTc

prolongation with moxifloxacin was 6 msec, ± 26 msec, 1.4 % compared to baseline.

Medication that can reduce potassium levels should be used with caution in patients receiving moxifloxacin.

Moxifloxacin should be used with caution in patients with ongoing proarrhythmic conditions, such as acute myocardial ischaemia.

QT prolongation may lead to an increased risk of ventricular arrhythmias, including torsade de pointes. The magnitude of QT prolongation may increase with increasing concentrations of the drug. Therefore, the recommended dose should not be exceeded.

The benefit of moxifloxacin treatment especially in infections with a low degree of severity should be balanced with the information contained in the warnings and precautions section.

If signs of cardiac arrhythmia occur during treatment with Avelox, treatment should be stopped and an ECG should be performed.

• Liver function tests/investigations should be performed in cases where indications of liver dysfunction occur.

• Pseudomembranous colitis has been reported in association with the use of broad spectrum antibiotics including moxifloxacin; therefore it is important to consider this diagnosis in patients who develop serious diarrhoea during or after the use of Avelox. In this situation adequate therapeutic measures should be initiated immediately. Drugs inhibiting peristalsis are contra-indicated in this situation.

• Patients with a family history of, or actual defects in glucose-6-phosphate dehydrogenase deficiency are prone to haemolytic reactions when treated with quinolones. Therefore, Avelox should be used with caution in these patients.

• Quinolones have been shown to cause photosensitivity reactions in patients. However, studies have shown that moxifloxacin has a lower risk to induce photosensitivity. Nevertheless patients should be advised to avoid exposure to either UV irradiation or extensive and/or strong sunlight during treatment with moxifloxacin.

• Very rarely hypersensitivity and allergic reactions have been reported including after first administration. Anaphylactic reactions in very rare instances can progress to life threatening shock, in some instances after the first administration. In these cases moxifloxacin should be discontinued and suitable treatment (e.g. treatment for shock) initiated.

• Patients with rare hereditary problems of galactose intolerance, the Lapp lactase deficiency or glucose-galactose malabsorption should not take this medicine.

4.5 Interaction with other medicinal products and other forms of Interaction

Interactions with medicinal products

An additive effect on QT interval prolongation between moxifloxacin and the following drugs cannot be excluded: antiarrhythmics class IA (e.g. quinidine, hydroquinidine, disopyramide) or antiarrhythmics class III (e.g. amiodarone, sotalol, dofetilide, ibutilide), neuroleptics (e.g. phenothiazines, pimozide, sertindole, haloperidol, sultopride), tricyclic antidepressive agents, certain antimicrobials (sparfloxacin, erythromycin IV, pentamidine, antimalarials particularly halofantrine), certain antihistaminics (terfenadine, astemizole, mizolastine), others (cisapride, vincamine IV, bepridil, diphemanil). This effect might lead to an increased risk of ventricular arrhythmias, notably torsade de pointes. Therefore moxifloxacin is contraindicated in patients treated with these drugs (see also Section 4.3).

An interval of about 6 hours should be left between administration of agents containing bivalent or trivalent cations (e.g. antacids containing magnesium or aluminium, didanosine tablets, sucralfate and agents containing iron or zinc) and administration of Avelox.

Concomitant administration of charcoal with an oral dose of 400 mg moxifloxacin leads to a pronounced prevention of drug absorption and a reduced systemic availability of the drug by more than 80%. Therefore, the concomitant use of these two drugs is not recommended (except for overdose cases, see also section 4.9).

After repeated dosing in healthy volunteers moxifloxacin increased Cmax of digoxin approximately 30 % without affecting AUC or trough levels. No precaution is required for use with digoxin.

In studies conducted in diabetic volunteers, concomitant administration of Avelox with glibenclamide resulted in a decrease of approximately 21 % in the peak plasma concentrations of glibenclamide. The combination of glibenclamide and moxifloxacin could theoretically result in a mild and transient hyperglycaemia. However, the observed pharmacokinetic changes for glibenclamide did not result in changes of the pharmacodynamic parameters (blood glucose, insulin). Therefore no clinically relevant interaction was observed between moxifloxacin and glibenclamide.

Changes in INR

A large number of cases showing an increase in oral anticoagulant activity have been reported in patients receiving antibiotics, especially fluoroquinolones, macrolides, tetracyclines, cotrimoxazole and some cephalosporins. The infectious and inflammatory conditions, age and general status of the patient appear to be risk factors. Under these circumstances, it is difficult to evaluate whether the infection or the antibiotic therapy cause the INR (international normalised ratio) disorder. A precautionary measure would be to more frequently monitor the INR. If necessary, the oral anticoagulant dosage should be adjusted as appropriate. Even if during an interaction study performed in healthy volunteers between moxifloxacin and warfarin, negative results have been observed, the precautionary measures as above stated should apply to warfarin as for other anticoagulants.

No interactions have occurred following concomitant administration of moxifloxacin with: ranitidine, probenecid, oral contraceptives, calcium supplements, morphine administered parenterally, theophylline or itraconazole.

In vitro studies with human P-450 enzymes support this data. Considering these results a metabolic interaction via P-450 enzymes is unlikely.

Note: The theophylline interaction study was conducted using a moxifloxacin dosage of 2 × 200 mg.

Interaction with food

Moxifloxacin has no clinically relevant interaction with food including dairy products.

4.6 Pregnancy and lactation

The safety of use of moxifloxacin in human pregnancy has not been evaluated. Reproduction studies performed in rats and monkeys did not reveal any evidence of teratogenicity or impairment of fertility. However, as with other quinolones, moxifloxacin has been shown to cause lesions in the cartilage of the weight bearing joints of immature animals. Preclinical data indicate that moxifloxacin passes into milk. The use of moxifloxacin in pregnancy and nursing mothers is contra-indicated.

4.7 Effects on ability to drive and use machines

Fluoroquinolones may result in an impairment of the patient's ability to drive or operate machinery due to CNS reactions (e.g. dizziness). Patients should be advised to see how they react to moxifloxacin before driving or operating machinery.

4.8 Undesirable effects

The following undesirable effects have been reported following treatment with Avelox.

The frequencies are shown below:

Common:	⩾ 1%	to	< 10%
Uncommon:	⩾ 0.1%	to	< 1%
Rare:	⩾ 0.01%	to	< 0.1%
Very rare:			< 0.01%

Apart from nausea and diarrhoea all adverse drug reactions were observed at frequencies below 3 %.

General:

Common:	Abdominal pain, headache
Uncommon:	Asthenia, pain, back pain, malaise, chest pain, allergic reaction, leg pain
Very rare:	Hypersensitivity: anaphylactic reaction, anaphylactic shock (possibly life threatening), angioedema (including laryngeal edema; potentially life-threatening)

Nervous system:

Common:	Dizziness
Uncommon:	Insomnia, vertigo, nervousness, somnolence, anxiety, tremor, paraesthesia, confusion, depression
Rare:	Hallucination, depersonalisation, incoordination, agitation, sleep disorders, abnormal dreams, convulsion
Very rare:	Psychotic reaction

Gastro-intestinal system:

Common:	Nausea, diarrhoea, vomiting, dyspepsia
Uncommon:	Dry mouth, nausea and vomiting, flatulence, constipation, oral moniliasis, anorexia, stomatitis, glossitis
Very rare:	Pseudomembranous colitis (in very rare cases associated with life threatening complications), hepatitis (predominantly cholestatic)

Cardiovascular system:

Common:	In patients with concomitant hypokalaemia: prolongation of the QT
Uncommon:	Tachycardia, peripheral oedema, hypertension, palpitation, atrial fibrillation, angina pectoris, in patients with normokalaemia: QT prolongation.
Rare:	Vasodilatation, hypotension, syncope
Very rare:	Ventricular arrhythmias, torsade de pointes and cardiac arrest especially in patients with severe underlying proarrhythmic conditions (see Section 4.4)

Respiratory system:

Uncommon:	Dyspnoea

Musculo-skeletal system:

Uncommon:	Arthralgia, myalgia
Rare:	Tendinitis
Very rare:	Tendon rupture

Skin:

Uncommon:	Rash, pruritus, sweating, urticaria
Rare:	Dry skin
Very rare:	Stevens-Johnson-Syndrome

Sensory organs:

Common:	Taste perversion
Uncommon:	Amblyopia
Rare:	Tinnitus, abnormal vision in the course of CNS reactions (e.g. dizziness or confusion), parosmia (including smell perversion, decreased smell and in rare cases loss of smell and/or taste)

Urogenital system:

Uncommon:	Vaginal moniliasis, vaginitis

Laboratory findings:

Common:	Abnormal liver function tests (mostly moderate increases of AST / ALT and / or bilirubin)
Uncommon:	Gamma-GT increase, amylase increase, leucopenia, prothrombin decrease / International Normalized Ratio (INR) increase, eosinophilia, thrombocythaemia, thrombopenia, anaemia
Rare:	Hyperglycaemia, hyperlipidaemia, prothrombin increase / International Normalized Ratio (INR) decrease, icterus (predominantly cholestatic), LDH increase (in connection with abnormal liver function), increase in creatinine or urea

The current clinical experience with Avelox does not allow for a final assessment of its adverse drug reaction profile. There have been isolated cases of the following side effects reported following treatment with other fluoroquinolones, which might possibly also occur during treatment with Avelox: transient loss of vision, balance disorders including ataxia, hypernatraemia, hypercalcaemia, neutropenia, haemolysis.

4.9 Overdose

No specific countermeasures after accidental overdosage are recommended. General symptomatic therapy should be initiated. Concomitant administration of charcoal with a dose of 400 mg oral moxifloxacin will reduce systemic availability of the drug by more than 80%. The use of charcoal early during absorption may be useful to prevent excessive increase in the systemic exposure to moxifloxacin in cases of oral overdose.

5. PHARMACOLOGICAL PROPERTIES

5.1 Pharmacodynamic properties

Moxifloxacin is a fluoroquinolone antibacterial (ATC Code JO1MA 14).

Mechanism of action

In vitro, moxifloxacin has been shown to have activity against a wide range of Gram-positive and Gram-negative pathogens.

The bactericidal action results from the interference with topoisomerase II (DNA Gyrase) and IV. Topoisomerases are essential enzymes which play a crucial part in the replication, transcription and repair of bacterial DNA. Topoisomerase IV is also known to influence bacterial chromosome division.

Kinetic investigations have demonstrated that moxifloxacin exhibits a concentration dependent killing rate. Minimum bactericidal concentrations (MBC) were found to be in the range of the minimum inhibitory concentrations (MIC).

Interference with culture test

Moxifloxacin therapy may give false negative culture results for *Mycobacterium spp.* by suppression of mycobacterial growth.

Effect on the intestinal flora in humans

The following changes in the intestinal flora were seen in volunteers following administration of moxifloxacin: *E. coli*, *Bacillus spp.*, *Enterococci*, and *Klebsiella spp.* were reduced, as were the anaerobes *Bacteroides vulgatus*, *Bifidobacterium*, *Eubacterium*, and *Peptostreptococcus*. For *B. fragilis* there was an increase. These changes returned to normal within two weeks. There was no selection of *Clostridium difficile* (MIC_{90} 2 mg/l) and its toxin under the administration of moxifloxacin. Moxifloxacin is not indicated for the treatment of *Clostridium difficile*.

The following MIC breakpoints separating susceptible from resistant organisms are suggested.

In vitro Susceptibility Data

Breakpoints S $\leqslant$ 1 mg/l, R > 2 mg/l

The prevalence of acquired resistance may vary geographically and with time for selected species and local information of resistance is desirable, particularly when treating severe infections. This information gives only approximate guidance on probabilities whether micro-organisms will be susceptible to moxifloxacin. Where resistance patterns for particular species are known to vary within the European Union, this is shown below.

Organism	Prevalence of acquired resistance
Sensitive:	
Gram-positive bacteria	
Staphylococcus aureus (methicillin sensitive)*	
Streptococcus agalactiae	
Streptococcus milleri	
Streptococcus mitior	
Streptococcus pneumoniae (including penicillin and macrolide resistant strains)*	<1%
Streptococcus pyogenes (group A)*	
Gram-negative bacteria	
Branhamella (Moraxella) catarrhalis (including β-lactamase negative and positive strains)*	
*Enterobacter cloacae**	0-13%
Escherichia coli*	0-10%
Haemophilus influenzae (including β-lactamase negative and positive strains)*	<1%
*Haemophilus parainfluenzae**	
Klebsiella oxytoca	0-10%
*Klebsiella pneumoniae**	2-13%
Anaerobes	
Fusobacterium spp.	
Peptostreptococcus spp.	
Prevotella spp.	
Others	
*Chlamydia pneumoniae**	
Coxiella burnettii	
Legionella pneumophila	
*Mycoplasma pneumoniae**	
Resistant:	
Gram-positive bacteria	
Staphylococcus aureus (methicillin resistant)	
Gram-negative bacteria	
Burkholderia cepacia	
Pseudomonas aeruginosa	
Pseudomonas fluorescens	
Stenotrophomonas maltophilia	

* Clinical efficacy has been demonstrated for susceptible isolates in approved clinical indications.

Resistance

Resistance mechanisms which inactivate penicillins, cephalosporins, aminoglycosides, macrolides and tetracyclines do not interfere with the antibacterial activity of moxifloxacin. Other resistance mechanisms such as permeation barriers (common, for example, in *Pseudomonas aeruginosa*) and efflux mechanisms may, however, also affect the sensitivity of corresponding bacteria to moxifloxacin. Apart from this there is no cross resistance between moxifloxacin and the aforementioned compound classes. Plasmid-mediated resistance has not been observed. Laboratory tests on the development of resistance against moxifloxacin in Gram-positive bacteria revealed that resistance develops slowly by multiple step mutations and is mediated by target site modifications (i.e. in topoisomerase II and IV) and efflux mechanisms. The frequency of resistance development is low (rate 10^{-7}-10^{-10}).

Parallel resistance is observed with other quinolones. However, as moxifloxacin inhibits both topoisomerases (II and IV) in Gram-positive organisms, some Gram-positive bacteria and anaerobes that are resistant to other quinolones may be susceptible to moxifloxacin.

5.2 Pharmacokinetic properties

Absorption and Bioavailability: Following oral administration moxifloxacin is rapidly and almost completely absorbed. The absolute bioavailability amounts to approximately 91 %.

Pharmacokinetics are linear in the range of 50 - 800 mg single dose and up to 600 mg once daily dosing over 10 days. Following a 400 mg oral dose peak concentrations of 3.1 mg/l are reached within 0.5 - 4 h post administration. Peak and trough plasma concentrations at steady-state (400 mg once daily) were 3.2 and 0.6 mg/l, respectively. At steady-state the exposure within the dosing interval is approximately 30 % higher than after the first dose.

Distribution: Moxifloxacin is distributed to extravascular spaces rapidly; after a dose of 400 mg an AUC of 35 mg.h/l is observed. The steady-state volume of distribution (Vss) is approximately 2 l/kg. *In vitro* and *ex vivo* experiments showed a protein binding of approximately 40-42 % independent of the concentration of the drug. Moxifloxacin is mainly bound to serum albumin.

The following peak concentrations (geometric mean) were observed following administration of a single oral dose of 400 mg moxifloxacin:

(see Table 1 below)

Metabolism: Moxifloxacin undergoes Phase II biotransformation and is excreted via renal and biliary/faecal pathways as unchanged drug as well as in the form of a sulphocompound (M1) and a glucuronide (M2). M1 and M2 are the only metabolites relevant in humans, both are microbiologically inactive.

In clinical Phase I and *in vitro* studies no metabolic pharmacokinetic interactions with other drugs undergoing Phase I biotransformation involving Cytochrome P-450 enzymes were observed. There is no indication of oxidative metabolism.

Elimination: Moxifloxacin is eliminated from plasma with a mean terminal half life of approximately 12 hours. The mean apparent total body clearance following a 400 mg dose ranges from 179 to 246 ml/min. Renal clearance amounted to about 24 - 53 ml/min suggesting partial tubular reabsorption of the drug from the kidneys. After a 400 mg dose, recovery from urine (approx. 19 % for unchanged drug, approx. 2.5 % for M1, and approx. 14 % for M2) and faeces (approx. 25 % of unchanged drug, approx. 36 % for M1, and no recovery for M2) totalled to approximately 96 %.

Concomitant administration of moxifloxacin with ranitidine or probenecid did not alter renal clearance of the parent drug.

Higher plasma concentrations are observed in healthy volunteers with low body weight (such as women) and in elderly volunteers.

The pharmacokinetic properties of moxifloxacin are not significantly different in patients with renal impairment (including creatinine clearance >20 ml/min/1.73 m^2). As renal function decreases, concentrations of the M2 metabolite (glucuronide) increase by up to a factor of 2.5 (with a creatinine clearance of <30 ml/min/1.73 m^2).

On the basis of the pharmacokinetic studies carried out so far in patients with liver failure (Child-Pugh A, B), it is not possible to determine whether there are any differences compared with healthy volunteers. Impaired liver function was associated with higher exposure to M1 in plasma, whereas exposure to parent drug was comparable to exposure in healthy volunteers. There is insufficient experience in the clinical use of moxifloxacin in patients with impaired liver function.

5.3 Preclinical safety data

Effects on the haematopoetic system (slight decreases in the number of erythrocytes and platelets) were seen in rats and monkeys. As with other quinolones, hepatotoxicity (elevated liver enzymes and vacuolar degeneration) was seen in rats, monkeys and dogs. In monkeys CNS toxicity (convulsions) occurred. These effects were seen only after treatment with high doses of moxifloxacin or after prolonged treatment.

Moxifloxacin, like other quinolones, was genotoxic in *in vitro* tests using bacteria or mammalian cells. Since these effects can be explained by an interaction with the gyrase in bacteria and - at higher concentrations - by an interaction with the topoisomerase II in mammalian cells, a threshold concentration for genotoxicity can be assumed. In *in vivo* tests, no evidence of genotoxicity was found despite the fact that very high moxifloxacin doses were used. Thus, a sufficient margin of safety to the therapeutic dose in man can be provided. Moxifloxacin was non-carcinogenic in an initiation-promotion study in rats.

Many quinolones are photo-reactive and can induce phototoxic, photomutagenic and photocarcinogenic effects. In contrast, moxifloxacin was proven to be devoid of phototoxic and photogenotoxic properties when tested in a comprehensive programme of *in vitro* and *in vivo* studies. Under the same conditions other quinolones induced effects.

At high concentrations, moxifloxacin is an inhibitor of the rapid component of the delayed rectifier potassium current of the heart and may thus cause prolongations of the QT-interval. Toxicological studies performed in dogs using oral doses of $\geqslant$ 90 mg/kg leading to plasma concentrations $\geqslant$ 16 mg/l caused QT-prolongations, but no arrhythmias. Only after very high cumulative intravenous administration of more than 50fold the human dose > 300 mg/kg), leading to plasma concentrations of $\geqslant$ 200 mg/l (more than 40fold the therapeutic level), reversible, non-fatal ventricular arrhythmias were seen.

Quinolones are known to cause lesions in the cartilage of the major diarthrodial joints in immature animals. The lowest oral dose of moxifloxacin causing joint toxicity in juvenile dogs was four times the maximum recommended therapeutic dose of 400 mg (assuming a 50 kg bodyweight) on a mg/kg basis, with plasma concentrations two to three times higher than those at the maximum therapeutic dose.

Toxicity tests in rats and monkeys (repeated dosing up to six months) revealed no indication regarding an oculotoxic risk. In dogs, high oral doses ($\geqslant$ 60 mg/kg) leading to plasma concentrations $\geqslant$ 20 mg/l caused changes in the electroretinogram and in isolated cases an atrophy of the retina.

Reproductive studies performed in rats, rabbits and monkeys indicate that placental transfer of moxifloxacin occurs. Studies in rats (p.o. and i.v.) and monkeys (p.o.) did not show evidence of teratogenicity or impairment of fertility following administration of moxifloxacin. A slightly increased incidence of vertebral and rib malformations was observed in foetuses of rabbits but only at a dose (20 mg/kg i.v.) which was associated with severe maternal toxicity. There was an increase in the incidence of abortions in monkeys at human therapeutic plasma concentrations. In rats, decreased foetal weights, an increased prenatal loss, a slightly increased duration of pregnancy and an increased spontaneous activity of some male and female offspring was observed at doses which were 63 times the maximum recommended dose on a mg/kg basis with plasma concentrations in the range of the human therapeutic dose.

6. PHARMACEUTICAL PARTICULARS

6.1 List of excipients

Microcrystalline cellulose, Croscarmellose sodium, Lactose monohydrate, Magnesium stearate.

The tablets are film-coated with a mixture of Hypromellose, Macrogol 4000, Ferric oxide (E172) and Titanium dioxide (E171).

6.2 Incompatibilities

Not applicable

Table 4

Tissue	Concentration		Site: Plasma ratio
Plasma	3.1	mg/L	–
Saliva	3.6	mg/L	0.75-1.3
Blister fluid	1.6[1]	mg/L	1.7[1]
Bronchial mucosa	5.4	mg/kg	1.7 - 2.1
Alveolar Macrophages	56.7	mg/kg	18.6 - 70.0
Epithelial lining fluid	20.7	mg/L	5 - 7
Maxillary sinus	7.5	mg/kg	2.0
Ethmoid sinus	8.2	mg/kg	2.1
Nasal Polyps	9.1	mg/kg	2.6
Interstitial fluid	1.0[2]	mg/L	0.8-1.4[2,3]

[1] 10 h after administration
[2] unbound concentration
[3] from 3 h up to 36 h post dose

6.3 Shelf life
5 years

6.4 Special precautions for storage
Polypropylene/aluminium blisters:

Do not store above 25 °C.

Store in the original package.

Aluminium/aluminium blisters:

No special storage condition.

6.5 Nature and contents of container
Cartons containing colourless or white opaque polypropylene/aluminium blisters:

The film-coated tablets are available in packs of 5, 7, and 10 tablets.

Hospital packs containing 25 (5x5), 50 (5x10), 70 (7x10) film-coated tablets or bundled containing 80 (5 × 16) or 100 (10x10) film-coated tablets.

Aluminium/aluminium blisters, pack size one tablet in a carton.

6.6 Instructions for use and handling
No special requirements.

7. MARKETING AUTHORISATION HOLDER
Bayer plc, T/A Pharmaceutical Division, Bayer House, Strawberry Hill, Newbury,

Berkshire RG14 1JA.

8. MARKETING AUTHORISATION NUMBER(S)
PL 00010/0291

9. DATE OF FIRST AUTHORISATION/RENEWAL OF THE AUTHORISATION
30.11.2003

10. DATE OF REVISION OF THE TEXT
07.04.2005

11. LEGAL CATEGORY
POM

Avloclor Tablets

(AstraZeneca UK Limited)

1. NAME OF THE MEDICINAL PRODUCT
Avloclor Tablets

2. QUALITATIVE AND QUANTITATIVE COMPOSITION
Tablets containing 250mg chloroquine phosphate Ph. Eur. which is equivalent to 155mg chloroquine base.

3. PHARMACEUTICAL FORM
Tablets.

4. CLINICAL PARTICULARS

4.1 Therapeutic indications
a) Treatment of malaria.

b) Prophylaxis and suppression of malaria.

c) Treatment of amoebic hepatitis and abscess.

d) Treatment of discoid and systemic lupus erythematosus.

e) Treatment of rheumatoid arthritis.

4.2 Posology and method of administration
The dose should be taken after food.

a) Treatment of malaria

i) P. falciparum and P. malariae infections

Adults: A single dose of four tablets, followed by two tablets six hours later and then two tablets a day for two days.

Children: A single dose of 10mg base/kg, followed by 5mg base/kg six hours later and then 5mg base/kg a day for two days.

(see Table 1)

ii) P. vivax and P. ovale infections

Adults: A single dose of four tablets, followed by two tablets six hours later and then two tablets a day for two days. Follow with a course of treatment with primaquine if a radical cure is required.

Children: A single dose of 10mg base/kg, followed by 5mg base/kg six hours later and then 5mg base/kg a day for two days. Follow with a course of treatment with primaquine if a radical cure is required.

Elderly Patients: There are no special dosage recommendations for the elderly, but it may be advisable to monitor elderly patients so that optimum dosage can be individually determined.

Hepatic or Renally Impaired Patients: Caution is necessary when giving Avloclor to patients with renal disease or hepatic disease.

b) Prophylaxis and suppression of malaria

Adults: Two tablets taken once a week, on the same day each week. Start one week before exposure to risk and continue until four weeks after leaving the malarious area.

Children: A single dose of 5mg chloroquine base/kg per week on the same day each week. Start one week before exposure to risk and continue until four weeks after leaving the malarious area.

For practical purposes, children aged over 14 years may be treated as adults. The dose given to infants and children should be calculated on their body weight and must not exceed the adult dose regardless of weight.

1 - 4 years ½ tablet

5 - 8 years 1 tablet

9 - 15 years 1 ½ tablets

Elderly Patients: There are no special dosage recommendations for the elderly, but it may be advisable to monitor elderly patients so that optimum dosage can be individually determined.

Hepatic or Renally Impaired Patients: Caution is necessary when giving Avloclor to patients with renal disease or hepatic disease.

c) Amoebic hepatitis

Adults: Four tablets daily for two days followed by one tablet twice daily for two or three weeks.

Elderly Patients: There are no special dosage recommendations for the elderly, but it may be advisable to monitor elderly patients so that optimum dosage can be individually determined.

Hepatic or Renally Impaired Patients: Caution is necessary when giving Avloclor to patients with renal disease or hepatic disease.

d) Lupus erythematosus

Adults: One tablet twice daily for one to two weeks followed by a maintenance dosage of one tablet daily.

Elderly Patients: There are no special dosage recommendations for the elderly, but it may be advisable to monitor elderly patients so that optimum dosage can be individually determined.

Hepatic or Renally Impaired Patients: Caution is necessary when giving Avloclor to patients with renal disease or hepatic disease.

e) Rheumatoid arthritis

Adults: The usual dosage is one tablet daily.

Elderly Patients: There are no special dosage recommendations for the elderly, but it may be advisable to monitor elderly patients so that optimum dosage can be individually determined.

Hepatic or Renally Impaired Patients: Caution is necessary when giving Avloclor to patients with renal disease or hepatic disease.

4.3 Contraindications
Known hypersensitivity to chloroquine or any other ingredients of the formulation.

4.4 Special warnings and special precautions for use
When used as malaria prophylaxis official guidelines and local information on prevalence of resistance to anti-malarial drugs should be taken into consideration.

Caution is necessary when giving Avloclor to patients with impaired hepatic function, particularly when associated with cirrhosis.

Caution is also necessary in patients with porphyria. Avloclor may precipitate severe constitutional symptoms and an increase in the amount of porphyrins excreted in the urine. This reaction is especially apparent in patients with high alcohol intake.

Caution is necessary when giving Avloclor to patients with renal disease.

Avloclor should be used with care in patients with a history of epilepsy. Potential risks and benefits should be carefully evaluated before use in subjects on anticonvulsant therapy or with a history of epilepsy as rare cases of convulsions have been reported in association with chloroquine.

Considerable caution is needed in the use of Avloclor for long-term high dosage therapy and such use should only be considered when no other drug is available. Patients on long-term therapy should also be monitored for cardiomyopathy.

Irreversible retinal damage and corneal changes may develop during long term therapy and after the drug has been discontinued. Ophthalmic examination prior to and at 3 – 6 monthly intervals during use is required if patients are receiving chloroquine

- at continuous high doses for longer than 12 months
- as weekly treatment for longer than 3 years
- when total consumption exceeds 1.6g/kg (cumulative dose 100g)

Full blood counts should be carried out regularly during extended treatment as bone marrow suppression may occur rarely. Caution is required if drugs known to induce blood disorders are used concurrently.

The use of Avloclor in patients with psoriasis may precipitate a severe attack.

Caution is advised in patients with glucose-6-phosphate dehydrogenase deficiency, as there may be a risk of haemolysis.

4.5 Interaction with other medicinal products and other forms of Interaction
If the patient is taking cyclosporin then chloroquine may cause an increase in cyclosporin levels.

Pre-exposure intradermal human diploid-cell rabies vaccine should not be administered to patients taking chloroquine as this may suppress the antibody response. When vaccinated against rabies, that vaccine should precede the start of the antimalarial dosing, otherwise the effectiveness of the vaccine might be reduced.

Chloroquine significantly reduces levels of praziquantel. Caution is therefore advised during co-administration. Prescribers may consider increasing the dose of praziquantel if the patient does not respond to the initial dose.

Antacids (aluminium, calcium and magnesium salts) may reduce the absorption of chloroquine, so antacids should be taken well separated from Avloclor (at least two hours before or after).

Amiodarone:	chloroquine and hydroxchloroquine increase the risk of cardiac arrhythmias including ventricular arrhythmias bradycardias and cardiac conduction defect. Concurrent use is contra-indicated.
Other antimalarials:	increased risk of convulsion with mefloquine.
Cardiac glycosides:	hydroxychloroquine and possibly chloroquine increase plasma concentration of digoxin.
Parasympathomimetics:	chloroquine and hydroxychloroquine have potential to increase symptoms of myasthenia gravis and thus diminish effect of neostigmine and pyridostigmine.
Ulcer healing drugs:	cimetidine inhibits metabolism of chloroquine (increased plasma concentration).

4.6 Pregnancy and lactation

Pregnancy

Avloclor should not be used during pregnancy unless, in the judgement of the physician, potential benefit outweighs the risk.

Short-term malaria prophylaxis:

Malaria in pregnant women increases the risk of maternal death, miscarriage, still-birth and low birth weight with the associated risk of neonatal death. Travel to malarious areas should be avoided during pregnancy but, if this is not possible, women should receive effective prophylaxis.

Long-term high dose:

There is evidence to suggest that Avloclor given to women in high doses throughout pregnancy can give rise to foetal abnormalities including visual loss, ototoxicity and cochlear-vestibular dysfunction.

Lactation

Although Avloclor is excreted in breast milk, the amount is too small to be harmful when used for malaria prophylaxis but as a consequence is insufficient to confer any benefit on the infant. Separate chemoprophylaxis for the infant is required. However, when long-term high doses are used for rheumatoid disease, breast feeding is not recommended.

4.7 Effects on ability to drive and use machines
Defects in visual accommodation may occur on first taking Avloclor and patients should be warned regarding driving or operating machinery.

4.8 Undesirable effects
The adverse reactions which may occur at doses used in the prophylaxis or treatment of malaria are generally not of a serious nature. Where prolonged high dosage is required,

Table 1

Age (years)	Initial dose	Second dose 6 hours after first	Dose on each of the two subsequent days
1 – 4	1 Tablet	½ Tablet	½Tablet
5 – 8	2 Tablets	1 Tablet	1 Tablet
9 -14	3 Tablets	1 ½ Tablets	1 ½ Tablets

i.e. in the treatment of rheumatoid arthritis, adverse reactions can be of a more serious nature.

Cardiovascular: hypotension and ECG changes (at high doses) cardiomyopathy.

Central nervous system: convulsions and psychotic reactions including hallucinations (rare), anxiety, personality changes.

Eye disorders: retinal degeneration, macular defects of colour vision, pigmentation, optic atrophy scotomas, field defects, blindness, corneal opacities and pigmented deposits, blurring of vision, difficulty in accommodation, diplopia.

Gastro-intestinal: gastro-intestinal disturbances, nausea, vomiting, diarrhoea, abdominal cramps.

General: headache.

Haematological: bone marrow depression, aplastic anaemia, agranulocytosis, thrombocytopenia, neutropenia.

Hepatic: Changes in liver function, including hepatitis and abnormal liver function tests, have been reported rarely.

Hypersensitivity: allergic and anaphylactic reactions, including urticaria, angioedema and vasculitis.

Hearing disorders: tinnitus, reduced hearing, nerve deafness.

Muscular: neuromyopathy and myopathy.

Skin: macular, urticarial and purpuric skin eruptions, occasional depigmentation or loss of hair, erythema multiforme, Stevens-Johnson syndrome, toxic epidermal necrolysis, precipitation of psoriasis, pruritus, photosensitivity, lichen-planus type reaction, pigmentation of the skin and mucous membranes (long term use).

4.9 Overdose

Chloroquine is highly toxic in overdose and children are particularly susceptible. The chief symptoms of overdosage include circulatory collapse due to a potent cardiotoxic effect, respiratory arrest and coma. Symptoms may progress rapidly after initial nausea and vomiting. Cardiac complications may occur without progressively deepening coma.

Death may result from circulatory or respiratory failure or cardiac arrhythmia. If there is no demonstrable cardiac output due to arrhythmias, asystole or electromechanical dissociation, external chest compression should be persisted with for as long as necessary, or until adrenaline and diazepam can be given (see below).

Gastric lavage should be carried out urgently, first protecting the airway and instituting artificial ventilation where necessary. There is a risk of cardiac arrest following aspiration of gastric contents in more serious cases. Activated charcoal left in the stomach may reduce absorption of any remaining chloroquine from the gut. Circulatory status (with central venous pressure measurement), respiration, plasma electrolytes and blood gases should be monitored, with correction of hypokalaemia and acidosis if indicated. Cardiac arrhythmias should not be treated unless life threatening; drugs with quinidine-like effects should be avoided. Intravenous sodium bicarbonate 1-2mmol/kg over 15 minutes may be effective in conduction disturbances, and DC shock is indicated for ventricular tachycardia and ventricular fibrillation.

Early administration of the following has been shown to improve survival in cases of serious poisoning:

1. Adrenaline infusion 0.25micrograms/kg/min initially, with increments of 0.25micrograms/kg/min until adequate systolic blood pressure (more than 100mg/Hg) is restored; adrenaline reduces the effects of chloroquine on the heart through its inotropic and vasoconstrictor effects.

2. Diazepam infusion (2mg/kg over 30 minutes as a loading dose, followed by 1-2mg/kg/day for up to 2-4 days). Diazepam may minimise cardiotoxicity.

Acidification of the urine, haemodialysis, peritoneal dialysis or exchange transfusion have not been shown to be of value in treating chloroquine poisoning. Chloroquine is excreted very slowly, therefore cases of overdosage require observation for several days.

5. PHARMACOLOGICAL PROPERTIES

5.1 Pharmacodynamic properties

The mode of action of chloroquine on plasmodia has not been fully elucidated. Chloroquine binds to and alters the properties of DNA. Chloroquine also binds to ferriprotoporphyrin IX and this leads to lysis of the plasmodial membrane.

In suppressive treatment, chloroquine inhibits the erythrocytic stage of development of plasmodia. In acute attacks of malaria, it interrupts erythrocytic schizogony of the parasite. Its ability to concentrate in parasitised erythrocytes may account for the selective toxicity against the erythrocytic stages of plasmodial infection.

5.2 Pharmacokinetic properties

Studies in volunteers using single doses of chloroquine phosphate equivalent to 300mg base have found peak plasma levels to be achieved within one to six hours. These levels are in the region of 54 - 102microgram/litre, the concentration in whole blood being some 4 to 10 times higher. Following a single dose, chloroquine may be detected in plasma for more than four weeks. Mean bioavailability from tablets of chloroquine phosphate is 89%. Chloroquine is widely distributed in body tissues such as the eyes, kidneys, liver, and lungs where retention is prolonged. The elimination of chloroquine is slow, with a multi exponential decline in plasma concentration. The initial distribution phase has a half-life of 2-6 days while the terminal elimination phase is 10-60 days. Approximately 50-70% of chloroquine in plasma is bound to the plasma proteins.

The principal metabolite is monodesethylchloroquine, which reaches a peak concentration of 10-20 microgram/litre within a few hours. Mean urinary recovery, within 3-13 weeks, is approximately 50% of the administered dose, most being unchanged drug and the remainder as metabolite. Chloroquine may be detected in urine for several months.

5.3 Preclinical safety data

Avloclor has been widely used for many years in clinical practice. There is no animal data which adds significant information relevant to the prescriber, to that covered elsewhere in this document.

6. PHARMACEUTICAL PARTICULARS

6.1 List of excipients

Magnesium stearate Ph. Eur.

Maize starch Ph. Eur.

6.2 Incompatibilities

None have been reported or are known.

6.3 Shelf life

5 years.

6.4 Special precautions for storage

Do not store above 30°C. Protect from light and moisture.

6.5 Nature and contents of container

HDPE bottle of 100's and PVC/Aluminium Foil Blister Pack of 20's

6.6 Instructions for use and handling

No special instructions.

7. MARKETING AUTHORISATION HOLDER

AstraZeneca UK Limited

600 Capability Green,

Luton, LU1 3LU, UK

8. MARKETING AUTHORISATION NUMBER(S)

PL 17901/0003

9. DATE OF FIRST AUTHORISATION/RENEWAL OF THE AUTHORISATION

18th June 2000/4th June 2005

10. DATE OF REVISION OF THE TEXT

4th June 2005

Avodart 0.5 mg soft capsules

(GlaxoSmithKline UK)

1. NAME OF THE MEDICINAL PRODUCT

Avodart 0.5 mg soft capsules.

2. QUALITATIVE AND QUANTITATIVE COMPOSITION

Each capsule contains 0.5 mg dutasteride. For excipients, see 6.1

3. PHARMACEUTICAL FORM

Capsules, soft.

The capsules are opaque, yellow, oblong soft gelatin capsules imprinted with GX CE2 on one side in red ink.

4. CLINICAL PARTICULARS

4.1 Therapeutic indications

Treatment of moderate to severe symptoms of benign prostatic hyperplasia (BPH).

Reduction in the risk of acute urinary retention (AUR) and surgery in patients with moderate to severe symptoms of BPH.

For information on effects of treatment and patient populations studied in clinical trials please see 5.1 Pharmacodynamic Properties, 'clinical studies'.

4.2 Posology and method of administration

Adults (including elderly):

The recommended dose of Avodart is one capsule (0.5 mg) taken orally once a day. The capsules should be swallowed whole and may be taken with or without food. Although an improvement may be observed at an early stage, it can take up to 6 months before a response to the treatment can be achieved. No dose adjustment is necessary in the elderly.

Renal impairment

The effect of renal impairment on dutasteride pharmacokinetics has not been studied. No adjustment in dosage is anticipated for patients with renal impairment (see 5.2 Pharmacokinetic Properties).

Hepatic impairment

The effect of hepatic impairment on dutasteride pharmacokinetics has not been studied so caution should be used in patients with mild to moderate hepatic impairment (see 4.4 Special Warnings and Precautions for Use and 5.2 Pharmacokinetic Properties). In patients with severe hepatic impairment, the use of dutasteride is contraindicated (See section 4.3 Contraindications).

4.3 Contraindications

Avodart is contraindicated for use in women and children and adolescents (see 4.6 Pregnancy and Lactation).

Avodart is contraindicated in patients with hypersensitivity to dutasteride, other 5-alpha reductase inhibitors, or any of the excipients.

Avodart is contraindicated in patients with severe hepatic impairment.

4.4 Special warnings and special precautions for use

Digital rectal examination, as well as other evaluations for prostate cancer, must be performed on patients with BPH prior to initiating therapy with Avodart and periodically thereafter.

Dutasteride is absorbed through the skin, therefore, women, children and adolescents must avoid contact with leaking capsules (see 4.6 Pregnancy and Lactation). If contact is made with leaking capsules, the contact area should be washed immediately with soap and water.

Dutasteride was not studied in patients with liver disease. Caution should be used in the administration of dutasteride to patients with mild to moderate hepatic impairment (see 4.2 Posology and Method of Administration, 4.3 Contraindications and 5.2 Pharmacokinetic Properties).

Serum prostate-specific antigen (PSA) concentration is an important component in the detection of prostate cancer. Generally, a total serum PSA concentration greater than 4 ng/mL (Hybritech) requires further evaluation and consideration of prostate biopsy. Physicians should be aware that a baseline PSA less than 4 ng/mL in patients taking Avodart does not exclude a diagnosis of prostate cancer. Avodart causes a decrease in serum PSA levels by approximately 50%, after 6 months, in patients with BPH, even in the presence of prostate cancer. Although there may be individual variation, the reduction in PSA by approximately 50% is predictable as it was observed over the entire range of baseline PSA values (1.5 to 10 ng/mL). Therefore to interpret an isolated PSA value in a man treated with Avodart for six months or more, PSA values should be doubled for comparison with normal ranges in untreated men. This adjustment preserves the sensitivity and specificity of the PSA assay and maintains its ability to detect prostate cancer. Any sustained increases in PSA levels while on Avodart should be carefully evaluated, including consideration of noncompliance to therapy with Avodart.

Total serum PSA levels return to baseline within 6 months of discontinuing treatment. The ratio of free to total PSA remains constant even under the influence of Avodart. If clinicians elect to use percent free PSA as an aid in the detection of prostate cancer in men undergoing Avodart therapy, no adjustment to its value appears necessary.

4.5 Interaction with other medicinal products and other forms of Interaction

For information on the decrease of serum PSA levels during treatment with dutasteride and guidance concerning prostate cancer detection, please see section 4.4.

Effects of other drugs on the pharmacokinetics of dutasteride

Use together with CYP3A4 and/or P-glycoprotein-inhibitors:

Dutasteride is mainly eliminated via metabolism. *In vitro* studies indicate that this metabolism is catalysed by CYP3A4 and CYP3A5. No formal interaction studies have been performed with potent CYP3A4 inhibitors. However, in a population pharmacokinetic study, dutasteride serum concentrations were on average 1.6 to 1.8 times greater, respectively, in a small number of patients treated concurrently with verapamil or diltiazem (moderate inhibitors of CYP3A4 and inhibitors of P-glycoprotein) than in other patients.

Long-term combination of dutasteride with drugs that are potent inhibitors of the enzyme CYP3A4 (e.g. ritonavir, indinavir, nefazodone, itraconazole, ketoconazole administered orally) may increase serum concentrations of dutasteride. Further inhibition of 5-alpha reductase at increased dutasteride exposure, is not likely. However, a reduction of the dutasteride dosing frequency can be considered if side effects are noted. It should be noted that in the case of enzyme inhibition, the long half-life may be further prolonged and it can take more than 6 months of concurrent therapy before a new steady state is reached.

Administration of 12g cholestyramine one hour before a 5mg single dose of dutasteride did not affect the pharmacokinetics of dutasteride.

Effects of dutasteride on the pharmacokinetics of other drugs

Dutasteride has no effect on the pharmacokinetics of warfarin or digoxin. This indicates that dutasteride does not inhibit/induce CYP2C9 or the transporter P-glycoprotein. *In vitro* interaction studies indicate that dutasteride does not inhibit the enzymes CYP1A2, CYP2D6, CYP2C9, CYP2C19 or CYP3A4.

In a small study (N=24) of two weeks duration in healthy men, no pharmacokinetic or pharmacodynamic interaction was observed between dutasteride and tamsulosin or terazosin.

There was no evidence of an interaction when dutasteride was co-administered with tamsulosin in a clinical trial of 327 patients for up to 9 months.

4.6 Pregnancy and lactation
Avodart is contraindicated for use by women.

Pregnancy

As with other 5 alpha reductase inhibitors, dutasteride inhibits the conversion of testosterone to dihydrotestosterone and may, if administered to a woman carrying a male foetus, inhibit the development of the external genitalia of the foetus (see 4.4 Special Warnings and Precautions for Use). Small amounts of dutasteride have been recovered from the semen in subjects receiving Avodart 0.5mg day. Based on studies in animals, it is unlikely that a male foetus will be adversely affected if his mother is exposed to the semen of a patient being treated with Avodart (the risk of which is greatest during the first 16 weeks of pregnancy). However, as with all 5 alpha reductase inhibitors, when the patient's partner is or may potentially be pregnant it is recommended that the patient avoids exposure of his partner to semen by use of a condom.

Lactation

It is not known whether dutasteride is excreted in human milk.

4.7 Effects on ability to drive and use machines
Based on the pharmacodynamic properties of dutasteride, treatment with dutasteride would not be expected to interfere with the ability to drive or operate machinery.

4.8 Undesirable effects
Approximately 19% of the 2167 patients who received dutasteride in the Phase III placebo-controlled trials developed adverse reactions. The majority of events were mild to moderate and occurred in the reproductive system.

The following adverse reactions have been reported with a higher incidence than in the placebo groups during the first year of treatment in controlled clinical trials:

Organ system	Adverse reaction	Incidence
Reproductive system and breast disorders	Impotence	6.0%
	Altered (decreased) libido	3.7%
	Ejaculation disorders	1.8%
	Gynaecomastia*	1.3%

* Includes breast enlargement and/or breast tendernessThe incidence of adverse events is decreasing with time.

The incidence of more rare adverse reactions or adverse reactions that may occur after long term treatment is currently unknown.

4.9 Overdose
In volunteer studies of Avodart, single daily doses of dutasteride up to 40 mg/day (80 times the therapeutic dose) have been administered for 7 days without significant safety concerns. In clinical studies, doses of 5mg daily have been administered to subjects for 6 months with no additional adverse effects to those seen at therapeutic doses of 0.5 mg. There is no specific antidote for Avodart, therefore, in suspected overdosage symptomatic and supportive treatment should be given as appropriate.

5. PHARMACOLOGICAL PROPERTIES

5.1 Pharmacodynamic properties
Pharmacotherapeutic group: testosterone-5-alpha-reductase inhibitors.

ATC code: G04C B02.

Dutasteride reduces circulating levels of dihydrotestosterone (DHT) by inhibiting both type 1 and type 2, 5α-reductase isoenzymes which are responsible for the conversion of testosterone to 5α-DHT.

Effects on DHT/Testosterone:

Effect of daily doses of Avodart on the reduction on DHT is dose dependant and is observed within 1-2 weeks (85% and 90% reduction, respectively).

In patients with BPH treated with dutasteride 0.5 mg/day, the median decrease in serum DHT was 94% at 1 year and 93% at 2 years and the median increase in serum testosterone was 19% at both 1 and 2 years.

Effect on Prostate Volume:

Significant reductions in prostate volume have been detected as early as one month after initiation of treatment and reductions continued through Month 24 ($p < 0.001$). Avodart led to a mean reduction of total prostate volume of 23.6% (from 54.9cc at baseline to 42.1cc) at Month 12 compared with a mean reduction of 0.5% (from 54.0cc to 53.7cc) in the placebo group. Significant ($p < 0.001$) reductions also occurred in prostate transitional zone volume as early as one month continuing through Month 24, with a mean reduction in prostate transitional zone volume of 17.8% (from 26.8cc at baseline to 21.4cc) in the Avodart group compared to a mean increase of 7.9% (from 26.8cc to 27.5cc) in the placebo group at Month 12. Reduction of the size of prostate leads to improvement of symptoms and a decreased risk for AUR and BPH-related surgery.

CLINICAL STUDIES

Avodart 0.5 mg/day or placebo was evaluated in 4325 male subjects with moderate to severe symptoms of BPH who had prostates ≥30cc and a PSA value within the range 1.5 - 10 ng/mL in three primary efficacy 2-year multicenter, multinational, placebo-controlled, double-blind studies. Results from pooled analyses of these study data are presented.

The most important clinical efficacy parameters were American Urological Association Symptom Index (AUA-SI), maximum urinary flow (Qmax) and the incidence of acute urinary retention and BPH-related surgery.

AUA-SI is a seven-item questionnaire about BPH-related symptoms with a maximum score of 35. At baseline the average score was approx. 17. After six months, one and two years treatment the placebo group had an average improvement of 2.5, 2.5 and 2.3 points respectively while the Avodart group improved 3.2, 3.8 and 4.5 points respectively. The differences between the groups were statistically significant.

Qmax (maximum urine flow):

Mean baseline Qmax for the studies was approx 10 ml/sec (normal Qmax ≥15 ml/sec). After one and two years treatment the flow in the placebo group had improved by 0.8 and 0.9 ml/sec respectively and 1.7 and 2.0 ml/sec respectively in the Avodart group. The difference between the groups was statistically significant from Month 1 to Month 24.

Acute Urinary Retention and Surgical Intervention

After two years of treatment, the incidence of AUR was 4.2% in the placebo group against 1.8% in the Avodart group (57% risk reduction). This difference is statistically significant and means that 42 patients (95% CI 30-73) need to be treated for two years to avoid one case of AUR.

The incidence of BPH-related surgery after two years was 4.1% in the placebo group and 2.2% in the Avodart group (48% risk reduction). This difference is statistically significant and means that 51 patients (95% CI 33-109) need to be treated for two years to avoid one surgical intervention.

Hair distribution

The effect of dutasteride on hair distribution was not formally studied during the phase III programme, however, 5 alpha-reductase inhibitors could reduce hair loss and may induce hair growth in subjects with male pattern hair loss (male androgenetic alopecia).

Thyroid function:

Thyroid function was evaluated in a one year study in healthy men. Free thyroxine levels were stable on dutasteride treatment but TSH levels were mildly increased (by 0.4 MCIU/mL) compared to placebo at the end of one year's treatment. However, as TSH levels were variable, median TSH ranges (1.4 - 1.9 MCIU/mL) remained within normal limits (0.5 - 5/6 MCIU/mL), free thyroxine levels were stable within the normal range and similar for both placebo and dutasteride treatment, the changes in TSH were not considered clinically significant. In all the clinical studies, there has been no evidence that dutasteride adversely affects thyroid function.

Breast neoplasia:

In the 2 year clinical trials, providing 3374 patient years of exposure to dutasteride, and at the time of registration in the 2 year open label extension, there were 2 cases of breast cancer reported in dutasteride-treated patients and 1 case in a patient who received placebo.

However, the relationship between breast cancer and dutasteride is not clear.

5.2 Pharmacokinetic properties

Absorption

Following oral administration of a single 0.5 mg dutasteride dose, the time to peak serum concentrations of dutasteride is 1 to 3 hours. The absolute bioavailability is approximately 60%. The bioavailability of dutasteride is not affected by food.

Distribution

Dutasteride has a large volume of distribution (300 to 500 L) and is highly bound to plasma proteins >99.5%). Following daily dosing, dutasteride serum concentrations achieve 65% of steady state concentration after 1 month and approximately 90% after 3 months.

Steady state serum concentrations (C_{ss}) of approximately 40 ng/mL are achieved after 6 months of dosing 0.5mg once a day. Dutasteride partitioning from serum into semen averaged 11.5%.

Elimination

Dutasteride is extensively metabolized *in vivo*. *In vitro*, dutasteride is metabolized by the cytochrome P450 3A4 and 3A5 to three monohydroxylated metabolites and one dihydroxylated metabolite.

Following oral dosing of dutasteride 0.5 mg/day to steady state, 1.0% to 15.4% (mean of 5.4%) of the administered dose is excreted as unchanged dutasteride in the faeces. The remainder is excreted in the faeces as 4 major metabolites comprising 39%, 21%, 7%, and 7% each of drug-related material and 6 minor metabolites (less than 5% each). Only trace amounts of unchanged dutasteride (less than 0.1% of the dose) are detected in human urine.

The elimination of dutasteride is dose dependent and the process appears to be described by two elimination pathways in parallel, one that is saturable at clinically relevant concentrations and one that is non saturable.

At low serum concentrations (less than 3ng/mL), dutasteride is cleared rapidly by both the concentration dependent and concentration independent elimination pathways. Single doses of 5 mg or less showed evidence of rapid clearance and a short half-life of 3 to 9 days.

At therapeutic concentrations, following repeat dosing of 0.5 mg/day, the slower, linear elimination pathway is dominating and the half-life is approx. 3-5 weeks.

Elderly

Dutasteride pharmacokinetics were evaluated in 36 healthy male subjects between the ages of 24 and 87 years following administration of a single 5mg dose of dutasteride. No significant influence of age was seen on the exposure of dutasteride but the half-life was shorter in men under 50 years of age. Half-life was not statistically different when comparing the 50-69 year old group to the greater than 70 years old.

Renal impairment

The effect of renal impairment on dutasteride pharmacokinetics has not been studied. However, less than 0.1% of a steady-state 0.5 mg dose of dutasteride is recovered in human urine, so no clinically significant increase of the dutasteride plasma concentrations is anticipated for patients with renal impairment (see 4.2 Posology and Method of Administration).

Hepatic impairment

The effect on the pharmacokinetics of dutasteride in hepatic impairment has not been studied (see section 4.3 Contraindications). Because dutasteride is eliminated mainly through metabolism the plasma levels of dutasteride are expected to be elevated in these patients and the half-life of dutasteride be prolonged (see 4.2 Posology and Method of Administration and 4.4 Special Warnings and Precautions for Use).

5.3 Preclinical safety data
Current studies of general toxicity, genotoxicity and carcinogenicity did not show any particular risk to humans.

Reproduction toxicity studies in male rats have shown a decreased weight of the prostate and seminal vesicles, decreased secretion from accessory genital glands and a reduction in fertility indices (caused by the pharmacological effect of dutasteride). The clinical relevance of these findings is unknown.

As with other 5 alpha reductase inhibitors, feminisation of male foetuses in rats and rabbits has been noted when dutasteride was administered during gestation. Dutasteride has been found in blood from female rats after mating with dutasteride treated males. When dutasteride was administered during gestation to primates, no feminisation of male foetuses was seen at blood exposures sufficiently in excess of those likely to occur via human semen. It is unlikely that a male foetus will be adversely affected following seminal transfer of dutasteride.

6. PHARMACEUTICAL PARTICULARS

6.1 List of excipients

Capsule contents:

mono- and diglycerides of caprylic/capric acid

butylhydroxytoluene (E321).

Capsule shell:

gelatin

glycerol

titanium dioxide (E171)

iron oxide yellow (E172)

triglycerides, medium chain

lecithin.

Red printing ink containing iron oxide red (E172) as the colourant, polyvinyl acetate phthalate, propylene glycol and polyethylene glycol.

6.2 Incompatibilities
Not applicable.

6.3 Shelf life
4 years.

6.4 Special precautions for storage
Do not store above 30°C.

6.5 Nature and contents of container
Blisters of opaque PVC/PVDC film containing 10 soft gelatin capsules packed into containers of 10, 30 and 90 capsules.

6.6 Instructions for use and handling
Dutasteride is absorbed through the skin, therefore contact with leaking capsules must be avoided. If contact is made with leaking capsules, the contact area should be washed immediately with soap and water (see 4.4 Special Warnings and Precautions for Use).

Administrative Data

7. MARKETING AUTHORISATION HOLDER

GlaxoSmithKline UK Limited

980 Great West Road

Brentford

Middlesex

TW8 9GS

United Kingdom

Trading as:

GlaxoSmithKline UK Ltd

Stockley Park West

Uxbridge

Middlesex,

UB11 1BT

8. MARKETING AUTHORISATION NUMBER(S)

19494/0006

9. DATE OF FIRST AUTHORISATION/RENEWAL OF THE AUTHORISATION

17 January 2003

10. DATE OF REVISION OF THE TEXT

26 May 2005

11. Legal Status

POM

AVONEX 30 micrograms powder and solvent for solution for injection

(Biogen Idec Ltd)

1. NAME OF THE MEDICINAL PRODUCT

AVONEX 30 micrograms powder and solvent for solution for injection

2. QUALITATIVE AND QUANTITATIVE COMPOSITION

Each vial of AVONEX BIO-SET contains 30 micrograms (6 million IU) of interferon beta-1a.

Following reconstitution with the water for injections the vial contains 1.0 ml of solution. The concentration is 30 micrograms per ml.

Using the World Health Organisation (WHO) natural interferon beta standard, Second International Standard for Interferon, Human Fibroblast (Gb-23-902-531), 30 micrograms of AVONEX contains 6 million IU of antiviral activity. The activity against other standards is not known.

For excipients, see section 6.1.

3. PHARMACEUTICAL FORM

Powder and solvent for solution for injection.

The vial contains a white to off-white cake.

4. CLINICAL PARTICULARS

4.1 Therapeutic indications

AVONEX is indicated for the treatment of ambulatory patients with relapsing multiple sclerosis (MS) characterised by at least two recurrent attacks of neurological dysfunction (relapses) over the preceding three-year period without evidence of continuous progression between relapses. AVONEX slows the progression of disability and decreases the frequency of relapses.

AVONEX is also indicated for the treatment of patients who have experienced a single demyelinating event with an active inflammatory process if it is severe enough to warrant treatment with intravenous corticosteroids, if alternative diagnoses have been excluded, and if they are determined to be at high risk of developing clinically definite MS (see section 5.1).

AVONEX should be discontinued in patients who develop progressive MS.

4.2 Posology and method of administration

Treatment should be initiated under supervision of a physician experienced in the treatment of the disease.

Adults: The recommended dosage of AVONEX - for the treatment of relapsing MS is 30 micrograms (1 ml solution), administered by intramuscular (IM) injection once a week (see section 6.6). No additional benefit has been shown by administering a higher dose (60 micrograms) once a week.

Children and adolescents: There is no experience with AVONEX in patients aged 16 years or less. Therefore, AVONEX should not be used in children and adolescents.

Elderly: Clinical studies of AVONEX did not include a sufficient number of patients aged 65 and over to determine whether they respond differently than younger patients. However, based on the mode of clearance of the active substance there are no theoretical reasons for any requirement for dose adjustments in the elderly.

The intramuscular injection site should be varied each week (see section 5.3).

Prior to injection and for an additional 24 hours after each injection, an antipyretic analgesic is advised to decrease flu-like symptoms associated with AVONEX administration. These symptoms are usually present during the first few months of treatment.

At the present time, it is not known for how long patients should be treated. Patients should be clinically evaluated after two years of treatment and longer-term treatment should be decided on an individual basis by the treating physician. Treatment should be discontinued if the patient develops chronic progressive MS.

4.3 Contraindications

AVONEX is contraindicated in:

- Patients with hypersensitivity to natural or recombinant interferon beta, human serum albumin or to any of the other excipients

- Pregnant patients (see section 4.6-)

- Patients with severe depressive disorders and/or suicidal ideation

- Epileptic patients with a history of seizures not adequately controlled by treatment.

4.4 Special warnings and special precautions for use

AVONEX, as other interferons, should be used with caution in patients with depression or other mood disorders, conditions that are common with MS. Depression has been reported in association with AVONEX use and it may occur at any time during treatment. Patients treated with AVONEX should be advised to immediately report any symptom of depression and/or suicidal ideation to their prescribing physician. Patients exhibiting depression should be monitored closely during therapy with AVONEX and treated appropriately. Cessation of therapy should be considered.

Caution should be exercised when administering AVONEX to patients with pre-existing seizure disorder. For patients without a pre-existing seizure disorder who develop seizures during therapy with AVONEX, an etiologic basis should be established and appropriate anti-convulsant therapy instituted prior to resuming AVONEX treatment.

Caution should be used and close monitoring considered when administering AVONEX to patients with severe renal and hepatic failure and to patients with severe myelosuppression.

Hepatic injury including elevated serum hepatic enzyme levels, hepatitis, autoimmune hepatitis and hepatic failure has been reported with interferon beta in post-marketing. In some cases, these reactions have occurred in the presence of other medicinal products that have been associated with hepatic injury. The potential of additive effects from multiple medicinal products or other hepatotoxic agents (e.g. alcohol) has not been determined. Patients should be monitored for signs of hepatic injury and caution exercised when interferons are used concomitantly with other medicinal products associated with hepatic injury.

Patients with cardiac disease, such as angina, congestive heart failure or arrhythmia, should be closely monitored for worsening of their clinical condition during treatment with AVONEX. Flu-like symptoms associated with AVONEX therapy may prove stressful to patients with underlying cardiac conditions.

Laboratory abnormalities are associated with the use of interferons. Therefore, in addition to those laboratory tests normally required for monitoring patients with MS, complete and differential white blood cell counts, platelet counts, and blood chemistry, including liver function tests, are recommended during AVONEX therapy. Patients with myelosuppression may require more intensive monitoring of complete blood cell counts, with differential and platelet counts.

Patients may develop antibodies to AVONEX. The antibodies of some of those patients reduce the activity of interferon beta-1a *in vitro* (neutralising antibodies). Neutralising antibodies are associated with a reduction in the *in vivo* biological effects of AVONEX and may potentially be associated with a reduction of clinical efficacy. It is estimated that the plateau for the incidence of neutralising antibody formation is reached after 12months of treatment. Data from patients treated up to two years with AVONEX suggests that approximately 8% develop neutralising antibodies.

The use of various assays to detect serum antibodies to interferons limits the ability to compare antigenicity among different products.

4.5 Interaction with other medicinal products and other forms of Interaction

No formal drug interaction studies have been conducted with AVONEX in humans.

The interaction of AVONEX with corticosteroids or adrenocorticotropic hormone (ACTH) has not been studied systematically. The clinical studies indicate that MS patients can receive AVONEX and corticosteroids or ACTH during relapses.

Interferons have been reported to reduce the activity of hepatic cytochrome P450-dependent enzymes in humans and animals. The effect of high-dose AVONEX administration on P450-dependent metabolism in monkeys was evaluated and no changes in liver metabolising capabilities were observed. Caution should be exercised when AVONEX is administered in combination with medicinal products that have a narrow therapeutic index and are largely dependent on the hepatic cytochrome P450 system for clearance, e.g. antiepileptics and some classes of antidepressants.

4.6 Pregnancy and lactation

Because of the potential hazards to the foetus, AVONEX - is contraindicated in pregnancy. There are no studies of interferon beta-1a in pregnant women. At high doses, in rhesus monkeys, abortifacient effects were observed. It cannot be excluded that such effects will be observed in humans.

Fertile women receiving AVONEX should take appropriate contraceptive measures. Patients planning for pregnancy and those becoming pregnant should be informed of the potential hazards and AVONEX should be discontinued.

Breast-feeding:

It is not known whether AVONEX is excreted in human milk. Because of the potential for serious adverse reactions in breast-fed infants, a decision should be made either to discontinue breast-feeding or to discontinue AVONEX therapy.

4.7 Effects on ability to drive and use machines

Studies of the effects of AVONEX on the ability to drive and use machinery have not been performed. Central nervous system-related adverse reactions may have a minor influence on the ability to drive and use machines in susceptible patients (see section 4.8).

4.8 Undesirable effects

The highest incidence of adverse reactions associated with AVONEX therapy is related to flu-like symptoms. The most commonly reported flu-like symptoms are myalgia, fever, chills, sweating, asthenia, headache and nausea. Flu-like symptoms tend to be most prominent at the initiation of therapy and decrease in frequency with continued treatment.

Transient neurological symptoms that may mimic MS exacerbations may occur following injections. Transient episodes of hypertonia and/or severe muscular weakness that prevent voluntary movements may occur at any time during treatment. These episodes are of limited duration, temporally related to the injections and may recur after subsequent injections. In some cases these symptoms are associated with flu-like symptoms.

The frequencies of adverse reactions are expressed in patient-years, according to the following categories:

Very common (>1/10 patient-years);

Common (>1/100, <1/10 patient-years);

Uncommon (>1/1, 000, <1/100 patient-years);

Rare (>1/10, 000, <1/1,000 patient-years);

Very rare (<1/10,000 patient-years);

Patient-time is the sum of individual units of time that the patient in the study has been exposed to AVONEX before experiencing the adverse reaction. For example, 100 person-years could be observed in 100 patients who were on treatment for one year or in 200 patients who were on treatment for half a year.

EXPERIENCE FROM STUDIES (clinical trials and observational studies, with a period of follow-up ranging from two years to six years)

Metabolism and nutrition disorders	
common	Anorexia
Psychiatric disorders	
common	insomnia, depression (see section 4.4)
Nervous system disorders	
very common	headache*
common	hypoesthesia, muscle spasticity
Vascular disorders	
common	flushing
Respiratory disorders	
common	rhinorrhoea
rare	dyspnoea
Gastrointestinal disorders	
common	vomiting, diarrhoea, nausea*
Skin and subcutaneous tissue disorders	
common	rash, sweating increased, contusion
uncommon	alopecia

Musculoskeletal, connective tissue and bone disorders	
common	muscle cramp, neck pain, myalgia*, arthralgia, pain in extremity, back pain, muscle stiffness, musculoskeletal stiffness
Reproductive system disorders	
uncommon	metrorrhagia, menorrhagia
General disorders and administration site conditions	
very common	flu-like symptoms, pyrexia*, chills*, sweating*
common	injection site pain, injection site erythema, injection site bruising, asthenia*, pain, fatigue*, malaise, night sweats
uncommon	injection site burning
Investigations	
common	lymphocyte count decreased, white blood cells count decreased, neutrophil count decreased, hematocrit decreased, blood potassium increased, blood urea nitrogen increased
uncommon	platelet count decreased

*The frequency of occurrence is higher at the beginning of treatment.

Other adverse reactions identified through spontaneous reporting, with unknown frequency are:

Blood and lymphatic system disorders	pancytopenia, thrombocytopenia
Endocrine disorders	hypothyroidism, hyperthyroidism
Psychiatric disorders	anxiety, suicide, psychosis, confusion, emotional lability
Nervous system disorders	neurological symptoms, syncope (1), hypertonia, dizziness, paraesthesia, seizures, migraine
Cardiac disorders	palpitations, tachycardia, arrythmia, cardiomyopathy, congestive heart failure (see section 4.4)
Vascular disorders	vasodilatation
Hepatobiliary disorders	hepatitis, autoimmune hepatitis, hepatic failure (see section 4.4)
Skin and subcutaneous tissue disorders	pruritus, rash vesicular, urticaria, aggravation of psoriasis, angioneurotic oedema
Musculoskeletal disorders	muscle weakness, arthritis, systemic lupus erythematosus
General disorders and administration site conditions	injection site reaction, injection site inflammation, injection site cellulitis (2), injection site necrosis, injection site bleeding, chest pain
Immune system disorders	Hypersensitivity reactions (angioedema, dyspnoea, urticaria, rash and pruritic rash), anaphylactic reaction, anaphylactic shock
Investigations	weight decreased, weight increased, liver function tests abnormal
Infections and infestations	injection site abscess (2)

(1) A syncope episode may occur after AVONEX injection, it is normally a single episode that usually appears at the beginning of the treatment and does not recur with subsequent injections.

(2) Injection site reactions including pain, inflammation and very rare cases of abscess or cellulitis that may require surgical intervention have been reported.

4.9 Overdose

No case of overdose has been reported. However, in case of overdose, patients should be hospitalised for observation and appropriate supportive treatment given.

5. PHARMACOLOGICAL PROPERTIES

5.1 Pharmacodynamic properties

Pharmacotherapeutic Group: Interferons, ATC code: L03 AB07.

Interferons are a family of naturally occurring proteins that are produced by eukaryotic cells in response to viral infection and other biological inducers. Interferons are cytokines that mediate antiviral, antiproliferative and immunomodulatory activities. Three major forms of interferons have been distinguished: alpha, beta and gamma. Interferons alpha and beta are classified as Type I interferons and interferon gamma is a Type II interferon. These interferons have overlapping but clearly distinguishable biological activities. They can also differ with respect to their cellular sites of synthesis.

Interferon beta is produced by various cell types including fibroblasts and macrophages. Natural interferon beta and AVONEX (interferon beta-1a) are glycosylated and have a single N-linked complex carbohydrate moiety. Glycosylation of other proteins is known to affect their stability, activity, biodistribution, and half-life in blood. However, the effects of interferon beta that are dependent on glycosylation are not fully defined.

AVONEX exerts its biological effects by binding to specific receptors on the surface of human cells. This binding initiates a complex cascade of intracellular events that leads to the expression of numerous interferon-induced gene products and markers. These include MHC Class I, Mx protein, 2' / 5'-oligoadenylate synthetase, β_2-microglobulin, and neopterin. Some of these products have been measured in the serum and cellular fractions of blood collected from patients treated with AVONEX. After a single intramuscular dose of AVONEX, serum levels of these products remain elevated for at least four days and up to one week.

Whether the mechanism of action of AVONEX in MS is mediated by the same pathway as the biological effects described above is not known because the pathophysiology of MS is not well established.

The effects of AVONEX in the treatment of MS were demonstrated in a placebo-controlled study of 301 patients (AVONEX n=158, placebo n=143) with relapsing MS. Due to the design of the study, patients were followed for variable lengths of time. One hundred and fifty AVONEX-treated patients completed one year on study and 85 completed two years on study. In the study, the cumulative percentage of patients who developed disability progression (by Kaplan-Meier life table analysis) by the end of two years was 35% for placebo-treated patients and 22% for AVONEX-treated patients. Disability progression was measured as an increase in the Expanded Disability Status Scale (EDSS) of 1.0 point, sustained for at least six months. It was also shown that there was a one-third reduction in annual relapse rate. This latter clinical effect was observed after more than one year of treatment.

A double-blind randomised dose comparison study of 802 relapsing MS patients (AVONEX 30 micrograms n=402, AVONEX 60 micrograms n=400) has shown no statistically significant differences or trends between the 30 micrograms and the 60 micrograms doses of AVONEX in clinical and general MRI parameters.

The effects of AVONEX in the treatment of MS were also demonstrated in a randomised double-blind study performed with 383 patients (AVONEX n=193, placebo n=190) with a single demyelinating event associated with at least two compatible brain MRI lesions. A reduction of the risk of experiencing a second event was noted in the AVONEX treatment group. An effect on MRI parameters was also seen. The estimated risk of a second event was 50% in three years and 39% in two years in the placebo group and 35% (three years) and 21% (two years) in the AVONEX group. In a post-hoc analysis, those patients with a baseline MRI with at least one Gd-enhancing lesion and nine T2 lesions had a two-year risk of suffering a second event of 56% in the placebo group and 21% in the AVONEX treatment group. However, the impact of early treatment with AVONEX is unknown even in this high-risk subgroup as the study was mainly designed to assess the time to the second event rather than the long term evolution of the disease. Furthermore, for the time-being there is no well established definition of a high risk patient although a more conservative approach is to accept at least nine T2 hyperintense lesions on the initial scan and at least one new T2 or one new Gd-enhancing lesion on a follow-up scan taken at least three months after the initial scan. In any case, treatment should only be considered for patients classified at high risk.

5.2 Pharmacokinetic properties

The pharmacokinetic profile of AVONEX -has been investigated indirectly with an assay that measures interferon antiviral activity. This assay is limited in that it is sensitive for interferon but lacks specificity for interferon beta. Alternative assay techniques are not sufficiently sensitive.

Following intramuscular administration of AVONEX, serum antiviral activity levels peak between five and 15 hours post-dose and decline with a half-life of approximately ten hours. With appropriate adjustment for the rate of absorption from the injection site, the calculated bioavailability is approximately 40%. The calculated bioavailability is greater without such adjustments. Intramuscular bioavailability is three-fold higher than subcutaneous bioavailability. Subcutaneous administration cannot be substituted for intramuscular administration.

5.3 Preclinical safety data

Carcinogenesis: No carcinogenicity data for interferon beta-1a are available in animals or humans.

Chronic Toxicity: In a 26-week, repeated-dose toxicity study in rhesus monkey by intramuscular route once per week, administered in combination with another immune modulating agent, an anti CD40 ligand monoclonal antibody, no immune response toward interferon beta-1a and no signs of toxicity were demonstrated.

Local Tolerance: Intramuscular irritation has not been evaluated in animals following repeated administration to the same injection site.

Mutagenesis: Limited but relevant mutagenesis tests have been carried out. The results have been negative.

Impairment of Fertility: Fertility and developmental studies in rhesus monkeys have been carried out with a related form of interferon beta-1a. At very high doses, anovulatory and abortifacient effects in test animals were observed. Similar reproductive dose-related effects have also been observed with other forms of alpha and beta interferons. No teratogenic effects or effects on foetal development have been observed, but the available information on the effects of interferon beta-1a in the peri- and postnatal periods is limited.

No information is available on the effects of interferon beta-1a on male fertility.

6. PHARMACEUTICAL PARTICULARS

6.1 List of excipients

Human serum albumin

Dibasic sodium phosphate

Monobasic sodium phosphate

Sodium chloride.

6.2 Incompatibilities

Not applicable.

6.3 Shelf life

2 years.

AVONEX should be administered as soon as possible after reconstitution. However, the reconstituted solution can be stored at 2 °C-8 °C for up to six hours, prior to injection.

6.4 Special precautions for storage

Store below 25 °C.

DO NOT FREEZE lyophilised or reconstituted product.

See section 6.3 for shelf life and storage conditions after reconstitution.

6.5 Nature and contents of container

AVONEX is available as a package of four individual doses. Each dose is supplied in a 3 ml clear glass vial with BIO-SET device and a 13 mm bromobutyl rubber stopper. It is provided with a 1 ml pre-filled glass syringe of solvent for reconstitution (water for injections) and one needle.

6.6 Instructions for use and handling

Use the supplied pre-filled syringe of solvent to reconstitute AVONEX for injection. Do not use any other solvent. Inject the content of the syringe into the vial of AVONEX by connecting the pre-filled syringe to the BIO-SET device. Gently swirl the contents in the vial until all materials are dissolved; DO NOT SHAKE. Inspect the reconstituted product: If it contains particulate matter or is other than colourless to slightly yellow in colour, the vial must not be used. After reconstitution, draw all the liquid (1 ml) from the vial back into the syringe for the administration of 30 microgramsAVONEX. The needle for intramuscular injection is provided. The formulation does not contain a preservative. Each vial of AVONEX contains a single dose only. Discard the unused portion of any vial.

7. MARKETING AUTHORISATION HOLDER

BIOGEN IDEC LIMITED
5 Roxborough Way
Foundation Park
Maidenhead
Berkshire
SL6 3UD
United Kingdom

8. MARKETING AUTHORISATION NUMBER(S)

EU/1/97/033/002

9. DATE OF FIRST AUTHORISATION/RENEWAL OF THE AUTHORISATION

22.01.2001

10. DATE OF REVISION OF THE TEXT

31st August 2005

AVONEX 30 micrograms/0.5 ml solution for injection.

(Biogen Idec Ltd)

1. NAME OF THE MEDICINAL PRODUCT

AVONEX 30 micrograms/0.5 ml solution for injection.

2. QUALITATIVE AND QUANTITATIVE COMPOSITION

Each 0.5 ml pre-filled syringe contains 30 micrograms (6 million IU) of interferon beta-1a.

The concentration is 30 micrograms per 0.5 ml

Using the World Health Organisation (WHO) natural interferon beta standard, Second International Standard for Interferon, Human Fibroblast (Gb-23-902-531), 30 micrograms of AVONEX contains 6 million IU of antiviral activity. The activity against other standards is not known.

For excipients, see section 6.1.

3. PHARMACEUTICAL FORM

Solution for injection.

Clear and colourless solution.

4. CLINICAL PARTICULARS

4.1 Therapeutic indications

AVONEX is indicated for the treatment of ambulatory patients with relapsing multiple sclerosis (MS) characterised by at least two recurrent attacks of neurological dysfunction (relapses) over the preceding three-year period without evidence of continuous progression between relapses. AVONEX slows the progression of disability and decreases the frequency of relapses.

AVONEX is also indicated for the treatment of patients who have experienced a single demyelinating event with an active inflammatory process if it is severe enough to warrant treatment with intravenous corticosteroids, if alternative diagnoses have been excluded, and if they are determined to be at high risk of developing clinically definite MS (see section 5.1).

AVONEX should be discontinued in patients who develop progressive MS.

4.2 Posology and method of administration

Treatment should be initiated under supervision of a physician experienced in the treatment of the disease.

Adults: The recommended dosage of AVONEX for the treatment of relapsing MS is 30 micrograms (0.5 ml solution) administered by intramuscular injection (IM) once a week (see section 6.6). No additional benefit has been shown by administering a higher dose (60 micrograms) once a week.

Children and adolescents: There is no experience with AVONEX in patients aged 16 years or less. Therefore, AVONEX should not be used in children and adolescents.

Elderly: Clinical studies of AVONEX did not include a sufficient number of patients aged 65 and over to determine whether they respond differently than younger patients. However, based on the mode of clearance of the active substance there are no theoretical reasons for any requirement for dose adjustments in the elderly.

The intramuscular injection site should be varied each week (see section 5.3).

Prior to injection and for an additional 24 hours after each injection, an antipyretic analgesic is advised to decrease flu-like symptoms associated with AVONEX administration. These symptoms are usually present during the first few months of treatment.

At the present time, it is not known for how long patients should be treated. Patients should be clinically evaluated after two years of treatment and longer-term treatment should be decided on an individual basis by the treating physician. Treatment should be discontinued if the patient develops chronic progressive MS.

4.3 Contraindications

AVONEX is contraindicated in:

- Patients with hypersensitivity to natural or recombinant interferon beta, or to any of the excipients
- Pregnant patients (see section 4.6)
- Patients with severe depressive disorders and/or suicidal ideation.
- Epileptic patients with a history of seizures not adequately controlled by treatment.

4.4 Special warnings and special precautions for use

AVONEX, as other interferons, should be used with caution in patients with depression or other mood disorders, conditions that are common with MS. Depression has been reported in association with AVONEX use and it may occur at any time during treatment. Patients treated with AVONEX should be advised to immediately report any symptom of depression and/or suicidal ideation to their prescribing physician. Patients exhibiting depression should be monitored closely during therapy with AVONEX and treated appropriately. Cessation of therapy should be considered.

Caution should be exercised when administering AVONEX to patients with pre-existing seizure disorder. For patients without a pre-existing seizure disorder who develop seizures during therapy with AVONEX, an etiologic basis should be established and appropriate anti-convulsant therapy instituted prior to resuming AVONEX treatment.

Caution should be used and close monitoring considered when administering AVONEX to patients with severe renal and hepatic failure and to patients with severe myelosuppression.

Hepatic injury including elevated serum hepatic enzyme levels, hepatitis, autoimmune hepatitis and hepatic failure has been reported with interferon beta in post-marketing. In some cases, these reactions have occurred in the presence of other medicinal products that have been associated with hepatic injury. The potential of additive effects from multiple medicinal products or other hepatotoxic agents (e.g. alcohol) has not been determined. Patients should be monitored for signs of hepatic injury and caution exercised when interferons are used concomitantly with other medicinal products associated with hepatic injury.

Patients with cardiac disease, such as angina, congestive heart failure or arrhythmia, should be closely monitored for worsening of their clinical condition during treatment with AVONEX. Flu-likesymptoms associated with AVONEX therapy may prove stressful to patients with underlying cardiac conditions.

Laboratory abnormalities are associated with the use of interferons. Therefore, in addition to those laboratory tests normally required for monitoring patients with MS, complete and differential white blood cell counts, platelet counts, and blood chemistry, including liver function tests, are recommended during AVONEX therapy. Patients with myelosuppression may require more intensive monitoring of complete blood cell counts, with differential and platelet counts.

Patients may develop antibodies to AVONEX. The antibodies of some of those patients reduce the activity of interferon beta-1a *in vitro* (neutralising antibodies). Neutralising antibodies are associated with a reduction in the *in vivo* biological effects of AVONEX and may potentially be associated with a reduction of clinical efficacy. It is estimated that the plateau for the incidence of neutralising antibody formation is reached after 12 months of treatment. Recent clinical studies with patients treated up to three years with AVONEX suggest that approximately 5% to 8% develop neutralising antibodies.

The use of various assays to detect serum antibodies to interferons limits the ability to compare antigenicity among different products.

The tip-cap of the pre-filled syringe contains dry natural rubber, which may cause allergic reactions.

4.5 Interaction with other medicinal products and other forms of Interaction

No formal drug interaction studies have been conducted with AVONEX in humans.

The interaction of AVONEX with corticosteroids or adrenocorticotropic hormone (ACTH) has not been studied systematically. The clinical studies indicate that MS patients can receive AVONEX and corticosteroids or ACTH during relapses.

Interferons have been reported to reduce the activity of hepatic cytochrome P450-dependent enzymes in humans and animals. The effect of high-dose AVONEX administration on P450-dependent metabolism in monkeys was evaluated and no changes in liver metabolising capabilities were observed. Caution should be exercised when AVONEX is administered in combination with medicinal products that have a narrow therapeutic index and are largely dependent on the hepatic cytochrome P450 system for clearance, e.g. antiepileptics and some classes of antidepressants.

4.6 Pregnancy and lactation

Because of the potential hazards to the foetus, AVONEX is contraindicated in pregnancy. There are no studies of interferon beta-1a in pregnant women. At high doses, in rhesus monkeys, abortifacient effects were observed. It cannot be excluded that such effects will be observed in humans.

Fertile women receiving AVONEX should take appropriate contraceptive measures. Patients planning for pregnancy and those becoming pregnant should be informed of the potential hazards and AVONEX should be discontinued.

Breast-feeding:

It is not known whether AVONEX is excreted in human milk. Because of the potential for serious adverse reactions in breast-fed infants, a decision should be made either to discontinue breast-feeding or to discontinue AVONEX therapy.

4.7 Effects on ability to drive and use machines

Studies of the effects of AVONEX on the ability to drive and use machinery have not been performed. Central nervous system-related adverse reactions may have a minor influence on the ability to drive and use machines in susceptible patients (see section 4.8).

4.8 Undesirable effects

The highest incidence of adverse reactions associated with AVONEX therapy is related to flu-like symptoms. The most commonly reported flu-like symptoms are myalgia, fever, chills, sweating, asthenia, headache and nausea. Flu-like symptoms tend to be most prominent at the initiation of therapy and decrease in frequency with continued treatment.

Transient neurological symptoms that may mimic MS exacerbations may occur following injections. Transient episodes of hypertonia and/or severe muscular weakness that prevent voluntary movements may occur at any time during treatment. These episodes are of limited duration, temporally related to the injections and may recur after subsequent injections. In some cases these symptoms are associated with flu-like symptoms.

The frequencies of adverse reactions are expressed in patient-years, according to the following categories:

Very common (>1/10 patient-years);
Common (>1/100, <1/10 patient-years);
Uncommon (>1/1, 000, <1/100 patient-years);
Rare (>1/10, 000, <1/1,000 patient-years);
Very rare (<1/10,000 patient-years);

Patient-time is the sum of individual units of time that the patient in the study has been exposed to AVONEX before experiencing the adverse reaction. For example, 100 person-years could be observed in 100 patients who were on treatment for one year or in 200 patients who were on treatment for half a year.

EXPERIENCE FROM STUDIES (clinical trials and observational studies, with a period of follow-up ranging from two years to six years)

Metabolism and nutrition disorders	
common	Anorexia
Psychiatric disorders	
common	insomnia, depression (see section 4.4)
Nervous system disorders	
very common	headache*
common	hypoesthesia, muscle spasticity
Vascular disorders	
common	flushing
Respiratory disorders	
common	rhinorrhoea
rare	dyspnoea
Gastrointestinal disorders	
common	vomiting, diarrhoea, nausea*
Skin and subcutaneous tissue disorders	
common	rash, sweating increased, contusion
uncommon	alopecia

Musculoskeletal, connective tissue and bone disorders	
common	muscle cramp, neck pain, myalgia*, arthralgia, pain in extremity, back pain, muscle stiffness, musculoskeletal stiffness
Reproductive system disorders	
uncommon	metrorrhagia, menorrhagia
General disorders and administration site conditions	
very common	flu-like symptoms, pyrexia*, chills*, sweating*
common	injection site pain, injection site erythema, injection site bruising, asthenia*, pain, fatigue*, malaise, night sweats
uncommon	injection site burning
Investigations	
common	lymphocyte count decreased, white blood cells count decreased, neutrophil count decreased, hematocrit decreased, blood potassium increased, blood urea nitrogen increased
uncommon	platelet count decreased

*The frequency of occurrence is higher at the beginning of treatment.

Other adverse reactions identified through spontaneous reporting, with unknown frequency are:

Blood and lymphatic system disorders	pancytopenia, thrombocytopenia
Endocrine disorders	hypothyroidism, hyperthyroidism
Psychiatric disorders	anxiety, suicide, psychosis, confusion, emotional lability
Nervous system disorders	neurological symptoms, syncope (1), hypertonia, dizziness, paraesthesia, seizures, migraine
Cardiac disorders	palpitations, tachycardia, arrythmia, cardiomyopathy, congestive heart failure (see section 4.4)
Vascular disorders	vasodilatation
Hepatobiliary disorders	hepatitis, autoimmune hepatitis, hepatic failure (see section 4.4)
Skin and subcutaneous tissue disorders	pruritus, rash vesicular, urticaria, aggravation of psoriasis, angioneurotic oedema
Musculoskeletal disorders	muscle weakness, arthritis, systemic lupus erythematosus
General disorders and administration site conditions	injection site reaction, injection site inflammation, injection site cellulitis (2), injection site necrosis, injection site bleeding, chest pain
Immune system disorders	Hypersensitivity reactions (angioedema, dyspnoea, urticaria, rash and pruritic rash), anaphylactic reaction, anaphylactic shock
Investigations	weight decreased, weight increased, liver function tests abnormal
Infections and infestations	injection site abscess (2)

(1) A syncope episode may occur after AVONEX injection, it is normally a single episode that usually appears at the beginning of the treatment and does not recur with subsequent injections.

(2) Injection site reactions including pain, inflammation and very rare cases of abscess or cellulitis that may require surgical intervention have been reported.

4.9 Overdose

No case of overdose has been reported. However, in case of overdose, patients should be hospitalised for observation and appropriate supportive treatment given.

5. PHARMACOLOGICAL PROPERTIES

5.1 Pharmacodynamic properties

Pharmacotherapeutic Group: Interferons, ATC code: L03 AB07.

Interferons are a family of naturally occurring proteins that are produced by eukaryotic cells in response to viral infection and other biological inducers. Interferons are cytokines that mediate antiviral, antiproliferative, and immunomodulatory activities. Three major forms of interferons have been distinguished: alpha, beta, and gamma. Interferons alpha and beta are classified as Type I interferons, and interferon gamma is a Type II interferon. These interferons have overlapping but clearly distinguishable biological activities. They can also differ with respect to their cellular sites of synthesis.

Interferon beta is produced by various cell types including fibroblasts and macrophages. Natural interferon beta and AVONEX (interferon beta-1a) are glycosylated and have a single N-linked complex carbohydrate moiety. Glycosylation of other proteins is known to affect their stability, activity, biodistribution, and half-life in blood. However, the effects of interferon beta that are dependent on glycosylation are not fully defined.

AVONEX exerts its biological effects by binding to specific receptors on the surface of human cells. This binding initiates a complex cascade of intracellular events that leads to the expression of numerous interferon-induced gene products and markers. These include MHC Class I, Mx protein, 2' / 5'-oligoadenylate synthetase, β_2-microglobulin, and neopterin. Some of these products have been measured in the serum and cellular fractions of blood collected from patients treated with AVONEX. After a single intramuscular dose of AVONEX, serum levels of these products remain elevated for at least four days and up to one week.

Whether the mechanism of action of AVONEX in MS is mediated by the same pathway as the biological effects described above is not known because the pathophysiology of MS is not well established.

The effects of lyophilised AVONEX in the treatment of MS were demonstrated in a placebo-controlled study of 301 patients (AVONEX n=158, placebo n=143) with relapsing MS. Due to the design of the study, patients were followed for variable lengths of time. One hundred and fifty AVONEX-treated patients completed one year on study and 85 completed two years on study. In the study, the cumulative percentage of patients who developed disability progression (by Kaplan-Meier life table analysis) by the end of two years was 35% for placebo-treated patients and 22% for AVONEX-treated patients. Disability progression was measured as an increase in the Expanded Disability Status Scale (EDSS) of 1.0 point, sustained for at least six months. It was also shown that there was a one-third reduction in annual relapse rate. This latter clinical effect was observed after more than one year of treatment.

A double-blind randomised dose comparison study of 802 relapsing MS patients (AVONEX 30 micrograms n=402, AVONEX 60 micrograms n=400) has shown no statistically significant differences or trends between the 30 micrograms and the 60 micrograms doses of AVONEX in clinical and general MRI parameters.

The effects of AVONEX in the treatment of MS were also demonstrated in a randomised double-blind study performed with 383 patients (AVONEX n=193, placebo n=190) with a single demyelinating event associated with at least two compatible brain MRI lesions. A reduction of the risk of experiencing a second event was noted in the AVONEX treatment group. An effect on MRI parameters was also seen. The estimated risk of a second event was 50% in three years and 39% in two years in the placebo group and 35% (three years) and 21% (two years) in the AVONEX group. In a post-hoc analysis, those patients with a baseline MRI with at least one Gd-enhancing lesion and nine T2 lesions had a two-year risk of suffering a second event of 56% in the placebo group and 21% in the AVONEX treatment group. However, the impact of early treatment with AVONEX is unknown even in this high-risk subgroup as the study was mainly designed to assess the time to the second event rather than the long term evolution of the disease. Furthermore, for the time-being there is no well established definition of a high risk patient although a more conservative approach is to accept at least nine T2 hyperintense lesions on the initial scan and at least one new T2 or one new Gd-enhancing lesion on a follow-up scan taken at least three months after the initial scan. In any case, treatment should only be considered for patients classified at high risk.

5.2 Pharmacokinetic properties

The pharmacokinetic profile of AVONEX has been investigated indirectly with an assay that measures interferon antiviral activity. This assay is limited in that it is sensitive for interferon but lacks specificity for interferon beta. Alternative assay techniques are not sufficiently sensitive.

Following intramuscular administration of AVONEX, serum antiviral activity levels peak between five and 15 hours post-dose and decline with a half-life of approximately ten hours. With appropriate adjustment for the rate of absorption from the injection site, the calculated bioavailability is approximately 40%. The calculated bioavailability is greater without such adjustments. Intramuscular bioavailability is three-fold higher than subcutaneous bioavailability. Subcutaneous administration cannot be substituted for intramuscular administration.

5.3 Preclinical safety data

Carcinogenesis: No carcinogenicity data for interferon beta-1a are available in animals or humans.

Chronic Toxicity: In a 26-week repeated dose toxicity study in rhesus monkey by intramuscular route once per week, administered in combination with another immunomodulating agent, an anti CD40 ligand monoclonal antibody, no immune response toward interferon beta-1a and no signs of toxicity were demonstrated.

Local Tolerance: Intramuscular irritation has not been evaluated in animals following repeated administration to the same injection site.

Mutagenesis: Limited but relevant mutagenesis tests have been carried out. The results have been negative.

Impairment of Fertility: Fertility and developmental studies in rhesus monkeys have been carried out with a related form of interferon beta-1a. At very high doses, anovulatory and abortifacient effects in test animals were observed. Similar reproductive dose-related effects have also been observed with other forms of alpha and beta interferons. No teratogenic effects or effects on foetal development have been observed, but the available information on the effects of Interferon beta-1a in the peri- and postnatal periods is limited.

No information is available on the effects of interferon beta-1a on male fertility.

6. PHARMACEUTICAL PARTICULARS

6.1 List of excipients

Sodium acetate trihydrate,

Acetic acid, glacial,

Arginine hydrochloride,

Polysorbate 20,

Water for injections

6.2 Incompatibilities

Not applicable.

6.3 Shelf life

18 months.

6.4 Special precautions for storage

Store in a refrigerator (2 °C-8 °C).

DO NOT FREEZE.

Store in the original package (sealed plastic tray) in order to protect from light (see section 6.5).

6.5 Nature and contents of container

1 ml pre-filled syringe made of glass (Type I) with tip cap (approximately 10% Dry Natural Rubber) and plunger stopper (bromobutyl) containing 0.5 ml of solution.

Pack size: box of four pre-filled syringes of 0.5 ml. Each syringe is packed in a sealed plastic tray which also contains one injection needle for intramuscular use.

6.6 Instructions for use and handling

AVONEX is provided as ready to use solution for injection in a pre-filled syringe.

Once removed from the refrigerator, AVONEX in a pre-filled syringe should be allowed to warm to room temperature (15-30°C) for about 30 minutes and used within 12 hours.

Do not use external heat sources such as hot water to warm AVONEX 30 micrograms solution for injection.

If the solution for injection contains particulate matter or if it is any colour other than clear colourless, the pre-filled syringe must not be used. The injection needle for intramuscular injection is provided. The formulation does not contain a preservative. Each pre-filled syringe of AVONEX contains a single dose only. Discard the unused portion of any pre-filled syringe.

7. MARKETING AUTHORISATION HOLDER

BIOGEN IDEC LIMITED
5 Roxborough Way
Foundation Park
Maidenhead
Berkshire
SL6 3UD
United Kingdom

8. MARKETING AUTHORISATION NUMBER(S)

EU/1/97/033/003

9. DATE OF FIRST AUTHORISATION/RENEWAL OF THE AUTHORISATION

24 June 2003

10. DATE OF REVISION OF THE TEXT

31st August 2005

Axid Capsules

(Flynn Pharma Ltd)

1. NAME OF THE MEDICINAL PRODUCT

Axid*.

2. QUALITATIVE AND QUANTITATIVE COMPOSITION

Axid 150mg capsules: Each capsule contains 150mg of nizatidine.

Axid 300mg capsules: Each capsule contains 300mg of nizatidine.

3. PHARMACEUTICAL FORM

Hard capsule.

Axid 150mg capsules: Size 2 capsule with an opaque dark yellow cap and opaque pale yellow body, imprinted with 'Flynn 3144' in black ink.

Axid 300mg capsules: Size 1 capsule with an opaque brown cap and opaque pale yellow body, imprinted with 'Flynn 3145' in black ink.

4. CLINICAL PARTICULARS

4.1 Therapeutic indications

For the treatment of the following diseases where reduction of gastric acid is indicated:

Duodenal ulcer

Benign gastric ulcer

Prevention of duodenal or benign gastric ulcer recurrence

Gastric oesophageal reflux disease (including erosions, ulcerations and associated heartburn)

Gastric and/or duodenal ulcer associated with concomitant use of non-steroidal anti-inflammatory drugs

4.2 Posology and method of administration

For oral administration.

Adults: For treatment of duodenal ulcer, the recommended daily dose is 300mg in the evening. Treatment should continue for four weeks, although this period may be reduced if healing is confirmed earlier by endoscopy. Most ulcers will heal within four weeks, but if complete ulcer healing has not occurred after four weeks therapy, patients should continue therapy for a further four weeks.

For the treatment of benign gastric ulcer, the recommended daily dose is 300mg in the evening for four or, if necessary, eight weeks. Prior to treatment with nizatidine, care should be taken to exclude the possibility of gastric cancer.

If preferred, the 300mg daily dose for the treatment of duodenal or benign gastric ulcer may be given as two divided doses of 150mg in the morning and evening.

For the prevention of duodenal or benign gastric ulcer recurrence (prophylactic maintenance therapy), the recommended daily dose is 150mg in the evening.

For the treatment of gastric oesophageal reflux disease, the recommended dosage is from 150mg twice daily, up to 300mg twice daily. Therapy for up to 12 weeks is indicated for erosions and ulcerations, and associated heartburn.

For the treatment of gastric and/or duodenal ulcer associated with concomitant use of non-steroidal anti-inflammatory drugs, the recommended daily dose is 300mg daily (either 300mg at bedtime or 150mg twice daily, in the morning and in the evening) for up to 8 weeks. In most patients, the ulcers will heal within 4 weeks. During treatment, the use of non-steroidal anti-inflammatory drugs may continue.

The elderly: Age does not significantly influence efficacy or safety. Normally dosage modification is not required, except in patients who have moderate to severe renal impairment (creatinine clearance less than 50ml/min).

Children: Not recommended, as safety and efficacy have not been established.

Patients with impaired renal function: For patients who have moderate renal impairment (creatinine clearance less than 50ml/min) or patients who have severe renal impairment (creatinine clearance less than 20ml/min), the dosage should be reduced as follows:

DOSAGE RECOMMENDED

No Renal Impairment	Moderate Renal Impairment	Severe Renal Impairment
600mg	150mg twice daily	150mg daily
300mg	150mg in the evening	150mg on alternate days
150mg	150mg on alternate days	150mg every third day

4.3 Contraindications

Known hypersensitivity to H_2-receptor antagonists.

4.4 Special warnings and special precautions for use

As nizatidine is partially metabolised by the liver and principally excreted by the kidneys, patients with impaired liver or kidney function should be treated with caution. (See section 4.2.)

Symptomatic response to nizatidine therapy does not preclude the presence of gastric malignancy.

4.5 Interaction with other medicinal products and other forms of Interaction

There is evidence that oral nizatidine does not affect the serum levels of concomitantly administered aminophylline, theophylline, chlordiazepoxide, diazepam, lignocaine, phenytoin, ibuprofen, metoprolol, warfarin, or lorazepam. Nizatidine does not inhibit the hepatic cytochrome P450-linked drug metabolising enzyme system, but may increase absorption of salicylates when they are used in very high dosage. However, nizatidine and other histamine H_2-receptor antagonists can reduce the gastric absorption of drugs whose absorption is dependent on an acidic gastric pH. Approximately 35% of nizatidine is bound to plasma protein. Warfarin, diazepam, paracetamol, propantheline, phenobarbitone, and propranolol did not affect plasma protein binding of nizatidine *in vitro.*

Absorption of nizatidine is not clinically significantly affected by food intake, anticholinergic agents, or antacids.

4.6 Pregnancy and lactation

Usage in pregnancy: The safety of nizatidine for use during pregnancy has not been established. Animal studies have shown no evidence of impaired fertility or teratogenicity attributable to nizatidine. Nizatidine should only be used in pregnant women, or in those planning pregnancy, if considered absolutely necessary, and then with caution.

Usage in lactation: Studies conducted in lactating women have shown that 0.1% of the administered oral dose of nizatidine is secreted in human milk in proportion to plasma concentrations. Because of the growth depression in pups reared by lactating rats treated with nizatidine, Axid should be administered to nursing mothers only if considered absolutely necessary.

4.7 Effects on ability to drive and use machines

None stated.

4.8 Undesirable effects

In large scale clinical trials, sweating and urticaria were significantly more common in patients treated with oral nizatidine when compared with placebo. In these trials, 1.9% of treated patients experienced somnolence, compared to 1.6% of placebo patients (non-significant).

In the same trials, patients treated with both nizatidine and placebo had mild, transient, asymptomatic elevations of transaminases or alkaline phosphatase; rare instances of marked elevations >500iu/l) occurred in nizatidine-treated patients. The overall rate of occurrences of elevated liver enzymes and elevations to 3-times the upper limit of normal, however, did not differ significantly from placebo. All abnormalities were reversible after discontinuation of nizatidine. Since introduction, hepatitis and jaundice have been reported. Rare cases of cholestatic or mixed hepatocellular and cholestatic injury with jaundice have been reported, with reversal of the abnormalities after discontinuation.

The following effects have also been rarely reported, although a causal relationship has not always been established: thrombocytopenic purpura, fatal thrombocytopenia, exfoliative dermatitis, vasculitis, arthralgia, myalgia, gynaecomastia, impotence, hyperuricaemia, fever, nausea, and reversible mental confusion.

Rare episodes of hypersensitivity reactions (eg, bronchospasm, laryngeal oedema, rash, pruritus, and eosinophilia), serum sickness, and anaphylaxis have been reported.

4.9 Overdose

There is little experience of overdose in humans. Tested at very high doses in animals, nizatidine has been shown to be relatively non-toxic. Animal studies suggest that cholinergic-type effects, including lacrimation, salivation, emesis, miosis, and diarrhoea, may occur following very large oral doses.

Treatment: Symptomatic and supportive therapy is recommended. Activated charcoal, emesis, or lavage may reduce nizatidine absorption. The ability of haemodialysis to remove nizatidine from the body has not been conclusively demonstrated. However, this method is not expected to be efficient, since nizatidine has a large volume of distribution.

5. PHARMACOLOGICAL PROPERTIES

5.1 Pharmacodynamic properties

Nizatidine is a potent, selective, competitive and fully reversible histamine H_2-receptor antagonist. Nizatidine significantly decreased basal and stimulated gastric acid and pepsin concentration, in addition to the volume of gastric secretion.

In various clinical trials, nizatidine, administered as either a single daily dose (at bedtime) or in two divided doses (morning and evening), significantly inhibited gastric acid secretion, and ulcer pain was usually rapidly abolished.

Nizatidine has no significant effect on the serum concentrations of gastrin, gonadotrophins, prolactin, growth hormone, antidiuretic hormone, cortisol, testosterone, 5-alpha-dihydrotestosterone, or oestradiol.

Nizatidine has no antiandrogenic action.

5.2 Pharmacokinetic properties

Absorption of nizatidine after oral administration is rapid and peak plasma concentrations (700-1800ng/ml after 150mg; 1400-3600ng/ml after 300mg dose) are usually achieved within two hours of administration (range 0.5-3 hours). Oral bioavailability exceeds 70%, and the elimination half-life is approximately 1.6 hours. Minor (6%) first pass hepatic metabolism occurs, but nizatidine is principally excreted via the kidneys, about 60% as unchanged drug, renal clearance is about 500ml/min. Metabolites include desmethyl nizatidine (7%), sulphoxide (6%), and N-oxide (5%). Desmethyl nizatidine is an active metabolite of limited potency. More than 90% of an oral dose of nizatidine (including metabolites) is excreted in the urine within 12 hours.

5.3 Preclinical safety data

There are no preclinical data of relevance to the prescriber in addition to that summarised in other sections of the Summary of Product Characteristics.

6. PHARMACEUTICAL PARTICULARS

6.1 List of excipients

Starch flowable powder

Starch

Silicone fluid 350 cs

Magnesium stearate (Axid 150mg)

Povidone (Axid 300mg)

Carboxymethyl cellulose sodium cross-linked (Axid 300mg)

Talc (Axid 300mg)

Capsules shell:

Yellow iron oxide

Red iron oxide (Axid 300mg)

Titanium dioxide

Gelatin

Colorcon black ink S-1-8100

6.2 Incompatibilities

None known.

6.3 Shelf life

24 months unopened.

6.4 Special precautions for storage

Do not store above 25°C.

6.5 Nature and contents of container

Opaque or transparent PVC/aluminium foil blisters.

Packs contain 28 or 30 capsules.

6.6 Instructions for use and handling

None.

7. MARKETING AUTHORISATION HOLDER

Flynn Pharma Limited
Alton House
4 Herbert Street
Dublin
Ireland

8. MARKETING AUTHORISATION NUMBER(S)

Axid 150mg capsules: PL 13621/0027

Axid 300mg capsules: PL 13621/0028

9. DATE OF FIRST AUTHORISATION/RENEWAL OF THE AUTHORISATION

Date of first authorisation: 11 August 1987

Date of last renewal of authorisation: 24 March 2000

10. DATE OF REVISION OF THE TEXT

February 2003

Axsain

(Zeneus Pharma Ltd)

1. NAME OF THE MEDICINAL PRODUCT
Axsain

2. QUALITATIVE AND QUANTITATIVE COMPOSITION
Capsaicin 0.075% w/w

3. PHARMACEUTICAL FORM
Cream for topical application.

4. CLINICAL PARTICULARS

4.1 Therapeutic indications
1. For the symptomatic relief of neuralgia associated with and following Herpes Zoster infections (post-herpetic neuralgia) after open skin lesions have healed.

2. For the symptomatic management of painful diabetic peripheral polyneuropathy.

4.2 Posology and method of administration
Adults and the elderly:

For topical administration to unbroken skin. Apply only a small amount of cream (pea size) to the affected area 3 or 4 times daily. These applications should be evenly spaced throughout the waking hours and not more often than every 4 hours. The cream should be gently rubbed in, there should be no residue left on the surface. Hands should be washed immediately after application of Axsain with the fingers. Do not apply near the eyes.

Patients using Axsain for the treatment of painful diabetic peripheral polyneuropathy should only do so under the direct supervision of a hospital consultant who has access to specialist resources. The recommended duration of use in the first instance is 8 weeks, since there is no clinical trial evidence of efficacy for treatment of more than 8 weeks duration. After this time, it is recommended that the patient's condition should be fully clinically assessed prior to continuation of treatment, and regularly re-evaluated thereafter, by the supervising consultant.

Not suitable for use in children.

4.3 Contraindications
Axsain cream is contra-indicated for use on broken or irritated skin.

Axsain Cream is contra-indicated in patients with known hypersensitivity to capsaicin or any of the excipients used in this product.

4.4 Special warnings and special precautions for use
Keep away from the eyes.

After applying Axsain cream with the fingers, hands should be washed immediately. Patients should avoid taking a hot bath or shower just before or after applying Axsain, as it can enhance the burning sensation.

Patients and carers should avoid inhalation of vapours from the cream, as transient irritation of the mucous membranes of the eyes and respiratory tract (including exacerbation of asthma) has been reported.

If the condition worsens, seek medical advice.

4.5 Interaction with other medicinal products and other forms of Interaction
Not applicable.

4.6 Pregnancy and lactation
The safety of Axsain during pregnancy or lactation has not been established in either humans or animals. However, in the small amounts absorbed transdermally from Axsain Cream, it is considered unlikely that capsaicin will cause any adverse effects in humans.

4.7 Effects on ability to drive and use machines
Not applicable.

4.8 Undesirable effects
Axsain may cause transient burning on application. This burning is observed more frequently when application schedules of less than 3-4 times daily are utilised. The burning can be enhanced if too much cream is used and if it is applied just before or after a bath or shower.

Irritation of the mucous membranes of the eyes and respiratory tract (such as coughing, sneezing, runny eyes) on application of Axsain cream has been reported rarely. These events are usually mild and self-limiting. There have been a few reports of dyspnea, wheezing and exacerbation of asthma.

4.9 Overdose
Not applicable.

5. PHARMACOLOGICAL PROPERTIES

5.1 Pharmacodynamic properties
Although the precise mechanism of action of capsaicin is not fully understood, current evidence suggests that capsaicin renders skin insensitive to pain by depleting and preventing reaccumulation of substance P in peripheral sensory neurons. Substance P is thought to be the principal chemomediator of pain impulses from the periphery to the Central Nervous System.

5.2 Pharmacokinetic properties
Absorption after topical application is unknown. Average consumption of dietary spice from capsicum fruit has been estimated as 2.5g/person/day in India and 5.0g/person/day in Thailand. Capsaicin content in capsicum fruit is approximately 1% therefore daily dietary intake of capsaicin may range from 0.5 - 1mg/kg/day for a 50kg person. Application of two tubes of Axsain Cream 0.075% (90g) each week results in a 9.6mg/day topical exposure. Assuming 100% absorption in a 50kg person, daily exposure would be 0.192mg/kg which is approximately one third to one quarter of the above mentioned dietary intake.

5.3 Preclinical safety data
The available animal toxicity data relating to capsicum, capsicum extracts and capsaicin do not suggest that, in usual doses, they pose any significant toxicity hazard to man. Thus, in both single and repeat dosing studies which have been reported, capsicum extracts and capsicum are generally well tolerated at many times even the highest estimated human intakes. The safety of Axsain for use in human pregnancy has not been established since no formal reproduction studies have been performed on either animals or man. However, there is no reason to suspect from human or animal studies currently available that any adverse effects in humans are likely.

Studies reported in the published literature, which relate to potential genotoxic and carcinogenic action of capsaicin have produced inconclusive and conflicting data. However, it is unlikely that capsaicin, in the quantities absorbed transdermally from Axsain Cream, will pose any significant hazard to humans.

6. PHARMACEUTICAL PARTICULARS

6.1 List of excipients
Purified water

Sorbitol solution

Isopropyl myristate

Cetyl alcohol

White Soft Paraffin

Glyceryl stearate and PEG-100 stearate (Arlacel 165)

Benzyl alcohol

6.2 Incompatibilities
Not applicable.

6.3 Shelf life
3 years

6.4 Special precautions for storage
Store below 25°C.

6.5 Nature and contents of container
Aluminium tubes with epoxyphenolic lining and polypropylene spiked cap containing 45g Axsain Cream, or 7.5g for use as professional sample.

6.6 Instructions for use and handling
Not applicable.

7. MARKETING AUTHORISATION HOLDER
Elan Pharma International Ltd

W.I.L. House

Shannon Business Park

Shannon

Co. Clare

Ireland

8. MARKETING AUTHORISATION NUMBER(S)
PL 16804/0020

9. DATE OF FIRST AUTHORISATION/RENEWAL OF THE AUTHORISATION
19 February 2003

10. DATE OF REVISION OF THE TEXT
February 2005

11. Legal Category
POM

Azactam for Injection

(E. R. Squibb & Sons Limited)

1. NAME OF THE MEDICINAL PRODUCT
Azactam for Injection

2. QUALITATIVE AND QUANTITATIVE COMPOSITION
Azactam for Injection vials contain 500mg, 1g or 2g aztreonam.

3. PHARMACEUTICAL FORM
Powder for solution for injection or infusion.

4. CLINICAL PARTICULARS

4.1 Therapeutic indications
The treatment of the following infections caused by susceptible aerobic Gram-negative micro-organisms:

Urinary tract infections: including pyelonephritis and cystitis (initial and recurrent) and asymptomatic bacteriuria, including those due to pathogens resistant to the aminoglycosides, cephalosporins or penicillins.

Gonorrhoea: acute uncomplicated urogenital or anorectal infections due to beta-lactamase producing or non-producing strains of *N. gonorrhoeae*.

Lower respiratory tract infections: including pneumonia, bronchitis and lung infections in patients with cystic fibrosis.

Bacteraemia/septicaemia.

Meningitis caused by *Haemophilus influenza* or *Neisseria meningitidis*. Since Azactam provides only Gram negative cover, it should not be given alone as initial blind therapy, but may be used with an antibiotic active against gram positive organisms until the results of sensitivity tests are known.

Bone and joint infections.

Skin and soft tissue infections: including those associated with postoperative wounds, ulcers and burns.

Intra-abdominal infections: peritonitis.

Gynaecological infections: pelvic inflammatory disease, endometritis and pelvic cellulitis.

Azactam is indicated for adjunctive therapy to surgery in the management of infections caused by susceptible organisms, including abscesses, infections complicating hollow viscus perforations, cutaneous infections and infections of serous surfaces.

Bacteriological studies to determine the causative organism(s) and their sensitivity to aztreonam should be performed. Therapy may be instituted prior to receiving the results of sensitivity tests.

In patients at risk of infections due to non-susceptible pathogens, additional antibiotic therapy should be initiated concurrently with Azactam to provide broad-spectrum coverage before identification and susceptibility testing results of the causative organism(s) are known. Based on these results, appropriate antibiotic therapy should be continued.

Patients with serious *Pseudomonas* infections may benefit from concurrent use of Azactam and an aminoglycoside because of their synergistic action. If such concurrent therapy is considered in these patients, susceptibility tests should be performed *in vitro* to determine the activity in combination. The usual monitoring of serum levels and renal function during aminoglycoside therapy applies.

4.2 Posology and method of administration
Intramuscular or intravenous injection, or intravenous infusion.

Adults:

The dose range of Azactam is 1 to 8g daily in equally divided doses. The usual dose is 3 to 4g daily. The maximum recommended dose is 8g daily. The dosage and route of administration should be determined by the susceptibility of the causative organisms, severity of infection and the condition of the patient.

Dosage Guide: Adults (see table on next page)

(see Table 1 on next page)

The intravenous route is recommended for patients requiring single doses greater than 1g, or those with bacterial septicaemia, localised parenchymal abscess (e.g. intra-abdominal abscess), peritonitis, meningitis or other severe systemic or life-threatening infections.

Elderly:

In the elderly, renal status is the major determinant of dosage. Estimated creatinine clearance should be used to determine appropriate dosage, since serum creatinine is not an accurate measurement of renal function in these patients.

Elderly patients normally have a creatinine clearance in excess of 30ml/min and therefore would receive the normal recommended dose. If renal function is below this level, the dosage schedule should be adjusted (see Renal Impairment).

Renal Impairment:

In patients with impaired renal function, the normal recommended initial dose should be given. This should be followed by maintenance doses as shown in the following table:

Estimated Creatinine Clearance (ml/min)	Maintenance Dose
10 - 30	Half the initial dose
Less than 10	One quarter of the initial dose

The normal dose interval should not be altered.

In patients on haemodialysis, a supplementary one eighth of the initial dose should be given after each dialysis.

Children:

The usual dosage for patients older than one week is 30mg/kg/dose every 6 or 8 hours. For severe infections in patients 2 years of age or older, 50mg/kg/dose every 6 or 8 hours is recommended. The total daily dose should not exceed 8g. Dosage information is not yet available for newborns less than 1 week old.

Reconstitution

Azactam for Injection is supplied in 15ml vials.

Upon the addition of the diluent the contents should be shaken immediately and vigorously. Vials of reconstituted Azactam are not intended for multi-dose use, and any unused solution from a single dose must be discarded. Depending on the type and amount of diluent, the pH

Table 1 Dosage Guide: Adults

Type of Infection[1]	Dosage (g)	Frequency (hr.)	Route
Urinary tract	0.5 - 1	8 - 12	IM or IV
Gonorrhoea / cystitis	1	single dose	IM
Cystic fibrosis	2	6 - 8	IV
Severe or life-threatening infections	2	6 - 8	IV
Other infections either	1	8	IM or IV
or	2	12	IV

[1]Because of the serious nature of infections due to *Pseudomonas aeruginosa*, a dose of 2g every 6 or 8 hours is recommended, at least for initial therapy in systemic infections caused by this organism.

ranges from 4.5 to 7.5, and the colour may vary from colourless to light straw-yellow, which may develop a slight pink tint on standing; however this does not affect the potency.

For intramuscular injection: For each gram of aztreonam add at least 3ml Water for Injections Ph. Eur. or 0.9% Sodium Chloride Injection B.P. and shake well.

Single Dose Vial Size	Volume of Diluent to be Added
0.5g	1.5ml
1.0g	3.0ml

Azactam is given by deep injection into a large muscle mass, such as the upper quadrant of the gluteus maximus or the lateral part of the thigh.

For intravenous injection: To the contents of the vial add 6 to 10ml of Water for Injections Ph. Eur. and shake well. Slowly inject directly into the vein over a period of 3 to 5 minutes.

For intravenous infusion:

Vials: For each gram of aztreonam add at least 3ml of Water for Injections Ph. Eur. and shake well.

Dilute this initial solution with an appropriate infusion solution to a final concentration less than 2% w/v (at least 50ml solution per gram of aztreonam). The infusion should be administered over 20-60 minutes.

Appropriate infusion solutions include:

0.9% Sodium Chloride Injection B.P.

5% Glucose Intravenous Infusion B.P.

5% or 10% Mannitol Intravenous Infusion B.P.

Sodium Lactate Intravenous Infusion B.P.

0.9%, 0.45% or 0.2% Sodium Chloride and 5% Glucose Intravenous Infusion B.P.

Compound Sodium Chloride Injection B.P.C. 1959 (Ringer's Solution for Injection)

Compound Sodium Lactate Intravenous Infusion B.P. (Hartmann's Solution for Injection).

A volume control administration set may be used to deliver the initial solution of Azactam into a compatible infusion solution being administered. With use of a Y-tube administration set, careful attention should be given to the calculated volume of Azactam solution required so that the entire dose will be infused.

Reconstitution:

Intravenous infusion solutions of Azactam for Injection prepared with 0.9% Sodium Chloride Injection B.P. or 5% Glucose Intravenous B.P., in PVC or glass containers, to which clindamycin phosphate, gentamicin sulphate, tobramycin sulphate, or cephazolin sodium have been added at concentrations usually used clinically, are stable for up to 24 hours in a refrigerator (2-8°C). Ampicillin sodium admixtures with aztreonam in 0.9% Sodium Chloride Injection B.P. are stable for 24 hours in a refrigerator (2-8°C); stability in 5% Glucose Intravenous Infusion B.P. is eight hours under refrigeration.

If aztreonam and metronidazole are to be used together, they should be administered separately as a cherry red colour has been observed after storage of solutions containing combinations of the two products.

4.3 Contraindications

Patients with a known hypersensitivity to aztreonam and L-arginine.

Aztreonam is contraindicated in pregnancy. Aztreonam crosses the placenta and enters the foetal circulation.

4.4 Special warnings and special precautions for use

Specific studies have not shown significant cross-reactivity between Azactam and antibodies to penicillins or cephalosporins. The incidence of hypersensitivity to Azactam in clinical trials has been low but caution should be exercised in patients with a history of hypersensitivity to beta-lactam antibiotics until further experience is gained.

Experience in patients with impaired hepatic function is limited. Appropriate liver function monitoring in these patients is recommended.

Concurrent therapy with other antimicrobial agents and Azactam is recommended as initial therapy in patients who are at risk of having an infection due to pathogens that are not susceptible to aztreonam.

As with other antibiotics, in the treatment of acute pulmonary exacerbations in patients with cystic fibrosis, while clinical improvement is usually noted, lasting bacterial eradications may not be achieved.

Therapy with Azactam may result in overgrowth of non-susceptible organisms which may require additional antimicrobial therapy. In comparative studies, the number of patients treated for superinfections was similar to that of the control drugs used.

It is recommended that prothrombin times should be monitored if the patient is on concomitant anticoagulant therapy.

4.5 Interaction with other medicinal products and other forms of Interaction

Single-dose pharmacokinetic studies have not shown any significant interaction between aztreonam and gentamicin, cephradine, clindamycin or metronidazole.

Unlike broad spectrum antibiotics, aztreonam produces no effects on the normal anaerobic intestinal flora. No disulfuram-like reactions with alcohol ingestion have been reported.

4.6 Pregnancy and lactation

Aztreonam is contraindicated in pregnancy. Aztreonam crosses the placenta and enters the foetal circulation.

Aztreonam is excreted in breast milk in concentrations that are less than 1% of those in simultaneously obtained maternal serum. Lactating mothers should refrain from breast feeding during the course of therapy.

4.7 Effects on ability to drive and use machines

None known

4.8 Undesirable effects

The following side effects have been reported with Azactam therapy:

Dermatological: rash, pruritus, urticaria, erythema, petechia, exfoliative dermatitis, flushing; very rarely toxic epidermal necrolysis.

Haematological: eosinophilia, increases in prothrombin and partial thromboplastin time have occurred. There have been isolated reports of thrombocytopenia, neutropenia, anaemia, bleeding and pancytopenia.

Hepatobiliary: Jaundice and hepatitis: transient elevations of hepatic transaminases and alkaline phosphatase (without overt signs or symptoms of hepatobiliary dysfunction).

Hypersensitivity: anaphylaxis, angioedema, bronchospasm.

Gastrointestinal: Diarrhoea, very rarely pseudomembranous colitis or gastrointestinal bleeding, nausea and/or vomiting, abdominal cramps, mouth ulcer and altered taste.

Local reactions: phlebitis and discomfort at the i.v. injection site: discomfort at the i.m. injection site.

Rare instances of the following events have been reported:-

vaginitis, candidosis, seizures, dyspnoea, hypotension, weakness, confusion, dizziness, vertigo, sweating, headache, breast tenderness, halitosis, muscle aches, fever, malaise, sneezing and nasal congestion; transient increases in serum creatinine.

4.9 Overdose

There have been no reported cases of overdosage.

5. PHARMACOLOGICAL PROPERTIES

5.1 Pharmacodynamic properties

Aztreonam is a monocyclic beta-lactam antibiotic with potent bactericidal activity against a wide spectrum of gram-negative aerobic pathogens.

Unlike the majority of beta-lactam antibiotics, it is not an inducer *in vitro* of beta-lactamase activity. Aztreonam is usually active *in vitro* against those resistant aerobic organisms whose beta-lactamases hydrolyse other antibiotics.

5.2 Pharmacokinetic properties

Single 30-minute i.v. infusions of 0.5g, 1.0g and 2.0g in healthy volunteers produced peak serum levels of 54, 90 and 204 mg/l, and single 3-minute i.v. injections of the same doses produced peak levels of 58, 125 and 242 mg/l. Peak levels of aztreonam are achieved at about one hour after i.m. administration. After identical single i.m. or i.v. doses, the serum concentrations are comparable at 1 hour (1.5 hours from the start of i.v. infusion), with similar slopes of serum concentrations thereafter.

The serum half-life of aztreonam averaged 1.7 hours in subjects with normal renal function, independent of the dose and route. In healthy subjects 60-70% of a single i.m. or i.v. dose was recovered in the urine by 8 hours, and urinary excretion was essentially complete by 12 hours.

5.3 Preclinical safety data

Aztreonam was well tolerated in a comprehensive series of preclinical toxicity and safety studies.

6. PHARMACEUTICAL PARTICULARS

6.1 List of excipients

L-arginine (780mg per g of aztreonam).

6.2 Incompatibilities

Azactam should not be physically mixed with any other drug, antibiotic or diluent, except those listed in the Posology and Method of Administration section under Reconstitution for Intravenous infusion.

With intermittent infusion of Azactam and another drug via a common delivery tube, the tube should be flushed before and after delivery of Azactam with any appropriate infusion solution compatible with both drug solutions. The drugs should not be delivered simultaneously.

6.3 Shelf life

(a) Product unopened: 36 months

(b) Reconstituted product: 24 hours (2-8°C)

6.4 Special precautions for storage

(a) Storage before reconstitution:

Do not store above 25°C.

(b) Stability after reconstitution:

Store at 2-8°C for not more than 24 hours.

Discard any unused solution.

6.5 Nature and contents of container

Pack of 5 × 15 ml glass vials

6.6 Instructions for use and handling

Any content of product remaining after use should be discarded.

7. MARKETING AUTHORISATION HOLDER

E.R. Squibb & Sons Ltd

Uxbridge Business Park

Sanderson Road

Uxbridge

Middlesex

UB8 1DH

8. MARKETING AUTHORISATION NUMBER(S)

Azactam for Injection 500mg vial: PL 0034/0250

Azactam for Injection 1g vial: PL 0034/0251

Azactam for Injection 2g vial: PL 0034/0252

9. DATE OF FIRST AUTHORISATION/RENEWAL OF THE AUTHORISATION

15th October 1986 / 22nd November 1991 / 13th August 1998

10. DATE OF REVISION OF THE TEXT

June 2005

Bactroban Cream

(GlaxoSmithKline UK)

1. NAME OF THE MEDICINAL PRODUCT
Bactroban® Cream.

2. QUALITATIVE AND QUANTITATIVE COMPOSITION
1g Cream contains: 21.5mg Mupirocin calcium equivalent to 20.0mg mupirocin.

For excipients, see Section 6.1.

3. PHARMACEUTICAL FORM
Cream.

Bactroban Cream is presented as a white cream of homogeneous appearance.

4. CLINICAL PARTICULARS
4.1 Therapeutic indications
Bactroban Cream is indicated for the topical treatment of secondarily infected traumatic lesions such as small lacerations, sutured wounds or abrasions (up to 10cm in length or 100cm^2 in area), due to susceptible strains of *Staphylococcus aureus* and *Streptococcus pyogenes*.

4.2 Posology and method of administration
Dosage
Adults/children/elderly
Three times a day for up to 10 days, depending on the response.

Patients not showing a clinical response within 3 to 5 days should be re-evaluated.

The duration of treatment should not exceed 10 days.

Hepatic impairment: No dosage adjustment is necessary.

Renal impairment: No dosage adjustment is necessary.

Method of administration
A thin layer of cream should be applied to the affected area with a piece of clean cotton wool or gauze swab.

The treated area may be covered by a dressing.

Do not mix with other preparations, as there is a risk of dilution, resulting in a reduction in the antibacterial activity and potential loss of stability of the mupirocin in the cream.

4.3 Contraindications
Bactroban Cream should not be given to patients with a history of hypersensitivity to mupirocin or any of the excipients. (See Excipients, Section 6.1)

4.4 Special warnings and special precautions for use
Avoid contact with the eyes.

Should a possible sensitisation reaction or severe local irritation occur with the use of Bactroban Cream, treatment should be discontinued, the product should be washed off and appropriate alternative therapy for the infection instituted.

As with other antibacterial products, prolonged use may result in overgrowth of non-susceptible organisms.

Bactroban Cream has not been studied in infants under 1 year old and therefore it should not be used in these patients until further data become available.

Bactroban Cream contains cetyl alcohol and stearyl alcohol. These inactive ingredients may cause local skin reactions (e.g. contact dermatitis).

4.5 Interaction with other medicinal products and other forms of Interaction
No drug interactions have been identified.

4.6 Pregnancy and lactation
Use in pregnancy:
Reproduction studies on mupirocin in animals have revealed no evidence of harm to the foetus. As there is no clinical experience on its use during pregnancy, mupirocin should only be used in pregnancy when the potential benefits outweigh the possible risks of treatment.

Use in lactation:
There is no information on the excretion of mupirocin in milk. If a cracked nipple is to be treated, it should be thoroughly washed prior to breast feeding.

4.7 Effects on ability to drive and use machines
No adverse effects on the ability to drive or operate machinery have been identified.

4.8 Undesirable effects
Data from clinical trials was used to determine the frequency of very common to rare undesirable effects.

The following convention has been used for the classification of frequency:-
very common $\geq$1/10, common $\geq$1/100 and <1/10, uncommon $\geq$1/1000 and <1/100, rare $\geq$1/10,000 and <1/1000, very rare <1/10,000.

Skin and subcutaneous tissue disorders:

Common: Application site hypersensitivity reactions including urticaria, pruritus, erythema, burning sensation, contact dermatitis, rash

Skin dryness and erythema have been reported in irritancy studies in volunteers.

4.9 Overdose
The toxicity of mupirocin is very low. In the event of accidental ingestion of the cream symptomatic treatment should be given.

5. PHARMACOLOGICAL PROPERTIES
5.1 Pharmacodynamic properties
Properties
ATC-code: D06A X09

Mupirocin is an antibiotic produced through fermentation by *Pseudomonas fluorescens*. Mupirocin inhibits isoleucyl transfer-RNA synthetase, thereby arresting bacterial protein synthesis. Due to this particular mode of action and its unique chemical structure, mupirocin does not show any cross-resistance with other clinically available antibiotics.

Mupirocin has bacteriostatic properties at minimum inhibitory concentrations and bactericidal properties at the higher concentrations reached when applied locally.

Activity
Mupirocin is a topical antibacterial agent showing *in vivo* activity against *Staphylococcus aureus* (including methicillin-resistant strains), *S. epidermidis* and beta-haemolytic *Streptococcus* species.

The in-vitro spectrum of activity includes but is not limited to the following bacteria which are most often implicated in skin infections:

- Staphylococcus aureus (including beta-lactamase-producing strains and methicillin resistant strains).
- Staphylococcus epidermidis (including beta-lactamase-producing strains and methicillin-resistant strains).
- Other coagulase-negative staphylococci (including methicillin-resistant strains).
- Streptococcus species.

5.2 Pharmacokinetic properties
Absorption
Systemic absorption of mupirocin through intact human skin is low although it may occur through broken/diseased skin. However, clinical trials have shown that when given systemically, it is metabolised to the microbiologically inactive metabolite monic acid and rapidly excreted.

Excretion
Mupirocin is rapidly eliminated from the body by metabolism to its inactive metabolite monic acid which is rapidly excreted by the kidney.

5.3 Preclinical safety data
Pre-clinical effects were seen only at exposures which give no cause for concern for man under normal conditions of clinical use. Mutagenicity studies revealed no risks to man.

6. PHARMACEUTICAL PARTICULARS
6.1 List of excipients
Xanthan gum, liquid paraffin, cetomacrogol 1000, stearyl alcohol, cetyl alcohol, phenoxyethanol, benzyl alcohol, purified water.

6.2 Incompatibilities
None known

6.3 Shelf life
18 months

6.4 Special precautions for storage
Do not store above 25°C. Do not freeze.

6.5 Nature and contents of container
Squeezable aluminium tubes with a screw cap containing 1 g, 15 g or 30 g of white cream.

6.6 Instructions for use and handling
Any product remaining at the end of treatment should be discarded.

Administrative Data
7. MARKETING AUTHORISATION HOLDER
Beecham Group plc

980 Great West Road, Brentford

Middlesex TW8 9GS

Trading as:

GlaxoSmithKline UK

Stockley Park West,

Uxbridge,

Middlesex, UB11 1BT

8. MARKETING AUTHORISATION NUMBER(S)
PL 00038/0372

9. DATE OF FIRST AUTHORISATION/RENEWAL OF THE AUTHORISATION
28 October 1998

10. DATE OF REVISION OF THE TEXT
May 2005

11. Legal category
POM

Bactroban Nasal Ointment

(GlaxoSmithKline UK)

1. NAME OF THE MEDICINAL PRODUCT
Bactroban® Nasal Ointment

2. QUALITATIVE AND QUANTITATIVE COMPOSITION
Mupirocin 2.0% w/w as mupirocin calcium.

3. PHARMACEUTICAL FORM
White soft paraffin based ointment containing a glycerin ester.

4. CLINICAL PARTICULARS
4.1 Therapeutic indications
The elimination of nasal carriage of staphylococci, including methicillin resistant *Staphylococcus aureus* (MRSA).

4.2 Posology and method of administration
Dosage: Adults (including the elderly) and children:

Bactroban Nasal Ointment should be applied to the anterior nares two to three times a day as follows:

A small amount of the ointment about the size of a match head is placed on the little finger and applied to the inside of each nostril. The nostrils are closed by pressing the sides of the nose together; this will spread the ointment throughout the nares. A cotton bud may be used instead of the little finger for the application in particular to infants or patients who are very ill.

Nasal carriage should normally clear within 5-7 days of commencing treatment.

Administration: Topical.

4.3 Contraindications
Bactroban Nasal Ointment should not be given to patients with a history of hypersensitivity to any of the constituents.

4.4 Special warnings and special precautions for use
As with all topical preparations care should be taken to avoid the eyes.

In the rare event of a possible sensitisation reaction or severe local irritation occurring with the use of Bactroban Nasal Ointment, treatment should be discontinued, the product should be wiped off and appropriate alternative therapy for the infection instituted.

4.5 Interaction with other medicinal products and other forms of Interaction
The product is not known to interact with other medicaments.

4.6 Pregnancy and lactation
This product should not be used during pregnancy and lactation unless considered essential by the physician.

Pregnancy: Adequate human data on use during pregnancy are not available. However animal studies have not identified any risk to pregnancy or embryo-foetal development.

Lactation: Adequate human and animal data on use during lactation are not available.

4.7 Effects on ability to drive and use machines
None known.

4.8 Undesirable effects
Adverse reactions are listed below by system organ class and frequency. Frequencies are defined as: very common ($\geq$1/10), common ($\geq$1/100, <1/10), uncommon ($\geq$1/1000, <1/100), rare ($\geq$1/10,000, <1/1000), very rare (<1/10,000), including isolated reports. Uncommon adverse reactions were determined from pooled safety data from a clinical trial population of 422 treated patients encompassing 12 clinical studies. Very rare adverse reactions were primarily determined from post-marketing experience data and therefore refer to reporting rate rather than true frequency.

Immune system disorders
Very rare: Cutaneous hypersensitivity reactions.

Respiratory, thoracic and mediastinal disorders
Uncommon: Nasal mucosa reactions.

4.9 Overdose
The toxicity of mupirocin is very low. In the event of overdose, symptomatic treatment should be given.

5. PHARMACOLOGICAL PROPERTIES

5.1 Pharmacodynamic properties

Mupirocin is a novel antibiotic formulated for topical application only. Its spectrum of *in-vitro* antibacterial activity includes *Staphylococcus aureus* (including methicillin resistant strains), *Staphylococcus epidermidis*, *Streptococcus* species and certain Gram-negative bacteria, particularly *Haemophilus influenzae* and *Escherichia coli*. Other Gram-negative bacteria are less susceptible and Pseudomonas aeruginosa is resistant.

Mupirocin is the major antibacterial compound of a group of structurally related metabolites produced by submerged fermentation of Ps. Fluorescens. Mupirocin has a novel mode of action, inhibiting bacterial iso-leucyl transfer-RNA synthetase and thus cross-resistance with other antibiotics is not experienced.

5.2 Pharmacokinetic properties

Studies have shown that following topical application of mupirocin there is very little systemic absorption of drug-related material. To mimic possible enhanced systemic penetration of mupirocin by application to damaged skin or a vascular site such as the mucous membrane, intravenous studies have been performed. Mupirocin was rapidly eliminated from the plasma by metabolism to monic acid, which in turn was excreted mainly in the urine.

5.3 Preclinical safety data

No further information of relevance.

6. PHARMACEUTICAL PARTICULARS

6.1 List of excipients

White soft paraffin and Softisan 649.

6.2 Incompatibilities

None known.

6.3 Shelf life

Bactroban Nasal Ointment has a shelf-life of three years.

6.4 Special precautions for storage

Store at room temperature (below 25°C).

6.5 Nature and contents of container

Lacquered aluminium tube fitted with a nozzle and screw cap - 3 g ointment.

6.6 Instructions for use and handling

None stated.

Administrative Data

7. MARKETING AUTHORISATION HOLDER

Beecham Group plc

980 Great West Road

Brentford

Middlesex TW8 9GS

trading as:

GlaxoSmithKline UK,

Stockley Park West,

Uxbridge,

Middlesex, UB11 1BT

8. MARKETING AUTHORISATION NUMBER(S)

PL 00038/0347

9. DATE OF FIRST AUTHORISATION/RENEWAL OF THE AUTHORISATION

15 October 1998

10. DATE OF REVISION OF THE TEXT

22 April 2004

11. Legal Status

POM

Bactroban Ointment

(GlaxoSmithKline UK)

1. NAME OF THE MEDICINAL PRODUCT

Bactroban® Ointment

2. QUALITATIVE AND QUANTITATIVE COMPOSITION

Mupirocin 2.0% w/w

3. PHARMACEUTICAL FORM

Ointment in a white, translucent, water-soluble, polyethylene glycol base. For topical administration.

4. CLINICAL PARTICULARS

4.1 Therapeutic indications

Bactroban is a topical antibacterial agent, active against those organisms responsible for the majority of skin infections, e.g. *Staphylococcus aureus*, including methicillin-resistant strains, other staphylococci, streptococci. It is also active against Gram-negative organisms such as *Escherichia coli* and *Haemophilus influenzae*. Bactroban Ointment is used for skin infections, e.g. impetigo, folliculitis, furunculosis.

4.2 Posology and method of administration

Dosage:

Adults (including elderly) and children:

Bactroban Ointment should be applied to the affected area up to three times a day for up to 10 days.

The area may be covered with a dressing or occluded if desired.

Administration:

Topical.

Do not mix with other preparations as there is a risk of dilution, resulting in a reduction of the antibacterial activity and potential loss of stability of the mupirocin in the ointment.

4.3 Contraindications

Bactroban ointment should not be given to patients with a history of hypersensitivity to any of its constituents.

This Bactroban Ointment formulation is not suitable for ophthalmic or intranasal use.

4.4 Special warnings and special precautions for use

When Bactroban Ointment is used on the face, care should be taken to avoid the eyes.

Polyethylene glycol can be absorbed from open wounds and damaged skin and is excreted by the kidneys. In common with other polyethylene glycol-based ointments, Bactroban Ointment should be used with caution if there is evidence of moderate or severe renal impairment.

In the rare event of a possible sensitisation reaction or severe local irritation occurring with the use of Bactroban ointment, treatment should be discontinued, the product should be rinsed off and appropriate alternative therapy for the infection instituted.

4.5 Interaction with other medicinal products and other forms of Interaction

None stated.

4.6 Pregnancy and lactation

This product should not be used during pregnancy and lactation unless considered essential by the physician.

Pregnancy: Adequate human data on use during pregnancy are not available. However animal studies have not identified any risk to pregnancy or embryo-foetal development.

Lactation: Adequate human and animal data on use during lactation are not available.

4.7 Effects on ability to drive and use machines

None stated.

4.8 Undesirable effects

Adverse reactions are listed below by system organ class and frequency. Frequencies are defined as: very common (≥1/10), common (≥1/100, <1/10), uncommon (≥1/1000, <1/100), rare (≥1/10,000, <1/1000), very rare (<1/10,000), including isolated reports. Common and uncommon adverse reactions were determined from pooled safety data from a clinical trial population of 1573 treated patients encompassing 12 clinical studies. Very rare adverse reactions were primarily determined from post-marketing experience data and therefore refer to reporting rate rather than true frequency.

Immune system disorders:

Very rare: Systemic allergic reactions have been reported with Bactroban Ointment.

Skin and subcutaneous tissue disorders:

Common: Burning localised to the area of application.

Uncommon: Itching, erythema, stinging and dryness localised to the area of application.

Uncommon: Cutaneous sensitisation reactions to mupirocin or the ointment base.

4.9 Overdose

The toxicity of mupirocin is very low. In the event of overdose, symptomatic treatment should be given.

5. PHARMACOLOGICAL PROPERTIES

5.1 Pharmacodynamic properties

Bactroban (mupirocin) potently inhibits bacterial protein and RNA synthesis by inhibition of isoleucyl-transfer RNA synthetase.

5.2 Pharmacokinetic properties

After topical application of Bactroban Ointment, mupirocin is only very minimally absorbed systemically and that which is absorbed is rapidly metabolised to the antimicrobially inactive metabolite, monic acid. Penetration of mupirocin into the deeper epidermal and dermal layers of the skin is enhanced in traumatised skin and under occlusive dressings.

5.3 Preclinical safety data

None stated.

6. PHARMACEUTICAL PARTICULARS

6.1 List of excipients

Polyethylene Glycol 400 USNF

Polyethylene Glycol 3350 USNF

6.2 Incompatibilities

None stated.

6.3 Shelf life

Bactroban Ointment has a shelf-life of two years.

6.4 Special precautions for storage

Store at room temperature (below 25°C).

6.5 Nature and contents of container

Original pack of 5 and 15 g* (sealed tube in a carton) with Patient Information Leaflet.

6.6 Instructions for use and handling

No special instructions.

Administrative Data

7. MARKETING AUTHORISATION HOLDER

Beecham Group plc

980 Great West Road,

Brentford,

Middlesex TW8 9GS

Trading as:

GlaxoSmithKine UK,

Stockley Park West,

Uxbridge,

Middlesex UB11 1BT

8. MARKETING AUTHORISATION NUMBER(S)

PL 00038/0319

9. DATE OF FIRST AUTHORISATION/RENEWAL OF THE AUTHORISATION

7 November 2002

10. DATE OF REVISION OF THE TEXT

22 April 2004

11. Legal Status

POM

* At time of printing only the details relevant to marketed packs will be included.

Balmosa Cream

(Forest Laboratories UK Limited)

1. NAME OF THE MEDICINAL PRODUCT

BALMOSA CREAM

2. QUALITATIVE AND QUANTITATIVE COMPOSITION

Active ingredients:

Menthol BP 2.0% w/w

Camphor BP 4.0% w/w

Methyl Salicylate Ph.Eur. 4.0% w/w

Capsicum Oleoresin BPC 0.035% w/w

3. PHARMACEUTICAL FORM

Cream for cutaneous use.

4. CLINICAL PARTICULARS

4.1 Therapeutic indications

Analgesic/rubefacient cream for the symptomatic relief of muscular rheumatism, fibrositis, lumbago, sciatica and unbroken chilblains.

4.2 Posology and method of administration

Adults and the elderly:

Apply topically. Massage gently into the affected area as required. Wash hands immediately after use.

Children under 12 years:

Not generally recommended.

4.3 Contraindications

Hypersensitivity to aspirin, other non-steroidal anti-inflammatory drugs, or any of the ingredients listed.

4.4 Special warnings and special precautions for use

For external use only.

If skin sensitivity reactions occur, discontinue use. Do not apply to inflamed or broken skin. Avoid contact with the eye and mucous membranes. Do not apply to the nostrils of infants. Do not use with occlusive dressings.

After use avoid exposing the affected area to excessive sunlight.

4.5 Interaction with other medicinal products and other forms of Interaction

None stated.

4.6 Pregnancy and lactation

With all salicylates there is animal evidence of teratogenicity. Use should be avoided during pregnancy and breast feeding.

4.7 Effects on ability to drive and use machines

None stated.

4.8 Undesirable effects

Skin sensitivity reactions are possible although rare. Topical applications of large amounts of Balmosa Cream may result in systemic effects, including hypersensitivity and worsening of asthma.

4.9 Overdose

Overdosage is extremely unlikely from topical use.

5. PHARMACOLOGICAL PROPERTIES

5.1 Pharmacodynamic properties

Capsicum oleoresin is a rubefacient. Camphor exhibits counter-irritant and weak local anaesthetic activity. Menthol and methyl salicylate impart analgesic properties to the formulation.

5.2 Pharmacokinetic properties
Not applicable

5.3 Preclinical safety data
There are no preclinical data of relevance to the prescriber which are additional to that already included in other sections of the SPC.

6. PHARMACEUTICAL PARTICULARS

6.1 List of excipients
Methylcellulose
White soft paraffin
Emulsifying wax
Liquid paraffin
Lanolin (anhydrous)
Phenonip
Purified Water

6.2 Incompatibilities
None stated.

6.3 Shelf life
3 years

6.4 Special precautions for storage
Do not store above 25°C.

6.5 Nature and contents of container
Aluminium tube with a polyethylene cap containing 20g or 40g of the product.

6.6 Instructions for use and handling
None stated.

7. MARKETING AUTHORISATION HOLDER
Forest Laboratories UK Limited
Bourne Road
Bexley
Kent DA5 1NX

8. MARKETING AUTHORISATION NUMBER(S)
PL 0108/5000R

9. DATE OF FIRST AUTHORISATION/RENEWAL OF THE AUTHORISATION
18 March 1983 / 22 May 2003

10. DATE OF REVISION OF THE TEXT
April 2003.

11. Legal Category
GSL

Bambec Tablets 10mg

(AstraZeneca UK Limited)

1. NAME OF THE MEDICINAL PRODUCT
Bambec Tablets 10 mg

2. QUALITATIVE AND QUANTITATIVE COMPOSITION
Each tablet contains 10 mg Bambuterol hydrochloride

For excipients, see Section 6.1

3. PHARMACEUTICAL FORM
Tablet

4. CLINICAL PARTICULARS

4.1 Therapeutic indications
Management of asthma, bronchospasm and/or reversible airways obstruction.

4.2 Posology and method of administration
Bambec is formulated as a tablet and should be taken once daily, shortly before bedtime. The dose should be individualised.

Adults: The recommended starting doses are 10 mg–20 mg. The 10 mg dose may be increased to 20 mg if necessary after 1–2 weeks, depending on the clinical effect.

In patients who have previously tolerated β_2-agonists well, the recommended starting dose, as well as maintenance dose, is 20 mg.

Children: Until the clinical documentation has been completed, Bambec should not be used in children.

Elderly: Dose adjustment is not required in the elderly.

Significant hepatic dysfunction: Not recommended because of unpredictable conversion to terbutaline.

Moderate to severely impaired renal function (GFR < 50ml/min): It is recommended that the starting dose of Bambec should be halved in these patients.

4.3 Contraindications
Bambec tablets are contraindicated in patients with a history of hypersensitivity to any of their ingredients. Bambec is presently not recommended for children due to limited clinical data in this age group.

4.4 Special warnings and special precautions for use
As terbutaline is excreted mainly via the kidneys, the dose of Bambec should be halved in patients with moderately to severely impaired renal function (GFR ⩽ 50 mL/min).

Care should be taken with patients suffering from myocardial insufficiency or thyrotoxicosis.

Due to the hyperglycaemic effects of β_2-stimulants, additional blood glucose measurements are recommended initially when Bambec therapy is commenced in diabetic patients.

Due to the positive inotropic effects of β_2-agonists these drugs should not be used in patients with hypertrophic cardiomyopathy.

β_2-agonists may be arrhythmogenic and this must be considered in the treatment of the individual patient.

Unpredictable inter-individual variation in the metabolism of bambuterol to terbutaline has been shown in subjects with liver cirrhosis. The use of an alternative β_2-agonist is recommended in patients with cirrhosis and other forms of severely impaired liver function.

Potentially serious hypokalaemia may result from β_2-agonist therapy mainly from parenteral or nebulised administration. Particular caution is advised in acute severe asthma as this effect may be augmented by hypoxia. The hypokalaemic effect may be potentiated by concomitant treatment with xanthine derivatives, corticosteroids and/or diuretics. It is recommended that serum potassium levels are monitored in such situations.

If a previously effective dosage regimen no longer gives the same symptomatic relief, the patient should urgently seek further medical advice. Consideration should be given to the requirements for additional therapy (including increased dosages of anti-inflammatory medication). Severe exacerbations of asthma should be treated as an emergency in the usual manner.

4.5 Interaction with other medicinal products and other forms of Interaction
Bambuterol may interact with suxamethonium (succinylcholine). A prolongation of the muscle-relaxing effect of suxamethonium of up to 2-fold has been observed in some patients after taking Bambec 20 mg on the evening prior to surgery. The interaction is dose-dependent. It is due to the fact that plasma cholinesterase, which inactivates suxamethonium, is partly, but fully reversibly, inhibited by bambuterol. In extreme situations, the interaction may result in a prolonged apnoea time which may be of clinical importance.

Bambuterol may also interact with other muscle relaxants metabolised by plasma cholinesterase.

Beta-receptor blocking agents including eyedrops, especially non-selective ones, may partly or totally inhibit the effect of beta-stimulants. Therefore, Bambec tablets and non-selective β-blockers should not normally be administered concurrently. Bambec should be used with caution in patients receiving other sympathomimetics.

Hypokalemia may result from β_2-agonist therapy and may be potentiated by concomitant treatment with xanthine derivatives, corticosteroids and diuretics (see Section 4.4, Warnings and Precautions).

4.6 Pregnancy and lactation
Unless there are compelling reasons, avoid in pregnancy, lactation and women of child-bearing potential who are not taking adequate contraceptive precautions. Although no teratogenic effects have been observed in animals after administration of bambuterol, there is no experience of use in human pregnancy. Terbutaline, the active metabolite of bambuterol, has been in widespread clinical use for many years and may be considered in such patients. Terbutaline should be used with caution in the first trimester of pregnancy. Maternal β_2-agonist treatment may result in transient hypoglycaemia in pre-term newborn infants.

It is not known whether bambuterol or intermediary metabolites pass into breast milk. Terbutaline does pass into breast milk, but an effect on the infant is unlikely at therapeutic doses.

4.7 Effects on ability to drive and use machines
None stated.

4.8 Undesirable effects
Side effects which have been reported e.g. tremor, headache, nausea, cramps, tachycardia and palpitations are all characteristic of sympathomimetic amines. The intensity of the side effects is dose-dependent and the majority of these effects have reversed spontaneously within the first 1–2 weeks of treatment.

Hypersensitivity reactions including angioedema, urticaria, exanthema, bronchospasm, hypotension and collapse have been very rarely reported with β_2-agonist therapy.

Potentially serious hypokalaemia may result from β_2-agonist therapy (see Section 4.4, Special Warnings and Special Precautions for Use).

Cardiac arrhythmias including atrial fibrillation, supraventricular tachycardia and extrasystoles have been reported in association with β_2-agonists, usually in susceptible patients.

Sleep disturbances and behavioural disturbances, such as agitation, hyperactivity and restlessness, have been observed.

4.9 Overdose
Overdosing may result in high levels of terbutaline.

Symptoms
The signs and symptoms described here have been recorded after terbutaline overdose.

Possible signs and symptoms: Headache, anxiety, tremor, nausea, cramps, palpitations, tachycardia, cardiac arrhythmias. A fall in blood pressure sometimes occurs.

Laboratory findings: Hypokalaemia, hyperglycaemia and lactic acidosis sometimes occur.

Overdose of Bambec is also likely to cause a prolonged inhibition of plasma cholinesterase.

Management
Mild and moderate cases: Reduce the dose.

Severe cases: Administration of activated charcoal if ingestion is recent. Determination of acid-base balance, blood sugar and electrolytes. Monitoring of heart rate and rhythm and blood pressure.

Metabolic changes should be corrected. A cardioselective β-blocker (e.g. metoprolol) is recommended for the treatment of haemodynamically significant cardiac arrhythmias. The β-blocker should be used with care because of the possibility of inducing bronchoconstriction. Serum potassium levels should be monitored. If the β_2-mediated vasodilation contributes significantly to the fall in blood pressure, a volume expander should be given.

5. PHARMACOLOGICAL PROPERTIES

5.1 Pharmacodynamic properties
Pharmacotherapeutic group: selective β_2-agonists, bambuterol, ATC code: R03C C12.

Bambuterol is an active precursor of the selective β_2-adrenergic agonist terbutaline. Bambuterol is the bis-dimethylcarbamate of terbutaline, and is present in the formulation as a 1:1 racemate.

Pharmacodynamic studies have shown that after oral administration of bambuterol to guinea pigs, a sustained protective effect was achieved against histamine-induced bronchoconstriction. At equipotent doses, the duration of the relaxing activity was more prolonged than after plain terbutaline. Bambuterol, or the monocarbamate ester, did not exert any smooth muscle relaxing properties. The bronchoprotective effects seen after oral administration of bambuterol are related to the generation of terbutaline, as were the secondary effects (effects on other organs).

Pharmacodynamic studies have been conducted in asthmatics and healthy volunteers. The effects observed were bronchodilation, tremor and increases in heart rate. The metabolic effects included a small increase in blood glucose, while the effect on serum potassium was negligible. In short-term studies on lipoprotein metabolism, an increase in HDL cholesterol has been observed. In conclusion, all pharmacodynamic effects observed can be ascribed to the active metabolite terbutaline.

5.2 Pharmacokinetic properties
On average, 17.5% of an oral dose is absorbed. Approximately 70–90% of the absorption occurs in the first 24 hours.

Bambuterol is metabolised in the liver and terbutaline is formed by both hydrolysis and oxidation. After absorption from the gut, about 2/3 of terbutaline is first-pass metabolised, bambuterol escapes this first-pass metabolism. Of the absorbed amount, about 65% reaches the circulation. Bambuterol therefore has a bioavailability of about 10%.

Protein binding of bambuterol is low, 40–50% at therapeutic concentrations.

The terminal half-life of bambuterol after an oral dose is 9–17 hours.

Studies on the effects on plasma cholinesterase showed that bambuterol inhibited activity, but that this was reversible.

All categories of subjects studied were able to form terbutaline in a predictive way except for liver cirrhotics.

5.3 Preclinical safety data
Bambuterol has not revealed any adverse effects which pose a risk to man at therapeutic dosages in the toxicity studies.

Bambuterol is given as a racemate: (-)-bambuterol is responsible for the pharmacodynamic effects via generation of (-)-terbutaline. (+)-bambuterol generates the pharmacodynamic inactive (+)-terbutaline. Both (+) and (-)-bambuterol are equally active as plasma cholinesterase inhibitors. This inhibition is reversible.

The toxicity studies showed that bambuterol has β_2-stimulatory effects, expressed as cardiotoxicity in dogs, and at high doses, observed in the acute toxicity studies, cholinergic effects.

There is no evidence from the preclinical safety data to indicate that bambuterol cannot be used in man for the intended indications with sufficient safety.

6. PHARMACEUTICAL PARTICULARS

6.1 List of excipients
Lactose monohydrate; maize starch; povidone; microcrystalline cellulose; magnesium stearate; water, purified.

6.2 Incompatibilities
Not applicable.

6.3 Shelf life
3 years.

6.4 Special precautions for storage
Do not store above 30°C.

6.5 Nature and contents of container
Amber glass bottle with LD-polyethene cap: 7, 14, 28, 30, 56 or 100 tablets.

HDPE container with LD-polyethene cap: 7, 14, 28, 30, 56 or 100 tablets.

HDPE container with polypropylene cap: 7, 14, 28, 30, 56 or 100 tablets.

PVC blisters: 7, 14, 28, 30, 56 or 100 tablets.

6.6 Instructions for use and handling
None.

7. MARKETING AUTHORISATION HOLDER
AstraZeneca UK Ltd.,

600 Capability Green,

Luton, LU1 3LU, UK.

8. MARKETING AUTHORISATION NUMBER(S)
PL 17901/0103

9. DATE OF FIRST AUTHORISATION/RENEWAL OF THE AUTHORISATION
21st May 2002

10. DATE OF REVISION OF THE TEXT
29th July 2005

Bambec Tablets 20mg

(AstraZeneca UK Limited)

1. NAME OF THE MEDICINAL PRODUCT
Bambec Tablets 20 mg

2. QUALITATIVE AND QUANTITATIVE COMPOSITION
Each tablet contains 20 mg Bambuterol hydrochloride

For excipients, see Section 6.1

3. PHARMACEUTICAL FORM
Tablet

4. CLINICAL PARTICULARS

4.1 Therapeutic indications
Management of asthma, bronchospasm and/or reversible airways obstruction.

4.2 Posology and method of administration
Bambec is formulated as a tablet and should be taken once daily, shortly before bedtime. The dose should be individualised.

Adults: The recommended starting doses are 10 mg–20 mg. The 10 mg dose may be increased to 20 mg if necessary after 1–2 weeks, depending on the clinical effect.

In patients who have previously tolerated β_2-agonists well, the recommended starting dose, as well as maintenance dose, is 20 mg.

Children: Until the clinical documentation has been completed, Bambec should not be used in children.

Elderly: Dose adjustment is not required in the elderly.

Significant hepatic dysfunction: Not recommended because of unpredictable conversion to terbutaline.

Moderate to severely impaired renal function (GFR < 50ml/min): It is recommended that the starting dose of Bambec should be halved in these patients.

4.3 Contraindications
Bambec tablets are contraindicated in patients with a history of hypersensitivity to any of their ingredients. Bambec is presently not recommended for children due to limited clinical data in this age group.

4.4 Special warnings and special precautions for use
As terbutaline is excreted mainly via the kidneys, the dose of Bambec should be halved in patients with moderately to severely impaired renal function (GFR ⩽ 50 mL/min).

Care should be taken with patients suffering from myocardial insufficiency or thyrotoxicosis.

Due to the hyperglycaemic effects of β_2-stimulants, additional blood glucose measurements are recommended initially when Bambec therapy is commenced in diabetic patients.

Due to the positive inotropic effects of β_2-agonists these drugs should not be used in patients with hypertrophic cardiomyopathy.

β_2-agonists may be arrhythmogenic and this must be considered in the treatment of the individual patient.

Unpredictable inter-individual variation in the metabolism of bambuterol to terbutaline has been shown in subjects with liver cirrhosis. The use of an alternative β_2-agonist is recommended in patients with cirrhosis and other forms of severely impaired liver function.

Potentially serious hypokalaemia may result from β_2-agonist therapy mainly from parenteral or nebulised administration. Particular caution is advised in acute severe asthma as this effect may be augmented by hypoxia. The hypokalaemic effect may be potentiated by concomitant treatment with xanthine derivatives, corticosteroids and/or diuretics. It is recommended that serum potassium levels are monitored in such situations.

If a previously effective dosage regimen no longer gives the same symptomatic relief, the patient should urgently seek further medical advice. Consideration should be given to the requirements for additional therapy (including increased dosages of anti-inflammatory medication). Severe exacerbations of asthma should be treated as an emergency in the usual manner.

4.5 Interaction with other medicinal products and other forms of Interaction
Bambuterol may interact with suxamethonium (succinylcholine). A prolongation of the muscle-relaxing effect of suxamethonium of up to 2-fold has been observed in some patients after taking Bambec 20 mg on the evening prior to surgery. The interaction is dose-dependent. It is due to the fact that plasma cholinesterase, which inactivates suxamethonium, is partly, but fully reversibly, inhibited by bambuterol. In extreme situations, the interaction may result in a prolonged apnoea time which may be of clinical importance.

Bambuterol may also interact with other muscle relaxants metabolised by plasma cholinesterase.

Beta-receptor blocking agents including eyedrops, especially non-selective ones, may partly or totally inhibit the effect of beta-stimulants. Therefore, Bambec tablets and non-selective β-blockers should not normally be administered concurrently. Bambec should be used with caution in patients receiving other sympathomimetics.

Hypokalemia may result from β_2-agonist therapy and may be potentiated by concomitant treatment with xanthine derivatives, corticosteroids and diuretics (see Section 4.4, Warnings and Precautions).

4.6 Pregnancy and lactation
Unless there are compelling reasons, avoid in pregnancy, lactation and women of child-bearing potential who are not taking adequate contraceptive precautions. Although no teratogenic effects have been observed in animals after administration of bambuterol, there is no experience of use in human pregnancy. Terbutaline, the active metabolite of bambuterol, has been in widespread clinical use for many years and may be considered in such patients. Terbutaline should be used with caution in the first trimester of pregnancy. Maternal β_2-agonist treatment may result in transient hypoglycaemia in pre-term newborn infants.

It is not known whether bambuterol or intermediary metabolites pass into breast milk. Terbutaline does pass into breast milk, but an effect on the infant is unlikely at therapeutic doses.

4.7 Effects on ability to drive and use machines
None stated.

4.8 Undesirable effects
Side effects which have been reported e.g. tremor, headache, nausea, cramps, tachycardia and palpitations are all characteristic of sympathomimetic amines. The intensity of the side effects is dose-dependent and the majority of these effects have reversed spontaneously within the first 1–2 weeks of treatment.

Hypersensitivity reactions including angioedema, urticaria, exanthema, bronchospasm, hypotension and collapse have been very rarely reported with β_2-agonist therapy.

Potentially serious hypokalaemia may result from β_2-agonist therapy (see Section 4.4, Special Warnings and Special Precautions for Use).

Cardiac arrhythmias including atrial fibrillation, supraventricular tachycardia and extrasystoles have been reported in association with β_2-agonists, usually in susceptible patients.

Sleep disturbances and behavioural disturbances, such as agitation, hyperactivity and restlessness, have been observed.

4.9 Overdose
Overdosing may result in high levels of terbutaline.

Symptoms

The signs and symptoms described here have been recorded after terbutaline overdose.

Possible signs and symptoms: Headache, anxiety, tremor, nausea, cramps, palpitations, tachycardia, cardiac arrhythmias. A fall in blood pressure sometimes occurs.

Laboratory findings: Hypokalaemia, hyperglycaemia and lactic acidosis sometimes occur.

Overdose of Bambec is also likely to cause a prolonged inhibition of plasma cholinesterase.

Management

Mild and moderate cases: Reduce the dose.

Severe cases: Administration of activated charcoal if ingestion is recent. Determination of acid-base balance, blood sugar and electrolytes. Monitoring of heart rate and rhythm and blood pressure.

Metabolic changes should be corrected. A cardioselective β-blocker (e.g. metoprolol) is recommended for the treatment of haemodynamically significant cardiac arrhythmias. The β-blocker should be used with care because of the possibility of inducing bronchoconstriction. Serum potassium levels should be monitored. If the β_2-mediated vasodilation contributes significantly to the fall in blood pressure, a volume expander should be given.

5. PHARMACOLOGICAL PROPERTIES

5.1 Pharmacodynamic properties
Pharmacotherapeutic group: selective β_2-agonists, bambuterol, ATC code: R03C C12.

Bambuterol is an active precursor of the selective β_2-adrenergic agonist terbutaline. Bambuterol is the bis-dimethylcarbamate of terbutaline, and is present in the formulation as a 1:1 racemate.

Pharmacodynamic studies have shown that after oral administration of bambuterol to guinea pigs, a sustained protective effect was achieved against histamine-induced bronchoconstriction. At equipotent doses, the duration of the relaxing activity was more prolonged than after plain terbutaline. Bambuterol, or the monocarbamate ester, did not exert any smooth muscle relaxing properties. The bronchoprotective effects seen after oral administration of bambuterol are related to the generation of terbutaline, as were the secondary effects (effects on other organs).

Pharmacodynamic studies have been conducted in asthmatics and healthy volunteers. The effects observed were bronchodilation, tremor and increases in heart rate. The metabolic effects included a small increase in blood glucose, while the effect on serum potassium was negligible. In short-term studies on lipoprotein metabolism, an increase in HDL cholesterol, has been observed. In conclusion, all pharmacodynamic effects observed can be ascribed to the active metabolite terbutaline.

5.2 Pharmacokinetic properties
On average, 17.5% of an oral dose is absorbed. Approximately 70–90% of the absorption occurs in the first 24 hours.

Bambuterol is metabolised in the liver and terbutaline is formed by both hydrolysis and oxidation. After absorption from the gut, about 2/3 of terbutaline is first-pass metabolised, bambuterol escapes this first-pass metabolism. Of the absorbed amount, about 65% reaches the circulation. Bambuterol therefore has a bioavailability of about 10%.

Protein binding of bambuterol is low, 40–50% at therapeutic concentrations.

The terminal half-life of bambuterol after an oral dose is 9–17 hours.

Studies on the effects on plasma cholinesterase showed that bambuterol inhibited activity, but that this was reversible.

All categories of subjects studied were able to form terbutaline in a predictive way except for liver cirrhotics.

5.3 Preclinical safety data
Bambuterol has not revealed any adverse effects which pose a risk to man at therapeutic dosages in the toxicity studies.

Bambuterol is given as a racemate: (-)-bambuterol is responsible for the pharmacodynamic effects via generation of (-)-terbutaline. (+)-bambuterol generates the pharmacodynamic inactive (+)-terbutaline. Both (+) and (-)-bambuterol are equally active as plasma cholinesterase inhibitors. This inhibition is reversible.

The toxicity studies showed that bambuterol has β_2-stimulatory effects, expressed as cardiotoxicity in dogs, and at high doses, observed in the acute toxicity studies, cholinergic effects.

There is no evidence from the preclinical safety data to indicate that bambuterol cannot be used in man for the intended indications with sufficient safety.

6. PHARMACEUTICAL PARTICULARS

6.1 List of excipients
Lactose monohydrate; maize starch; povidone; microcrystalline cellulose; magnesium stearate; water, purified.

6.2 Incompatibilities
Not applicable.

6.3 Shelf life
3 years.

6.4 Special precautions for storage
Do not store above 30°C.

6.5 Nature and contents of container
Amber glass bottle with LD-polyethene cap: 7, 14, 28, 30, 56 or 100 tablets.

HDPE container with LD-polyethene cap: 7, 14, 28, 30, 56 or 100 tablets.

HDPE container with polypropylene cap: 7, 14, 28, 30, 56 or 100 tablets.

PVC blisters: 7, 14, 28, 30, 56 or 100 tablets.

6.6 Instructions for use and handling
None.

7. MARKETING AUTHORISATION HOLDER
AstraZeneca UK Ltd.,

600 Capability Green,

Luton, LU1 3LU, UK.

8. MARKETING AUTHORISATION NUMBER(S)
PL 17901/0104

9. DATE OF FIRST AUTHORISATION/RENEWAL OF THE AUTHORISATION

21st May 2002

10. DATE OF REVISION OF THE TEXT

29th July 2005

Baratol Tablets 25mg

(Shire Pharmaceuticals Limited)

1. NAME OF THE MEDICINAL PRODUCT

Baratol™ Tablets 25mg

2. QUALITATIVE AND QUANTITATIVE COMPOSITION

Each tablet contains Indoramin Hydrochloride 27.63mg HSE equivalent to 25mg of indoramin base.

3. PHARMACEUTICAL FORM

Blue film coated tablets with shallow convex faces. "MPL 020" imprinted on one, "25" on the other.

4. CLINICAL PARTICULARS

4.1 Therapeutic indications

Treatment of all grades of essential hypertension and conditions for which alpha blockade is indicated.

4.2 Posology and method of administration

Route of administration

The tablet is taken orally.

Adults

Dose Range: 50 mg - 200 mg daily.

Initial Dose: 25 mg twice daily for all patients.

Dose Titration: The dose of Baratol should be titrated as necessary to control blood pressure to a maximum of 200mg daily in two or three divided doses. The daily dose may be increased by the progressive addition of 25mg or 50mg. This may be done at intervals of two weeks. Many patients may be stabilised with doses up to 100mg daily, especially those already being treated with diuretics. When unequal doses are used, the largest dose should be given at night in order to avoid day time sedation.

Elderly

Initial Dose: 25mg twice daily.

Clearance of indoramin may be affected in the elderly. A reduced dose and/or frequency of dosing may be sufficient for effective control of blood pressure in some elderly patients.

Children

Baratol is not recommended for children.

Combination with other anti-hypertensive agents:

The anti-hypertensive effect of Baratol is enhanced by concomitant administration of a thiazide diuretic or a β-adrenoceptor blocking drug.

When Baratol is used in combination with other anti-hypertensive agents, the dose of Baratol should be titrated in the same way as when it is used alone.

4.3 Contraindications

Baratol is contraindicated in patients:

- Who are currently receiving monoamine oxidase inhibitors.
- With established heart failure.

4.4 Special warnings and special precautions for use

Drowsiness is sometimes seen in the initial stages of treatment with Baratol or when dosage is increased too rapidly. Patients should be warned not to drive or operate machinery until it is established that they do not become drowsy while taking Baratol.

Incipient cardiac failure should be controlled with diuretics and digitalis before treatment with Baratol.

Caution should be observed in prescribing Baratol for patients with hepatic or renal insufficiency.

A few cases of extrapyramidal disorders have been reported in patients treated with Baratol. Caution should be observed in prescribing Baratol in patients with Parkinson's Disease.

In animals and in the one reported overdose in humans, convulsions have occurred. Due consideration should be given and great caution exercised in the use of Baratol in patients with epilepsy.

Caution should be observed in prescribing Baratol for patients with a history of depression.

Clearance of indoramin may be affected in the elderly. A reduced dose and/or frequency of dosing may be sufficient for effective control of blood pressure.

4.5 Interaction with other medicinal products and other forms of Interaction

The following, when administered at the same time as Baratol, result in an enhanced hypotensive effect:

- Anaesthetics
- Antidepressants, especially MAOIs
- Antihypertensives
- Beta-blockers
- Calcium-channel blockers
- Diuretics, especially thiazide diuretics

Moxisylyte, when administered at the same time as Baratol, may cause possible severe postural hypotension.

The ingestion of ethanol has been shown to increase both the rate and the extent of absorption of Baratol, and patients should be cautioned to avoid the ingestion of alcohol.

4.6 Pregnancy and lactation

Animal experiments indicate no teratogenic effects but Baratol Tablets should not be prescribed for pregnant women unless considered essential by the physician.

There is no data available on the excretion of Baratol in human milk but the drug should not be administered during lactation unless in the judgement of the physician such administration is clinically justifiable.

4.7 Effects on ability to drive and use machines

Baratol may cause drowsiness. See " Special warnings and precautions for use".

4.8 Undesirable effects

The most commonly reported adverse drug reactions are drowsiness, sedation or somnolence occurring in >10% of patients. This effect is often seen in the initial stages of treatment or when the dose is increased too rapidly.

Cardiac disorders

- Palpitations

Gastrointestinal disorders

- Diarrhoea
- Dry mouth
- Nausea

General disorders and administration site conditions

- Hypersensitivity reactions such as rash and pruritus
- Lack of energy
- Weakness

Investigations

- Weight increased

Nervous system disorders

- Dizziness
- Drowsiness
- Extrapyramidal disorder
- Headache
- Sedation
- Somnolence

Psychiatric disorders

- Depression

Renal and urinary disorders

- Urinary frequency
- Urinary incontinence

Reproductive system and breast disorders

- Ejaculation failure
- Priapism

Respiratory, thoracic and mediastinal disorders

- Nasal congestion

Vascular disorders

- Hypotension
- Postural hypotension

4.9 Overdose

The information available at present of the effects of acute overdosage in humans with Baratol is limited to one case. Effects seen in this case included deep sedation leading to coma, hypotension and fits. Results of animal work suggest that hypothermia may occur.

The suggested therapy is along the following lines:

- Recent ingestion of large numbers of tablets would require gastric lavage or a dose of Ipecacuanha to remove any of the product still in the stomach of the conscious patient.
- Ventilation should be monitored and assisted if necessary.
- Circulatory support and control of hypotension should be maintained.
- If convulsions occur, diazepam may be tried.
- Temperature should be closely monitored. If hypothermia occurs, rewarming should be carried out very slowly to avoid possible convulsions.

5. PHARMACOLOGICAL PROPERTIES

5.1 Pharmacodynamic properties

Baratol is an alpha-adrenoceptor blocking agent which acts selectively and competitively on post-synaptic alpha$_1$-adrenoceptors, causing a decrease in peripheral resistance.

5.2 Pharmacokinetic properties

Baratol tablets are rapidly absorbed and have a half-life of about 5 hours. There is little accumulation during long-term treatment. When three volunteers and four hypertensive patients were treated with radiolabelled indoramin at doses of 40-60mg daily for up to 3 days, plasma concentrations reached a peak 1-2 hours after administration of single doses. Over 90% of plasma indoramin was protein bound. After 2 or 3 days, 35% of the radioactivity was excreted in the urine and 46% in the faeces. Extensive first pass metabolism was suggested.

5.3 Preclinical safety data

None applicable.

6. PHARMACEUTICAL PARTICULARS

6.1 List of excipients

Amberlite IRP 88

Avicel PH 101

Lactose

Magnesium Stearate

Coating:

Hydroxypropylmethyl Cellulose 2010

Polyethylene Glycol 400

Opaspray M-1-20972

6.2 Incompatibilities

Not applicable.

6.3 Shelf life

36 months.

6.4 Special precautions for storage

Do not store above 25°C. Store in the original container.

6.5 Nature and contents of container

Pack sizes of 10, 28, 56, 84 100 and 112 in amber glass bottles with suitable closures, aluminium/polyethylene foil strip and securitainers.

Not all pack sizes may be marketed.

6.6 Instructions for use and handling

None

7. MARKETING AUTHORISATION HOLDER

Monmouth Pharmaceuticals Limited

Hampshire International Business Park

Chineham

Basingstoke

Hampshire RG24 8EP

United Kingdom

8. MARKETING AUTHORISATION NUMBER(S)

PL 10536/0015

9. DATE OF FIRST AUTHORISATION/RENEWAL OF THE AUTHORISATION

23 April 1993

10. DATE OF REVISION OF THE TEXT

March 2004

LEGAL CATEGORY

POM

Baxan Capsules and Suspension

(Bristol-Myers Pharmaceuticals)

1. NAME OF THE MEDICINAL PRODUCT

Baxan Capsules 500mg

Baxan Suspension 125mg/5ml, 250mg/5ml and 500mg/5ml

2. QUALITATIVE AND QUANTITATIVE COMPOSITION

Baxan Capsules: contain Cefadroxil Monohydrate equivalent to 500mg cefadroxil activity.

Baxan Suspension: contains Cefadroxil Monohydrate equivalent to 125mg, 250mg or 500mg cefadroxil activity per 5ml.

3. PHARMACEUTICAL FORM

Capsule.

Oral suspension.

4. CLINICAL PARTICULARS

4.1 Therapeutic indications

Baxan is indicated in the treatment of the following infections when due to susceptible micro-organisms:

Respiratory tract infections:

Tonsillitis, pharyngitis, lobar and bronchopneumonia, acute and chronic bronchitis, pulmonary abscess, empyema, pleurisy, sinusitis, laryngitis, otitis media.

Skin and soft-tissue infections:

Lymphadenitis, abscesses, cellulitis, decubitus ulcers, mastitis, furunculosis, erysipelas.

Genitourinary tract infections:

Pyelonephritis, cystitis, urethritis, gynaecological infections.

Other infections:

Osteomyelitis, septic arthritis.

4.2 Posology and method of administration

The bioavailability and consequent chemotherapeutic effects of cefadroxil are unaffected by food. It may, therefore, be taken with meals or on an empty stomach.

Adults and Children Weighing More Than 40kg (88lbs):

500mg to 1g twice a day, depending upon the severity of infection.

Alternatively, in skin and soft tissue and uncomplicated urinary tract infections, 1g once a day.

In the treatment of beta-haemolytic streptococcal infections, Baxan should be administered for at least 10 days.

Children Weighing Less Than 40kg (88lbs):

Under 1 Year: 25mg/kg daily in divided doses, e.g. 2.5ml of the 125mg per 5ml suspension twice a day for a 6 month old infant weighing 5kg, or 5ml of the 125ml per 5ml suspension twice a day for a 1 year old infant weighing 10kg.

1-6 years: 250mg twice a day.

Over 6 years: 500mg twice a day.

Elderly:

No specific dosage recommendations or precautions for use in the elderly except to monitor those patients with impaired renal function.

The bioavailability and consequent chemotherapeutic effects of cefadroxil are unaffected by food. It may, therefore, be taken with meals or on an empty stomach.

Renal Impairment:

In patients with renal impairment, the dosage should be adjusted according to creatinine clearance rates to prevent drug accumulation and serum levels should be monitored. A modified dosage schedule is unnecessary in patients with creatinine clearance rates of greater than 50ml/min. In those patients with creatinine clearance rates of 50ml/min or less, the following dosage schedule is recommended as a guideline, based upon the creatinine clearance rate (ml/min: 1.73 m^2).

Patients with renal insufficiency may be treated with an initial dose of 500mg to 1000mg of Baxan. Subsequent doses may be administered according to the following table:

Creatinine Clearance	Dose	Dose Interval
0 - 10 ml/min / 1.73 m^2	500 - 1000 mg	36 hrs
11 - 25 ml/min / 1.73 m^2	500 - 1000 mg	24 hrs
26 - 50 ml/min / 1.73 m^2	500 - 1000 mg	12 hrs

Baxan can be removed from the body by haemodialysis.

4.3 Contraindications
Baxan is contra-indicated in patients with a history of hypersensitivity to any of the ingredients.

4.4 Special warnings and special precautions for use
In patients with a history of penicillin allergy, Baxan should be used with caution. There is evidence of partial cross-allergenicity between the penicillins and the cephalosporins. Should an allergic reaction to Baxan occur, the drug should be discontinued and the patient treated with the usual agents (pressor amines, corticosteroids and/or antihistamines), depending on the severity of the reaction.

As experience in premature infants and neonates is limited, the use of Baxan in these patients should only be undertaken with caution.

As with all antibiotics, prolonged use may result in overgrowth of non-susceptible organisms.

As with other broad spectrum antibiotics, pseudomembranous colitis has been reported. It is important to consider its diagnosis in patients who develop diarrhoea in association with Baxan therapy.

4.5 Interaction with other medicinal products and other forms of Interaction
There are not sufficient data available to indicate whether the concurrent use of Baxan and potential nephrotoxic agents such as aminoglycosides causes any alteration in their nephrotoxic effects.

A false-positive Coombs' reaction may occur in some patients receiving Baxan.

Urine from patients treated with Baxan may give a false-positive glycosuria reaction when tested with Benedict's or Fehling's solutions. This does not occur with enzyme based tests.

4.6 Pregnancy and lactation
Although animal studies and clinical experience have not shown any evidence of teratogenicity, the safe use of Baxan during pregnancy has not been established. Baxan is excreted in breast milk and should be used with caution in lactating mothers.

4.7 Effects on ability to drive and use machines
None known.

4.8 Undesirable effects
The most commonly reported side-effects are gastrointestinal disturbances and hypersensitivity phenomena. Rash, pruritus, urticaria, angioneurotic oedema have been observed infrequently. Serum sickness, erythema multiforme and anaphylaxis have been reported rarely. Side-effects, including nausea, vomiting, diarrhoea, dyspepsia, abdominal discomfort, fever, dizziness, headache, arthralgia and genital moniliasis may also occur. Reversible neutropenia may occur rarely, as may leucopenia, thrombocytopenia, agranulocytosis and minor elevations in serum transaminase and Stevens-Johnson syndrome. Colitis, including rare instances of pseudo-membraneous colitis, has been reported.

4.9 Overdose
Ingestion of < 250 mg/kg in children under six years of age was not associated with significant outcomes. The patient should be observed and treated symptomatically. For amounts > 250 mg/kg gastric lavage or stimulation of vomiting is appropriate.

5. PHARMACOLOGICAL PROPERTIES
5.1 Pharmacodynamic properties
Baxan is a cephalosporin antibiotic, bactericidal *in vitro* against a wide range of Gram-positive and Gram-negative micro-organisms. Baxan inhibits mucopeptide synthesis in the bacterial cell wall, making it defective and osmotically unstable. The action *in vivo* is usually bactericidal, depending on organism susceptibility, dose, tissue concentrations and the rate at which organisms are multiplying. It is more effective against rapidly growing organisms forming cell walls. *In vitro*, Baxan is bactericidal against a wide range of organisms. Sensitive Gram-positive organisms include: penicillinase and non-penicillinase-producing *Staphylococci*, beta-haemolytic *Streptococci*, *Streptococcus pneumoniae* and *Streptococcus pyogenes*. Sensitive Gram-negative organisms include *Escherichia coli, Klebsiella* species, *Proteus mirabilis, Moraxella (Branhamella) catarrhalis* and *Bacteroides* spp. (excluding *Bacteroides fragilis*) and some strains of *Haemophilus influenzae*.

5.2 Pharmacokinetic properties
Baxan is rapidly absorbed after oral administration. The bioavailability is unaffected by food. Following single doses of 500 and 1,000mg, average peak serum levels were approximately 16 and 28 μg/ml, respectively. Measurable levels were present 12 hours after administration. Over 90% of the drug is excreted unchanged in the urine within 24 hours. Peak urine concentrations are approximately 1,800 μg/ml after a 500mg dose. Increases in dose generally produce a proportionate increase in Baxan urinary concentration. Oral dosing produces effective tissue penetration in lungs, tonsils, liver, gall bladder, bile duct, prostate, bone, muscle and synovial capsule as well as saliva, sputum, pleural exudate, bile and synovial fluid. The half-life is approximately 80-120 minutes and protein binding is approximately 20%. In addition, Baxan is soluble in lipids (0.19 mg/ml ether) and in water (12.79 mg/ml).

5.3 Preclinical safety data
No additional relevant data.

6. PHARMACEUTICAL PARTICULARS
6.1 List of excipients
Baxan Capsules:

Colloidal silicon dioxide, lactose, magnesium stearate; gelatin capsules contain gelatin and titanium dioxide.

Baxan Suspensions:

Flavours, polysorbate 40, sodium benzoate, sucrose, titanium dioxide and xanthan gum.

6.2 Incompatibilities
None known.

6.3 Shelf life
Capsules and Suspensions:

36 months

6.4 Special precautions for storage
Baxan Capsules:

Store below 30°C.

Baxan Suspensions:

Product unopened: Store below 30°C.

After reconstitution: The product may be stored for 7 days below 30°C or for 14 days in a refrigerator (2-8°C).

6.5 Nature and contents of container
Baxan Capsules:

Blister packs consisting of PVC/PVDC laminate and aluminium foil containing 20 capsules.

Baxan Suspensions:

HDPE bottles with polyethylene closures containing 60ml.

6.6 Instructions for use and handling
None.

7. MARKETING AUTHORISATION HOLDER
Bristol-Myers Squibb Holdings Limited
t/a Bristol-Myers Pharmaceuticals
Uxbridge Business Park
Sanderson Road
Uxbridge
Middlesex
UB8 1DH

8. MARKETING AUTHORISATION NUMBER(S)
Baxan Capsules 500mg:	PL 00125/0107
Baxan Suspension 125mg/5ml:	PL 0125/0110
Baxan Suspension 250mg/5ml:	PL 0125/0111
Baxan Suspension 500mg/5m:	PL 0125/0112

9. DATE OF FIRST AUTHORISATION/RENEWAL OF THE AUTHORISATION
Baxan Capsules:

2nd November 1979 / 9th July 2001

Baxan Suspensions:

11th December 1979 / 8th July 2001

10. DATE OF REVISION OF THE TEXT
Baxan Capsules:

July 2005

Baxan Suspensions:

July 2005

Becloforte Inhaler
(Allen & Hanburys)

1. NAME OF THE MEDICINAL PRODUCT
Becloforte™ Inhaler.

2. QUALITATIVE AND QUANTITATIVE COMPOSITION
250 micrograms Beclometasone Dipropionate BP per actuation. Each canister delivers 80 or 200 actuations.

3. PHARMACEUTICAL FORM
Aerosol.

4. CLINICAL PARTICULARS
4.1 Therapeutic indications
Beclometasone dipropionate given by inhalation offers preventative treatment for asthma. It provides effective anti-inflammatory action in the lungs with a lower incidence and severity of adverse effects than those observed when corticosteroids are administered systemically.

Becloforte Inhaler is indicated in the prophylactic management of severe asthma in adults.

Severe asthma: Patients with severe chronic asthma and those who are dependent on systemic corticosteroids for adequate control of symptoms. Many patients who are dependent on systemic corticosteroids for adequate control of symptoms may be able to reduce significantly, or eliminate, their requirement for oral corticosteroids when they are transferred to high dose inhaled beclometasone dipropionate.

4.2 Posology and method of administration
Becloforte Inhaler is for oral inhalation use only.

Some patients find difficulty in co-ordinating the firing of an inhaler with inspiration and therefore fail to maximise the potential benefit offered by treatment. Becloforte Inhaler may be used with a spacer device in patients who find it difficult to synchronise aerosol actuation with inspiration.

Patients should be given a starting dose of inhaled beclometasone dipropionate appropriate to the severity of their disease. Those demonstrating a need for high dose inhaled steroid therapy should start on 1,000 micrograms daily. The dose may then be adjusted until control is achieved and should be titrated to the lowest dose at which effective control of asthma is maintained.

Adults (including the elderly): 1,000 micrograms daily which may be increased to 2,000 micrograms daily. This may then be reduced when the patient's asthma has stabilised. The total daily dose may be administered as two, three, or four divided doses

For optimum results Becloforte Inhaler should be used regularly, even when patients are asymptomatic.

Children: Not recommended.

4.3 Contraindications
Hypersensitivity to any of the components.

Special care is necessary in patients with active or quiescent pulmonary tuberculosis.

4.4 Special warnings and special precautions for use
Patients' inhaler technique should be checked to make sure that aerosol actuation is synchronised with inspiration of breath for optimum delivery of drug to the lungs.

Patients should be made aware of the prophylactic nature of therapy with Becloforte and that, for optimum benefits, they should use it regularly, every day, even when they are asymptomatic.

Becloforte Inhaler is not designed to relieve acute asthmatic symptoms for which an inhaled short-acting bronchodilator is required. Patients should be advised to have such rescue medication available.

Severe asthma requires regular medical assessment, including lung function testing, as patients are at risk of severe attacks and even death.

Increasing use of bronchodilators, in particular short-acting inhaled Beta 2 agonists to relieve symptoms indicates deterioration of asthma control. If patients find that short acting relief bronchodilator treatment becomes less effective or they need more inhalations than usual, medical attention must be sought. In this situation patient should be reassessed and consideration given to the need for increased anti-inflammatory therapy (e.g. higher doses of inhaled corticosteroids or a course of oral corticosteroids). Severe exacerbations of asthma must be treated in the normal way.

Systemic effects of inhaled corticosteroids may occur, particularly at high doses prescribed for prolonged periods. These effects are much less likely to occur than with oral corticosteroids. Possible systemic effects include Cushing's syndrome, Cushingoid features, adrenal suppression, growth retardation in children and adolescents, decrease in bone mineral density, cataract and glaucoma. It is important therefore that the dose of inhaled corticosteroid is titrated to the lowest dose at which effective control of asthma is maintained.

It is recommended that the height of children receiving prolonged treatment with inhaled corticosteroids is regularly monitored. If growth is slowed, therapy should be reviewed with the aim of reducing the dose of inhaled corticosteroid, if possible, to the lowest dose at which effective control of asthma is maintained. In addition, consideration should be given to referring the patient to a paediatric respiratory specialist.

Prolonged treatment with high doses of inhaled corticosteroids, particularly higher than recommended doses, may result in clinically significant adrenal suppression. Additional systemic corticosteroid cover should be considered during periods of stress or elective surgery.

Lack of response of severe exacerbations of asthma should be treated by increasing the dose of inhaled beclometasone dipropionate and, if necessary, by giving a systemic steroid and/or an antibiotic if there is an infection, and with Beta-agonist therapy.

For the transfer of patients being treated with oral corticosteroids

The transfer of oral steroid-dependent patients to inhaled beclometasone dipropionate and their subsequent management needs special care as recovery from impaired adrenocortical function caused by prolonged systemic steroid therapy, may take a considerable time.

Patients who have been treated with systemic steroids for long periods of time or at a high dose may have adrenocortical suppression. With these patients adrenocortical function should be monitored regularly and their dose of systemic steroid reduced cautiously.

After approximately a week, gradual withdrawal of the systemic steroid is commenced. Decrements in dosages should be appropriate to the level of maintenance systemic steroid, and introduced at not less than weekly intervals. For maintenance doses of prednisolone (or equivalent) of 10mg daily or less, the decrements in dose should not be greater than 1mg per day, at not less than weekly intervals. For maintenance doses of predisolone in excess of 10mg daily, it may be appropriate to employ cautiously, larger decrements in dose at weekly intervals.

Some patients feel unwell in a non-specific way during the withdrawal phase despite maintenance or even improvement of the respiratory function. They should be encouraged to persevere with inhaled beclometasone dipropionate and to continue withdrawal of systemic steroid, unless there are objective signs of adrenal insufficiency.

Patients weaned off oral steroids whose adrenocortical function is impaired should carry a steroid warning card indicating that they may need supplementary systemic steroid during periods of stress e.g. worsening asthma attacks, chest infections, major intercurrent illness, surgery, trauma etc.

Replacement of systemic steroid treatment with inhaled therapy sometimes unmasks allergies such as allergic rhinitis or eczema previously controlled by the systemic drug. These allergies should be treated with antihistamine and/or topical preparations, including topical steroids.

Treatment with Becloforte Inhaler should not be stopped abruptly.

As with all inhaled corticosteroids, special care is necessary in patients with active quiescent pulmonary tuberculosis.

4.5 Interaction with other medicinal products and other forms of Interaction

None reported.

4.6 Pregnancy and lactation

There is inadequate evidence of safety in human pregnancy. Administration of corticosteroids to pregnant animals can cause abnormalities of fetal development including cleft palate and intra-uterine growth retardation. There may therefore be a very small risk of such effects in the human fetus. It should be noted, however, that the fetal changes in animals occur after relatively high systemic exposure. Becloforte Inhaler delivers the drug directly to the lungs by the inhaled route and so avoids the high level of exposure that occurs when corticosteroids are given by systemic routes.

The use of beclometasone dipropionate in pregnancy requires that the possible benefits of the drug be weighed against the possible hazards.

No specific studies examining the transference of beclometasone dipropionate into the milk of lactating animals have been performed. It is reasonable to assume that beclometasone dipropionate is secreted in milk, but at the dosages used for direct inhalation there is low potential for significant levels in breast milk.

The use of beclometasone dipropionate in mothers breast feeding their babies requires that the therapeutic benefits of the drug be weighed against the potential hazards to the mother and baby.

4.7 Effects on ability to drive and use machines

None reported.

4.8 Undesirable effects

Systemic effects of inhaled corticosteroids may occur, particularly at high doses prescribed for prolonged periods. These may include Cushing's syndrome, Cushingoid features, adrenal suppression, growth retardation in children and adolescents, decrease in bone mineral density, cataract and glaucoma.

As with other inhalation therapy, paradoxical bronchospasm may occur with an immediate increase in wheezing after dosing. This responds to a fast-acting inhaled bronchodilator. The preparation should be discontinued immediately, the patient assessed, and if necessary alternative therapy instituted.

Hypersensitivity reactions including rashes, urticaria, pruritus and erythema, and oedema of the eyes, face, lips and throat, have been reported.

There have been very rare reports of anxiety, sleep disorders and behavioural changes, including hyperactivity and irritability (predominantly in children).

Candidiasis of the mouth and throat (thrush) occurs in some patients, the incidence increasing with doses greater than 400 micrograms beclometasone dipropionate per day. Patients with high blood levels of *Candida precipitins*, indicating a previous infection, are most likely to develop this complication. Patients may find it helpful to rinse their mouth thoroughly with water after using Becloforte Inhaler. Symptomatic candidiasis can be treated with topical antifungal therapy whilst still continuing with the treatment.

In some patients inhaled beclometasone dipropionate may cause hoarseness or throat irritation. It may be helpful to rinse out the mouth with water immediately after inhalation. The use of a spacer device may also be considered.

4.9 Overdose

Acute: Inhalation of the drug in doses in excess of those recommended may lead to temporary suppression of adrenal function. This does not require emergency action. In these patients treatment should be continued at a dose sufficient to control asthma; adrenal function recovers in a few days and can be verified by measuring plasma cortisol.

Chronic: Use of inhaled beclometasone dipropionate in daily doses in excess of 1,500 micrograms over prolonged periods may lead to adrenal suppression. Monitoring of adrenal reserve may be indicated. Treatment should be continued at a dose sufficient to control asthma.

5. PHARMACOLOGICAL PROPERTIES

5.1 Pharmacodynamic properties

BDP is a pro-drug with weak glucocorticoid receptor binding activity. It is hydrolysed via esterase enzymes to the active metabolite beclometasone-17-monopropionate (B-17-MP), which has high topical anti-inflammatory activity.

5.2 Pharmacokinetic properties

Absorption

When administered via inhalation, there is extensive conversion of BDP to active metabolite B-17-MP within the lungs prior to systemic absorption. In healthy male volunteers the absolute bioavailability following inhalation is approximately 2%(95% CI 1-5%) and 62%(95% CI 47-83%) of the nominal dose for unchanged BDP and B-17-MP respectively. The systemic absorption of B-17-MP arises from both lung deposition (approximately 36%) and oral absorption of the swallowed dose (approximately 26%). BDP is absorbed rapidly with peak plasma concentrations first being observed (t_{max}) at 0.3h. B-17-MP appears more slowly with a t_{max} of 1h. There is an approximately linear increase in systemic exposure with increasing inhaled dose. When administered orally the bioavailability of BDP is negligible but pre-systemic conversion to B-17-MP results in 41% (95% CI 27-62%) of the dose being available as B-17-MP.

Metabolism

BDP is cleared very rapidly from the systemic circulation, owing to extensive first pass metabolism. The main product of metabolism is the active metabolite (B-17-MP). Minor inactive metabolites, beclometasone-21-monopropionate (B-21-MP) and beclometasone (BOH), are also formed but these contribute little to systemic exposure.

Distribution

The tissue distribution at steady-state for BDP is moderate (20l) but more extensive for B-17-MP (424l). Plasma protein binding is moderately high (87%).

Elimination

The elimination of BDP and B-17-MP are characterised by high plasma clearance (150 and 120L/h) with corresponding terminal elimination half-lives of 0.5h and 2.7h. Following oral administration of titrated BDP, approximately 60% of the dose was excreted in the faeces within 96 hours mainly as free and conjugated polar metabolites. Approximately 12% of the dose was excreted as free and conjugated polar metabolites in the urine.

5.3 Preclinical safety data

There are no pre-clinical data of relevance to the prescriber which are additional to that already included in other sections of the SPC.

6. PHARMACEUTICAL PARTICULARS

6.1 List of excipients

Oleic Acid.

Dichlorodifluoromethane.

Trichlorofluoromethane.

6.2 Incompatibilities

None reported.

6.3 Shelf life

3 years when not stored above 30°C.

3 years when not stored above 25°C. (80 actuations only).

6.4 Special precautions for storage

Do not store above 30°C.

Do not store above 25°C. (80 actuations only).

As with most inhaled medicines in aerosol canisters, the therapeutic effect may decrease when the canister is cold.

Protect from frost and direct sunlight.

The canister should not be broken, punctured or burnt, even when apparently empty.

6.5 Nature and contents of container

An inhaler comprising an aluminium can sealed with a metering valve, with an actuator and dust cap. Each canister provides 200 (Hospital packs 80) metered actuations of 250 micrograms beclometasone dipropionate.

6.6 Instructions for use and handling

The aerosol spray is inhaled through the mouth into the lungs. After shaking the inhaler, the mouthpiece is placed in the mouth and the lips closed around it. The actuator is depressed to release a spray, which must coincide with inspiration of breath.

For detailed instructions for use refer to the Patient Information Leaflet in every pack.

Administrative Data

7. MARKETING AUTHORISATION HOLDER

Glaxo Wellcome UK Limited

Trading as Allen & Hanburys,

Stockley Park West,

Uxbridge,

Middlesex, UB11 1BT.

8. MARKETING AUTHORISATION NUMBER(S)

PL 10949/0065

9. DATE OF FIRST AUTHORISATION/RENEWAL OF THE AUTHORISATION

14 March 2003

10. DATE OF REVISION OF THE TEXT

23 December 2004

11. Legal Status

POM.

Becloforte is a trade mark of the Glaxo Wellcome Group of Companies.

Becodisks 100mcg

(Allen & Hanburys)

1. NAME OF THE MEDICINAL PRODUCT

Becodisks 100 Micrograms

2. QUALITATIVE AND QUANTITATIVE COMPOSITION

Beclometasone Dipropionate 100 micrograms

3. PHARMACEUTICAL FORM

Dry Powder for Inhalation via Diskhaler Device

4. CLINICAL PARTICULARS

4.1 Therapeutic indications

Clinical Indications

Beclometasone dipropionate provides effective anti-inflammatory action in the lungs, with a lower incidence and severity of adverse effects than those observed when corticosteroids are administered systemically. It also offers preventive treatment of asthma.

Becodisks are indicated for the following:

Adults

Prophylactic management in:

Mild asthma (PEF values greater than 80% predicted at baseline with less than 20% variability):

Patients requiring intermittent symptomatic bronchodilator asthma medication on more than an occasional basis.

Moderate asthma (PEF values 60-80% predicted at baseline with 20-30% variability):

Patients requiring regular asthma medication and patients with unstable or worsening asthma on other prophylactic therapy or bronchodilator alone.

Severe asthma (PEF values less than 60% predicted at baseline with greater than 30% variability):

Patients with severe chronic asthma. On transfer to high dose inhaled beclometasone dipropionate, many patients who are dependent on systemic corticosteroids for adequate control of symptoms may be able to reduce significantly or eliminate their requirement for oral corticosteroids.

4.2 Posology and method of administration

Becodisks are for administration by the inhalation route only using a Diskhaler device.

Patients should be made aware of the prophylactic nature of therapy with inhaled beclometasone dipropionate and that it should be taken regularly everyday even when they are asymptomatic.

Patients should be given a starting dose of inhaled beclometasone dipropionate which is appropriate for severity of their disease. The dose may then be adjusted until control is achieved and should be titrated to the lowest dose at which effective control of asthma is maintained.

Adults

400 microgram twice daily is the usual starting dose. One 400 microgram blister or two 200 micrograms blisters twice daily is the usual maintenance dose. Alternatively, 200 micrograms may be administered three or four times daily.

Children

100 micrograms two, three or four times a day, according to the response. Alternatively, the usual starting dose of 200 micrograms twice daily may be administered.

Special Patient Groups

There is no need to adjust the dose in elderly patients or in those with hepatic or renal impairment.

4.3 Contraindications

Hypersensitivity to Becodisks or any of its compnents is a contraindication. (See Pharmaceutical Particulars – List of Excipients).

Special care is necessary in patients with active or quiescent pulmonary tuberculosis.

4.4 Special warnings and special precautions for use

Patients should be instructed in the proper use of the Diskhaler to ensure that the drug reaches the target areas within the lungs. They should be made aware that Becodisks have to be used regularly everyday for optimum benefit. Patients should be made aware of the prophylactic nature of therapy with Becodisks and that they should be used regularly, even when they are asymptomatic.

Becodisks are not designed to relieve acute asthmatic symptoms for which an inhaled short-acting bronchodilator is required. Patients should be advised to have such rescue medication available.

Severe asthma requires regular medical assessment including lung function testing as patients are at risk of severe attacks and even death.

Increasing use of bronchodilators, in particular short-acting inhaled beta$_2$ agonists to relieve symptoms indicates deterioration of asthma control. If patients find that short acting relief bronchodilator treatment becomes less effective or they need more inhalations than usual, medical attention must be sought.

In this situation patients should be reassessed and consideration given to the need for increased anti-inflammatory therapy (e.g. Higher doses of inhaled corticosteroids or a course of oral corticosteroids). Severe exacerbations of asthma must be treated in the normal way.

Systemic effects of inhaled corticosteroids may occur, particularly at high doses prescribed for prolonged periods. These effects are much less likely to occur than with oral corticosteroids. Possible systemic effects include Cushing's syndrome, Cushingoid features, adrenal suppression, growth retardation in children and adolescents, decrease in bone mineral density, cataract and glaucoma. It is important therefore that the dose of inhaled corticosteroid is titrated to the lowest dose at which effective control of asthma is maintained.

It is recommended that the height of children receiving prolonged treatment with inhaled corticosteroids is regularly monitored. If growth is slowed, therapy should be reviewed with the aim of reducing the dose of inhaled corticosteroid, if possible, to the lowest dose at which effective control of asthma is maintained. In addition, consideration should be given to referring the patient to a paediatric respiratory specialist.

Prolonged treatment with high doses of inhaled corticosteroids, particularly higher than recommended doses, may result in clinically significant adrenal suppression. Additional systemic corticosteroid cover should be considered during periods of stress or elective surgery.

Lack of response or severe exacerbations of asthma should be treated by increasing the dose of inhaled beclometasone dipropionate and, if necessary, by giving a systemic steroid and/or antibiotic if there is an infection, and by use of beta-agonist therapy.

For the transfer of patients being treated with oral corticosteroids:

The transfer of oral steroid-dependent patients to Becodisks and their subsequent management needs special care as recovery from impaired adrenocortical function, caused by prolonged systemic steroid therapy, may take a considerable time.

Patients who have been treated with systemic steroids for long periods of time or at a high dose may have adrenocortical suppression. With these patients adrenocortical function should be monitored regularly and their dose of systemic steroid reduced cautiously.

After approximately a week, gradual withdrawal of the systemic steroid is commenced. Decrements in dosages should be appropriate to the level of maintenance systemic steroid, and introduced at not less than weekly intervals. For maintenance doses of prednisolone (or equivalent) of 10mg daily or less, the decrements in dose should not be greater than 1mg per day, at not less than weekly intervals. For maintenance doses of prednisolone in excess of 10mg daily, it may be appropriate to employ cautiously, larger decrements in dose at weekly intervals.

Some patients feel unwell in a non-specific way during the withdrawal phase despite maintenance or even improvement of the respiratory function. They should be encouraged to persevere with the Diskhaler and withdrawal of systemic steroid continued, unless there are objective signs of adrenal insufficiency.

Patients weaned off oral steroids whose adrenocortical function is impaired should carry a steroid warning card indicating that they may need supplementary systemic steroid during periods of stress, e.g. Worsening asthma attacks, chest infections, major intercurrent illness, surgery, trauma, etc.

Replacement of systemic steroid treatment with inhaled therapy sometimes unmasks allergies such as allergic rhinitis or eczema previously controlled by the systemic drug. These allergies should be symptomatically treated with antihistamine and/or topical preparations, including topical steroids.

Treatment with Becodisks should not be stopped abruptly.

As with all inhaled corticosteroids, special care is necessary in patients with active or quiescent pulmonary tuberculosis

4.5 Interaction with other medicinal products and other forms of Interaction

No interactions have been reported.

4.6 Pregnancy and lactation

There is inadequate evidence of safety in human pregnancy. Administration of corticosteroids to pregnant animals can cause abnormalities of foetal development including cleft palate and intra-uterine growth retardation. There may therefore be a very small risk of such effects in the human foetus. It should be noted, however, that the foetal changes in animals occur after relatively high systemic exposure. Because beclometasone dipropionate is delivered directly to the lungs by the inhaled route it avoids the high level of exposure that occurs when corticosteroids are given by systemic routes.

The use of beclometasone dipropionate in pregnancy requires that the possible benefits of the drug be weighed against the possible hazards. It should be noted that the drug has been in widespread use for many years without apparent ill consequence.

No specific studies examining the transference of beclometasone dipropionate into the milk of lactating animals have been performed. It is reasonable to assume that beclometasone dipropionate is secreted in milk but at the dosages used for direct inhalation, there is low potential for significant levels in breast milk. The use of beclometasone dipropionate in mothers breast feeding their babies requires that the therapeutic benefits of the drug be weighed against the potential hazards to the mother and baby.

4.7 Effects on ability to drive and use machines

No adverse effect has been reported.

4.8 Undesirable effects

Systemic effects of inhaled corticosteroids may occur, particularly at high doses prescribed for prolonged periods. These may include Cushing's syndrome, Cushingoid features, adrenal suppression, growth retardation in children and adolescents, decrease in bone mineral density, cataract and glaucoma.

There have been very rare reports of anxiety, sleep disorders and behavioural changes, including hyperactivity and irritability (predominantly in children).

Candidiasis of the mouth and throat (thrush) occurs in some patients, the incidence of which is increased with doses greater than 400 micrograms beclometasone dipropionate per day. Patients with high blood levels of candida precipitins, indicating a previous infection, are most likely to develop this complication. Patients may find it helpful to rinse their mouth with water after using the Diskhaler. Symptomatic candidiasis can be treated with topical anti-fungal therapy whilst still continuing with the Becodisks.

In some patients inhaled beclometasone dipropionate may cause hoarseness or throat irritation. It may be helpful to rinse out the mouth with water immediately after inhalation.

As with other inhalation therapy, paradoxical bronchospasm may occur with an immediate increase in wheezing after dosing. This responds to a fast-acting inhaled bronchodilator. The preparation should be discontinued immediately, the patient assessed, and if necessary, alternative therapy instituted.

Hypersensitivity reactions including rashes, urticaria, pruritus and erythema, and oedema of the eyes, face, lips and throat, have been reported.

4.9 Overdose

Acute - inhalation of the drug in doses in excess of those recommended may lead to temporary suppression of adrenal function. This does not necessitate emergency action being taken. In these patients treatment with beclometasone dipropionate by inhalation should be continued at a dose sufficient to control asthma; adrenal function recovers in a few days and can be verified by measuring plasma cortisol.

Chronic - use of inhaled beclometasone dipropionate in daily doses in excess of 1500 micrograms over prolonged periods may lead to adrenal suppression. Monitoring of adrenal reserve may be indicated. Treatment with inhaled beclometasone dipropionate should be continued at a dose sufficient to control asthma.

5. PHARMACOLOGICAL PROPERTIES

5.1 Pharmacodynamic properties

BDP is a pro-drug with weak glucocorticoid receptor binding activity. It is hydrolysed via esterase enzymes to the active metabolite beclometasone-17-monopropionate (B-17-MP), which has high topical anti-inflammatory activity.

5.2 Pharmacokinetic properties

Absorption

When administered via inhalation (via metered dose inhaler) there is extensive conversion of BDP to the active metabolite B-17-MP within the lungs prior to systemic absorption. The systemic absorption of B-17-MP arises from both lung deposition and oral absorption of the swallowed dose. When administered orally, in healthy male volunteers, the bioavailability of BDP is negligible but pre-systemic conversion to B-17-MP results in 41% (95% CI 27- 62 %) of the dose being available as B-17-MP.

Metabolism

BDP is cleared very rapidly from the systemic circulation, owing to extensive first pass metabolism. The main product of metabolism is the active metabolite (B-17-MP). Minor inactive metabolites, beclometasone-21-monopropionate (B-21-MP) and beclometasone (BOH), are also formed but these contribute little to systemic exposure.

Distribution

The tissue distribution at steady state for BDP is moderate (20L) but more extensive for B-17-MP (424L). Plasma protein binding is moderately high (87%).

Elimination

The elimination of BDP and B-17-MP are characterised by high plasma clearance (150 and 120L/h) with corresponding terminal elimination half lives of 0.5h and 2.7h. Following oral administration of tritiated BDP, approximately 60% of the dose was excreted in the faeces within 96 hours mainly as free and conjugated polar metabolites. Approximately 12% of the dose was excreted as free and conjugated polar metabolites in the urine.

5.3 Preclinical safety data

No clinically relevant findings were observed in preclinical studies.

6. PHARMACEUTICAL PARTICULARS

6.1 List of excipients

Lactose (which contains milk protein)

6.2 Incompatibilities

No incompatibilities have been reported.

6.3 Shelf life

36 months

6.4 Special precautions for storage

Do not store above 30°C

6.5 Nature and contents of container

Circular double foil blister pack consisting of:

A) Lidding material (i) polyester over-lacquer/hard tempered aluminium foil/heat seal lacquer of total thickness = 39.4 - 48.6microns or (ii) nitrocellulose over-lacquer/hard tempered aluminium foil/heat seal lacquer of total thickness = 37.0 - 42.0microns.

Blister material - pvc film/aluminium foil/orientated polyamide. Becodisks are supplied as 8 blisters per Becodisk as follows:

Carton containing 14 disks plus a Diskhaler

Carton containing 15 disks plus a Diskhaler

Carton containing 5 disks plus a Diskhaler (Hospital pack)

Refill packs of 14 disks

Refill packs of 15 disks

Not all pack sizes may be marketed

6.6 Instructions for use and handling
See Patient Information Leaflet

Administrative Data

7. MARKETING AUTHORISATION HOLDER
Glaxo Wellcome UK Ltd.
Trading as Allen & Hanburys,
Stockley Park West,
Uxbridge
Middlesex, UB11 1BT

8. MARKETING AUTHORISATION NUMBER(S)
PL 10949/0055

9. DATE OF FIRST AUTHORISATION/RENEWAL OF THE AUTHORISATION
1 October 1993/11 December 1997

10. DATE OF REVISION OF THE TEXT
22 December 2004

11. Legal Status
POM

Becodisks 200mcg

(Allen & Hanburys)

1. NAME OF THE MEDICINAL PRODUCT
Becodisks 200 Micrograms

2. QUALITATIVE AND QUANTITATIVE COMPOSITION
Beclometasone Dipropionate 200micrograms

3. PHARMACEUTICAL FORM
Dry Powder for Inhalation via Diskhaler Device

4. CLINICAL PARTICULARS

4.1 Therapeutic indications

Clinical Indications

Beclometasone dipropionate provides effective anti-inflammatory action in the lungs, with a lower incidence and severity of adverse effects than those observed when corticosteroids are administered systemically. It also offers preventive treatment of asthma.

Becodisks are indicated for the following:

Adults

Prophylactic management in:

Mild asthma (PEF values greater than 80% predicted at baseline with less than 20% variability):

Patients requiring intermittent symptomatic bronchodilator asthma medication on more than an occasional basis.

Moderate asthma (PEF values 60-80% predicted at baseline with 20-30% variability):

Patients requiring regular asthma medication and patients with unstable or worsening asthma on other prophylactic therapy or bronchodilator alone.

Severe asthma (PEF values less than 60% predicted at baseline with greater than 30% variability):

Patients with severe chronic asthma. On transfer to high dose inhaled beclometasone dipropionate, many patients who are dependent on systemic corticosteroids for adequate control of symptoms may be able to reduce significantly or eliminate their requirement for oral corticosteroids.

4.2 Posology and method of administration
Becodisks are for administration by the inhalation route only using a Diskhaler device.

Patients should be made aware of the prophylactic nature of therapy with inhaled beclometasone dipropionate and that it should be taken regularly everyday even when they are asymptomatic.

Patients should be given a starting dose of inhaled beclometasone dipropionate which is appropriate for severity of their disease. The dose may then be adjusted until control is achieved and should be titrated to the lowest dose at which effective control of asthma is maintained.

Adults

400 microgram twice daily is the usual starting dose. One 400 microgram blister or two 200 micrograms blisters twice daily is the usual maintenance dose. Alternatively, 200 micrograms may be administered three or four times daily.

Children

100 micrograms two, three or four times a day, according to the response. Alternatively, the usual starting dose of 200 micrograms twice daily may be administered.

Special Patient Groups

There is no need to adjust the dose in elderly patients or in those with hepatic or renal impairment.

4.3 Contraindications
Hypersensitivity to Becodisks or any of its compnents is a contraindication. (See Pharmaceutical Particulars – List of Excipients).

Special care is necessary in patients with active or quiescent pulmonary tuberculosis.

4.4 Special warnings and special precautions for use
Patients should be instructed in the proper use of the Diskhaler to ensure that the drug reaches the target areas within the lungs. They should be made aware that Becodisks have to be used regularly everyday for optimum benefit. Patients should be made aware of the prophylactic nature of therapy with Becodisks and that they should be used regularly, even when they are asymptomatic.

Becodisks are not designed to relieve acute asthmatic symptoms for which an inhaled short-acting bronchodilator is required. Patients should be advised to have such rescue medication available.

Severe asthma requires regular medical assessment including lung function testing as patients are at risk of severe attacks and even death.

Increasing use of bronchodilators, in particular short-acting inhaled beta$_2$ agonists to relieve symptoms indicates deterioration of asthma control. If patients find that short acting relief bronchodilator treatment becomes less effective or they need more inhalations than usual, medical attention must be sought.

In this situation patients should be reassessed and consideration given to the need for increased anti-inflammatory therapy (e.g. Higher doses of inhaled corticosteroids or a course of oral corticosteroids). Severe exacerbations of asthma must be treated in the normal way.

Systemic effects of inhaled corticosteroids may occur, particularly at high doses prescribed for prolonged periods. These effects are much less likely to occur than with oral corticosteroids. Possible systemic effects include Cushing's syndrome, Cushingoid features, adrenal suppression, growth retardation in children and adolescents, decrease in bone mineral density, cataract and glaucoma. It is important therefore that the dose of inhaled corticosteroid is titrated to the lowest dose at which effective control of asthma is maintained.

It is recommended that the height of children receiving prolonged treatment with inhaled corticosteroids is regularly monitored. If growth is slowed, therapy should be reviewed with the aim of reducing the dose of inhaled corticosteroid, if possible, to the lowest dose at which effective control of asthma is maintained. In addition, consideration should be given to referring the patient to a paediatric respiratory specialist.

Prolonged treatment with high doses of inhaled corticosteroids, particularly higher than recommended doses, may result in clinically significant adrenal suppression. Additional systemic corticosteroid cover should be considered during periods of stress or elective surgery.

Lack of response or severe exacerbations of asthma should be treated by increasing the dose of inhaled beclometasone dipropionate and, if necessary, by giving a systemic steroid and/or antibiotic if there is an infection, and by use of beta-agonist therapy.

For the transfer of patients being treated with oral corticosteroids:

The transfer of oral steroid-dependent patients to Becodisks and their subsequent management needs special care as recovery from impaired adrenocortical function, caused by prolonged systemic steroid therapy, may take a considerable time.

Patients who have been treated with systemic steroids for long periods of time or at a high dose may have adrenocortical suppression. With these patients adrenocortical function should be monitored regularly and their dose of systemic steroid reduced cautiously.

After approximately a week, gradual withdrawal of the systemic steroid is commenced. Decrements in dosages should be appropriate to the level of maintenance systemic steroid, and introduced at not less than weekly intervals. For maintenance doses of prednisolone (or equivalent) of 10mg daily or less, the decrements in dose should not be greater than 1mg per day, at not less than weekly intervals. For maintenance doses of prednisolone in excess of 10mg daily, it may be appropriate to employ cautiously, larger decrements in dose at weekly intervals.

Some patients feel unwell in a non-specific way during the withdrawal phase despite maintenance or even improvement of the respiratory function. They should be encouraged to persevere with the Diskhaler and withdrawal of systemic steroid continued, unless there are objective signs of adrenal insufficiency.

Patients weaned off oral steroids whose adrenocortical function is impaired should carry a steroid warning card indicating that they may need supplementary systemic steroid during periods of stress, e.g. Worsening asthma attacks, chest infections, major intercurrent illness, surgery, trauma, etc.

Replacement of systemic steroid treatment with inhaled therapy sometimes unmasks allergies such as allergic rhinitis or eczema previously controlled by the systemic drug. These allergies should be symptomatically treated with antihistamine and/or topical preparations, including topical steroids.

Treatment with Becodisks should not be stopped abruptly.

As with all inhaled corticosteroids, special care is necessary in patients with active or quiescent pulmonary tuberculosis

4.5 Interaction with other medicinal products and other forms of Interaction
No interactions have been reported

4.6 Pregnancy and lactation
There is inadequate evidence of safety in human pregnancy. Administration of corticosteroids to pregnant animals can cause abnormalities of foetal development including cleft palate and intra-uterine growth retardation. There may therefore be a very small risk of such effects in the human foetus. It should be noted, however, that the foetal changes in animals occur after relatively high systemic exposure. Because beclometasone dipropionate is delivered directly to the lungs by the inhaled route it avoids the high level of exposure that occurs when corticosteroids are given by systemic routes.

The use of beclometasone dipropionate in pregnancy requires that the possible benefits of the drug be weighed against the possible hazards. It should be noted that the drug has been in widespread use for many years without apparent ill consequence.

No specific studies examining the transference of beclometasone dipropionate into the milk of lactating animals have been performed. It is reasonable to assume that beclometasone dipropionate is secreted in milk but at the dosages used for direct inhalation, there is low potential for significant levels in breast milk. The use of beclometasone dipropionate in mothers breast feeding their babies requires that the therapeutic benefits of the drug be weighed against the potential hazards to the mother and baby.

4.7 Effects on ability to drive and use machines
No adverse effect has been reported.

4.8 Undesirable effects
Systemic effects of inhaled corticosteroids may occur, particularly at high doses prescribed for prolonged periods. These may include Cushing's syndrome, Cushingoid features, adrenal suppression, growth retardation in children and adolescents, decrease in bone mineral density, cataract and glaucoma.

There have been very rare reports of anxiety, sleep disorders and behavioural changes, including hyperactivity and irritability (predominantly in children).

Candidiasis of the mouth and throat (thrush) occurs in some patients, the incidence of which is increased with doses greater than 400 micrograms beclometasone dipropionate per day. Patients with high blood levels of candida precipitins, indicating a previous infection, are most likely to develop this complication. Patients may find it helpful to rinse their mouth with water after using the Diskhaler. Symptomatic candidiasis can be treated with topical anti-fungal therapy whilst still continuing with the Becodisks.

In some patients inhaled beclometasone dipropionate may cause hoarseness or throat irritation. It may be helpful to rinse out the mouth with water immediately after inhalation.

As with other inhalation therapy, paradoxical bronchospasm may occur with an immediate increase in wheezing after dosing. This responds to a fast-acting inhaled bronchodilator. The preparation should be discontinued immediately, the patient assessed, and if necessary, alternative therapy instituted.

Hypersensitivity reactions including rashes, urticaria, pruritus and erythema, and oedema of the eyes, face, lips and throat, have been reported.

4.9 Overdose
Acute - inhalation of the drug in doses in excess of those recommended may lead to temporary suppression of adrenal function. This does not necessitate emergency action being taken. In these patients treatment with beclometasone dipropionate by inhalation should be continued at a dose sufficient to control asthma; adrenal function recovers in a few days and can be verified by measuring plasma cortisol.

Chronic - use of inhaled beclometasone dipropionate in daily doses in excess of 1500 micrograms over prolonged periods may lead to adrenal suppression. Monitoring of adrenal reserve may be indicated. Treatment with inhaled beclometasone dipropionate should be continued at a dose sufficient to control asthma.

5. PHARMACOLOGICAL PROPERTIES

5.1 Pharmacodynamic properties
BDP is a pro-drug with weak glucocorticoid receptor binding activity. It is hydrolysed via esterase enzymes to the active metabolite beclometasone-17-monopropionate (B-17-MP), which has high topical anti-inflammatory activity.

5.2 Pharmacokinetic properties

Absorption

When administered via inhalation (via metered dose inhaler) there is extensive conversion of BDP to the active metabolite B-17-MP within the lungs prior to systemic absorption. The systemic absorption of B-17-MP arises from both lung deposition and oral absorption of the swallowed dose. When administered orally, in healthy male volunteers, the bioavailability of BDP is negligible but pre-systemic conversion to B-17-MP results in 41% (95% CI 27- 62 %) of the dose being available as B-17-MP.

Metabolism

BDP is cleared very rapidly from the systemic circulation, owing to extensive first pass metabolism. The main product of metabolism is the active metabolite (B-17-MP). Minor inactive metabolites, beclometasone-21-monopropionate (B-21-MP) and beclometasone (BOH), are also formed but these contribute little to systemic exposure.

Distribution

The tissue distribution at steady state for BDP is moderate (20L) but more extensive for B-17-MP (424L). Plasma protein binding is moderately high (87%).

Elimination

The elimination of BDP and B-17-MP are characterised by high plasma clearance (150 and 120L/h) with corresponding terminal elimination half lives of 0.5h and 2.7h. Following oral administration of tritiated BDP, approximately 60% of the dose was excreted in the faeces within 96 hours mainly as free and conjugated polar metabolites. Approximately 12% of the dose was excreted as free and conjugated polar metabolites in the urine.

5.3 Preclinical safety data

No clinically relevant findings were observed in preclinical studies.

6. PHARMACEUTICAL PARTICULARS

6.1 List of excipients

Lactose(which contains milk protein)

6.2 Incompatibilities

No incompatibilities have been reported.

6.3 Shelf life

36 months

6.4 Special precautions for storage

Do not store above 30°C.

6.5 Nature and contents of container

Circular double foil blister pack consisting of:

A) Lidding material (i) polyester over-lacquer/hard tempered aluminium foil/heat seal lacquer of total thickness = 39.4 - 48.6microns or (ii) nitrocellulose over-lacquer/hard tempered aluminium foil/heat seal lacquer of total thickness = 37.0 - 42.0microns.

B) Blister material - pvc film/aluminium foil/orientated polyamide.

Becodisks are supplied as 8 blisters per Becodisk as follows:

- Carton containing 14 disks plus a Diskhaler
- Carton containing 15 disks plus a Diskhaler
- Carton containing 5 disks plus a Diskhaler (Hospital pack)
- Refill packs of 14 disks
- Refill packs of 15 disks

Not all pack sizes may be marketed

6.6 Instructions for use and handling

See Patient Information Leaflet

Administrative Data

7. MARKETING AUTHORISATION HOLDER

Glaxo Wellcome UK Ltd.

Trading as Allen & Hanburys,

Stockley Park West,

Uxbridge

Middlesex,

UB11 1BT

8. MARKETING AUTHORISATION NUMBER(S)

PL 10949/0056

9. DATE OF FIRST AUTHORISATION/RENEWAL OF THE AUTHORISATION

27 September 1993/11 December 1997

10. DATE OF REVISION OF THE TEXT

22 December 2004

11. Legal Status

POM

Becodisks 400mcg

(Allen & Hanburys)

1. NAME OF THE MEDICINAL PRODUCT

Becodisks 400 Micrograms

2. QUALITATIVE AND QUANTITATIVE COMPOSITION

Beclometasone Dipropionate Monohydrate (Micronised) 414μg equivalent to 400μg Beclometasone Dipropionate

3. PHARMACEUTICAL FORM

Dry Powder for Inhalation via Diskhaler Device

4. CLINICAL PARTICULARS

4.1 Therapeutic indications

Clinical Indications

Beclometasone dipropionate provides effective anti-inflammatory action in the lungs, with a lower incidence and severity of adverse effects than those observed when corticosteroids are administered systemically. It also offers preventive treatment of asthma.

Becodisks are indicated for the following:

Adults

Prophylactic management in:

Mild asthma (PEF values greater than 80% predicted at baseline with less than 20% variability):

Patients requiring intermittent symptomatic bronchodilator asthma medication on more than an occasional basis.

Moderate asthma (PEF values 60-80% predicted at baseline with 20-30% variability):

Patients requiring regular asthma medication and patients with unstable or worsening asthma on other prophylactic therapy or bronchodilator alone.

Severe asthma (PEF values less than 60% predicted at baseline with greater than 30% variability):

Patients with severe chronic asthma. On transfer to high dose inhaled beclometasone dipropionate, many patients who are dependent on systemic corticosteroids for adequate control of symptoms may be able to reduce significantly or eliminate their requirement for oral corticosteroids.

4.2 Posology and method of administration

Becodisks are for administration by the inhalation route only using a Diskhaler device.

Patients should be made aware of the prophylactic nature of therapy with inhaled beclometasone dipropionate and that it should be taken regularly everyday even when they are asymptomatic.

Patients should be given a starting dose of inhaled beclometasone dipropionate which is appropriate for the severity of their disease. The dose may then be adjusted until control is achieved and should be titrated to the lowest dose at which effective control of asthma is maintained.

Adults

The contents of one blister (400 micrograms) twice daily is the usual maintenance dose. This may be increased to two blisters (800 micrograms) twice daily in patients for whom there is a clinical need.

Children

Not recommended in children.

Special Patient Groups

There is no need to adjust the dose in elderly patients or in those with hepatic or renal impairment.

4.3 Contraindications

Hypersensitivity to Becodisks or any of its components is a contraindication. (See Pharmaceutical Particulars – List of Excipients).

Special care is necessary in patients with active or quiescent pulmonary tuberculosis

4.4 Special warnings and special precautions for use

Patients should be instructed in the proper use of the Diskhaler to ensure that the drug reaches the target areas within the lungs. They should be made aware that Becodisks have to be used regularly everyday for optimum benefit. Patients should be made aware of the prophylactic nature of therapy with Becodisks and that they should be used regularly, even when they are asymptomatic.

Becodisks are not designed to relieve acute asthmatic symptoms for which an inhaled short-acting bronchodilator is required. Patients should be advised to have such rescue medication available.

Severe asthma requires regular medical assessment including lung function testing as patients are at risk of severe attacks and even death.

Increasing use of bronchodilators, in particular short-acting inhaled beta$_2$ agonists to relieve symptoms indicates deterioration of asthma control. If patients find that short acting relief bronchodilator treatment becomes less effective or they need more inhalations than usual, medical attention must be sought.

In this situation patients should be reassessed and consideration given to the need or increased anti-inflammatory therapy (e.g. Higher doses of inhaled corticosteroids or a course of oral corticosteroids). Severe exacerbations of asthma must be treated in the normal way.

Systemic effects of inhaled corticosteroids may occur, particularly at high doses prescribed for prolonged periods. These effects are much less likely to occur than with oral corticosteroids. Possible systemic effects include Cushing's syndrome, Cushingoid features, adrenal suppression, growth retardation in children and adolescents, decrease in bone mineral density, cataract and glaucoma. It is important therefore that the dose of inhaled corticosteroid is titrated to the lowest dose at which effective control of asthma is maintained.

It is recommended that the height of children receiving prolonged treatment with inhaled corticosteroids is regularly monitored. If growth is slowed, therapy should be reviewed with the aim of reducing the dose of inhaled corticosteroid, if possible, to the lowest dose at which effective control of asthma is maintained. In addition, consideration should be given to referring the patient to a paediatric respiratory specialist.

Prolonged treatment with high doses of inhaled corticosteroids, particularly higher than recommended doses, may result in clinically significant adrenal suppression. Additional systemic corticosteroid cover should be considered during periods of stress or elective surgery.

Lack of response or severe exacerbations of asthma should be treated by increasing the dose of inhaled beclometasonedipropionate and, if necessary, by giving a systemic steroid and/or antibiotic if there is an infection, and by use of beta-agonist therapy.

For the transfer of patients being treated with oral corticosteroids:

The transfer of oral steroid-dependent patients to Becodisks and their subsequent management needs special care as recovery from impaired adrenocortical function, caused by prolonged systemic steroid therapy, may take a considerable time.

Patients who have been treated with systemic steroids for long periods of time or at a high dose may have adrenocortical suppression. With these patients adrenocortical function should be monitored regularly and their dose of systemic steroid reduced cautiously.

After approximately a week, gradual withdrawal of the systemic steroid is commenced. Decrements in dosages should be appropriate to the level of maintenance systemic steroid, and introduced at not less than weekly intervals. For maintenance doses of prednisolone (or equivalent) of 10mg daily or less, the decrements in dose should not be greater than 1mg per day, at not less than weekly intervals. For maintenance doses of prednisolone in excess of 10mg daily, it may be appropriate to employ cautiously, larger decrements in dose at weekly intervals.

Some patients feel unwell in a non-specific way during the withdrawal phase despite maintenance or even improvement of the respiratory function. They should be encouraged to persevere with the Diskhaler and withdrawal of systemic steroid continued, unless there are objective signs of adrenal insufficiency.

Patients weaned off oral steroids whose adrenocortical function is impaired should carry a steroid warning card indicating that they may need supplementary systemic steroid during periods of stress, e.g. Worsening asthma attacks, chest infections, major intercurrent illness, surgery, trauma, etc.

Replacement of systemic steroid treatment with inhaled therapy sometimes unmasks allergies such as allergic rhinitis or eczema previously controlled by the systemic drug. These allergies should be symptomatically treated with antihistamine and/or topical preparations, including topical steroids.

Treatment with Becodisks should not be stopped abruptly.

As with all inhaled corticosteroids, special care is necessary in patients with active or quiescent pulmonary tuberculosis.

4.5 Interaction with other medicinal products and other forms of Interaction

No interactions have been reported

4.6 Pregnancy and lactation

There is inadequate evidence of safety in human pregnancy. Administration of corticosteroids to pregnant animals can cause abnormalities of foetal development including cleft palate and intra-uterine growth retardation. There may therefore be a very small risk of such effects in the human foetus. It should be noted, however, that the foetal changes in animals occur after relatively high systemic exposure. Because beclometasone dipropionate is delivered directly to the lungs by the inhaled route it avoids the high level of exposure that occurs when corticosteroids are given by systemic routes.

The use of beclometasone dipropionate in pregnancy requires that the possible benefits of the drug be weighed against the possible hazards. It should be noted that the drug has been in widespread use for many years without apparent ill consequence.

No specific studies examining the transference of beclometasone dipropionate into the milk of lactating animals have been performed. It is reasonable to assume that beclometasone dipropionate is secreted in milk but at the dosages used for direct inhalation, there is low potential for significant levels in breast milk. The use of beclometasone dipropionate in mothers breast feeding their babies requires that the therapeutic benefits of the drug be weighed against the potential hazards to the mother and baby.

4.7 Effects on ability to drive and use machines

No adverse effect has been reported.

4.8 Undesirable effects

Systemic effects of inhaled corticosteroids may occur, particularly at high doses prescribed for prolonged periods. These may include Cushing's syndrome, Cushingoid features, adrenal suppression, growth retardation in children and adolescents, decrease in bone mineral density, cataract and glaucoma.

There have been very rare reports of anxiety, sleep disorders and behavioural changes, including hyperactivity and irritability (predominantly in children).

Candidiasis of the mouth and throat (thrush) occurs in some patients, the incidence of which is increased with doses greater than 400 micrograms beclometasone dipropionate per day. Patients with high blood levels of candida precipitins, indicating a previous infection, are most likely to develop this complication. Patients may find it helpful to rinse out their mouth with water after using the Diskhaler. Symptomatic candidiasis can be treated with topical antifungal therapy whilst still continuing with the Becodisks.

In some patients inhaled beclometasone dipropionate may cause hoarseness or throat irritation. It may be helpful to rinse out the mouth with water immediately after inhalation.

As with other inhalation therapy, paradoxical bronchospasm may occur with an immediate increase in wheezing after dosing. This responds to a fast-acting inhaled bronchodilator. The preparation should be discontinued immediately, the patient assessed, and if necessary, alternative therapy instituted.

Hypersensitivity reactions including rashes, urticaria, pruritus and erythema, and oedema of the eyes, face, lips and throat, have been reported.

4.9 Overdose

Acute - inhalation of the drug in doses in excess of those recommended may lead to temporary suppression of adrenal function. This does not necessitate emergency action being taken. In these patients treatment with beclometasone dipropionate by inhalation should be continued at a dose sufficient to control asthma; adrenal function recovers in a few days and can be verified by measuring plasma cortisol.

Chronic - use of inhaled beclometasone dipropionate in daily doses in excess of 1500 micrograms over prolonged periods may lead to adrenal suppression. Monitoring of adrenal reserve may be indicated. Treatment with inhaled beclometasone dipropionate should be continued at a dose sufficient to control asthma.

5. PHARMACOLOGICAL PROPERTIES

5.1 Pharmacodynamic properties

BDP is a pro-drug with weak glucocorticoid receptor binding activity. It is hydrolysed via esterase enzymes to the active metabolite beclometasone -17-monopropionate (B-17-MP), which has high topical anti-inflammatory activity.

5.2 Pharmacokinetic properties

Absorption

When administered via inhalation (via metered dose inhaler) there is extensive conversion of BDP to the active metabolite B-17-MP within the lungs prior to systemic absorption. The systemic absorption of B-17-MP arises from both lung deposition and oral absorption of the swallowed dose. When administered orally, in healthy male volunteers, the bioavailability of BDP is negligible but pre-systemic conversion to B-17-MP results in 41% (95% CI 27- 62 %) of the dose being available as B-17-MP.

Metabolism

BDP is cleared very rapidly from the systemic circulation, owing to extensive first pass metabolism. The main product of metabolism is the active metabolite (B-17-MP). Minor inactive metabolites, beclometasone-21-monopropionate (B-21-MP) and beclometasone (BOH), are also formed but these contribute little to systemic exposure.

Distribution

The tissue distribution at steady state for BDP is moderate (20L) but more extensive for B-17-MP (424L). Plasma protein binding is moderately high (87%).

Elimination

The elimination of BDP and B-17-MP are characterised by high plasma clearance (150 and 120L/h) with corresponding terminal elimination half lives of 0.5h and 2.7h. Following oral administration of titrated BDP, approximately 60% of the dose was excreted in the faeces within 96 hours mainly as free and conjugated polar metabolites. Approximately 12% of the dose was excreted as free and conjugated polar metabolites in the urine.

5.3 Preclinical safety data

No clinically relevant findings were observed in preclinical studies.

6. PHARMACEUTICAL PARTICULARS

6.1 List of excipients

Lactose(which contains milk protein)

6.2 Incompatibilities

No incompatibilities have been reported.

6.3 Shelf life

36 months

6.4 Special precautions for storage

Do not store above 30°C

6.5 Nature and contents of container

Circular double foil blister pack consisting of:

A) Lidding material (i) polyester over-lacquer/hard tempered aluminium foil/heat seal lacquer of total thickness = 39.4 - 48.6μ or (ii) nitrocellulose over-lacquer/hard tempered aluminium foil/heat seal lacquer of total thickness = 37.0 - 42.0μ.

B) Blister material - pvc film/aluminium foil/orientated polyamide.

Becodisks are supplied as 8 blisters per Becodisk as follows:

- Carton containing 7 disks plus a Diskhaler
- Carton containing 15 disks plus a Diskhaler
- Carton containing 2 disks plus a Diskhaler
- Refill pack of 7 disks
- Refill pack of 15 disks
- A starter pack consisting of a Diskhaler pre-load with one disk

Not all pack sizes may be marketed

6.6 Instructions for use and handling

See Patient Information Leaflet

Administrative Data

7. MARKETING AUTHORISATION HOLDER

Glaxo Wellcome UK Ltd.

Trading as Allen & Hanburys,

Stockley Park West,

Uxbridge

Middlesex,

UB11 1BT

8. MARKETING AUTHORISATION NUMBER(S)

PL10949/0057

9. DATE OF FIRST AUTHORISATION/RENEWAL OF THE AUTHORISATION

1 October 1993/31 March 2005

10. DATE OF REVISION OF THE TEXT

22 December 2004

11. Legal Status

POM

Beconase Aqueous Nasal Spray

(Allen & Hanburys)

1. NAME OF THE MEDICINAL PRODUCT

Beconase Aqueous Nasal Spray

2. QUALITATIVE AND QUANTITATIVE COMPOSITION

Beclometasone Dipropionate 50μg (as monohydrate, micronised)

3. PHARMACEUTICAL FORM

Aqueous suspension for intranasal inhalation via metered dose atomising pump.

4. CLINICAL PARTICULARS

4.1 Therapeutic indications

Beconase Aqueous Nasal Spray is indicated for the prophylaxis and treatment of perennial and seasonal allergic rhinitis including hayfever, and vasomotor rhinitis. Beclometasone dipropionate has a potent anti-inflammatory effect within the respiratory tract, with a lower incidence and severity of adverse events than those observed when corticosteroids are administered systemically.

4.2 Posology and method of administration

Beconase Aqueous Nasal Spray is for administration by the intranasal route only.

Adults and children over six years of age:

The recommended dosage is two sprays into each nostril twice daily (400 micrograms/day). Once control has been established it may be possible to maintain control with fewer sprays. A dosage regimen of one spray into each nostril morning and evening has been shown to be efficacious in some patients. However, should symptoms recur, patients should revert to the recommended dosage of two sprays into each nostril morning and evening. The minimum dose should be used at which effective control of symptoms is maintained. Total daily administration should not normally exceed eight sprays.

For full therapeutic benefit regular usage is essential. The co-operation of the patient should be sought to comply with the regular dosage schedule and it should be explained that maximum relief may not be obtained within the first few applications.

For children under six years old, there are insufficient clinical data to recommend use.

4.3 Contraindications

Beconase Aqueous Nasal Spray is contra-indicated in patients with a history of hypersensitivity to any of its components.

4.4 Special warnings and special precautions for use

Systemic effects of nasal corticosteroids may occur, particularly at high doses prescribed for prolonged periods. Growth retardation has been reported in children receiving nasal corticosteroids at licensed doses.

It is recommended that the height of children receiving prolonged treatment with nasal corticosteroids is regularly monitored. If growth is slowed, therapy should be reviewed with the aim of reducing the dose of nasal corticosteroid, if possible to the lowest dose at which effective control of symptoms is maintained. In addition, consideration should be given to referring the patient to a paediatric specialist.

Treatment with higher than recommended doses may result in clinically significant adrenal suppression. If there is evidence for higher than recommended doses being used then additional systemic corticosteroid cover should be considered during periods of stress or elective surgery.

Care must be taken while transferring patients from systemic steroid treatment to Beconase Aqueous Nasal Spray if there is any reason to suppose that their adrenal function is impaired.

Infections of the nasal passages and paranasal sinuses should be appropriately treated but do not constitute a specific contra-indication to treatment with Beconase Aqueous Nasal Spray.

Although Beconase Aqueous Nasal Spray will control seasonal allergic rhinitis in most cases, an abnormally heavy challenge of summer allergens may in certain instances necessitate appropriate additional therapy particularly to control eye symptoms.

4.5 Interaction with other medicinal products and other forms of Interaction

Not applicable

4.6 Pregnancy and lactation

There is inadequate evidence of safety in human pregnancy. Administration of corticosteroids to pregnant animals can cause abnormalities of foetal development including cleft palate and intra-uterine growth retardation. There may therefore be a very small risk of such effects in the human foetus. It should be noted, however, that the foetal changes in animals occur after relatively high systemic exposure. Beconase Aqueous Nasal Spray delivers beclometasone dipropionate directly to the nasal mucosa and so minimises systemic exposure.

The use of beclometasone dipropionate should be avoided during pregnancy unless thought essential by the doctor.

No specific studies examining the transference of beclometasone dipropionate into the milk of lactating animals have been performed. It is reasonable to assume that beclometasone dipropionate is secreted in milk but at the dosages used for direct intranasal administration there is low potential for significant levels in breast milk. The use of beclometasone dipropionate in mothers breast feeding their babies requires that the therapeutic benefits of the drug be weighed against the potential hazards to the mother and baby.

4.7 Effects on ability to drive and use machines

Not applicable

4.8 Undesirable effects

Systemic effects of nasal corticosteroids may occur particularly when used at high doses for prolonged periods.

Rare cases of nasal septal perforation have been reported following the use of intranasal corticosteroids.

As with other nasal sprays, dryness and irritation of the nose and throat, unpleasant taste and smell and epistaxis have been reported rarely.

Very rare cases of glaucoma, raised intraocular pressure or cataract in association with intranasal formulations of beclometasone have been reported.

Hypersensitivity reactions including rashes, urticaria, pruritus and erythema, and oedema of the eyes, face, lips and throat, have been reported.

4.9 Overdose

The only harmful effect that follows inhalation of large amounts of the drug over a short time period is suppression of Hypothalamic-Pituitary-Adrenal (HPA) function. No special emergency action need be taken. Treatment with Beconase Aqueous Nasal Spray should be continued at the recommended dose. HPA function recovers in a day or two.

5. PHARMACOLOGICAL PROPERTIES

5.1 Pharmacodynamic properties

Following topical administration beclometasone 17,21-dipropionate (BDP) produces potent anti-inflammatory and vasoconstrictor effects.

BDP is a pro-drug with weak corticosteroid receptor binding affinity. It is hydrolysed via esterase enzymes to the highly active metabolite beclometasone-17-monopropionate (B-17-MP), which has high topical anti-inflammatory activity.

Beclometasone dipropionate offers a preventative background treatment for hayfever when taken prior to allergen challenge. After which with regular use, BDP can continue to prevent allergy symptoms from reappearing.

5.2 Pharmacokinetic properties

Absorption

Following intranasal administration of BDP in healthy males, the systemic absorption was assessed by measuring the plasma concentrations of its active metabolite B-17-MP, for which the absolute bioavailability following intranasal administration is 44% (95% CI 28%, 70%). After intranasal administration, <1% of the dose is absorbed by the nasal mucosa. The remainder after being cleared from the nose, either by drainage or mucocilary clearance, is available for absorption from the gastrointestinal tract. Plasma B-17-MP is almost entirely due to conversion of BDP absorbed from the swallowed dose.

Following oral administration of BDP in healthy males, the systemic absorption was also assessed by measuring the plasma concentrations of its active metabolite B-17-MP, for which the absolute bioavailability following oral administration is 41% (95% CI 27%, 62%).

Following an oral dose, B-17-MP is absorbed slowly with peak plasma levels reached 3-5 hours after dosing.

Metabolism

BDP is cleared very rapidly from the circulation and plasma concentrations are undetectable (< 50pg/ml) following oral or intranasal dosing. There is rapid metabolism of the majority of the swallowed portion of BDP during its first passage through the liver. The main product of metabolism is the active metabolite (B-17-MP). Minor inactive metabolites, beclometasone-21-monopropionate (B-21-MP) and beclometasone (BOH), are also formed but these contribute little to systemic exposure.

Distribution

The tissue distribution at steady-state for BDP is moderate (20l) but more extensive for B-17-MP (424l). Plasma protein binding of BDP is moderately high (87%).

Elimination

The elimination of BDP and B-17-MP are characterised by high plasma clearance (150 and 120l/h) with corresponding terminal elimination half-lives of 0.5h and 2.7h. Following oral administration of tritiated BDP, approximately 60% of the dose was excreted in the faeces within 96 hours mainly as free and conjugated polar metabolites. Approximately 12% of the dose was excreted as free and conjugated polar metabolites in the urine.

5.3 Preclinical safety data

No clinically relevant findings were observed in preclinical studies.

6. PHARMACEUTICAL PARTICULARS

6.1 List of excipients

Avicel RC 591 (Microcrystalline Cellulose And Carboxymethylcellulose Sodium) US NF

Anhydrous Dextrose BP

Benzalkonium Chloride BP

Phenylethyl Alcohol USP

Polysorbate 80 BP

Purified Water BP

6.2 Incompatibilities

Not applicable

6.3 Shelf life

24 months when not stored above 30°C

6.4 Special precautions for storage

Beconase Aqueous Nasal Spray should not be stored above 30°C. Keepcontainer in the outer carton. Do not refrigerate.

6.5 Nature and contents of container

A 25ml amber neutral glass bottle fitted with a metering atomising pump, or a 30ml polypropylene bottle fitted with a tamper-resistant metering atomising pump. The pumps are manufactured by: Valois S.A. Le Prieure BPG, 27110 Le Neubourg, France.

Pack size: 200 Metered Spray.

6.6 Instructions for use and handling

Refer to Patient Information Leaflet.

Administrative Data

7. MARKETING AUTHORISATION HOLDER

Glaxo Wellcome UK Ltd.

Trading as Allen and Hanburys,

Stockley Park West,

Uxbridge

Middlesex, UB11 1BT

8. MARKETING AUTHORISATION NUMBER(S)

PL 10949/0104

9. DATE OF FIRST AUTHORISATION/RENEWAL OF THE AUTHORISATION

12th April 2003

10. DATE OF REVISION OF THE TEXT

22 December 2004

11. Legal Status

POM

Becotide 50, 100, 200 Inhaler

(Allen & Hanburys)

1. NAME OF THE MEDICINAL PRODUCT

Becotide® 50 Inhaler.

Becotide® 100 Inhaler.

Becotide® 200 Inhaler.

2. QUALITATIVE AND QUANTITATIVE COMPOSITION

50, 100 or 200 micrograms Beclometasone Dipropionate BP per actuation. Each canister delivers 80 or 200 actuations.

3. PHARMACEUTICAL FORM

Pressurised metered-dose aerosol.

4. CLINICAL PARTICULARS

4.1 Therapeutic indications

Beclometasone dipropionate given by inhalation offers preventative treatment for asthma. It provides effective anti-inflammatory action in the lungs with a lower incidence and severity of adverse effects than those observed when corticosteroids are administered systemically.

Becotide® Inhaler is indicated in the prophylactic management of mild, moderate, or severe asthma in adults or children.

Mild asthma: Patients requiring symptomatic bronchodilator asthma medication on a regular basis.

Moderate asthma: Patients with unstable or worsening asthma despite prophylactic therapy or bronchodilator alone.

Severe asthma: Patients with severe chronic asthma and those who are dependent on systemic corticosteroids for adequate control of symptoms. Many patients who are dependent on systemic corticosteroids for adequate control of symptoms may be able to reduce significantly, or eliminate, their requirement for oral corticosteroids when they are transferred to high dose inhaled beclometasone dipropionate.

4.2 Posology and method of administration

Becotide® Inhaler is for oral inhalation use only. A spacer device may be used in patients who find it difficult to synchronise aerosol actuation with inspiration of breath.

Patients should be given a starting dose of inhaled beclometasone dipropionate appropriate to the severity of their disease. The dose may then be adjusted until control is achieved, or reduced to the minimum effective dose according to individual response.

Adults (including the elderly): The usual starting dose is 200 micrograms twice a day. In more severe cases the starting dose may need to increase to 600 to 800 micrograms per day which may then be reduced when the patient's asthma has stabilised. The total daily dose may be administered as two, three, or four divided doses

Children: 50 to 100 micrograms should be given two, three or four times daily in accordance to the response. Alternatively, 100 micrograms or 200 micrograms twice daily should be given. The usual starting dose is 100 micrograms twice daily

Becotide 200 Inhaler is not recommended for children.

There is no need to increase the dose in patients with hepatic or renal impairment.

4.3 Contraindications

Hypersensitivity to any of the components.

Special care is necessary in patients with active or quiescent pulmonary tuberculosis.

4.4 Special warnings and special precautions for use

Patients should be instructed in the proper use of the inhaler, and their technique checked, to ensure that the drug reaches the target areas within the lungs. They should also be made aware that Becotide Inhaler has to be used regularly, every day, even when they are asymptomatic, for optimum benefit.

Becotide Inhaler is not designed to relieve acute asthma symptoms for which an inhaled short-acting bronchodilator is required. Patients should be advised to have such relief medication available.

Severe asthma requires regular medical assessment, including lung-function testing, as patients are at risk of severe attacks and even death. Patients must be instructed to seek medical attention if short-acting relief bronchodilator treatment becomes less effective, or more inhalations than usual are required as this may indicate deterioration of asthma control. In this situation, patients should be assessed and the need for increased anti-inflammatory therapy (e.g. higher doses of inhaled corticosteroid or a course of oral corticosteroid) considered.

Severe exacerbations of asthma must be treated in the normal way, e.g. by increasing the dose of inhaled beclometasone dipropionate and, if necessary by giving a systemic steroid, and/or an antibiotic if there is an infection, and by use of β-agonist therapy.

Treatment with Becotide Inhaler should not be stopped abruptly.

Systemic effects of inhaled corticosteroids may occur, particularly at high doses prescribed for prolonged periods. These effects are much less likely to occur than with oral corticosteroids. Possible systemic effects include Cushing's syndrome, Cushingoid features, adrenal suppression, growth retardation in children and adolescents, decrease in bone mineral density, cataract and glaucoma. It is important therefore that the dose of inhaled corticosteroid is titrated to the lowest dose at which effective control of asthma is maintained.

It is recommended that the height of children receiving prolonged treatment with inhaled corticosteroids is regularly monitored. If growth is slowed, therapy should be reviewed with the aim of reducing the dose of inhaled corticosteroid, if possible, to the lowest dose at which effective control of asthma is maintained. In addition, consideration should be given to referring the patient to a paediatric respiratory specialist.

Prolonged treatment with high doses of inhaled corticosteroids, particularly higher than recommended doses, may result in clinically significant adrenal suppression. Additional systemic corticosteroid cover should be considered during periods of stress or elective surgery.

The transfer to Becotide Inhaler of patients who have been treated with systemic steroids for long periods of time, or at a high dose, needs special care, since recovery from any adrenocortical suppression sustained may take a considerable time. Approximately one week after initiating treatment with Becotide Inhaler, reduction of the dose of systemic steroid can be commenced. The size of the reduction should correspond to the maintenance dose of systemic steroid. Reductions in dose of not more than 1mg are suitable for patients receiving maintenance doses of 10mg daily or less of prednisolone or its equivalent. Larger reductions in dose may be appropriate for higher maintenance doses. The reductions in dose should be introduced at not less than weekly intervals. Adrenocortical function should be monitored regularly as the dose of systemic steroid is gradually reduced.

Some patients feel unwell in a non-specific way during the withdrawal phase despite maintenance or even improvement of the respiratory function. They should be encouraged to persevere with inhaled beclometasone dipropionate and to continue withdrawal of systemic steroid, unless there are objective signs of adrenal insufficiency.

Patients weaned off oral steroids whose adrenocortical function is impaired should carry a steroid warning card indicating that they may need supplementary systemic steroid during periods of stress, e.g. worsening asthma attacks, chest infections, major intercurrent illness, surgery, trauma, etc.

Replacement of systemic steroid treatment with inhaled therapy sometimes unmasks allergies such as allergic rhinitis or eczema previously controlled by the systemic drug. These allergies should be symptomatically treated with antihistamine and/or topical preparations, including topical steroids.

As with all inhaled corticosteroids, special care is necessary in patients with active or quiescent pulmonary tuberculosis.

4.5 Interaction with other medicinal products and other forms of Interaction

None reported.

4.6 Pregnancy and lactation

There is inadequate evidence of safety in human pregnancy. Administration of corticosteroids to pregnant animals can cause abnormalities of fetal development including cleft palate and intra-uterine growth retardation. There may therefore be a very small risk of such effects in the human fetus. It should be noted, however, that the fetal changes in animals occur after relatively high systemic exposure. Becotide Inhaler delivers the drug directly to the lungs by the inhaled route and so avoids the high level of exposure that occurs when corticosteroids are given by systemic routes.

The use of Becotide Inhaler in pregnancy requires that the possible benefits of the drug be weighed against the possible hazards.

No specific studies examining the transference of beclometasone dipropionate into the milk of lactating animals have been performed. It is reasonable to assume that beclometasone dipropionate is secreted in milk, but at the dosages used for direct inhalation there is low potential for significant levels in breast milk.

The use of Becotide Inhaler in mothers breast feeding their babies requires that the therapeutic benefits of the drug be weighed against the potential hazards to the mother and baby.

4.7 Effects on ability to drive and use machines

None reported.

4.8 Undesirable effects

Systemic effects of inhaled corticosteroids may occur, particularly at high doses prescribed for prolonged periods. These may include Cushing's syndrome, Cushingoid features, adrenal suppression, growth retardation in children and adolescents, decrease in bone mineral density, cataract and glaucoma.

As with other inhalation therapy, paradoxical bronchospasm may occur with an immediate increase in wheezing after dosing. This should be treated immediately with a fast-acting inhaled bronchodilator. The Becotide Inhaler should be discontinued immediately, the patient assessed and, if necessary, alternative therapy instituted.

Hypersensitivity reactions including rashes, urticaria, pruritus and erythema, and oedema of the eyes, face, lips and throat, have been reported.

There have been very rare reports of anxiety, sleep disorders and behavioural changes, including hyperactivity and irritability (predominantly in children).

Candidiasis of the mouth and throat (thrush) occurs in some patients, the incidence increasing with doses greater than 400 micrograms beclometasone dipropionate per day. Patients with high blood levels of *Candida precipitins,* indicating a previous infection, are most likely to develop this complication. Patients may find it helpful to rinse their mouth thoroughly with water after using the inhaler. Symptomatic candidiasis can be treated with topical anti-fungal therapy whilst still continuing with Becotide Inhaler

In some patients inhaled beclometasone dipropionate may cause hoarseness or throat irritation. It may be helpful to rinse the mouth out with water immediately after inhalation. The use of a spacer device may be considered.

4.9 Overdose
Acute: Inhalation of the drug in doses in excess of those recommended may lead to temporary suppression of adrenal function. This does not require emergency action. In these patients treatment should be continued at a dose sufficient to control asthma; adrenal function recovers in a few days and can be verified by measuring plasma cortisol.

Chronic: Use of inhaled beclometasone dipropionate in daily doses in excess of 1,500 micrograms over prolonged periods may lead to adrenal suppression. Monitoring of adrenal reserve may be indicated. Treatment should be continued at a dose sufficient to control asthma.

5. PHARMACOLOGICAL PROPERTIES
5.1 Pharmacodynamic properties
BDP is a pro-drug with weak glucocorticoid receptor binding activity. It is hydrolysed via esterase enzymes to the active metabolite beclometasone-17-monopropionate (B-17-MP), which has high topical anti-inflammatory activity.

5.2 Pharmacokinetic properties
Absorption
When administered via inhalation, there is extensive conversion of BDP to active metabolite B-17-MP within the lungs prior to systemic absorption. In healthy male volunteers the absolute bioavailability following inhalation is approximately 2%(95% CI 1-5%) and 62%(95% CI 47-83%) of the nominal dose for unchanged BDP and B-17-MP respectively. The systemic absorption of B-17-MP arises from both lung deposition (approximately 36%) and oral absorption of the swallowed dose (approximately 26%). BDP is absorbed rapidly with peak plasma concentrations first being observed (t_{max}) at 0.3h. B-17-MP appears more slowly with a t_{max} of 1h. There is an approximately linear increase in systemic exposure with increasing inhaled dose. When administered orally the bioavailability of BDP is negligible but pre-systemic conversion to B-17-MP results in 41% (95% CI 27-62%) of the dose being available as B-17-MP.

Metabolism
BDP is cleared very rapidly from the systemic circulation, owing to extensive first pass metabolism. The main product of metabolism is the active metabolite (B-17-MP). Minor inactive metabolites, beclometasone-21-monopropionate (B-21-MP) and beclometasone (BOH), are also formed but these contribute little to systemic exposure.

Distribution
The tissue distribution at steady-state for BDP is moderate (20l) but more extensive for B-17-MP (424l). Plasma protein binding is moderately high (87%).

Elimination
The elimination of BDP and B-17-MP are characterised by high plasma clearance (150 and 120L/h) with corresponding terminal elimination half-lives of 0.5h and 2.7h. Following oral administration of titrated BDP, approximately 60% of the dose was excreted in the faeces within 96 hours mainly as free and conjugated polar metabolites. Approximately 12% of the dose was excreted as free and conjugated polar metabolites in the urine.

5.3 Preclinical safety data
None relevant to the prescriber additional to data already included in other sections.

6. PHARMACEUTICAL PARTICULARS
6.1 List of excipients
Oleic Acid.

Dichlorodifluoromethane.

Trichlorofluoromethane.

6.2 Incompatibilities
None reported.

6.3 Shelf life
3 years when not stored above 30°C.

6.4 Special precautions for storage
Do not store above 30°C.

As with most inhaled medicines in aerosol canisters, the therapeutic effect may decrease when the canister is cold.

Protect from frost and direct sunlight.

The canister should not be broken, punctured or burnt, even when apparently empty.

6.5 Nature and contents of container
An inhaler comprising an aluminium can fitted with a metering valve, actuator and dust cap. Each canister contains either 80 or 200 metered actuations of 50, 100 or 200 micrograms beclometasone dipropionate.

6.6 Instructions for use and handling
The aerosol spray is inhaled through the mouth into the lungs. After shaking the inhaler, the mouthpiece is placed in the mouth and the lips closed around it. The actuator is depressed to release a spray, which must coincide with inspiration of breath.

For detailed instructions for use refer to the Patient Information Leaflet in every pack.

Administrative Data
7. MARKETING AUTHORISATION HOLDER
Allen & Hanburys, Stockley Park West, Uxbridge, Middlesex, UB11 1BT

8. MARKETING AUTHORISATION NUMBER(S)
Becotide™ 50 Inhaler PL10949/0058
Becotide™ 100 Inhaler PL10949/0059
Becotide™ 200 Inhaler PL10949/0060

9. DATE OF FIRST AUTHORISATION/RENEWAL OF THE AUTHORISATION

Product	Licence Number	Renewal Date
Becotide™ 50 Inhaler	PL10949/0058	08/04/03
Becotide™ 100 Inhaler	PL10949/0059	04/03/99
Becotide™ 200 Inhaler	PL10949/0060	14/03/03

10. DATE OF REVISION OF THE TEXT
23 December 2004

11. Legal Category
POM.

Benadryl Allergy Oral Solution
(Pfizer Consumer Healthcare)

1. NAME OF THE MEDICINAL PRODUCT
Zirtek Allergy Solution 1mg/ml.
Benadryl Allergy Oral Solution.

2. QUALITATIVE AND QUANTITATIVE COMPOSITION
Cetirizine hydrochloride 1 mg/ml

3. PHARMACEUTICAL FORM
Solution for oral administration.

4. CLINICAL PARTICULARS
4.1 Therapeutic indications
Cetirizine is indicated for the symptomatic treatment of seasonal allergic rhinitis, perennial rhinitis and chronic idiopathic urticaria in adults and children aged six years and over, and additionally for the symptomatic treatment of seasonal allergic rhinitis in children between two to five years of age.

4.2 Posology and method of administration
Adults and children 6 years and above: 10mg daily.

Adults and children aged 12 years and above: 10ml once daily.

Children aged between 6 to 11 years: Either 5ml twice daily or 10ml once daily.

Children aged between 2-5 years: 5mg daily. Either 5ml once daily or 2.5ml twice daily.

At present there is insufficient clinical data to recommend the use of cetirizine in children under 2 years of age.

There is no data to suggest that the dose should be reduced in elderly patients.

In patients with renal insufficiency the dosage should be reduced to half the normal recommended daily dose.

4.3 Contraindications
A history of hypersensitivity to any of the constituents of the formulation.

4.4 Special warnings and special precautions for use
Do not exceed the recommended dose.

In patients with renal insufficiency the dosage should be reduced to half the usual recommended dose.

For patients whose symptoms persist, it is advised to consult a doctor or pharmacist.

4.5 Interaction with other medicinal products and other forms of Interaction
To date there are no known interactions with other drugs. Studies with diazepam and cimetidine have revealed no evidence of interactions. As with other antihistamines it is advisable to avoid excessive alcohol consumption.

4.6 Pregnancy and lactation
No adverse effects have been reported from animal studies. There has been little or no use of cetirizine during pregnancy. As with other drugs the use of cetirizine in pregnancy should be avoided.

Cetirizine is contraindicated in lactating women as it is excreted in breast milk.

4.7 Effects on ability to drive and use machines
Studies in healthy volunteers at 20 and 25 mg/day have not revealed effects on alertness or reaction time; however patients are advised not to exceed the recommended dose if driving or operating machinery.

4.8 Undesirable effects
In objective tests of psychomotor function the incidence of sedation with cetirizine was similar to that of placebo. There have been occasional reports of mild and transient side effects such as drowsiness, headache, dizziness, agitation, dry mouth and gastro-intestinal discomfort. If desired the dose might be taken as 5mg in the morning and 5 mg in the evening.

Convulsions have very rarely been reported.

4.9 Overdose
Drowsiness can be a symptom of overdosage. In children agitation can occur. In the case of massive overdosage, gastric lavage should be performed together with the usual supportive measures. To date there is no specific antidote.

5. PHARMACOLOGICAL PROPERTIES
5.1 Pharmacodynamic properties
Cetirizine is a potent antihistamine with a low potential for drowsiness at pharmacologically active doses and which has additional anti-allergic properties. It is a selective H_1 -antagonist with negligible effects on other receptors and so is virtually free from anti-cholinergic and anti-serotonin effects. Cetirizine inhibits the histamine-mediated "early" phase of the allergic reaction and also reduces the migration of inflammatory cells and the release of certain mediators associated with the "late" allergic response.

5.2 Pharmacokinetic properties
Peak blood levels in the order of 0.3 micrograms / ml are attained between 30 and 60 minutes following the administration of a 10 mg oral dose of cetirizine.

The terminal half-life is approximately ten hours in adults and six hours in children aged between 6 to 12 years. This is consistent with the urinary excretion half-life of the drug. The cumulative urinary excretion represents about two thirds of the dose given for both adults and children.

The apparent plasma clearance in children is higher than that measured in adults. A high proportion of cetirizine is bound to human plasma proteins.

5.3 Preclinical safety data
None stated.

6. PHARMACEUTICAL PARTICULARS
6.1 List of excipients
Sorbitol solution, glycerol, propylene glycol, saccharin sodium, methyl parahydroxybenzoate, propyl parahydroxybenzoate, banana flavouring, sodium acetate, acetic acid and purified water.

6.2 Incompatibilities
None.

6.3 Shelf life
3 years.

6.4 Special precautions for storage
Store below 30°C.

6.5 Nature and contents of container
75 ml, 100 ml or 200 ml in a Type III amber glass bottle.

6.6 Instructions for use and handling
No special requirements.

Administrative Data
7. MARKETING AUTHORISATION HOLDER
UCB Pharma Limited
3 George Street
Watford
Hertfordshire WD18 0UH

8. MARKETING AUTHORISATION NUMBER(S)
PL 08972/0033

9. DATE OF FIRST AUTHORISATION/RENEWAL OF THE AUTHORISATION
5th May 2000 / 31st October 2001

10. DATE OF REVISION OF THE TEXT
January 2003

Benadryl Allergy Relief
(Pfizer Consumer Healthcare)

1. NAME OF THE MEDICINAL PRODUCT
Benadryl Allergy Relief

2. QUALITATIVE AND QUANTITATIVE COMPOSITION
Benadryl Allergy Relief contains 8 mg Acrivastine per capsule.

3. PHARMACEUTICAL FORM
Capsules

4. CLINICAL PARTICULARS
4.1 Therapeutic indications
Benadryl Allergy Relief is indicated for the symptomatic relief of allergic rhinitis, including hay fever. Benadryl Allergy Relief is also indicated for chronic idiopathic urticaria.

4.2 Posology and method of administration
Adults and children 12 -65 years:

Oral. One 8 mg capsule, as necessary up to three times a day.

Use in the Elderly (over 65 years)

As yet, no specific studies have been carried out in the elderly. Until further information is available, Benadryl Allergy Relief should not be given to elderly patients.

4.3 Contraindications
Benadryl Allergy Relief is contraindicated in individuals with known hypersensitivity to acrivastine or triprolidine. Renal excretion is the principal route of elimination of acrivastine. Until specific studies have been carried out Benadryl Allergy Relief should not be given to patients with significant renal impairment.

4.4 Special warnings and special precautions for use
The following statements will appear on the pack:

Do not store above 30°C. Store in the original package. Keep out of the reach and sight of children.

4.5 Interaction with other medicinal products and other forms of Interaction
It is usual to advise patients not to undertake tasks requiring mental alertness whilst under the influence of alcohol and other CNS depressants. Concomitant administration of acrivastine may, in some individuals, produce additional impairment.

There are no data to demonstrate an interaction between acrivastine and ketoconazole, erythromycin or grapefruit juice. However, due to known interactions between these compounds and other non-sedating antihistamines, caution is advised.

4.6 Pregnancy and lactation
No information is available on the effects of administration of Benadryl Allergy Relief during human pregnancy or lactation. Acrivastine, like most medicines, should not be used during pregnancy or lactation unless the potential benefit of treatment to the mother outweighs any possible risk to the developing foetus/nursing infant.

Systemic administration of acrivastine in animal reproductive studies did not produce embryotoxic or teratogenic effects and did not impair fertility.

There is no information on the levels of acrivastine which may appear in human breast milk after administration of Benadryl Allergy Relief.

4.7 Effects on ability to drive and use machines
Most patients do not experience drowsiness with Benadryl Allergy Relief. Nevertheless, as there is individual variation in response to all medication, it is sensible to caution all patients about engaging activities requiring mental alertness, such as driving a car or operating machinery, until patients are familiar with their own response to the drug.

4.8 Undesirable effects
Reports of drowsiness directly attributable to Benadryl Allergy Relief are extremely rare. Indeed for the great majority of patients, treatment with Benadryl Allergy Relief is not associated with clinically significant anti-cholinergic or sedative side effects.

4.9 Overdose
There is no experience of overdose with Benadryl Allergy Relief. Appropriate supportive therapy, including gastric lavage should be initiated if indicated.

5. PHARMACOLOGICAL PROPERTIES

5.1 Pharmacodynamic properties
Acrivastine provides symptomatic relief in conditions believed to depend wholly or partly upon the triggered release of histamine.

It is a potent competitive histamine H_1 antagonist which lacks significant anti-cholinergic effects, and has a low potential to penetrate the central nervous system.

After oral administration of a single dose of 8 mg acrivastine to adults, the onset of actions, as determined by the ability to antagonise histamine induced weals and flares in the skin, is 15 minutes. Peak effects occur at 2 hours, and although activity declines slowly thereafter, significant inhibition of histamine induced weals and flares still occur 8 hours after dose.

In patients, relief from the symptoms of allergic rhinitis is apparent within 1 hour after the systemic administration of the drug.

5.2 Pharmacokinetic properties
Acrivastine is well absorbed from the gut. In healthy adult volunteers, the peak plasma concentration (Cmax) is approximately 150 NG/ML, occurring at about 1.5 hours (Tmax) after the administration of 8 mg acrivastine. The plasma half-life is approximately 1.5 hours. In multiple dose studies over 6 days, no accumulation of acrivastine was observed. Renal excretion is the principal route of elimination of acrivastine.

5.3 Preclinical safety data
There are no pre-clinical data of relevance to the prescriber which are additional to that already included in other sections of the SPC.

6. PHARMACEUTICAL PARTICULARS

6.1 List of excipients
Lactose

Sodium starch glycollate

Magnesium stearate

The capsule shell contains the following constituents:

Gelatin

Purified water

Titanium Dioxide

6.2 Incompatibilities
None known.

6.3 Shelf life
36 months.

6.4 Special precautions for storage
Do not store above 30°C. Store in the original package.

6.5 Nature and contents of container
PVC/aluminium foil blister packs - 7 (sample pack), 12, 21, 24 capsules.

6.6 Instructions for use and handling
None applicable.

Administrative Data

7. MARKETING AUTHORISATION HOLDER
Pfizer Consumer Healthcare

Alternative Trading Style:

Warner Lambert Consumer Healthcare

Walton Oaks

Dorking Road

Walton-on-the-Hill

Surrey KT20 7NS

United Kingdom

8. MARKETING AUTHORISATION NUMBER(S)
PL 15513/0035

9. DATE OF FIRST AUTHORISATION/RENEWAL OF THE AUTHORISATION
17th September 1997

10. DATE OF REVISION OF THE TEXT
February 2005

Benadryl One A Day Relief

(Pfizer Consumer Healthcare)

1. NAME OF THE MEDICINAL PRODUCT
Benadryl One A Day Relief

2. QUALITATIVE AND QUANTITATIVE COMPOSITION
Cetirizine hydrochloride: 10 mg per tablet. Cetirizine dihydrochloride Ph.Eur is also known as cetirizine hydrochloride as per the INNM/BANM.

For excipients, see section 6.1.

3. PHARMACEUTICAL FORM
Film-coated tablet.

4. CLINICAL PARTICULARS

4.1 Therapeutic indications
Cetirizine is indicated for the symptomatic treatment of perennial rhinitis, seasonal allergic rhinitis and chronic idiopathic urticaria.

4.2 Posology and method of administration
Adults and Children aged 12 years and over: 10 mg once daily

At present there are insufficient clinical data to recommend use of cetirizine in children under the age of 6.

For the time being, there is no data to suggest that the dose needs to be reduced in elderly patients.

In patients with renal insufficiency the dosage should be reduced to half the usual recommended daily dose.

4.3 Contraindications
A history of hypersensitivity to any of the constituents of the formulation.

4.4 Special warnings and special precautions for use
Do not exceed the stated dose. If symptoms persist consult your doctor.

4.5 Interaction with other medicinal products and other forms of Interaction
To date, there are no known interactions with other drugs. Studies with diazepam and cimetidine have revealed no evidence of interactions. As with other antihistamines it is advisable to avoid excessive alcohol consumption.

4.6 Pregnancy and lactation
No adverse effects have been reported from animal studies. There has been little or no clinical experience of cetirizine in pregnancy. As with other drugs, the use of cetirizine in pregnancy should be avoided.

Cetirizine is contraindicated in lactating women since it is excreted in breast milk.

4.7 Effects on ability to drive and use machines
Antihistamines can cause drowsiness in some patients. Although this has not been reported with cetirizine at the recommended dose, please be cautious whilst driving or operating machinery.

4.8 Undesirable effects
In objective tests of psychomotor function the incidence of sedation with cetirizine was similar to that of placebo. There have been occasional reports of mild and transient side effects such as headache, dizziness, drowsiness, agitation, dry mouth, and gastrointestinal discomfort. If affected the dose may be taken as 5 mg in the morning and 5 mg in the evening.

Convulsions have very rarely been reported.

4.9 Overdose
Drowsiness can be a symptom of overdosage. In children agitation can occur. In the case of massive overdosage, lavage should be performed together with the usual supportive measures. To date there is no specific antidote.

5. PHARMACOLOGICAL PROPERTIES

5.1 Pharmacodynamic properties
Cetirizine is a potent antihistamine with a low potential for drowsiness at normal therapeutic doses which has additional anti-allergic properties. It is a selective H_1 antagonist with negligible effects on other receptors and so is virtually free from anti-cholinergic and anti-serotonin effects. Cetirizine inhibits the histamine-mediated early phase of the allergic reaction and also reduces the migration of certain inflammatory cells and the release of certain mediators associated with the late allergic response.

5.2 Pharmacokinetic properties
Peak blood levels of the order of 0.3 micrograms/ml are reached between 30 and 60 minutes after the oral administration of a 10 mg dose of cetirizine. The terminal half-life is approximately ten hours in adults and six hours in children aged 6 - 12 years. This is consistent with the urinary excretion half-life of the drug. The cumulative urinary excretion represents about two thirds of the administered dose for both adults and children.

The apparent plasma clearance in children is higher than that measured in adults. A high proportion of cetirizine is bound to human plasma proteins.

5.3 Preclinical safety data
None stated.

6. PHARMACEUTICAL PARTICULARS

6.1 List of excipients
Tablet core:

Microcrystalline cellulose

Lactose

Colloidal anhydrous silica

Magnesium stearate

Film coating:

Opadry Y-1-7000

- Hydroxypropylmethylcellulose (E464)
- Titanium dioxide (E171)
- Polyethylene glycol

6.2 Incompatibilities
None.

6.3 Shelf life
60 months.

6.4 Special precautions for storage
No special precautions for storage.

6.5 Nature and contents of container
Aluminium / PVC blister packs:

Packs containing 4, 5, or 7 tablets.

Not all the packs may be marketed.

6.6 Instructions for use and handling
No special requirements.

Administrative Data

7. MARKETING AUTHORISATION HOLDER
Pfizer Consumer Healthcare

Walton Oaks

Dorking Road

Walton-on-the-Hill

Surrey KT20 7NS

8. MARKETING AUTHORISATION NUMBER(S)
PL 15513/0118

9. DATE OF FIRST AUTHORISATION/RENEWAL OF THE AUTHORISATION
20th February 2003

10. DATE OF REVISION OF THE TEXT
January 2004

Benadryl Plus Capsules

(Pfizer Consumer Healthcare)

1. NAME OF THE MEDICINAL PRODUCT
BENADRYL Plus Capsules

2. QUALITATIVE AND QUANTITATIVE COMPOSITION
BENADRYL Plus Capsules contain 8 mg acrivastine and 60 mg pseudoephedrine hydrochloride.

3. PHARMACEUTICAL FORM
Capsules.

4. CLINICAL PARTICULARS

4.1 Therapeutic indications
BENADRYL Plus Capsules are indicated for the symptomatic relief of allergic rhinitis.

4.2 Posology and method of administration
Adults and children 12 years and over:

Oral. One capsule as necessary, up to three times a day.

Children under 12 years:

BENADRYL Plus Capsules are not currently recommended for use in children under 12 years of age.

The Elderly:

BENADRYL Plus Capsules are not currently recommended for use in the elderly.

4.3 Contraindications
BENADRYL Plus Capsules are contra-indicated in individuals with known hypersensitivity to the product, any of its components or triprolidine.

BENADRYL Plus Capsules are contra-indicated in individuals with known intolerance to the product, any of its components or triprolidine.

BENADRYL Plus Capsules are contra-indicated in patients with severe hypertension or severe coronary artery disease.

The concomitant use of a pseudoephedrine-containing product and monoamine oxidase inhibitors can occasionally cause a rise in blood pressure. BENADRYL Plus Capsules are therefore contra-indicated in patients who are taking, or have taken, monoamine oxidase within the preceding two weeks.

The antibacterial agent furazolidone is known to cause a dose-related inhibition of monoamine oxidase. Although there are no reports of hypertensive crises having occurred, it should not be administered concurrently with BENADRYL Plus Capsules.

Renal excretion is the principal route of elimination of acrivastine. Until specific studies have been carried out, BENADRYL Plus Capsules should not be given to patients with significant renal impairment.

4.4 Special warnings and special precautions for use
It is usual to advise patients not to undertake tasks requiring mental alertness whilst under the influence of alcohol or other CNS depressants. Concomitant administration of BENADRYL Plus Capsules may, in some individuals, produce additional impairment.

Although pseudoephedrine has virtually no pressor effects in patients with normal blood pressure, BENADRYL Plus Capsules should be used with caution in patients taking antihypertensive agents, tricyclic antidepressants or other sympathomimetic agents such as decongestants, appetite suppressants and amfetamine-like psychostimulants. The effects of a single dose on the blood pressure of these patients should be observed before recommending repeated or unsupervised treatment.

As with other sympathomimetic agents, BENADRYL Plus Capsules should be used with caution in patients with hypertension, heart disease, diabetes, hyperthyroidism, elevated intra-ocular pressure or prostatic enlargement.

4.5 Interaction with other medicinal products and other forms of Interaction
Concomitant use of pseudoephedrine with tricyclic antidepressants, other sympathomimetic agents (such as decongestants, appetite suppressants and amfetamine-like psychostimulants) or with monoamine oxidase inhibitors (including furazolidone), which interfere with the catabolism of sympathomimetic amines, may occasionally cause a rise in blood pressure (see Contraindications).

The effect of antihypertensive agents, which interfere with sympathetic activity, may be partially reversed by BENADRYL Plus Capsules, e.g. bretylium, betanidine, guanethidine, debrisoquine, methyldopa, alpha- and beta-adrenergic blocking agents.

4.6 Pregnancy and lactation
No information is available on the effects of administration of BENADRYL Plus Capsules during human pregnancy. BENADRYL Plus Capsules, like most medicines, should not be used during pregnancy unless the potential benefit of treatment to the mother outweighs any possible risk to the developing foetus.

No information is available on levels of acrivastine which may appear in human breast milk following administration of BENADRYL Plus Capsules.

It has been estimated that approximately 0.5 to 0.7% of a single 60 mg dose of pseudoephedrine ingested by a nursing mother will be excreted in the breast milk over 24 hours, but the effect of this on breast-fed infants is not known.

4.7 Effects on ability to drive and use machines
Most patients do not experience drowsiness with BENADRYL Plus Capsules. Nevertheless as there is individual variation in response to all medication, it is recommended that patients are advised not to engage in activities requiring mental alertness, such as driving a car or operating machinery, until they have established their own response to the drug (see Special warnings and precautions for use).

It is recommended that patients are advised not to undertake tasks requiring mental alertness whilst under the influence of alcohol or other C.N.S. depressants. Concomitant administration of BENADRYL Plus Capsules may, in some patients, produce additional impairment.

4.8 Undesirable effects
In clinical trials with BENADRYL Plus Capsules, the incidence of somnolence and dizziness was no greater than that from placebo. Reports of drowsiness directly attributable to BENADRYL Plus Capsules are extremely rare. For the great majority of patients, treatment with BENADRYL Plus Capsules is not associated with clinically significant anticholinergic or sedative side effects.

Serious adverse effects associated with the use of pseudoephedrine are extremely rare. Symptoms of central nervous system excitation may occur including sleep disturbance, and, rarely, hallucinations.

Skin rashes, with or without irritation, have occasionally been reported with pseudoephedrine. Urinary retention has been reported occasionally in men receiving pseudoephedrine; prostatic enlargement could have been an important predisposing factor.

4.9 Overdose
There have been no reported cases of acute overdosage with BENADRYL Plus Capsules. It may be expected that as with other sympathomimetic drugs, the symptoms and signs of overdosage may include irritability, restlessness, tremor, convulsions, palpitations, hypertension and difficulty with micturition.

Patients should receive necessary supportive treatment in the event of overdosage. Gastric lavage should be performed if indicated. If desired, the elimination of pseudoephedrine can be accelerated by acid diuresis or by dialysis.

5. PHARMACOLOGICAL PROPERTIES

5.1 Pharmacodynamic properties
Acrivastine is a potent, competitive H_1-receptor antagonist that lacks significant anticholinergic effects and has a low potential to penetrate the central nervous system. Acrivastine provides symptomatic relief in conditions believed to depend wholly, or partly, upon the triggered release of histamine.

Pseudoephedrine has direct and indirect sympathomimetic activity and is an effective upper respiratory decongestant. Pseudoephedrine is less potent than ephedrine in producing both tachycardia and elevation of systolic blood pressure and is less potent in causing stimulation of the central nervous system. Pseudoephedrine produces its decongestant effect within 30 minutes, persisting for at least 4 hours.

After oral administration of a single dose of 8 mg acrivastine to adult volunteers, the onset of action, as determined by the ability to antagonise histamine induced weals and flares in the skin, is within 1 hour. Peak effects occur at 2 hours, and although activity declines slowly thereafter, significant inhibition of histamine induced weals and flares still occur 8 hours after dose.

Relief from the histamine-mediated symptoms of allergic rhinitis is apparent within 1 hour of systemic administration of the drug and lasts for up to 8 hours.

5.2 Pharmacokinetic properties
After the administration of one BENADRYL Plus Capsule to healthy adult volunteers, the peak plasma concentration (C_{max}) for acrivastine is approximately 140 ng/ml, occurring at about 1.3 hours (T_{max}) after drug administration. The plasma half-life is approximately 1.6 hours. The peak plasma concentration for pseudoephedrine is approximately 210 ng/ml, with T_{max} approximately 2 hours after drug administration. The plasma half-life is approximately 5.5 hours (urine pH maintained between 5.0 - 7.0). The plasma half-life of pseudoephedrine is markedly decreased by acidification of urine and increased by alkalination. Renal excretion is the principal route of elimination of both acrivastine and pseudoephedrine.

5.3 Preclinical safety data
Pre-clinical safety data do not add anything of further significance to the prescriber.

6. PHARMACEUTICAL PARTICULARS

6.1 List of excipients
Lactose

Sodium starch glycollate

Magnesium stearate

Gelatin

Titanium dioxide (E171)

Patent Blue V (E131)

6.2 Incompatibilities
None known.

6.3 Shelf life
36 months.

6.4 Special precautions for storage
Do not store above 25°C.

Store in the original package to protect from moisture.

6.5 Nature and contents of container
6, 21, 12, 24 or 84 capsules in PVC/PVDC Aluminium foil blister packs.

6 or 100 capsules in polypropylene containers with polyethylene snap-fitting lids.

6.6 Instructions for use and handling
None known.

7. MARKETING AUTHORISATION HOLDER
Pfizer Consumer Healthcare

Alternative Trading Style:

Warner Lambert Consumer Healthcare

Walton Oaks

Dorking Road

Walton-on-the-Hill

Surrey

KT20 7NS

United Kingdom

8. MARKETING AUTHORISATION NUMBER(S)
PL 15513/0017

9. DATE OF FIRST AUTHORISATION/RENEWAL OF THE AUTHORISATION
24th March 1998

10. DATE OF REVISION OF THE TEXT
October 2004

Benadryl Skin Allergy Relief Cream

(Pfizer Consumer Healthcare)

1. NAME OF THE MEDICINAL PRODUCT
Benadryl Skin Allergy Relief Cream

2. QUALITATIVE AND QUANTITATIVE COMPOSITION
Benadryl Skin Allergy Relief Cream contains:

1% w/v diphenhydramine hydrochloride Ph Eur

8% w/v zinc oxide Ph Eur

0.1% w/v racemic camphor Ph Eur.

3. PHARMACEUTICAL FORM
Cream.

4. CLINICAL PARTICULARS

4.1 Therapeutic indications
Benadryl Skin Allergy Relief Cream is indicated for the relief of irritation associated with urticaria, herpes zoster and other minor skin affections and alleviate the discomforts of sunburn, prickly heat, insect bites and nettle stings. In infants it may be used for hives.

4.2 Posology and method of administration
Adults:

Topical. Benadryl Skin Allergy Relief Cream may be applied to the affected area, three or four times daily.

Children and Infants:

Topical. As for adults.

The Elderly:

Topical. As for adults.

4.3 Contraindications
Do not use on chicken pox or measles or exudative dermatoses, unless supervised by a doctor. Do not use on extensive areas of the skin except as directed by a doctor. Do not use any other drugs containing diphenhydramine while using this product.

4.4 Special warnings and special precautions for use
Benadryl Skin Allergy Relief Cream should not be applied to raw, or broken surfaces or mucous membranes as this may result in percutaneous absorption giving rise to systemic effects. Avoid contact with the eyes. If a burning sensation or rash develops or if the condition persists, treatment should be discontinued. If necessary, remove by washing with soap and water.

4.5 Interaction with other medicinal products and other forms of Interaction
None known.

4.6 Pregnancy and lactation
The safety of Benadryl Skin Allergy Relief Cream in pregnancy and lactation has not been established. Like any medicine, Benadryl Skin Allergy Relief Cream should only be used if the possible benefits outweigh the potential risks involved. Diphenhydramine is known to be absorbed through the skin. Diphenhydramine crosses the placental barrier and is secreted in breast milk.

4.7 Effects on ability to drive and use machines
None known.

4.8 Undesirable effects

Rarely, sensitivity, eczematous reactions and photosensitivity have been reported after topical application of antihistamines. If this occurs, treatment should be discontinued.

4.9 Overdose

Symptoms and signs

Accidental ingestion or excessive absorption of Benadryl Skin Allergy Relief Cream may lead to dose-related signs of diphenhydramine toxicity. These include drowsiness and sedation with anti-cholinergic symptoms prevailing. Camphor may produce nausea, vomiting and dizziness. At higher doses, delirium leading to coma, ataxia, increased muscle reflexes and cloniform convulsions may appear.

Treatment

The stomach should be emptied by lavage and aspiration. In cases of acute poisoning, activated charcoal may be useful. A sodium sulphate purgative may be given. Convulsions may be controlled with diazepam or thiopental sodium. In the case of camphor poisoning, lipid haemodialysis or resin haemoperfusion may be useful.

5. PHARMACOLOGICAL PROPERTIES

5.1 Pharmacodynamic properties

Benadryl Skin Allergy Relief Cream contains diphenhydramine hydrochloride, zinc oxide and camphor. Diphenhydramine is a powerful antihistamine and local anaesthetic (antipruritic). In concentrations of between 0.1 – 3.0 %, camphor depresses cutaneous receptors and is an effective analgesic, anaesthetic and antipruritic, which provides a feeling of coolness when applied topically.

5.2 Pharmacokinetic properties

Benadryl Skin Allergy Relief Cream is intended only for topical application to the skin. At the recommended dose little of the active ingredients will be absorbed. Percutaneous penetration of diphenhydramine and camphor has been demonstrated during inappropriate use of these compounds separately, but has not been quantified.

5.3 Preclinical safety data

There are no preclinical data of relevance to the prescriber which are additional to that already included in other sections of the SPC.

6. PHARMACEUTICAL PARTICULARS

6.1 List of excipients

White ceresin

Cetostearyl alcohol

Ferric oxide red (E172)

Ferric oxide yellow (E172)

Sorbitan stearate

Propyl hydroxybenzoate

Propylene glycol

Polysorbate 60

Perfume oil soleil 78087

Purified water

6.2 Incompatibilities

None known.

6.3 Shelf life

3 years.

6.4 Special precautions for storage

Do not store above 25°C.

6.5 Nature and contents of container

Benadryl Allergy Relief Cream is stored in a 42 g epoxy phenolic-based lacquered aluminium tube with a white, polyethylene cap.

6.6 Instructions for use and handling

None applicable.

Administrative Data

7. MARKETING AUTHORISATION HOLDER

Pfizer Consumer Healthcare

Alternative Trading Style:

Warner Lambert Consumer Healthcare

Walton Oaks

Dorking Road

Walton-on-the-Hill

Surrey

KT20 7NS

United Kingdom

8. MARKETING AUTHORISATION NUMBER(S)

PL 15513/0078

9. DATE OF FIRST AUTHORISATION/RENEWAL OF THE AUTHORISATION

5th January 2000

10. DATE OF REVISION OF THE TEXT

March 2004

Benylin Chesty Coughs (Non-Drowsy)

(Pfizer Consumer Healthcare)

1. NAME OF THE MEDICINAL PRODUCT

BENYLIN Chesty Coughs (Non-drowsy)

2. QUALITATIVE AND QUANTITATIVE COMPOSITION

BENYLIN Chesty Coughs (Non-drowsy) contains 100 mg guaifenesin and 1.1 mg levomenthol in each 5 ml.

3. PHARMACEUTICAL FORM

Clear red syrup

4. CLINICAL PARTICULARS

4.1 Therapeutic indications

BENYLIN Chesty Coughs (Non-drowsy) is indicated for the symptomatic relief of cough.

4.2 Posology and method of administration

Adults and children over 12 years:

Oral. Two 5 ml spoonfuls four times a day.

Children aged 6 to 12 years:

Oral. One 5 ml spoonful four times a day.

Children under 6 years:

Not recommended.

The Elderly:

As for adults.

Hepatic/renal dysfunction

Experience with the use of this product suggests that normal adult dosage is appropriate for mild to moderate dysfunction. Caution should be exercised in severe hepatic and severe renal impairment. [See Pharmacokinetics].

4.3 Contraindications

BENYLIN Chesty Coughs (Non-drowsy) is contraindicated in individuals with known hypersensitivity to the product, or any of its components.

4.4 Special warnings and special precautions for use

BENYLIN Chesty Coughs (Non-drowsy) should be not used for persistent or chronic cough, such as occurs with asthma, or where cough is accompanied by excessive secretions, unless directed by a physician.

Caution should be exercised when using the product in the presence of severe renal or severe hepatic impairment, [See Pharmacokinetics].

4.5 Interaction with other medicinal products and other forms of Interaction

If urine is collected within 24 hours of a dose of BENYLIN Chesty Coughs (Non-drowsy) a metabolite of guaifenesin may cause a colour interference with laboratory determinations of urinary 5-hydroxyindoleacetic acid (5-HIAA) and vanillylmandelic acid (VMA).

4.6 Pregnancy and lactation

Insufficient information is available on the effects of administration of BENYLIN Chesty Coughs (Non-drowsy) during human pregnancy. BENYLIN Chesty Coughs (Non-drowsy), like most medicines, should not be used during pregnancy unless the potential benefit of treatment to the mother outweighs the possible risks to the developing foetus.

Guaifenesin is excreted in breast milk in small amounts with no effect expected on the infant.

4.7 Effects on ability to drive and use machines

No special comment - unlikely to produce an effect

4.8 Undesirable effects

Side effects resulting from guaifenesin administration are very rare.

Adverse reactions to menthol at the low concentration present in BENYLIN Chesty Coughs (Non-drowsy) are not anticipated.

4.9 Overdose

Symptoms and signs

The symptoms and signs of overdose may include gastro-intestinal discomfort, nausea and drowsiness.

Treatment

Treatment should be symptomatic and supportive.

5. PHARMACOLOGICAL PROPERTIES

5.1 Pharmacodynamic properties

Guaifenesin is thought to exert its pharmacological action by stimulating receptors in the gastric mucosa. This increases the output from secretory glands of the gastro-intestinal system and reflexly increases the flow of fluids from glands lining the respiratory tract. The result is an increase in volume and decrease in viscosity of bronchial secretions. Other actions may include stimulating vagal nerve endings in bronchial secretory glands and stimulating certain centres in the brain which in turn enhance respiratory fluid flow. Guaifenesin produces its expectorant action within 24 hours.

Menthol has mild local anaesthetic and decongestant properties.

5.2 Pharmacokinetic properties

Absorption

Guaifenesin is well absorbed from the gastro-intestinal tract following oral administration, although limited information is available on its pharmacokinetics. After the administration of 600 mg guaifenesin to healthy adult volunteers, the C_{max} was approximately 1.4 ug/ml, with t_{max} occurring approximately 15 minutes after drug administration.

Distribution

No information is available on the distribution of guaifenesin or menthol in humans.

Metabolism and elimination

Guaifenesin appears to undergo both oxidation and demethylation. Following an oral dose of 600 mg guaifenesin to 3 healthy male volunteers, the $t\frac{1}{2}$ was approximately 1 hour and the drug was not detectable in the blood after approximately 8 hours.

Menthol is hydroxylated in the liver by microsomal enzymes to p-methane -3,8 diol. This is then conjugated with glucuronide and excreted both in urine and bile as the glucuronide.

Pharmacokinetics inRenal/Hepatic Impairment

There have been no specific studies of BENYLIN Chesty Coughs (Non drowsy), menthol or guaifenesin in hepatic or renal impairment.

Pharmacokinetics in the Elderly

There have been no specific studies in the use of BENYLIN Chesty Coughs (Non-drowsy), menthol or guaifenesin in the elderly.

5.3 Preclinical safety data

Carcinogenicity

There is insufficient information available to determine whether guaifenesin or menthol have carcinogenic potential.

Mutagenicity

There is insufficient information available to determine whether guaifenesin has mutagenic potential.

The results of a range of tests suggest that menthol does not have a mutagenic potential.

Teratogenicity

There is insufficient information available to determine whether guaifenesin has teratogenic potential.

The results of a number of studies suggest that the administration of menthol does not produce any statistically significant teratogenic effects in rats, rabbits and mice.

Fertility

There is insufficient information available to determine whether guaifenesin or menthol have the potential to impair fertility.

6. PHARMACEUTICAL PARTICULARS

6.1 List of excipients

Sodium benzoate

Sucrose

Liquid glucose

Glycerol

Citric acid monohydrate

Sodium citrate

Saccharin sodium

Ethanol 96%

Caramel T12

Ponceau 4R (E124)

Concentrated raspberry essence double strength

Natural sweetness enhancer

Carbomer

Purified water

6.2 Incompatibilities

None known

6.3 Shelf life

3 years (bottles)

2 years (sachets)

6.4 Special precautions for storage

Do not store above 30°C.

6.5 Nature and contents of container

BENYLIN Chesty Coughs (Non-drowsy) is stored in a 30 ml, 125 ml or 300 ml amber glass bottle with an aluminium ROPP cap with melinex-faced pulpboard wad or with a 3 piece plastic child resistant, tamper evident closure fitted with a polyester faced wad or polyethylene/expanded polyethylene laminated wad.

and 10 × 5ml aluminium foil laminate sachets

A spoon with a 5ml measure is supplied with the sachet pack.

6.6 Instructions for use and handling

None applicable.

Administrative Data

7. MARKETING AUTHORISATION HOLDER

Pfizer Consumer Healthcare

Alternative Trading Style:

Warner-Lambert Consumer Healthcare

Walton Oaks

Dorking Road

Walton-on-the-Hill

Surrey KT20 7NS

United Kingdom

8. MARKETING AUTHORISATION NUMBER(S)
PL 15513/0056

9. DATE OF FIRST AUTHORISATION/RENEWAL OF THE AUTHORISATION
15 December 1997

10. DATE OF REVISION OF THE TEXT
May 2004

Benylin Chesty Coughs (Original)

(Pfizer Consumer Healthcare)

1. NAME OF THE MEDICINAL PRODUCT
Benylin Chesty Coughs (Original)

2. QUALITATIVE AND QUANTITATIVE COMPOSITION
Each 5 ml contains:-

Diphenhydramine hydrochloride	14.0	mg
L-menthol	2.0	mg

3. PHARMACEUTICAL FORM
Syrup.

A clear red syrup

4. CLINICAL PARTICULARS

4.1 Therapeutic indications
BENYLIN CHESTY COUGHS (ORIGINAL) is indicated for the relief of cough and associated congestive symptoms.

4.2 Posology and method of administration
For oral use

Adults and Children over 12 years

One 10 ml dose of syrup 4 times a day.

Maximum daily dose: 40 ml syrup.

Children aged 6 to 12 years:

One 5 ml dose of syrup 4 times a day.

Maximum daily dose: 20 ml syrup.

Children under 6 years:

BENYLIN Chesty Coughs (Original) is not suitable for administration to children under 6 years of age. BENYLIN for Children's Coughs is recommended for children aged 1 to 5 years.

The Elderly:

As for adults above (see Pharmacokinetics - The elderly).

Hepatic dysfunction

Caution should be exercised if moderate to severe hepatic dysfunction is present (see Pharmacokinetics - Hepatic dysfunction).

Renal dysfunction

It may be prudent to increase the dosage interval in subjects with moderate to severe renal failure (see Pharmacokinetics - Renal dysfunction).

4.3 Contraindications
BENYLIN CHESTY COUGHS (ORIGINAL) is contraindicated in individuals with known hypersensitivity to the product or any of its constituents.

Benylin Chesty Coughs (Original) is contraindicated in individuals with chronic or persistent cough, such as occurs with asthma, or where cough is accompanied by excessive secretions, unless directed by the physician.

Benylin Chesty Coughs (Original) should not be administered to patients currently receiving monoamine oxidase inhibitors (MAOI) or those patients who have received treatment with MAOIs within the last two weeks.

4.4 Special warnings and special precautions for use
This product may cause drowsiness. If affected individuals should not drive or operate machinery.

Subjects with moderate to severe renal or hepatic dysfunction or urinary retention should exercise caution when using this product (see Pharmacokinetics - Renal/Hepatic Dysfunction).

This product contains diphenhydramine and therefore should not be taken by individuals with narrow-angle glaucoma or symptomatic prostatic hypertrophy.

4.5 Interaction with other medicinal products and other forms of Interaction
This product contains diphenhydramine and therefore may potentiate the effects of alcohol, codeine, antihistamines and other CNS depressants.

As diphenhydramine possesses some anticholinergic activity, the effects of anticholinergics (eg, some psychotropic drugs and atropine) may be potentiated by this product. This may result in tachycardia, dry mouth, gastrointestinal disturbances (eg, colic), urinary retention and headache.

4.6 Pregnancy and lactation
Although diphenhydramine has been in widespread use for many years without ill consequence, it is known to cross the placenta and has been detected in breast milk. BENYLIN CHESTY COUGHS (ORIGINAL) should therefore only be used when the potential benefit of treatment to the mother exceeds any possible hazards to the developing foetus or suckling infant.

4.7 Effects on ability to drive and use machines
This product may cause drowsiness. If affected, the patient should not drive or operate machinery.

4.8 Undesirable effects
Side effects associated with the use of BENYLIN CHESTY COUGHS (ORIGINAL) are uncommon.

Diphenhydramine may cause drowsiness; dizziness; gastrointestinal disturbance; dry mouth; nose and throat; difficulty in urination or blurred vision.

Less frequently it may cause palpitations, tremor, convulsions or parasthesia.

Hypersensitivity reactions have been reported, in particular, skin rashes, erythema, urticaria and angiodema.

Adverse reactions to menthol at the low concentration present in BENYLIN CHESTY COUGHS (ORIGINAL) are not anticipated.

4.9 Overdose
Symptoms and signs

The symptoms and signs of BENYLIN CHESTY COUGHS (ORIGINAL) overdose may include drowsiness, hyperpyrexia and anticholinergic effects. With higher doses, and particularly in children, symptoms of CNS excitation including hallucinations and convulsions may appear; with massive doses, coma or cardiovascular collapse may follow.

Treatment

Treatment of overdose should be symptomatic and supportive. Measures to promote rapid gastric emptying (with Syrup of Ipecac-induced emesis or gastric lavage) and, in cases of acute poisoning, the use of activated charcoal may be useful. Seizures may be controlled with Diazepam or Thiopental Sodium. The intravenous use of Physostigmine may be efficacious in antagonising severe anticholinergic symptoms.

5. PHARMACOLOGICAL PROPERTIES

5.1 Pharmacodynamic properties
Diphenhydramine possesses antitussive, antihistaminic and anticholinergic properties. Experiments have shown that the antitussive effect (resulting from an action on the brainstem) is discrete from its antihistaminic effect.

The duration of activity of diphenhydramine is between 4 and 8 hours.

Menthol has mild local anaesthetic and decongestant properties.

5.2 Pharmacokinetic properties
Absorption

Diphenhydramine and menthol are well absorbed from the gut following oral administration. Peak serum levels of diphenhydramine following a 50 mg oral dose are reached at between 2 and 2.5 hours.

Distribution

Diphenhydramine is widely distributed throughout the body, including the CNS. Following a 50 mg oral dose of diphenhydramine, the volume of distribution is in the range 3.3 - 6.8 l/kg, and it is some 78% bound to plasma proteins.

Metabolism and Elimination

Diphenhydramine undergoes extensive first pass metabolism. Two successive N-demethylations occur, with the resultant amine being oxidised to a carboxylic acid. Values for plasma clearance of a 50 mg oral dose of diphenhydramine lie in the range 600-1300 ml/min and the terminal elimination half-life lies in the range 3.4 - 9.3 hours. Little unchanged drug is excreted in the urine. Menthol is hydroxylated in the liver by microsomal enzymes to p-methane-3,8 diol. This is then conjugated with glucuronide and excreted both in urine and bile as the Glucuronide.

The Elderly

Pharmacokinetic studies indicate no major differences in distribution or elimination of Diphenhydramine compared to younger adults.

Renal Dysfunction

The results of a review on the use of Diphenhydramine in renal failure suggest that in moderate to severe renal failure, the dose interval should be extended by a period dependent on Glomerular filtration rate (GFR).

Hepatic Dysfunction

After intravenous administration of 0.8 mg/kg Diphenhydramine, a prolonged half-life was noted in patients with chronic liver disease which correlated with the severity of the disease. However, the mean plasma clearance and apparent volume of distribution were not significantly affected.

5.3 Preclinical safety data
Mutagenicity

The results of a range of tests suggest that neither diphenhydramine nor menthol have mutagenic potential.

Carcinogenicity

There is insufficient information to determine the carcinogenic potential of diphenhydramine or menthol, although such effects have not been associated with these drugs in animal studies.

Teratogenicity

The results of a number of studies suggest that the administration of either diphenhydramine or menthol does not produce any statistically significant teratogenic effects in rats, rabbits and mice.

Fertility

There is insufficient information to determine whether diphenhydramine has the potential to impair fertility, although a diminished fertility rate has been observed in mice in one study.

6. PHARMACEUTICAL PARTICULARS

6.1 List of excipients
Ammonium chloride

Liquid glucose

Sucrose

Ethanol 96%

Glycerol

Sodium citrate

Saccharin sodium

Citric acid monohydrate

Sodium benzoate

Caramel T12

Raspberry flavour 503.850/T

Carbomer

Ponceau 4R (E124)

Purified water

6.2 Incompatibilities
None known

6.3 Shelf life
3 years

6.4 Special precautions for storage
Do not store above 25°C

6.5 Nature and contents of container
BENYLIN CHESTY COUGHS (ORIGINAL) is supplied in a round amber glass bottle of 30 ml, 125 ml, 300 ml with ROPP aluminium cap or a 3 piece plastic child resistant, tamper evident closure fitted with a polyester faced wad or polyethylene/expanded polyethylene laminated wad.

6.6 Instructions for use and handling
None applicable

Administrative Data

7. MARKETING AUTHORISATION HOLDER
PFIZER CONSUMER HEALTHCARE

Alternative Trading Style:

WARNER LAMBERT CONSUMER HEALTHCARE

Walton Oaks

Dorking Road

Walton-on-the-Hill

Surrey KT20 7NS

United Kingdom

8. MARKETING AUTHORISATION NUMBER(S)
PL 15513/0048

9. DATE OF FIRST AUTHORISATION/RENEWAL OF THE AUTHORISATION
16 June 1997 / 11 December 2000

10. DATE OF REVISION OF THE TEXT
January 2004

Benylin Children's Tickly Coughs

(Pfizer Consumer Healthcare)

1. NAME OF THE MEDICINAL PRODUCT
Infant Simple Cough Linctus 3 Months Plus or Infant Sugar Free Simple Cough Linctus or Children's 3 Months Plus Simple Cough Linctus

Boots Cough Syrup 3 Months Plus or Benylin Children's Tickly Coughs

2. QUALITATIVE AND QUANTITATIVE COMPOSITION

Active ingredient	% v/v	ml/5ml
Glycerol Ph Eur	15.00	0.75

3. PHARMACEUTICAL FORM
Syrup

4. CLINICAL PARTICULARS

4.1 Therapeutic indications
For the relief of dry tickly coughs.

4.2 Posology and method of administration
For oral administration.

Children 3 months – 1 year: One 5ml spoonful three to four times a day.

Children 1 to 5 years: Two 5ml spoonfuls three to four times a day.

Children under 3 months: Not recommended.

4.3 Contraindications
Hypersensitivity to any of the ingredients.

4.4 Special warnings and special precautions for use
Not recommended for children under 3 months.

If symptoms persist for more than 3 days consult your doctor.

Keep all medicines out of the reach of children.

4.5 Interaction with other medicinal products and other forms of Interaction
No clinically significant drug interactions.

4.6 Pregnancy and lactation
The safety of this product during pregnancy and lactation has not been established but is not thought to constitute a hazard.

4.7 Effects on ability to drive and use machines
No adverse effects known.

4.8 Undesirable effects
No adverse effects known.

4.9 Overdose
Overdosage with this product may possibly cause diarrhoea. Treatment should be symptomatic.

5. PHARMACOLOGICAL PROPERTIES

5.1 Pharmacodynamic properties
Glycerin has demulcent properties and may possibly block sensory cough receptors in the respiratory tract.

5.2 Pharmacokinetic properties
None stated.

5.3 Preclinical safety data
Not applicable

6. PHARMACEUTICAL PARTICULARS

6.1 List of excipients
Maltitol liquid

Hydroxyethylcellulose

Sodium benzoate

Citric acid monohydrate

Sodium citrate

Apple flavouring 5112OIE

Purified water

6.2 Incompatibilities
None stated

6.3 Shelf life
36 months.

6.4 Special precautions for storage
Keep tightly closed.

Do not store above 25°C.

6.5 Nature and contents of container
1) Bottle amber PET with polypropylene child resistant closure fitted with expanded polythene liner.

Pack size: 100ml and 150 ml

2) Bottle amber glass with polypropylene child resistant closure fitted with an expanded polyethylene liner.

Pack size 100, 125ml or 150ml.

6.6 Instructions for use and handling
Not applicable.

Administrative Data

7. MARKETING AUTHORISATION HOLDER
The Boots Company PLC

1 Thane Road West

Nottingham NG2 3AA

Trading as: BCM

8. MARKETING AUTHORISATION NUMBER(S)
PL 00014/0500

9. DATE OF FIRST AUTHORISATION/RENEWAL OF THE AUTHORISATION
Not applicable.

10. DATE OF REVISION OF THE TEXT
May 2003

Benylin Childrens Chesty Coughs

(Pfizer Consumer Healthcare)

1. NAME OF THE MEDICINAL PRODUCT
BENYLIN Children's Chesty Coughs

2. QUALITATIVE AND QUANTITATIVE COMPOSITION
BENYLIN Children's Chesty Coughs contains 50 mg guaifenesin in each 5 ml.

3. PHARMACEUTICAL FORM
Syrup

4. CLINICAL PARTICULARS

4.1 Therapeutic indications
BENYLIN Children's Chesty Coughs is indicated for the symptomatic relief of productive coughs which benefit from the administration of an expectorant.

4.2 Posology and method of administration
Adults and children over 12 years:

Not applicable.

Children aged 6 to 12 years:

Oral. 10 ml syrup four times daily.

Maximum daily dose: 40 ml syrup (400 mg guaifenesin)

Children aged 1 to 5 years:

Oral. 5 ml syrup four times daily.

Maximum daily dose: 20 ml syrup (200 mg guaifenesin)

Children under 1 year:

BENYLIN Children's Chesty Coughs is not recommended for administration to children under 1 year of age, except on the advice of a physician.

The Elderly

Not applicable.

4.3 Contraindications
BENYLIN Children's Chesty Coughs is contraindicated in individuals with known hypersensitivity to the product, or any of its components.

4.4 Special warnings and special precautions for use
BENYLIN Children's Chesty Coughs should be not used for persistent or chronic cough, such as occurs with asthma, or where cough is accompanied by excessive secretions, unless directed by a physician.

Caution should be exercised in the presence of severe renal or severe hepatic impairment.

4.5 Interaction with other medicinal products and other forms of Interaction
If urine is collected within 24 hours of a dose of BENYLIN Children's Chesty Coughs a metabolite of guaifenesin may cause a colour interference with laboratory determinations of urinary 5-hydroxyindoleacetic acid (5-HIAA) and vanillylmandelic acid (VMA).

4.6 Pregnancy and lactation
This product has been formulated specifically for children, and would therefore not normally be taken during pregnancy and lactation.

Insufficient information is available on the effects of BENYLIN Children's Chesty Coughs during human pregnancy. BENYLIN Children's Chesty Coughs, like most medicines, should not be used during pregnancy unless the potential benefit of treatment to the mother outweighs the possible risks to the developing foetus.

Guaifenesin is excreted in breast milk in small amounts with no effect expected on the infant.

4.7 Effects on ability to drive and use machines
Not applicable.

4.8 Undesirable effects
Side effects resulting from guaifenesin administration are very rare.

4.9 Overdose
Symptoms and signs

The effects of acute toxicity from guaifenesin may include gastrointestinal discomfort, nausea and drowsiness.

Treatment

Treatment should be symptomatic and supportive.

5. PHARMACOLOGICAL PROPERTIES

5.1 Pharmacodynamic properties
Guaifenesin is thought to exert its pharmacological action by stimulating receptors in the gastric mucosa. This increases the output from secretory glands of the gastrointestinal system and reflexly increases the flow of fluids from glands lining the respiratory tract. The result is an increase in volume and decrease in viscosity of bronchial secretions. Other actions may include stimulating vagal nerve endings in bronchial secretory glands and stimulating certain centres in the brain, which in turn enhance respiratory fluid flow. Guaifenesin produces its expectorant action within 24 hours.

5.2 Pharmacokinetic properties
Absorption

Guaifenesin is well absorbed from the gastro-intestinal tract following oral administration, although limited information regarding its pharmacokinetics is available. After the administration of 600 mg guaifenesin to healthy adult volunteers, the C_{max} was approximately 1.4 ug/ml, with t_{max} occurring approximately 15 minutes after drug administration.

Distribution

No information is available on the distribution of guaifenesin in humans.

Metabolism and elimination

Guaifenesin appears to undergo both oxidation and demethylation. Following an oral dose of 600 mg guaifenesin to 3 healthy male volunteers, the $t_{1/2}$ was approximately 1 hour and the drug was not detectable in the blood after approximately 8 hours.

Pharmacokinetics in Renal/Hepatic Impairment

There have been no specific studies of BENYLIN Children's Chesty Coughs or guaifenesin in subjects with renal or hepatic impairment.

Caution is therefore recommended when administering this product to subjects with severe renal or hepatic impairment.

Pharmacokinetics in the Elderly

Not applicable.

5.3 Preclinical safety data
Mutagenicity

There is insufficient information available to determine whether guaifenesin has mutagenic potential.

Carcinogenicity

There is insufficient information available to determine whether guaifenesin has carcinogenic potential.

Teratogenicity

There is insufficient information available to determine whether guaifenesin has teratogenic potential.

Fertility

There is insufficient information available to determine whether guaifenesin has the potential to impair fertility.

6. PHARMACEUTICAL PARTICULARS

6.1 List of excipients
Glycerol

Sorbitol liquid(non-crystallising)

Sodium citrate

Citric acid monohydrate

Sodium saccharin

Sodium benzoate

Carmellose Sodium

Strawberry 580.193/T

Purified water

6.2 Incompatibilities
None known

6.3 Shelf life
3 years (bottles)

2 years (sachets)

6.4 Special precautions for storage
Do not store above 25°C. Store in the original package.

6.5 Nature and contents of container
BENYLIN Children's Chesty Coughs is stored in 125 ml, 300 ml or 30 ml amber glass bottles with a polyester wadded white aluminium ROPP cap or a 3 piece plastic child resistant, tamper evident closure fitted with a polyester faced wad, or polyethylene/expanded polyethylene laminated wad.

and 10 × 5ml aluminium foil laminate sachets

A spoon with a 5ml measure is supplied with the sachet pack.

6.6 Instructions for use and handling
None applicable.

Administrative Data

7. MARKETING AUTHORISATION HOLDER
Pfizer Consumer Healthcare

Alternative Trading Style:

Warner-Lambert Consumer Healthcare

Walton Oaks

Dorking Road

Walton-on-the-Hill

Surrey KT20 7NS

United Kingdom

8. MARKETING AUTHORISATION NUMBER(S)
PL 15513/0052

9. DATE OF FIRST AUTHORISATION/RENEWAL OF THE AUTHORISATION
16/6/97

10. DATE OF REVISION OF THE TEXT
June 2004

Benylin Children's Coughs & Colds

(Pfizer Consumer Healthcare)

1. NAME OF THE MEDICINAL PRODUCT
Benylin Children's Coughs and Colds

2. QUALITATIVE AND QUANTITATIVE COMPOSITION
Benylin Children's Coughs and Colds contains:

Triprolidine hydrochloride	0.625 mg
Dextromethorphan hydrobromide	5.000 mg

3. PHARMACEUTICAL FORM
Oral solution

4. CLINICAL PARTICULARS

4.1 Therapeutic indications
Benylin Children's Coughs and Colds is indicated for the symptomatic relief of dry unproductive cough and other histamine-related symptoms associated with colds in children, thus permitting undisturbed sleep.

4.2 Posology and method of administration

Adults and children over 12 years
Older patients may find Actifed Compound Linctus formulation to be more suitable.

Children aged 6 to 12 years
Oral 10 ml three or four times a day - maximum daily dose: 40 ml

Children aged 2 years to 5 years
Oral. 5 ml three or four times a day - maximum daily dose: 20 ml

Children aged 1 year to less than 2 years
Oral. 2.5 ml three or four times a day - maximum daily dose: 10 ml

Use in the Elderly
Not applicable

4.3 Contraindications
Contraindicated in patients with a known hypersensitivity to triprolidine or dextromethorphan.

4.4 Special warnings and special precautions for use
Alcohol or other potentially sedating medicines should not be used concurrently with Benylin Children's Coughs and Colds.

Caution should be exercised in the presence of severe hepatic or renal impairment.

The packs will carry the following statements:

Store below 30°C.

Keep out of reach of children.

Warning: may cause drowsiness. If affected do not drive or operate machinery. Avoid alcoholic drink.

As with all medicines, if your child is currently taking any other medicine, consult your doctor or pharmacist before this product is taken.

If symptoms persist consult your doctor.

Do not exceed the stated dose.

4.5 Interaction with other medicinal products and other forms of Interaction
None known.

4.6 Pregnancy and lactation
Not applicable.

4.7 Effects on ability to drive and use machines
Triprolidine may cause drowsiness and impair performance in tests of auditory vigilance.

4.8 Undesirable effects
Skin rashes, with or without irritation, have occasionally been reported in association with administration of triprolidine.

Side effects attributed to dextromethorphan are uncommon; occasionally nausea, vomiting or gastro-intestinal disturbances may occur.

4.9 Overdose
The effects of acute toxicity from Benylin Children's Coughs and Colds may include drowsiness, lethargy, dizziness, ataxia, weakness, hypotonicity, respiratory depression, dryness of the skin and mucous membranes, tachycardia, nystagmus, hyperpyrexia, hyperactivity, nausea and vomiting.

Although there have been no reports of convulsions with Actidil Elixir (triprolidine HCl 2 mg/5 ml), either in therapeutic doses or in overdose, central excitation is a feature of poisoning with antihistamines and can result in convulsions, particularly in infants.

Necessary measures should be taken to maintain and support respiration and control convulsions. Gastric lavage should be performed if indicated.

Naloxone has been successful as a specific antagonist to dextromethorphan toxicity in a child.

5. PHARMACOLOGICAL PROPERTIES

5.1 Pharmacodynamic properties
Dextromethorphan provides antitussive activity by acting on the medullary cough centre. Triprolidine provides antihistamine activity by antagonising H_1-receptors.

5.2 Pharmacokinetic properties
In common with other antihistamines, triprolidine hydrochloride is rapidly absorbed, peak plasma levels being observed 2 hours after oral dose. It is metabolised in the liver and excreted mainly as metabolites in the urine. The plasma half-life is approximately 3 hours.

Dextromethorphan is well absorbed following oral administration, with peak plasma levels (after a 30 mg dose) being seen after 2 hours. Metabolism in the liver by N- and O- demethylation is followed by sulphate or glucuronic acid conjugation. It is excreted in the urine, up to 56% as metabolites and remainder as unchanged drug.

5.3 Preclinical safety data
Not applicable.

6. PHARMACEUTICAL PARTICULARS

6.1 List of excipients
Maltitol solution

Glycerol

Methyl hydroxybenzoate

Sodium benzoate

Saccharin sodium

Flavour

Purified water

6.2 Incompatibilities
None known.

6.3 Shelf life
36 months.

6.4 Special precautions for storage
Store below 30°C.

6.5 Nature and contents of container
30 ml, 40 ml, 50 ml 100 ml and 125 ml amber glass bottles with polypropylene screw caps fitted with PVDC faced wads or a 3 piece plastic child resistant, tamper evident closure fitted with a polyvinylidene chloride (PVDC) faced wad or polyethylene/expanded polyethylene laminated wad

The nature of the bottle and wad will be identical to the 30 ml and 100 ml pack sizes.

A double-ended spoon, with 2.5 ml and 5 ml measures will be included in each pack.

6.6 Instructions for use and handling
None applicable.

Administrative Data

7. MARKETING AUTHORISATION HOLDER
Pfizer Consumer Healthcare

Alternative Trading Style:

Warner-Lambert Consumer Healthcare

Walton Oaks

Dorking Road

Walton-on-the-Hill

Surrey

KT20 7NS

8. MARKETING AUTHORISATION NUMBER(S)
PL 15513/0012

9. DATE OF FIRST AUTHORISATION/RENEWAL OF THE AUTHORISATION
28th February 1997

10. DATE OF REVISION OF THE TEXT
January 2004

Benylin Childrens Dry Coughs

(Pfizer Consumer Healthcare)

1. NAME OF THE MEDICINAL PRODUCT
Benylin Children's Dry Coughs

2. QUALITATIVE AND QUANTITATIVE COMPOSITION
Active ingredient: Pholcodine 2.0 mg/5ml

3. PHARMACEUTICAL FORM
Oral solution

4. CLINICAL PARTICULARS

4.1 Therapeutic indications
For the symptomatic relief of dry, ticklish and unproductive coughs.

4.2 Posology and method of administration
For oral use.

Children 1-5 years: One 5ml spoonful three times a day.

Children under 1 year: Not recommended.

Children 6 -12 years: Two to three 5 ml spoonfuls three times a day.

4.3 Contraindications
Hypersensitivity to any of the ingredients. Patients with renal or hepatic failure. Should not be given to patients receiving MAOI therapy or within 14 days of stopping such treatment.

4.4 Special warnings and special precautions for use
Cough suppressants should be avoided in chronic obstructive airways disease as they may depress respiration. Cough suppression may cause sputum retention and this may be harmful in patients with chronic bronchitis and bronchiolitis.

Not recommended for children under 1 year.

Do not exceed the stated dose.

If symptoms persist consult your doctor.

Keep all medicines out of the reach of children.

4.5 Interaction with other medicinal products and other forms of Interaction
No clinically significant interactions known.

4.6 Pregnancy and lactation
The safety of pholcodine during pregnancy and lactation has not been established. Based on the available data for morphine, it would seem likely that use of pholcodine during pregnancy would not be associated with congenital defects and that use of pholcodine during lactation would not be contraindicated. However, its use should be carefully assessed by consideration of small benefits versus potential risk to the foetus or neonate.

4.7 Effects on ability to drive and use machines
No adverse effects known.

4.8 Undesirable effects
Nausea, drowsiness and constipation may occasionally occur.

4.9 Overdose
Symptoms of overdose may include nausea, drowsiness, restlessness, excitement, ataxia and respiratory depression. Treatment consists of emptying the stomach by aspiration and lavage. In cases of severe poisoning the specific narcotic antagonist naloxone may be used. Otherwise treatment should be symptomatic and supportive.

5. PHARMACOLOGICAL PROPERTIES

5.1 Pharmacodynamic properties
Pholcodine is a cough suppressant with mild sedative but little analgesic activity.

5.2 Pharmacokinetic properties
Maximum plasma concentrations are attained at 4 to 8 hours after an oral dose. The elimination of half-life ranges from 32 to 43 hours and volume of distribution is 36-49l/kg.

Pholcodine is protein bound to the extent of 23.5%.

Pholcodine is metabolised in the liver but undergoes little conjugation.

There is little or no metabolism of pholcodine to morphine and this may account for the lack of analgesic activity, morphine-like side effects and addictive potential.

5.3 Preclinical safety data
Not applicable.

6. PHARMACEUTICAL PARTICULARS

6.1 List of excipients
Lycasin 80/55

Sodium citrate

Citric acid monohydrate

Sodium benzoate

Blackcurrant flavour DA 13624

Vanilla bean extract AD17342

Water purified

Hydroxyethylcellulose

Glycerin

Acesulfame k

6.2 Incompatibilities
None stated.

6.3 Shelf life
24 months.

6.4 Special precautions for storage
Store below 30°C.

6.5 Nature and contents of container
150 ml amber PET bottle with a polypropylene cap fitted with an expanded polyethylene liner or a 125 ml amber glass bottle with a 3 piece plastic child resistant, tamper evident closure fitted with a polyethylene/polyvinylidene chloride/polyethylene laminate faced wad.

6.6 Instructions for use and handling
Not applicable.

Administrative Data

7. MARKETING AUTHORISATION HOLDER
Pfizer Consumer Healthcare

Alternative Trading Style:

Warner-Lambert Consumer Healthcare

Walton Oaks

Dorking Road

Walton-on-the-Hill

Surrey KT20 7NS

United Kingdom

8. MARKETING AUTHORISATION NUMBER(S)
15513/0054

9. DATE OF FIRST AUTHORISATION/RENEWAL OF THE AUTHORISATION
17th April 1997

10. DATE OF REVISION OF THE TEXT
January 2004

Benylin Childrens Night Coughs

(Pfizer Consumer Healthcare)

1. NAME OF THE MEDICINAL PRODUCT
BENYLIN CHILDREN'S NIGHT COUGHS

2. QUALITATIVE AND QUANTITATIVE COMPOSITION
BENYLIN CHILDREN'S NIGHT COUGHS contains -

Active Ingredient	Mg/5 ml
Diphenhydramine Hydrochloride	7.0 mg
Levomenthol	0.55 mg

3. PHARMACEUTICAL FORM
A clear colourless syrup with no insoluble matter.

4. CLINICAL PARTICULARS

4.1 Therapeutic indications
BENYLIN CHILDREN'S NIGHT COUGHS is indicated for the relief of cough and its congestive symptoms and in the treatment of hay fever and other allergic conditions affecting the upper respiratory tract. It is specially formulated for children and contains no artificial dyes or sucrose.

4.2 Posology and method of administration
Route of Administration: Oral

Children under 1 year Not recommended

Children 1-5 years: One 5 ml spoonful every 6 hours

6 to 12 years: Two 5 ml spoonfuls every 6 hours

No more than four doses should be given in any 24 hours.

4.3 Contraindications
BENYLIN CHILDREN'S NIGHT COUGHS is contraindicated in individuals with known hypersensitivity to the product or any of its constituents.

BENYLIN CHILDREN'S NIGHT COUGHS is contraindicated in individuals with chronic or persistent cough, such as occurs with asthma, or where cough is accompanied by excessive secretions, unless directed by the physician.

BENYLIN CHILDREN'S NIGHT COUGHS should not be administered to patients currently receiving monoamine oxidase inhibitors (MAOI) or those patients who have received treatment with MAOIs within the last two weeks.

4.4 Special warnings and special precautions for use
Diphenhydramine should not be taken by patients with narrow-angle glaucoma or symptomatic prostatic hypertrophy unless directed by a doctor.

Alcohol or other potential sedating medicines should not be used concurrently with Benylin Children's Night Coughs

Patients with moderate to severe renal or hepatic dysfunction or urinary retention should exercise caution when using this product (see Pharmacokinetics - Renal/Hepatic Dysfunction).

4.5 Interaction with other medicinal products and other forms of Interaction
This product may potentiate the effect of alcohol, codeine, antihistamines and other CNS depressants. The effects of anticholinergics eg. some psychotropic drugs and atropine may be potentiated by this product giving rise to tachycardia, mouth dryness, gastrointestinal disturbances eg., colic, urinary retention and headache.

4.6 Pregnancy and lactation
Diphenhydramine crosses the placenta and has been detected in breast milk. BENYLIN CHILDREN'S NIGHT COUGHS should only be used when the potential benefit of treatment to the mother exceeds any possible hazards to the developing foetus or suckling infant.

4.7 Effects on ability to drive and use machines
This preparation may cause drowsiness, dizziness or blurred vision. If affected, the patient should not drive or operate machinery.

4.8 Undesirable effects
Diphenhydramine may cause drowsiness, dizziness, gastrointestinal disturbance, dry mouth, nose and throat, difficulty in urination or blurred vision.

Less frequently it may cause palpitations, tremor, convulsions or parasthesia.

Hypersensitivity reactions have been reported, in particular, skin rashes, erythema, urticaria and angiodema.

Adverse reactions to menthol at the low concentration present in BENYLIN CHILDREN'S NIGHT COUGHS are not anticipated.

4.9 Overdose

Signs and Symptoms:
Drowsiness, hyperpyrexia and anticholinergic effects. In children, CNS excitation, including hallucinations and convulsions may appear; with larger doses, coma or cardiovascular collapse may follow.

Treatment
Treatment of overdose with BENYLIN CHILDREN'S NIGHT COUGHS is likely to involve supportive care and rapid gastric emptying with Syrup of Ipecac induced emesis or gastric lavage. In cases of acute poisoning, activated charcoal may be useful. Seizures may be controlled with Diazepam or Thiopental Sodium. In addition to supportive care, the intravenous use of Physostigmine may be efficacious in antagonising severe anticholinergic symptoms.

5. PHARMACOLOGICAL PROPERTIES

5.1 Pharmacodynamic properties
Diphenhydramine is a potent antihistamine and antitussive with anticholinergic properties. Recent experiments have shown that the antitussive action is discrete from H_1-receptor blockade and is located in the brain stem.

Menthol has mild local anaesthetic and decongestant properties.

5.2 Pharmacokinetic properties
Diphenhydramine is well absorbed from the gastro-intestinal tract. Peak serum levels are reached at between 2-2.5 hours after an oral dose. Duration of activity is between 4 - 8 hours. The drug is widely distributed throughout the body, including the CNS, and some 78% is bound to plasma proteins. Estimates of the volume of distribution lie in the range 3.3 - 6.8 l/kg.

Diphenhydramine experiences extensive first-pass metabolism, undergoing two successive N-Demethylations; the resultant amine is then oxidised to a carboxylic acid. Values for plasma clearance lie in the range 600 - 1300 ml/min and the terminal elimination half life lies in the range 3.4 - 9.3 hours. Little unchanged drug is excreted in the urine.

Pharmacokinetic studies in elderly subjects indicate no major differences in drug distribution or elimination compared with younger adults.

Menthol: After absorption, menthol is conjugated in the liver and excreted both in urine and bile as the glucuronide.

Renal Dysfunction
The results of a review on the use of diphenhydramine in renal failure suggest that in moderate to severe renal failure, the dose interval should be extended by a period dependent on Glomerular filtration rate (GFR).

Hepatic Dysfunction
After intravenous administration of 0.8 mg/kg diphenhydramine, a prolonged half-life was noted in patients with chronic liver disease which correlated with the severity of the disease. However, the mean plasma clearance and apparent volume of distribution were not significantly affected.

5.3 Preclinical safety data
Not applicable

6. PHARMACEUTICAL PARTICULARS

6.1 List of excipients
Sodium benzoate

Citric acid monohydrate

Sodium citrate

Saccharin sodium

Sodium carboxymethylcellulose 7MXF

Glycerol

Sorbitol 70% (non crystalline)

Concentrated raspberry essence

Ethanol 96%

Purified water

6.2 Incompatibilities
None stated

6.3 Shelf life
36 months unopened

6.4 Special precautions for storage
Store below 30°C

6.5 Nature and contents of container
125.000 ml, 30.000 ml Round amber glass bottles with roll-on-pilfer-proof (ROPP) aluminium caps containing melinex-faced pulpboard wad or 3 piece plastic child resistant, tamper evident closure fitted with a polyester faced wad or polyethylene/expanded polyethylene laminated wad.

6.6 Instructions for use and handling
Not applicable

Administrative Data

7. MARKETING AUTHORISATION HOLDER
Pfizer Consumer Healthcare

Alternative Trading Style:

Warner-Lambert Consumer Healthcare

Walton Oaks

Dorking Road

Walton-on-the-Hill

Surrey

KT20 7NS

United Kingdom

8. MARKETING AUTHORISATION NUMBER(S)
PL 15513/0044

9. DATE OF FIRST AUTHORISATION/RENEWAL OF THE AUTHORISATION
Date granted: 16 June 1997

10. DATE OF REVISION OF THE TEXT
March 2004

Benylin Cough & Congestion

(Pfizer Consumer Healthcare)

1. NAME OF THE MEDICINAL PRODUCT
BENYLIN COUGH & CONGESTION

2. QUALITATIVE AND QUANTITATIVE COMPOSITION
Each 5ml of BENYLIN COUGH & CONGESTION contains:
Diphenhydramine hydrochloride 14 mg

Dextromethorphan hydrobromide 6.5 mg

Pseudoephedrine hydrochloride 22.5 mg

Levomenthol 1.75 mg.

3. PHARMACEUTICAL FORM
Clear green syrup with a menthol taste and odour.

4. CLINICAL PARTICULARS

4.1 Therapeutic indications
BENYLIN COUGH & CONGESTION is indicated for the relief of cough and its congestive symptoms and is particularly suitable for those coughs associated with colds.

4.2 Posology and method of administration
Adults and children over 12 years:

Oral. 10 ml syrup to be taken four times a day.

Maximum daily dose: 40 ml

Elderly (over 65 years):

As for adults

Children aged 6 to 12 years:

Oral. 5 ml syrup to be taken four times daily.

Maximum daily dose: 20 ml

Children under 6 years:

BENYLIN COUGH & CONGESTION is not suitable for administration to children under 6 years of age.

4.3 Contraindications
BENYLIN COUGH & CONGESTION is contraindicated in individuals with known hypersensitivity to any of the active constituents, and in those receiving monoamine oxidase inhibitors or having received them within the previous fourteen days.

Caution may be necessary in patients with cardiovascular disease, hepatic dysfunction, hyperthyroidism and prostate enlargement.

4.4 Special warnings and special precautions for use
None known.

4.5 Interaction with other medicinal products and other forms of Interaction
Alcoholic drink should be avoided as this product potentiates the effects of alcohol and other CNS depressants.

4.6 Pregnancy and lactation
As with other medication care should be taken during pregnancy.

4.7 Effects on ability to drive and use machines
This preparation may cause drowsiness. If affected, the patient should not drive or operate machinery.

4.8 Undesirable effects
Dextromethorphan hydrobromide occasionally causes drowsiness, dizziness and gastro-intestinal upsets.

4.9 Overdose
Treatment: Gastric lavage in the conscious patient and intensive supportive therapy when necessary as with cases of overdosage with antihistaminic drugs.

5. PHARMACOLOGICAL PROPERTIES

5.1 Pharmacodynamic properties
Dextromethorphan hydrobromide

Dextromethorphan is the non-addictive d-isomer of the codeine analog of levorphanol. With antitussive doses, the cough threshold is elevated centrally without appreciable effects on the respiratory, cardiovascular or gastro-intestinal systems or sedation. The effectiveness of dextromethorphan has been demonstrated in controlled studies, its potency is nearly equal to that of codeine.

Diphenhydramine hydrochloride

Diphenhydramine hydrochloride is an ethanolamine derivative and has been demonstrated to have antihistamine, antitussive, local anaesthetic and anticholinergic activity.

Histamine acts on histamine H_1 receptors to contract smooth muscle and dilate and increase the permeability of the capillaries. The antihistamine action brought about by the histamine H_1 receptor antagonism of diphenhydramine helps provide relief from distressing symptoms such as nasal discharge and congestion, nasal irritation with sneezing and watering of the eyes.

Diphenhydramine hydrochloride provides significant antitussive effect by suppressing the cough reflex in the central nervous system.

Pseudoephedrine hydrochloride

Pseudoephedrine hydrochloride is a sterioisomer of ephedrine and has a similar action. That is a sympathomimetic agent with direct and indirect effects on adrenergic receptors. It has alpha- and beta- adrenergic activities and has stimulating effects on the central nervous system. It has a more prolonged, though less potent action than adrenaline. However, psuedoephedrine has been stated to have less pressor activity and central nervous system effects than ephedrine.

It is used as a nasal and bronchial decongestant.

Menthol

Menthol is chiefly used to relieve symptoms of bronchitis, sinusitis and similar conditions. Taken internally it has carminative and irritant effects and has been used as a mild expectorant.

5.2 Pharmacokinetic properties

Dextromethorphan hydrobromide

Dextromethorphan is well absorbed from the gastrointestinal tract, peak serum levels being achieved some two hours after oral administration.

Plasma levels of unmetabolised dextromethorphan following therapeutic doses are very low due to extensive biotransformation and tissue distribution which rapidly remove drug from the blood.

The drug is metabolised in the liver and excreted as unchanged dextromethorphan and demethylated morphinan compounds.

Diphenhydramine hydrochloride

Absorption

Diphenhydramine hydrochloride is readily absorbed from the gastro-intestinal tract after oral administration.

Distribution

98% is bound to plasma proteins. Maximum plasma levels of diphenhydramine hydrochloride in normal subjects ranging from 81 to 159 ng/ml were obtained two to four hours after administration of a single 100 mg oral dose. The plasma half life calculated over the period 4 to 24 hours after administration ranged from about 5 to 8 hours.

Following administration of diphenhydramine hydrochloride 50 mg four times daily for 13 doses to 4 subjects, plasma diphenhydramine concentrations reached a plateau after 2 or 3 days with a mean peak level of approximately 110 ng/ml. After the last dose the plasma half life was about 6 hours for diphenhydramine.

Metabolisms

Extensively metabolised; about 50% of an oral dose is metabolised in the liver before reaching the general circulation. Reactions include N-Dealkylation and Deamination.

Excretion

In the urine up to 3% of a dose is excreted unchanged, up to 13% as basic amines and up to 65% diphenhydramine metabolites. The major urinary metabolite appears to be diphenylmethoxyacetic acid in free or conjugated form.

Pseudoephedrine hydrochloride

Absorption

Pseudoephedrine hydrochloride is rapidly and completely absorbed from the gastrointestinal tract after oral administration; aluminium hydroxide increases and kaoline decreases the rate of absorption.

Distribution

After an oral dose of 180 mg, peak plasma concentrations of 500 to 900 ng/ml are attained in 1 to 3 hours.

The plasma half life after an oral dose is between 5 and 8 hours which may be increased in subjects with alkaline urine and decreased in subjects with acid urine.

The volume of distribution is 2 to 3 litres/kg body weight.

Excretion

About 70% of a dose is excreted in the urine in 36 hours with less than 1% as norpseudoephedrine and the remainder as unchanged drug. Elimination is enhanced in acid urine and reduced with alkaline urine.

Menthol

After absorption, menthol is excreted in the urine and bile as a glucuronide.

5.3 Preclinical safety data

The active ingredients of BENYLIN COUGH & CONGESTION are well known constituents of medicinal products and their safety profiles are well documented. The results of pre-clinical studies do not add anything of relevance for therapeutic purposes.

6. PHARMACEUTICAL PARTICULARS

6.1 List of excipients

Liquid glucose

Sucrose

Ethanol 96%

Glycerol

Sodium citrate

Saccharin sodium

Citric acid monohydrate

Carbomer

Quinoline yellow (E104)

Patent Blue V (E131)

Purified water

6.2 Incompatibilities

None known.

6.3 Shelf life

36 months.

6.4 Special precautions for storage

Do not store above 30°C.

6.5 Nature and contents of container

30 ml or 125 ml Amber glass bottles sealed with a ROPP cap or a 3 piece plastic child resistant, tamper evident closure fitted with a polyester faced wad.

6.6 Instructions for use and handling

None applicable.

7. MARKETING AUTHORISATION HOLDER

Pfizer Consumer Healthcare

Alternative Trading Style:

Warner-Lambert Consumer Healthcare

Walton Oaks

Dorking Road

Walton-on-the-Hill

Surrey KT20 7NS

United Kingdom

8. MARKETING AUTHORISATION NUMBER(S)

PL 15513/0061

9. DATE OF FIRST AUTHORISATION/RENEWAL OF THE AUTHORISATION

3rd October 1997

10. DATE OF REVISION OF THE TEXT

February 2004

Benylin Day & Night Tablets

(Pfizer Consumer Healthcare)

1. NAME OF THE MEDICINAL PRODUCT

Benylin Day and Night Tablets

2. QUALITATIVE AND QUANTITATIVE COMPOSITION

Blue (Night) Tablets

Paracetamol 500.00 mg

Diphenhydramine hydrochloride 25.00 mg

White (Day) Tablet

Paracetamol 500.00 mg

Pseudoephedrine hydrochloride 60.00 mg

3. PHARMACEUTICAL FORM

Tablet

White, biconvex oblong tablet with bisecting score on one side and "AC7" engraved on both sides of the score.

Film-coated Tablet

Blue, round, biconvex tablet.

4. CLINICAL PARTICULARS

4.1 Therapeutic indications

For the relief of the symptoms associated with colds and influenza.

4.2 Posology and method of administration

For oral use.

Adults and Children over 12 years

Four tablets should be taken daily:

One white tablet to be taken every 4 to 6 hours during the day (no more than three white tablets a day).

One blue tablet to be taken at night.

Take only one tablet at a time and only at the times of day indicated on the pack. Do not take the nighttime tablets during the day.

Elderly

As for adults (see Pharmacokinetics).

Children

Not recommended for children under 12 years of age.

4.3 Contraindications

Use in individuals with known hypersensitivity to the product or any of its constituents.

Use in individuals with severe hypertension or coronary artery disease.

Use in individuals who are taking or, have taken monoamine oxidase inhibitors within the preceding two weeks. The concomitant use of pseudoephedrine and this type of product may occasionally cause a rise in blood pressure.

4.4 Special warnings and special precautions for use

Although pseudoephedrine has virtually no pressor effects in normotensive patients, Benylin Day and Night Tablets should be used with caution in patients suffering with mild to moderate hypertension. The product should also be used with caution in patients with heart disease, diabetes, hyperthyroidism, elevated intraocular pressure and prostatic enlargement.

Caution should be exercised when using the product in the presence of severe hepatic impairment or moderate to severe renal impairment (particularly if accompanied by cardiovascular disease). The hazards of overdose are greater in those with non-cirrhotic alcoholic liver disease.

Concomitant use of other products containing paracetamol or decongestants with Benylin Day and Night Tablets could lead to overdosage and should, therefore, be avoided.

The labels will contain the following statements:

Nighttime tablets only: May cause drowsiness. If affected, do not drive or operate machinery. Avoid alcoholic drink.

Keep medicines out of the reach and sight of children.

If symptoms persist consult your doctor.

Do not exceed the stated dose.

Not to be taken during pregnancy or if breast-feeding.

Immediate medical advice should be sought in the event of an overdose, even if you feel well (label).

Immediate medical advice should be sought in the event of an overdose, even if you feel well, because of the risk of delayed, serious liver damage (leaflet).

Do not take with any other paracetamol containing products.

4.5 Interaction with other medicinal products and other forms of Interaction

Concomitant use of Benylin Day and Night Tablets with tricyclic antidepressants, sympathomimetic agents (such as decongestants, appetite suppressants and amfetamine-like stimulants) or with monoamine oxidase inhibitors, which interfere with the catabolism of sympathomimetic amines, and may occasionally cause a rise in blood pressure.

Because of the pseudoephedrine contents, Benylin Day and Night Tablets may partially reverse the hypotensive action of drugs which interfere with sympathetic activity including bretylium betanidine, guanethidine, debrisoquine, methyldopa, alpha- and beta-adrenergic blocking agents.

The use of drugs that induce hepatic microsomal enzymes, such as anticonvulsants and oral contraceptives, may increase the extent of metabolism of paracetamol, resulting in reduced plasma concentrations of the drug and a faster elimination rate.

The speed of absorption of paracetamol may be increased by metoclopramide or domperidone, and absorption reduced by colestyramine.

The anticoagulant effect of warfarin and other coumarins may be enhanced by prolonged regular use of paracetamol with increased risk of bleeding; occasional doses have no significant effect.

Chronic alcohol intake can increase the hepatotoxicity of paracetamol overdose and may have contributed to the acute pancreatitis reported in one patient who had taken an overdose of paracetamol. Acute alcohol intake may diminish an individual's ability to metabolise large doses of paracetamol, the plasma half-life of which can be prolonged.

Diphenhydramine may potentiate the effects of alcohol and other CNS depressants. The effects of anticholinergics (such as atropine and some psychotropic drugs) may be potentiated by this product.

4.6 Pregnancy and lactation

Benylin Day and Night Tablets, like most medicines, should not be used during pregnancy unless the potential benefit of treatment to the mother outweighs any possible risk to the developing foetus.

Paracetamol, pseudoephedrine and diphenhydramine have been in widespread use for many years without any apparent ill consequence. Epidemiological studies in human pregnancy have shown no ill effects due to paracetamol used in the recommended dosage, but patients should follow the advice of their doctor regarding its use. The safety of pseudoephedrine in pregnancy has not been established. Diphenhydramine is known to cross the placenta and, therefore, should only be used during pregnancy if considered essential by a doctor.

Pseudoephedrine is excreted in breast milk in small amounts, but the effect of this on breast-fed infants is not known. It has been estimated that approximately 0.4 to 0.7% of a single 60mg dose pseudoephedrine ingested by a nursing mother will be excreted in the breast milk over 24 hours.

Paracetamol is excreted in breast milk, but not in a clinically significant amount. Available published data do not contra-indicate breast-feeding. A pharmacokinetic study of paracetamol in 12 nursing mothers revealed that less than 1% of a 650mg oral dose of paracetamol appeared in the breast-milk. Similar findings have been reported in other studies, therefore maternal ingestion of therapeutic doses of paracetamol does not appear to present a risk to the infant.

Diphenhydramine is excreted into human breast-milk, but levels have not been reported. Although the levels are not thought to be sufficiently high enough after therapeutic doses to affect the infant, the use of diphenhydramine during breast-feeding is not recommended.

4.7 Effects on ability to drive and use machines
May cause drowsiness. If affected, do not drive or operate machinery.

4.8 Undesirable effects
Serious side effects associated with the use of pseudoephedrine are extremely rare. Symptoms of central nervous system excitation may occur, including sleep disturbances and rarely hallucinations have been reported. Urinary retention has been reported occasionally in men receiving pseudoephedrine, prostatic enlargement could have been a predisposing factor. Skin rashes, with or without irritation, have occasionally been reported with pseudoephedrine.

Adverse effects of paracetamol are rare but hypersensitivity including skin rash may occur. There have been reports of blood dyscrasias including thrombocytopenia and agranulocytosis following paracetamol use, but these were not necessarily causality related to the drug.

Side effects of diphenhydramine include drowsiness, dizziness, blurred vision, gastrointestinal disturbances, dry mouth, nose and throat, or urinary retention. Hypersensitivity reactions have been reported, in particular, itching and skin rashes, erythema and urticaria.

4.9 Overdose
Paracetamol:

Liver damage is possible in adults who have taken 10g or more of paracetamol. Ingestion of 5g or more of paracetamol may lead to liver damage if the patient has risk factors (see below).

Risk Factors:

If the patient

§ Is on long term treatment with carbamazepine, phenobarbital, phenytoin, primidone, rifampicin, St John's Wort or other drugs that induce liver enzymes.

Or

§ Regularly consumes ethanol in excess of recommended amounts.

Or

§ Is likely to be glutathione deplete e.g. eating disorders, cystic fibrosis, HIV infection, starvation, cachexia.

Symptoms of paracetamol overdosage in the first 24 hours are pallor, nausea, vomiting, anorexia and abdominal pain. Liver damage may become apparent 12 to 48 hours after ingestion. Abnormalities of glucose metabolism and metabolic acidosis may occur. In severe poisoning, hepatic failure may progress to encephalopathy, haemorrhage, hypoglycaemia, cerebral oedema, and death. Acute renal failure with acute tubular necrosis, strongly suggested by loin pain, haematuria and proteinuria, may develop even in the absence of severe liver damage. Cardiac arrhythmias and pancreatitis have been reported.

Immediate treatment is essential in the management of paracetamol overdose. Despite a lack of significant early symptoms, patients should be referred to hospital urgently for immediate medical attention. Symptoms may be limited to nausea or vomiting and may not reflect the severity of overdose or the risk of organ damage. Management should be in accordance with established treatment guidelines, see BNF overdose section.

Treatment with activated charcoal should be considered if the overdose has been taken within 1 hour. Plasma paracetamol concentration should be measured at 4 hours or later after ingestion (earlier concentrations unreliable). Treatment with N-acetylcysteine may be used up to 24 hours after ingestion of paracetamol, however, the maximum protective effect is obtained up to 8 hours post-ingestion. The effectiveness of the antidote declines sharply after this time. If required the patient should be given intravenous N-acetylcysteine, in line with the established dosage schedule. If vomiting is not a problem, oral methionine may be a suitable alternative for remote areas, outside hospital. Management of patients who present with serious hepatic dysfunction beyond 24h from ingestion should be discussed with the NPIS or a liver unit.

Pseudoephedrine:

As with other sympathomimetic agents, symptoms of overdose include irritability, restlessness, tremor, convulsions, palpitations, hypertension and difficulty in micturition.

Necessary measures should be taken to maintain and support respiration and control convulsions. Gastric lavage should be performed if indicated. Catheterisation of the bladder may be necessary. If desired, the elimination of pseudoephedrine can be accelerated by acid diuresis or by dialysis.

Diphenhydramine:

Symptoms of overdose may include drowsiness, hyperpyrexia and anticholinergic effects. With higher doses, and particularly in children, symptoms of CNS excitation include insomnia, nervousness, tremors and epileptiform convulsions. With massive overdose, coma or cardiovascular collapse may follow.

Treatment of overdosage should be symptomatic and supportive. Measures to promote rapid gastric emptying (such as induced emesis or gastric lavage) and in cases of acute poisoning activated charcoal, may be useful. The intravenous use of physostigmine may be efficacious in antagonising severe anticholinergic symptoms.

5. PHARMACOLOGICAL PROPERTIES

5.1 Pharmacodynamic properties
Paracetamol:

Paracetamol is an analgesic and antipyretic. The therapeutic effects of paracetamol are thought to be related to inhibition of prostaglandin synthesis, as a result of the inhibition of cyclo-oxygenase. There is some evidence that it is a more effective inhibitor of central as opposed to peripheral cyclo-oxygenase. Paracetamol has only weak anti-inflammatory properties. The antipyretic action of paracetamol appears to stem from a direct action on the hypothalamic heat-regulating centres, producing peripheral vasodilation, and consequent loss of heat.

Pseudoephedrine:

Pseudoephedrine has direct and indirect sympathomimetic activity and is an orally effective upper respiratory tract decongestant. Pseudoephedrine is less potent than ephedrine in producing both tachycardia and elevation in systolic blood pressure and less potent in causing stimulation of the central nervous system.

Diphenhydramine:

Diphenhydramine is an antihistamine that competes with histamine for receptor sites on effector cells. The compound also possesses antispasmodic, antitussive, antiemetic, sedative and secretolytic effects.

5.2 Pharmacokinetic properties
Paracetamol:

Paracetamol is rapidly absorbed from the gastrointestinal tract, with peak plasma concentrations occurring approximately 30 to 90 minutes following oral administration. Paracetamol is incompletely available to the systemic circulation after oral administration since a variable proportion is lost through first pass metabolism. Oral bioavailability in adults appears to depend on the amount of paracetamol administered, increasing from 63% following a 500mg dose, to nearly 90% after 1 or 2 g. Effects are apparent within 30 minutes and last for between 4 and 8 hours. Less than 50% is protein bound. The compound is extensively metabolised in the liver to inactive conjugates of glucuronic and sulphonic acids (saturable) and to a hepatotoxic intermediate metabolite (first order) by P450 mixed function oxidase. The intermediate is detoxified by glutathione (saturable). Less than 4% is excreted unchanged in the urine.

Half-life for the drug usually lies in the range 2.75-3.25 hours although this may be mildly increased in chronic liver disease, or extended in acute paracetamol poisoning.

There is some evidence to suggest that serum half-life is markedly increased, and clearance of paracetamol is decreased in frail, immobile, elderly subjects when compared to fit young individuals. However, differences in pharmacokinetic parameters observed between fit young and fit elderly subjects are not thought to be of clinical significance.

Pseudoephedrine:

Pseudoephedrine is rapidly and completely absorbed after oral administration. After the administration of an oral dose of 60mg to healthy adults, a peak plasma concentration of 180ng/ml was obtained approximately 2 hours post dose. The plasma half-life is approximately 5.5 hours. Urinary elimination is accelerated, and half-life consequently decreased, when the urine is acidified. Conversely, as the urine pH increases, the urinary elimination is reduced and half-life is increased. Pseudoephedrine is partly metabolised in the liver by N-demethylation to an active metabolite. Excretion of pseudoephedrine and its metabolite is mainly in the urine.

Diphenhydramine:

Diphenhydramine is well absorbed from the gastrointestinal tract. Peak serum levels are reached between 2 and 2.5 hours after an oral dose. Duration of activity is between 4 and 8 hours. The drug is widely distributed throughout the body, including the CNS and some 78% is bound to plasma proteins. Estimates of the volume of distribution lie in the range 3.3-6.8L/kg

Diphenhydramine experiences extensive first-pass metabolism, two successive N-demethylations, and the resultant amine is then oxidised to a carboxylic acid. Values for plasma clearance lie in the range 600-1300ml/min and the terminal elimination half-life lies in the range 3.4-9.3 hours. Little unchanged drug is excreted in the urine.

5.3 Preclinical safety data
Preclinical data, where available, reveal no special hazard for humans based on conventional studies of safety pharmacology, repeat dose toxicity, genotoxicity, carcinogenic potential, and toxicity to reproduction.

6. PHARMACEUTICAL PARTICULARS

6.1 List of excipients
Each white (DAY) tablet is formulated to contain:

Pregelatinised maize starch

Povidone

Crospovidone

Stearic acid

Microcrystalline cellulose

Croscarmellose sodium

Magnesium stearate

Each blue (NIGHT) tablet is formulated to contain:

Core

Microcrystalline cellulose

Maize starch

Sodium starch glycollate

Hydroxypropylcellulose

Pregelatinised maize starch

Croscarmellose sodium

Stearic acid (powder)

Magnesium stearate

Film coating:

Methocel E5 (E5 Premium)

Propylene glycol

Opaspray M-1F-4315B

6.2 Incompatibilities
None known.

6.3 Shelf life
36 months.

6.4 Special precautions for storage
Do not store above 25°C. Store in the original package.

6.5 Nature and contents of container
Carton containing 20 tablets (15 'DAY' tablets and 5 'NIGHT' tablets).

Each blister strip consists of a white, opaque PVC/PE/PVdC film and either:

Aluminium foil blister lidding

Or

Paper/aluminium foil child resistant blister lidding

6.6 Instructions for use and handling
Not applicable.

Administrative Data

7. MARKETING AUTHORISATION HOLDER
Pfizer Consumer Healthcare
Walton Oaks
Dorking Road
Walton-on-the-Hill
Surrey KT20 7NS
United Kingdom

8. MARKETING AUTHORISATION NUMBER(S)
PL 15513/0108

9. DATE OF FIRST AUTHORISATION/RENEWAL OF THE AUTHORISATION
12th March 2002

10. DATE OF REVISION OF THE TEXT
April 2005

Benylin dry Coughs (Non-Drowsy)

(Pfizer Consumer Healthcare)

1. NAME OF THE MEDICINAL PRODUCT
BENYLIN DRY COUGHS (NON DROWSY)

2. QUALITATIVE AND QUANTITATIVE COMPOSITION
BENYLIN DRY COUGHS (NON DROWSY) contains -

Dextromethorphan hydrobromide Ph Eur 7.5 mg in each 5 ml

3. PHARMACEUTICAL FORM
Pale brown coloured, peach flavoured syrup.

4. CLINICAL PARTICULARS

4.1 Therapeutic indications
BENYLIN DRY COUGHS (NON DROWSY) is indicated as an antitussive, for the relief of persistent, dry, irritating cough.

4.2 Posology and method of administration
Adults and Children over 12 years:

Oral. 10 ml syrup (15 mg dextromethorphan) 4 times a day.

Maximum daily dose: 40 ml syrup (60 mg dextromethorphan)

Children aged 6 to 12 years:

Oral. 5 ml syrup (7.5 mg dextromethorphan) 4 times a day.

Maximum daily dose: 20 ml syrup (30 mg dextromethorphan)

The Elderly (over 65 years)

As for adults above.

BENYLIN DRY COUGHS (NON DROWSY) is not suitable for administration to children under 6 years of age. Benylin for Children's Cough's is recommended for children aged 1 to 5 years.

Hepatic/renal dysfunction

Due to the extensive hepatic metabolism of dextromethorphan, caution should be exercised in the presence of moderate to severe hepatic impairment (see Pharmacokinetics).

4.3 Contraindications
BENYLIN DRY COUGHS (NON DROWSY) is contraindicated in individuals with known hypersensitivity to the product or any of its components.

BENYLIN DRY COUGHS (NON DROWSY) is contraindicated in individuals who are taking, or have taken, monoamine oxidase inhibitors within the preceding two weeks. The concomitant use of a dextromethorphan-containing product and monoamine oxidase inhibitors, can occasionally result in symptoms such as hyperpyrexia, hallucinations, gross excitation or coma.

Dextromethorphan, in common with other centrally acting antitussive agents, should not be given to subjects in, or at risk of developing respiratory failure.

4.4 Special warnings and special precautions for use
BENYLIN DRY COUGHS (NON DROWSY) should not be administered to patients with chronic or persistent cough, such as occurs with asthma, or where cough is accompanied by excessive secretions, unless directed by a physician.

There have been no specific studies of BENYLIN Dry Coughs (Non Drowsy) in renal or hepatic dysfunction. Due to the extensive hepatic metabolism of dextromethorphan, caution should be exercised in the presence of hepatic impairment.

4.5 Interaction with other medicinal products and other forms of Interaction
The concomitant use of a dextromethorphan-containing product and monoamine oxidase inhibitors can occasionally result in symptoms such as hyperpyrexia, hallucinations, gross excitation or coma.

4.6 Pregnancy and lactation
Although dextromethorphan has been in widespread use for many years without apparent ill consequence, there is insufficient information on the effects of administration during human pregnancy. In addition, it is not known whether dextromethorphan or its metabolites are excreted in breast milk.

BENYLIN DRY COUGHS (NON DROWSY) should therefore only be used when the potential benefit of treatment to the mother exceeds any possible hazards to the developing foetus or suckling infant.

4.7 Effects on ability to drive and use machines
Unlikely to produce an effect.

4.8 Undesirable effects
Side effects attributed to dextromethorphan are uncommon; occasionally dizziness, nausea, vomiting, or gastrointestinal disturbance may occur.

4.9 Overdose
Signs and symptoms

The effects of acute toxicity from BENYLIN DRY COUGHS (NON DROWSY) overdose may include drowsiness, lethargy, nystagmus, ataxia, respiratory depression, nausea, vomiting, hyperactivity.

Treatment

Treatment should be symptomatic and supportive. Gastric lavage may be of use. Naloxone has been used successfully as a specific antagonist to dextromethorphan toxicity in children.

5. PHARMACOLOGICAL PROPERTIES
5.1 Pharmacodynamic properties
Dextromethorphan is a non-opioid antitussive drug. It exerts its antitussive activity by acting on the cough centre in the medulla oblongata, raising the threshold for the cough reflex. A single oral dose of 10-20 mg dextromethorphan produces its antitussive action within 1 hour and lasts for at least 4 hours.

5.2 Pharmacokinetic properties
Absorption

Dextromethorphan is well absorbed from the gut following oral administration. Due to individual differences in the metabolism of dextromethorphan, pharmacokinetic values are highly variable. After the administration of a 20 mg dose of dextromethorphan to healthy volunteers, the C_{max} varied from < 1 mg/l to 8 mg/l, occurring within 2.5 hours of administration.

Distribution

Due to extensive pre-systemic metabolism by the liver, detailed analysis of the distribution of orally administered dextromethorphan is not possible.

Metabolism and Elimination

Dextromethorphan undergoes rapid and extensive first-pass metabolism in the liver after oral administration. Genetically controlled O-demethylation is the main determinant of dextromethorphan pharmacokinetics in human volunteers. It appears that there are distinct phenotypes for this oxidation process resulting in highly variable pharmacokinetics between subjects. Unmetabolised dextromethorphan, together with the three demethylated morphinan metabolites dextrophan (also known as 3-hydroxy-N-methylmorphinan) 3-hydroxymorphinan and 3-methoxymorphinan have been identified as conjugated products in the urine. Dextrorphan, which also has antitussive action, is the main metabolite.

5.3 Preclinical safety data
Mutagenicity

There is insufficient information to determine whether dextromethorphan has mutagenic potential.

Carcinogenicity

There is insufficient information to determine whether dextromethorphan has carcinogenic potential, although such effects have not been associated with these drugs in animal studies.

Teratogenicity

There is insufficient information to determine whether dextromethorphan has teratogenic potential.

Fertility

There is insufficient information to determine whether dextromethorphan has potential to impair fertility.

6. PHARMACEUTICAL PARTICULARS
6.1 List of excipients
Liquid glucose

Sucrose

Sorbitol solution 70% non crystallising

Ethanol 96%

Glycerol

Saccharin sodium

Citric acid monohydrate

Sodium benzoate

Caramel T12

Imitation peach flavour

Levomenthol

Carbomer

Purified Water

6.2 Incompatibilities
None known

6.3 Shelf life
3 years

6.4 Special precautions for storage
Store below 30°C

6.5 Nature and contents of container
BENYLIN Dry Coughs (Non Drowsy) is presented in an amber glass bottle containing 125 ml syrup or 30 ml (sample) with ROPP aluminium caps or a 3 piece plastic child resistant, tamper evident closure fitted with a polyester faced wad or polyethylene/expanded polyethylene laminated wad.

6.6 Instructions for use and handling
None applicable

Administrative Data
7. MARKETING AUTHORISATION HOLDER
Pfizer Consumer Healthcare

Alternative Trading Style:

Warner-Lambert Consumer Healthcare

Walton Oaks

Dorking Road

Walton-on-the-Hill

Surrey KT20 7NS

United Kingdom

8. MARKETING AUTHORISATION NUMBER(S)
15513/0051

9. DATE OF FIRST AUTHORISATION/RENEWAL OF THE AUTHORISATION
Date Granted: 16 June 1997

10. DATE OF REVISION OF THE TEXT
January 2004

Benylin Dry Coughs (Original)

(Pfizer Consumer Healthcare)

1. NAME OF THE MEDICINAL PRODUCT
BENYLIN Dry Coughs (Original)

2. QUALITATIVE AND QUANTITATIVE COMPOSITION
BENYLIN Dry Coughs (Original) contains diphenhydramine hydrochloride 14 mg, L-menthol 2 mg and dextromethorphan hydrobromide 6.5 mg in each 5 ml.

3. PHARMACEUTICAL FORM
Clear red syrup

4. CLINICAL PARTICULARS
4.1 Therapeutic indications
BENYLIN Dry Coughs (Original) is indicated as an antitussive, for the relief of persistent, dry, irritating cough.

4.2 Posology and method of administration
Adults and children 12 years and over:
Oral. 10 ml syrup 4 times a day.

Children aged 6 to 12 years:
Oral. 5 ml syrup 4 times a day.

Children under 6 years:
Not recommended.

The Elderly:
Normal adult dosage is appropriate, [See Pharmacokinetics in the Elderly].

4.3 Contraindications
BENYLIN Dry Coughs (Original) is contraindicated in individuals with known hypersensitivity to the product or any of its components.

BENYLIN Dry Coughs (Original) is contraindicated in individuals who are taking, or have taken, monoamine oxidase inhibitors within the preceding two weeks. The concomitant use of a dextromethorphan-containing product and monoamine oxidase inhibitors, can occasionally result in symptoms such as hyperpyrexia, hallucinations, gross excitation or coma.

Dextromethorphan, in common with other centrally acting antitussive agents, should not be given to subjects in, or at risk of developing respiratory failure.

4.4 Special warnings and special precautions for use
This product may cause drowsiness, if affected, individuals should not drive or operate machinery.

Diphenhydramine should not be taken by individuals with narrow-angle glaucoma or symptomatic prostatic hypertrophy. Subjects with moderate to severe renal or hepatic dysfunction should exercise caution when using this this product (see pharmacokinetics).

4.5 Interaction with other medicinal products and other forms of Interaction
The concomitant use of a dextromethorphan-containing product and monoamine oxidase inhibitors, can occasionally result in symptoms such as hyperpyrexia, hallucinations, gross excitation or coma. [See Contraindications]

This product contains diphenhydramine and therefore may potentiate the effects of alcohol, and other CNS depressants.

As diphenhydramine possess some anticholinergic activity, the effects of anticholinergics (e.g. some psychotrophic drugs and atropine) may be potentiated by this product. This may result in tachycardia, mouth dryness, gastrointestinal disturbances (e.g. colic), urinary retention and headache.

4.6 Pregnancy and lactation
Both diphenhydramine and dextromethorphan have been in widespread use for many years without apparent ill consequence. However, there is insufficient information on the effects of the administration of dextromethorphan during human pregnancy. In addition, it is not known whether dextromethorphan or its metabolites are excreted in breast milk. Diphenhydramine is known to cross the placenta and has also been detected in breast milk.

BENYLIN Dry Coughs (Original) should therefore only be used when the potential benefit of treatment to the mother exceeds any possible hazards to the developing foetus or suckling infant.

4.7 Effects on ability to drive and use machines
This product may cause drowsiness, if affected, individuals should not drive or operate machinery.

4.8 Undesirable effects
Diphenhydramine may cause: drowsiness; dizziness; gastrointestinal disturbance; dry mouth, nose and throat; difficulty in urination or blurred vision.

Dextromethorphan: dizziness, nausea, vomiting, or gastrointestinal disturbance may occur.

Adverse reactions to menthol at the low concentration present in BENYLIN Dry Coughs (Original) are not anticipated.

4.9 Overdose
Symptoms and signs

The effects of acute toxicity from of BENYLIN Dry Coughs (Original) may include drowsiness, hyperpyrexia, anticholinergic effects, lethargy, nystagmus, ataxia, respiratory depression, nausea, vomiting, hyperactivity. With higher doses, and particularly in children, symptoms of CNS excitation including hallucinations and convulsions may appear; with massive doses, coma or cardiovascular collapse may follow.

Treatment

Treatment of overdose should be symptomatic and supportive. Measures to promote rapid gastric emptying (with syrup of ipecac-induced emesis or gastric lavage) and, in cases of acute poisoning, the use of activated charcoal, may be useful. The intravenous use of physostigmine may be efficacious in antagonising severe anticholinergic symptoms. Naloxone has been used successfully as a specific antagonist to dextromethorphan toxicity in children. Convulsions may be controlled with diazepam and thiopental sodium.

5. PHARMACOLOGICAL PROPERTIES
5.1 Pharmacodynamic properties
Dextromethorphan

Dextromethorphan is a non-opioid antitussive drug. It exerts its antitussive activity by acting on the cough centre in the *medulla oblongata*, raising the threshold for the cough reflex. A single oral dose of 10-20 mg dextromethorphan produces its antitussive action within 1 hour and lasts for at least 4 hours.

Diphenhydramine

Diphenhydramine possesses antitussive, antihistaminic, and anticholinergic properties. Experiments have shown that the antitussive effect (resulting from an action on the brainstem) is discrete from its antihistaminic effect. The duration of activity of diphenhydramine is between 4 and 8 hours.

Menthol has mild local anaesthetic and decongestant properties.

5.2 Pharmacokinetic properties

Absorption

Diphenhydramine, dextromethorphan and menthol are well absorbed from the gut following oral administration. Peak serum levels of diphenhydramine following a 50 mg oral dose are reached at between 2 and 2.5 hrs after an oral dose. Due to individual differences in the metabolism of dextromethorphan [See Metabolism and Elimination], pharmacokinetic values are highly variable. After the administration of a 20 mg dose of dextromethorphan to healthy volunteers, the C_{max} varied from $< 1\mu g/l$ to $8\mu g/l$, occurring within 2.5 hrs of administration.

Distribution

Diphenhydramine

Diphenhydramine is widely distributed throughout the body, including the CNS. Following a 50 mg oral dose of diphenhydramine, the volume of distribution is in the range 3.3 - 6.8 L/kg and it is some 78% bound to plasma proteins.

Dextromethorphan

Due to extensive pre-systemic metabolism by the liver, detailed analysis of the distribution of orally administered dextromethorphan is not possible.

Metabolism and elimination

Diphenhydramine

Diphenhydramine undergoes extensive first pass metabolism. Two successive N-demethylations occur, with the resultant amine being oxidised to a carboxylic acid. Values for plasma clearance of a 50 mg oral dose of diphenhydramine lie in the range 600 - 1300 ml/min, and the terminal elimination half-life lies in the range 3.4 - 9.3 hours. Little unchanged drug is excreted in the urine.

Dextromethorphan

Dextromethorphan undergoes rapid and extensive first-pass metabolism in the liver after oral administration. Genetically controlled O-demethylation is the main determinant of dextromethorphan pharmacokinetics in human volunteers. It appears that there are distinct phenotypes for this oxidation process resulting in highly variable pharmacokinetics between subjects. Unmetabolised dextromethorphan, together with the three demethylated morphinan metabolites; dextrorphan (also known as 3-hydroxy-N-methylmorphinan), 3-hydroxymorphinan and 3-methoxymorphinan have been identified as conjugated products in the urine. Dextrorphan, which also has antitussive action, is the main metabolite.

Menthol

Menthol is hydroxylated in the liver by microsomal enzymes to p-methane -3,8 diol. This is then conjugated with glucuronide and excreted both in urine and bile as the glucuronide.

Pharmacokinetics in Renal Impairment

The results of a review on the use of diphenhydramine in renal failure suggest that in moderate to severe renal failure, the dose interval should be extended by a period dependent on the glomerular filtration rate (GFR).

There have been no specific studies of BENYLIN Dry Coughs (Original) or dextromethorphan in renal impairment.

Pharmacokinetics in Hepatic Impairment

After intravenous administration of 0.8 mg/kg diphenhydramine, a prolonged half-life was noted in patients with chronic liver disease which correlated with the severity of the disease. However, the mean plasma clearance and apparent volume of distribution were not significantly affected.

There have been no specific studies of BENYLIN Dry Coughs (Original) or dextromethorphan in hepatic impairment.

Pharmacokinetics in the Elderly

Pharmacokinetic studies indicate no major differences in distribution or elimination of diphenhydramine compared to younger adults.

There have been no specific studies of BENYLIN Dry Coughs (Original) or dextromethorphan in the elderly.

5.3 Preclinical safety data

The active ingredients of Benylin Dry Coughs (Original) are well-known constituents of medicinal products and their safety profiles are well documented. The results of pre-clinical studies do not add anything of relevance for therapeutic purposes.

6. PHARMACEUTICAL PARTICULARS

6.1 List of excipients

Liquid glucose

Sucrose

Ethanol (96%)

Glycerol

Sodium citrate

Saccharin sodium

Citric acid monohydrate

Sodium benzoate

Caramel T12

Raspberry flavour 503.850/T

Carbomer

Ponceau 4R (E124)

Purified water

6.2 Incompatibilities

None known

6.3 Shelf life

3 years.

6.4 Special precautions for storage

Do not store above 30°C. Store in the original container

6.5 Nature and contents of container

BENYLIN Dry Coughs (Original) is presented in a 30 or 125 ml round amber glass bottle with ropp aluminium cap or a 3 piece plastic child resistant, tamper evident closure fitted with a polyester faced wad or polyethylene/ expanded polyethylene laminated wad.

6.6 Instructions for use and handling

None applicable.

7. MARKETING AUTHORISATION HOLDER

Pfizer Consumer Healthcare

Alternative Trading Style:

Warner-Lambert Consumer Healthcare

Walton Oaks

Dorking Road

Walton-on-the-Hill

Surrey KT20 7NS

United Kingdom

8. MARKETING AUTHORISATION NUMBER(S)

PL 15513/0053

9. DATE OF FIRST AUTHORISATION/RENEWAL OF THE AUTHORISATION

15 December 1997

10. DATE OF REVISION OF THE TEXT

January 2004

Benylin Four Flu Liquid

(Pfizer Consumer Healthcare)

1. NAME OF THE MEDICINAL PRODUCT

Benylin Four Flu liquid

2. QUALITATIVE AND QUANTITATIVE COMPOSITION

Each 20 ml contains:

Diphenhydramine hydrochloride 25 mg

Paracetamol 1000 mg

Pseudoephedrine hydrochloride 45 mg

3. PHARMACEUTICAL FORM

Oral solution

A clear orange to brown oral solution

4. CLINICAL PARTICULARS

4.1 Therapeutic indications

For the relief of symptoms associated with colds and flu; including coughing, fever, headache, muscular aches and pains and congestion.

4.2 Posology and method of administration

For oral use

Adults, the elderly and children over 12 years

One 20 ml dose up to four times daily, as required. Do not take more frequently than every four hours.

Children 6 to 12 years

One 10 ml dose up to four times daily, as required. Do not take more frequently than every four hours.

Children under 6 years

Not recommended

4.3 Contraindications

Known hypersensitivity to any of the ingredients, severe hypertension or severe hyperthyroidism.

4.4 Special warnings and special precautions for use

This product should be used with caution by patients with cardiovascular disease, hypertension, hyperthyroidism, prostatic enlargement, liver disease, renal disease, glaucoma or diabetes.

The hazard of overdose is greater in those with non-cirrhotic alcoholic liver disease.

Patients should be advised not to exceed the recommended dose.

This preparation may cause urinary retention in patients with prostatic hypertrophy.

The product labelling will contain the following advice:-

Immediate medical advice should be sought in the event of an overdose, even if you feel well, because of the risk of delayed, serious liver damage.

Do not take with any other paracetamol-containing products.

If symptoms persist, consult your doctor or pharmacist.

Keep out of the reach of children.

4.5 Interaction with other medicinal products and other forms of Interaction

Diphenhydramine may potentiate the effects of other CNS depressants such as anti-depressants, minor tranquilisers, neuroleptics, barbiturates and alcohol, and other drugs with anti-cholinergic properties such as tricyclic anti-depressants.

Pseudoephedrine may reverse the effect of antihypertensive agents which modify sympathetic activity, and concomitant use with other sympathomimetic agents such as decongestants, tricyclic anti-depressants and appetite supressants or with monoamineoxidase inhibitors, which interfere with the catabolism of sympathomimetic amines may cause a rise in blood pressure. Concomitant use of monoamine oxidase inhibitors, or use of this class of drug within the previous 14 days should be avoided.

The speed of absorption of paracetamol may be increased by metoclopramide or domperidone, and absorption reduced by colestyramine.

The anticoagulant effect of warfarin and other coumarins may be enhanced by prolonged regular use of paracetamol with increased risk of bleeding; occasional doses have no significant effect.

The use of drugs which induce hepatic microsomal enzymes, such as anticonvulsants and oral contraceptive steroids, may increase the extent of metabolism of paracetamol, resulting in reduced plasma concentrations of the drug and a faster elimination rate.

4.6 Pregnancy and lactation

The active ingredients in Benylin Four Flu have not been conclusively associated with adverse effects on the developing foetus; but as with all drugs, care should be exercised in use of the product, particularly during the first trimester.

All of the actives are excreted into breast milk, although few adverse effects have been reported as a result of ingestion, cautious use of Benylin Four Flu is advised during lactation.

4.7 Effects on ability to drive and use machines

Benylin Four Flu may cause drowsiness. If patients are affected they should not drive or use machinery.

4.8 Undesirable effects

Adverse effects of paracetamol are rare but hypersensitivity reactions including skin rashes may occur. There have been reports of blood dyscrasias including thrombocytopoenia and agranulocytosis following paracetamol use, but these were not necessarily causally related to the drug.

Serious side-effects associated with the use of pseudoephedrine are extremely rare. The use of pseudoephedrine has been associated with tachycardia. Symptoms of central nervous system excitation may occur, including sleep disturbances and rarely hallucinations have been reported. Urinary retention has been reported occasionally in men receiving pseudoephedrine, prostatic enlargement could have been a predisposing factor. Skin rashes, with or without irritation, have occasionally been reported with pseudoephedrine.

Side effects of diphenhydramine include drowsiness, dizziness, headache, blurred vision, gastrointestinal disturbances, dry mouth, nose and throat, or urinary retention.

Hypersensitivity reactions have been reported, in particular, itching and skin rashes, erythema and urticaria.

4.9 Overdose

Paracetamol: Immediate treatment is essential in the management of paracetamol overdose. In view of the lack of significant early symptoms, any patient who is suspected of consuming an overdose of paracetamol should be referred to hospital for immediate medical attention. Administration of antidotes, such as oral methionine or intravenous N-acetylcysteine, may be required and activated charcoal should be considered if paracetamol in excess of 150 mg/ kg or 12 g (whichever is the smaller) is thought to have been ingested within the previous hour. General supportive measures must be available. Acetylcysteine may have a beneficial effect up to, and possibly beyond, 24 hours.

Symptoms of paracetamol overdose in the first 24 hours are pallor, nausea, vomiting, anorexia and abdominal pain. Liver damage may become apparent 12 to 48 hours after ingestion. Abnormalities of glucose metabolism and metabolic acidosis may occur. In severe poisoning, hepatic failure may progress to encephalopathy, coma and death. Acute renal failure with acute tubular necrosis may develop even in the absence of severe liver damage. Cardiac arrhythmias and pancreatitis have been reported.

As little as 10-15g or 150 mg/ kg of paracetamol taken within 24 hours may cause severe liver damage. It is considered that this is due to excess quantities of toxic metabolite (usually detoxified by glutathione when normal doses of paracetamol are ingested), becoming irreversibly bound to liver tissue.

Diphenhydramine: Symptoms of overdose may include drowsiness, hyperpyrexia and anticholinergic effects. With higher doses, and particularly in children, symptoms of CNS excitation include insomnia, nervousness, tremors and epileptiform convulsions. With massive overdose, coma or cardiovascular collapse may follow.

Treatment of overdose should be symptomatic and supportive. Measures to promote gastric emptying (such as induced emesis or gastric lavage), and in cases of acute poisoning activated charcoal, may be useful.

Pseudoephedrine: As with other sympathomimetic agents, symptoms of overdose include irritability, restlessness, tremor, convulsions, palpitations, hypertension and difficulty in micturition.

Necessary measures should be taken to maintain and support respiration and control convulsions. Gastric lavage should be performed if indicated. Catheterisation of the bladder may be necessary. If desired, the elimination of pseudoephedrine can be accelerated by acid diuresis or by dialysis.

5. PHARMACOLOGICAL PROPERTIES

5.1 Pharmacodynamic properties

Diphenhydramine has a potent antihistaminic action although the actions most beneficial in influenza are its antitussive and to a lesser extent anticholinergic properties, which may alleviate mucus hypersecretion. Paracetamol has central analgesic and antipyretic actions and pseudoephedrine is an indirectly acting sympathomimetic which has vasoconstrictor, bronchodilator and decongestant effects.

5.2 Pharmacokinetic properties

Diphenhydramine is well absorbed after oral administration with peak plasma levels at 2.5 hours and is subject to extensive first pass metabolism. The drug is 75% bound to plasma proteins, but binding decreases with chronic liver disease. Metabolism is by 2 successive N-demethylations followed by oxidation to a carboxylic acid. The terminal half life lies between 3.4 and 9.3 hours.

Paracetamol is rapidly and completely absorbed with peak plasma levels seen within 30 to 60 minutes. Less than 50% is protein bound and the drug is uniformly distributed throughout the body fluids. Paracetamol is eliminated by metabolism to inactive conjugates followed by urinary excretion. The half life is 2.75- 3.25 hours.

Pseudoephedrine is rapidly absorbed, with peak serum levels after approximately 2.6 hours and onset of effect within about 30 minutes. It is well distributed throughout body fluids and tissues. Approximately 50% of the drug is excreted unchanged, the remainder undergoes metabolism to inactive metabolites. About 6% is converted to the active metabolite norpseudoephedrine.

5.3 Preclinical safety data

The active ingredients of Benylin Four Flu liquid are well known constituents of medicinal products and their safety profile is well documented. The results of preclinical studies do not therefore add anything of relevance for therapeutic purposes.

6. PHARMACEUTICAL PARTICULARS

6.1 List of excipients

Polyethylene glycol, glycerol, propylene glycol, saccharin sodium, citric acid monohydrate, sodium benzoate, eucalyptol, menthol, sodium carboxymethylcellulose, sodium citrate, ethanol 10% v/v, colourings: Quinoline Yellow E 104, Ponceau 4R (E 124), Patent Blue V (E 131), flavourings: honey, lemon and cream. Water

6.2 Incompatibilities

None

6.3 Shelf life

3 years.

6.4 Special precautions for storage

Do not store above 30°C. Keep container in the outer carton.

6.5 Nature and contents of container

30 ml and 200 ml round amber glass bottles with aluminium screw cap.

30 ml and 200 ml round amber glass bottles with a plastic child resistant, tamper evident closure fitted with a polyester faced wad or polyethylene/expanded polyethylene laminated wad.

A polypropylene measuring cup is supplied with each 200 ml bottle.

6.6 Instructions for use and handling

Keep bottle tightly closed.

Administrative Data

7. MARKETING AUTHORISATION HOLDER

Pfizer Consumer Healthcare

Alternative Trading Style:

Warner-Lambert Consumer Healthcare
Walton Oaks
Dorking Road
Walton-on-the-Hill
Surrey
KT20 7NS
United Kingdom

8. MARKETING AUTHORISATION NUMBER(S)

PL 15513/0057

9. DATE OF FIRST AUTHORISATION/RENEWAL OF THE AUTHORISATION

15.09.97

10. DATE OF REVISION OF THE TEXT

October 2004

Benylin Four Flu tablets

(Pfizer Consumer Healthcare)

1. NAME OF THE MEDICINAL PRODUCT

Benylin Four Flu tablets

2. QUALITATIVE AND QUANTITATIVE COMPOSITION

Each tablet contains:

Diphenhydramine hydrochloride 12.5 mg
Paracetamol 500 mg
Pseudoephedrine hydrochloride 22.5 mg

3. PHARMACEUTICAL FORM

Orange film coated tablets

4. CLINICAL PARTICULARS

4.1 Therapeutic indications

For the relief of symptoms associated with colds and flu; including coughing, fever, headache, muscular aches and pains and congestion.

4.2 Posology and method of administration

For oral use

Adults, the elderly and children over 12 years

Two tablets, up to four times daily, as required. Do not take more frequently than every four hours.

Children 6 to 12 years

One tablet, up to four times daily, as required. Do not take more frequently than every four hours.

Children under 6 years

Not recommended

4.3 Contraindications

Known hypersensitivity to any of the ingredients, severe hypertension or severe hyperthyroidism.

4.4 Special warnings and special precautions for use

This product should be used with caution by patients with cardiovascular disease, hypertension, hyperthyroidism, liver disease, renal disease, glaucoma or diabetes.

The hazard of overdose is greater in those with non-cirrhotic alcoholic liver disease.

Patients should be advised not to exceed the recommended dose.

This preparation may cause urinary retention in patients with prostatic hypertrophy.

The product labelling will contain the following advice:-

Immediate medical advice should be sought in the event of an overdose, even if you feel well, because of the risk of delayed, serious liver damage.

Do not take with any paracetamol-containing products.

If symptoms persist, consult your doctor or pharmacist.

Keep out of the reach of children

4.5 Interaction with other medicinal products and other forms of Interaction

Diphenhydramine may potentiate the effects of other CNS depressants such as anti-depressants, minor tranquilisers, neuroleptics, barbiturates and alcohol, and other drugs with anti-cholinergic properties such as tricyclic anti-depressants. Pseudoephedrine may reverse the effect of antihypertensive agents which modify sympathetic activity, and concomitant use with other sympathomimetic agents such as decongestants, tricyclic anti-depressants and appetite supressants or with monoamine oxidase inhibitors, which interfere with the catabolism of sympathomimetic amines may cause a rise in blood pressure. Concomitant use of monoamine oxidase inhibitors, or use of this class of drug within the previous 14 days should be avoided.

The speed of absorption of paracetamol may be increased by metoclopramide or domperidone, and absorption reduced by colestyramine.

The anticoagulant effect of warfarin and other coumarins may be enhanced by prolonged regular use of paracetamol with increased risk of bleeding; occasional doses have no significant effect.

The use of drugs which induce hepatic microsomal enzymes, such as anticonvulsants and oral contraceptive steroids, may increase the extent of metabolism of paracetamol, resulting in reduced plasma concentrations of the drug and a faster elimination rate.

4.6 Pregnancy and lactation

The active ingredients in Benylin Four Flu have not been conclusively associated with adverse effects on the developing foetus; but as with all drugs, care should be exercised in use of the product, particularly during the first trimester.

All of the actives are excreted into breast milk, although few adverse effects have been reported as a result of ingestion, cautious use of Benylin Four Flu is advised during lactation.

4.7 Effects on ability to drive and use machines

Benylin Four Flu may cause drowsiness. If patients are affected they should not drive or use machinery.

4.8 Undesirable effects

Adverse effects of paracetamol are rare but hypersensitivity reactions including skin rashes may occur. There have been reports of blood dyscrasias including thrombocytopoenia and agranulocytosis following paracetamol use, but these were not necessarily causally related to the drug.

Serious side-effects associated with the use of pseudoephedrine are extremely rare. The use of pseudoephedrine has been associated with tachycardia. Symptoms of central nervous system excitation may occur, including sleep disturbances and rarely hallucinations have been reported. Urinary retention has been reported occasionally in men receiving pseudoephedrine, prostatic enlargement could have been a predisposing factor. Skin rashes, with or without irritation, have occasionally been reported with pseudoephedrine.

Side effects of diphenhydramine include drowsiness, dizziness, headache, blurred vision, gastrointestinal disturbances, dry mouth, nose and throat, or urinary retention.

Hypersensitivity reactions have been reported, in particular, itching and skin rashes, erythema and urticaria.

4.9 Overdose

Paracetamol: Immediate treatment is essential in the management of paracetamol overdose. In view of the lack of significant early symptoms, any patient who is suspected of consuming an overdose of paracetamol should be referred to hospital for immediate medical attention. Administration of antidotes, such as oral methionine or intravenous N-acetylcysteine, may be required and activated charcoal should be considered if paracetamol in excess of 150 mg/ kg or 12 g (whichever is the smaller) is thought to have been ingested within the previous hour. General supportive measures must be available. Acetylcysteine may have a beneficial effect up to, and possibly beyond, 24 hours.

Symptoms of paracetamol overdosage in the first 24 hours are pallor, nausea, vomiting, anorexia and abdominal pain. Liver damage may become apparent 12 to 48 hours after ingestion. Abnormalities of glucose metabolism and metabolic acidosis may occur. In severe poisoning, hepatic failure may progress to encephalopathy, coma and death. Acute renal failure with acute tubular necrosis may develop even in the absence of severe liver damage. Cardiac arrhythmias and pancreatitis have been reported.

As little as 10-15g or 150 mg/ kg of paracetamol taken within 24 hours may cause severe liver damage. It is considered that this is due to excess quantities of toxic metabolite (usually detoxified by glutathione when normal doses of paracetamol are ingested), becoming irreversibly bound to liver tissue.

Diphenhydramine: Symptoms of overdose may include drowsiness, hyperpyrexia and anticholinergic effects. With higher doses, and particularly in children, symptoms of CNS excitation include insomnia, nervousness, tremors and epileptiform convulsions. With massive overdose, coma or cardiovascular collapse may follow.

Treatment of overdosage should be symptomatic and supportive. Measures to promote gastric emptying (such as induced emesis or gastric lavage), and in cases of acute poisoning activated charcoal, may be useful.

Pseudoephedrine: As with other sympathomimetic agents, symptoms of overdose include irritability, restlessness, tremor, convulsions, palpitations, hypertension and difficulty in micturition.

Necessary measures should be taken to maintain and support respiration and control convulsions. Gastric lavage should be performed if indicated. Catheterisation of the bladder may be necessary. If desired, the elimination of pseudoephedrine can be accelerated by acid diuresis or by dialysis.

5. PHARMACOLOGICAL PROPERTIES

5.1 Pharmacodynamic properties

Diphenhydramine has a potent antihistaminic action although the actions most beneficial in influenza are its antitussive and to a lesser extent anticholinergic properties, which may alleviate mucus hypersecretion.

Paracetamol has central analgesic and antipyretic actions and pseudoephedrine is an indirectly acting sympathomimetic which has vasoconstrictor, bronchodilator and decongestant effects.

5.2 Pharmacokinetic properties

Diphenhydramine is well absorbed after oral administration with peak plasma levels at 2.5 hours and is subject to extensive first pass metabolism. The drug is 75% bound to plasma proteins, but binding decreases with chronic liver disease. Metabolism is by 2 successive N-demethylations followed by oxidation to a carboxylic acid. The terminal half life lies between 3.4 and 9.3 hours.

Paracetamol is rapidly and completely absorbed with peak plasma levels seen within 30 to 60 minutes. Less than 50% is protein bound and the drug is uniformly distributed throughout the body fluids. Paracetamol is eliminated by metabolism to inactive conjugates followed by urinary excretion. The half life is 2.75 - 3.25 hours.

Pseudoephedrine is rapidly absorbed, with peak serum levels after approximately 2.6 hours and onset of effect within about 30 minutes. It is well distributed throughout body fluids and tissues. Approximately 50% of the drug is excreted unchanged, the remainder undergoes metabolism to inactive metabolites. About 6% is converted to the active metabolite norpseudoephedrine.

5.3 Preclinical safety data

The active ingredients of Benylin Four Flu tablets are well known constituents of medicinal products and their safety profile is well documented. The results of preclinical studies do not add anything of relevance for therapeutic purposes.

6. PHARMACEUTICAL PARTICULARS

6.1 List of excipients

Pregelatinized maize starch

Povidone

Crospovidone

Stearic acid

Cellulose microcrystalline

Pregelatinised maize starch

Croscarmellose Sodium

Magnesium stearate

Film-coating material

Hypromellose Macrogol 6000 Talc

Titanium dioxide

Quinoline yellow lake Sunset yellow E110

Quinoline yellow

6.2 Incompatibilities

Not applicable.

6.3 Shelf life

3 years

6.4 Special precautions for storage

Do not store above 25°C. Store in the original package.

Keep container in the outer carton

6.5 Nature and contents of container

Blister pack containing 24 tablets (three strips of 8 tablets)

Each blister strip consists of a white, opaque PVC/PVdC film and either:

Aluminium foil blister lidding

Or

Paper/aluminium foil child resistant blister lidding

6.6 Instructions for use and handling

No special requirements

7. MARKETING AUTHORISATION HOLDER

Pfizer Consumer Healthcare

Alternative Trading Style:

Warner-Lambert Consumer Healthcare

Walton Oaks

Dorking Road

Walton-on-the-Hill

Surrey KT20 7NS

8. MARKETING AUTHORISATION NUMBER(S)

PL 15513/0058

9. DATE OF FIRST AUTHORISATION/RENEWAL OF THE AUTHORISATION

1/9/97

10. DATE OF REVISION OF THE TEXT

February 2005

Benylin Tickly Coughs Non-Drowsy

(Pfizer Consumer Healthcare)

1. NAME OF THE MEDICINAL PRODUCT

Nirolex Dry syrup or Nirolex Dry Cough Linctus or Benylin Tickly Coughs Non-Drowsy

2. QUALITATIVE AND QUANTITATIVE COMPOSITION

Active ingredient	per 5 ml
Glycerin	0.75 ml
Liquid sugar de-mineralised (Equivalent to sucrose 1.70 g)	1.93 ml

3. PHARMACEUTICAL FORM

Liquid

4. CLINICAL PARTICULARS

4.1 Therapeutic indications

For the relief of irritating, tickling dry coughs and sore throats.

4.2 Posology and method of administration

Adults and children over 5 years: 10 ml

Children 1 - 5 years: 5 ml

The dose may be repeated three or four times a day.

Children under one year: Not to be given to children under 1 year.

Elderly: There is no need for dosage reduction in the elderly.

For oral administration.

4.3 Contraindications

Hypersensitivity or intolerance to any of the ingredients.

4.4 Special warnings and special precautions for use

Diabetics should take note of the carbohydrate content of this product.

Do not give to children under one year.

Keep all medicines out of the reach of children.

4.5 Interaction with other medicinal products and other forms of Interaction

No clinically significant interactions known.

4.6 Pregnancy and lactation

The safety of Nirolex Dry Syrup during pregnancy and lactation has not been established, but is not considered to constitute a hazard during these periods.

4.7 Effects on ability to drive and use machines

Not applicable.

4.8 Undesirable effects

No adverse effects would be anticipated.

4.9 Overdose

Overdosage would not be expected to cause any problems and treatment would be merely symptomatic and supportive.

5. PHARMACOLOGICAL PROPERTIES

5.1 Pharmacodynamic properties

Glycerin and sucrose have demulcent properties and will soothe irritated sore throats and possibly block sensory cough receptors within the respiratory tract.

5.2 Pharmacokinetic properties

Glycerin is readily absorbed from the gastrointestinal tract and undergoes extensive metabolism principally in the liver. It may be used in the synthesis of lipids, and is metabolised to glucose or glycogen or oxidised to carbon dioxide and water. It may also be excreted in the urine unchanged.

Sucrose is hydrolysed in the small intestine by the enzyme sucrase to glucose and fructose which are then absorbed.

5.3 Preclinical safety data

There are no preclinical data of relevance to the prescriber which are additional to that already included.

6. PHARMACEUTICAL PARTICULARS

6.1 List of excipients

Citric acid monohydrate

Sodium benzoate

Cough Syrup 513277

Black Treacle

Liquid glucose

Purified water

6.2 Incompatibilities

Not applicable.

6.3 Shelf life

36 months.

6.4 Special precautions for storage

None.

6.5 Nature and contents of container

A white flint glass bottle with an aluminium roll-on pilfer proof cap with a flowed in liner, or a triseal (LDPE/EPE/LDPE) liner.

Alternative cap: A wadless polypropylene tamper evident cap.

Pack size: 200ml.

or

An amber glass bottle with an aluminium roll-on pilfer proof cap with a triseal LDPE/EPE/LDPE) liner.

Pack size: 125ml.

or

An amber PET bottle with a child resistant polypropylene cap fitted with an expanded polyethylene liner.

Pack size: 150ml

6.6 Instructions for use and handling

None.

Administrative Data

7. MARKETING AUTHORISATION HOLDER

The Boots Company PLC

1 Thane Road West

Nottingham

NG2 3AA

Trading as: BCM

8. MARKETING AUTHORISATION NUMBER(S)

PL 00014/0550

9. DATE OF FIRST AUTHORISATION/RENEWAL OF THE AUTHORISATION

13th December 1995 / 12th December 2000

10. DATE OF REVISION OF THE TEXT

May 2003

Benylin with Codeine

(Pfizer Consumer Healthcare)

1. NAME OF THE MEDICINAL PRODUCT

Benylin with Codeine

2. QUALITATIVE AND QUANTITATIVE COMPOSITION

BENYLIN WITH CODEINE contains -

Diphenhydramine Hydrochloride	Ph Eur 14.0 mg
Codeine Phosphate	Ph Eur 5.7 mg
L-menthol	Ph Eur 1.1 mg

3. PHARMACEUTICAL FORM

Clear red syrup.

4. CLINICAL PARTICULARS

4.1 Therapeutic indications

BENYLIN WITH CODEINE is indicated for the relief of persistent, dry, irritating cough.

4.2 Posology and method of administration

For oral use.

Adults and children over 12 years:

Two 5 ml spoonfuls four times a day. Maximum daily dose: 40ml syrup

Children:

6-12 years: One 5 ml spoonful four times a day. Maximum daily dose: 20 ml syrup

Under 6 years: Not recommended

The Elderly

Experience suggests that normal adult dosage is appropriate (see Pharmacokinetics – The Elderly)

Hepatic Dysfunction/respiratory failure

BENYLIN with Codeine is not suitable for administration to subjects with hepatic or respiratory failure.

Renal dysfunction

It may be prudent to increase the dosage interval in subjects with moderate to severe renal failure (see Pharmacokinetics – Renal dysfunction).

4.3 Contraindications

Contraindicated in patients with known hypersensitivity to the product or any of its constituents.

This product is contraindicated in individuals with hepatic or respiratory failure.

4.4 Special warnings and special precautions for use

May cause drowsiness. If affected do not drive or operate machinery.

Subjects with moderate to severe renal dysfunction should exercise caution when using this product (see Pharmacokinetics – Renal dysfunction).

Diphenhydramine should not be taken by individuals with narrow-angle glaucoma or symptomatic prostatic hypertrophy.

Codeine is a narcotic analgesic and tolerance, psychological dependence and constipation may occur with high doses.

4.5 Interaction with other medicinal products and other forms of Interaction

This product contains diphenhydramine and therefore may potentiate the effects of alcohol and other CNS depressants.

As diphenhydramine possesses some anticholinergic activity, the effects of anticholinergics (e.g. some psychotropic drugs and atropine) may be potentiated by this product. This may result in tachycardia, dry mouth, gastrointestinal disturbances, (e.g. colic), urinary retention and headache.

4.6 Pregnancy and lactation

Although diphenhydramine and codeine have been in widespread use for many years without ill consequence, both are known to cross the placenta and have been detected in breast milk. Consequently BENYLIN WITH CODEINE should only be used when the potential benefit of treatment to the mother exceeds any possible hazards to the developing foetus or suckling infant.

4.7 Effects on ability to drive and use machines
This product may cause drowsiness. If affected, individuals should not drive or operate machinery.

4.8 Undesirable effects
Side effects associated with the use of BENYIN with Codeine are uncommon.

Diphenhydramine may cause drowsiness, dizziness, gastrointestinal disturbance, dry mouth, nose and throat, difficulty in urination and blurred vision.

Codeine may cause constipation, nausea, dizziness and drowsiness.

Adverse reactions to menthol at the low concentration present in BENYLIN WITH CODEINE are not anticipated.

4.9 Overdose
Symptoms and signs
The signs and symptoms of BENYLIN with Codeine overdose may include drowsiness, hyperpyrexia and anticholinergic effects. With higher doses and particularly in children, symptoms of CNS excitation including hallucinations and convulsions may appear; with massive doses, coma or cardiovascular collapse may follow.

The effects in codeine overdosage will be potentiated by simultaneous ingestion of alcohol and psychotropic drugs.

Codeine overdose associated with central nervous system depression, including respiratory depression, may develop but is unlikely to be severe unless other sedative agents have been co-ingested, including alcohol, or the overdose is very large. The pupils may be pin-point in size; nausea and vomiting are common. Hypotension and tachycardia are possible but unlikely.

Treatment
Treatment of overdose should be symptomatic and supportive. The intravenous use of physostigmine may be efficacious in antagonising severe anticholinergic symptoms.

Management of codeine overdose include general symptomatic and supportive measures including a clear airway and monitoring of vital signs until stable. Consider activated charcoal if an adult presents within one hour of ingestion of more than 350 mg or a child more than 5 mg/kg. Give naloxone if coma or respiratory depression is present. Naloxone is a competitive antagonist and has a short half-life so large and repeated doses may be required in a seriously poisoned patient. Observe for at least four hours after ingestion, or eight hours if sustained release preparation has been taken.

5. PHARMACOLOGICAL PROPERTIES
5.1 Pharmacodynamic properties
Diphenhydramine possesses antitussive, antihistaminic and anticholinergic properties. Experiments have shown that the antitussive effect (resulting from an action on the brainstem) is discrete from its antihistaminic effect. The duration of activity is between 4 and 8 hours.

Codeine is an opiate agonist, having narcotic antitussive and analgesic properties.

Menthol has mild local anaesthetic and decongestant properties.

5.2 Pharmacokinetic properties
Absorption
Diphenhydramine, codeine and menthol are well absorbed from the gut following oral administration. Peak serum levels of diphenhydramine following a 50 mg oral dose are reached at between 2 and 2.5 hours. Peak plasma levels of codeine phosphate are attained within 2 hours following an oral dose.

Distribution
Diphenhydramine is widely distributed throughout the body, including the CNS. Following a 50 mg oral dose of diphenhydramine, the volume of distribution is in the range 3.3 - 6.8 l/kg and it is some 78% bound to plasma proteins. Codeine is widely distributed throughout the body and is some 25% bound to plasma proteins.

Metabolism and Elimination
Diphenhydramine undergoes extensive first pass metabolism. Two successive N-demethylations occur, with the resultant amine being oxidised to a carboxylic acid. Values for plasma clearance of a 50 mg oral dose of diphenhydramine lie in the range 600-1300 ml/min and the terminal elimination half-life lies in the range 3.4 - 9.3 hours. Little unchanged drug is excreted in the urine.

The plasma half-life of codeine has been reported to be between 3 and 4 hours. Metabolism takes place in the liver by O-demethylation to form morphine (approximately 10%), N-demethylation to form norcodeine, and conjugation to form glucuronides and sulphates of both unchanged drug and its metabolites. Codeine and its metabolites are excreted almost entirely by the kidney, mainly as conjugates with glucuronic acid. Menthol is conjugated in the liver and excreted both in urine and bile as the glucuronide.

Menthol is hydroxylated in the liver by microsomal enzymes to P-methane -3,8 diol. This is then conjugated with glucuronide and excreted both in urine and bile as the glucuronide.

The Elderly
Pharmacokinetic studies indicate no major differences in distribution or elimination of diphenhydramine compared to younger adults. There is insufficient information to determine the effects of old age on the pharmacokinetics of codeine (see pharmacokinetics - hepatic dysfunction).

Renal Dysfunction
The results of a review on the use of a variety of drugs in renal failure suggest that, for diphenhydramine, in moderate to severe renal failure, the dose interval should be extended by a period dependent on glomerular filtration rate (GFR). No dosage adjustments are suggested when administering codeine.

Hepatic Dysfunction
After intravenous administration of 0.8 mg/kg diphenhydramine, a prolonged half-life was noted in patients with chronic liver disease which correlated with the severity of the disease. However, the mean plasma clearance and apparent volume of distribution were not significantly affected. As codeine is metabolised in the liver, hepatic dysfunction may affect the pharmacokinetics of codeine.

5.3 Preclinical safety data
Mutagencity
The results of a range of tests suggest that neither diphenhydramine or menthol have mutagenic potential. There is insufficient information available to determine if codeine has mutagenic potential.

Carcinogenicity
There is insufficient information to determine the carcinogenic potential of diphenhydramine, menthol or codeine, although such effects have not been associated with these drugs in animal studies.

Teratogenicity
The results of a number of studies suggest that the administration of either diphenhydramine or menthol does not produce any statistically significant teratogenic effects in rats, rabbits and mice. There is insufficient information to determine whether codeine has teratogenic potential.

Fertility
There is insufficient information to determine whether diphenhydramine, codeine or menthol have the potential to impair fertility, although a diminished fertility rate has been observed in mice administered diphenhydramine in one study.

6. PHARMACEUTICAL PARTICULARS
6.1 List of excipients
Liquid glucose

Sucrose

Sodium Citrate

Ethanol 96%

Citric Acid Monohydrate

Glycerol

Saccharin Sodium

Sodium Benzoate

Ponceau 4R (E124)

Caramel T12

Raspberry Essence Double Strength

Purified Water

6.2 Incompatibilities
None known

6.3 Shelf life
36 months unopened

6.4 Special precautions for storage
Store below 30°C

6.5 Nature and contents of container
300 ml round amber glass bottles with roll on pilfer proof (ROPP) aluminium caps or 3 piece plastic child resistant, tamper evident closure fitted with a polyester faced wad or polyethylene/expanded polyethylene laminated wad.

6.6 Instructions for use and handling
None applicable

Administrative Data
7. MARKETING AUTHORISATION HOLDER
Pfizer Consumer Healthcare

Alternative Trading Style:

Warner-Lambert Consumer Healthcare

Walton Oaks

Dorking Road

Walton-on-the-Hill

Surrey KT20 7NS

United Kingdom

8. MARKETING AUTHORISATION NUMBER(S)
PL 15513/0046

9. DATE OF FIRST AUTHORISATION/RENEWAL OF THE AUTHORISATION
16 June 1997/ 8 May 2000

10. DATE OF REVISION OF THE TEXT
July 2004

Benzamycin Gel

(SCHWARZ PHARMA Limited)

1. NAME OF THE MEDICINAL PRODUCT
Benzamycin Gel.

2. QUALITATIVE AND QUANTITATIVE COMPOSITION
Benzoyl Peroxide 5% w/w.

Erythromycin 3% w/w.

For excipients, see 6.1.

3. PHARMACEUTICAL FORM
Gel after reconstitution

Three components before reconstitution: Gel, Powder, Diluent

4. CLINICAL PARTICULARS
4.1 Therapeutic indications
For the topical treatment of acne vulgaris.

4.2 Posology and method of administration
Benzamycin Gel should be applied twice daily, morning and evening, to areas usually affected by acne or as directed by the physician. These areas should first be gently washed, rinsed with lukewarm water, and gently patted dry. Benzamycin should be applied in a thin layer with the fingertips until dry and the hands washed after application.

It is not recommended for children.

4.3 Contraindications
Benzamycin is contraindicated in persons who have shown hypersensitivity to benzoyl peroxide, erythromycin or any of the other ingredients.

4.4 Special warnings and special precautions for use
For external use only. Keep away from the eyes, nose, mouth and other mucous membranes. Very fair skinned individuals should begin with a single application at bedtime allowing overnight medication.

May bleach hair or dyed fabrics.

4.5 Interaction with other medicinal products and other forms of Interaction
Concomitant topical acne therapy should be used with caution to avoid a possible cumulative irritancy effect. Antagonism has been demonstrated between clindamycin and erythromycin.

4.6 Pregnancy and lactation
The safe use of Benzamycin Gel during pregnancy or lactation has not been established and should only be used if considered essential by the physician.

4.7 Effects on ability to drive and use machines
None known.

4.8 Undesirable effects
Reported adverse reactions have been dryness of the skin, urticaria and face oedema.

4.9 Overdose
Due to the topical administration of this product overdose is unlikely to occur.

5. PHARMACOLOGICAL PROPERTIES
5.1 Pharmacodynamic properties
ATC Classification: D10AE 01 Peroxides (Benzoyl Peroxide); D10AF 02 Anti-infectives for treatment of acne (Erythromycin)

Benzamycin Gel provides an antimicrobial agent with mild keratolytic properties plus antibiotic effects and anti-seborrhoeic properties.

Erythromycin inhibits lipase production whilst benzoyl peroxide reduces the comedone count and has antibacterial action.

5.2 Pharmacokinetic properties
Not applicable.

5.3 Preclinical safety data
Little pre-clinical safety data is available for Benzamycin Gel, as there is sufficient knowledge of the two active ingredients without the need for further studies.

It is highly unlikely that the combination of erythromycin and benzoyl peroxide in a product for topical use will cause any greater risk to the patient than the topical application of these compounds individually.

6. PHARMACEUTICAL PARTICULARS
6.1 List of excipients
Carbomer 980

Sodium Hydroxide

SD Alcohol

Lemon Fragrance Oil

Methyl Salicylate

Docusate Sodium 75% Solution

Purified Water

Ethanol 70 HSE*

* Added by the pharmacist during reconstitution.

6.2 Incompatibilities
None known.

6.3 Shelf life
2 years as packaged for sale.

3 months following reconstitution.

6.4 Special precautions for storage
Prior to reconstitution store at or below 25°C (avoid storage in cold areas). After reconstitution store between 2 and 8°C. Do not freeze.

6.5 Nature and contents of container
Benzamycin Gel Base: 40g white polypropylene jar.

Erythro-pak: 1.6g white polypropylene vial.

Ethanol 70 HSE: 6.5ml plastic capped bottle.

Benzamycin Gel is dispensed in a plastic jar containing 46.6g of gel.

6.6 Instructions for use and handling
Reconstitution Instructions for the Pharmacist:

Prior to dispensing, tap the erythromycin vial to loosen the powder. Add 6ml of the ethanol 70 HSE provided to the powder. Shake to fully dissolve the erythromycin. Disperse the solution into the benzoyl peroxide by stirring for 60 to 90 seconds. Cold storage of the gel prior to reconstitution may cause the gel to thicken and hinder mixing.

Place a 3-month expiry date on the jar.

7. MARKETING AUTHORISATION HOLDER
SCHWARZ PHARMA Limited
Schwarz House
East Street
Chesham
Buckinghamshire HP5 1DG
England

8. MARKETING AUTHORISATION NUMBER(S)
PL 4438/0063

9. DATE OF FIRST AUTHORISATION/RENEWAL OF THE AUTHORISATION
24 January 2003

10. DATE OF REVISION OF THE TEXT
December 2004

Beta-Adalat

(Bayer plc)

1. NAME OF THE MEDICINAL PRODUCT
Beta-Adalat

2. QUALITATIVE AND QUANTITATIVE COMPOSITION
One capsule contains 20 mg nifedipine and 50 mg atenolol.

For excipients see Section 6.1.

3. PHARMACEUTICAL FORM
Capsule, hard

Brown-reddish, opaque gelatin capsules overprinted with "BETA-ADALAT" and the Bayer cross.

4. CLINICAL PARTICULARS

4.1 Therapeutic indications
Management of hypertension and of chronic stable angina pectoris where therapy with either a calcium channel blocker or a beta-blocker prove inadequate.

4.2 Posology and method of administration

Adults:

Hypertension: One capsule daily swallowed with water. If necessary, the dosage may be increased to one capsule dosed every 12 hours. Patients can be transferred to the combination from other antihypertensive treatments with the exception of clonidine (see Section 4.4).

Angina: One capsule every 12 hours swallowed with water. Where additional efficacy is necessary, prophylactic nitrate therapy or additional nifedipine may be of benefit.

Elderly:

Dosage should not exceed one capsule daily in hypertension or one capsule twice daily in angina.

The pharmacokinetics of nifedipine are altered in the elderly so that lower maintenance doses of nifedipine may be required compared to younger patients.

Children:

There is no paediatric experience with Beta-Adalat and therefore this preparation should not be used in children.

General:

Patients with renal or hepatic insufficiency may require lower dosages of Beta-Adalat, (see Section 4.4).

Beta-Adalat should not be taken with grapefruit juice (see Section 4.5).

4.3 Contraindications
Beta-Adalat should not be administered to patients with known hypersensitivity to atenolol, nifedipine or other dihydropyridines because of the theoretical risk of cross-reactivity.

Beta-Adalat should not be administered to patients with a history of wheezing or asthma or a tendency to bronchospasm (obstructive respiratory disease/bronchial asthma). (Label warning: Do not use if you have a history of wheezing or asthma.)

Beta-Adalat must not be administered to women capable of child-bearing or to nursing mothers.

Beta-Adalat must not be used in the presence of second or third degree heart block, sick sinus syndrome, sino-atrial block, in patients with evidence of overt heart failure or inadequately treated heart failure or decompensated heart failure, NYHA grades III and IV.

Beta-Adalat should not be used in cardiogenic shock, clinically significant aortic stenosis, unstable angina pectoris, or during or within one month of a myocardial infarction.

Beta-Adalat should not be used for the treatment of acute attacks of angina.

The safety of Beta-Adalat in malignant hypertension has not been established.

Beta-Adalat should not be used for secondary prevention of myocardial infarction.

Beta-Adalat must not be used in conjunction with other drugs with a cardio-depressant action, e.g. verapamil, as conduction disturbances may ensue.

Beta-Adalat should not be administered concomitantly with rifampicin since effective plasma levels of nifedipine may not be achieved owing to enzyme induction (see Section 4.5).

Beta-Adalat should not be used in pronounced bradycardia (resting heart rate before treatment less than 50 beats/min), hypotension with systolic pressure less than 90 mm Hg, or in the late stages of circulatory disturbances in the hands and legs or in severe peripheral arterial circulatory disturbances.

Beta-Adalat should not be used in patients with a decline in the pH of the blood (acidosis).

In patients with phaeochromocytoma, Beta-Adalat must be administered only after prior therapy with alpha-blockers.

Beta-Adalat must not be given with simultaneous administration of monoamine oxidase inhibitors (MAO inhibitors).

Beta-Adalat must not be used in patients with marked renal impairment (i.e. creatine clearance below 15 ml/min/1.73m^2, serum creatine greater than 600 micromol/litre).

4.4 Special warnings and special precautions for use Cardiac

Particular care should be taken with patients with conduction defects or whose cardiac reserve is poor. However, in patients already treated with a beta-adrenoceptor antagonist, and/or where signs of cardiac failure have been controlled, Beta-Adalat may be substituted with care if necessary.

Beta-Adalat should only be used with caution in patients with controlled congestive heart failure. Evidence of this condition worsening should be regarded as an indication to discontinue therapy.

Beta-Adalat may be used in combination with beta-blocking drugs and other antihypertensive agents but the possibility of an additive effect resulting in postural hypotension should be borne in mind. Beta-Adalat will not prevent possible rebound effects after cessation of other antihypertensive therapy, (see Section 4.5).

In patients with peripheral circulatory disorders (Raynaud's disease or syndrome, intermittent claudication), beta-blockers should be used with caution as aggravation of these disorders may occur.

Care should be taken in prescribing a beta-adrenoceptor blocking drug with Class I anti-dysrhythmic agents such as disopyramide.

One of the pharmacological actions of beta-adrenoceptor blocking drugs is to reduce heart rate. In the rare instances where symptoms may be attributable to the slow heart rate at a dose of one capsule daily, the drug should be discontinued.

Ischaemic pain has been reported in a small proportion of patients within one to four hours of the introduction of nifedipine therapy. Although a "steal" effect has not been demonstrated, patients experiencing this effect should discontinue Beta-Adalat.

Cessation of therapy with a beta-adrenoceptor blocking drug in patients with ischaemic heart disease should be gradual, if necessary initiating replacement therapy at the same time, to prevent exacerbation of angina pectoris.

Caution should be exercised when transferring patients from clonidine to beta-adrenoceptor blocking drugs. If beta-adrenoceptor blocking drugs are given concurrently, clonidine should not be discontinued until several days after withdrawal of the beta-adrenoceptor blocking drug.

Caution should be exercised in patients with severe hypotension (systolic pressure <90 mm Hg).

Caution should be exercised in cases of first degree heart block or mild heart failure, NYHA grade II.

Beta-blockers may increase the number and duration of anginal attacks in patients with Prinzmetal's angina due to unopposed alpha-receptor mediated coronary artery vasoconstriction. Therefore, beta$_1$ selective blockers such as atenolol should be used with care.

Obstructive airways disease

Although cardioselective (beta$_1$) beta-blockers may have less effect on lung function than non-selective beta-blockers, as with all beta-blockers, these should not be administered to patients with reversible obstructive airways disease.

Renal impairment

Dosage should not exceed one capsule daily in patients with renal dysfunction. The use of the combination is contra-indicated in patients with marked renal impairment, (see Section 4.3).

In dialysis patients with malignant hypertension and hypovolaemia, a marked decrease in blood pressure can occur.

Hepatic impairment

Care should be taken in patients with marked hepatic impairment. Although no dosage adjustment is suggested from the systemic availability of the monocomponents in patients with cirrhosis, hypertensive patients with clinically significant liver disease have not been studied. Nifedipine is metabolised primarily by the liver and therefore patients with liver dysfunction should be carefully monitored.

Anaesthesia

It is not advisable to withdraw beta-adrenoceptor blocking drugs prior to surgery in the majority of patients. However, care should be taken when using anaesthetic agents such as ether, cyclopropane and trichloroethylene. Vagal dominance, if it occurs, may be corrected with atropine (1-2 mg intravenously).

Diabetes

The use of nifedipine in diabetic patients may require adjustment of their control.

Beta-Adalat modifies the tachycardia of hypoglycaemia.

Beta-Adalat may mask the signs of thyrotoxicosis.

General

The benefits and risks must be carefully considered before drugs containing beta-receptor blockers (such as Beta-Adalat) are used in patients with a history or family history of psoriasis, patients with a history of severe hypersensitivity reactions and patients on desensitisation therapy (decreased adrenergic counter-regulation).

Whilst nifedipine is contra-indicated in pregnancy, particular care must be exercised when administering nifedipine in combination with i.v. magnesium sulphate to pregnant women.

4.5 Interaction with other medicinal products and other forms of Interaction

Known Interactions

As with other dihydropyridines, nifedipine should not be taken with grapefruit juice as elevated plasma concentrations occur, due to a decreased first pass metabolism. As a consequence, the blood pressure lowering effect of nifedipine may be increased. After regular intake of grapefruit juice, this effect may last for at least three days after the last ingestion of grapefruit juice.

The antihypertensive effect of nifedipine can be potentiated by simultaneous administration of cimetidine.

When used in combination with nifedipine, serum quinidine levels may be suppressed regardless of dosage of quinidine. Therefore, monitoring of quinidine plasma levels and if necessary adjustment of the quinidine dosage are recommended. The pharmacokinetics of nifedipine may also be altered when used in combination with quinidine. It is therefore recommended to monitor blood pressure, and if necessary reduce the nifedipine dosage.

Phenytoin induces the cytochrome P450 3A4 system. Upon co-administration with phenytoin, the bioavailability of nifedipine is reduced and thus its efficacy weakened. When both drugs are concomitantly administered, the clinical response to nifedipine should be monitored and, if necessary, an increase of the nifedipine dose considered. If the dose of nifedipine is increased during co-administration of both drugs, a reduction of the nifedipine dose should be considered when the treatment with phenytoin is discontinued.

Beta-Adalat should not be administered concomitantly with rifampicin since effective plasma levels of nifedipine may not be achieved owing to enzyme induction (see Section 4.3).

Concomitant use of prostaglandin synthease inhibiting drugs (e.g. ibuprofen, indomethacin) may decrease the hypotensive effects of beta-blockers. When Beta-Adalat is administered simultaneously with reserpine, alpha-methyldopa, clonidine, guanethidine, guanfacine, or cardiac glycosides, the heart rate may decline more markedly, and stimulus conduction may be delayed.

Beta-Adalat can increase the plasma levels of digoxin and theophylline. Monitoring is therefore recommended, and in some cases a reduction of the dose may be necessary.

Beta-Adalat should be used with great caution in patients who are receiving concomitant myocardial depressants such as chloroform, lignocaine, procainamide, beta-adrenoceptor stimulants such as isoprenaline, or alpha-adrenoceptor stimulants such as noradrenaline.

If Beta-Adalat is administered simultaneously with another beta-blocker, in addition to a more marked decrease in the blood pressure, heart failure may develop. Simultaneous administration of intravenous beta -receptor blockers must therefore be avoided.

In patients with a hypoglycaemic metabolic disorder simultaneously treated with Beta-Adalat and insulin or oral anti-diabetics, normalisation of the condition may be delayed, and the symptom of hypoglycaemia, tachycardia, be masked. Regular monitoring of the blood glucose is therefore necessary.

When Beta-Adalat is administered simultaneously with calcium antagonists of the verapamil or diltiazem type or antiarrhythmics, there may be a more marked decrease in the blood pressure, a decline in the heart rate, and disturbances of heart rhythm. Careful monitoring of the blood pressure and ECG is therefore necessary. Concomitant intravenous administration of calcium antagonists must be avoided during treatment with Beta-Adalat.

As diltiazem decreases the clearance of nifedipine, the combination of both drugs should be administered with caution.

Simultaneous therapy with noradrenaline or adrenaline as well as the administration of MAO-inhibitors can lead to an excessive increase in blood pressure.

Since simultaneous therapy with narcotics or antiarrhythmics adversely affects cardiac output, the anaesthetist should be informed that the patient is being treated with Beta-Adalat. If possible, Beta-Adalat should not be discontinued before the operation. However, it must be borne in mind that in the course of interaction of atenolol with narcotics or antiarrhythmics, cardiac output may be reduced more markedly, since the cardiac depressant effects (negative inotropism) of atenolol with narcotics or antiarrhythmics may be additive.

The action of non-depolarising muscle relaxant drugs may be potentiated by Beta-Adalat.

Nifedipine may increase the spectrophotometric values of urinary vanillylmandelic acid falsely. However, HPLC measurements are unaffected.

Simultaneous administration of cisapride and nifedipine or quinupristin/dalfopristin and nifedipine may lead to increased plasma concentrations of nifedipine. Consequently, the blood pressure should be monitored and, if necessary, the nifedipine dose reduced.

Potentiation of the blood pressure-lowering action must be anticipated when Beta-Adalat is used in combination with other antihypertensives or with diuretics, vasodilators, nitrates, narcotics, tricyclic antidepressants, barbiturates or phenothiazines, (see Section 4.4).

Theoretical Interactions

Nifedipine is metabolised via the cytochrome P450 3A4 system and, therefore, there are theoretical interactions for drugs which are known to inhibit this enzyme system (e.g. erythromycin, ketoconazole, itraconazole, fluconazole, fluoxetine, indinavir, nelfinavir, ritonavir, amprenavir and saquinavir). Although no formal *in vivo* interaction studies have been performed with these drugs, co-administration can be expected to lead to an increase in plasma concentrations of nifedipine. Blood pressure should therefore be monitored and, if necessary, a reduction in the nifedipine dose considered.

A clinical study investigating the potential of a drug interaction between nifedipine and nefazodone has not yet been performed. Nefazodone is known to inhibit the cytochrome P450 3A4 mediated metabolism of other drugs. Therefore an increase in nifedipine plasma concentrations upon co-administration of both drugs cannot be excluded. When nefazodone is given together with nifedipine, the blood pressure should be monitored and, if necessary, a reduction in the nifedipine dose considered.

Tacrolimus has been shown to be metabolised via the cytochrome P450 3A4 system. Upon co-administration of both drugs, the tacrolimus plasma concentrations should be monitored and, if necessary, a reduction in the tacrolimus dose considered.

Although no formal interaction studies have been performed between nifedipine and carbamazepine, phenobarbitone or valproic acid, these drugs have been shown to alter the plasma concentrations of a structurally similar calcium channel blocker. A decrease (carbamazepine, phenobarbitone) or an increase (valproic acid) in nifedipine plasma concentrations and hence an alteration in efficacy cannot be excluded.

4.6 Pregnancy and lactation

Beta-Adalat is contra-indicated in women capable of childbearing.

The safety of nifedipine for use in human pregnancy has not been established. Evaluation of experimental animal studies has shown reproductive toxicity consisting of embryotoxicity and teratogenic effects at maternally toxic doses.

Beta-Adalat is contra-indicated in nursing mothers, as nifedipine and atenolol may be present in breast milk.

In single cases of *in vitro* fertilisation calcium antagonists like nifedipine have been associated with reversible biochemical changes in the spermatozoa's head section that may result in impaired sperm function. In those men who are repeatedly unsuccessful in fathering a child by *in vitro* fertilisation, and where no other explanation can be found, calcium antagonists like nifedipine should be considered as possible causes.

Theoretically, beta-blockers such as atenolol cause a decrease in placental blood flow, which can result in intrauterine foetal death, and immature and premature deliveries. In addition, adverse effects (especially hypoglycaemia and bradycardia) may occur in foetus and neonates. There is an increased risk of cardiac and pulmonary complications in the neonate in the postnatal period.

4.7 Effects on ability to drive and use machines

Reactions to the drug, which vary in intensity from individual to individual, may impair the ability to drive or to operate machinery. This applies particularly at the start of treatment, on changing the medication and in combination with alcohol.

4.8 Undesirable effects

Beta-Adalat is well tolerated. Side effects occur predominantly at the beginning of treatment or at high doses, and are generally mild and transient. In clinical studies, the undesired events reported are usually attributed to the pharmacological actions of its components. The following undesired events, listed by body system, have been reported:

Beta-Adalat

Cardiovascular:	flushing; oedema
CNS:	headache; dizziness
Digestive system:	gastrointestinal disturbance
Others:	fatigue

Atenolol monotherapy

Cardiovascular:	disturbances of AV conduction; bradycardia; heart failure deterioration; postural hypotension which may be associated with syncope; cold and cyanotic extremities; in susceptible patients: precipitation of heart block, intermittent claudication, Raynaud's phenomenon (cold extremities)
CNS:	confusion; mood changes; nightmares; psychosis and hallucinations; sleep disturbances of the type noted with other beta-blockers
Digestive system:	dry mouth
Metabolic:	hyperglycaemia which may cause latent diabetes mellitus to become manifest, or lead to deterioration in pre-existing diabetes; should a hypoglycaemic metabolic disorder develop in a patient with diabetes, it must be borne in mind that, under treatment with Beta-Adalat, normalisation of the condition may be delayed and the symptom of hypoglycaemia, tachycardia, be masked
Haematological:	purpura; thrombocytopenia
Skin:	alopecia; psoriasiform skin reactions; exacerbation of psoriasis; skin rashes
Musculo-skeletal:	joint reactions (lupus erythematosus-like syndrome)
Neurological:	paraesthesia; myasthenia
Respiratory:	bronchospasm may occur in patients with bronchial asthma or a history of asthmatic complaints
Special senses:	visual disturbances; dry eyes
Urogenital:	impotence
Others:	an increase in ANA (antinuclear antibodies) has been observed, however the clinical relevance of this is not clear

Nifedipine monotherapy

Most side-effects are consequences of the vasodilatory effects of nifedipine and usually regress on withdrawal of therapy. Side-effects of nifedipine such as flushing and headache may occur at the beginning of the treatment. They are, however, mostly slight and diminish with continuous use. Other undesirable effects reported were:

Cardiovascular:	palpitations; tachycardia; syncopal episodes with initial dose due to blood pressure decrease; gravitational oedema; vasodilatation (flush, sensation of warmth, erythromelalgia); hypotension
CNS:	headache; dizziness; asthenia; lethargy; vertigo
Neurological:	paraesthesia; nervousness; tremor; mood changes
Digestive system:	altered bowel habit; nausea; feeling of repletion; gingival hyperplasia which usually regresses on withdrawal of therapy; disturbances of liver function such as increased transaminase or intra-hepatic cholestasis; rare cases of hypersensitivity-type jaundice have been reported
Metabolic:	initial hyperglycaemia
Skin:	pruritus; urticaria; exanthema; erythema; exfoliative dermatitis and photosensitive dermatitis; gynaecomastia in older men on long term therapy, which usually regresses on withdrawal of therapy
Hypersensitivity:	systemic allergic reactions
Musculo-skeletal:	myalgia
Respiratory:	dyspnoea
Special senses:	visual disturbances
Urogenital:	increased frequency of micturition; impotence may occur rarely
Haemic and lymphatic system:	purpura; agranulocytosis

As with other sustained release dihydropyridines, exacerbation of angina pectoris may occur rarely at the start of treatment with sustained release formulations of nifedipine. The occurrence of myocardial infarction has been described although it is not possible to distinguish such an event from the natural course of ischaemic heart disease.

4.9 Overdose

Clinical effects

As far as treatment is concerned, elimination of active substances and the restoration of stable cardiovascular conditions have priority.

The symptoms of overdosage may include bradycardia, hypotension, hypoglycaemia, acute cardiac insufficiency and bronchospasm.

These signs may not be fully manifested until several hours after ingestion.

Treatment

General treatment should include close supervision, treatment in an intensive care ward, the use of gastric lavage, activated charcoal and a laxative to prevent absorption of any drug still present in the gastrointestinal tract, the use of plasma and plasma substitutes to treat hypotension and shock.

Excessive bradycardia can be countered with atropine 1-2 mg intravenously. If necessary, this may be followed by a bolus dose of glucagon 10 mg intravenously. If required, this may be repeated or followed by an intravenous infusion of glucagon 1-10 mg/hour depending on response. Intravenous calcium gluconate combined with metaraminol may be beneficial for hypotension induced by nifedipine. If no response to glucagon occurs or if glucagon is unavailable, a beta-adrenoceptor stimulant such as dobutamine 2.5 – 10 microgram/kg/minute by intravenous infusion may be given. Dobutamine, due to its positive inotropic effects could also be used to treat hypotension and acute cardiac insufficiency. It is likely that these doses would be inadequate to reverse the cardiac effects of beta-blockade if a large overdose has been taken. The dose of dobutamine should therefore be increased if necessary to achieve the required response according to the clinical condition of the patient.

For bronchospasm: inhalation of $beta_2$ – stimulants such as salbutamol (2 puffs), or orciprenaline sulphate (0.5-1.0 mg) slowly iv. For generalised convulsions, administration of diazepam slowly intravenously is recommended.

Other possible treatments in cases of life-threatening intoxication are:

Pacemaker therapy, artificial ventilation and haemodialysis (atenolol) or plasma separation (nifedipine).

5. PHARMACOLOGICAL PROPERTIES

5.1 Pharmacodynamic properties

ATC codes:

C08C A55

Selective calcium channel blocker (dihydropyridine derivative) with mainly vascular effects.

Nifedipine, combinations.

C07F B03

Beta blocking agents, selective, and other antihypertensives.

Atenolol with other antihypertensives.

Atenolol is classified as a $beta_1$-selective (cardioselective) beta-adrenoceptor antagonist with no membrane-stabilising activity and no partial agonist activity. It is clearly the most hydrophilic of the currently available beta-blockers, and thus demonstrates poor penetration of cell membrane lipids. Atenolol has marked negative inotropic and chronotropic effects, thereby reducing cardiac output, myocardial oxygen demand, and blood pressure, particularly during exercise.

Nifedipine is a calcium antagonist of the 1,4-dihydropyridine type. Calcium antagonists reduce the transmembrane influx of calcium ions through the L-type calcium channels into the cell. Nifedipine acts particularly on the cells of the myocardium and the smooth muscle cells of the coronary arteries and the peripheral resistance vessels.

The fixed combination of nifedipine 20 mg and atenolol 50 mg is designed for the antihypertensive treatment of patients whose blood pressure is inadequately controlled on monotherapy. This combination of a cardioselective, hydrophilic $beta_1$-adrenoceptor antagonist (atenolol), and a potent, specific calcium antagonist (nifedipine) lowers blood pressure to a greater extent than either of its individual components.

Nifedipine's tendency to increase heart rate and plasma renin activity is counteracted by beta-adrenoceptor blockade, while the tendency of atenolol to increase peripheral resistance is counterbalanced by the vasodilatation and reflex increase in sympathetic tone induced by the calcium antagonist.

There is no evidence of clinically significant negative inotropic, dromotropic or chronotropic effects with the combined use of nifedipine and atenolol in man compared with treatment with atenolol alone. Similarly, the chronic renal pharmacodynamic effects of the fixed combination are not dissimilar to the use of atenolol alone; the acute natriuretic, uricosuric and diuretic effects of nifedipine alone are not seen following chronic use of the fixed combination in man.

5.2 Pharmacokinetic properties

The fixed combination of nifedipine 20 mg (slow release) and atenolol 50 mg is bioequivalent to its individual drug components, and there is no evidence of pharmacokinetic interaction between the two drugs.

In the elderly, the half life of nifedipine alone is increased from approximately 5½ hours to 9 hours, but peak plasma levels are unchanged.

The pharmacokinetics of atenolol 50 mg when dosed in free combination with nifedipine 20 mg (slow release) in the elderly were consistent with the published atenolol experience in demonstrating an approximately 45% increase in systemic bioavailability, with increased blood levels 24 hours after dosing in the elderly.

5.3 Preclinical safety data

There are no preclinical data of relevance to the prescriber which are additional to those already included in other sections of the Summary of Product Characteristics.

6. PHARMACEUTICAL PARTICULARS

6.1 List of excipients

Nifedipine tablets: microcrystalline cellulose, maize starch, lactose, polysorbate 80, magnesium stearate, hypromellose, macrogol 4000, titanium dioxide (E171) and red iron oxide (E172).

Atenolol granules: heavy magnesium carbonate, maize starch, sodium lauryl sulphate, gelatin, magnesium stearate.

Capsule shell: red iron oxide (E172), titanium dioxide (E171) and gelatin.

6.2 Incompatibilities

Not applicable.

6.3 Shelf life

Blister packs composed of PVC/PVDC foil backed with aluminium foil: 36 months.

Blister packs composed of PP foil backed with aluminium foil: 24 months.

6.4 Special precautions for storage

This medicinal product does not require any special storage conditions

6.5 Nature and contents of container

Blister packs composed of PVC/PVDC foil, backed with aluminium foil, each containing 28 capsules.

Blister packs composed of PP foil, backed with aluminium foil, each containing 28 capsules.

6.6 Instructions for use and handling

No additional information

7. MARKETING AUTHORISATION HOLDER

Bayer plc,

Bayer House,

Strawberry Hill,

Newbury

Berkshire RG14 1JA

United Kingdom

Trading as Bayer plc, Pharmaceutical Division or Baypharm or Baymet.

8. MARKETING AUTHORISATION NUMBER(S)

PL 0010/0155

9. DATE OF FIRST AUTHORISATION/RENEWAL OF THE AUTHORISATION

Date of first authorisation: 25 July 1988

Date of last renewal: 19 September 2001

10. DATE OF REVISION OF THE TEXT

April 2005

LEGAL CATEGORY

POM

Betacap Scalp Application

(Dermal Laboratories Limited)

1. NAME OF THE MEDICINAL PRODUCT

BETACAP® SCALP APPLICATION

2. QUALITATIVE AND QUANTITATIVE COMPOSITION

Betamethasone (as valerate) 0.1% w/w.

3. PHARMACEUTICAL FORM

Cutaneous solution.

Transparent, slightly gelled, emollient, scalp application.

4. CLINICAL PARTICULARS

4.1 Therapeutic indications

For the topical treatment of dermatoses of the scalp, such as psoriasis and seborrhoeic dermatitis, which are unresponsive to less potent corticosteroids.

4.2 Posology and method of administration

For adults, including the elderly, and children over the age of one year: Betacap Scalp Application should be applied sparingly to the scalp night and morning until improvement is noticeable. It may then be possible to sustain improvement by applying once a day, or less frequently.

For the treatment of seborrhoeic dermatitis in children, the product should not be used for longer than 5 to 7 days.

4.3 Contraindications

Not to be used where there is bacterial, fungal or viral infection of the scalp. Not to be used in cases of sensitivity to any of the ingredients. Not to be used in children under the age of one year.

4.4 Special warnings and special precautions for use

Keep away from the eyes. Betacap is highly flammable. Do not use near a fire or naked flame. Allow the treated scalp to dry naturally. Long-term continuous topical therapy should be avoided where possible, particularly in infants and children, as adrenal suppression can occur even without occlusion. Complications sometimes associated with the use of topical corticosteroids in psoriasis include the possibility of rebound relapses, development of tolerance, risk of generalised pustular psoriasis and development of local or systemic toxicity due to impaired barrier function of the skin. If used in psoriasis, careful patient supervision is important. For external use only.

4.5 Interaction with other medicinal products and other forms of Interaction

None known.

4.6 Pregnancy and lactation

There is inadequate evidence of safety in human pregnancy. Topical administration of corticosteroids to pregnant animals can cause abnormalities of foetal development including cleft palate and intra-uterine growth retardation. There may therefore be a very small risk of such effects in the human foetus.

4.7 Effects on ability to drive and use machines

None known.

4.8 Undesirable effects

Betamethasone valerate preparations are usually well tolerated, but if signs of hypersensitivity appear, application should be stopped immediately. As with other topical corticosteroids, prolonged use of large amounts or treatment of extensive areas can result in sufficient systemic absorption to produce the features of hypercorticism and suppression of the HPA axis. These effects are more likely to occur in infants and children, and if occlusive dressings are used. Local atrophy may occur after prolonged treatment, particularly under occlusion.

4.9 Overdose

Acute overdosage is very unlikely to occur. However, in the case of chronic overdosage or misuse, the features of hypercorticism may appear and in this situation treatment with Betacap Scalp Application should be discontinued.

5. PHARMACOLOGICAL PROPERTIES

5.1 Pharmacodynamic properties

Betamethasone (as valerate) is a well-established example of a corticosteroid which is used in dermatological therapy in pharmacological doses for its anti-inflammatory and immuno-suppressive glucocorticoid properties. It suppresses the clinical manifestations of a wide range of inflammatory dermatoses and is frequently used at the concentration of 0.1% (as valerate). Betacap Scalp Application complies with the specification given in the monograph for Betamethasone Valerate Scalp Application BP. Betacap Scalp Application includes a coconut-oil related emollient ingredient to reduce the drying effect that a standard alcoholic vehicle may otherwise have on the scalp. The vehicle also contains isopropyl alcohol, which has antiseptic activity.

5.2 Pharmacokinetic properties

For clinical usage, the betamethasone valerate is presented as a slightly thickened evaporative solution which allows drug availability over the affected area, whilst reducing the propensity to spread onto uninvolved skin. In addition, after rapidly drying, the drug substance is thus deposited uniformly in a micronised crystalline form for efficient absorption into the skin. The lipid characteristics of the drug substance ensure that these micro-fine crystals rapidly dissolve in skin lipids to enhance molecular diffusion through the outer epidermal tissue and to encourage permeation into the deeper layers where it reverses the pathological processes responsible for the inflammation.

5.3 Preclinical safety data

No relevant information additional to that contained elsewhere in this SPC.

6. PHARMACEUTICAL PARTICULARS

6.1 List of excipients

Macrogol 7 Glyceryl Cocoate (a water dispersible derivative of coconut oil); Isopropyl Alcohol; Carbomer; Sodium Hydroxide; Purified Water.

6.2 Incompatibilities

None known.

6.3 Shelf life

36 months.

6.4 Special precautions for storage

Do not store above 25°C. Protect from light. Return bottle to carton between use.

6.5 Nature and contents of container

100 ml plastic squeeze bottle with integral nozzle applicator for convenient direct application to the scalp through the hair, and tamper-evident replaceable cap. This is supplied as an original pack (OP).

6.6 Instructions for use and handling

Not applicable.

7. MARKETING AUTHORISATION HOLDER

Dermal Laboratories

Tatmore Place, Gosmore

Hitchin, Herts SG4 7QR, UK.

8. MARKETING AUTHORISATION NUMBER(S)

0173/0149.

9. DATE OF FIRST AUTHORISATION/RENEWAL OF THE AUTHORISATION

22 June 2004.

10. DATE OF REVISION OF THE TEXT

April 2005.

Beta-Cardone Tablets 40, 80, 200mg

(UCB Pharma Limited)

1. NAME OF THE MEDICINAL PRODUCT

Beta-Cardone Tablets 40mg, 80mg or 200mg

2. QUALITATIVE AND QUANTITATIVE COMPOSITION

Sotalol Hydrochloride 40mg, 80mg or 200mg

For excipients see 6.1.

3. PHARMACEUTICAL FORM

Tablet

40mg: Green, circular, flat-faced tablets with bevelled edges, with "Evans/BC4" on one face.

80mg: Pink, circular, flat-faced tablets with bevelled edges, with "Evans/BC8" on one face.

200mg: White, circular, flat-faced tablets with bevelled edges, with "Evans/BC20" one face.

4. CLINICAL PARTICULARS

4.1 Therapeutic indications

Ventricular arrhythmias: Treatment of life-threatening ventricular tachyarrhythmias and symptomatic non-sustained ventricular tachyarrhythmias.

Supraventricular arrhythmias: Prophylaxis of paroxysmal atrial tachycardia, paroxysmal atrial fibrillation, paroxysmal A-V nodal re-entrant tachycardia, paroxysmal A-V re-entrant tachycardia using accessory pathways, and paroxysmal supraventricular tachycardia after cardiac surgery. Maintenance of normal sinus rhythm following conversion of atrial fibrillation or atrial flutter.

4.2 Posology and method of administration

Oral administration in adults:

When administering Beta-Cardone to a patient for the first time, it is desirable to start with a low dose and gradually increase the dose until the desired response is obtained; this is especially important in the elderly, as a general rule the heart rate should not be reduced to less than 55 beats per minute.

Before starting treatment or increasing the dose the corrected QT interval should be measured and renal function, electrolyte balance, and concomitant medications assessed. Treatment with sotalol should be initiated and doses increased in a facility capable of monitoring and assessing cardiac rhythm. The dosage must be individualised and based on the patient's response. Proarrhythmic events can occur not only at initiation of therapy, but also with each upward dosage adjustment.

Treatment with Beta-Cardone should not be discontinued suddenly, especially in patients with ischaemic heart disease (angina pectoris, prior acute myocardial infarction) or hypertension, to prevent exacerbation of the disease (see section "abrupt withdrawal" under Special Warnings).

The following are guidelines for oral administration.

The initial dose is 80mg, as one or two divided doses. Oral dosage should be adjusted gradually allowing 2-3 days between dosing increments in order to attain steady-state, and to allow monitoring of QT intervals. Most patients respond to 160 to 320mg per day, in two divided doses.

The dosage should be reduced in renal impairment. Creatinine clearance: 60-30ml/min.: 1/2 recommended dose. Creatinine clearance 30-10ml/min.: 1/4 recommended dose.

Administration in children:

Beta-Cardone is not intended for administration to children.

4.3 Contraindications

Sick sinus syndrome; long QT syndromes, Torsades de Pointes; symptomatic sinus bradycardia; uncontrolled congestive heart failure; cardiogenic shock; anaesthesia that produces myocardial depression; untreated phaeochromocytoma; hypotension (except due to arrhythmia); Raynaud's phenomenon and severe peripheral circulatory disturbances; chronic obstructive airway disease or bronchial asthma; renal failure (creatinine clearance < 10 ml/min.).

Beta-Cardone should not be given to patients suffering from heart block or patients with Prinzmetal's angina and those who have a history of bronchospasm,

In patients with poor cardiac reserve beta-blockade can precipitate heart failure; in such cases, sotalol hydrochloride therapy should not be commenced until the patient has been controlled by therapy (ACE inhibitors, cardiac glycosides or, if necessary, diuretic therapy - see Interactions).

Diabetic ketoacidosis and metabolic acidosis: Sotalol hydrochloride should not be given to patients suffering from diabetic ketoacidosis or metabolic acidosis; therapy with sotalol hydrochloride can be commenced or resumed when the metabolic condition has been corrected.

Beta-Cardone should not be given to patients hypersensitive to sotalol.

4.4 Special warnings and special precautions for use

Beta-Cardone should not be given to patients who have a history of asthma or bronchospasm.

Beta-blockers may increase the sensitivity towards allergens and the seriousness of anaphylactic reactions.

Patients with a history of psoriasis should take beta-blockers only after careful consideration.

Abrupt withdrawal: Patients should be carefully monitored when discontinuing chronically administered sotalol, particularly those with ischaemic heart disease. If possible the dosage should be gradually reduced over a period of 1 to 2 weeks, if necessary at the same time initiating replacement therapy. Hypersensitivity to catecholamines is observed in patients withdrawn from beta-blocker therapy. Occasional cases of exacerbation of angina pectoris, arrhythmias and in some cases myocardial infarction have been reported after abrupt discontinuation of therapy. Abrupt discontinuation may unmask latent coronary insufficiency. In addition, hypertension may develop.

Proarrhythmias: Rarely, Beta-Cardone causes aggravation of pre-existing arrhythmias or the provocation of new arrhythmias.

Risk factors for Torsades de Pointes include prolongation of the QT interval, bradycardia, reduction in serum potassium and magnesium, and history of cardiomegaly or congestive heart failure, sustained ventricular tachycardia.

Proarrhythmic events can occur on initiating therapy and with every upward dose adjustment. The incidence of Torsades de Pointes is dose dependent.

Caution should be used if the QT_C exceeds 500 msec whilst on therapy. It is advisable to reduce dose or discontinue therapy when the QT_C interval exceeds 550 msec.

Electrolyte disturbances: Sotalol should not be used in patients with hypokalaemia or hypomagnesaemia. Potassium levels should be monitored. In conditions likely to provoke hypokalaemia/hypomagnesaemia, such as persistent diarrhoea, appropriate corrective clinical measures should be taken.

Heart failure: Beta-blockade may precipitate heart failure.

Following myocardial infarction careful monitoring and dose titration are critical during initiation and follow-up of therapy. Sotalol should be avoided in patients with left ventricular ejection fractions ⩽40% without serious ventricular arrhythmias.

Thyrotoxicosis: Beta-blockade may mask certain clinical signs of hyperthyroidism.

Treated diabetes: Beta-Cardone, like other beta-blocking agents, may reduce or mask the usual pre-hypoglycaemic warning signs. It may be necessary to adjust the dose of anti-diabetic therapy.

General anaesthesia: If desired, Beta-Cardone may be stopped four days prior to surgery. However, where sudden withdrawal might expose the patient to severe angina or arrhythmias, anaesthesia can proceed provided that the following precautions are taken.

1. Vagal dominance is counteracted by premedication with atropine sulphate (0.25 to 2.0mg) administered intravenously.

2. Anaesthetic agents such as ether, chloroform, cyclopropane, trichlorethylene, methoxyflurane and enflurane are not used.

Alcoholism: Beta-adrenoceptor blocking drugs may precipitate cardiac failure in alcoholic patients.

Upper respiratory infections: In these conditions patients without a history of airways obstruction may suffer bronchospasm from beta-blockade.

The product labelling will bear a statement warning against use in patients with a history of wheezing or asthma.

Patients with rare hereditary problems of galactose intolerance, the Lapp-lactose deficiency, or glucose-galactose malabsorption should not take this medicine.

4.5 Interaction with other medicinal products and other forms of Interaction

In combined therapy, clonidine should not be discontinued until several days after withdrawal of Beta-Cardone.

Use with great caution with drugs that also prolong QT interval, e.g. disopyramide, amiodarone, class I antiarrhythmic agents, calcium antagonists of the verapamil type or tricyclic antidepressants.

Concomitant potassium-depleting diuretics may increase the potential for Torsade de Pointes.

Proarrhythmic events are more common in patients also receiving digitalis glycosides.

Phenothiazines, terfenadine, astemizole, diltiazem and halofantrine.

Concomitant use of reserpine, guanethidine, or alpha methyldopa: Closely monitor for evidence of hypotension and/or marked bradycardia, syncope.

Tubocurarine: Neuromuscular blockade is prolonged by beta-blocking agents.

Calcium antagonists: Dihydropyridine derivatives such as nifedipine. The risk of hypotension may be increased. In patients with latent cardiac insufficiency, concomitant treatment with beta-blockers may lead to cardiac failure.

Prostaglandin synthetase inhibiting drugs may decrease the hypotensive effects of beta-blockers.

Sympathicomimetic agents: may counteract the effect of beta-adrenergic agents.

Concomitant administration of tricyclic antidepressants, barbiturates and phenothiazines as well as other antihypertensive agents may increase the blood pressure lowering effect.

Precautions for use:

Insulin and oral antidiabetic drugs, may intensify the blood sugar lowering effect (especially non-selective beta-blockers).

Beta-adrenergic blockade may prevent the appearance of signs of hypoglycaemia (tachycardia).

Cimetidine, hydralazine and alcohol induce increased levels of hepatically metabolised beta-blockers.

4.6 Pregnancy and lactation

Use in pregnancy should be avoided.

Pregnancy: Animal studies with sotalol hydrochloride have shown no evidence of teratogenicity or other harmful effects on the foetus. Nevertheless its use throughout pregnancy should be avoided unless it is absolutely necessary as it crosses the placenta and may cause foetal bradycardia.

Beta-blockers reduce placental perfusion which may result in intrauterine foetal death, immature and premature deliveries. In addition, adverse effects (especially hypoglycaemia and bradycardia) may occur in the foetus and neonate. There is an increased risk of cardiac and pulmonary complications in the neonate in the postnatal period. Most beta-blockers, particularly lipophilic compounds, will pass into breast milk although to a variable extent.

Lactation: Infants should not be fed with breast milk from mothers being treated with Beta-Cardone.

Newborns exposed near delivery should be closely observed for the first 24-48 hours for signs and symptoms of beta-blockade.

4.7 Effects on ability to drive and use machines

Side-effects such as dizziness and fatigue should be taken into account.

4.8 Undesirable effects

The most significant adverse effects are those due to proarrhythmia, including Torsades de Pointes. There is an increased risk of Torsades de Pointes in women.

Also bradycardia, dyspnoea, chest pain, palpitations, oedema, ECG abnormalities, hypotension, proarrhythmia, syncope, heart failure, presyncope. Nausea/vomiting, diarrhoea, dyspepsia, abdominal pain, flatulence, cramps, fatigue, dizziness, asthenia, lightheadedness, headache, sleep disturbances, depression, paraesthesia, mood changes, anxiety, sexual dysfunction, visual disturbances, taste abnormalities, hearing disturbances, fever, slowed AV-conduction or increase of an existing AV-block, cold and cyanotic extremities, Raynaud's phenomenon, increase of intermittent claudication.

Beta-blockers, even those with apparent cardioselectivity should not be used in patients with asthma or a history of obstructive airways disease unless no alternative treatment is available. In such cases, the risk of inducing bronchospasm should be appreciated and appropriate precautions taken. If bronchospasm should occur after the use of Beta-Cardone it can be treated with a $beta_2$-agonist by inhalation e.g. salbutamol (the dose of which may need to be greater than the usual dose in asthma) and, if necessary, intravenous atropine 1mg.

There have been reports of skin rashes and especially exacerbation of psoriasis disorders of lacrimation including dry eyes and conjunctivitis. In most cases the symptoms have cleared when the treatment was withdrawn. Discontinuance of the drug should be considered if any such reaction is not otherwise explicable. Cessation of therapy with a beta-blocker should be gradual.

An increase in Anti Nuclear Antibodies has been seen; its clinical relevance is not clear.

4.9 Overdose

Symptoms of overdose are: bradycardia, hypotension, bronchospasm and acute cardiac insufficiency.

After ingestion of an overdose or in the case of hypersensitivity, the patient should be kept under close supervision and treated in an intensive care ward. Absorption of any drug material still present in the gastro-intestinal tract can be prevented by gastric lavage, administration of activated charcoal and a laxative. Artificial respiration may be required. Bradycardia or extensive vagal reactions should be treated by administering atropine or methylatropine. Hypotension and shock should be treated with plasma/plasma substitutes and if necessary, catecholamines. The beta-blocking effect can be counteracted by slow intravenous administration of isoprenaline hydrochloride, starting with a dose of approximately 5 micrograms/minute, or dobutamine, starting with a dose of 2.5 micrograms/minute, until the required effect has been obtained.

In refractory cases isoprenaline can be combined with dopamine. If this does not produce the desired effect either, Intravenous administration of 8-10 mg of glucagon may be considered. If required the injection should be repeated within one hour, to be followed - if required - by an i.v. infusion of glucagon at an administration rate of 1-3 mg/hour. Administration of calcium ions, or the use of a cardiac pacemaker may also be considered. In patients intoxicated with hydrophylic beta-blocking agents hemodialysis or hemoperfusion may be considered.

Prolongation of the QT_c interval has been reported. Transvenous pacing may be required.

5. PHARMACOLOGICAL PROPERTIES

5.1 Pharmacodynamic properties

Sotalol has both beta-adrenoreceptor blocking (Vaughan Williams Class II) and cardiac action potential duration prolongation (Vaughan Williams Class III) antiarrhythmic properties. The d- and l-isomers of sotalol have similar Class III antiarrhythmic effects while the l-isomer is responsible for virtually all of the beta-blocking activity.

5.2 Pharmacokinetic properties

Sotalol is completely absorbed from the gastrointestinal tract and peak plasma concentrations are obtained about 2 or 3 hours after a dose. It is excreted unchanged in the urine. After oral administration the plasma half-life has been shown to be 17 hours. It is not bound to plasma proteins. The lipid solubility is very low.

5.3 Preclinical safety data

None stated.

6. PHARMACEUTICAL PARTICULARS

6.1 List of excipients

Lactose

Maize Starch

Pregelatinised Starch

Talc

Magnesium Stearate

Dispersed Blue 11076 and Quinoline Yellow Lake 19248 (40mg only)

Dispersed Red 11652 (80mg only)

6.2 Incompatibilities

None known.

6.3 Shelf life

36 months

6.4 Special precautions for storage

Beta-Cardone Tablets should be protected from light.

6.5 Nature and contents of container

Polypropylene securitainers containing 30 tablets (200mg only); 100 or 500 tablets (40mg, 80mg or 200mg).

PVC, PVdC and foil blister pack containing 56 tablets (40mg and 80mg only)

Polypropylene TraCeR pack containing 28 tablets (200mg only)

6.6 Instructions for use and handling

None stated.

7. MARKETING AUTHORISATION HOLDER

UCB Pharma Ltd
208 Bath Road
Slough
Berkshire
SL1 3WE
UK

8. MARKETING AUTHORISATION NUMBER(S)

40mg: PL 00039/0414

80mg: PL 00039/0415

200mg: PL00039/0416

9. DATE OF FIRST AUTHORISATION/RENEWAL OF THE AUTHORISATION
12 January 1993/11 May 2000

10. DATE OF REVISION OF THE TEXT
June 2005

11. Legal Category
POM

Betadine Alcoholic Solution

(Medlock Medical Ltd)

1. NAME OF THE MEDICINAL PRODUCT
Betadine Alcoholic Solution.

2. QUALITATIVE AND QUANTITATIVE COMPOSITION
Povidone iodine 10.0% w/v.

3. PHARMACEUTICAL FORM
Alcoholic solution.

4. CLINICAL PARTICULARS

4.1 Therapeutic indications
For use as an antiseptic skin cleanser for major and minor surgical procedures where a quick drying effect is desired.

4.2 Posology and method of administration
For topical administration.

4.3 Contraindications
Known or suspected iodine hypersensitivity. Regular use is contraindicated in patients and users with thyroid disorders (in particular nodular colloid goitre, endemic goitre and Hashimoto's thyroiditis).

4.4 Special warnings and special precautions for use
Special caution is needed when regular applications to broken skin are made to patients with pre-existing renal insufficiency.

4.5 Interaction with other medicinal products and other forms of Interaction
Absorption of iodine from povidone iodine through either intact or damaged skin may interfere with thyroid function tests. Contamination with povidone iodine of several types of tests for the detection of occult blood in faeces or blood in urine may produce false-positive results.

4.6 Pregnancy and lactation
Regular use of povidone iodine should be avoided in pregnant or lactating women as absorbed iodine can cross the placental barrier and can be secreted into breast milk. Although no adverse effects have been reported from limited use, caution should be recommended and therapeutic benefit must be balanced against possible effects of the absorption of iodine on foetal thyroid function and development.

4.7 Effects on ability to drive and use machines
None known.

4.8 Undesirable effects
Povidone iodine may produce local skin reactions, although it is considered to be less irritant than iodine. The application of povidone iodine to large wounds or severe burns may produce systemic adverse effects such as metabolic acidosis, hypernatraemia and impairment of renal function.

4.9 Overdose
Excess iodine can produce goitre and hypothyroidism or hyperthyroidism. Systemic absorption of iodine after repeated application of povidone iodine to large areas of wounds or burns may lead to a number of adverse effects: metallic taste in mouth, increased salivation, burning or pain in the throat or mouth, irritation and swelling of the eyes, pulmonary oedema, skin reactions, gastrointestinal upset and diarrhoea, metabolic acidosis, hypernatraemia and renal impairment. Treatment: In the case of accidental ingestion of large quantities of Betadine symptomatic and supportive treatment should be provided, with special attention to electrolyte balance and renal and thyroid function.

5. PHARMACOLOGICAL PROPERTIES

5.1 Pharmacodynamic properties
The active ingredient, povidone iodine, slowly liberates iodine when in contact with skin and mucous membranes. The activity of 'iodine' as a microbicide is then governed by a series of dissociations: $I_2 \leftrightarrow I^+ + I^-$; $I_2 + H_2O \leftrightarrow H_2OI^+ + I^-$; $I_2 + I^- \leftrightarrow I_3^-$. The microbicidal species H_2OI^+ preferentially displaces oxygen as the end electron acceptor in the microorganism's respiratory cycle. H_2OI^+ similarly interacts within the electron transport chain and reacts with the amino acids of the microbial cell membrane.

5.2 Pharmacokinetic properties
Betadine Alcoholic Solution is for topical application and therefore a consideration of the absorption, distribution, metabolism and excretion of povidone iodine is largely without relevance.

5.3 Preclinical safety data
Not applicable.

6. PHARMACEUTICAL PARTICULARS

6.1 List of excipients
Nonoxynol 9; dibasic sodium phosphate (anhydrous); citric acid monohydrate; glycerol; industrial methylated spirit; sodium hydroxide; purified water.

6.2 Incompatibilities
None.

6.3 Shelf life
36 months.

6.4 Special precautions for storage
To be stored at or below 25 degrees Celsius and protected from light.

6.5 Nature and contents of container
High-density polyethylene containers fitted with steran lined white polypropylene caps. Pack size: 500ml

6.6 Instructions for use and handling
None stated.

7. MARKETING AUTHORISATION HOLDER
Medlock Medical Limited, Tubiton House, Medlock Street, Oldham, OL1 3HS.

8. MARKETING AUTHORISATION NUMBER(S)
PL 21248/0002.

9. DATE OF FIRST AUTHORISATION/RENEWAL OF THE AUTHORISATION
14th March 2005.

10. DATE OF REVISION OF THE TEXT
March 2005.

Betadine Antiseptic Paint

(Medlock Medical Ltd)

1. NAME OF THE MEDICINAL PRODUCT
Betadine Antiseptic Paint.

2. QUALITATIVE AND QUANTITATIVE COMPOSITION
Povidone Iodine USP 10% w/v.

3. PHARMACEUTICAL FORM
Cutaneous solution.

4. CLINICAL PARTICULARS

4.1 Therapeutic indications
As a general antiseptic paint in the prevention and treatment of infections.

4.2 Posology and method of administration
For topical administration. Adults, children and the elderly: Apply Betadine Antiseptic Paint undiluted as necessary to the affected area and allow to dry. Rinse the brush thoroughly after use.

4.3 Contraindications
Hypersensitivity to iodine. History of abnormal thyroid function or goitre.

4.4 Special warnings and special precautions for use
If local irritation and hypersensitivity develop, then discontinue treatment.

4.5 Interaction with other medicinal products and other forms of Interaction
None stated.

4.6 Pregnancy and lactation
Use in pregnancy and lactation should be limited to minor lesions only. Although no adverse effects have been reported from limited use, caution should be recommended and therapeutic benefit must be balanced against possible effects of the absorption of iodine on foetal thyroid function and development.

4.7 Effects on ability to drive and use machines
None stated.

4.8 Undesirable effects
Rarely, local irritation may occur.

4.9 Overdose
In the case of deliberate or accidental ingestion of large quantities, symptomatic and supportive treatment should be provided with special attention to electrolyte balance and thyroid function.

5. PHARMACOLOGICAL PROPERTIES

5.1 Pharmacodynamic properties
Povidone iodine is a complex of iodine which shows all the broad-spectrum germicidal activity of elemental iodine. The germicidal activity is maintained in the presence of blood, pus, serum and necrotic tissue. It is effective in the treatment of infections caused by bacteria, fungi, yeasts and viruses (e.g. Herpes Virus Types I and II).

5.2 Pharmacokinetic properties
None stated.

5.3 Preclinical safety data
None stated.

6. PHARMACEUTICAL PARTICULARS

6.1 List of excipients
Glycerol; nonoxynol 9; disodium hydrogen phosphate (anhydrous); citric acid monohydrate; industrial methylated spirit; sodium hydroxide (5% solution); purified water.

6.2 Incompatibilities
None stated.

6.3 Shelf life
36 months unopened.

6.4 Special precautions for storage
Store below 25°C.

6.5 Nature and contents of container
Glass bottle with a white polypropylene cap and applicator brush containing 8ml of product.

6.6 Instructions for use and handling
None stated.

7. MARKETING AUTHORISATION HOLDER
Seton Healthcare Group plc, Tubiton House, Oldham, OL1 3HS.

8. MARKETING AUTHORISATION NUMBER(S)
PL 0223/0011.

9. DATE OF FIRST AUTHORISATION/RENEWAL OF THE AUTHORISATION
28th April 1993 / 8th November 2003.

10. DATE OF REVISION OF THE TEXT
November 2003.

Betadine Dry Powder Spray

(Medlock Medical Ltd)

1. NAME OF THE MEDICINAL PRODUCT
Betadine Dry Powder Spray.

2. QUALITATIVE AND QUANTITATIVE COMPOSITION
Povidone Iodine 2.5% w/w.

3. PHARMACEUTICAL FORM
Pressurised aerosol spray.

4. CLINICAL PARTICULARS

4.1 Therapeutic indications
Betadine Dry Powder Spray is an antiseptic for the treatment and prevention of infection in wounds including ulcers, burns, cuts and other minor injuries.

4.2 Posology and method of administration
For topical use only. Adults and children aged 2 years and over: Shake the can well before use. Spray the required area from a distance of 15-25cm (6-10 inches) until a dusting of powder is deposited. If necessary, the treated area may be covered with a dressing.

4.3 Contraindications
Hypersensitivity to iodine. Betadine Dry Powder Spray should not be used in serous cavities. Do not use this product regularly if the patient suffers from thyroid disorders or is receiving concurrent lithium therapy. Do not use on children under two years of age.

4.4 Special warnings and special precautions for use
Avoid inhaling or spraying into the eyes. Avoid use on patients with renal impairment. Should evidence of local irritation or sensitivity occur, use of the product should cease. If no improvement occurs, a doctor should be consulted.

4.5 Interaction with other medicinal products and other forms of Interaction
Use with concurrent lithium therapy has been shown to exhibit additive hypothyroidic effects.

4.6 Pregnancy and lactation
Use in pregnancy or lactation should be limited. Although no adverse effects are anticipated from such limited usage, caution is recommended and therapeutic benefit must be balanced against the possible effects of the absorption of iodine on foetal thyroid function and development.

4.7 Effects on ability to drive and use machines
None known.

4.8 Undesirable effects
Iodine is absorbed through burns and broken skin and to a lesser extent through intact skin. Following prolonged application of Betadine Dry Powder Spray to severe burns or large areas of denuded skin, systemic effects such as metabolic acidosis, parametrical renal impairment and thyroid dysfunction may occur.

4.9 Overdose
Excess iodine can produce goitre and hypothyroidism or hyperthyroidism. Systemic absorption of iodine after repeated application of povidone iodine to large areas of wounds or burns may lead to a number of adverse effects: metallic taste in mouth, increased salivation, burning or pain in the throat or mouth, irritation and swelling of the eyes, pulmonary oedema, skin reactions, gastrointestinal upset and diarrhoea, metabolic acidosis, hypernatraemia and renal impairment.

Treatment: In the case of deliberate or accidental ingestion of large quantities of Betadine, symptomatic and supportive treatment should be provided with special attention to electrolyte balance and renal and thyroid function.

5. PHARMACOLOGICAL PROPERTIES

5.1 Pharmacodynamic properties

Povidone iodine is a complex of iodine which retains the broad-spectrum germicidal activity of the elemental iodine without its disadvantages. The germicidal activity is maintained in the presence of blood, pus, serum and necrotic tissue.

5.2 Pharmacokinetic properties

Not applicable.

5.3 Preclinical safety data

None stated.

6. PHARMACEUTICAL PARTICULARS

6.1 List of excipients

Isopropyl myristate; n-pentane; butane 40; soya lecithin.

6.2 Incompatibilities

None known.

6.3 Shelf life

36 months unopened.

6.4 Special precautions for storage

Store at or below 25°C.

6.5 Nature and contents of container

Aerosol cans containing 100ml of product.

6.6 Instructions for use and handling

None.

7. MARKETING AUTHORISATION HOLDER

Seton Healthcare Group plc, Tubiton House, Oldham, OL1 3HS.

8. MARKETING AUTHORISATION NUMBER(S)

PL 0223/0013.

9. DATE OF FIRST AUTHORISATION/RENEWAL OF THE AUTHORISATION

17th August 1993 / 23rd October 2004.

10. DATE OF REVISION OF THE TEXT

October 2004.

Betadine Gargle & Mouthwash

(Medlock Medical Ltd)

1. NAME OF THE MEDICINAL PRODUCT

Betadine Gargle and Mouthwash.

2. QUALITATIVE AND QUANTITATIVE COMPOSITION

Povidone Iodine USP 1% w/v (equivalent to 0.1% w/v of available iodine).

3. PHARMACEUTICAL FORM

Solution.

4. CLINICAL PARTICULARS

4.1 Therapeutic indications

For the treatment of acute mucosal infections of the mouth and pharynx, for example gingivitis, and mouth ulcers. For oral hygiene prior to, during and after dental and oral surgery.

4.2 Posology and method of administration

For oral administration, as a gargle and mouthwash. The product should not be swallowed. *Adults and children over 6 years of age:* Use undiluted or diluted with an equal volume of warm water. Gargle or rinse with up to 10ml for up to 30 seconds without swallowing. Repeat up to four times daily, for up to 14 consecutive days, or as directed.

4.3 Contraindications

Not for use in children under 6 years of age and in patients with a known or suspected iodine hypersensitivity. Regular use is contraindicated in patients and users with thyroid disorders (in particular nodular colloid goitre, endemic goitre and Hashimoto's thyroiditis).

4.4 Special warnings and special precautions for use

Regular use should be avoided as prolonged use may lead to the absorption of a significant amount of iodine. Do not use for more than 14 days. If sores or ulcers in the mouth do not heal within 14 days, seek medical or dental advice. Regular use should be avoided in patients on concurrent lithium therapy.

4.5 Interaction with other medicinal products and other forms of Interaction

Absorption of iodine from povidone iodine may interfere with thyroid function tests. Contamination with povidone iodine of several types of tests for the detection of occult blood in faeces or blood in urine may produce false-positive results.

4.6 Pregnancy and lactation

Regular use of povidone iodine should be avoided in pregnant or lactating women as absorbed iodine can cross the placental barrier and be secreted into breast milk. Although no adverse effects have been reported from limited use, caution should be recommended and therapeutic benefit must be balanced against possible effects of the absorption of iodine on foetal thyroid function and development. The use of Betadine Gargle and Mouthwash in pregnant and lactating women should be limited to a single treatment session only.

4.7 Effects on ability to drive and use machines

None known.

4.8 Undesirable effects

Idiosyncratic mucosal irritation and hypersensitivity reactions may occur. Excessive absorption of iodine may produce systemic effects such as metabolic acidosis, hypernatraemia and impairment of renal function.

4.9 Overdose

Excessive iodine can produce goitre and hypothyroidism or hyperthyroidism. Acute overdose may result in symptoms of metallic taste in the mouth, increased salivation, burning or pain in the throat or mouth, irritation and swelling in the eyes, difficulty in breathing due to pulmonary oedema, skin reactions, gastrointestinal upset and diarrhoea. Metabolic acidosis, hypernatraemia and renal impairment may occur. Treatment: In the cases of deliberate or accidental ingestion of large quantities of Betadine, symptomatic and supportive treatment should be provided with special attention to electrolyte balance and renal and thyroid function.

5. PHARMACOLOGICAL PROPERTIES

5.1 Pharmacodynamic properties

Betadine Gargle and Mouthwash contains povidone iodine, a complex of iodine which shows all the broad spectrum germicidal activity of elemental iodine. The germicidal activity is maintained in the presence of blood, pus, serum and necrotic tissue. Betadine Gargle and Mouthwash kills bacteria, viruses, fungi, spores and protozoa.

5.2 Pharmacokinetic properties

The product is intended for topical application to the mouth and buccal cavity.

5.3 Preclinical safety data

None stated.

6. PHARMACEUTICAL PARTICULARS

6.1 List of excipients

Glycerol; menthol; methyl salicylate; ethanol 96%; saccharin sodium; purified water.

6.2 Incompatibilities

None stated.

6.3 Shelf life

36 months unopened.

6.4 Special precautions for storage

Store in a dry place below 25°C. Protect from light.

6.5 Nature and contents of container

Amber soda-lime-silica glass bottle (USP Type III) fitted with an externally ribbed white urea cap, with a steran faced wad or with a wadless polypropylene cap containing 250ml of product.

6.6 Instructions for use and handling

This product should not be swallowed.

7. MARKETING AUTHORISATION HOLDER

Seton Healthcare Group plc, Tubiton House, Oldham, OL1 3HS.

8. MARKETING AUTHORISATION NUMBER(S)

PL 0223/0014.

9. DATE OF FIRST AUTHORISATION/RENEWAL OF THE AUTHORISATION

28th April 1994 / 6th November 2003.

10. DATE OF REVISION OF THE TEXT

November 2003.

Betadine Ointment

(Medlock Medical Ltd)

1. NAME OF THE MEDICINAL PRODUCT

Betadine Ointment.

2. QUALITATIVE AND QUANTITATIVE COMPOSITION

Povidone Iodine 10% w/w.

3. PHARMACEUTICAL FORM

Ointment.

4. CLINICAL PARTICULARS

4.1 Therapeutic indications

Betadine Ointment is a broad-spectrum antiseptic for the topical treatment or prevention of infection in minor cuts and abrasions, minor surgical procedures and small areas of burns. Treatment of mycotic and bacterial skin infections and pyodermas. Treatment of infections in decubitus and stasis ulcers.

4.2 Posology and method of administration

Route of administration: Topical. For the treatment of infection: Apply once or twice daily for a maximum of 14 days. For the prevention of infection: Apply once or twice a week for as long as necessary. The affected skin should be cleaned and dried. Apply Betadine Ointment to the affected area. May be covered with a dressing or bandage. Not for use in children under two years of age.

4.3 Contraindications

Known or suspected iodine hypersensitivity. Regular use is contraindicated in patients and users with thyroid disorders (in particular nodular colloidal goitre, endemic goitre and Hashimoto's thyroiditis). Not for use in children under two years of age.

4.4 Special warnings and special precautions for use

Special caution is needed when regular applications to broken skin are made to patients with pre-existing renal insufficiency. Regular use should be avoided in patients on concurrent lithium therapy. Thyroid function tests should be performed during prolonged use.

4.5 Interaction with other medicinal products and other forms of Interaction

Absorption of iodine from povidone iodine through either intact or damaged skin may interfere with thyroid function tests. Contamination with povidone iodine of several types of tests for the detection of occult blood in faeces or blood in urine may produce false-positive results.

4.6 Pregnancy and lactation

Regular use of povidone iodine should be avoided in pregnant or lactating women as absorbed iodine can cross the placental barrier and can be secreted into breast milk. Although no adverse effects have been reported from limited use, caution should be recommended and therapeutic benefit must be balanced against possible effects of the absorption on foetal thyroid function and development.

4.7 Effects on ability to drive and use machines

None known.

4.8 Undesirable effects

Povidone iodine may produce local skin reactions although it is considered to be less irritant than iodine. The application of povidone iodine to large wounds or severe burns may produce systemic adverse effects such as metabolic acidosis, hypernatraemia and impairment of renal function.

4.9 Overdose

Excess iodine can produce goitre and hypothyroidism or hyperthyroidism. Systemic absorption of iodine after repeated application of povidone iodine to large areas of wounds or burns may lead to a number of adverse effects: metallic taste in mouth, increased salivation, burning or pain in the throat or mouth, irritation and swelling of the eyes, pulmonary oedema, skin reactions, gastrointestinal upset and diarrhoea, metabolic acidosis, hypernatraemia and renal impairment.

Treatment: In the case of deliberate or accidental ingestion of large quantities of Betadine, symptomatic and supportive treatment should be provided with special attention to electrolyte balance and renal and thyroid function.

5. PHARMACOLOGICAL PROPERTIES

5.1 Pharmacodynamic properties

Povidone iodine is a complex of iodine, which retains the broad-spectrum germicidal activity of elemental iodine without its disadvantages. The germicidal activity is maintained in the presence of blood, pus, serum and necrotic tissue.

5.2 Pharmacokinetic properties

Betadine Ointment is applied topically to the affected area.

5.3 Preclinical safety data

Not applicable.

6. PHARMACEUTICAL PARTICULARS

6.1 List of excipients

Polyethylene glycol 4000; polyethylene glycol 1000; polyethylene glycol 1500; purified water; sodium bicarbonate; polyethylene glycol 400.

6.2 Incompatibilities

None.

6.3 Shelf life

36 months unopened.

6.4 Special precautions for storage

Store at or below 25°C.

6.5 Nature and contents of container

Triple epoxy lacquered aluminium tubes with polyethylene closures containing 20 or 80g of product.

6.6 Instructions for use and handling

None stated.

7. MARKETING AUTHORISATION HOLDER

Seton Healthcare Group plc, Tubiton House, Oldham, OL1 3HS.

8. MARKETING AUTHORISATION NUMBER(S)

PL 0223/0015.

9. DATE OF FIRST AUTHORISATION/RENEWAL OF THE AUTHORISATION

21st July 1993 / 11th November 2003.

10. DATE OF REVISION OF THE TEXT

November 2003.

Betadine Shampoo

(Medlock Medical Ltd)

1. NAME OF THE MEDICINAL PRODUCT
Betadine Shampoo.

2. QUALITATIVE AND QUANTITATIVE COMPOSITION
Povidone Iodine 4.00% w/v.

3. PHARMACEUTICAL FORM
Shampoo for cutaneous use.

4. CLINICAL PARTICULARS

4.1 Therapeutic indications
Seborrhoeic conditions of the scalp associated with excessive dandruff, pruritis, scaling, exudation and erythema of the scalp, pityriasis capitis; infected lesions of the scalp - pyodermas (recurrent furunculosis, infective folliculitis and impetigo).

4.2 Posology and method of administration
Route of administration: topical use. Adults and children over 12 years: Having first wetted the hair, apply 2 or 3 capfuls of Betadine Shampoo, use warm water to lather. Rinse. Again, apply 2 or 3 capfuls of Betadine Shampoo and massage into the scalp with the tips of the fingers. Work up to a golden lather using warm water. Repeat treatment twice weekly until improvement is noted. Afterwards, use Betadine Shampoo once a week. Children aged 2 to 12 years: As for children over 12 years, substituting 1 or 2 capfuls of Betadine Shampoo. Children under 2 years: Contraindicated.

4.3 Contraindications
Known or suspected iodine hypersensitivity. Regular use is contra-indicated in patients and users with thyroid disorders (in particular nodular colloid goitre, endemic goitre and Hashimoto's thyroiditis). Not for use in children under two years.

4.4 Special warnings and special precautions for use
Special caution is needed when regular applications to broken skin are made to patients with pre-existing renal insufficiency. Regular use should be avoided in patients on concurrent lithium therapy.

4.5 Interaction with other medicinal products and other forms of Interaction
Absorption of iodine from povidone iodine through either intact or broken skin may interfere with thyroid function tests. Contamination with povidone iodine of several types of tests for the detection of occult blood in faeces or blood in urine may produce false-positive results.

4.6 Pregnancy and lactation
Regular use of povidone iodine should be avoided in pregnant or lactating women as absorbed iodine can cross the placental barrier and can be secreted into breast milk. Although no adverse effects have been reported from limited use, caution should be recommended and therapeutic benefit must be balanced against possible effects of the absorption of iodine on foetal thyroid function and development.

4.7 Effects on ability to drive and use machines
None known.

4.8 Undesirable effects
Povidone iodine may produce local skin reactions although it is considered to be less irritant than iodine.

4.9 Overdose
Excess iodine can produce goitre and hypothyroidism or hyperthyroidism. In the case of deliberate or accidental ingestion of large quantities of Betadine, symptomatic and supportive treatment should be provided with special attention to electrolyte balance and renal and thyroid function.

5. PHARMACOLOGICAL PROPERTIES

5.1 Pharmacodynamic properties
Betadine Shampoo contains povidone iodine, a complex of iodine which shows all the broad-spectrum germicidal activity of elemental iodine. The germicidal activity is maintained in the presence of blood, pus, serum and necrotic tissue. Povidone iodine kills bacteria, viruses, fungi, spores and protozoa.

5.2 Pharmacokinetic properties
The product is intended for topical application.

5.3 Preclinical safety data
None stated.

6. PHARMACEUTICAL PARTICULARS

6.1 List of excipients
Sulphated nonylphenoxypoly (oxyethylene) lauric diethanolamide; ethoxylated lanolin 50%; hydroxyethyl cellulose; perfume Vah Floral No 2; potassium iodate; sodium hydroxide; purified water.

6.2 Incompatibilities
None.

6.3 Shelf life
24 months unopened.

6.4 Special precautions for storage
Store in a dry place at or below 25°C and protected from light.

6.5 Nature and contents of container
White polypropylene containers fitted with white polypropylene lids, containing 250ml of product.

6.6 Instructions for use and handling
None stated.

7. MARKETING AUTHORISATION HOLDER
Seton Healthcare Group plc, Tubiton House, Oldham, OL1 3HS.

8. MARKETING AUTHORISATION NUMBER(S)
PL 0223/0021.

9. DATE OF FIRST AUTHORISATION/RENEWAL OF THE AUTHORISATION
16th September 1993 / 15th November 2003.

10. DATE OF REVISION OF THE TEXT
November 2003.

Betadine Skin Cleanser

(Medlock Medical Ltd)

1. NAME OF THE MEDICINAL PRODUCT
Betadine Skin Cleanser.

2. QUALITATIVE AND QUANTITATIVE COMPOSITION
Povidone Iodine USP 4.00% w/v.

3. PHARMACEUTICAL FORM
Topical aqueous solution.

4. CLINICAL PARTICULARS

4.1 Therapeutic indications
Acne vulgaris of the face and neck. For general disinfection of the skin (as a liquid soap).

4.2 Posology and method of administration
Route of administration: Topical. Adults, the elderly and children over 2 years: Apply directly or with moistened sponge to the affected areas and work up a rich lather. Allow to remain on the skin for 3-5 minutes then rinse off thoroughly with warm water and dry with a clean or sterile towel or gauze. Repeat twice daily. Infants under 2 years: Limit use to 2-3 days.

4.3 Contraindications
Hypersensitivity to iodine. History of abnormal thyroid function or goitre.

4.4 Special warnings and special precautions for use
Do not use on broken skin. Iodine is absorbed through burns and broken skin and, to a lesser extent, through intact skin. Restrict use in infants to 2-3 days.

4.5 Interaction with other medicinal products and other forms of Interaction
None known.

4.6 Pregnancy and lactation
Use in pregnancy and lactation should be limited and although no adverse effects are anticipated from such limited usage, caution is recommended and the therapeutic benefit must be balanced against the possible effects of the absorption of iodine on foetal thyroid function.

4.7 Effects on ability to drive and use machines
None known.

4.8 Undesirable effects
If local irritation or sensitivity develops, then discontinue treatment.

4.9 Overdose
Treatment: In the case of deliberate or accidental ingestion of large quantities of Betadine, symptomatic and supportive treatment should be provided with special attention to electrolyte balance and renal and thyroid function.

5. PHARMACOLOGICAL PROPERTIES

5.1 Pharmacodynamic properties
Betadine Skin Cleanser contains povidone iodine, a complex of iodine which shows all the broad-spectrum germicidal activity of elemental iodine. The germicidal activity is maintained in the presence of exfoliative debris and infected lesions whilst the colour persists. Betadine Skin Cleanser kills bacteria, viruses, fungi, spores and protozoa.

5.2 Pharmacokinetic properties
The product is intended for topical application.

5.3 Preclinical safety data
Not applicable.

6. PHARMACEUTICAL PARTICULARS

6.1 List of excipients
Purified water; potassium iodate; NPPE ester; lauric diethanolamide; hydroxyethylcellulose; Vah Floral Perfume No 2; sodium hydroxide.

6.2 Incompatibilities
None known.

6.3 Shelf life
36 months

6.4 Special precautions for storage
Store at a temperature not exceeding 25°C.

6.5 Nature and contents of container
Polypropylene container with polypropylene lid containing 250ml.

6.6 Instructions for use and handling
None stated.

7. MARKETING AUTHORISATION HOLDER
Medlock Medical Limited, Tubiton House, Medlock Street, Oldham, OL1 3HS.

8. MARKETING AUTHORISATION NUMBER(S)
PL 21248/0015.

9. DATE OF FIRST AUTHORISATION/RENEWAL OF THE AUTHORISATION
30th March 2005.

10. DATE OF REVISION OF THE TEXT
March 2005.

Betadine Standardised Antiseptic Solution

(Medlock Medical Ltd)

1. NAME OF THE MEDICINAL PRODUCT
Standardised Betadine Antiseptic Solution.

2. QUALITATIVE AND QUANTITATIVE COMPOSITION
Povidone Iodine 10.00% w/v.

3. PHARMACEUTICAL FORM
Aqueous solution.

4. CLINICAL PARTICULARS

4.1 Therapeutic indications
For use as a pre-operative and post-operative antiseptic skin cleanser for major and minor surgical procedures.

4.2 Posology and method of administration
Route of administration: Topical. Adults, the elderly and children: Apply full strength as a pre-operative and post-operative antiseptic skin cleanser. Avoid pooling both under the patient and in the skin folds. Wash off excess solution before using occlusive dressings. Povidone iodine is not recommended for regular use in neonates and is contraindicated in very low birth weight infants (below 1500 grams).

4.3 Contraindications
Known or suspected iodine hypersensitivity. Regular use is contraindicated in patients and users with thyroid disorders (in particular nodular colloid goitre, endemic goitre and Hashimoto's thyroiditis). Standardised Betadine Antiseptic Solution is not recommended for body cavity irrigation.

4.4 Special warnings and special precautions for use
Special caution is needed when regular applications to broken skin are made to patients with pre-existing renal insufficiency. Regular use should be avoided in patients on concurrent lithium therapy.

4.5 Interaction with other medicinal products and other forms of Interaction
Absorption of iodine from povidone iodine through either intact or damaged skin may interfere with thyroid function tests. Contamination with povidone iodine of several types of tests for the detection of occult blood in faeces or blood in urine may produce false-positive results.

4.6 Pregnancy and lactation
Regular use of povidone iodine should be avoided in pregnant or lactating women as absorbed iodine can cross the placental barrier and can be secreted into breast milk. Although no adverse effects have been reported from limited use, caution should be recommended and therapeutic benefit must be balanced against possible effects of the absorption on foetal thyroid function and development.

4.7 Effects on ability to drive and use machines
None known.

4.8 Undesirable effects
Povidone iodine may produce local skin reactions although it is considered to be less irritant than iodine. The application of povidone iodine to large wounds or severe burns may produce systemic adverse effects such as metabolic acidosis, hypernatraemia and impairment of renal function.

4.9 Overdose
Excess iodine can produce goitre and hypothyroidism or hyperthyroidism. Systemic absorption of iodine after repeated application of povidone iodine to large areas of wounds or burns may lead to a number of adverse effects: metallic taste in mouth, increased salivation, burning or pain in the throat or mouth, irritation and swelling of the eyes, pulmonary oedema, skin reactions, gastrointestinal upset and diarrhoea, metabolic acidosis, hypernatraemia and renal impairment.

In the case of deliberate or accidental ingestion of large quantities of Betadine, symptomatic and supportive treatment should be provided with special attention to electrolyte balance and renal and thyroid function.

5. PHARMACOLOGICAL PROPERTIES

5.1 Pharmacodynamic properties

Standardised Betadine Antiseptic Solution contains povidone iodine, a complex of iodine which shows all the broad spectrum germicidal activity of elemental iodine. The germicidal activity is maintained in the presence of blood, pus, serum and necrotic tissue. Standardised Betadine Antiseptic Solution kills bacteria, viruses, fungi, spores and protozoa.

5.2 Pharmacokinetic properties

The product is intended for topical application.

5.3 Preclinical safety data

None stated.

6. PHARMACEUTICAL PARTICULARS

6.1 List of excipients

Glycerol; nonoxynol 9; dibasic sodium phosphate (anhydrous); citric acid monohydrate; sodium hydroxide; potassium iodate; purified water.

6.2 Incompatibilities

None.

6.3 Shelf life

36 months unopened.

6.4 Special precautions for storage

Store at a temperature not exceeding 25°C.

6.5 Nature and contents of container

High-density polyethylene bottle containing 500ml of product, fitted with a white polypropylene cap with a steranlined wad.

6.6 Instructions for use and handling

None stated.

7. MARKETING AUTHORISATION HOLDER

Medlock Medical Limited, Tubiton House, Medlock Street, Oldham, OL1 3HS.

8. MARKETING AUTHORISATION NUMBER(S)

PL 21248/0002.

9. DATE OF FIRST AUTHORISATION/RENEWAL OF THE AUTHORISATION

30th March 2005.

10. DATE OF REVISION OF THE TEXT

March 2005.

Betadine Surgical Scrub

(Medlock Medical Ltd)

1. NAME OF THE MEDICINAL PRODUCT

Betadine Surgical Scrub.

2. QUALITATIVE AND QUANTITATIVE COMPOSITION

Povidone Iodine 7.5% w/v.

3. PHARMACEUTICAL FORM

Surgical scrub.

4. CLINICAL PARTICULARS

4.1 Therapeutic indications

For use as an antiseptic cleanser for pre-operative scrubbing and washing by surgeons and theatre staff, and pre-operative preparation of patients' skin.

4.2 Posology and method of administration

For topical administration. Adults, the elderly and children: Apply full strength as a pre-operative antiseptic skin cleanser. Povidone iodine is not recommended for regular use in neonates and is contraindicated in very low birth weight infants (below 1500grams).

4.3 Contraindications

Known or suspected iodine hypersensitivity. Regular use is contraindicated in patients and users with thyroid disorders (in particular nodular colloid goitre, endemic goitre and Hashimoto's thyroiditis).

4.4 Special warnings and special precautions for use

Special caution is needed when regular applications to broken skin are made to patients with pre-existing renal insufficiency. Regular use should be avoided in patients on concurrent lithium therapy.

4.5 Interaction with other medicinal products and other forms of Interaction

Absorption of iodine from povidone iodine through either intact or damaged skin may interfere with thyroid function tests. Contamination with povidone iodine of several types of tests for the detection of occult blood in faeces or blood in urine may produce false-positive results.

4.6 Pregnancy and lactation

Regular use of povidone iodine should be avoided in pregnant or lactating women as absorbed iodine can cross the placental barrier and can be secreted into breast milk. Although no adverse effects have been reported from limited use, caution should be recommended and therapeutic benefit must be balanced against possible effects of the absorption on foetal thyroid function and development.

4.7 Effects on ability to drive and use machines

None known.

4.8 Undesirable effects

Povidone iodine may produce local skin reactions although it is considered to be less irritant than iodine. The application of povidone iodine to large wounds or severe burns may produce systemic adverse effects such as metabolic acidosis, hypernatraemia and impairment of renal function.

4.9 Overdose

Excess iodine can produce goitre and hypothyroidism or hyperthyroidism. Systemic absorption of iodine after repeated application of povidone iodine to large areas of wounds or burns may lead to a number of adverse effects: metallic taste in mouth, irritation and swelling of the eyes, pulmonary oedema, skin reactions, gastrointestinal upset and diarrhoea, metabolic acidosis, hypernatraemia and impairment of renal function. In the case of accidental ingestion of large quantities of Betadine, symptomatic and supportive treatment should be provided with special attention to electrolyte balance and renal and thyroid function.

5. PHARMACOLOGICAL PROPERTIES

5.1 Pharmacodynamic properties

The active ingredient, povidone iodine, slowly liberates iodine when in contact with skin and mucous membranes. The activity of 'iodine' as a microbicide is then governed by a series of dissociations: $I_2 \leftrightarrow I^+ + I^-$; $I_2 + H_2O \leftrightarrow H_2O\,I^+ + I^-$; $I_2 + I^- \leftrightarrow I_3^-$. The microbicidal species $H_2O\,I^+$ preferentially displaces oxygen as the end electron acceptor in the microorganism's respiratory cycle. $H_2O\,I^+$ similarly interacts within the electron transport chain and reacts with the amino acids of the microbial cell membrane.

5.2 Pharmacokinetic properties

Betadine Surgical Scrub is intended for topical application and therefore a consideration of the absorption, distribution, metabolism and elimination of povidone iodine is largely without relevance.

5.3 Preclinical safety data

None stated.

6. PHARMACEUTICAL PARTICULARS

6.1 List of excipients

Sulphated nonylphenoxypoly(oxyethylene) ethanol ammonium salt; lauric diethanolamide;

ethoxylated lanolin 50%; hydroxyethylcellulose; sodium hydroxide; purified water.

6.2 Incompatibilities

None stated.

6.3 Shelf life

36 months unopened.

6.4 Special precautions for storage

Store below 25°C and protect from light.

6.5 Nature and contents of container

High density polyethylene containers fitted with steran lined white polypropylene caps containing 500ml of product.

6.6 Instructions for use and handling

None stated.

7. MARKETING AUTHORISATION HOLDER

Medlock Medical Limited, Tubiton House, Medlock Street, Oldham, OL1 3HS.

8. MARKETING AUTHORISATION NUMBER(S)

PL 21248/0009.

9. DATE OF FIRST AUTHORISATION/RENEWAL OF THE AUTHORISATION

14th March 2005.

10. DATE OF REVISION OF THE TEXT

March 2005.

Betadine Vaginal Cleansing (VC) Kit

(Medlock Medical Ltd)

1. NAME OF THE MEDICINAL PRODUCT

Betadine VC Kit 10% w/v.

2. QUALITATIVE AND QUANTITATIVE COMPOSITION

Povidone Iodine USP 10% w/v.

3. PHARMACEUTICAL FORM

Solution.

4. CLINICAL PARTICULARS

4.1 Therapeutic indications

As a vaginal cleanser in the treatment of vaginitis due to candidal, trichomonal, non-specific or mixed infections and for pre-operative preparation of the vagina.

4.2 Posology and method of administration

For intravaginal use. Adults and the elderly: Once a day (preferably in the morning) for a 14 day period, including days of menstruation. The Betadine VC Concentrate should be diluted 1:10 using the measuring cap, and used according to the patient instruction leaflet provided. The applicators should only be used for the administration of the diluted VC Kit solution. This product may be used in combination with Betadine Vaginal Pessaries. Children: Contra-indicated for use in pre-pubertal children.

4.3 Contraindications

Known or suspected iodine hypersensitivity. Regular use is contra-indicated in patients and users with thyroid disorders (in particular nodular colloid goitre, endemic goitre and Hashimoto's thyroiditis).

4.4 Special warnings and special precautions for use

Special caution is needed when regular applications to broken skin are made to patients with pre-existing renal insufficiency. Regular use should be avoided in patients on concurrent lithium therapy.

4.5 Interaction with other medicinal products and other forms of Interaction

Absorption of iodine from povidone iodine through either intact or broken skin may interfere with thyroid function tests. Contamination with povidone iodine of several types of tests for the detection of occult blood in faeces or blood in urine may produce false-positive results.

4.6 Pregnancy and lactation

Regular use of povidone iodine should be avoided in pregnant or lactating women as absorbed iodine can cross the placental barrier and can be secreted into breast milk. Although no adverse effects have been reported from limited use, caution should be recommended and therapeutic benefit must be balanced against possible effects of the absorption of iodine on foetal thyroid function and development.

4.7 Effects on ability to drive and use machines

None known.

4.8 Undesirable effects

If local irritation, redness or swelling develops, discontinue treatment. Iodine is absorbed from the vagina and following prolonged use, thyroid dysfunction may develop. The product may be spermicidal and should not be used when conception is desired.

4.9 Overdose

Excess iodine can produce goitre and hypothyroidism or hyperthyroidism. In the case of deliberate or accidental ingestion of large quantities of Betadine, symptomatic and supportive treatment should be provided with special attention to electrolyte balance and renal and thyroid function.

5. PHARMACOLOGICAL PROPERTIES

5.1 Pharmacodynamic properties

Povidone iodine is a complex of iodine which retains the broad spectrum germicidal activity of elemental iodine without its disadvantages. The germicidal activity is maintained in the presence of blood, pus, serum and necrotic tissue.

5.2 Pharmacokinetic properties

Betadine VC Concentrate is applied topically to the affected area.

5.3 Preclinical safety data

None stated.

6. PHARMACEUTICAL PARTICULARS

6.1 List of excipients

Nonoxynol 9; Fleuroma Bouquet 477; purified water.

6.2 Incompatibilities

Compatibility with barrier contraceptives has not been established. Therefore this product should not be used with such methods of contraception as their reliability may be affected.

6.3 Shelf life

36 months.

6.4 Special precautions for storage

Store at or below 25°C.

6.5 Nature and contents of container

Carton containing a white polypropylene container with a white polypropylene wadless cap containing 250ml Betadine VC Concentrate, an empty turquoise low density polypropylene squeeze bottle and a vaginal applicator.

6.6 Instructions for use and handling

None stated.

7. MARKETING AUTHORISATION HOLDER

Seton Healthcare Group plc, Tubiton House, Oldham, OL1 3HS.

8. MARKETING AUTHORISATION NUMBER(S)

PL 0223/0020.

9. DATE OF FIRST AUTHORISATION/RENEWAL OF THE AUTHORISATION

28th April 1993 / 17th November 1998.

10. DATE OF REVISION OF THE TEXT

April 2003.

Betadine Vaginal Pessaries

(Medlock Medical Ltd)

1. NAME OF THE MEDICINAL PRODUCT

Betadine Vaginal Pessaries.

2. QUALITATIVE AND QUANTITATIVE COMPOSITION

Povidone Iodine USP 200mg.

3. PHARMACEUTICAL FORM
Pessary.

4. CLINICAL PARTICULARS

4.1 Therapeutic indications
For the treatment of vaginitis due to candidal, trichomonal, non-specific or mixed infections and for pre-operative preparation of the vagina.

4.2 Posology and method of administration
For intravaginal use. Adults and the elderly: Using the applicator, insert 1 pessary night and morning for up to 14 days. Each pessary should be wetted with water immediately prior to insertion, thus ensuring maximum dispersion of the active constituent and avoiding risk of local irritation. If menstruation occurs during treatment, it is important to continue treatment during the days of the period. Children: Contra-indicated for use in pre-pubertal children.

4.3 Contraindications
Known or suspected iodine hypersensitivity. Regular use is contra-indicated in patients and users with thyroid disorders (in particular nodular colloid goitre, endemic goitre and Hashimoto's thyroiditis).

4.4 Special warnings and special precautions for use
Special caution is needed when regular applications to broken skin are made to patients with pre-existing renal insufficiency. Regular use should be avoided in patients on concurrent lithium therapy.

4.5 Interaction with other medicinal products and other forms of Interaction
Absorption of iodine from povidone iodine through either intact or broken skin may interfere with thyroid function tests. Contamination with povidone iodine of several types of tests for the detection of occult blood in faeces or blood in urine may produce false-positive results.

4.6 Pregnancy and lactation
Regular use of povidone iodine should be avoided in pregnant or lactating women as absorbed iodine can cross the placental barrier and can be secreted into breast milk. Although no adverse effects have been reported from limited use, caution should be recommended and therapeutic benefit must be balanced against possible effects of the absorption of iodine on foetal thyroid function and development.

4.7 Effects on ability to drive and use machines
None known.

4.8 Undesirable effects
If local irritation, redness or swelling develops, discontinue treatment. Iodine is absorbed from the vagina and following prolonged use, thyroid dysfunction may develop. The product may be spermicidal and should not be used when conception is desired.

4.9 Overdose
Excess iodine can produce goitre and hypothyroidism or hyperthyroidism. In the case of deliberate or accidental ingestion of large quantities of Betadine, symptomatic and supportive treatment should be provided with special attention to electrolyte balance and renal and thyroid function.

5. PHARMACOLOGICAL PROPERTIES

5.1 Pharmacodynamic properties
Povidone iodine is a complex of iodine which retains the broad-spectrum germicidal activity of elemental iodine without its disadvantages. The germicidal activity is maintained in the presence of blood, pus, serum and necrotic tissue.

5.2 Pharmacokinetic properties
Betadine Vaginal Pessaries are applied topically to the affected area.

5.3 Preclinical safety data
None stated.

6. PHARMACEUTICAL PARTICULARS

6.1 List of excipients
Polyethylene glycol 1000.

6.2 Incompatibilities
Compatibility with barrier contraceptives has not been established. Therefore this product should not be used with such methods of contraception as their reliability may be affected.

6.3 Shelf life
36 months.

6.4 Special precautions for storage
Store below 25°C.

6.5 Nature and contents of container
Strips of aluminium foil laminated to polyethylene; preformed PVC packaging with a polyethylene lining. Packs of 28.

6.6 Instructions for use and handling
None stated.

7. MARKETING AUTHORISATION HOLDER
Seton Healthcare Group plc, Tubiton House, Oldham, OL1 3HS.

8. MARKETING AUTHORISATION NUMBER(S)
PL 0223/0019.

9. DATE OF FIRST AUTHORISATION/RENEWAL OF THE AUTHORISATION
28th April 1993 / 18th November 1998.

10. DATE OF REVISION OF THE TEXT
November 1998.

Betaferon

(Schering Health Care Limited)

1. NAME OF THE MEDICINAL PRODUCT
Betaferon 250 microgram/ml, powder and solvent for solution for injection.

2. QUALITATIVE AND QUANTITATIVE COMPOSITION
Recombinant interferon beta-1b* 250 microgram (8.0 million IU) per ml when reconstituted.

Betaferon contains 300 microgram (9.6 million IU) of recombinant interferon beta-1b per vial.

For excipients, see 6.1.

3. PHARMACEUTICAL FORM
Powder and solvent for solution for injection.

4. CLINICAL PARTICULARS

4.1 Therapeutic indications
Betaferon is indicated for the treatment of patients with relapsing remitting multiple sclerosis and two or more relapses within the last two years. Betaferon is also indicated for patients with secondary progressive multiple sclerosis with active disease, evidenced by relapses.

4.2 Posology and method of administration
The treatment with Betaferon should be initiated under the supervision of a physician experienced in the treatment of the disease.

• Adult patients (⩾ 18 years):

The recommended dose of Betaferon in patients suffering from relapsing-remitting multiple sclerosis or from secondary progressive multiple sclerosis is 250 microgram (8.0 million IU), contained in 1 ml of the reconstituted solution (cf. 6.6 "Instructions for use, handling <,disposal>"), to be injected subcutaneously every other day.

The optimal dose has not been fully clarified.

At the present time, it is not known for how long the patient should be treated. The efficacy of treatment for longer than two years has not been sufficiently demonstrated for relapsing-remitting multiple sclerosis. For secondary progressive multiple sclerosis efficacy for a period of two years with limited data for a period of up to three years of treatment has been demonstrated under controlled clinical trial conditions.

Full clinical assessment should be made at two years in all patients.

A decision for longer-term treatment should be made on an individual basis by the treating physician.

Exposure data from clinical trials for longer than three years for patients with relapsing-remitting multiple sclerosis or longer than 4.5 years for patients with secondary-progressive multiple sclerosis are not available. Treatment is not recommended in patients with relapsing-remitting multiple sclerosis who have experienced less than 2 relapses in the previous 2 years or in patients with secondary-progressive multiple sclerosis who have had no active disease in the previous 2 years.

If the patient fails to respond, for example a steady progression in EDSS for 6 months occurs or treatment with at least 3 courses of ACTH or corticosteroids during a one year period is required despite Betaferon therapy, treatment with Betaferon should be stopped.

• Children and adolescents (< 18 years)

The efficacy and safety of Betaferon have not been investigated in children and adolescents of less than 18 years of age. Betaferon should therefore not be administered to this age group.

4.3 Contraindications

– Pregnancy (see section 4.6 "Pregnancy and lactation").

– Patients with a history of hypersensitivity to natural or recombinant interferon-β, human albumin or to any of the excipients.

– Patients with a history of severe depressive disorders and/or suicidal ideation. (see section 4.4 "Special warnings and special precautions for use" and 4.8 "Undesirable effects")

– Patients with decompensated liver disease. (see sections 4.4 "Special warnings and precautions for use", 4.5 "Interaction with other medicinal products and other forms of interaction", 4.8 "Undesirable effects")

– Patients with epilepsy not adequately controlled by treatment. (see sections 4.4 "Special warnings and precautions for use", 4.5 "Interaction with other medicinal products and other forms of interaction", 4.8 "Undesirable effects")

4.4 Special warnings and special precautions for use
Patients to be treated with Betaferon should be informed that depressive disorders and suicidal ideation may be an undesirable effect of the treatment and should report these symptoms immediately to the prescribing physician. In rare cases these symptoms may result in a suicide attempt. Patients exhibiting depressive disorders and suicidal ideation should be monitored closely and cessation of therapy should be considered.

Betaferon should be administered with caution to patients with previous or current depressive disorders, a history of seizures and to those receiving treatment with anti-epileptics (see section 4.5 "Interaction with other medicaments and other forms of interaction"). It should also be used with caution in patients who suffer from pre-existing cardiac disorders.

Serious hypersensitivity reactions (rare but severe acute reactions such as bronchospasm, anaphylaxis and urticaria) may occur. If reactions are severe, Betaferon should be discontinued and appropriate medical intervention instituted. Other moderate to severe adverse experiences may require modifications of the Betaferon dosage regimen or even discontinuation of the agent.

A full blood count and differential WBC should be obtained prior to initiation of Betaferon and regularly during therapy.

AST (SGOT), ALT (SGPT) and γ-GT levels should be obtained prior to initiation of Betaferon therapy and regularly during therapy. The occurrence of elevations in serum transaminases should lead to close monitoring and investigation with withdrawal of Betaferon if the levels become significantly increased or if there are associated symptoms suggesting the development of hepatitis. In the absence of clinical evidence for liver damage and after normalisation of liver enzymes a reintroduction of therapy could be considered with appropriate follow-up of hepatic functions.

In rare cases, pancreatitis was observed with Betaferon use, often associated with hypertriglyceridaemia.

There are no data on patients with renal impairment. Renal function should be monitored carefully when such patients receive Betaferon therapy.

In the multiple sclerosis studies, 29% (between 28% and 41% in different studies) of the patients developed serum interferon beta-1b neutralising activity confirmed by at least two consecutive positive titres; of these patients, 49% (between 37% and 55% in different studies) permanently lost their neutralising activity during the subsequent observational period of the respective study. Thedevelopment of neutralising activity is associated with a reduction in clinical efficacy only with regard to relapse activity. Some analyses suggest that this effect might be larger in patients with higher titre levels of neutralising activity. The decision to continue or discontinue treatment should be based on clinical disease activity rather than on neutralising activity status.

New adverse events have not been associated with the development of neutralising activity. It has been demonstrated *in vitro* that Betaferon cross reacts with natural interferon beta. However, this has not been investigated *in vivo* and its clinical significance is uncertain.

There are sparse and inconclusive data on patients who have developed neutralising activity and have completed Betaferon therapy.

Injection site necrosis has been reported in patients using Betaferon (see section 4.8 "Undesirable effects"). It can be extensive and may involve muscle fascia as well as fat and therefore can result in scar formation. Occasionally debridement and, less often, skin grafting are required and healing may take up to 6 months.

If the patient has multiple lesions Betaferon should be discontinued until healing has occurred. Patients with single lesions may continue on Betaferon provided the necrosis is not too extensive, as some patients have experienced healing of injection site necrosis whilst on Betaferon.

To minimise the risk of injection site necrosis patients should be advised to:

– use an aseptic injection technique

– rotate the injection sites with each dose

The procedure for the self-administration by the patient should be reviewed periodically especially if injection site reactions have occurred.

Caution should be exercised when administering Betaferon to patients with myelosuppression, anaemia or thrombocytopenia; patients who develop neutropenia should be monitored closely for the development of fever or infection. There have been reports of thrombocytopenia, with profound decreases in platelet count.

Rare cases of cardiomyopathy have been reported: If this occurs and a relationship to Betaferon is suspected, treatment should be discontinued.

The administration of cytokines to patients with a preexisting monoclonal gammopathy has been associated with the development of systemic capillary leak syndrome with shock-like symptoms and fatal outcome.

4.5 Interaction with other medicinal products and other forms of Interaction
No formal drug interaction studies have been carried out with Betaferon.

The effect of alternate-day administration of 250 microgram (8.0 million IU) of Betaferon on drug metabolism in multiple sclerosis patients is unknown. Corticosteroid or ACTH treatment of relapses for periods of up to 28 days has been well tolerated in patients receiving Betaferon.

Due to the lack of clinical experience in multiple sclerosis patients, the use of Betaferon together with immunomodulators other than corticoids or ACTH is not recommended.

Interferons have been reported to reduce the activity of hepatic cytochrome P450-dependent enzymes in humans and animals. Caution should be exercised when Betaferon is administered in combination with medicinal products that have a narrow therapeutic index and are largely dependent on the hepatic cytochrome P450 system for clearance, e.g. anti-epileptics. Additional caution should be exercised with any co-medication which has an effect on the haematopoetic system.

No interaction studies with anti-epileptics have been carried out.

4.6 Pregnancy and lactation

• Pregnancy

It is not known whether Betaferon can cause foetal harm when administered to a pregnant woman or can affect human reproductive capacity. Spontaneous abortions have been reported in subjects with multiple sclerosis in controlled clinical trials. Therefore, Betaferon is contraindicated during pregnancy. For preclinical results refer to section 5.3 "Preclinical safety data".

• Women of child-bearing potential

Women of child-bearing potential should take appropriate contraceptive measures. If the patient becomes pregnant or plans to become pregnant while taking Betaferon, she should be informed of the potential hazards and it should be recommended to discontinue therapy (for preclinical results refer to section 5.3 "Preclinical safety data").

• Lactation

It is not known whether interferon beta-1b is excreted in human milk. Because of the potential for serious adverse reactions to Betaferon in nursing infants a decision should be made whether nursing or Betaferon should be discontinued.

4.7 Effects on ability to drive and use machines

No studies on the effects on the ability to drive and use machines have been performed.

Central nervous system-related adverse events associated with the use of Betaferon might influence the ability to drive and use machines in susceptible patients.

4.8 Undesirable effects

a) At the beginning of treatment adverse reactions are common but in general they subside with further treatment. The most frequently observed adverse reactions are a flu-like symptom complex (fever, chills, headache, myalgia, arthralgia, malaise, or sweating) and injection site reactions.

b) The following side effects listing is based on reports from clinical trials *(table 1, adverse events with incidence rates ≥ 10% and the respective percentages under placebo; significantly associated side effects < 10%)* and from the post marketing surveillance *(table 2, reporting rates based on spontaneous adverse drug reaction reports classified as very common (≥ 10%), common (< 10% - ≥ 1%), uncommon (< 1% - ≥ 1‰), rare (< 1‰ - ≥ 1/10.000) and very rare (< 1/10.000))* of Betaferon use. Experience with Betaferon in patients with MS is limited, consequently those adverse events which occur very rarely may not yet have been observed:

Table 1 (adverse events with incidence rates ≥ 10% and the respective percentages under placebo; significantly associated side effects < 10%)

(see Table 1)

Table 2 (reporting rates based on spontaneous adverse drug reaction reports classified as very common (≥ 10%), common (< 10% - ≥ 1%), uncommon (< 1% - ≥ 1‰), rare (< 1‰ - ≥ 1/10.000) and very rare (< 1/10.000))

(see Table 2 on next page)

c) A flu-like symptom complex (fever, chills, headache, myalgia, arthralgia, malaise, or sweating) has been seen frequently and is mainly due to the pharmacological effects of the medicinal product.

Injection site reactions occurred frequently after administration of Betaferon. Redness, swelling, discoloration, inflammation, pain, hypersensitivity, necrosis, and non-specific reactions were significantly associated with 250 microgram (8 million IU) Betaferon treatment. Lymphadenopathy has also been reported. The incidence rate of injection site reactions usually decreased over time. If the patient experiences any break in the skin, which may be associated with swelling or drainage of fluid from the injection site, the patient should be advised to consult with their physician before continuing injections with Betaferon. (See 4.4 "Special warnings and special precautions for use").

4.9 Overdose

Interferon beta-1b has been given without serious adverse events compromising vital functions to adult cancer patients at individual doses as high as 5,500 microgram (176 million IU) i.v. three times a week.

Table 1 (adverse events with incidence rates ≥ 10% and the respective percentages under placebo; significantly associated side effects < 10%)

Adverse Event	Secondary Progressive Multiple Sclerosis (European Study)	Secondary Progressive Multiple Sclerosis (North American Study)	Relapsing Remitting Multiple Sclerosis
	Betaferon 250 microgram (Placebo) n=360 (n=358)	Betaferon 250 microgram (Placebo) n=317(n=308)	Betaferon 250 microgram (Placebo) n=124 (n=123)
Blood and the lymphatic system disorders			
Lymphocytes <1500/mm^3 °	53% (28%)	88% (68%)	82 % (67 %)
Abs.Neutr.Count. <1500/mm^3 *°	18% (5%)	4% (10%)	18 % (5 %)
White Blood Cells <3000/mm^3 *°	13% (4%)	13% (4%)	16 % (4) %
Lymphadenopathy	3% (1 %)	11% (5%)	14 % (11 %)
Metabolism and nutrition disorders			
ALT > 5 times baseline *°	14% (5%)	4% (2%)	19 % (6 %)
Glucose < 55 mg/dL	27% (27%)	5% (3%)	15 % (13 %)
Urine protein > 1+	14% (11%)	5% (5%)	5 % (3 %)
AST > 5 times baseline *°	4% (1%)	2% (1%)	4 % (0 %)
Peripheral edema	7% (7%)	21% (18%)	7% (8%)
Nervous system disorders			
Dizziness	14% (14 %)	28% (26%)	35 % (28 %)
Insomnia	12% (8 %)	26% (25%)	31 % (33 %)
Depression	24% (31%)	44% (41%)	25% (24%)
Hypertonia °	41% (31 %)	57% (57%)	26 % (24 %)
Anxiety	6% (5 %)	10% (11%)	15 % (13 %)
Eye disorders			
Conjunctivitis	2% (3 %)	6% (6%)	12 % (10 %)
Ear and labyrinth disorders			
Ear pain	<1% (1 %)	6% (8%)	16 % (15 %)
Cardiac disorders			
Palpitation *	2% (3 %)	5% (2%)	8 % (2 %)
Vascular disorders			
Migraine	4% (3 %)	5% (4%)	12 % (7 %)
Vasodilatation	6% (4%)	13% (8%)	18% (17%)
Hypertension °	4% (2 %)	9% (8%)	7 % (2 %)
Respiratory disorders			
Sinusitis	6 % (6%)	16% (18%)	36 % (26 %)
Cough increased	5% (10%)	11% (15%)	31% (23%)
Dyspnea *	3% (2 %)	8% (6%)	8 % (2 %)
Gastrointestinal disorders			
Diarrhoea	7% (10 %)	21% (19%)	35 % (29 %)
Constipation	12% (12 %)	22% (24%)	24 % (18 %)
Nausea	13% (13%)	32% (30%)	48% (49%)
Vomiting	4% (6 %)	10% (12%)	21 % (19 %)
Skin and subcutaneous tissue disorders			
Skin disorder	4% (4%)	19% (17%)	6% (8%)
Rash °	20% (12%)	26% (20%)	27% (32 %)
Sweating *	6% (6%)	10% (10%)	23% (11 %)
Musculoskeletal disorders			
Myalgia *°	23% (9 %)	19% (29%)	44% (28 %)
Myasthenia	39% (40 %)	57% (60%)	13% (10 %)
Renal and urinary disorders			
Urinary retention	4% (6%)	15% (13%)	-
Urinary frequency	6% (5%)	12% (11%)	3% (5%)
Urinary incontinence	8% (15%)	20% (19%)	2% (1%)
Urinary urgency	8% (7%)	21% (17%)	4% (2 %)
Reproductive system and breast disorders			
Dysmenorrhea	<1% (<1%)	6% (5%)	18% (11 %)
Menstrual disorder *	9% (13%)	10% (8%)	17% (8 %)

Metrorrhagia	12% (6%)	10% (10%)	15% (8 %)
Impotence	7% (4%)	10% (11%)	2% (1%)
General disorders and administration site conditions			
Injection site reaction * °	78% (20 %)	89% (37%)	85% (37 %)
Injection site necrosis * °	5% (0 %)	6% (0%)	5% (0 %)
Headache	47% (41 %)	55% (46%)	84 % (77 %)
Fever * °	40% (13 %)	29% (24%)	59 % (41 %)
Flu-like symptom complex * °	61% (40 %)	43% (33%)	52 % (48 %)
Pain	31% (25 %)	59% (59%)	52 % (48 %)
Chest pain °	5% (4%)	15% (8%)	15% (15%)
Back pain	26% (24%)	31% (32%)	36% (37%)
Asthenia *	63% (58 %)	64% (58%)	49 % (35 %)
Infection	13% (11%)	11% (10%)	14% (13%)
Chills * °	23% (7 %)	22% (12%)	46 % (19 %)
Abdominal pain °	11% (6 %)	18% (16%)	32 % (24 %)
Malaise *	8% (5 %)	6% (2%)	15 % (3 %)
Abscess °	4% (2 %)	4% (5%)	1 % (6 %)
Pain in extremity	14% (12 %)		0 % (0 %)

* Significantly associated with Betaferon treatment for RRMS, $p < 0.05$
° Significantly associated with Betaferon treatment for SPMS, $p < 0.05$

Table 2 (reporting rates based on spontaneous adverse drug reaction reports classified as very common (⩾ 10%), common (< 10% - ⩾ 1%), uncommon (< 1% - ⩾ 1‰), rare (< 1‰ - ⩾ 1/10.000) and very rare (< 1/10.000))

Blood and the lymphatic system disorders	Uncommon	Anaemia Thrombocytopenia Leucopenia
	Rare	Lymphadenopathy
Endocrine disorders	Rare	Hyperthyroidism Hypothyroidism Thyroid dysfunction
Metabolism and nutrition disorders	Uncommon	ALT increase AST increase
	Rare	Gamma GT increase Triglyceride increase
	Very rare	Hypocalcaemia Hyperuricaemia
Nervous system disorders	Uncommon	Hypertonia Depression
	Rare	Convulsion Confusion Anxiety Emotional lability
	Very rare	Depersonalisation
Cardiac disorders	Rare	Cardiomyopathy Tachycardia Palpitation
Vascular disorders	Uncommon	Hypertension
Respiratory disorders	Rare	Bronchospasm Dyspnea
Gastrointestinal disorders	Uncommon	Nausea Vomiting
	Rare	Pancreatitis
Hepatobiliary disorders	Rare	Hepatitis
Skin and subcutaneous tissue disorders	Uncommon	Alopecia Urticaria Puritus Rash
	Rare	Skin discoloration Sweating
Musculoskeletal disorders	Uncommon	Myalgia
Reproductive system disorders	Rare	Menstrual disorder
General disorders and administration site conditions	Very common	Flu-like symptom complex* Chills* Fever* Injection site reaction * Inflammation * Pain injection site *
	Common	Necrosis *
	Rare	Suicide attempt Anaphylactic reactions Malaise Chest pain

* frequencies based on clinical trials

5. PHARMACOLOGICAL PROPERTIES

5.1 Pharmacodynamic properties

Pharmacotherapeutic group: Interferons, ATC Code: L03A B

Interferons belong to the family of cytokines, which are naturally occurring proteins. Interferons have molecular weights ranging from 15,000 to 21,000 Daltons. Three major classes of interferons have been identified: alpha, beta, and gamma. Interferon alpha, interferon beta, and interferon gamma have overlapping yet distinct biologic activities. The activities of interferon beta-1b are species-restricted and therefore, the most pertinent pharmacological information on interferon beta-1b is derived from studies of human cells in culture or in human in vivo studies.

Interferon beta-1b has been shown to possess both antiviral and immunoregulatory activities. The mechanisms by which interferon beta-1b exerts its actions in multiple sclerosis are not clearly understood. However, it is known that the biologic response-modifying properties of interferon beta-1b are mediated through its interactions with specific cell receptors found on the surface of human cells. The binding of interferon beta-1b to these receptors induces the expression of a number of gene products that are believed to be the mediators of the biological actions of interferon beta-1b. A number of these products have been measured in the serum and cellular fractions of blood collected from patients treated with interferon beta-1b. Interferon beta-1b both decreases the binding affinity and enhances the internalisation and degradation of the interferon-gamma receptor. Interferon beta-1b also enhances the suppressor activity of peripheral blood mononuclear cells.

No separate investigations were performed regarding the influence of Betaferon on the cardiovascular system, respiratory system and the function of endocrine organs.

One controlled clinical trial with Betaferon in patients with relapsing remitting multiple sclerosis and able to walk unaided (baseline EDSS 0 to 5.5) was performed. Patients receiving Betaferon showed a reduction in frequency (30%) and severity of clinical relapses, as well as the number of hospitalisations due to disease. Furthermore, there was a prolongation of the relapse-free interval. There is no evidence of an effect of Betaferon on the duration of relapses or on symptoms in between relapses, and no significant effect was seen on the progression of the disease in relapsing remitting multiple sclerosis.

Two controlled clinical trials with Betaferon involving a total of 1657 patients with secondary progressive multiple sclerosis (baseline EDSS 3 to 6.5, i.e. patients were able to walk) were performed. Patients with mild disease and those unable to walk were not studied. The two studies showed inconsistent results for the primary endpoint time to confirmed progression, representing delay of disability progression:

One of the two studies demonstrated a statistically significant delay in the time to disability progression (Hazard Ratio = 0.69, 95% confidence interval (0.55, 0.86), p=0.0010, corresponding to a 31% risk reduction due to Betaferon) and in the time to becoming wheelchair bound (Hazard Ratio = 0.61, 95% confidence interval (0.44, 0.85), p=0.0036, corresponding to a 39% risk reduction due to Betaferon) in patients who received Betaferon. This effect continued over the observation period of up to 33 months. The treatment effect occurred in patients at all levels of disability investigated and independent of relapse activity.

In the second trial of Betaferon in secondary progressive multiple sclerosis, no delay in the time to disability progression was observed. There is evidence that the patients included in this study had overall less active disease than in the other study in secondary progressive multiple sclerosis.

In retrospective meta-analyses including the data of both studies, an overall treatment effect was found which was statistically significant (p=0.0076; 8 MIU Betaferon versus all placebo patients).

Retrospective analyses in subgroups showed that a treatment effect on disability progression is most likely in patients with active disease before treatment commences (Hazard Ratio 0.72, 95% confidence interval (0.59, 0.88), p=0.0011, corresponding to a 28 % risk reduction due to Betaferon in patients with relapses or pronounced EDSS progression, 8 MIU Betaferon versus all placebo patients). From these retrospective subgroup analyses there was evidence to suggest that relapses as well as pronounced EDSS progression (EDSS > 1 point or > 0.5 point for EDSS >=6 in the previous two years) can help to identify patients with active disease.

In both trials secondary progressive multiple sclerosis patients receiving Betaferon showed a reduction in frequency (30%) of clinical relapses. There is no evidence of Betaferon having an effect on the duration of relapses.

Betaferon was effective in all multiple sclerosis studies to reduce disease activity (acute inflammation in the central nervous system and permanent tissue alterations) as measured by magnetic resonance imaging (MRI). The relation of multiple sclerosis disease activity as measured by MRI and clinical outcome is currently not fully understood.

5.2 Pharmacokinetic properties

Betaferon serum levels were followed in patients and volunteers by means of a not completely specific bioassay. Maximum serum levels of about 40 IU/ml were found 1-8 hours after subcutaneous injection of 500 microgram (16.0 million IU) interferon beta-1b. From various studies mean clearance rates and half-lives of disposition phases from serum were estimated to be at most 30 ml·min^{-1}·kg^{-1} and 5 hours, respectively. Betaferon injections given every other day do not lead to serum level increases, and the pharmacokinetics does not seem to change during therapy.

The absolute bioavailability of subcutaneously administered interferon beta-1b was approximately 50%.

5.3 Preclinical safety data

No acute toxicity studies have been carried out. As rodents do not react to human interferon beta, repeated dose studies were carried out with rhesus monkeys. Transitory hyperthermia was observed, as well as a significant rise in lymphocytes and a significant decrease in thrombocytes and segmented neutrophils. No long-term studies have been conducted. Reproduction studies with rhesus monkeys revealed maternal and foetal toxicity, resulting in prenatal mortality. No malformations have been observed in the surviving animals. No investigations on fertility have been conducted. No influence on the monkey oestrous cycle has been observed. Experience with other interferons suggest a potential for impairment of male and female fertility.

In one single genotoxicity study (Ames test), no mutagenic effect has been observed. Carcinogenicity studies have not been performed. An in vitro cell transformation test gave no indication of tumorigenic potential. Local tolerance studies after subcutaneous administration were negative. However, in clinical studies local reactions have been observed following use of Betaferon.

6. PHARMACEUTICAL PARTICULARS

6.1 List of excipients

Human albumin

Mannitol

Solvent: sodium chloride solution (0.54% w/v)

6.2 Incompatibilities

This medicinal product must not be mixed with other medicinal products except for the supplied solvent mentioned in 6.6 "Instructions for use, handling <,disposal>"

6.3 Shelf life

2 years

After reconstitution an immediate use is recommended. However, the in-use stability has been demonstrated for 3 hours at 2-8 °C.

6.4 Special precautions for storage

Do not store above 25°C. Do not freeze.

6.5 Nature and contents of container

Powder for solution for injection in a 3 ml clear vial (type I glass) with a butyl rubber stopper (type I) and aluminium overseal and solvent in a 1.2 ml pre-filled syringe (type I glass).

Package containing 5 or 15 vials powder and 5 or 15 pre-filled solvent syringes.

6.6 Instructions for use and handling

To reconstitute lyophilised interferon beta-1b for injection, use the pre-filled solvent syringe and a needle to inject 1.2 ml of the solvent (sodium chloride solution, 0.54% w/v) into the Betaferon vial. Dissolve the powder completely without shaking. Inspect the reconstituted product visually before use. The reconstituted product is colourless to light yellow and slightly opalescent to opalescent. Discard the product before use if it contains particulate matter or is discoloured.

7. MARKETING AUTHORISATION HOLDER

Schering Aktiengesellschaft

D-13342 Berlin

Germany

8. MARKETING AUTHORISATION NUMBER(S)

EU/1/95/003/003

EU/1/95/003/004

9. DATE OF FIRST AUTHORISATION/RENEWAL OF THE AUTHORISATION

30.11.1995

26.11.1996

03.04.2001

10. DATE OF REVISION OF THE TEXT

12 July 2004

LEGAL CATEGORY

POM

* produced by genetic engineering from strain of *Escherichia coli*.

Betagan

(Allergan Ltd)

1. NAME OF THE MEDICINAL PRODUCT

Betagan®

Betagan® Eye Drops 0.5% w/v

2. QUALITATIVE AND QUANTITATIVE COMPOSITION

Levobunolol hydrochloride 0.5% w/v (equivalent to levobunolol 0.445% w/v)

3. PHARMACEUTICAL FORM

Eye Drops, Solution

4. CLINICAL PARTICULARS

4.1 Therapeutic indications

Reduction of intraocular pressure in chronic open-angle glaucoma and ocular hypertension.

4.2 Posology and method of administration

Adults (including the elderly)

The usual dose is one drop instilled in the affected eye(s) once or twice daily. In common with other topical ophthalmic beta-adrenergic blocking agents, full clinical response may take several weeks to occur. Intraocular pressure should therefore be measured approximately four weeks after starting treatment. Because of diurnal variations in intraocular pressure, satisfactory response is best determined by measuring the intraocular pressure at different times of the day.

Use in Children

Betagan is not currently recommended for use in children.

Concomitant administration

If the patient's intraocular pressure is not satisfactory on this regimen, concomitant therapy with dipivefrin or adrenaline and/or pilocarpine and other miotics, and/or systemically administered carbonic anhydrase inhibitors can be instituted.

4.3 Contraindications

Bronchial asthma; history of bronchial asthma; chronic obstructive pulmonary disease; sinus bradycardia; second and third degree atrioventricular block; cardiac failure; cardiogenic shock; hypersensitivity to any component; sick sinus syndrome (including sino-atrial block); Prinzmetal's angina; untreated phaeochromocytoma; metabolic acidosis; hypotension.

4.4 Special warnings and special precautions for use

As with other topically applied ophthalmic drugs, Betagan may be absorbed systemically and adverse reactions typical of oral beta-adrenoceptor agents may occur.

Respiratory and cardiac reactions have been reported including, rarely, death due to bronchospasm or associated with cardiac failure.

Congestive heart failure should be adequately controlled before commencing therapy with Betagan. In patients with a history of cardiac disease pulse rates should be monitored.

Diabetic control should be monitored during Betagan therapy in patients with labile diabetes. Beta-blockers may mask the symptoms of thyrotoxicosis.

Betagan has little or no effect on pupil size and if administered in angle-closure glaucoma, for reduction of intraocular pressure, must only be given in combination with a miotic.

Betagan contains benzalkonium chloride and should not be used in patients continuing to wear hydrophilic (soft) lenses.

Diminished response after prolonged therapy has been reported in some patients. If necessary, concomitant therapy with dipivefrin/ adrenaline, pilocarpine and/ or carbionic anhydrase inhibitors can be instituted.

In patients with peripheral circulatory disorders (Raynaud's disease or syndrome, intermittent claudication), beta-blockers should be used with great caution as aggravation of these disorders may occur.

Beta-blockers may induce bradycardia. If the pulse rate decreases to less than 50-55 beats per minute at rest and the patient experiences symptoms related to the bradycardia, review of intraocular pressure lowering therapy may be required.

Due to its negative effect on conduction time, beta-blockers should only be given with caution to patients with first degree heart block.

Beta-blockers may increase both the sensitivity towards allergens and the seriousness of anaphylactic reactions.

4.5 Interaction with other medicinal products and other forms of Interaction

Caution should be exercised when used concomitantly with oral beta-adrenergic blocking agents, because of the potential for additive effects on systemic blockade.

4.6 Pregnancy and lactation

Betagan has not been studied in human pregnancy. It is recommended that Betagan be avoided in pregnancy. If treatment with Betagan during lactation is considered necessary for the benefit of the mother, consideration should be given to the cessation of breast feeding.

4.7 Effects on ability to drive and use machines

There are no studies on the effect of this medicine on the ability to drive. When driving vehicles or operating machines it should be taken into account that occasionally dizziness or fatigue may occur.

4.8 Undesirable effects

Ocular: Transient burning and stinging on installation, conjunctival hyperaemia, eyelid oedema, impaired vision, blepharoconjunctivitis and iridocyclitis have been reported occasionally. Dry eye has been rarely reported. The pharmacological and physical properties of levobunolol indicate a potential for post-installation reduction in corneal sensitivity: this potential has not been confirmed in clinical studies with Betagan.

Cardiovascular: Bradycardia, hypotension, heart block and paraesthesia have been reported.

Respiratory: There have been reports of dyspnoea and asthma.

CNS: Headache, transient ataxia and dizziness, hallucinations, confusion, impotence, sleep disturbances, depression and lethargy have been reported occasionally.

Gastrointestinal: Nausea, vomiting, and diarrhoea have been reported occasionally.

Dermatological: Urticaria and pruritis have been rarely reported.

Immunological: Post-marketing reports of ocular and systemic hypersensitivity / allergic reactions have been received rarely.

4.9 Overdose

There are no data available on human overdosage with Betagan, which is unlikely to occur via the ocular route. Should accidental overdosage occur, flush the eye(s) with water or normal saline. If accidentally ingested, systemic symptoms of bradycardia, hypotension, bronchospasm and acute cardiac insufficiency may occur.

5. PHARMACOLOGICAL PROPERTIES

5.1 Pharmacodynamic properties

Levobunolol hydrochloride is a non-cardioselective beta-adrenoceptor blocking agent, equipotent at both beta-1 and beta-2 receptors. Levobunolol does not have significant local anaesthetic (membrane-stabilizing) or intrinsic sympathomimetic activity.

Because of levobunolol's affinity for beta-1 receptors there exists the theoretical possibility of a negative inotropic effect.

The primary mechanism of the ocular hypotensive activity of levobunolol hydrochloride is likely to be a decrease in aqueous humour production. There is little effect on pupil size or accommodation.

5.2 Pharmacokinetic properties

The onset of action of one drop of Betagan can be detected one hour after installation with the maximum effect seen between 2 and 6 hours. The half lives of orally ingested levobunolol and of its active metabolite dihydrolevobunolol are between 6 and 7 hours.

5.3 Preclinical safety data

Not applicable.

6. PHARMACEUTICAL PARTICULARS

6.1 List of excipients

Benzalkonium chloride Ph. Eur.

Disodium edetate Ph. Eur.

Polyvinyl alcohol USP

Sodium chloride Ph. Eur.

Sodium phosphate, dibasic, heptahydrate USP

Potassium phosphate, monobasic NF

Sodium metabisulphite BP

Sodium hydroxide or hydrochloride acid to adjust pH Ph. Eur.

Purified water Ph. Eur.

6.2 Incompatibilities

None known.

6.3 Shelf life

24 months unopened.

Discard 28 days after first opening.

6.4 Special precautions for storage

Do not store above 25°C.

Protect from light.

6.5 Nature and contents of container

10 ml white bottle and dropper tip made of low density polyethylene. The cap is either a "traditional" green, medium impact, polystyrene cap or a white medium impact polystyrene cap or a white, medium impact, polystyrene compliance cap (C-Cap) with an external rotating sleeve indicating daily dosage status. Each have a safety seal to ensure integrity. The bottle is filled with either 5 or 10 ml of Betagan.

6.6 Instructions for use and handling

No special instructions.

Administrative Data

7. MARKETING AUTHORISATION HOLDER

Allergan Limited
Coronation Road
High Wycombe
Bucks. HP12 3SH
UNITED KINGDOM

8. MARKETING AUTHORISATION NUMBER(S)

PL 00426/0060

9. DATE OF FIRST AUTHORISATION/RENEWAL OF THE AUTHORISATION

23rd March 1989/14th July 2005

10. DATE OF REVISION OF THE TEXT

14th July 2005

Betagan Unit Dose

(Allergan Ltd)

1. NAME OF THE MEDICINAL PRODUCT

Betagan Unit Dose

2. QUALITATIVE AND QUANTITATIVE COMPOSITION

Levobunolol hydrochloride 0.5% USP

3. PHARMACEUTICAL FORM

Sterile aqueous ophthalmic solution.

4. CLINICAL PARTICULARS

4.1 Therapeutic indications

Reduction of intraocular pressure in chronic open-angle glaucoma and ocular hypertension.

4.2 Posology and method of administration

Adults (including the elderly)

The recommended adult dose is one drop of Betagan Unit Dose once or twice daily in the affected eye(s). Discard product after use.

Children

Use in children is not currently recommended.

4.3 Contraindications

Bronchial asthma; history of bronchial asthma; chronic obstructive pulmonary disease; sinus bradycardia; second and third degree atrioventricular block; cardiac failure; cardiogenic shock; hypersensitivity to any component.

4.4 Special warnings and special precautions for use

As with other topically applied ophthalmic drugs, Betagan may be absorbed systemically.

4.5 Interaction with other medicinal products and other forms of Interaction

Betagan may have additive effects in patients taking systemic antihypertensive drugs. These possible additive effects may include hypotension, including orthostatic hypotension, bradycardia, dizziness, and/ or syncope. Conversely, systemic beta-adrenoceptor blocking agents may potentiate the ocular hypotensive effect of Betagan.

Betagan may potentially add to the effects of oral calcium antagonists, rauwolfia alkaloids or beta blockers to induce hypotension and/ or marked bradycardia.

4.6 Pregnancy and lactation

There are no adequate and well-controlled studies in pregnant women. Levobunolol should be used during pregnancy only if the potential benefit justifies the potential risk to the foetus.

It is not known whether this drug is excreted in human milk. Systemic beta-blockers and topical Timolol maleate are known to be excreted in human milk. Because similar drugs are excreted in human milk, caution should be exercised when Betagan is administered to a nursing woman.

4.7 Effects on ability to drive and use machines

None known.

4.8 Undesirable effects

Blepharoconjunctivitis, transient ocular burning, stinging, and decreases in heart rate and blood pressure have been reported occasionally with the use of Betagan. Urticaria has been reported rarely with the use of Betagan.

The following adverse effects have been reported rarely and a definite relationship with the use of Betagan has not been established: change in heart rhythm, iridocyclitis, browache, transient ataxia, lethargy, urticaria, elevated liver enzymes, eructation, dizziness and itching.

The following additional adverse reactions have been reported with ophthalmic use of $beta_1$ and $beta_2$ non selective blocking agents:

Special senses: conjunctivitis, blepharitis, keratitis and decreased corneal sensitivity, visual disturbances, including refractory changes, diplopia and ptosis.

Cardiovascular: bradycardia, hypotension, syncope, heartblock, cerebrovascular accident, cerebral ischaemia, congestive heart failure, palpitation and cardiac arrest.

Respiratory: bronchospasm, respiratory failure and dyspenea.

Body as a whole: asthenia, nausea and depression.

4.9 Overdose

There are no data available on human overdosage with Betagan which is unlikely to occur via the ocular route. Should accidental ocular overdosage occur, flush the eye(s) with water or normal saline. If accidentally ingested, efforts to decrease further absorption may be appropriate.

5. PHARMACOLOGICAL PROPERTIES

5.1 Pharmacodynamic properties

Levobunolol is a non-cardioselective beta-adrenoceptor blocking agent, equipotent at both $beta_1$ and $beta_2$ receptors. Levobunolol is greater than 60 times more potent than its dextro isomer in its beta-blocking activity. In order to obtain the highest degree of beta-blocking potential without increasing the potential for direct myocardial depression, the levo isomer, levobunolol, is used. Levobunolol does not have significant local anaesthetic (membrane-stabilising) or intrinsic sympathomimetic activity. Betagan has shown to be as effective as Timolol in lowering intraocular pressure.

Betagan when instilled in the eye will lower elevated intraocular pressure as well as normal intraocular pressure, whether or not accompanied by glaucoma. Elevated intraocular pressure presents a major risk factor in the pathogenesis of glaucomatous field loss. The higher the level of intraocular pressure, the likelihood of optic nerve damage and visual field loss.

The primary mechanism of action of levobunolol in reducing intraocular pressure is most likely a decrease in aqueous humor production. Betagan reduces intraocular pressure with little or no effect on pupil size in contrast to the miosis which cholinergic agents are known to produce.

The blurred vision and night blindness often associated with miotics would not be expected with the use of Betagan. Patients with cateracts avoid the inability to see around lenticular opacities caused by pupil constriction.

5.2 Pharmacokinetic properties

The onset of action with one drop of Betagan can be detected within one hour of treatment, with maximum effect seen between two and six hours. A significant decrease can be maintained for up to 24 hours following a single dose.

5.3 Preclinical safety data

Not applicable

6. PHARMACEUTICAL PARTICULARS

6.1 List of excipients

Polyvinyl alcohol USP
Sodium chloride EP
Disodium edetate EP
Sodium phosphate dibasic, heptahydrate USP
Potassium phosphate monobasic NF
Sodium hydroxide or hydrochloric acid (to adjust pH) EP
Purified water EP

6.2 Incompatibilities

No major incompatibilities have been reported from topical use of levobunolol.

6.3 Shelf life

24 months.

6.4 Special precautions for storage

Store at or below 25°.
Protect from light.
Discard after use.

6.5 Nature and contents of container

Low density polyethylene (LDPE) blow-fill-seal unit dose container (0.9 ml volume) filled with 0.4 ml solution.

Unit dose containers are packaged into a foil covered pouch (5 containers per pouch).

Pouches are packaged into cartons such that each carton contains 30 or 60 unit dose containers.

6.6 Instructions for use and handling

None.

7. MARKETING AUTHORISATION HOLDER

Allergan Limited
Coronation Road
High Wycombe
Bucks
HP12 3SH

8. MARKETING AUTHORISATION NUMBER(S)

PL 00426/0072

9. DATE OF FIRST AUTHORISATION/RENEWAL OF THE AUTHORISATION

26th July 2003

10. DATE OF REVISION OF THE TEXT

26th July 2003

Betaloc I.V. Injection

(AstraZeneca UK Limited)

1. NAME OF THE MEDICINAL PRODUCT

Betaloc I.V. Injection.

2. QUALITATIVE AND QUANTITATIVE COMPOSITION

Each ampoule of 5ml contains 5mg Metoprolol tartrate Ph. Eur.

3. PHARMACEUTICAL FORM

Solution for Injection.

4. CLINICAL PARTICULARS

4.1 Therapeutic indications

Control of tachyarrhythmias, especially supraventricular tachyarrhythmias.

Early intervention with Betaloc in acute myocardial infarction reduces infarct size and the incidence of ventricular fibrillation. Pain relief may also decrease the need for opiate analgesics.

Betaloc has been shown to reduce mortality when administered to patients with acute myocardial infarction.

4.2 Posology and method of administration

Control of Tachyarrhythmias: Initially up to 5mg injected I.V. at a rate of 1-2mg per minute. The injection can be repeated at 5 minute intervals until a satisfactory response has been obtained. A total dose of 10-15mg generally proves sufficient.

Because of the risk of a pronounced drop of blood pressure, the I.V. administration of Betaloc to patients with a systolic blood pressure below 100mmHg should only be given with special care.

During Anaesthesia: 2-4mg injected slowly I.V. at induction is usually sufficient to prevent the development of arrhythmias during anaesthesia. The same dosage can also be used to control arrhythmias developing during anaesthesia. Further injections of 2mg may be given as required to a maximum overall dose of 10mg.

Myocardial infarction: Early intervention. To achieve optimal benefits from intravenous Betaloc, suitable patients should present within 12 hours of the onset of chest pain. Therapy should commence with 5mg I.V. every 2 minutes to a maximum of 15mg total as determined by blood pressure and heart rate. The second or third dose should not be given if the systolic blood pressure is <90mmHg, the heart rate is <40 beats/min and the P-Q time is >0.26 seconds, or if there is any aggravation of dyspnoea or cold sweating. Oral therapy should commence 15 minutes after the injection with 50mg every 6 hours for 48 hours. Patients who fail to tolerate the full intravenous dose should be given half the suggested oral dose.

Elderly: Initially the lowest possible dose should be used, especially in the elderly.

Significant Hepatic Dysfunction: A reduction in dosage may be necessary.

4.3 Contraindications

AV Block. Uncontrolled heart failure. Severe bradycardia. Sick sinus syndrome. Cardiogenic shock. Severe peripheral arterial disease. Known hypersensitivity to β-blockers or to any of the constituents of Betaloc i.v. Metabolic acidosis. Untreated phaeochromocytoma.

Betaloc I.V. is also contra-indicated when acute myocardial infarction is complicated by significant bradycardia, first degree heart block, systolic hypotension (<100mmHg) and/or severe heart failure.

4.4 Special warnings and special precautions for use

If patients develop increasing bradycardia, Betaloc i.v. should be given in lower doses or gradually withdrawn. Symptoms of peripheral arterial circulatory disorders may be aggravated by Betaloc.

Abrupt interruption of β-blockers is to be avoided. During its withdrawal, patients should be kept under close surveillance, especially those with known ischaemic heart disease.

Betaloc i.v. may be administered when heart failure has been controlled. Digitalisation and/or diuretic therapy should also be considered for patients with a history of heart failure, or patients known to have a poor cardiac reserve. Betaloc i.v. should be used with caution in patients where cardiac reserve is poor.

Intravenous administration of calcium antagonists of the verapamil type should not be given to patients treated with β-blockers.

In patients with Prinzmetal's angina β_1 selective agents should be used with care.

Although cardioselective β-blockers may have less effect on lung function than non-selective β-blockers, as with all β-blockers these should be avoided in patients with reversible obstructive airways disease unless there are compelling clinical reasons for their use. When administration is necessary, use of a β_2-bronchodilator (e.g. terbutaline) may be advisable in some patients.

The label shall state - "Use with caution in patients who have a history of wheezing, asthma or any other breathing difficulties, see enclosed user leaflet."

In labile and insulin-dependent diabetes it may be necessary to adjust the hypoglycaemic therapy.

As with other β-blockers, Betaloc i.v. may mask the symptoms of thyrotoxicosis and the early signs of acute hypoglycaemia in patients with diabetes mellitus. However, the risk of this occurring is less than with non-selective β-blockers.

In patients with a phaeochromocytoma, an α-blocker should be given concomitantly.

The elderly should be treated with caution, starting with a lower dose.

Like all β-blockers, careful consideration should be given to patients with psoriasis before Betaloc i.v. is administered.

The administration of adrenaline to patients undergoing β-blockade can result in an increase in blood pressure and bradycardia although this is less likely to occur with β_1-selective drugs.

Betaloc i.v. therapy must be reported to the anaesthetist prior to general anaesthesia. If withdrawal of metoprolol is considered desirable, this should, if possible, be completed at least 48 hours before general anaesthesia. However, in some patients it may be desirable to employ a β-blocker as premedication. By shielding the heart against the effects of stress the β-blocker may prevent excessive sympathetic stimulation provoking cardiac arrhythmias or acute coronary insufficiency. If a β-blocker is given for this purpose, an anaesthetic with little negative inotropic activity should be selected to minimise the risk of myocardial depression.

Beta-blockers may increase both the sensitivity towards allergens and the seriousness of anaphylactic reactions.

4.5 Interaction with other medicinal products and other forms of Interaction

The effects of Betaloc i.v. and other drugs with an antihypertensive effect on blood pressure are usually additive, and care should be taken to avoid hypotension such as could be the result of concomitant administration with dihydropyridine derivatives, tricyclic antidepressant barbiturates and phenothiazines. However, combinations of antihypertensive drugs may often be used with benefit to improve control of hypertension.

Betaloc i.v. can reduce myocardial contractility and impair intracardiac conduction. Care should be exercised when drugs with similar activity, e.g. antiarrhythmic agents, general anaesthetics, are given concurrently. Like all other β-blockers, Betaloc i.v. should not be given in combination with verapamil, diltiazem or digitalis glycosides. A watch should be kept for possible negative effects when metoprolol is given in combination with calcium antagonists, since this may cause bradycardia, hypotension and asystole. Care should also be exercised when β-blockers are given in combination with sympathomimetic ganglion blocking agents, other β-blockers (i.e. eye drops) or MAO inhibitors.

If concomitant treatment with clonidine is to be discontinued, Betaloc i.v. should be withdrawn several days before clonidine.

As β-blockers may affect the peripheral circulation, care should be exercised when drugs with similar activity e.g. ergotamine are given concurrently.

Betaloc i.v. will antagonise the β_1-effects of sympathomimetic agents but should have little influence on the bronchodilator effects of β_2-agonists at normal therapeutic doses. Enzyme inducing agents (e.g. rifampicin) may reduce plasma concentrations of Betaloc i.v., whereas enzyme inhibitors (e.g. cimetidine, alcohol and hydralazine) may increase plasma concentrations. Metoprolol may impair the elimination of lidocaine (lignocaine).

The dosages of oral antidiabetic agents and also of insulin may have to be readjusted in patients receiving β-blockers.

Concomitant treatment with indomethacin and other prostaglandin synthetase inhibiting drugs may reduce the antihypertensive effect of β-blockers.

4.6 Pregnancy and lactation

Betaloc should not be used in pregnancy or nursing mothers unless the physician considers that the benefit outweighs the possible hazard to the foetus/infant. β-blockers reduce placental perfusion, which may result in intrauterine foetal death, immature and premature deliveries. As with all β-blockers, metoprolol may cause side-effects especially bradycardia and hypoglycaemia in the foetus, and in the newborn and breastfed infant. There is an increased risk of cardiac and pulmonary complications in the neonate. Metoprolol has, however, been used in pregnancy-associated hypertension under close supervision, after 20 weeks gestation. Although Betaloc crosses the placental barrier and is present in cord blood, no evidence of foetal abnormalities has been reported.

Use during lactation

Breast feeding is not recommended. The amount of metoprolol ingested via breast milk should not produce significant β-blocking effects in the neonate if the mother is treated with normal therapeutic doses.

4.7 Effects on ability to drive and use machines

When driving vehicles or operating machines, it should be taken into account that occasionally dizziness or fatigue may occur.

4.8 Undesirable effects

Metoprolol is usually well tolerated and adverse reactions have generally been mild and reversible. The following events have been reported as adverse events in clinical trials or reported from routine use.

As in the case of other β-blockers, a marked fall in blood pressure may sometimes occur following intravenous injection of Betaloc. Other side effects are usually mild and infrequent. The most common appear to be lassitude, GI disturbances (nausea, vomiting or abdominal pain) and disturbances of sleep pattern. In many cases these effects have been transient or have disappeared after a reduction in dosage.

Effects related to the CNS which have been reported occasionally are dizziness and headache and rarely paraesthesia, muscle cramps, depression, decreased mental alertness. There have also been isolated reports of personality disorderslike amnesia, memory impairment, confusion, hallucination, nervousness and anxiety.

Cardiovascular effects which have been reported occasionally are bradycardia, postural hypotension and rarely, heart failure, increased existing AV block, palpitations, cardiac arrhythmias, Raynauds phenomenon, peripheral oedema and precordial pain. There have also been isolated reports of cardiac conduction abnormalities, gangrene in patients with pre-existing severe peripheral circulatory disorders and increase of pre-existing intermittent claudication.

Common gastro-intestinal disturbances have been described above but rarely diarrhoea or constipation also occur and there have been isolated cases of dry mouth and abnormal liver function.

Skin rashes (urticaria, psoriasiform, dystrophic skin lesions) and positive anti-nuclear antibodies (not associated with SLE) occur rarely. Isolated cases of photosensitivity, psoriasis exacerbation, increased sweating and alopecia have been reported. Respiratory effects include occasional reports of dyspnoea on exertion and rare reports of bronchospasm and isolated cases of rhinitis.

Rarely impotence/sexual dysfunction. Isolated cases of weight gain, thrombocytopenia, disturbances of vision, conjunctivitis, tinnitus, dry or irritated eyes, taste disturbance and arthralgia have also been reported.

The reported incidence of skin rashes and/or dry eyes is small and in most cases the symptoms have cleared when treatment was withdrawn. Discontinuation of the drug should be considered if any such reaction is not otherwise explicable.

4.9 Overdose

Poisoning due to an overdose of Betaloc I.V. may lead to severe hypotension, sinus bradycardia, atrioventricular block, heart failure, cardiogenic shock, cardiac arrest, bronchospasm, impairment of consciousness, coma, nausea, vomiting, cyanosis, hypoglycaemia and, occasionally, hyperkalaemia.

Treatment should include close monitoring of cardiovascular, respiratory and renal function, and blood glucose and electrolytes. Cardiovascular complications should be treated symptomatically, which may require the use of sympathomimetic agents (e.g. noradrenaline, metaraminol), atropine or inotropic agents, (e.g. noradrenaline, metaraminol), atropine or inotropic agents, (e.g. dopamine, dobutamine). Temporary pacing may be required for AV block. Glucagon can reverse the effects of excessive β-blockade, given in a dose of 1-10mg intravenously.

Intravenous β_2-stimulants e.g. terbutaline may be required to relieve bronchospasm.

Betaloc I.V. cannot be effectively removed by haemodialysis.

5. PHARMACOLOGICAL PROPERTIES

5.1 Pharmacodynamic properties

Metoprolol is a competitive β-adrenoceptor antagonist. It acts preferentially to inhibit β-adrenoceptors (conferring some cardioselectivity), is devoid of intrinsic sympathomimetic activity (partial agonist activity) and possesses β-adrenoceptor blocking activity comparable in potency with propranolol.

A negative chronotrophic effect on the heart is a consistent feature of metoprolol administration. Thus, cardiac output and systolic blood pressure rapidly decrease following acute administration.

5.2 Pharmacokinetic properties

Metoprolol is eliminated mainly by hepatic metabolism, the average elimination half-life is 3.5 hours (range 1-9 hours). Rates of metabolism vary between individuals, with poor metabolisers (approximately 10%) showing higher plasma concentrations and slower elimination than extensive metabolisers. Within individuals, however, plasma concentrations are stable and reproducible.

5.3 Preclinical safety data

Pre-clinical information has not been included because the safety profile of metoprolol tartrate has been established after many years of clinical use. Please refer to section 4.

6. PHARMACEUTICAL PARTICULARS

6.1 List of excipients

Sodium chloride and water for injections.

6.2 Incompatibilities

None known.

6.3 Shelf life

4 years.

6.4 Special precautions for storage

Protect from light. Store below 25°C.

6.5 Nature and contents of container

5ml glass ampoule.

6.6 Instructions for use and handling

None.

7. MARKETING AUTHORISATION HOLDER

AstraZeneca UK Ltd.,

600 Capability Green,

Luton, LU1 3LU, UK.

8. MARKETING AUTHORISATION NUMBER(S)

PL 17901/0106

9. DATE OF FIRST AUTHORISATION/RENEWAL OF THE AUTHORISATION

28th May 2002

10. DATE OF REVISION OF THE TEXT

28th May 2002

Betaloc SA

(AstraZeneca UK Limited)

1. NAME OF THE MEDICINAL PRODUCT

Betaloc SA

2. QUALITATIVE AND QUANTITATIVE COMPOSITION

Metoprolol tartrate Ph. Eur.200mg

3. PHARMACEUTICAL FORM

Extended release formulation (Durules®)

4. CLINICAL PARTICULARS

4.1 Therapeutic indications

In the management of angina pectoris and hypertension. Prophylaxis of migraine.

4.2 Posology and method of administration

Angina Pectoris and Hypertension: One tablet daily, in the morning. In rare cases two tablets may be indicated.

Migraine Prophylaxis: One tablet daily, in the morning.

Betaloc SA tablets must not be chewed or crushed. They should be swallowed whole with half a glass of water.

Elderly: Initially the lowest possible dose should be used, especially in the elderly.

Significant Hepatic Dysfunction: A reduction in dosage may be necessary.

4.3 Contraindications

AV block. Uncontrolled heart failure. Severe bradycardia. Sick-sinus syndrome. Cardiogenic shock. Severe peripheral arterial disease. Known hypersensitivity to β-blockers or to any of the constituents of Belaloc SA. Metabolic acidosis. Untreated phaeochromocytoma.

Betaloc SA is also contra-indicated when acute myocardial infarction is complicated by significant bradycardia, first degree heart block, systolic hypotension (<100mmHg) and/or severe heart failure.

4.4 Special warnings and special precautions for use

If patients develop increasing bradycardia, Betaloc SA should be given in lower doses or gradually withdrawn. Symptoms of peripheral arterial circulatory disorders may be aggravated by Betaloc SA.

Abrupt interruption of β-blockers is to be avoided. When possible, Betaloc SA should be withdrawn gradually over a period of 10-14 days. During its withdrawal patients should be kept under close surveillance, especially those with known ischaemic heart disease.

Betaloc SA may be administered when heart failure has been controlled. Digitalisation and/or diuretic therapy should also be considered for patients with a history of heart failure, or patients known to have a poor cardiac reserve. Betaloc should be used with caution in patients where cardiac reserve is poor.

Intravenous administration of calcium antagonists of the verapamil type should not be given to patients treated with β-blockers.

In patients with Prinzmetal's angina β_1 selective agents should be used with care.

Although cardioselective β-blockers may have less effect on lung function than non-selective β-blockers, as with all β-blockers these should be avoided in patients with reversible obstructive airways disease unless there are compelling clinical reasons for their use. When administration is necessary, use of a β_2-bronchodilator (e.g. terbutaline) may be advisable in some patients.

The label shall state - "If you have a history of wheezing, asthma or any other breathing difficulties, you must tell your doctor before you take this medicine."

In labile and insulin-dependent diabetes it may be necessary to adjust the hypoglycaemic therapy.

As with other β-blockers, Betaloc SA may mask the symptoms of thyrotoxicosis and the early signs of acute hypoglycaemia in patients with diabetes mellitus. However, the risk of this occurring is less than with non-selective β-blockers.

In patients with a phaeochromocytoma, an alpha-blocker should be given concomitantly.

In the presence of liver cirrhosis the bioavailability of Betaloc SA may be increased and patients may need a lower dosage.

The elderly should be treated with caution, starting with a lower dose.

Like all β-blockers, careful consideration should be given to patients with psoriasis before Betaloc SA is administered.

The administration of adrenaline to patients undergoing β-blockade can result in an increase in blood pressure and bradycardia although this is less likely to occur with β_1-selective drugs.

Betaloc SA therapy must be reported to the anaesthetist prior to general anaesthesia. If withdrawal of metoprolol is considered desirable, this should if possible be completed at least 48 hours before general anaesthesia. However, in some patients it may be desirable to employ a β-blocker as premedication. By shielding the heart against the effects of stress the β-blocker may prevent excessive sympathetic stimulation provoking cardiac arrhythmias or acute coronary insufficiency.

If a β-blocker is given for this purpose, an anaesthetic with little negative inotropic activity should be selected to minimise the risk of myocardial depression.

Beta-blockers may increase both the sensitivity towards allergens and the seriousness of anaphylactic reactions.

4.5 Interaction with other medicinal products and other forms of Interaction

The effects of Betaloc SA and other drugs with an antihypertensive effect on blood pressure are usually additive, and care should be taken to avoid hypotension such as could be the result of concomitant administration with dihydropyridine derivatives, tricyclic antidepressant barbiturates and phenothiazines. However, combinations of antihypertensive drugs may often be used with benefit to improve control of hypertension.

Betaloc SA can reduce myocardial contractility and impair intracardiac conduction. Care should be exercised when drugs with similar activity, e.g. antiarrhythmic agents, general anaesthetics, are given concurrently. Like all other β-blockers, Betaloc SA should not be given in combination with verapamil, diltiazem or digitalis glycosides. A watch should be kept for possible negative effects when metoprolol is given in combination with calcium antagonists, since this may cause bradycardia, hypotension and asystole. Care should also be exercised when β-blockers are given in combination with sympathetic ganglion blocking agents, other β-blockers (i.e. eye drops) or MAO inhibitors.

If concomitant treatment with clonidine is to be discontinued, Betaloc SA should be withdrawn several days before clonidine.

As β-blockers may affect the peripheral circulation, care should be exercised when drugs with similar activity e.g. ergotamine are given concurrently.

Betaloc SA will antagonise the β_1-effects of sympathomimetic agents but should have little influence on the bronchodilator effects of β_2-agonists at normal therapeutic doses. Enzyme inducing agents (e.g. rifampicin) may reduce plasma concentrations of Betaloc SA, whereas enzyme inhibitors (e.g. cimetidine, alcohol and hydralazine) may increase plasma concentrations. Metoprolol may impair the elimination of lidocaine (lignocaine).

The dosages of oral antidiabetic agents and also of insulin may have to be readjusted in patients receiving β-blockers.

Concomitant treatment with indomethacin and other prostaglandin synthetase inhibiting drugs may reduce the antihypertensive effect of β-blockers.

4.6 Pregnancy and lactation

Betaloc SA should not be used in pregnancy or nursing mothers unless the physician considers that the benefit outweighs the possible hazard to the foetus/infant. β-blockers reduce placental perfusion, which may result in intrauterine foetal death, immature and premature deliveries, As with all β-blockers, metoprolol may cause side-effects especially bradycardia and hypoglycaemia in the foetus, and in the newborn and breastfed infant. There is an increased risk of cardiac and pulmonary complications in the neonate. Metoprolol has, however, been used in pregnancy-associated hypertension under close supervision, after 20 weeks gestation. Although Betaloc SA crosses the placental barrier and is present in cord blood, no evidence of foetal abnormalities has been reported.

Use during lactation

Breast feeding is not recommended. The amount of metoprolol ingested via breast milk should not produce significant β-blocking effects in the neonate if the mother is treated with normal therapeutic doses.

4.7 Effects on ability to drive and use machines

When driving vehicles or operating machines, it should be taken into account that occasionally dizziness or fatigue may occur.

4.8 Undesirable effects

Metoprolol is usually well tolerated and adverse reactions have generally been mild and reversible. The following events have been reported as adverse events in clinical trials or reported from routine use

These are usually mild and infrequent. The most common appear to be lassitude, GI disturbances (nausea, vomiting or abdominal pain) and disturbances of sleep pattern. In many cases these effects have been transient or have disappeared after a reduction in dosage.

Effects related to the CNS which have been reported occasionally are dizziness and headache and rarely paraesthesia, muscle cramps, depression, decreased mental alertness. There have also been isolated reports of personality disorders like amnesia, memory impairment, confusion, hallucination, nervousness and anxiety.

Cardiovascular effects which have been reported occasionally are bradycardia, postural hypotension and rarely, heart failure, ***increased existing AV block,*** palpitations, cardiac arrhythmias, Raynauds phenomenon, peripheral oedema and precordial pain. There have also been isolated reports of cardiac conduction abnormalities, gangrene in patients with pre-existing severe peripheral circulatory disorders and increase of pre-existing intermittent claudication.

Common gastro-intestinal disturbances have been described above but rarely diarrhoea or constipation also occur and there have been isolated cases of dry mouth and abnormal liver function.

Skin rashes (urticaria, psoriasiform, dystrophic skin lesions) and positive anti-nuclear antibodies (not associated with SLE) occur rarely. Isolated cases of photosensitivity, psoriasis exacerbation, increased sweating and alopecia have been reported. Respiratory effects include occasional reports of dyspnoea on exertion and rare reports of bronchospasm and isolated cases of rhinitis.

Rarely impotence/sexual dysfunction. Isolated cases of weight gain, thrombocytopenia, disturbances of vision, conjunctivitis, tinnitus, dry or irritated eyes, tastedisturbances and arthralgia have also been reported.

The reported incidence of skin rashes and/or dry eyes is small and in most cases the symptoms have cleared when treatment was withdrawn. Discontinuation of the drug should be considered if any such reaction is not otherwise explicable.

4.9 Overdose

Poisoning due to an overdose of Betaloc SA may lead to severe hypotension, sinus bradycardia, atrioventricular block, heart failure, cardiogenic shock, cardiac arrest, bronchospasm, impairment of consciousness, coma, nausea, vomiting, cyanosis, hypoglycaemia and, occasionally, hyperkalaemia. The first manifestations usually appear 20 minutes to 2 hours after drug ingestion.

Treatment should include close monitoring of cardiovascular, respiratory and renal function, and blood glucose and electrolytes. Further absorption may be prevented by induction of vomiting, gastric lavage or administration of activated-charcoal if ingestion is recent. Cardiovascular complications should be treated symptomatically, which may require the use of sympathomimetic agents (e.g. noradrenaline, metaraminol), atropine or inotropic agents (e.g. dopamine, dobutamine). Temporary pacing may be required for AV block. Glucagon can reverse the effects of excessive β-blockade, given in a dose of 1-10mg intravenously. Intravenous β_2-stimulants e.g. terbutaline may be required to relieve bronchospasm.

Metoprolol cannot be effectively removed by haemodialysis.

5. PHARMACOLOGICAL PROPERTIES

5.1 Pharmacodynamic properties

Metoprolol is a competitive β-adrenoceptor antagonist. It acts preferentially to inhibit β_1-adrenoceptors (conferring some cardioselectivity), is devoid of intrinsic sympathomimetic activity (partial agonist activity) and possesses β-adrenoceptor blocking activity comparable in potency with propranolol.

A negative chronotropic effect on the heart is a consistent feature of metoprolol administration. Thus cardiac output and systolic blood pressure rapidly decrease following acute administration.

5.2 Pharmacokinetic properties

Metoprolol is almost completely absorbed over a large part of the gastrointestinal tract, but bioavailability after oral administration is 40-50% of that after i.v. injection, because of hepatic first pass metabolism. The bioavailability of metoprolol after CR tablet administration is about 70% of that after plain tablets.

The steady state V_D of metoprolol is 3.2 L/kg and protein binding is about 12%.

Elimination half life of metoprolol is usually between about 3 and 5 hours. Elimination is by liver metabolism and metabolites are largely inactive. With metoprolol CR T_{max} is prolonged to about 8 hours. Mean C_{max} after Betaloc SA was 519nmol/L, achieved after 4 hours. Plasma levels at 24 hours were about 85nmol/L after Betaloc SA.

Initial absorption of metoprolol CR was more rapid and AUC increased when given together with food.

Urine recovery of unchanged drug was about 4% after metoprolol CR and metoprolol plain tablets. The pharmacokinetics and β-blocking effect of metoprolol are not significantly altered in patients with renal failure.

In healthy elderly volunteers there was no significant difference in the volume of distribution, elimination half life, total body clearance or bioavailability of metoprolol compared with young volunteers.

In patients with cirrhosis of the liver the bioavailability of metoprolol was increased and total body clearance reduced.

5.3 Preclinical safety data

There is no toxicity data that would indicate that metoprolol tartrate is unsafe for use in the indications given. Signs in rats and dogs indicate that metoprolol can exert a cardiopressive action at high plasma levels.

6. PHARMACEUTICAL PARTICULARS

6.1 List of excipients

Sodium aluminium silicate, paraffin, magnesium stearate, ethylcellulose, ethanol (used during manufacture), hydroxypropyl methylcellulose, polyethylene glycol, titanium dioxide (E171), hydrogen peroxide (30%) and water purified.

6.2 Incompatibilities

None known.

6.3 Shelf life

5 years.

6.4 Special precautions for storage

Store below 25°C.

6.5 Nature and contents of container

Blister strips (press through packs of thermoformed PVC) 7 tablets per strip - pack size 28.

Securitainers of 300 tablets.

6.6 Instructions for use and handling

Not applicable.

7. MARKETING AUTHORISATION HOLDER

AstraZeneca UK Ltd.,

600 Capability Green,

Luton, LU1 3LU, UK.

8. MARKETING AUTHORISATION NUMBER(S)

PL 17901/0107

9. DATE OF FIRST AUTHORISATION/RENEWAL OF THE AUTHORISATION

28th May 2002

10. DATE OF REVISION OF THE TEXT

28th May 2002

Betaloc Tablets 100mg

(AstraZeneca UK Limited)

1. NAME OF THE MEDICINAL PRODUCT

Betaloc Tablets 100mg.

2. QUALITATIVE AND QUANTITATIVE COMPOSITION

Metoprolol tartrate Ph. Eur. 100mg.

3. PHARMACEUTICAL FORM

Tablet.

4. CLINICAL PARTICULARS

4.1 Therapeutic indications

In the management of hypertension and angina pectoris. Cardiac arrhythmias, especially supraventricular tachyarrhythmias.

Adjunct to the treatment of hyperthyroidism.

Early intervention with Betaloc in acute myocardial infarction reduces infarct size and the incidence of ventricular fibrillation. Pain relief may also decrease the need for opiate analgesics.

Betaloc has been shown to reduce mortality when administered to patients with acute myocardial infarction.

Prophylaxis of migraine.

4.2 Posology and method of administration

The dose must always be adjusted to the individual requirements of the patient. The following are guidelines:

Hypertension: Total daily dosage Betaloc 100-400mg, to be given as a single or twice daily dose. The starting dose is 100mg per day. This may be increased by 100mg/day at weekly intervals. If full control is not achieved using a single daily dose, a b.d. regimen should be initiated. Combination therapy with a diuretic or other anti-hypertensive agent may also be considered.

Angina: Usually Betaloc 50-100mg twice or three times daily.

Cardiac Arrhythmias: Betaloc 50mg b.i.d. or t.i.d. should usually control the condition. If necessary the dose can be increased up to 300mg per day in divided doses.

Following the treatment of an acute arrhythmia with Betaloc injection, continuation therapy with Betaloc tablets should be initiated 4-6 hours later. The initial oral dose should not exceed 50mg t.i.d.

Hyperthyroidism: Betaloc 50mg four times a day. The dose should be reduced as the euthyroid state is achieved.

Myocardial Infarction: Early intervention - to achieve optimal benefits from intravenous Betaloc suitable patients should present within 12 hours of the onset of chest pain. Therapy should commence with 5mg i.v. every 2 minutes to a maximum of 15mg total as determined by blood pressure and heart rate. The second or third dose should not be given if the systolic blood pressure is $<$90mmHg, the heart rate is $<$40 beats/min and the P-Q time is $>$0.26 seconds, or if there is any aggravation of dyspnoea or cold sweating. Orally, therapy should commence 15 minutes after the last injection with 50mg every 6 hours for 48 hours. Patients who fail to tolerate the full intravenous dose should be given half the suggested oral dose.

Maintenance - the usual maintenance dose is 200mg daily, given in divided doses.

Migraine Prophylaxis: Betaloc 100-200mg daily, given in divided doses.

Elderly: Initially the lowest possible dose should be used, especially in the elderly.

Significant Hepatic Dysfunction: A reduction in dosage may be necessary.

4.3 Contraindications

AV block. Uncontrolled heart failure. Severe bradycardia. Sick-sinus syndrome. Cardiogenic shock. Severe peripheral arterial disease. Known hypersensitivity to β-blockers or to any of the constituents of Betaloc. Metabolic acidosis. Untreated phaeochromocytoma.

Betaloc is also contra-indicated when acute myocardial infarction is complicated by significant bradycardia, first degree heart block, systolic hypotension ($<$100mmHg) and/or severe heart failure.

4.4 Special warnings and special precautions for use

If patients develop increasing bradycardia, Betaloc should be given in lower doses or gradually withdrawn. Symptoms of peripheral arterial circulatory disorders, may be aggravated by Betaloc.

Abrupt interruption of β-blockers is to be avoided. When possible, Betaloc should be withdrawn gradually over a period of 10 -14 days, in diminishing doses to 25mg daily for the last 6 days. During its withdrawal patients should be kept under close surveillance, especially those with known ischaemic heart disease.

Betaloc may be administered when heart failure has been controlled.

Digitalisation and/or diuretic therapy should also be considered for patients with a history of heart failure, or patients known to have a poor cardiac reserve. Betaloc should be used with caution in patients where cardiac reserve is poor.

Intravenous administration of calcium antagonists of the verapamil type should not be given to patients treated with β-blockers.

In patients with Prinzmetal's angina β_1 selective agents should be used with care.

Although cardioselective β-blockers may have less effect on lung function than non-selective β-blockers, as with all β-blockers these should be avoided in patients with reversible obstructive airways disease unless there are compelling clinical reasons for their use. When administration is necessary, use of a β_2-bronchodilator (e.g. terbutaline) may be advisable in some patients.

The label shall state - "If you have a history of wheezing, asthma or any other breathing difficulties, you must tell your doctor before you take this medicine."

In labile and insulin-dependent diabetes it may be necessary to adjust the hypoglycaemic therapy.

As with other β-blockers, Betaloc may mask the symptoms of thyrotoxicosis and the early signs of acute hypoglycaemia in patients with diabetes mellitus. However, the risk of this occurring is less than with non-selective β-blockers.

In patients with a phaeochromocytoma, an α-blocker should be given concomitantly.

In the presence of liver cirrhosis the bioavailability of Betaloc may be increased and patients may need a lower dosage.

The elderly should be treated with caution, starting with a lower dose.

Like all β-blockers, careful consideration should be given to patients with psoriasis before Betaloc is administered.

The administration of adrenaline to patients undergoing β-blockade can result in an increase in blood pressure and bradycardia although this is less likely to occur with β_1-selective drugs.

Betaloc therapy must be reported to the anaesthetist prior to general anaesthesia. If withdrawal of metoprolol is considered desirable, this should if possible be completed at least 48 hours before general anaesthesia. However, in some patients it may be desirable to employ a β-blocker as premedication. By shielding the heart against the effects of stress the β-blocker may prevent excessive sympathetic stimulation provoking cardiac arrhythmias or acute coronary insufficiency. If a β-blocker is given for this purpose, an anaesthetic with little negative inotropic activity should be selected to minimise the risk of myocardial depression.

Beta-blockers may increase both the sensitivity towards allergens and the seriousness of anaphylactic reactions.

4.5 Interaction with other medicinal products and other forms of Interaction

The effects of Betaloc and other drugs with an antihypertensive effect on blood pressure are usually additive, and care should be taken to avoid hypotension such as could be the result of concomitant administration with dihydropyridine derivatives, tricyclic antidepressant, barbiturates and phenothiazines. However, combinations of antihypertensive drugs may often be used with benefit to improve control of hypertension.

Betaloc can reduce myocardial contractility and impair intracardiac conduction. Care should be exercised when drugs with similar activity, e.g. antiarrhythmic agents, general anaesthetics, are given concurrently. Like all other β-blockers, Betaloc should not be given in combination with verapamil, diltiazem or digitalis glycosides. A watch should be kept for possible negative effects when metoprolol is given in combination with calcium antagonists, since this may cause bradycardia, hypotension and asystole. Care should also be exercised when β-blockers are given in combination with sympathomimetic ganglion blocking agents, other β-blockers (i.e. eye drops) or MAO inhibitors.

If concomitant treatment with clonidine is to be discontinued, Betaloc should be withdrawn several days before clonidine.

As β-blockers may affect the peripheral circulation, care should be exercised when drugs with similar activity e.g. ergotamine are given concurrently.

Betaloc will antagonise the β_1-effects of sympathomimetic agents but should have little influence on the bronchodilator effects of β_2-agonists at normal therapeutic doses. Enzyme inducing agents (e.g. rifampicin) may reduce plasma concentrations of Betaloc, whereas enzyme inhibitors (e.g. cimetidine, alcohol and hydralazine) may increase plasma concentrations. Metoprolol may impair the elimination of lidocaine (lignocaine).

The dosages of oral antidiabetic agents and also of insulin may have to be readjusted in patients receiving β-blockers.

Concomitant treatment with indomethacin and other prostaglandin synthetase inhibiting drugs may reduce the antihypertensive effect of β-blockers.

4.6 Pregnancy and lactation

Betaloc should not be used in pregnancy or nursing mothers unless the physician considers that the benefit outweighs the possible hazard to the foetus/infant. β-blockers reduce placental perfusion, which may result in intrauterine foetal death, immature and premature deliveries. As with all β-blockers, metoprolol may cause side-effects especially bradycardia and hypoglycaemia in the foetus, and in the newborn and breastfed infant. There is an increased risk of cardiac and pulmonary complications in the neonate. Metoprolol has, however, been used in pregnancy-associated hypertension under close supervision, after 20 weeks gestation. Although Betaloc crosses the placental barrier and is present in cord blood, no evidence of foetal abnormalities has been reported.

Use during lactation

Breast feeding is not recommended. The amount of metoprolol ingested via breast milk should not produce significant β-blocking effects in the neonate if the mother is treated with normal therapeutic doses.

4.7 Effects on ability to drive and use machines

When driving vehicles or operating machines, it should be taken into account that occasionally dizziness or fatigue may occur.

4.8 Undesirable effects

Metoprolol is usually well tolerated and adverse reactions have generally been mild and reversible. The following events have been reported as adverse events in clinical trials or reported from routine use.

These are usually mild and infrequent. The most common appear to be lassitude, GI disturbances (nausea, vomiting or abdominal pain) and disturbances of sleep pattern. In many cases these effects have been transient or have disappeared after a reduction in dosage.

Effects related to the CNS which have been reported occasionally are dizziness and headache and rarely paraesthesia, muscle cramps, depression and decreased mental alertness. There have also been isolated reports of personality disorders like amnesia, memory impairment, confusion, hallucination, nervousness and anxiety.

Cardiovascular effects which have been reported occasionally are bradycardia, postural hypotension and rarely, heart failure, increased existing AV block, palpitations, cardiac arrhythmias, Raynauds phenomenon, peripheral oedema and precordial pain. There have also been isolated reports of cardiac conduction abnormalities, gangrene in patients with pre-existing severe peripheral circulatory disorders and increase of pre-existing intermittent claudication.

Common gastro-intestinal disturbances have been described above but rarely diarrhoea or constipation also occur and there have been isolated cases of dry mouth and abnormal liver function.

Skin rashes (urticaria, psoriasiform, dystrophic skin lesions) and positive anti-nuclear antibodies (not associated with SLE) occur rarely. Isolated cases of photosensitivity, psoriasis exacerbation, increased sweating and alopecia have been reported. Respiratory effects include occasional reports of dyspnoea on exertion and rare reports of bronchospasm and isolated cases of rhinitis. Rarely impotence/sexual dysfunction. Isolated cases of weight gain, thrombocytopenia, disturbances of vision, conjunctivitis, tinnitus, dry or irritated eyes, taste disturbance and arthralgia have also been reported.

The reported incidence of skin rashes and/or dry eyes is small and in most cases the symptoms have cleared when treatment was withdrawn. Discontinuation of the drug should be considered if any such reaction is not otherwise explicable.

4.9 Overdose

Poisoning due to an overdose of Betaloc may lead to severe hypotension, sinus bradycardia, atrioventricular block, heart failure, cardiogenic shock, cardiac arrest, bronchospasm, impairment of consciousness, coma, nausea, vomiting, cyanosis, hypoglycaemia and, occasionally, hyperkalaemia. The first manifestations usually appear 20 minutes to 2 hours after drug ingestion.

Treatment should include close monitoring of cardiovascular, respiratory and renal function, and blood glucose and electrolytes. Further absorption may be prevented by induction of vomiting, gastric lavage or administration of activated-charcoal if ingestion is recent. Cardiovascular complications should be treated symptomatically, which may require the use of sympathomimetic agents (e.g. noradrenaline, metaraminol), atropine or inotropic agents (e.g. dopamine, dobutamine). Temporary pacing may be required for AV block. Glucagon can reverse the effects of excessive β-blockade, given in a dose of 1-10mg intravenously. Intravenous β_2-stimulants e.g. terbutaline may be required to relieve bronchospasm.

Betaloc cannot be effectively removed by haemodialysis.

5. PHARMACOLOGICAL PROPERTIES

5.1 Pharmacodynamic properties

Metoprolol is a competitive β-adrenoceptor antagonist. It acts preferentially to inhibit β_1-adrenoceptors (conferring some cardioselectivity), is devoid of intrinsic sympathomimetic activity (partial agonist activity) and possesses β-adrenoceptor blocking activity comparable in potency with propranolol.

A negative chronotropic effect on the heart is a consistent feature of metoprolol administration. Thus, cardiac output and systolic blood pressure rapidly decrease following acute administration.

5.2 Pharmacokinetic properties

Metoprolol tablets dissolve rapidly which results in a rapid and complete absorption with t_{max} within 2 hours and consistent bioavailability data between different study populations.

Elimination is mainly via hepatic metabolism ($>$90%) terminal half-life is about 3-4 hours.

5.3 Preclinical safety data

The acute toxicity of metoprolol is low to moderate. Signs of toxicity are non-specific and do not indicate any target organ. Signs in rats and dogs indicate that metoprolol can exert a cardiopressive action at high plasma concentrations. Acute toxicity after oral administration is lower in rodents than in dogs.

There is no specific general toxicity after repeated administration to rats or dogs. Reproduction and mutagenicity studies have revealed no evidence of adverse effects. Carcinogenicity studies in rats and mice have shown no increased incidence of neoplasms related to metoprolol.

6. PHARMACEUTICAL PARTICULARS

6.1 List of excipients

Microcrystalline cellulose, lactose, sodium starch glycolate, magnesium stearate, colloidal silica, polyvidone.

6.2 Incompatibilities

None known.

6.3 Shelf life

5 years.

6.4 Special precautions for storage

Store below 25 °C.

6.5 Nature and contents of container

PVC/aluminium blister strips (10 tablets/strip) 50, 100 tablets in a cardboard outer.

Polypropylene securitainer 56, 100, 500 tablets with polyethylene cap.

6.6 Instructions for use and handling

Not applicable.

7. MARKETING AUTHORISATION HOLDER

AstraZeneca UK Ltd.,

600 Capability Green,

Luton, LU1 3LU, UK.

8. MARKETING AUTHORISATION NUMBER(S)

PL 17901/0108

9. DATE OF FIRST AUTHORISATION/RENEWAL OF THE AUTHORISATION

28th May 2002

10. DATE OF REVISION OF THE TEXT

28th May 2002

Betaloc Tablets 50mg

(AstraZeneca UK Limited)

1. NAME OF THE MEDICINAL PRODUCT
Betaloc Tablets 50mg.

2. QUALITATIVE AND QUANTITATIVE COMPOSITION
Metoprolol tartrate Ph. Eur. 50mg.

3. PHARMACEUTICAL FORM
Tablet.

4. CLINICAL PARTICULARS

4.1 Therapeutic indications
In the management of hypertension and angina pectoris. Cardiac arrhythmias, especially supraventricular tachyarrhythmias.

Adjunct to the treatment of hyperthyroidism.

Early intervention with Betaloc in acute myocardial infarction reduces infarct size and the incidence of ventricular fibrillation. Pain relief may also decrease the need for opiate analgesics.

Betaloc has been shown to reduce mortality when administered to patients with acute myocardial infarction.

Prophylaxis of migraine.

4.2 Posology and method of administration
The dose must always be adjusted to the individual requirements of the patient. The following are guidelines:

Hypertension: Total daily dosage Betaloc 100-400mg, to be given as a single or twice daily dose. The starting dose is 100mg per day. This may be increased by 100mg/day at weekly intervals. If full control is not achieved using a single daily dose, a b.d. regimen should be initiated. Combination therapy with a diuretic or other anti-hypertensive agent may also be considered.

Angina: Usually Betaloc 50-100mg twice or three times daily.

Cardiac Arrhythmias: Betaloc 50mg b.i.d. or t.i.d. should usually control the condition. If necessary the dose can be increased up to 300mg per day in divided doses.

Following the treatment of an acute arrhythmia with Betaloc injection, continuation therapy with Betaloc tablets should be initiated 4-6 hours later. The initial oral dose should not exceed 50mg t.i.d.

Hyperthyroidism: Betaloc 50mg four times a day. The dose should be reduced as the euthyroid state is achieved.

Myocardial Infarction: Early intervention - to achieve optimal benefits from intravenous Betaloc suitable patients should present within 12 hours of the onset of chest pain. Therapy should commence with 5mg i.v. every 2 minutes to a maximum of 15mg total as determined by blood pressure and heart rate. The second or third dose should not be given if the systolic blood pressure is <90mmHg, the heart rate is <40 beats/min and the P-Q time is >0.26 seconds, or if there is any aggravation of dyspnoea or cold sweating. Orally, therapy should commence 15 minutes after the last injection with 50mg every 6 hours for 48 hours. Patients who fail to tolerate the full intravenous dose should be given half the suggested oral dose.

Maintenance - the usual maintenance dose is 200mg daily, given in divided doses.

Migraine Prophylaxis: Betaloc 100-200mg daily, given in divided doses.

Elderly: Initially the lowest possible dose should be used, especially in the elderly.

Significant Hepatic Dysfunction: A reduction in dosage may be necessary.

4.3 Contraindications
AV block. Uncontrolled heart failure. Severe bradycardia. Sick-sinus syndrome. Cardiogenic shock. Severe peripheral arterial disease. Known hypersensitivity to β-blockers or to any of the constituents of Betaloc. Metabolic acidosis. Untreated phaeochromocytoma.

Betaloc is also contra-indicated when acute myocardial infarction is complicated by significant bradycardia, first degree heart block, systolic hypotension (<100mmHg) and/or severe heart failure.

4.4 Special warnings and special precautions for use
If patients develop increasing bradycardia, Betaloc should be given in lower doses or gradually withdrawn. Symptoms of peripheral arterial circulatory disorders may be aggravated by Betaloc.

Abrupt interruption of β-blockers is to be avoided. When possible, Betaloc should be withdrawn gradually over a period of 10 -14 days, in diminishing doses to 25mg daily for the last 6 days. During its withdrawal patients should be kept under close surveillance, especially those with known ischaemic heart disease.

Betaloc may be administered when heart failure has been controlled. Digitalisation and/or diuretic therapy should also be considered for patients with a history of heart failure, or patients known to have a poor cardiac reserve. Betaloc should be used with caution in patients where cardiac reserve is poor.

Intravenous administration of calcium antagonists of the verapamil type should not be given to patients treated with β-blockers.

In patients with Prinzmetal's angina β_1 selective agents should be used with care.

Although cardioselective β-blockers may have less effect on lung function than non-selective β-blockers, as with all β-blockers these should be avoided in patients with reversible obstructive airways disease unless there are compelling clinical reasons for their use. When administration is necessary, use of a β_2-bronchodilator (e.g. terbutaline) may be advisable in some patients.

The label shall state - "If you have a history of wheezing, asthma or any other breathing difficulties, you must tell your doctor before you take this medicine."

In labile and insulin-dependent diabetes it may be necessary to adjust the hypoglycaemic therapy.

As with other β-blockers, Betaloc may mask the symptoms of thyrotoxicosis and the early signs of acute hypoglycaemia in patients with diabetes mellitus. However, the risk of this occurring is less than with non-selective β-blockers.

In patients with a phaeochromocytoma, an α-blocker should be given concomitantly.

In the presence of liver cirrhosis the bioavailability of Betaloc may be increased and patients may need a lower dosage.

The elderly should be treated with caution, starting with a lower dose.

Like all β-blockers, careful consideration should be given to patients with psoriasis before Betaloc is administered.

The administration of adrenaline to patients undergoing β-blockade can result in an increase in blood pressure and bradycardia although this is less likely to occur with β_1-selective drugs.

Betaloc therapy must be reported to the anaesthetist prior to general anaesthesia. If withdrawal of metoprolol is considered desirable, this should if possible be completed at least 48 hours before general anaesthesia. However, in some patients it may be desirable to employ a β-blocker as premedication.

By shielding the heart against the effects of stress the β-blocker may prevent excessive sympathetic stimulation provoking cardiac arrhythmias or acute coronary insufficiency. If a β-blocker is given for this purpose, an anaesthetic with little negative inotropic activity should be selected to minimise the risk of myocardial depression.

Beta-blockers may increase both the sensitivity towards allergens and the seriousness of anaphylactic reactions.

4.5 Interaction with other medicinal products and other forms of Interaction
The effects of Betaloc and other drugs with an antihypertensive effect on blood pressure are usually additive, and care should be taken to avoid hypotension such as could be the result of concomitant administration with dihydropyridine derivatives, tricyclic antidepressants, barbiturates and phenothiazines. However, combinations of antihypertensive drugs may often be used with benefit to improve control of hypertension.

Betaloc can reduce myocardial contractility and impair intracardiac conduction. Care should be exercised when drugs with similar activity, e.g. antiarrhythmic agents, general anaesthetics, are given concurrently. Like all other β-blockers, Betaloc should not be given in combination with verapamil, diltiazem or digitalis glycosides. A watch should be kept for possible negative effects when metoprolol is given in combination with calcium antagonists, since this may cause bradycardia, hypotension and asystole. Care should also be exercised when β-blockers are given in combination with sympathomimetic ganglion blocking agents, other β-blockers (i.e. eye drops) or MAO inhibitors.

If concomitant treatment with clonidine is to be discontinued, Betaloc should be withdrawn several days before clonidine.

As β-blockers may affect the peripheral circulation, care should be exercised when drugs with similar activity e.g. ergotamine are given concurrently.

Betaloc will antagonise the β_1-effects of sympathomimetic agents but should have little influence on the bronchodilator effects of β_2-agonists at normal therapeutic doses. Enzyme inducing agents (e.g. rifampicin) may reduce plasma concentrations of Betaloc, whereas enzyme inhibitors (e.g. cimetidine, alcohol and hydralazine) may increase plasma concentrations. Metoprolol may impair the elimination of lidocaine (lignocaine).

The dosages of oral antidiabetic agents and also of insulin may have to be readjusted in patients receiving β-blockers.

Concomitant treatment with indomethacin and other prostaglandin synthetase inhibiting drugs may reduce the antihypertensive effect of β-blockers.

4.6 Pregnancy and lactation
Betaloc should not be used in pregnancy or nursing mothers unless the physician considers that the benefit outweighs the possible hazard to the foetus/infant. β-blockers reduce placental perfusion, which may result in intrauterine foetal death, immature and premature deliveries, As with all β-blockers, metoprolol may cause side-effects especially bradycardia and hypoglycaemia in the foetus, and in the newborn and breastfed infant. There is an increased risk of cardiac and pulmonary complications in the neonate. Metoprolol has, however, been used in pregnancy-associated hypertension under close supervision, after 20 weeks gestation. Although Betaloc crosses the placental barrier and is present in cord blood, no evidence of foetal abnormalities has been reported.

Use during lactation
Breast feeding is not recommended. The amount of metoprolol ingested via breast milk should not produce significant β-blocking effects in the neonate if the mother is treated with normal therapeutic doses.

4.7 Effects on ability to drive and use machines
When driving vehicles or operating machines, it should be taken into account that occasionally dizziness or fatigue may occur.

4.8 Undesirable effects
Metoprolol is usually well tolerated and adverse reactions have generally been mild and reversible. The following events have been reported as adverse events in clinical trials or reported from routine use.

These are usually mild and infrequent. The most common appear to be lassitude, GI disturbances (nausea, vomiting or abdominal pain) and disturbances of sleep pattern. In many cases these effects have been transient or have disappeared after a reduction in dosage.

Effects related to the CNS which have been reported occasionally are dizziness and headache and rarely paraesthesia, muscle cramps, depression and decreased mental alertness. There have also been isolated reports of personality disorders like amnesia, memory impairment, confusion, hallucination, nervousness and anxiety.

Cardiovascular effects which have been reported occasionally are bradycardia, postural hypotension and rarely, heart failure, increased existing AV block, palpitations, cardiac arrhythmias, Raynauds phenomenon, peripheral oedema and precordial pain. There have also been isolated reports of cardiac conduction abnormalities, gangrene in patients with pre-existing severe peripheral circulatory disorders and increase of pre-existing intermittent claudication.

Common gastro-intestinal disturbances have been described above but rarely diarrhoea or constipation also occur and there have been isolated cases of dry mouth and abnormal liver function.

Skin rashes (urticaria, psoriasiform, dystrophic skin lesions) and positive anti-nuclear antibodies (not associated with SLE) occur rarely. Isolated cases of photosensitivity, psoriasis exacerbation, increased sweating and alopecia have been reported. Respiratory effects include occasional reports of dyspnoea on exertion and rare reports of bronchospasm and isolated cases of rhinitis.

Rarely impotence/sexual dysfunction. Isolated cases of weight gain, thrombocytopenia, disturbances of vision, conjunctivitis, tinnitus, dry or irritated eyes, taste disturbance and arthralgia have also been reported.

The reported incidence of skin rashes and/or dry eyes is small and in most cases the symptoms have cleared when treatment was withdrawn. Discontinuation of the drug should be considered if any such reaction is not otherwise explicable.

4.9 Overdose
Poisoning due to an overdose of Betaloc may lead to severe hypotension, sinus bradycardia, atrioventricular block, heart failure, cardiogenic shock, cardiac arrest, bronchospasm, impairment of consciousness, coma, nausea, vomiting, cyanosis, hypoglycaemia and, occasionally, hyperkalaemia. The first manifestations usually appear 20 minutes to 2 hours after drug ingestion.

Treatment should include close monitoring of cardiovascular, respiratory and renal function, and blood glucose and electrolytes. Further absorption may be prevented by induction of vomiting, gastric lavage or administration of activated-charcoal if ingestion is recent. Cardiovascular complications should be treated symptomatically, which may require the use of sympathomimetic agents (e.g. noradrenaline, metaraminol), atropine or inotropic agents (e.g. dopamine, dobutamine). Temporary pacing may be required for AV block. Glucagon can reverse the effects of excessive β-blockade, given in a dose of 1-10mg intravenously. Intravenous β_2-stimulants e.g. terbutaline may be required to relieve bronchospasm.

Betaloc cannot be effectively removed by haemodialysis.

5. PHARMACOLOGICAL PROPERTIES

5.1 Pharmacodynamic properties
Metoprolol is a competitive β-adrenoceptor antagonist. It acts preferentially to inhibit β_1-adrenoceptors (conferring some cardioselectivity), is devoid of intrinsic sympathomimetic activity (partial agonist activity) and possesses β-adrenoceptor blocking activity comparable in potency with propranolol.

A negative chronotropic effect on the heart is a consistent feature of metoprolol administration. Thus, cardiac output and systolic blood pressure rapidly decrease following acute administration.

5.2 Pharmacokinetic properties

Metoprolol tablets dissolve rapidly which results in a rapid and complete absorption with t_{max} within 2 hours and consistent bioavailability data between different study populations.

Elimination is mainly via hepatic metabolism (>90%) terminal half life is about 3-4 hours.

5.3 Preclinical safety data

The acute toxicity of metoprolol is low to moderate. Signs of toxicity are non-specific and do not indicate any target organ. Signs in rats and dogs indicate that metoprolol can exert a cardiopressive action at high plasma concentrations. Acute toxicity after oral administration is lower in rodents than in dogs.

There is no specific general toxicity after repeated administration to rats or dogs. Reproduction and mutagenicity studies have revealed no evidence of adverse effects. Carcinogenicity studies in rats and mice have shown no increased incidence of neoplasms related to metoprolol.

6. PHARMACEUTICAL PARTICULARS

6.1 List of excipients

Microcrystalline cellulose, lactose, sodium starch glycolate, magnesium stearate, colloidal silica, polyvidone.

6.2 Incompatibilities

None known.

6.3 Shelf life

5 years.

6.4 Special precautions for storage

Store below 25 °C.

6.5 Nature and contents of container

PVC/aluminium blister strips (10 tablets/strip) 50, 100 tablets in a cardboard outer.

Polypropylene securitainer 56, 100, 500 tablets with polyethylene cap.

6.6 Instructions for use and handling

Not applicable.

7. MARKETING AUTHORISATION HOLDER

AstraZeneca UK Ltd.,

600 Capability Green,

Luton, LU1 3LU, UK.

8. MARKETING AUTHORISATION NUMBER(S)

PL 17901/0109

9. DATE OF FIRST AUTHORISATION/RENEWAL OF THE AUTHORISATION

28th May 2002

10. DATE OF REVISION OF THE TEXT

28th May 2002

Betim 10 mg Tablets

(Valeant Pharmaceuticals Ltd)

1. NAME OF THE MEDICINAL PRODUCT

Betim 10 mg Tablets

2. QUALITATIVE AND QUANTITATIVE COMPOSITION

Each tablet contains Timolol maleate Ph.Eur. 10 mg.

3. PHARMACEUTICAL FORM

Tablet.

4. CLINICAL PARTICULARS

4.1 Therapeutic indications

Betim is indicated in angina pectoris due to ischaemic heart disease, for the treatment of hypertension and to reduce mortality and reinfarction in patients surviving acute myocardial infarction. Betim is also indicated in the prophylactic treatment of migraine in order to reduce the number of attacks.

4.2 Posology and method of administration

For oral administration.

The lowest possible dosage should be given first in order to be able to identify cardiac decompensation or bronchial phenomena at an early stage; this is especially important in the elderly. Subsequent increases in dose should take place slowly, (e.g. once a week) under control or on the basis of clinical effect.

For angina:

The recommended dose range is 5-30 mg twice daily. The initial dose should be 5 mg twice daily, increasing the daily dose by 10 mg not more frequently than every 3-4 days to achieve optimum results.

Hypertension:

The recommended dose range is 10-60 mg daily. Most hypertensive patients will be controlled by 10-30 mg timolol which can be administered once daily or in two divided doses if preferred.

Doses in excess of 30 mg daily should be given in two equally divided doses. The dose of Betim may need adjustment when used in conjunction with other antihypertensive drugs.

After myocardial infarction:

Start with 5 mg (½ tablet) twice daily for two days. If there are no adverse effects, increase dosage to 10mg twice daily and maintain at this dose.

For the prophylactic treatment of migraine:

10 to 20 mg once daily or in two divided doses.

Dosage in the elderly:

Initiate treatment with lowest adult dose and thereafter adjust according to response.

Children:

Safety and efficacy in children has not been established.

4.3 Contraindications

Heart failure, unless adequately controlled, sinus bradycardia (<45 - 50 bpm) or heart block. Cardiogenic shock. History of bronchospasm and bronchial asthma. Chronic obstructive pulmonary disease. Patients receiving monoamine oxidase inhibitors. Pregnancy. Sick sinus syndrome (including sino-atrial block), severe peripheral vascular disease or Raynaud's disease. Prinzmetal's angina. Untreated phaeochromocytoma. Metabolic acidosis. Hypotension. Severe peripheral circulatory disturbances. Hypersensitivity to timolol or any other ingredients.

4.4 Special warnings and special precautions for use

Cardiovascular

Although Betim has no direct myocardial depressant activity, the continued depression of sympathetic drive through beta-blockade may lead to cardiac failure in patients with latent cardiac insufficiency. All patients should be observed for evidence of cardiac failure and, if it occurs, then treatment with beta blockers should be gradually withdrawn. If it is not possible to withdraw beta blocker treatment, then digitalisation and diuretic therapy should be considered.

Beta-blockers should not be used in patients with untreated congestive heart failure. This condition should first be stabilised.

In patients with ischaemic heart disease, treatment should not be discontinued suddenly. The dosage should gradually be reduced, i.e. over 1-2 weeks. If necessary, replacement therapy should be initiated at the same time, to prevent exacerbation of angina pectoris.

Beta-blockers may induce bradycardia. If the pulse rate decreases to less than 50-55 beats per minute at rest and the patient experiences symptoms related to the bradycardia, the dosage should be reduced.

In patients with peripheral circulatory disorders (Raynaud's disease or syndrome, intermittent claudication), beta-blockers should be used with great caution as aggravation of these disorders may occur.

Metabolic/endocrine

Betim should be administered with caution to patients with impaired renal function or impaired hepatic function. Patients with liver or kidney insufficiency may need a lower dosage.

Betim may be used safely in diabetes. It may, however, interfere with the cardiovascular and possibly the metabolic responses to hypoglycaemia and, therefore, should be used with caution in diabetic patients treated with insulin or oral hypoglycaemic agents as well as patients subject to spontaneous hypoglycaemia.

Beta-blockers may mask the symptoms of thyrotoxicosis or hypoglycaemia.

Other warnings

Patients with a history of psoriasis should take beta-blockers only after careful consideration.

Beta-blockers may increase sensitivity to allergens and the seriousness of anaphylactic reactions.

The following statement will appear on the label of this product: 'Do not take this medicine if you have a history of wheezing or asthma'.

4.5 Interaction with other medicinal products and other forms of Interaction

The depressant effect of beta-blocking drugs on myocardial contractility and on intracardiac conduction may be increased by concomitant use with other drugs having similar effects. Serious effects have been reported with verapamil, disopyramide, lignocaine and tocainide and may be anticipated with diltiazem, quinidine, amiodarone and any of the class 1 antiarrhythmic agents. Special care is necessary when any of these agents are given intravenously in patients who are beta blocked.

Concurrent administration of digitalis glycosides may increase the atrio-ventricular conduction time.

Beta-blockers increase the risk of 'rebound hypertension' when taken with clonidine. When clonidine is used in conjunction with non-selective beta-blockers such as timolol, treatment with clonidine should be continued for some time after treatment with the beta-blocker has been discontinued.

Concomitant administration of tricyclic antidepressants, barbiturates and phenothiazines, dihydropyridine derivatives such as nifedipine or antihypertensive agents may increase the blood pressure lowering effect.

Beta-blockers may intensify the blood sugar lowering effect of insulin and oral antidiabetic drugs.

Anaesthesia

The anaesthesiologist should be informed when the patient is receiving a beta-blocking agent. Concomitant use of beta blockers and anaesthetics may attenuate reflex tachycardia and increase the risk of hypotension.

The withdrawal of beta blocking drugs prior to surgery is not necessary in the majority of patients. If beta-blockade is interrupted in preparation for surgery, therapy should be discontinued at least 24 hours beforehand.

Continuation of beta-blockade reduces the risk of arrhythmias during induction and intubation, however the risk of hypertension may be increased. Anaesthetic agents such as ether, cyclopropane and trichloroethylene should not be used whereas halothane, isoflurane, nitrous oxide, intravenous induction agents, muscle relaxants, narcotic analgesics and local anaesthetic agents are all compatible with beta-adrenergic blockade. Local anaesthetics with added vasoconstrictors, e.g. adrenaline, should be avoided. The patient may be protected against vagal reactions by intravenous administration of atropine.

The bioavailability of Betim will be increased by co-administration with cimetidine or hydralazine and reduced with rifampicin.

Betim may be prescribed with vasodilation, but increased gastro-intestinal blood flow may affect absorption and metabolism of timolol.

Alcohol induces increased plasma levels of hepatically metabolised beta-blockers such as timolol.

Some prostaglandin synthetase inhibiting drugs have been shown to impair the antihypertensive effect of beta-blocking drugs.

The effect of sympathomimetic agents, e.g. isoprenaline, salbutamol, will be reduced by concomitant use of beta blockers. In addition, sympathomimetics may counteract the effect of beta-blocking agents.

The adverse vasoconstrictor effects of ergot preparations may be potentiated during the treatment of migraine with beta blocking drugs.

Caution is recommended when Betim is administered to patients on catecholamine depleting drugs such as reserpine or guanethidine.

4.6 Pregnancy and lactation

Betim is contra-indicated in pregnancy. Timolol maleate appears in breast milk (milk: plasma ratio 0.8). Breast feeding is therefore not recommended during administration of this product.

4.7 Effects on ability to drive and use machines

None known. When driving vehicles or operating machines it should be taken into account that occasionally dizziness or fatigue may occur.

4.8 Undesirable effects

General side effects: Betim is usually well tolerated in normal use. General symptoms resulting from beta blockade include fatigue and weakness.

Other potential side effects include:

Cardiovascular: bradycardia, heart failure, cold and cyanotic extremities, hypotension, heart block, a slowed AV-conduction or increase of an existing AV-block, Raynaud's phenomenon, paresthesia of the extremities, increase of an existing intermittent claudication, impotence.

Digestive: epigastric distress, nausea, vomiting and diarrhoea.

CNS: dizziness, disorientation, vertigo, paraesthesiae, headache, hallucinations, nightmares, insomnia, somnolence, depression, sleep disturbances, psychoses, confusion.

Respiratory: dyspnoea, broncho-spasm in patients with bronchial asthma or a history of asthmatic complaints.

Special senses: visual disturbance, dry eyes.

Retroperitoneal fibrosis, allergic skin reactions including erythematous or psoriaform rashes and arthralgia have been rarely reported.

An increase in anti-nuclear antibodies has been seen with beta-blocking agents; its clinical relevance is not clear.

Warning: There have been reports of skin rashes and/or dry eyes associated with the use of beta-adrenergic blocking drugs. The reported incidence is rare and in most cases the symptoms have cleared when treatment was withdrawn. Discontinuance of the drug should be considered if any such reaction is not otherwise explicable. Cessation of therapy with the beta blocker should be gradual although withdrawal symptoms with timolol are infrequent.

4.9 Overdose

Poisoning due to an overdose of Betim may lead to severe hypotension, sinus bradycardia, atrioventricular block, heart failure, cardiogenic shock, cardiac arrest, bronchospasm, impairment of consciousness, coma, occasionally hyperkalaemia. The first manifestations usually appear 20 minutes to 2 hours after drug ingestion.

Treatment should include close monitoring of cardiovascular, respiratory and renal function and blood glucose and electrolytes. Further absorption may be prevented by induction of vomiting, gastric lavage or administration of activated charcoal if ingestion is recent.

Cardiovascular complications should be treated symptomatically, which may require the use of sympathomimetic agents, (e.g. noradrenaline, metariminol), atropine or inotropic agents, (e.g. dopamine, dobutamine). Temporary pacing may be required for AV block. Glucagon can reverse the effects of excessive beta blockade, given in a dose of 1-10 mg intravenously. Intravenous B2-stimulants, e.g. terbutaline, may be required to relieve bronchospasm.

Timolol cannot be effectively removed by haemodialysis.

5. PHARMACOLOGICAL PROPERTIES

5.1 Pharmacodynamic properties

Betim is a beta-adrenergic receptor blocking agent. The competitive antagonism of adrenergic transmitters at beta receptors blocks beta-sympathomimetic activity particularly in the heart, the bronchi and blood vessels.

Betim has been shown to be a highly specific beta-adrenergic blocking drug and it does not block the chronotropic or inotropic effects of calcium, glucagon, theophylline or digitalis. It does not have significant local anaesthetic or direct myocardial depressant activity nor any significant intrinsic beta-adrenergic stimulant effect.

Betim reduces heart rate and force of myocardial contraction and, therefore, myocardial oxygen consumption. Modification of the cardiovascular responses to stress or exercise is therapeutically useful in the treatment of angina pectoris.

The beta-blocking action of Betim is also of therapeutic value in hypertension, although the exact mechanism of action is unclear.

5.2 Pharmacokinetic properties

Timolol maleate is rapidly and nearly completely absorbed following oral administration. Beta blocking activity is apparent within 30 minutes of administration and the duration of action, though dependent on dose, has been shown to last for up to 24 hours. Dose proportionality has been established. Plasma half-life is approximately 2.7-5.0 hours with a peak plasma concentration occurring approximately 2 hours post dose. Timolol undergoes significant hepatic metabolism, but "first pass metabolism" is low.

5% of timolol is excreted unchanged by the kidneys.

These pharmacokinetic parameters are unchanged in hypertensive patients and following multiple dosages.

The rate of timolol metabolism varies between individuals. Poor metabolisers (approximately 10%) show higher plasma levels and slower elimination of timolol than extensive metabolisers. Within individuals, however, plasma concentrations and half-life are reproducible. As the therapeutic response and some adverse effects are related to plasma concentrations of timolol, poor metabolisers may require lower than normal doses.

5.3 Preclinical safety data

Timolol has low toxicity and mutagenicity and reproduction and fertility studies have not demonstrated evidence of changes relevant to the dosage used in man.

6. PHARMACEUTICAL PARTICULARS

6.1 List of excipients

Microcrystalline cellulose, starch, magnesium stearate.

6.2 Incompatibilities

None known.

6.3 Shelf life

5 years.

6.4 Special precautions for storage

None.

6.5 Nature and contents of container

Glass bottle and blister packs of 30 and 100 tablets.

6.6 Instructions for use and handling

None.

Administrative Data

7. MARKETING AUTHORISATION HOLDER

ValeantPharmaceuticals Ltd.
Cedarwood
Chineham Business Park
Crockford Lane
Basingstoke
Hampshire
RG24 8WD

8. MARKETING AUTHORISATION NUMBER(S)

PL 15142/0024

9. DATE OF FIRST AUTHORISATION/RENEWAL OF THE AUTHORISATION

31 December 2000

10. DATE OF REVISION OF THE TEXT

November 2004

Legal Status

POM

Betnelan Tablets

(UCB Pharma Limited)

1. NAME OF THE MEDICINAL PRODUCT

Betnelan Tablets

2. QUALITATIVE AND QUANTITATIVE COMPOSITION

Each tablet contains 500 micrograms (0.5mg) betamethasone PhEur.

For excipients, see 6.1

3. PHARMACEUTICAL FORM

Tablet

Small white tablets engraved 'Betnelan Evans' on one side and scored on the reverse. The product complies with the specification for Betamethasone Tablets BP.

4. CLINICAL PARTICULARS

4.1 Therapeutic indications

Betamethasone is a glucocorticosteroid which is about eight to ten times as active as prednisolone on a weight-for-weight basis.

A wide variety of diseases may sometimes require corticosteroid therapy. Some of the principal indications are:

Bronchial asthma, severe hypersensitivity reactions, anaphylaxis;

Rheumatoid arthritis, systemic lupus erythematosus, dermatomyositis, mixed connective tissue disease (excluding systemic sclerosis), polyarteritis nodosa;

Inflammatory skin disorders, including pemphigus vulgaris, bullous pemphigoid and pyoderma gangrenosum;

Minimal change nephrotic syndrome, acute interstitial nephritis;

Ulcerative colitis, Crohn's disease;

Sarcoidosis;

Rheumatic carditis;

Haemolytic anaemia (autoimmune), acute and lymphatic leukaemia, malignant lymphoma, multiple myeloma, idiopathic thrombocytopenia purpura;

Immuno-suppression in transplantation.

4.2 Posology and method of administration

The lowest dosage that will produce an acceptable result should be used; when it is possible to reduce the dosage, this must be accomplished in stages. During prolonged therapy, dosage may need to be increased temporarily during periods of stress or in exacerbation of illness (see "Special Warnings and Precautions for Use").

Adults:

The dose used will depend upon the disease, its severity, and the clinical response obtained. The following regimens are for guidance only. Divided dosage is usually employed.

Short-term treatment:

2 to 3mg daily for the first few days, subsequently reducing the daily dosage by 250 or 500 micrograms (0.25 or 0.5mg) every two to five days, depending upon the response.

Rheumatoid arthritis:

500 micrograms (0.5mg) to 2mg daily. For maintenance therapy the lowest effective dosage is used.

Most other conditions:

1.5 to 5mg daily for one to three weeks, then reducing to the minimum effective dosage.

Larger doses may be needed for mixed connective tissue diseases and ulcerative colitis.

Children:

A proportion of the adult dosage may be used (e.g. 75% at twelve years, 50% at seven years and 25% at one year) but clinical factors must be given due consideration (see "Special Warnings and Precautions for Use").

Route of Administration: Oral

4.3 Contraindications

Systemic infections, unless specific anti-infective therapy is employed.

Hypersensitivity to any component of the tablets.

4.4 Special warnings and special precautions for use

A Patient Information Leaflet should be supplied with this product.

Undesirable effects may be minimised by using the lowest effective dose for the minimum period and by administering the daily requirement as a single morning dose, or as a single morning dose on alternate days whenever possible. Frequent patient review is required to appropriately titrate the dose against disease activity (see "Posology and Method of Administration").

Caution is advised with the use of corticosteroids in patients who have suffered a recent myocardial infarction because of the risk of myocardial rupture.

Caution is advised on the use of corticosteroids in patients with hypothyroidism.

Suppression of the inflammatory response and immune function increases the susceptibility to infections and their severity. The clinical presentation may often be atypical and serious infections such as septicaemia and tuberculosis may be masked and may reach an advanced stage before being recognised.

Chickenpox is of particular concern since this normally minor illness may be fatal in immunosuppressed patients. Patients (or parents of children) without a definite history of chickenpox should be advised to avoid close personal contact with chickenpox or herpes zoster and if exposed they should seek urgent medical attention. Passive immunisation with varicella/zoster immunoglobulin (VZIG) is needed by exposed non-immune patients who are receiving systemic corticosteroids or who have used them within the previous 3 months; this should be given within 10 days of exposure to chickenpox. If a diagnosis of chickenpox is confirmed, the illness warrants specialist care and urgent treatment. Corticosteroids should not be stopped and the dose may need to be increased

Corticosteriods may reduce immune function. Live vaccines should not be given to individuals with impaired immune responsiveness. The antibody response to other vaccines may be diminished.

Patients should be advised to take particular care to avoid exposure to measles and to seek immediate medical advice if exposure occurs. Prophylaxis with intramuscular normal immunoglobulin may be needed.

Adrenal suppression:

Adrenal cortical atrophy develops during prolonged therapy and may persist for years after stopping treatment.

In patients who have received more than physiological doses of systemic corticosteroids (approximately 1mg betamethasone or equivalent) for greater than 3 weeks, withdrawal should not be abrupt. How dose reduction should be carried out depends largely on whether the disease is likely to relapse as a dose of systemic corticosteroids is reduced. Clinical assessment of disease activity may be needed during withdrawal. If the disease is unlikely to relapse on withdrawal of systemic corticosteroids but there is uncertainty about hypothalamic-pituitary-adrenal (HPA) suppression, the dose of systemic corticosteroid may be reduced rapidly to physiological doses. Once a daily dose equivalent to 1mg betamethasone is reached, dose reduction should be slower to allow the HPA-axis to recover.

Abrupt withdrawal of systemic corticosteroid treatment, which has continued up to 3 weeks is appropriate if it is considered that the disease is unlikely to relapse. Abrupt withdrawal of doses of up to 6mg daily of betamethasone, or equivalent for 3 weeks is unlikely to lead to clinically relevant HPA-axis suppression, in the majority of patients. In the following patient groups, gradual withdrawal of systemic corticosteroid therapy should be ***considered*** even after courses lasting 3 weeks or less:

- Patients who have had repeated courses of systemic corticosteroids, particularly if taken for greater than 3 weeks,
- When a short course has been prescribed within one year of cessation of long-term therapy (months or years),
- Patients who have reasons for adrenocortical insufficiency other than exogenous corticosteroids therapy,
- Patients receiving doses of systemic corticosteroid greater than 6mg daily of betamethasone (or equivalent),
- Patients repeatedly taking doses in the evening.

During prolonged therapy any intercurrent illness, trauma or surgical procedure will require a temporary increase in dosage; if corticosteroids have been stopped following prolonged therapy they may need to be temporarily re-introduced.

Special precautions:

Particular care is required when considering the use of systemic corticosteroids in patients with the following conditions and frequent patient monitoring is necessary.

A. Osteoporosis (post-menopausal females are particularly at risk).

B. Hypertension or congestive heart failure.

C. Existing or previous history of severe affective disorders (especially previous steroid psychosis).

D. Diabetes mellitus (or a family history of diabetes).

E. History of, or active tuberculosis.

F. Glaucoma (or a family history of glaucoma).

G. Previous corticosteroid-induced myopathy.

H. Liver failure - blood levels of corticosteroid may be increased, (as with other drugs which are metabolised in the liver).

I. Renal insufficiency.

J. Epilepsy.

K. Peptic ulceration.

Patients should carry 'steroid treatment' cards which give clear guidance on the precautions to be taken to minimise risk and which provide details of prescriber, drug, dosage and the duration of treatment.

Use in children:

Corticosteroids cause dose-related growth retardation in infancy, childhood and adolescence, which may be irreversible. Treatment should be limited to the minimum dosage for the shortest possible time. In order to minimise suppression of the HPA axis and growth retardation, consideration should be given to administration of a single dose on alternate days.

Use in the elderly:

The common adverse effects of systemic corticosteroids may be associated with more serious consequences in old age, especially osteoporosis, hypertension, hypokalaemia, diabetes, susceptibility to infection and thinning of the skin. Close clinical supervision is required to avoid life-threatening reactions.

4.5 Interaction with other medicinal products and other forms of Interaction

Steroids may reduce the effects of anticholinesterases in myasthenia gravis, cholecystographic X-ray media and non-steroidal anti-inflammatory agents.

Rifampicin, rifabutin, carbamazepine, phenobarbitone, phenytoin, primidone, aminoglutethimide and ephedrine enhance the metabolism of corticosteroids; thus the corticosteroid therapeutic effect may be reduced.

The desired effects of hypoglycaemic agents (including insulin), anti-hypertensives and diuretics are antagonised by corticosteroids, and the hypokalaemic effects of acetazolamide, loop diuretics, thiazide diuretics and carbenoxolone are enhanced.

The efficacy of coumarin anticoagulants may be enhanced by concurrent corticosteroid therapy and close monitoring of the INR or prothrombin time is required to avoid spontaneous bleeding.

The renal clearance of salicylates is increased by corticosteroids and steroid withdrawal may result in salicylate intoxication.

The risk of hypokalaemia is increased with theophylline, ulcer healing drugs such as carbenoxolone and antifungals such as amphotericin B.

Increased toxicity may result if hypokalaemia occurs in patients on cardiac glycosides.

Ritonavir and oral contraceptives may result in increased plasma concentrations or corticosteroids.

The effect of corticosteroids may be reduced for 3-4 days after mifepristone.

The growth promoting effect of somatropin may be inhibited by corticosteroids.

An increase in the incidence of gastrointestinal bleeding may occur if NSAIDS are taken concomitantly with corticosteroids.

Corticosteroids may antagonise the effects of neuromuscular blocking drugs such as vecuronium.

4.6 Pregnancy and lactation

Pregnancy

The ability of corticosteroids to cross the placenta varies between individual drugs, however, betamethasone readily crosses the placenta. Administration of corticosteroids to pregnant animals can cause abnormalities of foetal development including cleft palate, intra-uterine growth retardation and effects on brain growth and development. There is no evidence that corticosteroids result in an increased incidence of congenital abnormalities, such as cleft palate/lip in man. However, when administered for prolonged periods or repeatedly during pregnancy, corticosteroids may increase the risk of intra-uterine growth retardation. Hypoadrenalism may, in theory, occur in the neonate following prenatal exposure to corticosteroids but usually resolves spontaneously following birth and is rarely clinically important. As with all drugs, corticosteroids should only be prescribed when the benefits to the mother and child outweigh the risks. When corticosteroids are essential however, patients with normal pregnancies may be treated as though they were in the non-gravid state. Patients with pre-eclampsia or fluid retention require close monitoring.

Betamethasone, systemically administered to a woman during pregnancy may result in a transient suppression of the foetal heart rate parameters and biophysical activities that are widely used for the assessment of foetal well – being. These characteristics can include a reduction in foetal breathing movements, body movements and heart rate.

Lactation

Corticosteroids may pass into breast milk, although no data are available for betamethasone. Infants of mothers taking high doses of systemic corticosteroids for prolonged periods may have a degree of adrenal suppression.

4.7 Effects on ability to drive and use machines

None known.

4.8 Undesirable effects

The incidence of predictable undesirable effects, including HPA axis suppression, correlates with the relative potency of the drug, dosage, timing of administration and the duration of treatment (see "Special Warnings and Precautions for Use").

Endocrine/metabolic:

Suppression of the hypothalamic-pituitary-adrenal axis, growth suppression in infancy, childhood and adolescence, menstrual irregularity and amenorrhoea. Cushingoid facies, hirsutism, weight gain, impaired carbohydrate tolerance with increased requirement for antidiabetic therapy. Negative protein, nitrogen and calcium balance. Increased appetite. Hyperhydrosis. Increased high – density lipoprotein and low – density lipoprotein concentrations in the blood.

Anti-inflammatory and immunosuppressive effects:

Increased susceptibility to and severity of infections with suppression of clinical symptoms and signs, opportunistic infections, recurrence of dormant tuberculosis (see "Special Warnings and Precautions for Use").

Musculoskeletal:

Osteoporosis, vertebral and long bone fractures, avascular osteonecrosis, tendon rupture, proximal myopathy.

Fluid and electrolyte disturbance:

Sodium and water retention, hypertension, potassium loss, hypokalaemic alkalosis.

Neuropsychiatric:

Euphoria, psychological dependence, depression, psychosis, insomnia, and aggravation of schizophrenia. Increased intra-cranial pressure with papilloedema in children (pseudotumour cerebri), usually after treatment withdrawal. Aggravation of epilepsy.

Ophthalmic:

Increased intra-ocular pressure, glaucoma, papilloedema, posterior subcapsular cataracts, corneal or scleral thinning, exacerbation of ophthalmic viral or fungal diseases.

Gastrointestinal:

Abdominal distension, oesophageal ulceration, nausea, dyspepsia, peptic ulceration with perforation and haemorrhage, acute pancreatitis, candidiasis.

Dermatological:

Impaired healing, skin atrophy, bruising, telangiectasia, striae, acne.

Other Side Effects:

Malaise, hiccups, myocardial rupture following recent myocardial infarction.

General:

Hypersensitivity including anaphylaxis, has been reported. Leucocytosis. Thrombo-embolism.

Withdrawal symptoms and signs:

Too rapid a reduction of corticosteroid dosage following prolonged treatment can lead to acute adrenal insufficiency, hypotension and death (see "Special Warnings and Precautions for Use").

A 'withdrawal syndrome' may also occur, including fever, myalgia, arthralgia, rhinitis, conjunctivitis, painful itchy skin nodules and loss of weight.

4.9 Overdose

Treatment is unlikely to be needed in cases of acute overdosage.

5. PHARMACOLOGICAL PROPERTIES

5.1 Pharmacodynamic properties

ATC Code: H02A B01

Betamethasone is a glucocorticoid which is about eight to ten times as active as prednisolone on a weight-for-weight basis.

5.2 Pharmacokinetic properties

Corticosteroids are bound to plasma proteins in varying degrees. Corticosteroids are metabolised primarily in the liver and are then excreted by the kidneys.

5.3 Preclinical safety data

None stated.

6. PHARMACEUTICAL PARTICULARS

6.1 List of excipients

Lactose

Starch Maize

Gelatin

Magnesium Stearate

Purified Water

6.2 Incompatibilities

None known.

6.3 Shelf life

3 years.

6.4 Special precautions for storage

Do not store above 30°C. Keep the container in the outer carton. Protect from light.

6.5 Nature and contents of container

Tubular glass vial with a polyurethane snap-plug closure containing 100 tablets

Tamper evident polypropylene container with a polyurethane foam wad and a low density polyethylene lid containing 500 tablets.

6.6 Instructions for use and handling

None stated.

7. MARKETING AUTHORISATION HOLDER

UCB Pharma Limited

208 Bath Road

Slough

Berkshire

SL1 3WE

UK

8. MARKETING AUTHORISATION NUMBER(S)

PL 00039/0392

9. DATE OF FIRST AUTHORISATION/RENEWAL OF THE AUTHORISATION

17th December 1992 / 21 January 1998

10. DATE OF REVISION OF THE TEXT

June 2005

POM

Betnesol Eye Ointment

(UCB Pharma Limited)

1. NAME OF THE MEDICINAL PRODUCT

Betnesol Eye Ointment

2. QUALITATIVE AND QUANTITATIVE COMPOSITION

Betamethasone sodium phosphate PhEur 0.1% w/w

For excipients, see 6.1

3. PHARMACEUTICAL FORM

Eye Ointment.

4. CLINICAL PARTICULARS

4.1 Therapeutic indications

Short-term treatment of steroid responsive inflammatory conditions of the eye after clinical exclusion of bacterial, viral and fungal infections.

4.2 Posology and method of administration

Adults and children (including the elderly)

The frequency of dosing depends on the clinical response. If there is no clinical response within 7 days of treatment, the ointment should be discontinued.

Treatment should be the lowest effective dose for the shortest possible time. After more prolonged treatment (over 6 to 8 weeks), the ointment should be withdrawn slowly to avoid relapse.

An extrusion of the ointment about 1/4 inch long may be introduced beneath the lower lid two or three times daily and/or at night.

4.3 Contraindications

Bacterial, viral, fungal, tuberculous or purulent conditions of the eye. Use is contraindicated if glaucoma is present, or where herpetic keratitis (e.g. dendritic ulcer) is considered a possibility. Use of topical steroids in the latter condition can lead to an extension of the ulcer and marked visual deterioration.

Hypersensitivity to any component of the preparation.

4.4 Special warnings and special precautions for use

A patient information leaflet should be supplied with this product.

Topical corticosteroids should never be given for an undiagnosed red eye as inappropriate use is potentially blinding.

Prolonged use may lead to the risk of adrenal suppression in infants.

Treatment with corticosteroid preparations should not be repeated or prolonged without regular review to exclude raised intraocular pressure, cataract formation or unsuspected infections.

4.5 Interaction with other medicinal products and other forms of Interaction

None relevant to topical use.

4.6 Pregnancy and lactation

Safety for use in pregnancy and lactation has not been established. There is inadequate evidence of safety in human pregnancy. Topical administration of corticosteroids to pregnant animals can cause abnormalities of foetal development including cleft palate and intrauterine growth retardation. There may therefore be a very small risk of such effects in the human foetus.

4.7 Effects on ability to drive and use machines

May cause transient blurring of vision on instillation. Patients should be warned not to drive or operate hazardous machinery unless vision is clear.

4.8 Undesirable effects

Hypersensitivity reactions, usually of the delayed type, may occur leading to irritation, burning, stinging, itching and dermatitis.

Topical corticosteroid use may result in corneal ulceration, increased intraocular pressure leading to optic nerve damage, reduced visual acuity and visual field defects.

Intensive or prolonged use of topical corticosteroids may lead to formation of posterior subcapsular cataracts.

In those diseases causing thinning of the cornea or sclera, corticosteroid therapy may result in thinning of the globe leading to perforation.

Mydriasis, ptosis and epithelial punctate keratitis have also been reported following ophthalmic use of corticosteroids.

4.9 Overdose

Oral ingestion of the contents of one tube (3g) of ointment is unlikely to lead to any serious adverse effects.

5. PHARMACOLOGICAL PROPERTIES

5.1 Pharmacodynamic properties

ATC Code: S01B A06

Betamethasone is a glucocorticoid which has topical anti-inflammatory activity.

5.2 Pharmacokinetic properties

Not applicable as the ointment is applied topically to the eye.

5.3 Preclinical safety data

None stated.

6. PHARMACEUTICAL PARTICULARS

6.1 List of excipients

White soft paraffin

Liquid paraffin

6.2 Incompatibilities

None known.

6.3 Shelf life

Unopened: 36 months

Opened: 4 weeks

6.4 Special precautions for storage

Store at a temperature below 30°C.

6.5 Nature and contents of container

Collapsible aluminium tubes with fine-bore extended nozzle tube fitted with a natural polyethylene cap containing 3 grams of ointment.

6.6 Instructions for use and handling

None stated.

7. MARKETING AUTHORISATION HOLDER

UCB Pharma Limited
208 Bath Road
Slough
Berkshire
SL1 3WE
UK

8. MARKETING AUTHORISATION NUMBER(S)

PL 00039/0388

9. DATE OF FIRST AUTHORISATION/RENEWAL OF THE AUTHORISATION

2 December 1992

10. DATE OF REVISION OF THE TEXT

June 2005

POM

Betnesol Eye, Ear, Nose Drops

(UCB Pharma Limited)

1. NAME OF THE MEDICINAL PRODUCT

Betnesol Eye, Ear and Nose Drops

2. QUALITATIVE AND QUANTITATIVE COMPOSITION

Betamethasone sodium phosphate PhEur 0.1% w/v.

For excipients, see 6.1

3. PHARMACEUTICAL FORM

Ear/Eye/Nose Drops, Solution

A clear and colourless aqueous solution.

4. CLINICAL PARTICULARS

4.1 Therapeutic indications

Short-term treatment of steroid responsive inflammatory conditions of the eye after clinical exclusion of bacterial, viral and fungal infections.

Non-infected inflammatory conditions of the ear or nose.

4.2 Posology and method of administration

The frequency of dosing depends on the clinical response. If there is no clinical response within 7 days of treatment, the drops should be discontinued.

Treatment should be the lowest effective dose for the shortest possible time. After more prolonged treatment (over 6 to 8 weeks), the drops should be withdrawn slowly to avoid relapse.

Eyes

1 or 2 drops instilled into the eye every one or two hours until control is achieved, when the frequency may be reduced.

Ears

2 or 3 drops instilled into the ear every two or three hours until control is achieved, when the frequency may be reduced.

Nose

2 or 3 drops instilled into each nostril two or three times daily.

4.3 Contraindications

Bacterial, viral, fungal, tuberculous or purulent conditions of the eye. Use is contraindicated if glaucoma is present or herpetic keratitis (e.g. dendritic ulcer) is considered a possibility. Use of topical steroids in the latter condition can lead to an extension of the ulcer and marked visual deterioration.

Corticosteroids should not be used in patients with a perforated tympanic membrane.

Hypersensitivity to any component of the preparation.

4.4 Special warnings and special precautions for use

A patient information leaflet should be supplied with this product.

Topical corticosteroids should never be given for an undiagnosed red eye as inappropriate use is potentially blinding. Ophthalmological treatment with corticosteroid preparations should not be repeated or prolonged without regular review to exclude raised intraocular pressure, cataract formation or unsuspected infections.

Nasal administration of corticosteroids is not advised if an untreated nasal infection is present, or if the patient has pulmonary tuberculosis or following nasal surgery (until healing has occurred).

Prolonged use may lead to the risk of adrenal suppression in infants.

4.5 Interaction with other medicinal products and other forms of Interaction

Betnesol Drops contain benzalkonium chloride as a preservative and therefore, should not be used to treat patients who wear soft contact lenses.

4.6 Pregnancy and lactation

Safety for use in pregnancy and lactation has not been established. There is inadequate evidence of safety in human pregnancy. Topical administration of corticosteroids to pregnant animals can cause abnormalities of foetal development including cleft palate and intrauterine growth retardation. There may therefore be a very small risk of such effects in the human foetus.

4.7 Effects on ability to drive and use machines

May cause transient blurring of vision on instillation. Patients should be warned not to drive or operate hazardous machinery unless vision is clear.

4.8 Undesirable effects

Hypersensitivity reactions, usually of the delayed type, may occur leading to irritation, burning, stinging, itching and dermatitis.

Topical corticosteroid use may result in corneal ulceration, increased intraocular pressure leading to optic nerve damage, reduced visual acuity and visual field defects.

Intensive or prolonged use of topical corticosteroids may lead to formation of posterior subcapsular cataracts.

In those diseases causing thinning of the cornea or sclera, corticosteroid therapy may result in thinning of the globe leading to perforation.

Mydriasis, ptosis and epithelial punctate keratitis have also been reported following ophthalmic use of corticosteroids.

Following nasal administration, the most common effects are nasal irritation and dryness, although sneezing, headache, lightheadedness, urticaria, nausea, epistaxis, rebound congestion, bronchial asthma, perforation of the nasal septum, ulceration of the nasal septum, anosmia, parosmia and disturbance to sense of taste have also been reported.

Systemic effects of nasal corticosteroids may occur, particularly at high doses prescribed for prolonged periods. Growth retardation has been reported in children receiving nasal corticosteroids at licensed doses.

It is recommended that the height of children receiving prolonged treatment with nasal corticosteroids is regularly monitored. If growth is slowed, therapy should be reviewed with the aim of reducing the dose of nasal corticosteroid, if possible, to the lowest dose at which effective control of symptoms is maintained. In addition, consideration should also be given to referring the patient to a paediatric specialist

4.9 Overdose

Oral ingestion of the contents of one bottle (up to 10ml) of drops, or one tube (3g) of ointment is unlikely to lead to any serious adverse effects. Long-term intensive topical use may lead to systemic effects.

Treatment with higher than recommended doses may result in clinically significant adrenal suppression. If there is evidence of higher than recommended doses being used then additional systemic corticosteroid cover should be considered during periods of stress or elective surgery.

5. PHARMACOLOGICAL PROPERTIES

5.1 Pharmacodynamic properties

ATC Code: S03B A

Not applicable.

5.2 Pharmacokinetic properties

Not applicable.

5.3 Preclinical safety data

None stated.

6. PHARMACEUTICAL PARTICULARS

6.1 List of excipients

Benzalkonium chloride solution

Disodium hydrogen phosphate anhydrous

Sodium chloride

Disodium edetate

Sodium hydroxide

Phosphoric acid

Water for Injection

6.2 Incompatibilities

None known.

6.3 Shelf life

Unopened: 24 months

Opened: 4 weeks

6.4 Special precautions for storage

Store at a temperature not exceeding 25°C. Avoid freezing. Always replace the bottle back in the carton after use to protect its contents from light. The sterility of the drops is assured until the cap seal is broken.

6.5 Nature and contents of container

5 or 10ml bottles with nozzle insert moulded in natural low density polyethylene closed with a tamper evident high density polyethylene cap.

6.6 Instructions for use and handling

None stated.

7. MARKETING AUTHORISATION HOLDER

UCB Pharma Limited
208 Bath Road
Slough
Berkshire
SL1 3WE
UK

8. MARKETING AUTHORISATION NUMBER(S)

PL 00039/0387

9. DATE OF FIRST AUTHORISATION/RENEWAL OF THE AUTHORISATION

17 December 1992

10. DATE OF REVISION OF THE TEXT

June 2005

POM

Betnesol Injection

(UCB Pharma Limited)

1. NAME OF THE MEDICINAL PRODUCT

Betnesol Injection

2. QUALITATIVE AND QUANTITATIVE COMPOSITION

Each ampoule contains 5.3mg of betamethasone sodium phosphate BP equivalent to 4mg betamethasone in 1ml of sterile aqueous solution.

For excipients, see 6.1

3. PHARMACEUTICAL FORM

Solution for Injection

1ml ampoules containing a clear colourless or pale yellow solution

4. CLINICAL PARTICULARS

4.1 Therapeutic indications

Betamethasone is a glucocorticosteroid which is about eight to ten times as active as prednisolone on a weight-for-weight basis. It may be indicated in the following conditions:

Status asthmaticus and acute allergic reactions, including anaphylactic reactions to drugs. Betnesol Injection supplements the action of adrenaline.

Severe shock arising from surgical or accidental trauma or overwhelming infection.

Acute adrenal crisis caused by abnormal stress in Addison's disease, Simmonds' disease, hypopituitarism following adrenalectomy, and when adrenocortical function has been suppressed by prolonged corticosteroid therapy.

Soft tissue lesions such as tennis elbow, tenosynovitis and bursitis.

NB. Betnesol Injection does not replace other forms of therapy for the treatment of shock and status asthmaticus.

4.2 Posology and method of administration

Betnesol Injection may be administered by slow intravenous injection, deep intramuscular injection or subconjunctival injection. Alternatively, Betnesol Injection may be given by intravenous infusion. Local injections of Betnesol Injection may be used when treating soft tissue lesions (see below).

The incidence of predictable undesirable effects, including hypothalamic-pituitary-adrenal (HPA) axis suppression correlates with the relative potency of the drug, dosage, timing of administration and the duration of treatment (see "Special Warnings and Precautions for Use").

Systemic therapy in adults

4 to 20mg betamethasone (1 to 5ml) administered by slow intravenous injection over half to one minute. This dose can be repeated three or four times in 24 hours, or as required, depending upon the condition being treated and the patient's response.

Alternatively, Betnesol Injection may be given by intravenous infusion. The same dose can be given by deep intramuscular injection but the response is likely to be less rapid, especially in shock. This dose can be repeated three or four times in 24 hours depending upon the condition being treated and the patient's response.

Systemic therapy in children

Infants up to 1 year may be given 1mg betamethasone intravenously; children aged 1 to 5 years, 2mg; 6 to 12 years, 4mg (1ml). This dose can be repeated three or four times in 24 hours, depending upon the condition being treated and the patient's response.

Other routes

Local injections of 4 to 8mg Betnesol may be used when treating soft tissue lesions in adults; children may require smaller doses. This dose can be repeated on two or three occasions depending upon the patient's response.

Betnesol Injection has also been administered sub-conjunctivally as a single injection of 0.5 to 1ml.

Intrathecal use is not recommended.

4.3 Contraindications

Systemic infections, unless specific anti-infective therapy is employed.

Betnesol injection contains sodium metabisulphite (0.1% w/v) as a preservative and therefore should not be used to treat patients with known hypersensitivity to bisulphite, metabisulphite or any other component of the injection.

Betnesol injection should not be injected directly into tendons.

4.4 Special warnings and special precautions for use

A patient information leaflet should be supplied with this product.

Undesirable effects may be minimised by using the lowest effective dose for the minimum period, and by administering the daily requirement as a single morning dose, or whenever possible as a single morning dose on alternate days. Frequent patient review is required to appropriately titrate the dose against disease activity (see "Posology and Method of Administration").

Caution is advised with the use of corticosteroids in patients who have suffered a recent myocardial infarction because of the risk of myocardial rupture.

Caution is advised on the use of corticosteroids in patients with hypothyroidism.

Suppression of the inflammatory response and immune function increases the susceptibility to infections and their severity. The clinical presentation may often be atypical and serious infections such as septicaemia and tuberculosis may be masked and may reach an advanced stage before being recognised.

Chickenpox is of particular concern since this normally minor illness may be fatal in immunosuppressed patients. Patients (or parents of children) without a definite history of chickenpox should be advised to avoid close personal contact with chickenpox or herpes zoster and if exposed they should seek urgent medical attention. Passive immunisation with varicella zoster immunoglobulin (VZIG) is needed by exposed non-immune patients who are receiving systemic corticosteroids or who have used them within the previous 3 months; this should be given within 10 days of exposure to chickenpox. If a diagnosis of chickenpox is confirmed, the illness warrants specialist care and urgent treatment. Corticosteroids should not be stopped and the dose may need to be increased.

Live vaccines should not be given to individuals with impaired immune responsiveness. The antibody response to other vaccines may be diminished.

Patients should be advised to take particular care to avoid exposure to measles and to seek immediate medical advice if exposure occurs. Prophylaxis with intramuscular normal immunoglobulin may be needed.

Corticosteroids should not be used for management of head injury or stroke because it is unlikely to be of benefit and may even be harmful.

In the treatment of cerebral oedema due to tumour, gastrointestinal bleeding may occur and stool examination may be helpful in diagnosis.

Adrenal suppression:

Adrenal cortical atrophy develops during prolonged therapy and may persist for years after stopping treatment.

In patients who have received more than physiological doses of systemic corticosteroids (approximately 1mg betamethasone or equivalent) for greater than 3 weeks, withdrawal should not be abrupt. How dose reduction should be carried out depends largely on whether the disease is likely to relapse as a dose of systemic corticosteroids is reduced. Clinical assessment of disease activity may be needed during withdrawal. If the disease is unlikely to relapse on withdrawal of systemic corticosteroids but there is uncertainty about HPA suppression, the dose of systemic corticosteroid may be reduced rapidly to physiological doses. Once a daily dose equivalent to 1mg betamethasone is reached, dose reduction should be slower to allow the HPA-axis to recover.

Abrupt withdrawal of systemic corticosteroid treatment, which has continued up to 3 weeks is appropriate if it is considered that the disease is unlikely to relapse. Abrupt withdrawal of doses of up to 6mg daily of betamethasone, or equivalent for 3 weeks is unlikely to lead to clinically relevant HPA-axis suppression, in the majority of patients. In the following patient groups, gradual withdrawal of systemic corticosteroid therapy should be ***considered*** even after courses lasting 3 weeks or less:

- Patients who have had repeated courses of systemic corticosteroids, particularly if taken for greater than 3 weeks,
- When a short course has been prescribed within one year of cessation of long-term therapy (months or years),
- Patients who have reasons for adrenocortical insufficiency other than exogenous corticosteroids therapy,
- Patients receiving doses of systemic corticosteroid greater than 6mg daily of betamethasone (or equivalent),
- Patients repeatedly taking doses in the evening.

During prolonged therapy any intercurrent illness, trauma or surgical procedure will require a temporary increase in dosage; if corticosteroids have been stopped following prolonged therapy they may need to be temporarily re-introduced.

Special precautions

Particular care is required when considering the use of systemic corticosteroids in patients with the following conditions and frequent patient monitoring is necessary.

A. Osteoporosis (post-menopausal females are particularly at risk).

B. Hypertension or congestive heart failure.

C. Existing or previous history of severe affective disorders (especially previous steroid psychosis).

D. Diabetes mellitus (or a family history of diabetes).

E. History of, or active, tuberculosis.

F. Glaucoma (or a family history of glaucoma).

G. Previous corticosteroid-induced myopathy.

H. Liver failure - blood levels of corticosteroid may be increased, as with other drugs which are metabolised in the liver.

I. Renal insufficiency.

J. Epilepsy.

K. History of, or active, peptic ulceration.

L. Herpes simplex keratitis.

M. Diverticulitis.

N. Thromboembolic tendencies.

Patients should carry 'steroid treatment' cards which give clear guidance on the precautions to be taken to minimise risk and which provide details of prescriber, drug, dosage and the duration of treatment.

Use in children

Corticosteroids cause dose-related growth retardation in infancy, childhood and adolescence, which may be irreversible. Treatment should be limited to the minimum dosage for the shortest possible time. In order to minimise suppression of the HPA axis and growth retardation, consideration should be given to administration of a single dose on alternate days.

Use in the elderly

The common adverse effects of systemic corticosteroids may be associated with more serious consequences in old age, especially osteoporosis, hypertension, hypokalaemia, diabetes, susceptibility to infection and thinning of the skin. Close clinical supervision is required to avoid life-threatening reactions.

4.5 Interaction with other medicinal products and other forms of Interaction

Steroids may reduce the effects of anticholinesterases in myasthenia gravis cholecystographic x-ray media and non-steroidal anti-inflammatory agents.

Rifampicin, rifabutin, carbamazepine, phenobarbitone, phenytoin, primidone, aminoglutethimide and ephedrine enhance the metabolism of corticosteroids and their therapeutic effects may be reduced.

The desired effects of hypoglycaemic agents (including insulin), anti-hypertensives and diuretics are antagonised by corticosteroids, and the hypokalaemic effects of acetazolamide, loop diuretics, thiazide diuretics and carbenoxolone are enhanced.

The efficacy of coumarin anticoagulants may be enhanced by concurrent corticosteroid therapy and close monitoring of the INR or prothrombin time is required to avoid spontaneous bleeding.

The renal clearance of salicylates is increased by corticosteroids and steroid withdrawal may result in salicylate intoxication.

The risk of hypokalaemia is increased with theophylline, ulcer healing drugs such as carbenoxolone and antifungals such as amphotericin B.

Increased toxicity may result if hypokalaemia occurs in patients on cardiac glycosides.

Ritonavir and oral contraceptives may result in increased plasma concentrations or corticosteroids.

The effect of corticosteroids may be reduced for 3-4 days after mifepristone.

The growth promoting effect of somatropin may be inhibited by corticosteroids.

An increase in the incidence of gastrointestinal bleeding may occur if NSAIDS are taken concomitantly with corticosteroids.

Corticosteroids may antagonise the effects of neuromuscular blocking drugs such as vecuronium.

4.6 Pregnancy and lactation

Pregnancy

The ability of corticosteroids to cross the placenta varies between individual drugs, however, betamethasone readily crosses the placenta. Administration of corticosteroids to pregnant animals can cause abnormalities of foetal development including cleft palate, intra-uterine growth retardation and effects on brain growth and development. There is no evidence that corticosteroids result in an increased incidence of congenital abnormalities, such as cleft palate/lip in man. However, when administered for prolonged periods or repeatedly during pregnancy, corticosteroids may increase the risk of intra-uterine growth retardation. Hypoadrenalism may, in theory, occur in the neonate following prenatal exposure to corticosteroids but usually resolves spontaneously following birth and is rarely clinically important. As with all drugs, corticosteroids should only be prescribed when the benefits to the mother and child outweigh the risks. When corticosteroids are essential however, patients with normal pregnancies may be treated as though they were in the non-gravid state. Patients with pre-eclampsia or fluid retention require close monitoring.

Betamethasone, systemically administered to a woman during pregnancy may result in a transient suppression of the foetal heart rate parameters and biophysical activities that are widely used for the assessment of foetal well – being. These characteristics can include a reduction in foetal breathing movements, body movements and heart rate.

Lactation

Corticosteroids may pass into breast milk, although no data is available for betamethasone. Infants of mothers taking high doses of systemic corticosteroids for prolonged periods may have a degree of adrenal suppression.

4.7 Effects on ability to drive and use machines

None known.

4.8 Undesirable effects

The incidence of predictable undesirable effects, including hypothalamic-pituitary-adrenal (HPA) axis suppression correlates with the relative potency of the drug, dosage, timing of administration and the duration of treatment (see "Special Warnings and Precautions for Use").

Endocrine/metabolic

Suppression of the hypothalamic-pituitary-adrenal (HPA) axis, growth suppression in infancy, childhood and adolescence, menstrual irregularity and amenorrhoea. Cushingoid facies, hirsutism, weight gain, impaired carbohydrate tolerance with increased requirement for antidiabetic therapy. Negative protein, nitrogen and calcium balance. Increased appetite. Hyperhydrosis. Increased high –density lipoprotein and low – density lipoprotein concentrations in the blood.

Anti-inflammatory and immunosuppressive effects

Increased susceptibility and severity of infections with suppression of clinical symptoms and signs, opportunistic infections, recurrence of dormant tuberculosis (see "Special Warnings and Precautions for Use").

Musculoskeletal

Osteoporosis, vertebral and long bone fractures, avascular osteonecrosis, tendon rupture, proximal myopathy.

Fluid and electrolyte disturbance

Sodium and water retention, hypertension, potassium loss, hypokalaemic alkalosis.

Neuropsychiatric

Euphoria, psychological dependence, depression, psychosis, insomnia, and aggravation of schizophrenia. Increased intra-cranial pressure with papilloedema in children (pseudotumour cerebri), usually after treatment withdrawal. Aggravation of epilepsy.

Ophthalmic

Increased intra-ocular pressure, glaucoma, papilloedema, posterior subcapsular cataracts, corneal or scleral thinning, exacerbation of ophthalmic viral or fungal diseases

Cardiac

Myocardial rupture following recent myocardial infarction.

Gastrointestinal

Abdominal distension, oesophageal ulceration, nausea, dyspepsia, peptic ulceration with perforation and haemorrhage, acute pancreatitis, candidiasis.

Dermatological

Impaired healing, skin atrophy, bruising, telangiectasia, striae, acne.

General

Hypersensitivity including anaphylaxis has been reported. Leucocytosis. Thrombo-embolism. Malaise. Hiccups.

Withdrawal symptoms and signs

Too rapid a reduction of corticosteroid dosage following prolonged treatment can lead to acute adrenal insufficiency, hypotension and death (see "Special Warnings and Precautions for Use").

A "withdrawal syndrome" may also occur including: fever, myalgia, arthralgia, rhinitis, conjunctivitis, painful itchy skin nodules and loss of weight.

4.9 Overdose

Should overdosage occur, the possibility of adrenal suppression should be minimised by a gradual reduction of dosage over a period of time. The patient may need support during any further trauma.

5. PHARMACOLOGICAL PROPERTIES

5.1 Pharmacodynamic properties

ATC Code: HO2A B01

Betamethasone is a glucocorticoid which is about eight to ten times as active as prednisolone on a weight-for-weight basis.

5.2 Pharmacokinetic properties

Corticosteroids are bound to plasma proteins in varying degrees. Corticosteroids are metabolised primarily by the liver and then excreted by the kidneys.

5.3 Preclinical safety data

None stated.

6. PHARMACEUTICAL PARTICULARS

6.1 List of excipients

Disodium edetate

Sodium metabisulphite

Sodium chloride

Sodium hydroxide

Hydrochloric acid

Water for injection

6.2 Incompatibilities

None known.

6.3 Shelf life

24 months.

6.4 Special precautions for storage

Store below 30°C and protect from light.

6.5 Nature and contents of container

1ml clear neutral glass ampoules in packs of five.

6.6 Instructions for use and handling

None stated.

7. MARKETING AUTHORISATION HOLDER

UCB Pharma Limited
208 Bath Road
Slough
Berkshire
SL1 3WE
UK

8. MARKETING AUTHORISATION NUMBER(S)

PL 00039/0391

9. DATE OF FIRST AUTHORISATION/RENEWAL OF THE AUTHORISATION

22nd December 1992

10. DATE OF REVISION OF THE TEXT

June 2005

POM

Betnesol Tablets

(UCB Pharma Limited)

1. NAME OF THE MEDICINAL PRODUCT

Betnesol Tablets

2. QUALITATIVE AND QUANTITATIVE COMPOSITION

Each tablet contains 500 micrograms (0.5mg) betamethasone as betamethasone sodium phosphate PhEur.

For excipients, see 6.1

3. PHARMACEUTICAL FORM

Soluble Tablet

Small, soluble, pink tablets engraved "Betnesol Evans" on one side and scored on the reverse.

The tablets comply with the specification for Betamethasone Sodium Phosphate Tablets BP.

4. CLINICAL PARTICULARS

4.1 Therapeutic indications

Betamethasone is a glucocorticoid which is about eight to ten times as active as prednisolone on a weight-for-weight basis.

Betamethasone sodium phosphate is very soluble in water, and is therefore less likely to cause local gastric irritation than corticosteroids which are only slightly soluble. This is important when high doses are required, as in immunosuppressive therapy.

Betnesol does not normally cause retention of salt and water and the risk of inducing oedema and hypertension is almost negligible.

A wide variety of diseases may sometimes require corticosteroid therapy. Some of the principal indications are:

Bronchial asthma, severe hypersensitivity reactions, anaphylaxis, rheumatoid arthritis, systemic lupus erythematosus, dermatomyositis, mixed connective tissue disease (excluding systemic sclerosis), polyarteritis nodosa;

Inflammatory skin disorders, including pemphigus vulgaris, bullous pemphigoid and pyoderma gangrenosum;

Minimal change nephrotic syndrome, acute interstitial nephritis;

Ulcerative colitis, Crohn's disease, sarcoidosis, rheumatic carditis;

Haemolytic anaemia (autoimmune), acute and lymphatic leukaemia, malignant lymphoma, multiple myeloma, idiopathic thrombocytopenic purpura;

Immunosuppression in transplantation.

4.2 Posology and method of administration

Betnesol Tablets are best taken dissolved in water, but they can be swallowed whole without difficulty. The lowest dosage that will produce an acceptable result should be used; when it is possible to reduce the dosage, this must be accomplished by stages. During prolonged therapy, dosage may need to be increased temporarily during periods of stress or in exacerbations of illness (see "Special Warnings and Precautions for Use").

Adults:

The dose used will depend on the disease, its severity, and the clinical response obtained. The following regimens are for guidance only. Divided dosage is usually employed.

Short term treatment:

2-3mg daily for the first few days, then reducing the daily dose by 250 or 500mcg (0.25 or 0.5mg) every two to five days, depending upon the response.

Rheumatoid arthritis:

500mcg (0.5mg) to 2mg daily. For maintenance therapy the lowest effective dosage is used.

Most other conditions:

1.5 to 5mg daily for one to three weeks, then reducing to the minimum effective dosage. Larger doses may be needed for mixed connective tissue diseases and ulcerative colitis.

Children:

A proportion of the adult dosage may be used (e.g. 75% at 12 years, 50% at 7 years and 25% at 1 year) but clinical factors must be given due weight (see "Special Warnings and Precautions for Use).

Route of Administration: Oral

4.3 Contraindications

Systemic infections, unless specific anti-infective therapy is employed.

Hypersensitivity to any component of the tablets.

4.4 Special warnings and special precautions for use

A patient information leaflet should be supplied with this product.

Undesirable effects may be minimised by using the lowest effective dose for the minimum period, and by administering the daily requirement as a single morning dose, or whenever possible as a single morning dose on alternate days. Frequent patient review is required to appropriately titrate the dose against disease activity (see "Posology and Method of Administration").

Caution is advised with the use of corticosteroids in patients who have suffered a recent myocardial infarction because of the risk of myocardial rupture.

Caution is advised on the use of corticosteroids in patients with hypothyroidism.

Suppression of the inflammatory response and immune function increases the susceptibility to infections and their severity. The clinical presentation may often be atypical and serious infections such as septicaemia and tuberculosis may be masked and may reach an advanced stage before being recognised.

Chickenpox is of particular concern since this normally minor illness may be fatal in immunosuppressed patients. Patients (or parents of children) without a definite history of chickenpox should be advised to avoid close personal contact with chickenpox or herpes zoster and if exposed they should seek urgent medical attention. Passive immunisation with varicella zoster immunoglobulin (VZIG) is needed by exposed non-immune patients who are receiving systemic corticosteroids or who have used them within the previous 3 months; this should be given within 10 days of exposure to chickenpox. If a diagnosis of chickenpox is confirmed, the illness warrants specialist care and urgent treatment. Corticosteroids should not be stopped and the dose may need to be increased.

Live vaccines should not be given to individuals with impaired immune responsiveness. The antibody response to other vaccines may be diminished.

Patients should be advised to take particular care to avoid exposure to measles and to seek immediate medical advice if exposure occurs. Prophylaxis with intramuscular normal immunoglobulin may be needed.

Adrenal suppression:

Adrenal cortical atrophy develops during prolonged therapy and may persist for years after stopping treatment.

In patients who have received more than physiological doses of systemic corticosteroids (approximately 1mg betamethasone or equivalent) for greater than 3 weeks, withdrawal should not be abrupt. How dose reduction should be carried out depends largely on whether the disease is likely to relapse as a dose of systemic corticosteroids is reduced. Clinical assessment of disease activity may be needed during withdrawal. If the disease is unlikely to relapse on withdrawal of systemic corticosteroids but there is uncertainty about hypothalamic-pituitary-adrenal (HPA) suppression, the dose of systemic corticosteroid may be reduced rapidly to physiological doses. Once a daily dose equivalent to 1mg betamethasone is reached, dose reduction should be slower to allow the HPA-axis to recover.

Abrupt withdrawal of systemic corticosteroid treatment, which has continued up to 3 weeks is appropriate if it is considered that the disease is unlikely to relapse. Abrupt withdrawal of doses of up to 6mg daily of betamethasone, or equivalent for 3 weeks is unlikely to lead to clinically relevant HPA-axis suppression, in the majority of patients. In the following patient groups, gradual withdrawal of systemic corticosteroid therapy should be ***considered*** even after courses lasting 3 weeks or less:

- Patients who have had repeated courses of systemic corticosteroids, particularly if taken for greater than 3 weeks,
- When a short course has been prescribed within one year of cessation of long-term therapy (months or years),
- Patients who have reasons for adrenocortical insufficiency other than exogenous corticosteroid therapy,
- Patients receiving doses of systemic corticosteroid greater than 6mg daily of betamethasone (or equivalent),
- Patients repeatedly taking doses in the evening.

During prolonged therapy any intercurrent illness, trauma or surgical procedure will require a temporary increase in dosage; if corticosteroids have been stopped following prolonged therapy they may need to be temporarily re-introduced.

Special precautions

Particular care is required when considering the use of systemic corticosteroids in patients with the following conditions and frequent patient monitoring is necessary.

A. Osteoporosis (post-menopausal females are particularly at risk).

B. Hypertension or congestive heart failure.

C. Existing or previous history of severe affective disorders (especially previous steroid psychosis).

D. Diabetes mellitus (or a family history of diabetes).

E. History of tuberculosis.

F. Glaucoma (or a family history of glaucoma).

G. Previous corticosteroid-induced myopathy.

H. Liver failure - blood levels of corticosteroid may be increased, (as with other drugs which are metabolised in the liver).

I. Renal insufficiency.

J. Epilepsy.

K. Peptic ulceration.

Patients should carry 'steroid treatment' cards which give clear guidance on the precautions to be taken to minimise risk and which provide details of prescriber, drug, dosage and the duration of treatment.

Use in children

Corticosteroids cause dose-related growth retardation in infancy, childhood and adolescence, which may be irreversible. Treatment should be limited to the minimum dosage for the shortest possible time. In order to minimise suppression of the HPA axis and growth retardation, consideration should be given to administration of a single dose on alternate days.

Use in the elderly

The common adverse effects of systemic corticosteroids may be associated with more serious consequences in old age, especially osteoporosis, hypertension, hypokalaemia, diabetes, susceptibility to infection and thinning of the skin. Close clinical supervision is required to avoid life-threatening reactions.

4.5 Interaction with other medicinal products and other forms of Interaction

Steroids may reduce the effects of anticholinesterases in myasthenia gravis cholecystographic X-ray media and non-steroidal anti-inflammatory agents.

Rifampicin, rifabutin, carbamazepine, phenobarbitone, phenytoin, primidone, aminoglutethimide and ephedrine enhance the metabolism of corticosteroids; thus the corticosteroid therapeutic effect may be reduced.

The desired effects of hypoglycaemic agents (including insulin), anti-hypertensives and diuretics are antagonised by corticosteroids, and the hypokalaemic effects of acetazolamide, loop diuretics, thiazide diuretics and carbenoxolone are enhanced.

The efficacy of coumarin anticoagulants may be enhanced by concurrent corticosteroid therapy and close monitoring of the INR or prothrombin time is required to avoid spontaneous bleeding.

The renal clearance of salicylates is increased by corticosteroids and steroid withdrawal may result in salicylate intoxication.

The risk of hypokalaemia is increased with theophylline, ulcer healing drugs such as carbenoxolone and antifungals such as amphotericin B.

Increased toxicity may result if hypokalaemia occurs in patients on cardiac glycosides.

Ritonavir and oral contraceptives may result in increased plasma concentrations or corticosteroids.

The effect of corticosteroids may be reduced for 3-4 days after mifepristone.

The growth promoting effect of somatropin may be inhibited by corticosteroids.

An increase in the incidence of gastrointestinal bleeding may occur if NSAIDS are taken concomitantly with corticosteroids.

Corticosteroids may antagonise the effects of neuromuscular blocking drugs such as vecuronium.

4.6 Pregnancy and lactation

Pregnancy

The ability of corticosteroids to cross the placenta varies between individual drugs, however, betamethasone readily crosses the placenta. Administration of corticosteroids to pregnant animals can cause abnormalities of foetal development including cleft palate, intra-uterine growth retardation and effects on brain growth and development. There is no evidence that corticosteroids result in an increased incidence of congenital abnormalities, such as cleft palate/lip in man. However, when administered for prolonged periods or repeatedly during pregnancy, corticosteroids may increase the risk of intra-uterine growth retardation. Hypoadrenalism may, in theory, occur in the neonate following prenatal exposure to corticosteroids but usually resolves spontaneously following birth and is rarely clinically important. As with all drugs, corticosteroids should only be prescribed when the benefits to the mother and child outweigh the risks. When corticosteroids are essential however, patients with normal pregnancies may be treated as though they were in the non-gravid state. Patients with pre-eclampsia or fluid retention require close monitoring.

Betamethasone, systemically administered to a woman during pregnancy may result in a transient suppression of the foetal heart rate parameters and biophysical activities that are widely used for the assessment of foetal well – being. These characteristics can include a reduction in foetal breathing movements, body movements and heart rate.

Lactation

Corticosteroids may pass into breast milk, although no data are available for betamethasone. Infants of mothers taking high doses of systemic corticosteroids for prolonged periods may have a degree of adrenal suppression.

4.7 Effects on ability to drive and use machines

None known.

4.8 Undesirable effects

The incidence of predictable undesirable effects, including hypothalamic-pituitary-adrenal (HPA) axis suppression correlates with the relative potency of the drug, dosage, timing of administration and the duration of treatment. (see "Special Warnings and Precautions for Use")

Endocrine/metabolic

Suppression of the hypothalamic-pituitary-adrenal axis, growth suppression in infancy, childhood and adolescence, menstrual irregularity and amenorrhoea. Cushingoid facies, hirsutism, weight gain, impaired carbohydrate tolerance with increased requirement for antidiabetic therapy. Negative protein, nitrogen and calcium balance. Increased appetite. Hyperhydrosis. Increased high –density lipoprotein and low – density lipoprotein concentrations in the blood.

Anti-inflammatory and immunosuppressive effects

Increased susceptibility to and severity of infections with suppression of clinical symptoms and signs, opportunistic infections, recurrence of dormant tuberculosis (see "Special Warnings and Precautions for Use").

Musculoskeletal

Osteoporosis, vertebral and long bone fractures, avascular osteonecrosis, tendon rupture, proximal myopathy.

Fluid and electrolyte disturbance

Sodium and water retention, hypertension, potassium loss, hypokalaemic alkalosis.

Neuropsychiatric

Euphoria, psychological dependence, depression, psychosis, insomnia, and aggravation of schizophrenia. Increased intra-cranial pressure with papilloedema in children (pseudotumour cerebri), usually after treatment withdrawal. Aggravation of epilepsy.

Ophthalmic

Increased intra-ocular pressure, glaucoma, papilloedema, posterior subcapsular cataracts, corneal or scleral thinning, exacerbation of ophthalmic viral or fungal diseases.

Cardiac

Myocardial rupture following recent myocardial infarction.

Gastrointestinal

Abdominal distension, oesophageal ulceration, nausea, dyspepsia, peptic ulceration with perforation and haemorrhage, acute pancreatitis, candidiasis.

Dermatological

Impaired healing, skin atrophy, bruising, telangiectasia, striae, acne.

General

Hypersensitivity including anaphylaxis, has been reported. Leucocytosis. Thrombo-embolism. Malaise. Hiccups.

Withdrawal symptoms and signs

Too rapid a reduction of corticosteroid dosage following prolonged treatment can lead to acute adrenal insufficiency, hypotension and death (see "Special Warnings and Precautions for Use").

A 'withdrawal syndrome' may also occur including; fever, myalgia, arthralgia, rhinitis, conjunctivitis, painful itchy skin nodules and loss of weight.

4.9 Overdose

Treatment is unlikely to be needed in cases of acute overdosage.

5. PHARMACOLOGICAL PROPERTIES

5.1 Pharmacodynamic properties

ATC: H02A B01

Betamethasone sodium phosphate is an active corticosteroid with topical anti-inflammatory activity.

5.2 Pharmacokinetic properties

The vast majority of corticosteroids, including betamethasone, are absorbed from the gastrointestinal tract.

Corticosteroids are metabolised mainly in the liver but also in the kidney, and are excreted in the urine.

Synthetic corticosteroids, such as prednisolone, have increased potency when compared to the natural corticosteroids, due to their slower metabolism and lower protein-binding affinity.

5.3 Preclinical safety data

None stated.

6. PHARMACEUTICAL PARTICULARS

6.1 List of excipients

Sodium Bicarbonate

Sodium Acid Citrate

Saccharin Sodium

Povidone

Erythrosine E127

Sodium Benzoate

6.2 Incompatibilities

None known.

6.3 Shelf life

3 years.

6.4 Special precautions for storage

Do not store above 25°C.

6.5 Nature and contents of container

The tablets are sealed into individual pockets in an aluminium/ polyethylene laminate (30 micron and 38 micron respectively). The tablets are strip-packed in cartons of 100.

6.6 Instructions for use and handling

None stated.

7. MARKETING AUTHORISATION HOLDER

UCB Pharma Limited

208 Bath Road

Slough

Berkshire

SL1 3WE

UK

8. MARKETING AUTHORISATION NUMBER(S)

PL 0039/0386

9. DATE OF FIRST AUTHORISATION/RENEWAL OF THE AUTHORISATION

14th December 1992.

10. DATE OF REVISION OF THE TEXT

June 2005

POM

Betnesol-N Eye Ointment

(UCB Pharma Limited)

1. NAME OF THE MEDICINAL PRODUCT

Betnesol-N Eye Ointment

2. QUALITATIVE AND QUANTITATIVE COMPOSITION

Betamethasone sodium phosphate PhEur	0.10% w/w
Neomycin sulphate PhEur	0.50% w/w

For Excipients, see 6.1

3. PHARMACEUTICAL FORM

Eye Ointment

4. CLINICAL PARTICULARS

4.1 Therapeutic indications

For the short-term treatment of steroid responsive inflammatory conditions of the eye when prophylactic antibiotic treatment is also required, after excluding the presence of viral and fungal disease.

4.2 Posology and method of administration

Adults (including the elderly) and children

The frequency of dosing depends on the clinical response. If there is no clinical response within 7 days of treatment, the ointment should be discontinued.

Treatment should be the lowest effective dose for the shortest possible time. Normally, Betnesol-N Ointment should not be given for more than 7 days, unless under expert supervision. After more prolonged treatment (over 6 to 8 weeks), the ointment should be withdrawn slowly to avoid relapse.

An extrusion of the ointment about 1/4 inch long may be introduced beneath the lower lid two or three times daily and/or at night.

4.3 Contraindications

Viral, fungal, tuberculous or purulent conditions of the eye. Use is contraindicated if glaucoma is present or herpetic keratitis (e.g. dendritic ulcer) is considered a possibility. Use of topical steroids in the latter condition can lead to an extension of the ulcer and marked visual deterioration.

Hypersensitivity to any component of the preparation.

4.4 Special warnings and special precautions for use

A patient information leaflet should be supplied with this product.

Topical corticosteroids should never be given for an undiagnosed red eye as inappropriate use is potentially blinding.

Treatment with corticosteroid/antibiotic combinations should not be continued for more than 7 days in the absence of any clinical improvement, since prolonged use may lead to occult extension of infection due to the masking effect of the steroid. Prolonged use may also lead to skin sensitisation and the emergence of resistant organisms.

Prolonged use may lead to the risk of adrenal suppression in infants.

Treatment with corticosteroid preparations should not be repeated or prolonged without regular review to exclude raised intraocular pressure, cataract formation or unsuspected infections.

Aminoglycoside antibiotics may cause irreversible, partial or total deafness when given systemically or when applied topically to open wounds or damaged skin. This effect is dose related and is enhanced by renal or hepatic impairment. Although this effect has not been reported following topical ocular use, the possibility should be considered when high dose topical treatment is given to small children or infants.

4.5 Interaction with other medicinal products and other forms of Interaction

None relevant to topical use.

4.6 Pregnancy and lactation

Safety for use in pregnancy and lactation has not been established. There is inadequate evidence of safety in human pregnancy. Topical administration of corticosteroids to pregnant animals can cause abnormalities of foetal development including cleft palate and intrauterine growth retardation. There may therefore be a very small risk of such effects in the human foetus.

There is a risk of foetal ototoxicity if aminoglycoside antibiotic preparations are administered during pregnancy.

4.7 Effects on ability to drive and use machines
May cause transient blurring of vision on instillation. Patients should be warned not to drive or operate hazardous machinery unless vision is clear.

4.8 Undesirable effects
Hypersensitivity reactions, usually of the delayed type, may occur leading to irritation, burning, stinging, itching and dermatitis.

Topical corticosteroid use may result in corneal ulceration, increased intraocular pressure leading to optic nerve damage, reduced visual acuity and visual field defects.

Intensive or prolonged use of topical corticosteroids may lead to formation of posterior subcapsular cataracts.

In those diseases causing thinning of the cornea or sclera, corticosteroid therapy may result in thinning of the globe leading to perforation.

Mydriasis, ptosis and epithelial punctate keratitis have also been reported following ophthalmic use of corticosteroids.

4.9 Overdose
Long-term intensive topical use may lead to systemic effects.

Oral ingestion of the contents of one tube (3g) of ointment is unlikely to lead to any serious adverse effects.

5. PHARMACOLOGICAL PROPERTIES
5.1 Pharmacodynamic properties
ATC Code: S01C A05
Betamethasone is a glucocorticoid which has topical anti-inflammatory activity. Neomycin is a broad spectrum aminoglycoside antibiotic.

5.2 Pharmacokinetic properties
Not applicable as the ointment is applied topically to the eye.

5.3 Preclinical safety data
None stated.

6. PHARMACEUTICAL PARTICULARS
6.1 List of excipients
White soft paraffin

Liquid paraffin

6.2 Incompatibilities
None known.

6.3 Shelf life

Unopened:	36 months
Opened:	4 weeks

6.4 Special precautions for storage
Store at a temperature not exceeding 25°C. Avoid freezing. Always replace the bottle back in the carton after use to protect its contents from light. The sterility of the ointment is assured until the cap seal is broken.

6.5 Nature and contents of container
Collapsible aluminium tubes with fine-bore extended nozzle tube fitted with a natural polyethylene cap containing 3 grams of ointment.

6.6 Instructions for use and handling
None stated.

7. MARKETING AUTHORISATION HOLDER
UCB Pharma Limited

208 Bath Road

Slough

Berkshire

SL1 3WE

UK

8. MARKETING AUTHORISATION NUMBER(S)
PL 00039/0390

9. DATE OF FIRST AUTHORISATION/RENEWAL OF THE AUTHORISATION
2 December 1992

10. DATE OF REVISION OF THE TEXT
June 2005

POM

Betnesol-N Eye, Ear, Nose Drops

(UCB Pharma Limited)

1. NAME OF THE MEDICINAL PRODUCT
Betnesol-N Eye, Ear and Nose Drops

2. QUALITATIVE AND QUANTITATIVE COMPOSITION

Betamethasone sodium phosphate PhEur 0.105% w/v.
(equivalent to 0.1% w/v betamethasone)

Neomycin sulphate PhEur 0.5% w/v.
(equivalent to 0.385% w/v neomycin base)

For excipients, see 6.1

3. PHARMACEUTICAL FORM
Ear/Eye/Nose Drops, Solution

A colourless to pale yellow solution.

4. CLINICAL PARTICULARS
4.1 Therapeutic indications
Eye

Short-term treatment of steroid responsive inflammatory conditions of the eye when prophylactic antibiotic treatment is also required, after excluding the presence of viral and fungal disease.

Ear

Otitis externa or other steroid responsive conditions where prophylactic antibiotic treatment is also required.

Nose

Steroid responsive inflammatory conditions where prophylactic antibiotic treatment is also required.

4.2 Posology and method of administration
The frequency of dosing depends on the clinical response. If there is no clinical response within 7 days of treatment, the drops should be discontinued.

Treatment should be the lowest effective dose for the shortest possible time. Normally, Betnesol-N Drops should not be given for more than 7 days, unless under expert supervision. After more prolonged treatment (over 6 to 8 weeks), the drops should be withdrawn slowly to avoid relapse.

Eyes

1 or 2 drops applied to each affected eye up to six times daily depending on clinical response.

Ears

2 or 3 drops instilled into the ear three or four times daily.

Nose

2 or 3 drops instilled into each nostril two or three times daily.

4.3 Contraindications
Viral, fungal, tuberculous or purulent conditions of the eye. Fungal infections of the nose or ear. Use is contraindicated if glaucoma is present or herpetic keratitis (e.g. dendritic ulcer) is considered a possibility. Use of topical steroids in the latter condition can lead to an extension of the ulcer and marked visual deterioration.

Otitis externa should not be treated when the eardrum is perforated because of the risk of ototoxicity.

Corticosteroids should not be used in patients with a perforated tympanic membrane.

Hypersensitivity to any component of the preparation.

4.4 Special warnings and special precautions for use
A patient information leaflet should be supplied with this product.

Topical corticosteroids should never be given for an undiagnosed red eye as inappropriate use is potentially blinding.

Treatment with corticosteroid/antibiotic combinations should not be continued for more than 7 days in the absence of any clinical improvement, since prolonged use may lead to occult extension of infection due to the masking effect of the steroid. Prolonged use may also lead to skin sensitisation and the emergence of resistant organisms.

Prolonged use may lead to the risk of adrenal suppression in infants.

Ophthalmological treatment with corticosteroid preparations should not be repeated or prolonged without regular review to exclude raised intraocular pressure, cataract formation or unsuspected infections.

Aminoglycoside antibiotics may cause irreversible, partial or total deafness when given systemically or when applied topically to open wounds or damaged skin. This effect is dose related and is enhanced by renal or hepatic impairment. Although this effect has not been reported following topical ocular use, the possibility should be considered when high dose topical treatment is given to small children or infants.

Nasal administration of corticosteroids is not advised if an untreated nasal infection is present or if the patient has pulmonary tuberculosis or following nasal surgery (until healing has occurred).

4.5 Interaction with other medicinal products and other forms of Interaction
Betnesol-N Drops contain benzalkonium chloride as a preservative and therefore should not be used as eye drops to treat patients who wear soft contact lenses.

4.6 Pregnancy and lactation
Safety for use in pregnancy and lactation has not been established. There is inadequate evidence of safety in human pregnancy. Topical administration of corticosteroids to pregnant animals can cause abnormalities of foetal development including cleft palate and intrauterine growth retardation. There may therefore be a very small risk of such effects in the human foetus.

There is a risk of foetal ototoxicity if aminoglycoside antibiotic preparations are administered during pregnancy.

4.7 Effects on ability to drive and use machines
May cause transient blurring of vision on instillation. Patients should be warned not to drive or operate hazardous machinery unless vision is clear.

4.8 Undesirable effects
Hypersensitivity reactions, usually of the delayed type, may occur leading to irritation, burning, stinging, itching and dermatitis.

Topical corticosteroid use may result in corneal ulceration, increased intraocular pressure leading to optic nerve damage, reduced visual acuity and visual field defects.

Intensive or prolonged use of topical corticosteroids may lead to formation of posterior subcapsular cataracts.

In those diseases causing thinning of the cornea or sclera, corticosteroid therapy may result in thinning of the globe leading to perforation.

Mydriasis, ptosis and epithelial punctate keratitis have also been reported following ophthalmic use of corticosteroids.

Following nasal administration, the most common effects are nasal irritation and dryness, although sneezing, headache, lightheadedness, urticaria, nausea, epistaxis, rebound congestion, bronchial asthma, perforation of the nasal septum, ulceration of the nasal septum, anosmia, parosmia and disturbance to sense of taste have also been reported.

Systemic effects of nasal corticosteroids may occur, particularly at high doses prescribed for prolonged periods. Growth retardation has been reported in children receiving nasal corticosteroids at licensed doses.

It is recommended that the height of children receiving prolonged treatment with nasal corticosteroids is regularly monitored. If growth is slowed, therapy should be reviewed with the aim of reducing the dose of nasal corticosteroid, if possible, to the lowest dose at which effective control of symptoms is maintained. In addition, consideration should also be given to referring the patient to a paediatric specialist.

4.9 Overdose
Long-term intensive topical use may lead to systemic effects.

Oral ingestion of the contents of one bottle (up to 10ml) is unlikely to lead to any serious adverse effects.

Treatment with higher than recommended doses may result in clinically significant adrenal suppression. If there is evidence of higher than recommended doses being used then additional systemic corticosteroid cover should be considered during periods of stress or elective surgery.

5. PHARMACOLOGICAL PROPERTIES
5.1 Pharmacodynamic properties
ATC Code: S03C A

Betamethasone has topical corticosteroid activity. The presence of neomycin should prevent the development of bacterial infection.

5.2 Pharmacokinetic properties
Not applicable as the drops are applied topically.

5.3 Preclinical safety data
None stated.

6. PHARMACEUTICAL PARTICULARS
6.1 List of excipients
Benzalkonium chloride (anhydrous equivalent)

Disodium edetate

Polyethylene glycol 300

Sodium formate

Anhydrous sodium sulphate

Disodium hydrogen phosphate anhydrous

Sodium acid phosphate

Sodium hydroxide or

Phosphoric acid

Water for injections

6.2 Incompatibilities
None known.

6.3 Shelf life

Unopened:	18 months
Opened:	4 weeks

6.4 Special precautions for storage
Store at a temperature not exceeding 25°C. Avoid freezing. Always replace the bottle back in the carton after use to protect its contents from light. The sterility of the drops is assured until the cap seal is broken.

6.5 Nature and contents of container
5 and 10ml bottles with nozzle insert moulded in natural low density polyethylene closed with a tamper evident high density polyethylene cap.

6.6 Instructions for use and handling
None stated.

7. MARKETING AUTHORISATION HOLDER
UCB Pharma Limited
208 Bath Road
Slough
Berkshire
SL1 3WE
UK

8. MARKETING AUTHORISATION NUMBER(S)
PL 00039/0389

9. DATE OF FIRST AUTHORISATION/RENEWAL OF THE AUTHORISATION
3 December 1992

10. DATE OF REVISION OF THE TEXT
June 2005

POM

Betnovate C Cream

(GlaxoSmithKline UK)

1. NAME OF THE MEDICINAL PRODUCT
Betnovate C Cream

2. QUALITATIVE AND QUANTITATIVE COMPOSITION
Betamethasone Valerate BP 0.122% $^{W}/_{W}$
Clioquinol BP 3.00% $^{W}/_{W}$

3. PHARMACEUTICAL FORM
Aqueous Cream

4. CLINICAL PARTICULARS
4.1 Therapeutic indications
Betamethasone valerate is an active topical corticosteroid which produces a rapid response in those inflammatory dermatoses that are normally responsive to topical corticosteroid therapy, and is often effective in the less responsive conditions such as psoriasis.

Clioquinol is an anti-infective agent which has both antibacterial and anticandidal activity.

Betnovate-C preparations are indicated for the treatment of the following conditions where secondary bacterial and/or fungal infection is present, suspected, or likely to occur: eczema in children and adults, including atopic and discoid eczemas, prurigo nodularis; psoriasis (excluding widespread plaque psoriasis); neurodermatoses; seborrhoeic dermatitis; contact sensitivity reactions and discoid lupus erythematosus.

Betnovate-C can also be used in the management of secondary infected insect bites and anal and genital intertrigo.

Betnovate-C cream is often appropriate for moist or weeping surfaces and Betnovate-C ointment for dry, lichenified or scaly lesions, but this is not invariably so.

4.2 Posology and method of administration
A small quantity should be applied gently to the affected area two or three times daily until improvement occurs. It may then be possible to maintain improvement by applying once a day, or even less often.

Children
Courses should be limited to five days if possible. Occlusion should not be used.

For topical application.

4.3 Contraindications
Rosacea, acne vulgaris and perioral dermatitis. Primary cutaneous viral infections (e.g. herpes simplex, chickenpox). Hypersensitivity to any component of the preparation or to iodine.

Use of Betnovate-C skin preparations is not indicated in the treatment of primary infected skin lesions caused by infection with fungi (e.g. candidiasis, tinea); or bacteria (e.g. impetigo); primary or secondary infections due to yeast; perianal or genital pruritus dermatoses in children under 1 years of age, including dermatitis and napkin eruptions.

4.4 Special warnings and special precautions for use
Long-term continuous topical therapy should be avoided where possible, particularly in infants and children, as adrenal suppression, with or without clinical features of Cushing's syndrome, can occur even without occlusion. In this situation, topical steroids should be discontinued gradually under medical supervision because of the risk of adrenal insufficiency (see section 4.8 Undesirable Effects and Section 4.9 Overdose).

The face, more than other areas of the body, may exhibit atrophic changes after prolonged treatment with potent topical corticosteroids. This must be borne in mind when treating such conditions as psoriasis, discoid lupus erythematosus and severe eczema with Betnovate. If applied to the eyelids, care is needed to ensure that the preparation does not enter the eye, as glaucoma might result.

If used in childhood, or on the face, courses should be limited to five days and occlusion should not be used.

Topical corticosteroids may be hazardous in psoriasis for a number of reasons including rebound relapses, development of tolerance, risk of generalised pustular psoriasis and development of local or systemic toxicity due to impaired barrier function of the skin. If used in psoriasis careful patient supervision is important.

If infection persists, systemic chemotherapy is required. Any spread of infection requires withdrawal of topical corticosteroid therapy. Bacterial infection is encouraged by the warm, moist conditions induced by occlusive dressings, and the skin should be cleansed before a fresh dressing is applied.

Do not continue for more than 7 days in the absence of clinical improvement, since occult extension of infection may occur due to the masking effect of the steroid.

Betnovate-C may stain hair, skin or fabric, and the application should be covered with a dressing to protect clothing.

Products which contain antimicrobial agents should not be diluted.

The least potent corticosteroid which will control the disease should be selected. These preparations do not contain lanolin or parabens.

There is a theoretical risk of neurotoxicity from the topical application of clioquinol, particularly when Betnovate-C is used for prolonged periods or under occlusion.

4.5 Interaction with other medicinal products and other forms of Interaction
None

4.6 Pregnancy and lactation
There is inadequate evidence of safety in human pregnancy. Topical administration of corticosteroids to pregnant animals can cause abnormalities of foetal development including cleft palate and intrauterine growth retardation. There may therefore be a very small risk of such effects in the human foetus.

4.7 Effects on ability to drive and use machines
None

4.8 Undesirable effects
Prolonged and intensive treatment with highly active corticosteroid preparations may cause local atrophic changes in the skin such as thinning, striae, and dilatation of the superficial blood vessels, particularly when occlusive dressings are used or when skin folds are involved.

As with other topical corticosteroids, prolonged use of large amounts or treatment of extensive areas can result in sufficient systemic absorption to produce suppression of the HPA axis and the clinical features of Cushing's syndrome (see Section 4.4 Special Warnings and Precautions for use). These effects are more likely to occur in infants and children, and if occlusive dressings are used. In infants the napkin may act as an occlusive dressing.

In rare instances, treatment of psoriasis with corticosteroids (or its withdrawal) is thought to have provoked the pustular form of the disease (see precautions).

There are reports of local skin burning, pruritus, pigmentation changes, allergic contact dermatitis and hypertrichosis with topical steroids.

The Betnovate preparations are usually well tolerated, but if signs of hypersensitivity appear, application should be stopped immediately.

Exacerbation of symptoms may occur.

4.9 Overdose
Acute overdosage is very unlikely to occur. However, in the case of chronic overdosage or misuse the features of Cushing's syndrome may appear and in this situation topical steroids should be discontinued gradually under medical supervision (see Section 4.4 Special Warnings and Precautions for use).

5. PHARMACOLOGICAL PROPERTIES
5.1 Pharmacodynamic properties
Betamethasone valerate is an active corticosteroid with topical anti-inflammatory activity.

Clioquinol is an anti-infective agent with has both antibacterial and anti-candidal activity.

5.2 Pharmacokinetic properties
The extent of percutaneous absorption of topical corticosteroid is determined by many factors including the vehicle, the integrity of the epidermal barrier, and the use of occlusive dressings.

Topical corticosteroids can be absorbed from normal intact skin. Inflammation and/or other disease processes in the skin increase percutaneous absorption. Occlusive dressings substantially increase the percutaneous absorption of topical corticosteroids.

Once absorbed through the skin, topical corticosteroids are handled through pharmacokinetic pathways similar to systematically administered corticosteroids. Corticosteroids are bound to plasma proteins in varying degrees. Corticosteroids are metabolised primarily by the liver and are then excreted by the kidneys.

5.3 Preclinical safety data
There are no preclinical data of relevance to the prescriber, which are additional to that in other sections of the SmPC.

6. PHARMACEUTICAL PARTICULARS
6.1 List of excipients

Chlorocresol	BP
Cetomacrogol 1000	BP
Cetostearyl Alcohol	BP
White Soft Paraffin	BP
Liquid Paraffin	BP
Sodium Acid Phosphate	BP
Phosphoric Acid	BP
Sodium Hydroxide	BP
Purified Water	BP

6.2 Incompatibilities
None known.

6.3 Shelf life
36 months.

6.4 Special precautions for storage
Store below 30°C.

6.5 Nature and contents of container
15 gm and 30 gm collapsible aluminium tubes coated with an epoxy resin based lacquer with an aluminium membrane seal and a polyethylene cap.

Not all pack sizes may be marketed

6.6 Instructions for use and handling
No special instructions.

Administrative Data
7. MARKETING AUTHORISATION HOLDER
Glaxo Wellcome UK Ltd.,
T/A GlaxoSmithKline UK
Stockley Park West,
Uxbridge,
Middlesex, UB11 1BT

8. MARKETING AUTHORISATION NUMBER(S)
PL 10949/0016

9. DATE OF FIRST AUTHORISATION/RENEWAL OF THE AUTHORISATION
3 September 1997

10. DATE OF REVISION OF THE TEXT
25th January 2005

11. Legal Status
POM

Betnovate -C Ointment

(GlaxoSmithKline UK)

1. NAME OF THE MEDICINAL PRODUCT
Betnovate C Ointment

2. QUALITATIVE AND QUANTITATIVE COMPOSITION
Betamethasone Valerate BP 0.122% $^{W}/_{W}$
Clioquinol BP 3.00% $^{W}/_{W}$

3. PHARMACEUTICAL FORM
Ointment

4. CLINICAL PARTICULARS
4.1 Therapeutic indications
Betamethasone valerate is an active topical corticosteroid which produces a rapid response in those inflammatory dermatoses that are normally responsive to topical corticosteroid therapy, and is often effective in the less responsive conditions such as psoriasis.

Clioquinol is an anti-infective agent which has both antibacterial and anticandidal activity.

Betnovate-C preparations are indicated for the treatment of the following conditions where secondary bacterial and/or fungal infection is present, suspected, or likely to occur: eczema in children and adults, including atopic and discoid eczemas, prurigo nodularis; psoriasis (excluding widespread plaque psoriasis); neurodermatoses; seborrhoeic dermatitis; contact sensitivity reactions and discoid lupus erythematosus.

Betnovate-C can also be used in the management of secondary infected insect bites and anal and genital intertrigo.

Betnovate-C ointment is often appropriate for dry, lichenified or scaly lesions, but this is not invariably so.

4.2 Posology and method of administration
A small quantity of Betnovate should be applied gently to the affected area two or three times daily until improvement occurs. It may then be possible to maintain improvement by applying once a day, or even less often.

Children
Courses should be limited to five days, if possible. Occlusion should not be used.

For topical application.

4.3 Contraindications
Rosacea, acne vulgaris and perioral dermatitis. Primary cutaneous viral infections (e.g. herpes simplex, chickenpox). Hypersensitivity to any component of the preparation or to iodine.

Use of Betnovate-C skin preparations is not indicated in the treatment of primary infected skin lesions caused by infection with fungi (e.g. candidiasis, tinea); or bacteria (e.g. impetigo); primary or secondary, infections due to yeast; perianal or genital pruritus; dermatoses in children under 1 years of age, including dermatitis and napkin eruptions.

4.4 Special warnings and special precautions for use
Long-term continuous topical therapy should be avoided where possible, particularly in infants and children, as adrenal suppression, with or without clinical features of Cushing's syndrome, can occur even without occlusion. In this situation, topical steroids should be discontinued gradually under medical supervision because of the risk of adrenal insufficiency (see section 4.8 Undesirable Effects and Section 4.9 Overdose).

The face, more than other areas of the body, may exhibit atrophic changes after prolonged treatment with potent topical corticosteroids. This must be borne in mind when treating such conditions as psoriasis, discoid lupus erythematosus and severe eczema with Betnovate. If applied to the eyelids, care is needed to ensure that the preparation does not enter the eye, as glaucoma might result.

If used in childhood, or on the face, courses should be limited to five days and occlusion should not be used.

Topical corticosteroids may be hazardous in psoriasis for a number of reasons including rebound relapses, development of tolerance, risk of generalised pustular psoriasis and development of local or systemic toxicity due to impaired barrier function of the skin. If used in psoriasis careful patient supervision is important.

If infection persists, systemic chemotherapy is required. Any spread of infection requires withdrawal of topical corticosteroid therapy. Bacterial infection is encouraged by the warm, moist conditions induced by occlusive dressings, and the skin should be cleansed before a fresh dressing is applied.

Do not continue for more than 7 days in the absence of clinical improvement, since occult extension of infection may occur due to the masking effect of the steroid.

Betnovate-C may stain hair, skin or fabric, and the application should be covered with a dressing to protect clothing.

Products which contain antimicrobial agents should not be diluted.

The least potent corticosteroid which will control the disease should be selected. These preparations do not contain lanolin or parabens.

There is a theoretical risk of neurotoxicity from the topical application of clioquinol, particularly when Betnovate-C is used for prolonged periods or under occlusion.

4.5 Interaction with other medicinal products and other forms of Interaction
None.

4.6 Pregnancy and lactation
There is inadequate evidence of safety in human pregnancy. Topical administration of corticosteroids to pregnant animals can cause abnormalities of foetal development including cleft palate and intrauterine growth retardation. There may therefore be a very small risk of such effects in the human foetus.

4.7 Effects on ability to drive and use machines
None.

4.8 Undesirable effects
Prolonged and intensive treatment with highly active corticosteroid preparations may cause local atrophic changes in the skin such as thinning, striae, and dilatation of the superficial blood vessels, particularly when occlusive dressings are used or when skin folds are involved.

As with other topical corticosteroids, prolonged use of large amounts or treatment of extensive areas can result in sufficient systemic absorption to produce suppression of the HPA axis and the clinical features of Cushing's syndrome (see Section 4.4 Special Warnings and Precautions for use). These effects are more likely to occur in infants and children, and if occlusive dressings are used. In infants the napkin may act as an occlusive dressing.

In rare instances, treatment of psoriasis with corticosteroids (or its withdrawal) is thought to have provoked the pustular form of the disease (see precautions)

There are reports of local skin burning, pruritus pigmentation changes, allergic contact dermatitis and hypertrichosis with topical steroids.

The Betnovate preparations are usually well tolerated, but if signs of hypersensitivity appear, application should be stopped immediately.

Exacerbation of symptoms may occur.

4.9 Overdose
Acute overdosage is very unlikely to occur. However, in the case of chronic overdosage or misuse the features of Cushing's syndrome may appear and in this situation topical steroids should be discontinued gradually under medical supervision (see Section 4.4 Special Warnings and Precautions for use).

5. PHARMACOLOGICAL PROPERTIES

5.1 Pharmacodynamic properties
Betamethasone valerate is an active corticosteroid with topical anti-inflammatory activity.

Clioquinol is an anti-infective agent which has both antibacterial and anti-candidal activity.

5.2 Pharmacokinetic properties
The extent of percutaneous absorption of topical corticosteroid is determined by many factors including the vehicle, the integrity of the epidermal barrier, and the use of occlusive dressings.

Topical corticosteroids can be absorbed from normal intact skin. Inflammation and/or other disease processes in the skin increase percutaneous absorption. Occlusive dressings substantially increase the percutaneous absorption of topical corticosteroids.

Once absorbed through the skin, topical corticosteroids are handled through pharmacokinetic pathways similar to systematically administered corticosteroids. Corticosteroids are bound to plasma proteins in varying degrees. Corticosteroids are metabolised primarily by the liver and are then excreted by the kidneys.

5.3 Preclinical safety data
There are no preclinical data of relevance to the prescriber which are additional to that in other sections of the SmPC.

6. PHARMACEUTICAL PARTICULARS

6.1 List of excipients

Liquid Paraffin	BP
White Soft Paraffin	BP

6.2 Incompatibilities
None known.

6.3 Shelf life
36 Months.

6.4 Special precautions for storage
Store below 30°C.

6.5 Nature and contents of container
15gm and 30gm collapsible aluminium tubes coated with an epoxy resin based lacquer with an aluminium membrane seal and a polyethylene cap.

Not all pack sizes may be marketed

6.6 Instructions for use and handling
No special instructions.

Administrative Data

7. MARKETING AUTHORISATION HOLDER
Glaxo Wellcome UK Ltd.,

T/A GlaxoSmithKline UK

Stockley Park West,

Uxbridge,

Middlesex UB11 1BT

8. MARKETING AUTHORISATION NUMBER(S)
PL 10949/0017

9. DATE OF FIRST AUTHORISATION/RENEWAL OF THE AUTHORISATION
24 October 1997

10. DATE OF REVISION OF THE TEXT
25th January 2005

11. Legal Status
POM

Betnovate Cream

(GlaxoSmithKline UK)

1. NAME OF THE MEDICINAL PRODUCT
Betnovate Cream

2. QUALITATIVE AND QUANTITATIVE COMPOSITION
Betamethasone Valerate BP 0.122% $^{w}/_{w}$

3. PHARMACEUTICAL FORM
Aqueous Cream

4. CLINICAL PARTICULARS

4.1 Therapeutic indications
Betamethasone valerate is an active topical corticosteroid which produces a rapid response in those inflammatory dermatoses that are normally responsive to topical corticosteroid therapy, and is often effective in the less responsive conditions such as psoriasis.

Betnovate preparations are indicated for the treatment of eczema in children and adults, including atopic and discoid eczemas, prurigo nodularis, psoriasis (excluding widespread plaque psoriasis); neurodermatoses, including lichen simplex, lichen planus; seborrhoeic dermatitis; contact sensitivity reactions; discoid lupus erythematosus and they may be used as an adjunct to systemic steroid therapy in generalised erythroderma.

4.2 Posology and method of administration
A small quantity of Betnovate should be applied gently to the affected area two or three times daily until improvement occurs. It may then be possible to maintain improvement by applying once a day, or even less often, or by using the appropriate ready-diluted (1 in 4) preparation Betnovate R.D. If no improvement is seen within two to four weeks, reassessment of the diagnosis, or referral, may be necessary.

Betnovate and Betnovate R.D. creams are especially appropriate for dry, lichenified or scaly lesions, but this is not invariably so.

In the more recent resistant lesions, such as the thickened plaques of psoriasis on elbows and knees, the effect of Betnovate can be enhanced, if necessary, by occluding the treatment area with polythene film. Overnight occlusion only is usually adequate to bring about a satisfactory response in such lesions; thereafter improvement can usually be maintained by regular application without occlusion.

Children

Courses should be limited to five days. Occlusion should not be used.

For topical administration.

4.3 Contraindications
Rosacea, acne and perioral dermatitis. Primary cutaneous viral infections (e.g. herpes simplex, chickenpox). Hypersensitivity to any component of the preparation.

The use of Betnovate skin preparations is not indicated in the treatment of primarily infected skin lesions caused by infections with fungi (e.g. candidiasis, tinea); or bacteria (e.g. impetigo); primary or secondary infections due to yeast; peri-anal and genital pruritus; dermatoses in children under 1 year of age, including dermatitis and napkin eruptions.

4.4 Special warnings and special precautions for use
Long-term continuous topical therapy should be avoided where possible, particularly in infants and children, as adrenal suppression, with or without clinical features of Cushing's syndrome, can occur even without occlusion. In this situation, topical steroids should be discontinued gradually under medical supervision because of the risk of adrenal insufficiency (see section 4.8 Undesirable Effects and Section 4.9 Overdose).

The face, more than other areas of the body, may exhibit atrophic changes after prolonged treatment with potent topical corticosteroids. This must be borne in mind when treating such conditions as psoriasis, discoid lupus erythematosus and severe eczema. If applied to the eyelids, care is needed to ensure that the preparation does not enter the eye, as glaucoma might result.

If used in childhood, or on the face, courses should be limited to five days and occlusion should not be used.

Topical corticosteroids may be hazardous in psoriasis for a number of reasons including rebound relapses, development of tolerance, risk of generalised pustular psoriasis and development of local or systemic toxicity due to impaired barrier function of the skin. If used in psoriasis careful patient supervision is important.

Appropriate antimicrobial therapy should be used whenever treating inflammatory lesions which have become infected. Any spread of infection requires withdrawal of topical corticosteroid therapy and systemic administration of antimicrobial agents. Bacterial infection is encouraged by the warm, moist conditions induced by occlusive dressings, and so the skin should be cleansed before a fresh dressing is applied.

Further Information

The least potent corticosteroid which will control the disease should be selected. None of these preparations contain lanolin. Betnovate Cream and Ointment and the corresponding RD preparations do not contain parabens. Betnovate Lotion contains parabens.

4.5 Interaction with other medicinal products and other forms of Interaction
None known.

4.6 Pregnancy and lactation
There is inadequate evidence of safety in human pregnancy. Topical administration of corticosteroids to pregnant animals can cause abnormalities of foetal development including cleft palate and intra-uterine growth retardation. There may therefore be a very small risk of such effects in the human foetus.

4.7 Effects on ability to drive and use machines
None known

4.8 Undesirable effects
Adverse events are listed below by system organ class and frequency. Frequencies are defined as: very common (≥1/10), common (≥1/100 and <1/10), uncommon (≥1/1000 and <1/100), rare (≥1/10,000 and <1/1000) and very rare (<1/10,000) including isolated reports. Very common, common and uncommon events were generally determined from clinical trial data. The background rates in placebo and comparator groups were not taken into account when assigning frequency categories to adverse events derived from clinical trial data, since these rates

were generally comparable to those in the active treatment group. Rare and very rare events were generally determined from spontaneous data.

Immune system disorders

Very rare: Hypersensitivity.

If signs of hypersensitivity appear, application should stop immediately.

Endocrine disorders

Very rare: Features of Cushing's syndrome

As with other topical corticosteroids, prolonged use of large amounts or treatment of extensive areas can result in sufficient systemic absorption to produce suppression of the HPA axis and the clinical features of Cushing's syndrome (see Section 4.4 Special Warnings and Precautions for use). These effects are more likely to occur in infants and children, and if occlusive dressings are used. In infants the napkin may act as an occlusive dressing.

Skin and subcutaneous tissue disorders

Common: Local skin burning and pruritus.

Very rare: Local atrophic changes in the skin such as thinning, striae and dilatation of the superficial blood vessels may be caused by prolonged and intensive treatment with highly active corticosteroid preparations, particularly when occlusive dressings are used or when skin folds are involved.

Pigmentation changes, hypertrichosis, allergic contact dermatitis, exacerbation of symptoms, pustular psoriasis (due to treatment of psoriasis with corticosteroids or its withdrawal: see Section 4.4. Special Warnings and Precautions for use)

4.9 Overdose

Acute overdosage is very unlikely to occur. However, in the case of chronic overdosage or misuse the features of Cushing's syndrome may appear and in this situation topical steroids should be discontinued gradually under medical supervision (see Section 4.4 Special Warnings and Precautions for use).

5. PHARMACOLOGICAL PROPERTIES

5.1 Pharmacodynamic properties

Betamethasone valerate is an active corticosteroid with topical anti-inflammatory activity.

5.2 Pharmacokinetic properties

The extent of percutaneous absorption of topical corticosteroids is determined by many factors including the vehicle, the integrity of the epidermal barrier, and the use of occlusive dressings.

Topical corticosteroids can be absorbed from normal intact skin. Inflammation and/or other disease processes in the skin increase percutaneous absorption. Occlusive dressings on the skin increase percutaneous absorption. Occlusive dressings substantially increase the percutaneous absorption of topical corticosteroids.

Once absorbed through the skin, topical corticosteroids are handled through pharmacokinetic pathways similar to systematically administered corticosteroids. Corticosteroids are bound to plasma proteins in varying degrees. Corticosteroids are metabolised primarily by the liver and are then excreted by the kidneys.

5.3 Preclinical safety data

There are no preclinical data of relevance to the prescriber which are additional to that in other sections of the SmPC.

6. PHARMACEUTICAL PARTICULARS

6.1 List of excipients

Chlorocresol	BP
Cetomacrogol 1000	BP
Cetostearyl Alcohol	BP
White Soft Paraffin	BP
Liquid Paraffin	BP
Sodium Acid Phosphate	BP
Phosphoric Acid	BP
Sodium Hydroxide	BP
Purified Water	BP

6.2 Incompatibilities

None known.

6.3 Shelf life

Tubes	36 Months
500gm pots	18 months

6.4 Special precautions for storage

Store below 25°C.

6.5 Nature and contents of container

15gm, 30gm and 100gm collapsible aluminium tubes internally coated with an epoxy resin based lacquer and closed with a cap.

500mg opaque high density polythene pots with black urea formaldehyde screw caps having a steran faced wad.

Not all pack sizes may be marketed

6.6 Instructions for use and handling

No special instructions.

Administrative Data

7. MARKETING AUTHORISATION HOLDER

Glaxo Wellcome UK Ltd.,

T/A GlaxoSmithKline UK

Stockley Park West,

Uxbridge,

Middlesex UB11 1BT

8. MARKETING AUTHORISATION NUMBER(S)

PL10949/0014

9. DATE OF FIRST AUTHORISATION/RENEWAL OF THE AUTHORISATION

24 October 1997

10. DATE OF REVISION OF THE TEXT

25th January 2005

Betnovate Lotion

(GlaxoSmithKline UK)

1. NAME OF THE MEDICINAL PRODUCT

Betnovate Lotion

2. QUALITATIVE AND QUANTITATIVE COMPOSITION

Betamethasone Valerate 0.122% $^{w}/_{w}$

3. PHARMACEUTICAL FORM

Lotion

4. CLINICAL PARTICULARS

4.1 Therapeutic indications

Betamethasone valerate is an active topical corticosteroid, which produces a rapid response in those inflammatory dermatoses that are normally responsive to topical corticosteroid therapy, and is often effective in the less responsive conditions such as psoriasis.

Betnovate preparations are indicated of the treatment of: eczema in children and adults; including atopic and discoid eczemas, prurigo nodularis; psoriasis (excluding widespread plaque psoriasis); neurodermatoses, including lichen simplex, lichen planus, seborrhoeic dermatitis; contact sensitivity reactions; discoid lupus erythematosus and they may be used as an adjunct to systemic steroid therapy in generalised erythroderma.

4.2 Posology and method of administration

A small quantity of Betnovate should be applied to the affected area two or three times daily until improvement occurs. It may then be possible to maintain improvement by applying once a day, or even less often. If no improvement is seen within two to four weeks, reassessment of the diagnosis or referral, may be necessary.

Betnovate lotion is particularly suitable when a minimal application to a large area is required.

In the more resistant lesions, such as the thickened plaques of psoriasis on elbows and knees, the effect of Betnovate can be enhanced, if necessary, by occluding the treatment area with polythene film. Overnight occlusion only is usually adequate to bring about a satisfactory response in such lesions. Thereafter improvement can usually be maintained by regular application without occlusion.

Children

Courses should be limited to five days if possible. Occlusion should not be used.

4.3 Contraindications

Rosacea, acne vulgaris and perioral dermatitis. Primary cutaneous viral infections (e.g. herpes simplex, chickenpox). Hypersensitivity to the preparation.

The use of Betnovate skin preparations is not indicated in the treatment of primarily infected skin lesions caused by infection with fungi (e.g. candidiasis, tinea); or bacteria (e.g. impetigo); primary or secondary infections due to yeast; perianal and genital pruritus; dermatoses in children under 1 year of age, including dermatitis and napkin eruptions.

4.4 Special warnings and special precautions for use

Long-term continuous topical therapy should be avoided where possible, particularly in infants and children, as adrenal suppression, with or without clinical features of Cushing's syndrome, can occur even without occlusion. In this situation, topical steroids should be discontinued gradually under medical supervision because of the risk of adrenal insufficiency (see section 4.8 Undesirable Effects and Section 4.9 Overdose).

The face, more than other areas of the body, may exhibit atrophic changes after prolonged treatment with potent topical corticosteroids. This must be borne in mind when treating such conditions as psoriasis, discoid lupus erythematosus and severe eczema. If applied to the eyelids, care is needed to ensure that the preparation does not enter the eye, as glaucoma might result.

If used in childhood, or on the face, courses should be limited to five days and occlusion should not be used.

Topical corticosteroids may be hazardous in psoriasis for a number of reasons including rebound relapses, development of tolerance, risk of generalised pustular psoriasis and development of local or systemic toxicity due to impaired barrier function of the skin. If used in psoriasis careful patient supervision is important.

Appropriate antimicrobial therapy should be used whenever treating inflammatory lesions, which have become infected. Any spread of infection requires withdrawal of topical corticosteroid therapy and systemic administration of antimicrobial agents.

Bacterial infection is encouraged by the warm moist conditions induced by occlusive dressings and so the skin should be cleansed before a fresh dressing is applied.

Further information:

The least potent corticosteroid, which will control the disease, should be selected. None of these preparations contain lanolin. Betnovate cream and ointment and the corresponding RD preparations do not contain parabens. Betnovate lotion contains parabens.

4.5 Interaction with other medicinal products and other forms of Interaction

None known

4.6 Pregnancy and lactation

There is inadequate evidence of safety in human pregnancy. Topical administration of corticosteroids to pregnant animals can cause abnormalities of foetal development including cleft palate and intrauterine growth retardation. There may therefore be a very small risk of such effects in the human foetus.

4.7 Effects on ability to drive and use machines

None known.

4.8 Undesirable effects

Adverse events are listed below by system organ class and frequency. Frequencies are defined as: very common (≥1/10), common (≥1/100 and <1/10), uncommon (≥1/1000 and <1/100), rare (≥1/10,000 and <1/1000) and very rare (<1/10,000) including isolated reports. Very common, common and uncommon events were generally determined from clinical trial data. The background rates in placebo and comparator groups were not taken into account when assigning frequency categories to adverse events derived from clinical trial data, since these rates were generally comparable to those in the active treatment group. Rare and very rare events were generally determined from spontaneous data.

Immune system disorders

Very rare: Hypersensitivity.

If signs of hypersensitivity appear, application should stop immediately.

Endocrine disorders

Very rare: Features of Cushing's syndrome

As with other topical corticosteroids, prolonged use of large amounts or treatment of extensive areas can result in sufficient systemic absorption to produce suppression of the HPA axis and the clinical features of Cushing's syndrome (see Section 4.4 Special Warnings and Precautions for use). These effects are more likely to occur in infants and children, and if occlusive dressings are used. In infants the napkin may act as an occlusive dressing.

Skin and subcutaneous tissue disorders

Common: Local skin burning and pruritus.

Very rare: Local atrophic changes in the skin such as thinning, striae and dilatation of the superficial blood vessels may be caused by prolonged and intensive treatment with highly active corticosteroid preparations, particularly when occlusive dressings are used or when skin folds are involved.

Pigmentation changes, hypertrichosis, allergic contact dermatitis, exacerbation of symptoms, pustular psoriasis (due to treatment of psoriasis with corticosteroids or its withdrawal: see Section 4.4. Special Warnings and Precautions for use)

4.9 Overdose

Acute overdosage is very unlikely to occur. However, in the case of chronic overdosage or misuse the features of Cushing's syndromemay appear and in this situation topical steroids should be discontinued gradually under medical supervision (see Section 4.4 Special Warnings and Precautions for use).

5. PHARMACOLOGICAL PROPERTIES

5.1 Pharmacodynamic properties

Betamethasone valerate is an active corticosteroid with topical anti-inflammatory activity.

5.2 Pharmacokinetic properties

The extent of percutaneous absorption of topical corticosteroid is determined by many factors including the vehicle, the integrity of the epidermal barrier, and the use of occlusive dressings.

Topical corticosteroids can be absorbed from normal intact skin. Inflammation and/or other disease processes in the skin increase percutaneous absorption. Occlusive dressings substantially increase the percutaneous absorption of topical corticosteroids.

Once absorbed through the skin, topical corticosteroids are handled through pharmacokinetic pathways similar to systemically administered corticosteroids. Corticosteroids are bound to plasma proteins in varying degrees.

Corticosteroids are metabolised primarily by the liver and are then excreted by the kidneys.

5.3 Preclinical safety data
There are no preclinical data of relevance to the prescriber which are additional to that in other sections of the SmPC.

6. PHARMACEUTICAL PARTICULARS

6.1 List of excipients
Methyl Hydroxybenzoate BP
Xanthan Gum USP
Cetostearyl Alcohol BP
Liquid Paraffin BP
Isopropyl Alcohol BP
Glycerol BP
Cetomacrogol 1000 BP
Sodium citrate BP
Citric Acid Monohydrate BP
Purified Water BP

6.2 Incompatibilities
None known.

6.3 Shelf life
36 months

6.4 Special precautions for storage
Store below 25°C

6.5 Nature and contents of container
Polyethylene squeeze bottle with a polyethylene nozzle and a polystyrene or polyethylene cap or

White High Density Polyethylene (HDPE) Hostalen GF4750 and Remafin white CEG 020 containerwith a polyethylene nozzle and a polystyrene or polyethylene cap.

Pack size: 20 ml; 100 ml

Not all pack sizes may be marketed

6.6 Instructions for use and handling
No special instructions

Administrative Data

7. MARKETING AUTHORISATION HOLDER
Glaxo Wellcome UK Limited
T/A GlaxoSmithKline UK
Stockley Park West
Uxbridge
Middlesex
UB11 1BT

8. MARKETING AUTHORISATION NUMBER(S)
PL 10949/0044

9. DATE OF FIRST AUTHORISATION/RENEWAL OF THE AUTHORISATION
10 September 1997

10. DATE OF REVISION OF THE TEXT
25th January 2005

Betnovate -N Cream

(GlaxoSmithKline UK)

1. NAME OF THE MEDICINAL PRODUCT
Betnovate - N Cream

2. QUALITATIVE AND QUANTITATIVE COMPOSITION
Betamethasone Valerate BP 0.122% $^{W}/_{w}$

Neomycin Sulphate BP 0.5% $^{W}/_{w}$

3. PHARMACEUTICAL FORM
Aqueous Cream

4. CLINICAL PARTICULARS

4.1 Therapeutic indications
Betnovate-N preparations are indicated for the treatment of the following conditions where secondary bacterial infection is present, suspected, or likely to occur: eczema in adults and children (aged 2 years and over), including atopic and discoid eczemas; prurigo nodularis; psoriasis (excluding widespread plaque psoriasis); neurodermatoses including lichen simplex and lichen planus; seborrhoeic dermatitis; contact sensitivity reactions; insect bite reactions; and anal and genital intertrigo.

4.2 Posology and method of administration
Betnovate-N Cream is especially appropriate for moist or weeping surfaces, and Betnovate-N Ointment for dry lichenified or scaly lesions, but this is not invariably so.

In adults, in the more resistant lesions, such as the thickened plaques of psoriasis on elbows and knees, the effect of Betnovate-N can be enhanced, if necessary, by occluding the treatment area with polythene film. Overnight occlusion only is usually adequate to bring about a satisfactory response in such lesions, thereafter Improvement can usually be maintained by regular application without occlusion.

Treatment should not be continued for more than 7 days without medical supervision.

Adults and children aged 2 years and over:

A small quantity should be applied to the affected area two or three times daily until improvement occurs. It may then be possible to maintain improvement by applying once a day or even less often.

Betnovate-N is suitable for use in children (2 years and over) at the same dose as adults. When used in children, courses should be limited to 5 days, if possible.

A possibility of increased absorption exists in very young children, thus Betnovate-N is not recommended for use in neonates and infants younger than 2 years of age (see 4.3 Contra-indications and 4.4 Special Warnings and Precautions for Use).

Dosage in renal impairment:

Dosage should be reduced in patients with reduced renal function (see 4.4 Special Warnings and Precautions for Use).

Elderly:

Betnovate-N is suitable for use in the elderly. Caution should be exercised in cases where a decrease in renal function exists and significant systemic absorption of neomycin sulphate may occur (see 4.4 Special Warnings and Precautions for Use).

For topical administration.

4.3 Contraindications

- Rosacea.
- Acne vulgaris.
- Perioral dermatitis.
- Perianal and genital pruritus.
- Primary cutaneous viral infections (e.g. herpes simplex, chickenpox).
- Hypersensitivity to any component of the preparation.
- Use is not indicated in treatment of primary infected skin lesions caused by infection with fungi or bacteria; primary or secondary infections due to yeast; or secondary infections due to *Pseudomonas* or *Proteus* species.
- Dermatoses in children under 2 years of age, including dermatitis and napkin eruptions. A possibility of increased absorption exists in very young children, thus Betnovate-N is not recommended for use in neonates and infants (up to 2 years). In neonates and infants, absorption by immature skin may be enhanced, and renal function may be immature.
- Preparations containing neomycin should not be used for the treatment of otitis externa when the ear-drum is perforated, because of the risk of ototoxicity.
- Due to the known ototoxic and nephrotoxic potential of neomycin sulphate, the use of Betnovate-N in large quantities or on large areas for prolonged periods of time is not recommended in circumstances where significant systemic absorption may occur.

4.4 Special warnings and special precautions for use
Long-term continuous topical therapy should be avoided where possible, particularly in infants and children, as adrenal suppression, with or without clinical features of Cushing's syndrome, can occur even without occlusion. In this situation, topical steroids should be discontinued gradually under medical supervision because of the risk of adrenal insufficiency (see section 4.8 Undesirable Effects and Section 4.9 Overdose).

If infection persists, systemic chemotherapy is required.

Withdraw topical corticosteroid if there is a spread of infection.

Bacterial infection is encouraged by the warm, moist conditions induced by occlusive dressings, and the skin should be cleansed before a fresh dressing is applied.

Avoid prolonged application to the face. The face, more than other areas of the body, may exhibit atrophic changes after prolonged treatment with potent topical corticosteroids. This must be borne in mind when treating such conditions as psoriasis, discoid lupus erythematosus and severe eczema.

If applied to the eyelids, care is needed to ensure that the preparation does not enter the eye, as glaucoma might result. If Betnovate-N Cream does enter the eye, the affected eye should be bathed in copious amounts of water.

Topical corticosteroids may be hazardous in psoriasis for a number of reasons including rebound relapses, development of tolerance, risk of generalised pustular psoriasis and development of local or systemic toxicity due to impaired barrier function of the skin. If used in psoriasis careful patient supervision is important.

Extended or recurrent application may increase the risk of contact sensitisation.

Extension of infection may occur due to the masking effect of the steroid.

Following significant systemic absorption, aminoglycosides such as neomycin can cause irreversible ototoxicity; and neomycin has nephrotoxic potential.

In renal impairment the plasma clearance of neomycin is reduced (see Dosage in renal impairment, Section 4.2 Posology and Method of Administration).

Products which contain antimicrobial agents should not be diluted.

4.5 Interaction with other medicinal products and other forms of Interaction
Following significant systemic absorption, neomycin sulphate can intensify and prolong the respiratory depressant effects of neuromuscular blocking agents.

4.6 Pregnancy and lactation
There is little information to demonstrate the possible effect of topically applied neomycin in pregnancy and lactation. However, neomycin present in maternal blood can cross the placenta and may give rise to a theoretical risk of foetal toxicity, thus use of Betnovate-N is not recommended in pregnancy or lactation.

4.7 Effects on ability to drive and use machines
None known.

4.8 Undesirable effects
Prolonged and intensive treatment with highly active corticosteroid preparations may cause local atrophic changes in the skin such as thinning, striae, and dilatation of the superficial blood vessels, particularly when occlusive dressings are used or when skin folds are involved

As with other topical corticosteroids, prolonged use of large amounts or treatment of extensive areas can result in sufficient systemic absorption to produce suppression of the HPA axis and the clinical features of Cushing's syndrome (see Section 4.4 Special Warnings and Precautions for use). These effects are more likely to occur in infants and children, and if occlusive dressings are used. In infants the napkin may act as an occlusive dressing.

In rare instances, treatment of psoriasis with corticosteroids (or its withdrawal) is thought to have provoked the pustular form of the disease.

There are reports of local skin burning, pruritus, pigmentation changes, allergic contact dermatitis and hypertrichosis with topical steroids.

The Betnovate preparations are usually well tolerated, but if signs of hypersensitivity appear, application should be stopped immediately.

Exacerbation of symptoms may occur.

4.9 Overdose
Acute overdosage is very unlikely to occur. However, in the case of chronic overdosage or misuse the features of Cushing's syndrome may appear and in this situation topical steroids should be discontinued gradually under medical supervision (see Section 4.4 Special Warnings and Precautions for use).

Also, consideration should be given to significant systemic absorption of neomycin sulphate (see 4.4 Special Warnings and Precautions for Use). If this is suspected, use of the product should be stopped and the patient's general status, hearing acuity, renal and neuromuscular functions should be monitored.

Blood levels of neomycin sulphate should also be determined. Haemodialysis may reduce the serum level of neomycin sulphate.

5. PHARMACOLOGICAL PROPERTIES

5.1 Pharmacodynamic properties
Betamethasone valerate is an active corticosteroid which produces a rapid response in those inflammatory dermatoses that are normally responsive to topical corticosteroid therapy, and is often effective in the less responsive conditions such as psoriasis.

Neomycin sulphate is a broad spectrum, bactericidal antibiotic effective against the majority of bacteria commonly associated with skin infections.

5.2 Pharmacokinetic properties
The extent of percutaneous absorption of topical corticosteroid is determined by many factors including the vehicle, the integrity of the epidermal barrier, and the use of occlusive dressings.

Topical corticosteroids can be absorbed from normal intact skin. Inflammation and/or other disease processes in the skin increase percutaneous absorption. Occlusive dressings substantially increase the percutaneous absorption of topical corticosteroids.

Once absorbed through the skin, topical corticosteroids are handled through pharmacokinetic pathways similar to systematically administered corticosteroids. Corticosteroids are bound to plasma proteins in varying degrees. Corticosteroids are metabolised primarily by the liver and are then excreted by the kidneys.

5.3 Preclinical safety data
There are no preclinical data of relevance to the prescriber which are additional to that in other sections of the SmPC.

6. PHARMACEUTICAL PARTICULARS

6.1 List of excipients
Chlorocresol
Cetomacrogol 1000
Cetostearyl Alcohol
White Soft Paraffin
Liquid Paraffin
Sodium Acid Phosphate
Phosphoric Acid
Sodium Hydroxide
Purified Water

6.2 Incompatibilities
None known.

6.3 Shelf life
36 Months.

6.4 Special precautions for storage
Store below 25°C.

6.5 Nature and contents of container
15 gm, 30 gm and 100 gm collapsible aluminium tubes internally coated with an epoxy resin based lacquer and closed with a wadless polypropylene cap.

Not all pack sizes may be marketed

6.6 Instructions for use and handling
Do not dilute

Administrative Data

7. MARKETING AUTHORISATION HOLDER
Glaxo Wellcome UK Ltd.,
trading as GlaxoSmithKline UK
Stockley Park West,
Uxbridge,
Middlesex UB11 1BT

8. MARKETING AUTHORISATION NUMBER(S)
PL 10949/0018

9. DATE OF FIRST AUTHORISATION/RENEWAL OF THE AUTHORISATION
7 November 1997

10. DATE OF REVISION OF THE TEXT
25th January 2005

11. Legal Status
POM

Betnovate -N Ointment

(GlaxoSmithKline UK)

1. NAME OF THE MEDICINAL PRODUCT
Betnovate-N Ointment

2. QUALITATIVE AND QUANTITATIVE COMPOSITION
Betamethasone Valerate BP 0.122% $^{W}/_{W}$

Neomycin Sulphate BP 0.5% $^{W}/_{W}$

3. PHARMACEUTICAL FORM
Ointment

4. CLINICAL PARTICULARS

4.1 Therapeutic indications
Betnovate-N preparations are indicated for the treatment of the following conditions where secondary bacterial infection is present, suspected or likely to occur: eczema in adults and children (aged 2 years and over), including atopic and discoid eczema; prurigo nodularis; psoriasis (excluding widespread plaque psoriasis); neurodermatoses including lichen simplex and lichen planus; seborrhoeic dermatitis; contact sensitivity reactions; insect bite reactions; and anal and genital intertrigo.

4.2 Posology and method of administration
Betnovate-N Cream is especially appropriate for moist or weeping surfaces, and Betnovate-N Ointment is especially appropriate for dry, lichenified or scaly lesions, but this is not invariably so.

In adults, in the more resistant lesions, such as the thickened plaques of psoriasis on elbows and knees, the effects of Betnovate-N can be enhanced, if necessary, by occluding the treatment area with polythene film. Overnight occlusion only is usually adequate to bring about a satisfactory response in such lesions, thereafter improvement can usually be maintained by regular application without occlusion.

Treatment should not be continued for more than 7 days without medical supervision.

Adults and children aged 2 years and over:

A small quantity should be applied to the affected area two or three times daily until improvement occurs. It may then be possible to maintain improvement by applying once a day, or even less often.

Betnovate-N is suitable for use in children (2 years and over) at the same dose as adults. When used in children, courses should be limited to 5 days, if possible.

A possibility of increased absorption exists in very young children, thus Betnovate-N is not recommended for use in neonates and infants younger than 2 years of age (see 4.3 Contra-indications and 4.4 Special Warnings and Precautions for Use).

Dosage in renal impairment:

Dosage should be reduced in patients with reduced renal function (see 4.4 Special Warnings and Precautions for Use).

Elderly:

Betnovate-N is suitable for use in the elderly. Caution should be exercised in cases where a decrease in renal function exists and significant systemic absorption of neomycin sulphate may occur (see 4.4 Special Warnings and Precautions for Use).

For topical administration.

4.3 Contraindications
- Rosacea.
- Acne vulgaris.
- Perioral dermatitis.
- Perianal and genital pruritus.
- Primary cutaneous viral infections (e.g. herpes simplex, chickenpox).
- Hypersensitivity to any component of the preparation.
- Use is not indicated in treatment of primary infected skin lesions caused by infection with fungi or bacteria; primary or secondary infections due to yeast; or secondary infections due to *Pseudomonas* or *Proteus* species.
- Dermatoses in children under 2 years of age, including dermatitis and napkin eruptions. A possibility of increased absorption exists in very young children, thus Betnovate-N is not recommended for use in neonates and infants (up to 2 years). In neonates and infants, absorption by immature skin may be enhanced, and renal function may be immature.
- Preparations containing neomycin should not be used for the treatment of otitis externa when the ear drum is perforated, because of the risk of ototoxicity.
- Due to the known ototoxic and nephrotoxic potential of neomycin sulphate, the use of Betnovate-N in large quantities or on large areas for prolonged periods of time is not recommended in circumstances where significant systemic absorption may occur.

4.4 Special warnings and special precautions for use
Long-term continuous topical therapy should be avoided where possible, particularly in infants and children, as adrenal suppression, with or without clinical features of Cushing's syndrome, can occur even without occlusion. In this situation, topical steroids should be discontinued gradually under medical supervision because of the risk of adrenal insufficiency (see section 4.8 Undesirable Effects and Section 4.9 Overdose).

If infection persists, systemic chemotherapy is required.

Withdraw topical corticosteroid if there is a spread of infection.

Bacterial infection is encouraged by the warm, moist conditions induced by occlusive dressings, and the skin should be cleansed before a fresh dressing is applied.

Avoid prolonged application to the face. The face, more than other areas of the body, may exhibit atrophic changes after prolonged treatment with potent topical corticosteroids. This must be borne in mind when treating such conditions as psoriasis, discoid lupus erythematosus and severe eczema.

If applied to the eyelids, care is needed to ensure that the preparation does not enter the eye, as glaucoma might result. If Betnovate-N Ointment does enter the eye, the affected eye should be bathed in copious amounts of water.

Topical corticosteroids may be hazardous in psoriasis for a number of reasons including rebound relapses, development of tolerance, risk of generalised pustular psoriasis and development of local or systemic toxicity due to impaired barrier function of the skin. If used in psoriasis careful patient supervision is important.

Extended or recurrent application may increase the risk of contact sensitisation.

Extension of infection may occur due to the masking effect of the steroid.

Following significant systemic absorption, aminoglycosides such as neomycin can cause irreversible ototoxicity; and neomycin has nephrotoxic potential.

In renal impairment the plasma clearance of neomycin is reduced (see Dosage in renal impairment, section 4.2 Posology and Method of Administration).

Products which contain antimicrobial agents should not be diluted.

4.5 Interaction with other medicinal products and other forms of Interaction
Following significant systemic absorption, neomycin sulphate can intensify and prolong the respiratory depressant effects of neuromuscular blocking agents.

4.6 Pregnancy and lactation
There is little information to demonstrate the possible effect of topically applied neomycin in pregnancy and lactation. However, neomycin present in maternal blood can cross the placenta and may give rise to a theoretical risk of foetal toxicity, thus use of Betnovate N is not recommended in pregnancy or lactation.

4.7 Effects on ability to drive and use machines
None known

4.8 Undesirable effects
Prolonged and intensive treatment with highly active corticosteroid preparations may cause local atrophic changes in the skin such as thinning, striae, and dilatation of the superficial blood vessels, particularly when occlusive dressings are used or when skin folds are involved.

As with other topical corticosteroids, prolonged use of large amounts or treatment of extensive areas can result in sufficient systemic absorption to produce suppression of the HPA axis and the clinical features of Cushing's syndrome (see Section 4.4 Special Warnings and Special Precautions for use). These effects are more likely to occur in infants and children, and if occlusive dressings are used. In infants the napkin may act as an occlusive dressing.

In rare instances, treatment of psoriasis with corticosteroids (or its withdrawal) is thought to have provoked the pustular form of the disease.

There are reports of local skin burning, pruritus, pigmentation changes allergic contact dermatitis and hypertrichosis with topical steroids.

The Betnovate preparations are usually well tolerated, but if signs of hypersensitivity appear, application should be stopped immediately.

Exacerbation of symptoms may occur.

4.9 Overdose
Acute overdosage is very unlikely to occur. However, in the case of chronic overdosage or misuse the features of Cushing's syndrome may appear and in this situation topical steroids should be discontinued gradually under medical supervision (see Section 4.4 Special Warnings and Special Precautions for use).

Also, consideration should be given to significant systemic absorption of neomycin sulphate (see 4.4 Special Warnings and Precautions for Use). If this is suspected, use of the product should be stopped and the patient's general status, hearing acuity, renal and neuromuscular functions should be monitored.

Blood levels of neomycin sulphate should also be determined. Haemodialysis may reduce the serum level of neomycin sulphate.

5. PHARMACOLOGICAL PROPERTIES

5.1 Pharmacodynamic properties
Betamethasone valerate is an active topical corticosteroid which produces a rapid response in those inflammatory dermatoses that are normally responsive to topical corticosteroid therapy, and is often effective in the less responsive conditions such as psoriasis.

Neomycin sulphate is a broad-spectrum bactericidal antibiotic affective against the majority of bacteria commonly associated with skin infections.

5.2 Pharmacokinetic properties
The extent of percutaneous absorption of topical corticosteroids is determined by many factors including the vehicle, the integrity of the epidermal barrier, and the use of occlusive dressings.

Topical corticosteroids can be absorbed from normal intact skin. Inflammation and/or other disease processes in the skin increase percutaneous absorption. Occlusive dressings substantially increase the percutaneous absorption of topical corticosteroids.

Once absorbed through the skin, topical corticosteroids are handled through pharmacokinetic pathways similar to systematically administered corticosteroids. Corticosteroids are bound to plasma proteins in varying degrees. Corticosteroids are metabolised primarily by the liver and are then excreted by the kidneys.

5.3 Preclinical safety data
There are no preclinical data of relevance to the prescriber which are additional to that in other sections of the SmPC.

6. PHARMACEUTICAL PARTICULARS

6.1 List of excipients
Liquid Paraffin

White Soft Paraffin

6.2 Incompatibilities
None known.

6.3 Shelf life
36 Months.

6.4 Special precautions for storage
Store at temperatures not exceeding 30°C.

6.5 Nature and contents of container
15 gm, 30 gm and 100 gm collapsible aluminium tubes internally coated with an epoxy resin based lacquer and closed with a wadless polypropylene cap.

Not all pack sizes may be marketed

6.6 Instructions for use and handling
Do not dilute

Administrative Data

7. MARKETING AUTHORISATION HOLDER
Glaxo Wellcome UK Ltd.,
T/A GlaxoSmithKline UK
Stockley Park West,
Uxbridge,
Middlesex UB11 1BT

8. MARKETING AUTHORISATION NUMBER(S)
PL 10949/0019

9. DATE OF FIRST AUTHORISATION/RENEWAL OF THE AUTHORISATION
3 December 1997

10. DATE OF REVISION OF THE TEXT
25th January 2005

11. Legal Status
POM

Betnovate Ointment

(GlaxoSmithKline UK)

1. NAME OF THE MEDICINAL PRODUCT
Betnovate Ointment

2. QUALITATIVE AND QUANTITATIVE COMPOSITION
Betamethasone Valerate B.P. 0.122% w/w

3. PHARMACEUTICAL FORM
Ointment

4. CLINICAL PARTICULARS

4.1 Therapeutic indications
Betamethasone valerate is an active topical corticosteroid which provides a rapid response in those inflammatory dermatoses that are often effective in the less responsive conditions such as psoriasis.

Betnovate preparations are indicated for the treatment of: eczema in children and adults; including atopic and discoid eczemas, prurigo nodularis; psoriasis (excluding widespread plaque psoriasis); neurodermatoses, including lichen simplex, lichen planus; seborrhoeic dermatitis; contact sensitivity reactions; discoid lupus erythematosus and they may be used as an adjunct to systemic steroid therapy in generalised erythroderma.

4.2 Posology and method of administration
A small quantity of Betnovate should be applied to the affected area two or three times daily until improvement occurs. It may then be possible to maintain improvement by applying once a day, or even less often, or by using the appropriate ready diluted (1 in 4) preparation, Betnovate RD. If no improvement is seen within two to four weeks, reassessment of the diagnosis, or referral, may be necessary.

Betnovate and Betnovate RD ointments are especially appropriate for dry, lichenified or scaly lesions, but this is not invariably so.

In the more resistant lesions, such as the thickened plaques of psoriasis on elbows and knees, the effect of Betnovate can be enhanced, if necessary, by occluding the treatment area with polythene film. Overnight occlusion only is usually adequate to bring about a satisfactory response in such lesions; thereafter improvement can usually be maintained by regular application without occlusion.

Children

Courses should be limited to five days. Occlusion should not be used.

For topical administration.

4.3 Contraindications
Rosacea, acne vulgaris, perioral dermatitis, primary cutaneous viral infections (e.g. herpes simplex, chickenpox). Hypersensitivity to any component of the preparation.

The use of Betnovate skin preparations is not indicated in the treatment of primarily infected skin lesions caused by infections with fungi (e.g. candidiasis, tinea); or bacteria (e.g. impetigo); primary or secondary infections due to yeast; peri-anal and genital pruritus; dermatoses in children under 1 year of age, including dermatitis and napkin eruptions.

4.4 Special warnings and special precautions for use
Long-term continuous topical therapy should be avoided where possible, particularly in infants and children, as adrenal suppression, with or without clinical features of Cushing's syndrome, can occur even without occlusion. In this situation, topical steroids should be discontinued gradually under medical supervision because of the risk of adrenal insufficiency (see section 4.8 Undesirable Effects and Section 4.9 Overdose).

The face, more than other areas of the body, may exhibit atrophic changes after prolonged treatment with potent topical corticosteroids. This must be borne in mind when treating such conditions as psoriasis, discoid lupus erythematosus and severe eczema. If applied to the eyelids, care is needed to ensure that the preparation does not enter the eye, as glaucoma might result.

If used in childhood, or on the face, courses should be limited to five days and occlusion should not be used.

Topical corticosteroids may be hazardous in psoriasis for a number of reasons including rebound relapses, development of tolerance, risk of generalised postural psoriasis and development of local or systemic toxicity due to impaired barrier function of the skin. If used in psoriasis careful patient supervision is important.

Appropriate antimicrobial therapy should be used whenever treating inflammatory lesions which have become infected. Any spread of infection requires withdrawal of topical corticosteroid therapy and systemic administration of antimicrobial agents. Bacterial infection is encouraged by the warm, moist conditions induced by occlusive dressings, and so the skin should be cleansed before a fresh dressing is applied.

4.5 Interaction with other medicinal products and other forms of Interaction
None known.

4.6 Pregnancy and lactation
There is inadequate evidence of safety in human pregnancy. Topical administration of corticosteroids to pregnant animals can cause abnormalities of foetal development including cleft palate and intrauterine growth retardation. There may therefore be a very small risk of such effects in the human foetus.

4.7 Effects on ability to drive and use machines
None known.

4.8 Undesirable effects
Adverse events are listed below by system organ class and frequency. Frequencies are defined as: very common (≥1/10), common (≥1/100 and <1/10), uncommon (≥1/1000 and <1/100), rare (≥1/10,000 and <1/1000) and very rare (<1/10,000) including isolated reports. Very common, common and uncommon events were generally determined from clinical trial data. The background rates in placebo and comparator groups were not taken into account when assigning frequency categories to adverse events derived from clinical trial data, since these rates were generally comparable to those in the active treatment group. Rare and very rare events were generally determined from spontaneous data.

Immune system disorders
Very rare: Hypersensitivity.

If signs of hypersensitivity appear, application should stop immediately.

Endocrine disorders
Very rare: Features of Cushing's syndrome.

As with other topical corticosteroids, prolonged use of large amounts or treatment of extensive areas can result in sufficient systemic absorption to produce suppression of the HPA axis and the clinical features of Cushing's syndrome (see Section 4.4 Special Warnings and Precautions for use). These effects are more likely to occur in infants and children, and if occlusive dressings are used. In infants the napkin may act as an occlusive dressing.

Skin and subcutaneous tissue disorders
Common: Local skin burning and pruritus.

Very rare: Local atrophic changes in the skin such as thinning, striae and dilatation of the superficial blood vessels may be caused by prolonged and intensive treatment with highly active corticosteroid preparations, particularly when occlusive dressings are used or when skin folds are involved. Pigmentation changes, hypertrichosis, allergic contact dermatitis, exacerbation of symptoms, pustular psoriasis (due to treatment of psoriasis with corticosteroids or its withdrawal: see Section 4.4. Special Warnings and Precautions for use)

4.9 Overdose
Acute overdosage is very unlikely to occur. However, in the case of chronic overdosage or misuse the features of Cushing's syndrome may appear and in this situation topical steroids should be discontinued gradually under medical supervision (see Section 4.4 Special Warnings and Precautions for use).

5. PHARMACOLOGICAL PROPERTIES

5.1 Pharmacodynamic properties
Bethamethasone valerate is an active corticosteroid with topical anti-inflammatory activity.

5.2 Pharmacokinetic properties
The extent of percutaneous absorption of topical corticosteroid is determined by many factors including the vehicle, the integrity of the epidermal barrier, and the use of occlusive dressings.

Topical corticosteroids can be absorbed from normal intact skin. Inflammation and/or other disease processes in the skin increase percutaneous absorption. Occlusive dressings substantially increase the percutaneous absorption of topical corticosteroids.

Once absorbed through the skin, topical corticosteroids are handled through pharmacokinetic pathways similar to systematically administered corticosteroids. Corticosteroids are bound to plasma proteins in varying degrees. Corticosteroids are metabolised primarily by the liver and are then excreted by the kidneys.

5.3 Preclinical safety data
There are no preclinical data of relevance to the prescriber which are additional to that in other sections of the SmPC.

6. PHARMACEUTICAL PARTICULARS

6.1 List of excipients

Liquid Paraffin	BP
White Soft Paraffin	BP

6.2 Incompatibilities
None known

6.3 Shelf life

Tubes	36 months
Pump Dispenser	24 months

6.4 Special precautions for storage

Tubes	Store below 30°C
Pump Dispenser	Store below 25°C

6.5 Nature and contents of container
30 gm and 100 gm collapsible aluminium tubes internally coated with an epoxy resin based lacquer and closed with a polypropylene cap.

100 gm polypropylene/polyethylene pump dispenser with natural (translucent) polypropylene body. The nozzle is sealed with a polyethylene acetyl tab. The pump is closed with an opaque polypropylene overcap and overwrapped with an opaque shrink-wrap.

Not all pack sizes may be marketed

6.6 Instructions for use and handling
No special instructions

Administrative Data

7. MARKETING AUTHORISATION HOLDER
Glaxo Wellcome UK Limited

trading as GlaxoSmithKline UK

Stockley Park West

Uxbridge

Middlesex

UB11 1BT

8. MARKETING AUTHORISATION NUMBER(S)
PL 10949/0020

9. DATE OF FIRST AUTHORISATION/RENEWAL OF THE AUTHORISATION
3 September 1997

10. DATE OF REVISION OF THE TEXT
25th January 2005

Betnovate RD Cream

(GlaxoSmithKline UK)

1. NAME OF THE MEDICINAL PRODUCT
Betnovate RD Cream

2. QUALITATIVE AND QUANTITATIVE COMPOSITION
Betamethasone Valerate B.P. Equivalent to Betamethasone 0.025%.

3. PHARMACEUTICAL FORM
Cream

4. CLINICAL PARTICULARS

4.1 Therapeutic indications
Betamethasone valerate is an active topical corticosteroid which produces a rapid response in those inflammatory dermatoses that are normally responsive to topical corticosteroid therapy, and is often effective in the less responsive conditions such as psoriasis.

Betnovate preparations are indicated for the treatment of: eczema in children and adults; including atopic and discoid eczemas; prurigo nodularis; psoriasis (excluding widespread plaque psoriasis); neurodermatoses, including lichen simplex, lichen planus; seborrhoeic dermatitis; contact sensitivity reactions; discoid lupus erythematosus and they may be used as an adjunct to systemic steroid therapy in generalised erythroderma.

Betnovate RD preparations are indicated for maintenance treatment when control has been achieved with Betnovate.

4.2 Posology and method of administration
A small quantity of Betnovate should be applied to the affected area two or three times daily until improvement occurs. It may then be possible to maintain improvement by applying once a day, or even less often, or by using the appropriate ready-diluted (1 in 4) preparation Betnovate RD. If no improvement is seen within two or four weeks, reassessment of the diagnosis, or referral, may be necessary.

Betnovate and Betnovate RD Creams are especially appropriate for moist or weeping surfaces but this is not invariably so.

In the more resistant lesions, such as the thickened plaques of psoriasis on elbows and knees, the effect of Betnovate can be enhanced, if necessary, by occluding the treatment area with polythene film. Overnight occlusion only is usually adequate to bring about a satisfactory response in such lesions; thereafter improvement can usually be maintained by regular application without occlusion.

Children

Courses should be limited to five days if possible. Occlusion should not be used.

4.3 Contraindications
Rosacea, acne vulgaris and peri-oral dermatitis. Primary cutaneous viral infections (e.g. herpes simplex, chickenpox). Hypersensitivity to the preparation.

The use of Betnovate skin preparations is not indicated in the treatment of primarily infected skin lesions caused by infection with fungi (e.g. candidiasis, tinea), or bacteria (e.g. impetigo); primary or secondary infections due to yeast; peri-anal and genital pruritus; dermatoses in children under 1 year of age, including dermatitis and napkin eruptions.

4.4 Special warnings and special precautions for use
Long-term continuous topical therapy should be avoided where possible, particularly in infants and children, as adrenal suppression, with or without clinical features of Cushing's syndrome, can occur even without occlusion. In this situation, topical steroids should be discontinued gradually under medical supervision because of the risk of adrenal insufficiency (see section 4.8 Undesirable Effects and Section 4.9 Overdose).

The face, more than other areas of the body, may exhibit atrophic changes after prolonged treatment with potent topical corticosteroids. This must be borne in mind when treating such conditions as psoriasis, discoid lupus erythematosus and severe eczema. If applied to the eyelids, care is needed to ensure that the preparation does not enter the eye, as glaucoma might result.

If used in childhood or on the face, courses should be limited if possible to five days and occlusion should not be used.

Topical corticosteroids may be hazardous in psoriasis for a number of reasons including rebound relapses, development of tolerance, risk of generalised pustular psoriasis and development of local or systemic toxicity due to impaired barrier function of the skin. If used in psoriasis careful patient supervision is important.

Appropriate antimicrobial therapy should be used whenever treating inflammatory lesions which have become infected. Any spread of infection requires withdrawal of topical corticosteroid therapy and systemic administration of antimicrobial agents. Bacterial infection is encouraged by the warm, moist conditions induced by occlusive dressings, and so the skin should be cleansed before a fresh dressing is applied.

In rare instances, treatment of psoriasis with corticosteroids (or its withdrawal) is thought to have provoked the pustular form of the disease. Betnovate RD is usually well tolerated but if signs of hypersensitivity appear, application should stop immediately.

4.5 Interaction with other medicinal products and other forms of Interaction
None known.

4.6 Pregnancy and lactation
Avoid extensive use in pregnancy. There is inadequate evidence of safety. Topical administration of corticosteroids to pregnant animals can cause abnormalities of foetal development including cleft palate and intrauterine growth retardation. There may therefore be a very small risk of such effects in the human foetus.

4.7 Effects on ability to drive and use machines
None known.

4.8 Undesirable effects
Adverse events are listed below by system organ class and frequency. Frequencies are defined as: very common (≥1/10), common (≥1/100 and <1/10), uncommon (≥1/1000 and <1/100), rare (≥1/10,000 and <1/1000) and very rare (<1/10,000) including isolated reports. Very common, common and uncommon events were generally determined from clinical trial data. The background rates in placebo and comparator groups were not taken into account when assigning frequency categories to adverse events derived from clinical trial data, since these rates were generally comparable to those in the active treatment group. Rare and very rare events were generally determined from spontaneous data.

Immune system disorders

Very rare: Hypersensitivity.

If signs of hypersensitivity appear, application should stop immediately.

Endocrine disorders

Very rare: Features of Cushing's syndrome

As with other topical corticosteroids, prolonged use of large amounts or treatment of extensive areas can result in sufficient systemic absorption to produce suppression of the HPA axis and the clinical features of Cushing's syndrome (see Section 4.4 Special Warnings and Precautions for Use). These effects are more likely to occur in infants and children, and if occlusive dressings are used. In infants the napkin may act as an occlusive dressing.

Skin and subcutaneous tissue disorders

Common: Local skin burning and pruritus.

Very rare: Local atrophic changes in the skin such as thinning, striae and dilatation of the superficial blood vessels may be caused by prolonged and intensive treatment with highly active corticosteroid preparations, particularly when occlusive dressings are used or when skin folds are involved.

Pigmentation changes, hypertrichosis, allergic contact dermatitis, exacerbation of symptoms, pustular psoriasis (due to treatment of psoriasis with corticosteroids or its withdrawal: see Section 4.4. Special Warnings and Precautions for use)

4.9 Overdose
Acute overdosage is very unlikely to occur. However, in the case of chronic overdosage or misuse the features of Cushing's syndromemay appear and in this situation topical steroids should be discontinued gradually under medical supervision (see Section 4.4 Special Warnings and Precautions for use).

5. PHARMACOLOGICAL PROPERTIES

5.1 Pharmacodynamic properties
Betamethasone is a corticosteroid with topical anti-inflammatory activity.

5.2 Pharmacokinetic properties
The extent of percutaneous absorption of topical corticosteroid is determined by many factors including the vehicle, the integrity of the epidermal barrier, and the use of occlusive dressings.

Topical corticosteroids can be absorbed from normal intact skin. Inflammation and/or other disease processes in the skin increase percutaneous absorption of topical corticosteroids.

Once absorbed through the skin, topical corticosteroids are handled through pharmacokinetic pathways similar to systematically administered corticosteroids. Corticosteroids are metabolised primarily by the liver and are then excreted by the kidneys.

5.3 Preclinical safety data
No additional data of relevance.

6. PHARMACEUTICAL PARTICULARS

6.1 List of excipients
Cetostearyl Alcohol B.P.

Cetomacrogol 1000 B.P.

White Soft Paraffin B.P.

Liquid Paraffin B.P.

Chlorocresol B.P.

Disodium Hydrogen Phosphate, Anhydrous

Citric Acid Monohydrate B.P.

Purified Water B.P.

6.2 Incompatibilities
None known.

6.3 Shelf life
36 months.

6.4 Special precautions for storage
Store below 25°C.

6.5 Nature and contents of container
100gm lacquered aluminium tubes with polypropylene screw caps.

6.6 Instructions for use and handling
No special instructions.

Administrative Data

7. MARKETING AUTHORISATION HOLDER
Glaxo Wellcome UK Ltd, trading as GlaxoSmithKline UK
Stockley Park West,
Uxbridge,
Middlesex UB11 1BT.

8. MARKETING AUTHORISATION NUMBER(S)
PL 10949/0021

9. DATE OF FIRST AUTHORISATION/RENEWAL OF THE AUTHORISATION
14 October 1996

10. DATE OF REVISION OF THE TEXT
25th January 2005

Betnovate RD Ointment

(GlaxoSmithKline UK)

1. NAME OF THE MEDICINAL PRODUCT
Betnovate RD Ointment

2. QUALITATIVE AND QUANTITATIVE COMPOSITION
Betamethasone Valerate B.P. 0.0305%. Equivalent to Betamethasone 0.025%.

3. PHARMACEUTICAL FORM
Ointment

4. CLINICAL PARTICULARS

4.1 Therapeutic indications
Betamethasone valerate is an active topical corticosteroid, which produces a rapid response in those inflammatory dermatoses that are normally responsive to topical corticosteroid therapy, and is often effective in the less responsive conditions such as psoriasis.

Betnovate preparations are indicated for the treatment of: eczema in children and adults; including atopic and discoid eczemas; prurigo nodularis; psoriasis (excluding widespread plaque psoriasis); neurodermatoses, including lichen simplex, lichen planus; seborrhoeic dermatitis; contact sensitivity reactions; discoid lupus erythematosus and they may be used as an adjunct to systemic steroid therapy in generalised erythroderma.

Betnovate RD preparations are indicated for maintenance treatment when control has been achieved with Betnovate.

4.2 Posology and method of administration
A small quantity of Betnovate should be applied to the affected area two or three times daily until improvement occurs. It may then be possible to maintain improvement by applying once a day, or even less often, or by using the appropriate ready-diluted (1 in 4) preparation Betnovate RD. If no improvement is seen within two or four weeks, reassessment of the diagnosis, or referral, may be necessary.

Betnovate and Betnovate RD ointments are especially appropriate for dry, lichenified or scaly lesions, but this is not invariably so.

In the more resistant lesions, such as the thickened plaques of psoriasis on elbows and knees, the effect of Betnovate can be enhanced, if necessary, by occluding the treatment area with polythene film. Overnight occlusion only is usually adequate to bring about a satisfactory response in such lesions; thereafter improvement can usually be maintained by regular application without occlusion.

Children

Courses should be limited to five days if possible. Occlusion should not be used.

4.3 Contraindications
Rosacea, acne vulgaris and peri-oral dermatitis. Primary cutaneous viral infections (e.g. herpes simplex, chickenpox). Hypersensitivity to the preparation.

The use of Betnovate skin preparations is not indicated in the treatment of primarily infected skin lesions caused by infection with fungi (e.g. candidiasis, tinea), or bacteria (e.g. impetigo); primary or secondary infections due to yeast; peri-anal and genital pruritus; dermatoses in children under 1 year of age, including dermatitis and napkin eruptions.

4.4 Special warnings and special precautions for use
Long-term continuous topical therapy should be avoided where possible, particularly in infants and children, as adrenal suppression, with or without clinical features of Cushing's syndrome, can occur even without occlusion. In this situation, topical steroids should be discontinued gradually under medical supervision because of the risk of adrenal insufficiency (see section 4.8 Undesirable Effects and Secion 4.9 Overdose).

The face, more than other areas of the body, may exhibit atrophic changes after prolonged treatment with potent topical corticosteroids. This must be borne in mind when treating such conditions as psoriasis, discoid lupus erythematosus and severe eczema. If applied to the eyelids, care is needed to ensure that the preparation does not enter the eye, as glaucoma might result.

If used in childhood or on the face, courses should be limited if possible to five days and occlusion should not be used.

Topical corticosteroids may be hazardous in psoriasis for a number of reasons including rebound relapses, development of tolerance, risk of generalised pustular psoriasis and development of local or systemic toxicity due to impaired barrier function of the skin. If used in psoriasis careful patient supervision is important.

Appropriate antimicrobial therapy should be used whenever treating inflammatory lesions, which have become infected. Any spread of infection requires withdrawal of topical corticosteroid therapy and systemic administration of antimicrobial agents. Bacterial infection is encouraged by the warm, moist conditions induced by occlusive dressings, and so the skin should be cleansed before a fresh dressing is applied.

In rare instances, treatment of psoriasis with corticosteroids (or its withdrawal) is thought to have provoked the pustular form of the disease. Betnovate RD is usually well tolerated but if signs of hypersensitivity appear, application should stop immediately.

4.5 Interaction with other medicinal products and other forms of Interaction
None known.

4.6 Pregnancy and lactation
Avoid extensive use in pregnancy. There is inadequate evidence of safety. Topical administration of corticosteroids to pregnant animals can cause abnormalities of foetal development including cleft palate and intrauterine growth retardation. There may therefore be a very small risk of such effects in the human foetus.

4.7 Effects on ability to drive and use machines
None known.

4.8 Undesirable effects
Adverse events are listed below by system organ class and frequency. Frequencies are defined as: very common (≥1/10), common (≥1/100 and <1/10), uncommon (≥1/1000 and <1/100), rare (≥1/10,000 and <1/1000) and very rare (<1/10,000) including isolated reports. Very common, common and uncommon events were generally determined from clinical trial data. The background rates in placebo and comparator groups were not taken into account when assigning frequency categories to adverse events derived from clinical trial data, since these rates were generally comparable to those in the active treatment group. Rare and very rare events were generally determined from spontaneous data.

Immune system disorders

Very rare: Hypersensitivity.

If signs of hypersensitivity appear, application should stop immediately.

Endocrine disorders

Very rare: Features of Cushing's syndrome

As with other topical corticosteroids, prolonged use of large amounts or treatment of extensive areas can result in sufficient systemic absorption to produce suppression of the HPA axis and the clinical features of Cushing's syndrome (see Section 4.4 Special Warnings and Precautions for use). These effects are more likely to occur in infants and children, and if occlusive dressings are used. In infants the napkin may act as an occlusive dressing.

Skin and subcutaneous tissue disorders

Common: Local skin burning and pruritus.

Very rare: Local atrophic changes in the skin such as thinning, striae and dilatation of the superficial blood vessels may be caused by prolonged and intensive treatment with highly active corticosteroid preparations, particularly when occlusive dressings are used or when skin folds are involved.

Pigmentation changes, hypertrichosis, allergic contact dermatitis, exacerbation of symptoms, pustular psoriasis (due to treatment of psoriasis with corticosteroids or its withdrawal: see Section 4.4. Special Warnings and Precautions for use)

4.9 Overdose

Acute overdosage is very unlikely to occur. However, in the case of chronic overdosage or misuse the features of Cushing's syndrome may appear and in this situation topical steroids should be discontinued gradually under medical supervision (see Section 4.4 Special Warnings and Precautions for use).

5. PHARMACOLOGICAL PROPERTIES

5.1 Pharmacodynamic properties

Betamethasone is a corticosteroid with topical anti-inflammatory activity.

5.2 Pharmacokinetic properties

The extent of percutaneous absorption of topical corticosteroid is determined by many factors including the vehicle, the integrity of the epidermal barrier, and the use of occlusive dressings.

Topical corticosteroids can be absorbed from normal intact skin. Inflammation and/or other disease processes in the skin increase percutaneous absorption of topical corticosteroids.

Once absorbed through the skin, topical corticosteroids are handled through pharmacokinetic pathways similar to systematically administered corticosteroids. Corticosteroids are metabolised primarily by the liver and are then excreted by the kidneys.

5.3 Preclinical safety data

No additional data of relevance.

6. PHARMACEUTICAL PARTICULARS

6.1 List of excipients

White Soft Paraffin	B.P.
Liquid Paraffin	B.P.

6.2 Incompatibilities

None known.

6.3 Shelf life

36 months.

6.4 Special precautions for storage

Store below 30°C.

6.5 Nature and contents of container

100gm lacquered aluminium tubes with polypropylene screw caps.

6.6 Instructions for use and handling

No special instructions.

Administrative Data

7. MARKETING AUTHORISATION HOLDER

Glaxo Wellcome UK Ltd,

trading as GlaxoSmithKline UK

Stockley Park West,

Uxbridge,

Middlesex

UB11 1BT.

8. MARKETING AUTHORISATION NUMBER(S)

PL 10949/0022

9. DATE OF FIRST AUTHORISATION/RENEWAL OF THE AUTHORISATION

17 January 2002

10. DATE OF REVISION OF THE TEXT

25th January 2005

11. Legal Category

POM

Betnovate Scalp Application

(GlaxoSmithKline UK)

1. NAME OF THE MEDICINAL PRODUCT

Betnovate Scalp Application.

2. QUALITATIVE AND QUANTITATIVE COMPOSITION

Betamethasone Valerate BP 0.122% w/w.

3. PHARMACEUTICAL FORM

Aqueous Suspension.

4. CLINICAL PARTICULARS

4.1 Therapeutic indications

Steroid responsive dermatoses of the scalp, such as psoriasis and seborrhoeic dermatitis.

4.2 Posology and method of administration

A small quantity of Betnovate Scalp Application should be applied to the scalp night and morning until improvement is noticeable. It may then be possible to sustain improvement by applying once a day, or less frequently.

For topical application.

4.3 Contraindications

Infections of the scalp. Hypersensitivity to the preparation. Dermatoses in children under one year of age, including dermatitis.

4.4 Special warnings and special precautions for use

Care must be taken to keep the preparation away from the eyes. Does not use near a naked flame.

Long-term continuous topical therapy should be avoided where possible, particularly in infants and children, as adrenal suppression, with or without clinical features of Cushing's syndrome, can occur even without occlusion. In this situation, topical steroids should be discontinued gradually under medical supervision because of the risk of adrenal insufficiency (see section 4.8 Undesirable Effects and Section 4.9 Overdose).

Topical corticosteroids may be hazardous in psoriasis for a number of reasons including rebound relapses, development of tolerance, risk of generalised pustular psoriasis and development of local or systemic toxicity due to impaired barrier function of the skin. If used in psoriasis careful patient supervision is important.

Development of secondary infection requires withdrawal of topical corticosteroid therapy and commencement of appropriate systemic antimicrobial therapy.

The least potent corticosteroid which will control the disease should be selected. The viscosity of the scalp application has been adjusted so that the preparation spreads easily without being too fluid. The specially-designed bottle and nozzle allow easy application direct to the scalp through the hair.

4.5 Interaction with other medicinal products and other forms of Interaction

None known.

4.6 Pregnancy and lactation

There is inadequate evidence of safety in human pregnancy. Topical administration of corticosteroids to pregnant animals can cause abnormalities of fetal development including cleft palate and intrauterine growth retardation. There may therefore be a very small risk of such effects in the human foetus.

4.7 Effects on ability to drive and use machines

None known.

4.8 Undesirable effects

Adverse events are listed below by system organ class and frequency. Frequencies are defined as: very common (≥1/10), common (≥1/100 and <1/10), uncommon (≥1/1000 and <1/100), rare (≥1/10,000 and <1/1000) and very rare (<1/10,000) including isolated reports. Very common, common and uncommon events were generally determined from clinical trial data. The background rates in placebo and comparator groups were not taken into account when assigning frequency categories to adverse events derived from clinical trial data, since these rates were generally comparable to those in the active treatment group. Rare and very rare events were generally determined from spontaneous data.

Immune system disorders

Very rare: Hypersensitivity.

If signs of hypersensitivity appear, application should be stopped immediately.

Endocrine disorders

Very rare: Features of Cushing's syndrome

As with other topical corticosteroids, prolonged use of large amounts or treatment of extensive areas can result in sufficient systemic absorption to produce suppression of the HPA axis and the clinical features of Cushing's syndrome (see Section 4.4 Special Warnings and Precautions for use). These effects are more likely to occur in infants and children, and if occlusive dressings are used.

Skin and subcutaneous tissue disorders

Common: Local skin burning and pruritus.

Very rare: Local atrophic changes in the skin such as thinning, striae and dilatation of the superficial blood vessels may be caused by prolonged and intensive treatment with highly active corticosteroid preparations, particularly when occlusive dressings are used or when skin folds are involved.

Pigmentation changes, hypertrichosis, allergic contact dermatitis, exacerbation of symptoms, pustular psoriasis (due to treatment of psoriasis with corticosteroids or its withdrawal: see Section 4.4. Special Warnings and Precautions for use)

4.9 Overdose

Acute overdosage is very unlikely to occur. However, in the case of chronic overdosage or misuse the features of Cushing's syndrome may appear and in this situation topical steroids should be discontinued gradually under medical supervision (see Section 4.4 Special Warnings and Precautions for use).

5. PHARMACOLOGICAL PROPERTIES

5.1 Pharmacodynamic properties

Betamethasone valerate is an active corticosteroid with topical anti-inflammatory activity.

5.2 Pharmacokinetic properties

The extent of percutaneous absorption of topical corticosteroids is determined by many factors including the vehicle, the integrity of the epidermal barrier, and the use of occlusive dressings.

Topical corticosteroids can be absorbed from normal intact skin. Inflammation and/or other disease processes in the skin increase percutaneous absorption.

Occlusive dressings substantially increase the percutaneous absorption of topical corticosteroids.

Once absorbed through the skin, topical corticosteroids are handled through pharmacokinetic pathways similar to systemically administered corticosteroids. Corticosteroids are bound to plasma proteins in varying degrees. Corticosteroids are metabolised primarily by the liver and are then excreted by the kidneys.

5.3 Preclinical safety data

There are no preclinical data of relevance to the prescriber which are additional to that in other sections of the SPC.

6. PHARMACEUTICAL PARTICULARS

6.1 List of excipients

Carbomer

Isopropyl Alcohol

Sodium Hydroxide

Purified Water

6.2 Incompatibilities

None known.

6.3 Shelf life

24 months.

6.4 Special precautions for storage

Store below 25°C

6.5 Nature and contents of container

Polyethylene squeeze bottle with a polyethylene nozzle and a polystyrene or polyethylene cap or white High Density Polyethylene (HDPE) Hostalen GF4750 and Remafin white CEG 020 container with a polyethylene nozzle and a polystyrene or polyethylene cap.

Pack size: 30ml; 100ml

Not all pack sizes may be marketed

6.6 Instructions for use and handling

No special instructions.

Administrative Data

7. MARKETING AUTHORISATION HOLDER

Glaxo Wellcome UK Limited

trading as GlaxoSmithKline UK

Stockley Park West

Uxbridge

Middlesex

UB11 1BT

8. MARKETING AUTHORISATION NUMBER(S)

PL 10949/0045.

9. DATE OF FIRST AUTHORISATION/RENEWAL OF THE AUTHORISATION

9 December 1997

10. DATE OF REVISION OF THE TEXT

25th January 2005

11. Legal Status

POM

Bettamousse

(UCB Pharma Limited)

1. NAME OF THE MEDICINAL PRODUCT

Bettamousse 1mg/g (0.1%) cutaneous foam

2. QUALITATIVE AND QUANTITATIVE COMPOSITION

Betamethasone 1mg/g (0.1%) as valerate.

For excipients, see 6.1.

3. PHARMACEUTICAL FORM

Cutaneous foam for use on the scalp.

Appearance: White, foam mousse

4. CLINICAL PARTICULARS

4.1 Therapeutic indications

Steroid responsive dermatoses of the scalp, such as psoriasis.

4.2 Posology and method of administration

Adults, the elderly and children (over the age of six years): No more than a "golf-ball" sized amount of mousse (containing approximately 3.5mg betamethasone), or proportionately less for children, to be massaged into the affected areas of the scalp twice daily (in the morning and evening) until the condition improves. If there is no improvement after 7 days, treatment should be discontinued. Once the condition has improved, application is reduced to once a day and after daily treatment it may be possible to maintain improvement by applying even less frequently. In children over the age of 6 years, this product should not, in general, be used for longer than 5 to 7 days.

Patients should be advised to use the product sparingly.

4.3 Contraindications

Bacterial, fungal, parasitic or viral infections of the scalp unless simultaneous treatment is initiated.

Hypersensitivity to any component of the preparation.

Dermatoses in children under six years of age.

4.4 Special warnings and special precautions for use

Avoid contact with the eyes, open wounds and mucosae. Do not use near a naked flame.

The least amount of mousse required to control the disease should be used for the shortest possible time. This should minimise the potential for long term side effects. This is particularly the case in children, as adrenal suppression can occur even without its use with an occlusive dressing.

As with other topical corticosteroids, at least monthly clinical review is recommended if treatment is prolonged, and it may be advisable to monitor for signs of systemic activity.

The use of topical corticosteroids in psoriasis requires careful supervision. Glucocorticoids can mask, activate and worsen a skin infection. Development of secondary infection requires appropriate antimicrobial therapy and may necessitate withdrawal of topical corticosteroid therapy. Occlusive treatment should be avoided when there are signs of secondary infection. There is a risk of the development of generalised pustular psoriasis or local or systemic toxicity due to impaired barrier function of the skin.

Tolerance may develop and rebound relapse may occur on withdrawal of treatment.

4.5 Interaction with other medicinal products and other forms of Interaction

Not relevant to topical use.

4.6 Pregnancy and lactation

There is inadequate evidence of safety in human pregnancy. Bettamousse should only be used in pregnancy or lactation if the potential benefit outweighs the risk. Topical administration of corticosteroids to pregnant animals can cause abnormalities of foetal development such as cleft palate, but the relevance of this in man is unknown. Reduced placental and birth weight have been recorded in animals and man after long-term treatment.

While betamethasone valerate passes over into the maternal milk, there appears to be little risk of therapeutic doses having an effect on the baby.

4.7 Effects on ability to drive and use machines

None known.

4.8 Undesirable effects

Prolonged use of large amounts, or treatment of extensive areas can result in sufficient systemic absorption to produce the features of hypercorticism and suppression of the hypothalamic-pituitary-adrenal axis. These effects are more likely to occur in children, and if occlusive dressings are used.

Individual cases of headache, stinging and pruritus have been described. If signs of hypersensitivity appear, application should be stopped immediately.

The following side effects can occur with topical use of steroids:

Less common: 1/100-1/1000. Skin atrophy, stria distensae. Secondary infection. Rosacea-like dermatitis (face). Ecchymoses.

Rare: <1/1000. Hypertrichosis. Hypersensitivity (steroid). Hypo-/hyper-pigmentation. Folliculitis. Telangiectases.

Other side effects include: purpura, acne (especially during prolonged application). Rarely, perioral dermatitis and systemic activity.

In rare instances, treatment of psoriasis with corticosteroids (or their withdrawal) is thought to have provoked the pustular form of the disease. (See Precautions).

4.9 Overdose

Acute overdosage is very unlikely to occur. However, in the case of chronic overdosage or misuse, the features of hypercorticism may appear. In this situation topical steroids should be discontinued under careful clinical supervision, with supportive therapy if appropriate.

5. PHARMACOLOGICAL PROPERTIES

5.1 Pharmacodynamic properties

Pharmacotherapeutic (ATC) code: DO7AC: Corticosteroids, dermatological preparations, potent (group III).

Betamethasone is a glucocorticosteroid which has topical anti-inflammatory activity.

5.2 Pharmacokinetic properties

Under conditions of normal use, topical administration of betamethasone is not associated with clinically significant systemic absorption.

5.3 Preclinical safety data

Topical administration of corticosteroids to pregnant animals has been associated with abnormalities of foetal development and growth retardation, although the relevance of this in humans is unknown.

6. PHARMACEUTICAL PARTICULARS

6.1 List of excipients

Cetyl alcohol

Stearyl alcohol

Polysorbate 60

Ethanol

Purified Water

Propylene glycol

Citric acid anhydrous

Potassium Citrate

Butane/Propane

6.2 Incompatibilities

None known.

6.3 Shelf life

Two years.

6.4 Special precautions for storage

Do not store above 25°C. Do not refrigerate.

6.5 Nature and contents of container

Pressurised container.

Aluminium EP-lined Cebal can with Precision valve and clear cover cap, with a net weight of 100g.

6.6 Instructions for use and handling

No special requirements

7. MARKETING AUTHORISATION HOLDER

Celltech Pharmaceuticals Limited

208 Bath Road

Slough

Berkshire SL1 3WE

UK

8. MARKETING AUTHORISATION NUMBER(S)

PL 00039/0488

9. DATE OF FIRST AUTHORISATION/RENEWAL OF THE AUTHORISATION

19 April 1996/19 April 2001

10. DATE OF REVISION OF THE TEXT

November 2001

Bezalip

(Roche Products Limited)

1. NAME OF THE MEDICINAL PRODUCT

Bezalip®

2. QUALITATIVE AND QUANTITATIVE COMPOSITION

Bezafibrate 200mg

3. PHARMACEUTICAL FORM

Tablet for oral use.

Bezalip is a round film-coated tablet with a white core and is imprinted BM/G6.

4. CLINICAL PARTICULARS

4.1 Therapeutic indications

Bezalip is indicated for use in hyperlipidaemias of Type IIa, IIb, III, IV and V (Fredrickson classification).

Bezalip should be employed only in patients with a fully defined and diagnosed lipid abnormality which is inadequately controlled by dietary means, or by other changes in life-style such as physical exercise and weight reduction, and in whom the long-term risks associated with the condition warrant treatment.

The rationale for the use of Bezalip is to control abnormalities of serum lipids and lipoproteins to reduce or prevent the long term effects which have been shown by many epidemiological studies to be positively and strongly correlated with such hyperlipidaemias.

4.2 Posology and method of administration

Adults

The recommended dosage for Bezalip tablets is three tablets daily, equivalent to 600mg bezafibrate. The tablets should be swallowed whole with a little fluid after each meal.

Elderly

No specific dosage reduction is necessary in elderly patients.

Children

At present there is inadequate information regarding an appropriate dosage in children.

Renal impairment

In patients with renal insufficiency the dose should be adjusted according to serum creatinine levels or creatinine clearance as shown in the following table;

Serum creatinine (μ mol/l)	Creatinine clearance (ml/min)	Dosage (tablets/day)
Up to 135	Over 60	3
136 – 225	60 – 40	2
226 – 530	40 – 15	1 every 1 or 2 days
Over 530	Less than 15	Contra-indicated

In dialysis patients the dosage must be further reduced. As a general rule a dosage of one Bezalip tablet every third day is recommended, to avoid overdosage. The patient should be carefully monitored.

The response to therapy is normally rapid, although a progressive improvement may occur over a number of weeks. Treatment should be withdrawn if an adequate response has not been achieved within 3 to 4 months.

4.3 Contraindications

Significant hepatic disease (other than fatty infiltration of the liver associated with raised triglyceride values), severe renal insufficiency (serum creatinine > 530μmol/l; creatinine clearance <15ml/min), gall bladder disease with or without cholelithiasis, nephrotic syndrome, known photo-allergic or phototoxic reactions to fibrates and hypersensitivity to bezafibrate or any component of the product or to other fibrates.

4.4 Special warnings and special precautions for use

See *Preclinical safety data.*

Bezafibrate could cause cholelithiasis, although there is no evidence of an increased frequency of gallstones in patients treated with Bezalip. Appropriate diagnostic procedures should be performed if cholelithic symptoms and signs occur (see section *4.8 Undesirable effects).*

Muscle effects: Bezafibrate and other fibrates may cause myopathy, manifested as muscle weakness or pain, often accompanied by a considerable increase in creatine kinase (CPK). In isolated cases severe muscle damage (rhabdomyolysis) may occur. The risk of rhabdomyolysis may be increased in patients with predisposing factors for myopathy, (including renal impairment, hypothyroidism, severe infection, trauma, surgery, disturbances of hormone or electrolyte imbalance and a high alcohol intake).

Bezafibrate should be used with caution in combination with HMG CoA reductase inhibitors as the combination of HMG CoA inhibitors and fibrates has been shown to increase the incidence and severity of myopathy. Patients should be monitored for signs of myopathy and increased CPK activity and combination therapy discontinued if signs of myopathy develop. Combination therapy should not be used in patients with predisposing factors for myopathy (see section *4.5 Interaction with other medicaments and other forms of interaction).*

4.5 Interaction with other medicinal products and other forms of Interaction

Care is required in administering Bezalip to patients taking coumarin-type anti-coagulants, the action of which may be potentiated. The dosage of anti-coagulant should be reduced by up to 50% and readjusted by monitoring blood coagulation.

As bezafibrate improves glucose utilisation the action of antidiabetic medication, including insulin, may be potentiated. Hypoglycaemia has not been observed although increased monitoring of the glycaemic status may be warranted for a brief period after introduction of Bezalip.

In isolated cases, a pronounced though reversible impairment of renal function (accompanied by a corresponding increase in serum creatinine level) has been reported in organ transplant patients receiving cyclosporin therapy and concomitant bezafibrate. Accordingly, renal function should be closely monitored in these patients and, in the event of relevant significant changes in laboratory parameters, bezafibrate, should if necessary, be discontinued.

Should combined therapy with an ion-exchange resin be considered necessary, there should be an interval of 2 hours between the intake of the resin and Bezalip as the absorption of bezafibrate otherwise may be impaired.

Concomitant therapy with HMG CoA reductase inhibitors and fibrates has been reported to increase the risk of myopathy (see section *4.4 Special warnings and precautions*). The underlying mechanism for this remains unclear; the available data do not suggest a pharmacokinetic interaction between bezafibrate and HMG CoA reductase inhibitors.

MAO-inhibitors (with hepatotoxic potential) should not be administered together with bezafibrate.

Since oestrogens may lead to a rise in lipid levels, the necessity for treatment with Bezalip in patients receiving oestrogens or oestrogen containing preparations should be considered on an individual basis.

4.6 Pregnancy and lactation
Although the drug substance has not been shown in animal studies to have any adverse effects on the foetus, it is recommended that Bezalip should not be administered to either pregnant women or to those who are breast feeding.

4.7 Effects on ability to drive and use machines
None known.

4.8 Undesirable effects
Gastro-intestinal system:

– occasionally gastro-intestinal symptoms such as loss of appetite, feelings of fullness in the stomach and nausea may occur. These side-effects are usually transient and generally do not require withdrawal of the drug. In susceptible patients a slowly increasing dosage over 5 to 7 days may help to avoid such symptoms.

Hepato-biliary system:

– in isolated cases, increase of transaminases, cholestasis and gallstones (see section *4.4 Special warnings and special precautions for use*).

Hypersensitivity:

– occasionally allergic skin reactions such as pruritus or urticaria.

– in isolated cases, photosensitivity or generalised hypersensitivity reactions may occur.

Haematology:

Isolated cases of:

– decreases in haemoglobin and leucocytes.

– thrombocytopenia, which may cause bleeding (e.g. purpura).

– pancytopenia.

Renal system:

– frequently slight increases in serum creatinine. In patients with existing impairment of renal function, if dosage recommendations are not followed, myopathy may develop (in extreme cases rhabdomyolysis).

Muscular system:

– Muscular weakness, myalgia and muscle cramps, often accompanied by a considerable increase in creatine kinase may occur. In isolated cases, severe muscular damage (rhabdomyolysis) has been observed. In cases of rhabdomyolysis, bezafibrate must be stopped immediately and renal function closely monitored.

Others:

– in rare cases, headache and dizziness, alopecia.

– isolated cases of potency disorders have been reported.

In general, most of the adverse drug reactions disappear after withdrawal of Bezalip.

4.9 Overdose
No specific effects of acute overdose are known. Rhabdomyolysis has occurred. In cases of rhabdomyolysis, bezafibrate must be stopped immediately and renal function carefully monitored.

5. PHARMACOLOGICAL PROPERTIES

5.1 Pharmacodynamic properties
Bezafibrate lowers elevated levels of serum cholesterol and triglycerides (i.e. lowers elevated low density lipoprotein and very low density lipoprotein levels, and raises lowered high density lipoprotein levels) by stimulating lipoprotein lipase and hepatic lipase, and by suppressing the activity of 3 HMGCo-A reductase resulting in stimulation of low density lipoprotein receptors on the cell surface.

Studies have shown bezafibrate to be effective in treating hyperlipidaemia in patients with diabetes mellitus. Some cases showed a beneficial reduction in fasting blood glucose.

Significant reductions in serum fibrinogen levels have been observed in hyperfibrinogenaemic patients treated with bezafibrate.

5.2 Pharmacokinetic properties
Maximum concentrations of bezafibrate appear around 2 hours after ingestion of Bezalip tablets. The protein-binding of bezafibrate in serum is approximately 95%. The elimination half-life is in the order of 2.1 hours although elimination is markedly slowed in the presence of limited renal function. Elimination may be increased in forced diuresis. The drug substance is non-dialysable (cuprophane filter).

5.3 Preclinical safety data
The chronic administration of a high dose of bezafibrate to rats was associated with hepatic tumour formation in females. This dosage was in the order of 30 to 40 times the human dosage. No such effect was apparent at reduced intake levels approximating more closely to the lipid-lowering dosage in humans.

6. PHARMACEUTICAL PARTICULARS

6.1 List of excipients
In addition to bezafibrate, the tablets contain maize starch, microcrystalline cellulose, colloidal silicon dioxide, sodium starch glycollate, magnesium stearate, polymethacrylic acid esters, lactose, polyethylene glycol, talc, kaolin, titanium dioxide (E171), polysorbate 80 and sodium citrate dihydrate.

6.2 Incompatibilities
Not applicable.

6.3 Shelf life
5 years.

6.4 Special precautions for storage
Bezalip tablets require no special storage conditions.

6.5 Nature and contents of container
Packs of 84 or 100 tablets in PVC/Aluminium blister strips.

6.6 Instructions for use and handling
Not applicable.

7. MARKETING AUTHORISATION HOLDER
Roche Products Limited, 40 Broadwater Road, Welwyn Garden City, Hertfordshire, AL7 3AY.

8. MARKETING AUTHORISATION NUMBER(S)
PL 00031/0523

9. DATE OF FIRST AUTHORISATION/RENEWAL OF THE AUTHORISATION
1 April 1999

10. DATE OF REVISION OF THE TEXT
November 2002

11. LEGAL STATUS
POM

Bezalip is a registered trade mark

P999685/1202

Bezalip Mono

(Roche Products Limited)

1. NAME OF THE MEDICINAL PRODUCT
Bezalip Mono

2. QUALITATIVE AND QUANTITATIVE COMPOSITION
Bezafibrate 400mg

3. PHARMACEUTICAL FORM
Modified release tablet for oral use.

Bezalip Mono is a round film-coated tablet with a white core and is imprinted BM/D9.

4. CLINICAL PARTICULARS

4.1 Therapeutic indications
Bezalip Mono is indicated for use in hyperlipidaemias of Type IIa, IIb, III, IV and V (Fredrickson classification).

Bezalip Mono should be employed only in patients with a fully defined and diagnosed lipid abnormality which is inadequately controlled by dietary means, or by other changes in life-style such as physical exercise and weight reduction, and in whom the long-term risks associated with the condition warrant treatment.

The rationale for the use of Bezalip Mono is to control abnormalities of serum lipids and lipoproteins to reduce or prevent the long term effects which have been shown by many epidemiological studies to be positively and strongly correlated with such hyperlipidaemias.

4.2 Posology and method of administration
Adults

The dosage for Bezalip Mono is one tablet daily, equivalent to 400mg bezafibrate. The tablets should be swallowed whole with a little fluid after a meal either at night or in the morning.

Elderly

No specific dosage reduction is necessary in elderly patients.

Children

At present there is inadequate information regarding an appropriate dosage in children.

Renal impairment

Bezalip Mono is contra-indicated in patients with renal impairment with serum creatinine> 135 micromol/l or creatinine clearance < 60ml/min. Such patients may be treated with conventional Bezalip tablets (200mg bezafibrate) using an appropriately reduced daily dosage.

The response to therapy is normally rapid, although a progressive improvement may occur over a number of weeks. Treatment should be withdrawn if an adequate response has not been achieved within 3 to 4 months.

4.3 Contraindications
Significant hepatic disease (other than fatty infiltration of the liver associated with raised triglyceride values), gall bladder disease with or without cholelithiasis, nephrotic syndrome or renal impairment (serum creatinine> 135 micromol/l or creatinine clearance < 60ml/min.) Patients undergoing dialysis, known photoallergic or phototoxic reactions to fibrates. Hypersensitivity to bezafibrate or any component of the product or to other fibrates.

4.4 Special warnings and special precautions for use
See *Preclinical safety data*.

Bezafibrate could cause cholelithiasis, although there is no evidence of an increased frequency of gallstones in patients treated with Bezalip Mono. Appropriate diagnostic procedures should be performed if cholelithic symptoms and signs occur (see section *4.8 Undesirable effects*).

Muscle effects: Bezafibrate and other fibrates may cause myopathy, manifested as muscle weakness or pain, often accompanied by a considerable increase in creatine kinase (CPK). In isolated cases severe muscle damage (rhabdomyolysis) may occur. The risk of rhabdomyolysis may be increased in patients with predisposing factors for myopathy, (including renal impairment, hypothyroidism, severe infection, trauma, surgery, disturbances of hormone or electrolyte imbalance and a high alcohol intake).

Bezafibrate should be used with caution in combination with HMG CoA reductase inhibitors as the combination of HMG CoA inhibitors and fibrates has been shown to increase the incidence and severity of myopathy. Patients should be monitored for signs of myopathy and increased CPK activity and combination therapy discontinued if signs of myopathy develop. Combination therapy should not be used in patients with predisposing factors for myopathy (see section *4.5 Interaction with other medicaments and other forms of interaction*).

4.5 Interaction with other medicinal products and other forms of Interaction
Care is required in administering Bezalip Mono to patients taking coumarin-type anti-coagulants, the action of which may be potentiated. The dosage of anti-coagulant should be reduced by up to 50% and readjusted by monitoring blood coagulation.

As bezafibrate improves glucose utilisation the action of antidiabetic medication, including insulin, may be potentiated. Hypoglycaemia has not been observed although increased monitoring of the glycaemic status may be warranted for a brief period after introduction of Bezalip Mono.

In isolated cases, a pronounced though reversible impairment of renal function (accompanied by a corresponding increase in serum creatinine level) has been reported in organ transplant patients receiving cyclosporin therapy and concomitant bezafibrate. Accordingly, renal function should be closely monitored in these patients and, in the event of relevant significant changes in laboratory parameters, bezafibrate, should if necessary, be discontinued.

Should combined therapy with an ion-exchange resin be considered necessary, there should be an interval of 2 hours between the intake of the resin and Bezalip Mono as the absorption of bezafibrate otherwise may be impaired.

Concomitant therapy with HMG CoA reductase inhibitors and fibrates has been reported to increase the risk of myopathy (see section *4.4 Special warnings and precautions*). The underlying mechanism for this remains unclear; the available data do not suggest a pharmacokinetic interaction between bezafibrate and HMG CoA reductase inhibitors.

MAO-inhibitors (with hepatotoxic potential) should not be administered together with bezafibrate.

Since oestrogens may lead to a rise in lipid levels, the necessity for treatment with Bezalip Mono in patients receiving oestrogens or oestrogen containing preparations should be considered on an individual basis.

4.6 Pregnancy and lactation
Although the drug substance has not been shown in animal studies to have any adverse effects on the foetus, it is recommended that Bezalip Mono should not be administered to either pregnant women or to those who are breast feeding.

4.7 Effects on ability to drive and use machines
None known.

4.8 Undesirable effects
Gastro-intestinal system:

– occasionally gastro-intestinal symptoms, such as loss of appetite, feelings of fullness in the stomach and nausea may occur. These side-effects are usually transient and generally do not require withdrawal of the drug. In susceptible patients a slowly increasing dosage over 5 to 7 days may help to avoid such symptoms.

Hepato-biliary system:

– in isolated cases, increase of transaminases, cholestasis and gallstones (see section *4.4 Special warnings and special precautions for use*).

Hypersensitivity:

– occasionally allergic skin reactions such as pruritus or urticaria.

– in isolated cases, photosensitivity or generalised hypersensitivity reactions may occur.

Haematology:

Isolated cases of:

– decreases in haemoglobin and leucocytes.

– thrombocytopenia, which may cause bleeding (e.g. purpura).

– pancytopenia.

Renal system:

– frequently slight increases in serum creatinine. In patients with existing impairment of renal function, if dosage recommendations are not followed, myopathy may develop (in extreme cases rhabdomyolysis).

Muscular system:

– Muscular weakness, myalgia and muscle cramps, often accompanied by a considerable increase in creatine kinase may occur. In isolated cases, severe muscular damage (rhabdomyolysis) has been observed. In cases of rhabdomyolysis, bezafibrate must be stopped immediately and renal function closely monitored.

Others:

– in rare cases, headache and dizziness, alopecia.

– isolated cases of potency disorders have been reported.

In general, most of the adverse drug reactions disappear after withdrawal of Bezalip Mono.

4.9 Overdose

No specific effects of acute overdose are known. Rhabdomyolysis has occurred. In cases of rhabdomyolysis bezafibrate must be stopped immediately and renal function carefully monitored.

5. PHARMACOLOGICAL PROPERTIES

5.1 Pharmacodynamic properties

Bezafibrate lowers elevated levels of serum cholesterol and triglycerides (i.e. lowers elevated low density lipoprotein and very low density lipoprotein levels, and raises lowered high density lipoprotein levels) by stimulating lipoprotein lipase and hepatic lipase, and by suppressing the activity of 3 HMGCo-A reductase resulting in stimulation of low density lipoprotein receptors on the cell surface.

Studies have shown bezafibrate to be effective in treating hyperlipidaemia in patients with diabetes mellitus. Some cases showed a beneficial reduction in fasting blood glucose.

Significant reductions in serum fibrinogen levels have been observed in hyperfibrinogenaemic patients treated with bezafibrate.

5.2 Pharmacokinetic properties

Maximum serum concentrations of bezafibrate appear around 4 hours after ingestion of Bezalip Mono tablets. The protein-binding of bezafibrate in serum is approximately 95%. The elimination half-life is in the order of 2.1 hours although elimination is markedly slowed in the presence of limited renal function.

5.3 Preclinical safety data

The chronic administration of a high dose of bezafibrate to rats was associated with hepatic tumour formation in females. This dosage was in the order of 30 to 40 times the human dosage. No such effect was apparent at reduced intake levels approximating more closely to the lipid-lowering dosage in humans.

6. PHARMACEUTICAL PARTICULARS

6.1 List of excipients

Lactose, povidone, sodium lauryl sulphate, hydroxypropyl methylcellulose, colloidal silicon dioxide, magnesium stearate, Eudragit E 30 D, polyethylene glycol, talc, titanium dioxide (E171), polysorbate 80 and sodium citrate dihydrate.

6.2 Incompatibilities

Not applicable.

6.3 Shelf life

5 years.

6.4 Special precautions for storage

Bezalip Mono requires no special storage conditions.

6.5 Nature and contents of container

Packs of 28 or 30 tablets in PVC/Aluminium blister strips. HDPE containers of 28 tablets.

6.6 Instructions for use and handling

Not applicable.

7. MARKETING AUTHORISATION HOLDER

Roche Products Limited, 40 Broadwater Road, Welwyn Garden City, Hertfordshire, AL7 3AY.

8. MARKETING AUTHORISATION NUMBER(S)

PL 00031/0524

9. DATE OF FIRST AUTHORISATION/RENEWAL OF THE AUTHORISATION

1 April 1999

10. DATE OF REVISION OF THE TEXT

November 2002

11. LEGAL STATUS

POM

Bezalip is a registered trade mark

P999684/1202

BiCNU Injection

(Bristol-Myers Pharmaceuticals)

1. NAME OF THE MEDICINAL PRODUCT

BiCNU Injection.

2. QUALITATIVE AND QUANTITATIVE COMPOSITION

100mg carmustine in a 30ml vial and 3ml ethanol diluent in a 5ml vial.

3. PHARMACEUTICAL FORM

Powder and solvent for solution for infusion.

4. CLINICAL PARTICULARS

4.1 Therapeutic indications

BiCNU is indicated as palliative therapy as a single agent or in established combination therapy with other approved chemotherapeutic agents in the following:

1. Brain tumours - lioblastoma, brainstem glioma, medullablastoma, astrocytoma, ependymoma, and metastatic brain tumours.

2. Multiple myeloma - In combination with prednisone.

3. Hodgkin's Disease - As secondary therapy in combination with other approved drugs in patients who relapse while being treated with primary therapy, or who fail to respond to primary therapy.

4. Non Hodgkin's lymphomas - As secondary therapy in combination with other approved drugs in patients who relapse while being treated with primary therapy, or who fail to respond to primary therapy.

4.2 Posology and method of administration

Adults:

Intravenous administration:

The recommended dose of BiCNU as single agent in previously untreated patients is 200mg/m^2 intravenously every six weeks. This may be given as a single dose or divided into daily injections such as 100mg/m^2 on two successive days.

When BiCNU is used in combination with other myelosuppressive drugs or in patients in whom bone marrow reserve is depleted the doses should be adjusted accordingly.

A repeat course of BiCNU should not be given until circulating blood elements have returned to acceptable levels (platelets above 100,000/mm^3; leucocytes above 4,000/mm^3) and this is usually in six weeks. Blood counts should be monitored frequently and repeat courses should not be given before six weeks because of delayed toxicity.

Doses subsequent to the initial dose should be adjusted according to the haematological response of the patient to the preceding dose. The following schedule is suggested as a guide to dosage adjustment.

Nadir after Prior Dose		*Percentage of prior dose to be given*
Leucocytes (mm^3)	*Platelets (mm^3)*	
>4000	>100,000	100
3000 - 3999	75,000 - 99,999	100
2000 - 2999	25,000 - 74,999	70
<2000	<25,000	50

Children:

BiCNU should be used with extreme caution in children due to the high risk of pulmonary toxicity (see Warnings).

Elderly:

No dosage adjustment is required on the grounds of age.

Route of administration: Following reconstitution with sterile absolute ethanol (3 ml vial provided) and dilution with water for injections, BiCNU should be administered by intravenous drip over a one to two hour period. The solution may be further diluted prior to administration with sodium chloride for injection or 5% dextrose for injection.

4.3 Contraindications

BiCNU should not be given to individuals who have demonstrated a previous hypersensitivity to it.

BiCNU should not be given to individuals with decreased circulating platelets, leucocytes, or erythrocytes either from previous chemotherapy or other causes.

4.4 Special warnings and special precautions for use

Pulmonary toxicity characterised by pulmonary infiltrates and/or fibrosis has been reported to occur with a frequency ranging up to 30%. This may occur within 3 years of therapy and appears to be dose related with total cumulative doses of 1200-1500mg/m^2 being associated with increased likelihood of lung fibrosis. Risk factors include smoking, the presence of a respiratory condition, pre-existing radiographic abnormalities, sequential or concomitant thoracic irradiation and association with other agents that cause lung damage.

Cases of late pulmonary fibrosis, occurring up to 17 years after treatment, have also been reported. In a long-term follow-up of 17 patients who survived childhood brain tumours eight (47%) died of lung fibrosis. Of these eight deaths, two occurred within 3 years of treatment and 6 occurred 8-13 years after treatment. Of the patients who died, the median age at treatment was 2.5 years (range 1-12); the median age of the long-term survivors was 10 years (5-16 years at treatment). All five patients treated under the age of 5 years have died of pulmonary fibrosis. In this study, the dose of BiCNU did not influence fatal outcome nor did co-administration of vincristine or spinal irradiation. Of the remaining survivors available for follow-up, evidence of lung fibrosis was detected in all patients. The risks and benefits of BiCNU therapy must be carefully considered especially in young patients, due to extremely high risk of pulmonary toxicity.

BiCNU is carcinogenic in rats and mice, producing a marked increase in tumour incidence in doses approximately those employed clinically.

BiCNU should be administered by individuals experienced in antineoplastic therapy. Bone marrow toxicity is a common and severe toxic effect of BiCNU. Complete blood counts should be monitored frequently for at least six weeks after a dose. Repeat doses of BiCNU should not be given more frequently than every six weeks.

The bone marrow toxicity of BiCNU is cumulative and therefore dosage adjustment must be considered on the basis of nadir blood counts from prior dose (see Dosage Adjustment Table under Dosage).

It is recommended that liver function, kidney function and pulmonary function also be monitored.

4.5 Interaction with other medicinal products and other forms of Interaction

None known.

4.6 Pregnancy and lactation

BiCNU should not normally be administered to patients who are pregnant or mothers who are breast feeding. Male patients should be advised to use adequate contraceptive measures.

Safe use in pregnancy has not been established and therefore the benefit to risk of toxicity must be carefully weighed. BiCNU is embryotoxic and teratogenic in rats and embryotoxic in rabbits at dose levels equivalent to the human dose. BiCNU also affects fertility in male rats at doses somewhat higher than the human dose.

4.7 Effects on ability to drive and use machines

None known.

4.8 Undesirable effects

Haematological:

Delayed myelosuppression is a frequent and serious adverse event associated with BiCNU administration. It usually occurs four to six weeks after drug administration and is dose related. Platelet nadirs occur at four to five weeks; leucocyte nadirs occur at five to six weeks post therapy. Thrombocytopenia is generally more severe than leucopenia. However both may be dose limiting toxicities. Anaemia also occurs, but is generally less severe. The occurrence of acute leukaemia and bone marrow dysplasias have been reported in patients following long term nitrosourea therapy.

Gastro-intestinal:

Nausea and vomiting after i.v. administration of BiCNU are noted frequently. This reaction appears within two hours of dosing, usually lasting four to six hours and is dose related. Prior administration of anti-emetics is effective in diminishing and sometimes preventing this side effect.

Hepatic:

When high doses of BiCNU have been employed, a reversible type of hepatic toxicity, manifested by increased transaminase, alkaline phosphatase and bilirubin levels, has been reported in a small percentage of patients.

Pulmonary:

See Warnings and Precautions (Section 4.4)

Renal:

Renal abnormalities consisting of decrease in kidney size, progressive azotaemia and renal failure have been reported in patients who receive large cumulative doses after prolonged therapy with BiCNU and related nitrosoureas. Kidney damage has also been reported in patients receiving lower total doses.

Cardiovascular:

Hypotension and tachycardia have been reported.

Local:

Burning at the site of injection is common but true thrombosis is rare.

Other:

Rapid i.v. infusion of BiCNU may produce intense flushing of the skin and suffusion of the conjunctiva within two hours, lasting about four hours.

Neuroretinitis, chest pain, headache, and allergic reactions have been reported.

4.9 Overdose
None known.

5. PHARMACOLOGICAL PROPERTIES

5.1 Pharmacodynamic properties
BiCNU alkylates DNA and RNA has also been shown to inhibit several enzymes by carbamoylation of amino acids in proteins. It is thought that the antineoplastic and toxic activities of BiCNU may be due to metabolites.

5.2 Pharmacokinetic properties
Intravenously administered BiCNU is rapidly degraded, with no intact drug detectable after 15 minutes. However, in studies with C^{14} labelled drug, prolonged levels of the isotope were observed in the plasma and tissue, probably representing radioactive fragments of the parent compound.

Approximately 60 to 70% of a total dose is excreted in the urine in 96 hours and about 10% as respiratory CO_2. The fate of the remainder is undetermined.

Because of the high lipid solubility and the relative lack of ionisation at a physiological pH, BiCNU crosses the blood brain barrier. Levels of radioactivity in the CSF are at least 50% higher than those measured concurrently in plasma.

5.3 Preclinical safety data
No further relevant data available.

6. PHARMACEUTICAL PARTICULARS

6.1 List of excipients
Ethanol.

6.2 Incompatibilities
Compatibility/Incompatibility with Containers

The intravenous solution is suitable for infusion in polythene or glass containers. Studies have shown carmustine to be incompatible with PVC containers as it is readily adsorbed on to the plastic.

6.3 Shelf life
3 Years.

6.4 Special precautions for storage
Unopened vials: Store at 2-8°C.

Reconstituted solution (diluted or undiluted): Store at 2-8°C for 24 hours and protect from light.

6.5 Nature and contents of container
Powder: Type I amber glass vial (30ml) sealed with a grey butyl lyophilising stopper and an aluminium seal/polypropelene cap.

Diluent: Type I glass vial (5ml) with an aluminium seal/ polypropylene cap.

6.6 Instructions for use and handling
IMPORTANT NOTE: The lyophilised dosage formulation contains no preservatives and is not intended as multiple dose vial. Reconstitutions and further dilutions should be carried out under aseptic conditions.

Preparation of intravenous solution:

Dissolve BiCNU with 3ml of the supplied sterile diluent (absolute ethanol) and then aseptically add 27ml of sterile water for injection to the alcohol solution. Each ml of the resulting solution will contain 3.3mg of BiCNU in 10% ethanol and has a pH of 5.6 to 6.0.

Reconstitution as recommended results in a clear colourless solution which may be further diluted to 500ml sodium chloride for injection, or 5% glucose for injection. The reconstituted solution must be given intravenously and should be administered by i.v. drip over a one- to two-hour period. Injection of BiCNU over shorter periods of time may produce intense pain and burning at the site of injection.

IMPORTANT NOTE: BiCNU has a low melting point (approximately 30.5-32.0°C or 86.9-89.6°F). Exposure of the drug to this temperature or above will cause the drug to liquefy and appear as an oil film in the bottom of the vials. This is a sign of decomposition and vials should be discarded.

Guidelines for the safe handling of antineoplastic agents:

1. Trained personnel should reconstitute the drug.
2. This should be performed in a designated area.
3. Adequate protective gloves should be worn.
4. Precautions should be taken to avoid the drug accidentally coming into contact with the eyes. In the event of contact with the eyes, flush with copious amounts of water and/or saline.
5. The cytotoxic preparation should not be handled by pregnant staff.
6. Adequate care and precaution should be taken in the disposal of items (syringes, needles etc) used to reconstitute cytotoxic drugs. Excess material and body waste may be disposed of by placing in double sealed polythene bags and incinerating at a temperature of 1,000°C. Liquid waste may be flushed with copious amounts of water.
7. The work surface should be covered with disposable plastic-backed absorbent paper.
8. Use Luer-Lock fittings on all syringes and sets. Large bore needles are recommended to minimise pressure and the possible formation of aerosols. The latter may also be reduced by the use of a venting needle.

7. MARKETING AUTHORISATION HOLDER
Bristol-Myers Squibb Holdings Ltd.
t/a Bristol-Myers Pharmaceuticals
Uxbridge Business Park
Sanderson Road
Uxbridge
Middlesex
UB8 1DH

8. MARKETING AUTHORISATION NUMBER(S)
PL 0125/0108

9. DATE OF FIRST AUTHORISATION/RENEWAL OF THE AUTHORISATION
6 March 1979 / 4 April 1995 / 30 April 2002

10. DATE OF REVISION OF THE TEXT
July 2005

Binovum Oral Contraceptive Tablets

(Janssen-Cilag Ltd)

1. NAME OF THE MEDICINAL PRODUCT
BINOVUM® Oral Contraceptive Tablets.

Recommended international non-proprietary name
norethisterone
ethinylestradiol

2. QUALITATIVE AND QUANTITATIVE COMPOSITION
Binovum are tablets for oral administration.

Each white tablet contains norethisterone PhEur 0.5 mg and ethinylestradiol PhEur 0.035 mg.

Each peach coloured tablet contains norethisterone PhEur 1.0 mg and ethinylestradiol PhEur 0.035 mg.

3. PHARMACEUTICAL FORM
Tablets.

The white tablets are small, round and engraved C 535 on both faces.

The peach-coloured tablets are small, round and engraved C 135 on both faces.

4. CLINICAL PARTICULARS

4.1 Therapeutic indications
Contraception and the recognised indications for such oestrogen/progestogen combinations.

4.2 Posology and method of administration
Adults
It is preferable that tablet intake from the first pack is started on the first day of menstruation in which case no extra contraceptive precautions are necessary.

If menstruation has already begun (that is 2, 3 or 4 days previously), tablet taking should commence on day 5 of the menstrual period. In this case, additional contraceptive precautions must be taken for the first 7 days of tablet taking.

If menstruation began more than 5 days previously then the patient should be advised to wait until her next menstrual period before starting to take Binovum.

How to take Binovum:

One tablet is taken daily at the same time (preferably in the evening) without interruption for 21 days, followed by a break of 7 tablet-free days. (A white tablet is taken every day for 7 days, then a peach coloured tablet is taken every day for 14 days, then 7 tablet-free days). Each subsequent pack is started after the 7 tablet-free days have elapsed. Additional contraceptive precautions are not then required.

Elderly:

Not applicable.

Children:

Not recommended.

4.3 Contraindications
Absolute contra-indications
– Pregnancy or suspected pregnancy (that cannot yet be excluded).

– Circulatory disorders (cardiovascular or cerebrovascular) such as thrombophlebitis and thrombo-embolic processes, or a history of these conditions (including history of confirmed venous thrombo-embolism (VTE), family history of idiopathic VTE and other known risk factors for VTE), moderate to severe hypertension, hyperlipoproteinaemia. In addition, the presence of more than one of the risk factors for arterial disease.

– Severe liver disease, cholestatic jaundice or hepatitis (viral or non-viral) or a history of these conditions if the results of liver function tests have failed to return to normal, and for 3 months after liver function tests have been found to be normal; a history of jaundice of pregnancy or jaundice due to the use of steroids, Rotor syndrome and Dubin-Johnson syndrome, hepatic cell tumours and porphyria.

– Cholelithiasis.

– Known or suspected oestrogen-dependent tumours; endometrial hyperplasia; undiagnosed vaginal bleeding.

– Systemic lupus erythematosus or a history of this condition.

– A history during pregnancy or previous use of steroids of:

- severe pruritus
- herpes gestationis
- a manifestation or deterioration of otosclerosis

Relative contra-indications:

If any relative contra-indication listed below are present, the benefits of oestrogen/progestogen containing preparations must be weighed against the possible risk for each individual case and the patient kept under close supervision. In case of aggravation or appearance of any of these conditions whilst the patient is taking the pill, its use should be discontinued.

– Conditions implicating an increasing risk of developing venous thrombo-embolic complications, eg severe varicose veins or prolonged immobilisation or major surgery. Disorders of coagulation.

– Presence of any risk factor for arterial disease e.g. smoking, hyperlipidaemia or hypertension.

– Other conditions associated with an increased risk of circulatory disease such as latent or overt cardiac failure, renal dysfunction, or a history of these conditions.

– Epilepsy or a history of this condition.

– Migraine or a history of this condition.

– A history of cholelithiasis.

– Presence of any risk factor for oestrogen-dependent tumours; oestrogen-sensitive gynaecological disorders such as uterine fibromyomata and endometriosis.

– Diabetes mellitus.

– Severe depression or a history of this condition. If this is accompanied by a disturbance in tryptophan metabolism, administration of vitamin B6 might be of therapeutic value.

– Sickle cell haemoglobinopathy, since under certain circumstances, e.g. during infections or anoxia, oestrogen containing preparations may induce thrombo-embolic process in patients with this condition.

– If the results of liver function tests become abnormal, use should be discontinued.

4.4 Special warnings and special precautions for use
Post partum administration
Following a vaginal delivery, oral contraceptive administration to non-breast-feeding mothers can be started 21 days post-partum provided the patient is fully ambulant and there are no puerperal complications. No additional contraceptive precautions are required. If post partum administration begins more than 21 days after delivery, additional contraceptive precautions are required for the first 7 days of pill-taking.

If intercourse has taken place post-partum, oral contraceptive use should be delayed until the first day of the first menstrual period.

After miscarriage or abortion, administration should start immediately, in which case no additional contraceptive precautions are required.

Changing from a 21 day pill or 22 day pill to Binovum
All tablets in the old pack should be finished. The first Binovum tablet is taken the next day i.e. no gap is left between taking tablets nor does the patient need to wait for her period to begin. Tablets should be taken as instructed in 'How to take Binovum' (see 4.2). Additional contraceptive precautions are not required. The patient will not have a period until the end of the first Binovum pack, but this is not harmful, nor does it matter if she experiences some bleeding on tablet-taking days.

Changing from a combined every day pill (28 day tablet) to Binovum
Binovum should be started after taking the last active tablet from the 'Every day Pill' pack (ie after taking 21 or 22 tablets). The first Binovum tablet is taken the next day, ie no gap is left between taking tablets nor does the patient need to wait for her period to begin. Tablets should be taken as instructed in 'How to take Binovum' (see 4.2). Additional contraceptive precautions are not required. Remaining tablets from the every day (ED) pack should be discarded.

The patient will not have a period until the end of the first Binovum pack, but this is not harmful, nor does it matter if she experiences some bleeding on tablet-taking days.

Changing from a progestogen-only pill (POP or mini pill) to Binovum
The first Binovum tablet should be taken on the first day of the period, even if the patient has already taken a mini pill on that day. Tablets should be taken as instructed in 'How to take Binovum' (see 4.2). Additional contraceptive precautions are not required. All the remaining progestogen-only pills in the mini pill pack should be discarded.

If the patient is taking a mini pill, then she may not always have a period, especially when she is breast-feeding. The first Binovum tablet should be taken on the day after stopping the mini pill. All remaining pills in the mini pill packet must be discarded. Additional contraceptive precautions must be taken for the first 7 days.

To skip a period

To skip a period, a new pack of Binovum should be started on the day after finishing the current pack (the patient skips the tablet-free days). Tablet-taking should be continued in the usual way.

During the use of the second pack, she may experience slight spotting or break-through bleeding but contraceptive protection will not be diminished provided there are no tablet omissions.

The next pack of Binovum is started after the usual 7 tablet-free days, regardless of whether the period has completely finished or not.

Reduced reliability

When Binovum is taken according to the directions for use the occurrence of pregnancy is highly unlikely. However the reliability of oral contraceptives may be reduced under the following circumstances:

i) Forgotten tablets

If the patient forgets to take a tablet, she should take it as soon as she remembers and take the next one at the normal time. This may mean that two tablets are taken in one day. Provided she is less than 12 hours late in taking her tablet, Binovum will still give contraceptive protection during this cycle and the rest of the pack should be taken as usual.

If she is more than 12 hours late in taking one or more tablets, then she should take the last missed pill as soon as she remembers but leave the other missed pills in the pack. She should continue to take the rest of the pack as usual but must use extra precautions (e.g. sheath, diaphragm, plus spermicide) and follow the '7-day rule' (see Further Information for the '7 day rule').

If there are 7 or more pills left in the pack after the missed and delayed pills then the usual 7-day break can be left before starting the next pack. If there are less than 7 pills left in the pack after the missed and delayed pills then when the pack is finished the next pack should be started the next day. If withdrawal bleeding does not occur at the end of the second pack then a pregnancy test should be performed.

ii) Vomiting or diarrhoea

If after tablet intake, vomiting or diarrhoea occurs, a tablet may not be absorbed properly by the body. If the symptoms disappear within 12 hours of tablet-taking, the patient should take an extra tablet from a spare pack and continue with the rest of the pack as usual.

However, if the symptoms continue beyond those 12 hours, additional contraceptive precautions are necessary for any sexual intercourse during the stomach or bowel upset and for the following 7 days (the patient must be advised to follow the '7-day rule').

iii) Change in bleeding pattern

If after taking Binovum for several months there is a sudden occurrence of spotting or breakthrough bleeding (not observed in previous cycles) or the absence of withdrawal bleeding, contraceptive effectiveness may be reduced. If withdrawal bleeding fails to occur and none of the above mentioned events has taken place, pregnancy is highly unlikely and oral contraceptive use can be continued until the end of the next pack. (If withdrawal bleeding fails to occur at the end of the second cycle, tablet intake should be discontinued and pregnancy excluded before oral contraceptive use can be resumed.) However, if withdrawal bleeding is absent and any of the above mentioned events has occurred, tablet intake should be discontinued and pregnancy excluded before oral contraceptive use can be resumed.

Medical examination/consultation

Assessment of women prior to starting oral contraceptives (and at regular intervals thereafter) should include a personal and family medical history of each woman. Physical examination should be guided by this and by the contra-indications (Section 4.3) and warnings (Section 4.4) for this product. The frequency and nature of these assessments should be based upon relevant guidelines and should be adapted to the individual woman, but should include measurement of blood pressure and, if judged appropriate by the clinician, breast, abdominal and pelvic examination including cervical cytology.

Caution should be observed when prescribing oral contraceptives to young women whose cycles are not yet stabilised.

Venous thrombo-embolic disease

An increased risk of venous thrombo-embolic disease (VTE) associated with the use of oral contraceptives is well established but is smaller than that associated with pregnancy, which has been estimated at 60 cases per 100,000 pregnancies. Some epidemiological studies have reported a greater risk of VTE for women using combined oral contraceptives containing desogestrel or gestodene (the so-called 'third generation' pills) than for women using pills containing levonorgestrel or norethisterone (the so-called 'second generation' pills).

The spontaneous incidence of VTE in healthy non-pregnant women (not taking any oral contraceptive) is about 5 cases per 100,000 per year. The incidence in users of second generation pills is about 15 per 100,000 women per year of use. The incidence in users of third generation pills is about 25 cases per 100,000 women per year of use; this excess incidence has not been satisfactorily explained by bias or confounding. The level of all of these risks of VTE increases with age and is likely to be further increased in women with other known risk factors for VTE such as obesity. The excess risk of VTE is highest during the first year a woman ever uses a combined oral contraceptive.

Surgery, varicose veins or immobilisation

In patients using oestrogen-containing preparations, the risk of deep vein thrombosis may be temporarily increased when undergoing a major operation (eg abdominal, orthopaedic), and surgery to the legs, medical treatment for varicose veins or prolonged immobilisation. Therefore, it is advisable to discontinue oral contraceptive use at least 4 to 6 weeks prior to these procedures if performed electively and to (re)start not less than 2 weeks after full ambulation. The latter is also valid with regard to immobilisation after an accident or emergency surgery. In case of emergency surgery, thrombotic prophylaxis is usually indicated, eg with subcutaneous heparin.

Chloasma

Chloasma may occasionally occur, especially in women with a history of chloasma gravidarum. Women with a tendency to chloasma should avoid exposure to the sun or ultraviolet radiation whilst taking this preparation. Chloasma is often not fully reversible.

Laboratory tests

The use of steroids may influence the results of certain laboratory tests. In the literature, at least a hundred different parameters have been reported to possibly be influenced by oral contraceptive use, predominantly by the oestrogenic component. Among these are: biochemical parameters of the liver, thyroid, adrenal and renal function, plasma levels of (carrier) proteins and lipid/lipoprotein fractions and parameters of coagulation and fibrinolysis.

Further information

Additional contraceptive precautions

When additional contraceptive precautions are required, the patient should be advised either not to have sex, or to use a cap plus spermicide or for her partner to use a condom. Rhythm methods should not be advised as the pill disrupts the usual cyclical changes associated with the natural menstrual cycle, eg changes in temperature and cervical mucus.

The 7-day rule

If any one tablet is forgotten for more than 12 hours.

If the patient has vomiting or diarrhoea for more than 12 hours.

If the patient is taking any of the drugs listed under 'Interactions'.

The patient should continue to take her tablets as usual and:

– Additional contraceptive precautions must be taken for the next 7 days.

But - if these 7 days run beyond the end of the current pack, the next pack must be started as soon as the current one is finished, ie no gap should be left between packs. (This prevents an extended break in tablet taking which may increase the risk of the ovaries releasing an egg and thus reducing contraceptive protection.) The patient will not have a period until the end of 2 packs but this is not harmful nor does it matter if she experiences some bleeding on tablet taking days.

4.5 Interaction with other medicinal products and other forms of Interaction

Irregular cycles and reduced reliability of oral contraceptives may occur when these preparations are used concomitantly with drugs such as anticonvulsants, barbiturates, antibiotics (eg tetracyclines, ampicillin, rifampicin, etc), griseofulvin, activated charcoal and certain laxatives. Special consideration should be given to patients being treated with antibiotics for acne. They should be advised to use a non-hormonal method of contraception, or to use an oral contraceptive containing a progestogen showing minimal androgenicity, which have been reported as helping to improve acne without using an antibiotic. Oral contraceptives may diminish glucose tolerance and increase the need for insulin or other antidiabetic drugs in diabetics.

The herbal remedy St John's Wort *(Hypericum perforatum)* should not be taken concomitantly with this medicine as this could potentially lead to a loss of contraceptive effect.

4.6 Pregnancy and lactation

Binovum is contra-indicated for use during pregnancy or suspected pregnancy, since it has been suggested that combined oral contraceptives, in common with many other substances, might be capable of affecting the normal development of the child in the early stages of pregnancy. It can be concluded, however, that, if a risk of abnormality exists at all, it must be very small.

Mothers who are breast-feeding should be advised not to use the combined pill since this may reduce the amount of breast milk, but may be advised instead to use a progestogen-only pill (POP).

4.7 Effects on ability to drive and use machines

Not applicable.

4.8 Undesirable effects

Various adverse reactions have been associated with oral contraceptive use. The first appearance of symptoms indicative of any one of these reactions necessitates immediate cessation of oral contraceptive use while appropriate diagnostic and therapeutic measures are undertaken.

Serious Adverse Reactions

– There is a general opinion, based on statistical evidence that users of combined oral contraceptives experience more often than non-users, various disorders of the coagulation. How often these disorders occur in users of modern low-oestrogen oral contraceptives is unknown, but there are reasons for suggesting that they may occur less often than with the older types of pill which contain more oestrogen.

Various reports have associated oral contraceptive use with the occurrence of deep venous thrombosis, pulmonary embolism and other embolisms. Other investigations of these oral contraceptives have suggested an increased risk of oestrogen and/or progestogen dose-dependent coronary and cerebrovascular accidents, predominantly in heavy smokers. Thrombosis has very rarely been reported to occur in other veins or arteries, eg hepatic, mesenteric, renal or retinal.

It should be noted that there is no consensus about often contradictory findings obtained in early studies. The physician should bear in mind the possibility of vascular accidents occurring and that there may not be full recovery from such disorders and they may be fatal. The physician should take into account the presence of risk factors for arterial disease and deep venous thrombosis when prescribing oral contraceptives. Risk factors for arterial disease include smoking, the presence of hyperlipidaemia, hypertension or diabetes.

Signs and symptoms of a thrombotic event may include: sudden severe pain in the chest, whether or not reaching to the left arm; sudden breathlessness; and unusual severe, prolonged headache, especially if it occurs for the first time or gets progressively worse, or is associated with any of the following symptoms: sudden partial or complete loss of vision or diplopia, aphasia, vertigo, a bad fainting attack or collapse with or without focal epilepsy, weakness or very marked numbness suddenly affecting one side or one part of the body, motor disturbances; severe pain in the calf of one leg; acute abdomen.

Cigarette smoking increases the risk of serious cardiovascular adverse reactions to oral contraceptive use. The risk increases with age and with heavy smoking and is more marked in women over 35 years of age. Women who use oral contraceptives should be strongly advised not to smoke.

– The use of oestrogen-containing oral contraceptives may promote growth of existing sex steroid dependent tumours. For this reason, the use of these oral contraceptives in patients with such tumours is contra-indicated. Numerous epidemiological studies have been reported on the risk of ovarian, endometrial, cervical and breast cancer in women using combined oral contraceptives.

The evidence is clear that combined oral contraceptives offer substantial protection against both ovarian and endometrial cancer. An increased risk of cervical cancer in long term users of combined oral contraceptives has been reported in some studies, but there continues to be controversy about the extent to which this is attributable to the confounding effects of sexual behaviour and other factors.

A meta-analysis from 54 epidemiological studies reported that there is a slightly increased relative risk (RR = 1.24) of having breast cancer diagnosed in women who are currently using combined oral contraceptives (COCs). The observed pattern of increased risk may be due to an earlier diagnosis of breast cancer in COC users, the biological effects of COCs or a combination of both. The additional breast cancers diagnosed in current users of COCs or in women who have used COCs in the last 10 years are more likely to be localised to the breast than those in women who never used COCs.

Breast cancer is rare among women under 40 years of age whether or not they take COCs. Whilst this background risk increases with age, the excess number of breast cancer diagnoses in current and recent COC users is small in relation to the overall risk of breast cancer (see bar chart).

The most important risk factor for breast cancer in COC users is the age women discontinue the COC; the older the age at stopping, the more breast cancers are diagnosed. Duration of use is less important and the excess risk gradually disappears during the course of the 10 years after stopping COC use such that by 10 years there appears to be no excess.

The possible increase in risk of breast cancer should be discussed with the user and weighed against the benefits of COCs taking into account the evidence that they offer substantial protection against the risk of developing certain other cancers (eg ovarian and endometrial cancer).

(see Figure 1 on next page)

Figure 1

Estimated number of breast cancers found in 10,000 women who took the Pill for 5 years then stopped, or who never took the Pill

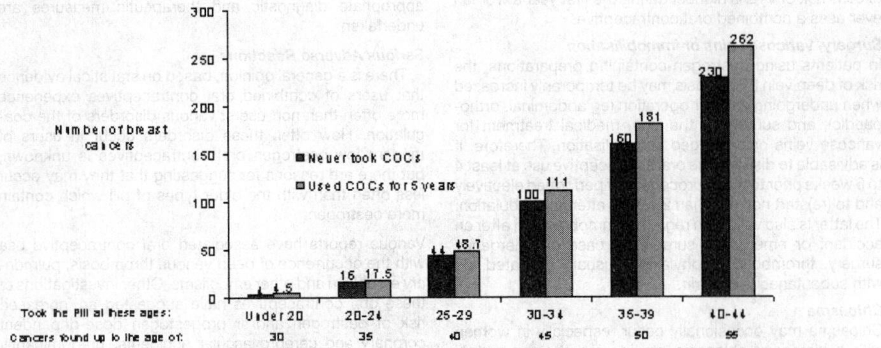

– Malignant hepatic tumours have been reported on rare occasions in long-term users of oral contraceptives. Benign hepatic tumours have also been associated with oral contraceptive usage. A hepatic tumour should be considered in the differential diagnosis when upper abdominal pain, enlarged liver or signs of intra-abdominal haemorrhage occur.

– The use of oral contraceptives may sometimes lead to the development of cholestatic jaundice or cholelithiasis.

– On rare occasions the use of oral contraceptives may trigger or reactivate systemic lupus erythematosus.

– A further rare complication of oral contraceptive use is the occurrence of chorea which can be reversed by discontinuing the pill. The majority of cases of oral contraceptive-induced chorea show a pre-existing predisposition which often relates to acute rheumatism.

Other Adverse Reactions

– Cardiovascular System

Rise of blood pressure. If hypertension develops, treatment should be discontinued.

– Genital Tract

Intermenstrual bleeding, post-medication amenorrhoea, changes in cervical secretion, increase in size of uterine fibromyomata, aggravation of endometriosis, certain vaginal infections, eg candidosis.

– Breast

Tenderness, pain, enlargement, secretion.

– Gastro-intestinal Tract

Nausea, vomiting, cholelithiasis, cholestatic jaundice.

– Skin

Erythema nodosum, rash, chloasma, erythema multiforme, hirsutism, loss of scalp hair.

– Eyes

Discomfort of the cornea if contact lenses are used.

– CNS

Headache, migraine, mood changes, depression.

– Metabolic

Fluid retention, change in body weight, reduced glucose tolerance.

– Other

Changes in libido, leg cramp, premenstrual-like syndrome.

4.9 Overdose

There have been no reports of serious ill-health from overdosage even when a considerable number of tablets has been taken by a small child. In general, it is therefore unnecessary to treat overdosage. However, if overdosage is discovered within two or three hours and is large, then gastric lavage can be safely used. There are no antidotes and further treatment should be symptomatic.

5. PHARMACOLOGICAL PROPERTIES

5.1 Pharmacodynamic properties

Binovum Oral Contraceptive Tablets act through the mechanism of gonadotrophin suppression by the oestrogenic and progestational actions of the ethinylestradiol and norethisterone. The primary mechanism of action is inhibition of ovulation, but alterations to the cervical mucus and to the endometrium may also contribute to the efficacy of the product.

5.2 Pharmacokinetic properties

Norethisterone and ethinylestradiol are absorbed from the gastro-intestinal tract and metabolised in the liver. To obtain maximal contraceptive effectiveness, the tablets should be taken as directed and at approximately the same time each day.

Because the active ingredients are metabolised in the liver, reduced contraceptive efficacy has been associated with concomitant use of oral contraceptives and rifampicin. A similar association has been suggested with oral contraceptives and barbiturates, phenytoin sodium, phenylbutazone, griseofulvin and ampicillin.

5.3 Preclinical safety data

The toxicology of norethisterone and ethinylestradiol has been extensively investigated in animal studies and through long term clinical experience with widespread use in contraceptives.

6. PHARMACEUTICAL PARTICULARS

6.1 List of excipients

Lactose

Magnesium stearate

Pregelatinised starch

Methanol (does not appear in final product)

Purified water (peach coloured tablets only; does not appear in final product)

FD & C yellow No. 6 (peach coloured tablets only)

6.2 Incompatibilities

Not applicable.

6.3 Shelf life

Three years.

6.4 Special precautions for storage

Store at room temperature (below 25°C). Protect from light.

6.5 Nature and contents of container

Cartons containing 3 PVC/foil blister strips of 21 tablets each.

6.6 Instructions for use and handling

Not applicable.

7. MARKETING AUTHORISATION HOLDER

Janssen-Cilag Limited
Saunderton
High Wycombe
Buckinghamshire
HP14 4HJ
UK

8. MARKETING AUTHORISATION NUMBER(S)

PL 0242/0208

9. DATE OF FIRST AUTHORISATION/RENEWAL OF THE AUTHORISATION

Renewal Application: October 1995

Renewal granted on: 18 March 1996

10. DATE OF REVISION OF THE TEXT

20th August 2004

Legal category POM

Biorphen

(Alliance Pharmaceuticals)

1. NAME OF THE MEDICINAL PRODUCT

Biorphen

2. QUALITATIVE AND QUANTITATIVE COMPOSITION

Orphenadrine Hydrochloride BP 25 mg/5mL

3. PHARMACEUTICAL FORM

An anise scented and flavoured clear colourless aqueous liquid.

4. CLINICAL PARTICULARS

4.1 Therapeutic indications

Parkinsonism, particularly with apathy and depression, and drug induced extrapyramidal syndrome.

4.2 Posology and method of administration

Oral dose

Adult and Elderly:

150 mg daily in divided doses. Maximum dose 400 mg daily. Optimal dose range 150 to 300 mg; this is usually achieved by raising the dose to 50 mg every two to three days.

Children:

Not recommended.

4.3 Contraindications

Glaucoma, prostatic hypertrophy, urinary retention, porphyria.

4.4 Special warnings and special precautions for use

Caution in renal and hepatic disease.

Antimuscarinic agents, including orphenadrine, should be used with caution in patients with pre-existing tachycardia, (e.g. in heart failure, thyrotoxicosis) as they may cause further acceleration of the heart rate.

Anti-muscarinic agents such as orphenadrine are not effective in the treatment of tardive dyskinesia which may be made worse, and should not be used in patients with this condition.

4.5 Interaction with other medicinal products and other forms of Interaction

May additionally increase anticholinergic activity.

As with other similar agents, the antimuscarinic effects of orphenadrine may be enhanced by the concomitant administration of other medications with antimuscarinic properties, such as antihistamines, antispasmodics, tricyclic antidepressants, phenothiazines, dopaminergic anti-parkinsonian drugs including amantandine, and anti-arrhythmics such as disopyramide. Although the additive effect may be minor, there is the potential for development of severe constipation and ileus, atropine-like psychoses and heat stroke.

Due to the anti-muscarinic effects of orphenadrine on the gastrointestinal tract, a reduction in gastric motility may occur which may affect the absorption of other orally administered drugs.

4.6 Pregnancy and lactation

No studies with Biorphen have been carried out, therefore the drug should only be used in pregnancy if there is no safer alternative.

It is not known whether orphenadrine passes into the breast milk, therefore mothers should refrain from breast feeding whilst taking Biorphen.

4.7 Effects on ability to drive and use machines

Patients should be warned of the potential hazards of driving or operating machinery if they experience blurred vision.

4.8 Undesirable effects

Occasionally dry mouth, disturbances of visual accomodation, gastro-intestinal disturbances, dizziness and micturition difficulties may occur; these usually disappear spontaneously or may be controlled by a slight reduction in dosage. Less commonly, tachycardia, hypersensitivity, nervousness, euphoria, hallucinations, confusion and co-ordination disturbances and insomnia may be seen.

4.9 Overdose

Effects seen on overdose are anti-cholinergic in nature and include agitation, confusion, hallucinations, inco-ordination, delirium, tachycardia and occasionally convulsions. Fatalities have been reported. Gastric lavage, emetic and high enema is recommended. Cholinergics may be useful.

5. PHARMACOLOGICAL PROPERTIES

5.1 Pharmacodynamic properties

Orphenadrine is a tertiary amine antimuscarinic agent.

5.2 Pharmacokinetic properties

Orphenadrine is readily absorbed from the gastro-intestinal tract and is almost completely metabolised, to at least 8 metabolites. It is mainly excreted in the urine.

5.3 Preclinical safety data

No formal preclinical studies have been undertaken with Biorphen, as its active ingredient is a well established pharmaceutical.

6. PHARMACEUTICAL PARTICULARS

6.1 List of excipients

Sorbitol, glycerol, anise water condensed, saccharin sodium, Tween 20, benzoic acid solution, water.

6.2 Incompatibilities

None known.

6.3 Shelf life

24 months.

6.4 Special precautions for storage

None.

6.5 Nature and contents of container

200 mL and 1000 mL amber glass bottles with polycone lined closures.

6.6 Instructions for use and handling

None stated.

Administrative Data

7. MARKETING AUTHORISATION HOLDER

Alliance Pharmaceuticals Ltd

Avonbridge House

Bath Road

Chippenham

Wiltshire

SN15 2BB

8. MARKETING AUTHORISATION NUMBER(S)

PL16853/0022

9. DATE OF FIRST AUTHORISATION/RENEWAL OF THE AUTHORISATION

04 April 2002

10. DATE OF REVISION OF THE TEXT

Feb 2003

11. Legal Status

POM

Alliance, Alliance Pharmaceuticals and associated devices are registered Trademarks of Alliance Pharmaceuticals Ltd.

Bisodol Extra Strong Mint Tablets

(Forest Laboratories UK Limited)

1. NAME OF THE MEDICINAL PRODUCT

Bisodol Extra Strong Mint Tablets

2. QUALITATIVE AND QUANTITATIVE COMPOSITION

Active ingredients per tablet:

Calcium Carbonate Ph.Eur.	522mg
Magnesium Carbonate Light Ph.Eur.	68mg
Sodium Bicarbonate Ph.Eur.	64mg

3. PHARMACEUTICAL FORM

Chewable tablet

4. CLINICAL PARTICULARS

4.1 Therapeutic indications

For relief from indigestion, dyspepsia, heartburn, acidity and flatulence.

4.2 Posology and method of administration

Adults, elderly and children over 12 years:

Take one or two tablets as required. Suck slowly or chew as preferred.

Children below 12 years:

Not recommended.

4.3 Contraindications

Hypophosphataemia, and avoid in patients with heart or renal failure.

4.4 Special warnings and special precautions for use

The label will contain the following statements:

1. If symptoms persist, consult your doctor.
2. Keep all medicines out of the reach of children.
3. Not to be taken during the first three months of pregnancy.

4.5 Interaction with other medicinal products and other forms of Interaction

Antacids are known to reduce the absorption of certain medicines including tetracyclines and iron salts.

4.6 Pregnancy and lactation

No clinical data on exposed pregnancies are available.

Animal studies do not indicate direct or indirect harmful effects with respect to pregnancy, embryonal/foetal development, parturition or postnatal development (see section 5.3).

Caution should be exercised when prescribing to pregnant women.

4.7 Effects on ability to drive and use machines

None stated

4.8 Undesirable effects

Calcium salts can have a constipating effect and magnesium salts can have a laxative effect. The mixture of antacids is intended to avoid the lower gastrointestinal effects seen with single antacid preparations. No side effects associated with sodium bicarbonate except when taken in excess.

Rebound hyperacidity may occur with prolonged dosage.

4.9 Overdose

Hypermagnesaemia – intravenous administration of calcium salts.

Hypernatraemia – give plenty of salt free liquids.

Hypercalcaemia – remove source of calcium.

5. PHARMACOLOGICAL PROPERTIES

5.1 Pharmacodynamic properties

Sodium bicarbonate, calcium carbonate and magnesium carbonate are antacids. They act by neutralising the hydrochloric acid produced by the stomach and thus reducing gastric and duodenal irritation.

Sodium Bicarbonate

Sodium bicarbonate is a rapid onset, short acting antacid which neutralises acid secretions in the gastrointestinal tract by reacting with hydrochloric acid to produce sodium chloride. During neutralisation carbon dioxide is released, facilitating erucation which provides a sense of relief.

Calcium Carbonate

Calcium carbonate is an antacid with a more prolonged effect than sodium bicarbonate. It rapidly reacts with gastric acid to produce calcium chloride.

Magnesium Carbonate

Magnesium carbonate reacts with gastric acid to form soluble magnesium chloride and carbon dioxide. Because of its crystalline structure it reacts less rapidly than sodium bicarbonate giving it a slower onset of action, and providing longer lasting relief.

5.2 Pharmacokinetic properties

Sodium Bicarbonate

Administration of sodium bicarbonate by mouth causes neutralisation of gastric acid with the production of carbon dioxide. Bicarbonate not involved in that reaction is absorbed and in the absence of a deficit of bicarbonate in the plasma, bicarbonate ions are excreted in the urine that is rendered alkaline with an accompanying diuresis.

Calcium Carbonate

Calcium carbonate is converted to calcium chloride by gastric acid. Some of the calcium is absorbed from the intestines but about 85% is reconverted to insoluble calcium salts, such as the carbonate and is excreted in the faeces.

Magnesium Carbonate

Magnesium carbonate reacts with gastric acid to form soluble magnesium chloride and carbon dioxide in the stomach. Some magnesium is absorbed but is usually excreted rapidly in the urine.

5.3 Preclinical safety data

The active ingredients in Bisodol Tablets have a well-established safety record.

6. PHARMACEUTICAL PARTICULARS

6.1 List of excipients

Saccharin Soluble

Starch

Sucrose

Calcium Stearate

Peppermint Essential Oil

6.2 Incompatibilities

None known

6.3 Shelf life

60 months

6.4 Special precautions for storage

Store at a temperature not exceeding 25°C.

6.5 Nature and contents of container

Tablets in a polypropylene container with polypropylene lid; 30 tablets.

6.6 Instructions for use and handling

None

7. MARKETING AUTHORISATION HOLDER

Forest Laboratories UK Limited

Bourne Road

Bexley

Kent DA5 1NX

8. MARKETING AUTHORISATION NUMBER(S)

PL 0108/0125

9. DATE OF FIRST AUTHORISATION/RENEWAL OF THE AUTHORISATION

22nd November 1993/26th May 2004

10. DATE OF REVISION OF THE TEXT

September 2004

11. Legal Category

GSL

Bisodol Heartburn Relief Tablets

(Forest Laboratories UK Limited)

1. NAME OF THE MEDICINAL PRODUCT

Bisodol Heartburn Relief Tablets

2. QUALITATIVE AND QUANTITATIVE COMPOSITION

Active ingredients per tablet:

Magaldrate BP	400mg
Alginic Acid Ph.Eur.	200mg
Sodium Bicarbonate Ph.Eur.	100mg

3. PHARMACEUTICAL FORM

Tablet for oral administration

4. CLINICAL PARTICULARS

4.1 Therapeutic indications

Bisodol Heartburn Relief provides relief of the symptoms of indigestion, and alleviates the painful conditions resulting from gastric reflux. It is indicated in heartburn, including heartburn of pregnancy, reflux oesophagitis, hiatus hernia, regurgitation and all cases of epigastric distress associated with gastric reflux.

4.2 Posology and method of administration

Adults, elderly and children over 12 years of age:

Suck or chew one or two tablets after meals and at bedtime.

Children under 12 years of age:

Not recommended.

4.3 Contraindications

Avoid in patients with heart failure or renal failure.

4.4 Special warnings and special precautions for use

Patients with renal impairment should not use this product except under the advice of a doctor.

If symptoms persist, consult your doctor.

Keep all medicines out of the reach of children.

Not to be taken during the first three months of pregnancy.

4.5 Interaction with other medicinal products and other forms of Interaction

Antacids are known to reduce the absorption of certain medicines including tetracyclines and iron salts.

4.6 Pregnancy and lactation

Animal studies do not indicate direct or indirect harmful effects with respect to pregnancy, embryonal/foetal development, parturition or postnatal development (see section 5.3).

Caution should be exercised when prescribing to pregnant women.

4.7 Effects on ability to drive and use machines

None

4.8 Undesirable effects

Abdominal distension and flatulence may occur.

4.9 Overdose

Abdominal distension and diarrhoea may occur.

Hypermagnesaemia – intravenous administration of calcium salts.

5. PHARMACOLOGICAL PROPERTIES

5.1 Pharmacodynamic properties

Magaldrate

Magaldrate rapidly neutralises acid and has sufficient buffering capacity to provide sustained activity. It reduces gastric and duodenal irritation and also binds bile salt and pepsin.

Alginic Acid

Alginic Acid forms a highly viscous solution (raft) that floats on the surface of gastric contents to act as a mechanical barrier to reflux or to serve as primary agent being refluxed.

Sodium Bicarbonate

Sodium Bicarbonate is a rapid onset, short-acting antacid which neutralises acid secretions in the gastro-intestinal tract by reacting with hydrochloric acid to produce sodium chloride. During neutralisation carbon dioxide is released, facilitating eructation which provides a sense of relief.

5.2 Pharmacokinetic properties

Magaldrate

Magaldrate reacts with acid in stages. The hydroxymagnesium is relatively rapidly converted to magnesium ion and the aluminate to hydrated aluminium hydroxide; the aluminium hydroxide then reacts more slowly to give a sustained antacid effect.

Anywhere from 15% to 30% of the magnesium ion is absorbed; however, in the normal person, magnesium ion is rapidly excreted by the kidney.

The reaction of magnesium hydroxide with hydrochloric acid produces magnesium chloride. Most of the magnesium chloride is converted to magnesium carbonate in the intestine and thus excreted.

In the stomach, aluminium hydroxide neutralises hydrochloric acid. After the aluminium chloride enters the intestine some of the chloride is reabsorbed, the insoluble aluminium hydroxide and aluminium phosphate are formed.

Alginic Acid

When ingested, almost all of the alginic acid remains undigested and is excreted either unchanged or as an alginate.

Sodium Bicarbonate

Sodium bicarbonate reacts with hydrochloric acid to form sodium chloride, and this together with any unreacted bicarbonate is absorbed and excreted in the urine.

5.3 Preclinical safety data
The active ingredients in Bisodol Heartburn Relief Tablets have a well established safety record.

6. PHARMACEUTICAL PARTICULARS
6.1 List of excipients
Compressible Sugar
Microcrystalline Cellulose
Maize Starch
Magnesium Stearate
Cherry Cream Flavour

6.2 Incompatibilities
None known

6.3 Shelf life
36 months

6.4 Special precautions for storage
Store at a temperature not exceeding 25°C.

6.5 Nature and contents of container
Blister packs of 250 micron/UPVC/20 micron aluminium foil with 6gsm heat seal coating. Packed in sleeve packs; 5 tablets or cartons; 10, 20, 40 tablets.

6.6 Instructions for use and handling
None

7. MARKETING AUTHORISATION HOLDER
Forest Laboratories UK Limited
Bourne Road
Bexley
Kent DA5 1NX

8. MARKETING AUTHORISATION NUMBER(S)
PL 0108/0124

9. DATE OF FIRST AUTHORISATION/RENEWAL OF THE AUTHORISATION
29th July 1993/24th May 2004

10. DATE OF REVISION OF THE TEXT
April 2004

11. Legal Category
GSL

Bisodol Indigestion Relief Powder
(Forest Laboratories UK Limited)

1. NAME OF THE MEDICINAL PRODUCT
Bisodol Indigestion Relief Powder

2. QUALITATIVE AND QUANTITATIVE COMPOSITION
Active ingredients:

Sodium Bicarbonate Ph.Eur.	532mg
Magnesium Carbonate Light Ph.Eur.	345mg
Magnesium Carbonate Heavy Ph.Eur.	18mg

3. PHARMACEUTICAL FORM
Powder for oral administration

4. CLINICAL PARTICULARS
4.1 Therapeutic indications
For relief of the symptoms of gastric hyperacidity, variously called indigestion, heartburn, dyspepsia and flatulence.

4.2 Posology and method of administration
Adults, the elderly and children over 12 years:

One level teaspoon (5 ml), well stirred in about one third of a tumbler of water (warm or cold) after meals or as required.

Children under 12 years:

Not recommended.

4.3 Contraindications
Hypophosphataemia, and avoid in patients with heart failure or renal failure.

4.4 Special warnings and special precautions for use
If symptoms persist, consult your doctor.

Keep all medicines out of the reach of children.

Not to be taken during the first 3 months of pregnancy.

4.5 Interaction with other medicinal products and other forms of Interaction
Antacids are known to reduce the absorption of certain medicines including tetracyclines and iron salts.

4.6 Pregnancy and lactation
Animal studies are insufficient with respect to effects on pregnancy/embryonal/foetal development/parturition and postnatal development.

Caution should be exercised when prescribing to pregnant women.

4.7 Effects on ability to drive and use machines
None stated

4.8 Undesirable effects
Magnesium salts can have a laxative effect. No side effects associated with sodium bicarbonate except when taken in excess.

Rebound hyperacidity may occur with prolonged dosage.

4.9 Overdose
Hypermagnesaemia – intravenous administration of calcium salts.

Hypernatraemia – give plenty of salt free fluids.

5. PHARMACOLOGICAL PROPERTIES
5.1 Pharmacodynamic properties
Sodium bicarbonate and magnesium carbonate are antacids. They act by neutralising the hydrochloric acid produced by the stomach, thus reducing gastric and duodenal irritation.

5.2 Pharmacokinetic properties
Magnesium Carbonate

Magnesium carbonate reacts with gastric acid to form soluble magnesium chloride and carbon dioxide in the stomach. Some magnesium is absorbed but is usually excreted rapidly in the urine.

Sodium Bicarbonate

Administration of sodium bicarbonate by mouth causes neutralisation of gastric acid with the production of carbon dioxide. Bicarbonate not involved in that reaction is absorbed and in the absence of a deficit of bicarbonate in the plasma, bicarbonate ions are excreted in the urine that is rendered alkaline with an accompanying diuresis.

5.3 Preclinical safety data
The active ingredients in Bisodol Indigestion Relief Powder have a well documented safety record.

6. PHARMACEUTICAL PARTICULARS
6.1 List of excipients
Peppermint Essential Oil Hanningtons White Diamond (374611E)

6.2 Incompatibilities
None stated

6.3 Shelf life
60 months

6.4 Special precautions for storage
Store at a temperature not exceeding 25°C.

6.5 Nature and contents of container
White polypropylene securitainers with blue polyethylene caps fitted with tamper evident tear-off retaining strips.

Pack sizes: 50g, 100g.

Amber glass bottle fitted with black plastic cap.

Pack size: 425g

6.6 Instructions for use and handling
None

7. MARKETING AUTHORISATION HOLDER
Forest Laboratories UK Limited
Bourne Road
Bexley
Kent DA5 1NX

8. MARKETING AUTHORISATION NUMBER(S)
PL 0108/0129

9. DATE OF FIRST AUTHORISATION/RENEWAL OF THE AUTHORISATION
29th January 1987 / 9th August 2003

10. DATE OF REVISION OF THE TEXT
June 2003

11. Legal Category
GSL

Bisodol Indigestion Relief Tablets
(Forest Laboratories UK Limited)

1. NAME OF THE MEDICINAL PRODUCT
Bisodol Indigestion Relief Tablets

2. QUALITATIVE AND QUANTITATIVE COMPOSITION
Active ingredients:

Sodium Bicarbonate Ph.Eur.	64mg/tablet
Calcium Carbonate Ph.Eur.	522mg/tablet
Magnesium Carbonate Light Ph.Eur.	68mg/tablet

3. PHARMACEUTICAL FORM
Chewable tablet for oral administration

4. CLINICAL PARTICULARS
4.1 Therapeutic indications
For relief of the symptoms of gastric hyperacidity, variously called indigestion, heartburn, dyspepsia and flatulence.

4.2 Posology and method of administration
Adults, elderly and children over 12 years of age:

Suck slowly or chew one or two tablets as required.

Children under 12 years of age:

Not recommended.

4.3 Contraindications
Hypophosphataemia, and avoid in patients with heart failure or renal failure.

4.4 Special warnings and special precautions for use
If symptoms persist, consult your doctor.

Keep all medicines out of the reach of children.

Not to be taken during the first three months of pregnancy.

4.5 Interaction with other medicinal products and other forms of Interaction
Antacids are known to reduce the absorption of certain medicines including tetracyclines and iron salts.

4.6 Pregnancy and lactation
Animal studies are insufficient with respect to effects on pregnancy/embryonal/foetal development/parturition and postnatal development.

Caution should be exercised when prescribing to pregnant women.

4.7 Effects on ability to drive and use machines
None stated

4.8 Undesirable effects
Calcium salts can have a constipating effect and magnesium salts can have a laxative effect. The specific mixture of antacids is intended to avoid the lower gastrointestinal effects seen with single antacid preparations. No side effects associated with sodium bicarbonate except when taken in excess.

Rebound hyperacidity may occur with prolonged dosage.

4.9 Overdose
Hypermagnesaemia – intravenous administration of calcium salts.

Hypernatraemia – give plenty of salt free fluids.Hypercalcaemia – remove source of calcium.

5. PHARMACOLOGICAL PROPERTIES
5.1 Pharmacodynamic properties
Sodium bicarbonate, calcium carbonate and magnesium carbonate are antacids. They act by neutralising the hydrochloric acid produced by the stomach and thus reducing gastric and duodenal irritation.

5.2 Pharmacokinetic properties
Calcium Carbonate

Calcium carbonate is converted to calcium chloride by gastric acid. Some of the calcium is absorbed from the intestines but about 85% is reconverted to insoluble calcium salts, such as the carbonate and is excreted in the faeces.

Magnesium Carbonate

Magnesium carbonate reacts with gastric acid to form soluble magnesium chloride and carbon dioxide in the stomach. Some magnesium is absorbed but is usually excreted rapidly in the urine.

Sodium Bicarbonate

Administration of sodium bicarbonate by mouth causes neutralisation of gastric acid with the production of carbon dioxide. Bicarbonate not involved in that reaction is absorbed and in the absence of a deficit of bicarbonate in the plasma, bicarbonate ions are excreted in the urine that is rendered alkaline with an accompanying diuresis.

5.3 Preclinical safety data
The active ingredients in Bisodol Indigestion Relief Tablets have a well documented safety record.

6. PHARMACEUTICAL PARTICULARS
6.1 List of excipients
Saccharin Soluble
Maize Starch
Sugar
Calcium Stearate
Peppermint Essential Oil Hanningtons White Diamond (374611E)

6.2 Incompatibilities
None stated

6.3 Shelf life

Polypropylene packs:	36 months
Other packs:	60 months

6.4 Special precautions for storage
Store at a temperature not exceeding 25°C.

6.5 Nature and contents of container
Cellulose over wrapped shell and slide cardboard cartons.

Pack sizes: 12, 30.

250 micron UPVC /20 micron coated aluminium blister packs in cardboard cartons.

Pack sizes: 24, 48.

Cellophane overwrapped carton of 5 rolls of 20 tablets in wax laminated foil with paper labels.

Pack size: 100.

Polypropylene roll holder with a polypropylene cap attached by a banding strip to the 100 tablet carton.

Amber glass bottle with black plastic cap.

Pack size: 250.

Rolls of 20 tablets in wax laminated foil with paper label.

Pack size: 20.

Polypropylene container and polypropylene lid.

Pack sizes: 30, 50.

Three rolls of 20 tablets in wax laminated foil packed together in cardboard carton.

Pack size: 60

6.6 Instructions for use and handling
None

7. MARKETING AUTHORISATION HOLDER
Forest Laboratories UK Limited

Bourne Road

Bexley

Kent DA5 1NX

8. MARKETING AUTHORISATION NUMBER(S)
PL 0108/0123

9. DATE OF FIRST AUTHORISATION/RENEWAL OF THE AUTHORISATION
29th January 1987 / 20th January 2004

10. DATE OF REVISION OF THE TEXT
December 2003

11. Legal Category
GSL

Bisodol Wind Relief

(Forest Laboratories UK Limited)

1. NAME OF THE MEDICINAL PRODUCT
Bisodol Wind Relief

2. QUALITATIVE AND QUANTITATIVE COMPOSITION
Active ingredients:

Calcium Carbonate Ph.Eur.	522mg/tablet
Magnesium Carbonate Ph.Eur.	68mg/tablet
Sodium Bicarbonate Ph.Eur.	63mg/tablet
Simethicone USP	100mg/tablet

3. PHARMACEUTICAL FORM
Tablet for oral administration.

4. CLINICAL PARTICULARS
4.1 Therapeutic indications
For the relief of indigestion, dyspepsia, heartburn, acidity and flatulence.

4.2 Posology and method of administration
Adults, the elderly and children over 12 years of age:

One or two tablets, sucked or chewed as required. To a maximum of 16 tablets daily.

Children under 12 years of age:

Not recommended.

4.3 Contraindications
Hypophosphataemia, and avoid in patients with heart or renal failure.

4.4 Special warnings and special precautions for use
The label will contain the following statements:

- If symptoms persist, consult your doctor.
- Keep all medicines out of the reach of children.
- Not to be taken during the first three months of pregnancy.

4.5 Interaction with other medicinal products and other forms of Interaction
Antacids are known to reduce the absorption of certain medicines including tetracyclines and iron salts.

4.6 Pregnancy and lactation
Do not use in the first trimester.

4.7 Effects on ability to drive and use machines
None stated

4.8 Undesirable effects
Magnesium salts can have a laxative effect. Calcium salts have a constipating effect. The mixture of antacids may prevent the lower gastrointestinal effects seen with single antacid preparations.

Belching may occur.

Rebound hyperacidity may occur with prolonged dosage.

4.9 Overdose
Hypermagnesaemia – intravenous administration of calcium salts.

Hypernatraemia – give plenty of salt free fluids.

Hypercalcaemia – remove source of calcium.

5. PHARMACOLOGICAL PROPERTIES
5.1 Pharmacodynamic properties
Simethicone is an anti-flatulence agent which acts by reducing surface tension of gas bubbles in the GI tract.

Sodium bicarbonate, calcium carbonate and magnesium carbonate are antacids. They act by neutralising the hydrochloric acid produced by the stomach and thus reducing gastric and duodenal irritation.

5.2 Pharmacokinetic properties
Calcium Carbonate

Calcium carbonate is converted to calcium chloride by gastric acid. Some of the calcium is absorbed from the intestines but about 85% is reconverted to insoluble calcium salts, such as the carbonate and is excreted in the faeces.

Magnesium Carbonate

Magnesium carbonate reacts with gastric acid to form soluble magnesium chloride and carbon dioxide in the stomach. Some magnesium is absorbed but is usually excreted rapidly in the urine.

Sodium Bicarbonate

Administration of sodium bicarbonate by mouth causes neutralisation of gastric acid with the production of carbon dioxide. Bicarbonate not involved in that reaction is absorbed and in the absence of a deficit of bicarbonate in the plasma, bicarbonate ions are excreted in the urine that is rendered alkaline with an accompanying diuresis.

5.3 Preclinical safety data
The active ingredients in Bisodol Wind Relief have a well documented safety record.

6. PHARMACEUTICAL PARTICULARS
6.1 List of excipients
Saccharin Sodium

Dextrose Monohydrate

Maize Starch

Emdex

Microcrystalline Cellulose

Spearmint Flavour EC180235

Patent Blue V Lake (E131)

Quinoline Yellow Lake (E104)

Magnesium Stearate

6.2 Incompatibilities
None stated

6.3 Shelf life
36 months

6.4 Special precautions for storage
Store at a temperature not exceeding 25°C.

6.5 Nature and contents of container
Blister packs of 250 micron UPVC/20 micron hard tempered aluminium foil.

Pack size: 12, 16, 20, 24, 36

Not all pack sizes may be marketed.

6.6 Instructions for use and handling
None

7. MARKETING AUTHORISATION HOLDER
Forest Laboratories UK Limited

Bourne Road

Bexley

Kent DA5 1NX

8. MARKETING AUTHORISATION NUMBER(S)
PL 0108/0126

9. DATE OF FIRST AUTHORISATION/RENEWAL OF THE AUTHORISATION
30 January 1989 / 11 March 1999

10. DATE OF REVISION OF THE TEXT
February 2005

11. Legal Category
GSL

Bleo-Kyowa

(Kyowa Hakko UK Ltd)

1. NAME OF THE MEDICINAL PRODUCT
Bleo-Kyowa™

2. QUALITATIVE AND QUANTITATIVE COMPOSITION
Bleomycin Sulphate equivalent to 15,000 IU (15 $\times$ 10^3 IU).

3. PHARMACEUTICAL FORM
Freeze dried powder in a glass vial for reconstitution and administration by infusion, injection or instillation.

4. CLINICAL PARTICULARS
4.1 Therapeutic indications
a) Squamous cell carcinoma affecting the mouth, nasopharynx and paranasal sinuses, larynx, oesophagus, external genitalia, cervix or skin. Well differentiated tumours usually respond better than anaplastic ones.

b) Hodgkin's disease and other malignant lymphomas, including mycosis fungoides.

c) Testicular teratoma.

d) Malignant effusions of serous cavities.

e) Secondary indications in which bleomycin has been shown to be of some value (alone or in combination with other drugs) include metastatic malignant melanoma, carcinoma of the thyroid, lung and bladder.

4.2 Posology and method of administration
Adults

Routes of administration
Bleomycin is usually administered intramuscularly but may be given intravenously (bolus or drip), intra-arterially, intrapleurally or intraperitoneally as a solution in physiological saline.

Local injection directly into the tumour may occasionally be indicated.

Recommended dose and dosage schedules
1. Squamous cell carcinoma and testicular teratoma:

Used alone the normal dosage is 15 $\times$ 10^3 IU (1 vial) three times a week or 30 $\times$ 10^3 IU (2 vials) twice a week, either intramuscularly or intravenously. Treatment may continue on consecutive weeks, or more usually at intervals of 3-4 weeks, up to a total cumulative dose of 500 $\times$ 10^3 IU although young men with testicular tumours have frequently tolerated twice this amount. Continuous intravenous infusion at a rate of 15 $\times$ 10^3 IU (1 vial) per 24 hours for up to 10 days, or 30 $\times$ 10^3 IU (2 vials) per 24 hours for up to 5 days may produce a therapeutic effect more rapidly. The development of stomatitis is the most useful guide to the determination of individual tolerance of maximum therapeutic response. The dose may need to be adjusted when bleomycin is used in combination chemotherapy. Use in elderly or children – see below.

2. Malignant lymphomas:

Used alone the recommended dosage regime is 15 $\times$ 10^3 IU (1 vial) once or twice a week, intramuscularly, to a total dose of 225 $\times$ 10^3 IU (15 vials). Dosage should be reduced in the elderly. The dose may need to be adjusted when bleomycin is used in combination chemotherapy. Use in elderly or children – see below.

3. Malignant effusions:

After drainage of the affected serous cavity 60 $\times$ 10^3 IU (4 vials) bleomycin dissolved in 100 ml physiological saline is introduced via the drainage needle or cannula. After instillation, the drainage needle or cannula may be withdrawn. Administration may be repeated if necessary subject to a total cumulative dose of 500 $\times$ 10^3 IU (about 33 vials). Use in the elderly or children – see below.

Combination therapy:

Bleomycin is commonly used in conjunction with radiotherapy, particularly in treatment of cancer of the head and neck region. Such a combination may enhance mucosal reactions if full doses of both forms of treatment are used and bleomycin dosage may require reduction, e.g. to 5 $\times$ 10^3 IU at the time of each radiotherapy fraction five days a week. Bleomycin is frequently used as one of the drugs in multiple chemotherapy regimes (e.g. squamous cell carcinoma, testicular teratoma, lymphoma). The mucosal toxicity of bleomycin should be borne in mind in the selection and dosage of drugs with similar toxic potential used in such combinations.

Elderly Patients:

The total dose of bleomycin used in the treatment of squamous cell carcinoma, testicular teratoma or malignant effusions should be reduced as indicated below

Age in years	Total Dose (IU)	Dose per week (IU)
80 and over	100 $\times$ 10^3	15 $\times$ 10^3
70 – 79	150 – 200 $\times$ 10^3	30 $\times$ 10^3
60 – 69	200 – 300 $\times$ 10^3	30 – 60 $\times$ 10^3
Under 60	500 $\times$ 10^3	30 – 60 $\times$ 10^3

Children
Until further data are available, administration of bleomycin to children should take place only under exceptional circumstances and in special centres. The dosage should be based on that recommended for adults and adjusted to body surface area or body weight.

Reduced kidney function
With serum creatinine values of 2-4 mg%, it is recommended to half the above dosages. With serum cretinine above 4 mg%, a further reduction in dose is indicated.

Preparation of solution
For intramuscular injections the required dose is dissolved in up to 5 ml of suitable solvents such as physiological

saline. If pain occurs at the site of injection a 1% solution of lignocaine may be used as a solvent.

For intravenous injections the dose required is dissolved in 5-200 ml of physiological saline and injected slowly or added to the reservoir of a running intravenous infusion. For intra-arterial administration a slow infusion in physiological saline is used. For intra-cavity injection 60 × 10^3 IU is dissolved in 100ml of normal saline.

For local injections bleomycin is dissolved in physiological saline to make a 1-3 × 10^3 IU/ml solution.

4.3 Contraindications
Bleomycin is contra-indicated in patients with acute pulmonary infection or greatly reduced lung function.

4.4 Special warnings and special precautions for use
Patients undergoing treatment with bleomycin should have chest X-rays weekly. These should continue to be taken for up to 4 weeks after completion of the course. If breathlessness of infiltrates appear, not obviously attributable to tumour or to co-existent lung disease, administration of the drug must be stopped immediately and patients should be treated with a corticosteriod and a broad spectrum antibiotic.

Lung function tests which use 100% oxygen should not be used in patients who have been treated with Bleomycin. Lung function tests using less than 21% oxygen are recommended as an alternative.

4.5 Interaction with other medicinal products and other forms of Interaction
When bleomycin is used as one of the drugs in multiple chemotherapy regimes the toxicity of bleomycin should be borne in mind in the selection and dosage of drugs with similar toxic potential. The addition of other cytotoxic drugs can necessitate changes and dose alterations.

Previous or concurrent radiotherapy to the chest is an important factor in increasing the incidence and severity of lung toxicity.

Because of bleomycin's sensitisation of lung tissue, patients who have received bleomycin pre-operatively are at greater risk of developing pulmonary toxicity when oxygen is administered at surgery and a reduction in inspired oxygen concentration during operation and post-operatively is recommended. (See section 4.4)

In patients treated for testicular cancer with a combination of bleomycin and vinca alkaloids a syndrome has been reported corresponding to morbus Raynaud, ischaemia which can lead to necrosis of peripheral parts of the body (fingers, toes, nose tip).

No specific clinical incompatibilities with other drugs or food have been encountered.

4.6 Pregnancy and lactation
Bleomycin should not normally be administered to patients who are pregnant or to mothers who are breast-feeding.

Animal experiences have revealed that bleomycin, like most cytotoxics, may have teratogenic and carcinogenic potential.

4.7 Effects on ability to drive and use machines
This depends on the patient's condition and should be considered in co-operation with the doctor.

4.8 Undesirable effects
Like most cytotoxic agents bleomycin can give rise to both to immediate and to delayed toxic effects. The most immediate effect is fever on the day of injection. Anorexia, tiredness or nausea also may occur. Pain at the injection site or in the region of the tumour has occasionally been reported, and other rare adverse effects are hypotension and local thrombophlebitis after intravenous administration.

The majority of patients who receive a full course of bleomycin develop lesions of the skin or oral mucosa. Induration, hyperkeratotis, reddening, tenderness and swelling of the tips of the fingers, ridging of the nails, bulla formation over pressure points such as elbows, loss of hair and stomatitis are rarely serious and usually disappear soon after completion of the course.

The most serious delayed effect is interstitial pneumonia, which may develop during, or occasionally after, a course of treatment. This condition may sometimes develop into fatal pulmonary fibrosis, although such an occurrence is rare at recommended doses. Previous or concurrent radiotherapy to the chest is an important factor in increasing the incidence and severity of lung toxicity.

A few cases of acute fulminant reactions with hyperpyrexia and cardiorespiratory collapse have been observed after intravenous injections of doses higher than those recommended. Hypotension, hyperpyrexia and drug-related deaths have been reported rarely following intra-cavitary instillation of bleomycin.

4.9 Overdose
The acute reaction to an overdosage of bleomycin would probably include hypotension, fever, rapid pulse and general symptoms of shock. Treatment is purely symptomatic. In the event of respiratory complications the patient should be treated with a corticosteroid and a broad-spectrum antibiotic. There is no specific antidote to bleomycin.

5. PHARMACOLOGICAL PROPERTIES

5.1 Pharmacodynamic properties
Bleomycin is a basic, water soluble glycopeptide with cytotoxic activity. The mechanism of action of bleomycin is believed to involve single-strand scission of DNA, leading to inhibition of cell division, of growth and of DNA synthesis in tumour cells.

Apart from its antibacterial and antitumour properties, bleomycin is relatively free from biological activity. When injected intravenously it may have a histamine-like effect on blood pressure and may cause a rise in body temperature.

5.2 Pharmacokinetic properties
Bleomycin is administered parenterally. After intravenous (IV) administration of a bolus dose of 15 × 10^3 IU/m^2 body surface, peak concentrations of 1 to 10 IU are achieved in plasma. Following the intramuscular (IM) injection of 15 × 10^3 IU peak plasma concentrations of about 1 IU/ml have been reported. The peak plasma concentration is reached 30 minutes after an IM injection. Continuous infusion of bleomycin 30 × 10^3 IU daily, for 4 to 5 days, resulted in an average steady state plasma concentration of 100-300 milli IU/ml. After IV injections of bleomycin in a dose of 15 × 10^3 IU/m^2 body surface, the area under the serum concentration curve is, on average, 300 milli IU × min × ml^{-1}.

Bleomycin is only bound to plasma proteins to a slight extent. Bleomycin is rapidly distributed in body tissues, with the highest concentrations in skin, lungs, peritoneum and lymph. Low concentrations are seen in the bone marrow. Bleomycin could not be detected in cerebrospinal fluid after intravenous injection. Bleomycin appears to cross the placental barrier.

The mechanism for bio-transformation is not yet fully known. Inactivation takes place during enzymatic breakdown by bleomycin hydrolase, primarily in plasma, liver and other organs and, to a much lesser degree, in skin and lungs. When bleomycin was administered as an IV bolus injection in a dose of 15 × 10^3 IU/m^2 body surface, initial and terminal half-lives were 0.5 and 4 hours respectively. Given as a continuous intravenous infusion in a dose of 30 × 10^3 IU daily for 4 to 5 days bleomycin disappears from plasma with initial and terminal half-lives of about 1.3 hours and 9 hours, respectively. About two thirds of the administered drug is excreted unchanged in the urine, probably by glomerular filtration. Approximately 50% is recovered in the urine in the 24 hours following an IV or IM injection. The rate of excretion, therefore, is highly influenced by renal function; concentrations in plasma are greatly elevated if usual doses are given to patients with renal impairment with only up to 20% excreted in 24 hours. Observations indicate that it is difficult to eliminate bleomycin from the body by dialysis.

5.3 Preclinical safety data
Animal experiences have revealed that bleomycin, like most cytotoxics, may have teratogenic and carcinogenic potential.

6. PHARMACEUTICAL PARTICULARS

6.1 List of excipients
None

6.2 Incompatibilities
Bleomycin solution should not be mixed with solutions of essential amino acids, riboflavine, ascorbic acid, dexamethasone, aminophylline or frusemide.

6.3 Shelf life
Three years.

6.4 Special precautions for storage
Protect from light. Store at 2-8° C.

6.5 Nature and contents of container
5 ml colourless glass vials with rubber closure and aluminium cap containing freeze dried bleomycin sulphate equivalent to 15,000 IU. Ten vials per carton.

6.6 Instructions for use and handling
Bleomycin should be handled with care. Precautions should be taken to avoid bleomycin coming into contact with skin, mucous membranes or eyes, but in the event of contamination the effected part should be washed with water.

Administrative Data

7. MARKETING AUTHORISATION HOLDER
Kyowa Hakko (UK) Ltd
258 Bath Road
Slough
Berkshire
SL1 4DX

8. MARKETING AUTHORISATION NUMBER(S)
PL 12196/0005

9. DATE OF FIRST AUTHORISATION/RENEWAL OF THE AUTHORISATION
14 April 1998

10. DATE OF REVISION OF THE TEXT
July 2000

Bondronat

(Roche Products Limited)

1. NAME OF THE MEDICINAL PRODUCT
Bondronat ▼2mg/2ml
Bondronat ▼6mg/6ml
Concentrate for solution for infusion

2. QUALITATIVE AND QUANTITATIVE COMPOSITION
Qualitative composition
Ibandronic acid, monosodium salt, monohydrate.

Quantitative composition
Bondronat 2mg/2ml
One vial with 2ml concentrate for solution for infusion (colourless, clear solution) contains 2.25mg ibandronic acid, monosodium salt, monohydrate corresponding to 2mg ibandronic acid.

1ml of solution contains 1.125mg ibandronic acid, monosodium salt, monohydrate, corresponding to 1mg ibandronic acid.

Bondronat 6mg/6ml
One vial with 6ml concentrate for solution for infusion (colourless, clear solution) contains 6.75mg ibandronic acid, monosodium salt, monohydrate corresponding to 6mg ibandronic acid.

1ml of solution contains 1.125mg ibandronic acid, monosodium salt, monohydrate, corresponding to 1mg ibandronic acid.

For excipients, see section *6.1*.

3. PHARMACEUTICAL FORM
Concentrate for solution for infusion.

4. CLINICAL PARTICULARS

4.1 Therapeutic indications
Bondronat is indicated for:

- Prevention of skeletal events (pathological fractures, bone complications requiring radiotherapy or surgery) in patients with breast cancer and bone metastases.

- Treatment of tumour-induced hypercalcaemia with or without metastases.

4.2 Posology and method of administration
Bondronat therapy should only be initiated by physicians experienced in the treatment of cancer.

For intravenous administration.

Prevention of Skeletal Events in Patients with Breast Cancer and Bone Metastases
The recommended dose for prevention of skeletal events in patients with breast cancer and bone metastases is 6mg IV given every 3 - 4 weeks. The dose should be infused over 1 hour. For infusion, the contents of the ampoule(s)/vials(s) should be added to 500ml isotonic sodium chloride solution (or 500ml 5% dextrose solution).

Treatment of Tumour-Induced Hypercalcaemia
Adults and elderly:
Prior to treatment with Bondronat the patient should be adequately rehydrated with 0.9% sodium chloride. Consideration should be given to the severity of the hypercalcaemia as well as the tumour type. In general patients with osteolytic bone metastases require lower doses than patients with the humoral type of hypercalcaemia. In most patients with severe hypercalcaemia (albumin-corrected serum calcium* ⩾ 3mmol/l or ⩾ 12mg/dl) 4mg is an adequate single dosage. In patients with moderate hypercalcaemia (albumin-corrected serum calcium < 3mmol/l or < 12mg/dl) 2mg is an effective dose. The highest dose used in clinical trials was 6mg but this dose does not add any further benefit in terms of efficacy.

*Note albumin-corrected serum calcium concentrations are calculated as follows:

Albumin-corrected serum calcium (mmol/l)
= serum calcium (mmol/l) - [0.02 × albumin (g/l)] + 0.8 **or**
Albumin-corrected serum calcium (mg/dl)
= serum calcium (mg/dl) + 0.8 × [4 - albumin (g/dl)]

To convert the albumin-corrected serum calcium in mmol/l value to mg/dl, multiply by 4.

In most cases a raised serum calcium level can be reduced to the normal range within 7 days. The median time to relapse (return of albumin-corrected serum calcium to levels above 3mmol/l) was 18 - 19 days for the 2mg and 4mg doses. The median time to relapse was 26 days with a dose of 6mg.

A limited number of patients (50 patients) have received a second infusion for hypercalcaemia. Repeated treatment may be considered in case of recurrent hypercalcaemia or insufficient efficacy.

Bondronat concentrate for solution for infusion should be administered as an intravenous infusion. For this purpose, the contents of the ampoules or vials are to be added to 500ml isotonic sodium chloride solution (or 500ml 5% dextrose solution) and infused over two hours.

As the inadvertent intra-arterial administration of preparations not expressly recommended for this purpose as well as paravenous administration can lead to tissue damage, care must be taken to ensure that Bondronat concentrate for solution for infusion is administered intravenously.

Special Dosage Instructions:

Patients with hepatic impairment

No dosage adjustment is expected to be necessary (see Section 5.2).

Patients with renal impairment

No dosage adjustment is necessary for patients with mild or moderate renal impairment where creatinine clearance is equal to or greater than 30ml/min.

Below 30ml/min creatinine clearance, the dose for prevention of skeletal events in patients with breast cancer and bone metastases should be reduced to 2mg every 3-4 weeks, infused over 1 hour.

Elderly

No dose adjustment is necessary.

Children and adolescents

Safety and efficacy have not been established in patients less than 18 years old.

4.3 Contraindications

Bondronat concentrate for solution for infusion must not be used in known hypersensitivity to the drug substance or to any of the excipients.

Caution is indicated in patients with known hypersensitivity to other bisphosphonates.

Bondronat concentrate for solution for infusion should not be used in children because of lack of clinical experience.

4.4 Special warnings and special precautions for use

Clinical studies have not shown any evidence of deterioration in renal function with long term Bondronat therapy. Nevertheless, according to clinical assessment of the individual patient, it is recommended that renal function, serum calcium, phosphate and magnesium should be monitored in patients treated with Bondronat.

As no clinical data are available, dosage recommendations cannot be given for patients with severe hepatic insufficiency.

Overhydration should be avoided in patients at risk of cardiac failure.

Hypocalcaemia and other disturbances of bone and mineral metabolism should be effectively treated before starting Bondronat therapy for metastatic bone disease. Adequate intake of calcium and vitamin D is important in all patients. Patients should receive supplemental calcium and/or vitamin D if dietary intake is inadequate.

4.5 Interaction with other medicinal products and other forms of Interaction

When co-administered with melphalan/prednisolone in patients with multiple myeloma, no interaction was observed.

Other interaction studies in postmenopausal women have demonstrated the absence of any interaction potential with tamoxifen or hormone replacement therapy (oestrogen).

In relation to disposition, no drug interactions of clinical significance are likely. Ibandronic acid is eliminated by renal secretion only and does not undergo any biotransformation. The secretory pathway does not appear to include known acidic or basic transport systems involved in the excretion of other active substances. In addition, ibandronic acid does not inhibit the major human hepatic P450 isoenzymes and does not induce the hepatic cytochrome P450 system in rats. Plasma protein binding is low at therapeutic concentrations and ibandronic acid is therefore unlikely to displace other active substances.

Caution is advised when bisphosphonates are administered with aminoglycosides, since both agents can lower serum calcium levels for prolonged periods. Attention should also be paid to the possible existence of simultaneous hypomagnesaemia.

In clinical studies, Bondronat has been administered concomitantly with commonly used anticancer agents, diuretics, antibiotics and analgesics without clinically apparent interactions occurring.

4.6 Pregnancy and lactation

There are no adequate data from the use of ibandronic acid in pregnant women. Studies in rats have shown reproductive toxicity (see section 5.3). The potential risk for humans is unknown. Therefore, Bondronat should not be used during pregnancy.

It is not known whether ibandronic acid is excreted in human milk. Studies in lactating rats have demonstrated the presence of low levels of ibandronic acid in the milk following intravenous administration. Consequently, caution should be exercised when prescribing Bondronat to breast-feeding women.

4.7 Effects on ability to drive and use machines

No studies on the effects on the ability to drive and use machines have been performed.

4.8 Undesirable effects

Adverse reactions are ranked under heading of frequency, the most frequent first, using the following convention: very common (≥ 10%), common (≥ 1% and < 10%), uncommon (≥ 0.1% and < 1%), rare (≥ 0.01% and < 0.1%), and very rare (≤ 0.01%).

Treatment of Tumour Induced Hypercalcaemia

The safety profile for Bondronat in tumour-induced hypercalcaemia is derived from controlled clinical trials in this indication and after the intravenous administration of Bondronat at the recommended doses. Treatment was most commonly associated with a rise in body temperature. Occasionally, a flu-like syndrome consisting of fever, chills, bone and/or muscle ache-like pain was reported. In most cases no specific treatment was required and the symptoms subsided after a couple of hours/days.

Table 1. Number (percentage) of Patients Reporting Adverse Events in Controlled Clinical Trials in Tumour-Induced Hypercalcaemia after treatment with Bondronat

Adverse Event		Frequency Number (%) (n=352)
Metabolism and nutrition disorders		
Common:	Hypocalcaemia	10 (2.8)
Musculoskeletal and connective tissue disorders:		
Common:	Bone Pain	6 (1.7)
Uncommon:	Myalgia	1 (0.3)
General disorders and administration site conditions:		
Very common:	Pyrexia	39 (11.1)
Uncommon:	Influenza-like illness	2 (0.6)
	Rigors	1 (0.3)

Note: Data for both the 2mg and 4mg doses of ibandronic acid are pooled. Events were recorded irrespective of a determination of causality.

Frequently, decreased renal calcium excretion is accompanied by a fall in serum phosphate levels not requiring therapeutic measures. The serum calcium level may fall to hypocalcaemic values.

Other adverse events reported at lower frequency are as follows:

Immune system disorders:

Very rare: Hypersensitivity NOS.

Skin and subcutaneous tissue disorders:

Very rare: Angioneurotic oedema

Respiratory, thoracic and mediastinal disorders:

Very rare: Bronchospasm NOS.

Administration of other bisphosphonates has been associated with broncho-constriction in acetylsalicylic acid-sensitive asthmatic patients.

Prevention of Skeletal Events in Patients with Breast Cancer and Bone Metastases

The safety profile of intravenous Bondronat in patients with breast cancer and bone metastases is derived from a controlled clinical trial in this indication and after the intravenous administration of Bondronat at the recommended dose.

Table 2 lists adverse events from the pivotal phase III study (152 patients treated with Bondronat 6mg), reported as remotely, possibly, or probably related to study medication, occurring commonly and more frequently in the active treatment group than in placebo.

Table 2 Related Adverse Events Occurring Commonly and Greater than Placebo in Patients with Metastatic Bone Disease due to Breast Cancer Treated with Bondronat 6mg i.v.

(see Table 2 on next page)

The following events occurred rarely (one patient in the Bondronat group): gastroenteritis NOS, oral candidiasis, vaginitis, benign skin neoplasm, anaemia NOS, blood dyscrasia NOS, hypophosphataemia, sleep disorder, anxiety, affect lability, amnesia, paraesthesia circumoral, hyperaesthesia, hypertonia, nerve root lesion NOS, neuralgia NOS, migraine, cerebrovascular disorder NOS, parosmia, deafness, cardiovascular disorder NOS, palpitations, myocardial ischaemia, hypertension, varicose veins NOS, lymphoedema, lung oedema, stridor, gastritis NOS, cheilitis, dysphagia, mouth ulceration, cholelithiasis, rash NOS, alopecia, cystitis NOS, renal cyst NOS, urinary retention, pelvic pain NOS, injection site pain, blood alkaline phosphatase increase, weight decreased, injury, hypothermia.

4.9 Overdose

Up to now there is no experience of acute poisoning with Bondronat concentrate for solution for infusion. Since both the kidney and the liver were found to be target organs for toxicity in preclinical studies with high doses, kidney and liver function should be monitored. Clinically relevant hypocalcaemia should be corrected by i.v. administration of calcium gluconate.

5. PHARMACOLOGICAL PROPERTIES

5.1 Pharmacodynamic properties

Pharmaco-therapeutic group: Bisphosphonate, *ATC Code:* M05B A06

Ibandronic acid belongs to the bisphosphonate group of compounds which act specifically on bone. Their selective action on bone tissue is based on the high affinity of bisphosphonates for bone mineral. Bisphosphonates act by inhibiting osteoclast activity, although the precise mechanism is still not clear.

In vivo, ibandronic acid prevents experimentally-induced bone destruction caused by cessation of gonadal function, retinoids, tumours or tumour extracts. The inhibition of endogenous bone resorption has also been documented by 45Ca kinetic studies and by the release of radioactive tetracycline previously incorporated into the skeleton.

At doses that were considerably higher than the pharmacologically effective doses, ibandronic acid did not have any effect on bone mineralisation.

Bone resorption due to malignant disease is characterised by excessive bone resorption that is not balanced with appropriate bone formation. Ibandronic acid selectively inhibits osteoclast activity, reducing bone resorption and thereby reducing skeletal complications of the malignant disease.

Clinical Studies in the Treatment of Tumour-Induced Hypercalcaemia

Clinical studies in hypercalcaemia of malignancy demonstrated that the inhibitory effect of ibandronic acid on tumour-induced osteolysis, and specifically on tumour-induced hypercalcaemia, is characterised by a decrease in serum calcium and urinary calcium excretion.

In the dose range recommended for treatment, the following response rates with the respective confidence intervals have been shown in clinical trials for patients with baseline albumin corrected serum calcium ≥ 3.0mmol/l after adequate rehydration.

(see Figure 1 below)

Figure 1

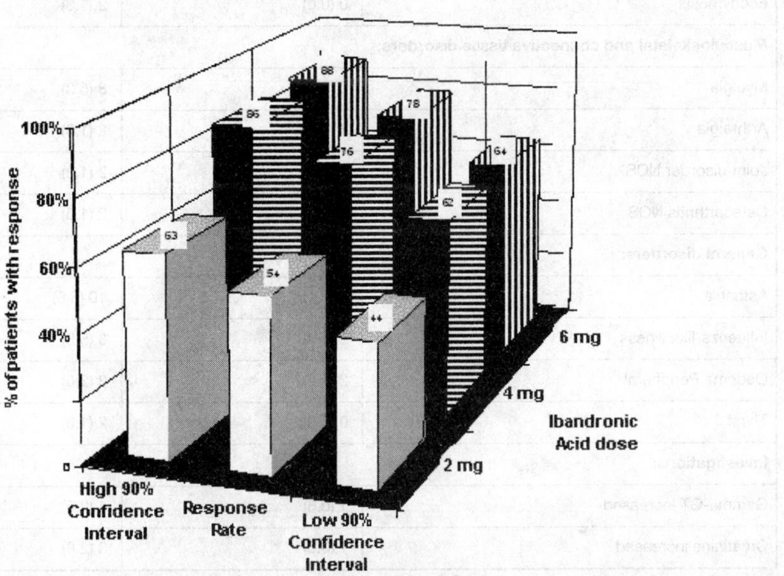

For these patients and dosages, the median time to achieve normocalcaemia was 4 to 7 days. The median time to relapse (return of albumin corrected serum calcium above 3.0mmol/l) was 18 to 26 days.

Clinical Studies in the Prevention of Skeletal Events in Patients with Breast Cancer and Bone Metastases

Clinical studies in patients with breast cancer and bone metastases have shown that there is a dose dependent inhibitory effect on bone osteolysis, expressed by markers of bone resorption, and a dose dependent effect on skeletal events.

Prevention of skeletal events in patients with breast cancer and bone metastases with Bondronat 6mg IV was assessed in one randomised placebo controlled phase III trial with duration of 96 weeks. Female patients with breast cancer and radiologically confirmed bone metastases were randomised to receive placebo (158 patients) or 6mg Bondronat (154 patients). The results from this trial are summarised below.

Primary Efficacy Endpoints

The primary endpoint of the trial was the skeletal morbidity period rate (SMPR). This was a composite endpoint which had the following skeletal related events (SREs) as sub-components:

- radiotherapy to bone for treatment of fractures/impending fractures
- surgery to bone for treatment of fractures
- vertebral fractures
- non-vertebral fractures.

The analysis of the SMPR was time-adjusted and considered that one or more events occurring in a single 12 week period could be potentially related. Multiple events were therefore counted only once for the purposes of the analysis. Data from this study demonstrated a significant advantage for Bondronat 6mg IV over placebo in the reduction in SREs measured by the time-adjusted SMPR (p=0.004). The number of SREs was also significantly reduced with Bondronat 6mg and there was a 40 % reduction in the risk of a SRE over placebo (relative risk 0.6, p = 0.003). Efficacy results are summarised in Table 3.

Table 2 Related Adverse Events Occurring Commonly and Greater than Placebo in Patients with Metastatic Bone Disease due to Breast Cancer Treated with Bondronat 6mg i.v.

Adverse Drug Reaction	Placebo (n = 157) No. (%)	Bondronat 6mg (n = 152) No. (%)
Infections and Infestations:		
Infection NOS	1 (0.6)	2 (1.3)
Endocrine disorders:		
Parathyroid disorder NOS	1 (0.6)	2 (1.3)
Nervous System disorders:		
Headache	4 (2.5)	9 (5.9)
Dizziness	2 (1.3)	4 (2.6)
Dysgeusia (taste perversion)	0 (0.0)	2 (1.3)
Eye disorders:		
Cataract	1 (0.6)	2 (1.3)
Cardiac disorders:		
Bundle branch block NOS	1 (0.6)	2 (1.3)
Respiratory, thoracic and mediastinal disorders:		
Pharyngitis	0 (0.0)	3 (2.0)
Gastrointestinal disorders:		
Diarrhoea NOS	1 (0.6)	8 (5.3)
Dyspepsia	5 (3.2)	6 (3.9)
Vomiting NOS	2 (1.3)	5 (3.3)
Gastrointestinal pain NOS	2 (1.3)	4 (2.6)
Tooth disorder NOS	0 (0.0)	3 (2.0)
Skin and subcutaneous tissue disorders:		
Skin disorder NOS	0 (0.0)	2 (1.3)
Ecchymosis	0 (0.0)	2 (1.3)
Musculoskeletal and connective tissue disorders:		
Myalgia	6 (3.8)	8 (5.3)
Arthralgia	1 (0.6)	2 (1.3)
Joint disorder NOS	0 (0.0)	2 (1.3)
Osteoarthritis NOS	0 (0.0)	2 (1.3)
General disorders:		
Asthenia	8 (5.1)	10 (6.6)
Influenza-like illness	2 (1.3)	8 (5.3)
Oedema Peripheral	2 (1.3)	3 (2.0)
Thirst	0 (0.0)	2 (1.3)
Investigations:		
Gamma-GT increased	1 (0.6)	4 (2.6)
Creatinine increased	1 (0.6)	3 (2.0)

Table 3 Efficacy Results (Breast Cancer Patients with Metastatic Bone Disease)

(see Table 3 on next page)

Secondary Efficacy Endpoints

A statistically significant improvement in bone pain score was shown for Bondronat 6mg IV compared to placebo. The pain reduction was consistently below baseline throughout the entire study and accompanied by a significantly reduced use of analgesics. The deterioration in Quality of Life was significantly less in Bondronat treated patients compared with placebo. A tabular summary of these secondary efficacy results is presented in Table 4.

Table 4 Secondary Efficacy Results (Breast cancer Patients with Metastatic Bone Disease)

(see Table 4 on next page)

There was a marked depression of urinary markers of bone resorption (pyridinoline and deoxypyridinoline) in patients treated with Bondronat that was statistically significant compared to placebo.

5.2 Pharmacokinetic properties

After a 2 hour infusion of 2, 4 and 6mg ibandronic acid pharmacokinetic parameters are dose proportional.

Distribution

After initial systemic exposure, ibandronic acid rapidly binds to bone or is excreted into urine. In humans, the apparent terminal volume of distribution is at least 90 l and the amount of dose reaching the bone is estimated to be 40 - 50% of the circulating dose. Protein binding in human plasma is approximately 87% at therapeutic concentrations, and thus drug-drug interaction due to displacement is unlikely.

Metabolism

There is no evidence that ibandronic acid is metabolised in animals or humans.

Elimination

The range of observed apparent half-lives is broad and dependent on dose and assay sensitivity, but the apparent terminal half-life is generally in the range of 10 - 60 hours. However, early plasma levels fall quickly, reaching 10% of peak values within 3 and 8 hours after intravenous or oral administration respectively. No systemic accumulation was observed when ibandronic acid was administered intravenously once every 4 weeks for 48 weeks to patients with metastatic bone disease.

Total clearance of ibandronic acid is low with average values in the range 84 - 160ml/min. Renal clearance (about 60ml/min in healthy postmenopausal females) accounts for 50 - 60% of total clearance and is related to creatinine clearance. The difference between the apparent total and renal clearances is considered to reflect the uptake by bone.

Pharmacokinetics in Special Populations

Gender

Bioavailability and pharmacokinetics of ibandronic acid are similar in both men and women.

Race

There is no evidence for clinically relevant interethnic differences between Asians and Caucasians in ibandronic acid disposition. There are only very few data available on patients with African origin.

Patients with renal impairment

Renal clearance of ibandronic acid in patients with various degrees of renal impairment is linearly related to creatinine clearance (CLcr). No dosage adjustment is necessary for patients with mild or moderate renal impairment (CLcr ≥ 30ml/min). After IV administration of 0.5mg, total, renal, and non-renal clearances decreased by 67%, 77% and 50%, respectively, in subjects with severe renal impairment. However, there was no reduction in tolerability associated with the increase in exposure. Reduction of the intravenous dose to 2mg infused over 1 hour every 3 - 4 weeks is recommended in patients with severe renal impairment (CLcr < 30ml/min) (see section *4.2*).

Patients with hepatic impairment

There are no pharmacokinetic data for ibandronic acid in patients who have hepatic impairment. The liver has no significant role in the clearance of ibandronic acid since it is not metabolised but is cleared by renal excretion and by uptake into bone. Therefore dosage adjustment is not necessary in patients with hepatic impairment. Further, as protein binding of ibandronic acid is approximately 87% at therapeutic concentrations, hypoproteinaemia in severe liver disease is unlikely to lead to clinically significant increases in free plasma concentration.

Elderly

In a multivariate analysis, age was not found to be an independent factor of any of the pharmacokinetic parameters studied. As renal function decreases with age, this is the only factor that should be considered (see renal impairment section).

Table 3 Efficacy Results (Breast Cancer Patients with Metastatic Bone Disease)

	All Skeletal Related Events (SREs)		
	Placebo n=158	Bondronat 6mg n=154	p-value
SMPR (per patient year)	1.48	1.19	p=0.004
Number of events (per patient)	3.64	2.65	p=0.025
SRE relative risk	-	0.60	p=0.003

Table 4 Secondary Efficacy Results (Breast cancer Patients with Metastatic Bone Disease)

	Placebo n=158	Bondronat 6mg n=154	p-value
Bone pain *	0.21	-0.28	p< 0.001
Analgesic use *	0.90	0.51	p=0.083
Quality of Life *	-45.4	-10.3	p=0.004

* Mean change from baseline to last assessment.

Children and adolescents

There are no data on the use of Bondronat in patients less than 18 years old.

5.3 Preclinical safety data

As with other bisphosphonates, the kidney was identified to be the primary target organ of systemic toxicity in animal studies. Toxic effects in animals were observed only at exposures sufficiently in excess of the maximum human exposure indicating little relevance to clinical use.

Mutagenicity/Carcinogenicity:

No indication of carcinogenic potential was observed. Tests for genotoxicity revealed no evidence of genetic activity for ibandronic acid.

Reproductive toxicity:

No evidence of direct foetal toxicity or teratogenic effects were observed for ibandronic acid in intravenously treated rats and rabbits. Adverse effects of ibandronic acid in reproductive toxicity studies in the rat were those expected for this class of drug (bisphosphonates). They include a decreased number of implantation sites, interference with natural delivery (dystocia), an increase in visceral variations (renal pelvis ureter syndrome) and teeth abnormalities in F1 offspring in rats.

6. PHARMACEUTICAL PARTICULARS

6.1 List of excipients

Sodium chloride

Acetic acid (99%)

Sodium acetate

Water for injections

6.2 Incompatibilities

To avoid potential incompatibilities Bondronat concentrate for solution for infusion should only be diluted with isotonic sodium chloride solution or 5% dextrose solution.

6.3 Shelf life

5 years.

After reconstitution: 24 hours.

6.4 Special precautions for storage

No special precautions for storage.

After reconstitution: Store at 2°C - 8°C (in a refrigerator).

From a microbiological point of view, the product should be used immediately. If not used immediately, in-use storage times and conditions prior to use are the responsibility of the user and would normally not be longer than 24 hours at 2 to 8°C, unless reconstitution has taken place in controlled and validated aseptic conditions.

6.5 Nature and contents of container

Bondronat 2mg/2ml is supplied as packs containing 1 vial (2ml glass vial, glass type I).

Bondronat 6mg/6ml is supplied as packs containing 1 and 5 vials (6ml glass vials, glass type 1). The vials are closed with rubber stoppers complying with Ph.Eur.

6.6 Instructions for use and handling

For single use only. Only clear solution without particles should be used.

Strict adherence to the intravenous route is recommended on parenteral administration of Bondronat concentrate for solution for infusion.

Use only isotonic saline or 5% dextrose solution as infusion solution.

Bondronat concentrate for solution for infusion should not be mixed with calcium containing solutions.

Unused solution should be discarded.

7. MARKETING AUTHORISATION HOLDER

Roche Registration Limited, 40 Broadwater Road, Welwyn Garden City, Hertfordshire, AL7 3AY, United Kingdom.

8. MARKETING AUTHORISATION NUMBER(S)

Bondronat 2mg/2ml

EU/1/96/012/004 - Packs of 1 vial

Bondronat 6mg/6ml

EU/1/96/012/012 - Packs of 5 vials

EU/1/96/012/011 - Packs of 1 vial

9. DATE OF FIRST AUTHORISATION/RENEWAL OF THE AUTHORISATION

Bondronat 2mg/2ml September 2001

Bondronat 6mg/6ml November 2003

10. DATE OF REVISION OF THE TEXT

October 2004

Bondronat is a registered trade mark

Bondronat 50mg Film-coated Tablets

(Roche Products Limited)

1. NAME OF THE MEDICINAL PRODUCT

Bondronat▼ 50 mg

Film Coated Tablets

2. QUALITATIVE AND QUANTITATIVE COMPOSITION

Qualitative composition

Ibandronic acid, monosodium salt, monohydrate.

Quantitative composition

Each film-coated tablet contains 50 mg of ibandronic acid (as ibandronic sodium monohydrate).

For excipients, see section 6.1.

3. PHARMACEUTICAL FORM

Film-coated tablets of oblong shape.

White to off-white in colour, engraved L2/IT.

4. CLINICAL PARTICULARS

4.1 Therapeutic indications

Bondronat is indicated for the prevention of skeletal events (pathological fractures, bone complications requiring radiotherapy or surgery) in patients with breast cancer and bone metastases.

4.2 Posology and method of administration

Bondronat should only be initiated by physicians experienced in the treatment of cancer.

For oral use.

Adults:

The recommended dose is one 50 mg film-coated tablet daily.

Dosing Instructions:

Bondronat tablets should be taken after an overnight fast (at least 6 hours) and before the first food or drink of the day. Medicinal products and supplements (including calcium) should similarly be avoided prior to taking Bondronat tablets. Fasting should be continued for at least 30 minutes after taking the tablet. Plain water may be taken at any time during the course of Bondronat treatment.

– The tablets should be swallowed whole with a full glass of plain water (180 to 240 ml) while the patient is standing or sitting in an upright position.

– Patients should not lie down for 60 minutes after taking Bondronat.

– Patients should not chew or suck the tablet because of a potential for oropharyngeal ulceration.

– Plain water is the only drink that should be taken with Bondronat. Please note that some mineral waters may have a higher concentration of calcium and therefore should not be used.

Special Dosage Instructions:

Patients with hepatic impairment

No dosage adjustment is expected to be necessary (see Section 5.2).

Patients with renal impairment

No dosage adjustment is necessary for patients with mild or moderate renal impairment where creatinine clearance is equal to or greater than 30 ml/min.

Below 30 ml/min creatinine clearance, the recommended dose is 50 mg once weekly. See dosing instructions, above.

Elderly

No dose adjustment is necessary.

Children and adolescents

Safety and efficacy have not been established in patients less than 18 years old.

4.3 Contraindications

Bondronat is contraindicated in patients with hypersensitivity to ibandronic acid or to any of the excipients.

4.4 Special warnings and special precautions for use

Caution is indicated in patients with known hypersensitivity to other bisphosphonates.

Hypocalcaemia and other disturbances of bone and mineral metabolism should be effectively treated before starting Bondronat therapy. Adequate intake of calcium and vitamin D is important in all patients. Patients should receive supplemental calcium and/or vitamin D if dietary intake is inadequate.

Oral bisphosphonates have been associated with dysphagia, oesophagitis and oesophageal or gastric ulcers. Therefore, patients should pay particular attention to the dosing instructions (see Section 4.2).

Physicians should be alert to signs or symptoms signalling a possible oesophageal reaction during therapy, and patients should be instructed to discontinue Bondronat and seek medical attention if they develop symptoms of oesophageal irritation such as new or worsening dysphagia, pain on swallowing, retrosternal pain, or heartburn.

Since NSAIDS are associated with gastrointestinal irritation, caution should be taken during concomitant oral medication with Bondronat.

Clinical studies have not shown any evidence of deterioration in renal function with long term Bondronat therapy. Nevertheless, according to clinical assessment of the individual patient, it is recommended that renal function, serum calcium, phosphate and magnesium should be monitored in patients treated with Bondronat.

Bondronat tablets contain lactose and should not be administered to patients with rare hereditary problems of galactose intolerance, Lapp lactase deficiency or glucose-galactose malabsorption.

4.5 Interaction with other medicinal products and other forms of Interaction

Drug-Food Interactions

Products containing calcium and other multivalent cations (such as aluminium, magnesium, iron), including milk and food, are likely to interfere with absorption of Bondronat tablets. Therefore, with such products, including food, intake must be delayed at least 30 minutes following oral administration.

Bioavailability was reduced by approximately 75% when Bondronat tablets were administered 2 hours after a standard meal. Therefore, it is recommended that the tablets should be taken after an overnight fast (at least 6 hours) and fasting should continue for at least 30 minutes after the dose has been taken (see Section 4.2).

Drug-Drug Interactions

When co-administered with melphalan/prednisolone in patients with multiple myeloma, no interaction was observed.

Other interaction studies in postmenopausal women have demonstrated the absence of any interaction potential with tamoxifen or hormone replacement therapy (oestrogen).

In healthy male volunteers and postmenopausal women, IV ranitidine caused an increase in ibandronic acid bioavailability of about 20% (which is within the normal variability of the bioavailability of ibandronic acid), probably as a result of reduced gastric acidity. However, no dosage adjustment is required when Bondronat is administered with H_2-antagonists or other drugs that increase gastric pH.

In relation to disposition, no drug interactions of clinical significance are likely. Ibandronic acid is eliminated by renal secretion only and does not undergo any biotransformation. The secretory pathway does not appear to include known acidic or basic transport systems involved in the excretion of other active substances. In addition, ibandronic acid does not inhibit the major human hepatic P450 isoenzymes and does not induce the hepatic cytochrome P450 system in rats. Plasma protein binding is low at therapeutic concentrations and ibandronic acid is therefore unlikely to displace other active substances.

Caution is advised when bisphosphonates are administered with aminoglycosides, since both agents can lower serum calcium levels for prolonged periods. Attention should also be paid to the possible existence of simultaneous hypomagnesaemia.

In clinical studies, Bondronat has been administered concomitantly with commonly used anticancer agents, diuretics, antibiotics and analgesics without clinically apparent interactions occurring.

4.6 Pregnancy and lactation

There are no adequate data from the use of ibandronic acid in pregnant women. Studies in rats have shown reproductive toxicity (see Section 5.3). The potential risk for humans is unknown. Therefore, Bondronat should not be used during pregnancy.

It is not known whether ibandronic acid is excreted in human milk. Studies in lactating rats have demonstrated the presence of low levels of ibandronic acid in the milk following intravenous administration. Consequently, caution should be exercised when prescribing Bondronat to breast-feeding women.

4.7 Effects on ability to drive and use machines

No studies on the effects on the ability to drive and use machines have been performed.

4.8 Undesirable effects

The safety profile of Bondronat film-coated tablets is derived from controlled clinical trials in the approved indication and after the oral administration of Bondronat at the recommended dose.

In the pooled database from the 2 pivotal phase III trials (286 patients treated with Bondronat 50 mg), the proportion of patients who experienced an adverse drug reaction with a possible or probable relationship to Bondronat was 27%.

Adverse reactions are ranked under heading of frequency, the most frequent first, using the following convention: very common (⩾ 10%), common (⩾ 1% and < 10%), uncommon (⩾ 0.1% and < 1%), rare (⩾ 0.01% and < 0.1%), and very rare (⩽ 0.01%).

Table 1 lists common adverse drug reactions from the pooled phase III trials. Adverse drug reactions that are equally frequent in both active and placebo or more frequent in placebo-treated patients are excluded.

Table 1: Related Adverse Events Reported Commonly and Greater than Placebo

Adverse drug reaction	Placebo p. o. daily (n=277 patients) No. (%)	Bondronat 50 mg p.o. daily (n=286 patients) No. (%)
Metabolism and Nutrition Disorders		
Hypocalcaemia	14 (5.1)	27 (9.4)
Gastrointestinal Disorders		
Dyspepsia	13 (4.7)	20 (7.0)
Nausea	4 (1.4)	10 (3.5)
Abdominal Pain Nos	2 (0.7)	6 (2.1)
Oesophagitis	2 (0.7)	6 (2.1)
General Disorders		
Asthenia	2 (0.7)	4 (1.4)

Adverse drug reactions occurring at a frequency < 1%:

The following list provides information on adverse drug reactions reported in study MF 4414 and MF 4434 occurring more frequently with Bondronat 50 mg than with placebo:

Uncommon:	
Blood and Lymphatic System Disorders	Anaemia
Nervous System Disorders	dysgeusia (taste perversion); paraesthesia
Gastrointestinal Disorders	abdominal pain, dry mouth, duodenal ulcer haemorrhage, dysphagia, gastritis
Skin and Subcutaneous Tissue Disorders	Pruritus
Renal & Urinary Disorders	Azotaemia (uraemia)
General Disorders:	chest pain, influenza-like illness, malaise, pain NOS
Investigations	Blood parathyroid hormone increased

4.9 Overdose

So far, no case of overdosing with Bondronat film-coated tablets has been reported.

No specific information is available on the treatment of overdosage with Bondronat. However, oral overdosage may result in upper gastrointestinal events, such as upset stomach, heartburn, oesophagitis, gastritis or ulcer. Milk or antacids should be given to bind Bondronat. Owing to the risk of oesophageal irritation, vomiting should not be induced and the patient should remain fully upright.

5. PHARMACOLOGICAL PROPERTIES

5.1 Pharmacodynamic properties

Pharmaco-therapeutic group: Bisphosphonate, ATC Code: M05B A 06

Ibandronic acid belongs to the bisphosphonate group of compounds which act specifically on bone. Their selective action on bone tissue is based on the high affinity of bisphosphonates for bone mineral. Bisphosphonates act by inhibiting osteoclast activity, although the precise mechanism is still not clear.

In vivo, ibandronic acid prevents experimentally-induced bone destruction caused by cessation of gonadal function, retinoids, tumours or tumour extracts. The inhibition of endogenous bone resorption has also been documented by ^{45}Ca kinetic studies and by the release of radioactive tetracycline previously incorporated into the skeleton.

At doses that were considerably higher than the pharmacologically effective doses, ibandronic acid did not have any effect on bone mineralisation.

Bone resorption due to malignant disease is characterised by excessive bone resorption that is not balanced with appropriate bone formation. Ibandronic acid selectively inhibits osteoclast activity, reducing bone resorption and thereby reducing skeletal complications of the malignant disease.

Clinical studies in patients with breast cancer and bone metastases have shown that there is a dose dependent inhibitory effect on bone osteolysis, expressed by markers of bone resorption, and a dose dependent effect on skeletal events.

Prevention of skeletal events in patients with breast cancer and bone metastases with Bondronat 50 mg tablets was assessed in two randomised placebo controlled phase III trials with duration of 96 weeks. Female patients with breast cancer and radiologically confirmed bone metastases were randomised to receive placebo (277 patients) or 50 mg Bondronat (287 patients). The results from these trials are summarised below.

Primary Efficacy Endpoints

The primary endpoint of the trials was the skeletal morbidity period rate (SMPR). This was a composite endpoint which had the following skeletal related events (SREs) as sub-components:

- radiotherapy to bone for treatment of fractures/impending fractures
- surgery to bone for treatment of fractures
- vertebral fractures
- non-vertebral fractures

The analysis of the SMPR was time-adjusted and considered that one or more events occurring in a single 12 week period could be potentially related. Multiple events were therefore, counted only once in any given 12 week period for the purposes of the analysis. Pooled data from these studies demonstrated a significant advantage for Bondronat 50 mg p.o. over placebo in the reduction in SREs measured by the SMPR (p=0.041). There was also a 38% reduction in the risk of developing an SRE for Bondronat treated patients when compared with placebo (relative risk 0.62, p=0.003). Efficacy results are summarised in Table 2.

Table 2 Efficacy Results (Breast Cancer Patients with Metastatic Bone Disease)

(see Table 2 below)

Secondary Efficacy Endpoints

A statistically significant improvement in bone pain score was shown for Bondronat 50 mg compared to placebo. The pain reduction was consistently below baseline throughout the entire study and accompanied by a significantly reduced use of analgesics compared to placebo. The deterioration in Quality of Life and WHO performance status was significantly less in Bondronat treated patients compared with placebo. Urinary concentrations of the bone resorption marker CTx (C-terminal telopeptide released from Type I collagen) were significantly reduced in the Bondronat group compared to placebo. This reduction in urinary CTx levels was significantly correlated with the primary efficacy endpoint SMPR (Kendall-tau-b (p< 0.001)). A tabular summary of the secondary efficacy results is presented in Table 3.

Table 3 Secondary Efficacy Results (Breast Cancer Patients with Metastatic Bone Disease)

(see Table 3 below)

5.2 Pharmacokinetic properties

Absorption

The absorption of ibandronic acid in the upper gastrointestinal tract is rapid after oral administration. Maximum observed plasma concentrations were reached within 0.5 to 2 hours (median 1 hour) in the fasted state and absolute bioavailability was about 0.6%. The extent of absorption is impaired when taken together with food or beverages (other than plain water). Bioavailability is reduced by about 90% when ibandronic acid is administered with a standard breakfast in comparison with bioavailability seen in fasted subjects. When taken 30 minutes before a meal, the reduction in bioavailability is approximately 30%. There is no meaningful reduction in bioavailability provided ibandronic acid is taken 60 minutes before a meal.

Bioavailability was reduced by approximately 75% when Bondronat tablets were administered 2 hours after a standard meal. Therefore, it is recommended that the tablets should be taken after an overnight fast (minimum 6 hours) and fasting should continue for at least 30 minutes after the dose has been taken (see Section 4.2).

Distribution

After initial systemic exposure, ibandronic acid rapidly binds to bone or is excreted into urine. In humans, the apparent terminal volume of distribution is at least 90 l and the amount of dose reaching the bone is estimated to be 40-50% of the circulating dose. Protein binding in human plasma is approximately 87% at therapeutic concentrations, and thus drug-drug interaction due to displacement is unlikely.

Metabolism

There is no evidence that ibandronic acid is metabolised in animals or humans.

Elimination

The absorbed fraction of ibandronic acid is removed from the circulation via bone absorption (estimated to be 40-50%) and the remainder is eliminated unchanged by the kidney. The unabsorbed fraction of ibandronic acid is eliminated unchanged in the faeces.

The range of observed apparent half-lives is broad and dependent on dose and assay sensitivity, but the apparent

Table 2 Efficacy Results (Breast Cancer Patients with Metastatic Bone Disease)

	All Skeletal Related Events (SREs)		
	Placebo n=277	Bondronat 50 mg n=287	p-value
SMPR (per patient year)	1.15	0.99	p=0.041
SRE relative risk	-	0.62	p=0.003

Table 3 Secondary Efficacy Results (Breast Cancer Patients with Metastatic Bone Disease)

	Placebo n=277	Bondronat 50 mg n=287	p-value
Bone pain *	0.20	-0.10	p=0.001
Analgesic use *	0.85	0.60	p=0.019
Quality of Life *	-26.8	-8.3	p=0.032
WHO performance score *	0.54	0.33	p=0.008
Urinary CTx **	10.95	-77.32	p=0.001

* Mean change from baseline to last assessment.

** Median change from baseline to last assessment.

terminal half-life is generally in the range of 10-60 hours. However, early plasma levels fall quickly, reaching 10% of peak values within 3 and 8 hours after intravenous or oral administration respectively.

Total clearance of ibandronic acid is low with average values in the range 84-160 ml/min. Renal clearance (about 60 ml/min in healthy postmenopausal females) accounts for 50-60% of total clearance and is related to creatinine clearance. The difference between the apparent total and renal clearances is considered to reflect the uptake by bone.

Pharmacokinetics in Special Populations

Gender

Bioavailability and pharmacokinetics of ibandronic acid are similar in both men and women.

Race

There is no evidence for clinically relevant interethnic differences between Asians and Caucasians in ibandronic acid disposition. There are only very few data available on patients with African origin.

Patients with renal impairment

Renal clearance of ibandronic acid in patients with various degrees of renal impairment is linearly related to creatinine clearance (CLcr). No dosage adjustment is necessary for patients with mild or moderate renal impairment (CLcr ⩾ 30 ml/min). Subjects with severe renal impairment (CLcr ⩽ 30 ml/min) receiving oral administration of 10 mg ibandronic acid daily for 21 days, had 2 - 3 fold higher plasma concentrations than subjects with normal renal function. Total clearance of ibandronic acid was reduced to 44 ml/min in the subjects with severe renal impairment. After IV administration of 0.5 mg, total, renal, and non-renal clearances decreased by 67%, 77% and 50%, respectively, in subjects with severe renal impairment. However, there was no reduction in tolerability associated with the increase in exposure. Reduction of the oral dose to one 50 mg tablet once weekly is recommended in patients with severe renal impairment (CLcr < 30 ml/min) (see Section 4.2).

Patients with hepatic impairment

There are no pharmacokinetic data for ibandronic acid in patients who have hepatic impairment. The liver has no significant role in the clearance of ibandronic acid since it is not metabolised but is cleared by renal excretion and by uptake into bone. Therefore dosage adjustment is not necessary in patients with hepatic impairment. Further, as protein binding of ibandronic acid is approximately 87% at therapeutic concentrations, hypoproteinaemia in severe liver disease is unlikely to lead to clinically significant increases in free plasma concentration.

Elderly

In a multivariate analysis, age was not found to be an independent factor of any of the pharmacokinetic parameters studied. As renal function decreases with age, this is the only factor to take into consideration (see renal impairment section).

Children and adolescents

There are no data on the use of Bondronat in patients less than 18 years old.

5.3 Preclinical safety data

As with other bisphosphonates, the kidney was identified to be the primary target organ of systemic toxicity in animal studies. Toxic effects in animals were observed only at exposures sufficiently in excess of the maximum human exposure indicating little relevance to clinical use.

Mutagenicity/Carcinogenicity:

No indication of carcinogenic potential was observed. Tests for genotoxicity revealed no evidence of genetic activity for ibandronic acid.

Reproductive toxicity:

No evidence of direct foetal toxicity or teratogenic effects was observed for ibandronic acid in intravenously or orally treated rats and rabbits. Adverse effects of ibandronic acid in reproductive toxicity studies in the rat were those expected for this class of drugs (bisphosphonates). They include a decreased number of implantation sites, interference with natural delivery (dystocia), an increase in visceral variations (renal pelvis ureter syndrome) and teeth abnormalities in F1 offspring in rats.

6. PHARMACEUTICAL PARTICULARS

6.1 List of excipients

Tablet core:

Lactose monohydrate

Povidone

Cellulose, microcrystalline

Crospovidone

Stearic acid

Silica, anhydrous colloidal

Tablet coat:

Hypromellose

Titanium dioxide E171

Talc

Macrogol 6000

6.2 Incompatibilities

Not applicable.

6.3 Shelf life

2 years.

6.4 Special precautions for storage

Store in the original package.

6.5 Nature and contents of container

Bondronat 50 mg film coated tablets are supplied in blisters (Aluminium) containing 7 tablets, which are presented as packs containing 28 or 84 tablets.

6.6 Instructions for use and handling

No special requirements.

7. MARKETING AUTHORISATION HOLDER

Roche Registration Limited

40 Broadwater Road

Welwyn Garden City

Hertfordshire, AL7 3AY

United Kingdom

8. MARKETING AUTHORISATION NUMBER(S)

EU/1/96/012/009

EU/1/96/012/010

9. DATE OF FIRST AUTHORISATION/RENEWAL OF THE AUTHORISATION

24 October 2003

10. DATE OF REVISION OF THE TEXT

June 2005

Bonviva 150mg Film-Coated Tablets

(Roche Products Limited)

1. NAME OF THE MEDICINAL PRODUCT

Bonviva® ▼150 mg film-coated tablets.

2. QUALITATIVE AND QUANTITATIVE COMPOSITION

Each film-coated tablet contains 150 mg ibandronic acid (as ibandronic sodium monohydrate).

For excipients, see section 6.1.

3. PHARMACEUTICAL FORM

Film-coated tablet.

White to off white film-coated tablets, of oblong shape marked "BNVA" on one side, and "150" on the other side.

4. CLINICAL PARTICULARS

4.1 Therapeutic indications

Treatment of osteoporosis in postmenopausal women in order to reduce the risk of vertebral fractures. Efficacy on femoral neck fractures has not been established.

4.2 Posology and method of administration

For oral use.

The recommended dose is one 150 mg film-coated tablet once a month. The tablet should preferably be taken on the same date each month.

Bonviva should be taken after an overnight fast (at least 6 hours) and 1 hour before the first food or drink (other than water) of the day (see section 4.5) or any other oral medicinal products or supplementation (including calcium):

• Tablets should be swallowed whole with a glass of plain water (180 to 240 ml) while the patient is sitting or standing in an upright position. Patients should not lie down for 1 hour after taking Bonviva.

• Plain water is the only drink that should be taken with Bonviva. Please note that some mineral waters may have a higher concentration of calcium and therefore, should not be used.

• Patients should not chew or suck the tablet because of a potential for oropharyngeal ulceration.

In case a dose is missed, patients should be instructed to take one Bonviva 150 mg tablet the morning after the tablet is remembered, unless the time to the next scheduled dose is within 7 days. Patients should then return to taking their dose once a month on their originally scheduled date.

If the next scheduled dose is within 7 days, patients should wait until their next dose and then continue taking one tablet once a month as originally scheduled.

Patients should not take two tablets within the same week.

Patients should receive supplemental calcium and / or vitamin D if dietary intake is inadequate (see section 4.4 and section 4.5).

Patients with renal impairment

No dosage adjustment is necessary for patients with mild or moderate renal impairment where creatinine clearance is equal to or greater than 30 ml/min.

Bonviva is not recommended for patients with a creatinine clearance below 30 ml/min due to limited clinical experience (see section 4.4 and section 5.2).

Patients with hepatic impairment

No dosage adjustment is required (see section 5.2).

Elderly

No dosage adjustment is required (see section 5.2).

Children and adolescents

Bonviva has not been tested in these age groups and should not be given to them.

4.3 Contraindications

- Hypocalcaemia (see section 4.4).

- Hypersensitivity to ibandronic acid or to any of the excipients.

4.4 Special warnings and special precautions for use

Hypocalcaemia must be corrected before starting Bonviva therapy. Other disturbances of bone and mineral metabolism should also be effectively treated. Adequate intake of calcium and vitamin D is important in all patients.

Bisphosphonates have been associated with dysphagia, oesophagitis and oesophageal or gastric ulcers. Therefore patients, especially those with a history of prolonged oesophageal transit time, should pay particular attention to and be able to comply with the dosing instructions (see section 4.2).

Physicians should be alert to signs or symptoms signalling a possible oesophageal reaction during therapy, and patients should be instructed to discontinue Bonviva and seek medical attention if they develop symptoms of oesophageal irritation such as new or worsening dysphagia, pain on swallowing, retrosternal pain or heartburn.

Since NSAIDS and bisphosphonates are both associated with gastrointestinal irritation, caution should be taken during concomitant administration.

Due to limited clinical experience, Bonviva is not recommended for patients with a creatinine clearance below 30 ml/min (see section 4.2 and section 5.2).

4.5 Interaction with other medicinal products and other forms of Interaction

Drug-Food Interactions

Oral bioavailability of ibandronic acid is generally reduced in the presence of food. In particular, products containing calcium and other multivalent cations (such as aluminium, magnesium, iron), including milk, are likely to interfere with absorption of Bonviva, which is consistent with findings in animal studies. Therefore, patients should fast overnight (at least 6 hours) before taking Bonviva and continue fasting for 1 hour following intake of Bonviva.

Drug-Drug Interactions

Calcium supplements, antacids and some oral medicinal products containing multivalent cations (such as aluminium, magnesium, iron) are likely to interfere with the absorption of Bonviva. Therefore, patients should not take other oral medicinal products for at least 6 hours before taking Bonviva and for 1 hour following intake of Bonviva.

Pharmacokinetic interaction studies in postmenopausal women have demonstrated the absence of any interaction potential with tamoxifen or hormone replacement therapy (oestrogen). No interaction was observed when co-administered with melphalan/prednisolone in patients with multiple myeloma.

In healthy male volunteers and postmenopausal women, intravenous administration of ranitidine caused an increase in ibandronic acid bioavailability of about 20 %, probably as a result of reduced gastric acidity. However, since this increase is within the normal variability of the bioavailability of ibandronic acid, no dosage adjustment is considered necessary when Bonviva is administered with H2-antagonists or other active substances which increase gastric pH.

Metabolic interactions are not considered likely, since ibandronic acid does not inhibit the major human hepatic P450 isoenzymes and has been shown not to induce the hepatic cytochrome P450 system in rats. Furthermore, plasma protein binding is approximately 85 % - 87 % (determined *in vitro* at therapeutic drug concentrations), and thus there is a low potential for drug-drug interaction due to displacement. Ibandronic acid is eliminated by renal excretion only and does not undergo any biotransformation. The secretory pathway appears not to include known acidic or basic transport systems involved in the excretion of other active substances.

In a two-year study in postmenopausal women with osteoporosis (BM 16549), the incidence of upper gastrointestinal events in patients concomitantly taking aspirin or NSAIDs was similar in patients taking Bonviva 2.5 mg daily or 150 mg once monthly after one and two years.

Of over 1500 patients enrolled in study BM 16549 comparing monthly with daily dosing regimens of ibandronic acid, 14 % and 18 % of patients used histamine (H2) blockers or proton pump inhibitors after one and two years, respectively. Among these patients, the incidence of upper gastrointestinal events in the patients treated with Bonviva 150 mg once monthly was similar to that in patients treated with Bonviva 2.5 mg daily.

4.6 Pregnancy and lactation

There are no adequate data from the use of ibandronic acid in pregnant women. Studies in rats have shown some reproductive toxicity (see section 5.3). The potential risk for humans is unknown.

Bonviva should not be used during pregnancy.

It is not known whether ibandronic acid is excreted in human milk. Studies in lactating rats have demonstrated the presence of low levels of ibandronic acid in the milk following intravenous administration.

Bonviva should not be used during lactation.

4.7 Effects on ability to drive and use machines

No studies on the effects on the ability to drive and use machines have been performed.

4.8 Undesirable effects

The safety of Bonviva 2.5 mg daily was evaluated in 1251 patients treated in 4 placebo-controlled clinical studies; 73 % of these patients came from the pivotal three-year treatment study (MF 4411). The overall safety profile of Bonviva 2.5 mg daily in all these studies was similar to that of placebo. The overall proportion of patients who experienced an adverse drug reaction, i.e. adverse event with a possible or probable relationship to trial medication, in the pivotal treatment study (MF 4411) was 19.8 % for Bonviva and 17.9 % for placebo.

In a two-year study in postmenopausal women with osteoporosis (BM 16549) the overall safety of Bonviva 150 mg once monthly and Bonviva 2.5 mg daily was similar. The overall proportion of patients who experienced an adverse drug reaction, i.e. adverse event with a possible or probable relationship to trial medication, was 22.7 % and 25.0 % for Bonviva 150 mg once monthly and 21.5 % and 22.5 % for Bonviva 2.5 mg daily after one and two years, respectively. The majority of adverse drug reactions were mild to moderate in intensity. Most cases did not lead to cessation of therapy.

Table 1 and Table 2 list adverse drug reactions occurring in more than 1 % of patients treated with Bonviva 150 mg monthly or 2.5 mg daily in study BM 16549 and in patients treated with Bonviva 2.5 mg daily in study MF 4411. The tables show the adverse drug reactions in the two studies that occurred with a higher incidence than in patients treated with placebo in study MF 4411.

Data at one year from BM 16549 are represented in Table 1 and cumulative data for the two years from BM 16549 are represented in Table 2.

(see Table 1 below)

(see Table 2 on next page)

Adverse drug reactions occurring at a frequency of less than or equal to 1 %

The following list provides information on adverse drug reactions reported in study MF 4411 occurring more frequently with Bonviva 2.5 mg daily than with placebo and study BM 16549 occurring more frequently with Bonviva 150 mg once monthly than with Bonviva 2.5 mg daily:

Uncommon (1/100 – 1/1,000)

Gastro-intestinal Disorders: dysphagia, vomiting gastritis, oesophagitis including oesophageal ulcerations or strictures

Nervous System Disorders: dizziness

Musculoskeletal and Connective Tissue Disorders: back pain

Rare (1/1,000 – 1/10,000)

Gastro-intestinal Disorders: duodenitis

Immune System Disorders: hypersensitivity reactions

Skin and Subcutaneous Tissue Disorders: angioedema, face oedema, urticaria

Patients with a previous history of gastrointestinal disease including patients with peptic ulcer without recent bleeding or hospitalisation and patients with dyspepsia or reflux controlled by medication were included in the once monthly treatment study. For these patients there was no difference in the incidence of upper gastrointestinal adverse events with the 150 mg once monthly regimen compared to the 2.5 mg daily regimen.

Laboratory test findings

In the pivotal three-year study with Bonviva 2.5 mg daily (MF 4411) there was no difference compared with placebo for laboratory abnormalities indicative of hepatic or renal dysfunction, an impaired haematologic system, hypocalcaemia or hypophosphataemia. Similarly, no differences were noted between the groups in study BM 16549 after one and two years.

4.9 Overdose

No specific information is available on the treatment of over dosage with Bonviva.

However, based on a knowledge of this class of compounds, oral over-dosage may result in upper gastrointestinal adverse reactions (such as upset stomach, dyspepsia, oesophagitis, gastritis, or ulcer) or hypocalcaemia. Milk or antacids should be given to bind Bonviva and any adverse reactions treated symptomatically. Owing to the risk of oesophageal irritation, vomiting should not be induced and the patient should remain fully upright.

5. PHARMACOLOGICAL PROPERTIES

5.1 Pharmacodynamic properties

Pharmacotherapeutic group: Bisphosphonates, ATC code: M05B A06

Mechanism of action

Ibandronic acid is a highly potent bisphosphonate belonging to the nitrogen-containing group of bisphosphonates, which act selectively on bone tissue and specifically inhibit osteoclast activity without directly affecting bone formation. It does not interfere with osteoclast recruitment. Ibandronic acid leads to progressive net gains in bone mass and a decreased incidence of fractures through the reduction of elevated bone turnover towards premenopausal levels in postmenopausal women.

Pharmacodynamic effects

The pharmacodynamic action of ibandronic acid is inhibition of bone resorption. *In vivo*, ibandronic acid prevents experimentally induced bone destruction caused by cessation of gonadal function, retinoids, tumours or tumour extracts. In young (fast growing) rats, the endogenous bone resorption is also inhibited, leading to increased normal bone mass compared with untreated animals.

Animal models confirm that ibandronic acid is a highly potent inhibitor of osteoclastic activity. In growing rats, there was no evidence of impaired mineralisation even at doses greater than 5,000 times the dose required for osteoporosis treatment.

Both daily and intermittent (with prolonged dose-free intervals) long-term administration in rats, dogs and monkeys was associated with formation of new bone of normal quality and maintained or increased mechanical strength even at doses in the toxic range. In humans, the efficacy of both daily and intermittent administration with a dose-free interval of 9-10 weeks of ibandronic acid was confirmed in a clinical trial (MF 4411), in which Bonviva demonstrated anti-fracture efficacy.

In animal models ibandronic acid produced biochemical changes indicative of dose-dependent inhibition of bone resorption, including suppression of urinary biochemical markers of bone collagen degradation (such as deoxypyridinoline, and cross-linked N-telopeptides of type I collagen (NTX)).

In a Phase 1 bioequivalence study conducted in 72 postmenopausal women receiving 150 mg orally every 28 days for a total of four doses, inhibition in serum CTX following the first dose was seen as early as 24 hours post-dose (median inhibition 28 %), with median maximal inhibition (69 %) seen 6 days later. Following the third and fourth dose, the median maximum inhibition 6 days post dose was 74 % with reduction to a median inhibition of 56 % seen 28 days following the fourth dose. With no further dosing, there is a loss of suppression of biochemical markers of bone resorption.

Clinical efficacy

Bonviva 150 mg once monthly

Bone mineral density (BMD)

Bonviva 150 mg once monthly was shown to be at least as effective as Bonviva 2.5 mg daily at increasing BMD in a two year, double-blind, multicentre study (BM 16549) of postmenopausal women with osteoporosis (lumbar spine BMD T score below -2.5 SD at baseline). This was demonstrated in both the primary analysis at one year and in the confirmatory analysis at two years endpoint (Table 3).

(see Table 3 on next page)

Furthermore, Bonviva 150 mg once monthly was proven superior to Bonviva 2.5 mg daily for increases in lumbar spine BMD in a prospectively planned analysis at one year, p=0.002, and at two years, p<0.001.

At one year (primary analysis), 91.3% (p=0.005) of patients receiving Bonviva 150 mg once monthly had a lumbar spine BMD increase above or equal to baseline (BMD responders), compared with 84.0% of patients receiving Bonviva 2.5 mg daily. At two years, 93.5 % (p=0.004) and 86.4% of patients receiving Bonviva 150 mg once monthly or Bonviva 2.5 mg daily, respectively, were responders.

For total hip BMD, 90.0% (p<0.001) of patients receiving Bonviva 150 mg once monthly and 76.7% of patients receiving Bonviva 2.5 mg daily had total hip BMD increases above or equal to baseline at one year. At two years 93.4% (p<0.001) of patients receiving Bonviva 150 mg once monthly and 78.4%, of patients receiving Bonviva 2.5 mg daily had total hip BMD increases above or equal to baseline.

When a more stringent criterion is considered, which combines both lumbar spine and total hip BMD, 83.9% (p<0.001) and 65.7% of patients receiving Bonviva 150 mg once monthly or Bonviva 2.5 mg daily, respectively, were responders at one year. At two years, 87.1% (p<0.001) and 70.5%, of patients met this criterion in the 150 mg monthly and 2.5 mg daily arms respectively.

Biochemical markers of bone turn-over

Clinically meaningful reductions in serum CTX levels were observed at all time points measured, i.e. months 3, 6, 12 and 24. After one year (primary analysis) the median relative change from baseline was -76% for Bonviva 150 mg once monthly and -67% for Bonviva 2.5 mg daily. At two years the median relative change was -68% and -62%, in the 150 mg monthly and 2.5 mg daily arms respectively.

At one year, 83.5% (p= 0.006) of patients receiving Bonviva 150 mg once monthly and 73.9% of patients receiving Bonviva 2.5 mg daily were identified as responders (defined as a decrease ≥ 50 % from baseline). At two years 78.7% (p=0.002) and 65.6% of patients were identi-

Table 1: Common adverse drug reactions >1/100, ≤ 1/10) in phase III osteoporosis studies that were considered by the investigator to be possibly or probably related to treatment - One year data from study BM 16549 and three year data from placebo-controlled fracture study MF 4411

	One year data in study BM 16549		Three year data in study MF 4411	
System Organ Class/ Adverse drug reaction	Bonviva 150 mg once monthly (N=396) (%)	Bonviva 2.5 mg daily (N=395) (%)	Bonviva 2.5 mg daily (N=977) (%)	Placebo (N=975) (%)
Gastrointestinal system				
Dyspepsia	3.3	5.8	4.3	2.9
Nausea	3.3	3.5	1.8	2.3
Abdominal pain	3.5	2.8	2.1	2.9
Diarrhoea	2.5	1.8	1.4	1.0
Flatulence	0.5	1.0	0.4	0.7
Gastro-oesophageal reflux disease	0.5	1.0	0.4	0.1
Nervous system				
Headache	0.8	1.5	0.8	0.6
General disorders				
Influenza like illness*	3.3	0.3	0.3	0.2
Fatigue	1.0	0.3	0.3	0.4
Musculoskeletal system				
Myalgia	1.5	0.3	1.8	0.8
Arthralgia	1.0	0.3	0.4	0.4
Skin disorders				
Rash	0.8	1.0	1.2	0.7

MedDRA version 6.1

* Transient, influenza-like symptoms have been reported with Bonviva 150 mg once monthly, typically in association with the first dose. Such symptoms were generally of short duration, mild or moderate in intensity and resolved during continuing treatment without requiring remedial measures. Influenza-like illness includes events reported as acute phase reaction or symptoms including myalgia, arthralgia, fever, chills, fatigue, nausea, loss of appetite, or bone pain.

Table 2: Cumulative common adverse drug reactions >1/100, ⩽ 1/10) in Phase III osteoporosis studies that were considered by the investigator to be possibly or probably related to treatment - Two year data from study BM 16549 and three year data from placebo-controlled fracture study MF 4411

	Two year cumulative data in study BM 16549		Three year data in study MF 4411	
System Organ Class/ Adverse drug reaction	Bonviva 150 mg once monthly (N=396) (%)	Bonviva 2.5 mg daily (N=395) (%)	Bonviva 2.5 mg daily (N=977) (%)	Placebo (N=975) (%)
Gastrointestinal system				
Dyspepsia	4.0	6.3	4.0	2.7
Nausea	3.0	3.5	1.8	2.3
Abdominal pain	4.0	3.0	2.1	2.9
Diarrhoea	2.5	2.0	1.4	1.0
Gastritis	1.0	0.3	0.7	0.5
Gastro-oesophageal reflux disease	0.8	1.0	0.5	0.1
Oesophagitis	0	1.0	0.5	0.4
Nervous system				
Headache	0.8	1.5	0.8	0.6
General disorders				
Influenza like illness*	3.3	0.3	0.3	0.2
Musculoskeletal system				
Myalgia	1.5	0.3	1.8	0.8
Arthralgia	1.0	0.5	0.4	0.4
Muscle cramp	0.5	1.0	0.1	0.4
Musculoskeletal pain	1.0	0.5	0	0
Musculoskeletal stiffness	1.0	0	0	0
Skin disorders				
Rash	0.8	1.0	1.2	0.7

MedDRA version 7.1

* Transient, influenza-like symptoms have been reported with Bonviva 150 mg once monthly, typically in association with the first dose. Such symptoms were generally of short duration, mild or moderate in intensity, and resolved during continuing treatment without requiring remedial measures. Influenza-like illness includes events reported as acute phase reaction or symptoms including myalgia, arthralgia, fever, chills, fatigue, nausea, loss of appetite, or bone pain.

Table 3: Mean relative change from baseline of lumbar spine, total hip, femoral neck and trochanter BMD after one year (primary analysis) and two years of treatment (Per-Protocol Population) in study BM 16549.

	One year data in study BM 16549		Two year data in study BM 16549	
Mean relative changes from baseline % [95% CI]	Bonviva 2.5 mg daily (N=318)	Bonviva 150 mg once monthly (N=320)	Bonviva 2.5 mg daily (N=294)	Bonviva 150 mg once monthly (N=291)
Lumbar spine L2-L4 BMD	3.9 [3.4, 4.3]	4.9 [4.4, 5.3]	5.0 [4.4, 5.5]	6.6 [6.0, 7.1]
Total hip BMD	2.0 [1.7, 2.3]	3.1 [2.8, 3.4]	2.5 [2.1, 2.9]	4.2 [3.8, 4.5]
Femoral neck BMD	1.7 [1.3, 2.1]	2.2 [1.9, 2.6]	1.9 [1.4, 2.4]	3.1 [2.7, 3.6]
Trochanter BMD	3.2 [2.8, 3.7]	4.6 [4.2, 5.1]	4.0 [3.5, 4.5]	6.2 [5.7, 6.7]

fied as responders in the 150 mg monthly and 2.5 mg daily arms respectively.

Based on the results of study BM 16549, Bonviva 150 mg once monthly is expected to be at least as effective in preventing fractures as Bonviva 2.5 mg daily.

Bonviva 2.5 mg daily

In the initial three-year, randomised, double-blind, placebo-controlled, fracture study (MF 4411), a statistically significant and medically relevant decrease in the incidence of new radiographic morphometric and clinical vertebral fractures was demonstrated (Table 4). In this study, Bonviva was evaluated at oral doses of 2.5 mg daily and 20 mg intermittently as an exploratory regimen. Bonviva was taken 60 minutes before the first food or drink of the day (post-dose fasting period). The study enrolled women aged 55 to 80 years, who were at least 5 years postmenopausal, who had a BMD at lumbar spine of 2 to 5 SD below the premenopausal mean (T-score) in at least one vertebra [L1-L4], and who had one to four prevalent vertebral fractures. All patients received 500 mg calcium and 400 IU vitamin D daily. Efficacy was evaluated in 2,928 patients. Bonviva 2.5 mg administered daily, showed a statistically significant and medically relevant reduction in the incidence of new vertebral fractures. This regimen reduced the occurrence of new radiographic vertebral fractures by 62 % (p=0.0001) over the three year duration of the study. A relative risk reduction of 61 % was observed after 2 years (p=0.0006). No statistically significant difference was attained after 1 year of treatment (p=0.056). The anti-fracture effect was consistent over the duration of the study. There was no indication of a waning of the effect over time.

The incidence of clinical vertebral fractures was also significantly reduced by 49 % (p=0.011). The strong effect on vertebral fractures was furthermore reflected by a statistically significant reduction of height loss compared to placebo (p<0.0001).

Table 4: Results from 3 years fracture study MF 4411 (%, 95 % CI)		
	Placebo (N=974)	Bonviva 2.5 mg daily (N=977)
Relative Risk Reduction New morphometric vertebral fractures		62 % (40.9, 75.1)
Incidence of new morphometric vertebral fractures	9.56 % (7.5, 11.7)	4.68 % (3.2,6.2)
Relative risk reduction of clinical vertebral fracture		49 % (14.03, 69.49)
Incidence of clinical vertebral fracture	5.33 % (3.73, 6.92)	2.75 % (1.61, 3.89)
BMD – mean change relative to baseline lumbar spine at year 3	1.26 % (0.8, 1.7)	6.54 % (6.1, 7.0)
BMD – mean change relative to baseline total hip at year 3	-0.69 % (-1.0, -0.4)	3.36 % (3.0, 3.7)

The treatment effect of Bonviva was further assessed in an analysis of the subpopulation of patients who at baseline had a lumbar spine BMD T-score below −2.5. The vertebral fracture risk reduction was very consistent with that seen in the overall population.

Table 5: Results from 3 years fracture study MF 4411 (%, 95 % CI) for patients with lumbar spine BMD T-score below −2.5 at baseline		
	Placebo (N=587)	Bonviva 2.5 mg daily (N=575)
Relative Risk Reduction New morphometric vertebral fractures		59 % (34.5, 74.3)
Incidence of new morphometric vertebral fractures	12.54 % (9.53, 15.55)	5.36 % (3.31, 7.41)
Relative risk reduction of clinical vertebral fracture		50 % (9.49, 71.91)
Incidence of clinical vertebral fracture	6.97 % (4.67, 9.27)	3.57 % (1.89, 5.24)
BMD – mean change relative to baseline lumbar spine at year 3	1.13 % (0.6, 1.7)	7.01 % (6.5, 7.6)
BMD – mean change relative to baseline total hip at year 3	-0.70 % (-1.1, -0.2)	3.59 % (3.1, 4.1)

No reduction was observed for non-vertebral fractures or femoral neck fractures in this study; however, the study was not specifically designed to demonstrate this.

Daily treatment with 2.5 mg resulted in progressive increases in BMD at vertebral and nonvertebral sites of the skeleton.

Three-year lumbar spine BMD increase compared to placebo was 5.3 % and 6.5 % compared to baseline. Increases at the hip compared to baseline were 2.8 % at the femoral neck, 3.4 % at the total hip, and 5.5 % at the trochanter.

Biochemical markers of bone turnover (such as urinary CTX and serum Osteocalcin) showed the expected pattern of suppression to premenopausal levels and reached maximum suppression within a period of 3-6 months.

A clinically meaningful reduction of 50 % of biochemical markers of bone resorption was observed as early as one month after start of treatment with Bonviva 2.5 mg.

Following treatment discontinuation, there is a reversion to the pathological pre-treatment rates of elevated bone resorption associated with postmenopausal osteoporosis.

The histological analysis of bone biopsies after two and three years of treatment of postmenopausal women showed bone of normal quality and no indication of a mineralisation defect.

5.2 Pharmacokinetic properties

The primary pharmacological effects of ibandronic acid on bone are not directly related to actual plasma concentrations, as demonstrated by various studies in animals and humans.

Absorption

The absorption of ibandronic acid in the upper gastrointestinal tract is rapid after oral administration and plasma concentrations increase in a dose-proportional manner up to 50 mg oral intake, with greater than dose-proportional increases seen above this dose. Maximum observed plasma concentrations were reached within 0.5 to 2 hours (median 1 hour) in the fasted state and absolute bioavailability was about 0.6 %. The extent of absorption is impaired when taken together with food or beverages (other than plain water). Bioavailability is reduced by about 90 % when Bonviva is administered with a standard breakfast in comparison with bioavailability seen in fasted subjects. There is no meaningful reduction in bioavailability provided ibandronic acid is taken 60 minutes before the first food of the day. Both bioavailability and BMD gains are reduced when food or beverage is taken less than 60 minutes after Bonviva is ingested.

Distribution

After initial systemic exposure, ibandronic acid rapidly binds to bone or is excreted into urine. In humans, the apparent terminal volume of distribution is at least 90 l and the amount of dose reaching the bone is estimated to be 40-50 % of the circulating dose. Protein binding in human plasma is approximately 85 % - 87 % (determined *in vitro* at therapeutic drug concentrations), and thus there is a low potential for drug-drug interaction due to displacement.

Metabolism

There is no evidence that ibandronic acid is metabolised in animals or humans.

Elimination

The absorbed fraction of ibandronic acid is removed from the circulation via bone absorption (estimated to be 40-50 % in postmenopausal women) and the remainder is eliminated unchanged by the kidney. The unabsorbed fraction of ibandronic acid is eliminated unchanged in the faeces.

The range of observed apparent half-lives is broad, the apparent terminal half-life is generally in the range of 10-72 hours. As the values calculated are largely a function of the duration of study, the dose used, and assay sensitivity, the true terminal half-life is likely to be substantially longer, in common with other bisphosphonates. Early plasma levels fall quickly reaching 10 % of peak values within 3 and 8 hours after intravenous or oral administration respectively.

Total clearance of ibandronic acid is low with average values in the range 84-160 ml/min. Renal clearance (about 60 mL/min in healthy postmenopausal females) accounts for 50-60 % of total clearance and is related to creatinine clearance. The difference between the apparent total and renal clearances is considered to reflect the uptake by bone.

Pharmacokinetics in special clinical situations

Gender

Bioavailability and pharmacokinetics of ibandronic acid are similar in men and women.

Race

There is no evidence for any clinically relevant inter-ethnic differences between Asians and Caucasians in ibandronic acid disposition. There are few data available on patients of African origin.

Patients with renal impairment

Renal clearance of ibandronic acid in patients with various degrees of renal impairment is linearly related to creatinine clearance.

No dosage adjustment is necessary for patients with mild or moderate renal impairment (CLcr equal or greater than 30 ml/min), as shown in study BM 16549 where the majority of patients had mild to moderate renal impairment.

Subjects with severe renal failure (CLcr less than 30 ml/min) receiving daily oral administration of 10 mg ibandronic acid for 21 days, had 2-3 fold higher plasma concentrations than subjects with normal renal function and total clearance of ibandronic acid was 44 ml/min. After intravenous administration of 0.5 mg, total, renal, and non-renal clearances decreased by 67 %, 77 % and 50 %, respectively, in subjects with severe renal failure but there was no reduction in tolerability associated with the increase in exposure. Due to the limited clinical experience, Bonviva is not recommended in patients with severe renal impairment (see section 4.2 and section 4.4). The pharmacokinetics of ibandronic acid was not assessed in patients with end-stage renal disease managed by other than haemodialysis. The pharmacokinetics of ibandronic acid in these patients is unknown, and ibandronic acid should not be used under these circumstances.

Patients with hepatic impairment

There are no pharmacokinetic data for ibandronic acid in patients who have hepatic impairment. The liver has no significant role in the clearance of ibandronic acid which is not metabolised but is cleared by renal excretion and by uptake into bone. Therefore dosage adjustment is not necessary in patients with hepatic impairment.

Elderly

In a multivariate analysis, age was not found to be an independent factor of any of the pharmacokinetic parameters studied. As renal function decreases with age this is the only factor to take into consideration (see renal impairment section).

Children and adolescents

There are no data on the use of Bonviva in these age groups.

5.3 Preclinical safety data

Toxic effects, e.g signs of renal damage, were observed in dogs only at exposures considered sufficiently in excess of the maximum human exposure indicating little relevance to clinical use.

Mutagenicity/Carcinogenicity:

No indication of carcinogenic potential was observed. Tests for genotoxicity revealed no evidence of genetic activity for ibandronic acid.

Reproductive toxicity:

There was no evidence for a direct foetal toxic or teratogenic effect of ibandronic acid in orally treated rats and rabbits and there were no adverse effects on the development in F_1 offspring in rats at an extrapolated exposure of at least 35 times above human exposure. Adverse effects of ibandronic acid in reproductive toxicity studies in the rat were those observed with bisphosphonates as a class. They include a decreased number of implantation sites, interference with natural delivery (dystocia), and an increase in visceral variations (renal pelvis ureter syndrome).

6. PHARMACEUTICAL PARTICULARS

6.1 List of excipients

Tablet core

Lactose monohydrate

Povidone

Cellulose, microcrystalline

Crospovidone

Stearic acid

Silica, colloidal anhydrous

Tablet coat

Hypromellose

Titanium dioxide E171

Talc

Macrogol 6,000

6.2 Incompatibilities

Not applicable.

6.3 Shelf life

2 years.

6.4 Special precautions for storage

This medicinal product does not require any special storage conditions.

6.5 Nature and contents of container

Bonviva 150 mg film-coated tablets are supplied in blisters (Aluminium/Aluminium) containing 1 or 3 tablets.

Not all pack sizes may be marketed.

6.6 Instructions for use and handling

No special requirements.

7. MARKETING AUTHORISATION HOLDER

Roche Registration Limited

40 Broadwater Road

Welwyn Garden City

Hertfordshire, AL7 3AY

United Kingdom

8. MARKETING AUTHORISATION NUMBER(S)

EU /1/03/265/003 (1 tablet)

EU/1/03/265/004 (3 tablets)

9. DATE OF FIRST AUTHORISATION/RENEWAL OF THE AUTHORISATION

September 2005

10. DATE OF REVISION OF THE TEXT

Not applicable

LEGAL STATUS

POM

P117215/905

BNV/SPC/05/21228/1 20801249

Botox

(Allergan Ltd)

1. NAME OF THE MEDICINAL PRODUCT

BOTOX®

2. QUALITATIVE AND QUANTITATIVE COMPOSITION

Clostridium botulinum type A neurotoxin complex (900 kD), 100 units.

3. PHARMACEUTICAL FORM

Powder for solution for injection.

4. CLINICAL PARTICULARS

4.1 Therapeutic indications

BOTOX® is indicated for the symptomatic relief of blepharospasm, hemifacial spasm and idiopathic cervical dystonia (spasmodic torticollis). It is indicated for the management of severe hyperhidrosis of the axillae, which does not respond to topical treatment with antiperspirants or antihidrotics.

BOTOX® is also indicated for focal spasticity, including the treatment of

- dynamic equinus foot deformity due to spasticity in ambulant paediatric cerebral palsy patients, two years of age or older

and

- wrist and hand disability due to upper limb spasticity associated with stroke in adults

The injections should be administered by appropriately trained personnel in hospital specialist centres.

The safety and effectiveness of BOTOX® in the treatment of blepharospasm, hemifacial spasm, or idiopathic cervical dystonia, or focal hyperhidrosis in children have not been demonstrated.

4.2 Posology and method of administration

Doses recommended for BOTOX® are not interchangeable with other preparations of botulinum toxin.

There is no difference in dose between adults and the elderly.

Blepharospasm

After reconstitution, BOTOX® is injected using a sterile, 27-30 gauge needle. Electromyographic guidance is not necessary. The initial recommended dose is 1.25-2.5 U (0.05-0.1 ml volume at each site) injected into the medial and lateral orbicularis oculi of the upper lid and the lateral orbicularis oculi of the lower lid. Additional sites in the brow area, the lateral orbicularis and in the upper facial area may also be injected if spasms here interfere with vision. In general, the initial effect of the injections is seen within three days and reaches a peak at one to two weeks post-treatment. Each treatment lasts approximately three months, following which the procedure can be repeated indefinitely. At repeat treatment sessions, the dose may be increased up to two-fold if the response from the initial treatment is considered insufficient - usually defined as an effect that does not last longer than two months. However, there appears to be little benefit obtainable from injecting more than 5.0 U per site. The initial dose should not exceed 25 U per eye. Normally no additional benefit is conferred by treating more frequently than every three months. It is rare for the effect to be permanent.

In the management of blepharospasm total dosing should not exceed 100 U every 12 weeks.

Hemifacial spasm

Patients with hemifacial spasm or VIIth nerve disorders should be treated as for unilateral blepharospasm, with other affected facial muscles being injected as needed. Electromyographic control may be necessary to identify affected small circumoral muscles.

Cervical dystonia

Several dosing regimens have been used in clinical trials for treatment of cervical dystonia with BOTOX®. Dosing must be tailored to the individual patient based on the patient's head and neck position, location of pain, muscle hypertrophy, patient's body weight, and patient response.

In practice, the maximum total dose is not usually more than 200 U. No more than 50 U should be given at any one injection site. The dilutions suggested are indicated in the following table:

Diluent added	Resulting dose in units per 0.1 ml
0.5 ml	20.0 U
1.0 ml	10.0 U
2.0 ml	5.0 U
4.0 ml	2.5 U
8.0 ml	1.25 U

The following doses are recommended:

(see Table 1 on next page)

The treatment of cervical dystonia typically may include injection of BOTOX® into the sternocleidomastoid, levator scapulae, scalene, splenius capitis, and/or the trapezius muscle(s). The muscle mass and the degree of hypertrophy are factors to be taken into consideration when selecting the appropriate dose.

The sternocleidomastoid muscle should not be injected bilaterally as there is an increased risk of adverse effects (in particular dysphagia) when bilateral injections or doses in excess of 100 U are administered to this muscle.

A 25, 27 or 30 gauge needle may be used for superficial muscles, and a 22 gauge needle may be used for deeper musculature. For cervical dystonia, localisation of the involved muscles with electromyographic guidance may be useful.

Multiple injection sites allow BOTOX® to have more uniform contact with the innervation areas of the dystonic muscle and are especially useful in larger muscles. The optimal number of injection sites is dependent upon the size of the muscle to be chemically denervated.

Table 1

Type I Head **rotated** toward side of shoulder elevation	Sternomastoid Levator scapulae Scalene Splenius capitis Trapezius	50 - 100 U; at least 2 sites 50 U; 1 - 2 sites 25 - 50 U; 1 - 2 sites 25 - 75 U; 1 - 3 sites 25 - 100 U; 1 - 8 sites
Type II Head rotation only	Sternomastoid	25 - 100 U; at least 2 sites if >25 U given
Type III Head **tilted** toward side of shoulder elevation	Sternomastoid Levator scapulae Scalene Trapezius	25 - 100 U at posterior border; at least 2 sites if >25 U given 25 - 100 U; at least 2 sites 25 - 75 U; at least 2 sites 25 - 100 U; 1 - 8 sites
Type IV Bilateral posterior cervical muscle spasm with elevation of the face	Splenius capitis and cervicis	50 - 200 U; 2 - 8 sites, treat bilaterally (This is the total dose and not the dose for each side of the neck)

Hyperhidrosis of the axillae

The recommended injection volume for intradermal injection in axillary hyperhidrosis is 0.1-0.2 ml. Reconstituted BOTOX® (100 U/4.0 mL) is injected using a 30 gauge needle. 50 U of BOTOX® is injected intradermally to each axilla, evenly distributed in multiple sites approximately 1-2 cm apart. The hyperhidrotic area to be injected may be defined by using standard staining techniques, e.g. Minor's iodine-starch test.

Clinical improvement generally occurs within the first week after injection. Repeat injections of axillary hyperhidrosis should be administered when effects from previous injections subside. Treatment response has been reported to persist for 4-7 months.

Paediatric cerebral palsy

Diluted BOTOX® is injected using a sterile 23-26 gauge needle. It is administered into each of two sites in the medial and lateral heads of the affected gastrocnemius muscle. The recommended total dose is 4 U/kg body weight. When both lower limbs are to be injected on the same occasion this dose should be divided between the two limbs.

Clinical improvement generally occurs within the first two weeks after injection. Repeat doses should be administered when the clinical effect of a previous injection diminishes but not more frequently than every two months.

Focal spasticity associated with stroke

Reconstituted BOTOX® is injected using a sterile 25, 27 or 30 gauge needle for superficial muscles, and a longer needle for deeper musculature. Localisation of the involved muscles with electromyographic guidance or nerve stimulation techniques may be useful. Multiple injection sites may allow BOTOX® to have more uniform contact with the innervation areas of the muscle and are especially useful in larger muscles.

The exact dosage and number of injection sites may be tailored to the individual based on the size, number and location of muscles involved, the severity of spasticity, and the presence of local muscle weakness.

In the controlled Phase 3 clinical trial the following doses were administered:

Muscle	Total Dose
Flexor digitorum profundus	50 U
Flexor digitorum sublimis	50 U
Flexor carpi radialis	50 U
Flexor carpi ulnaris	50 U
Adductor Pollicis	20 U
Flexor Pollicis Longus	20 U

In all clinical trials, the doses did not exceed 360 U divided among selected muscles at any treatment session.

Clinical improvement in muscle tone generally occurs within two weeks following treatment and the peak effect is generally seen within four to six weeks following treatment. Data on the repeated and long-term treatment are limited.

4.3 Contraindications

BOTOX® is contraindicated:

- in individuals with a known hypersensitivity to Clostridium botulinum type A neurotoxin complex (900 kD) or to any of the excipients,

- in the presence of myasthenia gravis or Eaton Lambert Syndrome

- in the presence of infection at the proposed injection site(s).

4.4 Special warnings and special precautions for use

The relevant anatomy, and any alterations to the anatomy due to prior surgical procedures, must be understood prior to administering BOTOX®. The recommended dosages and frequencies of administration of BOTOX® should not be exceeded.

An anaphylactic reaction may occur very rarely after injection of botulinum toxin. Epinephrine (adrenaline) and other anti-anaphylactic measures should therefore be available. Please see section 4.8c) for further information.

There have been rare spontaneous reports of death, sometimes associated with dysphagia, pneumonia and/or other significant debility, after treatment with botulinum toxin type A. Patients with a history of dysphagia should be treated with caution. Patients or caregivers should be advised to seek immediate medical care if swallowing, speech or respiratory disorders arise.

Dysphagia has also been reported following injection to sites other than the cervical musculature (see section 4.4 'Cervical Dystonia' for further information).

Clinical fluctuations during the repeated use of BOTOX® (as with all botulinum toxins) may be a result of different vial reconstitution procedures, injection intervals, muscles injected and slightly differing potency values given by the biological test method used.

Too frequent or excessive dosing can result in antibody formation, which may lead to resistance to treatment.

As with any treatment with the potential to allow previously-sedentary patients to resume activities, the sedentary patient should be cautioned to resume activity gradually.

Caution should be used when BOTOX® is used in the presence of inflammation at the proposed injection site(s) or when excessive weakness or atrophy is present in the target muscle. Caution should also be exercised when BOTOX® is used for treatment of patients with amyotrophic lateral sclerosis or disorders that produce peripheral neuromuscular dysfunction.

BOTOX® contains human serum albumin. When medicinal products derived from human blood or plasma are administered, the possibility of transmitting infectious agents cannot be totally excluded. To reduce the risk of transmission of infective agents, stringent controls are applied to the selection of blood donors and donations. In addition, virus inactivation procedures are included in the production process.

Blepharospasm

Reduced blinking following botulinum toxin injection into the orbicularis muscle can lead to corneal pathology. Careful testing of corneal sensation in eyes previously operated upon, avoidance of injection into the lower lid area to avoid ectropion, and vigorous treatment of any epithelial defect should be employed. This may require protective drops, ointment, therapeutic soft contact lenses, or closure of the eye by patching or other means.

Ecchymosis occurs easily in the soft eyelid tissues. This can be minimised by applying gentle pressure at the injection site immediately after injection.

Because of the anticholinergic activity of botulinum toxin, caution should be exercised when treating patients at risk for angle closure glaucoma.

Cervical dystonia

Patients with cervical dystonia should be informed of the possibility of experiencing dysphagia which may be very mild, but could be severe. Consequent to the dysphagia there is the potential for aspiration, dyspnoea and occasionally the need for tube feeding. In rare cases dysphagia followed by aspiration pneumonia and death has been reported. Dysphagia may persist for two to three weeks after injection, but has been reported to last up to five months post-injection.

Limiting the dose injected into the sternocleidomastoid muscle to less than 100 U may decrease the occurrence of dysphagia. Patients with smaller neck muscle mass, or patients who receive bilateral injections into the sternocleidomastoid muscle, have been reported to be at greater risk of dysphagia. Dysphagia is attributable to the spread of the toxin to the oesophageal musculature.

Hyperhidrosis of the axillae

Medical history and physical examination, along with specific additional investigations as required, should be performed to exclude potential causes of secondary hyperhidrosis (e.g. hyperthyroidism, phaeochromocytoma). This will avoid symptomatic treatment of hyperhidrosis without the diagnosis and/or treatment of underlying disease.

Focal spasticity associated with paediatric cerebral palsy and spasticity of the hand and wrist in adult post-stroke patients

BOTOX® is a treatment of focal spasticity that has only been studied in association with usual standard of care regimens, and is not intended as a replacement for these treatment modalities. BOTOX® is not likely to be effective in improving range of motion at a joint affected by a fixed contracture.

4.5 Interaction with other medicinal products and other forms of Interaction

Theoretically, the effect of botulinum toxin may be potentiated by aminoglycoside antibiotics or spectinomycin, or other medicinal products that interfere with neuromuscular transmission (e.g. tubocurarine-type muscle relaxants).

No specific tests have been carried out to establish the possibility of clinical interaction with other medicinal products. No interactions of clinical significance have been reported.

4.6 Pregnancy and lactation

Pregnancy

There are no adequate data from the use of botulinum toxin type A in pregnant women. Studies in animals have shown reproductive toxicity (see Section 5.3). The potential risk for humans is unknown. BOTOX® should not be used during pregnancy unless clearly necessary.

Lactation

There is no information on whether BOTOX® is excreted in human milk. The use of BOTOX® during lactation cannot be recommended.

4.7 Effects on ability to drive and use machines

The effects of BOTOX® on the ability to drive or to use machines can only be assessed after treatment.

4.8 Undesirable effects

a) General

Based on controlled clinical trial data patients would be expected to experience an adverse reaction after treatment with BOTOX® at the rates of 35% for blepharospasm, 28% for cervical dystonia, 17% for paediatric cerebral palsy and 11% for primary hyperhidrosis of the axillae. Sixteen percent (16%) of participants in clinical trials treated with BOTOX® for focal spasticity of the upper limb associated with stroke experienced an adverse reaction.

In general, adverse reactions occur within the first few days following injection and are transient.

Local muscle weakness represents the expected pharmacological action of botulinum toxin in muscle tissue.

As is expected for any injection procedure, localised pain, tenderness and/or bruising may be associated with the injection. Fever and flu syndrome have also been reported after injections of botulinum toxin.

b) Adverse reactions - frequency by indication

For each indication the frequency of adverse reactions arising from clinical experienceis given. The frequency is defined as follows:

Very Common (> 1/10); Common (>1/100, <1/10); Uncommon (>1/1,000, <1/100); Rare (>1/10,000, <1/1,000); Very Rare (<1/10,000).

Blepharospasm/hemifacial spasm

Very common:	Ptosis.
Common:	Superficial punctate keratitis, lagophthalmos, dry eye, irritation, photophobia, lacrimation, facial oedema.
Uncommon:	Keratitis, ectropion, diplopia, dizziness, diffuse skin rash/dermatitis, entropion, facial weakness, facial droop, tiredness, visual disturbance, blurring of vision.
Rare:	Eyelid swelling.
Very rare:	Angle closure glaucoma, corneal ulceration.

Cervical dystonia

Very common:	Dysphagia (See Section c) below.), local weakness, pain.
Common:	Dizziness, hypertonia, numbness, general weakness, drowsiness, flu syndrome, malaise, oral dryness, nausea, headache, stiffness, soreness, rhinitis, upper respiratory infection.
Uncommon:	Dyspnoea, diplopia, fever, ptosis, voice alteration.

Hyperhidrosis of the axillae

Common:	Non-axillary sweating, injection site reactions, pain, vasodilation (hot flushes).
Uncommon:	Weakness of the arms, pruritus, myalgia, joint disorder, arm pain.

Paediatric cerebral palsy

Very common: Viral infection, ear infection.

Common: Myalgia, muscle weakness, urinary incontinence, somnolence, gait abnormality, malaise, rash, tingling.

Focal upper limb spasticity associated with stroke

Common: Ecchymosis/purpura/injection site hemorrhage, arm pain, muscle weakness, hypertonia, injection site burning.

Uncommon: Hyperesthesia, arthralgia, asthenia, pain, bursitis, dermatitis, headache, injection site hypersensitivity, malaise, nausea, paresthesia, postural hypotension, pruritus, rash, incoordination, amnesia, circumoral paresthesia, depression, insomnia, peripheral oedema, vertigo (some of the uncommon events may be disease related).

c) Additional information

Dysphagia ranges in severity from mild to severe, with potential for aspiration, which occasionally may require medical intervention. See Section 4.4, Special Warnings and Special Precautions for Use.

There have been rare spontaneous reports of death, sometimes associated with dysphagia, pneumonia, and/or other significant debility, after treatment with botulinum toxin type A.

The following have been reported rarely since the medicinal product has been marketed; skin rash (including erythema multiforme, urticaria and psoriaform eruption), pruritus, and allergic reaction.

There have also been rare reports of adverse events involving the cardiovascular system, including arrhythmia and myocardial infarction, some with fatal outcomes. Some of these patients had risk factors including cardiovascular disease.

Rare reports of anaphylactic reactions associated with BOTOX use in conjunction with other agents known to cause similar reactions have been received.

A case of peripheral neuropathy has been reported in a large adult male after receiving four sets of BOTOX® injections, totalling 1800 U (for neck and back spasm, and severe pain) over an 11 week period.

Angle closure glaucoma has been reported very rarely following botulinum toxin treatment for blepharospasm.

A female patient developed brachial plexopathy two days after injection of 120 units of BOTOX® for the treatment of cervical dystonia, with recovery after five months.

In the management of primary axillary hyperhidrosis, increase in non-axillary sweating was reported in 4.5% of patients within 1 month after injection and showed no pattern with respect to anatomical sites affected. Resolution was seen in approximately 30% of the patients within four months. Weakness of the arm has been also reported uncommonly (0.7%) and was mild, transient, did not require treatment and recovered without sequelae. This adverse event may be related to treatment, injection technique, or both. In the uncommon event of muscle weakness being reported a neurological examination may be considered. In addition, a re-evaluation of injection technique prior to subsequent injection is advisable to ensure intradermal placement of injections.

There have been rare reports of seizures or convulsions, mostly in patients who are predisposed to experiencing these events. The exact relationship of these events to the botulinum toxin injection has not been established.

Needle-related pain and/or anxiety may result in vasovagal responses, e.g. syncope, hypotension, etc.

4.9 Overdose

There have not been any reported instances of systemic toxicity resulting from accidental injection of BOTOX®. Ingestion of BOTOX® is unknown. Signs of overdose are not apparent immediately post-injection. Should accidental injection or ingestion occur, the patient should be medically supervised for several days for signs and symptoms of systemic weakness or muscle paralysis.

Patients presenting with the symptoms of botulinum toxin type A poisoning (generalised weakness, ptosis, diplopia, swallowing and speech disorders, or paresis of the respiratory muscles) should be considered for admission to hospital.

With increasing dosage, generalised and profound muscular paralysis occurs. When the musculature of the oropharynx and oesophagus are affected, aspiration pneumonia may ensue. If the respiratory muscles become paralysed, intubation and assisted respiration will be required until recovery takes place.

5. PHARMACOLOGICAL PROPERTIES

5.1 Pharmacodynamic properties

ATC class M03A X01 and ATC class D11AX

The active constituent in BOTOX® is a protein complex derived from *Clostridium botulinum*. The protein consists of type A neurotoxin and several other proteins. Under physiological conditions it is presumed that the complex dissociates and releases the pure neurotoxin.

Clostridium botulinum toxin type A neurotoxin complex blocks peripheral acetyl choline release at presynaptic cholinergic nerve terminals.

Intramuscular injection of the neurotoxin complex blocks cholinergic transport at the neuromuscular junction by preventing the release of acetylcholine. The nerve endings of the neuromuscular junction no longer respond to nerve impulses and secretion of the chemotransmitter is prevented (chemical denervation). Re-establishment of impulse transmission is by newly formed nerve endings and motor end plates. Recovery after intramuscular injection takes place normally within 12 weeks of injection as nerve terminals sprout and reconnect with the endplates.

After intradermal injection, where the target is the eccrine sweat glands, the effect lasted for about 4-7 months in patients treated with 50 U per axilla.

5.2 Pharmacokinetic properties

a) General characteristics of the active substance:

Classical absorption, distribution, biotransformation and elimination studies on the active substance have not been performed due to the extreme toxicity of botulinum toxin type A.

b) Characteristics in patients:

Human ADME studies have not been performed due to the nature of the product. It is believed that little systemic distribution of therapeutic doses of BOTOX® occurs. BOTOX® is probably metabolised by proteases and the molecular components recycled through normal metabolic pathways.

5.3 Preclinical safety data

Acute toxicity

In monkeys receiving a single intramuscular (i.m.) injection of BOTOX®, the No Observed Effect Level (NOEL) ranged from 4 to 24 U/kg. The i.m. LD_{50} was reported to be 39 U/kg.

Toxicity on repeated injection

In three different studies (six months in rats; 20 weeks in juvenile monkeys; 1 year in monkeys) where the animals received i.m. injections, the NOEL was at the following respective BOTOX® dosage levels: < 4 U/kg, 8 U/kg and 4 U/kg. The main systemic effect was a transient decrease in body weight gain.

There was no indication of a cumulative effect in the animal studies when BOTOX® was given at dosage intervals of 1 month or greater.

Local toxicity

BOTOX® was shown not to cause ocular or dermal irritation, or give rise to toxicity when injected into the vitreous body in rabbits.

Allergic or inflammatory reactions in the area of the injection sites are rarely observed after BOTOX® administration. However, formation of haematoma may occur.

Reproduction toxicology

Teratogenic effects

When pregnant mice and rats were injected intramuscularly during the period of organogenesis, the developmental NOEL of BOTOX® was at 4 U/kg. Reductions in ossification were observed at 8 and 16 U/kg (mice) and reduced ossification of the hyoid bone at 16 U/kg (rats). Reduced foetal body weights were observed at 8 and 16 U/kg (rats).

In a range-finding study in rabbits, daily injections at dosages of 0.5 U/kg/day (days 6 to 18 of gestation), and 4 and 6 U/kg (administered on days 6 and 13 of gestation), caused death and abortions among surviving dams. External malformations were observed in one foetus each in the 0.125 U/kg/day and the 2 U/kg dosage groups. The rabbit appears to be a very sensitive species to BOTOX® treatment.

Impairment of fertility and reproduction

The reproductive NOEL following i.m. injection of BOTOX® was 4 U/kg in male rats and 8 U/kg in female rats. Higher dosages were associated with dose-dependent reductions in fertility. Provided impregnation occurred, there were no adverse effects on the numbers or viability of the embryos sired or conceived by treated male or female rats.

Pre- and post-natal developmental effects

In female rats, the reproductive NOEL was 16 U/kg. The developmental NOEL was 4 U/kg.

Mutagenicity

BOTOX® has been evaluated and shown to be non-mutagenic in a number of *in vitro* and *in vivo* systems including the Ames test, the AS52/XPRT Mammalian Cell Forward Gene Mutation assay and the CHO test, and non-clastogenic in the mouse PCE test.

Carcinogenicity

No animal studies have been conducted.

Antigenicity

BOTOX® showed antigenicity in mice only in the presence of adjuvant. BOTOX® was found to be slightly antigenic in the guinea pig.

Blood compatibility

No haemolysis was detected up to 100 U/ml of BOTOX® in normal human blood.

6. PHARMACEUTICAL PARTICULARS

6.1 List of excipients

Human serum albumin

Sodium chloride

6.2 Incompatibilities

None known, other than described in 4.5 above.

6.3 Shelf life

Unopened vial - 36 months.

Reconstituted vial - 4 hours.

6.4 Special precautions for storage

Unopened vials should be stored either at 2°C-8°C (in a refrigerator), or in a freezer at or below -5°C. After reconstitution BOTOX® may be stored in a refrigerator (2-8°C) for up to 4 hours prior to use.

6.5 Nature and contents of container

Clear glass vial, with rubber stopper and tamper-proof aluminium seal, containing white powder for solution for injection.

6.6 Instructions for use and handling

BOTOX® is reconstituted prior to use with sterile unpreserved normal saline (0.9% sodium chloride for injection). It is good practice to perform vial reconstitution and syringe preparation over plastic-lined paper towels to catch any spillage. An appropriate amount of diluent (see dilution table below) is drawn up into a syringe. The exposed portion of the rubber septum of the vial is cleaned with alcohol (70%) prior to insertion of the needle. Since BOTOX® is denatured by bubbling or similar violent agitation, the diluent should be injected gently into the vial. Discard the vial if a vacuum does not pull the diluent into the vial. Reconstituted BOTOX® is a clear colourless to slightly yellow solution free of particulate matter. When reconstituted, BOTOX® may be stored in a refrigerator (2-8°C) for up to 4 hours prior to use. After this period used or unused vials should be discarded.

Dilution table: Diluent added	Resulting dose in units per 0.1 ml
0.5 ml	20.0 U
1.0 ml	10.0 U
2.0 ml	5.0 U
4.0 ml	2.5 U
8.0 ml	1.25 U

The 'unit' by which the potency of preparations of BOTOX® is measured should be used to calculate dosages of BOTOX® only and is not transferable to other preparations of botulinum toxin.

An injection volume of approximately 0.1 ml is recommended. A decrease or increase in the BOTOX® dose is possible by administering a smaller or larger injection volume. The smaller the injection volume the less discomfort and less spread of toxin in the injected muscle occurs. This is of benefit in reducing effects on nearby muscles when small muscle groups are being injected.

For safe disposal, unused vials should be reconstituted with a small amount of water then autoclaved. Any used vials, syringes, and spillages etc. should be autoclaved, or the residual BOTOX® inactivated using dilute hypochlorite solution (0.5%).

Administrative Data

7. MARKETING AUTHORISATION HOLDER

Allergan Ltd., Coronation Road, High Wycombe, Bucks HP12 3SH

8. MARKETING AUTHORISATION NUMBER(S)

PL 00426/0074

9. DATE OF FIRST AUTHORISATION/RENEWAL OF THE AUTHORISATION

17 May 1994

10. DATE OF REVISION OF THE TEXT

April 2005

Brevinor Tablets

(Pharmacia Limited)

1. NAME OF THE MEDICINAL PRODUCT

Brevinor®

2. QUALITATIVE AND QUANTITATIVE COMPOSITION

Each tablet contains 0.5 milligrams norethisterone and 35 micrograms ethinyloestradiol.

3. PHARMACEUTICAL FORM

Blue, flat, circular, bevel-edged tablet inscribed 'SEARLE' on one side and 'BX' on the other side.

4. CLINICAL PARTICULARS

4.1 Therapeutic indications

Brevinor is indicated for oral contraception, with the benefit of a low intake of oestrogen.

4.2 Posology and method of administration

Oral Administration: The dosage of Brevinor for the initial cycle of therapy is 1 tablet taken at the same time each day from the first day of the menstrual cycle. For subsequent cycles, no tablets are taken for 7 days, then a new course is started of 1 tablet daily for the next 21 days. This sequence of 21 days on treatment, seven days off treatment is repeated for as long as contraception is required.

Patients unable to start taking Brevinor tablets on the first day of the menstrual cycle may start treatment on any day up to and including the 5th day of the menstrual cycle.

Patients starting on day 1 of their period will be protected at once. Those patients delaying therapy up to day 5 may not be protected immediately and it is recommended that another method of contraception is used for the first 7 days of tablet-taking. Suitable methods are condoms, caps plus spermicides and intra-uterine devices. The rhythm, temperature and cervical-mucus methods should not be relied upon.

Tablet omissions

Tablets must be taken daily in order to maintain adequate hormone levels and contraceptive efficacy.

If a tablet is missed within 12 hours of the correct dosage time then the missed tablet should be taken as soon as possible, even if this means taking 2 tablets on the same day, this will ensure that contraceptive protection is maintained. If one or more tablets are missed for more than 12 hours from the correct dosage time it is recommended that the patient takes the last missed tablet as soon as possible and then continues to take the rest of the tablets in the normal manner. In addition, it is recommended that extra contraceptive protection, such as a condom, is used for the next 7 days.

Patients who have missed one or more of the last 7 tablets in a pack should be advised to start the next pack of tablets as soon as the present one has finished (i.e. without the normal seven day gap between treatments). This reduces the risk of contraceptive failure resulting from tablets being missed close to a 7 day tablet free period.

Changing from another oral contraceptive

In order to ensure that contraception is maintained it is advised that the first dose of Brevinor tablets is taken on the day immediately after the patient has finished the previous pack of tablets.

Use after childbirth, miscarriage or abortion

Providing the patient is not breast-feeding the first dose of Brevinor tablets should be taken on the 21st day after childbirth. This will ensure the patient is protected immediately. If there is any delay in taking the first dose, contraception may not be established until 7 days after the first tablet has been taken. In these circumstances patients should be advised that extra contraceptive methods will be necessary.

After a miscarriage or abortion patients can take the first dose of Brevinor tablets on the next day; in this way they will be protected immediately.

4.3 Contraindications

As with all combined progestogen/oestrogen oral contraceptives, the following conditions should be regarded as contra-indications:

i. History of confirmed venous thromboembolic disease (VTE), family history of idiopathic VTE and other known risk factors of VTE

ii. Thrombophlebitis, cerebrovascular disorders, coronary artery disease, myocardial infarction, angina, hyperlipidaemia or a history of these conditions.

iii. Acute or severe chronic liver disease, including liver tumours, Dubin-Johnson or Rotor syndrome.

iv. History during pregnancy of idiopathic jaundice, severe pruritus or pemphigoid gestationis.

v. Known or suspected breast or genital cancer.

vi. Known or suspected oestrogen-dependent neoplasia.

vii. Undiagnosed abnormal vaginal bleeding.

viii. A history of migraines classified as classical focal or crescendo.

ix. Pregnancy.

4.4 Special warnings and special precautions for use

Assessment of women prior to starting oral contraceptives (and at regular intervals thereafter) should include a personal and family medical history of each woman. Physical examination should be guided by this and by the contra-indications (section 4.3) and warnings (section 4.4) for this product. The frequency and nature of these assessments should be based upon relevant guidelines and should be adapted to the individual woman, but should include measurement of blood pressure and, if judged appropriate by the clinician, breast, abdominal and pelvic examination including cervical cytology.

Women taking oral contraceptives require careful observation if they have or have had any of the following conditions: breast nodules; fibrocystic disease of the breast or an abnormal mammogram; uterine fibroids; a history of severe depressive states; varicose veins; sickle-cell anaemia; diabetes; hypertension; cardiovascular disease; migraine; epilepsy; asthma; otosclerosis; multiple sclerosis; porphyria; tetany; disturbed liver functions; gallstones; kidney disease; chloasma; any condition that is likely to worsen during pregnancy. The worsening or first appearance of any of these conditions may indicate that the oral contraceptive should be stopped. Discontinue treatment if there is a gradual or sudden, partial or complete loss of vision or any evidence of ocular changes, onset or aggravation of migraine or development of headache of a new kind, which is recurrent, persistent or severe.

Gastro-intestinal upsets, such as vomiting and diarrhoea, may interfere with the absorption of the tablets leading to a reduction in contraceptive efficacy. Patients should continue to take Brevinor, but they should also be encouraged to use another contraceptive method during the period of gastro-intestinal upset and for the next 7 days.

Progestogen oestrogen preparations should be used with caution in patients with a history of hepatic dysfunction or hypertension.

An increased risk of venous thromboembolic disease (VTE) associated with the use of oral contraceptives is well established but is smaller than that associated with pregnancy, which has been estimated at 60 cases per 100,000 pregnancies. Some epidemiological studies have reported a greater risk of VTE for women using combined oral contraceptives containing desogestrel or gestodene (the so-called 'third generation' pills) than for women using pills containing levonorgestrel or norethisterone (the so-called 'second generation' pills).

The spontaneous incidence of VTE in healthy non-pregnant women (not taking any oral contraceptive) is about 5 cases per 100,000 per year. The incidence in users of second generation pills is about 15 per 100,000 women per year of use. The incidence in users of third generation pills is about 25 cases per 100,000 women per year of use; this excess incidence has not been satisfactorily explained by bias or confounding. The level of all of these risks of VTE increases with age and is likely to be further increased in women with other known risk factors for VTE such as obesity. The excess risk of VTE is highest during the first year a woman ever uses a combined oral contraceptive.

Patients receiving oral contraceptives should be kept under regular surveillance, in view of the possibility of development of conditions such as thromboembolism.

The risk of coronary artery disease in women taking oral contraceptives is increased by the presence of other predisposing factors such as cigarette smoking, hypercholesterolaemia, obesity, diabetes, history of pre-eclamptic toxaemia and increasing age. After the age of thirty-five years, the patient and physician should carefully re-assess the risk/benefit ratio of using combined oral contraceptives as opposed to alternative methods of contraception.

Brevinor should be discontinued at least four weeks before, and for two weeks following, elective operations and during immobilisation. Patients undergoing injection treatment for varicose veins should not resume taking Brevinor until 3 months after the last injection.

Benign and malignant liver tumours have been associated with oral contraceptive use. The relationship between occurrence of liver tumours and use of female sex hormones is not known at present. These tumours may rupture causing intra-abdominal bleeding. If the patient presents with a mass or tenderness in the right upper quadrant or an acute abdomen, the possible presence of a tumour should be considered.

An increased risk of congenital abnormalities, including heart defects and limb defects, has been reported following the use of sex hormones, including oral contraceptives, in pregnancy. If the patient does not adhere to the prescribed schedule, the possibility of pregnancy should be considered at the time of the first missed period and further use of oral contraceptives should be withheld until pregnancy has been ruled out. It is recommended that for any patient who has missed two consecutive periods, pregnancy should be ruled out before continuing the contraceptive regimen. If pregnancy is confirmed the patient should be advised of the potential risks to the foetus and the advisability of continuing the pregnancy should be discussed in the light of these risks. It is advisable to discontinue Brevinor three months before a planned pregnancy.

The risk of arterial thrombosis associated with combined oral contraceptives increases with age, and this risk is aggravated by cigarette smoking. The use of combined oral contraceptives by women in the older age group, especially those who are cigarette smokers, should therefore be discouraged and alternative methods advised.

The use of this product in patients suffering from epilepsy, migraine, asthma or cardiac dysfunction may result in exacerbation of these disorders because of fluid retention. Caution should also be observed in patients who wear contact lenses.

Decreased glucose tolerance may occur in diabetic patients on this treatment, and their control must be carefully supervised.

The use of oral contraceptives has also been associated with a possible increased incidence of gall bladder disease.

Women with a history of oligomenorrhoea or secondary amenorrhoea or young women without regular cycles may have a tendency to remain anovulatory or to become amenorrhoeic after discontinuation of oral contraceptives. Women with these pre-existing problems should be advised of this possibility and encouraged to use other contraceptive methods.

Numerous epidemiological studies have been reported on the risks of ovarian, endometrial, cervical and breast cancer in women using combined oral contraceptives. The evidence is clear that combined oral contraceptives offer substantial protection against both ovarian and endometrial cancer.

An increased risk of cervical cancer in long-term users of combined oral contraceptives has been reported in some studies, but there continues to be controversy about the extent to which this is attributable to the confounding effects of sexual behaviour and other factors.

A meta-analysis from 54 epidemiological studies reported that there is a slightly increased relative risk (RR = 1.24) of having breast cancer diagnosed in women who are currently using combined oral contraceptives (COCs). The observed pattern of increased risk may be due to an earlier diagnosis of breast cancer in COC users, the biological effects of COCs or a combination of both. The additional breast cancers diagnosed in current users of COCs or in women who have used COCs in the last ten years are more likely to be localised to the breast than those in women who never used COCs.

Breast cancer is rare among women under 40 years of age whether or not they take COCs. Whilst this background risk increases with age, the excess number of breast cancer diagnoses in current and recent COC users is small in relation to the overall risk of breast cancer (see bar chart).

The most important risk factor for breast cancer in COC users is the age women discontinue the COC; the older the age at stopping, the more breast cancers are diagnosed. Duration of use is less important and the excess risk gradually disappears during the course of the 10 years after stopping COC use such that by 10 years there appears to be no excess.

The possible increase in risk of breast cancer should be discussed with the user and weighed against the benefits of COCs taking into account the evidence that they offer substantial protection against the risk of developing certain other cancers (e.g. ovarian and endometrial cancer).

Estimated cumulative numbers of breast cancers per 10,000 women diagnosed in 5 years of use and up to 10 years after stopping COCs, compared with numbers of breast cancer diagnosed in 10,000 women who had never used COCs.

(see Figure 1)

4.5 Interaction with other medicinal products and other forms of Interaction

The herbal remedy St John's wort (*Hypericum perforatum*) should not be taken concomitantly with this medicine as this could potentially lead to a loss of contraceptive effect.

Some drugs may modify the metabolism of Brevinor reducing its effectiveness; these include certain sedatives, antibiotics, anti-epileptic and anti-arthritic drugs. During the time such agents are used concurrently, it is advised that mechanical contraceptives also be used.

Figure 1

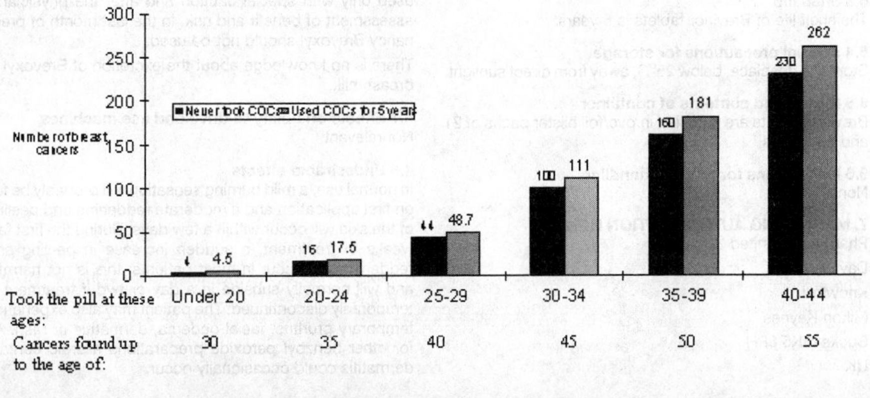

The results of a large number of laboratory tests have been shown to be influenced by the use of oestrogen containing oral contraceptives, which may limit their diagnostic value. Among these are: biochemical markers of thyroid and liver function; plasma levels of carrier proteins, triglycerides, coagulation and fibrinolysis factors.

4.6 Pregnancy and lactation
Contra-indicated in pregnancy.

Patients who are fully breast-feeding should not take Brevinor tablets since, in common with other combined oral contraceptives, the oestrogen component may reduce the amount of milk produced. In addition, active ingredients or their metabolites have been detected in the milk of mothers taking oral contraceptives. The effect of Brevinor on breast-fed infants has not been determined.

4.7 Effects on ability to drive and use machines
None.

4.8 Undesirable effects
As with all oral contraceptives, there may be slight nausea at first, weight gain or breast discomfort, which soon disappear.

Other side-effects known or suspected to occur with oral contraceptives include gastro-intestinal symptoms, changes in libido and appetite, headache, exacerbation of existing uterine fibroid disease, depression, and changes in carbohydrate, lipid and vitamin metabolism.

Spotting or bleeding may occur during the first few cycles. Usually menstrual bleeding becomes light and occasionally there may be no bleeding during the tablet-free days.

Hypertension, which is usually reversible on discontinuing treatment, has occurred in a small percentage of women taking oral contraceptives.

4.9 Overdose
Overdosage may be manifested by nausea, vomiting, breast enlargement and vaginal bleeding. There is no specific antidote and treatment should be symptomatic. Gastric lavage may be employed if the overdose is large and the patient is seen sufficiently early (within four hours).

5. PHARMACOLOGICAL PROPERTIES

5.1 Pharmacodynamic properties
The mode of action of Brevinor is similar to that of other progestogen/oestrogen oral contraceptives and includes the inhibition of ovulation, the thickening of cervical mucus so as to constitute a barrier to sperm and the rendering of the endometrium unreceptive to implantation. Such activity is exerted through a combined effect on one or more of the following: hypothalamus, anterior pituitary, ovary, endometrium and cervical mucus.

5.2 Pharmacokinetic properties
Norethisterone is rapidly and completely absorbed after oral administration, peak plasma concentrations occurring in the majority of subjects between 1 and 3 hours. Due to first-pass metabolism, blood levels after oral administration are 60% of those after i.v. administration. The half-life of elimination varies from 5 to 12 hours, with a mean of 7.6 hours. Norethisterone is metabolised mainly in the liver. Approximately 60% of the administered dose is excreted as metabolites in urine and faeces.

Ethinyloestradiol is rapidly and well absorbed from the gastro-intestinal tract but is subject to some first-pass metabolism in the gut-wall. Compared to many other oestrogens it is only slowly metabolised in the liver. Excretion is via the kidneys with some appearing also in the faeces.

5.3 Preclinical safety data
The toxicity of norethisterone is very low. Reports of teratogenic effects in animals are uncommon. No carcinogenic effects have been found even in long-term studies.

Long-term continuous administration of oestrogens in some animals increases the frequency of carcinoma of the breast, cervix, vagina and liver.

6. PHARMACEUTICAL PARTICULARS

6.1 List of excipients
Brevinor tablets contain:

Maize starch, polyvidone, magnesium stearate, lactose and E132.

6.2 Incompatibilities
None stated.

6.3 Shelf life
The shelf life of Brevinor tablets is 5 years.

6.4 Special precautions for storage
Store in a dry place, below 25°C, away from direct sunlight.

6.5 Nature and contents of container
Brevinor tablets are supplied in pvc/foil blister packs of 21 and 63 tablets.

6.6 Instructions for use and handling
None.

7. MARKETING AUTHORISATION HOLDER
Pharmacia Limited

Davy Avenue

Knowlhill

Milton Keynes

Bucks MK5 8PH

UK

8. MARKETING AUTHORISATION NUMBER(S)
PL 00032/0398

9. DATE OF FIRST AUTHORISATION/RENEWAL OF THE AUTHORISATION
27 June 2002

10. DATE OF REVISION OF THE TEXT
March 1996

February 1998

January 2000

April 2000

December 2000

February 2002

August 2002

Legal Category
POM.

Brevoxyl Cream

(Stiefel Laboratories (UK) Limited)

1. NAME OF THE MEDICINAL PRODUCT
Brevoxyl Cream

2. QUALITATIVE AND QUANTITATIVE COMPOSITION
Benzoyl peroxide 4%w/w as hydrous benzoyl peroxide Ph Eur

100g cream contains 4g benzoyl peroxide.

For excipients, see 6.1

3. PHARMACEUTICAL FORM
Cream

A white to off white cream.

4. CLINICAL PARTICULARS

4.1 Therapeutic indications
Brevoxyl is indicated for the treatment of moderate acne vulgaris.

4.2 Posology and method of administration
Adolescents and Adults:
Apply to the whole of the affected area once or twice daily. Wash with soap and water prior to application.

Paediatric use:
The safety and efficacy of Brevoxyl has not been established in children since acne vulgaris rarely presents in this age group.

Initial application of the product may be varied at the physician's instructions to reflect the patient's skin type and to avoid undesirable effects.

Improvement can generally be seen after 4-6 weeks of treatment. However, longer use may be necessary.

4.3 Contraindications
Patients with known hypersensitivity to any of the ingredients should not use the product.

4.4 Special warnings and special precautions for use
Avoid contact with the eyes, mouth and other mucous membranes. Care should be taken when applying the product to the neck and other sensitive areas.

It is recommended that exposure to sun or sunlamps should be minimised.

Simultaneous use of other keratolytics such as salicylates or sulphur may increase occurrence of skin irritation.

During the first few weeks of treatment, a sudden increase in peeling and reddening will occur in most patients; this is not harmful and will normally subside in a day or two if treatment is temporarily discontinued

The product may bleach hair and coloured or dyed fabrics.

4.5 Interaction with other medicinal products and other forms of Interaction
Simultaneous application of Brevoxyl and topical acne preparations containing vitamin A derivatives should be avoided.

4.6 Pregnancy and lactation
The safety of Brevoxyl in human pregnancy is not established. During pregnancy and lactation Brevoxyl should be used only with special caution and after the physician's assessment of benefit and risk. In the last month of pregnancy Brevoxyl should not be used.

There is no knowledge about the excretion of Brevoxyl in breast milk.

4.7 Effects on ability to drive and use machines
Not relevant

4.8 Undesirable effects
In normal use, a mild burning sensation will probably be felt on first application and a moderate reddening and peeling of the skin will occur within a few days. During the first few weeks of treatment, a sudden increase in peeling and reddening will occur in most patients; this is not harmful and will normally subside in a day or two if treatment is temporarily discontinued. The patient may also experience temporary pruritus, facial oedema, dermatitis or rash. As for other benzoyl peroxide preparations allergic contact dermatitis could occasionally occur.

4.9 Overdose
Not applicable.

5. PHARMACOLOGICAL PROPERTIES

5.1 Pharmacodynamic properties
ATC Code: D10A E01

Benzoyl peroxide is keratolytic and is an oxidising agent with antibacterial activity against *Propionibacterium acnes*, the organism implicated in acne vulgaris. It has keratolytic activity and is sebostatic, counteracting the hyperkeratinisation and excessive sebum production associated with acne.

5.2 Pharmacokinetic properties
After topical application, benzoyl peroxide is absorbed in varying quantities through the skin of man and animals.

Radio-labelled studies have shown that absorption of benzoyl peroxide through the skin can only occur following its conversion to benzoic acid. Benzoic acid is mostly conjugated to form hippuric acid which is excreted via the kidneys.

5.3 Preclinical safety data
Animal toxicity studies of benzoyl peroxide have shown that the compound is non-toxic when applied topically.

Benzoic acid, to which benzoyl peroxide is converted prior to absorption, has a wide margin of safety. Benzoic acid is an approved food additive.

Benzoyl peroxide is a free radical generating compound. The release of oxygen during its conversion to benzoic acid may be implicated in a tumour promoting effect seen in mouse skin.

Benzoyl peroxide at high doses (>20 times the normal human dose) has been shown to increase tumour growth initiated by dimethyl benzanthracene (DMBA) in mice. DMBA is a powerful chemical carcinogen to which patients are unlikely to be exposed. The relevance of these results to man is limited. Studies in mice have also shown that benzoyl peroxide does not increase the growth of tumours initiated by ultra violet light.

No reproductive toxicology studies have been performed. Up to date there are no indications that the topical use of Brevoxyl causes damage to the unborn child.

6. PHARMACEUTICAL PARTICULARS

6.1 List of excipients
Cetyl alcohol

Promulgen G (Stearyl alcohol and Macrogol cetostearyl ether)

Simethicone emulsion

Propylene glycol alginate

Dimethyl isosorbide

Fragrance X-23304

Purified water

6.2 Incompatibilities
Not applicable

6.3 Shelf life
2 years

6.4 Special precautions for storage
Do not store above 25°C.

6.5 Nature and contents of container
Lacquered aluminium or laminated tubes with white polypropylene screw caps.

Licensed pack sizes: 40g.

6.6 Instructions for use and handling
No special requirements.

7. MARKETING AUTHORISATION HOLDER
Stiefel Laboratories (UK) Ltd

Holtspur Lane

Wooburn Green

High Wycombe

Bucks HP10 0AU

8. MARKETING AUTHORISATION NUMBER(S)
PL 00174/0193

9. DATE OF FIRST AUTHORISATION/RENEWAL OF THE AUTHORISATION
29 May 2001

10. DATE OF REVISION OF THE TEXT
26 September 2005

Bricanyl Aerosol

(AstraZeneca UK Limited)

1. NAME OF THE MEDICINAL PRODUCT
Bricanyl Aerosol

2. QUALITATIVE AND QUANTITATIVE COMPOSITION
Terbutaline Sulphate 0.25mg/dose.

For excipients see Section 6.1.

3. PHARMACEUTICAL FORM
Pressurised inhalation suspension.

4. CLINICAL PARTICULARS

4.1 Therapeutic indications

Terbutaline is a selective β_2-adrenergic agonist recommended for the relief and prevention of bronchospasm in bronchial asthma and in chronic bronchitis and other bronchopulmonary disorders in which bronchospasm is a complicating factor.

4.2 Posology and method of administration

BRICANYL INHALER: Adults and children

Prophylaxis and relief of acute attacks: One or two inhalations as required, with a short interval between each inhalation at 6 hourly intervals. Not more than 8 inhalations should be necessary in any 24 hours, but medical advice should be sought and treatment reviewed if condition fails to improve.

BRICANYL SPACER INHALER: Adults and children

Prophylaxis and relief of acute attacks: One or two inhalations as required, with a short interval between each inhalation at 6 hourly intervals. Not more than 8 inhalations should be necessary in any 24 hours, but medical advice should be sought and treatment reviewed if condition fails to improve.

NEBUHALER: Adults and children

The dose must always be adjusted to patient response and severity of the bronchospasm.

Prophylaxis and relief of acute attacks: One or two inhalations as required, with a short interval between each inhalation at 6 hourly intervals. Not more than 8 inhalations should be necessary in any 24 hours, but medical advice should be sought and treatment reviewed if condition fails to improve.

Bricanyl via the Nebuhaler may also be used in conditions such as severe bronchospasm and severe acute asthma which are normally managed by administration of nebulised bronchodilators.

For hospital use in acute asthma:

Adults

The initial dose should be 2mg (8 actuations); this may be repeated up to a total dose of 8mg in one hour. Thereafter a dose of up to 4mg may be given four times daily.

A similar dose range may be used for domiciliary use, but patients should be warned that if either the usual relief or duration of action is diminished, they should seek medical advice immediately.

Children over 5 years

Dosage must be individualised but clinical studies have shown that when used for the management of acute asthma in children, the following dosages given over a 15 minute period have been as effective as equal doses administered by nebuliser.

Children under 25kg 1.25 - 2.5mg (5-10 puffs)

Children over 25kg 2.5 - 5.0mg (10-20 puffs)

Elderly

Dosage as for adults. Because of the difficulty experienced by many elderly patients, in co-ordinating inhalation with actuation, Bricanyl Spacer Inhaler or use via the Nebuhaler will provide a more certain delivery of drug.

Instructions for correct use.

On actuation of Bricanyl pressurised metered dose inhaler, a suspension of the substance is pumped out of the canister at high velocity.

When the patient inhales through the mouthpiece at the same time as releasing a dose, the substance will follow the inspired air into the airways.

NOTE: it is important to instruct the patient:

- To carefully read the instructions for use in the patient information leaflet packed together with each inhaler.
- To shake the inhaler thoroughly before each actuation, in order to mix the contents of the inhaler properly.
- To breathe in slowly and deeply through the mouthpiece and to release the dose while continuing to breath in.

Both the Bricanyl Spacer Inhaler and the Nebuhaler are recommended to enable patients with difficulty co-ordinating conventional aerosols to derive greater therapeutic benefit. A package insert is provided giving simple operating instructions.

Patients using the Nebuhaler must be instructed to actuate the aerosol and breathe in slowly and deeply through the mouthpiece. Ideally two inspirations per actuation are required to empty the Nebuhaler. For further doses, the procedure is repeated.

For young children who are unable to breathe through the mouthpiece, a face mask can be used. Compatible face masks are available separately and care should be taken to ensure a good fit is achieved.

4.3 Contraindications

Bricanyl preparations are contra-indicated in patients with a history of sensitivity to any of their constituents.

4.4 Special warnings and special precautions for use

Patients should be instructed in proper use and their inhalation technique checked regularly.

Care should be taken in patients suffering from myocardial insufficiency or thyrotoxicosis.

Due to the hyperglycaemic effects of β_2-stimulants, additional blood glucose measurements are initially recommended when Bricanyl therapy is commenced in diabetic patients.

If a previously effective dosage regimen no longer gives the same symptomatic relief, the patient should urgently seek further medical advice. Consideration should be given to the requirements for additional therapy (including increased dosages of anti-inflammatory medication). Severe exacerbations of asthma should be treated as an emergency in the usual manner.

Due to the positive inotropic effect of β_2-agonists, these drugs should not be used in patients with hypertrophic cardiomyopathy.

Potentially serious hypokalaemia may result from β_2-agonist therapy, mainly with parenteral or nebulised administration. Particular caution is advised in acute severe asthma as this effect may be augmented by hypoxia. The hypokalaemic effect may be potentiated by concomitant treatment with xanthine derivatives, corticosteroids and/or diuretics. It is recommended that serum potassium levels are monitored in such situations.

4.5 Interaction with other medicinal products and other forms of Interaction

Beta-blocking agents (including eye drops), especially the non-selective ones such as propranolol, may partially or totally inhibit the effect of beta-stimulants. Therefore, Bricanyl preparations and non-selective β-blockers should not normally be administered concurrently. Bricanyl should be used with caution in patients receiving other sympathomimetics.

Hypokalaemia may result from β_2-agonist therapy and may be potentiated by concomitant treatment with xanthine derivatives, corticosteroids and diuretics (see *Section 4.4, Special Warnings and Precautions for use*).

4.6 Pregnancy and lactation

Although no teratogenic effects have been observed in animals or in patients Bricanyl should only be administered with caution during the first trimester of pregnancy.

Terbutaline is secreted via breast milk but any effect on the infant is unlikely at therapeutic doses.

4.7 Effects on ability to drive and use machines

None.

4.8 Undesirable effects

The frequency of side-effects is low at the recommended doses. Side-effects which have been recorded such as tremor, nausea, headache, tonic cramp, mouth and throat irritation and palpitations are all characteristic of sympathomimetic amines. A few patients feel tense; this is also due to the effects on skeletal muscle and not to direct CNS stimulation. Whenever these side-effects have occurred, the majority have usually been spontaneously reversible within the first week of treatment. As with other β_2-agonists, tremor is dose related.

Tachycardia, with or without peripheral vasodilation, has been rarely reported during β_2-agonist therapy. Cardiac arrhythmias, including atrial fibrillation, supraventricular tachycardia and extrasystoles, have been reported in association with β_2-agonists, usually in susceptible patients.

In rare cases, through unspecified mechanisms, paradoxical bronchospasm may occur with wheezing immediately after inhalation. This should be immediately treated with a rapid-onset bronchodilator. Bricanyl therapy should be discontinued and, after assessment, an alternative therapy initiated.

The chlorofluorocarbons used as propellants may in some asthmatics cause a fall in FEV_1 immediately after exposure.

Potentially serious hypokalaemia may result from β_2-agonist therapy. (See also *Section 4.4, Special Warnings and Precautions for use.*)

Sleep disturbances and behavioural disturbances, such as agitation, hyperactivity and restlessness, have been observed.

Hypersensitivity reactions, including angioedema, urticaria, exanthema, bronchospasm, hypotension and collapse, have been very rarely reported with β_2-agonist therapy.

4.9 Overdose

i) **Possible symptoms and signs:** Headache, anxiety, tremor, nausea, tonic cramp, palpitations, tachycardia and arrhythmia. A fall in blood pressure sometimes occurs.

Laboratory findings: Hypokalaemia, hyperglycaemia and lactic acidosis sometimes occur.

ii) **Treatment:**

Mild and moderate cases: Reduce the dose.

Severe cases: Gastric lavage, administration of activated charcoal (where suspected that significant amounts have been swallowed). Determination of acid-base balance, blood sugar and electrolytes, particularly serum potassium levels. Monitoring of heart rate and rhythm and blood pressure. Metabolic changes should be corrected. A cardioselective β-blocker (e.g. metoprolol) is recommended for the treatment of arrhythmias causing haemodynamic deterioration. The β-blocker should be used with care because of the possibility of inducing bronchoconstriction: use with caution in patients with a history of bronchospasm. If the β_2-mediated reduction in peripheral vascular resistance significantly contributes to the fall in blood pressure, a volume expander should be given.

5. PHARMACOLOGICAL PROPERTIES

5.1 Pharmacodynamic properties

Pharmaco-therapeutic group: selective β_2-agonist, terbutaline, ATC code: R03A C03.

Terbutaline is a selective β_2-adrenergic stimulant having the following pharmacological effects:

i) **In the lung:** Bronchodilation; increase in mucociliary clearance; suppression of oedema and anti-allergic effects.

ii) **In skeletal muscle**: Stimulates Na^+/K^+ transport and also causes depression of subtetanic contractions in slow-contracting muscle.

iii) **In uterine muscle**: Inhibition of uterine contractions.

iv) **In the CNS:** Low penetration into the blood-brain barrier at therapeutic doses, due to the highly hydrophilic nature of the molecule.

v) **In the CVS**: Administration of terbutaline results in cardiovascular effects mediated through β_2-receptors in the peripheral arteries and in the heart e.g. in healthy subjects, 0.25 - 0.50mg injected S.C., is associated with an increase in cardiac output (up to 85% over controls) due to an increase in heart rate and a larger stroke volume. The increase in heart rate is probably due to a combination of a reflex tachycardia via a fall in peripheral resistance and a direct positive chronotropic effect of the drug.

5.2 Pharmacokinetic properties

Basic parameters have been evaluated in man after i.v. and oral administration of therapeutic doses, e.g.

I.V. single dose

Volume distribution (VSS)	- 114 L
Total body clearance (CL)	- 213 ml/min
Mean residence time (MRT)	- 9.0 h
Renal clearance (CLR)	- 149 ml/min (males)

Oral dose

Renal clearance (CLR)	- 1.925 ml/min (males)
Renal clearance (CLR)	- 2.32 ml/min (females)

The plasma concentration/time curve after i.v. administration is characterised by a fast distribution phase, an intermediate elimination phase and a late elimination phase.

Terminal half-life t½ has been determined after single and multiple dosing (mean values varied between 16-20 h).

Bioavailability

Food reduces bioavailability following oral dosing (10% on average). Fasting values of 14-15% have been obtained.

Metabolism

The main metabolite after oral dosing is the sulphate conjugate and also some glucoronide conjugate can be found in the urine.

5.3 Preclinical safety data

The major toxic effect of terbutaline, observed in toxicological studies in rats and dogs at exposures in excess of maximum human exposure, is focal myocardial necrosis. This type of cardiotoxicity is a well known pharmacological manifestation seen after the administration of high doses of β_2-agonists.

In rats, an increase in the incidence of benign uterine leiomyomas has been observed. This effect is looked upon as a class-effect observed in rodents after long term exposure to high doses of β_2-agonists

6. PHARMACEUTICAL PARTICULARS

6.1 List of excipients

Sorbitan trioleate, trichlorofluoromethane (propellant 11), dichlorotetrafluorethane (propellant 114), dichlorodifluoromethane (propellant 12).

6.2 Incompatibilities

None known.

6.3 Shelf life

36 months

6.4 Special precautions for storage

Do not store above 25°C.

Do not puncture or expose the canister to high temperatures (40°C) or direct sunlight, even when empty.

6.5 Nature and contents of container

Bricanyl Inhaler

Metered dose inhaler.

10 ml aluminium vial with 25 μl metering valve containing either 100 or 400 metered doses.

Bricanyl Spacer Inhaler

Metered dose aerosol with extended mouthpiece delivering 0.25mg terbutaline sulphate per actuation.

Nebuhaler

750ml plastic cone with a one-way valve.

6.6 Instructions for use and handling

None

7. MARKETING AUTHORISATION HOLDER

AstraZeneca UK Ltd.,

600 Capability Green,

Luton, LU1 3LU, UK.

8. MARKETING AUTHORISATION NUMBER(S)

PL 17901/0110

9. DATE OF FIRST AUTHORISATION/RENEWAL OF THE AUTHORISATION

28th May 2002

10. DATE OF REVISION OF THE TEXT

23rd April 2004

Bricanyl Injection, 0.5 mg/ml, solution for injection or infusion

(AstraZeneca UK Limited)

1. NAME OF THE MEDICINAL PRODUCT

Bricanyl® Injection, 0.5 mg/ml, solution for injection or infusion.

2. QUALITATIVE AND QUANTITATIVE COMPOSITION

Terbutaline sulphate 0.5 mg/ml.

For excipients see Section 6.1.

3. PHARMACEUTICAL FORM

Solution for injection or infusion.

A clear aqueous solution.

4. CLINICAL PARTICULARS

4.1 Therapeutic indications

Bronchodilation

Terbutaline is a selective β_2-adrenergic agonist recommended for the relief of bronchospasm in bronchial asthma and other bronchopulmonary disorders in which bronchospasm is a complicating factor.

For the management of uncomplicated premature labour

To arrest labour between 24 and 33 weeks of gestation in patients with no medical or obstetric contraindication to tocolytic therapy. The main effect of tocolytic therapy is a delay in delivery of up to 48 hours; no statistically significant effect on perinatal mortality or morbidity has as yet been observed in randomised, controlled trials. The greatest benefit from tocolytic therapy is gained by using the delay in delivery to administer glucocorticoids or to implement other measures known to improve perinatal health.

4.2 Posology and method of administration

Routes of administration

Parenteral - subcutaneous, intramuscular, intravenous.

The dosage should be individualised.

For bronchodilation

When a rapid therapeutic response is required, Bricanyl can be administered by any of the three standard parenteral routes: subcutaneous, intramuscular, or i.v. bolus. The preferred routes will usually be subcutaneous or intramuscular. When given as an i.v. bolus the injection must be made slowly noting patient response.

Adults: 0.5 - 1 ml (0.25 - 0.5 mg) up to four times a day.

Children 2 - 15 years: 0.01 mg/kg body weight to a maximum of 0.3 mg total.

Age	Average weight kg	(lb)	mg terbutaline	ml volume
<3	10	(22)	0.1	0.2
3	15	(33)	0.15	0.3
6	20	(44)	0.2	0.4
8	25	(55)	0.25	0.5
10+	30+	(66+)	0.3	0.6

By infusion: 3 - 5 ml (1.5 - 2.5 mg) in 500 ml 5% dextrose, saline or dextrose/saline given by continuous intravenous infusion at a rate of 10 - 20 drops (0.5 - 1 ml) per minute for 8 to 10 hours. A corresponding reduction in dosage should be made for children.

Elderly: Dosage as for adults.

For the management of premature labour

Procedure: To be administered as early as possible after the diagnosis of premature labour, and after evaluation of the patient to rule out contraindications to the use of terbutaline (*see Section 4.3, Contraindications*).

Initially, 5 mcg/min should be infused during the first 20 minutes increasing by 2.5 mcg/min at 20 minute intervals until the contractions stop. More than 10 mcg/min should seldom be given, 20 mcg/min should not be exceeded.

The infusion should be stopped if labour progresses despite treatment at the maximum dose.

If successful, the infusion should continue for 1 hour at the chosen rate and then be decreased by 2.5 mcg/min every 20 minutes to the lowest dose that produces suppression of contractions. Keep the infusion at this rate for 12 hours and then continue with oral maintenance therapy.

As an alternative, subcutaneous injections of 250 mcg should be given four times a day for a few days before oral treatment is commenced. Oral treatment may be continued for as long as the physician considers it desirable to prolong pregnancy.

Special cautions for infusion: The dose must be individually titrated with reference to suppression of contractions, increase in pulse rate and changes in blood pressure, which are limiting factors. These parameters should be carefully monitored during treatment. A maternal heart rate of more than 135 beats/min should be avoided.

Careful control of the level of hydration is essential to avoid the risk of maternal pulmonary oedema (*see Section 4.8, Undesirable effects*). The volume of fluid in which the drug is administered should thus be kept to a minimum. A controlled infusion device should be used, preferably a syringe pump.

Dilution:

The recommended infusion fluid is 5% dextrose. If a syringe pump is available, the concentration of the drug infused should be 0.1 mg/ml (10 ml Bricanyl Injection should be added to 40 ml of 5% dextrose).

At this dilution:

5 mcg/min ≡ 0.05 ml/min and

10 mcg/min ≡ 0.1 ml/min

If no syringe pump is available, the concentration of the drug should be 0.01 mg/ml (10 ml Bricanyl Injection should be added to 490 ml of 5% dextrose).

At this dilution:

5 mcg/min ≡ 0.5 ml/min and

10 mcg/min ≡ 1 ml/min.

4.3 Contraindications

Bricanyl preparations are contraindicated in patients with a history of hypersensitivity to any of their constituents.

Although Bricanyl Injection and oral preparations are used in the management of uncomplicated premature labour, their use in the following conditions is contra-indicated: any conditions of the mother or foetus in which prolongation of the pregnancy is hazardous e.g. severe toxaemia, antepartum haemorrhage, intra-uterine infection, abruptio placentae, threatened abortion during the first and second trimesters or cord compression.

4.4 Special warnings and special precautions for use

Care should be taken with patients suffering from myocardial insufficiency or thyrotoxicosis.

Due to the hyperglycaemic effects of β_2-stimulants, additional blood glucose measurements are initially recommended when Bricanyl therapy is commenced in diabetic patients.

If a previously effective dosage regimen no longer gives the same symptomatic relief, the patient should urgently seek further medical advice. Consideration should be given to the requirements for additional therapy (including increased dosages of anti-inflammatory medication). Severe exacerbations of asthma should be treated as an emergency in the usual manner.

Potentially serious hypokalaemia may result from β_2-agonist therapy, mainly with parenteral or nebulised administration. Particular caution is advised in acute severe asthma as this effect may be augmented by hypoxia. The hypokalaemic effect may be potentiated by concomitant treatment with xanthine derivatives, corticosteroids and/or diuretics. It is recommended that serum potassium levels are monitored in such situations.

Due to the positive inotropic effect of the β_2-agonists, these drugs should not be used in patients with hypertrophic cardiomyopathy.

In premature labour in a patient with known or suspected cardiac disease a physician experienced in cardiology should assess the suitability of treatment before i.v. infusion with Bricanyl.

In order to minimise the risk of hypotension associated with tocolytic therapy, special care should be taken to avoid caval compression by keeping the patient in the left or right lateral positions throughout the infusion.

In treatment of premature labour, hyperglycaemia and ketoacidosis have been found in pregnant women with diabetes after treatment with β_2-stimulants. It may therefore be necessary to adjust the insulin dose when β_2-stimulants are used in the treatment.

Increased tendency to uterine bleeding has been reported in connection with Caesarian section. However, this can be effectively stopped by propranolol 1-2 mg injected intravenously.

4.5 Interaction with other medicinal products and other forms of Interaction

Beta-blocking agents (including eye drops), especially the non-selective ones such as propranolol, may partially or totally inhibit the effect of β-stimulants. Therefore, Bricanyl preparations and non-selective β-blockers should not normally be administered concurrently. Bricanyl should be used with caution in patients receiving other sympathomimetics.

Hypokalaemia may result from β_2-agonist therapy and may be potentiated by concomitant treatment with xanthine derivatives, corticosteroids and diuretics (*see Section 4.4, Special Warnings and Precautions for use*).

4.6 Pregnancy and lactation

Although no teratogenic effects have been observed in animals or in patients, Bricanyl should only be administered with caution during the first trimester of pregnancy.

Terbutaline is secreted into breast milk, but any effects on the infant are unlikely at therapeutic doses.

Transient hypoglycaemia has been reported in newborn preterm infants after maternal β_2-agonist treatment.

4.7 Effects on ability to drive and use machines

Bricanyl does not affect the ability to drive or use machines.

4.8 Undesirable effects

When used as a bronchdilator, the frequency of side-effects is low. Side effects which have been recorded, such as tremor, headache, nausea, tonic cramp, mouth and throat irritation and palpitations, are all characteristic of sympathomimetic amines. A few patients feel tense; this is also due to effects on skeletal muscle and not to direct CNS stimulation. Whenever these side-effects have occurred, the majority have usually been spontaneously reversible within the first week of treatment. As with other β_2-agonists, tremor is dose related.

Sleep disturbances and behavioural disturbances, such as agitation, hyperactivity and restlessness, have been observed.

Tachycardia, with or without peripheral vasodilation, has been rarely reported during β_2-agonist therapy. Cardiac arrhythmias, including atrial fibrillation, supraventricular tachycardia and extrasystoles, have been reported in association with β_2-agonists, usually in susceptible patients.

Potentially serious hypokalaemia may result from β_2-agonist therapy. (See also *Section 4.4, Special Warnings and Precautions for use.*)

In rare cases, through unspecified mechanisms, paradoxical bronchospasm may occur, with wheezing immediately after inhalation. This should be immediately treated with a rapid-onset bronchodilator. Bricanyl therapy should be discontinued and, after assessment, an alternative therapy initiated.

Hypersensitivity reactions, including angioedema, urticaria, exanthema, bronchospasm, hypotension and collapse, have been very rarely reported with β_2-agonist therapy.

In common with other β_2-agonists, maternal pulmonary oedema has been reported in association with the use of terbutaline for the management of premature labour; in some cases this has proved fatal. Predisposing factors include fluid overload, multiple pregnancy, pre-existing cardiac disease and maternal infection. Close monitoring of the patient's state of hydration is essential. If signs of pulmonary oedema develop (e.g. cough, shortness of breath), treatment should be discontinued immediately and diuretic therapy instituted.

4.9 Overdose

i) Possible symptoms and signs: Headache, anxiety, tremor, nausea, tonic cramp, palpitations, tachycardia and arrhythmia. A fall in blood pressure sometimes occurs. Laboratory findings: hypokalaemia, hyperglycaemia and lactic acidosis sometimes occur.

ii) Treatment:

Mild and moderate cases: Reduce the dose.

Severe cases: Determination of acid-base balance, blood sugar and electrolytes, particularly serum potassium levels. Monitoring of heart rate and rhythm and blood pressure. Metabolic changes should be corrected. A cardioselective

β-blocker (e.g. metoprolol) is recommended for the treatment of arrhythmias causing haemodynamic deterioration. The β-blocker should be used with care because of the possibility of inducing bronchoconstriction: use with caution in patients with a history of bronchospasm. If the β_2-mediated reduction in peripheral vascular resistance significantly contributes to the fall in blood pressure, a volume expander should be given.

In preterm labour:

Pulmonary oedema: discontinue administration of Bricanyl. A normal dose of loop diuretic (e.g. frusemide) should be given intravenously.

Increased bleeding in connection with Caesarian section: propranolol, 1 - 2 mg intravenously.

5. PHARMACOLOGICAL PROPERTIES

5.1 Pharmacodynamic properties

Pharmaco-therapeutic group: selective β_2-agonist, terbutaline, ATC code: R03C C03.

Terbutaline is a selective β_2-adrenergic stimulant, having the following pharmacological effects:

i) In the lung: bronchodilation; increase in mucociliary clearance; suppression of oedema and anti-allergic effects.

ii) In skeletal muscle: stimulates Na^+/K^+ transport and also causes depression of subtetanic contractions in slow-contracting muscle.

iii) In uterine muscle: inhibition of uterine contractions.

iv) In the CNS: low penetration into the blood-brain barrier at therapeutic doses, due to the highly hydrophilic nature of the molecule.

v) In the CVS: administration of terbutaline results in cardiovascular effects mediated through β_2-receptors in the peripheral arteries and in the heart e.g. in healthy subjects, 0.25 - 0.5 mg injected s.c is associated with an increase in cardiac output (up to 85% over controls) due to an increase in heart rate and a larger stroke volume. The increase in heart rate is probably due to a combination of a reflex tachycardia, via a fall in peripheral resistance and a direct positive chronotropic effect of the drug.

5.2 Pharmacokinetic properties

Basic parameters have been evaluated in man after i.v. and oral administration of therapeutic doses, e.g.

i.v. single dose

Volume of distribution (VSS) - 114 L

Total body clearance (CL) - 213 ml/min

Mean residence time (MRT) - 9.0 h

Renal clearance (CLR) - 149 ml/min (males)

Oral dose

Renal clearance (CLR) - 1.925 ml/min (males)

Renal clearance (CLR) - 2.32 ml/min (females)

The plasma concentration/time curve after i.v. administration is characterised by a fast distribution phase, an intermediate elimination phase and a late elimination phase.

Terminal half-life ($t_{½}$) has been determined after single and multiple dosing (mean values varied between 16 - 20 h).

Bioavailability

Food reduces bioavailability following oral dosing (10% on average); fasting values of 14 - 15% have been obtained.

Metabolism

The main metabolite after oral dosing is the sulphate conjugate and also some glucuronide conjugate can be found in the urine.

5.3 Preclinical safety data

The major toxic effect of terbutaline, observed in toxicological studies in rats and dogs at exposures in excess of maximum human exposure, is focal myocardial necrosis. This type of cardiotoxicity is a well known pharmacological manifestation seen after the administration of high doses of β_2-agonists.

In rats, an increase in the incidence of benign uterine leiomyomas has been observed. This effect is looked upon as a class-effect observed in rodents after long term exposure to high doses of β_2-agonists

6. PHARMACEUTICAL PARTICULARS

6.1 List of excipients

Sodium chloride, hydrochloric acid and water for injection.

6.2 Incompatibilities

Bricanyl solution for injection should not be mixed with alkaline solutions, i.e. solutions with a pH higher than 7.0.

6.3 Shelf life

24 months

6.4 Special precautions for storage

Do not store above 25°C. Keep in the outer carton.

6.5 Nature and contents of container

Packs of 5 × 1ml glass ampoules

Packs of 10 × 5ml glass ampoules

6.6 Instructions for use and handling

Bronchodilation: the recommended diluent is 5% dextrose, saline or dextrose/saline.

In the management of premature labour, the recommended infusion fluid is 5% dextrose. Saline should be avoided due to the risk of pulmonary oedema. If saline is used, the patient should be carefully monitored.

7. MARKETING AUTHORISATION HOLDER

AstraZeneca UK Ltd.,

600 Capability Green,

Luton, LU1 3LU, UK.

8. MARKETING AUTHORISATION NUMBER(S)

PL 17901/0112

9. DATE OF FIRST AUTHORISATION/RENEWAL OF THE AUTHORISATION

7th May 2002

10. DATE OF REVISION OF THE TEXT

23rd April 2004

Bricanyl Respirator Solution, 10 mg/ml, nebuliser solution.

(AstraZeneca UK Limited)

1. NAME OF THE MEDICINAL PRODUCT

Bricanyl® Respirator Solution, 10 mg/ml, nebuliser solution.

2. QUALITATIVE AND QUANTITATIVE COMPOSITION

Terbutaline sulphate 10 mg/ml.

For excipients see Section 6.1.

3. PHARMACEUTICAL FORM

Nebuliser solution.

4. CLINICAL PARTICULARS

4.1 Therapeutic indications

Terbutaline is a selective β_2-adrenergic agonist recommended for the relief of severe bronchospasm in bronchial asthma and in chronic bronchitis and other bronchopulmonary disorders in which bronchospasm is a complicating factor.

4.2 Posology and method of administration

In most patients the use of terbutaline sulphate, based on the doses below, given 2 - 4 times daily will be sufficient to relieve bronchospasm. In acute severe asthma, additional doses may be necessary.

Adults: 0.5 to 1 ml (5 to 10 mg) diluted to required nebuliser volume with sterile physiological saline.

Elderly: Dosage as for adults.

Children: 0.2 to 0.5 ml (2 to 5 mg), see table, diluted to required nebuliser volume with sterile physiological saline.

Table illustrating ml undiluted solution required for administration to children

(see Table 1)

Chronic Usage: If Bricanyl Respirator Solution is to be used in a continuous ventilation system, a suitable dosage is 1 - 2 mg/hour at a dilution of 100 mcg/ml (1:100 dilution) for adults, with a pro rata reduction in dosage for children.

Bricanyl Respirator Solution must be used with a nebuliser. The mist produced is then inhaled through the mouthpiece of the mask.

To take your medicine, follow these steps:

1. Remove the screw cap from the Bricanyl Respirator Solution bottle and replace it with the graduated dropper, which is included in the pack.
2. Empty the prescribed volume of Bricanyl Respirator Solution into the nebuliser cup.
3. Next, dilute your Bricanyl Respirator Solution to the required nebuliser volume using sterile physiological saline. Your doctor may prescribe another drug to be used for the dilution instead of the sterile physiological saline, if so follow your doctor's instructions. Replace the nebuliser top on the nebuliser cup.
4. Connect one end of the cup to the mask or mouthpiece and the other end to the air pump, which should be connected to the compressor unit.
5. Start to nebulise. During nebulising, breathe in the mist of nebulised medicine calmly and deeply.
6. The length of nebulisation time will vary with the type of medicine or nebuliser you use, but, when no mist comes out of the mouthpiece or nebuliser, your treatment is completed.
7. You must wash the nebuliser cup and mouthpiece (or face mask) in warm soapy water and rinse well after each use. Then dry these parts by connecting up to the air outlet or compressor and blow air through them.

4.3 Contraindications

Bricanyl preparations are contraindicated in patients with a history of hypersensitivity to any of their constituents.

4.4 Special warnings and special precautions for use

Patients should be instructed in proper use and their inhalation technique checked regularly. (*See Section 4. 2, Posology and Method of Administration.*)

Care should be taken with patients suffering from myocardial insufficiency or thyrotoxicosis.

Due to the hyperglycaemic effects of β_2-stimulants, additional blood glucose measurements are initially recommended when Bricanyl therapy is commenced in diabetic patients.

If a previously effective dosage regimen no longer gives the same symptomatic relief, the patient should urgently seek further medical advice. Consideration should be given to the requirements for additional therapy (including increased dosages of anti-inflammatory medication). Severe exacerbations of asthma should be treated as an emergency in the usual manner.

Potentially serious hypokalaemia may result from β_2-agonist therapy, mainly with parenteral or nebulised administration. Particular caution is advised in acute severe asthma as this effect may be augmented by hypoxia. The hypokalaemic effect may be potentiated by concomitant treatment with xanthine derivatives, corticosteroids and/or diuretics. It is recommended that serum potassium levels are monitored in such situations.

Due to the positive inotropic effect of the β_2-agonists, these drugs should not be used in patients with hypertrophic cardiomyopathy.

4.5 Interaction with other medicinal products and other forms of Interaction

Beta blocking agents (including eye drops), especially the non-selective ones such as propranolol, may partially or totally inhibit the effect of β-stimulants. Therefore, Bricanyl preparations and non-selective β-blockers should not normally be administered concurrently. Bricanyl should be used with caution in patients receiving other sympathomimetics.

Hypokalaemia may result from β_2-agonist therapy and may be potentiated by concomitant treatment with xanthine derivatives, corticosteroids and diuretics (*see Section 4.4, Special Warnings and Precautions for use*).

4.6 Pregnancy and lactation

Although no teratogenic effects have been observed in animals or in patients, Bricanyl should only be administered with caution during the first trimester of pregnancy.

Terbutaline is secreted via breast milk but any effect on the infant is unlikely at therapeutic doses.

4.7 Effects on ability to drive and use machines

Bricanyl does not affect the ability to drive or use machines.

4.8 Undesirable effects

The frequency of side-effects is low. Side effects which have been recorded, such as tremor, headache, nausea, tonic cramp, mouth and throat irritation and palpitations, are all characteristic of sympathomimetic amines. A few patients feel tense; this is also due to effects on skeletal muscle and not to direct CNS stimulation. Whenever these side-effects have occurred, the majority have usually been spontaneously reversible within the first week of treatment. As with other β_2-agonists, tremor is dose related.

Sleep disturbances and behavioural disturbances, such as agitation, hyperactivity and restlessness, have been observed.

Tachycardia, with or without peripheral vasodilation, has been rarely reported during β_2-agonist therapy. Cardiac arrhythmias, including atrial fibrillation, supraventricular tachycardia and extrasystoles, have been reported in association with β_2-agonists, usually in susceptible patients.

Potentially serious hypokalaemia may result from β_2-agonist therapy. (See also *Section 4.4, Special Warnings and Precautions for use.*)

In rare cases, through unspecified mechanisms, paradoxical bronchospasm may occur, with wheezing immediately after inhalation. This should be immediately treated with a rapid-onset bronchodilator. Bricanyl therapy should be discontinued and, after assessment, an alternative therapy initiated.

Hypersensitivity reactions, including angioedema, urticaria, exanthema, bronchospasm, hypotension and collapse, have been very rarely reported with β_2-agonist therapy.

4.9 Overdose

i) Possible symptoms and signs

Headache, anxiety, tremor, nausea, tonic cramp, palpitations, tachycardia and arrhythmia. A fall in blood pressure sometimes occurs. Laboratory findings: Hypokalaemia, hyperglycaemia and metabolic acidosis sometimes occur.

ii) Treatment

Mild and moderate cases: Reduce the dose.

Severe cases: Gastric lavage, administration of activated charcoal (where suspected that significant amounts have been swallowed). Determination of acid-base balance, blood sugar and electrolytes, particularly serum potassium levels. Monitoring of heart rate and rhythm and blood pressure. Metabolic changes should be corrected. A cardioselective β-blocker (e.g. metoprolol) is recommended for the treatment of arrhythmias causing haemodynamic deterioration. The β-blocker should be used with care because of the possibility of inducing bronchoconstriction: use with caution in patients with a history of bronchospasm. If the β-mediated reduction in peripheral vascular resistance significantly contributes to the fall in blood pressure, a volume expander should be given.

5. PHARMACOLOGICAL PROPERTIES

5.1 Pharmacodynamic properties

Pharmaco-therapeutic group: selective β_2-agonist, terbutaline, ATC code: R03A C03.

Terbutaline is a selective β_2-adrenergic stimulant having the following pharmacological effects:

i) In the lung - bronchodilation, increase in mucociliary clearance, suppression of oedema and anti-allergic effects.

Table 1 Table illustrating ml undiluted solution required for administration to children

AGE	AVERAGE WEIGHT kg	lb	mg terbutaline	ml undiluted solution	drops undiluted solution
<3	10	22	2.0	0.2	6
3	15	33	3.0	0.3	8
6	20	44	4.0	0.4	11
8+	25+	55+	5.0	0.5	use mark on the dropper

ii) In skeletal muscle - stimulates Na^+/K^+ transport and also causes depression of subtetanic contractions in slow-contracting muscle.

iii) In uterine muscle - inhibition of uterine contractions.

iv) In the C.N.S. - low penetration into the blood-brain barrier at therapeutic doses, due to the highly hydrophilic nature of the molecule.

v) In the C.V.S. - administration of terbutaline results in cardiovascular effects mediated through β_2-receptors in the peripheral arteries and in the heart e.g. in healthy subjects, 0.25 - 0.5 mg injected s.c. is associated with an increase in cardiac output (up to 85% over controls) due to an increase in heart rate and a larger stroke volume. The increase in heart rate is probably due to a combination of a reflex tachycardia via a fall in peripheral resistance and a direct positive chronotropic effect of the drug.

5.2 Pharmacokinetic properties
Basic parameters have been evaluated in man after i.v. and oral administration of therapeutic doses, e.g.

I.V. single dose
Volume distribution (VSS) - 114 L.
Total body clearance (CL) - 213 ml/min.
Mean residence time (MRT) - 9.0 h.
Renal clearance (CLR) - 149 ml/min (males)

Oral dose
Renal clearance (CLR) - 1.925 ml/min (males)
Renal clearance (CLR - 2.32 ml/min (females)

The plasma concentration/time curve after i.v. administration is characterised by a fast distribution phase, an intermediate elimination phase and a late elimination phase. Terminal half-life life ($t_{½}$) has been determined after single and multiple dosing (mean values varied between 16 - 20 h).

Bioavailability
Food reduces bioavailability following oral dosing (10% on average) fasting values of 14 - 15% have been obtained.

Metabolism
The main metabolite after oral dosing is the sulphate conjugate and also some glucuronide conjugate can be found in the urine.

5.3 Preclinical safety data
The major toxic effect of terbutaline, observed in toxicological studies in rats and dogs at exposures in excess of maximum human exposure, is focal myocardial necrosis. This type of cardiotoxicity is a well known pharmacological manifestation seen after the administration of high doses of β_2-agonists.

In rats, an increase in the incidence of benign uterine leiomyomas has been observed. This effect is looked upon as a class-effect observed in rodents after long term exposure to high doses of β_2-agonists

6. PHARMACEUTICAL PARTICULARS

6.1 List of excipients
Sodium chloride, chlorobutanol hemihydrate, disodium edetate, hydrochloric acid and purified water.

6.2 Incompatibilities
None known.

6.3 Shelf life
3 years unopened.

The contents of the bottle should be used within 3 months of opening.

6.4 Special precautions for storage
Do not store above 25°C.

6.5 Nature and contents of container
20 ml amber, Type II (Ph.Eur.) glass bottles with a polypropylene screw cap.

A mounted plastic dropper is enclosed in the pack.

6.6 Instructions for use and handling
Bricanyl Respirator Solution in multidose bottles contains preservative and may be diluted before use with sterile physiological saline. Solution in nebulisers should be replaced daily. The pH of Bricanyl Respirator Solution is 2.5 - 3.5.

7. MARKETING AUTHORISATION HOLDER
AstraZeneca UK Ltd.,
600 Capability Green,
Luton, LU1 3LU, UK.

8. MARKETING AUTHORISATION NUMBER(S)
PL 17901/0113

9. DATE OF FIRST AUTHORISATION/RENEWAL OF THE AUTHORISATION
28th May 2002

10. DATE OF REVISION OF THE TEXT
23rd April 2004

Bricanyl Respules

(AstraZeneca UK Limited)

1. NAME OF THE MEDICINAL PRODUCT
Bricanyl® Respules®

2. QUALITATIVE AND QUANTITATIVE COMPOSITION
Terbutaline sulphate 2.5mg/ml.

Each single dose respule contains 2ml (5mg).

For excipients see Section 6.1.

3. PHARMACEUTICAL FORM
Nebuliser Solution.

A clear, aqueous, isotonic solution.

4. CLINICAL PARTICULARS

4.1 Therapeutic indications
Terbutaline is a selective β_2-adrenergic agonist recommended for the relief of severe bronchospasm in bronchial asthma and in chronic bronchitis and other bronchopulmonary disorders in which bronchospasm is a complicating factor.

4.2 Posology and method of administration
In most patients, the use of terbutaline sulphate, based on the doses below, given 2-4 times daily will be sufficient to relieve bronchospasm. In acute, severe asthma, additional doses may be necessary.

Bricanyl Respules:
Adults: 1 or 2 Respules (5 or 10mg)
Children: (>25kg) 1 Respule (5mg)
Children: (<25kg) use multidose bottles.

Multidose Bottles:
Adults: 0.5 to 1 ml (5 to 10mg) diluted to required nebuliser volume with sterile physiological saline.

Children: 0.2 to 0.5ml (2 to 5mg), see table, diluted to required nebuliser volume with sterile physiological saline.

Table illustrating ml undiluted solution from multidose bottle required for administration to children

Age	Average kg	weight lb	mg terbutaline	ml undiluted solution
<3	10	22	2.0	0.2
3	15	33	3.0	0.3
6	20	44	4.0	0.4
8+	25+	55+	5.0	0.5

Elderly: Dosage as for adults.

Instructions for use and cleaning are provided in the Patient Information Leaflet which can be found in each pack.

4.3 Contraindications
Bricanyl preparations are contra-indicated in patients with a history of hypersensitivity to any of their constituents.

4.4 Special warnings and special precautions for use
Patients should be instructed in proper use and their inhalation technique checked regularly.

Care should be taken with patients suffering from myocardial insufficiency or thyrotoxicosis.

Due to the hyperglycaemic effects of β_2-stimulants, additional blood glucose measurements are initially recommended when Bricanyl therapy is commenced in diabetic patients.

If a previously effective dosage regimen no longer gives the same symptomatic relief, the patient should urgently seek further medical advice. Consideration should be given to the requirements for additional therapy (including increased dosages of anti-inflammatory medication). Severe exacerbations of asthma should be treated as an emergency in the usual manner.

Potentially serious hypokalaemia may result from β_2-agonist therapy, mainly with parenteral or nebulised administration. Particular caution is advised in acute severe asthma as this effect may be augmented by hypoxia. The hypokalaemic effect may be potentiated by concomitant treatment with xanthine derivatives, corticosteroids and/or diuretics. It is recommended that serum potassium levels are monitored in such situations.

Due to the positive inotropic effect of the β_2-agonists, these drugs should not be used in patients with hypertrophic cardiomyopathy.

4.5 Interaction with other medicinal products and other forms of Interaction
Beta-blocking agents (including eye drops), especially the non-selective ones such as propranolol, may partially or totally inhibit the effect of β-stimulants. Therefore, Bricanyl preparations and non-selective β-blockers should not normally be administered concurrently. Bricanyl should be used with caution in patients receiving other sympathomimetics.

Hypokalaemia may result from β_2-agonist therapy and may be potentiated by concomitant treatment with xanthine derivatives, corticosteroids and diuretics (*see Section 4.4, Special Warnings and Precautions for use*).

4.6 Pregnancy and lactation
Although no teratogenic effects have been observed in animals or in patients, Bricanyl should only be administered with caution during the first trimester of pregnancy.

Terbutaline is secreted via breast milk, but effect on the infant is unlikely at therapeutic doses.

4.7 Effects on ability to drive and use machines
None Known

4.8 Undesirable effects
The frequency of side-effects is low. Side effects which have been recorded, such as tremor, headache, nausea, tonic cramp, mouth and throat irritation and palpitations, are all characteristic of sympathomimetic amines. A few patients feel tense; this is also due to effects on skeletal muscle and not to direct CNS stimulation. Whenever these side-effects have occurred, the majority have usually been spontaneously reversible within the first week of treatment. As with other β_2-agonists, tremor is dose related.

Sleep disturbances and behavioural disturbances, such as agitation, hyperactivity and restlessness, have been observed.

Tachycardia, with or without peripheral vasodilation, has been rarely reported during β_2-agonist therapy. Cardiac arrhythmias, including atrial fibrillation, supraventricular tacycardia and extrasystoles, have been reported in association with β_2-agonists, usually in susceptible patients.

Potentially serious hypokalaemia may result from β_2-agonist therapy. (See also *Section 4.4, Special Warnings and Precautions for use.*)

In rare cases, through unspecified mechanisms, paradoxical bronchospasm may occur, with wheezing immediately after inhalation. This should be immediately treated with a rapid onset bronchodilator. Bricanyl therapy should be discontinued and, after assessment, an alternative therapy initiated.

Hypersensitivity reactions, including angioedema, urticaria, exanthema, bronchospasm, hypotension and collapse, have been very rarely reported with β_2-agonist therapy.

4.9 Overdose
i) Possible symptoms and signs
Headache, anxiety, tremor, nausea, tonic cramp, palpitations, tachycardia and arrhythmia. A fall in blood pressure sometimes occurs. Laboratory findings; hypokalaemia, hyperglycaemia and metabolic acidosis sometimes occur.

ii) Treatment
Mild and moderate cases: Reduce the dose.

Severe cases: Gastric lavage, administration of activated charcoal, (where suspected that significant amounts have been swallowed). Determination of acid-base balance, blood sugar and electrolytes, particularly serum potassium levels. Monitoring of heart rate and rhythm and blood pressure. Metabolic changes should be corrected. A cardioselective β-blocker (e.g. metoprolol) is recommended for the treatment of arrhythmias causing haemodynamic deterioration. The β-blocker should be used with care because of the possibility of inducing bronchoconstriction: use with caution in patients with a history of bronchospasm. If the β-mediated reduction in peripheral vascular resistance significantly contributes to the fall in blood pressure, a volume expander should be given.

5. PHARMACOLOGICAL PROPERTIES

5.1 Pharmacodynamic properties
Pharmaco-therapeutic group: selective β_2-agonist, terbutaline, ATC code: R03A C03.

Terbutaline is a selective β_2-adrenergic stimulant, having the following pharmacological effects:-

i) In the lung: bronchodilation; increase in mucociliary clearance; suppression of oedema and anti-allergic effects.

ii) In skeletal muscle: stimulates Na^+/K^+ transport and also causes depression of subtetanic contractions in slow-contracting muscle.

iii) In uterine muscle: Inhibition of uterine contractions.

iv) In the C.N.S: Low penetration into the blood-brain barrier at therapeutic doses, due to the highly hydrophilic nature of the molecule.

v) In the C.V.S.: Administration of terbutaline results in cardiovascular effects mediated through β_2-receptors in the peripheral arteries and in the heart e.g. in healthy subjects, 0.25 - 0.5 mg injected s.c., is associated with an increase in cardiac output (up to 85% over controls) due to an increase in heart rate and a larger stroke volume. The increase in heart rate is probably due to a combination of a reflex tachycardia, via a fall in peripheral resistance, and a direct positive chronotropic effect of the drug.

5.2 Pharmacokinetic properties
Basic parameters have been evaluated in man after i.v. and oral administration of therapeutic doses, e.g.

I.V. single dose
Volume distribution (VSS) - 114L
Total body clearance (CL) - 213 ml/min.
Mean residence time (MRT) - 9.0 h.
Renal clearance (CLR) - 149 ml/min.(males)

Oral dose
Renal clearance (CLR) - 1.925 ml/min. (males)
Renal clearance (CLR) - 2.32 ml/min. (females)

The plasma concentration/time curve after i.v. administration is characterised by a fast distribution phase, an intermediate elimination phase and a late elimination phase.

Terminal half-life $t_{1/2}$ has been determined after single and multiple dosing (mean values varied between 16-20 h.).

Bioavailability

Food reduces bioavailability following oral dosing (10% on average) fasting values of 14-15% have been obtained.

Metabolism

The main metabolite after oral dosing is the sulphate conjugate and also some glucoronide conjugate can be found in the urine.

5.3 Preclinical safety data

The major toxic effect of terbutaline, observed in toxicological studies in rats and dogs at exposures in excess of maximum human exposure, is focal myocardial necrosis. This type of cardiotoxicity is a well known pharmacological manifestation seen after the administration of high doses of β_2-agonists.

In rats, an increase in the incidence of benign uterine leiomyomas has been observed. This effect is looked upon as a class-effect observed in rodents after long term exposure to high doses of β_2-agonists

6. PHARMACEUTICAL PARTICULARS

6.1 List of excipients

Sodium chloride, disodium edetate, hydrochloric acid, water for injections.

6.2 Incompatibilities

None known.

6.3 Shelf life

36 months

Single dose units in an opened foil envelope should be used within 3 months.

6.4 Special precautions for storage

Do not store above 30°C.

Store in the original container.

6.5 Nature and contents of container

Single dose, plastic units (Respules) in cartons of 20 Respules, as 4 strips of 5 units, each wrapped in a foil envelope.

6.6 Instructions for use and handling

Bricanyl Respules will not normally require dilution at recommended doses. The pH of Bricanyl Respules is 3-4.5.

If dilution is required use sterile normal saline.

7. MARKETING AUTHORISATION HOLDER

AstraZeneca UK Limited

600 Capability Green

Luton

LU1 3LU

United Kingdom

8. MARKETING AUTHORISATION NUMBER(S)

PL 17901/0114

9. DATE OF FIRST AUTHORISATION/RENEWAL OF THE AUTHORISATION

7th May 2002

10. DATE OF REVISION OF THE TEXT

23rd April 2004

Bricanyl SA, 7.5mg, Tablet

(AstraZeneca UK Limited)

1. NAME OF THE MEDICINAL PRODUCT

Bricanyl® SA, 7.5mg, Tablet

2. QUALITATIVE AND QUANTITATIVE COMPOSITION

Each tablet contains 7.5mg of terbutaline sulphate.

For excipients see Section 6.1.

3. PHARMACEUTICAL FORM

Prolonged-release tablet.

Off white, circular, biconvex tablet, engraved B^A^D on one side.

4. CLINICAL PARTICULARS

4.1 Therapeutic indications

Terbutaline is a selective β_2-adrenergic agonist recommended for relief and prevention of bronchospasm in bronchial asthma and in chronic bronchitis and other bronchopulmonary disorders in which bronchospasm is a complicating factor.

4.2 Posology and method of administration

Adults: 1 tablet morning and evening.

Elderly: Dosage as for adults.

The tablet may not be divided or chewed, but must be swallowed whole together with liquid.

The inactive components in Bricanyl SA form a matrix which is insoluble in the digestive juices. The empty matrix may sometimes pass through the digestive system unchanged and be excreted.

4.3 Contraindications

Bricanyl oral preparations are contraindicated in patients with a history of hypersensitivity to any of their constituents.

4.4 Special warnings and special precautions for use

Care should be taken with patients suffering from myocardial insufficiency or thyrotoxicosis.

Due to the hyperglycaemic effects of β_2-stimulants, additional blood glucose measurements are initially recommended when Bricanyl therapy is commenced in diabetic patients.

If a previously effective dosage regimen no longer gives the same symptomatic relief, the patient should urgently seek further medical advice. Consideration should be given to the requirements for additional therapy (including increased dosages of anti-inflammatory medication). Severe exacerbations of asthma should be treated as an emergency in the usual manner.

Potentially serious hypokalaemia may result from β_2-agonist therapy, mainly with parenteral or nebulised administration. Particular caution is advised in acute severe asthma as this effect may be augmented by hypoxia. The hypokalaemic effect may be potentiated by concomitant treatment with xanthine derivatives, corticosteroids and/or diuretics. It is recommended that serum potassium levels are monitored in such situations.

Due to the positive inotropic effect of β_2-agonists, these drugs should not be used in patients with hypertrophic cardiomyopathy.

4.5 Interaction with other medicinal products and other forms of Interaction

Beta-blocking agents (including eye drops), especially the non-selective ones such as propranolol, may partially or totally inhibit the effect of β-stimulants. Therefore, Bricanyl preparations and non-selective β-blockers should not normally be administered concurrently. Bricanyl should be used with caution in patients receiving other sympathomimetics.

Hypokalaemia may result from β_2-agonist therapy and may be potentiated by concomitant treatment with xanthine derivatives, corticosteroids and diuretics (*see Section 4.4, Special Warnings and Precautions for use*).

4.6 Pregnancy and lactation

Although no teratogenic effects have been observed in animals or in patients, terbutaline should only be administered with caution during the first trimester of pregnancy.

Terbutaline is secreted via breast milk, but any effect on the infant is unlikely at therapeutic doses.

Transient hypoglycaemia has been reported in newborn preterm infants after maternal β_2-agonist treatment.

4.7 Effects on ability to drive and use machines

Bricanyl does not affect the ability to drive or use machines.

4.8 Undesirable effects

The frequency of side-effects is low at the recommended doses. Side effects which have been recorded, such as tremor, headache, nausea, tonic cramp, mouth and throat irritation and palpitations, are all characteristic of sympathomimetic amines. A few patients feel tense; this is also due to effects on skeletal muscle and not to direct CNS stimulation. Whenever these side-effects have occurred, the majority have usually been spontaneously reversible within the first week of treatment. As with other β_2-agonists, tremor is dose related.

Sleep disturbances and behavioural disturbances, such as agitation, hyperactivity and restlessness, have been observed.

Tachycardia, with or without peripheral vasodilation, has been rarely reported during β_2-agonist therapy. Cardiac arrhythmias, including atrial fibrillation, supraventricular tachycardia and extrasystoles, have been reported in association with β_2-agonists, usually in susceptible patients.

Potentially serious hypokalaemia may result from β_2-agonist therapy. (See also *Section 4.4, Special Warnings and Precautions for use.*)

In rare cases, through unspecified mechanisms, paradoxical bronchospasm may occur, with wheezing immediately after inhalation. This should be immediately treated with a rapid-onset bronchodilator. Bricanyl therapy should be discontinued and, after assessment, an alternative therapy initiated.

Hypersensitivity reactions, including angioedema, urticaria, exanthema, bronchospasm, hypotension and collapse, have been very rarely reported with β_2-agonist therapy.

4.9 Overdose

Possible symptoms and signs: Headache, anxiety, tremor, nausea, tonic cramp, palpitations, tachycardia, arrhythmia. A fall in blood pressure sometimes occurs. Laboratory findings: hypokalaemia, hyperglycaemia and lactic acidosis sometimes occur.

Treatment:

a) Mild and moderate cases: Reduce the dose.

b) Severe cases: Gastric lavage, activated charcoal. Determination of acid-base balance, blood sugar and electrolytes, particularly serum potassium levels. Monitoring of heart rate and rhythm and blood pressure. Metabolic changes should be corrected. A cardioselective β-blocker (e.g. metoprolol) is recommended for the treatment of arrhythmias causing haemodynamic deterioration. The β-blocker should be used with care because of the possibility of inducing bronchoconstriction: use with caution in patients with a history of bronchospasm. If the β_2-mediated reduction in peripheral vascular resistance significantly contributes to the fall in blood pressure, a volume expander should be given.

5. PHARMACOLOGICAL PROPERTIES

5.1 Pharmacodynamic properties

Pharmaco-therapeutic group: selective β_2-agonist, terbutaline, ATC code: R03C C03.

Terbutaline is a selective β_2-adrenoceptor agonist.

5.2 Pharmacokinetic properties

In man, terbutaline and its metabolites are excreted predominantly in the urine.

In fasting subjects, 30 - 70% of an oral dose of terbutaline is absorbed. Bioavailability of terbutaline after oral administration is much lower than the amount absorbed, due to the first pass effect. Bioavailability of sustained release tablets is increased after fasting. Studies in healthy volunteers given repeat dose Bricanyl SA, 7.5mg to attain steady state show:

a) Peak plasma concentration reached in 4 - 8 hours.

b) Mean plasma concentration at steady state is 2.7mg/ml.

c) Single dose renal clearance - 63% (NB. Does not change at steady state).

5.3 Preclinical safety data

The major toxic effect of terbutaline, observed in toxicological studies in rats and dogs at exposures in excess of maximum human exposure, is focal myocardial necrosis. This type of cardiotoxicity is a well known pharmacological manifestation seen after the administration of high doses of β_2-agonists.

In rats, an increase in the incidence of benign uterine leiomyomas has been observed. This effect is looked upon as a class-effect observed in rodents after long term exposure to high doses of β_2-agonists

6. PHARMACEUTICAL PARTICULARS

6.1 List of excipients

Polyvinyl chloride, colloidal anhydrous silica, tartaric acid, ethyl cellulose and stearyl alcohol.

6.2 Incompatibilities

Not applicable

6.3 Shelf life

3 years.

6.4 Special precautions for storage

None

6.5 Nature and contents of container

Brown glass bottles containing 60 tablets.

6.6 Instructions for use and handling

None.

7. MARKETING AUTHORISATION HOLDER

AstraZeneca UK Ltd.,

600 Capability Green,

Luton, LU1 3LU, UK.

8. MARKETING AUTHORISATION NUMBER(S)

PL 17901/0115

9. DATE OF FIRST AUTHORISATION/RENEWAL OF THE AUTHORISATION

28th May 2002

10. DATE OF REVISION OF THE TEXT

23rd April 2004

Bricanyl Syrup

(AstraZeneca UK Limited)

1. NAME OF THE MEDICINAL PRODUCT

Bricanyl Syrup

2. QUALITATIVE AND QUANTITATIVE COMPOSITION

Terbutaline sulphate 0.3mg/ml.

For excipients see Section 6.1.

3. PHARMACEUTICAL FORM

Oral Solution.

Bricanyl syrup is a clear colourless raspberry flavoured oral solution.

4. CLINICAL PARTICULARS

4.1 Therapeutic indications

For bronchodilation

Terbutaline is a selective β_2-adrenergic agonist recommended for the relief and prevention of bronchospasm in bronchial asthma and other bronchopulmonary disorders in which bronchospasm is a complicating factor.

For the management of uncomplicated premature labour.

4.2 Posology and method of administration

Use in bronchospasm

Bricanyl Syrup has a duration of action of 7 to 8 hours. The minimum recommended dosage interval is therefore 7 hours.

Adults: The starting dose should be 2 × 5ml spoonfuls 3 times in 24 hours. The dose may then be increased to 3 × 5ml spoonfuls 3 times in 24 hours if necessary to achieve adequate bronchodilation.

Elderly: Dosage as for Adults.

Children:

The following dosage is recommended - 0.075mg (0.25ml)/kg body weight 3 times in a 24 hour period.

e.g.

Body weight (Kg)	Dosage
14	3.5 ml × 3
16	4 ml × 3
18	4.5 ml × 3
20	5 ml × 3
24	6 ml × 3
28	7 ml × 3
32	8 ml × 3
36	9 ml × 3
40	10 ml × 3

Use in the management of premature labour.

Oral treatment should not be used initially in an attempt to arrest premature labour. After uterine contractions have been controlled by intravenous infusion of Bricanyl Injection, (see Bricanyl Injection Summary of Product Characteristics) or subcutaneous injections (0.25mg, 4 times in a 24 hour period for a few days) maintenance therapy can be continued with oral treatment (5mg, 3 times in a 24 hour period). Oral treatment may be continued for as long as the physician considers it desirable to prolong pregnancy.

4.3 Contraindications

Bricanyl oral preparations are contra-indicated in patients with a history of hypersensitivity to any of their constituents.

Although Bricanyl Injection and oral preparations are used in the management of uncomplicated premature labour, their use in the following conditions is contra-indicated: - any condition of the mother or foetus in which prolongation of the pregnancy is hazardous, e.g. severe toxaemia, antipartum haemorrhage, intra-uterine infection, abruptio placentae, threatened abortion during the 1st and 2nd trimester, or cord compression.

4.4 Special warnings and special precautions for use

Care should be taken with patients suffering from myocardial insufficiency or thyrotoxicosis.

Due to the hyperglycaemic effects of β_2-stimulants, additional blood glucose measurements are initially recommended when Bricanyl therapy is commenced in diabetic patients.

If a previously effective dosage regimen no longer gives the same symptomatic relief, the patient should urgently seek further medical advice. Consideration should be given to the requirements for additional therapy (including increased dosages of anti-inflammatory medication). Severe exacerbations of asthma should be treated as an emergency in the usual manner.

Potentially serious hypokalaemia may result from β_2-agonist therapy, mainly with parenteral or nebulised administration. Particular caution is advised in acute severe asthma as this effect may be augmented by hypoxia. The hypokalaemic effect may be potentiated by concomitant treatment with xanthine derivatives, corticosteroids and/or diuretics. It is recommended that serum potassium levels are monitored in such situations.

Due to the positive inotropic effect of β_2-agonists, these drugs should not be used in patients with hypertrophic cardiomyopathy.

During infusion treatment in pregnant women with β_2-stimulants in combination with corticosteroids a rare complication with a pathological picture resembling pulmonary oedema, has been reported.

Increased tendency to uterine bleeding has been reported in connection with Caesarean section. However, this can be effectively stopped by propranolol 1-2mg injected intravenously.

4.5 Interaction with other medicinal products and other forms of Interaction

Beta-blocking agents (including eye drops), especially the non-selective ones such as propranolol, may partially or totally inhibit the effect of β-stimulants. Therefore Bricanyl preparations and non-selective β-blockers should not normally be administered concurrently. Bricanyl should be used with caution in patients receiving other sympathomimetics.

Hypokalaemia may result from β_2-agonist therapy and may be potentiated by concomitant treatment with xanthine derivatives, corticosteroids and diuretics (*see Section 4.4, Special Warnings and Precautions for use*).

4.6 Pregnancy and lactation

Although no teratogenic effects have been observed in animals or in patients, Bricanyl should only be administered with caution during the first trimester of pregnancy.

Terbutaline is secreted in breast milk, but effect on the infant is unlikely at therapeutic doses.

Transient hypoglycaemia has been reported in newborn preterm infants after maternal β_2-agonist treatment.

4.7 Effects on ability to drive and use machines

None Known.

4.8 Undesirable effects

The frequency of side-effects is low at the recommended doses. Side-effects which have been recorded such as tremor, headache, nausea, mouth and throat irritation, tonic cramp, and palpitations are all characteristic of sympathomimetic amines. A few patients feel tense; this is also due to the effects on skeletal muscle and not to direct CNS stimulation. Whenever these side-effects have occurred, the majority have usually been spontaneously reversible within the first week of treatment. As with other β_2-agonists, tremor is dose related.

Sleep disturbances and behavioural disturbances, such as agitation, hyperactivity and restlessness, have been observed.

Tachycardia, with or without peripheral vasodilation, has been rarely reported during β_2-agonist therapy. Cardiac arrhythmias, including atrial fibrillation, supraventricular tachycardia and extrasystoles, have been reported in association with β_2-agonists, usually in susceptible patients.

Potentially serious hypokalaemia may result from β_2-agonist therapy.

(See also *Section 4.4, Special Warnings and Precautions for use.*)

In rare cases, through unspecified mechanisms, paradoxical bronchospasm may occur, with wheezing immediately after inhalation. This should be immediately treated with a rapid-onset bronchodilator. Bricanyl therapy should be discontinued and, after assessment, an alternative therapy initiated.

Hypersensitivity reactions, including angioedema, urticaria, exanthema, bronchospasm, hypotension and collapse, have been very rarely reported with β_2-agonist therapy.

4.9 Overdose

Possible symptoms and signs

Headache, anxiety, tremor, nausea, tonic cramp, palpitations, tachycardia, arrhythmia. A fall in blood pressure sometimes occurs.

Laboratory findings; hypokalaemia, hyperglycaemia and lactic acidosis sometimes occur.

Treatment

Mild and moderate cases: Reduce the dose.

Severe cases: Gastric lavage, administration of activated charcoal. Determination of acid-base balance, blood sugar and electrolytes, particularly serum potassium levels. Monitoring of the heart rate and rhythm and blood pressure. Metabolic changes should be corrected.

A cardioselective β-blocker (e.g. metoprolol) is recommended for the treatment of arrhythmias causing haemodynamic deterioration. The β-blocker should be used with care because of the possibility of inducing bronchoconstriction: use with caution in patients with a history of bronchospasm. If the β_2-mediated reduction in the peripheral vascular resistance significantly contributes to the fall in blood pressure, a volume expander should be given.

Preterm labour: Pulmonary oedema: discontinue administration of Bricanyl. A normal dose of loop diuretic (e.g. frusemide) should be given intravenously.

Increased bleeding in connection with Caesarian section: propranolol, 1-2mg intravenously.

5. PHARMACOLOGICAL PROPERTIES

5.1 Pharmacodynamic properties

Pharmaco-therapeutic group: selective β_2-agonist, terbutaline ATC code:R03C C03.

Terbutaline is a selective β_2 -adrenergic stimulant having the following pharmacological effects:-

i) *In the lung*: bronchodilation; increase in mucociliary clearance; suppression of oedema and anti-allergic effects.

ii) *In skeletal muscle*: stimulates Na^+/K^+transport and also causes depression of subtetanic contractions in slow-contracting muscle.

iii) *In uterine muscle*: inhibition of uterine contractions.

iv) *In the CNS*: low penetration into the blood-brain barrier at therapeutic doses, due to the highly hydrophilic nature of the molecule.

v) *In the CVS*: administration of terbutaline results in cardiovascular effects mediated through β_2 -receptors in the peripheral arteries and in the heart e.g. in healthy subjects, 0.25 - 0.5mg injected s.c., is associated with an increase in cardiac output (up to 85% over controls) due to an increase in heart rate and a larger stroke volume. The increase in heart rate is probably due to a combination of a reflex tachycardia via a fall in peripheral resistance and a direct positive chronotropic effect of the drug.

5.2 Pharmacokinetic properties

Basic parameters have been evaluated in man after i.v and oral administration of therapeutic doses, e.g.

i.v. single dose

Volume distribution (VSS): 114 L

Total body clearance (CL): 213 ml/min

Mean residence time (MRT): 9.0 h

Renal clearance (CLR): 149 ml/min (males)

Oral dose

renal clearance (CLR): 1.925/ml/min (males)

renal clearance (CLR): 2.32ml/min (females)

The plasma concentration/time curve after iv administration is characterised by a fast distribution phase, an intermediate elimination phase and a late elimination phase.

Terminal half-life T ½ has been determined after single and multiple dosing (mean values varied between 16-20 h)

Bioavailability

Food reduces bioavailability following oral dosing (10% on average).

Fasting values of 14-15% have been obtained.

Metabolism

The main metabolite after oral dosing is the sulphate conjugate and also some glucoronide conjugate can be found in the urine.

5.3 Preclinical safety data

The major toxic effect of terbutaline, observed in toxicological studies in rats and dogs at exposures in excess of maximum human exposure, is focal myocardial necrosis. This type of cardiotoxicity is a well known pharmacological manifestation seen after the administration of high doses of β_2-agonists.

In rats, an increase in the incidence of benign uterine leiomyomas has been observed. This effect is looked upon as a class-effect observed in rodents after long term exposure to high doses of β_2-agonists

6. PHARMACEUTICAL PARTICULARS

6.1 List of excipients

Citric Acid, disodium edetate, ethanol, glycerol, sodium hydroxide, sorbitol, sodium benzoate, flavour lemon lime-tte, flavour raspberry, water.

6.2 Incompatibilities

None known.

6.3 Shelf life

4 years.

6.4 Special precautions for storage

Do not store above 25°C.

6.5 Nature and contents of container

Bottles of 100ml, 300ml and 1 litre.

6.6 Instructions for use and handling

Not applicable.

7. MARKETING AUTHORISATION HOLDER

AstraZeneca UK Ltd

600 Capability Green

Luton

LU1 3LU

United Kingdom

8. MARKETING AUTHORISATION NUMBER(S)

PL17901/0111

9. DATE OF FIRST AUTHORISATION/RENEWAL OF THE AUTHORISATION

7 May 2002

10. DATE OF REVISION OF THE TEXT

4 January 2005

Bricanyl Tablets 5mg

(AstraZeneca UK Limited)

1. NAME OF THE MEDICINAL PRODUCT

Bricanyl® Tablets 5mg

2. QUALITATIVE AND QUANTITATIVE COMPOSITION

Each tablet contains 5mg terbutaline sulphate.

For excipients see Section 6.1.

3. PHARMACEUTICAL FORM

Tablet.

Off white, circular, biconvex tablet, engraved A/BT and scored on one side, symbol '5' on the reverse.

4. CLINICAL PARTICULARS

4.1 Therapeutic indications

For bronchodilation: Terbutaline is a selective β_2-adrenergic agonist recommended for the relief and prevention of bronchospasm in bronchial asthma and other bronchopulmonary disorders in which bronchospasm is a complicating factor.

For the management of uncomplicated premature labour.

4.2 Posology and method of administration

Use in bronchospasm: Bricanyl Tablets have a duration of action of 7 to 8 hours. The minimum recommended dosage interval is therefore 7 hours.

Adults: During the first 1 - 2 weeks, 2.5mg (half a tablet) 3 times in a 24-hour period is recommended. The dose may then be increased to 5mg (1 tablet) 3 times in a 24-hour period to achieve adequate bronchodilation.

Elderly: Dosage as for Adults.

Children 7 - 15 years: The starting dose should normally be 2.5mg (half a tablet) 2 times in 24 hours. However, in some patients, the dose may need to be increased to 2.5mg 3 times in 24 hours.

Use in the management of premature labour: Oral treatment should not be used initially in an attempt to arrest premature labour. After uterine contractions have been controlled by intravenous infusion of Bricanyl Injection, (see Bricanyl Injection Summary of Product Characteristics) or subcutaneous injections (0.25mg, 4 times in a 24-hour period for a few days) maintenance therapy can be continued with oral treatment (5mg, 3 times in a 24-hour period). Oral treatment may be continued for as long as the physician considers it desirable to prolong pregnancy.

4.3 Contraindications

Bricanyl oral preparations are contraindicated in patients with a history of hypersensitivity to any of their constituents.

Although Bricanyl Injection and oral preparations are used in the management of uncomplicated premature labour, their use in the following conditions is contraindicated: any condition of the mother or foetus in which prolongation of the pregnancy is hazardous, e.g. severe toxaemia, antepartum haemorrhage, intra-uterine infection, abruptio placentae, threatened abortion during the 1st and 2nd trimesters, or cord compression.

4.4 Special warnings and special precautions for use

Care should be taken with patients suffering from myocardial insufficiency or thyrotoxicosis.

Due to the hyperglycaemic effects of β_2-stimulants, additional blood glucose measurements are initially recommended when Bricanyl therapy is commenced in diabetic patients.

If a previously effective dosage regimen no longer gives the same symptomatic relief, the patient should urgently seek further medical advice. Consideration should be given to the requirements for additional therapy (including increased dosages of anti-inflammatory medication). Severe exacerbations of asthma should be treated as an emergency in the usual manner.

Potentially serious hypokalaemia may result from β_2-agonist therapy, mainly with parenteral or nebulised administration. Particular caution is advised in acute severe asthma as this effect may be augmented by hypoxia. The hypokalaemic effect may be potentiated by concomitant treatment with xanthine derivatives, corticosteroids and/or diuretics. It is recommended that serum potassium levels are monitored in such situations.

Due to the positive inotropic effect of β_2-agonists, these drugs should not be used in patients with hypertrophic cardiomyopathy.

During infusion treatment in pregnant women with β_2-stimulants in combination with corticosteroids, a rare complication with a pathological picture resembling pulmonary oedema has been reported.

Increased tendency to uterine bleeding has been reported in connection with Caesarean section. However, this can be effectively stopped by propranolol 1 - 2mg injected intravenously.

4.5 Interaction with other medicinal products and other forms of Interaction

Beta-blocking agents (including eye drops), especially the non selective ones such as propranolol, may partially or totally inhibit the effect of β-stimulants. Therefore, Bricanyl preparations and non-selective β-blockers should not normally be administered concurrently. Bricanyl should be used with caution in patients receiving other sympathomimetics.

Hypokalaemia may result from β_2-agonist therapy and may be potentiated by concomitant treatment with xanthine derivatives, corticosteroids and diuretics (*see Section 4.4, Special Warnings and Precautions for use*).

4.6 Pregnancy and lactation

Although no teratogenic effects have been observed in animals or in patients, Bricanyl should only be administered with caution during the first trimester of pregnancy.

Terbutaline is secreted into breast milk, but any effect on the infant is unlikely at therapeutic doses.

Transient hypoglycaemia has been reported in newborn preterm infants after maternal β_2-agonist treatment.

4.7 Effects on ability to drive and use machines

None

4.8 Undesirable effects

The frequency of side-effects is low at the recommended doses. Side-effects which have been recorded, such as tremor, headache, nausea, tonic cramp, mouth and throat irritation and palpitations, are all characteristic of sympathomimetic amines. A few patients feel tense; this is also due to effects on skeletal muscle and not to direct CNS stimulation. Whenever these side-effects have occurred, the majority have usually been spontaneously reversible within the first week of treatment. As with other β_2-agonists, tremor is dose related.

Sleep disturbances and behavioural disturbances, such as agitation, hyperactivity and restlessness, have been observed.

Tachycardia, with or without peripheral vasodilation, has been rarely reported during β_2-agonist therapy. Cardiac arrhythmias, including atrial fibrillation, supraventricular tachycardia and extrasystoles, have been reported in association with β_2-agonists, usually in susceptible patients.

Potentially serious hypokalaemia may result from β_2-agonist therapy. (See also *Section 4.4, Special Warnings and Precautions for use.*)

In rare cases, through unspecified mechanisms, paradoxical bronchospasm may occur, with wheezing immediately after inhalation. This should be immediately treated with a rapid-onset bronchodilator. Bricanyl therapy should be discontinued and, after assessment, an alternative therapy initiated.

Hypersensitivity reactions, including angioedema, urticaria, exanthema, bronchospasm, hypotension and collapse, have been very rarely reported with β_2-agonist therapy.

4.9 Overdose

Possible symptoms and signs: Headache, anxiety, tremor, nausea, tonic cramp, palpitations, tachycardia, arrhythmia. A fall in blood pressure sometimes occurs. Laboratory findings: hypokalaemia, hyperglycaemia and lactic acidosis sometimes occur.

Treatment:

Mild and moderate cases: Reduce the dose.

Severe cases: Gastric lavage, administration of activated charcoal. Determination of acid-base balance, blood sugar and electrolytes, particularly serum potassium levels. Monitoring of the heart rate and rhythm and blood pressure. Metabolic changes should be corrected. A cardioselective β-blocker (e.g. metoprolol) is recommended for the treatment of arrhythmias causing haemodynamic deterioration. The β-blocker should be used with care because of the possibility of inducing bronchoconstriction: use with caution in patients with a history of bronchospasm. If the β_2-mediated reduction in the peripheral vascular resistance significantly contributes to the fall in blood pressure, a volume expander should be given.

Preterm labour: Pulmonary oedema: discontinue administration of Bricanyl. A normal dose of loop diuretic (e.g. frusemide) should be given intravenously.

Increased bleeding in connection with Caesarian section: propranolol, 1 - 2mg intravenously.

5. PHARMACOLOGICAL PROPERTIES

5.1 Pharmacodynamic properties

Pharmaco-therapeutic group: selective β_2-agonist, terbutaline, ATC code: R03C C03.

Terbutaline is a selective β_2-adrenergic stimulant having the following pharmacological effects:-

i) In the lung - bronchodilation; increased mucociliary clearance; suppression of oedema and anti-allergic effects.

ii) In skeletal muscle - stimulates Na^+/K^+ transport and also causes depression of subtetanic contractions in slow-contracting muscle.

iii) In uterine muscle - inhibition of uterine contractions.

iv) In the CNS - low penetration of the blood-brain barrier at therapeutic doses, due to the highly hydrophilic nature of the molecule.

v) In the CVS - administration of terbutaline results in cardiovascular effects mediated through β_2-receptors in the peripheral arteries and in the heart e.g. in healthy subjects, 0.25 - 0.5mg injected s.c. is associated with an increase in cardiac output (up to 85% over controls) due to an increase in heart rate and a larger stroke volume. The increase in heart rate is probably due to a combination of a reflex tachycardia via a fall in peripheral resistance and a direct positive chronotropic effect of the drug.

5.2 Pharmacokinetic properties

Basic parameters have been evaluated in man after i.v and oral administration of therapeutic doses, e.g.

i.v single dose

Volume distribution (vss): 114 L

Total body clearance (cl): 213 ml/min

Mean residence time (mrt): 9.0 h

Renal clearance (clr): 149 ml/min (males)

Oral dose

Renal clearance (clr): 1.925 ml/min (males)

Renal clearance (clr): 2.32 ml/min (females)

The plasma concentration/time curve after iv administration is characterised by a fast distribution phase, an intermediate elimination phase and a late elimination phase. Terminal half-life ($t_{½}$) has been determined after single and multiple dosing (mean values varied between 16 - 20 h).

Bioavailability

Food reduces bioavailability following oral dosing (10% on average).

Fasting values of 14 - 15% have been obtained.

Metabolism

The main metabolite after oral dosing is the sulphate conjugate and also some glucuronide conjugate can be found in the urine.

5.3 Preclinical safety data

The major toxic effect of terbutaline, observed in toxicological studies in rats and dogs at exposures in excess of maximum human exposure, is focal myocardial necrosis. This type of cardiotoxicity is a well known pharmacological manifestation seen after the administration of high doses of β_2-agonists.

In rats, an increase in the incidence of benign uterine leiomyomas has been observed. This effect is looked upon as a class-effect observed in rodents after long term exposure to high doses of β_2-agonists

6. PHARMACEUTICAL PARTICULARS

6.1 List of excipients

Lactose monohydrate, maize starch, povidone, microcrystalline cellulose and magnesium stearate.

6.2 Incompatibilities

None known.

6.3 Shelf life

4 years.

6.4 Special precautions for storage

Do not store above 25°C.

6.5 Nature and contents of container

Glass bottles and Securitainers of 100 and 500 tablets.

6.6 Instructions for use and handling

Not applicable

7. MARKETING AUTHORISATION HOLDER

AstraZeneca UK Ltd.,

600 Capability Green,

Luton, LU1 3LU, UK.

8. MARKETING AUTHORISATION NUMBER(S)

PL 17901/0116

9. DATE OF FIRST AUTHORISATION/RENEWAL OF THE AUTHORISATION

28th May 2002

10. DATE OF REVISION OF THE TEXT

23rd April 2004

Bricanyl Turbohaler, 0.5mg/dose, inhalation powder

(AstraZeneca UK Limited)

1. NAME OF THE MEDICINAL PRODUCT

Bricanyl® Turbohaler®, 0.5mg/dose, inhalation powder

2. QUALITATIVE AND QUANTITATIVE COMPOSITION

Terbutaline Sulphate 0.5mg/dose.

For excipients see Section 6.1.

3. PHARMACEUTICAL FORM

Inhalation powder.

Breath-actuated metered dose powder inhaler.

4. CLINICAL PARTICULARS

4.1 Therapeutic indications

Terbutaline is a selective β_2-adrenergic agonist recommended for the relief and prevention of bronchospasm in bronchial asthma and other bronchopulmonary disorders in which bronchospasm or reversible airways obstruction is a complicating factor.

4.2 Posology and method of administration

Adults and Children: One inhalation (0.5mg) as required. Not more than 4 inhalations should be required in any 24-hour period.

The duration of action of a single dose is up to 6 hours.

Elderly: Dosage as for adults.

Instructions for use and cleaning are provided in the Patient Information Leaflet, which can be found in each pack.

4.3 Contraindications

Bricanyl preparations are contraindicated in patients with a history of sensitivity to terbutaline sulphate.

4.4 Special warnings and special precautions for use

Patients should be instructed in proper use and their inhalation technique checked regularly.

Care should be taken in patients suffering from myocardial insufficiency or thyrotoxicosis.

Due to the hyperglycaemic effects of β_2-stimulants, additional blood glucose measurements are initially recommended when Bricanyl therapy is commenced in diabetic patients.

If a previously effective dosage regimen no longer gives the same symptomatic relief, the patient should urgently seek further medical advice. Consideration should be given to the requirements for additional therapy (including increased dosages of anti-inflammatory medication).

Severe exacerbations of asthma should be treated as an emergency in the usual manner.

Potentially serious hypokalaemia may result from β_2-agonist therapy, mainly with parenteral or nebulised administration. Particular caution is advised in acute severe asthma as this effect may be augmented by hypoxia. The hypokalaemic effect may be potentiated by concomitant treatment with xanthine derivatives, corticosteroids and/or diuretics. It is recommended that serum potassium levels are monitored in such situations.

Due to the positive inotropic effect of β_2-agonists, these drugs should not be used in patients with hypertrophic cardiomyopathy

4.5 Interaction with other medicinal products and other forms of Interaction

Beta-blocking agents (including eye drops), especially the non-selective ones such as propranolol, may partially or totally inhibit the effect of β-stimulants. Therefore, Bricanyl preparations and non-selective β-blockers should not normally be administered concurrently. Bricanyl should be used with caution in patients receiving other sympathomimetics.

Hypokalaemia may result from β_2-agonist therapy and may be potentiated by concomitant treatment with xanthine derivatives, corticosteroids and diuretics (*see Section 4.4, Special Warnings and Precautions for use*).

4.6 Pregnancy and lactation

Although no teratogenic effects have been observed in animals or in patients, Bricanyl should only be administered with caution during the first trimester of pregnancy.

Terbutaline is secreted via breast milk but any effect on the infant is unlikely at therapeutic doses.

4.7 Effects on ability to drive and use machines

None.

4.8 Undesirable effects

The frequency of side-effects is low. Side-effects which have been recorded such as tremor, headache, nausea, tonic cramp, mouth and throat irritation, and palpitations, are all characteristic of sympathomimetic amines. A few patients feel tense; this is also due to the effects on skeletal muscle and not to direct CNS stimulation. Whenever these side-effects have occurred, the majority have usually been spontaneously reversible within the first week of treatment. As with other β_2-agonists, tremor is dose related.

Sleep disturbances and behavioural disturbances, such as agitation, hyperactivity and restlessness, have been observed.

Tachycardia, with or without peripheral vasodilation, has been rarely reported during β_2-agonist therapy. Cardiac arrhythmias, including atrial fibrillation, supraventricular tachycardia and extrasystoles, have been reported in association with β_2-agonists, usually in susceptible patients.

Potentially serious hypokalaemia may result from β_2-agonist therapy. (See also *Section 4.4, Special Warnings and Precautions for use.*)

In rare cases, through unspecified mechanisms, paradoxical bronchospasm may occur, with wheezing immediately after inhalation. This should be immediately treated with a rapid-onset bronchodilator. Bricanyl therapy should be discontinued and, after assessment, an alternative therapy initiated.

Hypersensitivity reactions, including angioedema, urticaria, exanthema, bronchospasm, hypotension and collapse, have been very rarely reported with β_2-agonist therapy.

4.9 Overdose

i) Possible symptoms and signs:

Headache, anxiety, tremor, nausea, tonic cramp, palpitations, tachycardia and arrhythmia. A fall in blood pressure sometimes occurs. Laboratory findings: Hypokalaemia, hyperglycaemia and metabolic acidosis sometimes occur.

ii) Treatment:

Mild and moderate cases: Reduce the dose.

Severe cases: Gastric lavage, administration of activated charcoal (where suspected that significant amounts have been swallowed). Determination of acid-base balance, blood sugar and electrolytes, particularly serum potassium levels. Monitoring of heart rate and rhythm and blood pressure. Metabolic changes should be corrected. A cardioselective β-blocker (e.g. metoprolol) is recommended for the treatment of arrhythmias causing haemodynamic deterioration. The β-blocker should be used with care because of the possibility of inducing bronchoconstriction: use with caution in patients with a history of bronchospasm. If the β_2-mediated reduction in peripheral vascular resistance significantly contributes to the fall in blood pressure, a volume expander should be given.

5. PHARMACOLOGICAL PROPERTIES

5.1 Pharmacodynamic properties

Pharmaco-therapeutic group: selective β_2-agonist, terbutaline, ATC code: R03A C03.

Terbutaline sulphate is a selective β_2-adrenoceptor agonist, thus producing relaxation of bronchial smooth muscle, inhibition of the release of endogenous spasmogens, inhibitions of oedema caused by endogenous mediators, increased mucociliary clearance and relaxation of the uterine muscle.

5.2 Pharmacokinetic properties

Pharmacokinetic data from terbutaline inhaled from a pressurised aerosol reveal that less than 10% of the dose is absorbed from the airways. The remaining 90% is swallowed but is largely prevented from entering the systemic circulation due to extensive first pass metabolism.

Data suggest that inhaled terbutaline acts topically in the airways.

5.3 Preclinical safety data

The major toxic effect of terbutaline, observed in toxicological studies in rats and dogs at exposures in excess of maximum human exposure, is focal myocardial necrosis. This type of cardiotoxicity is a well known pharmacological manifestation seen after the administration of high doses of β_2-agonists.

In rats, an increase in the incidence of benign uterine leiomyomas has been observed. This effect is looked upon as a class-effect observed in rodents after long term exposure to high doses of β_2-agonists.

6. PHARMACEUTICAL PARTICULARS

6.1 List of excipients

None

6.2 Incompatibilities

None known.

6.3 Shelf life

24 months

6.4 Special precautions for storage

Do not store above 30°C.

6.5 Nature and contents of container

Bricanyl Turbohaler consists of a number of assembled plastic details, the main parts being the dosing mechanism, the drug substance store, the desiccant store and the mouthpiece. The inhaler is protected by an outer tubular cover screwed onto a bottom plate.

Each inhaler contains 100 doses.

6.6 Instructions for use and handling

None.

7. MARKETING AUTHORISATION HOLDER

AstraZeneca UK Ltd.,

600 Capability Green,

Luton, LU1 3LU, UK.

8. MARKETING AUTHORISATION NUMBER(S)

PL 17901/0117

9. DATE OF FIRST AUTHORISATION/RENEWAL OF THE AUTHORISATION

4th June 2002

10. DATE OF REVISION OF THE TEXT

23rd April 2004

BritLofex Tablets 0.2mg

(Britannia Pharmaceuticals Limited)

1. NAME OF THE MEDICINAL PRODUCT

BritLofex Tablets 0.2mg

2. QUALITATIVE AND QUANTITATIVE COMPOSITION

Lofexidine hydrochloride 0.2mg

3. PHARMACEUTICAL FORM

Film-coated tablet.

Peach coloured, round tablet.

4. CLINICAL PARTICULARS

4.1 Therapeutic indications

To relieve symptoms in patients undergoing opiate detoxification.

4.2 Posology and method of administration

The recommended route of administration is by mouth.

OPIATE DETOXIFICATION

Dosage should be adjusted according to the patient's response. Initial dosage should be one 0.2mg tablet twice daily, which may be increased by increments of 0.2-0.4mg/day up to a maximum of 2.4mg/day.

In cases where no opiate use occurs during detoxification, a duration of treatment of 7-10 days is recommended. In some cases the physician may consider longer treatment is warranted.

Concurrent medication to aid sleeping has been frequently used in withdrawal studies Chloral hydrate or anti-histamines are preferred, benzodiazepines may also suppress some of the withdrawal symptoms.

CHILDREN:

Safety and effectiveness in children has not been established.

ELDERLY:

There is no experience of dosing in the elderly from clinical studies. Should use in the elderly be necessary it is advised that special caution is observed in the presence of heart disease or anti-hypertensive therapy.

4.3 Contraindications

BritLofex tablets are contraindicated in patients who are allergic to lofexidine or to other imidazoline derivatives or to any excipients of BritLofex.

4.4 Special warnings and special precautions for use

As with other hypotensive agents, therapy with lofexidine should not be discontinued abruptly. Dosage should be reduced gradually over a period of 2-4 days or longer, to minimise blood pressure elevation and associated signs and symptoms. Lofexidine should be used with caution in patients with severe coronary insufficiency, recent myocardial infarction, cerebrovascular disease or chronic renal failure and in patients with marked bradycardia (55 beats per minute). Pulse rate should be assessed frequently. Patients with a history of depression should be carefully observed during long-term therapy with lofexidine.

There have been reports of asymptomatic QT prolongation during lofexidine treatment. Whilst the nature of the relationship between lofexidine and these ECG changes is not yet clear, it would be prudent to avoid the use of lofexidine in patients with known problems of QT prolongation and in patients taking other drugs known to cause QT prolongation.

4.5 Interaction with other medicinal products and other forms of Interaction

Lofexidine may enhance the CNS depressive effects of alcohol, barbiturates and other sedatives.

Lofexidine may enhance the effects of anti-hypertensive drug therapy.

Concomitant use of tricyclic antidepressants may reduce the efficacy of lofexidine

4.6 Pregnancy and lactation

The safety of lofexidine in pregnant women has not been established. High doses of lofexidine given to pregnant dogs and rabbits caused a reduction in foetal weight and increased abortions. Lofexidine should only be administered during pregnancy if the benefit outweighs the potential risk to mother and foetus. It is not known whether this drug is excreted in human milk and caution should be exercised when it is administered to a nursing woman.

4.7 Effects on ability to drive and use machines

Lofexidine may have a sedative effect. If affected, patients should be advised not to drive or operate machines.

4.8 Undesirable effects

The adverse effects of the drug are primarily related to its central alpha-adrenergic agonist effects and comprise drowsiness and related symptoms and dryness of mucous membranes especially mouth, throat and nose.

Hypotension and bradycardia may occur.

There have been reports of asymptomatic QT prolongation during lofexidine treatment.

4.9 Overdose

Overdosage may cause hypotension, bradycardia and sedation. Gastric lavage should be carried out where appropriate. In most cases, all that is required are general supportive measures.

5. PHARMACOLOGICAL PROPERTIES

5.1 Pharmacodynamic properties

Lofexidine hydrochloride is an orally active imidazoline adrenergic alpha-2-receptor agonist; and is believed to have a high affinity for 2A receptor subtypes resulting in less anti-hypertensive activity than clonidine, a non-selective alpha-2-receptor agonist. Hypotension may occur in susceptible subjects, accompanied by a decrease in heart rate.

Abrupt discontinuation of lofexidine has been, in some cases, associated with a transient increase in blood pressure to higher than pre-treatment levels.

5.2 Pharmacokinetic properties

Lofexidine is extensively absorbed and achieves peak plasma concentration at 3 hours after administration of a single dose. The elimination half-life is 11 hours with accumulation occurring up to four days with repeat dosing. Lofexidine undergoes extensive metabolism in the liver and excretion is mainly by the kidney.

5.3 Preclinical safety data

Animal toxicology. Lofexidine was tolerated at high dosage in singe dose toxicity studies in animals, the LD_{50} being > 77 mg/kg. With repeat dosing in mice, rats and dogs symptoms related to the pharmacology of the drug (ataxia, sedation, tremor, unkempt appearance and exhaustion) appeared.

Studies of mutagenicity are incomplete but lofexidine did not display mutagenicity in the Ames test. Long-term studies in rats showed no evidence of carcinogenicity.

High doses of lofexidine given to pregnant rats and rabbits caused a reduction in the foetal weight and increased abortions. No teratogenic effects were found.

6. PHARMACEUTICAL PARTICULARS

6.1 List of excipients

Lactose (monohydrate)

Citric acid

Povidone

Microcrystalline cellulose

Calcium stearate

Sodium lauryl sulphate

Purified water

Film Coat:

Opadry OY-S-9480 Brown

containing

Hydroxypropylmethyl cellulose

Titanium dioxide

Propylene glycol

Indigo Carmine (E132)

Sunset Yellow (E110)

6.2 Incompatibilities

None known.

6.3 Shelf life

36 months.

6.4 Special precautions for storage

Store below 25°C. Store in original package.

6.5 Nature and contents of container

Aluminium foil/aluminium foil blister strips

Aluminium foil/PVC blister strips

6.6 Instructions for use and handling

No special instructions.

7. MARKETING AUTHORISATION HOLDER

Britannia Pharmaceuticals Limited

41-51 Brighton Road

Redhill, Surrey RH1 6YS

8. MARKETING AUTHORISATION NUMBER(S)

PL 4483/0036

9. DATE OF FIRST AUTHORISATION/RENEWAL OF THE AUTHORISATION

June 1995

10. DATE OF REVISION OF THE TEXT

January 2004

Broflex Syrup 5mg/5ml

(Alliance Pharmaceuticals)

1. NAME OF THE MEDICINAL PRODUCT

Broflex syrup (5mg/5mL).

2. QUALITATIVE AND QUANTITATIVE COMPOSITION

Trihexyphenidyl hydrochloride BP 5mg/5mL.

3. PHARMACEUTICAL FORM

A blackcurrant scented and flavoured clear pink syrup.

4. CLINICAL PARTICULARS

4.1 Therapeutic indications

Parkinsonism and drug induced extrapyramidal syndrome.

4.2 Posology and method of administration

Adults and Elderly:

Initial dose 2mg. Subsequent doses up to 20mg as recommended by a physician.

Children:

Not recommended.

4.3 Contraindications

Incipient glaucoma may be precipitated. The following are not absolute contra-indications, nevertheless caution must be observed in patients with: hypertension, cardiac, liver or kidney dysfunction, glaucoma, obstructive disease of the gastro-intestinal or genito-urinary tracts and in males with a prostatic hypertrophy.

4.4 Special warnings and special precautions for use

Anticholinergic medications, including trihexyphenidyl, should not be withdrawn abruptly in patients on long-term therapy, to avoid recurrence of the original symptoms and possible anticholinergic rebound. Prescribers should be aware that trihexyphenidyl may be the subject of abuse due to its euphoric or hallucinogenic properties.

4.5 Interaction with other medicinal products and other forms of Interaction

Monoamine oxidase inhibitors (MAOI's), antihistamines, disopyramide, phenothiazines and tricyclic antidepressants increase the side effects of blurred vision and dry mouth, constipation, urinary retention. MAOI's, amantadine and some tricyclic antidepressants may also cause excitation, confusion and hallucination.

4.6 Pregnancy and lactation

Caution must be observed.

4.7 Effects on ability to drive and use machines

Patients should be warned of the potential hazards of driving or operating machinery if they experience blurred vision or a reduction in alertness.

4.8 Undesirable effects

Dry mouth, constipation and blurred vision may occur. This is more frequent in the elderly but reduces with tolerance. Psychiatric symptoms such as agitation, confusion, hallucinations, euphoria, insomnia, restlessness and very occasionally paranoid delusions have been reported. These are more likely to occur in patients receiving higher than recommended doses. There have been reports of abuse of trihexyphenidyl due to its euphoric and hallucinogenic properties.

Impairment of immediate and short-term memory functions has also been reported.

4.9 Overdose

There is no specific antidote. Gastric lavage, emetics and high enemas are recommended. Forced fluid intake and general supportive measures are necessary. Atropine antagonists may be helpful.

5. PHARMACOLOGICAL PROPERTIES

5.1 Pharmacodynamic properties

Trihexyphenidyl is a tertiary amine antimuscarinic. It also has a direct antispasmodic action on smooth muscle.

5.2 Pharmacokinetic properties

Trihexyphenidyl is well absorbed from the gastro-intestinal tract.

5.3 Preclinical safety data

No formal preclinical studies have been undertaken with Broflex, as its active ingredient is a well established pharmaceutical.

6. PHARMACEUTICAL PARTICULARS

6.1 List of excipients

Anhydrous citric acid, benzoic acid, propylene glycol, amaranth E123, glycerol, chloroform spirit, blackcurrant flavour A402, syrup, purified water.

6.2 Incompatibilities

None known.

6.3 Shelf life

24 months.

6.4 Special precautions for storage

None.

6.5 Nature and contents of container

200 mL pack size in amber glass bottle with polycone lined enclosure.

6.6 Instructions for use and handling

None stated.

Administrative Data

7. MARKETING AUTHORISATION HOLDER

Alliance Pharmaceuticals Ltd

Avonbridge House

Bath Road

Chippenham

Wiltshire

SN15 2BB

8. MARKETING AUTHORISATION NUMBER(S)

PL16853/0023

9. DATE OF FIRST AUTHORISATION/RENEWAL OF THE AUTHORISATION

30 June 1999

10. DATE OF REVISION OF THE TEXT

February 2004

11. Legal Status

POM

Alliance, Alliance Pharmaceuticals and associated devices are registered Trademarks of Alliance Pharmaceuticals Ltd.

Brufen 200 mg Tablets

(Abbott Laboratories Limited)

1. NAME OF THE MEDICINAL PRODUCT

Brufen Tablets 200 mg

2. QUALITATIVE AND QUANTITATIVE COMPOSITION

Active ingredientQuantity

Ibuprofen 200 mg

3. PHARMACEUTICAL FORM

A white, pillow-shaped, film-coated tablet with 'Brufen' printed in black on one face

4. CLINICAL PARTICULARS

4.1 Therapeutic indications

Brufen is indicated for its analgesic and anti-inflammatory effects in the treatment of rheumatoid arthritis (including juvenile rheumatoid arthritis or Still's disease), ankylosing spondylitis, osteoarthritis and other non-rheumatoid (seronegative) arthropathies.

In the treatment of non-articular rheumatic conditions, Brufen is indicated in periarticular conditions such as frozen shoulder (capsulitis), bursitis, tendonitis, tenosynovitis and low back pain; Brufen can also be used in soft tissue injuries such as sprains and strains.

Brufen is also indicated for its analgesic effect in the relief of mild to moderate pain such as dysmenorrhoea, dental and post-operative pain and for symptomatic relief of headache, including migraine headache.

4.2 Posology and method of administration

Adults: The recommended dosage of Brufen is 1200-1800 mg daily in divided doses. Some patients can be maintained on 600-1200 mg daily. In severe or acute conditions, it can be advantageous to increase the dosage until the acute phase is brought under control, provided that the total daily dose does not exceed 2400 mg in divided doses.

Children: The daily dosage of Brufen is 20 mg/kg of body weight in divided doses.

In Juvenile Rheumatoid Arthritis, up to 40 mg/kg of body weight daily in divided doses may be taken.

Not recommended for children weighing less than 7 kg.

Elderly: No special dosage modifications are required unless renal or hepatic function is impaired, in which case dosage should be assessed individually.

For oral administration.

4.3 Contraindications

Patients with a history of, or active, peptic ulceration. Patients who have previously shown hypersensitivity reactions (*e.g.* asthma, rhinitis or urticaria) in response to ibuprofen, aspirin or other nonsteroidal anti-inflammatory drugs.

4.4 Special warnings and special precautions for use

Caution is required if Brufen is administered to patients suffering from, or with a previous history of, bronchial asthma since ibuprofen has been reported to cause bronchospasm in such patients. Brufen should only be given with care to patients with a history of gastrointestinal disease.

Caution is required in patients with renal, hepatic or cardiac impairment since the use of NSAIDs may result in deterioration of renal function. The dose should be kept as low as possible and renal function should be monitored in these patients.

Brufen should be given with care to patients with a history of heart failure or hypertension since oedema has been reported in association with ibuprofen administration.

4.5 Interaction with other medicinal products and other forms of Interaction

Care should be taken in patients treated with any of the following drugs as interactions have been reported in some patients.

Antihypertensives: Reduced antihypertensive effect.

Diuretics: Reduced diuretic effect. Diuretics can increase the risk of nephrotoxicity of NSAIDs.

Cardiac glycosides: NSAIDs may exacerbate cardiac failure, reduce GFR and increase plasma cardiac glycoside levels.

Lithium: Decreased elimination of lithium.

Methotrexate: Decreased elimination of methotrexate.

Cyclosporin: Increased risk of nephrotoxicity with NSAIDs.

Mifepristone: NSAIDs should not be used for 8-12 days after mifepristone administration as NSAIDs can reduce the effects of mifepristone.

Other analgesics: Avoid concomitant use of two or more NSAIDs.

Corticosteroids: Increased risk of gastrointestinal bleeding.

Anticoagulants: Enhanced anticoagulant effect.

Quinolone antibiotics: Animal data indicate that NSAIDs can increase the risk of convulsions associated with quinolone antibiotics. Patients taking NSAIDs and quinolones may have an increased risk of developing convulsions.

4.6 Pregnancy and lactation

Whilst no teratogenic effects have been demonstrated in animal toxicity studies, the use of ibuprofen during pregnancy should, if possible, be avoided. Congenital abnormalities have been reported in association with ibuprofen administration in man; however, these are low in frequency and do not appear to follow any discernible pattern. In view of the known effects of NSAIDs on the foetal cardiovascular system (closure of ductus arteriosus), use in late pregnancy should be avoided.

In the limited studies so far available, ibuprofen appears in the breast milk in very low concentrations and is unlikely to adversely affect the breast-fed infant.

4.7 Effects on ability to drive and use machines

No adverse effects known.

4.8 Undesirable effects

Gastrointestinal: The most commonly-observed adverse events are gastrointestinal in nature. Nausea, vomiting, diarrhoea, dyspepsia, abdominal pain, melaena, haematemesis, ulcerative stomatitis and gastrointestinal haemorrhage have been reported following ibuprofen administration. Less frequently, gastritis, duodenal ulcer, gastric ulcer and gastrointestinal perforation have been observed. Epidemiological data indicate that of the seven most widely-used oral, non-aspirin NSAIDs, ibuprofen presents the lowest risk of upper gastrointestinal toxicity.

Hypersensitivity: Hypersensitivity reactions have been reported following treatment with ibuprofen. These may consist of (a) non-specific allergic reaction and anaphylaxis, (b) respiratory tract reactivity comprising asthma, aggravated asthma, bronchospasm or dyspnoea, or (c) assorted skin disorders, including rashes of various types, pruritus, urticaria, purpura, angioedema and, less commonly, bullous dermatoses (including epidermal necrolysis and erythema multiforme).

Cardiovascular: Oedema has been reported in association with ibuprofen treatment.

Other adverse events reported less commonly and for which causality has not necessarily been established include:

Renal: Nephrotoxicity in various forms, including interstitial nephritis, nephrotic syndrome and renal failure.

Hepatic: Abnormal liver function, hepatitis and jaundice.

Neurological and special senses: Visual disturbances, optic neuritis, headaches, paraesthesia, depression, confusion, hallucinations, tinnitus, vertigo, dizziness, malaise, fatigue and drowsiness.

Haematological: Thrombocytopenia, neutropenia, agranulocytosis, aplastic anaemia and haemolytic anaemia.

Dermatological: Photosensitivity (see 'Hypersensitivity' for other skin reactions).

4.9 Overdose
Symptoms include nausea, vomiting, dizziness and rarely, loss of consciousness. Large overdoses are generally well tolerated when no other drugs are involved.

Treatment consists of gastric lavage and, if necessary, correction of serum electrolytes and appropriate supportive measures.

There is no specific antidote to ibuprofen.

5. PHARMACOLOGICAL PROPERTIES
5.1 Pharmacodynamic properties
Ibuprofen is a propionic acid derivative with analgesic, anti-inflammatory and anti-pyretic activity. The drug's therapeutic effects as an NSAID are thought to result from its inhibitory effect on the enzyme cyclo-oxygenase, which results in a marked reduction in prostaglandin synthesis.

5.2 Pharmacokinetic properties
Ibuprofen is rapidly absorbed from the gastrointestinal tract, peak serum concentrations occurring 1-2 hours after administration. The elimination half-life is approximately 2 hours.

Ibuprofen is metabolised in the liver to two inactive metabolites and these, together with unchanged ibuprofen, are excreted by the kidney either as such or as conjugates. Excretion by the kidney is both rapid and complete.

Ibuprofen is extensively bound to plasma proteins.

5.3 Preclinical safety data
Not applicable.

6. PHARMACEUTICAL PARTICULARS
6.1 List of excipients
Microcrystalline cellulose

Croscarmellose sodium

Lactose monohydrate

Colloidal anhydrous silica

Sodium lauryl sulphate

Magnesium stearate

Opadry white

or

Hydroxypropylmethylcellulose *plus* Talc *plus* Opaspray white M-1-7111B

Opacode S-1-8152HV black

Butanol

or

Industrial methylated spirit

Purified water

6.2 Incompatibilities
None known.

6.3 Shelf life
36 months

6.4 Special precautions for storage
Do not store above 30°C

6.5 Nature and contents of container
White high-density polyethylene bottle with a white polypropylene screw cap fitted with a waxed aluminium-faced pulpboard liner - pack size 9, 12, 100, 250 or 500 tablets.

Not all pack sizes are marketed.

6.6 Instructions for use and handling
No special instructions.

7. MARKETING AUTHORISATION HOLDER
Abbott Laboratories Limited

Queenborough

Kent

ME11 5EL

United Kingdom

8. MARKETING AUTHORISATION NUMBER(S)
PL 00037/0333

9. DATE OF FIRST AUTHORISATION/RENEWAL OF THE AUTHORISATION
15 February 2002

10. DATE OF REVISION OF THE TEXT
12 March 2003

Brufen 400 mg Tablets
(Abbott Laboratories Limited)

1. NAME OF THE MEDICINAL PRODUCT
Brufen Tablets 400 mg

2. QUALITATIVE AND QUANTITATIVE COMPOSITION
Each Brufen tablet contains 400 mg Ibuprofen.

3. PHARMACEUTICAL FORM
A white, pillow-shaped, film-coated tablet with 'Brufen 400' printed in black on one face

4. CLINICAL PARTICULARS
4.1 Therapeutic indications
Brufen is indicated for its analgesic and anti-inflammatory effects in the treatment of rheumatoid arthritis (including juvenile rheumatoid arthritis or Still's disease), ankylosing spondylitis, osteoarthritis and other non-rheumatoid (seronegative) arthropathies.

In the treatment of non-articular rheumatic conditions, Brufen is indicated in periarticular conditions such as frozen shoulder (capsulitis), bursitis, tendonitis, tenosynovitis and low back pain; Brufen can also be used in soft tissue injuries such as sprains and strains.

Brufen is also indicated for its analgesic effect in the relief of mild to moderate pain such as dysmenorrhoea, dental and post-operative pain and for symptomatic relief of headache, including migraine headache.

4.2 Posology and method of administration
Adults: the recommended dosage of Brufen is 1200-1800 mg daily in divided doses. Some patients can be maintained on 600-1200 mg daily. In severe or acute conditions, it can be advantageous to increase the dosage until the acute phase is brought under control, provided that the total daily dose does not exceed 2400 mg in divided doses.

Children: the daily dosage of Brufen is 20 mg/kg of body weight in divided doses.

In juvenile rheumatoid arthritis, up to 40 mg/kg of body weight daily in divided doses may be taken.

Not recommended for children weighing less than 7 kg.

Elderly: no special dosage modifications are required unless renal or hepatic function is impaired, in which case dosage should be assessed individually.

For oral administration.

4.3 Contraindications
Patients with a history of, or active, peptic ulceration. Patients who have previously shown hypersensitivity reactions (*e.g.* asthma, rhinitis or urticaria) in response to ibuprofen, aspirin or other NSAIDs.

4.4 Special warnings and special precautions for use
Caution is required if Brufen is administered to patients suffering from, or with a previous history of, bronchial asthma since ibuprofen has been reported to cause bronchospasm in such patients. Brufen should only be given with care to patients with a history of gastrointestinal disease.

Caution is required in patients with renal, hepatic or cardiac impairment since the use of NSAIDs may result in deterioration of renal function. The dose should be kept as low as possible and renal function should be monitored in these patients.

Brufen should be given with care to patients with a history of heart failure or hypertension since oedema has been reported in association with ibuprofen administration.

4.5 Interaction with other medicinal products and other forms of Interaction
Care should be taken in patients treated with any of the following drugs as interactions have been reported in some patients.

Antihypertensives: reduced antihypertensive effect.

Diuretics: reduced diuretic effect. Diuretics can increase the risk of nephrotoxicity of NSAIDs.

Cardiac glycosides: NSAIDs may exacerbate cardiac failure, reduce GFR and increase plasma cardiac glycoside levels.

Lithium: decreased elimination of lithium.

Methotrexate: decreased elimination of methotrexate.

Cyclosporin: increased risk of nephrotoxicity with NSAIDs.

Mifepristone: NSAIDs should not be used for 8-12 days after mifepristone administration as NSAIDs can reduce the effects of mifepristone.

Other analgesics: avoid concomitant use of two or more NSAIDs.

Corticosteroids: increased risk of gastrointestinal bleeding.

Anticoagulants: enhanced anticoagulant effect.

Quinolone antibiotics: animal data indicate that NSAIDs can increase the risk of convulsions associated with quinolone antibiotics. Patients taking NSAIDs and quinolones may have an increased risk of developing convulsions.

4.6 Pregnancy and lactation
Whilst no teratogenic effects have been demonstrated in animal toxicology studies, the use of ibuprofen during pregnancy should, if possible, be avoided. Congenital abnormalities have been reported in association with ibuprofen administration in man; however, these are low in frequency and do not appear to follow any discernible pattern. In view of the known effects of NSAIDs on the foetal cardiovascular system (closure of ductus arteriosus), use in late pregnancy should be avoided.

In the limited studies so far available, ibuprofen appears in the breast milk in very low concentrations and is unlikely to adversely affect the breast-fed infant.

4.7 Effects on ability to drive and use machines
No adverse effects known.

4.8 Undesirable effects
Gastrointestinal: the most commonly-observed adverse events are gastrointestinal in nature. Nausea, vomiting, diarrhoea, dyspepsia, abdominal pain, melaena, haematemesis, ulcerative stomatitis and gastrointestinal haemorrhage have been reported following ibuprofen administration. Less frequently, gastritis, duodenal ulcer, gastric ulcer and gastrointestinal perforation have been observed. Epidemiological data indicate that of the seven most widely-used oral, non-aspirin NSAIDs, ibuprofen presents the lowest risk of upper gastrointestinal toxicity.

Hypersensitivity: hypersensitivity reactions have been reported following treatment with ibuprofen. These may consist of (a) non-specific allergic reaction and anaphylaxis, (b) respiratory tract reactivity comprising asthma, aggravated asthma, bronchospasm or dyspnoea, or (c) assorted skin disorders, including rashes of various types, pruritus, urticaria, purpura, angioedema and, less commonly, bullous dermatoses (including epidermal necrolysis and erythema multiforme).

Cardiovascular: oedema has been reported in association with ibuprofen treatment.

Other adverse events reported less commonly and for which causality has not necessarily been established include:

Renal: nephrotoxicity in various forms, including interstitial nephritis, nephrotic syndrome and renal failure.

Hepatic: abnormal liver function, hepatitis and jaundice.

Neurological and special senses: visual disturbances, optic neuritis, headaches, paraesthesia, depression, confusion, hallucinations, tinnitus, vertigo, dizziness, malaise, fatigue and drowsiness.

Haematological: thrombocytopenia, neutropenia, agranulocytosis, aplastic anaemia and haemolytic anaemia.

Dermatological: photosensitivity (see 'hypersensitivity' for other skin reactions).

4.9 Overdose
Symptoms include nausea, vomiting, dizziness and rarely, loss of consciousness. Large overdoses are generally well tolerated when no other drugs are involved.

Treatment consists of gastric lavage and, if necessary, correction of serum electrolytes and appropriate supportive measures.

There is no specific antidote to ibuprofen.

5. PHARMACOLOGICAL PROPERTIES
5.1 Pharmacodynamic properties
Ibuprofen is a propionic acid derivative with analgesic, anti-inflammatory and anti-pyretic activity. The drug's therapeutic effects as an NSAID are thought to result from its inhibitory effect on the enzyme cyclo-oxygenase, which results in a marked reduction in prostaglandin synthesis.

5.2 Pharmacokinetic properties
Ibuprofen is rapidly absorbed from the gastrointestinal tract, peak serum concentrations occurring 1-2 hours after administration. The elimination half-life is approximately 2 hours.

Ibuprofen is metabolised in the liver to two inactive metabolites and these, together with unchanged ibuprofen, are excreted by the kidney either as such or as conjugates. Excretion by the kidney is both rapid and complete.

Ibuprofen is extensively bound to plasma proteins.

5.3 Preclinical safety data
Not applicable.

6. PHARMACEUTICAL PARTICULARS

6.1 List of excipients

Microcrystalline cellulose

Croscarmellose sodium

Lactose monohydrate

Colloidal anhydrous silica

Sodium lauryl sulphate

Magnesium stearate

Opadry white

or

Hydroxypropylmethylcellulose *plus* Talc *plus* Opaspray white M-1-7111B

Opacode S-1-8152HV black

Butanol

or

Industrial methylated spirit

Purified water

6.2 Incompatibilities

Not applicable.

6.3 Shelf life

36 months.

6.4 Special precautions for storage

Do not store above 30°C.

6.5 Nature and contents of container

White high-density polyethylene bottle with a white polypropylene screw cap fitted with a waxed aluminium-faced pulpboard liner - pack size 9, 12, 100, 250 or 500 tablets.

Not all pack sizes are marketed.

6.6 Instructions for use and handling

None.

7. MARKETING AUTHORISATION HOLDER

Abbott Laboratories Limited

Queenborough

Kent

ME11 5EL

United Kingdom

8. MARKETING AUTHORISATION NUMBER(S)

PL 00037/0334

9. DATE OF FIRST AUTHORISATION/RENEWAL OF THE AUTHORISATION

15 February 2002

10. DATE OF REVISION OF THE TEXT

Brufen 600 mg Tablets

(Abbott Laboratories Limited)

1. NAME OF THE MEDICINAL PRODUCT

Brufen Tablets 600 mg

2. QUALITATIVE AND QUANTITATIVE COMPOSITION

Each Brufen Tablet contains 600 mg Ibuprofen.

3. PHARMACEUTICAL FORM

A white, pillow-shaped, film-coated tablet with 'Brufen 600' printed in black on one face.

4. CLINICAL PARTICULARS

4.1 Therapeutic indications

Brufen is indicated for its analgesic and anti-inflammatory effects in the treatment of rheumatoid arthritis (including juvenile rheumatoid arthritis or Still's disease), ankylosing spondylitis, osteoarthritis and other non-rheumatoid (seronegative) arthropathies.

In the treatment of non-articular rheumatic conditions, Brufen is indicated in periarticular conditions such as frozen shoulder (capsulitis), bursitis, tendinitis, tenosynovitis and low back pain; Brufen can also be used in soft tissue injuries such as sprains and strains.

Brufen is also indicated for its analgesic effect in the relief of mild to moderate pain such as dysmenorrhoea, dental and post-operative pain and for symptomatic relief of headache, including migraine headache.

4.2 Posology and method of administration

Adults: The recommended dosage of Brufen is 1200-1800 mg daily in divided doses. Some patients can be maintained on 600-1200 mg daily. In severe or acute conditions, it can be advantageous to increase the dosage until the acute phase is brought under control, provided that the total daily dose does not exceed 2400 mg in divided doses.

Children: The daily dosage of Brufen is 20 mg/kg of body weight in divided doses.

In juvenile rheumatoid arthritis, up to 40 mg/kg of body weight daily in divided doses may be taken.

Not recommended for children weighing less than 7 kg.

Elderly: No special dosage modifications are required unless renal or hepatic function is impaired, in which case dosage should be assessed individually.

For oral administration.

4.3 Contraindications

Patients with a history of, or active, peptic ulceration. Patients who have previously shown hypersensitivity reactions (*e.g.* asthma, rhinitis or urticaria) in response to ibuprofen, aspirin or other NSAIDs.

4.4 Special warnings and special precautions for use

Caution is required if Brufen is administered to patients suffering from, or with a previous history of, bronchial asthma since ibuprofen has been reported to cause bronchospasm in such patients. Brufen should only be given with care to patients with a history of gastrointestinal disease.

Caution is required in patients with renal, hepatic or cardiac impairment since the use of NSAIDs may result in deterioration of renal function. The dose should be kept as low as possible and renal function should be monitored in these patients.

Brufen should be given with care to patients with a history of heart failure or hypertension since oedema has been reported in association with ibuprofen administration.

4.5 Interaction with other medicinal products and other forms of Interaction

Care should be taken in patients treated with any of the following drugs as interactions have been reported in some patients.

Antihypertensives: Reduced antihypertensive effect.

Diuretics: Reduced diuretic effect. Diuretics can increase the risk of nephrotoxicity of NSAIDs.

Cardiac glycosides: NSAIDs may exacerbate cardiac failure, reduce GFR and increase plasma cardiac glycoside levels.

Lithium: Decreased elimination of lithium.

Methotrexate: Decreased elimination of methotrexate.

Cyclosporin: Increased risk of nephrotoxicity with NSAIDs.

Mifepristone: NSAIDs should not be used for 8-12 days after mifepristone administration as NSAIDs can reduce the effects of mifepristone.

Other analgesics: Avoid concomitant use of two or more NSAIDs.

Corticosteroids: Increased risk of gastrointestinal bleeding.

Anticoagulants: Enhanced anticoagulant effect.

Quinolone antibiotics: Animal data indicate that NSAIDs can increase the risk of convulsions associated with quinolone antibiotics. Patients taking NSAIDs and quinolones may have an increased risk of developing convulsions.

4.6 Pregnancy and lactation

Whilst no teratogenic effects have been demonstrated in animal toxicology studies, the use of ibuprofen during pregnancy should, if possible, be avoided. Congenital abnormalities have been reported in association with ibuprofen administration in man; however, these are low in frequency and do not appear to follow any discernible pattern. In view of the known effects of NSAIDs on the foetal cardiovascular system (closure of ductus arteriosus), use in late pregnancy should be avoided.

In the limited studies so far available, ibuprofen appears in the breast milk in very low concentrations and is unlikely to adversely affect the breast-fed infant.

4.7 Effects on ability to drive and use machines

No adverse effects known.

4.8 Undesirable effects

Gastrointestinal: The most commonly-observed adverse events are gastrointestinal in nature. Nausea, vomiting, diarrhoea, dyspepsia, abdominal pain, melaena, haematemesis, ulcerative stomatitis and gastrointestinal haemorrhage have been reported following ibuprofen administration. Less frequently, gastritis, duodenal ulcer, gastric ulcer and gastrointestinal perforation have been observed. Epidemiological data indicate that of the seven most widely-used oral, non-aspirin NSAIDs, ibuprofen presents the lowest risk of upper gastrointestinal toxicity.

Hypersensitivity: Hypersensitivity reactions have been reported following treatment with ibuprofen. These may consist of (a) non-specific allergic reaction and anaphylaxis, (b) respiratory tract reactivity comprising asthma, aggravated asthma, bronchospasm or dyspnoea, or (c) assorted skin disorders, including rashes of various types, pruritus, urticaria, purpura, angioedema and, less commonly, bullous dermatoses (including epidermal necrolysis and erythema multiforme).

Cardiovascular: Oedema has been reported in association with ibuprofen treatment.

Other adverse events reported less commonly and for which causality has not necessarily been established include:

Renal: Nephrotoxicity in various forms, including interstitial nephritis, nephrotic syndrome and renal failure.

Hepatic: Abnormal liver function, hepatitis and jaundice.

Neurological & special senses: Visual disturbances, optic neuritis, headaches, paraesthesia, depression, confusion, hallucinations, tinnitus, vertigo, dizziness, malaise, fatigue and drowsiness.

Haematological: Thrombocytopenia, neutropenia, agranulocytosis, aplastic anaemia and haemolytic anaemia.

Dermatological: Photosensitivity (see 'hypersensitivity' for other skin reactions).

4.9 Overdose

Symptoms include nausea, vomiting, dizziness and rarely, loss of consciousness. Large overdoses are generally well tolerated when no other drugs are involved.

Treatment consists of gastric lavage and, if necessary, correction of serum electrolytes and appropriate supportive measures.

There is no specific antidote to ibuprofen.

5. PHARMACOLOGICAL PROPERTIES

5.1 Pharmacodynamic properties

Ibuprofen is a propionic acid derivative with analgesic, anti-inflammatory and anti-pyretic activity. The drug's therapeutic effects as an NSAID are thought to result from its inhibitory effect on the enzyme cyclo-oxygenase, which results in a marked reduction in prostaglandin synthesis.

5.2 Pharmacokinetic properties

Ibuprofen is rapidly absorbed from the gastrointestinal tract, peak serum concentrations occurring 1-2 hours after administration. The elimination half-life is approximately 2 hours.

Ibuprofen is metabolised in the liver to two inactive metabolites and these, together with unchanged ibuprofen, are excreted by the kidney either as such or as conjugates. Excretion by the kidney is both rapid and complete.

Ibuprofen is extensively bound to plasma proteins.

5.3 Preclinical safety data

Not applicable.

6. PHARMACEUTICAL PARTICULARS

6.1 List of excipients

Microcrystalline cellulose

Croscarmellose sodium

Lactose monohydrate

Colloidal anhydrous silica

Sodium lauryl sulphate

Magnesium stearate

Opadry white

or

Hydroxypropylmethylcellulose *plus* Talc *plus* Opaspray white M-1-7111B

Opacode S-1-8152HV black

Butanol

or

Industrial methylated spirit

Purified water

6.2 Incompatibilities

None.

6.3 Shelf life

36 months.

6.4 Special precautions for storage

Do not store above 30°C

6.5 Nature and contents of container

White high-density polyethylene bottle with a white polypropylene screw cap fitted with a waxed aluminium-faced pulpboard liner - pack size 12, 30, 100 tablets.

Not all pack sizes are marketed.

6.6 Instructions for use and handling

None.

7. MARKETING AUTHORISATION HOLDER

Abbott Laboratories Limited

Queenborough

Kent

ME11 5EL

United Kingdom

8. MARKETING AUTHORISATION NUMBER(S)

PL 00037/0335

9. DATE OF FIRST AUTHORISATION/RENEWAL OF THE AUTHORISATION

15 February 2002

10. DATE OF REVISION OF THE TEXT

Brufen Granules

(Abbott Laboratories Limited)

1. NAME OF THE MEDICINAL PRODUCT

Brufen Granules

2. QUALITATIVE AND QUANTITATIVE COMPOSITION

Ibuprofen BP 600 mg

3. PHARMACEUTICAL FORM

Effervescent granules

4. CLINICAL PARTICULARS

4.1 Therapeutic indications

Brufen Granules are indicated for their analgesic and anti-inflammatory effects in the treatment of rheumatoid arthritis, ankylosing spondylitis, osteoarthritis and other non-rheumatoid (seronegative) arthropathies.

In the treatment of non-articular rheumatic conditions, Brufen Granules are indicated in peri-articular conditions such as frozen shoulder (capsulitis), bursitis, tendinitis, tenosynovitis and low back pain; Brufen Granules can also be used in soft-tissue injuries such as sprains and strains.

Brufen Granules are also indicated for their analgesic effect in the relief of mild to moderate pain such as dysmenorrhoea, dental and post-operative pain and for symptomatic relief of headache including migraine headache.

4.2 Posology and method of administration

For oral administration.

Adults: The recommended dosage of Brufen is 1200-1800 mg daily in divided doses. Some patients can be maintained on 600-1200 mg daily. Total daily dose should not exceed 2400 mg.

Children: Brufen Granules are not suitable for use in children.

Elderly: No special dosage modifications are required unless renal or hepatic function is impaired, in which case dosage should be assessed individually.

4.3 Contraindications

Patients with a history of, or active, peptic ulceration. Patients who have previously shown hypersensitivity reactions (*e.g.* asthma, rhinitis or urticaria) in response to ibuprofen, aspirin or other non-steroidal anti-inflammatory drugs.

4.4 Special warnings and special precautions for use

Caution is required if Brufen is administered to patients suffering from, or with a previous history of, bronchial asthma since ibuprofen has been reported to cause bronchospasm in such patients. Brufen should only be given with care to patients with a history of gastrointestinal disease.

Caution is required in patients with renal, hepatic or cardiac impairment since the use of NSAIDs may result in deterioration of renal function. The dose should be kept as low as possible and renal function should be monitored in these patients.

Brufen should be given with care to patients with a history of heart failure or hypertension since oedema has been reported in association with ibuprofen administration.

Each Brufen Granules sachet contains 197 mg (approximately 9 mEq) sodium. This should be considered in patients whose overall intake of sodium must be markedly restricted.

4.5 Interaction with other medicinal products and other forms of Interaction

Care should be taken in patients treated with any of the following drugs as interactions have been reported in some patients.

Antihypertensives: Reduced antihypertensive effect.

Diuretics: Reduced diuretic effect. Diuretics can increase the risk of nephrotoxicity of NSAIDs.

Cardiac glycosides: NSAIDs may exacerbate cardiac failure, reduce GFR and increase plasma cardiac glycoside levels.

Lithium: Decreased elimination of lithium.

Methotrexate: Decreased elimination of methotrexate.

Cyclosporin: Increased risk of nephrotoxicity with NSAIDs.

Mifepristone: NSAIDs should not be used for 8-12 days after mifepristone administration as NSAIDs can reduce the effects of mifepristone.

Other analgesics: Avoid concomitant use of two or more NSAIDs.

Corticosteroids: Increased risk of gastrointestinal bleeding.

Anticoagulants: Enhanced anticoagulant effect.

Quinolone antibiotics: Animal data indicate that NSAIDs can increase the risk of convulsions associated with quinolone antibiotics. Patients taking NSAIDs and quinolones may have an increased risk of developing convulsions.

4.6 Pregnancy and lactation

Whilst no teratogenic effects have been demonstrated in animal toxicology studies, the use of ibuprofen during pregnancy should, if possible, be avoided. Congenital abnormalities have been reported in association with ibuprofen administration in man; however, these are low in frequency and do not appear to follow any discernible pattern. In view of the known effects of NSAIDs on the foetal cardiovascular system (closure of ductus arteriosus), use in late pregnancy should be avoided.

In the limited studies so far available, ibuprofen appears in the breast milk in very low concentrations and is unlikely to adversely affect the breast-fed infant.

4.7 Effects on ability to drive and use machines

No adverse effects known.

4.8 Undesirable effects

Gastrointestinal: The most commonly-observed adverse events are gastrointestinal in nature. Nausea, vomiting, diarrhoea, dyspepsia, abdominal pain, melaena, haematemesis, ulcerative stomatitis and gastrointestinal haemorrhage have been reported following ibuprofen administration. Less frequently, gastritis, duodenal ulcer, gastric ulcer and gastrointestinal perforation have been observed. Epidemiological data indicate that of the seven most widely-used oral, non-aspirin NSAIDs, ibuprofen presents the lowest risk of upper gastrointestinal toxicity.

Hypersensitivity: Hypersensitivity reactions have been reported following treatment with ibuprofen. These may consist of (a) non-specific allergic reaction and anaphylaxis, (b) respiratory tract reactivity comprising asthma, aggravated asthma, bronchospasm or dyspnoea, or (c) assorted skin disorders, including rashes of various types, pruritus, urticaria, purpura, angioedema and, less commonly, bullous dermatoses (including epidermal necrolysis and erythema multiforme).

Cardiovascular: Oedema has been reported in association with ibuprofen treatment.

Other adverse events reported less commonly and for which causality has not necessarily been established include:

Renal: Nephrotoxicity in various forms, including interstitial nephritis, nephrotic syndrome and renal failure.

Hepatic: Abnormal liver function, hepatitis and jaundice.

Neurological & special senses: Visual disturbances, optic neuritis, headaches, paraesthesia, depression, confusion, hallucinations, tinnitus, vertigo, dizziness, malaise, fatigue and drowsiness.

Haematological: Thrombocytopenia, neutropenia, agranulocytosis, aplastic anaemia and haemolytic anaemia.

Dermatological: Photosensitivity (see 'hypersensitivity' for other skin reactions).

4.9 Overdose

Symptoms include nausea, vomiting, dizziness and rarely, loss of consciousness. Large overdoses are generally well tolerated when no other drugs are involved.

Treatment consists of gastric lavage and, if necessary, correction of serum electrolytes and appropriate supportive measures.

There is no specific antidote to ibuprofen.

5. PHARMACOLOGICAL PROPERTIES

5.1 Pharmacodynamic properties

Ibuprofen is a propionic acid derivative with analgesic, anti-inflammatory and anti-pyretic activity. The drug's therapeutic effects as a non-steroidal anti-inflammatory drug are thought to result from its inhibitory effect on the enzyme cyclo-oxygenase, which results in a marked reduction in prostaglandin synthesis.

5.2 Pharmacokinetic properties

Ibuprofen is rapidly absorbed from the gastrointestinal tract, peak serum concentrations occurring 1-2 hours after administration. The elimination half-life is approximately 2 hours.

Ibuprofen is metabolised in the liver to two inactive metabolites and these, together with unchanged ibuprofen are excreted by the kidney either as such or as conjugates. Excretion by the kidney is both rapid and complete.

Ibuprofen is extensively bound to plasma proteins.

5.3 Preclinical safety data

Not applicable.

6. PHARMACEUTICAL PARTICULARS

6.1 List of excipients

Anhydrous sodium carbonate

Microcrystalline cellulose

Croscarmellose sodium

Malic acid

Sodium saccharin (76% saccharin)

Pulverised sugar

Povidone (K29-32)

Sodium bicarbonate

Orange flavour 57.403/TP05.51 firme

Sodium lauryl sulphate

Isopropyl alcohol

6.2 Incompatibilities

Not applicable.

6.3 Shelf life

3 years.

6.4 Special precautions for storage

Store below 25°C.

6.5 Nature and contents of container

A heat-sealed sachet consisting of a paper/polythene/aluminium foil/polythene laminate.

Pack sizes: 2, 3, 20, 21, 50, 100.

6.6 Instructions for use and handling

None stated.

7. MARKETING AUTHORISATION HOLDER

Abbott Laboratories Limited

Queenborough

Kent

ME11 5EL

United Kingdom

8. MARKETING AUTHORISATION NUMBER(S)

PL 00037/0337

9. DATE OF FIRST AUTHORISATION/RENEWAL OF THE AUTHORISATION

15 February 2002

10. DATE OF REVISION OF THE TEXT

Brufen Retard

(Abbott Laboratories Limited)

1. NAME OF THE MEDICINAL PRODUCT

Brufen Retard

2. QUALITATIVE AND QUANTITATIVE COMPOSITION

Active Ingredient: Ibuprofen BP (800 mg)

3. PHARMACEUTICAL FORM

Sustained-release tablets.

4. CLINICAL PARTICULARS

4.1 Therapeutic indications

Brufen Retard is indicated for its analgesic and anti-inflammatory effects in the treatment of rheumatoid arthritis (including juvenile rheumatoid arthritis or Still's disease), ankylosing spondylitis, osteoarthritis and other non-rheumatoid (seronegative) arthropathies.

In the treatment of non-articular rheumatic conditions, Brufen Retard is indicated in periarticular conditions such as frozen shoulder (capsulitis), bursitis, tendinitis, tenosynovitis and low back pain; Brufen Retard can also be used in soft-tissue injuries such as sprains and strains.

Brufen Retard is also indicated for its analgesic effect in the relief of mild to moderate pain such as dysmenorrhoea, dental and post-operative pain and for symptomatic relief of headache including migraine headache.

4.2 Posology and method of administration

Adults: Two tablets taken as a single daily dose, preferably in the early evening well before retiring to bed. The tablets should be swallowed whole with plenty of fluid. In severe or acute conditions, total daily dosage may be increased to three tablets in two divided doses.

Children: Not recommended for children under 12 years.

Elderly: No special dosage modifications are required unless renal or hepatic function is impaired, in which case dosage should be assessed individually.

For oral administration.

4.3 Contraindications

Patients with a history of, or active, peptic ulceration. Patients who have previously shown hypersensitivity reactions (*e.g.* asthma, rhinitis or urticaria) in response to ibuprofen, aspirin or other non-steroidal anti-inflammatory drugs (NSAIDs).

4.4 Special warnings and special precautions for use

Caution is required if Brufen Retard is administered to patients suffering from, or with a previous history of, bronchial asthma since ibuprofen has been reported to cause bronchospasm in such patients. Brufen Retard should only be given with care to patients with a history of gastrointestinal disease.

Caution is required in patients with renal, hepatic or cardiac impairment since the use of NSAIDs may result in deterioration of renal function. The dose should be kept as low as possible and renal function should be monitored in these patients.

Brufen Retard should be given with care to patients with a history of heart failure or hypertension since oedema has been reported in association with ibuprofen administration.

4.5 Interaction with other medicinal products and other forms of Interaction

Care should be taken in patients treated with any of the following drugs as interactions have been reported in some patients.

Antihypertensives: Reduced antihypertensive effect.

Diuretics: Reduced diuretic effect. Diuretics can increase the risk of nephrotoxicity of NSAIDs.

Cardiac glycosides: NSAIDs may exacerbate cardiac failure, reduce GFR and increase plasma cardiac glycoside levels.

Lithium: Decreased elimination of lithium.

Methotrexate: Decreased elimination of methotrexate.

Cyclosporin: Increased risk of nephrotoxicity with NSAIDs.

Mifepristone: NSAIDs should not be used for 8-12 days after mifepristone administration as NSAIDs can reduce the effects of mifepristone.

Other analgesics: Avoid concomitant use of two or more NSAIDs.

Corticosteroids: Increased risk of gastrointestinal bleeding.

Anticoagulants: Enhanced anticoagulant effect.

Quinolone antibiotics: Animal data indicate that NSAIDs can increase the risk of convulsions associated with quinolone antibiotics. Patients taking NSAIDs and quinolones may have an increased risk of developing convulsions.

4.6 Pregnancy and lactation

Whilst no teratogenic effects have been demonstrated in animal toxicology studies, the use of ibuprofen during pregnancy should, if possible, be avoided. Congenital abnormalities have been reported in association with ibuprofen administration in man; however, these are low in frequency and do not appear to follow any discernible pattern. In view of the known effects of NSAIDs on the foetal cardiovascular system (closure of ductus arteriosus), use in late pregnancy should be avoided.

In the limited studies so far available, ibuprofen appears in the breast milk in very low concentrations and is unlikely to adversely affect the breast-fed infant.

4.7 Effects on ability to drive and use machines

No adverse effects known.

4.8 Undesirable effects

Gastrointestinal: The most commonly-observed adverse events are gastrointestinal in nature. Nausea, vomiting, diarrhoea, dyspepsia, abdominal pain, melaena, haematemesis, ulcerative stomatitis and gastrointestinal haemorrhage have been reported following ibuprofen administration. Less frequently, gastritis, duodenal ulcer, gastric ulcer and gastrointestinal perforation have been observed. Epidemiological data indicate that of the seven most widely-used oral, non-aspirin NSAIDs, ibuprofen presents the lowest risk of upper gastrointestinal toxicity.

Hypersensitivity: Hypersensitivity reactions have been reported following treatment with ibuprofen. These may consist of (a) non-specific allergic reaction and anaphylaxis, (b) respiratory tract reactivity comprising asthma, aggravated asthma, bronchospasm or dyspnoea, or (c) assorted skin disorders, including rashes of various types, pruritus, urticaria, purpura, angioedema and, less commonly, bullous dermatoses (including epidermal necrolysis and erythema multiforme).

Cardiovascular: Oedema has been reported in association with ibuprofen treatment.

Other adverse events reported less commonly and for which causality has not necessarily been established include:

Renal: Nephrotoxicity in various forms, including interstitial nephritis, nephrotic syndrome and renal failure.

Hepatic: Abnormal liver function, hepatitis and jaundice.

Neurological & special senses: Visual disturbances, optic neuritis, headaches, paraesthesia, depression, confusion, hallucinations, tinnitus, vertigo, dizziness, malaise, fatigue and drowsiness.

Haematological: Thrombocytopenia, neutropenia, agranulocytosis, aplastic anaemia and haemolytic anaemia.

Dermatological: Photosensitivity (see 'hypersensitivity' for other skin reactions).

4.9 Overdose

Symptoms include nausea, vomiting, dizziness and rarely, loss of consciousness. Large overdoses are generally well tolerated when no other drugs are involved.

Gastric lavage may be of value for a considerable time after ingestion. The tablets may not be totally retrieved. If necessary, correct serum electrolytes and implement appropriate supportive measures.

There is no specific antidote to ibuprofen.

5. PHARMACOLOGICAL PROPERTIES

5.1 Pharmacodynamic properties

Ibuprofen is a propionic acid derivative with analgesic, anti-inflammatory and antipyretic activity. The drug's therapeutic effect as a NSAID is thought to result from its inhibitory activity on prostaglandin synthetases.

5.2 Pharmacokinetic properties

The pharmacokinetic profile of Brufen Retard compared with that of conventional-release 400mg tablets showed that the sustained-release formulation reduced the peaks and troughs characteristic of the conventional-release tablets and gave higher levels at 5, 10, 15 and 24 hours. Compared with conventional-release tablets, the area under the plasma concentration time curve for sustained-release tablets was almost identical.

Both mean plasma profiles and the pre-dose plasma levels showed no major differences between the young and elderly age groups. In several studies, Brufen Retard produced a double peak plasma profile when taken under fasting conditions. The elimination half-life of ibuprofen is approximately 2 hours. Ibuprofen is metabolised in the liver to two inactive metabolites and these, together with unchanged ibuprofen, are excreted by the kidney either as such or as conjugates. Excretion by the kidney is both rapid and complete. Ibuprofen is extensively bound to plasma proteins.

5.3 Preclinical safety data

None stated.

6. PHARMACEUTICAL PARTICULARS

6.1 List of excipients

Colloidal Silicon Dioxide NF, Isopropyl Alcohol BP, Povidone BP, Stearic Acid BPC PDR BPC, Xanthan Gum NF.

French Chalk for tablets (Talc EP) EP, Hydroxypropylmethylcellulose USP, Purified Water EP, Opaspray White M-1-7111B (Solids), Opacode S-1-9005 HV Red (Solids), Industrial Methylated Spirit BP.

6.2 Incompatibilities

None.

6.3 Shelf life

All packs: 36 months.

6.4 Special precautions for storage

HDPE bottle and nylon/aluminium/PVC blister: store cool, dry, below 25°C.

PVC/PVDC blister: store cool, dry, below 25°C.

6.5 Nature and contents of container

1. White pigmented HDPE bottle with a white polypropylene screw cap with a waxed aluminium pulp-board liner. Pack size: 60.

2. A blister consisting of 250 μm opaque PVC/40 gsm PVDC bonded to

20 μm aluminium foil. The blisters are packed in a cardboard carton.

Pack size: 8 or 56.

3. A blister consisting of 25 μm polyamide/40 μm aluminium/60 μm PVC bonded to 20 μm aluminium foil. The blisters are packed in a cardboard carton. Pack size: 8 or 56.

6.6 Instructions for use and handling

None.

7. MARKETING AUTHORISATION HOLDER

Abbott Laboratories Limited

Queenborough

Kent

ME11 5EL

United Kingdom

8. MARKETING AUTHORISATION NUMBER(S)

PL 00037/0338

9. DATE OF FIRST AUTHORISATION/RENEWAL OF THE AUTHORISATION

31 December 2001

10. DATE OF REVISION OF THE TEXT

Brufen Syrup

(Abbott Laboratories Limited)

1. NAME OF THE MEDICINAL PRODUCT

Brufen Syrup

2. QUALITATIVE AND QUANTITATIVE COMPOSITION

Ibuprofen BP 100 mg/5 ml

3. PHARMACEUTICAL FORM

An orange-coloured, orange-flavoured, syrupy suspension.

4. CLINICAL PARTICULARS

4.1 Therapeutic indications

Brufen Syrup is indicated for its analgesic and anti-inflammatory effects in the treatment of rheumatoid arthritis (including juvenile rheumatoid arthritis or Still's disease), ankylosing spondylitis, osteoarthritis and other non-rheumatoid (seronegative) arthropathies.

In the treatment of non-articular rheumatic conditions, Brufen Syrup is indicated in peri-articular conditions such as frozen shoulder (capsulitis), bursitis, tendinitis, tenosynovitis and low back pain; Brufen Syrup can also be used in soft-tissue injuries such as sprains and strains.

Brufen Syrup is also indicated for its analgesic effect in the relief of mild to moderate pain such as dysmenorrhoea, dental and post-operative pain and for symptomatic relief of headache including migraine headache.

Brufen Syrup is indicated in short-term use for the treatment of pyrexia in children over one year of age.

4.2 Posology and method of administration

Adults: The recommended dosage of Brufen is 1200-1800 mg daily in divided doses. Some patients can be maintained on 600-1200 mg daily. Total daily dose should not exceed 2400 mg.

Children: The daily dosage of Brufen is 20 mg/kg of bodyweight in divided doses. This can be achieved as follows:

1-2 years: One 2.5 ml spoonful (50 mg) three to four times a day.

3-7 years: One 5 ml spoonful (100 mg) three to four times a day.

8-12 years: Two 5 ml spoonfuls (200 mg) three to four times a day.

Not recommended for children weighing less than 7 kg.

In juvenile rheumatoid arthritis, up to 40 mg/kg of bodyweight daily in divided doses may be taken.

Elderly: No special dosage modifications are required unless renal or hepatic function is impaired, in which case dosage should be assessed individually.

For oral administration.

4.3 Contraindications

Patients with a history of, or active, peptic ulceration. Patients who have previously shown hypersensitivity reactions (*e.g.* asthma, rhinitis or urticaria) in response to ibuprofen, aspirin or other non-steroidal anti-inflammatory drugs.

4.4 Special warnings and special precautions for use

Caution is required if Brufen is administered to patients suffering from, or with a previous history of, bronchial asthma since ibuprofen has been reported to cause bronchospasm in such patients. Brufen should only be given with care to patients with a history of gastrointestinal disease.

Caution is required in patients with renal, hepatic or cardiac impairment since the use of NSAIDs may result in deterioration of renal function. The dose should be kept as low as possible and renal function should be monitored in these patients.

Brufen should be given with care to patients with a history of heart failure or hypertension since oedema has been reported in association with ibuprofen administration.

4.5 Interaction with other medicinal products and other forms of Interaction

Care should be taken in patients treated with any of the following drugs as interactions have been reported in some patients.

Antihypertensives: Reduced antihypertensive effect.

Diuretics: Reduced diuretic effect. Diuretics can increase the risk of nephrotoxicity of NSAIDs.

Cardiac glycosides: NSAIDs may exacerbate cardiac failure, reduce GFR and increase plasma cardiac glycoside levels.

Lithium: Decreased elimination of lithium.

Methotrexate: Decreased elimination of methotrexate.

Cyclosporin: Increased risk of nephrotoxicity with NSAIDs.

Mifepristone: NSAIDs should not be used for 8-12 days after mifepristone administration as NSAIDs can reduce the effects of mifepristone.

Other analgesics: Avoid concomitant use of two or more NSAIDs.

Corticosteroids: Increased risk of gastrointestinal bleeding.

Anticoagulants: Enhanced anticoagulant effect.

Quinolone antibiotics: Animal data indicate that NSAIDs can increase the risk of convulsions associated with quinolone antibiotics. Patients taking NSAIDs and quinolones may have an increased risk of developing convulsions.

4.6 Pregnancy and lactation

Whilst no teratogenic effects have been demonstrated in animal toxicology studies, the use of ibuprofen during pregnancy should, if possible, be avoided. Congenital abnormalities have been reported in association with ibuprofen administration in man; however, these are low in frequency and do not appear to follow any discernible pattern. In view of the known effects of NSAIDs on the foetal cardiovascular system (closure of ductus arteriosus), use in late pregnancy should be avoided.

In the limited studies so far available, ibuprofen appears in the breast milk in very low concentrations and is unlikely to adversely affect the breast-fed infant.

4.7 Effects on ability to drive and use machines

No adverse effects known.

4.8 Undesirable effects

Gastrointestinal: The most commonly-observed adverse events are gastrointestinal in nature. Nausea, vomiting, diarrhoea, dyspepsia, abdominal pain, melaena, haematemesis, ulcerative stomatitis and gastrointestinal haemorrhage have been reported following ibuprofen administration. Less frequently, gastritis, duodenal ulcer, gastric ulcer and gastrointestinal perforation have been observed. Epidemiological data indicate that of the seven most widely-used oral, non-aspirin NSAIDs, ibuprofen presents the lowest risk of upper gastrointestinal toxicity.

Hypersensitivity: Hypersensitivity reactions have been reported following treatment with ibuprofen. These may consist of (a) non-specific allergic reaction and anaphylaxis, (b) respiratory tract reactivity comprising asthma, aggravated asthma, bronchospasm or dyspnoea, or (c) assorted skin disorders, including rashes of various types, pruritus, urticaria, purpura, angioedema and, less commonly, bullous dermatoses (including epidermal necrolysis and erythema multiforme).

Cardiovascular: Oedema has been reported in association with ibuprofen treatment.

Other adverse events reported less commonly and for which causality has not necessarily been established include:

Renal: Nephrotoxicity in various forms, including interstitial nephritis, nephrotic syndrome and renal failure.

Hepatic: Abnormal liver function, hepatitis and jaundice.

Neurological & special senses: Visual disturbances, optic neuritis, headaches, paraesthesia, depression, confusion, hallucinations, tinnitus, vertigo, dizziness, malaise, fatigue and drowsiness.

Haematological: Thrombocytopenia, neutropenia, agranulocytosis, aplastic anaemia and haemolytic anaemia.

Dermatological: Photosensitivity (see 'hypersensitivity' for other skin reactions).

4.9 Overdose
Symptoms include nausea, vomiting, dizziness and rarely, loss of consciousness. Large overdoses are generally well tolerated when no other drugs are involved.

Treatment consists of gastric lavage and, if necessary, correction of serum electrolytes and appropriate supportive measures.

There is no specific antidote to ibuprofen.

5. PHARMACOLOGICAL PROPERTIES

5.1 Pharmacodynamic properties
Ibuprofen is a propionic acid derivative, having analgesic, antiinflammatory and antipyretic activity. The drug's therapeutic effects as a nonsteroidal anti-inflammatory drug are thought to result from inhibitory activity on prostaglandin synthetase.

5.2 Pharmacokinetic properties
Ibuprofen is rapidly absorbed from the gastrointestinal tract, peak serum concentrations occurring 1-2 hours after administration. Elimination half-life is approximately 2 hours.

Ibuprofen is metabolised in the liver to two inactive metabolites and these together with unchanged ibuprofen are excreted by the kidney either as such or as conjugates. Excretion by the kidney is both rapid and complete.

Ibuprofen is extensively bound to plasma proteins.

5.3 Preclinical safety data
Not applicable.

6. PHARMACEUTICAL PARTICULARS

6.1 List of excipients
Methyl hydroxybenzoate

Propyl hydroxybenzoate

Refined sugar

Citric acid monohydrate granular

Sodium benzoate

Agar powder

Glycerin

Sorbitol solution 70% (non-crystallising)

Irradiated light kaolin

Polysorbate 80

Sunset yellow

Orange flavour D717

Purified water

6.2 Incompatibilities
None known.

6.3 Shelf life
36 months.

6.4 Special precautions for storage
Store below 25°C and protect from light.

6.5 Nature and contents of container
An amber glass bottle with either a wadless polypropylene cap or a thermoset cap with an expanded polythene liner.

or

Amber-coloured polyethylene terephthalate bottle with a pilfer-proof neck finish, with a thermoplastic or a thermoset screw cap fitted with a low density polythene cone liner.

or

An amber-coloured polyethylene terephthalate (PET) bottle with an aluminium roll-on pilfer-proof cap fitted with an expanded polyethylene liner lined with a film of low-density polyethylene.

Pack sizes of 150, 200, 500 or 1000 ml for each of the containers.

6.6 Instructions for use and handling
None stated.

7. MARKETING AUTHORISATION HOLDER
Abbott Laboratories Limited

Queenborough

Kent

ME11 5EL

United Kingdom

8. MARKETING AUTHORISATION NUMBER(S)
PL 00037/0339

9. DATE OF FIRST AUTHORISATION/RENEWAL OF THE AUTHORISATION
15 February 2002

10. DATE OF REVISION OF THE TEXT

Budenofalk 3mg

(Dr Falk Pharma UK Limited)

1. NAME OF THE MEDICINAL PRODUCT
Budenofalk® 3 mg

2. QUALITATIVE AND QUANTITATIVE COMPOSITION
Hard capsule containing 3 mg budesonide in gastro-resistant granules.

For excipients, see 6.1

3. PHARMACEUTICAL FORM
Capsule, hard, gelatine, pink colour containing white gastro-resistant granules.

The colour of the capsule is pink.

4. CLINICAL PARTICULARS

4.1 Therapeutic indications
- Induction of remission in patients with mild to moderate active Crohn's disease affecting the ileum and/or the ascending colon.

- Symptomatic relief of chronic diarrhoea due to collagenous colitis.

Please note:

Treatment with Budenofalk® 3 mg does not appear useful in patients with Crohn's disease affecting the upper gastrointestinal tract. Extraintestinal symptoms, e.g. involving the skin, eyes or joints, are unlikely to respond to Budenofalk 3 mg because of its local action.

4.2 Posology and method of administration
Posology

Adults age > 18 years:

The recommended daily dose is one capsule (containing 3 mg budesonide) three times daily (morning, midday and evening) about a half hour before meals.

Children:

Budenofalk® 3 mg should not be taken by children due to insufficient experience in this age group.

Method of Administration:

The capsules containing the gastro-resistant pellets should be taken before meals, swallowed whole with plenty of fluid (e.g. a glass of water). The duration of treatment in active Crohns disease and in collagenous colitis should be limited to 8 weeks. The treatment with Budenofalk®3 mg should not be stopped abruptly, but withdrawn gradually (tapering doses). In the first week, the dosage should be reduced to two capsules daily, one in the morning, one in the evening. In the second week, only one capsule should be taken in the morning. Afterwards treatment can be stopped.

4.3 Contraindications
Budenofalk® 3 mg must not be used in:

- hypersensitivity to budesonide or any of the ingredients

- hepatic cirrhosis with signs of portal hypertension, eg. Late-stage primary biliary cirrhosis.

4.4 Special warnings and special precautions for use
Treatment with Budenofalk® 3 mg results in lower systemic steroid levels than conventional oral steroid therapy. Transfer from other steroid therapy may result in symptoms relating to the change in systemic steroid levels.

Caution is required in patients with tuberculosis, hypertension, diabetes mellitus, osteoporosis, peptic ulcer, glaucoma, cataracts, family history of diabetes, family history of glaucoma.

Infection: Suppression of the inflammatory response and immune function increases the susceptibility to infections and their severity. The risk of deterioration of bacterial, fungal, amoebic, and viral infections during glucocorticoid treatment should be carefully considered. The clinical presentation may often be atypical and serious infections such as septicaemia and tuberculosis may be masked and may reach an advanced stage before being recognised.

Chickenpox: Chickenpox is of particular concern since this normally minor illness may be fatal in immunosuppressed patients. Patients without a definite history of chickenpox should be advised to avoid close personal contact with chickenpox or herpes zoster and if exposed they should seek urgent medical attention. If the patient is a child, parents must be given the above advice. Passive immunisation with varicella zoster immunoglobulin (VZIG) is needed by exposed non-immune patients who are receiving systemic corticosteroids or who have used them within the previous 3 months; this should be given within 10 days of exposure to chickenpox. If a diagnosis of chickenpox is confirmed, the illness warrants specialist care and urgent treatment. Corticosteroids should not be stopped and the dose may need to be increased.

Measles: Patients with compromised immunity who have come into contact with measles should, wherever possible, receive normal immunoglobulin as soon as possible after exposure.

Live vaccines: Live vaccines should not be given to individuals with impaired immune responsiveness. The antibody response to other vaccines may be diminished. In patients with severe liver function disorders, the elimination of glucocorticosteroids including Budenofalk will be reduced, and their systemic bioavailability will be increased.

Corticosteroids may cause suppression of the HPA axis and reduce the stress response. Where patients are subject to surgery or other stresses, supplementary systemic glucocorticoid treatment is recommended. Concomitant treatment with ketoconazole or other CYP3A4 inhibitors should be avoided (see section 4.5)

4.5 Interaction with other medicinal products and other forms of Interaction
Pharmacodynamic interactions

Cardiac glycosides: The action of the glycoside can be potentiated by potassiumdeficiency.

Saluretics: Potassium excretion can be enhanced.

-Pharmacokinetic interactions

–Cytochrome P450:

- *CYP3A4 inhibitors:*

Ketoconazole 200 mg once daily p.o. increased the plasma concentrations of budesonide (3 mg single dose) approximately 6-fold during concomitant administration. When ketoconazole was administered 12 hours after budesonide, the concentrations increased approximately 3-fold. As there are not enough data to give dose recommendations, the combination should be avoided. Other potent inhibitors of CYP3A4, such as ritonavir, itraconazole and clarithromycin, are also likely to give a marked increase of the plasma concentrations of budesonide. In addition, concomitant intake of grapefruit juice should be avoided.

- *CYP3A4 inducers:*

Compounds or drugs such as carbamazepine and rifampicin, which induce CYP3A4, might reduce the systemic but also the local exposure of budesonide at the gut mucosa. An adjustment of the budesonide dose might be necessary.

- *CYP3A4 substrates:*

Compounds or drugs which are metabolized by CYP3A4 might be in competition with budesonide. This might lead to an increased budesonide plasma concentration if the competing substance has a stronger affinity to CYP3A4, or - if budesonide binds stronger to CYP3A4 - the competing substance might be increased in plasma and a doseadaption/ reduction of this drug might be required. Elevated plasma concentrations and enhanced effects of corticosteroids have been reported in women also receiving oestrogens or oral contraceptives, but this has not been observed with oral low dose combination contraceptives.

Cimetidine at recommended doses in combination with budesonide has a small but insignificant effect on pharmacokinetics of budesonide. Omeprazole has no effect on the pharmacokinetics of budesonide.

- *Steroid-binding compounds*

In theory, potential interactions with steroid-binding synthetic resins such as colestyramine, and with antacids cannot be ruled out. If given at the same time as Budenofalk®3 mg, such interactions could result in a reduction in the effect of budesonide. Therefore these preparations should not be taken simultaneously, but at least two hours apart.

4.6 Pregnancy and lactation
Administration during pregnancy should be avoided unless there are compelling reasons for Budenofalk® 3 mg therapy. In pregnant animals, budesonide, like other glucocorticosteroids, has been shown to cause abnormalities of foetal development. The relevance of this to man has not been established. Since it is not known if budesonide passes into breast milk, the infant should not be breastfed during treatment with Budenofalk® 3 mg.

4.7 Effects on ability to drive and use machines
No effects are known.

4.8 Undesirable effects
The following undesirable effects and frequencies of Budenofalk®3 mg have been spontaneously reported:

Very rare (< 1/10,000), including isolated reports:

Metabolism and nutritional disorders: oedema of legs, Cushing's syndrome

Nervous system disorders: Pseudotumor cerebri (including papilloedema) in adolescents

Gastrointestinal disorders: Constipation

Musculoskeletal, connective tissue and bone disorders: diffuse muscle pain and weakness, osteoporosis

General disorders: tiredness, malaise.

Some of the undesired effects were reported after long-term use. Occasionally side effects may occur which are typical for systemic glucocorticosteroids. These side effects depend on the dosage, the period of treatment, concomitant or previous treatment with other glucocorticosteroids and the individual sensitivity. Clinical studies showed that the frequency of glucocorticosteroid associated side effects is lower with Budenofalk® 3 mg (approx. by half) than with oral treatment of equivalent dosages of prednisolone.

Immune system disorders:

Interference with the immune response (e.g. increase in risk of infections). An exacerbation or the reappearance of extraintestinal manifestations (especially affecting skin and joints) can occur on switching a patient from the systemically acting glucocorticosteroids to the locally acting budesonide.

Metabolism and nutrition disorders:

Cushing's syndrome: moon-face, truncal obesity, reduced glucose tolerance, diabetes mellitus, sodium retention with oedema formation, increased excretion of potassium, inactivity or atrophy of the adrenal cortex, growth retardation in children, disturbance of sex hormone secretion (e.g. amenorrhoea, hirsutism, impotence).

Nervous system disorders:

depression, irritability, euphoria

Eyes disorders:

glaucoma, cataract

Vascular disorders:

hypertension, increased risk of thrombosis, vasculitis (withdrawal syndrome after long-term therapy)

Gastro intestinal disorders:

stomach complaints, duodenal ulcer, pancreatitis

Skin and subcutaneous tissue disorders:

allergic exanthema, red striae, petechiae, ecchymosis, steroid acne, delayed wound healing, contact dermatitis

Musculoskeletal, connective tissue and bone disorders:

aseptic necrosis of bone (femur and head of the humerus)

4.9 Overdose
To date, no cases of overdosage with budesonide are known. In view of the properties of budesonide contained in Budenofalk® 3 mg, an overdose resulting in toxic damage is extremely unlikely.

5. PHARMACOLOGICAL PROPERTIES

5.1 Pharmacodynamic properties
Pharmacotherapeutic group: Glucocorticosteroid ATC code: A07EA06 The exact mechanism of budesonide in the treatment of Crohn's disease is not fully understood. Data from clinical pharmacology studies and controlled clinical trials strongly indicate that the mode of action of Budenofalk® 3 mg capsules is predominantly based on a local action in the gut. Budesonide is a glucocorticosteroid with a high local anti-inflammatory effect. At doses clinically equivalent to systemically acting glucocorticosteroids, budesonide gives significantly less HPA axis suppression and has a lower impact on inflammatory markers.

Budenofalk® 3 mg capsules show a dose-dependent influence on cortisol plasma levels which is at the recommended dose of 3 × 3 mg budesonide/day significantly smaller than that of clinically equivalent effective doses of systemic glucocorticosteroids.

5.2 Pharmacokinetic properties
Absorption:

Budenofalk® 3 mg capsules, which contain gastric juice resistant pellets, have - due to the specific coating of the pellets - a lag phase of 2 - 3 hours. In healthy volunteers, as well as in patients with Crohn's disease, mean maximal budesonide plasma concentrations of 1 – 2ng/ml were seen at about 5 hours following an oral dose of Budenofalk® 3 mg capsules at a single dose of 3 mg, taken before meals. The maximal release therefore occurs in the terminal ileum and caecum, the main area of inflammation in Crohn's disease.

In ileostomy patients, release of budesonide from Budenofalk® 3 mg is comparable to healthy subjects or Crohn's disease patients. In ileostomy patients it was demonstrated that about 30-40% of released budesonide is still found in the ileostomy bag, indicating that a substantial amount of budesonide from Budenofalk®3 mg will be transferred normally into the colon. Concomitant intake of food may delay release of pellets from stomach by 2-3 hours, prolonging the lag phase to about 4-6 hours, without change in absorption rates.

Distribution:

Budesonide has a high volume of distribution (about 3 l/kg). Plasma protein binding averages 85 -90%.

Biotransformation:

Budesonide undergoes extensive biotransformation in the liver (approximately 90 %) to metabolites of low glucocorticosteroid activity. The glucocorticosteroid activity of the major metabolites, 6β-hydroxybudesonide and 16α-hydroxyprednisolone, is less than 1 % of that of budesonide.

Elimination:

The average elimination half-life is about 3 - 4 hours. The systemic availability in healthy volunteers as well as in fasting patients with Crohn's disease is about 9 - 13%. The clearance rate is about 10 - 15 l/min for budesonide, determined by HPLC-based methods.

Specific patient populations (liver diseases):

Dependent on the type and severity of liver diseases and due to the fact that budesonide is metabolised by CYP3A4, the metabolization of budesonide might be decreased. Therefore, the systemic exposure of budesonide might be increased in patients with impaired hepatic functions, as has been shown for patients with autoimmune hepatitis (AIH). With improving the liver function and disease, metabolization of budesonide will normalize.

The bioavailability of budesonide has been found to be significantly higher in patients in the late stages of primary biliary cirrhosis (PBC Stage IV) than in patients in the early stages of primary biliary cirrhosis (PBC Stage I/II); on average, the areas under the plasma concentration-time curves were threefold greater in patients with late stage PBC, following repeated administration of budesonide 3 × 3mg daily, than in patients with earlystage PBC.

5.3 Preclinical safety data
Preclinical data in acute, subchronic and chronic toxicological studies with budesonide showed atrophies of the thymus gland and adrenal cortex and a reduction especially of lymphocytes. These effects were less pronounced or at the same magnitude as observed with other glucocorticosteroids. Like with other glucocorticosteroids, and in dependence of the dose and duration and in dependence of the diseases, these steroid effects might also be of relevance in man.

Budesonide had no mutagenic effects in a number of *in vitro* and *in vivo* tests.

A slightly increased number of basophilic hepatic foci were observed in chronic rat studies with budesonide, and in carcinogenicity studies an increased incidence of primary hepatocellular neoplasms, astrocytomas (in male rats) and mammary tumors (female rats) observed. These tumors are probably due to the specific steroid receptor action, increased metabolic burden on the liver and anabolic effects, effects which are also known from other glucocorticosteroids in rat studies and therefore represent a class effect. No similar effects have ever been observed in man for budesonide, neither in clinical trials nor from spontaneous reports.

In general, preclinical data reveal no special hazard for humans based on conventional studies of safety pharmacology, repeated dose toxicity, genotoxicity, carcinogenic potential. In pregnant animals, budesonide, like other glucocorticosteroids, has been shown to cause abnormalities of foetal development. But the relevance to man has not been established (see also section 4.6).

6. PHARMACEUTICAL PARTICULARS

6.1 List of excipients
Povidone K25, Lactose monohydrate, Sucrose, Talc, Maize starch, Methacrylic acid, methylmethacrylate copolymer (1:1) (Eudragit L 100), Methacrylic acid, methylmethacrylate copolymer (1:2) (Eudragit S 100), Poly(ethylacrylic acid, methylmethacrylate, trimethylammonium ethylmethacrylate chloride) (1:2:0.1) (Eudragit RS12.5), Poly (ethylacrylate, methylmethacrylate, trimethylammonium ethylmethacrylate chloride) (1:2:0.2) (Eudragit RL12.5), Dibutyl phthalate, Titanium dioxide (E 171), Water, Gelatin, Erythrosine (E127), Red iron oxide (E 172), Black iron oxide (E172), sodium laurilsulphate.

6.2 Incompatibilities
Not applicable

6.3 Shelf life
3 years.

This medicinal product must not be used after the expiry date.

6.4 Special precautions for storage
Do not store above 25 °C.

6.5 Nature and contents of container
Al/PVC/PVDC blister strips in cartons with 10, 50 and 90, 100, 120 capsules. Not all pack sizes may be marketed.

6.6 Instructions for use and handling
None

7. MARKETING AUTHORISATION HOLDER
Dr. Falk Pharma GmbH

Leinenweberstr. 5

D-79108 Freiburg

Postfach 6529

D-79041 Freiburg

8. MARKETING AUTHORISATION NUMBER(S)
PL 08637/0002

9. DATE OF FIRST AUTHORISATION/RENEWAL OF THE AUTHORISATION
January 4, 1999

10. DATE OF REVISION OF THE TEXT
April 2004

Bumetanide Injection 0.5mg/ml, solution for injection

(Leo Laboratories Limited)

1. NAME OF THE MEDICINAL PRODUCT
Bumetanide Injection 0.5 mg/ml, solution for injection.

2. QUALITATIVE AND QUANTITATIVE COMPOSITION
Bumetanide Ph Eur 0.5 mg/ml.

3. PHARMACEUTICAL FORM
Solution for injection.

4. CLINICAL PARTICULARS

4.1 Therapeutic indications
Bumetanide is indicated whenever diuretic therapy is required in the treatment of oedema, e.g. that associated with congestive heart failure, cirrhosis of the liver and renal disease including the nephrotic syndrome.

For those oedematous conditions where a prompt diuresis is required, Bumetanide Injection 0.5 mg/ml may be used, e.g. acute pulmonary oedema, acute and chronic renal failure. Bumetanide Injection 0.5 mg/ml can be given intravenously or intramuscularly to those patients who are unable to take Burinex Tablets or who fail to respond satisfactorily to oral therapy.

4.2 Posology and method of administration
Route of administration: parenteral.

Pulmonary oedema: Initially 1 - 2 mg by intravenous injection. This can be repeated, if necessary, 20 minutes later.

In those conditions in which an infusion is appropriate, 2 - 5 mg may be given in 500 ml infusion fluid over 30 - 60 minutes. (See Section 4.4, special warnings and precautions for use).

When intramuscular administration is considered appropriate, a dose of 1 mg should be given initially and the dose then adjusted according to diuretic response.

Children: not recommended for children under 12 years of age.

Dosage in the elderly: adjust dosage according to response. A dose of 0.5 mg bumetanide per day may be sufficient in some elderly patients.

4.3 Contraindications
Although bumetanide can be used to induce diuresis in renal insufficiency, any marked increase in blood urea or the development of oliguria or anuria during treatment of severe progressing renal disease are indications for stopping treatment with bumetanide.

Hypersensitivity to any of the ingredients. Bumetanide is contra-indicated in hepatic coma and care should be taken in states of severe electrolyte depletion.

As with other diuretics, bumetanide should not be administered concurrently with lithium salts. Diuretics can reduce lithium clearance resulting in high serum levels of lithium.

4.4 Special warnings and special precautions for use
Excessively rapid mobilisation of oedema, particularly in elderly patients, may give rise to sudden changes in cardiovascular pressure-flow relationships with circulatory collapse. This should be borne in mind when bumetanide is given in high doses intravenously or orally. Electrolyte disturbances may occur, particularly in those patients taking a low salt diet. Regular checks of serum electrolytes, in particular sodium, potassium, chloride and bicarbonate should be performed and replacement therapy instituted where indicated.

Like other diuretics, bumetanide shows a tendency to increase the excretion of potassium which can lead to an increase in the sensitivity of the myocardium to the toxic effects of digitalis. Thus the dose may need adjustment when given in conjunction with cardiac glycosides.

Bumetanide may potentiate the effects of antihypertensive drugs. Therefore, the dose of the latter may need adjustment when bumetanide is used to treat oedema in hypertensive patients.

As with other diuretics, bumetanide may cause an increase in blood uric acid. Periodic checks on urine and blood glucose should be made in diabetics and patients suspected of latent diabetes.

Patients with chronic renal failure on high doses of bumetanide should remain under constant hospital supervision.

Pharmaceutical precautions

Bumetanide Injection 0.5 mg/ml is presented in amber glass containers to protect against deterioration due to exposure to light.

When an intravenous infusion is required, Bumetanide Injection 0.5 mg/ml may be added to Dextrose Injection BP, Sodium Chloride Injection BP or Sodium Chloride and Dextrose Injection BP.

When 25 mg bumetanide (as Bumetanide Injection 0.5 mg/ml) was added to 1 litre of these infusion fluids, no evidence of precipitation was observed over a period of 72 hours. Higher concentrations of bumetanide in these infusion fluids may cause precipitation. It is good practice to inspect all infusion fluids containing bumetanide from time to time. Should cloudiness appear, the infusion should be discarded.

4.5 Interaction with other medicinal products and other forms of Interaction
See Section 4.4 above.

4.6 Pregnancy and lactation
Although tests in four animal species have shown no teratogenic effects, the ordinary precaution of avoiding use of bumetanide in the first trimester of pregnancy should at present be observed. Since it is not known whether bumetanide is distributed into breast milk, a nursing mother should either stop breast feeding or observe the infant for any adverse effects if the drug is absolutely necessary for the mother.

4.7 Effects on ability to drive and use machines
None known.

4.8 Undesirable effects
Reported reactions include skin rashes and muscular cramps in the legs, abdominal discomfort, thrombocytopenia and gynaecomastia. Bone marrow depression associated with the use of bumetanide has been reported rarely, but it has not been proven definitely to be attributed to the drug. Hearing disturbance after administration of bumetanide is rare and reversible. The possibility of hearing disturbance must be considered, particularly when bumetanide is injected too quickly and in high doses.

High Dose Therapy

In patients with severe chronic renal failure given high doses of bumetanide, there have been reports of severe, generalised, musculoskeletal pain sometimes associated with muscle spasm, occurring one to two hours after administration and lasting up to 12 hours. The lowest reported dose causing this type of adverse reaction was 5 mg by intravenous injection and the highest was 75 mg orally in a single dose. All patients recovered fully and there was no deterioration in their renal function.

The cause of this pain is uncertain but it may be a result of varying electrolyte gradients at the cell membrane level.

Experience suggests that the incidence of such reactions is reduced by initiating treatment at 5-10 mg daily and titrating upwards using a twice daily dosage regimen at doses of 20 mg per day or more.

4.9 Overdose
Symptoms would be those caused by excessive diuresis. General measures should be taken to restore blood volume, maintain blood pressure and correct electrolyte disturbance.

5. PHARMACOLOGICAL PROPERTIES

5.1 Pharmacodynamic properties
Mode of action: bumetanide is a potent high ceiling diuretic with a rapid onset and a short duration of action.

5.2 Pharmacokinetic properties
After intravenous injection, diuresis usually starts within a few minutes and ceases in about two hours.

In most patients, 1mg of bumetanide produces a similar diuretic effect to 40 mg frusemide. Bumetanide excretion in the urine shows a good correlation with the diuretic response. In patients with chronic renal failure, the liver takes more importance as an excretory pathway although the duration of action in such patients is not markedly prolonged.

5.3 Preclinical safety data
There are no pre-clinical data of relevance to the prescriber which are additional to that already included in other sections of the SPC.

6. PHARMACEUTICAL PARTICULARS

6.1 List of excipients
Xylitol, disodium hydrogen phosphate dihydrate, sodium dihydrogen phosphate dihydrate and water for injections.

6.2 Incompatibilities
None known

6.3 Shelf life
3 years.

6.4 Special precautions for storage
Do not store above 25°C.

6.5 Nature and contents of container
5 × 4 ml amber glass ampoules (OP), each ampoule containing 2mg bumetanide.

6.6 Instructions for use and handling
None.

7. MARKETING AUTHORISATION HOLDER
Leo Laboratories Limited

Longwick Road

Princes Risborough

Bucks HP27 9RR

UK

8. MARKETING AUTHORISATION NUMBER(S)
PL 0043/0060

9. DATE OF FIRST AUTHORISATION/RENEWAL OF THE AUTHORISATION
24 November 1978/13 January 1995.

10. DATE OF REVISION OF THE TEXT
April 2001.

LEGAL CATEGORY
POM

Bumetanide Liquid 0.2mg/ml oral solution

(Leo Laboratories Limited)

1. NAME OF THE MEDICINAL PRODUCT
Bumetanide Liquid 0.2 mg/ml oral solution

2. QUALITATIVE AND QUANTITATIVE COMPOSITION
Bumetanide Ph Eur 0.2 mg/ml

3. PHARMACEUTICAL FORM
Oral solution.

4. CLINICAL PARTICULARS

4.1 Therapeutic indications
Bumetanide is indicated whenever diuretic therapy is required in the treatment of oedema, e.g. that associated with congestive heart failure, cirrhosis of the liver and renal disease including the nephrotic syndrome.

4.2 Posology and method of administration
For oral administration.

Adults: Usually 1 mg (5 ml) as a single oral dose given morning or early evening. The dosage should be adjusted according to the patient's response.

Children: Not recommended for children under 12 years of age.

Elderly: Adjust dosage according to response: a dose of 0.5 mg bumetanide per day may be sufficient in some elderly patients.

4.3 Contraindications
Although bumetanide can be used to induce diuresis in renal insufficiency, any marked increase in blood urea or the development of oliguria or anuria during treatment of severe progressing renal disease are indications for stopping treatment with bumetanide.

Hypersensitivity to any of the ingredients. Bumetanide is contra-indicated in hepatic coma and care should be taken in states of severe electrolyte depletion.

As with other diuretics, bumetanide should not be administered concurrently with lithium salts. Diuretics can reduce lithium clearance resulting in high serum levels of lithium.

4.4 Special warnings and special precautions for use
Excessively rapid mobilisation of oedema particularly in elderly patients may give rise to sudden changes in cardiovascular pressure flow relationships with circulatory collapse. This should be borne in mind when bumetanide is given in high doses. Electrolyte disturbances may occur, particularly in those patients taking a low salt diet. Regular checks of serum electrolytes, in particular sodium, potassium, chloride and bicarbonate should be performed and replacement therapy instituted where indicated.

As with other diuretics, bumetanide may cause an increase in blood uric acid. Periodic checks on urine and blood glucose should be made in diabetics and patients suspected of latent diabetes.

Patients with chronic renal failure on high doses of bumetanide should remain under constant hospital supervision.

Bumetanide should be used with caution in patients already receiving nephrotoxic or ototoxic drugs.

4.5 Interaction with other medicinal products and other forms of Interaction
Like other diuretics, bumetanide shows a tendency to increase the excretion of potassium which can lead to an increase in the sensitivity of the myocardium to the toxic effects of digitalis. Thus the dose may need adjustment when given in conjunction with cardiac glycosides.

Bumetanide may potentiate the effects of antihypertensive drugs. Therefore, the dose of the latter may need adjustment when bumetanide is used to treat oedema in hypertensive patients.

Certain non-steroidal anti-inflammatory drugs have been shown to antagonise the action of diuretics.

4.6 Pregnancy and lactation
Although tests in four animal species have shown no teratogenic effects, the ordinary precaution of avoiding use of bumetanide in the first trimester of pregnancy should at present be observed.

4.7 Effects on ability to drive and use machines
None stated.

4.8 Undesirable effects
Reported reactions include skin rashes and muscular cramps in the legs, abdominal discomfort, thrombocytopenia and gynaecomastia. Bone marrow depression associated with the use of bumetanide has been reported rarely but it has not been proven definitely to be attributed to the drug. Hearing disturbance after administration of bumetanide is rare and reversible.

High Dose Therapy

In patients with severe chronic renal failure given high doses of bumetanide, there have been reports of severe, generalised, musculoskeletal pain sometimes associated with muscle spasm, occurring one or two hours after administration and lasting up to 12 hours. The lowest reported dose causing this type of adverse reaction was 5 mg by intravenous injection and the highest was 75 mg orally in a single dose. All patients recovered fully and there was no deterioration in their renal function. The cause of this pain is uncertain but it may be a result of varying electrolyte gradients at the cell membrane level.

Experience suggests that the incidence of such reactions is reduced by initiating treatment at 5-10 mg daily and titrating upwards using a twice daily dosage regimen at doses of 20 mg per day or more.

4.9 Overdose
Symptoms would be those caused by excessive diuresis. Empty stomach by gastric lavage or emesis. General measures should be taken to restore blood volume, maintain blood pressure and correct electrolyte disturbance.

5. PHARMACOLOGICAL PROPERTIES

5.1 Pharmacodynamic properties
Bumetanide is a potent, high ceiling diuretic with a rapid onset and a short duration of action.

5.2 Pharmacokinetic properties
After oral administration of 1 mg bumetanide, diuresis begins within 30 minutes with a peak effect between one and two hours. The diuretic effect is virtually complete in three hours after a 1 mg dose.

In most patients 1 mg of bumetanide produces a similar diuretic effect to 40 mg of furosemide.

Bumetanide is well absorbed after oral administration. Bumetanide excretion in the urine shows a good correlation with the diuretic response. In patients with chronic renal failure, the liver takes more importance as an excretory pathway, although the duration of action in such patients is not markedly prolonged.

5.3 Preclinical safety data
There are no preclinical data of relevance to the prescriber which are additional to that already included in other sections of the SPC.

6. PHARMACEUTICAL PARTICULARS

6.1 List of excipients
Methyl-para-hydroxybenzoate, propyl-para-hydroxybenzoate, sorbitol, xanthan gum, sodium citrate, patent blue V, quinoline yellow, peppermint flavour, purified water.

6.2 Incompatibilities
None known.

6.3 Shelf life
3 years.

6.4 Special precautions for storage
Store below 25°C.

6.5 Nature and contents of container
Amber glass bottles, with plastic screw caps, of 150 ml (OP) supplied with a polypropylene measuring cup with graduations at 2.5, 5, 10, 15 and 20 ml.

6.6 Instructions for use and handling
None.

7. MARKETING AUTHORISATION HOLDER
LEO Laboratories Limited

Longwick Road

Princes Risborough

Bucks. HP27 9RR.

8. MARKETING AUTHORISATION NUMBER(S)
PL 0043/0075

9. DATE OF FIRST AUTHORISATION/RENEWAL OF THE AUTHORISATION
29 July 1983 / 19 May 1999

10. DATE OF REVISION OF THE TEXT
January 2004.

LEGAL CATEGORY
POM

Burinex 1mg Tablets

(Leo Laboratories Limited)

1. NAME OF THE MEDICINAL PRODUCT
Burinex® 1 mg Tablets.

2. QUALITATIVE AND QUANTITATIVE COMPOSITION
Bumetanide Ph Eur 1 mg.

3. PHARMACEUTICAL FORM
Tablet.

4. CLINICAL PARTICULARS

4.1 Therapeutic indications
Burinex is indicated whenever diuretic therapy is required in the treatment of oedema, e.g. that associated with congestive heart failure, cirrhosis of the liver and renal disease including the nephrotic syndrome.

In oedema of cardiac or renal origin where high doses of a potent short acting diuretic are required, Burinex 5 mg tablets may be used.

4.2 Posology and method of administration
For oral administration.

Most patients require a daily dose of 1 mg which can be given as a single morning or early evening dose. Depending on the patient's response, a second dose can be given six to eight hours later. In refractory cases, the dose can be increased until a satisfactory diuretic response is obtained, or infusions of Burinex can be given.

Children: not recommended for children under 12 years of age.

Dosage in the elderly: adjust dosage according to response. A dose of 0.5 mg bumetanide per day may be sufficient in some elderly patients.

4.3 Contraindications
Although Burinex can be used to induce diuresis in renal insufficiency, any marked increase in blood urea or the development of oliguria or anuria during treatment of severe progressing renal disease are indications for stopping treatment with Burinex.

Hypersensitivity to Burinex. Burinex is contra-indicated in hepatic coma and care should be taken in states of severe electrolyte depletion.

As with other diuretics, Burinex should not be administered concurrently with lithium salts. Diuretics can reduce lithium clearance resulting in high serum levels of lithium.

4.4 Special warnings and special precautions for use

Excessively rapid mobilisation of oedema, particularly in elderly patients, may give rise to sudden changes in cardiovascular pressure-flow relationships with circulatory collapse. This should be borne in mind when Burinex is given in high doses intravenously or orally. Electrolyte disturbances may occur, particularly in those patients taking a low salt diet. Regular checks of serum electrolytes, in particular sodium, potassium, chloride and bicarbonate, should be performed and replacement therapy instituted where indicated.

Encephalopathy may be precipitated in patients with pre-existing hepatic impairment.

Burinex should be used with caution in patients already receiving nephrotoxic or ototoxic drugs.

4.5 Interaction with other medicinal products and other forms of Interaction

Like other diuretics, Burinex shows a tendency to increase the excretion of potassium which can lead to an increase in the sensitivity of the myocardium to the toxic effects of digitalis. Thus the dose may need adjustment when given in conjunction with cardiac glycosides.

Burinex may potentiate the effects of antihypertensive drugs. Therefore, the dose of the latter may need adjustment when Burinex is used to treat oedema in hypertensive patients.

As with other diuretics, Burinex may cause an increase in blood uric acid. Periodic checks on urine and blood glucose should be made in diabetics and patients suspected of latent diabetes.

Patients with chronic renal failure on high doses of Burinex should remain under constant hospital supervision.

Certain non-steroidal anti-inflammatory drugs have been shown to antagonise the action of diuretics.

4.6 Pregnancy and lactation

Although tests in four animal species have shown no teratogenic effects, the ordinary precaution of avoiding use of Burinex in the first trimester of pregnancy should at present be observed. Since it is not known whether bumetanide is distributed into breast milk, a nursing mother should either stop breast feeding or observe the infant for any adverse effects if the drug is absolutely necessary for the mother.

4.7 Effects on ability to drive and use machines

None known.

4.8 Undesirable effects

Reported reactions include abdominal pain, vomiting, dyspepsia, diarrhoea, stomach and muscle cramps, arthralgia, dizziness, fatigue, hypotension, headache, nausea, encephalopathy (in patients with pre-existing hepatic disease), fluid and electrolyte depletion, dehydration, hyperuricaemia, raised blood urea and serum creatinine, hyperglycaemia, abnormalities of serum levels of hepatic enzymes, skin rashes, pruritus, urticaria, thrombocytopenia, gynaecomastia and painful breasts. Bone marrow depression associated with the use of Burinex has been reported rarely but it has not been proven definitely to be attributed to the drug. Hearing disturbance after administration of Burinex is rare and reversible.

High dose therapy:

In patients with severe chronic renal failure given high doses of Burinex, there have been reports of severe, generalised musculoskeletal pain sometimes associated with muscle spasm, occurring one to two hours after administration and lasting up to 12 hours. The lowest reported dose causing this type of adverse reaction was 5 mg by intravenous injection and the highest was 75 mg orally in a single dose. All patients recovered fully and there was no deterioration in their renal function. The cause of this pain is uncertain but it may be a result of varying electrolyte gradients at the cell membrane level.

Experience suggests that the incidence of such reactions is reduced by initiating treatment at 5-10 mg daily and titrating upwards using a twice daily dosage regimen at doses of 20 mg per day or more.

4.9 Overdose

Symptoms would be those caused by excessive diuresis. Empty stomach by gastric lavage or emesis. General measures should be taken to restore blood volume, maintain blood pressure and correct electrolyte disturbance.

5. PHARMACOLOGICAL PROPERTIES

5.1 Pharmacodynamic properties

Burinex is a potent, high ceiling loop diuretic with a rapid onset and a short duration of action. The primary site of action is the ascending limb of the Loop of Henlé where it exerts inhibiting effects on electrolyte reabsorption causing the diuretic and natriuretic action observed.

After oral administration of 1 mg Burinex, diuresis begins within 30 minutes with a peak effect between one and two hours. The diuretic effect is virtually complete in three hours after a 1 mg dose.

5.2 Pharmacokinetic properties

Burinex is well absorbed after oral administration with the bioavailability reaching between 80 and 95%. The elimination half life ranges from between 0.75 to 2.6 hours. No active metabolites are known. Renal excretion accounts for approximately half the clearance with hepatic excretion responsible for the other half. There is an increase in half-life and a reduced plasma clearance in the presence of renal or hepatic disease. In patients with chronic renal failure the liver takes more importance as an excretory pathway although the duration of action is not markedly prolonged.

5.3 Preclinical safety data

There are no pre-clinical data of relevance to the prescriber which are additional to that already included in other sections of the SPC.

6. PHARMACEUTICAL PARTICULARS

6.1 List of excipients

Maize starch, lactose, colloidal anhydrous silica, polyvidone, polysorbate 80, agar powder, talc and magnesium stearate.

6.2 Incompatibilities

None known

6.3 Shelf life

5 years.

6.4 Special precautions for storage

None.

6.5 Nature and contents of container

Blister packs of 28 tablets (OP).

6.6 Instructions for use and handling

None.

7. MARKETING AUTHORISATION HOLDER

Leo Laboratories Limited

Longwick Road

Princes Risborough

Bucks HP27 9RR

UK

8. MARKETING AUTHORISATION NUMBER(S)

PL 0043/0021R

9. DATE OF FIRST AUTHORISATION/RENEWAL OF THE AUTHORISATION

27 June 1996.

10. DATE OF REVISION OF THE TEXT

February 2001.

LEGAL CATEGORY

POM

Burinex 5mg Tablets

(Leo Laboratories Limited)

1. NAME OF THE MEDICINAL PRODUCT

Burinex® 5 mg Tablets.

2. QUALITATIVE AND QUANTITATIVE COMPOSITION

Bumetanide Ph Eur 5 mg.

3. PHARMACEUTICAL FORM

Tablet.

4. CLINICAL PARTICULARS

4.1 Therapeutic indications

Burinex is indicated whenever diuretic therapy is required in the treatment of oedema, e.g. that associated with congestive heart failure, cirrhosis of the liver and renal disease including the nephrotic syndrome.

In oedema of cardiac or renal origin where high doses of a potent short acting diuretic are required, Burinex 5 mg tablets may be used.

4.2 Posology and method of administration

For oral administration.

The dose should be carefully titrated in each patient according to the patient's response and the required therapeutic activity. As a general rule, in patients not controlled on lower doses, dosage should be started at 5 mg daily and then increased by 5 mg increments every 12-24 hours until the required response is obtained or side-effects appear.

Consideration should be given to a twice daily dosage rather than once daily. Direct substitution of Burinex for frusemide in a 1:40 ratio at high doses should be avoided. Treatment should be initiated at a lower equivalent dose and gradually increased in 5 mg increments.

Children: not recommended for children under 12 years of age.

Dosage in the elderly: adjust dosage according to response. A dose of 0.5 mg bumetanide per day may be sufficient in some elderly patients.

4.3 Contraindications

Although Burinex can be used to induce diuresis in renal insufficiency, any marked increase in blood urea or the development of oliguria or anuria during treatment of severe progressing renal disease are indications for stopping treatment with Burinex.

Hypersensitivity to Burinex. Burinex is contra-indicated in hepatic coma and care should be taken in states of severe electrolyte depletion.

As with other diuretics, Burinex should not be administered concurrently with lithium salts. Diuretics can reduce lithium clearance resulting in high serum levels of lithium.

4.4 Special warnings and special precautions for use

Excessively rapid mobilisation of oedema, particularly in elderly patients, may give rise to sudden changes in cardiovascular pressure-flow relationships with circulatory collapse. This should be borne in mind when Burinex is given in high doses intravenously or orally. Electrolyte disturbances may occur, particularly in those patients taking a low salt diet. Regular checks of serum electrolytes, in particular sodium, potassium, chloride and bicarbonate, should be performed and replacement therapy instituted where indicated.

Encephalopathy may be precipitated in patients with pre-existing hepatic impairment.

Burinex should be used with caution in patients already receiving nephrotoxic or ototoxic drugs.

4.5 Interaction with other medicinal products and other forms of Interaction

Like other diuretics, Burinex shows a tendency to increase the excretion of potassium which can lead to an increase in the sensitivity of the myocardium to the toxic effects of digitalis. Thus the dose may need adjustment when given in conjunction with cardiac glycosides.

Burinex may potentiate the effects of antihypertensive drugs. Therefore, the dose of the latter may need adjustment when Burinex is used to treat oedema in hypertensive patients.

As with other diuretics, Burinex may cause an increase in blood uric acid. Periodic checks on urine and blood glucose should be made in diabetics and patients suspected of latent diabetes.

Patients with chronic renal failure on high doses of Burinex should remain under constant hospital supervision.

Certain non-steroidal anti-inflammatory drugs have been shown to antagonise the action of diuretics.

4.6 Pregnancy and lactation

Although tests in four animal species have shown no teratogenic effects, the ordinary precaution of avoiding use of Burinex in the first trimester of pregnancy should at present be observed. Since it is not known whether bumetanide is distributed into breast milk, a nursing mother should either stop breast feeding or observe the infant for any adverse effects if the drug is absolutely necessary for the mother.

4.7 Effects on ability to drive and use machines

None known.

4.8 Undesirable effects

Reported reactions include abdominal pain, vomiting, dyspepsia, diarrhoea, stomach and muscle cramps, arthralgia, dizziness, fatigue, hypotension, headache, nausea, encephalopathy (in patients with pre-existing hepatic disease), fluid and electrolyte depletion, dehydration, hyperuricaemia, raised blood urea and serum creatinine, hyperglycaemia, abnormalities of serum levels of hepatic enzymes, skin rashes, pruritus, urticaria, thrombocytopenia, gynaecomastia and painful breasts. Bone marrow depression associated with the use of Burinex has been reported rarely but it has not been proven definitely to be attributed to the drug. Hearing disturbance after administration of Burinex is rare and reversible.

High dose therapy:

In patients with severe chronic renal failure given high doses of Burinex, there have been reports of severe, generalised musculoskeletal pain sometimes associated with muscle spasm, occurring one to two hours after administration and lasting up to 12 hours. The lowest reported dose causing this type of adverse reaction was 5 mg by intravenous injection and the highest was 75 mg orally in a single dose. All patients recovered fully and there was no deterioration in their renal function. The cause of this pain is uncertain but it may be a result of varying electrolyte gradients at the cell membrane level.

Experience suggests that the incidence of such reactions is reduced by initiating treatment at 5-10 mg daily and titrating upwards using a twice daily dosage regimen at doses of 20 mg per day or more.

4.9 Overdose

Symptoms would be those caused by excessive diuresis. Empty stomach by gastric lavage or emesis. General measures should be taken to restore blood volume, maintain blood pressure and correct electrolyte disturbance.

5. PHARMACOLOGICAL PROPERTIES

5.1 Pharmacodynamic properties

Burinex is a potent, high ceiling loop diuretic with a rapid onset and a short duration of action. The primary site of action is the ascending limb of the Loop of Henlé where it exerts inhibiting effects on electrolyte reabsorption causing the diuretic and natriuretic action observed.

After oral administration of 1 mg Burinex, diuresis begins within 30 minutes with a peak effect between one and two hours. The diuretic effect is virtually complete in three hours after a 1 mg dose.

5.2 Pharmacokinetic properties

Burinex is well absorbed after oral administration with the bioavailability reaching between 80 and 95%. The elimination half life ranges from between 0.75 to 2.6 hours. No active metabolites are known. Renal excretion accounts for approximately half the clearance with hepatic excretion responsible for the other half. There is an increase in half-life and a reduced plasma clearance in the presence of renal or hepatic disease. In patients with chronic renal failure the liver takes more importance as an excretory pathway although the duration of action is not markedly prolonged.

5.3 Preclinical safety data
There are no pre-clinical data of relevance to the prescriber which are additional to that already included in other sections of the SPC.

6. PHARMACEUTICAL PARTICULARS

6.1 List of excipients
Maize starch, lactose, colloidal anhydrous silica, polyvidone, polysorbate 80, agar powder, talc and magnesium stearate.

6.2 Incompatibilities
None known

6.3 Shelf life
5 years.

6.4 Special precautions for storage
None.

6.5 Nature and contents of container
Blister packs of 28 tablets (OP).

6.6 Instructions for use and handling
None.

7. MARKETING AUTHORISATION HOLDER
Leo Laboratories Limited

Longwick Road

Princes Risborough

Bucks HP27 9RR

UK

8. MARKETING AUTHORISATION NUMBER(S)
PL 0043/0043R

9. DATE OF FIRST AUTHORISATION/RENEWAL OF THE AUTHORISATION
27 June 1996.

10. DATE OF REVISION OF THE TEXT
February 2001.

LEGAL CATEGORY
POM

Burinex A Tablets

(Leo Laboratories Limited)

1. NAME OF THE MEDICINAL PRODUCT
Burinex®A Tablets

2. QUALITATIVE AND QUANTITATIVE COMPOSITION
Each tablet contains Bumetanide Ph Eur 1mg and Amiloride Hydrochloride BP 5mg.

3. PHARMACEUTICAL FORM
Tablet

4. CLINICAL PARTICULARS

4.1 Therapeutic indications
Burinex A is indicated where a prompt diuresis is required. It is particularly of value in conditions where potassium conservation is important.

4.2 Posology and method of administration
For oral administration:

Adults: The normal adult dose is 1 to 2 tablets daily. The dose may be adjusted according to response.

Elderly: The dose should be adjusted according to needs and serum electrolytes and urea should be monitored carefully.

Children: Not recommended for use in children.

4.3 Contraindications
Hyperkalaemia (serum potassium > 5.3 mmol/litre), severe electrolyte imbalance, acute renal insufficiency, severe progressive renal disease, anuria, severe liver disease, adrenocortical insufficiency (Addison's Disease), precomatose states associated with cirrhosis, known sensitivity to bumetanide or amiloride or to Burinex A. Burinex A should not be given concurrently with potassium supplements or potassium-sparing agents. Burinex A is contra-indicated in children as safety in this age group has not been established.

Burinex A is contra-indicated in hepatic coma and care should be taken in states of severe electrolyte depletion.

4.4 Special warnings and special precautions for use
Serum uric acid levels may be increased and acute attacks of gout may be precipitated. Patients with prostatic hypertrophy or impaired micturition may be at risk of developing acute retention.

Burinex A should be discontinued before a glucose tolerance test. Burinex A may cause latent diabetes to become manifest. It may be necessary to increase the dose of hypoglycaemic agents in diabetic patients.

Burinex A should be used with caution in patients already receiving nephrotoxic or ototoxic drugs.

Patients who are being treated with this preparation require regular supervision with monitoring of fluid and electrolyte status to avoid excessive fluid loss.

In common with other potent diuretics, Burinex A should be used with caution in elderly patients or those with disorders rendering electrolyte balance precarious. Hyponatraemia, hypochloraemia and raised blood urea may occur during vigorous diuresis especially in seriously ill patients. Careful monitoring of serum electrolytes and urea should be undertaken in these patients.

4.5 Interaction with other medicinal products and other forms of Interaction
Hyperkalaemia has been observed in patients receiving amiloride and therefore concurrent use of Burinex A with potassium conserving diuretics is not recommended.

In common with other diuretics serum lithium levels may be increased when lithium is given concurrently with Burinex A necessitating adjustment of the lithium dosage.

As ACE Inhibitors may elevate serum potassium levels, especially in the presence of renal impairment, combination with Burinex A is best avoided in elderly patients or in those in whom renal function may be compromised. If use of the combination is considered essential the clinical condition and serum electrolytes must be carefully and continuously monitored.

The dose of cardiac glycosides or hypotensive agents may require adjustment.

Certain non-steroidal anti-inflammatory drugs have been shown to antagonise the action of diuretics.

4.6 Pregnancy and lactation
The safety of the use of Burinex A during pregnancy has not been established.

Since it is not known whether bumetanide or amiloride are distributed into breast milk, a nursing mother should either stop breast feeding or stop taking Burinex A. The decision depends on the importance of the drug to the mother.

4.7 Effects on ability to drive and use machines
None known.

4.8 Undesirable effects
Bumetanide and amiloride are generally well tolerated. Side effects which may occur include: abdominal pain, nausea and vomiting, dyspepsia, diarrhoea, stomach and muscle cramps, arthralgia, dizziness, fatigue, hypotension, headache, encephalopathy (in patients with pre-existing hepatic disease), fluid and electrolyte depletion, dehydration, hyperuricaemia, increased blood urea and serum creatinine, hyperglycaemia, abnormalities of serum levels of hepatic enzymes, skin rashes, pruritus, urticaria, thrombocytopenia, gynaecomastia and painful breasts. Bone marrow depression associated with the use of Burinex has been reported rarely but it has not been proven definitely to be attributed to the drug. Hearing disturbance after administration of Burinex is rare and reversible.

4.9 Overdose
Symptoms would be those caused by excessive diuresis such as dehydration, electrolyte imbalance, particularly hyperkalaemia, and hypotension and treatment should be aimed at reversing these. No specific antidote is available. Treatment is symptomatic and supportive. If hyperkalaemia is present appropriate measures must be instituted to reduce serum potassium.

5. PHARMACOLOGICAL PROPERTIES

5.1 Pharmacodynamic properties
Burinex A combines the potent loop diuretic bumetanide with the potassium sparing diuretic amiloride.

The action of bumetanide starts within 30 minutes and is virtually complete within 3 hours. The addition of amiloride will reduce any tendency towards hypokalaemia and its mild natriuretic effect will be additive to that of bumetanide.

5.2 Pharmacokinetic properties
The product contains a short acting diuretic and a potassium sparing diuretic with a more prolonged action.

After administration of one tablet containing bumetanide 1 mg and amiloride hydrochloride 5 mg to healthy volunteers, a C_{max} of 48.60 ± 19.08 ng/ml was found for bumetanide at T_{max} 0.91 ± 0.31 hours.

The corresponding data for amiloride hydrochloride was C_{max} 10.47 ± 4.02 ng/ml at T_{max} 2.92 ± 0.78 hours.

5.3 Preclinical safety data
There are no preclinical data of relevance to the prescriber which are additional to that already included in other sections of the SPC.

6. PHARMACEUTICAL PARTICULARS

6.1 List of excipients
Microcrystalline cellulose, lactose, magnesium stearate, maize starch.

6.2 Incompatibilities
None known.

6.3 Shelf life
3 years.

6.4 Special precautions for storage
None

6.5 Nature and contents of container
Blister packs of 28 tablets.

6.6 Instructions for use and handling
None.

7. MARKETING AUTHORISATION HOLDER
Leo Laboratories Limited, Longwick Road, Princes Risborough, Bucks HP27 9RR

8. MARKETING AUTHORISATION NUMBER(S)
PL 00043/0161

9. DATE OF FIRST AUTHORISATION/RENEWAL OF THE AUTHORISATION
25 July 1996

10. DATE OF REVISION OF THE TEXT
December 1999

Legal Category
POM

Burinex K Tablets

(Leo Laboratories Limited)

1. NAME OF THE MEDICINAL PRODUCT
Burinex® K Tablets

2. QUALITATIVE AND QUANTITATIVE COMPOSITION
Each tablet contains Bumetanide Ph Eur 0.5 mg and Potassium Chloride Ph.Eur. 573 mg.

3. PHARMACEUTICAL FORM
Tablet

4. CLINICAL PARTICULARS

4.1 Therapeutic indications
For the treatment of oedema where potassium supplementation is necessary.

4.2 Posology and method of administration
For oral administration.

Adults: The recommended initial dose is 2 tablets to be taken once daily (morning or evening). This may be increased up to 4 tablets daily (given as a single dose or in divided doses if preferred), or reduced to 1 tablet daily according to clinical response. If more than 4 tablets are to be taken daily, it is preferred to administer the diuretic and potassium supplement as 2 separate preparations.

Elderly: Adjust dosage according to response. A dose of 1 tablet per day may be sufficient in some elderly patients.

Burinex K tablets must be swallowed whole and never chewed. The tablets should be swallowed with at least 100ml of water.

Children: Not recommended in children under 12 years.

4.3 Contraindications
Burinex K should not be used with potassium sparing diuretics, (e.g. spironolactone, triamterene or amiloride) or in patients with renal insufficiency.

As with other diuretics, Burinex K should not be administered concurrently with lithium salts. Diuretics can reduce lithium clearance resulting in high serum levels of lithium.

All solid forms of potassium medication are contra-indicated in the presence of obstruction in the digestive tract (e.g. resulting from compression of the oesophagus due to dilation of the left atrium or from stenosis of the gut).

Anuria, Crohn's Disease, hyperkalaemia, precomatose states associated with liver cirrhosis, Addison's Disease, known hypersensitivity to bumetanide or Burinex.

4.4 Special warnings and special precautions for use
The 15.4 mmol of potassium included in the usual dose of Burinex K (2 tablets daily) should help to prevent hypokalaemia in many patients. Certain patients, however, as for example those with hepatic ascites or those on a very low potassium diet, may require considerably more potassium than this. Periodic checks should, therefore, be made on the serum potassium level in patients on long-term therapy.

The diuretic in Burinex K may increase blood uric acid and (though rarely) affect carbohydrate metabolism.

Non-specific small bowel lesions characterised by stenosis and possibly accompanied by ulceration have been associated with the oral administration of tablets and capsules containing potassium salts. Symptoms and signs which indicate ulceration or obstruction of the small bowel in patients taking tablets or capsules containing potassium salts are indications for stopping treatment with such preparations immediately.

Patients with prostatic hypertrophy or impairment of micturition have an increased risk of developing acute retention. Where indicated, steps should be taken to correct hypotension or hyperkalaemia before commencing therapy.

Excessively rapid mobilisation of oedema, particularly in elderly patients, may give rise to sudden changes in cardiovascular pressure-flow relationships with circulatory collapse. This should be borne in mind when Burinex K is given in high doses.

4.5 Interaction with other medicinal products and other forms of Interaction
For information on concomitant use of lithium salts or potassium-sparing diuretics, see Section 4.3.

ACE inhibitors should not be used with combination diuretic potassium products, such as Burinex K, as serum potassium levels may be increased.

The diuretic in Burinex K may potentiate the effect of antihypertensive drugs and other drugs with a hypotensive action. Patients taking tricyclic antidepressants concurrently with Burinex K may be at increased risk of postural hypotension. A dosage adjustment may be necessary.

The toxic effects of nephrotoxic or ototoxic drugs (e.g. non-steroidal anti-inflammatory drugs, aminoglycosides, cephalosporins) may be increased by concomitant administration of potent diuretics such as bumetanide.

Concomitant administration of certain non-steroidal anti-inflammatory drugs, or other drugs that can cause fluid retention, may antagonise the action of diuretics.

Bumetanide can cause hypokalaemia, which can increase the cardiac toxicity of anti-arrhythmics and digitalis glycosides.

Hypokalaemia can also antagonise the effect of certain drugs (e.g. lidocaine/lignocaine, mexiletine).

Loop diuretics may antagonise the effect of antidiabetics.

There is an increased risk of hypokalaemia when Burinex K is taken concurrently with other potassium-depleting drugs (e.g. corticosteroids, other diuretics, sympathomimetics). Plasma potassium should therefore be monitored in severe asthmatics.

Similarly, the risk of hyponatraemia may be increased when Burinex K is taken with sodium-depleting drugs.

Patients taking Burinex K with drugs that can cause ventricular arrhythmias are at increased risk of arrhythmias if electrolyte imbalance occurs.

4.6 Pregnancy and lactation

Although tests in four animal species have shown no teratogenic effects, the ordinary precaution of avoiding use of Burinex in the first trimester of pregnancy should at present be observed.

Since it is not known whether bumetanide is distributed into breast milk, a nursing mother should either stop breast feeding or observe the infant for any adverse effects if the drug is absolutely necessary for the mother.

4.7 Effects on ability to drive and use machines

When driving vehicles or operating machines it should be taken into account that occasionally dizziness, drowsiness, faintness or fatigue may occur. Patients who experience such effects should be advised not to drive or operate machines.

4.8 Undesirable effects

As with other diuretics, fluid and electrolyte balance may be disturbed as a result of diuresis after prolonged therapy. This may cause symptoms such as headache, hypotension and myalgia. Electrolyte disturbances which may occur include hyponatraemia, hypomagnesaemia and hypokalaemia. The hypokalaemic effect of bumetanide is counteracted by the potassium content but hypokalaemia may not be totally prevented.

Other reactions to bumetanide include gastrointestinal disorders (e.g. nausea, vomiting, diarrhoea or constipation, abdominal pain/cramps, dyspepsia), muscle cramps, dehydration, hypotension, dizziness or vertigo, fatigue, headache, encephalopathy (in patients with pre-existing hepatic disease), hyperuricaemia, raised blood urea and serum creatinine, hyperglycaemia, alkalosis, skin rashes, gynaecomastia or painful breasts, arthralgia, allergic reactions, vasculitis, thrombocytopenia, leucopenia.

Bone marrow depression associated with the use of Burinex has been reported rarely but it has not been proven definitely to be attributed to the drug. Hearing disturbance after administration of Burinex is rare and reversible.

4.9 Overdose

General measures should be taken to restore blood volume and maintain blood pressure. Any electrolyte imbalance should be corrected.

5. PHARMACOLOGICAL PROPERTIES

5.1 Pharmacodynamic properties

Burinex K combines the very potent high ceiling diuretic bumetanide with a slow release potassium chloride supplement. Bumetanide has a rapid onset and a short duration of action. As with most diuretics, long term therapy may be associated with potassium depletion.

5.2 Pharmacokinetic properties

The potassium supplement in Burinex K will help to maintain normal levels of potassium, especially in those patients whose dietary intake of potassium is inadequate.

The formulation of Burinex K presents the following advantages. The diuretic is coated around the tablet from which it is rapidly released. The diuretic and saluretic effects begin within 30 minutes after oral administration, peak at one to two hours and are largely complete within three hours. In contrast, the potassium chloride, which is included in an inert wax core, is released only slowly over a period of six hours after oral ingestion. This slow release minimises the risk of gastro-intestinal intolerance as well as that of ulceration and stenosis resulting from localised high concentrations of potassium salts in the small bowel.

5.3 Preclinical safety data

There are no pre-clinical data of relevance to the prescriber which are additional to that already included in other sections of the SPC.

6. PHARMACEUTICAL PARTICULARS

6.1 List of excipients

Ethyl cellulose, ferric oxide brown, glycerol, magnesium stearate, stearyl alcohol, hydroxypropylmethylcellulose, polyvidone K25, sucrose, talc, titanium dioxide.

6.2 Incompatibilities

None known.

6.3 Shelf life

3 years.

6.4 Special precautions for storage

Do not store above 25°C.

6.5 Nature and contents of container

Blister pack of 28 tablets.

6.6 Instructions for use and handling

None.

7. MARKETING AUTHORISATION HOLDER

Leo Laboratories Limited

Longwick Road

Princes Risborough

Bucks. HP27 9RR

8. MARKETING AUTHORISATION NUMBER(S)

PL 0043/0027R

9. DATE OF FIRST AUTHORISATION/RENEWAL OF THE AUTHORISATION

19 July 1995.

10. DATE OF REVISION OF THE TEXT

September 2000

LEGAL CATEGORY

POM

BurnEze Spray

(SSL International plc)

1. NAME OF THE MEDICINAL PRODUCT

BurnEze Spray.

2. QUALITATIVE AND QUANTITATIVE COMPOSITION

Benzocaine Ph Eur 1.0% w/w.

3. PHARMACEUTICAL FORM

Aerosol spray.

4. CLINICAL PARTICULARS

4.1 Therapeutic indications

For the symptomatic relief of pain from minor superficial burns and scalds where the skin is unbroken.

4.2 Posology and method of administration

For topical administration. Adults, the elderly, and children: To reduce pain and blistering, use BurnEze Spray as quickly as possible. Hold nozzle five inches from the skin and spray once for 2-3 seconds. Stop spraying immediately if a white frost deposit (frost) appears. If necessary, the application may be repeated once only after 15 minutes. If pain persists seek medical advice.

4.3 Contraindications

Do not use if you are sensitive to benzocaine.

4.4 Special warnings and special precautions for use

Patients with any known allergy should seek medical advice. Do not apply to large areas or to broken skin. Do not use in or near the mouth or eyes or under conditions in which significant inhalation is likely. Avoid freezing the skin by repeated or prolonged use. Seek medical advice immediately if burns are extensive (particularly in young children or if they affect fingers, toes or sensitive areas). For external use only. Keep out of the reach of children. Flammable. Do not use near fire or flame. Pressurised container. Protect from sunlight and do not expose to temperatures exceeding 50°C. Do not pierce or burn, even after use. Do not spray on a naked flame or any incandescent material. Do not use near or place container on polished or painted surfaces.

4.5 Interaction with other medicinal products and other forms of Interaction

None known.

4.6 Pregnancy and lactation

Safety of use in pregnancy and lactation has not been established.

4.7 Effects on ability to drive and use machines

None known.

4.8 Undesirable effects

May cause allergic dermatitis in sensitive individuals.

4.9 Overdose

An overdose is extremely unlikely with this type of preparation.

5. PHARMACOLOGICAL PROPERTIES

5.1 Pharmacodynamic properties

The active ingredient, benzocaine, is a local anaesthetic which relieves pain. The physical effects of the cooling propellants help reduce pain and blistering.

5.2 Pharmacokinetic properties

BurnEze Spray is applied topically to the affected area.

5.3 Preclinical safety data

Not applicable.

6. PHARMACEUTICAL PARTICULARS

6.1 List of excipients

Ethanol, Denatured; Isobutane; N-pentane.

6.2 Incompatibilities

None known.

6.3 Shelf life

Three years.

6.4 Special precautions for storage

Do not store above 25°C.

6.5 Nature and contents of container

Aluminium cans (60ml) internally coated with epoxyphenolic lacquer fitted with valve assembly and actuator button, protected by a plastic cap.

6.6 Instructions for use and handling

None.

7. MARKETING AUTHORISATION HOLDER

Seton Products Limited, Tubiton House, Oldham, OL1 3HS.

8. MARKETING AUTHORISATION NUMBER(S)

PL 11314/0038.

9. DATE OF FIRST AUTHORISATION/RENEWAL OF THE AUTHORISATION

15th December 1994 / 13th March 2000.

10. DATE OF REVISION OF THE TEXT

February 2002.

Buscopan Ampoules

(Boehringer Ingelheim Limited)

1. NAME OF THE MEDICINAL PRODUCT

Buscopan Ampoules

2. QUALITATIVE AND QUANTITATIVE COMPOSITION

Each 1ml ampoule contains hyoscine-N-butylbromide 20 mg.

3. PHARMACEUTICAL FORM

Solution for injection

4. CLINICAL PARTICULARS

4.1 Therapeutic indications

Buscopan Ampoules are indicated in acute spasm, as in renal or biliary colic, in radiology for differential diagnosis of obstruction and to reduce spasm and pain in pyelography, and in other diagnostic procedures where spasm may be a problem, e.g. gastro-duodenal endoscopy.

4.2 Posology and method of administration

Not recommended for children.

Adults:

One ampoule (20 mg) intramuscularly or intravenously, repeated after half an hour if necessary. Intravenous injection should be performed 'slowly' (in rare cases a marked drop in blood pressure and even shock may be produced by Buscopan). When used in endoscopy this dose may need to be repeated more frequently.

Maximum daily dose of 100mg.

Diluent:

Buscopan injection solution may be diluted with dextrose or with sodium chloride 0.9% injection solutions.

No specific information on the use of this product in the elderly is available. Clinical trials have included patients over 65 years and no adverse reactions specific to this age group have been reported.

4.3 Contraindications

Buscopan Ampoules should not be administered to patients with myasthenia gravis, megacolon, narrow angle glaucoma, tachycardia, prostatic enlargement with urinary retention, mechanical stenoses in the region of the gastro-intestinal tract or paralytic ileus.

In addition, Buscopan should not be used in patients with a known sensitivity to hyoscine-N-butylbromide or any other component of the product.

4.4 Special warnings and special precautions for use

Buscopan Ampoules should be used with caution in conditions characterised by tachycardia such as thyrotoxicosis, cardiac insufficiency or failure and in cardiac surgery where it may further accelerate the heart rate.

Because of the possibility that anticholinergics may reduce sweating, Buscopan should be administered with caution to patients with pyrexia.

Elevation of intraocular pressure may be produced by the administration of anticholinergic agents such as Buscopan in patients with undiagnosed and therefore untreated narrow angle glaucoma. Therefore, patients should seek urgent ophthalmological advice in case they should develop a painful, red eye with loss of vision after the injection of Buscopan.

After parenteral administration of Buscopan, cases of anaphylaxis including episodes of shock have been observed. As with all drugs causing such reactions, patients receiving Buscopan by injection should be kept under observation.

4.5 Interaction with other medicinal products and other forms of Interaction

The anticholinergic effect of tricyclic antidepressants, antihistamines, quinidine, amantadine, phenothiazines, butyrophenones and disopyramide may be intensified by Buscopan.

The tachycardic effects of beta-adrenergic agents may be enhanced by Buscopan.

Concomitant treatment with dopamine antagonists such as metoclopramide may result in diminution of the effects of both drugs on the gastrointestinal tract.

4.6 Pregnancy and lactation

Although Buscopan has been in wide general use for many years, there is no definitive evidence of ill-consequence during human pregnancy; animal studies have shown no hazard. Nevertheless, medicines should not be used in pregnancy, especially the first trimester, unless the expected benefit is thought to outweigh any possible risk to the foetus.

Safety during lactation has not yet been established.

4.7 Effects on ability to drive and use machines

Because of visual accommodation disturbances patients should not drive or operate machinery after parenteral administration of Buscopan until vision has normalised.

4.8 Undesirable effects

Anticholinergic side-effects including dry mouth, dyshidrosis, visual accommodation disturbances, tachycardia, dizziness, constipation and potentially urinary retention may occur but are generally mild and self-limiting.

There have been reports of hypotension and flushing.

Allergic reactions including skin reactions, anaphylactoid reactions and anaphylactic shock have been reported very rarely.

There have been extremely rare reports of dyspnoea in patients with a history of bronchial asthma or allergy.

Injection site pain, particularly after intramuscular use, occurs infrequently.

Hyoscine-N-butylbromide, the active ingredient of Buscopan, due to its chemical structure as a quaternary ammonium derivate, is not expected to enter the central nervous system. Hyoscine-N-butylbromide does not readily pass the blood-brain barrier. However, it cannot totally be ruled out that under certain circumstances psychiatric disorders (e.g. confusion) may also occur after administration of Buscopan.

4.9 Overdose

Symptoms

Serious signs of poisoning following acute overdosage have not been observed in man. In the case of overdosage, anticholinergic symptoms such as urinary retention, dry mouth, reddening of the skin, tachycardia, inhibition of gastrointestinal motility and transient visual disturbances may occur, and Cheynes-Stokes respiration has been reported.

Therapy

Symptoms of Buscopan overdosage respond to parasympathomimetics. For patients with glaucoma, pilocarpine should be given locally. Cardiovascular complications should be treated according to usual therapeutic principles. In case of respiratory paralysis, intubation and artificial respiration. Catheterisation may be required for urinary retention.

In addition, appropriate supportive measures should be used as required.

5. PHARMACOLOGICAL PROPERTIES

5.1 Pharmacodynamic properties

Buscopan is an antispasmodic agent which relaxes smooth muscle of the organs of the abdominal and pelvic cavities. It is believed to act predominantly on the intramural parasympathetic ganglia of these organs.

5.2 Pharmacokinetic properties

After intravenous administration hyoscine-N-butylbromide is rapidly distributed into the tissues. The volume of distribution (Vss) is 128 l. The half-life of the terminal elimination phase ($t_{½\gamma}$) is approximately 5 hours. The total clearance is 1.2 l/min, approximately half of the clearance is renal.

In rat, highest concentrations of hyoscine-N-butylbromide are found in the tissue of the gastrointestinal tract, liver and kidneys. Plasma protein binding of hyoscine-N-butylbromide is low.

Hyoscine-N-butylbromide does not readily pass the blood-brain barrier.

5.3 Preclinical safety data

None stated

6. PHARMACEUTICAL PARTICULARS

6.1 List of excipients

Sodium Chloride

Distilled Water

6.2 Incompatibilities

None

6.3 Shelf life

5 years

6.4 Special precautions for storage

Store below 30°C.

Protect from light.

6.5 Nature and contents of container

1ml colourless glass ampoules containing a clear colourless or almost colourless sterile solution, packed in cartons containing 10 ampoules.

6.6 Instructions for use and handling

None stated

7. MARKETING AUTHORISATION HOLDER

Boehringer Ingelheim Limited

Ellesfield Avenue

Bracknell

Berkshire

RG12 8YS

United Kingdom

8. MARKETING AUTHORISATION NUMBER(S)

PL 00015/5005R

9. DATE OF FIRST AUTHORISATION/RENEWAL OF THE AUTHORISATION

19 July 1985/11 December 1997

10. DATE OF REVISION OF THE TEXT

December 2002

Legal Category

POM

B10b/UK/SPC/7

Buscopan IBS Relief

(Boehringer Ingelheim Limited Self-Medication Division)

1. NAME OF THE MEDICINAL PRODUCT

Buscopan IBS Relief

2. QUALITATIVE AND QUANTITATIVE COMPOSITION

Each tablet contains hyoscine as 10mg of hyoscine butylbromide.

For excipients, see Section 6.1.

3. PHARMACEUTICAL FORM

Coated tablets.

4. CLINICAL PARTICULARS

4.1 Therapeutic indications

Buscopan IBS Relief tablets are indicated for the relief of gastro- intestinal tract spasm associated with medically confirmed Irritable Bowel Syndrome.

4.2 Posology and method of administration

Buscopan IBS Relief tablets should be swallowed whole with adequate water.

Adults and Children 12 years or over:

The recommended starting dose is 1 tablet three times daily; this can be increased up to 2 tablets four times daily if necessary.

Children under 12 years:

Not recommended.

No specific information on the use of this product in the elderly is available. Clinical trials have included patients over 65 years and no adverse reactions specific to this age group have been reported.

4.3 Contraindications

Buscopan IBS Relief tablets should not be administered to patients with myasthenia gravis, megacolon and narrow angle glaucoma. In addition, they should not be given to patients with a known sensitivity to hyoscine butylbromide or any other component of the product.

4.4 Special warnings and special precautions for use

Buscopan IBS Relief tablets should be used with caution in conditions characterised by tachycardia such as thyrotoxicosis, cardiac insufficiency or failure and in cardiac surgery where it may further accelerate the heart rate.

Due to the risk of anticholinergic complications, caution should also be used in patients susceptible to intestinal or urinary outlet obstructions.

Because of the possibility that anticholinergics may reduce sweating, Buscopan IBS Relief tablets should be administered with caution to patients with pyrexia.

Elevation of intraocular pressure may be produced by the administration of anticholinergic agents such as hyoscine butylbromide in patients with undiagnosed and therefore untreated narrow angle glaucoma. Therefore, patients should seek urgent ophthalmological advice if they develop a painful, red eye with loss of vision whilst, or after taking, Buscopan IBS Relief tablets.

Special warnings to be included in the Patient Information Leaflet:

Only take Buscopan IBS Relief if your doctor has diagnosed Irritable Bowel Syndrome.

If any of the following now apply to you, you must not use Buscopan IBS Relief without first discussing it with your doctor, even if you know you have IBS.

- if you are 40 years or over and it is some time since your last attack of IBS or the symptoms are different this time.
- if you have recently passed blood from the bowel
- if you suffer from severe constipation
- if you are feeling sick or vomiting
- if you have lost your appetite or lost weight
- if you have difficulty or pain passing urine
- if you have a fever
- if you have recently travelled abroad

Consult your doctor if you develop new symptoms, or if your symptoms worsen or have not improved over two weeks.

4.5 Interaction with other medicinal products and other forms of Interaction

The anticholinergic effect of other drugs, for example tricyclic antidepressants, antihistamines, quinidine, amantadine, butyrophenones, phenothiazines and disopyramide may be intensified by Buscopan IBS Relief tablets.

Concomitant treatment with dopamine antagonists such as metoclopramide may result in diminution of the effects of both drugs on the gastrointestinal tract.

The tachycardic effects of beta-adrenergic agents may be enhanced by Buscopan IBS Relief tablets.

4.6 Pregnancy and lactation

Although hyoscine butylbromide 10mg tablets have been in wide general use for many years, there is no definitive evidence of ill-consequence during human pregnancy; animal studies have shown no hazard.

Medicines should not be used in pregnancy, especially during the first trimester, unless the expected benefit is thought to outweigh any possible risk to the foetus.

Safety during lactation has not yet been established.

4.7 Effects on ability to drive and use machines

Because of possible visual accommodation disturbances patients should not drive or operate machinery if affected.

4.8 Undesirable effects

Adverse events have been ranked under headings of frequency using the following convention:

Very common ($\geq$ 1/10); common ($\geq$ 1/100, $<$ 1/10); uncommon ($\geq$ 1/1000, $<$1/100); rare ($\geq$ 1/10000, $<$1/1000); very rare ($<$1/10000).

<u>Immune system disorders</u>

Uncommon: hypersensitivity

Rare: anaphylactic reaction and anaphylactic shock

<u>Cardiac disorders</u>

Uncommon: tachycardia

<u>Respiratory, thoracic and mediastinal disorders</u>

Rare: dyspnoea

<u>Gastrointestinal disorders</u>

Common: dry mouth

<u>Skin and subcutaneous tissue disorders</u>

Uncommon: skin reactions

Rare: dyshidrosis

<u>Renal and urinary disorders</u>

Rare: urinary retention

4.9 Overdose

Symptoms:

Serious signs of poisoning following acute overdosage have not been observed in man. In the case of overdosage, anticholinergic effects such as urinary retention, dry mouth, reddening of the skin, tachycardia, inhibition of gastrointestinal motility and transient visual disturbances may occur, and Cheyne-Stokes respiration has been reported.

Therapy:

In the case of oral poisoning, gastric lavage with medicinal charcoal should be followed by magnesium sulphate (15%). Symptoms of Buscopan IBS Relief tablets overdosage respond to parasympathomimetics. For patients with glaucoma, pilocarpine should be given locally. Cardiovascular complications should be treated according to usual therapeutic principles. In case of respiratory paralysis, intubation and artificial respiration. Catheterisation may be required for urinary retention.

In addition, appropriate supportive measures should be administered as required.

5. PHARMACOLOGICAL PROPERTIES

5.1 Pharmacodynamic properties

Buscopan IBS Relief tablets exert a spasmolytic action on the smooth muscle of the gastrointestinal, biliary and genito-urinary tracts. Peripheral anticholinergic action results from a ganglion-blocking action within the visceral wall as well as from an anti-muscarinic activity.

5.2 Pharmacokinetic properties
Following oral and intravenous administration, hyoscine butylbromide concentrates in the tissue of the gastrointestinal tract, liver and kidneys. As a quaternary ammonium derivative, hyoscine butylbromide does not pass the blood-brain barrier or enter the central nervous system.

Following oral administration, hyoscine butylbromide is only partially absorbed. Nevertheless, despite the briefly measurable low blood levels, hyoscine butylbromide remains available at the site of action because of its high tissue affinity.

5.3 Preclinical safety data
There are no pre-clinical data of relevance to the prescriber which are additional to that already included in other sections of the SPC.

6. PHARMACEUTICAL PARTICULARS
6.1 List of excipients
Calcium Hydrogen Phosphate

Maize Starch

Starch, Soluble

Colloidal Silica

Tartaric Acid

Stearic Acid

Palmitic Acid

Sucrose

Talc

Acacia

Titanium Dioxide

Macrogol 6000

Carnauba Wax

White Beeswax

Povidone

6.2 Incompatibilities
None stated.

6.3 Shelf life
Five years

6.4 Special precautions for storage
Do not store above 25°C.

Keep in the original packaging.

6.5 Nature and contents of container
Buscopan IBS Relief tablets are in blister packs of 10, 12, 20 and 24.

Not all pack sizes may be marketed.

6.6 Instructions for use and handling
None stated.

7. MARKETING AUTHORISATION HOLDER
Boehringer Ingelheim Limited

Ellesfield Avenue

Bracknell

Berkshire

RG12 8YS

United Kingdom

Trading as:

Boehringer Ingelheim Consumer Healthcare

8. MARKETING AUTHORISATION NUMBER(S)
PL 00015/0253

9. DATE OF FIRST AUTHORISATION/RENEWAL OF THE AUTHORISATION
27th March 2001

10. DATE OF REVISION OF THE TEXT
September 2004

B14/UK/SPC/4

Busilvex

(Pierre Fabre Limited)

1. NAME OF THE MEDICINAL PRODUCT
Busilvex ▼6mg/ml concentrate for solution for infusion

2. QUALITATIVE AND QUANTITATIVE COMPOSITION
1 ml of concentrate contains 6 mg of busulfan (60 mg in 10 ml).

After dilution: 1 ml of solution contains 0.5 mg of busulfan.

For excipients see 6.1

3. PHARMACEUTICAL FORM
Concentrate for solution for infusion.

Clear, colourless solution.

4. CLINICAL PARTICULARS
4.1 Therapeutic indications
Busilvex followed by cyclophosphamide (BuCy2) is indicated as conditioning treatment prior to conventional haematopoietic progenitor cell transplantation (HPCT) in adult patients when the combination is considered the best available option.

4.2 Posology and method of administration
Busilvex administration should be supervised by a physician experienced in conditioning treatment prior to haematopoietic progenitor cell transplantation.

Dosage in adults
When followed by 2 cycles of 60 mg/kg body weight (BW) cyclophosphamide the recommended dosage and schedule is administration of 0.8 mg/kg BW of busulfan as a two-hour infusion every 6 hours over 4 consecutive days for a total of 16 doses prior to cyclophosphamide and conventional haematopoietic progenitor cell transplantation (HPCT)

It is recommended that cyclophosphamide dosing should not be initiated for at least 24 hours following the 16th dose of Busilvex (see 4.5).

Children and adolescents
The safety and efficacy of Busilvex in children and adolescents have not been established.

Administration
Busulfex must be diluted prior to administration (see 6.6). A final concentration of approximately 0.5 mg/ml busulfan should be achieved. Busilvex should be administered by intravenous infusion via central venous catheter.

Busilvex should not be given by rapid intravenous, *bolus* or peripheral injection.

All patients should be pre-medicated with anticonvulsant medicinal products to prevent seizures reported with the use of high dose busulfan. In the Busilvex studies, all patients received phenytoin for this purpose. There is no experience with other anticonvulsant agents such as benzodiazepines (see 4.4 and 4.5).

Antiemetics should be administered prior to the first dose of Busilvex and continued on a fixed schedule according to local practice through its administration.

Obese patients
For obese patients, dosing based on adjusted ideal body weight (AIBW) should be considered.

Ideal body weight (IBW) is calculated as follows:

IBW men (kg)=50 + 0.91x (height in cm-152);

IBW women (kg)=45 +0.91x (height in cm-152).

Adjusted ideal body weight (AIBW) is calculated as follows:

AIBW=IBW+0.25x (actual body weight – IBW).

Renally impaired patient
Studies in renally impaired patients have not be conducted, however, as busulfan is moderately excreted in the urine, dose modification is not recommended in these patients. However, caution is recommended (see 4.8 and 5.2).

Hepatically impaired patient
Busilvex as well as busulfan has not been studied in patients with hepatic impairment.

Caution is recommended, particularly in those patients with severe hepatic impairment (see 4.4).

Elderly patient
Patients older than 50 years of age (n=23) have been successfully treated with Busilvex without dose adjustment. However, for the safe use of Busilvex in patients older than 60 years only limited information is available. Same dose (see 5.2) for elderly as for adults (<50 years old) should be used.

4.3 Contraindications
Hypersensitivity to the active substance or to any of the excipients.

Pregnancy and lactation (see 4.6).

4.4 Special warnings and special precautions for use
The consequence of treatment with Busilvex at the recommended dose and schedule is profound myelosuppression, occurring in all patients. Severe granulocytopenia, thrombocytopenia, anaemia, or any combination thereof may develop. Frequent complete blood counts, including differential white blood cell counts, and platelet counts should be monitored during the treatment and until recovery is achieved. Absolute neutrophil counts $<0.5 \times 10^9/1$ at a median of 4 days post transplant occurred in 100% of patients and recovered at median day 10 and 13 days following autologous and allogeneic transplant respectively (median neutropenic period of 6 and 9 days respectively). Prophylactic or empiric use of anti-infectives (bacterial, fungal, viral) should be considered for the prevention and management of infections during the neutropenic period. Thrombocytopenia ($<25{,}000/mm^3$ or requiring platelet transfusion) occurred at a median of 5-6 days in 98% of patients. Anaemia (haemoglobin<8.0 g/dl) occurred in 69% of patients. Platelet and red blood cell support, as well as the use of growth factors such as G-CSF, should be employed as medically indicated.

Busilvex as well as busulfan has not been studied in patients with hepatic impairment. Since busulfan is mainly metabolized through the liver, caution should be observed when Busilvex is used in patients with pre-existing impairment of liver function, especially in those with severe hepatic impairment. It is recommended when treating these patients that serum transaminase, alkaline phosphatase, and bilirubin should be monitored regularly 28 days following transplant for early detection of hepatotoxicity.

Hepatic veno-occlusive disease is a major complication that can occur during treatment with Busilvex. Patients who have received prior radiation therapy, greater than or equal to three cycles of chemotherapy, or prior progenitor cell transplant may be at an increased risk (see 4.8).

Caution should be exercised when using paracetamol prior to (less than 72 hours) or concurrently with Busilvex due to a possible decrease in the metabolism of busulfan (see 4.5).

As documented in clinical studies, no treated patients experienced cardiac tamponade or other specific cardiac toxicities related to Busilvex. However cardiac function should be monitored regularly in patients receiving Busilvex (see 4.8).

Occurrence of acute respiratory distress syndrome with subsequent respiratory failure associated with interstitial pulmonary fibrosis was reported in Busilvex studies in one patient who died, although, no clear etiology was identified. In addition, busulfan might induce pulmonary toxicity that may be additive to the effects produced by other cytotoxic agents. Therefore, attention should be paid to this pulmonary issue in patients with prior history of mediastinal or pulmonary radiation (see 4.8).

Periodic monitoring of renal function should be considered during therapy with Busilvex (see 4.8).

Seizures have been reported with high dose busulfan treatment. Special caution should be exercised when administering the recommended dose of Busilvex to patients with a history of seizures. Patients should receive adequate anti-convulsant prophylaxis. All data with Busilvex were obtained using phenytoin. There are no data available on the use of other anticonvulsant agents such as benzodiazepines. Thus, the effect of anticonvulsant agents (other than phenytoin) on busulfan pharmacokinetics is not known (see 4.2 and 4.5).

The increased risk of a second malignancy should be explained to the patient. On the basis of human data, busulfan has been classified by the International Agency for Research on Cancer (IARC) as a human carcinogen. The World Health Association has concluded that there is a causal relationship between busulfan exposure and cancer. Leukaemia patients treated with busulfan developed many different cytological abnormalities, and some developed carcinomas. Busulfan is thought to be leukemogenic.

Fertility: busulfan can impair fertility. Therefore, men treated with Busilvex are advised not to father a child during and up to 6 months after treatment and to seek advice on cryo-conservation of sperm prior to treatment because of the possibility of irreversible infertility due to therapy with Busilvex. Ovarian suppression and amenorrhoea with menopausal symptoms commonly occur in pre-menopausal patients. Busulfan treatment in a pre-adolescent girl prevented the onset of puberty due to ovarian failure. Impotence, sterility, azoospermia, and testicular atrophy have been reported in male patients. The solvent dimethylacetamide (DMA) may also impair fertility. DMA decreases fertility in male and female rodents (see 4.6 and 5.3).

4.5 Interaction with other medicinal products and other forms of Interaction
No specific clinical trial was carried out to assess drug-drug interaction between i.v. busulfan and itraconazole. From published studies, administration of itraconazole to patients receiving high-dose busulfan may result in reduced busulfan clearance. Patients should be monitored for signs of busulfan toxicity when itraconazole is used as an antifungal prophylaxis with i.v. busulfan.

Published studies described that ketobemidone (analgesic) might be associated with high levels of plasma busulfan. Therefore special care is recommended with combining these two drugs.

For BuCy2 regimen it has been reported that the time interval between the last oral busulfan administration and the first cyclophosphamide administration may influence the development of toxicities. A reduced incidence of Hepatic Veino Occlusive Disease (HVOD) and other regimen-related toxicity have been observed in patients when the lag time between the last dose of oral busulfan and the first dose of cyclophosphamide is>24 hours.

Paracetemol is described to decrease glutathione levels in blood and tissues, and may therefore decrease busulfan clearance when used in combination (see 4.4).

Phenytoin was administered for seizure prophylaxis in all patients in the clinical trials conducted with i.v. busulfan. The concomitant systemic administration of phenytoin to patients receiving high-dose busulfan has been reported to increase busulfan clearance, due to induction of glutathion-S-transferase. However no evidence of this effect has been seen in i.v. data (see 4.4).

No interaction has been reported when benzodiazepines such as diazepam, clonazepam or lorazepam have been used to prevent seizures with high-dose busulfan (see 4.2 and 4.4).

No interaction was observed when busulfan was combined with fluconazole (antifungal agent) or

5 – HT_3 antiemetics such as ondansetron or granisetron.

4.6 Pregnancy and lactation
Pregnancy
HPCT is contraindicated in pregnant women; therefore, Busilvex is contraindicated during pregnancy. Busulfan

has caused embryofoetal lethality and malformations in pre-clinical studies (see 5.3).

There are no adequate and well-controlled studies of either busulfan or DMA in pregnant women. A few cases of congenital abnormalities have been reported with low-dose busulfan, not necessarily attributable to the drug, and third trimester exposure may be associated with impaired intrauterine growth.

Women of childbearing potential have to use effective contraception during and up to 6 months after treatment.

Lactation

Patients who are taking Busilvex would not breast-feed. It is not known whether busulfan and DMA are excreted in human milk. Because of the potential for tumorigenicity shown for busulfan in human and animal studies, breast-feeding should be discontinued at the start of therapy.

4.7 Effects on ability to drive and use machines

Not relevant

4.8 Undesirable effects

Adverse events informations are derived from two clinical trials (n=103) of Busilvex.

Serious toxicities involving the hematologic, hepatic and respiratory systems were considered as expected consequences of the conditioning regimen and transplant process. These include infection and Graft-versus host disease (GVHD) which although not directly related, were the major causes of morbidity and mortality, especially in allogeneic HPCT.

Blood and the lymphatic system disorders

Myelo-suppression and immuno-suppression were the desired therapeutic effects of the conditioning regimen. Therefore all patients experienced profound cytopenia: leukopoenia 96%, thrombocytopenia 94% and anemia 88%. The median time to neutropenia was 4 days for both autologous and allogeneic patients. The median duration of neutropenia was 6 days and 9 days for autologous and allogeneic patients.

Immune system disorders

The incidence of acute graft versus host disease (a-GVHD) data was collected in OMC-BUS-4 study (allogeneic) (n=61). A total of 11 patients (18%) experienced a-GVHD. The incidence of a-GVHD grades I-II was 13% (8/61), while the incidence of grade III-IV was 5% (3/61). Acute GVHD was rated as serious in 3 patients. Chronic GVHD (c-GVHD) was reported if serious or the cause of death, and was reported as the cause of death in 3 patients.

Infections and infestations

39% of patients (40/103) experienced one or more episodes of infection, of which 83% (33/40) were rated as mild or moderate. Pneumonia was fatal in 1% (1/103) and life-threatening in 3% of patients. Other infections were considered severe in 3% of patients. Fever was reported in 87% of patients and graded as mild/moderate in 84% and severe in 3%. 47% of patients experienced chills which were mild/moderate in 46% and severe in 1%.

Hepato—biliary disorders

15% of SAEs involved liver toxicity. HVOD is a recognised potential complication of conditioning therapy post-transplant. Six of 103 patients (6%) experienced HVOD. HVOD occurred in: 8.2% (5/61) allogeneic patients (fatal in 2 patients) and 2.5% (1/42) of autologous patients. Elevated bilirubine (n=3) and elevated AST (n=1) were also observed. Two of the above four patients with serious serum hepatotoxicity were among patients with diagnosed HVOD.

Respiratory, thoracic and mediastinal disorders

One patient experienced a fatal case of acute respiratory distress syndrome with subsequent respiratory failure associated with interstitial pulmonary fibrosis in the Busilvex studies.

In addition, the literature review reports alterations of cornea and lens of the eye with oral busulfan.

Adverse reactions reported as more than an isolated case are listed below, by system organ class and by frequency. Frequencies are defined as: very common (> 1/10), common (> 1/100, < 1/10), uncommon (> 1/1,000, < 1/100).

(see Table 1)

(see Table 2)

Table 1

System organ class	Very common	Common	Uncommon
Blood and lymphatic system disorders	Neutropenia Thrombocytopenia Anaemia Pancytopenia Febrile neutropenia		
Nervous system disorders	Insomnia Anxiety Dizziness Depression	Confusion	Delirium Nervousness Hallucination Agitation Encephalopathy Cerebral haemorrhage Seizure
Metabolism And nutrition disorders	Hyperglycaemia Hypomagnesaemia Hypokalaemia Hypocalcaemia Hypophosphatemia Oedema	Hyponatraemia	
Cardio vascular disorders	Tachycardia Hypertension Hypotension Vasodilatation Thrombosis	Arrhythmia Atrial fibrillation Cardiomegaly Pericardial effusion Pericarditis Decrease ejection fraction	Femoral artery thrombosis Ventricular extrasystoles Bradycardia Capillary leak syndrome

Table 2

Respiratory thoracic and mediastinal disorders	Dyspnoea Rhinitis Pharyngitis Cough Hiccup Epistaxis Abnormal breath sounds	Hyperventilation Respiratory failure Alveolar haemorrhages Asthma Atelectasis Pleural effusion	Hypoxia
Gastrointestinal disorders	Nausea Stomatitis Vomiting Anorexia Diarrhoea Constipation Dyspepsia Anus discomfort	Oesophagitis Ileus Haematemesis	Gastrointestinal haemorrhage
Hepato-biliary disorders	Hyperbilirubinaemia Jaundice, increased hepatic enzymes, blood alkaline phosphatase increased	Hepatomegaly	
Skin and subcutaneous tissue disorders	Rash Pruritis Alopecia		
Musculoskeletal connective tissue and bone disorders	Back pain Myalgia Arthralgia		
Renal and urinary disorders	Creatinine elevated Dysuria Oligurea	Bun increase Haematuria Moderate renal insufficiency	
General disorders and administration site conditions	Weight increase Fever Headache Abdominal pain Asthenia Chills Pain Allergic reaction Oedema general Pain or inflammation at injection site Chest pain		

4.9 Overdose

The principal toxic effect is profound myeloablation and pancytopenia but the central nervous system, liver, lungs and gastrointestinal tract may also be affected.

There is no known antidote to Busilvex other than haematopoietic progenitor cell transplantation. In the absence of haematopoietic progenitor cell transplantation, the recommended dosage of Busilvex would constitute an overdose of busulfan. The haematologic status should be closely monitored and vigorous supportive measures instituted as medically indicated.

There has been one report that busulfan is dialyzable, thus dialysis should be considered in the case of an overdose. Since busulfan is metabolized through conjugation with glutathione, administration of glutathione might be considered.

It must be considered that overdose of Busilvex will also increase exposure to DMA. In human the principal toxic effects were hepatotoxicity and central nervous system effects. CNS changes precede any of the more severe side effects. No specific antidote for DMA overdose is known. In case of overdose, management would include general supportive care.

5. PHARMACOLOGICAL PROPERTIES

5.1 Pharmacodynamic properties

Pharmacotherapeutic group: Cytotoxic agents (alkylating agents).

ATC code: L01AB01

Busulfan is a potent cytotoxic agent and a bifunctional alkylating agent. In aqueous media, release of the methanesulphonate groups produces carbonium ions which can alkylate DNA, thought to be an important biological mechanism for its cytotoxic effect.

Documentation of the safety and efficacy of Busilvex in combination with cyclophosphamide in the BuCy2 regimen prior to conventional allogeneic and/or autologous HPCT derive from two clinical trials (OMC-BUS-4 and OMC-BUS-3).

Two prospective, single arm, open-label, uncontrolled phase II studies were conducted in patients with haematological disease, the majority of whom had advanced disease.

Diseases included were acute leukaemia past first remission, in first or subsequent relapse, in first remission (high risk), or induction failures; chronic melogenous leukaemia in chronic or advanced phase; primary refractory or resistant relapsed Hodgkin's disease or non-Hodgkin's lymphoma, and myelodysplastic syndrome.

Patients received doses of 0.8 mg/kg busulfan every 6 hours infusion for a total 16 doses followed by cyclophosphamide at 60 mg/kg once per day for two days (BuCy2 regimen).

The primary efficacy parameters in these studies were myeloablation, engraftment, relapse, and survival.

In both studies, all patients received a 16/16 dose regimen of Busilvex. No patients were discontinued from treatment due to adverse reactions related to Busilvex.

All patients experienced a profound myelosuppression. The time to Absolute Neutrophil Count (ANC) greater than 0.5×10^6/1 was 13 days (range (9-29 days) in allogenic patients (OMC-BUS 4), and 10 days (range 8-19 days) in autologous patients (OMC-BUS 3). Overall mortality and non-relapse mortality at more than 100 days post-transplant was (8/61) 13% and (6/61) 10% in allotransplanted patients, respectively. During the same period there was no death in autologous recipients.

5.2 Pharmacokinetic properties
The pharmacokinetics of Busilvex has been investigated. The information presented on metabolism and elimination is based on oral busulfan.

Absorption
The pharmacokinetics of i.v. busulfan was studied in 124 evaluable patients following a 2-hour intravenous infusion for a total of 16 doses over four days. Immediate and complete availability of the dose is obtained after intravenous infusion of busulfan. Similar blood exposure was observed when comparing plasma concentrations in patients receiving oral and i.v. busulfan at 1 mg/kg and 0.8 mg/kg respectively. Low inter (CV=21%) and intra (CV=12%) patient variability on drug exposure was demonstrated through a population pharmacokinetic analysis, performed on 102 patients.

Distribution
Terminal volume of distribution V_z ranged between 0.62 and 0.85 1/kg.

Busulfan concentrations in the cerebrospinal fluid are comparable to those in plasma although these concentrations are probably insufficient for anti-neoplastic activity.

Reversible binding to plasma proteins was around 7% while irreversible binding, primarily to albumin, was about 32%.

Metabolism
Busulfan is metabolised mainly through conjugation with glutathione (spontaneous and glutathione-S-transferase mediated). The glutathione conjugate is then further metabolised in the liver by oxidation. None of the metabolites is thought to contribute significantly to either efficacy or toxicity.

Elimination
Total clearance in plasma ranged 2.25 – 2.74 ml/minute/kg. The terminal half-life ranged from 2.8 to 3.9 hours.

Approximately 30% of the administered dose is excreted into the urine over 48 hours with 1% as unchanged drug. Elimination in faeces is negligible. Irreversible protein binding may explain the incomplete recovery. Contribution of a long-lasting metabolites is not excluded.

Pharmacokinetic linearity
The dose proportional increase of drug exposure was demonstrated following intravenous busulfan up to 1 mg/kg.

Pharmacokinetic/pharmacodynamic relationships
The literature on busulfan suggests a therapeutic window between 900 and 1500 μMol.minute for AUC. During clinical trials with i.v. busulfan, 90% of patients AUCs were below the upper AUC limit (1500 μMol.minute) and at least 80% were within the targeted therapeutic window (900-1500 μMol.minute).

Special populations
The effects of renal dysfunction on i.v. busulfan disposition have not been assessed.

The effects of hepatic dysfunction on i.v. busulfan disposition have not been assessed. Nevertheless the risk of liver toxicity may be increased in this population.

No age effect on busulfan clearance was evidenced from available i.v. busulfan data in patients over 60 years.

5.3 Preclinical safety data
Busulfan is mutagenic and clastogenic. Busulfan was mutagenic in *Salmonella typhimurium*, *Drosophila melanogaster* and barley. Busulfan induced chromosomal aberrations *in vitro* (rodent and human cell) and *in vivo* (rodents and humans). Various chromosome aberrations have been observed in cells from patients receiving oral busulfan.

Busulfan belongs to a class of substances which are potentially carcinogenic based on their mechanism of action. On the basis of human data, busulfan has been classified by the IARC as a human carcinogen. WHO has concluded that there is a casual relationship between busulfan exposure and cancer. The available data in animals support the carcinogenic potential of busulfan. Intravenous administration of busulfan to mice significantly increased the incidences of thymic and ovarian tumours.

Busulfan is teratogen in rats, mice and rabbits. Malformations and anomalies included significant alterations in the musculoskeletal system, body weight gain, and size. In pregnant rats, busulfan produced sterility in both male and female offspring due to the absence of germinal cells in testes and ovaries. Busulfan was shown to cause sterility in rodents. Busulfan depleted oocytes of female rats, and induced sterility in male rats and hamster.

Repeated doses of DMA produced signs of liver toxicity, the first being increases in serum clinical enzymes followed by histopatological changes in the hepatocytes. Higher doses can product hepatic necrosis and liver damage can be seen following single high exposures.

DMA is teratogenic in rats. Doses of 400 mg/kg/day DMA administered during organogenesis caused significant developmental anomalies. The malformations included serious heart and/or major vessels anomalies: a common truncus arteriosis and no ductus arteriosis, coarctation of the pulmonary trunk and the pulmonary arteries, intraventricular defects of the heart. Other frequent anomalies included cleft palate, anasarca and skeletal anomalies of the vertebrae and ribs. DMA decreases fertility in male and female rodents. A single s.c. dose of 2.2 g/kg administered on gestation day 4 terminated pregnancy in 100% of tested hamsters. In rats, a DMA daily dose of 450 mg/kg given to rats for nine days caused inactive spermatogenesis.

6. PHARMACEUTICAL PARTICULARS

6.1 List of excipients
Dimethylacetamide, macrogol 400.

6.2 Incompatibilities
In the absence of compatibility studies, this medicinal product must not be mixed with other medicinal products except those mentioned in 6.6

Do not use polycarbonate syringes with Busilvex.

6.3 Shelf life
Ampoules: 2 years

Diluted solution
Chemical and physical in-use stability after dilution has been demonstrated for:

– 8 hours (including infusion time) after dilution in glucose 5% or sodium chloride 9 mg/ml (0.9%) solution for injection, stored at 20°C ± 5°C

– 12 hours after dilution in sodium chloride 9 mg/ml (0.9%) solution for injection stored at 2°C-8° C followed by 3 hours stored at 20°C ± 5°C (including infusion time).

From a microbiological point of view, the product should be used immediately after dilution. If not used immediately, in-use storage times and conditions prior to use are the responsibility of the user and would normally not be longer than the above mentioned conditions when dilution has taken place in controlled and validated aseptic conditions.

6.4 Special precautions for storage
Stored at 2°C-8°C (in a refrigerator).

Do not freeze.

6.5 Nature and contents of container
10 ml of concentrate for solution for infusion in clear glass ampoules (type 1)

Pack size: 8 ampoules per box

6.6 Instructions for use and handling
Preparation of Busilvex
Procedures for proper handling and disposal of anticancer drugs should be considered.

All transfer procedures require strict adherence to aseptic techniques, preferably employing a vertical laminar flow safety hood.

As with the other cytotoxic compounds, caution should be exercised in handling and preparing the Busilvex solution:

– The use of gloves and protective clothing is recommended

– If Busilvex or diluted Busilvex solution contacts the skin or mucosa, wash them thoroughly with water immediately.

Calculation of the quantity of Busilvex to be diluted and of the diluent
Busilvex must be diluted prior to use with either sodium chloride 9mg/ml (0.9%) solution for injection or glucose solution for injection 5%.

The quantity of the diluent must be 10 times the volume of Busilvex ensuring the final concentration of busulfan remains at approximately 0.5 mg/ml. By example:

The amount of Busilvex and the diluent to be administered would be calculated as follows:

For a patient with a Y kg body weight:

• Quantity of Busilvex

Y (kg) × 0.8 (mg/kg)

▪ = A ml of Busilvex to be diluted

6 (mg/ml)

Y: body weight of the patient in kg

• Quantity of diluent:

(A ml Busilvex) × (10) =B ml of diluent

To prepare the final solution for infusion, add (A) ml of Busilvex to (B) ml of diluent (sodium chloride 9 mg/ml (0.9%) solution for injection or glucose solution for injection 5%).

Preparation of the solution for infusion:

• Using sterile transfer techniques, break off the top of the ampoule

• Using a non polycarbonate syringe fitted with a needle:

– Remove the calculated volume of Busilvex from the ampoule

– Dispense the contents of the syringe into an intravenous bag (or syringe) which already contains the calculated amount of the selected diluent. Always add Busilvex to the diluent, not the diluent to Busilvex. Do not put Busilvex into an intravenous bag that does not contain sodium chloride 9 mg/ml (0.9%) solution for injection or glucose solution for injection (5%).

• Mix thoroughly by inverting several times.

After dilution, 1 ml of solution for infusion contains 0.5 mg of busulfan.

Diluted Busilvex is a clear colourless solution.

Instructions for use

Prior to and following each infusion, flush the indwelling catheter line with approximately 5 ml of sodium chloride 9 mg/ml (0.9%) solution for injection or glucose (5%) solution for injection.

Do not flush residual drug in the administration tubing as rapid infusion of Busilvex has not been tested and is not recommended.

The entire prescribed Busilvex dose should be delivered over two hours.

Do not infuse concomitantly with another intravenous solution.

Do not use polycarbonate syringes with Busilvex.

For single use only. A clear solution without any particles should be used.

Any unused product or waste should be disposed of in accordance with local requirements for cytotoxic drugs.

7. MARKETING AUTHORISATION HOLDER
Pierre Fabre Médicament
45, Place Abel Gance
F-92654 Boulogne Billancourt Cedex
France

8. MARKETING AUTHORISATION NUMBER(S)
EU/1/03/254/001

9. DATE OF FIRST AUTHORISATION/RENEWAL OF THE AUTHORISATION
09.07.2003

10. DATE OF REVISION OF THE TEXT

Buspar Tablets

(Bristol-Myers Pharmaceuticals)

1. NAME OF THE MEDICINAL PRODUCT
BUSPAR TABLETS.

2. QUALITATIVE AND QUANTITATIVE COMPOSITION
Each tablet contains either buspirone hydrochloride 5 mg or buspirone hydrochloride 10 mg.

3. PHARMACEUTICAL FORM
Oral tablet.

4. CLINICAL PARTICULARS

4.1 Therapeutic indications
Buspar is indicated for the short-term management of anxiety disorders and the relief of symptoms of anxiety with or without accompanying depression.

4.2 Posology and method of administration
Adults

Dosage should be adjusted according to response for maximum effect. The recommended initial dose is 5 mg two to three times daily and this may be increased every two to three days. The usual therapeutic dose is 15 to 30 mg daily in divided doses with a maximum recommended dose of 45mg daily in divided doses.

Elderly

Dosage should be adjusted according to response for maximum effect. The recommended initial dose is 5 mg two to three times daily and this may be increased as required. The usual therapeutic dose is 15 to 30 mg daily in divided doses with a maximum recommended dose of 45 mg daily in divided doses.

Renal and Hepatic Impairment
Dosage should be reduced in renal or hepatic impairment.

Children

Use in children has not been established.

4.3 Contraindications

Buspar should not be used in patients hypersensitive to any of the ingredients in the formulation. Buspar should not be used in patients with epilepsy. Buspar should not be used in patients with severe renal impairment, defined as creatinine clearance of 20 ml/minute or below, or a plasma creatinine above 200 micromoles/litre. Buspar should not be used in patients with severe hepatic disease.

4.4 Special warnings and special precautions for use

In controlled studies in healthy volunteers, Buspar in single doses up to 20 mg caused no significant impairment of cognitive or psychomotor functions, unlike the benzodiazepines, diazepam or lorazepam. In studies in healthy volunteers, Buspar did not potentiate the psychomotor impairment produced by alcohol, in contrast to a comparative benzodiazepine. However, no data are available on concomitant use of alcohol and Buspar at single doses greater than 20mg. It is prudent therefore to avoid alcohol while taking Buspar.

As Buspar does not exhibit cross-tolerance with benzodiazepines and other common sedative/hypnotic agents, it will not block the withdrawal syndrome often seen with cessation of therapy with these compounds. Before starting therapy with Buspar, it is advisable to withdraw patients gradually from prior chronic treatment with these agents.

In patients with a history of renal or hepatic impairment, Buspar should be used with caution.

4.5 Interaction with other medicinal products and other forms of Interaction

The occurrence of elevated blood pressure in patients receiving both buspirone and monoamine oxidase inhibitors (phenelzine and tranylcypromine) has been reported. It is therefore recommended that Buspar should not be used concomitantly with a monoamine oxidase inhibitor (MAOI).

In vitro studies have shown that buspirone does not displace warfarin, digoxin, phenytoin or propranolol from plasma proteins.

In a study in normal volunteers, no interaction with amitriptyline was seen. A similar study with diazepam showed a slight increase in metabolite (nordiazepam) levels.

Buspirone has been shown "in vitro" to be metabolised by Cytochrome P450 3A4(CYP3A4). This is consistent with the interaction observed between buspirone and substances that inhibit this isoenzyme, e.g. erythromycin, itraconazole, nefazodone, grapefruit juice, diltiazem and verapamil. In cases where Buspar is likely to be used with a potent inhibitor of CYP3A4 a lower dose of buspirone (e.g. 2.5mg b.i.d.) should be used.

Coadministration of rifampicin, a potent inducer of CYP3A4, with Buspar has been shown to considerably decrease the plasma concentration and pharmacodynamic effects of buspirone.

4.6 Pregnancy and lactation

In some studies, administration of high doses of buspirone to pregnant animals produced effects on survival, birth and weanling weights, although there was no effect on foetal development. Since the relevance of this finding in humans has not been established, Buspar is contraindicated in pregnancy and in lactation.

4.7 Effects on ability to drive and use machines

Since early and transient adverse events may occur, patients should be cautioned not to drive or operate machines until they are certain that buspar does not affect them adversely.

4.8 Undesirable effects

Buspar is generally well tolerated. If side-effects occur they are normally observed at the beginning of treatment and usually subside with continued use and/or decreased dosage.

In controlled trials, the only side-effects that occurred with significantly greater frequency with buspirone treatment than with placebo were dizziness, headache, nervousness, light-headedness, excitement and nausea. Tachycardia, palpitations, chest pain, drowsiness, confusion, seizures, dry mouth, fatigue and sweating/clamminess have also been reported rarely.

4.9 Overdose

There is no specific antidote to Buspar. Buspar is not removed by haemodialysis. The stomach should be emptied as quickly as possible. Treatment should be symptomatic and supportive. The ingestion of multiple agents should be suspected.

Death by deliberate or accidental overdose has not been observed. A dose of 375 mg per day in healthy volunteers produced no significant adverse effects. As maximum dose levels are reached symptoms most commonly observed are: nausea, vomiting, dizziness, drowsiness and miosis.

5. PHARMACOLOGICAL PROPERTIES

5.1 Pharmacodynamic properties

Buspar is an azaspirodecanedione. The exact mechanism of Buspar anxioselective action is not fully known. It does not act on benzodiazepine receptor sites and lacks sedative, anticonvulsant and muscle relaxant properties. From animal studies it is known to interact with serotonin, noradrenaline, acetylcholine and dopamine systems of the brain. Buspar enhances the activity of specific noradrenergic and dopaminergic pathways, whereas the activity of serotonin and acetylcholine are reduced.

5.2 Pharmacokinetic properties

Buspar is rapidly absorbed when given orally. It is then subject to considerable first-pass metabolism. Peak plasma levels occur 60-90 minutes after dosing. Plasma concentration is linearly related to dose. Following multiple dosing steady state plasma concentrations are achieved within 2 days. Buspar is 95% protein bound. Buspar is eliminated primarily by liver metabolism. In pharmacokinetic studies mean plasma half-lives varied from 2 to 11 hours.

5.3 Preclinical safety data

No further relevant information.

6. PHARMACEUTICAL PARTICULARS

6.1 List of excipients

Lactose anhydrous, sodium carboxymethyl starch, microcrystalline cellulose, silicon dioxide colloidal, magnesium stearate.

6.2 Incompatibilities

None known.

6.3 Shelf life

36 months.

6.4 Special precautions for storage

Store below 25°C

6.5 Nature and contents of container

The tablets are packaged in blisters packs containing 90 tablets.

6.6 Instructions for use and handling

None.

7. MARKETING AUTHORISATION HOLDER

Bristol-Myers Squibb Holdings Ltd

t/a Bristol-Myers Pharmaceuticals

Uxbridge Business Park

Sanderson Road

Uxbridge

Middlesex

UB8 1DH

8. MARKETING AUTHORISATION NUMBER(S)

Buspar Tablets 5mg: 0125/0162

Buspar Tablets 10mg: 0125/0163

9. DATE OF FIRST AUTHORISATION/RENEWAL OF THE AUTHORISATION

11th June 1987 / 11th June 1992.

10. DATE OF REVISION OF THE TEXT

July 2005

Cabaser Tablets 1mg

(Pharmacia Limited)

1. NAME OF THE MEDICINAL PRODUCT
Cabaser® Tablets 1 mg

2. QUALITATIVE AND QUANTITATIVE COMPOSITION
Cabergoline INN 1 mg.

For excipients, see 6.1

3. PHARMACEUTICAL FORM
Tablet

Cabaser 1 mg tablets are white, oval, 3.8 × 7.4mm and concave with one side scored and engraved '7' on the left and '01' on the right

4. CLINICAL PARTICULARS
4.1 Therapeutic indications
Treatment of Parkinson's disease
Cabaser is indicated for the treatment of symptoms of Parkinson's disease, as adjuvant therapy to levodopa plus dopa-decarboxylase inhibitor, in patients affected by "on-off" mobility problems with daily fluctuations in motor performance.

Controlled clinical studies have demonstrated that cabergoline administered once daily at an average dose of 4 mg/day following titration (up to 5-6 mg/day in the different studies) is effective in decreasing daily fluctuations in motor performance in Parkinsonian patients receiving levodopa/carbidopa therapy. Improvement of motor deficit has been demonstrated, while substantially decreasing the levodopa/carbidopa dose.

4.2 Posology and method of administration
The tablets are for oral administration.

Since the tolerability of dopaminergic agents is improved when administered with food, it is recommended that Cabaser be taken with meals.

Cabaser is intended for chronic, long term treatment.

Adults and elderly patients
As expected for dopamine agonists, dose response for both efficacy and side effects appears to be linked to individual sensitivity. Optimization of dose should be obtained through slow initial dose titration, from starting doses of 1 mg daily. The dosage of concurrent levodopa may be gradually decreased, while the dosage of Cabaser is increased, until the optimum balance is determined. In view of the long half-life of the compound, increments of the daily dose of 0.5-1 mg should be done at weekly (initial weeks) or bi-weekly intervals, up to optimal doses.

The recommended therapeutic dosage is 2 to 6 mg/day as adjuvant therapy to levodopa/carbidopa. Cabaser should be given as a single daily dose. Maximum doses higher than 6 mg/day and up to 20 mg/day have been administered in a small proportion of patients during clinical studies.

Use in children
The safety and efficacy of Cabaser have not been investigated in children as Parkinson's disease does not affect this population.

4.3 Contraindications
Hypersensitivity to any ergot alkaloid.

4.4 Special warnings and special precautions for use
While renal insufficiency has been shown not to modify cabergoline kinetics, hepatic insufficiency of severe degree > 10 Child-Pugh score, maximum score 12) has been shown to be associated with an increase of AUC, thus indicating that dose regimens in Parkinsonian patients with severe hepatic insufficiency should be modified accordingly.

Cabaser is an ergot derivative. Fibrotic and serosal inflammatory disorders such as pleuritis, pleural effusion, pleural fibrosis, pulmonary fibrosis, pericarditis, pericardial effusion and retroperitoneal fibrosis have occurred after prolonged usage of ergot derivatives. The factors predisposing patients to the risk of such disorders are not known, however, Parkinson's disease patients with a history of such disorders should not be treated with Cabaser, or any other ergot derivative, unless the potential clearly outweighs the risk.

Attention should be paid to the signs and symptoms of:

- Pleuro-pulmonary disease such as dyspnoea, shortness of breath, persistent cough or chest pain
- Renal insufficiency or ureteral/abdominal vascular obstruction that may occur with pain in the loin/flank and lower limb oedema as well as any possible abdominal masses or tenderness that may indicate retroperitoneal fibrosis
- Cardiac failure as cases of pericardial fibrosis have often manifested as cardiac failure. Constructive pericarditis should be excluded if such symptoms appear.

Appropriate investigations such as erythrocyte sedimentation rate, chest x-ray and serum creatinine measurements should be performed if necessary to support a diagnosis of a fibrotic disorder. It is also appropriate to perform baseline investigations of erythrocyte sedimentation rate or other inflammatory markers, lung function/chest x-ray and renal function prior to initiation of therapy.

These disorders can have an insidious onset and patients should be regularly and carefully monitored while taking Cabaser for manifestations of progressive fibrotic disorders. Cabaser should be withdrawn if fibrotic or serosal inflammatory changes are diagnosed or suspected.

In addition, by analogy with other ergot derivatives, Cabaser should be given with caution to patients suffering from severe cardiovascular disease, Raynaud's syndrome, peptic ulcer, gastrointestinal bleeding or a history of serious, particularly psychotic mental disease. Symptomatic hypotension can occur following adminstration of Cabaser: particular attention should be paid when administering Cabaser concomitantly with other drugs known to lower blood pressure.

Cabergoline has been associated with somnolence and episodes of sudden sleep onset, particularly in Patients with Parkinson's disease. Sudden onset of sleep during activities, in some cases without awareness or warning signs, has been reported uncommonly. Patients must be informed of this and advised to exercise caution while driving or operating machines during treatment with cabergoline. Patients who have experienced somnolence and/or an episode of sudden sleep onset must refrain from driving or operating machines. Furthermore a reduction of dosage or termination of therapy may be considered.

The effects of alcohol on overall tolerability of Cabaser are currently unknown.

4.5 Interaction with other medicinal products and other forms of Interaction
No pharmacokinetic interaction with L-Dopa or selegiline was observed in the studies carried out in parkinsonian patients. The concomitant use of other drugs, particularly other antiparkinsonian non-dopamine-agonist agents, was not associated with detectable interactions modifying the efficacy and safety of Cabaser.

No other information is available about possible interaction between Cabaser and other ergot alkaloids: therefore the concomitant use of these medications during long term treatment with Cabaser is not recommended.

Since Cabaser exerts its therapeutic effect by direct stimulation of dopamine receptors, it should not be concurrently administered with drugs which have dopamine antagonist activity (such as phenothiazines, butyrophenones, thioxanthenes, metoclopramide) since these might reduce the therapeutic effect of Cabaser.

By analogy with other ergot derivatives, Cabaser should not be used in association with macrolide antibiotics (e.g erythromycin) since the systemic bioavailability of Cabaser and adverse effects could increase.

4.6 Pregnancy and lactation
Cabaser has been shown to cross the placenta in rats: it is unknown whether this occurs also in humans.

Animal studies in rats and mice have not demonstrated any teratogenic effect or any effect of the compound on global reproductive performance. In clinical studies there have been over 100 pregnancies in women treated with cabergoline for hyperprolactinemic disorders. The compound was generally taken during the first 8 weeks after conception. Among the pregnancies evaluable so far, there were approximately 85% live births and about 10% spontaneous abortions. Three cases of congenital abnormalities (Down's syndrome, hydrocephalus, malformation of lower limbs) which led to therapeutic abortion and three cases of minor abnormalities in live births were observed.

These incidence rates are comparable with those quoted for normal populations and for women exposed to other ovulation-inducing drugs. Based on the above data, the use of the product does not appear to be associated with an increased risk of abortion, premature delivery, multiple pregnancy or congenital abnormalities.

Because clinical experience is still limited and the drug has a long half-life, as a precautionary measure it is recommended that women seeking pregnancy discontinue Cabaser one month before intended conception, in order to prevent possible foetal exposure to the drug. If conception occurs during therapy, treatment is to be discontinued as soon as pregnancy is confirmed, to limit foetal exposure to the drug.

In rats cabergoline and/or its metabolites are excreted in milk. Lactation is expected to be inhibited/suppressed by Cabaser, in view of its dopamine-agonist properties. Therefore, while no information on the excretion of cabergoline in maternal milk in humans is available, puerperal women should be advised not to breast-feed in case of failed lactation inhibition/suppression by the product.

4.7 Effects on ability to drive and use machines
Patients being treated with cabergoline and presenting with somnolence and/or sudden sleep onset episodes must be informed to refrain from driving or engaging in activities where impaired alertness may put themselves or others at risk of serious injury or death (e.g. operating machines) until such episodes and somnolence have resolved (see also Section 4.4).

4.8 Undesirable effects
About 1070 parkinsonian patients have received Cabaser as adjuvant therapy to L-dopa in clinical studies; of these 74% had at least one adverse event, mainly of mild to moderate severity and transient in nature, and requiring discontinuation in a small proportion of cases.

In the majority of cases (51%), events were related to the nervous system: most frequently reported events were dyskinesia, hyperkinesia, hallucinations or confusion. The gastrointestinal system was involved in 33% of cases: events most frequently reported were nausea, vomiting, dyspepsia and gastritis. The cardiovascular system was involved in 27% of cases, most frequently reported events being dizziness and hypotension.

There have been reports of fibrotic and serosal inflammatory conditions, such as pleuritis, pleural effusion, pleural fibrosis, pulmonary fibrosis, pericarditis, pericardial effusion and retroperitoneal fibrosis, in patients taking ergot derivatives such as Cabaser (see special warnings and special precautions for use).

Other adverse events expected for the pharmacological class, in view of the vasoconstrictive properties, include angina (reported in about 1% of the patients on cabergoline) and erythromelalgia (observed in 0.4% of the patients). Similarly expected for the pharmacological class, peripheral oedema occurred in 6% of patients.

Gastric upset was more frequent in female than in male patients, while CNS events were more frequent in the elderly.

A blood pressure decrease of clinical relevance was observed mainly on standing in a minority of patients. The effect was mainly evident in the first weeks of therapy. Neither modification of heart rate nor consistent changes of ECG tracing were observed during Cabaser treatment.

Cabergoline is associated with somnolence and has been associated uncommonly with excessive daytime somnolence and sudden sleep onset episodes.

Alterations in standard laboratory tests are uncommon during long term therapy with Cabaser.

4.9 Overdose
The acute toxicity studies carried out in animals indicate very low toxicity, with a wide safety margin with respect to pharmacologically active doses. Clinical signs and cause of death, if any, were related to CNS stimulation.

There is no experience in humans of overdosage with Cabaser in the proposed indication: it is likely to lead to symptoms due to over-stimulation of dopamine receptors. These might include nausea, vomiting, gastric complaints, hypotension, confusion/psychosis or hallucinations. The vomiting stimulating properties of dopamine agonists are expected to favour removal of unabsorbed drug. Supportive measures should be directed to maintain blood pressure, if necessary. In addition, in case of pronounced central nervous system effects (hallucinations) the administration of dopamine antagonist drugs may be advisable.

5. PHARMACOLOGICAL PROPERTIES
5.1 Pharmacodynamic properties
Cabaser is a dopaminergic ergoline derivative endowed with potent and long-lasting dopamine D2 receptor agonist properties. In rats the compound, acting at D2 dopamine receptors on pituitary lactotrophic cells, decreases PRL secretion at oral doses of 3-25 mcg/kg, and in vitro at a concentration of 45 pg/ml. In addition, Cabaser exerts a central dopaminergic effect via D2 receptor stimulation at doses higher than those effective in lowering serum PRL levels. Improvement of motor deficit in animal models of parkinson's disease was present at oral daily doses of 1-2.5 mg/kg in rats and at s.c. doses of 0.5-1 mg/kg in monkeys.

In healthy volunteers the administration of Cabaser at single oral doses of 0.3-2.5 mg was associated with a significant decrease in serum PRL levels. The effect is prompt (within 3 hours of administration) and persistent (up to 7-28 days). The PRL-lowering effect is dose-related both in terms of degree of effect and duration of action.

The pharmacodynamic actions of Cabaser not linked to the therapeutic effect relate only to blood pressure decrease. The maximal hypotensive effect of Cabaser as a single dose usually occurs during the first 6 hours after drug intake and is dose-dependent both in terms of maximal decrease and frequency.

5.2 Pharmacokinetic properties
The pharmacokinetic and metabolic profiles of Cabaser have been studied in healthy volunteers of both sexes, in female hyperprolactinemic patients and in parkinsonian patients. After oral administration of the labelled compound, radioactivity was rapidly absorbed from the gastro-intestinal tract as the peak of radioactivity in plasma was between 0.5 and 4 hours. Ten days after administration about 18/20% and 55/72% of the radioactive dose (^{3}H-cabergoline/^{14}C-cabergoline) was recovered in urine and faeces, respectively. Unchanged drug in urine accounted for 2-3% of the dose.

In urine, the main metabolite identified was 6-allyl-8b-carboxy-ergoline, which accounted for 4-6% of the dose. Three additional metabolites were identified in urine, which accounted overall for less than 3% of the dose. The metabolites have been found to be much less potent than Cabaser as D_2 dopamine receptor agonists "in vitro".

The low urinary excretion of unchanged Cabaser has been confirmed also in studies with non-radioactive product. The elimination half-life of Cabaser, estimated from urinary excretion rates, is long (63-68 hours in healthy volunteers, 79-115 hours in hyperprolactinemic patients).

The pharmacokinetics of Cabaser seem to be dose-independent both in healthy volunteers (doses of 0.5-1.5 mg) and parkinsonian patients (steady state of daily doses up to 7 mg/day).

On the basis of the elimination half-life, steady state conditions should be achieved after 4 weeks, as confirmed by the mean peak plasma levels of Cabaser obtained after a single dose (37±8 pg/ml) and after a 4 week multiple-regimen (101±43 pg/ml). "In vitro" experiments showed that the drug at concentrations of 0.1-10 ng/ml is 41-42% bound to plasma proteins.

Food does not appear to affect absorption and disposition of Cabaser.

While renal insufficiency has been shown not to modify cabergoline kinetics, hepatic insufficiency of severe degree > 10 Child-Pugh score, maximum score 12) has been shown to be associated with an increase of AUC.

5.3 Preclinical safety data
Almost all the findings noted throughout the series of preclinical safety studies are a consequence of the central dopaminergic effects or the long-lasting inhibition of PRL in rodents with a specific hormonal physiology different to man.

Preclinical safety studies of Cabaser indicate a consistent safety margin for this compound in rodents and in monkeys, as well as a lack of teratogenic, genotoxic or carcinogenic potential.

6. PHARMACEUTICAL PARTICULARS
6.1 List of excipients
Lactose anhydrous NF, USP
Leucine Ph Eur

6.2 Incompatibilities
Not applicable

6.3 Shelf life
24 months at room temperature (25°C).

6.4 Special precautions for storage
There are no special precautions for storage.

6.5 Nature and contents of container
The tablets are contained in Type I amber glass bottles with tamper resistant screw caps which contain silica gel desiccant.

Each bottle contains 20 or 30 tablets and is enclosed in an outer cardboard carton.

6.6 Instructions for use and handling
Bottles of Cabaser are supplied with desiccant in the caps. This desiccant must not be removed.

Administrative Data
7. MARKETING AUTHORISATION HOLDER
Pharmacia Laboratories Limited
Ramsgate Road
Sandwich
Kent
CT13 9NJ

8. MARKETING AUTHORISATION NUMBER(S)
PL 0022/0169

9. DATE OF FIRST AUTHORISATION/RENEWAL OF THE AUTHORISATION
14 February 1996

10. DATE OF REVISION OF THE TEXT
January 2005

Cabaser Tablets 2mg

(Pharmacia Limited)

1. NAME OF THE MEDICINAL PRODUCT
Cabaser® Tablets 2 mg

2. QUALITATIVE AND QUANTITATIVE COMPOSITION
Cabergoline INN 2 mg.

For excipients, see 6.1

3. PHARMACEUTICAL FORM
Tablet

Cabaser 2 mg tablets are white, oval, 5.1 × 10mm and concave with one side scored and engraved '7' on the left and '02' on the right

4. CLINICAL PARTICULARS
4.1 Therapeutic indications
Treatment of Parkinson's disease
Cabaser is indicated for the treatment of symptoms of Parkinson's disease, as adjuvant therapy to levodopa plus dopa-decarboxylase inhibitor, in patients affected by "on-off" mobility problems with daily fluctuations in motor performance.

Controlled clinical studies have demonstrated that cabergoline administered once daily at an average dose of 4 mg/day following titration (up to 5-6 mg/day in the different studies) is effective in decreasing daily fluctuations in motor performance in Parkinsonian patients receiving levodopa/carbidopa therapy. Improvement of motor deficit has been demonstrated, while substantially decreasing the levodopa/carbidopa dose.

4.2 Posology and method of administration
The tablets are for oral administration.

Since the tolerability of dopaminergic agents is improved when administered with food, it is recommended that Cabaser be taken with meals.

Cabaser is intended for chronic, long term treatment.

Adults and elderly patients
As expected for dopamine agonists, dose response for both efficacy and side effects appears to be linked to individual sensitivity. Optimization of dose should be obtained through slow initial dose titration, from starting doses of 1 mg daily. The dosage of concurrent levodopa may be gradually decreased, while the dosage of Cabaser is increased, until the optimum balance is determined. In view of the long half-life of the compound, increments of the daily dose of 0.5-1 mg should be done at weekly (initial weeks) or bi-weekly intervals, up to optimal doses.

The recommended therapeutic dosage is 2 to 6 mg/day as adjuvant therapy to levodopa/carbidopa. Cabaser should be given as a single daily dose. Maximum doses higher than 6 mg/day and up to 20 mg/day have been administered in a small proportion of patients during clinical studies.

Use in children
The safety and efficacy of Cabaser have not been investigated in children as Parkinson's disease does not affect this population.

4.3 Contraindications
Hypersensitivity to any ergot alkaloid.

4.4 Special warnings and special precautions for use
While renal insufficiency has been shown not to modify cabergoline kinetics, hepatic insufficiency of severe degree > 10 Child-Pugh score, maximum score 12) has been shown to be associated with an increase of AUC, thus indicating that dose regimens in Parkinsonian patients with severe hepatic insufficiency should be modified accordingly.

Cabaser is an ergot derivative. Fibrotic and serosal inflammatory disorders such as pleuritis, pleural effusion, pleural fibrosis, pulmonary fibrosis, pericarditis, pericardial effusion and retroperitoneal fibrosis have occurred after prolonged usage of ergot derivatives. The factors predisposing patients to the risk of such disorders are not known, however, Parkinson's disease patients with a history of such disorders should not be treated with Cabaser, or any other ergot derivative, unless the potential clearly outweighs the risk.

Attention should be paid to the signs and symptoms of:

- Pleuro-pulmonary disease such as dyspnoea, shortness of breath, persistent cough or chest pain

- Renal insufficiency or ureteral/abdominal vascular obstruction that may occur with pain in the loin/flank and lower limb oedema as well as any possible abdominal masses or tenderness that may indicate retroperitoneal fibrosis

- Cardiac failure as cases of pericardial fibrosis have often manifested as cardiac failure. Constructive pericarditis should be excluded if such symptoms appear.

Appropriate investigations such as erythrocyte sedimentation rate, chest x-ray and serum creatinine measurements should be performed if necessary to support a diagnosis of a fibrotic disorder. It is also appropriate to perform baseline investigations of erythrocyte sedimentation rate or other inflammatory markers, lung function/chest x-ray and renal function prior to initiation of therapy.

These disorders can have an insidious onset and patients should be regularly and carefully monitored while taking Cabaser for manifestations of progressive fibrotic disorders. Cabaser should be withdrawn if fibrotic or serosal inflammatory changes are diagnosed or suspected.

In addition, by analogy with other ergot derivatives, Cabaser should be given with caution to patients suffering from severe cardiovascular disease, Raynaud's syndrome, peptic ulcer, gastrointestinal bleeding or a history of serious, particularly psychotic mental disease. Symptomatic hypotension can occur following adminstration of Cabaser: particular attention should be paid when administering Cabaser concomitantly with other drugs known to lower blood pressure.

Cabergoline has been associated with somnolence and episodes of sudden sleep onset, particularly in Patients with Parkinson's disease. Sudden onset of sleep during activities, in some cases without awareness or warning signs, has been reported uncommonly. Patients must be informed of this and advised to exercise caution while driving or operating machines during treatment with cabergoline. Patients who have experienced somnolence and/or an episode of sudden sleep onset must refrain from driving or operating machines. Furthermore a reduction of dosage or termination of therapy may be considered.

The effects of alcohol on overall tolerability of Cabaser are currently unknown.

4.5 Interaction with other medicinal products and other forms of Interaction
No pharmacokinetic interaction with L-Dopa or selegiline was observed in the studies carried out in parkinsonian patients. The concomitant use of other drugs, particularly other antiparkinsonian non-dopamine-agonist agents, was not associated with detectable interactions modifying the efficacy and safety of Cabaser.

No other information is available about possible interaction between Cabaser and other ergot alkaloids: therefore the concomitant use of these medications during long term treatment with Cabaser is not recommended.

Since Cabaser exerts its therapeutic effect by direct stimulation of dopamine receptors, it should not be concurrently administered with drugs which have dopamine antagonist activity (such as phenothiazines, butyrophenones, thioxanthenes, metoclopramide) since these might reduce the therapeutic effect of Cabaser.

By analogy with other ergot derivatives, Cabaser should not be used in association with macrolide antibiotics (e.g. erythromycin) since the systemic bioavailability of Cabaser and adverse effects could increase.

4.6 Pregnancy and lactation
Cabaser has been shown to cross the placenta in rats: it is unknown whether this occurs also in humans.

Animal studies in rats and mice have not demonstrated any teratogenic effect or any effect of the compound on global reproductive performance. In clinical studies there have been over 100 pregnancies in women treated with cabergoline for hyperprolactinemic disorders. The compound was generally taken during the first 8 weeks after conception. Among the pregnancies evaluable so far, there were approximately 85% live births and about 10% spontaneous abortions. Three cases of congenital abnormalities (Down's syndrome, hydrocephalus, malformation of lower limbs) which led to therapeutic abortion and three cases of minor abnormalities in live births were observed.

These incidence rates are comparable with those quoted for normal populations and for women exposed to other ovulation-inducing drugs. Based on the above data, the use of the product does not appear to be associated with an increased risk of abortion, premature delivery, multiple pregnancy or congenital abnormalities.

Because clinical experience is still limited and the drug has a long half-life, as a precautionary measure it is recommended that women seeking pregnancy discontinue Cabaser one month before intended conception, in order to prevent possible foetal exposure to the drug. If conception occurs during therapy, treatment is to be discontinued as soon as pregnancy is confirmed, to limit foetal exposure to the drug.

In rats cabergoline and/or its metabolites are excreted in milk. Lactation is expected to be inhibited/suppressed by Cabaser, in view of its dopamine-agonist properties. Therefore, while no information on the excretion of cabergoline in maternal milk in humans is available, puerperal women should be advised not to breast-feed in case of failed lactation inhibition/suppression by the product.

4.7 Effects on ability to drive and use machines
Patients being treated with cabergoline and presenting with somnolence and/or sudden sleep onset episodes must be informed to refrain from driving or engaging in activities where impaired alertness may put themselves or others at risk of serious injury or death (e.g. operating machines) until such episodes and somnolence have resolved (see also Section 4.4).

4.8 Undesirable effects
About 1070 parkinsonian patients have received Cabaser as adjuvant therapy to L-dopa in clinical studies; of these 74% had at least one adverse event, mainly of mild to moderate severity and transient in nature, and requiring discontinuation in a small proportion of cases.

In the majority of cases (51%), events were related to the nervous system: most frequently reported events were dyskinesia, hyperkinesia, hallucinations or confusion. The gastrointestinal system was involved in 33% of cases: events most frequently reported were nausea, vomiting, dyspepsia and gastritis. The cardiovascular system was involved in 27% of cases, most frequently reported events being dizziness and hypotension.

There have been reports of fibrotic and serosal inflammatory conditions, such as pleuritis, pleural effusion, pleural fibrosis, pulmonary fibrosis, pericarditis, pericardial effusion and retroperitoneal fibrosis, in patients taking ergot derivatives such as Cabaser (see special warnings and special precautions for use).

Other adverse events expected for the pharmacological class, in view of the vasoconstrictive properties, include angina (reported in about 1% of the patients on cabergoline) and erythromelalgia (observed in 0.4% of the patients). Similarly expected for the pharmacological class, peripheral oedema occurred in 6% of patients.

Gastric upset was more frequent in female than in male patients, while CNS events were more frequent in the elderly.

A blood pressure decrease of clinical relevance was observed mainly on standing in a minority of patients. The effect was mainly evident in the first weeks of therapy. Neither modification of heart rate nor consistent changes of ECG tracing were observed during Cabaser treatment.

Cabergoline is associated with somnolence and has been associated uncommonly with excessive daytime somnolence and sudden sleep onset episodes.

Alterations in standard laboratory tests are uncommon during long term therapy with Cabaser.

4.9 Overdose

The acute toxicity studies carried out in animals indicate very low toxicity, with a wide safety margin with respect to pharmacologically active doses. Clinical signs and cause of death, if any, were related to CNS stimulation.

There is no experience in humans of overdosage with Cabaser in the proposed indication: it is likely to lead to symptoms due to over-stimulation of dopamine receptors. These might include nausea, vomiting, gastric complaints, hypotension, confusion/psychosis or hallucinations. The vomiting stimulating properties of dopamine agonists are expected to favour removal of unabsorbed drug. Supportive measures should be directed to maintain blood pressure, if necessary. In addition, in case of pronounced central nervous system effects (hallucinations) the administration of dopamine antagonist drugs may be advisable.

5. PHARMACOLOGICAL PROPERTIES

5.1 Pharmacodynamic properties

Cabaser is a dopaminergic ergoline derivative endowed with potent and long-lasting dopamine D2 receptor agonist properties. In rats the compound, acting at D2 dopamine receptors on pituitary lactotrophic cells, decreases PRL secretion at oral doses of 3-25 mcg/kg, and in vitro at a concentration of 45 pg/ml. In addition, Cabaser exerts a central dopaminergic effect via D2 receptor stimulation at doses higher than those effective in lowering serum PRL levels. Improvement of motor deficit in animal models of parkinson's disease was present at oral daily doses of 1-2.5 mg/kg in rats and at s.c. doses of 0.5-1 mg/kg in monkeys.

In healthy volunteers the administration of Cabaser at single oral doses of 0.3-2.5 mg was associated with a significant decrease in serum PRL levels. The effect is prompt (within 3 hours of administration) and persistent (up to 7-28 days). The PRL-lowering effect is dose-related both in terms of degree of effect and duration of action.

The pharmacodynamic actions of Cabaser not linked to the therapeutic effect relate only to blood pressure decrease. The maximal hypotensive effect of Cabaser as a single dose usually occurs during the first 6 hours after drug intake and is dose-dependent both in terms of maximal decrease and frequency.

5.2 Pharmacokinetic properties

The pharmacokinetic and metabolic profiles of Cabaser have been studied in healthy volunteers of both sexes, in female hyperprolactinemic patients and in parkinsonian patients. After oral administration of the labelled compound, radioactivity was rapidly absorbed from the gastrointestinal tract as the peak of radioactivity in plasma was between 0.5 and 4 hours. Ten days after administration about 18/20% and 55/72% of the radioactive dose (^{3}H-cabergoline/^{14}C-cabergoline) was recovered in urine and faeces, respectively. Unchanged drug in urine accounted for 2-3% of the dose.

In urine, the main metabolite identified was 6-allyl-8b-carboxy-ergoline, which accounted for 4-6% of the dose. Three additional metabolites were identified in urine, which accounted overall for less than 3% of the dose. The metabolites have been found to be much less potent than Cabaser as D_2 dopamine receptor agonists "in vitro".

The low urinary excretion of unchanged Cabaser has been confirmed also in studies with non-radioactive product. The elimination half-life of Cabaser, estimated from urinary excretion rates, is long (63-68 hours in healthy volunteers, 79-115 hours in hyperprolactinemic patients).

The pharmacokinetics of Cabaser seem to be dose-independent both in healthy volunteers (doses of 0.5-1.5 mg) and parkinsonian patients (steady state of daily doses up to 7 mg/day).

On the basis of the elimination half-life, steady state conditions should be achieved after 4 weeks, as confirmed by the mean peak plasma levels of Cabaser obtained after a single dose (37$\pm$8 pg/ml) and after a 4 week multiple-regimen (101$\pm$43 pg/ml). "In vitro" experiments showed that the drug at concentrations of 0.1-10 ng/ml is 41-42% bound to plasma proteins.

Food does not appear to affect absorption and disposition of Cabaser.

While renal insufficiency has been shown not to modify cabergoline kinetics, hepatic insufficiency of severe degree > 10 Child-Pugh score, maximum score 12) has been shown to be associated with an increase of AUC.

5.3 Preclinical safety data

Almost all the findings noted throughout the series of preclinical safety studies are a consequence of the central dopaminergic effects or the long-lasting inhibition of PRL in rodents with a specific hormonal physiology different to man.

Preclinical safety studies of Cabaser indicate a consistent safety margin for this compound in rodents and in monkeys, as well as a lack of teratogenic, genotoxic or carcinogenic potential.

6. PHARMACEUTICAL PARTICULARS

6.1 List of excipients

Lactose anhydrous NF, USP

Leucine Ph Eur

6.2 Incompatibilities

Not applicable

6.3 Shelf life

24 months at room temperature (25°C).

6.4 Special precautions for storage

There are no special precautions for storage.

6.5 Nature and contents of container

The tablets are contained in Type I amber glass bottles with tamper resistant screw caps which contain silica gel desiccant.

Each bottle contains 20 or 30 tablets and is enclosed in an outer cardboard carton.

6.6 Instructions for use and handling

Bottles of Cabaser are supplied with desiccant in the caps. This desiccant must not be removed.

Administrative Data

7. MARKETING AUTHORISATION HOLDER

Pharmacia Laboratories Limited

Ramsgate Road

Sandwich

Kent

CT13 9NJ

8. MARKETING AUTHORISATION NUMBER(S)

PL 0022/0170

9. DATE OF FIRST AUTHORISATION/RENEWAL OF THE AUTHORISATION

14 February 1996

10. DATE OF REVISION OF THE TEXT

January 2005

Cabaser Tablets 4mg

(Pharmacia Limited)

1. NAME OF THE MEDICINAL PRODUCT

Cabaser® Tablets 4 mg

2. QUALITATIVE AND QUANTITATIVE COMPOSITION

Cabergoline INN 4 mg.

For excipients, see 6.1

3. PHARMACEUTICAL FORM

Tablet

Cabaser 4 mg tablets are white, oval, 6.5 × 12.7mm and concave with one side scored and engraved '7' on the left and '03' on the right

4. CLINICAL PARTICULARS

4.1 Therapeutic indications

Treatment of Parkinson's disease

Cabaser is indicated for the treatment of symptoms of Parkinson's disease, as adjuvant therapy to levodopa plus dopa-decarboxylase inhibitor, in patients affected by "on-off" mobility problems with daily fluctuations in motor performance.

Controlled clinical studies have demonstrated that cabergoline administered once daily at an average dose of 4 mg/day following titration (up to 5-6 mg/day in the different studies) is effective in decreasing daily fluctuations in motor performance in Parkinsonian patients receiving levodopa/carbidopa therapy. Improvement of motor deficit has been demonstrated, while substantially decreasing the levodopa/carbidopa dose.

4.2 Posology and method of administration

The tablets are for oral administration.

Since the tolerability of dopaminergic agents is improved when administered with food, it is recommended that Cabaser be taken with meals.

Cabaser is intended for chronic, long term treatment.

Adults and elderly patients

As expected for dopamine agonists, dose response for both efficacy and side effects appears to be linked to individual sensitivity. Optimization of dose should be obtained through slow initial dose titration, from starting doses of 1 mg daily. The dosage of concurrent levodopa may be gradually decreased, while the dosage of Cabaser is increased, until the optimum balance is determined. In view of the long half-life of the compound, increments of the daily dose of 0.5-1 mg should be done at weekly (initial weeks) or bi-weekly intervals, up to optimal doses.

The recommended therapeutic dosage is 2 to 6 mg/day as adjuvant therapy to levodopa/carbidopa. Cabaser should be given as a single daily dose. Maximum doses higher than 6 mg/day and up to 20 mg/day have been administered in a small proportion of patients during clinical studies.

Use in children

The safety and efficacy of Cabaser have not been investigated in children as Parkinson's disease does not affect this population.

4.3 Contraindications

Hypersensitivity to any ergot alkaloid.

4.4 Special warnings and special precautions for use

While renal insufficiency has been shown not to modify cabergoline kinetics, hepatic insufficiency of severe degree > 10 Child-Pugh score, maximum score 12) has been shown to be associated with an increase of AUC, thus indicating that dose regimens in Parkinsonian patients with severe hepatic insufficiency should be modified accordingly.

Cabaser is an ergot derivative. Fibrotic and serosal inflammatory disorders such as pleuritis, pleural effusion, pleural fibrosis, pulmonary fibrosis, pericarditis, pericardial effusion and retroperitoneal fibrosis have occurred after prolonged usage of ergot derivatives. The factors predisposing patients to the risk of such disorders are not known, however, Parkinson's disease patients with a history of such disorders should not be treated with Cabaser, or any other ergot derivative, unless the potential clearly outweighs the risk.

Attention should be paid to the signs and symptoms of:

- Pleuro-pulmonary disease such as dyspnoea, shortness of breath, persistent cough or chest pain
- Renal insufficiency or ureteral/abdominal vascular obstruction that may occur with pain in the loin/flank and lower limb oedema as well as any possible abdominal masses or tenderness that may indicate retroperitoneal fibrosis
- Cardiac failure as cases of pericardial fibrosis have often manifested as cardiac failure. Constructive pericarditis should be excluded if such symptoms appear.

Appropriate investigations such as erythrocyte sedimentation rate, chest x-ray and serum creatinine measurements should be performed if necessary to support a diagnosis of a fibrotic disorder. It is also appropriate to perform baseline investigations of erythrocyte sedimentation rate or other inflammatory markers, lung function/chest x-ray and renal function prior to initiation of therapy.

These disorders can have an insidious onset and patients should be regularly and carefully monitored while taking Cabaser for manifestations of progressive fibrotic disorders. Cabaser should be withdrawn if fibrotic or serosal inflammatory changes are diagnosed or suspected.

In addition, by analogy with other ergot derivatives, Cabaser should be given with caution to patients suffering from severe cardiovascular disease, Raynaud's syndrome, peptic ulcer, gastrointestinal bleeding or a history of serious, particularly psychotic mental disease. Symptomatic hypotension can occur following adminstration of Cabaser: particular attention should be paid when administering Cabaser concomitantly with other drugs known to lower blood pressure.

Cabergoline has been associated with somnolence and episodes of sudden sleep onset, particularly in Patients with Parkinson's disease. Sudden onset of sleep during activities, in some cases without awareness or warning signs, has been reported uncommonly. Patients must be informed of this and advised to exercise caution while driving or operating machines during treatment with cabergoline. Patients who have experienced somnolence and/or an episode of sudden sleep onset must refrain from driving or operating machines. Furthermore a reduction of dosage or termination of therapy may be considered.

The effects of alcohol on overall tolerability of Cabaser are currently unknown.

4.5 Interaction with other medicinal products and other forms of Interaction

No pharmacokinetic interaction with L-Dopa or selegiline was observed in the studies carried out in parkinsonian patients. The concomitant use of other drugs, particularly other antiparkinsonian non-dopamine-agonist agents, was not associated with detectable interactions modifying the efficacy and safety of Cabaser.

No other information is available about possible interaction between Cabaser and other ergot alkaloids: therefore the concomitant use of these medications during long term treatment with Cabaser is not recommended.

Since Cabaser exerts its therapeutic effect by direct stimulation of dopamine receptors, it should not be concurrently administered with drugs which have dopamine antagonist activity (such as phenothiazines, butyrophenones, thioxanthenes, metoclopramide) since these might reduce the therapeutic effect of Cabaser.

By analogy with other ergot derivatives, Cabaser should not be used in association with macrolide antibiotics (e.g. erythromycin) since the systemic bioavailability of Cabaser and adverse effects could increase.

4.6 Pregnancy and lactation
Cabaser has been shown to cross the placenta in rats: it is unknown whether this occurs also in humans.

Animal studies in rats and mice have not demonstrated any teratogenic effect or any effect of the compound on global reproductive performance. In clinical studies there have been over 100 pregnancies in women treated with cabergoline for hyperprolactinemic disorders. The compound was generally taken during the first 8 weeks after conception. Among the pregnancies evaluable so far, there were approximately 85% live births and about 10% spontaneous abortions. Three cases of congenital abnormalities (Down's syndrome, hydrocephalus, malformation of lower limbs) which led to therapeutic abortion and three cases of minor abnormalities in live births were observed.

These incidence rates are comparable with those quoted for normal populations and for women exposed to other ovulation-inducing drugs. Based on the above data, the use of the product does not appear to be associated with an increased risk of abortion, premature delivery, multiple pregnancy or congenital abnormalities.

Because clinical experience is still limited and the drug has a long half-life, as a precautionary measure it is recommended that women seeking pregnancy discontinue Cabaser one month before intended conception, in order to prevent possible foetal exposure to the drug. If conception occurs during therapy, treatment is to be discontinued as soon as pregnancy is confirmed, to limit foetal exposure to the drug.

In rats cabergoline and/or its metabolites are excreted in milk. Lactation is expected to be inhibited/suppressed by Cabaser, in view of its dopamine-agonist properties. Therefore, while no information on the excretion of cabergoline in maternal milk in humans is available, puerperal women should be advised not to breast-feed in case of failed lactation inhibition/suppression by the product.

4.7 Effects on ability to drive and use machines
Patients being treated with cabergoline and presenting with somnolence and/or sudden sleep onset episodes must be informed to refrain from driving or engaging in activities where impaired alertness may put themselves or others at risk of serious injury or death (e.g. operating machines) until such episodes and somnolence have resolved (see also Section 4.4).

4.8 Undesirable effects
About 1070 parkinsonian patients have received Cabaser as adjuvant therapy to L-dopa in clinical studies; of these 74% had at least one adverse event, mainly of mild to moderate severity and transient in nature, and requiring discontinuation in a small proportion of cases.

In the majority of cases (51%), events were related to the nervous system: most frequently reported events were dyskinesia, hyperkinesia, hallucinations or confusion. The gastrointestinal system was involved in 33% of cases: events most frequently reported were nausea, vomiting, dyspepsia and gastritis. The cardiovascular system was involved in 27% of cases, most frequently reported events being dizziness and hypotension.

There have been reports of fibrotic and serosal inflammatory conditions, such as pleuritis, pleural effusion, pleural fibrosis, pulmonary fibrosis, pericarditis, pericardial effusion and retroperitoneal fibrosis, in patients taking ergot derivatives such as Cabaser (see special warnings and special precautions for use).

Other adverse events expected for the pharmacological class, in view of the vasoconstrictive properties, include angina (reported in about 1% of the patients on cabergoline) and erythromelalgia (observed in 0.4% of the patients). Similarly expected for the pharmacological class, peripheral oedema occurred in 6% of patients.

Gastric upset was more frequent in female than in male patients, while CNS events were more frequent in the elderly.

A blood pressure decrease of clinical relevance was observed mainly on standing in a minority of patients. The effect was mainly evident in the first weeks of therapy. Neither modification of heart rate nor consistent changes of ECG tracing were observed during Cabaser treatment.

Cabergoline is associated with somnolence and has been associated uncommonly with excessive daytime somnolence and sudden sleep onset episodes.

Alterations in standard laboratory tests are uncommon during long term therapy with Cabaser.

4.9 Overdose
The acute toxicity studies carried out in animals indicate very low toxicity, with a wide safety margin with respect to pharmacologically active doses. Clinical signs and cause of death, if any, were related to CNS stimulation.

There is no experience in humans of overdosage with Cabaser in the proposed indication: it is likely to lead to symptoms due to over-stimulation of dopamine receptors. These might include nausea, vomiting, gastric complaints, hypotension, confusion/psychosis or hallucinations. The vomiting stimulating properties of dopamine agonists are expected to favour removal of unabsorbed drug. Supportive measures should be directed to maintain blood pressure, if necessary. In addition, in case of pronounced central nervous system effects (hallucinations) the administration of dopamine antagonist drugs may be advisable.

5. PHARMACOLOGICAL PROPERTIES

5.1 Pharmacodynamic properties
Cabaser is a dopaminergic ergoline derivative endowed with potent and long-lasting dopamine D2 receptor agonist properties. In rats the compound, acting at D2 dopamine receptors on pituitary lactotrophic cells, decreases PRL secretion at oral doses of 3-25 mcg/kg, and in vitro at a concentration of 45 pg/ml. In addition, Cabaser exerts a central dopaminergic effect via D2 receptor stimulation at doses higher than those effective in lowering serum PRL levels. Improvement of motor deficit in animal models of parkinson's disease was present at oral daily doses of 1-2.5 mg/kg in rats and at s.c. doses of 0.5-1 mg/kg in monkeys.

In healthy volunteers the administration of Cabaser at single oral doses of 0.3-2.5 mg was associated with a significant decrease in serum PRL levels. The effect is prompt (within 3 hours of administration) and persistent (up to 7-28 days). The PRL-lowering effect is dose-related both in terms of degree of effect and duration of action.

The pharmacodynamic actions of Cabaser not linked to the therapeutic effect relate only to blood pressure decrease. The maximal hypotensive effect of Cabaser as a single dose usually occurs during the first 6 hours after drug intake and is dose-dependent both in terms of maximal decrease and frequency.

5.2 Pharmacokinetic properties
The pharmacokinetic and metabolic profiles of Cabaser have been studied in healthy volunteers of both sexes, in female hyperprolactinemic patients and in parkinsonian patients. After oral administration of the labelled compound, radioactivity was rapidly absorbed from the gastrointestinal tract as the peak of radioactivity in plasma was between 0.5 and 4 hours. Ten days after administration about 18/20% and 55/72% of the radioactive dose (^{3}H-cabergoline/^{14}C-cabergoline) was recovered in urine and faeces, respectively. Unchanged drug in urine accounted for 2-3% of the dose.

In urine, the main metabolite identified was 6-allyl-8b-carboxy-ergoline, which accounted for 4-6% of the dose. Three additional metabolites were identified in urine, which accounted overall for less than 3% of the dose. The metabolites have been found to be much less potent than Cabaser as D_2 dopamine receptor agonists "in vitro".

The low urinary excretion of unchanged Cabaser has been confirmed also in studies with non-radioactive product. The elimination half-life of Cabaser, estimated from urinary excretion rates, is long (63-68 hours in healthy volunteers, 79-115 hours in hyperprolactinemic patients).

The pharmacokinetics of Cabaser seem to be dose-independent both in healthy volunteers (doses of 0.5-1.5 mg) and parkinsonian patients (steady state of daily doses up to 7 mg/day).

On the basis of the elimination half-life, steady state conditions should be achieved after 4 weeks, as confirmed by the mean peak plasma levels of Cabaser obtained after a single dose (37 ± 8 pg/ml) and after a 4 week multiple-regimen (101 ± 43 pg/ml). "In vitro" experiments showed that the drug at concentrations of 0.1-10 ng/ml is 41-42% bound to plasma proteins.

Food does not appear to affect absorption and disposition of Cabaser.

While renal insufficiency has been shown not to modify cabergoline kinetics, hepatic insufficiency of severe degree > 10 Child-Pugh score, maximum score 12) has been shown to be associated with an increase of AUC.

5.3 Preclinical safety data
Almost all the findings noted throughout the series of preclinical safety studies are a consequence of the central dopaminergic effects or the long-lasting inhibition of PRL in rodents with a specific hormonal physiology different to man.

Preclinical safety studies of Cabaser indicate a consistent safety margin for this compound in rodents and in monkeys, as well as a lack of teratogenic, genotoxic or carcinogenic potential.

6. PHARMACEUTICAL PARTICULARS

6.1 List of excipients
Lactose anhydrous NF, USP

Leucine Ph Eur

6.2 Incompatibilities
Not applicable

6.3 Shelf life
24 months at room temperature (25°C).

6.4 Special precautions for storage
There are no special precautions for storage.

6.5 Nature and contents of container
The tablets are contained in Type I amber glass bottles with tamper resistant screw caps which contain silica gel desiccant.

Each bottle contains 20 or 30 tablets and is enclosed in an outer cardboard carton.

6.6 Instructions for use and handling
Bottles of Cabaser are supplied with desiccant in the caps. This desiccant must not be removed.

Administrative Data

7. MARKETING AUTHORISATION HOLDER
Pharmacia Laboratories Limited
Ramsgate Road
Sandwich
Kent
CT13 9NJ

8. MARKETING AUTHORISATION NUMBER(S)
PL 0022/0171

9. DATE OF FIRST AUTHORISATION/RENEWAL OF THE AUTHORISATION
14 February 1996

10. DATE OF REVISION OF THE TEXT
January 2005

CACIT D3 effervescent granules, 500 mg/440 IU.

(Procter & Gamble Pharmaceuticals UK Limited)

1. NAME OF THE MEDICINAL PRODUCT
CACIT D3 effervescent granules, 500 mg/440 IU.

2. QUALITATIVE AND QUANTITATIVE COMPOSITION
Cacit D3 500 mg/440IU contains 1250 mg of calcium carbonate (equivalent to 500mg of elemental calcium) and 440IU of cholecalciferol (vitamin D3) per sachet of 4 g.

3. PHARMACEUTICAL FORM
Effervescent granules for oral solution.

4. CLINICAL PARTICULARS

4.1 Therapeutic indications
For correction of vitamin D and calcium combined deficiency in elderly people.

Cacit D3 may be used as an adjunct to specific therapy for osteoporosis, in patients with either established vitamin D and calcium combined deficiencies or in those patients at high risk of needing such therapeutic supplements.

4.2 Posology and method of administration
Dosage:

One or two sachets of Cacit D3 effervescent granules, 500mg/440IU per day.

Method of administration:

Oral, after reconstitution.

Pour the contents of the sachet into a glass, add a large quantity of water, stir, then drink immediately the solution is obtained.

4.3 Contraindications
hypercalcaemia, hypercalciuria;

long-term immobilisation accompanied by hypercalciuria and/or hypercalcaemia;

calci-lithiasis;

hypersensitivity to one of the ingredients.

4.4 Special warnings and special precautions for use
With long-term treatment it is advisable to monitor serum and urinary calcium levels and kidney function, and reduce or interrupt treatment temporarily if urinary calcium exceeds 7.5 mmol/24 hours (300 mg/24 hours).

The product should be used with caution in patients with renal insufficiency and the effects on calcium and phosphate homeostasis should be monitored.

In the case of combined treatment with digitalis, bisphosphonate, sodium fluoride, thiazide diuretics, tetracyclines, see section 4.5 (interactions with other medicines).

Allowances should be made for vitamin D/calcium supplements from other sources. Additional administration of vitamin D or calcium should be carried out under strict medical supervision, with weekly monitoring of serum and urinary calcium.

The product should be prescribed with caution in patients with sarcoidosis because of possible increased metabolism of vitamin D to its active form. These patients should be monitored for serum and urinary calcium.

4.5 Interaction with other medicinal products and other forms of Interaction
The effects of digitalis and other cardiac glycosides may be accentuated with the oral administration of calcium

combined with vitamin D (increases the toxicity of digitalis and therefore the risk of dysrythmia). Strict medical supervision, and if necessary, monitoring ECG and calcaemia are necessary.

In case of concomitant treatment with a bisphosphonate or with sodium fluoride, it is advisable to allow a minimum period of two hours before taking the calcium (risk of reduction of the gastrointestinal absorption of bisphosphonate and sodium fluoride).

Thiazide diuretics increase the renal absorption of calcium, so the risk of hypercalcaemia should be considered. Strict medical supervision of calcaemia is recommended.

Concomitant treatment with phenytoin or barbiturates can decrease the effect of vitamin D because of metabolic inactivation.

Concomitant use of a glucocorticosteroid can decrease the effect of vitamin D.

Calcium salts reduce the absorption of tetracyclines. It is advisable to delay taking Cacit D3 by at least three hours.

Possible interactions with food (e.g. containing oxalic acid, phosphate or phytinic acid).

4.6 Pregnancy and lactation

The product may be used during pregnancy and lactation. However, the daily intake should not exceed 1500mg calcium and 600IU vitamin D.

Overdoses of vitamin D have shown teratogenic effects in pregnant animals. In humans overdoses of vitamin D must be avoided, as permanent hypercalcaemia can lead to physical and mental retardation, supravalvular aortic stenosis and retinopathy in the child. There are several case reports of administration of very high doses in hypoparathyroidism in the mother, where normal children were born.

Vitamin D and its metabolites pass into the breast milk.

4.7 Effects on ability to drive and use machines

No data are known about the effect of this product on driving capacity. However, an effect is unlikely.

4.8 Undesirable effects

Constipation, flatulence, nausea, gastric pain, diarrhoea.

Hypercalciuria and in rare cases hypercalcaemia with long-term treatment at high doses.

Skin reactions such as pruritus, rash, urticaria (especially in patients with a past history of allergy).

4.9 Overdose

The most serious consequence of acute or chronic overdose would be hypercalciuria and hypercalcaemia due to vitamin D toxicity. Symptoms include nausea, vomiting, thirst, polydipsia, polyuria and constipation. Chronic overdoses can lead to vascular and organ calcifications as a result of hypercalcaemia. Treatment would consist of stopping all intake of calcium and vitamin D and rehydration.

5. PHARMACOLOGICAL PROPERTIES

5.1 Pharmacodynamic properties

Vitamin D corrects an insufficient intake of vitamin D and increases intestinal absorption of calcium. The optimal amount of vitamin D in the elderly is 500 - 1000 IU/day.

Calcium corrects an insufficient intake of calcium in the diet.

The commonly accepted requirement of calcium in the elderly is 1500 mg/day.

Vitamin D and calcium correct secondary senile hyperparathyroidism.

In a double-blind placebo controlled study of 18 months, including 3270 women aged 84 ± 6 years with a low intake of calcium and living in nursing homes, had their diet supplemented with cholecalciferol (800 IU/day) + Calcium (1.2 g/day). A significant decrease in PTH secretion has been observed.

After 18 months, the results of the intent to treat analysis showed 80 hip fractures (5.7%) in the calcium vitamin D group and 110 hip fractures (7.9%) in the placebo group (p=0.004). Therefore, under these study conditions, the treatment of 1387 women prevented 30 hip fractures. After 36 months of follow-up, 137 women presented at least one hip fracture (11.6%) in the calcium-vitamin D group (n= 1176) and 178 (15.8%) in the placebo group (n= 1127) ($p \leqslant 0.02$).

5.2 Pharmacokinetic properties

During dissolution the calcium salt contained in Cacit D3 is transformed into calcium citrate. Calcium citrate is well absorbed, (approximately 30% to 40% of the ingested dose).

Calcium is eliminated in the urine and faeces and secreted in the sweat.

Vitamin D is absorbed in the intestine and transported by protein binding in the blood to the liver (first hydroxylation) then to the kidney (second hydroxylation).

The non-hydroxylated vitamin D is stored in reserve compartments such as adipose and muscle tissue. Its plasma half-life is several days; it is eliminated in the faeces and the urine.

5.3 Preclinical safety data

No remarkable findings.

6. PHARMACEUTICAL PARTICULARS

6.1 List of excipients

Citric acid, malic acid, gluconolactone, maltodextrin, sodium cyclamate, saccharin sodium, lemon flavouring (containing: sorbitol, mannitol, D-gluconolactone, dextrin, gum arabic, lemon oil), rice starch, corn starch, potassium carbonate, α-tocopherol, vegetable oils, gelatin, and sucrose.

One sachet of Cacit D3 500 mg/440IU contains a total of 0.22 mmol of sodium (5mg).

6.2 Incompatibilities

None known.

6.3 Shelf life

3 years.

6.4 Special precautions for storage

Do not store above 25°C

6.5 Nature and contents of container

Paper/aluminium/polyethylene sachets packed in boxes of 20*,28*, 30, 46*, 50* 56*, 60* or 100* and sample pack of 10 sachets

*** Not all pack sizes are intended for sale in all EU countries**

6.6 Instructions for use and handling

Pour the contents of the sachet into a glass, add a large quantity of water, stir, then drink immediately the solution is obtained.

7. MARKETING AUTHORISATION HOLDER

Procter & Gamble Pharmaceuticals UK Limited.
Rusham Park,
Whitehall Lane,
Egham,
Surrey.
TW20 9NW, UK.

8. MARKETING AUTHORISATION NUMBER(S)

PL0364/0060 and PA170/18/1 Cacit D3 500 mg/440IU

9. DATE OF FIRST AUTHORISATION/RENEWAL OF THE AUTHORISATION

March 1996

10. DATE OF REVISION OF THE TEXT

October 2002

Cacit Effervescent Tablets 500mg

(Procter & Gamble Pharmaceuticals UK Limited)

1. NAME OF THE MEDICINAL PRODUCT

Cacit Effervescent Tablets 500mg

2. QUALITATIVE AND QUANTITATIVE COMPOSITION

Each tablet contains 1.25g Calcium Carbonate Ph Eur which when dissolved in water provides 500mg of calcium as calcium citrate.

3. PHARMACEUTICAL FORM

Effervescent tablet

4. CLINICAL PARTICULARS

4.1 Therapeutic indications

1. Treatment of calcium deficiency states including osteomalacia, rickets and malabsorption syndromes affecting the upper gastrointestinal tract.

2. An adjunct to conventional therapy in the arrest or slowing down of bone demineralisation in osteoporosis.

3. In the arrest or slowing down of bone demineralisation in osteoporosis, where other effective treatment is contra-indicated.

4. As a therapeutic supplement during times when intake may be inadequate, particularly those associated with the increased demand of childhood, old age, pregnancy and lactation.

4.2 Posology and method of administration

The tablets must be dissolved in a glass of water and the solution should then be drunk immediately after complete dissolution of the tablets.

Adults and the Elderly

For calcium deficiency states including malabsorption, the dosage should be tailored to the individual patient's needs. A dose of 1.0 g to 2.5g per day is recommended.

For the treatment of osteoporosis a dose of up to 1.5g per day is normally required. In patients with adequate dietary calcium intake, 500mg daily may be sufficient.

Up to 1.5g of calcium per day is the recommended dosage for therapeutic supplementation.

Children

For calcium deficiency states including malabsorption and rickets, the dosage recommendation under adult dosage should be followed.

For therapeutic supplementation, a dose of up to 1.0g per day is recommended.

4.3 Contraindications

Hypercalcaemia (eg. due to hyperparathyroidism, hypervitaminosis D, decalcifying tumours, severe renal failure, bone metastases), severe hypercalciuria calci-lithiasis and renal calculi. Long term immobilisation accompanied by hypercalciuria and/or hypercalcaemia. Hypersensitivity to any of the ingredients.

4.4 Special warnings and special precautions for use

In mild hypercalciuria (exceeding 7.5 mmol/24 hours in adults or 0.12-0.15 mmol/kg/24 hours in children) or renal failure, or where there is evidence of stone formation in the urinary tract; adequate checks must be kept on urinary calcium excretion. If necessary the dosage should be reduced or calcium therapy discontinued. The product should be administered with caution in patients with sarcoidosis because of possible increased metabolism of vitamin D to its active form. These patients should be monitored for serum and urinary calcium.

4.5 Interaction with other medicinal products and other forms of Interaction

Concomitant administration with vitamin D causes an increase in calcium absorption and plasma levels may continue to rise after stopping vitamin D therapy.

The effects of digoxin and other cardiac glycosides may be accentuated by calcium and toxicity may be produced, especially in combination with vitamin D.

Calcium salts reduce the absorption of some drugs, in particular tetracyclines It is therefore recommended that administration of Cacit tablets be separated from these products by at least 3 hours.

Thiazide diuretics increase renal absorption of calcium, so the risk of hypercalcaemia should be considered.

Bisphosphonate, sodium fluoride: it is advisable to allow a two hour minimum period before taking Cacit (risk of reduction of the gastrointestinal absorption of bisphosphonate and sodium fluoride).

4.6 Pregnancy and lactation

Calcium supplements have been in wide use for many years without apparent ill consequence.

4.7 Effects on ability to drive and use machines

None

4.8 Undesirable effects

Mild gastrointestinal disturbances have occurred rarely (eg. nausea, abdominal pain, diarrhoea, constipation, flatulence and eructation). Hypercalciuria and, in rare cases, hypercalcaemia in cases of long-term treatment with high doses.

Skin reactions, such as pruritis, rash, and urticaria (especially urticaria in patients with a past history of allergy) have been reported. The colouring agent E110 can cause allergic type reactions including asthma. Allergy is more common in those people who are allergic to aspirin

4.9 Overdose

The amount of calcium absorbed will depend on the individuals calcium status. Deliberate overdosage is unlikely with effervescent preparations and acute overdosage has not been reported. It might cause gastrointestinal disturbance but would not be expected to cause hypercalcaemia, except in patients treated with excessive doses of vitamin D. Symptoms of overdose may include nausea, vomiting, polydipsia, polyuria and constipation. Treatment should be aimed at lowering serum calcium levels, eg. administration of oral phosphates and rehydration.

Chronic overdoses can lead to vascular and organ calcifications as a result of hypercalcaemia.

5. PHARMACOLOGICAL PROPERTIES

5.1 Pharmacodynamic properties

Calcium is an essential element of tissues and plasma.

5.2 Pharmacokinetic properties

When the tablets are added to water, insoluble calcium carbonate is converted into absorbable calcium citrate.

6. PHARMACEUTICAL PARTICULARS

6.1 List of excipients

Citric acid, sodium saccharin, sodium cyclamate, Sunset Yellow FCF (E110) and flavour. Cacit tablets contain no sugar and have a low sodium content.

6.2 Incompatibilities

None

6.3 Shelf life

Three years.

6.4 Special precautions for storage

Store in a dry place.

6.5 Nature and contents of container

Supplied in boxes of 76 tablets (4 polypropylene tubes with polyethylene stoppers each containing 19 tablets).

6.6 Instructions for use and handling

To be dissolved in water before administration as described in Section 4.2

7. MARKETING AUTHORISATION HOLDER
Procter & Gamble Pharmaceuticals UK Limited
Rusham Park
Whitehall Lane
Egham
Surrey
TW20 9NW
UK

8. MARKETING AUTHORISATION NUMBER(S)
PL 0364/0045

9. DATE OF FIRST AUTHORISATION/RENEWAL OF THE AUTHORISATION
2 October 1989

10. DATE OF REVISION OF THE TEXT
October 2002

Caelyx 2mg/ml concentrate for solution for infusion

(Schering-Plough Ltd)

1. NAME OF THE MEDICINAL PRODUCT
Caelyx 2 mg/ml concentrate for solution for infusion

2. QUALITATIVE AND QUANTITATIVE COMPOSITION
Caelyx contains 2 mg/ml doxorubicin hydrochloride in a pegylated liposomal formulation.

Caelyx, a liposome formulation, is doxorubicin hydrochloride encapsulated in liposomes with surface-bound methoxypolyethylene glycol (MPEG). This process is known as pegylation and protects liposomes from detection by the mononuclear phagocyte system (MPS), which increases blood circulation time.

For excipients, see section 6.1.

3. PHARMACEUTICAL FORM
Concentrate for solution for infusion

The suspension is sterile, translucent and red.

4. CLINICAL PARTICULARS

4.1 Therapeutic indications
Caelyx is indicated:

- As monotherapy for patients with metastatic breast cancer, where there is an increased cardiac risk.

- For treatment of advanced ovarian cancer in women who have failed a first-line platinum-based chemotherapy regimen.

- For treatment of AIDS-related Kaposi's sarcoma (KS) in patients with low CD_4 counts (< 200 CD_4 lymphocytes/mm^3) and extensive mucocutaneous or visceral disease.

Caelyx may be used as first-line systemic chemotherapy, or as second line chemotherapy in AIDS-KS patients with disease that has progressed with, or in patients intolerant to, prior combination systemic chemotherapy comprising at least two of the following agents: a vinca alkaloid, bleomycin and standard doxorubicin (or other anthracycline).

4.2 Posology and method of administration
Caelyx should only be administered under the supervision of a qualified oncologist specialised in the administration of cytotoxic agents.

Caelyx exhibits unique pharmacokinetic properties and must not be used interchangeably with other formulations of doxorubicin hydrochloride.

Breast cancer/Ovarian cancer:

Caelyx is administered intravenously at a dose of 50 mg/m^2 once every 4 weeks for as long as the disease does not progress and the patient continues to tolerate treatment.

For doses < 90 mg: dilute Caelyx in 250 ml 5 % (50 mg/ml) glucose solution for infusion.

For doses ⩾ 90 mg: dilute Caelyx in 500 ml 5 % (50 mg/ml) glucose solution for infusion.

To minimize the risk of infusion reactions, the initial dose is administered at a rate no greater than 1 mg/minute. If no infusion reaction is observed, subsequent Caelyx infusions may be administered over a 60 minute period.

In those patients who experience an infusion reaction, the method of infusion should be modified as follows:

5 % of the total dose should be infused slowly over the first 15 minutes. If tolerated without reaction, the infusion rate may then be doubled for the next 15 minutes. If tolerated, the infusion may then be completed over the next hour for a total infusion time of 90 minutes.

AIDS-related KS:

Caelyx is administered intravenously at 20 mg/m^2 every two-to-three weeks. Avoid intervals shorter than 10 days as medicinal product accumulation and increased toxicity cannot be ruled out. Treatment of patients for two-to-three months is recommended to achieve a therapeutic response. Continue treatment as needed to maintain a therapeutic response.

The dose of Caelyx is diluted in 250 ml 5 % (50 mg/ml) glucose solution for infusion and administered by intravenous infusion over 30 minutes.

For all patients:

If the patient experiences early symptoms or signs of infusion reaction (see sections 4.4 and 4.8), immediately discontinue the infusion, give appropriate premedications (antihistamine and/or short acting corticosteroid) and restart at a slower rate.

Do not administer Caelyx as a bolus injection or undiluted solution. It is recommended that the Caelyx infusion line be connected through the side port of an intravenous infusion of 5 % (50 mg/ml) glucose to achieve further dilution and minimise the risk of thrombosis and extravasation. The infusion may be given through a peripheral vein. Do not use with in-line filters. Caelyx must not be given by the intramuscular or subcutaneous route (see section 6.6).

To manage adverse events such as palmar-plantar erythrodysesthesia (PPE), stomatitis or haematological toxicity, the dose may be reduced or delayed. Guidelines for Caelyx dose modification secondary to these adverse effects are provided in the tables below. The toxicity grading in these tables is based on the National Cancer Institute Common Toxicity Criteria (NCI-CTC).

The tables for PPE (Table 1) and stomatitis (Table 2) provide the schedule followed for dose modification in clinical trials in the treatment of breast or ovarian cancer (modification of the recommended 4 week treatment cycle): if these toxicities occur in patients with AIDS related KS, the recommended 2 to 3 week treatment cycle can be modified in a similar manner.

The table for haematological toxicity (Table 3) provides the schedule followed for dose modification in clinical trials in the treatment of patients with breast or ovarian cancer only. Dose modification in patients with AIDS-KS is addressed in 4.8.

Guidelines For Caelyx Dose Modification

(see Table 1)

(see Table 2)

(see Table 3 on next page)

Patients with impaired hepatic function: Caelyx pharmacokinetics determined in a small number of patients with elevated total bilirubin levels do not differ from patients with normal total bilirubin; however, until further experience is gained, the Caelyx dosage in patients with impaired hepatic function should be reduced based on the experience from the breast and ovarian clinical trial programs as follows: at initiation of therapy, if the bilirubin is between 1.2 - 3.0 mg/dl, the first dose is reduced by 25 %. If the bilirubin is > 3.0 mg/dl, the first dose is reduced by 50 %. If the patient tolerates the first dose without an increase in serum bilirubin or liver enzymes, the dose for cycle 2 can be increased to the next dose level, i.e., if reduced by 25 % for the first dose, increase to full dose for cycle 2; if reduced by 50 % for the first dose, increase to 75 % of full dose for cycle 2. The dosage can be increased to full dose for subsequent cycles if tolerated. Caelyx can be administered to patients with liver metastases with concurrent elevation of bilirubin and liver enzymes up to 4 × the upper limit of the normal range. Prior to Caelyx administration, evaluate hepatic function using conventional clinical laboratory tests such as ALT/AST, alkaline phosphatase, and bilirubin.

Patients with impaired renal function: As doxorubicin is metabolised by the liver and excreted in the bile, dose modification should not be required. Population pharmacokinetic data (in the range of creatinine clearance tested of 30 - 156 ml/min) demonstrate that Caelyx clearance is not influenced by renal function. No pharmacokinetic data are available in patients with creatinine clearance of less than 30 ml/min.

AIDS-KS patients with splenectomy: As there is no experience with Caelyx in patients who have had splenectomy, treatment with Caelyx is not recommended.

Paediatric patients: Safety and effectiveness in patients less than 18 years of age have not been established.

Table 1 PALMAR – PLANTAR ERYTHRODYSESTHESIA

	Week After Prior Caelyx Dose		
Toxicity Grade At Current Assessment	**Week 4**	**Week 5**	**Week 6**
Grade 1 (mild erythema, swelling, or desquamation not interfering with daily activities)	**Redose unless** patient has experienced a previous Grade 3 or 4 skin toxicity, in which case wait an additional week	**Redose unless** patient has experienced a previous Grade 3 or 4 skin toxicity, in which case wait an additional week	**Decrease dose by 25 %; return to 4 week interval**
Grade 2 (erythema, desquamation, or swelling interfering with, but not precluding normal physical activities; small blisters or ulcerations less than 2 cm in diameter)	**Wait an additional week**	**Wait an additional week**	**Decrease dose by 25 %; return to 4 week interval**
Grade 3 (blistering, ulceration, or swelling interfering with walking or normal daily activities; cannot wear regular clothing)	**Wait an additional week**	**Wait an additional week**	**Withdraw patient**
Grade 4 (diffuse or local process causing infectious complications, or a bedridden state or hospitalization)	**Wait an additional week**	**Wait an additional week**	**Withdraw patient**

Table 2 STOMATITIS

	Week after Prior Caelyx Dose		
Toxicity Grade At Current Assessment	**4**	**5**	**6**
Grade 1 (painless ulcers, erythema, or mild soreness)	**Redose unless** patient has experienced a previous Grade 3 or 4 stomatitis in which case wait an additional week	**Redose unless** patient has experienced a previous Grade 3 or 4 stomatitis in which case wait an additional week	**Decrease dose by 25 %; return to 4 week interval** or withdraw patient per physician's assessment
Grade 2 (painful erythema, oedema, or ulcers, but can eat)	**Wait an additional week**	**Wait an additional week**	**Decrease dose by 25 %; return to 4 week interval** or withdraw patient per physician's assessment
Grade 3 (painful erythema, edema, or ulcers, but cannot eat)	**Wait an additional week**	**Wait an additional week**	**Withdraw patient**
Grade 4 (requires parenteral or enteral support)	**Wait an additional week**	**Wait an additional week**	**Withdraw patient**

Table 3 HAEMATOLOGICAL TOXICITY (ANC OR PLATELETS) – MANAGEMENT OF PATIENTS WITH BREAST OR OVARIAN CANCER

GRADE	ANC	PLATELETS	MODIFICATION
Grade 1	1,500 – 1,900	75,000 – 150,000	Resume treatment with no dose reduction.
Grade 2	1,000 – < 1,500	50,000 – < 75,000	Wait until ANC ⩾ 1,500 and platelets ⩾ 75,000; redose with no dose reduction.
Grade 3	500 – < 1,000	25,000 – < 50,000	Wait until ANC ⩾ 1,500 and platelets ⩾ 75,000; redose with no dose reduction.
Grade 4	< 500	< 25,000	Wait until ANC ⩾ 1,500 and platelets ⩾ 75,000; decrease dose by 25 % or continue full dose with growth factor support.

Elderly patients: Population based analysis demonstrates that age across the range tested

(21 – 75 years) does not significantly alter the pharmacokinetics of Caelyx.

4.3 Contraindications

- hypersensitivity to the active substance or to any of the excipients
- breast-feeding

Caelyx must not be used to treat AIDS-KS that may be treated effectively with local therapy or systemic alfa-interferon.

4.4 Special warnings and special precautions for use

Cardiac toxicity: It is recommended that all patients receiving Caelyx routinely undergo frequent ECG monitoring. Transient ECG changes such as T-wave flattening, S-T segment depression and benign arrhythmias are not considered mandatory indications for the suspension of Caelyx therapy. However, reduction of the QRS complex is considered more indicative of cardiac toxicity. If this change occurs, the most definitive test for anthracycline myocardial injury, i.e., endomyocardial biopsy, must be considered.

More specific methods for the evaluation and monitoring of cardiac functions as compared to ECG are a measurement of left ventricular ejection fraction by echocardiography or preferably by Multigated Angiography (MUGA). These methods must be applied routinely before the initiation of Caelyx therapy and repeated periodically during treatment. The evaluation of left ventricular function is considered to be mandatory before each additional administration of Caelyx that exceeds a lifetime cumulative anthracycline dose of 450 mg/m^2.

The evaluation tests and methods mentioned above concerning the monitoring of cardiac performance during anthracycline therapy are to be employed in the following order: ECG monitoring, measurement of left ventricular ejection fraction, endomyocardial biopsy. If a test result indicates possible cardiac injury associated with Caelyx therapy, the benefit of continued therapy must be carefully weighed against the risk of myocardial injury.

In patients with cardiac disease requiring treatment, administer Caelyx only when the benefit outweighs the risk to the patient.

Exercise caution in patients with impaired cardiac function who receive Caelyx.

Whenever cardiomyopathy is suspected, i.e., the left ventricular ejection fraction has substantially decreased relative to pre-treatment values and/or left ventricular ejection fraction is lower than a prognostically relevant value (e.g. < 45 %), endomyocardial biopsy may be considered and the benefit of continued therapy must be carefully evaluated against the risk of developing irreversible cardiac damage.

Congestive heart failure due to cardiomyopathy may occur suddenly, without prior ECG changes and may also be encountered several weeks after discontinuation of therapy.

Caution must be observed in patients who have received other anthracyclines. The total dose of doxorubicin hydrochloride must also take into account any previous (or concomitant) therapy with cardiotoxic compounds such as other anthracyclines/anthraquinones or e.g. 5-fluorouracil. Cardiac toxicity also may occur at cumulative anthracycline doses lower than 450 mg/m^2 in patients with prior mediastinal irradiation or in those receiving concurrent cyclophosphamide therapy.

The cardiac safety profile for the dosing schedule recommended for both breast and ovarian cancer (50 mg/m^2) is similar to the 20 mg/m^2 profile in patients with AIDS-KS (see section 4.8).

Myelosuppression: Many patients treated with Caelyx have baseline myelosuppression due to such factors as their pre-existing HIV disease or numerous concomitant or previous medications, or tumours involving bone marrow. In the pivotal trial in patients with ovarian cancer treated at a dose of 50 mg/m^2, myelosuppression was generally mild to moderate, reversible, and was not associated with episodes of neutropaenic infection or sepsis. Moreover, in a controlled clinical trial of Caelyx vs. topotecan, the incidence of treatment related sepsis was substantially less in the Caelyx-treated ovarian cancer patients as compared to the topotecan treatment group. A similar low incidence of myelosuppression was seen in patients with metastatic breast cancer receiving Caelyx in a first-line clinical trial. In contrast to the experience in patients with breast cancer or ovarian cancer, myelosuppression appears to be the dose-limiting adverse event in patients with AIDS-KS (see section 4.8). Because of the potential for bone marrow suppression, periodic blood counts must be performed frequently during the course of Caelyx therapy, and at a minimum, prior to each dose of Caelyx.

Persistent severe myelosuppression, may result in superinfection or haemorrhage.

In controlled clinical studies in patients with AIDS-KS against a bleomycin/vincristine regimen, opportunistic infections were apparently more frequent during treatment with Caelyx. Patients and doctors must be aware of this higher incidence and take action as appropriate.

As with other DNA-damaging antineoplastic agents, secondary acute myeloid leukemias and myelodysplasias have been reported in patients having received combined treatment with doxorubicin. Therefore, any patient treated with doxorubicin should be kept under haematological supervision.

Given the difference in pharmacokinetic profiles and dosing schedules, Caelyx should not be used interchangeably with other formulations of doxorubicin hydrochloride.

Infusion-associated reactions: Serious and sometimes life-threatening infusion reactions, which are characterised by allergic-like or anaphylactoid-like reactions, with symptoms including asthma, flushing, urticarial rash, chest pain, fever, hypertension, tachycardia, pruritus, sweating, shortness of breath, facial oedema, chills, back pain, tightness in the chest and throat and/or hypotension may occur within minutes of starting the infusion of Caelyx. Very rarely, convulsions also have been observed in relation to infusion reactions (see section 4.8). Temporarily stopping the infusion usually resolves these symptoms without further therapy. However, medications to treat these symptoms (e.g., antihistamines, corticosteroids, adrenaline, and anticonvulsants), as well as emergency equipment should be available for immediate use. In most patients treatment can be resumed after all symptoms have resolved, without recurrence. Infusion reactions rarely recur after the first treatment cycle. To minimise the risk of infusion reactions, the initial dose should be administered at a rate no greater than 1 mg/minute (see section 4.2).

Diabetic patients: Please note that each vial of Caelyx contains sucrose and the dose is administered in 5 % (50 mg/ml) glucose solution for infusion.

4.5 Interaction with other medicinal products and other forms of Interaction

No formal drug interaction studies have been conducted with Caelyx, although phase II combination trials with conventional chemotherapy agents have been conducted in patients with gynaecological malignancies. Exercise caution in the concomitant use of medicinal products known to interact with standard doxorubicin hydrochloride. Caelyx, like other doxorubicin hydrochloride preparations, may potentiate the toxicity of other anti-cancer therapies. During clinical trials in patients with solid tumours (including breast and ovarian cancer) who have received concomitant cyclophosphamide or taxanes, no new additive toxicities were noted. In patients with AIDS, exacerbation of cyclophosphamide-induced haemorrhagic cystitis and enhancement of the hepatotoxicity of 6-mercaptopurine have been reported with standard doxorubicin hydrochloride. Caution must be exercised when giving any other cytotoxic agents, especially myelotoxic agents, at the same time.

4.6 Pregnancy and lactation

Pregnancy: Doxorubicin hydrochloride is suspected to cause serious birth defects when administered during pregnancy. Therefore, Caelyx should not be used unless clearly necessary.

Women of child-bearing potential must be advised to avoid pregnancy while they or their male partner are receiving Caelyx and in the six months following discontinuation of Caelyx therapy (see section 5.3).

Lactation: It is not known whether Caelyx is excreted in human milk and because of the potential for serious adverse reactions in nursing infants, therefore mothers must discontinue nursing prior to beginning Caelyx treatment. Health experts recommend that HIV infected women do not breast-feed their infants under any circumstances in order to avoid transmission of HIV.

4.7 Effects on ability to drive and use machines

Caelyx has no or negligible influence on the ability to drive and use machines. However, in clinical studies to date, dizziness and somnolence were associated infrequently (< 5 %) with the administration of Caelyx. Patients who suffer from these effects must avoid driving and operating machinery.

4.8 Undesirable effects

The most common undesirable effect reported in breast/ovarian clinical trials (50 mg/m^2 every 4 weeks) was palmar-plantar erythrodysesthesia (PPE). The overall incidence of PPE reported was 44.0 % - 46.1 %. These effects were mostly mild, with severe (Grade III) cases reported in 17 % - 19.5 %. The reported incidence of life-threatening (Grade IV) cases was < 1 %. PPE infrequently resulted in permanent treatment discontinuation (3.7 % - 7.0 %). PPE is characterised by painful, macular reddening skin eruptions. In patients experiencing this event, it is generally seen after two or three cycles of treatment. Improvement usually occurs in one - two weeks, and in some cases, may take up to 4 weeks or longer for complete resolution. Pyridoxine at a dose of 50 - 150 mg per day and corticosteroids have been used for the prophylaxis and treatment of PPE, however, these therapies have not bee evaluated in phase III trials. Other strategies to prevent and treat PPE, which may be initiated for 4 to 7 days after treatment with Caelyx include keeping hands and feet cool, by exposing them to cool water (soaks, baths, or swimming), avoiding excessive heat/hot water and keeping them unrestricted (no socks, gloves, or shoes that are tight fitting). PPE appears to be primarily related to the dose schedule and can be reduced by extending the dose interval 1 - 2 weeks (see section 4.2). However, this reaction can be severe and debilitating in some patients and may require discontinuation of treatment. Stomatitis/mucositis and nausea were also commonly reported in breast/ovarian cancer patient populations, whereas the AIDS-KS Program (20 mg/m^2 every 2 weeks), myelosuppression (mostly leukopaenia) was the most common side effect (see AIDS-KS).

Breast Cancer Program: 509 patients with advanced breast cancer who had not received prior chemotherapy for metastatic disease were treated with Caelyx (n=254) at a dose of 50 mg/m^2 every 4 weeks, or doxorubicin (n=255) at a dose of 60 mg/m^2 every 3 weeks, in a phase III clinical trial (I97-328). The following common adverse events were reported more often with doxorubicin than with Caelyx: nausea (53 % vs. 37 %; Grade III/IV 5 % vs. 3 %), vomiting (31 % vs. 19 %; Grade III/IV 4 % vs. less than 1 %), any alopecia (66 % vs. 20 %), pronounced alopecia (54 % vs.7 %), and neutropaenia (10 % vs. 4 %; Grade III/IV 8 % vs. 2 %).

Mucositis (23 % vs. 13 %; Grade III/IV 4 % vs. 2 %), and stomatitis (22 % vs. 15 %; Grade III/IV 5 % vs. 2 %) were reported more commonly with Caelyx than with doxorubicin. The average duration of the most common severe (Grade III/IV) events for both groups was 30 days or less. See Table 4 for complete listing of undesirable effects reported in ⩾ 5 % of Caelyx-treated patients.

Anaemia, leukopaenia and thrombocytopaenia were infrequently reported among Caelyx patients at incidences of 5 %, 2 %, and 1 %, respectively. The incidence of life threatening (Grade IV) haematologic effects was < 1.0 % and sepsis was reported in 1 % of patients. Growth factor support or transfusion support was necessary in 5.1 % and 5.5 % of patients, respectively (see section 4.2).

Clinically significant laboratory abnormalities (Grades III and IV) in this group was low with elevated total bilirubin, AST and ALT reported in 2.4 %, 1.6 % and < 1 % of patients respectively. No clinically significant increases in serum creatinine were reported.

(see Table 4 on next page)

Undesirable effects reported between 1 % and 5 % in 404 Caelyx-treated breast cancer patients, not previously reported in Caelyx clinical trials were breast pain, leg cramps, oedema, leg oedema, peripheral neuropathy, oral pain, ventricular arrhythmia, folliculitis, bone pain, musculo-skeletal pain, thrombocythemia, cold sores (non-herpetic), fungal infection, epistaxis, upper respiratory tract infection, bullous eruption, dermatitis, erythematous rash, nail disorder, scaly skin, lacrimation, and blurred vision.

Ovarian cancer program: 512 patients with ovarian cancer (a subset of 876 solid tumour patients) were treated with Caelyx at a dose of 50 mg/m^2 in clinical trials. See Table 4 for undesirable effects reported in ⩾ 5 % of Caelyx-treated patients.

Myelosuppression was mostly mild or moderate and manageable. Leukopaenia was the most frequently reported haematological adverse effect, followed by anaemia, neutropaenia and thrombocytopaenia. Life threatening (Grade IV) haematological effects were reported at incidences of 1.6 %, 0.4 %, 2.9 %, 0.2 % respectively. Sepsis related to leukopaenia was observed infrequently (< 1 %). Growth

Table 4 Treatment Related Undesirable Effects Reported in Breast Cancer (I97-328) and Ovarian Cancer Clinical Trials (50 mg/m² every 4 weeks) (⩾ 5 % of Caelyx-treated patients) by Severity, Body System and Preferred Term

AE by body system	Breast Cancer All Severities % n=254	Breast Cancer Grades III/IV % n=254	Ovarian Cancer All Severities % n=512	Ovarian Cancer Grades III/IV % n=512
Blood and lymphatic system disorders				
Leukopaenia	*	*	33	9
Anaemia	5	1	32	6
Neutropaenia	*	*	32	12
Thrombocytopaenia	*	*	11	1
Nervous system disorders				
Paresthesia	*	*	8	< 1
Somnolence	*	*	5	< 1
Respiratory, thoracic and mediastinal disorders				
Pharyngitis	*	*	6	< 1
Skin and subcutaneous tissue disorders				
Alopecia	20	0	17	1
Dry skin	*	*	6	0
PPE**	48	17	46	20
Pigmentation abnormal	8	< 1	N/A	N/A
Rash	10	2	25	4
Skin Discolouration	*	*	6	0
Gastrointestinal disorders				
Abdominal pain	8	1	8	2
Anorexia	11	1	12	< 1
Constipation	8	< 1	13	< 1
Diarrhoea	7	1	12	2
Dyspepsia	*	*	6	< 1
Mouth ulceration	5	< 1	*	*
Mucositis NOS	23	4	N/A	N/A
Nausea	37	3	38	4
Stomatitis	22	5	39	9
Vomiting	19	< 1	24	5
General disorders and administration site conditions				
Asthenia	10	1	34	7
Erythema	7	< 1	N/A	N/A
Fatigue	12	< 1	N/A	N/A
Fever	8	0	9	< 1
Weakness	6	< 1	N/A	N/A
Mucous membrane disorder	N/A	N/A	15	3
Pain	*	*	7	1

* reported at an incidence of < 5 %

** palmar-plantar erythrodysesthesia (Hand- foot syndrome).

N/A Not applicable based on alternate dictionary term

factor support was required infrequently (< 5 %) and transfusion support was required in approximately 15 % of patients (see section 4.2).

Undesirable effects reported between 1 % and 5 % in Caelyx-treated patients were headache, allergic reaction, chills, infection, chest pain, back pain, malaise, vasodilatation, cardiovascular disorder, oral moniliasis, mouth ulceration, esophagitis, nausea and vomiting, gastritis, dysphagia, dry mouth, flatulence, gingivitis, hypochromic anaemia, peripheral oedema, weight loss, dehydration, cachexia, myalgia, dizziness, insomnia, anxiety, neuropathy, depression, hypertonia, dyspnoea, increased cough, vesiculobullous rash, pruritus, exfoliative dermatitis, skin disorder, maculopapular rash, sweating, acne, herpes zoster, skin ulcer, conjunctivitis, taste perversion, urinary tract infection, dysuria and vaginitis.

In a subset of 410 patients with ovarian cancer, clinically significant laboratory abnormalities occurring in clinical trials with Caelyx included increases in total bilirubin (usually in patients with liver metastases) (5 %) and serum creatinine levels (5 %). Increases in AST were less frequently (< 1 %) reported.

Solid tumour patients: in a larger cohort of 929 patients with solid tumours (including breast cancer and ovarian cancer) predominantly treated at a dose of 50 mg/m² every 4 weeks, the safety profile and incidence of adverse effects are comparable to those of the patients treated in the pivotal breast cancer and ovarian cancer trials.

AIDS-KS program: Clinical studies on AIDS-KS patients treated at 20 mg/m² with Caelyx show that myelosuppression was the most frequent undesirable effect considered related to Caelyx occurring in approximately one-half of the patients.

Leukopaenia is the most frequent undesirable effect experienced with Caelyx in this population; neutropaenia, anaemia and thrombocytopaenia have been observed. These effects may occur early on in treatment. Haematological toxicity may require dose reduction or suspension or delay of therapy. Temporarily suspend Caelyx treatment in patients when the ANC count is < 1,000/mm³ and/or the platelet count is < 50,000/mm³. G-CSF (or GM-CSF) may be given as concomitant therapy to support the blood count when the ANC count is < 1,000/mm³ in subsequent cycles. The haematological toxicity for ovarian cancer patients is less severe than in the AIDS-KS setting (see section for ovarian cancer patients above).

Other frequently (⩾ 5 %) observed undesirable effects were nausea, asthenia, alopecia, fever, diarrhoea, infusion-associated acute reactions, and stomatitis.

Respiratory undesirable effects frequently (⩾ 5 %) occurred in clinical studies of Caelyx and may be related to opportunistic infections in the AIDS population. Opportunistic infections (OI's) are observed in KS patients after administration with Caelyx, and are frequently observed in patients with HIV-induced immunodeficiency. The most frequently observed OI's in clinical studies were candidiasis, cytomegalovirus, herpes simplex, *Pneumocystis carinii* pneumonia, and mycobacterium avium complex.

Other less frequently (< 5 %) observed undesirable effects included palmar-plantar erythrodysesthesia, oral moniliasis, nausea and vomiting, vomiting, weight loss, rash, mouth ulceration, dyspnoea, abdominal pain, hypersensitivity reactions including anaphylactic reactions, vasodilatation, dizziness, anorexia, glossitis, constipation, paresthesia, retinitis and confusion. Following marketing, bullous eruption has been reported rarely in this population.

Clinically significant laboratory abnormalities frequently (⩾ 5 %) occurred including increases in alkaline phosphatase; AST and bilirubin which were believed to be related to the underlying disease and not Caelyx. Reduction in haemoglobin and platelets were less frequently (< 5 %) reported. Sepsis related to leukopaenia was rarely (< 1 %) observed. Some of these abnormalities may have been related to the underlying HIV infection and not Caelyx.

All patients: 100 out of 929 patients (10.8 %) with solid tumours were described as having an infusion-associated reaction during treatment with Caelyx as defined by the following Costart terms: allergic reaction, anaphylactoid reaction, asthma, face oedema, hypotension, vasodilatation, urticaria, back pain, chest pain, chills, fever, hypertension, tachycardia, dyspepsia, nausea, dizziness, dyspnoea, pharyngitis, rash, pruritus, sweating, injection site reaction and drug interaction. Permanent treatment discontinuation was infrequently reported at 2 %. A similar incidence of infusion reactions (12.4 %) and treatment discontinuation (1.5 %) was observed in the breast cancer program. In patients with AIDS-KS, infusion-associated reactions, were characterised by flushing, shortness of breath, facial oedema, headache, chills, back pain, tightness in the chest and throat and/or hypotension and can be expected at the rate of 5 % to 10 %. Very rarely, convulsions have been observed in relation to infusion reactions. In all patients, infusion associated reactions occurred primarily during the first infusion. Temporarily stopping the infusion usually resolves these symptoms without further therapy. In nearly all patients, Caelyx treatment can be resumed after all symptoms have resolved without recurrence. Infusion reactions rarely recur after the first treatment cycle with Caelyx (see section 4.2).

Stomatitis has been reported in patients receiving continuous infusions of conventional doxorubicin hydrochloride and was frequently reported in patients receiving Caelyx. It did not interfere with patients completing therapy and no dosage adjustments are generally required, unless stomatitis is affecting a patient's ability to eat. In this case, the dose interval may be extended by 1 - 2 weeks or the dose reduced (see section 4.2).

An increased incidence of congestive heart failure is associated with doxorubicin therapy at cumulative lifetime doses > 450 mg/m² or at lower doses for patients with cardiac risk factors. Endomyocardial biopsies on nine of ten AIDS-KS patients receiving cumulative doses of Caelyx greater than 460 mg/m² indicate no evidence of anthracycline-induced cardiomyopathy. The recommended dose of Caelyx for AIDS-KS patients is 20 mg/m² every two-to-three weeks. The cumulative dose at which cardiotoxicity would become a concern for these AIDS-KS patients (> 400 mg/m²) would require more than 20 courses of Caelyx therapy over 40 to 60 weeks.

In addition, endomyocardial biopsies were performed in 8 solid tumour patients with cumulative anthracycline doses of 509 mg/m² –1,680 mg/m². The range of Billingham cardiotoxicity scores was grades 0 - 1.5. These grading scores are consistent with no or mild cardiac toxicity.

In the pivotal phase III trial versus doxorubicin, 58/509 (11.4 %) randomized subjects (10 treated with Caelyx at a dose of 50 mg/m²/every 4 weeks versus 48 treated with doxorubicin at a dose of 60 mg/m²/every 3 weeks) met the protocol-defined criteria for cardiac toxicity during treatment and/or follow-up. Cardiac toxicity was defined as a decrease of 20 points or greater from baseline if the resting LVEF remained in the normal range or a decrease of 10 points or greater if the LVEF became abnormal (less than the lower limit for normal). None of the 10 Caelyx subjects who had cardiac toxicity by LVEF criteria developed signs and symptoms of CHF. In contrast, 10 of 48 doxorubicin subjects who had cardiac toxicity by LVEF criteria also developed signs and symptoms of CHF.

In patients with solid tumours, including a subset of patients with breast and ovarian cancers, treated at a dose of 50 mg/m²/cycle with lifetime cumulative anthracycline doses up to 1,532 mg/m², the incidence of clinically significant cardiac dysfunction was low. Of the 418 patients treated with Caelyx 50 mg/m²/cycle, and having a baseline measurement of left ventricular ejection fraction (LVEF) and at least one follow-up measurement assessed by MUGA scan, 88 patients had a cumulative anthracycline dose of > 400 mg/m², an exposure level associated with an increased risk of cardiovascular toxicity with conventional doxorubicin. Only 13 of these 88 patients (15 %) had at least one clinically significant change in their LVEF, defined as an LVEF value less than 45 % or a decrease of at least 20 points from baseline. Furthermore, only 1 patient (cumulative anthracycline dose of 944 mg/m²), discontinued study treatment because of clinical symptoms of congestive heart failure.

As with other DNA-damaging antineoplastic agents, secondary acute myeloid leukemias and myelodysplasias have been reported in patients having received combined treatment with doxorubicin. Therefore, any patient treated with doxorubicin should be kept under haematological supervision.

Although local necrosis following extravasation has been reported very rarely, Caelyx is considered to be an irritant. Animal studies indicate that administration of doxorubicin hydrochloride as a liposomal formulation reduces the potential for extravasation injury. If any signs or symptoms of extravasation occur (e.g., stinging, erythema) terminate the infusion immediately and restart in another vein. The application of ice over the site of extravasation for approximately 30 minutes may be helpful in alleviating the local reaction. Caelyx must not be given by the intramuscular or subcutaneous route.

Recall of skin reaction due to prior radiotherapy has rarely occurred with Caelyx administration.

4.9 Overdose

Acute overdosing with doxorubicin hydrochloride worsens the toxic effects of mucositis, leukopaenia and thrombocytopaenia. Treatment of acute overdose of the severely myelosuppressed patient consists of hospitalisation, antibiotics, platelet and granulocyte transfusions and symptomatic treatment of mucositis.

5. PHARMACOLOGICAL PROPERTIES

5.1 Pharmacodynamic properties

Pharmacotherapeutic group: Cytotoxic agents (anthracyclines and related substances), ATC code: L01DB.

The active ingredient of Caelyx is doxorubicin hydrochloride, a cytotoxic anthracycline antibiotic obtained from *Streptomyces peucetius* var. *caesius*. The exact mechanism of the antitumour activity of doxorubicin is not known. It is generally believed that inhibition of DNA, RNA and protein synthesis is responsible for the majority of the cytotoxic effects. This is probably the result of intercalation of the anthracycline between adjacent base pairs of the DNA double helix thus preventing their unwinding for replication.

A phase III randomized study of Caelyx versus doxorubicin in patients with metastatic breast cancer was completed in 509 patients. The protocol-specified objective of demonstrating non-inferiority between Caelyx and doxorubicin was met, the hazard ratio (HR) for progression-free survival (PFS) was 1.00 (95 % CI for HR=0.82 - 1.22). The treatment HR for PFS when adjusted for prognostic variables was consistent with PFS for the ITT population.

The primary analysis of cardiac toxicity showed the risk of developing a cardiac event as a function of cumulative anthracycline dose was significantly lower with Caelyx than with doxorubicin (HR=3.16, $p < 0.001$). At cumulative doses greater than 450 mg/m^2 there were no cardiac events with Caelyx.

A phase III comparative study of Caelyx versus topotecan in patients with epithelial ovarian cancer following the failure of first-line, platinum based chemotherapy was completed in 474 patients. There was a benefit in overall survival (OS) for Caelyx-treated patients over topotecan-treated patients as indicated by a hazard ratio (HR) of 1.216 (95 % CI; 1.000, 1.478), p=0.050. The survival rates at 1, 2 and 3 years were 56.3 %, 34.7 % and 20.2 % respectively on Caelyx, compared to 54.0 %, 23.6 % and 13.2 % on topotecan.

For the sub-group of patients with platinum-sensitive disease the difference was greater: HR of 1.432 (95 % CI; 1.066, 1.923), p=0.017. The survival rates at 1, 2 and 3 years were 74.1 %, 51.2 % and 28.4 % respectively on Caelyx, compared to 66.2 %, 31.0 % and 17.5 % on topotecan.

The treatments were similar in the sub-group of patients with platinum refractory disease: HR of 1.069 (95 % CI; 0.823, 1.387), p=0.618. The survival rates at 1, 2 and 3 years were 41.5 %, 21.1 % and 13.8 % respectively on Caelyx, compared to 43.2 %, 17.2 % and 9.5 % on topotecan.

5.2 Pharmacokinetic properties

Caelyx is a long-circulating pegylated liposomal formulation of doxorubicin hydrochloride. Pegylated liposomes contain surface-grafted segments of the hydrophilic polymer methoxypolyethylene glycol (MPEG). These linear MPEG groups extend from the liposome surface creating a protective coating that reduces interactions between the lipid bilayer membrane and the plasma components. This allows the Caelyx liposomes to circulate for prolonged periods in the blood stream. Pegylated liposomes are small enough (average diameter of approximately 100 nm) to pass intact (extravasate) through defective blood vessels supplying tumours. Evidence of penetration of pegylated liposomes from blood vessels and their entry and accumulation in tumours has been seen in mice with C-26 colon carcinoma tumours and in transgenic mice with KS-like lesions. The pegylated liposomes also have a low permeability lipid matrix and internal aqueous buffer system that combine to keep doxorubicin hydrochloride encapsulated during liposome residence time in circulation.

The plasma pharmacokinetics of Caelyx in humans differ significantly from those reported in the literature for standard doxorubicin hydrochloride preparations. At lower doses (10 mg/m^2 – 20 mg/m^2) Caelyx displayed linear pharmacokinetics. Over the dose range of 10 mg/m^2 – 60 mg/m^2 Caelyx displayed non-linear pharmacokinetics. Standard doxorubicin hydrochloride displays extensive tissue distribution (volume of distribution: 700 to 1,100 l/m^2) and a rapid elimination clearance (24 to 73 l/h/m^2). In contrast, the pharmacokinetic profile of Caelyx indicates that Caelyx is confined mostly to the vascular fluid volume and that the clearance of doxorubicin from the blood is dependent upon the liposomal carrier. Doxorubicin becomes available after the liposomes are extravasated and enter the tissue compartment.

At equivalent doses, the plasma concentration and AUC values of Caelyx which represent mostly pegylated liposomal doxorubicin hydrochloride (containing 90 % to 95 % of the measured doxorubicin) are significantly higher than those achieved with standard doxorubicin hydrochloride preparations.

Caelyx should not be used interchangeably with other formulations of doxorubicin hydrochloride.

Population pharmacokinetics

The pharmacokinetics of Caelyx was evaluated in 120 patients from 10 different clinical trials using the population pharmacokinetic approach. The pharmacokinetics of Caelyx over the dose range of 10 mg/m^2 to 60 mg/m^2 was best described by a two compartment non-linear model with zero order input and Michaelis-Menten elimination. The mean intrinsic clearance of Caelyx was 0.030 l/h/m^2 (range 0.008 to 0.152 l/h/m^2) and the mean central volume of distribution was 1.93 l/m^2 (range 0.96 – 3.85 l/m^2) approximating the plasma volume. The apparent half-life ranged from 24 – 231 hours, with a mean of 73.9 hours.

Breast Cancer Patients

The pharmacokinetics of Caelyx determined in 18 patients with breast carcinoma were similar to the pharmacokinetics determined in the larger population of 120 patients with various cancers. The mean intrinsic clearance was 0.016 l/h/m^2 (range 0.008 - 0.027 l/h/m^2), the mean central volume of distribution was 1.46 l/m^2 (range 1.10 - 1.64 l/m^2). The mean apparent half-life was 71.5 hours (range 45.2 - 98.5 hours).

Ovarian cancer patients

The pharmacokinetics of Caelyx determined in 11 patients with ovarian carcinoma were similar to the pharmacokinetics determined in the larger population of 120 patients with various cancers. The mean intrinsic clearance was 0.021 l/h/m^2 (range 0.009 – 0.041 l/h/m^2), the mean central volume of distribution was 1.95 l/m^2 (range 1.67 – 2.40 l/m^2). The mean apparent half-life was 75.0 hours (range 36.1 – 125 hours).

AIDS-KS patients

The plasma pharmacokinetics of Caelyx were evaluated in 23 patients with KS who received single doses of 20 mg/m^2 administered by a 30-minute infusion. The pharmacokinetic parameters of Caelyx (primarily representing pegylated liposomal doxorubicin hydrochloride and low levels of unencapsulated doxorubicin hydrochloride) observed after the 20 mg/m^2 doses are presented in Table 5.

Table 5. Pharmacokinetic Parameters in Caelyx-Treated AIDS-KS Patients

	Mean ± Standard Error
Parameter	20 mg/m^2 (n=23)
Maximum Plasma Concentration* (µg/ml)	8.34 ± 0.49
Plasma Clearance (l/h/m^2)	0.041 ± 0.004
Volume of Distribution (l/m^2)	2.72 ± 0.120
AUC (µg/ml>/>h)	590.00 ± 58.7
λ_1 half-life (hours)	5.2 ± 1.4
λ_2 half-life (hours)	55.0 ± 4.8

*Measured at the end of a 30-minute infusion

5.3 Preclinical safety data

In repeat dose studies conducted in animals, the toxicity profile of Caelyx appears very similar to that reported in humans who receive long-term infusions of standard doxorubicin hydrochloride. With Caelyx, the encapsulation of doxorubicin hydrochloride in pegylated liposomes results in these effects having a differing strength, as follows.

Cardiotoxicity: Studies in rabbits have shown that the cardiotoxicity of Caelyx is reduced compared with conventional doxorubicin hydrochloride preparations.

Dermal toxicity: In studies performed after the repeated administration of Caelyx to rats and dogs, serious dermal inflammations and ulcer formations were observed at clinically relevant dosages. In the study in dogs, the occurrence and severity of these lesions was reduced by lowering the dose or prolonging the intervals between doses. Similar dermal lesions, which are described as palmar-plantar erythrodysesthesia were also observed in patients after long-term intravenous infusion (see section 4.8).

Anaphylactoid response: During repeat dose toxicology studies in dogs, an acute response characterised by hypotension, pale mucous membranes, salivation, emesis and periods of hyperactivity followed by hypoactivity and lethargy was observed following administration of pegylated liposomes (placebo). A similar, but less severe response was also noted in dogs treated with Caelyx and standard doxorubicin.

The hypotensive response was reduced in magnitude by pretreatment with antihistamines. However, the response was not life-threatening and the dogs recovered quickly upon discontinuation of treatment.

Local toxicity: Subcutaneous tolerance studies indicate that Caelyx, as against standard doxorubicin hydrochloride, causes slighter local irritation or damage to the tissue after a possible extravasation.

Mutagenicity and carcinogenicity: Although no studies have been conducted with Caelyx, doxorubicin hydrochloride, the pharmacologically active ingredient of Caelyx, is mutagenic and carcinogenic. Pegylated placebo liposomes are neither mutagenic nor genotoxic.

Reproductive toxicity: Caelyx resulted in mild to moderate ovarian and testicular atrophy in mice after a single dose of 36 mg/kg. Decreased testicular weights and hypospermia were present in rats after repeat doses $\geqslant$ 0.25 mg/kg/day and diffuse degeneration of the seminiferous tubules and a marked decrease in spermatogenesis were observed in dogs after repeat doses of 1 mg/kg/day (see section 4.6).

6. PHARMACEUTICAL PARTICULARS

6.1 List of excipients

α-(2-[1,2-distearoyl-*sn*-glycero(3)phosphooxy]ethylcarbamoyl)-ω-methoxypoly(oxyethylen)-40 sodium salt (MPEG-DSPE), fully hydrogenated soy phosphatidylcholine (HSPC), cholesterol, ammonium sulphate, sucrose, histidine, water for injections, hydrochloric acid, sodium hydroxide.

6.2 Incompatibilities

This medicinal product must not be mixed with other medicinal products except those mentioned in 6.6.

6.3 Shelf life

20 months

After dilution:

- Chemical and physical in-use stability has been demonstrated for 24 hours at 2°C to 8°C.

- From a microbiological point of view, the product should be used immediately. If not used immediately, in-use storage times and conditions prior to use are the responsibility of the user and should not be longer than 24 hours at 2°C to 8°C.

- Partially used vials must be discarded.

6.4 Special precautions for storage

Store in a refrigerator (2°C - 8°C). Do not freeze.

6.5 Nature and contents of container

Type I glass vials, each with a siliconised grey bromobutyl stopper, and an aluminium seal, with a deliverable volume of 10 ml (20 mg) or 25 ml (50 mg).

Caelyx is supplied as a single pack or packs of ten vials.

Not all pack sizes may be marketed.

6.6 Instructions for use and handling

Do not use material that shows evidence of precipitation or any other particulate matter.

Caution must be exercised in handling Caelyx solution. The use of gloves is required. If Caelyx comes into contact with skin or mucosa, wash immediately and thoroughly with soap and water. Caelyx must be handled and disposed of in a manner consistent with that of other anticancer medicinal products in accordance with local requirements.

Determine the dose of Caelyx to be administered (based upon the recommended dose and the patient's body surface area). Take the appropriate volume of Caelyx up into a sterile syringe. Aseptic technique must be strictly observed since no preservative or bacteriostatic agent is present in Caelyx. The appropriate dose of Caelyx must be diluted in 5 % (50 mg/ml) glucose solution for infusion prior to administration. For doses < 90 mg, dilute Caelyx in 250 ml, and for doses $\geqslant$ 90 mg, dilute Caelyx in 500 ml. This can be infused over 60 or 90 minutes as detailed in 4.2.

The use of any diluent other than 5 % (50 mg/ml) glucose solution for infusion, or the presence of any bacteriostatic agent such as benzyl alcohol may cause precipitation of Caelyx.

It is recommended that the Caelyx infusion line be connected through the side port of an intravenous infusion of 5 % (50 mg/ml) glucose. Infusion may be given through a peripheral vein. Do not use with in-line filters.

7. MARKETING AUTHORISATION HOLDER

SP Europe

Rue de Stalle 73

BE – 1180 Bruxelles,

Belgium

8. MARKETING AUTHORISATION NUMBER(S)

EU/1/96/011/001

EU/1/96/011/002

EU/1/96/011/003

EU/1/96/011/004

9. DATE OF FIRST AUTHORISATION/RENEWAL OF THE AUTHORISATION

21 June 1996

10. DATE OF REVISION OF THE TEXT

17 February 2005

Caelyx/EU/2-05/7

Cafergot Suppositories 2mg

(Alliance Pharmaceuticals)

1. NAME OF THE MEDICINAL PRODUCT

Cafergot® Suppositories 2mg.

2. QUALITATIVE AND QUANTITATIVE COMPOSITION

Ergotamine tartrate PhEur 2mg and caffeine PhEur 100mg.

3. PHARMACEUTICAL FORM
2mg off-white suppositories, 3cm in length, 1cm in diameter.

4. CLINICAL PARTICULARS

4.1 Therapeutic indications
Acute attacks of migraine and migraine variants unresponsive to simple analgesics.

4.2 Posology and method of administration
Adults:

There is considerable inter-individual variation in the sensitivity of patients to ergotamine. Care should therefore be exercised in selecting the optimum therapeutic dose for an individual patient which will not give rise to unwanted effects, either acutely or chronically. The maximum recommended dosages should not be exceeded and ergotamine treatment should not be administered at intervals of less than 4 days.

For maximum efficacy, the optimal dose (in the preferred presentation) should be administered immediately prodromal symptoms are experienced.

One suppository should be administered at the first warning of an attack. This dose is normally sufficient, although some individuals may require higher dosages which should never exceed 2 suppositories (4mg ergotamine) in 24 hours. It is essential to use the minimum effective dose.

The maximum recommended weekly dosage of 4 suppositories (8mg ergotamine) should never be exceeded.

Children under 12 years: Not recommended.

Elderly: Whilst there is no evidence to suggest that the elderly require different dosages of Cafergot, the contra-indications of this drug are common in the elderly, eg. coronary heart disease, renal impairment, hepatic impairment and severe hypertension. Caution should therefore be exercised when prescribing for this age group.

4.3 Contraindications
Patients with peripheral vascular disease, coronary heart disease, temporal arteritis, obliterative vascular disease and Raynaud's Syndrome, in view of the increased risk of peripheral vasospasm secondary to ergotamine. Impaired hepatic or renal function, sepsis and severe hypertension, pregnancy or nursing mothers.

Cafergot should not be used for migraine prophylaxis nor should the recommended dosage be exceeded. Frequent attacks of migraine may be an indication for the use of a suitable prophylactic agent.

Cafergot should not be taken by patients who are undergoing treatment with potent CYP 3A4 inhibitors, including protease inhibitors and macrolide antibiotics. Inhibition of CYP 3A4 metabolism of ergotamine results in elevated serum levels, leading to increased risk of cerebral ishaemia and/or ischaemia of the extremities. Serious and life-threatening ergotism has been associated with concomitant use of CYP 3A4 and ergotamine derivatives.

4.4 Special warnings and special precautions for use
If symptoms such as tingling in the fingers or toes occur, the drug should be discontinued at once and the physician consulted.

4.5 Interaction with other medicinal products and other forms of Interaction
Concomitant treatment with ergotamine derivatives and inhibitors of CYP 3A4 may cause elevation of plasma ergotamine levels, leading to increased risk of vasospasm and cerebral or peripheral ischaemia.

Concomitant use of macrolide antibiotics, including erythromycin or clarithromycin, and ergotamine is contra-indicated, as this can result in an elevated concentration of ergotamine in the plasma.

As vasospastic reactions have been reported with beta-blockers alone and in a few patients treated concomitantly with ergotamine and propranolol, caution is advised in the concomitant use of these agents with Cafergot.

Isolated cases of severe ergotism characterised by peripheral vasospasm and ischaemia of the extremities have been reported in patients taking protease inhibitors such as ritonavir or indinavir and doses of ergotamine which are within the recommended safe dosage range.

Ergotamine should not be administered within six hours of therapy with 5-HT_1 receptor agonists. In addition, use of 5-HT_1 receptor agonists should be avoided for at least 24 hours after the last ergotamine dose.

4.6 Pregnancy and lactation
Ergotamine-containing products are contra-indicated in pregnancy due to oxytocic effects on the pregnant uterus, and in breast feeding mothers due to the risk of the infant developing ergotism. Repeated doses of ergotamine may inhibit lactation.

4.7 Effects on ability to drive and use machines
None known

4.8 Undesirable effects
The caffeine component of Cafergot may give rise to unwanted stimulant effects.

Side effects of Cafergot are related in the main to the ergotamine component. Acutely, these may include nausea, vomiting and abdominal pain. Paraesthesia and peripheral vasoconstriction or pain and weakness in the extremities may develop after both acute and chronic dosing. Numbness and tingling of the extremities can be indicative of peripheral vasospasm and treatment must be stopped immediately if signs of circulatory impairment appear. Failure to observe this precaution can lead to the development of ergotism. Due to its vasoconstrictor properties, ergotamine may cause precordial pain, myocardial ischaemia, or, in rare cases, infarction, even in patients with no known history of coronary heart disease. Rare cases of intestinal ischaemia have been associated with chronic use and overuse of ergotamine-containing preparations.

Excessive use of ergotamine-containing products for prolonged periods may result in fibrotic changes, in particular of the pleura and retroperitoneum. Rare cases of fibrosis of cardiac valves have also been reported.

Rare reports of rectal or anal stricture or ulceration, or rectovaginal fistula have occurred following chronic use of ergotamine-containing suppositories, usually at higher than recommended doses.

Rarely, headache may be provoked either by chronic over-dosage or by rapid withdrawal of the product.

4.9 Overdose
Symptoms: Nausea, vomiting, drowsiness, confusion, tachycardia, dizziness, tingling and numbness in the extremities due to ischaemia, respiratory depression, coma.

Treatment: Should be directed to the elimination of ingested material by aspiration and gastric lavage.

Caffeine is a weak stimulant and excessive use of Cafergot may lead to a state of arousal and anxiety.

If severe arteriospasms occur, vasodilators such as nitro-prusside sodium should be administered. General supportive measures should be applied with particular reference to the respiratory and cardiovascular systems.

5. PHARMACOLOGICAL PROPERTIES

5.1 Pharmacodynamic properties
Ergotamine is a highly vasoactive ergot alkaloid having characteristically complex pharmacological actions. It is a partial tryptaminic agonist in certain blood vessels and both a partial agonist and antagonist of α-adrenergic receptors of blood vessels.

Although its exact mode of action in migraine is not known, its therapeutic effects have been attributed to its ability to cause vasoconstriction, thereby eliminating the painful dilation/pulsation of branches of the external carotid artery.

5.2 Pharmacokinetic properties
There is great interindividual variation in the absorption of ergotamine in patients and volunteers. Bioavailability is of the order of 5% or less by oral or rectal administration. After im or iv administration, plasma concentrations decay in a bi-exponential fashion. The elimination half life is 2 to 2.5 hours and clearance is about 0.68L/h/kg. Metabolism occurs in the liver. The major enzyme involved in the metabolism of ergotamine is Cytochrome P450 (CYP) 3A4. The primary route of excretion is biliary.

5.3 Preclinical safety data
There are no pre-clinical data of relevance to the prescriber which are additional to those already included in other sections of the Summary of Product Characteristics.

6. PHARMACEUTICAL PARTICULARS

6.1 List of excipients
Tartaric acid, lactose, Suppocire AM.

6.2 Incompatibilities
None

6.3 Shelf life
3 years.

6.4 Special precautions for storage
Store below 25°C.

6.5 Nature and contents of container
Carton of 30 suppositories in an aluminium blister pack.

6.6 Instructions for use and handling
None.

Administrative Data

7. MARKETING AUTHORISATION HOLDER
Alliance Pharmaceuticals Ltd

Avonbridge House

Bath Road

Chippenham

Wiltshire

SN15 2BB

8. MARKETING AUTHORISATION NUMBER(S)
PL16853/0003

9. DATE OF FIRST AUTHORISATION/RENEWAL OF THE AUTHORISATION
25 June 1998

10. DATE OF REVISION OF THE TEXT
March 2003

11. Legal Status
POM

Alliance, Alliance Pharmaceuticals and associated devices are registered Trademarks of Alliance Pharmaceuticals Ltd.

Cafergot Tablets
(Alliance Pharmaceuticals)

1. NAME OF THE MEDICINAL PRODUCT
Cafergot® tablets 1mg

2. QUALITATIVE AND QUANTITATIVE COMPOSITION
Ergotamine tartrate PhEur 1.0mg and caffeine PhEur 100mg.

3. PHARMACEUTICAL FORM
White, round, sugar coated tablets

4. CLINICAL PARTICULARS

4.1 Therapeutic indications
Acute attacks of migraine and migraine variants unresponsive to simple analgesics.

4.2 Posology and method of administration
Adults:

There is considerable inter-individual variation in the sensitivity of patients to ergotamine. Care should therefore be exercised in selecting the optimum therapeutic dose for an individual patient which will not give rise to unwanted effects, either acutely or chronically. The maximum recommended dosages should not be exceeded and ergotamine treatment should not be administered at intervals of less than 4 days.

For maximum efficacy, the optimal dose (in the preferred presentation) should be administered immediately prodromal symptoms are experienced.

One or two tablets taken at the first warning of an attack are normally sufficient to obtain migraine relief. Some individuals may require higher dosages which should never exceed 4 tablets (4mg ergotamine) in 24 hours. It is essential to use the minimum effective dose.

The maximum recommended weekly dose of 8 tablets (8mg ergotamine) should not be exceeded.

Children under 12 years: Not recommended.

Elderly: Whilst there is no evidence to suggest that the elderly require different dosages of Cafergot, the contra-indications of this drug are common in the elderly, e.g. coronary heart disease, renal impairment, hepatic impairment and severe hypertension. Caution should therefore be exercised when prescribing for this age group.

4.3 Contraindications
Patients with peripheral vascular disease, coronary heart disease, temporal arteritis, obliterative vascular disease and Raynaud's syndrome, in view of the increased risk of peripheral vasospasm secondary to ergotamine. Impaired hepatic or renal function, sepsis and severe hypertension. Pregnancy or nursing mothers.

Cafergot should not be used for migraine prophylaxis nor should the recommended dosage be exceeded. Frequent attacks of migraine may be an indication for the use of a suitable prophylactic agent.

Cafergot should not be taken by patients who are undergoing treatment with potent CYP 3A4 inhibitors, including protease inhibitors and macrolide antibiotics. Inhibition of CYP 3A4 metabolism of ergotamine results in elevated serum levels, leading to increased risk of cerebral ishaemia and/or ischaemia of the extremities. Serious and life-threatening ergotism has been associated with concomitant use of CYP 3A4 and ergotamine derivatives.

4.4 Special warnings and special precautions for use
If symptoms such as tingling in the fingers or toes occur, the drug should be discontinued at once and the physician consulted.

4.5 Interaction with other medicinal products and other forms of Interaction
Concomitant treatment with ergotamine derivatives and inhibitors of CYP 3A4 may cause elevation of plasma ergotamine levels, leading to increased risk of vasospasm and cerebral or peripheral ischaemia.

Concomitant use of macrolide antibiotics, including erythromycin or clarithromycin, and ergotamine is contra-indicated, as this can result in an elevated concentration of ergotamine in the plasma.

As vasospastic reactions have been reported with beta-blockers alone and in a few patients treated concomitantly with ergotamine and propranolol, caution is advised in the concomitant use of these agents with Cafergot.

Isolated cases of severe ergotism characterised by peripheral vasospasm and ischaemia of the extremities have been reported in patients taking protease inhibitors such as ritonavir or indinavir and doses of ergotamine which are within the recommended safe dosage range.

Ergotamine should not be administered within six hours of therapy with 5-HT_1 receptor agonists. In addition, use of 5-HT_1 receptor agonists should be avoided for at least 24 hours after the last ergotamine dose.

4.6 Pregnancy and lactation
Ergotamine-containing products are contra-indicated in pregnancy due to oxytocic effects on the pregnant uterus, and in breast feeding mothers due to the risk of the infant developing ergotism. Repeated doses of ergotamine may inhibit lactation.

4.7 Effects on ability to drive and use machines
None known.

4.8 Undesirable effects
The caffeine component of Cafergot may give rise to unwanted stimulant effects.

Side effects of Cafergot are related in the main to the ergotamine component. Acutely, these may include nausea, vomiting and abdominal pain. Paraesthesia and peripheral vasoconstriction or pain and weakness in the extremities may develop after both acute and chronic dosing. Numbness and tingling of the extremities can be indicative of peripheral vasospasm and treatment must be stopped immediately if signs of circulatory impairment appear. Failure to observe this precaution can lead to the development of ergotism. Due to its vasoconstrictor properties, ergotamine may cause precordial pain, myocardial ischaemia, or, in rare cases, infarction, even in patients with no known history of coronary heart disease. Rare cases of intestinal ischaemia have been associated with chronic use and overuse of ergotamine-containing preparations.

Excessive use of ergotamine-containing products for prolonged periods may result in fibrotic changes, in particular of the pleura and retroperitoneum. Rare cases of fibrosis of cardiac valves have also been reported.

Rarely, headache may be provoked either by chronic overdosage or by rapid withdrawal of the product.

4.9 Overdose
Symptoms: Nausea, vomiting, drowsiness, confusion, tachycardia, dizziness, tingling and numbness in the extremities due to ischaemia, respiratory depression, coma.

Treatment: should be directed to the elimination of ingested material by aspiration and gastric lavage.

Caffeine is a weak stimulant and excessive use of Cafergot may lead to a state of arousal and anxiety.

If severe arteriospasms occur, vasodilators such as nitroprusside sodium should be administered. General supportive measures should be applied with particular reference to the respiratory and cardiovascular systems.

5. PHARMACOLOGICAL PROPERTIES

5.1 Pharmacodynamic properties
Ergotamine is a highly vasoactive ergot alkaloid having characteristically complex pharmacological actions. It is a partial tryptaminic agonist in certain blood vessels and both a partial agonist and antagonist of α-adrenergic receptors of blood vessels.

Although its exact mode of action in migraine is not known, its therapeutic effects have been attributed to its ability to cause vasoconstriction, thereby eliminating the painful dilation/pulsation of branches of the external carotid artery.

5.2 Pharmacokinetic properties
There is great interindividual variation in the absorption of ergotamine in patients and volunteers. Bioavailability is of the order of 5% or less by oral or rectal administration. After im or iv administration, plasma concentrations decay in a bi-exponential fashion. The elimination half life is 2 to 2.5 hours and clearance is about 0.68L/h/kg. Metabolism occurs in the liver. The major enzyme involved in the metabolism of ergotamine is Cytochrome P450 (CYP) 3A4. The primary route of excretion is biliary.

5.3 Preclinical safety data
There are no pre-clinical data of relevance to the prescriber which are additional to those already included in other sections of the Summary of Product Characteristics.

6. PHARMACEUTICAL PARTICULARS

6.1 List of excipients
Tartaric acid, gelatin, stearic acid, lactose, starch, talc, gum acacia, sugar, and carnauba wax.

6.2 Incompatibilities
None

6.3 Shelf life
2 years

6.4 Special precautions for storage
None

6.5 Nature and contents of container
Cartons of 30 tablets in opaque aluminium/PVdC blister packs.

6.6 Instructions for use and handling
None

Administrative Data

7. MARKETING AUTHORISATION HOLDER
Alliance Pharmaceuticals Ltd
Avonbridge House
Bath Road
Chippenham
Wiltshire
SN15 2BB

8. MARKETING AUTHORISATION NUMBER(S)
PL16853/0004

9. DATE OF FIRST AUTHORISATION/RENEWAL OF THE AUTHORISATION
25 June 1998

10. DATE OF REVISION OF THE TEXT
March 2003

11 Legal status
POM

Alliance, Alliance Pharmaceuticals and associated devices are registered Trademarks of Alliance Pharmaceuticals Ltd.

Calaband

(Medlock Medical Ltd)

1. NAME OF THE MEDICINAL PRODUCT
Calaband.

2. QUALITATIVE AND QUANTITATIVE COMPOSITION
Zinc Oxide BP 9.25% w/w; Calamine BP 5.75% w/w.

3. PHARMACEUTICAL FORM
Open-wove bleached cotton bandage impregnated with the paste formulation.

4. CLINICAL PARTICULARS

4.1 Therapeutic indications
For use in the management of leg ulcers, where venous insufficiency exists. The paste bandage should be adjunct to graduated pressure bandaging. For use in the treatment of chronic eczema/dermatitis, where occlusion is indicated.

4.2 Posology and method of administration
For topical administration only. Adults, the elderly and children: not applicable: the product is a medicated paste bandage. Frequency of dressing changes is at the discretion of the responsible physician (Differentiation between patients of differing age groups is less important when considering the 'dosage' regime than the apparent healing rate of the wound/condition).

4.3 Contraindications
Hypersensitivity to an ingredient of the paste and acute eczematous lesions.

4.4 Special warnings and special precautions for use
Avoid use on grossly macerated skin. The skin of leg ulcer patients is easily sensitised to topical medicaments including preservatives. Sensitisation should be suspected in patients, particularly where there is deterioration of the ulcer or surrounding skin. Such patients should be referred for special diagnosis including patch testing. One of the functions of occlusive bandages is to increase absorption. Care should therefore be taken if it is decided to apply topical steroid preparations under these bandages as their absorption may be significantly increased.

4.5 Interaction with other medicinal products and other forms of Interaction
None known.

4.6 Pregnancy and lactation
No special precautions required.

4.7 Effects on ability to drive and use machines
Not applicable.

4.8 Undesirable effects
None known.

4.9 Overdose
None known.

5. PHARMACOLOGICAL PROPERTIES

5.1 Pharmacodynamic properties
The product is a paste bandage with the active constituent presented in a glycerine, modified starch and castor oil based paste spread onto a cotton bandage. Zinc oxide and calamine (basic zinc carbonate) have astringent properties. Much of the therapeutic action of paste bandages is attributable to the bandaging technique, the physical support and protection provided, and to the maintenance of moist wound healing conditions.

5.2 Pharmacokinetic properties
The pharmacokinetics of the active ingredient are those relevant to topical application of the substances through whole or broken skin. Contemporary literature describes the biochemical properties but with the exception of zinc salts does not directly relate these properties to the disease states being treated.

5.3 Preclinical safety data
Not applicable.

6. PHARMACEUTICAL PARTICULARS

6.1 List of excipients
Phenosept; modified starch; citric acid; glycerine; castor oil; purified water; open wove cotton bandage.

6.2 Incompatibilities
None known.

6.3 Shelf life
30 months unopened.

6.4 Special precautions for storage
Do not store above 25°C. Store in the original package.

6.5 Nature and contents of container
Individually wrapped in waxed paper or polythene film and then placed in a nylon/foil/polythene laminate bag in a cardboard carton, or a sealed polythene bag in a cardboard carton. 12 cartons packed per corrugated cardboard carton.

6.6 Instructions for use and handling
Not applicable.

7. MARKETING AUTHORISATION HOLDER
Seton Healthcare Group plc, Tubiton House, Oldham, OL1 3HS.

8. MARKETING AUTHORISATION NUMBER(S)
PL 0223/5003R.

9. DATE OF FIRST AUTHORISATION/RENEWAL OF THE AUTHORISATION
19th October 1989 / 10th January 2002.

10. DATE OF REVISION OF THE TEXT
January 2004.

Calceos

(Provalis Healthcare)

1. NAME OF THE MEDICINAL PRODUCT
CALCEOS Chewable Tablets

2. QUALITATIVE AND QUANTITATIVE COMPOSITION
Calcium Carbonate 1250mg (i.e 500mg or 12.5mmol of elemental calcium), Colecalciferol (INN) (Vitamin D_3) 10μg (corresponding to 400 IU of Vitamin D_3)

3. PHARMACEUTICAL FORM
Chewable tablets, for oral administration

4. CLINICAL PARTICULARS

4.1 Therapeutic indications
Vitamin D and calcium deficiency correction in the elderly. Vitamin and calcium supplement as an adjunct to specific therapy for osteoporosis.

4.2 Posology and method of administration
Oral use. For adults only. One tablet, twice per day. Chew the tablets and drink a glass of water.

4.3 Contraindications
Hypersensitivity to one of the constituents. Hypercalcaemia as a result of hyperparathyroidism (primary or secondary), hypercalciuria, calcium lithiasis, tissue calcification (nephrocalcinosis). Vitamin D overdose. Myeloma and bone metastases. Renal insufficiency (creatinine clearance less than 20ml/min). Calceos tablets are also contra-indicated in patients where prolonged immobilisation is accompanied by hypercalcaemia and/or hypercalciuria. In these cases, treatments should only be resumed when the patient becomes mobile.

4.4 Special warnings and special precautions for use
Calculate the total vitamin D intake in case of treatment with another drug containing this vitamin.

The following may be important in patient monitoring: Plasma calcium and urinary calcium determinations.

Precautions: Plasma and urinary calcium levels should be monitored regularly. In the elderly, renal function must be monitored regularly. In patients with renal failure, dosage has to be adapted according to the creatinine clearance. In case of long term treatment, the urinary calcium excretion must be monitored and treatment must be reduced or momentarily suspended if urinary calcium exceeds 7.5 to 9 mmol/24h (300 to 360 mg/24h).

4.5 Interaction with other medicinal products and other forms of Interaction
In case of treatment with digitalis glycosides: risk of cardiac arrhythmias. Clinical surveillance is required and possibly electrocardiographic and plasma calcium monitoring are recommended.

Associations to be taken into account in the case of treatment with thiazide diuretics: Risk of hypercalcaemia by decreasing urinary calcium excretion. Calcium may impair the absorption of tetracyclines, etidronate, fluoride and iron. At least 3 hours should intervene between taking Calceos and these agents.

4.6 Pregnancy and lactation
Normal requirements for calcium and vitamin D are raised during pregnancy and lactation. If supplementation is necessary, it should be given at a different time to iron supplements. Calcium is excreted in breast milk but not sufficiently to produce an adverse effect in the infant.

4.7 Effects on ability to drive and use machines
None known.

4.8 Undesirable effects
- Hypercalciuria in cases of prolonged treatment at high doses, exceptionally hypercalcaemia.
- Hypophosphateamia
- Nausea
- Mild gastro-intestinal disturbances such as constipation can occur but are infrequent.

4.9 Overdose

Clinical signs: anorexia, intense thirst, nausea, vomiting, polyuria, polydipsia, dehydration, hypertension, vasomotor disorders, constipation.

Laboratory signs: hypercalcaemia, hypercalciuria, impaired renal function tests.

Emergency treatment:

- Stop all calcium and vitamin D supplements.

- Rehydration and, according to the severity of the intoxication, isolated or combined use of diuretics, corticosteroids, calcitonin, peritoneal dialysis.

5. PHARMACOLOGICAL PROPERTIES

5.1 Pharmacodynamic properties

Calceos is a fixed combination of Calcium and vitamin D. The high calcium and vitamin D concentration in each dose unit facilitates absorption of a sufficient quantity of calcium with a limited number of doses. Vitamin D is involved in calcium-phosphorus metabolism. It allows active absorption of calcium and phosphorus from the intestine and their uptake by bone.

5.2 Pharmacokinetic properties

Calcium carbonate:

Absorption: In the stomach, calcium carbonate releases calcium ion as a function of pH. Calcium is essentially absorbed in the proximal part of the small intestine. The rate of absorption of calcium in the gastrointestinal tract is of the order of 30% of the dose ingested.

Elimination: Calcium is eliminated in sweat and gastrointestinal secretions. The urinary calcium excretion depends on the glomerular filtration and rate of tubular resorption of calcium.

Vitamin D_3:

Vitamin D_3 is absorbed from the intestine and transported by protein binding in the blood to the liver (first hydroxylation) and to the kidney (2nd hydroxylation). Non-hydroxylated Vitamin D_3 is stored in reserve compartments such as muscle and adipose tissues. Its plasma half-life is of the order of several days; it is eliminated in faeces and urine.

5.3 Preclinical safety data

None Stated

6. PHARMACEUTICAL PARTICULARS

6.1 List of excipients

Xylitol, Sorbitol, Polyvinylpyrrolidone, Lemon Flavouring*, Magnesium stearate.

*compostion of the lemon flavouring: essential oils of lemon, orange, litsea cubeba, maltodextrin, acacia gum, sodium citrate.

6.2 Incompatibilities

None known

6.3 Shelf life

36 months

6.4 Special precautions for storage

None

6.5 Nature and contents of container

Polypropylene tubes containing 15, 30 and 60 tablets. Packs of 1,2 or 4 tubes in card outers.

6.6 Instructions for use and handling

None

Administrative Data

7. MARKETING AUTHORISATION HOLDER

Laboratoire Innotech International

7-9 Avenue Francois Vincent Raspail

BP 32 – 94111 Arcueil, Cedex

France

8. MARKETING AUTHORISATION NUMBER(S)

PL 19152/0001

9. DATE OF FIRST AUTHORISATION/RENEWAL OF THE AUTHORISATION

31 October 2001

10. DATE OF REVISION OF THE TEXT

Calcichew 500mg Chewable Tablets

(Shire Pharmaceuticals Limited)

1. NAME OF THE MEDICINAL PRODUCT

Calcichew 500mg Chewable Tablets

2. QUALITATIVE AND QUANTITATIVE COMPOSITION

Per tablet: Calcium carbonate 1250mg equivalent to 500mg of elemental calcium.

For excipients see section 6.1.

3. PHARMACEUTICAL FORM

Chewable tablet.

Round, white, uncoated and convex tablets. May have small specks.

4. CLINICAL PARTICULARS

4.1 Therapeutic indications

Calcichew 500mg chewable tablets are to be chewed as a supplemental source of calcium in the correction of dietary deficiencies or when normal requirements are high.

Calcichew 500mg chewable tablets may be used as an adjunct to conventional therapy in the prevention and treatment of osteoporosis. They may be used as a phosphate binding agent in the management of renal failure in patients on renal dialysis.

4.2 Posology and method of administration

Oral:

Adults and elderly:

Adjunct to osteoporosis therapy - 2 to 3 tablets daily.

Dietary deficiency - 2 to 3 tablets daily.

Osteomalacia - 2 to 6 tablets daily.

Children:

Dietary deficiency - 2 to 3 tablets daily.

Phosphate Binder:

Adults, children and elderly - Dose as required by the individual patient depending on serum phosphate level.

The tablets should be taken just before, during or just after each meal.

4.3 Contraindications

- Severe hypercalcaemia and hypercalciuria, for example in hyperparathyroidism, vitamin D overdosage, decalcifying tumours such as plasmocytoma and skeletal metastases, in severe renal failure untreated by renal dialysis and in osteoporosis due to immobilisation.
- Nephrolithiasis
- Hypersensitivity to the active substance or to any of the excipients.

4.4 Special warnings and special precautions for use

Calcichew 500mg chewable tablets contain aspartame and should be avoided by patients with phenylketonuria.

In renal insufficiency the tablets should be given only under controlled conditions for hyperphosphataemia. Caution should be exercised in patients with a history of renal calculi.

During high dose therapy and especially during concomitant treatment with vitamin D, there is a risk of hypercalcaemia with subsequent kidney function impairment. In these patients, serum calcium levels should be followed and renal function should be monitored.

4.5 Interaction with other medicinal products and other forms of Interaction

Thiazide diuretics reduce the urinary excretion of calcium. Due to increased risk of hypercalcaemia, serum calcium should be regularly monitored during concomitant use of thiazide diuretics.

Systemic corticosteroids reduce calcium absorption. During concomitant use, it may be necessary to increase the dose of Calcichew 500mg chewable tablets.

Calcium carbonate may interfere with the absorption of concomitantly administered tetracycline preparations. For this reason, tetracycline preparations should be administered at least two hours before, or four to six hours after, oral intake of calcium.

Hypercalcaemia may increase the toxicity of cardiac glycosides during treatment with calcium. Patients should be monitored with regard to electrocardiogram (ECG) and serum calcium levels.

If a bisphosphonate or sodium fluoride is used concomitantly, this preparation should be administered at least three hours before the intake of Calcichew 500mg chewable tablets since gastrointestinal absorption may be reduced.

Oxalic acid (found in spinach and rhubarb) and phytic acid (found in whole cereals) may inhibit calcium absorption through formation of insoluble calcium salts. The patient should not take calcium products within two hours of eating foods high in oxalic acid and phytic acid.

4.6 Pregnancy and lactation

The adequate daily intake (including food and supplementation) for normal pregnant and lactating women is 1000-1300 mg calcium. During pregnancy, the daily intake of calcium should not exceed 1500 mg. Significant amounts of calcium are secreted in milk during lactation. Calcichew 500mg chewable tablets can be used during pregnancy in case of a calcium deficiency.

4.7 Effects on ability to drive and use machines

There are no data about the effect of this product on driving capacity. An effect is, however, unlikely.

4.8 Undesirable effects

Adverse reactions are listed below, by system organ class and frequency. Frequencies are defined as: uncommon $>1/1,000$, $<1/100$) or rare $>1/10,000$, $<1/1,000$).

Metabolism and nutrition disorders

Uncommon: Hypercalcaemia and hypercalciuria.

Gastrointestinal disorders

Rare: Constipation, flatulence, nausea, abdominal pain and diarrhoea.

Skin and subcutaneous disorders

Rare: Pruritus, rash and urticaria.

4.9 Overdose

Overdose can lead to hypercalcaemia. Symptoms of hypercalcaemia may include anorexia, thirst, nausea, vomiting, constipation, abdominal pain, muscle weakness, fatigue, mental disturbances, polydipsia, polyuria, bone pain, nephrocalcinosis, nephrolithiasis and in severe cases, cardiac arrhythmias. Extreme hypercalcaemia may result in coma and death. Persistently high calcium levels may lead to irreversible renal damage and soft tissue calcification.

Treatment of hypercalcaemia: The treatment with calcium must be discontinued. Treatment with thiazide diuretics, lithium, vitamin A and cardiac glycosides must also be discontinued. Emptying of the stomach in patients with impaired consciousness. Rehydration, and, according to severity, isolated or combined treatment with loop diuretics, bisphosphonates, calcitonin and corticosteroids. Serum electrolytes, renal function and diuresis must be monitored. In severe cases, ECG and CVP should be followed.

5. PHARMACOLOGICAL PROPERTIES

5.1 Pharmacodynamic properties

Pharmacotherapeutic group: Calcium

ATC-code: A12A A04

An adequate intake of calcium is of importance during growth, pregnancy and breastfeeding.

5.2 Pharmacokinetic properties

Absorption: The amount of calcium absorbed through the gastrointestinal tract is approximately 30% of the swallowed dose.

Distribution and metabolism: 99% of the calcium in the body is concentrated in the hard structure of bones and teeth. The remaining 1% is present in the intra- and extracellular fluids. About 50% of the total blood-calcium content is in the physiologically active ionised form with approximately 10% being complexed to citrate, phosphate or other anions, the remaining 40% being bound to proteins, principally albumin.

Elimination: Calcium is eliminated through faeces, urine and sweat. Renal excretion depends on glomerular filtration and calcium tubular reabsorption.

5.3 Preclinical safety data

There is no information of relevance to the safety assessment in addition to what is stated in other parts of the SmPC.

6. PHARMACEUTICAL PARTICULARS

6.1 List of excipients

Sorbitol

Povidone

Isomalt

Orange oil

Magnesium stearate

Aspartame

Mono, di-fatty acid glycerides

6.2 Incompatibilities

Not applicable.

6.3 Shelf life

3 years.

6.4 Special precautions for storage

Do not store above 30°C.

Keep the container tightly closed in order to protect from moisture.

6.5 Nature and contents of container

Securitainer containing 100 tablets.

6.6 Instructions for use and handling

No special requirements.

7. MARKETING AUTHORISATION HOLDER

Shire Pharmaceuticals Limited

Hampshire International Business Park

Chineham

Basingstoke

Hampshire RG24 8EP

United Kingdom

8. MARKETING AUTHORISATION NUMBER(S)

PL 08557/0003

9. DATE OF FIRST AUTHORISATION/RENEWAL OF THE AUTHORISATION

27 November 1989/27 November 1997

10. DATE OF REVISION OF THE TEXT

April 2004

LEGAL CATEGORY

P

Calcichew D3

(Shire Pharmaceuticals Limited)

1. NAME OF THE MEDICINAL PRODUCT
Calcichew-D_3 Chewable Tablets

2. QUALITATIVE AND QUANTITATIVE COMPOSITION
Per tablet: Calcium carbonate 1250mg

(equivalent to 500mg of elemental calcium)

Cholecalciferol 200iu

(equivalent to 5 micrograms vitamin D_3)

For excipients see section 6.1.

3. PHARMACEUTICAL FORM
Chewable tablet.

Round, white, uncoated and convex tablets. May have small specks.

4. CLINICAL PARTICULARS

4.1 Therapeutic indications
Calcichew-D_3 chewable tablets should be used only as a therapeutic and not as a food supplement when the diet is deficient or when normal requirements of both components is increased.

Calcichew-D_3 chewable tablets may be used as an adjunct to specific therapy for osteoporosis or as a therapeutic supplement in established osteomalacia, pregnant patients at high risk of needing such a therapeutic supplementation or malnutrition when dietary intake is less than that required.

4.2 Posology and method of administration
Oral.

Adjunctive therapy in osteoporosis:

One chewable tablet 2-3 times per day

Calcium and vitamin D deficiency:

Adults - One chewable tablet 2-3 times per day.

Children - One chewable tablet 1-2 times per day.

Dosage in hepatic impairment:

No dose adjustment is required.

Dosage in renal impairment:

Calcichew-D_3 chewable tablets should not be used in patients with severe renal impairment.

4.3 Contraindications

- Diseases and/or conditions resulting in hypercalcaemia and/or hypercalciuria
- Nephrolithiasis
- Hypervitaminosis D
- Hypersensitivity to the active substances or to any of the excipients

4.4 Special warnings and special precautions for use
Calcichew-D_3 chewable tablets contain aspartame and should be avoided by patients with phenylketonuria.

During long-term treatment, serum calcium levels should be followed and renal function should be monitored through measurement of serum creatinine. Monitoring is especially important in elderly patients on concomitant treatment with cardiac glycosides or diuretics (see section 4.5) and in patients with a high tendency to calculus formation. In case of hypercalcaemia or signs of impaired renal function, the dose should be reduced or the treatment discontinued.

Vitamin D should be used with caution in patients with impairment of renal function and the effect on calcium and phosphate levels should be monitored. The risk of soft tissue calcification should be taken into account. In patients with severe renal insufficiency, vitamin D in the form of colecalciferol is not metabolised normally and other forms of vitamin D should be used (see section 4.3).

Calcichew-D_3 chewable tablets should be prescribed with caution to patients suffering from sarcoidosis because of the risk of increased metabolism of vitamin D to its active metabolite. In these patients, serum calcium levels and urinary calcium excretion must be monitored.

Calcichew-D_3 chewable tablets should be used with caution in immobilised patients with osteoporosis due to the increased risk of hypercalcaemia.

The dose of vitamin D (200 IU) in Calcichew-D_3 chewable tablets should be considered when prescribing other drugs containing vitamin D. Additional doses of calcium or vitamin D should be taken under close medical supervision. In such cases it is necessary to monitor serum calcium levels and urinary calcium excretion frequently.

4.5 Interaction with other medicinal products and other forms of Interaction
Thiazide diuretics reduce the urinary excretion of calcium. Due to increased risk of hypercalcaemia, serum calcium should be regularly monitored during concomitant use of thiazide diuretics.

Systemic corticosteroids reduce calcium absorption. During concomitant use, it may be necessary to increase the dose of Calcichew-D_3chewable tablets.

Simultaneous treatment with ion exchange resins such as cholestyramine or laxatives such as paraffin oil may reduce the gastrointestinal absorption of vitamin D.

Calcium carbonate may interfere with the absorption of concomitantly administered tetracycline preparations. For this reason, tetracycline preparations should be administered at least two hours before, or four to six hours after, oral intake of calcium.

Hypercalcaemia may increase the toxicity of cardiac glycosides during treatment with calcium and vitamin D. Patients should be monitored with regard to electrocardiogram (ECG) and serum calcium levels.

If a bisphosphonate or sodium fluoride is used concomitantly, this preparation should be administered at least three hours before the intake of Calcichew-D_3 chewable tablets since gastrointestinal absorption may be reduced.

Oxalic acid (found in spinach and rhubarb) and phytic acid (found in whole cereals) may inhibit calcium absorption through formation of insoluble calcium salts. The patient should not take calcium products within two hours of eating foods high in oxalic acid and phytic acid.

4.6 Pregnancy and lactation
Pregnancy

During pregnancy the daily intake should not exceed 1500 mg calcium and 600 IU colecalciferol (15μg vitamin D). Studies in animals have shown reproductive toxicity with high doses of vitamin D. In pregnant women, overdoses of calcium and vitamin D should be avoided as permanent hypercalcaemia has been related to adverse effects on the developing foetus. There are no indications that vitamin D at therapeutic doses is teratogenic in humans. Calcichew-D_3 chewable tabletscan be used during pregnancy, in case of a calcium and vitamin D deficiency.

Lactation

Calcichew-D_3 chewable tablets can be used during breastfeeding. Calcium and vitamin D_3 pass into breast milk. This should be considered when giving additional vitamin D to the child.

4.7 Effects on ability to drive and use machines
There are no data about the effect of this product on driving capacity. An effect is, however, unlikely.

4.8 Undesirable effects
Adverse reactions are listed below, by system organ class and frequency. Frequencies are defined as: uncommon $>1/1{,}000$, $<1/100$) or rare $>1/10{,}000$, $<1/1{,}000$).

Metabolism and nutrition disorders

Uncommon: Hypercalcaemia and hypercalciuria.

Gastrointestinal disorders

Rare: Constipation, flatulence, nausea, abdominal pain and diarrhoea.

Skin and subcutaneous disorders

Rare: Pruritus, rash and urticaria.

4.9 Overdose
Overdose can lead to hypervitaminosis D and hypercalcaemia. Symptoms of hypercalcaemia may include anorexia, thirst, nausea, vomiting, constipation, abdominal pain, muscle weakness, fatigue, mental disturbances, polydipsia, polyuria, bone pain, nephrocalcinosis, nephrolithiasis and in severe cases, cardiac arrhythmias. Extreme hypercalcaemia may result in coma and death. Persistently high calcium levels may lead to irreversible renal damage and soft tissue calcification.

Treatment of hypercalcaemia: The treatment with calcium must be discontinued. Treatment with thiazide diuretics, lithium, vitamin A and cardiac glycosides must also be discontinued. Emptying of the stomach in patients with impaired consciousness. Rehydration, and, according to severity, isolated or combined treatment with loop diuretics, bisphosphonates, calcitonin and corticosteroids. Serum electrolytes, renal function and diuresis must be monitored. In severe cases, ECG and CVP should be followed.

5. PHARMACOLOGICAL PROPERTIES

5.1 Pharmacodynamic properties
Pharmacotherapeutic group: Mineral supplements

ATC code: A12AX

Vitamin D increases the intestinal absorption of calcium.

Administration of calcium and vitamin D_3 counteracts the increase of parathyroid hormone (PTH) which is caused by calcium deficiency and which causes increased bone resorption.

A clinical study of institutionalised patients suffering from vitamin D deficiency indicated that a daily intake of two tablets of calcium 500mg/vitamin D 400iu for six months normalised the value of the 25-hydroxylated metabolite of vitamin D_3 and reduced secondary hyperparathyroidism and serum alkaline phosphatase.

5.2 Pharmacokinetic properties
Calcium

Absorption: The amount of calcium absorbed through the gastrointestinal tract is approximately 30% of the swallowed dose.

Distribution and metabolism: 99% of the calcium in the body is concentrated in the hard structure of bones and teeth. The remaining 1% is present in the intra- and extracellular fluids. About 50% of the total blood-calcium content is in the physiologically active ionised form with approximately 10% being complexed to citrate, phosphate or other anions, the remaining 40% being bound to proteins, principally albumin.

Elimination: Calcium is eliminated through faeces, urine and sweat. Renal excretion depends on glomerular filtration and calcium tubular reabsorption.

Vitamin D

Absorption: Vitamin D is easily absorbed in the small intestine.

Distribution and metabolism: Colecalciferol and its metabolites circulate in the blood bound to a specific globulin. Colecalciferol is converted in the liver by hydroxylation to the active form 25-hydroxycholecalciferol. It is then further converted in the kidneys to 1,25-hydroxycholecalciferol; 1,25-hydroxycholecalciferol is the metabolite responsible for increasing calcium absorption. Vitamin D, which is not metabolised, is stored in adipose and muscle tissues.

Elimination: Vitamin D is excreted in faeces and urine.

5.3 Preclinical safety data
At doses far higher than the human therapeutic range teratogenicity has been observed in animal studies. There is further no information of relevance to the safety assessment in addition to what is stated in other parts of the SmPC.

6. PHARMACEUTICAL PARTICULARS

6.1 List of excipients
Sorbitol

Povidone

Isomalt

Orange oil

Magnesium stearate

Aspartame

Mono, di-fatty acid glycerides

Sucrose

Gelatin

Vegetable fat

Tocopherol

Maize starch

6.2 Incompatibilities
Not applicable.

6.3 Shelf life
3 years.

6.4 Special precautions for storage
Do not store above 30°C. Keep the container tightly closed in order to protect from moisture.

6.5 Nature and contents of container
White HD Polyethylene containers with a primary tamper-evident seal and secondary re-sealable closure containing 60 and 100 tablets.

Not all pack sizes may be marketed.

6.6 Instructions for use and handling
No special requirements.

7. MARKETING AUTHORISATION HOLDER
Shire Pharmaceuticals Limited

Hampshire International Business Park

Chineham

Basingstoke

Hampshire RG24 8EP

United Kingdom

8. MARKETING AUTHORISATION NUMBER(S)
PL 8557/0021

9. DATE OF FIRST AUTHORISATION/RENEWAL OF THE AUTHORISATION
26 November 1991

10. DATE OF REVISION OF THE TEXT
April 2004

LEGAL CATEGORY
P

Calcichew D3 Forte Chewable Tablets

(Shire Pharmaceuticals Limited)

1. NAME OF THE MEDICINAL PRODUCT
Calcichew-D_3 Forte Chewable Tablets

2. QUALITATIVE AND QUANTITATIVE COMPOSITION
Per tablet:

Calcium carbonate 1250mg

(equivalent to 500mg of elemental calcium)

Colecalciferol 400 IU

(equivalent to 10 micrograms vitamin D_3)

For excipients, see Section 6.1.

3. PHARMACEUTICAL FORM
Chewable tablet.

Round, white, uncoated and convex tablets. May have small specks.

4. CLINICAL PARTICULARS

4.1 Therapeutic indications

The treatment and prevention of vitamin D/calcium deficiency (characterised by raised serum alkaline phosphatase levels associated with increased bone loss, raised levels of serum PTH and lowered 25-hydroxyvitamin D) particularly in the housebound and institutionalised elderly subjects.

The supplementation of vitamin D and calcium as an adjunct to specific therapy for osteoporosis, in pregnancy, in established vitamin D dependent osteomalacia, and in other situations requiring therapeutic supplementation of malnutrition.

4.2 Posology and method of administration

Oral

Adults and elderly:

2 chewable tablets per day, preferably one tablet morning and evening.

Dosage in hepatic impairment:

No dose adjustment is required.

Dosage in renal impairment:

Calcichew-D_3 Forte chewable tablets should not be used in patients with severe renal impairment.

4.3 Contraindications

- Diseases and/or conditions resulting in hypercalcaemia and/or hypercalciuria
- Nephrolithiasis
- Hypervitaminosis D
- Hypersensitivity to the active substances or to any of the excipients

4.4 Special warnings and special precautions for use

Calcichew-D_3 Forte chewable tablets contain aspartame and should be avoided by patients with phenylketonuria.

During long-term treatment, serum calcium levels should be followed and renal function should be monitored through measurements of serum creatinine. Monitoring is especially important in elderly patients on concomitant treatment with cardiac glycosides or diuretics (see section 4.5) and in patients with a high tendency to calculus formation. In case of hypercalcaemia or signs of impaired renal function the dose should be reduced or the treatment discontinued.

Vitamin D should be used with caution in patients with impairment of renal function and the effect on calcium and phosphate levels should be monitored. The risk of soft tissue calcification should be taken into account. In patients with severe renal insufficiency, vitamin D in the form of colecalciferol is not metabolised normally and other forms of vitamin D should be used (see section 4.3).

Calcichew-D_3 Forte chewable tablets should be prescribed with caution to patients suffering from sarcoidosis because of the risk of increased metabolism of vitamin D to its active metabolite. In these patients, serum calcium levels and urinary calcium excretion must be monitored.

Calcichew-D_3 Forte chewable tablets should be used with caution in immobilised patients with osteoporosis due to the increased risk of hypercalcaemia.

The dose of vitamin D (400 IU) in Calcichew-D_3 Forte chewable tablets should be considered when prescribing other drugs containing vitamin D. Additional doses of calcium or vitamin D should be taken under close medical supervision. In such cases it is necessary to monitor serum calcium levels and urinary calcium excretion frequently.

4.5 Interaction with other medicinal products and other forms of Interaction

Thiazide diuretics reduce the urinary excretion of calcium. Due to increased risk of hypercalcaemia, serum calcium should be regularly monitored during concomitant use of thiazide diuretics.

Systemic corticosteroids reduce calcium absorption. During concomitant use, it may be necessary to increase the dose of Calcichew-D_3 Forte chewable tablets.

Simultaneous treatment with ion exchange resins such as cholestyramine or laxatives such as paraffin oil may reduce the gastrointestinal absorption of vitamin D.

Calcium carbonate may interfere with the absorption of concomitantly administered tetracycline preparations. For this reason, tetracycline preparations should be administered at least two hours before, or four to six hours after, oral intake of calcium.

Hypercalcaemia may increase the toxicity of cardiac glycosides during treatment with calcium and vitamin D. Patients should be monitored with regard to electrocardiogram (ECG) and serum calcium levels.

If a bisphosphonate or sodium fluoride is used concomitantly, this preparation should be administered at least three hours before the intake of Calcichew-D_3 Forte chewable tablets since gastrointestinal absorption may be reduced.

Oxalic acid (found in spinach and rhubarb) and phytic acid (found in whole cereals) may inhibit calcium absorption through formation of insoluble calcium salts. The patient should not take calcium products within two hours of eating foods high in oxalic acid and phytic acid.

4.6 Pregnancy and lactation

Pregnancy

During pregnancy the daily intake should not exceed 1500 mg calcium and 600 IU colecalciferol (15μg vitamin D). Studies in animals have shown reproductive toxicity with high doses of vitamin D. In pregnant women, overdoses of calcium and vitamin D should be avoided as permanent hypercalcaemia has been related to adverse effects on the developing foetus. There are no indications that vitamin D at therapeutic doses is teratogenic in humans. Calcichew-D_3 Forte chewable tablets can be used during pregnancy, in case of a calcium and vitamin D deficiency.

Lactation

Calcichew-D_3 Forte chewable tablets can be used during breast-feeding. Calcium and vitamin D_3 pass into breast milk. This should be considered when giving additional vitamin D to the child.

4.7 Effects on ability to drive and use machines

There are no data about the effect of this product on driving capacity. An effect is, however, unlikely.

4.8 Undesirable effects

Adverse reactions are listed below, by system organ class and frequency. Frequencies are defined as: uncommon >1/1,000, <1/100) or rare >1/10,000, <1/1,000).

Metabolism and nutrition disorders

Uncommon: Hypercalcaemia and hypercalciuria.

Gastrointestinal disorders

Rare: Constipation, flatulence, nausea, abdominal pain and diarrhoea.

Skin and subcutaneous disorders

Rare: Pruritus, rash and urticaria.

4.9 Overdose

Overdose can lead to hypervitaminosis D and hypercalcaemia. Symptoms of hypercalcaemia may include anorexia, thirst, nausea, vomiting, constipation, abdominal pain, muscle weakness, fatigue, mental disturbances, polydipsia, polyuria, bone pain, nephrocalcinosis, nephrolithiasis and in severe cases, cardiac arrhythmias. Extreme hypercalcaemia may result in coma and death. Persistently high calcium levels may lead to irreversible renal damage and soft tissue calcification.

Treatment of hypercalcaemia: The treatment with calcium must be discontinued. Treatment with thiazide diuretics, lithium, vitamin A and cardiac glycosides must also be discontinued. Emptying of the stomach in patients with impaired consciousness. Rehydration, and, according to severity, isolated or combined treatment with loop diuretics, bisphosphonates, calcitonin and corticosteroids. Serum electrolytes, renal function and diuresis must be monitored. In severe cases, ECG and CVP should be followed.

5. PHARMACOLOGICAL PROPERTIES

5.1 Pharmacodynamic properties

Pharmacotherapeutic group: Mineral supplements

ATC code: A12AX

Vitamin D increases the intestinal absorption of calcium.

Administration of calcium and vitamin D_3 counteracts the increase of parathyroid hormone (PTH) which is caused by calcium deficiency and which causes increased bone resorption.

A clinical study of institutionalised patients suffering from vitamin D deficiency indicated that a daily intake of two tablets of Calcichew-D_3 Forte chewable tablets for six months normalised the value of the 25-hydroxylated metabolite of vitamin D_3 and reduced secondary hyperparathyroidism and serum alkaline phosphatase.

An 18 month double-blind, placebo controlled study including 3270 institutionalised women aged 84+/- 6 years who received supplementation of vitamin D (800 IU/day) and calcium phosphate (corresponding to 1200 mg/day of elemental calcium), showed a significant decrease of PTH secretion. After 18 months, an "intent-to treat" analysis showed 80 hip fractures in the calcium-vitamin D group and 110 hip fractures in the placebo group (p=0.004). A follow-up study after 36 months showed 137 women with at least one hip fracture in the calcium-vitamin D group (n=1176) and 178 in the placebo group (n=1127) (p≤0.02).

5.2 Pharmacokinetic properties

Calcium

Absorption: The amount of calcium absorbed through the gastrointestinal tract is approximately 30% of the swallowed dose.

Distribution and metabolism: 99% of the calcium in the body is concentrated in the hard structure of bones and teeth. The remaining 1% is present in the intra- and extracellular fluids. About 50% of the total blood-calcium content is in the physiologically active ionised form with approximately 10% being complexed to citrate, phosphate or other anions, the remaining 40% being bound to proteins, principally albumin.

Elimination: Calcium is eliminated through faeces, urine and sweat. Renal excretion depends on glomerular filtration and calcium tubular reabsorption.

Vitamin D

Absorption: Vitamin D is easily absorbed in the small intestine.

Distribution and metabolism: Colecalciferol and its metabolites circulate in the blood bound to a specific globulin. Colecalciferol is converted in the liver by hydroxylation to the active form 25-hydroxycholecalciferol. It is then further converted in the kidneys to 1,25-hydroxycholecalciferol; 1,25-hydroxycholecalciferol is the metabolite responsible for increasing calcium absorption. Vitamin D, which is not metabolised, is stored in adipose and muscle tissues.

Elimination: Vitamin D is excreted in faeces and urine.

5.3 Preclinical safety data

At doses far higher than the human therapeutic range teratogenicity has been observed in animal studies. There is further no information of relevance to the safety assessment in addition to what is stated in other parts of the SmPC.

6. PHARMACEUTICAL PARTICULARS

6.1 List of excipients

Sorbitol

Povidone

Isomalt

Lemon oil

Fatty acid mono- and diglycerides

Aspartame

Magnesium stearate

Sucrose

Gelatin

Vegetable fat

Tocopherol

Maize starch

6.2 Incompatibilities

Not applicable.

6.3 Shelf life

3 years.

6.4 Special precautions for storage

Do not store above 30°C. Keep the container tightly closed in order to protect from moisture.

6.5 Nature and contents of container

White, high density polyethylene bottles containing 20, 30, 60, 90 or 100 tablets with tamper-evident seal.

Not all pack sizes may be marketed.

6.6 Instructions for use and handling

No special requirements.

7. MARKETING AUTHORISATION HOLDER

Shire Pharmaceuticals Limited

Hampshire International Business Park

Chineham

Basingstoke

Hampshire RG24 8EP

United Kingdom

8. MARKETING AUTHORISATION NUMBER(S)

PL 08557/0029

9. DATE OF FIRST AUTHORISATION/RENEWAL OF THE AUTHORISATION

26 March 1996

10. DATE OF REVISION OF THE TEXT

April 2004

LEGAL CATEGORY

P

Calcichew Forte

(Shire Pharmaceuticals Limited)

1. NAME OF THE MEDICINAL PRODUCT

Calcichew Forte Chewable Tablets

2. QUALITATIVE AND QUANTITATIVE COMPOSITION

Per tablet: Calcium carbonate 2500mg equivalent to 1g of elemental calcium.

For excipients see Section 6.1.

3. PHARMACEUTICAL FORM

Chewable tablet.

Round, white, uncoated and convex tablets. May have small specks.

4. CLINICAL PARTICULARS

4.1 Therapeutic indications

Calcichew Forte chewable tablets are to be chewed as a supplemental source of calcium in the correction of dietary deficiencies or when normal requirements are high.

Calcichew Forte chewable tablets may be used as an adjunct to conventional therapy in the prevention and treatment of osteoporosis. They may be used as a phosphate binding agent in the management of renal failure in patients on renal dialysis.

4.2 Posology and method of administration
Oral.

Adults and elderly:

Adjunct to osteoporosis therapy - One tablet to be chewed daily.

Dietary deficiency - One tablet to be chewed daily.

Osteomalacia - 1-3g daily is recommended.

Children:

Dietary deficiency- One tablet to be chewed daily.

Phosphate Binder:

Adults, children and elderly - Dose as required by the individual patient depending on serum phosphate level.

The tablets should be taken just before, during or just after each meal.

4.3 Contraindications

• Severe hypercalcaemia and hypercalciuria, for example in hyperparathyroidism, vitamin D overdosage, decalcifying tumours such as plasmocytoma and skeletal metastases, in severe renal failure untreated by renal dialysis and in osteoporosis due to immobilisation.

• Nephrolithiasis

• Hypersensitivity to the active substance or to any of the excipients.

4.4 Special warnings and special precautions for use
Calcichew Forte chewable tablets contain aspartame and should be avoided by patients with phenylketonuria.

In renal insufficiency the tablets should be given only under controlled conditions for hyperphosphataemia. Caution should be exercised in patients with a history of renal calculi.

During high dose therapy and especially during concomitant treatment with vitamin D, there is a risk of hypercalcaemia with subsequent kidney function impairment. In these patients, serum calcium levels should be followed and renal function should be monitored.

4.5 Interaction with other medicinal products and other forms of Interaction
Thiazide diuretics reduce the urinary excretion of calcium. Due to increased risk of hypercalcaemia, serum calcium should be regularly monitored during concomitant use of thiazide diuretics.

Systemic corticosteroids reduce calcium absorption. During concomitant use, it may be necessary to increase the dose of Calcichew Forte chewable tablets.

Calcium carbonate may interfere with the absorption of concomitantly administered tetracycline preparations. For this reason, tetracycline preparations should be administered at least two hours before, or four to six hours after, oral intake of calcium.

Hypercalcaemia may increase the toxicity of cardiac glycosides during treatment with calcium. Patients should be monitored with regard to electrocardiogram (ECG) and serum calcium levels.

If a bisphosphonate or sodium fluoride is used concomitantly, this preparation should be administered at least three hours before the intake of Calcichew Forte chewable tablets since gastrointestinal absorption may be reduced.

Oxalic acid (found in spinach and rhubarb) and phytic acid (found in whole cereals) may inhibit calcium absorption through formation of insoluble calcium salts. The patient should not take calcium products within two hours of eating foods high in oxalic acid and phytic acid.

4.6 Pregnancy and lactation
The adequate daily intake (including food and supplementation) for normal pregnant and lactating women is 1000-1300 mg calcium. During pregnancy, the daily intake of calcium should not exceed 1500 mg. Significant amounts of calcium are secreted in milk during lactation. Calcichew Forte chewable tablets can be used during pregnancy in case of a calcium deficiency.

4.7 Effects on ability to drive and use machines
There are no data about the effect of this product on driving capacity. An effect is, however, unlikely.

4.8 Undesirable effects
Adverse reactions are listed below, by system organ class and frequency. Frequencies are defined as: uncommon >1/1,000, <1/100) or rare >1/10,000, <1/1,000).

Metabolism and nutrition disorders

Uncommon: Hypercalcaemia and hypercalciuria.

Gastrointestinal disorders

Rare: Constipation, flatulence, nausea, abdominal pain and diarrhoea.

Skin and subcutaneous disorders

Rare: Pruritus, rash and urticaria.

4.9 Overdose
Overdose can lead to hypercalcaemia. Symptoms of hypercalcaemia may include anorexia, thirst, nausea, vomiting, constipation, abdominal pain, muscle weakness, fatigue, mental disturbances, polydipsia, polyuria, bone pain, nephrocalcinosis, nephrolithiasis and in severe cases, cardiac arrhythmias. Extreme hypercalcaemia may result in coma and death. Persistently high calcium levels may lead to irreversible renal damage and soft tissue calcification.

Treatment of hypercalcaemia: The treatment with calcium must be discontinued. Treatment with thiazide diuretics, lithium, vitamin A and cardiac glycosides must also be discontinued. Emptying of the stomach in patients with impaired consciousness. Rehydration, and, according to severity, isolated or combined treatment with loop diuretics, bisphosphonates, calcitonin and corticosteroids. Serum electrolytes, renal function and diuresis must be monitored. In severe cases, ECG and CVP should be followed.

5. PHARMACOLOGICAL PROPERTIES

5.1 Pharmacodynamic properties
Pharmacotherapeutic group: Calcium

ATC-code: A12A A04

An adequate intake of calcium is of importance during growth, pregnancy and breastfeeding.

5.2 Pharmacokinetic properties
Absorption: The amount of calcium absorbed through the gastrointestinal tract is approximately 30% of the swallowed dose.

Distribution and metabolism: 99% of the calcium in the body is concentrated in the hard structure of bones and teeth. The remaining 1% is present in the intra- and extracellular fluids. About 50% of the total blood-calcium content is in the physiologically active ionised form with approximately 10% being complexed to citrate, phosphate or other anions, the remaining 40% being bound to proteins, principally albumin.

Elimination: Calcium is eliminated through faeces, urine and sweat. Renal excretion depends on glomerular filtration and calcium tubular reabsorption.

5.3 Preclinical safety data
There is no information of relevance to the safety assessment in addition to what is stated in other parts of the SmPC.

6. PHARMACEUTICAL PARTICULARS

6.1 List of excipients
Sorbitol

Povidone

Isomalt

Orange oil

Magnesium stearate

Aspartame

Mono, di-fatty acid glycerides

6.2 Incompatibilities
Not applicable.

6.3 Shelf life
3 years.

6.4 Special precautions for storage
Do not store above 30°C.

Keep the container tightly closed in order to protect from moisture.

6.5 Nature and contents of container
WiMo Box of 28, 30, 56, 60, 90 and 100 tablets. Not all pack sizes may be marketed.

It is a high density polyethylene cylindrical bottle with high density polyethylene screw cap and medium density polyethylene tamper-evident liner.

6.6 Instructions for use and handling
No special requirements.

7. MARKETING AUTHORISATION HOLDER
Shire Pharmaceuticals Limited

Hampshire International Business Park

Chineham

Basingstoke

Hampshire RG24 8EP

United Kingdom

8. MARKETING AUTHORISATION NUMBER(S)
PL 08557/0022

9. DATE OF FIRST AUTHORISATION/RENEWAL OF THE AUTHORISATION
2 January 1992

10. DATE OF REVISION OF THE TEXT
April 2004

LEGAL CATEGORY
P

Calcijex 1 microgram/ml Solution for Injection

(Abbott Laboratories Limited)

1. NAME OF THE MEDICINAL PRODUCT
Calcijex 1 microgram/ml Solution for Injection

2. QUALITATIVE AND QUANTITATIVE COMPOSITION
Calcitriol 1 microgram/ml

3. PHARMACEUTICAL FORM
Solution for Injection

4. CLINICAL PARTICULARS

4.1 Therapeutic indications
Calcijex is indicated in the management of hypocalcaemia in patients undergoing dialysis for chronic renal failure. It has been shown to significantly reduce elevated parathyroid hormone (PTH) levels. Reduction of PTH has been shown to result in an improvement in renal osteodystrophy.

4.2 Posology and method of administration

Use in Adults

The optimal dose of Calcijex must be carefully determined for each patient.

The effectiveness of Calcijex therapy is predicted on the assumption that each patient is receiving an adequate and appropriate daily intake of calcium. To ensure that each patient receives an adequate daily intake of calcium, the physician should either prescribe a calcium supplement, or instruct the patient in proper dietary measures.

The recommended initial dose of Calcijex is 0.50 microgram (approximately 0.01 microgram/kg) administered three times weekly, approximately every other day. Calcijex can be administered as a bolus dose intravenously through the catheter at the end of haemodialysis. If a satisfactory response in the biochemical parameters and clinical manifestations of the disease state is not observed, the dose may be increased by 0.25 to 0.50 microgram increments at two to four week intervals. During this titration period, serum calcium and phosphate levels should be obtained at least twice weekly, and if hypercalcaemia is noted, or a serum calcium times phosphate greater than 7-8 mmol/l is noted, the drug should be immediately discontinued until these parameters are normal. Then the Calcijex dose should be reinitiated at a lower dose. Most patients undergoing haemodialysis respond to doses of between 0.5 and 3.0 microgram three times per week. Incremental dosing must be individualised and commensurate with PTH, serum calcium and phosphorus levels.

Dialysis patients with moderate to severe secondary hyperparathyroidism

Based on limited data from clinical trials with dialysis patients with moderate to severe secondary hyperparathyroidism, an initial dose, depending on the severity of secondary hyperparathyroidism, of 1.0 to 2.0 microgram administered three times weekly approximately every other day may be considered in this group of patients. Doses as small as 0.5 microgram and as large as 4.0 microgram thrice weekly have been used as an initial dose in this group, depending on the severity of the hyperparathyroidism. If a satisfactory response in the biochemical parameters and clinical manifestations of the disease state is not observed, the dose may be increased by 0.25 to 0.5 microgram at two to four week intervals. Incremental dosing from 0.25 microgram to 2.0 microgram has been used and maximal doses up to 8 microgram three times per week have been reported in a small number of patients with severe secondary hyperparathyroidism. Close biochemical monitoring and other advice detailed above are essential during therapy, in particular during dose titration. Doses may need to be reduced as the PTH levels decrease in response to the therapy. Parathyroidectomy may be considered in patients with severe secondary hyperparathroidism, refractory to all standard treatment.

Higher doses of Calcijex may be required for patients taking barbiturates or anticonvulsants as these may reduce its effects. The effects of Calcijex may be counteracted by corticosteroids.

Parenteral drug products such as Calcijex should be inspected visually for particulate matter prior to administration. Although calcitriol itself is a colourless, crystalline compound, the sodium ascorbate added as an antioxidant in Calcijex is white or very faintly yellow, and can turn yellow as it combines with oxygen.

Calcijex should be drawn up into a plastic 1ml tuberculin syringe and administered at a bolus dose intravenously at the end of dialysis. It may be administered through the catheter at the end of haemodialysis.

Use in Children

Safety and efficacy of Calcijex in children have not be established.

Use in Elderly

As for adults.

4.3 Contraindications
Calcijex should not be given to patients with hypercalcaemia or evidence of vitamin D toxicity.

This drug is contraindicated in patients with previous hypersensitivity to calcitriol or any of its excipients.

4.4 Special warnings and special precautions for use

General

Excessive dosage of Calcijex induces hypercalcaemia, and in some instances hypercalciuria; therefore, early in treatment during dosage adjustment, serum calcium and phosphate should be determined at least twice weekly. Should hypercalcaemia develop, the drug should be discontinued immediately.

Calcijex should be given cautiously to patients on digitalis, because hypercalcaemia in such patients may precipitate cardiac arrhythmias.

Adynamic bone disease may develop if PTH levels are suppressed to abnormal levels. Monitoring of the development of adynamic bone disease can be performed using bone biopsies, or more simply via measurement of PTH levels. The use of bone biopsies to monitor the development of adynamic bone disease is appropriate if the biopsies are being performed primarily for other diagnostic reasons. Otherwise PTH levels may replace a bone biopsy for this purpose. It PTH levels fall below the recommended target range in patients treated with Calcijex, the Calcijex dose should be reduced or therapy discontinued. Discontinuation of Calcijex therapy may result in rebound effect, therefore, appropriate titration downward to a maintenance dose is recommended.

Since calcitriol is the most potent metabolite of vitamin D available, vitamin D and its derivatives should be withheld during treatment.

In patients undergoing dialysis who have high serum phosphate levels, appropriate serum phosphate binders should be used. Aluminium containing phosphate binders should not be used except in exceptional circumstances.

Low calcium dialysis fluids may be helpful in patients who develop hypercalcaemia whilst taking calcium-based phosphate binders in combination with vitamin D analogues.

Overdosage of any form of vitamin D is dangerous (see also Overdosage). Progressive hypercalcaemia due to overdosage of vitamin D and its metabolites may be so severe as to require emergency attention. Chronic hypercalcaemia can lead to generalised vascular calcification, nephrocalcinosis and other soft tissue calcification. The serum calcium times phosphate (Ca × P) product should not be allowed to exceed 7 - 8. Radiographic evaluation of suspects anatomical regions may be useful in the early detection of this condition.

Information for the Patient

The patient should be informed about adherence to instructions about diet and calcium supplementation and avoidance of the use of unapproved non-prescription drugs, including magnesium-containing antacids. Patients should be also be carefully informed about the symptoms of hypercalcaemia (see Undesirable Effects).

Essential Laboratory Tests

Serum calcium, phosphate, magnesium and alkaline phosphatase and 24-hour urinary calcium and phosphate should be determined periodically. During the initial phase of the medication, serum calcium and phosphate should be determined more frequently (twice weekly).

Renal Transplantation

The rate of bone loss can be excessive and may exceed 5% per year in the immediate post-transplant period. Recommendations for treating post-transplant bone loss with calcitriol have not been established.

4.5 Interaction with other medicinal products and other forms of Interaction

Magnesium-containing antacids and Calcijex should not be used concomitantly, because such use may lead to the development of hypermagnesaemia.

Concurrent use of vitamin D analogs and cardiac glycosides may result in cardiac arrhythmias.

The effects of vitamin D may be reduced in patients taking barbiturates or anticonvulsants.

Corticosteroids may counteract the effect of vitamin D analogs.

4.6 Pregnancy and lactation

There are no adequate and well-controlled studies in pregnant women. Calcijex should be used during pregnancy only if the potential benefit justifies the potential risk to the foetus.

It is not known whether this drug is excreted in human milk. Because of the potential for serious adverse reaction in nursing infants due to calcitriol, breast-feeding cannot be recommended.

4.7 Effects on ability to drive and use machines

None.

4.8 Undesirable effects

Adverse effects of Calcijex are, in general, similar to those encountered with excessive vitamin D intake. The early and late signs and symptoms of vitamin D intoxication associated with hypercalcaemia include:

Early

Weakness, headaches, somnolence, nausea, vomiting, dry mouth, constipation, muscle pain, bone pain and metallic taste.

Late

Polyuria, polydipsia, anorexia, weight loss, nocturia, conjunctivitis (calcific), pancreatitis, photophobia, rhinorrhea, pruritus, hyperthermia, decreased libido, elevated BUN, albuminuria, hypercholesterolaemia, elevated SGOT and SGPT, ectopic calcification, hypertension, cardiac arrhythmias and, rarely, overt psychosis.

Rare cases of hypersensitivity reactions have been reported including anaphylaxis and localised redness at the injection site.

4.9 Overdose

Administration of Calcijex to patients in excess of their requirements can cause hypercalcaemia, hypercalciuria and hyperphosphataemia. High intake of calcium and phosphate concomitant with Calcijex may lead to similar abnormalities.

Treatment of Hypercalcaemia and Overdose in Patients on Haemodialysis

General treatment of hypercalcaemia (greater than 1mg/dl above the upper limit of the normal range) consists of immediate discontinuation of Calcijex therapy, institution of a low calcium diet and withdrawal of calcium supplements. Serum calcium levels should be determined daily until normocalcaemia ensues. Hypercalcaemia usually resolves in two to seven days. When serum calcium levels have returned to within normal limits, Calcijex therapy may be reinstituted at a dose 0.5 microgram less than prior therapy. Serum calcium levels should be obtained at least twice weekly after all dosage changes.

Persistent or markedly elevated serum calcium levels may be corrected by dialysis against a calcium free dialysate.

Treatment of Accidental Overdosage of Calcitriol Injection

The treatment of acute accidental overdosage of Calcijex should consist of general supportive measures. Serial serum electrolyte determinations (especially calcium), rate of urinary calcium excretion and assessment of electrocardiographic abnormalities due to hypercalcaemia should be obtained. Such monitoring is critical in patients receiving digitalis. Discontinuation of supplemental calcium and initation of low calcium diet are also indicated in accidental overdosage. Due to the duration of the pharmacological action of calcitriol being only 3 to 5 days, further measures are probably unnecessary. Should, however, elevated serum calcium levels persist, there are a variety of therapeutic alternatives which may be considered, depending on the patients' underlying condition. These include the use of drugs such as bisphosphonates, mithramycin, calcitonin, gallium nitrate and corticosteroids as well as measures to induce an appropriate forced diuresis. The use of peritoneal dialysis and haemodialysis against a calcium-free dialysate has also been reported.

5. PHARMACOLOGICAL PROPERTIES

5.1 Pharmacodynamic properties

Calcitriol is the active form of vitamin D_3 (cholecalciferol). The natural or endogeneous supply of vitamin D in man mainly depends on ultraviolet light for conversion of 7-dehydrocholesterol to vitamin D_3 in the skin. Vitamin D_3 must be metabolically activated in the liver and kidney before it is fully active on its target tissues. The inital transformation is catalysed by vitamin D_3-25-hydroxylase enzyme present in the liver, and the product of this reaction is 25-(OH)D_3 (calcifediol). The latter undergoes hydroxylation in the mitochondria of kidney tissue, and this reaction is activated by the renal 25-hydroxyvitamin D_3-1- alphahydroxylase to produce 1-alpha-25- (OH) $_2D_3$ (calcitriol), the active form of vitamin D_3. A vitamin D resistant state may exist in uraemic patients because of the failure of the kidney to adequately convert precursors to the active compound, calcitriol.

The known sites of action of calcitiol are intestine, bone, kidney and parathyroid gland. Calcitriol is the most active form of vitamin D_3 in stimulating intestinal calcium transport. In acutely uraemic rats, calcitriol has been shown to stimulate intestinal calcium absorption. In bone, calcitriol, in conjunction with parathyroid hormone (PTH), stimulates resorption of calcium; and in the kidney, calcitriol increases the tubular reabsorption of calcium. In-vitro and in-vivo studies have shown that calcitriol directly suppresses secretion and synthesis of PTH.

Calcitriol when administered by bolus injection is rapidly available in the blood stream. Vitamin D metabolites are known to be transported in blood, bound in specific plasma proteins. The pharmacologic activity of an administered dose of calcitriol lasts about 3 to 5 days. Two metabolic pathways for calcitriol have been identified, conversion to 1,24,25-$(OH)_3$ D_3 and to calcitroic acid.

5.2 Pharmacokinetic properties

It is well established in the literature that regardless of the route of administration, the metabolic effects of calcitriol reach their peak and continue long after the plasma level of the hormone has returned to baseline values. Kinetic studies of calcitriol that would be useful in demonstrating that the administered hormone reaches the bloodstream and is eliminated in the same fashion as the endogenously synthesised compound would be of little value in determining the optimal therapeutic dosage. The optimal amount of calcitriol to be administered must be determined individually for each patient on the basis of the type, severity and duration of the calcium imbalance.

5.3 Preclinical safety data

None stated.

6. PHARMACEUTICAL PARTICULARS

6.1 List of excipients

Polysorbate 20, sodium chloride, sodium ascorbate (microcrystalline), sodium phoshate (dibasic, anhydrous), sodium phosphate (monobasic, monohydrate), editate disodium (dihydrate), water for injection.

6.2 Incompatibilities

Calcitriol is known to be adsorbed onto PVC containers and tubing. It should therefore not be infused with the dialysate during CAPD as the dose could be significantly reduced due to drug adsorption to the PVC bag and tubing. See Posology and Method of Administration for recommended dosing method.

6.3 Shelf life

The recommended shelf life is 30 months.

6.4 Special precautions for storage

Do not store above 25°C. Do not refrigerate. Store in the original container.

6.5 Nature and contents of container

Calcijex is supplied in USP Type 1ml amber glass ampoules containing calcitriol (1 microgram/ml).

6.6 Instructions for use and handling

Discard any unused solution immediately after use.

7. MARKETING AUTHORISATION HOLDER

Abbott Laboratories Ltd

Queenborough

Kent ME11 5EL

8. MARKETING AUTHORISATION NUMBER(S)

PL 0037/0245

9. DATE OF FIRST AUTHORISATION/RENEWAL OF THE AUTHORISATION

30 June 1994

10. DATE OF REVISION OF THE TEXT

March 2001

Calcijex 2 microgram/ml Solution for Injection

(Abbott Laboratories Limited)

1. NAME OF THE MEDICINAL PRODUCT

Calcijex 2 microgram/ml Solution for Injection

2. QUALITATIVE AND QUANTITATIVE COMPOSITION

Calcitriol 2 microgram/ml

3. PHARMACEUTICAL FORM

Solution for Injection

4. CLINICAL PARTICULARS

4.1 Therapeutic indications

Calcijex is indicated in the management of hypocalcaemia in patients undergoing dialysis for chronic renal failure. It has been shown to significantly reduce elevated parathyroid hormone (PTH) levels. Reduction of PTH has been shown to result in an improvement in renal osteodystrophy.

4.2 Posology and method of administration

Use in Adults

The optimal dose of Calcijex must be carefully determined for each patient.

The effectiveness of Calcijex therapy is predicted on the assumption that each patient is receiving an adequate and appropriate daily intake of calcium. To ensure that each patient receives an adequate daily intake of calcium, the physician should either prescribe a calcium supplement, or instruct the patient in proper dietary measures.

The recommended initial dose of Calcijex is 0.50 microgram (approximately 0.01 microgram/kg) administered three times weekly, approximately every other day. Calcijex can be administered as a bolus dose intravenously through the catheter at the end of haemodialysis. If a satisfactory response in the biochemical parameters and clinical manifestations of the disease state is not observed, the dose may be increased by 0.25 to 0.50 microgram increments at two to four week intervals. During this titration period, serum calcium and phosphate levels should be obtained at least twice weekly, and if hypercalcaemia is noted, or a serum calcium times phosphate greater than 7-8 mmol/l is noted, the drug should be immediately discontinued until these parameters are normal. Then the Calcijex dose should be reinitiated at a lower dose. Most patients undergoing haemodialysis respond to doses of between 0.5 and 3.0 microgram three times per week. Incremental dosing must be individualised and commensurate with PTH, serum calcium and phosphorus levels.

Dialysis patients with moderate to severe secondary hyperparathyroidism

Based on limited data from clinical trials with dialysis patients with moderate to severe secondary hyperparathyroidism, an initial dose, depending on the severity of secondary hyperparathyroidism, of 1.0 to 2.0 microgram administered three times weekly approximately every other day may be considered in this group of patients. Doses as small as 0.5 microgram and as large as 4.0 microgram thrice weekly have been used as an initial dose in this group, depending on the severity of the hyperparathyroidism. If a satisfactory response in the biochemical parameters and clinical manifestations of the disease state is not observed, the dose may be increased by 0.25 to 0.5 microgram at two to four week intervals. Incremental dosing from 0.25 microgram to 2.0 microgram has been used and maximal doses up to 8 microgram three times per week have been reported in a small number of patients with severe secondary hyperparathyroidism. Close biochemical monitoring and other advice detailed above are essential during therapy, in particular during dose titration. Doses may need to be reduced as the PTH levels decrease in response to the therapy. Parathyroidectomy may be considered in patients with severe secondary hyperparathroidism, refractory to all standard treatment.

Higher doses of Calcijex may be required for patients taking barbiturates or anticonvulsants as these may reduce its effects. The effects of Calcijex may be counteracted by corticosteroids.

Parenteral drug products such as Calcijex should be inspected visually for particulate matter prior to administration. Although calcitriol itself is a colourless, crystalline compound, the sodium ascorbate added as an antioxidant in Calcijex is white or very faintly yellow, and can turn yellow as it combines with oxygen.

Calcijex should be drawn up into a plastic 1ml tuberculin syringe and administered at a bolus dose intravenously at the end of dialysis. It may be administered through the catheter at the end of haemodialysis.

Use in Children
Safety and efficacy of Calcijex in children have not be established.

Use in Elderly
As for adults

4.3 Contraindications
Calcijex should not be given to patients with hypercalcaemia or evidence of vitamin D toxicity.

This drug is contraindicated in patients with previous hypersensitivity to calcitriol or any of its excipients.

4.4 Special warnings and special precautions for use
General
Excessive dosage of Calcijex induces hypercalcaemia, and in some instances hypercalciuria; therefore, early in treatment during dosage adjustment, serum calcium and phosphate should be determined at least twice weekly. Should hypercalcaemia develop, the drug should be discontinued immediately.

Calcijex should be given cautiously to patients on digitalis, because hypercalcaemia in such patients may precipitate cardiac arrhythmias.

Adynamic bone disease may develop if PTH levels are suppressed to abnormal levels. Monitoring of the development of adynamic bone disease can be performed using bone biopsies, or more simply via measurement of PTH levels. The use of bone biopsies to monitor the development of adynamic bone disease is appropriate if the biopsies are being performed primarily for other diagnostic reasons. Otherwise PTH levels may replace a bone biopsy for this purpose. It PTH levels fall below the recommended target range in patients treated with Calcijex, the Calcijex dose should be reduced or therapy discontinued. Discontinuation of Calcijex therapy may result in rebound effect, therefore, appropriate titration downward to a maintenance dose is recommended.

Since calcitriol is the most potent metabolite of vitamin D available, vitamin D and its derivatives should be withheld during treatment.

In patients undergoing dialysis who have high serum phosphate levels, appropriate serum phosphate binders should be used. Aluminium containing phosphate binders should not be used except in exceptional circumstances.

Low calcium dialysis fluids may be helpful in patients who develop hypercalcaemia whilst taking calcium-based phosphate binders in combination with vitamin D analogues.

Overdosage of any form of vitamin D is dangerous (see also Overdosage). Progressive hypercalcaemia due to overdosage of vitamin D and its metabolites may be so severe as to require emergency attention. Chronic hypercalcaemia can lead to generalised vascular calcification, nephrocalcinosis and other soft tissue calcification. The serum calcium times phosphate (Ca × P) product should not be allowed to exceed 7-8. Radiographic evaluation of suspects anatomical regions may be useful in the early detection of this condition.

Information for the Patient
The patient should be informed about adherence to instructions about diet and calcium supplementation and avoidance of the use of unapproved non-prescription drugs, including magnesium-containing antacids. Patients should be also be carefully informed about the symptoms of hypercalcaemia (see Undesirable Effects).

Essential Laboratory Tests
Serum calcium, phosphate, magnesium and alkaline phosphatase and 24-hour urinary calcium and phosphate should be determined periodically. During the initial phase of the medication, serum calcium and phosphate should be determined more frequently (twice weekly).

Renal Transplantation
The rate of bone loss can be excessive and may exceed 5% per year in the immediate post-transplant period. Recommendations for treating post-transplant bone loss with calcitriol have not been established.

4.5 Interaction with other medicinal products and other forms of Interaction
Magnesium-containing antacids and Calcijex should not be used concomitantly, because such use may lead to the development of hypermagnesaemia.

Concurrent use of vitamin D analogs and cardiac glycosides may result in cardiac arrhythmias.

The effects of vitamin D may be reduced in patients taking barbiturates or anticonvulsants.

Corticosteroids may counteract the effect of vitamin D analogs.

4.6 Pregnancy and lactation
There are no adequate and well-controlled studies in pregnant women. Calcijex should be used during pregnancy only if the potential benefit justifies the potential risk to the foetus.

It is not known whether this drug is excreted in human milk. Because of the potential for serious adverse reaction in nursing infants due to calcitriol, breast-feeding cannot be recommended.

4.7 Effects on ability to drive and use machines
None.

4.8 Undesirable effects
Adverse effects of Calcijex are, in general, similar to those encountered with excessive vitamin D intake. The early and late signs and symptoms of vitamin D intoxication associated with hypercalcaemia include:

Early
Weakness, headaches, somnolence, nausea, vomiting, dry mouth, constipation, muscle pain, bone pain and metallic taste.

Late
Polyuria, polydipsia, anorexia, weight loss, nocturia, conjunctivitis (calcific), pancreatitis, photophobia, rhinorrhea, pruritus, hyperthermia, decreased libido, elevated BUN, albuminuria, hypercholesterolaemia, elevated SGOT and SGPT, ectopic calcification, hypertension, cardiac arrhythmias and, rarely, overt psychosis.

Rare cases of hypersensitivity reactions have been reported including anaphylaxis and localised redness at the injection site.

4.9 Overdose
Administration of Calcijex to patients in excess of their requirements can cause hypercalcaemia, hypercalciuria and hyperphosphataemia. High intake of calcium and phosphate concomitant with Calcijex may lead to similar abnormalities.

Treatment of Hypercalcaemia and Overdose in Patients on Haemodialysis
General treatment of hypercalcaemia (greater than 1mg/dl above the upper limit of the normal range) consists of immediate discontinuation of Calcijex therapy, institution of a low calcium diet and withdrawal of calcium supplements. Serum calcium levels should be determined daily until normocalcaemia ensues. Hypercalcaemia usually resolves in two to seven days. When serum calcium levels have returned to within normal limits, Calcijex therapy may be reinstituted at a dose 0.5microgram less than prior therapy. Serum calcium levels should be obtained at least twice weekly after all dosage changes.

Persistent or markedly elevated serum calcium levels may be corrected by dialysis against a calcium free dialysate.

Treatment of Accidental Overdosage of Calcitriol Injection
The treatment of acute accidental overdosage of Calcijex should consist of general supportive measures. Serial serum electrolyte determinations (especially calcium), rate of urinary calcium excretion and assessment of electrocardiographic abnormalities due to hypercalcaemia should be obtained. Such monitoring is critical in patients receiving digitalis. Discontinuation of supplemental calcium and initation of low calcium diet are also indicated in accidental overdosage. Due to the duration of the pharmacological action of calcitriol being only 3 to 5 days, further measures are probably unnecessary. Should, however, elevated serum calcium levels persist, there are a variety of therapeutic alternatives which may be considered, depending on the patients' underlying condition. These include the use of drugs such as bisphosphonates, mithramycin, calcitonin, gallium nitrate and corticosteroids as well as measures to induce an appropriate forced diuresis. The use of peritoneal dialysis and haemodialysis against a calcium-free dialysate has also been reported.

5. PHARMACOLOGICAL PROPERTIES
5.1 Pharmacodynamic properties
Calcitriol is the active form of vitamin D_3 (cholecalciferol). The natural or endogeneous supply of vitamin D in man mainly depends on ultraviolet light for conversion of 7-dehydrocholesterol to vitamin D_3 in the skin. Vitamin D_3 must be metabolically activated in the liver and kidney before it is fully active on its target tissues. The inital transformation is catalysed by vitamin D_3-25-hydroxylase enzyme present in the liver, and the product of this reaction is 25-(OH)D_3 (calcifediol). The latter undergoes hydroxylation in the mitochondria of kidney tissue, and this reaction is activated by the renal 25-hydroxyvitamin D_3-1- alpha-hydroxylase to produce 1-alpha-25- (OH) $_2D_3$ (calcitrol), the active form of vitamin D_3. A vitamin D resistant state may exist in uraemic patients because of the failure of the kidney to adequately convert precursors to the active compound, calcitriol.

The known sites of action of calcitiol are intestine, bone, kidney and parathyroid gland. Calcitriol is the most active form of vitamin D_3 in stimulating intestinal calcium transport. In acutely uraemic rats, calcitriol has been shown to stimulate intestinal calcium absorption. In bone, calcitriol, in conjunction with parathyroid hormone (PTH), stimulates resorption of calcium; and in the kidney, calcitriol increases the tubular reabsorption of calcium. In-vitro and in-vivo studies have shown that calcitriol directly suppresses secretion and synthesis of PTH.

Calcitriol when administered by bolus injection is rapidly available in the blood stream. Vitamin D metabolites are known to be transported in blood, bound in specific plasma proteins. The pharmacologic activity of an administered dose of calcitriol lasts about 3 to 5 days. Two metabolic pathways for calcitriol have been identified, conversion to 1,24,25-$(OH)_3$ D_3 and to calcitroic acid.

5.2 Pharmacokinetic properties
It is well established in the literature that regardless of the route of administration, the metabolic effects of calcitriol reach their peak and continue long after the plasma level of the hormone has returned to baseline values. Kinetic studies of calcitriol that would be useful in demonstrating that the administered hormone reaches the bloodstream and is eliminated in the same fashion as the endogenously synthesised compound would be of little value in determining the optimal therapeutic dosage. The optimal amount of calcitriol to be administered must be determined individually for each patient on the basis of the type, severity and duration of the calcium imbalance.

5.3 Preclinical safety data
None stated.

6. PHARMACEUTICAL PARTICULARS
6.1 List of excipients
Polysorbate 20, sodium chloride, sodium ascorbate (microcrystalline), sodium phoshate (dibasic, anhydrous), sodium phosphate (monobasic, monohydrate), editate disodium (dihydrate), water for injection.

6.2 Incompatibilities
Calcitriol is known to be adsorbed onto PVC containers and tubing. It should therefore not be infused with the dialysate during CAPD as the dose could be significantly reduced due to drug adsorption to the PVC bag and tubing. See Posology and Method of Administration for recommended dosing method.

6.3 Shelf life
The recommended shelf life is 30 months.

6.4 Special precautions for storage
Do not store above 25°C. Do not refrigerate. Store in the original container.

6.5 Nature and contents of container
Calcijex is supplied in USP Type 1ml amber glass ampoules containing calcitriol (2 microgram/ml).

6.6 Instructions for use and handling
Discard any unused solution immediately after use.

7. MARKETING AUTHORISATION HOLDER
Abbott Laboratories Ltd
Queenborough
Kent ME11 5EL

8. MARKETING AUTHORISATION NUMBER(S)
PL 0037/0246

9. DATE OF FIRST AUTHORISATION/RENEWAL OF THE AUTHORISATION
30 June 1994

10. DATE OF REVISION OF THE TEXT
March 2001

Calciparine

(sanofi-aventis)

1. NAME OF THE MEDICINAL PRODUCT
Calciparine, 25,000 IU Heparin activity per ml.

2. QUALITATIVE AND QUANTITATIVE COMPOSITION
Heparin Calcium 25,000 IU/ml
For excipients, see 6.1.

3. PHARMACEUTICAL FORM
Solution for injection.

Sterile clear solution of 25,000 International Units of Heparin activity per ml as the calcium salt in water for injections.

4. CLINICAL PARTICULARS
4.1 Therapeutic indications
It is indicated for use as an anticoagulant for the prophylaxis and treatment of thromboembolic phenomena, especially myocardial infarction, acute arterial embolism or thrombosis, deep vein thrombosis, thrombophlebitis or pulmonary embolism.

4.2 Posology and method of administration
For subcutaneous administration only using a 26-gauge needle. The best site is the subcutaneous tissue of the lateral abdominal wall. The needle should be inserted perpendicularly into a pinched-up fold of skin and held

gently but firmly within the skinfold until injection has been completed. Do not rub the site of injection.

Calciparine is not intended for intramuscular use.

Adults

Prophylaxis:

A standard prophylactic dose regimen is 5,000 IU by subcutaneous injection 2 hours before operation, followed by 5,000 IU by subcutaneous injection every 8 to 12 hours for seven days. In patients still confined to bed at the end of this period, the same dosage should be continued until they are ambulant.

The standard prophylactic dose following myocardial infarction is 5,000 IU by subcutaneous injection twice daily for 10 days or until the patient is mobile.

In other medical conditions in which there is an associated increased risk of thromboembolic phenomena, the same dosage is recommended.

These standard prophylactic regimens do not require routine control in the absence of contra-indications or conditions listed under special warnings and precautions.

If a myocardial infarction is shown to be anterior and therefore has a risk of mural thrombosis of the left ventricle, a higher dose of 12,500 IU twice daily for at least 10 days is recommended. For this dosage regimen, regular monitoring should be considered.

Treatment:

For the treatment of existing thrombosis the standard dose is 0.1ml Calciparine (2,500 IU) per 10kg body weight 12 hourly. To enable dosage to be individually adjusted to maintain a coagulation time in a range of 1.5 to 3 times that of control it is recommended that the thrombin clotting time, whole blood clotting time or the activated partial thromboplastin time be measured on blood withdrawn 5 to 7 hours after the first injection and then at intervals until the patient is stabilised. During long term therapy the test should be repeated at least once each week.

Children

Dosage should be individually adjusted according to changes in whole blood clotting time and/or thrombin clotting time and/or APTT. The initial dose should be 0.1ml Calciparine (2,500 IU) by subcutaneous injection for each 10kg of body weight. The usual interval between doses is 12 hours, but this also may require individual adjustment.

Other special groups

For both prophylaxis and treatment, higher doses are likely to be required in patients of abnormally high body weight and in those suffering from cancer, diabetes mellitus or other diseases associated with marked hypercoagulability. Lower doses are usually indicated in the elderly and in those with low serum albumin or impaired renal or hepatic function. In such patients coagulation times should be checked frequently and dosage adjusted accordingly.

Use in pregnancy

Heparin does not cross the placental wall; no malformation or foetotoxicity have been reported in humans. Nonetheless, particular caution should be exercised due to uteroplacental haemorrhagic risks, particularly at the time of delivery. Calciparine should be discontinued if peridural anaesthesia is likely. Individual control is essential and the aim should be to maintain plasma heparin levels between 0.1 and 0.4 units/ml, as assessed by anti-XA assay, and a whole blood clotting time of 15 to 20 minutes.

The standard prophylactic dosage of 5,000 IU by subcutaneous injection every 8 hours is a suitable starting dose in the first 3 or 4 months of pregnancy but higher doses are needed as pregnancy progresses, 10,000 IU two or three times daily being usual in the last trimester. Dosage must be reduced during labour and standard prophylactic dosage is suitable post-partum.

Heparin is not excreted into breast milk.

4.3 Contraindications

- hypersensitivity to heparin.
- history of thrombocytopenia occurring with any kind of heparin
- active bleeding or increased risk of haemorrhage in relation to haemostasis disorders, except for disseminated intravascular coagulation not induced by heparin.
- organic lesion likely to bleed (including gastric and duodenal ulcer).
- threatened abortion
- sub-acute infectious endocarditis.
- post-operative period following surgery of the brain, spinal cord and eye.
- haemorrhagic cerebral vascular accident.
- in patients receiving Calciparine for treatment rather than prophylaxis, locoregional anaesthesia in elective surgical procedures is contra-indicated.
- Calciparine should not be used in patients with advanced renal or hepatic dysfunction, in severe hypertension or patients in shock.

4.4 Special warnings and special precautions for use

4.4.1 Special warnings

Platelet count monitoring:

Platelet count must be performed before the treatment, and subsequently twice weekly; if a prolonged treatment is found to be necessary, this monitoring program must be respected, at least during the first month; after that time, monitoring can be carried out less frequently.

Some rare cases of thrombocytopenia, occasionally severe, have been reported; they may be associated (or not) with arterial or venous thrombosis, and the treatment should be discontinued; such diagnosis should be considered in the following cases:

- thrombocytopenia or,
- any significant decrease in platelet count (30 - 50% of the baseline value),
- worsening of the initial thrombosis while on therapy,
- thrombosis occuring on treatment,
- disseminated intravascular coagulation.

These effects are probably of immuno-allergic nature and in case of a first treatment they occur mainly between the 5th and the 21st day of therapy.

When a thrombocytopenia occurs with standard heparin, the substitution with a low molecular weight heparin may be considered if continuing the heparin treatment is necessary. In such cases, monitoring should be performed at least daily, and the treatment should be discontinued as soon as possible: initial thrombocytopenia continuing after substitution have been described.

In vitro platelet aggregation tests are only of limited value.

The concomitant use of salicylates, NSAIDs or antiplatelet agents represents a relative contra-indication for heparin administration *(see 4.5, Interactions with Other Medicaments and Other Forms of Interactions).*

4.4.2 Special precautions

Patients should be warned of an increased risk of bruising.

Administer with care in cases of:

- hepatic failure,
- renal failure,
- hypertension
- history of digestive ulcer or any other organic lesion likely to bleed,
- vascular diseases of the chorio-retina.

Special care should be taken in elderly patients and pregnant women.

Heparin can suppress adrenal secretion of aldosterone leading to hyperkalaemia, particularly in patients with a raised plasma potassium or at risk of increased plasma potassium levels such as patients with diabetes mellitus, chronic renal failure, pre-existing metabolic acidosis or taking drugs that may increase plasma potassium (e.g. ACE inhibitors, NSAIDs).

The risk of hyperkalaemia appears to increase with duration of therapy but is usually reversible. Plasma potassium should be monitored in patients at risk.

In patients undergoing peridural or spinal anaesthesia or spinal puncture, the prophylactic use of Calciparine may be very rarely associated with epidural or spinal haematoma resulting in prolonged or permanent paralysis. The risk is increased by the use of a peridural or spinal catheter for anaesthesia, by the concomitant use of drugs affecting haemostasis such as nonsteroidal anti-inflammatory drugs (NSAIDs), platelet inhibitors or anticoagulants, and by traumatic or repeated puncture.

In decision-making on the interval between the last administration of Calciparine at prophylactic doses and the placement or removal of a peridural or spinal catheter, the product characteristics and the patient profile should be taken into account. Subsequent dose should not take place before at least four hours have elapsed. Re-administration should be delayed until the surgical procedure is completed.

Should a physician decide to administer anticoagulation in the context of peridural or spinal anaesthesia, extreme vigilance and frequent monitoring must be exercised to detect any signs and symptoms of neurologic impairment, such as back pain, sensory and motor deficits (numbness and weakness in lower limbs) and bowel or bladder dysfunction. Nurses should be trained to detect such signs and symptoms. Patients should be instructed to inform immediately a nurse or clinician if they experience any of these.

If signs or symptoms of epidural or spinal haematomas are suspected, urgent diagnosis and treatment including spinal cord decompression should be initiated.

4.5 Interaction with other medicinal products and other forms of Interaction

Concomitant use of aspirin (or other salicylates), non-steroidal anti-inflammatory drugs, or the use of antiplatelet agents (see 4.4.1, Special warnings) is not recommended, as they may increase the risk of bleeding.

Where such combination cannot be avoided, careful clinical and biological monitoring should be undertaken.

Calciparine should be administered with care in patients receiving oral anticoagulant agents (additive anticoagulant effect), systemic corticosteroids (gluco-) and dextrans (parenteral administration).

During transfer from heparin to oral anticoagulant therapy, clinical monitoring should be particularly vigilant.

4.6 Pregnancy and lactation

Pregnancy

Heparin does not cross the placental wall; no malformation or foetotoxicity have been reported in humans. Nonetheless, particular caution should be exercised due to uteroplacental haemorrhagic risks, particularly at the time of delivery. Calciparine should be discontinued if peridural anaesthesia is likely.

Lactation

Heparin is not excreted into breast milk.

4.7 Effects on ability to drive and use machines

None stated.

4.8 Undesirable effects

Adverse reactions have been ranked under heading of system-organ class and frequency using the following convention: very commonly (>= 1/10); commonly (>= 1/100, <1/10); uncommonly (>= 1/1,000, <1/100); rarely (>= 1/10,000, <1/1,000); very rarely (<1/10,000).

Haematological and bleeding disorders:

- Very commonly: haemorrhagic manifestations at various sites, more frequent in patients with other risk factors *(see Section 4.3 Contra-indications and Section 4.5 Interactions with Other Medicaments and Other Forms of Interaction).*
- Commonly: thrombocytopenia, usually reversible, sometimes thrombogenic *(see Section 4.4.1 Special warnings).*
- Rarely: eosinophilia, reversible following treatment discontinuation.
- Very rarely: epidural or spinal haematoma in the context of peridural or spinal anaesthesia and of spinal puncture. These haematomas have caused various degrees of neurological impairment, including prolonged and permanent paralysis. *(see Section 4.4.2 Special precautions).*

Cutaneous and subcutaneous disorders:

- Very commonly: small hematomas at the injection site. In some cases, the emergence of firm nodules which do not indicate an encystment of the heparin may be noted. These nodules usually disappear after a few days and are not an indication to withdraw treatment. Pain and bruising may also occur.
- Uncommonly: localised or generalized hypersensitivity reactions, including angioedema, erythema, rash, urticaria, pruritus.
- Rarely: cutaneous necrosis usually occuring at the injection site. It is preceded by purpura or infiltrated or painful erythematous blotches, with or without systemic signs. In such cases, treatment should be immediately discontinued.
- Very rarely: Alopecia, calcinosis at injection site, especially in patients with severe renal failure

Hepato-biliary disorders:

- Commonly: raised transaminases, usually transient.

Metabolism and nutrition disorders:

- Rarely: osteoporosis after several months of treatment, at high doses.
- Very rarely: hypoaldosteronism with hyperkaliemia and / or metabolic acidosis particularly in patients at risk (diabetes, renal failure) *(see Section 4.4 Special Warnings and Special Precautions for Use).*

Reproductive disorders:

- Rarely: priapism

4.9 Overdose

Haemorrhage is the major clinical sign of overdosage. In case of bleeding, the platelet count and APTT should be determined. Minor bleeding rarely requires specific therapy, and reducing and/or delaying subsequent doses of Calciparine is usually sufficient.

The anticoagulant effect of heparin can be reversed immediately by intravenous administration of a 1% protamine sulphate solution. The dose of protamine sulphate required for neutralisation should be determined accurately by titrating the patient's plasma.

It is important to avoid overdosage of protamine sulphate because protamine itself has anticoagulant properties. A single dose of protamine sulphate should never exceed 50mg. Intravenous injection of protamine may cause a sudden fall in blood pressure, bradycardia, dyspnoea and transitory flushing, but these may be avoided or diminished by slow and careful administration.

5. PHARMACOLOGICAL PROPERTIES

5.1 Pharmacodynamic properties

Pharmacotherapeutic group: Antithrombotic agent.

ATC Code: B01 AB01

Heparin calcium is a preparation containing the calcium salt of sulphated polysaccharide acid present in mammalian tissues. It is an anticoagulant which inhibits the clotting of blood in vitro and in vivo.

No further data are presented here as the pharmacodynamic properties of heparin calcium are well known and it is the subject of a European Pharmacopoeial monograph.

5.2 Pharmacokinetic properties

The slow and regular absorption kinetics of calciparine (or similar calcium heparins) given subcutaneously make it especially suitable for low dose prophylactic therapy.

Calciparine has been used effectively in the routine prophylaxis of postoperative thromboembolism.

No further data are presented here as the properties of heparin calcium are well known. Heparin calcium is the subject of a European Pharmacopoeial monograph.

5.3 Preclinical safety data

There is no pre-clinical data of relevance to the prescriber which are additional to that already included in other sections of the SPC.

6. PHARMACEUTICAL PARTICULARS

6.1 List of excipients

Water for injection, hydrochloric acid and calcium hydroxide solution.

6.2 Incompatibilities

Other preparations should not be mixed with Calciparine.

6.3 Shelf life

48 months.

6.4 Special precautions for storage

Do not store above 25°C. Do not freeze.

6.5 Nature and contents of container

Unit dose disposable syringe 5,000 IU in 0.2ml

6.6 Instructions for use and handling

Refer to Section 4.2 Posology and Method of Administration.

7. MARKETING AUTHORISATION HOLDER

Sanofi–Synthelabo Ltd

One Onslow Street

Guildford

Surrey GU1 4YS

8. MARKETING AUTHORISATION NUMBER(S)

11723/0011

9. DATE OF FIRST AUTHORISATION/RENEWAL OF THE AUTHORISATION

6th November 1998/23rd January 2003

10. DATE OF REVISION OF THE TEXT

September 2004

Calcium Chloride BP Sterile Solution

(UCB Pharma Limited)

1. NAME OF THE MEDICINAL PRODUCT

Calcium Chloride BP Sterile Solution

2. QUALITATIVE AND QUANTITATIVE COMPOSITION

Calcium Chloride Dihydrate BP 13.4% w/v

'For excipients, see 6.1'

3. PHARMACEUTICAL FORM

Sterile solution for slow intravenous injection.

4. CLINICAL PARTICULARS

4.1 Therapeutic indications

Calcium Chloride Sterile Solution is indicated for the treatment of acute hypocalcaemia where there is a requirement for the rapid replacement of calcium, e.g. severe hypocalcaemic tetany or hypoparathyroidism, or where the oral route is inappropriate due to malabsorption.

4.2 Posology and method of administration

Route of Administration: Slow intravenous injection.

Adults

A typical dose is 2.25 to 4.5 mmol of calcium given by slow intravenous injection not exceeding 1 ml per minute and repeated as necessary.

Children

The cause of the hypocalcaemia must be fully assessed before starting therapy including dietary review, measurement of vitamin D and PTH, together with regular serum calcium and phosphate levels. For children with hypocalcaemic tetany a dosage of 0.25 to 0.35 mmol/kg of calcium given by slow intravenous injection may be given, repeated every six to eight hours until a response is seen. For other hypocalcaemia conditions initial doses of 0.5 to 3.5 mmol of calcium may be given to elevate serum calcium concentrations.

Infants

Calcium chloride has been given to infants at doses of under 0.5 mmol of calcium, but calcium gluconate is usually preferred due to the irritancy of calcium chloride.

4.3 Contraindications

Parenteral calcium therapy is contraindicated in patients receiving cardiac glycosides. Unsuitable for the treatment of hypocalcaemia caused by renal insufficiencies.

Must not be given intramuscularly and subcutaneously as severe necrosis and sloughing may occur.

4.4 Special warnings and special precautions for use

Calcium chloride can cause gastro-intestinal irritation due to the stimulatory effects of calcium on gastric acid production. However, the effect would be most likely with oral administration.

Close monitoring of serum calcium levels is essential following IV administration of calcium.

Calcium salts should be used with caution in patients with impaired renal function, cardiac disease or sarcoidosis.

Because it is acidifying, calcium chloride should be used cautiously in patients with respiratory acidosis or respiratory failure.

4.5 Interaction with other medicinal products and other forms of Interaction

Calcium salts reduce the absorption of a number of drugs such as bisphosphonates, fluoride, some fluoroquinolones and tetracyclines; administration should be separated by at least 3 hours.

Calcium chloride infusion reduces the cardiotonic effects of dobutamine.

The effects of digitalis can be increased by increases in blood calcium levels, and the administration of intravenous calcium may result in the development of potentially life-threatening digitalis induced heart arrhythmias.

Thiazide diuretics decrease urinary calcium excretion, and caution is required if such drugs are administered with both calcium chloride and other calcium-containing preparations.

4.6 Pregnancy and lactation

Calcium chloride has no known effects on the foetus or infant, but as with all drugs it should not be administered during pregnancy or breast feeding unless considered essential.

4.7 Effects on ability to drive and use machines

None stated.

4.8 Undesirable effects

Rapid intravenous injection may cause vasodilation, decreased blood pressure, bradycardia and arrhythmias.

The patient may complain of tingling sensations, a chalky 'calcium' taste and a sense of oppression or 'heat wave'.

Irritation can occur after intravenous injection. Extravasation can cause burning, necrosis and sloughing of tissue, cellulitis and soft tissue calcification.

4.9 Overdose

Excessive administration of calcium salts leads to hypercalcaemia. Too rapid injection of calcium salts may also lead to many of the symptoms of hypercalcaemia as well as chalky taste, hot flushes and peripheral vasodilation. Treatment of hypercalcaemia is by the administration of sodium chloride by intravenous infusion.

5. PHARMACOLOGICAL PROPERTIES

5.1 Pharmacodynamic properties

ATC code:A12 A07

Calcium is an essential electrolyte involved in the function of nervous, muscular and skeletal systems, cell membrane and capillary permeability. The cation is also an important activator in many enzymatic reactions and plays a regulatory role in the release and storage of neurotransmitters and hormones.

5.2 Pharmacokinetic properties

Intravenously administered calcium will be absorbed directly into the blood system. Serum calcium levels will increase immediately and may return to normal values in thirty minutes to two hours depending on the rate of renal clearance.

5.3 Preclinical safety data

None stated.

6. PHARMACEUTICAL PARTICULARS

6.1 List of excipients

Sodium hydroxide

Hydrochloric acid

Water for injections

6.2 Incompatibilities

Calcium salts are incompatible with oxidising agents, citrates, soluble carbonates, bicarbonates, phosphates, tartrates and sulphates.

6.3 Shelf life

36 months.

6.4 Special precautions for storage

Store below 25°C.

6.5 Nature and contents of container

10ml neutral Type 1 glass ampoules in packs of 10.

6.6 Instructions for use and handling

None stated.

7. MARKETING AUTHORISATION HOLDER

UCB Pharma Limited

208 Bath Road

Slough

Berkshire

SL1 3 WE

UK

8. MARKETING AUTHORISATION NUMBER(S)

PL 00039/5888R

9. DATE OF FIRST AUTHORISATION/RENEWAL OF THE AUTHORISATION

18 February 1993, 17 February 2003

10. DATE OF REVISION OF THE TEXT

June 2005

11. Legal Category

POM

Calcium Chloride Injection

(International Medication Systems (UK) Ltd)

1. NAME OF THE MEDICINAL PRODUCT

Calcium Chloride Injection Minijet 10% w/v.

2. QUALITATIVE AND QUANTITATIVE COMPOSITION

Calcium Chloride Dihydrate USP 100mg in 1ml (0.68mmol/ml).

3. PHARMACEUTICAL FORM

Sterile aqueous solution for intracardiac or slow intravenous administration.

4. CLINICAL PARTICULARS

4.1 Therapeutic indications

Calcium Chloride Injection 10% w/v is indicated in the immediate treatment of hypocalcaemic tetany. Other therapy, such as parathyroid hormone and/or vitamin D, may be indicated according to the etiology of the tetany. It is also important to institute oral calcium therapy as soon as practicable.

In cardiac resuscitation, particularly after open heart surgery, calcium chloride has been used when adrenaline has failed to improve weak or ineffective myocardial contractions.

Calcium salts have been used as adjunctive therapy in a number of conditions, including the following:

1. In severe hyperkalaemia, calcium may be injected slowly while the ECG is monitoring the heart.

2. As an aid in the treatment of depression due to overdosage of magnesium sulphate (calcium is the antagonist of magnesium toxicity).

Routes of administration:

For intracardiac or slow intravenous use only.

4.2 Posology and method of administration

Intracardiac use:

In cardiac resuscitation, injection may be made into the ventricular cavity. Do not inject into the myocardium.

Adult dosage: 200-400mg (2-4ml)

Paediatric dosage: 0.2ml/kg of bodyweight.

Intravenous use:

Hypocalcaemic disorders

Adult dosage: 500mg to 1g (5-10ml) at intervals of 1 to 3 days, depending on response of the patient or serum calcium determinations. Repeated injection may be required.

Paediatric dosage: 0.2ml/kg of bodyweight. Maximum 1-10ml/day.

Magnesium Intoxication

Adult dosage: 500mg (5ml) administered promptly. Observe patient for signs of recovery before further doses are given.

Hyperkalaemic ECG disturbances of cardiac function

Adult dosage: Adjust dosage by constant monitoring of ECG changes during administration.

Geriatric patient dosage is the same as an adult.

4.3 Contraindications

In cardiac resuscitation, the use of calcium is contraindicated in the presence of ventricular fibrillation. Calcium chloride injection is contraindicated for injection into tissue (subcutaneous or intramuscular) as it may cause necrosis and sloughing.

Calcium chloride is also contraindicated in those patients with conditions associated with hypercalcaemia and hypercalcuria (e.g. some forms of malignant disease) or in those with conditions associated with elevated vitamin D levels (e.g. sarcoidosis) or in those with renal calculi or a history of calcium renal calculi.

4.4 Special warnings and special precautions for use

A moderate fall in blood pressure due to vasodilation may attend the injection. Since calcium chloride is an acidifying salt, it is usually undesirable in the treatment of hypocalcaemia of renal insufficiency.

Calcium chloride injection, 10% w/v is for intracardiac or slow intravenous injection only. Care should be taken not to infiltrate the perivascular tissue due to possible necrosis. Solutions should be warmed to body temperature. Injections should be made slowly through a small needle into a large vein to minimize venous irritation and avoid undesirable reactions.

It is particularly important to prevent a high concentration of calcium from reaching the heart because of danger of cardiac syncope. If injected into the ventricular cavity in cardiac resuscitation care must be taken to avoid injection into the myocardial tissue. Calcium chloride injection should never be given to infants orally because of severe irritation to the gastrointestinal tract. Infant injections should not be given through the scalp.

The use of calcium chloride is undesirable in patients with respiratory acidosis or respiratory failure due to the acidifying nature of the salt.

4.5 Interaction with other medicinal products and other forms of Interaction

Because of the danger involved in the simultaneous use of calcium salts and drugs of the digitalis group, a digitalized patient should not receive an intravenous injection of a calcium compound unless the indications are clearly defined. Calcium salts should not generally be mixed with carbonates, phosphates, sulphates or tartrate in parenteral mixtures.

Biphosphonates may interact with calcium chloride causing reduced absorption of biphosphates. Thiazide diuretics may increase the risk of hypercalcaemia.

4.6 Pregnancy and lactation

Studies on the effects of calcium chloride on pregnant women have not been carried out and problems have not been documented. Calcium crosses the placenta. The benefits of administration must outweigh any potential risk.

Calcium is excreted in breast milk but there are no data on the effects, if any, on the infant.

4.7 Effects on ability to drive and use machines

Not applicable.

4.8 Undesirable effects

Rapid intravenous injections may cause the patient to complain of tingling sensations, a calcium taste, a sense of oppression or "heat wave". Injections of calcium chloride are accompanied by peripheral vasodilation as well as a local burning sensation and there may be a moderate fall in blood pressure.

Necrosis and sloughing with subcutaneous or intramuscular administration or if extravasation occurs have been reported. Soft tissue calcification, bradycardia or arrhythmias have also been reported.

4.9 Overdose

Symptoms: anorexia, nausea, vomiting, constipation, abdominal pain, muscle weakness, mental disturbances, polydipsia, polyuria, bone pain, nephrocalcinosis, renal calculi and, in severe cases, cardiac arrhythmias and coma.

Treatment: withholding calcium administration will usually resolve mild hypercalcaemia in asymptomatic patients, provided renal function is adequate.

When serum calcium concentrations are greater than 12mg per 100ml, immediate measures may be required such as hydration, loop diuretics, chelating agents, calcitonin and corticosteroids. Serum calcium concentration should be determined at frequent intervals to guide therapy adjustments.

5. PHARMACOLOGICAL PROPERTIES

5.1 Pharmacodynamic properties

Calcium is essential for the functional integrity of the nervous and muscular systems. It is necessary for normal cardiac function. It is also one of the factors involved in the mechanism of blood coagulation.

Calcium ions increase the force of myocardial contraction. In response to electrical stimulation of muscle, calcium ions enter the sarcoplasm from the extracellular space. Calcium ions contained in the sarcoplasmic reticulum are rapidly transferred to the sites of interaction between the actin and myosin filaments of the sarcomere to initiate myofibril shortening. Thus, calcium increases myocardial function. Calcium's positive inotropic effects are modulated by its action on systemic vascular resistance. Calcium may either increase or decrease systemic vascular resistance. In the normal heart, calcium's positive inotropic and vasoconstricting effect produces a predictable rise in systemic arterial pressure.

5.2 Pharmacokinetic properties

The precise mechanism of action of calcium is not known.

Excretion is renal and varies directly with serum calcium ion concentration.

5.3 Preclinical safety data

Not applicable since calcium chloride has been used in clinical practice for many years and its effects in man are well known.

6. PHARMACEUTICAL PARTICULARS

6.1 List of excipients

Calcium Hydroxide

Hydrochloric Acid

Water for Injections

6.2 Incompatibilities

Calcium salts should not be mixed with carbonates, phosphates, sulphates, tartrates or tetracycline antibiotics in parenteral mixtures.

6.3 Shelf life

36 months.

6.4 Special precautions for storage

Store below 25°C.

6.5 Nature and contents of container

The solution is contained in a USP type I glass vial with an elastomeric closure which meets all the relevant USP specifications. The product is available as 10ml.

6.6 Instructions for use and handling

The container is specially designed for use with the IMS Minijet injector.

7. MARKETING AUTHORISATION HOLDER

International Medication Systems (UK) Limited

208 Bath Road

Slough

Berkshire

SL1 3WE

UK

8. MARKETING AUTHORISATION NUMBER(S)

PL 03265/0018

9. DATE OF FIRST AUTHORISATION/RENEWAL OF THE AUTHORISATION

Date first granted: PL 10 December 1976

Date renewed: PL 10 December 1996

10. DATE OF REVISION OF THE TEXT

April 2002

POM

Calcium Folinate 10mg/ml Injection ampoules

(Wockhardt UK Ltd)

1. NAME OF THE MEDICINAL PRODUCT

Calcium Folinate 10mg/ml Injection BP

2. QUALITATIVE AND QUANTITATIVE COMPOSITION

Each ml contains 12.71 mg of calcium folinate.$5H_2O$ equivalent to 10 mg of folinic acid.

For excipients, see 6.1.

3. PHARMACEUTICAL FORM

Solution for injection

4. CLINICAL PARTICULARS

4.1 Therapeutic indications

For calcium folinate rescue (folinate rescue) during intermediate and high-dose methotrexate therapy.

Treatment of metastatic colorectal cancer in combination with 5-fluorouracil.

4.2 Posology and method of administration

Calcium folinate can be administered parenterally (intramuscular or intravenous injection or intravenous infusion). Do not administer calcium folinate intrathecally.

As a rule calcium folinate rescue has to be performed by parenteral administration in patients with malabsorption syndromes or other gastrointestinal disorders (vomiting, diarrhoea, subileus etc.) where enteral absorption is not assured. Dosages above 50 mg should be given parenterally.

For intravenous infusion, calcium folinate injection may be diluted with Sodium Chloride 0.9% or Glucose 5% Intravenous Infusion before use.

Refer also to 6.6.

Dosage

Calcium Folinate Rescue

Since the calcium folinate rescue dosage regimen heavily depends on the posology and method of the intermediate or high dose methotrexate administration, the methotrexate protocol will dictate the calcium folinate rescue dosage regimen. For posology and method of administration of calcium folinate is therefore best referred to the applied intermediate or high dose methotrexate protocol.

The following guidelines may serve as an illustration for a calcium folinate rescue dosage regimen:

Calcium folinate rescue in intermediate and high-dose methotrexate therapy:

Folinic acid rescue is necessary when methotrexate is given at doses exceeding 500mg/m^2 body surface and should be considered with doses of 100mg - 500mg/m^2 body surface.

Since tolerance to folic acid antagonists depends on various factors, there are no strict guidelines for the calcium folinate dosage as a function of the methotrexate dose.

Dosage and duration of use of calcium folinate primarily depend on the type and dosage of methotrexate and/or the occurrence of toxicity symptoms. As a rule, the first dose of calcium folinate is 15 mg (6-12 mg/m^2) to be given 12-24 hours (24 hours at the latest) after the beginning of methotrexate infusion. The same dose is given every six hours throughout a period of 72 hours. After several parenteral doses treatment can be switched over to the oral form.

Forty-eight hours after the start of the methotrexate infusion, the residual methotrexate level should be measured. If the residual methotrexate-level > 0.5 μmol/l, calcium folinate dosages should be adapted according to the following table:

Residual methotrexate blood level 48 hours after the start of the methotrexate administration. Additional calcium folinate to be administered every six hours for 48 hours

μ 0.5 μmol/l 15 mg/m^2

μ 1.0 μmol/l 100 mg/m^2

μ 2.0 μmol/l 200 mg/m^2

Colorectal cancer

The doses and the dosing schedule of 5-Fluorouracil and calcium folinate vary between regimens.

Thefollowing regimens have been used in adults:

High dose regimen:

Calcium folinate is administered at 200 mg/m^2 by slow intravenous injection over a minimum of three minutes, followed by 5-fluorouracil at 370 mg/m^2 by intravenous injection.

Low dose regimen:

Calcium folinate is administered at 20 mg/m^2 by intravenous injection followed by 5-fluorouracil at 425 mg/m^2 by intravenous injection.

5-Fluorouracil and calcium folinate should be administered separately to avoid the formation of a precipitate.

Treatment is repeated daily for five days. This five-day treatment course may be repeated at 4 week (28 day) intervals, for two courses and then repeated at 4-5 weeks (28-35 day) intervals provided that the patient has completely recovered from the toxic effects of the prior treatment course. In subsequent treatment courses, the dosage of 5-Fluorouracil should be adjusted based on patient tolerance of the prior treatment course. (Please refer to the SPC of 5-Fluorouracil for dosage adjustments of 5-Fluorouracil in case of any toxicity.)

4.3 Contraindications

Hypersensitivity to one of the ingredients of the drug product.

Pernicious anaemia and other megaloblastic anaemias (since there is only haematological remission) and other anaemias due to vitamin B_{12} deficiency.

4.4 Special warnings and special precautions for use

Profound knowledge in this specific field of antineoplastic chemotherapy and the facilities necessary to take control and safety measures are obligatory.

Resistance to methotrexate as a result of decreased membrane transport implies also resistance to folinic acid rescue as both drugs share the same transport system.

Excessive calcium folinate doses must be avoided since this might impair the antitumour activity of methotrexate, especially in CNS tumours where calcium folinate accumulates after repeated courses.

For reduction of methotrexate toxicity is referred the Summary of Products Characteristics for methotrexate.

The use of folic acid or calcium folinate in megaloblastic anaemia due to vitamin B_{12} deficiency (e.g. pernicious anaemia) may lead to haematological remission along with progression of the underlying disease or neurological deficits.

Many cytotoxic drugs – direct or indirect DNA synthesis inhibitors – lead to a macrocytosis (hydroxycarbamide, cytarabine, mecaptourine, thioguanine). Such a macrocytosis is not considered to be treated by folinic acid.

Calcium folinate has no effect on non-haematological toxicities of methotrexate such as the nephrotoxicity resulting from drug and/or metabolite precipitation in the kidney.

Because of the high calcium concentration, intravenous administration of calcium folinate should not exceed 160 mg/minute.

In combination regimen with 5-fluorouracil, the toxicity risk of 5-fluorouracil is increased by calcium folinate, particularly in elderly or debilitated patients. The most common manifestations are leucopenia, mucositis, and/or diarrhoea which may be dose limiting. When calcium folinate and 5-flourouracil are used in the treatment of colorectal cancer, the 5-flourouracil dosage has to be reduced more in cases of toxicity than when 5-flourouracil is used alone. The toxicities observed in patients treated with the combination therapy are qualitatively similar to those observed in patients treated with 5- fluorouracil monotherapy. Gastrointestinal toxicity symptoms are more commonly and may be more severe and even life threatening. In severe cases the combination calcium folinate and 5-fluorouracil must be withdrawn.

4.5 Interaction with other medicinal products and other forms of Interaction

When calcium folinate is given in conjunction with a folic acid antagonist

(e.g. co-trimoxazole, pyrimethamine) the efficacy of the folic acid antagonist may either be reduced or completely neutralised.

Calcium folinate may diminish the effect of the antiepileptic substances phenobarbital, primidone and phenytoin, succinimides, and may increase the frequency of seizures. (A decrease of plasma levels of enzymatic-inductor anticonvulsant drugs may be observed because the hepatic metabolism is increased as folates are one of the cofactors)

Concomitant administration of calcium folinate with 5-fluorouracil has been shown to enhance the efficacy and toxicity of 5-fluorouracil.

4.6 Pregnancy and lactation
No formal animal reproductive toxicity studies have been conducted with calcium folinate, but indirect evidence from other studies suggests that it does not harm the foetus. No adequate or well-controlled studies have been conducted in pregnant women. Calcium folinate should only be used during pregnancy when the potential benefit to the mother outweighs any potential risk to the foetus.

It is not known whether calcium folinate is excreted in breast milk. Calcium folinate should be prescribed to breast-feeding mothers only when clearly needed.

4.7 Effects on ability to drive and use machines
No data available. However, an effect is not to be expected.

4.8 Undesirable effects
Very rarely allergic reactions.

Fever has been observed after administration of calcium folinate as solution for injection.

After high doses rarely gastrointestinal disorders, insomnia, excitation, depression.

4.9 Overdose
Concerning impaired methotrexate efficacy is referred to 4.4.

Should overdosage of the combination of 5-flourouracil with calcium folinate occur, follow the overdosages instructions for 5-flourouracil.

5. PHARMACOLOGICAL PROPERTIES

5.1 Pharmacodynamic properties
Pharmacotherapeutic group: Detoxifying agents for antineoplastic treatment, ATC-Code: V03A F03.

Folinic acid (5-formyl-tetrahydrofolic acid) (anti-anaemic) is the active form of folic acid, a nutritional factor essential for the human organism. It is involved in various metabolic processes, e.g. purine synthesis, pyrimidine nucleotide synthesis and amino acid metabolism.

Methotrexate competitively inhibits dihydrofolate reductase and thereby prevents the formation of reduced folates in the cell. As a consequence, it inhibits DNA, RNA and protein synthesis.

The folinic acid released from calcium folinate is rapidly converted into the active 5-methyl-tetrahydrofolic acid (calcium folinate rescue). Unlike folic acid, folinic acid (leucovorin) does not require a reduction by dihydrofolate reductase. Therefore, dihydrofolate reductase blockers have no effect on folinic acid.

The effect of methotrexate primarily depends on the rate of cell division and therefore it exerts its cytostatic effect on all rapidly growing tissues, i.e. in addition to tumour tissue also on other rapidly proliferating tissues (skin and mucosa, hematopoietic bone marrow, gonads). These vital tissues and organs can be protected from the cellular toxicity of methotrexate by calcium folinate (N^3- formyl –THF–folinic acid–citrovorum factor).

5.2 Pharmacokinetic properties
The major metabolic product of calcium folinate is 5-methyl-tetrahydrofolic acid, which is predominantly produced in the liver and intestinal mucosa.

The half-life of the active metabolites is about 6 hours (after intravenous and intramuscular administration).

The bioavailability of oral calcium folinate declines with increasing dosage due to saturation of folate absorption.

Excretion: 80-90% with the urine (5-and 10-formyl-tetrahydrofolates inactive metabolites), 5-8% with the faeces.

5.3 Preclinical safety data
Conventional studies of safety pharmacology, repeated dose toxicity, genotoxicity, carcinogenic potential and toxicity to reproduction have not been conducted with calcium folinate. There is extensive clinical experience, however, and anything of relevance to the prescriber is included in other sections of the SPC.

6. PHARMACEUTICAL PARTICULARS

6.1 List of excipients
Water for injections

Sodium Chloride

6.2 Incompatibilities
Calcium folinate solutions should not be mixed with infusion solutions containing hydrogen carbonate because of their chemical instability.

6.3 Shelf life
Unopened – 24 months.

The chemical and physical in-use stability of the solution diluted with Sodium Chloride 0.9% or Glucose 5% Intravenous Infusion has been demonstrated for 24 hours at a temperature not exceeding 25°C. From a microbiological point of view, the product should be used immediately. If not used immediately, in-use storage times and conditions prior to use are the responsibility of the user and would normally not be longer than 24 hours at 2 to 8°C, unless dilution has taken place in controlled and validated aseptic conditions.

6.4 Special precautions for storage
Store at 2°C-8°C. Keep container in the outer carton.

6.5 Nature and contents of container
Amber ampoules of hydrolytic type I glass, packed in a carton.

5 ampoules containing 30mg/3ml of Calcium folinate, each.

5 ampoules containing 50mg/5ml of Calcium folinate, each.

5 ampoules containing 100mg/10ml of Calcium folinate, each.

6.6 Instructions for use and handling
The product is for single use only.

Solutions should only be used if clear and particle free.

Any unused product or waste material should be disposed of in accordance with local requirements.

Calcium folinate for infusion may be prepared by dilution with Sodium Chloride 0.9% or Glucose 5% Intravenous Infusion. The concentration of calcium folinate solutions, diluted with Glucose 5%. Intravenous Infusion should not be less than 0.2 mg/ml (0.02% w/v).

7. MARKETING AUTHORISATION HOLDER
CP Pharmaceuticals Ltd

Ash Road North

Wrexham LL13 9UF

United Kingdom

8. MARKETING AUTHORISATION NUMBER(S)
PL 4543/0437

9. DATE OF FIRST AUTHORISATION/RENEWAL OF THE AUTHORISATION
16 May 2001

10. DATE OF REVISION OF THE TEXT

Calcium Folinate 10mg/ml Injection vials

(Wockhardt UK Ltd)

1. NAME OF THE MEDICINAL PRODUCT
Calcium Folinate 10mg/ml Injection BP

2. QUALITATIVE AND QUANTITATIVE COMPOSITION
Each ml contains 12.71 mg of calcium folinate.$5H_2O$ equivalent to 10 mg of folic acid.

For excipients, see 6.1.

3. PHARMACEUTICAL FORM
Solution for injection

4. CLINICAL PARTICULARS

4.1 Therapeutic indications
For calcium folinate rescue (folinate rescue) during intermediate and high-dose methotrexate therapy.

Treatment of metastatic colorectal cancer in combination with 5-fluorouracil.

4.2 Posology and method of administration
Calcium folinate can be administered parenterally (intramuscular or intravenous injection or intravenous infusion). Do not administer calcium folinate intrathecally.

As a rule calcium folinate rescue has to be performed by parenteral administration in patients with malabsorption syndromes or other gastrointestinal disorders (vomiting, diarrhoea, subileus etc.) where enteral absorption is not assured. Dosages above 50 mg should be given parenterally.

For intravenous infusion, calcium folinate injection may be diluted with Sodium Chloride 0.9% or Glucose 5% Intravenous Infusion before use.

Refer also to 6.6.

Dosage

Since the calcium folinate rescue dosage regimen heavily depends on the posology and method of the intermediate or high dose methotrexate administration, the methotrexate protocol will dictate the calcium folinate rescue dosage regimen. For posology and method of administration of calcium folinate is therefore best referred to the applied intermediate or high dose methotrexate protocol.

The following guidelines may serve as an illustration for a calcium folinate rescue dosage regimen:

Calcium folinate rescue in intermediate and high-dose methotrexate therapy:

Folinic acid rescue is necessary when methotrexate is given at doses exceeding 500mg/m^2 body surface and should be considered with doses of 100mg - 500mg/m^2 body surface.

Since tolerance to folic acid antagonists depends on various factors, there are no strict guidelines for the calcium folinate dosage as a function of the methotrexate dose.

Dosage and duration of use of calcium folinate primarily depend on the type and dosage of methotrexate and/or the occurrence of toxicity symptoms. As a rule, the first dose of calcium folinate is 15 mg (6-12 mg/m^2) to be given 12-24 hours (24 hours at the latest) after the beginning of methotrexate infusion. The same dose is given every six hours throughout a period of 72 hours. After several parenteral doses treatment can be switched over to the oral form.

Forty-eight hours after the start of the methotrexate infusion, the residual methotrexate level should be measured. If the residual methotrexate-level > 0.5 μmol/l, calcium folinate dosages should be adapted according to the following table:

Residual methotrexate blood level 48 hours after the start of the methotrexate administration. Additional calcium folinate to be administered every six hours for 48 hours

μ 0.5 μmol/l 15 mg/m^2

μ 1.0 μmol/l 100 mg/m^2

μ 2.0 μmol/l 200 mg/m^2

Colorectal cancer

The doses and the dosing schedule of 5-Fluorouracil and calcium folinate vary between regimens.

Thefollowing regimens have been used in adults:

High dose regimen:

Calcium folinate is administered at 200 mg/m^2 by slow intravenous injection over a minimum of three minutes, followed by 5-fluorouracil at 370 mg/m^2 by intravenous injection.

Low dose regimen:

Calcium folinate is administered at 20 mg/m^2 by intravenous injection followed by 5-fluorouracil at 425 mg/m^2 by intravenous injection.

5-Fluorouracil and calcium folinate should be administered separately to avoid the formation of a precipitate.

Treatment is repeated daily for five days. This five-day treatment course may be repeated at 4 week (28 day) intervals, for two courses and then repeated at 4-5 weeks (28-35 day) intervals provided that the patient has completely recovered from the toxic effects of the prior treatment course. In subsequent treatment courses, the dosage of 5-Fluorouracil should be adjusted based on patient tolerance of the prior treatment course. (Please refer to the SPC of 5-Fluorouracil for dosage adjustments of 5-Fluorouracil in case of any toxicity.)

4.3 Contraindications
Hypersensitivity to one of the ingredients of the drug product.

Pernicious anaemia and other megaloblastic anaemias (since there is only haematological remission) and other anaemias due to vitamin B_{12} deficiency.

4.4 Special warnings and special precautions for use
Profound knowledge in this specific field of antineoplastic chemotherapy and the facilities necessary to take control and safety measures are obligatory.

Resistance to methotrexate as a result of decreased membrane transport implies also resistance to folinic acid rescue as both drugs share the same transport system.

Excessive calcium folinate doses must be avoided since this might impair the antitumour activity of methotrexate, especially in CNS tumours where calcium folinate accumulates after repeated courses.

For reduction of methotrexate toxicity is referred the Summary of Products Characteristics for methotrexate.

The use of folic acid or calcium folinate in megaloblastic anaemia due to vitamin B_{12} deficiency (e.g. pernicious anaemia) may lead to haematological remission along with progression of the underlying disease or neurological deficits.

Many cytotoxic drugs – direct or indirect DNA synthesis inhibitors – lead to a macrocytosis (hydroxycarbamide, cytarabine, mecaptourine, thioguanine). Such a macrocytosis is not considered to be treated by folinic acid.

Calcium folinate has no effect on non-haematological toxicities of methotrexate such as the nephrotoxicity resulting from drug and/or metabolite precipitation in the kidney.

Because of the high calcium concentration, intravenous administration of calcium folinate should not exceed 160 mg/minute.

In combination regimen with 5-fluorouracil, the toxicity risk of 5-flourouracil is increased by calcium folinate, particularly in elderly or debilitated patients. The most common manifestations are leucopenia, mucositis, and/or diarrhoea which may be dose limiting. When calcium folinate and 5-flourouracil are used in the treatment of colorectal cancer, the 5-flourouracil dosage has to be reduced more in cases of toxicity than when 5-flourouracil is used alone. The toxicities observed in patients treated with the combination therapy are qualitatively similar to those observed in patients treated with 5- fluorouracil monotherapy. Gastrointestinal toxicity symptoms are more commonly and may be more severe and even life threatening. In severe cases the combination calcium folinate and 5-flourouracil must be withdrawn.

4.5 Interaction with other medicinal products and other forms of Interaction
When calcium folinate is given in conjunction with a folic acid antagonist (e.g. co-trimoxazole, pyrimethamine) the efficacy of the folic acid antagonist may either be reduced or completely neutralised.

Calcium folinate may diminish the effect of the antiepileptic substances phenobarbital, primidone and phenytoin, succinimides, and may increase the frequency of seizures. (A decrease of plasma levels of enzymatic-inductor anticonvulsant drugs may be observed because the hepatic metabolism is increased as folates are one of the cofactors)

Concomitant administration of calcium folinate with 5-fluorouracil has been shown to enhance the efficacy and toxicity of 5-fluorouracil.

4.6 Pregnancy and lactation

No formal animal reproductive toxicity studies have been conducted with calcium folinate, but indirect evidence from other studies suggests that it does not harm the foetus. No adequate or well-controlled studies have been conducted in pregnant women. Calcium folinate should only be used during pregnancy when the potential benefit to the mother outweighs any potential risk to the foetus.

It is not known whether calcium folinate is excreted in breast milk. Calcium folinate should be prescribed to breast-feeding mothers only when clearly needed.

4.7 Effects on ability to drive and use machines

No data available. However, an effect is not to be expected.

4.8 Undesirable effects

Very rarely allergic reactions.

Fever has been observed after administration of calcium folinate as solution for injection.

After high doses rarely gastrointestinal disorders, insomnia, excitation, depression.

4.9 Overdose

Concerning impaired methotrexate efficacy is referred to 4.4.

Should overdosage of the combination of 5-flourouracil with calcium folinate occur, follow the overdosages instructions for 5-flourouracil.

5. PHARMACOLOGICAL PROPERTIES

5.1 Pharmacodynamic properties

Pharmacotherapeutic group: Detoxifying agents for antineoplastic treatment, ATC-Code: V03A F03.

Folinic acid (5-formyl-tetrahydrofolic acid) (anti-anaemic) is the active form of folic acid, a nutritional factor essential for the human organism. It is involved in various metabolic processes, e.g. purine synthesis, pyrimidine nucleotide synthesis and amino acid metabolism.

Methotrexate competitively inhibits dihydrofolate reductase and thereby prevents the formation of reduced folates in the cell. As a consequence, it inhibits DNA, RNA and protein synthesis.

The folinic acid released from calcium folinate is rapidly converted into the active 5-methyl-tetrahydrofolic acid (calcium folinate rescue). Unlike folic acid, folinic acid (leucovorin) does not require a reduction by dihydrofolate reductase. Therefore, dihydrofolate reductase blockers have no effect on folinic acid.

The effect of methotrexate primarily depends on the rate of cell division and therefore it exerts its cytostatic effect on all rapidly growing tissues, i.e. in addition to tumour tissue also on other rapidly proliferating tissues (skin and mucosa, hematopoietic bone marrow, gonads). These vital tissues and organs can be protected from the cellular toxicity of methotrexate by calcium folinate (N^3- formyl –THF–folinic acid–citrovorum factor).

5.2 Pharmacokinetic properties

The major metabolic product of calcium folinate is 5-methyl-tetrahydrofolic acid, which is predominantly produced in the liver and intestinal mucosa.

The half-life of the active metabolites is about 6 hours (after intravenous and intramuscular administration).

The bioavailability of oral calcium folinate declines with increasing dosage due to saturation of folate absorption.

Excretion: 80-90 % with the urine (5-and 10-formyl-tetrahydrofolates inactive metabolites), 5-8% with the faeces.

5.3 Preclinical safety data

Conventional studies of safety pharmacology, repeated dose toxicity, genotoxicity, carcinogenic potential and toxicity to reproduction have not been conducted with calcium folinate. There is extensive clinical experience, however, and anything of relevance to the prescriber is included in other sections of the SPC.

6. PHARMACEUTICAL PARTICULARS

6.1 List of excipients

Water for injections

Sodium chloride

6.2 Incompatibilities

Calcium folinate solutions should not be mixed with infusion solutions containing hydrogen carbonate because of their chemical instability.

6.3 Shelf life

Unopened – 24 months.

The chemical and physical in-use stability of the solution diluted with Sodium Chloride 0.9% or Glucose 5% Intravenous Infusion has been demonstrated for 24 hours at a temperature not exceeding 25°C. From a microbiological point of view, the product should be used immediately. If not used immediately, in-use storage times and conditions prior to use are the responsibility of the user and would normally not be longer than 24 hours at 2 to 8°C, unless dilution has taken place in controlled and validated aseptic conditions.

6.4 Special precautions for storage

Store at 2°C- 8°C. Keep container in the outer carton.

6.5 Nature and contents of container

Amber vials of hydrolytic type I glass, packed in a carton.

Vials are closed with a rubber stopper with an aluminium crimp cap with flip-off.

Packs of 1 vial containing 100mg/10ml of calcium folinate

Packs of 1 vial containing 200mg/20ml of calcium folinate.

Packs of 1 vial containing 300mg/30ml of calcium folinate.

Packs of 1 vial containing 350mg/35ml of calcium folinate.

Packs of 1 vial containing 800mg/80ml of calcium folinate

6.6 Instructions for use and handling

The product is for single use only.

Solutions should only be used if clear and particle free.

Any unused product or waste material should be disposed of in accordance with local requirements.

Calcium folinate for infusion may be prepared by dilution with Sodium Chloride 0.9% or Glucose 5% Intravenous Infusion. The concentration of calcium folinate solutions, diluted with Glucose 5% Intravenous Infusion should not be less than 0.2 mg/ml (0.02% w/v).

7. MARKETING AUTHORISATION HOLDER

CP Pharmaceuticals Ltd

Ash Road North

Wrexham LL13 9UF

United Kingdom

8. MARKETING AUTHORISATION NUMBER(S)

PL 4543/0435

9. DATE OF FIRST AUTHORISATION/RENEWAL OF THE AUTHORISATION

16 May 2001

10. DATE OF REVISION OF THE TEXT

Calcium Leucovorin Powder for Injection

(Wyeth Pharmaceuticals)

1. NAME OF THE MEDICINAL PRODUCT

Calcium Leucovorin 30mg/vial Powder for solution for injection or infusion

2. QUALITATIVE AND QUANTITATIVE COMPOSITION

Each vial of powder contains 30mg of folinic acid provided as calcium folinate. After reconstitution with 3ml of Water for Injection, the concentration is 10mg/ml.

For excipients, see 6.1.

3. PHARMACEUTICAL FORM

Powder for Solution for Injection or Infusion

Pale yellow, fluffy powder or caked lumps

4. CLINICAL PARTICULARS

4.1 Therapeutic indications

Calcium folinate is indicated

- to diminish the toxicity and counteract the action of folic acid antagonists such as methotrexate in cytotoxic therapy and overdose in adults and children. In cytotoxic therapy, this procedure is commonly known as "Calcium Folinate Rescue"

- in combination with 5-fluorouracil in cytotoxic therapy.

4.2 Posology and method of administration

For intravenous and intramuscular administration only. In the case of intravenous administration, no more than 160 mg of calcium folinate should be injected per minute due to the calcium content of the solution.

For intravenous infusion, calcium folinate may be diluted with 0.9% sodium chloride solution or 5% glucose solution before use. Refer also to sections 6.3 and 6.6.

Calcium folinate rescue in methotrexate therapy:

Since the calcium folinate rescue dosage regimen depends heavily on the posology and method of the intermediate- or high-dose methotrexate administration, the methotrexate protocol will dictate the dosage regimen of calcium folinate rescue. Therefore, it is best to refer to the applied intermediate or high dose methotrexate protocol for posology and method of administration of calcium folinate.

The following guidelines may serve as an illustration of regimens used in adults, elderly and children:

Calcium folinate rescue has to be performed by parenteral administration in patients with malabsorption syndromes or other gastrointestinal disorders where enteral absorption is not assured. Dosages above 25-50 mg should be given parenterally due to saturable enteral absorption of calcium folinate.

Calcium folinate rescue is necessary when methotrexate is given at doses exceeding 500 mg/m^2 body surface and should be considered with doses of 100 mg – 500 mg/m^2 body surface.

Dosage and duration of calcium folinate rescue primarily depend on the type and dosage of methotrexate therapy, the occurrence of toxicity symptoms, and the individual excretion capacity for methotrexate. As a rule, the first dose of calcium folinate is 15 mg (6-12 mg/m^2) to be given 12-24 hours (24 hours at the latest) after the beginning of methotrexate infusion. The same dose is given every 6 hours throughout a period of 72 hours. After several parenteral doses treatment can be switched over to the oral form.

In addition to calcium folinate administration, measures to ensure the prompt excretion of methotrexate (maintenance of high urine output and alkalinisation of urine) are integral parts of the calcium folinate rescue treatment. Renal function should be monitored through daily measurements of serum creatinine.

Forty-eight hours after the start of the methotrexate infusion, the residual methotrexate-level should be measured. If the residual methotrexate-level is >0.5 μmol/l, calcium folinate dosages should be adapted according to the following table:

Residual methotrexate blood level 48 hours after the start of the methotrexate administration:	Additional calcium folinate to be administered every 6 hours for 48 hours or until levels of methotrexate are lower than 0.05 μmol/l:
≥ 0.5 μmol/l	15 mg/m^2
≥ 1.0 μmol/l	100 mg/m^2
≥ 2.0 μmol/l	200 mg/m^2

In combination with 5-fluorouracil in cytotoxic therapy:

Different regimens and different dosages are used, without any dosage having been proven to be the optimal one.

The following regimens have been used in adults and elderly in the treatment of advanced or metastatic colorectal cancer and are given as examples. There are no data on the use of these combinations in children:

Bimonthly regimen: Calcium folinate 200 mg/m^2 by intravenous infusion over two hours, followed by bolus 400 mg/m^2 of 5-FU and 22-hour infusion of 5-FU (600 mg/m^2) for 2 consecutive days, every 2 weeks on days 1 and 2.

Weekly regimen: Calcium folinate 20 mg/m^2 by bolus i.v. injection or 200 to 500 mg/m^2 as i.v. infusion over a period of 2 hours plus 500 mg/m^2 5-fluorouracil as i.v. bolus injection in the middle or at the end of the calcium folinate infusion.

Monthly regimen: Calcium folinate 20 mg/m^2 by bolus i.v. injection or 200 to 500 mg/m^2 as i.v. infusion over a period of 2 hours immediately followed by 425 or 370 mg/m^2 5-fluorouracil as i.v. bolus injection during five consecutive days.

For the combination therapy with 5-fluorouracil, modification of the 5-fluorouracil dosage and the treatment-free interval may be necessary depending on patient condition, clinical response and dose limiting toxicity as stated in the product information of 5-fluorouracil. A reduction of calcium folinate dosage is not required.

The number of repeat cycles used is at the discretion of the clinician.

Antidote to the folic acid antagonists trimetrexate, trimethoprime, and pyrimethamine:

Trimetrexate toxicity:

• Prevention: Calcium folinate should be administered every day during treatment with trimetrexate and for 72 hours after the last dose of trimetrexate. Calcium folinate can be administered either by the intravenous route at a dose of 20 mg/m^2 for 5 to 10 minutes every 6 hours for a total daily dose of 80 mg/m^2, or by oral route with four doses of 20 mg/m^2 administered at equal time intervals. Daily doses of calcium folinate should be adjusted depending on the haematological toxicity of trimetrexate.

• Overdosage (possibly occurring with trimetrexate doses above 90 mg/m^2 without concomitant administration of calcium folinate): after stopping trimetrexate, calcium folinate 40 mg/m^2 IV every 6 hours for 3 days.

Trimethoprime toxicity:

• After stopping trimethoprime, 3-10 mg/day calcium folinate until recovery of a normal blood count.

Pyrimethamine toxicity:

• In case of high dose pyrimethamine or prolonged treatment with low doses, calcium folinate 5 to 50 mg/day should be simultaneously administered, based on the results of the peripheral blood counts.

4.3 Contraindications

• Known hypersensitivity to calcium folinate, or to any of the excipients.

• Pernicious anaemia or other anaemias due to vitamin B_{12} deficiency.

Regarding the use of calcium folinate with methotrexate or 5-fluorouracil during pregnancy and lactation, see section

4.6, "Pregnancy and Lactation" and the summaries of product characteristics for methotrexate- and 5-fluorouracil- containing medicinal products".

4.4 Special warnings and special precautions for use

Calcium folinate should only be given by intramuscular or intravenous injection and must not be administered intrathecally. When folinic acid has been administered intrathecally following intrathecal overdose of methotrexate death has been reported.

General

Calcium folinate should be used with methotrexate or 5-fluorouracil only under the direct supervision of a clinician experienced in the use of cancer chemotherapeutic agents.

Calcium folinate treatment may mask pernicious anaemia and other anaemias resulting from vitamin B_{12} deficiency.

Many cytotoxic medicinal products – direct or indirect DNA synthesis inhibitors – lead to macrocytosis (hydroxycarbamide, cytarabine, mecaptopurine, thioguanine). Such macrocytosis should not be treated with folinic acid.

In epileptic patients treated with phenobarbital, phenytoine, primidone, and succinimides there is a risk to increase the frequency of seizures due to a decrease of plasma concentrations of anti-epileptic drugs. Clinical monitoring, possibly monitoring of the plasma concentrations and, if necessary, dose adaptation of the anti-epileptic drug during calcium folinate administration and after discontinuation is recommended (see also section 4.5 Interactions).

Calcium folinate/5-fluorouracil

Calcium folinate may enhance the toxicity risk of 5-fluorouracil, particularly in elderly or debilitated patients. The most common manifestations are leucopenia, mucositis, stomatitis and/or diarrhoea, which may be dose limiting. When calcium folinate and 5-fluorouracil are used in combination, the 5-fluorouracil dosage has to be reduced more in cases of toxicity than when 5-fluorouracil is used alone.

Combined 5-fluorouracil/calcium folinate treatment should neither be initiated nor maintained in patients with symptoms of gastrointestinal toxicity, regardless of the severity, until all of these symptoms have completely disappeared.

Because diarrhoea may be a sign of gastrointestinal toxicity, patients presenting with diarrhoea must be carefully monitored until the symptoms have disappeared completely, since a rapid clinical deterioration leading to death can occur. If diarrhoea and/or stomatitis occur, it is advisable to reduce the dose of 5-FU until symptoms have fully disappeared. Especially the elderly and patients with a low physical performance due to their illness are prone to these toxicities. Therefore, particular care should be taken when treating these patients.

In elderly patients and patients who have undergone preliminary radiotherapy, it is recommended to begin with a reduced dosage of 5-fluorouracil.

Calcium folinate must not be mixed with 5-fluorouracil in the same IV injection or infusion.

Calcium levels should be monitored in patients receiving combined 5-fluorouracil/calcium folinate treatment and calcium supplementation should be provided if calcium levels are low.

Calcium folinate/methotrexate

For specific details on reduction of methotrexate toxicity refer to the SPC of methotrexate.

Calcium folinate has no effect on non-haematological toxicities of methotrexate such as the nephrotoxicity resulting from methotrexate and/or metabolite precipitation in the kidney. Patients who experience delayed early methotrexate elimination are likely to develop reversible renal failure and all toxicities associated with methotrexate (please refer to the SPC for methotrexate). The presence of pre-existing- or methotrexate-induced renal insufficiency is potentially associated with delayed excretion of methotrexate and may increase the need for higher doses or more prolonged use of calcium folinate.

Excessive calcium folinate doses must be avoided since this might impair the antitumour activity of methotrexate, especially in CNS tumours where calcium folinate accumulates after repeated courses.

Resistance to methotrexate as a result of decreased membrane transport implies also resistance to folinic acid rescue as both medicinal products share the same transport system.

An accidental overdose with a folate antagonist, such as methotrexate, should be treated as a medical emergency. As the time interval between methotrexate administration and calcium folinate rescue increases, calcium folinate effectiveness in counteracting toxicity decreases.

The possibility that the patient is taking other medications that interact with methotrexate (eg, medications which may interfere with methotrexate elimination or binding to serum albumin) should always be considered when laboratory abnormalities or clinical toxicities are observed.

4.5 Interaction with other medicinal products and other forms of Interaction

When calcium folinate is given in conjunction with a folic acid antagonist (e.g. cotrimoxazole, pyrimethamine) the efficacy of the folic acid antagonist may either be reduced or completely neutralised.

Calcium folinate may diminish the effect of anti-epileptic substances: phenobarbital, primidone, phenytoine and succinimides, and may increase the frequency of seizures (a decrease of plasma levels of enzymatic inductor anticonvulsant drugs may be observed because the hepatic metabolism is increased as folates are one of the cofactors) (see also sections 4.4 and 4.8).

Concomitant administration of calcium folinate with 5-fluorouracil has been shown to enhance the efficacy and toxicity of 5-fluorouracil (see sections 4.2, 4.4 and 4.8).

4.6 Pregnancy and lactation

Pregnancy

There are no adequate and well-controlled clinical studies conducted in pregnant or breast-feeding women. No formal animal reproductive toxicity studies with calcium folinate have been conducted. There are no indications that folic acid induces harmful effects if administered during pregnancy.

During pregnancy, methotrexate should only be administered on strict indications, where the benefits of the drug to the mother should be weighed against possible hazards to the foetus. Should treatment with methotrexate or other folate antagonists take place despite pregnancy or lactation, there are no limitations as to the use of calcium folinate to diminish toxicity or counteract the effects.

5-fluorouracil use is generally contraindicated during pregnancy and contraindicated during breast-feeding; this applies also to the combined use of calcium folinate with 5-fluorouracil.

Please refer also to the summaries of product characteristics for methotrexate-, other folate antagonists and 5-fluorouracil- containing medicinal products.

Lactation

It is not known whether calcium folinate is excreted into human breast milk. Calcium folinate can be used during breast feeding when considered necessary according to the therapeutic indications.

4.7 Effects on ability to drive and use machines

There is no evidence that calcium folinate has an effect on the ability to drive or use machines.

4.8 Undesirable effects

Both therapeutic indications:

Immune system disorders

Very rare (<0.01%): allergic reactions, including anaphylactoid reactions and urticaria.

Psychiatric disorders

Rare (0.01-0.1%): insomnia, agitation and depression after high doses.

Gastrointestinal disorders

Rare (0.01-0.1%): gastrointestinal disorders after high doses.

Neurological disorders

Rare (0.01-0.1%): increase in the frequency of attacks in epileptics (see also section 4.5 Interactions.).

General disorders and administration site conditions

Uncommon (0.1-1%): fever has been observed after administration of calcium folinate as solution for injection.

Combination therapy with 5-fluorouracil:

Generally, the safety profile depends on the applied regimen of 5-fluorouracil due to enhancement of the 5-fluorouracil induced toxicities:

Monthly regimen:

Gastrointestinal disorders

Very common (>10%): vomiting and nausea

General disorders and administration site conditions

Very common (>10%): (severe) mucosal toxicity.

No enhancement of other 5-fluorouracil induced toxicities (e.g. neurotoxicity).

Weekly regimen:

Gastrointestinal disorders

Very common (>10%): diarrhoea with higher grades of toxicity, and dehydration, resulting in hospital admission for treatment and even death.

4.9 Overdose

There have been no reported sequelae in patients who have received significantly more calcium folinate than the recommended dosage. However, excessive amounts of calcium folinate may nullify the chemotherapeutic effect of folic acid antagonists.

Should overdosage of the combination of 5-fluorouracil and calcium folinate occur, the overdosage instructions for 5-FU should be followed.

5. PHARMACOLOGICAL PROPERTIES

5.1 Pharmacodynamic properties

Pharmacotherapeutic group: Detoxifying agents for antineoplastic treatment; ATC code: V03AF03

Calcium folinate is the calcium salt of 5-formyl tetrahydrofolic acid. It is an active metabolite of folinic acid and an essential coenzyme for nucleic acid synthesis in cytotoxic therapy.

Calcium folinate is frequently used to diminish the toxicity and counteract the action of folate antagonists, such as methotrexate. Calcium folinate and folate antagonists share the same membrane transport carrier and compete for transport into cells, stimulating folate antagonist efflux. It also protects cells from the effects of folate antagonist by repletion of the reduce folate pool. Calcium folinate serves as a pre-reduced source of H4 folate; it can therefore bypass folate antagonist blockage and provide a source for the various coenzyme forms of folic acid.

Calcium folinate is also frequently used in the biochemical modulation of fluoropyridine (5-FU) to enhance its cytotoxic activity. 5-FU inhibits thymidylate synthase (TS), a key enzyme involved in pyrimidine biosynthesis, and calcium folinate enhances TS inhibition by increasing the intracellular folate pool, thus stabilising the 5FU-TS complex and increasing activity.

Finally intravenous calcium folinate can be administered for the prevention and treatment of folate deficiency when it cannot be prevented or corrected by the administration of folic acid by the oral route. This may be the case during total parenteral nutrition and severe malabsorption disorders. It is also indicated for the treatment of megaloblastic anaemia due to folic acid deficiency, when oral administration is not feasible.

5.2 Pharmacokinetic properties

Absorption

Following intramuscular administration of the aqueous solution, systemic availability is comparable to an intravenous administration. However, lower peak serum levels (C_{max}) are achieved.

Metabolism

Calcium folinate is a racemate where the L-form (L-5-formyl-tetrahydrofolate, L-5-formyl-THF), is the active enantiomer.

The major metabolic product of folinic acid is 5-methyl-tetrahydrofolic acid (5-methyl-THF) which is predominantly produced in the liver and intestinal mucosa.

Distribution

The distribution volume of folinic acid is not known.

Peak serum levels of the parent substance (D/L-5-formyl-tetrahydrofolic acid, folinic acid) are reached 10 minutes after i.v. administration.

AUC for L-5-formyl-THF and 5-methyl-THF were 28.4±3.5 mg.min/l and 129±112 mg.min/l after a dose of 25 mg. The inactive D-isomer is present in higher concentration than L-5-formyl-tetrahydrofolate.

Elimination

The elimination half-life is 32 - 35 minutes for the active L-form and 352 - 485 minutes for the inactive D-form, respectively.

The total terminal half-life of the active metabolites is about 6 hours (after intravenous and intramuscular administration).

Excretion

80-90 % with the urine (5- and 10-formyl-tetrahydrofolates inactive metabolites), 5-8 % with the faeces.

5.3 Preclinical safety data

There are no preclinical data considered relevant to clinical safety beyond data included in other sections of the SPC.

6. PHARMACEUTICAL PARTICULARS

6.1 List of excipients

Sodium Chloride

Hydrochloric Acid

Sodium Hydroxide

6.2 Incompatibilities

Incompatibilities have been reported between injectable forms of calcium folinate and injectable forms of droperidol, fluorouracil, foscarnet and methotrexate.

Droperidol

1. Droperidol 1.25 mg/0.5 ml with calcium folinate 5 mg/0.5 ml, immediate precipitation in direct admixture in syringe for 5 minutes at 25° C followed by 8 minutes of centrifugation.

2. Droperidol 2.5 mg/0.5 ml with calcium folinate 10 mg/0.5 ml, immediate precipitation when the drugs were injected sequentially into a Y-site without flushing the Y-side arm between injections.

Fluorouracil

Calcium folinate must not be mixed in the same infusion as 5-fluorouracil because a precipitate may form. Fluorouracil 50 mg/ml with calcium folinate 20 mg/ml, with or without dextrose 5% in water, has been shown to be incompatible when mixed in different amounts and stored at 4° C, 23° C, or 32° C in polyvinyl chloride containers.

Foscarnet

Foscarnet 24 mg/ml with calcium folinate 20 mg/ml formation of a cloudy yellow solution reported.

6.3 Shelf life

36 months

6.4 Special precautions for storage

Do not store above 25°C. Do not refrigerate.

Chemical and physical in-use stability has been demonstrated for 24 hours at 2-8°C.

From a microbiological point of view, the product should be used immediately. If not used immediately, in-use storage times and conditions prior to use are the responsibility of the user and would normally not be longer than 24 hours at 2-8°C, unless reconstitution has taken place in controlled and validated aseptic conditions.

6.5 Nature and contents of container
Type I glass vials with a sterile rubber stopper sealed with a metal ring containing 30mg.

6.6 Instructions for use and handling
Prior to administration, calcium folinate should be inspected visually. The solution for injection or infusion should be a clear and yellowish solution. If cloudy in appearance or particles are observed, the solution should be discarded. Calcium folinate solution for injection or infusion is intended only for single use. Any unused portion of the solution should be disposed of in accordance with the local requirements.

7. MARKETING AUTHORISATION HOLDER
Cyanamid of Great Britain Limited
Fareham Road
Gosport
Hampshire PO13 0AS
UK

8. MARKETING AUTHORISATION NUMBER(S)
PL 0095/0087

9. DATE OF FIRST AUTHORISATION/RENEWAL OF THE AUTHORISATION
7 December 1981

10. DATE OF REVISION OF THE TEXT
January 2004

Calcium Leucovorin Tablets 15mg

(Wyeth Pharmaceuticals)

1. NAME OF THE MEDICINAL PRODUCT
Calcium Leucovorin Tablets 15mg

2. QUALITATIVE AND QUANTITATIVE COMPOSITION
Each tablet contains calcium folinate (calcium leucovorin) equivalent to 15mg folinic acid (leucovorin).
Excipients: See 6.1.

3. PHARMACEUTICAL FORM
Tablet
Yellowish white, circular, biconvex, scored tablets.

4. CLINICAL PARTICULARS
4.1 Therapeutic indications
Calcium Leucovorin Rescue
Calcium Leucovorin is used to diminish the toxicity and counteract the action of folic acid antagonists such as methotrexate in cytotoxic therapy. This procedure is commonly known as Calcium Leucovorin Rescue.
Treatment of Folate Deficiency
Calcium Leucovorin has also been demonstrated to be effective in producing amelioration of the blood picture in a number of megaloblastic anaemias due to folate deficiency.

4.2 Posology and method of administration
Method of administration:
Oral administration
Dosage: Adults, Children and the Elderly
Calcium Leucovorin Rescue
Calcium Leucovorin Rescue therapy should commence 24 hours after the beginning of methotrexate infusion. Dosage regimes vary depending upon the dose of methotrexate administered. In general, the Calcium Leucovorin should be administered at a dose of 15mg (approximately 10mg/m^2) every 6 hours for 10 doses, either parenterally by intramuscular injection, bolus intravenous injection or intravenous infusion or orally using Calcium Leucovorin tablets. Do not administer Calcium Leucovorin intrathecally.
Where overdosage of methotrexate is suspected, the dose of Calcium Leucovorin should be equal to or higher than the offending dose of methotrexate and should be administered in the first hour. In the presence of gastrointestinal toxicity, nausea or vomiting, Calcium Leucovorin should be administered parenterally. Do not administer Calcium Leucovorin intrathecally. Further, oral administration of doses greater than 50mg is not recommended since the absorption of Calcium Leucovoin is saturable. In the case of intravenous administration, no more than 160mg of Calcium Leucovorin should be injected per minute due to the calcium content of the solution.
In addition to Calcium Leucovorin administration, measures to ensure the prompt excretion of methotrexate are important as part of Calcium Leucovorin Rescue Therapy. These measures include:
a) Alkalinisation of urine so that the urinary pH is greater than 7.0 before methotrexate infusion (to increase solubility of methotrexate and its metabolites).
b) Maintenance of urine output of 1800-2000 cc/m^2/24hr by increased oral or intravenous fluids on days 2,3 and 4 following methotrexate therapy.
c) Plasma methotrexate concentration, BUN and creatinine should be measured on days 2,3 and 4.
These measures must be continued until the plasma methotrexate level is less than 10^{-7} molar (0.1μM).
Delayed methotrexate excretion may be seen in some patients. This may be caused by a third space accumulation (as seen in ascites or pleural effusion for example), renal insufficiency of inadequate hydration. Under such circumstances, higher doses of Calcium Leucovorin or prolonged administration may be indicated. Dosage and administration guidelines for these patients are given in Table 1. Patients who experience delayed early methotrexate elimination are likely to develop reversible renal failure.
Table 1: Dosage and Administration Guidelines for Calcium Leucovorin Rescue

Clinical Situation	Laboratory Findings	Leucovorin Dosage and Duration
Normal methotrexate elimination	Serum methotrexate level approx. 10μM 24 hours after administration, 1μM at 48 hours and less than 0.2μM at 72 hours.	15mg, PO, IM or IV every 6 hours for 60 hours (10 doses starting at 24 hours after start of methotrexate infusion).
Delayed late methotrexate elimination	Serum methotrexate level remaining above 0.2μM at 72 hours and more than 0.05μM at 96 hours after administration.	Continue 15mg PO, IM or IV every 6 hours, until methotrexate level is less than 0.05μM.
Delayed early methotrexate elimination and / or evidence of acute renal injury	Serum methotrexate level of 50μM or more at 24 hours or 5μM or more at 48 hours after administration, OR; a 100% or greater increase in serum creatinine level at 24 hours after methotrexate administration.	150mg IV every 3 hours until methotrexate level is less than 1 micromolar; then 15mg IV every 3 hours until methotrexate level is less than 0.05μM.

Treatment of Folate Deficiency

Children up to 12 years:	0.25mg/kg/day
Adults and the elderly:	10-20mg daily. Oral therapy with one tablet (15mg) of Calcium Leucovorin daily is more usual.

4.3 Contraindications
Calcium Leucovorin should not be used for the treatment of pernicious anaemia or other megaloblastic anaemias where Vitamin B_{12} is deficient.

4.4 Special warnings and special precautions for use
Calcium Leucovorin should only be used with methotrexate or 5-FU under the direct supervision of a clinician experienced in the use of cancer chemotherapeutic agents.
When Calcium Leucovorin has been administered intrathecally following intrathecal overdose of methotrexate, a death has been reported.
Seizures and/or syncope have been reported rarely in cancer patients receiving leucovorin, usually in association with fluoropyrimidine administration and most commonly in those with CNS metastases or other predisposing factors; however a causal relationship has not been established.
Patients with rare hereditary problems of galactose intolerance, the Lapp lactase deficiency or glucose-galactose malabsorption should not take this medicine, as one of the excipients in the tablets is lactose.

4.5 Interaction with other medicinal products and other forms of Interaction
Calcium Leucovorin should not be given simultaneously with an anti-neoplastic folic acid antagonist, e.g. methotrexate, to modify or abort clinical toxicity, as the therapeutic effect of the antagonist may be nullified. Concomitant Calcium Leucovorin will not inhibit the antibacterial activity of other folic acid antagonists such as trimethoprim and pyrimethamine.
Folinates given in large amounts may counteract the antiepileptic effect of phenobarbitone, phenytoin and primidone and increase the frequency of seizures in susceptible patients.

4.6 Pregnancy and lactation
Reproduction studies have been performed in rats and rabbits at doses of at least 50 times the human dose. These studies have revealed no evidence of harm to the foetus due to Calcium Leucovorin. There are, however, no adequate and well-controlled studies in pregnant women, because animal studies are not always predictive of human response. Calcium Leucovorin should only be used in pregnant women if the potential benefit justifies the potential risk to the foetus.
It is not known whether Calcium Leucovorin is excreted in human milk. As many drugs are excreted in human milk, caution should be exercised when Calcium Leucovorin is administered to a nursing mother.

4.7 Effects on ability to drive and use machines
None.

4.8 Undesirable effects
Adverse reactions to Calcium Leucovorin are rare, but occasional pyrexial reactions have been reported following parenteral administration.
Hypersensitivity, including anaphylactoid/anaphylactic reactions (including shock) and urticaria, has been reported following administration of both oral and parenteral leucovorin.

4.9 Overdose
There have been no reported sequelae in patients who have received significantly more Calcium Leucovorin than the recommended dosage. There is no specific antidote. In cases of overdosage, patients should be given appropriate supportive care. Should overdosage of the combination of 5-FU with Calcium Leucovorin occur, the overdosage instructions for 5-FU should be followed.

5. PHARMACOLOGICAL PROPERTIES
5.1 Pharmacodynamic properties

Pharmacotherapeutic Group:	*Detoxifying agents for antineoplastic treatment*
ATC Code:	J01A A20

Calcium Leucovorin is the calcium salt of a formyl tetrahydrofolic acid, the metabolite of folic acid and an essential coenzyme for nucleic acid synthesis. Calcium Leucovorin is used therefore to diminish the toxicity and counteract the action of folic acid antagonists such as methotrexate in cytotoxic therapy (Calcium Leucovorin Rescue).
Calcium Leucovorin is also effective in the treatment of megaloblastic anaemia.

5.2 Pharmacokinetic properties
Folinic acid is effectively absorbed when given by mouth and produces peak concentrations of folate in the serum after about 1 hour.

5.3 Preclinical safety data
Nothing of relevance to the prescriber.

6. PHARMACEUTICAL PARTICULARS
6.1 List of excipients
Lactose
Microcrystalline cellulose
Sodium starch glycollate
Pre-gelatinised maize starch
Magnesium stearate

6.2 Incompatibilities
None.

6.3 Shelf life
60 Months

6.4 Special precautions for storage
Do not store above 25°C. Do not refrigerate.

6.5 Nature and contents of container
Screw capped glass bottles or polypropylene bottles with plastic screw-on caps containing 10 tablets.

6.6 Instructions for use and handling
Not applicable

7. MARKETING AUTHORISATION HOLDER
Cyanamid of Great Britain
Fareham Rd
Gosport
Hants PO13 0AS
UK

8. MARKETING AUTHORISATION NUMBER(S)
PL 0095/0033

9. DATE OF FIRST AUTHORISATION/RENEWAL OF THE AUTHORISATION
24 May 2003

10. DATE OF REVISION OF THE TEXT
31 March 2004

Calcium Resonium

(sanofi-aventis)

1. NAME OF THE MEDICINAL PRODUCT
Calcium Resonium

2. QUALITATIVE AND QUANTITATIVE COMPOSITION
Contains Calcium Polystyrene Sulphonate 99.934% w/w

3. PHARMACEUTICAL FORM
An ion-exchange resin presented as a powder.

4. CLINICAL PARTICULARS

4.1 Therapeutic indications
Calcium Resonium is an ion-exchange resin that is recommended for the treatment of hyperkalaemia associated with anuria or severe oliguria. It is also used to treat hyperkalaemia in patients requiring dialysis and in patients on regular haemodialysis or on prolonged peritoneal dialysis.

4.2 Posology and method of administration
Calcium Resonium is to be taken either orally or rectally.

The dosage recommendations detailed below are a guide only; the precise requirements should be decided on the basis of regular serum electrolyte determinations.

Adults, including the elderly:

Oral
Usual dose 15g, three to four times a day. The resin is given by mouth in a little water, or it may be made into a paste with some sweetened vehicle.

Rectal
In cases where vomiting may make oral administration difficult, the resin may be given rectally as a suspension of 30g resin in 100ml 2% methylcellulose 450BP (medium viscosity) and 100ml water, as a daily retention enema. In the initial stages administration by this route as well as orally may help to achieve a rapid lowering of the serum potassium level.

The enema should if possible be retained for a least nine hours, then the colon should be irrigated to remove the resin. If both routes are used initially it is probably unnecessary to continue rectal administration once the oral resin has reached the rectum.

Children:

Oral
1g/kg body weight daily in divided doses in acute hyperkalaemia. Dosage may be reduced to 0.5g/kg body weight daily in divided doses for maintenance therapy.

The resin is given orally, preferably with a drink (not a fruit squash because of the high potassium content) or a little jam or honey.

Rectal
When refused by mouth it should be given rectally using a dose at least as great as that which would have been given orally, diluted in the same ratio as described for adults. Following retention of the enema, the colon should be irrigated to ensure adequate removal of the resin.

Neonates:

Calcium Resonium should not be given by the oral route. With rectal administration, the minimum effective dosage within the range 0.5g/kg to 1g/kg should be employed, diluted as for adults with adequate irrigation to ensure recovery of the resin.

4.3 Contraindications
- In patients with plasma potassium levels below 5mmol/litre.
- Conditions associated with hypercalcaemia (e.g. hyperparathyroidism, multiple myeloma, sarcoidosis or metastatic carcinoma).
- History of hypersensitivity to polystyrene sulphonate resins.
- Obstructive bowel disease.
- Calcium Resonium should not be administered orally to neonates and is contraindicated in neonates with reduced gut motility (post-operatively or drug-induced).

4.4 Special warnings and special precautions for use
Hypokalaemia: The possibility of severe potassium depletion should be considered and adequate clinical and biochemical control is essential during treatment, especially in patients on digitalis. Administration of the resin should be stopped when the serum potassium falls to 5mmol/litre.

Other electrolyte disturbances: Like all cation-exchange resins, calcium polystyrene sulphonate is not totally selective for potassium. Hypomagnesemia and/or hypercalcemia may occur. Accordingly, patients should be monitored for all applicable electrolyte disturbances. Serum calcium levels should be estimated at weekly intervals to detect the early development of hypercalcaemia, and the dose of resin adjusted to levels at which hypercalcaemia and hypokalaemia are prevented.

Other risks: In the event of clinically significant constipation, treatment should be discontinued until normal bowel movement has resumed. Magnesium-containing laxatives should not be used (see section 4.5 Interactions).

The patient should be positioned carefully when ingesting the resin, to avoid aspiration, which may lead to bronchopulmonary complications.

Children and neonates: In neonates, calcium polystyrene sulphonate should not be given by the oral route. In children and neonates, particular care is needed with rectal administration as excessive dosage or inadequate dilution could result in impaction of the resin. Due to the risk of digestive haemorrhage or colonic necrosis, particular care should be observed in premature infants or low birth weight infants.

4.5 Interaction with other medicinal products and other forms of Interaction

Concomitant use not recommended
Sorbitol (oral or rectal): Concomitant use of sorbitol with sodium polystyrene sulphonate may cause colonic necrosis. Therefore concomitant administration of sorbitol with calcium polystrene sulphonate is not recommended.

To be used with caution
Cation-donating agents: may reduce the potassium binding effectiveness of Calcium Resonium.

Non-absorbable cation-donating antacids and laxatives: There have been reports of systemic alkalosis following concurrent administration of cation-exchange resins and non-absorbable cation-donating antacids and laxatives such as magnesium hydroxide and aluminium carbonate.

Aluminium hydroxide: Intestinal obstruction due to concretions of aluminium hydroxide has been reported when aluminium hydroxide has been combined with the resin (sodium form).

Digitalis-like drugs: The toxic effects of digitalis on the heart, especially various ventricular arrhythmias and A-V nodal dissociation, are likely to be exaggerated if hypokalaemia and/or hypercalcaemia are allowed to develop (see 4.4 Special warnings and special precautions for use).

Lithium: Possible decrease of lithium absorption.

Levothyroxine: Possible decrease of levothyroxine absorption.

4.6 Pregnancy and lactation
No data are available regarding the use of polystyrene sulphonate resins in pregnancy and lactation. The administration of Calcium Resonium in pregnancy and during breast feeding therefore, is not advised unless, in the opinion of the physician, the potential benefits outweigh any potential risks.

4.7 Effects on ability to drive and use machines
There are no specific warnings.

4.8 Undesirable effects
In accordance with its pharmacological actions, the resin may give rise to hypokalaemia and hypercalcaemia and their related clinical manifestations (see Warnings and Precautions and Overdosage).

Hypercalcaemia has been reported in well dialysed patients receiving calcium resin, and in the occasional patient with chronic renal failure. Many patients in chronic renal failure have low serum calcium and high serum phosphate, but some, who cannot be screened out beforehand, show a sudden rise in serum calcium to high levels after therapy. The risk emphasises the need for adequate biochemical control.

- Gastrointestinal disorders

Gastric irritation, anorexia, nausea, vomiting, constipation and occasionally diarrhoea may occur. Faecal impaction following rectal administration particularly in children and gastrointestinal concretions (bezoars) following oral administration have been reported. Intestinal obstruction has also been reported although this has been extremely rare and, possibly, a reflection of co-existing pathology or inadequate dilution of resin.

Gastro-intestinal tract ulceration or necrosis which could lead to intestinal perforation have been reported following administration of sodium polystyrene sulphonate.

- **Respiratory disorders**

Some cases of acute bronchitis and/or bronchopneumonia associated with inhalation of particles of calcium polystyrene sulphonate have been described.

4.9 Overdose
Biochemical disturbances from overdosage may give rise to clinical signs of symptoms of hypokalaemia, including irritability, confusion, delayed thought processes, muscle weakness, hyporeflexia and eventual paralysis. Apnoea may be a serious consequence of this progression. Electrocardiographic changes may be consistent with hypokalaemia or hypercalcaemia; cardiac arrhythmia may occur. Appropriate measures should be taken to correct serum electrolytes and the resin should be removed from the alimentary tract by appropriate use of laxatives or enemas.

5. PHARMACOLOGICAL PROPERTIES

5.1 Pharmacodynamic properties
Ion-exchange resin

5.2 Pharmacokinetic properties
Not applicable as this product is not absorbed.

5.3 Preclinical safety data
There are no pre-clinical data of relevance to the prescriber which are additional to that already included in other sections of the SPC.

6. PHARMACEUTICAL PARTICULARS

6.1 List of excipients
Calcium Resonium also contains Vanillin and Saccharin.

6.2 Incompatibilities
There are no specific incompatibilities.

6.3 Shelf life
The shelf-life of Calcium Resonium is 5 years.

6.4 Special precautions for storage
Store in a dry place

6.5 Nature and contents of container
HDPE containers of 300g.

6.6 Instructions for use and handling
None

7. MARKETING AUTHORISATION HOLDER
Sanofi-Synthelabo
PO Box 597
Guildford
Surrey

8. MARKETING AUTHORISATION NUMBER(S)
PL 11723/0010

9. DATE OF FIRST AUTHORISATION/RENEWAL OF THE AUTHORISATION
2 April 2003

10. DATE OF REVISION OF THE TEXT
February 2005

Legal category: P

Calcium-Sandoz Syrup

(Alliance Pharmaceuticals)

1. NAME OF THE MEDICINAL PRODUCT
Calcium-Sandoz® Syrup

2. QUALITATIVE AND QUANTITATIVE COMPOSITION
Calcium glubionate 1.09g and calcium lactobionate USP 0.727g per 5ml.

3. PHARMACEUTICAL FORM
Colourless to pale straw coloured, fruit flavoured syrup.

4. CLINICAL PARTICULARS

4.1 Therapeutic indications
1. An adjunct to conventional therapy in the arrest or slowing down of bone demineralisation in osteoporosis.

2. In the arrest or slowing down of bone demineralisation in osteoporosis where other effective treatment is contra-indicated.

3. A supplemental source of calcium in the correction of dietary deficiencies or when normal requirements are high.

4. Neonatal hypocalcaemia.

4.2 Posology and method of administration
Treatment or therapeutic supplementation should aim to restore or maintain normal levels of calcium (2.25 to 2.75mmol/L or 4.5 to 5.5mEq/L).

Calcium Sandoz Syrup should be taken by mouth either as provided or after dilution with syrup BP.

Indication	Daily Dose Syrup (5ml spoonfuls)
Adults	
Osteoporosis	11-15
Therapeutic supplement (dose dependent upon severity)	3-15
Children	
Calcium deficiency	6-9
Dietary supplementation	2-6

Neonatal hypocalcaemia: Calcium-Sandoz Syrup may be given at a dose of 1mmol calcium/kg/24 hours in divided doses. Serum calcium levels should be monitored and the dosage adjusted if necessary. Doses may be mixed with the first (small) part of milk feeds. Note: 1mmol of calcium is equivalent to 1.85ml Calcium-Sandoz Syrup.

Elderly: No evidence exists that tolerance of Calcium-Sandoz is directly affected by advanced age; however, elderly patients should be supervised as factors sometimes associated with ageing, such as poor diet or impaired renal function, may indirectly affect tolerance and may require dosage reduction.

4.3 Contraindications
Hypercalcaemia (e.g., in hyperparathyroidism, vitamin D overdosage, decalcifying tumours such as plasmocytoma, severe renal failure, bone metastases), severe hypercalciuria, and renal calculi.

Due to its galactose component Calcium-Sandoz Syrup should not be given to patients with galactosaemia.

4.4 Special warnings and special precautions for use

In mild hypercalciuria (exceeding 300mg (7.5mmol)/24 hours) or renal failure, or where there is evidence of stone formation in the urinary tract, adequate checks must be kept on urinary calcium excretion; if necessary the dosage should be reduced or calcium therapy discontinued.

The sugar content of Calcium-Sandoz Syrup should be taken into account in diabetic patients.

4.5 Interaction with other medicinal products and other forms of Interaction

High vitamin D intake should be avoided during calcium therapy, unless especially indicated (see also Section 4.9, "Overdose").

Thiazide diuretics reduce urinary calcium excretion, so the risk of hypercalcaemia should be considered.

Oral calcium supplementation is aimed at restoring normal serum levels. Although it is extremely unlikely that high enough levels will be achieved to adversely affect digitalised patients, this theoretical possibility should be considered.

Oral calcium administration may reduce the absorption of oral tetracycline or fluoride preparations. An interval of 3 hours should be observed if the two are to be given.

4.6 Pregnancy and lactation

The likelihood of hypercalcaemia is increased in pregnant women in whom calcium and vitamin D are co-administered. Epidemiological studies with calcium have shown no increase in the teratogenic hazard to the foetus if used in the doses recommended. Although supplemental calcium may be excreted in breast milk, the concentration is unlikely to be sufficient to produce any adverse effect on the neonate.

4.7 Effects on ability to drive and use machines

None known.

4.8 Undesirable effects

Mild gastrointestinal disturbances (e.g., constipation, diarrhoea) have occurred rarely. Although hypercalcaemia would not be expected in patients unless their renal function were impaired, the following symptoms could indicate the possibility of hypercalcaemia: nausea, vomiting, anorexia, constipation, abdominal pain, bone pain, thirst, polyuria, muscle weakness, drowsiness or confusion.

4.9 Overdose

The amount of calcium absorbed following overdosage with Calcium-Sandoz Syrup will depend on the individual's calcium status. Deliberate overdosage is unlikely and acute overdosage has not been reported. It might cause gastrointestinal disturbances but would not be expected to cause hypercalcaemia except in patients treated with excessive doses of vitamin D. Treatment should be aimed at lowering serum calcium levels, e.g., administration of oral phosphates.

5. PHARMACOLOGICAL PROPERTIES

5.1 Pharmacodynamic properties

Calcium is an endogenous ion of the body essential for the maintenance of a number of physiologic processes. It participates as an integral factor in the maintenance of the functional integrity of the nervous system, in the contractile mechanisms of muscle tissue, in the clotting of blood, and in the formulation of the major structural material of the skeleton.

A dynamic equilibrium occurs between blood calcium and skeletal calcium, homeostasis being mainly regulated by the parathyroid hormone, by calcitonin and by vitamin D. Variations in the concentration of ionised calcium are responsible for the symptoms of hyper/hypocalcaemia. Soluble calcium salts are commonly used in the treatment of calcium deficiency and may be given by mouth or injection.

5.2 Pharmacokinetic properties

Concentrations of plasma calcium are determined chiefly by gastrointestinal absorption, bone metabolism and renal excretion, and levels are closely regulated within the normal limits of 4.5 – 5.5mEq/l (2.25-2.75mmol/L) of which 50-60% is present in ionized form. Up to 10% is present as diffusible complexes with organic acids; the remainder is present as non-diffusible complexes with proteins. More than 99% of the body calcium is deposited in bone as hydroxyapatite crystals, which are available for exchange with calcium in the extracellular fluids. In bone as a whole, about 1% of calcium is in a readily exchangeable pool. Bone therefore functions as the main reservoir of these ions from which they may be readily mobilised if the plasma concentration falls, or in which they may be deposited if the plasma level rises.

5.3 Preclinical safety data

There are no pre-clinical data of relevance to the prescriber which are additional to those already included in other sections of the Summary of Product Characteristics.

6. PHARMACEUTICAL PARTICULARS

6.1 List of excipients

Orange natural flavour, tamaris flavour, benzoic acid, formic acid, sugar and water.

6.2 Incompatibilities

None known.

6.3 Shelf life

Three years unopened. Up to 1 year once the bottle has been opened.

6.4 Special precautions for storage

None.

6.5 Nature and contents of container

Amber glass bottles of 300ml with a polythene closure (polythene wad faced with PP, PVDC or PET lining).

6.6 Instructions for use and handling

Calcium-Sandoz Syrup may be diluted with Syrup BP; the diluted syrup should be used within 14 days.

Administrative Data

7. MARKETING AUTHORISATION HOLDER

Alliance Pharmaceuticals Ltd

Avonbridge House

Bath Road

Chippenham

Wiltshire

SN15 2BB

8. MARKETING AUTHORISATION NUMBER(S)

PL16853/0005

9. DATE OF FIRST AUTHORISATION/RENEWAL OF THE AUTHORISATION

25 June 1998

10. DATE OF REVISION OF THE TEXT

March 1999

11. Legal status

Pharmacy

Alliance, Alliance Pharmaceuticals and associated devices are registered Trademarks of Alliance Pharmaceuticals Ltd.

Calcort 1mg, 6mg and 30 mg

(Shire Pharmaceuticals Limited)

1. NAME OF THE MEDICINAL PRODUCT

Calcort® 1mg, Calcort 6mg, Calcort 30mg.

2. QUALITATIVE AND QUANTITATIVE COMPOSITION

Active ingredient:

1mg tablet: deflazacort 1mg

6mg tablet: deflazacort 6mg

30mg tablet: deflazacort 30mg

3. PHARMACEUTICAL FORM

1mg tablets: Round, white, uncoated tablets, plain on one face with a 1 on the other face.

6mg tablets: Round, white, uncoated tablets, marked with a cross on one face and a 6 on the other face.

30mg tablets: Round, white, uncoated tablets, marked with a cross on one face and 30 on the other face.

4. CLINICAL PARTICULARS

4.1 Therapeutic indications

A wide range of conditions may sometimes need treatment with glucocorticoids. The indications include:

- Anaphylaxis, asthma, severe hypersensitivity reactions.
- Rheumatoid arthritis, juvenile chronic arthritis, polymyalgia rheumatica.
- Systemic lupus erythematosus, dermatomyositis, mixed connective tissue disease (other than systemic sclerosis), polyarteritis nodosa, sarcoidosis.
- Pemphigus, bullous pemphigoid, pyoderma gangrenosum.
- Minimal change nephrotic syndrome, acute interstitial nephritis.
- Rheumatic carditis.
- Ulcerative colitis, Crohn's disease.
- Uveitis, optic neuritis.
- Autoimmune haemolytic anaemia, idiopathic thrombocytopenic purpura.
- Acute and lymphatic leukaemia, malignant lymphoma, multiple myeloma.
- Immune suppression in transplantation.

4.2 Posology and method of administration

Deflazacort is a glucocorticoid derived from prednisolone and 6mg of deflazacort has approximately the same anti-inflammatory potency as 5mg prednisolone or prednisone.

Doses vary widely in different diseases and different patients. In more serious and life-threatening conditions, high doses of deflazacort may need to be given. When deflazacort is used long term in relatively benign chronic diseases, the maintenance dose should be kept as low as possible. Dosage may need to be increased during periods of stress or in exacerbation of illness.

The dosage should be individually titrated according to diagnosis, severity of disease and patient response and tolerance. The lowest dose that will produce an acceptable response should be used (see Warnings and Precautions).

Adults

For acute disorders, up to 120 mg/day deflazacort may need to be given initially. Maintenance doses in most conditions are within the range 3 - 18 mg/day. The following regimens are for guidance only.

Rheumatoid arthritis: The maintenance dose is usually within the range 3 - 18 mg/day. The smallest effective dose should be used and increased if necessary.

Bronchial asthma: In the treatment of an acute attack, high doses of 48 - 72 mg/day may be needed depending on severity and gradually reduced once the attack has been controlled. For maintenance in chronic asthma, doses should be titrated to the lowest dose that controls symptoms.

Other conditions: The dose of deflazacort depends on clinical need titrated to the lowest effective dose for maintenance. Starting doses may be estimated on the basis of ratio of 5mg prednisone or prednisolone to 6mg deflazacort.

Hepatic Impairment

In patients with hepatic impairment, blood levels of deflazacort may be increased. Therefore the dose of deflazacort should be carefully monitored and adjusted to the minimum effective dose.

Renal Impairment

In renally impaired patients, no special precautions other than those usually adopted in patients receiving glucocorticoid therapy are necessary.

Elderly

In elderly patients, no special precautions other than those usually adopted in patients receiving glucocorticoid therapy are necessary. The common adverse effects of systemic corticosteroids may be associated with more serious consequences in old age (see Warnings and Precautions).

Children

There has been limited exposure of children to deflazacort in clinical trials.

In children, the indications for glucocorticoids are the same as for adults, but it is important that the lowest effective dosage is used. Alternate day administration may be appropriate (see Warnings and Precautions).

Doses of deflazacort usually lie in the range 0.25 - 1.5 mg/kg/day. The following ranges provide general guidance:

Juvenile chronic arthritis: The usual maintenance dose is between 0.25 - 1.0 mg/kg/day.

Nephrotic syndrome: Initial dose of usually 1.5 mg/kg/day followed by down titration according to clinical need.

Bronchial asthma: On the basis of the potency ratio, the initial dose should be between 0.25 - 1.0 mg/kg deflazacort on alternate days.

Deflazacort withdrawal

In patients who have received more than physiological doses of systemic corticosteroids (approximately 9mg per day or equivalent) for greater than 3 weeks, withdrawal should not be abrupt. How dose reduction should be carried out depends largely on whether the disease is likely to relapse as the dose of systemic corticosteroids is reduced. Clinical assessment of disease activity may be needed during withdrawal. If the disease is unlikely to relapse on withdrawal of systemic corticosteroids but there is uncertainty about HPA suppression, the dose of systemic corticosteroids may be reduced rapidly to physiological doses. Once a daily dose equivalent to 9mg deflazacort is reached, dose reduction should be slower to allow the HPA-axis to recover.

Abrupt withdrawal of systemic corticosteroid treatment, which has continued up to 3 weeks, is appropriate if it is considered that the disease is unlikely to relapse. Abrupt withdrawal of doses up to 48 mg daily of deflazacort, or equivalent for 3 weeks is unlikely to lead to clinically relevant HPA-axis suppression, in the majority of patients. In the following patient groups, gradual withdrawal of systemic corticosteroid therapy should be *considered* even after courses lasting 3 weeks or less:

- Patients who have had repeated courses of systemic corticosteroids, particularly if taken for greater than 3 weeks.
- When a short course has been prescribed within one year of cessation of long-term therapy (months or years).
- Patients who may have reasons for adrenocortical insufficiency other than exogenous corticosteroid therapy.
- Patients receiving doses of systemic corticosteroid greater than 48 mg daily of deflazacort (or equivalent),
- Patients repeatedly taking doses in the evening.

4.3 Contraindications

Systemic infection unless specific anti-infective therapy is employed. Hypersensitivity to deflazacort or any of the ingredients. Patients receiving live virus immunisation.

4.4 Special warnings and special precautions for use

A patient information leaflet should be supplied with this product.

Patients with rare hereditary problems of galactose intolerance, the Lapp lactose deficiency or glucose-galactose malabsorption should not take this medicine.

Undesirable effects may be minimised by using the lowest effective dose for the minimum period, and by administering the daily requirement as a single morning dose or whenever possible as a single morning dose on alternate days. Frequent patient review is required to appropriately titrate the dose against disease activity (see Dosage section).

Adrenal suppression

Adrenal cortical atrophy develops during prolonged therapy and may persist for years after stopping treatment. Withdrawal of corticosteroids after prolonged therapy must therefore always be gradual to avoid acute adrenal insufficiency, being tapered off over weeks or months according to the dose and duration of treatment. During prolonged therapy, any intercurrent illness, trauma or surgical procedure will require a temporary increase in dosage; if corticosteroids have been stopped following prolonged therapy, they may need to be temporarily re-introduced.

Patients should carry 'Steroid treatment' cards, which give clear guidance on the precautions to be taken to minimise risk and which provide details of prescriber, drug, dosage and the duration of treatment.

Anti-inflammatory/immunosuppressive effects and infection

Suppression of the inflammatory response and immune function increases the susceptibility to infections and their severity. The clinical presentation may often be atypical and serious infections such as septicaemia and tuberculosis may be masked and may reach an advanced stage before being recognised.

Chickenpox is of particular concern since this normally minor illness may be fatal in immunosuppressed patients. Patients (or parents of children) without a definite history of chicken pox should be advised to avoid close personal contact with chickenpox or herpes zoster and, if exposed, they should seek urgent medical attention. Passive immunisation with varicella zoster immunoglobulin (VZIG) is needed by exposed non-immune patients who are receiving systemic corticosteroids or who have used them within the previous 3 months; this should be given within 10 days of exposure to chickenpox. If a diagnosis of chickenpox is confirmed, the illness warrants specialist care and urgent treatment. Corticosteroids should not be stopped and the dose may need to be increased.

Patients should be advised to take particular care to avoid exposure to measles and to seek immediate medical advice if exposure occurs. Prophylaxis with intramuscular normal immunoglobulin may be needed.

Live vaccines should not be given to individuals with impaired responsiveness. The antibody response to other vaccines may be diminished.

Prolonged use of glucocorticoids may produce posterior subcapsular cataracts, glaucoma with possible damage to the optic nerves and may enhance the establishment of secondary ocular infections due to fungi or viruses.

Use in active tuberculosis should be restricted to those cases of fulminating and disseminated tuberculosis in which deflazacort is used for management with appropriate antituberculosis regimen. If glucocorticoids are indicated in patients with latent tuberculosis or tuberculin reactivity, close observation is necessary as reactivation of the disease may occur. During prolonged glucocorticoid therapy, these patients should receive chemoprophylaxis.

Special precautions

The following clinical conditions require special caution and frequent patient monitoring is necessary: -

- Cardiac disease or congestive heart failure (except in the presence of active rheumatic carditis), hypertension, thromboembolic disorders. Glucocorticoids can cause salt and water retention and increased excretion of potassium. Dietary salt restriction and potassium supplementation may be necessary.
- Gastritis or oesophagitis, diverticulitis, ulcerative colitis if there is probability of impending perforation, abscess or pyogenic infections, fresh intestinal anastomosis, active or latent peptic ulcer.
- Diabetes mellitus or a family history, osteoporosis, myasthenia gravis, renal insufficiency.
- Emotional instability or psychotic tendency, epilepsy.
- Previous corticosteroid-induced myopathy.
- Liver failure.
- Hypothyroidism and cirrhosis, which may increase glucocorticoid effect.
- Ocular herpes simplex because of possible corneal perforation.

Use in Children

Corticosteroids cause dose-related growth retardation in infancy, childhood and adolescence, which may be irreversible.

Use in Elderly

The common adverse effects of systemic corticosteroids may be associated with more serious consequences in old age, especially osteoporosis, hypertension, hypokalaemia, diabetes, susceptibility to infection and thinning of the skin. Close clinical supervision is required to avoid life-threatening reactions.

Since complications of glucocorticoid therapy are dependent on dose and duration of therapy, the lowest possible dose must be given and a risk/benefit decision must be made as to whether intermittent therapy should be used.

4.5 Interaction with other medicinal products and other forms of Interaction

The same precautions should be exercised as for other glucocorticoids. Deflazacort is metabolised in the liver. It is recommended to increase the maintenance dose of deflazacort if drugs, which are liver enzyme inducers, are co-administered, e.g. rifampicin, rifabutin, carbamazepine, phenobarbitone, phenytoin, primidone and aminoglutethimide. For drugs, which inhibit liver enzymes, e.g. ketoconazole it may be possible to reduce the maintenance dose of deflazacort.

In patients taking estrogens, corticosteroid requirements may be reduced.

The desired effects of hypoglycaemic agents (including insulin), anti-hypertensives and diuretics are antagonised by corticosteroids and the hypokalaemic effects of acetazolamide, loop diuretics, thiazide diuretics and carbenoxolone are enhanced.

The efficacy of coumarin anticoagulants may be enhanced by concurrent corticosteroid therapy and close monitoring of the INR or prothrombin time is required to avoid spontaneous bleeding.

In patients treated with systemic corticosteroids, use of non-depolarising muscle relaxants can result in prolonged relaxation and acute myopathy. Risk factors for this include prolonged and high dose corticosteroid treatment, and prolonged duration of muscle paralysis. This interaction is more likely following prolonged ventilation (such as in the ITU setting).

The renal clearance of salicylates is increased by corticosteroids and steroid withdrawal may result in salicylate intoxication.

As glucocorticoids can suppress the normal responses of the body to attack by microorganisms, it is important to ensure that any anti-infective therapy is effective and it is recommended to monitor patients closely. Concurrent use of glucocorticoids and oral contraceptives should be closely monitored as plasma levels of glucocorticoids may be increased. This effect may be due to a change in metabolism or binding to serum proteins. Antacids may reduce bioavailability; leave at least 2 hours between administration of deflazacort and antacids.

4.6 Pregnancy and lactation

Pregnancy

The ability of corticosteroids to cross the placenta varies between individual drugs, however, deflazacort does cross the placenta.

Administration of corticosteroids to pregnant animals can cause abnormalities of foetal development including cleft palate, intra-uterine growth retardation and effects on brain growth and development. There is no evidence that corticosteroids result in an increased incidence of congenital abnormalities, such as cleft palate/lip in man. However, when administered for prolonged periods or repeatedly during pregnancy, corticosteroids may increase the risk of intra-uterine growth retardation. Hypoadrenalism may, in theory, occur in the neonate following prenatal exposure to corticosteroids but usually resolves spontaneously following birth and is rarely clinically important. As with all drugs, corticosteroids should only be prescribed when the benefits to the mother and child outweigh the risks. When corticosteroids are essential however, patients with normal pregnancies may be treated as though they were in the non-gravid state.

Lactation

Corticosteroids are excreted in breast milk, although no data are available for deflazacort. Doses of up to 50 mg daily of deflazacort are unlikely to cause systemic effects in the infant. Infants of mothers taking higher doses than this may have a degree of adrenal suppression but the benefits of breast-feeding are likely to outweigh any theoretical risk.

4.7 Effects on ability to drive and use machines

On the basis of the pharmacodynamic profile and reported adverse events, it is unlikely that deflazacort will produce an effect on the ability to drive and use machines.

4.8 Undesirable effects

The incidence of predictable undesirable effects, including hypothalamic-pituitary-adrenal suppression correlates with the relative potency of the drug, dosage, timing of administration and the duration of treatment (see Warnings and Precautions).

Endocrine/metabolic

Suppression of the hypothalamic-pituitary-adrenal axis, growth suppression in infancy, childhood and adolescence, menstrual irregularity and amenorrhoea. Cushingoid facies, hirsutism, weight gain, impaired carbohydrate tolerance with increased requirement for anti-diabetic therapy. Negative protein and calcium balance. Increased appetite.

Anti-inflammatory and immunosuppressive effects

Increased susceptibility and severity of infections with suppression of clinical symptoms and signs, opportunistic infections, recurrence of dormant tuberculosis (see Warnings and Precautions).

Musculoskeletal

Osteoporosis, vertebral and long bone fractures, avascular osteonecrosis, tendon rupture. Muscle wasting or myopathy (acute myopathy may be precipitated by non-depolarising muscle relaxants – see section 4.5), negative nitrogen balance.

Fluid and electrolyte disturbance

Sodium and water retention with hypertension, oedema and heart failure, potassium loss, hypokalaemic alkalosis.

Neuropsychiatric

Headache, vertigo, euphoria, psychological dependence, hypomania or depression, insomnia, restlessness and aggravation of schizophrenia. Increased intra-cranial pressure with papilloedema in children (pseudotumour cerebri), usually after treatment withdrawal. Aggravation of epilepsy.

Ophthalmic

Increased intra-ocular pressure, glaucoma, papilloedema, posterior subcapsular cataracts especially in children, corneal or scleral thinning, exacerbation of ophthalmic viral or fungal diseases.

Gastrointestinal

Dyspepsia, peptic ulceration with perforation and haemorrhage, acute pancreatitis (especially in children), candidiasis. Nausea.

Dermatological

Impaired healing, skin atrophy, bruising, telangiectasia, striae, acne.

General

Hypersensitivity including anaphylaxis has been reported. Leucocytosis. Thromboembolism. Rare incidence of benign intracranial hypertension.

Withdrawal symptoms and signs

Too rapid a reduction of corticosteroid dosage following prolonged treatment can lead to acute adrenal insufficiency, hypotension and death (see Warnings and Precautions).

A 'withdrawal syndrome' may also occur including fever, myalgia, arthralgia, rhinitis, conjunctivitis, painful itchy skin nodules and loss of weight. This may occur in patients even without evidence of adrenal insufficiency.

4.9 Overdose

It is unlikely that treatment is needed in cases of acute overdosage. The LD_{50} for the oral dose is greater than 4000 mg/kg in laboratory animals.

5. PHARMACOLOGICAL PROPERTIES

5.1 Pharmacodynamic properties

Deflazacort is a glucocorticoid. Its anti-inflammatory and immunosuppressive effects are used in treating a variety of diseases and are comparable to other anti-inflammatory steroids. Clinical studies have indicated that the average potency ratio of deflazacort to prednisolone is 0.69-0.89.

5.2 Pharmacokinetic properties

Orally administered deflazacort appears to be well absorbed and is immediately converted by plasma esterases to the pharmacologically active metabolite (D 21-OH), which achieves peak plasma concentrations in 1.5 to 2 hours. It is 40% protein-bound and has no affinity for corticosteroid binding globulin (transcortin). Its elimination plasma half-life is 1.1 to 1.9 hours. Elimination takes place primarily through the kidneys; 70% of the administered dose is excreted in the urine. The remaining 30% is eliminated in the faeces. Metabolism of D 21-OH is extensive; only 18% of urinary excretion represents D 21-OH. The metabolite of D 21-OH, deflazacort 6-beta-OH, represents one third of the urinary elimination.

5.3 Preclinical safety data

Safety studies have been carried out in the rat, dog, mouse and monkey. The findings are consistent with other glucocorticoids at comparable doses. Teratogenic effects demonstrated in rodents and rabbits are typical of those caused by other glucocorticoids. Deflazacort was not found to be carcinogenic in the mouse, but studies in the rat produced carcinogenic findings consistent with the findings with other glucocorticoids.

6. PHARMACEUTICAL PARTICULARS

6.1 List of excipients

1mg and 30mg tablets: Microcrystalline cellulose, lactose, maize starch and magnesium stearate.

6mg tablets: Microcrystalline cellulose, lactose, sucrose, maize starch and magnesium stearate.

6.2 Incompatibilities

None reported.

6.3 Shelf life

1mg tablets: 3 years

6mg and 30mg tablets: 5 years.

6.4 Special precautions for storage

Store in the original package. Do not store above 25°C.

6.5 Nature and contents of container
Deflazacort is packed in blister packs of polyvinylchloride and aluminium foil presented in cardboard cartons.

1mg tablets: 100 tablets per pack.

6mg tablets: 60 tablets per pack

30mg tablets: 30 tablets per pack

6.6 Instructions for use and handling
No special instructions for use or handling are required.

7. MARKETING AUTHORISATION HOLDER
Shire Pharmaceuticals Limited

Hampshire International Business Park

Chineham

Basingstoke

Hampshire RG24 8EP

United Kingdom

8. MARKETING AUTHORISATION NUMBER(S)
1mg tablets: 08557/0036

6mg tablets: 08557/0037

30mg tablets: 08557/0038

9. DATE OF FIRST AUTHORISATION/RENEWAL OF THE AUTHORISATION
1mg and 6mg tablets: 14 December 1997

30mg tablets: 31 October 1997

10. DATE OF REVISION OF THE TEXT
January 2005

LEGAL CATEGORY
POM

Calmurid Cream

(Galderma (U.K.) Ltd)

1. NAME OF THE MEDICINAL PRODUCT
Calmurid Cream

2. QUALITATIVE AND QUANTITATIVE COMPOSITION
A white cream containing Urea Ph.Eur 10.0 % w/w and Lactic Acid Ph.Eur 5.0% w/w in a stabilising emulsified base.

3. PHARMACEUTICAL FORM
Cream for topical (cutaneous) use.

4. CLINICAL PARTICULARS

4.1 Therapeutic indications
To be applied topically for the correction of hyperkeratosis and dryness in ichthyosis and allied conditions characterised by dry, rough, scaly skin.

4.2 Posology and method of administration
For external use only.

Adults, elderly and children:

A thick layer of Calmurid is applied twice daily after washing the affected area. The cream is left on the skin for 3-5 minutes and then rubbed lightly in. Excess cream should be wiped off the skin with a tissue, not washed off. Frequency of application can be reduced as the patient progresses. In hyperkeratosis of the feet apply Calmurid as above after soaking the feet in warm water for 15 minutes and drying with a rough towel.

4.3 Contraindications
Hypersensitivity to any constituent of the product.

4.4 Special warnings and special precautions for use
Calmurid is acidic and hypertonic and can cause smarting if applied to raw areas, fissures or mucous membranes. Where this is a barrier to therapy the use of Calmurid diluted 50% with aqueous cream B.P. for one week should result in freedom from smarting upon use of Calmurid.

4.5 Interaction with other medicinal products and other forms of Interaction
Low pH of cream might affect stability of other drugs.

4.6 Pregnancy and lactation
There is no specific data available regarding the use in pregnant women and during lactation.

4.7 Effects on ability to drive and use machines
None known.

4.8 Undesirable effects
Calmurid is acidic and hypertonic and can cause smarting if applied to raw areas, fissures or mucous membranes.

4.9 Overdose
Unlikely. In the case of smarting, wash the cream off.

5. PHARMACOLOGICAL PROPERTIES

5.1 Pharmacodynamic properties
Urea at a concentration of 10% has keratolytic, anti microbial, anti pruritic and hydrating effects on the skin. Lactic acid has keratolytic, hydrating and anti microbial properties also. Treatment of ichthyotic patients shows a parallel between clinical improvement and increase in the otherwise depressed binding capacity of the horny layer.

5.2 Pharmacokinetic properties
Not applicable.

5.3 Preclinical safety data
Urea and lactic acid are long established materials, whose pre-clinical profile is known.

6. PHARMACEUTICAL PARTICULARS

6.1 List of excipients
Glyceryl Monostearate Ph.Eur.

Betaine Monohydrate

Diethanolamine Cetylphosphate ("Amphisol")

Adeps Solidus (Hard Fat) Ph.Eur

Cholesterol USNF

Sodium chloride Ph.Eur

Purified water Ph.Eur.

6.2 Incompatibilities
The low pH due to lactic acid means care in choice of other packages or other drugs admixed.

6.3 Shelf life
30 months.

6.4 Special precautions for storage
Store below 25°C. Do not freeze. Do not put in alloy containers.

6.5 Nature and contents of container
Polythene tubes with polypropylene caps.

Package size: 100 g.

Plastic pump dispenser.

Package size: 500 g.

6.6 Instructions for use and handling
Not relevant.

7. MARKETING AUTHORISATION HOLDER
Galderma (UK) Limited

Galderma House

Church Lane

Kings Langley

Herts WD4 8JP

8. MARKETING AUTHORISATION NUMBER(S)
PL 10590/0009

9. DATE OF FIRST AUTHORISATION/RENEWAL OF THE AUTHORISATION
9 February 1993/24 March 1998

10. DATE OF REVISION OF THE TEXT
May 2001

11 Legal category
P

Calmurid HC Cream

(Galderma (U.K.) Ltd)

1. NAME OF THE MEDICINAL PRODUCT
Calmurid HC Cream

2. QUALITATIVE AND QUANTITATIVE COMPOSITION
Urea Ph. Eur. 10.0% w/w

Lactic Acid Ph. Eur. 5.0% w/w

Hydrocortisone Ph. Eur. 1.0% w/w

3. PHARMACEUTICAL FORM
Cream for topical (cutaneous) use.

4. CLINICAL PARTICULARS

4.1 Therapeutic indications
To be used topically for the treatment of atopic eczema, Besniers prurigo, acute and chronic allergic eczema, neurodermatitis and other hyperkeratotic skin conditions with accompanying inflammation.

4.2 Posology and method of administration
For external use only.

Adults, elderly and children:

Apply twice daily to the affected area after bathing or washing. Moist lesions should be treated as to dry them before using Calmurid HC.

4.3 Contraindications
Skin tuberculosis, viral infections accompanied by dermal manifestations e.g. herpes simplex, vaccinia, chicken pox and measles. Syphilitic skin lesions. In concurrent mycotic infections, the cream should be complemented with anti-mycotic treatment. Hypersensitivity to any constituent of the product.

4.4 Special warnings and special precautions for use
In infants, high surface area in relation to mass raises the likelihood of uptake of excessive amounts of steroid from the cream, even without occlusion, thus adrenal suppression is more likely. In infants, long term continuous topical therapy should be avoided.

4.5 Interaction with other medicinal products and other forms of Interaction
None known.

4.6 Pregnancy and lactation
There is no specific data available regarding the use in pregnant women and during lactation.

Pregnancy:

Evidence from animal studies suggests that prolonged intensive therapy with steroids during pregnancy should be avoided.

Lactation:

Given the slow uptake of hydrocortisone from the skin and the rapid destruction of hydrocortisone by the body, there would seem to be little risk of significant transfer at lactation.

4.7 Effects on ability to drive and use machines
None known.

4.8 Undesirable effects
If applied to open wounds or mucous membranes the hypertonic and acidic nature of the preparation may produce smarting. In such cases wash off with water. Where smarting is a barrier to therapy, dilute with an equal quantity of aqueous cream: after a week of treatment with this material, the normal strength should be tolerated.

4.9 Overdose
The barrier function in the skin to steroid uptake, the low toxicity of hydrocortisone and the nature mechanism for its rapid inactivation make overdose unlikely.

5. PHARMACOLOGICAL PROPERTIES

5.1 Pharmacodynamic properties
Urea at a concentration of 10% has keratolytic, anti microbial, anti pruritic and hydrating effects on the skin, properties also attributable to Lactic acid. Hydrocortisone 1% is the normal concentration of the drug used as a dermatological anti-inflammatory agent. In some patients with eczema, Calmurid HC cream may be as effective as fluorinated steroid creams.

5.2 Pharmacokinetic properties
Not applicable.

5.3 Preclinical safety data
Urea, lactic acid and hydrocortisone are long established materials, whose pre-clinical profile is known.

6. PHARMACEUTICAL PARTICULARS

6.1 List of excipients
Glyceryl Monostearate Ph. Eur.

Betaine Monohydrate

Diethanolamine Cetylphosphate ("Amphisol")

Adeps Solidus (Hard Fat) Ph. Eur.

Cholesterol USNF

Soduim Chloride Ph. Eur.

Purified Water Ph. Eur.

6.2 Incompatibilities
Do not mix with other preparations, as the effect on the stability of each is unknown. Do not pack in alloy containers as they may react with the lactic acid.

6.3 Shelf life
30 months.

6.4 Special precautions for storage
Store below 25°C.

6.5 Nature and contents of container
Polypropylene tubes.

Package sizes: 30 & 100 g.

6.6 Instructions for use and handling
Not relevant.

7. MARKETING AUTHORISATION HOLDER
Galderma (UK) Limited,

Galderma House,

Church Lane,

Kings Langley,

Hertfordshire, WD4 8JP,

England.

8. MARKETING AUTHORISATION NUMBER(S)
PL 10590/0010

9. DATE OF FIRST AUTHORISATION/RENEWAL OF THE AUTHORISATION
9 February 1993

10. DATE OF REVISION OF THE TEXT
September 2001

11. LEGAL STATUS
POM-Prescription only medicine

Calpol Infant Suspension

(Pfizer Consumer Healthcare)

1. NAME OF THE MEDICINAL PRODUCT
CALPOL Infant Suspension

2. QUALITATIVE AND QUANTITATIVE COMPOSITION
CALPOL Infant Suspension contains 120mg Paracetamol in each 5ml.

3. PHARMACEUTICAL FORM
Suspension

4. CLINICAL PARTICULARS

4.1 Therapeutic indications

CALPOL Infant Suspension is indicated for the treatment of mild to moderate pain (including teething pain) and as an antipyretic (including post immunisation fever).

4.2 Posology and method of administration

Children aged 1 to under 6 years:

Oral. 5 to 10ml (120mg to 240mg paracetamol). Repeat every 4 hours, if necessary, up to a maximum of 4 doses per 24 hours.

Infants 3 months to under 1 year:

Oral. 2.5 to 5 ml (60mg to 120mg paracetamol). Repeat every 4 hours, if necessary, up to a maximum of 4 doses per 24 hours.

Infants aged 2-3 months:

Oral. A 2.5ml (60 mg paracetamol) dose is suitable for babies who develop post vaccination fever at 2 months followed, if necessary, by a second dose 4 to 6 hours later. The same 2 doses may be given for other causes of fever or mild to moderate pain provided the infant weighs over 4 kg and was not born before 37 weeks gestation. Medical advice should be sought promptly if further doses are required or if the cause of the infant's fever or pain is not known,

The Elderly:

In the elderly, the rate and extent of paracetamol absorption is normal but plasma half-life is longer and paracetamol clearance is lower than in young adults.

4.3 Contraindications

CALPOL Infant Suspension is contra-indicated in patients with known hypersensitivity to paracetamol, or any of the other constituents.

4.4 Special warnings and special precautions for use

Care is advised in the administration of paracetamol to patients with severe renal or severe hepatic impairment.

The hazards of overdose are greater in those with non-cirrhotic alcoholic liver disease.

The label contains the following statements:

Do not exceed the recommended dose.

If symptoms persist consult your doctor.

Keep out of the reach and sight of children.

Leave at least 4 hours between doses.

Immediate advice should be sought in the event of an overdose, even if the child seems well. (label)

Immediate advice should be sought in the event of an overdose, even if the child seems well, because of the risk of delayed, serious liver damage. (leaflet)

Do not give with any other paracetamol containing products.

4.5 Interaction with other medicinal products and other forms of Interaction

The speed of absorption of paracetamol may be increased by metoclopramide or domperidone and absorption reduced by colestyramine.

The anticoagulant effect of warfarin and other coumarins may be enhanced by prolonged regular use of paracetamol with increased risk of bleeding; occasional doses have no significant effect.

Chronic alcohol intake can increase the hepatotoxicity of paracetamol overdose and may have contributed to the acute pancreatitis reported in one patient who had taken an overdose of paracetamol. Acute alcohol intake may diminish an individual's ability to metabolise large doses of paracetamol, the plasma half-life of which can be prolonged.

The use of drugs that induce hepatic microsomal enzymes, such as anticonvulsants and oral contraceptives, may increase the extent of metabolism of paracetamol, resulting in reduced plasma concentrations of the drug and a faster elimination rate.

4.6 Pregnancy and lactation

Epidemiological studies in human pregnancy have shown no ill effects due to paracetamol used in the recommended dosage, but patients should follow the advice of their doctor regarding its use.

Paracetamol is excreted in breast milk but not in a clinically significant amount. Available published data do not contra-indicate breast-feeding.

4.7 Effects on ability to drive and use machines

None known.

4.8 Undesirable effects

Adverse effects of paracetamol are rare but hypersensitivity including skin rash may occur. There have been reports of blood dyscrasias including thrombocytopenia and agranulocystosis but these were not necessarily causality related to paracetamol.

Most reports of adverse reactions to paracetamol relate to overdosage with the drug.

Chronic hepatic necrosis has been reported in a patient who took daily therapeutic doses of paracetamol for about a year and liver damage has been reported after daily ingestion of excessive amounts for shorter periods. A review of a group of patients with chronic active hepatitis failed to reveal differences in the abnormalities of liver function in those who were long-term users of paracetamol nor was the control of the disease improved after paracetamol withdrawal.

Nephrotoxicity following therapeutic doses of paracetamol is uncommon, but apillary necrosis has been reported after prolonged administration.

4.9 Overdose

Liver damage is possible in adults who have taken 10g or more of paracetamol. Ingestion of 5g or more of paracetamol may lead to liver damage if the patient has risk factors (see below).

Risk Factors:

If the patient

a, Is on long term treatment with carbamazepine, phenobarbital, phenytoin, primidone, rifampicin, St John's Wort or other drugs that induce liver enzymes.

Or

b, Regularly consumes ethanol in excess of recommended amounts

Or

c, Is likely to be glutathione deplete e.g. eating disorders, cystic fibrosis, HIV infection, starvation, cachexia.

Symptoms

Symptoms of paracetamol overdosage in the first 24 hours are pallor, nausea, vomiting, anorexia and abdominal pain. Liver damage may become apparent 12 to 48 hours after ingestion. Abnormalities of glucose metabolism and metabolic acidosis may occur. In severe poisoning, hepatic failure may progress to encephalopathy, haemorrhage, hypoglycaemia, cerebral oedema, and death. Acute renal failure with acute tubular necrosis, strongly suggested by loin pain, haematuria and proteinuria, may develop even in the absence of severe liver damage. Cardiac arrhythmias and pancreatitis have been reported.

Management

Immediate treatment is essential in the management of paracetamol overdose. Despite a lack of significant early symptoms, patients should be referred to hospital urgently for immediate medical attention. Symptoms may be limited to nausea or vomiting and may not reflect the severity of overdose or the risk of organ damage. Management should be in accordance with established treatment guidelines, see BNF overdose section.

Treatment with activated charcoal should be considered if the overdose has been taken within 1 hour. Plasma paracetamol concentration should be measured at 4 hours or later after ingestion (earlier concentrations are unreliable). Treatment with N-acetylcysteine may be used up to 24 hours after ingestion of paracetamol, however the maximum protective effect is obtained up to 8 hours post-ingestion. The effectiveness of the antidote declines sharply after this time. If required the patient should be given intravenous N-acetylcysteine, in line with the established dosage schedule. If vomiting is not a problem, oral methionine may be a suitable alternative for remote areas, outside hospital. Management of patients who present with serious hepatic dysfunction beyond 24h from ingestion should be discussed with the NPIS or a liver unit.

5. PHARMACOLOGICAL PROPERTIES

5.1 Pharmacodynamic properties

Paracetamol has analgesic and antipyretic effects that do not differ significantly from those of aspirin. However it has only weak anti-inflammatory effects. It is only a weak inhibitor of prostaglandin biosynthesis although there is some evidence to suggest it may be more effective against enzymes in the central nervous system than in the periphery. This may in part account for its activity profile.

5.2 Pharmacokinetic properties

Paracetamol is rapidly and almost completely absorbed from the gastrointestinal tract with peak plasma concentrations occurring 0.5-2 hours after dosing. The plasma half-life is approximately 2 hours after therapeutic doses in adults but is increased in neonates to about 5 hours. It is widely distributed through the body. Metabolism is principally by the hepatic microsomal enzymes and urinary excretion accounts for over 90% of the dose within 1 day. Virtually no paracetamol is excreted unchanged, the bulk being conjugated with glucoronic acid (60%), sulphuric acid (35%) or cysteine (3%). Children have less capacity for glucuronidation of the drug than adults.

5.3 Preclinical safety data

Mutagenicity

There are no studies relating to the mutagenic potential of CALPOL Infant Suspension.

In vivo mutagenicity tests of paracetamol in mammals are limited and show conflicting results. Therefore, there is insufficient information to determine whether paracetamol poses a mutagenic risk to man.

Paracetamol has been found to be non-mutagenic in bacterial mutagenicity assays, although a clear clastogenic effect has been observed in mammalian cells in vitro following exposure to paracetamol (3 and 10 mM for 2h).

Carcinogenicity

There are no studies to the carcinogenic potential of CALPOL Infant Suspension.

There is inadequate evidence to determine the carcinogenic potential of paracetamol in humans. A positive association between the use of paracetamol and cancer of the ureter (but not of other sites in the urinary tract) was observed in a case-control study in which approximate lifetime consumption of paracetamol (whether acute or chronic) was estimated. However, other similar studies have failed to demonstrate a statistically significant association between paracetamol and cancer of the urinary tract, or paracetamol and renal cell carcinoma.

There is limited evidence for the carcinogenicity of paracetamol in experimental animals. Liver cell tumours can be detected in rats following chronic feeding of 500 mg/kg/day paracetamol.

Teratogenicity

There is no information relating to the teratogenic potential of CALPOL Infant Suspension. In humans, paracetamol crosses the placenta and attains concentrations in the foetal circulation similar to those in the maternal circulation. Intermittent maternal ingestion of therapeutic doses of paracetamol are not associated with teratogenic effects in humans.

Paracetamol has been found to be foetotoxic to cultured rat embryo.

Fertility

There is no information relating to the effects of CALPOL Infant Suspension on fertility. A significant decrease in testicular weight was observed when male Sprague-Dawley rats were given daily high doses of paracetamol (500 mg/kg/body weight/day) orally for 70 days.

6. PHARMACEUTICAL PARTICULARS

6.1 List of excipients

Sucrose

Sorbitol Liquid (Non Crystallising)

Glycerol

Xanthan Gum

Dispersible Cellulose

Polysorbate 80

Acesulfame Potassium

Propyl Parahydroxybenzoate (E216)

Ethyl Parahydroxybenzoate (E214)

Strawberry Flavour 500018E

Methyl Hydroxybenzoate (E218)

Carmoisine (E122)

Purified Water

6.2 Incompatibilities

None known

6.3 Shelf life

36 months for the amber glass bottles and 24 months for the 5ml paper/foil/surlyn sachets.

6.4 Special precautions for storage

Do not store above 25°C. Store in the original container.

6.5 Nature and contents of container

10, 12 and 20 units of 5ml paper/foil/surlyn sachets.

200, 140 and 70ml amber glass bottle closed with a two-piece plastic child resistant, tamper evident closure fitted with a polyethylene/polvinylidine chloride (PVDC) polyethylene laminate faced wad

or

a three piece plastic child resistant, tamper evident closure fitted with a polyethylene/polyvinylidene chloride (PVDC) polyethylene laminate faced wad.

6.6 Instructions for use and handling

None applicable

7. MARKETING AUTHORISATION HOLDER

Pfizer Consumer Healthcare

Alternative Trading Style:

Warner-Lambert Consumer Healthcare

Walton Oaks

Dorking Road

Walton-on-the-Hill

Surrey KT20 7NS

United Kingdom

8. MARKETING AUTHORISATION NUMBER(S)

PL 15513/0004

9. DATE OF FIRST AUTHORISATION/RENEWAL OF THE AUTHORISATION

28 April 1997 / 31st March 2003

10. DATE OF REVISION OF THE TEXT

May 2005

Calpol Paediatric Suspension Sugar Free

(Pfizer Consumer Healthcare)

1. NAME OF THE MEDICINAL PRODUCT

CALPOL Paediatric Suspension Sugar Free

2. QUALITATIVE AND QUANTITATIVE COMPOSITION
CALPOL Paediatric Suspension Sugar Free contains 120 mg Paracetamol in each 5 ml.

3. PHARMACEUTICAL FORM
Suspension.

4. CLINICAL PARTICULARS

4.1 Therapeutic indications
CALPOL Paediatric Suspension Sugar Free is indicated for the treatment of pain (including teething pain), and as an antipyretic (including post immunisation fever).

4.2 Posology and method of administration

Children aged 1 to under 6 years:

Oral. 5 to 10 ml (120 mg to 240 mg paracetamol). Repeat every 4 hours, if necessary, up to a maximum of 4 doses per 24 hours.

Infants 3 months to under 1 year:

Oral. 2.5 to 5 ml (60 mg to 120 mg paracetamol). Repeat every 4 hours, if necessary, up to a maximum of 4 doses per 24 hours.

Infants aged 2 -3 months:

Oral. A 2.5 ml (60 mg paracetamol) dose is suitable for babies who develop post- vaccination fever at 2 months followed, if necessary, by a second dose 4 to 6 hours later. The same 2 doses may be given for other causes of fever or mild to moderate pain provided the infant weighs over 4 kg and was not born before 37 weeks gestation. Medical advice should be sought promptly if further doses are required or if the cause of the infant's fever or pain is not known.

The Elderly:

In the elderly, the rate and extent of paracetamol absorption is normal but plasma half-life is longer and paracetamol clearance is lower than in young adults.

4.3 Contraindications
CALPOL Paediatric Suspension Sugar Free is contraindicated in patients with known hypersensitivity to paracetamol, or any of the other components.

4.4 Special warnings and special precautions for use
CALPOL Paediatric Suspension Sugar Free should be used with caution in the presence of severe hepatic or renal impairment.

The hazards of overdose are greater in those with non-cirrhotic alcoholic liver disease.

Concomitant use of other paracetamol-containing products with CALPOL Infant Suspension Sugar/Colour Free could lead to paracetamol overdose and therefore should be avoided.

The label contains the following statements:

Shake the bottle thoroughly.

Dose up to 4 times a day as necessary.

Keep out of the reach and sight of children.

Do not exceed the stated dose.

Do not give more than 4 doses in 24 hours.

Leave at least 4 hours between doses.

Do not give for more than 3 days without consulting a doctor.

As with all medicines, if you are currently taking any medicine consult your doctor or pharmacist before taking this product.

If symptoms persist consult your doctor.

Contains paracetamol.

Immediate advice should be sought in the event of an overdose, even if the child seems well. (label)

Immediate advice should be sought in the event of an overdose, even if the child seems well, because of the risk of delayed, serious liver damage. (leaflet)

Do not give with any other paracetamol containing products.

4.5 Interaction with other medicinal products and other forms of Interaction
The speed of absorption of paracetamol may be increased by metoclopramide or domperidone and absorption reduced by colestyramine.

The anticoagulant effect of warfarin and other coumarins may be enhanced by prolonged regular use of paracetamol with increased risk of bleeding; occasional doses have no significant effect.

Chronic alcohol intake can increase the hepatotoxicity of paracetamol overdose and may have contributed to the acute pancreatitis reported in one patient who had taken an overdose of paracetamol. Acute alcohol intake may diminish an individual's ability to metabolise large doses of paracetamol, the plasma half-life of which can be prolonged.

The use of drugs that induce hepatic microsomal enzymes, such as anticonvulsants and oral contraceptives, may increase the extent of metabolism of paracetamol, resulting in reduced plasma concentrations of the drug and a faster elimination rate.

4.6 Pregnancy and lactation
Epidemiological studies in human pregnancy have shown no ill effects due to paracetamol used in the recommended dosage, but patients should follow the advice of their doctor regarding its use.

Paracetamol is excreted in breast milk but not in a clinically significant amount. Available published data do not contra-indicate breast feeding.

4.7 Effects on ability to drive and use machines
No special comment - unlikely to produce an effect.

4.8 Undesirable effects
Adverse effects of paracetamol are rare, but hypersensitivity including skin rash may occur. There have been reports of blood dyscrasias including thrombocytopenia and agranulocytosis, but these were not necessarily causality related to paracetamol.

Most reports of adverse reactions to paracetamol relate to overdose with the drug.

Chronic hepatic necrosis has been reported in a patient who took daily therapeutic doses of paracetamol for about a year and liver damage has been reported after daily ingestion of excessive amounts for shorter periods. A review of a group of patients with chronic active hepatitis failed to reveal differences in the abnormalities of liver function in those who were long-term users of paracetamol nor was the control of the disease improved after paracetamol withdrawal.

Nephrotoxicity following therapeutic doses of paracetamol are uncommon, but papillary necrosis has been reported after prolonged administration.

4.9 Overdose
Liver damage is possible in adults who have taken 10 g or more of paracetamol. Ingestion of 5g or more of paracetamol may lead to liver damage if the patient has risk factors (see below).

Risk Factors:
If the patient

a, Is on long term treatment with carbamazepine, phenobarbital, phenytoin, primidone, rifampicin, St John's Wort or other drugs that induce liver enzymes.

Or

b, Regularly consumes ethanol in excess of recommended amounts

Or

c, Is likely to be glutathione deplete e.g. eating disorders, cystic fibrosis, HIV infection, starvation, cachexia.

Symptoms
Symptoms of paracetamol overdosage in the first 24 hours are pallor, nausea, vomiting, anorexia and abdominal pain. Liver damage may become apparent 12 to 48 hours after ingestion. Abnormalities of glucose metabolism and metabolic acidosis may occur. In severe poisoning, hepatic failure may progress to encephalopathy, haemorrhage, hypoglycaemia, cerebral oedema and death. Acute renal failure with acute tubular necrosis, strongly suggested by loin pain, haematuria and proteinuria, may develop even in the absence of severe liver damage. Cardiac arrhythmias and pancreatitis have been reported.

Management
Immediate treatment is essential in the management of paracetamol overdose. Despite a lack of significant early symptoms, patients should be referred to hospital urgently for immediate medical attention. Symptoms may be limited to nausea or vomiting and may not reflect the severity of overdose or the risk of organ damage. Management should be in accordance with established treatment guidelines, see BNF overdose section.

Treatment with activated charcoal should be considered if the overdose has been taken within 1 hour. Plasma paracetamol concentration should be measured at 4 hours or later after ingestion (earlier concentrations are unreliable). Treatment with N-acetylcysteine may be used up to 24 hours after ingestion of paracetamol, however, the maximum protective effect is obtained up to 8 hours post-ingestion. The effectiveness of the antidote declines sharply after this time. If required the patient should be given intravenous N-acetylcysteine, in line with the established dosage schedule. If vomiting is not a problem, oral methionine may be a suitable alternative for remote areas, outside hospital. Management of patients who present with serious hepatic dysfunction beyond 24h from ingestion should be discussed with the NPIS or a liver unit.

5. PHARMACOLOGICAL PROPERTIES

5.1 Pharmacodynamic properties
Paracetamol has analgesic and antipyretic effects similar to those of aspirin and is useful in the treatment of mild to moderate pain. It has weak anti-inflammatory effects.

5.2 Pharmacokinetic properties
Paracetamol is rapidly and almost completely absorbed from the gastrointestinal tract. Peak plasma concentrations are reached 30-90 minutes post dose and the plasma half-life is in the range of 1 to 3 hours after therapeutic doses. Drug is widely distributed throughout most body fluids. Following therapeutic doses 90-100% of the drug is recovered in the urine within 24 hours almost entirely following hepatic conjugation with glucuronic acid (about 60%), sulphuric acid (about 35%) or cysteine (about 3%). Small amounts of hydroxylated and deacetylated metabolites have also been detected. Children have less capacity for glucuronidation of the drug than do adults. In overdose there is increased N-hydroxylation followed by glutathione conjugation. When the latter is exhausted, reaction with hepatic proteins is increased leading to necrosis.

5.3 Preclinical safety data
The active ingredient of this product is a well known constituent of medicinal products and its safety profile is well documented.

6. PHARMACEUTICAL PARTICULARS

6.1 List of excipients
Maltitol Liquid

Sorbitol solution (70% non crystallising)

Glycerol

Dispersible cellulose

Xanthan gum

Ethyl parahydroxybenzoate (E214)

Methyl parahydroxybenzoate (E218)

Propyl parahydroxybenzoate (E216)

Polysorbate 80

Strawberry flavour

Carmoisine (E122)

Purified water

6.2 Incompatibilities
None known

6.3 Shelf life
36 months bottles, 24 months sachets

6.4 Special precautions for storage
Do not store above 25°C. Store in the original container.

6.5 Nature and contents of container
5 ml paper/PE/foil/surlyn sachets.

Amber glass bottle with a plastic screw cap, a polyethylene or polyvinylidene chloride (PVDC) laminate faced wad.

or

Amber glassed bottle with a two-piece plastic child resistant, tamper evident closure fitted with a polyethylene or polyvinylidene chloride (PVDC) laminate faced wad.

or

Amber glass bottle with a three piece plastic child resistant, tamper evident closure fitted with a polyethylene or polyvinylidene chloride (PVDC) laminate faced wad.

Pack sizes

100 ml and 1000 ml

1000 ml amber glass bottle with an aluminium cap fitted with a polyethylene wad.

6.6 Instructions for use and handling
None applicable.

7. MARKETING AUTHORISATION HOLDER
Pfizer Consumer Healthcare

Alternative Trading Style:

Warner-Lambert Consumer Healthcare
Walton Oaks
Dorking Road
Walton-on-the-Hill
Surrey KT20 7NS
United Kingdom

8. MARKETING AUTHORISATION NUMBER(S)
PL 15513/0008

9. DATE OF FIRST AUTHORISATION/RENEWAL OF THE AUTHORISATION
28 April 1997 / 31st March 2003

10. DATE OF REVISION OF THE TEXT
May 2005

Calpol Six Plus Fastmelts

(Pfizer Consumer Healthcare)

1. NAME OF THE MEDICINAL PRODUCT
Calpol Six Plus Fastmelts (250 mg Orodispersible Tablets)

2. QUALITATIVE AND QUANTITATIVE COMPOSITION
Paracetamol 250 mg

For excipients, see 6.1.

3. PHARMACEUTICAL FORM
Orodispersible tablet

Round, white, bi-convex tablets with central concave depression.

4. CLINICAL PARTICULARS

4.1 Therapeutic indications
Calpol Six Plus Fastmelts are indicated for the treatment of mild to moderate pain such as headache, tooth pain and

sore throat, and as an antipyretic (e.g. fever associated with colds and flu).

4.2 Posology and method of administration

Oral:

Tablets should be placed in the mouth where they melt on the tongue. The tablet will rapidly disperse to a pleasant tasting paste that can be easily ingested. Alternatively the tablet can be dispersed in a teaspoonful of water or milk.

Adults and children

Over 12 years: 2 – 4 tablets (500 mg – 1000 mg paracetamol)

Repeat every 4-6 hours if necessary up to a maximum of 4 doses (4g)/24 hours.

6 to 12 years:

1 – 2 tablets (250 mg - 500 mg paracetamol)

Repeat every 4-6 hours if necessary up to a maximum of 4 doses (2g)/24 hours.

Under 6 years: Not recommended

Use in the Elderly

Normal adult dosage is appropriate. However, a reduction in dosing may be necessary in frail, elderly subjects (see Section 5.2).

4.3 Contraindications

Calpol Six Plus Fastmelts are contraindicated in patients with known hypersensitivity to paracetamol or any other ingredient and in subjects with phenylketonuria.

4.4 Special warnings and special precautions for use

Calpol Six Plus Fastmelts should be used with caution in the presence of severe hepatic or renal dysfunction. The hazards of overdose are greater in those with non-cirrhotic alcoholic liver disease.

Calpol Six Plus Fastmelts contain aspartame, which is a source of phenylalanine equivalent to 0.04 mg/250 mg tablet. The phenylalanine in the tablets may be harmful to people with phenylketonuria.

Calpol Six Plus Fastmelts contain mannitol, which may have a mild laxative effect.

The label shall contain the following statements:

Keep out of reach and sight of children.

Dose up to 4 times a day if necessary.

Do not exceed the recommended dose.

Do not give more than 4 doses in 24 hours.

Leave at least 4 hours between doses.

Do not give for more than 3 days without consulting a doctor.

As with all medicines, if your child is currently taking any other medicines consult your doctor or pharmacist before giving this product.

If symptoms persist consult your doctor.

Contains paracetamol.

Immediate medical advice should be sought in the event of an overdose, even if the child seems well. (label)

Immediate medical advice should be sought in the event of an overdose, even if the child seems well, because of the risk of delayed, serious liver damage (leaflet).

Do not give with any other paracetamol-containing products.

4.5 Interaction with other medicinal products and other forms of Interaction

The speed of absorption of paracetamol may be increased by metoclopramide or domperidone and absorption reduced by colestyramine.

The anticoagulant effect of warfarin and other coumarins may be enhanced by prolonged regular use of paracetamol with increased risk of bleeding; occasional doses have no significant effect.

Chronic alcohol intake can increase the hepatotoxicity of paracetamol overdose and may have contributed to the acute pancreatitis reported in one patient who had taken an overdose of paracetamol. Acute alcohol intake may diminish an individual's ability to metabolise large doses of paracetamol, the plasma half-life of which can be prolonged.

The use of drugs that induce hepatic microsomal enzymes, such as anticonvulsants and oral contraceptives, may increase the extent of metabolism of paracetamol, resulting in reduced plasma concentrations of the drug and a faster elimination rate.

4.6 Pregnancy and lactation

Epidemiological studies in human pregnancy have shown no ill effects due to paracetamol used in the recommended dosage, but patients should follow the advice of their doctor regarding its use.

Paracetamol is excreted in breast milk but not in a clinically significant amount. Available published data do not contra-indicate breast-feeding.

4.7 Effects on ability to drive and use machines

None known.

4.8 Undesirable effects

Adverse effects of paracetamol are rare but hypersensitivity including skin rash may occur. There have been reports of blood dyscrasias including thrombocytopenia and agranulocytosis, but these were not necessarily causality related to paracetamol.

Most reports of adverse reactions to paracetamol relate to overdose with the drug.

Nephrotoxicity following therapeutic doses of paracetamol is uncommon, but papillary necrosis has been reported after prolonged administration.

4.9 Overdose

Liver damage is possible in adults who have taken 10g or more of paracetamol. It is considered that excess quantities of a toxic metabolite (usually adequately detoxified by glutathione when normal doses of paracetamol are ingested) become irreversibly bound to liver tissue. Ingestion of 5g or more of paracetamol may lead to liver damage if the patient has risk factors (see below).

Risk Factors:

If the patient

a, Is on long term treatment with carbamezepine, Phenobarbital, phenytoin, primidone, rifampicin, St John's Wort or other drugs that induce liver enzymes.

Or

b, Regularly consumes ethanol in excess of recommended amounts.

Or

C, Is likely to be glutathione deplete e.g. eating disorders, cystic fibrosis, HIV infection, starvation, cachexia.

Symptoms

Symptoms of paracetamol overdose in the first 24 hours are pallor, nausea, vomiting, anorexia and abdominal pain. Liver damage may become apparent 12 to 48 hours after ingestion. Abnormalities of glucose metabolism and metabolic acidosis may occur. In severe poisoning, hepatic failure may progress to encephalopathy, haemorrhage, hypoglycaemia, cerebral oedema, and death. Acute renal failure with acute tubular necrosis, strongly suggested by loin pain, haematuria and proteinuria, may develop even in the absence of severe liver damage. Cardiac arrhythmias and pancreatitis have been reported

Managment

Immediate treatment is essential in the management of paracetamol overdose. Despite a lack of significant early symptoms, patients should be referred to hospital urgently for immediate medical attention. Symptoms may be limited to nausea or vomiting and may not reflct the severity of the overdose or the risk of organ damage. Management should be in accordance with established treatment guidelines, see BNF overdose section.

Treatment with activated charcoal should be considered if the overdose has been taken within 1 hour. Plasma paracetamol concentration should be measured at 4 hours or later after ingestion (earlier concentrations are unreliable). Treatment with N-acetylcysteine may be used up to 24 hours after ingestion of paracetamol, however, the maximum protective effect is obtained up to 8 hours post-ingestion. The effctiveness of the antidote declines sharply after this time. If required the patient should be given intravenous N-acetylcysteine, in line with the established dosage schedule. If vomiting is not a problem, oral methionine may be a suitable alternative for remote areas, outside hospital. Management of patients who present with serious hepatic dysfunction beyond 24h from ingestion should be discussed with the NPIS or a liver unit.

5. PHARMACOLOGICAL PROPERTIES

5.1 Pharmacodynamic properties

Paracetamol has analgesic and antipyretic effects similar to those of aspirin and is useful in the treatment of mild to moderate pain.

5.2 Pharmacokinetic properties

Paracetamol is rapidly and almost completely absorbed from the gastro-intestinal tract. Peak plasma concentrations are reached 30-90 minutes post dose.

Paracetamol is distributed rapidly throughout all tissues. Protein binding is low.

The plasma half-life is in the range of 1 to 4 hours after therapeutic doses.

Following therapeutic doses 90-100% of the drug is recovered in the urine within 24 hours almost entirely following hepatic conjugation with glucuronic acid (about 60%), sulphuric acid (about 35%) or cysteine (about 3%). Small amounts of hydroxylated and deacetylated metabolites have also been detected. Children have less capacity for glucuronidation of the drug than do adults. In overdose there is increased N-hydroxylation followed by glutathione conjugation. When the latter is exhausted reaction with hepatic proteins is increased leading to necrosis.

In the elderly, the rate and extent of paracetamol absorption is normal but plasma half-life is longer and paracetamol clearance is lower than in young adults.

5.3 Preclinical safety data

There are no preclinical data of relevance to the prescriber which are additional to those already included in other sections of the SPC.

6. PHARMACEUTICAL PARTICULARS

6.1 List of excipients

Mannitol

Crospovidone

Aspartame

Strawberry flavouring E. 9620941

Magnesium stearate

Polymethacrylate (Eudragit E 100)

Polyacrylate dispersion 30%

Colloidal anhydrous silica

6.2 Incompatibilities

Not applicable.

6.3 Shelf life

36 months.

6.4 Special precautions for storage

No special precautions for storage.

6.5 Nature and contents of container

Strip containing 12 tablets or 24 tablets.

The blister consists of a blister complex (Polyamide/PVC/Aluminium) and either:

an aluminium sealing sheet

or

a paper/aluminium child resistant sealing sheet.

6.6 Instructions for use and handling

None applicable.

7. MARKETING AUTHORISATION HOLDER

Pfizer Consumer Healthcare

Alternative Trading Style

Warner-Lambert Consumer Healthcare

Walton Oaks

Dorking Road

Walton-on-the-Hill

Surrey KT20 7NS

United Kingdom

8. MARKETING AUTHORISATION NUMBER(S)

PL 15513/0082

9. DATE OF FIRST AUTHORISATION/RENEWAL OF THE AUTHORISATION

19th March 2001

10. DATE OF REVISION OF THE TEXT

August 2005

Calpol Six Plus Sugar Free Suspension

(Pfizer Consumer Healthcare)

1. NAME OF THE MEDICINAL PRODUCT

Calpol Six Plus Sugar Free Suspension

2. QUALITATIVE AND QUANTITATIVE COMPOSITION

Calpol Six Plus Sugar Free Suspension contains 250 mg Paracetamol Ph Eur in each 5 ml.

3. PHARMACEUTICAL FORM

Suspension.

4. CLINICAL PARTICULARS

4.1 Therapeutic indications

Calpol Six Plus Sugar Free Suspension is indicated for the treatment of mild to moderate pain (including teething pain), and as an antipyretic.

4.2 Posology and method of administration

Posology

Adults and children 12 years and over:

Oral. The optimal dosage range is 500 mg to 1 g paracetamol, ie. 10 to 20 ml Calpol Six Plus Sugar Free Suspension (maximum 1 g), which may be repeated every 4 hours to a maximum of 4 g paracetamol/day (80 ml Calpol Six Plus Sugar Free Suspension).

Children aged 6 to 12 years:

Oral. 5 to 10 ml (250 mg to 500 mg paracetamol). Repeat every 4 hours, if necessary, up to a maximum of 4 doses per 24 hours.

Children under 6 years:

Not recommended.

Shake well before use.

The Elderly:

In the elderly, the rate and extent of paracetamol absorption is normal but plasma half-life is longer and paracetamol clearance is lower than in young adults.

4.3 Contraindications

Calpol Six Plus Sugar Free Suspension is contra-indicated in patients with known hypersensitivity to paracetamol, or any of the other components.

4.4 Special warnings and special precautions for use

Calpol Six Plus Sugar Free Suspension should be used with caution in moderate to severe renal impairment or severe hepatic impairment. The hazards of overdose are greater in those with non-cirrhotic alcoholic liver disease.

The label contains the following statements:

Keep out of reach of children.

Do not exceed the recommended dose.

Do not take more than 4 doses in 24 hours.

Leave at least 4 hours between doses

Do not give for more than 3 days without consulting a doctor.

As with all medicines, if you are currently taking any medicine consult your doctor or pharmacist before taking this product.

If symptoms persist consult your doctor.

Do not store above 25°C. Store in the original container.

Contains paracetamol.

Immediate advice should be sought in the event of an overdose, even if the child seems well. (label)

Immediate advice should be sought in the event of an overdose, even if the child seems well, because of the risk of delayed, serious liver damage. (leaflet)

Do not give with any other paracetamol-containing products.

4.5 Interaction with other medicinal products and other forms of Interaction

The speed of absorption of paracetamol may be increased by metoclopramide or domperidone and absorption reduced by colestyramine.

The anticoagulant effect of warfarin and other coumarins may be enhanced by prolonged regular use of paracetamol with increased risk of bleeding; occasional doses have no significant effect.

Chronic alcohol intake can increase the hepatotoxicity of paracetamol overdose and may have contributed to the acute pancreatitis reported in one patient who had taken an overdose of paracetamol. Acute alcohol intake may diminish an individual's ability to metabolise large doses of paracetamol, the plasma half-life of which can be prolonged.

The use of drugs that induce hepatic microsomal enzymes, such as anticonvulsants and oral contraceptives, may increase the extent of metabolism of paracetamol, resulting in reduced plasma concentrations of the drug and a faster elimination rate.

4.6 Pregnancy and lactation

Epidemiological studies in human pregnancy have shown no ill effects due to paracetamol used in the recommended dosage, but patients should follow the advice of the doctor regarding its use.

Paracetamol is excreted in breast milk but not in a clinically significant amount. Available published data do not contraindicate breast feeding.

4.7 Effects on ability to drive and use machines

None known.

4.8 Undesirable effects

Paracetamol has been widely used and, when taken at the usual recommended dosage, side effects are mild and infrequent and reports of adverse reactions are rare. Skin rash and other allergic reactions occur rarely.

There have been reports of blood dyscrasias including thrombocytopenia and agranulocystosis but these were not necessarily casually related to paracetamol.

Chronic hepatic necrosis has been reported in a patient who took daily therapeutic doses of paracetamol for about a year and liver damage has been reported after daily ingestion of excessive amounts for shorter periods. A review of a group of patients with chronic active hepatitis failed to reveal differences in the abnormalities of liver function in those who were long-term users of paracetamol nor was the control of the disease improved after paracetamol withdrawal.

Nephrotoxicity following therapeutic doses of paracetamol is uncommon. Papillary necrosis has been reported after prolonged administration.

4.9 Overdose

Immediate treatment is essential in the management of paracetamol overdose. Despite a lack of significant early symptoms, patients should be referred to hospital urgently for immediate medical attention and any patient who had ingested around 7.5 g or more of paracetamol in the preceding 4 hours should undergo gastric lavage.

Administration of oral methionine or intravenous N-acetylcysteine which may have beneficial effect up to at least 48 hours after overdose, may be required. General supportive measures must be available

Symptoms of paracetamol overdosage in the first 24 hours are pallor, nausea, vomiting, anorexia, and abdominal pain. Liver damage may become apparent 12 to 48 hours after ingestion. Abnormalities of glucose metabolism and metabolic acidosis may occur. In severe poisoning, hepatic failure may progress to encephalopathy, coma and death. Acute renal failure with acute tubular necrosis may develop even in the absence of severe liver damage. Cardiac arrhythmias and pancreatitis have been reported.

Liver damage is possible in adults who have taken 10 g or more of paracetamol.

5. PHARMACOLOGICAL PROPERTIES

5.1 Pharmacodynamic properties

Paracetamol has analgesic and antipyretic effects similar to those of aspirin and is useful in the treatment of mild to moderate pain. It has weak anti-inflammatory effects.

5.2 Pharmacokinetic properties

Paracetamol is rapidly and almost completely absorbed from the gastrointestinal tract. Peak plasma concentrations are reached 30-90 minutes post dose and the plasma half-life is in the range of 1 to 3 hours after therapeutic doses. Drug is widely distributed throughout most body fluids. Following therapeutic doses 90-100% of the drug is recovered in the urine within 24 hours almost entirely following hepatic conjugation with glucuronic acid (about 60%), sulphuric acid (about 35%) or cysteine (about 3%). Small amounts of hydroxylated and deacetylated metabolites have also been detected. Children have less capacity for glucuronidation of the drug than do adults. In overdosage there is increased N-hydroxylation followed by glutathione conjugation. When the latter is exhausted, reaction with hepatic proteins is increased leading to necrosis.

5.3 Preclinical safety data

The active constituent of this product is a well known constituent of medicinal products and its safety profile is well documented.

6. PHARMACEUTICAL PARTICULARS

6.1 List of excipients

Maltitol Liquid

Sorbitol Liquid (70% non crystallising)

Glycerol

Dispersible cellulose

Xanthan gum

Methyl parahydroxybenzoate

Propyl parahydroxybenzoate

Acesulfame potassium

Polysorbate 80

Saccharin Sodium

Strawberry flavour 500286E

Strawberry Cream 11407-33

Purified water

6.2 Incompatibilities

None known

6.3 Shelf life

24 months for the bottles.

24 months for the sachets.

6.4 Special precautions for storage

Do not store above 25°C. Store in the original container.

6.5 Nature and contents of container

10 × 5 ml aluminium foil/polyethylene laminate sachets.

70 ml, 100 ml, 140 ml, 200 ml, 500 ml and 1000 ml amber glassbottle closed with a two-piece plastic child resistant, tamper evident closure fitted with a polyethylene or polvinylidine chloride (PVDC) laminate faced wad

or

Amber glass bottle closed with a three piece plastic child resistant, tamper evident closure fitted with a polyethylene or polyvinylidene chloride (PVDC) laminate faced wad

or

Amber glass bottle closed with a plastic screw closure or metal roll-on pilfer proof closure fitted with a polyethylene or polyvinylidene chloride (PVDC) laminate faced wad.

A spoon with a 5ml measure is supplied with all packs of this product.

6.6 Instructions for use and handling

None applicable.

Administrative Data

7. MARKETING AUTHORISATION HOLDER

Pfizer Consumer Healthcare

Alternative Trading Style:

Warner-Lambert Consumer Healthcare

Walton Oaks

Dorking Road

Walton on the Hill

Surrey KT20 7NS

United Kingdom

8. MARKETING AUTHORISATION NUMBER(S)

PL 15513/0003

9. DATE OF FIRST AUTHORISATION/RENEWAL OF THE AUTHORISATION

28.04.97 / 25.05.00

10. DATE OF REVISION OF THE TEXT

January 2004

Calpol Six Plus Suspension

(Pfizer Consumer Healthcare)

1. NAME OF THE MEDICINAL PRODUCT

CALPOL SIX PLUS SUSPENSION

2. QUALITATIVE AND QUANTITATIVE COMPOSITION

CALPOL SIX PLUS SUSPENSION contains

Paracetamol Ph Eur 250 mg per 5 ml.

3. PHARMACEUTICAL FORM

Suspension for oral use.

4. CLINICAL PARTICULARS

4.1 Therapeutic indications

Calpol products are indicated for the treatment of mild to moderate pain and as an antipyretic.

4.2 Posology and method of administration

Adults: The optimal dosage range is 500 mg to 1g paracetamol, i.e. 10-20 ml

Calpol Six Plus Suspension (maximum 1g) which may be repeated every 4 hours to a maximum of 4 g paracetamol (80 ml Calpol Six Plus Suspension) per day.

6 to 12 years:

5 to 10 ml (250 mg - 500 mg paracetamol)

Children under 6 years: Not Recommended

Repeat every 4 hours if necessary up to a maximum of 4 doses per 24 hours.

Use in the Elderly

In the elderly the rate and extent of paracetamol absorption is normal but plasma half-life is longer and paracetamol clearance is lower than in young adults.

4.3 Contraindications

Calpol is contra-indicated in patients with known hypersensitivity to paracetamol and/or any other constituents.

4.4 Special warnings and special precautions for use

Care is advised in the administration of paracetamol to patients with severe renal or severe hepatic impairment. The hazards of overdose are greater in those with non-cirrhotic alcoholic liver disease.

CALPOL SIX PLUS suspension should not be diluted, where a dilution of CALPOL SIX PLUS suspension is prescribed, Calpol Infant suspension should be recommended.

The label shall contain the following statements:

Shake the bottle thoroughly.

Keep out of reach of children.

Dose 4 times a day.

Do not exceed the recommended dose.

Do not take more than 4 doses in 24 hours.

Leave at least 4 hours between doses.

Do not give for more than 3 days without consulting a doctor.

If you are currently taking any other medicine consult your doctor or pharmacist before taking this product.

If symptoms persist consult your doctor.

Do not store above 25°C.

Store in the original container.

Contains paracetamol.

Immediate medical advice should be sought in the event of an overdose, even if the child seems well. (label)

Immediate medical advice should be sought in the event of an overdose, even if the child seems well, because of the risk of delayed, serious liver damage (leaflet).

Do not give with any other paracetamol-containing products.

4.5 Interaction with other medicinal products and other forms of Interaction

The speed of absorption of paracetamol may be increased by metoclopramide or domperidone and absorption reduced by colestyramine.

The anticoagulant effect of warfarin and other coumarins may be enhanced by prolonged regular use of paracetamol with increased risk of bleeding; occasional doses have no significant effect.

Chronic alcohol intake can increase the hepatotoxicity of paracetamol overdose and may have contributed to the acute pancreatitis reported in one patient who had taken an overdose of paracetamol. Acute alcohol intake may diminish an individual's ability to metabolise large doses of paracetamol, the plasma half-life of which can be prolonged.

The use of drugs that induce hepatic microsomal enzymes, such as anticonvulsants and oral contraceptives, may increase the extent of metabolism of paracetamol, resulting in reduced plasma concentrations of the drug and a faster elimination rate.

4.6 Pregnancy and lactation

Epidemiological studies in human pregnancy have shown no ill effects due to paracetamol used in the recommended dosage, but patients should follow the advice of their doctor regarding its use.

Paracetamol is excreted in breast milk but not in a clinically significant amount. Available published data do not contra-indicate breast feeding.

4.7 Effects on ability to drive and use machines
None known

4.8 Undesirable effects
Adverse effects of paracetamol are rare but hypersensitivity including skin rash may occur. There have been reports of blood dyscreasis including thrombocytopenia and agranulocystosis but these were not necessarily causality related to paracetamol.

Most reports of adverse reactions to paracetamol relate to overdosage with the drug.

Chronic hepatic necrosis has been reported in a patient who took daily therapeutic doses of paracetamol for about a year and liver damage has been reported after daily ingestion of excessive amounts for shorter periods. A review of a group of patients with chronic active hepatitis failed to reveal differences in the abnormalities of liver function in those who were long-term users of paracetamol nor was the control of their disease improved after paracetamol withdrawal.

Nephrotoxicity following therapeutic doses of paracetamol is uncommon, but papillary necrosis has been reported after prolonged administration.

4.9 Overdose
Immediate treatment is essential in the management of paracetamol overdose. Despite a lack of significant early symptoms, patients should be referred to hospital urgently for immediate medical attention and any patient who had ingested around 7.5 g or more of paracetamol in the preceding 4 hours should undergo gastric lavage.

Administration of oral methionine or intravenous N-acetylcysteine which may have beneficial effect up to at least 48 hours after overdose, may be required. General supportive measures must be available

Symptoms of paracetamol overdosage in the first 24 hours are pallor, nausea, vomiting, anorexia, and abdominal pain. Liver damage may become apparent 12 to 48 hours after ingestion. Abnormalities of glucose metabolism and metabolic acidosis may occur. In severe poisoning, hepatic failure may progress to encephalopathy, coma and death. Acute renal failure with acute tubular necrosis may develop even in the absence of severe liver damage. Cardiac arrhythmias and pancreatitis have been reported.

Liver damage is possible in adults who have taken 10 g or more of paracetamol.

5. PHARMACOLOGICAL PROPERTIES

5.1 Pharmacodynamic properties
Paracetamol has analgesic and antipyretic effects similar to those of aspirin and is useful in the treatment of mild to moderate pain. It has only weak anti-inflammatory effects.

5.2 Pharmacokinetic properties
Paracetamol is rapidly and almost completely absorbed from the gastro-intestinal tract. Peak plasma concentrations are reached 30-90 minutes post dose and the plasma half-life is in the range of 1 to 3 hours after therapeutic doses. Drug is widely distributed throughout most body fluids following therapeutic doses 90-100% of the drug is recovered in the urine within 24 hours almost entirely following hepatic conjugation with glucuronic acid (about 60%), sulphuric acid (about 35%) or cysteine (about 3%). Small amounts of hydroxylated and deacetylated metabolites have also been detected. Children have less capacity for glucuronidation of the drug than do adults. In overdosage there is increased N-hydroxylation followed by glutathione conjugation. When the latter is exhausted reaction with hepatic proteins is increased leading to necrosis.

5.3 Preclinical safety data
The active ingredient of this product is a well known constituent of medicinal products and its safety profile is well documented.

6. PHARMACEUTICAL PARTICULARS

6.1 List of excipients
Sucrose
Sorbitol Solution
Glycerol
Dispersible Cellulose
Polysorbate 80
Flavour, white sugar DA 13780
Flavour, Orange 510652E
Methyl Hydroxybenzoate
F,D and C Yellow No. 6 Soluble/Sunset Yellow FCF, E110
Purified Water

6.2 Incompatibilities
None known

6.3 Shelf life
36 months unopened

6.4 Special precautions for storage
Do not store above 25C
Store in the original container.

6.5 Nature and contents of container
100 ml, 140 ml, 200 ml, 500 ml and 1000 ml amber glass bottle with plastic screw cap fitted with a polyethylene or polyvinylidene (PVDC) laminate faced wad,

or

amber glass bottle closed with a two-piece plastic child resistant, tamper evident closure fitted with a polyethylene or polyvinylidene chloride (PVDC) laminate faced wad,

or

Amber glass bottle closed with a three-piece plastic child resistant, tamper evident closure fitted with a polyethylene or polyvinylidene chloride (PVDC) laminate faced wad.

and

10 × 5 ml Paper /aluminium foil/surlyn sachets

A spoon with a 5 ml measure is supplied with all packs of this product.

6.6 Instructions for use and handling
None applicable

Administrative Data

7. MARKETING AUTHORISATION HOLDER
Pfizer Consumer Healthcare

Alternative Trading Style:
Warner-Lambert Consumer Healthcare
Walton Oaks
Dorking Road
Walton-on-the-Hill
Surrey KT20 7NS
United Kingdom

8. MARKETING AUTHORISATION NUMBER(S)
15513/0002

9. DATE OF FIRST AUTHORISATION/RENEWAL OF THE AUTHORISATION
28 April 1997 / 13 June 2000

10. DATE OF REVISION OF THE TEXT
August 2004

Calpol Sugar Free Infant Suspension

(Pfizer Consumer Healthcare)

1. NAME OF THE MEDICINAL PRODUCT
CALPOL Sugar Free Infant suspension

2. QUALITATIVE AND QUANTITATIVE COMPOSITION
CALPOL Sugar Free Infant suspension contains 120 mg Paracetamol in each 5 ml.

3. PHARMACEUTICAL FORM
Suspension.

4. CLINICAL PARTICULARS

4.1 Therapeutic indications
CALPOL Sugar Free Infant suspension is indicated for the treatment of mild to moderate pain (including teething pain), and as an antipyretic (including post immunisation fever).

4.2 Posology and method of administration

Children aged 1 to under 6 years:
Oral. 5 to 10 ml (120 mg to 240 mg paracetamol). Repeat every 4 hours, if necessary, up to a maximum of 4 doses per 24 hours.

Infants 3 months to under 1 year:
Oral. 2.5 to 5 ml (60 mg to 120 mg paracetamol). Repeat every 4 hours, if necessary, up to a maximum of 4 doses per 24 hours.

Infants aged 2 – 3 months:
Oral. A 2.5 ml (60 mg paracetamol) dose for babies who develop post-vaccination fever at 2 months followed, if necessary, by a second dose 4 to 6 hours later. The same 2 doses may be given for other causes of fever or mild to moderate pain provided the infant weighs over 4 kg and was not born before 37 weeks gestation. Medical advice should be sought promptly if further doses are required or if the cause of the infant's fever or pain is not known.

The Elderly:
In the elderly, the rate and extent of paracetamol absorption is normal but plasma half-life is longer and paracetamol clearance is lower than in young adults.

4.3 Contraindications
CALPOL Sugar Free Infant suspension is contra-indicated in patients with known hypersensitivity to paracetamol, or any of the other components.

4.4 Special warnings and special precautions for use
CALPOL Sugar Free Infant suspension should be used with caution in the presence of severe renal impairment or severe hepatic impairment.

The hazards of overdose are greater in those with non-cirrhotic alcoholic liver disease.

Concomitant use of other paracetamol-containing products should be avoided.

The label contains the following statements:
Shake the bottle thoroughly.
Keep out of the reach and sight of children.
Do not exceed the stated dose.
Do not take more than 4 doses in 24 hours.
Leave at least 4 hours between doses.
Do not give for more than 3 days without consulting a doctor.
If you are currently taking any medicine consult your doctor or pharmacist before taking this product.
If symptoms persist consult your doctor.
Do not store above 25°C. Keep container in outer carton.
Contains paracetamol.
Immediate medical advice should be sought in the event of an overdose, even if the child seems well. (label)
Immediate medical advice should be sought in the event of an overdose, even if the child seems well, because of the risk of delayed, serious liver damage. (leaflet)
Do not give with any other paracetamol-containing products.

4.5 Interaction with other medicinal products and other forms of Interaction
The speed of absorption of paracetamol may be increased by metoclopramide or domperidone and absorption reduced by colestyramine.

The anticoagulant effect of warfarin and other coumarins may be enhanced by prolonged regular use of paracetamol with increased risk of bleeding; occasional doses have no significant effect.

Chronic alcohol intake can increase the hepatotoxicity of paracetamol overdose and may have contributed to the acute pancreatitis reported in one patient who had taken an overdose of paracetamol. Acute alcohol intake may diminish an individual's ability to metabolise large doses of paracetamol, the plasma half-life of which can be prolonged.

The use of drugs that induce hepatic microsomal enzymes, such as anticonvulsants and oral contraceptives, may increase the extent of metabolism of paracetamol, resulting in reduced plasma concentrations of the drug and a faster elimination rate.

4.6 Pregnancy and lactation
Epidemiological studies in human pregnancy have shown no ill effects due to paracetamol used in the recommended dosage, but patients should follow the advice of their doctor regarding its use.

Paracetamol is excreted in breast milk but not in a clinically significant amount. Available published data do not contra-indicate breast feeding.

4.7 Effects on ability to drive and use machines
None known.

4.8 Undesirable effects
Adverse effects of paracetamol are rare but hypersensitivity including skin rash may occur. There have been reports of blood dyscrasias including thrombocytopenia and agranulocytosis but these were not necessarily causality related to paracetamol.

Most reports of adverse reactions to paracetamol relate to overdose with the drug.

Chronic hepatic necrosis has been reported in a patient who took daily therapeutic doses of paracetamol for about a year and liver damage has been reported after daily ingestion of excessive amounts for shorter periods. A review of a group of patients with chronic active hepatitis failed to reveal differences in the abnormalities of liver function in those who were long-term users of paracetamol nor was the control of their disease improved after paracetamol withdrawal.

Nephrotoxicity following therapeutic doses of paracetamol is uncommon, but papillary necrosis has been reported after prolonged administration.

4.9 Overdose
Liver damage is possible in adults who have taken 10 g or more of paracetamol. Ingestion of 5g or more of paracetamol may lead to liver damage if the patient has risk factors (see below).

Risk Factors:
If the patient

a, Is on long term treatment with carbamezipine, phenobarbital, phenytoin, primidone, rifampicin, St John's Wort or other drugs that induce liver enzymes.

Or

b, Regularly consumes ethanol in excess of recommended amounts.

Or

c, Is likely to be glutathione deplete e.g. eating disorders, cystic fibrosis, HIV infection, starvation, cachexia.

Symptoms
Symptoms of paracetamol overdosage in the first 24 hours are pallor, nausea, vomiting, anorexia, and abdominal pain. Liver damage may become apparent 12 to 48 hours after ingestion. Abnormalities of glucose metabolism and metabolic acidosis may occur. In severe poisoning, hepatic

failure may progress to encephalopathy, haemorrhage, hypoglycaemia, cerebral oedema, and death. Acute renal failure with acute tubular necrosis, strongly suggested by loin pain, haematuria and proteinuria, may develop even in the absence of severe liver damage. Cardiac arrhythmias and pancreatitis have been reported.

Management

Immediate treatment is essential in the management of paracetamol overdose. Despite a lack of significant early symptoms, patients should be referred to hospital urgently for immediate medical attention. Symptoms may be limited to nausea or vomiting and may not reflect the severity of overdose or the risk of organ damage. Management should be in accordance with established treatment guidelines, see BNF overdose section.

Treatment with activated charcoal should be considered if the overdose has been taken within 1 hour. Plasma paracetamol concentration should be measured at 4 hours or later after ingestion (earlier concentrations are unreliable). Treatment with N-acetylcysteine may be used up to 24 hours after ingestion of paracetamol, however, the maximum protective effect is obtained up to 8 hours post-ingestion. The effectiveness of the antidote declines sharply after this time. If required the patient should be given intravenous N-acetylcysteine, in line with the established dosage schedule. If vomiting is not a problem, oral methionine may be a suitable alternative for remote areas, outside hospital. Management of patients who present with serious hepatic dysfunction beyond 24h from ingestion should be discussed with the NPIS or a liver unit.

5. PHARMACOLOGICAL PROPERTIES

5.1 Pharmacodynamic properties

Paracetamol has analgesic and antipyretic effects similar to those of aspirin and is useful in the treatment of mild to moderate pain. It has only weak anti-inflammatory effects.

5.2 Pharmacokinetic properties

Paracetamol is rapidly and almost completely absorbed from the gastrointestinal tract. Peak plasma concentrations are reached 30-90 minutes post dose and the plasma half-life is in the range of 1 to 3 hours after therapeutic doses. Drug is widely distributed throughout most body fluids. Following therapeutic doses 90-100% of the drug is recovered in the urine within 24 hours almost entirely following hepatic conjugation with glucuronic acid (about 60%), sulphuric acid (about 35%) or cysteine (about 3%). Small amounts of hydroxylated and deacetylated metabolites have also been detected. Children have less capacity for glucuronidation of the drug than do adults. In overdosage there is increased N-hydroxylation followed by glutathione conjugation. When the latter is exhausted, reaction with hepatic proteins is increased leading to necrosis.

5.3 Preclinical safety data

The active ingredient of this product is a well known constituent of medicinal products and its safety profile is well documented.

6. PHARMACEUTICAL PARTICULARS

6.1 List of excipients

Maltitol liquid

Sorbitol solution (70% non crystallising)

Glycerol

Dispersible cellulose

Xanthan gum

Ethyl parahydroxybenzoate (E214)

Methyl parahydroxybenzoate (E218)

Propyl parahydroxybenzoate (E216)

Polysorbate 80

Strawberry flavour

Carmoisine (E122)

Purified water

6.2 Incompatibilities

None known

6.3 Shelf life

36 months for the amber glass bottles and 24 months for the 5 ml paper/PE/foil/surlyn sachets.

6.4 Special precautions for storage

Do not store above 25°C. Keep container in outer carton.

6.5 Nature and contents of container

5 ml sachet composed of a laminate made of paper/PE/Aluminium/Surlyn. Pack sizes 4, 6, 10, 12 or 20 sachets. A spoon with a 5 ml and 2.5 ml measure is supplied with this pack.

or

5 ml sachet composed of a laminate made of paper/PE/Aluminium/Surlyn. Pack sizes 4 or 6 sachets presented in a Polypropylene carry case. A spoon with a 5 ml and 2.5 ml measure is supplied with this pack.

Amber glass bottle with plastic screw cap, a polyethylene or polyvinylidene chloride (PVDC) laminate faced wad.

or

Amber glass bottle with a two-piece plastic child resistant, tamper evident closure fitted with a polyethylene or polyvinylidene chloride (PVDC) laminate faced wad.

or

Amber glass bottle with a three-piece plastic child resistant, tamper evident closure fitted with a polyethylene or polyvinylidene chloride (PVDC) laminate faced wad.

Pack sizes

30 ml, 70ml, 140 ml, 200 ml and 1000ml. A spoon with a 5 ml and 2.5 ml measure is supplied with this pack.

1000 ml amber glass bottle with an aluminium cap fitted with a polyethylene wad.

6.6 Instructions for use and handling

None applicable.

7. MARKETING AUTHORISATION HOLDER

Pfizer Consumer Healthcare

Alternative Trading Style:

Warner-Lambert Consumer Healthcare

Walton Oaks

Dorking Road

Walton-on-the-Hill

Surrey KT20 7NS

United Kingdom

8. MARKETING AUTHORISATION NUMBER(S)

PL 15513/0006

9. DATE OF FIRST AUTHORISATION/RENEWAL OF THE AUTHORISATION

28 April 1997 / 13th September 2004

10. DATE OF REVISION OF THE TEXT

May 2005

Calprofen

(Pfizer Consumer Healthcare)

1. NAME OF THE MEDICINAL PRODUCT

Fenpaed 100 mg/5 ml Oral Suspension

Calprofen

Enterprise Ibuprofen 100 mg/5 ml Oral Suspension

2. QUALITATIVE AND QUANTITATIVE COMPOSITION

Ibuprofen 100 mg / 5ml

For excipients - see section 6.1

3. PHARMACEUTICAL FORM

Oral Suspension

Sugar Free, Colour Free and Strawberry Flavour

4. CLINICAL PARTICULARS

4.1 Therapeutic indications

Prescription and OTC:

Ibuprofen 100 mg / 5 ml Oral Suspension is used as an analgesic for relief of mild to moderate muscular pain, symptomatic relief of headache, earache, dental pain and backache. It can also be used in minor injuries such as sprains and strains. Ibuprofen 100 mg / 5 ml Oral Suspension is effective in the relief of feverishness and symptoms of colds and influenza.

Prescription Only:

Ibuprofen 100 mg / 5 ml Oral Suspension is indicated for its analgesic and anti-inflammatory effects in the treatment of dysmenorrhoea, neuralgia, post-operative pain, rheumatoid arthritis (including juvenile rheumatoid arthritis or Still's disease), ankylosing spondylitis, osteoarthritis and other non-rheumatoid (seronegative) arthropathies.

In the treatment of non-articular rheumatic conditions, Ibuprofen 100 mg / 5 ml Oral Suspension is indicated for periarticular conditions such as frozen shoulder (capsulitis), bursitis, tendonitis, tenosynovitis and low back pain. Ibuprofen 100 mg / 5 ml Oral Suspension can also be used in soft tissue injuries such as sprains and strains.

4.2 Posology and method of administration

For oral administration.

Adults: The recommended dosage of Ibuprofen 100 mg / 5 ml Oral Suspension is 1200-1800 mg daily in divided doses. Some patients can be maintained on 600-1200 mg daily. In severe or acute conditions, it can be advantageous to increase the dosage until the acute phase is brought under control, provided the total daily dose does not exceed 2400mg in divided doses.

Children: Not recommended for children weighing less than 7 kg.

For pain and fever - 20mg/kg/day in divided doses (including OTC use).

Infants 6-12 months: 2.5ml three times a day.

Children 1-2 years: 2.5ml three to four times a day

Children 3-7 years: 5ml three to four times a day

Children 8-12 years: 10ml three to four times a day.

For Juvenile Rheumatoid Arthritis (prescription only use): Doses up to 30-40mg/kg/day may be taken in three or four divided doses.

Elderly: No special dosage modifications are required unless renal or hepatic function is impaired, in which case dosage should be assessed individually.

4.3 Contraindications

Hypersensitivity to Ibuprofen or any of the other constituents.

Patients with current or previous history of peptic ulceration.

Patients in whom Ibuprofen, Aspirin or other non-steroidal anti-inflammatory drugs induce symptoms of Asthma, Rhinitis or Urticaria.

4.4 Special warnings and special precautions for use

The elderly are at an increased risk of the serious consequences of adverse reactions.

Administration of NSAID'S such as Ibuprofen may cause dose dependent renal toxicity in patients with reduced renal blood flow or blood volume where renal prostaglandins support the maintainance of renal perfusion.

Patients at risk of this reaction include those with impaired renal function, heart failure or liver dysfunction. Caution is therefore required in the use of Ibuprofen in such patients. Ibuprofen inhibits platelet aggregation and prolongs bleeding time, although the effect is less pronounced than that seen with Aspirin. Ibuprofen should be used with caution in patients with coagulation defects and those on anticoagulant therapy.

Ibuprofen should be used with caution in patients with bronchial asthma or allergic disease, since such patients may have NSAID – sensitive asthma which has been associated with severe bronchospasm.

Additional Warnings for OTC use

If symptoms persist for more than 3 days, consult your doctor.

Do not exceed the stated dose.

Not recommended for children under 6 months.

4.5 Interaction with other medicinal products and other forms of Interaction

Care should be taken in patients treated with any of the following drugs as interactions have been reported in some patients.

Antihypertensives: reduced anti-hypertensive effect.

Diurectics: reduced diuretic effect. Diurectics can increase the risk of nephrotoxicity of NSAIDs.

Cardiac Glycosides: NSAIDs may exacerbate cardiac failure, reduce GFR and increase plasma cardiac glycoside levels.

Lithium: Decreased elimination of Lithium.

Methotrexate: decreased elimination of methotrexate.

Cyclosporin: increased risk of nephrotoxicity with NSAIDs.

Mifepristone: NSAIDs should not be used for 8-12 days after mifepristone administration as NSAIDs can reduce the effects of mifepristone.

Other analgesics: avoid concomitant use of two or more NSAIDs or concurrent use of asprin.

Corticosteroids: increased risk of gastrointestinal bleeding.

Anticoagulants: enhanced anticoagulant effect.

Quinolone antibiotics: animal data indicate that NSAIDs can increase the risk of convulsions associated with quinolone antibiotics. Patients taking NSAIDs and quinolones may have an increased risk of developing convulsions.

4.6 Pregnancy and lactation

The onset of labour may be delayed and the duration of labour increased.

Whilst no teratogenic effects have been demonstrated in animal experiments, the use of Ibuprofen during pregnancy should, if possible, be avoided. Congenital abnormalities have been reported in association with ibuprofen administration in man; however, these are low in frequency and do not appear to follow any discernible pattern. In view of the known side effects of NSAIDs on the foetal cardiovascular system (closure of ductus arteriosus), use in late pregnancy should be avoided.

In the limited studies so far available, ibuprofen appears in breast milk in very low concentrations and is unlikely to affect the breast-fed infant adversely.

4.7 Effects on ability to drive and use machines

No adverse effects known.

4.8 Undesirable effects

Adverse effects occurring most commonly with Ibuprofen are gastrointestinal disturbances such as abdominal pain, nausea, vomiting, diarrhoea, constipation, dyspepsia, melaena and haematemesis. Occasionally peptic ulceration and gastrointestinal bleeding and less frequently, gastritis, duodenal ulcer, gastric ulcer and gastrointestinal perforation have been reported. Epidemiological data indicate that ibuprofen presents the lowest risk of upper gastrointestinal toxicity of the seven most widely used oral NSAIDs.

Hypersensitivity reactions reported consist of

I. non-specific allergic reaction and anaphylaxis,

II. respiratory tract reactions of asthma, aggravated asthma, bronchospasm or dyspnoea

III. assorted skin disorders, including rashes of various types, pruritis, urticaria, purpura, angioedema and less commonly bullous dermatoses including exfoliative dermatitis, epidermal necrolysis and erythema multiforme.

Cardiovascular: Oedema has been reported following ibuprofen treatment.

Other adverse reactions for which the cause has not necessarily been established include the following.

Renal: Nephrotoxicity in various forms, including interstitial nephritis, papillary necrosis, nephrotic syndrome and renal failure.

Hepatic: Abnormal liver function, hepatitis and jaundice.

Neurological and sensory: Visual disturbance, optic neuritis, headaches, paraesthesia, depression, confusion, hallucinations, tinnitus, vertigo, dizziness, malaise, fatigue and drowsiness.

Hematological: thrombocytopenia, neutropenia, agranulocytosis, aplastic anaemia and haemolytic anaemia.

Dermatological: photosensitivity (for other skin reactions see 'hypersensitivity')

4.9 Overdose

Symptoms of overdose include headache, nausea, vomiting, drowsiness, hypotension and loss of conciousness.

Treatment of overdosage should include gastric lavage and, if necessary, correction of serum electrolytes and appropriate supportive measures.

There is no specific antidote to Ibuprofen.

5. PHARMACOLOGICAL PROPERTIES

5.1 Pharmacodynamic properties

Ibuprofen is a Phenylpropionic Acid derivative, which has analgesic anti-inflammatory and antipyretic actions. These actions are thought to be from its inhibitory effect on the enzyme cyclo-oxygenase which results in a reduction in prostaglandin synthesis.

5.2 Pharmacokinetic properties

Ibuprofen is absorbed from the gastro-intestinal tract and peak plasma concentrations occur about 1 to 2 hours after ingestion. The elimination half-life is about 2 hours.

It is metabolised to two inactive metabolites and these are rapidly excreted in urine. About 1 percent is excreted in urine as unchanged Ibuprofen and about 14 percent as conjugated Ibuprofen.

Ibuprofen is extensively bound to plasma proteins.

5.3 Preclinical safety data

No relevant information additional to that contained elsewhere in the SPC.

6. PHARMACEUTICAL PARTICULARS

6.1 List of excipients

Glycerol (E422), xanthan gum, maltitol syrup (Lycasin 80/55 (E965)), polysorbate 80, saccharin sodium (E954), citric acid monohydrate, sodium methylhydroxybenzoate, sodium propylhydroxybenzoate, purified water and strawberry flavour.

6.2 Incompatibilities

None stated except as in 'Interactions with other medicaments'.

6.3 Shelf life

24 months.

6.4 Special precautions for storage

Do not store above 25°C.

Keep out of reach and sight of children

6.5 Nature and contents of container

An amber glass bottle sealed with child resistant, tamper evident cap.

Pack sizes available: 50ml,100ml,150ml and 500 ml.

A HDPE bottle with tamper evident cap.

Pack size available: 500 ml.

6.6 Instructions for use and handling

Shake well before use. Return any left over medicine to the Pharmacist.

7. MARKETING AUTHORISATION HOLDER

Pinewood Laboratories Limited

Ballymacarbry,

Clonmel,

Co. Tipperary,

Ireland.

8. MARKETING AUTHORISATION NUMBER(S)

PL 04917/0044

9. DATE OF FIRST AUTHORISATION/RENEWAL OF THE AUTHORISATION

22nd March 2002

10. DATE OF REVISION OF THE TEXT

December 2002

Camcolit 250

(Norgine Limited)

1. NAME OF THE MEDICINAL PRODUCT

Camcolit 250mg, Lithium Carbonate

2. QUALITATIVE AND QUANTITATIVE COMPOSITION

The active ingredient is Lithium Carbonate; 250 mg/tablet.

3. PHARMACEUTICAL FORM

White film, coated tablets, engraved "CAMCOLIT" around one face and having a breakline on the reverse. For oral administration.

4. CLINICAL PARTICULARS

4.1 Therapeutic indications

The treatment and prophylaxis of mania, manic-depressive illness and recurrent depression, and the treatment of aggressive or self mutilating behaviour.

4.2 Posology and method of administration

Regular monitoring of plasma lithium concentration is always obligatory when lithium is used; lithium therapy should not be initiated unless adequate facilities for routine monitoring of plasma concentrations are available. On initiation of therapy plasma concentrations should be measured weekly until stabilisation is achieved, then weekly for one month and at monthly intervals thereafter. Additional measurements should be made if signs of lithium toxicity occur, on dosage alteration, development of significant intercurrent disease, signs of manic or depressive relapse and if significant change in sodium or fluid intake occurs. More frequent monitoring is required if patients are receiving any drug treatment that affects renal clearance of lithium e.g. diuretics and NSAID. As bioavailability may vary between formulations, should a change of preparation be made, blood levels should be monitored weekly until restabilisation is achieved.

Acute mania: Treatment should be initiated in hospital where regular monitoring of plasma lithium levels can be conducted. The dosage of Camcolit should be adjusted to produce a plasma lithium level between 0.6 and 1.0 mmol/l 12 hours after the last dose. The required plasma lithium level may be achieved in one of two ways but, whichever is adopted, regular estimations must be carried out to ensure maintenance of levels within the therapeutic range. For consistent results it is essential that the blood samples for plasma lithium estimations are taken 12 hours after the last dose of lithium.

1. 1,000-1,500 mg of lithium carbonate are administered daily for the first five days. A blood sample for plasma lithium estimation is taken 12 hours after the last dose on the fifth day, and the dosage of Camcolit is adjusted to keep the plasma lithium level within the therapeutic range. Subsequently, regular plasma lithium estimations must be carried out and, where necessary, the dosage of Camcolit adjusted accordingly. The precise initial dose of lithium should be decided in the light of the age and weight of the patient; young patients often require a dose higher than average and older patients a lower dose.

2. A lithium clearance test is carried out and the initial dosage calculated from the results. Even when the initial dosage is calculated in this way, it is still desirable that plasma lithium levels should be determined at weekly intervals during the first three weeks of treatment, and any necessary adjustments to dosage made as a result of the levels actually obtained.

Most of the above applies in the treatment of hypomania as well as mania, but the patient (if not too ill) can be started on treatment as an outpatient provided that facilities for regular plasma lithium monitoring are available, and assays are initiated within one week.

Prophylaxis of recurrent affective disorders: (Including unipolar mania & unipolar depressions and bipolar manic-depressive illness): A low dose of 300-400 mg of lithium carbonate can be administered daily for the first seven days. A blood sample for plasma lithium estimation is then taken 12 hours after the last dose, and the dosage of Camcolit is adjusted to keep the plasma lithium level within the range of 0.4-0.8 mmol/l. Toxic symptoms are usually associated with concentrations exceeding 1.5 mmol/l.

Use in elderly: As for prophylaxis above, but 12 hour lithium levels should be kept in the range of 0.4-0.7 mmol/l as toxic symptoms are likely with plasma concentrations above 1.0 mmol/l.

Use in children: Not recommended.

4.3 Contraindications

Patients with renal disease, cardiovascular disease, Addison's disease or those breast feeding.

4.4 Special warnings and special precautions for use

Pre-treatment and periodic routine clinical monitoring is essential. This should include assessment of renal function, urine analysis, assessment of thyroid function and cardiac function, especially in patients with cardiovascular disease.

Patients should be euthyroid before initiation of lithium therapy.

Clear instructions regarding the symptoms of impending toxicity should be given by the doctor to all patients receiving long-term lithium therapy.

Patients should also be warned to report if polyuria or polydipsia develop. Episodes of nausea and vomiting or other conditions leading to salt/water depletion (including severe dieting) should also be reported. Patients should be advised to maintain their usual salt and fluid intake.

Elderly patients are particularly liable to lithium toxicity.

4.5 Interaction with other medicinal products and other forms of Interaction

Lower doses of lithium may be required during diuretic therapy as lithium clearance is reduced.

Serum lithium concentrations may increase during concomitant therapy with non-steroidal anti-inflammatory drugs or tetracycline, possibly resulting in lithium toxicity. Serum lithium concentrations therefore should be monitored more frequently if NSAID or tetracycline therapy is initiated or discontinued.

Raised plasma levels of ADH may occur during treatment.

Symptoms of nephrogenic diabetes insipidus are particularly prevalent in patients receiving concurrent treatment with tricyclic or tetracyclic anti-depressants.

4.6 Pregnancy and lactation

Pregnancy: There is epidemiological evidence to suggest that the drug may be harmful during human pregnancy. Should the use of lithium be unavoidable, close monitoring of serum concentrations should be made throughout pregnancy and parturition.

Lactation: Infants of mothers on lithium should be bottle fed as lithium is present in the breast milk.

4.7 Effects on ability to drive and use machines

None known.

4.8 Undesirable effects

Long term treatment with lithium may result in permanent changes in the kidney and impairment of renal function. High serum concentrations of lithium, including episodes of acute lithium toxicity may enhance these changes. The minimum clinically effective dose of lithium should always be used. Patients should only be maintained on lithium after 3-5 years if, on assessment, benefit persists.

Renal function should be routinely monitored in patients with polyuria and polydipsia.

Side effects are usually related to serum lithium concentrations and are infrequent at levels below 1.0 mmol/l.

Mild gastro-intestinal effects, nausea, vertigo, muscle weakness and a dazed feeling may occur, but frequently disappear after stabilisation. Fine hand tremors, polyuria and mild thirst may persist. Some studies suggest that the tremor can be controlled by relatively small doses of propranolol.

Long term treatment with lithium is frequently associated with disturbances of thyroid function including goitre and hypothyroidism. These can be controlled by administration of small doses of thyroxine (0.05-0.2 mg daily) concomitantly with lithium. Thyrotoxicosis has also been reported.

Mild cognitive impairment may occur during long term use.

Hypercalcaemia, hypermagnesaemia, hyperparathyroidism and an increase in antinuclear antibodies have also been reported.

Exacerbation of psoriasis may occur.

Cardiovascular effects of lithium are rare and often benign. Reported effects are arrhythmia, oedema, and sinus node dysfunction. Any signs of cardiac disturbance e.g. syncope, heart rhythm or rate disturbances should be investigated further.

Oedema with weight gain can occur and may lead to an increased risk of lithium toxicity if treated incautiously with diuretic drugs.

4.9 Overdose

Appearance or aggravation of gasto-intestinal symptoms, muscle weakness, lack of co-ordination, drowsiness or lethargy may be early signs of intoxication. With increasing toxicity, ataxia, giddiness, tinnitus, blurred vision, coarse tremor, muscle twitching and a large output of dilute urine may be seen. At blood levels above 2-3 mmol/l, increasing disorientation, seizures, coma and death may occur.

There is no antidote to lithium poisoning. In the event, lithium treatment should be stopped immediately and serum lithium levels estimated every 6 hours. When ingestion is recent, gastric lavage should be carried out, together with general supportive measures. Special attention must be given to the maintenance of fluid and electrolyte balance, and also adequate renal function. Sodium-depleting diuretics should not be used in any circumstances. Forced alkaline diuresis may be used. If the serum lithium level is above 4.0 mmol/l, or if there is a deterioration in the patient's condition, or if the serum lithium concentration is not falling at a rate equivalent to a half-life of less than 30 hours, peritoneal dialysis or haemodialysis should be instituted promptly. This should be continued until the serum and dialysis fluid are free of lithium. Serum lithium levels should be monitored for at least another 7 days thereafter, as a rebound rise is possible due to delayed diffusion from the tissues.

5. PHARMACOLOGICAL PROPERTIES

5.1 Pharmacodynamic properties

The precise mechanism of action of lithium as a mood-stabilising agent remains unknown, although many cellular actions of lithium have been characterised.

5.2 Pharmacokinetic properties

The pharmacokinetics of lithium are extremely well documented. A single oral dose of CAMCOLIT 250 gives a peak plasma level approximately 2-3 hours later, with the level at 24 hours being approximately 40% of peak levels.

5.3 Preclinical safety data

There is no preclinical data of relevance to the prescriber.

6. PHARMACEUTICAL PARTICULARS

6.1 List of excipients

Maize Starch

Magnesium Stearate

Pregelatinised Maize Starch

Hypromellose

Macrogol 400

6.2 Incompatibilities

See 4.5 and 4.8 above.

6.3 Shelf life

The shelf life is 5 years.

6.4 Special precautions for storage

Do not store above 25°C. Keep container tightly closed. Keep out of reach and sight of children.

6.5 Nature and contents of container

Polypropylene containers of 100 or 1000 tablet capacity, and for hospital use only, screw-cap amber glass bottles of 50 or 100 tablet capacity.

6.6 Instructions for use and handling

None.

7. MARKETING AUTHORISATION HOLDER

Norgine Limited

Chaplin House, Widewater Place

Moorhall Road, Harefield

UXBRIDGE

Middlesex UB9 6NS, UK

8. MARKETING AUTHORISATION NUMBER(S)

PL 00322/5900R

9. DATE OF FIRST AUTHORISATION/RENEWAL OF THE AUTHORISATION

February 2003

10. DATE OF REVISION OF THE TEXT

25th January 2005

Legal Category: **POM**

Camcolit 400

(Norgine Limited)

1. NAME OF THE MEDICINAL PRODUCT

Camcolit 400 mg, controlled release Lithium Carbonate.

The product may also be sold as LITHONATE.

2. QUALITATIVE AND QUANTITATIVE COMPOSITION

The active ingredient is Lithium Carbonate; 400 mg/tablet.

3. PHARMACEUTICAL FORM

White film coated tablet, engraved "CAMCOLIT-S" around one face and having a breakline on the reverse. The tablet is a controlled release formulation. If sold as LITHONATE the tablet is engraved on one side "LIT 400".

For oral administration.

4. CLINICAL PARTICULARS

4.1 Therapeutic indications

The treatment and prophylaxis of mania, manic-depressive illness and recurrent depression, and the treatment of aggressive or self mutilating behaviour.

4.2 Posology and method of administration

Regular monitoring of plasma lithium concentration is always obligatory when lithium is used; lithium therapy should not be initiated unless adequate facilities for routine monitoring of plasma concentrations are available. On initiation of therapy plasma concentrations should be measured weekly until stabilisation is achieved, then weekly for one month and at monthly intervals thereafter. Additional measurements should be made if signs of lithium toxicity occur, on dosage alteration, development of significant intercurrent disease, signs of manic or depressive relapse and if significant change in sodium or fluid intake occurs. More frequent monitoring is required if patients are receiving any drug treatment that affects renal clearance of lithium e.g. diuretics and NSAID. As bioavailability may vary between formulations, should a change of preparation be made, blood levels should be monitored weekly until restabilisation is achieved.

Acute mania: Treatment should be initiated in hospital where regular monitoring of plasma lithium levels can be conducted. The dosage of Camcolit should be adjusted to produce a plasma lithium level between 0.6 and 1.0 mmol/l 12 hours after the last dose. The required plasma lithium level may be achieved in one of two ways but, whichever is adopted, regular estimations must be carried out to ensure maintenance of levels within the therapeutic range. For consistent results it is essential that the blood sample for plasma lithium estimations are taken 12 hours after the last dose of lithium.

1. 1,000-1,500 mg of lithium carbonate are administered daily for the first five days. A blood sample for plasma lithium estimation is taken 12 hours after the last dose on the fifth day, and the dosage of Camcolit is adjusted to keep the plasma lithium level within the therapeutic range. Subsequently, regular plasma lithium estimations must be carried out and, where necessary, the dosage of Camcolit adjusted accordingly. The precise initial dose of lithium should be decided in the light of the age and weight of the patient; young patients often require a dose higher than average and older patients a lower dose.

2. A lithium clearance test is carried out and the initial dosage calculated from the results. Even when the initial dosage is calculated in this way, it is still desirable that plasma lithium levels should be determined at weekly intervals during the first three weeks of treatment, and any necessary adjustments to dosage made as a result of the levels actually obtained.

Most of the above applies in the treatment of hypomania as well as mania, but the patient (if not too ill) can be started on treatment as an outpatient provided that facilities for regular plasma lithium monitoring are available, and assays are initiated within one week.

Prophylaxis of recurrent affective disorders: (Including unipolar mania & unipolar depressions and bipolar manic-depressive illness): A low dose of 300-400 mg of lithium carbonate can be administered daily for the first seven days. A blood sample for plasma lithium estimation is then taken 12 hours after the last dose, and the dosage of Camcolit is adjusted to keep the plasma lithium level within the range of 0.4-0.8 mmol/l. Toxic symptoms are usually associated with concentrations exceeding 1.5 mmol/l.

Use in elderly: As for prophylaxis above, but 12 hour lithium levels should be kept in the range of 0.4-0.7 mmol/l as toxic symptoms are likely with plasma concentrations above 1.0 mmol/l.

Use in children: Not recommended.

4.3 Contraindications

Patients with renal disease, cardiovascular disease, Addison's disease or those breast-feeding.

4.4 Special warnings and special precautions for use

Pre-treatment and periodic routine clinical monitoring is essential. This should include assessment of renal function, urine analysis, assessment of thyroid function and cardiac function, especially in patients with cardiovascular disease.

Patients should be euthyroid before initiation of lithium therapy.

Clear instructions regarding the symptoms of impending toxicity should be given by the doctor to all patients receiving long-term lithium therapy. Patients should also be warned to report if polyuria or polydipsia develop. Episodes of nausea and vomiting or other conditions leading to salt/water depletion (including severe dieting) should also be reported. Patients should be advised to maintain their usual salt and fluid intake.

Elderly patients are particularly liable to lithium toxicity.

4.5 Interaction with other medicinal products and other forms of Interaction

Lower doses of lithium may be required during diuretic therapy as lithium clearance is reduced.

Serum lithium concentrations may increase during concomitant therapy with non-steroidal anti-inflammatory drugs or tetracycline, possibly resulting in lithium toxicity. Serum lithium concentrations therefore should be monitored more frequently if NSAID or tetracycline therapy is initiated or discontinued.

Raised plasma levels of ADH may occur during treatment.

Symptoms of nephrogenic diabetes insipidus are particularly prevalent in patients receiving concurrent treatment with tricyclic or tetracyclic anti-depressants.

4.6 Pregnancy and lactation

Pregnancy: There is epidemiological evidence to suggest that the drug may be harmful during human pregnancy. Should the use of lithium be unavoidable, close monitoring of serum concentrations should be made throughout pregnancy and parturition.

Lactation: Infants of mothers on lithium should be bottle fed as lithium is present in the breast milk.

4.7 Effects on ability to drive and use machines

None known.

4.8 Undesirable effects

Long term treatment with lithium may result in permanent changes in the kidney and impairment of renal function. High serum concentrations of lithium, including episodes of acute lithium toxicity may enhance these changes. The minimum clinically effective dose of lithium should always be used. Patients should only be maintained on lithium after 3-5 years if, on assessment, benefit persists.

Renal function should be routinely monitored in patients with polyuria and polydipsia. Side effects are usually related to serum lithium concentrations and are infrequent at levels below 1.0 mmol/l.

Mild gastro-intestinal effects, nausea, vertigo, muscle weakness and a dazed feeling may occur, but frequently disappear after stabilisation. Fine hand tremors, polyuria and mild thirst may persist. Some studies suggest that the tremor can be controlled by relatively small doses of propranolol.

Long term treatment with lithium is frequently associated with disturbances of thyroid function including goitre and hypothyroidism. These can be controlled by administration of small doses of thyroxine (0.05-0.2 mg daily) concomitantly with lithium. Thyrotoxicosis has also been reported.

Mild cognitive impairment may occur during long term use.

Hypercalcaemia, hypermagnesaemia, hyperparathyroidism and an increase in antinuclear antibodies have also been reported.

Exacerbation of psoriasis may occur.

Cardiovascular effects of lithium are rare and often benign. Reported effects are arrhythmia, oedema, and sinus node dysfunction. Any signs of cardiac disturbance e.g. syncope, heart rhythm or rate disturbances should be investigated further.

Oedema with weight gain can occur and may lead to an increased risk of lithium toxicity if treated incautiously with diuretic drugs.

4.9 Overdose

Appearance or aggravation of gastro-intestinal symptoms, muscle weakness, lack of co-ordination, drowsiness or lethargy may be early signs of intoxication. With increasing toxicity, ataxia, giddiness, tinnitus, blurred vision, coarse tremor, muscle twitching and a large output of dilute urine may be seen. At blood levels above 2-3 mmol/l, increasing disorientation, seizures, coma and death may occur.

There is no antidote to lithium poisoning. In the event, lithium treatment should be stopped immediately and serum lithium levels estimated every 6 hours. When ingestion is recent, gastric lavage should be carried out, together with general supportive measures. Special attention must be given to the maintenance of fluid and electrolyte balance, and also adequate renal function. Sodium-depleting diuretics should not be used in any circumstances. Forced alkaline diuresis may be used. If the serum lithium level is above

4.0 mmol/l, or if there is a deterioration in the patient's condition, or if the serum lithium concentration is not falling at a rate equivalent to a half-life of less than 30 hours, peritoneal dialysis or haemodialysis should be instituted promptly. This should be continued until the serum and dialysis fluid are free of lithium. Serum lithium levels should be monitored for at least another 7 days thereafter, as a rebound rise is possible due to delayed diffusion from the tissues.

5. PHARMACOLOGICAL PROPERTIES

5.1 Pharmacodynamic properties

The precise mechanism of action of lithium as a mood-stabilising agent remains unknown, although many cellular actions of lithium have been characterised.

5.2 Pharmacokinetic properties

The pharmacokinetics of lithium are extremely well documented. A single oral dose of CAMCOLIT 400 gives a peak plasma level approximately 3-4 hours later, with the level at 24 hours being approximately 40% of peak levels.

5.3 Preclinical safety data

There is no preclinical data of relevance to the prescriber.

6. PHARMACEUTICAL PARTICULARS

6.1 List of excipients

Maize Starch

Acacia

Magnesium Stearate

Sodium Lauryl Sulphate

Hypromellose

Macrogol 400

Opaspray M-1-7111B

6.2 Incompatibilities

See 4.5 and 4.8 above.

6.3 Shelf life

The shelf life is 3 years.

6.4 Special precautions for storage

Do not store above 25°C.

Keep container tightly closed. Keep out of reach and sight of children.

6.5 Nature and contents of container

Polypropylene containers of 100 or 500 tablet capacity, and for hospital use only, screw-cap amber glass bottles of 50 or 100 tablet capacity.

6.6 Instructions for use and handling

None.

7. MARKETING AUTHORISATION HOLDER

Norgine Limited

Chaplin House

Widewater Place

Moorhall Road

Harefield

UXBRIDGE

Middlesex UB9 6NS, UK

8. MARKETING AUTHORISATION NUMBER(S)
PL 00322/0015

9. DATE OF FIRST AUTHORISATION/RENEWAL OF THE AUTHORISATION
June 1997

10. DATE OF REVISION OF THE TEXT
25 th January 2005

Legal category: **POM**

Campral EC

(Merck Pharmaceuticals)

1. NAME OF THE MEDICINAL PRODUCT
Campral EC

2. QUALITATIVE AND QUANTITATIVE COMPOSITION
Each tablet contains acamprosate (I.N.N.) calcium 333.0 mg as the active ingredient.

3. PHARMACEUTICAL FORM
Enterocoated tablets.

4. CLINICAL PARTICULARS
4.1 Therapeutic indications
Acamprosate is indicated as therapy to maintain abstinence in alcohol-dependent patients. It should be combined with counselling.

4.2 Posology and method of administration
Adults within the age range 18-65 years:

- 2 tablets three times daily with meals (2 tablets morning, noon and night) in subjects weighing 60kg or more.
- In subjects weighing less than 60kg, 4 tablets divided into three daily doses with meals (2 tablets in the morning, 1 at noon and 1 at night).

Children and the Elderly:

Acamprosate should not be administered to children and the elderly.

The recommended treatment period is one year. Treatment with acamprosate should be initiated as soon as possible after the withdrawal period and should be maintained if the patient relapses.

4.3 Contraindications
Acamprosate is contraindicated:

– in patients with a known hypersensitivity to the drug
– in pregnant women and lactating women
– in cases of renal insufficiency (serum creatinine >120 micromol/L)
– in cases with severe hepatic failure (Childs- Pugh Classification C)

4.4 Special warnings and special precautions for use
Acamprosate does not constitute treatment for the withdrawal period.

Acamprosate does not prevent the harmful effects of continuous alcohol abuse. Continued alcohol abuse negates the therapeutic benefit, therefore acamprosate treatment should only be initiated after weaning therapy, once the patient is abstinent from alcohol.

As mental co-morbidity is frequently reported in alcoholic patients, psychiatric disorders (mainly depression) could be attributed to the underlying condition of the patients undergoing therapy with acamprosate. Regular monitoring of patients is therefore required.

4.5 Interaction with other medicinal products and other forms of Interaction
The concomitant intake of alcohol and acamprosate does not affect the pharmacokinetics of either alcohol or acamprosate. Administering acamprosate with food diminishes the bioavailability of the drug compared with its administration in the fasting state. Pharmacokinetic studies have been completed and show no interaction between acamprosate and diazepam, disulfiram or imipramine. There is no information available on the concomitant administration of acamprosate with diuretics.

4.6 Pregnancy and lactation
Although animal studies have not shown any evidence of foetotoxicity or teratogenicity, the safety of acamprosate has not been established in pregnant women. Acamprosate should not be administered to pregnant women.

Acamprosate is excreted in the milk of lactating animals. Safe use of acamprosate has not been demonstrated in lactating women. Acamprosate should not be administered to breast feeding women.

4.7 Effects on ability to drive and use machines
Acamprosate should not impair the patient's ability to drive or operate machinery.

4.8 Undesirable effects
Adverse events associated with acamprosate tend to be mild and transient in nature. The adverse events are predominantly gastrointestinal or dermatological.

Diarrhoea, and less frequently nausea, vomiting and abdominal pain are the gastrointestinal adverse events. Pruritus is the predominant dermatological adverse event. An occasional maculopapular rash and rare cases of bullous skin reactions have been reported. Fluctuation in libido and psychiatric disorders, mainly depression, have been reported by patients receiving acamprosate as well as by patients receiving the placebo.

4.9 Overdose
Five cases of overdose associated with acamprosate therapy have been reported in humans, including one patient who ingested 43g of acamprosate. After gastric lavage all patients had an uneventful recovery. Diarrhoea was observed in two cases. No case of hypercalcaemia was reported in the course of these overdoses. However, should this occur, the patients should be treated for acute hypercalcaemia.

5. PHARMACOLOGICAL PROPERTIES
5.1 Pharmacodynamic properties
Acamprosate (calcium acetylhomotaurinate) has a chemical structure similar to that of amino acid neuromediators, such as taurine or gamma-amino-butyric acid (GABA), including an acetylation to permit passage across the blood brain barrier. Acamprosate may act by stimulating GABAergic inhibitory neurotransmission and antagonising excitatory amino-acids, particularly glutamate. Animal experimental studies have demonstrated that acamprosate affects alcohol dependence in rats, decreasing the voluntary intake of alcohol without affecting food and total fluid intake.

5.2 Pharmacokinetic properties
Acamprosate absorption across the gastrointestinal tract is moderate, slow and sustained and varies substantially from person to person. Food reduces the oral absorption of acamprosate. Steady state levels of acamprosate are achieved by the seventh day of dosing. Acamprosate is not protein bound.

Oral absorption shows considerable variability and is usually less than 10% of the ingested drug in the first 24 hours. The drug is excreted in the urine and is not metabolised significantly. There is a linear relationship between creatinine clearance values and total apparent plasma clearance, renal clearance and plasma half-life of acamprosate.

The kinetics of acamprosate are not modified in group A or B of the Child-Pugh classification of impaired liver function, a population which is likely to be part of the target population for acamprosate. This is in accordance with the absence of hepatic metabolism of the drug.

5.3 Preclinical safety data
In the preclinical studies, signs of toxicity are related to the excessive intake of calcium and not to acetylhomotaurine. Disorders of phosphorus/calcium metabolism have been observed including diarrhoea, soft tissue calcification, renal and cardiac lesions. Acamprosate had no mutagenic or carcinogenic effect, nor any teratogenic or adverse effects on the male or female reproductive systems of animals. Detailed *in vitro* and *in vivo* research on acamprosate to detect genetic and chromosomal mutations has not produced any evidence of potential genetic toxicity.

6. PHARMACEUTICAL PARTICULARS
6.1 List of excipients
Crospovidone (KOLLIDON CL)

Microcrystalline cellulose (AVICEL PH 101)

Magnesium silicate (COMPRESSIL)

Sodium starch glycolate (EXPLOTAB)

Anhydrous colloidal silica (AEROSIL 200)

Magnesium stearate

Anionic copolymer of methacrylic and acrylic acid ethyl ester (EUDRAGIT L30 D)

Talc

Propylene glycol

6.2 Incompatibilities
None known

6.3 Shelf life
3 years

6.4 Special precautions for storage
None

6.5 Nature and contents of container
Aluminium/PVC sheets of blisters presented in cartons of 168 tablets.

6.6 Instructions for use and handling
Not applicable.

7. MARKETING AUTHORISATION HOLDER
Merck Santé s.a.s

37 rue Saint Romain

69379 Lyon Cedex 08

France

8. MARKETING AUTHORISATION NUMBER(S)
MA 13466/0001

9. DATE OF FIRST AUTHORISATION/RENEWAL OF THE AUTHORISATION
18 December 1995 (first authorization)

10. DATE OF REVISION OF THE TEXT
14 April 2003

LEGAL CATEGORY POM

Campto 40mg/2ml and 100mg/5ml concentrate for solution for infusion

(Pfizer Limited)

1. NAME OF THE MEDICINAL PRODUCT
CAMPTO 40 mg/2 ml, concentrate for solution for infusion.

CAMPTO 100 mg/5 ml, concentrate for solution for infusion.

2. QUALITATIVE AND QUANTITATIVE COMPOSITION
The concentrate contains 20 mg/ml irinotecan hydrochloride, trihydrate (equivalent to 17.33 mg/ml irinotecan). Vials of CAMPTO contain 40 mg or 100 mg of irinotecan hydrochloride, trihydrate. For excipients, see « List of excipients ».

3. PHARMACEUTICAL FORM
Concentrate for solution for infusion.

4. CLINICAL PARTICULARS
4.1 Therapeutic indications
CAMPTO is indicated for the treatment of patients with advanced colorectal cancer:

- in combination with 5-fluorouracil and folinic acid in patients without prior chemotherapy for advanced disease,
- as a single agent in patients who have failed an established 5-fluorouracil containing treatment regimen.

4.2 Posology and method of administration
For adults only. CAMPTO solution for infusion should be infused into a peripheral or central vein.

Recommended dosage:

<u>In monotherapy (for previously treated patient):</u>

The recommended dosage of CAMPTO is 350 mg/m^2 administered as an intravenous infusion over a 30- to 90-minute period every three weeks (see « Instructions for Use/Handling » and « Special Warnings and Special Precautions for Use » sections).

<u>In combination therapy (for previously untreated patient):</u>

Safety and efficacy of CAMPTO in combination with 5-fluorouracil (5FU) and folinic acid (FA) have been assessed with the following schedule (see « Pharmacodynamic properties »):

- CAMPTO plus 5FU/FA in every 2 weeks schedule

The recommended dose of CAMPTO is 180 mg/m^2 administered once every 2 weeks as an intravenous infusion over a 30- to 90-minute period, followed by infusion with folinic acid and 5-fluorouracil.

Dosage adjustments:

CAMPTO should be administered after appropriate recovery of all adverse events to grade 0 or 1 NCI-CTC grading (National Cancer Institute Common Toxicity Criteria) and when treatment-related diarrhoea is fully resolved.

At the start of a subsequent infusion of therapy, the dose of CAMPTO, and 5FU when applicable, should be decreased according to the worst grade of adverse events observed in the prior infusion. Treatment should be delayed by 1 to 2 weeks to allow recovery from treatment-related adverse events.

With the following adverse events a dose reduction of 15 to 20 % should be applied for CAMPTO and/or 5FU when applicable:

- haematological toxicity (neutropenia grade 4, febrile neutropenia (neutropenia grade 3-4 and fever grade 2-4), thrombocytopenia and leukopenia (grade 4)),
- non haematological toxicity (grade 3-4).

Treatment Duration:

Treatment with CAMPTO should be continued until there is an objective progression of the disease or an unacceptable toxicity.

Special populations:

Patients with Impaired Hepatic Function: In monotherapy: Blood bilirubin levels (up to 3 times the upper limit of the normal range (UNL)) in patients with performance status ⩽ 2, should determine the starting dose of Campto. In these patients with hyperbilirubinemia and prothrombin time greater than 50%, the clearance of irinotecan is decreased (see "Pharmacokinetic properties" section) and therefore the risk of hematotoxicity is increased. Thus, weeklymonitoring of complete blood counts should be conducted in this patient population.

- In patients with bilirubin up to 1.5 times the upper limit of the normal range (ULN), the recommended dosage of CAMPTO is 350 mg/m^2,
- In patients with bilirubin ranging from 1.5 to 3 times the ULN, the recommended dosage of CAMPTO is 200 mg/m^2,
- Patients with bilirubin beyond to 3 times the ULN should not be treated with CAMPTO (see « Contraindications » and « Special Warnings and Special Precautions for Use » sections).

No data are available in patients with hepatic impairment treated by CAMPTO in combination.

Patients with Impaired Renal Function: CAMPTO is not recommended for use in patients with impaired renal function, as studies in this population have not been conducted. (See « Special Warnings and Special Precautions for Use » and « Pharmacokinetic Properties »).

Elderly: No specific pharmacokinetic studies have been performed in elderly. However, the dose should be chosen carefully in this population due to their greater frequency of decreased biological functions. This population should require more intense surveillance (see « Special Warnings and Special Precautions for Use »).

4.3 Contraindications

• Chronic inflammatory bowel disease and/or bowel obstruction (see « Special Warnings and Special Precautions for Use »).

• History of severe hypersensitivity reactions to irinotecan hydrochloride trihydrate or to one of the excipients of CAMPTO.

• Pregnancy and lactation (see « Pregnancy and Lactation » and « Special Warnings and Special Precautions for Use » sections).

• Bilirubin > 3 times the upper limit of the normal range (see « Special warnings and Special Precautions for Use » section).

• Severe bone marrow failure.

• WHO performance status > 2.

• Concomitant use with St John's Wort (see section 4.5)

4.4 Special warnings and special precautions for use

The use of CAMPTO should be confined to units specialised in the administration of cytotoxic chemotherapy and it should only be administered under the supervision of a physician qualified in the use of anticancer chemotherapy.

Given the nature and incidence of adverse events, CAMPTO will only be prescribed in the following cases after the expected benefits have been weighted against the possible therapeutic risks:

• in patients presenting a risk factor, particularly those with a WHO performance status = 2.

• in the few rare instances where patients are deemed unlikely to observe recommendations regarding management of adverse events (need for immediate and prolonged antidiarrhoeal treatment combined with high fluid intake at onset of delayed diarrhoea). Strict hospital supervision is recommended for such patients.

When CAMPTO is used in monotherapy, it is usually prescribed with the every-3-week-dosage schedule. However, the weekly-dosage schedule (see « Pharmacological properties ») may be considered in patients who may need a closer follow-up or who are at particular risk of severe neutropenia.

Delayed diarrhoea

Patients should be made aware of the risk of delayed diarrhoea occurring more than 24 hours after the administration of CAMPTO and at any time before the next cycle. In monotherapy, the median time of onset of the first liquid stool was on day 5 after the infusion of CAMPTO®. Patients should quickly inform their physician of its occurrence and start appropriate therapy immediately.

Patients with an increased risk of diarrhoea are those who had a previous abdominal/pelvic radiotherapy, those with baseline hyperleucocytosis, those with performance status ⩾ 2 and women. If not properly treated, diarrhoea can be life threatening, especially if the patient is concomitantly neutropenic.

As soon as the first liquid stool occurs, the patient should start drinking large volumes of beverages containing electrolytes and an appropriate antidiarrhoeal therapy must be initiated immediately. This antidiarrhoeal treatment will be prescribed by the department where CAMPTO has been administered. After discharge from the hospital, the patients should obtain the prescribed drugs so that they can treat the diarrhoea as soon as it occurs. In addition, they must inform their physician or the department administering CAMPTO when/if diarrhoea is occurring.

The currently recommended antidiarrhoeal treatment consists of high doses of loperamide (4 mg for the first intake and then 2 mg every 2 hours). This therapy should continue for 12 hours after the last liquid stool and should not be modified. In no instance should loperamide be administered for more than 48 consecutive hours at these doses, because of the risk of paralytic ileus, nor for less than 12 hours.

In addition to the anti-diarrhoeal treatment, a prophylactic broad-spectrum antibiotic should be given, when diarrhoea is associated with severe neutropenia (neutrophil count < 500 cells/mm^3).

In addition to the antibiotic treatment, hospitalisation is recommended for management of the diarrhoea, in the following cases:

- Diarrhoea associated with fever,
- Severe diarrhoea (requiring intravenous hydration),
- Diarrhoea persisting beyond 48 hours following the initiation of high-dose loperamide therapy.

Loperamide should not be given prophylactically, even in patients who experienced delayed diarrhoea at previous cycles.

In patients who experienced severe diarrhoea, a reduction in dose is recommended for subsequent cycles (see « Posology and Method of Administration » section).

Haematology

Weekly monitoring of complete blood cell counts is recommended during CAMPTO treatment. Patients should be aware of the risk of neutropenia and the significance of fever. Febrile neutropenia (temperature > 38°C and neutrophil count ⩽ 1,000 cells/mm^3) should be urgently treated in the hospital with broad-spectrum intravenous antibiotics.

In patients who experienced severe haematological events, a dose reduction is recommended for subsequent administration (see « Posology and Method of Administration » section).

There is an increased risk of infections and haematological toxicity in patients with severe diarrhoea. In patients with severe diarrhoea, complete blood cell counts should be performed.

Liver impairment

Liver function tests should be performed at baseline and before each cycle.

Weekly monitoring of complete blood counts should be conducted in patients with bilirubin ranging from 1.5 to 3 times ULN, due to decrease of the clearance of irinotecan (see "Pharmacokinetic properties" section) and thus increasing the risk of hematotoxicity in this population. For patients with a bilirubin > 3 times ULN (see « Contra-indications » section).

Nausea and vomiting

A prophylactic treatment with antiemetics is recommended before each treatment with CAMPTO. Nausea and vomiting have been frequently reported. Patients with vomiting associated with delayed diarrhoea should be hospitalised as soon as possible for treatment.

Acute cholinergic syndrome

If acute cholinergic syndrome appears (defined as early diarrhoea and various other symptoms such as sweating, abdominal cramping, lacrimation, myosis and salivation), atropine sulphate (0.25 mg subcutaneously) should be administered unless clinically contraindicated (see « Undesirable Effects » section). Caution should be exercised in patients with asthma. In patients who experienced an acute and severe cholinergic syndrome, the use of prophylactic atropine sulphate is recommended with subsequent doses of CAMPTO.

Respiratory disorders

Interstitial pulmonary disease presenting as pulmonary infiltrates is uncommon during irinotecan therapy. Interstitial pulmonary disease can be fatal. Risk factors possibly associated with the development of interstitial pulmonary disease include the use of pneumotoxic drugs, radiation therapy and colony stimulating factors. Patients with risk factors should be closely monitored for respiratory symptoms before and during irinotecan therapy.

Elderly

Due to the greater frequency of decreased biological functions, in particular hepatic function, in elderly patients, dose selection with CAMPTO should be cautious in this population (see « Posology and Method of Administration » section).

Patients with bowel obstruction

Patients must not be treated with CAMPTO until resolution of the bowel obstruction (see « Contraindications »).

Patients with Impaired Renal Function

Studies in this population have not been conducted. (see « Posology and Method of Administration » and « Pharmacokinetic Properties »).

Others

Since this medicinal contains sorbitol, it is unsuitable in hereditary fructose intolerance. Infrequent cases of renal insufficiency, hypotension or circulatory failure have been observed in patients who experienced episodes of dehydration associated with diarrhoea and/or vomiting, or sepsis. Contraceptive measures must be taken during and for at least three months after cessation of therapy.

Concomitant administration of irinotecan with a strong inhibitor (e.g. ketoconazole) or inducer (e.g. rifampicin, carbamazepine, phenobarbital, phenytoin, St John's Wort) of CYP3A4 may alter the metabolism of irinotecan and should be avoided (see section 4.5).

4.5 Interaction with other medicinal products and other forms of Interaction

Interaction between irinotecan and neuromuscular blocking agents cannot be ruled out. Since CAMPTO has anticholinesterase activity, drugs with anticholinesterase activity may prolong the neuromuscular blocking effects of suxamethonium and the neuromuscular blockade of non-depolarising drugs may be antagonised.

Several studies have shown that concomitant administration of CYP3A-inducing anticonvulsant drugs (e.g., carbamazepine, phenobarbital or phenytoin) leads to reduced exposure to irinotecan, SN-38 and SN-38 glucuronide and reduced pharmacodynamic effects. The effects of such anticonvulsant drugs was reflected by a decrease in AUC of SN-38 and SN-38G by 50% or more. In addition to induction of cytochrome P450 3A enzymes, enhanced glucuronidation and enhanced biliary excretion may play a role in reducing exposure to irinotecan and its metabolites.

A study has shown that the co-administration of ketoconazole resulted in a decrease in the AUC of APC of 87% and in an increase in the AUC of SN-38 of 109% in comparison to irinotecan given alone.

Caution should be exercised in patients concurrently taking drugs known to inhibit (e.g., ketoconazole) or induce (e.g., rifampicin, carbamazepine, phenobarbital or phenytoin) drug metabolism by cytochrome P450 3A4. Concurrent administration of irinotecan with an inhibitor/inducer of this metabolic pathway may alter the metabolism of irinotecan and should be avoided (see section 4.4).

In a small pharmacokinetic study (n=5), in which irinotecan 350 mg/m2 was co-administered with St. John's Wort (Hypericum perforatum) 900 mg, a 42% decrease in the active metabolite of irinotecan, SN-38, plasma concentrations was observed.

St. John's Wort decreases SN-38 plasma levels. As a result, St. John's Wort should not be administered with irinotecan (see section 4.3).

Coadministration of 5-fluorouracil/folinic acid in the combination regimen does not change the pharmacokinetics of irinotecan.

4.6 Pregnancy and lactation

Pregnancy:

There is no information on the use of CAMPTO in pregnant women.

CAMPTO has been shown to be embryotoxic, foetotoxic and teratogenic in rabbits and rats. Therefore, CAMPTO must not be used during pregnancy (see « Contraindications » and « Special Warnings and Special Precautions for Use »).

Women of childbearing potential:

Women of childbearing age receiving CAMPTO should be advised to avoid becoming pregnant, and to inform the treating physician immediately should this occur (see « Contraindications » and « Special Warnings and Special Precautions for Use »).

Lactation:

In lactating rats, ^{14}C-irinotecan was detected in milk. It is not known whether irinotecan is excreted in human milk. Consequently, because of the potential for adverse reactions in nursing infants, breast-feeding must be discontinued for the duration of CAMPTO therapy (see « Contraindications »).

4.7 Effects on ability to drive and use machines

Patients should be warned about the potential for dizziness or visual disturbances which may occur within 24 hours following the administration of CAMPTO, and advised not to drive or operate machinery if these symptoms occur.

4.8 Undesirable effects

The following adverse reactions considered to be possibly or probably related to the administration of CAMPTO have been reported from 765 patients at the recommended dose of 350 mg/m^2 in monotherapy, and from 145 patients treated by CAMPTO in combination therapy with 5FU/FA in every 2 weeks schedule at the recommended dose of 180 mg/m^2.

Gastrointestinal disorders

Delayed diarrhoea

Diarrhoea (occurring more than 24 hours after administration) is a dose-limiting toxicity of CAMPTO.

In monotherapy:

Severe diarrhoea was observed in 20 % of patients who follow recommendations for the management of diarrhoea. Of the evaluable cycles, 14 % have a severe diarrhoea. The median time of onset of the first liquid stool was on day 5 after the infusion of CAMPTO.

In combination therapy:

Severe diarrhoea was observed in 13.1 % of patients who follow recommendations for the management of diarrhoea. Of the evaluable cycles, 3.9 % have a severe diarrhoea.

Uncommon cases of pseudo-membranous colitis have been reported, one of which has been documented bacteriologically (*Clostridium difficile*).

Nausea and vomiting

In monotherapy:

Nausea and vomiting were severe in approximately 10 % of patients treated with antiemetics.

In combination therapy:

A lower incidence of severe nausea and vomiting was observed (2.1 % and 2.8 % of patients respectively).

Dehydration

Episodes of dehydration commonly associated with diarrhoea and/or vomiting have been reported.

Infrequent cases of renal insufficiency, hypotension or cardio-circulatory failure have been observed in patients who experienced episodes of dehydration associated with diarrhoea and/or vomiting.

Other gastrointestinal disorders

Constipation relative to CAMPTO and/or loperamide has been observed, shared between:

• in monotherapy: in less than 10 % of patients

• in combination therapy: 3.4 % of patients.

Infrequent cases of intestinal obstruction, ileus, or gastro-intestinal haemorrhage and rare cases of colitis, including typhlitis, ischemic and ulcerative colitis, were reported. Rare cases of intestinal perforation were reported. Other mild effects include anorexia, abdominal pain and mucositis.

Blood disorders

Neutropenia is a dose-limiting toxic effect. Neutropenia was reversible and not cumulative; the median day to nadir was 8 days whatever the use in monotherapy or in combination therapy.

In monotherapy:

Neutropenia was observed in 78.7 % of patients and was severe (neutrophil count < 500 cells/mm3) in 22.6 % of patients. Of the evaluable cycles, 18 % had a neutrophil count below 1,000 cells/mm^3 including 7.6 % with a neutrophil count < 500 cells/mm^3.

Total recovery was usually reached by day 22.

Fever with severe neutropenia was reported in 6.2 % of patients and in 1.7 % of cycles.

Infectious episodes occurred in about 10.3 % of patients (2.5 % of cycles) and were associated with severe neutropenia in about 5.3 % of patients (1.1 % of cycles), and resulted in death in 2 cases.

Anaemia was reported in about 58.7 % of patients (8 % with haemoglobin < 8 g/dl and 0.9 % with haemoglobin < 6.5 g/dl).

Thrombocytopenia (< 100,000 cells/mm^3) was observed in 7.4 % of patients and 1.8 % of cycles with 0.9 % with platelets count ≤ 50,000 cells/mm3 and 0.2 % of cycles.

Nearly all the patients showed a recovery by day 22.

In combination therapy:

Neutropenia was observed in 82.5 % of patients and was severe (neutrophil count < 500 cells/mm3) in 9.8 % of patients.

Of the evaluable cycles, 67.3 % had a neutrophil count below 1,000 cells/mm^3 including 2.7 % with a neutrophil count < 500 cells/mm^3.

Total recovery was usually reached within 7-8 days.

Fever with severe neutropenia was reported in 3.4 % of patients and in 0.9 % of cycles.

Infectious episodes occurred in about 2 % of patients (0.5 % of cycles) and were associated with severe neutropenia in about 2.1 % of patients (0.5 % of cycles), and resulted in death in 1 case.

Anaemia was reported in 97.2 % of patients (2.1 % with haemoglobin < 8 g/dl).

Thrombocytopenia (< 100,000 cells/mm^3) was observed in 32.6 % of patients and 21.8 % of cycles. No severe thrombocytopenia (< 50,000 cells/mm^3) has been observed.

One case of peripheral thrombocytopenia with antiplatelet antibodies has been reported in the post-marketing experience.

Infection and Infestation

Infrequent cases of renal insufficiency, hypotension or cardio-circulatory failure have been observed in patients who experienced sepsis.

General disorders and infusion site reactions

Acute cholinergic syndrome

Severe transient acute cholinergic syndrome was observed in 9 % of patients treated in monotherapy and in 1.4 % of patients treated in combination therapy. The main symptoms were defined as early diarrhoea and various other symptoms such as abdominal pain, conjunctivitis, rhinitis, hypotension, vasodilatation, sweating, chills, malaise, dizziness, visual disturbances, myosis, lachrimation and increased salivation occurring during or within the first 24 hours after the infusion of CAMPTO. These symptoms disappear after atropine administration (see « Special Warning and Special Precautions for Use »).

Asthenia was severe in less than 10 % of patients treated in monotherapy and in 6.2 % of patients treated in combination therapy. The causal relationship to CAMPTO has not been clearly established. Fever in the absence of infection and without concomitant severe neutropenia, occurred in 12 % of patients treated in monotherapy and in 6.2 % of patients treated in combination therapy.

Mild infusion site reactions have been reported although uncommonly.

Cardiac disorder

Rare cases of hypertension during or following the infusion have been reported.

Respiratory disorders

Interstitial pulmonary disease presenting as pulmonary infiltrates is uncommon during irinotecan therapy. Early effects such as dyspnoea have been reported (see section 4.4).

Skin and subcutaneous tissue disorders

Alopecia was very common and reversible. Mild cutaneous reactions have been reported although uncommonly.

Immune system disorders

Uncommon mild allergy reactions and rare cases of anaphylactic/anaphylactoid reactions have been reported.

Table 1

	Phases III CAMPTO versus supportive care			CAMPTO versus 5FU		
	CAMPTO	Supportive care	p values	CAMPTO	5FU	p values
	n=183	n=90		n=127	n=129	
Progression Free Survival at 6 months (%)	NA	NA		33.5 *	26.7	p=0.03
Survival at 12 months (%)	36.2 *	13.8	p=0.0001	44.8 *	32.4	p=0.0351
Median survival (months)	9.2*	6.5	p=0.0001	10.8*	8.5	p=0.0351

NA: Non Applicable

*: Statistically significant difference

Musculoskeletal disorders

Early effects such as muscular contraction or cramps and paresthesia have been reported.

Laboratory tests

In monotherapy, transient and mild to moderate increases in serum levels of either transaminases, alkaline phosphatase or bilirubin were observed in 9.2 %, 8.1 % and 1.8 % of the patients, respectively, in the absence of progressive liver metastasis.

Transient and mild to moderate increases of serum levels of creatinine have been observed in 7.3 % of the patients.

In combination therapy transient serum levels (grades 1 and 2) of either SGPT, SGOT, alkaline phosphatase or bilirubin were observed in 15 %, 11 %, 11 % and 10 % of the patients, respectively, in the absence of progressive liver metastasis. Transient grade 3 were observed in 0 %, 0%, 0 % and 1 % of the patients, respectively. No grade 4 was observed.

Increases of amylase and/or lipase have been very rarely reported.

Rare cases of hypokalemia and hyponatremia mostly related with diarrhoea and vomiting have been reported.

Nervous system disorders

There have been very rare postmarketing reports of transient speech disorders associated with CAMPTO infusions.

4.9 Overdose

There have been reports of overdosage at doses up to approximately twice the recommended therapeutic dose, which may be fatal. The most significant adverse reactions reported were severe neutropenia and severe diarrhoea. There is no known antidote for CAMPTO. Maximum supportive care should be instituted to prevent dehydration due to diarrhoea and to treat any infectious complications.

5. PHARMACOLOGICAL PROPERTIES

5.1 Pharmacodynamic properties

Cytostatic topoisomerase I inhibitor. ATC Code: L01XX19

Experimental data

Irinotecan is a semi-synthetic derivative of camptothecin. It is an antineoplastic agent which acts as a specific inhibitor of DNA topoisomerase I. It is metabolised by carboxylesterase in most tissues to SN-38, which was found to be more active than irinotecan in purified topoisomerase I and more cytotoxic than irinotecan against several murine and human tumour cell lines. The inhibition of DNA topoisomerase I by irinotecan or SN-38 induces single-strand DNA lesions which blocks the DNA replication fork and are responsible for the cytotoxicity. This cytotoxic activity was found time-dependent and was specific to the S phase.

In vitro, irinotecan and SN-38 were not found to be significantly recognised by the P -glycoprotein MDR, and displays cytotoxic activities against doxorubicin and vinblastine resistant cell lines.

Furthermore, irinotecan has a broad antitumor activity *in vivo* against murine tumour models (P03 pancreatic ductal adenocarcinoma, MA16/C mammary adenocarcinoma, C38 and C51 colon adenocarcinomas) and against human xenografts (Co-4 colon adenocarcinoma, Mx-1 mammary adenocarcinoma, ST-15 and SC-16 gastric adenocarcinomas). Irinotecan is also active against tumours expressing the P-glycoprotein MDR (vincristine- and doxorubicin-resistant P388 leukaemia's).

Beside the antitumor activity of CAMPTO, the most relevant pharmacological effect of irinotecan is the inhibition of acetyl cholinesterase.

Clinical data

In monotherapy:

Clinical phase II/III studies were performed in more than 980 patients in the every 3-week dosage schedule with metastatic colorectal cancer who failed a previous 5-FU regimen. The efficacy of CAMPTO was evaluated in 765 patients with documented progression on 5-FU at study entry.

(see Table 1 above)

In phase II studies, performed on 455 patients in the every 3-week dosage schedule, the progression free survival at 6 months was 30 % and the median survival was 9 months. The median time to progression was 18 weeks.

Additionally, non-comparative phase II studies were performed in 304 patients treated with a weekly schedule regimen, at a dose of 125 mg/m^2 administered as an intravenous infusion over 90 minutes for 4 consecutive weeks followed by 2 weeks rest. In these studies, the median time to progression was 17 weeks and median survival was 10 months. A similar safety profile has been observed in the weekly-dosage schedule in 193 patients at the starting dose of 125 mg/m^2, compared to the every 3-week-dosage schedule. The median time of onset of the first liquid stool was on day 11.

In combination therapy:

A phase III study was performed in 385 previously untreated metastatic colorectal cancer patients treated with either every 2 weeks schedule (see « Posology and method of administration ») or weekly schedule regimens. In the every 2 weeks schedule, on day 1, the administration of CAMPTO at 180 mg/m^2 once every 2 weeks is followed by infusion with folinic acid (200 mg/m^2 over a 2-hour intravenous infusion) and 5-fluorouracil (400 mg/m^2 as an intravenous bolus, followed by 600 mg/m^2 over a 22-hour intravenous infusion). On day 2, folinic acid and 5-fluorouracil are administered at the same doses and schedules. In the weekly schedule, the administration of CAMPTO at 80 mg/m^2 is followed by infusion with folinic acid (500 mg/m^2 over a 2-hour intravenous infusion) and then by 5-fluorouracil (2300 mg/m^2 over a 24-hour intravenous infusion) over 6 weeks.

In the combination therapy trial with the 2 regimens described above, the efficacy of CAMPTO was evaluated in 198 treated patients:

(see Table 2 on next page)

In the weekly schedule, the incidence of severe diarrhoea was 44.4% in patients treated by CAMPTO in combination with 5FU/FA and 25.6% in patients treated by 5FU/FA alone. The incidence of severe neutropenia (neutrophil count < 500 cells/mm^3) was 5.8% in patients treated by CAMPTO in combination with 5FU/FA and in 2.4% in patients treated by 5FU/FA alone.

Additionally, median time to definitive performance status deterioration was significantly longer in CAMPTO combination group than in 5FU/FA alone group (p=0.046).

Quality of life was assessed in this phase III study using the EORTC QLQ-C30 questionnaire. Time to definitive deterioration constantly occurred later in the CAMPTO groups. The evolution of the Global Health Status/Quality of life was slightly better in CAMPTO combination group although not significant; showing that efficacy of CAMPTO in combination could be reached without affecting the quality of life.

Pharmacokinetic/Pharmacodynamic data

The intensity of the major toxicities encountered with CAMPTO (e.g., leukoneutropenia and diarrhoea) is related to the exposure (AUC) to parent drug and metabolite SN-38. Significant correlations were observed between haematological toxicity (decrease in white blood cells and neutrophils at nadir) or diarrhoea intensity and both irinotecan and metabolite SN-38 AUC values in monotherapy.

5.2 Pharmacokinetic properties

In a phase I study in 60 patients with a dosage regimen of a 30-minute intravenous infusion of 100 to 750 mg/m^2 every three weeks, irinotecan showed a biphasic or triphasic elimination profile. The mean plasma clearance was 15 L/h/m^2 and the volume of distribution at steady state (Vss): 157 L/m^2. The mean plasma half-life of the first phase of the triphasic model was 12 minutes, of the second phase 2.5 hours, and the terminal phase half-life was 14.2 hours. SN-38 showed a biphasic elimination profile with a mean terminal elimination half-life of 13.8 hours. At the end of the infusion, at the recommended dose of 350 mg/m^2, the mean peak plasma concentrations of irinotecan and SN-38 were 7.7 μg/ml and 56 ng/ml, respectively, and the mean area under the curve (AUC) values were 34 μg.h/ml and 451 ng.h/ml, respectively. A large interindividual variability in pharmacokinetic parameters is generally observed for SN-38.

Table 2

	Combined regimens (n=198)		Weekly schedule (n=50)		Every 2 weeks schedule (n=148)	
	CAMPTO +5FU/FA	5FU/FA	CAMPTO +5FU/FA	5FU/FA	CAMPTO +5FU/FA	5FU/FA
Response rate (%)	40.8 *	23.1 *	51.2 *	28.6 *	37.5 *	21.6 *
p value	p<0.001		p=0.045		p=0.005	
Median time to progression (months)	6.7	4.4	7.2	6.5	6.5	3.7
p value	p<0.001		NS		p=0.001	
Median duration of response (months)	9.3	8.8	8.9	6.7	9.3	9.5
p value	NS		p=0.043		NS	
Median duration of response and stabilisation (months)	8.6	6.2	8.3	6.7	8.5	5.6
p value	p<0.001		NS		p=0.003	
Median time to treatment failure (months)	5.3	3.8	5.4	5.0	5.1	3.0
p value	p=0.0014		NS		p<0.001	
Median survival (months)	16.8	14.0	19.2	14.1	15.6	13.0
p value	p=0.028		NS		p=0.041	

5FU: 5-fluorouracil

FA: folinic acid

NS: Non Significant

*: As per protocol population analysis

A population pharmacokinetic analysis of irinotecan has been performed in 148 patients with metastatic colorectal cancer, treated with various schedules and at different doses in phase II trials. Pharmacokinetic parameters estimated with a three compartment model were similar to those observed in phase I studies. All studies have shown that irinotecan (CPT-11) and SN-38 exposure increase proportionally with CPT-11 administered dose; their pharmacokinetics are independent of the number of previous cycles and of the administration schedule.

In vitro, plasma protein binding for irinotecan and SN-38 was approximately 65 % and 95 % respectively.

Mass balance and metabolism studies with 14 C-labelled drug have shown that more than 50% of an intravenously administered dose of irinotecan is excreted as unchanged drug, with 33% in the faeces mainly via the bile and 22% in urine.

Two metabolic pathways account each for at least 12% of the dose:

• Hydrolysis by carboxylesterase into active metabolite SN-38, SN-38 is mainly eliminated by glucuronidation, and further by biliary and renal excretion (less than 0.5% of the irinotecan dose) The SN-38 glucuronite is subsequently probably hydrolysed in the intestine.

• Cytochrome P450 3A enzymes-dependent oxidations resulting in opening of the outer piperidine ring with formation of APC (aminopentanoic acid derivate) and NPC (primary amine derivate) (see section 4.5).

Unchanged irinotecan is the major entity in plasma, followed by APC, SN-38 glucuronide and SN-38. Only SN-38 has significant cytotoxic activity.

Irinotecan clearance is decreased by about 40% in patients with bilirubinemia between 1.5 and 3 times the upper normal limit. In these patients a 200 mg/m^2 irinotecan dose leads to plasma drug exposure comparable to that observed at 350 mg/m^2 in cancer patients with normal liver parameters.

5.3 Preclinical safety data

Irinotecan and SN-38 have been shown to be mutagenic *in vitro* in the chromosomal aberration test on CHO-cells as well as in the *in vivo* micronucleus test in mice.

However, they have been shown to be devoid of any mutagenic potential in the Ames test.

In rats treated once a week during 13 weeks at the maximum dose of 150 mg/m^2 (which is less than half the human recommended dose), no treatment related tumours were reported 91 weeks after the end of treatment.

Single- and repeated-dose toxicity studies with CAMPTO have been carried out in mice, rats and dogs. The main toxic effects were seen in the haematopoietic and lymphatic systems. In dogs, delayed diarrhoea associated with atrophy and focal necrosis of the intestinal mucosa was reported. Alopecia was also observed in the dog.

The severity of these effects was dose-related and reversible.

6. PHARMACEUTICAL PARTICULARS

6.1 List of excipients

Sorbitol, lactic acid, sodium hydroxide (to adjust to pH 3.5) and water for injections.

6.2 Incompatibilities

None known.

Do not admix with other medications.

6.3 Shelf life

The shelf-life of unopened vials is 36 months.

The CAMPTO solution should be used immediately after reconstitution, as it contains no antibacterial preservative. If reconstitution and dilution are performed under strict aseptic conditions (e.g. on Laminar Air Flow bench) CAMPTO solution should be used (infusion completed) within 12 hours at room temperature or 24 hours if stored 2°-8°C after the first breakage.

6.4 Special precautions for storage

Vials of CAMPTO concentrate for solution for infusion should be protected from light.

6.5 Nature and contents of container

CAMPTO 40 mg:

One 2-ml brown glass vial, with a halobutyl rubber closure coated with teflon on the inner side.

CAMPTO 100 mg:

One 5-ml brown glass vial, with a halobutyl rubber closure coated with teflon on the inner side.

6.6 Instructions for use and handling

As with other antineoplastic agents, CAMPTO must be prepared and handled with caution. The use of glasses, mask and gloves is required.

If CAMPTO solution or infusion solution should come into contact with the skin, wash immediately and thoroughly with soap and water. If CAMPTO solution or infusion solution should come into contact with the mucous membranes, wash immediately with water.

Preparation for the intravenous infusion administration:

As with any other injectable drugs, THE CAMPTO SOLUTION MUST BE PREPARED ASEPTICALLY (see « Shelf-life »).

If any precipitate is observed in the vials or after reconstitution, the product should be discarded according to standard procedures for cytotoxic agents.

Aseptically withdraw the required amount of CAMPTO solution from the vial with a calibrated syringe and inject into a 250 ml infusion bag or bottle containing either 0.9 % sodium chloride solution or 5 % dextrose solution. The infusion should then be thoroughly mixed by manual rotation.

Disposal:

All materials used for dilution and administration should be disposed of according to hospital standard procedures applicable to cytotoxic agents.

7. MARKETING AUTHORISATION HOLDER

Pfizer Limited

Ramsgate Road

Sandwich

Kent CT13 9NJ

8. MARKETING AUTHORISATION NUMBER(S)

CAMPTO 40 mg/2 ml, concentrate for solution for infusion – PL 00057/0626

CAMPTO 100 mg/5 ml, concentrate for solution for infusion – PL 00057/0627

9. DATE OF FIRST AUTHORISATION/RENEWAL OF THE AUTHORISATION

September 1995

10. DATE OF REVISION OF THE TEXT

21 February 2005

CANCIDAS (formerly Caspofungin MSD)

(Merck Sharp & Dohme Limited)

1. NAME OF THE MEDICINAL PRODUCT

CANCIDAS® 50 mg Powder for concentrate for solution for infusion

CANCIDAS® 70 mg Powder for concentrate for solution for infusion

2. QUALITATIVE AND QUANTITATIVE COMPOSITION

CANCIDAS 50 mg Powder for concentrate for solution for infusion: Each vial contains 50 mg Caspofungin equivalent to 55.5 mg caspofungin acetate.

CANCIDAS 70 mg Powder for concentrate for solution for infusion: Each vial contains 70 mg Caspofungin equivalent to 77.7 mg caspofungin acetate.

For excipients, see 6.1.

3. PHARMACEUTICAL FORM

Powder for concentrate for solution for infusion.

The vial contains a white to off-white compact, lyophilised powder.

4. CLINICAL PARTICULARS

4.1 Therapeutic indications

• Treatment of invasive candidiasis in adult patients.

• Treatment of invasive aspergillosis in adult patients who are refractory to or intolerant of amphotericin B, lipid formulations of amphotericin B and/or itraconazole. Refractoriness is defined as progression of infection or failure to improve after a minimum of 7 days of prior therapeutic doses of effective antifungal therapy.

• Empirical therapy for presumed fungal infections (such as *Candida* or *Aspergillus)* in febrile, neutropaenic adult patients.

4.2 Posology and method of administration

CANCIDAS should be initiated by a physician experienced in the management of invasive fungal infections.

After reconstitution and dilution, the solution should be administered by slow intravenous infusion over approximately 1 hour. Do not mix or co-infuse CANCIDAS with other medicines, as there are no data available on the compatibility of CANCIDAS with other intravenous substances, additives, or medicinal products. DO NOT USE DILUENTS CONTAINING GLUCOSE, as CANCIDAS is not stable in diluents containing glucose. For reconstitution directions see section 6.6.

Both 70 mg and 50 mg vials are available.

A single 70-mg loading dose should be administered on Day-1, followed by 50 mg daily thereafter. In patients weighing more than 80 kg, after the initial 70-mg loading dose, CANCIDAS 70 mg daily is recommended (see section 5.2). Doses higher than 70 mg daily have not been adequately studied.

Duration of empirical therapy should be based on the patient's clinical response. Therapy should be continued until up to 72 hours after resolution of neutropaenia (ANC≥500). Patients found to have a fungal infection should be treated for a minimum of 14 days and treatment should continue for at least 7 days after both neutropaenia and clinical symptoms are resolved.

Duration of treatment of invasive candidiasis should be based upon the patient's clinical and microbiological response. After signs and symptoms of invasive candidiasis have improved and cultures have become negative, a switch to oral antifungal therapy may be considered. In general, antifungal therapy should continue for at least 14 days after the last positive culture.

Duration of treatment of invasive aspergillosis is determined on a case by case basis and should be based upon the severity of the patient's underlying disease, recovery from immunosuppression, and clinical response. In general, treatment should continue for at least 7 days after resolution of symptoms.

In elderly patients (65 years of age or more), the area under the curve (AUC) is increased by approximately 30 %. However, no systematic dosage adjustment is required. There is limited treatment experience in patients 65 years of age and older.

No dosage adjustment is necessary based on gender, race, or renal impairment (see section 5.2).

For mild hepatic insufficiency (Child-Pugh score 5 to 6), no dosage adjustment is needed. For patients with moderate hepatic insufficiency (Child-Pugh score 7 to 9), CANCIDAS 35 mg daily is recommended. An initial 70-mg loading dose should be administered on Day-1. There is no clinical experience with severe hepatic insufficiency (Child-Pugh score greater than 9) (see section 4.4).

Caspofungin acetate has not been studied in paediatric patients. Use in patients under 18 years of age is not recommended.

Limited data suggest that an increase in the daily dose of CANCIDAS to 70 mg, following the 70-mg loading dose, should be considered when co-administering CANCIDAS with certain inducers of metabolic enzymes (see section 4.5).

4.3 Contraindications

Hypersensitivity to caspofungin acetate or to any of the excipients.

4.4 Special warnings and special precautions for use

Limited data suggest that less common non-*Candida* yeasts and non-*Aspergillus* moulds are not covered by caspofungin. The efficacy of caspofungin against these fungal pathogens has not been established.

Concomitant use of CANCIDAS with ciclosporin has been evaluated in healthy volunteers and in patients. Some healthy volunteers who received two 3 mg/kg doses of ciclosporin with caspofungin showed transient increases in alanine transaminase (ALT) and aspartate transaminase (AST) of less than or equal to 3-fold the upper limit of normal (ULN) that resolved with discontinuation of the treatment. In a retrospective study of 40 patients treated during marketed use with CANCIDAS and ciclosporin for 1 to 290 days (median 17.5 days), no serious hepatic adverse events were noted. These data suggest that CANCIDAS can be used in patients receiving ciclosporin when the potential benefit outweighs the potential risk. Close monitoring of liver enzymes should be considered if CANCIDAS and ciclosporin are used concomitantly.

In patients with mild and moderate hepatic impairment, the AUC is increased about 20 and 75 %, respectively. A reduction of the daily dose to 35 mg is recommended in moderate hepatic impairment. There is no clinical experience with severe hepatic insufficiency. A higher exposure than in moderate hepatic insufficiency is expected and CANCIDAS should be used with caution in these patients (see sections 4.2 and 5.2).

The safety information on treatment durations longer than 4 weeks is limited, however, available data suggest that caspofungin continues to be well tolerated with longer courses of therapy (up to 162 days).

4.5 Interaction with other medicinal products and other forms of Interaction

Studies *in vitro* show that caspofungin acetate is not an inhibitor of any enzyme in the cytochrome P450 (CYP) system. In clinical studies, caspofungin did not induce the CYP3A4 metabolism of other substances. Caspofungin is not a substrate for P-glycoprotein and is a poor substrate for cytochrome P450 enzymes. However, caspofungin has been shown to interact with other medicinal products in pharmacological and clinical studies (see below).

In two clinical studies performed in healthy subjects, ciclosporin A (one 4 mg/kg dose or two 3 mg/kg doses 12 hours apart) increased the AUC of caspofungin by approximately 35 %. These AUC increases are probably due to reduced uptake of caspofungin by the liver. CANCIDAS did not increase the plasma levels of ciclosporin. There were transient increases in liver ALT and AST of less than or equal to 3-fold the upper limit of normal (ULN) when CANCIDAS and ciclosporin were co-administered, that resolved with discontinuation of the medicinal products. In a retrospective study of 40 patients treated during marketed use with CANCIDAS and ciclosporin for 1 to 290 days (median 17.5 days), no serious hepatic adverse events were noted (see section 4.4). Close monitoring of liver enzymes should be considered if the two medicinal products are used concomitantly.

CANCIDAS reduced the trough concentration of tacrolimus by 26 %. For patients receiving both therapies, standard monitoring of tacrolimus blood concentrations and appropriate tacrolimus dosage adjustments are mandatory.

Rifampicin caused a 60 % increase in AUC and 170 % increase in trough concentration of caspofungin on the first day of co-administration when both medicinal products were initiated together. Caspofungin trough levels gradually decreased upon repeated administration. After two weeks' administration rifampicin had limited effect on AUC but trough levels were 30 % lower than in subjects who received caspofungin alone. The mechanism of interaction could possibly be due to an initial inhibition and subsequent induction of transport proteins. A similar effect could be expected for other medicinal products that induce metabolic enzymes. Limited data from population pharmacokinetics studies indicate that concomitant use of CANCIDAS with the inducers efavirenz, nevirapine, rifampicin, dexamethasone, phenytoin, or carbamazepine, may result in a decrease in caspofungin AUC. When co-administering inducers of metabolic enzymes, an increase in the daily dose of CANCIDAS to 70 mg, following the 70-mg loading dose, should be considered (see section 4.2).

Clinical studies in healthy volunteers show that the pharmacokinetics of CANCIDAS are not altered to a clinically relevant extent by itraconazole, amphotericin B, mycophenolate, nelfinavir, or tacrolimus. Caspofungin did not influence the pharmacokinetics of amphotericin B, itraconazole, rifampicin or mycophenolate mofetil. Although safety data are limited it appears that no special precautions are needed when amphotericin B, itraconazole, nelfinavir or mycophenolate mofetil are co-administered with caspofungin.

4.6 Pregnancy and lactation

For CANCIDAS, no clinical data on exposed pregnancies are available. Caspofungin should not be used during pregnancy unless clearly necessary. There are no adequate data from the use of caspofungin in pregnant women. Developmental studies in animals have shown adverse effects (see section 5.3). Caspofungin has been shown to cross the placental barrier in animal studies. The potential risk to the human foetus is unknown.

Caspofungin is excreted in milk of lactating animals. It is not known whether it is excreted in human milk. Women receiving caspofungin should not breast-feed.

4.7 Effects on ability to drive and use machines

No data are available on whether CANCIDAS impairs the ability to drive or operate machinery.

4.8 Undesirable effects

In clinical studies, 1440 individuals received single or multiple doses of CANCIDAS: 564 febrile neutropaenic patients (empirical therapy study), 125 patients with invasive candidiasis, 72 patients with invasive aspergillosis, 285 patients with localised *Candida* infections, and 394 individuals enrolled in Phase I studies. In the empirical therapy study patients had received chemotherapy for malignancy or had undergone hematopoietic stem-cell transplantation (including 39 allogeneic transplantations). In the studies involving patients with documented *Candida* infections, the majority of the patients with invasive *Candida* infections had serious underlying medical conditions (e.g., haematologic or other malignancy, recent major surgery, HIV) requiring multiple concomitant medications. Patients in the non-comparative *Aspergillus* study often had serious predisposing medical conditions (e.g., bone marrow or peripheral stem cell transplants, haematologic malignancy, solid tumours or organ transplants) requiring multiple concomitant medications.

Phlebitis was a commonly reported local injection-site adverse reaction in all patient populations. Other local reactions included erythema, pain/tenderness, itching, discharge, and a burning sensation.

Reported clinical and laboratory abnormalities among all patients treated with CANCIDAS (total 989) were typically mild and rarely led to discontinuation.

The following adverse events were reported:

[Very common (≥ 1/10), Common (≥ 1/100, < 1/10)]

Blood and lymphatic system disorders:

Common: anaemia

Nervous system disorders:

Common: headache

Cardiac disorders:

Common: tachycardia

Vascular disorders:

Common: phlebitis/thrombophlebitis, flushing

Respiratory, thoracic and mediastinal disorders:

Common: dyspnoea

Gastrointestinal disorders:

Common: abdominal pain, nausea, diarrhoea, vomiting

Skin and subcutaneous tissue disorders:

Common: rash, pruritus, sweating

General disorders and administration site conditions:

Very common: fever

Common: pain, chills, infused-vein complications

Investigations:

Common: elevated liver values (AST, ALT, alkaline phosphatase, direct and total bilirubin), increased serum creatinine, decreased haemoglobin, decreased haematocrit, blood potassium decreased, hypomagnesaemia, low albumin, decreased white blood cells, increased eosinophils, platelet count decreased, decreased neutrophils, increased urinary red blood cells, increased partial thromboplastin time, decreased total serum protein, increased urinary protein, increased prothrombin time, blood sodium decreased, increased urinary white blood cells and low calcium. High calcium has been reported as uncommon (≥1/1000, <1/100).

Possible histamine-mediated symptoms have been reported including reports of rash, facial swelling, pruritus, sensation of warmth, or bronchospasm. Anaphylaxis has been reported during administration of caspofungin.

Also reported in patients with invasive aspergillosis were pulmonary oedema, adult respiratory distress syndrome (ARDS), and radiographic infiltrates.

Post-Marketing experience:

The following post-marketing adverse events have been reported:

Hepatobiliary disorders:

Hepatic dysfunction

General disorders and administration site conditions:

Swelling and peripheral oedema

Investigations:

Hypercalcaemia

4.9 Overdose

Inadvertent administration of up to 140 mg of caspofungin in one day has been reported. These occurrences did not result in clinically important adverse experiences. Caspofungin is not dialysable.

5. PHARMACOLOGICAL PROPERTIES

5.1 Pharmacodynamic properties

Pharmacotherapeutic group: antimycotics for systemic use, ATC Code: J 02 AX 04

Caspofungin acetate is a semi-synthetic lipopeptide (echinocandin) compound synthesised from a fermentation product of *Glarea lozoyensis*. Caspofungin acetate inhibits the synthesis of beta (1,3)-D-glucan, an essential component of the cell wall of many filamentous fungi and yeast. Beta (1,3)-D-glucan is not present in mammalian cells.

Fungicidal activity with caspofungin has been demonstrated against *Candida* yeasts. Studies *in vitro* and *in vivo* demonstrate that exposure of *Aspergillus* to caspofungin results in lysis and death of hyphal apical tips and branch points where cell growth and division occur.

Caspofungin has *in vitro* activity against *Aspergillus* species (*Aspergillus fumigatus* [N = 75], *Aspergillus flavus* [N = 111], *Aspergillus niger* [N = 31], *Aspergillus nidulans* [N = 8], *Aspergillus terreus* [N = 52], and *Aspergillus candidus* [N = 3]). Caspofungin also has *in vitro* activity against *Candida* species (*Candida albicans* [N = 1032], *Candida dubliniensis* [N = 100], *Candida glabrata* [N = 151], *Candida guilliermondii* [N = 67], *Candida kefyr* [N = 62], *Candida krusei* [N = 147], *Candida lipolytica* [N = 20], *Candida lusitaniae* [N = 80], *Candida parapsilosis* [N = 215], *Candida rugosa* [N = 1], and *Candida tropicalis* [N = 258]), including isolates with multiple resistance transport mutations and those with acquired or intrinsic resistance to fluconazole, amphotericin B, and 5-flucytosine. Susceptibility testing was performed according to a modification of both the National Committee for Clinical Laboratory Standards (NCCLS) method M38-A (for *Aspergillus* species) and method M27-A (for *Candida* species). Mutants of *Candida* with reduced susceptibility to caspofungin have been identified in some patients during treatment. However, standardised techniques for susceptibility testing for antifungal agents, including beta (1,3)-D-glucan synthesis inhibitors, have not been established. MIC values for caspofungin should not be used to predict clinical outcome, since a correlation between MIC values and clinical outcome has not been established. Development of *in vitro* resistance to caspofungin by *Aspergillus* species has not been identified. In limited clinical experience, resistance to caspofungin in patients with invasive aspergillosis has not been observed. The incidence of resistance to caspofungin by various clinical isolates of *Candida* and *Aspergillus* is unknown.

Invasive Candidiasis: Two hundred thirty-nine patients were enrolled in a study to compare caspofungin and amphotericin B for the treatment of invasive candidiasis. Twenty-four patients had neutropaenia. The most frequent diagnoses were bloodstream infections (candidaemia) (77 %, n=186) and *Candida* peritonitis (8 %, n=19); patients with *Candida* endocarditis, osteomyelitis, or meningitis were excluded from this study. Caspofungin 50 mg once daily was administered following a 70-mg loading dose, while amphotericin B was administered at 0.6 to 0.7 mg/kg/day to non-neutropaenic patients or 0.7 to 1.0 mg/kg/day to neutropaenic patients. The mean duration of intravenous therapy was 11.9 days, with a range of 1 to 28 days. A favourable response required both symptom resolution and microbiological clearance of the *Candida* infection. Two hundred twenty-four patients were included in the primary efficacy analysis (MITT analysis) of response at the end of IV study therapy; favourable response rates for the treatment of invasive candidiasis were comparable for caspofungin (73 % [80/109]) and amphotericin B (62 % [71/115]) [% difference 12.7 (95.6 % CI -0.7, 26.0)]. Among patients with candidaemia, favourable response rates at the end of IV study therapy were comparable for caspofungin (72 % [66/92]) and amphotericin B (63 % [59/94]) in the primary efficacy analysis (MITT analysis) [% difference 10.0 (95.0 % CI -4.5, 24.5)]. Data in patients with non-blood sites of infection were more limited. Favourable response rates in neutropaenic patients were 7/14 (50 %) in the caspofungin group and 4/10 (40 %) in the amphotericin B group. These limited data are supported by the outcome of the empirical therapy study.

Invasive Aspergillosis: Sixty-nine adult patients (age 18-80) with invasive aspergillosis were enrolled in an open-label, non-comparative study to evaluate the safety, tolerability, and efficacy of caspofungin. Patients had to be either refractory to (disease progression or failure to improve with other antifungal therapies given for at least 7 days) (84 % of the enrolled patients) or intolerant of (16 % of enrolled patients) other standard antifungal therapies. Most patients had underlying conditions (haematologic malignancy [N = 24], allogeneic bone marrow transplant or stem cell transplant [N = 18], organ transplant [N = 8], solid tumour [N = 3], or other conditions [N = 10]). Stringent definitions, modelled after the Mycoses Study Group Criteria, were used for diagnosis of invasive aspergillosis and for response to therapy (favourable response required clinically significant improvement in radiographs as well as in signs and symptoms). The mean duration of therapy was 33.7 days, with a range of 1 to 162 days. An independent expert panel determined that 41 % (26/63) of patients receiving at least one dose of caspofungin had a favourable response. For those patients who received more than 7 days of therapy with caspofungin, 50 % (26/52) had a favourable response. The favourable response rates for patients who were either refractory to or intolerant of previous therapies were 36 % (19/53) and 70 % (7/10), respectively. Although the doses of prior antifungal therapies in 5 patients enrolled as refractory were lower than those often administered for invasive aspergillosis, the favourable response rate during therapy with caspofungin was similar in these patients to that seen in the remaining refractory patients (2/5 versus 17/48, respectively). The response rates among patients with pulmonary disease and extrapulmonary disease were 47 % (21/45) and 28 % (5/18), respectively. Among patients with extrapulmonary disease, 2 of 8 patients who also had definite, probable, or possible CNS involvement had a favourable response.

Empirical Therapy in Febrile, Neutropaenic Adult Patients: A total of 1111 patients with persistent fever and neutropaenia were enrolled in a clinical study and treated with either caspofungin 50 mg once daily following a 70-mg loading dose or liposomal amphotericin B 3.0 mg/kg/day. Eligible patients had received chemotherapy for malignancy or had undergone hematopoietic stem-cell transplantation, and presented with neutropaenia (<500 cells/mm^3 for 96 hours) and fever >38.0°C) not responding to ≥96 hours of parenteral antibacterial therapy. Patients were to be treated until up to 72 hours after resolution of neutropaenia, with a maximum duration of 28 days. However, patients found to have a documented fungal infection could be treated longer. If the drug was well tolerated but the patient's fever persisted and clinical condition deteriorated after 5 days of therapy, the dosage of study drug could be increased to 70 mg/day of caspofungin (13.3 % of patients treated) or to 5.0 mg/kg/day of liposomal amphotericin B (14.3 % of patients treated). There were 1095 patients included in the primary Modified Intention-To-Treat (MITT) efficacy analysis of overall favourable response; caspofungin (33.9 %) was as effective as liposomal amphotericin B (33.7 %) [% difference 0.2 (95.2 % CI –5.6, 6.0)]. An overall favourable response required meeting each of 5 criteria: (1) successful treatment of any baseline fungal infection (caspofungin 51.9 % [14/27], liposomal amphotericin B 25.9 % [7/27]), (2) no breakthrough fungal infections during administration of study drug or within 7 days after completion of treatment (caspofungin 94.8 % [527/556], liposomal amphotericin B 95.5 % [515/539]), (3) survival for 7 days after completion of study therapy (caspofungin 92.6 % [515/556], liposomal amphotericin B 89.2 % [481/539]), (4) no discontinuation from the study drug because of drug-related toxicity or lack of efficacy (caspofungin 89.7 % [499/556], liposomal amphotericin B 85.5 % [461/539]), and (5) resolution of fever during the period of neutropaenia (caspofungin 41.2 % [229/556], liposomal amphotericin B 41.4 % [223/539]). Response rates to caspofungin and liposomal amphotericin B for baseline infections caused by *Aspergillus* species were, respectively, 41.7 % (5/12) and 8.3 % (1/12), and by *Candida* species were 66.7 % (8/12) and 41.7 % (5/12). Patients in the caspofungin group experienced breakthrough infections due to the following uncommon yeasts and moulds: *Trichosporon* species (1), *Fusarium* species (1), *Mucor* species (1), and *Rhizopus* species (1).

5.2 Pharmacokinetic properties

Distribution

Caspofungin is extensively bound to albumin. The unbound fraction of caspofungin in plasma varies from 3.5 % in healthy volunteers to 7.6 % in patients with invasive candidiasis. Distribution plays the prominent role in caspofungin plasma pharmacokinetics and is the rate-controlling step in both the alpha- and beta-disposition phases. The distribution into tissues peaked at 1.5 to 2 days after dosing when 92 % of the dose was distributed into tissues. It is likely that only a small fraction of the caspofungin taken up into tissues later returns to plasma as parent compound. Therefore, elimination occurs in the absence of a distribution equilibrium, and a true estimate of the volume of distribution of caspofungin is currently impossible to obtain.

Metabolism

Caspofungin undergoes spontaneous degradation to an open ring compound. Further metabolism involves peptide hydrolysis and N-acetylation. Two intermediate products, formed during the degradation of caspofungin to this open ring compound, form covalent adducts to plasma proteins resulting in a low-level, irreversible binding to plasma proteins.

In vitro studies show that caspofungin is not an inhibitor of cytochrome P450 enzymes 1A2, 2A6, 2C9, 2C19, 2D6 or 3A4. In clinical studies, caspofungin did not induce or inhibit the CYP3A4 metabolism of other medicinal products. Caspofungin is not a substrate for P-glycoprotein and is a poor substrate for cytochrome P450 enzymes.

Elimination and excretion

The elimination of caspofungin from plasma is slow with a clearance of 10-12 ml/min. Plasma concentrations of caspofungin decline in a polyphasic manner following single 1-hour intravenous infusions. A short alpha-phase occurs immediately post-infusion, followed by a beta-phase with a half-life of 9 to 11 hours. An additional gamma-phase also occurs with a half-life of 45 hours. Distribution, rather than excretion or biotransformation, is the dominant mechanism influencing plasma clearance.

Approximately 75 % of a radioactive dose was recovered during 27 days: 41 % in urine and 34 % in faeces. There is little excretion or biotransformation of caspofungin during the first 30 hours after administration. Excretion is slow and the terminal half-life of radioactivity was 12 to 15 days. A small amount of caspofungin is excreted unchanged in urine (approximately 1.4 % of dose).

Caspofungin displays moderate non-linear pharmacokinetics with increased accumulation as the dose is increased, and a dose dependency in the time to reach steady state upon multiple-dose administration.

Special populations

Increased caspofungin exposure was seen in patients with renal impairment and mild liver impairment, in female subjects, and in the elderly. Generally the increase was modest and not large enough to warrant dosage adjustment. In patients with moderate liver impairment or in higher weight patients, a dosage adjustment may be necessary (see below).

Weight: Weight was found to influence caspofungin pharmacokinetics in the population pharmacokinetic analysis in candidiasis patients. The plasma concentrations decrease with increasing weight. The average exposure in a patient weighing 80 kg was predicted to be about 23 % lower than in a patient weighing 60 kg (see section 4.2).

Hepatic impairment: In patients with mild and moderate hepatic impairment, the AUC is increased about 20 and 75 %, respectively. There is no clinical experience with severe hepatic insufficiency. In a multiple-dose study, a dose reduction of the daily dose to 35 mg in moderate hepatic impairment has been shown to provide an AUC similar to that obtained in subjects with normal hepatic function receiving the standard regimen (see section 4.2).

Renal impairment: In a clinical study of single 70-mg doses, caspofungin pharmacokinetics were similar in volunteers with mild renal insufficiency (creatinine clearance 50 to 80 ml/min) and control subjects. Moderate (creatinine clearance 31 to 49 ml/min), advanced (creatinine clearance 5 to 30 ml/min), and end-stage (creatinine clearance <10 ml/min and dialysis dependent) renal insufficiency moderately increased caspofungin plasma concentrations after single-dose administration (range: 30 to 49 % for AUC). However, in patients with invasive candidiasis, oesophageal candidiasis, or invasive aspergillosis who received multiple daily doses of CANCIDAS 50 mg, there was no significant effect of mild to advanced renal impairment on caspofungin concentrations. No dosage adjustment is necessary for patients with renal insufficiency. Caspofungin is not dialysable, thus supplementary dosing is not required following haemodialysis.

Gender: Caspofungin plasma concentrations were on average 17-38 % higher in women than in men.

Elderly: A modest increase in AUC (28 %) and C_{24h} (32 %) was observed in elderly male subjects compared with young male subjects. In patients who were treated empirically or who had invasive candidiasis, a similar modest effect of age was seen in older patients relative to younger patients.

Race: Patient pharmacokinetic data indicated that no clinically significant differences in the pharmacokinetics of caspofungin were seen among Caucasians, Blacks, Hispanics, and Mestizos.

5.3 Preclinical safety data

Repeated dose toxicity studies in rat and monkey using doses up to 7-8 mg/kg given intravenously showed injection site reactions in rats and monkeys, signs of histamine release in rats, and evidence of adverse effects directed at the liver in monkey. Developmental toxicity studies in rats showed that caspofungin caused decreases in foetal body weights and an increase in the incidence of incomplete ossification of vertebra, sternebra, and skull bone at doses of 5 mg/kg that were coupled to adverse maternal effects such as signs of histamine release in pregnant rats. An increase in the incidence of cervical ribs was also noted. Caspofungin was negative in *in vitro* assays for potential genotoxicity as well as in the *in vivo* mouse bone marrow chromosomal test. No long-term studies in animals have been performed to evaluate the carcinogenic potential.

6. PHARMACEUTICAL PARTICULARS

6.1 List of excipients

Sucrose

Mannitol

Glacial acetic acid

Sodium hydroxide (to adjust the pH)

6.2 Incompatibilities

Do not mix with diluents containing glucose, as CANCIDAS is not stable in diluents containing glucose. Do not mix or co-infuse CANCIDAS with other medicinal products, as there are no data available on the compatibility of CANCIDAS with other intravenous substances, additives, or medicinal products.

6.3 Shelf life

2 years

Reconstituted concentrate: should be used immediately. Stability data have shown that the concentrate for solution for infusion can be stored for up to 24 hours when the vial is stored at 25°C or less and reconstituted with water for injections.

Dilute patient infusion solution: should be used immediately. Stability data have shown that the product can be used within 24 hours when stored at 25°C or less, or within 48 hours when the intravenous infusion bag (bottle) is stored refrigerated (2 to 8°C) and diluted with sodium chloride solution 9 mg/ml (0.9 %), 4.5 mg/ml (0.45 %), or 2.25 mg/ml (0.225 %) for infusion, or lactated Ringer's solution.

From a microbiological point of view, the product should be used immediately. If not used immediately, in use storage times and conditions prior to use are the responsibility of the user and would normally not be longer than 24 hours at 2 to 8°C, unless reconstitution and dilution have taken place in controlled validated aseptic conditions.

6.4 Special precautions for storage

Unopened vials: store at 2°C to 8°C (in a refrigerator).

Reconstituted concentrate: should be used immediately. Chemical and physical in-use stability has been demonstrated for 24 hours at 25°C.

Dilute patient infusion solution: should be used immediately. Chemical and physical in-use stability has been demonstrated for 24 hours at 25°C, and 48 hours under refrigeration (2 to 8°C).

CANCIDAS contains no preservatives. From a microbiological point of view, the product should be used immediately. If not used immediately, in-use storage times and conditions prior to use are the responsibility of the user and would normally not be longer than 24 hours at 2 to 8°C, unless reconstitution and dilution has taken place in controlled and validated aseptic conditions.

6.5 Nature and contents of container

CANCIDAS 50 mg Powder for concentrate for solution for infusion: 10 ml Type I glass vials with a grey butyl stopper

Table 1 PREPARATION OF THE SOLUTION FOR INFUSION

DOSE*	Volume of reconstituted CANCIDAS for transfer to intravenous bag or bottle	Standard preparation (reconstituted CANCIDAS added to 250 ml) final concentration	Reduced volume infusion (reconstituted CANCIDAS added to 100 ml) final concentration
50 mg	10 ml	0.19 mg/ml	-
50 mg at reduced volume	10 ml	-	0.45 mg/ml
35 mg for moderate hepatic insufficiency (from one 50 mg vial)	7 ml	0.14 mg/ml	-
35 mg for moderate hepatic insufficiency (from one 50 mg vial) at reduced volume	7 ml	-	0.33 mg/ml
70 mg	10 ml	0.27 mg/ml	Not recommended
70 mg (from two 50 mg vials)**	14 ml	0.27 mg/ml	Not recommended
35 mg for moderate hepatic insufficiency (from one 70-mg vial)	5 ml	0.14 mg/ml	0.33 mg/ml

* 10.5 ml should be used for reconstitution of all vials

**If 70 mg vial is not available, the 70 mg dose can be prepared from two 50 mg vials

and a plastic cap with a red aluminium band, for single use only.

CANCIDAS 70 mg Powder for concentrate for solution for infusion: 10 ml Type I glass vials with a grey butyl stopper and a plastic cap with a yellow/orange aluminium band, for single use only.

Supplied in packs of 1 vial.

6.6 Instructions for use and handling

Reconstitution of CANCIDAS

DO NOT USE ANY DILUENTS CONTAINING GLUCOSE as CANCIDAS is not stable in diluents containing glucose. DO NOT MIX OR CO-INFUSE CANCIDAS WITH ANY OTHER MEDICINES, as there are no data available on the compatibility of CANCIDAS with other intravenous substances, additives, or medicinal products. Visually inspect the infusion solution for particulate matter or discolouration.

Step 1 Reconstitution of conventional vials

To reconstitute the powder bring the vial to room temperature and aseptically add 10.5 ml of water for injections. The concentrations of the reconstituted vials will be: 5 mg/ml (50 mg vial) or 7 mg/ml (70 mg vial).

The white to off-white compact lyophilised powder will dissolve completely. Mix gently until a clear solution is obtained. Reconstituted solutions should be visually inspected for particulate matter or discolouration. This reconstituted solution may be stored for up to 24 hours at or below 25°C.

Step 2 Addition of Reconstituted CANCIDAS to patient infusion solution

Diluents for the final solution for infusion are: sodium chloride solution for injection, or lactated Ringer's solution. The solution for infusion is prepared by aseptically adding the appropriate amount of reconstituted concentrate (as shown in the table below) to a 250 ml infusion bag or bottle. Reduced volume infusions in 100 ml may be used, when medically necessary, for 50 mg or 35 mg daily doses. Do not use if the solution is cloudy or has precipitated. This infusion solution must be used within 24 hours if stored at or below 25°C, or within 48 hours if stored refrigerated at 2 to 8°C. Chemical and physical in-use stability of the diluted solution in sterile lactated Ringer's solution and sodium chloride solution 9 mg/ml (0.9 %), 4.5 mg/ml (0.45 %), and 2.25 mg/ml (0.225 %) for infusion has been demonstrated for 24 hours at 25°C and for 48 hours at 2 to 8°C. From a microbiological point of view, the solution must be used immediately. If not used immediately, in-use storage times and conditions prior to use are the responsibility of the user and would normally not be longer than 24 hours at 2 to 8°C, unless reconstitution and dilution has taken place in controlled and validated aseptic conditions.

PREPARATION OF THE SOLUTION FOR INFUSION

(see Table 1 on previous page)

7. MARKETING AUTHORISATION HOLDER

Merck Sharp & Dohme Ltd

Hertford Road, Hoddesdon

Hertfordshire EN11 9BU

United Kingdom

8. MARKETING AUTHORISATION NUMBER(S)

CANCIDAS 50 mg Powder for concentrate for solution for infusion: EU/1/01/196/001

CANCIDAS 70 mg Powder for concentrate for solution for infusion: EU/1/01/196/003

9. DATE OF FIRST AUTHORISATION/RENEWAL OF THE AUTHORISATION

24 October 2001

10. DATE OF REVISION OF THE TEXT

October 2004

SPC.CANC.04.UK/IRL.2109 (Var II/20)

Canesten 100mg Pessary

(Bayer plc)

1. NAME OF THE MEDICINAL PRODUCT

Canesten 100mg Pessary.

2. QUALITATIVE AND QUANTITATIVE COMPOSITION

Each pessary contains Clotrimazole Ph.Eur. 100mg.

3. PHARMACEUTICAL FORM

Pessaries.

4. CLINICAL PARTICULARS

4.1 Therapeutic indications

Canesten 100mg Pessaries are recommended for the treatment of candidal vaginitis.

4.2 Posology and method of administration

The pessaries should be inserted into the vagina using the applicator provided.

Adults:

Two pessaries should be inserted daily (preferably at night) for three consecutive days. Alternatively, one pessary may be inserted daily for six days, preferably at night. Treatment may be continued for 6, 12, or 18 days as necessary.

There is no separate dosage schedule for the elderly.

Children:

As this product is administered with an applicator, paediatric use is not recommended.

4.3 Contraindications

Hypersensitivity to clotrimazole.

4.4 Special warnings and special precautions for use

Medical advice should be sought if this is the first time the patient has experienced symptoms of candidal vaginitis.

Before using Canesten 100mg Pessaries, medical advice must be sought if any of the following are applicable:

- more than two infections of candidal vaginitis in the last six months.
- previous history of a sexually transmitted disease or exposure to partner with sexually transmitted disease.
- pregnancy or suspected pregnancy.
- aged under 16 or over 60 years.
- known hypersensitivity to imidazoles or other vaginal antifungal products.

Canesten 100mg Pessaries should not be used if the patient has any of the following symptoms whereupon medical advice should be sought:

- irregular vaginal bleeding.
- abnormal vaginal bleeding or a blood-stained discharge.
- vulval or vaginal ulcers, blisters or sores.
- lower abdominal pain or dysuria.
- any adverse events such as redness, irritation or swelling associated with the treatment.
- fever or chills.
- nausea or vomiting.
- diarrhoea.
- foul smelling vaginal discharge.

If no improvement in symptoms is seen after seven days the patient should consult a doctor.

4.5 Interaction with other medicinal products and other forms of Interaction

Laboratory tests have suggested that, when used together, this product may cause damage to latex contraceptives. Consequently the effectiveness of such contraceptives may be reduced. Patients should be advised to use alternative precautions for at least five days after using this product.

4.6 Pregnancy and lactation

In animal studies, clotrimazole has not been associated with teratogenic effects but following oral administration of high doses to rats, there was evidence of foetotoxicity. The relevance of this effect to topical application in humans is not known. However, clotrimazole has been used in pregnant patients for over a decade without attributable adverse effects. It is therefore recommended that clotrimazole should be used in pregnancy only when considered necessary by the clinician.

During pregnancy extra care should be taken when using the applicator to prevent the possibility of mechanical trauma.

4.7 Effects on ability to drive and use machines

Not applicable.

4.8 Undesirable effects

Rarely patients may experience local mild burning or irritation immediately after inserting the pessary. Very rarely the patient may find this irritation intolerable and stop treatment.

Hypersensitivity reactions may occur.

4.9 Overdose

In the event of accidental oral ingestion, routine measures such as gastric lavage should be performed as soon as possible after ingestion.

5. PHARMACOLOGICAL PROPERTIES

5.1 Pharmacodynamic properties

Clotrimazole has a broad-spectrum of activity (yeast, dermatophytes, moulds and a number of other fungi). It also exhibits activity against *Trichomonas vaginalis*, staphylococci, streptococci and *Bacteroides*.

5.2 Pharmacokinetic properties

Five female volunteers received one ^{14}C-clotrimazole 100mg pessary. Maximum equivalent concentrations of clotrimazole in the serum ranged between 0.016 and 0.05mcg/ml and were achieved 24-72 hours after administration.

5.3 Preclinical safety data

There are no pre-clinical data of relevance to the prescriber which are additional to the information included in other sections of the SPC.

6. PHARMACEUTICAL PARTICULARS

6.1 List of excipients

Calcium lactate pentahydrate

Maize starch

Crospovidone

Silica, colloidal anhydrous

Lactic acid

Lactose Monohydrate

Magnesium Stearate

Hypromellose

Cellulose, microcrystalline

6.2 Incompatibilities

None known.

6.3 Shelf life

48 months.

6.4 Special precautions for storage

There are no special storage requirements.

6.5 Nature and contents of container

Six pessaries are packed in a blister pack (foil 25μm PA + 45μm Al soft + 60μm PVC) sealed with aluminium backing foil (foil 20μm Al hard + 7g/m^2 HSL sealable to PVC/PVDC). An applicator is also provided.

The pessaries and applicator are enclosed in a cardboard carton.

6.6 Instructions for use and handling

1. Pull out plunger A until it stops.
Place pessary into the applicator.

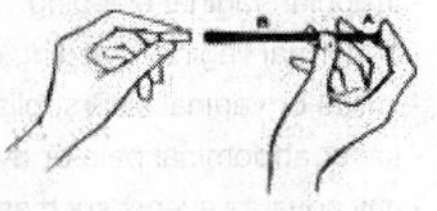

2. Insert applicator containing the pessary carefully as deeply as is comfortable into the vagina. (This is best done with the patient lying on her back with the knees bent up.)

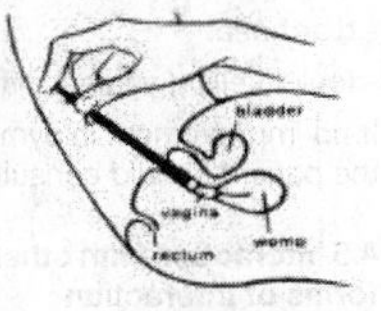

3. Push plunger A until it stops, thereby depositing the pessary into the vagina. Remove the applicator.

4. After use, remove plunger A completely by pulling it out of the applicator B.

Then wash it in warm (not boiling) soapy water, rinse and dry carefully.

7. MARKETING AUTHORISATION HOLDER

Bayer plc

Consumer Care Division

Bayer House

Strawberry Hill

Newbury, Berkshire

RG14 1JA

8. MARKETING AUTHORISATION NUMBER(S)

PL 0010/0015R

9. DATE OF FIRST AUTHORISATION/RENEWAL OF THE AUTHORISATION

Date of first authorisation: 18 August 1988.

Date of last renewal of authorisation: 17 February 1999.

10. DATE OF REVISION OF THE TEXT

August 2001

LEGAL CATEGORY:

P

Canesten 200mg Pessary

(Bayer plc)

1. NAME OF THE MEDICINAL PRODUCT

Canesten 200mg Pessary.

2. QUALITATIVE AND QUANTITATIVE COMPOSITION

Each pessary contains 200mg clotrimazole Ph.Eur.

3. PHARMACEUTICAL FORM

Pessaries.

4. CLINICAL PARTICULARS

4.1 Therapeutic indications

Canesten 200mg Pessaries are recommended for the treatment of candidal vaginitis.

4.2 Posology and method of administration

The pessaries should be inserted into the vagina using the applicator provided.

Adults:

One pessary should be inserted daily (preferably at night) for three consecutive days.

There is no separate dosage schedule for the elderly.

Children:

As this product is administered with an applicator, paediatric use is not recommended.

4.3 Contraindications

Hypersensitivity to clotrimazole.

4.4 Special warnings and special precautions for use

Medical advice should be sought if this is the first time the patient has experienced symptoms of candidal vaginitis.

Before using Canesten 200mg Pessaries, medical advice must be sought if any of the following are applicable:

- more than two infections of candidal vaginitis in the last six months.
- previous history of a sexually transmitted disease or exposure to partner with sexually transmitted disease.
- pregnancy or suspected pregnancy.
- aged under 16 or over 60 years.
- known hypersensitivity to imidazoles or other vaginal antifungal products.

Canesten 200mg Pessaries should not be used if the patient has any of the following symptoms whereupon medical advice should be sought:

- irregular vaginal bleeding.
- abnormal vaginal bleeding or a blood-stained discharge.
- vulval or vaginal ulcers, blisters or sores.
- lower abdominal pain or dysuria.
- any adverse events such as redness, irritation or swelling associated with the treatment.
- fever or chills.
- nausea or vomiting.
- diarrhoea.
- foul smelling vaginal discharge.

If no improvement in symptoms is seen after seven days, the patient should consult a doctor.

4.5 Interaction with other medicinal products and other forms of Interaction

Laboratory tests have suggested that, when used together, this product may cause damage to latex contraceptives. Consequently, the effectiveness of such contraceptives may be reduced. Patients should be advised to use alternative precautions for at least five days after using this product.

4.6 Pregnancy and lactation

In animal studies, clotrimazole has not been associated with teratogenic effects but following oral administration of high doses to rats, there was evidence of foetotoxicity. The relevance of this effect to topical application in humans is not known. However, clotrimazole has been used in pregnant patients for over a decade without attributable adverse effects. It is therefore recommended that clotrimazole should be used in pregnancy only when considered necessary by the clinician.

During pregnancy extra care should be taken when using the applicator to prevent the possibility of mechanical trauma.

4.7 Effects on ability to drive and use machines

Not applicable.

4.8 Undesirable effects

Rarely patients may experience local mild burning or irritation immediately after inserting the pessary. Very rarely the patient may find this irritation intolerable and stop treatment.

Hypersensitivity reactions may occur.

4.9 Overdose

In the event of accidental oral ingestion, routine measures such as gastric lavage should be performed as soon as possible after ingestion.

5. PHARMACOLOGICAL PROPERTIES

5.1 Pharmacodynamic properties

Clotrimazole has a broad-spectrum of activity (yeast, dermatophytes, moulds and a number of other fungi). It also exhibits activity against *Trichomonas vaginalis*, staphylococci and *Bacteroides*.

5.2 Pharmacokinetic properties

Five female volunteers received one ^{14}C-clotrimazole 100mg pessary. Maximum equivalent concentrations of clotrimazole in the serum ranged between 0.016 and 0.05 μg/ml and were achieved 24-72 hours after administration.

5.3 Preclinical safety data

There are no pre-clinical data of relevance to the prescriber which are additional to the information included in other sections of the SPC.

6. PHARMACEUTICAL PARTICULARS

6.1 List of excipients

Calcium lactate pentahydrate

Maize starch

Crospovidone

Silica, colloidal anhydrous

Lactic acid

Lactose Monohydrate

Magnesium Stearate

Hypromellose

Cellulose, microcrystalline

6.2 Incompatibilities

None known.

6.3 Shelf life

48 months.

6.4 Special precautions for storage

There are no special storage requirements.

6.5 Nature and contents of container

Three pessaries are packed in a blister pack (foil 25μm PA + 45μm Al soft + 60μm PVC) sealed with aluminium backing foil (foil 20μm Al hard + 7g/m^2 HSL sealable to PVC/PVDC). An applicator is also provided.

The pessaries and applicator are enclosed in a cardboard carton.

6.6 Instructions for use and handling

1. Pull out plunger A until it stops.
Place pessary into the applicator.

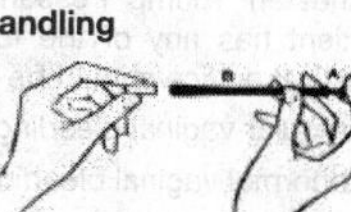

2. Insert applicator containing the pessary carefully as deeply as is comfortable into the vagina. (This is best done with the patient lying on her back with the knees bent up.)

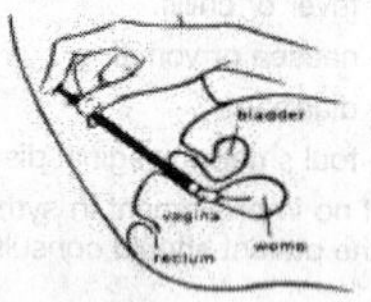

3. Push plunger A until it stops, thereby depositing the pessary into the vagina. Remove the applicator.

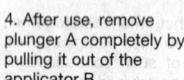

4. After use, remove plunger A completely by pulling it out of the applicator B.
Then wash it in warm (not boiling) soapy water, rinse and dry carefully.

7. MARKETING AUTHORISATION HOLDER

Bayer plc

Consumer Care Division

Bayer House

Strawberry Hill

Newbury, Berkshire

RG14 1JA

8. MARKETING AUTHORISATION NUMBER(S)

PL 0010/0072

9. DATE OF FIRST AUTHORISATION/RENEWAL OF THE AUTHORISATION

Date of first authorisation: 21 September 1979

Date of last renewal of authorisation: 10 November 1999

10. DATE OF REVISION OF THE TEXT

August 2001

LEGAL CATEGORY:

P

Canesten 500mg Vaginal Pessary

(Bayer plc)

1. NAME OF THE MEDICINAL PRODUCT

Canesten 500mg Vaginal Pessary.

2. QUALITATIVE AND QUANTITATIVE COMPOSITION

Clotrimazole 500mg.

For excipients, see 6.1.

3. PHARMACEUTICAL FORM

Pessary.

White convex pessary.

4. CLINICAL PARTICULARS

4.1 Therapeutic indications

Canesten 500mg Vaginal Pessary is recommended for the treatment of candidal vaginitis and mixed vaginal infections where *Trichomonas* is present or suspected. This product is not recommended as sole treatment for pure *Trichomoniasis* except in cases where systemic therapy is contra-indicated.

4.2 Posology and method of administration

The pessary should be inserted into the vagina using the applicator provided.

Adults: One 500mg pessary should be inserted at night. Using the applicator provided, the pessary should be inserted as deeply as possible into the vagina. This is best achieved when lying back with legs bent up.

Children: As the product is used with an applicator, paediatric usage is not recommended.

4.3 Contraindications

Known hypersensitivity to any of the ingredients in this product.

4.4 Special warnings and special precautions for use

None.

4.5 Interaction with other medicinal products and other forms of Interaction

Laboratory tests have suggested that, when used together, this product may cause damage to latex contraceptives. Consequently the effectiveness of such contraceptives may be reduced. Patients should be advised to use alternative precautions for at least five days after using this product.

4.6 Pregnancy and lactation

In animal studies clotrimazole has not been associated with teratogenic effects but following oral administration of high doses to rats there was evidence of foetotoxicity. The relevance of this effect to topical application in humans is not known. However, clotrimazole has been used in pregnant patients for over a decade without attributable adverse effects. It is, therefore, recommended that clotrimazole should be used in pregnancy only when considered necessary by the clinician. During pregnancy extra care should be taken when using the applicator to prevent the possibility of mechanical trauma.

4.7 Effects on ability to drive and use machines

Not applicable.

4.8 Undesirable effects

Rarely patients may experience local mild burning or irritation immediately after inserting the pessary. Very rarely the patient may find this irritation intolerable and stop treatment.

Hypersensitivity reactions may occur.

4.9 Overdose

In the event of accidental oral ingestion, routine measures such as gastric lavage should be performed as soon as possible after ingestion.

5. PHARMACOLOGICAL PROPERTIES

5.1 Pharmacodynamic properties

Clotrimazole has a broad spectrum of activity against yeast, dermatophytes, moulds and a number of other fungi. It also exhibits activity against *Trichomonas vaginalis, Staphylococci, Streptococci* and *Bacteroides*.

5.2 Pharmacokinetic properties

The vaginal availability of clotrimazole from 500mg pessaries was investigated in 8 volunteers. After 24 hours, samples of vaginal fluid gave an average of 68.1mg/ml clotrimazole (2.05mg/ml after 72 hours). In contrast the blood plasma concentrations of clotrimazole in the volunteers remained below the detection limit of 0.01μg/ml. Clotrimazole is absorbed vaginally and that which passes into the circulation undergoes extensive hepatic metabolism, the products of which are renally excreted.

5.3 Preclinical safety data

There are no pre-clinical data of relevance to the prescriber which are additional to the information included in other sections of the SmPC.

6. PHARMACEUTICAL PARTICULARS

6.1 List of excipients

Lactose Monohydrate

Cellulose, Microcrystalline

Lactic Acid

Maize Starch

Crospovidone

Calcium Lactate Pentahydrate

Magnesium Stearate

Silica, Colloidal Anhydrous

Hypromellose

6.2 Incompatibilities

Not applicable.

6.3 Shelf life

60 months.

6.4 Special precautions for storage

No special precautions for storage.

6.5 Nature and contents of container

Each pessary is packed into a blister consisting of 25μm PA (Polyamide) / 45μm Soft Aluminium / 60μm PVC and 20μm Hard Aluminium / 7 GSM HSL (Heat sealing lacquer). The blister and an applicator are enclosed in a cardboard carton.

The pessary is also available with a 10g tube of Canesten Thrush Cream as Canesten Combi 500mg Pessary and 2% Cream (Shelf life 36 months).

6.6 Instructions for use and handling
Not applicable.

7. MARKETING AUTHORISATION HOLDER
Bayer plc
Bayer House
Strawberry Hill
Newbury, Berkshire
RG14 1JA
United Kingdom
Trading as Bayer plc, Consumer Care Division.

8. MARKETING AUTHORISATION NUMBER(S)
PL 0010/0258

9. DATE OF FIRST AUTHORISATION/RENEWAL OF THE AUTHORISATION
11 July 2000

10. DATE OF REVISION OF THE TEXT
24 October 2001.

Canesten Combi Pessary & Cream

(Bayer plc)

1. NAME OF THE MEDICINAL PRODUCT
Canesten Combi Pessary & Cream

2. QUALITATIVE AND QUANTITATIVE COMPOSITION
Canesten Combi 500mg Pessary contains Clotrimazole 500mg.

Canesten Combi 2% Cream contains Clotrimazole 2% w/w.

For excipients, see 6.1.

3. PHARMACEUTICAL FORM
Pessary and cream

4. CLINICAL PARTICULARS
4.1 Therapeutic indications
The pessary is recommended for the treatment of candidal vaginitis.

The cream is recommended for the treatment of candidal vulvitis. It should be used as an adjunct to treatment of candidal vaginitis.

These products should only be used if candidal vulvovaginitis (thrush) was previously diagnosed by a doctor.

4.2 Posology and method of administration
Adults
One pessary should be inserted into the vagina at night. Using the applicator provided, the pessary should be inserted as deeply as possible into the vagina. This is best achieved when lying back with legs bent up.

The cream should be thinly applied to the vulva and surrounding area, two or three times daily and rubbed in gently.

Treatment with the cream should be continued until symptoms of the infection disappear. However, if after concomitant treatment of the vaginitis, the symptoms do not improve within seven days, the patient should consult a physician.

Children
Not for use in children under 16.

4.3 Contraindications
Hypersensitivity to clotrimazole or any of the other ingredients. Do not use to treat nail or scalp infections.

4.4 Special warnings and special precautions for use
This product contains cetostearyl alcohol, which may cause local skin reactions (e.g. contact dermatitis).

Before using Canesten Combi Pesasary & Cream, medical advice must be sought if any of the following are applicable:-

- more than two infections of candidal vaginitis in the last 6 months.
- previous history of sexually transmitted disease or exposure to partner with sexually transmitted disease.
- pregnancy or suspected pregnancy.
- aged under 16 or over 60 years.
- known hypersensitivity to imidazoles or other vaginal antifungal products.

The pessary and cream should not be used if the patient has any of the following symptoms where upon medical advice should be sought:-

- irregular vaginal bleeding.
- abnormal vaginal bleeding or a blood-stained discharge.
- vulval or vaginal ulcers, blisters or sores.
- lower abdominal pain or dysuria.
- any adverse events such as redness, irritation or swelling associated with the treatment.
- fever or chills.
- nausea or vomiting.
- diarrhoea.
- foul smelling vaginal discharge.

If no improvement in symptoms is seen after 7 days the patient should consult their doctor.

4.5 Interaction with other medicinal products and other forms of Interaction
Laboratory tests have suggested that, when used together, this product may cause damage to latex contraceptives. Consequently the effectiveness of such contraceptives may be reduced. Patients should be advised to use alternative precautions for at least five days after using this product.

4.6 Pregnancy and lactation
In animal studies clotrimazole has not been associated with teratogenic effects but following oral administration of high doses to rats there was evidence of foetotoxicity. The relevance of this effect to topical application in humans is not known. However, clotrimazole has been used in pregnant patients for over a decade without attributable adverse effects. It is, therefore, recommended that clotrimazole should be used in pregnancy only when considered necessary by the clinician. During pregnancy extra care should be taken when using the applicator to prevent the possibility of mechanical trauma.

4.7 Effects on ability to drive and use machines
Not applicable.

4.8 Undesirable effects
Rarely patients may experience local mild burning or irritation immediately after inserting the pessary or applying the cream. Very rarely the patient may find this irritation intolerable and stop treatment. Hypersensitivity reactions may occur.

4.9 Overdose
In the event of accidental oral ingestion, routine measures such as gastric lavage should be performed as soon as possible after ingestion.

5. PHARMACOLOGICAL PROPERTIES
5.1 Pharmacodynamic properties
ATC Code: G01A F18 Gynecological antiinfectives and antiseptics – imidazole derivatives

Clotrimazole has a broad spectrum of activity against yeast, dermatophytes, moulds and a number of other fungi. It is effective on yeasts, notably *Candida albicans* and *Torulopsis glabrata* as well as on *Trichomonas vaginalis* and some gram-positive and gram-negative bacteria (streptococci, staphylococci, *Gardnerella vaginalis*, *Bacteroides*).

5.2 Pharmacokinetic properties
The vaginal availability of clotrimazole from 500mg pessaries was investigated in 8 volunteers. After 24 hours, samples of vaginal fluid gave an average of 68.1mg/ml clotrimazole (2.05mg/ml after 72 hours). In contrast the blood plasma concentrations of clotrimazole in the volunteers remained below the detection limit of 0.01μg/ml. Clotrimazole is absorbed vaginally and that which passes into the circulation undergoes extensive hepatic metabolism, the products of which are renally excreted.

Studies in volunteers using radioactively labelled active substance applied as 1% vaginal cream indicated a rate of vaginal absorption between 3 and 10% of the dose applied. The concentrations of unchanged active substance in the plasma of volunteers following the application of 2% vaginal cream were below the limit of detection (10mg/ml). Since only very small amounts of active substance are absorbed by the vaginal skin and it is metabolised very quickly ($t½$ = 1-2 hours), concentrations in the blood plasma are always below the limit of detection.

5.3 Preclinical safety data
Toxicological studies in different animals with intravaginal or local application of clotrimazole showed good vaginal and local tolerability. No teratogenic or embryotoxic effects could be observed. Clotrimazole had no influence on the fertility and showed no mutagenic properties.

6. PHARMACEUTICAL PARTICULARS
6.1 List of excipients
The pessary contains:
Lactose monohydrate
Microcrystalline cellulose
Lactic acid
Maize Starch
Povidone
Calcium lactate pentahydrate
Magnesium stearate
Silica, colloidal anhydrous
Hypromellose

The cream contains:
Sorbitan stearate
Polysorbate 60
Cetyl palmitate
Cetostearyl alcohol
Octyldodecanol
Benzyl alcohol
Purified Water

6.2 Incompatibilities
None known

6.3 Shelf life
36 months.

6.4 Special precautions for storage
Do not store above 25°C.

6.5 Nature and contents of container
The pessary is packed into a blister consisting of 25μm PA (Polyamide) / 45μm Soft Aluminium / 60μm PVC and 20μm Hard Aluminium / 7 GSM HSL (Heat sealing lacquer) and is supplied with an applicator

The cream is filled into Aluminium tubes (10g) with internal lacquer coating, latex stopper and HDPE screw top.

The blister, an applicator and tube are enclosed in a cardboard carton.

6.6 Instructions for use and handling
The pessary is inserted as follows:

1.	Pull out plunger A until it stops. Place the pessary into the applicator B.	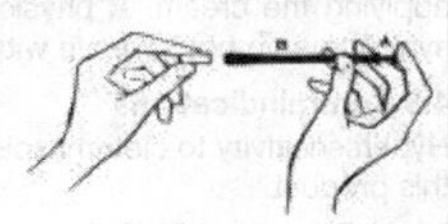
2.	Carefully insert the applicator containing the pessary as deeply as is comfortable into the vagina. This is best done with the patient lying on her back with the knees bent up.	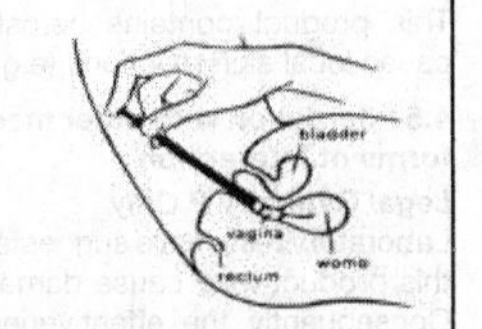
3.	Push plunger A until it stops, thereby depositing the pessary into the vagina. Withdraw the applicator and dispose of it hygienically.	

There are no special instructions for use of the cream

7. MARKETING AUTHORISATION HOLDER
Bayer plc
Bayer House
Strawberry Hill
Newbury, Berkshire
RG14 1JA
Trading as Bayer, plc, Consumer Care Division

8. MARKETING AUTHORISATION NUMBER(S)
PL 00010/0300

9. DATE OF FIRST AUTHORISATION/RENEWAL OF THE AUTHORISATION
18th March 2004.

10. DATE OF REVISION OF THE TEXT
November 2003

LEGAL CATEGORY
GSL

Canesten Cream / Canesten AF Cream

(Bayer plc)

1. NAME OF THE MEDICINAL PRODUCT
Canesten Cream (also available as Canesten AF Cream)

2. QUALITATIVE AND QUANTITATIVE COMPOSITION
Clotrimazole 1% w/w.

For excipients, see 6.1.

3. PHARMACEUTICAL FORM
A white cream for topical use.

4. CLINICAL PARTICULARS

4.1 Therapeutic indications

Legal Category P

Canesten is a broad-spectrum antifungal. It also exhibits activity against *Trichomonas,* staphylococci, streptococci and *Bacteroides.* It has no effect on lactobacilli.

It is indicated for the treatment of:

(i) All dermatomycoses due to moulds and other fungi, (e.g. *Trichophyton* species).

(ii) All dermatomycoses due to yeasts (*Candida* species).

(iii) Skin diseases showing secondary infection with these fungi.

(iv) Candidal nappy rash, vulvitis and balanitis.

Legal Category GSL

For the treatment of tinea pedis and tinea cruris.

4.2 Posology and method of administration

There is no separate dosage schedule for the young or elderly.

Legal Category P Only

Canesten Cream should be applied thinly 2-3 times daily and rubbed in gently. Treatment should be continued for at least one month for dermatophyte infections and at least two weeks for candidal infections.

If the feet are infected they should be washed and dried, especially between the toes, before applying the cream.

Legal Category GSL Only

Canesten Cream should be applied thinly 2-3 times daily and rubbed in gently. If the feet are infected they should be washed and dried, especially between the toes, before applying the cream. A physician should be consulted if symptoms do not improve within 7 days.

4.3 Contraindications

Hypersensitivity to clotrimazole or any of the excipients in this product.

Legal Category GSL Only

Do not use the cream to treat nail or scalp infections.

4.4 Special warnings and special precautions for use

This product contains cetostearyl alcohol, which may cause local skin reactions (e.g. contact dermatitis).

4.5 Interaction with other medicinal products and other forms of Interaction

Legal Category P Only

Laboratory tests have suggested that, when used together, this product may cause damage to latex contraceptives. Consequently the effectiveness of such contraceptives may be reduced. Patients should be advised to use alternative precautions for at least five days after using this product.

Legal Category GSL Only

No interactions.

4.6 Pregnancy and lactation

Data on a large number of exposed pregnancies indicate no adverse effects of Clotrimazole on pregnancy or on the health of the foetus/newborn child. To date, no other relevant epidemiological data available.

Clotrimazole can be used during pregnancy, but only under the supervision of a physician or midwife.

4.7 Effects on ability to drive and use machines

Not applicable.

4.8 Undesirable effects

Rarely patients may experience local mild burning or irritation immediately after applying the cream. Very rarely the patient may find this irritation intolerable and stop treatment.

Other undesirable effects:

Body as a whole: allergic reaction, pain

Skin and appendages: pruritis, rash

4.9 Overdose

In the event of accidental oral ingestion, gastric lavage is rarely required and should be considered only if a life-threatening amount of Clotrimazole has been ingested within the preceding hour or if clinical symptoms of overdose become apparent (e.g. dizziness, nausea or vomiting). It should be carried out only if the airway can be protected adequately.

5. PHARMACOLOGICAL PROPERTIES

5.1 Pharmacodynamic properties

ATC Code: D01A C01

Clotrimazole is an imidazole derivative with a broad spectrum of antimycotic activity.

Mechanism of Action

Clotrimazole acts against fungi by inhibiting ergosterol synthesis. Inhibition of ergosterol synthesis leads to structural and functional impairment of the cytoplasmic membrane.

Pharmacodynamic Effects

Clotrimazole has a broad antimycotic spectrum of action in vitro and in vivo, which includes dermatophytes, yeasts, moulds, etc.

The mode of action of clotrimazole is fungistatic or fungicidal depending on the concentration of clotrimazole at the site of infection. In-vitro activity is limited to proliferating fungal elements; fungal spores are only slightly sensitive.

Primarily resistant variants of sensitive fungal species are very rare; the development of secondary resistance by sensitive fungi has so far only been observed in very isolated cases under therapeutic conditions.

5.2 Pharmacokinetic properties

Pharmacokinetic investigations after dermal application have shown that clotrimazole is practically not absorbed from the intact or inflamed skin into the human blood circulation. The resulting peak serum concentrations of clotrimazole were below the detection limit of 0.001 mcg/ml, reflecting that clotrimazole applied topically does not lead to measurable systemic effects or side effects.

5.3 Preclinical safety data

There are no pre-clinical data of relevance to the prescriber which are additional to the information included in other sections of the SPC.

6. PHARMACEUTICAL PARTICULARS

6.1 List of excipients

Sorbitan stearate

Polysorbate 60

Cetyl palmitate

Cetostearyl alcohol

Octyldodecanol

Benzyl Alcohol

Purified water

6.2 Incompatibilities

Not applicable.

6.3 Shelf life

36 months.

6.4 Special precautions for storage

Do not store above 25°C.

6.5 Nature and contents of container

The cream is filled into aluminium tubes with internal lacquer coating and HDPE screw-on caps and enclosed in an outer carton. Pack sizes available are 15g (Canesten AF Cream), 20g and 50g.

6.6 Instructions for use and handling

No special requirements.

7. MARKETING AUTHORISATION HOLDER

Bayer plc

Bayer House

Strawberry Hill

Newbury, Berkshire

RG14 1JA

Trading as Bayer plc, Consumer Care Division

8. MARKETING AUTHORISATION NUMBER(S)

PL 0010/0016R

9. DATE OF FIRST AUTHORISATION/RENEWAL OF THE AUTHORISATION

Date of first authorisation: 18 August 1988

Date of last renewal of authorisation: 9 September 1999

10. DATE OF REVISION OF THE TEXT

September 2004

LEGAL CATEGORY

Canesten Cream P

Canesten AF Cream GSL

Canesten Cream Combi Internal & External Creams

(Bayer plc)

1. NAME OF THE MEDICINAL PRODUCT

Canesten Cream Combi Internal & External Creams

2. QUALITATIVE AND QUANTITATIVE COMPOSITION

Canesten Combi 10% Internal Cream contains Clotrimazole 10% w/w.

Canesten Combi 2% External Cream contains Clotrimazole 2% w/w.

For excipients, see 6.1

3. PHARMACEUTICAL FORM

Cream.

4. CLINICAL PARTICULARS

4.1 Therapeutic indications

The internal cream is recommended for the treatment of candidal vaginitis.

The external cream is recommended for the treatment of candidal vulvitis. It should be used as an adjunct to treatment of candidal vaginitis.

These products should only be used if candidal vulvovaginitis (thrush) was previously diagnosed by a doctor.

4.2 Posology and method of administration

Adults

The internal cream should be administered intravaginally using the applicator supplied.

The contents of the filled applicator (5g) should be inserted as deeply as possible into the vagina, preferably at night.

The external cream should be thinly applied to the vulva and surrounding area, two or three times daily and rubbed in gently.

Treatment with the external cream should be continued until symptoms of the infection disappear. However, if after concomitant treatment of the vaginitis, the symptoms do not improve within seven days, the patient should consult a physician.

Children

Not for use in children under 16.

4.3 Contraindications

Hypersensitivity to clotrimazole and any of the other ingredients. Do not use to treat nail or scalp infections.

4.4 Special warnings and special precautions for use

These products contain cetostearyl alcohol, which may cause local skin reactions (e.g. contact dermatitis).

Before using Canesten Cream Combi Internal & External Creams medical advice must be sought if any of the following are applicable: -

- more than two infections of candidal vaginitis in the last 6 months
- previous history of a sexually transmitted disease or exposure to partner with sexually transmitted disease
- pregnancy or suspected pregnancy
- aged under 16 or over 60 years
- known hypersensitivity to imidazoles or other vaginal antifungal products

The creams should not be used if the patient has any of the following symptoms whereupon medical advice should be sought: -

- irregular vaginal bleeding
- abnormal vaginal bleeding or a blood-stained discharge
- vulval or vaginal ulcers, blisters or sores
- lower abdominal pain or dysuria
- any adverse events such as redness, irritation or swelling associated with the treatment
- fever or chills
- nausea or vomiting
- diarrhoea
- foul smelling vaginal discharge

If no improvement in symptoms is seen after 7 days the patient should consult their doctor.

4.5 Interaction with other medicinal products and other forms of Interaction

Laboratory tests have suggested that this product may cause damage to latex contraceptives. Consequently the effectiveness of such contraceptives may be reduced. Patients should be advised to use alternative precautions for at least five days after using this product.

4.6 Pregnancy and lactation

In animal studies clotrimazole has not been associated with teratogenic effects but following oral administration of high doses to rats there was evidence of foetotoxicity. The relevance of this effect to topical application in humans is not known. However, clotrimazole has been used in pregnant patients for over a decade without attributable adverse effects. It is therefore recommended that clotrimazole should be used in pregnancy only when considered necessary by the clinician.

During pregnancy, extra care should be taken when using the applicator to prevent the possibility of mechanical trauma.

4.7 Effects on ability to drive and use machines

Not applicable.

4.8 Undesirable effects

Rarely, patients may experience local mild burning or irritation immediately after applying the cream. Very rarely the patient may find this intolerable and stop treatment.

Hypersensitivity reactions may occur.

4.9 Overdose

In the event of accidental oral ingestion, routine measures such as gastric lavage should be performed as soon as possible after ingestion.

5. PHARMACOLOGICAL PROPERTIES

5.1 Pharmacodynamic properties

ATC Code: G01A F18 Gynecological antiinfectives and antiseptics – imidazole derivatives

Clotrimazole has a broad spectrum of activity against yeasts, dermatophytes and a number of other fungi. It is effective on yeasts, notably *Candida albicans* and *Torulopsis glabrata* as well as on *Trichomonas vaginalis* and some gram-positive and gram-negative bacteria (streptococci, staphylococci, *Gardnerella vaginalis*, *Bacteroides*). It has no effect on lactobacilli.

5.2 Pharmacokinetic properties

External cream

Studies in volunteers using radioactively labelled active substance applied as 1% vaginal cream indicated a rate of vaginal absorption between 3 and 10% of the dose applied. The concentrations of unchanged active substance in the plasma of volunteers following the application of 2% vaginal cream were below the limit of detection (10mg/ml). Since only very small amounts of active substance are absorbed by the vaginal skin and it is metabolised very quickly ($t_{½}$ = 1-2 hours), concentrations in the blood plasma are always below the limit of detection.

Internal cream

A randomised double-blind study was conducted in 16 healthy, non-pregnant volunteers. Following administration of 5.0g of clotrimazole vaginal cream, the concentrations of active substance in the blood plasma and vaginal secretions were determined.

No active substance could be detected in the plasma samples by the microbiological determination method. However, microbiologically active clotrimazole concentrations were found in the vaginal secretions up to 48 hours after the application.

5.3 Preclinical safety data

Toxicological studies in different animals with intravaginal or local application of Canesten showed good vaginal and local tolerability. No teratogenic or embryotoxic effects could be observed. Canesten had no influence on the fertility and showed no mutagenic properties.

6. PHARMACEUTICAL PARTICULARS

6.1 List of excipients

Canesten Combi 10% Internal Cream contains:

Sorbitan stearate

Polysorbate 60

Cetyl palmitate

Cetostearyl alcohol

Isopropyl myristate

Benzyl alcohol

Purified water

Canesten Combi 2% External Cream contains:

Sorbitan stearate

Polysorbate 60

Cetyl palmitate

Cetostearyl alcohol

Octyldodecanol

Benzyl alcohol

Purified Water

6.2 Incompatibilities

None known.

6.3 Shelf life

24 months.

6.4 Special precautions for storage

Do not store above 25°C.

6.5 Nature and contents of container

Canesten Combi 10% Internal Cream:

A single dose applicator consisting of a body of HDPE (lupolene or hostalene), piston of LDPE, cap of LDPE, with a separate plunger of polystyrene. One applicator is contained in a blister pack. Pack size 5g.

Canesten Combi 2% External Cream:

The cream is filled into Aluminium tubes (10g) with internal lacquer coating, latex stopper and HDPE screw top.

The blister pack and tube are enclosed in a cardboard carton.

6.6 Instructions for use and handling

Canesten Combi 10% Internal Cream:

1. Remove applicator from package. Insert plunger (A) into applicator (B).

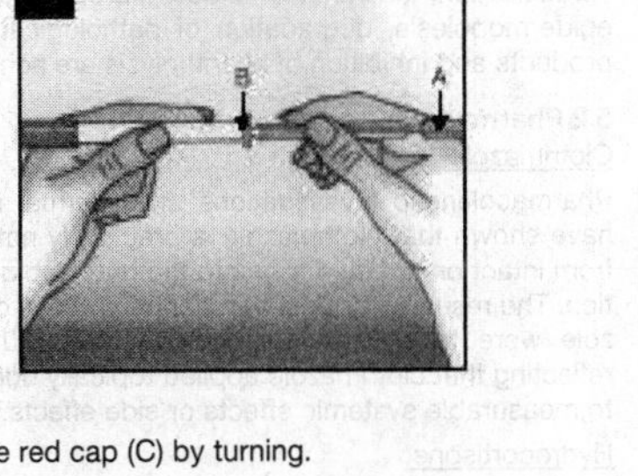

2. Remove red cap (C) by turning.

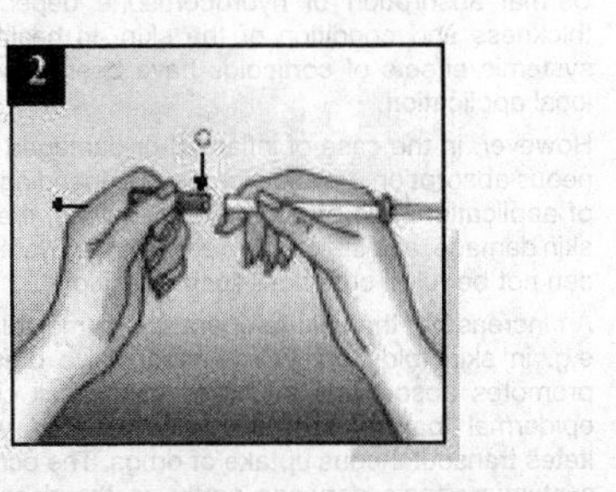

3. Introduce applicator (B) as deeply as possible into the vagina (this is best done with the patient lying on her back with the knees bent up) and empty its contents into the vagina by pushing the plunger (A).

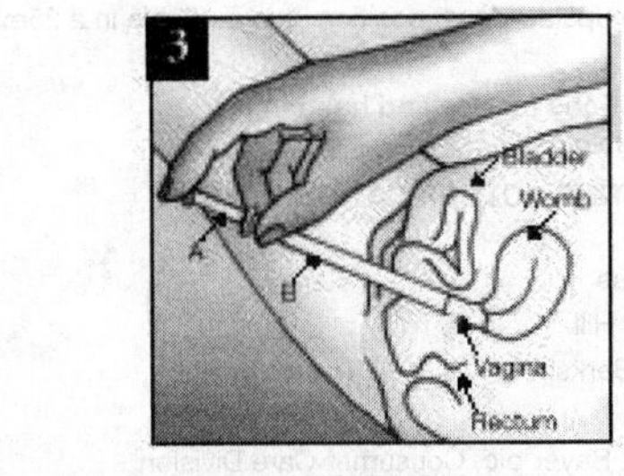

4. Remove the applicator and dispose of it hygienically.

Canesten Combi 2% External Cream:

There are no special instructions for use of the cream.

7. MARKETING AUTHORISATION HOLDER

Bayer plc

Bayer House

Strawberry Hill

Newbury, Berkshire

RG14 1JA.

Trading as Bayer plc, Consumer Care Division

8. MARKETING AUTHORISATION NUMBER(S)

PL 0010/0301

9. DATE OF FIRST AUTHORISATION/RENEWAL OF THE AUTHORISATION

08/12 2004

10. DATE OF REVISION OF THE TEXT

LEGAL CATEGORY

GSL

Canesten Dermatological Powder /Canesten AF Powder

(Bayer plc)

1. NAME OF THE MEDICINAL PRODUCT

Canesten Dermatological Powder (also available as Canesten AF Powder)

2. QUALITATIVE AND QUANTITATIVE COMPOSITION

The powder contains Clotrimazole Ph. Eur. 1% w/w.

3. PHARMACEUTICAL FORM

Powder for topical application.

4. CLINICAL PARTICULARS

4.1 Therapeutic indications

Legal Category P

Clotrimazole is a broad-spectrum antifungal. It also exhibits activity against *Trichomonas vaginalis*, staphylococci, streptococci and *Bacteroides*. It has no effect on lactobacilli.

Canesten Dermatological Powder should be used externally as an adjunct to treatment with Canesten Cream, Solution or Dermatological Spray and as a prophylactic against reinfection, particularly in infections involving skin folds, and where perspiration is a problem.

Legal Category GSL

Should be used as an adjunct to treatment with Canesten AF Cream or Canesten AF Spray and as a prophylactic against reinfection of tinea pedis (athlete's foot) only.

4.2 Posology and method of administration

Canesten Dermatological Powder should be sprinkled onto the affected areas two to three times daily after using Canesten Cream, Solution or Dermatological Spray. The powder may also be dusted inside articles of clothing and footwear which are in contact with the infected area.

4.3 Contraindications

Hypersensitivity to clotrimazole or the excipient rice starch.

Legal Category GSL Only

Do not use the powder to treat nail or scalp infections.

4.4 Special warnings and special precautions for use

None.

4.5 Interaction with other medicinal products and other forms of Interaction

None.

4.6 Pregnancy and lactation

In animal studies clotrimazole has not been associated with teratogenic effects but following oral administration of high doses to rats there was evidence of foetotoxicity. The relevance of this effect to topical application in humans is not known. However, clotrimazole has been used in pregnant patients for over a decade without attributable adverse effects. It is therefore recommended that clotrimazole should be used in pregnancy only when considered necessary by the clinician.

4.7 Effects on ability to drive and use machines

Not applicable.

4.8 Undesirable effects

Rarely, patients may experience local mild burning or irritation immediately after applying the powder. Very rarely the patient may find this intolerable and stop treatment.

Hypersensitivity reactions may occur.

4.9 Overdose

In the event of accidental oral ingestion, routine measures such as gastric lavage should be performed as soon as possible after ingestion.

5. PHARMACOLOGICAL PROPERTIES

5.1 Pharmacodynamic properties

Clotrimazole has a broad spectrum of activity (yeasts, dermatophytes, moulds and a number of other fungi). It also exhibits activity against *Trichomonas vaginalis*, staphylococci, streptococci and *Bacteroides*. It has no effect on lactobacilli.

5.2 Pharmacokinetic properties

Following the topical application of clotrimazole, absorption is minimal. This has been demonstrated when ^{14}C-clotrimazole was administered to three volunteers with normal skin, in the form of a 1% solution, at a dose of 0.5ml per 200cm^2 skin area, and with occlusive dressing for six hours. Less than 0.05% of applied activity was excreted with the urine within 48 hours and the serum activity remained below the detection limit of 0.001 mcg/ml.

5.3 Preclinical safety data

There are no preclinical data of relevance to the prescriber which are additional to those already included in other sections of the Summary of Product Characteristics.

6. PHARMACEUTICAL PARTICULARS

6.1 List of excipients

Canesten Dermatological Powder contains non-expandable rice starch Ph.Eur.

6.2 Incompatibilities

None known.

6.3 Shelf life

60 months.

6.4 Special precautions for storage

There are no special storage requirements.

6.5 Nature and contents of container

Polyethylene powder canister with a perforated conical plug for dusting and a screw cap. The canister contains 30g of powder.

6.6 Instructions for use and handling

Not applicable.

7. MARKETING AUTHORISATION HOLDER

Bayer plc

Bayer House

Strawberry Hill

Newbury, Berkshire

RG14 1JA.

Trading as Bayer plc, Consumer Care Division

8. MARKETING AUTHORISATION NUMBER(S)

PL 0010/0067

9. DATE OF FIRST AUTHORISATION/RENEWAL OF THE AUTHORISATION

Date of first authorisation: 27 July 1978

Date of last renewal: 8 January 1999

10. DATE OF REVISION OF THE TEXT

June 2001

LEGAL CATEGORY

Canesten Dermatological Powder P

Canesten AF Powder GSL

Canesten Dermatological Spray / Canesten AF Spray

(Bayer plc)

1. NAME OF THE MEDICINAL PRODUCT

Canesten Dermatological Spray (also available as Canesten AF Spray).

2. QUALITATIVE AND QUANTITATIVE COMPOSITION

The solution contains Clotrimazole Ph.Eur. 1% w/v.

3. PHARMACEUTICAL FORM

A colourless solution for topical administration by an atomiser.

4. CLINICAL PARTICULARS

4.1 Therapeutic indications

Legal Category P

Canesten is a broad-spectrum antifungal. It also exhibits activity against *Trichomonas*, staphylococci, streptococci and *Bacteroides*. It has no effect on lactobacilli.

It is recommended for the treatment of:

(i) All dermatomycoses due to moulds and other fungi, (e.g. *Trichophyton* species).

(ii) All dermatomycoses due to yeasts (*Candida* species).

(iii) Skin diseases showing secondary infection with these fungi.

Canesten Dermatological Spray is particularly suitable for infections covering large and/or hairy areas.

Legal Category GSL

For the treatment of tinea pedis (athlete's foot) and tinea cruris (jock itch).

4.2 Posology and method of administration

The spray should be applied thinly 2-3 times daily for at least one month for dermatophyte infections, and at least two weeks for candidal and *Pityriasis versicolor* infections.

If the feet are infected they should be washed and dried, especially between the toes, before applying.

There is no separate dosage schedule for the young or elderly.

4.3 Contraindications

Hypersensitivity to clotrimazole or any of the excipients in this product.

Legal Category GSL Only

Do not use the spray to treat nail or scalp infections.

4.4 Special warnings and special precautions for use

Canesten Dermatological Spray should not be used near a naked flame, should not be allowed to come into contact with the eyes, ears or mucous membranes and should not be inhaled.

4.5 Interaction with other medicinal products and other forms of Interaction

None known.

4.6 Pregnancy and lactation

In animal studies, clotrimazole has not been associated with teratogenic effects but following oral administration of high doses to rats, there was evidence of foetotoxicity. The relevance of this effect to topical application in humans is not known. However, clotrimazole has been used in pregnant patients for over a decade without attributable adverse effects. It is therefore recommended that clotrimazole should be used in pregnancy only when considered necessary by the clinician.

4.7 Effects on ability to drive and use machines

Not applicable.

4.8 Undesirable effects

Rarely patients may experience local mild burning or irritation immediately after applying the solution. Very rarely the patient may find this irritation intolerable and stop treatment.

Hypersensitivity reactions may occur.

4.9 Overdose

In the event of accidental oral ingestion, routine measures such as gastric lavage should be performed as soon as possible after ingestion.

5. PHARMACOLOGICAL PROPERTIES

5.1 Pharmacodynamic properties

Clotrimazole has a broad-spectrum of activity (yeast, dermatophytes, moulds and a number of other fungi). It also exhibits activity against *Trichomonas vaginalis*, staphylococci, streptococci and *Bacteroides*.

5.2 Pharmacokinetic properties

Clotrimazole ^{14}C was administered dermally to five volunteers with normal skin in the form of the 1% solution used in Canesten Dermatological Spray at a dose of 0.8ml/200cm ^{2} skin surface with occlusive dressing for 6 hours.

Maximum equivalent concentrations of approximately 0.004 to 0.0007mcg/ml were measured in the serum between 8 and 12 hours after administration.

Two days after administration the levels had fallen in all volunteers to <0.0004mcg/ml. Only 0.07 to 0.25 (mean value 0.16 ± 0.06) % of the activity administered was excreted in the urine within 5 days post dose.

5.3 Preclinical safety data

There are no pre-clinical data of relevance to the prescriber, which are additional to the information included in other sections of the SPC.

6. PHARMACEUTICAL PARTICULARS

6.1 List of excipients

Isopropanol

Macrogol 400

Propylene glycol

6.2 Incompatibilities

None known.

6.3 Shelf life

60 months.

6.4 Special precautions for storage

There are no special storage requirements.

6.5 Nature and contents of container

The solution is packaged in a white, high density polyethylene bottle and enclosed in a cardboard outer carton.

Canesten Dermatological Spray has an atomiser nozzle and screw-on cap. It is available in a 40ml pack size.

Canesten AF Spray has an atomiser nozzle with upside-down valve and lock cap. The valve enables the bottle to be used in the upside-down position. It is available in a 25ml pack size.

6.6 Instructions for use and handling

Not applicable.

7. MARKETING AUTHORISATION HOLDER

Bayer plc

Bayer House

Strawberry Hill

Newbury, Berkshire

RG14 1JA

Trading as: Bayer plc, Consumer Care Division

8. MARKETING AUTHORISATION NUMBER(S)

PL 0010/0060R

9. DATE OF FIRST AUTHORISATION/RENEWAL OF THE AUTHORISATION

Date of first authorisation: 18 August 1988.

Date of last renewal of authorisation: 14 January 1999.

10. DATE OF REVISION OF THE TEXT

June 2004

LEGAL CATEGORY

Canesten Dermatological Spray P

Canesten AF Spray GSL

Canesten HC Cream

(Bayer plc)

1. NAME OF THE MEDICINAL PRODUCT

Canesten HC Cream

2. QUALITATIVE AND QUANTITATIVE COMPOSITION

Clotrimazole 1% w/w and hydrocortisone 1% w/w

For excipients, see 6.1.

3. PHARMACEUTICAL FORM

Cream.

4. CLINICAL PARTICULARS

4.1 Therapeutic indications

Canesten HC is indicated for the treatment of the following skin infections where co-existing symptoms of inflammation, e.g. itching, require rapid relief:

a) All dermatomycoses due to dermatophytes (e.g. Trichophyton species), moulds and other fungi.

b) All dermatomycoses due to yeasts (Candida species).

c) Skin diseases showing secondary infection with these fungi.

d) The treatment of nappy rash where infection due to Candida albicans is present. Candidal vulvitis, candidal balanitis and candidal intertrigo.

Clotrimazole is a broad spectrum antifungal. It also exhibits activity against *Trichomonas*, staphylococci, streptococci and *Bacteroides*. It has no effect on lactobacilli.

4.2 Posology and method of administration

Canesten HC Cream should be thinly and evenly applied to the affected area twice daily and rubbed in gently. Treatment should be for a maximum of 7 days.

There is no separate dosage schedule for the elderly or the young. However, long-term therapy to extensive areas of skin should be avoided particularly in infants and children.

4.3 Contraindications

Hypersensitivity to Clotrimazole, hydrocortisone or any of the excipients in this product.

The following contra-indications apply to the hydrocortisone component: any untreated bacterial skin diseases, chicken pox, vaccination reactions, perioral dermatitis, viral skin diseases (e.g. herpes simplex, rosacea, shingles), use on broken skin, acne.

4.4 Special warnings and special precautions for use

Because of its corticosteroid content, Canesten HC should not be applied:

- to large areas (more than 5 - 10% of the body surface).
- in long term continuous therapy.
- under occlusive dressings.

These restrictions apply particularly in:

- Infants, where the nappy can act as an occlusive dressing and increase systemic absorption.

- Infants and children, where increased systemic absorption may occur resulting in adrenocortical suppression

4.5 Interaction with other medicinal products and other forms of Interaction

Laboratory tests have suggested that, when used together, this product may cause damage to latex contraceptives. Consequently, the effectiveness of such contraceptives may be reduced. To date this has not been reflected in clinical practice.

4.6 Pregnancy and lactation

Topical administration of corticosteroids to pregnant animals can cause abnormalities of foetal development. The relevance of this to humans has not been established. In animal studies, clotrimazole has not been associated with teratogenic effects but, following oral administration of high doses to rats, there was evidence of foetotoxicity. The relevance of this effect to topical administration in humans is not known.

However, clotrimazole has been used in pregnant patients for over a decade without attributable adverse effects.

It is therefore recommended that Canesten HC Cream should be used in pregnancy and lactation only when considered essential by the clinician.

4.7 Effects on ability to drive and use machines

None applicable.

4.8 Undesirable effects

Rarely, patients may experience local mild burning or irritation immediately after applying the cream. Very rarely, patients may find this irritation intolerable and stop treatment. Hypersensitivity reactions may occur.

After use on large areas (more than 10% of the body surface) and/or after long-term use (longer than 2-4 weeks) or use under occlusive dressings, local skin alterations such as skin atrophy, teleangiectasias, hypertrichosis, striations, hypopigmentation, secondary infection and acneiform symptoms may occur.

4.9 Overdose

In the event of accidental oral ingestion, gastric lavage is rarely required and should be considered only if a life-threatening amount of Clotrimazole has been ingested within the preceding hour or if clinical symptoms of overdose become apparent (e.g. dizziness, nausea or vomiting).

5. PHARMACOLOGICAL PROPERTIES

5.1 Pharmacodynamic properties

ATC Code: D01A C20

Canesten HC is a combination of clotrimazole, which is an imidazole derivative, and hydrocortisone, which is a glucocorticoid. Canesten HC is a broad spectrum antimycotic.

Mechanism of Action

Clotrimazole

Clotrimazole acts against fungi by inhibiting ergosterol synthesis. Inhibition of ergosterol synthesis leads to structural and functional impairment of the cytoplasmic membrane.

Hydrocortisone

Hydrocortisone is a weak corticosteroid with both glucocorticoid and to a lesser extent mineralocorticoid activity. As the active ingredient in a topical cream it exerts anti-inflammatory, antipruritic, antiexudative and antiallergic effects.

Pharmacodynamic Effects

Canesten HC has a broad antimycotic spectrum of action in vitro and in vivo, which includes dermatophytes, yeasts, moulds, etc.

The mode of action of clotrimazole is fungistatic or fungicidal depending on the concentration of clotrimazole at the site of infection. In-vitro activity is limited to proliferating fungal elements; fungal spores are only slightly sensitive.

Primary resistant variants of sensitive fungal species are very rare; the development of secondary resistance by sensitive fungi has so far only been observed in very isolated cases under therapeutic conditions.

Hydrocortisone exerts an anti-inflammatory, immunosuppressive, antimitotic (antiproliferative), antipruriginous and vasoconstrictive effect on the skin. Thus, in addition to the elimination of inflammation and pruritis, a normalisation of keratinisation, inhibition of excess fibroblast activity and epidermopoiesis, degradation of pathological metabolic products and inhibition of acantholysis are achieved.

5.2 Pharmacokinetic properties

Clotrimazole:

Pharmacokinetic investigations after dermal application have shown that clotrimazole is practically not absorbed from intact or inflamed skin into the human blood circulation. The resulting peak serum concentrations of clotrimazole were below the detection limit of 0.01 mcg/ml, reflecting that clotrimazole applied topically does not lead to measurable systemic effects or side effects.

Hydrocortisone:

Dermal absorption of hydrocortisone depends on the thickness and condition of the skin. In healthy skin no systemic effects of corticoids have been observed after local application.

However, in the case of inflamed or damaged skin, cutaneous absorption may be increased depending on the site of application, use of occlusive dressings, the degree of skin damage, and size of the treated area. Systemic effects can not be ruled out under such conditions.

An increase in the skin temperature or moisture content, e.g. in skin folds or under an occlusive dressing, also promotes absorption. In infants and small children the epidermal "barrier" is still poorly developed, which facilitates transcutaneous uptake of drugs. The occurrence of systemic effects depends partly on the dose and, to a much greater extent, on the duration of treatment.

More than 90% of the hydrocortisone absorbed is bound to plasma proteins. Hydrocortisone is metabolised in the liver and tissues, and the metabolites are excreted with urine. The biological half-life is approximately 100 minutes.

No relevant absorption of hydrocortisone is expected after its use for a short period on limited skin inflamed areas.

5.3 Preclinical safety data
There are no preclinical safety data of relevance to the prescriber which are additional to those already included in other sections of the Summary of Product Characteristics.

6. PHARMACEUTICAL PARTICULARS
6.1 List of excipients
Benzyl alcohol

Cetostearyl alcohol

Medium chain triglycerides

Triceteareth-4 phosphate

Purified water

6.2 Incompatibilities
Not applicable

6.3 Shelf life
30 months.

6.4 Special precautions for storage
Do not store above 25°C.

6.5 Nature and contents of container
Aluminium tube with internal lacquer coating and HDPE screw-on cap in cardboard carton.

Pack sizes available: 30g, 15g and 5g sample pack.

6.6 Instructions for use and handling
No special requirements

Administrative Data
7. MARKETING AUTHORISATION HOLDER
Bayer plc

Bayer House

Strawberry Hill

Newbury

Berkshire

RG14 1JA

United Kingdom

Trading as Bayer plc, Consumer Care Division

8. MARKETING AUTHORISATION NUMBER(S)
PL 0010/0120

9. DATE OF FIRST AUTHORISATION/RENEWAL OF THE AUTHORISATION
Date of first authorisation: 14 February 1984

Date of renewal of authorisation: 19 November 1999

10. DATE OF REVISION OF THE TEXT
September 2004

Canesten Hydrocortisone
(Bayer plc)

1. NAME OF THE MEDICINAL PRODUCT
Canesten Hydrocortisone

2. QUALITATIVE AND QUANTITATIVE COMPOSITION
Clotrimazole 1% w/w and hydrocortisone 1% w/w

For excipients, see 6.1.

3. PHARMACEUTICAL FORM
Cream

4. CLINICAL PARTICULARS
4.1 Therapeutic indications
Canesten Hydrocortisone is indicated for the treatment of the following skin infections where co-existing symptoms of inflammation, eg. itching, require rapid relief:

(i) Athlete's foot.

(ii) Candidal intertrigo.

Clotrimazole is a broad spectrum antifungal. It also exhibits activity against *Trichomonas*, staphylococci, streptococci and *Bacteroides.* It has no effect on lactobacilli.

4.2 Posology and method of administration
Adults, elderly and children age 10 years and over:

Canesten Hydrocortisone should be thinly and evenly applied to the affected area twice daily and rubbed in gently. The maximum period of treatment is seven days.

4.3 Contraindications
Canesten Hydrocortisone is contra-indicated in the following cases:

- Use on broken skin.
- Use on large areas of skin.
- Use for periods of longer than seven days.
- Hypersensitivity to any of the ingredients.
- To treat cold sores or acne.
- Use on the face, eyes, mouth or mucous membranes.
- Children under 10 years of age, unless prescribed by a doctor.
- Pregnancy and lactation, unless prescribed by a doctor.
- Use on the ano-genital area, unless prescribed by a doctor.
- To treat ringworm, unless prescribed by a doctor.
- To treat secondarily infected skin conditions, unless prescribed by a doctor.

The following contra-indications apply to the hydrocortisone component: any untreated bacterial skin diseases, chicken pox, vaccination reactions, perioral dermatitis, viral skin diseases (e.g. herpes simplex, rosacea, shingles).

4.4 Special warnings and special precautions for use
Because of its corticosteroid content, Canesten Hydrocortisone should not be applied:

- To large areas (more than 5 - 10% of the body surface).
- In long term continuous therapy.
- Under occlusive dressing

These restrictions apply particularly in children, where increased systemic absorption may occur resulting in adrenocortical suppression.

This product contains cetostearyl alcohol, which may cause local skin reactions (e.g. contact dermatitis).

4.5 Interaction with other medicinal products and other forms of Interaction
None.

4.6 Pregnancy and lactation
Topical administration of corticosteroids to pregnant animals can cause abnormalities of foetal development. The relevance of this to humans has not been established.

In animal studies, clotrimazole has not been associated with teratogenic effects but following oral administration of high doses to rats, there was evidence of foetotoxicity. The relevance of this effect to topical application in humans is not known. However, clotrimazole has been used in pregnant patients for over a decade without attributable adverse effects.

It is therefore recommended that Canesten Hydrocortisone should be used in pregnancy and lactation only when considered necessary by the clinician.

4.7 Effects on ability to drive and use machines
None applicable.

4.8 Undesirable effects
Rarely patients may experience local, mild burning or irritation immediately after applying the cream. Very rarely, patients may find this irritation intolerable and stop treatment. Hypersensitivity reactions may occur.

After use on large areas (more than 10% of the body surface) and/or after long-term use (longer than 2-4 weeks) or use under occlusive dressings, local skin alterations such as skin atrophy, teleangiectasias, hypertrichosis, striations, hypopigmentation, secondary infection and acneiform symptoms may occur.

4.9 Overdose
In the event of accidental oral ingestion, gastric lavage is rarely required and should be considered only if a life-threatening amount of clotrimazole has been ingested within the preceding hour or if clinical symptoms of overdose become apparent (e.g. dizziness, nausea or vomiting). It should be carried out only if the airway can be protected adequately.

5. PHARMACOLOGICAL PROPERTIES
5.1 Pharmacodynamic properties
ATC Code: D01A C20

Canesten Hydrocortisone is a combination of clotrimazole, which is an imidazole derivative, and hydrocortisone, which is a glucocorticoid. Canesten Hydrocortisone is a broad spectrum antimycotic.

Mechanism of Action

Clotrimazole

Clotrimazole acts against fungi by inhibiting ergosterol synthesis. Inhibition of ergosterol synthesis leads to structural and functional impairment of the cytoplasmic membrane.

Hydrocortisone

Hydrocortisone is a weak corticosteroid with both glucocorticoid and to a lesser extent mineralocorticoid activity. As the active ingredient in a topical cream it exerts anti-inflammatory, antipruritic, antiexudative and antiallergic effects.

Pharmacodynamic Effects
Canesten Hydrocortisone has a broad antimycotic spectrum of action in vitro and in vivo, which includes dermatophytes, yeasts, moulds, etc.

The mode of action of clotrimazole is fungistatic or fungicidal depending on the concentration of clotrimazole at the site of infection. In-vitro activity is limited to proliferating fungal elements; fungal spores are only slightly sensitive.

Primary resistant variants of sensitive fungal species are very rare; the development of secondary resistance by sensitive fungi has so far only been observed in very isolated cases under therapeutic conditions.

Hydrocortisone exerts an anti-inflammatory, immunosuppressive, antimitotic (antiproliferative), antipruriginous and vasoconstrictive effect on the skin. Thus, in addition to the elimination of inflammation and pruritis, a normalisation of keratinisation, inhibition of excess fibroblast activity and epidermopoiesis, degradation of pathological metabolic products and inhibition of acantholysis are achieved.

5.2 Pharmacokinetic properties
Clotrimazole:

Pharmacokinetic investigations after dermal application have shown that clotrimazole is practically not absorbed from intact or inflamed skin into the human blood circulation. The resulting peak serum concentrations of clotrimazole were below the detection limit of 0.01 mcg/ml, reflecting that clotrimazole applied topically does not lead to measurable systemic effects or side effects.

Hydrocortisone:

Dermal absorption of hydrocortisone depends on the thickness and condition of the skin. In healthy skin no systemic effects of corticoids have been observed after local application.

However, in the case of inflamed or damaged skin, cutaneous absorption may be increased depending on the site of application, use of occlusive dressings, the degree of skin damage, and size of the treated area. Systemic effects can not be ruled out under such conditions.

An increase in the skin temperature or moisture content, e.g. in skin folds or under an occlusive dressing, also promotes absorption. In infants and small children the epidermal "barrier" is still poorly developed, which facilitates transcutaneous uptake of drugs. The occurrence of systemic effects depends partly on the dose and, to a much greater extent, on the duration of treatment.

More than 90% of the hydrocortisone absorbed is bound to plasma proteins. Hydrocortisone is metabolised in the liver and tissues, and the metabolites are excreted with urine. The biological half-life is approximately 100 minutes.

No relevant absorption of hydrocortisone is expected after its use for a short period on limited skin inflamed areas.

5.3 Preclinical safety data
There are no preclinical safety data of relevance to the prescriber which are additional to those already included in other sections of the Summary of Product Characteristics.

6. PHARMACEUTICAL PARTICULARS
6.1 List of excipients
Triceteareth - 4 phosphate

Cetostearyl alcohol

Medium chain triglycerides

Benzyl alcohol

Purified water

6.2 Incompatibilities
Not applicable.

6.3 Shelf life
30 months.

6.4 Special precautions for storage
Do not store above 25°C.

6.5 Nature and contents of container
Aluminium tube with internal lacquer coating and HDPE screw-on cap containing 15g of cream.

6.6 Instructions for use and handling
No special requirements.

7. MARKETING AUTHORISATION HOLDER
Bayer plc

Bayer House

Strawberry Hill

Newbury, Berkshire

RG14 1JA

United Kingdom.

Trading as: Bayer plc, Consumer Care Division

8. MARKETING AUTHORISATION NUMBER(S)
PL 0010/0216

9. DATE OF FIRST AUTHORISATION/RENEWAL OF THE AUTHORISATION
Date of First Authorisation: 13 January 1997

Date of Last Renewal of Authorisation: 12 January 2002

10. DATE OF REVISION OF THE TEXT
September 2004

Legal Category
P

Canesten Internal Cream / Canesten 10% VC
(Bayer plc)

1. NAME OF THE MEDICINAL PRODUCT
Canesten Internal Cream

also available as Canesten 10% VC.

2. QUALITATIVE AND QUANTITATIVE COMPOSITION
5g vaginal cream containing 0.5g Clotrimazole Ph.Eur.

3. PHARMACEUTICAL FORM
Vaginal cream.

4. CLINICAL PARTICULARS

4.1 Therapeutic indications

Legal Category POM

Canesten 10% VC is recommended for the treatment of candidal vaginitis and mixed vaginal infections where *Trichomonas* is present or suspected. This product is not recommended as sole treatment for pure *Trichomoniasis* except in cases where systemic therapy is contra-indicated.

Legal Category P

Canesten Internal Cream is recommended for the treatment of candidal vaginitis.

4.2 Posology and method of administration

The cream should be administered intravaginally using the applicator supplied.

Adults:

The contents of the filled applicator (5g) should be inserted as deeply as possible into the vagina, preferably at night. A second treatment may be carried out if necessary.

Children:

As the product is used with an applicator, paediatric usage is not recommended.

4.3 Contraindications

Hypersensitivity to clotrimazole.

4.4 Special warnings and special precautions for use

Legal Category P Only

Medical advice should be sought if this is the first time the patient has experienced symptoms of candidal vaginitis.

Before using Canesten Internal Cream, medical advice must be sought if any of the following are applicable: -

- more than two infections of candidal vaginitis in the last 6 months.
- previous history of a sexually transmitted disease or exposure to partner with sexually transmitted disease
- pregnancy or suspected pregnancy
- aged under 16 or over 60 years
- known hypersensitivity to imidazoles or other vaginal antifungal products

Canesten Internal Cream should not be used if the patient has any of the following symptoms whereupon medical advice should be sought: -

- irregular vaginal bleeding
- abnormal vaginal bleeding or a blood-stained discharge
- vulval or vaginal ulcers, blisters or sores
- lower abdominal pain or dysuria
- any adverse events such as redness, irritation or swelling associated with the treatment
- fever or chills
- nausea or vomiting
- diarrhoea
- foul smelling vaginal discharge

If no improvement is seen after seven days, the patient should consult their doctor.

4.5 Interaction with other medicinal products and other forms of Interaction

Laboratory tests have suggested that, when used together, this product may cause damage to latex contraceptives. Consequently the effectiveness of such contraceptives may be reduced. Patients should be advised to use alternative precautions for at least five days after using this product.

4.6 Pregnancy and lactation

In animal studies, clotrimazole has not been associated with teratogenic effects but following oral administration of high doses to rats, there was evidence of foetotoxicity. The relevance of this effect to topical application in humans is not known. However, clotrimazole has been used in pregnant patients for over a decade without attributable adverse effects. It is, therefore, recommended that clotrimazole should be used in pregnancy only when considered necessary by the clinician. During pregnancy, extra care should be taken when using the applicator to prevent the possibility of mechanical trauma.

4.7 Effects on ability to drive and use machines

None applicable.

4.8 Undesirable effects

Rarely, patients may experience local mild burning or irritation immediately after applying the cream. Very rarely, the patient may find this intolerable and stop treatment.

Hypersensitivity reactions may occur.

4.9 Overdose

In the event of accidental oral ingestion, routine measures such as gastric lavage should be performed as soon as possible after ingestion.

5. PHARMACOLOGICAL PROPERTIES

5.1 Pharmacodynamic properties

Clotrimazole is a broad spectrum antifungal. It also exhibits activity against *Trichomonas*, staphylococci, streptococci and *Bacteroides*. It has no effect on lactobacilli.

5.2 Pharmacokinetic properties

A randomised double-blind study was conducted in 16 healthy, non-pregnant volunteers. Following administration of 5.0g of clotrimazole vaginal cream, the concentrations of active substance in the blood plasma and vaginal secretions were determined.

No active substance could be detected in the plasma samples by the microbiological determination method. However, microbiologically active clotrimazole concentrations were found in the vaginal secretions up to 48 hours after the application.

5.3 Preclinical safety data

Toxicological studies in different animals with intravaginal or local application showed good vaginal and local tolerability. No teratogenic or embryotoxic effects could be observed. Canesten had no influence on fertility and showed no mutagenic properties.

6. PHARMACEUTICAL PARTICULARS

6.1 List of excipients

Sorbitan stearate

Polysorbate 60

Cetyl palmitate

Cetostearyl alcohol

Isopropyl myristate

Benzyl alcohol

Purified water

6.2 Incompatibilities

None stated.

6.3 Shelf life

24 months.

6.4 Special precautions for storage

Do not store above 25°C.

6.5 Nature and contents of container

A single dose applicator consisting of a body of HDPE (lupolene or hostalene), piston of LDPE, cap of LDPE, with a separate plunger of polystyrene. One applicator is contained in a blister pack. Pack size 5gm.

The filled applicator of cream is also available in a combination pack with a 10 g tube of Canesten Thrush Cream as Canesten Complete Cream (Legal Category: P) and Canesten Cream Duo (Legal Category: POM).

6.6 Instructions for use and handling

1. Remove applicator from package. Insert plunger (A) into applicator (B).

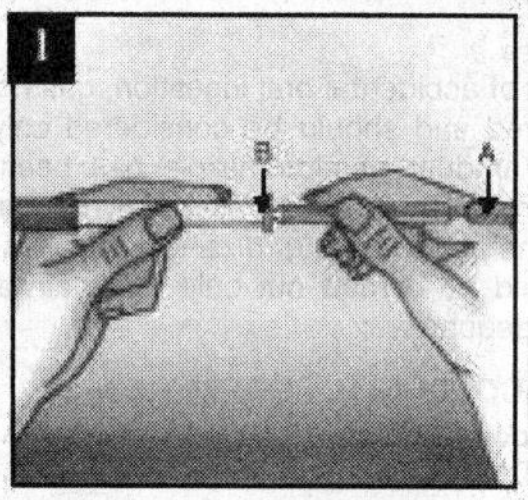

2. Remove red cap (C) by turning.

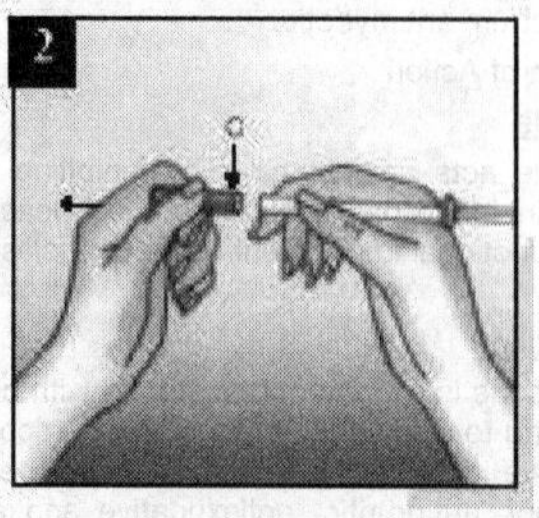

3. Introduce applicator (B) as deeply as possible into the vagina (this is best done with the patient lying on her back with the knees bent up) and empty its contents into the vagina by pushing the plunger (A).

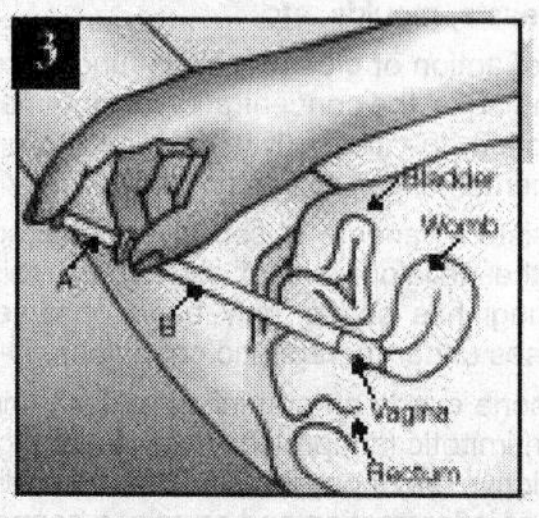

4. Remove the applicator and dispose of it.

Administrative Data

7. MARKETING AUTHORISATION HOLDER

Bayer plc

Consumer Care Division

Bayer House

Strawberry Hill

Newbury, Berkshire

RG14 1JA

8. MARKETING AUTHORISATION NUMBER(S)

PL 0010/0136

9. DATE OF FIRST AUTHORISATION/RENEWAL OF THE AUTHORISATION

Date of first authorisation: 30 January 1985

Date of last renewal of authorisation: 28 April 2000

10. DATE OF REVISION OF THE TEXT

June 2004

Legal Status

Canesten 10% VC and Canesten Cream Duo* POM

Canesten Internal Cream and Canesten Complete Cream P

*Not currently marketed.

Canesten Oral Capsule

(Bayer plc)

1. NAME OF THE MEDICINAL PRODUCT

Canesten® Oral Capsule (also available in the combination product Canesten Oral & Cream Duo)

2. QUALITATIVE AND QUANTITATIVE COMPOSITION

Fluconazole 150mg

For excipients, see 6.1

3. PHARMACEUTICAL FORM

Hard capsule

Opaque light blue capsule (size 1) printed "Canesten"

4. CLINICAL PARTICULARS

4.1 Therapeutic indications

Canesten Oral Capsule is recommended for the treatment of candidal vaginitis, acute or recurrent. It should also be used for the treatment of partners with associated candidal balanitis.

4.2 Posology and method of administration

Adults (16 to 60):

One capsule should be swallowed whole.

Children (under 16):

Paediatric use is not recommended.

Elderly:

Not recommended in patients over 60.

Renal Impairment:

There is no separate dosage schedule in patients with renal impairment for single dose therapy.

4.3 Contraindications

Known hypersensitivity to fluconazole, related azole compounds or any of the excipients in this product.

Fluconazole should not be administered concomitantly with terfenadine or cisapride (see 4.5).

4.4 Special warnings and special precautions for use

The product available from pharmacies without prescription will include a leaflet that advises the patient - *Do not use* Canesten Oral Capsule *without first consulting your doctor:*

If you are under 16 or over 60 years of age

If you are allergic to any of the ingredients in Canesten Oral Capsule or other antifungals and other thrush treatments (see section "After Taking Canesten Oral Capsule").

If you are taking any other medicine other than the Pill.

If you are taking the antihistamine terfenadine or the prescription medicine cisapride

If you have had thrush more than twice in the last six months

If you have any disease or illness affecting your liver or kidneys or have had unexplained jaundice.

If you suffer from any other chronic disease or illness.

If you or your partner have had exposure to a sexually transmitted disease.

If you are unsure of the cause of your symptoms.

Women only:

If you are pregnant, suspect you might be pregnant or are breast-feeding.

If you have any abnormal or irregular vaginal bleeding or a blood stained discharge

If you have vulval or vaginal sores, ulcers or blisters.

If you are experiencing lower abdominal pain or burning sensation on passing water.

Men only:

If your sexual partner does not have thrush.

If you have penile sores, ulcers or blisters.

If you have an abnormal penile discharge (leakage).

If your penis has started to smell.

If you have pain on passing urine.

The product should never be used again if the patient experiences a rash or anaphylaxis following the use of the drug.

Recurrent use (men and women): patients should be advised to consult their physician if the symptoms have not been relieved within one week of taking Canesten Oral Capsule. Canesten Oral Capsule can be used if the candidal infection returns after 7 days. However, if the candidal infection recurs more than twice within six months, patients should be advised to consult their physician.

4.5 Interaction with other medicinal products and other forms of Interaction

The drug interactions listed below relate to the use of multiple dose fluconazole. The relevance of this to a single dose of fluconazole 150mg has not been established.

Anticoagulants:

Fluconazole increased the prothrombin time after warfarin administration in healthy males during an interaction study. The change was small (12%) but bleeding events such as bruising, epistaxis, gastrointestinal bleeding, hematuria and melena have been reported in association with increases in prothrombin time in patients receiving fluconazole and warfarin concomitantly. Careful monitoring of prothrombin time in patients receiving coumarin type anticoagulants is recommended.

Sulphonylureas:

In healthy volunteers, fluconazole prolonged the serum half-life of oral sulphonylureas such as chlorpropamide, glibenclamide, glipizide and tolbutamide, when co-administered. Fluconazole and oral sulphonylureas may be concomitantly administered to diabetics but the possibility of an hypoglycaemic episode should be considered.

Hydrochlorothiazide:

Co-administration of fluconazole and multiple dose hydrochlorothiazide to healthy volunteers during a kinetic interaction study, increased plasma concentrations of fluconazole by 40%. However, although the prescriber should bear this in mind, the fluconazole dose in patients receiving concomitant diuretics should not need to be altered.

Benzodiazepines:

Substantial increases in midazolam concentrations and psychomotor effects are observed when oral midazolam and fluconazole (oral or intravenous) are co-administered. The effect on midazolam appears to be greater when fluconazole is administered orally than when fluconazole is administered intravenously. If concomitant administration of benzodiazepines and fluconazole is required then the prescriber should consider reducing the benzodiazepine dose and appropriate monitoring of the patient should be undertaken.

Phenytoin:

Levels of phenytoin may increase to a clinically significant degree during co-administration with fluconazole. Phenytoin levels should be monitored and the phenytoin dose adjusted to maintain therapeutic levels if co-administration is necessary.

Oral Contraceptives:

Studies on the use of combined oral contraceptives with multiple doses of fluconazole have been performed. No relevant effects on hormone levels occurred during a study with fluconazole 50mg, whilst the AUCs of ethinylestradiol and levonorgestrel were increased by 40% and 24% respectively during a study with fluconazole 200mg. It is therefore considered that multiple dose fluconazole is unlikely to affect the efficacy of the combined oral contraceptive.

Rifampicin:

A 25% decrease in the AUC and 20% shorter half-life of fluconazole occurred when fluconazole and rifampicin were administered concomitantly. An increase in the fluconazole dose should be considered in patients receiving concomitant rifampicin.

Endogenous Steroid:

No effect on endogenous steroid levels was observed in females when treated with fluconazole 50mg daily. No significant effect on endogenous steroid levels or on ACTH stimulated response was observed in healthy male volunteers when treated with fluconazole 200 to 400mg daily.

Ciclosporin:

In a kinetic study it was found that fluconazole 200mg daily slowly increases ciclosporin concentrations in renal transplant patients, but a multiple dose study with fluconazole 100mg daily showed no effect on ciclosporin levels in patients with bone marrow transplants. It is therefore recommended that ciclosporin plasma concentration is monitored in patients receiving fluconazole.

Theophylline:

Use of fluconazole 200mg for 14 days showed an 18% decrease in the mean plasma clearance of theophylline. Patients who require high doses of theophylline or who may be at increased risk of theophylline toxicity should be monitored for signs of theophylline toxicity when fluconazole is co-administered. The therapy should be modified if signs of toxicity occur.

Terfenadine:

Fluconazole 200mg daily did not show a prolongation in the QTc interval. Use of fluconazole (taken in multiple doses of 400mg and 800mg per day) and terfenadine concomitantly, significantly increased plasma levels of terfenadine. Spontaneous reports of palpitations, tachycardia, dizziness and chest pains have occurred in patients taking fluconazole and terfenadine concomitantly where the relationship of the reported adverse events to drug therapy or underlying medical condition is uncertain. It is recommended that terfenadine and fluconazole should not be administered concomitantly due to the potential seriousness of such an interaction. (See 4.3).

Cisapride:

Cardiac events including torsades de pointes have been reported in patients receiving fluconazole and cisapride concomitantly. Most of these patients appear to have been predisposed to arrhythmias or had serious underlying medical conditions, and the relationship of the reported events to a possible drug interaction is uncertain. Co-administration of cisapride is contra-indicated in patients receiving fluconazole. (See 4.3).

Zidovudine:

Zidovudine levels in AIDS or ARC patients were determined before and after daily treatment with fluconazole 200mg for 15 days. A significant increase in zidovudine AUC was observed (20%). A second study in HIV infected patients also showed a significant increase in zidovudine AUC (74%) when fluconazole was administered concomitantly. Patients received zidovudine 200mg every eight hours either with or without fluconazole 400mg for seven days on two occasions, 21 days apart. The increased zidovudine levels are most likely caused by a decrease in the conversion of zidovudine to its major metabolite. It is recommended that patients receiving fluconazole and zidovudine be monitored for zidovudine related adverse reactions.

Rifabutin:

Increased serum levels of rifabutin have been reported in patients receiving fluconazole and rifabutin concomitantly, suggesting a possible interaction. Uveitis has also been reported in patients receiving this combination. It is therefore recommended that patients are carefully monitored.

Tacrolimus:

Increased serum levels of tacrolimus have been reported in patients receiving fluconazole and tacrolimus concomitantly, suggesting a possible interaction. There have also been reports of nephrotoxicity in patients receiving this combination. It is recommended that patients receiving this combination are carefully monitored.

Astemizole or other drugs metabolised by the cytochrome P450 system taken concomitantly with fluconazole may be associated with elevations in serum levels of these drugs in patients. Fluconazole should be co-administered with caution in these circumstances and careful monitoring of patients should be undertaken.

Studies show that when fluconazole is taken orally with food, cimetidine, antacids or following total body irradiation for bone marrow transplantation, the absorption of fluconazole is not significantly impaired.

Drug – drug interaction studies with other medications have not been conducted but prescribers should be aware that such interactions may occur.

4.6 Pregnancy and lactation

Fluconazole should not be used during pregnancy or in women of childbearing potential unless adequate contraception is being used. Fluconazole is found in breast milk so it should not be used whilst breast-feeding.

4.7 Effects on ability to drive and use machines

Fluconazole is unlikely to affect the ability to drive or use machinery.

4.8 Undesirable effects

The more common side effects of Canesten Oral Capsule are gastrointestinal symptoms such as nausea, abdominal pain, diarrhoea and flatulence. Other adverse events such as rash are rarely encountered. Headache has been associated with Canesten Oral Capsule.

Rare cases of hepatotoxicity, usually reversible on discontinuation of therapy, have been reported.

Exfoliative skin disorders, seizures, leukopenia including neutropenia and agranulocytosis, thrombocytopenia and alopecia have occurred although a causal association is uncertain.

As with other azoles, in rare cases anaphylaxis has been reported.

4.9 Overdose

Supportive measures and symptomatic treatment, with gastric lavage if necessary, may be adequate.

Fluconazole is largely excreted in the urine and therefore, forced volume diuresis would probably increase the elimination rate. Plasma levels are decreased by approximately 50% during a 3-hour haemodialysis session.

5. PHARMACOLOGICAL PROPERTIES

5.1 Pharmacodynamic properties

Fluconazole is a triazole antifungal. It is a potent and selective inhibitor of fungal enzymes necessary for the synthesis of ergosterol.

Fluconazole shows little pharmacological activity in a wide range of animal studies. Some prolongation of pentabarbitone sleeping times in mice (p.o.), increased mean arterial and left ventricular blood pressure and increased heart rate in anaesthetised cats (i.v.) occurred. Inhibition of rat ovarian aromatase was observed at high concentrations.

Fluconazole was active in a variety of animal fungal infection models. Activity has been demonstrated against opportunistic mycoses, such as infections with *Candida* spp. including systemic candidiasis in immuno-compromised animals; with *Cryptococcus neoformans*, including intracranial infections; with *Microsporum* spp. and with *Trichophyton* spp. Fluconazole has also been shown to be active in animal models of endemic mycoses, including infections with *Blastomyces dermatitides*; with *Coccidoides immitis*, including intracranial infection and with *Histoplasma capsulatum* in normal and immuno-compromised animals.

There have been reports of cases of superinfection with *Candida* species other than *C. albicans*, which are often inherently not susceptible to fluconazole (e.g. *Candida krusei*). Such cases may require alternative antifungal therapy.

Fluconazole is highly specific for fungal cytochrome P-450 dependent enzymes. Fluconazole has been shown not to affect testosterone plasma concentrations in males or steroid concentrations in females of childbearing age when given 50mg daily for up to 28 days. No clinically significant effect has been seen on endogenous steroid levels or on ACTH stimulated response in healthy male volunteers taking fluconazole 200 – 400mg daily. Interaction studies with antipyrine indicate that single or multiple doses of fluconazole 50mg do not affect its metabolism.

5.2 Pharmacokinetic properties

The pharmacokinetic properties of fluconazole are similar whether administered orally or by the intravenous route. After oral administration, fluconazole is well absorbed and plasma levels (and systemic bioavailability) are over 90% of the levels achieved after intravenous administration. Concomitant food intake does not affect oral absorption. In the fasting state peak plasma concentrations occur between 0.5 and 1.5 hours post-dose with a plasma elimination half-life of approximately 30 hours. Plasma concentrations are proportional to dose. Ninety- percent steady state levels are reached by day 4 to 5 with multiple once daily dosing.

Administration of a loading dose (on day 1) of twice the usual daily dose enables plasma levels to approximate to 90% steady state levels by day 2. The apparent volume of distribution approximates to total body water. Plasma protein binding is low (11-12%).

Fluconazole achieves good penetration in all body fluids studied. The levels of fluconazole in saliva and sputum are similar to plasma levels. In patients with fungal meningitis, fluconazole levels in the CSF are approximately 80% of the corresponding plasma levels.

High skin concentrations of fluconazole, above serum concentrations, are achieved in the stratum corneum, epidermis-dermis and eccrine sweat. Fluconazole accumulates in the stratum corneum. At a dose of 50mg once daily, the concentration of fluconazole after 12 days was 73 mg/g and 7 days after cessation of treatment the concentration was still 5.8 mg/g.

Excretion is mainly renal, with approximately 80% of the administered dose appearing in the urine as unchanged drug. Fluconazole clearance is proportional to creatinine clearance. There is no evidence of circulating metabolites.

The long plasma elimination half-life provides the basis for single dose therapy for genital candidiasis.

A study compared the saliva and plasma concentrations of a single fluconazole 100mg dose administration in a capsule or in an oral suspension by rinsing and retaining in the mouth for 2 minutes and swallowing. The maximum concentration of fluconazole in saliva after the suspension was observed five minutes after ingestion and was 182 times higher than maximum saliva concentration after the capsule which occurred four hours after ingestion. After about four hours, the saliva concentrations of fluconazole were similar. The mean AUC (0-96) in saliva was significantly greater after the suspension compared to the capsule. There was no significant difference in the elimination rate from the saliva or the plasma pharmacokinetic parameters for the two formulations.

5.3 Preclinical safety data

Reproductive Toxicity:

At 25 and 50mg/kg and higher doses, increases in foetal anatomical variants (supernumerary ribs, renal pelvis dilation) and delays in ossification were observed. At doses ranging from 80mg/kg to 320mg/kg embryolethality in rats was increased and foetal abnormalities included wavy ribs, cleft palate and abnormal cranio-facial ossification. This may be a result of known effects of lowered oestrogen on pregnancy, organogenesis and parturition as it is consistent with the inhibition of oestrogen synthesis in rats.

Carcinogenesis:

No evidence of carcinogenic potential was observed in mice and rats treated orally with fluconazole for 24 months at doses of 2.5, 5 or 10mg/kg/day. The incidence of hepatocellular adenomas was increased in male rats treated with 5 and 10mg/kg/day.

Mutagenesis:

Fluconazole, with or without metabolic activation, was negative in tests for mutagenicity in 4 strains of *S.typhimurium* and in the mouse lymphoma L5178Y system. No evidence of chromosomal mutations was observed in cytogenetic studies *in vivo* (murine bone marrow cells, following oral administration of fluconazole) and *in vitro* (human lymphocytes exposed to fluconazole at 1000μg/ml).

Impairment of Fertility:

The fertility of male or female rats treated orally with daily doses of fluconazole at doses of 5, 10 or 20mg/kg or with parenteral doses of 5, 25 or 75mg/kg was not affected, although the onset of parturition was slightly delayed at 20mg/kg p.o. In an intravenous perinatal study in rats at 5, 20 and 40mg/kg, dystocia and prolongation of parturition were observed in a few dams at 20mg/kg and 40mg/kg, but not at 5mg/kg. The disturbances in parturition were reflected by a slight increase in the number of stillborn pups and decrease of neonatal survival at these dose levels. The effects on parturition in rats are consistent with the species specific oestrogen-lowering property produced by high doses of fluconazole. Such a hormone change has not been observed in women treated with fluconazole.

6. PHARMACEUTICAL PARTICULARS

6.1 List of excipients

Lactose monohydrate

Maize starch

Colloidal silicon dioxide

Magnesium stearate

Sodium lauryl sulphate

Capsule shells contain:

Brilliant blue FCF (E133)

Titanium dioxide (E171)

Gelatine

Printing ink contains:

Black iron oxide (E172)

Shellac

Soya lecithin

6.2 Incompatibilities

Not applicable.

6.3 Shelf life

24 months.

6.4 Special precautions for storage

No special precautions for storage.

6.5 Nature and contents of container

Opaque, white PVC/PVdC (60g/m^2) blister with 20μm aluminium foil backing containing one capsule.

The capsule is also available with a 10g tube of Canesten Thrush Cream as Canesten Oral & Cream Duo (Legal Category P).

6.6 Instructions for use and handling

Not applicable.

7. MARKETING AUTHORISATION HOLDER

Bayer plc

Bayer House

Strawberry Hill

Newbury

Berkshire

RG14 1JA

U.K.

Trading as Bayer plc, Consumer Care Division

8. MARKETING AUTHORISATION NUMBER(S)

PL 00010/0282

9. DATE OF FIRST AUTHORISATION/RENEWAL OF THE AUTHORISATION

25 September 2002

10. DATE OF REVISION OF THE TEXT

January2004

LEGAL STATUS

P

Canesten Pessary

(Bayer plc)

1. NAME OF THE MEDICINAL PRODUCT

Canesten Pessary (also available as Boots Thrush Relief Pessary).

2. QUALITATIVE AND QUANTITATIVE COMPOSITION

Clotrimazole 500mg.

For excipients, see 6.1

3. PHARMACEUTICAL FORM

Pessary

4. CLINICAL PARTICULARS

4.1 Therapeutic indications

Canesten Pessaries are recommended for the treatment of candidal vaginitis.

4.2 Posology and method of administration

The pessary should be inserted into the vagina, as high as possible, using the applicator provided.

Adults: One 500mg pessary should be inserted at night. Using the applicator provided, the pessary should be inserted as high as possible into the vagina. This is best achieved when lying back with legs bent up. A second treatment may be carried out if necessary.

Canesten pessaries need moisture in the vagina in order to dissolve completely, otherwise undissolved pieces of the pessary might crumble out of the vagina. Pieces of undissolved pessary may be noticed by women who experience vaginal dryness. To help prevent this it is important that the pessary is inserted as high as possible into the vagina at bedtime.

Generally:

treatment during the menstrual period should not be performed due to the risk of the pessary being washed out by the menstrual flow. The treatment should be finished before the onset of menstruation.

Children: As the product is used with an applicator, paediatric usage is not recommended.

4.3 Contraindications

Hypersensitivity to clotrimazole or any other ingredient in this medicine.

4.4 Special warnings and special precautions for use

Medical advice should be sought if this is the first time the patient has experienced symptoms of candidal vaginitis.

Before using Canesten Pessaries, medical advice must be sought if any of the following are applicable:

- more than two infections of candidal vaginitis in the last 6 months.

- previous history of sexually transmitted disease or exposure to partner with sexually transmitted disease.

- pregnancy or suspected pregnancy.

- aged under 16 or over 60 years.

- known hypersensitivity to imidazoles or other vaginal antifungal products.

Canesten Pessaries should not be used if the patient has any of the following symptoms where upon medical advice should be sought:

- irregular vaginal bleeding.

- abnormal vaginal bleeding or a blood-stained discharge.

- vulval or vaginal ulcers, blisters or sores.

- lower abdominal pain or dysuria.

- any adverse events such as redness, irritation or swelling associated with the treatment.

- fever or chills.

- nausea or vomiting.

- diarrhoea.

- foul smelling vaginal discharge.

Patients should be advised to consult their physician if the symptoms have not been relieved within one week of using Canesten Pessary. Canesten Pessary can be used again if the candidal infection returns after 7 days. However, if the candidal infection recurs more than twice within six months, patients should be advised to consult their physician.

4.5 Interaction with other medicinal products and other forms of Interaction

Laboratory tests have suggested that, when used together, this product may cause damage to latex contraceptives. Consequently the effectiveness of such contraceptives may be reduced. Patients should be advised to use alternative precautions for at least five days after using this product.

4.6 Pregnancy and lactation

Data on a large number of exposed pregnancies indicate no adverse effects of Clotrimazole on pregnancy or on the health of the foetus/newborn child. To date, no relevant epidemiological data are available.

Clotrimazole can be used during pregnancy, but only under the supervision of a physician or midwife.

During pregnancy extra care should be taken when using the applicator to prevent the possibility of mechanical trauma.

4.7 Effects on ability to drive and use machines

Not applicable.

4.8 Undesirable effects

Rarely patients may experience local mild burning or irritation immediately after inserting the pessary. Very rarely the patient may find this intolerable and stop treatment.

Other undesirable effects:

Body as a whole: allergic reaction (syncope, hypotension, dyspnea, gastrointestinal disorders), pain

Skin and appendages: pruritis, rash

4.9 Overdose

In the event of accidental oral ingestion, gastric lavage is rarely required and should be considered only if clinical symptoms of overdose become apparent (e.g. dizziness, nausea or vomiting). It should be carried out only if the airway can be protected adequately.

5. PHARMACOLOGICAL PROPERTIES

5.1 Pharmacodynamic properties

ATC Code: G01A F02

Clotrimazole is an imidazole derivative with a broad spectrum of antimycotic activity.

Mechanism of Action

Clotrimazole acts against fungi by inhibiting ergosterol synthesis. Inhibition of ergosterol synthesis leads to structural and functional impairment of the cytoplasmic membrane.

Pharmacodynamic Effects

Clotrimazole has a broad antimycotic spectrum of action in vitro and in vivo, which includes dermatophytes, yeasts, moulds, etc.

The mode of action of clotrimazole is fungistatic or fungicidal depending on the concentration of clotrimazole at the site of infection. In-vitro activity is limited to proliferating fungal elements; fungal spores are only slightly sensitive.

Primarily resistant variants of sensitive fungal species are very rare; the development of secondary resistance by sensitive fungi has so far only been observed in very isolated cases under therapeutic conditions.

5.2 Pharmacokinetic properties

Pharmacokinetic investigations after vaginal application have shown that only a small amount of clotrimazole (3 – 10% of the dose) is absorbed. Due to the rapid hepatic metabolism of absorbed clotrimazole into pharmacologically inactive metabolites the resulting peak plasma concentrations of clotrimazole after vaginal application of a 500mg dose were less than 10 mcg/ml, reflecting that clotrimazole applied intravaginally does not lead to measurable systemic effects or side effects.

5.3 Preclinical safety data

There are no pre-clinical data of relevance to the prescriber which are additional to the information included in other sections of the SPC.

6. PHARMACEUTICAL PARTICULARS

6.1 List of excipients

Lactose monohydrate

Microcrystalline cellulose

Lactic acid

Maize starch

Povidone

Calcium lactate pentahydrate

Magnesium stearate

Silica, colloidal anhydrous

Hypromellose

6.2 Incompatibilities

Not applicable.

6.3 Shelf life

60 months.

6.4 Special precautions for storage

No special precautions for storage.

6.5 Nature and contents of container

Each pessary is packed into a blister consisting of 25μm PA (Polyamide) / 45μm Soft Aluminium / 60μm PVC and 20μm Hard Aluminium / 7 GSM HSL (Heat sealing lacquer). The blister and an applicator are enclosed in a cardboard carton.

The pessary is also available with a 10g tube of Canesten Thrush Cream as Canesten Combi (Shelf-life 36 months). A Boots Thrush Relief Pessary is available with a 20g tube of Boots Thrush Cream as Boots Thrush Relief Combi.

6.6 Instructions for use and handling

1. Pull out plunger A until it stops. Place the pessary into the applicator B.

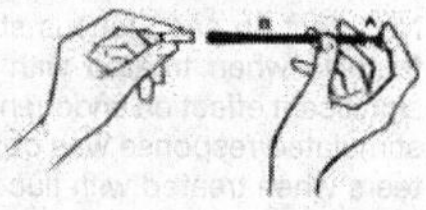

2. Carefully insert the applicator containing the pessary as deeply as is comfortable into the vagina.

This is best done with the patient lying on her back with the knees bent up.

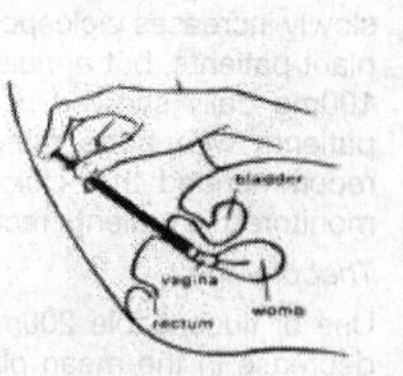

3. Push plunger A until it stops, thereby depositing the pessary into the vagina. Withdraw the applicator and dispose of it hygienically.

7. MARKETING AUTHORISATION HOLDER
Bayer plc
Bayer House
Strawberry Hill
Newbury, Berkshire
RG14 1JA
Trading as Bayer plc, Consumer Care Division

8. MARKETING AUTHORISATION NUMBER(S)
PL 0010/0083

9. DATE OF FIRST AUTHORISATION/RENEWAL OF THE AUTHORISATION
Date of first authorisation 4 January 1982.
Date of last renewal 31 July 2002.

10. DATE OF REVISION OF THE TEXT
September 2004

LEGAL CATEGORY
P

Canesten Solution

(Bayer plc)

1. NAME OF THE MEDICINAL PRODUCT
Canesten Solution

2. QUALITATIVE AND QUANTITATIVE COMPOSITION
Canesten Solution contains Clotrimazole Ph.Eur 1.0% w/v.

3. PHARMACEUTICAL FORM
A clear solution.

4. CLINICAL PARTICULARS

4.1 Therapeutic indications
Canesten Solution should be used to treat all fungal skin infections due to dermatophytes, yeasts, moulds and other fungi.

It is particularly suitable for use on hairy skin and in fungal infections of the outer ear (otitis externa) and middle ear (otomycoses).

4.2 Posology and method of administration
Canesten Solution should be thinly and evenly applied to the affected area 2 or 3 times daily. To prevent relapse, treatment should be continued for at least two weeks after the disappearance of all signs of infection.

There is no separate dosage schedule for the elderly or the young.

4.3 Contraindications
Hypersensitivity to clotrimazole.

4.4 Special warnings and special precautions for use
None known.

4.5 Interaction with other medicinal products and other forms of Interaction
There have been reports of a heat reaction when Canesten Solution is used concomitantly with Sofradex drops in the ear.

4.6 Pregnancy and lactation
In animal studies, clotrimazole has not been associated with teratogenic effects but following oral administration of high doses to rats, there was evidence of foetotoxicity. The relevance of this effect to topical application in humans is not known. However, clotrimazole has been used in pregnant patients for over a decade without attributable adverse effects. It is therefore recommended that clotrimazole should be used in pregnancy only when considered necessary by the physician.

4.7 Effects on ability to drive and use machines
Not applicable.

4.8 Undesirable effects
Rarely, patients may experience local mild burning or irritation immediately after applying the solution. Very rarely, the patient may find this irritation intolerable and stop treatment.

Hypersensitivity reactions may occur.

4.9 Overdose
In the event of accidental oral ingestion, routine measures such as gastric lavage should be performed as soon as possible after ingestion.

5. PHARMACOLOGICAL PROPERTIES

5.1 Pharmacodynamic properties
Clotrimazole is a broad-spectrum antifungal. It also exhibits activity against *Trichomonas*, staphylococci, streptococci, and *Bacteroides*.

5.2 Pharmacokinetic properties
^{14}C Clotrimazole in the form of a 1% solution was administered dermally to three volunteers with normal skin at a dose of 0.5ml per 200cm^2 skin area with an occlusive dressing for six hours.

Six hours after application, the equivalent concentrations were estimated to be:

(i) 50 - 100% per cm^3 in the stratum corneum

(ii) 3 - 6% per cm^3 in the stratum granulosum

(iii) 1.5 - 2% per cm^3 in the stratum basale and stratum papillare

(iv) 0.5 - 2% per cm^3 in the corium

There was no measurable radioactivity in the serum of any of the three test subjects 48 hours after treatment. (< 0.001 per ml serum.) Less than 0.05% of the activity applied to the skin was excreted in the urine.

5.3 Preclinical safety data
There are no pre-clinical data of relevance to the prescriber which are additional to the information included in other sections of the SPC.

6. PHARMACEUTICAL PARTICULARS

6.1 List of excipients
Macrogol 400.

6.2 Incompatibilities
None known.

6.3 Shelf life
36 months.

6.4 Special precautions for storage
Do not store above 25°C.

6.5 Nature and contents of container
HDPE bottles with dropper insert and screw-on cap.

Pack size: 20ml

6.6 Instructions for use and handling
Not applicable.

7. MARKETING AUTHORISATION HOLDER
Bayer plc
Consumer Care Division
Bayer House
Strawberry Hill
Newbury, Berkshire
RG14 1JA

8. MARKETING AUTHORISATION NUMBER(S)
PL 0010/0082

9. DATE OF FIRST AUTHORISATION/RENEWAL OF THE AUTHORISATION
Date of the first authorisation: 12 June 1981
Date of last renewal of authorisation: 28 May 2002

10. DATE OF REVISION OF THE TEXT
May 2002

Legal Category
P

Canesten Thrush Cream

(Bayer plc)

1. NAME OF THE MEDICINAL PRODUCT
Canesten Thrush Cream
(also available in the combination products Canesten Combi, Canesten 500mg Pessary and 2% Cream, Canesten Complete Cream, Canesten Cream Duo and Canesten Oral & Cream Duo)

2. QUALITATIVE AND QUANTITATIVE COMPOSITION
The cream contains Clotrimazole Ph.Eur 2% w/w.

3. PHARMACEUTICAL FORM
Cream for topical use.

4. CLINICAL PARTICULARS

4.1 Therapeutic indications
Canesten Thrush Cream is recommended for the treatment of candidal vulvitis. It should be used as an adjunct to treatment of candidal vaginitis.

It can also be used for treatment of the sexual partner's penis to prevent re-infection.

4.2 Posology and method of administration
Canesten Thrush Cream should be applied to the vulva and surrounding area.

It can also be applied to the sexual partner's penis to prevent re-infection.

Adults

The cream should be applied thinly two or three times daily and rubbed in gently.

Treatment should be continued until symptoms of the infection disappear. However, if after concomitant treatment of the vaginitis, the symptoms do not improve within seven days, the patient should consult a physician.

If the cream is being used for treatment of the sexual partner's penis it should be applied two or three times daily for two weeks.

Children

There is no clinical experience in the use of Canesten Thrush Cream in children.

4.3 Contraindications
Hypersensitivity to clotrimazole.

4.4 Special warnings and special precautions for use
Medical advice should be sought if this is the first time the patient has experienced symptoms of candidal vaginitis.

Before using Canesten Thrush Cream medical advice must be sought if any of the following are applicable: -

- more than two infections of candidal vaginitis in the last six months
- previous history of a sexually transmitted disease or exposure to partner with sexually transmitted disease
- pregnancy or suspected pregnancy
- aged under 16 or over 60 years
- known hypersensitivity to imidazoles or other vaginal antifungal products

Canesten Thrush Cream should not be used if the patient has any of the following symptoms whereupon medical advice should be sought: -

- irregular vaginal bleeding
- abnormal vaginal bleeding or a blood-stained discharge
- vulval or vaginal ulcers, blisters or sores
- lower abdominal pain or dysuria
- any adverse events such as redness, irritation or swelling associated with the treatment
- fever or chills
- nausea or vomiting
- diarrhoea
- foul smelling vaginal discharge

4.5 Interaction with other medicinal products and other forms of Interaction
Laboratory tests have suggested that, when used together, this product may cause damage to latex contraceptives. Consequently the effectiveness of such contraceptives may be reduced. Patients should be advised to use alternative precautions for at least five days after using this product.

4.6 Pregnancy and lactation
In animal studies clotrimazole has not been associated with teratogenic effects but following oral administration of high doses to rats there was evidence of foetotoxicity. The relevance of this effect to topical application in humans is not known. However, clotrimazole has been used in pregnant patients for over a decade without attributable adverse effects. It is therefore recommended that clotrimazole should be used in pregnancy only when considered necessary by the clinician.

4.7 Effects on ability to drive and use machines
Not applicable.

4.8 Undesirable effects
Rarely, patients may experience local mild burning or irritation immediately after applying the cream. Very rarely the patient may find this intolerable and stop treatment.

Hypersensitivity reactions may occur.

4.9 Overdose
In the event of accidental oral ingestion, routine measures such as gastric lavage should be performed as soon as possible after ingestion.

5. PHARMACOLOGICAL PROPERTIES

5.1 Pharmacodynamic properties
Canesten has a broad spectrum of activity (yeasts, dermatophytes and a number of other fungi). It is effective on yeasts, notably *Candida albicans* and *Torulopsis glabrata* as well as on *Trichomonas vaginalis* and some gram-positive and gram-negative bacteria (streptococci, staphylococci, *Gardnerella vaginalis*, *Bacteroides*).

5.2 Pharmacokinetic properties
Studies in volunteers using radioactively labelled active substance applied as 1% vaginal cream indicated a rate of vaginal absorption between 3 and 10% of the dose applied. The concentrations of unchanged active substance in the plasma of volunteers following the application of 2% vaginal cream were below the limit of detection (10mg/ml). Since only very small amounts of active substance are absorbed by the vaginal skin and it is metabolised very quickly ($t½$ = 1-2 hours), concentrations in the blood plasma are always below the limit of detection.

5.3 Preclinical safety data
Toxicological studies in different animals with intravaginal or local application of Canesten showed good vaginal and local tolerability. No teratogenic or embryotoxic effects could be observed. Canesten had no influence on the fertility and showed no mutagenic properties.

6. PHARMACEUTICAL PARTICULARS

6.1 List of excipients
Sorbitan stearate
Polysorbate 60
Cetyl palmitate
Cetostearyl alcohol
Octyldodecanol
Benzyl alcohol
Purified Water

6.2 Incompatibilities
None known.

6.3 Shelf life
36 months.

6.4 Special precautions for storage
Do not store above 25°C.

6.5 Nature and contents of container
Aluminium tubes (10g and 20g) with internal lacquer coating, latex stopper and HDPE screw top.

The 10g tube of cream is only available in combination packs as follows:

1) with a 500mg pessary as Canesten Combi (Legal Category: P) and Canesten Combi 500mg Pessary and 2% Cream (Legal Category: POM)

2) with a filled applicator (5g) of 10% cream as Canesten Complete Cream (Legal Category: P) and Canesten Cream Duo (Legal Category: POM)

3) with a fluconazole 150mg capsule as Canesten Oral & Cream Duo (Legal Category: P)

6.6 Instructions for use and handling
Not applicable.

7. MARKETING AUTHORISATION HOLDER
Bayer plc

Consumer Care Division

Bayer House

Strawberry Hill

Newbury

Berkshire

RG14 1JA

8. MARKETING AUTHORISATION NUMBER(S)
PL 0010/0077

9. DATE OF FIRST AUTHORISATION/RENEWAL OF THE AUTHORISATION
Date of first authorisation: 29 December 1980

Date of last renewal of authorisation: 17 April 2002

10. DATE OF REVISION OF THE TEXT
January 2004

LEGAL CATEGORY
Canesten Thrush Cream, Canesten Combi, Canesten Complete Cream, Canesten Oral & Cream Duo: P

Canesten Combi 500mg Pessary and 2% Cream, Canesten Cream Duo*: POM

*Not currently marketed

Canusal

(Wockhardt UK Ltd)

1. NAME OF THE MEDICINAL PRODUCT
Canusal

2. QUALITATIVE AND QUANTITATIVE COMPOSITION
Heparin sodium (mucous) 100 I.U./ml

For excipients see 6.1

3. PHARMACEUTICAL FORM
Solution for injection

A colourless or straw coloured liquid, free from turbidity and from matter that deposits on standing.

4. CLINICAL PARTICULARS

4.1 Therapeutic indications
Heparin is an anticoagulant and acts by potentiating the naturally occurring inhibitors of thrombin and factor X (Xa).

Canusal is indicated in any clinical circumstances in which it is desired to flush an intravenous catheter or cannula with a low concentration of heparin to ensure patency prior to administration of an intravenous injection.

4.2 Posology and method of administration
Not recommended for systemic use.

For cleaning indwelling cannulae.

Material to be used as an intravascular cannula or catheter flush in doses of 200 units every 4 hours or as required.

4.3 Contraindications
Do not use when there is established hypersensitivity to heparin.

4.4 Special warnings and special precautions for use
Caution should be exercised in patients with known hypersensitivity to low molecular weight heparins.

Rigorous aseptic technique should be observed at all times in its use.

Platelet counts should be measured in patients receiving heparin flushes for longer than seven days (or earlier in patients with previous exposure to heparin). In those who develop thrombocytopenia or paradoxical thrombosis, heparin should immediately be eliminated from all flushes and ports.

Repeated flushing of a catheter device with heparin may result in a systemic anticoagulant effect.

4.5 Interaction with other medicinal products and other forms of Interaction
When an indwelling device is used for repeated withdrawal of blood samples for laboratory analyses and the presence of heparin or saline is likely to interfere with or alter results of the desired blood tests, the in situ heparin flush solution should be cleared from the device by aspirating and discarding a volume of solution equivalent to that of the indwelling venipuncture device before the desired blood sample is taken.

4.6 Pregnancy and lactation
The safety of Canusal in pregnancy is not established, but the dose of heparin involved would not be expected to constitute a hazard.

Heparin does not appear in breast milk.

4.7 Effects on ability to drive and use machines
None stated.

4.8 Undesirable effects
Used as directed, it is extremely unlikely that the low levels of heparin reaching the blood will have any systemic effect. However, there have been rare reports of immune-mediated thrombocytopenia and thrombosis in patients receiving heparin flushes (see also Section 4.4, Special Warnings and Precautions for Use).

Hypersensitivity reactions to heparin are rare. They include urticaria, conjunctivitis, rhinitis, asthma, cyanosis, tachypnoea, feeling of oppression, fever, chills, angioneurotic oedema and anaphylactic shock.

4.9 Overdose
Not applicable

5. PHARMACOLOGICAL PROPERTIES

5.1 Pharmacodynamic properties
Canusal, containing only 200 I.U. of sodium heparin per ampoule (2ml), is used for flushing indwelling cannulae. This is unlikely to produce blood levels of heparin having any systemic effect.

5.2 Pharmacokinetic properties
None stated

5.3 Preclinical safety data
There are no pre-clinical data of relevance to the prescriber which are additional to those already included in other sections.

6. PHARMACEUTICAL PARTICULARS

6.1 List of excipients
Sodium chloride

Water for injections

Hydrochloric acid 3M

Sodium hydroxide 3M

6.2 Incompatibilities
Heparin and reteplase are incompatible when combined in solution.

If reteplase and heparin are to be given through the same line this, together with any Y-lines, must be thoroughly flushed with a 0.9% saline or a 5% glucose solution prior to and following the reteplase injection.

6.3 Shelf life
Unopened – 36 months

From a microbiological point of view, unless the method of opening precludes the risk of microbial contamination, the product should be used immediately.

If not used immediately, in-use storage times and conditions are the responsibility of the user.

6.4 Special precautions for storage
Do not store above 25°C

Store in the original package

6.5 Nature and contents of container
2ml clear glass ampoules

6.6 Instructions for use and handling
Not applicable

Administrative Data

7. MARKETING AUTHORISATION HOLDER
CP Pharmaceuticals Ltd

Ash Road North

Wrexham

LL13 9UF

UK.

8. MARKETING AUTHORISATION NUMBER(S)
4543/0322

9. DATE OF FIRST AUTHORISATION/RENEWAL OF THE AUTHORISATION
Date of first authorisation - 21 June 1991

Date of renewal - 28 November 1996

10. DATE OF REVISION OF THE TEXT
August 2001

Capasal Therapeutic Shampoo

(Dermal Laboratories Limited)

1. NAME OF THE MEDICINAL PRODUCT
CAPASAL™ THERAPEUTIC SHAMPOO

2. QUALITATIVE AND QUANTITATIVE COMPOSITION
Salicylic Acid 0.5% w/w; Coconut Oil 1.0% w/w; Distilled Coal Tar 1.0% w/w.

3. PHARMACEUTICAL FORM
Golden brown shampoo.

4. CLINICAL PARTICULARS

4.1 Therapeutic indications
For use as a shampoo in the treatment of dry, scaly scalp conditions such as seborrhoeic eczema, seborrhoeic dermatitis, pityriasis capitis, psoriasis, and cradle cap in children. It may also be used to remove previous scalp applications.

4.2 Posology and method of administration
For adults, children and the elderly: Use as a shampoo, daily if necessary. Wet the hair thoroughly. Massage a small amount of the shampoo into the scalp, leaving on for a few minutes before washing out. Repeat, producing a rich lather. Rinse hair well and dry.

4.3 Contraindications
Not to be used in cases of sensitivity to any of the ingredients.

4.4 Special warnings and special precautions for use
Keep away from the eyes. In case of irritation, discontinue treatment. For external use only.

4.5 Interaction with other medicinal products and other forms of Interaction
None known.

4.6 Pregnancy and lactation
No known side-effects.

4.7 Effects on ability to drive and use machines
None known.

4.8 Undesirable effects
None known.

4.9 Overdose
There are no known toxic effects resulting from excessive use of Capasal Therapeutic Shampoo.

5. PHARMACOLOGICAL PROPERTIES

5.1 Pharmacodynamic properties
The preparation has been designed for use in the treatment of dry, scaly scalp conditions by incorporating into a shampoo formulation three well known ingredients which have been established as safe and effective for use in this indication. They are as follows:

0.5% salicylic acid - mild keratolytic

1.0% coconut oil - emollient, softening agent and lubricant

1.0% distilled coal tar - anti-pruritic, keratoplastic

The preparation may also be used conveniently to remove any previous topical application.

5.2 Pharmacokinetic properties
The active ingredients of the formulation are readily available for intimate contact with the skin, as the shampoo is massaged into the scalp and left on for a few minutes before washing out. This is then repeated in order to produce a rich lather. The detergent effect of the shampoo will also remove any previous application to the scalp.

5.3 Preclinical safety data
No relevant information additional to that contained elsewhere in the SPC.

6. PHARMACEUTICAL PARTICULARS

6.1 List of excipients
Lauric Acid Diethanolamide; Coco Amido Propyl Dimethyl Betaine; Triethanolamine Lauryl Sulphate; Phenoxyethanol; Water.

6.2 Incompatibilities
None known.

6.3 Shelf life
36 months.

6.4 Special precautions for storage
Do not store above 25°C. Keep away from direct sunlight.

6.5 Nature and contents of container
Plastic 'flip top' bottle containing 250 ml. This is supplied as an original pack (OP).

6.6 Instructions for use and handling
Not applicable.

7. MARKETING AUTHORISATION HOLDER
Dermal Laboratories

Tatmore Place, Gosmore

Hitchin, Herts SG4 7QR, UK.

8. MARKETING AUTHORISATION NUMBER(S)
0173/0048.

9. DATE OF FIRST AUTHORISATION/RENEWAL OF THE AUTHORISATION
29 January 2001.

10. DATE OF REVISION OF THE TEXT
September 2000.

CAPASTAT

(King Pharmaceuticals Ltd)

1. NAME OF THE MEDICINAL PRODUCT
CAPASTAT Injection

2. QUALITATIVE AND QUANTITATIVE COMPOSITION
Each vial contains Capreomycin Sulphate (approximately equivalent to 1g Capreomycin base).

3. PHARMACEUTICAL FORM
Powder for injection

4. CLINICAL PARTICULARS

4.1 Therapeutic indications
Actions: Capreomycin is active against human strains of Mycobacterium tuberculosis.

Frequent cross-resistance occurs between capreomycin and viomycin. Varying degrees of cross-resistance between capreomycin and kanamycin and neomycin have been reported. No cross-resistance has been observed between capreomycin and isoniazid, aminosalicylic acid, cycloserine, streptomycin, ethionamide or ethambutol.

Indications: Capastat should be used concomitantly with other appropriate antituberculous agents for the treatment of pulmonary infections caused by capreomycin-susceptible strains of *Mycobacterium tuberculosis* when the primary agents (isoniazid, rifampicin, streptomycin and ethambutol) have been ineffective or cannot be used because of toxicity or the presence of resistant tubercle bacilli.

4.2 Posology and method of administration
The usual dose is 1g daily (but 20mg/kg/day should not be exceeded) given by deep intramuscular injection only for 60 to 120 days, followed by 1g intramuscularly two or three times a week. Capastat is always administered in combination with at least one other antituberculous agent to which the patient's strain of tubercle bacillus is susceptible.

Capastat should be dissolved in 2ml of 0.9% Sodium Chloride Intravenous Infusion BP or Water for Injections PhEur. Two to three minutes should be allowed for complete solution.

For administration of a 1g dose, the entire contents of the vial should be given. For dosages of less than 1g the following dilution table may be used:

Diluent to be added (ml)	Appropriate volume of Capastat solution (ml)	Approximate average concentration (mg/ml) in terms of mg of capreomycin activity
2.15	2.85	350
2.63	3.33	300
3.3	4.0	250
4.3	5.0	200

The elderly: As for adults. Reduce dosage if renal function is impaired.

Patients with reduced renal function: A reduced dosage should be given based on creatinine clearance using the guidance given in the following table. These dosages are designed to achieve a mean steady-state capreomycin level of 10 micrograms/ml, at various levels of renal function:

(see Table 1 below)

Infants and children: Not for paediatric use since the safety of capreomycin for use in infants and children has not been established.

4.3 Contraindications
Hypersensitivity to capreomycin

Table 1

Creatinine Clearance (ml/min)	Capreomycin clearance (l/kg/h × 10^2)	Half life (hours)	Dose for these dosing intervals (mg/kg) 24h	48h	72h
0	0.54	55.5	1.29	2.58	3.87
10	1.01	29.4	2.43	4.87	7.30
20	1.49	20.0	3.58	7.16	10.70
30	1.97	15.1	4.72	9.45	14.20
40	2.45	12.2	5.87	11.70	
50	2.92	10.2	7.01	14.00	
60	3.40	8.8	8.16		
80	4.35	6.8	10.40		
100	5.31	5.6	12.70		
110	5.78	5.2	13.90		

4.4 Special warnings and special precautions for use
Warnings

The use of capreomycin in patients with renal insufficiency or pre-existing auditory impairment must be undertaken with great caution, and the risk of additional eighth cranial nerve impairment or renal injury should be weighed against the benefits to be derived from treatment.

Capastat must be used only in conjunction with adequate doses of other antituberculous drugs. The use of Capastat alone allows the rapid development of strains resistant to it.

Precautions

As capreomycin is potentially ototoxic, audiometry and assessment of vestibular function should be performed before starting treatment and at regular intervals during treatment.

Regular tests of renal function should be made throughout the period of treatment, and reduced dosage should be used in patients known, or suspected, renal impairment (see ''Dosage and Administration'').

Since hypokalaemia may occur during capreomycin therapy, serum potassium levels should be determined frequently.

A partial neuromuscular block can occur after large doses of capreomycin.

Capreomycin should be administered cautiously to patients with a history of allergy, particularly to drugs.

4.5 Interaction with other medicinal products and other forms of Interaction
Simultaneous administration of other antituberculous drugs which also have ototoxic and nephrotoxic potential (e.g. streptomycin, viomycin) is not recommended. Also, use with other drugs that are not given for the treatment of tuberculosis but have ototoxic or nephrotoxic potential (e.g. polymyxin, colistin sulphate, amikacin, gentamicin, tobramycin, vancomycin, kanamycin and neomycin) should also be undertaken only with great caution.

4.6 Pregnancy and lactation
Pregnancy: The safety of capreomycin for use during pregnancy has not been established. Capreomycin has been shown to be teratogenic in rats when given at 3.5 times the human dose. There are no adequate and well controlled studies in pregnant women. Capastat should be used during pregnancy only if the potential benefit justifies the potential risk to the fetus.

Studies have not been performed to determine potential for carcinogenicity, mutagenicity, or impairment of fertility.

Nursing mothers: It is not known whether capreomycin is excreted in human milk. Caution should be exercised when administering to a nursing woman.

4.7 Effects on ability to drive and use machines
Not applicable

4.8 Undesirable effects
Renal: Elevation of serum creatinine or blood urea and abnormal urine sediment have been observed. Toxic nephritis was reported in one patient with tuberculosis and portal cirrhosis who was treated with capreomycin (1g) and aminosalicylic acid daily for one month. This patient developed renal insufficiency and oliguria and died. The post-mortem showed subsiding acute tubular necrosis.

Electrolyte disturbances resembling Bartter's syndrome have been reported in one patient.

Hepatic: A decrease in bromsulphthalein excretion without change in serum enzymes has been noted in the presence of pre-existing liver disease. Abnormal results in liver function tests have occurred in many patients receiving capreomycin in combination with other antituberculous agents which are also known to cause changes in hepatic function. Periodic determinations of liver function are recommended.

Haematological: Leucocytosis and leucopenia have been observed. Rare cases of thrombocytopenia have been reported. Most patients receiving daily capreomycin have had eosinophilia exceeding 5%, but this has subsided with the reduction of capreomycin dosage to two or three times weekly.

Hypersensitivity: Urticaria and maculopapular rashes associated in some cases with febrile reactions have been reported when capreomycin and other antituberculous drugs were given concomitantly.

Otic: Clinical and subclinical auditory loss has been noted. Some audiometric changes have proved reversible and others, with permanent loss have not been progressive following withdrawal of capreomycin. Tinnitus and vertigo have occurred.

Injection site reactions: Pain and induration at injection sites have been observed. Excessive bleeding and sterile abscesses have also been reported at these sites.

4.9 Overdose
Signs and symptoms: Hypokalaemia, hypocalcaemia, hypomagnesaemia and an electrolyte disturbance resembling Bartter's syndrome have been reported to occur in patients with capreomycin toxicity. Nephrotoxicity, including acute tubular necrosis; and ototoxicity, including dizziness, tinnitus, vertigo and loss of high-tone acuity (see 'Warnings' and 'Precautions'). Neuromuscular blockage or respiratory paralysis may occur following rapid intravenous administration.

If capreomycin is ingested, toxicity is unlikely because less than 1% is absorbed from an intact gastro-intestinal system.

Treatment: Symptomatic and supportive therapy is recommended. Activated charcoal may be more effective than emesis or lavage in reducing absorption.

Patients who have received an overdose of capreomycin and have normal renal function should be hydrated to maintain a urine output of 3-5ml/kg/hr. Fluid balance electrolytes and creatinine clearance should be monitored.

Haemodialysis is effective in patients with significant renal disease.

5. PHARMACOLOGICAL PROPERTIES

5.1 Pharmacodynamic properties
Capreomycin is active against human strains of Mycobacterium tuberculosis.

5.2 Pharmacokinetic properties
Capreomycin sulphate is not significantly absorbed from the gastrointestinal tract, and must be administered parenterally.

Following intramuscular injection of 1g of capreomycin in human subjects, peak serum concentrations in the range of 20-50μg/ml are achieved after 1-2 hours. Serum concentrations are low at 24 hours and daily injections of 1g for 30 days produced no significant accumulation in subjects with normal renal function.

Capreomycin is excreted in the urine, essentially unaltered, and approximately 50% of a 1g intramuscular dose is excreted within 12 hours.

5.3 Preclinical safety data
There are no preclinical data of relevance to the prescriber in addition to those summarised in other sections of the Summary of Product Characteristics.

6. PHARMACEUTICAL PARTICULARS

6.1 List of excipients
Not applicable

6.2 Incompatibilities
Not applicable

6.3 Shelf life
Two years.

Reconstituted product should be used within 24 hours.

6.4 Special precautions for storage
Store below 25°C

6.5 Nature and contents of container
Rubber stoppered, clear glass vial, with aluminium or plastic seal, containing 1g capreomycin base approximately) as sterile white powder.

6.6 Instructions for use and handling
Reconstituted solutions of Capastat may be stored below 25°C for 24 hours. Discard unused portion.

The solution may acquire a pale straw colour and darken with time, but this is not associated with loss of potency or the development of toxicity.

7. MARKETING AUTHORISATION HOLDER
King Pharmaceuticals Ltd
Donegal Street
Ballybofey
County Donegal
Ireland

8. MARKETING AUTHORISATION NUMBER(S)
PL 14385/0006

9. DATE OF FIRST AUTHORISATION/RENEWAL OF THE AUTHORISATION
19th November 1997

10. DATE OF REVISION OF THE TEXT
August 2003

Capoten Tablets 12.5mg, 25mg, 50mg

(E. R. Squibb & Sons Limited)

1. NAME OF THE MEDICINAL PRODUCT
Capoten Tablets 12.5mg, 25mg and 50mg

2. QUALITATIVE AND QUANTITATIVE COMPOSITION
Each tablet contains 12.5mg, 25mg or 50mg captopril.

For excipients, see 6.1

3. PHARMACEUTICAL FORM
Tablets

4. CLINICAL PARTICULARS

4.1 Therapeutic indications

Hypertension: Capoten is indicated for the treatment of hypertension.

Heart Failure: Capoten is indicated for the treatment of chronic heart failure with reduction of systolic ventricular function, in combination with diuretics and, when appropriate, digitalis and beta-blockers.

Myocardial Infarction:

- *short-term (4 weeks) treatment:* Capoten is indicated in any clinically stable patient within the first 24 hours of an infarction.

- *long-term prevention of symptomatic heart failure:* Capoten is indicated in clinically stable patients with asymptomatic left ventricular dysfunction (ejection fraction ⩽40%).

Type I Diabetic Nephropathy: Capoten is indicated for the treatment of macroproteinuric diabetic nephropathy in patients with type I diabetes.

(See Section 5.1).

4.2 Posology and method of administration

Dose should be individualised according to patient's profile (see 4.4) and blood pressure response. The recommended maximum daily dose is 150 mg.

Capoten may be taken before, during and after meals.

Hypertension: the recommended starting dose is 25-50 mg daily in two divided doses. The dose may be increased incrementally, with intervals of at least 2 weeks, to 100-150 mg/day in two divided doses as needed to reach target blood pressure. Captopril may be used alone or with other antihypertensive agents, especially thiazide diuretics. A once-daily dosing regimen may be appropriate when concomitant antihypertensive medication such as thiazide diuretics is added.

In patients with a strongly active renin-angiotensin-aldosterone system (hypovolaemia, renovascular hypertension, cardiac decompensation) it is preferable to commence with a single dose of 6.25 mg or 12.5 mg. The inauguration of this treatment should preferably take place under close medical supervision. These doses will then be administered at a rate of two per day. The dosage can be gradually increased to 50 mg per day in one or two doses and if necessary to 100 mg per day in one or two doses.

Heart failure: treatment with captopril for heart failure should be initiated under close medical supervision. The usual starting dose is 6.25 mg - 12.5 mg BID or TID. Titration to the maintenance dose (75 - 150 mg per day) should be carried out based on patient's response, clinical status and tolerability, up to a maximum of 150 mg per day in divided doses. The dose should be increased incrementally, with intervals of at least 2 weeks to evaluate patient's response.

Myocardial infarction:

- *short-term treatment:* Capoten treatment should begin in hospital as soon as possible following the appearance of the signs and/or symptoms in patients with stable haemodynamics. A 6.25 mg test dose should be administered, with a 12.5 mg dose being administered 2 hours afterwards and a 25 mg dose 12 hours later. From the following day, captopril should be administered in a 100 mg/day dose, in two daily administrations, for 4 weeks, if warranted by the absence of adverse haemodynamic reactions. At the end of the 4 weeks of treatment, the patient's state should be reassessed before a decision is taken concerning treatment for the post-myocardial infarction stage.

- *chronic treatment:* if captopril treatment has not begun during the first 24 hours of the acute myocardial infarction stage, it is suggested that treatment be instigated between the 3rd and 16th day post-infarction once the necessary treatment conditions have been attained (stable haemodynamics and management of any residual ischaemia). Treatment should be started in hospital under strict surveillance (particularly of blood pressure) until the 75 mg dose is reached. The initial dose must be low (see 4.4), particularly if the patient exhibits normal or low blood pressure at the initiation of therapy. Treatment should be initiated with a dose of 6.25 mg followed by 12.5 mg 3 times daily for 2 days and then 25 mg 3 times daily if warranted by the absence of adverse haemodynamic reactions. The recommended dose for effective cardioprotection during long-term treatment is 75 to 150 mg daily in two or three doses. In cases of symptomatic hypotension, as in heart failure, the dosage of diuretics and/or other concomitant vasodilators may be reduced in order to attain the steady state dose of captopril. Where necessary, the dose of captopril should be adjusted in accordance with the patient's clinical reactions. Captopril may be used in combination with other treatments for myocardial infarction such as thrombolytic agents, beta-blockers and acetylsalicylic acid.

Type I Diabetic nephropathy: in patients with type I diabetic nephropathy, the recommended daily dose of captopril is 75-100 mg in divided doses. If additional lowering of blood pressure is desired, additional antihypertensive medications may be added.

Renal impairment: since captopril is excreted primarily via the kidneys, dosage should be reduced or the dosage interval should be increased in patients with impaired renal function. When concomitant diuretic therapy is required, a loop diuretic (e.g. furosemide), rather than a thiazide diuretic, is preferred in patients with severe renal impairment.

In patients with impaired renal function, the following daily dose may be recommended to avoid accumulation of captopril.

Creatinine clearance (ml/min/1.73 m^2)	Daily starting dose (mg)	Daily maximum dose (mg)
>40	25-50	150
21-40	25	100
10-20	12.5	75
<10	6.25	37.5

Elderly patients: as with other antihypertensive agents, consideration should be given to initiating therapy with a lower starting dose (6.25 mg BID) in elderly patients who may have reduced renal function and other organ dysfunctions (see above and section 4.4).

Dosage should be titrated against the blood pressure response and kept as low as possible to achieve adequate control.

Children and adolescents: the efficacy and safety of captopril have not been fully established. The use of captopril in children and adolescents should be initiated under close medical supervision. The initial dose of captopril is about 0.3 mg/kg body weight. For patients requiring special precautions (children with renal dysfunction, premature infants, new-borns and infants, because their renal function is not the same with older children and adults) the starting dose should be only 0.15 mg captopril/kg weight. Generally, captopril is administered to children 3 times a day, but dose and interval of dose should be adapted individually according to patient's response.

4.3 Contraindications

1. History of hypersensitivity to captopril, to any of the excipients or any other ACE inhibitor.

2. History of angioedema associated with previous ACE inhibitor therapy.

3. Hereditary / idiopathic angioneurotic oedema.

4. Second and third trimester of pregnancy (see 4.6)

5. Lactation (see 4.6).

4.4 Special warnings and special precautions for use

Hypotension: rarely hypotension is observed in uncomplicated hypertensive patients. Symptomatic hypotension is more likely to occur in hypertensive patients who are volume and/or sodium depleted by vigorous diuretic therapy, dietary salt restriction, diarrhoea, vomiting or haemodialysis. Volume and/or sodium depletion should be corrected before the administration of an ACE inhibitor and a lower starting dose should be considered.

Patients with heart failure are at higher risk of hypotension and a lower starting dose is recommended when initiating therapy with an ACE inhibitor. Caution should be used whenever the dose of captopril or diuretic is increased in patients with heart failure.

As with any antihypertensive agent, excessive blood pressure lowering in patients with ischaemic cardiovascular or cerebrovascular disease may increase the risk of myocardial infarction or stroke. If hypotension develops, the patient should be placed in a supine position. Volume repletion with intravenous normal saline may be required.

Renovascular hypertension: there is an increased risk of hypotension and renal insufficiency when patients with bilateral renal artery stenosis or stenosis of the artery to a single functioning kidney are treated with ACE inhibitors. Loss of renal function may occur with only mild changes in serum creatinine. In these patients, therapy should be initiated under close medical supervision with low doses, careful titration and monitoring of renal function.

Renal impairment: in cases of renal impairment (creatinine clearance ⩽40 ml/min), the initial dosage of captopril must be adjusted according to the patient's creatinine clearance (se 4.2), and then as a function of the patient's response to treatment. Routine monitoring of potassium and creatinine are part of normal medical practice for these patients.

Angioedema: angioedema of the extremities, face, lips, mucous membranes, tongue, glottis or larynx may occur in patients treated with ACE inhibitors particularly during the first weeks of treatment. However, in rare cases, severe angioedema may develop after long-term treatment with an ACE inhibitor. Treatment should be discontinued promptly. Angioedema involving the tongue, glottis or larynx may be fatal. Emergency therapy should be instituted. The patient should be hospitalised and observed for at least 12 to 24 hours and should not be discharged until complete resolution of symptoms has occurred.

Cough: cough has been reported with the use of ACE inhibitors. Characteristically, the cough is non-productive, persistent and resolves after discontinuation of therapy.

Hepatic failure: rarely, ACE inhibitors have been associated with a syndrome that starts with cholestatic jaundice and progresses to fulminant hepatic necrosis and (sometimes) death. The mechanism of this syndrome is not understood. Patients receiving ACE inhibitors who develop jaundice or marked elevations of hepatic enzymes should discontinue the ACE inhibitor and receive appropriate medical follow-up.

Hyperkalaemia: elevations in serum potassium have been observed in some patients treated with ACE inhibitors, including captopril. Patients at risk for the development of hyperkalaemia include those with renal insufficiency, diabetes mellitus, or those using concomitant potassium-sparing diuretics, potassium supplements or potassium-containing salt substitutes; or those patients taking other drugs associated with increases in serum potassium (e.g. heparin). If concomitant use of the above mentioned agents is deemed appropriate, regular monitoring of serum potassium is recommended.

Lithium: the combination of lithium and captopril is not recommended (see 4.5)

Aortic and mitral valve stenosis/Obstructive hypertropic cardiomyopathy: ACE inhibitors should be used with caution in patients with left ventricular valvular and outflow tract obstruction and avoided in cases of cardiogenic shock and haemodynamically significant obstruction.

Neutropenia/Agranulocytosis: neutropenia/agranulocytosis, thrombocytopenia and anaemia have been reported in patients receiving ACE inhibitors, including captopril. In patients with normal renal function and no other complicating factors, neutropenia occurs rarely. Captopril should be used with extreme caution in patients with collagen vascular disease, immunosuppressant therapy, treatment with allopurinol or procainamide, or a combination of these complicating factors, especially if there is pre-existing impaired renal function. Some of these patients developed serious infections which in a few instances did not respond to intensive antibiotic therapy.

If captopril is used in such patients, it is advised that white blood cell count and differential counts should be performed prior to therapy, every 2 weeks during the first 3 months of captopril therapy, and periodically thereafter. During treatment all patients should be instructed to report any sign of infection (e.g. sore throat, fever) when a differential white blood cell count should be performed. Captopril and other concomitant medication (see 4.5) should be withdrawn if neutropenia (neutrophils less than 1000/mm^3) is detected or suspected.

In most patients neutrophil counts rapidly return to normal upon discontinuing captopril.

Proteinuria: proteinuria may occur particularly in patients with existing renal function impairment or on relatively high doses of ACE inhibitors.

Total urinary proteins greater than 1 g per day were seen in about 0.7% of patients receiving captopril. The majority of patients had evidence of prior renal disease or had received relatively high doses of captopril (in excess of 150 mg/day), or both. Nephrotic syndrome occurred in about one-fifth of proteinuric patients. In most cases, proteinuria subsided or cleared within six months whether or not captopril was continued. Parameters of renal function, such as BUN and creatinine, were seldom altered in the patients with proteinuria.

Patients with prior renal disease should have urinary protein estimations (dip-stick on first morning urine) prior to treatment, and periodically thereafter.

Anaphylactoid reactions during desensitisation: sustained life-threatening anaphylactoid reactions have been rarely reported for patients undergoing desensitising treatment with hymenoptera venom while receiving another ACE inhibitor. In the same patients, these reactions were avoided when the ACE inhibitor was temporarily withheld, but they reappeared upon inadvertent rechallenge. Therefore, caution should be used in patients treated with ACE inhibitors undergoing such desensitisation procedures.

Anaphylactoid reactions during high-flux dialysis / lipoprotein apheresis membrane exposure: anaphylactoid reactions have been reported in patients haemodialysed with high-flux dialysis membranes or undergoing low-density lipoprotein apheresis with dextran sulphate absorption. In these patients, consideration should be given to using a different type of dialysis, membrane or a different class of medication.

Surgery/Anaesthesia: hypotension may occur in patients undergoing major surgery or during treatment with anaesthetic agents that are known to lower blood pressure. If hypotension occurs, it may be corrected by volume expansion.

Diabetic patients: the glycaemia levels should be closely monitored in diabetic patients previously treated with oral antidiabetic drugs or insulin, namely during the first month of treatment with an ACE inhibitor.

Lactose: Capoten contains lactose, therefore it should not be used in cases of congenital galactosaemia, glucose and galactose malabsorption or lactase deficiency syndromes (rare metabolic diseases).

Ethnic differences: as with other angiotensin converting enzyme inhibitors, captopril is apparently less effective in lowering blood pressure in black people than in non-blacks, possibly because of a higher prevalence of low-renin states in the black hypertensive population.

4.5 Interaction with other medicinal products and other forms of Interaction

Potassium sparing diuretics or potassium supplements: ACE inhibitors attenuate diuretic induced potassium loss. Potassium sparing diuretics (e.g. spironolactone, triamterene or amiloride), potassium supplements, or potassium-containing salt substitutes may lead to significant increases in serum potassium. If concomitant use is indicated because of demonstrated hypokalaemia they should be used with caution and with frequent monitoring of serum potassium (see 4.4).

Diuretics (thiazide or loop diuretics): prior treatment with high dose diuretics may result in volume depletion and a risk of hypotension when initiating therapy with captopril (see 4.4). The hypotensive effects can be reduced by discontinuation of the diuretic, by increasing volume or salt intake or by initiating therapy with a low dose of captopril. However, no clinically significant drug interactions have been found in specific studies with hydrochlorothiazide or furosemide.

Other antihypertensive agents: captopril has been safely co-administered with other commonly used anti-hypertensive agents (e.g. beta-blockers and long-acting calcium channel blockers). Concomitant use of these agents may increase the hypotensive effects of captopril. Treatment with nitroglycerine and other nitrates, or other vasodilators, should be used with caution.

Treatments of acute myocardial infarction: captopril may be used concomitantly with acetylsalicylic acid (at cardiologic doses), thrombolytics, beta-blockers and/or nitrates in patients with myocardial infarction.

Lithium: reversible increases in serum lithium concentrations and toxicity have been reported during concomitant administration of lithium with ACE inhibitors. Concomitant use of thiazide diuretics may increase the risk of lithium toxicity and enhance the already increased risk of lithium toxicity with ACE inhibitors. Use of captopril with lithium is not recommended, but if the combination proves necessary, careful monitoring of serum lithium levels should be performed (see 4.4)

Tricyclic antidepressants / Antipsychotics: ACE inhibitors may enhance the hypotensive effects of certain tricyclic antidepressants and antipsychotics (see 4.4). Postural hypotension may occur.

Allopurinol, procainamide, cytostatic or immunosuppressive agents: concomitant administration with ACE inhibitors may lead to an increased risk for leucopenia especially when the latter are used at higher than currently recommended doses.

Non-steroidal anti-inflammatory medicinal products: it has been described that non-steroidal anti-inflammatory medicinal products (NSAIDs) and ACE inhibitors exert an additive effect on the increase in serum potassium whereas renal function may decrease. These effects are, in principle, reversible. Rarely, acute renal failure may occur, particularly in patients with compromised renal function such as the elderly or dehydrated. Chronic administration of NSAIDs may reduce the antihypertensive effect of an ACE inhibitor.

Sympathomimetics: may reduce the antihypertensive effects of ACE inhibitors; patients should be carefully monitored.

Antidiabetics: pharmacological studies have shown that ACE inhibitors, including captopril, can potentiate the blood glucose-reducing effects of insulin and oral antidiabetics such as sulphonylurea in diabetics. Should this very rare interaction occur, it may be necessary to reduce the dose of the antidiabetic during simultaneous treatment with ACE inhibitors.

Clinical Chemistry

Captopril may cause a false-positive urine test for acetone.

4.6 Pregnancy and lactation

Pregnancy: Capoten is not recommended during the first trimester of pregnancy. When a pregnancy is planned or confirmed, the switch to an alternative treatment should be initiated as soon as possible. Controlled studies with ACE inhibitors have not been done in humans, but limited number of cases of first trimester exposures have not shown malformations.

Capoten is contraindicated during the second and third trimesters of pregnancy. Prolonged captopril exposure during the second and third trimesters is known to induce toxicity in foetuses (decreased renal function, oligohydramnios, skull ossification retardation) and in neonates (neonatal renal failure, hypotension, hyperkalaemia) (see also 5.3).

Lactation: Capoten is contraindicated in the lactation period.

4.7 Effects on ability to drive and use machines

As with other antihypertensives, the ability to drive and use machines may be reduced, namely at the start of the treatment, or when posology is modified, and also when used in combination with alcohol, but these effects depend on the individual's susceptibility.

4.8 Undesirable effects

Undesirable effects reported for captopril and/or ACE inhibitor therapy include:

Blood and lymphatic disorders:

very rare: neutropenia/agranulocytosis (see 4.4), pancytopenia particularly in patients with renal dysfunction (see 4.4), anaemia (including aplastic and haemolytic), thrombocytopenia, lymphadenopathy, eosinophilia, autoimmune diseases and/or positive ANA-titres.

Metabolism and nutrition disorders:

rare: anorexia

very rare: hyperkalaemia, hypoglycaemia (see 4.4)

Psychiatric disorders:

common: sleep disorders

very rare: confusion, depression.

Nervous system disorders:

common: taste impairment, dizziness

rare: drowsiness, headache and paraesthesia

very rare: cerebrovascular incidents, including stroke, and syncope.

Eye disorders:

very rare: blurred vision

Cardiac disorders:

uncommon: tachycardia or tachyarrhythmia, angina pectoris, palpitations.

very rare: cardiac arrest, cardiogenic shock

Vascular disorders:

uncommon: hypotension (see 4.4), Raynaud syndrome, flush, pallor

Respiratory, thoracic and mediastinal disorders:

common: dry, irritating (non-productive) cough (see 4.4) and dyspnoea

very rare: bronchospasm, rhinitis, allergic alveolitis / eosinophilic pneumonia

Gastrointestinal disorders:

common: nausea, vomiting, gastric irritations, abdominal pain, diarrhoea, constipation, dry mouth.

rare: stomatitis/aphthous ulcerations

very rare: glossitis, peptic ulcer, pancreatitis.

Hepato-biliary disorders:

very rare: impaired hepatic function and cholestasis (including jaundice), hepatitis including necrosis, elevated liver enzymes and bilirubin.

Skin and subcutaneous tissue disorders:

common: pruritus with or without a rash, rash, and alopecia.

uncommon: angioedema (see 4.4)

very rare: urticaria, Stevens Johnson syndrome, erythema multiforme, photosensitivity, erythroderma, pemphigoid reactions and exfoliative dermatitis.

Musculoskeletal, connective tissue and bone disorders:

very rare: myalgia, arthralgia.

Renal and urinary disorders:

rare: renal function disorders including renal failure, polyuria, oliguria, increased urine frequency.

very rare: nephrotic syndrome.

Reproductive system and breast disorders:

very rare: impotence, gynaecomastia.

General disorders:

uncommon: chest pain, fatigue, malaise

very rare: fever

Investigations:

very rare: proteinuria, eosinophilia, increase of serum potassium, decrease of serum sodium, elevation of BUN, serum creatinine and serum bilirubin, decreases in haemoglobin, haematocrit, leucocytes, thrombocytes, positive ANA-titre, elevated ESR.

4.9 Overdose

Symptoms of overdosage are severe hypotension, shock, stupor, bradycardia, electrolyte disturbances and renal failure.

Measures to prevent absorption (e.g. gastric lavage, administration of adsorbents and sodium sulphate within 30 minutes after intake) and hasten elimination should be applied if ingestion is recent. If hypotension occurs, the patient should be placed in the shock position and salt and volume supplementations should be given rapidly. Treatment with angiotensin-II should be considered. Bradycardia or extensive vagal reactions should be treated by administering atropine. The use of a pacemaker may be considered.

Captopril may be removed from circulation by haemodialysis.

5. PHARMACOLOGICAL PROPERTIES

5.1 Pharmacodynamic properties

Pharmacotherapeutic group: ACE inhibitors, plain, ATC code: C09AA01.

Captopril is a highly specific, competitive inhibitor of angiotensin-I converting enzyme (ACE inhibitors).

The beneficial effects of ACE inhibitors appear to result primarily from the suppression of the plasma renin-angiotensin-aldosterone system. Renin is an endogenous enzyme synthesised by the kidneys and released into the circulation where it converts angiotensinogen to angiotensin-I a relatively inactive decapeptide. Angiotensin-I is then converted by angiotensin converting enzyme, a peptidyldipeptidase, to angiotensin-II. Angiotensin-II is a potent vasoconstrictor responsible for arterial vasoconstriction and increased blood pressure, as well as for stimulation of the adrenal gland to secrete aldosterone. Inhibition of ACE results in decreased plasma angiotensin-II, which leads to decreased vasopressor activity and to reduced aldosterone secretion. Although the latter decrease is small, small increases in serum potassium concentrations may occur, along with sodium and fluid loss. The cessation of the negative feedback of angiotensin-II on the renin secretion results in an increase of the plasma renin activity.

Another function of the converting enzyme is to degrade the potent vasodepressive kinin peptide bradykinin to inactive metabolites. Therefore, inhibition of ACE results in an increased activity of circulating and local kallikrein-kinin-system which contributes to peripheral vasodilation by activating the prostaglandin system; it is possible that this mechanism is involved in the hypotensive effect of ACE inhibitors and is responsible for certain adverse reactions.

Reductions of blood pressure are usually maximal 60 to 90 minutes after oral administration of an individual dose of captopril. The duration of effect is dose related. The reduction in blood pressure may be progressive, so to achieve maximal therapeutic effects, several weeks of therapy may be required. The blood pressure lowering effects of captopril and thiazide-type diuretics are additive.

In patients with hypertension, captopril causes a reduction in supine and erect blood pressure, without inducing any compensatory increase in heart rate, nor water and sodium retention.

In haemodynamic investigations, captopril caused a marked reduction in peripheral arterial resistance. In general there were no clinically relevant changes in renal plasma flow or glomerular filtration rate. In most patients, the antihypertensive effect began about 15 to 30 minutes after oral administration of captopril; the peak effect was achieved after 60 to 90 minutes. The maximum reduction in blood pressure of a defined captopril dose was generally visible after three to four weeks.

In the recommended daily dose, the antihypertensive effect persists even during long-term treatment. Temporary withdrawal of captopril does not cause any rapid, excessive increase in blood pressure (rebound). The treatment of hypertension with captopril leads also to a decrease in left ventricular hypertrophy.

Haemodynamic investigations in patients with heart failure, showed that captopril caused a reduction in peripheral systemic resistance and a rise in venous capacity. This resulted in a reduction in pre-load and after-load of the heart (reduction in ventricular filling pressure). In addition, rises in cardiac output, work index and exercise capacity have been observed during treatment with captopril. In a large, placebo-controlled study in patients with left ventricular dysfunction (LVEF $\leqslant$40%) following myocardial infarction, it was shown that captopril (initiated between the 3rd to the 16th day after infarction) prolonged the survival time and reduced cardiovascular mortality. The latter was manifested as a delay in the development of symptomatic heart failure and a reduction in the necessity for hospitalisation due to heart failure compared to placebo. There was also a reduction in re-infarction and in cardiac revascularisation procedures and/or in the need for additional medication with diuretics and/or digitalis or an increase in their dosage compared to placebo.

A retrospective analysis showed that captopril reduced recurrent infarcts and cardiac revascularisation procedures (neither were target criteria of the study).

Another large, placebo-controlled study in patients with myocardial infarction showed that captopril (given within 24 hours of the event and for a duration of one month) significantly reduced overall mortality after 5 weeks compared to placebo. The favourable effect of captopril on total mortality was still detectable even after one year. No indication of a negative effect in relation to early mortality on the first day of treatment was found.

Captopril cardioprotection effects are observed regardless of the patient's age or gender, location of the infarction and concomitant treatments with proven efficacy during the post-infarction period (thrombolytic agents, beta-blockers and acetylsalicylic acid).

Type I diabetic nephropathy

In a placebo-controlled, multicentre double blind clinical trial in insulin-dependent (Type I) diabetes with proteinuria, with or without hypertension (simultaneous administration of other antihypertensives to control blood pressure was allowed), captopril significantly reduced (by 51%) the time to doubling of the baseline creatinine concentration compared to placebo; the incidence of terminal renal failure (dialysis, transplantation) or death was also significantly less common under captopril than under placebo (51%). In patients with diabetes and microalbuminuria, treatment with captopril reduced albumin excretion within two years.

The effects of treatment with captopril on the preservation of renal function are in addition to any benefit that may have been derived from the reduction in blood pressure.

5.2 Pharmacokinetic properties
Captopril is an orally active agent that does not require biotransformation for activity. The average minimal absorption is approximately 75%. Peak plasma concentrations are reached within 60-90 minutes. The presence of food in the gastrointestinal tract reduces absorption by about 30-40%. Approximately 25-30% of the circulating drug is bound to plasma proteins.

The apparent elimination half-life of unchanged captopril in blood is about 2 hours. Greater than 95% of the absorbed dose is eliminated in the urine within 24 hours; 40-50% is unchanged drug and the remainder are inactive disulphide metabolites (captopril disulphide and captopril cysteine disulphide). Impaired renal function could result in drug accumulation. Therefore, in patients with impaired renal function the dose should be reduced and/or dosage interval prolonged (see 4.2).

Studies in animals indicate that captopril does not cross the blood-brain barrier to any significant extent.

5.3 Preclinical safety data
Animal studies performed during organogenesis with captopril have not shown any teratogenic effect but captopril has produced foetal toxicity in several species, including foetal mortality during late pregnancy, growth retardation and postnatal mortality in the rat. Preclinical data reveal no other specific hazard for humans based on conventional studies of safety pharmacology, repeated dose toxicology, genotoxicity and carcinogenicity.

6. PHARMACEUTICAL PARTICULARS

6.1 List of excipients
Lactose, maize starch, microcrystalline cellulose, stearic acid.

6.2 Incompatibilities
None.

6.3 Shelf life
48 Months.

6.4 Special precautions for storage
Store below 30°C.

Protect from moisture.

6.5 Nature and contents of container
The tablets are packaged in PVC/aluminium blisters.

Capoten Tablets 12.5mg:	Packs of 56 tablets.
Capoten Tablets 25mg and 50mg:	Packs of 56 or 84 tablets.

6.6 Instructions for use and handling
No special instructions.

7. MARKETING AUTHORISATION HOLDER
E.R. Squibb & Sons Limited
Uxbridge Business Park
Sanderson Road
Uxbridge
Middlesex UB8 1DH

8. MARKETING AUTHORISATION NUMBER(S)

Capoten Tablets 12.5mg:	PL 0034/0221
Capoten Tablets 25mg:	PL 0034/0193
Capoten Tablets 50mg:	PL 0034/0194

9. DATE OF FIRST AUTHORISATION/RENEWAL OF THE AUTHORISATION

Capoten Tablets 12.5mg:	20th September 1989
Capoten Tablets 25mg:	27th March 1981
Capoten Tablets 50mg:	27th March 1981

10. DATE OF REVISION OF THE TEXT
June 2005

Capozide LS Tablets

(E. R. Squibb & Sons Limited)

1. NAME OF THE MEDICINAL PRODUCT
Capozide LS Tablets

2. QUALITATIVE AND QUANTITATIVE COMPOSITION
Each tablet contains 25mg captopril and 12.5mg hydrochlorothiazide.

For excipients, see 6.1.

3. PHARMACEUTICAL FORM
Tablets.

4. CLINICAL PARTICULARS

4.1 Therapeutic indications
Treatment of essential hypertension.

This fixed dose combination is indicated in patients whose blood pressure is not adequately controlled by captopril alone or hydrochlorothiazide alone.

4.2 Posology and method of administration
Capozide LS can be administered in a single or two divided doses/day with or without food in patients whose blood pressure is not adequately controlled by captopril alone or hydrochlorothiazide alone. A maximum daily dose of 100 mg captopril/30 mg hydrochlorothiazide should not be exceeded. If satisfactory reduction of blood pressure has not been achieved, additional antihypertensive medication may be added (see 4.5).

Adults: The administration of the fixed combination of captopril and hydrochlorothiazide is usually recommended after dosage titration with the individual components. The usual maintenance dose is 50/25 mg, once a day, in the morning. When clinically appropriate a direct change from monotherapy to the fixed combination may be considered. The 25/25mg strength may be used once a day for patients whose blood pressure is not adequately controlled by hydrochlorothiazide 25 mg monotherapy and before titration of the captopril component. The 50/25mg and 25/25mg strengths are intended to be used once daily, as two tablets would result in an inappropriately high dose of hydrochlorothiazide (50mg/day). The 50/15 mg strength may be administered to start the fixed combination in patients whose blood pressure is not adequately controlled by 50 mg captopril monotherapy, and/or when a lower dose of hydrochlorothiazide is preferred.

The 25/25mg and 50/15mg tablet strengths are not available in the U.K.

Renal impairment: Creatinine clearance between 30 and 80 ml/min: the initial dose is usually 25/12.5 mg once a day, in the morning.

The combination captopril/hydrochlorothiazide is contraindicated in patients with severe renal impairment (creatinine clearance < 30 ml/min).

Special populations: In salt/volume depleted patients, elderly patients and diabetic patients, the usual starting dose is 25/12.5 mg once a day.

Children: The safety and efficacy of Capozide LS in children has not been established.

4.3 Contraindications
- History of hypersensitivity to captopril, to any of the excipients or any other ACE inhibitor.
- History of hypersensitivity to hydrochlorothiazide or other sulphonamide-derived drugs.
- History of angioedema associated with previous ACE inhibitor therapy.
- Hereditary/idiopathic angioneurotic oedema
- Severe renal impairment (creatinine clearance < 30 ml/min)
- Severe hepatic impairment.
- Second and third trimester of pregnancy (see 4.6)
- Lactation (see 4.6)

4.4 Special warnings and special precautions for use
CAPTOPRIL

Hypotension: Rarely hypotension is observed in uncomplicated hypertensive patients. Symptomatic hypotension is more likely to occur in hypertensive patients who are volume and/or sodium depleted by vigorous diuretic therapy, dietary salt restriction, diarrhoea, vomiting, or haemodialysis. Volume and/or sodium depletion should be corrected before the administration of an ACE inhibitor and a lower starting dose should be considered.

As with any antihypertensive agent, excessive blood pressure lowering in patients with ischaemic cardiovascular or cerebrovascular disease may increase the risk of myocardial infarction or stroke. If hypotension develops, the patient should be placed in a supine position. Volume repletion with intravenous normal saline may be required.

Renovascular hypertension: There is an increased risk of hypotension and renal insufficiency when patients with bilateral renal artery stenosis or stenosis of the artery to a single functioning kidney are treated with ACE inhibitors. Loss of renal function may occur with only mild changes in serum creatinine. In these patients, therapy should be initiated under close medical supervision with low doses, careful titration and monitoring of renal function.

Angioedema: Angioedema of the extremities, face, lips, mucous membranes, tongue, glottis or larynx may occur in patients treated with ACE inhibitors, particularly during the first weeks of treatment. However, in rare cases, severe angioedema may develop after long-term treatment with an ACE inhibitor. Treatment should be discontinued promptly. Angioedema involving the tongue, glottis or larynx may be fatal. Emergency therapy should be instituted. The patient should be hospitalised and observed for at least 12 to 24 hours and should not be discharged until complete resolution of symptoms has occurred.

Cough: Cough has been reported with the use of ACE inhibitors. Characteristically, the cough is non-productive, persistent and resolves after discontinuation of therapy.

Hepatic failure: Rarely, ACE inhibitors have been associated with a syndrome that starts with cholestatic jaundice and progresses to fulminant hepatic necrosis and (sometimes) death. The mechanism of this syndrome is not understood. Patients receiving ACE inhibitors who develop jaundice or marked elevations of hepatic enzymes should discontinue the ACE inhibitors and receive appropriate medical follow-up.

Hyperkalaemia: Elevations in serum potassium have been observed in some patients treated with ACE inhibitors, including captopril. Patients at risk for the development of hyperkalaemia include those with renal insufficiency, diabetes mellitus, or those using concomitant potassium-sparing diuretics, potassium supplements or potassium-containing salt substitutes; or those patients taking other drugs associated with increases in serum potassium (e.g. heparin). If concomitant use of the above mentioned agents is deemed appropriate, regular monitoring of serum potassium is recommended.

Aortic and mitral valve stenosis / Obstructive hypertrophic cardiomyopathy / Cardiogenic shock: ACE inhibitors should be used with caution in patients with left ventricular valvular and outflow tract obstruction and avoided in cases of cardiogenic shock and haemodynamically significant obstruction.

Neutropenia/Agranulocytosis: Neutropenia/agranulocytosis, thrombocytopenia and anaemia have been reported in patients receiving ACE inhibitors, including captopril. In patients with normal renal function and no other complicating factors, neutropenia occurs rarely. Captopril should be used with extreme caution in patients with collagen vascular disease, immunosuppressant therapy, treatment with allopurinol or procainamide, or a combination of these complicating factors, especially if there is pre-existing impaired renal function. Some of these patients developed serious infections which in a few instances did not respond to intensive antibiotic therapy.

If captopril is used in such patients, it is advised that white blood cell count and differential counts should be performed prior to therapy, every 2 weeks during the first 3 months of captopril therapy, and periodically thereafter. During treatment all patients should be instructed to report any sign of infection (e.g. sore throat, fever) when a differential white blood cell count should be performed. Captopril and other concomitant medication (see 4.5) should be withdrawn if neutropenia (neutrophils less than 1000/mm^3) is detected or suspected.

In most patients neutrophil counts rapidly return to normal upon discontinuing captopril.

Proteinurea: proteinuria may occur particularly in patients with existing renal function impairment or on relatively high doses of ACE inhibitors.

Total urinary proteins greater than 1 g per day were seen in about 0.7% of patients receiving captopril. The majority of patients had evidence of prior renal disease or had received relatively high doses of captopril (in excess of 150 mg/day), or both. Nephrotic syndrome occurred in about one-fifth of proteinuric patients. In most cases, proteinuria subsided or cleared within six months whether or not captopril was continued. Parameters of renal function, such as BUN and creatinine, were seldom altered in the patients with proteinuria.

Patients with prior renal disease should have urinary protein estimations (dip-stick on first morning urine) prior to treatment, and periodically thereafter.

Anaphylactoid reactions during desensitisation: sustained life-threatening anaphylactoid reactions have been rarely reported for patients undergoing desensitising treatment with hymenoptera venom while receiving another ACE inhibitor. In the same patients, these reactions were avoided when the ACE inhibitor was temporarily withheld, but they reappeared upon inadvertent rechallenge. Therefore, caution should be used in patients treated with ACE inhibitors undergoing such desensitisation procedures.

Anaphylactoid reactions during high-flux dialysis / lipoprotein apheresis membrane exposure: Anaphylactoid reactions have been reported in patients haemodialysed with high-flux dialysis membranes or undergoing low-density lipoprotein apheresis with dextran sulphate absorption. In these patients, consideration should be given to using a different type of dialysis membrane or a different class of medication.

Surgery/Anaesthesia: Hypotension may occur in patients undergoing major surgery or during treatment with anaesthetic agents that are known to lower blood pressure. If hypotension occurs, it may be corrected by volume expansion.

Diabetic patients: The glycaemia levels should be closely monitored in diabetic patients previously treated with oral antidiabetic drugs or insulin, namely during the first month of treatment with an ACE inhibitor.

As with other angiotensin converting enzyme inhibitors, Capozide LS is apparently less effective in lowering blood pressure in black people than in non-blacks, possibly because of higher prevalence of low-renin states in the black hypertensive population.

HYDROCHLOROTHIAZIDE

Renal impairment: In patients with renal disease, thiazides may precipitate azotaemia. Cumulative effects of the drug may develop in patients with impaired renal function.

If progressive renal impairment becomes evident, as indicated by a rising non-protein nitrogen, careful reappraisal of therapy is necessary, with consideration given to discontinuing diuretic therapy (see 4.3).

Hepatic impairment: Thiazides should be used with caution in patients with impaired hepatic function or progressive liver disease, since minor alterations of fluid and electrolyte balance may precipitate hepatic coma (see 4.3).

Metabolic and endocrine effects: Thiazide therapy may impair glucose tolerance. In diabetic patients dosage adjustments of insulin or oral hypoglycaemic agents may be required. Latent diabetes mellitus may become manifest during thiazide therapy.

Increases in cholesterol and triglyceride levels have been associated with thiazide diuretic therapy.

Hyperuricaemia may occur or frank gout may be precipitated in certain patients receiving thiazide therapy.

Electrolyte imbalance: As for any patient receiving diuretic therapy, periodic determination of serum electrolytes should be performed at appropriate intervals.

Thiazides, including hydrochlorothiazide, can cause fluid or electrolyte imbalance (hypokalaemia, hyponatraemia and hypochloraemic alkalosis). Warning signs of fluid or electrolyte imbalance are dryness of mouth, thirst, weakness, lethargy, drowsiness, restlessness, muscle pain or cramps, muscular fatigue, hypotension, oliguria, tachycardia and gastrointestinal disturbances such as nausea or vomiting.

Although hypokalaemia may develop with the use of thiazide diuretics, concurrent therapy with captopril may reduce diuretic-induced hypokalaemia. The risk of hypokalaemia is greatest in patients with cirrhosis of the liver, in patients experiencing brisk diuresis, in patients who are receiving inadequate oral intake of electrolytes and in patients receiving concomitant therapy with corticosteroids or ACTH (see 4.5).

Dilutional hyponatraemia may occur in oedematous patients in hot weather. Chloride deficit is generally mild and usually does not require treatment.

Thiazides may decrease urinary calcium excretion and cause an intermittent and slight elevation of serum calcium in the absence of known disorders of calcium metabolism. Marked hypercalcaemia may be evidence of hidden hyperparathyroidism. Thiazides should be discontinued before carrying out tests for parathyroid function.

Thiazides have been shown to increase the urinary excretion of magnesium, which may result in hypomagnesaemia.

Anti-doping test: hydrochlorothiazide contained in this medication could produce a positive analytical result in an anti-doping test.

Other: Sensitivity reactions may occur in patients with or without a history of allergy or bronchial asthma. The possibility of exacerbation or activation of systemic lupus erythematosus has been reported.

CAPTOPRIL/HYDROCHLOROTHIAZIDE COMBINATION

Pregnancy: Capozide LS is not recommended during the first trimester of pregnancy (see 4.6). If treatment is discontinued due to pregnancy, the prescriber should decide whether treatment of hypertension should be continued.

Risk of hypokalaemia: The combination of an ACE inhibitor with a thiazide diuretic does not rule out the occurrence of hypokalaemia. Regular monitoring of kalaemia should be performed.

Combination with lithium: Capozide LS is not recommended in association with lithium due to the potentiation of lithium toxicity (see 4.5).

Lactose: Capozide LS contains lactose. Therefore, it should not be used in cases of congenital galactosaemia, glucose and galactose malabsorption or lactase deficiency syndromes (rare metabolic diseases).

4.5 Interaction with other medicinal products and other forms of Interaction

CAPTOPRIL

Potassium sparing diuretics or potassium supplements: ACE inhibitors attenuate diuretic induced potassium loss. Potassium sparing diuretics (e.g. spironolactone, triamterene or amiloride), potassium supplements, or potassium-containing salt substitutes may lead to significant increases in serum potassium. If concomitant use is indicated because of demonstrated hypokalaemia they should be used with caution and with frequent monitoring of serum potassium (see 4.4).

Diuretics (thiazide or loop diuretics): Prior treatment with high dose diuretics may result in volume depletion and a risk of hypotension when initiating therapy with captopril (see 4.4). The hypotensive effects can be reduced by discontinuation of the diuretic, by increasing volume or salt intake or by initiating therapy with a low dose of captopril. However, no clinically significant drug interactions have been found in specific studies with hydrochlorothiazide or furosemide.

Other antihypertensive agents: Captopril has been safely co-administered with other commonly used anti-hypertensive agents (e.g. beta-blockers and long-acting calcium channel blockers). Concomitant use of these agents may increase the hypotensive effects of captopril. Nitroglycerine and other nitrates, or other vasodilators, should be used with caution.

Treatments of acute myocardial infarction: Captopril may be used concomitantly with acetylsalicylic acid (at cardiological doses), thrombolytics, beta-blockers and/or nitrates in patients with myocardial infarction.

Tricyclic antidepressants/Antipsychotics: ACE inhibitors may enhance the hypotensive effects of certain tricyclic antidepressants and antipsychotics (see 4.4). Postural hypotension may occur.

Allopurinol, procainamide, cytostatic or immuno-suppressant agents: Concomitant administration with ACE inhibitors may lead to an increased risk of leucopenia, especially when the latter are used at higher than currently recommended doses.

Sympathomimetics: may reduce the antihypertensive effects of ACE inhibitors; patients should be carefully monitored.

Antidiabetics: Pharmacological studies have shown that ACE inhibitors, including captopril, can potentiate the blood glucose-reducing effects of insulin and oral antidiabetics, such as sulphonylurea, in diabetics. Should this very rare interaction occur, it may be necessary to reduce the dose of the antidiabetic during simultaneous treatment with ACE inhibitors.

HYDROCHLOROTHIAZIDE

Amphotericin B (parenteral), carbenoxolone, corticosteroids, corticotropin (ACTH) or stimulant laxatives: hydrochlorothiazide may intensify electrolyte imbalance, particularly hypokalaemia.

Calcium salts: Increased serum calcium levels due to decreased excretion may occur when administered concurrently with thiazide diuretics.

Cardiac glycosides: Enhanced possibility of digitalis toxicity associated with thiazide induced hypokalaemia.

Cholestyramine resin and colestipol: may delay or decrease absorption of hydrochlorothiazide. Sulphonamide diuretics should be taken at least one hour before or four to six hours after these medications.

Nondepolarising muscle relaxants (e.g. tubocurarine chloride): effects of these agents may be potentiated by hydrochlorothiazide.

Drugs associated with torsades de pointes: Because of the risk of hypokalaemia, caution should be used when hydrochlorothiazide is coadministered with drugs associated with torsades de pointes, e.g. some anti-arrhythmics, some antipsychotics and other drugs known to induce torsades de pointes.

CAPTOPRIL/HYDROCHLOROTHIAZIDE COMBINATION

Lithium: Reversible increases in serum lithium concentrations and toxicity have been reported during concomitant administration of lithium with ACE inhibitors. Concomitant use of thiazide diuretics may increase the risk of lithium toxicity and enhance the already increased risk of lithium toxicity with ACE inhibitors. The combination of captopril and hydrochlorothiazide with lithium is therefore not recommended and careful monitoring of serum lithium levels should be performed if the combination proves necessary.

Non-steroidal anti-inflammatory medicinal products: It has been described that non-steroidal anti-inflammatory medicinal products (NSAIDs) and ACE inhibitors exert an additive effect on the increase in serum potassium, whereas renal function may decrease. These effects are, in principle, reversible. Rarely, acute renal failure may occur, particularly in patients with compromised renal function such as the elderly or dehydrated. Chronic administration of NSAIDs may reduce the antihypertensive effect of an ACE inhibitor. The administration of NSAIDs may reduce the diuretic, natriuretic and antihypertensive effects of thiazide diuretics.

Clinical Chemistry

Captopril may cause a false-positive urine test for acetone. Hydrochlorothiazide may cause diagnostic interference of the bentiromide test. Thiazides may decrease serum PBI (Protein Bound Iodine) levels without signs of thyroid disturbance.

4.6 Pregnancy and lactation

Pregnancy: Capozide LS is not recommended during the first trimester of pregnancy. When a pregnancy is planned or confirmed, an alternative treatment should be initiated as soon as possible. Controlled studies with ACE inhibitors have not been done in humans, but a limited number of cases of first trimester exposures has not shown malformations.

Capozide LS is contraindicated during the second and third trimesters of pregnancy. Prolonged captopril exposure during the second and third trimesters is known to induce toxicity in foetuses (decreased renal function, oligohydramnios, skull ossification retardation) and in neonates (neonatal renal failure, hypotension, hyperkalaemia) (see also 5.3).

Hydrochlorothiazide, in cases of prolonged exposure during the third trimester of pregnancy, may cause a foetoplacental ischaemia and risk of growth retardation. Moreover, rare cases of hypoglycaemia and thrombocytopenia in neonates have been reported in case of exposure near term.

Hydrochlorothiazide can reduce plasma volume as well as the uteroplacental blood flow.

Should exposure to Capozide have occurred from the second trimester of pregnancy, ultrasound check of renal function and skull is recommended.

Lactation: Capozide is contraindicated in the lactation period.

Both captopril and hydrochlorothiazide are excreted in human milk. Thiazides during breast feeding by lactating mothers have been associated with a decrease or even suppression of lactation. Hypersensitivity to sulphonamide-derived drugs, hypokalaemia and nuclear icterus might occur.

Because of the potential for serious adverse reactions in nursing infants from both drugs, a decision should be made whether to discontinue nursing or to discontinue therapy, taking into account the importance of this therapy to the mother.

4.7 Effects on ability to drive and use machines

As with other antihypertensives, the ability to drive and use machines may be reduced, e.g. at the start of the treatment or when the dose is modified, and also when used in combination with alcohol, but these effects depend on the individual's susceptibility.

4.8 Undesirable effects

CAPTOPRIL

Undesirable effects reported for captopril and/or ACE inhibitor therapy include:

Blood and lymphatic disorders:

very rare: neutropenia/agranulocytosis (see 4.4), pancytopenia, particularly in patients with renal dysfunction (see 4.4), anaemia (including aplastic and haemolytic), thrombocytopenia, lymphadenopathy, eosinophilia, autoimmune diseases and/or positive ANA-titres.

Metabolism and nutrition disorders:

rare: anorexia

very rare: hyperkalaemia, hypoglycaemia (see 4.4)

Psychiatric disorders:

common: sleep disorders

very rare: confusion, depression

Nervous system disorders:

common: taste impairment, dizziness

rare: drowsiness, headache and paraesthesia

very rare: cerebrovascular incidents, including stroke, and syncope

Eye disorders:

very rare: blurred vision.

Cardiac disorders:

uncommon: tachycardia or tachyarrhythmia, angina pectoris, palpitations

very rare: cardiac arrest, cardiogenic shock.

Vascular disorders:

uncommon: hypotension (see 4.4), Raynaud syndrome, flush, pallor

Respiratory, thoracic and mediastinal disorders:

common: dry, irritating (non-productive) cough (see 4.4) and dyspnoea

very rare: bronchospasm, rhinitis, allergic alveolitis/ eosinophilic pneumonia

Gastrointestinal disorders:

common: nausea, vomiting, gastric irritations, abdominal pain, diarrhoea, constipation, dry mouth

rare: stomatitis/aphthous ulcerations

very rare: glossitis, peptic ulcer, pancreatitis

Hepato-biliary disorders:

very rare: impaired hepatic function and cholestasis (including jaundice), hepatitis including necrosis, elevated liver enzymes and bilirubin.

Skin and subcutaneous tissue disorders:

common: pruritus with or without a rash, rash, and alopecia

uncommon: angioedema (see 4.4)

very rare: urticaria, Stevens Johnson syndrome, erythema multiforme, photo-sensitivity, erythroderma, pemphigoid reactions and exfoliative dermatitis.

Musculoskeletal, connective tissue and bone disorders:

very rare: myalgia, arthralgia

Renal and urinary disorders:

rare: renal function disorders, including renal failure, polyuria, oliguria, increased urine frequency

very rare: nephrotic syndrome

Reproductive system and breast disorders:

very rare: impotence, gynaecomastia

General disorders;

uncommon: chest pain, fatigue, malaise

very rare: fever

Investigations:

very rare: proteinuria, eosinophilia, increase of serum potassium, decrease of serum sodium, elevation of BUN, serum creatinine and serum bilirubin, decreases in haemoglobin, haematocrit, leucocytes, thrombocytes, positive ANA-titre, elevated ESR.

HYDROCHLOROTHIAZIDE

Infections and infestations: sialadenitis

Blood and lymphatic system disorders:

leucopenia, neutropenia/agranulocytosis, thrombocytopenia, aplastic anaemia, haemolytic anaemia, bone marrow depression

Metabolism and nutrition disorders:

anorexia, hyperglycaemia, glycosuria, hyperuricaemia, electrolyte imbalance (including hyponatraemia and hypokalaemia), increases in cholesterol and triglycerides.

Psychiatric disorders:

restlessness, depression, sleep disturbances

Nervous system disorders:

loss of appetite, paraesthesia, light-headedness

Eye disorders:

xanthopsia, transient blurred vision

Ear and labyrinth disorders:

vertigo

Cardiac disorders:

postural hypotension, cardiac arrhythmias

Vascular disorders:

necrotising angiitis (vasculitis, cutaneous vasculitis)

Respiratory, thoracic and mediastinal disorders:

respiratory distress (including pneumonitis and pulmonary oedema).

Gastrointestinal disorders:

gastric irritation, diarrhoea, constipation, pancreatitis

Hepato-biliary disorders:

jaundice (intrahepatic cholestatic jaundice)

Skin and subcutaneous tissue disorders:

photosensitivity reactions, rash, cutaneous lupus erythematosus-like reactions, reactivation of cutaneous lupus erythematosus, urticaria, anaphylactic reactions, toxic epidermal necrolysis.

Musculoskeletal, connective tissue and bone disorders:

muscle spasm

Renal and urinary disorders:

renal dysfunction, interstitial nephritis

General disorders

fever, weakness

4.9 Overdose

Symptoms of overdosage are: increased diuresis, electrolyte imbalance, severe hypotension, depression of consciousness (including coma), convulsions, paresis, cardiac arrhythmias, bradycardia, renal failure.

Measures to prevent absorption (e.g. gastric lavage, administration of absorbing agents and sodium sulphate within 30 minutes of intake) and to hasten elimination should be applied if ingestion is recent. If hypotension occurs, the patient should be placed in the shock position and sodium chloride and volume supplementation should be given rapidly. Treatment with angiotensin-II can be considered. Bradycardia or extensive vagal reactions should be treated by administering atropine. The use of a pacemaker may be considered. Constant monitoring of water, electrolyte and acid base balance, and blood glucose is essential. In the event of hypokalaemia, potassium substitution is necessary.

Captopril may be removed from circulation by haemodialysis. The degree to which hydrochloro-thiazide is removed by haemodialysis has not been established.

5. PHARMACOLOGICAL PROPERTIES

5.1 Pharmacodynamic properties

Pharmacotherapeutic group: ACE (Angiotensin-Converting-Enzyme) inhibitors, combinations, ATC code: C09BA01.

Capozide LS is a combination of an ACE inhibitor, captopril, and an antihypertensive diuretic, hydrochlorothiazide. The combination of these agents has an additive antihypertensive effect, reducing blood pressure to a greater degree than either component alone.

- Captopril is an angiotensin converting enzyme (ACE) inhibitor, i.e. it inhibits ACE, the enzyme involved in the conversion of angiotensin I to angiotensin II - a vasoconstrictor which also stimulates aldosterone secretion by the adrenal cortex.

Such inhibition leads to:

- reduced aldosterone secretion,

- increased plasma renin activity, since aldosterone no longer exerts negative feedback,

- a drop in total peripheral resistance (with a preferential effect on muscles and kidneys) which is not accompanied by water and sodium retention or reflex tachycardia during long-term treatment. Captopril also exerts its antihypertensive effect in subjects with low or normal renin concentrations.

Captopril is effective at all stages of hypertension, i.e. mild, moderate or severe. A reduction in supine and standing systolic and diastolic blood pressures is observed.

After a single dose, the antihypertensive effect is evident fifteen minutes post-dose and reaches a maximum between 1 h and 1.5 h after administration of the drug. Its duration of action is dose-dependent and varies from 6 to 12 hours.

Blood pressure becomes normalised (seated DBP <90mmHg) in patients after two weeks to one month of treatment and the drug retains its effectiveness over the course of time. Patients are also classified as responders if seated DBP decreased by 10% or more from baseline-BP.

Rebound hypertension does not occur when treatment is discontinued.

The treatment of hypertension with captopril leads to an increase in arterial compliance, a rise in renal blood flow without any significant drop in the glomerular filtration rate and a decrease in left ventricular hypertrophy.

- Hydrochlorothiazide is a thiazide diuretic which acts by inhibiting the reabsorption of sodium in the cortical diluting segment of renal tubules. It increases the excretion of sodium and chloride in urine and, to a lesser extent, the excretion of potassium and magnesium thereby increasing urinary output and exerting an antihypertensive effect.

The time to onset of diuretic activity is approximately 2 hours. Diuretic activity reaches a peak after 4 hours and is maintained for 6 to 12 hours. Above a certain dose, thiazide diuretics reach a plateau in terms of therapeutic effect whereas adverse reactions continue to multiply. When treatment is ineffective, increasing the dose beyond recommended doses serves no useful purpose and often gives rise to adverse reactions.

- The concomitant administration of captopril and hydrochlorothiazide in clinical trials led to greater reductions in blood pressure than when either of the products was administered alone.

The administration of captopril inhibits the renin angiotensin aldosterone system and tends to reduce hydrochlorothiazide-induced potassium loss.

Combination of an ACE inhibitor with a thiazide diuretic produces a synergistic effect and also lessens the risk of hypokalaemia provoked by the diuretic alone.

5.2 Pharmacokinetic properties

Captopril LS is quickly absorbed after oral administration and maximum serum concentrations are obtained around one hour after administration. Minimum mean absorption is approximately 75%. Peak plasma concentrations are reached within 60-90 minutes. The presence of food in the gastrointestinal tract reduces absorption by about 30-40%. Approximately 25-30% of the circulating drug is bound to plasma proteins. The apparent elimination half-life of unchanged captopril in blood is about 2 hours. Greater than 95% of the absorbed dose is eliminated in the urine within 24 hours; 40-50% is unchanged drug and the remainder are inactive disulphide metabolites (captopril disulphide and captopril cysteine disulphide). Impaired renal function could result in drug accumulation. Studies in animals indicate that captopril does not cross the blood-brain barrier to any significant extent.

Oral absorption of hydrochlorothiazide is relatively rapid. The mean plasma half-life in fasted individuals has been reported to be 5 to 15 hours. Hydrochloro-thiazide is eliminated rapidly by the kidney and excreted unchanged (>95%) in the urine.

5.3 Preclinical safety data

Animal studies performed during organogenesis with captopril and/or hydrochlorothiazide have not shown any teratogenic effect but captopril has produced foetal toxicity in several species, including foetal mortality during late pregnancy, growth retardation and postnatal mortality in the rat. Preclinical data reveal no other specific hazard for humans based on conventional studies of safety pharmacology, repeated dose toxicology, genotoxicity and carcinogenicity.

6. PHARMACEUTICAL PARTICULARS

6.1 List of excipients

Lactose, magnesium stearate, maize starch, microcrystalline cellulose, stearic acid.

6.2 Incompatibilities

None.

6.3 Shelf life

36 months.

6.4 Special precautions for storage

Store below 30°C. Protect from moisture.

6.5 Nature and contents of container

PVC/PVDC/aluminium foil blisters, containing 28 tablets per pack.

6.6 Instructions for use and handling

No special instructions.

7. MARKETING AUTHORISATION HOLDER

E.R. Squibb & Sons Ltd.
Uxbridge Business Park
Sanderson Road
Uxbridge
Middlesex UB8 1DH

8. MARKETING AUTHORISATION NUMBER(S)

0034/0279

9. DATE OF FIRST AUTHORISATION/RENEWAL OF THE AUTHORISATION

31st May 1990

10. DATE OF REVISION OF THE TEXT

June 2005

Capozide Tablets

(E. R. Squibb & Sons Limited)

1. NAME OF THE MEDICINAL PRODUCT

Capozide ™ Tablets

2. QUALITATIVE AND QUANTITATIVE COMPOSITION

Each tablet contains 50 mg captopril and 25 mg hydrochlorothiazide.

For excipients, see 6.1.

3. PHARMACEUTICAL FORM

Tablets

4. CLINICAL PARTICULARS

4.1 Therapeutic indications

Treatment of essential hypertension.

This fixed dose combination is indicated in patients whose blood pressure is not adequately controlled by captopril alone or hydrochlorothiazide alone.

4.2 Posology and method of administration

Capozide can be administered in a single or two divided doses/day with or without food in patients whose blood pressure is not adequately controlled by captopril alone or hydrochlorothiazide alone. A maximum daily dose of 100 mg captopril/50 mg hydrochlorothiazide should not be exceeded. If satisfactory reduction of blood pressure has not been achieved, additional antihypertensive medication may be added (see 4.5).

Adults: The administration of the fixed combination of captopril and hydrochlorothiazide is usually recommended after dosage titration with the individual components. The usual maintenance dose is 50/25 mg, once a day, in the morning. When clinically appropriate a direct change from monotherapy to the fixed combination may be considered. The 25/25mg strength may be used once a day for patients whose blood pressure is not adequately controlled by hydrochlorothiazide 25 mg monotherapy and before titration of the captopril component. The 50/25mg and 25/25mg strengths are intended to be used once daily, as two tablets would result in an inappropriately high dose of hydrochlorothiazide (50mg/day). The 50/15 mg strength may be administered to start the fixed combination in patients whose blood pressure is not adequately controlled by 50 mg captopril monotherapy, and/or when a lower dose of hydrochlorothiazide is preferred.

The 25/25mg and 50/15mg tablet strengths are not available in the U.K.

Renal impairment: Creatinine clearance between 30 and 80 ml/min: the initial dose is usually 25/12.5 mg once a day, in the morning.

The combination captopril/hydrochlorothiazide is contraindicated in patients with severe renal impairment (creatinine clearance < 30 ml/min).

Special populations: In salt/volume depleted patients, elderly patients and diabetic patients, the usual starting dose is 25/12.5 mg once a day.

Children: The safety and efficacy of Capozide in children has not been established.

4.3 Contraindications

- History of hypersensitivity to captopril, to any of the excipients or any other ACE inhibitor.

- History of hypersensitivity to hydrochlorothiazide or other sulphonamide-derived drugs.

- History of angioedema associated with previous ACE inhibitor therapy.

- Hereditary/idiopathic angioneurotic oedema

- Severe renal impairment (creatinine clearance < 30 ml/min)

- Severe hepatic impairment.

- Second and third trimester of pregnancy (see 4.6)

- Lactation (see 4.6)

4.4 Special warnings and special precautions for use

CAPTOPRIL

Hypotension: Rarely hypotension is observed in uncomplicated hypertensive patients. Symptomatic hypotension is more likely to occur in hypertensive patients who are volume and/or sodium depleted by vigorous diuretic therapy, dietary salt restriction, diarrhoea, vomiting, or haemodialysis. Volume and/or sodium depletion should be corrected before the administration of an ACE inhibitor and a lower starting dose should be considered.

As with any antihypertensive agent, excessive blood pressure lowering in patients with ischaemic cardiovascular or cerebrovascular disease may increase the risk of myocardial infarction or stroke. If hypotension develops, the patient should be placed in a supine position. Volume repletion with intravenous normal saline may be required.

Renovascular hypertension: There is an increased risk of hypotension and renal insufficiency when patients with bilateral renal artery stenosis or stenosis of the artery to a single functioning kidney are treated with ACE inhibitors. Loss of renal function may occur with only mild changes in serum creatinine. In these patients, therapy should be initiated under close medical supervision with low doses, careful titration and monitoring of renal function.

Angioedema: Angioedema of the extremities, face, lips, mucous membranes, tongue, glottis or larynx may occur in patients treated with ACE inhibitors, particularly during the first weeks of treatment. However, in rare cases, severe angioedema may develop after long-term treatment with an ACE inhibitor. Treatment should be discontinued promptly. Angioedema involving the tongue, glottis or larynx may be fatal. Emergency therapy should be instituted. The patient should be hospitalised and observed for at least 12 to 24 hours and should not be discharged until complete resolution of symptoms has occurred.

Cough: Cough has been reported with the use of ACE inhibitors. Characteristically, the cough is non-productive, persistent and resolves after discontinuation of therapy.

Hepatic failure: Rarely, ACE inhibitors have been associated with a syndrome that starts with cholestatic jaundice and progresses to fulminant hepatic necrosis and (sometimes) death. The mechanism of this syndrome is not understood. Patients receiving ACE inhibitors who develop jaundice or marked elevations of hepatic enzymes should discontinue the ACE inhibitors and receive appropriate medical follow-up.

Hyperkalaemia: Elevations in serum potassium have been observed in some patients treated with ACE inhibitors, including captopril. Patients at risk for the development of hyperkalaemia include those with renal insufficiency, diabetes mellitus, or those using concomitant potassium-sparing diuretics, potassium supplements or potassium-containing salt substitutes; or those patients taking other drugs associated with increases in serum potassium (e.g. heparin). If concomitant use of the above mentioned agents is deemed appropriate, regular monitoring of serum potassium is recommended.

Aortic and mitral valve stenosis / Obstructive hypertrophic cardiomyopathy / Cardiogenic shock: ACE inhibitors should be used with caution in patients with left ventricular valvular and outflow tract obstruction and avoided in cases of cardiogenic shock and haemodynamically significant obstruction.

Neutropenia/Agranulocytosis: Neutropenia/agranulocytosis, thrombocytopenia and anaemia have been reported in patients receiving ACE inhibitors, including captopril. In patients with normal renal function and no other complicating factors, neutropenia occurs rarely. Captopril should be used with extreme caution in patients with collagen vascular disease, immunosuppressant therapy, treatment with allopurinol or procainamide, or a combination of these complicating factors, especially if there is pre-existing impaired renal function. Some of these patients developed serious infections which in a few instances did not respond to intensive antibiotic therapy.

If captopril is used in such patients, it is advised that white blood cell count and differential counts should be performed prior to therapy, every 2 weeks during the first 3 months of captopril therapy, and periodically thereafter. During treatment all patients should be instructed to report any sign of infection (e.g. sore throat, fever) when a differential white blood cell count should be performed. Captopril and other concomitant medication (see 4.5) should be withdrawn if neutropenia (neutrophils less than 1000/mm^3) is detected or suspected.

In most patients neutrophil counts rapidly return to normal upon discontinuing captopril.

Proteinurea: proteinuria may occur particularly in patients with existing renal function impairment or on relatively high doses of ACE inhibitors.

Total urinary proteins greater than 1 g per day were seen in about 0.7% of patients receiving captopril. The majority of patients had evidence of prior renal disease or had received relatively high doses of captopril (in excess of 150 mg/day), or both. Nephrotic syndrome occurred in about one-fifth of proteinuric patients. In most cases, proteinuria subsided or cleared within six months whether or not captopril was continued. Parameters of renal function, such as BUN and creatinine, were seldom altered in the patients with proteinuria.

Patients with prior renal disease should have urinary protein estimations (dip-stick on first morning urine) prior to treatment, and periodically thereafter.

Anaphylactoid reactions during desensitisation: sustained life-threatening anaphylactoid reactions have been rarely reported for patients undergoing desensitising treatment with hymenoptera venom while receiving another ACE inhibitor. In the same patients, these reactions were avoided when the ACE inhibitor was temporarily withheld, but they reappeared upon inadvertent rechallenge. Therefore, caution should be used in patients treated with ACE inhibitors undergoing such desensitisation procedures.

Anaphylactoid reactions during high-flux dialysis / lipoprotein apheresis membrane exposure: Anaphylactoid reactions have been reported in patients haemodialysed with high-flux dialysis membranes or undergoing low-density lipoprotein apheresis with dextran sulphate absorption. In these patients, consideration should be given to using a different type of dialysis membrane or a different class of medication.

Surgery/Anaesthesia: Hypotension may occur in patients undergoing major surgery or during treatment with anaesthetic agents that are known to lower blood pressure. If hypotension occurs, it may be corrected by volume expansion.

Diabetic patients: The glycaemia levels should be closely monitored in diabetic patients previously treated with oral antidiabetic drugs or insulin, namely during the first month of treatment with an ACE inhibitor.

As with other angiotensin converting enzyme inhibitors, Capozide is apparently less effective in lowering blood pressure in black people than in non-blacks, possibly because of higher prevalence of low-renin states in the black hypertensive population.

HYDROCHLOROTHIAZIDE

Renal impairment: In patients with renal disease, thiazides may precipitate azotaemia. Cumulative effects of the drug may develop in patients with impaired renal function. If progressive renal impairment becomes evident, as indicated by a rising non-protein nitrogen, careful reappraisal of therapy is necessary, with consideration given to discontinuing diuretic therapy (see 4.3).

Hepatic impairment: Thiazides should be used with caution in patients with impaired hepatic function or progressive liver disease, since minor alterations of fluid and electrolyte balance may precipitate hepatic coma (see 4.3).

Metabolic and endocrine effects: Thiazide therapy may impair glucose tolerance. In diabetic patients dosage adjustments of insulin or oral hypoglycaemic agents may be required. Latent diabetes mellitus may become manifest during thiazide therapy.

Increases in cholesterol and triglyceride levels have been associated with thiazide diuretic therapy.

Hyperuricaemia may occur or frank gout may be precipitated in certain patients receiving thiazide therapy.

Electrolyte imbalance: As for any patient receiving diuretic therapy, periodic determination of serum electrolytes should be performed at appropriate intervals.

Thiazides, including hydrochlorothiazide, can cause fluid or electrolyte imbalance (hypokalaemia, hyponatraemia and hypochloraemic alkalosis). Warning signs of fluid or electrolyte imbalance are dryness of mouth, thirst, weakness, lethargy, drowsiness, restlessness, muscle pain or cramps, muscular fatigue, hypotension, oliguria, tachycardia and gastrointestinal disturbances such as nausea or vomiting.

Although hypokalaemia may develop with the use of thiazide diuretics, concurrent therapy with captopril may reduce diuretic-induced hypokalaemia. The risk of hypokalaemia is greatest in patients with cirrhosis of the liver, in patients experiencing brisk diuresis, in patients who are receiving inadequate oral intake of electrolytes and in patients receiving concomitant therapy with corticosteroids or ACTH (see 4.5).

Dilutional hyponatraemia may occur in oedematous patients in hot weather. Chloride deficit is generally mild and usually does not require treatment.

Thiazides may decrease urinary calcium excretion and cause an intermittent and slight elevation of serum calcium in the absence of known disorders of calcium metabolism. Marked hypercalcaemia may be evidence of hidden hyperparathyroidism. Thiazides should be discontinued before carrying out tests for parathyroid function.

Thiazides have been shown to increase the urinary excretion of magnesium, which may result in hypomagnesaemia.

Anti-doping test: hydrochlorothiazide contained in this medication could produce a positive analytical result in an anti-doping test.

Other: Sensitivity reactions may occur in patients with or without a history of allergy or bronchial asthma. The possibility of exacerbation or activation of systemic lupus erythematosus has been reported.

CAPTOPRIL/HYDROCHLOROTHIAZIDE COMBINATION

Pregnancy: Capozide is not recommended during the first trimester of pregnancy (see 4.6). If treatment is discontinued due to pregnancy, the prescriber should decide whether treatment of hypertension should be continued.

Risk of hypokalaemia: The combination of an ACE inhibitor with a thiazide diuretic does not rule out the occurrence of hypokalaemia. Regular monitoring of kalaemia should be performed.

Combination with lithium: Capozide is not recommended in association with lithium due to the potentiation of lithium toxicity (see 4.5).

Lactose: Capozide contains lactose. Therefore, it should not be used in cases of congenital galactosaemia, glucose and galactose malabsorption or lactase deficiency syndromes (rare metabolic diseases).

4.5 Interaction with other medicinal products and other forms of Interaction

CAPTOPRIL

Potassium sparing diuretics or potassium supplements: ACE inhibitors attenuate diuretic induced potassium loss. Potassium sparing diuretics (e.g. spironolactone, triamterene or amiloride), potassium supplements, or potassium-containing salt substitutes may lead to significant increases in serum potassium. If concomitant use is indicated because of demonstrated hypokalaemia they should be used with caution and with frequent monitoring of serum potassium (see 4.4).

Diuretics (thiazide or loop diuretics): Prior treatment with high dose diuretics may result in volume depletion and a risk of hypotension when initiating therapy with captopril (see 4.4). The hypotensive effects can be reduced by discontinuation of the diuretic, by increasing volume or salt intake or by initiating therapy with a low dose of captopril. However, no clinically significant drug interactions have been found in specific studies with hydrochlorothiazide or furosemide.

Other antihypertensive agents: captopril has been safely co-administered with other commonly used anti-hypertensive agents (e.g. beta-blockers and long-acting calcium channel blockers). Concomitant use of these agents may increase the hypotensive effects of captopril. Nitroglycerine and other nitrates, or other vasodilators, should be used with caution.

Treatments of acute myocardial infarction: Captopril may be used concomitantly with acetylsalicylic acid (at cardiological doses), thrombolytics, beta-blockers and/or nitrates in patients with myocardial infarction.

Tricyclic antidepressants/Antipsychotics: ACE inhibitors may enhance the hypotensive effects of certain tricyclic antidepressants and antipsychotics (see 4.4). Postural hypotension may occur.

Allopurinol, procainamide, cytostatic or immuno-suppressant agents: Concomitant administration with ACE inhibitors may lead to an increased risk of leucopenia, especially when the latter are used at higher than currently recommended doses.

Sympathomimetics: may reduce the antihypertensive effects of ACE inhibitors; patients should be carefully monitored.

Antidiabetics: Pharmacological studies have shown that ACE inhibitors, including captopril, can potentiate the blood glucose-reducing effects of insulin and oral antidiabetics, such as sulphonylurea, in diabetics. Should this very rare interaction occur, it may be necessary to reduce the dose of the antidiabetic during simultaneous treatment with ACE inhibitors.

HYDROCHLOROTHIAZIDE

Amphotericin B (parenteral), carbenoxolone, corticosteroids, corticotropin (ACTH) or stimulant laxatives: hydrochlorothiazide may intensify electrolyte imbalance, particularly hypokalaemia.

Calcium salts: Increased serum calcium levels due to decreased excretion may occur when administered concurrently with thiazide diuretics.

Cardiac glycosides: Enhanced possibility of digitalis toxicity associated with thiazide induced hypokalaemia.

Cholestyramine resin and colestipol: may delay or decrease absorption of hydrochlorothiazide. Sulphonamide diuretics should be taken at least one hour before or four to six hours after these medications.

Nondepolarising muscle relaxants (e.g. tubocurarine chloride): effects of these agents may be potentiated by hydrochlorothiazide.

Drugs associated with torsades de pointes: Because of the risk of hypokalaemia, caution should be used when hydrochlorothiazide is coadministered with drugs associated with torsades de pointes, e.g. some anti-arrhythmics, some antipsychotics and other drugs known to induce torsades de pointes.

CAPTOPRIL/HYDROCHLOROTHIAZIDE COMBINATION

Lithium: Reversible increases in serum lithium concentrations and toxicity have been reported during concomitant administration of lithium with ACE inhibitors. Concomitant use of thiazide diuretics may increase the risk of lithium toxicity and enhance the already increased risk of lithium toxicity with ACE inhibitors. The combination of captopril and hydrochlorothiazide with lithium is therefore not recommended and careful monitoring of serum lithium levels should be performed if the combination proves necessary.

Non-steroidal anti-inflammatory medicinal products: It has been described that non-steroidal anti-inflammatory medicinal products (NSAIDs) and ACE inhibitors exert an additive effect on the increase in serum potassium, whereas renal function may decrease. These effects are, in principle, reversible. Rarely, acute renal failure may occur, particularly in patients with compromised renal function such as the elderly or dehydrated. Chronic administration of NSAIDs may reduce the antihypertensive effect of an ACE inhibitor. The administration of NSAIDs may reduce the diuretic, natriuretic and antihypertensive effects of thiazide diuretics.

Clinical Chemistry

Captopril may cause a false-positive urine test for acetone. Hydrochlorothiazide may cause diagnostic interference of the bentiromide test. Thiazides may decrease serum PBI (Protein Bound Iodine) levels without signs of thyroid disturbance.

4.6 Pregnancy and lactation

Pregnancy: Capozide is not recommended during the first trimester of pregnancy. When a pregnancy is planned or confirmed, an alternative treatment should be initiated as soon as possible. Controlled studies with ACE inhibitors have not been done in humans, but a limited number of cases of first trimester exposures has not shown malformations.

Capozide is contraindicated during the second and third trimesters of pregnancy. Prolonged captopril exposure during the second and third trimesters is known to induce toxicity in foetuses (decreased renal function, oligohydramnios, skull ossification retardation) and in neonates (neonatal renal failure, hypotension, hyperkalaemia) (see also 5.3).

Hydrochlorothiazide, in cases of prolonged exposure during the third trimester of pregnancy, may cause a foetoplacental ischaemia and risk of growth retardation. Moreover, rare cases of hypoglycaemia and thrombocytopenia in neonates have been reported in case of exposure near term.

Hydrochlorothiazide can reduce plasma volume as well as the uteroplacental blood flow.

Should exposure to Capozide have occurred from the second trimester of pregnancy, ultrasound check of renal function and skull is recommended.

Lactation: Capozide is contraindicated in the lactation period.

Both captopril and hydrochlorothiazide are excreted in human milk. Thiazides during breast feeding by lactating mothers have been associated with a decrease or even suppression of lactation. Hypersensitivity to sulphonamide-derived drugs, hypokalaemia and nuclear icterus might occur.

Because of the potential for serious adverse reactions in nursing infants from both drugs, a decision should be made whether to discontinue nursing or to discontinue therapy, taking into account the importance of this therapy to the mother.

4.7 Effects on ability to drive and use machines

As with other antihypertensives, the ability to drive and use machines may be reduced, e.g. at the start of the treatment or when the dose is modified, and also when used in combination with alcohol, but these effects depend on the individual's susceptibility.

4.8 Undesirable effects

CAPTOPRIL

Undesirable effects reported for captopril and/or ACE inhibitor therapy include:

Blood and lymphatic disorders:

very rare: neutropenia/agranulocytosis (see 4.4), pancytopenia, particularly in patients with renal dysfunction (see 4.4), anaemia (including aplastic and haemolytic), thrombocytopenia, lymphadenopathy, eosinophilia, autoimmune diseases and/or positive ANA-titres.

Metabolism and nutrition disorders:

rare: anorexia

very rare: hyperkalaemia, hypoglycaemia (see 4.4)

Psychiatric disorders:

common: sleep disorders

very rare: confusion, depression

Nervous system disorders:

common: taste impairment, dizziness

rare: drowsiness, headache and paraesthesia

very rare: cerebrovascular incidents, including stroke, and syncope

Eye disorders:

very rare: blurred vision.

Cardiac disorders:

uncommon: tachycardia or tachyarrhythmia, angina pectoris, palpitations

very rare: cardiac arrest, cardiogenic shock.

Vascular disorders:

uncommon: hypotension (see 4.4), Raynaud syndrome, flush, pallor

Respiratory, thoracic and mediastinal disorders:

common: dry, irritating (non-productive) cough (see 4.4) and dyspnoea

very rare: bronchospasm, rhinitis, allergic alveolitis/ eosinophilic pneumonia

Gastrointestinal disorders:

common: nausea, vomiting, gastric irritations, abdominal pain, diarrhoea, constipation, dry mouth

rare: stomatitis/aphthous ulcerations

very rare: glossitis, peptic ulcer, pancreatitis

Hepato-biliary disorders:

very rare: impaired hepatic function and cholestasis (including jaundice), hepatitis including necrosis, elevated liver enzymes and bilirubin.

Skin and subcutaneous tissue disorders:

common: pruritus with or without a rash, rash, and alopecia

uncommon: angioedema (see 4.4)

very rare: urticaria, Stevens Johnson syndrome, erythema multiforme, photo-sensitivity, erythroderma, pemphigoid reactions and exfoliative dermatitis.

Musculoskeletal, connective tissue and bone disorders:

very rare: myalgia, arthralgia

Renal and urinary disorders:

rare: renal function disorders, including renal failure, polyuria, oliguria, increased urine frequency

very rare: nephrotic syndrome

Reproductive system and breast disorders:

very rare: impotence, gynaecomastia

General disorders;

uncommon: chest pain, fatigue, malaise

very rare: fever

Investigations:

very rare: proteinuria, eosinophilia, increase of serum potassium, decrease of serum sodium, elevation of BUN, serum creatinine and serum bilirubin, decreases in haemoglobin, haematocrit, leucocytes, thrombocytes, positive ANA-titre, elevated ESR.

HYDROCHLOROTHIAZIDE

Infections and infestations: sialadenitis

Blood and lymphatic system disorders:

leucopenia, neutropenia/agranulocytosis, thrombocytopenia, aplastic anaemia, haemolytic anaemia, bone marrow depression

Metabolism and nutrition disorders:

anorexia, hyperglycaemia, glycosuria, hyperuricaemia, electrolyte imbalance (including hyponatraemia and hypokalaemia), increases in cholesterol and triglycerides.

Psychiatric disorders:

restlessness, depression, sleep disturbances

Nervous system disorders:

loss of appetite, paraesthesia, light-headedness

Eye disorders:

xanthopsia, transient blurred vision

Ear and labyrinth disorders:

vertigo

Cardiac disorders:

postural hypotension, cardiac arrhythmias

Vascular disorders:

necrotising angiitis (vasculitis, cutaneous vasculitis)

Respiratory, thoracic and mediastinal disorders:

respiratory distress (including pneumonitis and pulmonary oedema).

Gastrointestinal disorders:

gastric irritation, diarrhoea, constipation, pancreatitis

Hepato-biliary disorders:

jaundice (intrahepatic cholestatic jaundice)

Skin and subcutaneous tissue disorders:

photosensitivity reactions, rash, cutaneous lupus erythematosus-like reactions, reactivation of cutaneous lupus erythematosus, urticaria, anaphylactic reactions, toxic epidermal necrolysis.

Musculoskeletal, connective tissue and bone disorders:

muscle spasm

Renal and urinary disorders:

renal dysfunction, interstitial nephritis

General disorders

fever, weakness

4.9 Overdose

Symptoms of overdosage are: increased diuresis, electrolyte imbalance, severe hypotension, depression of consciousness (including coma), convulsions, paresis, cardiac arrhythmias, bradycardia, renal failure.

Measures to prevent absorption (e.g. gastric lavage, administration of absorbing agents and sodium sulphate within 30 minutes of intake) and to hasten elimination should be applied if ingestion is recent. If hypotension occurs, the patient should be placed in the shock position and sodium chloride and volume supplementation should be given rapidly. Treatment with angiotensin-II can be considered. Bradycardia or extensive vagal reactions should be treated by administering atropine. The use of a pacemaker may be considered. Constant monitoring of water, electrolyte and acid base balance, and blood glucose is essential. In the event of hypokalaemia, potassium substitution is necessary.

Captopril may be removed from circulation by haemodialysis. The degree to which hydrochlorothiazide is removed by haemodialysis has not been established.

5. PHARMACOLOGICAL PROPERTIES

5.1 Pharmacodynamic properties

Pharmacotherapeutic group: ACE (Angiotensin-Converting-Enzyme) inhibitors, combinations, ATC code: C09BA01.

Capozide is a combination of an ACE inhibitor, captopril, and an antihypertensive diuretic, hydrochlorothiazide. The combination of these agents has an additive antihypertensive effect, reducing blood pressure to a greater degree than either component alone.

- Captopril is an angiotensin converting enzyme (ACE) inhibitor, i.e. it inhibits ACE, the enzyme involved in the conversion of angiotensin I to angiotensin II - a vasoconstrictor which also stimulates aldosterone secretion by the adrenal cortex.

Such inhibition leads to:

- reduced aldosterone secretion,

- increased plasma renin activity, since aldosterone no longer exerts negative feedback,

- a drop in total peripheral resistance (with a preferential effect on muscles and kidneys) which is not accompanied by water and sodium retention or reflex tachycardia during long-term treatment. Captopril also exerts its antihypertensive effect in subjects with low or normal renin concentrations.

Captopril is effective at all stages of hypertension, i.e. mild, moderate or severe. A reduction in supine and standing systolic and diastolic blood pressures is observed.

After a single dose, the antihypertensive effect is evident fifteen minutes post-dose and reaches a maximum between 1 h and 1.5 h after administration of the drug. Its duration of action is dose-dependent and varies from 6 to 12 hours.

Blood pressure becomes normalised (seated DBP <90mmHg) in patients after two weeks to one month of treatment and the drug retains its effectiveness over the course of time. Patients are also classified as responders if seated DBP decreased by 10% or more from baseline-BP.

Rebound hypertension does not occur when treatment is discontinued.

The treatment of hypertension with captopril leads to an increase in arterial compliance, a rise in renal blood flow without any significant drop in the glomerular filtration rate and a decrease in left ventricular hypertrophy.

- Hydrochlorothiazide is a thiazide diuretic which acts by inhibiting the reabsorption of sodium in the cortical diluting segment of renal tubules. It increases the excretion of sodium and chloride in urine and, to a lesser extent, the excretion of potassium and magnesium thereby increasing urinary output and exerting an antihypertensive effect.

The time to onset of diuretic activity is approximately 2 hours. Diuretic activity reaches a peak after 4 hours and is maintained for 6 to 12 hours. Above a certain dose, thiazide diuretics reach a plateau in terms of therapeutic effect whereas adverse reactions continue to multiply. When treatment is ineffective, increasing the dose beyond recommended doses serves no useful purpose and often gives rise to adverse reactions.

- The concomitant administration of captopril and hydrochlorothiazide in clinical trials led to greater reductions in blood pressure than when either of the products was administered alone.

The administration of captopril inhibits the renin angiotensin aldosterone system and tends to reduce hydrochlorothiazide-induced potassium loss.

Combination of an ACE inhibitor with a thiazide diuretic produces a synergistic effect and also lessens the risk of hypokalaemia provoked by the diuretic alone.

5.2 Pharmacokinetic properties

Captopril is quickly absorbed after oral administration and maximum serum concentrations are obtained around one hour after administration. Minimum mean absorption is approximately 75%. Peak plasma concentrations are reached within 60-90 minutes. The presence of food in the gastrointestinal tract reduces absorption by about 30-40%. Approximately 25-30% of the circulating drug is bound to plasma proteins. The apparent elimination half-life of unchanged captopril in blood is about 2 hours. Greater than 95% of the absorbed dose is eliminated in the urine within 24 hours; 40-50% is unchanged drug and the remainder are inactive disulphide metabolites (captopril disulphide and captopril cysteine disulphide). Impaired renal function could result in drug accumulation. Studies in animals indicate that captopril does not cross the blood-brain barrier to any significant extent.

Oral absorption of hydrochlorothiazide is relatively rapid. The mean plasma half-life in fasted individuals has been reported to be 5 to 15 hours. Hydrochlorothiazide is eliminated rapidly by the kidney and excreted unchanged (>95%) in the urine.

5.3 Preclinical safety data
Animal studies performed during organogenesis with captopril and/or hydrochlorothiazide have not shown any teratogenic effect but captopril has produced foetal toxicity in several species, including foetal mortality during late pregnancy, growth retardation and postnatal mortality in the rat. Preclinical data reveal no other specific hazard for humans based on conventional studies of safety pharmacology, repeated dose toxicology, genotoxicity and carcinogenicity.

6. PHARMACEUTICAL PARTICULARS
6.1 List of excipients
Lactose, magnesium stearate, pregelatinised starch, microcrystalline cellulose, stearic acid.

6.2 Incompatibilities
None.

6.3 Shelf life
36 months.

6.4 Special precautions for storage
Store at room temperature.

6.5 Nature and contents of container
PVC/PVDC/aluminium foil blisters, containing 28 tablets per pack.

6.6 Instructions for use and handling
No special instructions.

7. MARKETING AUTHORISATION HOLDER
E.R. Squibb & Sons Limited
Uxbridge Business Park
Sanderson Road
Uxbridge
Middlesex UB8 1DH

8. MARKETING AUTHORISATION NUMBER(S)
0034/0263

9. DATE OF FIRST AUTHORISATION/RENEWAL OF THE AUTHORISATION
12th May 1992

10. DATE OF REVISION OF THE TEXT
June 2005

Carace 10 Plus and Carace 20 Plus Tablets

(Bristol-Myers Squibb Pharmaceuticals Ltd)

1. NAME OF THE MEDICINAL PRODUCT
Carace 10 Plus and Carace 20 Plus

2. QUALITATIVE AND QUANTITATIVE COMPOSITION
Carace 10 Plus:

Each tablet contains 10 mg lisinopril and 12.5 mg hydrochlorothiazide.

Carace 20 Plus:

Each tablet contains 20 mg lisinopril and 12.5 mg hydrochlorothiazide.

3. PHARMACEUTICAL FORM
Tablets

Carace 10 Plus:

Blue, hexagonal, biconvex tablet with the product code '145' on one side.

Carace 20 Plus:

Yellow, hexagonal scored tablet with the product code 'MSD 140' on one side.

4. CLINICAL PARTICULARS
4.1 Therapeutic indications
For the management of mild to moderate hypertension in patients who have been stabilised on the individual components given in the same proportions.

4.2 Posology and method of administration
Route of administration: Oral

Adults

Essential hypertension: The usual dosage of Carace Plus is 1 tablet, administered once daily. If necessary, the dosage may be increased to 2 tablets, administered once daily.

Dosage in renal insufficiency: Thiazides may not be appropriate diuretics for use in patients with renal impairment and are ineffective at creatinine clearance values of 30 ml/min or below (i.e. moderate or severe renal insufficiency).

Carace Plus is not to be used as initial therapy in any patient with renal insufficiency.

In patients with creatinine clearance of >30 and <80 ml/min, Carace Plus may be used, but only after titration of the individual components.

Prior diuretic therapy:

Symptomatic hypotension may occur following the initial dose of Carace Plus: this is more likely in patients who are volume and/or salt depleted as a result of prior diuretic therapy. If possible, the diuretic therapy should be discontinued for 2-3 days prior to initiation of therapy with lisinopril alone, in a 2.5 mg dose.

Use in the elderly

Lisinopril was equally effective in elderly (65 years or older) and non-elderly hypertensive patients. In elderly hypertensive patients, monotherapy with lisinopril was as effective in reducing diastolic blood pressure as monotherapy with either hydrochlorothiazide or atenolol. In clinical studies, age did not affect the tolerability of lisinopril.

In clinical studies the eficacy and tolerability of lisinopril and hydrochlorothiazide, administered concomitantly, were similar in both elderly and younger hypertensive patients.

Paediatric Use

Safety and effectiveness in children have not been established.

4.3 Contraindications
Carace Plus is contraindicated in patients with anuria or aortic stenosis or hyperkalaemia.

Carace Plus is contraindicated in patients who are hypersensitive to any component of this product.

Carace Plus is contraindicated in patients with a history of angioneurotic oedema relating to previous treatment with an angiotensin-converting enzyme inhibitor and in patients with hereditary or idiopathic angioedema.

Carace Plus is contraindicated in patients who are hypersensitive to other sulphonamide-derived drugs.

The use of Carace Plus during pregnancy is not recommended. When pregnancy is detected Carace Plus should be discontinued as soon as possible, unless it is considered life-saving for the mother.

Carace Plus is contraindicated in lactating women who are breast-feeding infants. It is not known whether lisinopril is excreted in human milk. Thiazides do appear in human milk. See also 'Breast-feeding mothers' under '4.6 Pregnancy and Lactation'.

4.4 Special warnings and special precautions for use
Hypotension and electrolyte/fluid imbalance: As with all antihypertensive therapy, symptomatic hypotension may occur in some patients. This was rarely seen in uncomplicated hypertensive patients but is more likely in the presence of fluid or electrolyte imbalance, e.g. volume depletion, hyponatraemia, hypochloraemic alkalosis, hypomagnesaemia or hypokalaemia which may occur from prior diuretic therapy, dietary salt restriction, dialysis, or during intercurrent diarrhoea or vomiting. Periodic determination of serum electrolytes should be performed at appropriate intervals in such patients.

Particular consideration should be given when therapy is administered to patients with ischaemic heart or cerebrovascular disease, because an excessive fall in blood pressure could result in a myocardial infarction or cerebrovascular accident.

If hypotension occurs, the patient should be placed in the supine position and, if necessary, should receive an intravenous infusion of normal saline. A transient hypotensive response is not a contraindication to further doses. Following restoration of effective blood volume and pressure, reinstitution of therapy at reduced dosage may be possible; or either of the components may be used appropriately alone.

Aortic stenosis/Hypertrophic cardiomyopathy: As with all vasodilators, ACE inhibitors should be given with caution to patients with obstruction in the outflow tract of the left ventricle.

Renal function impairment: Thiazides may not be appropriate diuretics for use in patients with renal impairment and are ineffective at creatinine clearance values of 30 ml/min or below (i.e. moderate or severe renal insufficiency). Carace Plus should not be administered to patients with renal insufficiency (creatinine clearance <80 ml/min) until titration of the individual components has shown the need for the doses present in the combination tablet.

Some hypertensive patients, with no apparent pre-existing renal disease, have developed usually minor and transient increases in blood urea and serum creatinine when lisinopril has been given concomitantly with a diuretic. If this occurs during therapy with Carace Plus, the combination should be discontinued. Reinstitution of therapy at reduced dosage may be possible, or either of the components may be used appropriately alone.

In some patients, with bilateral renal artery stenosis or stenosis of the single artery to a solitary kidney, increases in blood urea and serum creatinine, usually reversible upon discontinuation of therapy, have been seen with angiotensin-converting enzyme (ACE) inhibitors.

Haemodialysis patients: The use of Carace Plus is not indicated in patients requiring dialysis for renal failure. A high incidence of anaphylactoid reactions has been reported in patients dialysed with high-flux membranes (e.g. AN 69) and treated concomitantly with an ACE inhibitor. In these patients consideration should be given to using a different type of dialysis membrane or a different class of antihypertensive agent.

Anaphylactoid reactions during LDL apheresis: Rarely, patients receiving ACE inhibitors during low-density lipoprotein (LDL) apheresis with dextran sulphate have experienced life-threatening anaphylactoid reactions. These reactions were avoided by temporarily withholding ACE inhibitor therapy prior to each apheresis.

Hepatic disease: Thiazides should be used with caution in patients with impaired hepatic function or progressive liver disease, since minor alterations of fluid and electrolyte balance may precipitate hepatic coma.

Surgery/anaesthesia: In patients undergoing major surgery or during anaesthesia with agents that produce hypotension, lisinopril may block angiotensin II formation secondary to compensatory renin release. If hypotension occurs and is considered to be due to this mechanism, it can be corrected by volume expansion.

Metabolic and endocrine effects: Thiazide therapy may impair glucose tolerance. Dosage adjustment of antidiabetic agents, including insulin, may be required.

Thiazides may decrease urinary calcium excretion and may cause intermittent and slight elevation of serum calcium. Marked hypercalcaemia may be evidence of hidden hyperparathyroidism. Thiazides should be discontinued before carrying out tests for parathyroid function.

Increases in cholesterol and triglyceride levels may be associated with thiazide diuretic therapy.

Thiazide therapy may precipitate hyperuricaemia and/or gout in certain patients. However, lisinopril may increase urinary uric acid and thus may attenuate the hyperuricaemic effect of hydrochlorothiazide.

Hypersensitivity/angioneurotic oedema: Angioneurotic oedema of the face, extremities, lips, tongue, glottis and/or larynx has been reported rarely in patients treated with angiotensin-converting enzyme inhibitors, including lisinopril. This may occur at anytime during treatment. In such cases, Carace Plus should be discontinued promptly, and appropriate monitoring should be instituted to ensure complete resolution of symptoms prior to dismissing the patient.

In those instances where swelling has been confined to the face and lips, the condition generally resolved without treatment, although antihistamines have been useful in relieving symptoms. Angioneurotic oedema associated with laryngeal oedema may be fatal. Where there is involvement of the tongue, glottis or larynx, likely to cause airway obstruction, appropriate therapy (which may include subcutaneous ephinephrine (adrenaline) solution 1:1,000 (0.3 ml to 0.5 ml) and/or measures to ensure a patent airway) should be administered promptly.

Black patients receiving ACE inhibitors have been reported to have a higher incidence of angioedema compared to non-blacks.

Patients with a history of angioedema unrelated to ACE-inhibitor therapy may be at increased risk of angioedema while receiving an ACE inhibitor. (See also 'Contraindications').

In patients receiving thiazides, sensitivity reactions may occur with or without a history of allergy or bronchial asthma. Exacerbation or activation of systemic lupus erythematosus has been reported with the use of thiazides.

Anaphylactoid Reactions during Hymenoptera Desensitisation: Rarely, patients receiving ACE inhibitors during desensitisation with hymenoptera venom (e.g. Bee or Wasp venom) have experienced life-threatening anaphylactoid reactions. These reactions were avoided by temporarily withholding ACE inhibitor therapy prior to each desensitisation.

Cough: Cough has been reported with the use of ACE inhibitors. Characteristically, the cough is non-productive, persistent, and resolves after discontinuation of therapy. ACE inhibitor-induced cough should be considered as part of the differential diagnosis of cough.

4.5 Interaction with other medicinal products and other forms of Interaction
Serum potassium: The potassium-losing effect of thiazide diuretics is usually attenuated by the potassium-conserving effect of lisinopril.

The use of potassium supplements, potassium-sparing agents or potassium-containing salt substitutes, particularly in patients with impaired renal function, may lead to a significant increase in serum potassium. If concomitant use of Carace Plus and any of these agents is deemed appropriate, they should be used with caution and with frequent monitoring of serum potassium.

Antidiabetic drugs: Epidemiological studies have suggested that concomitant administration of ACE-inhibitors and antidiabetic medicines (insulins, oral hypoglycaemic agents) may cause an increased blood-glucose-lowering effect with risk of hypoglycaemia. This phenomenon appeared to be more likely to occur during the first weeks of combined treatment and in patients with renal impairment. Long term controlled clinical trials with lisinopril have not confirmed these findings and do not preclude the use of lisinopril in diabetic patients. It is advised, however that these patients be monitored. (See below for information regarding antidiabetic drugs and thiazide diuretics.)

Lithium: Diuretic agents and ACE inhibitors reduce the renal clearance of lithium and add a high risk of lithium toxicity; concomitant use is not recommended. Refer to prescribing information for lithium preparations before use of such preparations.

Narcotic drugs/antipsychotics: Postural hypotension may occur with ACE inhibitors.

Alcohol: Alcohol may enhance the hypotensive effect of any antihypertensive.

Other agents: Indomethacin may diminish the antihypertensive effect of concomitantly administered Carace Plus. In some patients with compromised renal function who are being treated with non-steroidal anti-inflammatory drugs the co-administration of ACE inhibitors may result in further deterioration of renal function. These effects are usually reversible. The antihypertensive effect of Carace Plus may be potentiated when given concomitantly with other agents likely to cause postural hypotension.

Non-depolarising muscle relaxants: Thiazides may increase the responsiveness to tubocurarine.

Allopurinol, cytostatic or immunosuppressive agents, systemic corticosteroids, or procainamide: Concomitant administration with ACE inhibitors may lead to an increased risk of leucopenia.

Antacids: Induce decreased bioavailability of ACE inhibitors.

Sympathomimetics: May reduce the antihypertensive effects of ACE inhibitors; patients should be carefully monitored to confirm that the desired effect is being obtained.

Cyclosporin: Increase the risk of hyperkalaemia with ACE inhibitors.

When administered concurrently, the following drugs may interact with thiazide diuretics:

Barbiturates or narcotics: Potentiation of orthostatic hypotension may occur.

Antidiabetic drugs (oral agents and insulin): Dosage adjustment of the antidiabetic drug may be required. (See above for information regarding antidiabetic drugs and lisinopril).

Cholestyramine and colestipol resins: Absorption of hydrochlorothiazide is impaired in the presence of anionic exchange resins. Single doses of either cholestyramine or colestipol resins bind the hydrochlorothiazide and reduce its absorption from the gastrointestinal tract by up to 85 and 43 percent, respectively.

Corticosteroids, ACTH: Intensified electrolyte depletion, particularly hypokalaemia.

Pressor amines (e.g. epinephrine (adrenaline)): Possible decreased response to pressor amines but not sufficient to preclude their use.

Non-steroidal anti-inflammatory drugs: In some patients, the administration of a non-steroidal anti-inflammatory agent can reduce the diuretic, natriuretic, and antihypertensive effects of diuretics.

4.6 Pregnancy and lactation

Pregnancy

The use of Carace Plus during pregnancy is not recommended. When pregnancy is detected Carace Plus should be discontinued as soon as possible, unless it is considered life-saving for the mother.

ACE inhibitors can cause foetal and neonatal morbidity and mortality when administered to pregnant women during the second and third trimesters. Use of ACE inhibitors during this period has been associated with foetal and neonatal injury including hypotension, renal failure, hyperkalemia, and/or skull hypoplasia in the newborn. Maternal oligohydramnios, presumably representing decreased foetal renal function, has occurred and may result in limb contractures, craniofacial deformations and hypoplastic lung development.

These adverse effects to the embryo and foetus do not appear to have resulted from intrauterine ACE inhibitor exposure limited to the first trimester.

The routine use of diuretics in otherwise healthy pregnant women is not recommended and exposes mother and foetus to unnecessary hazard including foetal or neonatal jaundice, thrombocytopenia and possibly other adverse reactions which have occurred in the adult.

If Carace Plus is used during pregnancy, the patient should be apprised of the potential hazard to the foetus. In those rare cases where use during pregnancy is deemed essential, serial ultrasound examinations should be performed to assess the intraamniotic environment. If oligohydramnios is detected, Carace Plus should be discontinued unless it is considered life-saving for the mother. Patients and physicians should be aware, however, that oligohydramnios may not appear until after the foetus has sustained irreversible injury.

Infants whose mothers have taken Carace Plus should be closely observed for hypotension, oliguria and hyperkalaemia. Lisinopril, which crosses the placenta, has been removed from the neonatal circulation by peritoneal dialysis with some clinical benefit, and theoretically may be removed by exchange transfusion. There is no experience with the removal of hydrochlorothiazide, which also crosses the placenta, from the neonatal circulation.

Lactation

Breast-feeding mothers: It is not known whether lisinopril is secreted in human milk; however, thiazides do appear in human milk. Because of the potential for serious reactions in nursing infants, a decision should be made whether to discontinue breast-feeding or to discontinue Carace Plus, taking into account the importance of the drug to the mother.

4.7 Effects on ability to drive and use machines

Usually Carace Plus does not interfere with the ability to drive and to operate machinery. Patients should be instructed to first determine how they respond to Carace Plus before performing hazardous tasks.

4.8 Undesirable effects

Carace Plus is usually well tolerated. In clinical studies, side effects have usually been mild and transient, and in most instances have not required interruption of therapy. The side effects that have been observed have been limited to those reported previously with lisinopril or hydrochlorothiazide.

One of the most common clinical side effects was dizziness, which generally responded to dosage reduction and seldom required discontinuation of therapy. Other, less frequent, side effects were headache, dry cough, fatigue, and hypotension including orthostatic hypotension.

Still less common were diarrhoea, nausea, vomiting, pancreatitis, dry mouth, rash, gout, palpitation, chest discomfort, muscle cramps and weakness, paraesthesia, asthenia, and impotence.

Hypersensitivity/angioneurotic oedema: Angioneurotic oedema of the face, extremities, lips, tongue, glottis and/or larynx has been reported rarely (see 'Precautions').

A symptom complex has been reported which may include some or all of the following: fever, vasculitis, myalgia, arthralgia/arthritis, a positive ANA, elevated ESR, eosinophilia, and leucocytosis. Rash, photosensitivity, or other dermatological manifestations may occur.

Laboratory test findings: Laboratory side effects have rarely been of clinical importance. Occasional hyperglycaemia, hyperuricaemia and hyperkalaemia or hypokalaemia have been noted. Usually minor and transient increases in blood urea nitrogen and serum creatinine have been seen in patients without evidence of pre-existing renal impairment. If such increases persist, they are usually reversible upon discontinuation of Carace Plus. Small decreases in haemoglobin and haematocrit have been reported frequently in hypertensive patients treated with Carace Plus but were rarely of clinical importance unless another cause of anaemia co-existed. Rarely, elevation of liver enzymes and/or serum bilirubin have occurred, but a causal relationship to Carace Plus has not been established.

Other side effects reported with the individual components alone, and which may be potential side effects with Carace Plus, are:

Lisinopril: Myocardial infarction or cerebrovascular accident possibly secondary to excessive hypotension in high-risk patients (see 'Precautions'), tachycardia, abdominal pain, hepatitis - either hepatocellular or cholestatic jaundice), mood alterations, mental confusion, bronchospasm, urticaria, pruritis, diaphoresis, alopecia, uraemia, oliguria/anuria, renal dysfunction, acute renal failure, bone marrow depression manifest as anaemia and/or thrombocytopenia and/or leucopenia, hyponatraemia. Rare cases of neutropenia have been reported, although no causal relationship has been established. There have been reports of haemolytic anaemia in patients taking lisinopril, although no causal relationship has been established.

Hydrochlorothiazide: Anorexia, gastric irritation, constipation, jaundice (intrahepatic cholestatic jaundice), sialoadenitis, vertigo, xanthopsia, leucopenia, agranulocytosis, thrombocytopenia, aplastic anaemia, haemolytic anaemia, purpura, photosensitivity, urticaria, necrotising angiitis (vasculitis, cutaneous vasculitis), fever, respiratory distress including pneumonitis and pulmonary oedema, anaphylactic reactions, toxic epidermal necrolysis, hyperglycaemia, glycosuria, hyperuricaemia, electrolyte imbalance including hyponatraemia, muscle spasm, restlessness, transient blurred vision, renal failure, renal dysfunction, and interstitial nephritis.

4.9 Overdose

No specific information is available on the treatment of overdosage with Carace Plus. Treatment is symptomatic and supportive. Therapy with Carace Plus should be discontinued and the patient observed closely. Suggested measures include induction of emesis and/or gastric lavage, if ingestion is recent, and correction of dehydration, electrolyte imbalance and hypotension by established procedures.

Lisinopril: The most likely features of overdosage would be hypotension, for which the usual treatment would be intravenous infusion of normal saline solution, if available angiotensin II may be beneficial.

Lisinopril may be removed from the general circulation by haemodialysis. (See 'Special Warnings and Precautions, Haemodialysis Patients').

Hydrochlorothiazide: The most common signs and symptoms observed are those caused by electrolyte depletion (hypokalaemia, hypochloraemia, hyponatraemia) and dehydration resulting from excessive diuresis. If digitalis has also been administered, hypokalaemia may accentuate cardiac arrhythmias.

5. PHARMACOLOGICAL PROPERTIES

5.1 Pharmacodynamic properties

Carace Plus contains antihypertensive and diuretic activity. Lisinopril and hydrochlorothiazide have been used alone and concurrently for the treatment of hypertension where their effects are approximately additive.

Lisinopril is an inhibitor of the angiotensin-converting enzyme (ACE). Inhibition of the formation of angiotensin II results in vasodilation and a fall in blood pressure.

Hydrochlorothiazide is a diuretic and antihypertensive agent. Use of this agent alone results in increased renin secretion. Although lisinopril alone is antihypertensive, even in patients with low renin hypertension, concomitant administration with hydrochlorothiazide results in a greater reduction in blood pressure. Lisinopril attenuates the potassium loss associated with hydrochlorothiazide.

5.2 Pharmacokinetic properties

In clinical studies, peak serum concentrations of lisinopril occurred within about 6 to 8 hours following oral administration. Declining serum concentrations exhibited a prolonged terminal phase which did not contribute to drug accumulation. This terminal phase probably represents saturable binding to ACE and was not proportional to dose. Lisinopril did not appear to be bound to other plasma proteins.

Lisinopril does not undergo significant metabolism and is excreted unchanged predominantly in the urine. Based on urinary recovery in clinical studies, the extent of absorption of lisinopril was approximately 25%. Lisinopril absorption was not influenced by the presence of food in the gastrointestinal tract.

On multiple dosing, lisinopril exhibited an effective accumulation half-life of 12 hours.

In patients with renal insufficiency, disposition of lisinopril was similar to that in patients with normal renal function until glomerular filtration rate reached 30 ml/min or less; peak and trough lisinopril levels, and time to peak then increased and time to steady state was sometimes prolonged. Animal studies indicate lisinopril crosses the blood-brain barrier poorly. No clinically significant pharmacokinetic interactions occurred when lisinopril was used concomitantly with propranolol, digoxin or hydrochlorothiazide.

When plasma levels of hydrochlorothiazide have been followed for at least 24 hours the plasma half-life has been observed to vary between 5.6 and 14.8 hours. Hydrochlorothiazide is not metabolised but is eliminated rapidly by the kidney. At least 61% of the oral dose is eliminated unchanged within 24 hours. Hydrochlorothiazide crosses the placental but not the blood-brain barrier.

Concomitant multiple doses of lisinopril and hydrochlorothiazide have little or no effect on the bioavailability of these drugs. The combination tablet is bioequivalent to concomitant administration of the separate entities.

5.3 Preclinical safety data

Lisinopril and hydrochlorothiazide are well established in medical use. Preclinical data is broadly consistent with clinical experience. For reproduction toxicity, see section 4.6.

6. PHARMACEUTICAL PARTICULARS

6.1 List of excipients

Mannitol BP

Calcium Phosphate Dibasic Hydrous EP

Blue FD & C Aluminium Lake (E132) (Carace 10 Plus)

Yellow Ferric Oxide (E172) (Carace 20 Plus)

Starch EP

Pregelatinised Starch BP

Magnesium Stearate EP

6.2 Incompatibilities

Not applicable.

6.3 Shelf life

Carace 10 Plus	30 months
Carace 20 Plus	36 months

6.4 Special precautions for storage

Store in a dry place below 25°C.

6.5 Nature and contents of container

Blister packs of 28 tablets.

6.6 Instructions for use and handling

Not applicable.

7. MARKETING AUTHORISATION HOLDER

Bristol-Myers Squibb Pharmaceuticals Limited

Uxbridge Business Park

Sanderson Road

Uxbridge

Middlesex

UB8 1DH

8. MARKETING AUTHORISATION NUMBER(S)

Carace 10 Plus	PL 11184/0103
Carace 20 Plus	PL 11184/0102

9. DATE OF FIRST AUTHORISATION/RENEWAL OF THE AUTHORISATION

26th February 2002

10. DATE OF REVISION OF THE TEXT

June 2005

®denotes registered trademark of Merck & Co., Inc., Whitehouse Station, New Jersey, USA.

Carace 2.5 mg, 5 mg, 10mg and 20 mg Tablets

(Bristol-Myers Squibb Pharmaceuticals Ltd)

1. NAME OF THE MEDICINAL PRODUCT

'Carace' 2.5 mg, 5mg, 10mg and 20mg

2. QUALITATIVE AND QUANTITATIVE COMPOSITION

Each tablet contains either 2.5 mg, 5mg, 10mg or 20mg of lisinopril.

3. PHARMACEUTICAL FORM

Tablets.

'Carace' 2.5 mg: blue, half-scored, oval tablets, marked 'MSD 15'.

'Carace' 5 mg: white, half-scored, oval tablets, marked 'CARACE' and '5'.

'Carace' 10 mg: yellow, half-scored, oval tablets, marked 'CARACE' and '10'.

'Carace' 20 mg: orange, half-scored, oval tablets, marked 'CARACE' and '20'.

4. CLINICAL PARTICULARS

4.1 Therapeutic indications

Hypertension

All grades of essential hypertension and renovascular hypertension. 'Carace' may be used alone or with other antihypertensive agents.

Heart Failure

In heart failure, 'Carace' is indicated as an adjunctive therapy with non-potassium-sparing diuretics and, where appropriate, digitalis.

Severe Heart Failure

Treatment with 'Carace' should always be initiated in hospital under close medical supervision.

Mild to Moderate Heart Failure

Treatment with 'Carace' should always be initiated under close medical supervision.

Acute Myocardial Infarction

'Carace' is indicated for the treatment of haemodynamically stable patients, defined as patients not in cardiogenic shock and who have a systolic blood pressure greater than 100 mmHg. 'Carace' may be initiated within 24 hours of acute myocardial infarction to prevent the subsequent development of left ventricular dysfunction or heart failure and to improve survival. Patients should receive, as appropriate, the standard recommended treatments such as thrombolytics, aspirin and beta-blocker.

4.2 Posology and method of administration

Route of administration: oral

The absorption of 'Carace' is not affected by food. 'Carace' should be administered in a single daily dose. As with all single daily dose medications 'Carace' should be taken at approximately the same time each day.

Hypertension

The need for dosage titration should be determined by measurement of the blood pressure just before the next dose.

Essential and renovascular hypertension

Treatment should be started with 2.5 mg once daily, and titrated upwards to achieve optimal blood pressure control. For essential hypertension, in general, if the desired therapeutic effect cannot be achieved in a period of 2 to 4 weeks on a certain dose level, the dose can be further increased.

A 2.5 mg dose seldom achieves a therapeutic response. The usual effective dose range is 10-20 mg once daily.

The maximum recommended dose is 40 mg daily.

Diuretic-treated patients

Symptomatic hypotension can occur following the initial dose of 'Carace'; this is more likely when 'Carace' is added to previous diuretic therapy. Caution is recommended, therefore, since these patients may be volume or salt depleted.

If possible, the diuretic should be discontinued, or the dose reduced, two to three days before beginning therapy with 'Carace' (see 'Special Warnings and Precautions') and may be resumed later if required.

'Carace' reduces the development of thiazide-induced hypokalaemia and hyperuricaemia.

Use in the elderly

Age alone does not appear to affect the efficacy or safety profile of 'Carace'. Thus, elderly patients should start treatment with 'Carace' as directed above.

Congestive heart failure

'Carace' may be used as adjunctive therapy with non-potassium-sparing diuretics with or without digitalis.

Initial dosage: Therapy with 'Carace' should be initiated under close medical supervision (in hospital for severe heart failure) with a recommended starting dose of 2.5 mg once daily. If possible, the dose of diuretic should be reduced before beginning treatment.

Blood pressure and renal function should be monitored closely both before and during treatment because severe hypotension and, more rarely, consequent renal failure have been reported with angiotensin-converting enzyme (ACE) inhibitors (see 'Special Warnings and Precautions').

The appearance of hypotension after the initial dose of 'Carace' does not preclude subsequent careful dose adjustment with the drug, following effective treatment of the hypotension.

Some patients, other than those with severe heart failure, are considered to be at higher risk when started on an ACE inhibitor and are recommended for initiation of therapy in hospital. Research data have shown such patients to be: those on multiple or high-dose diuretics (e.g. >80 mg frusemide); patients with hypovolaemia; hyponatraemia (serum sodium <130 mEq/l); pre-existing hypotension (systolic blood pressure <90 mm Hg); patients with unstable cardiac failure; renal impairment (serum creatinine >150 micromol/l); those on high-dose vasodilator therapy; patients aged 70 years or over.

Maintenance dosage: The dose should be gradually increased, depending on the patient's response, to the usual maintenance dose (5-20 mg). This dose adjustment may be performed over a two- to four-week period, or more rapidly if clinically indicated.

Acute myocardial infarction

Treatment with 'Carace' may be started within 24 hours of the onset of symptoms. The first dose of 'Carace' is 5 mg given orally, followed by 5 mg after 24 hours, 10 mg after 48 hours and then 10 mg once daily thereafter. Patients with a low systolic blood pressure (120 mmHg or less) should be given a lower dose - 2.5 mg orally (see 'Special Warnings and Precautions'). If hypotension occurs (systolic blood pressure less than or equal to 100 mmHg) a daily maintenance dose of 5 mg may be given with temporary reductions to 2.5 mg if needed. If prolonged hypotension occurs (systolic blood pressure less than 90 mmHg for more than1 hour) 'Carace' should be withdrawn.

Dosing for patients with acute myocardial infarction should continue for six weeks. The benefit appears to be greatest in patients with large myocardial infarctions and evidence of impaired left ventricular function. For patients who develop symptoms of heart failure, see 'Posology and Method of Administration', congestive heart failure.

'Carace' is compatible with intravenous or transdermal glyceryl trinitrate.

Impaired renal function

'Carace' is excreted by the kidney, and should be used with caution in patients with renal insufficiency. The dose should be titrated against the response and should be kept as low as possible to maintain adequate control of blood pressure or heart failure.

'Carace' is dialysable. Dialysis patients may be given the usual dose of 'Carace' on dialysis days. On the days when patients are not on dialysis the dosage should be tailored to the blood pressure response.

Paediatric use

'Carace' has not been studied for use in children.

4.3 Contraindications

The use of 'Carace' during pregnancy is contraindicated. When pregnancy is determined 'Carace' should be discontinued as soon as possible unless it is considered life-saving for the mother. (See '4.6 Pregnancy and Lactation').

Hypersensitivity to 'Carace', and in patients with a history of angioneurotic oedema relating to previous treatment with an ACE inhibitor and in patients with hereditary or idiopathic angioedema.

4.4 Special warnings and special precautions for use

Assessment of renal function: Evaluation of the patient should include assessment of renal function prior to initiation of therapy, and during treatment.

Impaired renal function: 'Carace' should be used with caution in patients with renal insufficiency, as they may require reduced or less frequent doses (see 'Posology'). Close monitoring of renal function during therapy should be performed as deemed appropriate in those with renal insufficiency. In the majority, renal function will not alter, or may improve.

Renal failure has been reported in association with ACE inhibitors and has been mainly in patients with severe congestive heart failure or underlying renal disease, including renal artery stenosis. If recognised promptly and treated appropriately, renal failure is usually reversible.

Some hypertensive patients, with no apparent pre-existing renal disease, have developed increases in blood urea and creatinine when 'Carace' has been given concurrently with a diuretic. Dosage reduction of 'Carace' and/or discontinuation of the diuretic may be required. This situation should raise the possibility of underlying renal artery stenosis (see 'Renovascular hypertension').

Symptomatic hypotension was seen rarely in uncomplicated hypertensive patients. It is more likely to occur in patients who have been volume-depleted by diuretic therapy, dietary salt restriction, dialysis, diarrhoea, or vomiting. In these patients, by discontinuing diuretic therapy or significantly reducing the diuretic dose for two to three days prior to initiating 'Carace', the possibility of this occurrence is reduced.

Similar caution and close supervision may apply also to patients with ischaemic heart or cerebrovascular disease in whom severe hypotension could result in a myocardial infarct or cerebrovascular accident. (See 'Undesirable Effects').

Severe hypotension has been reported with ACE inhibitors, mainly in patients with severe heart failure. Many of these patients were on high doses of loop diuretics, and some had hyponatraemia or functional renal impairment. If hypotension develops, the patient should be placed in a supine position. Volume repletion with oral fluids or intravenous normal saline may be required. Intravenous atropine may be necessary if there is associated bradycardia. Treatment with 'Carace' may be restarted with careful dose titration following restoration of effective blood volume and pressure.

In some patients with congestive heart failure who have normal or low blood pressure, additional lowering of systemic blood pressure may occur with 'Carace'. This effect is anticipated and usually is not a reason to discontinue therapy. If such hypotension becomes symptomatic, a reduction of dose or discontinuation of 'Carace' may become necessary.

Hypotension In Acute Myocardial Infarction

Treatment with lisinopril must not be initiated in acute myocardial infarction patients who are at risk of further serious haemodynamic deterioration after treatment with a vasodilator. These are patients with systolic blood pressure of 100 mmHg or lower or cardiogenic shock. During the first 3 days following the infarction, the dose should be reduced if the systolic blood pressure is 120 mmHg or lower. Maintenance doses should be reduced to 5 mg or temporarily to 2.5 mg if systolic blood pressure is 100 mmHg or lower. If hypotension persists (systolic blood pressure less than 90 mmHg for more than 1 hour) then 'Carace' should be withdrawn.

Renovascular hypertension

'Carace' can be used when surgery is not indicated, or prior to surgery. In some patients with bilateral renal artery stenosis or stenosis of the artery to a solitary kidney, increases of blood urea and creatinine, usually reversible upon discontinuation of therapy, have been seen. This is especially likely in patients treated with diuretics and/or those with renal insufficiency.

In acute myocardial infarction, treatment with lisinopril should not be initiated in patients with evidence of renal dysfunction, defined as serum creatinine concentration exceeding 177 micromol/l and/or proteinuria exceeding 500mg / 24h. If renal dysfunction develops during treatment with 'Carace' (serum creatinine concentration exceeding 265 micromol/l or a doubling from the pre-treatment value) then the physician should consider withdrawal of 'Carace'.

Angioneurotic oedema: It has been reported with angiotensin-converting enzyme inhibitors, including 'Carace'. This may occur at any time during treatment. In such cases, 'Carace' should be discontinued promptly and appropriate monitoring should be instituted to ensure complete resolution of symptoms prior to dismissing the patient. Where swelling is confined to the face, lips and mouth, the condition will usually resolve without further treatment, although antihistamines may be useful in relieving symptoms. These patients should be followed carefully until the swelling has resolved. However, where there is involvement of the tongue, glottis or larynx likely to cause airways obstruction, appropriate therapy (which may include subcutaneous epinephrine (adrenaline) (0.5 ml 1:1,000) and/or measures to ensure a patent airway) should be administered promptly.

Black patients receiving ACE inhibitors have been reported to have a higher incidence of angioedema compared to non-blacks.

Patients with a history of angioedema unrelated to ACE-inhibitor therapy may be at increased risk of angioedema while receiving an ACE inhibitor (see also 'Contraindications').

Other hypersensitivity reactions have been reported.

Anaphylactoid reactions during hymenoptera desensitisation: Rarely, patients receiving ACE inhibitors during desensitisation with hymenoptera venom (e.g. Bee or Wasp venom) have experienced life-threatening anaphylactoid reactions. These reactions were avoided by temporarily withholding ACE inhibitor therapy prior to each desensitisation.

Haemodialysis patients: Anaphylactoid reactions have been reported in patients dialysed with high-flux membranes (e.g. AN 69) and treated concomitantly with an ACE inhibitor. In these patients, it is recommended that a different type of dialysis membrane or different class of antihypertensive agent is used.

Anaphylactoid reactions during LDL apheresis: Rarely, patients receiving ACE inhibitors during low-density lipoprotein (LDL) apheresis with dextran sulphate have experienced life-threatening anaphylactoid reactions. These reactions were avoided by temporarily withholding ACE inhibitor therapy prior to each apheresis.

Cough: Cough has been reported with the use of ACE-inhibitors. Characteristically, the cough is non-productive, persistent, and resolves after discontinuation of therapy. ACE-inhibitor-induced cough should be considered as part of the differential diagnosis of cough.

Surgery/anaesthesia: In patients undergoing major surgery or during anaesthesia with agents that produce hypotension, 'Carace' blocks angiotensin II formation secondary to compensatory renin release. This may lead to hypotension which can be corrected by volume expansion.

Aortic stenosis/Hypertrophic cardiomyopathy: As with all vasodilators, ACE inhibitors should be given with caution to patients with obstruction in the outflow tract of the left ventricle.

Neutropenia/Agranulocytosis: Agranulocytosis and bone marrow depression have been caused by ACE inhibitors. Several cases of agranulocytosis and neutropenia have been reported in which a causal relationship to lisinopril cannot be excluded. These cases generally involved patients with collagen vascular disease and renal disease.

General

'Carace' should not be used in patients with aortic stenosis, cor pulmonale or outflow tract obstruction.

Where 'Carace' is used as a single agent in hypertension, Afro-Caribbean patients may show a reduced therapeutic response.

4.5 Interaction with other medicinal products and other forms of Interaction

When 'Carace' is combined with other antihypertensive agents such as beta-blockers and diuretics, the antihypertensive effect is usually additive.

'Carace' reduces the development of thiazide induced hypokalaemia and hyperuricaemia.

'Carace' has been used with nitrates without significant clinical interaction.

Indomethacin may reduce the antihypertensive efficacy of 'Carace'.

In some patients with compromised renal function who are being treated with non-steroidal anti-inflammatory drugs, the co-administration of ACE inhibitors may result in further deterioration of renal function. These effects are usually reversible.

As 'Carace' may reduce the elimination of lithium, serum levels of lithium should be monitored if lithium salts are administered.

Plasma potassium usually remains within normal limits, although a few cases of hyperkalaemia have occurred. If 'Carace' is given with a diuretic, the likelihood of diuretic-induced hypokalaemia may be lessened. 'Carace' may elevate plasma potassium levels in patients with renal failure. Potassium supplements, potassium-sparing diuretics and potassium-containing salt substitutes are not recommended.

Epidemiological studies have suggested that concomitant administration of ACE-inhibitors and antidiabetic medicines (insulins, oral hypoglycaemic agents) may cause an increased blood-glucose-lowering effect with risk of hypoglycaemia. This phenomenon appeared to be more likely to occur during the first weeks of combined treatment and in patients with renal impairment. Long term controlled clinical trials with lisinopril have not confirmed these findings and do not preclude the use of lisinopril in diabetic patients. It is advised, however that these patients be monitored.

Alcohol may enhance the hypotensive effect of any antihypertensive.

Narcotic drugs/antipsychotics: Postural hypotension may occur with ACE inhibitors.

Allopurinol, cytostatic or immunosuppressive agents, systemic corticosteroids, or procainamide: Concomitant administration with ACE inhibitors may lead to an increased risk of leucopenia.

Antacids: induce decreased bioavailability of ACE inhibitors.

Sympathomimetics: may reduce the antihypertensive effects of ACE inhibitors; patients should be carefully monitored to confirm that the desired effect is being obtained.

Cyclosporin: increase the risk of hyperkalaemia with ACE inhibitors.

4.6 Pregnancy and lactation

The use of 'Carace' during pregnancy is contraindicated. When pregnancy is detected 'Carace' should be discontinued as soon as possible, unless it is considered life-saving for the mother.

ACE inhibitors can cause foetal and neonatal morbidity and mortality when administered to pregnant women during the second and third trimesters. Use of ACE inhibitors during this period has been associated with foetal and neonatal injury including hypotension, renal failure, hyperkalaemia, and/or skull hypoplasia in the newborn. Maternal oligohydramnios, presumably representing decreased foetal renal function, has occurred and may result in limb contractures, craniofacial deformations and hypoplastic lung development. If 'Carace' is used, the patient should be apprised of the potential hazard to the foetus.

These adverse effects to the embryo and foetus do not appear to have resulted from intrauterine ACE-inhibitor exposure limited to the first trimester.

In those rare cases where ACE inhibitor use during pregnancy is deemed essential, serial ultrasound examinations should be performed to assess the intraamniotic environment. If oligohydramnios is detected, 'Carace' should be discontinued unless it is considered life-saving for the mother. Patients and physicians should be aware, however, that oligohydramnios may not appear until after the foetus has sustained irreversible injury.

Infants whose mothers have taken 'Carace' should be closely observed for hypertension, oliguria and hyperkalaemia. Lisinopril, which crosses the placenta, has been removed from the neonatal circulation by peritoneal dialysis with some clinical benefit, and theoretically may be removed by exchange transfusion.

Nursing mothers

It is not known whether 'Carace' is excreted in human milk. Because many drugs are secreted in human milk, caution should be exercised if 'Carace' is given to a nursing mother.

4.7 Effects on ability to drive and use machines

No data are known about the effect on the ability to drive and to operate machinery.

4.8 Undesirable effects

Hypotension has occurred in association with therapy with 'Carace'. This appears to occur in certain specific subgroups (see 'Special Warnings and Precautions').

Hypersensitivity/angioneurotic oedema:

Angioneurotic oedema of the face, extremities, lips, tongue, glottis and/or larynx has been reported rarely (see 'Special Warnings and Precautions').

Other adverse reactions

Dizziness, headache, diarrhoea, fatigue, cough, and nausea are the most frequent. Other less frequent side effects include: orthostatic effects (including hypotension), rash, and asthenia.

Rare side effects include:

Cardiovascular: myocardial infarction or cerebrovascular accident possibly secondary to excessive hypotension in high risk patients (see 'Special Warnings and Precautions'), palpitation, tachycardia, angina pectoris, rhythm disturbances.

Gastrointestinal: pancreatitis, abdominal pain, dry mouth, hepatitis (hepatocellular or cholestatic), jaundice, constipation, dyspepsia, vomiting.

Nervous system/psychiatric: mood alterations, mental confusion, paraesthesia, depression, insomnia, somnolence, vertigo.

Respiratory: bronchospasm, bronchitis, dyspnoea, nasal congestion, rhinitis, sinusitis.

Skin: urticaria, pruritus, diaphoresis, alopecia, erythema multiforme, pemphigus, Stevens-Johnson syndrome, toxic epidermal necrolysis.

Urogenital: uraemia, oliguria/anuria, renal dysfunction, acute renal failure, impotence.

Other: syncope, blurred vision, taste disturbances.

There have been reports of haemolytic anaemia in patients taking lisinopril, although no causal relationship has been established.

A symptom complex has been reported which may include fever, vasculitits, myalgia, arthralgia/arthritis, a positive ANA, elevated erythrocyte sedimentation rate, eosinophilia and leucocytosis. Rash, photosensitivity, or other dermatological manifestations may occur.

Laboratory Test Findings

Increases in blood urea and creatinine, reversible on discontinuation of 'Carace', are most likely in the presence of bilateral renal artery stenosis, especially in patients with renal insufficiency (see 'Special Warnings and Precautions'). However, increases in blood urea and creatinine may occur without evidence of pre-existing renal impairment, especially in patients taking diuretics. In this event, undiagnosed renal artery stenosis should be suspected. Dosage reduction of 'Carace' and/or discontinuation of the diuretic should be considered. Rare cases of neutropenia have been reported, although no causal relationship has been shown.

Increases in liver enzymes and serum bilirubin have occurred which are usually reversible on discontinuation of 'Carace'.

Bone marrow depression, manifest as anaemia and/or thrombocytopenia and/or leucopenia, has been reported.

Decreases in haemoglobin and haematocrit have been reported in a few patients, but were rarely of clinical importance unless another cause of anaemia was present.

Hyperkalaemia has occurred frequently (incidence of 2% in clinical trials).

Hyponatraemia has occurred rarely.

4.9 Overdose

There are no data on overdosage in humans. The most likely manifestation of overdosage would be hypotension, for which the usual treatment would be intravenous infusion of normal saline solution. Lisinopril may be removed from the general circulation by haemodialysis. (See 'Special Warnings and Precautions', Haemodialysis Patients).

5. PHARMACOLOGICAL PROPERTIES

5.1 Pharmacodynamic properties

Lisinopril is a peptidyl dipeptidase inhibitor. It inhibits the angiotensin converting enzyme (ACE) that catalyses the conversion of angiotensin I to the vasoconstrictor peptide, angiotensin II. Angiotensin II also stimulates aldosterone secretion by the adrenal cortex. Inhibition of ACE results in decreased concentrations of angiotensin II which results in decreased vasopressor activity and reduced aldosterone secretion. The latter decrease may result in an increase in serum potassium concentration. While the mechanism through which lisinopril lowers blood pressure is believed to be primarily suppression of the renin-angiotensin-aldosterone system, lisinopril is antihypertensive even in patients with low-renin hypertension. ACE is identical to kininase II, an enzyme that degrades bradykinin. Whether increased levels of bradykinin, a potent vasodilatory peptide, play a role in the therapeutic effects of lisinopril remains to be elucidated.

5.2 Pharmacokinetic properties

In clinical studies, following oral administration of lisinopril, peak serum concentrations occur within about 6-8 hours. On multiple dosing lisinopril has an effective half-life accumulation of 12.6 hours.

Declining serum concentrations exhibited a prolonged terminal phase which did not contribute to drug accumulation. This terminal phase probably represents saturable binding to ACE and was not proportional to dose. Lisinopril did not appear to bound to other serum proteins.

The disposition of lisinopril in patients with renal insufficiency was similar to that in patients with normal renal function until the glomerular filtration rate reached 30 ml/min or less. Peak and trough lisinopril levels then increased, time to peak concentrations was increased and time to steady state was sometimes prolonged. Lisinopril can be removed by dialysis.

In elderly healthy subjects (65 years and above), a single dose of lisinopril 20 mg produced higher serum concentrations than those seen in young healthy adults given a similar dose. In another study, single daily doses of lisinopril 5 mg were given for 7 consecutive days to young and elderly healthy volunteers and to elderly patients with congestive heart failure. Maximum serum concentrations of lisinopril on Day 7 were higher in the elderly volunteers than in the young and still higher in the elderly patients with congestive heart failure. These findings are consistent with the concept that drugs of low lipid solubility (such as lisinopril) achieve a reduced volume of distribution in the elderly, who have decreased lean body mass/fat ratio: and renal clearance of lisinopril was decreased in the elderly, particularly in the presence of congestive heart failure.

Based on urinary recovery, the mean extent of absorption of lisinopril is approximately 25% with interpatient variability (6-60%) at all doses tested (5-80mg).

Lisinopril does not undergo metabolism and absorbed drug is excreted unchanged entirely in the urine. Lisinopril absorption is not affected by the presence of food in the gastrointestinal tract.

Studies in rats indicate that lisinopril crosses the blood-brain barrier poorly.

5.3 Preclinical safety data

No relevant information

6. PHARMACEUTICAL PARTICULARS

6.1 List of excipients

Calcium Hydrogen Phosphate BP

Magnesium Stearate BP

Pregelatinised Maize Starch BP

Mannitol BP

Maize Starch BP

'Carace' 2.5mg contains Indigo Carmine Aluminium Lake E132

'Carace' 10mg and 20mg contain Iron Oxides E172

6.2 Incompatibilities

Not applicable

6.3 Shelf life

36 months

6.4 Special precautions for storage

Do not store above 25°C. Store in the original package.

6.5 Nature and contents of container

Polyvinyl chloride/aluminium blister packs of 28 tablets.

6.6 Instructions for use and handling

Not applicable

7. MARKETING AUTHORISATION HOLDER

Bristol-Myers Squibb Pharmaceuticals Limited
Uxbridge Business Park
Sanderson Road
Uxbridge
Middlesex
UB8 1DH

8. MARKETING AUTHORISATION NUMBER(S)

'Carace' 2.5mg: PL 11184/0096

'Carace' 5mg: PL 11184/0097

'Carace' 10mg: PL 11184/0098

'Carace' 20mg: PL 11184/0099

9. DATE OF FIRST AUTHORISATION/RENEWAL OF THE AUTHORISATION

26 February 2002

10. DATE OF REVISION OF THE TEXT

June 2005

Carboplatin 10mg/ml Injection BP (150mg/15ml)

(Wockhardt UK Ltd)

1. NAME OF THE MEDICINAL PRODUCT

Carboplatin 10mg/ml Concentrate for Solution for Injection BP

2. QUALITATIVE AND QUANTITATIVE COMPOSITION

Carboplatin 150mg in 15ml (10mg/ml)

For excipients see 6.1

3. PHARMACEUTICAL FORM

Concentrate for solution for injection

Clear, colourless or almost colourless solution

4. CLINICAL PARTICULARS

4.1 Therapeutic indications

Carboplatin is indicated for the treatment of:

1. Advanced ovarian carcinoma of epithelial origin in:

(a) first line therapy

(b) second line therapy, after other treatments have failed.

2. Small cell carcinoma of the lung.

4.2 Posology and method of administration

Dosage and Administration:

Carboplatin should be used **by the intravenous route only**. The recommended dosage of carboplatin in previously untreated adult patients with normal kidney function is 400 mg/m^2 as a single i.v. dose administered by a 15 to 60 minutes infusion. Alternatively, see Calvert formula below:

Dose (mg) = target AUC (mg/ml × min) × [GFR ml/min + 25]

Patient treatment status	Planned chemotherapy	Target AUC
Previously untreated	Single agent carboplatin	5-7 mg/ml.min
Previously treated	Single agent carboplatin	4-6 mg/ml.min
Previously untreated	Carboplatin plus cyclophosphamide	4-6 mg/ml

Note: With the Calvert formula, the total dose of carboplatin is calculated in mg, not mg/m^2.

Therapy should not be repeated until four weeks after the previous carboplatin course and/or until the neutrophil count is at least 2,000 cells/mm^3 and the platelet count is at least 100,000 cells/mm^3.

Reduction of the initial dosage by 20-25% is recommended for those patients who present with risk factors such as prior myelosuppressive treatment and low performance status (ECOG-Zubrod 2-4 or Karnofsky below 80).

Determination of the haematological nadir by weekly blood counts during the initial courses of treatment with carboplatin is recommended for future dosage adjustment.

Impaired Renal Function:

The optimal use of carboplatin in patients presenting with impaired renal function requires adequate dosage adjustments and frequent monitoring of both haematological nadirs and renal function.

Combination Therapy:

The optimal use of carboplatin in combination with other myelosuppressive agents requires dosage adjustments according to the regimen and schedule to be adopted.

Paediatrics:

Sufficient usage of carboplatin in paediatrics has not occurred to allow specific dosage recommendations to be made.

Elderly:

Dosage adjustment, initially or subsequently, may be necessary, dependent on the physical condition of the patient.

Dilution & Reconstitution:

See 6.6 Instructions for Use / Handling

4.3 Contraindications

Carboplatin should not be used in patients with severe pre-existing renal impairment (creatinine clearance at or below 20ml/minute).

It should not be employed in severely myelosuppressed patients. It is also contraindicated in patients with a history of severe allergic reactions to carboplatin or other platinum containing compounds.

4.4 Special warnings and special precautions for use

Carboplatin should be administered by individuals experienced in the use of anti-neoplastic therapy.

Carboplatin myelosuppression is closely related to its renal clearance. Patients with abnormal kidney function or receiving concomitant therapy with other drugs with nephrotoxic potential are likely to experience more severe and prolonged myelotoxicity. Renal function parameters should therefore be carefully assessed before and during therapy. Carboplatin courses should not be repeated more frequently than monthly under normal circumstances. Thrombocytopenia, leukopenia and anaemia occur after administration of carboplatin. Frequent monitoring of peripheral blood counts is recommended throughout and following therapy with carboplatin. Carboplatin combination therapy with other myelosuppressive compounds must be planned very carefully with respect to dosages and timing in order to minimise additive effects. Supportive transfusional therapy may be required in patients who suffer severe myelosuppression.

Carboplatin can cause nausea and vomiting. Premedication with anti-emetics has been reported to be useful in reducing the incidence and intensity of these effects.

Renal and hepatic function impairment may be encountered with carboplatin. Very high doses of carboplatin (>5 times single agent recommended dose) have resulted in severe abnormalities in hepatic and renal function. Although no clinical evidence on compounding nephrotoxicity has been accumulated, it is recommended not to combine carboplatin with aminoglycosides or other nephrotoxic compounds.

Infrequent allergic reactions to carboplatin have been reported, e.g. erythematous rash, fever with no apparent cause or pruritus. Rarely anaphylaxis, angio-oedema and anaphylactoid reactions including bronchospasm, urticaria and facial oedema have occurred. These reactions are similar to those observed after administration of other platinum containing compounds and may occur within minutes. The incidence of allergic reactions may increase with previous exposure to platinum therapy; however, allergic reactions have been observed upon initial exposure to carboplatin. Patients should be observed carefully for possible allergic reactions and managed with appropriate supportive therapy.

The carcinogenic potential of carboplatin has not been studied but compounds with similar mechanisms of action and mutagenicity have been reported to be carcinogenic.

Precautions:

Peripheral blood counts and renal and hepatic function tests should be monitored closely. Blood counts at the beginning of the therapy and weekly to assess haematological nadir for subsequent dose adjustment are recommended. Neurological evaluations should also be performed on a regular basis.

4.5 Interaction with other medicinal products and other forms of Interaction

The use of carboplatin with nephrotoxic compounds is not recommended.

4.6 Pregnancy and lactation

The safe use of carboplatin during pregnancy has not been established: carboplatin has been shown to be an embryotoxin and teratogen in rats. If carboplatin is used during pregnancy the patient should be appraised of the potential hazard to the foetus. Women of child-bearing potential should be advised to avoid becoming pregnant.

Carboplatin has been shown to be mutagenic in vivo and in vitro.

Nursing Mothers:

It is not known whether carboplatin is excreted in human milk.

4.7 Effects on ability to drive and use machines

None reported.

4.8 Undesirable effects

Incidences of adverse reactions reported hereunder are based on cumulative data obtained in a large group of patients with various pretreatment prognostic features.

Haematological toxicity:

Myelosuppression is the dose-limiting toxicity of carboplatin. At maximum tolerated dosages of carboplatin administered as a single agent, thrombocytopenia, with nadir platelet counts of less than 50 × 10^9/L, occurs in about a quarter of the patients.

The nadir usually occurs between days 14 and 21, with recovery within 35 days from the start of therapy. Leukopenia has also occurred in approximately 14% of patients but its recovery from the day of nadir (day 14-28) may be slower and usually occurs within 42 days from the start of therapy. Neutropenia with granulocyte counts below 1 × 10^9/L occurs in approximately one fifth of patients. Anaemia with haemoglobin values below 11g/dL has been observed in more than two-thirds of patients with normal base-line values.

Myelosuppression may be more severe and prolonged in patients with impaired renal function, extensive prior treatment, poor performance status and age above 65. Myelosuppression is also worsened by therapy combining carboplatin with other compounds that are myelosuppressive.

Myelosuppression is usually reversible and not cumulative when carboplatin is used as a single agent and at the recommended dosages and frequencies of administration.

Infectious complications have occasionally been reported. Haemorrhagic complications, usually minor, have also been reported.

Nephrotoxicity:

Renal toxicity is usually not dose-limiting in patients receiving carboplatin, nor does it require preventive measures such as high volume fluid hydration or forced diuresis. Nevertheless, increasing blood urea or serum creatinine levels can occur. Renal function impairment, as defined by a decrease in the creatinine clearance below 60 ml/min, may also be observed. The incidence and severity of nephrotoxicity may increase in patients who have impaired kidney function before carboplatin treatment. It is not clear whether an appropriate hydration programme might overcome such an effect, but dosage reduction or discontinuation of therapy is required in the presence of severe alteration of renal function tests.

Decreases in serum electrolytes (sodium, magnesium, potassium and calcium) have been reported after treatment with carboplatin but have not been reported to be severe enough to cause the appearance of clinical signs or symptoms.

Cases of hyponatraemia have been reported. Haemolytic uraemic syndrome has been reported rarely.

Gastrointestinal toxicity:

Nausea without vomiting occurs in about 15% of patients receiving carboplatin; vomiting has been reported in over half of the patients and about one-fifth of these suffer severe emesis. Nausea and vomiting usually disappear within 24 hours after treatment and are usually responsive to (and may be prevented by) anti-emetic medication. A fifth of patients experience no nausea or vomiting.

Cases of anorexia have been reported.

Allergic reactions:

Infrequent allergic reactions to carboplatin have been reported, e.g., erythematous rash, fever with no apparent cause or pruritus. Rarely, anaphylaxis, angio-oedema and anaphylactoid reactions, including bronchospasm, urticaria and facial oedema have occurred. (See Warnings.)

Ototoxicity:

Subclinical decrease in hearing acuity, consisting of high-frequency (4000-8000 Hz) hearing loss determined by audiogram, has been reported in 15% of the patients treated with carboplatin. However, only 1% of patients present with clinical symptoms, manifested in the majority of cases by tinnitus. In patients who have been previously treated with cisplatin and have developed hearing loss related to such treatment, the hearing impairment may persist or worsen.

At higher than recommended doses in combination with other ototoxic agents, clinically significant hearing loss has been reported to occur in paediatric patients when carboplatin solution was administered.

Neurotoxicity:

The incidence of peripheral neuropathies after treatment with carboplatin is 4%. In the majority of the patients neurotoxicity is limited to paraesthesia and decreased deep tendon reflexes. The frequency and intensity of this side effect increases in elderly patients and those previously treated with cisplatin.

Paraesthesia present before commencing carboplatin therapy, particularly if related to prior cisplatin treatment, may persist or worsen during treatment with carboplatin.

Ocular toxicity:

Transient visual disturbances, sometimes including transient sight loss, have been reported rarely with platinum therapy. This is usually associated with high dose therapy in renally impaired patients.

Other:

Abnormalities of liver function tests (usually mild to moderate) have been reported with carboplatin in about one-third of the patients with normal baseline values. The alkaline phosphatase level is increased more frequently than SGOT, SGPT or total bilirubin. The majority of these abnormalities regress spontaneously during the course of treatment.

Infrequent events consisting of taste alteration, asthenia, alopecia, fever and chills without evidence of infection have occurred.

4.9 Overdose

There is no known antidote for carboplatin overdosage. The anticipated complications of overdosage would be related to myelosuppression as well as impairment of hepatic and renal function.

5. PHARMACOLOGICAL PROPERTIES

5.1 Pharmacodynamic properties

Carboplatin is an antineoplastic agent. Its activity has been demonstrated against several murine and human cell lines.

Carboplatin exhibited comparable activity to cisplatin against a wide range of tumours regardless of implant site.

Alkaline elution techniques and DNA binding studies have demonstrated the qualitatively similar modes of action of carboplatin and cisplatin. Carboplatin, like cisplatin, induces changes in the superhelical conformation of DNA which is consistent with a "DNA shortening effect".

5.2 Pharmacokinetic properties

Carboplatin has biochemical properties similar to those of cisplatin, thus producing predominantly interstrand and intrastrand DNA crosslinks. Following administration of carboplatin in man, linear relationships exist between dose and plasma concentrations of total and free ultrafilterable platinum. The area under the plasma concentration versus time curve for total platinum also shows a linear relationship with the dose when creatinine clearance exceeds 60ml/min.

Repeated dosing during four consecutive days did not produce an accumulation of platinum in plasma. Following the administration of carboplatin, reported values for the terminal elimination half-lives of free ultrafilterable platinum and carboplatin in man are approximately 6 hours and 1.5 hours respectively. During the initial phase, most of the free ultrafilterable platinum is present as carboplatin. The terminal half-life for total plasma platinum is 24 hours. Approximately 87% of plasma platinum is protein bound within 24 hours following administration. Carboplatin is excreted primarily in the urine, with recovery of approximately 70% of the administered platinum within 24 hours. Most of the drug is excreted in the first 6 hours. Total body and renal clearances of free ultrafilterable platinum correlate with the rate of glomerular filtration but not tubular secretion.

5.3 Preclinical safety data

Carboplatin has been shown to be embryotoxic and teratogenic in rats. (See para. 4.6, Pregnancy and Lactation.) It is mutagenic in vivo and in vitro and although the carcinogenic potential of carboplatin has not been studied, compounds with similar mechanisms of action and mutagenicity have been reported to be carcinogenic.

6. PHARMACEUTICAL PARTICULARS

6.1 List of excipients

Water for injections

Nitrogen

6.2 Incompatibilities

Needles or intravenous sets containing aluminium parts that may come into contact with carboplatin should not be used for preparation or administration of carboplatin.

6.3 Shelf life

18 months (unopened)

After dilution:

24 hours under refrigeration (2 - 8°C)

6.4 Special precautions for storage

Do not store above 25 °C. Keep container in the outer carton.

After dilution (see section 6.6.):

Chemical and physical in-use stability has been demonstrated for 24 hours at 25°C for solutions with a final concentration of carboplatin 0.4mg/ml or 2.0mg/ml after dilution of the carboplatin10mg/ml with glucose solution 5%.

From a microbiological point of view, the product should be used immediately. If not used immediately, in-use storage times and conditions prior to use are the responsibility of the user and would normally not be longer than 24 hours at 2 to 8°C, unless dilution has taken place in controlled and validated aseptic conditions.

6.5 Nature and contents of container

Amber vials of hydrolytic type I glass, packed in a carton.

Vials are closed with a rubber stopper with an aluminium crimp cap with flip-off.

Packs of 1 vial containing 150mg/15ml of carboplatin.

6.6 Instructions for use and handling

This product is for single dose use only.

Solutions should only be used if clear and particle free.

Trained personnel should prepare carboplatin for infusion in designated areas. Protective clothing (including gloves) should be worn. The eyes should be protected. In the event of contact with the eyes, wash with water and/or saline.

Pregnant staff should not handle cytotoxics.

Any unused product, syringes, containers, absorbent material or other waste material should be disposed of using adequate care and precautions. Excess material and body waste may be disposed of by placing in double sealed polythene bags and incinerating at a temperature of 1000°C. Liquid waste may be flushed with copious amounts of water.

Carboplatin for infusion may be prepared by dilution with Glucose 5% Solution.

Administrative Data

7. MARKETING AUTHORISATION HOLDER

CP Pharmaceuticals Ltd

Ash Road North

Wrexham LL13 9UF

United Kingdom

8. MARKETING AUTHORISATION NUMBER(S)

PL 04543/0460

9. DATE OF FIRST AUTHORISATION/RENEWAL OF THE AUTHORISATION

8th August 2003

10. DATE OF REVISION OF THE TEXT

Carboplatin 10mg/ml Injection BP (450mg/45ml)

(Wockhardt UK Ltd)

1. NAME OF THE MEDICINAL PRODUCT

Carboplatin 10mg/ml Concentrate for Solution for Injection BP

2. QUALITATIVE AND QUANTITATIVE COMPOSITION

Carboplatin 450mg in 45ml (10mg/ml)

For excipients see 6.1

3. PHARMACEUTICAL FORM

Concentrate for solution for injection

Clear, colourless or almost colourless solution

4. CLINICAL PARTICULARS

4.1 Therapeutic indications

Carboplatin is indicated for the treatment of:

1. Advanced ovarian carcinoma of epithelial origin in:

(a) first line therapy

(b) second line therapy, after other treatments have failed.

2. Small cell carcinoma of the lung.

4.2 Posology and method of administration

Dosage and Administration:

Carboplatin should be used **by the intravenous route only**. The recommended dosage of carboplatin in previously untreated adult patients with normal kidney function is 400 mg/m^2 as a single i.v. dose administered by a 15 to 60 minutes infusion. Alternatively, see Calvert formula below:

Dose (mg) = target AUC (mg/ml × min) × [GFR ml/min + 25]

Patient treatment status	Planned chemotherapy	Target AUC
Previously untreated	Single agent carboplatin	5-7 mg/ml.min
Previously treated	Single agent carboplatin	4-6 mg/ml.min
Previously untreated	Carboplatin plus cyclophosphamide	4-6 mg/ml

Note: With the Calvert formula, the total dose of carboplatin is calculated in mg, not mg/m^2.

Therapy should not be repeated until four weeks after the previous carboplatin course and/or until the neutrophil count is at least 2,000 cells/mm^3 and the platelet count is at least 100,000 cells/mm^3.

Reduction of the initial dosage by 20-25% is recommended for those patients who present with risk factors such as prior myelosuppressive treatment and low performance status (ECOG-Zubrod 2-4 or Karnofsky below 80).

Determination of the haematological nadir by weekly blood counts during the initial courses of treatment with carboplatin is recommended for future dosage adjustment.

Impaired Renal Function:

The optimal use of carboplatin in patients presenting with impaired renal function requires adequate dosage adjustments and frequent monitoring of both haematological nadirs and renal function.

Combination Therapy:

The optimal use of carboplatin in combination with other myelosuppressive agents requires dosage adjustments according to the regimen and schedule to be adopted.

Paediatrics:

Sufficient usage of carboplatin in paediatrics has not occurred to allow specific dosage recommendations to be made.

Elderly:

Dosage adjustment, initially or subsequently, may be necessary, dependent on the physical condition of the patient.

Dilution & Reconstitution:

See 6.6 Instructions for Use / Handling

4.3 Contraindications

Carboplatin should not be used in patients with severe pre-existing renal impairment (creatinine clearance at or below 20ml/minute).

It should not be employed in severely myelosuppressed patients. It is also contraindicated in patients with a history of severe allergic reactions to carboplatin or other platinum containing compounds.

4.4 Special warnings and special precautions for use

Carboplatin should be administered by individuals experienced in the use of anti-neoplastic therapy.

Carboplatin myelosuppression is closely related to its renal clearance. Patients with abnormal kidney function or receiving concomitant therapy with other drugs with nephrotoxic potential are likely to experience more severe and prolonged myelotoxicity. Renal function parameters should therefore be carefully assessed before and during therapy. Carboplatin courses should not be repeated more frequently than monthly under normal circumstances. Thrombocytopenia, leukopenia and anaemia occur after administration of carboplatin. Frequent monitoring of peripheral blood counts is recommended throughout and following therapy with carboplatin. Carboplatin combination therapy with other myelosuppressive compounds must be planned very carefully with respect to dosages and timing in order to minimise additive effects. Supportive transfusional therapy may be required in patients who suffer severe myelosuppression.

Carboplatin can cause nausea and vomiting. Premedication with anti-emetics has been reported to be useful in reducing the incidence and intensity of these effects.

Renal and hepatic function impairment may be encountered with carboplatin. Very high doses of carboplatin (>5 times single agent recommended dose) have resulted in severe abnormalities in hepatic and renal function. Although no clinical evidence on compounding nephrotoxicity has been accumulated, it is recommended not to combine carboplatin with aminoglycosides or other nephrotoxic compounds.

Infrequent allergic reactions to carboplatin have been reported, e.g. erythematous rash, fever with no apparent cause or pruritus. Rarely anaphylaxis, angio-oedema and anaphylactoid reactions including bronchospasm, urticaria and facial oedema have occurred. These reactions are similar to those observed after administration of other platinum containing compounds and may occur within minutes. The incidence of allergic reactions may increase with previous exposure to platinum therapy; however, allergic reactions have been observed upon initial exposure to carboplatin. Patients should be observed carefully for possible allergic reactions and managed with appropriate supportive therapy.

The carcinogenic potential of carboplatin has not been studied but compounds with similar mechanisms of action and mutagenicity have been reported to be carcinogenic.

Precautions:

Peripheral blood counts and renal and hepatic function tests should be monitored closely. Blood counts at the beginning of the therapy and weekly to assess haematological nadir for subsequent dose adjustment are recommended. Neurological evaluations should also be performed on a regular basis.

4.5 Interaction with other medicinal products and other forms of Interaction

The use of carboplatin with nephrotoxic compounds is not recommended.

4.6 Pregnancy and lactation

The safe use of carboplatin during pregnancy has not been established: carboplatin has been shown to be an embryotoxin and teratogen in rats. If carboplatin is used during pregnancy the patient should be appraised of the potential hazard to the foetus. Women of child-bearing potential should be advised to avoid becoming pregnant.

Carboplatin has been shown to be mutagenic in vivo and in vitro.

Nursing Mothers:

It is not known whether carboplatin is excreted in human milk.

4.7 Effects on ability to drive and use machines

None reported.

4.8 Undesirable effects

Incidences of adverse reactions reported hereunder are based on cumulative data obtained in a large group of patients with various pretreatment prognostic features.

Haematological toxicity:

Myelosuppression is the dose-limiting toxicity of carboplatin. At maximum tolerated dosages of carboplatin administered as a single agent, thrombocytopenia, with nadir platelet counts of less than 50 × 10^9/L, occurs in about a quarter of the patients.

The nadir usually occurs between days 14 and 21, with recovery within 35 days from the start of therapy. Leukopenia has also occurred in approximately 14% of patients but its recovery from the day of nadir (day 14-28) may be slower and usually occurs within 42 days from the start of therapy. Neutropenia with granulocyte counts below 1 × 10^9/L occurs in approximately one fifth of patients.

Anaemia with haemoglobin values below 11g/dL has been observed in more than two-thirds of patients with normal base-line values.

Myelosuppression may be more severe and prolonged in patients with impaired renal function, extensive prior treatment, poor performance status and age above 65. Myelosuppression is also worsened by therapy combining carboplatin with other compounds that are myelosuppressive.

Myelosuppression is usually reversible and not cumulative when carboplatin is used as a single agent and at the recommended dosages and frequencies of administration.

Infectious complications have occasionally been reported. Haemorrhagic complications, usually minor, have also been reported.

Nephrotoxicity:

Renal toxicity is usually not dose-limiting in patients receiving carboplatin, nor does it require preventive measures such as high volume fluid hydration or forced diuresis. Nevertheless, increasing blood urea or serum creatinine levels can occur. Renal function impairment, as defined by a decrease in the creatinine clearance below 60 ml/min, may also be observed. The incidence and severity of nephrotoxicity may increase in patients who have impaired kidney function before carboplatin treatment. It is not clear whether an appropriate hydration programme might overcome such an effect, but dosage reduction or discontinuation of therapy is required in the presence of severe alteration of renal function tests.

Decreases in serum electrolytes (sodium, magnesium, potassium and calcium) have been reported after treatment with carboplatin but have not been reported to be severe enough to cause the appearance of clinical signs or symptoms.

Cases of hyponatraemia have been reported. Haemolytic uraemic syndrome has been reported rarely.

Gastrointestinal toxicity:

Nausea without vomiting occurs in about 15% of patients receiving carboplatin; vomiting has been reported in over half of the patients and about one-fifth of these suffer severe emesis. Nausea and vomiting usually disappear within 24 hours after treatment and are usually responsive to (and may be prevented by) anti-emetic medication. A fifth of patients experience no nausea or vomiting.

Cases of anorexia have been reported.

Allergic reactions:

Infrequent allergic reactions to carboplatin have been reported, e.g., erythematous rash, fever with no apparent cause or pruritus. Rarely, anaphylaxis, angio-oedema and anaphylactoid reactions, including bronchospasm, urticaria and facial oedema have occurred. (See Warnings.)

Ototoxicity:

Subclinical decrease in hearing acuity, consisting of high-frequency (4000-8000 Hz) hearing loss determined by audiogram, has been reported in 15% of the patients treated with carboplatin. However, only 1% of patients present with clinical symptoms, manifested in the majority of cases by tinnitus. In patients who have been previously treated with cisplatin and have developed hearing loss related to such treatment, the hearing impairment may persist or worsen.

At higher than recommended doses in combination with other ototoxic agents, clinically significant hearing loss has been reported to occur in paediatric patients when carboplatin solution was administered.

Neurotoxicity:

The incidence of peripheral neuropathies after treatment with carboplatin is 4%. In the majority of the patients neurotoxicity is limited to paraesthesia and decreased deep tendon reflexes. The frequency and intensity of this side effect increases in elderly patients and those previously treated with cisplatin.

Paraesthesia present before commencing carboplatin therapy, particularly if related to prior cisplatin treatment, may persist or worsen during treatment with carboplatin.

Ocular toxicity:

Transient visual disturbances, sometimes including transient sight loss, have been reported rarely with platinum therapy. This is usually associated with high dose therapy in renally impaired patients.

Other:

Abnormalities of liver function tests (usually mild to moderate) have been reported with carboplatin in about one-third of the patients with normal baseline values. The alkaline phosphatase level is increased more frequently than SGOT, SGPT or total bilirubin. The majority of these abnormalities regress spontaneously during the course of treatment.

Infrequent events consisting of taste alteration, asthenia, alopecia, fever and chills without evidence of infection have occurred.

4.9 Overdose

There is no known antidote for carboplatin overdosage. The anticipated complications of overdosage would be related to myelosuppression as well as impairment of hepatic and renal function.

5. PHARMACOLOGICAL PROPERTIES

5.1 Pharmacodynamic properties

Carboplatin is an antineoplastic agent. Its activity has been demonstrated against several murine and human cell lines.

Carboplatin exhibited comparable activity to cisplatin against a wide range of tumours regardless of implant site.

Alkaline elution techniques and DNA binding studies have demonstrated the qualitatively similar modes of action of carboplatin and cisplatin. Carboplatin, like cisplatin, induces changes in the superhelical conformation of DNA which is consistent with a "DNA shortening effect".

5.2 Pharmacokinetic properties

Carboplatin has biochemical properties similar to those of cisplatin, thus producing predominantly interstrand and intrastrand DNA crosslinks. Following administration of carboplatin in man, linear relationships exist between dose and plasma concentrations of total and free ultrafilterable platinum. The area under the plasma concentration versus time curve for total platinum also shows a linear relationship with the dose when creatinine clearance exceeds 60ml/min.

Repeated dosing during four consecutive days did not produce an accumulation of platinum in plasma. Following the administration of carboplatin, reported values for the terminal elimination half-lives of free ultrafilterable platinum and carboplatin in man are approximately 6 hours and 1.5 hours respectively. During the initial phase, most of the free ultrafilterable platinum is present as carboplatin. The terminal half-life for total plasma platinum is 24 hours. Approximately 87% of plasma platinum is protein bound within 24 hours following administration. Carboplatin is excreted primarily in the urine, with recovery of approximately 70% of the administered platinum within 24 hours. Most of the drug is excreted in the first 6 hours. Total body and renal clearances of free ultrafilterable platinum correlate with the rate of glomerular filtration but not tubular secretion.

5.3 Preclinical safety data

Carboplatin has been shown to be embryotoxic and teratogenic in rats. (See para. 4.6, Pregnancy and Lactation.) It is mutagenic in vivo and in vitro and although the carcinogenic potential of carboplatin has not been studied, compounds with similar mechanisms of action and mutagenicity have been reported to be carcinogenic.

6. PHARMACEUTICAL PARTICULARS

6.1 List of excipients

Water for injections

Nitrogen

6.2 Incompatibilities

Needles or intravenous sets containing aluminium parts that may come into contact with carboplatin should not be used for preparation or administration of carboplatin.

6.3 Shelf life

18 months (unopened)

After dilution:

24 hours under refrigeration (2 - 8°C)

6.4 Special precautions for storage

Do not store above 25 °C. Keep container in the outer carton.

After dilution (see section 6.6.):

Chemical and physical in-use stability has been demonstrated for 24 hours at 25°C for solutions with a final concentration of carboplatin 0.4mg/ml or 2.0mg/ml after dilution of the carboplatin10mg/ml with glucose solution 5%.

From a microbiological point of view, the product should be used immediately. If not used immediately, in-use storage times and conditions prior to use are the responsibility of the user and would normally not be longer than 24 hours at 2 to 8°C, unless dilution has taken place in controlled and validated aseptic conditions.

6.5 Nature and contents of container

Amber vials of hydrolytic type I glass, packed in a carton.

Vials are closed with a rubber stopper with an aluminium crimp cap with flip-off.

Packs of 1 vial containing 450mg/45ml of carboplatin.

6.6 Instructions for use and handling

This product is for single dose use only.

Solutions should only be used if clear and particle free.

Trained personnel should prepare carboplatin for infusion in designated areas. Protective clothing (including gloves) should be worn. The eyes should be protected. In the event of contact with the eyes, wash with water and/or saline.

Pregnant staff should not handle cytotoxics.

Any unused product, syringes, containers, absorbent material or other waste material should be disposed of using adequate care and precautions. Excess material and body waste may be disposed of by placing in double sealed polythene bags and incinerating at a temperature of 1000°C. Liquid waste may be flushed with copious amounts of water.

Carboplatin for infusion may be prepared by dilution with Glucose 5% Solution.

Administrative Data

7. MARKETING AUTHORISATION HOLDER

CP Pharmaceuticals Ltd

Ash Road North

Wrexham LL13 9UF

United Kingdom

8. MARKETING AUTHORISATION NUMBER(S)

PL 04543/0461

9. DATE OF FIRST AUTHORISATION/RENEWAL OF THE AUTHORISATION

5th August 2003

10. DATE OF REVISION OF THE TEXT

Carboplatin 10mg/ml Injection BP (50mg/5ml)

(Wockhardt UK Ltd)

1. NAME OF THE MEDICINAL PRODUCT

Carboplatin 10mg/ml Concentrate for Solution for Injection BP

2. QUALITATIVE AND QUANTITATIVE COMPOSITION

Carboplatin 50mg in 5ml (10mg/ml)

For excipients see 6.1

3. PHARMACEUTICAL FORM

Concentrate for solution for injection.

Clear, colourless or almost colourless solution

4. CLINICAL PARTICULARS

4.1 Therapeutic indications

Carboplatin is indicated for the treatment of:

1. Advanced ovarian carcinoma of epithelial origin in:

(a) first line therapy

(b) second line therapy, after other treatments have failed.

2. Small cell carcinoma of the lung.

4.2 Posology and method of administration

Dosage and Administration:

Carboplatin should be used **by the intravenous route only**. The recommended dosage of carboplatin in previously untreated adult patients with normal kidney function is 400 mg/m^2 as a single i.v. dose administered by a 15 to 60 minutes infusion. Alternatively, see Calvert formula below:

Dose (mg) = target AUC (mg/ml × min) × [GFR ml/min + 25]

Patient treatment status	Planned chemotherapy	Target AUC
Previously untreated	Single agent carboplatin	5-7 mg/ml.min
Previously treated	Single agent carboplatin	4-6 mg/ml.min
Previously untreated	Carboplatin plus cyclophosphamide	4-6 mg/ml

Note: With the Calvert formula, the total dose of carboplatin is calculated in mg, not mg/m^2.

Therapy should not be repeated until four weeks after the previous carboplatin course and/or until the neutrophil count is at least 2,000 cells/mm^3 and the platelet count is at least 100,000 cells/mm^3.

Reduction of the initial dosage by 20-25% is recommended for those patients who present with risk factors such as prior myelosuppressive treatment and low performance status (ECOG-Zubrod 2-4 or Karnofsky below 80).

Determination of the haematological nadir by weekly blood counts during the initial courses of treatment with carboplatin is recommended for future dosage adjustment.

Impaired Renal Function:

The optimal use of carboplatin in patients presenting with impaired renal function requires adequate dosage adjustments and frequent monitoring of both haematological nadirs and renal function.

Combination Therapy:

The optimal use of carboplatin in combination with other myelosuppressive agents requires dosage adjustments according to the regimen and schedule to be adopted.

Paediatrics:

Sufficient usage of carboplatin in paediatrics has not occurred to allow specific dosage recommendations to be made.

Elderly:

Dosage adjustment, initially or subsequently, may be necessary, dependent on the physical condition of the patient.

<u>Dilution & Reconstitution:</u>

See 6.6 Instructions for Use / Handling

4.3 Contraindications

Carboplatin should not be used in patients with severe pre-existing renal impairment (creatinine clearance at or below 20ml/minute).

It should not be employed in severely myelosuppressed patients. It is also contraindicated in patients with a history of severe allergic reactions to carboplatin or other platinum containing compounds.

4.4 Special warnings and special precautions for use

Carboplatin should be administered by individuals experienced in the use of anti-neoplastic therapy.

Carboplatin myelosuppression is closely related to its renal clearance. Patients with abnormal kidney function or receiving concomitant therapy with other drugs with nephrotoxic potential are likely to experience more severe and prolonged myelotoxicity. Renal function parameters should therefore be carefully assessed before and during therapy. Carboplatin courses should not be repeated more frequently than monthly under normal circumstances. Thrombocytopenia, leukopenia and anaemia occur after administration of carboplatin. Frequent monitoring of peripheral blood counts is recommended throughout and following therapy with carboplatin. Carboplatin combination therapy with other myelosuppressive compounds must be planned very carefully with respect to dosages and timing in order to minimise additive effects. Supportive transfusional therapy may be required in patients who suffer severe myelosuppression.

Carboplatin can cause nausea and vomiting. Premedication with anti-emetics has been reported to be useful in reducing the incidence and intensity of these effects.

Renal and hepatic function impairment may be encountered with carboplatin. Very high doses of carboplatin (>5 times single agent recommended dose) have resulted in severe abnormalities in hepatic and renal function. Although no clinical evidence on compounding nephrotoxicity has been accumulated, it is recommended not to combine carboplatin with aminoglycosides or other nephrotoxic compounds.

Infrequent allergic reactions to carboplatin have been reported, e.g. erythematous rash, fever with no apparent cause or pruritus. Rarely anaphylaxis, angio-oedema and anaphylactoid reactions including bronchospasm, urticaria and facial oedema have occurred. These reactions are similar to those observed after administration of other platinum containing compounds and may occur within minutes. The incidence of allergic reactions may increase with previous exposure to platinum therapy; however, allergic reactions have been observed upon initial exposure to carboplatin. Patients should be observed carefully for possible allergic reactions and managed with appropriate supportive therapy.

The carcinogenic potential of carboplatin has not been studied but compounds with similar mechanisms of action and mutagenicity have been reported to be carcinogenic.

Precautions:

Peripheral blood counts and renal and hepatic function tests should be monitored closely. Blood counts at the beginning of the therapy and weekly to assess haematological nadir for subsequent dose adjustment are recommended. Neurological evaluations should also be performed on a regular basis.

4.5 Interaction with other medicinal products and other forms of Interaction

The use of carboplatin with nephrotoxic compounds is not recommended.

4.6 Pregnancy and lactation

The safe use of carboplatin during pregnancy has not been established: carboplatin has been shown to be an embryotoxin and teratogen in rats. If carboplatin is used during pregnancy the patient should be appraised of the potential hazard to the foetus. Women of child-bearing potential should be advised to avoid becoming pregnant.

Carboplatin has been shown to be mutagenic in vivo and in vitro.

Nursing Mothers:

It is not known whether carboplatin is excreted in human milk.

4.7 Effects on ability to drive and use machines

None reported.

4.8 Undesirable effects

Incidences of adverse reactions reported hereunder are based on cumulative data obtained in a large group of patients with various pretreatment prognostic features.

Haematological toxicity:

Myelosuppression is the dose-limiting toxicity of carboplatin. At maximum tolerated dosages of carboplatin administered as a single agent, thrombocytopenia, with nadir platelet counts of less than 50×10^9/L, occurs in about a quarter of the patients.

The nadir usually occurs between days 14 and 21, with recovery within 35 days from the start of therapy. Leukopenia has also occurred in approximately 14% of patients but its recovery from the day of nadir (day 14-28) may be slower and usually occurs within 42 days from the start of therapy. Neutropenia with granulocyte counts below 1×10^9/L occurs in approximately one fifth of patients.

Anaemia with haemoglobin values below 11g/dL has been observed in more than two-thirds of patients with normal base-line values.

Myelosuppression may be more severe and prolonged in patients with impaired renal function, extensive prior treatment, poor performance status and age above 65. Myelosuppression is also worsened by therapy combining carboplatin with other compounds that are myelosuppressive.

Myelosuppression is usually reversible and not cumulative when carboplatin is used as a single agent and at the recommended dosages and frequencies of administration.

Infectious complications have occasionally been reported. Haemorrhagic complications, usually minor, have also been reported.

Nephrotoxicity:

Renal toxicity is usually not dose-limiting in patients receiving carboplatin, nor does it require preventive measures such as high volume fluid hydration or forced diuresis. Nevertheless, increasing blood urea or serum creatinine levels can occur. Renal function impairment, as defined by a decrease in the creatinine clearance below 60 ml/min, may also be observed. The incidence and severity of nephrotoxicity may increase in patients who have impaired kidney function before carboplatin treatment. It is not clear whether an appropriate hydration programme might overcome such an effect, but dosage reduction or discontinuation of therapy is required in the presence of severe alteration of renal function tests.

Decreases in serum electrolytes (sodium, magnesium, potassium and calcium) have been reported after treatment with carboplatin but have not been reported to be severe enough to cause the appearance of clinical signs or symptoms.

Cases of hyponatraemia have been reported. Haemolytic uraemic syndrome has been reported rarely.

Gastrointestinal toxicity:

Nausea without vomiting occurs in about 15% of patients receiving carboplatin; vomiting has been reported in over half of the patients and about one-fifth of these suffer severe emesis. Nausea and vomiting usually disappear within 24 hours after treatment and are usually responsive to (and may be prevented by) anti-emetic medication. A fifth of patients experience no nausea or vomiting.

Cases of anorexia have been reported.

Allergic reactions:

Infrequent allergic reactions to carboplatin have been reported, e.g., erythematous rash, fever with no apparent cause or pruritus. Rarely, anaphylaxis, angio-oedema and anaphylactoid reactions, including bronchospasm, urticaria and facial oedema have occurred. (See Warnings.)

Ototoxicity:

Subclinical decrease in hearing acuity, consisting of high-frequency (4000-8000 Hz) hearing loss determined by audiogram, has been reported in 15% of the patients treated with carboplatin. However, only 1% of patients present with clinical symptoms, manifested in the majority of cases by tinnitus. In patients who have been previously treated with cisplatin and have developed hearing loss related to such treatment, the hearing impairment may persist or worsen.

At higher than recommended doses in combination with other ototoxic agents, clinically significant hearing loss has been reported to occur in paediatric patients when carboplatin solution was administered.

Neurotoxicity:

The incidence of peripheral neuropathies after treatment with carboplatin is 4%. In the majority of the patients neurotoxicity is limited to paraesthesia and decreased deep tendon reflexes. The frequency and intensity of this side effect increases in elderly patients and those previously treated with cisplatin.

Paraesthesia present before commencing carboplatin therapy, particularly if related to prior cisplatin treatment, may persist or worsen during treatment with carboplatin.

Ocular toxicity:

Transient visual disturbances, sometimes including transient sight loss, have been reported rarely with platinum therapy. This is usually associated with high dose therapy in renally impaired patients.

Other:

Abnormalities of liver function tests (usually mild to moderate) have been reported with carboplatin in about one-third of the patients with normal baseline values. The alkaline phosphatase level is increased more frequently than SGOT, SGPT or total bilirubin. The majority of these abnormalities regress spontaneously during the course of treatment.

Infrequent events consisting of taste alteration, asthenia, alopecia, fever and chills without evidence of infection have occurred.

4.9 Overdose

There is no known antidote for carboplatin overdosage. The anticipated complications of overdosage would be related to myelosuppression as well as impairment of hepatic and renal function.

5. PHARMACOLOGICAL PROPERTIES

5.1 Pharmacodynamic properties

Carboplatin is an antineoplastic agent. Its activity has been demonstrated against several murine and human cell lines.

Carboplatin exhibited comparable activity to cisplatin against a wide range of tumours regardless of implant site.

Alkaline elution techniques and DNA binding studies have demonstrated the qualitatively similar modes of action of carboplatin and cisplatin. Carboplatin, like cisplatin, induces changes in the superhelical conformation of DNA which is consistent with a "DNA shortening effect".

5.2 Pharmacokinetic properties

Carboplatin has biochemical properties similar to those of cisplatin, thus producing predominantly interstrand and intrastrand DNA crosslinks. Following administration of carboplatin in man, linear relationships exist between dose and plasma concentrations of total and free ultrafilterable platinum. The area under the plasma concentration versus time curve for total platinum also shows a linear relationship with the dose when creatinine clearance exceeds 60ml/min.

Repeated dosing during four consecutive days did not produce an accumulation of platinum in plasma. Following the administration of carboplatin, reported values for the terminal elimination half-lives of free ultrafilterable platinum and carboplatin in man are approximately 6 hours and 1.5 hours respectively. During the initial phase, most of the free ultrafilterable platinum is present as carboplatin. The terminal half-life for total plasma platinum is 24 hours. Approximately 87% of plasma platinum is protein bound within 24 hours following administration. Carboplatin is excreted primarily in the urine, with recovery of approximately 70% of the administered platinum within 24 hours. Most of the drug is excreted in the first 6 hours. Total body and renal clearances of free ultrafilterable platinum correlate with the rate of glomerular filtration but not tubular secretion.

5.3 Preclinical safety data

Carboplatin has been shown to be embryotoxic and teratogenic in rats. (See para. 4.6, Pregnancy and Lactation.) It is mutagenic in vivo and in vitro and although the carcinogenic potential of carboplatin has not been studied, compounds with similar mechanisms of action and mutagenicity have been reported to be carcinogenic.

6. PHARMACEUTICAL PARTICULARS

6.1 List of excipients

Water for injections

Nitrogen

6.2 Incompatibilities

Needles or intravenous sets containing aluminium parts that may come into contact with carboplatin should not be used for preparation or administration of carboplatin.

6.3 Shelf life

18 months (unopened)

After dilution:

24 hours under refrigeration (2 - 8°C)

6.4 Special precautions for storage

Do not store above 25 °C. Keep container in the outer carton.

After dilution (see section 6.6.):

Chemical and physical in-use stability has been demonstrated for 24 hours at 25°C for solutions with a final concentration of carboplatin 0.4mg/ml or 2.0mg/ml after dilution of the carboplatin10mg/ml with glucose solution 5%.

From a microbiological point of view, the product should be used immediately. If not used immediately, in-use storage times and conditions prior to use are the responsibility of the user and would normally not be longer than 24 hours at 2 to 8°C, unless dilution has taken place in controlled and validated aseptic conditions.

6.5 Nature and contents of container

Amber vials of hydrolytic type I glass, packed in a carton.

Vials are closed with a rubber stopper with an aluminium crimp cap with flip-off.

Packs of 1 vial containing 50mg/5ml of carboplatin.

6.6 Instructions for use and handling

This product is for single dose use only.

Solutions should only be used if clear and particle free.

Trained personnel should prepare carboplatin for infusion in designated areas. Protective clothing (including gloves) should be worn. The eyes should be protected. In the event of contact with the eyes, wash with water and/or saline.

Pregnant staff should not handle cytotoxics.

Any unused product, syringes, containers, absorbent material or other waste material should be disposed of using adequate care and precautions. Excess material and body waste may be disposed of by placing in double sealed polythene bags and incinerating at a temperature of 1000°C. Liquid waste may be flushed with copious amounts of water.

Carboplatin for infusion may be prepared by dilution with Glucose 5% Solution.

Administrative Data

7. MARKETING AUTHORISATION HOLDER

CP Pharmaceuticals Ltd

Ash Road North

Wrexham LL13 9UF

United Kingdom

8. MARKETING AUTHORISATION NUMBER(S)

PL 04543/0459

9. DATE OF FIRST AUTHORISATION/RENEWAL OF THE AUTHORISATION

5th August 2003

10. DATE OF REVISION OF THE TEXT

Cardene 20 and 30mg

(Astellas Pharma Limited)

1. NAME OF THE MEDICINAL PRODUCT

Cardene 20 mg

Cardene 30 mg

2. QUALITATIVE AND QUANTITATIVE COMPOSITION

Nicardipine hydrochloride 20 mg

Nicardipine hydrochloride 30 mg

3. PHARMACEUTICAL FORM

Capsules

4. CLINICAL PARTICULARS

4.1 Therapeutic indications

Cardene is indicated for the prophylaxis of patients with chronic stable angina. For the treatment of hypertension considered to be mild to moderate in severity.

4.2 Posology and method of administration

Nicardipine should be taken with a little water.

Prophylaxis of chronic stable angina:

Starting dose: 20 mg every 8 hours titrating upwards as required.

Usual effective dose: 30 mg every 8 hours (range of total dose 60 mg - 120 mg per day).

Allow at least 3 days before increasing the dose of Cardene to ensure steady state plasma levels have been achieved.

Hypertension:

Starting dose: 20 mg every 8 hours titrating upwards as required.

Usual effective dose: 30 mg every 8 hours (range of total dose 60 mg - 120 mg per day).

Use in elderly:

Starting dose is 20 mg 3 times a day. Titrate upwards with care as nicardipine may lower systolic pressure more than diastolic pressure in these patients.

Children:

Cardene is not recommended in patients under the age of 18.

Cardene capsules are for oral administration.

4.3 Contraindications

(1) Pregnancy and lactation.

(2) Hypersensitivity to nicardipine hydrochloride or other dihydropyridines because of the theoretical risk of cross reactivity.

(3) Because part of the effect of nicardipine is secondary to reduced afterload, the drug should not be given to patients with advanced aortic stenosis. Reduction of diastolic pressure in these patients may worsen rather than improve myocardial infarction.

(4) Cardene should not be used in cardiogenic shock, clinically significant aortic stenosis, unstable angina, and during or within one month of a myocardial infarction.

(5) Cardene should not be used for acute attacks of angina.

(6) Cardene should not be used for secondary prevention of myocardial infarction.

4.4 Special warnings and special precautions for use

If used in combination with diuretics or beta-blockers, careful titration of Cardene is advised to avoid excessive reduction in blood pressure.

If switching from beta-blockers to Cardene, gradually reduce the beta-blocker dose (preferably over 8 - 10 days) since nicardipine gives no protection against the dangers of abrupt beta-blocker withdrawal.

Stop Cardene in patients experiencing ischaemic pain within 30 minutes of starting therapy or after increasing the dose.

Use in patients with congestive heart failure or poor cardiac reserve:

Haemodynamic studies in patients with heart failure have shown that nicardipine reduces afterload and improves overall haemodynamics. In one study, intravenous nicardipine reduced myocardial contractility in patients with severe heart failure despite increases in cardiac index and ejection fraction noted in the same patients.

Since nicardipine has not been extensively studied in patients with severe left ventricular dysfunction and cardiac failure one must consider that worsening of cardiac failure may occur.

Use in patients with impaired hepatic or renal function:

Since Cardene is subject to first-pass metabolism, use with caution in patients with impaired liver function or reduced hepatic blood flow. Patients with severe liver disease showed elevated blood levels and the half-life of nicardipine was prolonged. Cardene blood levels may also be elevated in some renally impaired patients. Therefore the lowest starting dose and extending the dosing interval should be individually considered in these patients.

Use in patients following a stroke (infarction or haemorrhage):

Avoid inducing systemic hypotension when administering Cardene to these patients.

Laboratory tests:

Transient elevations of alkaline phosphatase, serum bilirubin, SGPT, SGOT and glucose, have been observed. BUN and creatinine may also become elevated. While out-of-range values were seen in T_3, T_4 and TSH, the lack of consistent alterations suggest that any changes were not drug-related.

Treatment with short acting nicardipine may induce an exaggerated fall in blood pressure and reflex tachycardia which can cause cardiovascular complications such as myocardial and cerebrovascular ischaemia.

There has been some concern about increased mortality and morbidity in the treatment of ischaemic heart disease using higher than recommended doses of some other short-acting dihydropyridines.

4.5 Interaction with other medicinal products and other forms of Interaction

Digoxin

Careful monitoring of serum digoxin levels is advised in patients also receiving Cardene as levels may be increased.

Propanolol, Dipyridamole, Warfarin, Quinidine, Naproxen:

Therapeutic concentrations of these drugs does not change the *in vitro* plasma protein binding of nicardipine.

Cimetidine:

Cimetidine increases nicardipine plasma levels. Carefully monitor patients receiving both drugs.

Fentanyl Anaesthesia:

Severe hypotension has been reported during fentanyl anaesthesia with concomitant use of a beta-blocker and calcium blockade. Even though such interactions have not been seen in clinical trials, such hypotensive episodes should be vigorously treated with conventional therapy such as intravenous fluids.

Cyclosporin:

Monitor cyclosporin plasma levels and reduce dosage accordingly in patients concomitantly receiving nicardipine as elevated cyclosporin levels have been reported.

Rifampicin:

Rifampicin can interact with other dihydropyridines to substantially reduce their plasma levels and so rifampicin and nicardipine should be used together with caution.

As with other dihydropyridines, nicardipine should not be taken with grapefruit juice because bioavailability may be increased.

Cardene may be used in combination with beta-blocking and other anti-hypertensive drugs but the possibility of an additive effect resulting in postural hypotension should be considered.

4.6 Pregnancy and lactation

See contra-indications.

4.7 Effects on ability to drive and use machines

None known.

4.8 Undesirable effects

Majority are not serious and are expected consequences of the vasodilator effects of Cardene.

The most frequent side-effects reported are headache, pedal oedema, heat sensation and/or flushing, palpitations, nausea and dizziness.

Other side-effects noted in clinical trials include the following:

Cardiovascular System: As with the use of other short-acting dihydropyridines in patients with ischaemic heart disease, exacerbation of angina pectoris may occur frequently at the start of treatment with nicardipine capsules. The occurrence of myocardial infarction has been reported although it is not possible to distinguish such an event from the natural course of ischaemic heart disease.

Central nervous system: Drowsiness, insomnia, tinnitus, paraesthesia, functional disorders.

Skin: Itching, rashes.

Hepato-Renal: Impairment, frequency of micturition.

Dyspnoea, gastro-intestinal upset and, rarely, depression, impotence and thrombocytopenia, have also been reported.

4.9 Overdose

Symptoms may include marked hypotension, bradycardia, palpitations, flushing, drowsiness, confusion and slurred speech. In laboratory animals, overdosage also resulted in reversible hepatic function abnormalities, sporadic focal hepatic necrosis and progressive atrioventricular conduction block.

For treatment of overdose, standard measures including monitoring of cardiac and respiratory functions should be implemented. The patient should be positioned so as to avoid cerebral anoxia. Frequent blood pressure determinations are essential. Vasopressors are clinically indicated for patients exhibiting profound hypotension. Intravenous calcium gluconate may help reverse the effects of calcium entry blockade.

5. PHARMACOLOGICAL PROPERTIES

5.1 Pharmacodynamic properties

Cardene is a potent calcium antagonist. Pharmacological studies demonstrate its preferential high selectivity for the peripheral vasculature over the myocardium which accounts for its minimal negative inotropic effects. Cardene produces smooth muscle relaxation and marked peripheral vasodilatation.

In man Cardene produces a significant decrease in systemic vascular resistance, the degree of vasodilatation being more predominant in hypertensive patients than in normotensive subjects. Haemodynamic studies in patients with coronary artery disease and normal left ventricular function have shown significant increases in cardiac index and coronary blood flow, with little if any increase in left ventricular end-diastolic pressure.

Electrophysiologic effects: Electrophysiological studies in man show that Cardene does not depress sinus node function or atrial or ventricular conduction in patients with either normal or decreased electrical conduction systems. Refractory periods of the His-Purkinje system were actually shortened slightly by nicardipine and SA conduction time was improved.

5.2 Pharmacokinetic properties

Pharmacokinetics and metabolism: Nicardipine is rapidly and completely absorbed with plasma levels detectable 20 minutes following an oral dose. Maximal plasma levels are observed within 30 minutes to two hours (mean T_{max} = 1 hour). When given with a high fat meal peak plasma levels are reduced by 30%. Nicardipine is subject to saturable first-pass metabolism and the bioavailability is about 35% following a 30 mg oral dose at steady state.

The pharmacokinetics of Cardene are non-linear due to saturable hepatic first pass metabolism.

Steady state plasma levels are achieved after about 3 days of dosing at 20 and 30 mg tds and remain relatively constant over 28 days of dosing at 30 mg tds. Considerable intersubject variability in plasma levels is observed. Following dosing to steady state using doses of 30 and 40 mg (tds), the terminal plasma half-life of nicardipine averaged 8.6 hours. Nicardipine is highly protein-bound ($>$99%) in human plasma over a wide concentration range.

Nicardipine does not induce its own metabolism and does not induce hepatic microsomal enzymes.

5.3 Preclinical safety data

Please refer to section 4.6 Pregnancy and Lactation.

6. PHARMACEUTICAL PARTICULARS

6.1 List of excipients

Starch, Pregelatinised

Magnesium Stearate

Cardene 20mg *Capsule shell body*

Titanium Dioxide E171

Gelatin

Cardene 30mg *Capsule shell body*

Indigotine E132

Titanium Dioxide E171

Gelatin

Cardene 20mg and 30mg *Capsule shell cap*

Indigotine E132

Titanium Dioxide E171

Gelatin

6.2 Incompatibilities

None known.

6.3 Shelf life

Cardene 20mg

Securitainer: 60 months.

Blister packs of 21, 100 and 200 capsules: 60 months.

Blister packs of 56 and 84 capsules: 36 months.

Cardene 30mg

Securitainer: 60 months

Blister packs of 21, 56, 60, 100 and 200 capsules: 60 months.

Blister packs of 84 capsules: 36 months.

6.4 Special precautions for storage

Do not store above 25°C.

6.5 Nature and contents of container

Cardene 20mg

Securitainer packs of 50 and 100.

PVC/aluminium foil blister strips of 21, 56, 84,100 and 200 capsules.

Cardene 30mg

Securitainer packs of 50 and 100.

PVC/aluminium foil blister strips of 21, 56, 60, 84,100 and 200 capsules.

6.6 Instructions for use and handling

Not applicable.

Administrative Data

7. MARKETING AUTHORISATION HOLDER

Yamanouchi Pharma Ltd

Yamanouchi House

Pyrford Road

West Byfleet

Surrey

KT14 6RA

United Kingdom

8. MARKETING AUTHORISATION NUMBER(S)

Cardene 20mg - PL 00166/0181

Cardene 30mg - PL 00166/0182

9. DATE OF FIRST AUTHORISATION/RENEWAL OF THE AUTHORISATION

15 May 1998/ 15 July 2002

10. DATE OF REVISION OF THE TEXT

Date of partial revision = 13 November 2003.

11. Legal category

POM

Cardene SR 30 and 45mg

(Astellas Pharma Limited)

1. NAME OF THE MEDICINAL PRODUCT

Cardene SR 30

Cardene SR 45

2. QUALITATIVE AND QUANTITATIVE COMPOSITION

Nicardipine hydrochloride 30 mg

Nicardipine hydrochloride 45 mg

3. PHARMACEUTICAL FORM

Sustained release capsules

4. CLINICAL PARTICULARS

4.1 Therapeutic indications

Treatment of mild to moderate hypertension.

4.2 Posology and method of administration

Adults

Starting dose: 30 mg every 12 hours titrating upwards as required.

Usual effective dose: 45 mg every 12 hours (range 30 mg to 60 mg every 12 hours).

Individually adjust the dose for each patient. Where appropriate Cardene SR may also be used in combination with beta-blockers and/or diuretics.

Use in the elderly:

Starting dose: 30 mg every 12 hours. Titrate upwards with care as nicardipine may lower systolic pressure more than diastolic pressure in these patients.

Children:

Cardene SR is not recommended for use in patients under the age of 18.

4.3 Contraindications

i) Use in pregnancy and lactation.

ii) Hypersensitivity to nicardipine hydrochloride or other dihydropyridines because of the theoretical risk of cross reactivity.

iii) As part of the effect of nicardipine is secondary to reduced afterload, the drug should not be given to patients with advanced aortic stenosis. Reduction in diastolic pressure in these patients may worsen rather than improve myocardial oxygen balance.

iv) Cardene should not be used in cardiogenic shock, clinically significant aortic stenosis and during or within one month of a myocardial infarction.

v) Cardene should not be used for secondary prevention of myocardial infarction.

4.4 Special warnings and special precautions for use

If used in combination with diuretics or beta-blockers, careful titration of Cardene SR is advised to avoid excessive reduction in blood pressure.

If switching from beta-blockers to Cardene SR, gradually reduce the beta-blocker dose (preferably over 8 – 10 days) since nicardipine gives no protection against the dangers of abrupt beta-blocker withdrawal.

Stop Cardene SR in patients experiencing ischaemic pain within 30 minutes of starting therapy or after increasing the dose.

Use in patients with congestive heart failure or poor cardiac reserve:

Haemodynamic studies in patients with heart failure have shown that nicardipine reduces afterload and improves overall haemodynamics. In one study, intravenous nicardipine reduced myocardial contractility in patients with severe heart failure despite increases in cardiac index and ejection fraction noted in the same patients.

Since nicardipine has not been extensively studied in patients with severe left ventricular dysfunction and cardiac failure, one must consider that worsening of cardiac failure may occur.

Use in patients with impaired hepatic or renal function:

Since Cardene is subject to first-pass metabolism, use with caution in patients with impaired liver function or reduced hepatic blood flow. Patients with severe liver disease showed elevated blood levels and the half-life of nicardipine was prolonged. Cardene blood levels may also be elevated in some renally impaired patients. Therefore the lowest starting dose and extending the dosing interval should be individually considered in these patients.

Use in patients following a stroke (infarction or haemorrhage):

Avoid inducing systemic hypotension when administering Cardene SR to these patients.

Laboratory tests:

Transient elevations of alkaline phosphatase, serum bilirubin, SGPT, SGOT and glucose, have been observed. BUN and creatinine may also become elevated. While out-of-range values were seen in T_3, T_4 and TSH, the lack of consistent alterations suggest that any changes were not drug-related.

Treatment with short acting nicardipine may induce an exaggerated fall in blood pressure and reflex tachycardia which can cause cardiovascular complications such as myocardial and cerebrovascular ischaemia.

There has been some concern about increased mortality and morbidity in the treatment of ischaemic heart disease using higher than recommended doses of some other short-acting dihydropyridines.

4.5 Interaction with other medicinal products and other forms of Interaction

Digoxin

Careful monitoring of serum digoxin levels is advised in patients also receiving Cardene as levels may be increased.

Propranolol, Dipyridamole, Warfarin, Quinidine, Naproxen:

Therapeutic concentrations of these drugs does not change the *in vitro* plasma protein binding of nicardipine.

Cimetidine:

Cimetidine increases nicardipine plasma levels. Carefully monitor patients receiving both drugs.

Fentanyl Anaesthesia:

Severe hypotension has been reported during fentanyl anaesthesia with concomitant use of a beta-blocker and calcium blockade. Even though such interactions have not been seen in clinical trials, such hypotensive episodes should be vigorously treated with conventional therapy such as intravenous fluids.

Cyclosporin:

Monitor cyclosporin plasma levels and reduce dosage accordingly in patients concomitantly receiving nicardipine as elevated cyclosporin levels have been reported.

Rifampicin:

Rifampicin can interact with other dihydropyridines to substantially reduce their plasma levels and so rifampicin and nicardipine should be used together with caution.

As with other dihydropyridines, nicardipine should not be taken with grapefruit juice because bioavailability may be increased.

Cardene may be used in combination with beta-blocking and other anti-hypertensive drugs but the possibility of an additive effect resulting in postural hypotension should be considered.

4.6 Pregnancy and lactation

See contra-indications.

4.7 Effects on ability to drive and use machines

None known.

4.8 Undesirable effects

Most are expected consequences of the vasodilator effects of Cardene SR.

The most frequent side-effects reported are headache, pedal oedema, heat sensation and/or flushing, palpitations, nausea and dizziness.

Other side-effects noted in clinical trials include the following:

Cardiovascular System: As with the use of other sustained release dihydropyridines in patients with ischaemic heart disease, exacerbation of angina pectoris may occur rarely at the start of treatment with Cardene SR. The occurrence of myocardial infarction has been reported although it is not possible to distinguish such an event from the natural course of ischaemic heart disease.

Central Nervous System: Drowsiness, insomnia, tinnitus, paraesthesia, functional disorders.

Skin: Itching, rashes.

Hepato-Renal: Impairment, frequency.

Dyspnoea, gastro-intestinal upset and, rarely, depression, impotence and thrombocytopenia, have also been reported.

4.9 Overdose

Symptoms may include marked hypotension, bradycardia, palpitations, flushing, drowsiness, confusion and slurred speech. In laboratory animals, overdosage also resulted in reversible hepatic function abnormalities, sporadic focal hepatic necrosis and progressive atrioventricular conduction block.

Use routine measures (eg gastric lavage) including monitoring of cardiac and respiratory functions. Position the patient to avoid cerebral anoxia. Frequent blood pressure determinations are essential. Vasopressors are clinically indicated for patients exhibiting the effects of calcium entry blockade.

5. PHARMACOLOGICAL PROPERTIES

5.1 Pharmacodynamic properties

Mode of action

Cardene is a potent calcium channel blocker. Pharmacological studies suggest it is highly selective for the peripheral vasculature over the myocardium accounting for its minimal negative inotropic effects and marked peripheral vasodilatation when used clinically.

In mild to moderate hypertensive patients Cardene SR has been shown to reduce blood pressure and maintain control over 24 hours, only if the doses are regularly administered exactly 12 hours apart.

Electrophysiologic effects:

Electrophysiological studies in man show that Cardene does not depress sinus node function or atrial or ventricular conduction in patients with either normal or decreased electrical conduction systems. Refractory periods of the His-Purkinje system were actually shortened slightly by nicardipine and SA conduction time was improved.

5.2 Pharmacokinetic properties

Cardene Capsules are completely absorbed with plasma levels detectable 20 minutes following an oral dose. Maximal plasma levels are generally achieved between one and four hours. Cardene SR is subject to saturable first pass metabolism with somewhat lower bioavailability than the standard capsule formulation of nicardipine (about 35% following a 30mg oral standard capsule at steady state) except at the 60mg dose. Minimum plasma levels produced by equivalent daily doses are similar. Cardene SR thus exhibits significantly reduced fluctuation in plasma levels in comparison to standard nicardipine capsules.

When Cardene SR is taken with a high fat meal, fluctuation in plasma levels are reduced.

Cardene is extensively metabolised by the liver; none of the metabolites possess significant biological activity.

5.3 Preclinical safety data

Please refer to section 4.6 Pregnancy and Lactation.

6. PHARMACEUTICAL PARTICULARS

6.1 List of excipients

Starch, Pregelatinised

Magnesium Stearate

Microcrystalline cellulose

Starch

Lactose

Methacrylic acid co-polymer

Cardene SR 30mg *Capsule shell body*

Titanium Dioxide E171

Gelatin

Cardene SR 45mg *Capsule shell body*

Titanium Dioxide E171

Gelatin

Indigotine E132

Cardene SR 30mg *Capsule shell cap*

Titanium Dioxide E171

Gelatin

Cardene SR 45mg *Capsule shell cap*

Titanium Dioxide E171

Gelatin

Indigotine E132

6.2 Incompatibilities

None known.

6.3 Shelf life

60 months.

6.4 Special precautions for storage

Protect from light and excessive humidity. Store below 25°C.

6.5 Nature and contents of container

Blister packs of 56

Blister packs of 14

Securitainers of 100

6.6 Instructions for use and handling
No special instructions required.

Administrative Data
7. MARKETING AUTHORISATION HOLDER
Yamanouchi Pharma Ltd
Yamanouchi House
Pyrford Road
West Byfleet
Surrey
KT14 6RA

8. MARKETING AUTHORISATION NUMBER(S)
Cardene SR 30mg - PL 00166/0183
Cardene SR 45mg - PL 00166/0184

9. DATE OF FIRST AUTHORISATION/RENEWAL OF THE AUTHORISATION
1 July 1998/ 15 July 2002

10. DATE OF REVISION OF THE TEXT
Date of partial revision = 8th April 2004

11. Legal Category
POM

Cardicor 1.25mg, 2.5mg, 3.75mg, 5mg, 7.5mg, 10mg Film Coated Tablets

(Merck Pharmaceuticals)

1. NAME OF THE MEDICINAL PRODUCT
Cardicor 1.25 mg film-coated tablets▼
Cardicor 2.5 mg film-coated tablets▼
Cardicor 3.75 mg film-coated tablets▼
Cardicor 5 mg film-coated tablets▼
Cardicor 7.5 mg film-coated tablets▼
Cardicor 10 mg film-coated tablets▼

2. QUALITATIVE AND QUANTITATIVE COMPOSITION
Each tablet contains 1.25, 2.5, 3.75, 5, 7.5 or 10 mg bisoprolol fumarate (2:1)

For excipients, see section 6.1.

3. PHARMACEUTICAL FORM
Film-coated tablet.

off-white, round film-coated tablets

4. CLINICAL PARTICULARS
4.1 Therapeutic indications
Treatment of stable chronic moderate to severe heart failure with reduced systolic ventricular function (ejection fraction ⩽ 35%, based on echocardiography) in addition to ACE inhibitors, and diuretics, and optionally cardiac glycosides (for additional information see section 5.1).

4.2 Posology and method of administration
The patients should have stable chronic heart failure without acute failure during the past six weeks and a mainly unchanged basic therapy during the past two weeks. They should be treated at optimal dose with an ACE inhibitor (or other vasodilator in case of intolerance to ACE inhibitors) and a diuretic, and optionally cardiac glycosides, prior to the administration of bisoprolol.

It is recommended that the treating physician should be experienced in the management of chronic heart failure.

Warning: The treatment of stable chronic heart failure with bisoprolol has to be initiated with a titration phase as given in the description below.

The treatment with bisoprolol is to be started with a gradual uptitration according to the following steps:

- 1.25 mg once daily for 1 week, if well tolerated increase to
- 2.5 mg once daily for a further week, if well tolerated increase to
- 3.75 mg once daily for a further week, if well tolerated increase to
- 5 mg once daily for the 4 following weeks, if well tolerated increase to
- 7.5 mg once daily for the 4 following weeks, if well tolerated increase to
- 10 mg once daily for the maintenance therapy.

After initiation of treatment with 1.25 mg, the patients should be observed over a period of approximately 4 hours (especially as regards blood pressure, heart rate, conduction disturbances, signs of worsening of heart failure).

The maximum recommended dose is 10 mg once daily.

Occurrence of adverse events may prevent all patients being treated with the maximum recommended dose. If necessary, the dose reached can also be decreased step by step. The treatment may be interrupted if necessary and reintroduced as appropriate. During the titration phase, in case of worsening of the heart failure or intolerance, it is recommended first to reduce the dose of bisoprolol, or to stop immediately if necessary (in case of severe hypotension, worsening of heart failure with acute pulmonary oedema, cardiogenic shock, symptomatic bradycardia or AV block).

Treatment of stable chronic heart failure with bisoprolol is generally a long-term treatment.

The treatment with bisoprolol is not recommended to be stopped abruptly since this might lead to a transitory worsening of heart failure. If discontinuation is necessary, the dose should be gradually decreased divided into halves weekly.

Bisoprolol tablets should be taken in the morning and can be taken with food. They should be swallowed with liquid and should not be chewed.

Renal or liver insufficiency
There is no information regarding pharmacokinetics of bisoprolol in patients with chronic heart failure and with impaired liver or renal function. Uptitration of the dose in these populations should therefore be made with additional caution.

Elderly
No dosage adjustment is required.

Children
There is no paediatric experience with bisoprolol, therefore its use cannot be recommended for children.

4.3 Contraindications
Bisoprolol is contraindicated in chronic heart failure patients with:

- acute heart failure or during episodes of heart failure decompensation requiring i.v. inotropic therapy
- cardiogenic shock
- AV block of second or third degree (without a pacemaker)
- sick sinus syndrome
- sinoatrial block
- bradycardia with less than 60 beats/min before the start of therapy
- hypotension (systolic blood pressure less than 100 mm Hg)
- severe bronchial asthma or severe chronic obstructive pulmonary disease
- late stages of peripheral arterial occlusive disease and Raynaud's syndrome
- untreated phaeochromocytoma (see 4.4)
- metabolic acidosis
- hypersensitivity to bisoprolol or to any of the excipients

4.4 Special warnings and special precautions for use
Bisoprolol must be used with caution in:

- bronchospasm (bronchial asthma, obstructive airways diseases)
- diabetes mellitus with large fluctuations in blood glucose values; symptoms of hypoglycaemia can be masked
- strict fasting
- ongoing desensitisation therapy
- AV block of first degree
- Prinzmetal's angina
- peripheral arterial occlusive disease (intensification of complaints might happen especially during the start of therapy)
- General anaesthesia

In patients undergoing general anaesthesia beta-blockade reduces the incidence of arrhythmias and myocardial ischemia during induction and intubation, and the post-operative period. It is currently recommended that maintenance beta-blockade be continued peri-operatively. The anaesthetist must be aware of beta-blockade because of the potential for interactions with other drugs, resulting in bradyarrhythmias, attenuation of the reflex tachycardia and the decreased reflex ability to compensate for blood loss. If it is thought necessary to withdraw beta-blocker therapy before surgery, this should be done gradually and completed about 48 hours before anaesthesia.

There is no therapeutic experience of bisoprolol treatment of heart failure in patients with the following diseases and conditions:

- NYHA class II heart failure
- insulin dependent diabetes mellitus (type I)
- impaired renal function (serum creatinine >300 micromol/l)
- impaired liver function
- patients older than 80 years
- restrictive cardiomyopathy
- congenital heart disease
- haemodynamically significant organic valvular disease
- myocardial infarction within 3 months

Combination of bisoprolol with calcium antagonists of the verapamil and diltiazem type, with Class I antiarrhythmic drugs and with centrally acting antihypertensive drugs is generally not recommended, for details please refer to section 4.5.

In bronchial asthma or other chronic obstructive lung diseases, which may cause symptoms, bronchodilating therapy should be given concomitantly. Occasionally an increase of the airway resistance may occur in patients with asthma, therefore the dose of beta2-stimulants may have to be increased.

As with other beta-blockers, bisoprolol may increase both the sensitivity towards allergens and the severity of anaphylactic reactions. Adrenaline treatment does not always give the expected therapeutic effect.

Patients with psoriasis or with a history of psoriasis should only be given beta-blockers (e.g. bisoprolol) after carefully balancing the benefits against the risks.

In patients with phaeochromocytoma bisoprolol must not be administered until after alpha-receptor blockade.

Under treatment with bisoprolol the symptoms of a thyreotoxicosis may be masked.

The initiation of treatment with bisoprolol necessitates regular monitoring. For the posology and method of administration please refer to section 4.2.

The cessation of therapy with bisoprolol should not be done abruptly unless clearly indicated. For further information please refer to section 4.2.

4.5 Interaction with other medicinal products and other forms of Interaction
Combinations not recommended
Calcium antagonists of the verapamil type and to a lesser extent of the diltiazem type: Negative influence on contractility and atrio-ventricular conduction. Intravenous administration of verapamil in patients on β-blocker treatment may lead to profound hypotension and atrioventricular block.

Class I antiarrhythmic drugs (e.g. quinidine, disopyramide; lidocaine, phenytoin; flecainide, propafenone): Effect on atrio-ventricular conduction time may be potentiated and negative inotropic effect increased.

Centrally acting antihypertensive drugs such as clonidine and others (e.g. methyldopa, moxonodine, rilmenidine): Concomitant use of centrally acting antihypertensive drugs may worsen heart failure by a decrease in the central sympathetic tonus (reduction of heart rate and cardiac output, vasodilation). Abrupt withdrawal, particularly if prior to beta-blocker discontinuation, may increase risk of "rebound hypertension".

Combinations to be used with caution
Calcium antagonists of the dihydropyridine type such as felodipine and amlodipine: Concomitant use may increase the risk of hypotension, and an increase in the risk of a further deterioration of the ventricular pump function in patients with heart failure cannot be excluded.

Class-III antiarrhythmic drugs (e.g. amiodarone): Effect on atrio-ventricular conduction time may be potentiated.

Topical beta-blockers (e.g. eye drops for glaucoma treatment) may add to the systemic effects of bisoprolol.

Parasympathomimetic drugs: Concomitant use may increase atrio-ventricular conduction time and the risk of bradycardia.

Insulin and oral antidiabetic drugs: Intensification of blood sugar lowering effect. Blockade of beta-adrenoreceptors may mask symptoms of hypoglycaemia.

Anaesthetic agents: Attenuation of the reflex tachycardia and increase of the risk of hypotension (for further information on general anaesthesia see also section 4.4.).

Digitalis glycosides: Reduction of heart rate, increase of atrio-ventricular conduction time.

Non-steroidal anti-inflammatory drugs (NSAIDs): NSAIDs may reduce the hypotensive effect of bisoprolol.

β-Sympathomimetic agents (e.g. isoprenaline, dobutamine): Combination with bisoprolol may reduce the effect of both agents.

Sympathomimetics that activate both β- and α-adrenoceptors (e.g. noradrenaline, adrenaline): Combination with bisoprolol may unmask the α-adrenoceptor-mediated vasoconstrictor effects of these agents leading to blood pressure increase and exacerbated intermittent claudication. Such interactions are considered to be more likely with nonselective β-blockers.

Concomitant use with antihypertensive agents as well as with other drugs with blood pressure lowering potential (e.g. tricyclic antidepressants, barbiturates, phenothiazines) may increase the risk of hypotension.

Combinations to be considered
Mefloquine: increased risk of bradycardia

Monoamine oxidase inhibitors (except MAO-B inhibitors): Enhanced hypotensive effect of the beta-blockers but also risk for hypertensive crisis.

4.6 Pregnancy and lactation
Pregnancy:
Bisoprolol has pharmacological effects that may cause harmful effects on pregnancy and/or the fetus/newborn. In general, beta-adrenoceptor blockers reduce placental perfusion, which has been associated with growth retardation, intrauterine death, abortion or early labour. Adverse effects (e.g. hypoglycaemia and bradycardia) may occur in the fetus and newborn infant. If treatment with beta-adrenoceptor blockers is necessary, beta1-selective adrenoceptor blockers are preferable.

Bisoprolol should not be used during pregnancy unless clearly necessary. If treatment with bisoprolol is considered necessary, the uteroplacental blood flow and the fetal growth should be monitored. In case of harmful effects on pregnancy or the fetus alternative treatment should be considered. The newborn infant must be closely monitored. Symptoms of hypoglycaemia and bradycardia are generally to be expected within the first 3 days.

Lactation:

It is not known whether this drug is excreted in human milk. Therefore, breastfeeding is not recommended during administration of bisoprolol.

4.7 Effects on ability to drive and use machines
In a study with coronary heart disease patients bisoprolol did not impair driving performance. However, due to individual variations in reactions to the drug, the ability to drive a vehicle or to operate machinery may be impaired. This should be considered particularly at start of treatment and upon change of medication as well as in conjunction with alcohol.

4.8 Undesirable effects
Clinical trial data

The table below shows incidences of adverse events reported from both the placebo and the bisoprolol cohort of the CIBIS II trial. Regardless of causal relationship all adverse events are included. Each patient is only counted once for each adverse event occurring in at least 5% of the study population.

(see Table 1)

Post-marketing data

The following data results from post-marketing experience with bisoprolol:

Common (>1% and <10%), uncommon (>0.1% and <1%), rare (>0.01% and <0.1%), very rare (<0.01%), single cases.

Cardiac disorders:

Uncommon: bradycardia, AV-stimulus disturbances, worsening of heart failure.

Ear and labyrinth disorders:

Rare: hearing impairment.

Eye disorders:

Rare: reduced tear flow (to be considered if the patient uses lenses).

Very rare: conjunctivitis.

Gastrointestinal disorders:

Common: Nausea, vomiting, diarrhoea, constipation.

General disorders:

Uncommon: Muscular weakness and cramps.

Hepatobiliary disorders:

Rare: increased liver enzymes (ALAT, ASAT), hepatitis.

Metabolism and nutrition disorders:

Rare: Increased triglycerides.

Nervous system disorders:

Common: Tiredness*, exhaustion*, dizziness*, headache*.

Uncommon: Sleep disturbances, depression.

Rare: Nightmares, hallucinations.

Reproductive system and breast disorders:

Rare: Potency disorders.

Respiratory, thoracic and mediastinal disorders:

Uncommon: Bronchospasm in patients with bronchial asthma or a history of obstructive airways disease.

Rare: allergic rhinitis.

Skin and subcutaneous tissue disorders:

Rare: hypersensitivity reactions (itching, flush, rash).

Very rare: beta-blockers may provoke or worsen psoriasis or induce psoriasis-like rash, alopecia.

Vascular disorders:

Common: Feeling of coldness or numbness in the extremities.

Uncommon: orthostatic hypotension.

*These symptoms especially occur at the beginning of the therapy. They are generally mild and usually disappear within 1-2 weeks.

4.9 Overdose
With overdose (e.g. daily dose of 15 mg instead of 7.5 mg) third degree AV-block, bradycardia, and dizziness have been reported. In general the most common signs expected with overdosage of a beta-blocker are bradycardia, hypotension, bronchospasm, acute cardiac insufficiency and hypoglycaemia. To date a few cases of overdose (maximum: 2000 mg) with bisoprolol have been reported in patients suffering from hypertension and/or coronary heart disease showing bradycardia and/or hypotension; all patients recovered. There is a wide interindividual variation in sensitivity to one single high dose of bisoprolol and patients with heart failure are probably very sensitive. Therefore it is mandatory to initiate the treatment of these patients with a gradual uptitration according to the scheme given in section 4.2.

If overdose occurs, bisoprolol treatment should be stopped and supportive and symptomatic treatment should be provided. Limited data suggest that bisoprolol is hardly dialysable. Based on the expected pharmacologic actions and recommendations for other beta-blockers, the following general measures should be considered when clinically warranted.

Bradycardia: Administer intravenous atropine. If the response is inadequate, isoprenaline or another agent with positive chronotropic properties may be given cautiously. Under some circumstances, transvenous pacemaker insertion may be necessary.

Hypotension: Intravenous fluids and vasopressors should be administered. Intravenous glucagon may be useful.

AV block (second or third degree): Patients should be carefully monitored and treated with isoprenaline infusion or transvenous cardiac pacemaker insertion.

Acute worsening of heart failure: Administer i.v. diuretics, inotropic agents, vasodilating agents.

Bronchospasm: Administer bronchodilator therapy such as isoprenaline, beta2-sympathomimetic drugs and/or aminophylline.

Hypoglycaemia: Administer i.v. glucose.

5. PHARMACOLOGICAL PROPERTIES

5.1 Pharmacodynamic properties
Pharmacotherapeutic group: Beta blocking agents, selective

ATC Code: C07AB07

Bisoprolol is a highly beta1-selective-adrenoceptor blocking agent, lacking intrinsic stimulating and relevant membrane stabilising activity. It only shows low affinity to the beta2-receptor of the smooth muscles of bronchi and vessels as well as to the beta2-receptors concerned with metabolic regulation. Therefore, bisoprolol is generally not to be expected to influence the airway resistance and beta2-mediated metabolic effects. Its beta1-selectivity extends beyond the therapeutic dose range.

In total 2647 patients were included in the CIBIS II trial. 83% (n = 2202) were in NYHA class III and 17% (n = 445) were in NYHA class IV. They had stable symptomatic systolic heart failure (ejection fraction <35%, based on echocardiography). Total mortality was reduced from 17.3% to 11.8% (relative reduction 34%). A decrease in sudden death (3.6% vs 6.3%, relative reduction 44%) and a reduced number of heart failure episodes requiring hospital admission (12% vs 17.6%, relative reduction 36%) was observed. Finally, a significant improvement of the functional status according to NYHA classification has been shown. During the initiation and titration of bisoprolol hospital admission due to bradycardia (0.53%), hypotension (0.23%), and acute decompensation (4.97%) were observed, but they were not more frequent than in the placebo-group (0%, 0.3% and 6.74%). The numbers of fatal and disabling strokes during the total study period were 20 in the bisoprolol group and 15 in the placebo group.

Bisoprolol is already used for the treatment of hypertension and angina.

In acute administration in patients with coronary heart disease without chronic heart failure bisoprolol reduces the heart rate and stroke volume and thus the cardiac output and oxygen consumption. In chronic administration the initially elevated peripheral resistance decreases.

5.2 Pharmacokinetic properties
Bisoprolol is absorbed and has a biological availability of about 90% after oral administration. The plasma protein binding of bisoprolol is about 30%. The distribution volume is 3.5 l/kg. Total clearance is approximately 15 l/h. The half-life in plasma of 10-12 hours gives a 24 hour effect after dosing once daily.

Bisoprolol is excreted from the body by two routes. 50% is metabolised by the liver to inactive metabolites which are then excreted by the kidneys. The remaining 50% is excreted by the kidneys in an unmetabolised form. Since the elimination takes place in the kidneys and the liver to the same extent a dosage adjustment is not required for patients with impaired liver function or renal insufficiency. The pharmacokinetics in patients with stable chronic heart failure and with impaired liver or renal function has not been studied.

The kinetics of bisoprolol are linear and independent of age.

In patients with chronic heart failure (NYHA stage III) the plasma levels of bisoprolol are higher and the half-life is prolonged compared to healthy volunteers. Maximum plasma concentration at steady state is 64+21 ng/ml at a daily dose of 10 mg and the half-life is 17+5 hours.

5.3 Preclinical safety data
Preclinical data reveal no special hazard for humans based on conventional studies of safety pharmacology, repeated dose toxicity, genotoxicity or carcinogenicity. Like other beta-blockers, bisoprolol caused maternal (decreased food intake and decreased body weight) and embryo/fetal toxicity (increased incidence of resorptions, reduced birth weight of the offspring, retarded physical development) at high doses but was not teratogenic.

6. PHARMACEUTICAL PARTICULARS

6.1 List of excipients
Tablet core: Silica, colloidal anhydrous; magnesium stearate, crospovidone, pregelatinised maize starch, maize starch, microcrystalline cellulose, calcium hydrogen phosphate, anhydrous.

Film coating: Dimethicone, talc, macrogol 400, titanium dioxide (E171), hypromellose.

6.2 Incompatibilities
Not applicable.

6.3 Shelf life
3 years.

6.4 Special precautions for storage
Do not store above 25 °C.

6.5 Nature and contents of container
The container is a blister, which is made of a polyvinylchloride base film and an aluminium cover foil.

Pack sizes: 20, 28, 30, 50, 56, 60, 90 and 100 tablets.

Not all pack sizes may be marketed.

6.6 Instructions for use and handling
No special requirements.

7. MARKETING AUTHORISATION HOLDER
E Merck Ltd
Harrier House
High Street
West Drayton
Middlesex
UB7 7QG
UK

8. MARKETING AUTHORISATION NUMBER(S)
PL 0493/0179-0184

9. DATE OF FIRST AUTHORISATION/RENEWAL OF THE AUTHORISATION
4 June 2004

10. DATE OF REVISION OF THE TEXT
16 May 2005

Table 1

Preferred Term WHO	Placebo (n=1321)		Bisoprolol (n=1328)	
	Pat. with AE	% Pat. with AE	Pat. with AE	% Pat. with AE
Cardiac failure	301	22.8	244	18.4
Dyspnoea	224	17.0	183	13.8
Dizziness	126	9.5	177	13.3
Cardiomyopathy	132	10.0	141	10.6
Bradycardia	60	4.5	202	15.2
Hypotension	96	7.3	152	11.4
Tachycardia	144	10.9	79	5.9
Fatigue	94	7.1	123	9.3
Viral infection	75	5.7	86	6.5
Pneumonia	69	5.2	65	4.9

AE = Adverse Events

Cardiolite

(Bristol-Myers Squibb Pharmaceuticals Ltd)

1. NAME OF THE MEDICINAL PRODUCT
CARDIOLITE®,

Kit for the preparation of Technetium Tc-99m Sestamibi.

2. QUALITATIVE AND QUANTITATIVE COMPOSITION
1 vial contains
Active ingredients

Tetrakis (2-methoxy isobutyl isonitrile) Copper (I) Tetrafluoroborate	1.00 mg
Stannous chloride dihydrate	0.075 mg
L-Cysteine hydrochloride monohydrate	1.0 mg

3. PHARMACEUTICAL FORM
Powder for injection.

4. CLINICAL PARTICULARS
4.1 Therapeutic indications
For intravenous injection after reconstitution with Sodium pertechnetate [^{99m} Tc] solution and may be used for:

Adjunct for diagnosis of ischaemic heart disease.

Adjunct for diagnosis and localisation of myocardial infarction.

Assessment of global ventricular function (first pass technique for determination of ejection fraction and/or regional wall motion).

A second line diagnostic aid in the investigation of patients with suspected breast cancer when the results of mammography are unsatisfactory or equivocal, particularly in patients with dense breasts.

Diagnostic aid in the investigation of patients with recurrent or persistent hyper-pararathyroidism.

4.2 Posology and method of administration
The vial is reconstituted with a maximum of 11.1 GBq (300mCi) of oxidant-free Sodium Pertechnetate Tc-99m Injection Ph. Eur. in 1-3 ml. Radiochemical purity should be checked prior to patient administration (see section 6.6).

The suggested dose range for intravenous administration to a patient of average weight

(70 kg) is:

Diagnosis of reduced coronary perfusion and myocardial infarction:

185 - 740 MBq

Assessment of global ventricular function:

600 - 800 MBq

Injected as a bolus

For diagnosis of ischaemic heart disease two injections (stress and rest) are required in order to differentiate transiently from persistently reduced myocardial uptake. Not more than a total of 925 MBq should be administered by these two injections which should be done at least six hours apart but may be performed in either order. After the stress injection, exercise should be encouraged for an additional one minute (if possible).

For diagnosis of myocardial infarction one injection at rest may be sufficient.

For breast imaging: 740 - 925 MBq
Injected as a bolus.

For parathyroid imaging: 185 - 740 MBq
Injected as a bolus

(The dose used should in every case be as low as reasonably practical).

Cardiac Imaging: If possible, patients should fast for **at least** four hours prior to the study. It is recommended that patients eat a light fatty meal or drink a glass or two of milk after each injection, prior to imaging. This will promote rapid hepatobiliary clearance of Technetium Tc-99m Sestamibi resulting in less liver activity in the image.

The heart to background ratio will increase with time but the ideal imaging time, reflecting the best compromise between heart count rate and contrast, is approximately 1-2 hours after rest injection and stress injection. There is no evidence for significant changes in myocardial tracer concentration or redistribution, therefore imaging for up to 6 hours post injection is possible.

Either planar or tomographic imaging can be performed for diagnosis of ischaemic heart disease and myocardial infarction. Both may be performed ECG gated.

For planar imaging the standard three view (anterior, LAO 45°, LAO 70° or LL) planar projections should be used (e.g. 5-10 minutes each).

For tomographic imaging each projection should be acquired for approximately 20-40 seconds depending on injected dose.

For assessment of **global ventricular function** the same standard techniques and projections can be used, as established for Tc-99m first pass ejection studies; data should be acquired in list or fast frame mode in a computer using a high count rate scintillation camera. Gated Blood Pool Imaging protocols may be used for assessment of regional wall motion, however, they must only be evaluated visually.

Breast imaging is optimally initiated 5 to 10 minutes post injection with the patient in the prone position with breast freely pendant. A 10 minute lateral image of the breast suspected of containing cancer should be obtained with the camera face as close to the breast as practical.

The patient should then be repositioned so that the contralateral breast is pendant and a lateral image of it should be obtained. An anterior supine image may then be obtained with the patient's arms behind her head.

Parathyroid imaging depends on whether subtraction technique or wash-out technique is used. For the subtraction technique, either sodium iodide (I-123) or Tc 99m pertechnetate can be used. When I-123 is used, 11 to 22 MBq of oral sodium iodide (I-123) are administered. Four hours after the administration of I-123, I-123 neck and thorax images are obtained. After I-123 image acquisition, 185 to 370 MBq of Tc 99m Sestamibi are injected and images acquired 10 minutes post injection. When pertechnetate is used, 37 to 148 MBq of sodium pertechnetate are injected and neck and thorax images are acquired 30 minutes later. After image acquisition, 185-370 MBq of Tc 99m Sestamibi are injected and images acquired 10 minutes post injection

If double-phase technique is used, 370 to 740 MBq of Tc-99m Sestamibi are injected and the first neck and thorax image obtained 10 minutes later. After a wash-out period of 1 to 2 hours, neck and thorax imaging is again performed.

4.3 Contraindications
Pregnancy.

4.4 Special warnings and special precautions for use
Radiopharmaceutical agents should be used only by qualified personnel with the appropriate government authorisation for use and manipulation of radionuclides.

This radiopharmaceutical may be received, used and administered only by authorised persons in designated clinical settings. Its receipt, storage, use, transfer and disposal are subject to the regulations and/or appropriate licences of the local competent official organisation.

Radiopharmaceuticals should be prepared by the user in a manner which satisfies both radiation safety and pharmaceutical quality requirements. Appropriate aseptic precautions should be taken, complying with the requirements of Good Manufacturing Practice for pharmaceuticals.

Contents of the vial are intended only for use in the preparation of Technetium Tc-99m Sestamibi and are not to be administered directly to the patient without first undergoing the preparative procedure.

Safety and efficacy in children below the age of 18 years have not been established.

PROPER HYDRATION AND FREQUENT URINATION ARE NECESSARY TO REDUCE BLADDER IRRADIATION.

IN CASE OF KIDNEY FAILURE, EXPOSURE TO IONISING RADIATION CAN BE INCREASED. THIS MUST BE TAKEN INTO ACCOUNT WHEN CALCULATING THE ACTIVITY TO BE ADMINISTERED.

4.5 Interaction with other medicinal products and other forms of Interaction
No drug interactions have been described to date.

4.6 Pregnancy and lactation
When it is necessary to administer radioactive products to women of childbearing potential, information should be sought about pregnancy. Any women who has missed a period should be assumed to be pregnant until proven otherwise. Where uncertainty exists it is important that radiation exposure should be the minimum consistent with obtaining the desired clinical information. Alternative techniques which do not involve ionising radiation should be considered.

The anticipated dose to the uterus from a 740 MBq rest injection would be 5.8 mGy. A radiation dose above 0.5 mGy (approximately equivalent to that exposure from annual background radiation) could potentially result in risk to the foetus. It is therefore contraindicated in women known to be pregnant.

Before administering a radioactive medicinal product to a mother who is breast feeding consideration should be given as to whether the investigation could be reasonably delayed until after the mother has ceased breast feeding and as to whether the most appropriate choice of radiopharmaceutical has been made, bearing in mind the secretion of activity in breast milk.

If the administration is considered necessary, breast feeding should be interrupted for 24 hours and the expressed feeds discarded. It is usual to advise that breastfeeding can be restarted when the level in the milk will not result in a radiation dose to the child greater than 1 mSv.

4.7 Effects on ability to drive and use machines
Effects on the ability to drive and use machines have not been described.

4.8 Undesirable effects
Immediately after injection of Technetium Tc-99m Sestamibi, a small percentage of patients experienced a metallic and bitter taste, transient headache, flushing and a non-itching rash. Few cases of oedema, injection site inflammation, dyspepsia, nausea, vomiting, pruritus, rash, urticaria, dry mouth, fever dizziness, fatigue, dyspnoea and hypotension have been attributed to administration of the agent. Seizures have been reported very rarely (<0.001%) after administration; a causal relationship to Cardiolite has not been established.

For each patient, exposure to ionising radiation must be justified on the basis of likely benefit. The activity administered must be such that the resulting radiation dose is as low as reasonably achievable bearing in mind the need to obtain the intended diagnostic or therapeutic result.

Exposure to ionising radiation is linked with cancer induction and a potential for development of hereditary defects. For diagnostic nuclear medicine investigations the current evidence suggests that these adverse effects will occur with low frequency because of the low radiation doses incurred.

For most diagnostic investigations using a nuclear medicine procedure the radiation dose delivered (effective dose/ EDE) is less than 20 mSv. Higher doses may be justified in some clinical circumstances.

4.9 Overdose
In the event of administration of a radiation overdose with Technetium Tc-99m Sestamibi the absorbed dose to the patient should be reduced where possible by increasing the elimination of the radionuclide from the body by frequent micturation and defaecation.

5. PHARMACOLOGICAL PROPERTIES
5.1 Pharmacodynamic properties
Pharmacodynamic effects are not expected after administration of Cardiolite.

5.2 Pharmacokinetic properties
After reconstitution with Sodium Pertechnetate Tc-99m Injection, Ph. Eur. solution, the following complex forms (Technetium Tc-99m Sestamibi):

Tc-99m $(MIBI)_6^+$ Where: MIBI = 2-methoxyisobutylisonitrile

Like Thallous Chloride T1 201, this cationic complex accumulates in the viable myocardial tissue proportional to the circulation. Scintigraphic pictures which were obtained after i.v. injection of Technetium Tc-99m Sestamibi to animals and man are comparable with those obtained with Thallous Chloride T1 201. This correlation applies to normal as well as infarcted and ischaemic cardiac tissue.

Technetium Tc-99m Sestamibi from the blood is rapidly distributed into the tissue: 5 minutes after injection only about 8% of the injected dose is still in circulation.

Animal experiments have shown that uptake is not dependent on the functional capability of the sodium-potassium pump.

Elimination

The major metabolic pathway for clearance of Technetium Tc-99m Sestamibi is the hepatobiliary system. Activity from the gallbladder appears in the intestine within one hour of injection. About twenty-seven percent of the injected dose is cleared through renal elimination after 24 hours and approximately thirty-three percent of the injected dose is cleared through the faeces in 48 hours. At five minutes post injection about 8% of the injected dose remains in circulation.

Half-Life

The biological myocardial T½ is approximately seven (7) hours at rest and stress. The effective T½ (which includes biological and physical half-lives) is approximately three (3) hours.

Myocardial uptake

Myocardial uptake which is coronary flow dependent is 1.5% of the injected dose at stress and 1.2% of the injected dose at rest.

5.3 Preclinical safety data
In acute intravenous toxicity studies in mice, rats and dogs, the lowest dose of the reconstituted Cardiolite kit that resulted in any deaths was 7 mg/kg (expressed as Cu $(MIBI)_4$ BF_4 content) in female rats. This corresponds to 500 times the maximal human dose (MHD) of 0.014 mg/kg for adults (70 kg). Neither rats nor dogs exhibited treatment related effects at reconstituted Cardiolite kit doses of 0.42 mg/kg (30 times MHD) and 0.07 mg/kg (5 times MHD) respectively for 28 days. Studies on reproductive toxicity have not been conducted. Cu $(MIBI)_4$ BF_4 showed no genotoxic activity in the Ames, CHO/HPRT and sister chromatid exchange tests. At cytotoxic concentrations, an increase in chromosome aberration was observed in the in vitro human lymphocyte assay. No genotoxic activity was observed in the in vivo mouse micronucleus test at 9 mg/kg. Studies to assess the carcinogenic potential of Cardiolite have not been conducted.

5.4 Radiation Dosimetry
The projected radiation doses to organs and tissues of a patient of average weight (70 kg) after intravenous injection of Technetium Tc-99m Sestamibi are given below:

Data adopted from ICRP-publication nr. 62 (Volume 22. nr. 3. 1993): "Radiological Protection in Biomedical Research."

Absorbed dose per unit administered activity (mGy/MBq) for adults

Organ	At rest	Stress
Pancreas	7.7E-03	6.9E-03
Uterus	7.8E-03	7.2E-03
Adrenals	7.5E-03	6.6E-03
Bladder wall	1.1E-02	9.8E-03
Breast	3.8E-03	3.4E-03
Bone surface	8.2E-03	7.8E-03
Gall bladder wall	3.9E-02	3.3E-02
Heart	6.3E-03	7.2E-03
Brains	5.2E-03	4.4E-03
Skin	3.1E-03	2.9E-03
Liver	1.1E-02	9.2E-03
Lungs	4.6E-03	4.4E-03
GI-tract		
Stomach	6.5E-03	5.9E-03
Small intestine	1.5E-02	1.2E-02
Upper large intestine	2.7E-02	2.2E-02
Lower large intestine	1.9E-02	1.6E-02
Spleen	6.5E-03	5.8E-03
Kidneys	3.6E-02	2.6E-02
Ovaries	9.1E-03	8.1E-03
Red marrow	5.5E-03	5.0E-03
Thyroid	5.3E-03	4.4E-03
Oesophagus	4.1E-03	4.0E-03
Salivary glands	1.4E-02	9.2E-03
Muscle	2.9E-03	3.2E-03
Testes	3.8E-03	3.7E-03
Thymus	4.1E-03	4.0E-03
Other organs	3.1E-03	3.3E-03
ED (mSv/MBq)	8.5E-03	7.5E-03

The effective dose resulting from an administered amount of 925 MBq in the adult is

7.9 mSv at rest and 6.9 mSv at stress.

6. PHARMACEUTICAL PARTICULARS

6.1 List of excipients

Sodium citrate dihydrate

Mannitol

6.2 Incompatibilities

The Technetium labelling reactions involved depend on maintaining the stannous level in the reduced state. Hence, Sodium Pertechnetate Tc-99m Injection, Ph. Eur., containing oxidants should not be employed.

6.3 Shelf life

Of the finished drug in an unopened container: 24 months

After preparation of the ready-to-use formulation: 10 hours

6.4 Special precautions for storage

Before and after preparation, the drug should be stored at 15-25°C and protected from light. The contents of the vial are not radioactive. However, after labelling with Sodium Pertechnetate Tc-99m Injection Ph. Eur. the contents are radioactive and the currently valid protection and safety regulations must be complied with.

6.5 Nature and contents of container

5 ml glass vials, type 1 borosilicate glass (Ph. Eur.) sealed with a halobutyl rubber stopper.

6.6 Instructions for use and handling

The contents of the kit before preparation are not radioactive. However, after Sodium Pertechnetate Tc-99m Injection, Ph. Eur. is added, adequate shielding of the final preparation must be maintained.

The administration of radiopharmaceuticals create risks for other persons from external radiation or contamination from spill of urine, vomiting etc. Radiation protection precautions in accordance with national regulations must therefore be taken.

The preparation contains no bacteriostatic preservative.

Technetium Tc-99m Sestamibi is to be used within ten (10) hours of reconstitution.

Reconstitute with oxidant-free Sodium Pertechnetate Tc-99m Injection, Ph. Eur.

As with any pharmaceutical product, if at any time in the preparation of this product the integrity of this vial is compromised it should not be used.

Instructions for Preparation of Technetium Tc-99m Sestamibi

A. Boiling procedure:

Preparation of Technetium Tc-99m Sestamibi from the Cardiolite Kit is to be done according to the following aseptic procedure:

1. Waterproof gloves should be worn during the preparation procedure. Remove the plastic disc from the Cardiolite Kit vial and swab the top of the vial closure with alcohol to disinfect the surface.
2. Place the vial in a suitable radiation shield appropriately labelled with date, time of preparation, volume and activity.
3. With a sterile shielded syringe, aseptically obtain additive-free, sterile, non-pyrogenic Sodium Pertechnetate Tc-99m solution (max. 11.1 GBq – 300 mCi) in approximately 1 to 3 ml.
4. Aseptically add the Sodium Pertechnetate Tc-99m solution to the vial in the lead shield. Without withdrawing the needle, remove an equal volume of headspace to maintain atmospheric pressure within the vial.
5. Shake vigorously, about 5 to 10 quick upward-downward motions.
6. Remove the vial from the lead shield and place **upright** in an appropriately shielded and contained boiling water bath, such that the vial is suspended above the bottom of the bath, and boil for 10 minutes. The bath must be shielded. Timing for the 10 minutes commences as soon as the water **begins to boil** again.
7. **Note:** The vial **must** remain upright during the boiling step. Use a water bath where the stopper will be above the level of the water.
8. Remove the shielded vial from the water bath and allow to cool for fifteen minutes.
9. Inspect visually for the absence of particulate matter and discoloration prior to administration.
10. Aseptically withdraw material using a sterile shielded syringe. Use within ten (10) hours of preparation.
11. Radiochemical purity should be checked prior to patient administration according to the Radio TLC Method as detailed below.

NOTE: The potential for cracking and significant contamination exists whenever vials containing radioactive material are heated.

B. Thermal Cycler procedure:

Preparation of Technetium Tc-99m Sestamibi from the Cardiolite Kit is to be done according to the following aseptic procedure:

1. Waterproof gloves should be worn during the preparation procedure. Remove the plastic disc from the Cardiolite Kit vial and swab the top of the vial closure with alcohol to disinfect the surface.
2. Place the vial in a suitable radiation shield appropriately labelled with date, time of preparation, volume and activity.
3. With a sterile shielded syringe, aseptically obtain additive-free, sterile, non-pyrogenic Sodium Pertechnetate Tc-99m solution (max. 11.1 GBq – 300 mCi) in approximately 1 to 3 ml.
4. Aseptically add the Sodium Pertechnetate Tc-99m solution to the vial in the lead shield. Without withdrawing the needle, remove an equal volume of headspace to maintain atmospheric pressure within the vial.
5. Shake vigorously, about 5 to 10 quick upward-downward motions.
6. Place the shield in the sample block. While slightly pressing downwards, give the shield a quarter turn to make certain there is a firm fit between the shield and the sample block.
7. Press the proceed button to initiate the program (the thermal cycler automatically heats & cools the vial and contents). Please see the Recon-o-stat Instruction Manual for further details.
8. Inspect visually for the absence of particulate matter and discoloration prior to administration.
9. Aseptically withdraw material using a sterile shielded syringe. Use within ten (10) hours of preparation.
10. Radiochemical purity should be checked prior to patient administration according to the Radio TLC Method as detailed below.

Radio-TLC Method for the Quantification of Technetium Tc-99m Sestamibi

1. Materials

1.1. Baker-Flex-Aluminium Oxide plate, # 1 B-F, pre-cut to 2.5 cm × 7.5 cm.

1.2. Ethanol >95%.

1.3. Capintec, or equivalent instrument for measuring radioactivity in the 0.74 - 11.12 GBq (20-300 mCi) range.

1.4. 1 ml syringe with a 22-26 gauge needle.

1.5. Small developing tank with cover, (100 ml beaker covered with Parafilm® is sufficient).

2. Procedure

2.1. Pour enough ethanol into the developing tank (beaker) to have a depth of 3-4 mm of solvent. Cover the tank (beaker) with Parafilm® and allow it to equilibrate for approximately 10 minutes.

2.2. Apply 1 drop of ethanol, using a 1 ml syringe with a 22-26 gauge needle on to the Aluminium Oxide TLC plate, 1.5 cm from the bottom. Do not allow the spot to dry.

2.3. Apply 1 drop of the kit solution on top of the ethanol spot. Dry the spot. Do not heat!

2.4. Develop the plate a distance of 5.0 cm from the spot.

2.5. Cut the strip 4.0 cm from the bottom, and measure each piece in your dose calibrator.

2.6. Calculate the % Radiochemical purity as: % Tc-99m Sestamibi = (Activity top portion)/(Activity both pieces) × 100.

2.7. % Tc-99m Sestamibi should be > 90%; otherwise the preparation should be discarded.

Note: Do not use material if the radiochemical purity is less than 90%.

After reconstitution the container and any unused contents should be disposed of in accordance with local requirements for radioactive materials.

7. MARKETING AUTHORISATION HOLDER

Bristol-Myers Squibb Pharma Belgium Sprl

100 Rue de la Fusée

1130 Brussels

Belgium

8. MARKETING AUTHORISATION NUMBER(S)

PL 14207/0019

9. DATE OF FIRST AUTHORISATION/RENEWAL OF THE AUTHORISATION

26 March 2002

10. DATE OF REVISION OF THE TEXT

November 2003

LEGAL STATUS

POM

Cardura

(Pfizer Limited)

1. NAME OF THE MEDICINAL PRODUCT

CARDURA®

2. QUALITATIVE AND QUANTITATIVE COMPOSITION

Doxazosin mesilate:

1.213mg equivalent to 1mg doxazosin

2.43mg equivalent to 2mg doxazosin

For excipients, see 6.1.

3. PHARMACEUTICAL FORM

Tablets for oral administration.

1mg pentagonal tablets marked DXP1 on one side and 'PFIZER' on the other.

2mg ovoid tablets marked DXP2 on one side and 'PFIZER' on the other.

4. CLINICAL PARTICULARS

4.1 Therapeutic indications

Hypertension: Cardura is indicated for the treatment of hypertension and can be used as the sole agent to control blood pressure in the majority of patients. In patients inadequately controlled on single antihypertensive therapy, Cardura may be used in combination with a thiazide diuretic, beta-adrenoceptor blocking agent, calcium antagonist or an angiotensin-converting enzyme inhibitor.

Benign prostatic hyperplasia: Cardura is indicated for the treatment of urinary outflow obstruction and symptoms associated with benign prostatic hyperplasia (BPH). Cardura may be used in BPH patients who are either hypertensive or normotensive.

4.2 Posology and method of administration

Cardura may be administered in the morning or the evening.

Hypertension: Cardura is used in a once daily regimen: the initial dose is 1mg, to minimise the potential for postural hypotension and/or syncope (see section 4.4 Special warnings and special precautions for use). Dosage may then be increased to 2mg after an additional one or two weeks of therapy and thereafter, if necessary to 4mg. The majority of patients who respond to Cardura will do so at a dose of 4mg or less. Dosage can be further increased if necessary to 8mg or the maximum recommended dose of 16mg.

Benign prostatic hyperplasia: The recommended initial dosage of Cardura is 1mg given once daily to minimise the potential for postural hypotension and/or syncope (see section 4.4 Special warnings and special precautions for use). Depending on the individual patient's urodynamics and BPH symptomatology dosage may then be increased to 2mg and thereafter to 4mg and up to the maximum recommended dose of 8mg. The recommended titration interval is 1-2 weeks. The usual recommended dose is 2-4mg daily.

Children: The safety and efficacy of Cardura in children have not been established.

Elderly: Normal adult dosage.

Patients with renal impairment: Since there is no change in pharmacokinetics in patients with impaired renal function, the usual adult dose of Cardura is recommended.

Cardura is not dialysable.

Patients with hepatic impairment: There are only limited data in patients with liver impairment and on the effect of drugs known to influence hepatic metabolism (e.g. cimetidine). As with any drug wholly metabolised by the liver, Cardura should be administered with caution to patients with evidence of impaired liver function (see section 4.4 Special warnings and special precautions for use, and section 5.2 Pharmacokinetic properties).

4.3 Contraindications

Cardura is contraindicated in patients with a known hypersensitivity to quinazolines, (e.g. doxazosin), or any of the inert ingredients.

Use during lactation: Animal studies have shown that doxazosin accumulates in breast milk. The clinical safety of Cardura during lactation has not been established, consequently Cardura is contra-indicated in nursing mothers.

4.4 Special warnings and special precautions for use

Postural Hypotension/Syncope: As with all alpha-blockers, a very small percentage of patients have experienced postural hypotension evidenced by dizziness and weakness, or rarely loss of consciousness (syncope), particularly with the commencement of therapy (see section 4.2 Posology and method of administration). When instituting therapy with any effective alpha-blocker, the patient should be advised how to avoid symptoms resulting from postural hypotension and what measures to take should they develop. The patient should be cautioned to avoid situations where injury could result, should dizziness or weakness occur during the initiation of Cardura therapy.

Impaired liver function: As with any drug wholly metabolised by the liver, Cardura should be administered with caution to patients with evidence of impaired hepatic function (see section 4.2 Posology and method of administration).

4.5 Interaction with other medicinal products and other forms of Interaction

Doxazosin is highly bound to plasma proteins (98%). *In vitro* data in human plasma indicates that doxazosin has no effect on protein binding of the drugs tested (digoxin, phenytoin, warfarin or indomethacin). No adverse drug interactions have been observed with thiazide diuretics, frusemide, beta-blocking agents, non-steroidal anti-inflammatory drugs, antibiotics, oral hypoglycaemic drugs, uricosuric agents, or anticoagulants.

4.6 Pregnancy and lactation

Use during pregnancy: Although no teratogenic effects were seen in animal testing, reduced foetal survival was observed in animals at extremely high doses. These doses were approximately 300 times the maximum recommended human dose. As there are no adequate and well-controlled studies in pregnant women, the safety of Cardura during pregnancy has not yet been established. Accordingly, Cardura should be used only when, in the opinion of the physician, the potential benefit outweighs the potential risk.

Use during lactation: Contraindicated. See section 4.3 Contraindications above.

4.7 Effects on ability to drive and use machines

The ability to drive or use machinery may be impaired, especially when initiating therapy.

4.8 Undesirable effects

Hypertension: In clinical trials involving patients with hypertension, the most common reactions associated with Cardura therapy were of a postural type (rarely associated with fainting) or non-specific and included:

Ear and Labyrinth Disorders: vertigo

Gastrointestinal Disorders: nausea

General Disorders and Administration Site Conditions: asthenia, oedema, fatigue, malaise

Nervous System Disorders: dizziness, headache, postural dizziness, somnolence, syncope

Respiratory, Thoracic and Mediastinal Disorders: rhinitis

Benign prostatic hyperplasia: Experience in controlled clinical trials in BPH indicates a similar adverse event profile to that seen in hypertension.

In post marketing experience, the following additional adverse events have been reported:

Blood and Lymphatic Disorders: leucopenia, thrombocytopenia

Ear and Labyrinth Disorders: tinnitus

Eye Disorders: blurred vision

Gastrointestinal Disorders: abdominal pain, constipation, diarrhoea, dyspepsia, flatulence, dry mouth, vomiting

General Disorders and Administration Site Conditions: pain

Hepatobiliary Disorders: cholestasis, hepatitis, jaundice

Immune System Disorders: allergic reaction

Investigations: abnormal liver function tests, weight increase

Metabolism and Nutrition: anorexia

Musculoskeletal and Connective Tissue Disorders: arthralgia, back pain, muscle cramps, muscle weakness, myalgia

Nervous System Disorders: hypoaesthesia, paraesthesia, tremor

Psychiatric Disorders: agitation, anxiety, depression, insomnia, nervousness

Renal and Urinary System Disorders: dysuria, haematuria,, micturition disorder, micturition frequency, nocturia, polyuria, urinary incontinence

Reproductive System and Breast Disorders: gynaecomastia, impotence, priapism

Respiratory, Thoracic and Mediastinal Disorders: aggravated bronchospasm, coughing, dyspnoea, epistaxis

Skin and Subcutaneous Tissue Disorders: alopecia, pruritus, purpura, skin rash, urticaria

Vascular Disorders: hot flushes, hypotension, postural hypotension

The following additional adverse events have been reported in marketing experience among patients treated for hypertension. In general, these are not distinguishable from symptoms that might have occurred in the absence of exposure to Cardura: bradycardia, tachycardia, palpitations, chest pain, angina pectoris, myocardial infarction, cerebrovascular accidents and cardiac arrhythmias.

4.9 Overdose

Should overdosage lead to hypotension, the patient should be immediately placed in a supine, head down position. Other supportive measures may be appropriate in individual cases. Since Cardura is highly protein bound, dialysis is not indicated.

5. PHARMACOLOGICAL PROPERTIES

5.1 Pharmacodynamic properties

Doxazosin is a potent and selective post-junctional alpha-1-adrenoceptor antagonist. This action results in a decrease in systemic blood pressure. Cardura is appropriate for oral administration in a once daily regimen in patients with essential hypertension.

Cardura has been shown to be free of adverse metabolic effects and is suitable for use in patients with coexistent diabetes mellitus, gout and insulin resistance.

Cardura is suitable for use in patients with co-existent asthma, left ventricular hypertrophy and in elderly patients. Treatment with Cardura has been shown to result in regression of left ventricular hypertrophy, inhibition of platelet aggregation and enhanced activity of tissue plasminogen activator. Additionally, Cardura improves insulin sensitivity in patients with impairment.

Cardura, in addition to its antihypertensive effect, has in long term studies produced a modest reduction in plasma total cholesterol, LDL-cholesterol and triglyceride concentrations and therefore may be of particular benefit to hypertensive patients with concomitant hyperlipidaemia.

Administration of Cardura to patients with symptomatic BPH results in a significant improvement in urodynamics and symptoms. The effect in BPH is thought to result from selective blockade of the alpha-adrenoceptors located in the muscular stroma and capsule of the prostate, and in the bladder neck.

5.2 Pharmacokinetic properties

Absorption: Following oral administration in humans (young male adults or the elderly of either sex), doxazosin is well absorbed and approximately two thirds of the dose is bioavailable.

Biotransformation/Elimination: Approximately 98% of doxazosin is protein-bound in plasma.

Doxazosin is extensively metabolised in man and in the animal species tested, with the faeces being the predominant route of excretion.

The mean plasma elimination half-life is 22 hours thus making the drug suitable for once daily administration.

After oral administration of Cardura the plasma concentrations of the metabolites are low. The most active (6' hydroxy) metabolite is present in man at one fortieth of the plasma concentration of the parent compound, which suggests that the antihypertensive activity is in the main due to doxazosin.

There are only limited data in patients with liver impairment and on the effects of drugs known to influence hepatic metabolism (e.g. cimetidine). In a clinical study in 12 subjects with moderate hepatic impairment, single dose administration of doxazosin resulted in an increase in AUC of 43% and a decrease in apparent oral clearance of 40%. As with any drug wholly metabolised by the liver, Cardura should be administered with caution to patients with impaired liver function (see section 4.4 Special warnings and special precautions for use).

5.3 Preclinical safety data

Preclinical data reveal no special hazard for humans based on conventional animal studies in safety pharmacology, repeated dose toxicity, genotoxicity and carcinogenicity. For further information see section 4.6 Pregnancy and lactation.

6. PHARMACEUTICAL PARTICULARS

6.1 List of excipients

Lactose, magnesium stearate, microcrystalline cellulose, sodium lauryl sulphate and sodium starch glycollate.

6.2 Incompatibilities

None stated.

6.3 Shelf life

5 years.

6.4 Special precautions for storage

Do not store above 30°C.

6.5 Nature and contents of container

Cardura 1mg and 2mg Tablets are available as calendar packs of 28 tablets. Aluminium/PVC/PVdC blister strips,

14 tablets/strip, 2 strips in a carton box.

6.6 Instructions for use and handling

No special requirements.

7. MARKETING AUTHORISATION HOLDER

Pfizer Limited

Ramsgate Road

Sandwich

Kent, CT13 9NJ

United Kingdom

8. MARKETING AUTHORISATION NUMBER(S)

Cardura 1mg PL 00057/0276

Cardura 2mg PL 00057/0277

9. DATE OF FIRST AUTHORISATION/RENEWAL OF THE AUTHORISATION

22 August 1988/20 January 1999

10. DATE OF REVISION OF THE TEXT

May 2003

11. LEGAL CATEGORY

POM

Ref:CR4_1 UK

Cardura XL

(Pfizer Limited)

1. NAME OF THE MEDICINAL PRODUCT

CARDURA® XL 4mg

CARDURA® XL 8mg

2. QUALITATIVE AND QUANTITATIVE COMPOSITION

Doxazosin mesilate:

4.85mg equivalent to 4mg doxazosin

9.70mg equivalent to 8mg doxazosin

For excipients, see 6.1.

3. PHARMACEUTICAL FORM

Modified release tablet

Cardura XL 4mg and 8mg tablets are white, round, biconvex shaped tablets with a hole in one side, marked CXL4 and CXL8.

4. CLINICAL PARTICULARS

4.1 Therapeutic indications

Hypertension: Cardura XL is indicated for the treatment of hypertension and can be used as the sole agent to control blood pressure in the majority of patients. In patients inadequately controlled on single antihypertensive therapy, Cardura XL may be used in combination with a thiazide diuretic, beta-adrenoceptor blocking agent, calcium antagonist or an angiotensin-converting enzyme inhibitor.

Benign prostatic hyperplasia: Cardura XL is indicated for the treatment of urinary outflow obstruction and symptoms associated with benign prostatic hyperplasia (BPH).

Cardura XL may be used in BPH patients who are either hypertensive or normotensive. While the blood pressure changes in normotensive patients with BPH are not usually clinically significant, patients with hypertension and BPH have had both conditions effectively treated with doxazosin monotherapy.

4.2 Posology and method of administration

Hypertension and benign prostatic hyperplasia: The initial dose of Cardura XL is 4mg once daily. Over 50% of patients with mild to moderate severity hypertension will be controlled on Cardura XL 4mg once daily. Optimal effect of Cardura XL may take up to 4 weeks. If necessary, the dosage may be increased following this period to 8mg once daily according to patient response.

The maximum recommended dose of Cardura XL is 8mg once daily.

Cardura XL can be taken with or without food.

The tablets should be swallowed whole with a sufficient amount of liquid.

Children: The safety and efficacy of Cardura XL in children have not been established.

Elderly: Normal adult dosage.

Patients with renal impairment: Since there is no change in pharmacokinetics in patients with impaired renal function the usual adult dose of Cardura XL is recommended. Doxazosin is not dialysable.

Patients with hepatic impairment: As with any drug wholly metabolised by the liver, Cardura XL should be administered with caution to patients with evidence of impaired hepatic function (see section 4.4 Special warnings and special precautions for use, and section 5.2 Pharmacokinetic properties).

4.3 Contraindications

Cardura XL is contraindicated in:

Patients with a history of gastro-intestinal obstruction, oesophageal obstruction, or any degree of decreased lumen diameter of the gastro-intestinal tract.

Patients with a known hypersensitivity to quinazolines, (e.g. doxazosin, prazosin, terazosin), or any of the inert ingredients of Cardura XL.

Use during lactation: Animal studies have shown that doxazosin accumulates in breast milk. The clinical safety of Cardura XL during lactation has not been established, consequently Cardura XL is contra-indicated in nursing mothers.

4.4 Special warnings and special precautions for use

Information for the patient: Patients should be informed that Cardura XL tablets should be swallowed whole. Patients should not chew, divide or crush the tablets.

In Cardura XL, the medication is contained within a non-absorbable shell that has been specially designed to slowly release the drug. When this process is completed the empty tablet is eliminated from the body. Patients should be advised that they should not be concerned if they occasionally observe in the stools something that looks like a tablet.

Postural hypotension / syncope: As with all alpha-blockers, a very small percentage of patients have experienced postural hypotension evidenced by dizziness and weakness, or rarely loss of consciousness (syncope), particularly with the commencement of therapy. When instituting therapy with any effective alpha-blocker, the patient should be advised how to avoid symptoms resulting from postural hypotension and what measures to take should they develop. The patient should be cautioned to avoid situations where injury could result should dizziness or weakness occur during the initiation of Cardura XL therapy.

Impaired liver function: As with any drug wholly metabolised by the liver, Cardura XL should be administered with caution to patients with evidence of impaired hepatic function (see section 4.2 Posology and method of administration, and section 5.2 Pharmacokinetic properties).

4.5 Interaction with other medicinal products and other forms of Interaction

Doxazosin is highly bound to plasma proteins (98%). *In vitro* data in human plasma indicates that doxazosin has no effect on protein binding of the drugs tested (digoxin, phenytoin, warfarin or indomethacin). No adverse drug interactions have been observed with thiazide diuretics, frusemide, beta-blocking agents, non-steroidal anti-inflammatory drugs, antibiotics, oral hypoglycaemic drugs, uricosuric agents, or anticoagulants.

4.6 Pregnancy and lactation

Use during pregnancy: Although no teratogenic effects were seen in animal testing, reduced foetal survival was observed in animals at extremely high doses. These doses were approximately 300 times the maximum recommended human dose. As there are no adequate and well-controlled studies in pregnant women, the safety of Cardura XL during pregnancy has not yet been established. Accordingly, Cardura XL should be used only when, in the opinion of the physician, the potential benefit outweighs the potential risk.

Use during lactation: Contraindicated. See section 4.3 Contraindications above.

4.7 Effects on ability to drive and use machines

The ability to drive or use machinery may be impaired, especially when initiating therapy.

4.8 Undesirable effects

Hypertension: In clinical trials, the most common reactions associated with Cardura XL therapy were of a postural type (rarely associated with fainting) or non-specific and included:

Cardiac Disorders: palpitation, tachycardia

Ear and Labyrinth Disorders: vertigo

Gastrointestinal Disorders: abdominal pain, dry mouth, nausea

General Disorders and Administration Site Conditions: asthenia, chest pain, peripheral oedema

Musculoskeletal and Connective Tissue Disorders: back pain, myalgia

Nervous System Disorders: dizziness, headache

Respiratory, Thoracic and Mediastinal Disorders: coughing

Skin and Subcutaneous Tissue Disorders: pruritis

Renal and Urinary Disorders: urinary incontinence

Vascular Disorders: postural hypotension

Benign Prostatic Hyperplasia: Experience in controlled clinical trials in BPH indicates a similar adverse event profile to that seen in hypertension.

Ear and Labyrinth Disorders: vertigo

Gastrointestinal Disorders: abdominal pain, nausea

General Disorders and Administration Site Conditions: asthenia, peripheral oedema

Infection and Infestations: respiratory tract infection

Musculoskeletal and Connective Tissue Disorders: back pain, myalgia

Nervous System Disorders: dizziness, headache, somnolence

Respiratory, Thoracic and Mediastinal Disorders: dyspnoea, rhinitis

Vascular Disorders: hypotension, postural hypotension

In post-marketing experience, the following additional adverse events have been reported:

Blood and Lymphatic Disorders: leucopenia, thrombocytopenia

Cardiac Disorders: bradycardia

Ear and Labyrinth Disorders: tinnitus

Eye Disorders: blurred vision

Gastrointestinal Disorders: constipation, diarrhoea, dyspepsia, flatulence, vomiting

General Disorders and Administration Site Conditions: fatigue, malaise, pain

Hepatobiliary Disorders: cholestasis, hepatitis, jaundice

Immune System Disorders: allergic reaction

Investigations: abnormal liver function tests, weight increase

Metabolism and Nutrition: anorexia

Musculoskeletal and Connective Tissue Disorders: arthralgia, muscle cramps, muscle weakness

Nervous System Disorders: postural dizziness, hypoaesthesia, paraesthesia, syncope, tremor

Psychiatric Disorders: agitation, anxiety, depression, insomnia, nervousness

Renal and Urinary Disorders: dysuria, haematuria, micturition disorder, micturition frequency, nocturia, polyuria

Reproductive System and Breast Disorders: gynaecomastia, impotence, priapism

Respiratory, Thoracic and Mediastinal Disorders: aggravated bronchospasm, epistaxis

Skin and Subcutaneous Tissue Disorders: alopecia, purpura, skin rash, urticaria

Vascular Disorders: hot flushes

The following additional adverse events have been reported in marketing experience with immediate release doxazosin tablets among patients treated for hypertension. In general, these are not distinguishable from symptoms of the underlying disease that might have occurred in the absence of exposure to Cardura: tachycardia, palpitations, chest pain, angina pectoris, myocardial infarction, cerebrovascular accidents and cardiac arrhythmias.

The adverse events for Cardura XL are similar to those with immediate release doxazosin tablets.

4.9 Overdose

Should overdosage lead to hypotension, the patient should be immediately placed in a supine, head down position. Other supportive measures may be appropriate in individual cases. Since doxazosin is highly protein bound, dialysis is not indicated.

5. PHARMACOLOGICAL PROPERTIES

5.1 Pharmacodynamic properties

Doxazosin is a potent and selective post-junctional alpha-1-adrenoceptor antagonist.

Administration of Cardura XL to hypertensive patients causes a clinically significant reduction in blood pressure as a result of a reduction in systemic vascular resistance. This effect is thought to result from selective blockade of the alpha-1-adrenoreceptors located in the vasculature. With once daily dosing, clinically significant reductions in blood pressure are present throughout the day and at 24 hours post dose. The majority of patients are controlled on the initial dose. In patients with hypertension, the decrease in blood pressure during treatment with Cardura XL was similar in both the sitting and standing position.

Subjects treated with immediate release doxazosin tablets can be transferred to Cardura XL 4mg and the dose titrated upwards as needed.

Doxazosin has been shown to be free of adverse metabolic effects and is suitable for use in patients with coexistent diabetes mellitus, gout and insulin resistance.

Doxazosin is suitable for use in patients with co-existent asthma, left ventricular hypertrophy and in elderly patients. Treatment with doxazosin has been shown to result in regression of left ventricular hypertrophy, inhibition of platelet aggregation and enhanced activity of tissue plasminogen activator. Additionally, doxazosin improves insulin sensitivity in patients with impairment.

Doxazosin, in addition to its antihypertensive effect, has in long term studies produced a modest reduction in plasma total cholesterol, LDL-cholesterol and triglyceride concentrations and therefore may be of particular benefit to hypertensive patients with concomitant hyperlipidaemia.

Administration of Cardura XL to patients with symptomatic BPH results in a significant improvement in urodynamics and symptoms. The effect in BPH is thought to result from selective blockade of the alpha-adrenoceptors located in the prostatic muscular stroma, capsule and bladder neck.

5.2 Pharmacokinetic properties

Absorption: After oral administration of therapeutic doses, Cardura XL is well absorbed with peak blood levels gradually reached at 8 to 9 hours after dosing. Peak plasma levels are approximately one third of those of the same dose of immediate release doxazosin tablets. Trough levels at 24 hours are, however, similar.

Peak/trough ratio of Cardura XL is less than half that of immediate release doxazosin tablets.

At steady-state, the relative bioavailability of doxazosin from Cardura XL compared to immediate release form was 54% at the 4mg dose and 59% at the 8mg dose.

Pharmacokinetic studies with Cardura XL in the elderly have shown no significant alterations compared to younger patients.

Biotransformation/elimination: The plasma elimination is biphasic with the terminal elimination half-life being 22 hours and hence this provides the basic for once daily dosing. Doxazosin is extensively metabolised with <5% excreted as unchanged drug.

Pharmacokinetic studies with doxazosin in patients with renal impairment also showed no significant alterations compared to patients with normal renal function.

There are only limited data in patients with liver impairment and on the effects of drugs known to influence hepatic metabolism (e.g. cimetidine). In a clinical study in 12 subjects with moderate hepatic impairment, single dose administration of doxazosin resulted in an increase in AUC of 43% and a decrease in apparent oral clearance of 40%.

Approximately 98% of doxazosin is protein-bound in plasma.

Doxazosin is primarily metabolised by O-demethylation and hydroxylation.

5.3 Preclinical safety data

Preclinical data reveal no special hazard for humans based on conventional animal studies in safety pharmacology, repeated dose toxicity, genotoxicity and carcinogenicity. For further information see section 4.6 Pregnancy and lactation.

6. PHARMACEUTICAL PARTICULARS

6.1 List of excipients

Polyethylene oxide, sodium chloride, hypromellose, red ferric oxide (E172), titanium dioxide (E171), magnesium stearate, cellulose acetate, Macrogol, pharmaceutical glaze, black iron oxide (E172) and ammonium hydroxide.

6.2 Incompatibilities

None stated.

6.3 Shelf life

2 years.

6.4 Special precautions for storage

Do not store above 30°C.

Store in the original package.

6.5 Nature and contents of container

Blister strips of aluminium foil/aluminium foil of 7 tablets in pack size of 28 tablets.

6.6 Instructions for use and handling

No special requirements.

7. MARKETING AUTHORISATION HOLDER

Pfizer Limited

Ramsgate Road

Sandwich

Kent, CT13 9NJ

United Kingdom

8. MARKETING AUTHORISATION NUMBER(S)

Cardura XL 4mg PL 00057/0417

Cardura XL 8mg PL 00057/0418

9. DATE OF FIRST AUTHORISATION/RENEWAL OF THE AUTHORISATION

15 January 2001

10. DATE OF REVISION OF THE TEXT

March 2004

11. LEGAL CATEGORY

POM

Ref: CX2_2 UK

Carnitor Injection 1g

(Shire Pharmaceuticals Limited)

1. NAME OF THE MEDICINAL PRODUCT
Carnitor® Injection 1g

2. QUALITATIVE AND QUANTITATIVE COMPOSITION
Contains L-carnitine inner salt 1g

3. PHARMACEUTICAL FORM
A clear, colourless or light straw- coloured liquid presented in 5ml Ph. Eur. type 1 clear glass ampoules.

4. CLINICAL PARTICULARS

4.1 Therapeutic indications
Indicated for the treatment of primary and secondary carnitine deficiency in adults, children, infants and neonates.

Secondary carnitine deficiency in haemodialysis patients.

Secondary carnitine deficiency should be suspected in long-term haemodialysis patients who have the following conditions:

1. Severe and persistent muscle cramps and/or hypotensive episodes during dialysis.

2. Lack of energy causing a significant negative effect on the quality of life.

3. Skeletal muscle weakness and/or myopathy.

4. Cardiomyopathy.

5. Anaemia of uraemia unresponsive to or requiring large doses of erythropoietin.

6. Muscle mass loss caused by malnutrition.

4.2 Posology and method of administration
Adults, Children, infants and neonates:

For slow intravenous administration over 2-3 minutes.

It is advisable to monitor therapy by measuring free and acyl carnitine levels in both plasma and urine.

The management of inborn errors of metabolism:
The dosage required depends upon the specific inborn error of metabolism concerned and the severity of presentation at the time of treatment. However, the following can be considered as a general guide.

In acute decompensation, dosages of up to 100 mg/kg/day in 3-4 divided doses are recommended. Higher doses have been used although an increase in adverse events, primarily diarrhoea, may occur.

Secondary carnitine deficiency in haemodialysis patients:
It is strongly recommended that, before initiating therapy with Carnitor, plasma carnitine is measured. Secondary carnitine deficiency is suggested by a plasma ratio of acyl to free carnitine of greater than 0.4 and/or when free carnitine concentrations are lower than 20 μmol/litre.

A dose of 20mg per kg should be administered as an intravenous bolus at the end of each dialysis session (assuming three sessions per week). The duration of intravenous treatment should be at least three months, which is the time usually required to restore normal muscle levels of free carnitine. The overall response should be assessed by monitoring plasma acyl to free carnitine levels and by evaluating the patient's symptoms. When carnitine supplementation has been stopped there will be a progressive decline in carnitine levels. The need for a repeat course of therapy can be assessed by plasma carnitine assays at regular intervals and by monitoring the patient's symptoms.

Haemodialysis - maintenance therapy:
If significant clinical benefit has been gained by the first course of intravenous Carnitor then maintenance therapy can be considered using 1g per day of Carnitor orally. On the day of the dialysis, oral Carnitor has to be administered at the end of the session.

4.3 Contraindications
Hypersensitivity to any of the constituents of the product.

4.4 Special warnings and special precautions for use
While improving glucose utilisation, the administration of L-carnitine to diabetic patients receiving either insulin or hypoglycaemic oral treatment may result in hypoglycaemia. Plasma glucose levels in these subjects must be monitored regularly in order to adjust the hypoglycaemic treatment immediately, if required.

Both the 30% oral solution and the chewable tablets contain sucrose. This must be considered when treating diabetics or patients who are following diets to reduce calorie intake.

The safety and efficacy of oral L-carnitine has not been evaluated in patients with renal insufficiency. Chronic administration of high doses of oral L-carnitine in patients with severely compromised renal function or in end stage renal disease (ESRD) patients on dialysis may result in an accumulation of the potentially toxic metabolites, trimethylamine (TMA) and trimethylamine-N-oxide (TMAO), since these metabolites are usually excreted in the urine. This situation has not been observed following intravenous administration of L-carnitine.

4.5 Interaction with other medicinal products and other forms of Interaction
There are no known interactions.

4.6 Pregnancy and lactation
Reproductive studies were performed in rats and rabbits. There was no evidence of a teratogenic effect in either species. In the rabbit but not in the rat, there was a statistically insignificant greater number of post implantation losses at the highest dose tested (600 mg/kg daily) as compared with control animals. The significance of these findings for man is unknown. There is no experience of use in pregnant patients with primary systemic carnitine deficiency.

Taking into account the serious consequences to a pregnant woman who has primary systemic carnitine deficiency stopping treatment, the risk to the mother of discontinuing treatment seems greater than the theoretical risk to the foetus if treatment is continued.

Levocarnitine is a normal component of human milk. Use of levocarnitine supplementation in nursing mothers has not been studied.

4.7 Effects on ability to drive and use machines
None known.

4.8 Undesirable effects
Various mild gastro-intestinal complaints have been reported during the long-term administration of oral levocarnitine, these include transient nausea and vomiting, abdominal cramps and diarrhoea.

Decreasing the dosage often diminishes or eliminates drug-related patient body odour or gastro-intestinal symptoms when present. Tolerance should be monitored very closely during the first week of administration and after any dosage increase.

4.9 Overdose
There have been no reports of toxicity from levocarnitine overdosage. Overdosage should be treated with supportive care.

5. PHARMACOLOGICAL PROPERTIES

5.1 Pharmacodynamic properties
L-Carnitine is present as a natural constituent in animal tissues, micro-organisms and plants. In man the physiological metabolic requirements are met both by the consumption of food containing carnitine and the endogenous synthesis in the liver and kidneys from lysine with methionine serving as the methyl donor. Only the L-isomer is biologically active, playing an essential role in lipid metabolism as well as in the metabolism of ketone bodies as branched chain-amino-acids. L-Carnitine as a factor is necessary in the transport of long-chain fatty acids into the mitochondria – facilitating the oxidation of fatty acids rather than their incorporation into triglycerides. By releasing CoA from its thioesters, through the action of CoA; carnitine acetyl transferase, L-carnitine also enhances the metabolic flux in the Kreb's cycle; with the same mechanism it stimulates the activity of pyruvate dehydrogenase and in skeletal muscle, the oxidation of branched chain-amino acids. L-Carnitine is thus involved, directly or indirectly in several pathways so that its availability should be an important factor controlling not only the oxidative utilisation of fatty acids and ketone bodies but also that of glucose and some amino acids.

5.2 Pharmacokinetic properties
The absorbed L-carnitine is transported to various organ systems via the blood. The presence of membrane-bound proteins in several tissues including red blood cells that bind carnitine, suggest that a transport system in the blood and a cellular system for the collective uptake is present in several tissues. Tissue and serum carnitine concentration depends on several metabolic processes, carnitine biosynthesis and dietary contributions, transport into and out of tissues, degradation and excretion may all affect tissue carnitine concentrations.

Absorption

L-Carnitine is absorbed by the mucosal cells of the small intestine and enters the blood stream relatively slowly; the absorption is probably associated with an active translumninal mechanism.

The apparent systemic availability after oral administration is limited (<10%) and variable.

Distribution

Absorbed L-carnitine is transported to various organ systems via the blood; it is thought that a transport system in the blood and a cellular system for selective uptake is involved.

Excretion

L-Carnitine is excreted mainly in the urine and is variable. The excretion is directly proportional to the blood levels.

Metabolism

L-Carnitine is metabolised to a very limited extent.

5.3 Preclinical safety data
L-Carnitine is a naturally occurring body substance in human beings, plants and animals. Carnitor products are used to bring the level of L-carnitine in the body up to those found naturally. Appropriate pre-clinical studies have been undertaken and show no signs of toxicity at normal therapeutic doses.

6. PHARMACEUTICAL PARTICULARS

6.1 List of excipients
Hydrochloric acid 10%

Water for injection

6.2 Incompatibilities
None known.

6.3 Shelf life
5 years.

6.4 Special precautions for storage
Store at a temperature not exceeding 25°C.

Protect from light.

6.5 Nature and contents of container
Ph.Eur. Type 1 clear glass ampoules of 5 ml capacity.

The ampoules are packed in cardboard outer cartons containing 5 ampoules.

6.6 Instructions for use and handling
None.

7. MARKETING AUTHORISATION HOLDER
Sigma-Tau Industrie Farmaceutiche Riunite SpA,

Viale Shakespeare 47-00144,

Rome, Italy.

8. MARKETING AUTHORISATION NUMBER(S)
PL 08381/0003

9. DATE OF FIRST AUTHORISATION/RENEWAL OF THE AUTHORISATION
30 November 1999

10. DATE OF REVISION OF THE TEXT
July 2002

Legal Category
POM

Carnitor Oral Single Dose 1g

(Shire Pharmaceuticals Limited)

1. NAME OF THE MEDICINAL PRODUCT
Carnitor® Oral Single Dose 1g

2. QUALITATIVE AND QUANTITATIVE COMPOSITION
L-Carnitine inner salt 1.0g

3. PHARMACEUTICAL FORM
Clear, colourless or light straw- coloured liquid.

4. CLINICAL PARTICULARS

4.1 Therapeutic indications
Indicated for the treatment of primary and secondary carnitine deficiency in adults and children over 12 years of age.

4.2 Posology and method of administration
For oral administration only.

Adults and children over 12 years of age

It is advisable to monitor therapy by measuring free and acyl carnitine levels in both plasma and urine.

The management of inborn errors of metabolism

The dosage required depends upon the specific inborn error of metabolism concerned and the severity of presentation at the time of treatment. However, the following can be considered as a general guide.

An oral dosage of up to 200mg/kg/day in divided doses (2 to 4) is recommended for chronic use in some disorders, with lower doses sufficing in other conditions. If clinical and biochemical symptoms do not improve, the dose may be increased on a short-term basis. Higher doses of up to 400mg/kg/day may be necessary in acute metabolic decompensation or the i.v. route may be required.

Haemodialysis - maintenance therapy

If significant clinical benefit has been gained by a first course of intravenous Carnitor then maintenance therapy can be considered using 1g per day of Carnitor orally. On the day of the dialysis oral Carnitor has to be administered at the end of the session.

The Oral Solution can be drunk directly or diluted further in water or fruit juices.

4.3 Contraindications
Hypersensitivity to any of the constituents of the product.

4.4 Special warnings and special precautions for use
While improving glucose utilisation, the administration of L-carnitine to diabetic patients receiving either insulin or hypoglycaemic oral treatment may result in hypoglycaemia. Plasma glucose levels in these subjects must be monitored regularly in order to adjust the hypoglycaemic treatment immediately, if required.

Both the 30% oral solution and the chewable tablets contain sucrose. This must be considered when treating diabetics or patients who are following diets to reduce calorie intake.

The safety and efficacy of oral L-carnitine has not been evaluated in patients with renal insufficiency. Chronic administration of high doses of oral L-carnitine in patients with severely compromised renal function or in end stage renal disease (ESRD) patients on dialysis may result in an accumulation of the potentially toxic metabolites, trimethylamine (TMA) and trimethylamine-N-oxide (TMAO), since these metabolites are usually excreted in the urine. This situation has not been observed following intravenous administration of L-carnitine.

4.5 Interaction with other medicinal products and other forms of Interaction
There are no known interactions.

4.6 Pregnancy and lactation
Reproductive studies were performed in rats and rabbits. There was no evidence of a teratogenic effect in either species. In the rabbit but not in the rat, there was a statistically insignificant greater number of post-implantation losses at the highest dose tested (600mg/kg daily) as compared with control animals. The significance of these findings in man is unknown. There is no experience of use in pregnant patients with primary systemic carnitine deficiency.

Taking into account the serious consequences in a pregnant woman who has primary systemic carnitine deficiency stopping treatment, the risk to the mother of discontinuing treatment seems greater than the theoretical risk to the foetus if treatment is continued.

Levocarnitine is a normal component of human milk. Use of levocarnitine supplementation in nursing mothers has not been studied.

4.7 Effects on ability to drive and use machines
None known.

4.8 Undesirable effects
Various mild gastro-intestinal complaints have been reported during the long-term administration of oral levocarnitine, these include transient nausea and vomiting, abdominal cramps and diarrhoea.

Decreasing the dosage often diminishes or eliminates drug related patient body odour or gastro-intestinal symptoms when present. Tolerance should be monitored very closely during the first week of administration and after any dosage increase.

4.9 Overdose
There have been no reports of toxicity from levocarnitine overdosage. Overdosage should be treated with supportive care.

5. PHARMACOLOGICAL PROPERTIES

5.1 Pharmacodynamic properties
L-Carnitine is present as a natural constituent in animal tissues, micro-organisms and plants. In man the physiological metabolic requirements are met both by the consumption of food containing carnitine and the endogenous synthesis in the liver and kidneys from lysine with methionine serving as the methyl donor. Only the L-isomer is biologically active, playing an essential role in lipid metabolism as well as in the metabolism of ketone bodies as branched-chain amino acids. L-Carnitine as a factor is necessary in the transport of long-chain fatty acids into the mitochondria - facilitating the oxidation of fatty acids rather than their incorporation into triglycerides. By releasing CoA from its thioesters, through the action of CoA; carnitine acetyl transferase, L-carnitine also enhances the metabolic flux in the Kreb's cycle; with the same mechanism it stimulates the activity of pyruvate dehydrogenase and in skeletal muscle, the oxidation of branched-chain amino acids. L-Carnitine is thus involved, directly or indirectly in several pathways so that its availability should be an important factor controlling not only the oxidative utilisation of fatty acids and ketone bodies but also that of glucose and some amino acids.

5.2 Pharmacokinetic properties
The absorbed L-carnitine is transported to various organ systems via the blood. The presence of membrane-bound proteins in several tissues including red blood cells that bind carnitine, suggest that a transport system in the blood and a cellular system for the collective uptake is present in several tissues. Tissue and serum carnitine concentration depend on several metabolic processes, carnitine biosynthesis and dietary contributions, transport into and out of tissues, degradation and excretion may all affect tissue carnitine concentrations.

It has been demonstrated that pharmacokinetic parameters increase significantly with dosage. Apparent bioavailability in healthy volunteers is about 10-16%. The data suggests a relationship between maximal plasma concentration/dosage, dosage, plasma AUC, dosage/urinary accumulation. Maximum concentration is reached about four hours after ingestion.

5.3 Preclinical safety data
L-Carnitine is a naturally occurring body substance in human beings, plants and animals. Carnitor products are used to bring the level of L-carnitine in the body up to those found naturally. Appropriate pre-clinical studies have been undertaken and show no signs of toxicity at normal therapeutic doses.

6. PHARMACEUTICAL PARTICULARS

6.1 List of excipients
Malic acid, saccharin sodium, sodium methyl hydroxybenzoate, sodium propyl hydroxybenzoate and purified water.

6.2 Incompatibilities
None known.

6.3 Shelf life
4 years.

6.4 Special precautions for storage
Store below 25°C. Protect from light.

6.5 Nature and contents of container
10ml amber glass bottles with a fully removable low density polyethylene cap.

6.6 Instructions for use and handling
None.

7. MARKETING AUTHORISATION HOLDER
Sigma-Tau Industrie Farmaceutiche Riunite SpA,
Viale Shakespeare 47-00144,
Rome, Italy.

8. MARKETING AUTHORISATION NUMBER(S)
PL 08381/0004

9. DATE OF FIRST AUTHORISATION/RENEWAL OF THE AUTHORISATION
16 October 1998

10. DATE OF REVISION OF THE TEXT
April 2003

LEGAL CATEGORY
POM

Carnitor Paediatric Solution 30%

(Shire Pharmaceuticals Limited)

1. NAME OF THE MEDICINAL PRODUCT
Carnitor™ Paediatric Solution 30%

2. QUALITATIVE AND QUANTITATIVE COMPOSITION
L-Carnitine inner salt 30% w/v

3. PHARMACEUTICAL FORM
Colourless or slightly yellow solution

4. CLINICAL PARTICULARS

4.1 Therapeutic indications
Indicated for the treatment of primary and secondary carnitine deficiency in children of under 12 years, infants and newborns.

4.2 Posology and method of administration
Children under 12 years, infants and newborns:
It is advisable to monitor therapy by measuring free and acyl carnitine levels in both plasma and urine.

The management of inborn errors of metabolism
The dosage required depends upon the specific inborn error of metabolism concerned and the severity of presentation at the time of treatment. However, the following can be considered as a general guide.

An oral dosage of up to 200mg/kg/day in divided doses (2 to 4) is recommended for chronic use in some disorders, with lower doses sufficing in other conditions. If clinical and biochemical symptoms do not improve, the dose may be increased on a short-term basis. Higher doses of up to 400mg/kg/day may be necessary in acute metabolic decompensation or the i.v. route may be required.

Haemodialysis - maintenance therapy
If significant clinical benefit has been gained by a first course of intravenous Carnitor then maintenance therapy can be considered using 1g per day of Carnitor orally. On the day of the dialysis oral Carnitor has to be administered at the end of the session.

The Paediatric Solution can be drunk directly or diluted further in water or fruit juices.

4.3 Contraindications
Hypersensitivity to any of the constituents of the product.

4.4 Special warnings and special precautions for use
While improving glucose utilisation, the administration of L-carnitine to diabetic patients receiving either insulin or hypoglycaemic oral treatment may result in hypoglycaemia. Plasma glucose levels in these subjects must be monitored regularly in order to adjust the hypoglycaemic treatment immediately, if required.

Both the 30% oral solution and the chewable tablets contain sucrose. This must be considered when treating diabetics or patients who are following diets to reduce calorie intake.

The safety and efficacy of oral L-carnitine has not been evaluated in patients with renal insufficiency. Chronic administration of high doses of oral L-carnitine in patients with severely compromised renal function or in end stage renal disease (ESRD) patients on dialysis may result in an accumulation of the potentially toxic metabolites, trimethylamine (TMA) and trimethylamine-N-oxide (TMAO), since these metabolites are usually excreted in the urine. This situation has not been observed following intravenous administration of L-carnitine.

4.5 Interaction with other medicinal products and other forms of Interaction
There are no known interactions.

4.6 Pregnancy and lactation
Reproductive studies were performed in rats and rabbits. There was no evidence of a teratogenic effect in either species. In the rabbit but not in the rat there was a statistically insignificant greater number of post implantation losses at the highest dose tested (600mg/kg daily) as compared with control animals. The significance of these findings in man is unknown. There is no experience of use in pregnant patients with primary systemic carnitine deficiency.

Taking into account the serious consequences in a pregnant woman who has primary systemic carnitine deficiency stopping treatment, the risk to the mother of discontinuing treatment seems greater than the theoretical risk to the foetus if treatment is continued.

Levocarnitine is a normal component of human milk. Use of levocarnitine supplementation in nursing mothers has not been studied.

4.7 Effects on ability to drive and use machines
None known.

4.8 Undesirable effects
Various mild gastro-intestinal complaints have been reported during the long term administration of oral levocarnitine, these include transient nausea and vomiting, abdominal cramps and diarrhoea.

Decreasing the dosage often diminishes or eliminates drug related patient body odour or gastro-intestinal symptoms when present. Tolerance should be monitored very closely during the first week of administration and after any dosage increase.

4.9 Overdose
There have been no reports of toxicity from levocarnitine overdosage. Overdosage should be treated with supportive care.

5. PHARMACOLOGICAL PROPERTIES

5.1 Pharmacodynamic properties
L-Carnitine is present as a natural constituent in animal tissues, micro-organisms and plants. In man the physiological metabolic requirements are met both by the consumption of food containing carnitine and the endogenous synthesis in the liver and kidneys from lysine with methionine serving as the methyl donor. Only the L-isomer is biologically active, playing an essential role in lipid metabolism as well as in the metabolism of ketone bodies as branched chain-amino-acids. L-Carnitine as a factor is necessary in the transport of long-chain fatty acids into the mitochondria - facilitating the oxidation of fatty acids rather than their incorporation into triglycerides. By releasing CoA from its thioesters, through the action of CoA; carnitine acetyl transferase, L-carnitine also enhances the metabolic flux in the Kreb's cycle; with the same mechanism it stimulates the activity of pyruvate dehydrogenase and in skeletal muscle, the oxidation of branched-chain amino acids. L-Carnitine is thus involved, directly or indirectly in several pathways so that its availability should be an important factor controlling not only the oxidative utilisation of fatty acids and ketone bodies but also that of glucose and some amino acids.

5.2 Pharmacokinetic properties
The absorbed L-carnitine is transported to various organ systems via the blood. The presence of membrane-bound proteins in several tissues including red blood cells that bind carnitine, suggest that a transport system in the blood and a cellular system for the collective uptake is present in several tissues. Tissue and serum carnitine concentration depend on several metabolic processes, carnitine biosynthesis and dietary contributions, transport into and out of tissues, degradation and excretion may all affect tissue carnitine concentrations.

It has been demonstrated that pharmacokinetic parameters increase significantly with dosage. Apparent bioavailability in healthy volunteers is about 10-16%. The data suggests a relationship between maximal plasma concentration/dosage, dosage, plasma AUC, dosage/urinary accumulation. Maximum concentration is reached about four hours after ingestion.

5.3 Preclinical safety data
L-Carnitine is a naturally occurring body substance in human beings, plants and animals. Carnitor products are used to bring the level of L-carnitine in the body up to those found naturally. Appropriate pre-clinical studies have been undertaken and show no signs of toxicity at normal therapeutic doses.

6. PHARMACEUTICAL PARTICULARS

6.1 List of excipients
Sorbitol solution (70%), tartaric acid, sodium propyl hydroxybenzoate, sodium methyl hydroxybenzoate, colourless cherry flavour, colourless sour black cherry flavour, saccharose and purified water.

6.2 Incompatibilities
None known.

6.3 Shelf life
3 years.

6.4 Special precautions for storage
Store at a temperature not exceeding 25°C in a dry place. Protect from light.

6.5 Nature and contents of container
20ml amber glass bottles with a polyethylene lined, polypropylene child proof cap.

6.6 Instructions for use and handling
None

7. MARKETING AUTHORISATION HOLDER
Sigma-Tau Industrie Farmaceutiche Riunite SpA,
Viale Shakespeare 47-00144,
Rome, Italy.

8. MARKETING AUTHORISATION NUMBER(S)
PL 08381/0005

9. DATE OF FIRST AUTHORISATION/RENEWAL OF THE AUTHORISATION
20 November 1998

10. DATE OF REVISION OF THE TEXT
July 2002

Legal Category
POM

Carylderm Liquid

(SSL International plc)

1. NAME OF THE MEDICINAL PRODUCT
Carylderm Liquid
CARYLDERM LIQUID.

2. QUALITATIVE AND QUANTITATIVE COMPOSITION
Carbaril 1.0% w/w.

3. PHARMACEUTICAL FORM
Liquid.

4. CLINICAL PARTICULARS

4.1 Therapeutic indications
For the eradication of head lice and their eggs.

4.2 Posology and method of administration
Adults, the elderly and children aged 6 months and above: For external use only. As this product does not contain alcohol, it may be more suitable for those with asthma and eczema. Keep the head upright and rub Carylderm Liquid well into the roots of the hair and scalp, paying particular attention to the partings, back of the neck, fringes and around the ears. Leave the hair to dry naturally and wash in ordinary shampoo the next day or after 12 hours. After shampoo wash, remove dead eggs with a metal nit comb while the hair is wet. Family members and close contacts should also be treated simultaneously, if infected. In the event of early re-infestation, Carylderm Liquid should be applied again, provided 7 days have elapsed since the first application. Not to be used on children under the age of 6 months except under medical supervision.

4.3 Contraindications
Known sensitivity to carbaril.

4.4 Special warnings and special precautions for use
Avoid contact with eyes. Not to be used on infants under 6 months of age, unless under medical supervision. Use in clinics: nursing staff involved in repeated applications should wear rubber gloves when carrying out treatment. For external use only. If Carylderm Liquid is inadvertently swallowed a doctor or casualty department should be contacted at once. Continued prolonged treatment with Carylderm Liquid should be avoided. It should not be used more than once a week for three weeks at a time. The feeding of carbaril to rats and mice throughout life led to an increased incidence of benign and malignant tumours only at very high doses. However, a range of in vivo and in vitro mutagenicity tests have indicated that carbaril is not genotoxic. These findings suggest that the use of carbaril to treat louse infestations is unlikely to pose a significant cancer risk in humans.

4.5 Interaction with other medicinal products and other forms of Interaction
None known.

4.6 Pregnancy and lactation
No evidence for safety of this product has been determined in pregnancy and lactation. It is not necessary to contraindicate this product in pregnancy and lactation provided caution is exercised and the directions for use are followed.

4.7 Effects on ability to drive and use machines
None stated.

4.8 Undesirable effects
None stated.

4.9 Overdose
Accidental ingestion: it is unlikely that a toxic dose of carbaril will be ingested. Treatment consists of gastric lavage, assisted respiration and, if necessary in the event of massive ingestion, administration of atropine.

5. PHARMACOLOGICAL PROPERTIES

5.1 Pharmacodynamic properties
The action of carbamates is to inhibit the acetyl cholinesterases present at synaptic junctions within the insects' nervous systems.

5.2 Pharmacokinetic properties
Carylderm Liquid is applied topically to the affected area.

5.3 Preclinical safety data
None stated.

6. PHARMACEUTICAL PARTICULARS

6.1 List of excipients
Potassium Citrate Ph Eur; Citric Acid Ph Eur; Lanette Wax SX; Propyl Hydroxybenzoate (E217) Ph Eur; Methyl Hydroxybenzoate (E219) Ph Eur; Diethylene Glycol; Dimethyl Phthalate BP; Colour Blue 1249 (E131); Bronopol BP; Water.

6.2 Incompatibilities
None stated.

6.3 Shelf life
Three years.

6.4 Special precautions for storage
Store at or below 25°C and do not refrigerate. Protect from sunlight.

6.5 Nature and contents of container
Clear or amber glass bottles with polyethylene caps and polypropylene faced wads. The clear glass bottles are contained in cartons. The product is available in bottles containing either 50 or 200 ml of product.

6.6 Instructions for use and handling
None stated.

7. MARKETING AUTHORISATION HOLDER
Seton Products Limited, Tubiton House, Oldham, OL1 3HS.

8. MARKETING AUTHORISATION NUMBER(S)
PL 11314/0044.

9. DATE OF FIRST AUTHORISATION/RENEWAL OF THE AUTHORISATION
2nd July 1997.

10. DATE OF REVISION OF THE TEXT
December 1996.

Carylderm Lotion

(SSL International plc)

1. NAME OF THE MEDICINAL PRODUCT
Carylderm Lotion.

2. QUALITATIVE AND QUANTITATIVE COMPOSITION
Carbaril 0.5% w/w.

3. PHARMACEUTICAL FORM
Lotion.

4. CLINICAL PARTICULARS

4.1 Therapeutic indications
For the eradication of head louse infestation.

4.2 Posology and method of administration
Adults, the elderly and children aged 6 months and above. For topical external use only. For head lice. Rub the lotion gently into the scalp until all the hair is thoroughly moistened. Allow to dry naturally in a well ventilated room. Do not use a hairdryer or other artificial heat. Live lice will be eradicated after a minimum treatment period of two hours. However, the lotion should be left on the head for a further period of 8-10 hours to ensure that all lice eggs are totally eradicated. Shampoo in the normal manner. Rinse and comb the hair while wet to remove the dead lice. In the event of early reinfestation, Carylderm Lotion may be applied again provided 7 days have elapsed since the first application. Residual protective effect is variable, of short duration and should not be relied upon. Not to be used on children under six months of age except on medical advice.

4.3 Contraindications
Not to be used on children under 6 months of age except under medical supervision. Known sensitivity to carbaril.

4.4 Special warnings and special precautions for use
Avoid contact with the eyes. Do not cover the head until the hair has dried completely. It is advisable that nursing staff involved in repeated applications should wear rubber gloves when carrying out treatment. Carylderm Lotion is for external use only and should be kept out of the reach of children. Keep away from exposed flame or lighted objects (e.g. cigarettes, gas and electric fires) during application and while hair is wet. Continued prolonged treatment with Carylderm Lotion should be avoided. It should not be used more than once a week for three weeks at a time. Alcohol based skin products may cause a stinging sensation on patients with sensitive skin and wheezing in asthmatic patients. The feeding of carbaril to rats and mice throughout life has led to an increased incidence of benign and malignant tumours only at very high doses. However, a range of in vivo and in vitro mutagenicity tests have indicted that carbaril is not genotoxic. These findings suggest that use of carbaril to treat louse infestations is unlikely to pose a significant cancer risk in humans.

4.5 Interaction with other medicinal products and other forms of Interaction
None known.

4.6 Pregnancy and lactation
No evidence of safety of this product has been determined in pregnancy and lactation. It is not necessary to contraindicate this product in pregnancy and lactation provided caution is exercised and the directions for use are followed. However, as with all medicines, the advice of a doctor should be sought before the product is used.

4.7 Effects on ability to drive and use machines
None known.

4.8 Undesirable effects
Very rarely, skin irritation has been reported with carbaril products. Carylderm Lotion contains isopropyl alcohol, which may cause wheezing in asthmatics.

4.9 Overdose
Accidental ingestion: gastric lavage, assisted respiration and, if necessary, administration of atropine.

5. PHARMACOLOGICAL PROPERTIES

5.1 Pharmacodynamic properties
The action of carbamates is to inhibit the acetyl cholinesterases present at synaptic junctions within the insect's nervous system.

5.2 Pharmacokinetic properties
Carylderm Lotion is applied topically to the affected area.

5.3 Preclinical safety data
None stated.

6. PHARMACEUTICAL PARTICULARS

6.1 List of excipients
Isopropyl alcohol IPSI BP; D-Limonene 17449; Terpineol 18689 BP; Shellsol T; Colour Blue 12401 (E131); Perfume Loxol P6160; Citric Acid EP.

6.2 Incompatibilities
None stated.

6.3 Shelf life
Two years.

6.4 Special precautions for storage
Store at or below 25°C. Protect from sunlight.

6.5 Nature and contents of container
Clear or amber glass bottles with LDPE caps with HDPE sprinkle plug inserts. The clear glass bottles will be marketed in cartons containing 50 or 200ml of product.

6.6 Instructions for use and handling
None stated.

7. MARKETING AUTHORISATION HOLDER
Seton Products Limited, Tubiton House, Oldham, OL1 3HS.

8. MARKETING AUTHORISATION NUMBER(S)
PL 11314/0053.

9. DATE OF FIRST AUTHORISATION/RENEWAL OF THE AUTHORISATION
1st July 1997.

10. DATE OF REVISION OF THE TEXT
March 1999.

Casodex 150 mg Film-coated Tablets.

(AstraZeneca UK Limited)

1. NAME OF THE MEDICINAL PRODUCT
Casodex® 150 mg Film-coated Tablets.

2. QUALITATIVE AND QUANTITATIVE COMPOSITION
Each tablet contains 150 mg Bicalutamide (INN)
For excipients, see Section 6.1.

3. PHARMACEUTICAL FORM
Film-coated tablet.
White.

4. CLINICAL PARTICULARS

4.1 Therapeutic indications
In patients with locally advanced prostate cancer (T3-T4, any N, MO; T1-T2, N+, MO), Casodex 150mg is indicated as immediate therapy either alone or as adjuvant to treatment by radical prostatectomy or radiotherapy. (See section 5.1 Pharmacodynamics).

Casodex 150 mg is also indicated for the management of patients with locally advanced, non-metastatic prostate cancer for whom surgical castration or other medical intervention is not considered appropriate or acceptable.

4.2 Posology and method of administration
Adult males including the elderly: The dosage is one 150 mg tablet to be taken orally once a day.

Casodex 150 mg should be taken continuously for at least 2 years or until disease progression.

Renal Impairment: no dosage adjustment is necessary for patients with renal impairment.

Hepatic Impairment: no dosage adjustment is necessary for patients with mild hepatic impairment. Increased accumulation may occur in patients with moderate to severe hepatic impairment (see Section 4.4).

4.3 Contraindications

Casodex 150 mg is contra-indicated in females and children.

Casodex 150 mg must not be given to any patient who has shown a hypersensitivity to the active substance or any of the excipients.

Co-administration of terfenadine, astemizole or cisapride with Casodex is contra-indicated (see Section 4.5).

4.4 Special warnings and special precautions for use

Bicalutamide is extensively metabolised in the liver. Data suggest that its elimination may be slower in subjects with severe hepatic impairment and this could lead to increased accumulation of Bicalutamide. Therefore, Casodex 150 mg should be used with caution in patients with moderate to severe hepatic impairment.

Periodic liver function testing should be considered due to the possibility of hepatic changes. The majority of cases are expected to occur within the first 6 months of Casodex therapy.

Severe hepatic changes have been observed rarely with Casodex 150 mg (see Section 4.8). Casodex 150 mg therapy should be discontinued if changes are severe.

For patients who have an objective progression of disease together with elevated PSA, cessation of Casodex therapy should be considered.

Bicalutamide has been shown to inhibit cytochrome P450 (CYP 3A4), as such, caution should be exercised when co-administered with drugs metabolised predominantly by CYP 3A4, see Sections 4.3 and 4.5.

Lactose sensitive patients should be aware that each Casodex 150 mg tablet contains 183 mg of lactose monohydrate.

4.5 Interaction with other medicinal products and other forms of Interaction

In vitro studies have shown that R- Bicalutamide is an inhibitor of CYP 3A4, with lesser inhibitory effects on CYP 2C9, 2C19 and 2D6 activity. Although clinical studies using antipyrine as a marker of cytochrome P450 (CYP) activity showed no evidence of a drug interaction potential with Casodex, mean midazolam exposure (AUC) was increased by up to 80%, after co-administration of Casodex for 28 days. For drugs with a narrow therapeutic index such an increase could be of relevance. As such, concomitant use of terfenadine, astemizole and cisapride is contra-indicated and caution should be exercised with the co-administration of Casodex with compounds such as cyclosporin and calcium channel blockers. Dosage reduction may be required for these drugs particularly if there is evidence of enhanced or adverse drug effect. For cyclosporin, it is recommended that plasma concentrations and clinical condition are closely monitored following initiation or cessation of Casodex therapy.

Caution should be exercised when prescribing Casodex with other drugs which may inhibit drug oxidation eg, cimetidine and ketoconazole. In theory, this could result in increased plasma concentrations of Bicalutamide which theoretically could lead to an increase in side effects.

In vitro studies have shown that Bicalutamide can displace the coumarin anticoagulant, warfarin, from its protein binding sites. It is therefore recommended that if Casodex 150 mg is started in patients who are already receiving coumarin anticoagulants, prothrombin time should be closely monitored.

4.6 Pregnancy and lactation

Bicalutamide is contra-indicated in females and must not be given to pregnant women or nursing mothers.

4.7 Effects on ability to drive and use machines

No effects on ability to drive and use machines have been observed during treatment with Casodex 150 mg.

4.8 Undesirable effects

The pharmacological action of Bicalutamide may give rise to certain undesirable effects. These include the following:

Very common (>10%):

Gynaecomastia, breast tenderness. The majority of patients receiving Casodex 150mg as monotherapy experience gynaecomastia and/or breast pain. In studies these symptoms were considered to be severe in up to 5% of the patients. Gynaecomastia may not resolve spontaneously following cessation of therapy, particularly after prolonged treatment.

Common or frequent (≥ 1% and <10%):

Hot flushes, pruritus, asthenia, alopecia, hair regrowth, dry skin, decreased libido, nausea, impotence and weight gain.

Uncommon or infrequent (≥ 0.1% to <1%):

Abdominal pain, depression, dyspepsia, haematuria and interstitial lung disease.

Hypersensitivity reactions, including angioneurotic oedema and urticaria.

Hepatic changes (elevated levels of transaminases, cholestasis and jaundice), which are rarely severe. The changes were frequently transient, resolving or improving with continued therapy or following cessation of therapy. Hepatic failure has occurred very rarely in patients treated with Bicalutamide but a causal relationship has not been established with certainty. Periodic liver function testing should be considered (see Section 4.4).

4.9 Overdose

There is no human experience of overdosage. There is no specific antidote; treatment should be symptomatic. Dialysis may not be helpful, since Bicalutamide is highly protein bound and is not recovered unchanged in the urine. General supportive care, including frequent monitoring of vital signs, is indicated.

5. PHARMACOLOGICAL PROPERTIES

5.1 Pharmacodynamic properties

Antiandrogen, ATC code L02 B B03

Bicalutamide is a non-steroidal antiandrogen, devoid of other endocrine activity. It binds to the wild type or normal androgen receptor without activating gene expression, and thus inhibits the androgen stimulus. Regression of prostatic tumours results from this inhibition. Clinically, discontinuation of Casodex can result in the 'antiandrogen withdrawal syndrome' in a subset of patients.

Casodex 150 mg was studied as a treatment for patients with localised (T1-T2, N0 or NX, M0) or locally advanced (T3-T4, any N, M0; T1-T2, N+, M0) non metastatic prostate cancer in a combined analysis of three placebo controlled, double-blind studies in 8113 patients, where Casodex was given as immediate hormonal therapy or as adjuvant to radical prostatectomy or radiotherapy. At 5.4 years median follow up, 19.7% and 23.6% of all Casodex and placebo treated patients, respectively, had experienced objective disease progression.

In the subgroup of patients with locally advanced prostate cancer who did not receive treatment with radical prostatectomy or radiotherapy, immediate therapy with Casodex 150mg significantly reduced the risk of objective disease progression (Hazard Ratio (HR)=0.53; 95% CI 0.42 to 0.65). A statistically significant reduction in the risk of objective disease progression was also seen in the subgroup of patients with locally advanced disease who received Casodex as adjuvant to radical prostatectomy or radiotherapy (HR=0. 67; 95% CI 0. 56 to.82).

A reduction in risk of objective disease progression was seen across most patients groups but was most evident in those at highest risk of disease progression. Therefore, clinicians may decide that the optimum medical strategy for a patient at low risk of disease progression may be to defer hormonal therapy until signs that the disease is progressing.

No overall survival difference was seen with 15.2% mortality (HR=1.03; 95% CI 0.92 to 1.15). However, some trends were apparent in exploratory subgroup analyses of those patients receiving Casodex as immediate therapy alone.

- Patients with localised disease receiving Casodex alone showed a trend toward decreased survival compared with placebo patients (HR=1.23; 95% CI 1.00 to1.50). In view of this, the benefit-risk profile for the use of Casodex is not considered favourable in this group of patients.
- Patients with locally advanced disease showed a trend toward improved survival with Casodex compared to placebo (HR=0.81; 95% CI 0.63 to 1.04).
- In the adjuvant group of patients, the survival data are immature. There was no difference evident after 5.4 years follow up.

In a separate programme, the efficacy of Casodex 150 mg for the treatment of patients with locally advanced non-metastatic prostate cancer for whom immediate castration was indicated, was demonstrated in a combined analysis of 2 studies with 480 previously untreated patients with non metastatic (M0) prostate cancer. At 56% mortality and a median follow-up of 6.3 years, there was no significant difference between Casodex and castration in survival (hazard ratio = 1.05 [CI 0.81 to 1.36]); however, equivalence of the two treatments could not be concluded statistically.

In a combined analysis of 2 studies with 805 previously untreated patients with metastatic (M1) disease at 43% mortality, Casodex 150mg was demonstrated to be less effective than castration in survival time (hazard ratio = 1.30 [CI 1.04 to 1.65]), with a numerical difference in estimated time to death of 42 days (6 weeks) over a median survival time of 2 years.

Bicalutamide is a racemate with its antiandrogen activity being almost exclusively in the R-enantiomer.

5.2 Pharmacokinetic properties

Bicalutamide is well absorbed following oral administration. There is no evidence of any clinically relevant effect of food on bioavailability.

The (S)-enantiomer is rapidly cleared relative to (R)-enantiomer, the latter having a plasma elimination half-life of about 1 week.

On daily administration of Casodex 150 mg, the (R)-enantiomer accumulates about 10-fold in plasma as a consequence of its long half-life.

Steady state plasma concentrations of the (R)-enantiomer, of approximately 22 microgram/ml are observed during daily administration of Casodex 150 mg. At steady state, the predominantly active (R)-enantiomer accounts for 99% of the total circulating enantiomers.

The pharmacokinetics of the (R)-enantiomer are unaffected by age, renal impairment or mild to moderate hepatic impairment. There is evidence that for subjects with severe hepatic impairment, the (R)-enantiomer is more slowly eliminated from plasma.

Bicalutamide is highly protein bound (racemate 96%, (R)-enantiomer > 99%) and extensively metabolised (oxidation and glucuronidation); its metabolites are eliminated via the kidneys and bile in approximately equal proportions.

5.3 Preclinical safety data

Bicalutamide is a potent antiandrogen and a mixed function oxidase enzyme inducer in animals. Target organ changes, including tumour induction (Leydig cells, thyroid, liver) in animals, are related to these activities. Enzyme induction has not been observed in man and none of these findings is considered to have relevance to the treatment of patients with prostate cancer. Atrophy of seminiferous tubules is a predicted class effect with antiandrogens and has been observed for all species examined. Full reversal of testicular atrophy was 24 weeks after a 12-month repeated dose toxicity study in rats, although functional reversal was evident in reproduction studies 7 weeks after the end of an 11 week dosing period. A period of subfertility or infertility should be assumed in man.

6. PHARMACEUTICAL PARTICULARS

6.1 List of excipients

Casodex 150 mg includes the following excipients:

Tablet core: Lactose Monohydrate, Magnesium Stearate, Povidone, Carboxymethyl amidon sodium.

Film-coating material: Hypromellose, Macrogol 300, Titanium Dioxide.

6.2 Incompatibilities

Not applicable.

6.3 Shelf life

4 years.

6.4 Special precautions for storage

Do not store above 30°C.

6.5 Nature and contents of container

PVC/Aluminium foil blister pack comprising strips of 5, 10 and 14 tablets to give pack sizes of 10, 20, 30, 40, 50, 80, 90, 100, 200 or 14, 28, 56, 84, 140 and 280 tablets.

Not all pack sizes may be marketed.

6.6 Instructions for use and handling

No special requirements.

7. MARKETING AUTHORISATION HOLDER

AstraZeneca UK Ltd

600 Capability Green,

Luton, LU1 3LU, UK.

8. MARKETING AUTHORISATION NUMBER(S)

PL 17901/0006

9. DATE OF FIRST AUTHORISATION/RENEWAL OF THE AUTHORISATION

18th June 2000

10. DATE OF REVISION OF THE TEXT

27th January 2004

Casodex Tablets 50mg

(AstraZeneca UK Limited)

1. NAME OF THE MEDICINAL PRODUCT

'Casodex' Tablets 50 mg

2. QUALITATIVE AND QUANTITATIVE COMPOSITION

Each tablet contains 50mg bicalutamide (INN)

3. PHARMACEUTICAL FORM

White film-coated tablet

4. CLINICAL PARTICULARS

4.1 Therapeutic indications

Treatment of advanced prostate cancer in combination with LHRH analogue therapy or surgical castration.

4.2 Posology and method of administration

Adult males including the elderly: one tablet (50mg) once a day.

Treatment with 'Casodex' should be started at least 3 days before commencing treatment with an LHRH analogue, or at the same time as surgical castration.

Children: 'Casodex' is contra-indicated in children.

Renal impairment: no dosage adjustment is necessary for patients with renal impairment.

Hepatic impairment: no dosage adjustment is necessary for patients with mild hepatic impairment. Increased accumulation may occur in patients with moderate to severe hepatic impairment (see Section 4.4).

4.3 Contraindications

'Casodex' is contra-indicated in females and children.

'Casodex' must not be given to any patient who has shown a hypersensitivity reaction to its use.

Co-administration of terfenadine, astemizole or cisapride with 'Casodex' is contra-indicated.

4.4 Special warnings and special precautions for use

'Casodex' is extensively metabolised in the liver. Data suggests that its elimination may be slower in subjects with severe hepatic impairment and this could lead to increased accumulation of 'Casodex'. Therefore, 'Casodex' should be used with caution in patients with moderate to severe hepatic impairment.

Periodic liver function testing should be considered due to the possibility of hepatic changes. The majority of changes are expected to occur within the first 6 months of 'Casodex' therapy.

Severe hepatic changes have been observed rarely with 'Casodex' (see Section 4.8). 'Casodex' therapy should be discontinued if changes are severe.

'Casodex' has been shown to inhibit Cytochrome P450 (CYP 3A4), as such caution should be exercised when co-administered with drugs metabolised predominantly by CYP 3A4, see Sections 4.3 and 4.5.

4.5 Interaction with other medicinal products and other forms of Interaction

There is no evidence of any pharmacodynamic or pharmacokinetic interactions between 'Casodex' and LHRH analogues.

In vitro studies have shown that R-bicalutamide is an inhibitor of CYP 3A4, with lesser inhibitory effects on CYP 2C9, 2C19 and 2D6 activity.

Although clinical studies using antipyrine as a marker of cytochrome P450 (CYP) activity showed no evidence of a drug interaction potential with 'Casodex', mean midazolam exposure (AUC) was increased by up to 80%, after co-administration of 'Casodex' for 28 days. For drugs with a narrow therapeutic index such an increase could be of relevance. As such, concomitant use of terfenadine, astemizole and cisapride is contra-indicated and caution should be exercised with the co-administration of 'Casodex' with compounds such as cyclosporin and calcium channel blockers. Dosage reduction may be required for these drugs particularly if there is evidence of enhanced or adverse drug effect. For cyclosporin, it is recommended that plasma concentrations and clinical condition are closely monitored following initiation or cessation of 'Casodex' therapy.

Caution should be exercised when prescribing 'Casodex' with other drugs which may inhibit drug oxidation e.g. cimetidine and ketoconazole. In theory, this could result in increased plasma concentrations of 'Casodex' which theoretically could lead to an increase in side effects.

In vitro studies have shown that 'Casodex' can displace the coumarin anticoagulant, warfarin, from its protein binding sites. It is therefore recommended that if 'Casodex' is started in patients who are already receiving coumarin anticoagulants, prothrombin time should be closely monitored.

4.6 Pregnancy and lactation

'Casodex' is contra-indicated in females and must not be given to pregnant women or nursing mothers.

4.7 Effects on ability to drive and use machines

'Casodex' is unlikely to impair the ability of patients to drive or operate machinery. However, it should be noted that occasionally somnolence may occur. Any affected patients should exercise caution.

4.8 Undesirable effects

'Casodex' in general, has been well tolerated with few withdrawals due to adverse events.

Table 1 Frequency of Adverse Reactions

Frequency	System Organ Class	Event
Very common (≥ 10%)	Reproductive system and breast disorders	Breast tenderness[1] Gynaecomastia[1]
	General disorders	Hot flushes[1]
Common (≥ 1% and <10%)	Gastrointestinal disorders	Diarrhoea Nausea
	Hepato-biliary disorders	Hepatic changes (elevated levels of transaminases, cholestasis and jaundice)[2]
	General disorders	Asthenia Pruritus
Uncommon (≥ 0.1% and <1%)	Immune system disorders	Hypersensitivity reactions, including angioneurotic oedema and urticaria
	Respiratory, thoracic and mediastinal disorders	Interstitial lung disease
Rare (≥ 0.01% and < 0.1%)	Gastrointestinal disorders	Vomiting
	Skin and subcutaneous tissue disorders	Dry skin
	Hepato- biliary disorders	Hepatic failure[3]

1. May be reduced by concomitant castration.

2. Hepatic changes are rarely severe and were frequently transient, resolving or improving with continued therapy or following cessation of therapy (see section 4.4 Special warnings and special precautions for use).

3. Hepatic failure has occurred very rarely in patients treated with 'Casodex', but a causal relationship has not been established with certainty. Periodic liver function testing should be considered (see also section 4.4).

Rare cardiovascular effects such as angina, heart failure, conduction defects including PR and QT interval prolongations, arrhythmias and non-specific ECG changes have been observed.

Thrombocytopenia has been reported rarely.

In addition, the following adverse experiences were reported in clinical trials (as possible adverse drug reactions in the opinion of investigating clinicians, with a frequency of ≥1%) during treatment with 'Casodex' plus an LHRH analogue. No causal relationship of these experiences to drug treatment has been made and some of the experiences reported are those that commonly occur in elderly patients:

Cardiovascular system: heart failure.

Gastrointestinal system: anorexia, dry mouth, dyspepsia, constipation, flatulence.

Central nervous system: dizziness, insomnia, somnolence, decreased libido.

Respiratory system: dyspnoea.

Urogenital: impotence, nocturia.

Haematological: anaemia.

Skin and appendages: alopecia, rash, sweating, hirsutism.

Metabolic and nutritional: diabetes mellitus, hyperglycaemia, oedema, weight gain, weight loss.

Whole body: abdominal pain, chest pain, headache, pain, pelvic pain, chills.

4.9 Overdose

There is no human experience of overdosage. There is no specific antidote; treatment should be symptomatic. Dialysis may not be helpful, since 'Casodex' is highly protein bound and is not recovered unchanged in the urine. General supportive care, including frequent monitoring of vital signs, is indicated.

5. PHARMACOLOGICAL PROPERTIES

5.1 Pharmacodynamic properties

'Casodex' is a non-steroidal antiandrogen, devoid of other endocrine activity. It binds to androgen receptors without activating gene expression, and thus inhibits the androgen stimulus. Regression of prostatic tumours results from this inhibition. Clinically, discontinuation of 'Casodex' can result in antiandrogen withdrawal syndrome in a subset of patients.

'Casodex' is a racemate with its antiandrogenic activity being almost exclusively in the (R)-enantiomer.

5.2 Pharmacokinetic properties

'Casodex' is well absorbed following oral administration. There is no evidence of any clinically relevant effect of food on bioavailability.

The (S)-enantiomer is rapidly cleared relative to the (R)-enantiomer, the latter having a plasma elimination half-life of about 1 week.

On daily administration of 'Casodex', the (R)-enantiomer accumulates about 10 fold in plasma as a consequence of its long half-life.

Steady state plasma concentrations of the (R)-enantiomer of approximately

9 microgram/ml are observed during daily administration of 50 mg doses of 'Casodex'. At steady state the predominantly active (R)-enantiomer accounts for 99% of the total circulating enantiomers.

The pharmacokinetics of the (R)-enantiomer are unaffected by age, renal impairment or mild to moderate hepatic impairment. There is evidence that for subjects with severe hepatic impairment, the (R)-enantiomer is more slowly eliminated from plasma.

'Casodex' is highly protein bound (racemate 96%, R-bicalutamide 99.6%) and extensively metabolised (via oxidation and glucuronidation): Its metabolites are eliminated via the kidneys and bile in approximately equal proportions.

5.3 Preclinical safety data

'Casodex' is a potent antiandrogen and a mixed function oxidase enzyme inducer in animals. Target organ changes, including tumour induction, in animals, are related to these activities. None of the findings in the preclinical testing is considered to have relevance to the treatment of advanced prostate cancer patients.

6. PHARMACEUTICAL PARTICULARS

6.1 List of excipients

'Casodex' includes the following excipients:

Lactose Ph. Eur, Magnesium Stearate Ph. Eur, Hypromellose Ph. Eur, Macrogol 300 Ph Eur, Povidone Ph. Eur, Carboxymethyl amidon sodium Ph. Eur and Titanium Dioxide Ph. Eur.

6.2 Incompatibilities

None known

6.3 Shelf life

5 years.

6.4 Special precautions for storage

Do not store above 30°C.

6.5 Nature and contents of container

PVC blister/aluminium foil packs.

6.6 Instructions for use and handling

No special precautions required.

7. MARKETING AUTHORISATION HOLDER

AstraZeneca UK Limited,

600 Capability Green,

Luton, LU1 3LU, UK.

8. MARKETING AUTHORISATION NUMBER(S)

17901/0005

9. DATE OF FIRST AUTHORISATION/RENEWAL OF THE AUTHORISATION

18th June 2000

10. DATE OF REVISION OF THE TEXT

27th January 2004

Catapres Ampoules

(Boehringer Ingelheim Limited)

1. NAME OF THE MEDICINAL PRODUCT

Catapres Ampoules 150 micrograms in 1 ml.

2. QUALITATIVE AND QUANTITATIVE COMPOSITION

Each 1 ml ampoule contains clonidine hydrochloride 150 micrograms.

For excipients, see 6.1.

3. PHARMACEUTICAL FORM

Solution for injection.

Clear, colourless solution.

4. CLINICAL PARTICULARS

4.1 Therapeutic indications

Catapres is indicated for the treatment of hypertensive crises.

4.2 Posology and method of administration

Adults, including the elderly

In hypertensive crises 1 or 2 Catapres Ampoules (150 to 300 micrograms) should be given by slow intravenous injection.

Up to 5 ampoules (750 micrograms) may be given in 24 hours to achieve and maintain the required blood pressure.

Patients undergoing anaesthesia should continue their Catapres treatment before, during and after anaesthesia using oral or intravenous administration according to individual circumstances.

Intravenous injection of Catapres should be given slowly over 10-15 minutes to avoid a possible transient pressor effect.

Catapres injection solution is compatible with 0.9% sodium chloride solution and with 5% Dextrose solution.

Children

Not recommended.

4.3 Contraindications

Catapres should not be used in children or in patients with known hypersensitivity to the active ingredient or other components of the product, and in patients with severe bradyarrhythmia resulting from either sick sinus syndrome or AV block of 2nd or 3rd degree.

4.4 Special warnings and special precautions for use

Clonidine should only be used with caution in patients with depression or a history thereof, with Raynaud's disease or other peripheral vascular occlusive disease.

The product should only be used with caution in patients with cerebrovascular or coronary insufficiency. Catapres should be used with caution in patients with mild to moderate bradyarrhythmia such as low sinus rhythm, and with polyneuropathy or constipation.

As with other antihypertensive drugs, treatment with Catapres should be monitored particularly carefully in patients with heart failure.

In hypertension caused by phaeochromocytoma no therapeutic effect of Catapres can be expected.

Clonidine, the active ingredient of Catapres, and its metabolites, are extensively excreted in urine. Dosage must be adjusted to the individual antihypertensive response, which can show high variability in patients with renal insufficiency: careful monitoring is required.

Since only a minimal amount of clonidine is removed during routine haemodialysis, there is no need to give supplemental clonidine following dialysis.

4.5 Interaction with other medicinal products and other forms of Interaction

The reduction in blood pressure induced by clonidine can be further potentiated by concurrent administration of other hypotensive agents. This can be of therapeutic use in the case of other antihypertensive agents such as diuretics, vasodilators, beta-receptor blockers, calcium antagonists and ACE-inhibitors, but the effect of alpha$_1$-blockers is unpredictable.

The antihypertensive effect of clonidine may be reduced or abolished and orthostatic hypotension may be provoked or aggravated by concomitant administration of tricyclic antidepressants or neuroleptics with alpha-receptor blocking properties.

Substances which raise blood pressure or induce a sodium ion (Na^+) and water retaining effect such as non-steroidal anti-inflammatory agents can reduce the therapeutic effect of clonidine.

Substances with alpha-receptor blocking properties may abolish the alpha$_2$-receptor mediated effects of clonidine in a dose-dependent manner.

Concomitant administration of substances with a negative chronotropic or dromotropic effect such as beta-receptor blockers or digitalis glycosides can cause or potentiate bradycardic rhythm disturbances.

It cannot be ruled out that concomitant administration of a beta-receptor blocker will cause or potentiate peripheral vascular disorder.

Based on observations in patients in a state of alcoholic delirium it has been suggested that high intravenous doses of clonidine may increase the arrhythmogenic potential (QT-prolongation, ventricular fibrillation) of high intravenous doses of haloperidol. Causal relationship and relevance for antihypertensive treatment have not been established.

The effects of centrally depressant substances or alcohol can be potentiated by clonidine.

4.6 Pregnancy and lactation

This product should only be used in pregnancy if considered essential by the physician.

Clonidine passes the placental barrier and may lower the heart rate of the foetus. Post partum a transient rise in blood pressure in the new born cannot be excluded.

The use of Catapres during lactation is not recommended due to a lack of supporting information.

4.7 Effects on ability to drive and use machines

This product may cause drowsiness. Patients who are affected should not drive or operate machinery.

4.8 Undesirable effects

Side effects include sedation and dry mouth and with withdrawal, agitation.

Occasionally constipation, nausea and vomiting, headache, malaise, impotence, decreased libido, gynaecomastia, orthostatic hypotension and associated dizziness, paraesthesia of the extremities, peripheral vasoconstriction, Raynaud's phenomenon, pain in the parotid gland, drying out of the nasal mucosa and reduced lachrymal flow (caution: contact lens wearers) as well as skin reactions with symptoms such as rash, urticaria, pruritus and alopecia have been observed. Sleep disturbances, nightmares, depression, perceptual disorders, hallucinations, confusion and disturbances of accommodation may occur. Fluid retention, ECG abnormalities and abnormal liver function tests have been reported occasionally. Two cases of hepatitis have also been reported.

In very rare cases, pseudo-obstruction of the large bowel has been observed.

Clonidine may cause or potentiate bradyarrhythmic conditions such as sinus bradycardia or AV-block.

Acute administration of clonidine hydrochloride in animals or in man has occasionally induced a transient elevation of blood sugar. This is believed to be due to the initial pharmacological effect of alpha-adrenergic stimulation. Investigators agree that this has no clinical significance. The inclusion of diabetic patients in many clonidine hydrochloride investigations has confirmed its suitability as an antihypertensive agent for such patients.

4.9 Overdose

Symptoms:

Manifestations of intoxication are due to a generalised sympathetic depression and include pupillary constriction, lethargy, bradycardia, hypotension, hypothermia, coma and apnoea. Paradoxical hypertension caused by stimulation of peripheral alpha$_1$-receptors may occur. Transient hypertension may be seen if the total dose is over 10 mg.

Treatment:

In most cases all that is required are general supportive measures. Where bradycardia is severe atropine will increase the heart rate.

5. PHARMACOLOGICAL PROPERTIES

5.1 Pharmacodynamic properties

Clonidine acts primarily on the central nervous system, resulting in reduced sympathetic outflow and a decrease in peripheral resistance, renal vascular resistance, heart rate and blood pressure. Renal blood flow and glomerular filtration rate remain essentially unchanged. Normal postural reflexes are intact and therefore orthostatic symptoms are mild and infrequent. During long-term therapy, cardiac output tends to return to control values, while peripheral resistance remains decreased. Slowing of the pulse has been observed in most patients given clonidine, but the drug does not alter normal haemodynamic response to exercise.

5.2 Pharmacokinetic properties

The pharmacokinetics of clonidine is dose proportional in the range of 100-600 micrograms. Clonidine, the active ingredient of Catapres, is well absorbed and no first pass effect exists. It is rapidly and extensively distributed into tissues and crosses the blood-brain barrier as well as the placental barrier. The plasma protein binding is 30-40%.

The mean plasma half-life of clonidine is 13 hours ranging between 10 and 20 hours. The half-life does not depend on the sex or race of the patient but can be prolonged in patients with severely impaired renal function up to 41 hours.

About 70% of the dose administered is excreted with the urine mainly in the form of the unchanged parent drug (40-60%). The main metabolite p-hydroxy-clonidine is pharmacologically inactive. Approximately 20% of the total amount is excreted with the faeces.

The antihypertensive effect is reached at plasma concentrations between about 0.2 and 1.5ng/ml in patients with normal excretory function. A further rise in the plasma levels will not enhance the antihypertensive effect.

5.3 Preclinical safety data

Not applicable

6. PHARMACEUTICAL PARTICULARS

6.1 List of excipients

Sodium chloride

1N hydrochloric acid

Water for injections

6.2 Incompatibilities

None known.

6.3 Shelf life

5 years.

Once opened, use immediately.

6.4 Special precautions for storage

Do not store above 30°C.

Keep container in the outer carton.

6.5 Nature and contents of container

1 ml colourless glass (Ph. Eur. Type I) ampoules, marketed in packs of 5.

6.6 Instructions for use and handling

None.

7. MARKETING AUTHORISATION HOLDER

Boehringer Ingelheim Limited

Ellesfield Avenue

Bracknell

Berkshire

RG12 8YS

United Kingdom

8. MARKETING AUTHORISATION NUMBER(S)

PL 00015/5008R

9. DATE OF FIRST AUTHORISATION/RENEWAL OF THE AUTHORISATION

18.07.85 / 10.08.00

10. DATE OF REVISION OF THE TEXT

November 2002

11. Legal Category

POM

C2a/UK/SPC/6

Catapres Tablets 300mcg

(Boehringer Ingelheim Limited)

1. NAME OF THE MEDICINAL PRODUCT

Catapres Tablets 300 micrograms.

2. QUALITATIVE AND QUANTITATIVE COMPOSITION

Each tablet contains 300 micrograms of clonidine hydrochloride.

For excipients see 6.1

3. PHARMACEUTICAL FORM

Tablet.

White compressed tablets impressed with the motif 03C / 03C on one side and with the Company symbol on the reverse.

4. CLINICAL PARTICULARS

4.1 Therapeutic indications

Catapres is indicated for the treatment of all grades of essential and secondary hypertension.

4.2 Posology and method of administration

Catapres Tablets are for oral administration only.

Oral treatment should commence with 50 - 100 micrograms three times daily. This dose should be increased gradually every second or third day until control is achieved. Most patients will be controlled on divided daily doses of 300 -1200 micrograms. However, some patients may require higher doses, e.g. 1800 micrograms or more.

Catapres may be added to an existing antihypertensive regimen where blood pressure control has not been satisfactorily achieved. If side effects with existing therapy are troublesome the concomitant use of Catapres may allow a lower dose of the established regimen to be employed. Patients changing treatment should have their existing therapy reduced gradually whilst Catapres is added to their regimen.

Patients undergoing anaesthesia should continue their Catapres treatment before, during and after anaesthesia using oral or intravenous administration according to individual circumstances.

No specific information on the use of this product in the elderly is available. Clinical trials have included patients over 65 years and no adverse reactions specific to this age group have been reported.

4.3 Contraindications

Catapres should not be used in patients with known hypersensitivity to the active ingredient or other components of the product and in patients with severe bradyarrhythmia resulting from either sick sinus syndrome or AV block of 2nd or 3rd degree.

4.4 Special warnings and special precautions for use

Caution should be exercised in patients with Raynaud's disease or other peripheral vascular disease. As with all drugs used in hypertension Catapres should be used with caution in patients with cerebrovascular or coronary insufficiency.

Catapres should also be used with caution in patients with mild to moderate bradyarrhythmia such as low sinus rhythm, and with polyneuropathy or constipation.

Patients with a known history of depression should be carefully supervised while under long-term treatment with Catapres as there have been occasional reports of further depressive episodes during oral treatment in such patients.

As with other antihypertensive drugs, treatment with Catapres should be monitored particularly carefully in patients with heart failure.

In hypertension caused by phaeochromocytoma no therapeutic effect of Catapres can be expected.

Clonidine, the active ingredient of Catapres, and its metabolites are extensively excreted in the urine. Dosage must be adjusted to the individual antihypertensive response, which can show high variability in patients with renal insufficiency; careful monitoring is required. Since only a minimal amount of clonidine is removed during routine haemodialysis there is no need to give supplemental clonidine following dialysis.

Sudden withdrawal of Catapres, particularly in those patients receiving high doses, may result in rebound hypertension. Cases of restlessness, palpitations, nervousness, tremor, headache and abdominal symptoms have also been reported. Patients should be instructed not to discontinue therapy without consulting their physician. When discontinuing therapy the physician should reduce the dose gradually. However, if withdrawal symptoms should nevertheless occur, these can usually be treated with reintroduction of clonidine or with alpha and beta adrenoceptor blocking agents.

If Catapres is being given concurrently with a beta-blocker, Catapres should not be discontinued until several days after the withdrawal of the beta-blocker.

There is as yet insufficient evidence to enable Catapres to be recommended for children.

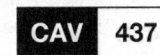

4.5 Interaction with other medicinal products and other forms of Interaction

The reduction in blood pressure induced by clonidine can be further potentiated by concurrent administration of other hypotensive agents. This can be of therapeutic use in the case of other antihypertensive agents such as diuretics, vasodilators, beta-receptor blockers, calcium antagonists and ACE-inhibitors, but the effect of alpha$_1$-blockers is unpredictable.

The antihypertensive effect of clonidine may be reduced or abolished and orthostatic hypotension may be provoked or aggravated by concomitant administration of tricyclic antidepressants or neuroleptics with alpha-receptor blocking properties.

Substances which raise blood pressure or induce a sodium ion (Na^+) and water retaining effect such as non-steroidal anti-inflammatory agents can reduce the therapeutic effect of clonidine.

Substances with alpha$_2$-receptor blocking properties may abolish the alpha$_2$-receptor mediated effects of clonidine in a dose-dependent manner.

Concomitant administration of substances with a negative chronotropic or dromotropic effect such as beta-receptor blockers or digitalis glycosides can cause or potentiate bradycardic rhythm disturbances.

It cannot be ruled out that concomitant administration of a beta-receptor blocker will cause or potentiate peripheral vascular disorders.

Based on observations in patients in a state of alcoholic delirium it has been suggested that high intravenous doses of clonidine may increase the arrhythmogenic potential (QT-prolongation, ventricular fibrillation) of high intravenous doses of haloperidol. Causal relationship and relevance for antihypertensive treatment have not been established.

The effects of centrally depressant substances or alcohol can be potentiated by clonidine.

4.6 Pregnancy and lactation

This product should only be used in pregnancy if considered essential by the physician. Careful monitoring of mother and child is recommended.

Clonidine passes the placental barrier and may lower the heart rate of the foetus. Post partum, a transient rise in blood pressure in the new born cannot be excluded.

During pregnancy the oral forms of Catapres should be preferred. Intravenous injection of clonidine should be avoided.

There is no adequate experience regarding the long-term effects of prenatal exposure.

The use of Catapres during lactation is not recommended due to a lack of supporting information.

4.7 Effects on ability to drive and use machines

This product may cause drowsiness. Patients who are affected should not drive or operate machinery. Sedation due to the drug may be increased by the concomitant use of other central nervous system depressants.

4.8 Undesirable effects

Initially, sedation or dry mouth are encountered in a few patients. These effects usually subside as treatment continues.

Other drug-related side effects which have been reported include constipation, nausea and vomiting, headache, malaise, impotence (rarely), decreased libido, gynaecomastia, orthostatic hypotension and associated dizziness, paresthesia of the extremities, Raynaud's phenomenon, pain in the parotid gland, drying out of the nasal mucosa and reduced lachrymal flow (caution: contact lens wearers), skin reactions with symptoms such as rash, urticaria, pruritus and alopecia, nocturnal unrest, nightmares, depression, perceptual disorders, hallucinations, confusion, disturbances of accommodation and also agitation on withdrawal of long term therapy may occur.

In very rare cases, pseudo-obstruction of the large bowel has been observed.

Clonidine may cause or potentiate bradycardia or bradyarrhythmic conditions such as AV block.

Acute administration in animals or man has occasionally induced a transient elevation of blood sugar. This is believed to be due to the initial pharmacological effect of alpha-adrenergic stimulation. Investigators agree that this has no clinical significance. The inclusion of diabetic patients in many Catapres investigations has confirmed its suitability as an antihypertensive agent for such patients.

There are occasional reports of fluid retention during initial stages of oral treatment. This is usually transitory and can be corrected by the addition of a diuretic.

Occasional reports of abnormal liver function tests and two cases of hepatitis have also been reported.

4.9 Overdose

Symptoms:

Manifestations of intoxication are due to a generalised sympathetic depression and include pupillary constriction, lethargy, bradycardia, hypotension, hypothermia, coma and apnoea. Paradoxical hypertension caused by stimulation of peripheral alpha$_1$-receptors may occur. Transient hypertension may be seen if the total dose is over 10 mg.

Treatment:

Gastric lavage should be performed where appropriate. In most cases all that is required are general supportive measures. Where bradycardia is severe atropine will increase the heart rate.

5. PHARMACOLOGICAL PROPERTIES

5.1 Pharmacodynamic properties

Catapres has been shown to have both central and peripheral sites of action. With long-term treatment Catapres reduces the responsiveness of peripheral vessels to vasoconstrictor and vasodilator substances and to sympathetic nerve stimulation. Early in treatment, however, blood pressure reduction is associated with a central reduction of sympathetic outflow and increased vagal tone.

Clinically, there may be reduced venous return and slight bradycardia resulting in reduced cardiac output. Although initially peripheral resistance may be unchanged, it tends to be reduced as treatment continues. There is no interference with myocardial contractility. Studies have shown that cardiovascular reflexes, as shown by the lack of postural hypotension and exercise hypotension, are preserved.

5.2 Pharmacokinetic properties

Clonidine is well absorbed from the GI tract. Peak plasma concentrations are observed 3-5 hours after administration, declining with a half life up to about 23 hours. Clonidine is metabolised in the liver. About 65% is excreted in the urine, partly as unchanged clonidine and about 20% is excreted in the faeces.

5.3 Preclinical safety data

There are no pre-clinical data of relevance to the prescriber which are additional to that already included in other sections of the SPC.

6. PHARMACEUTICAL PARTICULARS

6.1 List of excipients

Lactose monohydrate, fine

Calcium hydrogen phosphate (anhydrous)

Maize starch, dried

Colloidal silica (anhydrous)

Povidone

Starch, soluble

Stearic acid

6.2 Incompatibilities

Not applicable.

6.3 Shelf life

5 years.

6.4 Special precautions for storage

Do not store above 30°C.

Store in the original container (polypropylene securitainers)

Keep the container in the outer carton (PVC blisters)

6.5 Nature and contents of container

Polypropylene securitainers with polyethylene lids in packs of 84, 100 and 112 tablets.

PVC blister packs (foil 20 μm thick, PVC 200 μm thick) of 100 tablets (currently marketed).

6.6 Instructions for use and handling

None.

7. MARKETING AUTHORISATION HOLDER

Boehringer Ingelheim Limited

Ellesfield Avenue

Bracknell

Berkshire

RG12 8YS

United Kingdom

8. MARKETING AUTHORISATION NUMBER(S)

PL 00015/5041R

9. DATE OF FIRST AUTHORISATION/RENEWAL OF THE AUTHORISATION

18/07/85 and 23/08/00

10. DATE OF REVISION OF THE TEXT

November 2003

11. Legal Category

POM

C2d300/UK/SPC/7

Caverject Dual Chamber 10 micrograms

(Pharmacia Limited)

1. NAME OF THE MEDICINAL PRODUCT

Caverject® Dual Chamber 10 micrograms, Powder and solvent for solution for injection

2. QUALITATIVE AND QUANTITATIVE COMPOSITION

Each 0.5ml cartridge delivers a maximum dose of 10 micrograms of alprostadil.

For excipients see 6.1

3. PHARMACEUTICAL FORM

Powder and solvent for solution for injection

Dual chamber glass cartridge containing a white lyophilised powder and diluent for reconstitution.

4. CLINICAL PARTICULARS

4.1 Therapeutic indications

Caverject Dual Chamber is indicated for the symptomatic treatment of erectile dysfunction in adult males due to neurogenic, vasculogenic, psychogenic, or mixed etiology.

Caverject Dual Chamber may be a useful adjunct to other diagnostic tests in the diagnosis of erectile dysfunction.

4.2 Posology and method of administration

No formal studies with Caverject have been performed in patients younger than 18 years and older than 75 years.

General Information

Caverject Dual Chamber should be administered by direct intracavernosal injection using the 1/2-inch 29 gauge needle provided. The usual site of injection is along the dorsolateral aspect of the proximal third of the penis. Visible veins should be avoided. Both the side of the penis and the site of injection must be altered between injections.

The initial injections of Caverject Dual Chamber must be administered by medically trained personnel and after proper training, alprostadil may be injected at home. It is recommended that patients are regularly monitored (e.g. every 3 months) particularly in the initial stages of self injection therapy when dose adjustments may be needed.

The dose of Caverject Dual Chamber should be individualized for each patient by careful titration under a physician's supervision. The lowest, effective dose should be used that provides the patient with an erection that is satisfactory for sexual intercourse. It is recommended that the dose administered produces a duration of the erection not exceeding one hour. If the duration is longer, the dose should be reduced. The majority of patients achieve a satisfactory response with doses in the range of 5 to 20 micrograms.

The delivery device is designed to deliver a single dose which can be set at 25% increments of the nominal dose. Doses greater than 40 micrograms of alprostadil are not routinely justified. The following doses can be given using Caverject Dual Chamber:

Presentation	Dose Available
Caverject Dual Chamber 10 micrograms	2.5, 5, 7.5, 10 micrograms

A Treatment

The initial dose of alprostadil for erectile dysfunction of vasculogenic, psychogenic, or mixed aetiology is 2.5 micrograms. The second dose should be 5 micrograms if there is a partial response, and 7.5 micrograms if there is no response. Subsequent incremental increases of 5 - 10 micrograms should be given until an optimal dose is identified. If there is no response to the administered dose, then the next higher dose may be given within one hour. If there is a response, there should be a one day interval before the next dose is given.

For patients with erectile dysfunction of neurogenic origin requiring doses less than 2.5 micrograms, it should be considered to dose titrate with Caverject Powder for Injection. Starting with a dose of 1.25 micrograms, if this produces no response, the second dose should be 2.5 micrograms. Apart from the starting dose, it is possible to dose titrate with either Caverject Dual Chamber or Caverject Powder for Injection with similar increments to the treatment of non-neurogenic erectile dysfunction.

The maximum recommended frequency of injection is no more than once daily and no more than three times weekly.

B Adjunct to aetiologic diagnosis.

Subjects without evidence of neurological dysfunction: 10-20 micrograms alprostadil to be injected into the corpus cavernosum and massaged through the penis. Over 80% of subjects may be expected to respond to a single 20 micrograms dose of alprostadil.

Subjects with evidence of neurological dysfunction: These patients can be expected to respond to lower doses of alprostadil. In subjects with erectile dysfunction caused by neurologic disease/trauma the dose for diagnostic testing must not exceed 10 micrograms and an initial dose of 5 micrograms is likely to be appropriate.

Should an ensuing erection persist for more than one hour, detumescent therapy should be employed prior to the subject leaving the clinic to prevent a risk of priapism (please refer to Section 4.9 - Overdose). At the time of discharge from the clinic, the erection should have subsided entirely and the penis must be in a completely flaccid state.

In case of lack of erectile response during the titration phase, patients should be monitored for systemic adverse effects.

4.3 Contraindications

Caverject Dual Chamber should not be used in patients who have a known hypersensitivity to any of the constituents of the product; in patients who have conditions that might predispose them to priapism, such as sickle cell anaemia or trait, multiple myeloma, or leukaemia; or in patients with anatomical deformation of the penis, such as angulation, cavernosal fibrosis, or Peyronie's disease.

Patients with penile implants should not be treated with Caverject Dual Chamber.

Caverject Dual Chamber should not be used in men for whom sexual activity is inadvisable or contraindicated (e.g. patients suffering from severe heart disease).

4.4 Special warnings and special precautions for use

Prolonged erection and/or priapism may occur. Patients should be instructed to report to a physician any erection lasting for a prolonged time period, such as 4 hours or longer. Treatment of priapism should not be delayed more than 6 hours (please refer to Section 4.9 - Overdose).

Painful erection is more likely to occur in patients with anatomical deformations of the penis, such as angulation, phimosis, cavernosal fibrosis, Peyronie's disease or plaques. Penile fibrosis, including angulation, fibrotic nodules and Peyronie's disease may occur following the intracavernosal administration of Caverject Dual Chamber. The occurrence of fibrosis may increase with increased duration of use. Regular follow-up of patients, with careful examination of the penis, is strongly recommended to detect signs of penile fibrosis or Peyronie's disease. Treatment with Caverject Dual Chamber should be discontinued in patients who develop penile angulation, cavernosal fibrosis, or Peyronie's disease.

Patients on anticoagulants such as warfarin or heparin may have increased propensity for bleeding after the intracavernous injection. In some patients, injection of Caverject Dual Chamber can induce a small amount of bleeding at the site of injection. In patients infected with blood-born diseases, this could increase the transmission of such diseases to their partner.

Caverject should be used with care in patients who have experienced transient ischaemic attacks or those with unstable cardiovascular disorders.

Caverject Dual Chamber is not intended for co-administration with any other agent for the treatment of erectile dysfunction (see also 4.5).

The potential for abuse of caverject should be considered in patients with a history of psychiatric disorder or addiction.

Sexual stimulation and intercourse can lead to cardiac and pulmonary events in patients with coronary heart disease, congestive heart failure or pulmonary disease. Caverject should be used with care in these patients.

Reconstituted solutions of Caverject Dual Chamber are intended for single use only. Any unused contents of the syringe should be discarded.

4.5 Interaction with other medicinal products and other forms of Interaction

No known interactions.

Sympathomimetics may reduce the effect of alprostadil. Alprostadil may enhance the effects of antihypertensives, vasodilative agents, anticoagulants and platelet aggregation inhibitors.

The effects of combinations of alprostadil with other treatments for erectile dysfunction (e.g. sildenafil) or other drugs inducing erection (e.g. papaverine) have not been formally studied. Such agents should not be used in combination with Caverject due to the potential for inducing prolonged erections.

4.6 Pregnancy and lactation

Not applicable.

4.7 Effects on ability to drive and use machines

Not applicable.

4.8 Undesirable effects

The most frequent adverse effects following an intracavernous injection was pain in the penis. Thirty percent of patients reported pain at least once. Pain was associated with 11% of the injections administered. In most cases pain was assessed as mild or moderate. Three per cent of patients discontinued treatment because of pain.

Penile fibrosis, including angulation, fibrotic nodules, and Peyronie's disease, was reported in 3% of clinical trial patients overall. In one self-injection study in which the duration of use was up to 18 months, the incidence of penile fibrosis was higher, approximately 8%.

Haematoma and ecchymosis at the injection site, which is related with the injection technique rather than the effect of alprostadil, was reported by 3% and 2% of patients, respectively.

Prolonged erection (an erection for 4 - 6 h) developed in 4% of patients. Priapism (a painful erection for more than 6 hours) occurred in 0.4%. In most cases it disappeared spontaneously.

Adverse drug reactions reported during clinical trials and post marketing experience are presented in the following table:

Cardiac disorders *Uncommon*: Supraventricular extrasystole
Eye disorders *Uncommon*: Mydriasis
Gastrointestinal disorders *Uncommon* Nausea; dry mouth
General disorders and administration site conditions *Common*: Haematoma; ecchymosis *Uncommon*: Haematoma; haemorrhage; pruritis; inflammation; irritation; swelling; oedema; numbness and sensitivity in the injection site; sensation of warmth in the penis; venous bleeding; asthenia.
Investigations *Uncommon:* Urethral haemorrhage; haematuria; decrease blood pressure; increase in cardiac rate; elevated serum creatinine value.
Musculoskeletal, connective tissue and bone disorders *Common*: Connective tissue disorders (including penile fibrosis, angulation, and fibrotic nodules). *Uncommon:* Leg cramps
Infections and infestations *Uncommon:* Yeast infection, symptoms of common cold.
Nervous system disorders *Uncommon*: Vasovagal reactions; hypaesthesia
Renal and urinary disorders *Uncommon*: Impaired urination; increased urinary frequency; urinary urgency.
Reproductive system and breast disorders *Very Common:* Pain in the penis *Common*: Prolonged erection; Peyronie's disease *Uncommon*: Balanitis; priapism; phimosis; painful erection; abnormal ejaculation; pain in the testes, scrotum and the pelvic area; oedema of the testes and scrotum; spermatocele; testicular disorders;
Skin and subcutaneous tissue disorders *Uncommon:* Rash; local pruritus and irritation; erythema of the scrotum; diaphoresis; testicular thickening.
Vascular disorders *Uncommon:* Symptomatic hypotension; hypotension; vasodilation; peripheral vascular disorder

Very Common (≥1/10)	Common (≥1/100, <1/10)	Uncommon (≥1/1000, < 1/100)

Benzyl alcohol may cause hypersensitivity reactions.

4.9 Overdose

Overdosage was not observed in clinical trials with alprostadil. If intracavernous overdose of Caverject Dual Chamber occurs, the patient should be placed under medical supervision until any systemic effects have resolved and/or until penile detumescence has occurred. Symptomatic treatment of any systemic symptoms would be appropriate.

The treatment of priapism (prolonged erection) should not be delayed more than 6 hours. Initial therapy should be by penile aspiration. Using aseptic technique, insert a 19-21 gauge butterfly needle into the corpus cavernosum and aspirate 20-50 ml of blood. This may detumesce the penis. If necessary, the procedure may be repeated on the opposite side of the penis until a total of up to 100 ml blood has been aspirated. If still unsuccessful, intracavernous injection of alpha-adrenergic medication is recommended. Although the usual contra-indication to intrapenile administration of a vasoconstrictor does not apply in the treatment of priapism, caution is advised when this option is exercised. Blood pressure and pulse should be continuously monitored during the procedure. Extreme caution is required in patients with coronary heart disease, uncontrolled hypertension, cerebral ischaemia, and in subjects taking monoamine oxidase inhibitors. In the latter case, facilities should be available to manage a hypertensive crisis. A 200 microgram/ml solution of phenylephrine should be prepared, and 0.5 to 1.0 ml of the solution injected every 5 to 10 minutes. Alternatively, a 20 microgram/ml solution of epinephrine should be used. If necessary, this may be followed by further aspiration of blood through the same butterfly needle. The maximum dose of phenylephrine should be 1 mg, or epinephrine 100 micrograms (5 ml of the solution). As an alternative metaraminol may be used, but it should be noted that fatal hypertensive crises have been reported. If this still fails to resolve the priapism, urgent surgical referral for further management, which may include a shunt procedure is required.

5. PHARMACOLOGICAL PROPERTIES

5.1 Pharmacodynamic properties

Pharmacotherapeutic group: Drugs used in erectile dysfunction ATC code: G04B E01

Alprostadil is the naturally occurring form of prostaglandin E_1 (PGE_1). Alprostadil has a wide variety of pharmacological actions; vasodilation and inhibition of platelet aggregation are among the most notable of these effects. In most animal species tested, alprostadil relaxed retractor penis and corpus cavernosum urethrae in vitro. Alprostadil also relaxed isolated preparations of human corpus cavernosum and spongiosum, as well as cavernous arterial segments contracted by either phenylephrine or $PGF_{2\alpha}$ in vitro. In pigtail monkeys (Macaca nemestrina), alprostadil increased cavernous arterial blood flow in vivo. The degree and duration of cavernous smooth muscle relaxation in this animal model was dose-dependent.

Alprostadil induces erection by relaxation of trabecular smooth muscle and by dilation of cavernosal arteries. This leads to expansion of lacunar spaces and entrapment of blood by compressing the venules against the tunica albuginea, a process referred to as the corporal veno-occlusive mechanism. Erection usually occurs 5 to 15 minutes after injection. Its duration is dose dependent.

5.2 Pharmacokinetic properties

Caverject Dual Chamber contains alprostadil as the active ingredient in a complex with alfadex. At reconstitution, the complex is immediately dissociated into alprostadil and alfadex. The pharmacokinetics of alprostadil is therefore unchanged in Caverject Dual Chamber in comparison with Caverject Powder for Injection.

ADME

Absorption: For the treatment of erectile dysfunction, alprostadil is administered by injection into the corpora cavernosa.

Distribution: Following intracavernosal injection of 20 micrograms alprostadil, mean plasma concentrations of alprostadil increased 22 fold from the baseline endogenous levels approximately 5 minutes post-injection. Alprostadil concentrations then returned to endogenous levels within 2 hours after injection. Alprostadil is bound in plasma primarily to albumin (81% bound) and to a lesser extent α-globulin IV-4 fraction (55% bound). No significant binding to erythrocytes or white blood cells was observed.

Metabolism: Alprostadil is rapidly converted to compounds that are further metabolized prior to excretion. Following intravenous administration, approximately 80% of circulating alprostadil is metabolized in one pass through the lungs, primarily by beta- and omega-oxidation. Hence, any alprostadil entering the systemic circulation following intracavernosal injection is rapidly metabolized. The primary metabolites of alprostadil are 15-keto-PGE_1, 15-keto-13,14-dihydro-PGE_1, and 13,14-dihydro-PGE_1. In contrast to 15-keto-PGE_1 and 15-keto-13,14-dihydro-PGE_1, which lack almost completely biological activity, 13,14-dihydro-PGE_1 has been shown to lower blood pressure and inhibit platelet aggregation. Plasma concentrations of the major circulating metabolite (15-keto-13,14-dihydro-PGE_1) increased 34 fold from the baseline endogenous levels 10 minutes after the injection and returned to baseline levels 2 hours post-injection. Plasma concentrations of 13,14-dihydro-PGE_1 increased 7 fold, 20 minutes after injection.

Elimination: The metabolites of alprostadil are excreted primarily by the kidney, with almost 90% of an administered intravenous dose excreted in urine within 24 hours. The remainder of the dose is excreted in the faeces. There is no evidence of tissue retention of alprostadil or its metabolites following intravenous administration. In healthy volunteers, 70% to 90% of alprostadil is extensively extracted and metabolized in a single pass through the lungs, resulting in a short elimination half-life of less than one minute.

Pharmacokinetics in sub-populations

Effect of renal or hepatic impairment: Pulmonary first-pass metabolism is the primary factor influencing the systemic clearance of alprostadil. Although the pharmacokinetics of alprostadil have not been formally examined in patients with renal or hepatic insufficiency, alterations in renal or hepatic function would not be expected to have a major influence on the pharmacokinetics of alprostadil.

5.3 Preclinical safety data

Preclinical effects were observed only at exposures considered sufficiently in excess of the maximum human exposure indicating little relevance to clinical use.

Alprostadil at subcutaneous doses of up to 0.2 mg/kg/day had no adverse effect on the reproductive function in male rats

A standard battery of genotoxicity studies revealed no mutagenic potential of alprostadil or alprostadil/alfadex.

6. PHARMACEUTICAL PARTICULARS

6.1 List of excipients

Caverject Dual Chamber powder: Lactose Monohydrate

Sodium citrate

Alfadex

Hydrochloric acid

Sodium hydroxide

Diluent: Benzyl alcohol

Water for injections

6.2 Incompatibilities

Not applicable.

6.3 Shelf life

Shelf life of the medicinal product as packaged for sale

36 months.

Shelf life of the medicinal product after reconstitution

Chemical and physical in-use stability has been demonstrated for 24 hours at 25°C

6.4 Special precautions for storage

No special precautions for storage.

6.5 Nature and contents of container

Two or ten*, Type I, Ph. Eur, clear, borosilicate glass cartridges divided into two compartments and sealed with a bromobutyl rubber plunger. The cartridge is sealed with an aluminium cap containing a bromobutyl rubber disc.

Two or ten* 29 G injection needles.

Four or twenty*, pouches containing isopropyl cleansing tissues.

*Not all pack sizes may be marketed.

6.6 Instructions for use and handling

Instructions for use

To perform the reconstitution, attach the needle to the device by pressing the needle onto the tip of the device and turning clockwise until it stops. Remove the outer protective cap of the needle. Turn the white plunger rod clockwise until it stops to reconstitute the alprostadil powder. Invert the device twice in order to make sure the solution is evenly mixed. The solution should be clear. Carefully remove the inner protective cap from the needle. Holding the device upright, press the plunger rod as far as it will go. A few drops will appear at the needle tip. Turn the end of the plunger rod clockwise to select the desired dose.

The package insert provides full instructions on reconstitution, cleansing of the injection site, and also how to perform the injection.

Administrative Data

7. MARKETING AUTHORISATION HOLDER

Pharmacia Limited

Ramsgate Road

Sandwich

Kent

CT13 9NJ

United Kingdom

8. MARKETING AUTHORISATION NUMBER(S)

Caverject Dual Chamber 10 micrograms: PL 0032/0263

9. DATE OF FIRST AUTHORISATION/RENEWAL OF THE AUTHORISATION

13 July 2000

10. DATE OF REVISION OF THE TEXT

09 November 2004

Caverject Dual Chamber 20 micrograms

(Pharmacia Limited)

1. NAME OF THE MEDICINAL PRODUCT

Caverject® Dual Chamber 20 micrograms, Powder and solvent for solution for injection

2. QUALITATIVE AND QUANTITATIVE COMPOSITION

Each 0.5 ml cartridge delivers a maximum dose of 20 micrograms of alprostadil.

For excipients see 6.1

3. PHARMACEUTICAL FORM

Powder and solvent for solution for injection

Dual chamber glass cartridge containing a white lyophilised powder and diluent for reconstitution.

4. CLINICAL PARTICULARS

4.1 Therapeutic indications

Caverject Dual Chamber is indicated for the symptomatic treatment of erectile dysfunction in adult males due to neurogenic, vasculogenic, psychogenic, or mixed aetiology.

Caverject Dual Chamber may be a useful adjunct to other diagnostic tests in the diagnosis of erectile dysfunction.

4.2 Posology and method of administration

No formal studies with Caverject have been performed in patients younger than 18 years and older than 75 years. General Information

Caverject Dual Chamber should be administered by direct intracavernosal injection using the 1/2-inch 29 gauge needle provided. The usual site of injection is along the dorsolateral aspect of the proximal third of the penis. Visible veins should be avoided. Both the side of the penis and the site of injection must be altered between injections.

The initial injections of Caverject Dual Chamber must be administered by medically trained personnel and after proper training, alprostadil may be injected at home. It is recommended that patients are regularly monitored (e.g. every 3 months) particularly in the initial stages of self injection therapy when dose adjustments may be needed.

The dose of Caverject Dual Chamber should be individualized for each patient by careful titration under a physician's supervision. The lowest, effective dose should be used that provides the patient with an erection that is satisfactory for sexual intercourse. It is recommended that the dose administered produces a duration of the erection not exceeding one hour. If the duration is longer, the dose should be reduced. The majority of patients achieve a satisfactory response with doses in the range of 5 to 20 micrograms.

The delivery device is designed to deliver a single dose which can be set at 25% increments of the nominal dose.

Doses greater than 40 micrograms of alprostadil are not routinely justified. The following doses can be given using Caverject Dual Chamber:

PresentationDose Available	
Caverject Dual Chamber 20 micrograms	5, 10, 15, 20 micrograms

A Treatment

The initial dose of alprostadil for erectile dysfunction of vasculogenic, psychogenic, or mixed aetiology is 2.5 micrograms. The second dose should be 5 micrograms if there is a partial response, and 7.5 micrograms if there is no response. Subsequent incremental increases of 5 - 10 micrograms should be given until an optimal dose is identified. If there is no response to the administered dose, then the next higher dose may be given within one hour. If there is a response, there should be a one day interval before the next dose is given.

For patients with erectile dysfunction of neurogenic origin requiring doses less than 2.5 micrograms, it should be considered to dose titrate with Caverject Powder for Injection. Starting with a dose of 1.25 micrograms, if this produces no response, the second dose should be 2.5 micrograms. Apart from the starting dose, it is possible to dose titrate with either Caverject Dual Chamber or Caverject Powder for Injection with similar increments to the treatment of non-neurogenic erectile dysfunction.

The maximum recommended frequency of injection is no more than once daily and no more than three times weekly.

B Adjunct to aetiologic diagnosis.

Subjects without evidence of neurological dysfunction: 10-20 micrograms alprostadil to be injected into the corpus cavernosum and massaged through the penis. Over 80% of subjects may be expected to respond to a single 20 micrograms dose of alprostadil.

Subjects with evidence of neurological dysfunction: These patients can be expected to respond to lower doses of alprostadil. In subjects with erectile dysfunction caused by neurologic disease/trauma the dose for diagnostic testing must not exceed 10 micrograms and an initial dose of 5 micrograms is likely to be appropriate.

Should an ensuing erection persist for more than one hour, detumescent therapy should be employed prior to the subject leaving the clinic to prevent a risk of priapism (please refer to Section 4.9 - Overdose). At the time of discharge from the clinic, the erection should have subsided entirely and the penis must be in a completely flaccid state.

In case of lack of erectile response during the titration phase, patients should be monitored for systemic adverse effects.

4.3 Contraindications

Caverject Dual Chamber should not be used in patients who have a known hypersensitivity to any of the constituents of the product; in patients who have conditions that might predispose them to priapism, such as sickle cell anaemia or trait, multiple myeloma, or leukaemia; or in patients with anatomical deformation of the penis, such as angulation, cavernosal fibrosis, or Peyronie's disease. Patients with penile implants should not be treated with Caverject Dual Chamber.

Caverject Dual Chamber should not be used in men for whom sexual activity is inadvisable or contraindicated (e.g. patients suffering from severe heart disease).

4.4 Special warnings and special precautions for use

Prolonged erection and/or priapism may occur. Patients should be instructed to report to a physician any erection lasting for a prolonged time period, such as 4 hours or longer. Treatment of priapism should not be delayed more than 6 hours (please refer to Section 4.9 - Overdose).

Painful erection is more likely to occur in patients with anatomical deformations of the penis, such as angulation, phimosis, cavernosal fibrosis, Peyronie's disease or plaques. Penile fibrosis, including angulation, fibrotic nodules and Peyronie's disease may occur following the intracavernosal administration of Caverject Dual Chamber. The occurrence of fibrosis may increase with increased duration of use. Regular follow-up of patients, with careful examination of the penis, is strongly recommended to detect signs of penile fibrosis or Peyronie's disease. Treatment with Caverject Dual Chamber should be discontinued in patients who develop penile angulation, cavernosal fibrosis, or Peyronie's disease.

Patients on anticoagulants such as warfarin or heparin may have increased propensity for bleeding after the intracavernous injection. In some patients, injection of Caverject Dual Chamber can induce a small amount of bleeding at the site of injection. In patients infected with blood-born diseases, this could increase the transmission of such diseases to their partner.

Caverject should be used with care in patients who have experienced transient ischaemic attacks or those with unstable cardiovascular disorders.

Caverject Dual Chamber is not intended for co-administration with any other agent for the treatment of erectile dysfunction (see also 4.5).

The potential for abuse of caverject should be considered in patients with a history of psychiatric disorder or addiction.

Sexual stimulation and intercourse can lead to cardiac and pulmonary events in patients with coronary heart disease, congestive heart failure or pulmonary disease. Caverject should be used with care in these patients.

Reconstituted solutions of Caverject Dual Chamber are intended for single use only. Any unused contents of the syringe should be discarded.

4.5 Interaction with other medicinal products and other forms of Interaction

No known interactions.

Sympathomimetics may reduce the effect of alprostadil.

Alprostadil may enhance the effects of antihypertensives, vasodilative agent, anticoauglants and platelet aggregation inhibitors.

The effects of combinations of alprostadil with other treatments for erectile dysfunction (e.g. sildenafil) or other drugs inducing erection (e.g. papaverine) have not been formally studied. Such agents should not be used in combination with Caverject due to the potential for inducing prolonged erections.

4.6 Pregnancy and lactation

Not applicable.

4.7 Effects on ability to drive and use machines

Not applicable.

4.8 Undesirable effects

The most frequent adverse effects following an intracavernous injection was pain in the penis. Thirty percent of patients reported pain at least once. Pain was associated with 11% of the injections administered. In most cases pain was assessed as mild or moderate. Three per cent of patients discontinued treatment because of pain.

Penile fibrosis, including angulation, fibrotic nodules, and Peyronie's disease, was reported in 3% of clinical trial patients overall. In one self-injection study in which the duration of use was up to 18 months, the incidence of penile fibrosis was higher, approximately 8%.

Haematoma and ecchymosis at the injection site, which is related with the injection technique rather than the effect of alprostadil, was reported by 3% and 2% of patients, respectively.

Prolonged erection (an erection for 4 - 6 h) developed in 4% of patients. Priapism (a painful erection for more than 6 hours) occurred in 0.4%. In most cases it disappeared spontaneously.

Adverse drug reactions reported during clinical trials and post marketing experience are presented in the following table:

Cardiac disorders *Uncommon*: Supraventricular extrasystole
Eye disorders *Uncommon*:Mydriasis
Gastrointestinal disorders *Uncommon* Nausea; dry mouth
General disorders and administration site conditions *Common*: Haematoma; ecchymosis *Uncommon*: Haematoma; haemorrhage; pruritis; inflammation; irritation; swelling; oedema; numbness and sensitivity in the injection site; sensation of warmth in the penis; venous bleeding; asthenia.
Investigations *Uncommon:* Urethral haemorrhage; haematuria; decrease blood pressure; increase in cardiac rate; elevated serum creatinine value.
Musculoskeletal, connective tissue and bone disorders *Common*: Connective tissue disorders (including penile fibrosis, angulation, and fibrotic nodules). *Uncommon*: Leg cramps
Infections and infestations *Uncommon:* Yeast infection, symptoms of common cold.
Nervous system disorders *Uncommon:* Vasovagal reactions; hypaesthesia
Renal and urinary disorders *Uncommon:* Impaired urination; increased urinary frequency; urinary urgency.
Reproductive system and breast disorders *Very Common:* Pain in the penis *Common*: Prolonged erection; Peyronie's disease *Uncommon*: Balanitis; priapism; phimosis; painful erection; abnormal ejaculation; pain in the testes, scrotum and the pelvic area; oedema of the testes and scrotum; spermatocele; testicular disorders;
Skin and subcutaneous tissue disorders *Uncommon:* Rash; local pruritus and irritation; erythema of the scrotum; diaphoresis; testicular thickening.

Vascular disorders		
Uncommon: Symptomatic hypotension; hypotension; vasodilation; peripheral vascular disorder		
Very Common (≥1/10)	Common (≥1/100, <1/10)	Uncommon (≥1/1000, < 1/100)

Benzyl alcohol may cause hypersensitivity reactions.

4.9 Overdose

Overdosage was not observed in clinical trials with alprostadil. If intracavernous overdose of Caverject Dual Chamber occurs, the patient should be placed under medical supervision until any systemic effects have resolved and/or until penile detumescence has occurred. Symptomatic treatment of any systemic symptoms would be appropriate.

The treatment of priapism (prolonged erection) should not be delayed more than 6 hours. Initial therapy should be by penile aspiration. Using aseptic technique, insert a 19-21 gauge butterfly needle into the corpus cavernosum and aspirate 20-50 ml of blood. This may detumesce the penis. If necessary, the procedure may be repeated on the opposite side of the penis until a total of up to 100 ml blood has been aspirated. If still unsuccessful, intracavernous injection of alpha-adrenergic medication is recommended. Although the usual contra-indication to intrapenile administration of a vasoconstrictor does not apply in the treatment of priapism, caution is advised when this option is exercised. Blood pressure and pulse should be continuously monitored during the procedure. Extreme caution is required in patients with coronary heart disease, uncontrolled hypertension, cerebral ischaemia, and in subjects taking monoamine oxidase inhibitors. In the latter case, facilities should be available to manage a hypertensive crisis. A 200 microgram/ml solution of phenylephrine should be prepared, and 0.5 to 1.0 ml of the solution injected every 5 to 10 minutes. Alternatively, a 20 microgram/ml solution of epinephrine should be used. If necessary, this may be followed by further aspiration of blood through the same butterfly needle. The maximum dose of phenylephrine should be 1 mg, or epinephrine 100 micrograms (5 ml of the solution). As an alternative metaraminol may be used, but it should be noted that fatal hypertensive crises have been reported. If this still fails to resolve the priapism, urgent surgical referral for further management, which may include a shunt procedure is required.

5. PHARMACOLOGICAL PROPERTIES

5.1 Pharmacodynamic properties

Pharmacotherapeutic group: Drugs used in erectile dysfunction ATC code: G04B E01

Alprostadil is the naturally occurring form of prostaglandin E_1 (PGE_1). Alprostadil has a wide variety of pharmacological actions; vasodilation and inhibition of platelet aggregation are among the most notable of these effects. In most animal species tested, alprostadil relaxed retractor penis and corpus cavernosum urethrae in vitro. Alprostadil also relaxed isolated preparations of human corpus cavernosum and spongiosum, as well as cavernous arterial segments contracted by either phenylephrine or $PGF_{2\alpha}$ in vitro. In pigtail monkeys (Macaca nemestrina), alprostadil increased cavernous arterial blood flow in vivo. The degree and duration of cavernous smooth muscle relaxation in this animal model was dose-dependent.

Alprostadil induces erection by relaxation of trabecular smooth muscle and by dilation of cavernosal arteries. This leads to expansion of lacunar spaces and entrapment of blood by compressing the venules against the tunica albuginea, a process referred to as the corporal veno-occlusive mechanism. Erection usually occurs 5 to 15 minutes after injection. Its duration is dose dependent.

5.2 Pharmacokinetic properties

Caverject Dual Chamber contains alprostadil as the active ingredient in a complex with alfadex. At reconstitution, the complex is immediately dissociated into alprostadil and alfadex. The pharmacokinetics of alprostadil is therefore unchanged in Caverject Dual Chamber in comparison with Caverject Powder for Injection.

ADME

Absorption: For the treatment of erectile dysfunction, alprostadil is administered by injection into the corpora cavernosa.

Distribution: Following intracavernosal injection of 20 micrograms alprostadil, mean plasma concentrations of alprostadil increased 22 fold from the baseline endogenous levels approximately 5 minutes post-injection. Alprostadil concentrations then returned to endogenous levels within 2 hours after injection. Alprostadil is bound in plasma primarily to albumin (81% bound) and to a lesser extent α-globulin IV-4 fraction (55% bound). No significant binding to erythrocytes or white blood cells was observed.

Metabolism: Alprostadil is rapidly converted to compounds that are further metabolized prior to excretion. Following intravenous administration, approximately 80% of circulating alprostadil is metabolized in one pass through the lungs, primarily by beta- and omega-oxidation. Hence, any alprostadil entering the systemic circulation following intracavernosal injection is rapidly metabolized. The primary metabolites of alprostadil are 15-keto-PGE_1, 15-keto-13,14-dihydro-PGE_1, and 13,14-dihydro-PGE_1. In contrast to 15-keto-PGE_1 and 15-keto-13,14-dihydro-PGE_1, which lack almost completely biological activity, 13,14-dihydro-PGE_1 has been shown to lower blood pressure and inhibit platelet aggregation. Plasma concentrations of the major circulating metabolite (15-keto-13,14-dihydro-PGE_1) increased 34 fold from the baseline endogenous levels 10 minutes after the injection and returned to baseline levels 2 hours post-injection. Plasma concentrations of 13,14-dihydro-PGE_1 increased 7 fold, 20 minutes after injection.

Elimination: The metabolites of alprostadil are excreted primarily by the kidney, with almost 90% of an administered intravenous dose excreted in urine within 24 hours. The remainder of the dose is excreted in the faeces. There is no evidence of tissue retention of alprostadil or its metabolites following intravenous administration. In healthy volunteers, 70% to 90% of alprostadil is extensively extracted and metabolized in a single pass through the lungs, resulting in a short elimination half-life of less than one minute.

Pharmacokinetics in sub-populations

Effect of renal or hepatic impairment: Pulmonary first-pass metabolism is the primary factor influencing the systemic clearance of alprostadil. Although the pharmacokinetics of alprostadil have not been formally examined in patients with renal or hepatic insufficiency, alterations in renal or hepatic function would not be expected to have a major influence on the pharmacokinetics of alprostadil.

5.3 Preclinical safety data

Preclinical effects were observed only at exposures considered sufficiently in excess of the maximum human exposure indicating little relevance to clinical use.

Alprostadil at subcutaneous doses of up to 0.2 mg/kg/day had no adverse effect on the reproductive function in male rats

A standard battery of genotoxicity studies revealed no mutagenic potential of alprostadil or alprostadil/alfadex.

6. PHARMACEUTICAL PARTICULARS

6.1 List of excipients

Caverject Dual Chamber powder: Lactose Monohydrate

Sodium citrate

Alfadex

Hydrochloric acid

Sodium hydroxide

Diluent: Benzyl alcohol

Water for injections

6.2 Incompatibilities

Not applicable.

6.3 Shelf life

Shelf life of the medicinal product as packaged for sale

36 months.

Shelf life of the medicinal product after reconstitution

Chemical and physical in-use stability has been demonstrated for 24 hours at 25°C

6.4 Special precautions for storage

No special precautions for storage.

6.5 Nature and contents of container

Two or ten*, Type I, Ph. Eur, clear, borosilicate glass cartridges divided into two compartments and sealed with a bromobutyl rubber plunger. The cartridge is sealed with an aluminium cap containing a bromobutyl rubber disc.

Two or ten* 29 G injection needles.

Four or twenty*, pouches containing isopropyl cleansing tissues.

*Not all pack sizes may be marketed.

6.6 Instructions for use and handling

Instructions for use:

To perform the reconstitution, attach the needle to the device by pressing the needle onto the tip of the device and turning clockwise until it stops. Remove the outer protective cap of the needle. Turn the white plunger rod clockwise until it stops to reconstitute the alprostadil powder. Invert the device twice in order to make sure the solution is evenly mixed. The solution should be clear. Carefully remove the inner protective cap from the needle. Holding the device upright, press the plunger rod as far as it will go. A few drops will appear at the needle tip. Turn the end of the plunger rod clockwise to select the desired dose.

The package insert provides full instructions on reconstitution, cleansing the injection site, and also how to perform the injection.

Administrative Data

7. MARKETING AUTHORISATION HOLDER

Pharmacia Limited

Ramsgate Road

Sandwich

Kent

CT13 9NJ

United Kingdom

8. MARKETING AUTHORISATION NUMBER(S)

Caverject Dual Chamber 20 micrograms: PL 0032/0264

9. DATE OF FIRST AUTHORISATION/RENEWAL OF THE AUTHORISATION

13 July 2000

10. DATE OF REVISION OF THE TEXT

09 November 2004

Caverject Powder for Injection 5, 10, 20, 40 Micrograms

(Pharmacia Limited)

1. NAME OF THE MEDICINAL PRODUCT

Caverject 5, 10, 20 or 40 microgramspowder for solution for injection

2. QUALITATIVE AND QUANTITATIVE COMPOSITION

Alprostadil 5, 10, 20 or 40 micrograms.

When reconstituted, each 1ml delivers a dose of 5, 10, 20 or 40 micrograms of alprostadil.

For excipients, see section 6.1.

3. PHARMACEUTICAL FORM

Powder for Solution for Injection

Powder: A white to off-white powder.

4. CLINICAL PARTICULARS

4.1 Therapeutic indications

Caverject is indicated for the treatment of erectile dysfunction in adult males due to neurogenic, vasculogenic, psychogenic or mixed aetiology.

Caverject may be a useful adjunct to other diagnostic tests in the diagnosis of erectile dysfunction.

4.2 Posology and method of administration

Caverject is administered by direct intracavernous injection. A half inch, 27 to 30 gauge needle is generally recommended. The dose of Caverject should be individualised for each patient by careful titration under supervision by a physician.

The intracavernosal injection must be done under sterile conditions. The site of injection is usually along the dorsolateral aspect of the proximal third of the penis. Visible veins should be avoided. Both the side of the penis that is injected and the site of injection must be alternated; prior to the injection, the injection site must be cleansed with an alcohol swab.

To reconstitute Caverject using the prefilled diluent syringe: flip off the plastic cap from the vial, and use one of the swabs to wipe the rubber cap. Fit the 22 gauge needle to the syringe.

Inject the 1 ml of diluent into the vial, and shake to dissolve the powder entirely. Withdraw slightly more than the required dose of Caverject solution, remove the 22 gauge needle, and fit the 30 gauge needle. Adjust volume to the required dose for injection. Following administration, any unused contents of the vial or syringe should be discarded.

A. As an aid to aetiologic diagnosis.

i) Subjects without evidence of neurological dysfunction; 20 micrograms alprostadil to be injected into the corpus cavernosum and massaged through the penis. Should an ensuing erection persist for more than one hour detumescent therapy (please refer to Section 4.9 - Overdose) should be employed prior to the subject leaving the clinic to prevent a risk of priapism.

Over 80% of subjects may be expected to respond to a single 20 micrograms dose of alprostadil. At the time of discharge from the clinic, the erection should have subsided entirely and the penis must be in a completely flaccid state.

ii) Subjects with evidence of neurological dysfunction; these patients can be expected to respond to lower doses of alprostadil. In subjects with erectile dysfunction caused by neurologic disease/trauma the dose for diagnostic testing must not exceed 10 micrograms and an initial dose of 5 micrograms is likely to be appropriate. Should an ensuing erection persist for more than one hour detumescent therapy (please refer to Section 4.9 - Overdose) should be employed prior to the subject leaving the clinic to prevent a risk of priapism. At the time of discharge from the clinic, the erection should have subsided entirely and the penis must be in a completely flaccid state.

B. Treatment

The initial dose of alprostadil in patients with erectile dysfunction of neurogenic origin secondary to spinal cord injury is 1.25 micrograms, with a second dose of 2.5 micrograms, a third of 5 micrograms, and subsequent incremental increases of 5 micrograms until an optimal dose is achieved. For erectile dysfunction of vasculogenic, psychogenic, or mixed aetiology, the initial dose is 2.5 micrograms. The second dose should be 5 micrograms if there is a partial response, and 7.5 micrograms if there is no response. Subsequent incremental increases of 5-10 micrograms should be given until an optimal dose is achieved. If there is no response to the administered dose, then the next higher dose may be given within 1 hour. If there is a response, there should be at least a 1-day interval before the next dose is given. The usual maximum recommended frequency of injection is no more than once daily and no more than three times weekly.

The first injections of alprostadil must be done by medically trained personnel. After proper training and instruction, alprostadil may be injected at home. If self-administration is planned, the physician should make an assessment of the patient's skill and competence with the procedure. It is recommended that patients are regularly monitored (e.g. every 3 months) particularly in the initial stages of self injection therapy when dose adjustments may be needed.

The dose that is selected for self-injection treatment should provide the patient with an erection that is satisfactory for sexual intercourse. It is recommended that the dose administered produces a duration of the erection not exceeding one hour. If the duration is longer, the dose should be reduced. The majority of patients achieve a satisfactory response with doses in the range of 5 to 20 micrograms. Doses of greater than 60 micrograms of alprostadil are not recommended. The lowest effective dose should be used.

4.3 Contraindications

Caverject should not be used in patients who have a known hypersensitivity to any of the constituents of the product; in patients who have conditions that might predispose them to priapism, such as sickle cell anaemia or trait, multiple myeloma, or leukaemia; or in patients with anatomical deformation of the penis, such as angulation, cavernosal fibrosis, or Peyronie's disease. Patients with penile implants should not be treated with Caverject.

Caverject should not be used in men for whom sexual activity is inadvisable or contraindicated.

4.4 Special warnings and special precautions for use

Prolonged erection and/or priapism may occur. Patients should be instructed to report to a physician any erection lasting for a prolonged time period, such as 4 hours or longer. Treatment of priapism should not be delayed more than 6 hours (please refer to Section 4.9 - Overdose).

Painful erection is more likely to occur in patients with anatomical deformations of the penis, such as angulation, phimosis, cavernosal fibrosis, Peyronie's disease or plaques. Penile fibrosis, including angulation, fibrotic nodules and Peyronie's disease may occur following the intracavernosal administration of Caverject. The occurrence of fibrosis may increase with increased duration of use. Regular follow-up of patients, with careful examination of the penis, is strongly recommended to detect signs of penile fibrosis or Peyronie's disease. Treatment with Caverject should be discontinued in patients who develop penile angulation, cavernosal fibrosis, or Peyronie's disease.

Patients on anticoagulants such as warfarin or heparin may have increased propensity for bleeding after the intracavernous injection.

Underlying treatable medical causes of erectile dysfunction should be diagnosed and treated prior to initiation of therapy with Caverject.

Use of intracavernosal alprostadil offers no protection from the transmission of sexually transmitted diseases. Individuals who use alprostadil should be counselled about the protective measures that are necessary to guard against the spread of sexually transmitted diseases, including the human immunodeficiency virus (HIV). In some patients, injection of Caverject can induce a small amount of bleeding at the site of injection. In patients infected with blood-born diseases, this could increase the transmission of such diseases to their partner.

Reconstituted solutions of Caverject are intended for single use only, they should be used immediately and not stored.

4.5 Interaction with other medicinal products and other forms of Interaction

No known interactions. Caverject is not intended for co-administration with any other agent for the treatment of erectile dysfunction.

4.6 Pregnancy and lactation

Not applicable.

(High doses of alprostadil (0.5 to 2.0 mg/kg subcutaneously) had an adverse effect on the reproductive potential of male rats, although this was not seen with lower doses (0.05 to 0.2 mg/kg). Alprostadil did not affect rat spermatogenesis at doses 200 times greater than the proposed human intrapenile dose.

4.7 Effects on ability to drive and use machines

Not applicable.

4.8 Undesirable effects

The most frequent adverse reaction after intracavernosal injection of Caverject is penile pain. In studies, 37% of the patients reported penile pain at least once; however, this event was associated with only 11% of the administered injections. In the majority of the cases, penile pain was rated mild or moderate in intensity. 3% of patients discontinued treatment because of penile pain.

Prolonged erection (defined as an erection that lasts for 4 to 6 hours) after intracavernosal administration of Caverject was reported in 4% of patients. The frequency of priapism (defined as an erection that lasts 6 hours or longer) was 0.4%. (Please refer to Section 4.4 - Special warnings and precautions for use). In the majority of cases, spontaneous detumescence occurred.

Penile fibrosis, including angulation, fibrotic nodules and Peyronie's disease was reported in 3% of clinical trial patients overall, however, in one self-injection study in which the duration of use was up to 18 months, the incidence of penile fibrosis was 7.8% (please refer to Section 4.4).

Haematoma and ecchymosis at the site of injection, which is related to the injection technique rather than to the effects of alprostadil, occurred in 3% and 2% of patients, respectively. Penile oedema or rash was reported by 1% of alprostadil treated patients.

The following local adverse reactions were reported by fewer than 1% of patients in clinical studies following intracavernosal injection of Caverject: balanitis, injection site haemorrhage, injection site inflammation, injection site itching, injection site swelling, injection site oedema, urethral bleeding and penile warmth, numbness, yeast infection, irritation, sensitivity, phimosis, pruritus, erythema, venous leak, painful erection and abnormal ejaculation.

In terms of systemic events, 2 to 4% of alprostadil-treated patients reported headache, hypertension, upper respiratory infection, flu-like syndrome, prostatic disorder, localised pain (buttocks pain, leg pain, genital pain, abdominal pain), trauma, and sinusitis. One percent of patients reported each of the following: dizziness, back pain, nasal congestion and cough. The following were reported for less than 1% of patients in clinical trials and were judged to be possibly related to Caverject use: testicular pain, scrotal disorder (redness, pain, spermatocele), scrotal oedema, haematuria, testicular disorder (warmth, swelling, mass, thickening), impaired urination, urinary frequency, urinary urgency, pelvic pain, hypotension, vasodilatation, peripheral vascular disorder, supraventricular extrasystoles, vasovagal reactions, hypaesthesia, non-generalised weakness, diaphoresis, rash, non-application site pruritus, skin neoplasm, nausea, dry mouth, increased serum creatinine, leg cramps and mydriasis.

Haemodynamic changes, manifested as decreases in blood pressure and increases in pulse rate, were observed during clinical studies, principally at doses above 20 micrograms and above 30 micrograms of Caverject, respectively and appeared to be dose-dependent. However, these changes were usually clinically unimportant; only three patients (0.2%) discontinued the treatment because of symptomatic hypotension.

Caverject had no clinically important effect on serum or urine laboratory tests.

4.9 Overdose

The pharmacotoxic signs of alprostadil are similar in all animal species and include depression, soft stools or diarrhoea and rapid breathing. In animals, the lowest acute LD_{50} was 12 mg/kg which is 12,000 times greater than the maximum recommended human dose of 60 micrograms.

In man, prolonged erection and/or priapism are known to occur following intracavernous administration of vasoactive substances, including alprostadil. Patients should be instructed to report to a physician any erection lasting for a prolonged time period, such as 4 hours or longer.

The treatment of priapism (prolonged erection) should not be delayed more than 6 hours. Initial therapy should be by penile aspiration. Using aseptic technique, insert a 19-21 gauge butterfly needle into the corpus cavernosum and aspirate 20-50 ml of blood. This may detumesce the penis. If necessary, the procedure may be repeated on the opposite side of the penis until a total of up to 100 ml blood has been aspirated. If still unsuccessful, intracavernous injection of alpha-adrenergic medication is recommended. Although the usual contra-indication to intrapenile administration of a vasoconstrictor does not apply in the treatment of priapism, caution is advised when this option is exercised. Blood pressure and pulse should be continuously monitored during the procedure. Extreme caution is required in patients with coronary heart disease, uncontrolled hypertension, cerebral ischaemia, and in subjects taking monoamine oxidase inhibitors. In the latter case, facilities should be available to manage a hypertensive crisis. A 200 microgram/ml solution of phenylephrine should be prepared, and 0.5 to 1.0 ml of the solution injected every 5 to 10 minutes. Alternatively, a 20 microgram/ml solution of adrenaline should be used. If necessary, this may be followed by further aspiration of blood through the same butterfly needle. The maximum dose of phenylephrine should be 1 mg, or adrenaline 100 micrograms (5 ml of the solution). As an alternative metaraminol may be used, but it should be noted that fatal hypertensive crises have been reported. If this still fails to resolve the priapism, urgent surgical referral for further management, which may include a shunt procedure, is required.

5. PHARMACOLOGICAL PROPERTIES

5.1 Pharmacodynamic properties

Alprostadil is present in various mammalian tissues and fluids. It has a diverse pharmacologic profile, among which some of its more important effects are vasodilation, inhibition of platelet aggregation, inhibition of gastric secretion, and stimulation of intestinal and uterine smooth muscle. The pharmacologic effect of alprostadil in the treatment of erectile dysfunction is presumed to be mediated by inhibition of $alpha_1$-adrenergic activity in penile tissue and by its relaxing effect on cavernosal smooth muscle.

5.2 Pharmacokinetic properties

Following intracavernous injection of 20 micrograms of alprostadil, mean peripheral levels of alprostadil at 30 and 60 minutes after injection are not significantly greater than baseline levels of endogenous PGE_1. Peripheral levels of the major circulating metabolite, 15-oxo-13,14-dihydro-PGE_1, increase to reach a peak 30 minutes after injection and return to pre-dose levels by 60 minutes after injection. Any alprostadil entering the systemic circulation from the corpus cavernosum will be rapidly metabolized. Following intravenous administration, approximately 80% of the circulating alprostadil is metabolized in one pass through the lungs, primarily by beta- and omega-oxidation. The metabolites are excreted primarily by the kidney and excretion is essentially complete within 24 hours. There is no evidence of tissue retention of alprostadil or its metabolites following intravenous administration.

5.3 Preclinical safety data

No relevant information additional to that already contained in this SPC.

6. PHARMACEUTICAL PARTICULARS

6.1 List of excipients

Lactose, sodium citrate, hydrochloric acid, sodium hydroxide

6.2 Incompatibilities

Caverject is not intended to be mixed or coadministered with any other products.

6.3 Shelf life

24 months. Reconstituted solutions should be used immediately and not stored.

40 micrograms only: 24 months under refrigerated conditions (2-8°C). After dispensing, 3 months at room temperature (do not store above 25°C), included in 24 months shelf life. After reconstitution, the product may be stored for 6 hours below 25°C.

6.4 Special precautions for storage

Do not store above 25°C. Reconstituted solutions are intended for single use only, they should be used immediately and not stored.

40 micrograms only: Store at 2-8°C until dispensed. After dispensing, may be stored at room temperature (do not store above 25°C) for up to 3 months. After reconstitution, the product may be stored for 6 hours below 25°C. Do not refrigerate or freeze.

6.5 Nature and contents of container

Single pack containing a vial of Caverject 5, 10, 20 or 40 micrograms powder

Packs also each contain a syringe of solvent, a sterile 22G and a 30G needle plus pre-injection swab.

6.6 Instructions for use and handling

The presence of benzyl alcohol in the reconstitution vehicle decreases the degree of binding to package surfaces. Therefore, a more consistent product delivery is produced when Bacteriostatic Water for Injection containing benzyl alcohol is used.

5,10 & 20 micrograms only: Use immediately after reconstitution.

7. MARKETING AUTHORISATION HOLDER

Pharmacia Limited
Ramsgate Road
Sandwich
Kent, CT13 9NJ
United Kingdom

8. MARKETING AUTHORISATION NUMBER(S)

PL 00032/0214
PL 00032/0203
PL 00032/0188
PL 00032/0227

9. DATE OF FIRST AUTHORISATION/RENEWAL OF THE AUTHORISATION

25 March 1997 / 03 April 2003
08 February 1996 / 03 April 2003
15 March 1994 / 16 March 1999
23 June 1998 / 22 June 2003

10. DATE OF REVISION OF THE TEXT

February 2004

11. LEGAL CATEGORY

POM

Ref: CJ1_0UK

Cedocard Retard -20

(Pharmacia Limited)

1. NAME OF THE MEDICINAL PRODUCT

Cedocard Retard 20 Tablets

2. QUALITATIVE AND QUANTITATIVE COMPOSITION

Isosorbide Dinitrate BP 20.0 mg

3. PHARMACEUTICAL FORM

Uncoated sustained release tablets for oral administration.

4. CLINICAL PARTICULARS

4.1 Therapeutic indications

For the prophylaxis of angina pectoris.

4.2 Posology and method of administration
By oral administration, the tablets should be swallowed, with a little water without chewing.

Children:
There is no recommended dose for children.

Adults:
One tablet in the morning and one before retiring to sleep.

Elderly:
The dosage of nitrates in cardiovascular disease is usually determined by patient response and stabilisation. Clinical experience has not necessitated alternative advice for use in elderly patients. The pharmacokinetics of isosorbide dinitrate in patients with severe renal failure and liver cirrhosis are similar to those in normal subjects.

The onset of action is 20-30 minutes.

The duration of action is 10-12 minutes.

4.3 Contraindications
A history of sensitivity to the drug.

4.4 Special warnings and special precautions for use
Tolerance and cross-tolerance to other nitrates may occur.

4.5 Interaction with other medicinal products and other forms of Interaction
Alcohol may potentiate the effect of isosorbide dinitrate.

4.6 Pregnancy and lactation
No data have been reported which would indicate the possibility of adverse effects resulting from the use of isosorbide dinitrate in pregnancy. Safety in pregnancy however, has not been established. Isosorbide dinitrate should only be used in pregnancy if, in the opinion of the physician, the possible benefits of treatment outweigh the possible hazards. Lactation – there are no data available on the transfer of isosorbide dinitrate in breast milk or its effect on breast-fed children.

4.7 Effects on ability to drive and use machines
Side effects include throbbing headache and dizziness. Patients are advised not to drive or operate machinery is so affected.

4.8 Undesirable effects
Headaches may occur (common), these are usually temporary. Less frequent, cutaneous vasodilation with flushing. Transient episodes of dizziness and weakness and other signs of cerebral ischaemia may occur with postural hypotension.

4.9 Overdose
In rare cases of overdosage, gastric lavage is indicated. Passive exercise of the extremities of the recumbent patient will promote venous return.

5. PHARMACOLOGICAL PROPERTIES

5.1 Pharmacodynamic properties
Vasodilator.

5.2 Pharmacokinetic properties
After administration of one tablet of Cedocard Retard 20 at least two peak concentration of ISDN occurred in the plasma. The initial peak (mean 1.9 ng/ml), range 1.0-3.4 mg/ml) occurred during 0.5 to 2 hours, and then mean plasma concentrations declined to 1.3 ng/ml at 3 hours. The concentration then increased again to reach a major peak level (mean 6.2 ng/ml, range 1.6-12.3 ng/ml) during 4-6 hours after dosing.

Plasma concentrations of ISDN have been measured after administration of increasing doses in the range 20-100 mg (as Cedocard Retard 20 tablets).

Means of peak concentrations of 4.2 ng/ml, 13.1 ng/ml, 20.7 ng/ml, 36.8 ng/ml and 34.9 ng/ml were measured after doses of 20 mg, 40 mg, 60 mg, 80 mg and 100 mg respectively.

5.3 Preclinical safety data
There are no preclinical data of relevance to the prescriber which are additional to that already included in other sections of the SPC.

6. PHARMACEUTICAL PARTICULARS

6.1 List of excipients
Lactose
Talc
Magnesium Stearate
Polyvinyl Acetate
Quinoline Yellow (E104)
Yellow Orange S (E110)
Methylene Chloride
Water

6.2 Incompatibilities
None known.

6.3 Shelf life
60 months.

6.4 Special precautions for storage
Protect from heat and moisture.

6.5 Nature and contents of container
PVC/Aluminium foil blister strip.

Pack size: 60 tablets

6.6 Instructions for use and handling
There are no special instructions for handling.

Administrative Data

7. MARKETING AUTHORISATION HOLDER
Pharmacia Limited
Davy Avenue
Milton Keynes
Buckinghamshire
MK5 8PH
United Kingdom

8. MARKETING AUTHORISATION NUMBER(S)
PL 00032/0331

9. DATE OF FIRST AUTHORISATION/RENEWAL OF THE AUTHORISATION
30 September 2002

10. DATE OF REVISION OF THE TEXT

Cedocard Retard -40

(Pharmacia Limited)

1. NAME OF THE MEDICINAL PRODUCT
Cedocard Retard 40

2. QUALITATIVE AND QUANTITATIVE COMPOSITION
Isosorbide Dinitrate BP 40.0 mg

3. PHARMACEUTICAL FORM
Uncoated sustained release tablets for oral administration.

4. CLINICAL PARTICULARS

4.1 Therapeutic indications
Cedocard Retard is indicated for prophylactic treatment of angina pectoris.

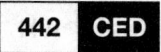

4.2 Posology and method of administration
Children:
There is no recommended dose for children.

Adults:
One or two tablets to be taken twice daily.

Elderly:
Dosage as for other adults.

4.3 Contraindications
Isosorbide dinitrate is contra-indicated in patients with a history of sensitivity to the drug. Sildenafil has been shown to potentiate the hypotensive effects of nitrates, and its co-administration with nitrates, or nitric oxide donors is therefore contra-indicated.

4.4 Special warnings and special precautions for use
Tolerance and cross-tolerance to other nitrates and nitrites may occur.

4.5 Interaction with other medicinal products and other forms of Interaction
Tolerance and cross-tolerance to other nitrates and nitrites may occur. The hypotensive effects of nitrates are potentiated by concurrent administration of sildenafil.

4.6 Pregnancy and lactation
No data have been reported which would indicate the possibility of adverse effects resulting from the use of isosorbide dinitrate in pregnancy. Safety in pregnancy however, has not been established. Isosorbide dinitrate should only be used in pregnancy if, in the opinion of the physician, the possible benefits of treatment outweigh the possible hazards. Lactation - there are no data available on the transfer of isosorbide dinitrate in breast milk or its effect on breast fed children.

4.7 Effects on ability to drive and use machines
Side effects include throbbing headache and dizziness. Patients are advised not to drive or operate machinery if so affected.

4.8 Undesirable effects
Side effects include throbbing headache and dizziness. Patients are advised not to drive or operate machinery if so affected.

4.9 Overdose
No available data.

5. PHARMACOLOGICAL PROPERTIES

5.1 Pharmacodynamic properties
Isosorbide dinitrate is a vasodilator. It relaxes vascular smooth muscle and produces coronary vasodilation, reduction in peripheral resistance and venous return, alteration of myocardial metabolism and reduction of the myocardial oxygen demand.

5.2 Pharmacokinetic properties
The mean plasma concentrations of ISDN at the end of each 12 hour dosage interval (Cmin) during the period of administration of 40 mg as the sustained release tablets were 0.6 ng/ml, 0.6 ng/ml, 0.9 ng/ml and 0.6 ng/ml after the first, second, third and fourth doses respectively and was 0.9 ng/ml at 12 hours after the last dose. At 1, 4 and 8 hours after the first dose the mean plasma levels of ISDN were 1.3 ng/ml, 4.0 ng/ml and 2.2 ng/ml respectively. At 1, 4 and 8 hours after the 3rd dose the mean plasma levels of ISDN were 2.1 ng/ml, 4.0 ng/ml and 2.0 ng/ml respectively at 14 after the last dose, the peak plasma concentrations of ISDN of 12.7 ng/ml occurred at 5 hours and thereafter mean concentrations of ISDN declined to 0.4 ng/ml at 14 hours after the last dose.

5.3 Preclinical safety data
Due to the age and well established safety nature of this product, preclinical data has not been included.

6. PHARMACEUTICAL PARTICULARS

6.1 List of excipients

Lactose	Ph. Eur
Talc	Ph. Eur
Magnesium stearate	Ph. Eur
Polyvinyl acetate	
Red (E124)	
Yellow-orange S (E110)	
Potato starch	Ph. Eur
Methylene chloride	USP
Water	
Sodium chloride	
Sodium sulphate	

6.2 Incompatibilities
None known.

6.3 Shelf life
60 months.

6.4 Special precautions for storage
Protect from heat and moisture.

6.5 Nature and contents of container
PVC/Aluminium blisters in packs of 60 or 1000 tablets.

6.6 Instructions for use and handling
There are no special instructions for handling.

7. MARKETING AUTHORISATION HOLDER
Pharmacia Limited
Davy Avenue
Milton Keynes
MK5 8PH
UK

8. MARKETING AUTHORISATION NUMBER(S)
PL 00032/0332

9. DATE OF FIRST AUTHORISATION/RENEWAL OF THE AUTHORISATION
12 December 2002

10. DATE OF REVISION OF THE TEXT

Cefotaxime for Injection

(Wockhardt UK Ltd)

1. NAME OF THE MEDICINAL PRODUCT
Cefotaxime for Injection 500mg
Cefotaxime for Injection 1g

2. QUALITATIVE AND QUANTITATIVE COMPOSITION
Cefotaxime sodium equivalent to 500mg of cefotaxime
Cefotaxime sodium equivalent to 1g of cefotaxime

3. PHARMACEUTICAL FORM
Powder for solution for injection/infusion.

Cefotaxime sodium is supplied as a white to slightly yellow powder.

4. CLINICAL PARTICULARS

4.1 Therapeutic indications
1. Cefotaxime is indicated in the treatment of serious infections, either before the infecting organism has been identified or when caused by bacteria of established sensitivity, including

osteomyelitis,

septicaemia,

bacterial endocarditis,

meningitis, and

peritonitis.

and other serious bacterial infections suitable for parenteral antibiotic therapy.

2. Cefotaxime may be used for pre-operative prophylaxis in patients undergoing surgical procedures, that may be classified as contaminated or potentially so.

4.2 Posology and method of administration
Cefotaxime may be administered intravenously or by bolus injection or infusion or intramuscularly. The dosage, route and frequency of administration should be determined by the severity of infection, the sensitivity of causative organisms and condition of the patient. Therapy may be initiated before the results of sensitivity tests are known.

Adults:
The recommended dosage for mild to moderate infections is 1g 12 hourly. However, dosage may be varied according

to the severity of the infection, sensitivity of causative organisms and condition of the patient. Therapy may be initiated before the results of sensitivity tests are known.

In severe infections dosage may be increased up to 12g daily given in 3 or 4 divided doses. For infections caused by sensitive *Pseudomonas* species daily doses of greater than 6g will usually be required.

Children:

The usual dosage range is 100-150mg/kg/day in 2 to 4 divided doses. However, in very severe infection doses of up to 200mg/kg/day may be required.

Neonates: The recommended dosage is 50mg/kg/day in 2 to 4 divided doses. In severe infections 150-200mg/kg/day, in divided doses, have been given.

Dosage in renal impairment: Because of extra-renal elimination, it is only necessary to reduce the dosage of cefotaxime in severe renal failure (GFR <5ml/min = serum creatinine approximately 751 micromol/litre). After an initial loading dose of 1g, daily dose should be halved without change in the frequency of dosing, i.e. 1g twelve hourly becomes 0.5g twelve hourly, 1g eight hourly becomes 0.5g eight hourly, 2g eight hourly becomes 1g eight hourly etc. As in all other patients, dosage may require further adjustment according to the course of the infection and the general condition of the patient.

Intravenous and Intramuscular Administration: Reconstitute cefotaxime with Water for Injections PhEur as directed in Section 6.6 (Instructions for use/handling). Shake well until dissolved and then withdraw the entire contents of the vial into the syringe.

Intravenous Infusion: Cefotaxime may be administered by intravenous infusion using the fluids stated in Section 6.6 (Instructions for use/handling). The prepared infusion may be administered over 20-60 minutes.

4.3 Contraindications

Known or suspected allergy to cephalosporins.

4.4 Special warnings and special precautions for use

Preliminary enquiry about hypersensitivity to penicillin and other β-Lactam antibiotics is necessary before prescribing cephalosporins since cross allergy occurs in 5–10% of cases.

Hypersensitivity reactions (anaphylaxis) occurring with the two types of antibiotics can be serious and occasionally fatal. Hypersensitivity requires that treatment be stopped.

Patients with severe renal dysfunction should be placed on the dosage schedule recommended under "Posology and Method of Administration".

As with other antibiotics, the use of cefotaxime, especially if prolonged, may result in overgrowth of non susceptible organisms, such as Enterococcus spp. Repeated evaluation of the condition of the patient is essential. If superinfection occurs during treatment with cefotaxime, specific anti-microbial therapy should be instituted if considered clinically necessary.

Cefotaxime constituted with lignocaine must never be used:

- by the intravenous route
- in infants under 30 months
- in subjects with a previous history of hypersensitivity to this product
- in patients who have an unpaced heart block
- in patients with severe heart failure.

The sodium content of cefotaxime (2.09mmol/g) should be taken into account when prescribing to patients requiring sodium restriction.

Cefotaxime may predispose patients to pseudomembranous colitis. Although any antibiotic may predispose to pseudomembranous colitis, the risk is higher with broad spectrum drugs, such as cephalosporins. This side effect, which may occur more frequently in patients receiving higher doses for prolonged periods, should be considered as potentially serious. The presence of C. difficile toxin should be investigated, and treatment with cefotaxime stopped in cases of suspected colitis. Diagnosis can be confirmed by toxin detection and specific antibiotic therapy (e.g. oral vancomycin or metronidazole) should be initiated if considered clinically necessary. The administration of products which cause faecal stasis should be avoided.

4.5 Interaction with other medicinal products and other forms of Interaction

Cephalosporin antibiotics at high dosage should be given with caution to patients receiving aminoglycoside antibiotics or potent diuretics such as frusemide as these combinations are suspected to adversely affect renal function. However, at the recommended doses, enhancement of nephrotoxicity is unlikely to be a problem with cefotaxime.

Probenecid interferes with renal tubular transfer of cefotaxime delaying its excretion and increasing the plasma concentration.

Interference with Laboratory Tests: A positive Coombs test may be seen during treatment with cephalosporins. This phenomenon may occur during treatment with cefotaxime.

A false positive reaction to glucose may occur with reducing substances but not with the use of specific glucose oxidase methods.

4.6 Pregnancy and lactation

Pregnancy: It is known that cefotaxime crosses the placental barrier. Although studies in animals have not shown an adverse effect on the developing foetus, the safety of cefotaxime in human pregnancy has not been established. Consequently, cefotaxime should not be administered during pregnancy especially during the first trimester, without carefully weighing the expected benefit against possible risks.

Lactation: Cefotaxime is excreted in the milk.

4.7 Effects on ability to drive and use machines

None known.

4.8 Undesirable effects

Adverse reactions to cefotaxime have occurred relatively infrequently and have generally been mild and transient. Effects reported include candidiasis, nausea, vomiting, abdominal pain, diarrhoea (diarrhoea may sometimes be a symptom of pseudomembranous colitis (see warnings)), transient rises in liver transaminases, alkaline phosphatase and/or bilirubin.

As with other cephalosporins, changes in renal function have been rarely observed with high doses of cefotaxime, particularly when co-prescribed with aminoglycosides. Rare cases of interstitial nephritis have been reported in patients treated with cefotaxime. Administration of high doses of cephalosporins, particularly in patients with renal insufficiency, may result in encephalopathy (e.g. impairment of consciousness, abnormal movements and convulsions).

Hypersensitivity reactions have been reported. These include skin rashes, pruritus and less frequently urticaria, drug fever and very rarely anaphylaxis (e.g. angioedema and bronchospasm possibly culminating in shock).

As with other cephalosporins, occasional cases of bullous reactions such as Stevens-Johnson syndrome, toxic epidermal necrolysis and erythema multiforme have also been reported.

As with other beta-lactam antibiotics, granulocytopenia and more rarely agranulocytosis may develop during treatment with cefotaxime, particularly if given over long periods. A few cases of eosinophilia and neutropenia have been observed, reversible when treatment is ceased. Some cases of rapidly reversible eosinophilia and thrombocytopenia on stopping treatment, have been reported. Rare cases of haemolytic anaemia have been reported. For cases of treatment lasting longer than 10 days, blood count should therefore be monitored.

Transient pain may be experienced at the site of injection. This is more likely to occur with higher doses. Occasionally, phlebitis has been reported in patients receiving intravenous cefotaxime. However, this has rarely been a cause for discontinuation of treatment.

A very small number of cases of arrhythmias have occurred following rapid bolus infusion through a central venous catheter.

The following symptoms have occurred after several weeks of treatment for borreliosis (Lyme's Disease): skin rash, itching, fever, leucopenia, increases in liver enzymes, difficulty of breathing, joint discomfort. To some extent these manifestations are consistent with the symptoms of the underlying disease, for which the patient is being treated.

4.9 Overdose

Serum levels of cefotaxime may be reduced by peritoneal dialysis or haemodialysis. In the case of overdosage, particularly in renal insufficiency, there is a risk of reversible encephalopathy.

5. PHARMACOLOGICAL PROPERTIES

5.1 Pharmacodynamic properties

Cefotaxime is a broad spectrum bactericidal cephalosporin antibiotic. Cefotaxime is exceptionally active in vitro against Gram-negative organisms sensitive or resistant to first or second generation cephalosporins. It is similar to other cephalosporins in activity against Gram-positive bacteria.

5.2 Pharmacokinetic properties

After a 1000mg intravenous bolus, mean peak plasma concentrations of cefotaxime usually range between 81 and 102 microgram/ml. Doses of 500mg and 2000mg produce plasma concentrations of 38 and 200 microgram/ml, respectively. There is no accumulation following administration of 1000mg intravenously or 500mg intramuscularly for 10 or 14 days.

The apparent volume of distribution at steady-state of cefotaxime is 21.6 litres/1.73m^2 after 1g intravenous 30 minute infusion.

Concentrations of cefotaxime (usually determined by non-selective assay) have been studied in a wide range of human body tissues and fluids. Cerebrospinal fluid concentrations are low when the meninges are not inflamed, but are between 3 and 30 microgram/ml in children with meningitis. Cefotaxime usually passes the blood-brain barrier in levels above the minimum inhibitory concentration of common sensitive pathogens when the meninges are inflamed. Concentrations (0.2-5.4 microgram/ml), inhibitory for most Gram-negative bacteria, are attained in purulent sputum, bronchial secretions and pleural fluid after doses of 1 or 2g. Concentrations likely to be effective against most sensitive organisms are similarly attained in female reproductive organs, otitis media effusions, prostatic tissue, interstitial fluid, renal tissue, peritoneal fluid and gall bladder wall, after usual therapeutic doses. High concentrations of cefotaxime and desacetyl-cefotaxime are attained in bile.

Cefotaxime is partially metabolised prior to excretion. The principal metabolite is the microbiologically active product, desacetyl-cefotaxime. Most of a dose of cefotaxime is excreted in the urine - about 60% as unchanged drug and a further 24% as desacetyl-cefotaxime. Plasma clearance is reported to be between 260 and 390ml/minute and renal clearance 145 to 217 ml/minute.

After intravenous administration of cefotaxime to healthy adults, the elimination half-life of the parent compound is 0.9 to 1.14 hours and that of the desacetyl metabolite, about 1.3 hours.

In neonates the pharmacokinetics are influenced by gestational and chronological age, the half-life being prolonged in premature and low birth weight neonates of the same age.

In severe renal dysfunction the elimination half-life of cefotaxime itself is increased minimally to about 2.5 hours, whereas that of desacetyl-cefotaxime is increased to about 10 hours. Total urinary recovery of cefotaxime and its principal metabolite decreases with reduction in renal function.

5.3 Preclinical safety data

There are no pre-clinical data of relevance to the prescriber that are additional to those included in other sections.

6. PHARMACEUTICAL PARTICULARS

6.1 List of excipients

None.

6.2 Incompatibilities

Cefotaxime sodium should not be mixed with alkaline solutions such as sodium bicarbonate injection or solutions containing aminophylline.

6.3 Shelf life

The unreconstituted dry powder is stable for 24 months. For the reconstituted solution, chemical and physical in-use stability has been demonstrated for 24 hours at 2-8°C. From a microbiological point of view, once opened, the product should be used immediately. If not used immediately, in-use storage times and conditions prior to use are the responsibility of the user and would normally not be longer than 24 hours at 2-8°C, unless reconstitution has taken place in controlled and validated aseptic conditions.

6.4 Special precautions for storage

Do not store above 25°C. Keep the container in the outer carton.

6.5 Nature and contents of container

Cefotaxime is supplied in Type III 10ml glass vials, closed with a Type I rubber stopper coated with Omniflex and sealed with an aluminium cap fitted with a detachable flip top.

The vials are boxed individually and in packs of 10, 25 or 50 vials.

6.6 Instructions for use and handling

When dissolved in Water for Injections PhEur, cefotaxime forms a straw-coloured solution suitable for intravenous and intramuscular injection. Variations in the intensity of colour of the freshly prepared solutions do not indicate a change in potency or safety.

Dilution table:

(see Table 1)

Reconstituted solution: Whilst it is preferable to use only freshly prepared solutions for both intravenous and intramuscular injection, cefotaxime is compatible with several commonly used intravenous infusion fluids and will retain satisfactory potency for up to 24 hours refrigerated in the following:

Water for Injection Ph Eur

Sodium Chloride Injection BP

5% Glucose Injection BP

Glucose and Sodium Chloride Injection BP

Table 1 Dilution table

Vial size	Diluent to be added	Approx available volume	Approx displacement volume
500mg	2ml	2.2ml	0.2ml
1g	4ml	4.5ml	0.5ml

Compound Sodium Lactate Injection BP (Ringer-lactate injection)

After 24 hours any unused solution should be discarded.

Cefotaxime is compatible with 1% lignocaine; however freshly prepared solutions should be used.

Cefotaxime is also compatible with metronidazole infusion (500mg/100ml) and both will maintain potency when refrigerated for up to 24 hours. Some increase in colour of prepared solutions may occur on storage. However, provided the recommended storage conditions are observed, this does not indicate change in potency or safety.

Administrative Data

7. MARKETING AUTHORISATION HOLDER

CP Pharmaceuticals Ltd

Ash Road North

Wrexham

LL13 9UF

United Kingdom

8. MARKETING AUTHORISATION NUMBER(S)

Cefotaxime for Injection 500mg – PL 04543/0419, PA 409/20/1

Cefotaxime for Injection 1g – PL 04543/0419, PA 409/20/2

9. DATE OF FIRST AUTHORISATION/RENEWAL OF THE AUTHORISATION

2 November 2000

10. DATE OF REVISION OF THE TEXT

4th August 2003

Cefotaxime for Injection 2g

(Wockhardt UK Ltd)

1. NAME OF THE MEDICINAL PRODUCT

Cefotaxime for Injection 2g

2. QUALITATIVE AND QUANTITATIVE COMPOSITION

Cefotaxime sodium equivalent to 2g of cefotaxime.

3. PHARMACEUTICAL FORM

Powder for solution for injection/infusion.

Cefotaxime sodium is supplied as a white to slightly yellow powder.

4. CLINICAL PARTICULARS

4.1 Therapeutic indications

1. Cefotaxime is indicated in the treatment of serious infections, either before the infecting organism has been identified or when caused by bacteria of established sensitivity, including

osteomyelitis,

septicaemia,

bacterial endocarditis,

meningitis, and

peritonitis.

and other serious bacterial infections suitable for parenteral antibiotic therapy.

2. Cefotaxime may be used for pre-operative prophylaxis in patients undergoing surgical procedures, that may be classified as contaminated or potentially so.

4.2 Posology and method of administration

Cefotaxime may be administered intravenously or by bolus injection or infusion or intramuscularly. The dosage, route and frequency of administration should be determined by the severity of infection, the sensitivity of causative organisms and condition of the patient. Therapy may be initiated before the results of sensitivity tests are known.

Adults:

The recommended dosage for mild to moderate infections is 1g 12 hourly. However, dosage may be varied according to the severity of the infection, sensitivity of causative organisms and condition of the patient. Therapy may be initiated before the results of sensitivity tests are known.

In severe infections dosage may be increased up to 12g daily given in 3 or 4 divided doses. For infections caused by sensitive *Pseudomonas* species daily doses of greater than 6g will usually be required.

Children:

The usual dosage range is 100-150mg/kg/day in 2 to 4 divided doses. However, in very severe infection doses of up to 200mg/kg/day may be required.

Neonates: The recommended dosage is 50mg/kg/day in 2 to 4 divided doses. In severe infections 150-200mg/kg/day, in divided doses, have been given.

Dosage in renal impairment: Because of extra-renal elimination, it is only necessary to reduce the dosage of cefotaxime in severe renal failure (GFR <5ml/min = serum creatinine approximately 751 micromol/litre). After an initial loading dose of 1g, daily dose should be halved without change in the frequency of dosing, i.e. 1g twelve hourly becomes 0.5g twelve hourly, 1g eight hourly becomes 0.5g eight hourly, 2g eight hourly becomes 1g eight hourly etc. As in all other patients, dosage may require further adjustment according to the course of the infection and the general condition of the patient.

Intravenous and Intramuscular Administration: Reconstitute cefotaxime with Water for Injections PhEur as directed in Section 6.6 (Instructions for use/handling). Shake well until dissolved and then withdraw the entire contents of the vial into the syringe.

Intravenous Infusion: Cefotaxime may be administered by intravenous infusion using the fluids stated in Section 6.6 (Instructions for use/handling). The prepared infusion may be administered over 20-60 minutes.

4.3 Contraindications

Known or suspected allergy to cephalosporins.

4.4 Special warnings and special precautions for use

Preliminary enquiry about hypersensitivity to penicillin and other β-Lactam antibiotics is necessary before prescribing cephalosporins since cross allergy occurs in 5–10% of cases.

Hypersensitivity reactions (anaphylaxis) occurring with the two types of antibiotics can be serious and occasionally fatal. Hypersensitivity requires that treatment be stopped.

Patients with severe renal dysfunction should be placed on the dosage schedule recommended under "Posology and Method of Administration".

As with other antibiotics, the use of cefotaxime, especially if prolonged, may result in overgrowth of non susceptible organisms, such as Enterococcus spp. Repeated evaluation of the condition of the patient is essential. If superinfection occurs during treatment with cefotaxime, specific anti-microbial therapy should be instituted if considered clinically necessary.

Cefotaxime constituted with lignocaine must never be used:

- by the intravenous route
- in infants under 30 months
- in subjects with a previous history of hypersensitivity to this product
- in patients who have an unpaced heart block
- in patients with severe heart failure.

The sodium content of cefotaxime (2.09mmol/g) should be taken into account when prescribing to patients requiring sodium restriction.

Cefotaxime may predispose patients to pseudomembranous colitis. Although any antibiotic may predispose to pseudomembranous colitis, the risk is higher with broad spectrum drugs, such as cephalosporins. This side effect, which may occur more frequently in patients receiving higher doses for prolonged periods, should be considered as potentially serious. The presence of C. difficile toxin should be investigated, and treatment with cefotaxime stopped in cases of suspected colitis. Diagnosis can be confirmed by toxin detection and specific antibiotic therapy (e.g. oral vancomycin or metronidazole) should be initiated if considered clinically necessary. The administration of products which cause faecal stasis should be avoided.

4.5 Interaction with other medicinal products and other forms of Interaction

Cephalosporin antibiotics at high dosage should be given with caution to patients receiving aminoglycoside antibiotics or potent diuretics such as frusemide as these combinations are suspected to adversely affect renal function. However, at the recommended doses, enhancement of nephrotoxicity is unlikely to be a problem with cefotaxime.

Probenecid interferes with renal tubular transfer of cefotaxime delaying its excretion and increasing the plasma concentration.

Interference with Laboratory Tests: A positive Coombs test may be seen during treatment with cephalosporins. This phenomenon may occur during treatment with cefotaxime.

A false positive reaction to glucose may occur with reducing substances but not with the use of specific glucose oxidase methods.

4.6 Pregnancy and lactation

Pregnancy: It is known that cefotaxime crosses the placental barrier. Although studies in animals have not shown an adverse effect on the developing foetus, the safety of cefotaxime in human pregnancy has not been established. Consequently, cefotaxime should not be administered during pregnancy especially during the first trimester, without carefully weighing the expected benefit against possible risks.

Lactation: Cefotaxime is excreted in the milk.

4.7 Effects on ability to drive and use machines

None known.

4.8 Undesirable effects

Adverse reactions to cefotaxime have occurred relatively infrequently and have generally been mild and transient. Effects reported include candidiasis, nausea, vomiting, abdominal pain, diarrhoea (diarrhoea may sometimes be a symptom of pseudomembranous colitis (see warnings)), transient rises in liver transaminases, alkaline phosphatase and/or bilirubin.

As with other cephalosporins, changes in renal function have been rarely observed with high doses of cefotaxime, particularly when co-prescribed with aminoglycosides. Rare cases of interstitial nephritis have been reported in patients treated with cefotaxime. Administration of high doses of cephalosporins, particularly in patients with renal insufficiency, may result in encephalopathy (e.g. impairment of consciousness, abnormal movements and convulsions).

Hypersensitivity reactions have been reported. These include skin rashes, pruritus and less frequently urticaria, drug fever and very rarely anaphylaxis (e.g. angioedema and bronchospasm possibly culminating in shock).

As with other cephalosporins, occasional cases of bullous reactions such as Stevens-Johnson syndrome, toxic epidermal necrolysis and erythema multiforme have also been reported.

As with other beta-lactam antibiotics, granulocytopenia and more rarely agranulocytosis may develop during treatment with cefotaxime, particularly if given over long periods. A few cases of eosinophilia and neutropenia have been observed, reversible when treatment is ceased. Some cases of rapidly reversible eosinophilia and thrombocytopenia on stopping treatment, have been reported. Rare cases of haemolytic anaemia have been reported. For cases of treatment lasting longer than 10 days, blood count should therefore be monitored.

Transient pain may be experienced at the site of injection. This is more likely to occur with higher doses. Occasionally, phlebitis has been reported in patients receiving intravenous cefotaxime. However, this has rarely been a cause for discontinuation of treatment.

A very small number of cases of arrhythmias have occurred following rapid bolus infusion through a central venous catheter.

The following symptoms have occurred after several weeks of treatment for borreliosis (Lyme's Disease): skin rash, itching, fever, leucopenia, increases in liver enzymes, difficulty of breathing, joint discomfort. To some extent these manifestations are consistent with the symptoms of the underlying disease, for which the patient is being treated.

4.9 Overdose

Serum levels of cefotaxime may be reduced by peritoneal dialysis or haemodialysis. In the case of overdosage, particularly in renal insufficiency, there is a risk of reversible encephalopathy.

5. PHARMACOLOGICAL PROPERTIES

5.1 Pharmacodynamic properties

Cefotaxime is a broad spectrum bactericidal cephalosporin antibiotic. Cefotaxime is exceptionally active in vitro against Gram-negative organisms sensitive or resistant to first or second generation cephalosporins. It is similar to other cephalosporins in activity against Gram-positive bacteria.

5.2 Pharmacokinetic properties

After a 1000mg intravenous bolus, mean peak plasma concentrations of cefotaxime usually range between 81 and 102 microgram/ml. Doses of 500mg and 2000mg produce plasma concentrations of 38 and 200 microgram/ml, respectively. There is no accumulation following administration of 1000mg intravenously or 500mg intramuscularly for 10 or 14 days.

The apparent volume of distribution at steady-state of cefotaxime is 21.6 litres/1.73m^2 after 1g intravenous 30 minute infusion.

Concentrations of cefotaxime (usually determined by non-selective assay) have been studied in a wide range of human body tissues and fluids. Cerebrospinal fluid concentrations are low when the meninges are not inflamed, but are between 3 and 30 microgram/ml in children with meningitis. Cefotaxime usually passes the blood-brain barrier in levels above the minimum inhibitory concentration of common sensitive pathogens when the meninges are inflamed. Concentrations (0.2-5.4 microgram/ml), inhibitory for most Gram-negative bacteria, are attained in purulent sputum, bronchial secretions and pleural fluid after doses of 1 or 2g. Concentrations likely to be effective against most sensitive organisms are similarly attained in female reproductive organs, otitis media effusions, prostatic tissue, interstitial fluid, renal tissue, peritoneal fluid and gall bladder wall, after usual therapeutic doses. High concentrations of cefotaxime and desacetyl-cefotaxime are attained in bile.

Cefotaxime is partially metabolised prior to excretion. The principal metabolite is the microbiologically active product, desacetyl-cefotaxime. Most of a dose of cefotaxime is excreted in the urine - about 60% as unchanged drug and a further 24% as desacetyl-cefotaxime. Plasma clearance is reported to be between 260 and 390ml/minute and renal clearance 145 to 217 ml/minute.

After intravenous administration of cefotaxime to healthy adults, the elimination half-life of the parent compound is 0.9 to 1.14 hours and that of the desacetyl metabolite, about 1.3 hours.

In neonates the pharmacokinetics are influenced by gestational and chronological age, the half-life being prolonged in premature and low birth weight neonates of the same age.

In severe renal dysfunction the elimination half-life of cefotaxime itself is increased minimally to about 2.5 hours, whereas that of desacetyl-cefotaxime is increased to

Table 1 Dilution table

Vial size	Diluent to be added	Approx available volume	Approx displacement volume
2g	10ml	11.2ml	1.2ml

about 10 hours. Total urinary recovery of cefotaxime and its principal metabolite decreases with reduction in renal function.

5.3 Preclinical safety data
There are no pre-clinical data of relevance to the prescriber that are additional to those included in other sections.

6. PHARMACEUTICAL PARTICULARS
6.1 List of excipients
None.

6.2 Incompatibilities
Cefotaxime sodium should not be mixed with alkaline solutions such as sodium bicarbonate injection or solutions containing aminophylline.

6.3 Shelf life
The unreconstituted dry powder is stable for 24 months. For the reconstituted solution, chemical and physical in-use stability has been demonstrated for 24 hours at 2-8°C. From a microbiological point of view, once opened, the product should be used immediately. If not used immediately, in-use storage times and conditions prior to use are the responsibility of the user and would normally not be longer than 24 hours at 2-8°C, unless reconstitution has taken place in controlled and validated aseptic conditions.

6.4 Special precautions for storage
Do not store above 25°C. Keep the container in the outer carton.

6.5 Nature and contents of container
Cefotaxime is supplied in Type III 10ml glass vials, closed with a Type I rubber stopper coated in Omniflex and sealed with an aluminium cap fitted with a detachable flip top.

The vials are boxed individually and in packs of 10, 25 or 50 vials.

6.6 Instructions for use and handling
When dissolved in Water for Injections PhEur, cefotaxime forms a straw-coloured solution suitable for intravenous and intramuscular injection. Variations in the intensity of colour of the freshly prepared solutions do not indicate a change in potency or safety.

Dilution table:

(see Table 1 above)

Reconstituted solution: Whilst it is preferable to use only freshly prepared solutions for both intravenous and intramuscular injection, cefotaxime is compatible with several commonly used intravenous infusion fluids and will retain satisfactory potency for up to 24 hours refrigerated in the following:

Water for Injection Ph Eur

Sodium Chloride Injection BP

5% Glucose Injection BP

Glucose and Sodium Chloride Injection BP

Compound Sodium Lactate Injection BP (Ringer-lactate injection)

After 24 hours any unused solution should be discarded.

Cefotaxime is compatible with 1% lignocaine; however freshly prepared solutions should be used.

Cefotaxime is also compatible with metronidazole infusion (500mg/100ml) and both will maintain potency when refrigerated for up to 24 hours. Some increase in colour of prepared solutions may occur on storage. However, provided the recommended storage conditions are observed, this does not indicate change in potency or safety.

Administrative Data
7. MARKETING AUTHORISATION HOLDER
CP Pharmaceuticals Ltd
Ash Road North
Wrexham
LL13 9UF
United Kingdom

8. MARKETING AUTHORISATION NUMBER(S)
PL 04543/0421
PA 409/20/3

9. DATE OF FIRST AUTHORISATION/RENEWAL OF THE AUTHORISATION
2 November 2000

10. DATE OF REVISION OF THE TEXT
4th August 2003

Ceftazidime for Injection

(Wockhardt UK Ltd)

1. NAME OF THE MEDICINAL PRODUCT
Ceftazidime for Injection 1g

Ceftazidime for Injection 2g

2. QUALITATIVE AND QUANTITATIVE COMPOSITION
Each vial contains ceftazidime 1g or 2g (as pentahydrate)

For excipients, see 6.1

3. PHARMACEUTICAL FORM
Powder for solution for injection or infusion

White to cream coloured, crystalline powder

4. CLINICAL PARTICULARS
4.1 Therapeutic indications
Ceftazidime is indicated for the treatment of the following infections when known or likely to be due to one or more susceptible microorganisms (see section 5. 1) and when parenteral therapy is required:

- Respiratory tract infections, including lower respiratory tract infections in patients with cystic fibrosis
- Urinary tract infections; ceftazidime may also be used for peri-operative prophylaxis during trans-urethral prostatectomy
- Skin and soft tissue infections
- Biliary tract infections
- Intra-abdominal infections
- Bone and joint infections
- Infections associated peritoneal dialysis and with continuous ambulatory peritoneal dialysis (CAPD)
- Meningitis due to aerobic gram-negative organisms

Whenever possible, it is recommended that the results of bacterial cultures and susceptibility tests are known before commencing treatment. This is especially important if ceftazidime is to be used as monotherapy. Ceftazidime should be used in combination with an additional antibacterial agent(s) when treating infections that are likely to be due to a mixture of susceptible and resistant bacterial species.

Consideration should be given to official guidance regarding the appropriate use of antibacterial agents.

4.2 Posology and method of administration
Posology

The range of usual dose regimens in patients with normal renal function for the age groups defined is as follows:

Age Group	Infection	Usual Dose
Adults	Most uses	1 g 8-hourly OR 2 g 12-hourly
	Severe infections and infections in neutropenic patients	2 g 8-hourly OR 3 g 12-hourly
	UTI	500 mg 12-hourly OR 1 g 12-hourly
	Prophylaxis for prostatectomy	1 g at induction ± 1g at catheter removal
	Cystic fibrosis	100-150 mg/kg/ day in three divided doses; not to exceed 9 g/day
Elderly	All infections, especially in those > 80 years	Not to exceed 3 g daily total
Infants > 2 months and children	Most uses	30-100 mg/kg/day in two or three divided doses
	Severe infections	up to 150 mg/kg/ day (max 6 g total per day) in three divided doses
Neonates and infants < 2 months	Most uses	25 – 60 mg/kg/day in two divided doses

Dosage in renal insufficiency:

Ceftazidime is almost exclusively excreted by glomerular filtration and the dose should be reduced when the glomerular filtration rate (GFR) is less than 50ml/min.

In adults with renal insufficiency, an initial loading dose of lg of ceftazidime may be given, followed by an appropriate maintenance dose as in the table:

Recommended maintenance doses of ceftazidime in adults with renal insufficiency

(see Table 1 on next page)

In patients with renal insufficiency and severe infections, especially in neutropenics, who would normally receive 6g of ceftazidime daily were it not for renal insufficiency, the unit dose given in the table above may be increased by 50% or the dosing frequency increased appropriately. In such patients it is recommended that ceftazidime serum levels should be monitored and trough levels should not exceed 40 mg/litre.

In children with renal insufficiency the creatinine clearance should be adjusted for body surface area or lean body mass and the dosing frequency reduced as for adults.

In patients on haemodialysis
The serum half-life of ceftazidime during haemodialysis ranges from 3 to 5 hours. The appropriate maintenance dose of ceftazidime should be repeated following each haemodialysis period.

For patients in renal failure on continuous arteriovenous haemodialysis or high-flux haemofiltration in intensive therapy units, it is recommended that the dosage should be lg daily in divided doses. For low-flux haemofiltration it is recommended that the dosage should be that suggested under impaired renal function.

In patients on peritoneal dialysis
Ceftazidime may also be used in patients who are undergoing peritoneal dialysis and continuous ambulatory peritoneal dialysis (CAPD) at a dose adjusted according to renal function. In such patients, a loading dose of lg of ceftazidime may be given, followed by 500mg every 24 hours. In addition, for intra-peritoneal infections, ceftazidime can be incorporated into the dialysis fluid (usually 125 to 250 mg for 2 L of dialysis fluid).

Dosage in hepatic insufficiency

No dose adjustment is required unless there is concomitant renal insufficiency.

Method of Administration

Ceftazidime may be given intravenously (by slow bolus injection over a few minutes or by infusion over 20-30 minutes) or by deep intramuscular injection into a large muscle mass, such as the upper outer quadrant of the gluteus maximus or lateral part of the thigh. See section 6 for information on preparation of solutions for intravenous or intramuscular administrations.

4.3 Contraindications
Hypersensitivity to ceftazidime, to any of the cephalosporins or to sodium carbonate.

Previous immediate and/or severe hypersensitivity reaction to a penicillin or to any other type of beta-lactam drug.

4.4 Special warnings and special precautions for use
Before therapy with ceftazidime is instituted, careful inquiry should be made to determine whether the patient has had any previous hypersensitivity reactions to ceftazidime, cephalosporins, penicillins, or other beta-lactam drugs.

Ceftazidime is contraindicated in patients who have had a previous hypersensitivity reaction to any cephalosporin. It is also contraindicated in patients who have had a previous immediate and/or any severe hypersensitivity reaction to any penicillin or to any other beta-lactam drug. Ceftazidime should be given with caution to patients who have had any other type of hypersensitivity reaction to a penicillin or any other beta-lactam drug.

Antibiotic-associated diarrhoea, colitis and pseudomembranous colitis have all been reported with the use of ceftazidime. These diagnoses should be considered in any patient who develops diarrhoea during or shortly after treatment. Ceftazidime should be discontinued if severe and/or bloody diarrhoea occurs during treatment and appropriate therapy instituted.

Ceftazidime should be used with caution in individuals with a previous history of gastro-intestinal disease, particularly colitis.

Ceftazidime has not been shown to be nephrotoxic. However, the total daily dosage should be reduced when ceftazidime is administered to patients with acute or chronic renal insufficiency in order to avoid potential clinical consequences, such as seizures (see section 4.2).

Cephalosporin antibiotics should be given with caution to patients receiving concurrent treatment with nephrotoxic drugs such as aminoglycoside antibiotics or potent diuretics (such as frusemide) as these combinations may have an adverse effect on renal function and have been associated with ototoxicity (see section 4.5).

As with other cephalosporins, prolonged use of ceftazidime may result in the overgrowth of non-susceptible organisms, such as enterococci and Candida *spp*.

Ceftazidime does not interfere with enzyme-based tests for glycosuria. Slight interference with copper reduction methods (Benedict's, Feliling's, Clinitest) may be observed.

Table 1 Recommended maintenance doses of ceftazidime in adults with renal insufficiency

Creatinine clearance ml/min	Approx. serum creatinine* µmol/l(mg/dl)	Recommended unit dose of ceftazidime (g)	Frequency of dosing (hourly)
50 – 31	150-200 (1.7-2.3)	1	12
30 – 16	200-350 (2.3-4.0)	1	24
15 – 6	350-500 (4.0-5.6)	0.5	24
<5	>500 >5.6)	0.5	48

* These values are guidelines and may not accurately predict renal function in all patients especially in the elderly in whom the serum creatinine concentration may overestimate renal function.

Ceftazidime does not interfere in the alkaline picrate assay for creatinine.

The development of a positive Coombs' test associated with the use of ceftazidime in about 5% of patients may interfere with the cross-matching of blood.

This vial contains 2.26mmol of sodium in total. The sodium content should be taken into consideration when prescribing to patients requiring sodium restriction.

4.5 Interaction with other medicinal products and other forms of Interaction

Nephrotoxicity has been reported following concomitant administration of cephalosporins and aminoglycoside antibiotics or potent diuretics, such as furosemide (frusemide). Renal function should be carefully monitored, especially if higher dosages of the aminoglycosides are to be administered or if therapy is prolonged, because of the potential nephrotoxicity and ototoxicity of aminoglycoside antibiotics.

In vitro, chloramphenicol has been shown to be antagonistic with respect to ceftazidime and other cephalosporins. The clinical relevance of this finding is unknown, but if concurrent administration of ceftazidime with chloramphenicol is proposed, the possibility of antagonism should be considered.

4.6 Pregnancy and lactation

Pregnancy

Reproduction studies have not revealed any evidence of impaired fertility or harm to the foetus due to ceftazidime. However, as animal reproduction studies are not always predictive of human response, this drug should be used during pregnancy only if clearly needed.

Lactation

Ceftazidime is excreted in human milk in low concentrations and consequently caution should be exercised when ceftazidime is administered to a nursing woman.

4.7 Effects on ability to drive and use machines

Dizziness can occur which can affect the ability to drive and to use machines.

4.8 Undesirable effects

The most common adverse reactions during ceftazidime treatment are local reactions following intravenous injection, allergic reactions, and effects on the gastro-intestinal tract.

Local effects: Phlebitis or thrombophlebitis, and pain and/or inflammation at the site of injection.

Hypersensitivity: Pruritus, rash, urticaria, erythema multiforme and fever. Toxic epidermal necrolysis and Stevens Johnson syndrome have been reported rarely. Angioedema and anaphylaxis (bronchospasm and/or hypotension) have been reported very rarely.

Gastro-intestinal: Diarrhoea, nausea, vomiting and abdominal pain. Very rarely, oral thrush and pseudomembranous colitis (see section 4.4 - 'Warnings').

Central nervous system: Headache, dizziness, paraesthesiae and bad taste. There have been reports of neurological sequelae, including tremor, myoclonia, convulsions, encephalopathy and coma in patients with renal impairment in whom the dose of ceftazidime has not been appropriately reduced.

Genito-urinary: Candidiasis and vaginitis.

Laboratory test changes (usually transient):

Eosinophilia, positive Coombs' test without haemolysis, haemolytic anaemia, thrombocytosis and very rarely leucopenia, neutropenia, agranulocytosis, thrombocytopenia and lymphocytosis.

Slight elevations in one or more hepatic enzymes: AST (SGOT), ALT (SGPT), LDH, GGT and alkaline phosphatase. Very rarely, clinically apparent jaundice has been reported.

Elevations of blood urea, blood urea nitrogen and/or serum creatinine have been observed occasionally.

4.9 Overdose

An overdose of ceftazidime may be associated with pain, inflammation and phlebitis at the injection site.

Overdose or the administration of inappropriately large doses in the presence of renal insufficiency can lead to neurological sequelae including dizziness, paraesthesiae, headache, encephalopathy, convulsion and coma.

Laboratory abnormalities that may occur after an overdose include elevations in creatinine, BUN, liver enzymes and bilirubin, a positive Coombs' test, thrombocytosis, thrombocytopenia, eosinophilia, leucopenia and prolongation of the prothrombin time.

General symptomatic and supportive measures should be instituted, together with specific measures to control any seizures. In cases of severe overdose, especially in a patient with renal failure, combined haemodialysis and haemoperfusion may be considered if response to more conservative therapy fails.

5. PHARMACOLOGICAL PROPERTIES

5.1 Pharmacodynamic properties

General properties

ATC classification: J01DA11

Mode of Action

Ceftazidime is a semi-synthetic bactericidal antibacterial agent of the cephalosporin class. Like other beta-lactam drugs, ceftazidime exerts antibacterial activity by binding to and inhibiting the action of certain bacterial cell wall synthetic enzymes (transpeptidases). Inhibition of one or more of these essential penicillin-binding proteins results in the interruption of cell wall biosynthesis at the final stage of peptidoglycan production, resulting in bacterial cell lysis and death.

Mechanisms of resistance

Bacterial resistance to ceftazidime may be due to one or more of the following mechanisms:

– hydrolysis by beta-lactamases. Ceftazidime may be efficiently hydrolysed by certain of the extended-spectrum beta-lactamases (ESBLs) and by the chromosomally-encoded (AmpC) enzymes that may be induced or stably derepressed in certain aerobic gram-negative bacterial species

– reduced affinity of penicillin-binding proteins for ceftazidime

– outer membrane impermeability, which restricts access of ceftazidime to penicillin binding proteins in gram-negative organisms

– drug efflux pumps

More than one of these mechanisms of resistance may co-exist in a single bacterial cell. Depending on the mechanism(s) present, bacteria may express cross-resistance to several or all other beta-lactams and/or antibacterial drugs of other classes.

Breakpoints

According to the National Committee for Clinical Laboratory Standards Guidelines (NCCLS), the MIC breakpoints for sensitive, intermediately sensitive or resistant organisms are as follows:

MIC (µg/mL) *Interpretation*

≤8 Sensitive

16

Intermediately Sensitive

≥32 mg/L Resistant

• *Haemophilus spp.* Susceptible ≤2 µg/mL

• *Neisseria gonorrhoeae* Susceptible <0.5 µg/mL

Susceptibility

The prevalence of acquired resistance may vary geographically and with time for selected species and local information on resistance is desirable, particularly when treating severe infections. As necessary, expert advice should be sought when the local prevalence of resistance is such that the utility of the agent in at least some types of infections is questionable.

Commonly susceptible species, i.e. resistance <10% in all EU Member States +
Gram-positive micro-organisms:
Streptococcus agalactiae (Group B)
Streptococcus pneumoniae, penicillin susceptible #
Streptococcus pyogenes
Gram-negative micro-organisms:
Escherichia coli
Haemophilus influenzae
Moraxella catarrhalis
Proteus mirabilis
Proteus vulgaris
Salmonella spp
Serratia spp.

Species for which acquired resistance may be a problem, i.e. resistance ≥ 10% in at least one of the EU Member States +
Gram-negative micro-organisms:
Acinetobacter spp.
Burkholderia cepacia
Citrobacter freundii
Citrobacter spp.
Enterobacter spp.
Klebsiella pneumoniae
Klebsiella spp.
Morganella morganii
Pseudomonas aeruginosa
Pseudomonas spp.

Inherently resistant organisms
Gram-positive micro-organisms:
Enterococcus spp.
Micrococcus spp.
Staphylococcus aureus, methicillin resistant (MRSA) *
Staphylococcus – coagulase negative, methicillin resistant*

+ Based on published data from several different sources

* Shows some in-vitro activity against methicillin-susceptible strains but should not be relied upon to treat staphylococcal infections.

Shows some in-vitro activity against penicillin-susceptible strains but should not be relied upon to treat pneumococcal infections

5.2 Pharmacokinetic properties

The approximate C_{max} cetazidime after different doses and modes of administration to subjects with normal renal function were as follows:

(see Table 2 below)

In general, plasma concentrations at 8 hours after intravenous or intramuscular administration of 500 mg or more ceftazidime are in excess of 2 mg/1. Following multiple

Table 2

	Intramuscular injection (after 1 hour)	Intravenous bolus-injection (after 5 min)	Intermittent infusion (after 20 – 30 minutes)
500mg	18mg/l	45mg/l	40mg/l
1g	39mg/l	90mg/l	70mg/l
2g		170mg/l	170mg/l

Table 3

Instructions for reconstitution: See table for addition volumes and solution concentrations, which may be useful when fractional doses are required.

PREPARATION OF SOLUTION

Vial size		Amount of Diluent to be added (ml)	Approximate Concentration (mg/ml)
1g	Intramuscular	3.0	260
1g	Intravenous	10.0	90
2g	Intravenous bolus	10.0	170
2g	Intravenous Infusion	50.0*	40‡

*Note: Addition should be in two stages.

‡Note: Use Sodium Chloride Injection 0.9%, Dextrose Injection 5% or other approved diluent, as Water for Injections produces hypotonic solutions at this concentration.

intravenous doses of 1 g and 2g every 8 hours for 10 days, there was no evidence of accumulation of ceftazidime in the serum of individuals with normal renal function.

Distribution

Less than 10% of ceftazidime is protein bound and the degree of protein binding is independent of concentration. Concentrations of ceftazidime in excess of the minimum inhibitory levels of common pathogens can be achieved in tissues such as bone, heart, bile, sputum, aqueous humour, synovial, pleural and peritoneal fluids. Transplacental transfer of the antibiotic readily occurs. Ceftazidime penetrates the intact blood-brain barrier poorly and low levels are achieved in the CSF in the absence of inflammation. Therapeutic levels of 4 to 20 mg/1 or more are achieved in the CSF when the meninges are inflamed.

Elimination

Approximately 80% to 90% of a dose of ceftazidime is excreted unchanged by the kidneys over a 24-hourperiod, resulting in high urinary concentrations.

In subjects with normal renal function, the half life of ceftazidime is approximately 2 hours after intravenous or intramuscular administration.

The presence of hepatic dysfunction had no effect on the pharmacokinetics of ceftazidime in individuals who received 2g intravenously every 8 hours for 5 days. Therefore dosage adjustment is not required for patients with hepatic dysfunction, unless renal function is also impaired.

5.3 Preclinical safety data

Long term studies in animals have not been performed to evaluate carcinogenic potential. However, a mouse micronucleus test and an Ames test were both negative for mutagenic effects.

6. PHARMACEUTICAL PARTICULARS

6.1 List of excipients

Sodium carbonate (anhydrous sterile)

6.2 Incompatibilities

Ceftazidime is less stable in Sodium Bicarbonate Injection than other intravenous fluids. It is not recommended as a diluent.

Ceftazidime and aminoglycosides should not be mixed in the same giving set or syringe.

Precipitation has been reported when vancomycin has been added to ceftazidime in solution. It is recommended that giving sets and intravenous lines are flushed between administration of these two agents.

6.3 Shelf life

Unopened - 24 months

For reconstituted solution, chemical and physical in-use stability has been demonstrated for eight hours at 25°C and 24 hours at 4°C. From a microbiological point of view, once opened, the product should be used immediately. If not used immediately, in-use storage times and conditions prior to use are the responsibility of the user and would normally not be longer than 24 hours at 2-8°C, unless reconstitution has taken place in controlled and validated aseptic conditions.

6.4 Special precautions for storage

Unopened: Do not store above 25°C. Keep container in the outer carton.

After reconstitution: Store at 2-8°C (see 6.3 Shelf Life).

6.5 Nature and contents of container

Packs of one or five Type III colourless glass 25ml vials stoppered with coated rubber stopper, capped with flip-off cap (1g)

Packs of one or five Type I colourless glass 50ml vials stoppered with coated rubber stopper, capped with flip-off cap (2g)

6.6 Instructions for use and handling

(see Table 3 above)

Ceftazidime (at the given concentration) has been shown to be compatible with the following diluent solutions:-

<u>Solvents for 40mg/ml ceftazidime concentration:</u>

Sodium Chloride 0.9%

Ringer Solution

Ringer Lactate Solution

Glucose 5%

Glucose 10%

Glucose 5% and Sodium Chloride 0.9%

Glucose 5% and Sodium Chloride 0.45%

Glucose 5% and Sodium Chloride 0.2%

Dextran 40%/10% and Sodium Chloride 0.9%

Dextran 70%/6% and Sodium Chloride 0.9%

Lidocaine Hydrochloride 0.5%

Lidocaine Hydrochloride 1%

Water for Injections

The reconstituted solution should appear clear and colourless.

All sizes of vials as supplied are under reduced pressure. As the product dissolves, carbon dioxide is released and a positive pressure develops. For ease of use, it is recommended that the following techniques of reconstitution are adopted.

1. Insert the syringe needle through the vial closure and inject the recommended volume of diluent. The vacuum may assist entry of the diluent. Remove the syringe needle.

2. Shake to dissolve: carbon dioxide is released and a clear solution will be obtained in about 1 to 2 minutes.

3. Invert the vial. With the syringe plunger fully depressed, insert the needle through the vial closure and withdraw the total volume of solution into the syringe (the pressure in the vial may aid withdrawal). Ensure that the needle remains within the solution and does not enter the head space. The withdrawn solution may contain small bubbles of carbon dioxide; they may be disregarded.

7. MARKETING AUTHORISATION HOLDER

CP Pharmaceuticals Ltd

Ash Road North

Wrexham LL13 9UF

United Kingdom

8. MARKETING AUTHORISATION NUMBER(S)

PL 04543/0480 (1g) PL 04543/0481 (2g)

9. DATE OF FIRST AUTHORISATION/RENEWAL OF THE AUTHORISATION

9th March 2004

10. DATE OF REVISION OF THE TEXT

9th January 2005

Ceftriaxone Sodium 1g for Injection BP

(Wockhardt UK Ltd)

1. NAME OF THE MEDICINAL PRODUCT

Ceftriaxone for Injection 1g

2. QUALITATIVE AND QUANTITATIVE COMPOSITION

Hydrated disodium ceftriaxone equivalent to 1g of ceftriaxone.

For excipients, see 6.1.

3. PHARMACEUTICAL FORM

Powder for solution for injection.

Ceftriaxone sodium is supplied as a white to pale yellow crystalline powder.

4. CLINICAL PARTICULARS

4.1 Therapeutic indications

Ceftriaxone sodium is a broad-spectrum bactericidal cephalosporin antibiotic. Ceftriaxone is active *in vitro* against a wide range of Gram-positive and Gram-negative organisms, which include β-lactamase producing strains.

Ceftriaxone is indicated in the treatment of the following infections either before the infecting organism has been identified or when known to be caused by bacteria of established sensitivity.

Pneumonia

Septicaemia

Meningitis

Skin and soft tissue infections

Infections in neutropenic patients

Gonorrhoea

Peri-operative prophylaxis of infections associated with surgery

Treatment may be started before the results of susceptibility tests are known.

Consideration should be given to official guidance on the appropriate use of antibacterial agents.

4.2 Posology and method of administration

Ceftriaxone may be administered by deep intramuscular injection or as a slow intravenous injection after reconstitution of the solution according to the directions given below. The dosage and mode of administration should be determined by the severity of the infection, susceptibility of the causative organism and the patient's condition. Under most circumstances a once-daily dose or, in the specified indications, one dose will give satisfactory therapeutic results.

Intramuscular injection: 1g ceftriaxone should be dissolved in 3.5ml of 1% Lignocaine Hydrochloride Injection BP. The solution should be administered by deep intramuscular injection. Doses greater than 1g should be divided and injected at more than one site.

Intravenous injection: 1g ceftriaxone should be dissolved in 10ml of Water for Injections BP. The injection should be administered over at least 2-4 minutes, directly into the vein or via the tubing of an intravenous infusion.

Adults and children 12 years and over:

Standard therapeutic dosage: 1g once daily.

Severe infections: 2-4 g daily, normally as a once daily dose.

The duration of therapy varies according to the course of the disease. As with antibiotic therapy in general, administration of ceftriaxone should be continued for a minimum of 48 to 72 hours after the patient has become afebrile or evidence of bacterial eradication has been obtained.

Acute, uncomplicated gonorrhoea: One dose of 250mg intramuscularly should be administered. Simultaneous administration of probenecid is not indicated.

Peri-operative prophylaxis: Usually one dose of 1g given by intramuscular or slow intravenous injection. In colorectal surgery, 2g should be given intramuscularly (in divided doses at different injection sites), by slow intravenous injection or by slow intravenous infusion, in conjunction with a suitable agent against anaerobic bacteria.

Elderly: These dosages do not require modification in elderly patients provided that renal and hepatic function are satisfactory (see below).

In the neonate, the intravenous dose should be given over 60 minutes to reduce the displacement of bilirubin from albumin, thereby reducing the potential risk of bilirubin encephalopathy (see *Special warning and precautions for use*).

Children under 12 years

Standard therapeutic dosage: 20-50mg/kg body-weight once daily.

Up to 80mg/kg body-weight daily may be given in severe infections, except in premature neonates where a daily dosage of 50mg/kg should not be exceeded. For children with body weights of 50kg or more, the usual dosage should be used. Doses of 50mg/kg or over should be given by slow intravenous infusion over at least 30 minutes. Doses greater than 80mg/kg body weight should be avoided because of the increased risk of biliary precipitates.

Renal and hepatic impairment: In patients with impaired renal function, there is no need to reduce the dosage of ceftriaxone provided liver function is intact. Only in cases of pre-terminal renal failure (creatinine clearance <10ml per minute) should the daily dosage be limited to 2g or less.

In patients with liver damage there is no need for the dosage to be reduced provided renal function is intact.

In severe renal impairment accompanied by hepatic insufficiency, the plasma concentration of ceftriaxone should be determined at regular intervals and dosage adjusted.

In patients undergoing dialysis, no additional supplementary dosage is required following the dialysis. Plasma concentrations should be monitored, however, to determine whether dosage adjustments are necessary, since the elimination rate in these patients may be reduced.

4.3 Contraindications

Solutions in lignocaine should not be administered intravenously.

Ceftriaxone should not be given to patients with a history of hypersensitivity to cephalosporin antibiotics.

Ceftriaxone should not be given to neonates with jaundice or those who are hypoalbuminaemic or acidotic or have other conditions, such as prematurity, in which bilirubin binding is likely to be impaired.

4.4 Special warnings and special precautions for use

The stated dosage should not be exceeded.

Care is required when administering ceftriaxone to patients who have previously shown hypersensitivity (especially anaphylactic reaction) to penicillins or other non-cephalosporin β-lactam antibiotics, as occasional instances of cross allergenicity between cephalosporins and these antibiotics have been recorded. Anaphylactic shock requires immediate counter measures.

In severe renal impairment accompanied by hepatic insufficiency, dosage reduction is required as outlined under *Posology and method of administration*.

In vivo and *in vitro* studies have shown that ceftriaxone, like some other cephalosporins, can displace bilirubin from serum albumin. Clinical data obtained in neonates have confirmed this finding. Ceftriaxone should therefore not be used in jaundiced newborns or in babies who are hypoalbuminaemic, acidotic or born prematurely, in whom bilirubin binding is likely to be impaired.

Ceftriaxone may precipitate in the gall bladder and then be detectable as shadows on ultrasound (see *Undesirable effects*). This can happen in patients of any age, but is more likely in infants and small children who are usually given a larger dose of ceftriaxone on a body weight basis. In children, doses greater than 80mg/kg body weight should be avoided because of the increased risk of biliary precipitates. There is no clear evidence of gallstones or of acute cholecystitis developing in children or infants treated with ceftriaxone, and conservative management of ceftriaxone precipitate in the gallbladder is recommended.

Cephalosporins as a class tend to be absorbed onto the surface of the red cell membranes and react with antibodies directed against the drug to produce a positive Coombs' test and occasionally a rather mild haemolytic anaemia. In this respect, there may be some cross-reactivity with penicillins.

During treatment, the blood count should be checked regularly (refer to Section 4.8).

Cases of pancreatitis, possibly of biliary obstruction aetiology, have been rarely reported in patients treated with ceftriaxone. Most patients presented with risk factors for biliary stasis and biliary sludge, e.g. preceding major therapy, severe illness and total parenteral nutrition. A trigger or cofactor role of ceftriaxone-related biliary precipitation can not be ruled out.

Each gram of ceftriaxone sodium contains approximately 3.6mmol sodium.

4.5 Interaction with other medicinal products and other forms of Interaction

No impairment of renal function has been observed in man after simultaneous administration of ceftriaxone with diuretics.

No interference with the action or increase in nephrotoxicity of aminoglycosides has been observed during simultaneous administration with ceftriaxone.

The ceftriaxone molecule does not contain the N-methylthio-tetrazole substituent, which has been associated with a disulfiram-like effect, when alcohol is taken during therapy with certain cephalosporins.

In an *in vitro* study, antagonistic effects have been observed with the combination of chloramphenicol and ceftriaxone.

In patients treated with ceftriaxone, the Coombs' test may rarely become false-positive. Ceftriaxone, like other antibiotics, may result in false-positive tests for galactosaemia. Likewise, non-enzymatic methods for glucose determination in urine may give false-positive results. For this reason, urine-glucose determination during therapy with ceftriaxone should be done enzymatically.

4.6 Pregnancy and lactation

Ceftriaxone has not been associated with adverse events on foetal development in laboratory animals but its safety in human pregnancy has not been established. Therefore it should not be used in pregnancy unless absolutely indicated. Only minimal amounts of ceftriaxone are excreted in breast milk. However, caution is advised in nursing mothers.

4.7 Effects on ability to drive and use machines

None known.

4.8 Undesirable effects

Ceftriaxone has been generally well tolerated. Adverse reactions are usually mild and transient.

The most common side-effects are gastrointestinal, consisting mainly of loose stools and diarrhoea or, occasionally, nausea and vomiting, stomatitis and glossitis. Cutaneous reactions, including maculopapular rash or exanthema, pruritus, urticaria, oedema and allergic dermatitis have occurred. Isolated cases of severe cutaneous adverse reactions (erythema multiforme, Stevens Johnson Syndrome and Lyell's Syndrome/toxic epidermal necrolysis) have been reported.

Haematological reactions have included anaemia (all grades), haemolytic anaemia, leucopenia, neutropenia, thrombocytopenia, eosinophilia, agranulocytosis and positive Coombs' test. Regular blood counts should be carried out during treatment. Ceftriaxone has rarely been associated with prolongation of prothrombin time.

Headache and dizziness, drug fever, shivering and transient elevations in liver function tests have been reported in a few cases. Other rarely observed adverse reactions include glycosuria, oliguria, haematuria, increase in serum creatinine, mycosis of the genital tract and anaphylactic-type reactions such as bronchospasm.

Very rarely, reversible symptomatic urinary precipitates of calcium ceftriaxone have occurred after ceftriaxone administration. Patients who are very young, immobilised or who are dehydrated are at increased risk. There have been a few reports of anuria and renal impairment following this reaction.

Shadows which have been mistaken for gallstones, but which are precipitates of calcium ceftriaxone, have been detected by sonograms. These abnormalities are commonly observed after an adult daily dose of two grams per day or more, or its equivalent in children. At doses of two grams a day or above these biliary precipitates may occasionally cause symptoms. Should patients develop symptoms, non-surgical management is recommended and discontinuation of ceftriaxone should be considered. The evidence suggests biliary precipitates usually disappear once ceftriaxone has been stopped. The risk of biliary precipitates may be increased by treatment duration greater than 14 days, renal failure, dehydration or total parenteral nutrition. There have been isolated reports of pancreatitis although a causal relationship to ceftriaxone has not been established.

Superinfections with yeasts, fungi or other resistant organisms may occur. A rare side-effect is pseudomembranous colitis which has resulted from infection with *Clostridium difficile* during treatment with ceftriaxone. Therefore it is important to consider this diagnosis in patients who present with diarrhoea subsequent to the administration of antibacterial agents.

Pain or discomfort may be experienced at the site of intramuscular injection immediately after administration but is usually well tolerated and transient. Local phlebitis has occurred rarely following intravenous administration but can be minimised by slow injection over at least 2-4 minutes.

4.9 Overdose

In the case of overdosage, drug concentrations would not be reduced by haemodialysis or peritoneal dialysis. There is no specific antidote. Treatment should be symptomatic.

5. PHARMACOLOGICAL PROPERTIES

5.1 Pharmacodynamic properties

Ceftriaxone (ATC code: JO1D A) has potent bactericidal activity against a wide range of Gram-positive and, especially, Gram-negative organisms. The spectrum of activity includes both aerobic and some anaerobic species. It has considerable resistance to degradation by most bacterial β-lactamases.

Microbiology:

Ceftriaxone is usually active against the following microorganisms *in vitro* and in clinical infections (see *Therapeutic indications*). The list is not exhaustive and focuses on those organisms of particular clinical interest.

Gram-positive aerobes:Staphylococcus aureus (including penicillinase-producing strains) *Streptococcus pneumoniae*, Streptococcus group A (*Streptococcus pyogenes*), Streptococcus group B (*Streptococcus agalactiae*), *Streptococcus viridans* and *Streptococcus bovis*.

Note: Methicillin-resistant *Staphylococcus* spp. are resistant to cephalosporins, including ceftriaxone. Most strains of enterococci (e.g. *Enterococcus faecalis*) are resistant. *Listeria monocytogenes* is also not susceptible to ceftriaxone.

Gram-negative aerobes: Acinetobacter lwoffi (some strains are resistant), *Aeromonas* spp., *Alcaligenes* spp., *Moraxella catarrhalis* (β-lactamase negative and positive), *Capnocytophaga* spp., *Citrobacter* spp., *Enterobacter* spp. (some strains are resistant), *Escherichia coli, Haemophilus ducreyi, Haemophilus influenzae* (including penicillinase-producing strains), *Haemophilus parainfluenzae, Hafnia alvei, Klebsiella* spp. (including *K.pneumoniae*), *Moraxella* spp., *Morganella morganii* (*=Proteus morganii*), *Neisseria gonorrhoeae* (including penicillinase-producing strains), *Neisseria meningitidis, Pasteurella multocida, Plesiomonas shigelloides, Proteus mirabilis, Proteus vulgaris, Providencia* spp., *Salmonella* spp., (including *S.typhi*), *Serratia* spp., (including *S. marcescens*), *Shigella* spp., *Vibrio* spp., (including *V.cholerae*), *Yersinia* spp., (including *Y. enterocolitica*).

Anaerobic organisms:Clostridium spp., (except *C. difficile*), *Fusobacterium* spp., (except *F.mortiferum* and *F. varium*), *Peptococcus* spp, *Peptostreptococcus* spp.

5.2 Pharmacokinetic properties

The pharmacokinetics of ceftriaxone are largely determined by its concentration-dependent binding to plasma albumin. The plasma free (unbound) fraction of the drug in man is approximately 5% over most of the therapeutic concentration range, increasing to 15% at concentrations of 300mg/l. Owing to the lower albumin content, the proportion of free ceftriaxone in interstitial fluid is correspondingly higher than in plasma.

Plasma concentrations: Mean peak concentrations after bolus intravenous injection are about 120mg/l following a 500mg dose and about 200mg/l following a 1g dose; mean levels of 250mg/l are achieved after infusion of 2g over 30 minutes. Intramuscular injection of 500mg ceftriaxone in 1% lignocaine produces mean peak plasma concentrations of 40-70 mg/l within one hour. Bioavailability after intramuscular injection is 100%.

Excretion: Ceftriaxone is eliminated mainly as unchanged drug, approximately 60% of the dose being excreted in the urine (almost exclusively by glomerular filtration) and the remainder via the biliary and intestinal tracts. The total plasma clearance is 10-22 ml/min. The renal clearance is 5-12 ml/min. A notable feature of ceftriaxone is its relatively long plasma elimination half-life of approximately eight hours which makes single or once daily dosage of the drug appropriate for most patients. The half-life is not significantly affected by the dose, the route of administration or by repeated administration.

Pharmacokinetics in special clinical situations: In the first week of life, 80% of the dose is excreted in the urine; over the first month, this falls to levels similar to those in the adult.

In elderly persons aged over 75 years, the average elimination half-life is usually two to three times longer that in the young adult group. As with all cephalosporins, a decrease in renal function in the elderly may lead to an increase in half-life. Evidence gathered to date with ceftriaxone however, suggests that no modification of the dosage regimen is needed.

In patients with *renal or hepatic dysfunction*, the pharmacokinetics of ceftriaxone are only minimally altered and the elimination half-life is only slightly increased. If kidney function alone is impaired, biliary elimination of ceftriaxone is increased; if liver function alone is impaired, renal elimination is increased.

Cerebrospinal fluid: Ceftriaxone crosses non-inflamed and inflamed meninges, attaining concentrations 4-17% of the simultaneous plasma concentration.

5.3 Preclinical safety data

There are no preclinical safety data of relevance to the prescriber that are additional to those included in other sections.

6. PHARMACEUTICAL PARTICULARS

6.1 List of excipients

None

6.2 Incompatibilities

Solutions containing ceftriaxone should not be mixed with or added to solutions containing other agents except 1% Lignocaine Hydrochloride Injection BP (for intramuscular injection only). In particular, ceftriaxone is not compatible with calcium-containing solutions such as Hartmann's solution and Ringer's solution. Based on literature reports, ceftriaxone is not compatible with amsacrine, vancomycin, fluconazole, aminoglycosides and labetalol.

6.3 Shelf life

Unopened – Three years.

For reconstituted solution, chemical and physical in-use stability has been demonstrated for 24 hours at 25°C and for four days at 2-8°C. From a microbiological point of view, once opened, the product should be used immediately. If not used immediately, in-use storage times and conditions prior to use are the responsibility of the user and would normally not be longer than 24 hours at 2-8°C, unless reconstitution has taken place in controlled and validated aseptic conditions

6.4 Special precautions for storage

Unopened: Do not store above 25°C. Keep container in the outer carton.

After reconstitution: Store at 2-8°C, see section 6.3 for complete storage instructions.

6.5 Nature and contents of container

Ceftriaxone is supplied in Type III 10ml clear glass vials, closed with a Type I rubber stopper uncoated/coated in Omniflex and sealed with an aluminium cap.

The vials are packed in boxes of 1, 5, 10, 25 or 50 vials. Not all pack sizes are marketed.

6.6 Instructions for use and handling

Reconstitution table:

(see Table 1)

Ceftriaxone should not be mixed in the same syringe with any drug other than 1% Lignocaine Hydrochloride Injection BP (for intramuscular injection only).

Ceftriaxone is compatible with several commonly used intravenous infusion fluids e.g. Sodium Chloride Injection BP, 5% or 10% Glucose Injection BP, Sodium Chloride and Glucose Injection BP (0.45% sodium chloride and 2.5% glucose), Dextran 6% in Glucose Injection BP 5% and isotonic hydroxyethylstarch 6-10% infusions.

The reconstituted solution should be clear. Do not use if particles are present.

Ceftriaxone sodium when dissolved in Water for Injections Ph Eur forms a pale yellow to amber solution. Variations in

Table 1 Reconstitution table

Vial size	Diluent to be added	Approx available volume	Approx displacement volume
1g	10ml	10.8ml	0.8ml

the intensity of colour of the freshly prepared solutions do not indicate a change in potency or safety.

For single patient use. Discard any unused solution.

Administrative Data

7. MARKETING AUTHORISATION HOLDER
CP Pharmaceuticals Ltd
Ash Road North
Wrexham
LL13 9UF
United Kingdom

8. MARKETING AUTHORISATION NUMBER(S)
PL 04543/0425
PA 409/21/1

9. DATE OF FIRST AUTHORISATION/RENEWAL OF THE AUTHORISATION
16 May 2001

10. DATE OF REVISION OF THE TEXT
3rd November 2003

Ceftriaxone Sodium 2g for Injection BP

(Wockhardt UK Ltd)

1. NAME OF THE MEDICINAL PRODUCT
Ceftriaxone for Injection 2g

2. QUALITATIVE AND QUANTITATIVE COMPOSITION
Hydrated disodium ceftriaxone equivalent to 2g of ceftriaxone.

For excipients, see 6.1

3. PHARMACEUTICAL FORM
Powder for solution for injection or infusion.

Ceftriaxone sodium is supplied as a white to pale yellow crystalline powder.

4. CLINICAL PARTICULARS

4.1 Therapeutic indications
Ceftriaxone sodium is a broad-spectrum bactericidal cephalosporin antibiotic. Ceftriaxone is active *in vitro* against a wide range of Gram-positive and Gram-negative organisms, which include β-lactamase producing strains.

Ceftriaxone is indicated in the treatment of the following infections either before the infecting organism has been identified or when known to be caused by bacteria of established sensitivity.

Pneumonia

Septicaemia

Meningitis

Skin and soft tissue infections

Infections in neutropenic patients

Gonorrhoea

Peri-operative prophylaxis of infections associated with surgery

Treatment may be started before the results of susceptibility tests are known.

Consideration should be given to official guidance on the appropriate use of antibacterial agents

4.2 Posology and method of administration
Ceftriaxone may be administered by deep intramuscular injection, slow intravenous injection, or as a slow intravenous infusion, after reconstitution of the solution according to the directions given below. The dosage and mode of administration should be determined by the severity of the infection, susceptibility of the causative organism and the patient's condition. Under most circumstances, a once-daily dose or, in the specified indications, one dose will give satisfactory therapeutic results.

Intramuscular injection: 2g ceftriaxone should be dissolved in 7.0ml of 1% Lignocaine Hydrochloride Injection BP. The solution should be administered by deep intramuscular injection. Doses greater than 1g should be divided and injected at more than one site.

Intravenous infusion: 2g of ceftriaxone should be dissolved in 40ml of one of the following calcium-free solutions; Glucose Injection BP 5% or 10%, Sodium Chloride Injection BP, Sodium Chloride and Glucose Injection BP (0.45% sodium chloride and 2.5% Glucose), dextran 6% in Glucose Injection BP 5%, isotonic hydroxyethylstarch 6-10% infusions. The infusion should be administered over at least 30 minutes.

Adults and children 12 years and over:

Standard therapeutic dosage: 1g once daily.

Severe infections: 2-4g daily, normally as a once-daily dose.

The duration of therapy varies according to the course of the disease. As with antibiotic therapy in general, administration of ceftriaxone should be continued for a minimum of 48 to 72 hours after the patient has become afebrile or evidence of bacterial eradication has been obtained.

Acute, uncomplicated gonorrhoea: One dose of 250mg intramuscularly should be administered. Simultaneous administration of probenecid is not indicated.

Peri-operative prophylaxis: Usually one dose of 1g given by intramuscular or slow intravenous injection. In colorectal surgery, 2g should be given intramuscularly (in divided doses at different injection sites), by slow intravenous injection or by slow intravenous infusion, in conjunction with a suitable agent against anaerobic bacteria.

Elderly: These dosages do not require modification in elderly patients provided that renal and hepatic function are satisfactory (see below).

In the neonate, the intravenous dose should be given over 60 minutes to reduce the displacement of bilirubin from albumin, thereby reducing the potential risk of bilirubin encephalopathy (see *Special warning and precautions for use*).

Children under 12 years

Standard therapeutic dosage: 20-50mg/kg body-weight once daily.

Up to 80mg/kg body-weight daily may be given in severe infections, except in premature neonates where a daily dosage of 50mg/kg should not be exceeded. For children with body weights of 50kg or more, the usual dosage should be used. Doses of 50mg/kg or over should be given by slow intravenous infusion over at least 30 minutes. Doses greater than 80mg/kg body weight should be avoided because of the increased risk of biliary precipitates.

Renal and hepatic impairment: In patients with impaired renal function, there is no need to reduce the dosage of ceftriaxone provided liver function is intact. Only in cases of pre-terminal renal failure (creatinine clearance <10ml per minute) should the daily dosage be limited to 2g or less.

In patients with liver damage there is no need for the dosage to be reduced provided renal function is intact.

In severe renal impairment accompanied by hepatic insufficiency, the plasma concentration of ceftriaxone should be determined at regular intervals and dosage adjusted.

In patients undergoing dialysis, no additional supplementary dosage is required following the dialysis. Plasma concentrations should be monitored, however, to determine whether dosage adjustments are necessary, since the elimination rate in these patients may be reduced.

4.3 Contraindications
Solutions in lignocaine should not be administered intravenously.

Ceftriaxone should not be given to patients with a history of hypersensitivity to cephalosporin antibiotics.

Ceftriaxone should not be given to neonates with jaundice or those who are hypoalbuminaemic or acidotic or have other conditions, such as prematurity, in which bilirubin binding is likely to be impaired.

4.4 Special warnings and special precautions for use
The stated dosage should not be exceeded.

Care is required when administering ceftriaxone to patients who have previously shown hypersensitivity (especially anaphylactic reaction) to penicillins or other non-cephalosporin β-lactam antibiotics, as occasional instances of cross allergenicity between cephalosporins and these antibiotics have been recorded. Anaphylactic shock requires immediate counter measures.

In severe renal impairment accompanied by hepatic insufficiency, dosage reduction is required as outlined under *Posology and method of administration.*

In vivo and *in vitro* studies have shown that ceftriaxone, like some other cephalosporins, can displace bilirubin from serum albumin. Clinical data obtained in neonates have confirmed this finding. Ceftriaxone should therefore not be used in jaundiced new-borns or in babies who are hypoalbuminaemic, acidotic or born prematurely, in whom bilirubin binding is likely to be impaired.

Ceftriaxone may precipitate in the gall bladder and then be detectable as shadows on ultrasound (see *Undesirable effects*). This can happen in patients of any age, but is more likely in infants and small children who are usually given a larger dose of ceftriaxone on a body weight basis. In children, doses greater than 80mg/kg body weight should be avoided because of the increased risk of biliary precipitates. There is no clear evidence of gallstones or of acute cholecystitis developing in children or infants treated with ceftriaxone, and conservative management of ceftriaxone precipitate in the gallbladder is recommended.

Cephalosporins as a class tend to be absorbed onto the surface of the red cell membranes and react with antibodies directed against the drug to produce a positive Coombs' test and occasionally a rather mild haemolytic anaemia. In this respect, there may be some cross-reactivity with penicillins.

During treatment, the blood count should be checked regularly (refer to Section 4.8).

Cases of pancreatitis, possibly of biliary obstruction aetiology, have been rarely reported in patients treated with ceftriaxone. Most patients presented with risk factors for biliary stasis and biliary sludge, e.g. preceding major therapy, severe illness and total parenteral nutrition. A trigger or cofactor role of ceftriaxone-related biliary precipitation can not be ruled out.

Each gram of ceftriaxone sodium contains approximately 3.6mmol sodium.

4.5 Interaction with other medicinal products and other forms of Interaction
No impairment of renal function has been observed in man after simultaneous administration of ceftriaxone with diuretics.

No interference with the action or increase in nephrotoxicity of aminoglycosides has been observed during simultaneous administration with ceftriaxone.

The ceftriaxone molecule does not contain the N-methylthio-tetrazole substituent, which has been associated with a disulfiram-like effect, when alcohol is taken during therapy with certain cephalosporins.

In an *in vitro* study, antagonistic effects have been observed with the combination of chloramphenicol and ceftriaxone.

In patients treated with ceftriaxone, the Coombs' test may rarely become false-positive. Ceftriaxone, like other antibiotics, may result in false-positive tests for galactosaemia. Likewise, non-enzymatic methods for glucose determination in urine may give false-positive results. For this reason, urine-glucose determination during therapy with ceftriaxone should be done enzymatically.

4.6 Pregnancy and lactation
Ceftriaxone has not been associated with adverse events on foetal development in laboratory animals but its safety in human pregnancy has not been established. Therefore, it should not be used in pregnancy unless absolutely indicated. Only minimal amounts of ceftriaxone are excreted in breast milk. However, caution is advised in nursing mothers.

4.7 Effects on ability to drive and use machines
None known.

4.8 Undesirable effects
Ceftriaxone has been generally well tolerated. Adverse reactions are usually mild and transient.

The most common side-effects are gastro-intestinal, consisting mainly of loose stools and diarrhoea or, occasionally, nausea and vomiting, stomatitis and glossitis. Cutaneous reactions, including maculopapular rash or exanthema, pruritus, urticaria, oedema and allergic dermatitis have occurred. Isolated cases of severe cutaneous adverse reactions (erythema multiforme, Stevens Johnson Syndrome and Lyell's Syndrome/toxic epidermal necrolysis) have been reported.

Haematological reactions have included anaemia (all grades), haemolytic anaemia, leucopenia, neutropenia, thrombocytopenia, eosinophilia, agranulocytosis and positive Coombs' test. Regular blood counts should be carried out during treatment. Ceftriaxone has rarely been associated with prolongation of prothrombin time.

Headache and dizziness, drug fever, shivering and transient elevations in liver function tests have been reported in a few cases. Other rarely observed adverse reactions include glycosuria, oliguria, haematuria, increase in serum creatinine, mycosis of the genital tract and anaphylactic-type reactions such as bronchospasm.

Very rarely, reversible symptomatic urinary precipitates of calcium ceftriaxone have occurred after ceftriaxone administration. Patients who are very young, immobilised or who are dehydrated are at increased risk. There have been a few reports of anuria and renal impairment following this reaction.

Shadows which have been mistaken for gallstones, but which are precipitates of calcium ceftriaxone, have been detected by sonograms. These abnormalities are commonly observed after an adult daily dose of two grams per day or more, or its equivalent in children. At doses of two grams a day or above these biliary precipitates may occasionally cause symptoms. Should patients develop symptoms, non-surgical management is recommended and discontinuation of ceftriaxone should be considered. The evidence suggests biliary precipitates usually disappear once ceftriaxone has been stopped. The risk of biliary precipitates may be increased by treatment duration greater than 14 days, renal failure, dehydration or total parenteral nutrition. There have been isolated reports of pancreatitis although a causal relationship to ceftriaxone has not been established.

Superinfections with yeasts, fungi or other resistant organisms may occur. A rare side-effect is pseudomembranous colitis which has resulted from infection with *Clostridium difficile* during treatment with ceftriaxone. Therefore it is important to consider this diagnosis in patients who present with diarrhoea subsequent to the administration of antibacterial agents.

Pain or discomfort may be experienced at the site of intramuscular injection immediately after administration but is usually well tolerated and transient. Local phlebitis has occurred rarely following intravenous administration but can be minimised by slow injection over at least 2-4 minutes.

4.9 Overdose
In the case of overdosage, drug concentrations would not be reduced by haemodialysis or peritoneal dialysis. There is no specific antidote. Treatment should be symptomatic.

Table 1 Reconstitution table

Vial size	Diluent to be added	Approx available volume	Approx displacement volume
2g	40ml	41.03ml	1.03ml

5. PHARMACOLOGICAL PROPERTIES

5.1 Pharmacodynamic properties

Ceftriaxone (ATC code: JO1D A) has potent bactericidal activity against a wide range of Gram-positive and, especially, Gram-negative organisms. The spectrum of activity includes both aerobic and some anaerobic species. It has considerable resistance to degradation by most bacterial β-lactamases.

Microbiology:

Ceftriaxone is usually active against the following micro-organisms *in vitro* and in clinical infections (see *Therapeutic Indications*). The list is not exhaustive and focuses on the organisms of particular clinical interest.

Gram-positive aerobes:Staphylococcus aureus (including penicillinase-producing strains) *Streptococcus pneumoniae*, Streptococcus group A (*Streptococcus pyogenes*), Streptococcus group B (*Streptococcus agalactiae*), *Streptococcus viridans* and *Streptococcus bovis*.

Note: Methicillin-resistant *Staphylococcus* spp. are resistant to cephalosporins, including ceftriaxone. Most strains of enterococci (e.g. *Enterococcus faecalis*) are resistant. *Listeria monocytogenes* is also not susceptible to ceftriaxone.

Gram-negative aerobes: Acinetobacter lwoffi (some strains are resistant), *Aeromonas* spp., *Alcaligenes* spp., *Moraxella catarrhalis* (β-lactamase negative and positive), *Capnocytophaga* spp., *Citrobacter* spp., *Enterobacter* spp. (some strains are resistant), *Escherichia coli, Haemophilus ducreyi, Haemophilus influenzae* (including β-lactamase producing strains), *Haemophilus parainfluenzae, Hafnia alvei, Klebsiella* spp. (including *K.pneumoniae*), *Moraxella* spp., *Morganella morganii* (=*Proteus morganii*), *Neisseria gonorrhoeae* (including penicillinase-producing strains), *Neisseria meningitidis, Pasteurella multocida, Plesiomonas shigelloides, Proteus mirabilis, Proteus vulgaris, Providencia* spp., *Salmonella* spp., (including *S.typhi*), *Serratia* spp., (including *S. marcescens*), *Shigella* spp., *Vibrio spp.*, (including *V.cholerae*), *Yersinia* spp., (including *Y. enterocolitica*).

Anaerobic organisms:Clostridium spp., (except *C. difficile*), *Fusobacterium* spp., (except *F.mortiferum* and *F. varium*), *Peptococcus* spp, *Peptostreptococcus* spp.

5.2 Pharmacokinetic properties

The pharmacokinetics of ceftriaxone are largely determined by its concentration-dependent binding to plasma albumin. The plasma free (unbound) fraction of the drug in man is approximately 5% over most of the therapeutic concentration range, increasing to 15% at concentrations of 300mg/l. Owing to the lower albumin content, the proportion of free ceftriaxone in interstitial fluid is correspondingly higher than in plasma.

Plasma concentrations: Mean peak concentrations after bolus intravenous injection are about 120mg/l following a 500mg dose and about 200mg/l following a 1g dose; mean levels of 250mg/l are achieved after infusion of 2g over 30 minutes. Intramuscular injection of 500mg ceftriaxone in 1% lignocaine produces mean peak plasma concentrations of 40-70 mg/l within one hour. Bioavailability after intramuscular injection is 100%.

Excretion: Ceftriaxone is eliminated mainly as unchanged drug, approximately 60% of the dose being excreted in the urine (almost exclusively by glomerular filtration) and the remainder via the biliary and intestinal tracts. The total plasma clearance is 10-22 ml/min. The renal clearance is 5-12 ml/min. A notable feature of ceftriaxone is its relatively long plasma elimination half-life of approximately eight hours which makes single or once daily dosage of the drug appropriate for most patients. The half-life is not significantly affected by the dose, the route of administration or by repeated administration.

Pharmacokinetics in special clinical situations: In the first week of life, 80% of the dose is excreted in the urine; over the first month, this falls to levels similar to those in the adult.

In elderly persons aged over 75 years, the average elimination half-life is usually two to three times longer that in the young adult group. As with all cephalosporins, a decrease in renal function in the elderly may lead to an increase in half-life. Evidence gathered to date with ceftriaxone, however, suggests that no modification of the dosage regimen is needed.

In patients with *renal* or *hepatic dysfunction*, the pharmacokinetics of ceftriaxone are only minimally altered and the elimination half-life is only slightly increased. If kidney function alone is impaired, biliary elimination of ceftriaxone is increased; if liver function alone is impaired, renal elimination is increased.

Cerebrospinal fluid: Ceftriaxone crosses non-inflamed and inflamed meninges, attaining concentrations 4-17% of the simultaneous plasma concentration.

5.3 Preclinical safety data

There are no preclinical safety data of relevance to the prescriber that are additional to those included in other sections.

6. PHARMACEUTICAL PARTICULARS

6.1 List of excipients

None

6.2 Incompatibilities

Solutions containing ceftriaxone should not be mixed with or added to solutions containing other agents except 1% Lignocaine Hydrochloride Injection BP (for intramuscular injection only). In particular, ceftriaxone is not compatible with calcium-containing solutions such as Hartmann's solution and Ringer's solution. Based on literature reports, ceftriaxone is not compatible with amsacrine, vancomycin, fluconazole, aminoglycosides and labetalol.

6.3 Shelf life

Unopened – Three years.

For reconstituted solution, chemical and physical in-use stability has been demonstrated for 24 hours at 25°C and for four days at 2-8°C. From a microbiological point of view, once opened, the product should be used immediately. If not used immediately, in-use storage times and conditions prior to use are the responsibility of the user and would normally not be longer than 24 hours at 2-8°C, unless reconstitution has taken place in controlled and validated aseptic conditions

6.4 Special precautions for storage

Unopened: Do not store above 25°C. Keep container in the outer carton.

After reconstitution: Store at 2-8°C, see section 6.3 for complete storage instructions.

6.5 Nature and contents of container

Ceftriaxone is supplied in moulded Type I 50 ml clear glass infusion bottles, closed with a Type I rubber stopper uncoated/coated in Omniflex and sealed with an aluminium cap.

The vials are packed in boxes of 1 vial with a plastic hanging device.

6.6 Instructions for use and handling

Reconstitution table:

(see Table 1 above)

Ceftriaxone is compatible with several commonly used intravenous infusion fluids e.g. Sodium Chloride Injection BP, 5% or 10% Glucose Injection BP, Sodium Chloride and Glucose Injection BP (0.45% sodium chloride and 2.5% glucose), Dextran 6% in Glucose Injection BP 5% and isotonic hydroxyethylstarch 6-10% infusions.

The reconstituted solution should be clear. Do not use if particles are present.

Ceftriaxone sodium when dissolved in Water for Injections Ph Eur forms a pale yellow to amber solution. Variations in the intensity of colour of the freshly prepared solutions do not indicate a change in potency or safety.

For single patient use. Discard any unused solution.

Administrative Data

7. MARKETING AUTHORISATION HOLDER

CP Pharmaceuticals Ltd

Ash Road North

Wrexham

LL13 9 UF

United Kingdom

8. MARKETING AUTHORISATION NUMBER(S)

PL 04543/0426

PA 409/21/2

9. DATE OF FIRST AUTHORISATION/RENEWAL OF THE AUTHORISATION

15 May 2001

10. DATE OF REVISION OF THE TEXT

3rd November 2003

Cefuroxime Sodium for Injection

(Flynn Pharma Ltd)

1. NAME OF THE MEDICINAL PRODUCT

Cefuroxime sodium for injection 250mg, cefuroxime sodium for injection 750mg and cefuroxime sodium for injection 1.5g.

2. QUALITATIVE AND QUANTITATIVE COMPOSITION

Each vial contains, as the active ingredient, cefuroxime sodium for injection equivalent to 250mg, 750mg or 1.5g of cefuroxime.

3. PHARMACEUTICAL FORM

Vials containing an off-white to slightly yellow sterile powder for solution for injection or infusion.

4. CLINICAL PARTICULARS

4.1 Therapeutic indications

Cefuroxime sodium for injection is indicated for the treatment of infections caused by susceptible strains of the designated micro-organisms, or before the infecting organism has been identified, in the diseases listed below.

Respiratory tract infections, for example, acute and chronic bronchitis, infected bronchiectasis, bacterial pneumonia, lung abscess and postoperative chest infections.

Ear, nose and throat infections, for example, sinusitis, tonsillitis and pharyngitis.

Urinary tract infections, for example, acute and chronic pyelonephritis, cystitis and asymptomatic bacteriuria.

Soft tissue infections, for example, cellulitis, erysipelas, peritonitis and wound infections.

Bone and joint infections, for example, osteomyelitis and septic arthritis.

Obstetric and gynaecological infections, pelvic inflammatory disease.

Gonorrhoea, particularly if penicillin is unsuitable.

Other infections, including septicaemia and meningitis.

Prophylaxis against infection in abdominal, pelvic, orthopaedic, cardiac, pulmonary, oesophageal and vascular surgery where there is increased risk from infection.

Consideration should be given to official local guidance (eg, national recommendations) on the appropriate use of antibacterial agents.

Susceptibility of the causative organism to the treatment should be tested (if possible), although therapy may be initiated before the results are available.

4.2 Posology and method of administration

Usually cefuroxime is effective when administered alone, but when appropriate it may be used in combination with metronidazole or an aminoglycoside.

General Dosage

Adults: Many infections will respond to 750mg three times daily by intramuscular or intravenous injection. For more severe infections this dose should be increased to 1.5g three times daily intravenously. The frequency of dosage may be increased to six-hourly injections, intramuscular or intravenous, giving total daily doses of 3g to 6g.

Infants and children: Doses of 30 to 100mg/kg/day given in three or four divided doses. A dose of 60mg/kg/day will be appropriate for most infections.

Neonates: Doses of 30 to 100mg/kg/day given in two or three divided doses. In the first weeks of life the serum half-life of cefuroxime can be three to five times that in adults.

Gonorrhoea

1.5g should be given as a single dose or as two 750mg injections into different sites, eg, each buttock.

Meningitis

Cefuroxime therapy is suitable for sole therapy of bacterial meningitis due to sensitive strains.

Infants and children: 200 to 240mg/kg/day intravenously in three or four divided doses. This dosage may be reduced to 100mg/kg/day after three days or when clinical improvement occurs.

Neonates: The initial dosage should be 100mg/kg/day intravenously. This dosage may be reduced to 50mg/kg/day after three days or when clinical improvement occurs.

Adults: 3g intravenously every eight hours. No data is currently available to recommend a dose for intrathecal administration.

Prophylaxis

The usual dose is 1.5g intravenously with induction of anaesthesia. For orthopaedic, pelvic and abdominal operations this may be followed with two 750mg doses 8 and 16 hours later. For vascular, cardiac, oesophageal and pulmonary operations this may be supplemented with 750mg intramuscularly three times a day for a further 24 to 48 hours.

In total joint replacement, 1.5g cefuroxime powder may be mixed dry with each pack of methyl methacrylate cement polymer before adding the liquid monomer.

Dosage in Impaired Renal Function

As cefuroxime is excreted by the kidneys, the dosage should be reduced to allow for slower excretion in patients with impaired renal function, once creatinine clearance falls below 20ml/min, as follows:

Marked impairment (creatinine clearance 10 to 20ml/min)	750mg twice daily
Severe impairment (creatinine clearance of less than 10ml/min)*	750mg once daily
Continuous peritoneal dialysis	750mg twice daily
Renal failure on continuous arteriovenous haemodialysis or high-flux haemofiltration in intensive therapy units	750mg twice daily
Low-flux haemofiltration	As for impaired renal function

*For patients on haemodialysis, a further 750mg should be given at the end of each dialysis session.

4.3 Contraindications

Contra-indicated in patients hypersensitive to the cephalosporin group of antibiotics.

4.4 Special warnings and special precautions for use

Cephalosporin antibiotics may, in general, be given safely to patients who are hypersensitive to penicillins, although cross-reactions have been reported. Special care is indicated in patients who have experienced an anaphylactic reaction to penicillin.

Cephalosporin antibiotics at high dosage should be given with caution to patients receiving potent diuretics or aminoglycosides, as these combinations are suspected of adversely affecting renal function. Clinical experience has shown that this is not likely to be a problem at the recommended dose levels.

4.5 Interaction with other medicinal products and other forms of Interaction

Concurrent administration of probenecid prolongs the excretion of cefuroxime and produces an elevated peak serum level.

Concurrent administration of potent diuretics, aminoglycosides may adversely affect renal function (see section 4.4).

Interference with Laboratory Tests

Slight interference may occur with the copper reduction methods (Fehling's, Benedict's) but this should not lead to false-positive results. Cefuroxime does not interfere with the enzyme based tests for glycosuria, or with the alkaline picrate method for creatinine. It is recommended that either the hexokinase or glucose oxidase methods are used for determination of blood/plasma glucose levels.

4.6 Pregnancy and lactation

Studies in animals revealed no evidence of embryopathic or teratogenic effects due to cefuroxime, but, as with all drugs, it should be used with caution during pregnancy.

Since cefuroxime is excreted in human milk, caution should be exercised when administering this antibiotic to a nursing mother.

4.7 Effects on ability to drive and use machines

Cefuroxime is not known to affect the ability to drive or use machines.

4.8 Undesirable effects

Hypersensitivity reactions: Including skin rashes (maculopapular and urticarial), interstitial nephritis, drug fever and, very rarely, anaphylaxis. As with any antibiotic, prolonged use may lead to overgrowth of non-susceptible organisms, eg, Candida.

As with other cephalosporins, there have been rare reports of erythema multiforme, Stevens-Johnson syndrome and toxic epidermal necrolysis.

Gastro-intestinal disturbance: Including, very rarely, pseudomembranous colitis, which has been reported with most broad spectrum antibiotics.

Haematological: A decrease in haemoglobin concentration, eosinophilia, leucopenia and neutropenia have been observed. Positive Coombs' tests have been reported. As with other cephalosporins, thrombocytopenia has been reported rarely.

Hepatic: Transient rises in liver enzymes or serum bilirubin have been observed, particularly in patients with pre-existing liver disease, but there is no evidence of hepatic involvement.

Renal: There may be some variation in the results of biochemical tests of renal function, but these results do not appear to be of clinical significance.

Other: Transient pain may be experienced at the site of intramuscular injection. Occasionally thrombophlebitis may occur at the site of intravenous injection. A burning sensation may be observed after intravenous injection. Mild to moderate hearing loss has been reported in some children treated for meningitis. Dizziness and headache has been reported in patients receiving cefuroxime.

4.9 Overdose

Overdosage of cephalosporins can lead to cerebral irritation and seizures. With seizures the drug should be discontinued and appropriate anticonvulsive and supportive therapy administered. Serum levels of cefuroxime can be reduced by haemodialysis or peritoneal dialysis.

5. PHARMACOLOGICAL PROPERTIES

5.1 Pharmacodynamic properties

Cefuroxime is a cephalosporin antibiotic, ATC code J01DA06 (Cephalosporins and Related Substances). All cephalosporins (β-lactam antibiotics) inhibit cell wall production and are selective inhibitors of peptidoglycan synthesis. The initial step in drug action consists of binding of the drug to cell receptors, called penicillin-binding proteins. After a β-lactam antibiotic has bound to these receptors, the transpeptidation reaction is inhibited and peptidoglycan synthesis is blocked. Bacterial lysis is the end result.

Susceptibility

The following MIC breakpoints separating susceptible from intermediately susceptible organisms and intermediately susceptible from resistant organisms are used.

Table 1: **Susceptibility Breakpoints**

Bacterial Breakpoints	Organism
NCCLS Breakpoints	
S: ≤8mg/l I: 16 R: ≥32mg/l	Enterobacteriaceae
S: ≤4mg/l I: 8 R: ≥16mg/l	Enterococcus
S: ≤4mg/l I: 8 R: ≥16mg/l	Haemophilus influenzae
S: ≤1mg/l I: 2 R: ≥4mg/l	*Neisseria gonorrhoeae*
S: ≤0.5mg/l I: 1 R: ≥2mg/l	Streptococcus pneumoniae
DIN Breakpoints	
S: ≤4mg/l I: 8 R: ≥16mg/l	All bacterial isolates
BSAC Breakpoints	
S: ≤1mg/l I: 2-16 R: ≥32mg/l	*Acinetobacter* spp. and Enterobacteriaceae
	Streptococcus pneumoniae
S: ≤1mg/l R: ≥2mg/l	Moraxella catarrhalis
	Neisseria gonorrhoeae
	Haemophilus influenzae

NCCLS: National Committee for Clinical Laboratory Standards
DIN: Deutches Institut fur Normung
BSAC: British Society for Antimicrobial Chemotherapy
S: Susceptible, I: Intermediately susceptible, R: Resistant

The prevalence of resistance may vary geographically and with time for selected species and local information is desirable, particularly when treating several infections. This information gives only an approximate guidance on probabilities whether organisms will be susceptible to cefuroxime or not.

Table 2: **Range of Bacterial Resistance to Cefuroxime in Europe**

Category	Range of Resistance in Europe
Susceptible	
Gram +ve Aerobes	
Staphylococcus aureus (methicillin-susceptible strains)	0-46%
Staphylococcus epidermidis (methicillin-susceptible strains)	
Streptococcus pneumoniae	
Streptococcus pyogenes	
Streptococcus viridans	
Gram -ve Aerobes	2-17%
Escherichia coli	0-29%
Haemophilus influenzae	6-21%
Klebsiella spp.	
Moraxella catarrhalis	
Neisseria spp.	0-17%
Proteus mirabilis	0-75%
Providencia spp., including	
Providencia rettgeri	
Providencia rettgeri only	
Anaerobes	
Clostridium perfringens	
Intermediate	
Gram -ve Aerobes	
Bordetella pertussis	
Citrobacter	21-52%
Enterobacter spp.	36-83%
Anaerobes	
Bacteroides fragilis	
Insusceptible	
Gram +ve Aerobes	
Enterococcus faecalis	
Staphylococcus aureus (methicillin-resistant strains)	
Staphylococcus epidermidis (methicillin-resistant strains)	
Gram -ve Aerobes	
Acinetobacter spp.	
Campylobacter spp.	
Legionella spp.	
Pseudomonas spp.	
Serratia spp.	70-94%
Morganella morganii	75-100%
Proteus vulgaris	
Anaerobes	
Clostridium difficile	

Cross-Reactivity Between Cefuroxime and Other Antibiotics

Cross-resistance between cefuroxime and several other β-lactam antibiotics, including amoxicillin, methicillin, penicillin and ampicillin and some cephalosporins, has been recorded.

Amoxicillin-sensitive *Haemophilus influenzae* are more likely to be susceptible to cefuroxime than amoxicillin-resistant *Haemophilus influenzae*. Similarly, methicillin-sensitive *Staphylococcus aureus* and *Staphylococcus epidermidis* are usually cefuroxime-susceptible, while methicillin-resistant *Staphylococcus aureus* and *Staphylococcus epidermidis* are resistant to cefuroxime.

Resistance of *Staphylococcus aureus* and *Staphylococcus pneumoniae* to penicillin can result in an increase in the cefuroxime MIC_{50} and MIC_{90} values for these organisms. In addition, resistance of *Escherichia coli* and *Haemophilus influenzae* to ampicillin may result in an increase of the cefuroxime MIC_{50} values for these organisms.

Mechanisms of Resistance to Cefuroxime

Known mechanisms of resistance in targeted pathogens are the following:

- Production of β-lactamases which are able to hydrolyse cefuroxime efficiently (eg, several of the extended-spectrum and chromosomally-mediated β-lactamases).
- Reduced affinity of penicillin-binding proteins for cefuroxime (eg, penicillin-resistant *Streptococcus pneumoniae*).
- Cell wall impermeability.
- Efflux pumps.

5.2 Pharmacokinetic properties

The serum half-life after either intramuscular or intravenous administration is approximately 70 minutes. After intramuscular injection the peak serum level occurs after about 45 minutes.

The antibiotic can be found in bone, synovial fluid and aqueous humour above the minimum inhibitory levels for common pathogens. The blood-brain barrier can be passed by cefuroxime when the meninges are inflamed.

Cefuroxime is excreted approximately 50% by glomerular filtration and 50% through the renal tubules. Cefuroxime is almost completely recovered unchanged in the urine within 24 hours, most being excreted within six hours.

5.3 Preclinical safety data

There is no experimental evidence of embryopathic or teratogenic effects attributable to cefuroxime.

6. PHARMACEUTICAL PARTICULARS

6.1 List of excipients

Each vial contains only the active ingredient, cefuroxime sodium.

6.2 Incompatibilities

Cefuroxime should not be mixed in the syringe with aminoglycoside antibiotics.

6.3 Shelf life

Before reconstitution: 18 months.

In keeping with good pharmaceutical practice, freshly constituted suspensions or solutions should be used immediately. If this is not practicable then solution may be stored at 2°C-8°C (in a refrigerator) for up to 24 hours.

6.4 Special precautions for storage

Protect from light. Before reconstitution do not store above 25°C. After reconstitution the product may be stored at 2°C-8°C (in a refrigerator) for up to 24 hours.

6.5 Nature and contents of container

Type III flint glass vial, stoppered with halobutyl closures and sealed with aluminium seals that may be combined with a polypropylene cap.

6.6 Instructions for use and handling

Intramuscular injection: Add 1ml of water for injections to 250mg or 3ml of water for injections to 750mg. Shake gently to produce a suspension.

Intravenous administration: Dissolve cefuroxime in water for injections using at least 2ml for 250mg, at least 6ml for 750mg and at least 15ml for 1.5g. For short intravenous infusion, 1.5g may be dissolved in 50ml of water for injections. Reconstituted solutions may be diluted with:

5% or 10% dextrose

5% dextrose containing 0.2%, 0.225%, 0.45% or 0.9% sodium chloride injection

5% dextrose containing 20mEq potassium chloride

0.9% sodium chloride injection

M/6 sodium lactate injection

Ringer's injection

Lactated Ringer's injection

Heparin (10 and 50 units/ml) in 0.9% sodium chloride injection

10mEq potassium chloride in 0.9% sodium chloride injection

These solutions may be given directly into a vein or introduced into the tubing of the giving set if the patient is receiving parenteral fluids.

7. MARKETING AUTHORISATION HOLDER

Flynn Pharma Ltd

Alton House

4 Herbert Street

Dublin 2

Ireland

8. MARKETING AUTHORISATION NUMBER(S)

Cefuroxime sodium for injection 250mg: PL 13621/0017

Cefuroxime sodium for injection 750mg: PL 13621/0018

Cefuroxime sodium for injection 1.5g: PL 13621/0019

9. DATE OF FIRST AUTHORISATION/RENEWAL OF THE AUTHORISATION

Date of first authorisation: 1st June 2005

10. DATE OF REVISION OF THE TEXT

Legal Category POM

Package Quantities

1.5g × 1, 20ml vial

250mg × 1, 10ml vial

750mg × 1, 10ml vial

CFX2M

Celebrex 100 mg & 200 mg

(Pharmacia Limited)

1. NAME OF THE MEDICINAL PRODUCT

Celebrex 100 mg capsule, hard.

Celebrex 200 mg capsule, hard.

2. QUALITATIVE AND QUANTITATIVE COMPOSITION

Each capsule contains 100 mg or 200 mg celecoxib.

For excipients, see 6.1.

3. PHARMACEUTICAL FORM

Capsule, hard.

Opaque, white with two blue bands marked 7767 and 100 (Celebrex 100 mg).

Opaque, white with two gold bands marked 7767 and 200 (Celebrex 200 mg).

4. CLINICAL PARTICULARS

4.1 Therapeutic indications

Symptomatic relief in the treatment of osteoarthritis or rheumatoid arthritis.

The decision to prescribe a selective COX-2 inhibitor should be based on an assessment of the individual patient's overall risks (see sections 4.3, 4.4).

4.2 Posology and method of administration

As the cardiovascular risks of celecoxib may increase with dose and duration of exposure, the shortest duration possible and the lowest effective daily dose should be used. The patient's need for symptomatic relief and response to therapy should be re-evaluated periodically, especially in patients with osteoarthritis (4.3, 4.4, 4.8 and 5.1).

Osteoarthritis: The usual recommended daily dose is 200 mg taken once daily or in two divided doses. In some patients, with insufficient relief from symptoms, an increased dose of 200 mg twice daily may increase efficacy. In the absence of an increase in therapeutic benefit after two weeks, other therapeutic options should be considered.

Rheumatoid arthritis: The initial recommended daily dose is 200mg taken in two divided doses. The dose may, if needed, later be increased to 200 mg twice daily. In the absence of an increase in therapeutic benefit after two weeks, other therapeutic options should be considered.

The maximum recommended daily dose is 400 mg for both indications.

Celebrex may be taken with or without food.

Elderly: >65 years) As in younger adults, 200 mg per day should be used initially. The dose may, if needed, later be increased to 200 mg twice daily. Particular caution should be exercised in elderly with a body weight less than 50 kg (see 4.4 and 5.2).

Hepatic impairment: Treatment should be initiated at half the recommended dosein patients with establishedmoderate liver impairment with a serumalbumin of25-35 g/l. Experience in such patients is limited to cirrhotic patients (see 4.3, 4.4 and 5.2).

Renal impairment: Experience with celecoxib in patients with mild or moderate renal impairment is limited, therefore such patients should be treated with caution. (see 4.3, 4.4 and 5.2).

Children: Celecoxib is not indicated for use in children.

4.3 Contraindications

History of hypersensitivity to the active substance or to any of the excipients (see 6.1).

Known hypersensitivity to sulphonamides.

Active peptic ulceration or gastrointestinal (GI) bleeding.

Patients who have experienced asthma, acute rhinitis, nasal polyps, angioneurotic oedema, urticaria or other allergic-type reactions after taking acetylsalicylic acid or NSAIDs including COX-2 (cyclooxygenase-2) inhibitors.

In pregnancy and in women of childbearing potential unless using an effective method of contraception (See 4.5). Celecoxib has been shown to cause malformations in the two animal species studied (See 4.6 and 5.3). The potential for human risk in pregnancy is unknown, but cannot be excluded.

Breast feeding (See 4.6 and 5.3).

Severe hepatic dysfunction (serum albumin <25 g/l or Child-Pugh score ≥10).

Patients with estimatedcreatinine clearance <30 ml/min.

Inflammatory bowel disease.

Congestive heart failure (NYHA II-IV).

Established ischaemic heart disease and/or cerebrovascular disease.

4.4 Special warnings and special precautions for use

Upper gastrointestinal complications [perforations, ulcers or bleedings (PUBs)], some of them resulting in fatal outcome, have occurred in patients treated with celecoxib. Caution is advised with treatment of patients most at risk of developing a gastrointestinal complication with NSAIDs; the elderly, patients using any other NSAID or acetylsalicylic acid concomitantly or patients with a prior history of gastrointestinal disease, such as ulceration and GI bleeding.

There is further increase in the risk of gastrointestinal adverse effects for celecoxib (gastrointestinal ulceration or other gastrointestinal complications), when celecoxib is taken concomitantly with acetylsalicylic acid (even at low doses). A significant difference in GI safety between selective COX-2 inhibitors + acetylsalicylic acid *vs.* NSAIDs + acetylsalicylic acid has not been demonstrated in long-term clinical trials (see 5.1).

Increased number of serious cardiovascular events, mainly myocardial infarction, has been found in a long-term placebo-controlled study in subjects with sporadic adenomatous polyps treated with celecoxib at doses of 200mg BID and 400mg BID compared to placebo (see 5.1).

As the cardiovascular risks of celecoxib may increase with dose and duration of exposure, the shortest duration possible and the lowest effective daily dose should be used. The patient's need for symptomatic relief and response to therapy should be re-evaluated periodically, especially in patients with osteoarthritis (4.2, 4.3, 4.8 and 5.1).

Patients with significant risk factors for cardiovascular events (e.g. hypertension, hyperlipidaemia, diabetes mellitus, smoking) or peripheral arterial disease should only be treated with celecoxib after careful consideration (see 5.1).

COX-2 selective inhibitors are not a substitute for acetylsalicylic acid for prophylaxis of cardiovascular thromboembolic diseases because of their lack of antiplatelet effects. Therefore, antiplatelet therapies should not be discontinued (see section 5.1).

As with other drugs known to inhibit prostaglandin synthesis fluid retention and oedema have been observed in patients taking celecoxib. Therefore, celecoxib should be used with caution in patients with history of cardiac failure, left ventricular dysfunction or hypertension, and in patients with pre-existing oedema from any other reason, since prostaglandin inhibition may result in deterioration of renal function and fluid retention. Caution is also required in patients taking diuretic treatment or otherwise at risk of hypovolaemia.

Compromised renal or hepatic function and especially cardiac dysfunction are more likely in the elderly and therefore medically appropriate supervision should be maintained. Clinical trials with celecoxib have shown renal effects similar to those observed with comparator NSAIDs.

If during treatment, patients deteriorate in any of the organ system functions described above, appropriate measures should be taken and discontinuation of celecoxib therapy should be considered.

Celecoxib inhibits CYP2D6. Although it is not a strong inhibitor of this enzyme, a dose reduction may be necessary for individually dose-titrated drugs that are metabolised by CYP2D6 (See 4.5).

Patients known to be CYP2C9 poor metabolisers should be treated with caution (see 5.2.).

Serious skin reactions, including exfoliative dermatitis, Stevens-Johnson syndrome, and toxic epidermal necrolysis, have been reported in association with the use of NSAIDs including celecoxib during postmarketing surveillance (see 4.8). Hypersensitivity reactions (anaphylaxis and angioedema) have been reported in patients receiving celecoxib (see 4.8). Patients with a history of sulphonamide allergy may be at greater risk of hypersensitivity reactions (see 4.3). Celecoxib should be discontinued at the first sign of hypersensitivity.

Celecoxib may mask fever and other signs of inflammation.

In patients on concurrent therapy with warfarin, serious bleeding events have occurred. Caution should be exercised when combining celecoxib with warfarin and other oral anticoagulants (See 4.5).

Celebrex 100 mg and 200 mg capsules contain lactose (149.7 mg and 49.8 mg, respectively). Patients with rare hereditary problems of galactose intolerance, the Lapp lactose deficiency or glucose-galactose malabsorption should not take this medicine.

4.5 Interaction with other medicinal products and other forms of Interaction

Pharmacodynamic interactions

Anticoagulant activity should be monitored particularly in the first few days after initiating or changing the dose of celecoxib in patients receiving warfarin or other anticoagulants since these patients have an increased risk of bleeding complications. Therefore, patients receiving oral anticoagulants should be closely monitored for their prothrombin time INR, particularly in the first few days when therapy with celecoxib is initiated or the dose of celecoxib is changed. (see 4.4). Bleeding events in association with increases in prothrombin time have been reported, predominantly in the elderly, in patients receiving celecoxib concurrently with warfarin, some of them fatal.

NSAIDs may reduce the effect of diuretics and antihypertensive medicinal products. As for NSAIDs, the risk of acute renal insufficiency, which is usually reversible, may be increased in some patients with compromised renal function (e.g. dehydrated patients or elderly patients) when ACE inhibitors or angiotensin II receptor antagonists are combined with NSAIDs, including celecoxib. Therefore, the combination should be administered with caution, especially in the elderly. Patients should be adequately hydrated and consideration should be given to monitoring of renal function after initiation of concomitant therapy, and periodically thereafter.

Co-administration of NSAIDs and cyclosporin or tacrolimus have been suggested to increase the nephrotoxic effect of cyclosporin and tacrolimus. Renal function should be monitored when celecoxib and any of these drugs are combined.

Celecoxib can be used with low dose acetylsalicylic acid but is not a substitute for acetylsalicylic acid for cardiovascular prophylaxis. In the submitted studies, as with other NSAIDs, an increased risk of gastrointestinal ulceration or other gastrointestinal complications compared to use of celecoxib alone was shown for concomitant administration of low-dose acetylsalicylic acid. (see 5.1)

Pharmacokinetic interactions

Effects of celecoxib on other drugs

Celecoxib is an inhibitor of CYP2D6. During celecoxib treatment, the plasma concentrations of the CYP2D6 substrate dextromethorphan were increased by 136%. The plasma concentrations of drugs that are substrates of this enzyme may be increased when celecoxib is used concomitantly. Examples of drugs which are metabolised by CYP2D6 are antidepressants (tricyclics and SSRIs), neuroleptics, anti-arrhythmic drugs, etc. The dose of individually dose-titrated CYP2D6 substrates may need to be reduced when treatment with celecoxib is initiated or increased if treatment with celecoxib is terminated.

In vitro studies have shown some potential for celecoxib to inhibit CYP2C19 catalysed metabolism. The clinical significance of this *in vitro* finding is unknown. Examples of drugs which are metabolised by CYP2C19 are diazepam, citalopram and imipramine.

In an interaction study, celecoxib had no clinically relevant effects on the pharmacokinetics of oral contraceptives (1 mg norethisterone /35 microg ethinylestradiol).

Celecoxib does not affect the pharmacokinetics of tolbutamide (CYP2C9 substrate), or glibenclamideto a clinically relevant extent.

In patients with rheumatoid arthritis celecoxib had no statistically significant effect on the pharmacokinetics (plasma or renal clearance) of methotrexate (in rheumatologic doses). However, adequate monitoring for methotrexate-related toxicity should be considered when combining these two drugs.

In healthy subjects, co-administration of celecoxib 200 mg twice daily with 450 mg twice daily of lithium resulted in a mean increase in C_{max} of 16% and in AUC of 18% of lithium. Therefore, patients on lithium treatment should be closely monitored when celecoxib is introduced or withdrawn.

Effects of other drugs on celecoxib

Since celecoxib is predominantly metabolised by CYP2C9 it should be used at half the recommended dose in patients receiving fluconazole. Concomitant use of 200 mg single dose of celecoxib and 200 mg once daily of fluconazole, a potent CYP2C9 inhibitor, resulted in a mean increase in celecoxib C_{max} of 60% and in AUC of 130%. Concomitant use of inducers of CYP2C9 such as rifampicin, carbamazepine and barbiturates may reduce plasma concentrations of celecoxib.

Ketoconazole or antacids have not been observed to affect the pharmacokinetics of celecoxib.

4.6 Pregnancy and lactation

No clinical data on exposed pregnancies are available for celecoxib. Studies in animals (rats and rabbits) have shown reproductive toxicity, including malformations (see 4.3 and 5.3). The potential for human risk in pregnancy is unknown, but cannot be excluded. Celecoxib, as with other drugs inhibiting prostaglandin synthesis, may cause uterine inertia and premature closure of the ductus arteriosus during the last trimester. Celecoxib is contraindicated in pregnancy and in women who can become pregnant (see 4.3 and 4.4). If a woman becomes pregnant during treatment, celecoxib should be discontinued.

There are no studies on the excretion of celecoxib in human milk. Celecoxib is excreted in the milk of lactating rats at concentrations similar to those in plasma. Women who take celecoxib should not breastfeed.

4.7 Effects on ability to drive and use machines

Patients who experience dizziness, vertigo or somnolence while taking celecoxib should refrain from driving or operating machinery.

4.8 Undesirable effects

Approximately 7400 patients were treated with celecoxib in controlled trials and of those approximately 2300 have received it for 1 year or longer. The following events have been reportedin patients receiving celecoxib in 12 placebo and/oractivecontrolled trials. Side-effects listed havea rate equal or greater than placebo, and the discontinuation rate due to side-effects was 7.1% in patients receiving celecoxib and 6.1% in patients receiving placebo.

[Very Common >1/10), Common (⩾1/100, <1/10), Uncommon (⩾1/1000, <1/100), Rare (⩾1/10,000, <1/1000), Very rare (<1/10,000 including isolated cases)]

Infections and infestations

Common: sinusitis, upper respiratory tract infection

Uncommon: urinary tract infection

Blood and the lymphatic system disorders

Uncommon: anaemia.

Rare: leucopenia, thrombocytopenia

Metabolism and nutrition disorders

Uncommon: hyperkalaemia

Psychiatric disorders

Common: insomnia

Uncommon: anxiety, depression, tiredness.

Nervous system disorders

Common: dizziness

Uncommon: blurred vision, hypertonia, paraesthesia

Rare: ataxia, taste alteration

Ear and labyrinth disorders

Uncommon: tinnitus

Cardiac disorders

Uncommon: myocardial infarction*, heart failure, palpitations

Vascular disorders

Uncommon: hypertension, hypertension aggravated,

Rare: ischaemic stroke*

Respiratory, thoracic and mediastinal disorders

Common: pharyngitis, rhinitis

Uncommon: cough, dyspnoea

Gastrointestinal disorders

Common: abdominal pain, diarrhoea, dyspepsia, flatulence

Uncommon: constipation, eructation, gastritis, stomatitis, vomiting, aggravation of gastrointestinal inflammation.

Rare: duodenal, gastric, oesophageal, intestinal and colonic ulceration, dysphagia, intestinal perforation, oesophagitis, melaena.

Hepato-biliary disorders

Uncommon: abnormal hepatic function

Skin and subcutaneous tissue disorders

Common: rash.

Uncommon: urticaria.

Rare: alopecia, photosensitivity

Musculoskeletal and connective tissue disorders

Uncommon: leg cramps

General disorders and administration site conditions

Common: peripheral oedema/ fluid retention.

Investigations

Uncommon: increased SGOT and SGPT, increased creatinine, BUN increased

Reports from post-marketing experience include headache, nausea and arthralgia, also the following very rare (<1/10,000, including isolated cases):

Blood and lymphatic system disorders: pancytopenia.

Immune system disorders: serious allergic reactions, anaphylactic shock.

Psychiatric disorders: confusion, hallucinations.

Nervous system disorders: aggravated epilepsy, meningitis aseptic, ageusia, anosmia

Ear and labyrinth disorders: decreased hearing.

Vascular disorders: vasculitis

Respiratory, thoracic and mediastinal disorders: bronchospasm

Reproductive system and breast disorders: menstrual disorder NOS

Gastrointestinal disorders: gastrointestinal haemorrhage, acute pancreatitis, colitis/colitis aggravated.

Hepatobiliary disorders: hepatitis, jaundice, hepatic failure.

Skin and subcutaneous tissue disorders: angioedema, skin exfoliation including: Stevens-Johnson syndrome, epidermal necrolysis, erythema multiforme.

Musculoskeletal and connective tissue disorders: myositis

Renal and urinary disorders: acute renal failure, interstitial nephritis.

*Foot Note: Data on myocardial infarction are available from the following two sources while the information on ischaemic stroke is only available from the second source:

1). Based on a meta-analysis of placebo-controlled trials with celecoxib in OA and RA with duration up to 1 year reported by Dec 2004, that included 6847 patients taking 200 mg or 400mg of celecoxib daily and 5683 patients taking placebo, the excess rate over placebo of myocardial infarction was: (9/6847)-(3/5683)=0.08% (Rare).

2). The excess rate over placebo of myocardial infarction was estimated based on preliminary data from two long-term studies in patients with colorectal polyps treated with celecoxib 400mg daily for up to 3 years. It was 1.6-0.4=1.2% in one study; and 0.9-0.6=0.3% in the other; pooled: 1.2-0.5=0.7% (Uncommon). In the same studies, the excess for ischaemic stroke for 400 mg daily dose is: 0.43-0.38=0.05% (Rare).

4.9 Overdose

There is no clinical experience of overdose. Single doses up to 1200 mg and multiple doses up to 1200 mg twice daily have been administered to healthy subjects for nine days without clinically significant adverse effects. In the event of suspected overdose, appropriate supportive medical care should be provided e.g. by eliminating the gastric contents, clinical supervision and, if necessary, the institution of symptomatic treatment. Dialysis is unlikely to be an efficient method of drug removal due to high protein binding.

5. PHARMACOLOGICAL PROPERTIES

5.1 Pharmacodynamic properties

Pharmacotherapeutic group: ATC code: M01AH01.

Celecoxib is an oral, selective, cyclooxygenase-2 (COX-2) inhibitor within the clinical dose range (200-400 mg daily). No statistically significant inhibition of COX-1 (assessed as *ex vivo* inhibition of thromboxane B2 [TxB2] formation) was observed in this dose range in healthy volunteers.

Cyclooxygenase is responsible for generation of prostaglandins. Two isoforms, COX-1 and COX-2, have been identified. COX-2 is the isoform of the enzyme that has been shown to be induced by pro-inflammatory stimuli and has been postulated to be primarily responsible for the synthesis of prostanoid mediators of pain, inflammation, and fever. COX-2 is also involved in ovulation, implantation and closure of the ductus arteriosus, regulation of renal function, and central nervous system functions (fever induction, pain perception and cognitive function). It may also play a role in ulcer healing. COX-2 has been identified in tissue around gastric ulcers in man but its relevance to ulcer healing has not been established.

The difference in antiplatelet activity between some COX-1 inhibiting NSAIDs and COX-2 selective inhibitors may be of clinical significance in patients at risk of thrombo-embolic reactions. COX-2 selective inhibitors reduce the formation of systemic (and therefore possibly endothelial) prostacyclin without affecting platelet thromboxane.

Celecoxib is a diaryl-substituted pyrazole, chemically similar to other non-arylamine sulfonamides (e.g. thiazides, furosemide) but differs from arylamine sulfonamides (e.g. sulfamethoxizole and other sulfonamide antibiotics).

A dose dependent effect on TxB2 formation has been observed after high doses of celecoxib. However, in healthy subjects, in small multiple dose studies with 600 mg BID (three times the highest recommended dose) celecoxib had no effect on platelet aggregation and bleeding time compared to placebo.

Several clinical studies have been performed confirming efficacy and safety in osteoarthritis and rheumatoid arthritis. Celecoxib was evaluated for the treatment of the inflammation and pain of OA of the knee and hip in approximately 4200 patients in placebo and active controlled trials of up to 12 weeks duration. It was also evaluated for treatment of the inflammation and pain of RA in approximately 2100 patients in placebo and active controlled trials of up to 24 weeks duration. Celecoxib at daily doses of 200 mg - 400 mg provided pain relief within 24 hours of dosing. Five randomised double-blind controlled studies have been conducted including scheduled upper gastrointestinal endoscopy in approximately 4500 patients free from initial ulceration (celecoxib doses from 50 mg - 400 mg BID). In twelve week endoscopy studies celecoxib (100 - 800 mg per day) was associated with a significantly lower risk of gastroduodenal ulcers compared with naproxen (1000 mg per day) and ibuprofen (2400 mg per day). The data were inconsistent in comparison with diclofenac (150 mg per day). In two of the 12-week studies the percentage of patients with endoscopic gastroduodenal ulceration were not significantly different between placebo and celecoxib 200 mg BID and 400 mg BID.

In a prospective long-term safety outcome study (6 to 15 month duration, CLASS study), 5,800 OA and 2, 200 RA patients received celecoxib 400 mg BID (4-fold and 2-fold the recommended OA and RA doses, respectively), ibuprofen 800 mg TID or diclofenac 75 mg BID (both at therapeutic doses). Twenty-two percent of enrolled patients took concomitant low-dose acetylsalicylic acid (⩽325 mg/day), primarily for cardiovascular prophylaxis. For the primary endpoint complicated ulcers (defined as gastrointestinal bleeding, perforation or obstruction) celecoxib was not significantly different than either ibuprofen or diclofenac individually. Also for the combined NSAID group there was no statistically significant difference for complicated ulcers (relative risk 0.77, 95 % CI 0.41-1.46, based on entire study duration). For the combined endpoint, complicated and symptomatic ulcers, the incidence was significantly lower in the celecoxib group compared to the NSAID group, relative risk 0.66, 95% CI 0.45-0.97 but not between celecoxib and diclofenac. Those patients on celecoxib and concomitant low-dose acetylsalicylic acid experienced 4 fold higher rates of complicated ulcers as compared to those on celecoxib alone. The incidence of clinically significant decreases in haemoglobin >2 g/dL), confirmed by repeat testing, was significantly lower in patients on celecoxib compared to the NSAID group, relative risk 0.29, 95% CI 0.17- 0.48. The significantly lower incidence of this event with celecoxib was maintained with or without acetylsalicylic acid use.

Ongoing clinical Trials: Preliminary safety information from three long-term studies in Sporadic Adenomatous Polyps and Alzheimer's disease with celecoxib is available. In one of the three studies, there was a dose-related increase in cardiovascular events (mainly myocardial infarction, MI) at doses of 200mg BID and 400mg BID compared to placebo. The increased risk persisted throughout the study period (33 months). The relative risk for the composite endpoint (cardiovascular death, MI or stroke) was 3.2 (95% CI 1.3 – 8.0) for the higher dose and 2.5 (95% CI 1.0 – 6.3) for the lower dose of celecoxib, respectively, compared to placebo. Preliminary data from the other two long-term studies did not show a significantly increased cardiovascular risk with celecoxib 200mg BID and 400mg QD compared to placebo. This information will be updated as final data become available.

5.2 Pharmacokinetic properties

Celecoxib is well absorbed reaching peak plasma concentrations after approximately 2-3 hours. Dosing with food (high fat meal) delays absorption by about 1 hour.

Celecoxib is mainly eliminated by metabolism. Less than 1% of the dose is excreted unchanged in urine. The inter-subject variability in the exposure of celecoxib is about 10-fold. Celecoxib exhibits dose- and time-independent pharmacokinetics in the therapeutic dose range. Plasma protein binding is about 97% at therapeutic plasma concentrations and the drug is not preferentially bound to erythrocytes. Elimination half-life is 8-12 hours. Steady state plasma concentrations are reached within5 days of treatment. Pharmacological activity resides in the parent drug. The main metabolites found in the circulation have no detectable COX-1 or COX-2 activity.

Celecoxib is metabolised in the liver by hydroxylation, oxidation and some glucuronidation. The phase I metabolism is mainly catalysed by CYP2C9. There is a genetic polymorphism of this enzyme. Less than 1% of the population are poor metabolisers and have an enzyme with decreased activity. Plasma concentrations of celecoxib are probably markedly increased in such patients. Patients known to be CYP2C9 poor metabolisers should be treated with caution.

No clinically significant differences were found in PK parameters of celecoxib between elderly African-Americans and Caucasians.

The plasma concentration of celecoxib is approximately 100% increased in elderly women >65 years).

Compared to subjects with normal hepatic function, patients with mild hepatic impairment had a mean increase in C_{max} of 53% and in AUC of 26% of celecoxib. The corresponding values in patients with moderate hepatic impairment were 41% and 146% respectively. The metabolic capacity in patients with mild to moderate impairment was best correlated to their albumin values. Treatment should be initiated at half therecommended dose in patients with moderate liver impairment (with serum albumin 25-35g/L). Patients with severe hepatic impairment (serum albumin <25 g/l) have not been studied and celecoxib is contraindicated in this patient group.

There is little experience of celecoxib in renal impairment. The pharmacokinetics of celecoxib has not been studied in patients with renal impairment but is unlikely to be markedly changed in these patients. Thus caution is advised when treating patients with renal impairment. Severe renal impairment is contraindicated.

5.3 Preclinical safety data

Conventional embryo-fetaltoxicity studies resulted in dose dependent occurrences of diaphragmatic hernia in rat fetusesand of cardiovascular malformations in rabbit fetusesat systemic exposures to free drugapproximately 5X (rat) and 3X (rabbit) higher than those achieved atthe maximum recommended daily human dose (400 mg). Diaphragmatic hernia was also seen in a peri-post natal toxicity study in rats, which included exposure during the organogenetic period. In the latter study, at the lowest systemic exposure where this anomaly occurred in a single animal, the estimated margin relative to the maximum recommended daily human dose was 3X.

In animals, exposure to celecoxib during early embryonic development resulted in pre-implantation and post-implantation losses. These effects are expected following inhibition of prostaglandin synthesis.

Celecoxib was excreted in rat milk. In a peri-post natal study in rats, pup toxicity was observed.

Based on conventional studies, genotoxicity or carcinogenicity, no special hazard for humans was observed, beyond those addressed in other sections of the SmPC.

In a two-year toxicity study an increase in nonadrenal thrombosis was observed in male rat at high doses.

6. PHARMACEUTICAL PARTICULARS

6.1 List of excipients

Capsules 100 mg contain lactose monohydrate, sodium lauryl sulphate, povidone K30, croscarmellose sodium and magnesium stearate. Capsule shells contain gelatin, titanium dioxide E171; ink contains indigotine E132.

Capsules 200 mg contain lactose monohydrate, sodium lauryl sulphate, povidone K30, croscarmellose sodium and magnesium stearate. Capsule shells contain gelatin, titanium dioxide E171; ink contains iron oxide E172.

6.2 Incompatibilities

Not applicable.

6.3 Shelf life

3 years.

6.4 Special precautions for storage

Do not store above 30°C.

6.5 Nature and contents of container

Clear or opaque PVC blisters or aluminium cold-formed blisters. Pack of 2, 5, 6, 10, 20, 30, 40, 50, 60, 100, 10x10, 10x30, 10x50, 1x50 unit dose, 1x100 unit dose.

6.6 Instructions for use and handling

No special requirements.

7. MARKETING AUTHORISATION HOLDER

Pharmacia Limited

Ramsgate Road

Sandwich

Kent

CT13 9NJ

United Kingdom

8. MARKETING AUTHORISATION NUMBER(S)

Celebrex 100 mg: PL 00032/0399

Celebrex 200 mg: PL 00032/0400

9. DATE OF FIRST AUTHORISATION/RENEWAL OF THE AUTHORISATION

1st September 2002

10. DATE OF REVISION OF THE TEXT

17th February 2005

11 LEGAL CATEGORY

POM

Celectol 200 and 400 Tablets

(sanofi-aventis)

1. NAME OF THE MEDICINAL PRODUCT

Celectol 200 Tablets

Celectol 400 Tablets

2. QUALITATIVE AND QUANTITATIVE COMPOSITION

Celectol 200 Tablets: Celiprolol Hydrochloride 200mg.

Celectol 400 Tablets: Celiprolol Hydrochloride 400mg.

3. PHARMACEUTICAL FORM

Celectol 200 Tablets: White film coated biconvex heart shaped tablets engraved with 200 and a breakline on one face and the Celectol logo on the other face.

Celectol 400 Tablets: White film coated biconvex heart shaped tablets engraved with the Celectol logo on one face with 400 on the other.

4. CLINICAL PARTICULARS

4.1 Therapeutic indications

The management of mild to moderate hypertension.

4.2 Posology and method of administration

Route of Administration: Oral

Adults:

The initial dose is 200mg orally taken once daily with a glass of water. Celectol should be taken on rising, half an hour before food. If response is inadequate, the dose may be increased to 400 mg once daily.

Elderly patients:

Dosage as for adults.

Children:

Not recommended.

4.3 Contraindications

As with other beta-adrenoceptor antagonists, celiprolol should not be used in cases of cardiogenic shock, uncontrolled heart failure, sick-sinus syndrome, second or third degree heart block, severe bradycardia, severe renal impairment with creatinine clearance less than 15ml per minute, acute episodes of asthma, untreated phaeochromocytoma, metabolic acidosis, hypotension, hypersensitivity to the substance, or severe peripheral arterial circulatory disturbances.

Although cardio selective beta blockers may have less effect on lung function than non selective beta blockers, as with all beta blockers these should be avoided in patients with chronic obstructive airways disease, and in patients with a history of bronchospasm or bronchial asthma, unless there are compelling clinical reasons for their use. Where such reasons exist, celiprolol may be used but with the utmost caution. The label will carry the following warning: *If you have a history of asthma or wheezing, please ask your doctor before taking this medicine.*

Celectol tablets should not be prescribed for patients being treated with theophylline.

4.4 Special warnings and special precautions for use

The pharmacokinetics are not significantly different in the elderly, however these patients should be regularly monitored and due regard made for decreased renal and liver function in this age group.

Celectol may be used in patients with mild to moderate degrees of reduced renal function as celiprolol is cleared by both renal and non-renal excretory pathways. A reduction in dosage by half may be appropriate in patients with creatinine clearances in the range of 15 to 40ml per minute. However, careful surveillance of such patients is recommended until steady state blood levels are achieved which typically would be within one week. Celectol is not recommended for patients with creatinine clearance less than 15ml per minute. Patients with hepatic impairment should also be carefully monitored after commencing therapy and a reduced dosage should be considered.

Sudden withdrawal of beta-adrenoceptor blocking agents in patients with ischemic heart disease may result in the appearance of anginal attacks of increased frequency or severity or deterioration in cardiac state. Although no adverse effects due to abrupt cessation of Celectol have been seen in clinical trials, therapy should be gradually reduced over 1-2 weeks, at the same time, if necessary, initiating replacement therapy to prevent exacerbation of angina pectoris.

Celectol therapy must be reported to the anaesthetist prior to general anaesthesia. If it is decided to withdraw the drug before surgery, 48 hours should be allowed to elapse between the last dose and anaesthesia. Continuation of beta blockade reduces the risk of arrhythmias during induction and intubation, although reflex tachycardia may be attenuated and the risk of hypotension may be increased (see "Interactions"). In the event of continuation of Celectol treatment special care should be exercised when using anaesthetic agents such as ether, cyclopropane or trichloroethylene. The patient may be protected against vagal reactions by the intravenous administration of atropine.

Celectol should only be used with caution in patients with controlled congestive cardiac failure. Evidence of decompensation should be regarded as a signal to discontinue therapy.

In patients with peripheral circulatory disorders (Raynaud's disease or syndrome, intermittent claudication), beta blockers should be used with great caution as aggravation of these disorders may occur.

Celiprolol may induce bradycardia. If the pulse rate decreases to less than 50-55 beats per minute at rest and the patient experiences symptoms related to the bradycardia, the dosage should be reduced.

Due to its negative effect on conduction time, celiprolol should only be given with caution to patients with first degree heart block.

Beta blockers may increase the number and the duration of anginal attacks in patients with Prinzmetal's angina, due to unopposed alpha-receptor mediated coronary artery vasoconstriction. The use of beta-i selective adrenoceptor blocking drugs such as celiprolol may be considered in these patients, but the utmost care should be exercised.

Beta blockers have been reported to exacerbate psoriasis, and patients with a history of psoriasis should take celiprolol only after careful consideration.

In patients with a history of anaphylactic reactions, beta blockers may increase the sensitivity to allergens and the seriousness of the reactions.

Beta blockers may mask the symptoms of thyrotoxicosis or hypoglycaemia (in particular, tachycardia).

4.5 Interaction with other medicinal products and other forms of Interaction

Not recommended association

It has been shown that the bioavailability of celiprolol is impaired when it is given with food. Co-administration of chlorthalidone and hydrochlorothiazide also reduces the bioavailability of celiprolol.

Calcium channel antagonists such as verapamil (and to a lesser extent diltiazem) and beta blockers both slow A-V conduction and depress myocardial contractility through different mechanisms. When changing from verapamil to celiprolol and vice versa, a period between stopping one and starting the other is recommended. Concomitant administration of both drugs is not recommended and should only be initiated with ECG monitoring. Patients with pre existing conduction abnormalities should not be given the two drugs together.

Digitalis glycosides, in association with beta-adrenoceptor blocking drugs, may increase
A-V conduction time.

Beta blockers may exacerbate the rebound hypertension which can follow the withdrawal of clonidine. If the two drugs are co-administered, the beta-adrenoceptor blocking drug should be withdrawn several days before discontinuing clonidine. There is a theoretical risk that concurrent administration of monoamine oxidase inhibitors and high doses of beta-adrenoceptor blockers, even if they are cardio selective, can produce hypertension.

Precautions for use

Care should be taken in prescribing beta-adrenoceptor blockers with Class I antiarrhythmic agents (e.g. disopyramide, quinidine) and amiodarone, since these agents may potentiate the negative effects on A-V conduction and myocardial contractility.

Beta blockers may intensify the blood sugar lowering effects of insulin and oral antidiabetic drugs, and the dosage of antidiabetics may therefore require adjustment. In addition, beta-adrenoceptor blockers may mask the symptoms of thyrotoxicosis or hypoglycaemia (in particular, tachycardia).

Therapy with beta-adrenoceptor blockers must be reported to the anaesthetist prior to general anaesthesia (see "Special warnings and special precautions for use"). Continuation of beta blockade reduces the risk of arrhythmias during induction and intubation, but reflex tachycardia may be attenuated and the risk of hypotension may be increased. Anaesthetic agents causing myocardial depression (e.g. ether, cyclopropane, trichloroethylene) are best avoided.

Take into account

Concomitant therapy with dihydropyridine calcium channel antagonists, such as nifedipine, may increase the risk of hypotension, and cardiac failure may occur in patients with latent cardiac insufficiency.

Drugs inhibiting prostaglandin synthetase, such as ibuprofen or indomethacin, may decrease the hypotensive effects of beta-adrenoceptor blocking drugs.

Sympathomimetic agents, such as adrenaline, may counteract the effects of beta blockers.

Concomitant use of other antihypertensive agents, or of tricyclic antidepressants, barbiturates or phenothiazines, may potentiate the hypotensive effects of beta blockers.

4.6 Pregnancy and lactation

The safety of this medicinal product for use in human pregnancy have not been established. An evaluation of experimental animal studies does not indicate direct or indirect harmful effects with respect to reproduction, development of the embryo or foetus, the course of gestation and peri- and post-natal development.

However, beta-adrenoceptor blocking drugs in general have been associated with reduced placental perfusion, which may result in intrauterine foetal death, immature and premature deliveries. In addition, adverse effects (especially hypoglycaemia and bradycardia) may occur in foetus and neonate, together with an increased risk of cardiac and pulmonary complications in the neonate in the post natal period. Most beta blockers will pass into breast milk, although to variable extents. The use of Celectol is not recommended in breast-feeding mothers.

4.7 Effects on ability to drive and use machines

It has been shown that driving ability is unlikely to be impaired in patients taking Celectol. However, it should be taken into account that occasional dizziness or fatigue may occur.

4.8 Undesirable effects

Beta-adrenoceptor blockers may mask the symptoms of thyrotoxicosis or hypoglycaemia (in particular, tachycardia).

Occasional side effects, which are usually mild and transient have occurred. These include headache, dizziness, fatigue, nausea, somnolence and insomnia (sleep disturbances). Additional side effects associated with beta-2 agonist activity, tremor and palpitations, have been reported. These effects usually do not require withdrawal of therapy. Depression and hypersensitivity pneumonitis have been reported rarely.

Bronchospasm, skin rashes and/or visual disturbances have been reported in association with the use of beta blockers. Celectol should be discontinued if these effects occur.

In addition, the following undesirable effects, listed by body system, are generally attributable to the pharmacological activity of beta-adrenergic blockers:

Cardiovascular: bradycardia, slowed A-V conduction, hypotension, heart failure, cold and cyanotic extremities. In susceptible patients: precipitation of existing A-V block, exacerbation of intermittent claudication, Raynaud's disease or syndrome.

CNS: confusion, hallucinations, psychoses, nightmares.

Neurological: paraesthesia.

Respiratory: bronchospasm may occur in patients with bronchial asthma or with a history of bronchial complaints.

Gastro-intestinal: vomiting, diarrhoea.

Integumentary: skin disorders (especially rash), dry eyes.

Others: disturbances of libido and potency. An increase in ANA (antinuclear antibodies) has been reported, although its clinical relevance is not clear.

4.9 Overdose

No data are available regarding celiprolol overdose in humans.

The most common symptoms to be expected following overdosage with a beta-adrenoceptor blocking drug are bradycardia, hypotension, bronchospasm and acute cardiac insufficiency.

General treatment should include close supervision, with the use of gastric lavage, activated charcoal and a laxative to prevent absorption of any drug still present in the gastrointestinal tract. Haemodyalysis or haemoperfusion may be considered.

Bradycardia or extensive vagal reactions should be treated with intravenous atropine, 1-2mg. Cardiac pacing should be considered in refractory bradycardia and heart block. Hypotension should be treated with plasma or plasma substitutes and, if necessary, intravenous catecholamines including dopamine and dobutamine.

The effects of excessive beta blockade can be counteracted by the slow intravenous infusion of a beta-adrenoceptor stimulant such as isoprenaline, starting with a dose of approximately 5 micrograms per minute with close cardiac monitoring, or dobutamine, starting with a dose of 2.5 micrograms per kilogram per minute, until the required effect has been obtained. In severe overdosage, intravenous glucagon may be considered: an initial bolus dose of 10mg may be repeated within one hour, if required, or followed by intravenous infusion of glucagon at a rate of 1-10mg per hour, depending on response.

5. PHARMACOLOGICAL PROPERTIES

5.1 Pharmacodynamic properties

Celiprolol is a vasoactive beta-l selective adrenoceptor antagonist with partial beta-2 agonist activity indicated in mild to moderate hypertension. The beta-2 agonist activity is thought to account for its mild vasodilating properties. It lowers blood pressure in hypertensive patients at rest and on exercise. The effects on heart rate and cardiac output are dependant on the pre-existing background level of sympathetic tone.

Under conditions of stress such as exercise celiprolol attenuates chronotropic and inotropic responses to sympathetic stimulation. However, at rest minimal impairment of cardiac function is seen.

Celectol therapy has not been shown to adversely effect plasma lipid profiles.

5.2 Pharmacokinetic properties

Celiprolol is a hydrophilic compound that is incompletely absorbed from the gastrointestinal tract. Plasma half-life is approximately 5-6 hours and pharmacodynamic effects are present for at least 24 hours. After once daily administration celiprolol is only slightly metabolised before excretion in the bile and urine in almost equal quantities.

It has been shown that the bioavailability of celiprolol is impaired when it is given with food. Co-administration of chlorthalidone, hydrochlorothiazide and theophylline also reduces the bioavailability of celiprolol.

5.3 Preclinical safety data

There are no preclinical data of relevance to the prescriber which are additional to that already included in other sections of the SPC.

6. PHARMACEUTICAL PARTICULARS

6.1 List of excipients

Mannitol BP

Microcrystalline Cellulose BP

Croscarmellose Sodium NF

Magnesium Stearate BP

Demineralised Water

Film coating:

Opadry YS-l-7006 (clear) contains E464 and polyethylene glycol.

Opadry Y-1-7000 (white) contains E171, E464 and polyethylene glycol.

6.2 Incompatibilities

None stated.

6.3 Shelf life

36 months.

6.4 Special precautions for storage

Store below 25°C.

6.5 Nature and contents of container

Container	Pack size
Blister packs 250μ clear opaque rigid UPVC with 20μ hard temper aluminium foil	28

6.6 Instructions for use and handling

No special instructions.

7. MARKETING AUTHORISATION HOLDER

Aventis Pharma Ltd

50 Kings Hill Avenue

Kings Hill

West Malling

Kent

ME19 4AH

United Kingdom

8. MARKETING AUTHORISATION NUMBER(S)

Celectol 200 Tablets: PL 04425/0361

Celectol 400 Tablets: PL 04425/0362

9. DATE OF FIRST AUTHORISATION/RENEWAL OF THE AUTHORISATION

15 September 2004

10. DATE OF REVISION OF THE TEXT

September 2004

Legal classification: POM

Celevac Tablets

(Shire Pharmaceuticals Limited)

1. NAME OF THE MEDICINAL PRODUCT

Celevac 500mg Tablets

2. QUALITATIVE AND QUANTITATIVE COMPOSITION

Each tablet contains 500mg of methylcellulose.

For excipients, see 6.1.

3. PHARMACEUTICAL FORM

Tablet.

Pink, biconvex tablet marked with a breakline on one face and Celevac on the other.

4. CLINICAL PARTICULARS

4.1 Therapeutic indications

Methylcellulose is a hydrophilic colloid which absorbs water causing it to swell to a soft gel of uniform consistency.

- Recommended clinical use

- In the control of colostomy, ileostomy and simple diarrhoea.

- In the management of diverticular disease and ulcerative colitis.

- In the management of simple constipation.

- As an aid to appetite control and the treatment of obesity.

Route of administration

Oral.

4.2 Posology and method of administration

It is recommended that the tablets should be broken in the mouth before swallowing. Celevac tablets swell in contact with water and should therefore be swallowed carefully. It is not recommended that these tablets be taken before going to bed.

Colostomy and ileostomy control and for simple diarrhoea: 3-6 tablets twice daily with the minimum of liquid. Liquids should be avoided for 30 minutes before and after each dose. Dosage should be adjusted to give stools of the required consistency.

Diverticular disease and ulcerative colitis: 3-6 tablets twice daily adjusted according to the degree of constipation (with 300 ml of liquid), diarrhoea (with a little liquid) or spastic pain.

Simple constipation: 3-6 tablets twice daily to be taken with at least 300ml of liquid. The dose may be reduced as normal bowel function is restored.

As an aid to appetite control and the treatment of obesity: 3 tablets with at least 300ml of warm liquid, half an hour before each meal and between meals when hunger pangs are severe.

4.3 Contraindications

Celevac tablets are contraindicated in patients:

- hypersensitive to methylcellulose or to any of the excipients
- with imminent or threatened intestinal obstruction
- with faecal impaction
- who have difficulty in swallowing
- with colonic atony
- with infective bowel disease
- with severe dehydration

4.4 Special warnings and special precautions for use

Adequate fluid intake should be maintained to avoid intestinal obstruction. Guidance on fluid intake is stated in Section 4.2 Posology and method of administration.

Supervision may be necessary for patients who:

- are elderly
- are debilitated
- have intestinal narrowing
- have decreased intestinal motility.

Bowel obstruction is a rare complication of treatment with any bulk-forming hydrophilic colloid (refer also to Section 4.8 Undesirable Effects).

Patients with rare hereditary problems of galactose intolerance, the Lapp lactase deficiency or glucose-galactose malabsorption should not take this medicine.

4.5 Interaction with other medicinal products and other forms of Interaction

None listed.

4.6 Pregnancy and lactation

Although Celevac has been in wide general use for many years there is no evidence of ill consequence during human pregnancy. Medicines should not be used in pregnancy, especially the first trimester, unless the expected benefit is thought to outweigh any possible risk to the foetus.

4.7 Effects on ability to drive and use machines

None listed.

4.8 Undesirable effects

The most commonly reported reactions with methylcellulose are of a gastrointestinal nature:

Flatulence and abdominal distension.

Reactions not already stated, which are attributable to bulk-forming laxatives include gastrointestinal obstruction, faecal impaction and hypersensitivity.

4.9 Overdose

Methylcellulose is not absorbed. The features to be expected would be abdominal distension which may be followed by intestinal obstruction.

Gastric lavage should be employed where appropriate. The patient should be observed and fluid given. If obstruction develops, appropriate measures such as rectal washout must be taken.

5. PHARMACOLOGICAL PROPERTIES

5.1 Pharmacodynamic properties

Pharmacotherapeutic group:	Alimentary Tract and Metabolism; Laxatives; Bulk producers - Methylcellulose
ATC Code:	A06AC 06

The active ingredient is a simple bulking agent.

5.2 Pharmacokinetic properties

The active ingredient is not absorbed and hence the product cannot be described in terms of pharmacokinetics.

5.3 Preclinical safety data

None listed.

6. PHARMACEUTICAL PARTICULARS

6.1 List of excipients

Lactose monohydrate

Saccharin sodium

Povidone

Erythrosine (E127)

Strawberry flavour 52.318 AP

Talc

Magnesium stearate

6.2 Incompatibilities

None listed.

6.3 Shelf life

3 years

6.4 Special precautions for storage

Do not store above 25°C.

6.5 Nature and contents of container

Polypropylene securitainer, containing 112 tablets with polyethylene cap.

6.6 Instructions for use and handling

None given.

7. MARKETING AUTHORISATION HOLDER

Monmouth Pharmaceuticals Ltd

Hampshire International Business Park

Chineham

Basingstoke

Hampshire RG24 8EP

United Kingdom

8. MARKETING AUTHORISATION NUMBER(S)

PL 10536/0017

9. DATE OF FIRST AUTHORISATION/RENEWAL OF THE AUTHORISATION

11 November 1992

10. DATE OF REVISION OF THE TEXT

August 2004

Legal Category

GSL

Cellcept 250mg Capsules

(Roche Products Limited)

1. NAME OF THE MEDICINAL PRODUCT

CellCept 250mg capsules▼.

2. QUALITATIVE AND QUANTITATIVE COMPOSITION

Each capsule contains 250mg mycophenolate mofetil.

For excipients, see section 6.1.

3. PHARMACEUTICAL FORM

CellCept capsules:Oblong, blue/brown, branded with black "CellCept 250" on the capsule cap and "Company logo" on the capsule body.

4. CLINICAL PARTICULARS

4.1 Therapeutic indications

CellCept is indicated in combination with ciclosporin and corticosteroids for the prophylaxis of acute transplant rejection in patients receiving allogeneic renal, cardiac or hepatic transplants.

4.2 Posology and method of administration

Treatment with CellCept should be initiated and maintained by appropriately qualified transplant specialists.

Use in renal transplant:

Adults: oral CellCept should be initiated within 72 hours following transplantation. The recommended dose in renal transplant patients is 1.0g administered twice daily (2g daily dose).

Children and adolescents (aged 2 to 18 years): the recommended dose of mycophenolate mofetil is 600mg/m^2 administered orally twice daily (up to a maximum 2g daily). Cellcept capsules should only be prescribed to patients with a body surface area of at least 1.25m^2. Patients with a body surface area of 1.25 to 1.5m^2 may be prescribed CellCept capsules at a dose of 750mg twice daily (1.5g daily dose). Patients with a body surface area greater than 1.5m^2 may be prescribed CellCept capsules at a dose of 1g twice daily (2g daily dose). As some adverse reactions occur with greater frequency in this age group (see section 4.8 Undesirable effects) compared with adults, temporary dose reduction or interruption may be required; these will need to take into account relevant clinical factors including severity of reaction.

Children (< 2 years): there are limited safety and efficacy data in children below the age of 2 years. These are insufficient to make dosage recommendations and therefore use in this age group is not recommended.

Use in cardiac transplant:

Adults: oral CellCept should be initiated within 5 days following transplantation. The recommended dose in cardiac transplant patients is 1.5g administered twice daily (3g daily dose).

Children: no data are available for paediatric cardiac transplant patients.

Use in hepatic transplant:

Adults: IV CellCept should be administered for the first 4 days following hepatic transplant, with oral CellCept initiated as soon after this as it can be tolerated. The recommended oral dose in hepatic transplant patients is 1.5g administered twice daily (3g daily dose).

Children: no data are available for paediatric hepatic transplant patients.

Use in elderly (≥ 65 years): the recommended dose of 1.0g administered twice a day for renal transplant patients and 1.5g twice a day for cardiac or hepatic transplant patients is appropriate for the elderly.

Use in renal impairment: in renal transplant patients with severe chronic renal impairment (glomerular filtration rate < 25ml•min^{-1}•1.73 m^{-2}), outside the immediate post-transplant period, doses greater than 1g administered twice a day should be avoided. These patients should also be carefully observed. No dose adjustments are needed in patients experiencing delayed renal graft function post-operatively (see section 5.2 Pharmacokinetic properties). No data are available for cardiac or hepatic transplant patients with severe chronic renal impairment.

Use in severe hepatic impairment: no dose adjustments are needed for renal transplant patients with severe hepatic parenchymal disease. No data are available for cardiac transplant patients with severe hepatic parenchymal disease.

Treatment during rejection episodes: MPA (mycophenolic acid) is the active metabolite of mycophenolate mofetil. Renal transplant rejection does not lead to changes in MPA pharmacokinetics; dosage reduction or interruption of CellCept is not required. There is no basis for CellCept dose adjustment following cardiac transplant rejection. No pharmacokinetic data are available during hepatic transplant rejection.

4.3 Contraindications

Hypersensitivity reactions to CellCept have been observed (see section 4.8 Undesirable effects). Therefore, CellCept is contraindicated in patients with a hypersensitivity to mycophenolate mofetil or mycophenolic acid.

CellCept is contraindicated in women who are breastfeeding (see section 4.6 Pregnancy and lactation).

For information on use in pregnancy and contraceptive requirements see section 4.6 Pregnancy and lactation.

4.4 Special warnings and special precautions for use

Patients receiving immunosuppressive regimens involving combinations of drugs, including CellCept, are at increased risk of developing lymphomas and other malignancies, particularly of the skin (see section 4.8 Undesirable effects). The risk appears to be related to the intensity and duration of immunosuppression rather than to the use of any specific agent. As general advice to minimise the risk for skin cancer, exposure to sunlight and UV light should be limited by wearing protective clothing and using a sunscreen with a high protection factor.

Patients receiving CellCept should be instructed to report immediately any evidence of infection, unexpected bruising, bleeding or any other manifestation of bone marrow depression.

Oversuppression of the immune system increases the susceptibility to infection including opportunistic infections, fatal infections and sepsis (see section 4.8 Undesirable effects).

Patients receiving CellCept should be monitored for neutropenia, which may be related to CellCept itself, concomitant medications, viral infections, or some combination of these causes. Patients taking CellCept should have complete blood counts weekly during the first month, twice monthly for the second and third months of treatment, then monthly through the first year. If neutropenia develops (absolute neutrophil count < 1.3 × 10^3/μl) it may be appropriate to interrupt or discontinue CellCept.

Patients should be advised that during treatment with CellCept vaccinations may be less effective and the use of live attenuated vaccines should be avoided (see section 4.5 Interaction with other medicinal products and other forms of interaction). Influenza vaccination may be of value. Prescribers should refer to national guidelines for influenza vaccination.

Because CellCept has been associated with an increased incidence of digestive system adverse events, including infrequent cases of gastrointestinal tract ulceration, haemorrhage and perforation, CellCept should be administered with caution in patients with active serious digestive system disease.

CellCept is an IMPDH (inosine monophosphate dehydrogenase) inhibitor. On theoretical grounds therefore, it should be avoided in patients with rare hereditary deficiency of hypoxanthine-guanine phosphoribosyl-transferase (HGPRT) such as Lesch-Nyhan and Kelley-Seegmiller syndrome.

It is recommended that CellCept not be administered concomitantly with azathioprine because such concomitant administration has not been studied.

In view of the significant reduction in the AUC of MPA by colestyramine, caution should be used in the concomitant administration of CellCept with drugs that interfere with enterohepatic recirculation because of the potential to reduce the efficacy of CellCept.

The risk:benefit of mycophenolate mofetil in combination with tacrolimus has not been established (see also section 4.5 Interaction with other medicinal products and other forms of interaction).

4.5 Interaction with other medicinal products and other forms of Interaction

Aciclovir: higher MPAG and aciclovir plasma concentrations were observed when mycophenolate mofetil was administered with aciclovir in comparison to the administration of each drug alone. The changes in MPAG pharmacokinetics (MPAG increased by 8%) were minimal and are not considered clinically significant. Because MPAG plasma concentrations are increased in the presence of renal impairment, as are aciclovir concentrations, the potential exists for mycophenolate mofetil and aciclovir, or its prodrugs, e.g. valaciclovir, to compete for tubular secretion and further increases in concentrations of both drugs may occur.

Antacids with magnesium and aluminium hydroxides: absorption of mycophenolate mofetil was decreased when administered with antacids.

Colestyramine: following single dose administration of 1.5g of mycophenolate mofetil to normal healthy subjects pre-treated with 4g TID of colestyramine for 4 days, there was a 40% reduction in the AUC of MPA. (see section 4.4 Special warnings and special precautions for use, and section 5.2 Pharmacokinetic properties). Caution should be used during concomitant administration because of the potential to reduce efficacy of CellCept.

Drugs that interfere with enterohepatic circulation: caution should be used with drugs that interfere with enterohepatic circulation because of their potential to reduce the efficacy of CellCept.

Ciclosporin A: ciclosporin A pharmacokinetics were unaffected by mycophenolate mofetil.

Several studies have demonstrated that ciclosporin A reduces MPA plasma AUC levels by 19 – 38%, possibly as a result of inhibiting biliary secretion with consequent reduction of the entero-hepatic recirculation. However, as efficacy studies were carried out using CellCept combined with ciclosporin A and corticosteroids, these findings do not affect the recommended dose requirements (see section 4.2 Posology and method of administration).

Ganciclovir: based on the results of a single dose administration study of recommended doses of oral mycophenolate and IV ganciclovir and the known effects of renal impairment on the pharmacokinetics of CellCept (see section 4.2 Posology and method of administration) and ganciclovir, it is anticipated that co-administration of these agents (which compete for mechanisms of renal tubular secretion) will result in increases in MPAG and ganciclovir concentration. No substantial alteration of MPA pharmacokinetics are anticipated and CellCept dose adjustment is not required. In patients with renal impairment in which CellCept and ganciclovir or its prodrugs, e.g. valganciclovir, are co-administered the dose recommendations for ganciclovir should be observed and patients monitored carefully.

Oral contraceptives: the pharmacokinetics and pharmacodynamics of oral contraceptives were unaffected by coadministration of CellCept (see also section 5.2 Pharmacokinetic properties).

Trimethoprim/sulfamethoxazole: no effect on the bioavailability of MPA was observed.

Tacrolimus: *in renal transplant patients*: stable renal transplant patients receiving ciclosporin and CellCept (1g BID) showed about a 30% increase in MPA plasma AUC and about a 20% decrease in MPAG plasma AUC when ciclosporin was replaced with tacrolimus. MPA C_{max} was not affected, while MPAG C_{max} was reduced by approximately 20%. The mechanism of this finding is not well understood. Increased biliary secretion of MPAG accompanied with increased enterohepatic recirculation of MPA may be partly responsible for the finding, since the elevation of MPA concentrations associated with tacrolimus administration was more pronounced in the later portions of the concentration-time profile (4 – 12 hours after dosing). In another study in renal transplant patients it was shown that the tacrolimus concentration did not appear to be altered by CellCept.

In hepatic transplant patients: very limited pharmacokinetic data on MPA AUC are available in hepatic transplant patients treated with CellCept in combination with tacrolimus. In a study designed to evaluate the effect of CellCept on the pharmacokinetics of tacrolimus in stable hepatic transplant patients, there was an increase of approximately 20% in tacrolimus AUC when multiple doses of CellCept (1.5g BID) were administered to patients taking tacrolimus.

Other interactions: co-administration of probenecid with mycophenolate mofetil in monkeys raises plasma AUC of MPAG by 3-fold. Thus, other drugs known to undergo renal tubular secretion may compete with MPAG and thereby raise plasma concentrations of MPAG or the other drug undergoing tubular secretion.

Live vaccines: live vaccines should not be given to patients with an impaired immune response. The antibody response to other vaccines may be diminished (see also section 4.4 Special warnings and special precautions for use).

4.6 Pregnancy and lactation

It is recommended that CellCept therapy should not be initiated until a negative pregnancy test has been obtained. Effective contraception must be used before beginning CellCept therapy, during therapy, and for six weeks following discontinuation of therapy (see section 4.5 Interaction with other medicinal products and other forms of interaction). Patients should be instructed to consult their physician immediately should pregnancy occur.

The use of CellCept is not recommended during pregnancy and should be reserved for cases where no more suitable alternative treatment is available. CellCept should be used in pregnant women only if the potential benefit outweighs the potential risk to the foetus. There are no adequate data from the use of CellCept in pregnant women. Studies in animals have shown reproductive toxicity (see section 5.3 Preclinical safety data). The potential risk for humans is unknown.

Mycophenolate mofetil has been shown to be excreted in the milk of lactating rats. It is not known whether this drug is excreted in human milk. Because of the potential for serious adverse reactions to mycophenolate mofetil in breast-fed infants, CellCept is contraindicated in nursing mothers (see section 4.3 Contraindications).

4.7 Effects on ability to drive and use machines

No specific studies have been performed. The pharmacodynamic profile and the reported adverse reactions indicate that an effect is unlikely.

4.8 Undesirable effects

The following undesirable effects cover adverse drug reactions from clinical trials:

The principal adverse drug reactions associated with the administration of CellCept in combination with ciclosporin and corticosteroids include diarrhoea, leucopenia, sepsis and vomiting and there is evidence of a higher frequency of certain types of infections (see section 4.4 Special warnings and special precautions for use).

Malignancies:

Patients receiving immunosuppressive regimens involving combinations of drugs, including CellCept, are at increased risk of developing lymphomas and other malignancies, particularly of the skin (see section 4.4 Special warnings and special precautions for use). Lymphoproliferative disease or lymphoma developed in 0.6% of patients receiving CellCept (2g or 3g daily) in combination with other immunosuppressants in controlled clinical trials of renal (2g data), cardiac and hepatic transplant patients followed for at least 1 year. Non-melanoma skin carcinomas occurred in 3.6% of patients; other types of malignancy occurred in 1.1% of patients. Three-year safety data in renal and cardiac transplant patients did not reveal any unexpected changes in incidence of malignancy compared to the 1-year data. Hepatic transplant patients were followed for at least 1 year, but less than 3 years.

Opportunistic infections:

All transplant patients are at increased risk of opportunistic infections; the risk increased with total immunosuppressive load (see section 4.4 Special warnings and special precautions for use). The most common opportunistic infections in patients receiving CellCept (2g or 3g daily) with other immunosuppressants in controlled clinical trials of renal (2g data), cardiac and hepatic transplant patients followed for at least 1 year were candida mucocutaneous, CMV viraemia/syndrome and Herpes simplex. The proportion of patients with CMV viraemia/syndrome was 13.5%.

Children and adolescents (aged 2 to 18 years):

The type and frequency of adverse drug reactions in a clinical study, which recruited 92 paediatric patients aged 2 to 18 years who were given 600 mg/m^2 mycophenolate mofetil orally twice daily, were generally similar to those observed in adult patients given 1 g CellCept twice daily. However, the following treatment-related adverse events were more frequent in the paediatric population, particularly in children under 6 years of age, when compared to adults: diarrhoea, sepsis, leucopenia, anaemia and infection.

Elderly patients (⩾ 65 years):

Elderly patients (⩾ 65 years) may generally be at increased risk of adverse drug reactions due to immunosuppression. Elderly patients receiving CellCept as part of a combination immunosuppressive regimen, may be at increased risk of certain infections (including cytomegalovirus tissue invasive disease) and possibly gastrointestinal haemorrhage and pulmonary oedema, compared to younger individuals.

Other adverse drug reactions:

Adverse drug reactions, probably or possibly related to CellCept, reported in ⩾ 10% and in 1 - < 10% of patients treated with CellCept in the controlled clinical trials of renal (2g data), cardiac and hepatic transplant patients are listed in the following table.

Adverse Drug Reactions, Probably or Possibly Related to CellCept, Reported in Patients Treated with CellCept in Renal, Cardiac and Hepatic Clinical Trials when Used in Combination with Ciclosporin and Corticosteroids

Body System		Adverse drug reactions
Body as a whole	⩾ 10%	Sepsis
	1 - < 10%	Moniliasis, infection, fever, chills, malaise, headache, flu syndrome, pain, asthenia, weight loss, oedema
Blood and lymphatic	⩾ 10%	Leucopenia, thrombocytopenia, anaemia
	1 - < 10%	Pancytopenia, leucocytosis
Renal and urogenital	⩾ 10%	Urinary tract infection
	1 - < 10%	Vaginal moniliasis, abnormal kidney function, increased creatinine, increased BUN
Cardio-vascular	⩾10%	
	1 - < 10%	Hypotension, hypertension, tachycardia, vasodilatation
Metabolic/nutritional	⩾ 10%	
	1 - < 10%	Hyperkalaemia, acidosis, hypokalaemia, hypomagnesaemia, hypocalcaemia, hypercholesterolaemia, gout, hyperlipaemia, increased alkaline phosphatase, hyperglycaemia, hypophosphataemia, hyperuricaemia, increased lactate dehydrogenase
Gastro-intestinal	⩾ 10%	Moniliasis, vomiting, diarrhoea, nausea, abdominal pain
	1 - < 10%	Gastrointestinal haemorrhage, peritonitis, gastric ulcer, duodenal ulcer, colitis, infection, ileus, stomatitis, gastritis, gastroenteritis, anorexia, oesophagitis, dyspepsia, constipation, flatulence, eructation
Hepatic	⩾ 10%	-
	1 - < 10%	Hepatitis, jaundice, bilirubinaemia, elevation of enzymes
Respiratory	⩾ 10%	-
	1 - < 10%	Pneumonia, infection, moniliasis, dyspnoea, sinusitis, bronchitis, pharyngitis, pleural effusion, increased cough, rhinitis
Skin and appendages	⩾ 10%	Herpes simplex, herpes zoster
	1 - < 10%	Carcinoma, moniliasis, fungal dermatitis, acne, rash, alopecia, hypertrophy, benign neoplasia
Nervous	⩾ 10%	-
	1 - < 10%	Convulsion, depression, confusion, agitation, anxiety, hypertonia, dizziness, abnormal thinking, tremor, paraesthesia, insomnia, somnolence
Musculo-skeletal	⩾ 10%	-
	1 - < 10%	Myasthenia, arthralgia
Special senses	⩾ 10%	-
	1 - < 10%	Dysgeusia

Note: 501 (2g CellCept daily), 289 (3g CellCept daily) and 277 (2g IV / 3g oral CellCept daily) patients were treated in Phase III studies for the prevention of rejection in renal, cardiac and hepatic transplantation, respectively.

The following undesirable effects cover adverse reactions from post-marketing experience:

The types of adverse drug reactions reported during post-marketing with CellCept are similar to those seen in the controlled renal, cardiac and hepatic transplant studies. Additional adverse drug reactions reported during post-marketing are described below.

Gastrointestinal: colitis (including CMV colitis), pancreatitis, isolated cases of intestinal villous atrophy.

Disorders related to immunosuppression: serious life-threatening infections including meningitis, infectious endocarditis, tuberculosis and atypical mycobacterial infection. Some cases of agranulocytosis have been reported. Neutropenia has been reported in some patients, therefore regular monitoring of patients taking CellCept is advised (see section 4.4. Special warnings and special precautions for use).

Hypersensitivity: Hypersensitivity reactions, including angioedema and anaphylaxis, have been reported very rarely.

4.9 Overdose

The experience with overdose of CellCept in humans is very limited. The events received from reports of overdose fall within the known safety profile of the drug.

Haemodialysis would not be expected to remove clinically significant amounts of MPA or MPAG. By interfering with enterohepatic circulation of the drug, bile acid sequestrants, such as colestyramine, reduce the MPA AUC.

5. PHARMACOLOGICAL PROPERTIES

5.1 Pharmacodynamic properties

Pharmacotherapeutic group: immunosuppressant ATC code LO4AA06.

Mycophenolate mofetil is the 2-morpholinoethyl ester of MPA. MPA is a potent, selective, uncompetitive and reversible inhibitor of inosine monophosphate dehydrogenase, and therefore inhibits the *de novo* pathway of guanosine nucleotide synthesis without incorporation into DNA. Because T- and B-lymphocytes are critically dependent for their proliferation on *de novo* synthesis of purines whereas other cell types can utilise salvage pathways, MPA has more potent cytostatic effects on lymphocytes than on other cells.

5.2 Pharmacokinetic properties

Following oral administration, mycophenolate mofetil undergoes rapid and extensive absorption and complete presystemic metabolism to the active metabolite, MPA. As evidenced by suppression of acute rejection following renal transplantation, the immunosuppressant activity of CellCept is correlated with MPA concentration. The mean bioavailability of oral mycophenolate mofetil, based on MPA AUC, is 94% relative to IV mycophenolate mofetil. Food had no effect on the extent of absorption (MPA AUC) of mycophenolate mofetil when administered at doses of 1.5g BID to renal transplant patients. However, MPA C_{max} was decreased by 40% in the presence of food. Mycophenolate mofetil is not measurable systemically in plasma following oral administration. MPA at clinically relevant concentrations, is 97% bound to plasma albumin.

As a result of enterohepatic recirculation, secondary increases in plasma MPA concentration are usually observed at approximately 6 – 12 hours post-dose. A reduction in the AUC of MPA of approximately 40% is associated with the co-administration of colestyramine (4g TID), indicating that there is a significant amount of enterohepatic recirculation.

MPA is metabolised principally by glucuronyl transferase to form the phenolic glucuronide of MPA (MPAG), which is not pharmacologically active.

A negligible amount of drug is excreted as MPA (< 1% of dose) in the urine. Orally administered radiolabelled mycophenolate mofetil results in complete recovery of the administered dose; with 93% of the administered dose recovered in the urine and 6% recovered in the faeces. Most (about 87%) of the administered dose is excreted in the urine as MPAG.

At clinically encountered concentrations, MPA and MPAG are not removed by haemodialysis. However, at high MPAG plasma concentrations (> 100μg/ml), small amounts of MPAG are removed.

In the early post-transplant period (< 40 days post-transplant), renal, cardiac and hepatic transplant patients had mean MPA AUCs approximately 30% lower and C_{max} approximately 40% lower compared to the late post-transplant period (3 – 6 months post-transplant).

Renal impairment:

In a single dose study (6 subjects/group), mean plasma MPA AUC observed in subjects with severe chronic renal impairment (glomerular filtration rate < 25ml•min^{-1}•1.73m^{-2}) were 28 – 75% higher relative to the means observed in normal healthy subjects or subjects with lesser degrees of renal impairment. However, the mean single dose MPAG AUC was 3 – 6 fold higher in subjects with severe renal impairment than in subjects with mild renal impairment or normal healthy subjects, consistent with the known renal elimination of MPAG. Multiple dosing of mycophenolate mofetil in patients with severe chronic renal impairment has not been studied. No data are available for cardiac or hepatic transplant patients with severe chronic renal impairment.

Delayed renal graft function:

In patients with delayed renal graft function post-transplant, mean MPA AUC(0-12h) was comparable to that seen in post-transplant patients without delayed graft function. Mean plasma MPAG AUC(0-12h) was 2 – 3-fold higher than in post-transplant patients without delayed graft function. There may be a transient increase in the free fraction and concentration of plasma MPA in patients with delayed renal graft function. Dose adjustment of CellCept does not appear to be necessary.

Hepatic impairment:

In volunteers with alcoholic cirrhosis, hepatic MPA glucuronidation processes were relatively unaffected by hepatic parenchymal disease. Effects of hepatic disease on this process probably depend on the particular disease. However, hepatic disease with predominantly biliary damage, such as primary biliary cirrhosis, may show a different effect.

Children and adolescents (aged 2 to 18 years):

Pharmacokinetic parameters were evaluated in 49 paediatric renal transplant patients given 600 mg/m^2 mycophenolate mofetil orally twice daily. This dose achieved MPA AUC values similar to those seen in adult renal transplant patients receiving CellCept at a dose of 1 g bid in the early and late post-transplant period. MPA AUC values across age groups were similar in the early and late post-transplant period.

Elderly patients (⩾ 65 years):

Pharmacokinetic behaviour of CellCept in the elderly has not been formally evaluated.

Oral contraceptives:

The pharmacokinetics of oral contraceptives were unaffected by coadministration of CellCept (see also section 4.5 Interaction with other medicinal products and other forms of interaction). A study of the coadministration of CellCept (1g bid) and combined oral contraceptives containing ethinylestradiol (0.02mg to 0.04mg) and levonorgestrel (0.05mg to 0.15mg), desogestrel (0.15mg) or gestodene (0.05mg to 0.10mg) conducted in 18 non-transplant women (not taking other immunosupressants) over 3 consecutive menstrual cycles showed no clinically relevant influence of CellCept on the ovulation suppressing action of the oral contraceptives. Serum levels of LH, FSH and progesterone were not significantly affected.

5.3 Preclinical safety data

In experimental models, mycophenolate mofetil was not tumourigenic. The highest dose tested in the animal carcinogenicity studies resulted in approximately 2 – 3 times the systemic exposure (AUC or C_{max}) observed in renal transplant patients at the recommended clinical dose of 2g/day and 1.3 – 2 times the systemic exposure (AUC or C_{max})

observed in cardiac transplant patients at the recommended clinical dose of 3g/day.

Two genotoxicity assays (*in vitro* mouse lymphoma assay and *in vivo* mouse bone marrow micronucleus test) showed a potential of mycophenolate mofetil to cause chromosomal aberrations. These effects can be related to the pharmacodynamic mode of action, i.e. inhibition of nucleotide synthesis in sensitive cells. Other *in vitro* tests for detection of gene mutation did not demonstrate genotoxic activity.

Mycophenolate mofetil had no effect on fertility of male rats at oral doses up to 20mg•kg^{-1}•day^{-1}. The systemic exposure at this dose represents 2 to 3 times the clinical exposure at the recommended clinical dose of 2g/day in renal transplant patients and 1.3 – 2 times the clinical exposure at the recommended clinical dose of 3g/day in cardiac transplant patients. In a female fertility and reproduction study conducted in rats, oral doses of 4.5mg•kg^{-1}•day^{-1} caused malformations (including anophthalmia, agnathia, and hydrocephaly) in the first generation offspring in the absence of maternal toxicity. The systemic exposure at this dose was approximately 0.5 times the clinical exposure at the recommended clinical dose of 2g/day for renal transplant patients and approximately 0.3 times the clinical exposure at the recommended clinical dose of 3g/day for cardiac transplant patients. No effects on fertility or reproductive parameters were evident in the dams or in the subsequent generation.

In teratology studies in rats and rabbits, foetal resorptions and malformations occurred in rats at 6mg•kg^{-1}•day^{-1} (including anophthalmia, agnathia, and hydrocephaly) and in rabbits at 90mg•kg^{-1}•day^{-1} (including cardiovascular and renal anomalies, such as ectopia cordis and ectopic kidneys, and diaphragmatic and umbilical hernia), in the absence of maternal toxicity. The systemic exposure at these levels are approximately equivalent to or less than 0.5 times the clinical exposure at the recommended clinical dose of 2g/day for renal transplant patients and approximately 0.3 times the clinical exposure at the recommended clinical dose of 3g/day for cardiac transplant patients.

Refer to section 4.6 Pregnancy and lactation.

The haematopoietic and lymphoid systems were the primary organs affected in toxicology studies conducted with mycophenolate mofetil in the rat, mouse, dog and monkey. These effects occurred at systemic exposure levels that are equivalent to or less than the clinical exposure at the recommended dose of 2g/day for renal transplant recipients. Gastrointestinal effects were observed in the dog at systemic exposure levels equivalent to or less than the clinical exposure at the recommended doses. Gastrointestinal and renal effects consistent with dehydration were also observed in the monkey at the highest dose (systemic exposure levels equivalent to or greater than clinical exposure). The nonclinical toxicity profile of mycophenolate mofetil appears to be consistent with adverse events observed in human clinical trials which now provide safety data of more relevance to the patient population (see section 4.8 Undesirable effects).

6. PHARMACEUTICAL PARTICULARS

6.1 List of excipients

Excipients of CellCept capsules are pregelatinised maize starch, croscarmellose sodium, polyvidone (K-90) and magnesium stearate. The capsule shells contain gelatin, indigo carmine (E132), yellow iron oxide (E172), red iron oxide (E172), titanium dioxide (E171), black iron oxide (E172), potassium hydroxide, shellac.

6.2 Incompatibilities

Not applicable.

6.3 Shelf life

3 years.

6.4 Special precautions for storage

Do not store above 30°C.

Store in the original package.

6.5 Nature and contents of container

CellCept 250mg capsules:1 carton contains 100 capsules (in blister packs of 10).

1 carton contains 300 capsules (in blister packs of 10).

6.6 Instructions for use and handling

Because mycophenolate mofetil has demonstrated teratogenic effects in rats and rabbits, CellCept capsules should not be opened or crushed. Avoid inhalation or direct contact with skin or mucous membranes of the powder contained in CellCept capsules. If such contact occurs, wash thoroughly with soap and water; rinse eyes with plain water.

Any unused product or waste material should be disposed of in accordance with local requirements.

7. MARKETING AUTHORISATION HOLDER

Roche Registration Limited, 40 Broadwater Road, Welwyn Garden City, Hertfordshire AL7 3AY, United Kingdom.

8. MARKETING AUTHORISATION NUMBER(S)

EU/1/96/005/001 CellCept (100 capsules)

EU/1/96/005/003 CellCept (300 capsules)

9. DATE OF FIRST AUTHORISATION/RENEWAL OF THE AUTHORISATION

3 May 2001

10. DATE OF REVISION OF THE TEXT

April 2005

CellCept is a registered trade mark

Cellcept 500mg Powder

(Roche Products Limited)

1. NAME OF THE MEDICINAL PRODUCT

CellCept® ▼500mg powder for concentrate for solution for infusion.

2. QUALITATIVE AND QUANTITATIVE COMPOSITION

Each vial contains the equivalent of 500mg mycophenolate mofetil (as hydrochloride salt).

For excipients, see section 6.1.

3. PHARMACEUTICAL FORM

Powder for concentrate for solution for infusion.

CellCept 500mg powder for concentrate for solution for infusion must be reconstituted and further diluted with glucose intravenous infusion 5% prior to administration to the patient (see section 6.6 Instructions for use and handling, and disposal).

4. CLINICAL PARTICULARS

4.1 Therapeutic indications

CellCept 500mg powder for concentrate for solution for infusion is indicated in combination with ciclosporin and corticosteroids for the prophylaxis of acute transplant rejection in patients receiving allogeneic renal or hepatic transplants.

4.2 Posology and method of administration

Treatment with CellCept should be initiated and maintained by appropriately qualified transplant specialists.

CAUTION:

CELLCEPT I.V. SOLUTION SHOULD NEVER BE ADMINISTERED BY RAPID OR BOLUS INTRAVENOUS INJECTION.

CellCept 500mg powder for concentrate for solution for infusion is an alternative dosage form to CellCept oral forms (capsules, tablets and powder for oral suspension) that may be administered for up to 14 days. The initial dose of CellCept 500mg powder for concentrate for solution for infusion should be given within 24 hours following transplantation.

Following reconstitution to a concentration of 6mg/ml, CellCept 500mg powder for concentrate for solution for infusion must be administered by slow intravenous infusion over a period of 2 hours by either a peripheral or a central vein (see section 6.6 Instructions for use and handling, and disposal).

Use in renal transplant: the recommended dose in renal transplant patients is 1.0g administered twice daily (2g daily dose).

Use in hepatic transplant: the recommended dose of CellCept for infusion in hepatic transplant patients is 1.0g administered twice daily (2g daily dose). IV CellCept should continue for the first 4 days following hepatic transplant, with oral CellCept initiated as soon after this as it can be tolerated. The recommended dose of oral CellCept in hepatic transplant patients is 1.5g administered twice daily (3g daily dose).

Use in children:safety and efficacy of CellCept for infusion in paediatric patients have not been established. No pharmacokinetic data with CellCept for infusion are available for paediatric renal transplant patients. No pharmacokinetic data are available for paediatric patients following hepatic transplants.

Use in elderly (≥ 65 years): the recommended dose of 1.0g administered twice a day for renal or hepatic transplant patients is appropriate for the elderly.

Use in renal impairment: in renal transplant patients with severe chronic renal impairment (glomerular filtration rate < 25ml•min^{-1}•1.73 m^{-2}), outside the immediate post-transplant period, doses greater than 1g administered twice a day should be avoided. These patients should also be carefully observed. No dose adjustments are needed in patients experiencing delayed renal graft function post-operatively (see section 5.2 Pharmacokinetic properties). No data are available for hepatic transplant patients with severe chronic renal impairment.

Use in severe hepatic impairment: no dose adjustments are needed for renal transplant patients with severe hepatic parenchymal disease.

Treatment during rejection episodes: MPA (mycophenolic acid) is the active metabolite of mycophenolate mofetil. Renal transplant rejection does not lead to changes in MPA pharmacokinetics; dosage reduction or interruption of CellCept is not required. No pharmacokinetic data are available during hepatic transplant rejection.

4.3 Contraindications

Hypersensitivity reactions to CellCept have been observed (see section 4.8 Undesirable effects). Therefore, CellCept is contraindicated in patients with a hypersensitivity to mycophenolate mofetil or mycophenolic acid. CellCept 500mg powder for concentrate for solution for infusion is contraindicated in patients who are allergic to polysorbate 80.

CellCept is contraindicated in women who are breastfeeding (see section 4.6 Pregnancy and lactation).

For information on use in pregnancy and contraceptive requirements, see section 4.6 Pregnancy and lactation.

4.4 Special warnings and special precautions for use

Patients receiving immunosuppressive regimens involving combinations of drugs, including CellCept are at increased risk of developing lymphomas and other malignancies, particularly of the skin (see section 4.8 Undesirable effects). The risk appears to be related to the intensity and duration of immunosuppression rather than to the use of any specific agent. As general advice to minimise the risk for skin cancer, exposure to sunlight and UV light should be limited by wearing protective clothing and using a sunscreen with a high protection factor.

Patients receiving CellCept should be instructed to report immediately any evidence of infection, unexpected bruising, bleeding or any other manifestation of bone marrow depression.

Oversuppression of the immune system increases the susceptibility to infection including opportunistic infections, fatal infections and sepsis (see section 4.8 Undesirable effects).

Patients receiving CellCept should be monitored for neutropenia, which may be related to CellCept itself, concomitant medications, viral infections, or some combination of these causes. Patients taking CellCept should have complete blood counts weekly during the first month, twice monthly for the second and third months of treatment, then monthly through the first year. If neutropenia develops (absolute neutrophil count < $1.3 \times 10^3/\mu l$) it may be appropriate to interrupt or discontinue CellCept.

Patients should be advised that during treatment with CellCept vaccinations may be less effective and the use of live attenuated vaccines should be avoided (see section 4.5 Interaction with other medicinal products and other forms of interaction). Influenza vaccination may be of value. Prescribers should refer to national guidelines for influenza vaccination.

Because CellCept has been associated with an increased incidence of digestive system adverse events, including infrequent cases of gastrointestinal tract ulceration, haemorrhage and perforation. CellCept should be administered with caution in patients with active serious digestive system disease.

CellCept is an IMPDH (inosine monophosphate dehydrogenase) inhibitor. On theoretical grounds, therefore, it should be avoided in patients with rare hereditary deficiency of hypoxanthine-guanine phosphoribosyl-transferase (HGPRT) such as Lesch-Nyhan and Kelley-Seegmiller syndrome.

It is recommended that CellCept not be administered concomitantly with azathioprine because such concomitant administration has not been studied.

In view of the significant reduction in the AUC of MPA by colestyramine, caution should be used in the concomitant administration of CellCept with drugs that interfere with enterohepatic recirculation because of the potential to reduce the efficacy of CellCept. Some degree of enterohepatic recirculation is anticipated following intravenous administration of CellCept.

The risk: benefit of mycophenolate mofetil in combination with tacrolimus has not been established (see also section 4.5 Interaction with other medicinal products and other forms of interaction).

4.5 Interaction with other medicinal products and other forms of Interaction

Aciclovir: higher MPAG and aciclovir plasma concentrations were observed when mycophenolate mofetil was administered with aciclovir in comparison to the administration of each drug alone. The changes in MPAG pharmacokinetics (MPAG increased by 8%) were minimal and are not considered clinically significant. Because MPAG plasma concentrations are increased in the presence of renal impairment, as are aciclovir concentrations, the potential exists for mycophenolate mofetil and aciclovir, or its prodrugs, e.g. valaciclovir, to compete for tubular secretion and further increases in concentrations of both drugs may occur.

Colestyramine: following single dose, oral administration of 1.5g of mycophenolate mofetil to normal healthy subjects pre-treated with 4g TID of colestyramine for 4 days, there was a 40% reduction in the AUC of MPA. (see section 4.4 Special warnings and special precautions for use and section 5.2 Pharmacokinetic properties). Caution should be used during concomitant administration because of the potential to reduce efficacy of CellCept.

Drugs that interfere with enterohepatic circulation: caution should be used with drugs that interfere with enterohepatic circulation because of their potential to reduce the efficacy of CellCept.

Ciclosporin A: ciclosporin A pharmacokinetics were unaffected by mycophenolate mofetil.

Several studies have demonstrated that ciclosporin A reduces MPA plasma AUC levels by 19 – 38%, possibly as a result of inhibiting biliary secretion with consequent reduction of the entero-hepatic recirculation. However, as efficacy studies were carried out using CellCept combined with ciclosporin A and corticosteroids, these findings do not affect the recommended dose requirements (see section 4.2 Posology and method of administration).

Ganciclovir: based on the results of a single dose administration study of recommended doses of oral mycophenolate and IV ganciclovir and the known effects of renal impairment on the pharmacokinetics of CellCept (see section 4.2 Posology and method of administration) and ganciclovir, it is anticipated that co-administration of these agents (which compete for mechanisms of renal tubular secretion) will result in increases in MPAG and ganciclovir concentration. No substantial alteration of MPA pharmacokinetics are anticipated and CellCept dose adjustment is not required. In patients with renal impairment in which CellCept and ganciclovir or its prodrugs, e.g. valganciclovir, are co-administered the dose recommendations for ganciclovir should be observed and patients monitored carefully.

Oral contraceptives: the pharmacokinetics and pharmacodynamics of oral contraceptives were unaffected by co-administration of CellCept (see also section 5.2 Pharmacokinetic properties).

Trimethoprim/sulfamethoxazole: no effect on the bioavailability of MPA was observed.

Tacrolimus: *in renal transplant patients*:stable renal transplant patients receiving ciclosporin and CellCept (1g BID) showed about a 30% increase in MPA plasma AUC and about a 20% decrease in MPAG plasma AUC when ciclosporin was replaced with tacrolimus. MPA C_{max} was not affected, while MPAG C_{max} was reduced by approximately 20%. The mechanism of this finding is not well understood. Increased biliary secretion of MPAG accompanied with increased enterohepatic recirculation of MPA may be partly responsible for the finding, since the elevation of MPA concentrations associated with tacrolimus administration was more pronounced in the later portions of the concentration-time profile (4 – 12 hours after dosing). In another study in renal transplant patients it was shown that the tacrolimus concentration did not appear to be altered by CellCept.

In hepatic transplant patients: very limited pharmacokinetic data on MPA AUC are available in hepatic transplant patients treated with CellCept in combination with tacrolimus. In a study designed to evaluate the effect of CellCept on the pharmacokinetics of tacrolimus in stable hepatic transplant patients, there was an increase of approximately 20% in tacrolimus AUC when multiple doses of CellCept (1.5g BID) were administered to patients taking tacrolimus.

Other interactions: co-administration of probenecid with mycophenolate mofetil in monkeys raises plasma AUC of MPAG by 3-fold. Thus, other drugs known to undergo renal tubular secretion may compete with MPAG and thereby raise plasma concentrations of MPAG or the other drug undergoing tubular secretion.

Live vaccines: live vaccines should not be given to patients with an impaired immune response. The antibody response to other vaccines may be diminished, (see also section 4.4 Special warnings and special precautions for use).

4.6 Pregnancy and lactation

It is recommended that CellCept therapy should not be initiated until a negative pregnancy test has been obtained. Effective contraception must be used before beginning CellCept therapy, during therapy, and for six weeks following discontinuation of therapy (see section 4.5 Interaction with other medicinal products and other forms of interaction). Patients should be instructed to consult their physician immediately should pregnancy occur.

The use of CellCept is not recommended during pregnancy and should be reserved for cases where no more suitable alternative treatment is available. CellCept should be used in pregnant women only if the potential benefit outweighs the potential risk to the foetus. There are no adequate data from the used of CellCept in pregnant women. Studies in animals have shown reproductive toxicity (see section 5.3 Preclinical safety data). The potential risk for humans is unknown.

Mycophenolate mofetil has been shown to be excreted in the milk of lactating rats. It is not known whether this drug is excreted in human milk. Because of the potential for serious adverse reactions to mycophenolate mofetil in breast-fed infants, CellCept is contraindicated in nursing mothers (see section 4.3 Contraindications).

4.7 Effects on ability to drive and use machines

No specific studies have been performed. The pharmacodynamic profile and the reported adverse reactions indicate that an effect is unlikely.

4.8 Undesirable effects

The following undesirable effects cover adverse drug reactions from clinical trials:

The principal adverse drug reactions associated with the administration of CellCept in combination with ciclosporin and corticosteroids include diarrhoea, leucopenia, sepsis and vomiting and there is evidence of a higher frequency of certain types of infections (see section 4.4 Special warnings and special precautions for use). The adverse drug reaction profile associated with the administration of CellCept 500mg powder for concentrate for solution for infusion has been shown to be similar to that observed after oral administration.

Malignancies:

Patients receiving immunosuppressive regimens involving combinations of drugs, including CellCept, are at increased risk of developing lymphomas and other malignancies, particularly of the skin (see section 4.4 Special warnings and special precautions for use). Lymphoproliferative disease or lymphoma developed in 0.6% of patients receiving CellCept (2g or 3g daily) in combination with other immunosuppressants in controlled clinical trials of renal (2g data), cardiac and hepatic transplant patients followed for at least 1 year. Non-melanoma skin carcinomas occurred in 3.6% of patients; other types of malignancy occurred in 1.1% of patients. Three-year safety data in renal and cardiac transplant patients did not reveal any unexpected changes in incidence of malignancy compared to the 1-year data. Hepatic transplant patients were followed for at least 1 year, but less than 3 years.

Opportunistic infections:

All transplant patients are at increased risk of opportunistic infections; the risk increased with total immunosuppressive load (see section 4.4 Special warnings and special precautions for use). The most common opportunistic infections in patients receiving CellCept (2g or 3g daily) with other immunosuppressants in controlled clinical trials of renal (2g data), cardiac and hepatic transplant patients followed for at least 1 year were candida mucocutaneous, CMV viraemia/syndrome and Herpes simplex. The proportion of patients with CMV viraemia/syndrome was 13.5%.

Elderly patients (≥ 65 years):

Elderly patients (≥ 65 years) may generally be at increased risk of adverse drug reactions due to immunosuppression. Elderly patients receiving CellCept as part of a combination immunosuppressive regimen, may be at increased risk of certain infections (including cytomegalovirus tissue invasive disease) and possibly gastrointestinal haemorrhage and pulmonary oedema, compared to younger individuals.

Other adverse drug reactions:

The following data refer to the safety experience of oral CellCept in renal transplant patients. Data in hepatic transplant patients are based on i.v. dosing of CellCept for up to 14 days followed by oral dosing. Adverse drug reactions, probably or possibly related to CellCept, reported in ≥ 10% and in 1 - < 10% of patients treated with CellCept in the controlled clinical trials of renal (2g data) and hepatic transplant patients are listed in the following table.

Adverse Drug Reactions, Probably or Possibly Related to CellCept, Reported in Patients Treated with CellCept in Renal and Hepatic Clinical Trials when Used in Combination with Ciclosporin and Corticosteroids

Body System		Adverse drug reaction
Body as a whole	≥10%	Sepsis
	1 - < 10%	Moniliasis, infection, fever, chills, malaise, headache, flu syndrome, pain, asthenia, weight loss, oedema
Blood and lymphatic	≥10%	Leucopenia, thrombocytopenia, anaemia
	1 - < 10%	Pancytopenia, leucocytosis
Renal and urogenital	≥10%	Urinary tract infection
	1 - < 10%	Vaginal moniliasis, abnormal kidney function, increased creatinine
Cardio-vascular	≥10%	-
	1 - < 10%	Hypotension, hypertension, tachycardia
Metabolic/ nutritional	≥10%	-
	1 - < 10%	Hyperkalaemia, acidosis, hypokalaemia, hypomagnesaemia, hypocalcaemia, hypercholesterolaemia, hyperlipaemia, increased alkaline phosphatase, hyperglycaemia, hypophosphataemia, increased lactate dehydrogenase
Gastro-intestinal	≥10%	Moniliasis, vomiting, diarrhoea, nausea, abdominal pain
	1 - < 10%	Gastrointestinal haemorrhage, peritonitis, gastric ulcer, duodenal ulcer, colitis, infection, ileus, gastritis, gastroenteritis, anorexia, oesophagitis, dyspepsia, constipation, flatulence, stomatitis
Hepatic	≥ 10%	-
	1 - < 10%	Hepatitis, elevation of enzymes
Respiratory	≥10%	-
	1 - < 10%	Pneumonia, infection, moniliasis, dyspnoea, sinusitis, bronchitis, pharyngitis, pleural effusion, increased cough, rhinitis
Skin and appendages	≥10%	Herpes simplex, herpes zoster
	1 - < 10%	Carcinoma, fungal dermatitis, acne, rash, alopecia, benign neoplasia
Nervous	≥10%	-
	1 - < 10%	Convulsion, depression, hypertonia, abnormal thinking, tremor, paraesthesia, insomnia, somnolence
Musculo-skeletal	≥10%	-
	1 - < 10%	Arthralgia

Note: 501 (2g CellCept daily) and 277 (2g IV / 3g oral CellCept daily) patients were treated in Phase III studies for the prevention of rejection in renal and hepatic transplantation, respectively.

Adverse drug reactions attributable to peripheral venous infusion were phlebitis and thrombosis, both observed at 4% in patients treated with CellCept 500mg powder for concentrate for solution for infusion.

The following undesirable effects cover adverse drug reactions from post-marketing experience:

Adverse drug reactions reported during post-marketing with CellCept are similar to those seen in the controlled renal and hepatic transplant studies. Additional adverse drug reactions reported during post-marketing experience with CellCept are described below.

Gastrointestinal: colitis (including CMV colitis), pancreatitis, isolated cases of intestinal villous atrophy.

Disorders related to immunosuppression: serious life-threatening infections including meningitis, infectious endocarditis, tuberculosis and atypical mycobacterial infection. Some cases of agranulocytosis have been reported. Neutropenia has been reported in some patients, therefore regular monitoring of patients taking CellCept is advised (see section 4.4. Special warnings and special precautions for use).

Hypersensitivity: Hypersensitivity reactions, including angioedema and anaphylaxis, have been reported very rarely.

4.9 Overdose

The experience with overdose of CellCept in humans is very limited. The events received from reports of overdose fall within the known safety profile of the drug.

Haemodialysis would not be expected to remove clinically significant amounts of MPA or MPAG. By interfering with enterohepatic circulation of the drug, bile acid sequestrants, such as colestyramine, reduce the MPA AUC.

5. PHARMACOLOGICAL PROPERTIES

5.1 Pharmacodynamic properties

Pharmacotherapeutic group: immunosuppressant, ATC code L04AA06.

Mycophenolate mofetil is the 2-morpholinoethyl ester of MPA. MPA is a potent, selective, uncompetitive and reversible inhibitor of inosine monophosphate dehydrogenase, and therefore inhibits the *de novo* pathway of guanosine nucleotide synthesis without incorporation into DNA. Because T- and B-lymphocytes are critically dependent for their proliferation on *de novo* synthesis of purines whereas other cell types can utilise salvage pathways, MPA has more potent cytostatic effects on lymphocytes than on other cells.

5.2 Pharmacokinetic properties

Following intravenous administration, mycophenolate mofetil undergoes rapid and complete metabolism to the active metabolite, MPA. MPA at clinically relevant concentrations is 97% bound to plasma albumin. The parent drug mycophenolate mofetil can be measured systemically during intravenous infusion; however, after oral administration it is below the limit of quantitation (0.4μg/ml).

As a result of enterohepatic recirculation, secondary increases in plasma MPA concentration are usually observed at approximately 6 – 12 hours post-dose. A reduction in the AUC of MPA of approximately 40% is associated with the co-administration of colestyramine (4g TID), indicating that there is a significant amount of enterohepatic recirculation.

MPA is metabolised principally by glucuronyl transferase to form the phenolic glucuronide of MPA (MPAG), which is not pharmacologically active.

A negligible amount of drug is excreted as MPA (< 1% of dose) in the urine. Orally administered radiolabelled mycophenolate mofetil results in complete recovery of the administered dose; with 93% of the administered dose recovered in the urine and 6% recovered in faeces. Most (about 87%) of the administered dose is excreted in the urine as MPAG.

At clinically encountered concentrations, MPA and MPAG are not removed by haemodialysis. However, at high MPAG plasma concentrations (> 100μg/ml), small amounts of MPAG are removed.

In the early post-transplant period (< 40 days post-transplant), renal, cardiac and hepatic transplant patients had mean MPA AUCs approximately 30% lower and C_{max} approximately 40% lower compared to the late post-transplant period (3 – 6 months post-transplant). MPA AUC values obtained following administration of 1g BID intravenous CellCept to renal transplant patients in the early post-transplant phase are comparable to those observed following 1g BID oral CellCept. In hepatic transplant patients, administration of 1g BID intravenous CellCept followed by 1.5g BID oral CellCept resulted in MPA AUC values similar to those found in renal transplant patients administered 1g CellCept BID.

Renal impairment:

In a single dose study (6 subjects/group), mean plasma MPA AUC observed in subjects with severe chronic renal impairment (glomerular filtration rate < 25ml•min^{-1}•1.73m^{-2}) were 28 – 75% higher relative to the means observed in normal healthy subjects or subjects with lesser degrees of renal impairment. However, the mean single dose MPAG AUC was 3 – 6 fold higher in subjects with severe renal impairment than in subjects with mild renal impairment or normal healthy subjects, consistent with the known renal elimination of MPAG. Multiple dosing of mycophenolate mofetil in patients with severe chronic renal impairment has not been studied. No data are available for hepatic transplant patients with severe chronic renal impairment.

Delayed renal graft function:

In patients with delayed renal graft function post-transplant, mean MPA AUC(0-12h) was comparable to that seen in post-transplant patients without delayed graft function. Mean plasma MPAG AUC(0-12h) was 2 – 3 fold higher than in post-transplant patients without delayed graft function. There may be a transient increase in the free fraction and concentration of plasma MPA in patients with delayed renal graft function. Dose adjustment of CellCept does not appear to be necessary.

Hepatic impairment:

In volunteers with alcoholic cirrhosis, hepatic MPA glucuronidation processes were relatively unaffected by hepatic parenchymal disease. Effects of hepatic disease on this process probably depend on the particular disease. However, hepatic disease with predominantly biliary damage, such as primary biliary cirrhosis, may show a different effect.

Elderly patients (≥ 65 years):

Pharmacokinetic behaviour of CellCept in the elderly has not been formally evaluated.

Oral contraceptives:

The pharmacokinetics of oral contraceptives were unaffected by coadministration of CellCept (see also section 4.5 Interaction with other medicinal products and other forms of interaction). A study of the coadministration of CellCept (1g bid) and combined oral contraceptives containing ethinylestradiol (0.02mg to 0.04mg) and levonorgestrel (0.05mg to 0.15mg), desogestrel (0.15mg) or gestodene (0.05mg to 0.10mg) conducted in 18 non-transplant women (not taking other immunosupressants) over 3 consecutive menstrual cycles showed no clinically relevant influence of CellCept on the ovulation suppressing action of the oral contraceptives. Serum levels of LH, FSH and progesterone were not significantly affected.

5.3 Preclinical safety data

In experimental models, mycophenolate mofetil was not tumourigenic. The highest dose tested in the animal carcinogenicity studies resulted in approximately 2 – 3 times the systemic exposure (AUC or C_{max}) observed in renal transplant patients at the recommended clinical dose of 2g/day.

Two genotoxicity assays (*in vitro* mouse lymphoma assay and *in vivo* mouse bone marrow micronucleus test) showed a potential of mycophenolate mofetil to cause chromosomal aberrations. These effects can be related to the pharmacodynamic mode of action, i.e. inhibition of nucleotide synthesis in sensitive cells. Other *in vitro* tests for detection of gene mutation did not demonstrate genotoxic activity.

Mycophenolate mofetil had no effect on fertility of male rats at oral doses up to 20mg•kg^{-1}•day^{-1}. The systemic exposure at this dose represents 2 – 3 times the clinical exposure at the recommended clinical dose of 2g/day. In a female fertility and reproduction study conducted in rats, oral doses of 4.5mg•kg^{-1}•day^{-1} caused malformations (including anophthalmia, agnathia, and hydrocephaly)in the first generation offspring in the absence of maternal toxicity. The systemic exposure at this dose was approximately 0.5 times the clinical exposure at the recommended clinical dose of 2g/day. No effects on fertility or reproductive parameters were evident in the dams or in the subsequent generation.

In teratology studies in rats and rabbits, foetal resorptions and malformations occurred in rats at 6mg•kg^{-1}•day^{-1} (including anophthalmia, agnathia, and hydrocephaly) and in rabbits at 90mg•kg^{-1}•day^{-1} (including cardiovascular and renal anomalies, such as ectopia cordis and ectopic kidneys, and diaphragmatic and umbilical hernia), in the absence of maternal toxicity. The systemic exposure at these levels are approximately equivalent to or less than 0.5 times the clinical exposure at the recommended clinical dose of 2g/day.

Refer to section 4.6 Pregnancy and lactation.

The haematopoietic and lymphoid systems were the primary organs affected in toxicology studies conducted with mycophenolate mofetil in the rat, mouse, dog and monkey. These effects occurred at systemic exposure levels that are equivalent to or less than the clinical exposure at the recommended dose of 2g/day. Gastrointestinal effects were observed in the dog at systemic exposure levels equivalent to or less than the clinical exposure at the recommended dose. Gastrointestinal and renal effects consistent with dehydration were also observed in the monkey at the highest dose (systemic exposure levels equivalent to or greater than clinical exposure). The nonclinical toxicity profile of mycophenolate mofetil appears to be consistent with adverse events observed in human clinical trials which now provide safety data of more relevance to the patient population (see section 4.8 Undesirable effects).

6. PHARMACEUTICAL PARTICULARS

6.1 List of excipients

Polysorbate 80, citric acid, hydrochloric acid and sodium chloride.

6.2 Incompatibilities

CellCept 500mg powder for concentrate for solution for infusion infusion solution should not be mixed or administered concurrently via the same catheter with other intravenous drugs or infusion admixtures.

This medicinal product must not be mixed with other medicinal products except those mentioned in section 6.6.

6.3 Shelf life

Powder for concentrate for solution for infusion: 3 years.

Reconstituted solution and infusion solution: if the infusion solution is not prepared immediately prior to administration, the commencement of administration of the infusion solution should be within 3 hours from reconstitution and dilution of the drug product.

6.4 Special precautions for storage

Powder for concentrate for solution for infusion: Do not store above 30°C.

Reconstituted solution and infusion solution: Store at 15 - 30°C.

6.5 Nature and contents of container

20ml type I clear glass vials with grey butyl rubber stopper and aluminium seals with plastic flip-off caps. CellCept 500mg powder for concentrate for solution for infusion is available in packs containing 4 vials.

6.6 Instructions for use and handling

Preparation of Infusion Solution (6mg/ml)

CellCept 500mg powder for concentrate for solution for infusion does not contain an antibacterial preservative; therefore, reconstitution and dilution of the product must be performed under aseptic conditions.

CellCept 500mg powder for concentrate for solution for infusion must be prepared in two steps: the first step is a reconstitution step with glucose intravenous infusion 5% and the second step is a dilution step with glucose intravenous infusion 5%. A detailed description of the preparation is given below:

Step 1

a. Two vials of CellCept 500mg powder for concentrate for solution for infusion are used for preparing each 1g dose, Reconstitute the content of each vial by injecting 14ml of glucose intravenous infusion 5%.

b. Gently shake the vial to dissolve the drug yielding a slightly yellow solution.

c. Inspect the resulting solution for particulate matter and discoloration prior to further dilution. Discard the vial if particulate matter or discoloration is observed.

Step 2

a. Further dilute the content of the two reconstituted vials (approx. 2 × 15ml) into 140ml of glucose intravenous infusion 5%. The final concentration of the solution is 6mg/ml mycophenolate mofetil.

b. Inspect the infusion solution for particulate matter or discoloration. Discard the infusion solution if particulate matter or discoloration is observed.

If the infusion solution is not prepared immediately prior to administration, the commencement of administration of the infusion solution should be within 3 hours from reconstitution and dilution of the drug product. Keep solutions at 15 – 30°C.

Because mycophenolate mofetil has demonstrated teratogenic effects in rats and rabbits, avoid direct contact of prepared solutions of CellCept 500mg powder for concentrate for solution for infusion with skin or mucous membranes. If such contact occurs, wash thoroughly with soap and water; rinse eyes with plain water.

Any unused product or waste material should be disposed of in accordance with local requirements.

7. MARKETING AUTHORISATION HOLDER

Roche Registration Limited, 40 Broadwater Road, Welwyn Garden City, Hertfordshire, AL7 3AY, United Kingdom.

8. MARKETING AUTHORISATION NUMBER(S)

EU/1/96/005/005 CellCept (4 vials)

9. DATE OF FIRST AUTHORISATION/RENEWAL OF THE AUTHORISATION

3 May 2001

10. DATE OF REVISION OF THE TEXT

April 2005

CellCept is a registered trade mark

Cellcept 500mg Tablets

(Roche Products Limited)

1. NAME OF THE MEDICINAL PRODUCT

CellCept 500mg tablets▼.

2. QUALITATIVE AND QUANTITATIVE COMPOSITION

Each tablet contains 500mg mycophenolate mofetil.

For excipients, see section 6.1.

3. PHARMACEUTICAL FORM

CellCept tablets: lavender coloured caplet-shaped tablet, engraved with "CellCept 500" on one side and "Company logo" on the other.

4. CLINICAL PARTICULARS

4.1 Therapeutic indications

CellCept is indicated in combination with ciclosporin and corticosteroids for the prophylaxis of acute transplant rejection in patients receiving allogeneic renal, cardiac or hepatic transplants.

4.2 Posology and method of administration

Treatment with CellCept should be initiated and maintained by appropriately qualified transplant specialists.

Use in renal transplant:

Adults: oral CellCept should be initiated within 72 hours following transplantation. The recommended dose in renal transplant patients is 1.0g administered twice daily (2g daily dose).

Children and adolescents (aged 2 to 18 years): the recommended dose of mycophenolate mofetil is 600mg/m^2 administered orally twice daily (up to a maximum of 2g daily). CellCept tablets should only be prescribed to patients with a body surface area greater than 1.5 m^2, at a dose of 1g twice daily (2g daily dose). As some adverse reactions occur with greater frequency in this age group (see section 4.8 Undesirable effects) compared with adults, temporary dose reduction or interruption may be required; these will need to take into account relevant clinical factors including severity of reaction.

Children (< 2 years): there are limited safety and efficacy data in children below the age of 2 years. These are insufficient to make dosage recommendations and therefore use in this age group is not recommended.

Use in cardiac transplant:

Adults: oral CellCept should be initiated within 5 days following transplantation. The recommended dose in cardiac transplant patients is 1.5g administered twice daily (3g daily dose).

Children: no data are available for paediatric cardiac transplant patients.

Use in hepatic transplant:

Adults: IV CellCept should be administered for the first 4 days following hepatic transplant, with oral CellCept initiated as soon after this as it can be tolerated. The recommended oral dose in hepatic transplant patients is 1.5g administered twice daily (3g daily dose).

Children: no data are available for paediatric hepatic transplant patients.

Use in elderly (⩾ 65 years): the recommended dose of 1.0g administered twice a day for renal transplant patients and 1.5g twice a day for cardiac or hepatic transplant patients is appropriate for the elderly.

Use in renal impairment: in renal transplant patients with severe chronic renal impairment (glomerular filtration rate < 25ml•min^{-1}•1.73m^{-2}), outside the immediate post-transplant period, doses greater than 1g administered twice a day should be avoided. These patients should also be carefully observed. No dose adjustments are needed in patients experiencing delayed renal graft function post-operatively (see section 5.2 Pharmacokinetic properties). No data are available for cardiac or hepatic transplant patients with severe chronic renal impairment.

Use in severe hepatic impairment: no dose adjustments are needed for renal transplant patients with severe hepatic parenchymal disease. No data are available for cardiac transplant patients with severe hepatic parenchymal disease.

Treatment during rejection episodes: MPA (mycophenolic acid) is the active metabolite of mycophenolate mofetil. Renal transplant rejection does not lead to changes in MPA pharmacokinetics; dosage reduction or interruption of CellCept is not required. There is no basis for CellCept dose adjustment following cardiac transplant rejection. No pharmacokinetic data are available during hepatic transplant rejection.

4.3 Contraindications

Hypersensitivity reactions to CellCept have been observed (see section 4.8 Undesirable effects). Therefore, CellCept is contra-indicated in patients with a hypersensitivity to mycophenolate mofetil or mycophenolic acid.

CellCept is contraindicated in women who are breastfeeding (see section 4.6 Pregnancy and lactation).

For information on use in pregnancy and contraceptive requirements see section 4.6 Pregnancy and lactation.

4.4 Special warnings and special precautions for use

Patients receiving immunosuppressive regimens involving combinations of drugs, including CellCept, are at increased risk of developing lymphomas and other malignancies, particularly of the skin (see section 4.8 Undesirable effects). The risk appears to be related to the intensity and duration of immunosuppression rather than to the use of any specific agent. As general advice to minimise the risk for skin cancer, exposure to sunlight and UV light should be limited by wearing protective clothing and using a sunscreen with a high protection factor.

Patients receiving CellCept should be instructed to report immediately any evidence of infection, unexpected bruising, bleeding or any other manifestation of bone marrow depression.

Oversuppression of the immune system increases the susceptibility to infection including opportunistic infections, fatal infections and sepsis (see section 4.8 Undesirable effects).

Patients receiving CellCept should be monitored for neutropenia, which may be related to CellCept itself, concomitant medications, viral infections, or some combination of these causes. Patients taking CellCept should have complete blood counts weekly during the first month, twice monthly for the second and third months of treatment, then monthly through the first year. If neutropenia develops (absolute neutrophil count < 1.3 × 10^3/μl) it may be appropriate to interrupt or discontinue CellCept.

Patients should be advised that during treatment with CellCept vaccinations may be less effective and the use of live attenuated vaccines should be avoided (see section 4.5 Interaction with other medicinal products and other forms of interaction). Influenza vaccination may be of value. Prescribers should refer to national guidelines for influenza vaccination.

Because CellCept has been associated with an increased incidence of digestive system adverse events, including infrequent cases of gastrointestinal tract ulceration, haemorrhage and perforation, CellCept should be administered with caution in patients with active serious digestive system disease.

CellCept is an IMPDH (inosine monophosphate dehydrogenase) inhibitor. On theoretical grounds therefore it should be avoided in patients with rare hereditary deficiency of hypoxanthine-guanine phosphoribosyl-transferase (HGPRT) such as Lesch-Nyhan and Kelley-Seegmiller syndrome.

It is recommended that CellCept not be administered concomitantly with azathioprine because such concomitant administration has not been studied.

In view of the significant reduction in the AUC of MPA by colestyramine, caution should be used in the concomitant administration of CellCept with drugs that interfere with enterohepatic recirculation because of the potential to reduce the efficacy of CellCept.

The risk: benefit of mycophenolate mofetil in combination with tacrolimus has not been established (see also section 4.5 Interaction with other medicinal products and other forms of interaction).

4.5 Interaction with other medicinal products and other forms of Interaction

Aciclovir: higher MPAG and aciclovir plasma concentrations were observed when mycophenolate mofetil was administered with aciclovir in comparison to the administration of each drug alone. The changes in MPAG pharmacokinetics (MPAG increased by 8%) were minimal and are not considered clinically significant. Because MPAG plasma concentrations are increased in the presence of renal impairment, as are aciclovir concentrations, the potential exists for mycophenolate mofetil and aciclovir, or its prodrugs, e.g. valaciclovir, to compete for tubular secretion and further increases in concentrations of both drugs may occur.

Antacids with magnesium and aluminium hydroxides: absorption of mycophenolate mofetil was decreased when administered with antacids.

Colestyramine: following single dose administration of 1.5g of mycophenolate mofetil to normal healthy subjects pretreated with 4g TID of colestyramine for 4 days, there was a 40% reduction in the AUC of MPA (see section 4.4 Special warnings and special precautions for use and section 5.2 Pharmacokinetic properties) Caution should be used during concomitant administration because of the potential to reduce efficacy of CellCept.

Drugs that interfere with enterohepatic circulation: caution should be used with drugs that interfere with enterohepatic circulation because of their potential to reduce the efficacy of CellCept.

Ciclosporin A: ciclosporin A pharmacokinetics were unaffected by mycophenolate mofetil.

Several studies have demonstrated that ciclosporin A reduces MPA plasma AUC levels by 19 – 38%, possibly as a result of inhibiting biliary secretion with consequent reduction of the entero-hepatic recirculation. However, as efficacy studies were carried out using CellCept combined with ciclosporin A and corticosteroids, these findings do not affect the recommended dose requirements (see section 4.2 Posology and method of administration).

Ganciclovir: based on the results of a single dose administration study of recommended doses of oral mycophenolate and IV ganciclovir and the known effects of renal impairment on the pharmacokinetics of CellCept (see section 4.2 Posology and method of administration) and ganciclovir, it is anticipated that co-administration of these agents (which compete for mechanisms of renal tubular secretion) will result in increases in MPAG and ganciclovir concentration. No substantial alteration of MPA pharmacokinetics are anticipated and CellCept dose adjustment is not required. In patients with renal impairment in which CellCept and ganciclovir or its prodrugs, e.g. valganciclovir, are co-administered the dose recommendations for ganciclovir should be observed and patients monitored carefully.

Oral contraceptives: the pharmacokinetics and pharmacodynamics of oral contraceptives were unaffected by co-administration of CellCept (see also section 5.2 Pharmacokinetic properties).

Trimethoprim/sulfamethoxazole: no effect on the bioavailability of MPA was observed.

Tacrolimus: *In renal transplant patients*: stable renal transplant patients receiving ciclosporin and CellCept (1g BID) showed about a 30% increase in MPA plasma AUC and about a 20% decrease in MPAG plasma AUC when ciclosporin was replaced with tacrolimus. MPA C_{max} was not affected, while MPAG C_{max} was reduced by approximately 20%. The mechanism of this finding is not well understood. Increased biliary secretion of MPAG accompanied with increased enterohepatic recirculation of MPA may be partly responsible for the finding, since the elevation of MPA concentrations associated with tacrolimus administration was more pronounced in the later portions of the concentration-time profile (4 – 12 hours after dosing). In another study in renal transplant patients it was shown that the tacrolimus concentration did not appear to be altered by CellCept.

In hepatic transplant patients: very limited pharmacokinetic data on MPA AUC are available in hepatic transplant patients treated with CellCept in combination with tacrolimus. In a study designed to evaluate the effect of CellCept on the pharmacokinetics of tacrolimus in stable hepatic transplant patients, there was an increase of approximately 20% in tacrolimus AUC when multiple doses of CellCept (1.5g BID) were administered to patients taking tacrolimus.

Other interactions: co-administration of probenecid with mycophenolate mofetil in monkeys raises plasma AUC of MPAG by 3-fold. Thus, other drugs known to undergo renal tubular secretion may compete with MPAG and thereby raise plasma concentrations of MPAG or the other drug undergoing tubular secretion.

Live vaccines: live vaccines should not be given to patients with an impaired immune response. The antibody response to other vaccines may be diminished (see also 4.4 Special warnings and special precautions for use).

4.6 Pregnancy and lactation

It is recommended that CellCept therapy should not be initiated until a negative pregnancy test has been obtained. Effective contraception must be used before beginning CellCept therapy, during therapy, and for six weeks following discontinuation of therapy (see section 4.5 Interaction with other medicinal products and other forms of interaction). Patients should be instructed to consult their physician immediately should pregnancy occur.

The use of CellCept is not recommended during pregnancy and should be reserved for cases where no more suitable alternative treatment is available. CellCept should be used in pregnant women only if the potential benefit outweighs the potential risk to the foetus. There are no adequate data from the use of CellCept in pregnant women. Studies in animals have shown reproductive toxicity (see section 5.3 Preclinical safety data). The potential risk for humans is unknown.

Mycophenolate mofetil has been shown to be excreted in the milk of lactating rats. It is not known whether this drug is excreted in human milk. Because of the potential for serious adverse reactions to mycophenolate mofetil in breast-fed infants. CellCept is contraindicated in nursing mothers (see section 4.3 Contraindications).

4.7 Effects on ability to drive and use machines

No specific studies have been performed. The pharmacodynamic profile and the reported adverse reactions indicate that an effect is unlikely.

4.8 Undesirable effects

The following undesirable effects cover adverse drug reactions from clinical trials:

The principal adverse drug reactions associated with the administration of CellCept in combination with ciclosporin and corticosteroids include diarrhoea, leucopenia, sepsis and vomiting and there is evidence of a higher frequency of certain types of infections (see section 4.4 Special warnings and special precautions for use).

Malignancies:

Patients receiving immunosuppressive regimens involving combinations of drugs, including CellCept, are at increased risk of developing lymphomas and other malignancies, particularly of the skin (see section 4.4 Special warnings and special precautions for use). Lymphoproliferative disease or lymphoma developed in 0.6% of patients receiving CellCept (2g or 3g daily) in combination with other immunosuppressants in controlled clinical trials of renal (2g data), cardiac and hepatic transplant patients followed for at least 1 year. Non-melanoma skin carcinomas occurred in 3.6% of patients; other types of malignancy occurred in 1.1% of patients. Three-year safety data in renal and cardiac transplant patients did not reveal any unexpected changes in incidence of malignancy compared to the 1-year data. Hepatic transplant patients were followed for at least 1 year, but less than 3 years.

Opportunistic infections:

All transplant patients are at increased risk of opportunistic infections; the risk increased with total immunosuppressive load (see section 4.4 Special warnings and special precautions for use) The most common opportunistic infections in patients receiving CellCept (2g or 3g daily) with other immunosuppressants in controlled clinical trials of renal (2g data), cardiac and hepatic transplant patients followed for at least 1 year were candida mucocutaneous, CMV viraemia/syndrome and Herpes simplex. The proportion of patients with CMV viraemia/syndrome was 13.5%.

Children and adolescents (aged 2 to 18 years):

The type and frequency of adverse drug reactions in a clinical study, which recruited 92 paediatric patients aged 2 to 18 years who were given 600mg/m^2 mycophenolate mofetil orally twice daily, were generally similar to those observed in adult patients given 1g CellCept twice daily. However, the following treatment-related adverse events were more frequent in the paediatric population, particularly in children under 6 years of age, when compared to adults: diarrhoea, sepsis, leucopenia, anaemia and infection.

Elderly patients (⩾ 65 years):

Elderly patients (⩾ 65 years) may generally be at increased risk of adverse drug reactions due to immunosuppression. Elderly patients receiving CellCept as part of a combination immunosuppressive regimen, may be at increased risk of certain infections (including cytomegalovirus tissue invasive disease) and possibly gastrointestinal haemorrhage and pulmonary oedema, compared to younger individuals.

Other adverse drug reactions:

Adverse drug reactions, probably or possibly related to CellCept, reported in ⩾ 10% and in 1 – < 10% of patients treated with CellCept in the controlled clinical trials of renal (2g data), cardiac and hepatic transplant patients are listed in the following table.

Adverse Drug Reactions, Probably or Possibly Related to CellCept, Reported in Patients Treated with CellCept in Renal, Cardiac and Hepatic Clinical Trials when Used in Combination with Ciclosporin and Corticosteroids

Body System		Adverse drug reactions
Body as a whole	⩾ 10%	Sepsis
	1 - < 10%	Moniliasis, infection, fever, chills, malaise, headache, flu syndrome, pain, asthenia, weight loss, oedema

Blood and lymphatic	⩾ 10%	Leucopenia, thrombocytopenia, anaemia
	1 - < 10%	Pancytopenia, leucocytosis
Renal and urogenital	⩾ 10%	Urinary tract infection
	1 - < 10%	Vaginal moniliasis, abnormal kidney function, increased creatinine, increased BUN
Cardio-vascular	⩾10%	-
	1 - < 10%	Hypotension, hypertension, tachycardia, vasodilatation
Metabolic/ nutritional	⩾ 10%	-
	1 - < 10%	Hyperkalaemia, acidosis, hypokalaemia, hypomagnesaemia, hypocalcaemia, hypercholesterolaemia, gout, hyperlipaemia, increased alkaline phosphatase, hyperglycaemia, hypophosphataemia, hyperuricaemia, increased lactate dehydrogenase
Gastro-intestinal	⩾ 10%	Moniliasis, vomiting, diarrhoea, nausea, abdominal pain
	1 - < 10%	Gastrointestinal haemorrhage, peritonitis, gastric ulcer, duodenal ulcer, colitis, infection, ileus, stomatitis, gastritis, gastroenteritis, anorexia, oesophagitis, dyspepsia, constipation, flatulence, eructation
Hepatic	⩾ 10%	-
	1 - < 10%	Hepatitis, jaundice, bilirubinaemia, elevation of enzymes
Respiratory	⩾ 10%	-
	1 - < 10%	Pneumonia, infection, moniliasis, dyspnoea, sinusitis, bronchitis, pharyngitis, pleural effusion, increased cough, rhinitis
Skin and appendages	⩾ 10%	Herpes simplex, herpes zoster
	1 - < 10%	Carcinoma, moniliasis, fungal dermatitis, acne, rash, alopecia, hypertrophy, benign neoplasia
Nervous	⩾ 10%	-
	1 - < 10%	Convulsion, depression, confusion, agitation, anxiety, hypertonia, dizziness, abnormal thinking, tremor, paraesthesia, insomnia, somnolence
Musculo-skeletal	⩾ 10%	-
	1 - < 10%	Myasthenia, arthralgia
Special senses	⩾ 10%	-
	1 - < 10%	Dysgeusia

Note: 501 (2g CellCept daily), 289 (3g CellCept daily) and 277 (2g IV / 3g oral CellCept daily) patients were treated in Phase III studies for the prevention of rejection in renal, cardiac and hepatic transplantation, respectively.

The following undesirable effects cover adverse drug reactions from post-marketing experience:

The types of adverse drug reactions reported during post-marketing with CellCept are similar to those seen in the controlled renal, cardiac and hepatic transplant studies. Additional adverse drug reactions reported during post-marketing are described below.

Gastrointestinal: colitis (including CMV colitis), pancreatitis, isolated cases of intestinal villous atrophy.

Disorders related to immunosuppression: serious life-threatening infections including meningitis, infectious endocarditis, tuberculosis and atypical mycobacterial infection. Some cases of agranulocytosis have been reported. Neutropenia has been reported in some patients, therefore regular monitoring of patients taking CellCept is advised (see section 4.4 Special warnings and special precautions for use.)

Hypersensitivity: Hypersensitivity reactions, including angioedema and anaphylaxis, have been reported very rarely.

4.9 Overdose

The experience with overdose of CellCept in humans is very limited. The events received from reports of overdose fall within the known safety profile of the drug.

Haemodialysis would not be expected to remove clinically significant amounts of MPA or MPAG. By interfering with enterohepatic circulation of the drug, bile acid sequestrants, such as colestyramine reduce the MPA AUC.

5. PHARMACOLOGICAL PROPERTIES

5.1 Pharmacodynamic properties

Pharmacotherapeutic group: immunosuppressant ATC code LO4AA06

Mycophenolate mofetil is the 2-morpholinoethyl ester of MPA. MPA is a potent, selective, uncompetitive and reversible inhibitor of inosine monophosphate dehydrogenase, and therefore inhibits the *de novo* pathway of guanosine nucleotide synthesis without incorporation into DNA. Because T- and B-lymphocytes are critically dependent for their proliferation on *de novo* synthesis of purines whereas other cell types can utilise salvage pathways, MPA has more potent cytostatic effects on lymphocytes than on other cells.

5.2 Pharmacokinetic properties

Following oral administration, mycophenolate mofetil undergoes rapid and extensive absorption and complete presystemic metabolism to the active metabolite, MPA. As evidenced by suppression of acute rejection following renal transplantation, the immunosuppressant activity of CellCept is correlated with MPA concentration. The mean bioavailability of oral mycophenolate mofetil, based on MPA AUC, is 94% relative to IV mycophenolate mofetil. Food had no effect on the extent of absorption (MPA AUC) of mycophenolate mofetil when administered at doses of 1.5g BID to renal transplant patients. However, MPA C_{max} was decreased by 40% in the presence of food. Mycophenolate mofetil is not measurable systemically in plasma following oral administration. MPA at clinically relevant concentrations, is 97% bound to plasma albumin.

As a result of enterohepatic recirculation, secondary increases in plasma MPA concentration are usually observed at approximately 6 – 12 hours post-dose. A reduction in the AUC of MPA of approximately 40% is associated with the co-administration of colestyramine (4g TID), indicating that there is a significant amount of enterohepatic recirculation.

MPA is metabolised principally by glucuronyl transferase to form the phenolic glucuronide of MPA (MPAG), which is not pharmacologically active.

A negligible amount of drug is excreted as MPA (< 1 % of dose) in the urine. Orally administered radiolabelled mycophenolate mofetil results in complete recovery of the administered dose; with 93% of the administered dose recovered in the urine and 6% recovered in the faeces. Most (about 87%) of the administered dose is excreted in the urine as MPAG.

At clinically encountered concentrations, MPA and MPAG are not removed by haemodialysis. However, at high MPAG plasma concentrations (> 100μg/ml), small amounts of MPAG are removed.

In the early post-transplant period (< 40 days post-transplant), renal, cardiac and hepatic transplant patients had mean MPA AUCs approximately 30% lower and C_{max} approximately 40% lower compared to the late post-transplant period (3 – 6 months post-transplant).

Renal impairment:

In a single dose study (6 subjects/group), mean plasma MPA AUC observed in subjects with severe chronic renal impairment (glomerular filtration rate < $25ml\bullet min^{-1}\bullet 1.73m^{-2}$) were 28 – 75% higher relative to the means observed in normal healthy subjects or subjects with lesser degrees of renal impairment. However, the mean single dose MPAG AUC was 3 – 6 fold higher in subjects with severe renal impairment than in subjects with mild renal impairment or normal healthy subjects, consistent with the known renal elimination of MPAG. Multiple dosing of mycophenolate mofetil in patients with severe chronic renal impairment has not been studied. No data are available for cardiac or hepatic transplant patients with severe chronic renal impairment.

Delayed renal graft function:

In patients with delayed renal graft function post-transplant, mean MPA AUC(0-12h) was comparable to that seen in post-transplant patients without delayed graft function. Mean plasma MPAG AUC(0-12h) was 2 – 3-fold higher than in post-transplant patients without delayed graft function. There may be a transient increase in the free fraction and concentration of plasma MPA in patients with delayed renal graft function. Dose adjustment of CellCept does not appear to be necessary.

Hepatic impairment:

In volunteers with alcoholic cirrhosis, hepatic MPA glucuronidation processes were relatively unaffected by hepatic parenchymal disease. Effects of hepatic disease on this process probably depend on the particular disease. However, hepatic disease with predominantly biliary damage, such as primary biliary cirrhosis, may show a different effect.

Children and adolescents (aged 2 to 18 years):

Pharmacokinetic parameters were evaluated in 49 paediatric renal transplant patients given 600mg/m^2 mycophenolate mofetil orally twice daily. This dose achieved MPA AUC values similar to those seen in adult renal transplant patients receiving CellCept at a dose of 1g bid in the early and late post-transplant period. MPA AUC values across age groups were similar in the early and late post-transplant period.

Elderly patients (⩾ 65 years):

Pharmacokinetic behaviour of CellCept in the elderly has not been formally evaluated.

Oral contraceptives:

The pharmacokinetics of oral contraceptives were unaffected by coadministration of CellCept (see also section 4.5 Interaction with other medicinal products and other forms of interaction). A study of the coadministration of CellCept (1g bid) and combined oral contraceptives containing ethinylestradiol (0.02mg to 0.04mg) and levonorgestrel (0.05mg to 0.15mg), desogestrel (0.15mg) or gestodene (0.05mg to 0.10mg) conducted in 18 non-transplant women (not taking other immunosupressants) over 3 consecutive menstrual cycles showed no clinically relevant influence of CellCept on the ovulation suppressing action of the oral contraceptives. Serum levels of LH, FSH and progesterone were not significantly affected.

5.3 Preclinical safety data

In experimental models, mycophenolate mofetil was not tumourigenic. The highest dose tested in the animal carcinogenicity studies resulted in approximately 2 – 3 times the systemic exposure (AUC or C_{max}) observed in renal transplant patients at the recommended clinical dose of 2g/day and 1.3 – 2 times the systemic exposure (AUC or C_{max}) observed in cardiac transplant patients at the recommended clinical dose of 3g/day.

Two genotoxicity assays (*in vitro* mouse lymphoma assay and *in vivo* mouse bone marrow micronucleus test) showed a potential of mycophenolate mofetil to cause chromosomal aberrations. These effects can be related to the pharmacodynamic mode of action, i.e. inhibition of nucleotide synthesis in sensitive cells. Other *in vitro* tests for detection of gene mutation did not demonstrate genotoxic activity.

Mycophenolate mofetil had no effect on fertility of male rats at oral doses up to $20mg\bullet kg^{-1}\bullet day^{-1}$. The systemic exposure at this dose represents 2 – 3 times the clinical exposure at the recommended clinical dose of 2g/day in renal transplant patients and 1.3 – 2 times the clinical exposure at the recommended clinical dose of 3g/day in cardiac transplant patients. In a female fertility and reproduction study conducted in rats, oral doses of $4.5mg\bullet kg^{-1}\bullet day^{-1}$ caused malformations (including anophthalmia, agnathia, and hydrocephaly) in the first generation offspring in the absence of maternal toxicity. The systemic exposure at this dose was approximately 0.5 times the clinical exposure at the recommended clinical dose of 2g/day for renal transplant patients and approximately 0.3 times the clinical exposure at the recommended clinical dose of 3g/day for cardiac transplant patients. No effects on fertility or reproductive parameters were evident in the dams or in the subsequent generation.

In teratology studies in rats and rabbits, foetal resorptions and malformations occurred in rats at $6mg\bullet kg^{-1}\bullet day^{-1}$ (including anophthalmia, agnathia, and hydrocephaly) and in rabbits at $90mg\bullet kg^{-1}\bullet day^{-1}$ (including cardiovascular and renal anomalies, such as ectopia cordis and ectopic kidneys, and diaphragmatic and umbilical hernia), in the absence of maternal toxicity. The systemic exposure at these levels are approximately equivalent to or less than 0.5 times the clinical exposure at the recommended clinical dose of 2g/day for renal transplant patients and approximately 0.3 times the clinical exposure at the recommended clinical dose of 3g/day for cardiac transplant patients.

Refer to section 4.6 Pregnancy and lactation.

The haematopoietic and lymphoid systems were the primary organs affected in toxicology studies conducted with mycophenolate mofetil in the rat, mouse, dog and monkey. These effects occurred at systemic exposure levels that are equivalent to or less than the clinical exposure at the recommended dose of 2g/day for renal transplant recipients. Gastrointestinal effects were observed in the dog at systemic exposure levels equivalent to or less than the clinical exposure at the recommended doses. Gastrointestinal and renal effects consistent with dehydration were also observed in the monkey at the highest dose (systemic exposure levels equivalent to or greater than clinical exposure). The nonclinical toxicity profile of mycophenolate mofetil appears to be consistent with adverse events observed in human clinical trials which now provide safety data of more relevance to the patient population (see section 4.8 Undesirable effects).

6. PHARMACEUTICAL PARTICULARS

6.1 List of excipients

Excipients of CellCept tablets are microcrystalline cellulose, polyvidone (K-90), croscarmellose sodium and magnesium stearate. The tablet coating consists of hydroxypropyl methylcellulose, hydroxypropyl cellulose, titanium dioxide (E171), polyethylene glycol 400, indigo carmine aluminium lake (E132) and red iron oxide (E172).

6.2 Incompatibilities

Not applicable.

6.3 Shelf life

3 years.

6.4 Special precautions for storage

Do not store above 30°C. Keep in the outer carton.

6.5 Nature and contents of container

CellCept 500mg tablets: 1 carton contains 50 tablets (in blister packs of 10).

1 carton contains 150 tablets (in blister packs of 10).

6.6 Instructions for use and handling

Because mycophenolate mofetil has demonstrated teratogenic effects in rats and rabbits, CellCept tablets should not be crushed.

Any unused product or waste material should be disposed of in accordance with local requirements.

7. MARKETING AUTHORISATION HOLDER

Roche Registration Limited, 40 Broadwater Road, Welwyn Garden City, Hertfordshire, AL7 3AY, United Kingdom.

8. MARKETING AUTHORISATION NUMBER(S)

EU/1/96/005/002 CellCept (50 tablets)

EU/1/96/005/004 CellCept (150 tablets)

9. DATE OF FIRST AUTHORISATION/RENEWAL OF THE AUTHORISATION

3 May 2001

10. DATE OF REVISION OF THE TEXT

April 2005

CellCept is a registered trade mark

CellCept Suspension

(Roche Products Limited)

1. NAME OF THE MEDICINAL PRODUCT

CellCept▼ 1g/5ml powder for oral suspension

2. QUALITATIVE AND QUANTITATIVE COMPOSITION

Each bottle contains 35g mycophenolate mofetil in 110g powder for oral suspension. 5ml of the constituted suspension contains 1g of mycophenolate mofetil.

For excipients, see section 6.1.

3. PHARMACEUTICAL FORM

Powder for oral suspension.

4. CLINICAL PARTICULARS

4.1 Therapeutic indications

CellCept 1g/5ml powder for oral suspension is indicated in combination with ciclosporin and corticosteroids for the prophylaxis of acute transplant rejection in patients receiving allogeneic renal, cardiac or hepatic transplants.

4.2 Posology and method of administration

Treatment with CellCept should be initiated and maintained by appropriately qualified transplant specialists.

Use in renal transplant:

Adults: oral CellCept 1g/5ml powder for oral suspension should be initiated within 72 hours following transplantation. The recommended dose in renal transplant patients is 1.0g administered twice daily (2g daily dose), i.e. 5ml oral suspension twice daily.

Children and adolescents (aged 2 to 18 years): the recommended dose of CellCept 1g/5mL powder for oral suspension is 600mg/m^2 administered twice daily (up to a maximum of 2g/10mL oral suspension daily). As some adverse reactions occur with greater frequency in this age group (see section 4.8 Undesirable effects) compared with adults, temporary dose reduction or interruption may be required; these will need to take into account relevant clinical factors including severity of reaction.

Children (< 2 years): there are limited safety and efficacy data in children below the age of 2 years. These are insufficient to make dosage recommendations and therefore use in this age group is not recommended.

Use in cardiac transplant:

Adults:oral CellCept should be initiated within 5 days following transplantation. The recommended dose in cardiac transplant patients is 1.5g administered twice daily (3g daily dose).

Children: no data are available for paediatric cardiac transplant patients.

Use in hepatic transplant:

Adults: IV CellCept should be administered for the first 4 days following hepatic transplant, with oral CellCept initiated as soon after this as it can be tolerated. The recommended oral dose in hepatic transplant patients is 1.5g administered twice daily (3g daily dose).

Children: no data are available for paediatric hepatic transplant patients.

Use in elderly (≥ 65 years): the recommended dose of 1.0g administered twice a day for renal transplant patients and 1.5g twice a day for cardiac or hepatic transplant patients is appropriate for the elderly.

Use in renal impairment: in renal transplant patients with severe chronic renal impairment (glomerular filtration rate $< 25 ml \bullet min^{-1} \bullet 1.73 m^{-2}$), outside the immediate post-transplant period, doses greater than 1g administered twice a day should be avoided. These patients should also be carefully observed. No dose adjustments are needed in patients experiencing delayed renal graft function post-operatively, (see section 5.2 Pharmacokinetic properties). No data are available for cardiac or hepatic transplant patients with severe chronic renal impairment.

Use in severe hepatic impairment: no dose adjustments are needed for renal transplant patients with severe hepatic parenchymal disease. No data are available for cardiac transplant patients with severe hepatic parenchymal disease.

Treatment during rejection episodes: MPA (mycophenolic acid) is the active metabolite of mycophenolate mofetil. Renal transplant rejection does not lead to changes in MPA pharmacokinetics; dosage reduction or interruption of CellCept is not required. There is no basis for CellCept dose adjustment following cardiac transplant rejection. No pharmacokinetic data are available during hepatic transplant rejection.

Note

If required, CellCept 1g/5ml powder for oral suspension can be administered via a nasogastric tube with a minimum size of 8 French (minimum 1.7mm interior diameter).

4.3 Contraindications

Hypersensitivity reactions to CellCept have been observed (see section 4.8 Undesirable effects). Therefore, CellCept is contra-indicated in patients with a hypersensitivity to mycophenolate mofetil or mycophenolic acid.

Cellcept is contraindicated in women who are breastfeeding (see section 4.6 Pregnancy and lactation).

For information on use in pregnancy and contraceptive requirements, see section 4.6 Pregnancy and lactation.

4.4 Special warnings and special precautions for use

Patients receiving immunosuppressive regimens involving combinations of drugs, including CellCept, are at increased risk of developing lymphomas and other malignancies, particularly of the skin (see section 4.8 Undesirable effects). The risk appears to be related to the intensity and duration of immunosuppression rather than to the use of any specific agent. As general advice to minimise the risk for skin cancer, exposure to sunlight and UV light should be limited by wearing protective clothing and using a sunscreen with a high protection factor.

Patients receiving CellCept should be instructed to report immediately any evidence of infection, unexpected bruising, bleeding or any other manifestation of bone marrow depression.

Oversuppression of the immune system increases the susceptibility to infection including opportunistic infections, fatal infections and sepsis (see section 4.8 Undesirable effects).

Patients receiving CellCept should be monitored for neutropenia, which may be related to CellCept itself, concomitant medications, viral infections, or some combination of these causes. Patients taking CellCept should have complete blood counts weekly during the first month, twice monthly for the second and third months of treatment, then monthly through the first year. If neutropenia develops (absolute neutrophil count $< 1.3 \times 10^3/\mu l$) it may be appropriate to interrupt or discontinue CellCept.

Patients should be advised that during treatment with CellCept vaccinations may be less effective and the use of live attenuated vaccines should be avoided (see section 4.5 Interaction with other medicinal products and other forms of interaction). Influenza vaccination may be of value. Prescribers should refer to national guidelines for influenza vaccination.

Because CellCept has been associated with an increased incidence of digestive system adverse events, including infrequent cases of gastrointestinal tract ulceration, haemorrhage and perforation, CellCept should be administered with caution in patients with active serious digestive system disease.

CellCept is an IMPDH (inosine monophosphate dehydrogenase) inhibitor. On theoretical grounds therefore, it should be avoided in patients with rare hereditary deficiency of hypoxanthine-guanine phosphoribosyl-transferase (HGPRT) such as Lesch-Nyhan and Kelley-Seegmiller syndrome.

It is recommended that CellCept not be administered concomitantly with azathioprine because such concomitant administration has not been studied.

In view of the significant reduction in the AUC of MPA by colestyramine, caution should be used in the concomitant administration of CellCept with drugs that interfere with enterohepatic recirculation because of the potential to reduce the efficacy of CellCept.

CellCept 1g/5ml powder for oral suspension contains aspartame. Therefore care should be taken if CellCept 1g/5ml powder for oral suspension is administered to patients with phenylketonuria (see section 6.1 List of excipients).

The risk: benefit of mycophenolate mofetil in combination with tacrolimus has not been established (see also section 4.5 Interaction with other medicinal products and other forms of interaction).

4.5 Interaction with other medicinal products and other forms of Interaction

Aciclovir: higher MPAG and aciclovir plasma concentrations were observed when mycophenolate mofetil was administered with aciclovir in comparison to the administration of each drug alone. The changes in MPAG pharmacokinetics (MPAG increased by 8%) were minimal and are not considered clinically significant. Because MPAG plasma concentrations are increased in the presence of renal impairment, as are aciclovir concentrations, the potential exists for mycophenolate mofetil and aciclovir, or its prodrugs, e.g. valaciclovir, to compete for tubular secretion and further increases in concentrations of both drugs may occur.

Antacids with magnesium and aluminium hydroxides: absorption of mycophenolate mofetil was decreased when administered with antacids.

Colestyramine: following single dose administration of 1.5g of mycophenolate mofetil to normal healthy subjects pre-treated with 4g TID of colestyramine for 4 days, there was a 40% reduction in the AUC of MPA. (see section 4.4 Special warnings and special precautions for use, and section 5.2 Pharmacokinetic properties). Caution should be used during concomitant administration because of the potential to reduce efficacy of CellCept.

Drugs that interfere with enterohepatic circulation: caution should be used with drugs that interfere with enterohepatic circulation because of their potential to reduce the efficacy of CellCept.

Ciclosporin A: ciclosporin A pharmacokinetics were unaffected by mycophenolate mofetil.

Several studies have demonstrated that ciclosporin A reduces MPA plasma AUC levels by 19 – 38%, possibly as a result of inhibiting biliary secretion with consequent reduction of the entero-hepatic recirculation. However, as efficacy studies were carried out using CellCept combined with ciclosporin A and corticosteroids, these findings do not affect the recommended dose requirements (see section 4.2 Posology and method of administration).

Ganciclovir: based on the results of a single dose administration study of recommended doses of oral mycophenolate and IV ganciclovir and the known effects of renal impairment on the pharmacokinetics of CellCept (see section 4.2 Posology and method of administration) and ganciclovir, it is anticipated that co-administration of these agents (which compete for mechanisms of renal tubular secretion) will result in increases in MPAG and ganciclovir concentration. No substantial alteration of MPA pharmacokinetics are anticipated and CellCept dose adjustment is not required. In patients with renal impairment in which CellCept and ganciclovir or its prodrugs, e.g. valganciclovir, are co-administered, the dose recommendations for ganciclovir should be observed and patients monitored carefully.

Oral contraceptives: the pharmacokinetics and pharmacodynamics of oral contraceptives were unaffected by co-administration of CellCept (see also section 5.2 Pharmacokinetic properties).

Trimethoprim/sulfamethoxazole: no effect on the bioavailability of MPA was observed.

Tacrolimus:*in renal transplant patients*: stable renal transplant patients receiving ciclosporin and CellCept (1g BID) showed about a 30% increase in MPA plasma AUC and about a 20% decrease in MPAG plasma AUC when ciclosporin was replaced with tacrolimus. MPA C_{max} was not affected, while MPAG C_{max} was reduced by approximately 20%. The mechanism of this finding is not well understood. Increased biliary secretion of MPAG accompanied with increased enterohepatic recirculation of MPA may be partly responsible for the finding, since the elevation of MPA concentrations associated with tacrolimus administration was more pronounced in the later portions of the concentration-time profile (4 – 12 hours after dosing). In another study in renal transplant patients it was shown that the tacrolimus concentration did not appear to be altered by CellCept.

In hepatic transplant patients: very limited pharmacokinetic data on MPA AUC are available in hepatic transplant patients treated with CellCept in combination with tacrolimus. In a study designed to evaluate the effect of CellCept on the pharmacokinetics of tacrolimus in stable hepatic transplant patients, there was an increase of approximately 20% in tacrolimus AUC when multiple doses of CellCept (1.5g BID) were administered to patients taking tacrolimus.

Other interactions: co-administration of probenecid with mycophenolate mofetil in monkeys raises plasma AUC of MPAG by 3-fold. Thus, other drugs known to undergo renal tubular secretion may compete with MPAG and thereby raise plasma concentrations of MPAG or the other drug undergoing tubular secretion.

Live vaccines: live vaccines should not be given to patients with an impaired immune response. The antibody response to other vaccines may be diminished (see also section 4.4 Special warnings and special precautions for use).

4.6 Pregnancy and lactation

It is recommended that CellCept therapy should not be initiated until a negative pregnancy test has been obtained. Effective contraception must be used before beginning CellCept therapy, during therapy, and for six weeks following discontinuation of therapy (see section 4.5 Interaction with other medicinal products and other forms of interaction). Patients should be instructed to consult their physician immediately should pregnancy occur.

The use of Cellcept is not recommended during pregnancy and should be reserved for cases where no more suitable alternative treatment is available. CellCept should be used in pregnant women only if the potential benefit outweighs the potential risk to the foetus. There are no adequate data from the use of CellCept in pregnant women. Studies in animals have shown reproductive toxicity (see section 5.3 Preclinical safety data). The potential risk for humans is unknown.

Mycophenolate mofetil has been shown to be excreted in the milk of lactating rats. It is not known whether this drug is excreted in human milk. Because of the potential for serious adverse reactions to mycophenolate mofetil in breast-fed infants, Cellcept is contraindicated in nursing mothers (see section 4.3 Contraindications).

4.7 Effects on ability to drive and use machines

No specific studies have been performed. The pharmacodynamic profile and the reported adverse reactions indicate that an effect is unlikely.

4.8 Undesirable effects

The following undesirable effects cover adverse drug reactions from clinical trials:

The principal adverse drug reactions associated with the administration of CellCept in combination with ciclosporin and corticosteroids include diarrhoea, leucopenia, sepsis and vomiting and there is evidence of a higher frequency of certain types of infections (see section 4.4 Special warnings and special precautions for use).

Malignancies:

Patients receiving immunosuppressive regimens involving combinations of drugs, including CellCept, are at increased risk of developing lymphomas and other malignancies, particularly of the skin (see section 4.4 Special warnings and special precautions for use). Lymphoproliferative disease or lymphoma developed in 0.6% of patients receiving CellCept (2g or 3g daily) in combination with other immunosuppressants in controlled clinical trials of renal (2g data), cardiac and hepatic transplant patients followed for at least 1 year. Non-melanoma skin carcinomas occurred in 3.6% of patients; other types of malignancy occurred in 1.1% of patients. Three-year safety data in renal and cardiac transplant patients did not reveal any unexpected changes in incidence of malignancy compared to the 1-year data. Hepatic transplant patients were followed for at least 1 year, but less than 3 years.

Opportunistic Infections:

All transplant patients are at increased risk of opportunistic infections; the risk increased with total immunosuppressive load (see section 4.4 Special warnings and special precautions for use). The most common opportunistic infections in patients receiving CellCept (2g or 3g daily) with other immunosuppressants in controlled clinical trials of renal (2g data), cardiac and hepatic transplant patients followed for at least 1 year were candida mucocutaneous, CMV viraemia/syndrome and Herpes simplex. The proportion of patients with CMV viraemia/syndrome was 13.5%.

Children and adolescents (aged 2 to 18 years):

The type and frequency of adverse drug reactions in a clinical study, which recruited 92 paediatric patients aged 2 to 18 years who were given 600mg/m^2 mycophenolate mofetil orally twice daily, were generally similar to those observed in adult patients given 1g CellCept twice daily. However, the following treatment-related adverse events were more frequent in the paediatric population, particularly in children under 6 years of age, when compared to adults: diarrhoea, sepsis, leucopenia, anaemia and infection.

Elderly patients (⩾ 65 years):

Elderly patients (⩾ 65 years) may generally be at increased risk of adverse drug reactions due to immunosuppression. Elderly patients receiving CellCept as part of a combination immunosuppressive regimen, may be at increased risk of certain infections (including cytomegalovirus tissue invasive disease) and possibly gastrointestinal haemorrhage and pulmonary oedema, compared to younger individuals.

Other Adverse Drug Reactions:

Adverse drug reactions, probably or possibly related to CellCept, reported in ⩾ 10% and in 1 - < 10% of patients treated with CellCept in the controlled clinical trials of renal (2g data), cardiac and hepatic transplant patients are listed in the following table.

Adverse Drug Reactions, Probably or Possibly Related to CellCept, Reported in Patients Treated with CellCept in Renal, Cardiac and Hepatic Clinical Trials when Used in Combination with Ciclosporin and Corticosteroids

Body System		Adverse drug reactions
Body as a whole	⩾ 10%	Sepsis
	1 - < 10%	Moniliasis, infection, fever, chills, malaise, headache, flu syndrome, pain, asthenia, weight loss, oedema
Blood and lymphatic	⩾ 10%	Leucopenia, thrombocytopenia, anaemia
	1 - < 10%	Pancytopenia, leucocytosis
Renal and urogenital	⩾ 10%	Urinary tract infection
	1 - < 10%	Vaginal moniliasis, abnormal kidney function, increased creatinine, increased BUN
Cardio-vascular	⩾10%	-
	1 - < 10%	Hypotension, hypertension, tachycardia, vasodilatation
Metabolic/ nutritional	⩾ 10%	-
	1 - < 10%	Hyperkalaemia, acidosis, hypokalaemia, hypomagnesaemia, hypocalcaemia, hypercholesterolaemia, gout, hyperlipaemia, increased alkaline phosphatase, hyperglycaemia, hypophosphataemia, hyperuricaemia, increased lactate dehydrogenase
Gastro-intestinal	⩾ 10%	Moniliasis, vomiting, diarrhoea, nausea, abdominal pain
	1 - < 10%	Gastrointestinal haemorrhage, peritonitis, gastric ulcer, duodenal ulcer, colitis, infection, ileus, stomatitis, gastritis, gastroenteritis, anorexia, oesophagitis, dyspepsia, constipation, flatulence, eructation
Hepatic	⩾ 10%	-
	1 - < 10%	Hepatitis, jaundice, bilirubinaemia, elevation of enzymes
Respiratory	⩾ 10%	-
	1 - < 10%	Pneumonia, infection, moniliasis, dyspnoea, sinusitis, bronchitis, pharyngitis, pleural effusion, increased cough, rhinitis
Skin and appendages	⩾ 10%	Herpes simplex, herpes zoster
	1 - < 10%	Carcinoma, moniliasis, fungal dermatitis, acne, rash, alopecia, hypertrophy, benign neoplasia
Nervous	⩾ 10%	-
	1 - < 10%	Convulsion, depression, confusion, agitation, anxiety, hypertonia, dizziness, abnormal thinking, tremor, paraesthesia, insomnia, somnolence
Musculo-skeletal	⩾ 10%	-
	1 - < 10%	Myasthenia, arthralgia
Special senses	⩾ 10%	-
	1 - < 10%	Dysgeusia

Note: 501 (2g CellCept daily), 289 (3g CellCept daily) and 277 (2g IV / 3g oral CellCept daily) patients were treated in Phase III studies for the prevention of rejection in renal, cardiac and hepatic transplantation, respectively.

The following undesirable effects cover adverse drug reactions from post-marketing experience:

The types of adverse drug reactions reported during post-marketing with CellCept are similar to those seen in the controlled renal, cardiac and hepatic transplant studies. Additional adverse drug reactions reported during post-marketing are described below.

Gastrointestinal: colitis (including CMV colitis), pancreatitis, isolated cases of intestinal villous atrophy.

Disorders related to immunosuppression: serious life-threatening infections including meningitis, infectious endocarditis, tuberculosis and atypical mycobacterial infection. Some cases of agranulocytosis have been reported. Neutropenia has been reported in some patients, therefore regular monitoring of patients taking CellCept is advised (see section 4.4 Special warnings and special precautions for use).

Hypersensitivity: Hypersensitivity reactions, including angioedema and anaphylaxis, have been reported very rarely.

4.9 Overdose

The experience with overdose of CellCept in humans is very limited. The events received from reports of overdose fall within the known safety profile of the drug.

Haemodialysis would not be expected to remove clinically significant amounts of MPA or MPAG. By interfering with enterohepatic circulation of the drug, bile acid sequestrants, such as colestyramine, reduce the MPA AUC.

5. PHARMACOLOGICAL PROPERTIES

5.1 Pharmacodynamic properties

Pharmacotherapeutic group: immunosuppressant ATC code L04AA06.

Mycophenolate mofetil is the 2-morpholinoethyl ester of MPA. MPA is a potent, selective, uncompetitive and reversible inhibitor of inosine monophosphate dehydrogenase, and therefore inhibits the *de novo* pathway of guanosine nucleotide synthesis without incorporation into DNA. Because T- and B-lymphocytes are critically dependent for their proliferation on *de novo* synthesis of purines whereas other cell types can utilise salvage pathways, MPA has more potent cytostatic effects on lymphocytes than on other cells.

5.2 Pharmacokinetic properties

Following oral administration, mycophenolate mofetil undergoes rapid and extensive absorption and complete pre-systemic metabolism to the active metabolite, MPA. As evidenced by suppression of acute rejection following renal transplantation, the immunosuppressant activity of CellCept is correlated with MPA concentration. The mean bioavailability of oral mycophenolate mofetil, based on MPA AUC, is 94% relative to IV mycophenolate mofetil. Food had no effect on the extent of absorption (MPA AUC) of mycophenolate mofetil when administered at doses of 1.5 g BID to renal transplant patients. However, MPA C_{max} was decreased by 40% in the presence of food. Mycophenolate mofetil is not measurable systemically in plasma following oral administration. MPA at clinically relevant concentrations is 97% bound to plasma albumin.

As a result of enterohepatic recirculation, secondary increases in plasma MPA concentration are usually observed at approximately 6 – 12 hours post-dose. A reduction in the AUC of MPA of approximately 40% is associated with the co-administration of colestyramine (4g TID), indicating that there is a significant amount of enterohepatic recirculation.

MPA is metabolised principally by glucuronyl transferase to form the phenolic glucuronide of MPA (MPAG), which is not pharmacologically active.

A negligible amount of drug is excreted as MPA (< 1% of dose) in the urine. Orally administered radiolabelled mycophenolate mofetil results in complete recovery of the administered dose; with 93% of the administered dose recovered in the urine and 6% recovered in the faeces. Most (about 87%) of the administered dose is excreted in the urine as MPAG.

At clinically encountered concentrations, MPA and MPAG are not removed by haemodialysis. However, at high MPAG plasma concentrations (> 100μg/ml), small amounts of MPAG are removed.

In the early post-transplant period (< 40 days post-transplant), renal, cardiac and hepatic transplant patients had mean MPA AUCs approximately 30% lower and C_{max} approximately 40% lower compared to the late post-transplant period (3 – 6 months post-transplant).

Renal impairment:

In a single dose study (6 subjects/group), mean plasma MPA AUC observed in subjects with severe chronic renal impairment (glomerular filtration rate < $25ml\bullet min^{-1}\bullet 1.73m^{-2}$) were 28 – 75% higher relative to the means observed in normal healthy subjects or subjects with lesser degrees of renal impairment. However, the mean single dose MPAG AUC was 3 - 6-fold higher in subjects with severe renal impairment than in subjects with mild renal impairment or normal healthy subjects, consistent with the known renal elimination of MPAG. Multiple dosing of mycophenolate mofetil in patients with severe chronic renal impairment has not been studied. No data are available for cardiac or hepatic transplant patients with severe chronic renal impairment.

Delayed renal graft function:

In patients with delayed renal graft function post-transplant, mean MPA AUC(0-12h) was comparable to that seen in post-transplant patients without delayed graft function. Mean plasma MPAG AUC(0-12h) was 2 – 3-fold higher than in post-transplant patients without delayed graft function. There may be a transient increase in the free fraction and concentration of plasma MPA in patients with delayed renal graft function. Dose adjustment of CellCept does not appear to be necessary.

Hepatic impairment:

In volunteers with alcoholic cirrhosis, hepatic MPA glucuronidation processes were relatively unaffected by hepatic parenchymal disease. Effects of hepatic disease on this process probably depend on the particular disease. However, hepatic disease with predominantly biliary damage, such as primary biliary cirrhosis, may show a different effect.

Children and adolescents (aged 2 to 18 years):

Pharmacokinetic parameters were evaluated in 49 paediatric renal transplant patients given 600 mg/m^2 mycophenolate mofetil orally twice daily. This dose achieved MPA AUC values similar to those seen in adult renal transplant patients receiving CellCept at a dose of 1 g bid in the early and late post-transplant period. MPA AUC values across age groups were similar in the early and late post-transplant period.

Elderly patients (≥ 65 years):

Pharmacokinetic behaviour of CellCept in the elderly has not been formally evaluated.

Oral contraceptives:

The pharmacokinetics of oral contraceptives were unaffected by co-administration of CellCept (see also section 4.5 Interaction with other medicinal products and other forms of interaction). A study of the coadministration of CellCept (1g bid) and combined oral contraceptives containing ethinylestradiol (0.02mg to 0.04mg) and levonorgestrel (0.05mg to 0.15mg), desogestrel (0.15mg) or gestodene (0.05mg to 0.10mg) conducted in 18 non-transplant women (not taking other immunosupressants) over 3 consecutive menstrual cycles showed no clinically relevant influence of CellCept on the ovulation suppressing action of the oral contraceptives. Serum levels of LH, FSH and progesterone were not significantly affected.

5.3 Preclinical safety data

In experimental models, mycophenolate mofetil was not tumourigenic. The highest dose tested in the animal carcinogenicity studies resulted in approximately 2 – 3 times the systemic exposure (AUC or C_{max}) observed in renal transplant patients at the recommended clinical dose of 2g/day and 1.3 – 2 times the systemic exposure (AUC or C_{max}) observed in cardiac transplant patients at the recommended clinical dose of 3g/day.

Two genotoxicity assays (*in vitro* mouse lymphoma assay and *in vivo* mouse bone marrow micronucleus test) showed a potential of mycophenolate mofetil to cause chromosomal aberrations. These effects can be related to the pharmacodynamic mode of action, i.e. inhibition of nucleotide synthesis in sensitive cells. Other *in vitro* tests for detection of gene mutation did not demonstrate genotoxic activity.

Mycophenolate mofetil had no effect on fertility of male rats at oral doses up to $20mg\bullet kg^{-1}\bullet day^{-1}$. The systemic exposure at this dose represents 2 – 3 times the clinical exposure at the recommended clinical dose of 2g/day in renal transplant patients and 1.3 – 2 times the clinical exposure at the recommended clinical dose of 3g/day in cardiac transplant patients. In a female fertility and reproduction study conducted in rats, oral doses of $4.5mg\bullet kg^{-1}\bullet day^{-1}$ caused malformations (including anophthalmia, agnathia, and hydrocephaly)in the first generation offspring in the absence of maternal toxicity. The systemic exposure at this dose was approximately 0.5 times the clinical exposure at the recommended clinical dose of 2g/day for renal transplant patients and approximately 0.3 times the clinical exposure at the recommended clinical dose of 3g/day for cardiac transplant patients. No effects on fertility or reproductive parameters were evident in the dams or in the subsequent generation.

In teratology studies in rats and rabbits, foetal resorptions and malformations occurred in rats at $6mg\bullet kg^{-1}\bullet day^{-1}$ (including anophthalmia, agnathia, and hydrocephaly) and in rabbits at $90mg\bullet kg^{-1}\bullet day^{-1}$ (including cardiovascular and renal anomalies, such as ectopia cordis and ectopic kidneys, and diaphragmatic and umbilical hernia), in the absence of maternal toxicity. The systemic exposure at these levels are approximately equivalent to or less than 0.5 times the clinical exposure at the recommended clinical dose of 2g/day for renal transplant patients and approximately 0.3 times the clinical exposure at the recommended clinical dose of 3g/day for cardiac transplant patients.

Refer to section 4.6 Pregnancy and lactation.

The haematopoietic and lymphoid systems were the primary organs affected in toxicology studies conducted with mycophenolate mofetil in the rat, mouse, dog and monkey. These effects occurred at systemic exposure levels that are equivalent to or less than the clinical exposure at the recommended dose of 2g/day for renal transplant recipients. Gastrointestinal effects were observed in the dog at systemic exposure levels equivalent to or less than the clinical exposure at the recommended dose. Gastrointestinal and renal effects consistent with dehydration were also observed in the monkey at the highest dose (systemic exposure levels equivalent to or greater than clinical exposure). The nonclinical toxicity profile of mycophenolate mofetil appears to be consistent with adverse events observed in human clinical trials which now provide safety data of more relevance to the patient population (see section 4.8 Undesirable effects).

6. PHARMACEUTICAL PARTICULARS

6.1 List of excipients

Excipients of CellCept 1g/5ml powder for oral suspension are sorbitol; silica, colloidal anhydrous; sodium citrate; soybean lecithin; mixed fruit flavour; xanthan gum; aspartame (E951); methyl parahydroxybenzoate (E218); and citric acid, anhydrous.

Aspartame contains phenylalanine equivalent to 2.78mg/5ml of suspension.

6.2 Incompatibilities

This medicinal product must not be mixed with other medicinal products except those mentioned in section 6.6.

6.3 Shelf life

The shelf-life of the powder for oral suspension is 2 years.

The shelf-life of the constituted suspension is 2 months.

6.4 Special precautions for storage

Powder for oral suspension and constituted suspension: Do not store above 30°C.

6.5 Nature and contents of container

Each bottle contains 110g of powder for oral suspension. When constituted, the volume of the suspension is 175ml, providing a usable volume of 160 – 165ml.

A bottle adapter and 2 oral dispensers are also provided.

6.6 Instructions for use and handling

Because mycophenolate mofetil has demonstrated teratogenic effects in rats and rabbits, avoid inhalation or direct contact with skin or mucous membranes of the dry powder as well as direct contact of the constituted suspension with the skin. If such contact occurs, wash thoroughly with soap and water; rinse eyes with plain water.

Any unused product or waste material should be disposed of in accordance with local requirements.

It is recommended that CellCept 1g/5ml powder for oral suspension be constituted by the pharmacist prior to dispensing to the patient.

Preparation of suspension

1. Tap the closed bottle several times to loosen the powder.

2. Measure 94ml of purified water in a graduated cylinder.

3. Add approximately half of the total amount of purified water to the bottle and shake the closed bottle well for about 1 minute.

4. Add the remainder of water and shake the closed bottle well for about 1 minute.

5. Remove child-resistant cap and push bottle adapter into neck of bottle.

6. Close bottle with child-resistant cap tightly. This will assure the proper seating of the bottle adapter in the bottle and child-resistant status of the cap.

7. Write the date of expiration of the constituted suspension on the bottle label. (The shelf-life of the constituted suspension is two months).

7. MARKETING AUTHORISATION HOLDER

Roche Registration Limited, 40 Broadwater Road, Welwyn Garden City, Hertfordshire AL7 3AY, United Kingdom.

8. MARKETING AUTHORISATION NUMBER(S)

EU/1/96/005/006 CellCept (1 bottle 110g).

9. DATE OF FIRST AUTHORISATION/RENEWAL OF THE AUTHORISATION

3 May 2001

10. DATE OF REVISION OF THE TEXT

April 2005

CellCept is a registered trade mark

Celluvisc

(Allergan Ltd)

1. NAME OF THE MEDICINAL PRODUCT

Celluvisc▼ 1.0% w/v Eye drops, solution

2. QUALITATIVE AND QUANTITATIVE COMPOSITION

1 ml contains 10 mg carmellose sodium.

One drop (≈ 0.05 ml) contains 0.5 mg of carmellose sodium.

For excipients, see 6.1.

3. PHARMACEUTICAL FORM

Eye drops, solution.

A clear, colourless to slightly yellow viscous solution.

4. CLINICAL PARTICULARS

4.1 Therapeutic indications

Treatment of the symptoms of dry eye.

4.2 Posology and method of administration

Do not contaminate the open-end of the ampoule when in use. Twist-off tab and apply drops topically as follows:

Instil one to two drops as required or directed into conjunctival sac.

4.3 Contraindications

Hypersensitivity to any of the ingredients.

4.4 Special warnings and special precautions for use

If irritation, pain, redness and changes in vision occur or worsen, treatment should be discontinued and a new assessment considered.

Contact lenses should be removed before each application and may be inserted after 15 minutes.

Concomitant ocular medication should be administered 15 minutes prior to the instillation of Celluvisc.

To avoid contamination, do not touch the tip to the eye or any surface. Discard open ampoule after use.

4.5 Interaction with other medicinal products and other forms of Interaction

1. No interactions have been observed with Celluvisc. Given the formulation of Celluvisc, no interactions are anticipated.

2. If this product is used concomitantly with other topical eye medications there must be an interval of at least 15 minutes between the two medications.

4.6 Pregnancy and lactation

The constituents of Celluvisc have been used as pharmaceutical agents for many years with no untoward effects. No special precautions are necessary for the use of Celluvisc in pregnancy and lactation.

4.7 Effects on ability to drive and use machines

May cause transient blurring of vision. Do not drive or use machinery unless vision is clear.

4.8 Undesirable effects

Ocular evens (transient – typically lasting 1 to 15 minutes):

Ocular irritation, burning or stinging sensation

Blurring of vision

Tearing.

4.9 Overdose

Accidental overdosage will present no hazard.

5. PHARMACOLOGICAL PROPERTIES

5.1 Pharmacodynamic properties

Celluvisc exerts a physical, not a pharmacological action. Carmellose sodium is a viscosity enhancer which increases the retention time of the product.

5.2 Pharmacokinetic properties

Carmellose sodium has a large molecular weight and is unlikely to penetrate the cornea. The period of retention on the cornea is approximately 22 minutes in healthy eyes.

5.3 Preclinical safety data

No additional information of relevance for the doctor has been obtained from the preclinical testing.

6. PHARMACEUTICAL PARTICULARS

6.1 List of excipients

Sodium chloride

Sodium lactate

Potassium chloride

Calcium chloride

Purified Water

6.2 Incompatibilities

Not applicable.

6.3 Shelf life

2 years. The eye drop solution should be used immediately after opening. Any unused solution should be discarded.

6.4 Special precautions for storage

Do not store above 25°C.

6.5 Nature and contents of container

Clear, single-dose containers made from low density polyethylene formed with a twist-off tab.

Each unit is filled with 0.4 ml of solution.

Pack sizes may include: 5, 10, 20, 30, 40, 60 or 90 single-dose containers.

Not all pack sizes may be marketed.

6.6 Instructions for use and handling
Ensure that ampoule is intact before use. Discard any unused solution (i.e. once opened do not re-use container for subsequent doses).

7. MARKETING AUTHORISATION HOLDER
Allergan Pharmaceuticals Ireland
Castlebar Road
Westport
County Mayo
IRELAND

8. MARKETING AUTHORISATION NUMBER(S)
PL 05179/0001

9. DATE OF FIRST AUTHORISATION/RENEWAL OF THE AUTHORISATION
29th January 2001 / 29th September 2003

10. DATE OF REVISION OF THE TEXT
10th September 2004

Cerazette 75 microgram film-coated tablet

(Organon Laboratories Limited)

1. NAME OF THE MEDICINAL PRODUCT
Cerazette® 75 microgram film-coated tablet.

2. QUALITATIVE AND QUANTITATIVE COMPOSITION
Each tablet contains 75 microgram desogestrel.

For excipients, see 6.1.

3. PHARMACEUTICAL FORM
Film-coated tablet.

The tablet is white, round, biconvex and 5 mm in diameter. On one side it is coded KV above 2 and on the reverse side Organon *.

4. CLINICAL PARTICULARS

4.1 Therapeutic indications
Contraception.

4.2 Posology and method of administration
Tablets must be taken every day at about the same time so that the interval between two tablets always is 24 hours. The first tablet should be taken on the first day of menstrual bleeding. Thereafter one tablet each day is to be taken continuously, without taking any notice on possible bleeding. A new blister is started directly the day after the previous one.

How to start Cerazette

No preceding hormonal contraceptive use [in the past month]

Tablet-taking has to start on day 1 of the woman's natural cycle (day 1 is the first day of her menstrual bleeding). Starting on days 2-5 is allowed, but during the first cycle a barrier method is recommended for the first 7 days of tablet-taking.

Following first-trimester abortion

After first-trimester abortion it is recommended to start immediately. In that case there is no need to use an additional method of contraception.

Following delivery or second-trimester abortion

Contraceptive treatment with Cerazette after delivery can be initiated before the menstruations have returned. If more than 21 days have elapsed pregnancy ought to be ruled out and an additional method of contraception should be used for the first week.

For additional information for breastfeeding women see Section 4.6.

How to start Cerazette when changing from other contraceptive methods

Changing from a combined oral contraceptive (COC)

The woman should start with Cerazette on the day after the last active tablet of her COC. In this case, the use of an additional contraceptive is not necessary.

Changing from a progestogen-only-method (minipill, injection, implant or from a progestogen-releasing intrauterine system [IUS])

The woman may switch any day from the minipill (from an implant or the IUS on the day of its removal, from an injectable when the next injection would be due).

Missed tablet

Contraceptive protection may be reduced if more than 36 hours have elapsed between two tablets. If the user is less than 12 hours late in taking any tablet, the missed tablet should be taken as soon as it is remembered and the next tablet should be taken at the usual time. If she is more than 12 hours late, she should use an additional method of contraception for the next 7 days. If tablets were missed in the first week and intercourse took place in the week before the tablets were missed, the possibility of a pregnancy should be considered. If vomiting occurs within 3-4 hours after tablet-taking, the same advice is applicable as for a missed tablet.

Treatment surveillance

Before prescription, a thorough case history should be taken and a thorough gynaecological examination is recommended to exclude pregnancy. Bleeding disturbances, such as oligomenorrhoea and amenorrhoea should be investigated before prescription. The interval between check-ups depends on the circumstances in each individual case. If the prescribed product may conceivably influence latent or manifest disease (see Section 4.4), the control examinations should be timed accordingly.

Despite the fact that Cerazette is taken regularly, bleeding disturbances may occur. If bleeding is very frequent and irregular, another contraceptive method should be considered. If the symptoms persist, an organic cause should be ruled out.

Management of amenorrhoea during treatment depends on whether or not the tablets have been taken in accordance with the instructions and may include a pregnancy test.

The treatment should be stopped if a pregnancy occurs.

4.3 Contraindications

- Known or suspected pregnancy.
- Active venous thromboembolic disorder.
- Presence or history of severe hepatic disease as long as liver function values have not returned to normal.
- Progestogen-dependent tumours.
- Undiagnosed vaginal bleeding.
- Hypersensitivity to any of the ingredients of Cerazette.

4.4 Special warnings and special precautions for use
The risk for breast cancer increases in general with increasing age. During the use of oral contraceptives (OCs) the risk of having breast cancer diagnosed is slightly increased. This increased risk disappears gradually within 10 years after discontinuation of OC use and is not related to the duration of use, but to the age of the woman when using the OC. The expected number of cases diagnosed per 10 000 women who use combined OCs (up to 10 years after stopping) relative to never users over the same period have been calculated for the respective age groups to be: 4.5/4 (16-19 years), 17.5/16 (20-24 years), 48.7/44 (25-29 years), 110/100 (30-34 years), 180/160 (35-39 years) and 260/230 (40-44 years). The risk in POP users is possibly of similar magnitude as that associated with combined OCs. However, for POPs the evidence is less conclusive. Compared to the risk of getting breast cancer ever in life, the increased risk associated with OCs is low. The cases of breast cancer diagnosed in OC users tend to be less advanced than in those who have not used OCs. The increased risk in OC users may be due to an earlier diagnosis, biological effects of the pill or a combination of both. Since a biological effect cannot be excluded, an individual benefit/risk assessment should be made in women with pre-existing breast cancer and in women in whom breast cancer is diagnosed while using Cerazette.

Since a biological effect of progestogens on liver cancer cannot be excluded an individual benefit/risk assessment should be made in women with liver cancer.

Epidemiological investigations have associated the use of combined OCs with an increased incidence of venous thromboembolism (VTE, deep venous thrombosis and pulmonary embolism). Although the clinical relevance of this finding for desogestrel used as a contraceptive in the absence of an oestrogenic component is unknown, Cerazette should be discontinued in the event of a thrombosis. Discontinuation of Cerazette should also be considered in case of long-term immobilisation due to surgery or illness. Women with a history of thrombo-embolic disorders should be made aware of the possibility of a recurrence.

Although progestogens may have an effect on peripheral insulin resistance and glucose tolerance, there is no evidence for a need to alter the therapeutic regimen in diabetics using progestogen-only pills. However, diabetic patients should be carefully observed during the first months of use.

Treatment with Cerazette leads to decreased estradiol serum levels, to a level corresponding with the early follicular phase. It is as yet unknown whether the decrease has any clinically relevant effect on bone mineral density.

The protection with traditional progestogen-only pills against ectopic pregnancies is not as good as with combined oral contraceptives, which has been associated with the frequent occurrence of ovulations during the use of progestogen-only pills. Despite the fact that Cerazette consistently inhibits ovulation, ectopic pregnancy should be taken into account in the differential diagnosis if the woman gets amenorrhoea or abdominal pain.

Chloasma may occasionally occur, especially in women with a history of chloasma gravidarum. Women with a tendency to chloasma should avoid exposure to the sun or ultraviolet radiation whilst taking Cerazette.

4.5 Interaction with other medicinal products and other forms of Interaction
Drug interactions may reduce the efficacy of oral contraceptives (OCs). The data are primarily based on reports with combined OCs; however, reports on progestogen-only contraceptives also exist. Interactions have been established with hydantoins, barbiturates, primidone, carbamazepine and rifampicin; and probably also for oxcarbazepine, rifabutin, felbamate, ritonavir, griseofulvin and products containing St. John's wort (Hypericum perforatum). The mechanism of these interactions appears to be based on the hepatic enzyme-inducing properties of these drugs. Maximal enzyme induction is not seen for 2-3 weeks, but may then be sustained for at least 4 weeks after the cessation of drug therapy. In women treated with enzyme-inducing drugs it is recommended to advise the additional temporary use of a barrier method or prescribe another non-hormonal contraceptive method.

During treatment with medical charcoal, the absorption of the steroid in the tablet may be reduced and thereby the contraceptive efficacy. Under these circumstances the advice as given for missed tablets is applicable.

4.6 Pregnancy and lactation
Animal studies have shown that very high doses of progestogenic substances may cause masculinisation of female foetuses.

Extensive epidemiological studies have revealed neither an increased risk of birth defects in children born to women who used OCs prior to pregnancy, nor a teratogenic effect when OCs were taken inadvertently during early pregnancy. Pharmacovigilance data collected with various desogestrel-containing combined OCs also do not indicate an increased risk.

Cerazette does not influence the production or the quality of breast milk. However, small amounts of etonogestrel are excreted with the milk. As a result, 0.01 - 0.05 microgram etonogestrel per kg body weight per day may be ingested by the child (based on an estimated milk ingestion of 150 ml/kg/day). Whilst long-term follow-up data are not available, 7-month data for Cerazette do not indicate a risk to the nursing infant. Nevertheless, development and growth of the child should be carefully observed.

4.7 Effects on ability to drive and use machines
Not applicable.

4.8 Undesirable effects
The most commonly reported undesirable effect in the clinical trials is bleeding irregularity. Some kind of bleeding irregularity has been reported in up to 50% of women using Cerazette. Since Cerazette causes ovulation inhibition close to 100%, in contrast to other progestogen-only pills, irregular bleeding is more common than with other progestogen-only pills. In 20 - 30% of the women, bleeding

Table 1

Body system	Frequency of adverse reactions Common ⩾ 1/100	Uncommon < 1/100, ⩾ 1/1000	**Rare** (<1/1000)
Skin and appendages disorders	Acne	Alopecia	Rash, urticaria, erythema nodosum
Psychiatric disorders	Mood changes, decreased libido	Fatigue	
Eye disorders		Difficulties in wearing contact lenses	
Gastro-intestinal system disorders	Nausea	Vomiting	
Reproductive disorders, female	Breast pain, irregular bleeding, amenorrhoea	Vaginitis, dysmenorrhoea, ovarian cysts	
Body as a whole	Headache, weight increase		

may become more frequent, whereas in another 20% bleeding may become less frequent or totally absent. Vaginal bleeding may also be of longer duration. After a couple of months of treatment, bleedings tend to become less frequent. Information, counselling and a bleeding diary can improve the woman's acceptance of the bleeding pattern.

The most commonly reported other undesirable effects in the clinical trials with Cerazette > 2.5%) were acne, mood changes, breast pain, nausea and weight increase. The undesirable effects mentioned in the table below have been judged, by the investigators, as having an established, probable or possible link to the treatment.

(see Table 1 on previous page)

In women using (combined) oral contraceptives a number of (serious) undesirable effects have been reported, which are discussed in more detail in Section 4.4 Special warnings and precautions for use. These include venous thromboembolic disorders, arterial thromboembolic disorders, hormone-dependent tumours (e.g. liver tumours, breast cancer) and chloasma.

4.9 Overdose

There have been no reports of serious deleterious effects from overdose. Symptoms that may occur in this case are nausea, vomiting and, in young girls, slight vaginal bleeding. There are no antidotes and further treatment should be symptomatic.

5. PHARMACOLOGICAL PROPERTIES

5.1 Pharmacodynamic properties

Cerazette is a progestogen-only pill, which contains the progestogen desogestrel (ATC class G03AC09). Like other progestogen-only pills, Cerazette is best suited for use during breast feeding and for women who may not or do not want to use oestrogens. In contrast to traditional progestogen-only pills, the contraceptive effect of Cerazette is achieved primarily by inhibition of ovulation. Other effects include increased viscosity of the cervical mucus.

When studied for 2 cycles, using a definition of ovulation as a progesterone level greater than

16 nmol/L for 5 consecutive days, the ovulation incidence was found to be 1 % (1/103) with a 95% confidence interval of 0.02%- 5.29% in the ITT group (user and method failures). Ovulation inhibition was achieved from the first cycle of use. In this study, when Cerazette was discontinued after 2 cycles (56 continuous days), ovulation occurred on average after 17 days (range 7 - 30 days).

In a comparative efficacy trial (which allowed a maximum time of 3 hours for missed pills) the overall ITT Pearl-Index found for Cerazette was 0.4 (95% confidence interval 0.09 - 1.20), compared to 1.6 for 30 μg levonorgestrel (95% confidence interval 0.42 - 3.96).

The Pearl-Index for Cerazette is comparable to the one historically found for combined OCs in the general OC-using population.

Treatment with Cerazette leads to decreased estradiol levels, to a level corresponding to the early follicular phase. No clinically relevant effects on carbohydrate metabolism, lipid metabolism and haemostasis have been observed.

5.2 Pharmacokinetic properties

ABSORPTION

After oral dosing of Cerazette desogestrel (DSG) is rapidly absorbed and converted into etonogestrel (ENG). Under steady-state conditions, peak serum levels are reached 1.8 hours after tablet-intake and the absolute bioavailability of ENG is approximately 70%.

DISTRIBUTION

ENG is 95.5-99% bound to serum proteins, predominantly to albumin and to a lesser extent to SHBG.

METABOLISM

DSG is metabolised via hydroxylation and dehydrogenation to the active metabolite ENG. ENG is metabolised via sulphate and glucuronide conjugation.

ELIMINATION

ENG is eliminated with a mean half-life of approximately 30 hours, with no difference between single and multiple dosing. Steady-state levels in plasma are reached after 4-5 days. The serum clearance after i.v. administration of ENG is approximately 10 l per hour. Excretion of ENG and its metabolites either as free steroid or as conjugates, is with urine and faeces (ratio 1.5:1). In lactating women, ENG is excreted in breast milk with a milk/serum ratio of 0.37-0.55. Based on these data and an estimated milk intake of 150 ml/kg/day, 0.01 - 0.05 microgram etonogestrel maybe ingested by the infant.

5.3 Preclinical safety data

Toxicological studies did not reveal any effects other than those, which can be explained from the hormonal properties of desogestrel.

6. PHARMACEUTICAL PARTICULARS

6.1 List of excipients

TABLET CORE

Silica, colloidal anhydrous; α-tocopherol; lactose monohydrate; maize starch; povidone; stearic acid.

FILM COATING

Hypromellose; macrogol 400; talc; titanium dioxide (E 171).

6.2 Incompatibilities

Not applicable

6.3 Shelf life

3 Years.

6.4 Special precautions for storage

No special storage conditions.

6.5 Nature and contents of container

Blister of 28 tablets each. PVC/Aluminium foil push-through blister (1, 3 or 6 strips per box). Each blister is enveloped in aluminium laminate sachets, packed in a printed cardboard box.

6.6 Instructions for use and handling

Not applicable.

7. MARKETING AUTHORISATION HOLDER

Organon Laboratories Ltd, Cambridge Science Park, Milton Road, Cambridge, CB4 0FL, UK

8. MARKETING AUTHORISATION NUMBER(S)

PL0065/0159

9. DATE OF FIRST AUTHORISATION/RENEWAL OF THE AUTHORISATION

9 November 1998 / 8 January 2004

10. DATE OF REVISION OF THE TEXT

May 2004

Ref. UK SmPC 03 Cera v1.4 Printed Version

Cerumol Ear Drops

(Laboratories for Applied Biology Limited)

1. NAME OF THE MEDICINAL PRODUCT

Cerumol Ear Drops

2. QUALITATIVE AND QUANTITATIVE COMPOSITION

Active Drug Substances

Arachis Oil (Peanut Oil)	BP	57.3%
Chlorobutanol (Chlorbutol)	BP	5.0%
p-Dichlorobenzene	BPC 1949	2.0%

3. PHARMACEUTICAL FORM

Ear drops: Oily drops for topical application.

4. CLINICAL PARTICULARS

4.1 Therapeutic indications

To loosen wax causing occlusion or partial occlusion of the external auditory meatus. (Either a collection of soft wax or a harder wax plug.)

4.2 Posology and method of administration

At home: With the head inclined, 5 drops are put into the ear. This may cause a harmless tingling sensation. A plug of cotton wool moistened with Cerumol or smeared with petroleum jelly should then be applied to retain the liquid. One hour later, or the next morning, the plug is removed. The procedure is repeated twice a day for three days; the loosened wax may then come out on its own making syringing unnecessary. If any wax remains the doctor should be consulted so that syringing of the softened residue may be carried out.

At the surgery: If there has been no prior treatment with Cerumol, 5 drops are instilled as described above and left for at least 20 minutes. Then syringing or a probe tipped with cotton wool may be employed.

4.3 Contraindications

Otitis externa, seborrhoeic dermatitis and eczema affecting the outer ear. Perforated ear drums.

4.4 Special warnings and special precautions for use

Not to be taken internally. Do not use for more than three days without consulting your doctor. Cerumol contains Arachis oil (peanut oil) and should not be taken by patients known to be allergic to peanut. As there is a possible relationship between allergy to peanut and allergy to soya, patients with soya allergy should also avoid Cerumol.

4.5 Interaction with other medicinal products and other forms of Interaction

None known.

4.6 Pregnancy and lactation

No side effects have been reported.

4.7 Effects on ability to drive and use machines

None known, but the actual wax plug may cause deafness.

4.8 Undesirable effects

Local reaction is extremely rare.

4.9 Overdose

As the product is applied topically, overdosage as such is not possible. In the case of accidental ingestion, the amounts of the majority of the ingredients in the bottle are too small to give rise to toxic effects. The 550 mg of Chlorobutanol in the whole bottle might cause excessive sedation in a child.

5. PHARMACOLOGICAL PROPERTIES

5.1 Pharmacodynamic properties

The drug is applied topically to aid the removal of cerumen. Thus normal pharmacological criteria cannot be applied.

The action is thought to be due to the loosening and lubricating properties of the solvent mixture, rather than its solvent properties. This is intrinsic to the solvent mixture.

Arachis Oil: is an oily substance to aid lubrication of the cerumen plug (water based solvents cause swelling of cerumen). It is however too viscous to be used on its own.

Chlorobutanol: This is an anti-bacterial and anti-fungal, but its main purpose in this product is to reduce the viscosity of the mixture, giving better penetrating characteristics to the oil.

p-Dichlorobenzene: is an insecticide whose presence also reduces viscosity.

5.2 Pharmacokinetic properties

The rate of loosening or dissolution of the cerumen is extremely variable. Trials have shown that Cerumol is the only one of a number of agents that was significantly better than sodium bicarbonate in aiding the removal of wax.*

*J Fraser, J Laryng. and Otology, 1970, 84, (10), 1055.

5.3 Preclinical safety data

None stated.

6. PHARMACEUTICAL PARTICULARS

6.1 List of excipients

Oil of Turpentine	BP	10.0%
3-methoxy butyl acetate (Butoxyl Hoechst)	House	10.0%
o-Dichlorobenzene	House	14.5%

6.2 Incompatibilities

None known.

6.3 Shelf life

5 years. Use within 6 months of opening.

6.4 Special precautions for storage

No special precautions necessary.

6.5 Nature and contents of container

11ml contained in a 12.5ml amber glass bottle. Packaged together with a separate dropper.

6.6 Instructions for use and handling

None

7. MARKETING AUTHORISATION HOLDER

Laboratories for Applied Biology Ltd

91 Amhurst Park

London N 16 5 DR ML 0118/01

8. MARKETING AUTHORISATION NUMBER(S)

UK 0118/0013R

9. DATE OF FIRST AUTHORISATION/RENEWAL OF THE AUTHORISATION

Granted 10 December 1971.

Renewed 07 July 1999.

10. DATE OF REVISION OF THE TEXT

April 1998 (correction of omissions)

January 1999 (correction of Posology)

June 1999 (correction of section 4.4 AND in section 5.1 change of Chlorbutol to Chlorobutanol)

July 1999 (renewal)

March 2003 (change in 4.4 and addition of allergy to soya warning)

Cetrotide 0.25 mg

(Serono Ltd)

1. NAME OF THE MEDICINAL PRODUCT

Cetrotide 0.25 mg powder and solvent for solution for injection

2. QUALITATIVE AND QUANTITATIVE COMPOSITION

1 vial contains:

0.26 - 0.27 mg cetrorelix acetate equivalent to 0.25 mg cetrorelix.

After reconstitution with the solvent provided, the concentration of cetrorelix is 0.25 mg/ml.

For excipients, see section 6.1.

3. PHARMACEUTICAL FORM

Powder and solvent for solution for injection.

Appearance of the powder: white lyophilised pellet.

Appearance of the solvent: clear colourless solution.

4. CLINICAL PARTICULARS

4.1 Therapeutic indications

Prevention of premature ovulation in patients undergoing a controlled ovarian stimulation, followed by oocyte pick-up and assisted reproductive techniques.

In clinical trials Cetrotide 0.25 mg was used with human menopausal gonadotropin (HMG), however, limited experience with recombinant FSH suggested similar efficacy.

4.2 Posology and method of administration

Cetrotide 0.25 mg should only be prescribed by a specialist experienced in this field.

Cetrotide 0.25 mg is for subcutaneous injection into the lower abdominal wall.

The first administration of Cetrotide should be performed under the supervision of a physician and under conditions where treatment of possible pseudo-allergic reactions is immediately available. The following injections may be self-administered as long as the patient is made aware of the signs and symptoms that may indicate hypersensitivity, the consequences of such a reaction and the need for immediate medical intervention.

The contents of 1 vial (0.25 mg cetrorelix) are to be administered once daily, at 24 h intervals, either in the morning or in the evening. Following the first administration, it is advised that the patient be kept under medical supervision for 30 minutes to ensure there is no allergic/pseudo-allergic reaction to the injection. Facilities for the treatment of such reactions should be immediately available.

Administration in the morning: Treatment with Cetrotide 0.25 mg should commence on day 5 or 6 of ovarian stimulation (approximately 96 to 120 hours after start of ovarian stimulation) with urinary or recombinant gonadotropins and is to be continued throughout the gonadotropin treatment period including the day of ovulation induction.

Administration in the evening: Treatment with Cetrotide 0.25 mg should commence on day 5 of ovarian stimulation (approximately 96 to 108 hours after start of ovarian stimulation) with urinary or recombinant gonadotropins and is to be continued throughout the gonadotropin treatment period until the evening prior to the day of ovulation induction.

For instructions for use and handling, see section 6.6.

4.3 Contraindications

• Hypersensitivity to cetrorelix acetate or any structural analogues of GnRH, extrinsic peptide hormones or mannitol.

• Pregnancy and lactation.

• Postmenopausal women.

• Patients with moderate and severe renal and hepatic impairment.

4.4 Special warnings and special precautions for use

Special care should be taken in women with signs and symptoms of active allergic conditions or known history of allergic predisposition. Treatment with Cetrotide is not advised in women with severe allergic conditions.

During or following ovarian stimulation an ovarian hyperstimulation syndrome can occur. This event must be considered as an intrinsic risk of the stimulation procedure with gonadotropins.

An ovarian hyperstimulation syndrome should be treated symptomatically, e.g. with rest, intravenous electrolytes/colloids and heparin therapy.

Luteal phase support should be given according to the reproductive medical centrés practice.

There is limited experience up to now with the administration of Cetrotide 0.25 mg during a repeated ovarian stimulation procedure. Therefore Cetrotide 0.25 mg should be used in repeated cycles only after a careful risk/benefit evaluation.

4.5 Interaction with other medicinal products and other forms of Interaction

In vitro investigations have shown that interactions are unlikely with medications that are metabolised by cytochrome P450 or glucuronised or conjugated in some other way. However, interactions with commonly used medicinal products, including products that may induce histamine release in susceptible individuals, may occur.

4.6 Pregnancy and lactation

Cetrotide 0.25 mg is not intended to be used during pregnancy and lactation (see section 4.3 "Contra-indications").

Studies in animals have indicated that cetrorelix exerts a dose related influence on fertility, reproductive performance and pregnancy. No teratogenic effects occurred when the drug was administered during the sensitive phase of gestation.

4.7 Effects on ability to drive and use machines

Due to its pharmacological profile cetrorelix is unlikely to impair the patient's ability to drive or to operate machinery.

4.8 Undesirable effects

Local reactions at the injection site (e.g. erythema, swelling and pruritis) have been reported. Usually they were transient in nature and mild intensity. The frequency as reported in clinical trials was 9.4% following multiple injections of 0.25 mg cetrorelix. Rare cases of hypersensitivity reactions including pseudo-allergic/anaphylactoid reactions have also been reported.

Common

Mild to moderate ovarian hyperstimulation syndrome (WHO grade I or II) can occur which is an intrinsic risk of the stimulation procedure (see section 4.4 "Special warnings and precautions for use").

Uncommon

Severe ovarian hyperstimulation syndrome (WHO grade III)

Nausea and headache

4.9 Overdose

Overdosage in humans may result in a prolonged duration of action but is unlikely to be associated with acute toxic effects.

In acute toxicity studies in rodents non-specific toxic symptoms were observed after intraperitoneal administration of cetrorelix doses more than 200 times higher than the pharmacologically effective dose after subcutaneous administration.

5. PHARMACOLOGICAL PROPERTIES

5.1 Pharmacodynamic properties

Pharmacotherapeutic group: LHRH-Antagonist, ATC code: H01CC02.

Cetrorelix is a luteinising hormone releasing hormone (LHRH) antagonist. LHRH binds to membrane receptors on pituitary cells. Cetrorelix competes with the binding of endogenous LHRH to these receptors. Due to this mode of action, cetrorelix controls the secretion of gonadotropins (LH and FSH).

Cetrorelix dose-dependently inhibits the secretion of LH and FSH from the pituitary gland. The onset of suppression is virtually immediate and is maintained by continuous treatment, without initial stimulatory effect.

In females, cetrorelix delays the LH surge and consequently ovulation. In women undergoing ovarian stimulation the duration of action of cetrorelix is dose dependent. Following a single dose of 3 mg of cetrorelix a duration of action of at least 4 days has been evaluated. On day 4 the suppression was approximately 70%. At a dose of 0.25 mg per injection repeated injections every 24 hours will maintain the effect of cetrorelix.

In animals as well as in humans, the antagonistic hormonal effects of cetrorelix were fully reversible after termination of treatment.

5.2 Pharmacokinetic properties

The absolute bioavailability of cetrorelix after subcutaneous administration is about 85%.

The total plasma clearance and the renal clearance are 1.2 ml × min^{-1} × kg^{-1} and 0.1 ml × min^{-1} × kg^{-1}, respectively. The volume of distribution ($V_{d,area}$) is 1.1 l × kg^{-1}. The mean terminal half-lives following intravenous and subcutaneous administration are about 12 h and 30 h, respectively, demonstrating the effect of absorption processes at the injection site. The subcutaneous administration of single doses (0.25 mg to 3 mg cetrorelix) and also daily dosing over 14 days show linear kinetics.

5.3 Preclinical safety data

No target organ toxicity could be observed from acute, subacute and chronic toxicity studies in rats and dogs following subcutaneous administration of cetrorelix. No signs of drug-related local irritation or incompatibility were noted in dogs after intravenous, intra-arterial and paravenous injection when cetrorelix was administered in doses clearly above the intended clinical use in man.

Cetrorelix showed no mutagenic or clastogenic potential in gene and chromosome mutation assays.

6. PHARMACEUTICAL PARTICULARS

6.1 List of excipients

Mannitol, water for injections

6.2 Incompatibilities

As cetrorelix is incompatible with several substances of common parenteral solutions it should be dissolved only by using water for injections.

6.3 Shelf life

2 years.

The solution should be used immediately after preparation.

6.4 Special precautions for storage

Do not store above 25 °C. Keep the container in the outer carton.

6.5 Nature and contents of container

Packs with 1 or 7 Type I glass vials each containing 55.7 mg powder for solution for injection sealed with a rubber stopper.

Additionally for each vial the packs contain:

1 pre-filled syringe (Type I glass cartridge closed with rubber stoppers) with 1 ml solvent for parenteral use

1 injection needle (20 gauge)

1 hypodermic injection needle (27 gauge)

2 alcohol swabs.

6.6 Instructions for use and handling

Cetrotide 0.25 mg should only be reconstituted with the solvent provided, using a gentle, swirling motion. Vigorous shaking with bubble formation should be avoided.

The reconstitution solution is without particles and clear. Do not use if the solution contains particles or if the solution is not clear.

Withdraw the entire contents of the vial. This ensures a delivery to the patient of a dose of at least 0.23 mg cetrorelix.

The solution should be used immediately after reconstitution.

The injection site should be varied daily.

7. MARKETING AUTHORISATION HOLDER

Serono Europe Limited
56 Marsh Wall
London E14 9TP
United Kingdom

8. MARKETING AUTHORISATION NUMBER(S)

EU/1/99/100/001
EU/1/99/100/002

9. DATE OF FIRST AUTHORISATION/RENEWAL OF THE AUTHORISATION

Granted: 13 April 1999 Renewed: 17 August 2004

10. DATE OF REVISION OF THE TEXT

17th August 2004

LEGAL STATUS

POM

NAME AND ADDRESS OF DISTRIBUTOR IN UK

Serono Ltd
Bedfont Cross
Stanwell Road
Feltham
Middlesex
TW14 8NX

NAME AND ADDRESS OF DISTRIBUTOR IN IRELAND

Allphar Services Limited
Pharmaceutical Agents and Distributors
Belgard Road
Tallaght
Dublin 24

Cetrotide 3 mg

(Serono Ltd)

1. NAME OF THE MEDICINAL PRODUCT

Cetrotide 3 mg powder and solvent for solution for injection

2. QUALITATIVE AND QUANTITATIVE COMPOSITION

1 vial contains:

3.12 - 3.24 mg cetrorelix acetate equivalent to 3 mg cetrorelix.

After reconstitution with the solvent provided, the concentration of cetrorelix is 1 mg/ml.

For excipients, see section 6.1.

3. PHARMACEUTICAL FORM

Powder and solvent for solution for injection

Appearance of the powder: white lyophilised pellet

Appearance of the solvent: clear colourless solution

4. CLINICAL PARTICULARS

4.1 Therapeutic indications

Prevention of premature ovulation in patients undergoing a controlled ovarian stimulation, followed by oocyte pick-up and assisted reproductive techniques.

In clinical trials Cetrotide 3 mg was used with human menopausal gonadotropin (HMG), however, limited experience with recombinant FSH suggested similar efficacy.

4.2 Posology and method of administration

Cetrotide 3 mg should only be prescribed by a specialist experienced in this field.

Cetrotide 3 mg is for subcutaneous injection into the lower abdominal wall.

The first administration of Cetrotide should be performed under the supervision of a physician and under conditions where treatment of possible pseudo-allergic reactions is immediately available. The following injections may be self-administered as long as the patient is made aware of the signs and symptoms that may indicate hypersensitivity, the consequences of such a reaction and the need for immediate medical intervention.

The contents of 1 vial (3 mg cetrorelix) are to be administered on day 7 of ovarian stimulation (approximately 132 to 144 hours after start of ovarian stimulation) with urinary or recombinant gonadotropins. Following the first administration, it is advised that the patient be kept under medical supervision for 30 minutes to ensure there is no allergic/pseudo-allergic reaction to the injection. Facilities for the treatment of such reactions should be immediately available.

If the follicle growth does not allow ovulation induction on the fifth day after injection of Cetrotide 3 mg, additionally 0.25 mg cetrorelix (Cetrotide 0.25 mg) should be administered once daily beginning 96 hours after the injection of Cetrotide 3 mg until the day of ovulation induction.

For instructions for use and handling, see section 6.6.

4.3 Contraindications

- Hypersensitivity to cetrorelix acetate or any structural analogue of GnRH, extrinsic peptide hormones or mannitol.
- Pregnancy, and lactation.
- Postmenopausal women.
- Patients with moderate and severe renal and hepatic impairment.

4.4 Special warnings and special precautions for use

Special care should be taken in women with signs and symptoms of active allergic conditions or known history of allergic predisposition. Treatment with Cetrotide is not advised in women with severe allergic conditions.

During or following ovarian stimulation an ovarian hyperstimulation syndrome can occur. This event must be considered as an intrinsic risk of the stimulation procedure with gonadotropins.

An ovarian hyperstimulation syndrome should be treated symptomatically, e.g. with rest, intravenous electrolytes/colloids and heparin therapy.

Luteal phase support should be given according to the reproductive medical centrés practice.

There is limited experience up to now with the administration of Cetrotide 3 mg during a repeated ovarian stimulation procedure. Therefore Cetrotide 3 mg should be used in repeated cycles only after a careful risk/benefit evaluation.

4.5 Interaction with other medicinal products and other forms of interaction

In vitro investigations have shown that interactions are unlikely with medications that are metabolised by cytochrome P450 or glucuronised or conjugated in some other way. However, interactions with commonly used medicinal products, including products that may induce histamine release in susceptible individuals, may occur.

4.6 Pregnancy and lactation

Cetrotide 3 mg is not intended to be used during pregnancy and lactation (see section 4.3 "Contra-indications").

Studies in animals have indicated that cetrorelix exerts a dose related influence on fertility, reproductive performance and pregnancy. No teratogenic effects occurred when the drug was administered during the sensitive phase of gestation.

4.7 Effects on ability to drive and use machines

Due to its pharmacological profile cetrorelix is unlikely to impair the patient's ability to drive or to operate machinery.

4.8 Undesirable effects

Local reactions at the injection site (e.g. erythema, swelling and pruritis) have been reported. Usually they were transient in nature and mild intensity. The frequency as observed in a clinical trial was 8%. Rare cases of hypersensitivity reactions including pseudo-allergic/anaphylactoid reactions have also been reported.

Common

Mild to moderate ovarian hyperstimulation syndrome (WHO grade I or II) can occur which is an intrinsic risk of the stimulation procedure (see section 4.4 "Special warnings and precautions for use").

Uncommon

Severe ovarian hyperstimulation syndrome (WHO grade III)

Nausea and headache

4.9 Overdose

Overdosage in humans may result in a prolonged duration of action but is unlikely to be associated with acute toxic effects.

In acute toxicity studies in rodents non-specific toxic symptoms were observed after intraperitoneal administration of cetrorelix doses more than 200 times higher than the pharmacologically effective dose after subcutaneous administration.

5. PHARMACOLOGICAL PROPERTIES

5.1 Pharmacodynamic properties

Pharmacotherapeutic group: LHRH-Antagonist, ATC code: H01CC02.

Cetrorelix is a luteinising hormone releasing hormone (LHRH) antagonist. LHRH binds to membrane receptors on pituitary cells. Cetrorelix competes with the binding of endogenous LHRH to these receptors. Due to this mode of action, cetrorelix controls the secretion of gonadotropins (LH and FSH).

Cetrorelix dose-dependently inhibits the secretion of LH and FSH from the pituitary gland. The onset of suppression is virtually immediate and is maintained by continuous treatment, without initial stimulatory effect.

In females, cetrorelix delays the LH surge and consequently ovulation.

In women undergoing ovarian stimulation the duration of action of cetrorelix is dose dependent. Following a single dose of 3 mg of cetrorelix a duration of action of at least 4 days has been evaluated. On day 4 the suppression was approximately 70%. At a dose of 0.25 mg per injection repeated injections every 24 hours will maintain the effect of cetrorelix.

In animals as well as in humans, the antagonistic hormonal effects of cetrorelix were fully reversible after termination of treatment.

5.2 Pharmacokinetic properties

The absolute bioavailability of cetrorelix after subcutaneous administration is about 85%.

The total plasma clearance and the renal clearance are 1.2 ml × min^{-1} × kg^{-1} and 0.1 ml × min^{-1} × kg^{-1}, respectively. The volume of distribution ($V_{d,area}$) is 1.1 l × kg^{-1}. The mean terminal half-lives following intravenous and subcutaneous administration are about 12 h and 30 h, respectively, demonstrating the effect of absorption processes at the injection site. The subcutaneous administration of single doses (0.25 mg to 3 mg cetrorelix) and also daily dosing over 14 days show linear kinetics.

5.3 Preclinical safety data

No target organ toxicity could be observed from acute, subacute and chronic toxicity studies in rats and dogs following subcutaneous administration of cetrorelix. No signs of drug-related local irritation or incompatibility were noted in dogs after intravenous, intra-arterial and paravenous injection when cetrorelix was administered in doses clearly above the intended clinical use in man.

Cetrorelix showed no mutagenic or clastogenic potential in gene and chromosome mutation assays.

6. PHARMACEUTICAL PARTICULARS

6.1 List of excipients

Mannitol, water for injections

6.2 Incompatibilities

As cetrorelix is incompatible with several substances of common parenteral solutions it should be dissolved only by using water for injections.

6.3 Shelf life

2 years.

The solution should be used immediately after preparation.

6.4 Special precautions for storage

Do not store above 25 °C. Keep the container in the outer carton.

6.5 Nature and contents of container

Pack with 1 Type I glass vial containing 167.7 mg powder for solution for injection sealed with a rubber stopper.

Additionally the pack contains:

1 pre-filled syringe (Type I glass cartridge closed with rubber stoppers) with 3 ml

solvent for parenteral use

1 injection needle (20 gauge)

1 hypodermic injection needle (27 gauge)

2 alcohol swabs.

6.6 Instructions for use and handling

Cetrotide 3 mg should only be reconstituted with the solvent provided, using a gentle, swirling motion. Vigorous shaking with bubble formation should be avoided.

The reconstituted solution is without particles and clear. Do not use if the solution contains particles or if the solution is not clear.

Withdraw the entire contents of the vial. This ensures a delivery to the patient of a dose of at least 2.82 mg cetrorelix.

The solution should be used immediately after reconstitution.

7. MARKETING AUTHORISATION HOLDER

Serono Europe Limited

56 Marsh Wall

London E14 9TP

United Kingdom

8. MARKETING AUTHORISATION NUMBER(S)

EU/1/99/100/003

9. DATE OF FIRST AUTHORISATION/RENEWAL OF THE AUTHORISATION

Granted: 13 April 1999 Renewed: 17 August 2004

10. DATE OF REVISION OF THE TEXT

17th August 2004

LEGAL STATUS

POM

NAME AND ADDRESS OF DISTRIBUTOR IN UK

Serono Ltd

Bedfont Cross

Stanwell Road

Feltham

Middlesex

TW14 8NX

NAME AND ADDRESS OF DISTRIBUTOR IN IRELAND

Allphar Services Limited

Pharmaceutical Agents and Distributors

Belgard Road

Tallaght

Dublin 24

Charcodote

(Pliva Pharma Ltd)

1. NAME OF THE MEDICINAL PRODUCT

Charcodote

2. QUALITATIVE AND QUANTITATIVE COMPOSITION

Activated charcoal 200mg/ml

3. PHARMACEUTICAL FORM

Oral suspension

4. CLINICAL PARTICULARS

4.1 Therapeutic indications

Charcodote is indicated for oral use as an emergency antidote in the treatment of poisoning or drug overdosage by most drugs and chemicals. It can be used either before or after gastric lavage where this is indicated. Charcodote adsorbs toxic substances and reduces or prevents systemic absorption.

4.2 Posology and method of administration

Adult: Single dose:- 250ml (equivalent to 50g of activated charcoal) as soon as possible after ingestion or suspected ingestion of the potential poison. Charcodote may also be administered after emesis or gastric lavage via intragastric intubation. Dosage may be repeated as recommended by a physician.

Children: Children aged under 12 years should be given half of the contents of one bottle (125ml; 25g of activated charcoal) unless a large quantity of intoxicant has been ingested, and where there is a risk to life. In these circumstances, the administration of the full 50g dose is indicated.

Repeated dosing at intervals of four hours should be considered in the case of poisoning with phenobarbitone, carbamazepine, theophylline, quinine, dapsone or salicylate, but should only be undertaken where appropriate patient monitoring is available.

4.3 Contraindications

None

4.4 Special warnings and special precautions for use

Charcodote should only be administered to unconscious patients who have a cuffed endotracheal tube in place in order to protect the airway.

Although not contraindicated in poisoning by caustic or corrosive substances, Charcodote has limited value as a detoxicant for these substances and the presence of activated charcoal may hinder the visualisation of oesophageal erosions or burns.

Activated charcoal does not adsorb cyanide and is relatively ineffective in adsorbing lithium salts, caustic or corrosive alkalis and acids, ethanol, methanol, ethylene glycol, iron salts, sodium chloride, lead, boric acid, other mineral acids and petroleum distillates.

If other oral antidotes are to be used (eg methionine for paracetamol poisoning) care must be taken as activated charcoal will reduce the effectiveness of such compounds.

4.5 Interaction with other medicinal products and other forms of Interaction

Ice-cream or other foods should not be used as a vehicle for the administration of activated charcoal as they reduce the adsorptive capacity of the activated charcoal.

When used as an antidote for oral poisoning, simultaneous administration of ipecac syrup with activated charcoal is not recommended since the ipecac syrup is adsorbed by the charcoal thus preventing emesis. If both ipecac syrup and activated charcoal are to be used, it is recommended that the charcoal be administered only after vomiting has been induced and completed.

4.6 Pregnancy and lactation

There is no evidence to suggest that Charcodote should not be used in pregnant or breast-feeding women.

4.7 Effects on ability to drive and use machines

Activated charcoal should not affect the ability of patients to drive or operate machinery.

4.8 Undesirable effects

Activated charcoal has been associated with bezoar formation, intestinal obstruction, and rarely intestinal perforation following multiple dosing - although a direct causative association has not been demonstrated. Charcodote will colour stools black which may be alarming to the patient but is medically insignificant.

4.9 Overdose

Not applicable.

5. PHARMACOLOGICAL PROPERTIES

5.1 Pharmacodynamic properties

Activated charcoal can adsorb a wide range of plant and inorganic poisons and many drugs. Thus, when administered by mouth it reduces their systemic absorption from the gastrointestinal tract and is used in the treatment of acute oral poisoning. However, activated charcoal does not adsorb cyanide and is relatively ineffective in adsorbing lithium salts, caustic or corrosive alkalis and acids, ethanol, methanol, ethylene glycol, iron salts, sodium chloride, lead, boric acid, other mineral acids and petroleum distillates.

5.2 Pharmacokinetic properties
Following oral administration, activated charcoal does not get absorbed from the gastrointestinal tract and does not undergo metabolism. It is excreted in the faeces.

5.3 Preclinical safety data
None

6. PHARMACEUTICAL PARTICULARS
6.1 List of excipients
Purified water

6.2 Incompatibilities
None known

6.3 Shelf life
2 years. Use immediately upon opening. Any remaining unused suspension should be discarded after first use.

6.4 Special precautions for storage
Do not store above 25°C. Do not freeze.

6.5 Nature and contents of container
Low density polyethylene bottle with screw cap designed for administration either directly or via an intragastric tube. Each bottle contains 250ml (50g activated charcoal).

6.6 Instructions for use and handling
Shake well before use.

Administrative Data
7. MARKETING AUTHORISATION HOLDER
PLIVA Pharma Limited
Vision House
Bedford Road
Petersfield
Hampshire
GU32 3QB

8. MARKETING AUTHORISATION NUMBER(S)
PL 10622/0033

9. DATE OF FIRST AUTHORISATION/RENEWAL OF THE AUTHORISATION
24th August 1999

10. DATE OF REVISION OF THE TEXT
23 September 2002

Pharmaceutical Classification P

Chemydur 60XL

(Sovereign Medical)

1. NAME OF THE MEDICINAL PRODUCT
Chemydur 60XL

2. QUALITATIVE AND QUANTITATIVE COMPOSITION
Isosorbide-5-Mononitrate 60mg.

International non-proprietary name (INN): Isosorbide mononitrate

Chemical name: 1,4: 3,6 dianhydro-D-glucitol-5-nitrate.

For excipients, see 6.1

3. PHARMACEUTICAL FORM
Tablets (modified release).

4. CLINICAL PARTICULARS
4.1 Therapeutic indications
Prophylactic treatment of angina pectoris

4.2 Posology and method of administration
Adults: one tablet (60mg) once daily given in the morning. The dose may be increased to two tablets (120mg), the whole doses to be given together.

The dose can be titrated to minimise the possibility of headache by initiating treatment with half a tablet (30mg) for the first two to four days.

The tablets should not be chewed or crushed and should be swallowed with half a glass of fluid.

Children: The safety and efficacy of Isosorbide mononitrate modified release tablets have not been established.

Elderly: No need for routine dosage adjustment in the elderly has been found, but special care may be needed in those with increased susceptibility to hypotension or marked hepatic or renal insufficiency.

The lowest effective dose should be used.

Attenuation of effect has occurred in some patients being treated with sustained release preparations. In such patients intermittent therapy may be more appropriate. (see section 4.4).

As with other drugs for the treatment of angina pectoris, abrupt discontinuation of therapy may lead to exacerbation of symptoms. When discontinuing long term treatment, the dosage should be reduced gradually over several days, and the patient carefully monitored (see section 4.4).

4.3 Contraindications
Hypersensitivity to any of the components.

Hypertrophic obstructive cardiomyopathy and constrictive pericarditis, aortic stenosis, cardiac tamponade, mitral stenosis and severe anaemia, hypovolaemia, cerebral haemorrhage, head trauma, closed-angle glaucoma.

Severe cerebrovascular insufficiency or hypotension are relative contra-indications to the use of Isosorbide mononitrate modified release tablets.

Sildenafil has been shown to potentiate the hypotensive effects of nitrates, and its co-administration with nitrates or nitric oxide donors is therefore contraindicated.

4.4 Special warnings and special precautions for use
The lowest effective dose should be used.

Attenuation of effect has occurred in some patients being treated with sustained release preparations. In such patients intermittent therapy may be more appropriate. (see section 4.2).

Therapy should not be discontinued suddenly. Both dosage and frequency should be tapered gradually (see section 4.2).

Caution should be exercised in patients suffering from hypothyroidism, malnutrition, hypothermia, and recent history of myocardial infarction.

Hypotension induced by nitrates may be accompanied by paradoxical bradycardia and increased angina.

Severe postural hypotension with light-headedness and dizziness is frequently observed after the consumption of alcohol.

Isosorbide mononitrate modified release tablets are not indicated for relief of acute anginal attacks: in the event of an acute attack, sublingual or buccal glyceryl trinitrate tablets should be used.

The administration of Isosorbide mononitrate causes a decrease of ERPF (Effective Renal Plasma Flow) in cirrhotic patients and its use in patients with renal impairment should be considered cautiously.

4.5 Interaction with other medicinal products and other forms of Interaction
The hypotensive effect of nitrates are potentiated by concurrent administration of sildenafil (see contra-indications), sublingual apomorphine and alcohol. There is a possibility that ISMN may enhance the hypotensive effect of 'hydralazine.

4.6 Pregnancy and lactation
The safety and efficacy of Isosorbide mononitrate modified release tablets during pregnancy or lactation has not been established.

4.7 Effects on ability to drive and use machines
The patient should be warned not to drive or operate machinery if hypotension or dizziness occurs.

4.8 Undesirable effects
Most of the adverse reactions are pharmacodynamically mediated and dose dependent.

Headache may occur when treatment is initiated, but usually disappears after 1-2 weeks of treatment. Flushing, dizziness, postural hypotension, tachycardia and paradoxical bradycardia have been reported. Hypotension with symptoms such as dizziness or nausea had occasionally been reported. These symptoms generally disappear during long-term treatment.

Rash and pruritus have been reported rarely. Myalgia has been reported very rarely.

4.9 Overdose
Symptoms

Pulsing headache. More serious symptoms are excitation, flushing, cold perspiration, nausea, vomiting, vertigo, syncope, tachycardia and a fall in blood pressure. A rise in intracranial pressure with confusion and neurological deficits can sometimes occur.

Management

Induction of emesis, activated charcoal. In case of pronounced hypotension the patient should first be placed in the supine position with legs raised. If necessary, fluids should be administrated intravenously.

Consider oral activated charcoal if ingestion of a potentially toxic amount has occurred within 1 hour. Observe for at least 12 hours after the overdose. Monitor blood pressure and pulse.

5. PHARMACOLOGICAL PROPERTIES
5.1 Pharmacodynamic properties
Organic nitrates (including GTN, ISDN, and ISMN) are potent relaxers of smooth muscle. They have a powerful effect on vascular smooth muscle with less effect on bronchiolar, gastrointestinal, ureteral and uterine smooth muscle. Low concentrations dilate both arteries and veins.

Venous dilation pools blood in the periphery leading to a decrease in venous return, central blood volume, and ventricular filling volumes and pressures. Cardiac output may remain unchanged or it may decline as a result of the decrease in venous return. Arterial blood pressure usually declines secondary to a decrease in cardiac output or arteriolar vasodilatation, or both. A modest reflex increase in heart rate results from the decrease in arterial blood pressure. Nitrates can dilate epicardial coronary arteries including atherosclerotic stenoses.

The cellular mechanism of nitrate-induced smooth muscle relaxation has become apparent in recent years. Nitrates enter the smooth muscle cell and are cleaved to inorganic nitrate and eventually to nitric oxide. This cleavage requires the presence of sulphydryl groups, which apparently come from the amino acid cysteine. Nitric oxide undergoes further reduction to nitrosothiol by further interaction with sulphydryl groups. Nitrosothiol activates guanylate cyclase in the vascular smooth muscle cells, thereby generating cyclic guanosine monophosphate (CGMP). It is this latter compound, CGMP, that produces smooth muscle relaxation by accelerating the release of calcium from these cells.

5.2 Pharmacokinetic properties
Absorption
Isosorbide-5-Mononitrate is readily absorbed from the gastro-intestinal tract.

Distribution
Following oral administration of conventional tablets, peak plasma levels are reached in about 1 hour. Unlike isosorbide dinitrate, ISMN does not undergo first pass hepatic metabolism and bioavailability is 100%. ISMN has a volume of distribution of about 40 litres and is not significantly protein bound.

Elimination
ISMN is metabolised to inactive metabolites including isosorbide and isosorbide glucuronide. The pharmacokinetics are unaffected by the presence of heart failure, renal or hepatic insufficiency. Only 20% of ISMN are excreted unchanged in the urine. An elimination half-life of about 4-5 hours has been reported.

5.3 Preclinical safety data
No relevant information additional to that already included elsewhere in the SPC.

6. PHARMACEUTICAL PARTICULARS
6.1 List of excipients
Stearic acid, carnauba wax, hydroxypropylmethylcellulose, lactose, magnesium stearate, talc, purified siliceous earth, polyethylene glycol 4000, E171, E172.

6.2 Incompatibilities
Not known.

6.3 Shelf life
3 years.

6.4 Special precautions for storage
Store in a dry place at or below 25°C. Protect from sunlight.

6.5 Nature and contents of container
The tablets are packed in aluminium foil/PVC blisters packed in boxes of 28, 30, 56, 60 and 100 oval, cream-coloured tablets, half-scored on both sides and marked ISMN on one side.

6.6 Instructions for use and handling
The tablets should be swallowed whole with half a glass of water. They must not be chewed or crushed.

Administrative Data
7. MARKETING AUTHORISATION HOLDER
Waymade PLC
t/a Sovereign Medical
Sovereign House
Miles Gray Road
Basildon
Essex, SS14 3FR

8. MARKETING AUTHORISATION NUMBER(S)
PL 06464/0506

9. DATE OF FIRST AUTHORISATION/RENEWAL OF THE AUTHORISATION
12 March 1998

10. DATE OF REVISION OF THE TEXT
April 2003

Chirocaine 0.625 mg/ml solution for infusion

(Abbott Laboratories Limited)

1. NAME OF THE MEDICINAL PRODUCT
Chirocaine 0.625 mg/ml solution for infusion

2. QUALITATIVE AND QUANTITATIVE COMPOSITION
Levobupivacaine hydrochloride corresponding to 0.625 mg/ml Levobupivacaine. For excipients, see section 6.1.

3. PHARMACEUTICAL FORM
Solution for infusion
Clear solution

4. CLINICAL PARTICULARS
4.1 Therapeutic indications
Adults
Pain management
Continuous epidural infusion, for the management of post operative pain and labour analgesia.

4.2 Posology and method of administration
Levobupivacaine should be administered only by, or under the supervision of, a clinician having the necessary training and experience.

Chirocaine Solution for Infusion is for epidural use only. It must not be used for intravenous administration.

(see Table 1 on next page)

Careful aspiration before infusion is recommended to prevent intravascular injection. If toxic symptoms occur, the injection should be stopped immediately.

Table 1

Type of Block	Concentration mg/ml	Infusion Rate Per Hour	
		ml	mg
Continuous Infusion: Post operative pain management	0.625	20-30	12.5-18.75
Lumbar epidural (analgesia in labour)	0.625	8-20	5-12.5

Maximum dose

The maximum dosage must be determined by evaluating the size and physical status of the patient. The maximum recommended dose during a 24 hour period is 400 mg.

For post-operative pain management, the dose should not exceed 18.75 mg/hour, however the accumulated dose for a 24 hour period should not exceed 400 mg. For labour analgesia by epidural infusion, the dose should not exceed 12.5 mg/ hour.

Children

The safety and efficacy of levobupivacaine in children for pain management has not been established.

Special Populations

Debilitated, elderly or acutely ill patients should be given reduced doses of levobupivacaine commensurate with their physical status.

In the management of post-operative pain, the dose given during surgery must be taken into account.

There are no relevant data in patients with hepatic impairment (see sections 4.4 and 5.2).

4.3 Contraindications

General contra-indications related to regional anaesthesia, regardless of the local anaesthetic used, should be taken into account.

Levobupivacaine solutions are contra-indicated in patients with a known hypersensitivity to levobupivacaine, local anaesthetics of the amide type or any of the excipients.

Levobupivacaine solutions are contra-indicated for intravenous regional anaesthesia (Bier's block).

Levobupivacaine solutions are contra-indicated in patients with severe hypotension such as cardiogenic or hypovolaemic shock.

Levobupivacaine solutions are contra-indicated for use in paracervical block in obstetrics (see section 4.6).

4.4 Special warnings and special precautions for use

All forms of local and regional anaesthesia with levobupivacaine should be performed in well-equipped facilities and administered by staff trained and experienced in the required anaesthetic techniques and able to diagnose and treat any unwanted adverse effects that may occur.

The introduction of local anesthetics via epidural administration into the central nervous system in patients with preexisting CNS diseases may potentially exacerbate some of these disease states. Therefore, clinical judgment should be exercised when contemplating epidural anesthesia in such patients.

During epidural administration of levobupivacaine, concentrated solutions (0.5-0.75%) should be administered in incremental doses of 3 to 5 ml with sufficient time between doses to detect toxic manifestations of unintentional intravascular or intrathecal injection. When a large dose is to be injected, e.g. in epidural block, a test dose of 3-5 ml lidocaine with adrenaline is recommended. An inadvertent intravascular injection may then be recognised by a temporary increase in heart rate and accidental intrathecal injection by signs of a spinal block. Syringe aspirations should also be performed before and during each supplemental injection in continuous (intermittent) catheter techniques. An intravascular injection is still possible even if aspirations for blood are negative. During the administration of epidural anesthesia, it is recommended that a test dose be administered initially and the effects monitored before the full dose is given.

Epidural anaesthesia with any local anaesthetic may cause hypotension and bradycardia. All patients must have intravenous access established. The availability of appropriate fluids, vasopressors, anaesthetics with anticonvulsant properties, myorelaxants, and atropine, resuscitation equipment and expertise must be ensured (see section 4.9).

Special populations

Debilitated, elderly or acutely ill patients: levobupivacaine should be used with caution in debilitated, elderly or acutely ill patients (see section 4.2).

Hepatic impairment: since levobupivacaine is metabolised in the liver, it should be used cautiously in patients with liver disease or with reduced liver blood flow e.g. alcoholics or cirrhotics (see section 5.2).

4.5 Interaction with other medicinal products and other forms of Interaction

In vitro studies indicate that the CYP3A4 isoform and CYP1A2 isoform mediate the metabolism of levobupivacaine. Although no clinical studies have been conducted, metabolism of levobupivacaine may be affected by CYP3A4 inhibitors eg: ketoconazole, and CYP1A2 inhibitors eg: methylxanthines.

Levobupivacaine should be used with caution in patients receiving anti-arrhythmic agents with local anaesthetic activity, e.g., mexiletine, or class III anti-arrhythmic agents since their toxic effects may be additive.

No clinical studies have been completed to assess levobupivacaine in combination with adrenaline.

4.6 Pregnancy and lactation

Pregnancy

Levobupivacaine solutions are contraindicated for use in paracervical block in obstetrics. Based on experience with bupivacaine foetal bradycardia may occur following paracervical block (see section 4.3).

For levobupivacaine, there are no clinical data on first trimester-exposed pregnancies. Animal studies do not indicate teratogenic effects but have shown embryo-foetal toxicity at systemic exposure levels in the same range as those obtained in clinical use (see section 5.3). The potential risk for human is unknown. Levobupivacaine should therefore not be given during early pregnancy unless clearly necessary.

Nevertheless, to date, the clinical experience of bupivacaine for obstetrical surgery (at the term of pregnancy or for delivery) is extensive and has not shown a foetotoxic effect.

Lactation

Levobupivacaine excretion in breast milk is unknown. However, levobupivacaine is likely to be poorly transmitted in the breast milk, as for bupivacaine. Thus breast feeding is possible after local anaesthesia.

4.7 Effects on ability to drive and use machines

Levobupivacaine can have a major influence on the ability to drive or use machines. Patients should be warned not to drive or operate machinery until all the effects of the anaesthesia and the immediate effects of surgery are passed.

4.8 Undesirable effects

Adverse reactions with local anaesthetics of the amide type are rare, but they may occur as a result of overdosage or unintentional intravascular injection and may be serious.

Accidental intrathecal injection of local anaesthetics can lead to very high spinal anaesthesia possibly with apnoea, severe hypotension and loss of consciousness.

Central nervous system effects: Numbness of the tongue, light headedness, dizziness, blurred vision and muscle twitch followed by drowsiness, convulsions, unconsciousness and possible respiratory arrest.

Cardiovascular effects are related to depression of the conduction system of the heart and a reduction in myocardial excitability and contractility. This results in decreased cardiac output, hypotension and ECG changes indicative of either heart block, bradycardia or ventricular tachyarrythmias that may lead to cardiac arrest. Usually these will be preceded by major CNS toxicity, i.e. convulsions, but in rare cases, cardiac arrest may occur without prodromal CNS effects.

SOC	FREQUENCY	ADVERSE EVENT
Blood and the lymphatic system disorders	Very Common	Anaemia
Nervous system disorders	Common Common	Dizziness Headache
Cardiac disorders	Very Common	Hypotension
Gastrointestinal disorders	Very Common Common	Nausea Vomiting
Pregnancy, puerperium and perinatal conditions	Common	Foetal distress
General disorders and administration site conditions	Common Common Common	Back pain Fever Post-operative pain

The most frequent adverse events reported in clinical trials irrespective of causality are listed in the table above.

Neurological damage is a rare but well recognised consequence of regional and particularly epidural and spinal anaesthesia. It may be due to direct injury to the spinal cord or spinal nerves, anterior spinal artery syndrome, injection of an irritant substance or an injection of a non-sterile solution. These may result in localised areas of paraesthesia or anaesthesia, motor weakness, loss of sphincter control and paraplegia. Rarely, these may be permanent.

Postmarketing reports

Very rare reports of convulsions have occurred following accidental intravenous administration.

4.9 Overdose

Accidental intravascular injection of local anaesthetics may cause immediate toxic reactions. In the event of overdose, peak plasma concentrations may not be reached until 2 hours after administration depending upon the injection site and, therefore, signs of toxicity may be delayed. The effects of the drug may be prolonged.

Systemic adverse reactions following overdose or accidental intravascular injection reported with long acting local anaesthetic agents involve both CNS and cardiovascular effects.

CNS Effects

Convulsions should be treated immediately with intravenous thiopentone or diazepam titrated as necessary. Thiopentone and diazepam also depress central nervous system, respiratory and cardiac function. Therefore, their use may result in apnoea. Neuro-muscular blockers may be used only if the clinician is confident ofmaintaining a patient airway and managing a fully paralysed patient.

If not treated promptly, convulsions with subsequent hypoxia and hypercarbia plus myocardial depression from the effects of the local anaesthetic on the heart, may result in cardiac arrhythmias, ventricular fibrillation or cardiac arrest.

Cardiovascular Effects

Hypotension may be prevented or attenuated by pre-treatment with a fluid load and/or the use of vasopressors. If hypotension occurs it should be treated with intravenous crystalloids or colloids and/or incremental doses of a vasopressor such as ephedrine 5-10 mg. Any coexisting causes of hypotension should be rapidly treated.

If severe bradycardia occurs, treatment with atropine 0.3-1.0 mg will normally restore the heart rate to an acceptable level.

Cardiac arrhythmia should be treated as required and ventricular fibrillation should be treated by cardioversion.

5. PHARMACOLOGICAL PROPERTIES

5.1 Pharmacodynamic properties

Pharmacotherapeutic group: Local anaesthetics, amide

ATC Code N01B B10

Levobupivacaine is a long acting local anaesthetic and analgesic. It blocks nerve conduction in sensory and motor nerves largely by interacting with voltage sensitive sodium channels on the cell membrane, but also potassium and calcium channels are blocked. In addition, levobupivacaine interferes with impulse transmission and conduction in other tissues where effects on the cardiovascular and central nervous systems are most important for the occurrence of clinical adverse reactions.

The dose of levobupivacaine is expressed as base, whereas, in the racemate bupivacaine the dose is expressed as hydrochloride salt. This gives rise to approximately 13% more active substance in levobupivacaine solutions compared to bupivacaine. In clinical studies at the same nominal concentrations levobupivacaine showed similar clinical effect to bupivacaine.

In a clinical pharmacology study using the ulnar nerve block model, levobupivacaine was equipotent with bupivacaine.

5.2 Pharmacokinetic properties

In human studies, the distribution kinetics of levobupivacaine following i.v. administration are essentially the same as bupivacaine. The plasma concentration of levobupivacaine following therapeutic administration depends on dose and, as absorption from the site of administration is affected by the vascularity of the tissue, on route of administration.

There are no relevant data in patients with hepatic impairment (see section 4.4).

There are no data in patients with renal impairment. Levobupivacaine is extensively metabolised and unchanged levobupivacaine is not excreted in urine.

Plasma protein binding of levobupivacaine in man was evaluated *in vitro* and was found to be > 97% at concentrations between 0.1 and 1.0 μg/ml.

In a clinical pharmacology study where 40 mg levobupivacaine was given by intravenous administration, the mean half-life was approximately 80 $\pm$ 22 minutes, C_{max} 1.4 $\pm$ 0.2 μg/ml and AUC 70 $\pm$ 27 μg•min/ml.

The mean C_{max} and AUC(0-24h) of levobupivacaine were approximately dose-proportional following epidural administration of 75 mg (0.5%) and 112.5 mg (0.75%) and following doses of 1 mg/kg (0.25%) and 2 mg/kg (0.5%) used for brachial plexus block. Following epidural administration of 112.5 mg (0.75%) the mean C_{max} and

AUC values were 0.58 μg/ml and 3.56 μg•h/ml respectively.

The mean total plasma clearance and terminal half-life of levobupivacaine after intravenous infusion were 39 litres/hour and 1.3 hours, respectively. The volume of distribution after intravenous administration was 67 litres.

Levobupivacaine is extensively metabolised with no unchanged levobupivacaine detected in urine or faeces. 3-hydroxylevobupivacaine, a major metabolite of levobupivacaine, is excreted in the urine as glucuronic acid and sulphate ester conjugates. *In vitro* studies showed that CYP3A4 isoform and CYP1A2 isoform mediate the metabolism of levobupivacaine to desbutyl-levobupivacaine and 3-hydroxylevobupivacaine respectively. These studies indicate that the metabolism of levobupivacaine and bupivacaine are similar.

Following intravenous administration, recovery of levobupivacaine was quantitative with a mean total of about 95% being recovered in urine (71%) and faeces (24%) in 48 hours.

There is no evidence of *in vivo* racemisation of levobupivacaine.

5.3 Preclinical safety data

In an embryo-foetal toxicity study in rats, an increased incidence of dilated renal pelvis, dilated ureters, olfactory ventricle dilatation and extra thoraco-lumbar ribs was observed at systemic exposure levels in the same range as those obtained at clinical use. There were no treatment-related malformations.

Levobupivacaine was not genotoxic in a standard battery of assays for mutagenicity and clastogenicity. No carcinogenicity testing has been conducted.

6. PHARMACEUTICAL PARTICULARS

6.1 List of excipients

Sodium Chloride

Sodium Hydroxide

Hydrochloric acid

Water for Injections

6.2 Incompatibilities

Levobupivacaine may precipitate if diluted with alkaline solutions and should not be diluted or co-administered with sodium bicarbonate injections. This medicinal product must not be mixed with other medicinal products except those mentioned in section 6.6.

6.3 Shelf life

Shelf life as packaged for sale: 2 years

Shelf life after first opening: The product should be used immediately after opening.

Chemical and physical in-use stability has been demonstrated for both levobupivacaine 0.625 mg/ml and 1.25 mg/ml with 8.3-8,4 μg/ml clonidine, 50 μg /ml morphine and 2 μg /ml fentanyl, respectively, stored for 30 days at either 2-8°C or 20–22°C. Chemical and physical in-use stability has been demonstrated for both levobupivacaine 0.625 mg/ml and 1.25 mg/ml with sufentanil added in the concentration of 0.4 μg /ml and stored for 30 days at 2-8°C or 7 days at 20–22°C.

From a microbiological point of view, the product should be used immediately after opening. If not used immediately, in-use storage times and conditions prior to use are the responsibility of the user and would normally not be longer than 24 hours at 2-8°C, unless the admix has been prepared in controlled and validated aseptic conditions.

6.4 Special precautions for storage

This medicinal product does not require any special storage conditions

6.5 Nature and contents of container

Chirocaine is available in two presentations;

• 100 ml solution in a 100 ml flexible polyester bag with an aluminium foil overpouch.

• 200 ml solution in a 250 ml flexible polyester bag with an aluminium foil overpouch.

Each polyester bag contains one PVC admixture port and one PVC administration port.

Pack sizes: 5 bags of the 100 ml solution.

5 bags of the 200 ml solution.

24 bags of the 100 ml solution.

12 bags of the 200 ml solution.

60 bags of the 100 ml solution.

32 bags of the 200 ml solution.

Not all pack sizes may be marketed.

6.6 Instructions for use and handling

For single epidural use only. Do not use unless the solution is clear and container is undamaged. Discard any unused solution.

The solution/dilution should be inspected visually prior to use. Only clear solutions without visible particles should be used.

7. MARKETING AUTHORISATION HOLDER

Abbott Laboratories limited

Queenborough

Kent

ME11 5EL

United Kingdom

8. MARKETING AUTHORISATION NUMBER(S)

Chirocaine 0.625 mg/ml: PL 00037/0404

9. DATE OF FIRST AUTHORISATION/RENEWAL OF THE AUTHORISATION

20 August 2003/ 13 October 2004

10. DATE OF REVISION OF THE TEXT

13 October 2004

Chirocaine 1.25 mg/ml solution for infusion

(Abbott Laboratories Limited)

1. NAME OF THE MEDICINAL PRODUCT

Chirocaine 1.25 mg/ml solution for infusion

2. QUALITATIVE AND QUANTITATIVE COMPOSITION

Levobupivacaine hydrochloride corresponding to 1.25 mg/ml Levobupivacaine. For excipients, see section 6.1.

3. PHARMACEUTICAL FORM

Solution for infusion

Clear solution

4. CLINICAL PARTICULARS

4.1 Therapeutic indications

Adults

Pain management

Continuous epidural infusion, for the management of post operative pain and labour analgesia.

4.2 Posology and method of administration

Levobupivacaine should be administered only by, or under the supervision of, a clinician having the necessary training and experience.

Chirocaine Solution for Infusion is for epidural use only. It must not be used for intravenous administration.

(see Table 1)

Careful aspiration before infusion is recommended to prevent intravascular injection. If toxic symptoms occur, the injection should be stopped immediately.

Maximum dose

The maximum dosage must be determined by evaluating the size and physical status of the patient. The maximum recommended dose during a 24 hour period is 400 mg.

For post-operative pain management, the dose should not exceed 18.75 mg/hour, however the accumulated dose for a 24 hour period should not exceed 400 mg. For labour analgesia by epidural infusion, the dose should not exceed 12.5 mg/ hour.

Children

The safety and efficacy of levobupivacaine in children for pain management has not been established.

Special Populations

Debilitated, elderly or acutely ill patients should be given reduced doses of levobupivacaine commensurate with their physical status.

In the management of post-operative pain, the dose given during surgery must be taken into account.

There are no relevant data in patients with hepatic impairment (see sections 4.4 and 5.2).

4.3 Contraindications

General contra-indications related to regional anaesthesia, regardless of the local anaesthetic used, should be taken into account.

Levobupivacaine solutions are contra-indicated in patients with a known hypersensitivity to levobupivacaine, local anaesthetics of the amide type or any of the excipients.

Levobupivacaine solutions are contra-indicated for intravenous regional anaesthesia (Bier's block).

Levobupivacaine solutions are contra-indicated in patients with severe hypotension such as cardiogenic or hypovolaemic shock.

Levobupivacaine solutions are contra-indicated for use in paracervical block in obstetrics (see section 4.6).

4.4 Special warnings and special precautions for use

All forms of local and regional anaesthesia with levobupivacaine should be performed in well-equipped facilities and administered by staff trained and experienced in the required anaesthetic techniques and able to diagnose and treat any unwanted adverse effects that may occur.

The introduction of local anesthetics via epidural administration into the central nervous system in patients with preexisting CNS diseases may potentially exacerbate some of these disease states. Therefore, clinical judgment should be exercised when contemplating epidural anesthesia in such patients.

During epidural administration of levobupivacaine, concentrated solutions (0.5-0.75%) should be administered in incremental doses of 3 to 5 ml with sufficient time between doses to detect toxic manifestations of unintentional intravascular or intrathecal injection. When a large dose is to be injected, e.g. in epidural block, a test dose of 3-5 ml lidocaine with adrenaline is recommended. An inadvertent intravascular injection may then be recognised by a temporary increase in heart rate and accidental intrathecal injection by signs of a spinal block. Syringe aspirations should also be performed before and during each supplemental injection in continuous (intermittent) catheter techniques. An intravascular injection is still possible even if aspirations for blood are negative. During the administration of epidural anesthesia, it is recommended that a test dose be administered initially and the effects monitored before the full dose is given.

Epidural anaesthesia with any local anaesthetic may cause hypotension and bradycardia. All patients must have intravenous access established. The availability of appropriate fluids, vasopressors, anaesthetics with anticonvulsant properties, myorelaxants, and atropine, resuscitation equipment and expertise must be ensured (see section 4.9).

Special populations

Debilitated, elderly or acutely ill patients: levobupivacaine should be used with caution in debilitated, elderly or acutely ill patients (see section 4.2).

Hepatic impairment: since levobupivacaine is metabolised in the liver, it should be used cautiously in patients with liver disease or with reduced liver blood flow e.g. alcoholics or cirrhotics (see section 5.2).

4.5 Interaction with other medicinal products and other forms of Interaction

In vitro studies indicate that the CYP3A4 isoform and CYP1A2 isoform mediate the metabolism of levobupivacaine. Although no clinical studies have been conducted, metabolism of levobupivacaine may be affected by CYP3A4 inhibitors eg: ketoconazole, and CYP1A2 inhibitors eg: methylxanthines.

Levobupivacaine should be used with caution in patients receiving anti-arrhythmic agents with local anaesthetic activity, e.g., mexiletine, or class III anti-arrhythmic agents since their toxic effects may be addictive.

No clinical studies have been completed to assess levobupivacaine in combination with adrenaline.

4.6 Pregnancy and lactation

Pregnancy

Levobupivacaine solutions are contraindicated for use in paracervical block in obstetrics. Based on experience with bupivacaine foetal bradycardia may occur following paracervical block (see section 4.3).

For levobupivacaine, there are no clinical data on first trimester-exposed pregnancies. Animal studies do not indicate teratogenic effects but have shown embryo-foetal toxicity at systemic exposure levels in the same range as those obtained in clinical use (see section 5.3). The potential risk for human is unknown. Levobupivacaine should therefore not be given during early pregnancy unless clearly necessary.

Nevertheless, to date, the clinical experience of bupivacaine for obstetrical surgery (at the term of pregnancy or for delivery) is extensive and has not shown a foetotoxic effect.

Lactation

Levobupivacaine excretion in breast milk is unknown. However, levobupivacaine is likely to be poorly transmitted in the breast milk, as for bupivacaine. Thus breast feeding is possible after local anaesthesia.

4.7 Effects on ability to drive and use machines

Levobupivacaine can have a major influence on the ability to drive or use machines. Patients should be warned not to drive or operate machinery until all the effects of the anaesthesia and the immediate effects of surgery are passed.

4.8 Undesirable effects

Adverse reactions with local anaesthetics of the amide type are rare, but they may occur as a result of overdosage or unintentional intravascular injection and may be serious.

Accidental intrathecal injection of local anaesthetics can lead to very high spinal anaesthesia possibly with apnoea, severe hypotension and loss of consciousness.

Table 1

Type of Block	Concentration mg/ml	Infusion Rate Per Hour	
		ml	mg
Continuous Infusion: Post operative pain management	1.25	10-15	12.5-18.75
Lumbar epidural (analgesia in labour)	1.25	4-10	5–12.5

Central nervous system effects: Numbness of the tongue, light headedness, dizziness, blurred vision and muscle twitch followed by drowsiness, convulsions, unconsciousness and possible respiratory arrest.

Cardiovascular effects are related to depression of the conduction system of the heart and a reduction in myocardial excitability and contractility. This results in decreased cardiac output, hypotension and ECG changes indicative of either heart block, bradycardia or ventricular tachyarrythmias that may lead to cardiac arrest. Usually these will be preceded by major CNS toxicity, i.e. convulsions, but in rare cases, cardiac arrest may occur without prodromal CNS effects.

SOC	FREQUENCY	ADVERSE EVENT
Blood and the lymphatic system disorders	Very Common	Anaemia
Nervous system disorders	Common	Dizziness Headache
Cardiac disorders	Very Common	Hypotension
Gastrointestinal disorders	Very Common Common	Nausea Vomiting
Pregnancy, puerperium and perinatal conditions	Common	Foetal distress
General disorders and administration site conditions	Common Common Common	Back pain Fever Post-operative pain

The most frequent adverse events reported in clinical trials irrespective of causality are listed in the table above.

Neurological damage is a rare but well recognised consequence of regional and particularly epidural and spinal anaesthesia. It may be due to direct injury to the spinal cord or spinal nerves, anterior spinal artery syndrome, injection of an irritant substance or an injection of a non-sterile solution. These may result in localised areas of paraesthesia or anaesthesia, motor weakness, loss of sphincter control and paraplegia. Rarely, these may be permanent.

Postmarketing reports

Very rare reports of convulsions have occurred following accidental intravenous administration.

4.9 Overdose

Accidental intravascular injection of local anaesthetics may cause immediate toxic reactions. In the event of overdose, peak plasma concentrations may not be reached until 2 hours after administration depending upon the injection site and, therefore, signs of toxicity may be delayed. The effects of the drug may be prolonged.

Systemic adverse reactions following overdose or accidental intravascular injection reported with long acting local anaesthetic agents involve both CNS and cardiovascular effects.

CNS Effects

Convulsions should be treated immediately with intravenous thiopentone or diazepam titrated as necessary. Thiopentone and diazepam also depress central nervous system, respiratory and cardiac function. Therefore their use may result in apnoea. Neuro-muscular blockers may be used only if the clinician is confident ofmaintaining a patent airway and managing a fully paralysed patient.

If not treated promptly, convulsions with subsequent hypoxia and hypercarbia plus myocardial depression from the effects of the local anaesthetic on the heart, may result in cardiac arrhythmias, ventricular fibrillation or cardiac arrest.

Cardiovascular Effects

Hypotension may be prevented or attenuated by pre-treatment with a fluid load and/or the use of vasopressors. If hypotension occurs it should be treated with intravenous crystalloids or colloids and/or incremental doses of a vasopressor such as ephedrine 5-10 mg. Any coexisting causes of hypotension should be rapidly treated.

If severe bradycardia occurs, treatment with atropine 0.3-1.0 mg will normally restore the heart rate to an acceptable level.

Cardiac arrhythmia should be treated as required and ventricular fibrillation should be treated by cardioversion.

5. PHARMACOLOGICAL PROPERTIES

5.1 Pharmacodynamic properties

Pharmacotherapeutic group: Local anaesthetics, amide

ATC Code N01B B10

Levobupivacaine is a long acting local anaesthetic and analgesic. It blocks nerve conduction in sensory and motor nerves largely by interacting with voltage sensitive sodium channels on the cell membrane, but also potassium and calcium channels are blocked. In addition, levobupivacaine interferes with impulse transmission and conduction in other tissues where effects on the cardiovascular and central nervous systems are most important for the occurrence of clinical adverse reactions.

The dose of levobupivacaine is expressed as base, whereas, in the racemate bupivacaine the dose is expressed as hydrochloride salt. This gives rise to approximately 13% more active substance in levobupivacaine solutions compared to bupivacaine. In clinical studies at the same nominal concentrations levobupivacaine showed similar clinical effect to bupivacaine.

In a clinical pharmacology study using the ulnar nerve block model, levobupivacaine was equipotent with bupivacaine.

5.2 Pharmacokinetic properties

In human studies, the distribution kinetics of levobupivacaine following i.v. administration are essentially the same as bupivacaine. The plasma concentration of levobupivacaine following therapeutic administration depends on dose and, as absorption from the site of administration is affected by the vascularity of the tissue, on route of administration.

There are no relevant data in patients with hepatic impairment (see section 4.4).

There are no data in patients with renal impairment. Levobupivacaine is extensively metabolised and unchanged levobupivacaine is not excreted in urine.

Plasma protein binding of levobupivacaine in man was evaluated *in vitro* and was found to be $> 97\%$ at concentrations between 0.1 and 1.0 μg/ml.

In a clinical pharmacology study where 40 mg levobupivacaine was given by intravenous administration, the mean half-life was approximately 80 $\pm$ 22 minutes, C_{max} 1.4 $\pm$ 0.2 μg/ml and AUC 70 $\pm$ 27 μg•min/ml.

The mean C_{max} and AUC(0-24h) of levobupivacaine were approximately dose-proportional following epidural administration of 75 mg (0.5%) and 112.5 mg (0.75%) and following doses of 1 mg/kg (0.25%) and 2 mg/kg (0.5%) used for brachial plexus block. Following epidural administration of 112.5 mg (0.75%) the mean C_{max} and AUC values were 0.58 μg/ml and 3.56 μg•h/ml respectively.

The mean total plasma clearance and terminal half-life of levobupivacaine after intravenous infusion were 39 litres/hour and 1.3 hours, respectively. The volume of distribution after intravenous administration was 67 litres.

Levobupivacaine is extensively metabolised with no unchanged levobupivacaine detected in urine or faeces. 3-hydroxylevobupivacaine, a major metabolite of levobupivacaine, is excreted in the urine as glucuronic acid and sulphate ester conjugates. *In vitro* studies showed that CYP3A4 isoform and CYP1A2 isoform mediate the metabolism of levobupivacaine to desbutyl-levobupivacaine and 3-hydroxylevobupivacaine respectively. These studies indicate that the metabolism of levobupivacaine and bupivacaine are similar.

Following intravenous administration, recovery of levobupivacaine was quantitative with a mean total of about 95% being recovered in urine (71%) and faeces (24%) in 48 hours.

There is no evidence of *in vivo* racemisation of levobupivacaine.

5.3 Preclinical safety data

In an embryo-foetal toxicity study in rats, an increased incidence of dilated renal pelvis, dilated ureters, olfactory ventricle dilatation and extra thoraco-lumbar ribs was observed at systemic exposure levels in the same range as those obtained at clinical use. There were no treatment-related malformations.

Levobupivacaine was not genotoxic in a standard battery of assays for mutagenicity and clastogenicity. No carcinogenicity testing has been conducted.

6. PHARMACEUTICAL PARTICULARS

6.1 List of excipients

Sodium Chloride

Sodium Hydroxide

Hydrochloric acid

Water for Injections

6.2 Incompatibilities

Levobupivacaine may precipitate if diluted with alkaline solutions and should not be diluted or co-administered with sodium bicarbonate injections. This medicinal product must not be mixed with other medicinal products except those mentioned in section 6.6.

6.3 Shelf life

Shelf life as packaged for sale: 2 years

Shelf life after first opening: The product should be used immediately after opening.

Chemical and physical in-use stability has been demonstrated for both levobupivacaine 0.625 mg/ml and 1.25 mg/ml with 8.3-8.4 μg/ml clonidine, 50 μg/ml morphine and 2 μg/ml fentanyl, respectively, stored for 30 days at either 2-8°C or 20–22°C. Chemical and physical in-use stability has been demonstrated for both levobupivacaine 0.625 mg/ml and 1.25 mg/ml with sufentanil added in the concentration of 0.4 μg/ml and stored for 30 days at 2-8°C or 7 days at 20–22°C.

From a microbiological point of view, the product should be used immediately after opening. If not used immediately, in-use storage times and conditions prior to use are the responsibility of the user and would normally not be longer than 24 hours at 2-8°C, unless the admix has been prepared in controlled and validated aseptic conditions.

6.4 Special precautions for storage

This medicinal product does not require any special storage conditions

6.5 Nature and contents of container

Chirocaine is available in two presentations;

- 100 ml solution in a 100 ml flexible polyester bag with an aluminium foil overpouch.
- 200 ml solution in a 250 ml flexible polyester bag with an aluminium foil overpouch.

Each polyester bag contains one PVC admixture port and one PVC administration port.

Pack sizes: 5 bags of the 100 ml solution.

5 bags of the 200 ml solution.

24 bags of the 100 ml solution.

12 bags of the 200 ml solution.

60 bags of the 100 ml solution.

32 bags of the 200 ml solution.

Not all pack sizes may be marketed.

6.6 Instructions for use and handling

For single epidural use only. Do not use unless the solution is clear and container is undamaged. Discard any unused solution.

The solution/dilution should be inspected visually prior to use. Only clear solutions without visible particles should be used.

7. MARKETING AUTHORISATION HOLDER

Abbott Laboratories limited

Queenborough

Kent

ME11 5EL

United Kingdom

8. MARKETING AUTHORISATION NUMBER(S)

PL 00037/0405

9. DATE OF FIRST AUTHORISATION/RENEWAL OF THE AUTHORISATION

20 August 2003/ 13 October 2004

10. DATE OF REVISION OF THE TEXT

13 October 2004

Chirocaine 2.5, 5.0 & 7.5 mg/ml

(Abbott Laboratories Limited)

1. NAME OF THE MEDICINAL PRODUCT

Chirocaine 2.5 mg/ml, 5 mg/ml and 7.5 mg/ml solution for injection/concentrate

for solution for infusion.

2. QUALITATIVE AND QUANTITATIVE COMPOSITION

One ml contains 2.5 mg, 5 mg or 7.5 mg levobupivacaine as levobupivacaine hydrochloride.

Each ampoule contains 25 mg, 50 mg or 75 mg in 10 ml. For excipients, see section 6.1.

3. PHARMACEUTICAL FORM

Solution for injection/concentrate for solution for infusion.

Clear colourless solution, practically free of particles.

4. CLINICAL PARTICULARS

4.1 Therapeutic indications

Adults

Surgical anaesthesia

–Major, e.g. epidural (including for caesarean section), intrathecal, peripheral nerve block.

–Minor, e.g. local infiltration, peribulbar block in ophthalmic surgery.

Pain management

–Continuous epidural infusion, single or multiple bolus epidural administration for the management of pain especially post-operative pain or labour analgesia.

Children

Analgesia (ilioinguinal/iliohypogastric blocks).

4.2 Posology and method of administration

Levobupivacaine should be administered only by, or under the supervision of, a clinician having the necessary training and experience.

The table below is a guide to dosage for the more commonly used blocks. For analgesia (e.g. epidural administration for pain management), the lower concentrations and doses are recommended. Where profound or prolonged anaesthesia is required with dense motor block (e.g. epidural or peribulbar block), the higher concentrations may be used. Careful aspiration before and during injection is recommended to prevent intravascular injection.

Aspiration should be repeated before and during administration of a bolusdose, which should be injected slowly andin incremental doses, at a rate of 7.5–30 mg/min, while closely observing the patient's vital functions and maintaining verbal contact.

If toxic symptoms occur, the injection should be stopped immediately.

Maximum dose

The maximum dosage must be determined by evaluating the size and physical status of the patient, together with the concentration of the agent and the area and route of administration. Individual variation in onset and duration of block does occur. Experience from clinical studies shows onset of sensory block adequate for surgery in 10-15 minutes following epidural administration, with a time to regression in the range of 6-9 hours.

The recommended maximum single dose is 150 mg. Where sustained motor and sensory block are required for a prolonged procedure, additional doses may be required. The maximum recommended dose during a 24 hour period is 400 mg. For post-operative pain management, the dose should not exceed 18.75 mg/hour.

Obstetrics

For caesarean section, higher concentrations than the 5.0 mg/ml solution should not be used (See section 4.3). The maximum recommended dose is 150 mg.

For labour analgesia by epidural infusion, the dose should not exceed 12.5 mg/hour.

Children

In children, the maximum recommended dose for analgesia (ilioinguinal/iliohypogastric blocks) is 1.25 mg/kg/side.

The safety and efficacy of levobupivacaine in children for other indications have not been established.

Special populations

Debilitated, elderly or acutely ill patients should be given reduced doses of levobupivacaine commensurate with their physical status.

In the management of post-operative pain, the dose given during surgery must be taken into account.

There are no relevant data in patients with hepatic impairment (see sections 4.4 and 5.2).

Table of Doses

(see Table 1)

4.3 Contraindications

General contra-indications related to regional anaesthesia, regardless of the local anaesthetic used, should be taken into account.

Levobupivacaine solutions are contra-indicated in patients with a known hypersensitivity to levobupivacaine, local anaesthetics of the amide type or any of the excipients.

Levobupivacaine solutions are contra-indicated for intravenous regional anaesthesia (Bier's block).

Levobupivacaine solutions are contra-indicated in patients with severe hypotension such as cardiogenic or hypovolaemic shock.

Levobupivacaine solutions are contra-indicated for use in paracervical block in obstetrics (see section 4.6).

4.4 Special warnings and special precautions for use

All forms of local and regional anaesthesia with levobupivacaine should be performed in well-equipped facilities and administered by staff trained and experienced in the required anaesthetic techniques and able to diagnose and treat any unwanted adverse effects that may occur.

Levobupivacaine should be used with caution for regional anaesthesia in patients with impaired cardiovascular function e.g. serious cardiac arrhythmias.

The introduction of local anesthetics via either intrathecal or epidural administration into the central nervous system in patients with preexisting CNS diseases may potentially exacerbate some of these disease states. Therefore, clinical judgment should be exercised when contemplating epidural or intrathecal anesthesia in such patients.

Epidural Anesthesia

During epidural administration of levobupivacaine, concentrated solutions (0.5-0.75%) should be administered in incremental doses of 3 to 5 ml with sufficient time between doses to detect toxic manifestations of unintentional intravascular or intrathecal injection. When a large dose is to be injected, e.g. in epidural block, a test dose of 3-5 ml lidocaine with adrenaline is recommended. An inadvertent intravascular injection may then be recognised by a temporary increase in heart rate and accidental intrathecal injection by signs of a spinal block.

Syringe aspirations should also be performed before and during each supplemental injection in continuous (intermittent) catheter techniques. An intravascular injection is still possible even if aspirations for blood are negative. During the administration of epidural anesthesia, it is recommended that a test dose be administered initially and the effects monitored before the full dose is given.

Epidural anaesthesia with any local anaesthetic may cause hypotension and bradycardia. All patients must have intravenous access established. The availability of appropriate fluids, vasopressors, anaesthetics with anticonvulsant properties, myorelaxants, and atropine, resuscitation equipment and expertise must be ensured (see section 4.9).

Major regional nerve blocks

The patient should have I.V. fluids running via an indwelling catheter to assure a functioning intravenous pathway. The lowest dosage of local anesthetic that results in effective anesthesia should be used to avoid high plasma levels and serious adverse effects. The rapid injection of a large volume of local anesthetic solution should be avoided and fractional (incremental) doses should be used when feasible.

Table 1 Table of Doses

	Concentration (mg/ml)[1]	Dose	Motor Block
Surgical Anaesthesia			
Epidural (slow) bolus[2] for surgery - Adults	5.0-7.5	10-20 ml (50-150 mg)	Moderate to complete
Epidural slow injection[3] for Caesarean Section	5.0	15-30 ml (75-150 mg)	Moderate to complete
Intrathecal	5.0	3 ml (15 mg)	Moderate to complete
Peripheral Nerve	2.5-5.0	1-40 ml (2.5-150 mg max.)	Moderate to complete
Ilioinguinal/Iliohypogastric blocks in children < 12 years	2.5-5.0	0.25-0.5 ml/kg (0.625-2.5 mg/kg)	Not applicable
Ophthalmic (peribulbar block)	7.5	5–15 ml (37.5-112.5 mg)	Moderate to complete
Local Infiltration - Adults	2.5	1-60 ml (2.5-150 mg max.)	Not applicable
Pain Management[4]			
Labour Analgesia (epidural bolus[5])	2.5	6-10 ml (15-25 mg)	Minimal to moderate
Labour Analgesia (epidural infusion)	1.25[6]	4-10 ml/h (5-12.5 mg/h)	Minimal to moderate
Post-operative pain	1.25[6] 2.5	10-15ml/h (12.5-18.75mg/h) 5-7.5ml/h (12.5 –18.75mg/h)	Minimal to moderate

[1] Levobupivacaine solution for injection/concentration for solution for infusion is available in 2.5, 5.0 and 7.5 mg/ml solutions.

[2] Spread over 5 minutes (see also text).

[3] Given over 15-20 minutes.

[4] In cases where levobupivacaine is combined with other agents e.g. opioids in pain management, the levobupivacaine dose should be reduced and use of a lower concentration (e.g. 1.25 mg/ml) is preferable.

[5] The minimum recommended interval between intermittent injections is 15 minutes.

[6] For information on dilution, see section 6.6.

Use in Head and Neck Area

Small doses of local anesthetics injected into the head and neck area, including retrobulbar, dental and stellate ganglion blocks, may produce adverse reactions similar to systemic toxicity seen with unintentional intravascular injections of larger doses. The injection procedures require the utmost care. Reactions may be due to intraarterial injection of the local anesthetic with retrograde flow to the cerebral circulation. They may also be due to puncture of the dural sheath of the optic nerve during retrobulbar block with diffusion of any local anesthetic along the subdural space to the midbrain. Patients receiving these blocks should have their circulation and respiration monitored and be constantly observed. Resuscitative equipment and personnel for treating adverse reactions should be immediately available.

Use in Ophthalmic Surgery

Clinicians who perform retrobulbar blocks should be aware that there have been reports of respiratory arrest following local anesthetic injection. Prior to retrobulbar block, as with all other regional procedures, the immediate availability of equipment, drugs, and personnel to manage respiratory arrest or depression, convulsions, and cardiac stimulation or depression should be assured. As with other anesthetic procedures, patients should be constantly monitored following ophthalmic blocks for signs of these adverse reactions.

Special populations

Debilitated, elderly or acutely ill patients: levobupivacaine should be used with caution in debilitated, elderly or acutely ill patients (see section 4.2).

Hepatic impairment: since levobupivacaine is metabolised in the liver, it should be used cautiously in patients with liver disease or with reduced liver blood flow e.g. alcoholics or cirrhotics (see section 5.2).

4.5 Interaction with other medicinal products and other forms of Interaction

In vitro studies indicate that the CYP3A4 isoform and CYP1A2 isoform mediate the metabolism of levobupivacaine. Although no clinical studies have been conducted, metabolism of levobupivacaine may be affected by CYP3A4 inhibitors eg: ketoconazole, and CYP1A2 inhibitors eg: methylxanthines.

Levobupivacaine should be used with caution in patients receiving anti-arrhythmic agents with local anaesthetic activity, e.g., mexiletine, or class III anti-arrhythmic agents since their toxic effects may be additive.

No clinical studies have been completed to assess levobupivacaine in combination with adrenaline.

4.6 Pregnancy and lactation

Pregnancy

Levobupivacaine solutions are contraindicated for use in paracervical block in obstetrics. Based on experience with bupivacaine foetal bradycardia may occur following paracervical block (see section 4.3).

For levobupivacaine, there are no clinical data on first trimester-exposed pregnancies. Animal studies do not indicate teratogenic effects but have shown embryo-foetal toxicity at systemic exposure levels in the same range as those obtained in clinical use (see section 5.3). The potential risk for human is unknown. Levobupivacaine should therefore not be given during early pregnancy unless clearly necessary.

Nevertheless, to date, the clinical experience of bupivacaine for obstetrical surgery (at the term of pregnancy or for delivery) is extensive and has not shown a foetotoxic effect.

Lactation

Levobupivacaine excretion in breast milk is unknown. However, levobupivacaine is likely to be poorly transmitted in the breast milk, as for bupivacaine. Thus breast feeding is possible after local anaesthesia.

4.7 Effects on ability to drive and use machines

Levobupivacaine can have a major influence on the ability to drive or use machines. Patients should be warned not to drive or operate machinery until all the effects of the anaesthesia and the immediate effects of surgery are passed.

4.8 Undesirable effects

Adverse reactions with local anaesthetics of the amide type are rare, but they may occur as a result of overdosage or unintentional intravascular injection and may be serious.

Accidental intrathecal injection of local anaesthetics can lead to very high spinal anaesthesia possibly with apnoea, severe hypotension and loss of consciousness.

Central nervous system effects: Numbness of the tongue, light headedness, dizziness, blurred vision and muscle twitch followed by drowsiness, convulsions, unconsciousness and possible respiratory arrest.

Cardiovascular effects are related to depression of the conduction system of the heart and a reduction in myocardial excitability and contractility. This results in decreased cardiac output, hypotension and ECG changes indicative of either heart block, bradycardia or ventricular tachyarrythmias that may lead to cardiac arrest. Usually these will be preceded by major CNS toxicity, i.e. convulsions, but in rare cases, cardiac arrest may occur without prodromal CNS effects.

SOC	FREQUENCY	ADVERSE EVENT
Blood and the lymphatic system disorders	Very Common	Anaemia
Nervous system disorders	Common	Dizziness Headache
Cardiac disorders	Very Common	Hypotension
Gastrointestinal disorders	Very Common Common	Nausea Vomiting
Pregnancy, puerperium and perinatal conditions	Common	Foetal distress
General disorders and administration site conditions	Common Common Common	Back pain Fever Post-operative pain

The most frequent adverse events reported in clinical trials irrespective of causality are listed in the table above.

Neurological damage is a rare but well recognised consequence of regional and particularly epidural and spinal anaesthesia. It may be due to direct injury to the spinal cord or spinal nerves, anterior spinal artery syndrome, injection of an irritant substance or an injection of a non-sterile solution. These may result in localised areas of paraesthesia or anaesthesia, motor weakness, loss of sphincter control and paraplegia. Rarely, these may be permanent.

Postmarketing reports

Very rare reports of convulsions have occurred following accidental intravenous administration.

4.9 Overdose

Accidental intravascular injection of local anaesthetics may cause immediate toxic reactions. In the event of overdose, peak plasma concentrations may not be reached until 2 hours after administration depending upon the injection site and, therefore, signs of toxicity may be delayed. The effects of the drug may be prolonged.

Systemic adverse reactions following overdose or accidental intravascular injection reported with long acting local anaesthetic agents involve both CNS and cardiovascular effects.

CNS Effects

Convulsions should be treated immediately with intravenous thiopentone or diazepam titrated as necessary. Thiopentone and diazepam also depress central nervous system, respiratory and cardiac function. Therefore their use may result in apnoea. Neuro-muscular blockers may be used only if the clinician is confident ofmaintaining a patent airway and managing a fully paralysed patient.

If not treated promptly, convulsions with subsequent hypoxia and hypercarbia plus myocardial depression from the effects of the local anaesthetic on the heart, may result in cardiac arrhythmias, ventricular fibrillation or cardiac arrest.

Cardiovascular Effects

Hypotension may be prevented or attenuated by pre-treatment with a fluid load and/or the use of vasopressors. If hypotension occurs it should be treated with intravenous crystalloids or colloids and/or incremental doses of a vasopressor such as ephedrine 5-10 mg. Any coexisting causes of hypotension should be rapidly treated.

If severe bradycardia occurs, treatment with atropine 0.3-1.0 mg will normally restore the heart rate to an acceptable level.

Cardiac arrhythmia should be treated as required and ventricular fibrillation should be treated by cardioversion.

5. PHARMACOLOGICAL PROPERTIES

5.1 Pharmacodynamic properties

Pharmacotherapeutic group: Local anaesthetics, amide

ATC Code N01B B10

Levobupivacaine is a long acting local anaesthetic and analgesic. It blocks nerve conduction in sensory and motor nerves largely by interacting with voltage sensitive sodium channels on the cell membrane, but also potassium and calcium channels are blocked. In addition, levobupivacaine interferes with impulse transmission and conduction in other tissues where effects on the cardiovascular and central nervous systems are most important for the occurrence of clinical adverse reactions.

The dose of levobupivacaine is expressed as base, whereas, in the racemate bupivacaine the dose is expressed as hydrochloride salt. This gives rise to approximately 13% more active substance in levobupivacaine solutions compared to bupivacaine. In clinical studies at the same nominal concentrations levobupivacaine showed similar clinical effect to bupivacaine.

In a clinical pharmacology study using the ulnar nerve block model, levobupivacaine was equipotent with bupivacaine.

5.2 Pharmacokinetic properties

In human studies, the distribution kinetics of levobupivacaine following i.v. administration are essentially the same as bupivacaine. The plasma concentration of levobupivacaine following therapeutic administration depends on dose and, as absorption from the site of administration is affected by the vascularity of the tissue, on route of administration.

There are no relevant data in patients with hepatic impairment (see section 4.4).

There are no data in patients with renal impairment. Levobupivacaine is extensively metabolised and unchanged levobupivacaine is not excreted in urine.

Plasma protein binding of levobupivacaine in man was evaluated *in vitro* and was found to be > 97% at concentrations between 0.1 and 1.0 μg/ml.

In a clinical pharmacology study where 40 mg levobupivacaine was given by intravenous administration, the mean half-life was approximately 80 ± 22 minutes, C_{max} 1.4 ± 0.2 μg/ml and AUC 70 ± 27 μg•min/ml.

The mean C_{max} and AUC(0-24h) of levobupivacaine were approximately dose-proportional following epidural administration of 75 mg (0.5%) and 112.5 mg (0.75%) and following doses of 1 mg/kg (0.25%) and 2 mg/kg (0.5%) used for brachial plexus block. Following epidural administration of 112.5 mg (0.75%) the mean C_{max} and AUC values were 0.58 μg/ml and 3.56 μg•h/ml respectively.

The mean total plasma clearance and terminal half-life of levobupivacaine after intravenous infusion were 39 litres/hour and 1.3 hours, respectively. The volume of distribution after intravenous administration was 67 litres.

Levobupivacaine is extensively metabolised with no unchanged levobupivacaine detected in urine or faeces. 3-hydroxylevobupivacaine, a major metabolite of levobupivacaine, is excreted in the urine as glucuronic acid and sulphate ester conjugates. *In vitro* studies showed that CYP3A4 isoform and CYP1A2 isoform mediate the metabolism of levobupivacaine to desbutyl-levobupivacaine and 3-hydroxylevobupivacaine respectively. These studies indicate that the metabolism of levobupivacaine and bupivacaine are similar.

Following intravenous administration, recovery of levobupivacaine was quantitative with a mean total of about 95% being recovered in urine (71%) and faeces (24%) in 48 hours.

There is no evidence of *in vivo* racemisation of levobupivacaine.

5.3 Preclinical safety data

In an embryo-foetal toxicity study in rats, an increased incidence of dilated renal pelvis, dilated ureters, olfactory ventricle dilatation and extra thoraco-lumbar ribs was observed at systemic exposure levels in the same range as those obtained at clinical use. There were no treatment-related malformations.

Levobupivacaine was not genotoxic in a standard battery of assays for mutagenicity and clastogenicity. No carcinogenicity testing has been conducted.

6. PHARMACEUTICAL PARTICULARS

6.1 List of excipients

Sodium Chloride

Sodium Hydroxide

Hydrochloric acid

Water for Injections

6.2 Incompatibilities

Levobupivacaine may precipitate if diluted with alkaline solutions and should not be diluted or co-administered with sodium bicarbonate injections. This medicinal product must not be mixed with other medicinal products except those mentioned in section 6.3.

6.3 Shelf life

Shelf life as packaged for sale: 3 years

Shelf life after first opening: The product should be used immediately

Shelf life after dilution in sodium chloride solution 0.9%: Chemical and physical in-use stability has been demonstrated for 7 days at 20-22°C. Chemical and physical in-use stability with clonidine, morphine or fentanyl has been demonstrated for 40 hours at 20-22°C.

From a microbiological point of view, the product should be used immediately. If not used immediately, in-use storage times and conditions prior to use are the responsibility of the user.

6.4 Special precautions for storage

Polypropylene ampoules: polypropylene ampoules do not require any special storage conditions.

6.5 Nature and contents of container

Chirocaine is available in two presentations;

10 ml polypropylene ampoule in packs of 5, 10 & 20

10 ml polypropylene ampoule, in sterile blister packs of 5, 10 & 20

Not all pack sizes may be marketed.

6.6 Instructions for use and handling

For single use only. Discard any unused solution.

The solution/dilution should be inspected visually prior to use. Only clear solutions without visible particles should be used.

A sterile blistercontainer should be chosen when a sterile ampoule surface is required. Ampoule surface is not sterile if sterile blisteris pierced.

Dilutions of levobupivacaine standard solutions should be made with sodium chloride 9 mg/ml (0.9%) solution for injection using aseptic techniques.

Clonidine 8.4 μg/ml, morphine 0.05 mg/ml and fentanyl 4 μg/ml have been shown to be compatible with levobupivacaine in sodium chloride 9 mg/ml (0.9%) solution for injection.

7. MARKETING AUTHORISATION HOLDER

Abbott Laboratories limited

Queenborough

Kent

ME11 5EL

United Kingdom

8. MARKETING AUTHORISATION NUMBER(S)

Chirocaine 2.5 mg/ml: PL 00037/0300

Chirocaine 5 mg/ml: PL 00037/0301

Chirocaine 7.5 mg/ml: PL 00037/0302

9. DATE OF FIRST AUTHORISATION/RENEWAL OF THE AUTHORISATION

06/01/2000, 13/10/2004

10. DATE OF REVISION OF THE TEXT

13/10/2004

Chloroquine sulphate injection

(sanofi-aventis)

1. NAME OF THE MEDICINAL PRODUCT

Chloroquine Sulphate Injection

2. QUALITATIVE AND QUANTITATIVE COMPOSITION

Chloroquine Sulphate BP 54.5 mg per ml.

3. PHARMACEUTICAL FORM

Injection.

4. CLINICAL PARTICULARS

4.1 Therapeutic indications

Treatment of all types of human malaria by intramuscular or intravenous injection when oral administration is impracticable.

4.2 Posology and method of administration

Adults and children:

Slow intravenous infusion: 10 mg/kg bodyweight chloroquine base to be administered in sodium chloride 0.9% injection by slow intravenous infusion over eight hours followed by three further 8 hour infusions containing 5 mg base per kg (total dose 25 mg base per kg over 32 hours). The dose should be modified in renal or hepatic disease.

Exceptionally, where intravenous administration is not possible, chloroquine may be given by intramuscular or subcutaneous injection in small divided doses of 3.5 mg chloroquine base per kg bodyweight every 6 hours or 2.5 mg base per kg every 4 hours.

4.3 Contraindications

The use of chloroquine is contraindicated in patients with known hypersensitivity to 4-aminoquinoline compounds.

Chloroquine is generally contraindicated in pregnancy. However, clinicians may decide to administer chloroquine to pregnant women for the prevention or treatment of malaria. Ocular or inner ear damage may occur in infants born of mothers who receive high doses of chloroquine throughout pregnancy.

4.4 Special warnings and special precautions for use

Chloroquine should be used with care in patients with a history of epilepsy as it has been reported to provoke seizures. Caution is advised in cases of porphyria (precipitated disease may be especially apparent in patients with a high alcohol intake), hepatic disease (particularly cirrhosis) or renal disease, severe gastrointestinal, neurological and blood disorders and in patients receiving anticoagulant therapy.

Chloroquine should be used with care in patients with psoriasis as the condition may be exacerbated.

Although chloroquine may have a temporary effect on visual accommodation during short term treatment, irreversible retinal damage may occur with prolonged treatment (see sections 4.7 and 4.8, below). Therefore, patients should be advised to discontinue the medication and seek immediate medical advice if they notice any deterioration in their vision which persists for more than 48 hours. Ophthalmological examination should always be carried out before and regularly (3-6 monthly intervals) during prolonged treatment. Retinal damage is particularly likely to occur if treatment has been given for longer than one year, or if the total dosage has exceeded 1.6 g/kg bodyweight. These precautions also apply to patients receiving chloroquine continuously at weekly intervals as a prophylactic against malarial attack for more than three years.

Bone marrow depression, including aplastic anaemia occurs rarely. Full blood counts should therefore be carried out regularly during extended treatment. Caution is required if drugs known to induce blood disorders are used concurrently.

Resistance of Plasmodium falciparum to chloroquine is well documented. When used as malaria prophylaxis official guidelines and local information on prevalence of resistance to anti-malarial drugs should be taken into consideration.

4.5 Interaction with other medicinal products and other forms of Interaction

Concomitant administration of chloroquine with magnesium-containing antacids or kaolin may result in reduced absorption of chloroquine. Chloroquine should, therefore, be administered at least two hours apart from antacids or kaolin.

Concomitant use of cimetidine and chloroquine may result in an increased half-life and a decreased clearance of chloroquine.

Chloroquine and mefloquine can lower the convulsive threshold. Co-administration of chloroquine and mefloquine may increase the risk of convulsions. Also, the activity of antiepileptic drugs might be impaired if co-administered with chloroquine.

There have been isolated case reports of an increased plasma ciclosporin level when ciclosporin and chloroquine were co-administered.

Chloroquine may affect the antibody response to rabies vaccine (HDCV).

Caution is advised in patients receiving anticoagulant therapy.

Co-administration of chloroquine and other drugs that have arrhythmogenic potential (e.g. amiodarone) may increase the risk of cardiac arrhythmias.

Concomitant administration of chloroquine and digoxin may increase plasma concentrations of digoxin.

Concomitant use of chloroquine with neostigmine or pyridostigmine has the potential to increase the symptoms of myasthenia gravis and thus diminish the effects of neostigmine and pyridostigmine.

4.6 Pregnancy and lactation

Chloroquine is generally contraindicated in pregnancy. However, clinicians may decide to administer chloroquine to pregnant women for the prevention or treatment of malaria. Ocular or inner ear damage may occur in infants born of mothers who receive high doses of chloroquine throughout pregnancy.

Although chloroquine is excreted in breast milk, the amount is insufficient to confer any benefit on the infant. Separate chemoprophylaxis for the infant is required.

When used for rheumatoid disease breast feeding is not recommended.

4.7 Effects on ability to drive and use machines

Chloroquine has a temporary effect on visual accommodation and patients should be warned that they should not drive or operate machinery if they are affected.

4.8 Undesirable effects

Cardiovascular

- cardiomyopathy has been reported during long term therapy at high doses,

- cardiac dysrhythmias at high doses can occur,

- hypotension.

Central Nervous System (See Section 4.4)

- seizures,

- convulsions have been reported rarely (these may result from cerebral malaria. Such patients should receive an injections of phenobarbitone to prevent seizures, in a dose of 3.5mg/kg in addition to intravenous administration of chloroquine),

- psychiatric disorders such as anxiety, confusion, hallucinations, delirium.

Eye disorders (See Sections 4.4 and 4.7)

- transient blurred vision and reversible corneal opacity,

- cases of retinopathy as well as cases of irreversible retinal damage have damage have been reported during long term, high dose therapy.

- macular defects of colour vision, optic atrophy, scotomas, field defects, blindness and pigmented deposits, difficult in focusing, diplopia.

Gastro-intestinal

- gastrointestinal disturbances such as nausea, vomiting, diarrhoea, abdominal cramps.

General

- headache.

Haematological (See Section 4.4)

- bone marrow depression, including aplastic anaemia, agranulocytosis, thrombocytopenia, neutropenia occurs rarely.

Hepatic

- changes in liver function, including hepatitis and abnormal liver function tests, have been reported rarely.

Hypersensitivity

- allergic and anaphylactic reactions, urticaria and angiodema have occurred rarely.

Hearing disorders

- ototoxicity such as tinnitus, reduced hearing, nerve deafness.

Muscular

- neuropathy, myopathy.

Skin (See Section 4.4)

- skin eruptions, pruritis, depigmentation, loss of hair, exacerbation of psoriasis, photosensitivity, pigmentation of the nails and mucosae (long term use).

- Rare reports of erythema multiforme, Stevens-Johnson syndrome, toxic epidermal necrolysis, exfoliative dermatitis and similar desquamation-type events.

4.9 Overdose

Chloroquine is highly toxic in overdosage; children are particularly susceptible to toxic doses of chloroquine. The chief symptoms of overdose include circulatory collapse due to a potent cardiotoxic effect, respiratory arrest and coma. Symptoms may progress rapidly after initial headache, drowsiness, visual disturbances nausea and vomiting. Death may result from circulatory or respiratory failure or cardiac dysrhythmia.

Gastric lavage should be carried out urgently, first protecting the airways and instituting artificial ventilation where necessary. There is a risk of cardiac arrest following aspiration of gastric contents in more serious cases. Activated charcoal left in the stomach may reduce absorption of any remaining chloroquine from the gut. Circulatory status (with central venous pressure measurement), respiration, plasma electrolytes and blood gases should be monitored, with correction of hypokalaemia and acidosis if indicated. Cardiac arrhythmias should not be treated unless life threatening; drugs with quinidine-like effects should be avoided.

Early administration of the following has been shown to improve survival in cases of serious poisoning:

1) Adrenaline infusion (0.25 micrograms/kg/min initially, with increments of 0.25 micrograms/kg/min until adequate systolic blood pressure (more than 100 mm mercury) is restored; adrenaline reduces the effects of chloroquine on the heart through its inotropic and vasoconstrictor effects.

2) Diazepam infusion (2 mg/kg over 30 minutes as a loading dose, followed by 1-2 mg/kg/day for up to 2-4 days). Diazepam may minimise cardiotoxicity.

Acidification of the urine, haemodialysis, peritoneal dialysis or exchange transfusions have not been shown to be of value in treating chloroquine poisoning. Chloroquine is excreted very slowly, therefore symptomatic cases merit observation for several days.

5. PHARMACOLOGICAL PROPERTIES

5.1 Pharmacodynamic properties

Chloroquine is used for the suppression and treatment of malaria. It has rapid schizonticidal effect and appears to affect cell growth by interfering with DNA; its activity also seems to depend on preferential accumulation in the infected erythrocyte. Chloroquine kills the erythrocytic forms of malaria parasites at all stages of development.

5.2 Pharmacokinetic properties

Chloroquine is readily absorbed from the gastro-intestinal tract and about 55% in the circulation is bound to plasma proteins. It accumulates in high concentrations in some tissues, such as kidneys, liver, lungs and spleen and is strongly bound in melanin containing cells such as those in the eyes and the skin; it is also bound to double stranded DNA, present in red blood cells containing schizonts. Chloroquine is eliminated very slowly from the body and it may persist in tissues for a long period. Up to 70% of a dose may be excreted unchanged in urine and up to 25% may be excreted also in the urine as the desethyl metabolite. The rate of urinary excretion of chloroquine is increased at low pH values.

5.3 Preclinical safety data

No additional preclinical data of relevance to the prescriber.

6. PHARMACEUTICAL PARTICULARS

6.1 List of excipients

Water for injections BP.

6.2 Incompatibilities

None known.

6.3 Shelf life

60 months.

6.4 Special precautions for storage

Protect from light.

6.5 Nature and contents of container

Cartons containing 10 clear glass ampoules holding 5 ml of injection solution.

6.6 Instructions for use and handling

None stated.

7. MARKETING AUTHORISATION HOLDER

Aventis Pharma Limited
50 Kings Hill Avenue
Kings Hill
West Malling
Kent ME19 4AH

8. MARKETING AUTHORISATION NUMBER(S)

PL 04425/0352

9. DATE OF FIRST AUTHORISATION/RENEWAL OF THE AUTHORISATION

28 July 2003

10. DATE OF REVISION OF THE TEXT

January 2005

LEGAL CLASSIFICATION: POM

Chlorphenamine injection

(Link Pharmaceuticals Ltd)

1. NAME OF THE MEDICINAL PRODUCT

Chlorphenamine injection.

2. QUALITATIVE AND QUANTITATIVE COMPOSITION

Each 1ml of solution contains: Chlorphenamine Maleate Ph. Eur. 10mg.

Chlorphenamine is the International Non-proprietary Name and chlorpheniramine is the British Approved Name for the active ingredient of chlorphenamine injection.

3. PHARMACEUTICAL FORM

Clear, colourless sterile solution for injection.

4. CLINICAL PARTICULARS

4.1 Therapeutic indications

Chlorphenamine injection is indicated for acute urticaria, control of allergic reactions to insect bites and stings, angioneurotic oedema, drug and serum reactions, desensitisation reactions, hayfever, vasomotor rhinitis, severe pruritus of non-specific origin.

4.2 Posology and method of administration

Adults:

The usual dose of chlorphenamine injection for adults is 10mg to 20mg, but not more than 40mg should be given within a 24-hour period. The injection may be given by the subcutaneous, intramuscular or intravenous route.

When a rapid effect is desired, as in anaphylactic reactions, the intravenous route is recommended in addition to emergency therapy with adrenaline (epinephrine), corticosteroids, oxygen and supportive therapy as required. In this case chlorphenamine injection should be injected slowly over a period of one minute, using the smallest adequate syringe. Any drowsiness, giddiness or hypotension which may follow is usually transitory.

In the event of a blood transfusion reaction, a dose of 10mg to 20mg of chlorphenamine injection should be given by the subcutaneous route. This can be repeated to a total of 40mg within a 24-hour period, or oral forms of chlorphenamine may be given until the symptoms subside.

Chlorphenamine injection may be helpful in the prevention of delayed reactions to penicillin and other drugs when given separately by intramuscular injection immediately prior to administration of the other drug. The usual dose is 10mg.

Chlorphenamine injection cannot, however, be relied on to prevent anaphylactic reactions in patients known to be allergic to a particular drug.

Children:

The dose for children should be calculated, based on either the child's age or their body weight, using the following table:

(see Table 1 on next page)

Extra care should be taken when preparing the injection for children under 1 year due to the small volumes that are required. Dilution of chlorphenamine injection with sodium chloride intravenous infusion (0.9% w/v) should facilitate preparation. For example, diluting 0.2ml chlorphenamine injection to 2ml with sodium chloride 0.9% injection produces a solution containing chlorphenamine 1mg/ml. The diluted product should be used immediately.

4.3 Contraindications

Chlorphenamine injection is contraindicated in patients who are hypersensitive to antihistamines or to any of the other ingredients.

The anticholinergic properties of chlorphenamine are intensified by monoamine oxidase inhibitors (MAOIs). Chlorphenamine injection is therefore contraindicated in patients who have been treated with MAOIs within the last fourteen days.

4.4 Special warnings and special precautions for use

Chlorphenamine, in common with other drugs having anticholinergic effects, should be used with caution in epilepsy; raised intra-ocular pressure including glaucoma; prostatic hypertrophy; severe hypertension or cardiovascular disease; bronchitis; bronchiectasis and asthma;

Table 1

Age	Dose		
1 month to 1 year			0.25mg/kg
1 to 5 years	2.5mg to 5mg	OR	0.20mg/kg
6 to 12 years	5mg to 10mg	OR	0.20mg/kg
12 to 18 years	10mg to 20mg	OR	0.20mg/kg

hepatic disease and thyrotoxicosis. Children and the elderly are more likely to experience the neurological anticholinergic effects.

4.5 Interaction with other medicinal products and other forms of Interaction

Concurrent use of chlorphenamine and hypnotics or anxiolytics may potentiate drowsiness. Concurrent use of alcohol may have a similar effect.

Chlorphenamine inhibits phenytoin metabolism and can lead to phenytoin toxicity.

The anticholinergic effects of chlorphenamine are intensified by MAOIs (see section 4.3 *Contraindications*).

4.6 Pregnancy and lactation

There is inadequate evidence of safety in human pregnancy. Chlorphenamine injection should only be used during pregnancy when clearly needed and when the potential benefits outweigh the potential unknown risks to the foetus. Use during the third trimester may result in reactions in neonates.

It is reasonable to assume that chlorphenamine may inhibit lactation and may be secreted in breast milk. The use of chlorphenamine injection in mothers breast-feeding their babies requires that the therapeutic benefits of the drug should be weighed against the potential hazards to the mother and baby.

4.7 Effects on ability to drive and use machines

The anticholinergic properties of chlorphenamine may cause drowsiness, blurred vision and psychomotor impairment, which can seriously hamper the patient's ability to drive and use machinery.

4.8 Undesirable effects

The most common side-effect is sedation varying from slight drowsiness to deep sleep. The following may also occasionally occur: inability to concentrate; lassitude; blurred vision; gastro-intestinal disturbances such as nausea, vomiting and diarrhoea.

Urinary retention; headaches; dry mouth; dizziness; palpitation; painful dyspepsia; anorexia; hepatitis including jaundice; thickening of bronchial secretions; haemolytic anaemia and other blood dyscrasias; allergic reactions including exfoliative dermatitis, photosensitivity, skin reactions and urticaria; twitching, muscular weakness and incoordination; tinnitus; depression; irritability and nightmares infrequently occur.

Paradoxical excitation in children and confusional psychosis in the elderly can occur.

Some patients have reported a stinging or burning sensation at the site of injection. Rapid intravenous injection may cause transitory hypotension or CNS stimulation.

4.9 Overdose

The estimated lethal dose of chlorphenamine is 25mg to 50mg/kg body weight. Symptoms and signs include sedation, paradoxical stimulation of the CNS, toxic psychosis, seizures, apnoea, convulsions, anticholinergic effects, dystonic reactions and cardiovascular collapse including arrhythmias.

Symptomatic and supportive measures should be provided with special attention to cardiac, respiratory, renal and hepatic functions, and fluid and electrolytic balance. If overdosage is by the oral route, treatment should include gastric lavage or induced emesis using syrup of ipecacuanha. Following these measures activated charcoal and cathartics may be administered to minimise absorption.

Treat hypotension and arrhythmias vigorously. CNS convulsions may be treated with iv diazepam. Haemoperfusion may be used in severe cases.

5. PHARMACOLOGICAL PROPERTIES

5.1 Pharmacodynamic properties

Antihistamines, including chlorphenamine, used in the treatment of allergy act by competing with histamine for H_1-receptor sites on cells and tissues. Chlorphenamine also has anticholinergic activity.

The mechanism by which chlorphenamine exerts its antiemetic, anti-motion sickness and anti-vertigo effects is not precisely known but may be related to its central actions. Further, most antihistamines, including chlorphenamine, cross the blood-brain barrier and probably produce sedation largely by occupying H_1-receptors in the brain.

5.2 Pharmacokinetic properties

Following iv administration, the apparent steady-state volume of distribution of chlorphenamine is approximately 3L/kg in adults and 3.8L/kg in children.

Chlorphenamine is approximately 70% bound to plasma proteins.

In adults with normal renal and hepatic function, the terminal elimination half-life of chlorphenamine reportedly ranges from 12 to 43 hours.

The systemic exposure per mg dose is lower in children than adults and the elimination half-life may be shorter.

5.3 Preclinical safety data

There are no preclinical data of relevance to the prescriber which are additional to that already included in other sections of the Summary of Product Characteristics.

6. PHARMACEUTICAL PARTICULARS

6.1 List of excipients

Sodium chloride, Water for Injections.

6.2 Incompatibilities

In the absence of incompatibility studies, this product must not be mixed with other medicinal products.

6.3 Shelf life

3 years.

6.4 Special precautions for storage

Do not store above 25°C. Keep the container in the outer carton in order to protect from light.

6.5 Nature and contents of container

Chlorphenamine injection is presented in 1ml neutral glass ampoules. It is supplied in boxes of 5 ampoules.

6.6 Instructions for use and handling

No special requirements.

7. MARKETING AUTHORISATION HOLDER

Link Pharmaceuticals Limited, Bishops Weald House, Albion Way, Horsham, West Sussex, RH12 1AH, UK

8. MARKETING AUTHORISATION NUMBER(S)

PL 12406/0013.

9. DATE OF FIRST AUTHORISATION/RENEWAL OF THE AUTHORISATION

16 December 1999.

10. DATE OF REVISION OF THE TEXT

October 2003.

11. LEGAL CATEGORY

POM

Choragon 5000 U and Choragon Solvent

(Ferring Pharmaceuticals Ltd)

1. NAME OF THE MEDICINAL PRODUCT

Choragon® 5000U and Choragon Solvent

2. QUALITATIVE AND QUANTITATIVE COMPOSITION

Active Ingredient:

Each ampoule with dry substance contains chorionic gonadotrophin EP corresponding to 5000 units.

3. PHARMACEUTICAL FORM

Powder for injection and solvent for parenteral use.

4. CLINICAL PARTICULARS

4.1 Therapeutic indications

In the female

In the management of anovulatory infertility.

In the male

In the management of delayed puberty, undescended testes and oligospermia.

4.2 Posology and method of administration

Treatment should only commence after expert assessment.

In the female

Induction of ovulation: 10000 units mid-cycle if plasma oestrogen levels are favourable following follicular stimulation.

In the male

Delayed puberty: Dose should be titrated against plasma testosterone, starting with 500 units twice weekly. Treatment should be continued for 4 - 6 weeks.

Undescended testes: Treatment should begin before puberty, the optimum age range being 7 - 10 years. 500 units three times weekly is a suitable starting dose. This may be increased to 4000 units if necessary. Treatment should continue for 6 - 10 weeks. In males over 17 years of age a commencing dose of 1000 units twice weekly can be given. Treatment should be continued for one or two months after testicular descent.

Oligospermia: Dose should be titrated against seminal analysis starting with 500 units two or three times weekly. Treatment should be continued for 16 weeks.

Choragon® is given by intramuscular injection.

4.3 Contraindications

hCG should not be given to patients with disorders that might be exacerbated by androgen release.

4.4 Special warnings and special precautions for use

hCG should be given with care to patients in whom fluid retention might be a hazard, as in asthma, epilepsy, migraine or cardiac or renal disorders.

Allergic reactions may occur and patients thought to be susceptible should be given skin tests before treatment.

hCG preparations should only be used under the supervision of a specialist having available adequate facilities for appropriate laboratory monitoring.

In the female - Use in induction of ovulation may result in ovarian enlargement or cysts, acute abdominal pain, superovulation or multiple pregnancies, particularly if endocrine monitoring is inadequate.

In the male - Treatment for undescended testes may produce precocious puberty; use should cease immediately. Gynaecomastia has been reported. A growth spurt may also be associated with use and this should be kept in mind particularly where epiphyseal growth is still potentially active.

4.5 Interaction with other medicinal products and other forms of Interaction

None known.

4.6 Pregnancy and lactation

Not applicable as only recommended in females for infertility.

4.7 Effects on ability to drive and use machines

None known.

4.8 Undesirable effects

Headache, tiredness and mood changes have been described.

4.9 Overdose

See "Warnings".

5. PHARMACOLOGICAL PROPERTIES

5.1 Pharmacodynamic properties

Gonadotrophin.

5.2 Pharmacokinetic properties

hCG is not effective when taken orally and is administered by intramuscular injection.

5.3 Preclinical safety data

There are no preclinical data of relevance to the Prescriber which are additional to those already included in other sections of the SPC.

6. PHARMACEUTICAL PARTICULARS

6.1 List of excipients

Dry substance:	mannitol, sodium hydroxide for pH-adjustment
Diluent:	Isotonic sodium chloride solution (0.9% w/w), dilute hydrochloric acid for pH adjustment.

6.2 Incompatibilities

None stated.

6.3 Shelf life

36 months as packaged for sale.

6.4 Special precautions for storage

Protect from light and store below 20°C.

6.5 Nature and contents of container

Each pack contains ampoule(s) with 5000 units of hCG powder for solution for injection packaged together with ampoule(s) of 1ml Choragon® solvent. Ampoules are assembled in boxes containing either 1 pair, 3 pairs or 5 pairs of ampoules and solvents.

6.6 Instructions for use and handling

The dry substance must be reconstituted with the solvent prior to use.

7. MARKETING AUTHORISATION HOLDER

Ferring Pharmaceuticals Limited, The Courtyard, Waterside Drive, Langley, Berkshire SL3 6EZ

8. MARKETING AUTHORISATION NUMBER(S)

PL 03194/0065

9. DATE OF FIRST AUTHORISATION/RENEWAL OF THE AUTHORISATION

15th August 1996

10. DATE OF REVISION OF THE TEXT

August 1999

11. Legal Category

POM

Cialis 10mg film-coated tablets, Cialis 20mg film-coated tablets

(Eli Lilly and Company Limited)

1. NAME OF THE MEDICINAL PRODUCT

Cialis*▼ 10mg film-coated tablets.

Cialis▼ 20mg film-coated tablets.

2. QUALITATIVE AND QUANTITATIVE COMPOSITION

Each 10mg tablet contains 10mg tadalafil.

Each 20mg tablet contains 20mg tadalafil.

For excipients, see section 6.1.

3. PHARMACEUTICAL FORM

Film-coated tablet.

The 10mg tablets are light yellow and almond shaped, marked 'C 10' on one side.

The 20mg tablets are yellow and almond shaped, marked 'C 20' on one side.

4. CLINICAL PARTICULARS

4.1 Therapeutic indications

Treatment of erectile dysfunction.

In order for Cialis to be effective, sexual stimulation is required.

Cialis is not indicated for use by women.

4.2 Posology and method of administration

For oral use.

Use in adult men

The recommended dose is 10mg taken prior to anticipated sexual activity and without regard to food. In those patients in whom tadalafil 10mg does not produce an adequate effect, 20mg might be tried. It may be taken at least 30 minutes prior to sexual activity.

The maximum dosing frequency is once per day.

Continuous daily use of the medication is strongly discouraged because the long-term safety after prolonged daily dosing has not been established and also because the effect of tadalafil usually lasts for longer than one day. See section 4.4, last paragraph, and section 5.1.

Use in elderly men

Dosage adjustments are not required in elderly patients.

Use in men with impaired renal function

Dosage adjustments are not required in patients with mild to moderate renal impairment. For patients with severe renal impairment, 10mg is the maximum recommended dose. (See section 5.2.)

Use in men with impaired hepatic function

The recommended dose of Cialis is 10mg taken prior to anticipated sexual activity and without regard to food. There is limited clinical data on the safety of Cialis in patients with severe hepatic insufficiency (Child-Pugh class C); if prescribed, a careful individual benefit/risk evaluation should be undertaken by the prescribing physician. There are no available data about the administration of doses higher than 10mg of tadalafil to patients with hepatic impairment. (See sections 4.4 and 5.2.)

Use in men with diabetes

Dosage adjustments are not required in diabetic patients.

Use in children and adolescents

Cialis should not be used in individuals below 18 years of age.

4.3 Contraindications

In clinical studies, tadalafil was shown to augment the hypotensive effects of nitrates. This is thought to result from the combined effects of nitrates and tadalafil on the nitric oxide/cGMP pathway. Therefore, administration of Cialis to patients who are using any form of organic nitrate is contra-indicated. (See section 4.5.)

Agents for the treatment of erectile dysfunction, including Cialis, should not be used in men with cardiac disease for whom sexual activity is inadvisable. Physicians should consider the potential cardiac risk of sexual activity in patients with pre-existing cardiovascular disease.

The following groups of patients with cardiovascular disease were not included in clinical trials and the use of tadalafil is therefore contra-indicated:

- Patients with myocardial infarction within the last 90 days.
- Patients with unstable angina or angina occurring during sexual intercourse.
- Patients with New York Heart Association class 2 or greater heart failure in the last 6 months.
- Patients with uncontrolled arrhythmias, hypotension (<90/50mmHg), or uncontrolled hypertension.
- Patients with a stroke within the last 6 months.

Cialis should not be used in patients with hypersensitivity to tadalafil or to any of the excipients.

4.4 Special warnings and special precautions for use

A medical history and physical examination should be undertaken to diagnose erectile dysfunction and determine potential underlying causes, before pharmacological treatment is considered.

Prior to initiating any treatment for erectile dysfunction, physicians should consider the cardiovascular status of their patients, since there is a degree of cardiac risk associated with sexual activity. Tadalafil has vasodilator properties, resulting in mild and transient decreases in blood pressure (see section 5.1), and as such potentiates the hypotensive effect of nitrates (see section 4.3).

Serious cardiovascular events, including myocardial infarction, unstable angina pectoris, ventricular arrhythmia, strokes, and transient ischaemic attacks, occurred during clinical studies of Cialis. In addition, hypertension and hypotension (including postural hypotension) were also seen infrequently in clinical trials. Most of the patients in whom these events have been observed had pre-existing cardiovascular risk factors. However, it is not possible to definitively determine whether these events are related directly to these risk factors.

There is limited clinical data on the safety of Cialis in patients with severe hepatic insufficiency (Child-Pugh class C); if prescribed, a careful individual benefit/risk evaluation should be undertaken by the prescribing physician.

Patients who experience erections lasting 4 hours or more should be instructed to seek immediate medical assistance. If priapism is not treated immediately, penile tissue damage and permanent loss of potency may result.

Agents for the treatment of erectile dysfunction, including Cialis, should be used with caution in patients with anatomical deformation of the penis (such as angulation, cavernosal fibrosis, or Peyronie's disease) or in patients who have conditions which may predispose them to priapism (such as sickle cell anaemia, multiple myeloma, or leukaemia).

The evaluation of erectile dysfunction should include a determination of potential underlying causes and the identification of appropriate treatment following an appropriate medical assessment. It is not known if Cialis is effective in patients with spinal cord injuries and patients who have undergone pelvic surgery or radical non-nerve-sparing prostatectomy.

Cialis should not be administered to patients with hereditary problems of galactose intolerance, the Lapp lactase deficiency, or glucose-galactose malabsorption.

In patients who are taking $alpha_1$-blockers, such as doxazosin, concomitant administration of Cialis may lead to symptomatic hypotension in some patients (see section 4.5). Therefore, the combination of tadalafil and alpha-blockers is not recommended.

Caution should be exercised when prescribing Cialis to patients using potent CYP3A4 inhibitors (ritonavir, saquinavir, ketoconazole, itraconazole, and erythromycin), as increased tadalafil exposure (AUC) has been observed if the drugs are combined (see section 4.5).

The safety and efficacy of combinations of Cialis and other treatments for erectile dysfunction have not been studied. Therefore, the use of such combinations is not recommended.

In dogs given tadalafil daily for 6 to 12 months at doses of 25mg/kg/day (resulting in at least a 3-fold greater exposure [range 3.7-18.6] than seen in humans at a 20mg single dose) and above, there was regression of the seminiferous tubular epithelium that resulted in a decrease in spermatogenesis in some dogs. Results from two 6-month studies in volunteers suggest that this effect is unlikely in humans (see section 5.1). The effects of longer-term daily dosing have not been established. Therefore, daily use of the medication is strongly discouraged.

4.5 Interaction with other medicinal products and other forms of Interaction

Interaction studies were conducted with 10 and/or 20mg tadalafil, as indicated below. With regard to those interaction studies where only the 10mg tadalafil dose was used, clinically relevant interactions at higher doses cannot be completely ruled out.

Effects of other medicinal products on tadalafil

Tadalafil is principally metabolised by CYP3A4. A selective inhibitor of CYP3A4, ketoconazole (200mg daily), increased tadalafil (10mg) exposure (AUC) 2-fold and C_{max} by 15%, relative to the AUC and C_{max} values for tadalafil alone. Ketoconazole (400mg daily) increased tadalafil (20mg) exposure (AUC) 4-fold and C_{max} by 22%. Ritonavir, a protease inhibitor (200mg dose given twice daily), which is an inhibitor of CYP3A4, CYP2C9, CYP2C19, and CYP2D6, increased tadalafil (20mg) exposure (AUC) 2-fold with no change in C_{max}. Although specific interactions have not been studied, other protease inhibitors, such as saquinavir, and other CYP3A4 inhibitors, such as erythromycin, clarithromycin, itraconazole, and grapefruit juice, should be co-administered with caution, as they would be expected to increase plasma concentrations of tadalafil. Consequently, the incidence of the undesirable effects listed in section 4.8 might be increased.

The role of transporters (for example, p-glycoprotein) in the disposition of tadalafil is not known. There is thus the potential of drug interactions mediated by inhibition of transporters.

A CYP3A4 inducer, rifampicin, reduced tadalafil AUC by 88%, relative to the AUC values for tadalafil alone (10mg dose). It can be expected that concomitant administration of other CYP3A4 inducers, such as phenobarbital, phenytoin, and carbamazepine, will also decrease plasma concentrations of tadalafil.

Effects of tadalafil on other medicinal products

In clinical studies, tadalafil (10 and 20mg) was shown to augment the hypotensive effects of nitrates. Therefore, administration of Cialis to patients who are using any form of organic nitrate is contra-indicated (see section 4.3). Based on the results of a clinical study in which 150 subjects receiving daily doses of tadalafil 20mg for 7 days and 0.4mg sublingual nitroglycerin at various times, this interaction lasted for more than 24 hours and was no longer detectable when 48 hours had elapsed after the last tadalafil dose. Thus, in a patient prescribed Cialis, where nitrate administration is deemed medically necessary in a life-threatening situation, at least 48 hours should have elapsed after the last dose of Cialis before nitrate administration is considered. In such circumstances, nitrates should only be administered under close medical supervision with appropriate haemodynamic monitoring.

Tadalafil is not expected to cause clinically significant inhibition or induction of the clearance of drugs metabolised by CYP450 isoforms. Studies have confirmed that tadalafil does not inhibit or induce CYP450 isoforms, including CYP3A4, CYP1A2, CYP2D6, CYP2E1, CYP2C9, and CYP2C19.

Tadalafil (10 and 20mg) had no clinically significant effect on exposure (AUC) to S-warfarin or R-warfarin (CYP2C9 substrate), nor did tadalafil affect changes in prothrombin time induced by warfarin.

Tadalafil (10 and 20mg) did not potentiate the increase in bleeding time caused by acetylsalicylic acid.

In clinical pharmacology studies, the potential for tadalafil to augment the hypotensive effects of antihypertensive agents was examined. Major classes of antihypertensive agents were studied, including calcium channel blockers (amlodipine), angiotensin converting enzyme (ACE) inhibitors (enalapril), beta-adrenergic receptor blockers (metoprolol), thiazide diuretics (bendrofluazide), and angiotensin II receptor blockers (various types and doses, alone or in combination with thiazides, calcium channel blockers, beta-blockers, and/or alpha-blockers). Tadalafil (10mg, except for studies with angiotensin II receptor blockers and amlodipine in which a 20mg dose was applied) had no clinically significant interaction with any of these classes. In another clinical pharmacology study, tadalafil (20mg) was studied in combination with up to 4 classes of antihypertensives. In subjects taking multiple antihypertensives, the ambulatory blood pressure changes appeared to relate to the degree of blood pressure control. In this regard, in study subjects whose blood pressure was well controlled, the reduction was minimal and similar to that seen in healthy subjects. In study subjects whose blood pressure was not controlled, the reduction was greater, although this reduction was not associated with hypotensive symptoms in the majority of subjects. In patients receiving concomitant antihypertensive medications, tadalafil 20mg may induce a blood pressure decrease, which (with the exception of alpha-blockers - see below) is, in general, minor and not likely to be clinically relevant. Analysis of Phase 3 clinical trial data showed no difference in adverse events in patients taking tadalafil with or without antihypertensive medications. However, appropriate clinical advice should be given to patients regarding a possible decrease in blood pressure when they are treated with antihypertensive medications.

In subjects receiving concomitant tadalafil (20mg) and doxazosin (8mg daily), an $alpha_1$-adrenergic receptor blocker, there was an augmentation of the blood pressure lowering effect of doxazosin. This effect was still present at 12 hours post dose and had generally disappeared at 24 hours. The number of subjects with potentially clinically significant standing blood pressure decreases was greater for the combination. Some subjects experienced dizziness, but no cases of syncope were reported. Lower doses of doxazosin have not been studied. Therefore, the combination of tadalafil and alpha-blockers is not recommended. In a single study in 18 healthy volunteers, tadalafil (10 and 20mg) had no clinically significant effect on blood pressure changes due to tamsulosin, a selective $alpha_{1A}$-adrenergic receptor blocking agent. It is not known how this extrapolates to other $alpha_{1A}$-adrenergic receptor blocking agents.

Alcohol concentrations (mean maximum blood concentration 0.08%) were not affected by co-administration with tadalafil (10 or 20mg). In addition, no changes in tadalafil concentrations were seen 3 hours after co-administration with alcohol. Alcohol was administered in a manner to maximise the rate of alcohol absorption (overnight fast with no food until 2 hours after alcohol). Tadalafil (20mg) did not augment the mean blood pressure decrease produced by alcohol (0.7g/kg or approximately 180ml of 40% alcohol [vodka] in an 80 kg male) but, in some subjects, postural dizziness and orthostatic hypotension were observed. When tadalafil was administered with lower doses of alcohol (0.6g/kg), hypotension was not observed and dizziness occurred with similar frequency to alcohol alone. The effect of alcohol on cognitive function was not augmented by tadalafil (10mg).

Tadalafil has been demonstrated to produce an increase in the oral bioavailability of ethinyloestradiol; a similar increase may be expected with oral administration of terbutaline, although the clinical consequence of this is uncertain.

When tadalafil 10mg was administered with theophylline (a non-selective phosphodiesterase inhibitor) in a clinical pharmacology study, there was no pharmacokinetic interaction. The only pharmacodynamic effect was a small (3.5 bpm) increase in heart rate. Although this effect is minor and was of no clinical significance in this study, it should be considered when co-administering these medications.

Specific interaction studies with antidiabetic agents were not conducted.

4.6 Pregnancy and lactation

Cialis is not indicated for use by women. There are no studies of tadalafil in pregnant women.

There was no evidence of teratogenicity, embryotoxicity, or foetotoxicity in rats or mice that received up to 1,000mg/kg/day.

4.7 Effects on ability to drive and use machines

Cialis is expected to have no or negligible influence on the ability to drive and/or use machines. No specific studies have been performed to evaluate a potential effect. Although the frequency of reports of dizziness in placebo and tadalafil arms in clinical trials was similar, patients should be aware of how they react to Cialis, before driving or operating machinery.

4.8 Undesirable effects

The most commonly reported adverse reactions are headache and dyspepsia, see tables below.

Table 1

Very common adverse reactions (>1/10)

System Organ Class	Adverse Reaction	Cialis 10-20mg (%) n = 724	Placebo (%) n = 379
Nervous system	Headache	14.5	5.5
Gastro-intestinal	Dyspepsia	12.3	1.8

Table 2

Common adverse reactions (>1/100, <1/10)

System Organ Class	Adverse Reaction	Cialis 10-20mg (%) n = 724	Placebo (%) n = 379
Nervous system	Dizziness	2.3	1.8
Vascular	Flushing	4.1	1.6
Respiratory, thoracic, and mediastinal	Nasal congestion	4.3	3.2
Musculoskeletal and connective tissue	Back pain Myalgia	6.5 5.7	4.2 1.8

Swelling of eyelids, sensations described as eye pain and conjunctival hyperaemia are uncommon adverse reactions.

The adverse events reported with tadalafil were transient, and generally mild or moderate.

Adverse event data are limited in patients over 75 years of age.

In postmarketing surveillance, prolonged erection and priapism have been reported very rarely.

4.9 Overdose

Single doses of up to 500mg have been given to healthy subjects, and multiple daily doses up to 100mg have been given to patients. Adverse events were similar to those seen at lower doses.

In cases of overdose, standard supportive measures should be adopted, as required. Haemodialysis contributes negligibly to tadalafil elimination.

5. PHARMACOLOGICAL PROPERTIES

5.1 Pharmacodynamic properties

Pharmacotherapeutic group: Drugs used in erectile dysfunction (ATC code: G04B E).

Tadalafil is a selective, reversible inhibitor of cyclic guanosine monophosphate (cGMP)-specific phosphodiesterase type 5 (PDE5). When sexual stimulation causes the local release of nitric oxide, inhibition of PDE5 by tadalafil produces increased levels of cGMP in the corpus cavernosum. This results in smooth muscle relaxation and inflow of blood into the penile tissues, thereby producing an erection. Tadalafil has no effect in the absence of sexual stimulation.

Studies *in vitro* have shown that tadalafil is a selective inhibitor of PDE5. PDE5 is an enzyme found in corpus cavernosum smooth muscle, vascular and visceral smooth muscle, skeletal muscle, platelets, kidney, lung, and cerebellum. The effect of tadalafil is more potent on PDE5 than on other phosphodiesterases. Tadalafil is >10,000-fold more potent for PDE5 than for PDE1, PDE2, and PDE4, enzymes which are found in the heart, brain, blood vessels, liver, and other organs. Tadalafil is >10,000-fold more potent for PDE5 than for PDE3, an enzyme found in the heart and blood vessels. This selectivity for PDE5 over PDE3 is important because PDE3 is an enzyme involved in cardiac contractility. Additionally, tadalafil is approximately 700-fold more potent for PDE5 than for PDE6, an enzyme which is found in the retina and is responsible for phototransduction. Tadalafil is also >10,000-fold more potent for PDE5 than for PDE7 through PDE10.

Three clinical studies were conducted in 1,054 patients in an at-home setting to define the period of responsiveness to Cialis. Cialis demonstrated statistically significant improvement in erectile function and the ability to have successful sexual intercourse up to 36 hours following dosing, as well as patients' ability to attain and maintain erections for successful intercourse compared to placebo as early as 16 minutes following dosing.

Cialis administered to healthy subjects produced no significant difference compared to placebo in supine systolic and diastolic blood pressure (mean maximal decrease of 1.6/0.8mmHg, respectively), in standing systolic and diastolic blood pressure (mean maximal decrease of 0.2/4.6mmHg, respectively), and no significant change in heart rate.

In a study to assess the effects of tadalafil on vision, no impairment of colour discrimination (blue/green) was detected using the Farnsworth-Munsell 100-hue test. This finding is consistent with the low affinity of tadalafil for PDE6 compared to PDE5. Across all clinical studies, reports of changes in colour vision were rare (<0.1%).

Two studies were conducted in men to assess the potential effect of Cialis 10mg and 20mg administered daily for 6 months on spermatogenesis. The results of these studies demonstrate no difference from placebo with respect to the proportion of men showing a 50% or greater decrease in sperm concentration. In addition, in comparison with placebo, there were no adverse effects observed with respect to mean change in sperm count, sperm morphology, or sperm motility at either dose. However, in the study of 10mg Cialis taken daily for 6 months, results showed a decrease in mean sperm concentration relative to placebo. This effect was not seen in the study where the higher dose, 20mg, Cialis was taken daily for 6 months. In addition, there was no effect on mean concentrations of testosterone, luteinizing hormone, or follicle stimulating hormone with either 10 or 20mg of Cialis compared to placebo. The effects of longer-term daily dosing have not been established. See also sections 4.4 and 5.3.

Tadalafil at doses of 2 to 100mg has been evaluated in 16 clinical studies involving 3,250 patients, including patients with erectile dysfunction of various severities (mild, moderate, severe), aetiologies, ages (range 21-86 years), and ethnicities. Most patients reported erectile dysfunction of at least 1 year in duration. In the primary efficacy studies of general populations, 81% of patients reported that Cialis improved their erections as compared to 35% with placebo. Also, patients with erectile dysfunction in all severity categories reported improved erections whilst taking Cialis (86%, 83%, and 72% for mild, moderate, and severe, respectively, as compared to 45%, 42%, and 19% with placebo). In the primary efficacy studies, 75% of intercourse attempts were successful in Cialis-treated patients as compared to 32% with placebo.

5.2 Pharmacokinetic properties

Absorption

Tadalafil is readily absorbed after oral administration and the mean maximum observed plasma concentration (C_{max}) is achieved at a median time of 2 hours after dosing. Absolute bioavailability of tadalafil following oral dosing has not been determined.

The rate and extent of absorption of tadalafil are not influenced by food, thus Cialis may be taken with or without food. The time of dosing (morning versus evening) had no clinically relevant effects on the rate and extent of absorption.

Distribution

The mean volume of distribution is approximately 63 litres, indicating that tadalafil is distributed into tissues. At therapeutic concentrations, 94% of tadalafil in plasma is bound to proteins. Protein binding is not affected by impaired renal function.

Less than 0.0005% of the administered dose appeared in the semen of healthy subjects.

Biotransformation

Tadalafil is predominantly metabolised by the cytochrome P450 (CYP) 3A4 isoform. The major circulating metabolite is the methylcatechol glucuronide. This metabolite is at least 13,000-fold less potent than tadalafil for PDE5. Consequently, it is not expected to be clinically active at observed metabolite concentrations.

Elimination

The mean oral clearance for tadalafil is 2.5 l/h and the mean half-life is 17.5 hours in healthy subjects.

Tadalafil is excreted predominantly as inactive metabolites, mainly in the faeces (approximately 61% of the dose) and to a lesser extent in the urine (approximately 36% of the dose).

Linearity/non-linearity

Tadalafil pharmacokinetics in healthy subjects are linear with respect to time and dose. Over a dose range of 2.5 to 20mg, exposure (AUC) increases proportionally with dose. Steady-state plasma concentrations are attained within 5 days of once daily dosing.

Pharmacokinetics determined with a population approach in patients with erectile dysfunction are similar to pharmacokinetics in subjects without erectile dysfunction.

Special populations

Elderly

Healthy elderly subjects (65 years or over) had a lower oral clearance of tadalafil, resulting in 25% higher exposure (AUC) relative to healthy subjects aged 19 to 45 years. This effect of age is not clinically significant and does not warrant a dose adjustment.

Renal insufficiency

In clinical pharmacology studies using single dose tadalafil (5-20mg), tadalafil exposure (AUC) approximately doubled in subjects with mild (creatinine clearance 51 to 80ml/min) or moderate (creatinine clearance 31 to 50ml/min) renal impairment and in subjects with end-stage renal disease on dialysis. In haemodialysis patients, C_{max} was 41% higher than that observed in healthy subjects. Haemodialysis contributes negligibly to tadalafil elimination.

Hepatic insufficiency

Tadalafil exposure (AUC) in subjects with mild and moderate hepatic impairment (Child-Pugh class A and B) is comparable to exposure in healthy subjects when a dose of 10mg is administered. There is limited clinical data on the safety of Cialis in patients with severe hepatic insufficiency (Child-Pugh class C); if prescribed, a careful individual benefit/risk evaluation should be undertaken by the prescribing physician. There are no available data about the administration of doses higher than 10mg of tadalafil to patients with hepatic impairment.

Patients with diabetes

Tadalafil exposure (AUC) in patients with diabetes was approximately 19% lower than the AUC value for healthy subjects. This difference in exposure does not warrant a dose adjustment.

5.3 Preclinical safety data

Preclinical data reveal no special hazard for humans based on conventional studies of safety pharmacology, genotoxicity, carcinogenic potential, and toxicity to reproduction.

There was no evidence of teratogenicity, embryotoxicity, or foetotoxicity in rats or mice that received up to 1,000mg/kg/day. In a rat prenatal and postnatal development study, the no observed effect dose was 30mg/kg/day. In the pregnant rat the AUC for calculated free drug at this dose was approximately 18-times the human AUC at a 20mg dose.

There was no impairment of fertility in male and female rats. In dogs given tadalafil daily for 6 to 12 months at doses of 25mg/kg/day (resulting in at least a 3-fold greater exposure [range 3.7-18.6] than seen in humans given a single 20mg dose) and above, there was regression of the seminiferous tubular epithelium that resulted in a decrease in spermatogenesis in some dogs. See also sections 4.4 and 5.1.

6. PHARMACEUTICAL PARTICULARS

6.1 List of excipients

Tablet core:

Lactose monohydrate

Croscarmellose sodium

Hydroxypropylcellulose

Microcrystalline cellulose

Sodium laurilsulfate

Magnesium stearate

Film-coat:

Lactose monohydrate

Hypromellose

Triacetin

Titanium dioxide (E171)

Iron oxide yellow (E172)

Talc

6.2 Incompatibilities

Not applicable.

6.3 Shelf life

3 years (10mg tablets)

2 years (20mg tablets).

6.4 Special precautions for storage

Store in the original package.

6.5 Nature and contents of container

Aluminium/PVC/PE/Aclar blisters in cartons of 4 tablets 10mg.

Aluminium/PVC/PE/Aclar blisters in cartons of 4 or 8 tablets 20mg.

6.6 Instructions for use and handling

No special requirements.

7. MARKETING AUTHORISATION HOLDER
Lilly ICOS Limited
St Bride's House
10 Salisbury Square
London
EC4Y 8EH
United Kingdom

8. MARKETING AUTHORISATION NUMBER(S)
EU/1/02/237/001: 4 × 10mg tablets
EU/1/02/237/003: 4 × 20mg tablets
EU/1/02/237/004: 8 × 20mg tablets

9. DATE OF FIRST AUTHORISATION/RENEWAL OF THE AUTHORISATION
12 November 2002

10. DATE OF REVISION OF THE TEXT
1 October 2004

LEGAL CATEGORY
POM

*CIALIS (tadalafil) is a trademark of Lilly ICOS LLC.

CI4M

Cicatrin Cream

(GlaxoSmithKline UK)

1. NAME OF THE MEDICINAL PRODUCT
Cicatrin Cream

2. QUALITATIVE AND QUANTITATIVE COMPOSITION

Neomycin Sulphate EP	3,300 units/g
Bacitracin zinc BP	250 units/g
Glycine BP	1.0% w/w
L-Cysteine	0.2% w/w
DL-Threonine USP	0.1% w/w

3. PHARMACEUTICAL FORM
Cream

4. CLINICAL PARTICULARS
4.1 Therapeutic indications
Topical broad-spectrum antibacterial. Superficial bacterial infection of the skin, such as impetigo, varicose ulcers, pressure sores, trophic ulcers and burns.

4.2 Posology and method of administration
Administration and dosage in adults
Before use, the area for application should be cleaned gently. Debris such as pus or crusts should be removed from the affected area.
A thin film of the cream should be applied to the affected area up to three times/day, depending on the clinical condition. Treatment should not be continued for more than seven days without medical supervision (see Precautions and Warnings).

Dosage in children
Cicatrin Cream is suitable for use in children (2 years and over) at the same dose as adults. A possibility of increased absorption exists in very young children, thus Cicatrin is not recommended for use in neonates and infants (<2 years) (see 4.3 Contra-Indications and 4.4 Special Warnings and Special Precautions for Use).

Dosage in the elderly
No specific studies have been carried out in the elderly however, Cicatrin Cream is suitable for use in the elderly. Caution should be exercised in cases where a decrease in renal function exists and significant systemic absorption of neomycin sulphate may occur (See Dosage in Renal Impairment and Precautions and Warnings).

Dosage in renal impairment
Dosage should be reduced in patients with reduced renal function (see Precautions and Warnings).

Route of Administration
Topical

4.3 Contraindications
The use of Cicatrin Cream is contra-indicated in patients who have demonstrated allergic hypersensitivity to the product or any of its constituents, or to cross-sensitizing substances such as framycetin, kanamycin, gentamicin and other related antibiotics.

Due to known ototoxic and nephrotoxic potential of neomycin sulphate, the use of Cicatrin in large quantities or on large areas for prolonged periods of time is not recommended in circumstances where significant systemic absorption may occur.

A possibility of increased absorption exists in very young children, therefore Cicatrin Cream is not recommended for use in neonates and infants (up to 2 years). In neonates and infants, absorption by immature skin may be enhanced, and renal function may be immature.

The presence of pre-existing nerve deafness is a contraindication to the use of Cicatrin Cream in circumstances in which significant systemic absorption could occur.

Cicatrin Cream should not be applied to the eyes.

4.4 Special warnings and special precautions for use
Caution should be exercised so that the recommended dosage is not exceeded (see Dosage and Administration and Contra-indications).

Following significant systemic absorption, aminoglycosides such as neomycin can cause irreversible ototoxicity (and exacerbate existing partial nerve deafness); both neomycin sulphate and bacitracin zinc have nephrotoxic potential.

After a treatment course, administration should not be repeated for at least three months.

In renal impairment the plasma clearance of neomycin is reduced, this is associated with an increased risk of ototoxicity; therefore, a reduction in dose should be made that relates to the degree of renal impairment.

As with other antibacterial preparations, prolonged use may result in overgrowth by non-susceptible organisms, including fungi.

Concurrent administration of other aminoglycosides is not recommended.

4.5 Interaction with other medicinal products and other forms of Interaction
Following significant systemic absorption, neomycin sulphate can intensify and prolong the respiratory depressant effect of neuromuscular blocking agents.

4.6 Pregnancy and lactation
Pregnancy
There is little information to demonstrate the possible effect of topically applied neomycin in pregnancy and lactation, therefore the use of Cicatrin is not recommended.

Lactation
No information is available regarding the excretion of the active ingredients in human milk.

4.7 Effects on ability to drive and use machines
None known.

4.8 Undesirable effects
The incidence of allergic hypersensitivity to neomycin sulphate in the general population is low. However, there is an increased incidence of sensitivity to neomycin in certain selected groups of patients in dermatological practice, particularly those with venous stasis eczema and ulceration.

Allergic hypersensitivity to neomycin following topical application may manifest itself as a reddening and scaling of the affected skin, as an eczematous exacerbation of the lesion, or as a failure of the lesion to heal.

Allergic hypersensitivity following topical application of bacitracin zinc has been reported but is rare.

Anaphylactic reactions following the topical administration of bacitracin zinc have been reported but are rare.

4.9 Overdose
Symptoms and signs
No specific symptoms or signs have been associated with excessive use of Cicatrin Cream. However, consideration should be given to significant systemic absorption (see Precautions and Warnings).

Management
Use of the product should be stopped and the patient's general status, hearing acuity, renal and neuromuscular functions should be monitored. Blood levels of neomycin sulphate and bacitracin zinc should be determined, and haemodialysis may reduce the serum level of neomycin sulphate.

5. PHARMACOLOGICAL PROPERTIES
5.1 Pharmacodynamic properties
Not available.

5.2 Pharmacokinetic properties
Not applicable.

5.3 Preclinical safety data
A. Mutagenicity
There is insufficient information available to determine whether the active ingredients have mutagenic potential.

B. Carcinogenicity
There is insufficient information available to determine whether the active ingredients have carcinogenic potential.

C. Teratogenicity
There is insufficient information available to determine whether the active ingredients have teratogenic potential.

Neomycin present in maternal blood can cross the placenta and may give rise to a theoretical risk of foetal ototoxicity.

D. Fertility
There is insufficient information available to determine whether any of the active ingredients can affect fertility.

6. PHARMACEUTICAL PARTICULARS
6.1 List of excipients
Sorbitan Trioleate
Wool Alcohols
Macrogol (4) Lauryl Ether
Liquid Paraffin
Polysorbate 85
Hard Paraffin
White Soft Paraffin

6.2 Incompatibilities
Cicatrin Cream should not be diluted.

6.3 Shelf life
2 years.

6.4 Special precautions for storage
Store below 25°C.

6.5 Nature and contents of container
Internally lacquered aluminium collapsible tubes with polypropylene screw caps.
Pack Size: 15g and 30g

6.6 Instructions for use and handling
No special instructions.

Administrative Data
7. MARKETING AUTHORISATION HOLDER
The Wellcome Foundation Ltd
Glaxo Wellcome House
Berkeley Avenue
Greenford
Middlesex UB6 ONN
Trading as
GlaxoSmithKline UK
Stockley Park West
Uxbridge
Middlesex UB11 1BT

8. MARKETING AUTHORISATION NUMBER(S)
PL 00003/5082R

9. DATE OF FIRST AUTHORISATION/RENEWAL OF THE AUTHORISATION
18 September 1998

10. DATE OF REVISION OF THE TEXT
2 April 2003

Cicatrin Powder

(GlaxoSmithKline UK)

1. NAME OF THE MEDICINAL PRODUCT
Cicatrin Powder

2. QUALITATIVE AND QUANTITATIVE COMPOSITION

Neomycin Sulphate	3,300 units/g
Bacitracin zinc	250 units/g
Glycine	1% w/w
L-Cysteine	0.2% w/w
DL-Threonine	0.1% w/w

3. PHARMACEUTICAL FORM
Powder

4. CLINICAL PARTICULARS
4.1 Therapeutic indications
Topical broad-spectrum antibacterial. Superficial bacterial infection of the skin, such as impetigo, varicose ulcers, pressure sores, trophic ulcers and burns.

4.2 Posology and method of administration
Administration and dosage in adults
Before use, the area for application should be cleaned gently. Debris such as pus or crusts should be removed from the affected area.

A light dusting of the powder should be applied to the affected area up to three times/day, depending on the clinical condition. Treatment should not be continued for more than seven days without medical supervision (see Precautions and Warnings).

Dosage in children
Cicatrin Powder is suitable for use in children (2 years and over) at the same dose as adults. A possibility of increased absorption exists in very young children, thus Cicatrin is not recommended for use in neonates and infants (<2 years) (see 4.3 Contra-Indications and 4.4 Special Warnings and Special Precautions for Use).

Dosage in the elderly
No specific studies have been carried out in the elderly however, Cicatrin Powder is suitable for use in the elderly. Caution should be exercised in cases where a decrease in renal function exists and significant systemic absorption of neomycin sulphate may occur (See Dosage in Renal Impairment and Precautions and Warnings).

Dosage in renal impairment

Dosage should be reduced in patients with reduced renal function (see Precautions and Warnings).

Route of Administration

Topical

4.3 Contraindications

The use of Cicatrin Powder is contra-indicated in patients who have demonstrated allergic hypersensitivity to the product or any of its constituents, or to cross-sensitizing substances such as framycetin, kanamycin, gentamicin and other related antibiotics.

Due to known ototoxic and nephrotoxic potential of neomycin sulphate, the use of Cicatrin in large quantities or on large areas for prolonged periods of time is not recommended in circumstances where significant systemic absorption may occur.

A possibility of increased absorption exists in very young children, therefore Cicatrin Powder is not recommended for use in neonates and infants (up to 2 years). In neonates and infants, absorption by immature skin may be enhanced, and renal function may be immature.

The presence of pre-existing nerve deafness is a contra-indication to the use of Cicatrin Powder in circumstances in which significant systemic absorption could occur.

Cicatrin Powder should not be applied to the eyes.

4.4 Special warnings and special precautions for use

Caution should be exercised so that the recommended dosage is not exceeded (see Dosage and Administration and Contra-indications).

Following significant systemic absorption, aminoglycosides such as neomycin can cause irreversible ototoxicity (and exacerbate existing partial nerve deafness); both neomycin sulphate and bacitracin zinc have nephrotoxic potential.

After a treatment course, administration should not be repeated for at least three months.

In renal impairment the plasma clearance of neomycin is reduced, this is associated with an increased risk of ototoxicity; therefore, a reduction in dose should be made that relates to the degree of renal impairment.

As with other antibacterial preparations, prolonged use may result in overgrowth by non-susceptible organisms, including fungi.

Concurrent administration of other aminoglycosides is not recommended.

4.5 Interaction with other medicinal products and other forms of Interaction

Following significant systemic absorption, neomycin sulphate can intensify and prolong the respiratory depressant effect of neuromuscular blocking agents.

4.6 Pregnancy and lactation

Pregnancy

There is little information to demonstrate the possible effect of topically applied neomycin in pregnancy and lactation, therefore the use of Cicatrin is not recommended.

Lactation

No information is available regarding the excretion of the active ingredients in human milk.

4.7 Effects on ability to drive and use machines

None known.

4.8 Undesirable effects

The incidence of allergic hypersensitivity to neomycin sulphate in the general population is low. However, there is an increased incidence of sensitivity to neomycin in certain selected groups of patients in dermatological practice, particularly those with venous stasis eczema and ulceration.

Allergic hypersensitivity to neomycin following topical application may manifest itself as a reddening and scaling of the affected skin, as an eczematous exacerbation of the lesion, or as a failure of the lesion to heal.

Allergic hypersensitivity following topical application of bacitracin zinc has been reported but is rare.

Anaphylactic reactions following the topical administration of bacitracin zinc have been reported but are rare.

4.9 Overdose

Symptoms and signs

No specific symptoms or signs have been associated with excessive use of Cicatrin powder. However, consideration should be given to significant systemic absorption (see Precautions and Warnings).

Management

Use of the product should be stopped and the patient's general status, hearing acuity, renal and neuromuscular functions should be monitored. Blood levels of neomycin sulphate and bacitracin zinc should be determined, and haemodialysis may reduce the serum level of neomycin sulphate.

5. PHARMACOLOGICAL PROPERTIES

5.1 Pharmacodynamic properties

Not available.

5.2 Pharmacokinetic properties

Not applicable.

5.3 Preclinical safety data

A. Mutagenicity

There is insufficient information available to determine whether the active ingredients have mutagenic potential.

B. Carcinogenicity

There is insufficient information available to determine whether the active ingredients have carcinogenic potential.

C. Teratogenicity

There is insufficient information available to determine whether the active ingredients have teratogenic potential.

Neomycin present in maternal blood can cross the placenta and may give rise to a theoretical risk of foetal ototoxicity.

D. Fertility

There is insufficient information available to determine whether any of the active ingredients can affect fertility.

6. PHARMACEUTICAL PARTICULARS

6.1 List of excipients

Sterilised Maize Starch

6.2 Incompatibilities

Cicatrin Powder should not be diluted.

6.3 Shelf life

2 years.

6.4 Special precautions for storage

Store below 25°C.

6.5 Nature and contents of container

Low density polyethylene bottles with nozzle inserts and urea formaldehyde screw caps.

Pack Size: 15g and 50g

6.6 Instructions for use and handling

No special instructions.

Administrative Data

7. MARKETING AUTHORISATION HOLDER

The Wellcome Foundation Ltd
Glaxo Wellcome House
Berkeley Avenue
Greenford
Middlesex
UB6 ONN
Trading as
GlaxoSmithKline UK
Stockley Park West
Uxbridge
Middlesex UB11 1BT

8. MARKETING AUTHORISATION NUMBER(S)

PL 00003/5081R

9. DATE OF FIRST AUTHORISATION/RENEWAL OF THE AUTHORISATION

25 May 2004

10. DATE OF REVISION OF THE TEXT

25 May 2004

Cidomycin Adult Injectable 80mg/2ml

(sanofi-aventis)

1. NAME OF THE MEDICINAL PRODUCT

Cidomycin™ Adult Injectable 80mg/2ml.

2. QUALITATIVE AND QUANTITATIVE COMPOSITION

Each ampoule or vial (2ml) contains Gentamicin Sulphate Ph Eur equivalent to 80mg Gentamicin base.

For excipients, see section 6.1

3. PHARMACEUTICAL FORM

Solution for Injection.

Clear, colourless solution.

4. CLINICAL PARTICULARS

4.1 Therapeutic indications

Gentamicin is an aminoglycoside antibiotic with broad-spectrum bactericidal activity. It is usually active against most strains of the following organisms: Escherichia coli, Klebsiella spp., Proteus spp. (indole positive and indole negative), Pseudomonas aeruginosa, Staphylococci, Enterobacter spp., Citrobacter spp and Providencia spp.

Gentamicin injection and gentamicin paediatric injection are indicated in urinary-tract infections, chest infections, bacteraemia, septicaemia, severe neonatal infections and other systemic infections due to sensitive organisms.

4.2 Posology and method of administration

ADULTS:

Serious infections: If renal function is not impaired, 5mg/kg/daily in divided doses at six or eight hourly intervals. The total daily dose may be subsequently increased or decreased as clinically indicated.

Systemic infections: If renal function is not impaired, 3-5mg/kg/day in divided doses according to severity of infection, adjusting according to clinical response and body weight.

Urinary tract infections: As "Systemic infections". Or, if renal function is not impaired, 160mg once daily may be used.

CHILDREN:

Premature infants or full term neonates up to 2 weeks or age: 3mg/kg 12 hourly. 2 weeks to 12 years: 2mg/kg 8 hourly.

THE ELDERLY:

There is some evidence that elderly patients may be more susceptible to aminoglycoside toxicity whether secondary to previous eighth nerve impairment or borderline renal dysfunction. Accordingly, therapy should be closely monitored by frequent determination of gentamicin serum levels, assessment of renal function and signs of ototoxicity.

RENAL IMPAIRMENT:

Gentamicin is excreted by simple glomerular filtration and therefore reduced dosage is necessary where renal function is impaired. Nomograms are available for the calculation of dose, which depends on the patient's age, weight and renal function. The following table may be useful when treating adults.

(see Table 1)

The recommended dose and precautions for intramuscular and intravenous administration are identical. Gentamicin when given intravenously should be injected directly into a vein or into the drip set tubing over no less than three minutes. If administered by infusion, this should be over no longer than 20 minutes and in no greater volume of fluid than 100ml.

4.3 Contraindications

Hypersensitivity; Myasthenia Gravis.

4.4 Special warnings and special precautions for use

Ototoxicity has been recorded following the use of gentamicin. Groups at special risk include patients with impaired renal function, infants and possibly the elderly. Consequently, renal, auditory and vestibular functions should be monitored in these patients and serum levels determined so as to avoid peak concentrations above 10mg/l and troughs above 2mg/l. As there is some evidence that risk of both ototoxicity and nephrotoxicity is related to the level of total exposure, duration of therapy should be the shortest possible compatible with clinical recovery. In some patients with impaired renal function there has been a transient rise in blood-urea-nitrogen which has usually reverted to normal during or following cessation of therapy. It is important to adjust the frequency of dosage according to the degree of renal function.

Gentamicin should only be used in pregnancy if considered essential by the physician (see section 4.6 Pregnancy and Lactation.)

Gentamicin should be used with care in conditions characterised by muscular weakness.

Table 1

Blood Urea (mg/100ml)	(mmol/l)	Creatinine clearance (GFR) (ml/min)	Dose & frequency of administration
< 40	6 - 7	> 70	80mg* 8 hourly
40 - 100	6 - 17	30 - 70	80mg* 12 hourly
100 - 200	17 - 34	10 - 30	80mg* daily
> 200	> 34	5 - 10	80mg* every 48 hours
Twice weekly intermittent haemodialysis		< 5	80mg* after dialysis

*60mg if body weight <60kg. Frequency of dosage in hours may also be approximated as serum creatinine (mg%) × eight or in si units, as serum creatinine (umol/l) divided by 11. If these dosage guides are used peak serum levels must be measured. Peak levels of gentamicin occur approximately one hour after intra muscular injection and intravenous injection. Trough levels are measured just prior to the next injection. Assay of peak serum levels gives confirmation of adequacy of dosage and also serves to detect levels above 10mg/l, at which the possibility of ototoxicity should be considered. One hour concentrations of gentamicin should not exceed 10mg/l (but should reach 4mg/l), while the pre dose trough concentration should be less than 2mg/l.

In cases of significant obesity gentamicin serum concentrations should be closely monitored and a reduction in dose should be considered.

4.5 Interaction with other medicinal products and other forms of Interaction
Concurrent administration of gentamicin and other potentially ototoxic or nephrotoxic drugs should be avoided. Potent diuretics such as etacrynic acid and furosemide are believed to enhance the risk of ototoxicity whilst amphotericin B, cisplatin and ciclosporin are potential enhancers of nephrotoxicity.

Any potential nephrotoxicity of cephalosporins, and in particular cephaloridine, may also be increased in the presence of gentamicin. Consequently, if this combination is used monitoring of kidney function is advised.

Neuromuscular blockade and respiratory paralysis have been reported from administration of aminoglycosides to patients who have received curare-type muscle relaxants during anaesthesia.

Indometacin possibly increases plasma concentrations of gentamicin in neonates.

Concurrent use with oral anticoagulants may increase the hypothrombinanaemic effect.

Concurrent use of bisphosphonates may increase the risk of hypocalcaemia.

Concurrent use of the Botulinum Toxin and gentamicin may increase the risk of toxicity due to enhanced neuromuscular block.

Antagonism of effect may occur with concomitant administration of gentamicin with either neostigmine or pyridostigmine.

4.6 Pregnancy and lactation
There are no proven cases of intrauterine damage caused by gentamicin. However, in common with most drugs known to cross the placenta, usage in pregnancy should only be considered in life threatening situations where expected benefits outweigh possible risks. In the absence of gastro-intestinal inflammation, the amount of gentamicin ingested from the milk is unlikely to result in significant blood levels in breast-fed infants.

4.7 Effects on ability to drive and use machines
Not known.

4.8 Undesirable effects
Side-effects include vestibular damage or hearing loss, particularly after exposure to ototoxic drugs or in the presence of renal dysfunction. Nephrotoxicity (usually reversible) and occasionally acute renal failure, hypersensitivity, anaemia, blood dycrasias, purpura, stomatitis, convulsions and effects on liver function occur occasionally.

Rarely hypomagnesia on prolonged therapy and antibiotic–associated colitis have been reported.

Nausea, vomiting and rash have also been reported.

Central neurotoxicity, including encephalopathy, confusion, lethargy, mental depression and hallucinations, has been reported in association with gentamicin therapy but this is extremely rare.

4.9 Overdose
Haemodialysis and peritoneal dialysis will aid the removal from blood but the former is probably more efficient. Calcium salts given intravenously have been used to counter the neuromuscular blockade caused by gentamicin.

5. PHARMACOLOGICAL PROPERTIES
5.1 Pharmacodynamic properties
Gentamicin is a mixture of antibiotic substances produced by the growth of micromonospora purpurea. It is bactericidal with greater antibacterial activity than streptomycin, neomycin or kanamycin.

Gentamicin exerts a number of effects on cells of susceptible bacteria. It affects the integrity of the plasma membrane and the metabolism of RNA, but its most important effects is inhibition of protein synthesis at the level of the 30s ribosomal subunit.

5.2 Pharmacokinetic properties
Gentamicin is not readily absorbed from the gastro-intestinal tract. Gentamicin is 70-85% bound to plasma albumin following administration and is excreted 90% unchanged in urine. The half-life for its elimination in normal patients is 2 to 3 hours.

Effective plasma concentration is 4-8 μg/ml.

The volume of distribution (vd) is 0.3 l/kg.

The elimination rate constant is:

0.02 hr^{-1} for anuric patients *

0.30 hr^{-1} normal

* Therefore in those with anuria care must be exercised following the usual initial dose, any subsequent administration being reduced in-line with plasma concentrations of gentamicin.

5.3 Preclinical safety data
Not applicable.

6. PHARMACEUTICAL PARTICULARS
6.1 List of excipients
Methyl parahydroxybenzoate (E218)
Propyl parahydroxybenzoate (E216)
Disodium Edetate
Water for Injections
2M Sodium Hydroxide
1M Sulphuric Acid

6.2 Incompatibilities
In general, gentamicin injection should not be mixed. In particular the following are incompatible in mixed solution with gentamicin injection: penicillins, cephalosporins, erythromycin, heparins, sodium bicarbonate. * Dilution in the body will obviate the danger of physical and chemical incompatibility and enable gentamicin to be given concurrently with the drugs listed above either as a bolus injection into the drip tubing, with adequate flushing, or at separate sites. In the case of carbenicillin, administration should only be at a separate site.

* Carbon dioxide may be liberated on addition of the two solutions. Normally this will dissolve in the solution but under some circumstances small bubbles may form.

6.3 Shelf life
3 years

6.4 Special precautions for storage
Do not store above 25°C. Do not refrigerate or freeze.

6.5 Nature and contents of container
Cidomycin Adult Injectable is supplied in ampoules and vials.

6.6 Instructions for use and handling
Not applicable.

7. MARKETING AUTHORISATION HOLDER
Aventis Pharma
Broadwater Park
Denham
Uxbridge
Middlesex UB9 5HP

8. MARKETING AUTHORISATION NUMBER(S)
PL 0109/5065R

9. DATE OF FIRST AUTHORISATION/RENEWAL OF THE AUTHORISATION
24th January 1991

10. DATE OF REVISION OF THE TEXT
July 2005

Legal category: POM

Cilest

(Janssen-Cilag Ltd)

1. NAME OF THE MEDICINAL PRODUCT
Cilest®

2. QUALITATIVE AND QUANTITATIVE COMPOSITION
Cilest are tablets for oral administration.

Each tablet contains norgestimate 0.25 mg and ethinylestradiol PhEur 0.035 mg.

3. PHARMACEUTICAL FORM
Tablets (small, round, dark blue, engraved 'C 250' on both faces).

4. CLINICAL PARTICULARS
4.1 Therapeutic indications
Contraception and the recognised indications for such oestrogen/progestogen combinations.

4.2 Posology and method of administration
For oral administration.

Adults
It is preferable that tablet intake from the first pack is started on the first day of menstruation in which case no extra contraceptive precautions are necessary.

If menstruation has already begun (that is 2, 3 or 4 days previously), tablet taking should commence on day 5 of the menstrual period. In this case additional contraceptive precautions must be taken for the first 7 days of tablet taking.

If menstruation began more than 5 days previously then the patient should be advised to wait until her next menstrual period before starting to take Cilest.

How to take Cilest:

One tablet is taken daily at the same time (preferably in the evening) without interruption for 21 days, followed by a break of 7 tablet-free days. Each subsequent pack is started after the 7 tablet-free days have elapsed. Additional contraceptive precautions are not then required.

Elderly:

Not applicable.

Children:

Not recommended.

4.3 Contraindications
Absolute contra-indications
– Pregnancy or suspected pregnancy (that cannot yet be excluded).

– Circulatory disorders (cardiovascular or cerebrovascular) such as thrombophlebitis and thrombo-embolic processes, or a history of these conditions (including history of confirmed venous thrombo-embolism (VTE), family history of idiopathic VTE and other known risk factors for VTE), moderate to severe hypertension, hyperlipoproteinaemia. In addition the presence of more than one of the risk factors for arterial disease.

– Severe liver disease, cholestatic jaundice or hepatitis (viral or non-viral) or a history of these conditions if the results of liver function tests have failed to return to normal, and for 3 months after liver function tests have been found to be normal; a history of jaundice of pregnancy or jaundice due to the use of steroids, Rotor syndrome and Dubin-Johnson syndrome, hepatic cell tumours and porphyria.

– Cholelithiasis

– Known or suspected oestrogen-dependent tumours; endometrial hyperplasia; undiagnosed vaginal bleeding.

– Systemic lupus erythematosus or a history of this condition.

– A history during pregnancy or previous use of steroids of:

- severe pruritus
- herpes gestationis
- a manifestation or deterioration of otosclerosis

Relative contra-indications:

If any relative contra-indications listed below are present, the benefits of oestrogen/progestogen-containing preparations must be weighed against the possible risk for each individual case and the patient kept under close supervision. In case of aggravation or appearance of any of these conditions whilst the patient is taking the pill, its use should be discontinued.

– Conditions implicating an increasing risk of developing venous thrombo-embolic complications, eg severe varicose veins or prolonged immobilisation or major surgery. Disorders of coagulation.

– Presence of any risk factor for arterial disease eg smoking, hyperlipidaemia or hypertension.

– Other conditions associated with an increased risk of circulatory disease such as latent or overt cardiac failure, renal dysfunction, or a history of these conditions.

– Epilepsy or a history of this condition.

– Migraine or a history of this condition.

– A history of cholelithiasis.

– Presence of any risk factor for oestrogen-dependent tumours; oestrogen-sensitive gynaecological disorders such as uterine fibromyomata and endometriosis.

– Diabetes mellitus.

– Severe depression or a history of this condition. If this is accompanied by a disturbance in tryptophan metabolism, administration of vitamin B6 might be of therapeutic value.

– Sickle cell haemoglobinopathy, since under certain circumstances, eg during infections or anoxia, oestrogen-containing preparations may induce thrombo-embolic process in patients with this condition.

– If the results of liver function tests become abnormal, use should be discontinued.

4.4 Special warnings and special precautions for use
Post-partum administration
Following a vaginal delivery, oral contraceptive administration to non-breast-feeding mothers can be started 21 days post-partum provided the patient is fully ambulant and there are no puerperal complications. No additional contraceptive precautions are required. If post-partum administration begins more than 21 days after delivery, additional contraceptive precautions are required for the first 7 days of pill-taking.

If intercourse has taken place post-partum, oral contraceptive use should be delayed until the first day of the first menstrual period.

After miscarriage or abortion administration should start immediately in which case no additional contraceptive precautions are required.

Changing from a 21 day pill or another 22 day pill to Cilest:

All tablets in the old pack should be finished. The first Cilest tablet is taken the next day, ie no gap is left between taking tablets nor does the patient need to wait for her period to begin. Tablets should be taken as instructed in 'How to take Cilest' (see 4.2). Additional contraceptive precautions are not required. The patient will not have a period until the end of the first Cilest pack, but this is not harmful, nor does it matter if she experiences some bleeding on tablet-taking days.

Changing from a combined every day pill (28 day tablets) to Cilest:

Cilest should be started after taking the last active tablet from the 'Every day Pill' pack (ie after taking 21 or 22 tablets). The first Cilest tablet is taken the next day ie no gap is left between taking tablets nor does the patient need to wait for her period to begin. Tablets should be taken as instructed in 'How to take Cilest' (see 4.2). Additional contraceptive precautions are not required. Remaining tablets from the every day (ED) pack should be discarded.

The patient will not have a period until the end of the first Cilest pack, but this is not harmful, nor does it matter if she experiences some bleeding on tablet-taking days.

Changing from a progestogen-only pill (POP or mini pill) to Cilest:

The first Cilest tablet should be taken on the first day of the period, even if the patient has already taken a mini pill on that day. Tablets should be taken as instructed in 'How to take Cilest' (see 4.2). Additional contraceptive precautions are not required. All the remaining progestogen-only pills in the mini pill pack should be discarded.

If the patient is taking a mini pill, then she may not always have a period, especially when she is breast feeding. The first Cilest tablet should be taken on the day after stopping the mini pill. All remaining pills in the mini pill packet must be discarded. Additional contraceptive precautions must be taken for the first 7 days.

To skip a period

To skip a period, a new pack of Cilest should be started on the day after finishing the current pack (the patient skips the tablet-free days). Tablet-taking should be continued in the usual way.

During the use of the second pack she may experience slight spotting or break-through bleeding but contraceptive protection will not be diminished provided there are no tablet omissions.

The next pack of Cilest is started after the usual 7 tablet-free days, regardless of whether the period has completely finished or not.

Reduced reliability

When Cilest is taken according to the directions for use the occurrence of pregnancy is highly unlikely. However, the reliability of oral contraceptives may be reduced under the following circumstances:

(i) Forgotten tablets

If the patient forgets to take a tablet, she should take it as soon as she remembers and take the next one at the normal time. This may mean that two tablets are taken in one day. Provided she is less than 12 hours late in taking her tablet, Cilest will still give contraceptive protection during this cycle and the rest of the pack should be taken as usual.

If she is more than 12 hours late in taking one or more tablets then she should take the last missed pill as soon as she remembers but leave the other missed pills in the pack. She should continue to take the rest of the pack as usual but must use extra precautions (eg sheath, diaphragm, plus spermicide) and follow the '7-day rule' (see Further Information for the 7-day rule).

If there are 7 or more pills left in the pack after the missed and delayed pills then the usual 7-day break can be left before starting the next pack. If there are less than 7 pills left in the pack after the missed and delayed pills then when the pack is finished the next pack should be started the next day. If withdrawal bleeding does not occur at the end of the second pack then a pregnancy test should be performed.

(ii) Vomiting or diarrhoea

If after tablet intake vomiting or diarrhoea occurs, a tablet may not be absorbed properly by the body. If the symptoms disappear within 12 hours of tablet-taking, the patient should take an extra tablet from a spare pack and continue with the rest of the pack as usual.

However, if the symptoms continue beyond those 12 hours, additional contraceptive precautions are necessary for any sexual intercourse during the stomach or bowel upset and for the following 7 days (the patient must be advised to follow the '7-day rule').

(iii) Change in bleeding pattern

If after taking Cilest for several months there is a sudden occurrence of spotting or breakthrough bleeding (not observed in previous cycles) or the absence of withdrawal bleeding, contraceptive effectiveness may be reduced. If withdrawal bleeding fails to occur and none of the above mentioned events has taken place, pregnancy is highly unlikely and oral contraceptive use can be continued until the end of the next pack. (If withdrawal bleeding fails to occur at the end of the second cycle, tablet intake should be discontinued and pregnancy excluded before oral contraceptive use can be resumed.) However, if withdrawal bleeding is absent and any of the above mentioned events has occurred, tablet intake should be discontinued and pregnancy excluded before oral contraceptive use can be resumed.

Medical examination/consultation

Assessment of women prior to starting oral contraceptives (and at regular intervals thereafter) should include a personal and family medical history of each woman. Physical examination should be guided by this and by the contra-indications (Section 4.3) and warnings (Section 4.4) for this product. The frequency and nature of these assessments should be based upon relevant guidelines and should be adapted to the individual woman, but should include measurement of blood pressure and, if judged appropriate by the clinician, breast, abdominal and pelvic examination including cervical cytology.

Caution should be observed when prescribing oral contraceptives to young women whose cycles are not yet stabilised.

Venous thrombo-embolic disease

The use of any combined oral contraceptive (COCs) carries an increased risk for venous thrombo-embolism (VTE), including deep venous thrombosis and pulmonary embolism, compared with no use. The excess risk of VTE is highest during the first year a woman ever uses a combined oral contraceptive. This increased risk is less than the risk of VTE associated with pregnancy, which is estimated as 60 per 100,000 pregnancies. VTE is fatal in 1-2% of cases.

It is not known how Cilest influences the risk of VTE compared with other combined oral contraceptives.

However, epidemiological studies have shown that the incidence of VTE in users of oral contraceptives with low estrogen content (<50 μg ethinyl estradiol) ranges from about 20-40 cases per 100,000 women years, but this risk estimate varies according to the progestogen. This compares with 5-10 cases per 100,000 women years for non-users.

Epidemiological studies have also associated the use of combined oral contraceptives with an increased risk for arterial thrombo-embolism (eg myocardial infarction, transient ischaemic attack).

Surgery, varicose veins or immobilisation

In patients using oestrogen-containing preparations the risk of deep vein thrombosis may be temporarily increased when undergoing a major operation (eg abdominal, orthopaedic), and surgery to the legs, medical treatment for varicose veins or prolonged immobilisation. Therefore, it is advisable to discontinue oral contraceptive use at least 4 to 6 weeks prior to these procedures if performed electively and to (re)start not less than 2 weeks after full ambulation. The latter is also valid with regard to immobilisation after an accident or emergency surgery. In case of emergency surgery, thrombotic prophylaxis is usually indicated eg with subcutaneous heparin.

Chloasma

Chloasma may occasionally occur, especially in women with a history of chloasma gravidarum. Women with a tendency to chloasma should avoid exposure to the sun or ultraviolet radiation whilst taking this preparation. Chloasma is often not fully reversible.

Laboratory tests

The use of steroids may influence the results of certain laboratory tests. In the literature, at least a hundred different parameters have been reported to possibly be influenced by oral contraceptive use, predominantly by the oestrogenic component. Among these are: biochemical parameters of the liver, thyroid, adrenal and renal function, plasma levels of (carrier) proteins and lipid/lipoprotein fractions and parameters of coagulation and fibrinolysis.

Further information

Additional contraceptive precautions

When additional contraceptive precautions are required, the patient should be advised either not to have sex, or to use a cap plus spermicide or for her partner to use a condom. Rhythm methods should not be advised as the pill disrupts the usual cyclical changes associated with the natural menstrual cycle, eg changes in temperature and cervical mucus.

The 7-day rule

If any one tablet is forgotten for more than 12 hours.

If the patient has vomiting or diarrhoea for more than 12 hours.

If the patient is taking any of the drugs listed under 'Interactions':

The patient should continue to take her tablets as usual and:

– Additional contraceptive precautions must be taken for the next 7 days.

But - if these 7 days run beyond the end of the current pack, the next pack must be started as soon as the current one is finished, ie no gap should be left between packs. (This prevents an extended break in tablet taking which may increase the risk of the ovaries releasing an egg and thus reducing contraceptive protection). The patient will not have a period until the end of 2 packs but this is not harmful nor does it matter if she experiences some bleeding on tablet taking days.

4.5 Interaction with other medicinal products and other forms of Interaction

Irregular cycles and reduced reliability of oral contraceptives may occur when these preparations are used concomitantly with drugs such as anticonvulsants, barbiturates, antibiotics, (eg tetracyclines, ampicillin, rifampicin, etc), griseofulvin, activated charcoal and certain laxatives. Special consideration should be given to patients being treated with antibiotics for acne. They should be advised to use a non-hormonal method of contraception, or to use an oral contraceptive containing a progestogen showing minimal androgenicity, which have been reported as helping to improve acne without using an antibiotic. Oral contraceptives may diminish glucose tolerance and increase the need for insulin or other antidiabetic drugs in diabetics.

The herbal remedy St John's Wort *(Hypericum perforatum)* should not be taken concomitantly with this medicine as this could potentially lead to a loss of contraceptive effect.

4.6 Pregnancy and lactation

Cilest is contra-indicated for use during pregnancy or suspected pregnancy, since it has been suggested that combined oral contraceptives, in common with many other substances, might be capable of affecting the normal development of the child in the early stages of pregnancy. It can be definitely concluded, however, that, if a risk of abnormality exists at all, it must be very small.

Mothers who are breast-feeding should be advised not to use the combined pill since this may reduce the amount of breast-milk, but may be advised instead to use a progestogen-only pill (POP).

4.7 Effects on ability to drive and use machines

Not applicable.

4.8 Undesirable effects

Various adverse reactions have been associated with oral contraceptive use. The first appearance of symptoms indicative of any one of these reactions necessitates immediate cessation of oral contraceptive use while appropriate diagnostic and therapeutic measures are undertaken.

Serious Adverse Reactions

There is a general opinion, based on statistical evidence, that users of combined oral contraceptives experience more often than non-users various disorders of the coagulation. How often these disorders occur in users of modern low-oestrogen oral contraceptives is unknown, but there are reasons for suggesting that they may occur less often than with the older types of pill which contain more oestrogen.

Various reports have associated oral contraceptive use with the occurrence of deep venous thrombosis, pulmonary embolism and other embolisms. Other investigations of these oral contraceptives have suggested an increased risk of oestrogen and/or progestogen dose-dependent coronary and cerebrovascular accidents, predominantly in heavy smokers. Thrombosis has very rarely been reported to occur in other veins or arteries, eg hepatic, mesenteric, renal or retinal.

It should be noted that there is no consensus about often contradictory findings obtained in early studies. The physician should bear in mind the possibility of vascular accidents occurring and that there may not be full recovery from such disorders and they may be fatal. The physician should take into account the presence of risk factors for arterial disease and deep venous thrombosis when prescribing oral contraceptives. Risk factors for arterial disease include smoking, the presence of hyperlipidaemia, hypertension or diabetes.

Signs and symptoms of a thrombotic event may include: sudden severe pain in the chest, whether or not reaching to the left arm; sudden breathlessness; and unusual severe, prolonged headache, especially if it occurs for the first time or gets progressively worse, or is associated with any of the following symptoms: sudden partial or complete loss of vision or diplopia, aphasia, vertigo, a bad fainting attack or collapse with or without focal epilepsy, weakness or very marked numbness suddenly affecting one side or one part of the body, motor disturbances; severe pain in the calf of one leg; acute abdomen.

Cigarette smoking increases the risk of serious cardiovascular adverse reactions to oral contraceptive use. The risk increases with age and with heavy smoking and is more marked in women over 35 years of age. Women who use oral contraceptives should be strongly advised not to smoke.

The use of oestrogen-containing oral contraceptives may promote growth of existing sex steroid dependent tumours. For this reason, the use of these oral contraceptives in patients with such tumours is contra-indicated. Numerous epidemiological studies have been reported on the risk of ovarian, endometrial, cervical and breast cancer in women using combined oral contraceptives. The evidence is clear that combined oral contraceptives offer substantial protection against both ovarian and endometrial cancer. An increased risk of cervical cancer in long term users of combined oral contraceptives has been reported in some studies, but there continues to be controversy about the extent to which this is attributable to the confounding effects of sexual behaviour and other factors.

A meta-analysis from 54 epidemiological studies reported that there is a slightly increased relative risk (RR = 1.24) of having breast cancer diagnosed in women who are currently using combined oral contraceptives (COCs). The observed pattern of increased risk may be due to an earlier diagnosis of breast cancer in COC users, the biological effects of COCs or a combination of both. The additional breast cancers diagnosed in current users of COCs or in women who have used COCs in the last 10 years are more likely to be localised to the breast than those in women who never used COCs.

Breast cancer is rare among women under 40 years of age whether or not they take COCs. Whilst this background risk increases with age, the excess number of breast cancer diagnoses in current and recent COC users is small in relation to the overall risk of breast cancer (see bar chart).

Figure 1

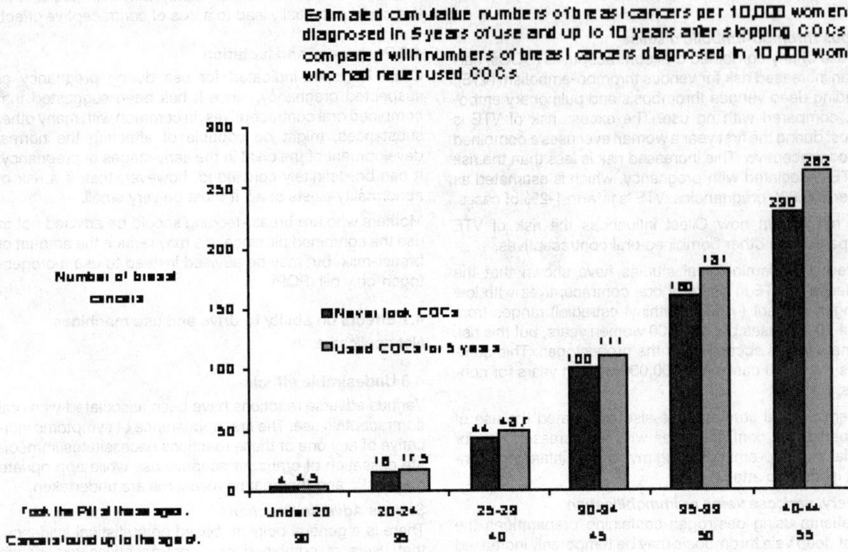

The most important risk factor for breast cancer in COC users is the age women discontinue the COC; the older the age at stopping, the more breast cancers are diagnosed. Duration of use is less important and the excess risk gradually disappears during the course of the 10 years after stopping COC use such that by 10 years there appears to be no excess.

The possible increase in risk of breast cancer should be discussed with the user and weighed against the benefits of COCs taking into account the evidence that they offer substantial protection against the risk of developing certain other cancers (e.g. ovarian and endometrial cancer).

(see Figure 1 above)

Malignant hepatic tumours have been reported on rare occasions in long-term users of oral contraceptives. Benign hepatic tumours have also been associated with oral contraceptive usage. A hepatic tumour should be considered in the differential diagnosis when upper abdominal pain, enlarged liver or signs of intra-abdominal haemorrhage occur.

The use of oral contraceptives may sometimes lead to the development of cholestatic jaundice or cholelithiasis.

On rare occasions the use of oral contraceptives may trigger or reactivate systemic lupus erythematosus.

A further rare complication of oral contraceptive use is the occurrence of chorea which can be reversed by discontinuing the pill. The majority of cases of oral contraceptive-induced chorea shows a pre-existing predisposition which often relates to acute rheumatism.

Other Adverse Reactions

Cardiovascular System

Rise of blood pressure. If hypertension develops, treatment should be discontinued.

Genital Tract

Intermenstrual bleeding, post-medication amenorrhoea, changes in cervical secretion, increase in size of uterine fibromyomata, aggravation of endometriosis, certain vaginal infections, eg candidiasis.

Breast

Tenderness, pain, enlargement, secretion.

Gastro-intestinal Tract

Nausea, vomiting, cholelithiasis, cholestatic jaundice.

Skin

Erythema nodosum, rash, chloasma, erythema multiforme.

Eyes

Discomfort of the cornea if contact lenses are used.

CNS

Headache, migraine, mood changes, depression.

Metabolic

Fluid retention, change in body weight, reduced glucose tolerance.

Other

Changes in libido.

4.9 Overdose

There have been no reports of serious ill-health from overdosage even when a considerable number of tablets has been taken by a small child. In general, it is therefore unnecessary to treat overdosage. However, if overdosage is discovered within two or three hours and is large, then gastric lavage can be safely used. There are no antidotes and further treatment should be symptomatic.

5. PHARMACOLOGICAL PROPERTIES

5.1 Pharmacodynamic properties

Cilest acts through the mechanism of gonadotrophin suppression by the oestrogenic and progestational actions of ethinylestradiol and norgestimate. The primary mechanism of action is inhibition of ovulation, but alterations to the cervical mucus and to the endometrium may also contribute to the efficacy of the product.

5.2 Pharmacokinetic properties

Norgestimate and ethinylestradiol are absorbed from the gastro-intestinal tract and metabolised in the liver. To obtain maximal contraceptive effectiveness the tablets should be taken as directed and at approximately the same time each day. Because the active ingredients are metabolised in the liver, reduced contraceptive efficacy has been associated with concomitant use of oral contraceptives and rifampicin. A similar association has been suggested with oral contraceptives and barbiturates, phenytoin sodium, phenylbutazone, griseofulvin and ampicillin.

5.3 Preclinical safety data

The toxicology of norgestimate and ethinylestradiol has been extensively investigated in animal studies and through long term clinical experience with widespread use in contraceptives.

6. PHARMACEUTICAL PARTICULARS

6.1 List of excipients

Lactose (anhydrous)

Magnesium Stearate

Pregelatinised Starch

F.D. & C. Blue No. 2 Lake

Methanol (does not appear in final product)

6.2 Incompatibilities

Not applicable.

6.3 Shelf life

Three years.

6.4 Special precautions for storage

Store at room temperature (below 25°C). Protect from light.

6.5 Nature and contents of container

Cartons containing 1 (Starter Pack), 3 and 6 PVC/foil blister strips of 21 tablets each.

6.6 Instructions for use and handling

Not applicable.

Administrative Data

7. MARKETING AUTHORISATION HOLDER

Janssen-Cilag Limited

Saunderton

High Wycombe

Buckinghamshire

HP14 4HJ

UK

8. MARKETING AUTHORISATION NUMBER(S)

0242/0209

9. DATE OF FIRST AUTHORISATION/RENEWAL OF THE AUTHORISATION

1 July 1995

10. DATE OF REVISION OF THE TEXT

19th August 2004

Legal category POM

CIPRALEX 5, 10 and 20 mg Film-Coated Tablets

(Lundbeck Limited)

1. NAME OF THE MEDICINAL PRODUCT

CIPRALEX® 5, 10 and 20 mg film-coated tablets▼

2. QUALITATIVE AND QUANTITATIVE COMPOSITION

Cipralex 5 mg: Each tablet contains 5 mg escitalopram (as oxalate)

Cipralex 10 mg: Each tablet contains 10 mg escitalopram (as oxalate)

Cipralex 20 mg: Each tablet contains 20 mg escitalopram (as oxalate)

For excipients, see section 6.1 List of excipients

3. PHARMACEUTICAL FORM

Film-coated tablet.

Cipralex 5 mg: Round, white, film-coated tablet marked with "EK" on one side.

Cipralex 10 mg: Oval, white, scored, film-coated tablet marked with "EL" on one side.

Cipralex 20 mg: Oval, white, scored, film-coated tablet marked with "EN" on one side.

4. CLINICAL PARTICULARS

4.1 Therapeutic indications

Treatment of major depressive episodes.

Treatment of panic disorder with or without agoraphobia.

Treatment of social anxiety disorder (social phobia).

4.2 Posology and method of administration

Safety of daily doses above 20 mg has not been demonstrated.

Cipralex is administered as a single daily dose and may be taken with or without food.

Major depressive episodes

Usual dosage is 10 mg once daily. Depending on individual patient response, the dose may be increased to a maximum of 20 mg daily.

Usually 2-4 weeks are necessary to obtain antidepressant response. After the symptoms resolve, treatment for at least 6 months is required for consolidation of the response.

Panic disorder with or without agoraphobia

An initial dose of 5 mg is recommended for the first week before increasing the dose to 10 mg daily. The dose may be further increased, up to a maximum of 20 mg daily, dependent on individual patient response.

Maximum effectiveness is reached after about 3 months. The treatment lasts several months.

Social anxiety disorder

Usual dosage is 10 mg once daily. Usually 2-4 weeks are necessary to obtain symptom relief. The dose may subsequently, depending on individual patient response, be decreased to 5 mg or increased to a maximum of 20 mg daily.

Social anxiety disorder is a disease with a chronic course, and treatment for 12 weeks is recommended to consolidate response. Long-term treatment of responders has been studied for 6 months and can be considered on an individual basis to prevent relapse; treatment benefits should be re-evaluated at regular intervals.

Social anxiety disorder is a well-defined diagnostic terminology of a specific disorder, which should not be confounded with excessive shyness. Pharmacotherapy is only indicated if the disorder interferes significantly with professional and social activities.

The place of this treatment compared to cognitive behavioural therapy has not been assessed. Pharmacotherapy is part of an overall therapeutic strategy.

Elderly patients (> 65 years of age)

Initial treatment with half the usually recommended dose and a lower maximum dose should be considered (see section 5.2 Pharmacokinetic properties).

The efficacy of Cipralex in social anxiety disorder has not been studied in elderly patients.

Children and adolescents (< 18 years)

Not recommended, since safety and efficacy have not been investigated in this population.

Reduced renal function

Dosage adjustment is not necessary in patients with mild or moderate renal impairment. Caution is advised in patients with severely reduced renal function (CL_{CR} less than 30 ml/min.) (see section 5.2 Pharmacokinetic properties).

Reduced hepatic function

An initial dose of 5 mg daily for the first two weeks of treatment is recommended. Depending on individual patient response, the dose may be increased to 10 mg (see section 5.2 Pharmacokinetic properties).

Poor metabolisers of CYP2C19

For patients who are known to be poor metabolisers with respect to CYP2C19, an initial dose of 5 mg daily during the first two weeks of treatment is recommended. Depending on individual patient response, the dose may be increased to 10 mg (see section 5.2 Pharmacokinetic properties).

Discontinuation

When stopping treatment with Cipralex the dose should be gradually reduced over a period of one or two weeks in order to avoid possible withdrawal reactions (see section 4.4 Special warnings and precautions for use).

4.3 Contraindications

Hypersensitivity to escitalopram or to any of the excipients.

Concomitant treatment with non-selective, irreversible monoamine oxidase inhibitors (MAO-inhibitors) (see section 4.5. Interactions with other medicinal products and other forms of interaction).

4.4 Special warnings and special precautions for use

The use in children and adolescents under age of 18 is not recommended due to the lack of studies.

The following special warnings and precautions apply to the therapeutic class of SSRIs (Selective Serotonin Reuptake Inhibitors).

Paradoxical anxiety

Some patients with panic disorder may experience increased anxiety symptoms at the beginning of treatment with antidepressants. This paradoxical reaction usually subsides within two weeks during continued treatment. A low starting dose is advised to reduce the likelihood of an anxiogenic effect (see section 4.2 Posology and method of administration).

Seizures

The medicinal product should be discontinued in any patient who develops seizures. SSRIs should be avoided in patients with unstable epilepsy and patients with controlled epilepsy should be carefully monitored. SSRIs should be discontinued if there is an increase in seizure frequency.

Mania

SSRIs should be used with caution in patients with a history of mania/hypomania. SSRIs should be discontinued in any patient entering a manic phase.

Diabetes

In patients with diabetes, treatment with an SSRI may alter glycaemic control. Insulin and/or oral hypoglycaemic dosage may need to be adjusted.

Suicide

It is general clinical experience with SSRIs that the risk of suicide may increase during the first weeks of therapy. Close monitoring of the patient during this period is important.

Hyponatraemia

Hyponatraemia, probably due to inappropriate antidiuretic hormone secretion (SIADH), has been reported rarely with the use of SSRIs and generally resolves on discontinuation of therapy. Caution should be exercised in patients at risk, such as elderly, cirrhotic patients or patients concomitantly treated with medications known to cause hyponatraemia.

Haemorrhage

There have been reports of cutaneous bleeding abnormalities, such as ecchymoses and purpura, with SSRIs. Caution is advised in patients taking SSRIs, particularly in concomitant use with oral anticoagulants, with medicinal products known to affect platelet function (e.g. atypical antipsychotics and phenothiazines, most tricyclic antidepressants, acetylsalicylic acid and non-steroidal anti-inflammatory medicinal products (NSAIDs), ticlopidin and dipyridamol) and in patients with known bleeding tendencies.

ECT(electroconvulsive therapy)

There is limited clinical experience of concurrent administration of SSRIs and ECT, therefore caution is advisable.

Reversible, selective MAO-A inhibitors

The combination of escitalopram with MAO-A inhibitors is generally not recommended due to the risk of onset of a serotonin syndrome (see section 4.5 Interactions with other medicinal products and other forms of interaction).

Concomitant treatment with non-selective, irreversible MAO-inhibitors see section 4.5 Interactions with other medicinal products and other forms of interaction.

Serotonin syndrome

Caution is advisable if escitalopram is used concomitantly with medicinal products with serotonergic effects such as sumatriptan or other triptans, tramadol and tryptophan. In rare cases, serotonin syndrome has been reported in patients using SSRIs concomitantly with serotonergic medicinal products. A combination of symptoms, such as agitation, tremor, myoclonus and hyperthermia may indicate the development of this condition. If this occurs treatment with the SSRI and the serotonergic medicinal product should be discontinued immediately and symptomatic treatment initiated.

St. John's Wort

Concomitant use of SSRIs and herbal remedies containing St. John's Wort (*Hypericum perforatum*) may result in an increased incidence of adverse reactions (see section 4.5 Interactions with other medicinal products and other forms of interaction).

Withdrawal reactions

When stopping therapy with Cipralex, the dose should be gradually reduced over a period of one or two weeks in order to avoid possible withdrawal reactions (see section 4.2 Posology and method of administration).

Coronary heart disease

Due to limited clinical experience, caution is advised in patients with coronary heart disease (see section 5.3 Preclinical safety data).

4.5 Interaction with other medicinal products and other forms of Interaction

Pharmacodynamic interactions

Contra-indicated combinations:

Non-selective MAOIs

Cases of serious reactions have been reported in patients receiving an SSRI in combination with a non-selective monoamine oxidase inhibitor (MAOI), and in patients who have recently discontinued SSRI treatment and have been started on MAOI treatment (see section 4.3 Contra indications). In some cases, the patient developed serotonin syndrome (see section 4.8 Undesirable effects).

Escitalopram is contra-indicated in combination with non-selective MAOIs. Escitalopram may be started 14 days after discontinuing treatment with an irreversible MAOI and at least one day after discontinuing treatment with the reversible MAOI (RIMA), moclobemide. At least 7 days should elapse after discontinuing escitalopram treatment, before starting a non-selective MAOI.

Inadvisable combinations:

Reversible, selective MAO-A inhibitor (moclobemide)

Due to the risk of serotonin syndrome, the combination of escitalopram with a MAO-A inhibitor is not recommended (see section 4.4 Special warnings and precautions for use). If the combination proves necessary, it should be started at the minimum recommended dosage and clinical monitoring should be reinforced.

Combinations requiring precautions for use:

Selegiline

In combination with selegiline (irreversible MAO-B inhibitor), caution is required due to the risk of developing serotonin syndrome. Selegiline doses up to 10 mg/day have been safely co-administered with racemic citalopram.

Serotonergic medicinal products

Co-administration with serotonergic medicinal products (e.g. tramadol, sumatriptan and other triptans) may lead to serotonin syndrome.

Medicinal products lowering the seizure threshold

SSRIs can lower the seizure threshold. Caution is advised when concomitantly using other medicinal products capable of lowering the seizure threshold.

Lithium, tryptophan

There have been reports of enhanced effects when SSRIs have been given together with lithium or tryptophan, therefore concomitant use of SSRIs with these medicinal products should be undertaken with caution.

St. John's Wort

Concomitant use of SSRIs and herbal remedies containing St. John's Wort (*Hypericum perforatum*) may result in an increased incidence of adverse reactions (see section 4.4 Special warnings and precautions for use).

Haemorrhage

Altered anti-coagulant effects may occur when escitalopram is combined with oral anticoagulants. Patients receiving oral anticoagulant therapy should receive careful coagulation monitoring when escitalopram is started or stopped (see section 4.4 Special warnings and precautions for use).

Alcohol

No pharmacodynamic or pharmacokinetic interactions are expected between escitalopram and alcohol. However, as with other psychotropic medicinal products, the combination with alcohol is not advisable.

Pharmacokinetic interactions

Influence of other medicinal products on the pharmacokinetics of escitalopram

The metabolism of escitalopram is mainly mediated by CYP2C19. CYP3A4 and CYP2D6 may also contribute to the metabolism although to a smaller extent. The metabolism of the major metabolite S-DCT (demethylated escitalopram) seems to be partly catalysed by CYP2D6.

Co-administration of medicinal products that inhibit CYP2C19 can result in elevated plasma concentrations of escitalopram. Caution is recommended in concomitant use of such medicinal products, e.g. omeprazole. A reduction in the dose of escitalopram may be necessary.

Co-administration of racemic citalopram with cimetidine (moderately potent general enzyme-inhibitor) resulted in increased plasma concentrations of the racemate (<45% increase). Thus, caution should be exercised at the upper end of the dose range of escitalopram when used concomitantly with high doses of cimetidine. Citalopram was measured non-stereoselectively and, therefore, the magnitude of the increase of the pharmacologically active S-enantiomer (escitalopram) is unknown. Thus, these data should be interpreted with caution.

Effect of escitalopram on the pharmacokinetics of other medicinal products

Escitalopram is an inhibitor of the enzyme CYP2D6. Caution is recommended when escitalopram is co-administered with medicinal products that are mainly metabolised by this enzyme, and that have a narrow therapeutic index, e.g. flecainide, propafenone and metoprolol (when used in cardiac failure), or some CNS acting medicinal products that are mainly metabolised by CYP2D6, e.g. antidepressants such as desipramine, clomipramine and nortryptyline or antipsychotics like risperidone, thioridazine and haloperidol. Dosage adjustment may be warranted.

Co-administration with desipramine or metoprolol resulted in both cases in a twofold increase in the plasma levels of these two CYP2D6 substrates.

In vitro studies have demonstrated that escitalopram may also cause weak inhibition of CYP2C19. Caution is recommended with concomitant use of medicinal products that are metabolised by CYP2C19.

4.6 Pregnancy and lactation

Pregnancy

For escitalopram no clinical data are available regarding exposed pregnancies. In rat reproductive toxicity studies performed with escitalopram, embryo-fetotoxic effects, but no increased incidence of malformations, were observed (see section 5.3 Preclinical safety data). The risk for humans is unknown. Therefore, Cipralex should not be used during pregnancy unless clearly necessary and only after careful consideration of the risk/benefit.

Lactation

It is expected that escitalopram will be excreted into human milk. Breast-feeding women should not be treated with escitalopram or breast-feeding should be discontinued.

4.7 Effects on ability to drive and use machines

Although escitalopram has been shown not to affect intellectual function or psychomotor performance, any psychoactive medicinal product may impair judgement or skills. Patients should be cautioned about the potential risk of an influence on their ability to drive a car and operate machinery.

4.8 Undesirable effects

Adverse reactions are most frequent during the first or second week of treatment and usually decrease in intensity and frequency with continued treatment.

After prolonged administration abrupt cessation of SSRIs may produce withdrawal reactions in some patients. Although withdrawal reactions may occur on stopping therapy, the available preclinical and clinical evidence does not suggest that SSRIs cause dependence.

Withdrawal symptoms (dizziness, headache and nausea) have been observed in some patients after abrupt discontinuation of escitalopram treatment. Most symptoms were mild and self-limiting. In order to avoid withdrawal reactions, tapered discontinuation over 1-2 weeks is recommended.

The following adverse reactions have occurred more frequently with escitalopram than with placebo in double-blind placebo-controlled studies. The frequencies listed are not placebo-corrected.

Metabolism And Nutrition Disorders	Common (>1/100, <1/10):	appetite decreased
Psychiatric Disorders	Common (>1/100, <1/10):	libido decreased, anorgasmia (female)
Nervous System Disorders	Common (>1/100, <1/10): Uncommon (>1/1000, <1/100):	insomnia, somnolence, dizziness taste disturbance, sleep disorder
Respiratory, Thoracic And Mediastinal Disorders	Common (>1/100, <1/10):	sinusitis, yawning
Gastrointestinal Disorders	Very common (>1/10): Common (>1/100, <1/10):	nausea diarrhoea, constipation
Skin And Subcutaneous Tissue Disorders	Common (>1/100, <1/10):	sweating increased
Reproductive System And Breast Disorders	Common (>1/100, <1/10):	ejaculation disorder, impotence
General Disorders And Administration Site Conditions	Common (>1/100, <1/10):	fatigue, pyrexia

The following adverse reactions apply to the therapeutic class of SSRIs.

Cardiovascular disorders – Postural hypotension

Disorders of metabolism and nutrition – Hyponatraemia, inappropriate ADH secretion

Disorders of the eye - Abnormal vision

Gastrointestinal disorders - Nausea, vomiting, dry mouth, diarrhoea, anorexia

General disorders - Insomnia, dizziness, fatigue, drowsiness, anaphylactic reactions

Hepato-biliary disorders - Abnormal liver function tests

Musculoskeletal disorders - Arthralgia, myalgia

Neurological disorders - Seizures, tremor, movement disorders, serotonin syndrome

Psychiatric disorders - Hallucinations, mania, confusion, agitation, anxiety, depersonalisation, panic attacks, nervousness

Renal and Urinary disorders - Urinary retention

Reproductive disorders - Galactorrhoea, sexual dysfunction terms including impotence, ejaculation disorder, anorgasmia

Skin disorders - Rash, ecchymoses, pruritus, angioedema, sweating

4.9 Overdose

Toxicity

Clinical data on escitalopram overdose are limited. However, it has been observed that doses of 190 mg of escitalopram have been taken without any serious symptoms being reported.

Symptoms

Symptoms of overdose with racemic citalopram (>600 mg): Dizziness, tremor, agitation, somnolence, unconsciousness, seizures, tachycardia, changes in the ECG with ST-T changes, broadening of the QRS complex, prolonged QT interval, arrhythmias, respiratory depression, vomiting, rhabdomyolysis, metabolic acidosis, hypokalaemia. It is anticipated that overdoses with escitalopram would result in similar symptoms.

Treatment

There is no specific antidote. Establish and maintain an airway, ensure adequate oxygenation and respiratory function. Gastric lavage should be carried out as soon as possible after oral ingestion. The use of activated charcoal should be considered. Cardiac and vital signs monitoring are recommended along with general symptomatic supportive measures.

5. PHARMACOLOGICAL PROPERTIES

5.1 Pharmacodynamic properties

Pharmacotherapeutic group: antidepressants, selective serotonin reuptake inhibitors

ATC-code: N 06 AB 10

Mechanism of action

Escitalopram is a selective inhibitor of serotonin (5-HT) re-uptake. The inhibition of 5-HT re-uptake is the only likely mechanism of action explaining the pharmacological and clinical effects of escitalopram.

Escitalopram has no or low affinity for a number of receptors including $5\text{-}HT_{1A}$, $5\text{-}HT_2$, DA D_1 and D_2 receptors, α_1-, α_2-, β-adrenoceptors, histamine H_1, muscarine cholinergic, benzodiazepine, and opioid receptors.

Clinical efficacy

Major Depressive Episodes

Escitalopram has been found to be effective in the acute treatment of major depressive episodes in three out of four double-blind, placebo controlled short-term (8-weeks) studies. In a long-term relapse prevention study, 274 patients who had responded during an initial 8-week open label treatment phase with escitalopram 10 or 20 mg/day, were randomised to continuation with escitalopram at the same dose, or to placebo, for up to 36 weeks. In this study, patients receiving continued escitalopram experienced a significantly longer time to relapse over the subsequent 36 weeks compared to those receiving placebo.

Social Anxiety Disorder

Escitalopram was effective in both three short-term (12-week) studies and in responders in a 6 months relapse prevention study in social anxiety disorder. In a 24-week dose-finding study, efficacy of 5, 10 and 20 mg escitalopram has been demonstrated.

5.2 Pharmacokinetic properties

Absorption

Absorption is almost complete and independent of food intake. (Mean time to maximum concentration (mean T_{max}) is 4 hours after multiple dosing). As with racemic citalopram, the absolute bio-availability of escitalopram is expected to be about 80%.

Distribution

The apparent volume of distribution ($V_{d,\beta}/F$) after oral administration is about 12 to 26 L/kg. The plasma protein binding is below 80% for escitalopram and its main metabolites.

Biotransformation

Escitalopram is metabolised in the liver to the demethylated and didemethylated metabolites. Both of these are pharmacologically active. Alternatively, the nitrogen may be oxidised to form the N-oxide metabolite. Both parent and metabolites are partly excreted as glucuronides. After multiple dosing the mean concentrations of the demethyl and didemethyl metabolites are usually 28-31% and <5%, respectively, of the escitalopram concentration. Biotransformation of escitalopram to the demethylated metabolite is mediated primarily by CYP2C19. Some contribution by the enzymes CYP3A4 andCYP2D6 is possible.

Elimination

The elimination half-life ($t_{½\,\beta}$) after multiple dosing is about 30 hours and the oral plasma clearance (Cl_{oral}) is about 0.6 L/min. The major metabolites have a significantly longer half-life. Escitalopram and major metabolites are assumed to be eliminated by both the hepatic (metabolic) and the renal routes, with the major part of the dose excreted as metabolites in the urine.

There is linear pharmacokinetics. Steady-state plasma levels are achieved in about 1 week. Average steady-state concentrations of 50 nmol/L (range 20 to 125 nmol/L) are achieved at a daily dose of 10 mg.

Elderly patients (> 65 years)

Escitalopram appears to be eliminated more slowly in elderly patients compared to younger patients. Systemic exposure (AUC) is about 50 % higher in elderly compared to young healthy volunteers (see section 4.2 Posology and method of administration).

Reduced hepatic function

Escitalopram has not been studied in patients with reduced hepatic function. For racemic citalopram the half-life was about twice as long (83 vs 37 hours) and the steady-state concentration was on average about 60% higher in patients with reduced hepatic function than in subjects with normal liver function. The pharmacokinetics of the metabolites have not been studied in this population. Citalopram was measured non-stereoselectively and, therefore, the magnitude of the increase of the pharmacologically active S-enantiomer (escitalopram) is unknown. Thus, these data should be interpreted with caution (see section 4.2 Posology and method of administration).

Reduced renal function

With racemic citalopram, a longer half-life and a minor increase in exposure have been observed in patients with reduced kidney function (CL_{cr} 10-53 ml/min). Plasma concentrations of the metabolites have not been studied, but they may be elevated (see section 4.2 Posology and method of administration).

Polymorphism

It has been observed that poor metabolisers with respect to CYP2C19 have twice as high a plasma concentration of escitalopram as extensive metabolisers. No significant change in exposure was observed in poor metabolisers with respect to CYP2D6 (see section 4.2 Posology and method of administration).

5.3 Preclinical safety data

No complete conventional battery of preclinical studies was performed with escitalopram since the bridging toxicokinetic and toxicological studies conducted in rats with escitalopram and citalopram showed a similar profile. Therefore, all the citalopram information can be extrapolated to escitalopram.

In comparative toxicological studies in rats, escitalopram and citalopram caused cardiac toxicity, including congestive heart failure, after treatment for some weeks, when using dosages that caused general toxicity. The cardiotoxicity seemed to correlate with peak plasma concentrations rather than to systemic exposures (AUC). Peak plasma concentrations at no-effect-level were in excess (8-fold) of those achieved in clinical use, while AUC for escitalopram was only 3- to 4-fold higher than the exposure achieved in clinical use. For citalopram AUC values for the S-enantiomer were 6- to 7-fold higher than exposure achieved in clinical use. The findings are probably related to an exaggerated influence on biogenic amines i.e. secondary to the primary pharmacological effects, resulting in hemodynamic effects (reduction in coronary flow) and ischemia. However, the exact mechanism of cardiotoxicity in rats is not clear. Clinical experience with citalopram, and the clinical trial experience with escitalopram, do not indicate that these findings have a clinical correlate.

Increased content of phospholipids has been observed in some tissues e.g. lung, epididymides and liver after treatment for longer periods with escitalopram and citalopram in rats. Findings in the epididymides and liver were seen at exposures similar to that in man. The effect is reversible after treatment cessation. Accumulation of phospholipids (phospholipidosis) in animals has been observed in connection with many cationic amphiphilic medicines. It is not known if this phenomenon has any significant relevance for man.

In the developmental toxicity study in the rat embryotoxic effects (reduced foetal weight and reversible delay of ossification) were observed at exposures in terms of AUC in excess of the exposure achieved during clinical use. No increased frequency of malformations was noted. A pre- and postnatal study showed reduced survival during the lactation period at exposures in terms of AUC in excess of the exposure achieved during clinical use.

6. PHARMACEUTICAL PARTICULARS

6.1 List of excipients

Tablet core:

Microcrystalline cellulose, Colloidal anhydrous silica, Talc, Croscarmellose sodium, Magnesium stearate

Coating:

Hypromellose, Macrogol 400, Titanium dioxide (E 171)

6.2 Incompatibilities

Not applicable.

6.3 Shelf life

3 years.

6.4 Special precautions for storage

No special precautions for storage.

6.5 Nature and contents of container

Blister: Transparent; PVC/PE/PVdC/Aluminium blister, pack with an outer carton; 14, 28, 56, 98 tablets - Unit dose; 49x1, 100x1, 500x1 tablets (5, 10 and 20 mg)

Blister: White; PVC/PE/PVdC/Aluminium blister, pack with an outer carton; 14, 20, 28, 50, 100, 200 tablets (5, 10 and 20 mg)

Polypropylene tablet container; 100 (5, 10 and 20 mg), 200 (5 and 10 mg) tablets

Not all pack sizes may be marketed

6.6 Instructions for use and handling

No special requirements

7. MARKETING AUTHORISATION HOLDER

H. Lundbeck A/S

Ottiliavej 7-9

DK-2500 Copenhagen-Valby

Denmark

8. MARKETING AUTHORISATION NUMBER(S)

Cipralex 5 mg PL 13761/0008

Cipralex 10 mg PL 13761/0009

Cipralex 20 mg PL 13761/0011

9. DATE OF FIRST AUTHORISATION/RENEWAL OF THE AUTHORISATION

10 June 2002

10. DATE OF REVISION OF THE TEXT

19 March 2004

Cipramil Drops 40 mg/ml

(Lundbeck Limited)

1. NAME OF THE MEDICINAL PRODUCT

Cipramil® Drops 40 mg/ml

2. QUALITATIVE AND QUANTITATIVE COMPOSITION

Oral drops 40 mg/ml (44.48 mg citalopram hydrochloride corresponding to 40 mg citalopram base per ml).

3. PHARMACEUTICAL FORM

Oral drops, solution.

4. CLINICAL PARTICULARS

4.1 Therapeutic indications

Treatment of depressive illness in the initial phase and as maintenance against potential relapse/recurrence.

Cipramil is also indicated in the treatment of panic disorder with or without agoraphobia.

4.2 Posology and method of administration

4.2.1 Posology

Treating Depression

Citalopram drops should be administered as a single oral dose of 16 mg (8 drops) daily. Dependent on individual patient response this may be increased to a maximum of 48 mg (24 drops) daily. The dose may be taken in the morning or evening without regard for food.

A treatment period of at least 6 months is usually necessary to provide adequate maintenance against the potential for relapse.

Treating Panic Disorder

In common with other pharmacotherapy used in this patient group, a low starting dose is advised to reduce the likelihood of a paradoxical initial anxiogenic effect. A single oral dose of 8 mg (4 drops) is recommended for the first week before increasing the dose to 16 mg (8 drops) daily. The dose may be further increased, up to a maximum of 48 mg (24 drops) daily dependent on individual patient response, however an optimum dose of 20-30 mg tablets (drops equivalent – 16 to 24 mg/8 to 12 drops) daily was indicated in a clinical study.

Maximum effectiveness of citalopram in treating panic disorder is reached after about 3 months and the response is maintained during continued treatment. Dependent on individual patient response it may be necessary to continue treatment for several months.

Elderly patients

The recommended daily dose is 16 mg (8 drops). Dependent on individual patient response this may be increased to a maximum of 32 mg (16 drops) daily.

Children

Not recommended, as safety and efficacy have not been established in this population.

Reduced hepatic function

Dosage should be restricted to the lower end of the dose range.

Reduced renal function

Dosage adjustment is not necessary in cases of mild or moderate renal impairment. No information is available in cases of severe renal impairment (creatinine clearance <20 mL / min).

4.2.2 Method of administration

For oral administration after mixing with water, orange juice or apple juice.

Cipramil Oral Drops can be taken as a single daily dose, at any time of day, without regard to food intake.

Citalopram oral drops have approximately 25% increased bioavailability compared to tablets. The tablet corresponds to the number of drops as follows:

Tablets / dose Equivalent	Drops
10 mg	8 mg (4 drops)
20 mg	16 mg (8 drops)
30 mg	24 mg (12 drops)
40 mg	32 mg (16 drops)
60 mg	48 mg (24 drops)

4.3 Contraindications

Hypersensitivity to citalopram.

Monoamine Oxidase Inhibitors. Cases of serious and sometimes fatal reactions have been reported in patients receiving an SSRI in combination with monoamine oxidase inhibitor (MAOI), including the selective MAOI selegiline and the reversible MAOI (RIMA), moclobemide and in patients who have recently discontinued an SSRI and have been started on a MAOI.

Some cases presented with features resembling serotonin syndrome. Symptoms of a drug interaction with a MAOI include: hyperthermia, rigidity, myoclonus, autonomic instability with possible rapid fluctuations of vital signs, mental status changes that include confusion, irritability and extreme agitation progressing to delirium and coma.

Citalopram should not be used in combination with a MAOI. Citalopram may be started 14 days after discontinuing treatment with an irreversible MAOI and at least one day after discontinuing treatment with the reversible MAOI (RIMA), moclobemide. At least 7 days should elapse after discontinuing citalopram treatment before starting a MAOI or RIMA.

4.4 Special warnings and special precautions for use

Diabetes - In patients with diabetes, treatment with an SSRI may alter glycaemic control, possibly due to improvement of depressive symptoms. Insulin and or oral hypoglycaemic dosage may need to be adjusted.

Seizures – Seizures are a potential risk with antidepressant drugs. The drug should be discontinued in any patient who develops seizures. Citalopram should be avoided in patients with unstable epilepsy and patients with controlled epilepsy should be carefully monitored. Citalopram should be discontinued if there is an increase in seizure frequency.

ECT – There is little clinical experience of concurrent administration of citalopram and ECT, therefore caution is advisable.

Mania – Citalopram should be used with caution in patients with a history of mania/hypomania. Citalopram should be discontinued in any patient entering a manic phase.

Suicide – As improvement may not occur during the first few weeks or more of treatment, patients should be closely monitored during this period. The possibility of a suicide attempt is inherent in depression and may persist until significant therapeutic effect is achieved and it is general clinical experience with all antidepressant therapies that the risk of suicide may increase in the early stages of recovery.

Haemorrhage – There have been reports of cutaneous bleeding abnormalities such as ecchymoses and purpura, as well as haemorrhagic manifestations e.g. gastrointestinal haemorrhage with SSRIs. The risk of gastrointestinal haemorrhage may be increased in elderly people during treatment with SSRIs. Caution is advised in patients taking SSRIs, particularly in concomitant use with drugs known to affect platelet function (e.g. atypical antipsychotics and phenothiazines, most tricyclic antidepressants, aspirin and non-steroidal anti-inflammatory drugs (NSAIDs) as well as in patients with a history of bleeding disorders.

Experience with citalopram has not revealed any clinically relevant interactions with neuroleptics. However, as with other SSRIs, the possibility of a pharmacodynamic interaction cannot be excluded.

Consideration should be given to factors which may affect the disposition of a minor metabolite of citalopram (didemethylcitalopram) since increased levels of this metabolite could theoretically prolong the QTc interval in susceptible individuals. However, in ECG monitoring of 2500 patients in clinical trials, including 277 patients with pre-existing cardiac conditions, no clinically significant changes were noted.

As with most antidepressants, citalopram should be discontinued if the patient enters a manic phase. There is little clinical experience of concurrent use of citalopram and ECT.

Some patients with panic disorder experience an initial anxiogenic effect when starting pharmacotherapy. A low starting dose (see Posology) reduces the likelihood of this effect.

4.5 Interaction with other medicinal products and other forms of Interaction

Monoamine Oxidase Inhibitors (MAOIs) should not be used in combination with SSRIs (see 4.3 Contraindications).

The metabolism of citalopram is only partly dependent on the hepatic cytochrome P450 isozyme CYP2D6 and, unlike some other SSRIs, citalopram is only a weak inhibitor of this important enzyme system which is involved in the metabolism of many drugs (including antiarrhythmics, neuroleptics, beta-blockers, TCAs and some SSRIs). Protein binding is relatively low (<80%). These properties give citalopram a low potential for clinically significant drug interactions.

Alcohol – The combination of citalopram and alcohol is not advisable. However clinical studies have revealed no adverse pharmacodynamic interactions between citalopram and alcohol.

Serotonergic drugs – Co administration with serotonergic drugs (e.g. tramadol, sumatriptan) may lead to enhancement of 5-HT associated effects.

Lithium & tryptophan – There is no pharmacokinetic interaction between lithium and citalopram. However, there have been reports of enhanced serotonergic effects when SSRIs have been given with lithium or tryptophan and therefore the concomitant use of citalopram with these drugs should be undertaken with caution. Routine monitoring of lithium levels need not be adjusted.

In a pharmacokinetic study no effect was demonstrated on either citalopram or imipramine levels, although the level of desipramine, the primary metabolite of imipramine, was increased. In animal studies cimetidine had little or no influence on citalopram kinetics.

Dynamic interactions between citalopram and herbal remedy St John's Wort (Hypericum perforatum) can occur, resulting in an increase in undesirable effects.

No pharmacodynamic interactions have been noted in clinical studies in which citalopram has been given concomitantly with benzodiazepines, neuroleptics, analgesics, lithium, alcohol, antihistamines, antihypertensive drugs, beta-blockers and other cardiovascular drugs.

4.6 Pregnancy and lactation

Pregnancy - Animal studies did not show any evidence of teratogenicity, however the safety of citalopram during human pregnancy has not been established. As with all drugs citalopram should only be used in pregnancy if the potential benefits of treatment to the mother outweigh the possible risks to the developing foetus.

Lactation – Citalopram is known to be excreted in breast milk. Its effects on the nursing infant have not been established. If treatment with citalopram is considered necessary, discontinuation of breast feeding should be considered.

4.7 Effects on ability to drive and use machines

Citalopram does not impair intellectual function and psychomotor performance. However, patients who are prescribed psychotropic medication may be expected to have some impairment of general attention and concentration either due to the illness itself, the medication or both and should be cautioned about their ability to drive a car and operate machinery.

4.8 Undesirable effects

Adverse effects observed with citalopram are in general mild and transient. They are most prominent during the first one or two weeks of treatment and usually attenuate as the depressive state improves.

The most commonly observed adverse events associated with the use of citalopram and not seen at an equal incidence among placebo-treated patients were: nausea, somnolence, mouth dry, sweating increased and tremor. The incidence of each in excess over placebo is low (<10%).

In comparative clinical trials with tricyclic antidepressants the incidence of adverse events occurring with citalopram was found to be lower in all cases.

Withdrawal reactions have been reported in association with selective serotonin reuptake inhibitors (SSRIs), including Cipramil. Common symptoms include dizziness, paraesthesia, headache, anxiety and nausea. Abrupt discontinuation of treatment with Cipramil should be avoided. The majority of symptoms experienced on withdrawal of SSRIs are non-serious and self-limiting.

Treatment emergent adverse events reported in clinical trials (N=2985):

<u>Frequent:</u> (⩾ 5 - 20%)

Skin and appendages disorders: Sweating increased (13%).

Central and peripheral nervous system disorders: Headache (19%), tremor (12%), dizziness (8%).

Vision disorders: Accommodation abnormal (5%).

Psychiatric disorders: Somnolence (17%), insomnia (12%), agitation (6%), nervousness (6%).

Gastro-intestinal system disorders: Nausea (20%), mouth dry (18%), constipation (10%), diarrhoea (7%).

Heart rate and rhythm disorders: Palpitation (6%).

Body as a whole: Asthenia (11%).

<u>Less frequent:</u> (1 - <5%)

Skin and appendages disorders: Rash, pruritus.

Central and peripheral nervous system disorders: Paraesthesia, migraine.

Vision disorders: Vision abnormal.

Special senses other, disorder: Taste perversion.

Psychiatric disorders: Sleep disorder, libido decreased, concentration impaired, dreaming abnormal, amnesia, anxiety, appetite increased, anorexia, apathy, impotence, suicide attempt, confusion, yawning.

Gastrointestinal system disorders: Dyspepsia, vomiting, abdominal pain, flatulence, saliva increased.

Metabolic and nutritional disorders: Weight decrease, weight increase.

Cardiovascular disorders, general: Hypotension postural.

Heart rate and rhythm disorders: Tachycardia.

Respiratory system disorders: Rhinitis.

Urinary system disorders: Micturition disorder, polyuria.

Reproductive disorders, male: Ejaculation failure.

Reproductive disorders, female: Anorgasmia female.

Body as a whole: Fatigue

<u>Rare:</u>(<1%)

Musculo-skeletal system disorder: Myalgia.

Central and peripheral nervous system disorders: Exrapyramidal disorder, convulsions.

Hearing and vestibular disorders: Tinnitus.

Psychiatric disorders: Euphoria, libido increased.

Respiratory system disorder: Coughing.

Body as a whole: Malaise.

<u>Post Marketing</u>

- The following adverse reactions apply to the therapeutic class of SSRIs

Skin Disorders: Angiodema; ecchymoses. Photosensitivity reactions have been reported very rarely.

Disorders of metabolism and nutrition: Rare cases of hyponatraemia and inappropriate ADH secretion have been reported and appear to be reversible on discontinuation. The majority of the reports were associated with older patients.

Gastrointestinal disorders: Gastrointestinal bleeding.

General disorders: Anaphylactoid reactions.

Hepato-billiary disorders: Abnormal LFT's.

Musculoskeletal disorders: Arthralgia.

Neurological disorders: Serotonin syndrome.

Psychiatric disorders: Hallucinations; mania; depersonalisation; panic attacks (these symptoms may be due to the underlying disease).

Reproductive disorders: Galactorrhoea.

4.9 Overdose

Citalopram is given to patients at potential risk of suicide and some reports of attempted suicide have been received. Detail is often lacking regarding precise dose or combination with other drugs and/or alcohol.

Symptoms

Experience from 8 cases considered due to citalopram alone has recorded the following symptoms/signs: somnolence, coma, stiffened expression, episode of grand mal convulsion, sinus tachycardia, occasional nodal rhythm, sweating, nausea, vomiting, cyanosis, hyperventilation. No case was fatal. The clinical picture was inconsistent, no observation being made in more than two individuals.

Six fatalities have been reported. In one overdose was suspected; high post mortem plasma levels were seen although it is not technically possible to interpret these with confidence.

In the remaining five a combination with other drugs had been taken. The clinical syndrome observed prior to death in three of these cases where citalopram was taken with moclobemide was interpreted as that of serotonin syndrome. No clinical details are available on the other two.

Treatment

There is no specific antidote. Treatment is symptomatic and supportive. Gastric lavage should be carried out as soon as possible after oral ingestion. Medical surveillance is advisable.

5. PHARMACOLOGICAL PROPERTIES

5.1 Pharmacodynamic properties

ATC-code: N 06 AB 04

Biochemical and behavioural studies have shown that citalopram is a potent inhibitor of the serotonin (5-HT)-uptake. Tolerance to the inhibition of 5-HT-uptake is not induced by long-term treatment with citalopram.

Citalopram is the most Selective Serotonin Reuptake Inhibitor (SSRI) yet described, with no, or minimal, effect on noradrenaline (NA), dopamine (DA) and gamma aminobutyric acid (GABA) uptake.

In contrast to many tricyclic antidepressants and some of the newer SSRI's, citalopram has no or very low affinity for a series of receptors including 5-HT $_{1A}$, 5-HT$_2$, DA D$_1$ and D$_2$ receptors, α_1-, α_2-, β-adrenoceptors, histamine H$_1$, muscarine cholinergic, benzodiazepine, and opioid receptors. A series of functional *in vitro* tests in isolated organs as well as functional *in vivo* tests have confirmed the lack of receptor affinity. This absence of effects on receptors could explain why citalopram produces fewer of the traditional side effects such as dry mouth, bladder and gut disturbance, blurred vision, sedation, cardiotoxicity and orthostatic hypotension.

Suppression of rapid eye movement (REM) sleep is considered a predictor of antidepressant activity. Like tricyclic antidepressants, other SSRI's and MAO inhibitors, citalopram suppresses REM-sleep and increases deep slow-wave sleep.

Although citalopram does not bind to opioid receptors it potentiates the anti-nociceptive effect of commonly used opioid analgesics. There was potentiation of d-amphetamine-induced hyperactivity following administration of citalopram.

The main metabolites of citalopram are all SSRIs although their potency and selectivity ratios are lower than those of citalopram. However, the selectivity ratios of the metabolites are higher than those of many of the newer SSRIs. The metabolites do not contribute to the overall antidepressant effect.

In humans citalopram does not impair cognitive (intellectual function) and psychomotor performance and has no or minimal sedative properties, either alone or in combination with alcohol.

Citalopram did not reduce saliva flow in a single dose study in human volunteers and in none of the studies in healthy volunteers did citalopram have significant influence on cardiovascular parameters. Citalopram has no effect on the serum levels of prolactin and growth hormone.

5.2 Pharmacokinetic properties

Absorption

Absorption is almost complete and independent of food intake (T_{max} mean 2 hours) after ingestion of drops and T_{max} mean 3 hours after intake of tablets. Oral bioavailability is about 80% after ingestion of tablets. Relative bioavailability of drops is approximately 25% greater than the tablets.

Distribution

The apparent volume of distribution $(V_d)_\beta$ is about 12.3 L/kg. The plasma protein binding is below 80% for citalopram and its main metabolites.

Biotransformation

Citalopram is metabolized to the active demethylcitalopram, didemethylcitalopram, citalopram-N-oxide and an inactive deaminated propionic acid derivative. All the active metabolites are also SSRIs, although weaker than the parent compound. Unchanged citalopram is the predominant compound in plasma.

Elimination

The elimination half-life ($T_{½, \beta}$) is about 1.5 days and the systemic citalopram plasma clearance (Cl_s) is about 0.33 L/min, and oral plasma clearance (Cl_{oral}) is about 0.41 L/min.

Citalopram is excreted mainly via the liver (85%) and the remainder (15%) via the kidneys. About 12% of the daily dose is excreted in urine as unchanged citalopram. Hepatic (residual) clearance is about 0.35 L/min and renal clearance about 0.068 L/min.

The kinetics are linear. Steady state plasma levels are achieved in 1-2 weeks. Average concentrations of 250 nmol/L (100-500 nmol/L) are achieved at a daily dose of 40 mg. There is no clear relationship between citalopram plasma levels and therapeutic response or side effects.

Elderly patients (⩾ 65 years)

Longer half-lives and decreased clearance values due to a reduced rate of metabolism have been demonstrated in elderly patients.

Reduced hepatic function

Citalopram is eliminated more slowly in patients with reduced hepatic function. The half-life of citalopram is about twice as long and steady state citalopram concentrations at a given dose will be about twice as high as in patients with normal liver function.

Reduced renal function

Citalopram is eliminated more slowly in patients with mild to moderate reduction of renal function, without any major impact on the pharmacokinetics of citalopram. At present no information is available for treatment of patients with severely reduced renal function (creatinine clearance <20 mL / min).

5.3 Preclinical safety data

Citalopram has low acute toxicity. In chronic toxicity studies there were no findings of concern for the therapeutic use of citalopram. Based on data from reproduction toxicity studies (segment I, II and III) there is no reason to have special concern for the use of citalopram in women of child-bearing potential. Citalopram has no mutagenic or carcinogenic potential.

6. PHARMACEUTICAL PARTICULARS

6.1 List of excipients

Methyl-parahydroxybenzoate, Propyl-parahydroxybenzoate, Ethyl alcohol 9% v/v, Hydroxyethylcellulose, Purified water.

6.2 Incompatibilities

Cipramil Drops should only be mixed with water, orange juice or apple juice.

6.3 Shelf life

24 months (there is a "use by" date on the label).

A bottle may be used for 16 weeks after first use, if stored below 25°.

6.4 Special precautions for storage

None

6.5 Nature and contents of container

Brown glass bottle containing 15 mL with screw cap and polyethylene dropper. One bottle per carton.

6.6 Instructions for use and handling

Nil.

7. MARKETING AUTHORISATION HOLDER

Lundbeck Limited
Lundbeck House
Caldecotte Lake Business Park
Caldecotte
Milton Keynes
MK7 8LF

8. MARKETING AUTHORISATION NUMBER(S)

PL 0458/0071

9. DATE OF FIRST AUTHORISATION/RENEWAL OF THE AUTHORISATION

4 August 1998

10. DATE OF REVISION OF THE TEXT

April 2003

Cipramil Tablets

(Lundbeck Limited)

1. NAME OF THE MEDICINAL PRODUCT

Cipramil® Tablets 10, 20 & 40 mg

2. QUALITATIVE AND QUANTITATIVE COMPOSITION

Tablets of 10, 20 or 40 mg (12.49, 24.98 or 49.96 mg citalopram hydrobromide corresponding to 10, 20 or 40 mg citalopram base).

3. PHARMACEUTICAL FORM

Tablet

4. CLINICAL PARTICULARS

4.1 Therapeutic indications

Treatment of depressive illness in the initial phase and as maintenance against potential relapse/recurrence.

Cipramil is also indicated in the treatment of panic disorder with or without agoraphobia.

4.2 Posology and method of administration

4.2.1 Posology

Treating Depression

Citalopram should be administered as a single oral dose of 20 mg daily. Dependent on individual patient response this may be increased to a maximum of 60 mg daily. The dose may be taken in the morning or evening without regard for food.

A treatment period of at least 6 months is usually necessary to provide adequate maintenance against the potential for relapse.

Treating Panic Disorder

In common with other pharmacotherapy used in this patient group, a low starting dose is advised to reduce the likelihood of a paradoxical initial anxiogenic effect. A single oral dose of 10 mg daily is recommended for the first week before increasing the dose to 20 mg daily. The dose may be further increased, up to a maximum of 60 mg daily dependent on individual patient response, however an optimum dose of 20-30 mg daily was indicated in a clinical study.

Maximum effectiveness of citalopram in treating panic disorder is reached after about 3 months and the response is maintained during continued treatment. Dependent on individual patient response it may be necessary to continue treatment for several months.

Elderly patients

The recommended daily dose is 20 mg. Dependent on individual patient response this may be increased to a maximum of 40 mg daily.

Children

Not recommended, as safety and efficacy have not been established in this population.

Reduced hepatic function

Dosage should be restricted to the lower end of the dose range.

Reduced renal function

Dosage adjustment is not necessary in cases of mild or moderate renal impairment. No information is available in cases of severe renal impairment (creatinine clearance <20 mL / min).

4.2.2 Method of administration

Citalopram tablets are administered as a single daily dose. Citalopram tablets can be taken any time of the day without regard to food intake.

4.3 Contraindications

Hypersensitivity to citalopram.

Monoamine Oxidase Inhibitors: Cases of serious and sometimes fatal reactions have been reported in patients receiving an SSRI in combination with monoamine oxidase inhibitor (MAOI), including the selective MAOI selegiline and the reversible MAOI (RIMA), moclobemide and in patients who have recently discontinued an SSRI and have been started on a MAOI.

Some case presented with features resembling serotonin syndrome. Symptoms of a drug interaction with a MAOI include: hyperthermia, rigidity, myoclonus, autonomic instability with possible rapid fluctuations of vital signs, mental status changes that include confusion, irritability and extreme agitation progressing to delirium and coma.

Citalopram should not be used in combination with a MAOI. Citalopram may be started 14 days after discontinuing treatment with an irreversible MAOI and at least one day after discontinuing treatment with the reversible MAOI (RIMA), moclobemide. At least 7 days should elapse after discontinuing citalopram treatment before starting a MAOI or RIMA.

4.4 Special warnings and special precautions for use

Diabetes - In patients with diabetes, treatment with an SSRI may alter glycaemic control, possibly due to improvement of depressive symptoms. Insulin and or oral hypoglycaemic dosage may need to be adjusted.

Seizures – Seizures are a potential risk with antidepressant drugs. The drug should be discontinued in any patient who develops seizures. Citalopram should be avoided in patients with unstable epilepsy and patients with controlled epilepsy should be carefully monitored. Citalopram should be discontinued if there is an increase in seizure frequency.

ECT – There is little clinical experience of concurrent administration of citalopram and ECT, therefore caution is advisable.

Mania – Citalopram should be used with caution in patients with a history of mania/hypomania. Citalopram should be discontinued in any patient entering a manic phase.

Suicide – As improvement may not occur during the first few weeks or more of treatment, patients should be closely monitored during this period. The possibility of a suicide attempt is inherent in depression and may persist until significant therapeutic effect is achieved and it is general clinical experience with all antidepressant therapies that the risk of suicide may increase in the early stages of recovery.

Haemorrhage – There have been reports of cutaneous bleeding abnormalities such as ecchymoses and purpura, as well as haemorrhagic manifestations e.g. gastrointestinal haemorrhage with SSRIs. The risk of gastrointestinal haemorrhage may be increased in elderly people during treatment with SSRIs. Caution is advised in patients taking SSRIs, particularly in concomitant use with drugs known to affect platelet function (e.g. atypical antipsychotics and phenothiazines, most tricyclic antidepressants, aspirin and non-steroidal anti-inflammatory drugs (NSAIDs) as well as in patients with a history of bleeding disorders.

Experience with citalopram has not revealed any clinically relevant interactions with neuroleptics. However, as with other SSRIs, the possibility of a pharmacodynamic interaction cannot be excluded.

Consideration should be given to factors which may affect the disposition of a minor metabolite of citalopram (didemethylcitalopram) since increased levels of this metabolite could theoretically prolong the QTc interval in susceptible individuals. However, in ECG monitoring of 2500 patients in clinical trials, including 277 patients with pre-existing cardiac conditions, no clinically significant changes were noted.

As with most antidepressants, citalopram should be discontinued if the patient enters a manic phase. There is little clinical experience of concurrent use of citalopram and ECT.

Some patients with panic disorder experience an initial anxiogenic effect when starting pharmacotherapy. A low starting dose (see Posology) reduces the likelihood of this effect.

4.5 Interaction with other medicinal products and other forms of Interaction

Monoamine Oxidase Inhibitors (MAOIs) should not be used in combination with SSRIs (see Contraindications)

The metabolism of citalopram is only partly dependent on the hepatic cytochrome P450 isozyme CYP2D6 and, unlike some other SSRIs, citalopram is only a weak inhibitor of this important enzyme system which is involved in the metabolism of many drugs (including antiarrhythmics, neuroleptics, beta-blockers, TCAs and some SSRIs). Protein binding is relatively low (<80%). These properties give citalopram a low potential for clinically significant drug interactions.

Alcohol – The combination of citalopram and alcohol is not advisable. However clinical studies have revealed no adverse pharmacodynamic interactions between citalopram and alcohol.

Serotonergic drugs – Co administration with serotonergic drugs (e.g. tramadol, sumatriptan) may lead to enhancement of 5-HT associated effects.

Lithium & tryptophan – There is no pharmacokinetic interaction between lithium and citalopram. However there are have been reports of enhanced effects when SSRIs have been given with lithium or tryptophan and therefore the concomitant use of citalopram with these drugs should be undertaken with caution. Routine monitoring of lithium levels need not be adjusted.

In a pharmacokinetic study no affect was demonstrated on either citalopram or imipramine levels, although the level of desipramine, the primary metabolite of imipramine, was increased. In animal studies cimetidine had little or no influence on citalopram kinetics.

Dynamic interactions between citalopram and herbal remedy St John's Wort (Hypericum perforatum) can occur, resulting in an increase in undesirable effects.

No pharmacodynamic interactions have been noted in clinical studies in which citalopram has been given concomitantly with benzodiazepines, neuroleptics, analgesics, lithium, alcohol, antihistamines, antihypertensive drugs, beta-blockers and other cardiovascular drugs.

4.6 Pregnancy and lactation

Pregnancy – Animal studies did not provide any evidence of teratogenicity, however the safety of citalopram during human pregnancy has not been established. As with all drugs citalopram should only be used in pregnancy if the potential benefits of treatment to the mother outweigh the possible risks to the developing foetus.

Lactation – Citalopram is known to be excreted in breast milk. Its effects on the nursing infant have not been established. If treatment with citalopram is considered necessary, discontinuation of breast feeding should be considered.

4.7 Effects on ability to drive and use machines

Citalopram does not impair intellectual function and psychomotor performance. However, patients who are prescribed psychotropic medication may be expected to have some impairment of general attention and concentration either due to the illness itself, the medication or both and should be cautioned about their ability to drive a car and operate machinery.

4.8 Undesirable effects

Adverse effects observed with citalopram are in general mild and transient. They are most prominent during the first one or two weeks of treatment and usually attenuate as the depressive state improves.

The most commonly observed adverse events associated with the use of citalopram and not seen at an equal incidence among placebo-treated patients were: nausea, somnolence, dry mouth, increased sweating and tremor. The incidence of each in excess over placebo is low (<10%).

In comparative clinical trials with tricyclic antidepressants the incidence of adverse events occurring with citalopram was found to be lower in all cases.

Withdrawal reactions have been reported in association with selective serotonin reuptake inhibitors (SSRIs), including Cipramil. Common symptoms include dizziness, paraesthesia, headache, anxiety and nausea. Abrupt discontinuation of treatment with Cipramil should be avoided. The majority of symptoms experienced on withdrawal of SSRIs are non-serious and self-limiting.

Treatment emergent adverse events reported in clinical trials (N=2985):

Frequent (⩾5 - 20%)

Increased sweating, headache, tremor, dizziness, abnormal accommodation, somnolence, insomnia, agitation, nervousness, nausea, dry mouth, constipation, diarrhoea, palpitation, asthenia.

Less frequent (1 - <5%)

Rash, pruritus, paraesthesia, migraine, abnormal vision, taste perversion, sleep disorder, decreased libido, impaired concentration, abnormal dreaming, amnesia, anxiety, increased appetite, anorexia, apathy, impotence, suicide attempt, confusion, dyspepsia, vomiting, abdominal pain, flatulence, increased salivation, weight decrease, weight increase, postural hypotension, tachycardia, rhinitis, micturition disorder, polyuria, ejaculation failure, female anorgasmia, fatigue.

Rare (<1%)

Myalgia, movement disorders, convulsions, tinnitus, euphoria, increased libido, coughing, malaise.

Post Marketing

- The following adverse reactions apply to the therapeutic class of SSRIs

Skin Disorders: Angiodema; ecchymoses. Photosensitivity reactions have been reported very rarely.

Disorders of metabolism and nutrition: Rare cases of hyponatraemia and inappropriate ADH secretion have been reported and appear to be reversible on discontinuation. The majority of the reports were associated with the older patients.

Gastrointestinal disorders : Gastrointestinal bleeding.

General disorders: Anaphylactoid reactions.

Hepato-billiary disorders: Abnormal LFT's.

Musculoskeletal disorders: Arthralgia.

Neurological disorders: Serotonin syndrome.

Psychiatric disorders: Hallucinations; mania; depersonalisation; panic attacks (these symptoms may be due to the underlying disease).

Reproductive disorders: Galactorrhoea.

4.9 Overdose

Citalopram is given to patients at potential risk of suicide and some reports of attempted suicide have been received. Detail is often lacking regarding precise dose or combination with other drugs and/or alcohol.

Symptoms

Experience from 8 cases considered due to citalopram alone has recorded the following symptoms/signs: somnolence, coma, stiffened expression, episode of grand mal convulsion, sinus tachycardia, occasional nodal rhythm, sweating, nausea, vomiting, cyanosis, hyperventilation. No case was fatal. The clinical picture was inconsistent, no observation being made in more than two individuals.

Six fatalities have been reported. In one overdose was suspected; high post mortem plasma levels were seen although it is not technically possible to interpret these with confidence.

In the remaining five a combination with other drugs had been taken. The clinical syndrome observed prior to death in three of these cases where citalopram was taken with moclobemide was interpreted as that of serotonin syndrome. No clinical details are available on the other two.

Treatment

There is no specific antidote. Treatment is symptomatic and supportive. Gastric lavage should be carried out as soon as possible after oral ingestion. Medical surveillance is advisable.

5. PHARMACOLOGICAL PROPERTIES

5.1 Pharmacodynamic properties

ATC-code: N 06 AB 04

Biochemical and behavioural studies have shown that citalopram is a potent inhibitor of the serotonin (5-HT)-uptake. Tolerance to the inhibition of 5-HT-uptake is not induced by long-term treatment with citalopram.

Citalopram is the most Selective Serotonin Reuptake Inhibitor (SSRI) yet described, with no, or minimal, effect on noradrenaline (NA), dopamine (DA) and gamma aminobutyric acid (GABA) uptake.

In contrast to many tricyclic antidepressants and some of the newer SSRI's, citalopram has not or very low affinity for a series of receptors including 5-HT $_{1A}$, 5-HT$_2$, DA D$_1$ and D$_2$ receptors, α_1-, α_2-, β-adrenoceptors, histamine H$_1$, muscarine cholinergic, benzodiazepine, and opioid receptors. A series of functional *in vitro* tests in isolated organs as well as functional *in vivo* tests have confirmed the lack of receptor affinity. This absence of effects on receptors could explain why citalopram produces fewer of the traditional side effects such as dry mouth, bladder and gut disturbance, blurred vision, sedation, cardiotoxicity and orthostatic hypotension.

Suppression of rapid eye movement (REM) sleep is considered a predictor of antidepressant activity. Like tricyclic antidepressants, other SSRI's and MAO inhibitors, citalopram suppresses REM-sleep and increases deep slow-wave sleep.

Although citalopram does not bind to opioid receptors it potentiates the anti-nociceptive effect of commonly used opioid analgesics. There was potentiation of d-amphetamine-induced hyperactivity following administration of citalopram.

The main metabolites of citalopram are all SSRIs although their potency and selectivity ratios are lower than those of citalopram. However, the selectivity ratios of the metabolites are higher than those of many of the newer SSRIs. The metabolites do not contribute to the overall antidepressant effect.

In humans citalopram does not impair cognitive (intellectual function) and psychomotor performance and has no or minimal sedative properties, either alone or in combination with alcohol.

Citalopram did not reduce saliva flow in a single dose study in human volunteers and in none of the studies in healthy volunteers did citalopram have significant influence on cardiovascular parameters. Citalopram has no effect on the serum levels of prolactin and growth hormone.

5.2 Pharmacokinetic properties

Absorption

Absorption is almost complete and independent of food intake (T_{max} average/mean 3.8 hours). Oral bioavailability is about 80%.

Distribution

The apparent volume of distribution $(V_d)_\beta$ is about 12.3 L/kg. The plasma protein binding is below 80% for citalopram and its main metabolites.

Biotransformation

Citalopram is metabolized to the active demethylcitalopram, didemethylcitalopram, citalopram-N-oxide and an inactive deaminated propionic acid derivative. All the active metabolites are also SSRIs, although weaker than the parent compound. Unchanged citalopram is the predominant compound in plasma.

Elimination

The elimination half-life ($T_{½\beta}$) is about 1.5 days and the systemic citalopram plasma clearance (Cl_s) is about 0.33 L/min, and oral plasma clearance (Cl_{oral}) is about 0.41 L/min.

Citalopram is excreted mainly via the liver (85%) and the remainder (15%) via the kidneys. About 12% of the daily dose is excreted in urine as unchanged citalopram. Hepatic (residual) clearance is about 0.35 L/min and renal clearance about 0.068 L/min.

The kinetics are linear. Steady state plasma levels are achieved in 1-2 weeks. Average concentrations of 250 nmol/L (100-500 nmol/L) are achieved at a daily dose of 40 mg. There is no clear relationship between citalopram plasma levels and therapeutic response or side effects.

Elderly patients (⩾ 65 years)

Longer half-lives and decreased clearance values due to a reduced rate of metabolism have been demonstrated in elderly patients.

Reduced hepatic function

Citalopram is eliminated more slowly in patients with reduced hepatic function. The half-life of citalopram is about twice as long and steady state citalopram concentrations at a given dose will be about twice as high as in patients with normal liver function.

Reduced renal function

Citalopram is eliminated more slowly in patients with mild to moderate reduction of renal function, without any major impact on the pharmacokinetics of citalopram. At present no information is available for treatment of patients with severely reduced renal function (creatinine clearance <20 mL/min).

5.3 Preclinical safety data

Citalopram has low acute toxicity. In chronic toxicity studies there were no findings of concern for the therapeutic use of citalopram. Based on data from reproduction toxicity studies (segment I, II and III) there is no reason to have special concern for the use of citalopram in women of child-bearing potential. Citalopram has no mutagenic or carcinogenic potential.

6. PHARMACEUTICAL PARTICULARS

6.1 List of excipients

Tablets: Maize starch, Lactose, Microcystalline-cellulose, Copolyvidone, Glycerol, Croscarmellose Sodium Type A, Magnesium stearate, Methylhydroxypropyl-cellulose, Macrogol, Titanium dioxide.

6.2 Incompatibilities

Nil.

6.3 Shelf life

Each pack has an expiry date.

Citalopram tablets are valid for 5 years

6.4 Special precautions for storage

Do not store above 25°C

6.5 Nature and contents of container

Press through packs (UPVC/PVdC with aluminium closure) 28 tablets.

6.6 Instructions for use and handling

Nil.

Administrative Data

7. MARKETING AUTHORISATION HOLDER

Lundbeck Limited

Lundbeck House

Caldecotte Lake Business Park

Caldecotte

Milton Keynes

MK7 8LF

(Manufacturer: H. Lundbeck A/S, DK-2500 Copenhagen-Valby, Denmark)

8. MARKETING AUTHORISATION NUMBER(S)
10 mg tablet: PL 0458/0057

20 mg tablet: PL 0458/0058

40 mg tablet: PL 0458/0059

9. DATE OF FIRST AUTHORISATION/RENEWAL OF THE AUTHORISATION
First authorisation: 17 March 1995

Renewal of authorisation: 24 August 2001

10. DATE OF REVISION OF THE TEXT
April 2003

Ciproxin Infusion

(Bayer plc)

1. NAME OF THE MEDICINAL PRODUCT
Ciproxin Infusion

2. QUALITATIVE AND QUANTITATIVE COMPOSITION
Qualitative composition: Ciprofloxacin (INN)

Quantitative composition:

Each presentation of Ciproxin Infusion in glass bottles contains the following:

50ml pack size: 100mg Ciprofloxacin Ph.Eur. as 127.2mg ciprofloxacin lactate.

100ml pack size: 200mg Ciprofloxacin Ph.Eur. as 254.4mg ciprofloxacin lactate.

200ml pack size: 400mg Ciprofloxacin Ph.Eur. as 508.8mg ciprofloxacin lactate.

3. PHARMACEUTICAL FORM
Sterile solution for intravenous infusion.

4. CLINICAL PARTICULARS

4.1 Therapeutic indications
Ciprofloxacin is indicated for the treatment of the following infections caused by sensitive bacteria:

Adults:

Severe systemic infections: e.g. septicaemia, bacteraemia, peritonitis, infections in immunosuppressed patients with haematological or solid tumours and in patients in intensive care units with specific problems such as infected burns.

Respiratory tract infections: e.g. lobar and bronchopneumonia, acute and chronic bronchitis, acute exacerbation of cystic fibrosis, bronchiectasis, empyema. Ciprofloxacin is not recommended as first-line therapy for the treatment of pneumococcal pneumonia. Ciprofloxacin may be used for treating Gram-negative pneumonia.

Ear, nose and throat infections: e.g. mastoiditis, otitis media and sinusitis, especially if due to Gram-negative bacteria (including *Pseudomonas* spp.). Ciprofloxacin is not recommended for the treatment of acute tonsillitis.

Eye infections: e.g. bacterial conjunctivitis.

Urinary tract infections: e.g. uncomplicated and complicated urethritis, cystitis, pyelonephritis, prostatitis, epididymitis.

Skin and soft tissue infections: e.g. infected ulcers, wound infections, abscesses, cellulitis, otitis externa, erysipelas, infected burns.

Bone and joint infections: e.g. osteomyelitis, septic arthritis

Intra-abdominal infections: e.g. peritonitis, intra-abdominal abscesses.

Infections of the biliary tract: e.g. cholangitis, cholecystitis, empyema of the gall bladder.

Gastro-intestinal infections: e.g. enteric fever, infective diarrhoea.

Pelvic infections: e.g. salpingitis, endometritis, pelvic inflammatory disease.

Gonorrhoea: including urethral, rectal and pharyngeal gonorrhoea caused by β-lactamase producing organisms or organisms moderately sensitive to penicillin.

Children:

For the treatment of acute pulmonary exacerbation of cystic fibrosis associated with *P. aeruginosa* infection in paediatric patients aged 5 – 17 years.

Inhalation Anthrax in Adults and Children: To reduce the incidence or progression of disease following confirmed or suspected exposure to aerosolised *Bacillus anthracis*.

4.2 Posology and method of administration
The dosage of intravenous ciprofloxacin is determined by the severity and type of infection, the sensitivity of the causative organism(s) and the age, weight and renal function of the patient.

The dosage range for adults is 100-400mg twice daily. The product may be infused directly and administered by short-term infusion over periods of 30-60 minutes. The 400mg dose should be administered over a period of 60 minutes. Initial intravenous administration may be followed by oral treatment.

<u>Adults</u>

The following dosages for specific types of infection are recommended:

<u>Table 1: Recommended Adult Dosage</u>

Indication	Dosage i.v. (mg ciprofloxacin)
<u>Treatment</u>	
Gonorrhoea	100mg single dose
Upper and lower urinary tract infections	100mg b.d.
Upper and lower respiratory tract infections (depending on severity and sensitivity of causative organism)	200-400mg b.d.
Pneumococcal pneumonia (second-line PL 0010/0148)	No recommended i.v. dosage, 750mg p.o. b.d.
Cystic fibrosis patients with pseudomonal lower RTI*	400mg b.d.
Other infections as detailed under 4.1	200-400mg b.d.
Inhalation Anthrax	400mg b.d.

* Although the pharmacokinetics of ciprofloxacin remains unchanged in patients with cystic fibrosis, the low body-weight of these patients should be taken into consideration when determining dosage.

<u>Impaired Renal Function</u>

Dosage adjustments are not usually required, except in patients with severe renal impairment (serum creatinine >265 micromole/l or creatinine clearance <20ml/minute). If adjustment is necessary, this may be achieved by reducing the total daily dose by half, although monitoring of drug serum levels provides the most reliable basis for dose adjustment.

<u>Impaired Hepatic Function</u>

No adjustment of dosage is necessary.

<u>Elderly</u>

Although higher ciprofloxacin serum levels are found in the elderly, no adjustment of dosage is necessary.

<u>Adolescents and Children</u>

As with other drugs in its class, ciprofloxacin has been shown to cause arthropathy in weight-bearing joints of immature animals. Although analysis of available safety data from ciprofloxacin use in patients less than 18 years of age, the majority of whom had cystic fibrosis, did not disclose any evidence of drug related cartilage or articular damage, its use in the paediatric patient population is generally not recommended.

Clinical and pharmacokinetic data support the use of ciprofloxacin in paediatric cystic fibrosis patients (aged 5-17 years) with acute pulmonary exacerbation associated with *P. aeruginosa* infection, at a dose of 10mg/kg iv three times daily (maximum daily dose 1200mg). The infusion should be administered over 60 minutes.

Sequential therapy can also be used. Dosage as follows: 10mg/kg iv three times daily (maximum daily dose 1200mg) followed by 20mg/kg orally twice daily (maximum daily dose 1500mg).

For the indication of inhalation anthrax, the risk-benefit assessment indicates that administration of ciprofloxacin to paediatric patients at a dose of 10 mg/kg i.v. twice daily (maximum daily dose of 800 mg) is appropriate.

For indications other than the treatment of pulmonary exacerbation in cystic fibrosis and inhalation anthrax, ciprofloxacin may be used in children and adolescents where the benefit is considered to outweigh the potential risks. In these cases a dosage of 4 – 8 mg/kg iv twice daily or 5 – 15mg/kg orally twice daily should be administered depending upon the severity of the infection.

Dosing in children with impaired renal and/or hepatic function has not been studied.

<u>Duration of Treatment</u>

The duration of treatment depends upon the severity of infection, clinical response and bacteriological findings. The usual treatment period for acute infections is 5-7 days.

Generally, acute and chronic infections (e.g. osteomyelitis and prostatitis, etc), where the causative organism is known to be sensitive to ciprofloxacin, should be treated for at least three days after the signs and symptoms of the infection have disappeared.

For acute pulmonary exacerbation of cystic fibrosis associated with *P. aeruginosa* infection in paediatric patients (aged 5 – 17 years), the duration of treatment is 10 – 14 days.

For inhalation anthrax, drug administration should begin as soon as possible after confirmed or suspected exposure and should be continued for 60 days.

4.3 Contraindications
Ciprofloxacin is contra-indicated in patients who have shown hypersensitivity to ciprofloxacin or other quinolone anti-infectives.

Except in cases of exacerbation of cystic fibrosis associated with *P. aeruginosa* (in patients aged 5- 17 years) and inhalation anthrax, ciprofloxacin is contra-indicated in children and growing adolescents unless the benefits of treatment are considered to outweigh the risks.

4.4 Special warnings and special precautions for use
Ciprofloxacin should be used with caution in epileptics and patients with a history of CNS disorders and only if the benefits of treatment are considered to outweigh the risk of possible CNS side-effects. CNS side-effects have been reported after first administration of ciprofloxacin in some patients. Treatment should be discontinued if the side-effects, depression or psychoses lead to self-endangering behaviour (see also Section 4.8).

Crystalluria related to the use of ciprofloxacin has been reported. Patients receiving ciprofloxacin should be well hydrated and excessive alkalinity of the urine should be avoided.

Patients with a family history of or actual defects in glucose-6-phosphate dehydrogenase activity are prone to haemolytic reactions with quinolones, and so ciprofloxacin should be used with caution in these patients.

Tendon inflammation and rupture may occur with quinolone antibiotics. Such reactions have been observed particularly in older patients and in those treated concurrently with corticosteroids. At the first sign of pain or inflammation, patients should discontinue ciprofloxacin and rest the affected limbs.

There is a risk of pseudomembranous colitis with broad-spectrum antibiotics possibly leading to a fatal outcome. It is important to consider this in patients suffering from severe, persistent diarrhoea. With ciprofloxacin this effect has been reported rarely. If pseudomembranous colitis is suspected treatment with ciprofloxacin should be stopped and appropriate treatment given (e.g. oral vancomycin).

As with other quinolones, patients should avoid prolonged exposure to strong sunlight or UV radiation during treatment.

Laboratory tests may give abnormal findings if performed whilst patients are receiving ciprofloxacin, e.g. increased alkaline phosphatase; increases in liver function tests, e.g. transaminases and cholestatic jaundice, especially in patients with previous liver damage.

4.5 Interaction with other medicinal products and other forms of Interaction
Increased plasma levels of theophylline have been observed following concurrent administration with ciprofloxacin. It is recommended that the dose of theophylline should be reduced and plasma levels of theophylline monitored. The reaction between theophylline and ciprofloxacin is potentially life-threatening. Therefore, where monitoring of plasma levels is not possible, the use of ciprofloxacin should be avoided in patients receiving theophylline. Particular caution is advised in those patients with convulsive disorders.

Phenytoin levels may be altered when Ciproxin is used concomitantly.

Prolongation of bleeding time has been reported during concomitant administration of ciprofloxacin and oral anticoagulants.

Animal data have shown that high doses of quinolones in combination with some non-steroidal anti-inflammatory drugs, (e.g. fenbufen, but not acetylsalicylic acid) can lead to convulsions.

Transient increases in serum creatinine have been seen following concomitant administration of ciprofloxacin and cyclosporin. Therefore, monitoring of serum creatinine levels is advisable.

The simultaneous administration of quinolones and glibenclamide can on occasion potentiate the effect of glibenclamide resulting in hypoglycaemia.

Renal tubular transport of methotrexate may be inhibited by concomitant administration of ciprofloxacin potentially leading to increased plasma levels of methotrexate. This may increase the risk of methotrexate associated toxic reactions. Therefore, patients receiving methotrexate therapy should be carefully monitored when concomitant ciprofloxacin therapy is indicated.

Concomitant use with probenecid reduces the renal clearance of ciprofloxacin, resulting in increased quinolone plasma levels.

4.6 Pregnancy and lactation
Reproduction studies performed in mice, rats and rabbits using parenteral and oral administration did not reveal any evidence of teratogenicity, impairment of fertility or impairment of peri-/post-natal development. However, as with other quinolones, ciprofloxacin has been shown to cause arthropathy in immature animals, and therefore its use during pregnancy is not recommended. Studies have indicated that ciprofloxacin is secreted in breast milk. Administration to nursing mothers is thus not recommended.

4.7 Effects on ability to drive and use machines

Ciprofloxacin could result in impairment of the patient's ability to drive or operate machinery, particularly in conjunction with alcohol.

4.8 Undesirable effects

Ciprofloxacin is generally well tolerated. The most frequently reported adverse reactions are: nausea, diarrhoea and rash.

The following adverse reactions have been observed:

Hypersensitivity/skin, e.g. rash, pruritus, urticaria, photosensitivity, drug-induced fever, anaphylactic/anaphylactoid reactions including angioedema and dyspnoea. Rarely, erythema nodosum and erythema multiforme. Very rarely, petechiae, haemorrhagic bullae, vasculitis, serum sickness-like reaction, fixed drug reactions, Stevens-Johnson Syndrome and Lyells Syndrome. Treatment with ciprofloxacin should be discontinued if any of the above occur upon first administration.

General, e.g. moniliasis, asthenia, hyperglycaemia and abnormal gait, pain, pain in extremeties, back pain, chest pain. Thrombophlebitis.

CNS, e.g. headache, restlessness, depression, dizziness, tremor, convulsions, confusion, hallucinations, somnolence, sleep disorders, insomnia. Rarely, hypesthesia. Very rarely, migraine, hyperesthesia, ataxia, hypertonia, twitching or anxiety states. Isolated cases of ciprofloxacin-induced psychoses have been reported, which may progress to self-endangering behaviour. There are isolated reports of intracranial hypertension associated with quinolone therapy. Paraesthesia has been reported.

Gastro-intestinal, e.g. nausea, diarrhoea, vomiting, dyspepsia, abdominal pain, anorexia, flatulence, dysphagia. Rarely, pancreatitis or pseudomembranous colitis.

Cardiovascular, e.g. tachycardia, oedema, fainting, hot flushes, hypotension and sweating.

Effects on haematological parameters, e.g. anaemia, eosinophilia, increases or decreases in white cell and/or platelet count, altered prothrombin levels, and, very rarely, haemolytic anaemia, agranulocytosis, pancytopenia or bone marrow depression. Pancytopenia and bone marrow depression may be potentially life-threatening.

Hepatic, e.g. transient increases in liver enzymes or serum bilirubin (particularly in patients with previous liver damage), hepatitis, jaundice/cholestasis and major liver disorders including hepatic necrosis, which may rarely progress to life-threatening hepatic failure.

Renal, e.g. transient increases in blood urea or serum creatinine, renal failure, crystalluria, haematuria, nephritis.

Musculoskeletal, e.g. reversible arthralgia, joint swelling and myalgia. Rarely, myasthenia or tenosynovitis. Tendon inflammation (predominantly of the Achilles tendon) has been reported which may lead to tendon rupture. Treatment should be discontinued immediately if these symptoms occur.

Rarely, exacerbation of the symptoms of myasthenia gravis have been reported.

Special senses, e.g. very rarely, visual disturbances including diplopia and colour disturbances, impaired taste and smell usually reversible upon discontinuation of treatment, tinnitus, transient impairment of hearing particularly at high frequencies.

Abnormal laboratory findings, e.g. increased alkaline phosphatase, amylase and lipase; increases in liver function tests, e.g transaminases, and cholestatic jaundice, especially in patients with previous liver damage.

Injection site reaction associated with irritation and pain may sometimes occur. In a small number of patients this may be accompanied by phlebitis or thrombophlebitis.

4.9 Overdose

Based on the limited information available in two cases of ingestion of over 18g of ciprofloxacin, reversible renal toxicity has occurred. Therefore, apart from routine emergency measures, it is recommended to monitor renal function, including urinary pH and acidify, if required, to prevent crystalluria. Patients must be kept well hydrated, and in the case of renal damage resulting in prolonged oliguria, dialysis should be initiated.

Serum levels of ciprofloxacin are reduced by dialysis.

5. PHARMACOLOGICAL PROPERTIES

ATC Code J01 MA 02

5.1 Pharmacodynamic properties

Ciprofloxacin is a synthetic 4-quinolone derivative, with bactericidal activity. It acts via inhibition of bacterial DNA gyrase, ultimately resulting in interference with DNA function. Ciprofloxacin is highly active against a wide range of Gram-positive and Gram-negative organisms and has shown activity against some anaerobes, *Chlamydia* spp. and *Mycoplasma* spp. Killing curves demonstrate the rapid bactericidal effect against sensitive organisms and it is often found that minimum bactericidal concentrations are in the range of minimum inhibitory concentrations. Ciprofloxacin has been shown to have no activity against *Treponema pallidum* and *Ureaplasma urealyticum*, *Nocardia asteroides*, and *Enterococcus faecium* are resistant.

Breakpoints

S ⩽ 1 μg/ml, R ⩾ 4 μg/ml

Susceptibility

The prevalence of resistance may vary geographically and with time for selected species and local area information on resistance is desirable, particularly when treating severe infections. This information gives only an approximate guidance on probabilities whether micro-organisms will be susceptible to ciprofloxacin or not.

ORGANISM	PREVALENCE OF RESISTANCE
Sensitive:	
Gram-positive bacteria	
Corynebacterium diphtheriae	0%
Corynebacterium spp.	-
Staphylococcus aureus (methicillin sensitive)	0 - 14%
Staphylococcus aureus (methicillin resistant)	48 - 90%
Streptococcus agalactiae	0 – 17%
Bacillus anthracis	-
Gram-negative bacteria	
Acinetobacter baumanii	6 - 93%
Acinetobacter spp.	14 – 70%
Aeromonas hydrophilia	0%
Aeromonas spp.	
Bordetella pertussis	0%
Brucella melitensis	0%
Campylobacter jejuni/coli	0 – 82%
Campylobacter spp.	0%
Citrobacter freundii	0 – 4%
Citrobacter spp.	0%
Edwardsiella tarda	0%
Enterobacter aerogenes	0%
Enterobacter cloacae	0 - 3%
Enterobacter spp.	3 - 13%
Escherichia coli	2 -7%
Escherichia coli, EHEC and EPEC	-
Haemophilus influenzae	0 – 1%
Haemophilus influenzae (β-lactam negative)	0%
Haemophilus influenzae (β-lactam positive)	0%
Haemophilus parainfluenzae	0%
Hafnia alvei	0%
Klebsiella oxytoca	0%
Klebsiella pneumoniae	2 – 5.8%
Klebsiella spp.	2 – 21%
Legionella pneumophila	0%
Legionella spp.	0%
Moraxella catarrhalis	0%
Morganella morganii	1 – 2%
Neisseria gonorrhoeae	0%
Neisseria gonorrhoeae, β-lactamase	0%
Neisseria gonorrhoeae, β-lactamase positive	0%
Neisseria meningitidis	0%
Neisseria meningitidis, β-lactamase negative	0%
Plesiomonas shigelloides	0%
Proteus mirabilis	0 – 10%
Proteus vulgaris	4%
Providencia rettgeri	
Providencia spp.	4%
Providencia stuartii	-
Pseudomonas aeruginosa	1 – 28%
Salmonella spp.	0%
Salmonella typhi	0 - 2%
Serratia liquefaciens	-
Serratia marcescens	23%
Serratia spp.	0 – 21%
Shigella spp.	0%
Vibrio cholerae	0%
Vibrio parahaemolyticus	0%
Vibrio spp.	0%
Yersinia enterocolitica	0%
Anaerobes	
Bacteroides ureolyticus	0%
Clostridium perfringens	-
Peptococcus spp.	0%
Peptostreptococcus spp.	-
Peptostreptococcus magnus	0%
Veillonella parvula	0%
Other pathogens	
Chlamydia spp.	-
Helicobacter pylori	
Mycobacterium fortuitum	0%
Mycobacterium tuberculosis	0%
Mycoplasma hominis	16%
Intermediate	
Gram-positive aerobes	
Enterococci	5%
Enterococcus faecalis	9 – 34%
Staphylococcus epidermis, methicillin sensitive	10 - 16%
Staphylococcus epidermis, methicillin resistant	26 - 56%
Staphylococcus haemolyticus	-
Staphylococcus haemolyticus, methicillin sensitive	8%
Staphylococcus haemolyticus, methicillin resistant	73%
Streptococcus anginosus	9%
Streptococcus bovis	-
Streptococcus milleri	5%
Streptococcus mitis	-
Streptococcus pneumoniae, penicillin sensitive	0 – 1%
Streptococcus pneumoniae, penicillin intermediate	

Streptococcus pneumoniae, penicillin intermediate and resistant	2.8%
Streptococcus pneumoniae, penicillin resistant	-
Streptococcus pyogenes	0 - 28%
Streptococcus, viridans group	-
Streptococcus viridans, penicillin sensitive	-
Streptococcus viridans, penicillin resistant	-
Streptococcus, β-haemolytic groups A, C, and G	0%
Gram-negative aerobes	
Alcaligenes spp.	-
Listeria monocytogenes	0%
Listeria spp.	0%
Anaerobes	
Fusobacterium spp.	-
Gardnerella vaginalis	0%
Prevotella spp.	-
Other pathogens	
Ureaplasma urealyticum	11%
Resistant	
Gram-positive aerobes	
Enterococcus faecium	-
Stenotrophomonas maltophilia	94%
Streptococcus sanguis	
Gram-negative aerobes	
Flavobacterium meningosepticum	-
Nocardia asteroides	-
Anaerobes	
Bacteroides fragilis	-
Bacteroides thetaiotaomicron	-
Clostridium difficile	-

Plasmid-related transfer of resistance has not been observed with ciprofloxacin and the overall frequency of development of resistance is low (10^{-9} - 10^{-7}). Cross-resistance to penicillins, cephalosporins, aminoglycosides and tetracyclines has not been observed and organisms resistant to these antibiotics are generally sensitive to ciprofloxacin. Ciprofloxacin is also suitable for use in combination with these antibiotics, and additive behaviour is usually observed.

5.2 Pharmacokinetic properties

Absorption of oral doses of ciprofloxacin 250mg, 500mg and 750mg tablet formulation occurs rapidly, mainly from the small intestine, the half-life of absorption being 2-15 minutes. Plasma levels are dose-related and peak 0.5-2.0 hours after oral dosing. The AUC also increases dose proportionately after administration of both single and repeated oral (tablet) and intravenous doses. The pharmacokinetic profile of intravenous ciprofloxacin was shown to be linear over the dose range (100mg-400mg). Following intravenous administration of ciprofloxacin, the mean maximum plasma concentrations were achieved at the end of the infusion period. That is, for a 100mg or 200mg dose, 30 minutes, and for a 400mg dose, 60 minutes. Reported plasma levels at this time point were 1.8mg/l, 3.4mg/l and 3.9mg/l, respectively. The absolute bioavailability is reported to be 52-83% and ciprofloxacin is subject to only slight first-pass metabolism.

Distribution of ciprofloxacin within tissues is wide and the volume of distribution high, though slightly lower in the elderly. Protein binding is low (between 19-40%). Ciprofloxacin is present in plasma largely in a non-ionised form.

Only 10-20% of a single oral or intravenous dose is eliminated as metabolites (which exhibit lower activity than the parent drug). Four different antimicrobially active metabolites have been reported, desethyleneciprofloxacin (M1), sulphociprofloxacin (M2), oxaciprofloxacin (M3) and formylciprofloxacin (M4). M2 and M3 account for one third each of metabolised substance and M1 is found in small amounts (1.3-2.6% of the dose). M4 has been found in very small quantities (<0.1% of the dose). M1-M3 have antimicrobial activity comparable to nalidixic acid and M4 found in the smallest quantity has antimicrobial activity similar to that of norfloxacin.

Elimination of ciprofloxacin and its metabolites occurs rapidly, primarily by the kidney. After single oral and intravenous doses of ciprofloxacin, 55% and 75% respectively are eliminated by the kidney and 39% and 14% in the faeces within 5 days. Renal elimination takes place mainly during the first 12 hours after dosing and renal clearance levels suggest that active secretion by the renal tubules occurs in addition to normal glomerular filtration. Renal clearance is between 0.18-0.3 l/h.kg and total body clearance between 0.48-0.60 l/h.kg. The elimination kinetics are linear and after repeated dosing at 12 hourly intervals, no further accumulation is detected after the distribution equilibrium is attained (at 4-5 half-lives). The elimination half-life of unchanged ciprofloxacin over a period of 24-48 hours post-dose is 3.1-5.1 hours. A total body clearance of approximately 35l/h was observed after intravenous administration.

Some studies carried out with ciprofloxacin in severely renally impaired patients (serum creatinine >265 micromole/l or creatinine clearance <20ml/minute) demonstrated either a doubling of the elimination half-life, or fluctuations in half-life in comparison with healthy volunteers, whereas other studies showed no significant correlation between elimination half-life and creatinine clearance. However, it is recommended that in severely renally impaired patients, the total daily dose should be reduced by half, although monitoring of drug serum levels provides the most reliable basis for dose adjustment as necessary.

Results of pharmacokinetic studies in paediatric cystic fibrosis patients have shown dosages of 20mg/kg orally twice daily or 10mg/kg iv three times daily are recommended to achieve plasma concentration/time profiles comparable to those achieved in the adult population at the currently recommended dosage regimen.

Inhalation anthrax: Ciprofloxacin serum concentrations achieved in humans serve as a surrogate endpoint reasonably likely to predict clinical benefit and provide the basis for the recommended doses.

5.3 Preclinical safety data

Following extensive oral and intravenous toxicology testing with ciprofloxacin, only two findings which may be considered relevant to the use of ciprofloxacin in man were observed. Crystalluria was noted in those species of animals which had a normally alkaline urine. Kidney damage without the presence of crystalluria was not observed. This effect is considered a secondary inflammatory foreign-body reaction, due to the precipitation of a crystalline complex of ciprofloxacin, magnesium and protein in the distal tubule system of the kidneys. This is considered not to be a problem in man, because the urine is normally acidic. However, to avoid the occurrence of crystalluria, patients should be well hydrated and excessive alkalinity of the urine avoided.

As with other quinolones, damage to the weight-bearing joints of only juvenile rats and dogs treated with ciprofloxacin was noted in repeat dose toxicity testing. This was more noticeable in the dog. Although analysis of available safety data from ciprofloxacin use in paediatric patients did not disclose any evidence of drug related cartilage or articular damage, the use of ciprofloxacin in children and growing adolescents is generally not recommended (with the exception of treatment of cystic fibrosis), unless the benefits are considered to outweigh the potential risks. Additionally, because of the potential of arthropathy, the use of ciprofloxacin during pregnancy and lactation is not recommended.

6. PHARMACEUTICAL PARTICULARS

6.1 List of excipients

Lactic Acid Ph.Eur. (0.01%), Sodium Chloride Ph.Eur. (900mg/100ml equivalent to 154mmol sodium per litre), concentrated Hydrochloric Acid Ph.Eur. and Water for Injections Ph.Eur.

6.2 Incompatibilities

Ciproxin Infusion is incompatible with injection solutions (e.g. penicillins, heparin solutions) which are chemically or physically unstable at its pH of 3.9-4.5. Unless compatibility is proven, the infusion should always be administered separately. For compatible co-infusion solutions see Section 6.6.

6.3 Shelf life

For all pack sizes (50ml, 100ml, 200ml), the shelf-life is four years.

6.4 Special precautions for storage

Since Ciproxin Infusion is light-sensitive, the bottles should always be stored in the cardboard outer container. No special precautions are required during the normal 30-60 minute infusion period.

Do not refrigerate Ciproxin Infusion. If the product is inadvertently refrigerated, crystals may form. Do not use if crystals are present. These crystals will, however, redissolve at room temperature and do not adversely affect the quality of the product.

6.5 Nature and contents of container

Type II, internally siliconised, colourless glass infusion bottles with a matt grey teflon-coated chlorobutyl rubber stopper, containing 50ml, 100ml or 200ml of Ciproxin Infusion solution, with a cardboard outer.

6.6 Instructions for use and handling

Ciproxin Infusion should be infused directly and be administered by short-term intravenous infusion over a period of 30-60 minutes. The 400mg/200ml dose should be administered over 60 minutes. The product should not be mixed with other drug products which are chemically or physically unstable at its pH of 3.9-4.5 (see Section 6.2). However, Ciproxin Infusion has been shown to be compatible with Ringer's solution, 0.9% sodium chloride solution, 5% and 10% glucose solutions, glucose/saline and fructose 10% solution. Unless compatibility is proven, the infusion solution should always be administered separately. In addition, discard any unused portion of product immediately after use.

7. MARKETING AUTHORISATION HOLDER

	Trading as:
Bayer plc	Bayer plc
Bayer House	Pharmaceutical Division
Strawberry Hill	Bayer House
Newbury, Berkshire	Strawberry Hill
RG14 1JA	Newbury, Berkshire
	RG14 1JA
	or BAYPHARM or BAYMET

8. MARKETING AUTHORISATION NUMBER(S)

PL 0010/0150

9. DATE OF FIRST AUTHORISATION/RENEWAL OF THE AUTHORISATION

3rd February 1987/21st July 1999

10. DATE OF REVISION OF THE TEXT

July 2003

Ciproxin Suspension

(Bayer plc)

1. NAME OF THE MEDICINAL PRODUCT

Ciproxin Suspension

2. QUALITATIVE AND QUANTITATIVE COMPOSITION

Qualitative composition: Ciprofloxacin (INN)

Quantitative composition:

(i) Per presentation

5 g/100ml (5% w/v)

1 bottle containing 7.95g of film-coated granules containing 5.0g ciprofloxacin (base form).

1 bottle containing 99.20g of a non-aqueous diluent to prepare 100ml of ready-to-use suspension.

(ii) Per standard 5ml dosage

Each nominal 5ml graduated measuring spoon (supplied with the product) contains 250mg of ciprofloxacin.

3. PHARMACEUTICAL FORM

Gastro-resistant granules and non-aqueous diluent for reconstitution as a ready-to-use suspension for oral administration.

4. CLINICAL PARTICULARS

4.1 Therapeutic indications

Ciprofloxacin is indicated for the treatment of the following infections caused by sensitive bacteria:

Adults:

Respiratory tract infections: e.g. lobar and bronchopneumonia, acute and chronic bronchitis, acute exacerbation of cystic fibrosis, bronchiectasis, empyema. Ciprofloxacin is not recommended as first-line therapy for the treatment of pneumococcal pneumonia. Ciprofloxacin may be used for treating Gram-negative pneumonia.

Ear, nose and throat infections: e.g. mastoiditis, otitis media and sinusitis, especially if due to Gram-negative bacteria (including *Pseudomonas* spp.). Ciprofloxacin is not recommended for the treatment of acute tonsillitis.

Eye infections: e.g. bacterial conjunctivitis.

Urinary tract infections: e.g. uncomplicated and complicated urethritis, cystitis, pyelonephritis, prostatitis, epididymitis.

Skin and soft tissue infections: e.g. infected ulcers, wound infections, abscesses, cellulitis, otitis externa, erysipelas, infected burns.

Bone and joint infections: e.g. osteomyelitis, septic arthritis.

Intra-abdominal infections: e.g. peritonitis, intra-abdominal abscesses.

Infections of the biliary tract: e.g. cholangitis, cholecystitis, empyema of the gall bladder.

Gastro-intestinal infections: e.g. enteric fever, infective diarrhoea.

Pelvic infections: e.g. salpingitis, endometritis, pelvic inflammatory disease.

Severe systemic infections: e.g. septicaemia, bacteraemia, peritonitis, infections in immuno-suppressed patients.

Gonorrhoea: including urethral, rectal and pharyngeal gonorrhoea caused by β-lactamase producing organisms or organisms moderately sensitive to penicillin.

Ciprofloxacin is also indicated for prophylaxis against infection in elective upper gastro-intestinal tract surgery and endoscopic procedures, where there is an increased risk of infection.

Children:

For the treatment of acute pulmonary exacerbation of cystic fibrosis associated with *P. aeruginosa* infection in paediatric patients aged 5-17 years.

Inhalation Anthrax in Adults and Children: To reduce the incidence or progression of disease following confirmed or suspected exposure to aerosolised *Bacillus anthracis*.

4.2 Posology and method of administration

The dosage of Ciproxin Suspension is determined by the severity and type of infection, the sensitivity of the causative organism(s) and the age, weight and renal function of the patient.

If Ciproxin Suspension is taken on an empty stomach, the active substance is absorbed more rapidly. In this case, the suspension should not be taken concurrently with dairy products or with mineral fortified drinks alone (e.g. milk, yoghurt, calcium fortified orange juice). However, a normal diet that will contain small amounts of calcium, does not significantly affect ciprofloxacin absorption.

The reconstituted suspension should be swallowed whole and the granules should not be chewed. A glass of water may be taken after dosing.

The dosage range for adults is 250-750mg twice daily. The reconstituted suspension should always be dosed with the graduated measuring spoon provided. Each nominal 5.0ml spoonful will deliver 250mg ciprofloxacin. The ½ marking on the spoon will dose a nominal 2.5ml of product. The 1/1 marking on the spoon will dose a nominal 5.0ml of product.

Adults

The following dosages for specific types of infection are recommended:

Table 1: Recommended Adult Dosage

Indication	Dosage (mg ciprofloxacin)	No. of Spoonfuls (5ml) of Reconstituted Ciproxin Suspension*
Treatment		
Gonorrhoea	250mg single dose	1 s.d.
Acute, uncomplicated cystitis	250mg b.d.	1 b.d.
Upper and lower urinary tract infections (depending on severity)	250-500mg b.d.	1 or 2 b.d.
Upper and lower respiratory tract infections (depending on severity	250-750mg b.d.	1, 2 or 3 b.d.
Pneumococcal pneumonia (second-line)	750mg b.d.	3 b.d.
Cystic fibrosis patients with pseudomonal lower RTI**	750mg b.d.	3 b.d.
Other infections as detailed under 4.1	500-750mg b.d.	2 or 3 b.d.
Severe infections, particularly due to Pseudomonas, staphylococci and streptococci	750mg b.d.	3 b.d.
Inhalation anthrax	500mg b.d.	2 b.d.
Prophylaxis		
Elective upper gastro-intestinal surgical and endoscopic procedures	750mg single dose 60-90 minutes prior to the procedure. If gastro-oesophageal obstructive lesions are suspected use with an anti-infective effective against anaerobes	3 s.d.

* For correct dosing always use the graduated measuring spoon supplied with the product.

** Although the pharmacokinetics of ciprofloxacin remains unchanged in patients with cystic fibrosis, the low bodyweight of these patients should be taken into consideration when determining dosage.

Impaired Renal Function

Dosage adjustments are not usually required, except in patients with severe renal impairment (serum creatinine >265 micromole/l or creatinine clearance <20ml/minute). If adjustment is necessary, this may be achieved by reducing the total daily dose by half, although monitoring of drug serum levels provides the most reliable basis for dose adjustment.

Impaired Hepatic Function

No adjustment of dosage is necessary.

Elderly

Although higher ciprofloxacin serum levels are found in the elderly, no adjustment of dosage is necessary.

Adolescents and children

As with other drugs in its class, ciprofloxacin has been shown to cause arthropathy in weight-bearing joints of immature animals. Although analysis of available safety data from ciprofloxacin use in patients less than 18 years of age, the majority of whom had cystic fibrosis, did not disclose any evidence of drug related cartilage or articular damage, its use in the paediatric patient population is generally not recommended.

Clinical and pharmacokinetic data support the use of ciprofloxacin in paediatric cystic fibrosis patients (aged 5-17 years) with acute pulmonary exacerbation associated with *P. aeruginosa* infection, at a dose of 20mg/kg orally twice daily (maximum daily dose 1500mg).

For the indication of inhalation anthrax, the risk-benefit assessment indicates that administration of ciprofloxacin to paediatric patients at a dose of 15 mg/kg orally twice daily (maximum daily dose of 1000 mg) is appropriate.

For indications other than treatment of pulmonary exacerbations in cystic fibrosis and inhalation anthrax, ciprofloxacin may be used in children and adolescents where the benefit is considered to outweigh the potential risks. In these cases a dosage of 4-8mg/kg iv twice daily or 5-15mg/kg orally twice daily should be administered, depending upon the severity of infection. N.B. Ciproxin Suspension should not be used in children of less than two years of age (see Section 4.4).

Dosing in children with impaired renal and/or hepatic function has not been studied.

Duration of Treatment

The duration of treatment depends upon the severity of infection, clinical response and bacteriological findings.

In acute, uncomplicated cystitis the treatment period is three days.

In other acute infections the usual treatment period is 5-10 days. Generally, acute and chronic infections (e.g. osteomyelitis and prostatitis, etc), where the causative organism is known to be sensitive to ciprofloxacin, should be treated for at least three days after the signs and symptoms of the infection have disappeared.

For acute pulmonary exacerbation of cystic fibrosis associated with *P. aeruginosa* infection in paediatric patients (aged 5-17 years), the duration of treatment is 10-14 days.

For inhalation anthrax, drug administration should begin as soon as possible after confirmed or suspected exposure and should be continued for 60 days.

4.3 Contraindications

Ciprofloxacin is contra-indicated in patients who have shown hypersensitivity to ciprofloxacin or other quinolone anti-infectives.

Except in cases of exacerbation of cystic fibrosis associated with *P. aeruginosa* (in patients aged 5-17 years) and inhalation anthrax, ciprofloxacin is contra-indicated in children and growing adolescents unless the benefits of treatment are considered to outweigh the risks.

Ciproxin Suspension should not be used in children of less than two years of age (see Section 4.4).

4.4 Special warnings and special precautions for use

Ciprofloxacin should be used with caution in epileptics and patients with a history of CNS disorders and only if the benefits of treatment are considered to outweigh the risk of possible CNS side-effects. CNS side-effects have been reported after first administration of ciprofloxacin in some patients. Treatment should be discontinued if the side-effects, depression or psychoses lead to self-endangering behaviour (see also Section 4.8).

Crystalluria related to the use of ciprofloxacin has been reported. Patients receiving ciprofloxacin should be well hydrated and excessive alkalinity of the urine should be avoided.

Patients with a family history of or actual defects in glucose-6-phosphate dehydrogenase activity are prone to haemolytic reactions with quinolones, and so ciprofloxacin should be used with caution in these patients.

Tendon inflammation and rupture may occur with quinolone antibiotics. Such reactions have been observed particularly in older patients and in those treated concurrently with corticosteroids. At the first sign of pain or inflammation, patients should discontinue ciprofloxacin and rest the affected limbs.

The tolerability of Ciproxin Suspension has not been investigated in children or adolescents. In addition, owing to the presence of lecithin in the suspension formulation, there is a theoretical possibility of increased gastro-intestinal side-effects in children of less than two years of age. Therefore, the product is not recommended for use in this patient group.

There is a risk of pseudomembranous colitis with broad-spectrum antibiotics possibly leading to a fatal outcome. It is important to consider this in patients suffering from severe, persistent diarrhoea. With ciprofloxacin this effect has been reported rarely. If pseudomembranous colitis is suspected treatment with ciprofloxacin should be stopped and appropriate treatment given (e.g. oral vancomycin).

As with other quinolones, patients should avoid prolonged exposure to strong sunlight or UV radiation during treatment.

Laboratory tests may give abnormal findings if performed whilst patients are receiving ciprofloxacin, e.g. increased alkaline phosphatase; increases in liver function tests, e.g. transaminases and cholestatic jaundice, especially in patients with previous liver damage.

4.5 Interaction with other medicinal products and other forms of Interaction

Increased plasma levels of theophylline have been observed following concurrent administration with ciprofloxacin. It is recommended that the dose of theophylline should be reduced and plasma levels of theophylline monitored. The reaction between theophylline and ciprofloxacin is potentially life-threatening. Therefore, where monitoring of plasma levels is not possible, the use of ciprofloxacin should be avoided in patients receiving theophylline. Particular caution is advised in those patients with convulsive disorders.

Phenytoin levels may be altered when Ciproxin is used concomitantly.

Ciproxin Suspension should not be administered within four hours of multivalent cationic drugs and mineral supplements (e.g. calcium, magnesium, aluminium or iron), sucralfate or antacids and highly buffered drugs (e.g. didanosine) as interference with absorption may occur. When appropriate, patients should be advised not to self-medicate with preparations containing these compounds during therapy with ciprofloxacin. This restriction does not apply to the class of H2 receptor blocker drugs.

The concurrent administration of dairy products or fortified drinks alone (e.g. milk, yoghurt, calcium fortified orange juice) and ciprofloxacin should be avoided because absorption of ciprofloxacin may be reduced. However a normal diet, that will contain small amounts of calcium, does not significantly affect ciprofloxacin absorption.

Prolongation of bleeding time has been reported during concomitant administration of ciprofloxacin and oral anticoagulants.

Animal data have shown that high doses of quinolones in combination with some non-steroidal anti-inflammatory drugs, (e.g. fenbufen, but not acetylsalicylic acid) can lead to convulsions.

Transient increases in serum creatinine have been seen following concomitant administration of ciprofloxacin and cyclosporin. Therefore, monitoring of serum creatinine levels is advisable.

The simultaneous administration of quinolones and glibenclamide can on occasion potentiate the effect of glibenclamide resulting in hypoglycaemia.

Renal tubular transport of methotrexate may be inhibited by concomitant administration of ciprofloxacin potentially leading to increased plasma levels of methotrexate. This may increase the risk of methotrexate associated toxic reactions. Therefore, patients receiving methotrexate therapy should be carefully monitored when concomitant ciprofloxacin therapy is indicated.

Concomitant use with probenecid reduces the renal clearance of ciprofloxacin, resulting in increased quinolone plasma levels.

The use of metoclopramide with ciprofloxacin may accelerate the absorption of ciprofloxacin.

When Ciproxin Suspension is used for surgical prophylaxis, it is recommended that opiate premedicants, (e.g. papaveretum) or opiate premedicants used with anticholinergic premedicants, (e.g. atropine or hyoscine) are not used, as the serum levels of ciprofloxacin are reduced and adequate cover may not be obtained during surgery. Co-administration of ciprofloxacin and benzodiazepine premedicants has been shown not to affect ciprofloxacin plasma levels.

4.6 Pregnancy and lactation

Reproduction studies performed in mice, rats and rabbits using parenteral and oral administration did not reveal any evidence of teratogenicity, impairment of fertility or impairment of peri-/post-natal development. However, as with other quinolones, ciprofloxacin has been shown to cause arthropathy in immature animals, and therefore its use during pregnancy is not recommended. Studies have indicated that ciprofloxacin is secreted in breast milk. Administration to nursing mothers is thus not recommended.

4.7 Effects on ability to drive and use machines

Ciprofloxacin could result in impairment of the patient's ability to drive or operate machinery, particularly in conjunction with alcohol.

4.8 Undesirable effects

Ciprofloxacin is generally well tolerated. The most frequently reported adverse reactions are nausea, diarrhoea and rash.

The following adverse reactions have been observed:

Hypersensitivity/skin, e.g. rash, pruritus, urticaria, photosensitivity, drug-induced fever, anaphylactic/anaphylactoid reactions including angioedema and dyspnoea. Rarely, erythema nodosum and erythema multiforme. Very rarely, petechiae, haemorrhagic bullae, vasculitis, serum sickness-like reaction, fixed drug reactions, Stevens-Johnson Syndrome and Lyells Syndrome. Treatment with ciprofloxacin should be discontinued if any of the above occur upon first administration.

General, e.g. moniliasis, asthenia, hyperglycaemia and abnormal gait, pain, pain in extremeties, back pain, chest pain. Thrombophlebitis.

CNS, e.g. headache, restlessness, depression, dizziness, tremor, convulsions, confusion, hallucinations, somnolence, sleep disorders, insomnia. Rarely, hypesthesia. Very rarely, migraine, hyperesthesia, ataxia, hypertonia, twitching or anxiety states. Isolated cases of ciprofloxacin-induced psychoses have been reported, which may progress to self-endangering behaviour. There are isolated reports of intracranial hypertension associated with quinolone therapy. Paraesthesia has been reported.

Gastro-intestinal, e.g. nausea, diarrhoea, vomiting, dyspepsia, abdominal pain, anorexia, flatulence, dysphagia. Rarely, pancreatitis or pseudomembranous colitis.

Cardiovascular, e.g. tachycardia, oedema, fainting, hot flushes, hypotension and sweating.

Effects on haematological parameters, e.g. anaemia, eosinophilia, increases or decreases in white cell and/or platelet count, altered prothrombin levels, and, very rarely, haemolytic anaemia, agranulocytosis, pancytopenia or bone marrow depression. Pancytopenia and bone marrow depression may be potentially life-threatening.

Hepatic, e.g. transient increases in liver enzymes or serum bilirubin (particularly in patients with previous liver damage), hepatitis, jaundice/cholestasis and major liver disorders including hepatic necrosis, which may rarely progress to life-threatening hepatic failure.

Renal, e.g. transient increases in blood urea or serum creatinine, renal failure, crystalluria, haematuria, nephritis.

Musculoskeletal, e.g. reversible arthralgia, joint swelling and myalgia. Rarely, myasthenia or tenosynovitis. Tendon inflammation (predominantly of the Achilles tendon) has been reported which may lead to tendon rupture. Treatment should be discontinued immediately if these symptoms occur.

Rarely, exacerbation of the symptoms of myasthenia gravis have been reported.

Special senses, e.g. very rarely, visual disturbances including diplopia and colour disturbances, impaired taste and smell usually reversible upon discontinuation of treatment, tinnitus, transient impairment of hearing particularly at high frequencies.

Abnormal laboratory findings, e.g. increased alkaline phosphatase, amylase and lipase; increases in liver function tests, e.g transaminases, and cholestatic jaundice, especially in patients with previous liver damage.

4.9 Overdose

Based on the limited information available in two cases of ingestion of over 18g of ciprofloxacin, reversible renal toxicity has occurred. Therefore, apart from routine emergency measures, it is recommended to monitor renal function, including urinary pH and acidify, if required, to prevent crystalluria. Patients must be kept well hydrated, and in the case of renal damage resulting in prolonged oliguria, dialysis should be initiated.

Calcium or magnesium antacids may be administered as soon as possible after ingestion of Ciproxin Suspension in order to reduce the absorption of ciprofloxacin.

Serum levels of ciprofloxacin are reduced by dialysis.

5. PHARMACOLOGICAL PROPERTIES

ATC Code J01 MA 02

5.1 Pharmacodynamic properties

Ciprofloxacin is a synthetic 4-quinolone derivative, with bactericidal activity. It acts via inhibition of bacterial DNA gyrase, ultimately resulting in interference with DNA function. Ciprofloxacin is highly active against a wide range of Gram-positive and Gram-negative organisms and has shown activity against some anaerobes, *Chlamydia* spp. and *Mycoplasma* spp. Killing curves demonstrate the rapid bactericidal effect against sensitive organisms and it is often found that minimum bactericidal concentrations are in the range of minimum inhibitory concentrations. Ciprofloxacin has been shown to have no activity against *Treponema pallidum* and *Ureaplasma urealyticum. Nocardia asteroides*, and *Enterococcus faecium* are resistant.

Breakpoints

$S \leqslant 1\ \mu g/ml$, $R \geqslant 4\ \mu g/ml$

Susceptibility

The prevalence of resistance may vary geographically and with time for selected species and local area information on resistance is desirable, particularly when treating severe infections. This information gives only an approximate guidance on probabilities whether micro-organisms will be susceptible to ciprofloxacin or not.

Organism	Prevalence of Resistance
Sensitive:	
Gram-positive bacteria	
Corynebacterium diphtheriae	0%
Corynebacterium spp.	-
Staphylococcus aureus (methicillin sensitive)	0 - 14%
Staphylococcus aureus (methicillin resistant)	48 - 90%
Streptococcus agalactiae	0 - 17%
Bacillus anthracis	
Gram-negative bacteria	
Acinetobacter baumanii	6 - 93%
Acinetobacter spp.	14 - 70%
Aeromonas hydrophilia	0%
Aeromonas spp.	
Bordetella pertussis	0%
Brucella melitensis	0%
Campylobacter jejuni/coli	0 - 82%
Campylobacter spp.	0%
Citrobacter freundii	0 - 4%
Citrobacter spp.	0%
Edwardsiella tarda	0%
Enterobacter aerogenes	0%
Enterobacter cloacae	0 - 3%
Enterobacter spp.	3 - 13%
Escherichia coli	2 -7%
Escherichia coli, EHEC and EPEC	-
Haemophilus influenzae	0 - 1%
Haemophilus influenzae (β -lactam negative)	0%
Haemophilus influenzae (β -lactam positive)	0%
Haemophilus parainfluenzae	0%
Hafnia alvei	0%
Klebsiella oxytoca	0%
Klebsiella pneumoniae	2 - 5.8%
Klebsiella spp.	2 - 21%
Legionella pneumophila	0%
Legionella spp.	0%
Moraxella catarrhalis	0%
Morganella morganii	1 - 2%
Neisseria gonorrhoeae	0%
Neisseria gonorrhoeae, β -lactamase	0%
Neisseria gonorrhoeae, β -lactamase positive	0%
Neisseria meningitidis	0%
Neisseria meningitidis, β -lactamase negative	0%
Plesiomonas shigelloides	0%
Proteus mirabilis	0 - 10%
Proteus vulgaris	4%
Providencia rettgeri	
Providencia spp.	4%
Providencia stuartii	
Pseudomonas aeruginosa	1 - 28%
Salmonella spp.	0%
Salmonella typhi	0 - 2%
Serratia liquefaciens	-
Serratia marcescens	23%
Serratia spp.	0 - 21%
Shigella spp.	0%
Vibrio cholerae	0%
Vibrio parahaemolyticus	0%
Vibrio spp.	0%
Yersinia enterocolitica	0%
Anaerobes	
Bacteroides ureolyticus	0%
Clostridium perfringens	-
Peptococcus spp.	0%
Peptostreptococcus spp.	-
Peptostreptococcus magnus	0%
Veillonella parvula	0%
Other pathogens	
Chlamydia spp.	-
Helicobacter pylori	-
Mycobacterium fortuitum	0%
Mycobacterium tuberculosis	0%
Mycoplasma hominis	16%
Intermediate	
Gram-positive aerobes	
Enterococci	5%
Enterococcus faecalis	9 - 34%
Staphylococcus epidermis, methicillin sensitive	10 - 16%
Staphylococcus epidermis, methicillin resistant	26 - 56%

Staphylococcus haemolyticus	-
Staphylococcus haemolyticus, methicillin sensitive	8%
Staphylococcus haemolyticus, methicillin resistant	73%
Streptococcus anginosus	9%
Streptococcus bovis	-
Streptococcus milleri	5%
Streptococcus mitis	-
Streptococcus pneumoniae, penicillin sensitive	0 - 1%
Streptococcus pneumoniae, penicillin intermediate	-
Streptococcus pneumoniae, penicillin intermediate and resistant	2.8%
Streptococcus pneumoniae, penicillin resistant	-
Streptococcus pyogenes	0 - 28%
Streptococcus, *viridans group*	-
Streptococcus viridans, penicillin sensitive	-
Streptococcus viridans, penicillin resistant	-
Streptococcus, *β*-haemolytic groups A, C, and G	0%
Gram-negative aerobes	
Alcaligenes spp.	-
Listeria monocytogenes	0%
Listeria spp.	0%
Anaerobes	
Fusobacterium spp.	-
Gardnerella vaginalis	0%
Prevotella spp.	-
Other pathogens	
Ureaplasma urealyticum	11%
Resistant	
Gram-positive aerobes	
Enterococcus faecium	-
Stenotrophomonas maltophilia	94%
Streptococcus sanguis	-
Gram-negative aerobes	
Flavobacterium meningosepticum	-
Nocardia asteroides	-
Anaerobes	
Bacteroides fragilis	-
Bacteroides thetaiotaomicron	-
Clostridium difficile	-

Plasmid-related transfer of resistance has not been observed with ciprofloxacin and the overall frequency of development of resistance is low (10^{-9} - 10^{-7}). Cross-resistance to penicillins, cephalosporins, aminoglycosides and tetracyclines has not been observed and organisms resistant to these antibiotics are generally sensitive to ciprofloxacin. Ciprofloxacin is also suitable for use in combination with these antibiotics, and additive behaviour is usually observed.

5.2 Pharmacokinetic properties

Absorption of oral doses of ciprofloxacin 250mg, 500mg and 750mg tablet formulation occurs rapidly, mainly from the small intestine, the half-life of absorption being 2-15 minutes. Plasma levels are dose-related and peak 0.5-2.0 hours after dosing. The AUC also increases dose proportionately after administration of both single and repeated oral (tablet) and intravenous doses. Bioequivalence of the same dose of the tablet formulation with that of the suspension formulation has been demonstrated. Plasma levels peak approximately 1.5-2.5 hours after dosing and the $AUC_{0-\infty}$ is in the range of 5-12mg.h/l. The absolute bioavailability is reported to be 52-83% and ciprofloxacin is subject to only slight first pass metabolism. The oral bioavailability is approximately 70-80%.

The intake of food at the same time as administration of oral ciprofloxacin (tablet or suspension) has a marginal but clinically not relevant effect on the pharmacokinetic parameters C_{max} and AUC. In a food effect study with the suspension formulation, C_{max} was decreased by 11% and the AUC increased by 13% after administration of the suspension with food. However, there was no significant decrease in the rate and extent of absorption compared with administration of the suspension without food. Therefore, no specific recommendations are necessary with regard to time of administration of the suspension relative to food intake.

Distribution of ciprofloxacin within tissues is wide and the volume of distribution high, though slightly lower in the elderly. Protein binding is low (between 19-40%).

Only 10-20% of a single oral or intravenous dose is eliminated as metabolites (which exhibit lower activity than the parent drug). Four different antimicrobially active metabolites have been reported, desethyleneciprofloxacin (M1), sulphociprofloxacin (M2), oxaciprofloxacin (M3) and formylciprofloxacin (M4). M2 and M3 account for one third each of metabolised substance and M1 is found in small amounts (1.3-2.6% of the dose). M4 has been found in very small quantities (<0.1% of the dose). M1-M3 have antimicrobial activity comparable to nalidixic acid and M4 found in the smallest quantity has antimicrobial activity similar to that of norfloxacin.

Elimination of ciprofloxacin and its metabolites occurs rapidly, primarily by the kidney. After single oral and intravenous doses of ciprofloxacin, 55% and 75% respectively are eliminated by the kidney and 39% and 14% in the faeces within 5 days. Renal elimination takes place mainly during the first 12 hours after dosing and renal clearance levels suggest that active secretion by the renal tubules occurs in addition to normal glomerular filtration. Renal clearance is between 0.18-0.3 l/h.kg and total body clearance between 0.48-0.60 l/h.kg. Approximately 1% of a ciprofloxacin dose is excreted via the biliary route. The elimination kinetics are linear and after repeated dosing at 12 hourly intervals, no further accumulation is detected after the distribution equilibrium is attained (at 4-5 half-lives). The elimination half-life of unchanged ciprofloxacin over a period of 24-48 hours post-dose is 3.1-5.1 hours.

Some studies carried out with ciprofloxacin in severely renally impaired patients (serum creatinine >265 micromole/l or creatinine clearance <20ml/minute) demonstrated either a doubling of the elimination half-life, or fluctuations in half-life in comparison with healthy volunteers, whereas other studies showed no significant correlation between elimination half-life and creatinine clearance. However, it is recommended that in severely renally impaired patients, the total daily dose should be reduced by half, although monitoring of drug serum levels provides the most reliable basis for dose adjustment as necessary.

Results of pharmacokinetic studies in paediatric cystic fibrosis patients have shown dosages of 20mg/kg orally twice daily or 10mg/kg iv three times daily are recommended to achieve plasma concentration/time profiles comparable to those achieved in the adult population at the currently recommended dosage regimen.

Inhalation anthrax: Ciprofloxacin serum concentrations achieved in humans serve as a surrogate endpoint reasonably likely to predict clinical benefit and provide the basis for the recommended doses.

5.3 Preclinical safety data

Following extensive oral and intravenous toxicology testing with ciprofloxacin, only two findings which may be considered relevant to the use of ciprofloxacin in man were observed. Crystalluria was noted in those species of animals which had a normally alkaline urine. Kidney damage without the presence of crystalluria was not observed. This effect is considered a secondary inflammatory foreign-body reaction, due to the precipitation of a crystalline complex of ciprofloxacin, magnesium and protein in the distal tubule system of the kidneys. This is considered not to be a problem in man, because the urine is normally acidic. However, to avoid the occurrence of crystalluria, patients should be well hydrated and excessive alkalinity of the urine avoided.

As with other quinolones, damage to the weight-bearing joints of only juvenile rats and dogs treated with ciprofloxacin was noted in repeat dose toxicity testing. This was more noticeable in the dog. Although analysis of available safety data from ciprofloxacin use in paediatric patients did not disclose any evidence of drug related cartilage or articular damage, the use of ciprofloxacin in children and growing adolescents is generally not recommended (with the exception of treatment of cystic fibrosis), unless the benefits are considered to outweigh the potential risks. Additionally, because of the potential of arthropathy, the use of ciprofloxacin during pregnancy and lactation is not recommended.

6. PHARMACEUTICAL PARTICULARS

6.1 List of excipients

(i) Film-coated Granules

Copolymer of ethyl acrylate and methyl methacrylate, magnesium stearate, hypromellose, polysorbate 20, polyvidone 25.

(ii) Diluent

Lecithin, medium chain triglycerides, sucrose, purified water, strawberry flavours.

6.2 Incompatibilities

No other products should be added to the reconstituted suspension.

6.3 Shelf life

(i) Shelf-life of packaged product

Film-coated granules: 3 years.

Diluent: 2 years.

(ii) Shelf-life of re-constituted suspension

In a refrigerator (2-8°C), 14 days.

At room temperature (up to 30°C), 14 days.

6.4 Special precautions for storage

(i) Packaged Product

Film-coated granules: Do not store above 25°C.

Diluent: Protect from freezing. Do not store above 25°C. Avoid inverted storage. Occasionally a slight yellow layer is observed on the surface of the sucrose in the diluent prior to resuspending. However upon shaking, this layer is dispersed and has been shown to have no influence on the quality of the product.

(ii) Re-constituted Suspension

Avoid inverted storage.

6.5 Nature and contents of container

(i) Film-coated granules: Brown glass Type III narrow-necked bottle with a PP/PE child resistant closure.

(ii) Diluent: Plastic PE white transparent bottle with sealing insert and white opaque PP child resistant screw cap.

(iii) Re-constituted suspension: This is the same container as is used for the diluent prior to reconstitution.

(iv) Measuring spoon: Blue opaque PE with graduation marks.

The above (iii) contains a nominal 100ml of re-constituted ready-to-use suspension. For quantities of (i) and (ii) see Section 2.

6.6 Instructions for use and handling

(i) Preparation of the Re-constituted Suspension

The re-constituted suspension is prepared for use as follows:

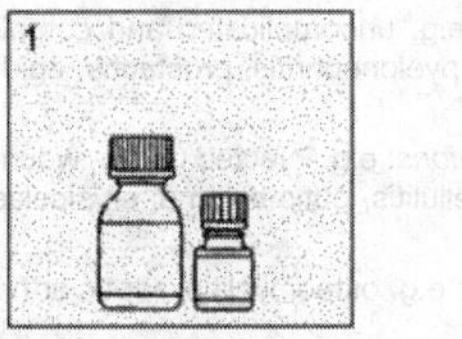

The product is packed in two bottles. The small bottle contains film-coated granules containing the active substance, and the larger bottle contains the diluent.

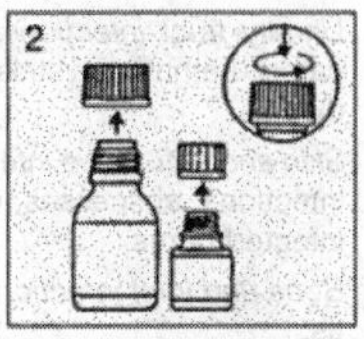

Open both bottles. The child-resistant cap is opened by pressing down and turning it to the left.

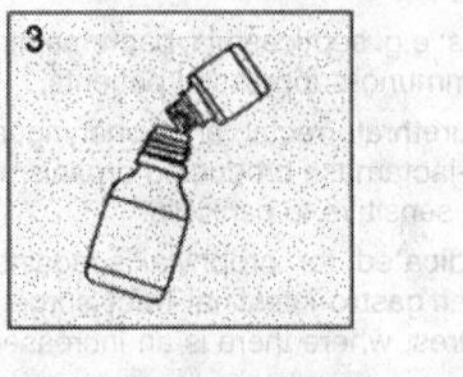

Empty the bottle containing the granules into the large bottle containing the diluent. **Do not pour water into the suspension.**

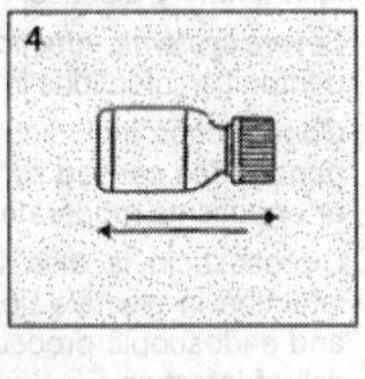

Re-close the large bottle and shake it vigorously **horizontally** for approx. 15 seconds. The suspension is now ready for use.

(ii) Dosing the Re-constituted Suspension

The re-constituted suspension should be shaken vigorously for approx. 15 seconds prior to each dosage. In order to ensure correct dosing, each dose should be measured into the graduated measuring spoon provided with the product. The ½ marking will dose a nominal 2.5ml of product, the 1/1 marking will dose a nominal 5.0ml of product. The re-constituted suspension should be swallowed whole and the granules should not be chewed. A glass of water may be taken after dosing of the suspension. Reclose the bottle properly after use according to the instructions on the cap.

After the treatment period, the reconstituted suspension should not be stored and re-used. It should be disposed of.

7. MARKETING AUTHORISATION HOLDER

	Trading as:
Bayer plc	Bayer plc
Bayer House	Pharmaceutical Division
Strawberry Hill	Bayer House
Newbury, Berkshire	Strawberry Hill
RG14 1JA	Newbury, Berkshire
	RG14 1JA
	or BAYPHARM or BAYMET

8. MARKETING AUTHORISATION NUMBER(S)
PL 0010/0211

9. DATE OF FIRST AUTHORISATION/RENEWAL OF THE AUTHORISATION
19 April 1996.

10. DATE OF REVISION OF THE TEXT
June 2003

Ciproxin Tablets 100mg

(Bayer plc)

1. NAME OF THE MEDICINAL PRODUCT
Ciproxin Tablets 100mg

2. QUALITATIVE AND QUANTITATIVE COMPOSITION
Each tablet contains 116.4mg ciprofloxacin hydrochloride equivalent to 100mg Ciprofloxacin (INN).

3. PHARMACEUTICAL FORM
Immediate release film-coated tablet for oral administration.

4. CLINICAL PARTICULARS

4.1 Therapeutic indications
Ciprofloxacin is indicated for the treatment of the following infections caused by sensitive bacteria:

Adults:

Respiratory tract infections: e.g. lobar and bronchopneumonia, acute and chronic bronchitis, acute exacerbation of cystic fibrosis, bronchiectasis, empyema. Ciprofloxacin is not recommended as first-line therapy for the treatment of pneumococcal pneumonia. Ciprofloxacin may be used for treating Gram-negative pneumonia.

Ear, nose and throat infections: e.g. mastoiditis, otitis media and sinusitis, especially if due to Gram-negative bacteria (including *Pseudomonas* spp.). Ciprofloxacin is not recommended for the treatment of acute tonsillitis.

Eye infections: e.g. bacterial conjunctivitis.

Urinary tract infections: e.g. uncomplicated and complicated urethritis, cystitis, pyelonephritis, prostatitis, epididymitis.

Skin and soft tissue infections: e.g. infected ulcers, wound infections, abscesses, cellulitis, otitis externa, erysipelas, infected burns.

Bone and joint infections: e.g. osteomyelitis, septic arthritis.

Intra-abdominal infections: e.g. peritonitis, intra-abdominal abscesses.

Infections of the biliary tract: e.g. cholangitis, cholecystitis, empyema of the gall bladder.

Gastro-intestinal infections: e.g. enteric fever, infective diarrhoea.

Pelvic infections: e.g. salpingitis, endometritis, pelvic inflammatory disease.

Severe systemic infections: e.g. septicaemia, bacteraemia, peritonitis, infections in immuno-suppressed patients.

Gonorrhoea: including urethral, rectal and pharyngeal gonorrhoea caused by β-lactamase producing organisms or organisms moderately sensitive to penicillin.

Ciprofloxacin is also indicated for prophylaxis against infection in elective upper gastro-intestinal tract surgery and endoscopic procedures, where there is an increased risk of infection.

Children:

For the treatment of acute pulmonary exacerbation of cystic fibrosis associated with *P. aeruginosa* infection in paediatric patients aged 5-17 years.

Inhalation Anthrax in Adults and Children: To reduce the incidence or progression of disease following confirmed or suspected exposure to aerosolised *Bacillus anthracis*.

4.2 Posology and method of administration

General dosage recommendations: The dosage of Ciproxin tablets is determined by the severity and type of infection, the sensitivity of the causative organism(s) and the age, weight and renal function of the patient. Ciproxin tablets should be swallowed whole with an adequate amount of liquid.

If Ciproxin Tablets are taken on an empty stomach, the active substance is absorbed more rapidly. In this case, the tablets should not be taken concurrently with dairy products or with mineral fortified drinks alone (e.g. milk, yoghurt, calcium fortified orange juice). However, a normal diet that will contain small amounts of calcium, does not significantly affect ciprofloxacin absorbtion.

Adults

The dosage range for adults is 100-750mg twice daily. The following dosages for specific types of infection are recommended:

Table 1: Recommended Adult Dosage

Indication	Dosage (mg ciprofloxacin)
Treatment	
Gonorrhoea	250mg single dose
Acute, uncomplicated cystitis in women	100mg b.d.
Upper and lower urinary tract infections (depending on severity)	250-500mg b.d.
Upper and lower respiratory tract infections (depending on severity)	250-750mg b.d.
Pneumococcal pneumonia (second-line)	750mg b.d.
Cystic fibrosis patients with pseudomonal lower RTI*	750mg b.d.
Other infections as detailed under 4.1	500-750mg b.d.
Severe infections, particularly due to Pseudomonas, staphylococci and streptococci	750mg b.d.
Inhalation Anthrax	500mg b.d.
Prophylaxis	
Elective upper gastro-intestinal surgical and endoscopic procedures	750mg single dose 60-90 minutes prior to the procedure**. If gastro-oesophageal obstructive lesions are suspected use with an anti-infective effective against anaerobes

* Although the pharmacokinetics of ciprofloxacin remains unchanged in patients with cystic fibrosis, the low bodyweight of these patients should be taken into consideration when determining dosage.

** The tablet may be given with an oral pre-medicant, but see Section 4.5

Impaired Renal Function

Dosage adjustments are not usually required, except in patients with severe renal impairment (serum creatinine >265 micromole/l or creatinine clearance <20ml/minute). If adjustment is necessary, this may be achieved by reducing the total daily dose by half, although monitoring of drug serum levels provides the most reliable basis for dose adjustment.

Impaired Hepatic Function

No adjustment of dosage is necessary.

Elderly

Although higher ciprofloxacin serum levels are found in the elderly, no adjustment of dosage is necessary.

Adolescents and children

As with other drugs in its class, ciprofloxacin has been shown to cause arthropathy in weight-bearing joints of immature animals. Although analysis of available safety data from ciprofloxacin use in patients less than 18 years of age, the majority of whom had cystic fibrosis, did not disclose any evidence of drug-related cartilage or articular damage, its use in the paediatric population is generally not recommended.

Clinical and pharmacokinetic data support the use of ciprofloxacin in paediatric cystic fibrosis patients (aged 5 - 17 years) with acute pulmonary exacerbations associated with *P. aeruginosa* infection, at a dose of 20mg/kg orally twice daily (maximum daily dose 1500mg).

For the indication of inhalation anthrax, the risk-benefit assessment indicates that administration of ciprofloxacin to paediatric patients at a dose of 15 mg/kg orally twice daily (maximum daily dose of 1000 mg) is appropriate.

For indications other than treatment of pulmonary exacerbations in cystic fibrosis and inhalation anthrax, ciprofloxacin may be used in children and adolescents where the benefit is considered to outweigh the potential risks. In these cases a dosage of 5-15mg/kg orally twice daily should be administered depending upon the severity of infection.

Dosing in children with impaired renal and/or hepatic function has not been studied.

Duration of Treatment

The duration of treatment depends upon the severity of infection, clinical response and bacteriological findings.

In acute, uncomplicated cystitis the treatment period is three days.

In other acute infections the usual treatment period is 5-10 days. Generally, acute and chronic infections (e.g. osteomyelitis and prostatitis, etc), where the causative organism is known to be sensitive to ciprofloxacin, should be treated for at least three days after the signs and symptoms of the infection have disappeared.

For acute pulmonary exacerbations of cystic fibrosis associated with *P. aeruginosa* infection in paediatric patients (aged 5-17 years), the duration of treatment is 10 - 14 days.

For inhalation anthrax, drug administration should begin as soon as possible after confirmed or suspected exposure and should be continued for 60 days.

4.3 Contraindications

Ciprofloxacin is contra-indicated in patients who have shown hypersensitivity to ciprofloxacin or other quinolone anti-infectives.

Except in cases of exacerbations of cystic fibrosis associated with *P. aeruginosa* (in patients aged 5-17 years) and inhalation anthrax, ciprofloxacin is contra-indicated in children and growing adolescents unless the benefits of treatment are considered to outweigh the risks.

4.4 Special warnings and special precautions for use

Ciprofloxacin should be used with caution in epileptics and patients with a history of CNS disorders and only if the benefits of treatment are considered to outweigh the risk of possible CNS side-effects. CNS side-effects have been reported after first administration of ciprofloxacin in some patients. Treatment should be discontinued if the side-effects, depression or psychoses lead to self-endangering behaviour (see also Section 4.8).

Crystalluria related to the use of ciprofloxacin has been reported. Patients receiving ciprofloxacin should be well hydrated and excessive alkalinity of the urine should be avoided.

Patients with a family history of or actual defects in glucose-6-phosphate dehydrogenase activity are prone to haemolytic reactions with quinolones, and so ciprofloxacin should be used with caution in these patients.

Tendon inflammation and rupture may occur with quinolone antibiotics. Such reactions have been observed particularly in older patients and in those treated concurrently with corticosteroids. At the first sign of pain or inflammation, patients should discontinue ciprofloxacin and rest the affected limbs.

There is a risk of pseudomembranous colitis with broad-spectrum antibiotics possibly leading to a fatal outcome. It is important to consider this in patients suffering from severe, persistent diarrhoea. With ciprofloxacin this effect has been reported rarely. If pseudomembranous colitis is suspected treatment with ciprofloxacin should be stopped and appropriate treatment given (e.g. oral vancomycin).

As with other quinolones, patients should avoid prolonged exposure to strong sunlight or UV radiation during treatment.

Laboratory tests may give abnormal findings if performed whilst patients are receiving ciprofloxacin e.g. increased alkaline phosphatase; increases in liver function tests e.g. transaminases and cholestatic jaundice, especially in patients with previous liver damage.

4.5 Interaction with other medicinal products and other forms of Interaction

Increased plasma levels of theophylline have been observed following concurrent administration with ciprofloxacin. It is recommended that the dose of theophylline should be reduced and plasma levels of theophylline monitored. The reaction between theophylline and ciprofloxacin is potentially life-threatening. Therefore, where monitoring of plasma levels is not possible, the use of ciprofloxacin should be avoided in patients receiving theophylline. Particular caution is advised in those patients with convulsive disorders.

Phenytoin levels may be altered when Ciproxin is used concomitantly.

Ciproxin Tablets should not be administered within four hours of multivalent cationic drugs and mineral supplements (e.g. calcium, magnesium, aluminium or iron), sucralfate or antacids and highly buffered drugs (e.g. didanosine) as interference with absorption may occur. When appropriate, patients should be advised not to self-medicate with preparations containing these compounds during therapy with ciprofloxacin. This restriction does not apply to the class of H2 receptor blocker drugs.

The concurrent administration of dairy products or fortified drinks alone (e.g. milk, yoghurt, calcium fortified orange juice) and ciprofloxacin should be avoided because absorption of ciprofloxacin may be reduced. However a normal diet, that will contain small amounts of calcium, does not significantly affect ciprofloxacin absorption.

Prolongation of bleeding time has been reported during concomitant administration of ciprofloxacin and oral anti-coagulants.

Animal data have shown that high doses of quinolones in combination with some non-steroidal anti-inflammatory drugs, (e.g. fenbufen, but not acetylsalicylic acid) can lead to convulsions.

Transient increases in serum creatinine have been seen following concomitant administration of ciprofloxacin and cyclosporin. Therefore, monitoring of serum creatinine levels is advisable.

The simultaneous administration of quinolones and glibenclamide can on occasion potentiate the effect of glibenclamide resulting in hypoglycaemia.

Renal tubular transport of methotrexate may be inhibited by concomitant administration of ciprofloxacin potentially leading to increased plasma levels of methotrexate. This may increase the risk of methotrexate associated toxic reactions. Therefore, patients receiving methotrexate therapy should be carefully monitored when concomitant ciprofloxacin therapy is indicated.

Concomitant use with probenecid reduces the renal clearance of ciprofloxacin, resulting in increased quinolone plasma levels.

The use of metoclopramide with ciprofloxacin may accelerate the absorption of ciprofloxacin.

When ciprofloxacin is used for surgical prophylaxis, it is recommended that opiate premedicants, (e.g. papaveretum) or opiate premedicants used with anticholinergic premedicants, (e.g. atropine or hyoscine) are not used, as the serum levels of ciprofloxacin are reduced and adequate cover may not be obtained during surgery. Co-administration of ciprofloxacin and benzodiazepine premedicants has been shown not to affect ciprofloxacin plasma levels.

4.6 Pregnancy and lactation

Reproduction studies performed in mice, rats and rabbits using parenteral and oral administration did not reveal any evidence of teratogenicity, impairment of fertility or impairment of peri-/post-natal development. However, as with other quinolones, ciprofloxacin has been shown to cause arthropathy in immature animals, and therefore its use during pregnancy is not recommended. Studies have indicated that ciprofloxacin is secreted in breast milk. Administration to nursing mothers is thus not recommended.

4.7 Effects on ability to drive and use machines

Ciprofloxacin could result in impairment of the patient's ability to drive or operate machinery, particularly in conjunction with alcohol.

4.8 Undesirable effects

Ciprofloxacin is generally well tolerated. The most frequently reported adverse reactions are nausea, diarrhoea and rash.

The following adverse reactions have been observed:

Hypersensitivity/skin, e.g. rash, pruritus, urticaria, photosensitivity, drug-induced fever, anaphylactic/anaphylactoid reactions including angioedema and dyspnoea. Rarely, erythema nodosum and erythema multiforme. Very rarely, petechiae, haemorrhagic bullae, vasculitis, serum sickness-like reaction, fixed drug reactions, Stevens-Johnson Syndrome and Lyells Syndrome. Treatment with ciprofloxacin should be discontinued if any of the above occur upon first administration.

General, e.g. moniliasis, asthenia, hyperglycaemia and abnormal gait, pain, pain in extremeties, back pain, chest pain. Thrombophlebitis.

CNS, e.g. headache, restlessness, depression, dizziness, tremor, convulsions, confusion, hallucinations, somnolence, sleep disorders, insomnia. Rarely, hypesthesia. Very rarely, migraine, hyperesthesia, ataxia, hypertonia, twitching or anxiety states. Isolated cases of ciprofloxacin-induced psychoses have been reported, which may progress to self-endangering behaviour. There are isolated reports of intracranial hypertension associated with quinolone therapy. Paraesthesia has been reported.

Gastro-intestinal, e.g. nausea, diarrhoea, vomiting, dyspepsia, abdominal pain, anorexia, flatulence, dysphagia. Rarely, pancreatitis or pseudomembranous colitis.

Cardiovascular, e.g. tachycardia, oedema, fainting, hot flushes, hypotension and sweating.

Effects on haematological parameters, e.g. anaemia, eosinophilia, increases or decreases in white cell and/or platelet count, altered prothrombin levels, and, very rarely, haemolytic anaemia, agranulocytosis, pancytopenia or bone marrow depression. Pancytopenia and bone marrow depression may be potentially life-threatening.

Hepatic, e.g. transient increases in liver enzymes or serum bilirubin (particularly in patients with previous liver damage), hepatitis, jaundice/cholestasis and major liver disorders including hepatic necrosis, which may rarely progress to life-threatening hepatic failure.

Renal, e.g. transient increases in blood urea or serum creatinine, renal failure, crystalluria, haematuria, nephritis.

Musculoskeletal, e.g. reversible arthralgia, joint swelling and myalgia. Rarely, myasthenia or tenosynovitis. Tendon inflammation (predominantly of the Achilles tendon) has been reported which may lead to tendon rupture. Treatment should be discontinued immediately if these symptoms occur.

Rarely, exacerbation of the symptoms of myasthenia gravis have been reported.

Special senses, e.g. very rarely, visual disturbances including diplopia and colour disturbances, impaired taste and smell usually reversible upon discontinuation of treatment, tinnitus, transient impairment of hearing particularly at high frequencies.

Abnormal laboratory findings, e.g. increased alkaline phosphatase, amylase and lipase; increases in liver function tests, e.g transaminases, and cholestatic jaundice, especially in patients with previous liver damage.

4.9 Overdose

Based on the limited information available in two cases of ingestion of over 18g of ciprofloxacin, reversible renal toxicity has occurred. Therefore, apart from routine emergency measures, it is recommended to monitor renal function, including urinary pH and acidify, if required, to prevent crystalluria. Patients must be kept well hydrated, and in the case of renal damage resulting in prolonged oliguria, dialysis should be initiated.

Calcium or magnesium antacids may be administered as soon as possible after ingestion of Ciproxin tablets in order to reduce the absorption of ciprofloxacin.

Serum levels of ciprofloxacin are reduced by dialysis.

5. PHARMACOLOGICAL PROPERTIES

ATC Code J01 MA 02

5.1 Pharmacodynamic properties

Ciprofloxacin is a synthetic 4-quinolone derivative, with bactericidal activity. It acts via inhibition of bacterial DNA gyrase, ultimately resulting in interference with DNA function. Ciprofloxacin is highly active against a wide range of Gram-positive and Gram-negative organisms and has shown activity against some anaerobes, *Chlamydia* spp. and *Mycoplasma* spp. Killing curves demonstrate the rapid bactericidal effect against sensitive organisms and it is often found that minimum bactericidal concentrations are in the range of minimum inhibitory concentrations. Ciprofloxacin has been shown to have no activity against *Treponema pallidum* and *Ureaplasma urealyticum*. *Nocardia asteroides* and *Enterococcus faecium* are resistant.

Breakpoints

$S \leqslant 1\ \mu g/ml$, $R \geqslant 4\ \mu g/ml$

Susceptibility

The prevalence of resistance may vary geographically and with time for selected species and local area information on resistance is desirable, particularly when treating severe infections. This information gives only an approximate guidance on probabilities whether micro-organisms will be susceptible to ciprofloxacin or not.

Organism	Prevalence of Resistance
Sensitive:	
Gram-positive bacteria	
Corynebacterium diphtheriae	0%
Corynebacterium spp.	-
Staphylococcus aureus (methicillin sensitive)	0 - 14%
Staphylococcus aureus (methicillin resistant)	48 - 90%
Streptococcus agalactiae	0 – 17%
Bacillus anthracis	-
Gram-negative bacteria	
Acinetobacter baumanii	6 - 93%
Acinetobacter spp.	14 – 70%
Aeromonas hydrophilia	0%
Aeromonas spp.	-
Bordetella pertussis	0%
Brucella melitensis	0%
Campylobacter jejuni/coli	0 – 82%
Campylobacter spp.	0%
Citrobacter freundii	0 – 4%
Citrobacter spp.	0%
Edwardsiella tarda	0%
Enterobacter aerogenes	0%
Enterobacter cloacae	0 - 3%
Enterobacter spp.	3 - 13%
Escherichia coli	2 -7%
Escherichia coli, EHEC and EPEC	-
Haemophilus influenzae	0 – 1%
Haemophilus influenzae (β–lactam negative)	0%
Haemophilus influenzae (β–lactam positive)	0%
Haemophilus parainfluenzae	0%
Hafnia alvei	0%
Klebsiella oxytoca	0%
Klebsiella pneumoniae	2 – 5.8%
Klebsiella spp.	2 – 21%
Legionella pneumophila	0%
Legionella spp.	0%
Moraxella catarrhalis	0%
Morganella morganii	1 – 2%
Neisseria gonorrhoeae	0%
Neisseria gonorrhoeae, β-lactamase	0%
Neisseria gonorrhoeae, β-lactamase positive	0%
Neisseria meningitidis	0%
Neisseria meningitidis, β-lactamase negative	0%
Plesiomonas shigelloides	0%
Proteus mirabilis	0 – 10%
Proteus vulgaris	4%
Providencia rettgeri	-
Providencia spp.	4%
Providencia stuartii	-
Pseudomonas aeruginosa	1 – 28%
Salmonella spp.	0%
Salmonella typhi	0 - 2%
Serratia liquefaciens	-
Serratia marcescens	23%
Serratia spp.	0 – 21%
Shigella spp.	0%
Vibrio cholerae	0%
Vibrio parahaemolyticus	0%
Vibrio spp.	0%
Yersinia enterocolitica	0%
Anaerobes	
Bacteroides ureolyticus	0%
Clostridium perfringens	
Peptococcus spp.	0%
Peptostreptococcus spp.	-
Peptostreptococcus magnus	0%
Veillonella parvula	0%
Other pathogens	
Chlamydia spp.	-
Helicobacter pylori	-
Mycobacterium fortuitum	0%
Mycobacterium tuberculosis	0%
Mycoplasma hominis	16%

Intermediate	
Gram-positive aerobes	
Enterococci	5%
Enterococcus faecalis	9 - 34%
Staphylococcus epidermis, methicillin sensitive	10 - 16%
Staphylococcus epidermis, methicillin resistant	26 - 56%
Staphylococcus haemolyticus	-
Staphylococcus haemolyticus, methicillin sensitive	8%
Staphylococcus haemolyticus, methicillin resistant	73%
Streptococcus anginosus	9%
Streptococcus bovis	-
Streptococcus milleri	5%
Streptococcus mitis	-
Streptococcus pneumoniae, penicillin sensitive	0 – 1%
Streptococcus pneumoniae, penicillin intermediate	-
Streptococcus pneumoniae, penicillin intermediate and resistant	2.8%
Streptococcus pneumoniae, penicillin resistant	-
Streptococcus pyogenes	0 - 28%
Streptococcus, viridans group	-
Streptococcus viridans, penicillin sensitive	-
Streptococcus viridans, penicillin resistant	-
Streptococcus, β-haemolytic groups A, C, and G	0%
Gram-negative aerobes	
Alcaligenes spp.	-
Listeria monocytogenes	0%
Listeria spp.	0%
Anaerobes	
*Fusobacterium*spp.	-
Gardnerella vaginalis	0%
Prevotella spp.	-
Other pathogens	
Ureaplasma urealyticum	11%
Resistant	
Gram-positive aerobes	
Enterococcus faecium	-
Stenotrophomonas maltophilia	94%
Streptococcus sanguis	-
Gram-negative aerobes	
Flavobacterium meningosepticum	-
Nocardia asteroides	-
Anaerobes	
Bacteroides fragilis	-
Bacteroides thetaiotaomicron	-
Clostridium difficile	-

Plasmid-related transfer of resistance has not been observed with ciprofloxacin and the overall frequency of development of resistance is low (10^{-9} - 10^{-7}). Cross-resistance to penicillins, cephalosporins, aminoglycosides and tetracyclines has not been observed and organisms resistant to these antibiotics are generally sensitive to ciprofloxacin. Ciprofloxacin is also suitable for use in combination with these antibiotics, and additive behaviour is usually observed.

5.2 Pharmacokinetic properties

Absorption of oral doses of ciprofloxacin tablet formulation occurs rapidly, mainly from the small intestine, the half-life of absorption being 2-15 minutes. Plasma levels are dose-related and peak 0.5-2.0 hours after dosing. The AUC also increases dose proportionately after administration of both single and repeated oral (tablet) and intravenous doses. The absolute bioavailability is reported to be 52-83% and ciprofloxacin is subject to only slight first pass metabolism. The oral bioavailability is approximately 70-80%.

The intake of food at the same time as administration of oral ciprofloxacin has a marginal but clinically not relevant effect on the pharmacokinetic parameters C_{max} and AUC. No specific recommendations are necessary with regard to time of administration of oral ciprofloxacin relative to food intake.

Distribution of ciprofloxacin within tissues is wide and the volume of distribution high, though slightly lower in the elderly. Protein binding is low (between 19-40%).

Only 10-20% of a single oral or intravenous dose is eliminated as metabolites (which exhibit lower activity than the parent drug). Four different antimicrobially active metabolites have been reported, desethyleneciprofloxacin (M1), sulphociprofloxacin (M2), oxaciprofloxacin (M3) and formylciprofloxacin (M4). M2 and M3 account for one third each of metabolised substance and M1 is found in small amounts (1.3-2.6% of the dose). M4 has been found in very small quantities (<0.1% of the dose). M1-M3 have antimicrobial activity comparable to nalidixic acid and M4 found in the smallest quantity has antimicrobial activity similar to that of norfloxacin.

Elimination of ciprofloxacin and its metabolites occurs rapidly, primarily by the kidney. After single oral and intravenous doses of ciprofloxacin, 55% and 75% respectively are eliminated by the kidney and 39% and 14% in the faeces within 5 days. Renal elimination takes place mainly during the first 12 hours after dosing and renal clearance levels suggest that active secretion by the renal tubules occurs in addition to normal glomerular filtration. Renal clearance is between 0.18 – 0.3 l/h.kg and total body clearance between 0.48 – 0.60 l/h.kg. Approximately 1% of a ciprofloxacin dose is excreted via the biliary route. The elimination kinetics are linear and after repeated dosing at 12 hourly intervals, no further accumulation is detected after the distribution equilibrium is attained (at 4-5 half-lives). The elimination half-life of unchanged ciprofloxacin over a period of 24-48 hours post-dose is 3.1-5.1 hours.

Some studies carried out with ciprofloxacin in severely renally impaired patients (serum creatinine >265 micromole/l or creatinine clearance <20ml/minute) demonstrated either a doubling of the elimination half-life, or fluctuations in half-life in comparison with healthy volunteers, whereas other studies showed no significant correlation between elimination half-life and creatinine clearance. However, it is recommended that in severely renally impaired patients, the total daily dose should be reduced by half, although monitoring of drug serum levels provides the most reliable basis for dose adjustment as necessary.

Results of pharmacokinetic studies in paediatric cystic fibrosis patients have shown dosages of 20mg/kg orally twice daily or 10mg/kg iv three times daily are recommended to achieve plasma concentration/time profiles comparable to those achieved in the adult population at the currently recommended dosage regimen.

Inhalation anthrax: Ciprofloxacin serum concentrations achieved in humans serve as a surrogate endpoint reasonably likely to predict clinical benefit and provide the basis for the recommended doses.

5.3 Preclinical safety data

Following extensive oral and intravenous toxicology testing with ciprofloxacin, only two findings which may be considered relevant to the use of ciprofloxacin in man were observed. Crystalluria was noted in those species of animals which had a normally alkaline urine. Kidney damage without the presence of crystalluria was not observed. This effect is considered a secondary inflammatory foreign-body reaction, due to the precipitation of a crystalline complex of ciprofloxacin, magnesium and protein in the distal tubule system of the kidneys. This is considered not to be a problem in man, because the urine is normally acidic. However, to avoid the occurrence of crystalluria, patients should be well hydrated and excessive alkalinity of the urine avoided.

As with other quinolones, damage to the weight-bearing joints of only juvenile rats and dogs treated with ciprofloxacin was noted in repeat dose toxicity testing. This was more noticeable in the dog. Although analysis of available safety data from ciprofloxacin use in paediatric patients did not disclose any evidence of drug related cartilage or articular damage, the use of ciprofloxacin in children and growing adolescents is generally not recommended, unless the benefits are considered to outweigh the potential risks (with the exception of treatment of cystic fibrosis). Additionally, because of the potential of arthropathy, the use of ciprofloxacin during pregnancy and lactation is not recommended.

6. PHARMACEUTICAL PARTICULARS

6.1 List of excipients

Each tablet contains microcrystalline cellulose, maize starch, crospovidone, colloidal silicon dioxide, magnesium stearate and purified water. The tablet film-coat consists of a mixture of hypromellose, Macrogol 4000, titanium dioxide and purified water.

6.2 Incompatibilities

None known.

6.3 Shelf life

5 years.

6.4 Special precautions for storage

No special storage precautions are necessary.

6.5 Nature and contents of container

Blister strips in cardboard outers comprising:

a) 250μm, 40g/m² PVC/PVDC foil with 20μm hard aluminium backing foil.

Pack sizes 10, 20, 100 tablets.

b) 300μm polypropylene foil with 20μm hard aluminium backing foil with a 3.5g/m²

heat seal polypropylene coating.

Pack sizes: 6, 10, 20, 100 tablets.

6.6 Instructions for use and handling

Not applicable.

7. MARKETING AUTHORISATION HOLDER

Bayer plc	Trading as:
Bayer House	Bayer plc
Strawberry Hill	Pharmaceutical Division
Newbury	Bayer House
Berkshire	Strawberry Hill
RG14 1JA	Newbury
	Berkshire
	RG14 1JA
	BAYPHARM or BAYMET

8. MARKETING AUTHORISATION NUMBER(S)

PL 0010/0145

9. DATE OF FIRST AUTHORISATION/RENEWAL OF THE AUTHORISATION

3 February 1987/25 February 1999

10. DATE OF REVISION OF THE TEXT

June 2003

Ciproxin Tablets 250mg

(Bayer plc)

1. NAME OF THE MEDICINAL PRODUCT

Ciproxin Tablets 250mg

2. QUALITATIVE AND QUANTITATIVE COMPOSITION

Each tablet contains 291.0mg ciprofloxacin hydrochloride equivalent to 250mg Ciprofloxacin (INN).

3. PHARMACEUTICAL FORM

Immediate release film-coated tablet for oral administration.

4. CLINICAL PARTICULARS

4.1 Therapeutic indications

Ciprofloxacin is indicated for the treatment of the following infections caused by sensitive bacteria:

Adults:

Respiratory tract infections: e.g. lobar and bronchopneumonia, acute and chronic bronchitis, acute exacerbation of cystic fibrosis, bronchiectasis, empyema. Ciprofloxacin is not recommended as first-line therapy for the treatment of pneumococcal pneumonia. Ciprofloxacin may be used for treating Gram-negative pneumonia.

Ear, nose and throat infections: e.g. mastoiditis, otitis media and sinusitis, especially if due to Gram-negative bacteria (including *Pseudomonas* spp.). Ciprofloxacin is not recommended for the treatment of acute tonsillitis.

Eye infections: e.g. bacterial conjunctivitis.

Urinary tract infections: e.g. uncomplicated and complicated urethritis, cystitis, pyelonephritis, prostatitis, epididymitis.

Skin and soft tissue infections: e.g. infected ulcers, wound infections, abscesses, cellulitis, otitis externa, erysipelas, infected burns.

Bone and joint infections: e.g. osteomyelitis, septic arthritis.

Intra-abdominal infections: e.g. peritonitis, intra-abdominal abscesses.

Infections of the biliary tract: e.g. cholangitis, cholecystitis, empyema of the gall bladder.

Gastro-intestinal infections: e.g. enteric fever, infective diarrhoea.

Pelvic infections: e.g. salpingitis, endometritis, pelvic inflammatory disease.

Severe systemic infections: e.g. septicaemia, bacteraemia, peritonitis, infections in immuno-suppressed patients.

Gonorrhoea: including urethral, rectal and pharyngeal gonorrhoea caused by β-lactamase producing organisms or organisms moderately sensitive to penicillin.

Ciprofloxacin is also indicated for prophylaxis against infection in elective upper gastro-intestinal tract surgery and endoscopic procedures, where there is an increased risk of infection.

Children:

For the treatment of acute pulmonary exacerbation of cystic fibrosis associated with *P. aeruginosa* infection in paediatric patients aged 5-17 years.

Inhalation Anthrax in Adults and Children: To reduce the incidence or progression of disease following confirmed or suspected exposure to aerosolised *Bacillus anthracis*.

4.2 Posology and method of administration

General dosage recommendations: The dosage of Ciproxin tablets is determined by the severity and type of infection, the sensitivity of the causative organism(s) and the age, weight and renal function of the patient. Ciproxin tablets should be swallowed whole with an adequate amount of liquid.

If Ciproxin Tablets are taken on an empty stomach, the active substance is absorbed more rapidly. In this case, the tablets should not be taken concurrently with dairy products or with mineral fortified drinks alone (e.g. milk, yoghurt, calcium fortified orange juice). However, a normal diet that will contain small amounts of calcium, does not significantly affect ciprofloxacin absorbtion.

Adults

The dosage range for adults is 100-750mg twice daily. The following dosages for specific types of infection are recommended:

Table 1: Recommended Adult Dosage

Indication	Dosage (mg ciprofloxacin)
Treatment	
Gonorrhoea	250mg single dose
Acute, uncomplicated cystitis	100mg b.d.
Upper and lower urinary tract infections (depending on severity)	250-500mg b.d.
Upper and lower respiratory tract infections (depending on severity)	250-750mg b.d.
Pneumococcal pneumonia (second-line)	750mg b.d.
Cystic fibrosis patients with pseudomonal lower RTI*	750mg b.d.
Other infections as detailed under 4.1	500-750mg b.d.
Severe infections, particularly due to Pseudomonas, staphylococci and streptococci	750mg b.d.
Inhalation Anthrax	500mg b.d.
Prophylaxis	
Elective upper gastro-intestinal surgical and endoscopic procedures	750mg single dose 60-90 minutes prior to the procedure**. If gastro-oesophageal obstructive lesions are suspected use with an anti-infective effective against anaerobes

* Although the pharmacokinetics of ciprofloxacin remains unchanged in patients with cystic fibrosis, the low body-weight of these patients should be taken into consideration when determining dosage.

** The tablet may be given with an oral pre-medicant, but see Section 4.5

Impaired Renal Function

Dosage adjustments are not usually required, except in patients with severe renal impairment (serum creatinine >265 micromole/l or creatinine clearance <20ml/minute). If adjustment is necessary, this may be achieved by reducing the total daily dose by half, although monitoring of drug serum levels provides the most reliable basis for dose adjustment.

Impaired Hepatic Function

No adjustment of dosage is necessary.

Elderly

Although higher ciprofloxacin serum levels are found in the elderly, no adjustment of dosage is necessary.

Adolescents and children

As with other drugs in its class, ciprofloxacin has been shown to cause arthropathy in weight-bearing joints of immature animals. Although analysis of available safety data from ciprofloxacin use in patients less than 18 years of age, the majority of whom had cystic fibrosis, did not disclose any evidence of drug-related cartilage or articular damage, its use in the paediatric population is generally not recommended.

Clinical and pharmacokinetic data support the use of ciprofloxacin in paediatric cystic fibrosis patients (aged 5 - 17 years) with acute pulmonary exacerbations associated with *P. aeruginosa* infection, at a dose of 20mg/kg orally twice daily (maximum daily dose 1500mg).

For the indication of inhalation anthrax, the risk-benefit assessment indicates that administration of ciprofloxacin to paediatric patients at a dose of 15 mg/kg orally twice daily (maximum daily dose of 1000 mg) is appropriate.

For indications other than treatment of pulmonary exacerbations in cystic fibrosis and inhalation anthrax, ciprofloxacin may be used in children and adolescents where the benefit is considered to outweigh the potential risks. In these cases a dosage of 5-15mg/kg orally twice daily should be administered depending upon the severity of infection.

Dosing in children with impaired renal and/or hepatic function has not been studied.

Duration of Treatment

The duration of treatment depends upon the severity of infection, clinical response and bacteriological findings.

In acute, uncomplicated cystitis the treatment period is three days.

In other acute infections the usual treatment period is 5-10 days. Generally, acute and chronic infections (e.g. osteomyelitis and prostatitis, etc), where the causative organism is known to be sensitive to ciprofloxacin, should be treated for at least three days after the signs and symptoms of the infection have disappeared.

For acute pulmonary exacerbations of cystic fibrosis associated with *P. aeruginosa* infection in paediatric patients (aged 5-17 years), the duration of treatment is 10 - 14 days.

For inhalation anthrax, drug administration should begin as soon as possible after confirmed or suspected exposure and should be continued for 60 days.

4.3 Contraindications

Ciprofloxacin is contra-indicated in patients who have shown hypersensitivity to ciprofloxacin or other quinolone anti-infectives.

Except in cases of exacerbations of cystic fibrosis associated with *P. aeruginosa* (in patients aged 5-17 years) and inhalation anthrax, ciprofloxacin is contra-indicated in children and growing adolescents unless the benefits of treatment are considered to outweigh the risks.

4.4 Special warnings and special precautions for use

Ciprofloxacin should be used with caution in epileptics and patients with a history of CNS disorders and only if the benefits of treatment are considered to outweigh the risk of possible CNS side-effects. CNS side-effects have been reported after first administration of ciprofloxacin in some patients. Treatment should be discontinued if the side-effects, depression or psychoses lead to self-endangering behaviour (see also Section 4.8).

Crystalluria related to the use of ciprofloxacin has been reported. Patients receiving ciprofloxacin should be well hydrated and excessive alkalinity of the urine should be avoided.

Patients with a family history of or actual defects in glucose-6-phosphate dehydrogenase activity are prone to haemolytic reactions with quinolones, and so ciprofloxacin should be used with caution in these patients.

Tendon inflammation and rupture may occur with quinolone antibiotics. Such reactions have been observed particularly in older patients and in those treated concurrently with corticosteroids. At the first sign of pain or inflammation, patients should discontinue ciprofloxacin and rest the affected limbs.

There is a risk of pseudomembranous colitis with broad-spectrum antibiotics possibly leading to a fatal outcome. It is important to consider this in patients suffering from severe, persistent diarrhoea. With ciprofloxacin this effect has been reported rarely. If pseudomembranous colitis is suspected treatment with ciprofloxacin should be stopped and appropriate treatment given (e.g. oral vancomycin).

As with other quinolones, patients should avoid prolonged exposure to strong sunlight or UV radiation during treatment.

Laboratory tests may give abnormal findings if performed whilst patients are receiving ciprofloxacin e.g. increased alkaline phosphatase; increases in liver function tests e.g. transaminases and cholestatic jaundice, especially in patients with previous liver damage.

4.5 Interaction with other medicinal products and other forms of Interaction

Increased plasma levels of theophylline have been observed following concurrent administration with ciprofloxacin. It is recommended that the dose of theophylline should be reduced and plasma levels of theophylline monitored. The reaction between theophylline and ciprofloxacin is potentially life-threatening. Therefore, where monitoring of plasma levels is not possible, the use of ciprofloxacin should be avoided in patients receiving theophylline. Particular caution is advised in those patients with convulsive disorders.

Phenytoin levels may be altered when Ciproxin is used concomitantly.

Ciproxin Tablets should not be administered within four hours of multivalent cationic drugs and mineral supplements (e.g. calcium, magnesium, aluminium or iron), sucralfate or antacids and highly buffered drugs (e.g. didanosine) as interference with absorption may occur. When appropriate, patients should be advised not to self-medicate with preparations containing these compounds during therapy with ciprofloxacin. This restriction does not apply to the class of H2 receptor blocker drugs.

The concurrent administration of dairy products or fortified drinks alone (e.g. milk, yoghurt, calcium fortified orange juice) and ciprofloxacin should be avoided because absorption of ciprofloxacin may be reduced. However a normal diet, that will contain small amounts of calcium, does not significantly affect ciprofloxacin absorption.

Prolongation of bleeding time has been reported during concomitant administration of ciprofloxacin and oral anti-coagulants.

Animal data have shown that high doses of quinolones in combination with some non-steroidal anti-inflammatory drugs, (e.g. fenbufen, but not acetylsalicylic acid) can lead to convulsions.

Transient increases in serum creatinine have been seen following concomitant administration of ciprofloxacin and cyclosporin. Therefore, monitoring of serum creatinine levels is advisable.

The simultaneous administration of quinolones and glibenclamide can on occasion potentiate the effect of glibenclamide resulting in hypoglycaemia.

Renal tubular transport of methotrexate may be inhibited by concomitant administration of ciprofloxacin potentially leading to increased plasma levels of methotrexate. This may increase the risk of methotrexate associated toxic reactions. Therefore, patients receiving methotrexate therapy should be carefully monitored when concomitant ciprofloxacin therapy is indicated.

Concomitant use with probenecid reduces the renal clearance of ciprofloxacin, resulting in increased quinolone plasma levels.

The use of metoclopramide with ciprofloxacin may accelerate the absorption of ciprofloxacin.

When ciprofloxacin is used for surgical prophylaxis, it is recommended that opiate premedicants, (e.g. papaveretum) or opiate premedicants used with anticholinergic premedicants, (e.g. atropine or hyoscine) are not used, as the serum levels of ciprofloxacin are reduced and adequate cover may not be obtained during surgery. Co-administration of ciprofloxacin and benzodiazepine premedicants has been shown not to affect ciprofloxacin plasma levels.

4.6 Pregnancy and lactation

Reproduction studies performed in mice, rats and rabbits using parenteral and oral administration did not reveal any evidence of teratogenicity, impairment of fertility or impairment of peri-/post-natal development. However, as with other quinolones, ciprofloxacin has been shown to cause arthropathy in immature animals, and therefore its use during pregnancy is not recommended. Studies have indicated that ciprofloxacin is secreted in breast milk. Administration to nursing mothers is thus not recommended.

4.7 Effects on ability to drive and use machines

Ciprofloxacin could result in impairment of the patient's ability to drive or operate machinery, particularly in conjunction with alcohol.

4.8 Undesirable effects

Ciprofloxacin is generally well tolerated. The most frequently reported adverse reactions are nausea, diarrhoea and rash.

The following adverse reactions have been observed:

Hypersensitivity/skin, e.g. rash, pruritus, urticaria, photosensitivity, drug-induced fever, anaphylactic/anaphylactoid reactions including angioedema and dyspnoea. Rarely, erythema nodosum and erythema multiforme. Very rarely, petechiae, haemorrhagic bullae, vasculitis, serum sickness-like reaction, fixed drug reactions, Stevens-Johnson Syndrome and Lyells Syndrome. Treatment with ciprofloxacin should be discontinued if any of the above occur upon first administration.

General, e.g. moniliasis, asthenia, hyperglycaemia and abnormal gait, pain, pain in extremeties, back pain, chest pain. Thrombophlebitis.

CNS, e.g. headache, restlessness, depression, dizziness, tremor, convulsions, confusion, hallucinations, somnolence, sleep disorders, insomnia. Rarely, hypesthesia. Very rarely, migraine, hyperesthesia, ataxia, hypertonia, twitching or anxiety states. Isolated cases of ciprofloxacin-induced psychoses have been reported, which may progress to self-endangering behaviour. There are isolated reports of intracranial hypertension associated with quinolone therapy. Paraesthesia has been reported.

Gastro-intestinal, e.g. nausea, diarrhoea, vomiting, dyspepsia, abdominal pain, anorexia, flatulence, dysphagia. Rarely, pancreatitis or pseudomembranous colitis.

Cardiovascular, e.g. tachycardia, oedema, fainting, hot flushes, hypotension and sweating.

Effects on haematological parameters, e.g. anaemia, eosinophilia, increases or decreases in white cell and/or platelet count, altered prothrombin levels, and, very rarely, haemolytic anaemia, agranulocytosis, pancytopenia or bone marrow depression. Pancytopenia and bone marrow depression may be potentially life-threatening.

Hepatic, e.g. transient increases in liver enzymes or serum bilirubin (particularly in patients with previous liver damage), hepatitis, jaundice/cholestasis and major liver disorders including hepatic necrosis, which may rarely progress to life-threatening hepatic failure.

Renal, e.g. transient increases in blood urea or serum creatinine, renal failure, crystalluria, haematuria, nephritis.

Musculoskeletal, e.g. reversible arthralgia, joint swelling and myalgia. Rarely, myasthenia or tenosynovitis. Tendon inflammation (predominantly of the Achilles tendon) has been reported which may lead to tendon rupture. Treatment should be discontinued immediately if these symptoms occur.

Rarely, exacerbation of the symptoms of myasthenia gravis have been reported.

Special senses, e.g. very rarely, visual disturbances including diplopia and colour disturbances, impaired taste and smell usually reversible upon discontinuation of treatment, tinnitus, transient impairment of hearing particularly at high frequencies.

Abnormal laboratory findings, e.g. increased alkaline phosphatase, amylase and lipase; increases in liver function tests, e.g transaminases, and cholestatic jaundice, especially in patients with previous liver damage.

4.9 Overdose

Based on the limited information available in two cases of ingestion of over 18g of ciprofloxacin, reversible renal toxicity has occurred. Therefore, apart from routine emergency measures, it is recommended to monitor renal function, including urinary pH and acidify, if required, to prevent crystalluria. Patients must be kept well hydrated, and in the case of renal damage resulting in prolonged oliguria, dialysis should be initiated.

Calcium or magnesium antacids may be administered as soon as possible after ingestion of Ciproxin tablets in order to reduce the absorption of ciprofloxacin.

Serum levels of ciprofloxacin are reduced by dialysis.

5. PHARMACOLOGICAL PROPERTIES

ATC Code J01 MA 02

5.1 Pharmacodynamic properties

Ciprofloxacin is a synthetic 4-quinolone derivative, with bactericidal activity. It acts via inhibition of bacterial DNA gyrase, ultimately resulting in interference with DNA function. Ciprofloxacin is highly active against a wide range of Gram-positive and Gram-negative organisms and has shown activity against some anaerobes, *Chlamydia* spp. and *Mycoplasma* spp. Killing curves demonstrate the rapid bactericidal effect against sensitive organisms and it is often found that minimum bactericidal concentrations are in the range of minimum inhibitory concentrations. Ciprofloxacin has been shown to have no activity against *Treponema pallidum* and *Ureaplasma urealyticum. Nocardia asteroides* and *Enterococcus faecium* are resistant.

Breakpoints

S $\leqslant 1\ \mu g/ml$, R $\geqslant 4\ \mu g/ml$

Susceptibility

The prevalence of resistance may vary geographically and with time for selected species and local area information on resistance is desirable, particularly when treating severe infections. This information gives only an approximate guidance on probabilities whether micro-organisms will be susceptible to ciprofloxacin or not.

Organism	Prevalence of Resistance
Sensitive:	
Gram-positive bacteria	
Corynebacterium diphtheriae	0%
Corynebacterium spp.	-
Staphylococcus aureus (methicillin sensitive)	0 - 14%
Staphylococcus aureus (methicillin resistant)	48 - 90%
Streptococcus agalactiae	0 – 17%
Bacillus anthracis	
Gram-negative bacteria	
Acinetobacter baumanii	6 - 93%
Acinetobacter spp.	14 – 70%
Aeromonas hydrophilia	0%
Aeromonas spp.	-
Bordetella pertussis	0%
Brucella melitensis	0%
Campylobacter jejuni/coli	0 – 82%
Campylobacter spp.	0%
Citrobacter freundii	0 – 4%
Citrobacter spp.	0%
Edwardsiella tarda	0%
Enterobacter aerogenes	0%
Enterobacter cloacae	0 - 3%
Enterobacter spp.	3 - 13%
Escherichia coli	2 -7%
Escherichia coli, EHEC and EPEC	
Haemophilus influenzae	0 – 1%
Haemophilus influenzae (β-lactam negative)	0%
Haemophilus influenzae (β-lactam positive)	0%
Haemophilus parainfluenzae	0%
Hafnia alvei	0%
Klebsiella oxytoca	0%
Klebsiella pneumoniae	2 – 5.8%
Klebsiella spp.	2 – 21%
Legionella pneumophila	0%
Legionella spp.	0%
Moraxella catarrhalis	0%
Morganella morganii	1 – 2%
Neisseria gonorrhoeae	0%
Neisseria gonorrhoeae, β-lactamase	0%
Neisseria gonorrhoeae, β-lactamase positive	0%
Neisseria meningitidis	0%
Neisseria meningitidis, β-lactamase negative	0%
Plesiomonas shigelloides	0%
Proteus mirabilis	0 – 10%
Proteus vulgaris	4%
Providencia rettgeri	0%
Providencia spp.	4%
Providencia stuartii	0%
Pseudomonas aeruginosa	1 – 28%
Salmonella spp.	0%
Salmonella typhi	0 - 2%
Serratia liquefaciens	-
Serratia marcescens	23%
Serratia spp.	0 – 21%
Shigella spp.	0%
Vibrio cholerae	0%
Vibrio parahaemolyticus	0%
Vibrio spp.	0%
Yersinia enterocolitica	0%
Anaerobes	
Bacteroides ureolyticus	0%
Clostridium perfringens	-
Peptococcus spp.	0%
Peptostreptococcus spp.	-
Peptostreptococcus magnus	0%
Veillonella parvula	0%
Other pathogens	
Chlamydia spp.	0%
Helicobacter pylori	-
Mycobacterium fortuitum	0%
Mycobacterium tuberculosis	0%
Mycoplasma hominis	16%
Intermediate	
Gram-positive aerobes	
Enterococci	5%
Enterococcus faecalis	9 – 34%
Staphylococcus epidermis, methicillin sensitive	10 - 16%
Staphylococcus epidermis, methicillin resistant	26 - 56%
Staphylococcus haemolyticus	-
Staphylococcus haemolyticus, methicillin sensitive	8%
Staphylococcus haemolyticus, methicillin resistant	73%
Streptococcus anginosus	9%
Streptococcus bovis	-
Streptococcus milleri	5%
Streptococcus mitis	-
Streptococcus pneumoniae, penicillin sensitive	0 – 1%
Streptococcus pneumoniae, penicillin intermediate	
Streptococcus pneumoniae, penicillin intermediate and resistant	2.8%
Streptococcus pneumoniae, penicillin resistant	-
Streptococcus pyogenes	0 - 28%
Streptococcus, viridans group	
Streptococcus viridans, penicillin sensitive	-
Streptococcus viridans, penicillin resistant	

Streptococcus, *β*-haemolytic groups A, C, and G	0%
Gram-negative aerobes	
Alcaligenes spp.	
Listeria monocytogenes	0%
Listeria spp.	
Anaerobes	
Fusobacterium spp.	
Gardnerella vaginalis	0%
Prevotella spp.	
Other pathogens	
Ureaplasma urealyticum	11%
Resistant	
Gram-positive aerobes	
Enterococcus faecium	-
Stenotrophomonas maltophilia	94%
Streptococcus sanguis	
Gram-negative aerobes	
Flavobacterium meningosepticum	-
Nocardia asteroides	-
Anaerobes	
Bacteroides fragilis	-
Bacteroides thetaiotaomicron	-
Clostridium difficile	-

Plasmid-related transfer of resistance has not been observed with ciprofloxacin and the overall frequency of development of resistance is low (10^{-9} - 10^{-7}). Cross-resistance to penicillins, cephalosporins, aminoglycosides and tetracyclines has not been observed and organisms resistant to these antibiotics are generally sensitive to ciprofloxacin. Ciprofloxacin is also suitable for use in combination with these antibiotics, and additive behaviour is usually observed.

5.2 Pharmacokinetic properties

Absorption of oral doses of ciprofloxacin tablet formulation occurs rapidly, mainly from the small intestine, the half-life of absorption being 2-15 minutes. Plasma levels are dose-related and peak 0.5-2.0 hours after dosing. The AUC also increases dose proportionately after administration of both single and repeated oral (tablet) and intravenous doses. The absolute bioavailability is reported to be 52-83% and ciprofloxacin is subject to only slight first pass metabolism. The oral bioavailability is approximately 70-80%.

The intake of food at the same time as administration of oral ciprofloxacin has a marginal but clinically not relevant effect on the pharmacokinetic parameters C_{max} and AUC. No specific recommendations are necessary with regard to time of administration of oral ciprofloxacin relative to food intake.

Distribution of ciprofloxacin within tissues is wide and the volume of distribution high, though slightly lower in the elderly. Protein binding is low (between 19-40%).

Only 10-20% of a single oral or intravenous dose is eliminated as metabolites (which exhibit lower activity than the parent drug). Four different antimicrobially active metabolites have been reported, desethyleneciprofloxacin (M1), sulphociprofloxacin (M2), oxaciprofloxacin (M3) and formylciprofloxacin (M4). M2 and M3 account for one third each of metabolised substance and M1 is found in small amounts (1.3-2.6% of the dose). M4 has been found in very small quantities (<0.1% of the dose). M1-M3 have antimicrobial activity comparable to nalidixic acid and M4 found in the smallest quantity has antimicrobial activity similar to that of norfloxacin.

Elimination of ciprofloxacin and its metabolites occurs rapidly, primarily by the kidney. After single oral and intravenous doses of ciprofloxacin, 55% and 75% respectively are eliminated by the kidney and 39% and 14% in the faeces within 5 days. Renal elimination takes place mainly during the first 12 hours after dosing and renal clearance levels suggest that active secretion by the renal tubules occurs in addition to normal glomerular filtration. Renal clearance is between 0.18 – 0.3 l/h.kg and total body clearance between 0.48 – 0.60 l/h.kg. Approximately 1% of a ciprofloxacin dose is excreted via the biliary route. The elimination kinetics are linear and after repeated dosing at 12 hourly intervals, no further accumulation is detected after the distribution equilibrium is attained (at 4-5 half-lives). The elimination half-life of unchanged ciprofloxacin over a period of 24-48 hours post-dose is 3.1-5.1 hours.

Some studies carried out with ciprofloxacin in severely renally impaired patients (serum creatinine >265 micromole/l or creatinine clearance <20ml/minute) demonstrated either a doubling of the elimination half-life, or fluctuations in half-life in comparison with healthy volunteers, whereas other studies showed no significant correlation between elimination half-life and creatinine clearance. However, it is recommended that in severely renally impaired patients, the total daily dose should be reduced by half, although monitoring of drug serum levels provides the most reliable basis for dose adjustment as necessary.

Results of pharmacokinetic studies in paediatric cystic fibrosis patients have shown dosages of 20mg/kg orally twice daily or 10mg/kg iv three times daily are recommended to achieve plasma concentration/time profiles comparable to those achieved in the adult population at the currently recommended dosage regimen.

Inhalation anthrax: Ciprofloxacin serum concentrations achieved in humans serve as a surrogate endpoint reasonably likely to predict clinical benefit and provide the basis for the recommended doses.

5.3 Preclinical safety data

Following extensive oral and intravenous toxicology testing with ciprofloxacin, only two findings which may be considered relevant to the use of ciprofloxacin in man were observed. Crystalluria was noted in those species of animals which had a normally alkaline urine. Kidney damage without the presence of crystalluria was not observed. This effect is considered a secondary inflammatory foreign-body reaction, due to the precipitation of a crystalline complex of ciprofloxacin, magnesium and protein in the distal tubule system of the kidneys. This is considered not to be a problem in man, because the urine is normally acidic. However, to avoid the occurrence of crystalluria, patients should be well hydrated and excessive alkalinity of the urine avoided.

As with other quinolones, damage to the weight-bearing joints of only juvenile rats and dogs treated with ciprofloxacin was noted in repeat dose toxicity testing. This was more noticeable in the dog. Although analysis of available safety data from ciprofloxacin use in paediatric patients did not disclose any evidence of drug related cartilage or articular damage, the use of ciprofloxacin in children and growing adolescents is generally not recommended, unless the benefits are considered to outweigh the potential risks (with the exception of treatment of cystic fibrosis). Additionally, because of the potential of arthropathy, the use of ciprofloxacin during pregnancy and lactation is not recommended.

6. PHARMACEUTICAL PARTICULARS

6.1 List of excipients

Each tablet contains microcrystalline cellulose, maize starch, crospovidone, colloidal silicon dioxide, magnesium stearate and purified water. The tablet film-coat consists of a mixture of hypromellose, macrogol 4000, titanium dioxide and purified water.

6.2 Incompatibilities

None known.

6.3 Shelf life

5 years.

6.4 Special precautions for storage

No special storage precautions are necessary.

6.5 Nature and contents of container

Blister strips in cardboard outers comprising:

a) 250μm, 40g/m^2 PVC/PVDC foil with 20μm hard aluminium backing foil.

Pack sizes 10, 20, 100 tablets.

b) 300μm polypropylene foil with 20μm hard aluminium backing foil with a 3.5g/m^2

heat seal polypropylene coating.

Pack sizes: 10, 20, 100 tablets.

c) 130μm PA/aluminium/PVC foil with 20μm hard aluminium backing foil.

Pack size: 2 tablets (sample pack).

6.6 Instructions for use and handling

Not applicable.

7. MARKETING AUTHORISATION HOLDER

Bayer plc
Bayer House
Strawberry Hill
Newbury
Berkshire
RG14 1JA

Trading as:
Bayer plc
Pharmaceutical Division
Bayer House
Strawberry Hill
Newbury
Berkshire
RG14 1JA
Or BAYPHARM or BAYMET

8. MARKETING AUTHORISATION NUMBER(S)

PL 0010/0146

9. DATE OF FIRST AUTHORISATION/RENEWAL OF THE AUTHORISATION

3 February 1987/25 February 1999

10. DATE OF REVISION OF THE TEXT

June 2003

Ciproxin Tablets 500mg

(Bayer plc)

1. NAME OF THE MEDICINAL PRODUCT

Ciproxin Tablets 500mg

2. QUALITATIVE AND QUANTITATIVE COMPOSITION

Each tablet contains 582.0mg ciprofloxacin hydrochloride equivalent to 500mg Ciprofloxacin (INN).

3. PHARMACEUTICAL FORM

Immediate release film-coated tablet for oral administration.

4. CLINICAL PARTICULARS

4.1 Therapeutic indications

Ciprofloxacin is indicated for the treatment of the following infections caused by sensitive bacteria:

Adults:

Respiratory tract infections: e.g. lobar and bronchopneumonia, acute and chronic bronchitis, acute exacerbation of cystic fibrosis, bronchiectasis, empyema. Ciprofloxacin is not recommended as first-line therapy for the treatment of pneumococcal pneumonia. Ciprofloxacin may be used for treating Gram-negative pneumonia.

Ear, nose and throat infections: e.g. mastoiditis, otitis media and sinusitis, especially if due to Gram-negative bacteria (including *Pseudomonas* spp.). Ciprofloxacin is not recommended for the treatment of acute tonsillitis.

Eye infections: e.g. bacterial conjunctivitis.

Urinary tract infections: e.g. uncomplicated and complicated urethritis, cystitis, pyelonephritis, prostatitis, epididymitis.

Skin and soft tissue infections: e.g. infected ulcers, wound infections, abscesses, cellulitis, otitis externa, erysipelas, infected burns.

Bone and joint infections: e.g. osteomyelitis, septic arthritis.

Intra-abdominal infections: e.g. peritonitis, intra-abdominal abscesses.

Infections of the biliary tract: e.g. cholangitis, cholecystitis, empyema of the gall bladder.

Gastro-intestinal infections: e.g. enteric fever, infective diarrhoea.

Pelvic infections: e.g. salpingitis, endometritis, pelvic inflammatory disease.

Severe systemic infections: e.g. septicaemia, bacteraemia, peritonitis, infections in immuno-suppressed patients.

Gonorrhoea: including urethral, rectal and pharyngeal gonorrhoea caused by *β*-lactamase producing organisms or organisms moderately sensitive to penicillin.

Ciprofloxacin is also indicated for prophylaxis against infection in elective upper gastro-intestinal tract surgery and endoscopic procedures, where there is an increased risk of infection.

Children:

For the treatment of acute pulmonary exacerbation of cystic fibrosis associated with *P. aeruginosa* infection in paediatric patients aged 5-17 years.

Inhalation Anthrax in Adults and Children: To reduce the incidence or progression of disease following confirmed or suspected exposure to aerosolised *Bacillus anthracis*.

4.2 Posology and method of administration

General dosage recommendations: The dosage of Ciproxin tablets is determined by the severity and type of infection, the sensitivity of the causative organism(s) and the age, weight and renal function of the patient. Ciproxin tablets should be swallowed whole with an adequate amount of liquid.

If Ciproxin Tablets are taken on an empty stomach, the active substance is absorbed more rapidly. In this case, the tablets should not be taken concurrently with dairy products or with mineral fortified drinks alone (e.g. milk, yoghurt, calcium fortified orange juice). However, a normal diet that will contain small amounts of calcium, does not significantly affect ciprofloxacin absorption.

Adults

The dosage range for adults is 100-750mg twice daily. The following dosages for specific types of infection are recommended:

Table 1: Recommended Adult Dosage

Indication	Dosage (mg ciprofloxacin)
Treatment	
Gonorrhoea	250mg single dose

Acute, uncomplicated cystitis	100mg b.d.
Upper and lower urinary tract infections (depending on severity)	250-500mg b.d.
Upper and lower respiratory tract infections (depending on severity)	250-750mg b.d.
Pneumococcal pneumonia (second-line)	750mg b.d.
Cystic fibrosis patients with pseudomonal lower RTI*	750mg b.d.
Other infections as detailed under 4.1	500-750mg b.d.
Severe infections, particularly due to Pseudomonas, staphylococci and streptococci	750mg b.d.
Inhalation Anthrax	500mg b.d.
Prophylaxis	
Elective upper gastro-intestinal surgical and endoscopic procedures	750mg single dose 60-90 minutes prior to the procedure**. If gastro-oesophageal obstructive lesions are suspected use with an anti-infective effective against anaerobes

* Although the pharmacokinetics of ciprofloxacin remains unchanged in patients with cystic fibrosis, the low body-weight of these patients should be taken into consideration when determining dosage.

** The tablet may be given with an oral pre-medicant, but see Section 4.5

Impaired Renal Function

Dosage adjustments are not usually required, except in patients with severe renal impairment (serum creatinine >265 micromole/l or creatinine clearance <20ml/minute). If adjustment is necessary, this may be achieved by reducing the total daily dose by half, although monitoring of drug serum levels provides the most reliable basis for dose adjustment.

Impaired Hepatic Function

No adjustment of dosage is necessary

Elderly

Although higher ciprofloxacin serum levels are found in the elderly, no adjustment of dosage is necessary.

Adolescents and children

As with other drugs in its class, ciprofloxacin has been shown to cause arthropathy in weight-bearing joints of immature animals. Although analysis of available safety data from ciprofloxacin use in patients less than 18 years of age, the majority of whom had cystic fibrosis, did not disclose any evidence of drug-related cartilage or articular damage, its use in the paediatric population is generally not recommended.

Clinical and pharmacokinetic data support the use of ciprofloxacin in paediatric cystic fibrosis patients (aged 5 - 17 years) with acute pulmonary exacerbations associated with *P. aeruginosa* infection, at a dose of 20mg/kg orally twice daily (maximum daily dose 1500mg).

For the indication of inhalation anthrax, the risk-benefit assessment indicates that administration of ciprofloxacin to paediatric patients at a dose of 15 mg/kg orally twice daily (maximum daily dose of 1000 mg) is appropriate.

For indications other than treatment of pulmonary exacerbations in cystic fibrosis and inhalation anthrax, ciprofloxacin may be used in children and adolescents where the benefit is considered to outweigh the potential risks. In these cases a dosage of 5-15mg/kg orally twice daily should be administered depending upon the severity of infection.

Dosing in children with impaired renal and/or hepatic function has not been studied.

Duration of Treatment

The duration of treatment depends upon the severity of infection, clinical response and bacteriological findings.

In acute, uncomplicated cystitis the treatment period is three days.

In other acute infections the usual treatment period is 5-10 days. Generally, acute and chronic infections (e.g. osteomyelitis and prostatitis, etc), where the causative organism is known to be sensitive to ciprofloxacin, should be treated for at least three days after the signs and symptoms of the infection have disappeared.

For acute pulmonary exacerbations of cystic fibrosis associated with *P. aeruginosa* infection in paediatric patients (aged 5-17 years), the duration of treatment is 10 - 14 days.

For inhalation anthrax, drug administration should begin as soon as possible after confirmed or suspected exposure and should be continued for 60 days.

4.3 Contraindications

Ciprofloxacin is contra-indicated in patients who have shown hypersensitivity to ciprofloxacin or other quinolone anti-infectives.

Except in cases of exacerbations of cystic fibrosis associated with *P. aeruginosa* (in patients aged 5-17 years) and inhalation anthrax, ciprofloxacin is contra-indicated in children and growing adolescents unless the benefits of treatment are considered to outweigh the risks.

4.4 Special warnings and special precautions for use

Ciprofloxacin should be used with caution in epileptics and patients with a history of CNS disorders and only if the benefits of treatment are considered to outweigh the risk of possible CNS side-effects. CNS side-effects have been reported after first administration of ciprofloxacin in some patients. Treatment should be discontinued if the side-effects, depression or psychoses lead to self-endangering behaviour (see also Section 4.8).

Crystalluria related to the use of ciprofloxacin has been reported. Patients receiving ciprofloxacin should be well hydrated and excessive alkalinity of the urine should be avoided.

Patients with a family history of or actual defects in glucose-6-phosphate dehydrogenase activity are prone to haemolytic reactions with quinolones, and so ciprofloxacin should be used with caution in these patients.

Tendon inflammation and rupture may occur with quinolone antibiotics. Such reactions have been observed particularly in older patients and in those treated concurrently with corticosteroids. At the first sign of pain or inflammation, patients should discontinue ciprofloxacin and rest the affected limbs.

There is a risk of pseudomembranous colitis with broad-spectrum antibiotics possibly leading to a fatal outcome. It is important to consider this in patients suffering from severe, persistent diarrhoea. With ciprofloxacin this effect has been reported rarely. If pseudomembranous colitis is suspected treatment with ciprofloxacin should be stopped and appropriate treatment given (e.g. oral vancomycin).

As with other quinolones, patients should avoid prolonged exposure to strong sunlight or UV radiation during treatment.

Laboratory tests may give abnormal findings if performed whilst patients are receiving ciprofloxacin e.g. increased alkaline phosphatase; increases in liver function tests e.g. transaminases and cholestatic jaundice, especially in patients with previous liver damage.

4.5 Interaction with other medicinal products and other forms of Interaction

Increased plasma levels of theophylline have been observed following concurrent administration with ciprofloxacin. It is recommended that the dose of theophylline should be reduced and plasma levels of theophylline monitored. The reaction between theophylline and ciprofloxacin is potentially life-threatening. Therefore, where monitoring of plasma levels is not possible, the use of ciprofloxacin should be avoided in patients receiving theophylline. Particular caution is advised in those patients with convulsive disorders.

Phenytoin levels may be altered when Ciproxin is used concomitantly.

Ciproxin Tablets should not be administered within four hours of multivalent cationic drugs and mineral supplements (e.g. calcium, magnesium, aluminium or iron), sucralfate or antacids and highly buffered drugs (e.g. didanosine) as interference with absorption may occur. When appropriate, patients should be advised not to self-medicate with preparations containing these compounds during therapy with ciprofloxacin. This restriction does not apply to the class of H2 receptor blocker drugs.

The concurrent administration of dairy products or fortified drinks alone (e.g. milk, yoghurt, calcium fortified orange juice) and ciprofloxacin should be avoided because absorption of ciprofloxacin may be reduced. However a normal diet, that will contain small amounts of calcium, does not significantly affect ciprofloxacin absorption.

Prolongation of bleeding time has been reported during concomitant administration of ciprofloxacin and oral anticoagulants.

Animal data have shown that high doses of quinolones in combination with some non-steroidal anti-inflammatory drugs, (e.g. fenbufen, but not acetylsalicylic acid) can lead to convulsions.

Transient increases in serum creatinine have been seen following concomitant administration of ciprofloxacin and cyclosporin. Therefore, monitoring of serum creatinine levels is advisable.

The simultaneous administration of quinolones and glibenclamide can on occasion potentiate the effect of glibenclamide resulting in hypoglycaemia.

Renal tubular transport of methotrexate may be inhibited by concomitant administration of ciprofloxacin potentially leading to increased plasma levels of methotrexate. This may increase the risk of methotrexate associated toxic reactions. Therefore, patients receiving methotrexate therapy should be carefully monitored when concomitant ciprofloxacin therapy is indicated.

Concomitant use with probenecid reduces the renal clearance of ciprofloxacin, resulting in increased quinolone plasma levels.

The use of metoclopramide with ciprofloxacin may accelerate the absorption of ciprofloxacin.

When ciprofloxacin is used for surgical prophylaxis, it is recommended that opiate premedicants, (e.g. papaveretum) or opiate premedicants used with anticholinergic premedicants, (e.g. atropine or hyoscine) are not used, as the serum levels of ciprofloxacin are reduced and adequate cover may not be obtained during surgery. Co-administration of ciprofloxacin and benzodiazepine premedicants has been shown not to affect ciprofloxacin plasma levels.

4.6 Pregnancy and lactation

Reproduction studies performed in mice, rats and rabbits using parenteral and oral administration did not reveal any evidence of teratogenicity, impairment of fertility or impairment of peri-/post-natal development. However, as with other quinolones, ciprofloxacin has been shown to cause arthropathy in immature animals, and therefore its use during pregnancy is not recommended. Studies have indicated that ciprofloxacin is secreted in breast milk. Administration to nursing mothers is thus not recommended.

4.7 Effects on ability to drive and use machines

Ciprofloxacin could result in impairment of the patient's ability to drive or operate machinery, particularly in conjunction with alcohol.

4.8 Undesirable effects

Ciprofloxacin is generally well tolerated. The most frequently reported adverse reactions are nausea, diarrhoea and rash.

The following adverse reactions have been observed:

Hypersensitivity/skin, e.g. rash, pruritus, urticaria, photosensitivity, drug-induced fever, anaphylactic/anaphylactoid reactions including angioedema and dyspnoea. Rarely, erythema nodosum and erythema multiforme. Very rarely, petechiae, haemorrhagic bullae, vasculitis, serum sickness-like reaction, fixed drug reactions, Stevens-Johnson Syndrome and Lyells Syndrome. Treatment with ciprofloxacin should be discontinued if any of the above occur upon first administration.

General, e.g. moniliasis, asthenia, hyperglycaemia and abnormal gait, pain, pain in extremeties, back pain, chest pain. Thrombophlebitis.

CNS, e.g. headache, restlessness, depression, dizziness, tremor, convulsions, confusion, hallucinations, somnolence, sleep disorders, insomnia. Rarely, hypesthesia. Very rarely, migraine, hyperesthesia, ataxia, hypertonia, twitching or anxiety states. Isolated cases of ciprofloxacin-induced psychoses have been reported, which may progress to self-endangering behaviour. There are isolated reports of intracranial hypertension associated with quinolone therapy. Paraesthesia has been reported.

Gastro-intestinal, e.g. nausea, diarrhoea, vomiting, dyspepsia, abdominal pain, anorexia, flatulence, dysphagia. Rarely, pancreatitis or pseudomembranous colitis.

Cardiovascular, e.g. tachycardia, oedema, fainting, hot flushes, hypotension and sweating.

Effects on haematological parameters, e.g. anaemia, eosinophilia, increases or decreases in white cell and/or platelet count, altered prothrombin levels, and, very rarely, haemolytic anaemia, agranulocytosis, pancytopenia or bone marrow depression. Pancytopenia and bone marrow depression may be potentially life-threatening.

Hepatic, e.g. transient increases in liver enzymes or serum bilirubin (particularly in patients with previous liver damage), hepatitis, jaundice/cholestasis and major liver disorders including hepatic necrosis, which may rarely progress to life-threatening hepatic failure.

Renal, e.g. transient increases in blood urea or serum creatinine, renal failure, crystalluria, haematuria, nephritis.

Musculoskeletal, e.g. reversible arthralgia, joint swelling and myalgia. Rarely, myasthenia or tenosynovitis. Tendon inflammation (predominantly of the Achilles tendon) has been reported which may lead to tendon rupture. Treatment should be discontinued immediately if these symptoms occur.

Rarely, exacerbation of the symptoms of myasthenia gravis have been reported.

Special senses, e.g. very rarely, visual disturbances including diplopia and colour disturbances, impaired taste and smell usually reversible upon discontinuation of treatment, tinnitus, transient impairment of hearing particularly at high frequencies.

Abnormal laboratory findings, e.g. increased alkaline phosphatase, amylase and lipase; increases in liver function tests, e.g transaminases, and cholestatic jaundice, especially in patients with previous liver damage.

4.9 Overdose

Based on the limited information available in two cases of ingestion of over 18g of ciprofloxacin, reversible renal toxicity has occurred. Therefore, apart from routine emergency measures, it is recommended to monitor renal function, including urinary pH and acidify, if required, to prevent crystalluria. Patients must be kept well hydrated, and in the case of renal damage resulting in prolonged oliguria, dialysis should be initiated.

Calcium or magnesium antacids may be administered as soon as possible after ingestion of Ciproxin tablets in order to reduce the absorption of ciprofloxacin.

Serum levels of ciprofloxacin are reduced by dialysis.

5. PHARMACOLOGICAL PROPERTIES

ATC Code J01 MA 02

5.1 Pharmacodynamic properties

Ciprofloxacin is a synthetic 4-quinolone derivative, with bactericidal activity. It acts via inhibition of bacterial DNA gyrase, ultimately resulting in interference with DNA function. Ciprofloxacin is highly active against a wide range of Gram-positive and Gram-negative organisms and has shown activity against some anaerobes, *Chlamydia* spp. and *Mycoplasma* spp. Killing curves demonstrate the rapid bactericidal effect against sensitive organisms and it is often found that minimum bactericidal concentrations are in the range of minimum inhibitory concentrations. Ciprofloxacin has been shown to have no activity against *Treponema pallidum* and *Ureaplasma urealyticum*. *Nocardia asteroides* and *Enterococcus faecium* are resistant.

Breakpoints

S $\leqslant 1\ \mu g/ml$, R $\geqslant 4\ \mu g/ml$

Susceptibility

The prevalence of resistance may vary geographically and with time for selected species and local area information on resistance is desirable, particularly when treating severe infections. This information gives only an approximate guidance on probabilities whether micro-organisms will be susceptible to ciprofloxacin or not.

Organism	Prevalence of Resistance
Sensitive:	
Gram-positive bacteria	
Corynebacterium diphtheriae	0%
Corynebacterium spp.	-
Staphylococcus aureus (methicillin sensitive)	0 - 14%
Staphylococcus aureus (methicillin resistant)	48 - 90%
Streptococcus agalactiae	0 – 17%
Bacillus anthracis	-
Gram-negative bacteria	
Acinetobacter baumanii	6 - 93%
Acinetobacter spp.	14 – 70%
Aeromonas hydrophilia	0%
Aeromonas spp.	-
Bordetella pertussis	0%
Brucella melitensis	0%
Campylobacter jejuni/coli	0 – 82%
Campylobacter spp.	0%
Citrobacter freundii	0 – 4%
Citrobacter spp.	0%
Edwardsiella tarda	0%
Enterobacter aerogenes	0%
Enterobacter cloacae	0 - 3%
Enterobacter spp.	3 - 13%
Escherichia coli	2 -7%
Escherichia coli, EHEC and EPEC	-
Haemophilus influenzae	0 – 1%
Haemophilus influenzae (β-lactam negative)	0%
Haemophilus influenzae (β-lactam positive)	0%
Haemophilus parainfluenzae	0%
Hafnia alvei	0%
Klebsiella oxytoca	0%
Klebsiella pneumoniae	2 – 5.8%
Klebsiella spp.	2 – 21%
Legionella pneumophila	0%
Legionella spp.	0%
Moraxella catarrhalis	0%
Morganella morganii	1 – 2%
Neisseria gonorrhoeae	0%
Neisseria gonorrhoeae, β-lactamase	0%
Neisseria gonorrhoeae, β-lactamase positive	0%
Neisseria meningitidis	0%
Neisseria meningitidis, β-lactamase negative	0%
Plesiomonas shigelloides	0%
Proteus mirabilis	0 – 10%
Proteus vulgaris	4%
Providencia rettgeri	-
Providencia spp.	4%
Providencia stuartii	-
Pseudomonas aeruginosa	1 – 28%
Salmonella spp.	0%
Salmonella typhi	0 - 2%
Serratia liquefaciens	
Serratia marcescens	23%
Serratia spp.	0 – 21%
Shigella spp.	0%
Vibrio cholerae	0%
Vibrio parahaemolyticus	0%
Vibrio spp.	0%
Yersinia enterocolitica	0%
Anaerobes	
Bacteroides ureolyticus	0%
Clostridium perfringens	-
Peptococcus spp.	0%
Peptostreptococcus spp.	-
Peptostreptococcus magnus	0%
Veillonella parvula	0%
Other pathogens	
Chlamydia spp.	-
Helicobacter pylori	-
Mycobacterium fortuitum	0%
Mycobacterium tuberculosis	0%
Mycoplasma hominis	16%
Intermediate	
Gram-positive aerobes	
Enterococci	5%
Enterococcus faecalis	9 – 34%
Staphylococcus epidermis, methicillin sensitive	10 - 16%
Staphylococcus epidermis, methicillin resistant	26 - 56%
Staphylococcus haemolyticus	-
Staphylococcus haemolyticus, methicillin sensitive	8%
Staphylococcus haemolyticus, methicillin resistant	73%
Streptococcus anginosus	9%
Streptococcus bovis	-
Streptococcus milleri	5%
Streptococcus mitis	-
Streptococcus pneumoniae, penicillin sensitive	0 – 1%
Streptococcus pneumoniae, penicillin intermediate	-
Streptococcus pneumoniae, penicillin intermediate and resistant	2.8%
Streptococcus pneumoniae, penicillin resistant	-
Streptococcus pyogenes	0 - 28%
Streptococcus, viridans group	-
Streptococcus viridans, penicillin sensitive	-
Streptococcus viridans, penicillin resistant	-
Streptococcus, b-haemolytic groups A, C, and G	0%
Gram-negative aerobes	
Alcaligenes spp.	-
Listeria monocytogenes	0%
Listeria spp.	0%
Anaerobes	
Fusobacterium spp.	-
Gardnerella vaginalis	0%
Prevotella spp.	-
Other pathogens	
Ureaplasma urealyticum	11%
Resistant	
Gram-positive aerobes	
Enterococcus faecium	-
Stenotrophomonas maltophilia	94%
Streptococcus sanguis	-
Gram-negative aerobes	
Flavobacterium meningosepticum	-
Nocardia asteroides	-
Anaerobes	
Bacteroides fragilis	-
Bacteroides thetaiotaomicron	-
Clostridium difficile	-

Plasmid-related transfer of resistance has not been observed with ciprofloxacin and the overall frequency of development of resistance is low (10^{-9} - 10^{-7}). Cross-resistance to penicillins, cephalosporins, aminoglycosides and tetracyclines has not been observed and organisms resistant to these antibiotics are generally sensitive to ciprofloxacin. Ciprofloxacin is also suitable for use in combination with these antibiotics, and additive behaviour is usually observed.

5.2 Pharmacokinetic properties

Absorption of oral doses of ciprofloxacin tablet formulation occurs rapidly, mainly from the small intestine, the half-life of absorption being 2-15 minutes. Plasma levels are dose-related and peak 0.5-2.0 hours after dosing. The AUC also increases dose proportionately after administration of both single and repeated oral (tablet) and intravenous doses. The absolute bioavailability is reported to be 52-83% and ciprofloxacin is subject to only slight first pass metabolism. The oral bioavailability is approximately 70-80%.

The intake of food at the same time as administration of oral ciprofloxacin has a marginal but clinically not relevant effect on the pharmacokinetic parameters C_{max} and AUC. No specific recommendations are necessary with regard to time of administration of oral ciprofloxacin relative to food intake.

Distribution of ciprofloxacin within tissues is wide and the volume of distribution high, though slightly lower in the elderly. Protein binding is low (between 19-40%).

Only 10-20% of a single oral or intravenous dose is eliminated as metabolites (which exhibit lower activity than the parent drug). Four different antimicrobially active metabolites have been reported, desethyleneciprofloxacin (M1), sulphociprofloxacin (M2), oxaciprofloxacin (M3) and formylciprofloxacin (M4). M2 and M3 account for one third each of metabolised substance and M1 is found in small amounts (1.3-2.6% of the dose). M4 has been found in very small quantities (<0.1% of the dose). M1-M3 have antimicrobial activity comparable to nalidixic acid and M4 found in the smallest quantity has antimicrobial activity similar to that of norfloxacin.

Elimination of ciprofloxacin and its metabolites occurs rapidly, primarily by the kidney. After single oral and intravenous doses of ciprofloxacin, 55% and 75% respectively are eliminated by the kidney and 39% and 14% in the faeces within 5 days. Renal elimination takes place mainly during the first 12 hours after dosing and renal clearance levels suggest that active secretion by the renal tubules occurs in addition to normal glomerular filtration. Renal clearance is between 0.18 – 0.3 l/h.kg and total body clearance between 0.48 – 0.60 l/h.kg. Approximately 1% of a ciprofloxacin dose is excreted via the biliary route. The elimination kinetics are linear and after repeated dosing at 12 hourly intervals, no further accumulation is detected after the distribution equilibrium is attained (at 4-5 half-lives). The elimination half-life of unchanged ciprofloxacin over a period of 24-48 hours post-dose is 3.1-5.1 hours.

Some studies carried out with ciprofloxacin in severely renally impaired patients (serum creatinine >265 micromole/l or creatinine clearance <20ml/minute) demonstrated either a doubling of the elimination half-life, or fluctuations in half-life in comparison with healthy volunteers, whereas other studies showed no significant correlation between elimination half-life and creatinine clearance. However, it is recommended that in severely renally impaired patients, the total daily dose should be reduced by half, although monitoring of drug serum levels provides the most reliable basis for dose adjustment as necessary.

Results of pharmacokinetic studies in paediatric cystic fibrosis patients have shown dosages of 20mg/kg orally twice daily or 10mg/kg iv three times daily are recommended to achieve plasma concentration/time profiles comparable to those achieved in the adult population at the currently recommended dosage regimen.

Inhalation anthrax: Ciprofloxacin serum concentrations achieved in humans serve as a surrogate endpoint reasonably likely to predict clinical benefit and provide the basis for the recommended doses.

5.3 Preclinical safety data

Following extensive oral and intravenous toxicology testing with ciprofloxacin, only two findings which may be considered relevant to the use of ciprofloxacin in man were observed. Crystalluria was noted in those species of animals which had a normally alkaline urine. Kidney damage without the presence of crystalluria was not observed. This effect is considered a secondary inflammatory foreign-body reaction, due to the precipitation of a crystalline complex of ciprofloxacin, magnesium and protein in the distal tubule system of the kidneys. This is considered not to be a problem in man, because the urine is normally acidic. However, to avoid the occurrence of crystalluria, patients should be well hydrated and excessive alkalinity of the urine avoided.

As with other quinolones, damage to the weight-bearing joints of only juvenile rats and dogs treated with ciprofloxacin was noted in repeat dose toxicity testing. This was more noticeable in the dog. Although analysis of available safety data from ciprofloxacin use in paediatric patients did not disclose any evidence of drug related cartilage or articular damage, the use of ciprofloxacin in children and growing adolescents is generally not recommended, unless the benefits are considered to outweigh the potential risks (with the exception of treatment of cystic fibrosis). Additionally, because of the potential of arthropathy, the use of ciprofloxacin during pregnancy and lactation is not recommended.

6. PHARMACEUTICAL PARTICULARS

6.1 List of excipients

Each tablet contains microcrystalline cellulose, maize starch, crospovidone, colloidal silicon dioxide, magnesium stearate and purified water. The tablet film-coat consists of a mixture of hypromellose, Macrogol 4000, titanium dioxide and purified water.

6.2 Incompatibilities

None known.

6.3 Shelf life

5 years.

6.4 Special precautions for storage

No special storage precautions are necessary.

6.5 Nature and contents of container

Blister strips in cardboard outers comprising:

a) 250μm, 40g/m^2 PVC/PVDC foil with 20μm hard aluminium backing foil.

Pack sizes 10, 20, 100 tablets.

b) 300μm polypropylene foil with 20μm hard aluminium backing foil with a 3.5g/m^2

heat seal polypropylene coating.

Pack sizes: 10, 20, 100 tablets.

c) 130μm PA/aluminium/PVC foil with 20μm hard aluminium backing foil.

Pack size: 2 tablets (sample pack).

6.6 Instructions for use and handling

Not applicable.

7. MARKETING AUTHORISATION HOLDER

Bayer plc Bayer House Strawberry Hill Newbury Berkshire RG14 1JA	Trading as: Bayer plc Pharmaceutical Division Bayer House Strawberry Hill Newbury Berkshire RG14 1JA Or BAYPHARM or BAYMET

8. MARKETING AUTHORISATION NUMBER(S)

PL 0010/0147

9. DATE OF FIRST AUTHORISATION/RENEWAL OF THE AUTHORISATION

3 February 1987/25 February 1999

10. DATE OF REVISION OF THE TEXT

June 2003

Ciproxin Tablets 750mg

(Bayer plc)

1. NAME OF THE MEDICINAL PRODUCT

Ciproxin Tablets 750mg

2. QUALITATIVE AND QUANTITATIVE COMPOSITION

Each tablet contains 873.0mg ciprofloxacin hydrochloride equivalent to 750mg Ciprofloxacin (INN).

3. PHARMACEUTICAL FORM

Immediate release film-coated tablet for oral administration.

4. CLINICAL PARTICULARS

4.1 Therapeutic indications

Ciprofloxacin is indicated for the treatment of the following infections caused by sensitive bacteria:

Adults:

Respiratory tract infections: e.g. lobar and bronchopneumonia, acute and chronic bronchitis, acute exacerbation of cystic fibrosis, bronchiectasis, empyema. Ciprofloxacin is not recommended as first-line therapy for the treatment of pneumococcal pneumonia. Ciprofloxacin may be used for treating Gram-negative pneumonia.

Ear, nose and throat infections: e.g. mastoiditis, otitis media and sinusitis, especially if due to Gram-negative bacteria (including *Pseudomonas* spp.). Ciprofloxacin is not recommended for the treatment of acute tonsillitis.

Eye infections: e.g. bacterial conjunctivitis.

Urinary tract infections: e.g. uncomplicated and complicated urethritis, cystitis, pyelonephritis, prostatitis, epididymitis.

Skin and soft tissue infections: e.g. infected ulcers, wound infections, abscesses, cellulitis, otitis externa, erysipelas, infected burns.

Bone and joint infections: e.g. osteomyelitis, septic arthritis.

Intra-abdominal infections: e.g. peritonitis, intra-abdominal abscesses.

Infections of the biliary tract: e.g. cholangitis, cholecystitis, empyema of the gall bladder.

Gastro-intestinal infections: e.g. enteric fever, infective diarrhoea.

Pelvic infections: e.g. salpingitis, endometritis, pelvic inflammatory disease.

Severe systemic infections: e.g. septicaemia, bacteraemia, peritonitis, infections in immuno-suppressed patients.

Gonorrhoea: including urethral, rectal and pharyngeal gonorrhoea caused by β-lactamase producing organisms or organisms moderately sensitive to penicillin.

Ciprofloxacin is also indicated for prophylaxis against infection in elective upper gastro-intestinal tract surgery and endoscopic procedures, where there is an increased risk of infection.

Children:

For the treatment of acute pulmonary exacerbation of cystic fibrosis associated with *P. aeruginosa* infection in paediatric patients aged 5-17 years.

Inhalation Anthrax in Adults and Children: To reduce the incidence or progression of disease following confirmed or suspected exposure to aerosolised *Bacillus anthracis*.

4.2 Posology and method of administration

General dosage recommendations: The dosage of Ciproxin tablets is determined by the severity and type of infection, the sensitivity of the causative organism(s) and the age, weight and renal function of the patient. Ciproxin tablets should be swallowed whole with an adequate amount of liquid.

If Ciproxin Tablets are taken on an empty stomach, the active substance is absorbed more rapidly. In this case, the tablets should not be taken concurrently with dairy products or with mineral fortified drinks alone (e.g. milk, yoghurt, calcium fortified orange juice). However, a normal diet that will contain small amounts of calcium, does not significantly affect ciprofloxacin absorption.

Adults

The dosage range for adults is 100-750mg twice daily. The following dosages for specific types of infection are recommended:

Table 1: Recommended Adult Dosage

Indication	Dosage (mg ciprofloxacin)
Treatment	
Gonorrhoea	250mg single dose
Acute, uncomplicated cystitis	100mg b.d.
Upper and lower urinary tract infections (depending on severity)	250-500mg b.d.
Upper and lower respiratory tract infections (depending on severity)	250-750mg b.d.
Pneumococcal pneumonia (second-line)	750mg b.d.
Cystic fibrosis patients with pseudomonal lower RTI*	750mg b.d.
Other infections as detailed under 4.1	500-750mg b.d.
Severe infections, particularly due to Pseudomonas, staphylococci and streptococci	750mg b.d.
Inhalation Anthrax	500mg b.d.
Prophylaxis	
Elective upper gastro-intestinal surgical and endoscopic procedures	750mg single dose 60-90 minutes prior to the procedure**. If gastro-oesophageal obstructive lesions are suspected use with an anti-infective effective against anaerobes

* Although the pharmacokinetics of ciprofloxacin remains unchanged in patients with cystic fibrosis, the low body-weight of these patients should be taken into consideration when determining dosage.

** The tablet may be given with an oral pre-medicant, but see Section 4.5

Impaired Renal Function

Dosage adjustments are not usually required, except in patients with severe renal impairment (serum creatinine >265 micromole/l or creatinine clearance <20ml/minute). If adjustment is necessary, this may be achieved by reducing the total daily dose by half, although monitoring of drug serum levels provides the most reliable basis for dose adjustment.

Impaired Hepatic Function

No adjustment of dosage is necessary.

Elderly

Although higher ciprofloxacin serum levels are found in the elderly, no adjustment of dosage is necessary.

Adolescents and children

As with other drugs in its class, ciprofloxacin has been shown to cause arthropathy in weight-bearing joints of immature animals. Although analysis of available safety data from ciprofloxacin use in patients less than 18 years of age, the majority of whom had cystic fibrosis, did not disclose any evidence of drug-related cartilage or articular damage, its use in the paediatric population is generally not recommended.

Clinical and pharmacokinetic data support the use of ciprofloxacin in paediatric cystic fibrosis patients (aged 5 - 17 years) with acute pulmonary exacerbations associated with *P. aeruginosa* infection, at a dose of 20mg/kg orally twice daily (maximum daily dose 1500mg).

For the indication of inhalation anthrax, the risk-benefit assessment indicates that administration of ciprofloxacin to paediatric patients at a dose of 15 mg/kg orally twice daily (maximum daily dose of 1000 mg) is appropriate.

For indications other than treatment of pulmonary exacerbations in cystic fibrosis and inhalation anthrax, ciprofloxacin may be used in children and adolescents where the benefit is considered to outweigh the potential risks. In these cases a dosage of 5-15mg/kg orally twice daily should be administered depending upon the severity of infection.

Dosing in children with impaired renal and/or hepatic function has not been studied.

Duration of Treatment

The duration of treatment depends upon the severity of infection, clinical response and bacteriological findings.

In acute, uncomplicated cystitis the treatment period is three days.

In other acute infections the usual treatment period is 5-10 days. Generally, acute and chronic infections (e.g. osteomyelitis and prostatitis, etc), where the causative organism is known to be sensitive to ciprofloxacin, should be treated for at least three days after the signs and symptoms of the infection have disappeared.

For acute pulmonary exacerbations of cystic fibrosis associated with *P. aeruginosa* infection in paediatric patients (aged 5-17 years), the duration of treatment is 10 - 14 days.

For inhalation anthrax, drug administration should begin as soon as possible after confirmed or suspected exposure and should be continued for 60 days.

4.3 Contraindications

Ciprofloxacin is contra-indicated in patients who have shown hypersensitivity to ciprofloxacin or other quinolone anti-infectives.

Except in cases of exacerbations of cystic fibrosis associated with *P. aeruginosa* (in patients aged 5-17 years) and inhalation anthrax, ciprofloxacin is contra-indicated in children and growing adolescents unless the benefits of treatment are considered to outweigh the risks.

4.4 Special warnings and special precautions for use

Ciprofloxacin should be used with caution in epileptics and patients with a history of CNS disorders and only if the benefits of treatment are considered to outweigh the risk of possible CNS side-effects. CNS side-effects have been reported after first administration of ciprofloxacin in some patients. Treatment should be discontinued if the side-effects, depression or psychoses lead to self-endangering behaviour (see also Section 4.8).

Crystalluria related to the use of ciprofloxacin has been reported. Patients receiving ciprofloxacin should be well hydrated and excessive alkalinity of the urine should be avoided.

Patients with a family history of or actual defects in glucose-6-phosphate dehydrogenase activity are prone to haemolytic reactions with quinolones, and so ciprofloxacin should be used with caution in these patients.

Tendon inflammation and rupture may occur with quinolone antibiotics. Such reactions have been observed particularly in older patients and in those treated concurrently with corticosteroids. At the first sign of pain or inflammation, patients should discontinue ciprofloxacin and rest the affected limbs.

There is a risk of pseudomembranous colitis with broad-spectrum antibiotics possibly leading to a fatal outcome. It is important to consider this in patients suffering from severe, persistent diarrhoea. With ciprofloxacin this effect has been reported rarely. If pseudomembranous colitis is suspected treatment with ciprofloxacin should be stopped and appropriate treatment given (e.g. oral vancomycin).

As with other quinolones, patients should avoid prolonged exposure to strong sunlight or UV radiation during treatment.

Laboratory tests may give abnormal findings if performed whilst patients are receiving ciprofloxacin e.g. increased alkaline phosphatase; increases in liver function tests e.g. transaminases and cholestatic jaundice, especially in patients with previous liver damage.

4.5 Interaction with other medicinal products and other forms of Interaction

Increased plasma levels of theophylline have been observed following concurrent administration with ciprofloxacin. It is recommended that the dose of theophylline should be reduced and plasma levels of theophylline monitored. The reaction between theophylline and ciprofloxacin is potentially life-threatening. Therefore, where monitoring of plasma levels is not possible, the use of ciprofloxacin should be avoided in patients receiving theophylline. Particular caution is advised in those patients with convulsive disorders.

Phenytoin levels may be altered when Ciproxin is used concomitantly.

Ciproxin Tablets should not be administered within four hours multivalent cationic drugs and mineral supplements (e.g. calcium, magnesium, aluminium or iron), sucralfate or antacids and highly buffered drugs (e.g. didanosine) as interference with absorption may occur. When appropriate, patients should be advised not to self-medicate with preparations containing these compounds during therapy with ciprofloxacin. This restriction does not apply to the class of H2 receptor blocker drugs.

The concurrent administration of dairy products or fortified drinks alone (e.g. milk, yoghurt, calcium fortified orange juice) and ciprofloxacin should be avoided because absorption of ciprofloxacin may be reduced. However a normal diet, that will contain small amounts of calcium, does not significantly affect ciprofloxacin absorption.

Prolongation of bleeding time has been reported during concomitant administration of ciprofloxacin and oral anticoagulants.

Animal data have shown that high doses of quinolones in combination with some non-steroidal anti-inflammatory drugs, (e.g. fenbufen, but not acetylsalicylic acid) can lead to convulsions.

Transient increases in serum creatinine have been seen following concomitant administration of ciprofloxacin and cyclosporin. Therefore, monitoring of serum creatinine levels is advisable.

The simultaneous administration of quinolones and glibenclamide can on occasion potentiate the effect of glibenclamide resulting in hypoglycaemia.

Renal tubular transport of methotrexate may be inhibited by concomitant administration of ciprofloxacin potentially leading to increased plasma levels of methotrexate. This may increase the risk of methotrexate associated toxic reactions. Therefore, patients receiving methotrexate therapy should be carefully monitored when concomitant ciprofloxacin therapy is indicated.

Concomitant use with probenecid reduces the renal clearance of ciprofloxacin, resulting in increased quinolone plasma levels.

The use of metoclopramide with ciprofloxacin may accelerate the absorption of ciprofloxacin.

When ciprofloxacin is used for surgical prophylaxis, it is recommended that opiate premedicants, (e.g. papaveretum) or opiate premedicants used with anticholinergic premedicants, (e.g. atropine or hyoscine) are not used, as the serum levels of ciprofloxacin are reduced and adequate cover may not be obtained during surgery. Co-administration of ciprofloxacin and benzodiazepine premedicants has been shown not to affect ciprofloxacin plasma levels.

4.6 Pregnancy and lactation

Reproduction studies performed in mice, rats and rabbits using parenteral and oral administration did not reveal any evidence of teratogenicity, impairment of fertility or impairment of peri-/post-natal development. However, as with other quinolones, ciprofloxacin has been shown to cause arthropathy in immature animals, and therefore its use during pregnancy is not recommended. Studies have indicated that ciprofloxacin is secreted in breast milk. Administration to nursing mothers is thus not recommended.

4.7 Effects on ability to drive and use machines

Ciprofloxacin could result in impairment of the patient's ability to drive or operate machinery, particularly in conjunction with alcohol.

4.8 Undesirable effects

Ciprofloxacin is generally well tolerated. The most frequently reported adverse reactions are nausea, diarrhoea and rash.

The following adverse reactions have been observed:

Hypersensitivity/skin, e.g. rash, pruritus, urticaria, photosensitivity, drug-induced fever, anaphylactic/anaphylactoid reactions including angioedema and dyspnoea. Rarely, erythema nodosum and erythema multiforme. Very rarely, petechiae, haemorrhagic bullae, vasculitis, serum sickness-like reaction, fixed drug reactions, Stevens-Johnson Syndrome and Lyells Syndrome. Treatment with ciprofloxacin should be discontinued if any of the above occur upon first administration.

General, e.g. moniliasis, asthenia, hyperglycaemia and abnormal gait pain, pain in extremeties, back pain, chest pain. Thrombophlebitis.

CNS, e.g. headache, restlessness, depression, dizziness, tremor, convulsions, confusion, hallucinations, somnolence, sleep disorders, insomnia. Rarely, hypesthesia. Very rarely, migraine, hyperesthesia, ataxia, hypertonia, twitching or anxiety states. Isolated cases of ciprofloxacin-induced psychoses have been reported, which may progress to self-endangering behaviour. There are isolated reports of intracranial hypertension associated with quinolone therapy. Paraesthesia has been reported.

Gastro-intestinal, e.g. nausea, diarrhoea, vomiting, dyspepsia, abdominal pain, anorexia, flatulence, dysphagia. Rarely, pancreatitis or pseudomembranous colitis.

Cardiovascular, e.g. tachycardia, oedema, fainting, hot flushes, hypotension and sweating.

Effects on haematological parameters, e.g. anaemia, eosinophilia, increases or decreases in white cell and/or platelet count, altered prothrombin levels, and, very rarely, haemolytic anaemia, agranulocytosis, pancytopenia or bone marrow depression. Pancytopenia and bone marrow depression may be potentially life-threatening.

Hepatic, e.g. transient increases in liver enzymes or serum bilirubin (particularly in patients with previous liver damage), hepatitis, jaundice/cholestasis and major liver disorders including hepatic necrosis, which may rarely progress to life-threatening hepatic failure.

Renal, e.g. transient increases in blood urea or serum creatinine, renal failure, crystalluria, haematuria, nephritis.

Musculoskeletal, e.g. reversible arthralgia, joint swelling and myalgia. Rarely, myasthenia or tenosynovitis. Tendon inflammation (predominantly of the achilles tendon) has been reported which may lead to tendon rupture. Treatment should be discontinued immediately if these symptoms occur.

Rarely, exacerbation of the symptoms of myasthenia gravis have been reported.

Special senses, e.g. very rarely, visual disturbances including diplopia and colour disturbances, impaired taste and smell usually reversible upon discontinuation of treatment, tinnitus, transient impairment of hearing particularly at high frequencies.

Abnormal laboratory findings, e.g. increased alkaline phosphatase, amylase and lipase; increases in liver function tests, e.g transaminases, and cholestatic jaundice, especially in patients with previous liver damage.

4.9 Overdose

Based on the limited information available in two cases of ingestion of over 18g of ciprofloxacin, reversible renal toxicity has occurred. Therefore, apart from routine emergency measures, it is recommended to monitor renal function, including urinary pH and acidify, if required, to prevent crystalluria. Patients must be kept well hydrated, and in the case of renal damage resulting in prolonged oliguria, dialysis should be initiated.

Calcium or magnesium antacids may be administered as soon as possible after ingestion of Ciproxin tablets in order to reduce the absorption of ciprofloxacin.

Serum levels of ciprofloxacin are reduced by dialysis.

5. PHARMACOLOGICAL PROPERTIES

ATC Code J01 MA 02

5.1 Pharmacodynamic properties

Ciprofloxacin is a synthetic 4-quinolone derivative, with bactericidal activity. It acts via inhibition of bacterial DNA gyrase, ultimately resulting in interference with DNA function. Ciprofloxacin is highly active against a wide range of Gram-positive and Gram-negative organisms and has shown activity against some anaerobes, *Chlamydia* spp. and *Mycoplasma* spp. Killing curves demonstrate the rapid bactericidal effect against sensitive organisms and it is often found that minimum bactericidal concentrations are in the range of minimum inhibitory concentrations. Ciprofloxacin has been shown to have no activity against *Treponema pallidum* and *Ureaplasma urealyticum. Nocardia asteroides* and *Enterococcus faecium* are resistant.

Breakpoints

S $\leqslant$ 1 μg/ml, R $\geqslant$ 4 μg/ml

Susceptibility

The prevalence of resistance may vary geographically and with time for selected species and local area information on resistance is desirable, particularly when treating severe infections. This information gives only an approximate guidance on probabilities whether micro-organisms will be susceptible to ciprofloxacin or not.

Organism	Prevalence of Resistance
Sensitive:	
Gram-positive bacteria	
Corynebacterium diphtheriae	0%
Corynebacterium spp.	-
Staphylococcus aureus (methicillin sensitive)	0 - 14%

Staphylococcus aureus (methicillin resistant)	48 - 90%
Streptococcus agalactiae	0 – 17%
Bacillus anthracis	-
Gram-negative bacteria	
Acinetobacter baumanii	6 - 93%
Acinetobacter spp.	14 – 70%
Aeromonas hydrophilia	0%
Aeromonas spp.	-
Bordetella pertussis	0%
Brucella melitensis	0%
Campylobacter jejuni/coli	0 – 82%
Campylobacter spp.	0%
Citrobacter freundii	0 – 4%
Citrobacter spp.	0%
Edwardsiella tarda	0%
Enterobacter aerogenes	0%
Enterobacter cloacae	0 - 3%
Enterobacter spp.	3 - 13%
Escherichia coli	2 -7%
Escherichia coli, EHEC and EPEC	-
Haemophilus influenzae	0 – 1%
Haemophilus influenzae (b-lactam negative)	0%
Haemophilus influenzae (b-lactam positive)	0%
Haemophilus parainfluenzae	0%
Hafnia alvei	0%
Klebsiella oxytoca	0%
Klebsiella pneumoniae	2 – 5.8%
Klebsiella spp.	2 – 21%
Legionella pneumophila	0%
Legionella spp.	0%
Moraxella catarrhalis	0%
Morganella morganii	1 – 2%
Neisseria gonorrhoeae	0%
Neisseria gonorrhoeae, β-lactamase	0%
Neisseria gonorrhoeae, β-lactamase positive	0%
Neisseria meningitidis	0%
Neisseria meningitidis, β-lactamase negative	0%
Plesiomonas shigelloides	0%
Proteus mirabilis	0 – 10%
Proteus vulgaris	4%
Providencia rettgeri	-
Providencia spp.	4%
Providencia stuartii	-
Pseudomonas aeruginosa	1 – 28%
Salmonella spp.	0%
Salmonella typhi	0 - 2%
Serratia liquefaciens	-
Serratia marcescens	23%
Serratia spp.	0 – 21%
Shigella spp.	0%
Vibrio cholerae	0%
Vibrio parahaemolyticus	0%
Vibrio spp.	0%
Yersinia enterocolitica	0%
Anaerobes	
Bacteroides ureolyticus	0%
Clostridium perfringens	-
Peptococcus spp.	0%
Peptostreptococcus spp.	-
Peptostreptococcus magnus	0%
Veillonella parvula	0%
Other pathogens	
Chlamydia spp.	-
Helicobacter pylori	-
Mycobacterium fortuitum	0%
Mycobacterium tuberculosis	0%
Mycoplasma hominis	16%
Intermediate	
Gram-positive aerobes	
Enterococci	5%
Enterococcus faecalis	9 - 34%
Staphylococcus epidermis, methicillin sensitive	10 - 16%
Staphylococcus epidermis, methicillin resistant	26 - 56%
Staphylococcus haemolyticus	-
Staphylococcus haemolyticus, methicillin sensitive	8%
Staphylococcus haemolyticus, methicillin resistant	73%
Streptococcus anginosus	9%
Streptococcus bovis	-
Streptococcus milleri	5%
Streptococcus mitis	-
Streptococcus pneumoniae, penicillin sensitive	0 – 1%
Streptococcus pneumoniae, penicillin intermediate	-
Streptococcus pneumoniae, penicillin intermediate and resistant	2.8%
Streptococcus pneumoniae, penicillin resistant	-
Streptococcus pyogenes	0 - 28%
Streptococcus, viridans group	-
Streptococcus viridans, penicillin sensitive	-
Streptococcus viridans, penicillin resistant	-
Streptococcus, β-haemolytic groups A, C, and G	0%
Gram-negative aerobes	
Alcaligenes spp.	-
Listeria monocytogenes	0%
Listeria spp.	0%
Anaerobes	
Fusobacterium spp.	-
Gardnerella vaginalis	0%
Prevotella spp.	-
Other pathogens	
Ureaplasma urealyticum	11%
Resistant	
Gram-positive aerobes	
Enterococcus faecium	-
Stenotrophomonas maltophilia	94%
Streptococcus sanguis	-
Gram-negative aerobes	
Flavobacterium meningosepticum	-
Nocardia asteroides	-
Anaerobes	
Bacteroides fragilis	-
Bacteroides thetaiotaomicron	-
Clostridium difficile	-

Plasmid-related transfer of resistance has not been observed with ciprofloxacin and the overall frequency of development of resistance is low (10^{-9} - 10^{-7}). Cross-resistance to penicillins, cephalosporins, aminoglycosides and tetracyclines has not been observed and organisms resistant to these antibiotics are generally sensitive to ciprofloxacin. Ciprofloxacin is also suitable for use in combination with these antibiotics, and additive behaviour is usually observed.

5.2 Pharmacokinetic properties

Absorption of oral doses of ciprofloxacin tablet formulation occurs rapidly, mainly from the small intestine, the half-life of absorption being 2-15 minutes. Plasma levels are dose-related and peak 0.5-2.0 hours after dosing. The AUC also increases dose proportionately after administration of both single and repeated oral (tablet) and intravenous doses. The absolute bioavailability is reported to be 52-83% and ciprofloxacin is subject to only slight first pass metabolism. The oral bioavailability is approximately 70-80%.

The intake of food at the same time as administration of oral ciprofloxacin has a marginal but clinically not relevant effect on the pharmacokinetic parameters C_{max} and AUC. No specific recommendations are necessary with regard to time of administration of oral ciprofloxacin relative to food intake.

Distribution of ciprofloxacin within tissues is wide and the volume of distribution high, though slightly lower in the elderly. Protein binding is low (between 19-40%).

Only 10-20% of a single oral or intravenous dose is eliminated as metabolites (which exhibit lower activity than the parent drug). Four different antimicrobially active metabolites have been reported, desethyleneciprofloxacin (M1), sulphociprofloxacin (M2), oxaciprofloxacin (M3) and formylciprofloxacin (M4). M2 and M3 account for one third each of metabolised substance and M1 is found in small amounts (1.3-2.6% of the dose). M4 has been found in very small quantities (<0.1% of the dose). M1-M3 have antimicrobial activity comparable to nalidixic acid and M4 found in the smallest quantity has antimicrobial activity similar to that of norfloxacin.

Elimination of ciprofloxacin and its metabolites occurs rapidly, primarily by the kidney. After single oral and intravenous doses of ciprofloxacin, 55% and 75% respectively are eliminated by the kidney and 39% and 14% in the faeces within 5 days. Renal elimination takes place mainly during the first 12 hours after dosing and renal clearance levels suggest that active secretion by the renal tubules occurs in addition to normal glomerular filtration. Renal clearance is between 0.18 – 0.3 l/h.kg and total body clearance between 0.48 – 0.60 l/h.kg. Approximately 1% of a ciprofloxacin dose is excreted via the biliary route. The elimination kinetics are linear and after repeated dosing at 12 hourly intervals, no further accumulation is detected after the distribution equilibrium is attained (at 4-5 half-lives). The elimination half-life of unchanged ciprofloxacin over a period of 24-48 hours post-dose is 3.1-5.1 hours.

Some studies carried out with ciprofloxacin in severely renally impaired patients (serum creatinine >265 micromole/l or creatinine clearance <20ml/minute) demonstrated either a doubling of the elimination half-life, or fluctuations in half-life in comparison with healthy volunteers, whereas other studies showed no significant correlation between elimination half-life and creatinine clearance. However, it is recommended that in severely renally impaired patients, the total daily dose should be reduced by half, although monitoring of drug serum levels provides the most reliable basis for dose adjustment as necessary.

Results of pharmacokinetic studies in paediatric cystic fibrosis patients have shown dosages of 20mg/kg orally twice daily or 10mg/kg iv three times daily are recommended to achieve plasma concentration/time profiles comparable to those achieved in the adult population at the currently recommended dosage regimen.

Inhalation anthrax: Ciprofloxacin serum concentrations achieved in humans serve as a surrogate endpoint reasonably likely to predict clinical benefit and provide the basis for the recommended doses.

5.3 Preclinical safety data
Following extensive oral and intravenous toxicology testing with ciprofloxacin, only two findings which may be considered relevant to the use of ciprofloxacin in man were observed. Crystalluria was noted in those species of animals which had a normally alkaline urine. Kidney damage without the presence of crystalluria was not observed. This effect is considered a secondary inflammatory foreign-body reaction, due to the precipitation of a crystalline complex of ciprofloxacin, magnesium and protein in the distal tubule system of the kidneys. This is considered not to be a problem in man, because the urine is normally acidic. However, to avoid the occurrence of crystalluria, patients should be well hydrated and excessive alkalinity of the urine avoided.

As with other quinolones, damage to the weight-bearing joints of only juvenile rats and dogs treated with ciprofloxacin was noted in repeat dose toxicity testing. This was more noticeable in the dog. Although analysis of available safety data from ciprofloxacin use in paediatric patients did not disclose any evidence of drug related cartilage or articular damage, the use of ciprofloxacin in children and growing adolescents is generally not recommended, unless the benefits are considered to outweigh the potential risks (with the exception of treatment of cystic fibrosis). Additionally, because of the potential of arthropathy, the use of ciprofloxacin during pregnancy and lactation is not recommended.

6. PHARMACEUTICAL PARTICULARS
6.1 List of excipients
Each tablet contains microcrystalline cellulose, maize starch, crospovidone, colloidal silicon dioxide, magnesium stearate and purified water. The tablet film-coat consists of a mixture of hypromellose, Macrogol 4000, titanium dioxide and purified water.

6.2 Incompatibilities
None known.

6.3 Shelf life
5 years.

6.4 Special precautions for storage
No special storage precautions are necessary.

6.5 Nature and contents of container
Blister strips in cardboard outers comprising:

a) 250μm, 40g/m^2 PVC/PVDC foil with 20μm hard aluminium backing foil.

Pack sizes 10, 20, 100 tablets.

b) 300μm polypropylene foil with 20μm hard aluminium backing foil with a 3.5g/m^2

heat seal polypropylene coating.

Pack sizes: 10, 20, 100 tablets.

c) 130μm PA/aluminium/PVC foil with 20μm hard aluminium backing foil.

Pack sizes: 1, 2 tablets (sample packs).

6.6 Instructions for use and handling
Not applicable.

7. MARKETING AUTHORISATION HOLDER

Bayer plc Bayer House Strawberry Hill Newbury Berkshire RG14 1JA	Trading as: Bayer plc Pharmaceutical Division Bayer House Strawberry Hill Newbury Berkshire RG14 1JA Or BAYPHARM or BAYMET

8. MARKETING AUTHORISATION NUMBER(S)
PL 0010/0148

9. DATE OF FIRST AUTHORISATION/RENEWAL OF THE AUTHORISATION
3 February 1987/ 25 February 1999

10. DATE OF REVISION OF THE TEXT
June 2003

Cisplatin 1mg/ml Injection BP
(Wockhardt UK Ltd)

1. NAME OF THE MEDICINAL PRODUCT
Cisplatin 1mg/ml Injection BP

2. QUALITATIVE AND QUANTITATIVE COMPOSITION
1 ml contains 1.0 mg cisplatin

For excipients, see section 6.1.

3. PHARMACEUTICAL FORM
Concentrate for solution for infusion

The concentrate is a clear and colourless solution.

4. CLINICAL PARTICULARS
4.1 Therapeutic indications
To be used as mono-therapy, or as part of an existing chemotherapy for advanced or metastatic tumours: testicular carcinoma (palliative and curative poly-chemotherapy) and ovary carcinoma (stages III and IV), and head and neck squamous-cell epithelioma (palliative therapy).

4.2 Posology and method of administration
Cisplatin 1mg/ml concentrate for solution for infusion is to be diluted before use (see section 6.6.).

The diluted solution should be administered only intravenously by infusion (see below).

For administration, any device containing aluminium that may come in contact with cisplatin (sets for intravenous infusion, needles, catheters, syringes) must be avoided (see section 6.2.).

Adults and children:

The cisplatin dosage depends on the primary disease, the expected reaction, and on whether cisplatin is used for monotherapy or as a component of a combination chemotherapy. The dosage directions are applicable for both adults and children.

For monotherapy, the following two dosage regimens are recommended:

- Single dose of 50 to 120 mg/m^2 body surface every 3 to 4 weeks;

- 15 to 20 mg/m^2/day for five days, every 3 to 4 weeks.

If cisplatin is used in combination chemotherapy, the dose of cisplatin must be reduced. A typical dose is 20 mg/m^2 or more once every 3 to 4 weeks.

For warnings and precautions to be considered prior to the start of the next treatment cycle, see section 4.4.

In patients with renal dysfunction or bone marrow depression, the dose should be reduced adequately.

The cisplatin solution for infusion prepared according to instructions (see section 6.6.) should be administered by intravenous infusion over a period of 6 to 8 hours.

Adequate hydration must be maintained from 2 to 12 hours prior to administration until a minimum of 6 hours after the administration of cisplatin.

Hydration is necessary to cause sufficient diuresis during and after treatment with cisplatin. It is realised by intravenous infusion of one of the following solutions:

- sodium chloride solution 0.9%;

- mixture of sodium chloride solution 0.9% and glucose solution 5% (1:1).

Hydration prior to treatment with cisplatin:

Intravenous infusion of 100 to 200ml/hour for a period of 6 to 12 hours.

Hydration after termination of the administration of cisplatin:

Intravenous infusion of another 2 litres at a rate of 100 to 200 ml per hour for a period of 6 to 12 hours.

Forced diuresis may be required should the urine secretion be less than 100 to 200 ml/hour after hydration. Forced diuresis may be realised by intravenously administering 37.5g mannitol as a 10% solution (375 ml mannitol solution 10%), or by administration of a diuretic if the kidney functions are normal. The administration of mannitol or a diuretic is also required when the administrated cisplatin dose is higher than 60 mg/m^2 of body surface.

It is necessary that the patient drinks large quantities of liquids for 24 hours after the cisplatin infusion to ensure adequate urine secretion.

4.3 Contraindications
Cisplatin is contraindicated in patients:

- with hypersensitivity to the active substance or other platinum containing medicinal products;

- with renal dysfunction;

- in dehydrated condition (pre- and post-hydration is required to prevent serious renal dysfunction);

- with myelosuppression;

- with a hearing impairment;

- with neuropathy caused by cisplatin and

- who are pregnant or breastfeeding (see section 4.6. Pregnancy and lactation).

4.4 Special warnings and special precautions for use
Cisplatin may only be administered under the supervision of a physician qualified in oncology with experience in the use of antineoplastic chemotherapy.

Cisplatin is proven to be cumulative ototoxic, nephrotoxic, and neurotoxic. The toxicity caused by cisplatin may be amplified by the combined use with other medicinal products, which are toxic for the said organs or systems.

Audiograms must be made before starting treatment with cisplatin and always before starting another treatment cycle.

Nephrotoxicity can be prevented by maintaining adequate hydration before, during and after the intravenous infusion of cisplatin.

Before, during and after administration of cisplatin, the following parameters resp. organ functions must be determined:

– renal function;

– hepatic function;

– hematopoiesis functions (number of red and white blood cellsand blood platelets);

– serum electrolytes (calcium, sodium, potassium, magnesium).

These examinations must be repeated every week over the entire duration of the treatment with cisplatin.

Repeating administration of cisplatin must be delayed until normal values are achieved for the following parameters:

Serum creatinine:	$\leqslant$130 μmol/l rsp. 1.5 mg/dl
Urea:	< 25 mg/dl
White blood cells:	> 4.000/μl resp. > 4.0 × 10^9/l
Blood platelets:	>100.000/μl resp. > 100 × 10^9/l
Audiogram:	Results within the normal range.

Special caution must be exercised for patients with peripheral neuropathy not caused by cisplatin.

Special care is required for patients with acute bacterial or viral infections.

In cases of extravasation:

- immediately end the infusion of cisplatin;

- do not move the needle, aspirate the extravasate from the tissue, and rinse with sodium chloride solution 0.9% (if solutions with cisplatin concentrations higher than recommended were used; see section 6.6.).

Nausea, vomiting and diarrhoea often occur after administration of cisplatin (see section 4.8.). Prophylactic administration of an anti-emetic may be effective in alleviating or preventing nausea and vomiting. The liquid loss caused by vomiting and diarrhoea must be compensated.

Both male and female patients must use contraceptive methods to prevent conception and/or reproduction during and for at least 6 months after treatment with cisplatin. Genetic consultation is recommended if the patient wishes to have children after ending the treatment. Since a treatment with cisplatin may cause irreversible infertility, it is recommended that men, who wish to become fathers in the future, ask for advice regarding cryo-conservation of their sperm prior to the treatment.

4.5 Interaction with other medicinal products and other forms of Interaction
Simultaneous use of myelosuppressives or radiation will boost the effects of cisplatin's myelosuppressive activity.

The occurrence of nephrotoxicity caused by cisplatin may be intensified by concomitant treatment with antihypertensives containing furosemide, hydralazine, diazoxide, and propranolol.

It may be required to adjust the dosage of allopurinol, colchicine, probenecid, or sulfinpyrazone if used together with cisplatin, since cisplatin causes an increase in serum uric acid concentration.

Except for patients receiving doses of cisplatin exceeding 60 mg/m^2, whose urine secretion is less than 1000 ml per 24 hours, no forced diuresis with loop diuretics should be applied in view of possible damage to the kidney tract and ototoxicity.

Simultaneous use of antihistamines, buclizine, cyclizine, loxapine, meclozine, phenothiazines, thioxanthenes or trimethobenzamides may mask ototoxicity symptoms (such as dizziness and tinnitus).

Concomitant administration of nephrotoxic (e.g. cephalosporins, aminoglycosides) or ototoxic (e.g. aminoglycosides) medicinal products will potentiate the toxic effect of cisplatin on these organs. During or after treatment with cisplatin caution is advised with predominantly renally eliminated substances, e.g. cytostatic agents such as bleomycin and methotrexate, because of potentially reduced renal elimination.

Simultaneous use of ifosfamide causes increased protein excretion. The ototoxicity of cisplatin was reportedly enhanced by concomitant use of ifosfamide, an agent which is not ototoxic when given alone.

In a randomised trial in patients with advanced ovarian carcinoma the response to therapy was influenced negatively by concomitant administration of pyridoxine and hexamethylmelamine.

Evidence has been established that the treatment with cisplatin prior to an infusion with paclitaxel may reduce the clearance of paclitaxel by 70-75%.

Reduction of the blood's lithium values was noticed in a few cases after treatment with cisplatin combined with bleomycinand etoposide. It is therefore recommended to monitor the lithium values.

Cisplatin may reduce the absorption of phenytoin resulting in reduced epilepsy control.

Chelating agents like penicillamine may diminish the effectiveness of cisplatin.

No living virus vaccinations should be given within three months following the end of the cisplatin treatment.

4.6 Pregnancy and lactation

Cisplatin is suspected to cause serious birth defects when used during pregnancy. Cisplatin is contraindicated during the pregnancy period.

Women of child-bearing age should take contraceptives to prevent conception and/or reproduction during and for at least 6 months after treatment with cisplatin. Genetic consultation is recommended if the patient wishes to have children after ending the treatment. For male patients please refer to Section 4.4. Special warnings and precautions for use.

Cisplatin was found in the milk of milk producing animals. Breastfeeding during the therapy is contraindicated.

4.7 Effects on ability to drive and use machines

The profiles of undesirable effects (central nervous system and special senses) may reduce the patients' driving skills and abilities to operate machinery.

4.8 Undesirable effects

Undesirable effects depend on the used dose and may have cumulative effects.

Nephrotoxicity: a light and reversible renal dysfunction may be noticed after singleuse of an intermediary dose (20 mg/m^2 to < 50 mg/m^2). The use of a single high dose (50-120 mg/m^2), or repeated daily use of cisplatin, may cause kidney insufficiency with tubular necrosis revealed as uremia or anuria. The kidney insufficiency may be irreversible.

The nephrotoxicity is cumulative and may occur 2-3 days, or two weeks after the first dose of cisplatin was used. The serum creatinine and urea concentrations may increase. However, the forced diuresis by hydration before and after the cisplatin administration decreases the nephrotoxicity risk. Nephrotoxicity was noticed in 28-36% of patients without sufficient hydration after a single dose of 50 mg/m^2 of cisplatin.

Hyperuricaemia may occur asymptomatically or as gout. Hyperuricaemia has been reported in 25-30% of patients in conjunction with nephrotoxicity.

Myelosuppression: dose dependent, cumulative and mostly reversible leukopenia, trombocytopenia and anemia have been noticed. Cases were reported of Coombs positive hemolytic anemia, which is reversible when the use of cisplatin is ended. Literature has been published regarding hemolysis possibly caused by cisplatin. Serious bone marrow depression (including agranulocytosis and/or aplastic anemia) may occur after using high doses of cisplatin. A considerable decrease in the number of white blood cellsis often noticed approximately 14 days after the use (less than 1.5 × 10^9/l for 5% of the patients). A decrease in the number of blood platelets is noticed after approximately 21 days (less than 10% of the patients showed a total inferior to 50 × 10^9/l) (the recovery period is approximately 39 days).

Gastro-intestinal toxicity: anorexia, nausea, vomiting, stomach-aches, and diarrhoea often occur between 1 and 4 hours after the use. These symptoms disappear for most patients after 24 hours. Less serious nausea and anorexia may continue to occur up to seven days after the treatment. (See section 4.4.) Oral mucositis rarely occurs.

Ototoxicity: has been documented for approximately 30% of the patients treated with 50 mg/m^2 cisplatin. The defect is cumulative, may be irreversible, and is sometimes limited to one ear. Ototoxicity manifests itself as tinnitus and/or hearing impairment at higher frequencies (4,000-8,000 Hz). Hearing impairment at frequencies of 250-2000Hz (normal hearing range) was noticed for 10 to 15% of the patients. Also deafness and vestibular toxicity combined with vertigo may occur. Earlier or simultaneous cranial radiation increases the risk of hearing loss. It rarely occurs that a patient loses the ability to conduct a normal conversation. Ototoxicity for children may be serious. (See section 4.4.)

Ocular toxicity: loss of eyesight rarely occurs in the course of a combination treatment with cisplatin. A papiledema with visual defects has been incidentally noticed, but is reversible after ending the treatment. Only one case of unilateral retrobulbar neuritis with loss of vision sharpness has been reported after poly-chemotherapy followed by a cisplatin treatment.

Neurotoxicity: neurotoxicity caused by cisplatin is characterised by peripheral neuropathy (typically bilateral and sensory), and rarely by the loss of taste or tactile function, or by retrobulbar neuritis with loss of sight and cerebral dysfunction (confusion, unclear speech, individual cases of cortical blindness, loss of memory, paralysis). Lhermitte's signs, autonomous neuropathy and myelopathy of the spinal cordhave been noticed. Loss of the vital brain functions were reported (including one report of acute cerebrovascular complications, cerebral arteriitis, occlusion of the carotid artery, encephalopathy). The use of cisplatin should end immediately if one of the last mentioned cerebral symptoms occurs. Neurotoxicity caused by cisplatin may be reversible. However, the process is irreversible for 30-50% of the patients, even after ending the treatment. Neurotoxicity may occur after the first dose of cisplatin, or after a long-term therapy.

Serum electrolytes: hypomagnesemia, hypocalcemia, hyponatremia, hypophosphatemia and hypokalemia with muscle cramps and/or changes to the ECG rarely occur as a result of damage to the kidney tract caused by cisplatin, reducing the tubular resorption of these actions.

Allergic reactions: rare cases of anaphylactic reactions have been reported. They may occur as rashes, urticaria, erythema, or pruritus. Rare cases of hypotension, tachycardia, dyspnoea, bronchospasms, facial oedema and fever have been reported. Treatment with antihistamines, epinephrine (adrenaline) and steroids may be required.

Hepatic: liver dysfunction with increased serum transaminases rarely occurs and is reversible. Reduced albumin levels were rarely noticed and may be linked to the treatment with cisplatin.

Cardiac: cardiac rhythm disorders including bradycardia and tachycardia, and arrhythmia rarely occur. Changes of the ECG have rarely been observed. Cardiac arrest has been reported in extremely rare cases after a treatment with cisplatin combined with other cytostatic medicinal products.

Immune system: immunosuppression has been evidenced.

Other

Local oedema and pain, erythema, skin ulceration and phlebitis may occur in the area of the injection after intravenous administration.

A metallic setting on the gums has been noticed.

Alopecia, dysfunctional spermatogenesis and ovulation, and painful gynaecomastia may occur.

The development of secondary non-lymphatic leukaemia has been linked to the use of cisplatin.

Independent descriptions link vascular disorders (cerebral or coronary ischemia, impairment of the peripheral blood circulation related to the Raynaud's syndrome) to cisplatin including chemotherapy.

Carcinogenicity is theoretically possible, (based on cisplatin's mechanism of action), but not proven.

Hypercholesterolemia (rarely), inadequate ADH secretion (individual cases), increased amylasein the serum (rarely), thrombotic microangiopathy combined with hemolytic-uremic syndrome (individual cases).

Increased iron concentrations have incidentally been registered.

4.9 Overdose

Overdoses are expected to cause the toxic activities as described hereinbefore to an excessive extent. Efficient hydration and osmotic diuresis may contribute to the reduction of the cisplatin toxicity, if used immediately after the overdose.

An overdose (⩾ 200 mg/m^2) may directly affect the respiratory centre, which may cause fatal respiratory dysfunction and upsetting of the acid/base balance resulting from passing the blood-brain barrier.

5. PHARMACOLOGICAL PROPERTIES

5.1 Pharmacodynamic properties

Pharmacotherapeutic group: Antineoplastic agents / Platinum compounds ATC code: L01XA01

Cisplatin is an anorganic substance containing a heavy metal (cis-diamminedichlorophlatinum(II)). This substance inhibits the DNA synthesis by realising transverse connections within and between the DNA strings. The protein and RNA synthesis is inhibited to a lesser extent.

Although the primary activity of cisplatin seems to be the inhibition of DNA synthesis, the antineoplastic process includes other activities, such as enlargement of the tumour immunogenicity. Cisplatin's oncolytic functions can be compared to the functions of alkylating substances. Cisplatin also offers immunosuppressive, radiosensitising and antibacterial features.

Cisplatin does not seem to be cell cycle specific.

The cytotoxic activities of cisplatin are caused by binding all DNA bases, with a preference for the N-7 position of guanine and adenosine.

5.2 Pharmacokinetic properties

After intravenous administration, cisplatin is rapidly distributed among all tissues. Following cisplatin doses of 20 to 120 mg/m^2, the concentrations of platinum are highest in liver, prostate and kidney, somewhat lower in bladder, muscles, testicles, pancreas and spleen and lowest in bowel, adrenal, heart, lung, cerebrum and cerebellum.

Over 90% of the total plasma cisplatin is bounded with protein after two hours following the administration. This process may be irreversible. The protein-bounded part is not antineoplastic active. Cisplatin is non-linearly pharmacokinetic. Cisplatin is converted by a non-enzymatic process into one or more metabolites. Elimination from the plasma is realised in two phases after intravenous bolus injection of 50-100 mg/m^2 of cisplatin. The following half-life periodhave been registered for humans:

t ½ (distribution): 10-60 minutes

t ½ (terminal): approximately 2-5 days

The considerable protein binding of the total platinum contents results in an extended or incomplete excretion phase with cumulative urine secretion ranging from 27 to 45% of the administered dose in a period from 84 to 120 hours. An extended infusion results in the urine secretion of a larger part of the dose. The faecal secretion is minimal, and small amounts of platinum can be traced in the gall-bladder and the large intestine. Dysfunctional kidneys increase the plasma half-life period, which may also increase theoretically in the presence of ascites caused by the highly protein binding activities of cisplatin.

5.3 Preclinical safety data

Chronic toxicity:

Chronic toxicity models indicate kidney damage, bone marrow depression, gastro-intestine disorders and ototoxicity.

Mutagenity and carcinogenity:

Cisplatin is mutagenic in numerous *in vitro* and *in vivo* tests (bacterial test systems and chromosome defects in animal cells and tissue cultures). Long term studies of cisplatin on mice and rats evidenced the carcinogenic effects.

Reproductive toxicity:

Fertility: Gonadal suppression resulting in amenorrhoea or azoospermia may be irreversible and cause definitive infertility.

Pregnancy and lactation: Cisplatin is embryotoxic and teratogenic for mice and rats, and defects have been reported for both species. Cisplatin was found in the milk.

6. PHARMACEUTICAL PARTICULARS

6.1 List of excipients

Sodium chloride

Hydrochloric acid 10% m/m

Water for injections

6.2 Incompatibilities

Cisplatin reacts with aluminium which results in production of a black platinum precipitate. Therefore any device containing aluminium that may come in contact with cisplatin (sets for intravenous infusion, needles, catheters, syringes) must be avoided.

This medicinal product must not be mixed with other medicinal products except those mentioned in section 6.6.

The cisplatin 1 mg/ml concentrate must not be diluted with glucose solution 5% alone or mannitol solution 5% alone, but only with the mixtures containing additionally sodium chloride as stated in section 6.6.

Antioxidants (such as sodium metabisulphite), bicarbonates (sodium bicarbonate), sulphates, fluorouracil and paclitaxel may inactivate cisplatin in infusion systems.

6.3 Shelf life

2 years

After dilution (see section 6.6. and 6.4.): 48 hours at 2-8°C

6.4 Special precautions for storage

Do not store above 25 °C. Do not refrigerate or freeze. Keep container in the outer carton.

After dilution (see section 6.6.):

Chemical and physical in-use stability has been demonstrated for 24 hours at 25 °C for solutions with a final cisplatin 0.1 mg/ml after dilution of the cisplatin 1 mg/ml with one of the following solutions:

- sodium chloride solution 0.9%;
- mixture of sodium chloride solution 0.9% and glucose solution 5% (1:1);
- mixture of sodium chloride solution 0.9% and mannitol solution 5% (1:1).

From a microbiological point of view, the product should be used immediately. If not used immediately, in-use storage times and conditions prior to use are the responsibility of the user and would normally not be longer than 24 hours at 2 to 8 °C, unless dilution has taken place in controlled and validated aseptic conditions. In this case stability for 48 hours at 2-8°C has been demonstrated.

6.5 Nature and contents of container

Amber type I glass vial (100 ml) with chlorobutyl rubber stopper with aluminium overseal.

Packs of 1 vial containing with 100 ml solution for infusion each.

6.6 Instructions for use and handling

Cisplatin 1 mg/ml solution for infusion is to be diluted before use. For preparation of solution for infusion, any device containing aluminium that may come in contact with cisplatin (sets for intravenous infusion, needles, catheters, syringes) must be avoided (see section 6.2.).

Preparation of solution for infusion must take place in aseptic conditions.

For dilution of the concentrate, one of the following solutions should be used:

- sodium chloride solution 0.9%;
- mixture of sodium chloride solution 0.9% and glucose solution 5% (1:1) (resulting final concentrations: sodium chloride 0.45%, glucose 2.5%).

Should hydration prior to the treatment with cisplatin be impossible, the concentrate may be diluted with:

- mixture of sodium chloride solution 0.9% and mannitol solution 5% (1:1) (resulting final concentrations: sodium chloride 0.45%, mannitol 2.5%).

Preparation of cisplatin solution for infusion:

The required amount (dose) of the cisplatin 1 mg/ml calculated according to the instructions in section 4.2. should be diluted in 1-2 litres of one of the above mentioned solutions.

The diluted solution should be administered only by intravenous infusion (see section 4.2.).

Only clear and colourless solutions without visible particles should be used.

For single use only.

As any other cytotoxic agent, cisplatin should be used with extreme caution: gloves, face masks and protective clothing are required and vital. Cisplatin should be processed under a protective hood, if possible. Contact with skin and/or mucous membranes must be avoided. Pregnant hospital employees should not work with cisplatin.

Skin contact: Rinse with large quantities of water. Apply an ointment if you have a temporary burning feeling. (Note: Some persons are sensitive to platinum and may experience a skin reaction).

Any unused product or waste material should be disposed of in accordance with local requirements.

7. MARKETING AUTHORISATION HOLDER
CP Pharmaceuticals Ltd
Ash Road North
Wrexham
LL13 9UF

8. MARKETING AUTHORISATION NUMBER(S)
PL 04543/0438

9. DATE OF FIRST AUTHORISATION/RENEWAL OF THE AUTHORISATION
14 December 2001

10. DATE OF REVISION OF THE TEXT
March 2003

Cisplatin 50mg Freeze Dried Powder for Injection

(Pharmacia Limited)

1. NAME OF THE MEDICINAL PRODUCT
Cisplatin 50

2. QUALITATIVE AND QUANTITATIVE COMPOSITION
Cisplatin 50.0mg

3. PHARMACEUTICAL FORM
Yellowish-white, freeze-dried cake in vials containing 50mg Cisplatin.

4. CLINICAL PARTICULARS
4.1 Therapeutic indications
Cisplatin has antitumour activity either as a single agent or in combination chemotherapy particularly in the treatment of testicular and metastatic ovarian tumours, also cervical tumours, lung carcinoma and bladder cancer.

4.2 Posology and method of administration
Route of administration: Intravenous infusion.

Cisplatin should be dissolved in water for injections such that the reconstituted solution contains 1 mg/ml of Cisplatin. This solution should then be diluted in 2 litres of 0.9% saline or a dextrose/saline solution (to which 37.5 g of mannitol may be added) and administration should be over a 6-8 hour period.

Adults and children

Single agent therapy

The usual dose regimen given as a single agent is 50 - 120 mg/m^2 by infusion once every 3 - 4 weeks or 15 - 20 mg/m^2 by infusion daily for 5 consecutive days, every 3 - 4 weeks.

Combination chemotherapy

Dosage may be adjusted if the drug is used in combination with other antitumour chemotherapy.

With multiple drug treatment schedules Cisplatin is usually given in doses 20 mg/m^2 upwards every 3 - 4 weeks.

Dosage should be reduced for patients with renal impairment or depressed bone marrow function.

Pre-treatment hydration with 1 - 2 litres of fluid infused for 8 - 12 hours prior to the Cisplatin will initiate diuresis. Adequate subsequent hydration should maintain diuresis during the 24 hours following administration.

Aluminium containing equipment should not be used for administration of Cisplatin as it may react with metal aluminium to form a black precipitate of platinum.

4.3 Contraindications
Cisplatin is contra-indicated in patients who have previous allergic reactions to Cisplatin or other platinum compounds as anaphylactic-like reactions have been reported. Relative contra-indications are pre-existing renal impairment, hearing disorders and depressed bone marrow function which may increase toxicity.

4.4 Special warnings and special precautions for use
This agent should only be administered under the direction of physicians experienced in cancer chemotherapy.

Renal function: Cisplatin produces cumulative nephrotoxicity. Renal function and serum electrolyte (magnesium, sodium, potassium and calcium) should be evaluated prior to initiating cisplatin treatment and prior to each subsequent course of therapy.

To maintain urine output and reduce renal toxicity it is recommended that Cisplatin be administered as an intravenous infusion over 6-8 hours, as indicated in section 4.2 'Posology and method of administration'. Moreover, pretreatment intravenous hydration with 1-2 litres of fluid over 8-12 hours followed by adequate hydration for the next 24 hours is recommended.

Repeat courses of Cisplatin should not be given unless levels of serum creatinine are below 1.5 mg/100 ml (100 mcmol/l) or blood urea below 55 mg/100 ml (9 mmol/l) and circulating blood elements are at an acceptable level.

Special care has to be taken when cisplatin-treated patients are given concomitant therapies with other potentially nephrotoxic drugs (See also section 4.5 'Interaction with other medicinal products and other forms of Interaction').

In addition, adequate post-treatment hydration and urinary output should be monitored. Concomitant use of nephrotoxic drugs may seriously impair kidney function.

Bone marrow function: Peripheral blood counts should be monitored frequently in patients receiving Cisplatin. Although the haematologic toxicity is usually moderate and reversible, severe thrombocytopenia and leucopenia may occur. In patients who develop thrombocytopenia special precautions are recommended: care in performing invasive procedures; search for signs of bleeding or bruising; test of urine, stools and emesis for occult blood, avoiding aspirin and other NSAIDs. Patients who develop leucopenia should be observed carefully for signs of infection and might require antibiotic support and blood product transfusions.

Hearing function: Cisplatin may produce cumulative ototoxicity, which is more likely to occur with high-dose regimens. Audiometry should be performed prior to initiating therapy, and repeated audiograms should be performed when auditory symptoms occur or clinical hearing changes become apparent. Clinically important deterioration of auditive function may require dosage modifications or discontinuation of therapy.

CNS functions: Cisplatin is known to induce neurotoxicity; therefore, neurologic examination is warranted in patients receiving a cisplatin-containing treatment. Since neurotoxicity may result in irreversible damage, it is recommended to discontinue therapy with Cisplatin when neurologic toxic signs or symptoms become apparent.

Anaphylactic-like reactions to Cisplatin have been observed. These reactions can be controlled by administration of antihistamines, adrenaline and/or glucocorticoids.

Neurotoxicity secondary to Cisplatin administration has been reported and therefore neurological examinations are recommended. Cisplatin has been shown to be mutagenic. It may also have an anti-fertility effect. Other antineoplastic substances have been shown to be carcinogenic and this possibility should be borne in mind in long term use of Cisplatin.

Liver function should also be monitored periodically.

4.5 Interaction with other medicinal products and other forms of Interaction
Cisplatin is mostly used in combination with antineoplastic drugs having similar cytotoxic effects. In these circumstances additive toxicity is likely to occur.

Nephrotoxic drugs: Aminoglycoside antibiotics, when given concurrently or within 1-2 weeks after cisplatin administration, may potentiate its nephrotoxic effects. Concomitant use of other potentially nephrotoxic drugs (e.g. amphotericin B) is not recommended during Cisplatin therapy.

Ototoxic drugs: Concurrent and/or sequential administration of ototoxic drugs such as aminoglycoside antibiotics or loop diuretics may increase the potential of Cisplatin to cause ototoxicity, especially in the presence of renal impairment.

Renally excreted drugs: Literature data suggest that Cisplatin may alter the renal elimination of bleomycin and methotrexate (possibly as a result of cisplatin-induced nephrotoxicity) and enhance their toxicity.

Anticonvulsant agents: In patients receiving Cisplatin and phenytoin, serum concentrations of the latter may be decreased, possibly as a result of decreased absorption and/or increased metabolism. In these patients, serum levels of phenytoin should be monitored and dosage adjustments made as necessary.

Antigout agents: Cisplatin may raise the concentration of blood uric acid. Thus, in patients concurrently receiving antigout agents such as allopurinol, colchicine, probenecid or sulfinpyrazone, dosage adjustment of these drugs may be necessary to control hyperuricemia and gout.

4.6 Pregnancy and lactation
Cisplatin has been shown to be teratogenic and embryotoxic in animals. The use of the drug should be avoided in pregnant of nursing women if possible.

4.7 Effects on ability to drive and use machines
There are no known effects of Cisplatin on the ability to drive or operate machinery. However, the profile of undesirable effects (central nervous system and special sense) may reduce the patient's driving skills and abilities to operate machinery.

4.8 Undesirable effects
Nephrotoxicity: Acute renal toxicity, which was highly frequent in the past and represented the major dose-limiting toxicity of Cisplatin, has been greatly reduced by the use of 6 to 8-hour infusions as well as by concomitant intravenous hydration and forced diuresis. Cumulative toxicity, however, remains a problem and may be severe. Renal impairment, which is associated with tubular damage, may be first noted during the second week after a dose and is manifested by an increase in serum creatinine, blood urea nitrogen, serum uric acid and/or a decrease in creatinine clearance. Renal insufficiency is generally mild to moderate and reversible at the usual doses of the drug (recovery occurring as a rule within 2-4 weeks); however, high or repeated Cisplatin doses can increase the severity and duration of renal impairment and may produce irreversible renal insufficiency (sometimes fatal). Renal failure has been reported also following intraperitoneal instillation of the drug.

Cisplatin may also cause serious electrolyte disturbances, mainly represented by hypomagnesemia, hypocalcemia, and hypokalemia, and associated with renal tubular dysfunction. Hypomagnesemia and/or hypocalcemia may become symptomatic, with muscle irritability or cramps, clonus, tremor, carpopedal spasm, and/or tetany.

Gastrointestinal toxicity: Nausea and vomiting occur in the majority of Cisplatin-treated patients, usually starting within 1 hour of treatment and lasting up to 24 hours or longer. These side effects are only partially relieved by standard antiemetics. The severity of these systems may be reduced by dividing the total dose per cycle into smaller doses given once daily for five days.

Haematologic toxicity: Myelosuppression often occurs during Cisplatin therapy, but is mostly mild to moderate and reversible at the usual doses. Leucopenia is dose-related, possibly cumulative, and usually reversible. The onset of leucopenia occurs usually between days 6 and 26 and the time of recovery ranges from 21 to 45 days. Thrombocytopenia is also a dose-limiting effect of Cisplatin but is usually reversible. The onset of thrombocytopenia is usually from days 10 to 26 and the time of recovery ranges from about 28 to 45 days.

The incidence of Cisplatin-induced anaemia (haemoglobin drop of 2 g/100 ml) ranges from 9% to 40%, although this is a difficult toxic effect to assess because it may have a complex aetiology in cancer patients.

There have been rare reports of acute myelogenous leukemias and myelodysplastic syndromes arising in patients who have been treated with Cisplatin, mostly when given in combination with other potentially leukomogenic agents.

Ototoxicity: Unilateral or bilateral tinnitus, with or without hearing loss, occurs in about 10% of Cisplatin-treated patients and is usually reversible. The damage to the hearing system appears to be dose-related and cumulative, and it is reported more frequently in very young and very old patients.

The overall incidence of audiogram abnormalities is 24%, but large variations exist. These abnormalities usually appear within 4 days after drug administration and consist of at least a 15 decibel loss in pure tone threshold. The audiogram abnormalities are most common in the 4000-8000 Hz frequencies.

Neurotoxicity: Peripheral neuropathies occur infrequently with usual doses of the drug. These are generally sensory in nature (e.g. paresthesia of the upper and lower extremities) but can also include motor difficulties, reduced reflexes and leg weakness. Autonomic neuropathy, seizures, slurred speech, loss of taste and memory loss have also been reported. These neuropathies usually appear after prolonged therapy, but have also developed after a single drug dose. Peripheral neuropathy may be irreversible in some patients; however, it has been partially or completely reversible in others following discontinuance of Cisplatin therapy.

Hypersensitivity: Anaphylactic and anaphylactic-like reactions, such as flushing, facial oedema, wheezing, tachycardia and hypotension, have been occasionally reported. These reactions may occur within a few minutes after intravenous administration. Antihistamine, adrenaline and/or glucocorticoids control all these reactions. Rarely, urticarial or maculopapular skin rashes have also been observed.

Ocular toxicity: Optic neuritis, papilloedema, and cortical blindness have been reported rarely in patients receiving Cisplatin. These events are usually reversible after drug withdrawal.

Hepatotoxicity: Mild and transient elevations of serum AST and ALT levels may occur infrequently.

Other toxicities: Other reported toxicities are:

cardiovascular abnormalities (coronary artery disease, congestive heart failure, arrhythmias, postural hypotension, thrombotic microangiopathy, etc), hyponatremia / syndrome of inappropriate antidiuretic hormone (SIADH)), mild alopecia, myalgia, pyrexia and gingival platinum line. Pulmonary toxicity has been reported in patients treated with Cisplatin in combination with bleomycin or 5-fluorouracil.

Hyperuricaemia: Hyperuricaemia occurring with Cisplatin is more pronounced with doses greater than 50 mg/m^2. Allopurinol effectively reduces uric acid levels.

Hypomagnesemia: Asymptomatic hypomagnesemia has been documented in a certain number of patients treated with Cisplatin, symptomatic hypomagnesemia has been observed in a limited number of cases.

Convulsions: Seizures have also been reported with the use of this product.

Cardiotoxicity: Isolated cases of tachycardia and arrhythmia have been reported with Cisplatin chemotherapy.

Thromboembolism: Cancer patients are generally at an increased risk for thromboembolic events. Cerebrovascular accidents (e.g. haemorrhagic and ischaemic stroke, amaurosis fugax, sagittal sinus thrombosis) have been observed in patients receiving Cisplatin therapy.

Local effects such as phlebitis, cellulitis and skin necrosis (following extravasation of the drug) may also occur.

Cisplatin can affect male fertility. Impairment of spermatogenesis and azoospermia have been reported. Although the impairment of spermatogenesis can be reversible, males undergoing Cisplatin treatment should be warned about the possible adverse effects on male fertility.

4.9 Overdose
There are no special instructions.

5. PHARMACOLOGICAL PROPERTIES

5.1 Pharmacodynamic properties
In vitro studies indicate that DNA is the principal target molecule of cis-platinum.

The basis for the selectivity of the cis-isomer may reside in its ability to react in a specifically defined configuration with DNA.

Modification of the DNA template results in the selective inhibition of DNA synthesis. The drug is cell cycle non-specific.

5.2 Pharmacokinetic properties
A biphasic plasma-decay pattern occurs in man after bolus administration. The initial plasma half-life in man is 25 - 49 minutes and the terminal half-life 3 - 4 days. In addition, a third excretory phase with a longer half-life may be postulated from the high plasma platinum concentration found after 21 days. During the terminal phase more than 90% of the drug is bound to plasma proteins.

The urinary elimination of the drug is incomplete: the 5-day recovery of platinum in the urine being only 27 to 45%.

Studies in man measuring free platinum species have shown a mean terminal half-life of 48 minutes after bolus injection, which probably corresponds to the initial half-life (25 - 49 minutes) seen when total platinum is monitored and reflects the distribution of the drug. Urinary excretion of filterable platinum was greater after 6 hours infusion (75%) than after a 15 minute injection (40%) of the same dose of cis-platinum.

Diuresis induced by high-volume hydration or mannitol infusion was associated with a reduction in the concentration of platinum excreted in the urine. The reduced concentration of platinum caused by the high urine volume may play a role in renal protection.

5.3 Preclinical safety data
No further preclinical safety data are available.

6. PHARMACEUTICAL PARTICULARS

6.1 List of excipients
Sodium chloride

Mannitol

6.2 Incompatibilities
None known.

6.3 Shelf life
36 months.

6.4 Special precautions for storage
The unopened vials should be stored at room temperature, protected from light.

The reconstituted solution must not be cooled or refrigerated, as cooling may result in precipitation. It should be kept at room temperature and protected from light, also during intravenous infusion. Any unused solution should be discarded.

Keep out of the reach and sight of children.

6.5 Nature and contents of container
Colourless glass vials (Type II) with bromobutyl rubber stoppers and aluminium snap-caps.

6.6 Instructions for use and handling
Cisplatin powder should be dissolved in sterile Water for Injections such that the reconstituted solution contains 1mg/ml of Cisplatin. The reconstituted solution should be diluted in 2 litres of 0.9% saline or a dextrose/saline solution (to which 37.5g of mannitol may be added).

Personnel should be trained in good technique for reconstitution and handling. Pregnant staff should be excluded from working with Cisplatin.

Care should be taken to prevent inhaling particles and exposing the skin to Cisplatin. Adequate protective clothing should be worn, such as PVC gloves, safety glasses, disposable gowns and masks.

In the event of contact with eyes, wash with water or saline. If the skin comes into contact with the drug wash thoroughly with water and in both cases seek medical advice. Seek immediate medical attention if the drug is ingested or inhaled.

All used materials, needles, syringes, vials and other items which have come into contact with cytotoxic drugs should be incinerated. Contaminated surfaces should be washed with copious amounts of water.

7. MARKETING AUTHORISATION HOLDER
Pharmacia Limited
Ramsgate Road
Sandwich
Kent
CT13 9NJ
United Kingdom

8. MARKETING AUTHORISATION NUMBER(S)
PL 00032/0334

9. DATE OF FIRST AUTHORISATION/RENEWAL OF THE AUTHORISATION
25 March 2002

10. DATE OF REVISION OF THE TEXT
13 June 2005

11. LEGAL CATEGORY
POM

Citanest 1%

(AstraZeneca UK Limited)

1. NAME OF THE MEDICINAL PRODUCT
Citanest 1%

2. QUALITATIVE AND QUANTITATIVE COMPOSITION
Each ml of sterile, clear, aqueous solution contains Prilocaine Hydrochloride 10mg.

For excipients, see 6.1

3. PHARMACEUTICAL FORM
Solution for injection.

4. CLINICAL PARTICULARS

4.1 Therapeutic indications
Citanest is a local anaesthetic for use in infiltration anaesthesia and nerve blocks.

4.2 Posology and method of administration
Care should be taken to prevent toxic reactions by avoiding intravascular injection. Careful aspiration before and during the injection is recommended. When a large dose is to be injected, e.g. in epidural block, a test dose of 3-5 ml of prilocaine containing adrenaline is recommended. An accidental intravascular injection may be recognised by a temporary increase in heart rate. The main dose should be injected slowly, at a rate of 100-200 mg/min, or in incremental doses, while keeping in constant verbal contact with the patient. If toxic symptoms occur, the injection should be stopped immediately.

The dose is adjusted according to the response of the patient and the site of administration.

The lowest concentration and smallest dose producing the required effect should be given.

The maximum dose of Citanest for healthy adults should not exceed 400mg.

Elderly or debilitated patients require smaller doses, commensurate with age and physical status.

In children above the age of 6 months the dosage can be calculated on a weight basis up to 5mg/kg.

Prilocaine for injection is not recommended in children under 6 months of age and for use in paracervical (PCB) block and pudendal block in the obstetric patient. There is an increased risk of methaemoglobin formation in children and in the neonate after delivery.

4.3 Contraindications
Known hypersensitivity to anaesthetics of the amide type or to any component of the solution.

Citanest should be avoided in patients with anaemia or congenital or acquired methaemoglobinaemia.

4.4 Special warnings and special precautions for use
Regional or local anaesthetic procedures, except those of the most trivial nature, should always be performed in a properly equipped and staffed area, with the equipment and drugs necessary for monitoring an emergency resuscitation immediately available. When performing major blocks, an i.v. cannula should be inserted before the local anaesthetic is injected. Clinicians should have received adequate and appropriate training in the procedure to be performed and should be familiar with the diagnosis and treatment of side effects, systemic toxicity or other complications, see Section 4.9.

Great caution must be exercised to avoid accidental intravascular injection of this compound, since it may give rise to the rapid onset of toxicity, with marked restlessness, twitching, or convulsions, followed by coma with apnoea and cardiovascular collapse.

In common with other local anaesthetics, Citanest should be used cautiously in the elderly, patients in poor health, patients with epilepsy, severe or untreated hypertension, impaired cardiac conduction, severe heart disease, impaired respiratory function, and in patients with liver or kidney damage, if the dose or site of administration is likely to result in high blood levels.

Certain local anaesthetic procedures may be associated with serious adverse reactions, regardless of the local anaesthetic drug used, e.g:

- Central nerve blocks may cause cardiovascular depression, especially in the presence of hypovolaemia. Epidural anaesthesia should be used with caution in patients with impaired cardiovascular function.

- Retrobulbar injections may rarely reach the cranial subarachnoid space causing serious / severe reactions, including cardiovascular collapse, apnoea, convulsions and temporary blindness.

- Retro- and peribulbar injections of local anaesthetics carry a low risk of persistent ocular muscle dysfunction. The primary causes include trauma and/or local toxic effects on muscles and/or nerves.

The severity of such tissue reactions is related to the degree of trauma, the concentration of the local anaesthetic and the duration of exposure of the tissue to the local anaesthetic. For this reason, as with all local anaesthetics, the lowest effective concentration and dose of local anaesthetic should be used.

- Injections in the head and neck regions may be made inadvertently into an artery, causing cerebral symptoms even at low doses.

- Paracervical block can sometimes cause fetal bradycardia/tachycardia, and careful monitoring of the foetal heart rate is necessary

Epidural anaesthesia may lead to hypotension and bradycardia. This risk can be reduced either by preloading the circulation with crystalloidal or colloidal solutions. Hypotension should be treated promptly with e.g. ephedrine 5-10 mg intravenously and repeated as necessary.

To reduce the risk of dangerous side effects, children below the age of 6 months require special attention due to the risk of methaemoglobinaemia. Paracervical block (PCB) or pudendal block in the obstetric patient may lead to methaemoglobinaemia in the neonate.

Local anaesthetics should be avoided when there is inflammation at the site of the proposed injection.

4.5 Interaction with other medicinal products and other forms of Interaction
Drugs which may predispose to methaemoglobin formation, e.g. sulfonamides (eg cotrimoxazole), antimalarials and certain nitric compounds, could potentiate this adverse effect of prilocaine.

Prilocaine should be used with caution in patients receiving other local anaesthetics or agents structurally related to amide-type anaesthetics, since the toxic effects are additive.

4.6 Pregnancy and lactation

Pregnancy

Although there is no evidence from animal studies of harm to the foetus, as with all drugs Citanest should not be given in early pregnancy unless the benefits are considered to outweigh the risks.

Neonatal methaemoglobinaemia has been reported after paracervical block (PCB) or pudendal block in the obstetric patient.

Foetal adverse effects due to local anaesthetics, such as foetal bradycardia, seem to be most apparent in paracervical block anaesthesia. Such effects may be due to high concentrations of anaesthetic reaching the foetus.

Lactation

Prilocaine enters the mothers milk but there is generally no risk of effects on the infant at recommended doses.

4.7 Effects on ability to drive and use machines
Depending on dosage, local anaesthetics may have a very mild effect on mental function and may temporarily impair locomotion and co-ordination.

4.8 Undesirable effects
In common with other local anaesthetics, adverse reactions to Citanest are extremely rare and are usually the result of excessively high blood concentrations due to inadvertent intravascular injection, excessive dosage, rapid absorption or occasionally to hypersensitivity, idiosyncrasy or diminished tolerance on the part of the patient. In such circumstances systemic effects occur involving the central nervous system and/or the cardiovascular system.

CNS reactions are excitatory and/or depressant and may be characterised by nervousness, dizziness, blurred vision and tremors, followed by drowsiness, convulsions, unconsciousness and possibly respiratory arrest. The excitatory reactions may be very brief or may not occur at all, in which case the first manifestations of toxicity may be drowsiness, merging into unconsciousness and respiratory arrest.

Cardiovascular reactions are depressant and may be characterised by hypotension, myocardial depression, bradycardia and possibly cardiac arrest.

Allergic reactions to local anaesthetics of the amide type are extremely rare. They may be characterised by cutaneous lesions, urticaria, oedema or anaphylactoid reactions. However, other constituents of the solutions, e.g. methylparahydroxybenzoate, may cause this type of reaction. Detection of sensitivity by skin testing is of doubtful value.

Neurological complications for example nerve trauma, neuropathy, anterior spinal artery occlusion, arachnoiditis etc., have been associated with regional anaesthetic techniques, regardless of the local anaesthetic drug used.

Hypotension may occur as a physiological response to central nerve blocks.

This product gives rise to methaemoglobinaemia in a dose related fashion.

Clinically significant levels occur with cyanosis when doses of prilocaine exceed 600mg.

Methaemoglobinaemia may occur at lower doses of prilocaine in patients suffering from anaemia, from congenital or acquired haemoglobinopathy (including methaemoglobinaemia), or in patients receiving concomitant therapy e.g. sulphonamides, known to cause such conditions. Infants are particularly susceptible, due to a lower activity of the enzyme which reduces methaemoglobin to haemoglobin. Hence prilocaine is not recommended for paracervical block (PCB) or pudendal block in the obstetric patient and in children under the age of 6 months.

Methaemoglobinaemia may be treated by the intravenous administration of a 1% solution of methylene blue in a dose of 1mg/kg, over a 5 minute period.

Even low concentrations of methaemoglobin may interfere with pulse oximetry readings, indicating a false low oxygen saturation.

4.9 Overdose
Acute systemic toxicity

Central nervous system toxicity is a graded response with symptoms and signs of escalating severity. The first symptoms are circumoral paraesthesia, numbness of the tongue, light-headedness, hyperacusis and tinnitus. Visual disturbance and muscular tremors are more serious and precede the onset of generalized convulsions. These signs must not be mistaken for a neurotic behaviour. Unconsciousness and grand mal convulsions may follow which may last from a few seconds to several minutes. Hypoxia and hypercarbia occur rapidly following convulsions due to the increased muscular activity, together with the interference with normal respiration and loss of the airway. In severe cases apnoea may occur. Acidosis increases the toxic effects of local anaesthetics.

Effects on the cardiovascular system may be seen in severe cases. Hypotension, bradycardia, arrhythmia and even cardiac arrest may occur as a result of high systemic concentrations.

Cardiovascular toxic effects are generally preceded by signs of toxicity in the central nervous system, unless the patient is receiving a general anaesthetic or is heavily sedated with drugs such as benzodiazepine or barbiturate.

Recovery is due to redistribution of the local anaesthetic drug from the central nervous system and metabolism. Recovery may be rapid unless large amounts of the drug have been injected.

Treatment of acute toxicity

Treatment of a patient with systemic toxicity consists of arresting convulsions and ensuring adequate ventilation with oxygen, if necessary by assisted or controlled ventilation (respiration). If convulsions occur they must be treated promptly by intravenous injection of thiopentone 100 to 200mg or diazepam 5 to 10mg. Alternatively succinylcholine 50 to 100mg i.v. may be used providing the clinician is capable of performing endotracheal intubation and managing a fully paralysed patient. If cardiac arrest occurs effective cardiopulmonary resuscitation must be instituted. This should include external cardiac compression, artificial ventilation with oxygen, adrenaline and sodium bicarbonate.

If cardiovascular depression is evident (hypotension, bradycardia), ephedrine 5-10 mg i.v. should be given and repeated, if necessary, after 2-3 min.

Should circulatory arrest occur, immediate cardiopulmonary resuscitation should be instituted. Optimal oxygenation and ventilation and circulatory support as well as treatment of acidosis are of vital importance, since hypoxia and acidosis will increase the systemic toxicity of local anaesthetics.

5. PHARMACOLOGICAL PROPERTIES

5.1 Pharmacodynamic properties
ATC code: NO1B B04

Prilocaine is a local anaesthetic of the amide type. Local anaesthetics act by preventing transmission of impulses along nerve fibres and at nerve endings; depolarisation and ion-exchange are inhibited. The effects are reversible.

5.2 Pharmacokinetic properties
Prilocaine hydrochloride is absorbed more slowly than lidocaine (lignocaine) because of its slight vasoconstrictor action but its half life in blood is less than that of lidocaine (lidocaine half life approximately 10 minutes, elimination half life approximately 2 hours).

Amidases in the liver and kidney metabolise prilocaine directly.

5.3 Preclinical safety data
Prilocaine hydrochloride is a well established active ingredient.

6. PHARMACEUTICAL PARTICULARS

6.1 List of excipients
Sodium chloride, sodium hydroxide/hydrochloric acid for pH adjustment, methyl parahydroxybenzoate and water for injections.

6.2 Incompatibilities
None known

6.3 Shelf life
The shelf-life is 3 years

6.4 Special precautions for storage
Do not store above 25°C.

6.5 Nature and contents of container
Multi-dose glass vials of 20ml and 50ml

6.6 Instructions for use and handling
None stated

7. MARKETING AUTHORISATION HOLDER
AstraZeneca UK Ltd

600 Capability Green,

Luton, LU1 3LU, UK.

8. MARKETING AUTHORISATION NUMBER(S)
PL 17901/0118

9. DATE OF FIRST AUTHORISATION/RENEWAL OF THE AUTHORISATION
14th May 2002

10. DATE OF REVISION OF THE TEXT
28th January 2004

Claforan

(sanofi-aventis)

1. NAME OF THE MEDICINAL PRODUCT
Claforan™ Injection 500mg, 1g and 2g.

2. QUALITATIVE AND QUANTITATIVE COMPOSITION

500mg vial:	Contains Cefotaxime sodium Ph. Eur equivalent to 500mg cefotaxime base.
1g vial:	Contains Cefotaxime sodium Ph. Eur equivalent to 1g cefotaxime base.
2g vial:	Contains Cefotaxime sodium Ph. Eur equivalent to 2g cefotaxime base.

Each gram of Claforan contains approximately 48mg (2.09mmol) of sodium.

3. PHARMACEUTICAL FORM
Vials containing powder for injection or infusion.

Claforan is supplied as a white to slightly creamy powder, which when dissolved in Water for Injections Ph. Eur. forms a straw-coloured solution suitable for IV or IM injection. Variations in the intensity of colour of the freshly prepared solution do not indicate a change in potency or safety.

4. CLINICAL PARTICULARS

4.1 Therapeutic indications
Properties: Claforan is a broad-spectrum bactericidal cephalosporin antibiotic. Claforan is exceptionally active *in vitro* against Gram-negative organisms sensitive or resistant to first or second generation cephalosporins. It is similar to other cephalosporins in activity against Gram-positive organisms.

Indications: Claforan is indicated in the treatment of the following infections either before the infecting organism has been identified or when caused by bacteria of established sensitivity.

Septicaemias

Respiratory Tract Infections such as acute and chronic bronchitis, bacterial pneumonia, infected bronchiectasis, lung abscess and post-operative chest infections.

Urinary Tract Infections such as acute and chronic pyelonephritis, cystitis and asymptomatic bacteriuria.

Soft-Tissue Infections such as cellulitis, peritonitis and wound infections.

Bone and Joint Infections such as osteomyelitis, septic arthritis.

Obstetric and Gynaecological Infections such as pelvic inflammatory disease.

Gonorrhoea particularly when penicillin has failed or is unsuitable.

Other Bacterial Infections meningitis and other sensitive infections suitable for parenteral antibiotic therapy.

Prophylaxis:

The administration of Claforan prophylactically may reduce the incidence of certain post-operative infections in patients undergoing surgical procedures that are classified as contaminated or potentially contaminated or in clean operations where infection would have serious effects.

Protection is best ensured by achieving adequate local tissue concentrations at the time contamination is likely to occur. Claforan should therefore be administered immediately prior to surgery and if necessary continued in the immediate post-operative period.

Administration should usually be stopped within 24 hours since continuing use of any antibiotic in the majority of surgical procedures does not reduce the incidence of subsequent infection.

Bacteriology:

The following organisms have shown *in vitro* sensitivity to Claforan.

Gram-positive: Staphylococci, including coagulase-positive, coagulase-negative and penicillinase-producing strains.

Beta-haemolytic and other streptococci such as *Streptococcus mitis* (*viridans*) (many strains of enterococci, e.g. *Streptococcus faecalis*, are relatively resistant).

Streptococcus (Diplococcus) pneumoniae.

Clostridium spp.

Gram-negative:

Escherichia coli.

Haemophilus influenzae including ampicillin resistant strains.

Klebsiella spp.

Proteus spp. (both indole positive and indole negative).

Enterobacter spp.

Neisseria spp. (including β-lactamase producing strains of *N. gonorrhoea*).

Salmonella spp. (including *Sal. typhi*).

Shigella spp.

Providencia spp.

Serratia spp.

Citrobacter spp.

Claforan has frequently exhibited useful *in vitro* activity against *Pseudomonas* and *Bacteroides* species although some strains of *Bacteroides fragilis* are resistant.

There is *in vitro* evidence of synergy between Claforan and aminoglycoside antibiotics such as gentamicin against some species of Gram-negative bacteria including some strains of *Pseudomonas*. No *in vitro* antagonism has been noted. In severe infections caused by *Pseudomonas* spp. the addition of an aminoglycoside antibiotic may be indicated.

4.2 Posology and method of administration
DOSAGE:

Claforan may be administered intravenously, by bolus injection, by infusion or intramuscularly. The dosage, route and frequency of administration should be determined by the severity of infection, the sensitivity of causative organisms and condition of the patient. Therapy may be initiated before the results of sensitivity tests are known.

Adults: The recommended dosage for mild to moderate infections is 1g 12 hourly. However, dosage may be varied according to the severity of the infection, sensitivity of causative organisms and condition of the patient. Therapy may be initiated before the results of sensitivity tests are known.

In severe infections dosage may be increased up to 12g daily given in 3 or 4 divided doses. For infections caused by sensitive *Pseudomonas* spp. daily doses of greater than 6g will usually be required.

Children: The usual dosage range is 100-150mg/kg/day in 2 to 4 divided doses. However, in very severe infections doses of up to 200mg/kg/day may be required.

Neonates: The recommended dosage is 50mg/kg/day in 2 to 4 divided doses. In severe infections 150-200mg/kg/day, in divided doses, have been given.

Dosage in Gonorrhoea: A single injection of 1g may be administered intramuscularly or intravenously.

Dosage in Renal Impairment: Because of extra-renal elimination, it is only necessary to reduce the dosage of Claforan in severe renal failure (GFR < 5ml/min = serum creatinine approximately 751 micromol/l). After an initial loading dose of 1g, daily dose should be halved without change in the frequency of dosing, i.e. 1g in 12 hourly becomes 0.5g 12 hourly, 1g 8 hourly becomes 0.5g 8 hourly, 2g 8 hourly becomes 1g 8 hourly etc. As in all other patients, dosage may require further adjustment according to the course of the infection and the general condition of the patient.

ADMINISTRATION:

Intravenous and Intramuscular Administration: Reconstitute Claforan with Water for Injection Ph.Eur as given in the Dilution Table. Shake well until dissolved and then withdraw the entire contents of the vial into the syringe and use immediately.

Dilution Table:

Vial size	Diluent to be added
500mg	2ml
1g	4ml
2g	10ml

Intravenous Infusion: Claforan may be administered by intravenous infusion. 1-2g are dissolved in 40–100ml of Water for Injection Ph.Eur or in the infusion fluids listed under "Pharmaceutical Particulars". The prepared infusion may be administered over 20-60 minutes. To produce an infusion using vials with an infusion connector, remove the safety cap and directly connect the infusion bag. The needle in the closure will automatically pierce the vial stopper. Pressing the infusion bag will transfer solvent into the vial. Reconstitute by shaking the vial and finally, transfer the reconstituted solution back to the infusion bag ready for use.

4.3 Contraindications

Known or suspected hypersensitivity to cephalosporins.

4.4 Special warnings and special precautions for use

Preliminary enquiry about hypersensitivity to penicillin and other β-Lactam antibiotics is necessary before prescribing cephalosporins since cross allergy occurs in 5–10% of cases.

Hypersensitivity reactions (anaphylaxis) occurring with the two types of antibiotics can be serious and occasionally fatal. Hypersensitivity requires that treatment be stopped.

Patients with severe renal dysfunction should be placed on the dosage schedule recommended under "Posology and Method of Administration".

As with other antibiotics, the use of Claforan, especially if prolonged, may result in overgrowth of non susceptible organisms, such as *Enterococcus* spp. Repeated evaluation of the condition of the patient is essential. If superinfection occurs during treatment with Claforan, specific anti-microbial therapy should be instituted if considered clinically necessary.

Claforan constituted with lignocaine must never be used:

- by the intravenous route
- in infants under 30 months
- in subjects with a previous history of hypersensitivity to this product
- in patients who have an unpaced heart block
- in patients with severe heart failure.

The sodium content of Claforan (2.09mmol/g) should be taken into account when prescribing to patients requiring sodium restriction.

Claforan may predispose patients to pseudomembranous colitis. Although any antibiotic may predispose to pseudomembranous colitis, the risk is higher with broad spectrum drugs, such as cephalosporins. This side effect, which may occur more frequently in patients receiving higher doses for prolonged periods, should be considered as potentially serious. The presence of *C. difficile* toxin should be investigated, and treatment with Claforan stopped in cases of suspected colitis. Diagnosis can be confirmed by toxin detection and specific antibiotic therapy (e.g. oral vancomycin or metronidazole) should be initiated if considered clinically necessary. The administration of products which cause faecal stasis should be avoided.

4.5 Interaction with other medicinal products and other forms of Interaction

Cephalosporin antibiotics at high dosage should be given with caution to patients receiving aminoglycoside antibiotics or potent diuretics such as frusemide as these combinations are suspected to adversely affect renal function. However, at the recommended doses, enhancement of nephrotoxicity is unlikely to be a problem with Claforan.

Probenecid interferes with renal tubular transfer of Claforan delaying its excretion and increasing the plasma concentration.

Interference with Laboratory Tests: A positive Coombs test may be seen during treatment with cephalosporins. This phenomenon may occur during treatment with cefotaxime.

A false positive reaction to glucose may occur with reducing substances but not with the use of specific glucose oxidase methods.

4.6 Pregnancy and lactation

Pregnancy: It is known that Claforan crosses the placental barrier. Although studies in animals have not shown an adverse effect on the developing foetus, the safety of Claforan in human pregnancy has not been established. Consequently, Claforan should not be administered during pregnancy especially during the first trimester, without carefully weighing the expected benefit against possible risks.

Lactation: Claforan is excreted in the milk.

4.7 Effects on ability to drive and use machines

There is no evidence that Claforan directly impairs the ability to drive or to operate machines.

4.8 Undesirable effects

Adverse reactions to Claforan have occurred relatively infrequently and have generally been mild and transient. Effects reported include candidiasis, nausea, vomiting, abdominal pain, diarrhoea (diarrhoea may sometimes be a symptom of pseudomembranous colitis (see warnings)), transient rises in liver transaminases, alkaline phosphatase and/or bilirubin.

As with other cephalosporins, changes in renal function have been rarely observed with high doses of Claforan, particularly when co-prescribed with aminoglycosides. Rare cases of interstitial nephritis have been reported in patients treated with Claforan. Administration of high doses of cephalosporins, particularly in patients with renal insufficiency, may result in encephalopathy (e.g. impairment of consciousness, abnormal movements and convulsions).

Hypersensitivity reactions have been reported. These include skin rashes, pruritus and less frequently urticaria, drug fever and very rarely anaphylaxis (e.g. angioedema and bronchospasm possibly culminating in shock).

As with other cephalosporins, occasional cases of bullous reactions such as Stevens-Johnson syndrome, toxic epidermal necrolysis and erythema multiforme have also been reported.

As with other beta-lactam antibiotics, granulocytopenia and more rarely agranulocytosis may develop during treatment with Claforan, particularly if given over long periods. A few cases of eosinophilia and neutropenia have been observed, reversible when treatment is ceased. Some cases of rapidly reversible eosinophilia and thrombocytopenia on stopping treatment, have been reported. Rare cases of haemolytic anaemia have been reported. For cases of treatment lasting longer than 10 days, blood count should therefore be monitored.

Transient pain may be experienced at the site of injection. This is more likely to occur with higher doses. Occasionally, phlebitis has been reported in patients receiving intravenous Claforan. However, this has rarely been a cause for discontinuation of treatment.

A very small number of cases of arrhythmias have occurred following rapid bolus infusion through a central venous catheter.

The following symptoms have occurred after several weeks of treatment for borreliosis (Lyme's Disease): skin rash, itching, fever, leucopenia, increases in liver enzymes, difficulty of breathing, joint discomfort. To some extent these manifestations are consistent with the symptoms of the underlying disease, for which the patient is being treated.

4.9 Overdose

Serum levels of Claforan may be reduced by peritoneal dialysis or haemodialysis. In the case of overdosage, particularly in renal insufficiency there is a risk of reversible encephalopathy.

5. PHARMACOLOGICAL PROPERTIES

5.1 Pharmacodynamic properties

Claforan is a broad spectrum bactericidal cephalosporin antibiotic. Claforan is exceptionally active *in vitro* against Gram-negative organisms sensitive or resistant to first or second generation cephalosporins. It is similar to other cephalosporins in activity against Gram-positive bacteria.

5.2 Pharmacokinetic properties

After a 1000mg intravenous bolus, mean peak plasma concentrations of cefotaxime usually range between 81 and 102μg/ml. Doses of 500mg and 2000mg produce plasma concentrations of 38 and 200μg/ml, respectively. There is no accumulation following administration of 1000mg intravenously or 500mg intramuscularly for 10 or 14 days.

The apparent volume of distribution at steady-state of cefotaxime is 21.6L/1.73m^2 after 1g intravenous 30 minute infusion.

Concentrations of cefotaxime (usually determined by non-selective assay) have been studied in a wide range of human body tissues and fluids. Cerebrospinal fluid concentrations are low when the meninges are not inflamed, but are between 3 and 30μg/ml in children with meningitis. Cefotaxime usually passes the blood-brain barrier in levels above the MIC of common sensitive pathogens when the meninges are inflamed. Concentrations (0.2-5.4μg/ml), inhibitory for most Gram-negative bacteria, are attained in purulent sputum, bronchial secretions and pleural fluid after doses of 1 or 2g. Concentrations likely to be effective against most sensitive organisms are similarly attained in female reproductive organs, otitis media effusions, prostatic tissue, interstitial fluid, renal tissue, peritoneal fluid and gall bladder wall, after usual therapeutic doses. High concentrations of cefotaxime and desacetyl-cefotaxime are attained in bile.

Cefotaxime is partially metabolised prior to excretion. The principal metabolite is the microbiologically active product, desacetyl-cefotaxime. Most of a dose of cefotaxime is excreted in the urine about 60% as unchanged drug and a further 24% as desacetyl-cefotaxime. Plasma clearance is reported to be between 260 and 390ml/minute and renal clearance 145 to 217ml/minute.

After intravenous administration of cefotaxime to healthy adults, the elimination half-life of the parent compound is 0.9 to 1.14 hours and that of the desacetyl metabolite, about 1.3 hours.

In neonates the pharmacokinetics are influenced by gestational and chronological age, the half-life being prolonged in premature and low birth weight neonates of the same age.

In severe renal dysfunction the elimination half-life of cefotaxime itself is increased minimally to about 2.5 hours, whereas that of desacetyl-cefotaxime is increased to about 10 hours. Total urinary recovery of cefotaxime and its principal metabolite decreases with reduction in renal function.

5.3 Preclinical safety data

Not applicable.

6. PHARMACEUTICAL PARTICULARS

6.1 List of excipients

None.

6.2 Incompatibilities

None stated.

6.3 Shelf life

Finished product: 24 months.

Reconstituted solution: 24 hours.

6.4 Special precautions for storage

Finished Product: Store below 25°C. Protect from light.

Reconstituted Solution: Whilst it is preferable to use only freshly prepared solutions for both intravenous and intramuscular injection, Claforan is compatible with several commonly used intravenous infusion fluids and will retain satisfactory potency for up to 24 hours refrigerated (2-8°C) in the following:

- Water for Injections Ph. Eur.
- Sodium Chloride Injection BP.
- 5% Dextrose Injection BP.
- Dextrose and Sodium Chloride Injection BP.
- Compound Sodium Lactate Injection BP (Ringer-lactate Injection).

After 24 hours any unused solution should be discarded.

Claforan is also compatible with 1% lignocaine, however freshly prepared solutions should be used.

Claforan is also compatible with metronidazole infusion (500mg/100ml) and both will maintain potency when refrigerated (2-8°C) for up to 24 hours. Some increase in colour of prepared solutions may occur on storage. However, provided the recommended storage conditions are observed, this does not indicate change in potency or safety.

6.5 Nature and contents of container

Claforan is supplied in tubular or moulded glass vials Ph. Eur, closed with a grey elastomer stopper and sealed with either an aluminium cap fitted with a detachable flip top, or an infusion connector closure.

The bottles are boxed individually and in packs of 10.

6.6 Instructions for use and handling

Not applicable.

7. MARKETING AUTHORISATION HOLDER

Aventis Pharma Ltd

50 Kings Hill Avenue

West Malling

Kent

ME19 4AH

United Kingdom

8. MARKETING AUTHORISATION NUMBER(S)

PL 04425/0188

9. DATE OF FIRST AUTHORISATION/RENEWAL OF THE AUTHORISATION

31 October 2002

10. DATE OF REVISION OF THE TEXT

11. Legal Category

POM

Clexane

(sanofi-aventis)

1. NAME OF THE MEDICINAL PRODUCT

Clexane Syringes

Clexane Forte Syringes

2. QUALITATIVE AND QUANTITATIVE COMPOSITION

Clexane pre-filled syringes:

20 mg Injection Enoxaparin sodium 20 mg (equivalent to 2,000 IU anti-Xa activity) in 0.2 mL Water for Injections

40 mg Injection Enoxaparin sodium 40 mg (equivalent to 4,000 IU anti-Xa activity) in 0.4 mL Water for Injections

60 mg Injection Enoxaparin sodium 60 mg (equivalent to 6,000 IU anti-Xa activity) in 0.6 mL Water for Injections

80 mg Injection Enoxaparin sodium 80 mg (equivalent to 8,000 IU anti-Xa activity) in 0.8 mL Water for Injections

100 mg Injection Enoxaparin sodium 100mg (equivalent to 10,000 IU anti-Xa activity) in 1.0 mL Water for Injections

Clexane Forte pre-filled syringes

120 mg Injection Enoxaparin sodium 120 mg (equivalent to 12,000 IU anti-Xa activity) in 0.8 mL Water for Injections

150 mg Injection Enoxaparin sodium 150 mg (equivalent to 15,000 IU anti-Xa activity) in 1.0 mL Water for Injections

3. PHARMACEUTICAL FORM

Solution for injection.

4. CLINICAL PARTICULARS

4.1 Therapeutic indications

The prophylaxis of thromboembolic disorders of venous origin, in particular those which may be associated with orthopaedic or general surgery.

The prophylaxis of venous thromboembolism in medical patients bedridden due to acute illness.

The treatment of venous thromboembolic disease presenting with deep vein thrombosis, pulmonary embolism or both.

The treatment of unstable angina and non-Q-wave myocardial infarction, administered concurrently with aspirin.

The prevention of thrombus formation in the extracorporeal circulation during haemodialysis.

4.2 Posology and method of administration

Adults:

Prophylaxis of venous thromboembolism:

In patients with a low to moderate risk of venous thromboembolism the recommended dosage is 20 mg (2,000 IU) once daily for 7 to 10 days, or until the risk of thromboembolism has diminished. In patients undergoing surgery, the initial dose should be given approximately 2 hours pre-operatively.

In patients with a higher risk, such as in orthopaedic surgery, the dosage should be 40 mg (4,000 IU) daily with the initial dose administered approximately 12 hours before surgery.

Prophylaxis of venous thromboembolism in medical patients:

The recommended dose of enoxaparin sodium is 40 mg (4,000 IU) once daily. Treatment with enoxaparin sodium is prescribed for a minimum of 6 days and continued until the return to full ambulation, for a maximum of 14 days.

Treatment of venous thromboembolism:

Clexane should be administered subcutaneously as a single daily injection of 1.5 mg/kg (150 IU/kg). Clexane treatment is usually prescribed for at least 5 days and until adequate oral anticoagulation is established.

Treatment of unstable angina and non-Q-wave myocardial infarction

The recommended dose is 1 mg/kg Clexane every 12 hours by subcutaneous injection, administered concurrently with oral aspirin (100 to 325mg once daily)

Treatment with Clexane in these patients should be prescribed for a minimum of 2 days and continued until clinical stabilisation. The usual duration of treatment is 2 to 8 days.

Prevention of extracorporeal thrombus formation during haemodialysis:

A dose equivalent to 1 mg/kg (100 IU/kg) introduced into the arterial line at the beginning of a dialysis session is usually sufficient for a 4 hour session. If fibrin rings are found, such as after a longer than normal session, a further dose of 0.5 to 1mg/kg (50 to 100 IU/kg) may be given. For patients at a high risk of haemorrhage the dose should be reduced to 0.5 mg/kg (50 IU/kg) for double vascular access or 0.75 mg/kg (75 IU/kg) for single vascular access.

Elderly: No dosage adjustments are necessary in the elderly, unless kidney function is impaired (see also Posology and method of administration: *Renal impairment*; Special warnings and precautions for use: *Haemorrhage in the elderly*; *Renal impairment and Monitoring*; Pharmacokinetic properties).

Children: Not recommended, as dosage not established.

Renal impairment: (See also Special warnings and precautions for use: *Renal impairment and Monitoring*; Pharmacokinetic properties).

Severe renal impairment:

A dosage adjustment is required for patients with severe renal impairment (creatinine clearance < 30 ml/min), according to the following tables, since enoxaparin sodium exposure is significantly increased in this patient population:

Dosage adjustments for therapeutic dosage ranges

Standard dosing	Severe renal impairment
1 mg/kg twice daily	1 mg/kg once daily
1.5 mg/kg once daily	1 mg/kg once daily

Dosage adjustments for prophylactic dosage ranges

Standard dosing	Severe renal impairment
40 mg once daily	20 mg once daily
20 mg once daily	20 mg once daily

The recommended dosage adjustments do not apply to the haemodialysis indication.

Moderate and mild renal impairment:

Although no dosage adjustments are recommended in patients with moderate renal impairment (creatinine clearance 30-50 ml/min) or mild renal impairment (creatinine clearance 50-80 ml/min), careful clinical monitoring is advised.

Hepatic impairment: In the absence of clinical studies, caution should be exercised.

Body weight:

No dosage adjustments are recommended in obesity or low body weight (see also Special warnings and precautions for use: *Low body weight and Monitoring*; Pharmacokinetic properties).

Clexane is administered by subcutaneous injection for the prevention of venous thromboembolic disease, treatment of deep vein thrombosis or for the treatment of unstable angina and non-Q-wave myocardial infarction; and through the arterial line of a dialysis circuit for the prevention of thrombus formation in the extra-corporeal circulation during haemodialysis. It must not be administered by the intramuscular route.

Subcutaneous injection technique. The prefilled disposable syringe is ready for immediate use.

Clexane should be administered when the patient is lying down by deep subcutaneous injection. The administration should be alternated between the left and right anterolateral or posterolateral abdominal wall. The whole length of the needle should be introduced vertically into a skin fold held between the thumb and index finger. The skin fold should not be released until the injection is complete. Do not rub the injection site after administration.

4.3 Contraindications

Contraindicated in patients with acute bacterial endocarditis; major bleeding disorders; thrombocytopenia in patients with a positive in-vitro aggregation test in the presence of enoxaparin; active gastric or duodenal ulceration; hypersensitivity to enoxaparin; stroke (unless due to systemic emboli); other patients with an increased risk of haemorrhage; in patients receiving heparin for treatment rather than prophylaxis, locoregional anaesthesia in elective surgical procedures is contra-indicated.

4.4 Special warnings and special precautions for use

As different low molecular weight heparins may not be equivalent, alternative products should not be substituted during a course of treatment.

Enoxaparin is to be used with extreme caution in patients with a history of heparin-induced thrombocytopenia with or without thrombosis.

As there is a risk of antibody-mediated heparin-induced thrombocytopenia also occurring with low molecular weight heparins, regular platelet count monitoring should be considered prior to and during therapy with these agents. Thrombocytopenia, should it occur, usually appears between the 5th and the 21st day following the beginning of therapy. If platelet count is significantly reduced (30 to 50 % of the initial value), therapy must be discontinued immediately and an alternative therapy initiated.

Enoxaparin injection, as with any other anticoagulant therapy, should be used with caution in conditions with increased potential for bleeding, such as: impaired haemostasis, history of peptic ulcer, recent ischaemic stroke, uncontrolled severe arterial hypertension, diabetic retinopathy, recent neuro- or ophthalmologic surgery.

Heparin can suppress adrenal secretion of aldosterone leading to hyperkalaemia, particularly in patients such as those with diabetes mellitus, chronic renal failure, pre-existing metabolic acidosis, a raised plasma potassium or taking potassium sparing drugs. The risk of hyperkalaemia appears to increase with duration of therapy but is usually reversible. Plasma potassium should be measured in patients at risk before starting heparin therapy and monitored regularly thereafter particularly if treatment is prolonged beyond about 7 days.

As with other anti-coagulants, there have been cases of intra-spinal haematomas reported with the concurrent use of enoxaparin sodium and spinal/epidural anaesthesia or spinal punctureresulting in long term or permanent paralysis. These events are rare with enoxaparin sodium dosage regimens 40 mg od or lower. The risk is greater with higher enoxaparin sodium dosage regimens, use of post-operative indwelling catheters or the concomitant use of additional drugs affecting haemostasis such as NSAID's (see Interactions with other medicinal products or other forms of interaction). The risk also appears to be increased by traumatic or repeated neuraxial puncture.

To reduce the potential risk of bleeding associated with the concurrent use of enoxaparin sodium and epidural anaesthesia/analgesia, the pharmacokinetic profile of the drug should be considered (see Pharmacokinetic properties). Placement and removal of the catheter is best performed when the anticoagulation effect of enoxaparin is low.

Placement or removal of a catheter should be delayed for 10 - 12 hours after administration of DVT prophylactic doses of enoxaparin sodium, whereas patients receiving higher doses of enoxaparin sodium (1.5 mg/kg once daily) will require longer delays (24 hours). The subsequent enoxaparin sodium dose should be given no sooner than 4 hours after catheter removal.

Should the physician decide to administer anticoagulation in the context of epidural/spinal anaesthesia, extreme vigilance and frequent monitoring must be exercised to detect any signs and symptoms of neurological impairment such as midline back pain, sensory and motor deficits (numbness or weakness in lower limbs), bowel and/or bladder dysfunction. Patients should be instructed to inform their nurse or physician immediately if they experience any of the above signs or symptoms. If signs or symptoms of spinal haematoma are suspected, urgent diagnosis and treatment including spinal cord decompression should be initiated.

Percutaneous coronary revascularisation procedures:

To minimise the risk of bleeding following the vascular instrumentation during the treatment of unstable angina, the vascular sheath should remain in place for 6 to 8 hours following a dose of enoxaparin sodium. The next scheduled dose should be given no sooner than 6 to 8 hours after sheath removal. The site of the procedure should be observed for signs of bleeding or haematoma formation.

For some patients with pulmonary embolism (e.g. those with severe haemodynamic instability) alternative treatment such as thrombolysis or surgery may be indicated.

Prosthetic Heart Valves

There have been no adequate studies to assess the safe and effective use of enoxaparin sodium in preventing valve thrombosis in patients with prosthetic heart valves. Prophylactic doses of enoxaparin are not sufficient to prevent valve thrombosis in patients with prosthetic heart valves. Therapeutic failures have been reported in pregnant women with prosthetic heart valves on full anti-coagulant doses (see Use during Pregnancy and Lactation). The use of enoxaparin sodium cannot be recommended for this purpose.

Haemorrhage in the elderly: No increased bleeding tendency is observed in the elderly within the prophylactic dosage ranges. Elderly patients (especially patients aged eighty years and above) may be at an increased risk for bleeding complications within the therapeutic dosage ranges. Careful clinical monitoring is advised (see also Posology and method of administration: Elderly; Pharmacokinetic properties).

Renal impairment: In patients with renal impairment, there is an increase in enoxaparin exposure which increases the risk of bleeding. Since enoxaparin exposure is significantly increased in patients with severe renal impairment (creatinine clearance < 30 ml/min) dosage adjustments are recommended in therapeutic and prophylactic dosage ranges. Although no dosage adjustments are recommended in patients with moderate (creatinine clearance 30-50 ml/min) and mild (creatinine clearance 50-80 ml/min) renal impairment, careful clinical monitoring is advised (see also Posology and method of administration: Renal impairment; Pharmacokinetic properties).

Low body weight: In low-weight women (< 45 kg) and low-weight men (< 57 kg), an increase in enoxaparin exposure has been observed within the prophylactic dosage ranges (non-weight adjusted), which may lead to a higher risk of bleeding. Therefore, careful clinical monitoring is advised in these patients (see also Pharmacokinetic properties).

Monitoring: Risk assessment and clinical monitoring are the best predictors of the risk of potential bleeding. Routine anti-Xa activity monitoring is usually not required. However, anti-Xa activity monitoring might be considered in those patients treated with LMWH who also have either an increased risk of bleeding (such as those with renal impairment, elderly and extremes of weight) or are actively bleeding.

4.5 Interaction with other medicinal products and other forms of Interaction

It is recommended that agents which affect haemostasis should be discontinued prior to enoxaparin therapy unless their use is essential, such as: systemic salicylates, acetylsalicylic acid, NSAIDs including ketorolac, dextran and ticlopidine, systemic glucocorticoids, thrombolytics and anticoagulants. If the combination cannot be avoided, enoxaparin should be used with careful clinical and laboratory monitoring.

4.6 Pregnancy and lactation

Pregnancy: Animal studies have not shown any evidence of foetotoxicity or teratogenicity. In the pregnant rat, the transfer of ^{35}S-enoxaparin across the maternal placenta to the foetus is minimal.

In humans, there is no evidence that enoxaparin crosses the placental barrier during the second trimester of pregnancy. There is no information available concerning the first and the third trimesters.

As there are no adequate and well-controlled studies in pregnant women and because animal studies are not always predictive of human response, this drug should not be used in pregnant patients unless no safer alternative is available.

Lactation: In lactating rats, the concentration of ^{35}S-enoxaparin or its labelled metabolites in milk is very low.

It is not known whether unchanged enoxaparin is excreted in human breast milk. The oral absorption of enoxaparin is unlikely. However, as a precaution, lactating mothers receiving enoxaparin should be advised to avoid breast-feeding.

Prosthetic Heart Valves:

In a South African clinical study of pregnant women with prosthetic heart valves given enoxaparin sodium (1mg/1kg/b.i.d.) to prevent valve thrombosis, two women developed clots resulting in blockage of the valve and leading to death. In the absence of clear dosing, efficacy and safety information in this circumstance, enoxaparin sodium is not recommended for use in pregnant women with prosthetic heart valves.

4.7 Effects on ability to drive and use machines

Enoxaparin has no effect on the ability to drive and operate machines

4.8 Undesirable effects

As with other anticoagulants bleeding may occur during enoxaparin therapy in the presence of associated risk factors such as: organic lesions liable to bleed or the use of medications affecting haemostasis (see Interaction section). The origin of the bleeding should be investigated and appropriate treatment instituted.

Major haemorrhage including retroperitoneal and intracranial bleeding have been reported, in rare instances these have been fatal.

Mild, transient, asymptomatic thrombocytopenia has been reported during the first days of therapy. Immuno-allergic thrombocytopenia, with or without thrombosis, has rarely been reported.

Pain, haematoma and mild local irritation may follow the subcutaneous injection of enoxaparin. Rarely, hard inflammatory nodules which are not cystic enclosures of enoxaparin, have been observed at the injection site. They resolve after a few days and should not cause therapy discontinuation.

Exceptional cases of skin necrosis at the injection site have been reported with heparins and low molecular weight heparins. These phenomena are usually preceded by purpura or erythematous plaques, infiltrated and painful. Enoxaparin must be discontinued.

Although rare, cutaneous or systemic allergic reactions may occur. In some cases discontinuation of therapy may be necessary.

Asymptomatic and reversible increases in platelet counts and liver enzyme levels have been reported.

Long term therapy with heparin has been associated with a risk of osteoporosis. Although this has not been observed with enoxaparin the risk of osteoporosis cannot be excluded.

Heparin products can cause hypoaldosteronism which may result in an increase in plasma potassium. Rarely, clinically significant hyperkalaemia may occur particularly in patients with chronic renal failure and diabetes mellitus (see Special Warnings and Precautions for Use).

There have been very rare reports of intra-spinal haematomas with the concurrent use of enoxaparin and spinal/epidural anaesthesia, spinal puncture and post-operative indwelling catheters. These events have resulted in varying degrees of neurological injuries including long term or permanent paralysis (see Special Warnings and Precautions for Use).

Valve thrombosis in patients with prosthetic heart valves have been reported rarely, usually associated with inadequate dosing (see Special Warnings and Precautions for Use).

4.9 Overdose

Orally administered enoxaparin is poorly absorbed and even large oral doses should not lead to any serious consequences. This may be checked by plasma assays of anti-Xa and anti-IIa activities.

Accidental overdose following parenteral administration may produce haemorrhagic complications. These may be largely neutralised by slow intravenous injection of protamine sulphate or hydrochloride. The dose of protamine should be equal to the dose of enoxaparin injected, that is, 100 anti-heparin units of protamine should neutralise the anti-IIa activity generated by 1mg (100 IU) of enoxaparin. However, even with high doses of protamine, the anti-Xa activity of enoxaparin is never completely neutralised (maximum about 60%).

5. PHARMACOLOGICAL PROPERTIES

5.1 Pharmacodynamic properties

Enoxaparin is a low molecular weight heparin which has antithrombotic activity. It is characterised by a higher ratio of antithrombotic activity to anticoagulant activity than unfractionated heparin. At recommended doses, it does not significantly influence platelet aggregation, binding of fibrinogen to platelets or global clotting tests such as APTT and prothrombin time.

5.2 Pharmacokinetic properties

Enoxaparin is rapidly and completely absorbed following subcutaneous injection. The maximum plasma anti-Xa activity occurs 1 to 4 hours after injection with peak activities in the order of 0.16 IU/ml and 0.38 IU/ml after doses of 20 mg or 40 mg respectively. The anti-Xa activity generated is localised within the vascular compartments and elimination is characterised by a half life of 4 to 5 hours. Following a 40 mg dose, anti-Xa activity may persist in the plasma for 24 hours.

A linear relationship between anti-Xa plasma clearance and creatinine clearance at steady-state has been observed, which indicates decreased clearance of enoxaparin sodium in patients with reduced renal function. In patients with severe renal impairment (creatinine clearance < 30 ml/min), the AUC at steady state is significantly increased by an average of 65% after repeated, once daily subcutaneous doses of 40mg.

Hepatic metabolism by desulphation and depolymerisation also contributes to elimination. The elimination half life may be prolonged in elderly patients although no dosage adjustment is necessary.

A study of repeated, once daily subcutaneous doses of 1.5 mg/kg in healthy volunteers suggests that no dosage adjustment is necessary in obese subjects (BMI 30-48 kg/m^2) compared to non-obese subjects.

Enoxaparin, as detected by anti-Xa activity, does not cross the placental barrier during the second trimester of pregnancy.

5.3 Preclinical safety data

There are no pre-clinical data of relevance to the prescriber which are additional to that already included in other sections of the SPC

6. PHARMACEUTICAL PARTICULARS

6.1 List of excipients

Water for Injections BP

6.2 Incompatibilities

Clexane should not be mixed with any other injections or infusions

6.3 Shelf life

Clexane syringes - 36 months.

Clexane Forte Syringes – 24 months

6.4 Special precautions for storage

Do not store above 25°C. Do not refrigerate or freeze.

Clexane pre-filled syringes are single dose containers - discard any unused product.

6.5 Nature and contents of container

Solution for injection in Type I glass pre-filled syringes fitted with injection needle in packs of 10.

6.6 Instructions for use and handling

See "Posology and method of administration "

7. MARKETING AUTHORISATION HOLDER

May & Baker Limited

trading as Aventis Pharma, or Rhône Poulenc Rorer

50 Kings Hill Avenue

West Malling

Kent

ME19 4AH

8. MARKETING AUTHORISATION NUMBER(S)

Clexane Syringes PL 0012/0196

Clexane Forte syringes PL 0012/0339

9. DATE OF FIRST AUTHORISATION/RENEWAL OF THE AUTHORISATION

Clexane Syringes August 2002

Clexane Forte Syringes December 1999

10. DATE OF REVISION OF THE TEXT

Clexane Syringes November 2004

Clexane Forte Syringes August 2004

11. LEGAL STATUS

POM

Climagest 1mg, film coated tablet, 2mg, film coated tablet

(Novartis Pharmaceuticals UK Ltd)

1. NAME OF THE MEDICINAL PRODUCT

Climagest® 1mg, film coated tablet

Climagest® 2mg, film coated tablet

2. QUALITATIVE AND QUANTITATIVE COMPOSITION

16 tablets each containing 1 mg or 2 mg estradiol valerate USP, 12 tablets each containing 1 mg or 2 mg estradiol valerate USP and 1 mg norethisterone Ph Eur.

For excipients, see 6.1.

3. PHARMACEUTICAL FORM

Film-coated tablet.

Estradiol valerate 1mg tablets: grey-blue tablet, coded OC on one side, CG on the other.

Combination tablets: white tablet, coded OE on one side, CG on the other.

Estradiol valerate 2 mg tablets: blue tablet, coded OD on one side, CG on the other

Combination tablets: yellow-white tablet, coded OF on one side, CG on the other

4. CLINICAL PARTICULARS

4.1 Therapeutic indications

Hormone replacement therapy for the treatment of menopausal symptoms.

The experience treating women older than 65 years is limited.

4.2 Posology and method of administration

Climagest provides continuous estrogen and sequential progestagen to women.

Treatment commences with one grey-blue tablet daily for the first 16 days followed by one white tablet daily for the next 12 days, as directed on the 28 day calendar pack. Women not menstruating may start therapy at any time. However, if the patient is menstruating regularly it is advised that the patient starts therapy on the first day of bleeding. Menstrual bleeding during initial Climagest therapy may be irregular. Pregnancy should be excluded before starting therapy. For the initiation and continuation of treatment of postmenopausal symptoms, the lowest effective dose for the shortest duration (see also Section 4.4) should be used.

Climagest may be taken continuously by women with an intact uterus as it provides both estrogen and progestogen to reduce endometrial hyperstimulation.

Unless there is a previous diagnosis of endometriosis, it is not recommended to add a progestagen in hysterectomised women.

Patients changing from another continuous sequential or cyclical preparation should complete the cycle and may then change to Climagest without a break in therapy. Patients changing from a continuous combined preparation may start therapy at any time if amenorrhoea is established, or otherwise start on the first day of bleeding.

Missed tablet: If a tablet is missed it should be taken within 12 hours of when normally taken; otherwise the tablet should be discarded, and the usual tablet should be taken the following day. Forgetting or missing a dose may increase the likelihood of breakthrough bleeding.

Use in the elderly

Climagest should only be used in the elderly for the indications listed.

Use in children

Climagest should not be used in children.

4.3 Contraindications

- Known, past or suspected breast cancer.
- Known or suspected estrogen-dependent malignant tumours. (e.g. endometrial cancer)
- Undiagnosed genital bleeding.
- Untreated endometrial hyperplasia.
- Severe renal disease.
- Acute liver disease, or a history of liver disease as long as liver function tests have failed to return to normal.
- Previous idiopathic or current venous thromboembolism (deep venous thrombosis, pulmonary embolism).
- Active or recent arterial thromboembolic disease (e.g. angina, myocardial infarction).
- Known hypersensitivity to the active substance or to any of the excipients.
- Porphyria.

4.4 Special warnings and special precautions for use

As Climagest is not an oral contraceptive adequate non-hormonal measures should be taken to exclude pregnancy.

For the treatment of postmenopausal symptoms, HRT should only be initiated for symptoms that adversely affect quality of life. In all cases, a careful appraisal of the risks and benefits should be undertaken at least annually and HRT should only be continued as long as the benefit outweighs the risk.

Medical Examination / follow-up

Before initiating or reinstituting HRT, a complete personal and family medical history should be taken. Physical (including pelvic and breast) examination should be guided by this and by the contraindications and warnings for use. During treatment, periodic check-ups are recommended of a frequency and nature adapted to the individual woman. Women should be advised what changes in their breasts should be reported to their doctor or nurse (see 'Breast cancer' below). Investigations, including mammography, should be carried out in accordance with currently accepted screening practices, modified according to the clinical needs of the individual.

Conditions which need supervision

If any of the following conditions are present, have occurred previously, and/or have been aggravated during pregnancy or previous hormone treatment, the patient should be closely supervised. It should be taken into account that these conditions may recur or be aggravated during treatment with Climagest, in particular:

- Leiomyoma (uterine fibroids) or endometriosis
- A history of, or risk factors for, thromboembolic disorders (see below)
- Risk factors for estrogen dependent tumours, e.g. 1st degree heredity for breast cancer
- Hypertension
- Liver disorders (eg liver adenoma) – patients with mild chronic disease should have their liver function checked every 8-12 weeks.
- Diabetes mellitus with or without vascular involvement
- Cholelithiasis
- Migraine or (severe) headache
- Systemic lupus erythematosus
- A history of endometrial hyperplasia (see below)
- Epilepsy
- Asthma
- Otosclerosis

Reasons for immediate withdrawal of therapy:

Therapy should be discontinued in case a contra-indication is discovered and in the following situations:

- Jaundice or deterioration in liver function
- Significant increase in blood pressure
- New onset of migraine-type headache, or any other symptoms that are a possible prodromata of vascular occlusion
- Pregnancy

Endometrial hyperplasia

- The risk of endometrial hyperplasia and carcinoma is increased when estrogens are administered alone for prolonged periods (see Section 4.8). The addition of a progestagen for at least 12 days per cycle in non-hysterectomised women greatly reduces this risk.
- Break-through bleeding and spotting may occur during the first months of treatment. If break through bleeding or spotting appears after some time on therapy, or continues after treatment has been discontinued, the reason should be investigated, which may include endometrial biopsy to exclude endometrial malignancy.

Breast cancer

A randomised placebo-controlled trial, the Women's Health Initiative study (WHI) and epidemiological studies, including the Million Women Study (MWS), have reported an increased risk of breast cancer in women taking estrogens or estrogen-progestagen combinations or tibolone for HRT for several years (see Section 4.8).

For all HRT, an excess risk becomes apparent within a few years of use and increases with duration of intake but returns to baseline within a few (at most five) years after stopping treatment.

In the MWS, the relative risk of breast cancer with conjugated equine estrogens (CEE) or estradiol (E2) was greater when a progestagen was added, either sequentially or continuously, and regardless of type of progestagen. There was no evidence of a difference in risk between the different routes of administration.

In the WHI study, the continuous combined conjugated equine estrogen and medroxyprogesterone acetate (CEE + MPA) product used was associated with breast cancers that were slightly larger in size and more frequently had local lymph node metastases compared to placebo.

HRT, especially estrogen-progestagen combined treatment, increases the density of mammographic images which may adversely affect the radiological detection of breast cancer.

Venous thromboembolism

HRT is associated with a higher relative risk of developing venous thromboembolism (VTE), i.e. deep vein thrombosis or pulmonary embolism. One randomised controlled trial and epidemiological studies found a 2-3 fold higher risk for users compared with non-users. For non-users, it is estimated that the number of cases of VTE that will occur over a 5 year period is about 3 per 1000 women aged 50-59 years and 8 per 1000 women aged between 60-69 years. It is estimated that in healthy women who use HRT for 5 years, the number of additional cases of VTE over a 5 year period will be between 2 and 6 (best estimate=4) per 1000 women aged 50-59 years and between 5 and 15 (best estimate=9) per 1000 women aged 60-69 years. The occurrence of such an event is more likely in the first year of HRT than later.

Generally recognised risk factors for VTE include a personal history or family history, severe obesity (Body Mass Index > 30kg/m²) and systemic lupus erythematosus (SLE). There is no consensus about the role of varicose veins in VTE.

Patients with a history of VTE or known thrombophilic states have an increased risk of VTE. HRT may add to this risk. Personal or strong family history of thromboembolism or recurrent spontaneous abortion should be investigated in order to exclude a thrombophilic predisposition. Until a thorough evaluation of thrombophilic factors has been made or anticoagulant treatment initiated, use of HRT in such patients should be viewed as contra-indicated. Those women already on anticoagulant treatment require careful consideration of the benefit-risk of use of HRT.

The risk of VTE may be temporarily increased with prolonged immobilisation, major trauma or major surgery. As in all post-operative patients scrupulous attention should be given to prophylactic measures to prevent VTE following surgery. Where prolonged immobilisation is liable to follow elective surgery, particularly abdominal or orthopaedic surgery to the lower limbs, consideration should be given to temporarily stopping HRT four to six weeks earlier, if possible. Treatment should not be restarted until the woman is completely mobilised.

If VTE develops after initiating therapy, the drug should be discontinued. Patients should be told to contact their doctors immediately when they are aware of a potential thromboembolic symptom (e.g. painful swelling of a leg, sudden pain in the chest, dyspnoea).

Coronary artery disease (CAD)

There is no evidence from randomised controlled trials of cardiovascular benefit with continuous combined conjugated estrogens and medroxyprogesterone acetate (MPA). Two large clinical trials (WHI and HERS i.e. Heart and Estrogen/progestin Replacement Study) showed a possible increased risk of cardiovascular morbidity in the first year of use and no overall benefit. For other HRT products there are only limited data from randomised controlled trials to date examining effects in cardiovascular morbidity or mortality. Therefore, it is uncertain whether these findings also extend to other HRT products.

Stroke

One large randomised clinical trial (WHI-trial) found, as a secondary outcome, an increased risk of ischaemic stroke in healthy women during treatment with continuous combined conjugated estrogens and MPA. For women who do not use HRT, it is estimated that the number of cases of stroke that will occur over a 5 year period is about 3 per 1000 women aged 50-59 years and 11 per 1000 women aged 60-69 years. It is estimated that for women who use conjugated estrogens and MPA for 5 years, the number of additional cases will be between 0 and 3 (best estimate=1) per 1000 users aged 50-59 years and between 1 and 9 (best estimate=4) per 1000 users aged 60-69 years. It is unknown whether the increased risk also extends to other HRT products.

Ovarian cancer

Long-term (at least 5 to 10 years) use of estrogen-only HRT products in hysterectomised women has been associated with an increased risk of ovarian cancer in some epidemiological studies. It is uncertain whether long-term use of combined HRT confers a different risk than estrogen-only products.

Other conditions

Estrogens may cause fluid retention, and therefore patients with cardiac or renal dysfunction should be carefully observed. Patients with terminal renal insufficiency should be closely observed, since it is expected that the level of circulating active ingredients in Climagest is increased.

Women with pre-existing hypertriglyceridemia should be followed closely during estrogen replacement or hormone replacement therapy, since rare cases of large increases of plasma triglycerides leading to pancreatitis have been reported with estrogen therapy in this condition.

Estrogens increase thyroid binding globulin (TBG), leading to increased circulating total thyroid hormone, as measured by protein-bound iodine (PBI), T4 levels (by column or by radio-immunoassay) or T3 levels (by radio-immunoassay). T3 resin uptake is decreased, reflecting the elevated TBG. Free T4 and free T3 concentrations are unaltered. Other binding proteins may be elevated in serum, ie corticoid binding globulin (CBG), sex-hormone-binding globulin (SHBG) leading to increased circulating corticosteroidsand sex steroids, respectively. Free or biological active hormone concentrations are unchanged. Other plasma proteins may be increased (angiotensinogen/renin substrate, alpha-I-antitrypsin, ceruloplasmin).

There is no conclusive evidence for improvement of cognitive function. There is some evidence from the WHI trial of increased risk of probable dementia in women who start using continuous combined CEE and MPA after the age of 65. It is unknown whether the findings apply to younger post-menopausal women or other HRT products.

4.5 Interaction with other medicinal products and other forms of Interaction

The metabolism of estrogens and progestagens may be increased by concomitant use of substances known to induce drug-metabolising enzymes, specifically cytochrome P450 enzymes, such as anticonvulsants (e.g. phenobarbital, phenytoin, carbamazepine) and anti-infectives (e.g. rifampicin, rifabutin, nevirapine, efavirenz).

Ritonavir and nelfinavir, although known as strong inhibitors, by contrast exhibit inducing properties when used concomitantly with steroid hormones.

Herbal preparations containing St John's wort (*Hypericum perforatum*) may induce the metabolism of estrogens.

Clinically, an increased metabolism of estrogens and progestogens may lead to decreased effect and changes in the uterine bleeding profile.

4.6 Pregnancy and lactation

Climagest is not indicated during pregnancy. If pregnancy occurs during medication with Climagest treatment should be withdrawn immediately.

Data on a limited number of exposed pregnancies indicate adverse effects of norethisterone on the foetus. At doses higher than normally used in OC and HRT formulations, masculinisation of the female foetus was observed.

The results of most epidemiological studies to date relevant to inadvertent foetal exposure to combinations of estrogens and progestagens indicate no teratogenic or foetotoxic effects.

Climagest is not indicated during lactation.

4.7 Effects on ability to drive and use machines

No adverse effects on the ability to drive or operate machines have been recorded.

4.8 Undesirable effects

Reproductive and urogenital tract: Breast tension and pain, breast cancer*, mucous vaginal discharge

Central Nervous System: Headaches, dizziness, vertigo, changes in libido, depressive mood

Cardiovascular system: Hypertension, palpitations, thrombophlebitis, oedema, epistaxis,

Gastrointestinal tract: Dyspepsia, flatulence, nausea, vomiting, abdominal pain and bloating, biliary stasis

Skin and appendages: General pruritus, alopecia, urticaria and other rashes

Endocrine system: Decrease in glucose tolerance

Miscellaneous: Weight gain

*Breast cancer

According to evidence from a large number of epidemiological studies and one randomised placebo-controlled trial, the Women's Health Initiative (WHI), the overall risk of breast cancer increases with increasing duration of HRT use in current or recent HRT users.

For *estrogen-only* HRT, estimates of relative risk (RR) from a reanalysis of original data from 51 epidemiological studies (in which >80% of HRT use was estrogen-only HRT) and from the epidemiological Million Women Study (MWS) are similar at 1.35 (95%CI 1.21 – 1.49) and 1.30 (95%CI 1.21 – 1.40), respectively.

For *estrogen plus progestagen* combined HRT, several epidemiological studies have reported an overall higher risk for breast cancer than with estrogens alone.

The MWS reported that, compared to never users, the use of various types of estrogen-progestagen combined HRT was associated with a higher risk of breast cancer (RR = 2.00, 95%CI: 1.88 – 2.12) than use of estrogens alone (RR = 1.30, 95%CI: 1.21 – 1.40) or use of tibolone (RR=1.45; 95%CI 1.25-1.68).

The WHI trial reported a risk estimate of 1.24 (95%CI 1.01 – 1.54) after 5.6 years of use of estrogen-progestagen combined HRT (CEE + MPA) in all users compared with placebo.

The absolute risks calculated from the MWS and the WHI trial are presented below:

The MWS has estimated, from the known average incidence of breast cancer in developed countries, that:

– For women not using HRT, about 32 in every 1000 are expected to have breast cancer diagnosed between the ages of 50 and 64 years.

– For 1000 current or recent users of HRT, the number of *additional* cases during the corresponding period will be

– For users of *estrogen-only* replacement therapy

- between 0 and 3 (best estimate = 1.5) for 5 years' use
- between 3 and 7 (best estimate = 5) for 10 years' use.

– For users of *estrogen plus progestagen* combined HRT,

- between 5 and 7 (best estimate = 6) for 5 years' use

between 18 and 20 (best estimate = 19) for 10 years' use.

The WHI trial estimated that after 5.6 years of follow-up of women between the ages of 50 and 79 years, an *additional* 8 cases of invasive breast cancer would be due to *estrogen-progestagen combined* HRT (CEE + MPA) per 10,000 women years.

According to calculations from the trial data, it is estimated that:

– For 1000 women in the placebo group,

• about 16 cases of invasive breast cancer would be diagnosed in 5 years.

– For 1000 women who used estrogen + progestagen combined HRT (CEE + MPA), the number of *additional* cases would be

• between 0 and 9 (best estimate = 4) for 5 years' use.

The number of additional cases of breast cancer in women who use HRT is broadly similar for women who start HRT irrespective of age at start of use (between the ages of 45-65) (see Section 4.4).

Endometrial cancer

In women with an intact uterus, the risk of endometrial hyperplasia and endometrial cancer increases with increasing duration of use of unopposed estrogens. According to data from epidemiological studies, the best estimate of the risk is that for women not using HRT, about 5 in every 1000 are expected to have endometrial cancer diagnosed between the ages of 50 and 65. Depending on the duration of treatment and estrogen dose, the reported increase in endometrial cancer risk among unopposed estrogen users varies from 2-to 12-fold greater compared with non-users. Adding a progestagen to estrogen-only therapy greatly reduces this increased risk.

Other adverse reactions have been reported in association with estrogen/progestagen treatment:

• Estrogen-dependent neoplasms benign and malignant (e.g. endometrial cancer)

• Venous thromboembolism, i.e. deep leg or pelvic venous thrombosis and pulmonary embolism, is more frequent among hormone replacement therapy users than among non-users. For further information, see Section 4.3 Contraindications and 4.4 Special warnings and precautions for use.

• Myocardial infarction and stroke.

• Gall bladder disease.

• Skin and subcutaneous disorders: chloasma, erythema multiforme, erythema nodosum, vascular purpura.

• Probable dementia (see Section 4.4).

4.9 Overdose

There have been no reports of ill-effects from overdosage. There are no specific antidotes, and further treatment should be symptomatic.

5. PHARMACOLOGICAL PROPERTIES

5.1 Pharmacodynamic properties

Estradiol

The active ingredient, synthetic 17β-estradiol, is chemically and biologically identical to endogenous human estradiol. It substitutes for the loss of estrogen production in menopausal women, and alleviates menopausal symptoms.

Estradiol valerate is used in estrogen deficiency states. Treatment with estrogens relieves menopausal vasomotor symptoms. Estrogens cross the placenta.

Progestagen

As estrogens promote the growth of the endometrium, unopposed estrogens increase the risk of endometrial hyperplasia and cancer. The addition of progestagen reduces but does not eliminate the estrogen induced risk of endometrial hyperplasia in non hysterectomised women.

Norethisterone is a progestogen added to prevent endometrial hyperplasia and increased risk of endometrial carcinoma which can be induced by unopposed estrogen use.

5.2 Pharmacokinetic properties

Estradiol valerate, like most natural estrogens, is readily and fully absorbed from the GI tract, is 50% bound to plasma proteins and is rapidly metabolised in the liver to oestriol and oestrone. When given orally in doses of 1-2 mg, peak levels of estradiol are generally observed 3-6 hours after ingestion, but by 24 hours (range 6-48 hours) concentrations have returned to baseline (ie pre-treatment concentrations).

Estradiol undergoes first-pass effect in the liver. There is some enterohepatic recycling. It is excreted via the kidney in the urine as water soluble esters (sulphate and glucuronide) together with a small proportion of unchanged estradiol. Other metabolites have been identified.

Norethisterone is absorbed from the GI tract and its effects last for at least 24 hours. When a dose of 1 mg is given, there are wide variations in serum norethisterone levels at any particular time point after dosing (100-1700 pg/mL). Norethisterone undergoes first pass effects with a resulting loss of 36% of the dose. When injected, it is detectable in the plasma after 2 days and it not completely excreted in the urine after 5 days. There are large inter-subject variations in elimination half-life and bioavailability. The most important metabolites are several isomers of 5α-dihydro-norethisterone and tetrahydro-norethisterone which are excreted mainly as glucuronides.

5.3 Preclinical safety data

Acute toxicity of estrogens is low. Because of marked differences between animal species and between animals and humans preclinical results possess a limited predictive value for the application of estrogens in humans.

In experimental animals estradiol or estradiol valerate displayed an embryolethal effect already at relatively low oral doses; malformations of the urogenital and feminisation of male fetuses were observed.

Norethisterone, like other progestagens, caused virilisation of female fetuses in rats and monkeys. After high oral doses of norethisterone embryolethal effects were observed.

Preclinical data based on conventional studies of repeated dose toxicity, genotoxicity and carcinogenic potential revealed no particular human risks beyond those discussed in other sections of the SmPC.

6. PHARMACEUTICAL PARTICULARS

6.1 List of excipients

1mg Tablet:

Estradiol only tablets:

Tablet core: lactose monohydrate, maize starch, povidone, talc, magnesium stearate, FD &C blue no.2 lake (E132), purified water.

Tablet coat: hypromellose, propylene glycol, opaspray blue M-1-6516 (E171, E464, E132), purified water.

Combination tablets:

1mg Tablet: *Tablet core:* lactose monohydrate, maize starch, povidone, talc, magnesium stearate, purified water

Tablet coat: hypromellose, propylene glycol, Opaspray white M-1-7-111B (E171 and E464), purified water.

2mg Tablet:

Estradiol only tablets:

Tablet core: lactose monohydrate, maize starch, povidone, talc, magnesium stearate, FD &C blue no.2 lake (E132), purified water.

Tablet coat: hypromellose, propylene glycol, opaspray blue M-1-6517 (E171, E464, E132), purified water.

Combination tablets:

Tablet core: lactose monohydrate, maize starch, povidone, talc, magnesium stearate, iron oxide yellow (E172), purified water

Tablet coat: hypromellose, propylene glycol, Opaspray yellow M-1-8462 (E171, E464 and E172), purified water.

6.2 Incompatibilities

Not applicable

6.3 Shelf life

3 years

6.4 Special precautions for storage

Do not store above 25°C. Store in the original package.

6.5 Nature and contents of container

Blister strips of aluminium foil/UPVC (20μm/250μm), in cardboard cartons, each blister contains 28 tablets and cartons will contain 1 or 3 blisters

6.6 Instructions for use and handling

There are no special instructions for handling.

7. MARKETING AUTHORISATION HOLDER

Novartis Pharmaceuticals UK Limited

Trading as Sandoz Pharmaceuticals

Frimley Business Park

Frimley

Camberley

Surrey

GU16 7SR

8. MARKETING AUTHORISATION NUMBER(S)

1mg Tablet: PL 00101/0328

2mg Tablet: PL 00101/0366

9. DATE OF FIRST AUTHORISATION/RENEWAL OF THE AUTHORISATION

18 September 1997

10. DATE OF REVISION OF THE TEXT

1mg Tablet: 21 June 2004

2mg Tablet: 10 June 2004

LEGAL CATEGORY

POM

Climaval 1mg, Climaval 2mg

(Novartis Pharmaceuticals UK Ltd)

1. NAME OF THE MEDICINAL PRODUCT

Climaval® 1mg

Climaval® 2mg

2. QUALITATIVE AND QUANTITATIVE COMPOSITION

Climaval tablets contain 1 mg or 2 mg estradiol valerate. For excipients, see 6.1.

3. PHARMACEUTICAL FORM

Film-coated tablet

1mg: Grey-blue tablet, coded OC on one side, CG on the other.

2mg: Blue tablet, coded OD on one side, CG on the other.

4. CLINICAL PARTICULARS

4.1 Therapeutic indications

Hormone replacement therapy (HRT) for estrogen deficiency symptoms in postmenopausal women who have been hysterectomised.

The experience treating women older than 65 years is limited.

4.2 Posology and method of administration

1 mg to 2 mg daily. Dosage may be adjusted according to severity of symptoms or clinical response. Climaval may be taken continuously in hysterectomised patients. For initiation and continuation of treatment of postmenopausal symptoms, the lowest effective dose for the shortest duration (see also Section 4.4) should be used. HRT should only be continued as long as the benefit in alleviation of severe symptoms outweighs the risks of HRT.

Unless there is a previous diagnosis of endometriosis, it is not recommended to add a progestagen in hysterectomised women.

Missed tablet: If a tablet is missed it should be taken within 12 hours of when normally taken; otherwise the tablet should be discarded, and the usual tablet should be taken the following day.

Use in children

Not to be used in children

Use in the elderly

In the elderly, Climaval should only be used for the control of post-menopausal symptoms.

4.3 Contraindications

• Known, past or suspected breast cancer.

• Known or suspected estrogen-dependent malignant tumours. (e.g. endometrial cancer)

• Undiagnosed genital bleeding.

• Untreated endometrial hyperplasia.

• Severe renal disease.

• Acute liver disease, or a history of liver disease as long as liver function tests have failed to return to normal.

• Previous idiopathic or current venous thromboembolism (deep venous thrombosis, pulmonary embolism).

• Active or recent arterial thromboembolic disease (e.g. angina, myocardial infarction).

• Known hypersensitivity to the active substance or to any of the excipients.

• Porphyria.

4.4 Special warnings and special precautions for use

For the treatment of postmenopausal symptoms, HRT should only be initiated for symptoms that adversely affect quality of life. In all cases, a careful appraisal of the risks and benefits should be undertaken at least annually and HRT should only be continued as long as the benefit outweighs the risk.

Medical Examination / follow-up

Before initiating or reinstituting HRT, a complete personal and family medical history should be taken. Physical (including pelvic and breast) examination should be guided by this and by the contraindications and warnings for use. During treatment, periodic check-ups are recommended of a frequency and nature adapted to the individual woman. Women should be advised what changes in their breasts should be reported to their doctor or nurse (see 'Breast cancer' below). Investigations, including mammography, should be carried out in accordance with currently accepted screening practices, modified according to the clinical needs of the individual.

Conditions which need supervision

If any of the following conditions are present, have occurred previously, and/or have been aggravated during pregnancy or previous hormone treatment, the patient should be closely supervised. It should be taken into account that these conditions may recur or be aggravated during treatment with Climaval, in particular:

• Endometriosis

• A history of, or risk factors for, thromboembolic disorders (see below)

• Risk factors for estrogen dependent tumours, e.g. 1st degree heredity for breast cancer

• Hypertension

• Liver disorders (eg liver adenoma) – patients with mild chronic disease should have their liver function checked every 8-12 weeks

• Diabetes mellitus with or without vascular involvement

• Cholelithiasis

• Migraine or (severe) headache

• Systemic lupus erythematosus

• A history of endometrial hyperplasia (see below)

• Epilepsy

• Asthma

• Otosclerosis

Reasons for immediate withdrawal of therapy:

Therapy should be discontinued in case a contra-indication is discovered and in the following situations:

- Jaundice or deterioration in liver function
- Significant increase in blood pressure
- New onset of migraine-type headache, or any other symptoms that are a possible prodromata of vascular occlusion

Endometriosis

Unopposed estrogen stimulation may lead to premalignant or malignant transformation in the residual foci of endometriosis. Therefore, the addition of progestagens to estrogen replacement therapy should be considered in women who have undergone hysterectomy because of endometriosis, if they are known to have residual endometriosis.

Breast cancer

A randomised placebo-controlled trial, the Women's Health Initiative study (WHI) and epidemiological studies, including the Million Women Study (MWS), have reported an increased risk of breast cancer in women taking estrogens or estrogen-progestagen combinations or tibolone for HRT for several years (see Section 4.8).

For all HRT, an excess risk becomes apparent within a few years of use and increases with duration of intake but returns to baseline within a few (at most five) years after stopping treatment.

In the MWS, the relative risk of breast cancer with conjugated equine estrogens (CEE) or estradiol (E2) was greater when a progestagen was added, either sequentially or continuously, and regardless of type of progestagen. There was no evidence of a difference in risk between the different routes of administration.

In the WHI study, the continuous combined conjugated equine estrogen and medroxyprogesterone acetate (CEE + MPA) product used was associated with breast cancers that were slightly larger in size and more frequently had local lymph node metastases compared to placebo.

HRT, especially estrogen-progestagen combined treatment, increases the density of mammographic images which may adversely affect the radiological detection of breast cancer.

Venous thromboembolism

HRT is associated with a higher relative risk of developing venous thromboembolism (VTE), i.e. deep vein thrombosis or pulmonary embolism. One randomised controlled trial and epidemiological studies found a 2-3 fold higher risk for users compared with non-users For non-users, it is estimated that the number of cases of VTE that will occur over a 5 year period is about 3 per 1000 women aged 50-59 years and 8 per 1000 women aged between 60-69 years. It is estimated that in healthy women who use HRT for 5 years, the number of additional cases of VTE over a 5 year period will be between 2 and 6 (best estimate=4) per 1000 women aged 50-59 years and between 5 and 15 (best estimate=9) per 1000 women aged 60-69 years. The occurrence of such an event is more likely in the first year of HRT than later.

Generally recognised risk factors for VTE include a personal history or family history, severe obesity (Body Mass Index > 30kg/m^2) and systemic lupus erythematosus (SLE). There is no consensus about the role of varicose veins in VTE.

Patients with a history of VTE or known thrombophilic states have an increased risk of VTE. HRT may add to this risk. Personal or strong family history of thromboembolism or recurrent spontaneous abortion should be investigated in order to exclude a thrombophilic predisposition. Until a thorough evaluation of thrombophilic factors has been made or anticoagulant treatment initiated, use of HRT in such patients should be viewed as contra-indicated. Those women already on anticoagulant treatment require careful consideration of the benefit-risk of use of HRT.

The risk of VTE may be temporarily increased with prolonged immobilisation, major trauma or major surgery. As in all post-operative patients scrupulous attention should be given to prophylactic measures to prevent VTE following surgery. Where prolonged immobilisation is liable to follow elective surgery, particularly abdominal or orthopaedic surgery to the lower limbs, consideration should be given to temporarily stopping HRT four to six weeks earlier, if possible. Treatment should not be restarted until the woman is completely mobilised.

If VTE develops after initiating therapy, the drug should be discontinued. Patients should be told to contact their doctors immediately when they are aware of a potential thromboembolic symptom (e.g. painful swelling of a leg, sudden pain in the chest, dyspnoea).

Coronary artery disease (CAD)

There is no evidence from randomised controlled trials of cardiovascular benefit with continuous combined conjugated estrogens and medroxyprogesterone acetate (MPA). Two large clinical trials (WHI and HERS i.e. Heart and Estrogen/progestin Replacement Study) showed a possible increased risk of cardiovascular morbidity in the first year of use and no overall benefit. For other HRT products there are only limited data from randomised controlled trials to date examining effects in cardiovascular morbidity or mortality. Therefore, it is uncertain whether these findings also extend to other HRT products.

Stroke

One large randomised clinical trial (WHI-trial) found, as a secondary outcome, an increased risk of ischaemic stroke in healthy women during treatment with continuous combined conjugated estrogens and MPA. For women who do not use HRT, it is estimated that the number of cases of stroke that will occur over a 5 year period is about 3 per 1000 women aged 50-59 years and 11 per 1000 women aged 60-69 years. It is estimated that for women who use conjugated estrogens and MPA for 5 years, the number of additional cases will be between 0 and 3 (best estimate=1) per 1000 users aged 50-59 years and between 1 and 9 (best estimate=4) per 1000 users aged 60-69 years. It is unknown whether the increased risk also extends to other HRT products.

Ovarian cancer

Long-term (at least 5 to 10 years) use of estrogen-only HRT products in hysterectomised women has been associated with an increased risk of ovarian cancer in some epidemiological studies. It is uncertain whether long-term use of combined HRT confers a different risk than estrogen-only products.

Other conditions

Estrogens may cause fluid retention, and therefore patients with cardiac or renal dysfunction should be carefully observed. Patients with terminal renal insufficiency should be closely observed, since it is expected that the level of circulating active ingredients in Climaval is increased.

Women with pre-existing hypertriglyceridemia should be followed closely during estrogen replacement or hormone replacement therapy, since rare cases of large increases of plasma triglycerides leading to pancreatitis have been reported with estrogen therapy in this condition.

Estrogens increase thyroid binding globulin (TBG), leading to increased circulating total thyroid hormone, as measured by protein-bound iodine (PBI), T4 levels (by column or by radio-immunoassay) or T3 levels (by radio-immunoassay). T3 resin uptake is decreased, reflecting the elevated TBG. Free T4 and free T3 concentrations are unaltered. Other binding proteins may be elevated in serum, ie corticoid binding globulin (CBG), sex-hormone-binding globulin (SHBG) leading to increased circulating corticosteroids and sex steroids, respectively. Free or biological active hormone concentrations are unchanged. Other plasma proteins may be increased (angiotensinogen/renin substrate, alpha-I-antitrypsin, ceruloplasmin).

There is no conclusive evidence for improvement of cognitive function. There is some evidence from the WHI trial of increased risk of probable dementia in women who start using continuous combined CEE and MPA after the age of 65. It is unknown whether the findings apply to younger post-menopausal women or other HRT products.

4.5 Interaction with other medicinal products and other forms of Interaction

The metabolism of estrogens may be increased by concomitant use of substances known to induce drug-metabolising enzymes, specifically cytochrome P450 enzymes, such as anticonvulsants (e.g. phenobarbital, phenytoin, carbamazepine) and anti-infectives (e.g. rifampicin, rifabutin, nevirapine, efavirenz).

Ritonavir and nelfinavir, although known as strong inhibitors, by contrast exhibit inducing properties when used concomitantly with steroid hormones.

Herbal preparations containing St John's wort (*Hypericum perforatum*) may induce the metabolism of estrogens.

4.6 Pregnancy and lactation

Not application, because Climaval is only indicated in women without a uterus.

4.7 Effects on ability to drive and use machines

No adverse effects on the ability to drive or operate machines have been recorded.

4.8 Undesirable effects

Reproductive and urogenital tract: Breast tension and pain, breast cancer*, mucous vaginal discharge

Central Nervous System: Headaches, dizziness, vertigo, changes in libido, depressive mood

Cardiovascular system: Hypertension, palpitations, cardiac symptoms, thrombophlebitis, oedema, epistaxis

Gastrointestinal tract: Dyspepsia, flatulence, nausea, vomiting, abdominal pain and bloating, biliary stasis

Skin and appendages: General pruritus, alopecia, urticaria and other rashes

Endocrine system: Decrease in glucose tolerance

Miscellaneous: Weight gain

*Breast cancer

According to evidence from a large number of epidemiological studies and one randomised placebo-controlled trial, the Women's Health Initiative (WHI), the overall risk of breast cancer increases with increasing duration of HRT use in current or recent HRT users.

For *estrogen-only* HRT, estimates of relative risk (RR) from a reanalysis of original data from 51 epidemiological studies (in which > 80% of HRT use was estrogen-only HRT) and from the epidemiological Million Women Study (MWS) are similar at 1.35 (95%CI 1.21 – 1.49) and 1.30 (95%CI 1.21 – 1.40), respectively.

For *estrogen plus progestagen* combined HRT, several epidemiological studies have reported an overall higher risk for breast cancer than with estrogens alone.

The MWS reported that, compared to never users, the use of various types of estrogen-progestagen combined HRT was associated with a higher risk of breast cancer (RR = 2.00, 95%CI: 1.88 – 2.12) than use of estrogens alone (RR = 1.30, 95%CI: 1.21 – 1.40) or use of tibolone (RR=1.45; 95%CI 1.25-1.68).

The WHI trial reported a risk estimate of 1.24 (95%CI 1.01 – 1.54) after 5.6 years of use of estrogen-progestagen combined HRT (CEE + MPA) in all users compared with placebo.

The absolute risks calculated from the MWS and the WHI trial are presented below:

The MWS has estimated, from the known average incidence of breast cancer in developed countries, that:

- For women not using HRT, about 32 in every 1000 are expected to have breast cancer diagnosed between the ages of 50 and 64 years.

- For 1000 current or recent users of HRT, the number of *additional* cases during the corresponding period will be

- For users of *estrogen-only* replacement therapy

- between 0 and 3 (best estimate = 1.5) for 5 years' use
- between 3 and 7 (best estimate = 5) for 10 years' use.

- For users of *estrogen plus progestagen* combined HRT,

- between 5 and 7 (best estimate = 6) for 5 years' use
- between 18 and 20 (best estimate = 19) for 10 years' use.

The WHI trial estimated that after 5.6 years of follow-up of women between the ages of 50 and 79 years, an *additional* 8 cases of invasive breast cancer would be due to *estrogen-progestagen combined* HRT (CEE + MPA) per 10,000 women years.

According to calculations from the trial data, it is estimated that:

- For 1000 women in the placebo group, about 16 cases of invasive breast cancer would be diagnosed in 5 years.

- For 1000 women who used estrogen + progestagen combined HRT (CEE + MPA), the number of *additional* cases would be between 0 and 9 (best estimate = 4) for 5 years' use.

The number of additional cases of breast cancer in women who use HRT is broadly similar for women who start HRT irrespective of age at start of use (between the ages of 45-65) (see Section 4.4).'

Endometrial cancer

In women with an intact uterus, the risk of endometrial hyperplasia and endometrial cancer increases with increasing duration of use of unopposed estrogens. According to data from epidemiological studies, the best estimate of the risk is that for women not using HRT, about 5 in every 1000 are expected to have endometrial cancer diagnosed between the ages of 50 and 65. Depending on the duration of treatment and estrogen dose, the reported increase in endometrial cancer risk among unopposed estrogen users varies from 2-to 12-fold greater compared with non-users. Adding a progestagen to estrogen-only therapy greatly reduces this increased risk.

Other adverse reactions have been reported in association with estrogen/progestagen treatment:

- Estrogen-dependent neoplasms benign and malignant (e.g. endometrial cancer)
- Venous thromboembolism, i.e. deep leg or pelvic venous thrombosis and pulmonary embolism, is more frequent among hormone replacement therapy users than among non-users. For further information, see Section 4.3 Contra-indications and 4.4 Special warnings and special precautions for use.
- Myocardial infarction and stroke.
- Gall bladder disease.
- Skin and subcutaneous disorders: chloasma, erythema multiforme, erythema nodosum, vascular purpura.
- Probable dementia (see Section 4.4).

4.9 Overdose

There have been no reports of ill-effects from overdose. There are no specific antidotes, and further treatment should be symptomatic.

5. PHARMACOLOGICAL PROPERTIES

5.1 Pharmacodynamic properties

The active ingredient, synthetic 17β-estradiol, is chemically and biologically identical to endogenous human estradiol. It substitutes for the loss of estrogen production in menopausal women, and alleviates menopausal symptoms.

Estradiol valerate is used in estrogen deficiency states.

After the menopause the protective effects which endogenous estrogens appear to have on the female cardiovascular system are lost, therefore the risk of women developing cardiovascular disease rises to become similar to that of men.

5.2 Pharmacokinetic properties

Estradiol valerate, like most natural estrogens, is readily and fully absorbed from the GI tract, is 50% bound to plasma proteins and is rapidly metabolised in the liver to oestriol and oestrone. When given orally in doses of 1-2 mg, peak levels of estradiol are generally observed 3-6 hours after ingestion, but by 24 hours (range 6-48 hours) concentrations have returned to baseline (ie pre-treatment concentrations). The average half-life of estradiol in plasma is about one hour.

Estradiol undergoes first-pass effect in the liver. There is some enterohepatic recycling. It is excreted via the kidney in the urine as sulphate and glucuronide esters together with a small proportion of unchanged oestradiol. Other metabolites have been identified.

5.3 Preclinical safety data

Acute toxicity of estrogens is low. Because of marked differences between animal species and between animals and humans preclinical results possess a limited predictive value for the application of estrogens in humans.

Preclinical data based on conventional studies of repeated dose toxicity, genotoxicity and carcinogenic potential revealed no particular human risks beyond those discussed in other sections of the SmPC.

6. PHARMACEUTICAL PARTICULARS

6.1 List of excipients

Tablet core:

Lactose monohydrate, maize starch, FD & C blue no. 2 lake (E132), povidone (grade 30), purified water, talc (sterilised, white), magnesium stearate.

Tablet coat:

Hypromellose, propylene glycol, Opaspray blue M-1-6517 (E171, E464, E132).

6.2 Incompatibilities

No incompatibilities have been described.

6.3 Shelf life

3 years.

6.4 Special precautions for storage

Do not store above 25°C. Store in the original package.

6.5 Nature and contents of container

Blister strips of 28 tablets packed in cardboard cartons. Two sizes are available; cartons containing one blister strip or three blister strips.

Blister consists of 20μm layer of aluminium foil on a 250μm UPVC blister.

6.6 Instructions for use and handling

The pack was designed to help patients take the tablets correctly. The arrows on the foil should be followed and the tablets taken on the days shown.

7. MARKETING AUTHORISATION HOLDER

Novartis Pharmaceuticals UK Limited

Trading as Sandoz Pharmaceuticals

Frimley Business Park

Frimley

Camberley

Surrey

GU16 7SR

8. MARKETING AUTHORISATION NUMBER(S)

PL 00101/0307 – 1 mg

PL 00101/0308 – 2 mg

9. DATE OF FIRST AUTHORISATION/RENEWAL OF THE AUTHORISATION

25 March 1997.

10. DATE OF REVISION OF THE TEXT

10 June 2004

LEGAL CATEGORY:

POM

Climesse 2 mg film coated tablets

(Novartis Pharmaceuticals UK Ltd)

1. NAME OF THE MEDICINAL PRODUCT

Climesse® 2 mg film coated tablets

2. QUALITATIVE AND QUANTITATIVE COMPOSITION

28 tablets each containing 2 mg estradiol valerate USP and 0.7 mg norethisterone Ph Eur.

For excipients, see Section 6.1

3. PHARMACEUTICAL FORM

Film-coated tablet

Pink biconvex tablet coated OG on one side CG on the other.

4. CLINICAL PARTICULARS

4.1 Therapeutic indications

Hormone replacement therapy (HRT) for estrogen deficiency symptoms in postmenopausal women.

Prevention of osteoporosis in postmenopausal women at high risk of future fractures who are intolerant of, or contraindicated for, other medicinal products approved for the prevention of osteoporosis.

(See also section 4.4.)

The experience treating women older than 65 years is limited.

4.2 Posology and method of administration

Climesse is a continuous combined hormone replacement therapy.

One tablet to be taken daily, as directed on the 28 day calendar pack. Climesse should be taken continuously without a break between packs.

It is recommended that Climesse should not be taken by women until at least 12 months after their last natural menstrual bleed. Irregular bleeding during tablet taking may occur during the first few months of therapy but is usually transient, and amenorrhoea will develop in a majority of women. Amenorrhoea is most likely to occur in women who are more than 2 years post-menopausal but may also be achieved before that in a significant proportion of women. After 3-4 months treatment, some women may experience continued unacceptable bleeding and in these cases Climesse should be discontinued. If bleeding subsides within three weeks then no further investigation is needed.

Pregnancy should be excluded before starting therapy.

For initiation and continuation of treatment of postmenopausal symptoms, the lowest effective dose for the shortest duration (see also section 4.4) should be used.

Unless there is a previous diagnosis of endometriosis, it is not recommended to add a progestagen in hysterectomised women.

Patients changing from another continuous sequential or cyclical preparation should complete the cycle and may then change to Climesse without a break in therapy. Patients changing from a continuous combined preparation may start therapy at any time if amenorrhoea is established, or otherwise start on the first day of bleeding.

Climesse should normally be used only in women more than 12 months postmenopausal. When changing from sequential therapy menopausal status may not be known, and in some women endogenous estrogens may still be being produced. This could result in unpredictable bleeding patterns.

If a tablet is missed, it should be taken within 12 hours of when normally taken; otherwise the tablet should be discarded, and the usual tablet should be taken the following day. Forgetting or missing a dose may increase the likelihood of breakthrough bleeding.

Use in the elderly

Climesse should only be used in the elderly for the indications listed.

Use in children

Climesse should not to be used in children

4.3 Contraindications

- Known, past or suspected breast cancer
- Known or suspected estrogen-dependent malignant tumours (e.g. endometrial cancer)
- Undiagnosed genital bleeding
- Untreated endometrial hyperplasia
- Severe renal disease
- Previous idiopathic or current venous thromboembolism (deep venous thrombosis, pulmonary embolism)
- Active or recent arterial thromboembolic disease (e.g. angina, myocardial infarction)
- Acute liver disease, or a history of liver disease as long as liver function tests have failed to return to normal
- Known hypersensitivity to the active substance or to any of the excipients
- Porphyria

4.4 Special warnings and special precautions for use

For the treatment of postmenopausal symptoms, HRT should only be initiated for symptoms that adversely affect quality of life. In all cases, a careful appraisal of the risks and benefits should be undertaken at least annually and HRT should only be continued as long as the benefit outweighs the risk.

Medical Examination / follow-up

Before initiating or reinstituting HRT, a complete personal and family medical history should be taken. Physical (including pelvic and breast) examination should be guided by this and by sections 4.3 Contraindications and 4.4 Special warnings and special precautions for use. During treatment, periodic check-ups are recommended of a frequency and nature adapted to the individual woman. Women should be advised what changes in their breasts should be reported to their doctor or nurse (see 'Breast cancer' below). Investigations, including mammography, should be carried out in accordance with currently accepted screening practices, modified according to the clinical needs of the individual.

Conditions which need supervision

If any of the following conditions are present, have occurred previously, and/or have been aggravated during pregnancy or previous hormone treatment, the patient should be closely supervised. It should be taken into account that these conditions may recur or be aggravated during treatment with Climesse, in particular:

- Leiomyoma (uterine fibroids) or endometriosis
- A history of, or risk factors for, thromboembolic disorders (see below)
- Risk factors for estrogen dependent tumours, e.g. 1st degree heredity for breast cancer
- Hypertension
- Liver disorders (eg liver adenoma) – patients with mild chronic disease should have their liver function checked every 8-12 weeks
- Diabetes mellitus with or without vascular involvement
- Cholelithiasis
- Migraine or (severe) headache
- Systemic lupus erythematosus (SLE)
- A history of endometrial hyperplasia (see below)
- Epilepsy
- Asthma
- Otosclerosis.

Reasons for immediate withdrawal of therapy:

Therapy should be discontinued in case a contra-indication is discovered and in the following situations:

- Jaundice or deterioration in liver function
- Significant increase in blood pressure
- New onset of migraine-type headache, or any other symptoms that are a possible prodromata of vascular occlusion
- Pregnancy.

Endometrial hyperplasia

The risk of endometrial hyperplasia and carcinoma is increased when estrogens are administered alone for prolonged periods (see section 4.8). The addition of a progestagen for at least 12 days per cycle in non-hysterectomised women greatly reduces this risk.

Break-through bleeding and spotting may occur during the first months of treatment. If break through bleeding or spotting appears after some time on therapy, or continues after treatment has been discontinued, the reason should be investigated, which may include endometrial biopsy to exclude endometrial malignancy.

Bleeding after a period of amenorrhoea or heavy bleeding after a period of light bleeding may occur.

Breast cancer

A randomised placebo- controlled trial, the Women's Health Initiative study (WHI), and epidemiological studies, including the Million Women Study (MWS) have reported an increased risk of breast cancer in women taking estrogens, estrogen-progestagen combinations or tibolone for HRT for several years (see section 4.8).

For all HRT, an excess risk becomes apparent within a few years of use and increases with duration of intake of HRT but returns to baseline within a few (at most five) years after stopping treatment.

In the MWS, the relative risk of breast cancer with conjugated equine estrogens (CEE) or estradiol (E2) was greater when a progestagen was added, either sequentially or continuously, and regardless of type of progestagen. There was no evidence of a difference in risk between the different routes of administration.

In the WHI study, the continuous combined conjugated equine estrogen and medroxyprogesterone acetate (CEE + MPA) product used was associated with breast cancers that were slightly larger in size and more frequently had local lymph node metastases compared to placebo.

HRT, especially estrogen-progestagen combined treatment, increases the density of mammographic images which may adversely affect the radiological detection of breast cancer.

Venous thromboembolism

HRT is associated with a higher relative risk of developing venous thromboembolism (VTE), i.e. deep vein thrombosis or pulmonary embolism. One randomised controlled trial and epidemiological studies found a 2-3 fold higher risk for users compared with non-users. For non-users, it is estimated that the number of cases of VTE that will occur over a 5 year period is about 3 per 1000 women aged 50-59 years and 8 per 1000 women aged between 60-69 years. It is estimated that in healthy women who use HRT for 5 years, the number of additional cases of VTE over a 5 year period will be between 2 and 6 (best estimate=4) per 1000 women aged 50-59 years and between 5 and 15 (best estimate=9) per 1000 women aged 60-69 years. The occurrence of such an event is more likely in the first year of HRT than later.

Generally recognised risk factors for VTE include a personal history or family history, severe obesity (Body Mass Index > 30kg/m^2) and systemic lupus erythematosus (SLE). There is no consensus about the possible role of varicose veins in VTE.

Patients with a history of VTE or known thrombophilic states have an increased risk of VTE. HRT may add to this risk. Personal or strong family history of thromboembolism or recurrent spontaneous abortion should be investigated in order to exclude a thrombophilic predisposition. Until a thorough evaluation of thrombophilic factors has been made or anticoagulant treatment initiated, use of HRT in such patients should be viewed as contra-indicated. Those women already on anticoagulant treatment require careful consideration of the benefit-risk of use of HRT.

The risk of VTE may be temporarily increased with prolonged immobilisation, major trauma or major surgery. As in all post-operative patients scrupulous attention should be given to prophylactic measures to prevent VTE following surgery. Where prolonged immobilisation is liable to follow elective surgery, particularly abdominal or orthopaedic surgery to the lower limbs, consideration should be given to temporarily stopping HRT four to six weeks earlier, if possible. Treatment should not be restarted until the woman is completely mobilised.

If VTE develops after initiating therapy, the drug should be discontinued. Patients should be told to contact their doctors immediately when they are aware of a potential thromboembolic symptom (e.g. painful swelling of a leg, sudden pain in the chest, dyspnoea).

Coronary artery disease (CAD)

There is no evidence from randomised controlled trials of cardiovascular benefit with continuous combined conjugated estrogens and medroxyprogesterone acetate (MPA). Two large clinical trials (WHI and HERS i.e. Heart and Estrogen/progestin Replacement Study) showed a possible increased risk of cardiovascular morbidity in the first year of use and no overall benefit. For other HRT products there are only limited data from randomised controlled trials examining effects in cardiovascular morbidity or mortality. Therefore, it is uncertain whether these findings also extend to other HRT products.

Stroke

One large randomised clinical trial (WHI-trial) found, as a secondary outcome, an increased risk of ischaemic stroke in healthy women during treatment with continuous combined conjugated estrogens and MPA. For women who do not use HRT, it is estimated that the number of cases of stroke that will occur over a 5 year period is about 3 per 1000 women aged 50-59 years and 11 per 1000 women aged 60-69 years. It is estimated that for women who use conjugated estrogens and MPA for 5 years, the number of additional cases will be between 0 and 3 (best estimate=1) per 1000 users aged 50-59 years and between 1 and 9 (best estimate=4) per 1000 users aged 60-69 years. It is unknown whether the increased risk also extends to other HRT products.

Ovarian cancer

Long-term (at least 5 to 10 years) use of estrogen-only HRT products in hysterectomised women has been associated with an increased risk of ovarian cancer in some epidemiological studies. It is uncertain whether long-term use of combined HRT confers a different risk than estrogen-only products.

Other conditions

Estrogens may cause fluid retention, and therefore patients with cardiac or renal dysfunction should be carefully observed. Patients with terminal renal insufficiency should be closely observed, since it is expected that the level of circulating active ingredients in Climesse is increased.

Women with pre-existing hypertriglyceridemia should be followed closely during estrogen replacement or hormone replacement therapy, since rare cases of large increases of plasma triglycerides leading to pancreatitis have been reported with estrogen therapy in this condition.

Estrogens increase thyroid binding globulin (TBG), leading to increased circulating total thyroid hormone, as measured by protein-bound iodine (PBI), T4 levels (by column or by radio-immunoassay) or T3 levels (by radio-immunoassay). T3 resin uptake is decreased, reflecting the elevated TBG. Free T4 and free T3 concentrations are unaltered. Other binding proteins may be elevated in serum, i.e. corticoid binding globulin (CBG), sex-hormone-binding globulin (SHBG) leading to increased circulating corticosteroids and sex steroids, respectively. Free or biological active hormone concentrations are unchanged. Other plasma proteins may be increased (angiotensinogen/renin substrate, alpha-I-antitrypsin, ceruloplasmin).

There is no conclusive evidence for improvement of cognitive function. There is some evidence from the WHI trial of increased risk of probable dementia in women who start using continuous combined conjugated estrogens and MPA after the age of 65. It is unknown whether the findings apply to younger post-menopausal women or other HRT products.

Climesse is designed to prevent stimulation of the endometrium in postmenopausal women, usually resulting in amenorrhoea. Irregular bleeding may occur in the first few months of therapy but this will usually settle completely. A certain proportion of women, particularly those closer to the menopause, may fail to develop amenorrhoea and for these women an alternative form of hormone replacement therapy may be more suitable. Certain conditions may predispose to persistent irregular bleeding, such as uterine polyps and fibroids and this may warrant further investigation. As for all postmenopausal bleeding, appropriate investigations, including endometrial assessment should be carried out in all women who experience prolonged bleeding or who begin to bleed after initiation of therapy following a period of amenorrhoea.

Premenopausal women should not receive Climesse therapy because it may inhibit ovulation, disturb cycle regularity and result in unpredictable bleeding patterns. Climesse is not intended to be an oral contraceptive and should not be used to prevent pregnancy.

4.5 Interaction with other medicinal products and other forms of Interaction

The metabolism of estrogens and progestagens may be increased by concomitant use of substances known to induce drug-metabolising enzymes, specifically cytochrome P450 enzymes, such as anticonvulsants (e.g. phenobarbital, phenytoin, carbamazepine) and anti-infectives (e.g. rifampicin, rifabutin, nevirapine, efavirenz).

Ritonavir and nelfinavir, although known as strong inhibitors, by contrast exhibit inducing properties when used concomitantly with steroid hormones.

Herbal preparations containing St John's wort (*Hypericum perforatum*) may induce the metabolism of estrogens.

Clinically, an increased metabolism of estrogens and progestagens may lead to decreased effect and changes in the uterine bleeding profile.

4.6 Pregnancy and lactation

Pregnancy

Climesse is not indicated during pregnancy. If pregnancy occurs during medication with Climesse treatment should be withdrawn immediately.

Data on a limited number of exposed pregnancies indicate adverse effects of norethisterone on the foetus. At doses higher than normally used in OC and HRT formulations, masculinisation of the female foetus was observed.

The results of most epidemiological studies to date relevant to inadvertent foetal exposure to combinations of estrogens and progestagens indicate no teratogenic or foetotoxic effects.

Lactation

Climesse is not indicated during lactation.

4.7 Effects on ability to drive and use machines

No adverse effects on the ability to drive or operate machines have been recorded.

4.8 Undesirable effects

Urogenital tract

During the first few months of therapy irregular bleeding or spotting may occur; this is usually transient. Mucous vaginal discharge, dysmenorrhoea.

Central nervous system

Headaches, dizziness, vertigo, fatigue, irritability, depressive mood, changes in libido.

Cardiovascular system

Hypertension, palpitations, thrombophlebitis, oedema, epistaxis.

Gastrointestinal tract

Dyspepsia, flatulence, nausea, vomiting, abdominal pain and bloating, biliary stasis.

Skin and appendages

General pruritus, urticaria and other rashes, acne, alopecia.

Endocrine system

Breast tension and pain, enlargement of the breasts/breast cancer*, decrease in glucose tolerance.

Miscellaneous

Weight gain, leg cramps.

*Breast cancer

According to evidence from a large number of epidemiological studies and one randomised placebo-controlled trial, the Women's Health Initiative (WHI), the overall risk of breast cancer increases with increasing duration of HRT use in current or recent HRT users.

For *estrogen-only* HRT, estimates of relative risk (RR) from a reanalysis of original data from 51 epidemiological studies (in which >80% of HRT use was estrogen-only HRT) and from the epidemiological Million Women Study (MWS) are similar at 1.35 (95%CI 1.21 – 1.49) and 1.30 (95%CI 1.21 – 1.40), respectively.

For *estrogen plus progestagen* combined HRT, several epidemiological studies have reported an overall higher risk for breast cancer than with estrogens alone.

The MWS reported that, compared to never users, the use of various types of estrogen-progestagen combined HRT was associated with a higher risk of breast cancer (RR = 2.00, 95%CI: 1.88 – 2.12) than use of estrogens alone (RR = 1.30, 95%CI: 1.21 – 1.40) or use of tibolone (RR=1.45; 95%CI 1.25-1.68).

The WHI trial reported a risk estimate of 1.24 (95%CI 1.01 – 1.54) after 5.6 years of use of estrogen-progestagen combined HRT (CEE + MPA) in all users compared with placebo.

The absolute risks calculated from the MWS and the WHI trial are presented below:

The MWS has estimated, from the known average incidence of breast cancer in developed countries, that:

- For women not using HRT, about 32 in every 1000 are expected to have breast cancer diagnosed between the ages of 50 and 64 years.

- For 1000 current or recent users of HRT, the number of *additional* cases during the corresponding period will be:

- For users of *estrogen-only* replacement therapy

• between 0 and 3 (best estimate = 1.5) for 5 years' use,

• between 3 and 7 (best estimate = 5) for 10 years' use.

- For users of *estrogen plus progestagen* combined HRT

• between 5 and 7 (best estimate = 6) for 5 years' use,

• between 18 and 20 (best estimate = 19) for 10 years' use.

The WHI trial estimated that after 5.6 years of follow-up of women between the ages of 50 and 79 years, an *additional* 8 cases of invasive breast cancer would be due to *estrogen-progestagen combined* HRT (CEE + MPA) per 10,000 women years.

According to calculations from the trial data, it is estimated that:

- For 1000 women in the placebo group, about 16 cases of invasive breast cancer would be diagnosed in 5 years.

- For 1000 women who used estrogen + progestagen combined HRT (CEE + MPA), the number of *additional* cases would be between 0 and 9 (best estimate = 4) for 5 years' use.

The number of additional cases of breast cancer in women who use HRT is broadly similar for women who start HRT irrespective of age at start of use (between the ages of 45-65) (see section 4.4).

Endometrial cancer

In women with an intact uterus, the risk of endometrial hyperplasia and endometrial cancer increases with increasing duration of use of unopposed estrogens. According to data from epidemiological studies, the best estimate of the risk is that for women not using HRT, about 5 in every 1000 are expected to have endometrial cancer diagnosed between the ages of 50 and 65. Depending on the duration of treatment and estrogen dose, the reported increase in endometrial cancer risk among unopposed estrogen users varies from 2- to 12- fold greater compared with non-users. Adding a progestagen to estrogen-only therapy greatly reduces this increased risk.

Other adverse reactions have been reported in association with estrogen/progestagen treatment:

• Estrogen-dependent neoplasms benign and malignant (e.g. endometrial cancer).

• Venous thromboembolism, i.e. deep leg or pelvic venous thrombosis and pulmonary embolism, is more frequent among hormone replacement therapy users than among non-users. For further information, see section 4.3 Contra-indications and 4.4 Special warnings and special precautions for use.

• Myocardial infarction and stroke.

• Gall bladder disease.

• Skin and subcutaneous disorders: chloasma, erythema multiforme, erythema nodosum, vascular purpura.

• Probable dementia (see section 4.4)

4.9 Overdose

No reports of ill-effects from overdosage have been reported. There are no specific antidotes for overdosage and if further treatment is required it should be symptomatic.

5. PHARMACOLOGICAL PROPERTIES

5.1 Pharmacodynamic properties

Estradiol

The active ingredient, synthetic 17β-estradiol, is chemically and biologically identical to endogenous human estradiol. It substitutes for the loss of estrogen production in menopausal women, and alleviates menopausal symptoms. Estrogens prevent bone loss following menopause or ovariectomy.

Estradiol valerate is used in estrogen deficient states. Treatment with estrogens relieves menopausal vasomotor symptoms. Estrogens cross the placenta.

Progestagen

As estrogens promote the growth of the endometrium, unopposed estrogens increase the risk of endometrial hyperplasia and cancer. The addition of progestagen reduces but does not eliminate the estrogen induced risk of endometrial hyperplasia in non-hysterectomised women.

Norethisterone is a progestagen added to prevent endometrial hyperplasia and increased risk of endometrial carcinoma which can be induced by unopposed estrogen use.

-Prevention of osteoporosis

- Estrogen deficiency at menopause is associated with an increasing bone turnover and decline in bone mass. The effect of estrogens on the bone mineral density is dose-dependent. Protection appears to be effective for as long as treatment is continued.

After discontinuation of HRT, bone mass is lost at a rate similar to that in untreated women.

- Evidence from the WHI trial and meta-analysed trials shows that current use of HRT, alone or in combination with a progestagen – given to predominantly healthy women – reduces the risk of hip, vertebral, and other osteoporotic fractures. HRT may also prevent fractures in women with low bone density and/or established osteoporosis, but the evidence for that is limited.

5.2 Pharmacokinetic properties

Estradiol valerate, like most natural estrogens, is readily and fully absorbed from the GI tract is 50% bound to plasma proteins and is rapidly metabolised in the liver to oestriol and oestrone. When given orally in doses of 1-2 mg, peak levels of estradiol are generally observed 3-6 hours after ingestion, but by 24 hours (range 6-48 hours) concentrations have returned to baseline (i.e. pre-treatment concentrations).

Estradiol undergoes first-pass effect in the liver. There is some enterohepatic recycling. It is excreted via the kidney in the urine as water soluble esters (sulphate and glucuronide) together with a small proportion of unchanged estradiol. Other metabolites have been identified.

Norethisterone is absorbed from the GI tract and its effects last for at least 24 hours. When a dose of 1 mg is given, there are wide variations in serum norethisterone levels at any particular time point after dosing (100-1700 pg/mL). Norethisterone undergoes first pass effect with a resulting loss of 36% of the dose. When injected, it is detectable in the plasma after 2 days and is not completely excreted in the urine after 5 days. There are large inter-subject variations in elimination half-life and bioavailability. The most important metabolites are several isomers of 5-α-dihydronorethisterone and of tetrahydronorethisterone which are excreted mainly as glucuronides.

5.3 Preclinical safety data

Acute toxicity of estrogens is low. Because of marked differences between animal species and between animals and humans, preclinical results possess a limited predictive value for the application of estrogens in humans.

In experimental animals, estradiol or estradiol valerate displayed an embryolethal effect already at relatively low oral doses; malformations of the urogenital tract and feminisation of male foetus were observed.

Norethisterone, like other progestagens, caused virilisation of the female foetuses in rats and monkeys. After high oral doses of norethisterone, embryolethal effects were observed.

Preclinical data based on conventional studies of repeated dose toxicity, genotoxicity and carcinogenic potential revealed no particular human risks beyond those discussed in other sections of the SPC.

6. PHARMACEUTICAL PARTICULARS

6.1 List of excipients

Tablet core

Lactose monohydrate, maize starch, povidone, purified water, talc, magnesium stearate.

Tablet coat

Hypromellose, polyethylene glycol, iron oxide red (E172), titanium dioxide (E171), purified water.

6.2 Incompatibilities

Not applicable.

6.3 Shelf life

3 years

6.4 Special precautions for storage

Do not store above 25°C. Store in the original package.

6.5 Nature and contents of container

Blister strips of aluminum foil/UPVC (20μm/250μm), in cardboard cartons. Each blister contains 28 tablets and cartons will contain 1 or 3 blisters.

6.6 Instructions for use and handling

There are no special instructions for handling.

7. MARKETING AUTHORISATION HOLDER

Novartis Pharmaceuticals UK Limited

Trading as Sandoz Pharmaceuticals

Frimley Business Park

Frimley

Camberley

Surrey

GU16 7SR

8. MARKETING AUTHORISATION NUMBER(S)

PL 00101/0396

9. DATE OF FIRST AUTHORISATION/RENEWAL OF THE AUTHORISATION

17th November 2001

10. DATE OF REVISION OF THE TEXT

8th March 2004.

LEGAL CATEGORY

POM

Clinoril Tablets

(Merck Sharp & Dohme Limited)

1. NAME OF THE MEDICINAL PRODUCT

CLINORIL®

2. QUALITATIVE AND QUANTITATIVE COMPOSITION

'Clinoril' 100 mg Tablets contain 100 mg of sulindac

'Clinoril' 200 mg Tablets contain 200 mg of sulindac.

3. PHARMACEUTICAL FORM

Brilliant yellow, hexagonal-shaped tablets, with one side scored. The 200 mg tablets are marked 'MSD 942' and the 100 mg tablets are marked 'MSD 943'.

4. CLINICAL PARTICULARS

4.1 Therapeutic indications

'Clinoril' is a non-steroidal, analgesic/anti-inflammatory agent with antipyretic properties.

Indicated in osteoarthritis, rheumatoid arthritis, ankylosing spondylitis, acute gouty arthritis, peri-articular disorders such as bursitis, tendinitis, and tenosynovitis.

4.2 Posology and method of administration

The dosage should be taken twice a day and adjusted to the severity of the disease.

The usual dosage is 400 mg a day. However, the dosage may be lowered depending on the response. Doses above 400 mg per day are not recommended.

In the treatment of acute gouty arthritis, therapy for seven days is usually adequate.

In peri-articular disorders, treatment should be limited to seven to ten days.

'Clinoril' should be administered with fluids or food.

Children: The use of 'Clinoril' in children is contra-indicated.

Use in the elderly: The dosage does not require modification for the elderly patient.

4.3 Contraindications

Hypersensitivity to any component of this product.

The use of 'Clinoril is contra-indicated in patients with hepatic insufficiency. Poor liver function may alter the blood levels of circulating metabolites of 'Clinoril'.

'Clinoril' should not be used in patients in whom acute asthmatic attacks, urticaria or rhinitis have been precipitated by aspirin or other non-steroidal anti-inflammatory agents.

The drug should not be administered to patients with active gastro-intestinal bleeding.

The use of 'Clinoril' should be avoided in patients with active peptic ulcer.

Since paediatric indications and dosage have not yet been established, 'Clinoril' should not be given to children.

4.4 Special warnings and special precautions for use

Platelet aggregation

'Clinoril' has less effect on platelet function and bleeding time than aspirin; however, since 'Clinoril' is an inhibitor of platelet function, patients who may be adversely affected should be carefully observed when 'Clinoril' is administered.

Gastro-intestinal effects

'Clinoril' should be used with caution in patients having a history of gastro-intestinal haemorrhage or ulcers.

Hypersensitivity syndrome

A potentially life-threatening, apparent hypersensitivity syndrome has been reported. In cases where the syndrome is suspected, therapy should be discontinued immediately, and not recontinued. This syndrome may include constitutional symptoms (fever, chills, diaphoresis, flushing), cutaneous findings (rash or other dermatological reactions - see 4.8 Undesirable Effects), conjunctivitis, involvement of major organs (changes in liver-function tests, hepatic failure, jaundice, pancreatitis, pneumonitis with or without pleural effusion, leucopenia, leucocytosis, eosinophilia, disseminated intravascular coagulation, anaemia, renal impairment, including renal failure), and other less specific findings (adenitis, arthralgia, arthritis, myalgia, fatigue, malaise, hypotension, chest pain, tachycardia).

Infections

Non-steroidal anti-inflammatory drugs, including 'Clinoril', may mask the usual signs and symptoms of infection; therefore, the physician must be continually on the alert for this and should use the drug with extra care in the presence of existing infection.

Ocular effects

Because of reports of adverse eye findings with agents of this class it is recommended that patients who develop eye complaints during treatment with 'Clinoril' have ophthalmological evaluations.

Cardiovascular effects

Peripheral oedema has been observed in some patients taking 'Clinoril'. Therefore, as with other drugs in this class, 'Clinoril' should be used with caution in patients with compromised cardiac function, hypertension, or other conditions predisposed to fluid retention.

Hepatic effects

A patient with signs and/or symptoms suggesting liver dysfunction, or in whom an abnormal liver-function test has occurred, should be evaluated for evidence of a more severe hepatic reaction while on therapy. Significant elevations of AST (SGOT) and ALT (SGPT) (three times higher than normal) were seen in less than 1% of patients in controlled clinical trials.

Cases of hepatitis, jaundice, or both, with or without fever, may occur within the first three months of therapy. In some patients, the findings are consistent with those of cholestatic hepatitis.

Fever or other evidence of hypersensitivity, including abnormalities in one or more liver-function tests and skin reactions, have occurred during therapy. Some fatalities have occurred.

Whenever a patient develops unexplained fever, rash or other dermatological reactions, or constitutional symptoms, 'Clinoril' should be permanently stopped and liver function investigated. Fever and abnormal liver function are reversible.

Renal effects

As with other non-steroidal anti-inflammatory drugs, there have been reports of acute interstitial nephritis with haematuria, proteinuria and, occasionally, nephrotic syndrome in patients receiving sulindac.

In patients with reduced renal blood flow where renal prostaglandins play a major role in maintaining renal perfusion, administration of a non-steroidal anti-inflammatory agent may precipitate overt renal decompensation. Patients at greatest risk of this reaction are those with renal or hepatic dysfunction, diabetes mellitus, advanced age, extracellular volume depletion, congestive heart failure, sepsis, or concomitant use of any nephrotoxic drug. A non-steroidal anti-inflammatory drug should be given with caution and renal function should be monitored in any patient who may have reduced renal reserve. Discontinuation of non-steroidal anti-inflammatory therapy is usually followed by recovery to the pre-treatment state.

Since 'Clinoril' is eliminated primarily by the kidneys, patients with significantly impaired renal function should be closely monitored; a lower daily dosage should be used to avoid excessive drug accumulation.

Sulindac metabolites have been reported rarely as the major, or a minor, component in renal stones in association with other calculus components. 'Clinoril' should be used with caution in patients with a history of renal lithiasis and they should be kept well hydrated while receiving 'Clinoril'. In patients with renal functional impairment, since the major route of excretion of the drug is via the kidney, the dosage may need to be reduced.

4.5 Interaction with other medicinal products and other forms of Interaction

Dimethyl sulphoxide

Dimethyl sulphoxide should not be used with 'Clinoril'. Concomitant use has been reported to reduce plasma levels of the active metabolite of 'Clinoril', and also cause peripheral neuropathy.

Methotrexate

Caution should be used if 'Clinoril' is administered concomitantly with methotrexate. Non-steroidal anti-inflammatory drugs have been reported to decrease the tubular secretion of methotrexate and potentiate the toxicity.

Cyclosporin

Administration of non-steroidal anti-inflammatory drugs concomitantly with cyclosporin has been associated with an increase in cyclosporin-induced toxicity, possibly due to the decreased synthesis of renal prostacyclin. NSAIDs should be used with caution in patients taking cyclosporin, and renal function should be monitored carefully.

Oral anticoagulants and hypoglycaemic agents

Although sulindac and its sulphide metabolite are highly bound to protein, studies (in which 'Clinoril' was given at a dose of 400 mg daily) have shown no clinically significant interaction with oral anticoagulants or oral hypoglycaemic agents. However, patients should be monitored carefully until it is certain that no change in their anticoagulant or hypoglycaemic dose is required.

Aspirin

Concomitant administration with aspirin in normal volunteers significantly depressed plasma levels of the active sulphide metabolite. Clinical study of the combination showed an increase in GI side effects with no improvement in the therapeutic response to 'Clinoril'. The combination is not recommended.

Diflunisal

Concomitant administration with diflunisal in normal volunteers reduced the plasma level of active sulphide metabolite by approximately one-third.

Other NSAIDS

The concomitant use of 'Clinoril' with other NSAIDs is not recommended due to the increased possibility of gastrointestinal toxicity, with little or no increase in efficacy.

Probenecid

Probenecid given concomitantly with sulindac had only a slight effect on plasma sulphide levels, while plasma levels of sulindac and sulphone were increased. Sulindac was shown to produce a modest reduction in the uricosuric action of probenecid which probably is not usually significant.

Dextropropoxyphene hydrochloride/paracetamol

Neither dextropropoxyphene hydrochloride nor paracetamol had any effect on the plasma levels of sulindac or its sulphide metabolite.

Antacids

In a drug interaction study, an antacid (magnesium and aluminium hydroxides in suspension) was administered with 'Clinoril' with no significant difference in absorption.

Antihypertensive agents

In contrast to most other non-steroidal anti-inflammatory drugs, 'Clinoril' does not reduce the antihypertensive effect of thiazides and a variety of other agents used to treat mild to moderate hypertension. However, the blood pressure of patients taking 'Clinoril' with antihypertensive agents should be closely monitored.

4.6 Pregnancy and lactation

Use in pregnancy

'Clinoril' should be used during the first two trimesters of pregnancy only if the potential benefit justifies the potential risk to the fetus.

The known effects of drugs of this class on the human fetus during the third trimester of pregnancy include: constriction of the ductus arteriosus prenatally, tricuspid incompetence, and pulmonary hypertension; non-closure of the ductus arteriosus postnatally which may be resistant to medical management; myocardial degenerative changes, platelet dysfunction with resultant bleeding, intracranial bleeding, renal dysfunction or failure, renal injury/dysgenesis which may result in prolonged or permanent renal failure, oligohydramnios, gastro-intestinal bleeding or perforation and increased risk of necrotising enterocolitis. Use of 'Clinoril' during the third trimester of pregnancy is not recommended.

Use in breast-feeding

It is not known whether sulindac is excreted in human milk. Because other drugs of this class are excreted in human milk, a decision should be made whether to discontinue breast-feeding or discontinue the drug, taking into account the importance of the drug to the mother.

4.7 Effects on ability to drive and use machines

'Clinoril' may cause dizziness in some people. Patients taking the product should not drive or operate machinery unless it has been shown not to interfere with their physical or mental ability.

4.8 Undesirable effects

'Clinoril' is generally well tolerated. Those side effects experienced are usually mild and may often respond to a reduction in dosage.

Side effects reported frequently

Gastro-intestinal: the most frequent types of side effects occurring with 'Clinoril' are gastro-intestinal; these include gastro-intestinal pain, dyspepsia, nausea with or without vomiting, diarrhoea, constipation, flatulence, anorexia, and gastro-intestinal cramps.

Dermatological: rash, pruritus.

Central nervous system: dizziness, headache, nervousness.

Special senses: tinnitus.

Miscellaneous: oedema.

Side effects reported less frequently

The following side effects were reported less frequently. The probability exists of a causal relationship between 'Clinoril' and these side effects:

Gastro-intestinal: stomatitis, gastritis or gastro-enteritis. Peptic ulcer, colitis, as well as gastro-intestinal bleeding and gastro-intestinal perforations have been reported rarely. Fatalities have occurred. Pancreatitis, ageusia, glossitis, and intestinal strictures (diaphragms).

It has also been reported that a probable sulindac metabolite has been found in biliary sludge in patients with symptoms of cholecystitis who underwent a cholecystectomy.

Hepatic: Liver-function-test abnormalities, jaundice sometimes with fever, cholestasis, hepatitis, hepatic failure.

Dermatological: sore or dry mucous membranes, alopecia, photosensitivity, erythema multiforme, toxic epidermal necrolysis, Stevens-Johnson syndrome, exfoliative dermatitis.

Cardiovascular: congestive heart failure, especially in patients with marginal cardiac function; palpitation, hypertension.

Haematological: thrombocytopenia; ecchymosis; purpura; leucopenia; agranulocytosis; neutropenia; bone-marrow depression, including aplastic anaemia; haemolytic anaemia, increased prothrombin time in patients on oral anticoagulants.

Genito-urinary: urine discoloration, dysuria, vaginal bleeding, haematuria, proteinuria, crystalluria, renal impairment including renal failure, interstitial nephritis, nephrotic syndrome.

Nervous system: vertigo, somnolence, insomnia, sweating, asthenia, paraesthesia, convulsions, syncope, depression, psychic disturbances including acute psychosis, aseptic meningitis.

Metabolic: Hyperkalaemia.

Musculoskeletal: Muscle weakness.

Special senses: visual disturbances including blurred vision, decreased hearing, metallic or bitter taste.

Respiratory: epistaxis.

Hypersensitivity reactions: anaphylaxis and angioneurotic oedema. Bronchial spasm, dyspnoea, hypersensitivity vasculitis, hypersensitivity syndrome (see 4.4 Special Warnings And Precautions For Use).

Causal relationship unknown: other reactions have been reported in clinical trials or since the drug was marketed, but occurred under circumstances where a causal relationship could not be established. However, in these rarely reported events, that possibility cannot be excluded. Therefore, these observations are listed to serve as alerting information to physicians.

Cardiovascular: arrhythmia.

Metabolic: hyperglycaemia.

Nervous system: neuritis.

Special senses: disturbances of the retina and its vasculature.

Miscellaneous: gynaecomastia.

Rarely, occurrences of fulminant necrotising fasciitis, particularly in association with Group A β-haemolytic streptococcus, has been described in persons treated with non-steroidal anti-inflammatory agents, sometimes with fatal outcome (see 4.4 Special Warnings And Precautions For Use).

4.9 Overdose

Cases of overdosage have been reported and, rarely, fatalities have occurred. The following signs and symptoms may be observed following overdosage: stupor, coma, diminished urine output and hypotension. In isolated cases patients have received up to 600 mg a day without adverse consequences being reported.

In the event of acute overdosage, if ingestion is recent, the stomach should be emptied by inducing vomiting or by gastric lavage, and the patient carefully observed and given symptomatic and supportive treatment.

Animal studies show that absorption is decreased by the prompt administration of activated charcoal, and excretion is enhanced by alkalinisation of the urine.

The readiness of sulindac and its metabolites to dialyse is unknown at present. But because they are highly bound to plasma proteins, dialysis is not likely to be effective.

The mean half-life of sulindac is 7.8 hours while the mean half-life of the active sulphide metabolite is 16.4 hours.

5. PHARMACOLOGICAL PROPERTIES

5.1 Pharmacodynamic properties

'Clinoril' is a non-steroidal, antirheumatic agent with anti-inflammatory analgesic and antipyretic properties. It is not a salicylate, propionic acid, pyrazolone or corticosteroid.

Prostaglandin synthetase inhibition has been hypothesised to be the mechanism of action of non-steroidal anti-inflammatory agents. Following absorption, sulindac undergoes two major biotransformations: reversible reduction to the sulphide metabolite, and irreversible oxidation to the inactive sulphone metabolite. The sulphide metabolite is a potent inhibitor of prostaglandin synthesis, and available evidence indicates that the biological activity of 'Clinoril' resides with the sulphide metabolite, thus the sulphoxide form (sulindac) is a prodrug.

5.2 Pharmacokinetic properties

Sulindac is approximately 90% absorbed in man after oral administration. The peak plasma concentrations of the biologically active sulphide metabolite are achieved in about two hours when sulindac is administered in the fasting state; and in about three to four hours when sulindac is administered with food. The mean half-life of sulindac is 7.8 hours, while the mean half-life of the sulphide metabolite is 16.4 hours. Sustained plasma levels of the sulphide metabolite are consistent with a prolonged anti-inflammatory action.

Sulindac and its sulphone metabolite undergo extensive enterohepatic circulation relative to the sulphide metabolite. The enterohepatic circulation together with the reversible metabolism are probably major contributors to sustained plasma levels of the active drug.

The primary route of excretion in man is via the urine as both sulindac and its sulphone metabolite and glucoronide conjugates. Approximately 50% of an oral dose is excreted in the urine, with the conjugated sulphone metabolite accounting for the major portion. Approximately 25% of an oral dose is found in the faeces, primarily as the sulphone and sulphide metabolites.

The bioavailability of sulindac and the active sulphide metabolite from the oral liquid is greater than 90% of that of the tablet.

5.3 Preclinical safety data

No relevant information.

6. PHARMACEUTICAL PARTICULARS

6.1 List of excipients

Cellulose microcrystalline, pregelatinised maize starch, magnesium stearate. (An alternative method of manufacture uses maize starch instead of pregelatinised maize starch.)

6.2 Incompatibilities

None known.

6.3 Shelf life

36 months.

6.4 Special precautions for storage

Do not store above 25°C. Store in the original package. Keep in outer carton.

6.5 Nature and contents of container

Bottles containing 100 tablets or blister packs containing 60 tablets

6.6 Instructions for use and handling

None.

7. MARKETING AUTHORISATION HOLDER

Merck Sharp & Dohme Limited

Hertford Road, Hoddesdon, Hertfordshire, EN11 9BU, UK

8. MARKETING AUTHORISATION NUMBER(S)

100 mg, PL 0025/0121

200 mg, PL 0025/0122

9. DATE OF FIRST AUTHORISATION/RENEWAL OF THE AUTHORISATION

5 January 1977 / 17 June 1997.

10. DATE OF REVISION OF THE TEXT

November 2003.

11. LEGAL CATEGORY

POM

® denotes registered trademark of Merck & Co., Inc., Whitehouse Station, NJ, USA.

SPC.COR.03.UK.1028

Clomid

(sanofi-aventis)

1. NAME OF THE MEDICINAL PRODUCT

Clomid™ 50mg Tablets

2. QUALITATIVE AND QUANTITATIVE COMPOSITION

Clomifene Citrate 50mg.

3. PHARMACEUTICAL FORM

Tablet.

4. CLINICAL PARTICULARS

4.1 Therapeutic indications

Clomid 50mg Tablets (Clomifene citrate BP) is indicated for the treatment of ovulatory failure in women desiring pregnancy. Clomid 50mg Tablets is indicated only for patients in whom ovulatory dysfunction is demonstrated. Other causes of infertility must be excluded or adequately treated before giving Clomid 50mg Tablets

4.2 Posology and method of administration

Route of Administration:

Oral.

Adults Only:

The recommended dose for the first course of Clomid 50mg Tablets (Clomifene citrate BP) is 50mg (1 tablet) daily for 5 days. Therapy may be started at any time in the patient who has had no recent uterine bleeding. If progestin-induced bleeding is planned, or if spontaneous uterine bleeding occurs before therapy, the regimen of 50mg daily for 5 days should be started on or about the fifth day of the cycle. When ovulation occurs at this dosage, there is no advantage to increasing the dose in subsequent cycles of treatment.

If ovulation appears not to have occurred after the first course of therapy, a second course of 100mg daily (two 50mg tablets given as a single daily dose) for 5 days should be given. This course may be started as early as 30 days after the previous one. Increase of the dosage or duration of therapy beyond 100mg/day for 5 days should not be undertaken.

The majority of patients who are going to respond will respond to the first course of therapy, and 3 courses should constitute an adequate therapeutic trial. If ovulatory menses have not yet occurred, the diagnosis should be re-evaluated. Treatment beyond this is not recommended in the patient who does not exhibit evidence of ovulation.

Long-term cyclic therapy:

Not recommended.

The relative safety of long-term cyclic therapy has not been conclusively demonstrated and, since the majority of patients will ovulate following 3 courses, long-term cyclic therapy is not recommended, i.e. beyond a total of about 6 cycles (including 3 ovulatory cycles).

4.3 Contraindications

Pregnancy: See "Pregnancy and Lactation".

Liver disease: Clomid 50mg Tablets (Clomifene citrate BP) therapy is contraindicated in patients with liver disease or a history of liver dysfunction.

Abnormal uterine bleeding: Clomid 50mg Tablets is contraindicated in patients with hormone-dependent tumours or in patients with abnormal uterine bleeding of undetermined origin.

Ovarian cyst: Clomid 50mg Tablets should not be given in the presence of an ovarian cyst, except polycystic ovary, since further enlargement of the cyst may occur. Patients should be evaluated for the presence of ovarian cyst prior to each course of treatment.

4.4 Special warnings and special precautions for use
Warnings:

General: Good levels of endogenous oestrogen (as estimated from vaginal smears, endometrial biopsy, assay of urinary oestrogen, or endometrial bleeding in response to progesterone) provide a favourable prognosis for ovulatory response induced by Clomid 50mg Tablets. A low level of oestrogen, although clinically less favourable, does not preclude successful outcome of therapy. Clomid 50mg Tablets therapy is ineffective in patients with primary pituitary or primary ovarian failure. Clomid 50mg Tablets therapy cannot be expected to substitute for specific treatment of other causes of ovulatory failure, such as thyroid or adrenal disorders. For hyperprolactinaemia there is other preferred specific treatment. Clomid 50mg Tablets is not first line treatment for low weight related amenorrhoea, with infertility, and has no value if a high FSH blood level is observed following an early menopause.

Ovarian Hyperstimulation Syndrome: Ovarian Hyperstimulation Syndrome (OHSS) has been reported in patients receiving Clomid 50mg Tablets therapy for ovulation induction. In some cases, OHSS occurred following the cyclic use of Clomid 50mg Tablets therapy or when Clomid 50mg Tablets was used in combination with gonadotropins. The following symptoms have been reported in association with this syndrome during Clomid 50mg Tablets therapy: pericardial effusion, anasarca, hydrothorax, acute abdomen, renal failure, pulmonary oedema, ovarian haemorrhage, deep venous thrombosis, torsion of the ovary and acute respiratory distress. If conception results, rapid progression to the severe form of the syndrome may occur.

To minimise the hazard of the abnormal ovarian enlargement associated with Clomid 50mg Tablets therapy, the lowest dose consistent with expectation of good results should be used. The patient should be instructed to inform the physician of any abdominal or pelvic pain, weight gain, discomfort or distension after taking Clomid 50mg Tablets. Maximal enlargement of the ovary may not occur until several days after discontinuation of the course of Clomid 50mg Tablets. Some patients with polycystic ovary syndrome who are unusually sensitive to gonadotropin may have an exaggerated response to usual doses of Clomid 50mg Tablets.

The patient who complains of abdominal or pelvic pain, discomfort, or distension after taking Clomid 50mg Tablets should be examined because of the possible presence of an ovarian cyst or other cause. Due to fragility of enlarged ovaries in severe cases, abdominal and pelvic examination should be performed very cautiously. If abnormal enlargement occurs Clomid 50mg Tablets should not be given until the ovaries have returned to pre-treatment size. Ovarian enlargement and cyst formation associated with Clomid 50mg Tablets therapy usually regress spontaneously within a few days or weeks after discontinuing treatment. Most of these patients should be managed conservatively. The dosage and/or duration of the next course of treatment should be reduced.

Visual Symptoms: Patients should be advised that blurring or other visual symptoms may occasionally occur during or shortly after therapy with Clomid 50mg Tablets. Patients should be warned that visual symptoms may render such activities as driving a car or operating machinery more hazardous than usual, particularly under conditions of variable lighting. The significance of these visual symptoms is not understood. If the patient has any visual symptoms, treatment should be discontinued and ophthalmologic evaluation performed.

Precautions:

Multiple Pregnancy: There is an increased chance of multiple pregnancy when conception occurs in relationship to Clomid 50mg Tablets therapy. During the clinical investigation studies, the incidence of multiple pregnancy was 7.9% (186 of 2369 Clomid 50mg Tablets associated pregnancies on which outcome was reported). Among these 2369 pregnancies, 165 (6.9%) twin, 11 (0.5%) triplet, 7 (0.3%) quadruplet and 3 (0.13%) quintuplet. Of the 165 twin pregnancies for which sufficient information was available, the ratio of monozygotic twins was 1:5.

Ectopic Pregnancy: There is an increased chance of ectopic pregnancy (including tubal and ovarian sites) in women who conceive following Clomid 50mg Tablets therapy. Ectopic pregnancy associated with Clomid 50mg Tablets involves a multiple pregnancy with coexisting extrauterine and intrauterine gestations.

Uterine Fibroids: Caution should be exercised when using Clomid 50mg Tablets in patients with uterine fibroids due to potential for further enlargement of the fibroids.

Pregnancy Wastage and Birth Anomalies: The overall incidence of reported birth anomalies from pregnancies associated with maternal Clomid 50mg Tablets ingestion (before or after conception) during the investigational studies was within the range of that reported in the published references for the general population. Among the birth anomalies spontaneously reported in the published literature as individual cases, the proportion of neural tube defects has been high among pregnancies associated with ovulation induced by Clomid 50mg Tablets, but this has not been supported by data from population based studies.

The physician should explain so that the patient understands the assumed risk of any pregnancy whether the ovulation was induced with the aid of Clomid 50mg Tablets or occurred naturally.

The patient should be informed of the greater pregnancy risks associated with certain characteristics or conditions of any pregnant woman: e.g. age of female and male partner, history of spontaneous abortions, Rh genotype, abnormal menstrual history, infertility history (regardless of cause), organic heart disease, diabetes, exposure to infectious agents such as rubella, familial history of birth anomaly, and other risk factors that may be pertinent to the patient for whom Clomid 50mg Tablets is being considered. Based upon the evaluation of the patient, genetic counselling may be indicated.

Population based reports have been published on possible elevation of risk of Down's Syndrome in ovulation induction cases and of increase in trisomy defects among spontaneously aborted foetuses from subfertile women receiving ovulation inducing drugs (no women with Clomid 50mg Tablets alone and without additional inducing drug). However, as yet, the reported observations are too few to confirm or not confirm the presence of an increased risk that would justify amniocentesis other than for the usual indications because of age and family history.

The experience from patients of all diagnosis during clinical investigation of Clomid 50mg Tablets shows a pregnancy (single and multiple) wastage or foetal loss rate of 21.4% (abortion rate of 19.0%), ectopic pregnancies, 1.18%, hydatidiform mole, 0.17%, foetus papyraceous, 0.04% and of pregnancies with one or more stillbirths, 1.01%.

Clomid 50mg Tablets therapy after conception was reported for 158 of the 2369 delivered and reported pregnancies in the clinical investigations. Of these 158 pregnancies 8 infants (born of 7 pregnancies) were reported to have birth defects.

There was no difference in reported incidence of birth defects whether Clomid 50mg Tablets was given before the 19th day after conception or between the 20th and 35th day after conception. This incidence is within the anticipated range of general population.

Ovarian Cancer: There have been rare reports of ovarian cancer with fertility drugs; infertility itself is a primary risk factor. Epidemiological data suggest that prolonged use of Clomid 50mg Tablets may increase this risk. Therefore the recommended duration of treatment should not be exceeded (see "Posology and Method of Administration").

4.5 Interaction with other medicinal products and other forms of Interaction

None stated.

4.6 Pregnancy and lactation

Clomid 50mg Tablets is not indicated during pregnancy. Although there is no evidence that Clomid 50mg Tablets has a harmful effect on the human foetus, there is evidence that Clomid 50mg Tablets has a deleterious effect on rat and rabbit foetuses when given in high doses to the pregnant animal. To avoid inadvertent Clomid 50mg Tablets administration during early pregnancy, appropriate tests should be utilised during each treatment cycle to determine whether ovulation occurs. The patient should have a pregnancy test before the next course of Clomid 50mg Tablets therapy.

It is not known whether Clomifene citrate is excreted in human milk. Clomiphene may reduce lactation.

4.7 Effects on ability to drive and use machines

Patients should be warned that visual symptoms may render such activities as driving a car or operating machinery more hazardous than usual, particularly under conditions of variable lighting (see "Special Warnings and Special Precautions for Use").

4.8 Undesirable effects

Symptoms/Signs/Conditions: Adverse effects appeared to be dose-related, occurring more frequently at the higher dose and with the longer courses of treatment used in investigational studies. At recommended dosage, adverse effects are not prominent and infrequently interfere with treatment.

During the investigational studies, the more common reported adverse effects included ovarian enlargement (13.6%), vasomotor flushes (10.4%), abdominal-pelvic discomfort (distension, bloating) (5.5%), nausea and vomiting (2.2%), breast discomfort (2.1%), visual symptoms (1.5%), headache (1.3%) and intermenstrual spotting or menorrhagia (1.3%).

Ovarian Enlargement: At recommended dosage, abnormal ovarian enlargement is infrequent although the usual cyclic variation in ovarian size may be exaggerated. Similarly, cyclic ovarian pain (mittelschmerz) may be accentuated. With higher or prolonged dosage, more frequent ovarian enlargement and cyst formation may occur, and the luteal phase of the cycle may be prolonged.

Rare instances of massive ovarian enlargement are recorded. Such an instance has been described in a patient with polycystic ovary syndrome whose Clomid 50mg Tablets therapy consisted of 100mg daily for 14 days. Abnormal ovarian enlargement usually regresses spontaneously; most of the patients with this condition should be treated conservatively.

Eye/Visual Symptoms: Symptoms described usually as "blurring" or spots or flashes (scintillating scotomata) increase in incidence with increasing total dose and usually disappear within periods ranging from a few days to a few weeks after Clomid 50mg Tablets is discontinued.

These symptoms appear to be due to intensification and prolongation of after-images. After-images as such have also been reported. Symptoms often first appear or are accentuated with exposure to bright-light environment.

Ophthalmologically definable scotomata, phosphenes and reduced visual acuity have been reported.

There are rare reports of cataracts and optic neuritis.

Genitourinary: There are reports of new cases of endometriosis and exacerbation of pre-existing endometriosis during Clomid 50mg Tablets therapy.

Multiple pregnancies, including simultaneous intrauterine and extrauterine pregnancies, have been reported.

Tumours/Neoplasms: Isolated reports have been received on the occurrence of endocrine-related or dependent neoplasms or their aggravation. Ovarian cancer: see "Special Warnings and Special Precautions for Use".

Central Nervous System: Convulsions have been reported; patients with a history of seizures may be predisposed. In investigational patients, CNS symptoms/signs, conditions of dizziness, light-headedness/vertigo (0.9%), nervous tension/insomnia (0.8%) and fatigue/depression (0.7%) were reported. After prescription availability, there were isolated additional reports of these conditions and also reports of other conditions such as syncope/fainting, cerebrovascular accident, cerebral thrombosis, psychotic reactions including paranoid psychosis, neurologic impairment, disorientation and speech disturbance.

Dermatoses: Dermatitis and rash were reported by investigational patients. Conditions such as rash and urticaria were the most common ones reported after prescription availability but also reported were conditions such as allergic reaction, erythema multiforme, ecchymosis and angioneurotic oedema. Hair thinning has been reported very rarely.

Liver Function: Bromsulphalein (BSP) retention of greater than 5% was reported in 32 of 141 patients in whom it was measured, including 5 of 43 patients who took approximately the dose of Clomid 50mg Tablets now recommended. Retention was usually minimal unless associated with prolonged continuous Clomid 50mg Tablets administration or with apparently unrelated liver disease. Other liver function tests were usually normal. In a later study in which patients were given 6 consecutive monthly courses of Clomid 50mg Tablets (50 or 100mg daily for 3 days) or matching placebo, BSP tests were done on 94 patients. Values in excess of 5% retention were recorded in 11 patients, 6 of whom had taken drug and 5 placebo.

In a separate report, one patient taking 50mg of Clomid 50mg Tablets daily developed jaundice on the 19th day of treatment; liver biopsy revealed bile stasis without evidence of hepatitis.

4.9 Overdose

Toxic effects of acute overdosage of Clomid 50mg Tablets have not been reported but the number of overdose cases recorded is small. In the event of overdose, appropriate supportive measures should be employed.

5. PHARMACOLOGICAL PROPERTIES

5.1 Pharmacodynamic properties

Clomid 50mg Tablets is a triarylethylene compound (related to chlorotrianisene and triparanol). It is a non-steroidal agent which stimulates ovulation in a high percentage of appropriately selected anovulatory women.

5.2 Pharmacokinetic properties

Orally administered ^{14}C labelled Clomifene citrate was readily absorbed when administered to humans. Cumulative excretion of the ^{14}C label by way of urine and faeces averaged about 50% of the oral dose after 5 days in 6 subjects, with mean urinary excretion of 7.8% and mean faecal excretion of 42.4%. A mean rate of excretion of 0.73% per day of the ^{14}C dose after 31 days to 35 days and 0.45% per day of the ^{14}C dose after 42 days to 45 days was seen in faecal and urine samples collected from 6 subjects for 14 to 53 days after Clomifene citrate ^{14}C administration. The remaining drug/metabolites may be slowly excreted from a sequestered enterohepatic recirculation pool.

5.3 Preclinical safety data

None stated.

6. PHARMACEUTICAL PARTICULARS

6.1 List of excipients

Sucrose

Lactose

Soluble starch

Maize starch

Magnesium stearate

Iron oxide yellow E172

Purified Water

6.2 Incompatibilities
Not applicable.

6.3 Shelf life
5 years.

6.4 Special precautions for storage
Store in original container, do not store above 25°C.

6.5 Nature and contents of container
Blister pack:

Base: 250 micron PVC

Foil: 20 micron hard-tempered aluminium

(in cardboard cartons)

Pack sizes: 30 and 100 tablets

6.6 Instructions for use and handling
None.

7. MARKETING AUTHORISATION HOLDER
Aventis Pharma Ltd
50 Kings Hill Avenue
Kings Hill
West Malling
Kent ME19 4AH

8. MARKETING AUTHORISATION NUMBER(S)
PL 04425/5900R

9. DATE OF FIRST AUTHORISATION/RENEWAL OF THE AUTHORISATION
29 September 1995/ 6th November 2003

10. DATE OF REVISION OF THE TEXT
May 2003

11 LEGAL CLASSIFICATION
POM

Clomifene Tablets BP

(Wockhardt UK Ltd)

1. NAME OF THE MEDICINAL PRODUCT
Clomifene Tablets BP 50mg

2. QUALITATIVE AND QUANTITATIVE COMPOSITION
Clomifene citrate 50mg

For excipients, see 6.1

3. PHARMACEUTICAL FORM
Tablet

White, round tablets with HG C50 on one side and a breakline on the other side.

4. CLINICAL PARTICULARS

4.1 Therapeutic indications
The treatment of anovulatory infertility in women.

4.2 Posology and method of administration
Route of administration: Oral

(i) Dosage Schedule

The recommended dose for the first course of treatment is 50mg (one tablet) daily for five days, starting within the first five days of spontaneous or induced menstrual bleeding. Therapy may be started as an arbitrary time in patients who have had no recent menstrual bleeding.

If ovulation occurs but is not followed by pregnancy, subsequent courses at the same dosage may be given up to a maximum of three cycles.

The majority of patients who are going to respond will respond to the first course of therapy, and three courses should constitute an adequate therapeutic trial. If ovulatory menses have not yet occurred, the diagnosis should be re-evaluated. Treatment beyond this is not recommended in the patient who does not exhibit evidence of ovulation.

Long-term cyclic therapy:

Not recommended.

The relative safety of long-term cyclic therapy has not been conclusively demonstrated and, since the majority of patients will ovulate following three courses, long-term cyclic therapy is not recommended, i.e. beyond a total of about six cycles (including three ovulatory cycles).

(ii) Types of Patient

Not intended for children.

Not intended for elderly patients.

Only for women of reproductive age with anovulatory infertility.

4.3 Contraindications
Pregnancy

Liver disease or a history of liver dysfunction

Abnormal uterine bleeding until the cause has been determined

Pituitary or ovarian tumours

4.4 Special warnings and special precautions for use
Causes of infertility other than ovarian dysfunction should be excluded before the start of treatment.

Hyperstimulation of the ovary, with excessive ovarian enlargement, may occur rarely; pelvic examination, which should be carried out with care, will reveal the diagnosis. The dose of clomifene should be reduced. Further courses should not be given until the ovaries have returned to pre-treatment size.

The incidence of multiple pregnancy is increased when conception takes place during a clomifene-stimulated cycle.

In order to avoid inadvertant administration of clomifene in early pregnancy, the basal body temperature should be monitored. In the absence of expected menses, a sensitive pregnancy test should be performed and only if negative should the patient be given the course of clomifene.

4.5 Interaction with other medicinal products and other forms of Interaction
None known.

4.6 Pregnancy and lactation
Use during pregnancy is contraindicated.

4.7 Effects on ability to drive and use machines
Drowsiness or sedation do not occur, but patients should be warned that visual symptoms particularly blurring or vision occasionally occur. Its onset is gradual.

4.8 Undesirable effects
Side effects, when they occur, are generally mild. They are dose related.

Side effects are reversible on drug withdrawal.

Among those reported, which are of low frequency at the recommended doses are ovarian enlargement, abdominal pelvic discomfort, hot flushes, nausea/vomiting, breast tenderness or discomfort and visual blurring. Very rarely and only at much higher doses than those recommended, massive ovarian enlargement has been reported.

Convulsions have been reported. Patients with a history of seizures may be predisposed.

There have been rare reports of ovarian cancer with fertility drugs. Epidemiological data have shown that there was no increase in risk of ovarian cancer with clomifene when used for the recommended duration of treatment. However, prolonged use of clomifene (for example, 12 cycles or more) may be associated with an increased risk. Therefore the recommended duration of treatment should not be exceeded (see Dosage and Administration).

4.9 Overdose
There is no experience with overdosage

5. PHARMACOLOGICAL PROPERTIES

5.1 Pharmacodynamic properties
Clomifene is used to induce ovulation in women with anovulatory cycles. This agent is an anti-oestrogen and is believed to act by binding to oestrogen receptors in the hypothalamus and allowing follicle stimulating hormone (FSH) to rise in order to stimulate follicular development and ultimately result in ovulation.

It is probable that clomifene additionally exerts a direct effect on ovarian function.

5.2 Pharmacokinetic properties
Clomifene is absorbed from the gastrointestinal tract and slowly excreted through the liver into the bile. The biological half life is reported to be about five days. Enterohepatic recirculation takes place.

5.3 Preclinical safety data
Nothing of relevance to the prescriber which dose not appear elsewhere in the SPC.

6. PHARMACEUTICAL PARTICULARS

6.1 List of excipients
Magnesium stearate

Maize starch

Lactose

6.2 Incompatibilities
Not applicable

6.3 Shelf life
Five years

6.4 Special precautions for storage
Do not store above 25°C.

Store in original packaging.

6.5 Nature and contents of container
Blister packs of 10 tablets manufactured from 250 micron white opaque PVC and 20 micron hard temper aluminium foil

Pack Sizes: 10, 20, 30, 100 tablets (1,2,3 or 10 strips) in an outer carton.

6.6 Instructions for use and handling
None

Administrative Data

7. MARKETING AUTHORISATION HOLDER
CP Pharmaceuticals Ltd
Ash Road North
Wrexham
LL13 9UF
UK.

8. MARKETING AUTHORISATION NUMBER(S)
PL 4543/0424

9. DATE OF FIRST AUTHORISATION/RENEWAL OF THE AUTHORISATION
30 April 2000

10. DATE OF REVISION OF THE TEXT
December 2002

Clopixol Acuphase Injection

(Lundbeck Limited)

1. NAME OF THE MEDICINAL PRODUCT
CLOPIXOL ACUPHASE

2. QUALITATIVE AND QUANTITATIVE COMPOSITION
Zuclopenthixol acetate 5.0% w/v equivalent to 4.526% w/v of zuclopenthixol base.

3. PHARMACEUTICAL FORM
Oily solution for deep intramuscular injection.

4. CLINICAL PARTICULARS

4.1 Therapeutic indications
For the initial treatment of acute psychoses including mania and exacerbation of chronic psychoses, particularly where a rapid onset of action, and a duration of effect of 2-3 days is desirable.

4.2 Posology and method of administration

Dosage

Adults:

Dosage should be adjusted according to the severity of the patient's illness. CLOPIXOL ACUPHASE is administered by deep intramuscular injection, into the upper outer buttock or lateral thigh.

The usual dosage is 50-150 mg (1-3 mL), repeated if necessary after 2 or 3 days. Some patients may need an additional injection between 1 and 2 days after the first injection.

CLOPIXOL ACUPHASE is not intended for long-term use and duration of treatment should not be more than two weeks. The maximum accumulated dosage in a course should not exceed 400 mg and the number of injections should not exceed four.

Patients with compromised hepatic function should receive half the recommended dosages for normal patients. Where there is reduced renal function, it is not necessary to reduce the dosage but where there is renal failure dosage should be reduced to half the normal dosage.

Elderly:

The dosage may need to be reduced in the elderly owing to reduced rates of metabolism and elimination. Maximum dosage per injection should be 100 mg.

Children:

Not recommended for children.

Maintenance Therapy:

CLOPIXOL ACUPHASE is not intended for long-term use.

A single injection of CLOPIXOL ACUPHASE has an onset of sedative action shortly after injection and an antipsychotic action persisting for 2 to 3 days. In this period, maintenance treatment with tablets or a longer acting depot neuroleptic can be initiated. The possible side-effects of long-term maintenance treatment with a neuroleptic, including tardive dyskinesia, should be considered.

Maintenance treatment where required can be continued with CLOPIXOL tablets, CLOPIXOL injection or CLOPIXOL CONC. injection, according to the following guidelines:

1. Introduce CLOPIXOL tablets at a dosage of 20-60 mg/day in divided doses, 2 to 3 days after the last injection of CLOPIXOL ACUPHASE. If necessary increase the tablet dosage by 10-20 mg each day up to a maximum of 150 mg/day.

or

2. Concomitantly with the last injection of CLOPIXOL ACUPHASE, administer 200-500 mg of CLOPIXOL injection or CLOPIXOL CONC. injection by deep intramuscular injection and repeat the CLOPIXOL injection or CLOPIXOL CONC. injection at intervals of 2 to 4 weeks. Higher dosages or a shorter interval may be necessary.

Route of Administration:

Deep intramuscular injection, into the upper outer buttock or lateral thigh.

4.3 Contraindications
Comatose states, including acute alcohol, barbiturate, and opiate intoxication.

4.4 Special warnings and special precautions for use
Like other neuroleptics zuclopenthixol acetate should be used with caution in patients with convulsive disorders or advanced hepatic, renal or cardiovascular disease.

Zuclopenthixol is not suitable for patients who do not tolerate oral neuroleptic drugs or for patients suffering from Parkinson's disease.

The possibility of development of neuroleptic malignant syndrome (hyperthermia, rigidity, fluctuating consciousness, instability of the autonomous nervous system) exists with any neuroleptic. The risk is possibly greater with the more potent agents. Patients with pre-existing organic brain syndrome, mental retardation, opiate and alcohol abuse are over represented among fatal cases

Treatment: Discontinuation of the neuroleptic. Symptomatic treatment and use of general supportive measures. Dantrolene and bromocriptine may be helpful. Symptoms may persist for more than a week after oral neuroleptics are discontinued and somewhat longer when associated with the depot forms of the drugs.

4.5 Interaction with other medicinal products and other forms of Interaction

Zuclopenthixol enhances the response to alcohol and the effects of barbiturates and other CNS depressants. Potentiation of the effects of general anaesthetics may occur. Zuclopenthixol acetate should not be given concomitantly with guanethidine or similarly acting compounds, since neuroleptics may block the antihypertensive effect of these compounds. Tricyclic antidepressants and neuroleptics mutually inhibit the metabolism of each other. Zuclopenthixol may reduce the effect of levodopa and the effect of adrenergic drugs. Concomitant use of metoclopramide and piperazine increases the risk of extrapyramidal symptoms.

The possibility of interaction with lithium salts should be borne in mind.

4.6 Pregnancy and lactation

Animal tests have not revealed any evidence that zuclopenthixol causes an increased incidence of foetal damage. Nevertheless, zuclopenthixol acetate should not be administered during pregnancy or to women of childbearing potential, unless they are taking adequate contraceptive precautions or unless the expected benefit to the patient outweighs the potential risk to the foetus.

Zuclopenthixol is found in very low concentrations in the breast milk of mothers receiving CLOPIXOL treatment. It is recommended that mothers treated with CLOPIXOL ACUPHASE should not breast feed.

4.7 Effects on ability to drive and use machines

The ability to drive a car or operate machinery may be affected and patients should be warned of this risk.

4.8 Undesirable effects

The frequency of unwanted effects is in general low and the severity of the symptoms is most often mild. The frequency and severity are most pronounced the day after the first injection and then decrease rapidly.

Extrapyramidal symptoms, including dystonia, rigidity, motor akathisia, hypokinesia and tremor, have been reported. These side effects can be satisfactorily controlled by antiparkinson drugs.

Orthostatic dizziness occurs rarely and only occasionally to a severe degree.

Reduced salivation of a mild degree has been observed.

Other reported undesirable effects include tachycardia, abnormalities of visual accommodation, paraesthesia and convulsions.

4.9 Overdose

Symptoms: somnolence, coma, extrapyramidal symptoms, convulsions, hypotension, shock, hyper or hypothermia. ECG changes have been reported when administered in overdose together with drugs known to affect the heart.

Treatment: treatment is symptomatic and supportive. Measures aimed at supporting the respiratory and cardiovascular systems should be instituted. Adrenaline (epinephrine) must not be used in these patients. There is no specific antidote.

5. PHARMACOLOGICAL PROPERTIES

5.1 Pharmacodynamic properties

Zuclopenthixol is a potent neuroleptic of the thioxanthene series with a piperazine side-chain. The antipsychotic effect of neuroleptics is related to their dopamine receptor blocking effect. The thioxanthenes have a high affinity for both the adenylate cyclase coupled dopamine D1 receptors and for the dopamine D2 receptors; in the phenothiazine group the affinity for D1 receptors is much lower than that for D2 receptors, whereas butyrophenones, diphenylbutylpiperidines and benzamides only have affinity for D2 receptors.

In the traditional tests for antipsychotic effect, eg antagonism of stereotypic behaviour induced by dopamine agonists, the chemical groups of neuroleptics mentioned reveal equal but dosage dependent activity. However, the antistereotypic effect of phenothiazines, butyrophenones, diphenylbutylpiperidines, and benzamindes is strongly counteracted by the anticholinergic drug, scopolamine, while the antisteriotypic effect of the thioxanthenes, eg zuclopenthixol, is not, or only very slightly, influenced by concomitant treatment with anticholinergics.

5.2 Pharmacokinetic properties

By esterification of zuclopenthixol with acetic acid, zuclopenthixol has been converted to a more lipophilic substance, zuclopenthixol acetate. When dissolved in oil and injected intramuscularly this substance diffuses slowly into the surrounding body water, where enzymatic breakdown occurs releasing the active component zuclopenthixol.

Maximum serum concentrations of zuclopenthixol are usually reached 36 hours after an injection, after which the serum levels decline slowly. The average maximum serum level corresponding to the 100 mg dose is 41 ng/mL. Three days after the injection the serum level is about one third of the maximum.

Zuclopenthixol is distributed in the body in a similar way to other neuroleptics; with the higher concentrations of drug and metabolites in liver, lungs, intestines and kidneys and lower concentrations in heart, spleen, brain and blood. The apparent volume of distribution is about 20 L/kg and the protein binding about 98%.

Zuclopenthixol crosses the placental barrier in small amounts. Zuclopenthixol is excreted in small amounts with the milk - the ratio milk concentration/serum concentration in women is on average 0.3.

The metabolism of zuclopenthixol proceeds via three main routes - sulphoxidation, side chain N-dealkylation and glucuronic acid conjugation. The metabolites are devoid of psychopharmacolical activity. The excretion proceeds mainly with the faeces but also to some degree with the urine. The systemic clearance is about 0.9 L/min.

The kinetics seem to be linear, since highly significant correlation exist between the dose and the area under the serum concentration curve.

5.3 Preclinical safety data

Zuclopenthixol has no mutagenic potential. In a rat oncogeneticity study, 30 mg/kg/day resulted in slight non statistical increases in the incidence of mammary adenocarcinomas and pancreatic islet cell adenomas and carcinomas in females and of thyroid parafollicular carcinomas. This is a common finding for D_2 antagonists which increase prolactin secretion when administered to rats. The physiological differences between rats and humans suggest that these changes are not predictive of an oncogenic risk in patients.

Local muscle damage is less pronounced with oily solutions of zuclopenthixol (including Clopixol Acuphase) then with aqueous solutions of zuclopenthixol and other neuroleptics.

6. PHARMACEUTICAL PARTICULARS

6.1 List of excipients

Thin vegetable oil (derived from coconuts).

6.2 Incompatibilities

Zuclopenthixol acetate should not be mixed with other injection fluids.

6.3 Shelf life

2 years as packaged for sale.

6.4 Special precautions for storage

Store at room temperature (at or below 25°C). Protect from light.

6.5 Nature and contents of container

Clear glass ampoules containing either 1 or 2 mL of zuclopenthixol acetate 5% w/v in thin vegetable oil.

The ampoules are packed in boxes of 5.

6.6 Instructions for use and handling

Nil.

7. MARKETING AUTHORISATION HOLDER

Lundbeck Ltd

Lundbeck House

Caldecotte Lake Business Park

Caldecotte

Milton Keynes

MK7 8LF

8. MARKETING AUTHORISATION NUMBER(S)

PL 0458/0063

9. DATE OF FIRST AUTHORISATION/RENEWAL OF THE AUTHORISATION

First authorised in UK: 16 March 1990

Renewal due: 8 May 2006

10. DATE OF REVISION OF THE TEXT

18 March 2003

Clopixol Conc Injection

(Lundbeck Limited)

1. NAME OF THE MEDICINAL PRODUCT

Clopixol® Conc. Injection

2. QUALITATIVE AND QUANTITATIVE COMPOSITION

Zuclopenthixol Decanoate 50.0% w/v (equivalent to zuclopenthixol base 36.1% w/v).

3. PHARMACEUTICAL FORM

Solution for injection.

4. CLINICAL PARTICULARS

4.1 Therapeutic indications

The maintenance treatment of schizophrenia and paranoid psychoses.

4.2 Posology and method of administration

Route of administration: by deep intramuscular injection into the upper outer buttock or lateral thigh.

Note: As with all oil based injections it is important to ensure, by aspiration before injection, that inadvertent intravascular entry does not occur.

Adults: Dosage and dosage interval should be adjusted according to the patient's symptoms and response to treatment.

The usual dosage range of zuclopenthixol decanoate is 200-500 mg every one to four weeks, depending on response, but some patients may require up to 600 mg per week. In patients who have not previously received depot antipsychotics, treatment is usually started with a small dose (eg 100 mg) to assess tolerance. An interval, of at least one week should be allowed before the second injection is given at a dose consistent with the patient's condition.

Adequate control of severe psychotic symptoms may take up to 4 to 6 months at high enough dosage. Once stabilised lower maintenance doses may be considered, but must be sufficient to prevent relapse.

Injection volumes of greater than 2 ml should be distributed between two injection sites.

Elderly: In accordance with standard medical practice, initial dosage may need to be reduced to a quarter or half the normal starting dose in the frail or elderly.

Children: Not indicated for children.

4.3 Contraindications

Comatose states, including alcohol, barbiturate, or opiate intoxication.

4.4 Special warnings and special precautions for use

Caution should be exercised in patients having: liver disease; cardiac disease, or arrhythmias; severe respiratory disease; renal failure; epilepsy (and conditions predisposing to epilepsy, eg alcohol withdrawal or brain damage); Parkinson's disease; narrow angle glaucoma; prostatic hypertrophy; hypothyroidism; hyperthyroidism; myasthenia gravis; phaeochromocytoma and patients who have shown hypersensitivity to thioxanthenes or other antipsychotics.

The elderly require close supervision because they are especially prone to experience such adverse effects as sedation, hypotension, confusion and temperature changes.

Acute withdrawal symptoms, including nausea, vomiting, sweating and insomnia have been described after abrupt cessation of antipsychotic drugs. Recurrence of psychotic symptoms may also occur, and the emergence of involuntary movement disorders (such as akathisia, dystonia and dyskinesia) has been reported. Therefore, gradual withdrawal is usually advisable. The plasma concentrations of Clopixol Conc Injection 500mg/ml gradually decrease over several weeks which make gradual dosage tapering unnecessary.

When transferring patients from oral to depot antipsychotic treatment, the oral medication should not be discontinued immediately, but gradually withdrawn over a period of several days after administering the first injection.

4.5 Interaction with other medicinal products and other forms of Interaction

In common with other antipsychotics zuclopenthixol enhances the response to alcohol, the effects of barbiturates and other CNS depressants. Zuclopenthixol may potentiate the effects of general anaesthetics and anticoagulants and prolong the action of neuromuscular blocking agents.

The anticholinergic effects of atropine or other drugs with anticholinergic properties may be increased. Concomitant use of drugs such as metoclopramide, piperazine or antiparkinson drugs may increase the risk of extrapyramidal effects such as tardive dyskinesia. Combined use of antipsychotics and lithium or sibutramine has been associated with an increased risk of neurotoxicity.

Antipsychotics may enhance the cardiac depressant effects of quinidine; the absorption of corticosteroids and digoxin. The hypotensive effect of vasodilator antihypertensive agents such as hydralazine and α-blockers (e.g. doxazosin), or methyl-dopa may be enhanced. Concomitant use of zuclopenthixol and drugs known to cause QT prolongation or cardiac arrhythmias, such as tricyclic antidepressants, other antipsychotics or terfenadine should be avoided.

Antipsychotics may antagonise the effects of adrenaline and other sympathomimetic agents, and reverse the antihypertensive effects of guanethidine and similar adrenergic-blocking agents. Antipsychotics may also impair the effect of levodopa, adrenergic drugs and anticonvulsants.

The metabolism of tricyclic antidepressants may be inhibited and the control of diabetes may be impaired.

4.6 Pregnancy and lactation

As the safety of this drug during pregnancy has not been established, use during pregnancy, especially the first and last trimesters, should be avoided. Unless the expected benefit to the patient outweighs the potential risk to the foetus.

Zuclopenthixol is excreted into breast milk. If the use of Clopixol is considered essential, nursing mothers should be advised to stop breast feeding.

The newborn of mothers treated with antipsychotics in late pregnancy, or labour, may show signs of intoxication such as lethargy, tremor and hyperexcitability, and have a low apgar score.

4.7 Effects on ability to drive and use machines

Alertness may be impaired, especially at the start of treatment, or following the consumption of alcohol; patients should be warned of this risk and advised not to drive or operate machinery until their susceptibility is known. Patients should not drive if they have blurred vision.

4.8 Undesirable effects

Drowsiness and sedation may occur but are more often seen with high dosage and at the start of treatment, particularly in the elderly. Other adverse effects include blurring of vision, tachycardia and urinary incontinence and frequency. Dose-related postural hypotension may occur, particular in the elderly.

Because Clopixol may impair alertness, especially at the start of treatment or following the consumption of alcohol, patients should be warned of this risk and advised not to drive or operate machinery, until their susceptibility is known.

Extrapyramidal reactions in the form of acute dystonias (including oculogyric crisis), parkinsonian rigidity, tremor, akinesia and akathisia have been reported and may occur even at lower dosage in susceptible patients. Such effects would usually be encountered early in treatment, but delayed reactions may also occur. Antiparkinson agents should not be prescribed routinely because of the possible risk of precipitating toxic-confusional states, impairing therapeutic efficacy or causing anticholinergic side-effects. They should only be given if required and their requirement reassessed at regular intervals.

Tardive dyskinesia can occur with antipsychotic treatment. It is more common at high doses for prolonged periods and has been reported at lower dosage for short periods. The risk seems to be greater in the elderly, especially females. It has been reported that fine vermicular movements of the tongue are an early sign. It has been observed occasionally in patients receiving Clopixol. The concurrent use of anticholinergic antiparkinson drugs may exacerbate this effect. The potential irreversibility and seriousness, as well as the unpredictability of the syndrome, requires especially careful assessment of the risk versus benefit, and the lowest possible dosage and duration of treatment consistent with therapeutic efficacy. Short-lived dyskinesia may occur after abrupt withdrawal of the drug (see section 4.4).

The neuroleptic malignant syndrome has rarely been reported in patients receiving antipsychotics including zuclopenthixol. This potentially fatal syndrome is characterised by hyperthermia, a fluctuating level of consciousness, muscular rigidity and autonomic dysfunction with pallor, tachycardia, labile blood pressure, sweating and urinary incontinence. Antipsychotic therapy should be discontinued immediately and vigorous symptomatic treatment implemented.

Epileptic fits have occasionally been reported. Confusional states can occur.

The hormonal effects of antipsychotic drugs include hyperprolactinaemia, which may be associated with galactorrhoea, gynaecomastia, oligomenorrhoea or amenorrhoea. Sexual function, including erection and ejaculation may be impaired, but increased libido has also been reported.

ECG changes with prolongation of the QT interval and T-wave changes may occur with moderate to high doses; they are reversible on reducing the dose.

Zuclopenthixol may impair body temperature control, and cases of hyperthermia have occurred rarely. The possible development of hypothermia, particularly in the elderly and hypothyroid, should be borne in mind.

Blood dyscrasias have occasionally been reported. Blood counts should be carried out if a patient develops signs of persistent infection. Jaundice and other liver abnormalities have been reported rarely.

Weight gain and less commonly weight loss have been reported.

Occasionally local reactions such as erythema, swelling or tender fibrous nodules have been reported.

Oedema has occasionally been reported and has been considered to be allergic in origin. Rashes have occurred rarely. Although less likely than with phenothiazines, zuclopenthixol can rarely cause increased susceptibility to sunburn.

Zuclopenthixol, even in low doses, in susceptible (especially non-psychotic) individuals may unusually cause nausea, dizziness or headache, excitement, agitation, insomnia, or unpleasant subjective feeling of being mentally dulled or slowed down.

4.9 Overdose

Symptoms: somnolence, coma, extrapyramidal symptoms, convulsions, hypotension, shock, hyper or hypothermia. ECG changes have been reported when administered in overdose together with drugs known to affect the heart.

Treatment: treatment is symptomatic and supportive. Measures aimed at supporting the respiratory and cardiovascular systems should be instituted. Adrenaline (epinephrine) must not be used in these patients. There is no specific antidote.

5. PHARMACOLOGICAL PROPERTIES

5.1 Pharmacodynamic properties

The action of zuclopenthixol, as with other antipsychotics is mediated through dopamine receptor blockade. Zuclopenthixol has a high affinity for D_1 and D_2 receptors and activity has been demonstrated in standard animal models used to assess antipsychotic action. Serotonergic blocking properties, a high affinity for alpha-adrenoreceptors and slight antihistamine properties have been observed.

5.2 Pharmacokinetic properties

After deep intramuscular injection of Clopixol, serum levels of zuclopenthixol increase during the first week and decline slowly thereafter. A linear relationship has been observed between Clopixol dosage and serum level. Metabolism proceeds by sulphoxidation, dealkylation and glucuronic acid conjugation. Sulphoxide metabolites are mainly excreted in the urine while unchanged drug and the dealkylated form tend to be excreted in the faeces.

5.3 Preclinical safety data

Nil of relevance

6. PHARMACEUTICAL PARTICULARS

6.1 List of excipients

Thin vegetable oil.

6.2 Incompatibilities

This product may be mixed in the same syringe with other products in the Clopixol Injection range, including Clopixol Acuphase Injection (zuclopenthixol acetate 50 mg/ml).

It should not be mixed with any other injection fluids.

6.3 Shelf life

48 months.

6.4 Special precautions for storage

Store at or below 25°C. Protect from light.

6.5 Nature and contents of container

Ampoules containing 1 ml of 500 mg/ml zuclopenthixol decanoate in thin vegetable oil. Pack size: 5 ampoules per box.

6.6 Instructions for use and handling

Nil.

7. MARKETING AUTHORISATION HOLDER

Lundbeck Limited

Lundbeck House

Caldecotte Lake Business Park

Caldecotte

Milton Keynes

MK7 8LF

8. MARKETING AUTHORISATION NUMBER(S)

PL 0458/0060

9. DATE OF FIRST AUTHORISATION/RENEWAL OF THE AUTHORISATION

First Authorisation November 1988

Renewal of Authorisation May 2004

10. DATE OF REVISION OF THE TEXT

4 September 2004

® Registered trademark

Clopixol Injection

(Lundbeck Limited)

1. NAME OF THE MEDICINAL PRODUCT

Clopixol® Injection

2. QUALITATIVE AND QUANTITATIVE COMPOSITION

Zuclopenthixol Decanoate 20.0% w/v (equivalent to zuclopenthixol base 14.445% w/v).

3. PHARMACEUTICAL FORM

Solution for Injection.

4. CLINICAL PARTICULARS

4.1 Therapeutic indications

The maintenance treatment of schizophrenia and paranoid psychoses.

4.2 Posology and method of administration

Route of administration: by deep intramuscular injection into the upper outer buttock or lateral thigh.

Note: As with all oil based injections it is important to ensure, by aspiration before injection, that inadvertent intravascular entry does not occur.

Adults

Dosage and dosage interval should be adjusted according to the patients' symptoms and response to treatment.

The usual dosage range of zuclopenthixol decanoate is 200-500 mg every one to four weeks, depending on response, but some patients may require up to 600 mg per week. In patients who have not previously received depot neuroleptics, treatment is usually started with a small dose (eg 100 mg) to assess tolerance. An interval, of at least one week should be allowed before the second injection is given at a dose consistent with the patients condition.

Adequate control of severe psychotic symptoms may take up to 4 to 6 months at high enough dosage. Once stabilised lower maintenance doses may be considered, but must be sufficient to prevent relapse.

Injection volumes of greater than 2 ml should be distributed between two injection sites.

Elderly

In accordance with standard medical practice initial dosage may need to be reduced to a quarter or half the normal starting dose in the frail or elderly.

Children

Not indicated for children.

4.3 Contraindications

Comatose states including acute alcohol, barbiturate or opiate intoxication.

4.4 Special warnings and special precautions for use

Caution should be exercised in patients having: liver disease; cardiac disease, or arrhythmias; severe respiratory disease; renal failure; epilepsy (and conditions predisposing to epilepsy, eg alcohol withdrawal or brain damage); Parkinson's disease; narrow angle glaucoma; prostatic hypertrophy; hypothyroidism; hyperthyroidism; myasthenia gravis; phaeochromocytoma and patients who have shown hypersensitivity to thioxanthenes or other antipsychotics.

The elderly require close supervision because they are specially prone to experience such adverse effects as sedation, hypotension, confusion and temperature changes.

Acute withdrawal symptoms, including nausea, vomiting, sweating and insomnia have been described after abrupt cessation of antipsychotic drugs. Recurrence of psychotic symptoms may also occur, and the emergence of involuntary movement disorders (such as akathisia, dystonia and dyskinesia) has been reported. Therefore, gradual withdrawal is usually advisable. The plasma concentrations of the Clopixol Injection 200mg/ml gradually decrease over several weeks which make gradual dosage tapering unnecessary.

When transferring patients from oral to depot antipsychotic treatment, the oral medication should not be discontinued immediately, but gradually withdrawn over a period of several days after administering the first injection.

4.5 Interaction with other medicinal products and other forms of Interaction

In common with other antipsychotics, zuclopenthixol enhances the response to alcohol, the effects of barbiturates and other CNS depressants. Zuclopentixol may potentiate the effects of general anaesthetics and anticoagulants and prolong the action of neuromuscular blocking agents.

The anticholinergic effects of atropine or other drugs with anticholinergic properties may be increased. Concomitant use of drugs such as metoclopramide, piperazine or antiparkinson drugs may increase the risk of extrapyramidal effects such as tardive dyskinesia. Combined use of antipsychotics and lithium or sibutramine has been associated with an increased risk of neurotoxicity.

Antipsychotics may enhance the cardiac depressant effects of quinidine; the absorption of corticosteroids and digoxin. The hypotensive effect of vasodilator antihypertensive agents such as hydralazine and α-blockers (e.g. doxazosin), or methyl-dopa may be enhanced. Concomitant use of zuclopenthixol and drugs known to cause QT prolongation or cardiac arrhythmias, such as tricyclic antidepressants, other antipsychotics or terfenadine should be avoided.

Antipsychotics may antagonise the effects of adrenaline and other sympathomimetic agents, and reverse the antihypertensive effects of guanethidine and similar adrenergic-blocking agents. Antipsychotics may also impair the effect of levodopa, adrenergic drugs and anticonvulsants.

The metabolism of tricyclic antidepressants may be inhibited and the control of diabetes may be impaired.

4.6 Pregnancy and lactation

As the safety of this drug during pregnancy has not been established, use during pregnancy, especially the first and last trimesters, should be avoided. Unless the expected benefit to the patient outweighs the potential risk to the foetus.

Zuclopenthixol is excreted into breast milk. If the use of Clopixol is considered essential, nursing mothers should be advised to stop breast feeding.

The newborn of mothers treated with antipsychotics in late pregnancy, or labour, may show signs of intoxication such as lethargy, tremor and hyperexcitability, and have a low apgar score.

4.7 Effects on ability to drive and use machines
Alertness may be impaired, especially at the start of treatment, or following the consumption of alcohol; patients should be warned of this risk and advised not to drive or operate machinery until their susceptibility is known. Patients should not drive if they have blurred vision.

4.8 Undesirable effects
Drowsiness and sedation may occur but are more often seen with high dosage and at the start of treatment, particularly in the elderly. Other adverse effects include blurring of vision, tachycardia and urinary incontinence and frequency. Dose-related postural hypotension may occur, particular in the elderly.

Because Clopixol may impair alertness, especially at the start of treatment or following the consumption of alcohol, patients should be warned of this risk and advised not to drive or operate machinery, until their susceptibility is known.

Extrapyramidal reactions in the form of acute dystonias (including oculogyric crisis), parkinsonian rigidity, tremor, akinesia and akathisia have been reported and may occur even at lower dosage in susceptible patients. Such effects would usually be encountered early in treatment, but delayed reactions may also occur. Antiparkinson agents should not be prescribed routinely because of the possible risk of precipitating toxic-confusional states, impairing therapeutic efficacy or causing anticholinergic side-effects. They should only be given if required and their requirement reassessed at regular intervals.

Tardive dyskinesia can occur with antipsychotic treatment. It is more common at high doses for prolonged periods and has been reported at lower dosage for short periods. The risk seems to be greater in the elderly, especially females. It has been reported that fine vermicular movements of the tongue are an early sign. It has been observed occasionally in patients receiving Clopixol. The concurrent use of anticholinergic antiparkinson drugs may exacerbate this effect. The potential irreversibility and seriousness, as well as the unpredictability of the syndrome, requires especially careful assessment of the risk versus benefit, and the lowest possible dosage and duration of treatment consistent with therapeutic efficacy. Short-lived dyskinesia may occur after abrupt withdrawal of the drug (see section 4.4).

The neuroleptic malignant syndrome has rarely been reported in patients receiving antipsychotics including zuclopenthixol. This potentially fatal syndrome is characterised by hyperthermia, a fluctuating level of consciousness, muscular rigidity and autonomic dysfunction with pallor, tachycardia, labile blood pressure, sweating and urinary incontinence. Antipsychotic therapy should be discontinued immediately and vigorous symptomatic treatment implemented.

Epileptic fits have occasionally been reported. Confusional states can occur.

The hormonal effects of antipsychotic drugs include hyperprolactinaemia, which may be associated with galactorrhoea, gynaecomastia, oligomenorrhoea or amenorrhoea.

Sexual function, including erection and ejaculation may be impaired, but increased libido has also been reported.

ECG changes with prolongation of the QT interval and T-wave changes may occur with moderate to high doses; they are reversible on reducing the dose.

Zuclopenthixol may impair body temperature control, and cases of hyperthermia have occurred rarely. The possible development of hypothermia, particularly in the elderly and hypothyroid, should be borne in mind.

Blood dyscrasias have occasionally been reported. Blood counts should be carried out if a patient develops signs of persistent infection. Jaundice and other liver abnormalities have been reported rarely.

Weight gain and less commonly weight loss have been reported.

Occasionally local reactions such as erythema, swelling or tender fibrous nodules have been reported.

Oedema has occasionally been reported and has been considered to be allergic in origin. Rashes have occurred rarely. Although less likely than with phenothiazines, zuclopenthixol can rarely cause increased susceptibility to sunburn.

Zuclopenthixol, even in low doses, in susceptible (especially non-psychotic) individuals may unusually cause nausea, dizziness or headache, excitement, agitation, insomnia, or unpleasant subjective feeling of being mentally dulled or slowed down.

4.9 Overdose
Overdosage may cause somnolence, or even coma, extrapyramidal symptoms, convulsions, hypotension, shock, hyper- or hypothermia. Treatment is symptomatic and supportive, with measures aimed at supporting the respiratory and cardiovascular systems. The following specific measures may be employed if required.

- Anticholinergic antiparkinson drugs if extrapyramidal symptoms occur
- Sedation (with benzodiazepines) in the unlikely event of agitation or excitement or convulsions
- Noradrenaline in saline intravenous drip if the patient is in shock. Adrenaline must not be given.

5. PHARMACOLOGICAL PROPERTIES

5.1 Pharmacodynamic properties
The action of zuclopenthixol, as with other antipsychotics is mediated through dopamine receptor blockade. Zuclopenthixol has a high affinity for D_1 and D_2 receptors and activity has been demonstrated in standard animal models used to assess antipsychotic action. Serotonergic blocking properties, a high affinity for alpha-adrenoreceptors and slight antihistamine properties have been observed.

5.2 Pharmacokinetic properties
After deep intramuscular injection of Clopixol, serum levels of zuclopenthixol increase during the first week and decline slowly thereafter. A linear relationship has been observed between Clopixol dosage and serum level. Metabolism proceeds by sulphoxidation, dealkylation and glucuronic acid conjugation. Sulphoxide metabolites are mainly excreted in the urine while unchanged drug and the dealkylated form tend to be excreted in the faeces.

5.3 Preclinical safety data
Nil of relevance.

6. PHARMACEUTICAL PARTICULARS

6.1 List of excipients
Thin vegetable oil

6.2 Incompatibilities
This product may be mixed in the same syringe with other products in the Clopixol Injection range, including Clopixol Acuphase Injection (zuclopenthixol acetate 50 mg/ml).

It should not be mixed with any other injection fluids.

6.3 Shelf life
1 ml ampoules: 36 months.

10 ml vials: 36 months (unopened), shelf life after opening vials: 1 day

6.4 Special precautions for storage
Store at or below 25°C. Protect from light.

6.5 Nature and contents of container
Ampoules containing 1 ml of 200 mg/ml zuclopenthixol decanoate in thin vegetable oil. Pack size: 10 ampoules per box.

10 ml clear glass vials with a rubber stopper secured with an aluminium collar having a flip-top cap. Pack size: 1 vial per box.

6.6 Instructions for use and handling
Nil.

7. MARKETING AUTHORISATION HOLDER
Lundbeck Limited

Lundbeck House

Caldecotte Lake Business Park

Caldecotte

Milton Keynes

MK7 8LF

8. MARKETING AUTHORISATION NUMBER(S)
PL 0458/0017

9. DATE OF FIRST AUTHORISATION/RENEWAL OF THE AUTHORISATION
Date of First Authorisation May 1978

Renewal of Authorisation January 2002

10. DATE OF REVISION OF THE TEXT
September 2002

® Trademark Clopixol is made by H Lundbeck A/S, Denmark

Clopixol Tablets

(Lundbeck Limited)

1. NAME OF THE MEDICINAL PRODUCT
Clopixol® Tablets 2 mg, 10 mg and 25 mg

2. QUALITATIVE AND QUANTITATIVE COMPOSITION
2, 10 or 25 mg tablets (containing 2.36, 11.9 or 29.7 mg zuclopenthixol dihydrochloride equivalent to 2, 10 or 25 mg zuclopenthixol base respectively).

3. PHARMACEUTICAL FORM
Round, biconvex, pale red, film-coated tablets.

4. CLINICAL PARTICULARS

4.1 Therapeutic indications
The treatment of psychoses, especially schizophrenia.

4.2 Posology and method of administration
Route of administration: Oral.

Adults: The dosage range is 4-150 mg/day in divided doses. The usual initial dose is 20-30 mg/day (sometimes with higher dosage requirements in acute cases), increasing as necessary. The usual maintenance dose is 20-50 mg/day.

When transferring patients from oral to depot antipsychotic treatment, the oral medication should not be discontinued immediately, but gradually withdrawn over a period of several days after administering the first injection.

Elderly: In accordance with standard medical practice, initial dosage may need to be reduced to a quarter or half the normal starting dose in the frail or elderly.

Children: Not indicated for children.

4.3 Contraindications
Comatose states, including acute alcohol, barbiturate, or opiate intoxication.

4.4 Special warnings and special precautions for use
Caution should be exercised in patients having: liver disease; cardiac disease or arrhythmias; severe respiratory disease; renal failure; epilepsy (and conditions predisposing to epilepsy e.g. alcohol withdrawal or brain damage); Parkinson's disease; narrow angle glaucoma; prostatic hypertrophy; hypothyroidism; hyperthyroidism; myasthenia gravis; phaeochromocytoma and patients who have shown hypersensitivity to thioxanthenes or other antipsychotics.

The elderly require close supervision because they are specially prone to experience such adverse effects as sedation, hypotension, confusion and temperature changes.

Acute withdrawal symptoms, including nausea, vomiting, sweating and insomnia have been described after abrupt cessation of antipsychotic drugs. Recurrence of psychotic symptoms may also occur, and the emergence of involuntary movement disorders (such as akathisia, dystonia and dyskinesia) has been reported. Therefore, gradual withdrawal is advisable.

4.5 Interaction with other medicinal products and other forms of Interaction
In common with other antipsychotics, zuclopenthixol enhances the response to alcohol, the effects of barbiturates and other CNS depressants. Zuclopentixol may potentiate the effects of general anaesthetics and anticoagulants and prolong the action of neuromuscular blocking agents.

The anticholinergic effects of atropine or other drugs with anticholinergic properties may be increased. Concomitant use of drugs such as metoclopramide, piperazine or antiparkinson drugs may increase the risk of extrapyramidal effects such as tardive dyskinesia. Combined use of antipsychotics and lithium or sibutramine has been associated with an increased risk of neurotoxicity.

Antipsychotics may enhance the cardiac depressant effects of quinidine; the absorption of corticosteroids and digoxin. The hypotensive effect of vasodilator antihypertensive agents such as hydralazine and α-blockers (e.g. doxazosin), or methyl-dopa may be enhanced. Concomitant use of zuclopenthixol and drugs known to cause QT prolongation or cardiac arrhythmias, such as tricyclic antidepressants, other antipsychotics or terfenadine should be avoided.

Antipsychotics may antagonise the effects of adrenaline and other sympathomimetic agents, and reverse the antihypertensive effects of guanethidine and similar adrenergic-blocking agents. Antipsychotics may also impair the effect of levodopa, adrenergic drugs and anticonvulsants.

The metabolism of tricyclic antidepressants may be inhibited and the control of diabetes may be impaired.

4.6 Pregnancy and lactation
As the safety of this drug during pregnancy has not been established, use during pregnancy, especially the first and last trimesters, should be avoided, unless the expected benefit to the patient outweighs the potential risk to the foetus.

Zuclopenthixol is excreted into the breast milk. If the use of Clopixol is considered essential, nursing mothers should be advised to stop breast feeding.

The newborn of mothers treated with antipsychotics in late pregnancy, or labour, may show signs of intoxication such as lethargy, tremor and hyperexcitability, and have a low apgar score.

4.7 Effects on ability to drive and use machines
Alertness may be impaired, especially at the start of treatment, or following the consumption of alcohol; patients should be warned of this risk and advised not to drive or operate machinery until their susceptibility is known. Patients should not drive if they have blurred vision.

4.8 Undesirable effects
Drowsiness and sedation may occur but are more often seen with high dosage and at the start of treatment, particularly in the elderly. Other adverse effects include blurring of vision, tachycardia and urinary incontinence and frequency. Dose-related postural hypotension may occur, particularly in the elderly.

Because Clopixol may impair alertness, especially at the start of treatment or following the consumption of alcohol, patients should be warned of the risk and advised not to drive or operate machinery, until their susceptibility is known.

Extrapyramidal reactions in the form of acute dystonias (including oculogyric crisis), parkinsonian rigidity, tremor, akinesia and akathisia have been reported and may occur even at lower dosage in susceptible patients. Such effects would usually be encountered early in treatment, but delayed reactions may also occur. Antiparkinson agents should not be prescribed routinely because of the possible risk of precipitating toxic-confusional states, impairing therapeutic efficacy or causing anticholinergic side-effects. They should only be given if required and their requirement reassessed at regular intervals.

Tardive dyskinesia can occur with antipsychotic treatment. It is more common at high doses for prolonged periods but has been reported at lower dosage for short periods. The risk seems to be greater in the elderly, especially females. It has been reported that fine vermicular movements of the tongue are an early sign. It has been observed occasionally in patients receiving Clopixol. The concurrent use of anticholinergic antiparkinson drugs may exacerbate this effect. The potential irreversibility and seriousness, as well as the unpredictability of the syndrome, requires especially careful assessment of the risk versus benefit, and the lowest possible dosage and duration of treatment consistent with therapeutic efficacy. Short-lived dyskinesia may occur after abrupt withdrawal of the drug (see section 4.4).

The neuroleptic malignant syndrome has rarely been reported in patients receiving antipsychotics, including zuclopenthixol. This potentially fatal syndrome is characterised by hyperthermia, a fluctuating level of consciousness, muscular rigidity and autonomic dysfunction with pallor, tachycardia, labile blood pressure, sweating and urinary incontinence. Antipsychotic therapy should be discontinued immediately and vigorous symptomatic treatment implemented.

Epileptic fits have occasionally been reported. Confusional states can occur.

The hormonal effects of antipsychotic drugs include hyperprolactinaemia, which may be associated with galactorrhoea, gynaecomastia, oligomenorrhoea or amenorrhoea. Sexual function, including erection and ejaculation may be impaired; but increased libido has also been reported.

ECG changes with prolongation of the QT interval and T-wave changes may occur with moderate to high doses; they are reversible on reducing the dose.

Zuclopenthixol may impair body temperature control, and cases of hyperthermia have occurred rarely. The possible development of hypothermia, particularly in the elderly and hypothyroid, should be borne in mind.

Blood dyscrasias have occasionally been reported. Blood counts should be carried out if a patient develops signs of persistent infection. Jaundice and other liver abnormalities have been reported rarely.

Weight gain and less commonly weight loss have been reported; oedema has occasionally been reported and has been considered to be allergic in origin. Rashes have occurred rarely. Although less likely than with phenothiazines, zuclopenthixol can rarely cause increased susceptibility to sunburn.

Zuclopenthixol, even in low doses, in susceptible (especially non-psychotic) individuals may unusually cause nausea, dizziness or headache, excitement, agitation, insomnia, or unpleasant subjective feelings of being mentally dulled or slowed down.

4.9 Overdose

Overdosage may cause somnolence, or even coma, extrapyramidal symptoms, convulsions, hypotension, shock, hyper-or hypothermia. Treatment is symptomatic and supportive, with measures aimed at supporting the respiratory and cardiovascular systems. The following specific measures may be employed if required.

- anticholinergic antiparkinson drugs if extrapyramidal symptoms occur.
- sedation (with benzodiazepines) in the unlikely event of agitation or excitement or convulsions.
- noradrenaline in saline intravenous drip if the patient is in shock. Adrenaline must not be given
- Gastric lavage should be considered.

5. PHARMACOLOGICAL PROPERTIES

5.1 Pharmacodynamic properties

The action of zuclopenthixol as with other antipsychotics is mediated through dopamine receptor blockage. Zuclopenthixol has a high affinity for D_1 and D_2 receptors and activity has been demonstrated in standard animal models used to assess antipsychotic action. Serotonergic blocking properties, a high affinity for alpha-adrenoreceptors and slight antihistaminergic properties have been observed.

5.2 Pharmacokinetic properties

Zuclopenthixol given orally in man is relatively quickly absorbed and maximum serum concentrations are reached in 3-6 hours. There is good correlation between the dose of zuclopenthixol and the concentrations achieved in serum. The biological half-life in man is about one day. Zuclopenthixol is distributed in the liver, lungs, intestines and kidney, with somewhat lower concentration in the brain. Small amounts of drug or metabolites cross the placenta and are excreted in milk.

Zuclopenthixol is metabolised by sulphoxidation, N-Dealkylation and glucuronic acid conjugation.

The faecal route of excretion predominates and mostly unchanged zuclopenthixol and N-dealkylated metabolite are excreted in this way.

5.3 Preclinical safety data

Nil of relevance

6. PHARMACEUTICAL PARTICULARS

6.1 List of excipients

Potato starch, Lactose, Microcrystalline cellulose, Copolyvidone, Glycerol, Talc, Caster oil, hydrogenated, Magnesium Stearate, Methylhydroxypropyl Cellulose, Macrogol, Titanium Dioxide (E171) and Red Iron Oxide (E172).

6.2 Incompatibilities

None known.

6.3 Shelf life

Clopixol Tablets 2 mg are stable for 2 years. Clopixol Tablets 10 mg and 25 mg are stable for 5 years. Each container has an expiry date.

6.4 Special precautions for storage

Store in original container, protected from light and moisture, below 25°C.

6.5 Nature and contents of container

Grey polypropylene container with desiccant capsule or glass bottle.

Contents: 100 tablets.

6.6 Instructions for use and handling

Nil.

7. MARKETING AUTHORISATION HOLDER

Lundbeck Ltd

Lundbeck House

Caldecotte Lake Business Park

Caldecotte

Milton Keynes

MK7 8LF

8. MARKETING AUTHORISATION NUMBER(S)

2 mg tablets	PL 0458/0027
10 mg tablets	PL 0458/0028
25 mg tablets	PL 0458/0029

9. DATE OF FIRST AUTHORISATION/RENEWAL OF THE AUTHORISATION

First Authorisation: March 1982

Renewal of Authorisation: January 2002

10. DATE OF REVISION OF THE TEXT

September 2002

®Trademark Clopixol is made by H Lundbeck A/S, Denmark

Clotam Rapid

(Provalis Healthcare)

1. NAME OF THE MEDICINAL PRODUCT

Clotam® Rapid.

2. QUALITATIVE AND QUANTITATIVE COMPOSITION

Tolfenamic acid 200mg.

3. PHARMACEUTICAL FORM

Tablets.

4. CLINICAL PARTICULARS

4.1 Therapeutic indications

Acute migraine.

4.2 Posology and method of administration

Method of Administration:

Adults: Migraine – acute attacks: 200mg when the first symptoms of migraine appear. The treatment can be repeated once after 1-2 hours if a satisfactory response is not obtained.

Children: A paediatric dosage regimen has not yet been established.

Elderly: Normal adult dose.

4.3 Contraindications

Active peptic ulceration. Significantly impaired kidney or liver function.

Tolfenamic acid is contraindicated in patients in whom attacks of asthma, urticaria or acute rhinitis are precipitated by aspirin or other non-steroidal anti-inflammatory agents.

4.4 Special warnings and special precautions for use

As is the case with other NSAIDs, tolfenamic acid should be used with caution in patients with a history of gastrointestinal ulceration, or impaired liver or kidney function.

4.5 Interaction with other medicinal products and other forms of Interaction

Anticoagulants: In patients treated with anticoagulants, close monitoring of blood coagulation is recommended. *Diuretics:* The effect of loop diuretics may be reduced. *Lithium*: The effect of lithium may be increased.

4.6 Pregnancy and lactation

Pregnancy: Reproduction studies in animals have not shown any signs of foetal damage. Controlled studies in pregnant women are not available. As is the case with the use of other NSAIDs, tolfenamic acid should not be given in the last trimester, due to risks of premature closure of the ductus arteriosus and prolonged parturition.

Lactation: Tolfenamic acid is excreted to such a very small extent in mothers' milk that it should be without risk to the breast-fed baby.

4.7 Effects on ability to drive and use machines

None.

4.8 Undesirable effects

Tolfenamic acid is well tolerated at the recommended dosage. The following side effects have been observed:

Gastrointestinal tract: Diarrhoea, nausea, epigastric pain, vomiting, dyspepsia, isolated reports of gastric ulceration.

Allergic skin reactions: Drug exanthema, erythema, pruritus, urticaria.

Urinary tract: Harmless dysuria in the form of smarting during urina-tion may occur occasionally, most commonly in males. The occurrence is correlated with the concentration of a metabolite and is most probably due to local irritation of the urethra. Increased consumption of liquid or reduction of the dose diminishes the risk of smarting. The urine may, due to coloured metabolites, become a little more lemon-coloured.

As is the case with the use of other NSAIDs, the side effects listed below have occasionally been observed: *Central nervous system*: Headache, vertigo, tremor, euphoria, fatigue. *Respiratory tract:* Isolated cases of dyspnoea, pulmonary infiltration, bronchospasm and asthma attack. *Haematolgoy:* Isolated cases of thrombocytopenia, anaemia and leu-copenia. *Liver:* Isolated cases of reversible liver function disturbances and toxic hepatitis.

4.9 Overdose

No symptoms of overdosage are known in man. In cases where treatment is required, this should be symptomatic. There is no specific antidote to tolfenamic acid.

5. PHARMACOLOGICAL PROPERTIES

5.1 Pharmacodynamic properties

NSAID with anti-inflammatory, analgesic and antipyretic effects. Tolfenamic acid is a prostaglandin synthesis inhibitor and a leukotriene synthesis inhibitor.

5.2 Pharmacokinetic properties

Tolfenamic acid is absorbed quickly and almost completely after oral administration. Hepatic first pass metabolism is a low as 15% (bio-availability 85%). Maximum plasma concentrations are reached after about 1-1½ hours. The half-life in plasma is about two hours. Tolfenamic acid is extensively bound to plasma proteins (99%). It is metabolised in the liver and tolfenamic acid, as well as the metabolites are conjugated with glucuronic acid. About 90% of a given dose of tolfenamic acid is excreted in the urine as glucuronic acid conjugates, and about 10% is excreted in the faeces. Enterohepatic circulation exists.

5.3 Preclinical safety data

The therapeutic index for tolfenamic acid is high, and gastrointestinal ulceration and kidney changes have only been seen with oral doses approximately 6-10 times the maximum therapeutic dose recommended for tolfenamic acid. In human volunteers, tolfenamic acid did not affect renal function.

6. PHARMACEUTICAL PARTICULARS

6.1 List of excipients

Maize starch; Sodium starch glycollate (Type A); Macrogol 6000; Alginic acid; Cellulose, microcrystalline; Croscarmellose sodium; Silica, colloidal anhydrous; Sodium stearyl fumarate.

6.2 Incompatibilities

None known.

6.3 Shelf life

Five years

6.4 Special precautions for storage

Store below 25°C.

6.5 Nature and contents of container

Al/PVC foil blister, HDPE tablet container with LDPE closure. Pack sizes:

3, 10 and 30 capsules.

6.6 Instructions for use and handling

None.

7. MARKETING AUTHORISATION HOLDER

A/S GEA Farmaceutisk Fabrik,

Holger Danskes Vej 89,

DK-2000 Frederiksberg,

Denmark.

8. MARKETING AUTHORISATION NUMBER(S)

PL 4012/0043.

9. DATE OF FIRST AUTHORISATION/RENEWAL OF THE AUTHORISATION

25th April 1997

10. DATE OF REVISION OF THE TEXT

22nd June 1999

Clozaril

(Novartis Pharmaceuticals UK Ltd)

1. NAME OF THE MEDICINAL PRODUCT

CLOZARIL ® 25 mg Tablets

CLOZARIL ® 100 mg Tablets

UK Clozaril Official Recommendations

The UK Clozaril Patient Monitoring Service (CPMS) was developed in order to manage the risk of agranulocytosis associated with clozapine. It is available 24 hours a day. When a monitoring service is not used, evidence suggests a mortality rate from agranulocytosis of 0.3%[1]. This is compared to a mortality rate when Clozaril is used in conjunction with the Clozaril Patient Monitoring Service, of 0.01%[2].

The Clozaril Patient Monitoring Service provides for the centralised monitoring of leucocyte and neutrophil counts which is a mandatory requirement for all patients in the UK who are treated with Clozaril. The use of Clozaril is restricted to patients who are registered with the Clozaril Patient Monitoring Service. In addition to registering their patients, prescribing physicians must register themselves and a nominated pharmacist with the Clozaril Patient Monitoring Service. All Clozaril-treated patients must be under the supervision of an appropriate specialist and supply of Clozaril is restricted to hospital and retail pharmacies registered with the Clozaril Patient Monitoring Service. Clozaril is not sold to, or distributed through wholesalers.

In the UK, a white cell count with a differential count must be monitored:

- At least weekly for the first 18 weeks of treatment
- At least at 2 week intervals between weeks 18 and 52
- After 1 year of treatment with stable neutrophil counts, patients may be monitored at least at 4 week intervals
- Monitoring must continue throughout treatment and for at least 4 weeks after discontinuation

The Clozaril Patient Monitoring Service maintains a database which includes all patients who have developed abnormal leucocyte or neutrophil findings and who should not be re-exposed to Clozaril.

Prescribers and pharmacists should adhere to brand prescribing and dispensing of clozapine in order to prevent the disruption to effective monitoring that may be caused if patients switch brands. Furthermore, in order to protect patient safety, at any one time patients should only be prescribed one brand of clozapine and only registered with the monitoring service connected to that brand.

For further information regarding Clozaril and the Clozaril Patient Monitoring Service please call 08457 698269.

[1] De la Chapelle A, et al. *Clozapine-induced agranulocytosis: a genetic and epidemiologic study.* Hum Genet, 1977. 37: p. 183-194.

[2] Clozaril Patient Monitoring Service, data on file

Clozaril can cause agranulocytosis. Its use should be limited to patients:

- **with schizophrenia who are non-responsive to or intolerant of antipsychotic drug treatment, or with psychosis in Parkinson's disease when other treatment strategies have failed (see point 4.1)**
- **who have initially normal leukocyte findings (white blood cell count ⩾ 3500/mm³ (3.5x10⁹/L), and ANC ⩾ 2000/mm³ (2.0x10⁹/L)), and**
- **in whom regular white blood cell (WBC) counts and absolute neutrophil counts (ANC) can be performed as follows: weekly during the first 18 weeks of therapy, and at least every 4 weeks thereafter throughout treatment. Monitoring must continue throughout treatment and for 4 weeks after complete discontinuation of Clozaril.**

Prescribing physicians should comply fully with the required safety measures. At each consultation, a patient receiving Clozaril should be reminded to contact the treating physician immediately if any kind of infection begins to develop. Particular attention should be paid to flu-like complaints such as fever or sore throat and to other evidence of infection, which may be indicative of neutropenia.

Clozaril must be dispensed under strict medical supervision in accordance with official recommendations.

Myocarditis

Clozapine is associated with an increased risk of myocarditis which has, in rare cases, been fatal. The increased risk of myocarditis is greatest in the first 2 months of treatment. Fatal cases of cardiomyopathy have also been reported rarely.

Myocarditis or cardiomyopathy should be suspected in patients who experience persistent tachycardia at rest, especially in the first 2 months of treatment, and/or palpitations, arrhythmias, chest pain and other signs and symptoms of heart failure (e.g. unexplained fatigue, dyspnoea, tachypnoea) or symptoms that mimic myocardial infarction.

If myocarditis or cardiomyopathy are suspected, Clozaril treatment should be promptly stopped and the patient immediately referred to a cardiologist.

Patients who develop clozapine-induced myocarditis or cardiomyopathy should not be re-exposed to clozapine.

2. QUALITATIVE AND QUANTITATIVE COMPOSITION

Each tablet contains 25 mg or 100 mg clozapine.

For excipients, see section 6.1 List of excipients

3. PHARMACEUTICAL FORM

Tablet.

25 mg tablet:

Yellow, circular, flat, bevelled edged tablet. Coded "CLOZ 25" in circular on one side with a break score on the reverse.

100 mg tablet:

Yellow, circular, flat, bevelled edged tablet. Coded "CLOZARIL 100" in circular on one side.

4. CLINICAL PARTICULARS

4.1 Therapeutic indications

Clozaril is indicated in treatment-resistant schizophrenic patients and in schizophrenia patients who have severe, untreatable neurological adverse reactions to other antipsychotic agents, including atypical antipsychotics.

Treatment resistance is defined as a lack of satisfactory clinical improvement despite the use of adequate doses of at least two different antipsychotic agents, including an atypical antipsychotic agent, prescribed for adequate duration.

Clozaril is also indicated in psychotic disorders occurring during the course of Parkinson's disease, in cases where standard treatment has failed.

4.2 Posology and method of administration

The dosage must be adjusted individually. For each patient the lowest effective dose should be used.

Initiation of Clozaril treatment must be restricted to those patients with a WBC count ⩾ 3500/mm³ (3.5x10⁹/L) and an ANC ⩾ 2000/mm³ (2.0x10⁹/L) within standardised normal limits.

Dose adjustment is indicated in patients who are also receiving medicinal products that have pharmacodynamic and pharmacokinetic interactions with Clozaril, such as benzodiazepines or selective serotonin re-uptake inhibitors (see section 4.5 Interaction with other medicinal products and other forms of interaction).

The following dosages are recommended:

Treatment-resistant schizophrenic patients

Starting therapy

12.5 mg (half a 25 mg tablet) once or twice on the first day, followed by one or two 25 mg tablets on the second day. If well tolerated, the daily dose may then be increased slowly in increments of 25 to 50 mg in order to achieve a dose level of up to 300 mg/day within 2 to 3 weeks. Thereafter, if required, the daily dose may be further increased in increments of 50 to 100 mg at half-weekly or, preferably, weekly intervals.

Use in the elderly

Initiation of treatment is recommended at a particularly low dose (12.5 mg given once on the first day), with subsequent dose increments restricted to 25 mg/day.

Use in children

Safety and efficacy of Clozaril in children under the age of 16 have not been established. It should not be used in this group until further data become available.

Therapeutic dose range

In most patients, antipsychotic efficacy can be expected with 200 to 450 mg/day given in divided doses. The total daily dose may be divided unevenly, with the larger portion at bedtime. For maintenance dose, see below.

Maximum dose

To obtain full therapeutic benefit, a few patients may require larger doses, in which case judicious increments (i.e. not exceeding 100 mg) are permissible up to 900 mg/day. The possibility of increased adverse reactions (in particular seizures) occurring at doses over 450 mg/day must be borne in mind.

Maintenance dose

After achieving maximum therapeutic benefit, many patients can be maintained effectively on lower doses. Careful downward titration is therefore recommended. Treatment should be maintained for at least 6 months. If the daily dose does not exceed 200 mg, once daily administration in the evening may be appropriate.

Ending therapy

In the event of planned termination of Clozaril therapy, a gradual reduction in dose over a 1- to 2-week period is recommended. If abrupt discontinuation is necessary, the patient should be carefully observed for the occurrence of withdrawal reactions (see section 4.4 Special warnings and special precautions for use)

Restarting therapy

In patients in whom the interval since the last dose of Clozaril exceeds 2 days, treatment should be re-initiated with 12.5 mg (half a 25 mg tablet) given once or twice on the first day. If this dose is well tolerated, it may be feasible to titrate the dose to the therapeutic level more quickly than is recommended for initial treatment. However, in any patient who has previously experienced respiratory or cardiac arrest with initial dosing (see section 4.4 Special warnings and special precautions for use), but was then able to be successfully titrated to a therapeutic dose, re-titration should be carried out with extreme caution.

Switching from a previous antipsychotic therapy to Clozaril

It is generally recommended that Clozaril should not be used in combination with other antipsychotics. When Clozaril therapy is to be initiated in a patient undergoing oral antipsychotic therapy, it is recommended that the other antipsychotic should first be discontinued by tapering the dosage downwards.

Psychotic disorders occurring during the course of Parkinson's disease, in cases where standard treatment has failed

The starting dose must not exceed 12.5 mg/day (half a 25 mg tablet), taken in the evening. Subsequent dose increases must be by 12.5 mg increments, with a maximum of two increments a week up to a maximum of 50 mg, a dose that cannot be reached until the end of the second week. The total daily amount should preferably be given as a single dose in the evening.

The mean effective dose is usually between 25 and 37.5 mg/day. In the event that treatment for at least one week with a dose of 50 mg fails to provide a satisfactory therapeutic response, dosage may be cautiously increased by increments of 12.5 mg/week.

The dose of 50 mg/day should only be exceeded in exceptional cases, and the maximum dose of 100 mg/day must never be exceeded.

Dose increases should be limited or deferred if orthostatic hypotension, excessive sedation or confusion occurs. Blood pressure should be monitored during the first weeks of treatment.

When there has been complete remission of psychotic symptoms for at least 2 weeks, an increase in anti-parkinsonian medication is possible if indicated on the basis of motor status. If this approach results in the recurrence of psychotic symptoms, Clozaril dosage may be increased by increments of 12.5 mg/week up to a maximum of 100 mg/day, taken in one or two divided doses (see above).

Ending therapy: A gradual reduction in dose by steps of 12.5 mg over a period of at least one week (preferably two) is recommended.

Treatment must be discontinued immediately in the event of neutropenia or agranulocytosis as indicated in section 4.4 (Special warnings and precautions for use). In this situation, careful psychiatric monitoring of the patient is essential since symptoms may recur quickly.

4.3 Contraindications

- Hypersensitivity to the active substance or to any of the excipients.
- Patients unable to undergo regular blood tests.
- History of toxic or idiosyncratic granulocytopenia/agranulocytosis (with the exception of granulocytopenia/agranulocytosis from previous chemotherapy).
- History of Clozaril -induced agranulocytosis.
- Impaired bone marrow function.
- Uncontrolled epilepsy.
- Alcoholic and other toxic psychoses, drug intoxication, comatose conditions.
- Circulatory collapse and/or CNS depression of any cause.
- Severe renal or cardiac disorders (e.g. myocarditis).
- Active liver disease associated with nausea, anorexia or jaundice; progressive liver disease, hepatic failure.
- Paralytic ileus.
- Clozaril treatment must not be started concurrently with drugs known to have a substantial potential for causing agranulocytosis; concomitant use of depot antipsychotics is to be discouraged.

4.4 Special warnings and special precautions for use

Clozaril can cause agranulocytosis. The incidence of agranulocytosis and the fatality rate in those developing agranulocytosis have decreased markedly since the institution of WBC counts and ANC monitoring. The following precautionary measures are therefore mandatory and should be carried out in accordance with official recommendations.

Because of the risks associated with Clozaril, its use is limited to patients in whom therapy is indicated as set out in section 4.1 (Therapeutic indications) and:

- who have initially normal leukocyte findings (WBC count ⩾ 3500/mm³ (3.5x10⁹/L) and ANC ⩾ 2000/mm³ (2.0x10⁹/L), and
- in whom regular WBC counts and ANC can be performed weekly for the first 18 weeks and at least 4-week intervals thereafter. Monitoring must continue throughout treatment and for 4 weeks after complete discontinuation of Clozaril.

Before initiating clozapine therapy patients should have a blood test (see "agranulocytosis") and a history and physical examination. Patients with history of cardiac illness or abnormal cardiac findings on physical examination should be referred to a specialist for other examinations that might include an ECG, and the patient treated only if the expected benefits clearly outweigh the risks (see Section 4.3). The treating physician should consider performing a pre-treatment ECG.

Prescribing physicians should comply fully with the required safety measures.

Prior to treatment initiation, physicians must ensure, to the best of their knowledge, that the patient has not previously experienced an adverse haematological reaction to clozapine that necessitated its discontinuation. Prescriptions should not be issued for periods longer than the interval between two blood counts.

Immediate discontinuation of Clozaril is mandatory if either the WBC count is less than 3000/mm^3 (3.0x10^9/L) or the ANC is less than 1500/mm^3 (1.5x10^9/L) at any time during Clozaril treatment. Patients in whom Clozaril has been discontinued as a result of either WBC or ANC deficiencies must not be re-exposed to Clozaril.

At each consultation, a patient receiving Clozaril should be reminded to contact the treating physician immediately if any kind of infection begins to develop. Particular attention should be paid to flu-like complaints such as fever or sore throat and to other evidence of infection, which may be indicative of neutropenia. Patients and their caregivers must be informed that, in the event of any of these symptoms, they must have a blood cell count performed immediately. Prescribers are encouraged to keep a record of all patients' blood results and to take any steps necessary to prevent these patients from accidentally being rechallenged in the future.

Patients with a history of primary bone marrow disorders may be treated only if the benefit outweighs the risk. They should be carefully reviewed by a haematologist prior to starting Clozaril.

Patients who have low WBC counts because of benign ethnic neutropenia should be given special consideration and may be started on Clozaril with the agreement of a haematologist.

WBC counts and ANC monitoring

WBC and differential blood counts must be performed within 10 days prior to initiating Clozaril treatment to ensure that only patients with normal WBC counts and ANC (WBC count ⩾ 3500/mm^3 (3.5x10^9/L) and ANC ⩾ 2000/mm^3 (2.0x10^9/L)) will receive the drug. After the start of Clozaril treatment the WBC count and ANC must be monitored weekly for the first 18 weeks, and at least at four-week intervals thereafter.

Monitoring must continue throughout treatment and for 4 weeks after complete discontinuation of Clozaril or until haematological recovery has occurred (see below Low WBC count/ANC). At each consultation, the patient should be reminded to contact the treating physician immediately if any kind of infection, fever, sore throat or other flu-like symptoms develop. WBC and differential blood counts must be performed immediately if any symptoms or signs of an infection occur.

Low WBC count/ANC

If, during Clozaril therapy, either the WBC count falls to between 3500/mm^3 (3.5x10^9/L) and 3000/mm^3 (3.0x10^9/L) or the ANC falls to between 2000/mm^3 (2.0x10^9/L) and 1500/mm^3 (1.5x10^9/L), haematological evaluations must be performed at least twice weekly until the patient's WBC count and ANC stabilise within the range 3000-3500/mm^3 (3.0-3.5x10^9/L) and 1500-2000/mm^3 (1.5-2.0x10^9/L), respectively, or higher.

Immediate discontinuation of Clozaril treatment is mandatory if either the WBC count is less than 3000/mm^3 (3.0x10^9/L) or the ANC is less than 1500/mm^3 (1.5x10^9/L) during Clozaril treatment. WBC counts and differential blood counts should then be performed daily and patients should be carefully monitored for flu-like symptoms or other symptoms suggestive of infection. Confirmation of the haematological values is recommended by performing two blood counts on two consecutive days; however, Clozaril should be discontinued after the first blood count.

Following discontinuation of Clozaril, haematological evaluation is required until haematological recovery has occurred.

Blood cell count		Action required
WBC/mm^3 (/L)	ANC/mm^3 (/L)	
⩾ 3500 (⩾ 3.5x10^9)	⩾ 2000 (⩾ 2.0x10^9)	Continue Clozaril treatment
3000-3500 (3.0x10^9 -3.5x10^9)	1500-2000 (1.5x10^9 -2.0x10^9)	Continue Clozaril treatment, sample blood twice weekly until counts stabilise or increase
< 3000 (<3.0x10^9)	< 1500 (< 1.5x10^9)	Immediately stop Clozaril treatment, sample blood daily until haematological abnormality is resolved, monitor for infection. Do not re-expose the patient.

If Clozaril has been withdrawn and either a further drop in the WBC count below 2000/mm^3 (2.0x10^9/L) occurs or the ANC falls below 1000/mm^3 (1.0x10^9/L), the management of this condition must be guided by an experienced haematologist.

Discontinuation of therapy for haematological reasons

Patients in whom Clozaril has been discontinued as a result of either WBC or ANC deficiencies (see above) must not be re-exposed to Clozaril.

Prescribers are encouraged to keep a record of all patients' blood results and to take any steps necessary to prevent the patient being accidentally rechallenged in the future.

Discontinuation of therapy for other reasons

Patients who have been on Clozaril for more than 18 weeks and have had their treatment interrupted for more than 3 days but less than 4 weeks should have their WBC count and ANC monitored weekly for an additional 6 weeks. If no haematological abnormality occurs, monitoring at intervals not exceeding 4 weeks may be resumed. If Clozaril treatment has been interrupted for 4 weeks or longer, weekly monitoring is required for the next 18 weeks of treatment and the dose should be re-titrated (see section 4.2 Posology and method of administration).

Other precautions

Patients with rare hereditary problems of galactose intolerance, the Lapp lactase deficiency or glucose-galactose malabsorption should not take this medicine

In the event of **eosinophilia**, discontinuation of Clozaril is recommended if the eosinophil count rises above 3000/mm^3 (3.0x10^9/L); therapy should be restarted only after the eosinophil count has fallen below 1000/mm^3 (1.0x10^9/L).

In the event of **thrombocytopenia**, discontinuation of Clozaril therapy is recommended if the platelet count falls below 50 000/mm^3 (50x10^9/L).

Orthostatic hypotension, with or without syncope, can occur during Clozaril treatment. Rarely, collapse can be profound and may be accompanied by cardiac and/or respiratory arrest. Such events are more likely to occur with concurrent use of benzodiazepine or any other psychotropic agent (see section 4.5 Interaction with other medicinal products and other forms of interaction) and during initial titration in association with rapid dose escalation; on very rare occasions they may occur even after the first dose. Therefore, patients commencing Clozaril treatment require close medical supervision. Monitoring of standing and supine blood pressure is necessary during the first weeks of treatment in patients with Parkinson's disease.

Analysis of safety databases suggests that the use of Clozaril is associated with an increased risk of **myocarditis** especially during, but not limited to, the first two months of treatment. Some cases of myocarditis have been fatal. **Pericarditis/pericardial effusion** and **cardiomyopathy** have also been reported in association with Clozaril use; these reports also include fatalities. Myocarditis or cardiomyopathy should be suspected in patients who experience persistent tachycardia at rest, especially in the first two months of treatment, and/or palpitations, arrhythmias, chest pain and other signs and symptoms of heart failure (e.g. unexplained fatigue, dyspnoea, tachypnoea), or symptoms that mimic myocardial infarction. Other symptoms which may be present in addition to the above include flu-like symptoms. If myocarditis or cardiomyopathy are suspected, Clozaril treatment should be promptly stopped and the patient immediately referred to a cardiologist.

Patients with clozapine-induced myocarditis or cardiomyopathy should not be re-exposed to Clozaril.

Patients with a history of epilepsy should be closely observed during Clozaril therapy since dose-related convulsions have been reported. In such cases, the dose should be reduced (see section 4.2 Posology and method of administration) and, if necessary, an anti-convulsant treatment should be initiated.

Patients with stable pre-existing liver disorders may receive Clozaril, but need regular liver function tests. Liver function tests should be performed in patients in whom symptoms of possible **liver dysfunction**, such as nausea, vomiting and/or anorexia, develop during Clozaril therapy. If the elevation of the values is clinically relevant (more than 3 times the UNL) or if symptoms of jaundice occur, treatment with Clozaril must be discontinued. It may be resumed (see "Re-starting therapy" under section 4.2) only when the results of liver function tests are normal. In such cases, liver function should be closely monitored after re-introduction of the drug.

Clozaril exerts anticholinergic activity, which may produce undesirable effects throughout the body. Careful supervision is indicated in the presence of **prostatic enlargement** and **narrow-angle glaucoma**. Probably on account of its anticholinergic properties, Clozaril has been associated with varying degrees of **impairment of intestinal peristalsis**, ranging from **constipation** to **intestinal obstruction**, **faecal impaction** and **paralytic ileus** (see section 4.8 Undesirable effects). On rare occasions these cases have been fatal. Particular care is necessary in patients who are receiving concomitant medications known to cause constipation (especially those with anticholinergic properties such as some antipsychotics, antidepressants and antiparkinsonian treatments), have a history of colonic disease or a history of lower abdominal surgery as these may exacerbate the situation. It is vital that constipation is recognised and actively treated.

During Clozaril therapy, patients may experience transient **temperature elevations** above 38°C, with the peak incidence within the first 3 weeks of treatment. This fever is generally benign. Occasionally, it may be associated with an increase or decrease in the WBC count. Patients with fever should be carefully evaluated to rule out the possibility of an underlying infection or the development of agranulocytosis. In the presence of high fever, the possibility of **neuroleptic malignant syndrome** (NMS) must be considered.

Impaired glucose tolerance and/or development or exacerbation of diabetes mellitus has been reported rarely during treatment with clozapine. A mechanism for this possible association has not yet been determined. Cases of severe hyperglycaemia with ketoacidosis or hyperosmolar coma have been reported very rarely in patients with no prior history of hyperglycaemia, some of which have been fatal. When follow-up data were available, discontinuation of clozapine resulted mostly in resolution of the impaired glucose tolerance, and reinstitution of clozapine resulted in its reoccurrence. The discontinuation of clozapine should be considered in patients where active medical management of their hyperglycaemia has failed.

Since Clozaril may be associated with **thromboembolism**, immobilisation of patients should be avoided.

Acute withdrawal reactions have been reported following abrupt cessation of clozapine therefore gradual withdrawal is recommended. If abrupt discontinuation is necessary (e.g. because of leucopenia), the patient should be carefully observed for the recurrence of psychotic symptoms and symptoms related to cholinergic rebound such as profuse sweating, headache, nausea, vomiting and diarrhoea

Use in the elderly

Initiation of treatment in the elderly is recommended at a lower dose (see section 4.2 Posology and method of administration).

Orthostatic hypotension can occur with Clozaril treatment and there have been reports of tachycardia, which may be sustained. Elderly patients, particularly those with compromised cardiovascular function, may be more susceptible to these effects.

Elderly patients may also be particularly susceptible to the anticholinergic effects of Clozaril, such as urinary retention and constipation.

4.5 Interaction with other medicinal products and other forms of Interaction

Contraindication of concomitant use

Drugs known to have a substantial potential to depress bone marrow function should not be used concurrently with Clozaril (see section 4.3. Contraindications).

Long-acting depot antipsychotics (which have myelosuppressive potential) should not be used concurrently with Clozaril because these cannot be rapidly removed from the body in situations where this may be required, e.g. neutropenia (see section 4.3 Contraindications).

Alcohol should not be used concomitantly with Clozaril due to possible potentiation of sedation.

Precautions including dose adjustment

Clozaril may enhance the central effects of CNS depressants such as narcotics, antihistamines, and benzodiazepines. Particular caution is advised when Clozaril therapy is initiated in patients who are receiving a benzodiazepine or any other psychotropic drug. These patients may have an increased risk of circulatory collapse, which, on rare occasions, can be profound and may lead to cardiac and/or respiratory arrest. It is not clear whether cardiac or respiratory collapse can be prevented by dose adjustment.

Because of the possibility of additive effects, caution is essential in the concomitant administration of drugs possessing anticholinergic, hypotensive, or respiratory depressant effects.

Owing to its anti-α-adrenergic properties, Clozaril may reduce the blood-pressure-increasing effect of norepinephrine or other predominantly α-adrenergic agents and reverse the pressor effect of epinephrine.

Concomitant administration of drugs known to inhibit the activity of some cytochrome P450 isozymes may increase the levels of clozapine, and the dose of clozapine may need to be reduced to prevent undesirable effects. This is more important for CYP 1A2 inhibitors such as caffeine (see below) and the selective serotonin reuptake inhibitors fluvoxamine and (more controversial) paroxetine. Some of the other serotonin reuptake inhibitors such as fluoxetine and sertraline are CYP 2D6 inhibitors and, as a consequence, major pharmacokinetic interactions with clozapine are less likely. Similarly, pharmacokinetic interactions with CYP 3A4 inhibitors such as azole antimycotics, cimetidine, erythromycin, and protease inhibitors are unlikely, although some have been reported. Because the plasma concentration of clozapine is increased by caffeine intake and decreased by nearly 50% following a 5-day caffeine-free period, dosage changes of clozapine may be necessary when there is a change in caffeine-drinking habit. In cases of sudden cessation of smoking, the plasma clozapine concentration may be increased, thus leading to an increase in adverse effects.

Concomitant administration of drugs known to induce cytochrome P450 enzymes may decrease the plasma

Table 1 Reference to the most common drug interactions with Clozaril

Drug	Interactions	Comments
Bone marrow suppressants (e.g. carbamazepine, chloramphenicol, sulphonamides (e.g. co-trimoxazole), pyrazolone analgesics (e.g. phenylbutazone), penicillamine, cytotoxic agents and long-acting depot injections of antipsychotics	Interact to increase the risk and/or severity of bone marrow suppression	Clozaril **should not be used** concomitantly with other agents having a well known potential to suppress bone marrow function (see Section 4.3 Contraindications)
Benzodiazepines	Concomitant use may increase risk of circulatory collapse, which may lead to cardiac and/or respiratory arrest	Whilst the occurrence is rare, caution is advised when using these drugs together. Reports suggest that respiratory depression and collapse are more likely to occur at the start of this combination or when Clozaril is added to an established benzodiazepine regimen.
Anticholinergics	Clozaril potentiates the action of these drugs through additive anticholinergic activity	Observe patients for anticholinergic side –effects, e.g. constipation, especially when using to help control hypersalivation
Antihypertensives	Clozaril can potentiate the hypotensive effects of these drugs due to its sympathomimetic antagonistic effects	Caution is advised if Clozaril is used concomitantly with antihypertensive agents. Patients should be advised of the risk of hypotension, especially during the period of initial dose titration
Alcohol, MAOIs, CNS depressants, including narcotics and benzodiazepines	Enhanced central effects. Additive CNS depression and cognitive and motor performance interference when used in combination with these drugs	Caution is advised if Clozaril is used concomitantly with other CNS active agents. Advise patients of the possible additive sedative effects and caution them not to drive or operate machinery
Highly protein bound drugs (e.g. warfarin and digoxin)	Clozaril may cause an increase in plasma concentration of these drugs due to displacement from plasma proteins	Patients should be monitored for the occurrence of side effects associated with these drugs, and doses of the protein bound drug adjusted, if necessary
Phenytoin	Addition of phenytoin to Clozaril drug regimen may cause a decrease in the clozapine plasma concentrations	If phenytoin must be used, the patient should be monitored closely for a worsening or recurrence of psychotic symptoms
Lithium	Concomitant use can increase the risk of development of neuroleptic malignant syndrome (NMS)	Observe for signs and symptoms of NMS

levels of clozapine, leading to reduced efficacy. Drugs known to induce the activity of cytochrome P450 enzymes and with reported interactions with clozapine include, for instance, carbamazepine (not to be used concomitantly with clozapine, due to its myelosuppresive potential), phenytoin and rifampicin. Known inducers of CYP1A2 such as omeprazole, may lead to decreased clozapine levels. The potential for reduced efficacy of clozapine should be considered when it is used in combination with these drugs

Others

Concomitant use of lithium or other CNS-active agents may increase the risk of development of neuroleptic malignant syndrome (NMS).

Rare but serious reports of seizures, including onset of seizures in non-epileptic patients, and isolated cases of delirium where Clozaril was co-administered with valproic acid have been reported. These effects are possibly due to a pharmacodynamic interaction, the mechanism of which has not been determined.

Caution is called for in patients receiving concomitant treatment with other drugs which are either inhibitors or inducers of the cytochrome P450 isozymes. With tricyclic antidepressants, phenothiazines and type 1_C anti-arrhythmics, which are known to bind to cytochrome P450 2D6, no clinically relevant interactions have been observed thus far.

An outline of drug interactions believed to be most important with Clozaril is given in Table 1 below (this is not an exhaustive list).

(see Table 1 above)

4.6 Pregnancy and lactation

Pregnancy

For Clozaril, there are only limited clinical data on exposed pregnancies. Animal studies do not indicate direct or indirect harmful effects with respect to pregnancy, embryonal/foetal development, parturition or postnatal development (see 5.3). Caution should be exercised when prescribing to pregnant women.

Lactation

Animal studies suggest that clozapine is excreted in breast milk and has an effect in the nursing infant; therefore, mothers receiving Clozaril should not breast-feed.

Women of child-bearing potential

A return to normal menstruation may occur as a result of switching from other antipsychotics to Clozaril. Adequate contraceptive measures must therefore be ensured in women of childbearing potential.

4.7 Effects on ability to drive and use machines

Owing to the ability of Clozaril to cause sedation and lower the seizure threshold, activities such as driving or operating machinery should be avoided, especially during the initial weeks of treatment.

4.8 Undesirable effects

For the most part, the adverse event profile of clozapine is predictable from its pharmacological properties. An important exception is its propensity to cause agranulocytosis (see section 4.4 Special warnings and special precautions for use). Because of this risk, its use is restricted to treatment-resistant schizophrenia and psychosis occurring during the course of Parkinson's disease in cases where standard treatment has failed. While blood monitoring is an essential part of the care of patients receiving clozapine, the physician should be aware of other rare but serious adverse events, which may be diagnosed in the early stages only by careful observation and questioning of the patient in order to prevent morbidity and mortality.

Blood and lymphatic system

Development of granulocytopenia and agranulocytosis is a risk inherent to Clozaril treatment. Although generally reversible on withdrawal of treatment, agranulocytosis may result in sepsis and can prove fatal. Because immediate withdrawal of the drug is required to prevent the development of life-threatening agranulocytosis, monitoring of the WBC count is mandatory (see section 4.4 Special warnings and special precautions for use). Table 2 below summarises the estimated incidence of agranulocytosis for each Clozaril treatment period.

Table 2: Estimated incidence of agranulocytosis[1]

Treatment period	Incidence of agranulocytosis per 100,000 person-weeks[2] of observation
Weeks 0-18	32.0
Weeks 19-52	2.3
Weeks 53 and higher	1.8

[1] From the UK Clozaril Patient Monitoring Service lifetime registry experience between 1989 and 2001.

[2] Person-time is the sum of individual units of time that the patients in the registry have been exposed to Clozaril before experiencing agranulocytosis. For example, 100,000 person-weeks could be observed in 1,000 patients who were in the registry for 100 weeks (100*1000=100,000), or in 200 patients who were in the registry for 500 weeks (200*500=100,000) before experiencing agranulocytosis.

The cumulative incidence of agranulocytosis in the UK Clozaril Patient Monitoring Service lifetime registry experience (0 - 11.6 years between 1989 and 2001) is 0.78%. The majority of cases (approximately 70%) occur within the first 18 weeks of treatment.

Metabolic and Nutritional Disorders

Impaired glucose tolerance and/or development or exacerbation of diabetes mellitus has been reported rarely during treatment with clozapine. On very rare occasions, severe hyperglycaemia, sometimes leading to ketoacidosis/hyperosmolar coma, has been reported in patients on Clozaril treatment with no prior history of hyperglycaemia. Glucose levels normalised in most patients after discontinuation of Clozaril and in a few cases hyperglycaemia recurred when treatment was reinitiated. Although most patients had risk factors for non-insulin-dependent diabetes mellitus, hyperglycaemia has also been documented in patients with no known risk factors(see section 4.4. Special warnings and special precautions for use).

Nervous System Disorders

The very common adverse events observed include drowsiness/sedation, and dizziness.

Clozaril can cause EEG changes, including the occurrence of spike and wave complexes. It lowers the seizure threshold in a dose-dependent manner and may induce myoclonic jerks or generalised seizures. These symptoms are more likely to occur with rapid dose increases and in patients with pre-existing epilepsy. In such cases the dose should be reduced and, if necessary, anticonvulsant treatment initiated. Carbamazepine should be avoided because of its potential to depress bone marrow function, and with other anticonvulsant drugs the possibility of a pharmacokinetic interaction should be considered. In rare cases, patients treated with Clozaril may experience delirium.

Very rarely, tardive dyskinesia has been reported in patients on Clozaril who had been treated with other antipsychotic agents. Patients in whom tardive dyskinesia developed with other antipsychotics have improved on Clozaril.

Cardiac Disorders

Tachycardia and postural hypotension with or without syncope may occur, especially in the initial weeks of treatment. The prevalence and severity of hypotension is influenced by the rate and magnitude of dose titration. Circulatory collapse as a result of profound hypotension, in particular related to aggressive titration of the drug, with the possible serious consequences of cardiac or pulmonary arrest, has been reported with Clozaril.

A minority of Clozaril -treated patients experience ECG changes similar to those seen with other antipsychotic drugs, including S-T segment depression and flattening or inversion of T waves, which normalise after discontinuation of Clozaril. The clinical significance of these changes is unclear. However, such abnormalities have been observed in patients with myocarditis, which should therefore be considered.

Isolated cases of cardiac arrhythmias, pericarditis/pericardial effusion and myocarditis have been reported, some of which have been fatal. The majority of the cases of myocarditis occurred within the first 2 months of initiation of therapy with Clozaril. Cardiomyopathy generally occurred later in the treatment.

Eosinophilia has been co-reported with some cases of myocarditis (approximately 14%) and pericarditis/pericardial effusion; it is not known, however, whether eosinophilia is a reliable predictor of carditis.

Signs and symptoms of myocarditis or cardiomyopathy include persistent tachycardia at rest, palpitations, arrhythmias, chest pain and other signs and symptoms of heart failure (e.g. unexplained fatigue, dyspnoea, tachypnoea), or symptoms that mimic myocardial infarction. Other symptoms which may be present in addition to the above include flu-like symptoms.

Sudden, unexplained deaths are known to occur among psychiatric patients who receive conventional antipsychotic medication but also among untreated psychiatric patients. Such deaths have been reported very rarely in patients receiving Clozaril.

Vascular Disorders

Rare cases of thromboembolism have been reported.

Respiratory System

Respiratory depression or arrest has occurred very rarely, with or without circulatory collapse (see sections 4.4 Special warnings and special precautions for use and 4.5 Interaction with other medicinal products and other forms of interaction).

Gastrointestinal System

Constipation and hypersalivation have been observed very frequently, and nausea and vomiting frequently. Very rarely ileus may occur (see section 4.4 Special warnings and special precautions for use). Rarely Clozaril treatment may be associated with dysphagia. Aspiration of ingested food may occur in patients presenting with dysphagia or as a consequence of acute overdosage.

Hepatobiliary Disorders

Transient, asymptomatic elevations of liver enzymes and rarely, hepatitis and cholestatic jaundice may occur. Very rarely, fulminant hepatic necrosis has been reported. If jaundice develops, Clozaril should be discontinued (see section 4.4. Special warnings and special precautions for use). In rare cases, acute pancreatitis has been reported.

Renal Disorders

Isolated cases of acute interstitial nephritis have been reported in association with Clozaril therapy.

Reproductive and Breast Disorders

Very rare reports of priapism have been received.

General Disorders

Cases of neuroleptic malignant syndrome (NMS) have been reported in patients receiving Clozaril either alone or in combination with lithium or other CNS-active agents.

Acute withdrawal reactions have been reported (see section 4.4 Special warnings and special precautions for use)

The table below (Table 3) summarises the adverse reactions accumulated from reports made spontaneously and during clinical studies.

Table 3: Treatment-Emergent Adverse Experience Frequency Estimate from Spontaneous and Clinical Trial Reports

Adverse reactions are ranked under headings of frequency, using the following convention: Very common ($\geq$ 1/10), common ($\geq$ 1/100, < 1/10), uncommon ($\geq$ 1/1,000, < 1/100), rare ($\geq$ 1/10,000, < 1/1,000), very rare (< 1/10,000), including isolated reports.

Blood and lymphatic system disorders	
Common	Leukopenia/decreased WBC/neutropenia, eosinophilia, leukocytosis
Uncommon	Agranulocytosis
Very rare	Thrombocytopenia, thrombocythaemia
Metabolism and nutrition disorders	
Common	Weight gain
Rare	Impaired glucose tolerance, diabetes mellitus
Very rare	Ketoacidosis, hyperosmolar coma, severe hyperglycaemia, hypertriglyceridaemia, hypercholesterolaemia
Psychiatric disorders	
Rare	Restlessness, agitation
Nervous system disorders	
Very common	Drowsiness/sedation, dizziness
Common	Blurred vision, headache, tremor, rigidity, akathisia, extrapyramidal symptoms, seizures/convulsions/myoclonic jerks
Rare	Confusion, delirium
Very rare	Tardive dyskinesia
Cardiac disorders	
Very common	Tachycardia
Common	ECG changes
Rare	Circulatory collapse, arrhythmias, myocarditis, pericarditis/pericardial effusion
Very rare	Cardiomyopathy, cardiac arrest
Vascular disorders	
Common	Hypertension, postural hypotension, syncope
Rare	Thromboembolism
Respiratory disorders	
Rare	Aspiration of ingested food
Very rare	Respiratory depression/arrest
Gastrointestinal disorders	
Very common	Constipation, hypersalivation
Common	Nausea, vomiting, anorexia, dry mouth
Rare	Dysphagia
Very rare	Parotid gland enlargement, intestinal obstruction/paralytic ileus/faecal impaction
Hepatobiliary disorders	
Common	Elevated liver enzymes
Rare	Hepatitis, cholestatic jaundice, pancreatitis
Very rare	Fulminant hepatic necrosis
Skin and subcutaneous tissue disorders	
Very rare	Skin reactions
Renal and urinary disorders	
Common	Urinary incontinence, urinary retention
Very rare	Interstitial nephritis
Reproductive system disorders	
Very rare	Priapism
General disorders	
Common	Fatigue, fever, benign hyperthermia, disturbances in sweating/temperature regulation
Uncommon	Neuroleptic malignant syndrome
Very rare	Sudden unexplained death
Investigations	
Rare	Increased CPK

4.9 Overdose

In cases of acute intentional or accidental Clozaril overdosage for which information on the outcome is available, mortality to date is about 12%. Most of the fatalities were associated with cardiac failure or pneumonia caused by aspiration and occurred at doses above 2000 mg. There have been reports of patients recovering from an overdose in excess of 10 000 mg. However, in a few adult individuals, primarily those not previously exposed to Clozaril, the ingestion of doses as low as 400 mg led to life-threatening comatose conditions and, in one case, to death. In young children, the intake of 50 to 200 mg resulted in strong sedation or coma without being lethal.

Signs and symptoms

Drowsiness, lethargy, areflexia, coma, confusion, hallucinations, agitation, delirium, extrapyramidal symptoms, hyperreflexia, convulsions; hypersalivation, mydriasis, blurred vision, thermolability; hypotension, collapse, tachycardia, cardiac arrhythmias; aspiration pneumonia, dyspnoea, respiratory depression or failure.

Treatment

Gastric lavage and/or administration of activated charcoal within the first 6 hours after the ingestion of the drug. Peritoneal dialysis and haemodialysis are unlikely to be effective. Symptomatic treatment under continuous cardiac monitoring, surveillance of respiration, monitoring of electrolytes and acid-base balance. The use of epinephrine should be avoided in the treatment of hypotension because of the possibility of a 'reverse epinephrine' effect.

Close medical supervision is necessary for at least 5 days because of the possibility of delayed reactions.

5. PHARMACOLOGICAL PROPERTIES

5.1 Pharmacodynamic properties

Pharmacotherapeutic group: Antipsychotic agent (ATC code NO5A H02)

Clozaril has been shown to be an antipsychotic agent that is different from classic antipsychotics.

In pharmacological experiments, the compound does not induce catalepsy or inhibit apomorphine- or amphetamine-induced stereotyped behaviour. It has only weak dopamine-receptor-blocking activity at D_1, D_2, D_3 and D_5 receptors, but shows high potency for the D_4 receptor, in addition to potent anti-alpha-adrenergic, anticholinergic, antihistaminic, and arousal-reaction-inhibiting effects. It has also been shown to possess antiserotoninergic properties.

Clinically Clozaril produces rapid and marked sedation and exerts antipsychotic effects in schizophrenic patients resistant to other drug treatment. In such cases, Clozaril has proven effective in relieving both positive and negative schizophrenic symptoms mainly in short-term trials. In an open clinical trial performed in 319 treatment resistant patients treated for 12 months, a clinically relevant improvement was observed in 37% of patients within the first week of treatment and in an additional 44% by the end of 12 months. The improvement was defined as about 20% reduction from baseline in Brief Psychiatric Rating Scale Score. In addition, improvement in some aspects of cognitive dysfunction has been described.

Compared to classic antipsychotics, Clozaril produces fewer major extrapyramidal reactions such as acute dystonia, parkinsonian-like side effects and akathisia. In contrast to classic antipsychotics, Clozaril produces little or no prolactin elevation, thus avoiding adverse effects such as gynaecomastia, amenorrhoea, galactorrhoea, and impotence.

A potentially serious adverse reaction caused by Clozaril therapy is granulocytopenia and agranulocytosis occurring at an estimated incidence of 3% and 0.7%, respectively. In view of this risk, the use of Clozaril should be limited to patients who are treatment-resistant or patients with psychosis in Parkinson's disease when other treatment strategies have failed (see section 4.1 Therapeutic indications) and in whom regular haematological examinations can be performed (see sections 4.4 Special warnings and special precautions for use and 4.8 Undesirable effects).

5.2 Pharmacokinetic properties

The absorption of orally administered Clozaril is 90 to 95%; neither the rate nor the extent of absorption is influenced by food.

Clozaril is subject to moderate first-pass metabolism, resulting in an absolute bioavailability of 50 to 60%. In steady-state conditions, when given twice daily, peak blood levels occur on an average at 2.1 hours (range: 0.4 to 4.2 hours), and the volume of distribution is 1.6 l/kg. Clozaril is approximately 95% bound to plasma proteins. Its elimination is biphasic, with a mean terminal half-life of 12 hours (range: 6 to 26 hours). After single doses of 75 mg the mean terminal half-life was 7.9 hours; it increased to 14.2 hours when steady-state conditions were reached by administering daily doses of 75 mg for at least 7 days. Dosage increases from 37.5 mg to 75 mg and 150 mg given twice daily were found to result during steady state in linearly dose-proportional increases in the area under the plasma concentration/time curve (AUC), and in the peak and minimum plasma concentrations.

Clozaril is almost completely metabolised before excretion. Of the main metabolites only the demethyl metabolite was found to be active. Its pharmacological actions resemble those of clozapine, but are considerably weaker and of short duration. Only trace amounts of unchanged drug are detected in the urine and faeces, approximately 50% of the administered dose being excreted as metabolites in the urine and 30% in the faeces.

5.3 Preclinical safety data

Preclinical data reveal no special hazard for humans based on conventional studies of safety pharmacology, repeated dose toxicity, genotoxicity and carcinogenic potential (for reproductive toxicity, see section 4.6).

6. PHARMACEUTICAL PARTICULARS

6.1 List of excipients

Magnesium stearate

Silica, colloidal anhydrous

Povidone

Talc

Maize starch

Lactose monohydrate

6.2 Incompatibilities

Not applicable

6.3 Shelf life

5 years

6.4 Special precautions for storage

No special precautions for storage.

6.5 Nature and contents of container

25 mg and 100 mg tablets:

PVC/PVDC/Aluminium blister packs containing 7, 14, 20, 28, 30, 40, 50, 60, 84, 98, 100, 500 or 5000 tablets.

Amber glass bottles (class III) containing 100 tablets

Not all pack sizes may be marketed.

6.6 Instructions for use and handling

No special requirements

7. MARKETING AUTHORISATION HOLDER

Novartis Pharmaceuticals UK Limited

Trading as Sandoz Pharmaceuticals

Frimley Business Park

Frimley

Camberley

Surrey

GU16 7SR

8. MARKETING AUTHORISATION NUMBER(S)

CLOZARIL 25 mg Tablets: PL 00101/0228

CLOZARIL 100 mg Tablets: PL 00101/0229

9. DATE OF FIRST AUTHORISATION/RENEWAL OF THE AUTHORISATION

Date of Licence Granted: 22/12/89

Date of Last Renewal: 09/07/2003

10. DATE OF REVISION OF THE TEXT

10th September 2004

Legal category

POM

Co-amoxiclav for Injection 1000/200mg

(Wockhardt UK Ltd)

1. NAME OF THE MEDICINAL PRODUCT

Co-amoxiclav for Injection 1000/200mg.

2. QUALITATIVE AND QUANTITATIVE COMPOSITION

Each vial contains 1000mg amoxicillin (as sodium salt) and 200mg clavulanic acid (as potassium salt).

Each 1.2g vial of co-amoxiclav contains 1.0mmol of potassium and 3.1 mmol of sodium (approx).

3. PHARMACEUTICAL FORM

Powder for solution for injection or infusion.

4. CLINICAL PARTICULARS

4.1 Therapeutic indications

Treatment of the following bacterial infections when caused by amoxicillin-resistant but amoxicillin-clavulanate susceptible organisms (see section 5.1):

Upper and Lower Respiratory Tract Infections, including:

- otitis media
- acute sinusitis
- acute exacerbations of chronic bronchitis
- community-acquired pneumonia

Upper and Lower Urinary Tract Infections

Skin and Soft Tissue Infections

Genito-Urinary Tract Infections including septic abortion, pelvic or puerperal sepsis, intra-abdominal sepsis

Consideration should be given to the official guidance on the appropriate use of antibacterial agents.

4.2 Posology and method of administration

Dosages for the treatment of infection

Adults and children over 12 years

Usually 1.2g eight hourly. In more serious infections, increase frequency to six-hourly intervals.

Children 3 months – 12 years

Usually 30mg/kg* co-amoxiclav eight hourly. In more serious infections, increase frequency to six-hourly intervals.

Children 0-3 months

30mg/kg* co-amoxiclav every 12 hours in premature infants and in full-term infants during the perinatal period, increasing to eight hours thereafter.

*Each 30mg co-amoxiclav provides 25mg of amoxicillin and 5mg of clavulanic acid.

Each 1.2g vial of co-amoxiclav contains 1.0mmol of potassium and 3.1 mmol of sodium (approx).

Adult dosage for surgical prophylaxis

The usual dose is 1.2g co-amoxiclav injection given at the induction of anaesthesia. Operations where there is a high risk of infection, e.g. colorectal surgery, may require three, and up to four doses of 1.2g of co-amoxiclav injection in a 24 hour period. These doses are usually given at 0, 8, 16 (and 24) hours. This regimen can be continued for several days if the procedure has a significantly increased risk of infection.

Clear clinical signs of infection at operation will require a normal course of intravenous or oral co-amoxiclav therapy post-operatively.

Dosage in renal impairment

Adults

Mild impairment (creatinine clearance >30 ml/min): No change in dosage.

Moderate impairment (creatinine clearance 10-30 ml/min): 1.2g IV stat., followed by 600mg IV 12 hourly.

Severe impairment (creatinine clearance <10 ml/min): 1.2g IV stat., followed by 600mg IV 24 hourly. Dialysis decreases serum concentrations of co-amoxiclav and an additional 600mg IV dose may need to be given during dialysis and at the end of dialysis.

Children

Similar reductions in dosage should be made for children.

Dosage in hepatic impairment

Dose with caution. Monitor hepatic function at regular intervals. There are, as yet, insufficient data on which to base a dosage recommendation.

Each 1.2g vial of co-amoxiclav contains 1.0mmol of potassium and 3.1 mmol of sodium (approx).

Co-amoxiclav may not be used in patients with severe hepatic impairment and in patients in whom hepatic functional impairment has occurred on previous therapy with co-amoxiclav (see section 4.3 and 4.4). Liver function parameters should be checked at regular intervals in patients with signs of hepatic lesions and a change of therapy should be given considerations if these parameters exacerbate on treatment.

Administration

Co-amoxiclav injection may be administered either by intravenous injection or by intermittent infusion. Therapy can be started parenterally and continued with an oral preparation.

Co-amoxiclav Injection should be given by slow intravenous injection over a period of three to four minutes and used within 20 minutes of reconstitution. It may be injected directly into a vein or via a drip tube.

Alternatively, co-amoxiclav intravenous may be infused in Water for Injections Ph Eur or Sodium Chloride Intravenous Injection BP (0.9% w/v). Add, without delay, 600 mg reconstituted solution to 50 ml infusion fluid or 1.2 g reconstituted solution to 100 ml infusion fluid (e.g. using a minibag or in-line burette). Infuse over 30-40 minutes and complete within four hours of reconstitution.

Any residual antibiotic solutions should be discarded.

Co-amoxiclav Injection is less stable in infusions containing glucose, dextran or bicarbonate. Reconstituted solution should, therefore, not be added to such infusions but may be injected into the drip tubing over a period of three to four minutes.

It is not suitable for intramuscular administration. Duration of therapy should be appropriate to the indication and should not exceed 14 days without review.

4.3 Contraindications

Hypersensitivity to the constituents, amoxicillin and clavulanic acid. Penicillin hypersensitivity. Attention should be paid to possible cross-sensitivity with other β-lactam antibiotics, e.g. penicillins, cephalosporins, carbapenems, monobactams due to the danger of anaphylactic shock. Consequently a careful history should be taken in regard to allergic reaction before commencing treatment. Co-amoxiclav should not be given to patients with a verified hypersensitivity to any beta-lactam drug.

A previous history of co-amoxiclav or penicillin-associated jaundice/hepatic dysfunction.

Co-amoxiclav may not be used in patients with severe hepatic impairment and in patients in whom hepatic functional impairment has occurred on previous therapy with co-amoxiclav, for example cholestatic jaundice induced by co-amoxiclav or penicillin.

Patients with infectious mononucleosis (glandular fever) and patients with lymphatic leukaemia have a higher risk of exanthema and consequently co-amoxiclav injection should not be administered during these diseases to treat concomitant bacterial infections.

4.4 Special warnings and special precautions for use

Although severe allergic reactions are more likely in patients who have experienced beta-lactam hypersensitivity, these may occur in the absence of any such history. In such cases treatment should be discontinued immediately and appropriate management instituted.

Co-amoxiclav should be used with caution in patients with allergic diathesis, including asthma, since such patients may have a higher risk of allergic reactions to co-amoxiclav.

Patients with evidence of hepatic dysfunction should be treated with caution. Liver function parameters should be monitored in patients with signs or symptoms of hepatic impairment. Discontinuation of therapy should be considered in case of deterioration of liver function parameters during treatment.

In long term use (more than 10-14 days), regular monitoring of renal and hepatic function is recommended.

Prolonged use of co-amoxiclav, or other broadspectrum antibiotics, may lead to superinfections due to an overgrowth of non-susceptible organisms and yeasts.

In case of severe and persistent diarrhoea, the possibility of pseudomembraneous colitis must be considered, in which case therapy should be discontinued.

In patients with renal impairment, excretion of co-amoxiclav will be delayed and depending on the degree of the impairment, it may be necessary to reduce the total daily dosage (see section 4.2).

The presence of high urinary concentrations of amoxicillin can cause precipitation of the product in urinary catheters. Therefore, catheters should be visually inspected at intervals.

At high doses, adequate fluid intake and urinary output must be maintained to minimise the possibility of amoxicillin crystalluria.

4.5 Interaction with other medicinal products and other forms of Interaction

Other bacterial agents: There is a possibility that the antibacterial action of amoxicillin could be antagonised on co-administration with macrolides, tetracyclines, sulphonamides or chloramphenicol.

Probenecid: By inhibiting the renal elimination of amoxicillin (but not clavulanic acid) the concomitant administration of probenecid leads to an increase in the concentrations of amoxicillin in serum and bile.

Allopurinol: Concomitant administration of allopurinol may promote the occurrence of allergic cutaneous reactions.

Digoxin: An increase in the absorption of digoxin is possible on concurrent administration with amoxicillin.

Co-amoxiclav / disulfiram: Co-amoxiclav should not be used concurrently with disulfiram.

Methotrexate: Concomitant administration with methotrexate may lead to an increase in toxicity of methotrexate.

Anticoagulants: Concomitant administration of amoxicillin and coumarin anticoagulants, such as warfarin, may increase the incidence of bleeding.

Oral hormonal contraceptives: Administration of amoxicillin can transiently decrease the plasma level of oestrogens and progesterone and may reduce the efficacy of oral contraceptives. Patients should be advised to use supplemental non-hormonal contraceptive measures.

Other forms of interaction: Amoxicillin may produce false positive results in glucose determination tests and tests for urobilinogen performed with nonenzymatic methods. Likewise the urobilinogen test can be affected.

Amoxicillin may decrease the amount of urinary estriol in pregnant women. Diarrhoea may decrease the absorption of other drugs and consequently have a negative influence on their effectivity.

Forced diuresis will lead to an increased elimination of amoxicillin resulting in decreased serum concentrations.

4.6 Pregnancy and lactation

Reproduction studies in animals (mice and rats) with orally and parenterally administered co-amoxiclav have shown no teratogenic effects. There is limited experience of the use of co-amoxiclav in human pregnancy. As with all medicines, use should be avoided in pregnancy, especially during the first trimester, unless considered essential by the physician.

Co-amoxiclav may be administered during the period of lactation. With the exception of the risk of sensitisation, associated with the excretion of trace quantities in breast milk, there are no known detrimental effects for the breast-fed infant.

4.7 Effects on ability to drive and use machines

Co-amoxiclav may sometimes be associated with side effects (such as rarely dizziness and even less often convulsions) that may impair the ability to drive a vehicle, to operate machinery and/or work safely (see section 4.8).

4.8 Undesirable effects

The most commonly reported adverse drug reactions are hypersensitivity reactions:

Common (⩾ 1% but < 10%)

- Cutaneous reactions such as exanthema, pruritus, urticaria; the typical morbilliform exanthema occurs 5-11 days after start of therapy. Immediate appearance of urticaria indicates an allergic reaction to amoxicillin and therapy should therefore be discontinued.

Rare (⩾ 0.01% but < 0.1%): (see also section 4.4)

- Angioneurotic oedema (Quincke's oedema)
- Erythema multiforme syndrome
- Stevens-Johnson syndrome
- Eosinophilia
- Drug fever
- Laryngeal oedema
- Serum sickness
- Haemolytic anaemia
- Allergic vasculitis
- Interstitial nephritis
- Anaphylactic shock

Other possible side effects

Blood disorders:

There have been isolated reports of leucopenia, granulocytopenia, thrombocytopenia, pancytopenia, anaemia, myelosuppression, agranulocytosis, prolongation of bleeding time and prolongation of prothrombin time. However, these changes were reversible on discontinuation of therapy.

Gastrointestinal disorders:

Common (≥ 1% but < 10%):

Gastric complaints, nausea, loss of appetite, vomiting, flatulence, soft stools, diarrhoea, enanthemas (particularly in the region of the mouth), dry mouth, taste disturbances. These effects on the gastrointestinal system are mostly mild and frequently disappear either during the treatment or very soon after completion of therapy. The occurrence of these side-effects can generally be reduced by taking amoxicillin during meals or with some food. If severe and persistent diarrhoea occurs, the rare possibility of pseudomembraneouscolitisshould be considered. The administration of anti-peristaltic drug is contraindicated.

Very rare (< 0.01%)

Development of a black tongue.

Liver disorders:

Uncommon (≥ 0.1% but < 1%):

Moderate and transient increase of liver enzymes. Rare reports of hepatitis and cholestatic jaundice.

Renal disorders:

Uncommon (≥ 0.01% but < 0.1%):

Acute interstitial nephritis may occur in rare cases.

CNS disorders:

CNS effects have been seen rarely. They include hyperkinesia, dizziness and convulsions. Convulsions may occur in patients with impaired renal function or in those receiving high doses.

Other undesirable effects

Prolonged and repeated use of the preparation can result in superinfections and colonisation with resistant organisms or yeasts such as oral and vaginal candidiasis.

4.9 Overdose

Symptoms of overdosage

In the event of overdosage, gastrointestinal symptoms, such as nausea, vomiting and diarrhoea and disturbances of the fluid and electrolyte balance are possible. Also, convulsions may exist.

Management of overdosage

There is no specific antidote for overdose. Treatment consists of haemodialysis and symptomatic measures paying particular attention to the water and electrolyte balance, especially if there are any gastro-intestinal symptoms. Administration of medicinal charcoal and gastric lavage are useful only in cases of very high overdose (> 250mg/kg). In case of severe renal insufficiency, Co-amoxiclav can be eliminated from the circulation via haemodialysis.

5. PHARMACOLOGICAL PROPERTIES

5.1 Pharmacodynamic properties

Antibiotic/chemotherapeutic (penicillin with broad spectrum of action) (JOICR).

Mechanism of Action

Amoxicillin:

Amoxicillin is an acid-stable aminopenicillin that is susceptible to hydrolysis by common β-lactamase enzymes.

Clavulanic acid:

Clavulanic acid is a β-lactam molecule that is able to inhibit many of the most commonly occurring β-lactamases such as staphylococcal penicillinases and enzymes of the TEM, OXA, SHV families (including many of the extended spectrum β-lactamases of these groups). Thus, combination of amoxicillin with clavulanic acid maintains the activity of the aminopenicillin against organisms that produce sufficient quantities of these enzymes that would otherwise render inactive.

However, clavulanic acid is not able to inhibit the AmpC (Class 1) β-lactamases that may be produced by certain Gram-negative bacilli or the metallo-β-lactamases (such as carbapenemases). Therefore, organisms that are normally susceptible to amoxicillin but have acquired the ability to produce any if these enzymes in amounts sufficient to render amoxicillin inactive would not be susceptible to Co-amoxiclav.

Antibacterial Spectrum

MIC Breakpoints

The MIC breakpoints according to the NCCLS criteria and methodology that separates susceptible (S) organisms from those that are immediately susceptible (I) or resistant (R) are:

- Enterobacteriaceae: S ≤ 8/4 mg/L; I = 16/8 mg/L; R ≥ 32/16 mg/L
- Staphylococci: S ≤ 4/2 mg/L; R ≥ 8/4 mg/L
- Haemophilus influenzae: S ≤ 4/2 mg/L; R ≥ 8/4 mg/L
- Streptococcus pneumoniae: S ≤ 0.5/0.25 mg/L; I = 1/0.5 mg/L; R ≥ 2/1 mg/L

BSAC criteria are as follows (Expressed as amoxicillin):

- Enterobacteriaceae: S ≤ 8mg/L; R ≥ 16 mg/L
- In UTI: S ≤ 32mg/L; R ≥ 64 mg/L
- Haemophilus influenzae, Moraxella catarrhalis: S ≤ 1 mg/L; R ≥ 2 mg/L

Spectrum of action of Co-amoxiclav

The prevalence of resistance may vary geographically and with time for selected species and local information on resistance is desirable, particularly when treating severe infections. This information gives only approximate guidance on the probabilities whether micro-organisms will be susceptible to Co-amoxiclav or not. As far as possible the information on the European range of acquired resistance for the individual micro-organism is indicated in brackets.

Micro-organisms	Resistance prevalence in the EU*
SUSCEPTIBLE	
Gram-positive aerobes	
E.faecalis	
S.aureus methicillin-susceptible	
S.pneumoniae	0% - 26%*
S.pyogenes	
Gram-negative organisms	
E.coli	5 – 20% *
K.pneumoniae	7% *
H.influenzae	2%
M.catarrhalis	
P.mirabilis *N.gonorrhoeae*	Up to 34% *
Anaerobes	
B.fragilis	
C.perfringens	
Peptostreptococcus spp	
RESISTANT	
Gram-positive organisms	
E.faecium	
S.aureus methicillin-resistant	
Gram-negative organisms	
E.aerogenes	
E.cloacae	
M.morganii	
P.aeroginosa	
Serratia spp.	
P.rettgeri	
Others	
Legionellae	
Chlamydia spp.	
Mycoplasma spp.	
Ricketsia spp.	

* It is recommended that local information on the epidemiology of resistant micro-organisms should be consulted.

Resistance

Organisms that are normally resistant to amoxicillin by non-beta-lactamase-mediated mechanisms (such as impermability, altered penicillin-binding proteins or drug efflux pumps) or via the manufacture of enzymes that are not inhibited by clavulanic acid would also be resistant to amoxicillin/clavulanate.

5.2 Pharmacokinetic properties

Amoxicillin:

The absolute bioavailability of amoxicillin depends on the dose and ranges between approximately 72 and 94%. Absorption is not affected by intake of food. Peak plasma concentrations are present about 1 to 2 hours after administration of amoxicillin. The apparent distribution volume ranges between approximately 0.3 and 0.4 l/kg and binding to serum proteins is approximately 17 – 20%. Amoxicillin diffuses through the placental barrier and a small fraction is excreted into breast milk.

Amoxicillin is largely excreted through the kidneys (52 ± 15% of a dose in unchanged form within 7 hours) and a small fraction is excreted in the bile. Total clearance ranges between approximately 250 and 370 ml/min. The serum half-life of amoxicillin in subjects with intact renal function is approximately 1 hour (0.9 – 1.2h), in patients with creatinine clearance ranging between 10 and 30ml/min it is about 6 hours and in anuria it ranges between 10 and 15 hours.

Clavulanic acid:

The absolute bioavailability of clavulanic acid of approximately 60% differs markedly from individual to individual. Absorption is not affected by intake of food. Peal concentrations of clavulanic acid are present after approximately 1 to 2 hours. The apparent distribution volume is about 0.2 l/kg and the serum protein binding rate is approximately 22%. Clavulanic acid diffuses through the placental barrier. No exact data are as yet available in regard to excretion into breast milk.

The substance is partly metabolised (approximately 50 – 70%) and is about 40% is eliminated through the kidneys (18 – 38% of the dose is unchanged form). The total clearance is approximately 260 ml/min. The serum half-life of clavulanic acid in subjects with intact renal function is approximately 1 hour, in patients with creatinine clearance ranging from 20 and 70ml/min it is approximately 2.6 hours and in anuria it ranges between 3 and 4 hours.

Pharmacologically relevant pharmacokinetic interaction between amoxicillin and clavulanic acid have not been observed so far. Both amoxicillin and clavulanic acid are haemodialysable.

5.3 Preclinical safety data

a) Acute toxicity

Investigations of the acute toxicity (LD_{50}) of amoxicillin and clavulanic acid in adult animals and neonates have confirmed very low toxicity potential. The LD_{50} of clavulanic acid (potassium salt) is determined by the potassium content.

Administration of clavulanic acid (potassium salt) together with amoxicillin does not result in any unexpected or synergistic toxicity.

b) Chronic toxicity / subchronic toxicity

Extensive studies of the chronic toxicity have been carried out based on international standards. Solely after high doses (corresponding to 20- to 50- fold the maximal human dose) were mild haematological and blood-chemical changes observed which regressed completely following discontinuation of the therapy.

c) Mutagenic and tumorigenic potential

In-vitro and in-vivo studies did not reveal any signs of any mutagenic effects of the combination of amoxicillin and clavulanic acid.

d) Reproductive toxicity

After treatment of various infections in pregnant women (approximately 560 pregnancies) with Co-amoxiclav no increased occurrence of malformations was observed. Amoxicillin and clavulanic acid diffuse through the placenta and are excreted into breast milk (probable elimination of clavulanic acid into breast milk).

6. PHARMACEUTICAL PARTICULARS

6.1 List of excipients

None

6.2 Incompatibilities

Co-amoxiclav Injection should not be mixed with blood products, other proteinaceous fluids such as protein hydrolysates or with intravenous lipid emulsions.

If co-amoxiclav is prescribed concurrently with an aminoglycoside, the antibiotics should not be mixed in the syringe, intravenous fluid container or giving set because loss of activity of the aminoglycoside can occur under these conditions.

6.3 Shelf life

Two years

6.4 Special precautions for storage

Do not store above 25°C.

Keep container in the outer carton.

6.5 Nature and contents of container

Clear 20ml glass vials (Ph.Eur Type II) with a red chlorobutyl stopper and aluminium-propylene flip-off cap.

6.6 Instructions for use and handling

To reconstitute dissolve in 20 ml Water for Injections Ph Eur.

(Final volume 20.9 ml.)

Administrative Data

7. MARKETING AUTHORISATION HOLDER

CP Pharmaceuticals Ltd
Ash Road North
Wrexham
LL13 9UF
UK

8. MARKETING AUTHORISATION NUMBER(S)

04543/0473

9. DATE OF FIRST AUTHORISATION/RENEWAL OF THE AUTHORISATION

29 October 2003

10. DATE OF REVISION OF THE TEXT

Co-amoxiclav for Injection 500/100mg

(Wockhardt UK Ltd)

1. NAME OF THE MEDICINAL PRODUCT

Co-amoxiclav for Injection 500/100mg.

2. QUALITATIVE AND QUANTITATIVE COMPOSITION

Each vial contains 500mg amoxicillin (as sodium salt) and 100mg clavulanic acid (as potassium salt).

Each 600mg vial of co-amoxiclav contains 0.5mmol of potassium and 1.55mmol of sodium (approx).

3. PHARMACEUTICAL FORM

Powder for solution for injection or infusion.

4. CLINICAL PARTICULARS

4.1 Therapeutic indications

Treatment of the following bacterial infections when caused by amoxicillin-resistant but amoxicillin-clavulanate susceptible organisms (see section 5.1):

Upper and Lower Respiratory Tract Infections, including:

- otitis media
- acute sinusitis
- acute exacerbations of chronic bronchitis
- community-acquired pneumonia

Upper and Lower Urinary Tract Infections

Skin and Soft Tissue Infections

Genito-Urinary Tract Infections including septic abortion, pelvic or puerperal sepsis, intra-abdominal sepsis

Consideration should be given to the official guidance on the appropriate use of antibacterial agents.

4.2 Posology and method of administration

Dosages for the treatment of infection

Adults and children over 12 years

Usually 1.2g eight hourly. In more serious infections, increase frequency to six-hourly intervals.

Children 3 months – 12 years

Usually 30mg/kg* co-amoxiclav eight hourly. In more serious infections, increase frequency to six-hourly intervals.

Children 0-3 months

30mg/kg* co-amoxiclav every 12 hours in premature infants and in full-term infants during the perinatal period, increasing to eight hours thereafter.

*Each 30mg co-amoxiclav provides 25mg of amoxicillin and 5mg of clavulanic acid.

Each 600mg vial of co-amoxiclav contains 0.5mmol of potassium and 1.55mmol of sodium (approx).

Adult dosage for surgical prophylaxis

The usual dose is 1.2g co-amoxiclav injection given at the induction of anaesthesia. Operations where there is a high risk of infection, e.g. colorectal surgery, may require three, and up to four doses of 1.2g of co-amoxiclav injection in a 24 hour period. These doses are usually given at 0, 8, 16 (and 24) hours. This regimen can be continued for several days if the procedure has a significantly increased risk of infection.

Clear clinical signs of infection at operation will require a normal course of intravenous or oral co-amoxiclav therapy post-operatively.

Dosage in renal impairment

Adults

Mild impairment (creatinine clearance >30 ml/min): No change in dosage.

Moderate impairment (creatinine clearance 10-30 ml/min): 1.2g IV stat., followed by 600mg IV 12 hourly.

Severe impairment (creatinine clearance <10 ml/min): 1.2g IV stat., followed by 600mg IV 24 hourly. Dialysis decreases serum concentrations of co-amoxiclav and an additional 600mg IV dose may need to be given during dialysis and at the end of dialysis.

<u>Children</u>

Similar reductions in dosage should be made for children.

Dosage in hepatic impairment

Dose with caution. Monitor hepatic function at regular intervals. There are, as yet, insufficient data on which to base a dosage recommendation.

Each 600mg vial of co-amoxiclav contains 1.0mmol of potassium and 3.1 mmol of sodium (approx).

Co-amoxiclav may not be used in patients with severe hepatic impairment and in patients in whom hepatic functional impairment has occurred on previous therapy with Co-amoxiclav (see section 4.3 and 4.4). Liver function parameters should be checked at regular intervals in patients with signs of hepatic lesions and a change of therapy should be given considerations if these parameters exacerbate on treatment.

<u>Administration</u>

Co-amoxiclav injection may be administered either by intravenous injection or by intermittent infusion. Therapy can be started parenterally and continued with an oral preparation.

Co-amoxiclav injection should be given by slow intravenous injection over a period of three to four minutes and used within 20 minutes of reconstitution. It may be injected directly into a vein or via a drip tube.

Alternatively, co-amoxiclav intravenous may be infused in Water for Injections Ph Eur or Sodium Chloride Intravenous Injection BP (0.9% w/v). Add, without delay, 600 mg reconstituted solution to 50 ml infusion fluid or 1.2 g reconstituted solution to 100 ml infusion fluid (e.g. using a minibag or in-line burette). Infuse over 30-40 minutes and complete within four hours of reconstitution.

Any residual antibiotic solutions should be discarded.

Co-amoxiclav Injection is less stable in infusions containing glucose, dextran or bicarbonate. Reconstituted solution should, therefore, not be added to such infusions but may be injected into the drip tubing over a period of three to four minutes.

It is not suitable for intramuscular administration. Duration of therapy should be appropriate to the indication and should not exceed 14 days without review.

4.3 Contraindications

Hypersensitivity to the constituents, amoxicillin and clavulanic acid. Penicillin hypersensitivity. Attention should be paid to possible cross-sensitivity with other β-lactam antibiotics, e.g. penicillins, cephalosporins, carbapenems, monobactams due to the danger of anaphylactic shock. Consequently a careful history should be taken in regard to allergic reaction before commencing treatment. Co-amoxiclav should not be given to patients with a verified hypersensitivity to any beta-lactam drug.

A previous history of co-amoxiclav or penicillin-associated jaundice/hepatic dysfunction.

Co-amoxiclav may not be used in patients with severe hepatic impairment and in patients in whom hepatic functional impairment has occurred onprevioustherapy with co-amoxiclav, for example cholestatic jaundice induced by co-amoxiclav or penicillin.

Patients with infectious mononucleosis (glandular fever) and patients with lymphatic leukaemia have a higher risk of exanthema and consequently co-amoxiclav injection should not be administered during these diseases to treat concomitant bacterial infections.

4.4 Special warnings and special precautions for use

Although severe allergic reactions are more likely in patients who have experienced beta-lactam hypersensitivity, these may occur in the absence of any such history. In such cases treatment should be discontinued immediately and appropriate management instituted.

Co-amoxiclav should be used with caution in patients with allergic diathesis, including asthma, since such patients may have a higher risk of allergic reactions to co-amoxiclav.

Patients with evidence of hepatic dysfunction should be treated with caution. Liver function parameters should be monitored in patients with signs or symptoms of hepatic impairment. Discontinuation of therapy should be considered in case of deterioration of liver function parameters during treatment.

In long term use (more than 10-14 days), regular monitoring of renal and hepatic function is recommended.

Prolonged use of co-amoxiclav, or other broadspectrum antibiotics, may lead to superinfections due to an overgrowth of non-susceptible organisms and yeasts.

In case of severe and persistent diarrhoea, the possibility of pseudomembraneous colitis must be considered, in which case therapy should be discontinued.

In patients with renal impairment, excretion of co-amoxiclav will be delayed and depending on the degree of the impairment, it may be necessary to reduce the total daily dosage (see section 4.2).

The presence of high urinary concentrations of amoxicillin can cause precipitation of the product in urinary catheters. Therefore, catheters should be visually inspected at intervals.

At high doses, adequate fluid intake and urinary output must be maintained to minimise the possibility of amoxicillin crystalluria.

4.5 Interaction with other medicinal products and other forms of Interaction

Other bacterial agents: There is a possibility that the antibacterial action of amoxicillin could be antagonised on co-administration with macrolides, tetracyclines, sulphonamides or chloramphenicol.

Probenecid: By inhibiting the renal elimination of amoxicillin (but not clavulanic acid) the concomitant administration of probenecid leads to an increase in the concentrations of amoxicillin in serum and bile.

Allopurinol: Concomitant administration of allopurinol may promote the occurrence of allergic cutaneous reactions.

Digoxin: An increase in the absorption of digoxin is possible on concurrent administration with amoxicillin.

Co-amoxiclav / disulfiram: Co-amoxiclav should not be used concurrently with disulfiram.

Methotrexate: Concomitant administration with methotrexate may lead to an increase in toxicity of methotrexate.

Anticoagulants: Concomitant administration of amoxicillin and coumarin anticoagulants, such as warfarin, may increase the incidence of bleeding.

Oral hormonal contraceptives: Administration of amoxicillin can transiently decrease the plasma level of oestrogens and progesterone and may reduce the efficacy of oral contraceptives. Patients should be advised to use supplemental non-hormonal contraceptive measures.

Other forms of interaction: Amoxicillin may produce false positive results in glucose determination tests and tests for urobilinogen performed with nonenzymatic methods. Likewise the urobilinogen test can be affected.

Amoxicillin may decrease the amount of urinary estriol in pregnant women. Diarrhoea may decrease the absorption of other drugs and consequently have a negative influence on their effectivity.

Forced diuresis will lead to an increased elimination of amoxicillin resulting in decreased serum concentrations.

4.6 Pregnancy and lactation

Reproduction studies in animals (mice and rats) with orally and parenterally administered co-amoxiclav have shown no teratogenic effects. There is limited experience of the use of co-amoxiclav in human pregnancy. As with all medicines, use should be avoided in pregnancy, especially during the first trimester, unless considered essential by the physician.

Co-amoxiclav may be administered during the period of lactation. With the exception of the risk of sensitisation, associated with the excretion of trace quantities in breast milk, there are no known detrimental effects for the breast-fed infant.

4.7 Effects on ability to drive and use machines

Co-amoxiclav may sometimes be associated with side effects (such as rarely dizziness and even less often convulsions) that may impair the ability to drive a vehicle, to operate machinery and/or work safely (see section 4.8).

4.8 Undesirable effects

<u>The most commonly reported adverse drug reactions are hypersensitivity reactions:</u>

Common (⩾ 1% but < 10%)

- Cutaneous reactions such as exanthema, pruritus, urticaria; the typical morbilliform exanthema occurs 5-11 days after start of therapy. Immediate appearance of urticaria indicates an allergic reaction to amoxicillin and therapy should therefore be discontinued.

Rare (⩾ 0.01% but < 0.1%): (see also section 4.4)

- Angioneurotic oedema (Quincke's oedema)
- Erythema multiforme syndrome
- Stevens-Johnson syndrome
- Eosinophilia
- Drug fever
- Laryngeal oedema
- Serum sickness
- Haemolytic anaemia
- Allergic vasculitis
- Interstitial nephritis
- Anaphylactic shock

<u>Other possible side effects</u>

<u>Blood disorders:</u>

There have been isolated reports of leucopenia, granulocytopenia, thrombocytopenia, pancytopenia, anaemia, myelosuppression, agranulocytosis, prolongation of bleeding time and prolongation of prothrombin time. However, these changes were reversible on discontinuation of therapy.

Gastrointestinal disorders:

Common (⩾ 1% but < 10%):

Gastric complaints, nausea, loss of appetite, vomiting, flatulence, soft stools, diarrhoea, enanthemas (particularly in the region of the mouth), dry mouth, taste disturbances. These effects on the gastrointestinal system are mostly mild and frequently disappear either during the treatment or very soon after completion of therapy. The occurrence of these side-effects can generally be reduced by taking amoxicillin during meals or with some food. If severe and persistent diarrhoea occurs, the rare possibility of pseudomembraneous colitis should be considered. The administration of anti-peristaltic drug is contraindicated.

Very rare (< 0.01%)

Development of a black tongue.

Liver disorders:

Uncommon (⩾ 0.1% but < 1%):

Moderate and transient increase of liver enzymes. Rare reports of hepatitis and cholestatic jaundice.

Renal disorders:

Uncommon (⩾ 0.01% but < 0.1%):

Acute interstitial nephritis may occur in rare cases.

CNS disorders:

CNS effects have been seen rarely. They include hyperkinesia, dizziness and convulsions. Convulsions may occur in patients with impaired renal function or in those receiving high doses.

Other undesirable effects

Prolonged and repeated use of the preparation can result in superinfections and colonisation with resistant organisms or yeasts such as oral and vaginal candidiasis.

4.9 Overdose

Symptoms of overdosage

In the event of overdosage, gastrointestinal symptoms, such as nausea, vomiting and diarrhoea and disturbances of the fluid and electrolyte balance are possible. Also, convulsions may exist.

Management of overdosage

There is no specific antidote for overdose. Treatment consists of haemodialysis and symptomatic measures paying particular attention to the water and electrolyte balance, especially if there are any gastro-intestinal symptoms. Administration of medicinal charcoal and gastric lavage are useful only in cases of very high overdose (> 250mg/kg). In case of severe renal insufficiency, Co-amoxiclav can be eliminated from the circulation via haemodialysis.

5. PHARMACOLOGICAL PROPERTIES

5.1 Pharmacodynamic properties

Antibiotic/chemotherapeutic (penicillin with broad spectrum of action) (JOICR).

Mechanism of Action

Amoxicillin:

Amoxicillin is an acid-stable aminopenicillin that is susceptible to hydrolysis by common β-lactamase enzymes.

Clavulanic acid:

Clavulanic acid is a β-lactam molecule that is able to inhibit many of the most commonly occurring β-lactamases such as staphylococcal penicillinases and enzymes of the TEM, OXA, SHV families (including many of the extended spectrum β-lactamases of these groups). Thus, combination of amoxicillin with clavulanic acid maintains the activity of the aminopenicillin against organisms that produce sufficient quantities of these enzymes that would otherwise render inactive.

However, clavulanic acid is not able to inhibit the AmpC (Class 1) β-lactamases that may be produced by certain Gram-negative bacilli or the metallo-β-lactamases (such as carbapenemases). Therefore, organisms that are normally susceptible to amoxicillin but have acquired the ability to produce any if these enzymes in amounts sufficient to render amoxicillin inactive would not be susceptible to Co-amoxiclav.

Antibacterial Spectrum

MIC Breakpoints

The MIC breakpoints according to the NCCLS criteria and methodology that separates susceptible (S) organisms from those that are immediately susceptible (I) or resistant (R) are:

• Enterobacteriaceae:	S ⩽ 8/4 mg/L
	I = 16/8 mg/L
	R ⩾ 32/16 mg/L
• Staphylococci:	S ⩽ 4/2 mg/L
	R ⩾ 8/4 mg/L
• Haemophilus influenzae:	S ⩽ 4/2 mg/L
	R ⩾ 8/4 mg/L
• Streptococcus pneumoniae:	S ⩽ 0.5/0.25 mg/L
	I = 1/0.5 mg/L
	R ⩾ 2/1 mg/L

BSAC criteria are as follows (Expressed as amoxicillin):

• Enterobacteriaceae:	S ⩽ 8mg/L
	R ⩾ 16 mg/L
• In UTI:	S ⩽ 32mg/L
	R ⩾ 64 mg/L
• Haemophilus influenzae, Moraxella catarrhalis:	S ⩽ 1 mg/L
	R ⩾ 2 mg/L

Spectrum of action of Co-amoxiclav

The prevalence of resistance may vary geographically and with time for selected species and local information on resistance is desirable, particularly when treating severe infections. This information gives only approximate guidance on the probabilities whether micro-organisms will be susceptible to Co-amoxiclav or not. As far as possible the information on the European range of acquired resistance for the individual micro-organism is indicated in brackets.

Micro-organisms	Resistance prevalence in the EU*
SUSCEPTIBLE	
Gram-positive aerobes	
E.faecalis	
S.aureus methicillin-susceptible	
S.pneumoniae	0% - 26%*
S.pyogenes	
Gram-negative organisms	
E.coli	5 – 20% *
K.pneumoniae	7% *
H.influenzae	2%
M.catarrhalis	
P.mirabilis *N.gonorrhoeae*	Up to 34% *
Anaerobes	
B.fragilis	
C.perfringens	
Peptostreptococcus spp	
RESISTANT	
Gram-positive organisms	
E.faecium	
S.aureus methicillin-resistant	
Gram-negative organisms	
E.aerogenes	
E.cloacae	
M.morganii	
P.aeroginosa	
Serratia spp.	
P.rettgeri	
Others	
Legionellae	
Chlamydia spp.	
Mycoplasma spp.	
Ricketsia spp.	

* It is recommended that local information on the epidemiology of resistant micro-organisms should be consulted.

Resistance

Organisms that are normally resistant to amoxicillin by non-beta-lactamase-mediated mechanisms (such as impermeability, altered penicillin-binding proteins or drug efflux pumps) or via the manufacture of enzymes that arenot inhibited by clavulanic acid would also be resistant to amoxicillin/clavulanate.

5.2 Pharmacokinetic properties

Amoxicillin:

The absolute bioavailability of amoxicillin depends on the dose and ranges between approximately 72 and 94%. Absorption is not affected by intake of food. Peak plasma concentrations are present about 1 to 2 hours after administration of amoxicillin. The apparent distribution volume ranges between approximately 0.3 and 0.4 l/kg and binding to serum proteins is approximately 17 – 20%. Amoxicillin diffuses through the placental barrier and a small fraction is excreted into breast milk.

Amoxicillin is largely excreted through the kidneys (52 ± 15% of a dose in unchanged form within 7 hours) and a small fraction is excreted in the bile. Total clearance ranges between approximately 250 and 370 ml/min. The serum half-life of amoxicillin in subjects with intact renal function is approximately 1 hour (0.9 – 1.2h), in patients with creatinine clearance ranging between 10 and 30ml/min it is about 6 hours and in anuria it ranges between 10 and 15 hours.

Clavulanic acid:

The absolute bioavailability of clavulanic acid of approximately 60% differs markedly from individual to individual. Absorption is not affected by intake of food. Peal concentrations of clavulanic acid are present after approximately 1 to 2 hours. The apparent distribution volume is about 0.2 l/kg and the serum protein binding rate is approximately 22%. Clavulanic acid diffuses through the placental barrier. No exact data are as yet available in regard to excretion into breast milk.

The substance is partly metabolised (approximately 50 – 70%) and is about 40% is eliminated through the kidneys (18 – 38% of the dose is unchanged form). The total clearance is approximately 260 ml/min. The serum half-life of clavulanic acid in subjects with intact renal function is approximately 1 hour, in patients with creatinine clearance ranging from 20 and 70ml/min it is approximately 2.6 hours and in anuria it ranges between 3 and 4 hours.

Pharmacologically relevant pharmacokinetic interaction between amoxicillin and clavulanic acid have not been observed so far. Both amoxicillin and clavulanic acid are haemodialysable.

5.3 Preclinical safety data

a) Acute toxicity

Investigations of the acute toxicity (LD_{50}) of amoxicillin and clavulanic acid in adult animals and neonates have confirmed very low toxicity potential. The LD_{50} of clavulanic acid (potassium salt) is determined by the potassium content.

Administration of clavulanic acid (potassium salt) together with amoxicillin does not result in any unexpected or synergistic toxicity.

b) Chronic toxicity / subchronic toxicity

Extensive studies of the chronic toxicity have been carried out based on international standards. Solely after high doses (corresponding to 20- to 50- fold the maximal human dose) were mild haematological and blood-chemical changes observed which regressed completely following discontinuation of the therapy.

c) Mutagenic and tumorigenic potential

In-vitro and in-vivo studies did not reveal any signs of any mutagenic effects of the combination of amoxicillin and clavulanic acid.

d) Reproductive toxicity

After treatment of various infections in pregnant women (approximately 560 pregnancies) with Co-amoxiclav no increased occurrence of malformations was observed. Amoxicillin and clavulanic acid diffuse through the placenta and are excreted into breast milk (probable elimination of clavulanic acid into breast milk).

6. PHARMACEUTICAL PARTICULARS

6.1 List of excipients

None

6.2 Incompatibilities

Co-amoxiclav Injection should not be mixed with blood products, other proteinaceous fluids such as protein hydrolysates or with intravenous lipid emulsions.

If co-amoxiclav is prescribed concurrently with an aminoglycoside, the antibiotics should not be mixed in the syringe, intravenous fluid container or giving set because loss of activity of the aminoglycoside can occur under these conditions.

6.3 Shelf life

Two years

6.4 Special precautions for storage

Do not store above 25°C.

Keep container in the outer carton.

6.5 Nature and contents of container

Clear 10ml glass vials (Ph.Eur. Type II) with a grey bromobutyl stopper and aluminium-propylene flip-off cap.

6.6 Instructions for use and handling

To reconstitute dissolve in 10 ml Water for Injections Ph Eur.

(Final volume 10.5 ml.)

Administrative Data

7. MARKETING AUTHORISATION HOLDER

CP Pharmaceuticals Ltd

Ash Road North

Wrexham

LL13 9UF

UK

8. MARKETING AUTHORISATION NUMBER(S)

04543/0472

9. DATE OF FIRST AUTHORISATION/RENEWAL OF THE AUTHORISATION

29 October 2003.

10. DATE OF REVISION OF THE TEXT

CoAprovel 150/12.5 mg and 300/12.5 mg Film-Coated Tablets

(Bristol-Myers Squibb Pharmaceuticals Ltd)

1. NAME OF THE MEDICINAL PRODUCT

CoAprovel 150/12.5 mg film-coated tablets

CoAprovel 300/12.5 mg film-coated tablets

2. QUALITATIVE AND QUANTITATIVE COMPOSITION

Each film-coated tablet contains either 150 mg irbesartan and 12.5 mg hydrochlorothiazide or 300mg irbesartan with 12.5 mg hydrochlorothiazide.

For excipients, see 6.1.

3. PHARMACEUTICAL FORM

Film-coated tablet.

Peach, biconvex, oval-shaped, with a heart debossed on one side. On the other side, the number 2875 is engraved on the 150/12.5mg tablet and the number 2876 on the 300/12.5mg tablet.

4. CLINICAL PARTICULARS

4.1 Therapeutic indications

Treatment of essential hypertension.

This fixed dose combination is indicated in patients whose blood pressure is not adequately controlled on irbesartan or hydrochlorothiazide alone.

4.2 Posology and method of administration

CoAprovel can be used once daily, with or without food in patients whose blood pressure is not adequately controlled by irbesartan or hydrochlorothiazide alone.

Dose titration with the individual components (i.e. irbesartan and hydrochlorothiazide) can be recommended.

When clinically appropriate direct change from monotherapy to the fixed combinations may be considered:

- CoAprovel 150/12.5 mg may be administered in patients whose blood pressure is not adequately controlled with hydrochlorothiazide or irbesartan 150 mg alone;

- CoAprovel 300/12.5 mg may be administered in patients insufficiently controlled by irbesartan 300 mg or by CoAprovel 150/12.5 mg.

- CoAprovel 300/25 mg may be administered in patients insufficiently controlled by CoAprovel 300/12.5 mg.

Doses higher than 300 mg irbesartan / 25 mg hydrochlorothiazide once daily are not recommended.

When necessary, CoAprovel may be administered with another antihypertensive drug (see 4.5).

Renal impairment: Due to the hydrochlorothiazide component, CoAprovel is not recommended for patients with severe renal dysfunction (creatinine clearance < 30 ml/min). Loop diuretics are preferred to thiazides in this population. No dosage adjustment is necessary in patients with renal impairment whose renal creatinine clearance is ⩾ 30 ml/min (see 4.3 and 4.4).

Intravascular volume depletion: Volume and/or sodium depletion should be corrected prior to administration of CoAprovel.

Hepatic impairment: CoAprovel is not indicated in patients with severe hepatic impairment. Thiazides should be used with caution in patients with impaired hepatic function. No dosage adjustment of CoAprovel is necessary in patients with mild to moderate hepatic impairment (see 4.3).

Elderly patients: No dosage adjustment of CoAprovel is necessary in elderly patients.

Children: Safety and efficacy of CoAprovel have not been established in children (< 18 years).

4.3 Contraindications

Second and third trimester of pregnancy (see 4.6).

Lactation (see 4.6).

Hypersensitivity to the active substances, to any of the excipients (see 6.1), or to other sulfonamide-derived substances (hydrochlorothiazide is a sulfonamide-derived substance).

The following contraindications are associated with hydrochlorothiazide:

- severe renal impairment (creatinine clearance < 30 ml/min),

- refractory hypokalaemia, hypercalcaemia,

- severe hepatic impairment, biliary cirrhosis and cholestasis.

4.4 Special warnings and special precautions for use

Hypotension - Volume-depleted patients: CoAprovel has been rarely associated with symptomatic hypotension in hypertensive patients without other risk factors for hypotension. Symptomatic hypotension may be expected to occur in patients who are volume and/or sodium depleted by vigorous diuretic therapy, dietary salt restriction, diarrhoea or vomiting. Such conditions should be corrected before initiating therapy with CoAprovel.

Renal artery stenosis - Renovascular hypertension: There is an increased risk of severe hypotension and renal insufficiency when patients with bilateral renal artery stenosis or stenosis of the artery to a single functioning kidney are treated with angiotensin converting enzyme inhibitors or angiotensin-II receptor antagonists. While this is not documented with CoAprovel, a similar effect should be anticipated.

Renal impairment and kidney transplantation: When CoAprovel is used in patients with impaired renal function, a periodic monitoring of potassium, creatinine and uric acid serum levels is recommended. There is no experience regarding the administration of CoAprovel in patients with a recent kidney transplantation. CoAprovel should not be used in patients with severe renal impairment (creatinine clearance < 30 ml/min) (see 4.3). Thiazide diuretic-associated azotaemia may occur in patients with impaired renal function. No dosage adjustment is necessary in patients with renal impairment whose creatinine clearance is ⩾ 30 ml/min. However, in patients with mild to moderate renal impairment (creatinine clearance ⩾ 30 ml/min but < 60 ml/min) this fixed dose combination should be administered with caution.

Hepatic impairment: Thiazides should be used with caution in patients with impaired hepatic function or progressive liver disease, since minor alterations of fluid and electrolyte balance may precipitate hepatic coma. There is no clinical experience with CoAprovel in patients with hepatic impairment.

Aortic and mitral valve stenosis, obstructive hypertrophic cardiomyopathy: As with other vasodilators, special caution is indicated in patients suffering from aortic or mitral stenosis, or obstructive hypertrophic cardiomyopathy.

Primary aldosteronism: Patients with primary aldosteronism generally will not respond to anti-hypertensive drugs acting through inhibition of the renin-angiotensin system. Therefore, the use of CoAprovel is not recommended.

Metabolic and endocrine effects: Thiazide therapy may impair glucose tolerance. In diabetic patients dosage adjustments of insulin or oral hypoglycaemic agents may be required. Latent diabetes mellitus may become manifest during thiazide therapy.

Increases in cholesterol and triglyceride levels have been associated with thiazide diuretic therapy; however at the 12.5 mg dose contained in CoAprovel, minimal or no effects were reported.

Hyperuricaemia may occur or frank gout may be precipitated in certain patients receiving thiazide therapy.

Electrolyte imbalance: As for any patient receiving diuretic therapy, periodic determination of serum electrolytes should be performed at appropriate intervals.

Thiazides, including hydrochlorothiazide, can cause fluid or electrolyte imbalance (hypokalaemia, hyponatraemia, and hypochloraemic alkalosis). Warning signs of fluid or electrolyte imbalance are dryness of mouth, thirst, weakness, lethargy, drowsiness, restlessness, muscle pain or cramps, muscular fatigue, hypotension, oliguria, tachycardia and gastrointestinal disturbances such as nausea or vomiting.

Although hypokalaemia may develop with the use of thiazide diuretics, concurrent therapy with irbesartan may reduce diuretic-induced hypokalaemia. The risk of hypokalaemia is greatest in patients with cirrhosis of the liver, in patients experiencing brisk diuresis, in patients who are receiving inadequate oral intake of electrolytes and in patients receiving concomitant therapy with corticosteroids or ACTH. Conversely, due to the irbesartan component of CoAprovel, hyperkalaemia might occur, especially in the presence of renal impairment and/or heart failure, and diabetes mellitus. Adequate monitoring of serum potassium in patients at risk is recommended. Potassium-sparing diuretics, potassium supplements or potassium-containing salts substitutes should be co-administered cautiously with CoAprovel (see 4.5).

There is no evidence that irbesartan would reduce or prevent diuretic-induced hyponatraemia. Chloride deficit is generally mild and usually does not require treatment.

Thiazides may decrease urinary calcium excretion and cause an intermittent and slight elevation of serum calcium in the absence of known disorders of calcium metabolism. Marked hypercalcaemia may be evidence of hidden hyperparathyroidism. Thiazides should be discontinued before carrying out tests for parathyroid function.

Thiazides have been shown to increase the urinary excretion of magnesium, which may result in hypomagnasaemia.

Lithium: The combination of lithium and CoAprovel is not recommended (see 4.5).

Anti-doping test: Hydrochlorothiazide contained in this medication could produce a positive analytic result in an anti-doping test.

General: In patients whose vascular tone and renal function depend predominantly on the activity of the renin-angiotensin-aldosterone system (e.g. patients with severe congestive heart failure or underlying renal disease, including renal artery stenosis), treatment with angiotensin converting enzyme inhibitors or angiotensin-II receptor antagonists that affect this system has been associated with acute hypotension, azotaemia, oliguria, or rarely acute renal failure. As with any anti-hypertensive agent, excessive blood pressure decrease in patients with ischaemic cardiopathy or ischaemic cardiovascular disease could result in a myocardial infarction or stroke.

Hypersensitivity reactions to hydrochlorothiazide may occur in patients with or without a history of allergy or bronchial asthma, but are more likely in patients with such a history.

Exacerbation or activation of systemic lupus erythematosus has been reported with the use of thiazide diuretics.

In the first trimester of pregnancy, CoAprovel is not recommended (see 4.6).

4.5 Interaction with other medicinal products and other forms of Interaction

Other antihypertensive agents The antihypertensive effect of CoAprovel may be increased with the concomitant use of other antihypertensive agents. Irbesartan and hydrochlorothiazide (at doses up to 300 mg irbesartan / 25 mg hydrochlorothiazide) have been safely administered with other antihypertensive agents including calcium channel blockers and beta-adrenergic blockers. Prior treatment with high dose diuretics may result in volume depletion and a risk of hypotension when initiating therapy with irbesartan with or without thiazide diuretics unless the volume depletion is corrected first (see 4.4).

Lithium

Reversible increases in serum lithium concentrations and toxicity have been reported during concomitant administration of lithium with angiotensin converting enzyme inhibitors. Similar effects have been very rarely reported with irbesartan. Furthermore, renal clearance of lithium is reduced by thiazides so the risk of lithium toxicity could be increased with CoAprovel. Therefore, the combination of lithium and CoAprovel is not recommended (see 4.4). If the combination proves necessary, careful monitoring of serum lithium is recommended.

Medicinal products affecting potassium: The potassium-depleting effect of hydrochlorothiazide is attenuated by the potassium-sparing effect of irbesartan. However, this effect of hydrochlorothiazide on serum potassium would be expected to be potentiated by other drugs associated with potassium loss and hypokalaemia (e.g. other kaliuretic diuretics, laxatives, amphotericin, carbenoxolone, penicillin G sodium). Conversely, based on the experience with the use of other drugs that blunt the renin-angiotensin system, concomitant use of potassium-sparing diuretics, potassium supplements, salt substitutes containing potassium or other drugs that may increase serum potassium levels (e.g. heparin sodium) may lead to increases in serum potassium. Adequate monitoring of serum potassium in patients at risk is recommended (see 4.4).

Medicinal products affected by serum potassium disturbances: Periodic monitoring of serum potassium is recommended when CoAprovel is administered with drugs affected by serum potassium disturbances (e.g. digitalis glycosides, antiarrhythmics).

Non-steroidal anti-inflammatory drugs: When angiotensin II antagonists are administered simultaneously with non-steroidal anti-inflammatory drugs (i.e. selective COX-2 inhibitors, acetylsalicylic acid >3 g/day) and non-selective NSAIDs), attenuation of the antihypertensive effect may occur.

As with ACE inhibitors, concomitant use of angiotensin II antagonists and NSAIDs may lead to an increased risk of worsening of renal failure, including possible acute renal failure, and an increase in serum potassium, especially in patients with poor pre-existing renal function. The combination should be administered with caution, especially in the elderly. Patients should be adequately hydrated and consideration should be given to monitoring renal function after initiation of concomitant therapy, and periodically thereafter.

Additional information on irbesartan interactions: In clinical studies, the pharmacokinetics of irbesartan are not affected by hydrochlorothiazide. Irbesartan is mainly metabolised by CYP2C9 and to a lesser extent by glucuronidation. No significant pharmacokinetic or pharmacodynamic interactions were observed when irbesartan was co-administered with warfarin, a drug metabolised by CYP2C9. The effects of *CYP*2C9 inducers such as rifampicin on the pharmacokinetics of irbesartan have not been evaluated. The pharmacokinetics of digoxin were not altered by co-administration of irbesartan.

Additional information on hydrochlorothiazide interactions: When administered concurrently, the following drugs may interact with thiazide diuretics:

- *Alcohol:* potentiation of orthostatic hypotension may occur;

- *Antidiabetic drugs (oral agents and insulins):* dosage adjustment of the antidiabetic drug may be required (see 4.4);

- *Colestyramine and Colestipol resins:* absorption of hydrochlorothiazide is impaired in the presence of anionic exchange resins;

- *Corticosteroids, ACTH:* electrolyte depletion, particularly hypokalaemia, may be increased;

- *Digitalis glycosides:* thiazide induced hypokalaemia or hypomagnesaemia favour the onset of digitalis-induced cardiac arrhythmias (see 4.4);

- *Non-steroidal anti-inflammatory drugs:* the administration of a non-steroidal anti-inflammatory drug may reduce the diuretic, natriuretic and antihypertensive effects of thiazide diuretics in some patients;

- *Pressor amines (e.g. noradrenaline):* the effect of pressor amines may be decreased, but not sufficiently to preclude their use;

- *Nondepolarizing skeletal muscle relaxants (e.g. tubocurarine):* the effect of nondepolarizing skeletal muscle relaxants may be potentiated by hydrochlorothiazide;

- *Anti-gout medication:* dosage adjustments of antigout medications may be necessary as hydrochlorothiazide may raise the level of serum uric acid. Increase in dosage of probenecid or sulfinpyrazone may be necessary. Co-administration of thiazide diuretics may increase the incidence of hypersensitivity reactions to allopurinol;

- *Calcium salts:* thiazide diuretics may increase serum calcium levels due to decreased excretion. If calcium supplements or calcium sparing drugs (e.g. Vitamin D therapy) must be prescribed, serum calcium levels should be monitored and calcium dosage adjusted accordingly;

- *Other interactions:* the hyperglycaemic effect of beta-blockers and diazoxide may be enhanced by thiazides. Anticholinergic agents (e.g. atropine, beperiden) may increase the bioavailability of thiazide-type diuretics by decreasing gastrointestinal motility and stomach emptying rate. Thiazides may increase the risk of adverse effects caused by amantadine. Thiazides may reduce the renal excretion of cytotoxic drugs (e.g. cyclophosphamide, methotrexate) and potentiate their myelosuppressive effects.

4.6 Pregnancy and lactation

Pregnancy: See sections 4.3 and 4.4.

Thiazides cross the placental barrier and appear in cord blood. They may cause decreased placental perfusion, foetal electrolyte disturbances and possibly other reactions that have occurred in the adults. Cases of neonatal thrombocytopenia, or foetal or neonatal jaundice have been reported with maternal thiazide therapy. Since CoAprovel contains hydrochlorothiazide, it is not recommended during the first trimester of pregnancy. A switch to a suitable alternative treatment should be carried out in advance of a planned pregnancy.

In the second and third trimesters, substances that act directly on the renin-angiotensin-system can cause foetal or neonatal renal failure, foetal skull hypoplasia and even foetal death. Therefore, CoAprovel is contra-indicated in the second and third trimesters of pregnancy. If pregnancy is diagnosed, CoAprovel should be discontinued as soon as possible, skull and renal function should be checked with echography if, inadvertently, the treatment was taken for a long period.

Lactation: because of the potential adverse effects on the nursing infant, CoAprovel is contraindicated during lactation (see 4.3). It is not known if irbesartan is excreted in human milk. It is excreted in the milk of lactating rats. Thiazides appear in human milk and may inhibit lactation.

4.7 Effects on ability to drive and use machines

The effect of CoAprovel on ability to drive and use machines has not been studied, but based on its pharmacodynamic properties, CoAprovel is unlikely to affect this ability. When driving vehicles or operating machines, it should be taken into account that occasionally dizziness or weariness may occur during treatment of hypertension.

4.8 Undesirable effects

The frequency of adverse reactions listed below is defined using the following convention: very common ($\geqslant$ 1/10); common ($\geqslant$ 1/100, < 1/10); uncommon ($\geqslant$ 1/1,000, < 1/100); rare ($\geqslant$ 1/10,000, < 1/1,000); very rare (< 1/10,000).

Irbesartan/hydrochlorothiazide combination:

In placebo-controlled trials in patients with hypertension, the overall incidence of adverse events did not differ between the irbesartan / hydrochlorothiazide and the placebo groups. Discontinuation due to any clinical or laboratory adverse event was less frequent for irbesartan / hydrochlorothiazide-treated patients than for placebo-treated patients. The incidence of adverse events was not related to gender, age, race, or dose within the recommended dose range. In placebo-controlled trials in which 898 hypertensive patients received various doses (range: 37.5mg/6.25mg to 300 mg/25mg irbesartan / hydrochlorothiazide), the following adverse reactions were reported:

Nervous system disorders:

Common: dizziness

Uncommon: orthostatic dizziness

Cardiac disorders:

Uncommon: hypotension, oedema, syncope, tachycardia

Vascular disorders:

Uncommon: flushing

Gastrointestinal disorders:

Common: nausea/vomiting

Uncommon: diarrhoea

Musculoskeletal, connective tissue and bone disorders:

Uncommon: swelling extremity

Renal and urinary disorders:

Common: abnormal urination

Reproductive system and breast disorders:

Uncommon: libido changes, sexual dysfunction

General disorders and administration site conditions:

Common: fatigue

Investigations: patients treated with irbesartan / hydrochlorothiazide had changes in laboratory test parameters which were rarely clinically significant

Common: increases in BUN, creatinine and creatine kinase

Uncommon: decreases in serum potassium and sodium

In addition, since introduction of irbesartan / hydrochlorothiazide in the market the following adverse reactions have also been reported:

Immune system disorders:

Rare: as with other angiotensin-II receptor antagonists, rare cases of hypersensitivity reactions such as angioedema, rash, urticaria have been reported

Metabolism and nutrition disorders:

Very rare: hyperkalaemia

Nervous system disorders:

Very rare: headache

Ear and labyrinth disorders:

Very rare: tinnitus

Respiratory, thoracic and mediastinal disorders:

Very rare: cough

Gastrointestinal disorders:

Very rare: dysgeusia, dyspepsia

Hepato-biliary disorders:

Very rare: abnormal liver function, hepatitis

Musculoskeletal, connective tissue and bone disorders:

Very rare: arthralgia, myalgia

Renal and urinary disorders:

Very rare: impaired renal function including isolated cases of renal failure in patients at risk (see 4.4)

Additional information on individual components: in addition to the adverse reactions listed above for the combination product, other undesirable effects previously reported with one of the individual components may be potential undesirable effects with CoAprovel.

Irbesartan:

General disorders and administration site conditions:

Uncommon: chest pain

Hydrochlorothiazide:

Adverse events (regardless of relationship to drug) reported with the use of hydrochlorothiazide alone include:

Blood and lymphatic system:

aplastic anaemia, bone marrow depression, haemolytic anaemia, leucopenia, neutropenia/agranulocytosis, thrombocytopenia

Psychiatric disorders:

depression, sleep disturbances

Nervous system disorders:

light-headedness, paraesthesia, restlessness, vertigo

Eye disorders:

transient blurred vision, xanthopsia

Cardiac disorders:

cardiac arrhythmias

Vascular disorders:

postural hypotension

Respiratory, thoracic and mediastinal disorders:

respiratory distress (including pneumonitis and pulmonary oedema)

Gastrointestinal disorders:

pancreatitis, anorexia, constipation, diarrhoea, gastric irritation, loss of appetite, sialadenitis

Hepatobiliary disorders:

jaundice (intrahepatic cholestatic jaundice)

Skin and subcutaneous tissue disorders:

anaphylactic reactions, toxic epidermal necrolysis, cutaneous lupus erythematosus-like reactions, necrotizing angiitis (vasculitis, cutaneous vasculitis), photosensitivity reactions, rash, reactivation of cutaneous lupus erythematosus, urticaria

Musculoskeletal, connective tissue and bone disorders:

muscle spasm, weakness

Renal and urinary disorders:

interstitial nephritis, renal dysfunction

General disorders and administration site conditions:

fever

Investigations:

electrolyte imbalance (including hypokalaemia and hyponatraemia, see 4.4), glycosuria, hyperglycaemia, hyperuricaemia, increases in cholesterol and triglycerides

The dose dependent side effects of hydrochlorothiazide (particularly electrolyte disturbances) may increase when titrating the hydrochlorothiazide.

4.9 Overdose

No specific information is available on the treatment of overdosage with CoAprovel. The patient should be closely monitored, and the treatment should be symptomatic and supportive. Management depends on the time since ingestion and the severity of the symptoms. Suggested measures include induction of emesis and/or gastric lavage. Activated charcoal may be useful in the treatment of overdosage. Serum electrolytes and creatinine should be monitored frequently. If hypotension occurs, the patient should be placed in a supine position, with salt and volume replacements given quickly.

The most likely manifestations of irbesartan overdosage are expected to be hypotension and tachycardia; bradycardia might also occur.

Overdosage with hydrochlorothiazide is associated with electrolyte depletion (hypokalaemia, hypochloraemia, hyponatraemia) and dehydration resulting from excessive diuresis. The most common signs and symptoms of overdosage are nausea and somnolence. Hypokalaemia may result in muscle spasms and/or accentuate cardiac arrhythmias associated with the concomitant use of digitalis glycosides or certain anti-arrhythmic drugs.

Irbesartan is not removed by haemodialysis. The degree to which hydrochlorothiazide is removed by haemodialysis has not been established.

5. PHARMACOLOGICAL PROPERTIES

5.1 Pharmacodynamic properties

Pharmacotherapeutic group: angiotensin-II antagonists, combinations: ATC code C09D A04.

CoAprovel is a combination of an angiotensin-II receptor antagonist, irbesartan, and a thiazide diuretic, hydrochlorothiazide. The combination of these ingredients has an additive antihypertensive effect, reducing blood pressure to a greater degree than either component alone.

Irbesartan is a potent, orally active, selective angiotensin-II receptor (AT_1 subtype) antagonist. It is expected to block all actions of angiotensin-II mediated by the AT_1 receptor, regardless of the source or route of synthesis of angiotensin-II. The selective antagonism of the angiotensin-II (AT_1) receptors results in increases in plasma renin levels and angiotensin-II levels, and a decrease in plasma aldosterone concentration. Serum potassium levels are not significantly affected by irbesartan alone at the recommended doses in patients without risk of electrolyte imbalance (see 4.4 and 4.5). Irbesartan does not inhibit ACE (kininase-II), an enzyme which generates angiotensin-II and also degrades bradykinin into inactive metabolites. Irbesartan does not require metabolic activation for its activity.

Hydrochlorothiazide is a thiazide diuretic. The mechanism of antihypertensive effect of thiazide diuretics is not fully known. Thiazides affect the renal tubular mechanisms of electrolyte reabsorption, directly increasing excretion of sodium and chloride in approximately equivalent amounts. The diuretic action of hydrochlorothiazide reduces plasma volume, increases plasma renin activity, increases aldosterone secretion, with consequent increases in urinary potassium and bicarbonate loss, and decreases in serum potassium. Presumably through blockade of the renin-angiotensin-aldosterone system, co-administration of irbesartan tends to reverse the potassium loss associated with these diuretics. With hydrochlorothiazide, onset of diuresis occurs in 2 hours, and peak effect occurs at about 4 hours, while the action persists for approximately 6-12 hours.

The combination of hydrochlorothiazide and irbesartan produces dose-related additive reductions in blood pressure across their therapeutic dose ranges. The addition of 12.5 mg hydrochlorothiazide to 300 mg irbesartan once daily in patients not adequately controlled on 300 mg irbesartan alone resulted in further placebo-corrected diastolic blood pressure reductions at trough (24 hours post-dosing) of 6.1 mm Hg. The combination of 300 mg irbesartan and 12.5 mg hydrochlorothiazide resulted in an overall placebo-subtracted systolic/diastolic reduction of up to 13.6/11.5 mm Hg.

Limited clinical data (7 out of 22 patients) suggest that patients not controlled with the 300/12.5 combination may respond when uptitrated to 300/25. In these patients, an incremental blood pressure lowering effect was observed for both SBP and DBP (13.3 and 8.3 mm Hg, respectively).

Once daily dosing with 150 mg irbesartan and 12.5 mg hydrochlorothiazide gave systolic/diastolic mean placebo-adjusted blood pressure reductions at trough (24 hours post-dosing) of 12.9/6.9 mm Hg in patients with mild-to-moderate hypertension. Peak effects occurred at 3-6 hours. When assessed by ambulatory blood pressure monitoring, the combination 150 mg irbesartan and 12.5 mg hydrochlorothiazide once daily produced consistent reduction in blood pressure over the 24 hours period with mean 24-hour placebo-subtracted systolic/diastolic reductions of 15.8/10.0 mm Hg. When measured by ambulatory blood pressure monitoring, the trough to peak effects of CoAprovel 150/12.5 mg were 100%. The trough to peak effects measured by cuff during office visits were 68% and 76% for CoAprovel 150/12.5 mg and CoAprovel 300/12.5 mg, respectively. These 24-hour effects were observed without excessive blood pressure lowering at peak and are consistent with safe and effective blood-pressure lowering over the once-daily dosing interval.

In patients not adequately controlled on 25 mg hydrochlorothiazide alone, the addition of irbesartan gave an added placebo-subtracted systolic/diastolic mean reduction of 11.1/7.2 mm Hg.

The blood pressure lowering effect of irbesartan in combination with hydrochlorothiazide is apparent after the first dose and substantially present within 1-2 weeks, with the maximal effect occurring by 6-8 weeks. In long-term follow-up studies, the effect of irbesartan / hydrochlorothiazide was maintained for over one year. Although not specifically studied with the CoAprovel, rebound hypertension has not been seen with either irbesartan or hydrochlorothiazide.

The effect of the combination of irbesartan and hydrochlorothiazide on morbidity and mortality has not been studied. Epidemiological studies have shown that long term treatment with hydrochlorothiazide reduces the risk of cardiovascular mortality and morbidity.

There is no difference in response to CoAprovel, regardless of age or gender. When irbesartan is administered concomitantly with a low dose of hydrochlorothiazide (e.g. 12.5 mg daily), the antihypertensive response in black patients approaches that of non-black patients.

5.2 Pharmacokinetic properties
Concomitant administration of hydrochlorothiazide and irbesartan has no effect on the pharmacokinetics of either drug.

Irbesartan and hydrochlorothiazide are orally active agents and do not require biotransformation for their activity. Following oral administration of CoAprovel, the absolute oral bioavailability is 60-80% and 50-80% for irbesartan and hydrochlorothiazide, respectively. Food does not affect the bioavailability of CoAprovel. Peak plasma concentration occurs at 1.5-2 hours after oral administration for irbesartan and 1-2.5 hours for hydrochlorothiazide.

Plasma protein binding of irbesartan is approximately 96%, with negligible binding to cellular blood components. The volume of distribution for irbesartan is 53-93 litres. Hydrochlorothiazide is 68% protein-bound in the plasma, and its apparent volume of distribution is 0.83-1.14 l/kg.

Irbesartan exhibits linear and dose proportional pharmacokinetics over the dose range of 10 to 600 mg. A less than proportional increase in oral absorption at doses beyond 600 mg was observed; the mechanism for this is unknown. The total body and renal clearance are 157-176 and 3.0-3.5 ml/min, respectively. The terminal elimination half-life of irbesartan is 11-15 hours. Steady-state plasma concentrations are attained within 3 days after initiation of a once-daily dosing regimen. Limited accumulation of irbesartan (< 20%) is observed in plasma upon repeated once-daily dosing. In a study, somewhat higher plasma concentrations of irbesartan were observed in female hypertensive patients. However, there was no difference in the half-life and accumulation of irbesartan. No dosage adjustment is necessary in female patients. Irbesartan AUC and C_{max} values were also somewhat greater in elderly subjects (⩾ 65 years) than those of young subjects (18-40 years). However the terminal half-life was not significantly altered. No dosage adjustment is necessary in elderly patients. The mean plasma half-life of hydrochlorothiazide reportedly ranges from 5-15 hours.

Following oral or intravenous administration of ^{14}C irbesartan, 80-85% of the circulating plasma radioactivity is attributable to unchanged irbesartan. Irbesartan is metabolised by the liver via glucuronide conjugation and oxidation. The major circulating metabolite is irbesartan glucuronide (approximately 6%). *In vitro* studies indicate that irbesartan is primarily oxidised by the cytochrome P450 enzyme *CYP2C9*; isoenzyme *CYP3A4* has negligible effect. Irbesartan and its metabolites are eliminated by both biliary and renal pathways. After either oral or IV administration of ^{14}C irbesartan, about 20% of the radioactivity is recovered in the urine, and the remainder in the faeces. Less than 2% of the dose is excreted in the urine as unchanged irbesartan. Hydrochlorothiazide is not metabolized but is eliminated rapidly by the kidneys. At least 61% of the oral dose is eliminated unchanged within 24 hours. Hydrochlorothiazide crosses the placental but not the blood-brain barrier, and is excreted in breast milk.

Renal impairment: In patients with renal impairment or those undergoing haemodialysis, the pharmacokinetic parameters of irbesartan are not significantly altered. Irbesartan is not removed by haemodialysis. In patients with creatinine clearance < 20 ml/min, the elimination half-life of hydrochlorothiazide was reported to increase to 21 hours.

Hepatic impairment: In patients with mild to moderate cirrhosis, the pharmacokinetic parameters of irbesartan are not significantly altered. Studies have not been performed in patients with severe hepatic impairment.

5.3 Preclinical safety data
Irbesartan/hydrochlorothiazide: The potential toxicity of the irbesartan / hydrochlorothiazide combination after oral administration was evaluated in rats and macaques in studies lasting up to 6 months. There were no toxicological findings observed of relevance to human therapeutic use.

The following changes, observed in rats and macaques receiving the irbesartan / hydrochlorothiazide combination at 10/10 and 90/90 mg/kg/day, were also seen with one of the two drugs alone and/or were secondary to decreases in blood pressure (no significant toxicological interactions were observed):

- kidney changes, characterized by slight increases in serum urea and creatinine, and hyperplasia / hypertrophy of the juxtaglomerular apparatus, which are a direct consequence of the interaction of irbesartan with the renin-angiotensin system;

- slight decreases in erythrocyte parameters (erythrocytes, haemoglobin, haematocrit);

- stomach discoloration, ulcers and focal necrosis of gastric mucosa were observed in few rats in a 6 months toxicity study at irbesartan 90 mg/kg/day, hydrochlorothiazide 90 mg/kg/day, and irbesartan / hydrochlorothiazide 10/10 mg/kg/day. These lesions were not observed in macaques;

- decreases in serum potassium due to hydrochlorothiazide and partly prevented when hydrochlorothiazide was given in combination with irbesartan.

Most of the above mentioned effects appear to be due to the pharmacological activity of irbesartan (blockade of angiotensin-II-induced inhibition of renin release, with stimulation of the renin-producing cells) and occur also with angiotensin converting enzyme inhibitors. These findings appear to have no relevance to the use of therapeutic doses of irbesartan / hydrochlorothiazide in humans.

No teratogenic effects were seen in rats given irbesartan and hydrochlorothiazide in combination at doses that produced maternal toxicity. The effects of the irbesartan / hydrochlorothiazide combination on fertility have not been evaluated in animal studies, as there is no evidence of adverse effect on fertility in animals or humans with either irbesartan or hydrochlorothiazide when administered alone. However, another angiotensin-II antagonist affected fertility parameters in animal studies when given alone. These findings were also observed with lower doses of this other angiotensin-II antagonist when given in combination with hydrochlorothiazide.

There was no evidence of mutagenicity or clastogenicity with the irbesartan / hydrochlorothiazide combination. The carcinogenic potential of irbesartan and hydrochlorothiazide in combination has not been evaluated in animal studies.

Irbesartan: There was no evidence of abnormal systemic or target organ toxicity at clinically relevant doses. In preclinical safety studies, high doses of irbesartan (⩾ 250 mg/kg/day in rats and ⩾ 100 mg/kg/day in macaques) caused a reduction of red blood cell parameters (erythrocytes, haemoglobin, haematocrit). At very high doses (⩾ 500 mg/kg/day) degenerative changes in the kidneys (such as interstitial nephritis, tubular distension, basophilic tubules, increased plasma concentrations of urea and creatinine) were induced by irbesartan in the rat and the macaque and are considered secondary to the hypotensive effects of the drug which led to decreased renal perfusion. Furthermore, irbesartan induced hyperplasia / hypertrophy of the juxtaglomerular cells (in rats at ⩾ 90 mg/kg/day, in macaques at ⩾ 10 mg/kg/day). All of these changes were considered to be caused by the pharmacological action of irbesartan. For therapeutic doses of irbesartan in humans, the hyperplasia / hypertrophy of the renal juxtaglomerular cells does not appear to have any relevance.

There was no evidence of mutagenicity, clastogenicity or carcinogenicity.

Animal studies with irbesartan showed transient toxic effects (increased renal pelvic cavitation, hydroureter or subcutaneous oedema) in rat foetuses, which were resolved after birth. In rabbits, abortion or early resorption was noted at doses causing significant maternal toxicity, including mortality. No teratogenic effects were observed in the rat or rabbit.

Hydrochlorothiazide: Although equivocal evidence for a genotoxic or carcinogenic effect was found in some experimental models, the extensive human experience with hydrochlorothiazide has failed to show an association between its use and an increase in neoplasms.

6. PHARMACEUTICAL PARTICULARS

6.1 List of excipients
Tablet core: lactose monohydrate, microcrystalline cellulose, croscarmellose sodium, hypromellose, silicon dioxide, magnesium stearate.

Film-coating: lactose monohydrate, hypromellose, titanium dioxide (E171), macrogol, red and yellow ferric oxides (E172) carnauba wax.

6.2 Incompatibilities
Not applicable.

6.3 Shelf life
3 years.

6.4 Special precautions for storage
Do not store above 30°C.

Store in the original package.

6.5 Nature and contents of container
CoAprovel film-coated tablets are packaged in cartons containing 28 tablets in PVC/PVDC/aluminium blisters.

6.6 Instructions for use and handling
No special requirements.

7. MARKETING AUTHORISATION HOLDER
SANOFI PHARMA BRISTOL-MYERS SQUIBB SNC

174 avenue de France

F-75013 Paris - France

8. MARKETING AUTHORISATION NUMBER(S)

CoAprovel 150/12.5mg film-coated tablets: EU/1/98/086/012

CoAprovel 300/12.5mg film-coated tablets: EU/1/98/086/017

9. DATE OF FIRST AUTHORISATION/RENEWAL OF THE AUTHORISATION
02 March 2004

10. DATE OF REVISION OF THE TEXT
28 October 2004

CoAprovel Film-Coated Tablets

(sanofi-aventis)

1. NAME OF THE MEDICINAL PRODUCT
CoAprovel 150/12.5 mg film-coated tablets

CoAprovel 300/12.5 mg film-coated tablets

2. QUALITATIVE AND QUANTITATIVE COMPOSITION
Each film-coated tablet contains either 150 mg irbesartan and 12.5 mg hydrochlorothiazide or 300mg irbesartan with 12.5 mg hydrochlorothiazide.

For excipients, see 6.1.

3. PHARMACEUTICAL FORM
Film-coated tablet.

Peach, biconvex, oval-shaped, with a heart debossed on one side. On the other side, the number 2875 is engraved on the 150/12.5mg tablet and the number 2876 on the 300/12.5mg tablet.

4. CLINICAL PARTICULARS

4.1 Therapeutic indications
Treatment of essential hypertension.

This fixed dose combination is indicated in patients whose blood pressure is not adequately controlled on irbesartan or hydrochlorothiazide alone.

4.2 Posology and method of administration
CoAprovel can be used once daily, with or without food in patients whose blood pressure is not adequately controlled by irbesartan or hydrochlorothiazide alone.

Dose titration with the individual components (i.e. irbesartan and hydrochlorothiazide) can be recommended.

When clinically appropriate direct change from monotherapy to the fixed combinations may be considered:

- CoAprovel 150/12.5 mg may be administered in patients whose blood pressure is not adequately controlled with hydrochlorothiazide or irbesartan 150 mg alone;

- CoAprovel 300/12.5 mg may be administered in patients insufficiently controlled by irbesartan 300 mg or by CoAprovel 150/12.5 mg.

- CoAprovel 300/25 mg may be administered in patients insufficiently controlled by CoAprovel 300/12.5 mg.

Doses higher than 300 mg irbesartan / 25 mg hydrochlorothiazide once daily are not recommended.

When necessary, CoAprovel may be administered with another antihypertensive drug (see 4.5).

Renal impairment: Due to the hydrochlorothiazide component, CoAprovel is not recommended for patients with severe renal dysfunction (creatinine clearance < 30 ml/min). Loop diuretics are preferred to thiazides in this population. No dosage adjustment is necessary in patients with renal impairment whose renal creatinine clearance is ⩾ 30 ml/min (see 4.3 and 4.4).

Intravascular volume depletion: Volume and/or sodium depletion should be corrected prior to administration of CoAprovel.

Hepatic impairment: CoAprovel is not indicated in patients with severe hepatic impairment. Thiazides should be used with caution in patients with impaired hepatic function. No dosage adjustment of CoAprovel is necessary in patients with mild to moderate hepatic impairment (see 4.3).

Elderly patients: No dosage adjustment of CoAprovel is necessary in elderly patients.

Children: Safety and efficacy of CoAprovel have not been established in children (< 18 years).

4.3 Contraindications
Second and third trimester of pregnancy (see 4.6).

Lactation (see 4.6).

Hypersensitivity to the active substances, to any of the excipients (see 6.1), or to other sulfonamide-derived substances (hydrochlorothiazide is a sulfonamide-derived substance).

The following contraindications are associated with hydrochlorothiazide:

- severe renal impairment (creatinine clearance < 30 ml/min),

- refractory hypokalaemia, hypercalcaemia,

- severe hepatic impairment, biliary cirrhosis and cholestasis.

4.4 Special warnings and special precautions for use

Hypotension - Volume-depleted patients: CoAprovel has been rarely associated with symptomatic hypotension in hypertensive patients without other risk factors for hypotension. Symptomatic hypotension may be expected to occur in patients who are volume and/or sodium depleted by vigorous diuretic therapy, dietary salt restriction, diarrhoea or vomiting. Such conditions should be corrected before initiating therapy with CoAprovel.

Renal artery stenosis - Renovascular hypertension: There is an increased risk of severe hypotension and renal insufficiency when patients with bilateral renal artery stenosis or stenosis of the artery to a single functioning kidney are treated with angiotensin converting enzyme inhibitors or angiotensin-II receptor antagonists. While this is not documented with CoAprovel, a similar effect should be anticipated.

Renal impairment and kidney transplantation: When CoAprovel is used in patients with impaired renal function, a periodic monitoring of potassium, creatinine and uric acid serum levels is recommended. There is no experience regarding the administration of CoAprovel in patients with a recent kidney transplantation. CoAprovel should not be used in patients with severe renal impairment (creatinine clearance < 30 ml/min) (see 4.3). Thiazide diuretic-associated azotaemia may occur in patients with impaired renal function. No dosage adjustment is necessary in patients with renal impairment whose creatinine clearance is ⩾ 30 ml/min. However, in patients with mild to moderate renal impairment (creatinine clearance ⩾ 30 ml/min but < 60 ml/min) this fixed dose combination should be administered with caution.

Hepatic impairment: Thiazides should be used with caution in patients with impaired hepatic function or progressive liver disease, since minor alterations of fluid and electrolyte balance may precipitate hepatic coma. There is no clinical experience with CoAprovel in patients with hepatic impairment.

Aortic and mitral valve stenosis, obstructive hypertrophic cardiomyopathy: As with other vasodilators, special caution is indicated in patients suffering from aortic or mitral stenosis, or obstructive hypertrophic cardiomyopathy.

Primary aldosteronism: Patients with primary aldosteronism generally will not respond to anti-hypertensive drugs acting through inhibition of the renin-angiotensin system. Therefore, the use of CoAprovel is not recommended.

Metabolic and endocrine effects: Thiazide therapy may impair glucose tolerance. In diabetic patients dosage adjustments of insulin or oral hypoglycaemic agents may be required. Latent diabetes mellitus may become manifest during thiazide therapy.

Increases in cholesterol and triglyceride levels have been associated with thiazide diuretic therapy; however at the 12.5 mg dose contained in CoAprovel, minimal or no effects were reported.

Hyperuricaemia may occur or frank gout may be precipitated in certain patients receiving thiazide therapy.

Electrolyte imbalance: As for any patient receiving diuretic therapy, periodic determination of serum electrolytes should be performed at appropriate intervals.

Thiazides, including hydrochlorothiazide, can cause fluid or electrolyte imbalance (hypokalaemia, hyponatraemia, and hypochloraemic alkalosis). Warning signs of fluid or electrolyte imbalance are dryness of mouth, thirst, weakness, lethargy, drowsiness, restlessness, muscle pain or cramps, muscular fatigue, hypotension, oliguria, tachycardia and gastrointestinal disturbances such as nausea or vomiting.

Although hypokalaemia may develop with the use of thiazide diuretics, concurrent therapy with irbesartan may reduce diuretic-induced hypokalaemia. The risk of hypokalaemia is greatest in patients with cirrhosis of the liver, in patients experiencing brisk diuresis, in patients who are receiving inadequate oral intake of electrolytes and in patients receiving concomitant therapy with corticosteroids or ACTH. Conversely, due to the irbesartan component of CoAprovel, hyperkalaemia might occur, especially in the presence of renal impairment and/or heart failure, and diabetes mellitus. Adequate monitoring of serum potassium in patients at risk is recommended. Potassium-sparing diuretics, potassium supplements or potassium-containing salts substitutes should be co-administered cautiously with CoAprovel (see 4.5).

There is no evidence that irbesartan would reduce or prevent diuretic-induced hyponatraemia. Chloride deficit is generally mild and usually does not require treatment.

Thiazides may decrease urinary calcium excretion and cause an intermittent and slight elevation of serum calcium in the absence of known disorders of calcium metabolism. Marked hypercalcaemia may be evidence of hidden hyperparathyroidism. Thiazides should be discontinued before carrying out tests for parathyroid function.

Thiazides have been shown to increase the urinary excretion of magnesium, which may result in hypomagnasaemia.

Lithium: The combination of lithium and CoAprovel is not recommended (see 4.5).

Anti-doping test: Hydrochlorothiazide contained in this medication could produce a positive analytic result in an anti-doping test.

General: In patients whose vascular tone and renal function depend predominantly on the activity of the renin-angiotensin-aldosterone system (e.g. patients with severe congestive heart failure or underlying renal disease, including renal artery stenosis), treatment with angiotensin converting enzyme inhibitors or angiotensin-II receptor antagonists that affect this system has been associated with acute hypotension, azotaemia, oliguria, or rarely acute renal failure. As with any anti-hypertensive agent, excessive blood pressure decrease in patients with ischaemic cardiopathy or ischaemic cardiovascular disease could result in a myocardial infarction or stroke.

Hypersensitivity reactions to hydrochlorothiazide may occur in patients with or without a history of allergy or bronchial asthma, but are more likely in patients with such a history.

Exacerbation or activation of systemic lupus erythematosus has been reported with the use of thiazide diuretics.

In the first trimester of pregnancy, CoAprovel is not recommended (see 4.6).

4.5 Interaction with other medicinal products and other forms of Interaction

Other antihypertensive agents The antihypertensive effect of CoAprovel may be increased with the concomitant use of other antihypertensive agents. Irbesartan and hydrochlorothiazide (at doses up to 300 mg irbesartan / 25 mg hydrochlorothiazide) have been safely administered with other antihypertensive agents including calcium channel blockers and beta-adrenergic blockers. Prior treatment with high dose diuretics may result in volume depletion and a risk of hypotension when initiating therapy with irbesartan with or without thiazide diuretics unless the volume depletion is corrected first (see 4.4).

Lithium

Reversible increases in serum lithium concentrations and toxicity have been reported during concomitant administration of lithium with angiotensin converting enzyme inhibitors. Similar effects have been very rarely reported with irbesartan. Furthermore, renal clearance of lithium is reduced by thiazides so the risk of lithium toxicity could be increased with CoAprovel. Therefore, the combination of lithium and CoAprovel is not recommended (see 4.4). If the combination proves necessary, careful monitoring of serum lithium is recommended.

Medicinal products affecting potassium: The potassium-depleting effect of hydrochlorothiazide is attenuated by the potassium-sparing effect of irbesartan. However, this effect of hydrochlorothiazide on serum potassium would be expected to be potentiated by other drugs associated with potassium loss and hypokalaemia (e.g. other kaliuretic diuretics, laxatives, amphotericin, carbenoxolone, penicillin G sodium). Conversely, based on the experience with the use of other drugs that blunt the renin-angiotensin system, concomitant use of potassium-sparing diuretics, potassium supplements, salt substitutes containing potassium or other drugs that may increase serum potassium levels (e.g. heparin sodium) may lead to increases in serum potassium. Adequate monitoring of serum potassium in patients at risk is recommended (see 4.4).

Medicinal products affected by serum potassium disturbances: Periodic monitoring of serum potassium is recommended when CoAprovel is administered with drugs affected by serum potassium disturbances (e.g. digitalis glycosides, antiarrhythmics).

Non-steroidal anti-inflammatory drugs: When angiotensin II antagonists are administered simultaneously with non-steroidal anti-inflammatory drugs (i.e. selective COX-2 inhibitors, acetylsalicylic acid >3 g/day) and non-selective NSAIDs), attenuation of the antihypertensive effect may occur.

As with ACE inhibitors, concomitant use of angiotensin II antagonists and NSAIDs may lead to an increased risk of worsening of renal failure, including possible acute renal failure, and an increase in serum potassium, especially in patients with poor pre-existing renal function. The combination should be administered with caution, especially in the elderly. Patients should be adequately hydrated and consideration should be given to monitoring renal function after initiation of concomitant therapy, and periodically thereafter.

Additional information on irbesartan interactions: In clinical studies, the pharmacokinetics of irbesartan are not affected by hydrochlorothiazide. Irbesartan is mainly metabolised by CYP2C9 and to a lesser extent by glucuronidation. No significant pharmacokinetic or pharmacodynamic interactions were observed when irbesartan was co-administered with warfarin, a drug metabolised by CYP2C9. The effects of *CYP2C9* inducers such as rifampicin on the pharmacokinetics of irbesartan have not been evaluated. The pharmacokinetics of digoxin were not altered by co-administration of irbesartan.

Additional information on hydrochlorothiazide interactions: When administered concurrently, the following drugs may interact with thiazide diuretics:

- *Alcohol:* potentiation of orthostatic hypotension may occur;

- *Antidiabetic drugs (oral agents and insulins):* dosage adjustment of the antidiabetic drug may be required (see 4.4);

- *Colestyramine and Colestipol resins:* absorption of hydrochlorothiazide is impaired in the presence of anionic exchange resins;

- *Corticosteroids, ACTH:* electrolyte depletion, particularly hypokalaemia, may be increased;

- *Digitalis glycosides:* thiazide induced hypokalaemia or hypomagnesaemia favour the onset of digitalis-induced cardiac arrhythmias (see 4.4);

- *Non-steroidal anti-inflammatory drugs:* the administration of a non-steroidal anti-inflammatory drug may reduce the diuretic, natriuretic and antihypertensive effects of thiazide diuretics in some patients;

- *Pressor amines (e.g. noradrenaline):* the effect of pressor amines may be decreased, but not sufficiently to preclude their use;

- *Nondepolarizing skeletal muscle relaxants (e.g. tubocurarine):* the effect of nondepolarizing skeletal muscle relaxants may be potentiated by hydrochlorothiazide;

- *Anti-gout medication:* dosage adjustments of antigout medications may be necessary as hydrochlorothiazide may raise the level of serum uric acid. Increase in dosage of probenecid or sulfinpyrazone may be necessary. Co-administration of thiazide diuretics may increase the incidence of hypersensitivity reactions to allopurinol;

- *Calcium salts:* thiazide diuretics may increase serum calcium levels due to decreased excretion. If calcium supplements or calcium sparing drugs (e.g. Vitamin D therapy) must be prescribed, serum calcium levels should be monitored and calcium dosage adjusted accordingly;

- *Other interactions:* the hyperglycaemic effect of beta-blockers and diazoxide may be enhanced by thiazides. Anticholinergic agents (e.g. atropine, beperiden) may increase the bioavailability of thiazide-type diuretics by decreasing gastrointestinal motility and stomach emptying rate. Thiazides may increase the risk of adverse effects caused by amantadine. Thiazides may reduce the renal excretion of cytotoxic drugs (e.g. cyclophosphamide, methotrexate) and potentiate their myelosuppressive effects.

4.6 Pregnancy and lactation

Pregnancy: See sections 4.3 and 4.4.

Thiazides cross the placental barrier and appear in cord blood. They may cause decreased placental perfusion, foetal electrolyte disturbances and possibly other reactions that have occurred in the adults. Cases of neonatal thrombocytopenia, or foetal or neonatal jaundice have been reported with maternal thiazide therapy. Since CoAprovel contains hydrochlorothiazide, it is not recommended during the first trimester of pregnancy. A switch to a suitable alternative treatment should be carried out in advance of a planned pregnancy.

In the second and third trimesters, substances that act directly on the renin-angiotensin-system can cause foetal or neonatal renal failure, foetal skull hypoplasia and even foetal death. Therefore, CoAprovel is contra-indicated in the second and third trimesters of pregnancy. If pregnancy is diagnosed, CoAprovel should be discontinued as soon as possible, skull and renal function should be checked with echography if, inadvertently, the treatment was taken for a long period.

Lactation: because of the potential adverse effects on the nursing infant, CoAprovel is contraindicated during lactation (see 4.3). It is not known if irbesartan is excreted in human milk. It is excreted in the milk of lactating rats. Thiazides appear in human milk and may inhibit lactation.

4.7 Effects on ability to drive and use machines

The effect of CoAprovel on ability to drive and use machines has not been studied, but based on its pharmacodynamic properties, CoAprovel is unlikely to affect this ability. When driving vehicles or operating machines, it should be taken into account that occasionally dizziness or weariness may occur during treatment of hypertension.

4.8 Undesirable effects

The frequency of adverse reactions listed below is defined using the following convention: very common (⩾ 1/10); common (⩾ 1/100, < 1/10); uncommon (⩾ 1/1,000, < 1/100); rare (⩾ 1/10,000, < 1/1,000); very rare (< 1/10,000).

Irbesartan/hydrochlorothiazide combination:

In placebo-controlled trials in patients with hypertension, the overall incidence of adverse events did not differ between the irbesartan / hydrochlorothiazide and the placebo groups. Discontinuation due to any clinical or laboratory adverse event was less frequent for irbesartan / hydrochlorothiazide-treated patients than for placebo-treated patients. The incidence of adverse events was not related to gender, age, race, or dose within the recommended dose range. In placebo-controlled trials in which 898 hypertensive patients received various doses (range: 37.5mg/6.25mg to 300 mg/25mg irbesartan / hydrochlorothiazide), the following adverse reactions were reported:

<u>Nervous system disorders:</u>

Common: dizziness

Uncommon: orthostatic dizziness

Cardiac disorders:

Uncommon: hypotension, oedema, syncope, tachycardia

Vascular disorders:

Uncommon: flushing

Gastrointestinal disorders:

Common: nausea/vomiting

Uncommon: diarrhoea

Musculoskeletal, connective tissue and bone disorders:

Uncommon: swelling extremity

Renal and urinary disorders:

Common: abnormal urination

Reproductive system and breast disorders:

Uncommon: libido changes, sexual dysfunction

General disorders and administration site conditions:

Common: fatigue

Investigations: patients treated with irbesartan / hydrochlorothiazide had changes in laboratory test parameters which were rarely clinically significant

Common: increases in BUN, creatinine and creatine kinase

Uncommon: decreases in serum potassium and sodium

In addition, since introduction of irbesartan / hydrochlorothiazide in the market the following adverse reactions have also been reported:

Immune system disorders:

Rare: as with other angiotensin-II receptor antagonists, rare cases of hypersensitivity reactions such as angioedema, rash, urticaria have been reported

Metabolism and nutrition disorders:

Very rare: hyperkalaemia

Nervous system disorders:

Very rare: headache

Ear and labyrinth disorders:

Very rare: tinnitus

Respiratory, thoracic and mediastinal disorders:

Very rare: cough

Gastrointestinal disorders:

Very rare: dysgeusia, dyspepsia

Hepato-biliary disorders:

Very rare: abnormal liver function, hepatitis

Musculoskeletal, connective tissue and bone disorders:

Very rare: arthralgia, myalgia

Renal and urinary disorders:

Very rare: impaired renal function including isolated cases of renal failure in patients at risk (see 4.4)

Additional information on individual components: in addition to the adverse reactions listed above for the combination product, other undesirable effects previously reported with one of the individual components may be potential undesirable effects with CoAprovel.

Irbesartan:

General disorders and administration site conditions:

Uncommon: chest pain

Hydrochlorothiazide:

Adverse events (regardless of relationship to drug) reported with the use of hydrochlorothiazide alone include:

Blood and lymphatic system:

aplastic anaemia, bone marrow depression, haemolytic anaemia, leucopenia, neutropenia/agranulocytosis, thrombocytopenia

Psychiatric disorders:

depression, sleep disturbances

Nervous system disorders:

light-headedness, paraesthesia, restlessness, vertigo

Eye disorders:

transient blurred vision, xanthopsia

Cardiac disorders:

cardiac arrhythmias

Vascular disorders:

postural hypotension

Respiratory, thoracic and mediastinal disorders:

respiratory distress (including pneumonitis and pulmonary oedema)

Gastrointestinal disorders:

pancreatitis, anorexia, constipation, diarrhoea, gastric irritation, loss of appetite, sialadenitis

Hepatobiliary disorders:

jaundice (intrahepatic cholestatic jaundice)

Skin and subcutaneous tissue disorders:

anaphylactic reactions, toxic epidermal necrolysis, cutaneous lupus erythematosus-like reactions, necrotizing angiitis (vasculitis, cutaneous vasculitis), photosensitivity reactions, rash, reactivation of cutaneous lupus erythematosus, urticaria

Musculoskeletal, connective tissue and bone disorders:

muscle spasm, weakness

Renal and urinary disorders:

interstitial nephritis, renal dysfunction

General disorders and administration site conditions:

fever

Investigations:

electrolyte imbalance (including hypokalaemia and hyponatraemia, see 4.4), glycosuria, hyperglycaemia, hyperuricaemia, increases in cholesterol and triglycerides

The dose dependent side effects of hydrochlorothiazide (particularly electrolyte disturbances) may increase when titrating the hydrochlorothiazide.

4.9 Overdose

No specific information is available on the treatment of overdosage with CoAprovel. The patient should be closely monitored, and the treatment should be symptomatic and supportive. Management depends on the time since ingestion and the severity of the symptoms. Suggested measures include induction of emesis and/or gastric lavage. Activated charcoal may be useful in the treatment of overdosage. Serum electrolytes and creatinine should be monitored frequently. If hypotension occurs, the patient should be placed in a supine position, with salt and volume replacements given quickly.

The most likely manifestations of irbesartan overdosage are expected to be hypotension and tachycardia; bradycardia might also occur.

Overdosage with hydrochlorothiazide is associated with electrolyte depletion (hypokalaemia, hypochloraemia, hyponatraemia) and dehydration resulting from excessive diuresis. The most common signs and symptoms of overdosage are nausea and somnolence. Hypokalaemia may result in muscle spasms and/or accentuate cardiac arrhythmias associated with the concomitant use of digitalis glycosides or certain anti-arrhythmic drugs.

Irbesartan is not removed by haemodialysis. The degree to which hydrochlorothiazide is removed by haemodialysis has not been established.

5. PHARMACOLOGICAL PROPERTIES

5.1 Pharmacodynamic properties

Pharmacotherapeutic group: angiotensin-II antagonists, combinations: ATC code C09D A04.

CoAprovel is a combination of an angiotensin-II receptor antagonist, irbesartan, and a thiazide diuretic, hydrochlorothiazide. The combination of these ingredients has an additive antihypertensive effect, reducing blood pressure to a greater degree than either component alone.

Irbesartan is a potent, orally active, selective angiotensin-II receptor (AT_1 subtype) antagonist. It is expected to block all actions of angiotensin-II mediated by the AT_1 receptor, regardless of the source or route of synthesis of angiotensin-II. The selective antagonism of the angiotensin-II (AT_1) receptors results in increases in plasma renin levels and angiotensin-II levels, and a decrease in plasma aldosterone concentration. Serum potassium levels are not significantly affected by irbesartan alone at the recommended doses in patients without risk of electrolyte imbalance (see 4.4 and 4.5). Irbesartan does not inhibit ACE (kininase-II), an enzyme which generates angiotensin-II and also degrades bradykinin into inactive metabolites. Irbesartan does not require metabolic activation for its activity.

Hydrochlorothiazide is a thiazide diuretic. The mechanism of antihypertensive effect of thiazide diuretics is not fully known. Thiazides affect the renal tubular mechanisms of electrolyte reabsorption, directly increasing excretion of sodium and chloride in approximately equivalent amounts. The diuretic action of hydrochlorothiazide reduces plasma volume, increases plasma renin activity, increases aldosterone secretion, with consequent increases in urinary potassium and bicarbonate loss, and decreases in serum potassium. Presumably through blockade of the renin-angiotensin-aldosterone system, co-administration of irbesartan tends to reverse the potassium loss associated with these diuretics. With hydrochlorothiazide, onset of diuresis occurs in 2 hours, and peak effect occurs at about 4 hours, while the action persists for approximately 6-12 hours.

The combination of hydrochlorothiazide and irbesartan produces dose-related additive reductions in blood pressure across their therapeutic dose ranges. The addition of 12.5 mg hydrochlorothiazide to 300 mg irbesartan once daily in patients not adequately controlled on 300 mg irbesartan alone resulted in further placebo-corrected diastolic blood pressure reductions at trough (24 hours post-dosing) of 6.1 mm Hg. The combination of 300 mg irbesartan and 12.5 mg hydrochlorothiazide resulted in an overall placebo-subtracted systolic/diastolic reduction of up to 13.6/11.5 mm Hg.

Limited clinical data (7 out of 22 patients) suggest that patients not controlled with the 300/12.5 combination may respond when uptitrated to 300/25. In these patients, an incremental blood pressure lowering effect was observed for both SBP and DBP (13.3 and 8.3 mm Hg, respectively).

Once daily dosing with 150 mg irbesartan and 12.5 mg hydrochlorothiazide gave systolic/diastolic mean placebo-adjusted blood pressure reductions at trough (24 hours post-dosing) of 12.9/6.9 mm Hg in patients with mild-to-moderate hypertension. Peak effects occurred at 3-6 hours. When assessed by ambulatory blood pressure monitoring, the combination 150 mg irbesartan and 12.5 mg hydrochlorothiazide once daily produced consistent reduction in blood pressure over the 24 hours period with mean 24-hour placebo-subtracted systolic/diastolic reductions of 15.8/10.0 mm Hg. When measured by ambulatory blood pressure monitoring, the trough to peak effects of CoAprovel 150/12.5 mg were 100%. The trough to peak effects measured by cuff during office visits were 68% and 76% for CoAprovel 150/12.5 mg and CoAprovel 300/12.5 mg, respectively. These 24-hour effects were observed without excessive blood pressure lowering at peak and are consistent with safe and effective blood-pressure lowering over the once-daily dosing interval.

In patients not adequately controlled on 25 mg hydrochlorothiazide alone, the addition of irbesartan gave an added placebo-subtracted systolic/diastolic mean reduction of 11.1/7.2 mm Hg.

The blood pressure lowering effect of irbesartan in combination with hydrochlorothiazide is apparent after the first dose and substantially present within 1-2 weeks, with the maximal effect occurring by 6-8 weeks. In long-term follow-up studies, the effect of irbesartan / hydrochlorothiazide was maintained for over one year. Although not specifically studied with the CoAprovel, rebound hypertension has not been seen with either irbesartan or hydrochlorothiazide.

The effect of the combination of irbesartan and hydrochlorothiazide on morbidity and mortality has not been studied. Epidemiological studies have shown that long term treatment with hydrochlorothiazide reduces the risk of cardiovascular mortality and morbidity.

There is no difference in response to CoAprovel, regardless of age or gender. When irbesartan is administered concomitantly with a low dose of hydrochlorothiazide (e.g. 12.5 mg daily), the antihypertensive response in black patients approaches that of non-black patients.

5.2 Pharmacokinetic properties

Concomitant administration of hydrochlorothiazide and irbesartan has no effect on the pharmacokinetics of either drug.

Irbesartan and hydrochlorothiazide are orally active agents and do not require biotransformation for their activity. Following oral administration of CoAprovel, the absolute oral bioavailability is 60-80% and 50-80% for irbesartan and hydrochlorothiazide, respectively. Food does not affect the bioavailability of CoAprovel. Peak plasma concentration occurs at 1.5-2 hours after oral administration for irbesartan and 1-2.5 hours for hydrochlorothiazide.

Plasma protein binding of irbesartan is approximately 96%, with negligible binding to cellular blood components. The volume of distribution for irbesartan is 53-93 litres. Hydrochlorothiazide is 68% protein-bound in the plasma, and its apparent volume of distribution is 0.83-1.14 l/kg.

Irbesartan exhibits linear and dose proportional pharmacokinetics over the dose range of 10 to 600 mg. A less than proportional increase in oral absorption at doses beyond 600 mg was observed; the mechanism for this is unknown. The total body and renal clearance are 157-176 and 3.0-3.5 ml/min, respectively. The terminal elimination half-life of irbesartan is 11-15 hours. Steady-state plasma concentrations are attained within 3 days after initiation of a once-daily dosing regimen. Limited accumulation of irbesartan ($< 20\%$) is observed in plasma upon repeated once-daily dosing. In a study, somewhat higher plasma concentrations of irbesartan were observed in female hypertensive patients. However, there was no difference in the half-life and accumulation of irbesartan. No dosage adjustment is necessary in female patients. Irbesartan AUC and C_{max} values were also somewhat greater in elderly subjects ($\geqslant$ 65 years) than those of young subjects (18-40 years). However the terminal half-life was not significantly altered. No dosage adjustment is necessary in elderly patients. The mean plasma half-life of hydrochlorothiazide reportedly ranges from 5-15 hours.

Following oral or intravenous administration of ^{14}C irbesartan, 80-85% of the circulating plasma radioactivity is attributable to unchanged irbesartan. Irbesartan is metabolised by the liver via glucuronide conjugation and oxidation. The major circulating metabolite is irbesartan glucuronide (approximately 6%). *In vitro* studies indicate that irbesartan is primarily oxidised by the cytochrome P450 enzyme *CYP2C9*; isoenzyme *CYP3A4* has negligible effect. Irbesartan and its metabolites are eliminated by both biliary and renal pathways. After either oral or IV administration of ^{14}C irbesartan, about 20% of the radioactivity is recovered in the urine, and the remainder in the faeces. Less than 2% of the dose is excreted in the urine as unchanged irbesartan. Hydrochlorothiazide is not metabolized but is eliminated rapidly by the kidneys. At least 61% of the oral dose is eliminated unchanged within 24 hours. Hydrochlorothiazide crosses the placental but not the blood-brain barrier, and is excreted in breast milk.

Renal impairment: In patients with renal impairment or those undergoing haemodialysis, the pharmacokinetic parameters of irbesartan are not significantly altered. Irbesartan is not removed by haemodialysis. In patients with creatinine clearance < 20 ml/min, the elimination half-life of hydrochlorothiazide was reported to increase to 21 hours.

Hepatic impairment: In patients with mild to moderate cirrhosis, the pharmacokinetic parameters of irbesartan are not significantly altered. Studies have not been performed in patients with severe hepatic impairment.

5.3 Preclinical safety data

Irbesartan/hydrochlorothiazide: The potential toxicity of the irbesartan / hydrochlorothiazide combination after oral administration was evaluated in rats and macaques in studies lasting up to 6 months. There were no toxicological findings observed of relevance to human therapeutic use.

The following changes, observed in rats and macaques receiving the irbesartan / hydrochlorothiazide combination at 10/10 and 90/90 mg/kg/day, were also seen with one of the two drugs alone and/or were secondary to decreases in blood pressure (no significant toxicological interactions were observed):

- kidney changes, characterized by slight increases in serum urea and creatinine, and hyperplasia / hypertrophy of the juxtaglomerular apparatus, which are a direct consequence of the interaction of irbesartan with the renin-angiotensin system;

- slight decreases in erythrocyte parameters (erythrocytes, haemoglobin, haematocrit);

- stomach discoloration, ulcers and focal necrosis of gastric mucosa were observed in few rats in a 6 months toxicity study at irbesartan 90 mg/kg/day, hydrochlorothiazide 90 mg/kg/day, and irbesartan / hydrochlorothiazide 10/10 mg/kg/day. These lesions were not observed in macaques;

- decreases in serum potassium due to hydrochlorothiazide and partly prevented when hydrochlorothiazide was given in combination with irbesartan.

Most of the above mentioned effects appear to be due to the pharmacological activity of irbesartan (blockade of angiotensin-II-induced inhibition of renin release, with stimulation of the renin-producing cells) and occur also with angiotensin converting enzyme inhibitors. These findings appear to have no relevance to the use of therapeutic doses of irbesartan / hydrochlorothiazide in humans.

No teratogenic effects were seen in rats given irbesartan and hydrochlorothiazide in combination at doses that produced maternal toxicity. The effects of the irbesartan / hydrochlorothiazide combination on fertility have not been evaluated in animal studies, as there is no evidence of adverse effect on fertility in animals or humans with either irbesartan or hydrochlorothiazide when administered alone. However, another angiotensin-II antagonist affected fertility parameters in animal studies when given alone. These findings were also observed with lower doses of this other angiotensin-II antagonist when given in combination with hydrochlorothiazide.

There was no evidence of mutagenicity or clastogenicity with the irbesartan / hydrochlorothiazide combination. The carcinogenic potential of irbesartan and hydrochlorothiazide in combination has not been evaluated in animal studies.

Irbesartan: There was no evidence of abnormal systemic or target organ toxicity at clinically relevant doses. In preclinical safety studies, high doses of irbesartan (⩾ 250 mg/kg/day in rats and ⩾ 100 mg/kg/day in macaques) caused a reduction of red blood cell parameters (erythrocytes, haemoglobin, haematocrit). At very high doses (⩾ 500 mg/kg/day) degenerative changes in the kidneys (such as interstitial nephritis, tubular distension, basophilic tubules, increased plasma concentrations of urea and creatinine) were induced by irbesartan in the rat and the macaque and are considered secondary to the hypotensive effects of the drug which led to decreased renal perfusion. Furthermore, irbesartan induced hyperplasia / hypertrophy of the juxtaglomerular cells (in rats at ⩾ 90 mg/kg/day, in macaques at ⩾ 10 mg/kg/day). All of these changes were considered to be caused by the pharmacological action of irbesartan. For therapeutic doses of irbesartan in humans, the hyperplasia / hypertrophy of the renal juxtaglomerular cells does not appear to have any relevance.

There was no evidence of mutagenicity, clastogenicity or carcinogenicity.

Animal studies with irbesartan showed transient toxic effects (increased renal pelvic cavitation, hydroureter or subcutaneous oedema) in rat foetuses, which were resolved after birth. In rabbits, abortion or early resorption was noted at doses causing significant maternal toxicity, including mortality. No teratogenic effects were observed in the rat or rabbit.

Hydrochlorothiazide: Although equivocal evidence for a genotoxic or carcinogenic effect was found in some experimental models, the extensive human experience with hydrochlorothiazide has failed to show an association between its use and an increase in neoplasms.

6. PHARMACEUTICAL PARTICULARS

6.1 List of excipients

Tablet core: lactose monohydrate, microcrystalline cellulose, croscarmellose sodium, hypromellose, silicon dioxide, magnesium stearate.

Film-coating: lactose monohydrate, hypromellose, titanium dioxide (E171), macrogol, red and yellow ferric oxides (E172) carnauba wax.

6.2 Incompatibilities

Not applicable.

6.3 Shelf life

3 years.

6.4 Special precautions for storage

Do not store above 30°C.

Store in the original package.

6.5 Nature and contents of container

CoAprovel film-coated tablets are packaged in cartons containing 28 tablets in PVC/PVDC/aluminium blisters.

6.6 Instructions for use and handling

No special requirements.

7. MARKETING AUTHORISATION HOLDER

SANOFI PHARMA BRISTOL-MYERS SQUIBB SNC

174 avenue de France

F-75013 Paris - France

8. MARKETING AUTHORISATION NUMBER(S)

CoAprovel 150/12.5mg film-coated tablets: EU/1/98/086/012

CoAprovel 300/12.5mg film-coated tablets: EU/1/98/086/017

9. DATE OF FIRST AUTHORISATION/RENEWAL OF THE AUTHORISATION

02 March 2004

10. DATE OF REVISION OF THE TEXT

28 October 2004

Legal Category: POM

CoAprovel Film-Coated Tablets

(Sanofi Pharma Bristol-Myers Squibb SNC)

1. NAME OF THE MEDICINAL PRODUCT

CoAprovel 150/12.5 mg film-coated tablets

CoAprovel 300/12.5 mg film-coated tablets

2. QUALITATIVE AND QUANTITATIVE COMPOSITION

Each film-coated tablet contains either 150 mg irbesartan and 12.5 mg hydrochlorothiazide or 300mg irbesartan with 12.5 mg hydrochlorothiazide.

For excipients, see 6.1.

3. PHARMACEUTICAL FORM

Film-coated tablet.

Peach, biconvex, oval-shaped, with a heart debossed on one side. On the other side, the number 2875 is engraved on the 150/12.5mg tablet and the number 2876 on the 300/12.5mg tablet.

4. CLINICAL PARTICULARS

4.1 Therapeutic indications

Treatment of essential hypertension.

This fixed dose combination is indicated in patients whose blood pressure is not adequately controlled on irbesartan or hydrochlorothiazide alone.

4.2 Posology and method of administration

CoAprovel can be used once daily, with or without food in patients whose blood pressure is not adequately controlled by irbesartan or hydrochlorothiazide alone.

Dose titration with the individual components (i.e. irbesartan and hydrochlorothiazide) can be recommended.

When clinically appropriate direct change from monotherapy to the fixed combinations may be considered:

- CoAprovel 150/12.5 mg may be administered in patients whose blood pressure is not adequately controlled with hydrochlorothiazide or irbesartan 150 mg alone;

- CoAprovel 300/12.5 mg may be administered in patients insufficiently controlled by irbesartan 300 mg or by CoAprovel 150/12.5 mg.

- CoAprovel 300/25 mg may be administered in patients insufficiently controlled by CoAprovel 300/12.5 mg.

Doses higher than 300 mg irbesartan / 25 mg hydrochlorothiazide once daily are not recommended.

When necessary, CoAprovel may be administered with another antihypertensive drug (see 4.5).

Renal impairment: Due to the hydrochlorothiazide component, CoAprovel is not recommended for patients with severe renal dysfunction (creatinine clearance < 30 ml/min). Loop diuretics are preferred to thiazides in this population. No dosage adjustment is necessary in patients with renal impairment whose renal creatinine clearance is ⩾ 30 ml/min (see 4.3 and 4.4).

Intravascular volume depletion: Volume and/or sodium depletion should be corrected prior to administration of CoAprovel.

Hepatic impairment: CoAprovel is not indicated in patients with severe hepatic impairment. Thiazides should be used with caution in patients with impaired hepatic function. No dosage adjustment of CoAprovel is necessary in patients with mild to moderate hepatic impairment (see 4.3).

Elderly patients: No dosage adjustment of CoAprovel is necessary in elderly patients.

Children: Safety and efficacy of CoAprovel have not been established in children (< 18 years).

4.3 Contraindications

Second and third trimester of pregnancy (see 4.6).

Lactation (see 4.6).

Hypersensitivity to the active substances, to any of the excipients (see 6.1), or to other sulfonamide-derived substances (hydrochlorothiazide is a sulfonamide-derived substance).

The following contraindications are associated with hydrochlorothiazide:

- severe renal impairment (creatinine clearance < 30 ml/min),

- refractory hypokalaemia, hypercalcaemia,

- severe hepatic impairment, biliary cirrhosis and cholestasis.

4.4 Special warnings and special precautions for use

Hypotension - Volume-depleted patients: CoAprovel has been rarely associated with symptomatic hypotension in hypertensive patients without other risk factors for hypotension. Symptomatic hypotension may be expected to occur in patients who are volume and/or sodium depleted by vigorous diuretic therapy, dietary salt restriction, diarrhoea or vomiting. Such conditions should be corrected before initiating therapy with CoAprovel.

Renal artery stenosis - Renovascular hypertension: There is an increased risk of severe hypotension and renal insufficiency when patients with bilateral renal artery stenosis or stenosis of the artery to a single functioning kidney are treated with angiotensin converting enzyme inhibitors or angiotensin-II receptor antagonists. While this is not documented with CoAprovel, a similar effect should be anticipated.

Renal impairment and kidney transplantation: When CoAprovel is used in patients with impaired renal function, a periodic monitoring of potassium, creatinine and uric acid serum levels is recommended. There is no experience regarding the administration of CoAprovel in patients with a recent kidney transplantation. CoAprovel should not be used in patients with severe renal impairment (creatinine clearance < 30 ml/min) (see 4.3). Thiazide diuretic-associated azotaemia may occur in patients with impaired renal function. No dosage adjustment is necessary in patients with renal impairment whose creatinine clearance is ⩾ 30 ml/min. However, in patients with mild to moderate renal impairment (creatinine clearance ⩾ 30 ml/min but < 60 ml/min) this fixed dose combination should be administered with caution.

Hepatic impairment: Thiazides should be used with caution in patients with impaired hepatic function or progressive liver disease, since minor alterations of fluid and electrolyte balance may precipitate hepatic coma. There is no clinical experience with CoAprovel in patients with hepatic impairment.

Aortic and mitral valve stenosis, obstructive hypertrophic cardiomyopathy: As with other vasodilators, special caution is indicated in patients suffering from aortic or mitral stenosis, or obstructive hypertrophic cardiomyopathy.

Primary aldosteronism: Patients with primary aldosteronism generally will not respond to anti-hypertensive drugs acting through inhibition of the renin-angiotensin system. Therefore, the use of CoAprovel is not recommended.

Metabolic and endocrine effects: Thiazide therapy may impair glucose tolerance. In diabetic patients dosage adjustments of insulin or oral hypoglycaemic agents may be required. Latent diabetes mellitus may become manifest during thiazide therapy.

Increases in cholesterol and triglyceride levels have been associated with thiazide diuretic therapy; however at the 12.5 mg dose contained in CoAprovel, minimal or no effects were reported.

Hyperuricaemia may occur or frank gout may be precipitated in certain patients receiving thiazide therapy.

Electrolyte imbalance: As for any patient receiving diuretic therapy, periodic determination of serum electrolytes should be performed at appropriate intervals.

Thiazides, including hydrochlorothiazide, can cause fluid or electrolyte imbalance (hypokalaemia, hyponatraemia, and hypochloraemic alkalosis). Warning signs of fluid or electrolyte imbalance are dryness of mouth, thirst, weakness, lethargy, drowsiness, restlessness, muscle pain or cramps, muscular fatigue, hypotension, oliguria, tachycardia and gastrointestinal disturbances such as nausea or vomiting.

Although hypokalaemia may develop with the use of thiazide diuretics, concurrent therapy with irbesartan may reduce diuretic-induced hypokalaemia. The risk of hypokalaemia is greatest in patients with cirrhosis of the liver, in patients experiencing brisk diuresis, in patients who are receiving inadequate oral intake of electrolytes and in patients receiving concomitant therapy with corticosteroids or ACTH. Conversely, due to the irbesartan component of CoAprovel, hyperkalaemia might occur, especially in the presence of renal impairment and/or heart failure, and diabetes mellitus. Adequate monitoring of serum potassium in patients at risk is recommended. Potassium-sparing diuretics, potassium supplements or potassium-containing salts substitutes should be co-administered cautiously with CoAprovel (see 4.5).

There is no evidence that irbesartan would reduce or prevent diuretic-induced hyponatraemia. Chloride deficit is generally mild and usually does not require treatment.

Thiazides may decrease urinary calcium excretion and cause an intermittent and slight elevation of serum calcium in the absence of known disorders of calcium metabolism. Marked hypercalcaemia may be evidence of hidden hyperparathyroidism. Thiazides should be discontinued before carrying out tests for parathyroid function.

Thiazides have been shown to increase the urinary excretion of magnesium, which may result in hypomagnasaemia.

Lithium: The combination of lithium and CoAprovel is not recommended (see 4.5).

Anti-doping test: Hydrochlorothiazide contained in this medication could produce a positive analytic result in an anti-doping test.

General: In patients whose vascular tone and renal function depend predominantly on the activity of the renin-angiotensin-aldosterone system (e.g. patients with severe congestive heart failure or underlying renal disease, including renal artery stenosis), treatment with angiotensin converting enzyme inhibitors or angiotensin-II receptor antagonists that affect this system has been associated with acute hypotension, azotaemia, oliguria, or rarely acute renal failure. As with any anti-hypertensive agent, excessive blood pressure decrease in patients with ischaemic cardiopathy or ischaemic cardiovascular disease could result in a myocardial infarction or stroke.

Hypersensitivity reactions to hydrochlorothiazide may occur in patients with or without a history of allergy or bronchial asthma, but are more likely in patients with such a history.

Exacerbation or activation of systemic lupus erythematosus has been reported with the use of thiazide diuretics.

In the first trimester of pregnancy, CoAprovel is not recommended (see 4.6).

4.5 Interaction with other medicinal products and other forms of Interaction

Other antihypertensive agents The antihypertensive effect of CoAprovel may be increased with the concomitant use of other antihypertensive agents. Irbesartan and hydrochlorothiazide (at doses up to 300 mg irbesartan / 25 mg hydrochlorothiazide) have been safely administered with other antihypertensive agents including calcium channel blockers and beta-adrenergic blockers. Prior treatment with high dose diuretics may result in volume depletion and a risk of hypotension when initiating therapy with irbesartan with or without thiazide diuretics unless the volume depletion is corrected first (see 4.4).

Lithium

Reversible increases in serum lithium concentrations and toxicity have been reported during concomitant administration of lithium with angiotensin converting enzyme inhibitors. Similar effects have been very rarely reported with irbesartan. Furthermore, renal clearance of lithium is reduced by thiazides so the risk of lithium toxicity could be increased with CoAprovel. Therefore, the combination of lithium and CoAprovel is not recommended (see 4.4). If the combination proves necessary, careful monitoring of serum lithium is recommended.

Medicinal products affecting potassium: The potassium-depleting effect of hydrochlorothiazide is attenuated by the potassium-sparing effect of irbesartan. However, this effect of hydrochlorothiazide on serum potassium would be expected to be potentiated by other drugs associated with potassium loss and hypokalaemia (e.g. other kaliuretic diuretics, laxatives, amphotericin, carbenoxolone, penicillin G sodium). Conversely, based on the experience with the use of other drugs that blunt the renin-angiotensin system, concomitant use of potassium-sparing diuretics, potassium supplements, salt substitutes containing potassium or other drugs that may increase serum potassium levels (e.g. heparin sodium) may lead to increases in serum potassium. Adequate monitoring of serum potassium in patients at risk is recommended (see 4.4).

Medicinal products affected by serum potassium disturbances: Periodic monitoring of serum potassium is recommended when CoAprovel is administered with drugs affected by serum potassium disturbances (e.g. digitalis glycosides, antiarrhythmics).

Non-steroidal anti-inflammatory drugs: When angiotensin II antagonists are administered simultaneously with non-steroidal anti-inflammatory drugs (i.e. selective COX-2 inhibitors, acetylsalicylic acid >3 g/day) and non-selective NSAIDs), attenuation of the antihypertensive effect may occur.

As with ACE inhibitors, concomitant use of angiotensin II antagonists and NSAIDs may lead to an increased risk of worsening of renal failure, including possible acute renal failure, and an increase in serum potassium, especially in patients with poor pre-existing renal function. The combination should be administered with caution, especially in the elderly. Patients should be adequately hydrated and consideration should be given to monitoring renal function after initiation of concomitant therapy, and periodically thereafter.

Additional information on irbesartan interactions: In clinical studies, the pharmacokinetics of irbesartan are not affected by hydrochlorothiazide. Irbesartan is mainly metabolised by CYP2C9 and to a lesser extent by glucuronidation. No significant pharmacokinetic or pharmacodynamic interactions were observed when irbesartan was co-administered with warfarin, a drug metabolised by CYP2C9. The effects of *CYP2C9* inducers such as rifampicin on the pharmacokinetics of irbesartan have not been evaluated. The pharmacokinetics of digoxin were not altered by co-administration of irbesartan.

Additional information on hydrochlorothiazide interactions: When administered concurrently, the following drugs may interact with thiazide diuretics:

- *Alcohol:* potentiation of orthostatic hypotension may occur;

- *Antidiabetic drugs (oral agents and insulins):* dosage adjustment of the antidiabetic drug may be required (see 4.4);

- *Colestyramine and Colestipol resins:* absorption of hydrochlorothiazide is impaired in the presence of anionic exchange resins;

- *Corticosteroids, ACTH:* electrolyte depletion, particularly hypokalaemia, may be increased;

- *Digitalis glycosides:* thiazide induced hypokalaemia or hypomagnesaemia favour the onset of digitalis-induced cardiac arrhythmias (see 4.4);

- *Non-steroidal anti-inflammatory drugs:* the administration of a non-steroidal anti-inflammatory drug may reduce the diuretic, natriuretic and antihypertensive effects of thiazide diuretics in some patients;

- *Pressor amines (e.g. noradrenaline):* the effect of pressor amines may be decreased, but not sufficiently to preclude their use;

- *Nondepolarizing skeletal muscle relaxants (e.g. tubocurarine):* the effect of nondepolarizing skeletal muscle relaxants may be potentiated by hydrochlorothiazide;

- *Anti-gout medication:* dosage adjustments of antigout medications may be necessary as hydrochlorothiazide may raise the level of serum uric acid. Increase in dosage of probenecid or sulfinpyrazone may be necessary. Co-administration of thiazide diuretics may increase the incidence of hypersensitivity reactions to allopurinol;

- *Calcium salts:* thiazide diuretics may increase serum calcium levels due to decreased excretion. If calcium supplements or calcium sparing drugs (e.g. Vitamin D therapy) must be prescribed, serum calcium levels should be monitored and calcium dosage adjusted accordingly;

- *Other interactions:* the hyperglycaemic effect of beta-blockers and diazoxide may be enhanced by thiazides. Anticholinergic agents (e.g. atropine, beperiden) may increase the bioavailability of thiazide-type diuretics by decreasing gastrointestinal motility and stomach emptying rate. Thiazides may increase the risk of adverse effects caused by amantadine. Thiazides may reduce the renal excretion of cytotoxic drugs (e.g. cyclophosphamide, methotrexate) and potentiate their myelosuppressive effects.

4.6 Pregnancy and lactation

Pregnancy: See sections 4.3 and 4.4.

Thiazides cross the placental barrier and appear in cord blood. They may cause decreased placental perfusion, foetal electrolyte disturbances and possibly other reactions that have occurred in the adults. Cases of neonatal thrombocytopenia, or foetal or neonatal jaundice have been reported with maternal thiazide therapy. Since CoAprovel contains hydrochlorothiazide, it is not recommended during the first trimester of pregnancy. A switch to a suitable alternative treatment should be carried out in advance of a planned pregnancy.

In the second and third trimesters, substances that act directly on the renin-angiotensin-system can cause foetal or neonatal renal failure, foetal skull hypoplasia and even foetal death. Therefore, CoAprovel is contra-indicated in the second and third trimesters of pregnancy. If pregnancy is diagnosed, CoAprovel should be discontinued as soon as possible, skull and renal function should be checked with echography if, inadvertently, the treatment was taken for a long period.

Lactation: because of the potential adverse effects on the nursing infant, CoAprovel is contraindicated during lactation (see 4.3). It is not known if irbesartan is excreted in human milk. It is excreted in the milk of lactating rats. Thiazides appear in human milk and may inhibit lactation.

4.7 Effects on ability to drive and use machines

The effect of CoAprovel on ability to drive and use machines has not been studied, but based on its pharmacodynamic properties, CoAprovel is unlikely to affect this ability. When driving vehicles or operating machines, it should be taken into account that occasionally dizziness or weariness may occur during treatment of hypertension.

4.8 Undesirable effects

The frequency of adverse reactions listed below is defined using the following convention: very common (⩾ 1/10); common (⩾ 1/100, < 1/10); uncommon (⩾ 1/1,000, < 1/100); rare (⩾ 1/10,000, < 1/1,000); very rare (< 1/10,000).

Irbesartan/hydrochlorothiazide combination:

In placebo-controlled trials in patients with hypertension, the overall incidence of adverse events did not differ between the irbesartan / hydrochlorothiazide and the placebo groups. Discontinuation due to any clinical or laboratory adverse event was less frequent for irbesartan / hydrochlorothiazide-treated patients than for placebo-treated patients. The incidence of adverse events was not related to gender, age, race, or dose within the recommended dose range. In placebo-controlled trials in which 898 hypertensive patients received various doses (range: 37.5mg/6.25mg to 300 mg/25mg irbesartan / hydrochlorothiazide), the following adverse reactions were reported:

Nervous system disorders:

Common: dizziness

Uncommon: orthostatic dizziness

Cardiac disorders:

Uncommon: hypotension, oedema, syncope, tachycardia

Vascular disorders:

Uncommon: flushing

Gastrointestinal disorders:

Common: nausea/vomiting

Uncommon: diarrhoea

Musculoskeletal, connective tissue and bone disorders:

Uncommon: swelling extremity

Renal and urinary disorders:

Common: abnormal urination

Reproductive system and breast disorders:

Uncommon: libido changes, sexual dysfunction

General disorders and administration site conditions:

Common: fatigue

*Investigations:*patients treated with irbesartan / hydrochlorothiazide had changes in laboratory test parameters which were rarely clinically significant

Common: increases in BUN, creatinine and creatine kinase

Uncommon: decreases in serum potassium and sodium

In addition, since introduction of irbesartan / hydrochlorothiazide in the market the following adverse reactions have also been reported:

Immune system disorders:

Rare: as with other angiotensin-II receptor antagonists, rare cases of hypersensitivity reactions such as angioedema, rash, urticaria have been reported

Metabolism and nutrition disorders:

Very rare: hyperkalaemia

Nervous system disorders:

Very rare: headache

Ear and labyrinth disorders:

Very rare: tinnitus

Respiratory, thoracic and mediastinal disorders:

Very rare: cough

Gastrointestinal disorders:

Very rare: dysgeusia, dyspepsia

Hepato-biliary disorders:

Very rare: abnormal liver function, hepatitis

Musculoskeletal, connective tissue and bone disorders:

Very rare: arthralgia, myalgia

Renal and urinary disorders:

Very rare: impaired renal function including isolated cases of renal failure in patients at risk (see 4.4)

Additional information on individual components: in addition to the adverse reactions listed above for the combination product, other undesirable effects previously reported with one of the individual components may be potential undesirable effects with CoAprovel.

Irbesartan:

General disorders and administration site conditions:

Uncommon: chest pain

Hydrochlorothiazide:

Adverse events (regardless of relationship to drug) reported with the use of hydrochlorothiazide alone include:

Blood and lymphatic system:

aplastic anaemia, bone marrow depression, haemolytic anaemia, leucopenia, neutropenia/agranulocytosis, thrombocytopenia

Psychiatric disorders:

depression, sleep disturbances

Nervous system disorders:

light-headedness, paraesthesia, restlessness, vertigo

Eye disorders:

transient blurred vision, xanthopsia

Cardiac disorders:

cardiac arrhythmias

Vascular disorders:

postural hypotension

Respiratory, thoracic and mediastinal disorders:

respiratory distress (including pneumonitis and pulmonary oedema)

Gastrointestinal disorders:

pancreatitis, anorexia, constipation, diarrhoea, gastric irritation, loss of appetite, sialadenitis

Hepatobiliary disorders:

jaundice (intrahepatic cholestatic jaundice)

Skin and subcutaneous tissue disorders:

anaphylactic reactions, toxic epidermal necrolysis, cutaneous lupus erythematosus-like reactions, necrotizing angiitis (vasculitis, cutaneous vasculitis), photosensitivity reactions, rash, reactivation of cutaneous lupus erythematosus, urticaria

Musculoskeletal, connective tissue and bone disorders:

muscle spasm, weakness

Renal and urinary disorders:

interstitial nephritis, renal dysfunction

General disorders and administration site conditions:

fever

Investigations:

electrolyte imbalance (including hypokalaemia and hyponatraemia, see 4.4), glycosuria, hyperglycaemia, hyperuricaemia, increases in cholesterol and triglycerides

The dose dependent side effects of hydrochlorothiazide (particularly electrolyte disturbances) may increase when titrating the hydrochlorothiazide.

4.9 Overdose

No specific information is available on the treatment of overdosage with CoAprovel. The patient should be closely monitored, and the treatment should be symptomatic and supportive. Management depends on the time since ingestion and the severity of the symptoms. Suggested measures include induction of emesis and/or gastric lavage. Activated charcoal may be useful in the treatment of overdosage. Serum electrolytes and creatinine should be monitored frequently. If hypotension occurs, the patient should be placed in a supine position, with salt and volume replacements given quickly.

The most likely manifestations of irbesartan overdosage are expected to be hypotension and tachycardia; bradycardia might also occur.

Overdosage with hydrochlorothiazide is associated with electrolyte depletion (hypokalaemia, hypochloraemia, hyponatraemia) and dehydration resulting from excessive diuresis. The most common signs and symptoms of overdosage are nausea and somnolence. Hypokalaemia may result in muscle spasms and/or accentuate cardiac arrhythmias associated with the concomitant use of digitalis glycosides or certain anti-arrhythmic drugs.

Irbesartan is not removed by haemodialysis. The degree to which hydrochlorothiazide is removed by haemodialysis has not been established.

5. PHARMACOLOGICAL PROPERTIES

5.1 Pharmacodynamic properties

Pharmacotherapeutic group: angiotensin-II antagonists, combinations: ATC code C09D A04.

CoAprovel is a combination of an angiotensin-II receptor antagonist, irbesartan, and a thiazide diuretic, hydrochlorothiazide. The combination of these ingredients has an additive antihypertensive effect, reducing blood pressure to a greater degree than either component alone.

Irbesartan is a potent, orally active, selective angiotensin-II receptor (AT_1 subtype) antagonist. It is expected to block all actions of angiotensin-II mediated by the AT_1 receptor, regardless of the source or route of synthesis of angiotensin-II. The selective antagonism of the angiotensin-II (AT_1) receptors results in increases in plasma renin levels and angiotensin-II levels, and a decrease in plasma aldosterone concentration. Serum potassium levels are not significantly affected by irbesartan alone at the recommended doses in patients without risk of electrolyte imbalance (see 4.4 and 4.5). Irbesartan does not inhibit ACE (kininase-II), an enzyme which generates angiotensin-II and also degrades bradykinin into inactive metabolites. Irbesartan does not require metabolic activation for its activity.

Hydrochlorothiazide is a thiazide diuretic. The mechanism of antihypertensive effect of thiazide diuretics is not fully known. Thiazides affect the renal tubular mechanisms of electrolyte reabsorption, directly increasing excretion of sodium and chloride in approximately equivalent amounts. The diuretic action of hydrochlorothiazide reduces plasma volume, increases plasma renin activity, increases aldosterone secretion, with consequent increases in urinary potassium and bicarbonate loss, and decreases in serum potassium. Presumably through blockade of the renin-angiotensin-aldosterone system, co-administration of irbesartan tends to reverse the potassium loss associated with these diuretics. With hydrochlorothiazide, onset of diuresis occurs in 2 hours, and peak effect occurs at about 4 hours, while the action persists for approximately 6-12 hours.

The combination of hydrochlorothiazide and irbesartan produces dose-related additive reductions in blood pressure across their therapeutic dose ranges. The addition of 12.5 mg hydrochlorothiazide to 300 mg irbesartan once daily in patients not adequately controlled on 300 mg irbesartan alone resulted in further placebo-corrected diastolic blood pressure reductions at trough (24 hours post-dosing) of 6.1 mm Hg. The combination of 300 mg irbesartan and 12.5 mg hydrochlorothiazide resulted in an overall placebo-subtracted systolic/diastolic reduction of up to 13.6/11.5 mm Hg.

Limited clinical data (7 out of 22 patients) suggest that patients not controlled with the 300/12.5 combination may respond when uptitrated to 300/25. In these patients, an incremental blood pressure lowering effect was observed for both SBP and DBP (13.3 and 8.3 mm Hg, respectively).

Once daily dosing with 150 mg irbesartan and 12.5 mg hydrochlorothiazide gave systolic/diastolic mean placebo-adjusted blood pressure reductions at trough (24 hours post-dosing) of 12.9/6.9 mm Hg in patients with mild-to-moderate hypertension. Peak effects occurred at 3-6 hours. When assessed by ambulatory blood pressure monitoring, the combination 150 mg irbesartan and 12.5 mg hydrochlorothiazide once daily produced consistent reduction in blood pressure over the 24 hours period with mean 24-hour placebo-subtracted systolic/diastolic reductions of 15.8/10.0 mm Hg. When measured by ambulatory blood pressure monitoring, the trough to peak effects of CoAprovel 150/12.5 mg were 100%. The trough to peak effects measured by cuff during office visits were 68% and 76% for CoAprovel 150/12.5 mg and CoAprovel 300/12.5 mg, respectively. These 24-hour effects were observed without excessive blood pressure lowering at peak and are consistent with safe and effective blood-pressure lowering over the once-daily dosing interval.

In patients not adequately controlled on 25 mg hydrochlorothiazide alone, the addition of irbesartan gave an added placebo-subtracted systolic/diastolic mean reduction of 11.1/7.2 mm Hg.

The blood pressure lowering effect of irbesartan in combination with hydrochlorothiazide is apparent after the first dose and substantially present within 1-2 weeks, with the maximal effect occurring by 6-8 weeks. In long-term follow-up studies, the effect of irbesartan / hydrochlorothiazide was maintained for over one year. Although not specifically studied with the CoAprovel, rebound hypertension has not been seen with either irbesartan or hydrochlorothiazide.

The effect of the combination of irbesartan and hydrochlorothiazide on morbidity and mortality has not been studied. Epidemiological studies have shown that long term treatment with hydrochlorothiazide reduces the risk of cardiovascular mortality and morbidity.

There is no difference in response to CoAprovel, regardless of age or gender. When irbesartan is administered concomitantly with a low dose of hydrochlorothiazide (e.g. 12.5 mg daily), the antihypertensive response in black patients approaches that of non-black patients.

5.2 Pharmacokinetic properties

Concomitant administration of hydrochlorothiazide and irbesartan has no effect on the pharmacokinetics of either drug.

Irbesartan and hydrochlorothiazide are orally active agents and do not require biotransformation for their activity. Following oral administration of CoAprovel, the absolute oral bioavailability is 60-80% and 50-80% for irbesartan and hydrochlorothiazide, respectively. Food does not affect the bioavailability of CoAprovel. Peak plasma concentration occurs at 1.5-2 hours after oral administration for irbesartan and 1-2.5 hours for hydrochlorothiazide.

Plasma protein binding of irbesartan is approximately 96%, with negligible binding to cellular blood components. The volume of distribution for irbesartan is 53-93 litres. Hydrochlorothiazide is 68% protein-bound in the plasma, and its apparent volume of distribution is 0.83-1.14 l/kg.

Irbesartan exhibits linear and dose proportional pharmacokinetics over the dose range of 10 to 600 mg. A less than proportional increase in oral absorption at doses beyond 600 mg was observed; the mechanism for this is unknown. The total body and renal clearance are 157-176 and 3.0-3.5 ml/min, respectively. The terminal elimination half-life of irbesartan is 11-15 hours. Steady-state plasma concentrations are attained within 3 days after initiation of a once-daily dosing regimen. Limited accumulation of irbesartan (< 20%) is observed in plasma upon repeated once-daily dosing. In a study, somewhat higher plasma concentrations of irbesartan were observed in female hypertensive patients. However, there was no difference in the half-life and accumulation of irbesartan. No dosage adjustment is necessary in female patients. Irbesartan AUC and C_{max} values were also somewhat greater in elderly subjects (⩾ 65 years) than those of young subjects (18-40 years). However the terminal half-life was not significantly altered. No dosage adjustment is necessary in elderly patients. The mean plasma half-life of hydrochlorothiazide reportedly ranges from 5-15 hours.

Following oral or intravenous administration of ^{14}C irbesartan, 80-85% of the circulating plasma radioactivity is attributable to unchanged irbesartan. Irbesartan is metabolised by the liver via glucuronide conjugation and oxidation. The major circulating metabolite is irbesartan glucuronide (approximately 6%). *In vitro* studies indicate that irbesartan is primarily oxidised by the cytochrome P450 enzyme *CYP2C9*; isoenzyme *CYP3A4* has negligible effect. Irbesartan and its metabolites are eliminated by both biliary and renal pathways. After either oral or IV administration of ^{14}C irbesartan, about 20% of the radioactivity is recovered in the urine, and the remainder in the faeces. Less than 2% of the dose is excreted in the urine as unchanged irbesartan. Hydrochlorothiazide is not metabolized but is eliminated rapidly by the kidneys. At least 61% of the oral dose is eliminated unchanged within 24 hours. Hydrochlorothiazide crosses the placental but not the blood-brain barrier, and is excreted in breast milk.

Renal impairment: In patients with renal impairment or those undergoing haemodialysis, the pharmacokinetic parameters of irbesartan are not significantly altered. Irbesartan is not removed by haemodialysis. In patients with creatinine clearance < 20 ml/min, the elimination half-life of hydrochlorothiazide was reported to increase to 21 hours.

Hepatic impairment: In patients with mild to moderate cirrhosis, the pharmacokinetic parameters of irbesartan are not significantly altered. Studies have not been performed in patients with severe hepatic impairment.

5.3 Preclinical safety data

Irbesartan/hydrochlorothiazide: The potential toxicity of the irbesartan / hydrochlorothiazide combination after oral administration was evaluated in rats and macaques in studies lasting up to 6 months. There were no toxicological findings observed of relevance to human therapeutic use.

The following changes, observed in rats and macaques receiving the irbesartan / hydrochlorothiazide combination at 10/10 and 90/90 mg/kg/day, were also seen with one of the two drugs alone and/or were secondary to decreases in blood pressure (no significant toxicological interactions were observed):

- kidney changes, characterized by slight increases in serum urea and creatinine, and hyperplasia / hypertrophy of the juxtaglomerular apparatus, which are a direct consequence of the interaction of irbesartan with the renin-angiotensin system;
- slight decreases in erythrocyte parameters (erythrocytes, haemoglobin, haematocrit);
- stomach discoloration, ulcers and focal necrosis of gastric mucosa were observed in few rats in a 6 months toxicity study at irbesartan 90 mg/kg/day, hydrochlorothiazide 90 mg/kg/day, and irbesartan / hydrochlorothiazide 10/10 mg/kg/day. These lesions were not observed in macaques;
- decreases in serum potassium due to hydrochlorothiazide and partly prevented when hydrochlorothiazide was given in combination with irbesartan.

Most of the above mentioned effects appear to be due to the pharmacological activity of irbesartan (blockade of angiotensin-II-induced inhibition of renin release, with stimulation of the renin-producing cells) and occur also with angiotensin converting enzyme inhibitors. These findings appear to have no relevance to the use of therapeutic doses of irbesartan / hydrochlorothiazide in humans.

No teratogenic effects were seen in rats given irbesartan and hydrochlorothiazide in combination at doses that produced maternal toxicity. The effects of the irbesartan / hydrochlorothiazide combination on fertility have not been evaluated in animal studies, as there is no evidence of adverse effect on fertility in animals or humans with either irbesartan or hydrochlorothiazide when administered alone. However, another angiotensin-II antagonist affected fertility parameters in animal studies when given alone. These findings were also observed with lower doses of this other angiotensin-II antagonist when given in combination with hydrochlorothiazide.

There was no evidence of mutagenicity or clastogenicity with the irbesartan / hydrochlorothiazide combination. The carcinogenic potential of irbesartan and hydrochlorothiazide in combination has not been evaluated in animal studies.

Irbesartan: There was no evidence of abnormal systemic or target organ toxicity at clinically relevant doses. In preclinical safety studies, high doses of irbesartan (⩾ 250 mg/kg/day in rats and ⩾ 100 mg/kg/day in macaques) caused a reduction of red blood cell parameters (erythrocytes, haemoglobin, haematocrit). At very high doses (⩾ 500 mg/kg/day) degenerative changes in the kidneys (such as interstitial nephritis, tubular distension, basophilic tubules, increased plasma concentrations of urea and creatinine) were induced by irbesartan in the rat and the macaque and are considered secondary to the hypotensive effects of the drug which led to decreased renal perfusion. Furthermore, irbesartan induced hyperplasia / hypertrophy of the juxtaglomerular cells (in rats at ⩾ 90 mg/kg/day, in macaques at ⩾ 10 mg/kg/day). All of these changes were considered to be caused by the pharmacological action of irbesartan. For therapeutic doses of irbesartan in humans, the hyperplasia / hypertrophy of the renal juxtaglomerular cells does not appear to have any relevance.

There was no evidence of mutagenicity, clastogenicity or carcinogenicity.

Animal studies with irbesartan showed transient toxic effects (increased renal pelvic cavitation, hydroureter or subcutaneous oedema) in rat foetuses, which were resolved after birth. In rabbits, abortion or early resorption was noted at doses causing significant maternal toxicity, including mortality. No teratogenic effects were observed in the rat or rabbit.

Hydrochlorothiazide: Although equivocal evidence for a genotoxic or carcinogenic effect was found in some experimental models, the extensive human experience with hydrochlorothiazide has failed to show an association between its use and an increase in neoplasms.

6. PHARMACEUTICAL PARTICULARS

6.1 List of excipients

Tablet core: lactose monohydrate, microcrystalline cellulose, croscarmellose sodium, hypromellose, silicon dioxide, magnesium stearate.

Film-coating: lactose monohydrate, hypromellose, titanium dioxide (E171), macrogol, red and yellow ferric oxides (E172) carnauba wax.

6.2 Incompatibilities

Not applicable.

6.3 Shelf life

3 years.

6.4 Special precautions for storage

Do not store above 30°C.

Store in the original package.

6.5 Nature and contents of container

CoAprovel film-coated tablets are packaged in cartons containing 28 tablets in PVC/PVDC/aluminium blisters.

6.6 Instructions for use and handling

No special requirements.

7. MARKETING AUTHORISATION HOLDER

SANOFI PHARMA BRISTOL-MYERS SQUIBB SNC

174 avenue de France

F-75013 Paris - France

8. MARKETING AUTHORISATION NUMBER(S)

CoAprovel 150/12.5mg film-coated tablets: EU/1/98/086/012

CoAprovel 300/12.5mg film-coated tablets: EU/1/98/086/017

9. DATE OF FIRST AUTHORISATION/RENEWAL OF THE AUTHORISATION

02 March 2004

10. DATE OF REVISION OF THE TEXT

28 October 2004

Legal Category: POM

Cobalin-H injection

(Link Pharmaceuticals Ltd)

1. NAME OF THE MEDICINAL PRODUCT

Cobalin-H®

2. QUALITATIVE AND QUANTITATIVE COMPOSITION

Anhydrous hydroxocobalamin 1000mcg/ml

3. PHARMACEUTICAL FORM

Injection

4. CLINICAL PARTICULARS

4.1 Therapeutic indications

Treatment of Addisonian pernicious anaemia.

Prophylaxis and treatment of other macrocytic anaemias due to vitamin B_{12} deficiency.

Treatment of tobacco amblyopia.

Treatment of Leber's atrophy.

4.2 Posology and method of administration

The following dosages are suitable for children and adults.

Addisonian pernicious anaemia and other macrocytic anaemias without neurological involvement:

Initially:	250 micrograms to 1000 micrograms intramuscularly on alternate days for one or two weeks then 250 micrograms weekly until blood count is normal.
Maintenance:	1000 micrograms every two or three months.

Addisonian pernicious anaemia and other macrocytic anaemias with neurological involvement:

Initially:	1000 micrograms by intramuscular injection on alternate days as long as improvement continues.
Maintenance:	1000 micrograms every two months.

Prophylaxis of macrocytic anaemias associated with vitamin B12 deficiency resulting from gastrectomy, ileal resection, certain malabsorption states and vegetarianism:

1000 micrograms every two or three months.

Tobacco amblyopia and Leber's optic atrophy:

Initially:	1000 micrograms daily by intramuscular injection for two weeks then twice weekly as long as improvement is maintained.
Maintenance:	1000 micrograms every three months or as required

4.3 Contraindications

Sensitivity to hydroxocobalamin / vitamin B_{12}.

4.4 Special warnings and special precautions for use

Cobalin-H should not be given before a megaloblastic marrow has been demonstrated. Regular monitoring of the blood is advisable. Doses of hydroxocobalamin greater than 10 micrograms daily may produce a haematological response in patients with folate deficiency. Indiscriminate use may mask the exact diagnosis. Cardiac arrhythmias secondary to hypokalaemia have been reported during initial therapy and plasma potassium should, therefore, be monitored during this period.

4.5 Interaction with other medicinal products and other forms of Interaction

The serum concentration of hydroxocobalamin may be reduced by concurrent administration of oral contraceptives. Chloramphenicol-treated patients may respond poorly to hydroxocobalamin. Vitamin B_{12} assays by microbiological techniques are invalidated by antimetabolites and most antibiotics.

4.6 Pregnancy and lactation

Hydroxocobalamin should not be used to treat megaloblastic anaemia of pregnancy.

4.7 Effects on ability to drive and use machines

None stated.

4.8 Undesirable effects

Allergic hypersensitivity reactions have occurred rarely following the administration of hydroxocobalamin.

4.9 Overdose

Treatment is unlikely to be needed in cases of overdosage.

5. PHARMACOLOGICAL PROPERTIES

5.1 Pharmacodynamic properties

Vitamin B_{12}

ATC classification: B03B A03

5.2 Pharmacokinetic properties

Vitamin B_{12} is extensively bound to specific plasma proteins called transcobalamins; transcobalamin II appears to be involved in the rapid transport of the cobalamins to tissues. It is stored in the liver, excreted in the bile, and undergoes enterohepatic recycling; part of a dose is excreted in the urine, most of it in the first 8 hours.

5.3 Preclinical safety data

There are no pre-clinical data of relevance to the prescriber which are additional to that already included in other sections of the Summary of Product Characteristics.

6. PHARMACEUTICAL PARTICULARS

6.1 List of excipients

Sodium dihydrogen orthophosphate, Sodium chloride, Water for Injections

6.2 Incompatibilities

None stated.

6.3 Shelf life

60 months.

6.4 Special precautions for storage

Store below 25°C and protect from light.

6.5 Nature and contents of container

Cobalin-H is supplied in clear 1ml Type I glass ampoules in cartons of 5.

6.6 Instructions for use and handling

None stated.

7. MARKETING AUTHORISATION HOLDER

Link Pharmaceuticals Limited, Bishops Weald House, Albion Way, Horsham, West Sussex RH12 1AH

8. MARKETING AUTHORISATION NUMBER(S)

PL 12406/0001

9. DATE OF FIRST AUTHORISATION/RENEWAL OF THE AUTHORISATION

November 1998

10. DATE OF REVISION OF THE TEXT

April 2000

® Cobalin-H is a registered trade mark

Co-Betaloc Tablets

(Pharmacia Limited)

1. NAME OF THE MEDICINAL PRODUCT

Co-Betaloc® Tablets

2. QUALITATIVE AND QUANTITATIVE COMPOSITION

Metoprolol tartrate Ph. Eur. 100mg.

Hydrochlorothiazide Ph. Eur. 12.5mg.

3. PHARMACEUTICAL FORM

Tablet.

4. CLINICAL PARTICULARS

4. Clinical Particulars

4.1 Therapeutic indications

In the management of mild or moderate hypertension. Co-Betaloc may be suitable for use when satisfactory control of arterial blood pressure cannot be obtained with either a diuretic or a beta-adrenoreceptor blocking drug used alone.

4.2 Posology and method of administration

The dose will depend on patient response. Usually 1-3 tablets per day as a single or divided dose.

Elderly: Initially the lowest possible dose should be used, especially in the elderly.

Significant Hepatic Dysfunction: A reduction in dosage may be necessary.

4.3 Contraindications

AV block. Uncontrolled heart failure. Severe bradycardia. Sick-sinus syndrome. Cardiogenic shock. Severe peripheral arterial disease. Known hypersensitivity to other β-blockers or any of the constituents of Co-Betaloc. Metabolic acidosis. Untreated phaeochromocytoma.

Co-Betaloc is also contra-indicated when acute myocardial infarction is complicated by significant bradycardia, first-degree heart block, systolic hypotension (<100mmHg) and/or severe heart failure.

Severe kidney and liver failure. Therapy resistant hypokalaemia and hyponatraemia. Hypercalcaemia, symptomatic hyperuricaemia. Anuria. Known hypersensitivity to hydrochlorothiazide or other sulphonamide derivatives.

An anti-diuretic effect has been reported following concomitant treatment with diuretics and lithium. As with all products which contain diuretics, Co-Betaloc is contra-indicated during lithium therapy.

4.4 Special warnings and special precautions for use

If patients develop increasing bradycardia, Co-Betaloc should be given in lower doses or gradually withdrawn. Symptoms of peripheral arterial circulatory disorders may be aggravated by Co-Betaloc.

Abrupt interruption of β-blockers is to be avoided. When possible, Co-Betaloc should be withdrawn gradually over a period of 10-14 days. During its withdrawal patients should be kept under close surveillance, especially those with known ischaemic heart disease.

Co-Betaloc may be administered when heart failure has been controlled. Digitalisation and/or additional diuretic therapy should also be considered for patients with a history of heart failure, or patients known to have a poor cardiac reserve. Co-Betaloc should be used with caution in patients where cardiac reserve is poor.

Intravenous administration of calcium antagonists of the verapamil type should not be given to patients treated with β-blockers.

In patients with Prinzmetal's angina β_1 selective agents should be used with care.

Although cardioselective β-blockers may have less effect on lung function than non-selective β-blockers, as with all β-blockers these should be avoided in patients with reversible obstructive airways disease unless there are compelling clinical reasons for their use. When administration is necessary, use of a β_2-bronchodilator (e.g. terbutaline) may be advisable in some patients.

The label shall state - "If you have a history of wheezing, asthma or any other breathing difficulties, you must tell your doctor before you take this medicine."

In labile and insulin-dependent diabetes it may be necessary to adjust the hypoglycaemic therapy.

As with other β-blockers, Co-Betaloc may mask the symptoms of thyrotoxicosis and the early signs of acute hypoglycaemia in patients with diabetes mellitus. However, the risk of this occurring is less than with non-selective β-blockers.

In patients with a phaeochromocytoma, an α-blocker should be given concomitantly.

In the presence of liver cirrhosis the bioavailability of metoprolol may be increased and patients may need a lower dosage.

The elderly should be treated with caution, starting with a lower dose.

Like all β-blockers, careful consideration should be given to patients with psoriasis before Co-Betaloc is administered.

The administration of adrenaline to patients undergoing β-blockade can result in an increase in blood pressure and bradycardia although this is less likely to occur with β_1-selective drugs.

Co-Betaloc therapy must be reported to the anaesthetist prior to general anaesthesia. If withdrawal of metoprolol is considered desirable, this should if possible be completed at least 48 hours before general anaesthesia. However, in some patients it may be desirable to employ a β-blocker as premedication. By shielding the heart against the effects of stress the β-blocker may prevent excessive sympathetic stimulation provoking cardiac arrhythmias or acute coronary insufficiency. If a β-blocker is given for this purpose, an anaesthetic with little negative inotropic activity should be selected to minimise the risk of myocardial depression.

Co-Betaloc does not interfere with potassium balance. However, at higher doses of hydrochlorothiazide disturbances in the electrolyte and water balance may be experienced. Hyperuricaemia may occur or frank gout may be precipitated in certain patients receiving higher doses of thiazide therapy. Latent diabetes may become manifest during thiazide therapy.

Diuretics in higher doses may precipitate azotemia in patients with renal disease. Cumulative effects of hydrochlorothiazide may develop in patients with impaired renal function. If renal impairment becomes evident metoprolol/hydrochlorothiazide therapy should be discontinued.

Beta-blockers may increase both the sensitivity towards allergens and the seriousness of anaphylactic reactions.

4.5 Interaction with other medicinal products and other forms of Interaction

The effects of metoprolol and other drugs with an antihypertensive effect on blood pressure are usually additive, and care should be taken to avoid hypotension such as could be the result of concomitant administration with dihydropyridine derivatives, tricyclic antidepressant barbiturates and phenothiazines. However, combinations of antihypertensive drugs may often be used with benefit to improve control of hypertension.

Metoprolol can reduce myocardial contractility and impair intracardiac conduction. Care should be exercised when drugs with similar activity, e.g. antiarrhythmic agents, general anaesthetics, are given concurrently. Like all other β-blockers, metoprolol should not be given in combination with verapamil, diltiazem or digitalis glycosides. A watch should be kept for possible negative effects when metoprolol is given in combination with calcium antagonists, since this may cause bradycardia, hypotension and asystole. Care should also be exercised when β-blockers are given in combination with sympathomimetic ganglion blocking agents, other β-blockers (i.e. eye drops) or MAO inhibitors.

If concomitant treatment with clonidine is to be discontinued, metoprolol should be withdrawn several days before clonidine.

As β-blockers may affect the peripheral circulation, care should be exercised when drugs with similar activity e.g. ergotamine are given concurrently.

Metoprolol will antagonise the β_1-effects of sympathomimetic agents but should have little influence on the bronchodilator effects of β_2-agonists at normal therapeutic doses. Enzyme inducing agents (e.g. rifampicin) may reduce plasma concentrations of metoprolol, whereas enzyme inhibitors (e.g. cimetidine, alcohol and hydralazine) may increase plasma concentrations. Metoprolol may impair the elimination of lidocaine (lignocaine).

The dosages of oral antidiabetic agents and also of insulin may have to be readjusted in patients receiving β-blockers. Concomitant treatment with indomethacin and other prostaglandin synthetase inhibiting drugs may reduce the antihypertensive effect of β-blockers.

In general, reported interactions have occurred with doses of hydrochlorothiazide higher than those used in this combination. Insulin requirements in diabetic patients may be altered and lithium renal clearance is reduced, increasing the risk of lithium toxicity. Responsiveness to tubocurarine may be increased and arterial responsiveness to noradrenaline may be decreased, but not enough to preclude effectiveness of the pressor agent for therapeutic use. Hypokalaemia may develop during concomitant use of steroids or ACTH, and may sensitise or exaggerate the response of the heart to toxic effects of digitalis.

4.6 Pregnancy and lactation

Use During Pregnancy

Co-Betaloc should not be used in pregnancy or nursing mothers unless the physician considers that the benefit outweighs the possible hazard to the foetus/infant. β-blockers reduce placental perfusion, which may result in intrauterine foetal death, immature and premature deliveries. As with all β-blockers, metoprolol may cause side effects especially bradycardia and hypoglycaemia in the foetus, and in the newborn and breastfed infant. There is an increased risk of cardiac and pulmonary complications in the neonate. Metoprolol has, however, been used in pregnancy associated hypertension under close supervision, after 20 weeks gestation. Although Betaloc crosses the placental barrier and is present in cord blood, no evidence of foetal abnormalities has been reported.

Hydrochlorothiazide can reduce the plasma volume as well as the uteroplacental blood circulation.

Use During Lactation

Breast-feeding is not recommended. The amount of metoprolol ingested via breast milk should not produce significant β-blocking effects in the neonate if the mother is treated with normal therapeutic doses.

As hydrochlorothiazide passes into breast milk, consideration should be given to withdrawal of Co-Betaloc, replacement by metoprolol in monotherapy or breast-feeding stopped.

4.7 Effects on ability to drive and use machines

When driving vehicles or operating machines, it should be taken into account that occasionally dizziness or fatigue may occur.

4.8 Undesirable effects

Metoprolol is usually well tolerated and adverse reactions have generally been mild and reversible. The following events have been reported as adverse events in clinical trials or reported from routine use.

Side effects to metoprolol are usually mild and infrequent. The most common appear to be lassitude, GI disturbances (nausea, vomiting or abdominal pain) and disturbances of sleep pattern. In many cases these effects have been transient or have disappeared after a reduction in dosage.

Effects related to the CNS which have been reported occasionally are dizziness and headache and rarely paraesthesia, muscle cramps, depression and decreased mental alertness. There have also been isolated reports of personality disorders like amnesia, memory impairment, confusion, hallucination, nervousness and anxiety.

Cardiovascular effects which have been reported occasionally are bradycardia, postural hypotension and rarely, heart failure, increased existing AV block, palpitations, cardiac arrhythmias, Raynauds phenomenon, peripheral oedema and precordial pain. There have also been isolated reports of cardiac conduction abnormalities, gangrene in patients with pre-existing severe peripheral circulatory disorders and increase of pre-existing intermittent claudication.

Common gastro-intestinal disturbances have been described above but rarely diarrhoea or constipation also occur and there have been isolated cases of dry mouth and abnormal liver function.

Skin rashes (urticaria, psoriasiform, dystrophic skin lesions) and positive anti-nuclear antibodies (not associated with SLE) occur rarely. Isolated cases of photosensitivity, psoriasis exacerbation, increased sweating and alopecia have been reported. Respiratory effects include occasional reports of dyspnoea on exertion and rare reports of bronchospasm and isolated cases of rhinitis.

Rarely impotence/sexual dysfunction. Isolated cases of weight gain, thrombocytopenia, disturbances of vision, conjunctivitis, tinnitus, dry or irritated eyes, taste disturbance and arthralgia have also been reported.

The reported incidence of skin rashes and/or dry eyes is small and in most cases the symptoms have cleared when treatment was withdrawn. Discontinuation of the drug should be considered if any such reaction is not otherwise explicable.

Hydrochlorothiazide is generally well tolerated at the dose used (12.5mg) in the combination. However, the familiar side-effects of thiazide diuretics may be expected e.g. gastro-intestinal disturbances, metabolic and electrolyte changes, disturbances in sleep pattern, skin rashes and effects relating to the CNS.

4.9 Overdose

Poisoning due to an overdose of Co-Betaloc may lead to severe hypotension, sinus bradycardia, atrioventricular block, heart failure, cardiogenic shock, cardiac arrest, bronchospasm, impairment of consciousness, coma, nausea, vomiting, cyanosis, hypoglycaemia and, occasionally, hyperkalaemia. The first manifestations usually appear 20 minutes to 2 hours after drug ingestion.

The most prominent feature of poisoning due to hydrochlorothiazide is acute loss of fluid and electrolytes. The following symptoms may also be observed: dizziness, sedation/impairment of consciousness, hypotension and muscle cramps.

Treatment should include close monitoring of cardiovascular, respiratory and renal function, and blood glucose and electrolytes. Further absorption may be prevented by induction of vomiting, gastric lavage or administration of activated charcoal if ingestion is recent. Cardiovascular complications should be treated symptomatically, which may require the use of sympathomimetic agents (e.g. noradrenaline, metaraminol), atropine or inotropic agents (e.g. dopamine, dobutamine). Temporary pacing may be required for AV block. Glucagon can reverse the effects of excessive β-blockade, given in a dose of 1-10mg intravenously. Intravenous β_2-stimulants e.g. terbutaline may be required to relieve bronchospasm.

Intravenous volume and electrolyte-replacement may be necessary.

Metoprolol cannot be effectively removed by haemodialysis.

5. PHARMACOLOGICAL PROPERTIES

5.1 Pharmacodynamic properties

Metoprolol is a cardioselective β-adrenoceptor blocking agent. The stimulant effect of catecholamine on the heart is reduced or inhibited by metoprolol. This leads to a decrease in heart rate, cardiac output cardiac contractility and blood pressure.

Hydrochlorothiazide is a thiazide diuretic which reduces the reabsorption of electrolytes from the renal tubules, thereby increasing the excretion of sodium and chloride ions and consequently of water. Potassium is excreted to a lesser extent. The thiazides have a slight lowering effect on blood pressure and enhance the effects of other antihypertensive agents.

5.2 Pharmacokinetic properties

Metoprolol is well absorbed after oral administration, peak plasma concentrations occurring 1.5-2 hours after dosing. The bioavailability of a single dose is approximately 50%, increasing to approximately 70% during repeated administration. The bioavailability also increases if metoprolol is given with food.

Elimination is mainly by hepatic metabolism and the average elimination half-life is 3.5 hours (range 1 to 9 hours). Rates of metabolism vary between individuals, with poor metabolisers (approximately 10%) showing higher plasma concentrations and slower elimination than extensive metabolisers. Within individuals, however, plasma concentrations are stable and reproducible. Because of variation in rates of metabolism, the dose of metoprolol should always be adjusted to the individual requirements of the patient. As the therapeutic response, adverse effects and relative cardioselectivity are related to plasma concentration, poor metabolisers may require lower than normal doses. Dosage adjustment is not routinely required in the elderly or in patients with renal failure, but dosage may need to be reduced in patients with significant hepatic dysfunction when metoprolol elimination may be impaired.

5.3 Preclinical safety data

There are no toxicity data that would indicate that metoprolol tartrate or hydrochlorothiazide are unsafe for use in the indication given. Signs in rats and dogs indicate that metoprolol can exert a cardiopressive action at high plasma concentrations.

6. PHARMACEUTICAL PARTICULARS

6.1 List of excipients

Lactose, Microcrystalline cellulose, Sodium starch glycollate, Polyvinyl pyrrolidone, Colloidal silicon dioxide, Magnesium stearate.

6.2 Incompatibilities

None known.

6.3 Shelf life

3 years.

6.4 Special precautions for storage

Store below 25°C in a dry place.

6.5 Nature and contents of container

PVC blister strips in an outer carton

Pack size 28

Securitainers- Pack size 300

6.6 Instructions for use and handling

7. MARKETING AUTHORISATION HOLDER

Pharmacia Limited

Davy Avenue

Knowlhill

Milton Keynes

MK5 8PH

8. MARKETING AUTHORISATION NUMBER(S)

PL 00032/0403

9. DATE OF FIRST AUTHORISATION/RENEWAL OF THE AUTHORISATION

15 April 2002

10. DATE OF REVISION OF THE TEXT

Legal Category

POM.

Cocois Coconut Oil Compound

(UCB Pharma Limited)

1. NAME OF THE MEDICINAL PRODUCT

Cocois (Coconut Oil Compound Ointment).

2. QUALITATIVE AND QUANTITATIVE COMPOSITION

Active ingredients % w/w

Coal Tar Solution BP 12.0

Precipitated Sulphur BP 4.0

Salicylic Acid Ph.Eur 2.0

3. PHARMACEUTICAL FORM

Ointment for topical application.

4. CLINICAL PARTICULARS

4.1 Therapeutic indications

Cocois has mild, antipruritic, antiseptic and keratolytic properties. It is indicated in the treatment of scaly skin disorders of the scalp such as psoriasis, eczema, seborrhoeic dermatitis and dandruff.

4.2 Posology and method of administration

Adults, children over 12 years and the elderly

Mild dandruff

To be used intermittently as an adjunctive treatment to be applied approximately once a week.

Psoriasis, eczema, seborrhoeic dermatitis and severe dandruff

To be used daily for three to seven days until improvement has been achieved. Intermittent repeated applications may be necessary to maintain improvement.

In all cases, the affected area should be treated and shampooed off using warm water approximately one hour later.

Children 6-12 years

To be used under medical supervision only.

Children under 6 years

Not recommended.

4.3 Contraindications

The product is contraindicated in patients known to be sensitive to any of the ingredients including sulphur and salicylates, in the presence of acute local infections, or acute pustular psoriasis.

4.4 Special warnings and special precautions for use

Avoid contact with the eyes and wash hands immediately after use. Discontinue use if irritation develops.

If symptoms persist after four weeks, a doctor should be consulted.

Coal tar may stain bed linen and jewellery.

4.5 Interaction with other medicinal products and other forms of Interaction

None.

4.6 Pregnancy and lactation

To be used at the discretion of the physician.

4.7 Effects on ability to drive and use machines

None.

4.8 Undesirable effects

Coal tar may cause skin irritation, folliculitis and rarely photosensitivity.

4.9 Overdose

Overdose is extremely unlikely. Treat symptomatically, if necessary.

5. PHARMACOLOGICAL PROPERTIES

5.1 Pharmacodynamic properties

Coal Tar is antipuritic, keratoplastic and a weak antiseptic

Salicylic acid has keratolytic properties.

Sulphur is a keratolytic, with weak antiseptic and parasiticide properties.

Combinations of coal tar, salicylic acid and sulphur are widely used in the treatment of hyperkeratotic and scaling skin conditions.

5.2 Pharmacokinetic properties

No data is available for the proposed formulation

5.3 Preclinical safety data

None stated.

6. PHARMACEUTICAL PARTICULARS

6.1 List of excipients

Coconut Oil BP

White Soft Paraffin BP

Cetostearyl Alcohol BP

Glycerol Ph.Eur

Liquid Paraffin Ph.Eur

Polyoxyethylene Glycerol Monostearate HSE

Hard Paraffin BP

6.2 Incompatibilities

None known.

6.3 Shelf life

2 years.

6.4 Special precautions for storage

Store between 10°C and 25°C.

6.5 Nature and contents of container

Cocois is packed into internally lacquered, membrane sealed, aluminium tubes (5g, 15g, 40g and 100g) fitted with a polyurethane cap.

6.6 Instructions for use and handling

None stated.

7. MARKETING AUTHORISATION HOLDER

UCB Pharma Limited

208 Bath Road

Slough

Berkshire SL1 3WE

UK

8. MARKETING AUTHORISATION NUMBER(S)

PL 00039/0499

9. DATE OF FIRST AUTHORISATION/RENEWAL OF THE AUTHORISATION

Date of first Authorisation: 09/06/1997

10. DATE OF REVISION OF THE TEXT

June 2005

Co-danthramer capsules and Strong Co-danthramer capsules

(Napp Pharmaceuticals Limited)

1. NAME OF THE MEDICINAL PRODUCT

Co-danthramer capsules

Strong Co-danthramer capsules

2. QUALITATIVE AND QUANTITATIVE COMPOSITION

Co-danthramer capsules contain Dantron BP 25 mg and Poloxamer 188 BP 200 mg.

Strong Co-danthramer capsules contain Dantron BP 37.5 mg and Poloxamer 188 BP 500 mg.

3. PHARMACEUTICAL FORM

Capsule, hard

Co-danthramer capsules have light brown bodies, opaque orange caps and are marked CX and Napp.

Strong Co-danthramer capsules have light brown bodies, opaque green caps and are marked CXF and Napp.

4. CLINICAL PARTICULARS

4.1 Therapeutic indications

Constipation in terminally ill patients

4.2 Posology and method of administration

Adults

One or two capsules at bedtime.

Children under 12 years of age

Co-danthramer capsules: One capsule at bedtime or as recommended by the physician.

Strong Co-danthramer capsules: Not recommended.

Elderly

As recommended by the physician.

4.3 Contraindications

In common with other gastro-intestinal evacuants, Co-danthramer capsules should not be given when acute or painful conditions of the abdomen are present or when the cause of the constipation is thought to be an intestinal obstruction. Pregnancy and lactation.

4.4 Special warnings and special precautions for use

Oral administration of dantron has been reported to cause liver or intestinal tumours in rats and mice. There is no sound evidence to conclude a no effect dose and therefore there may be a risk of such effects in humans.

Co-danthramer use should therefore be restricted to the licensed indications.

In babies, children and patients wearing nappies there may be staining of the buttocks. This may lead to superficial sloughing of the skin. Therefore, Co-danthramer should not be given to infants in nappies and should be used with caution in all incontinent patients.

4.5 Interaction with other medicinal products and other forms of Interaction

None stated.

4.6 Pregnancy and lactation

Co-danthramer capsules are contraindicated in pregnant women and nursing mothers.

4.7 Effects on ability to drive and use machines

None stated.

4.8 Undesirable effects

Dantron may cause temporary harmless pink or red colouring of the urine and peri-anal skin. With prolonged high dosage the mucosa of the large intestine may become coloured.

4.9 Overdose

In case of overdosage, patients should be given plenty of fluids. An anti-cholinergic preparation such as atropine sulphate may be given to offset the excessive intestinal motility.

5. PHARMACOLOGICAL PROPERTIES

5.1 Pharmacodynamic properties

Dantron is an anthraquinone derivative which acts on the nerve endings of the myenteric plexus and stimulates the muscles of the large intestine.

Poloxamer 188 is a wetting agent which increases the penetration of water into faecal material. The surface activity of the poloxamer has a lubricant effect on the gut contents.

5.2 Pharmacokinetic properties

Like other anthraquinone compounds, dantron is partially absorbed from the small intestine. Because it does not affect the small intestine, griping and cramping do not occur. Dantron begins to act between 6-12 hours after administration.

Poloxamer 188 is not absorbed and is fully recovered in the faeces.

5.3 Preclinical safety data

There are no pre-clinical data of relevance to the prescriber which are additional to that already included in other sections of the SPC.

6. PHARMACEUTICAL PARTICULARS

6.1 List of excipients

Butylhydroxytoluene (E321)

Capsule shell

Gelatin

(contains E127, E172, E132, E171)

Sodium dodecylsulphate

Printing ink

Opacode S-1-7020 HV white 005

(containing shellac, soya, lecithin, 2-ethoxyethanol, dimethicone, E171)

6.2 Incompatibilities

None stated.

6.3 Shelf life

Three years

6.4 Special precautions for storage

Do not store above 30°C.

6.5 Nature and contents of container

Clear or pale yellow blister packs (aluminium foil sealed to 250μm PVC with a PVdC coating of at least 40 gsm thickness), containing 60 capsules.

6.6 Instructions for use and handling

None

7. MARKETING AUTHORISATION HOLDER

Napp Pharmaceuticals Ltd

Cambridge Science Park

Milton Road

Cambridge CB4 0GW

8. MARKETING AUTHORISATION NUMBER(S)

PL 16950/0017-0018

9. DATE OF FIRST AUTHORISATION/RENEWAL OF THE AUTHORISATION

19 October 1994/15 September 2000

10. DATE OF REVISION OF THE TEXT

July 2002

11. Legal category

POM

Co-danthramer suspension and Strong Co-danthramer suspension

(Napp Pharmaceuticals Limited)

1. NAME OF THE MEDICINAL PRODUCT

Co-danthramer suspension

Strong Co-danthramer suspension

2. QUALITATIVE AND QUANTITATIVE COMPOSITION

Each 5 ml of Co-danthramer suspension contains Dantron BP 25 mg and Poloxamer 188 BP 200 mg.

Each 5 ml of Strong Co-danthramer suspension contains Dantron BP 75 mg and Poloxamer 188 BP 1.0 g.

3. PHARMACEUTICAL FORM

Viscous, orange-yellow coloured suspension.

4. CLINICAL PARTICULARS

4.1 Therapeutic indications

Constipation in terminally ill patients.

4.2 Posology and method of administration

Adults and elderly

Suspension: 5 – 10 ml at bedtime.

Strong suspension: One 5 ml spoonful at bedtime.

Children

Suspension: Half to one 5 ml spoonful at bedtime as recommended by a medical practitioner.

Strong suspension: Not recommended for children under twelve years of age.

4.3 Contraindications

In common with other gastro-intestinal evacuants, Co-danthramer should not be given when acute or painful conditions of the abdomen are present or when the cause of the constipation is thought to be an intestinal obstruction. Pregnancy and lactation.

4.4 Special warnings and special precautions for use

Oral administration of dantron has been reported to cause liver or intestinal tumours in rats and mice. There is no sound evidence to conclude a no effect dose and therefore there may be a risk of such effects in humans. Co-danthramer use should therefore be restricted to the licensed indication.

In babies, children and patients wearing nappies there may be staining of the buttocks. This may lead to superficial sloughing of the skin. Therefore, Co-danthramer should not be given to infants in nappies and should be used with caution in all incontinent patients.

4.5 Interaction with other medicinal products and other forms of Interaction
None stated.

4.6 Pregnancy and lactation
Co-danthramer is contraindicated in pregnant women and nursing mothers.

4.7 Effects on ability to drive and use machines
None stated.

4.8 Undesirable effects
Dantron may cause temporary harmless pink or red colouring of the urine and peri-anal skin. With prolonged or high dosage the mucosa of the large intestine may become coloured.

4.9 Overdose
In case of overdosage, patients should be given plenty of fluids. An anti-cholinergic preparation such as atropine sulphate may be given to offset the excessive intestinal motility.

5. PHARMACOLOGICAL PROPERTIES

5.1 Pharmacodynamic properties
Co-danthramer suspension owes its laxative action to the mild purgative dantron, which is the subject of a monograph in the British Pharmacopoeia. This is an anthraquinone derivative chemically related to emodin, the active principle of cascara and other naturally occurring products such as senna, aloes and rhubarb. It acts on the nerve endings of the myenteric plexus and stimulates the muscles of the large intestine.

Poloxamer 188 is a wetting agent which increases the penetration of water into faecal material. The surface activity of the poloxamer has a lubricant effect on the gut contents.

5.2 Pharmacokinetic properties
Like other anthraquinone compounds, dantron is partially absorbed from the small intestine. Because it does not affect the small intestine, griping and cramping do not occur. Dantron begins to act between 6 to 12 hours after administration.

Poloxamer 188, a non-ionic surfactant is not absorbed and is fully recovered in the faeces.

5.3 Preclinical safety data
There are no pre-clinical data of relevance to the prescriber which are additional to that already included in other sections of the SPC.

6. PHARMACEUTICAL PARTICULARS

6.1 List of excipients
Magnesium aluminium silicate
Potassium sorbate
Saccharin sodium
Glyceryl mono/di-oleate
Sorbitol solution (70%)
Citric acid monohydrate
Sodium phosphate
Ethanol
Propylene glycol
Peach flavour
Nipasept sodium
Butylhydroxytoluene (E321)
Water

Strong Co-danthramer suspension also contains capsicum oleoresin flavour.

6.2 Incompatibilities
None stated

6.3 Shelf life
Two years

6.4 Special precautions for storage
Do not store above 25°C

6.5 Nature and contents of container
Amber PET bottles containing:
Co-danthramer suspension: 300 ml
Strong Co-danthramer suspension: 300 ml

6.6 Instructions for use and handling
None

7. MARKETING AUTHORISATION HOLDER
Napp Pharmaceuticals Ltd
Cambridge Science Park
Milton Road
Cambridge CB4 0GW

8. MARKETING AUTHORISATION NUMBER(S)
PL 16950/0015-0016

9. DATE OF FIRST AUTHORISATION/RENEWAL OF THE AUTHORISATION
13th August 1993/15 September 2000

10. DATE OF REVISION OF THE TEXT
July 2002

11. Legal category
POM

® The Napp Device is a Registered Trade Mark
© Napp Pharmaceuticals Ltd 2002.

Co-Diovan 80/12.5 mg, 160/12.5 mg, 160/25 mg Tablets

(Novartis Pharmaceuticals UK Ltd)

1. NAME OF THE MEDICINAL PRODUCT
▼Co-Diovan® 80/12.5 mg Tablets.
▼Co-Diovan® 160/12.5 mg Tablets.
▼Co-Diovan® 160/25 mg Tablets.

2. QUALITATIVE AND QUANTITATIVE COMPOSITION
Co-Diovan 80/12.5 mg Tablets: One tablet contains 80 mg valsartan and 12.5 mg hydrochlorothiazide.

Co-Diovan 160/12.5 mg Tablets: One tablet contains 160 mg valsartan and 12.5 mg hydrochlorothiazide.

Co-Diovan 160/25 mg Tablets: One tablet contains 160 mg valsartan and 25 mg hydrochlorothiazide.

For excipients, see 6.1.

3. PHARMACEUTICAL FORM
Co-Diovan 80/12.5 mg Tablets:
Oval, non-divisible, film-coated tablets measuring approx. 10.2 to 5.4 mm in diameter and 3.7 mm in thickness, and weighing approx. 156 mg. The tablets are coloured light orange and imprinted with HGH on one side and CG on the other side.

Co-Diovan 160/12.5 mg Tablets:
Oval, non-divisible, film-coated tablets measuring approximately 15.2 mm by 6.2 mm and 4.4 mm in thickness, and weighing approximately 312 mg. The tablets are coloured dark red and imprinted with HHH on one side and CG on the other side.

Co-Diovan 160/25 mg Tablets:
Oval, non-divisible, film-coated tablets measuring approximately 14.2 mm by 5.7 mm and 4.5 mm in thickness, and weighing approximately 310 mg. The tablets are coloured brown orange and imprinted with HXH on one side and NVR on the other side.

4. CLINICAL PARTICULARS

4.1 Therapeutic indications
Treatment of essential hypertension.

Co-Diovan fixed dose combination (80 mg valsartan and 12.5mg hydrochlorothiazide or 160 mg valsartan and 12.5 mg hydrochlorothiazide or 160 mg valsartan and 25 mg hydrochlorothiazide) is indicated in patients whose blood pressure is not adequately controlled on valsartan or hydrochlorothiazide monotherapy.

4.2 Posology and method of administration
The recommended dose of Co-Diovan® is one coated tablet per day. When clinically appropriate, either 80 mg valsartan and 12.5 mg hydrochlorothiazide or 60 mg valsartan and 12.5 mg hydrochlorothiazide may be used. When necessary, 160 mg valsartan and 25 mg hydrochlorothiazide may be used. The maximum antihypertensive effect is seen within 2-4 weeks.

Doses higher than valsartan 160 mg/hydrochlorothiazide 25 mg once daily have not been investigated and are therefore not recommended.

Renal Impairment:
Due to the HCTZ component, Co-Diovan is not recommended for use in patients with significant renal impairment (creatinine clearance < 30 mL/min). No dosage adjustment is required for patients with mild to moderate renal impairment (creatinine clearance > 30 mL/min).

Hepatic Impairment:
Patients with severe hepatic impairment, cirrhosis or biliary obstruction should not use Co-Diovan (see Section 4.3 Contra-indications). No dosage adjustment is required in patients with mild to moderate hepatic insufficiency of non biliary origin and without cholestasis (see Section 4.4 Special Warnings and Precautions for use).

Use in children:
The safety and efficacy of Co-Diovan have not been established in children under the age of 18.

Elderly:
Use in patients over 65 years: The exposure to valsartan may be increased by over 50% in the elderly. However, no dose adjustment is required in the elderly patients.

4.3 Contraindications
Contraindications for the use of Co-Diovan are as follows:-

Hypersensitivity to any of the components of Co-Diovan or other sulphonamide-derived products.

Pregnancy and lactation (See section 4.6 Pregnancy and lactation).

In addition, there are contraindications to the use of the individual components of Co-Diovan. These are as follows:

Valsartan is contraindicated in the following conditions:

- severe hepatic impairment
- cirrhosis and
- biliary obstruction.

Hydrochlorothiazide is contraindicated in the following conditions:

- Anuria
- creatinine clearance < 30 mL/min
- conditions involving enhanced potassium loss e.g. salt losing nephropathies and pre-renal (cardiogenic) impairment of kidney function
- hepatic failure
- refractory hypokalaemia
- hyponatraemia
- hypercalcaemia
- hyperuricaemia
- history of gout and uric acid calculi
- hypertension during pregnancy
- untreated Addison's disease and
- concomitant lithium therapy.

4.4 Special warnings and special precautions for use

Serum electrolyte changes:
Concomitant use with potassium supplements, potassium sparing diuretics, salt substitutes containing potassium, or other drugs that may increase potassium levels (heparin, etc.) should be used with caution. Hypokalaemia has been reported under treatment with thiazide diuretics. Frequent monitoring of serum potassium is recommended.

Treatment with thiazide diuretics has been associated with hyponatraemia and hypochloroaemic alkalosis. Thiazides increase the urinary excretion of magnesium, which may result in hypomagnesaemia. Calcium excretion is decreased by thiazide diuretics. This may result in hypercalcaemia. Thiazides should be discontinued before carrying out tests for parathyroid function.

Sodium, and/or volume-depleted patients:
Patients should be observed for clinical signs of fluid or electrolyte imbalance e.g. when the patient is vomiting excessively or receiving parenteral fluids as this may precipitate sudden worsening of hepatic function. Warning signs of fluid or electrolyte imbalance are dryness of mouth, thirst, weakness, lethargy, drowsiness, restless muscle pains or cramps, muscular fatigue, hypotension, oliguria, tachycardia, gastrointestinal disturbances such as nausea or vomiting.

In severely sodium-depleted and/or volume-depleted patients such as those receiving high doses of diuretics, there is a risk symptomatic hypotension may occur in rare cases after initiation of therapy with Co-Diovan. Sodium and/or volume depletion should be corrected before starting treatment with Co-Diovan.

If hypotension occurs, the patient should be placed in a supine position and, if necessary, given an intravenous infusion of normal saline. Treatment can be continued once the blood pressure has stabilised.

Renal impairment:
No dosage adjustment is required for patients with renal impairment (creatinine clearance >30 mL/min).

Renal artery stenosis:
In patients with unilateral or bilateral renal artery stenosis or stenosis to a solitary kidney, the safe use of Co-Diovan has not been established. Thus Co-Diovan should not be used to treat hypertension in these patients.

Hepatic impairment:
In patients with mild to moderate hepatic impairment without cholestasis, no dosage adjustment is required. However, Co-Diovan® should be used with caution. Liver disease does not significantly alter the pharmacokinetics of hydrochlorothiazide (see section 4.3 Contraindications).

Systemic Lupus Erythematosus:
Thiazide diuretics have been reported to exacerbate or activate Systemic Lupus Erythematosus.

Other metabolic disturbances:
Thiazide diuretics may alter glucose tolerance (see section 4.5 Interaction with other medicinal products and other forms of interaction) and raise serum levels of cholesterol, triglycerides and uric acid.

Thiazides may decrease serum protein bound iodine levels without signs of thyroid disturbance.

Sensitivity reactions may occur in patients receiving thiazides with or without any previous history of allergy or bronchial asthma.

4.5 Interaction with other medicinal products and other forms of Interaction

Potential drug interactions due to the combination of valsartan and hydrochlorothiazide:
The antihypertensive effect may be increased with concomitant use of other antihypertensive drugs.

Concomitant use with potassium supplements, potassium-sparing diuretics, salt substitutes containing potassium, or other drugs that may alter potassium levels (heparin, etc.) should be used with caution and with frequent monitoring of potassium.

Reversible increases in serum lithium concentrations and toxicity have been reported during concurrent use of ACE inhibitors and thiazides. There is no experience with concomitant use of valsartan and lithium. Therefore, monitoring of serum lithium concentrations is recommended during concurrent use.

Potential drug interactions due to valsartan:

In monotherapy with valsartan, no drug interactions of clinical significance have been found with cimetidine, warfarin, furosemide, digoxin, atenolol, indometacin, hydrochlorothiazide, amlodipine and glibenclamide.

As valsartan is not metabolised to a significant extent, clinically relevant drug-drug interactions in the form of metabolic induction or inhibition of the cytochrome P450 system are not expected with valsartan. Although valsartan is highly bound to plasma proteins, in vitro studies have not shown any interaction at this level with a range of molecules which are also highly protein-bound, such as diclofenac, furosemide, and warfarin.

Potential drug interactions due to hydrochlorothiazide:

Thiazides potentiate the action of curare derivatives.

Concomitant administration of NSAIDs (e.g. salicylic acid derivative, indometacin) may weaken the diuretic and antihypertensive activity of the thiazide component of Co-Diovan. Concurrent hypovolemia may induce acute renal failure.

The hypokalaemic effect of diuretics may be increased by kaliuretic diuretics, corticosteroids, ACTH, amphotericin, carbenoxolone, penicillin G and salicylic acid derivatives.

Thiazide-induced hypokalaemia or hypomagnesaemia may occur as unwanted effects, favouring the onset of digitalis-induced cardiac arrhythmias.

It may prove necessary to readjust the dosage of insulin and of oral antidiabetic agents.

Co-administration of thiazide diuretics may increase the incidence of hypersensitivity reactions to allopurinol, may increase the risk of adverse effects caused by amantadine, may enhance the hyperglycaemic effect of diazoxide, and may reduce the renal excretion of cytotoxic drugs (e.g. cyclophosphamide and methotrexate) and potentiate their myelosuppressive effects.

The bioavailability of thiazide-type diuretics may be increased by anticholinergic agents (e.g. atropine and biperiden) due to a decrease in gastrointestinal motility and the stomach emptying rate.

There have been reports in the literature of haemolytic anaemia occurring with concomitant use of hydrochlorothiazide and methyldopa.

Absorption of thiazide diuretics is decreased by cholestyramine.

Administration of thiazide diuretics with vitamin D or with calcium salts may potentiate the rise in serum calcium.

Concomitant treatment with ciclosporin may increase the risk of hyperuricaemia and gout-type complications.

Co-administration with alcohol, barbiturates or narcotics may potentiate orthostatic hypotension.

Absorption of hydrochlorothiazide is impaired in the presence of anionic exchange resins. Single doses of cholestyramine or cholestipol resins bind hydrochlorothiazide and reduce their absorption from the gastrointestinal tract.

Pressor amines such as adrenaline may show decreased arterial responsiveness when used with hydrochlorothiazide but this reaction is not enough to preclude therapeutic usefulness.

4.6 Pregnancy and lactation

Valsartan:

Due to the mechanism of action of angiotensin II antagonists, a risk factor for the foetus cannot be excluded. In-utero exposure to angiotensin converting enzyme (ACE) inhibitors given to pregnant women during the second and third trimesters has been reported to cause injury and death to the developing foetus.

It is not known whether valsartan is excreted in human milk. Valsartan was excreted in the milk of lactating rats.

Hydrochlorothiazide:

Intrauterine exposure to thiazide diuretics is associated with fetal or neonatal thrombocytopenia, and may be associated with other adverse reactions that have occurred in adults.

Hydrochlorothiazide crosses the placenta and is excreted in human milk. Thus it is not advisable to use Co-Diovan in lactating mothers.

As for any drug that also acts directly on the renin-angiotensin-aldosterone system (RAAS), Co-Diovan should not be used during pregnancy or lactation. If pregnancy is detected during therapy, Co-Diovan should be discontinued as soon as possible.

4.7 Effects on ability to drive and use machines

As with other antihypertensive agents, it is advisable to exercise caution when driving or operating machinery.

4.8 Undesirable effects

Co-Diovan has been evaluated for safety in more than 2159 patients. Adverse experiences have generally been mild and transient in nature.

The following table of adverse experiences is based on three controlled trials involving a total of 2159 patients. Of the 2159 patients, 2066 received valsartan in combination with hydrochlorothiazide. The overall incidence of adverse experiences with Co-Diovan was similar to placebo. All adverse experiences showing an incidence of 1% or more in the Co-Diovan group are included in the following table, irrespective of their causal association with the study drug.

	[1]Co-Diovan N = 2066 %	Placebo N = 93 %
Headache (not otherwise specified)	5.1	17.2
Dizziness (excluding vertigo)	3.9	6.5
Nasopharyngitis[2]	2.7	1.1
Fatigue	2.0	1.1
Back pain	1.5	3.2
Cough	1.4	0.0
Upper respiratory tract infection	1.4	2.2
Sinusitis (not otherwise specified)	1.3	3.2
Diarrhoea (not otherwise classified)	1.2	0.0
Chest pain (not elsewhere classified)	1.1	1.1
Pain in limb[3]	1.1	0.0
Nausea	1.0	1.1

[1] Includes all combinations of valsartan 80 and 160 mg with hydrochlorothiazide 12.5 and 25 mg

[2] Nasopharyngitis including pharyngitis + rhinitis

[3] Pain in limb including arm pain + leg pain

Other adverse experiences with a frequency below 1% included abdominal pain, abnormal vision, anxiety, arthralgia, arthritis, bronchitis, dyspepsia, impotence, insomnia, leg cramps, micturition frequency, palpitations, rash, sprains and strains, urinary tract infection, viral infection, oedema, asthenia and vertigo. It is unknown whether these effects were causally related to the therapy.

Post marketing data revealed very rare cases of angioedema, rash, pruritus and other hypersensitivity or allergic reactions including serum sickness and vasculitis. Very rare cases of impaired renal function have also been reported.

Laboratory findings:

A greater than 20% decrease in serum potassium was observed in 2.2% of patients receiving Co-Diovan® as compared to placebo (3.3%), (see 4.4 Special Warnings and Precautions).

Elevation in creatinine occurred in 1.4% of patients taking Co-Diovan and 1.1% given placebo in controlled clinical trials.

Valsartan:

Other additional adverse experiences reported in clinical trials with valsartan monotherapy, irrespective of their causal association with the study drug were: With a frequency greater than 1%: arthralgia; With a frequency below 1%: oedema, asthenia, insomnia, rash, decreased libido and vertigo.

Hydrochlorothiazide:

Hydrochlorothiazide has been extensively prescribed for many years, frequently in higher doses than those contained in Co-Diovan. The following adverse reactions have been reported in patients treated with thiazide diuretics alone, including hydrochlorothiazide.

Electrolytes and metabolic disorders:

Electrolyte disorders: hypokalaemia, hyponatraemia, hypomagnesaemia, hypochloroaemic alkalosis, hypercalcaemia.

Metabolic disorders: altered glucose tolerance, rise in serum levels of cholesterol, triglycerides and uric acid.

Others:

Common: urticaria and other forms of rash, loss of appetite, mild nausea and vomiting, postural hypotension which may be aggravated by alcohol, anaesthetics or sedatives, and impotence.

Rare: photosensitisation, abdominal distress, constipation, diarrhoea and gastrointestinal discomfort, intrahepatic cholestasis or jaundice, cardiac arrhythmias, headache, dizziness or lightheadedness, sleep disturbances, depression, paraesthesia, disturbances of vision, thrombocytopenia, sometimes with purpura.

Very rare: necrotising vasculitis and toxic epidermal necrolysis, cutaneous lupus erythematosis-like reactions, reactivation of cutaneous lupus erythematosis, pancreatitis, leucopenia, agranulocytosis, bone marrow depression, haemolytic anaemia, hypersensitivity reactions, respiratory distress including pneumonitis and pulmonary oedema.

4.9 Overdose

Although there is no experience of overdosage with Co-Diovan, the major sign that might be expected is marked hypotension. If the ingestion is recent, vomiting should be induced. Otherwise, the usual treatment would be intravenous infusion of normal saline solution.

Valsartan cannot be eliminated by means of haemodialysis because of its strong plasma binding behaviour whereas clearance of hydrochlorothiazide will be achieved by dialysis.

5. PHARMACOLOGICAL PROPERTIES

5.1 Pharmacodynamic properties

Pharmacotherapeutic group: angiotensin II antagonists combination (valsartan) with diuretics (hydrochlorothiazide).

ATC Code: C09D A03.

The active hormone of the RAAS is angiotensin II, which is formed from angiotensin I through ACE. Angiotensin II binds to specific receptors located in the cell membranes of various tissues. It has a wide variety of physiological effects, including in particular both direct and indirect involvement in the regulation of blood pressure. As a potent vasoconstrictor angiotensin II exerts a direct pressor response. In addition, it promotes sodium retention and stimulation of aldosterone secretion.

Valsartan is an orally active and specific angiotensin II (Ang II) receptor antagonist. It acts selectively on the AT_1 receptor subtype, which is responsible for the known actions of angiotensin II. The increased plasma levels of Ang II following AT_1 receptor blockade with valsartan may stimulate the unblocked AT_2 receptor, which appears to counterbalance the effect of the AT_1 receptor. Valsartan does not exhibit any partial agonist activity at the AT_1 receptor and has much (about 20,000 fold) greater affinity for the AT_1 receptor than for the AT_2 receptor.

Valsartan does not inhibit ACE, also known as kininase II, which converts Ang I to Ang II and degrades bradykinin. No potentiation of bradykinin related side effects should be expected. In clinical trials where valsartan was compared with an ACE inhibitor, the incidence of dry cough was significantly ($P < 0.05$) less in patients treated with valsartan than in those treated with an ACE inhibitor (2.6% versus 7.9% respectively). In a clinical trial of patients with a history of dry cough during ACE inhibitor therapy, 19.5% of trial subjects receiving valsartan and 19.0% of those receiving a thiazide diuretic experienced cough compared to 68.5% of those treated with an ACE inhibitor ($p < 0.05$). Valsartan does not bind to or block other hormone receptors or ion channels known to be important in cardiovascular regulation.

Administration of valsartan to patients with hypertension results in reduction of blood pressure without affecting pulse rate.

In most patients, after administration of a single oral dose, onset of antihypertensive activity occurs within 2 hours, and the peak reduction of blood pressure is achieved within 4-6 hours. The antihypertensive effect persists over 24 hours after dosing. During repeated dosing, the maximum reduction in blood pressure with any dose is generally attained within 2-4 weeks and is sustained during long-term therapy. Combined with hydrochlorothiazide, a significant additional reduction in blood pressure is achieved.

The site of action of thiazide diuretics is primarily in the renal distal convoluted tubule. It has been shown that there is a high affinity receptor in the renal cortex with the primary binding site for the thiazide diuretic action and inhibition of NaC1 transport in the distal convoluted tubule. The mode of action of thiazides is through inhibition of the Na^+C1^- symporter perhaps by competing as the $C1^-$ site affecting mechanisms of electrolyte reabsorption:- directly increasing excretion of sodium and chloride in approximately equivalent amounts – indirectly of diuretic action reducing plasma volume, with consequent increases in plasma renin activity increases in aldosterone secretion, increases in urinary potassium loss, and decreases in serum potassium. The renin-aldosterone link is mediated by angiotensin II, so co-administration of an angiotensin II receptor antagonist tends to reverse the potassium with these diuretics.

5.2 Pharmacokinetic properties

Valsartan:

Absorption of valsartan after oral administration is rapid, although the amount absorbed varies widely. Mean absolute bioavailability for Diovan is 23%. Valsartan shows multi-exponential decay kinetics ($t_{1/2\alpha} < 1$ hour and $t_{1/2\beta}$ about 9 hours).

The pharmacokinetics of valsartan are linear in the dose range tested. There is no change in the kinetics of valsartan on repeated administration and little accumulation when dosed once daily. Plasma concentrations were observed to be similar in males and females.

Valsartan is highly bound to serum protein (94 – 97%), mainly serum albumin. Steady-state volume of distribution is low (about 17 L). Plasma clearance is relatively slow (about 2 L/h) when compared with hepatic blood flow (about 30 L/h). Of the absorbed dose of valsartan, 70% is excreted in the faeces and 30% in the urine, mainly as unchanged compound.

When valsartan is given with food, the area under the plasma concentration curve (AUC) of valsartan is reduced by 48%, although from about 8 hours post dosing plasma valsartan concentrations are similar for the fed and fasted group. This reduction in AUC, however, is not accompanied by a clinically significant reduction in the therapeutic effect.

Hydrochlorothiazide:

The absorption of hydrochlorothiazide, after an oral dose, is rapid (t_{max} about 2 hours), with similar absorption characteristics for both suspension and tablet formulations. The distribution and elimination kinetics have generally been described by a bi-exponential decay function, with a terminal half-life of 6-15 hours.

The increase in mean AUC is linear and dose proportional in the therapeutic range. There is no change in the kinetics of hydrochlorothiazide on repeated dosing, and accumulation is minimal when dosed once daily.

Absolute bioavailability of hydrochlorothiazide is 60-80% after oral administration, with >95% of the absorbed dose being excreted as unchanged compound in the urine, and about 4% as the hydrolysate, 2-amino-4-cholor-*m*-benezenedisulfoamide.

Concomitant administration with food has been reported to both increase and decrease the system availability of hydrochlorothiazide compared with the fasted state. The magnitude of these effects is small and has little clinical importance.

Valsartan/hydrochlorothiazide:

The systemic availability of hydrochlorothiazide is reduced by about 30% when co-administered with valsartan. The kinetics of valsartan are not markedly affected by the co-administration of hydrochlorothiazide. This observed interaction has no impact on the combined use of valsartan and hydrochlorothiazide, since controlled clinical trials have shown a clear anti-hypertensive effect, greater than that obtained with drug given alone, or placebo.

Special populations

Elderly:

A higher systemic exposure to valsartan was observed in some elderly subjects than in young subjects. However, this has not been shown to have any clinical significance.

Limited data suggest that the systemic clearance of hydrochlorothiazide is reduced in both healthy and hypertensive elderly subjects compared to young healthy volunteers.

Renal impairment:

No dose adjustment is required for patients with a creatinine clearance of 30-70 mL/min.

In patients with severe renal impairment (creatinine clearance <30 mL/min) and patients undergoing dialysis, no data are available for Co-Diovan. Valsartan is highly bound to plasma protein and is not to be removed by dialysis, whereas clearance of hydrochlorothiazide will be achieved by dialysis.

Renal clearance of hydrochlorothiazide is composed of passive filtration and active secretion into the renal tubule. As expected for a compound which is cleared almost exclusively via the kidneys, renal function has a marked effect on the kinetics of hydrochlorothiazide (see Section 4.3 Contraindications).

Hepatic impairment:

In a pharmacokinetics trial in patients with mild (n=6) to moderate (n=5) hepatic dysfunction, exposure to valsartan was increased approximately twofold compared with healthy volunteers. There are no data available on the use of valsartan in patients with severe hepatic dysfunction.

Hepatic disease does not significantly affect the pharmacokinetics of hydrochlorothiazide, and no dose reduction is considered necessary.

5.3 Preclinical safety data

Preclinical safety data reveal no special hazard for humans based on conventional studies of repeated dose toxicity and toxicity to reproduction (foetotoxicity at maternal toxic doses). Preclinical effects were observed only at exposures considered sufficiently in excess of the maximum human exposure indicating little relevance to clinical use.

Both valsartan and hydrochlorothiazide have been tested individually for mutagenicity, clastogenicity and carcinogenicity with negative results. The tests were not repeated for the combination of valsartan and hydrochlorothiazide, as there is no evidence for an interaction between the two compounds.

6. PHARMACEUTICAL PARTICULARS

6.1 List of excipients

Co-Diovan 80/12.5 mg Tablets:

Core:

Colloidal anhydrous silica
Crospovidone
Magnesium stearate
Microcrystalline cellulose

Coating:

Hypromellose
Macrogol 8000
Talc
Red iron oxide (E172)
Yellow iron oxide (E172)
Titanium dioxide (E171).

Co-Diovan 160/12.5 mg Tablets:

Core:

Colloidal anhydrous silica
Crospovidone
Magnesium stearate
Microcrystalline cellulose

Coating:

Hypromellose,
Macrogol 8000
Talc
Titanium dioxide (E171)
Red iron oxide (E172)

Co-Diovan 160/25 mg Tablets:

Core:

Colloidal anhydrous silica
Crospovidone
Magnesium stearate
Microcrystalline cellulose

Coating:

Hypromellose
Macrogol 4000
Talc
Titanium dioxide (E171)
Red iron oxide (E172)
Black iron oxide (E172)
Yellow iron oxide (E172)

6.2 Incompatibilities

Not applicable.

6.3 Shelf life

Co-Diovan 80/12.5 mg Tablets: 3 years
Co-Diovan 160/12.5 mg Tablets: 3 years
Co-Diovan 160/25 mg Tablets: 2 years

6.4 Special precautions for storage

Do not store above 30°C.
Store in the original package.

6.5 Nature and contents of container

PVC/PE/PVDC aluminium blister packs containing 28, 56 and 98 tablets per pack.

6.6 Instructions for use and handling

No specific instructions for use or handling.

7. MARKETING AUTHORISATION HOLDER

Novartis Pharmaceuticals UK Limited
Trading as: Ciba Laboratories
Frimley Business Park
Frimley
Camberley
Surrey
GU16 7SR

8. MARKETING AUTHORISATION NUMBER(S)

Co-Diovan 80/12.5 mg Tablets: PL 00101/0480
Co-Diovan 160/12.5 mg Tablets: PL 00101/0650
Co-Diovan 160/25 mg Tablets: PL 00101/0651

9. DATE OF FIRST AUTHORISATION/RENEWAL OF THE AUTHORISATION

Co-Diovan 80/12.5 mg Tablets: 29 January 2003
Co-Diovan 160/12.5 mg Tablets: 23 June 2004
Co-Diovan 160/25 mg Tablets: 23 June 2004

10. DATE OF REVISION OF THE TEXT

29 July 2005

LEGAL CATEGORY

POM

Cogentin Injection

(Merck Sharp & Dohme Limited)

1. NAME OF THE MEDICINAL PRODUCT

COGENTIN® Injection

2. QUALITATIVE AND QUANTITATIVE COMPOSITION

Each sterile injection of 'Cogentin' contains 0.1% w/v benztropine mesylate BP.

3. PHARMACEUTICAL FORM

'Cogentin' Injection is supplied as a colourless, sterile solution for injection.

4. CLINICAL PARTICULARS

4.1 Therapeutic indications

'Cogentin' is an anti—parkinsonian agent with powerful anticholinergic effects.

It is indicated for symptomatic treatment of all types of 'classical' parkinsonism including arteriosclerotic, post—encephalitic, and idiopathic parkinsonism, and of extra-pyramidal reactions induced by phenothiazines or reserpine.

'Cogentin' is particularly effective in the relief of rigidity and tremor. Among other symptoms which it can ameliorate are: sialorrhoea, drooling, mask—like facies, oculogyric crises, speech and writing difficulties, gait disturbances, dysphagia, and pain and insomnia due to muscle spasm and cramps.

'Cogentin' often is helpful in patients who have become unresponsive to other agents. Therapy is directed toward control of disturbing symptoms to permit the patient maximum integration of function with minimum discomfort. In non—drug—induced parkinsonism, partial control of symptoms is usually achieved.

'Cogentin' Injection is only to be used in an emergency or when a patient is unable to swallow tablets.

4.2 Posology and method of administration

As 'Cogentin' is cumulative in action, treatment should begin with a low dosage, which can be increased by amounts of 0.5 mg at intervals of five to six days, to the smallest dosage necessary for optimal relief without excessive side—effects. Maximum dosage, 6 mg a day.

'Cogentin' Injection may be used intramuscularly or intravenously in emergencies, or for patients unable to swallow tablets. (As there is no significant difference in time of onset of effect between intramuscular and intravenous administration, the intravenous route is not usually necessary.)

In emergencies, 1—2 ml (1—2 mg) of 'Cogentin' Injection will normally provide quick relief. If signs of parkinsonism begin to return, the dose can be repeated.

'Classical' parkinsonism:

Usual dosage: 1—2 mg a day, with a range of 0.5—6 mg a day. Dosage must be adjusted on an individual basis, taking into consideration the age and weight of the patient, and the type of parkinsonism. Older patients, thin patients and those with arteriosclerotic parkinsonism usually cannot tolerate large dosages. Most patients with post—encephalitic parkinsonism need and indeed tolerate fairly large dosages. Patients with a poor mental outlook may respond poorly. In arteriosclerotic and idiopathic parkinsonism, therapy may be initiated with a single daily dose of 0.5—1 mg at bedtime. This dosage will be adequate in some patients, whereas 4—6 mg a day may be required by others. In post—encephalitic parkinsonism, therapy may be initiated in most patients with 2 mg a day in one or more doses. In highly sensitive individuals, therapy may be initiated with 0.5 mg at bedtime, and increased as necessary.

Some patients obtain greatest relief by taking the entire dose at bedtime; others react more favourably to divided dosage, two to four times a day. One dose a day frequently is sufficient; divided doses may be unnecessary or even undesirable.

Drug—induced parkinsonism: Usual dosage range: 1—4 mg once or twice a day.

Acute dystonic reactions: 1—2 ml (1—2 mg) by intravenous injection followed usually by 1—2 mg orally twice a day.

Extrapyramidal reactions appearing soon after starting phenothiazine or reserpine therapy are likely to be temporary, and are usually controlled in one or two days by 1—2 mg of 'Cogentin' two or three times a day. 'Cogentin' should be withdrawn after one or two weeks to determine if it is still needed. It can be reinstated if necessary.

Certain extrapyramidal reactions which develop slowly (e.g. tardive dyskinesia) do not usually respond to 'Cogentin'.

Paediatric use: Use with caution in children over 3 years old (see 'Contra—indications').

Use in the elderly: As with younger patients, dosage should be the smallest possible for optimum relief of symptoms. Initial dosage should be 0.5—1 mg preferably at night, increasing until optimum effect is seen. Older patients usually cannot tolerate large doses.

4.3 Contraindications

Because of the atropine—like side effects, 'Cogentin' is contra—indicated in children under 3 years old and should be used with caution in older children. 'Cogentin' is contra—indicated in patients who are hypersensitive to this product.

4.4 Special warnings and special precautions for use

Continued supervision of patients is recommended as 'Cogentin' has a cumulative action. Patients with a tendency towards tachycardia and those with prostatic hypertrophy, should be closely observed.

Patients with mental disorders should be carefully supervised when 'Cogentin' is used to control drug—induced extrapyramidal reactions, especially when therapy is started or the dosage of 'Cogentin' is increased. Intensification of mental symptoms may occasionally occur. 'Cogentin' should be temporarily withdrawn if the reactions are severe.

'Cogentin' has anticholinergic effects, and glaucoma is a possibility. Although 'Cogentin' does not appear to have any adverse effect on simple glaucoma, its use is probably not advisable in narrow—angle glaucoma. It may cause anhidrosis; this should be borne in mind, particularly in hot weather, especially when given concomitantly with other atropine—like drugs to the chronically ill, alcoholics, or patients with a central nervous system disease and those who do manual labour in a hot environment. 'Cogentin' should be used cautiously in patients with or prone to abnormalities of sweating.

If there is evidence of anhidrosis, the possibility of hyperthermia should be considered. Dosage should be decreased as necessary to maintain body heat equilibrium by the action of perspiration. Severe anhidrosis and fatal hyperthermia have occurred.

4.5 Interaction with other medicinal products and other forms of Interaction

Extra care should be taken when 'Cogentin' is given concomitantly with phenothiazines, haloperidol or other drugs with anticholinergic or antidopaminergic activity. Patients should be advised to report gastro—intestinal complaints, fever or heat intolerance promptly. Paralytic ileus, sometimes fatal, has occurred in patients taking anticholinergic—type anti—parkinsonian drugs, including 'Cogentin', in combination with phenothiazines and/or tricyclic antidepressants.

Tardive dyskinesia may appear in some patients on long—term therapy with phenothiazines or related agents, or after discontinuation of such therapy. Anti—parkinsonian agents do not usually alleviate symptoms of tardive dyskinesia, and in some cases may aggravate or unmask them. 'Cogentin' is not recommended in tardive dyskinesia.

4.6 Pregnancy and lactation

It is not known whether 'Cogentin' can cause foetal harm when administered to a pregnant woman or can affect reproductive capacity. 'Cogentin' should be given to a pregnant woman only if clearly needed.

Breast-feeding mothers: it is not known whether this drug is excreted in human milk. Because many drugs are excreted in human milk, caution should be exercised when 'Cogentin' is administered to a breast—feeding mother.

4.7 Effects on ability to drive and use machines

'Cogentin' may impair the mental alertness and physical ability required for the performance of such hazardous tasks as driving a car or operating machinery.

4.8 Undesirable effects

Side effects, most of which are anticholinergic or antihistaminic in nature are listed below by body system in order of decreasing severity.

Cardiovascular
Tachycardia.

Digestive
Constipation, dry mouth, nausea, vomiting.

If dry mouth is so severe that there is difficulty in swallowing or speaking, or loss of appetite and weight occur, reduce dosage, or discontinue the drug temporarily.

Slight reduction in dosage may control nausea and still give sufficient relief of symptoms. Vomiting may be controlled by temporary discontinuation, followed by resumption at a lower dosage.

Nervous system
Toxic psychosis, including confusion, disorientation, memory impairment, visual hallucinations; exacerbation of pre—existing psychotic symptoms; nervousness; depression; listlessness; numbness of fingers.

Special Senses
Blurred vision, dilated pupils.

Urogenital
Urinary retention, dysuria.

Metabolic/Immune and Skin
Occasionally, an allergic reaction, e.g., skin rash, develops. If this cannot be controlled by dosage reduction, the medication should be discontinued.

Other
Heat stroke, hyperthermia, fever.

4.9 Overdose

Symptoms may be any of those seen in atropine poisoning or antihistamine overdosage: CNS depression, preceded or followed by stimulation; confusion; nervousness; listlessness; intensification of mental symptoms or toxic psychosis in patients with mental illness being treated with neuroleptic drugs (e.g. phenothiazines); hallucinations (especially visual); dizziness; muscle weakness; ataxia; dry mouth; mydriasis; blurred vision; palpitations; tachycardia; nausea; vomiting; dysuria; numbness of fingers; dysphagia, allergic reactions, e.g. skin rash; headache; hot, dry, flushed skin; delirium; coma; shock; convulsions; respiratory arrest; anhidrosis; hyperthermia; glaucoma; constipation.

Physostigmine salicylate (1—2 mg, subcutaneously or intravenously) is reported to reverse symptoms of anticholinergic intoxication. A second injection may be given after two hours if needed. Otherwise, treatment is symptomatic and supportive.

A short—acting barbiturate may be used for CNS excitement, but with caution to avoid subsequent depression. Supportive care for CNS depression may be required (such convulsant stimulants as picrotoxin, leptazol or bemegride should be avoided). In severe respiratory depression, artificial respiration may be required. Also needed may be a local miotic for mydriasis and cycloplegia, ice bags or other cold applications and alcohol sponges for hyperpyrexia, a vasopressor and fluids for circulatory collapse, and a darkened room for photophobia.

Data on the metabolism of benztropine maleate are not available at present; but a death was recorded 1½ hours after ingestion.

5. PHARMACOLOGICAL PROPERTIES

5.1 Pharmacodynamic properties

Anticholinergic drugs exert their anti-parkinsonian effect by correcting the relating cholinergic excess which is thought to occur in parkinsonism as a result of dopamine deficiency.

The deficiency of dopamine in the striatum of patients with parkinsonism intensifies the excitatory effects of the cholinergic system within the striatum. Anticholinergics aid such patients by blunting this component of the nigrostriated pathway.

5.2 Pharmacokinetic properties

Following i.m. injection, the clinical effects of benztropine are apparent within 10 minutes and the maximum effect is seen within 30 minutes.

Benztropine has a cumulative effect and a prolonged duration of action when compared with other anticholinergic agents used in the treatment of Parkinson's disease such as trihexyphenidyl. In patients on long-term maintenance therapy, it may take up to seven days before all evidence of drug-related effects have ceased.

5.3 Preclinical safety data

No relevant information.

6. PHARMACEUTICAL PARTICULARS

6.1 List of excipients

Sodium chloride Ph Eur, and water for injection Ph Eur.

6.2 Incompatibilities

None known.

6.3 Shelf life

36 months.

6.4 Special precautions for storage

Store below 25°C, protected from light and freezing.

6.5 Nature and contents of container

Type I glass ampoules of 2 ml.

6.6 Instructions for use and handling

None.

7. MARKETING AUTHORISATION HOLDER

Merck Sharp & Dohme Limited
Hertford Road, Hoddesdon, Hertfordshire EN11 9BU, UK

8. MARKETING AUTHORISATION NUMBER(S)

PL 0025/5024R

9. DATE OF FIRST AUTHORISATION/RENEWAL OF THE AUTHORISATION

Reviewed Licence: 25 September 1986.

Renewal: 12 December 1996.

10. DATE OF REVISION OF THE TEXT

April 2000

LEGAL CATEGORY

POM

® denotes registered trademark of Merck & Co., Inc., Whitehouse Station, NJ, USA.

MSD (logo)
Merck Sharp & Dohme Limited
Hertford Road, Hoddesdon, Hertfordshire EN11 9BU, UK.
SPC.CGTI.00.GB.0496.
04 APRIL 2000
(CGTI-03)

Colazide

(Shire Pharmaceuticals Limited)

1. NAME OF THE MEDICINAL PRODUCT

COLAZIDE®

2. QUALITATIVE AND QUANTITATIVE COMPOSITION

Balsalazide disodium 750 mg

INN: balsalazide

Each capsule contains balsalazide disodium 750 mg corresponding to balsalazide 612.8 mg and to mesalazine 262.5 mg.

3. PHARMACEUTICAL FORM

Capsule, hard.

Size 00 beige gelatin capsules.

4. CLINICAL PARTICULARS

4.1 Therapeutic indications

Colazide is indicated for:

Treatment of mild-to-moderate active ulcerative colitis and maintenance of remission.

4.2 Posology and method of administration

To be swallowed whole with or after food.

Adults

Treatment of active disease:

2.25g Balsalazide disodium (3 capsules) three times daily (6.75g daily) until remission or for 12 weeks maximum.

Rectal or oral steroids can be given concomitantly if necessary.

Maintenance treatment:

The recommended starting dose is 1.5g Balsalazide disodium (2 capsules) twice daily (3g daily). The dose can be adjusted based on each patient's response; there may be an additional benefit with a dose up to 6g daily.

Elderly No dose adjustment is anticipated.

Children Colazide is not recommended in children.

4.3 Contraindications

Hypersensitivity to any component of the product or its metabolites, including mesalazine. History of hypersensitivity to salicylates.

Severe hepatic impairment, moderate-severe renal impairment.

Pregnant and breast feeding women.

4.4 Special warnings and special precautions for use

Colazide should be used with caution in patients with asthma, bleeding disorders, active ulcer disease, mild renal impairment or those with established hepatic disease.

During treatment with Colazide blood counts, BUN/creatinine and urine analysis should be performed. Patients receiving balsalazide should be advised to report any unexplained bleeding, bruising, purpura, sore throat, fever or malaise that occurs during treatment. A blood count should be performed and the drug stopped immediately if there is suspicion of a blood dyscrasia.

4.5 Interaction with other medicinal products and other forms of Interaction

Formal interaction studies have not been performed with Colazide. Available data suggest that the systemically available amounts of balsalazide and its metabolites may be increased if Colazide is administered in the fasting as compared with the fed state. Therefore, Colazide should preferably be administered with food.

The acetylated metabolites of balsalazide are actively secreted in the renal tubule to a high degree. Therefore, plasma levels of co-prescribed drugs also eliminated by this route may be raised and this should be noted in the case of those with a narrow therapeutic range, such as methotrexate.

Pharmacodynamic interactions have not been studied. However, while balsalazide, mesalazine, and N-acetylmesalazine are salicylates chemically, their properties and kinetics make classical salicylate interactions such as those found with acetylsalicylic acid very unlikely.

The uptake of digoxin has been impaired in some individuals by concomitant treatment with sulphasalazine. Even if it is not known whether this would occur also during treatment with balsalazide, it is recommended that plasma levels of digoxin should be monitored in digitalised patients starting Colazide.

4.6 Pregnancy and lactation

Animal studies on fertility and reproductive function did not reveal adverse effects of balsalazide. Human experience with balsalazide is limited, therefore Colazide should not be given to pregnant women. Colazide should not be given to breast feeding women as the active metabolite mesalazine has produced adverse effects in nursing infants.

4.7 Effects on ability to drive and use machines

No evidence of any relevant effect. Presumed to be safe.

4.8 Undesirable effects

The adverse effects are expected to be those of mesalazine.

Reactions reported during treatment with oral mesalazine are listed in the table below.

Organ group	Adverse Event
Blood and lymphatic system disorders	Blood dyscrasias Aplastic anaemia Leucopenia Neutropenia Agranulocytosis Thrombocytopenia
Nervous system disorders	Headache Neuropathy
Cardiac disorders	Myocarditis Pericarditis

Respiratory, thoracic and mediastinal disorders	Bronchospasm Allergic alveolitis
Gastrointestinal disorders	Abdominal pain Diarrhoea Nausea, vomiting Aggravation of ulcerative colitis Acute pancreatitis
Hepatobiliary disorders	Hepatitis Cholelithiasis
Skin and subcutaneous tissue disorders	Alopecia Rash
Musculoskeletal and connective tissue disorders	Systemic lupus erythematosus-like syndrome Arthralgia Myalgia
Renal and urinary disorders	Interstitial nephritis

See Section 4.4 Special warnings and special precautions for use

4.9 Overdose

To date, there are no reports of overdosage with mesalazine-releasing products. Overdose with large amounts of balsalazide may result in symptoms resembling mild salicylate intoxication. Treatment should be symptomatic.

5. PHARMACOLOGICAL PROPERTIES

5.1 Pharmacodynamic properties

ATC-code: A07 EC.

Balsalazide consists of mesalazine linked to a carrier molecule (4-aminobenzoyl-β-alanine) via an azo bond.

Bacterial azo-reduction releases mesalazine as an active metabolite in the colon. Mesalazine is an intestinal anti-inflammatory agent acting locally on the colonic mucosa. Its precise mechanism of action is unknown. Balsalazide and the carrier do not contribute to the pharmacodynamic action.

5.2 Pharmacokinetic properties

The pharmacokinetics of balsalazide and its metabolites have been studied in healthy subjects and patients in remission. The systemic uptake of balsalazide itself is low (<1%) and the major part of the dose is split in the colon by bacterial azoreductase. This cleavage results in the primary metabolites 5-aminosalicylic acid (5-ASA), responsible for the anti-inflammatory action, and 4-aminobenzoyl-beta-alanine (4-ABA), considered to be an inert carrier.

Most of the dose is eliminated via the faeces but about 25% of the released 5-ASA appears systemically predominantly as the N-acetylated metabolite (NASA) after inactivation in the colonic mucosa and liver. The systemic uptake of 4-ABA is only 10-15% of that of 5-ASA and also this metabolite is grossly N-acetylated (to NABA) in the first pass.

In urine, virtually only NASA and NABA are recovered and their renal clearances are high: 0.2-0.3 L/min and 0.4-0.5 L/min, respectively. The half-life of NASA is in the order of 6-9 hours. The half-life of 5-ASA itself is very short: about 1 hour.

Because of the great importance of renal clearance for the elimination, Colazide should be used with caution in renal impairment. No studies have been performed in patients with hepatic disease.

Protein binding of 5-ASA is about 40% and that of NASA about 80%. Available data suggest that the pharmacokinetics of balsalazide is not affected by genetic polymorphism, nor does age seem to be an important factor. Fasting slightly increases the systemic uptake of balsalazide and its metabolites.

5.3 Preclinical safety data

Preclinical data reveal no special hazard for humans based on conventional studies of genotoxicity, carcinogenic potential, toxicity to reproduction, safety pharmacology and validating kinetics and metabolism. In repeated dose toxicity studies, nephrotoxicity, an effect known to occur following mesalazine, was observed particularly in rats.

6. PHARMACEUTICAL PARTICULARS

6.1 List of excipients

Magnesium stearate, colloidal anhydrous silica, gelatin, shellac, titanium dioxide (E171), yellow, red and black iron oxide (E172).

6.2 Incompatibilities

Not relevant.

6.3 Shelf life

3 years.

6.4 Special precautions for storage

No special precautions for storage.

6.5 Nature and contents of container

High density polyethylene container fitted with tamper-evident, child-resistant, high density polyethylene screw caps.

Pack size: 130 capsules.

6.6 Instructions for use and handling

None.

7. MARKETING AUTHORISATION HOLDER

Shire Pharmaceuticals Ltd
Hampshire International Business Park
Chineham
Basingstoke
Hampshire RG24 8EP
United Kingdom

8. MARKETING AUTHORISATION NUMBER(S)

PL 08557/0044

9. DATE OF FIRST AUTHORISATION/RENEWAL OF THE AUTHORISATION

1 August 2000 / 17 December 2002

10. DATE OF REVISION OF THE TEXT

December 2002

LEGAL CATEGORY

POM

Colchicine Tablets BP 500mcg

(Celltech Manufacturing Services Limited)

1. NAME OF THE MEDICINAL PRODUCT

Colchicine Tablets BP 500 mcg

2. QUALITATIVE AND QUANTITATIVE COMPOSITION

Colchicine BP 0.50 mg

3. PHARMACEUTICAL FORM

White or faintly yellow biconvex uncoated tablets. Engraved Evans 126 on one side, plain on the other.

4. CLINICAL PARTICULARS

4.1 Therapeutic indications

Colchicine is used for the treatment of acute gout.

Colchicine is also used for the prophylaxis of recurrent gout and to prevent acute attacks during the initial treatment with allopurinol or uricosuric drugs.

4.2 Posology and method of administration

Oral administration in Adults.

Treatment for acute gout

1 mg initially, followed by 500 mcg every 2-3 hours until relief of pain is obtained or vomiting or diarrhoea occurs, or until a total dose of 10 mg has been reached. The course should not be repeated within 3 days.

Prophylaxis

500 mcg weekly or up to 2-3 times daily.

Prophylaxis of recurrent gout and prevention of acute attacks during initial treatment with allopurinol or uricosuric drugs, 500 mcg 2-3 times daily.

Administration in Elderly

The adult dose should apply, but with caution in patients with renal impairment, where the dosage should be reduced by up to 50%.

Administration in Children

There is no special dosage schedule for children, the safety and efficacy for use in children has not been established.

4.3 Contraindications

Hypersensitivity to Colchicine, serious gastro-intestinal, renal, hepatic, cardiac disorders, and blood dyscrasias.

4.4 Special warnings and special precautions for use

Other special warnings and precautions

Colchicine should be given with great care to elderly or debilitated patients and those with cardiac, hepatic, renal or gastro-intestinal disease. Colchicine has adversely affected spermatogenesis in humans under certain conditions of therapy. Periodic blood counts should be done in patients receiving long term therapy. Notify physician if skin rash, sore throat, fever, unusual bleeding, bruising, tiredness or weakness, numbness or tingling occurs. Discontinue medication as soon as gout pain is relieved or at the first sign of nausea, vomiting, stomach pain, or diarrhoea. If symptoms persist, notify physician.

4.5 Interaction with other medicinal products and other forms of Interaction

Colchicine has been shown to induce reversible malabsorption of vitamin B12, apparently by altering the function of ileal mucosa. Colchicine may impair the absorption of fat, sodium, potassium, nitrogen, xylose and other actively transported sugars. This may lead to decreased serum cholesterol and carotene concentrations.

Colchicine is inhibited by acidifying agents but is potentiated by alkalinizing agents.

Colchicine may increase sensitivity to CNS depressants and enhance the response to sympathomimetic agents.

Colchicine may cause false-positive results when testing urine for RBC or haemoglobin.

Colchicine may react with cyclosporin leading to an increased risk of nephrotoxicity and increased plasma-cyclosporin concentration.

Colchicine has been reported to interfere with urinary determinations of 17-hydroxycorticoids using the Reddy, Jenkins and Thorn procedure.

4.6 Pregnancy and lactation

Colchicine has been shown to be teratogenic in animals and there is a risk of teratogenicity or of foetal chromosomal damage in humans. Colchicine should not be used during the first trimester of pregnancy and only used in late stages of pregnancy where the risk/benefit ratio has been considered as Colchicine may be excreted in breast milk. It should not be given to lactating mother because of the risk of cytotoxic effects.

4.7 Effects on ability to drive and use machines

No specific statement.

4.8 Undesirable effects

Colchicine therapy may cause elevated alkaline phosphatase and SGOT values.

Decreased thrombocyte values may be obtained during therapy.

Bone marrow depression with aplastic anaemic, agranulocytosis, leukopenia or thrombocytopenia may occur in patients receiving long term therapy. Loss of hair, rashes, vesicular dermatitis, peripheral neuritis or neuropathy, myopathy, anuria, renal damage, haematuria and purpura have been reported with prolonged administration of colchicine.

Vomiting, diarrhoea, abdominal pain and nausea may occur, especially when maximum doses are necessary for a therapeutic effect. These may be particularly troublesome in the presence of peptic ulcer or spastic colon.

At toxic doses colchicine may cause severe diarrhoea, generalised vascular damage and renal damage with haematuria and oliguria. To avoid more serious toxicity, discontinue use when these symptoms appear, regardless of whether joint pain has been relieved. Dermatoses have been reported; hypersensitivity reactions may occur infrequently.

4.9 Overdose

Symptoms do not appear for at least several hours. The first symptoms are nausea, vomiting and diarrhoea. The diarrhoea may be severe and haemorrhagic and can lead to metabolic acidosis, dehydration, hypotension and shock. A burning sensation of the throat, stomach and skin may also occur. Extensive vascular damage and acute renal toxicity with oliguria and haematuria have been reported. Bone marrow depression with leukopenia may be followed by rebound leukocytosis. The patient may develop convulsions, delerium, muscle weakness, neuropathy and ascending paralysis of the CNS. Death may be due to respiratory depression, cardiovascular collapse or bone marrow depression.

Other symptoms are stomatitis, arthralgia, malaise, hypocalcemia, fever and rashes including scarlatiniform rash. Tender hepatomegaly with elevated serum concentrations of AST (SGOT) and alkaline phosphatase may occur. Hematological manifestations of colchicine toxicity, other than leucopenia, include thrombocytopenia, granulocytopenia, immature leucocytes, pancytopenia, anaemia with anisocytosis, polychromasia, and basophilic stippling. Deep tendon reflexes may be lost and a positive Babinski's reflex may be found.

Treatment

Patients should be monitored carefully for some time to take account of the delayed onset of symptoms. In acute poisoning the stomach should be emptied by aspiration and lavage. Respiration may require assistance. The circulation should be maintained and fluid and electrolyte imbalance corrected. Morphine or atropine may be given to treat other symptoms. Haemodialysis or peritoneal dialysis may be of value when kidney function is compromised.

5. PHARMACOLOGICAL PROPERTIES

5.1 Pharmacodynamic properties

The exact mechanism of action of Colchicine in gout is not known. It is involved in leukocyte migration inhibition; reduction of lactic acid production by leukocytes which results in a decreased deposition of uric acid; interference with kinin formation and reduction of phagocytosis with inflammatory response abatement.

Colchicine apparently exerts its effect by reducing the inflammatory response to the deposited crystals and also by diminishing phagocytosis.

Colchicine diminishes lactic acid production by leukocytes directly and by diminishing phagocytosis and thereby interrupts the cycle of urate crystal deposition and inflammatory response that sustains the acute attack.

The oxidation of glucose in phagocytizing as well as in nonphagocytizing leukocytes in vitro is suppressed by Colchicine.

Colchicine is not an analgesic, although it relieves pain in acute attacks. It is not a uricosuric agent and will not prevent the progression of gout to chronic gouty arthritis.

It has a prophylactic, suppressive effect which helps reduce the incidence of acute attacks and relieve the patients occasional residual pain and mild discomfort.

Colchicine can produce a temporary leukopenia which is followed by leukocytosis.

5.2 Pharmacokinetic properties

Absorption

Readily absorbed after oral administration, peak concentrations in plasma after 2 hours.

Half-Life

Plasma half-life about 1 hour, but 60 hours in leucocytes, which is increased in renal function impairment and decreased in hepatic function impairment.

Distribution

Colchicine does not appear to be specifically localised in any tissues except the liver leucocytes, spleen and kidneys; it undergoes enterohepatic circulation.

Metabolic Reactions

Deacetylated in the liver.

Excretion

Colchicine is mainly excreted in the faeces, with 10-20% in the urine. The percentage excreted in the urine rises in patients with hepatic disease.

5.3 Preclinical safety data

Colchicine has been shown to be teratogenic in animals and there is a risk of teratogenicity or of foetal damage in humans.

6. PHARMACEUTICAL PARTICULARS

6.1 List of excipients

Lactose BP

Starch Maize BP

Purified Water BP

Magnesium Stearate BP

6.2 Incompatibilities

None stated

6.3 Shelf life

36 months

6.4 Special precautions for storage

Protect from light

Store below 25°C

Keep well closed

6.5 Nature and contents of container

Pigmented polypropylene with tamper-evident closure of low density polyethylene.

Pack size 20, 28, 30, 50, 60 and 100.

6.6 Instructions for use and handling

As directed by physician.

Administrative Data

7. MARKETING AUTHORISATION HOLDER

Celltech Manufacturing Services Limited

Vale of Bardsley

Ashton-under-Lyne

Lancashire

OL7 9RR

United Kingdom

8. MARKETING AUTHORISATION NUMBER(S)

PL 18816/0004

9. DATE OF FIRST AUTHORISATION/RENEWAL OF THE AUTHORISATION

18 July 2001

10. DATE OF REVISION OF THE TEXT

COLESTID granules for oral suspension

(Pharmacia Limited)

1. NAME OF THE MEDICINAL PRODUCT

Colestid granules for oral suspension 5g

2. QUALITATIVE AND QUANTITATIVE COMPOSITION

Each level scoopful or sachet contains 5.0 grams of Colestipol hydrochloride BP.

For excipients see 6.1

3. PHARMACEUTICAL FORM

Granules for oral suspension.

Light yellow, tasteless and odourless granules.

4. CLINICAL PARTICULARS

4.1 Therapeutic indications

Colestid is indicated as adjunctive therapy to diet in the management of patients with elevated cholesterol levels who have not responded adequately to diet. It may be used alone or in combination with additional lipid lowering agents.

Dietary therapy specific for the type of hypercholesterolaemia should be the initial treatment of choice. Excess body weight may be an important factor and weight reduction should be attempted prior to drug therapy in the overweight. The use of drugs should be considered only when reasonable attempts have been made to obtain satisfactory results with non-drug method. When drug therapy is begun, the patient should be instructed of the importance of adhering to the correct diet.

Although Colestid is effective in all types of hypercholesterolaemia, it is medically most appropriate in patients with Fredrickson's type II hyperlipoproteinaemia.

4.2 Posology and method of administration

Route of administration: Oral, mixed with water or other fluids.

Adults:

The recommended initial daily adult dosage of colestipol hydrochloride is 5 grams either once or twice daily.

For adults colestipol hydrochloride is recommended in doses of 5 - 30 grams taken as one dose or two divided doses. Initiation of therapy is recommended at 5 grams either once or twice daily with 5 gram increments at one month intervals. Appropriate use of lipid profiles including LDL-cholesterol and triglycerides is advised so that optimal, but not excessive doses are used to obtain the desired therapeutic effect on LDL-cholesterol level. If the desired therapeutic effect is not obtained at a dose of 5 - 30 grams/day with good compliance and acceptable side-effects, combined therapy or alternate treatment should be considered.

Patients should take other drugs at least one hour before or four hours after Colestid to minimise possible interference with their absorption. However, Colestid and Gemfibrozil may be used in the same patient when administered 2 hours apart (see Interactions).

Preparation:

Colestid Granules should always be taken mixed in a liquid such as orange or tomato juice, water, skimmed milk or non-carbonated beverage. The contents of the sachet or level scoopful should be added to 100 ml or more of the preferred aqueous vehicle and mixed thoroughly until dispersed. Colestid may also be taken in soups or with cereals, pulpy fruits with a higher water content or yoghurt.

Elderly Patients:

At present there are no extensive clinical studies with colestipol in patients over the age of 65. Review of available data does not suggest that the elderly are more predisposed to side effects attributable to colestipol than the general population; however, therapy should be individualised and based on each patient's clinical characteristics and tolerance to the medication.

Children:

Dosage in children has not been established.

4.3 Contraindications

Colestipol is contra-indicated in individuals who have previously demonstrated hypersensitivity to its use.

4.4 Special warnings and special precautions for use

Warnings:

Before instituting therapy with Colestid, diseases contributing to increased blood cholesterol such as hypothyroidism, diabetes mellitus, nephrotic syndrome, dysproteinaemias and obstructive liver disease should be looked for and specifically treated.

To avoid accidental inhalation or oesophageal distress, Colestid should not be taken in its dry form.

Colestid may elevate serum triglyceride levels when used as sole therapy. This elevation is generally transient but may persist in some individuals. A significant rise in triglyceride level should be considered as an indication for dose reduction, drug discontinuation, or combined or alternate therapy.

The use of Colestid in children has been limited; however, it does appear to be effective in lowering serum cholesterol in older children and young adults. Because bile acid sequestrants may interfere with the absorption of fat soluble vitamins, appropriate monitoring of growth and development is essential. Dosage and long term safety in children has not been established.

Precautions:

Because it sequesters bile acids, Colestid may interfere with normal fat absorption and thus may alter absorption of fat soluble vitamins such as A, D, E and K. A study in humans found only one patient in whom a prolonged prothombin time was noted. Most studies did not show a decrease in vitamin A, D or E levels during the administration of Colestid; however, if Colestid is to be given for a long period these vitamin levels should be monitored and supplements given if necessary.

Both clinical usage and animal studies with Colestid have provided no evidence of drug related intestinal neoplasms. Colestid is not mutagenic in the Ames test.

4.5 Interaction with other medicinal products and other forms of Interaction

In man, Colestid may delay or reduce the absorption of certain concomitant oral drugs (digitalis and its glycosides, propranolol, chlorothiazide and hydrochlorothiazide, tetracycline hydrochloride, penicillin G, gemfibrozil). Particular caution should be taken with digitalis preparations since conflicting results have been obtained for the effect of Colestid on the availability of digoxin and digitoxin. Colestid has been shown not to interfere with the absorption of clindamycin, clofibrate, asparin, tolbutamide, warfarin, methyldopa and phenytoin. The clinical response to concomitant medication should be closely monitored and appropriate adjustments made.

Repeated doses of Colestid given prior to a single dose of propranolol in human trials have been reported to decrease propranolol absorption. However, in a follow-up study in normal subjects, single dose administration of Colestid and propranolol or multiple dose administration of both agents did not affect the extent of propranolol absorption. Effects on the absorption of other beta-blockers have not been determined. Patients on propranolol should be observed when Colestid is either added or deleted from a therapeutic regimen.

4.6 Pregnancy and lactation

Safety for use in pregnant women has not been established. The use of Colestid in pregnancy or lactation or by women of childbearing age requires that the potential benefits of treatment be weighed against the possible hazards to the mother and child.

4.7 Effects on ability to drive and use machines

No adverse effect has been reported.

4.8 Undesirable effects

Side-effects

The most common adverse reactions reported with Colestid have been of a functional gastro-intestinal nature. The most frequent is constipation which is usually mild, transient and responsive to the usual adjunctive measures. At times, constipation can be severe and may be accompanied by impaction. As such, haemorrhoids can be aggravated, and infrequent blood in the stools has been reported. Less frequent gastro-intestinal complaints are abdominal discomfort, belching, flatulence, indigestion, nausea, vomiting and diarrhoea. Rarely, peptic ulceration and bleeding, cholelithiasis and cholecystitis have been reported, although these are not necessarily drug related.

Transient and modest elevation of SGOT and alkaline phosphatase have been observed. No medical significance is attached to these observed changes.

Although not necessarily drug-related, the following non gastro-intestinal medical events have been reported during clinical trials at a similar incidence to placebo.

Cardiovascular: Chest pain, angina and tachycardia have been infrequently reported.

Hypersensitivity: Rash has been infrequently reported. Urticaria and dermatitis have been rarely noted.

Musculoskeletal: Musculoskeletal pain, aches and pains in the extremities, joint pain and arthritis, and backache have been reported.

Neurological: Headache, migraine headache and sinus headache have been reported. Other infrequently reported complaints include dizziness, light-headedness, and insomnia.

Miscellaneous: Anorexia, fatigue, weakness, shortness of breath, and swelling of the hands or feet, have been infrequently reported.

4.9 Overdose

No toxic effects due to overdosage have been reported. Should overdosage occur, obstruction of the gastro-intestinal tract would be expected to occur. Treatment would be determined by the location and degree of obstruction.

5. PHARMACOLOGICAL PROPERTIES

5.1 Pharmacodynamic properties

Ion exchange resin which lowers plasma cholesterol through binding with bile acids in the intestinal lumen.

5.2 Pharmacokinetic properties

Colestid is not absorbed; its action is limited to the lumen of the gastro-intestinal tract, and it is passed in the faeces. It binds bile acids in the intestinal lumen and causes them to be excreted in the faeces together with the polymer. When the enterohepatic circulation of bile acids is interrupted, cholesterol conversion to bile acids is enhanced and plasma cholesterol levels are thereby lowered.

5.3 Preclinical safety data

Both clinical and animal studies with Colestid have provided no evidence of drug related intestinal neospasms. Colestid is not mutagenic in the Ames test.

6. PHARMACEUTICAL PARTICULARS

6.1 List of excipients

Colloidal Anhydrous Silica Ph.Eur

6.2 Incompatibilities

None

6.3 Shelf life

4 years

6.4 Special precautions for storage

None

6.5 Nature and contents of container

Paper/Aluminium foil/vinyl sachets of 5 gm in packs of 30 sachets

6.6 Instructions for use and handling

None

Administrative Data

7. MARKETING AUTHORISATION HOLDER

Pharmacia Limited

Davy Avenue

Milton Keynes

MK5 8PH

UK

8. MARKETING AUTHORISATION NUMBER(S)

PL 0032/0055

9. DATE OF FIRST AUTHORISATION/RENEWAL OF THE AUTHORISATION

26 October 1992

10. DATE OF REVISION OF THE TEXT

September 2002

Company Reference: CL2_0

COLESTID Orange

(Pharmacia Limited)

1. NAME OF THE MEDICINAL PRODUCT

Colestid Orange

2. QUALITATIVE AND QUANTITATIVE COMPOSITION

Colestipol Hydrochloride USP 5.0 gram

3. PHARMACEUTICAL FORM

Granules for oral administration.

4. CLINICAL PARTICULARS

4.1 Therapeutic indications

Colestid is indicated as adjunctive therapy to diet in the management of patients with elevated cholesterol levels who have not responded adequately to diet. It may be used alone or in combination with additional lipid lowering agents.

Dietary therapy specific for the type of hypercholesterolaemia should be the initial treatment of choice. Excess body weight may be an important factor and weight reduction should be attempted prior to drug therapy in the overweight. The use of drugs should be considered only when reasonable attempts have been made to obtain satisfactory results with non-drug methods. When drug therapy is begun, the patient should be instructed of the importance of adhering to the correct diet.

Although Colestid is effective in all types of hypercholesterolaemia, it is medically most appropriate in patients with Fredrickson's type II hyperlipoproteinaemia.

4.2 Posology and method of administration

Route of administration: Oral, mixed with water or other fluids.

Adults:

The recommended initial daily adult dosage of colestipol hydrochloride is 5 grams either once or twice daily.

For adults colestipol hydrochloride is recommended in doses of 5-30 grams taken as one dose or two divided doses. Initiation of therapy is recommended at 5 grams either once or twice daily with 5 gram increments at one month intervals. Appropriate use of lipid profiles including LDL-cholesterol and triglycerides is advised so that optimal, but not excessive doses are used to obtain the desired therapeutic effect on LDL-cholesterol level. If the desired therapeutic effect is not obtained at a dose of 5-30 grams/day with good compliance and acceptable side-effects, combined therapy or alternate treatment should be considered.

Patients should take other drugs at least one hour before or four hours after Colestid to minimise possible interference with their absorption. However, Colestid and gemfibrozil may be used in the same patient when administered 2 hours apart. (See interactions).

Preparation:

Colestid should always be taken mixed in a liquid such as orange or tomato juice, water, skimmed milk or non-carbonated beverage. The contents of the sachet or level scoopful should be added to 100 ml or more of the preferred aqueous vehicle and mixed thoroughly until dispersed. Colestid may also be taken in soups or with cereals, pulpy fruits with a high water content or yoghurt.

Elderly patients:

At present there are no extensive clinical studies with colestipol in patients over the age of 65. Review of available data does not suggest that the elderly are more predisposed to side-effects attributable to colestipol than the general population; however, therapy should be individualised and based on each patient's clinical characteristics and tolerance to the medication.

Children:

Dosage in children has not been established.

4.3 Contraindications

Colestipol is contra-indicated in individuals who have previously demonstrated hypersensitivity to its use.

4.4 Special warnings and special precautions for use

Warnings:

Before instituting therapy with Colestid, diseases contributing to increased blood cholesterol such as hypothyroidism, diabetes mellitus, nephrotic syndrome, dysproteinaemias and obstructive liver diseases should be looked for and specifically treated.

To avoid accidental inhalation or oesophageal distress, Colestid should not be taken in its dry form.

Colestid Orange contains 0.0325 g aspartame per sachet or level scoopful. This should be taken into consideration in patients suffering from phenylketonuria since excessive amounts of aspartame may interfere with the control of this condition.

Colestid may elevate serum triglyceride levels when used as sole therapy. This elevation is generally transient but may persist in some individuals. A significant rise in triglyceride level should be considered as an indication for dose reduction, drug discontinuation, or combined or alternate therapy.

The use of Colestid in children has been limited; however, it does appear to be effective in lowering serum cholesterol in older children and young adults. Because bile acid sequestrants may interfere with the absorption of fat-soluble vitamins, appropriate monitoring of growth and development is essential. Dosage and long term safety in children have not been established.

Precautions:

Because it sequesters bile acids, Colestid may interfere with normal fat absorption and thus may alter absorption of fat soluble vitamins such as A, D, E and K. A study in humans found only one patient in whom a prolonged prothombin time was noted. Most studies did not show a decrease in vitamin A, D or E levels during the administration of Colestid; however, if Colestid is to be given for a long period these vitamin levels should be monitored and supplements given if necessary.

4.5 Interaction with other medicinal products and other forms of Interaction

In man, Colestid may delay or reduce the absorption of certain concomitant oral drugs (digitalis and its glycosides, propranolol, chlorothiazide and hydrochlorothiazide, tetracycline hydrochloride, penicillin G, gemfibrozil and furosemide). Particular caution should be taken with digitalis preparations since conflicting results have been obtained for the effect of Colestid on the availability of digoxin and digitoxin. Colestid has been shown not to interfere with the absorption of clindamycin, clofibrate, aspirin, tolbutamide, warfarin, methyldopa and phenytoin. The clinical response to concomitant medication should be closely monitored and appropriate adjustments made.

Repeated doses of Colestid given prior to a single dose of propranolol in human trials have been reported to decrease propranolol absorption. However, in a follow-up study in normal subjects, single dose administration of Colestid and propranolol or multiple dose administration of both agents did not affect the extent of propranolol absorption. Effects on the absorption of other beta-blockers have not been determined. Patients on propranolol should be observed when Colestid is either added or deleted from a therapeutic regimen.

4.6 Pregnancy and lactation

Safety for use in pregnant women has not been established. The use of Colestid in pregnancy or lactation or by women of childbearing age requires that the potential benefits of treatment be weighed against the possible hazards to the mother and child.

4.7 Effects on ability to drive and use machines

No adverse effect has been reported.

4.8 Undesirable effects

Side-effects:

The most common adverse reactions reported with Colestid have been of a functional gastro-intestinal nature. The most frequent is constipation which is usually mild, transient and responsive to the usual adjunctive measures. At times, constipation can be severe and may be accompanied by impaction. As such, haemorrhoids can be aggravated, and infrequent blood in the stools has been reported. Less frequent gastro-intestinal complaints are abdominal discomfort, belching, flatulence, indigestion, nausea, vomiting and diarrhoea. Rarely, peptic ulceration and bleeding, cholelithiasis and cholecystitis have been reported, although these are not necessarily drug related.

Transient and modest elevation of SGOT and alkaline phosphatase have been observed. No medical significance is attached to these observed changes.

Although not necessarily drug-related, the following non-gastro-intestinal medical events have been reported during clinical trials at a similar incidence to placebo.

Cardiovascular: Chest pain, angina, and tachycardia have been infrequently reported.

Hypersensitivity: Rash has been infrequently reported. Urticaria and dermatitis have been rarely noted.

Musculoskeletal: Musculoskeletal pain, aches and pains in the extremities, joint pain and arthritis, and backache have been reported.

Neurological: Headache, migraine headache and sinus headache have been reported. Other infrequently reported complaints include dizziness, light-headedness, and insomnia.

Miscellaneous: Anorexia, fatigue, weakness, shortness of breath, and swelling of the hands or feet, have been infrequently reported.

4.9 Overdose

No toxic effects due to overdosage have been reported. Should overdosage occur, obstruction of the gastro-intestinal tract would be expected to occur. Treatment should be determined by the location and degree of obstruction.

5. PHARMACOLOGICAL PROPERTIES

5.1 Pharmacodynamic properties

Ion exchange resin which lowers plasma cholesterol through binding with bile acids in the intestinal lumen.

5.2 Pharmacokinetic properties

Colestid is not absorbed; its action is limited to the lumen of the gastro-intestinal tract, and it is passed in the faeces. It binds bile acids in the intestinal lumen and causes them to be excreted in the faeces together with the polymer. When the enterohepatic circulation of bile acids is interrupted, cholesterol conversion to bile acids is enhanced and plasma cholesterol levels are thereby lowered.

5.3 Preclinical safety data

Both clinical usage and animal studies with Colestid have provided no evidence of drug related intestinal neoplasms. Colestid is not mutagenic in the ames test.

6. PHARMACEUTICAL PARTICULARS

6.1 List of excipients

Mannitol Ph. Eur.

Methylcellulose (15CPS) Ph. Eur.

Citric Acid Ph. Eur.

Orange Durarome Wonf HSE

Aspartame Powder NF

Maltol HSE

Ethyl Vanillin NF

Beta Carotene 1% HSE

Glycerol Ph. Eur.

Purified Water Ph. Eur.

6.2 Incompatibilities

None.

6.3 Shelf life

24 months.

6.4 Special precautions for storage

Store at controlled room temperature (15-30°C).

6.5 Nature and contents of container

Foil sachets in packs 30 sachets.

6.6 Instructions for use and handling

None.

7. MARKETING AUTHORISATION HOLDER

Pharmacia Limited

Davy Avenue

Milton Keynes

MK5 8PH

UK

8. MARKETING AUTHORISATION NUMBER(S)

PL 0032/0172

9. DATE OF FIRST AUTHORISATION/RENEWAL OF THE AUTHORISATION

Date of Grant: 25 February 1992

Date of Renewal: 30 Oct 2002

10. DATE OF REVISION OF THE TEXT

5 March 2003

Legal Category POM

Company Reference: CL2_0

Colifoam

(Meda Pharmaceuticals)

1. NAME OF THE MEDICINAL PRODUCT

Colifoam.

2. QUALITATIVE AND QUANTITATIVE COMPOSITION

Hydrocortisone Acetate 10% w/w.

3. PHARMACEUTICAL FORM

Aerosol foam.

4. CLINICAL PARTICULARS

4.1 Therapeutic indications

Ulcerative colitis, proctosigmoiditis and granular proctitis.

4.2 Posology and method of administration

All ages:

One applicatorful inserted into the rectum once or twice daily for two to three weeks and every second day thereafter.

4.3 Contraindications
Local contra-indications to the use of intrarectal steroids include obstruction, abscess, perforation, peritonitis, fresh intestinal anastomoses, extensive fistulae, and tuberculous, fungal or viral infections.

4.4 Special warnings and special precautions for use
General precautions common to all corticosteroid therapy should be observed during treatment with Colifoam, especially in the case of young children. Treatment should be administered with caution in patients with severe ulcerative disease because of their predisposition to perforation of the bowel wall. Although uncommon at this dosage local irritation may occur.

4.5 Interaction with other medicinal products and other forms of Interaction
None known.

4.6 Pregnancy and lactation
Systemic and topical administration of corticosteroids to pregnant animals can cause abnormalities of foetal development. The relevance of this finding to human beings has not been established but at present steroids should not be used extensively in pregnancy, that is in large amounts or for prolonged periods.

4.7 Effects on ability to drive and use machines
None known.

4.8 Undesirable effects
Although uncommon at this dosage, irritation may occur.

Side effects are very unusual with Colifoam, but long term frequent use may cause problems in some people. This is particularly so if the medicine is not used as directed. Although uncommon at this dosage, the following side effects may occur; unexpected fattening of the face, neck and body, periods may stop unexpectedly and hair starts to grow on the face (in women), dusky complexion with purple markings, local irritation.

4.9 Overdose
Not applicable.

5. PHARMACOLOGICAL PROPERTIES
5.1 Pharmacodynamic properties
The use of topically applied steroids in the treatment of ulcerative colitis, proctosigmoiditis and granular proctitis is well known.

5.2 Pharmacokinetic properties
The topically applied steroid acts locally and so pharmacokinetics are not relevant to its activity.

5.3 Preclinical safety data
None stated.

6. PHARMACEUTICAL PARTICULARS
6.1 List of excipients
Propylene Glycol

Emulsifying Wax

Polyoxyethylene (10) Stearyl Ether

Cetyl Alcohol

Methyl Hydroxybenzoate

Propyl Hydroxybenzoate

Triethanolamine

Water Purified

Propellant HP-70

6.2 Incompatibilities
None known.

6.3 Shelf life
60 months.

6.4 Special precautions for storage
Pressurised container containing flammable propellant. Protect from sunlight and do not expose to temperatures about 50°C. Store below 25°C. Do not refrigerate. Do not spray on naked flame or any incandescent material. Keep away from sources of ignition - no smoking. Do not pierce or burn even after use.

6.5 Nature and contents of container
Aerosol canister containing 20.8g of foam, plus a plastic applicator.

6.6 Instructions for use and handling
SEE LEAFLET.

1. Shake the canister vigorously before each use.

2. Fill applicator so that the foam fills about ¼ of the applicator body. Only a short press is needed to do this.

3. Wait until foam has stopped expanding.

4. Repeat step 2 until the foam expands to just reach the "Fill" line. This normally takes 2 - 4 short press/waits.

5. Stand with one leg raised on a chair, or lie down on your left side. Insert gently into back passage and push plunger fully into the applicator.

7. MARKETING AUTHORISATION HOLDER
Meda Pharmaceuticals Ltd

Sherwood House

7 Gregory Boulevard

Nottingham

NG7 6LB

United Kingdom

Trading as: Meda Pharmaceuticals, Regus House, Herald Way, Pegasus Business Park, Castle Donington, Derbyshire, DE74 2TZ, UK.

8. MARKETING AUTHORISATION NUMBER(S)
PL 19477/0009.

9. DATE OF FIRST AUTHORISATION/RENEWAL OF THE AUTHORISATION
5th July 1973/18th September 2001.

10. DATE OF REVISION OF THE TEXT
30th November 2003.

Colofac MR
(Solvay Healthcare Limited)

1. NAME OF THE MEDICINAL PRODUCT
Colofac® MR

2. QUALITATIVE AND QUANTITATIVE COMPOSITION
Mebeverine hydrochloride BP 200 mg.

3. PHARMACEUTICAL FORM
White, opaque, modified release capsule imprinted S 245

4. CLINICAL PARTICULARS
4.1 Therapeutic indications
For the symptomatic relief of irritable bowel syndrome.

4.2 Posology and method of administration
Adults (including the elderly): One capsule twice a day, preferably 20 minutes before meals.

Children: Not recommended.

4.3 Contraindications
Paralytic ileus.

Hypersensitivity to any of the components of the capsule.

4.4 Special warnings and special precautions for use
Porphyria.

4.5 Interaction with other medicinal products and other forms of Interaction
None known.

4.6 Pregnancy and lactation
Pregnancy: Animal experiments have failed to show any teratogenic effects. However, the usual precautions concerning the administration of any drug during pregnancy should be observed.

Lactation: Mebeverine is excreted in milk of lactating women after therapeutic doses.

4.7 Effects on ability to drive and use machines
None.

4.8 Undesirable effects
In very rare cases allergic reactions have been reported, in particular erythematous rash, urticaria and angioedema.

4.9 Overdose
On theoretical grounds it may be predicted that CNS excitability will occur in cases of overdosage. No specific antidote is known; gastric lavage and symptomatic treatment is recommended.

5. PHARMACOLOGICAL PROPERTIES
5.1 Pharmacodynamic properties
Mebeverine is a musculotropic antispasmodic with a direct action on the smooth muscle of the gastrointestinal tract, relieving spasm without affecting normal gut motility.

5.2 Pharmacokinetic properties
Mebeverine is rapidly and completely absorbed after oral administration in the form of tablets or suspension. Mebeverine is not excreted as such, but metabolised completely. The first step in the metabolism is hydrolysis, leading to veratric acid and mebeverine alcohol. Both veratric acid and mebeverine alcohol are excreted into the urine, the latter partly as the corresponding carboxylic acid and partly as the demethylated carboxylic acid.

6. PHARMACEUTICAL PARTICULARS
6.1 List of excipients
Magnesium stearate, copolymer of ethyl acrylate and methyl methacrylate, talc, methylhydroxypropylcellulose, methacrylic acid-ethyl acrylate copolymer (1:1) and glycerol triacetate.

Capsule shell: gelatin and titanium dioxide (E171).

Printing inks: shellac (E904), black iron oxide (E172), soya lecithin (E322) and Antifoam DC.

6.2 Incompatibilities
Not applicable.

6.3 Shelf life
3 years when stored in the original container.

6.4 Special precautions for storage
Do not store above 30°C. Do not refrigerate or freeze. Store in the original package.

6.5 Nature and contents of container
Boxes containing 10 or 60 capsules in PVC-Al press through strips.

6.6 Instructions for use and handling
None.

Administrative Data
7. MARKETING AUTHORISATION HOLDER
Solvay Healthcare Limited

Mansbridge Road

West End

Southampton

SO18 3JD

8. MARKETING AUTHORISATION NUMBER(S)
PL 00512/0155

9. DATE OF FIRST AUTHORISATION/RENEWAL OF THE AUTHORISATION
14 August 1998

10. DATE OF REVISION OF THE TEXT
July 2002

Legal Category
POM

Colofac Tablets 135mg
(Solvay Healthcare Limited)

1. NAME OF THE MEDICINAL PRODUCT
Colofac Tablets 135 mg

2. QUALITATIVE AND QUANTITATIVE COMPOSITION
Mebeverine hydrochloride 135mg.

For excipients, see section 6.1

3. PHARMACEUTICAL FORM
Coated tablets.

Round white sugar coated tablets, with no superficial markings.

4. CLINICAL PARTICULARS
4.1 Therapeutic indications
For the symptomatic treatment of irritable bowel syndrome and other conditions usually included in this grouping, such as: chronic irritable colon, spastic constipation, mucous colitis, spastic colitis. Colofac is effectively used to treat the symptoms of these conditions, such as: colicky abdominal pain and cramps, persistent, non-specific diarrhoea (with or without alternating constipation) and flatulence.

4.2 Posology and method of administration
Adults (including the elderly) and children 10 years and over:

One tablet three times a day, preferably 20 minutes before meals. After a period of several weeks, when the desired effect has been obtained, the dosage may be gradually reduced.

Children under 10 years: Not applicable.

4.3 Contraindications
Hypersensitivity to any component of the product.

4.4 Special warnings and special precautions for use
None.

4.5 Interaction with other medicinal products and other forms of Interaction
None known.

4.6 Pregnancy and lactation
Animal experiments have failed to show any teratogenic effects. However, the usual precautions concerning the administration of any drug during pregnancy should be observed.

4.7 Effects on ability to drive and use machines
None.

4.8 Undesirable effects
In very rare cases allergic reactions have been reported, in particular erythematous rash, urticaria and angioedema.

4.9 Overdose
On theoretical grounds it may be predicted that CNS excitability will occur in cases of overdosage. No specific antidote is known; gastric lavage and symptomatic treatment is recommended.

5. PHARMACOLOGICAL PROPERTIES
5.1 Pharmacodynamic properties
Mebeverine is a musculotropic antispasmodic with a direct action on the smooth muscle of the gastrointestinal tract, relieving spasm without affecting normal gut motility.

5.2 Pharmacokinetic properties
Mebeverine is rapidly and completely absorbed after oral administration in the form of tablets or suspension. Mebeverine is not excreted as such, but metabolised completely. The first step in the metabolism is hydrolysis, leading to veratric acid and mebeverine alcohol. Both veratric acid and mebeverine alcohol are excreted into the urine, the latter partly as the corresponding carboxylic acid and partly as the demethylated carboxylic acid.

5.3 Preclinical safety data
Not applicable.

6. PHARMACEUTICAL PARTICULARS
6.1 List of excipients
Lactose, starch (potato or maize), povidone, talc, magnesium stearate, sucrose, gelatin, acacia, carnauba wax.

6.2 Incompatibilities
Not applicable.

6.3 Shelf life
5 years.

6.4 Special precautions for storage
Do not store above 30°C. Store in the original package.

6.5 Nature and contents of container
Boxes containing 10, 15, 84 or 100 tablets in blister strips.

HDPE tamper-evident tablet container with snap on cap containing 500 tablets.

6.6 Instructions for use and handling
None.

7. MARKETING AUTHORISATION HOLDER
Solvay Healthcare Limited
Mansbridge Road
West End
Southampton
SO18 3JD

8. MARKETING AUTHORISATION NUMBER(S)
PL 00512/0044

9. DATE OF FIRST AUTHORISATION/RENEWAL OF THE AUTHORISATION
14 March 1978/21 April 2005

10. DATE OF REVISION OF THE TEXT
April 2004

Legal Status
POM

Colomycin Injection

(Forest Laboratories UK Limited)

1. NAME OF THE MEDICINAL PRODUCT
COLOMYCIN INJECTION 500,000, 1 million or 2 million International Units.

Powder for solution for injection or inhalation.

2. QUALITATIVE AND QUANTITATIVE COMPOSITION
Each vial contains either 500,000, 1 million or 2 million International Units Colistimethate Sodium.

For excipients, see 6.1

3. PHARMACEUTICAL FORM
Powder for solution for injection or inhalation.

500,000 IU/vial: Sterile white powder in a 10ml colourless glass vial with a blue 'flip-off' cap.

1 million IU/vial: Sterile white powder in a 10ml colourless glass vial with a red 'flip-off' cap.

2 million IU/vial: Sterile white powder in a 10ml colourless glass vial with a lilac 'flip-off' cap.

4. CLINICAL PARTICULARS
4.1 Therapeutic indications
Colomycin is indicated in the treatment of the following infections where sensitivity testing suggests that they are caused by susceptible bacteria:

Treatment by inhalation of *Pseudomonas aeruginosa* lung infection in patients with cystic fibrosis (CF).

Intravenous administration for the treatment of some serious infections caused by Gram-negative bacteria, including those of the lower respiratory tract and urinary tract, when more commonly used systemic antibacterial agents may be contra-indicated or may be ineffective because of bacterial resistance.

4.2 Posology and method of administration
SYSTEMIC TREATMENT

Colomycin can be given as a 50ml intravenous infusion over a period of 30 minutes. Patients with a totally implantable venous access device (TIVAD) in place may tolerate a bolus injection of up to 2 million units in 10ml given over a minimum of 5 minutes (see section 6.6).

The dose is determined by the severity and type of infection and the age, weight and renal function of the patient. Should clinical or bacteriological response be slow the dose may be increased as indicated by the patient's condition.

Serum level estimations are recommended especially in renal impairment, neonates and cystic fibrosis patients. Levels of 10–15 mg/l (approximately 125-200 units/ml) colistimethate sodium should be adequate for most infections.

A minimum of 5 days treatment is generally recommended. For the treatment of respiratory exacerbations in cystic fibrosis patients, treatment should be continued for up to 12 days.

Children and adults (including the elderly):

Up to 60kg: 50,000 units/kg/day to a maximum of 75,000 units/kg/day. The total daily dose should be divided into three doses given at approximately 8-hour intervals.

Over 60kg: 1-2 million units three times a day. The maximum dose is 6 million units in 24 hours.

Anomalous distribution in patients with cystic fibrosis may require higher doses in order to maintain therapeutic serum levels.

Renal impairment: In moderate to severe renal impairment, excretion of colistimethate sodium is delayed. Therefore, the dose and dose interval should be adjusted in order to prevent accumulation. The table below is a guide to dose regimen modifications in patients of 60kg bodyweight or greater. It is emphasised that further adjustments may have to be made based on blood levels and evidence of toxicity.

SUGGESTED DOSAGE ADJUSTMENT IN RENAL IMPAIRMENT

Grade	Creatinine clearance (ml/min)	Over 60kg bodyweight
Mild	20-50	1-2 million units every 8hr
Moderate	10-20	1 million units every 12-18 hr
Severe	<10	1 million units every 18-24 hr

AEROSOL INHALATION

For local treatment of lower respiratory tract infections Colomycin powder is dissolved in 2-4 ml of water for injections or 0.9% sodium chloride intravenous infusion for use in a nebuliser attached to an air/oxygen supply (see section 6.6).

In small, uncontrolled clinical trials, doses of from 500,000 units twice daily up to 2 million units three times daily have been found to be safe and effective in patients with cystic fibrosis.

The following recommended doses are for guidance only and should be adjusted according to clinical response:

Children <2 years: 500,000-1 million units twice daily

Children >2 years and adults: 1-2 million units twice daily

4.3 Contraindications
Hypersensitivity to colistimethate sodium (colistin) or to polymyxin B.

Patients with myasthenia gravis.

4.4 Special warnings and special precautions for use
Use with extreme caution in patients with porphyria.

Nephrotoxicity or neurotoxicity may occur if the recommended parenteral dose is exceeded.

Use with caution in renal impairment (see Section 4.2 - Posology and method of administration). It is advisable to assess baseline renal function and to monitor during treatment. Serum colistimethate sodium concentrations should be monitored.

Bronchospasm may occur on inhalation of antibiotics. This may be prevented or treated with appropriate use of beta$_2$-agonists. If troublesome, treatment should be withdrawn.

4.5 Interaction with other medicinal products and other forms of Interaction
Concomitant use of colistimethate sodium with other medicinal products of neurotoxic and/or nephrotoxic potential should be avoided. These include the aminoglycoside antibiotics such as gentamicin, amikacin, netilmicin and tobramycin. There may be an increased risk of nephrotoxicity if given concomitantly with cephalosporin antibiotics.

Neuromuscular blocking drugs and ether should be used with extreme caution in patients receiving colistimethate sodium.

4.6 Pregnancy and lactation
There are no adequate data from the use of colistimethate sodium in pregnant women. Single dose studies in human pregnancy show that colistimethate sodium crosses the placental barrier and there may be a risk of foetal toxicity if repeated doses are given to pregnant patients. Animal studies are insufficient with respect to the effect of colistimethate sodium on reproduction and development (see Section 5.3 – Preclinical safety data). Colistimethate sodium should be used in pregnancy only if the benefit to the mother outweighs the potential risk to the fetus.

Colistimethate sodium is secreted in breast milk. Colistimethate sodium should be administered to breastfeeding women only when clearly needed.

4.7 Effects on ability to drive and use machines
During parenteral treatment with colistimethate sodium neurotoxicity may occur with the possibility of dizziness, confusion or visual disturbance. Patients should be warned not to drive or operate machinery if these effects occur.

4.8 Undesirable effects
Systemic treatment

The likelihood of adverse events may be related to the age, renal function and condition of the patient.

In cystic fibrosis patients neurological events have been reported in up to 27% of patients. These are generally mild and resolve during or shortly after treatment.

Neurotoxicity may be associated with overdose, failure to reduce the dose in patients with renal insufficiency and concomitant use of either neuromuscular blocking drugs or other drugs with similar neurological effects. Reducing the dose may alleviate symptoms. Effects may include apnoea, transient sensory disturbances (such as facial paraesthesia and vertigo) and, rarely, vasomotor instability, slurred speech, visual disturbances, confusion or psychosis.

Adverse effects on renal function have been reported, usually following use of higher than recommended doses in patients with normal renal function, or failure to reduce the dosage in patients with renal impairment or during concomitant use of other nephrotoxic drugs. The effects are usually reversible on discontinuation of therapy.

In cystic fibrosis patients treated within the recommended dosage limits, nephrotoxicity appears to be rare (less than 1%). In seriously ill hospitalised non-CF patients, signs of nephrotoxicity have been reported in approximately 20% of patients.

Hypersensitivity reactions including skin rash and drug fever have been reported. If these occur treatment should be withdrawn.

Local irritation at the site of injection may occur.

Inhalation treatment

Inhalation may induce coughing or bronchospasm.

Sore throat or mouth has been reported and may be due to *Candida albicans* infection or hypersensitivity. Skin rash may also indicate hypersensitivity, if this occurs treatment should be withdrawn.

4.9 Overdose
Overdose can result in neuromuscular blockade that can lead to muscular weakness, apnoea and possible respiratory arrest. Overdose can also cause acute renal failure characterised by decreased urine output and increased serum concentrations of BUN and creatinine.

There is no specific antidote, manage by supportive treatment. Measures to increase the rate of elimination of colistin e.g. mannitol diuresis, prolonged haemodialysis or peritoneal dialysis may be tried, but effectiveness is unknown.

5. PHARMACOLOGICAL PROPERTIES
5.1 Pharmacodynamic properties
Pharmacotherapeutic group: Antibacterials for systemic use.

ATC Code: JOIX B01

Mode of action

Colistimethate sodium is a cyclic polypeptide antibiotic derived from *Bacillus polymyxa var. colistinus* and belongs to the polymyxin group. The polymyxin antibiotics are cationic agents that work by damaging the cell membrane. The resulting physiological affects are lethal to the bacterium. Polymyxins are selective for Gram-negative bacteria that have a hydrophobic outer membrane.

Resistance

Resistant bacteria are characterised by modification of the phosphate groups of lipopolysaccharide that become substituted with ethanolamine or aminoarabinose. Naturally resistant Gram-negative bacteria, such as *Proteus mirabilis* and *Burkholderia cepacia*, show complete substitution of their lipid phosphate by ethanolamine or aminoarabinose.

Cross resistance

Cross resistance between colistimethate sodium and polymyxin B would be expected. Since the mechanism of action of the polymyxins is different from that of other antibiotics, resistance to colistin and polymyxin by the above mechanism alone would not be expected to result in resistance to other drug classes.

Breakpoints

The suggested general MIC breakpoint to identify bacteria susceptible to colistimethate sodium is ≤ 4mg/l.

Bacteria for which the MIC of colistimethate sodium is ≥ 8mg/l should be considered resistant.

Susceptibility

The prevalence of acquired resistance may vary geographically and with time for selected species and local information on resistance is desirable, particularly when treating severe infections. As necessary, expert advice should be sought when the local prevalence of resistance is such that the utility of the agent in at least some types of infections is questionable.

Commonly susceptible species
Acinetobacter species* *Citrobacter* species *Escherichia coli* *Haemophilus influenzae* *Pseudomonas aeruginosa*
Species for which acquired resistance may be a problem
Enterobacter species *Klebsiella* species
Inherently resistant organisms
Brucella species *Burkholderia cepacia* and related species. *Neisseria* species *Proteus* species *Providencia* species *Serratia* species
Anaerobes All Gram positive organisms

*In-vitro results may not correlate with clinical responses in the case of Acinetobacter spp.

5.2 Pharmacokinetic properties

Absorption

Absorption from the gastrointestinal tract does not occur to any appreciable extent in the normal individual.

When given by nebulisation, variable absorption has been reported that may depend on the aerosol particle size, nebuliser system and lung status. Studies in healthy volunteers and patients with various infections have reported serum levels from nil to potentially therapeutic concentrations of 4mg/l or more. Therefore, the possibility of systemic absorption should always be borne in mind when treating patients by inhalation.

Distribution

After the administration to patients with cystic fibrosis of 7.5 mg/kg/day in divided doses given as 30-min intravenous infusions to steady state the C max was determined to be 23±6 mg/l and C min at 8 h was 4.5±4 mg/l. In another study in similar patients given 2 million units every 8 hours for 12 days the C max was 12.9 mg/l (5.7 - 29.6 mg/l) and the C min was 2.76 mg/l (1.0 - 6.2 mg/l). In healthy volunteers given a bolus injection of 150mg (2 million units approx.) peak serum levels of 18 mg/l were observed 10 minutes after injection.

Protein binding is low. Polymyxins persist in the liver, kidney, brain, heart and muscle. One study in cystic fibrosis patients gives the steady-state volume of distribution as 0.09 L/kg.

Biotransformation

Colistimethate sodium is converted to the base *in vivo*. As 80% of the dose can be recovered unchanged in the urine, and there is no biliary excretion, it can be assumed that the remaining drug is inactivated in the tissues. The mechanism is unknown.

Elimination

The main route of elimination after parenteral administration is by renal excretion with 40% of a parenteral dose recovered in the urine within 8 hours and around 80% in 24 hours. Because colistimethate sodium is largely excreted in the urine, dose reduction is required in renal impairment to prevent accumulation. Refer to the table in Section 4.2.

After intravenous administration to healthy adults the elimination half-life is around 1.5 hrs. In a study in cystic fibrosis patients given a single 30-minute intravenous infusion the elimination half-life was 3.4 ± 1.4 hrs.

The elimination of colistimethate sodium following inhalation has not been studied. A study in cystic fibrosis patients failed to detect any colistimethate sodium in the urine after 1 million units were inhaled twice daily for 3 months.

Colistimethate sodium kinetics appear to be similar in children and adults, including the elderly, provided renal function is normal. Limited data are available on use in neonates which suggest kinetics are similar to children and adults but the possibility of higher peak serum levels and prolonged half-life in these patients should be considered and serum levels monitored.

5.3 Preclinical safety data

Data on potential genotoxicity are limited and carcinogenicity data for colistimethate sodium are lacking. Colistimethate sodium has been shown to induce chromosomal aberrations in human lymphocytes, in vitro. This effect may be related to a reduction in mitotic index, which was also observed.

Reproductive toxicity studies in rats and mice do not indicate teratogenic properties. However, colistimethate sodium given intramuscularly during organogenesis to rabbits at 4.15 and 9.3 mg/kg resulted in talipes varus in 2.6 and 2.9% of fetuses respectively. These doses are 0.5 and 1.2 times the maximum daily human dose. In addition, increased resorption occurred at 9.3 mg/kg.

There are no other preclinical safety data of relevance to the prescriber which are additional to safety data derived from patient exposure and already included in other sections of the SPC.

6. PHARMACEUTICAL PARTICULARS

6.1 List of excipients

None

6.2 Incompatibilities

Mixed infusions, injections and nebuliser solutions involving colistimethate sodium should be avoided.

6.3 Shelf life

Before opening: 3 years

Reconstituted solutions: Solutions for infusion or injection:

Chemical and physical in-use stability for 28 days at 4°C has been demonstrated.

From a microbiological point of view, solutions should be used immediately. If not used immediately in-use storage times and conditions prior to use are the responsibility of the user. They would normally be no longer than 24 hours at 2 to 8°C, unless reconstituted and diluted under controlled and validated aseptic conditions.

Solutions for nebulisation:

Solutions for nebulisation have similar in-use stability and should be treated as above. Patients self-treating with nebulised antibiotic should be advised to use solutions immediately after preparation. If this is not possible, solutions should not be stored for longer than 24hrs in a refrigerator.

6.4 Special precautions for storage

Do not store above 25°C. Keep the vials in the outer carton.

6.5 Nature and contents of container

Type I glass vials in outer cartons of 10.

6.6 Instructions for use and handling

Parenteral administration

The normal adult dose of 2 million units should be dissolved in 10-50ml of 0.9% sodium chloride intravenous infusion or water for injections to form a clear solution. The solution is for single use only and any remaining solution should be discarded.

Inhalation

The required amount of powder is dissolved preferably in 2-4ml 0.9% sodium chloride solution and poured into the nebuliser. Alternatively, water for injections may be used. The solution will be slightly hazy and may froth if shaken. Usually jet or ultrasonic nebulisers are preferred for antibiotic delivery. These should produce the majority of their output in the respirable particle diameter range of 0.5-5.0 microns when used with a suitable compressor. The instructions of the manufacturers should be followed for the operation and care of the nebuliser and compressor.

The output from the nebuliser may be vented to the open air or a filter may be fitted. Nebulisation should take place in a well ventilated room.

The solution is for single use only and any remaining solution should be discarded.

7. MARKETING AUTHORISATION HOLDER

Forest Laboratories UK Limited

Bourne Road

Bexley

Kent DA5 1NX

U.K.

8. MARKETING AUTHORISATION NUMBER(S)

500,000 IU/vial:	PL 0108/5005R
1 million IU/vial:	PL 0108/5006R
2 million IU/vial:	PL 0108/0122

9. DATE OF FIRST AUTHORISATION/RENEWAL OF THE AUTHORISATION

500,000 IU/vial:	May 1986 / November 2001
1 million IU/vial:	June 1986 / November 2001
2 million IU/vial:	June 2003

10. DATE OF REVISION OF THE TEXT

October 2004

11. LEGAL CATEGORY

POM

Colomycin Syrup

(Forest Laboratories UK Limited)

1. NAME OF THE MEDICINAL PRODUCT

COLOMYCIN SYRUP

2. QUALITATIVE AND QUANTITATIVE COMPOSITION

Each bottle contains 4,000,000 units Colistin Sulphate BP, equivalent to 250,000 units/5ml when dispensed.

3. PHARMACEUTICAL FORM

Powder for syrup

4. CLINICAL PARTICULARS

4.1 Therapeutic indications

For the treatment of gastrointestinal infections caused by sensitive Gram negative organisms. Also for bowel preparation.

Colistin sulphate is not absorbed from the gastrointestinal tract except in infants under the age of 6 months, and must not be given orally for the treatment of systemic infections in any age group.

4.2 Posology and method of administration

After reconstitution, the following doses are taken orally:

Adults over 30kg (including the elderly):

1,500,000 to 3,000,000 units every 8 hours.

Colomycin Tablets may be more suitable for adults.

Children (up to 15kg):

250,000 to 500,000 units (i.e. 5-10ml syrup) every 8 hours.

Children (15-30kg):

750,000 to 1,500,000 (15-30ml syrup) units every 8 hours.

A minimum of 5 days treatment is recommended. Dosage may be increased when clinical or bacteriological response is slow. For bowel preparation, a 24-hour course at the normal dosage above is given. Treatment should preferably finish 12 hours before surgery.

4.3 Contraindications

The preparation is contra-indicated in patients with known sensitivity to colistin and those with myasthenia gravis.

4.4 Special warnings and special precautions for use

Colistin is subject to limited and unpredictable absorption from the gastrointestinal tract in infants under six months. Studies in older children and in adults have demonstrated no systemic absorption of colistin following oral administration.

Nevertheless, caution should be employed in the use of the preparation in patients with renal failure and in patients receiving curari-form muscle relaxants and patients with porphyria.

4.5 Interaction with other medicinal products and other forms of Interaction

Neurotoxicity has been reported in association with the concomitant use of either curari-form agents or antibiotics with similar neurotoxic effects. Therapy need not be discontinued and reduction of dosage may alleviate symptoms.

4.6 Pregnancy and lactation

Safety in human pregnancy has not been established. Animal studies do not indicate teratogenic properties; however, parenteral single dose studies in human pregnancy show that Colomycin crosses the placental barrier and there is a risk of foetal toxicity if repeated doses are given to pregnant patients. Colomycin should only be used in pregnancy if the potential benefit justifies the potential risk.

Colomycin is secreted in breast milk and patients to whom the drug is administered should not breast-feed an infant.

4.7 Effects on ability to drive and use machines

No specific warnings

4.8 Undesirable effects

No significant systemic absorption has been found to occur in older children and adults following oral administration nor have any systemic side effects been reported.

However, since the use of colistin may be associated with unpredictable, albeit limited, absorption in infants under 6 months, the potential adverse effects of systemic administration should be noted for this patient population. These adverse effects may include transient sensory disturbances such as perioral paraesthesia and vertigo.

Neurotoxicity and adverse effects on renal function have been reported in association with systemic over-dosage, failure to reduce dosage in patients with renal insufficiency and the concomitant use of either curariform agents or antibiotics with similar neurotoxic effects.

Therapy need not be discontinued and reduction of dosage may alleviate symptoms. Permanent nerve damage such as deafness or vestibular damage has not been reported.

4.9 Overdose

No symptoms of overdosage have been reported following oral use of colistin. However, following systemic administration overdosage can result in renal insufficiency, muscle weakness and apnoea and this should be borne in mind in the oral therapy of infants under 6 months old (see 'Undesirable effects' above).

There is no specific antidote. Manage by supportive treatment and measures to increase the rate of elimination of colistin, e.g. mannitol diuresis, prolonged haemodialysis or peritoneal dialysis.

5. PHARMACOLOGICAL PROPERTIES

5.1 Pharmacodynamic properties

Colistin is a polymyxin antibiotic derived from Bacillus polymyxin var. colistinus. It has a bactericidal action on most Gram negative bacilli, including Pseudomonas aeruginosa, and use is largely free from the development or transference of resistance. It is not recommended for Proteus spp.

5.2 Pharmacokinetic properties

In adults and older children, colistin sulphate taken orally is not absorbed from the G.I. tract. However, in small infants less than 6 months old, some very limited and unpredictable absorption may occur.

Following oral administration of colistin sulphate, excretion is through faecal matter in both children and adults. Assuming minimal absorption in the intestine, only 1 to 10% of colistin is found in faeces, to that estimated from the dose administered and stool volume. Colistin faecal levels in man average 128μg/g when daily oral doses of 5-20mg/kg are administered (1mg Colistin Sulphate BP contains approx. 19,500 units).

Control studies have indicated that colistin is bound by the stool. When greater concentrations of colistin were assayed, significantly less activity, percentage-wise, was lost. This suggests that the 'binding sites' in the stool were saturated.

5.3 Preclinical safety data

There are no preclinical data of relevance to the prescriber that might add to the safety data provided in other sections of this SPC.

6. PHARMACEUTICAL PARTICULARS

6.1 List of excipients

Sucrose

Sodium Citrate

Cherry Trusil flavour

Benzoic Acid

Sodium Methylhydroxybenzoate

6.2 Incompatibilities

None stated

6.3 Shelf life

Three years

6.4 Special precautions for storage

Store below 25°C in a dry place, protected from light.

6.5 Nature and contents of container

Colomycin Syrup powder is presented in a 4oz amber glass Winchester bottle fitted with a white polypropylene cap.

6.6 Instructions for use and handling

Colomycin Syrup powder is reconstituted by adding 58ml of water, and shaking the bottle until the powder is dissolved.

7. MARKETING AUTHORISATION HOLDER

Forest Laboratories UK Limited

Bourne Road

Bexley

Kent DA5 1NX

8. MARKETING AUTHORISATION NUMBER(S)

PL 0108/5009R

9. DATE OF FIRST AUTHORISATION/RENEWAL OF THE AUTHORISATION

21 March 1991 / 24 September 1996

10. DATE OF REVISION OF THE TEXT

June 2001

11. Legal Category

POM

Colomycin Tablets

(Forest Laboratories UK Limited)

1. NAME OF THE MEDICINAL PRODUCT

COLOMYCIN TABLETS

2. QUALITATIVE AND QUANTITATIVE COMPOSITION

Colistin Sulphate BP 1.5MU per tablet.

3. PHARMACEUTICAL FORM

Tablet

4. CLINICAL PARTICULARS

4.1 Therapeutic indications

For the treatment of gastrointestinal infections caused by sensitive Gram negative organisms. Also for bowel preparation.

Colistin sulphate is not absorbed from the gastrointestinal tract and must not, therefore, be used for systemic infections.

4.2 Posology and method of administration

To be taken orally.

Adults (including the elderly) (over 30kg):

1,500,000 to 3,000,000 units every 8 hours.

Children (up to 15kg):

250,000 to 500,000 units every 8 hours.

Children (15-30kg):

750,000 to 1,500,000 units every 8 hours.

A minimum of five days treatment is recommended. Dosage may be increased when clinical or bacteriological response is slow.

For bowel preparation, a 24 hour course at the normal dosage above is given. Treatment should preferably finish 12 hours before surgery.

4.3 Contraindications

Contra-indicated in patients with known sensitivity to colistin and those with myasthenia gravis.

4.4 Special warnings and special precautions for use

Colistin is subject to limited and unpredictable absorption from the GI tract in infants under six months. Studies in older children and in adults have demonstrated no systemic absorption of colistin following oral administration.

Nevertheless, caution should be employed in the use of the preparation in patients with renal failure, patients receiving curari-form muscle relaxants and patients with porphyria.

4.5 Interaction with other medicinal products and other forms of Interaction

Neurotoxicity has been reported in association with the concomitant use of either curariform agents or antibiotics with similar neurotoxic effects.

Therapy need not be discontinued and reduction of dosage may alleviate symptoms.

4.6 Pregnancy and lactation

Safety in human pregnancy has not been established. Animal studies do not indicate teratogenic properties; however, parenteral single dose studies in human pregnancy show that Colomycin crosses the placental barrier and there is a risk of foetal toxicity if repeated doses are given to pregnant patients. Colomycin should only be used in pregnancy if the potential benefit justifies the potential risk.

Colomycin is secreted in breast milk and patients to whom the drug is administered should not breast-feed an infant.

4.7 Effects on ability to drive and use machines

No specific warnings

4.8 Undesirable effects

No significant systemic absorption has been found to occur in older children and adults following oral administration nor have any systemic side effects been reported. However, since the use of colistin may be associated with unpredictable, albeit limited, absorption in infants under 6 months the potential adverse effects of systemic administration should be noted for this patient population. These adverse effects may include transient sensory disturbances such as perioral parasthesia and vertigo.

Neuro-toxicity and adverse effects on renal function have been reported in association with systemic over-dosage, failure to reduce dosage in patients with renal insufficiency and the concomitant use of either curariform agents or antibiotics with similar neurotoxic effects. Therapy need not be discontinued and reduction of dosage may alleviate symptoms. Permanent nerve damage such as deafness or vestibular damage has not been reported.

4.9 Overdose

No symptoms of overdosage have been reported following oral use of colistin. However, following systemic administration overdosage can result in renal insufficiency, muscle weakness and apnoea and this should be borne in mind in the oral therapy of infants under 6 months old (see 'Undesirable Effects' above).

There is no specific antidote. Manage by supportive treatment and measures to increase the rate of elimination of colistin, e.g. mannitol diuresis, prolonged haemodialysis or peritoneal dialysis.

5. PHARMACOLOGICAL PROPERTIES

5.1 Pharmacodynamic properties

Colistin is a polypeptide antibiotic derived from Bacillus polymyxa var. colistinus.

It possesses a rapid bactericidal activity against a number of Gram-negative organisms, including Pseudomonas aeruginosa and is largely free from the development or transference of resistance.

5.2 Pharmacokinetic properties

Studies on the gastrointestinal absorption of colistin have shown no significant systemic absorption following oral administration in adults and older children.

Limited and unpredictable absorption is, however, evident in infants under 6 months.

5.3 Preclinical safety data

There are no preclinical data of relevance to the prescriber which are additional to that already included in other sections of the SPC.

6. PHARMACEUTICAL PARTICULARS

6.1 List of excipients

Microcrystalline cellulose

Starch (maize)

Colloidal silicon dioxide

Cutina HR.

6.2 Incompatibilities

None stated.

6.3 Shelf life

5 years

6.4 Special precautions for storage

Do not store above 25°C. Store in the original container.

6.5 Nature and contents of container

Plastic container of 50 tablets

6.6 Instructions for use and handling

None stated

7. MARKETING AUTHORISATION HOLDER

Forest Laboratories UK Limited

Bourne Road

Bexley

Kent DA5 1NX

8. MARKETING AUTHORISATION NUMBER(S)

PL 0108/5008R

9. DATE OF FIRST AUTHORISATION/RENEWAL OF THE AUTHORISATION

30 May 1986 / 11 July 1996

10. DATE OF REVISION OF THE TEXT

July 1996

11. Legal Category

POM

Colpermin

(Pharmacia Ltd - (Consumer Products))

1. NAME OF THE MEDICINAL PRODUCT

COLPERMIN

2. QUALITATIVE AND QUANTITATIVE COMPOSITION

Peppermint Oil BP 0.2ml

3. PHARMACEUTICAL FORM

Sustained release enteric coated capsule, size 1. Body opaque light blue, cap opaque blue, with a blue band between body and cap.

4. CLINICAL PARTICULARS

4.1 Therapeutic indications

For the relief of the symptoms of Irritable Bowel Syndrome.

4.2 Posology and method of administration

For oral use.

Adults:

One capsule three times a day. This dosage may be increased to two capsules three times a day if discomfort is severe.

The capsules should be taken until symptoms resolve which would normally be within one or two weeks. The treatment can be continued for longer periods of between 2 to 3 months, when symptoms are more persistent.

Elderly:

As adult dose.

Children:

There is no experience in the use of these capsules in children under the age of 15.

4.3 Contraindications

None

4.4 Special warnings and special precautions for use

The capsules should be swallowed whole, ie not broken or chewed. Patients who already suffer from heartburn sometimes have an exacerbation of this symptom after taking Colpermin. Treatment should be discontinued in these patients.

Colpermin contains Arachis oil (peanut oil) and should not be taken by patients known to be allergic to peanut. As there is a possible relationship between allergy to peanut and allergy to Soya, patients with Soya allergy should also avoid Colpermin.

The patient should be advised to consult a doctor before use in the following circumstances:

- first presentation of these symptoms for confirmation of IBS
- aged 40 years or over and it is some time since the last attack,

or the symptoms have changed

- blood has been passed from the bowel
- there is a feeling of sickness or there is vomiting
- loss of appetite or loss of weight
- paleness and tiredness
- severe constipation
- fever
- recent foreign travel
- pregnancy or planning a pregnancy or possibly pregnant
- abnormal vaginal bleeding or discharge
- difficulty or pain in passing urine

If there are new symptoms or worsening of the condition or failure to improve over two weeks, the patient should consult their doctor.

4.5 Interaction with other medicinal products and other forms of Interaction
The capsules should not be taken immediately after food. Indigestion remedies should not be taken at the same time as Colpermin.

4.6 Pregnancy and lactation
There are no data available to establish the safety of Colpermin in pregnancy, therefore it should be used only if, in the opinion of the physician, the possible benefits of treatment outweighs the possible hazards. Levels of menthol were not detectable in plasma or saliva following administration of Colpermin indicating rapid first pass metabolism. Significant levels of menthol in breast milk are thought to be unlikely.

4.7 Effects on ability to drive and use machines
None

4.8 Undesirable effects
Occasional heartburn, perianal irritation; allergic reactions to menthol, which are rare, include erythematous rash, headache, bradycardia, muscle tremor and ataxia, which may occur in conjunction with alcohol.

4.9 Overdose
In the event of overdosage, the stomach should be emptied by gastric lavage. Observations should be carried out with symptomatic treatment if necessary.

5. PHARMACOLOGICAL PROPERTIES

5.1 Pharmacodynamic properties
Antispasmodic and carminative.

The mode of action is local rather than systemic. The enteric coating delays opening of the capsule until it reaches the distal small bowel. Peppermint oil is then slowly released as the matrix passes along the gut. The oil exerts a local effect of colonic relaxation and a fall of intra-colonic pressure.

Pharmacological studies have demonstrated that peppermint oil exerts its inhibitory effect on gastrointestinal smooth muscle by interference with the mobilisation of calcium ions.

5.2 Pharmacokinetic properties
Not relevant.

5.3 Preclinical safety data
Not relevant.

6. PHARMACEUTICAL PARTICULARS

6.1 List of excipients
White beeswax

Arachis oil

Colloidal Silica

Gelatin, Titanium dioxide

Indigotine (E132)

Eudragit S100

Eudragit L30 D55

Triethyl citrate,

Ammonia solution 10%

Monostearin

Polyethyleneglycol 4000

Talc

Purified Water

6.2 Incompatibilities
None

6.3 Shelf life
36 months

6.4 Special precautions for storage
Store below 25°C, avoid direct sunlight.

6.5 Nature and contents of container
Aluminium foil/PVC blister pack containing 10 capsules (250μm PVC, 20μm Al).

Marketed packs 20 and 100. 10 and 60 packs are also registered.

6.6 Instructions for use and handling
Not applicable

7. MARKETING AUTHORISATION HOLDER
Pfizer Consumer Healthcare

Walton Oaks

Dorking Road

Walton-on-the-Hill

Surrey KT20 7NS

United Kingdom

8. MARKETING AUTHORISATION NUMBER(S)
PL 15513/0141

9. DATE OF FIRST AUTHORISATION/RENEWAL OF THE AUTHORISATION
01st May 2005

10. DATE OF REVISION OF THE TEXT
18th April 2003

Combigan

(Allergan Ltd)

1. NAME OF THE MEDICINAL PRODUCT
Combigan eye drops, solution ▼

2. QUALITATIVE AND QUANTITATIVE COMPOSITION
One ml solution contains:

2.0 mg brimonidine tartrate, equivalent to 1.3 mg of brimonidine

5.0 mg timolol, equivalent to 6.8 mg of timolol maleate

For excipients, see 6.1

3. PHARMACEUTICAL FORM
Eye drops, solution.

Clear, greenish-yellow solution

4. CLINICAL PARTICULARS

4.1 Therapeutic indications
Reduction of intraocular pressure (IOP) in patients with chronic open-angle glaucoma or ocular hypertension who are insufficiently responsive to topical beta-blockers.

4.2 Posology and method of administration
Recommended dosage in adults (including the elderly)

The recommended dose is one drop of Combigan in the affected eye(s) twice daily, approximately

12 hours apart. If more than one topical ophthalmic product is to be used, the different products should be instilled at least 5 minutes apart.

Use in renal and hepatic impairment

Combigan has not been studied in patients with hepatic or renal impairment. Therefore, caution should be used in treating such patients.

Use in children and adolescents

Combigan should not be used in neonates (see Section 4.3 Contraindications and Section 4.9 Overdose).

The safety and effectiveness of Combigan in children and adolescents have not been established and therefore, its use is not recommended in children or adolescents.

4.3 Contraindications

• Reactive airway disease including bronchial asthma or a history of bronchial asthma, severe chronic obstructive pulmonary disease.

• Sinus bradycardia, second or third degree atrioventricular block, overt cardiac failure, cardiogenic shock.

• Use in neonates

• Patients receiving monoamine oxidase (MAO) inhibitor therapy.

• Patients on antidepressants which affect noradrenergic transmission (e.g. tricyclic antidepressants and mianserin)

• Hypersensitivity to the active substances or any of the excipients.

4.4 Special warnings and special precautions for use
Like other topically applied ophthalmic agents, Combigan may be absorbed systemically. No enhancement of the systemic absorption of the individual active substances has been observed.

Due to the beta-adrenergic component, timolol, the same types of cardiovascular and pulmonary adverse reactions as seen with systemic beta-blockers may occur.

Caution should be exercised in treating patients with severe or unstable and uncontrolled cardiovascular disease. Cardiac failure should be adequately controlled before beginning therapy. Patients with a history of severe cardiac disease should be watched for signs of cardiac failure and have their pulse rates checked. Cardiac and respiratory reactions, including death due to bronchospasm in patients with asthma, and, rarely, death in association with cardiac failures have been reported following administration of timolol maleate.

Beta-blockers may also mask the signs of hyperthyroidism and cause worsening of Prinzmetal angina, severe peripheral and central circulatory disorders and hypotension.

Beta-adrenergic blocking agents should be administered with caution in patients subject to spontaneous hypoglycaemia or to diabetic patients (especially those with labile diabetes) as beta- blockers may mask the signs and symptoms of acute hypoglycaemia.

Combigan should be used with caution in patients with depression, cerebral or coronary insufficiency, Raynaud's phenomenon, orthostatic hypotension, or thromboangiitis obliterans.

While taking beta-blockers, patients with a history of atopy or a history of severe anaphylactic reaction to a variety of allergens may be unresponsive to the usual dose of adrenaline used to treat anaphylactic reactions.

As with systemic beta-blockers, if discontinuation of treatment is needed in patients with coronary heart disease, therapy should be withdrawn gradually to avoid rhythm disorders, myocardial infarct or sudden death.

The preservative in Combigan, benzalkonium chloride, may cause eye irritation. Remove contact lenses prior to application and wait at least 15 minutes before reinsertion. Benzalkonium chloride is known to discolour soft contact lenses.

4.5 Interaction with other medicinal products and other forms of Interaction
Although specific drug interactions studies have not been conducted with Combigan, the theoretical possibility of an additive or potentiating effect with CNS depressants (alcohol, barbiturates, opiates, sedatives, or anaesthetics) should be considered.

There is potential for additive effects resulting in hypotension, and/or marked bradycardia when eye drops with timolol are administered concomitantly with oral calcium channel blockers, guanethidine, or beta-blocking agents, anti-arrhythmics, digitalis glycosides or parasympathomimetics. After the application of brimonidine, very rare (<1 in 10,000) cases of hypotension have been reported. Caution is therefore advised when using Combigan with systemic antihypertensives.

Beta-blockers may increase the hypoglycaemic effect of antidiabetic agents. Beta-blockers can mask the signs and symptoms of hypoglycaemia (see 4.4 Special warnings and precautions for use)

The hypertensive reaction to sudden withdrawal of clonidine can be potentiated when taking beta-blockers.

Potentiated systemic beta-blockade (e.g., decreased heart rate) has been reported during combined treatment with quinidine and timolol, possibly because quinidine inhibits the metabolism of timolol via the P450 enzyme, CYP2D6.

No data on the level of circulating catecholamines after Combigan administration are available. Caution, however, is advised in patients taking medication which can affect the metabolism and uptake of circulating amines e.g. chlorpromazine, methylphenidate, reserpine.

Caution is advised when initiating (or changing the dose of) a concomitant systemic agent (irrespective of pharmaceutical form) which may interact with α-adrenergic agonists or interfere with their activity i.e. agonists or antagonists of the adrenergic receptor e.g. (isoprenaline, prazosin).

Although specific drug interactions studies have not been conducted with Combigan, the theoretical possibility of an additive IOP lowering effect with prostamides, prostaglandins, carbonic anhydrase inhibitors and pilocarpine should be considered.

4.6 Pregnancy and lactation
Pregnancy

There are no adequate data for the use of Combigan in pregnant women.

Brimonidine tartrate

In animal studies, brimonidine tartrate did not cause any teratogenic effects. Brimonidine tartrate has been shown to cause abortion in rabbits and postnatal growth reduction in rats at systemic exposures approximately 37-times and 134-times those obtained during therapy in humans, respectively.

Timolol

Teratogenicity studies in mice, rats and rabbits, at oral doses up to 4200 times the human daily dose of Combigan, show no evidence of foetal malformation.

However, epidemiological studies suggest that a risk of intra uterine growth retardation may exist following exposure to systemic beta-blockers. In addition, some signs and symptoms of beta-blockade (eg bradycardia) have been observed in both the foetus and the neonate.

Consequently, Combigan should not be used during pregnancy unless clearly necessary.

Lactation

Timolol is excreted in human milk. It is not known if brimonidineis excreted in human milk but is excreted in the milk of the lactating rat. Therefore, Combigan should not be used by women breast-feeding infants.

4.7 Effects on ability to drive and use machines
Combigan may cause transient blurring of vision, fatigue and/or drowsiness which may impair the ability to drive or operate machines.

4.8 Undesirable effects
Based on 12 month clinical data, the most commonly reported ADRs were conjunctival hyperaemia (approximately 15% of patients) and burning sensation in the eye (approximately 11% of patients). The majority of cases were mild and led to discontinuation rates of only 3.4% and 0.5% respectively.

The following adverse drug reactions were reported during clinical trials with Combigan:

Eye disorders

Very Common (>1/10): conjunctival hyperaemia, burning sensation

Common (>1/100, <1/10): stinging sensation in the eye, eye pruritus, allergic conjunctivitis, conjunctival folliculosis, visual disturbance, blepharitis, epiphora, corneal erosion, superficial punctuate keratitis, eye dryness, eye discharge, eye pain, eye irritation, foreign body sensation

Uncommon (>1/1000, <1/100): visual acuity worsened, conjunctival oedema, follicular conjunctivitis, conjunctivitis, vitreous floater, asthenopia, photophobia, papillary hypertrophy, eyelid pain, conjunctival blanching, corneal oedema, corneal infiltrates, vitreous detachment

Psychiatric disorders

Common (>1/100, <1/10): depression

Nervous system disorders

Common (>1/100, <1/10): somnolence, headache

Uncommon (>1/1000, <1/100): dizziness, syncope

Cardiac disorders:

Uncommon (>1/1000, <1/100): congestive heart failure, palpitations

Vascular disorders

Common (>1/100, <1/10): hypertension

Respiratory, thoracic and mediastinal disorders

Uncommon (>1/1000, <1/100): rhinitis, nasal dryness

Gastrointestinal disorders

Common (>1/100, <1/10): oral dryness

Uncommon (>1/1000, <1/100): taste perversion

Skin and subcutaneous tissue disorders

Common (>1/100, <1/10): eyelid oedema, eyelid pruritus, eyelid erythema

Uncommon (>1/1000, <1/100): allergic contact dermatitis

General disorders and administration site conditions

Common (>1/100, <1/10): asthenic conditions

Investigations:

Common (>1/100, <1/10): LFTs abnormal

Additional adverse events that have been seen with one of the components and may potentially occur also with Combigan:

Brimonidine

Eye disorders: iritis, miosis

Psychiatric disorders: insomnia

Cardiac disorders: arrhythmias (including bradycardia and tachycardia)

Vascular disorders: hypotension

Respiratory, thoracic and mediastinal disorders: upper respiratory symptoms, dyspnoea

Gastrointestinal disorders: Gastrointestinal symptoms

General disorders and administration site conditions: systemic allergic reactions

Timolol

Eye disorders: decreased corneal sensitivity, diplopia, ptosis, choroidal detachment (following filtration surgery), refractive changes (due to withdrawal of miotic therapy in some cases)

Psychiatric disorders: insomnia, nightmares, decreased libido

Nervous system disorders: memory loss, increase in signs and symptoms of myasthenia gravis, paresthaesia, cerebral ischaemia

Ear and labyrinth disorders: tinnitus

Cardiac disorders: heart block, cardiac arrest, arrhythmia

Vascular disorders: hypotension, cerebrovascular accident, claudication, Raynaud's phenomenon, cold hands and feet

Respiratory, thoracic and mediastinal disorders: bronchospasm (predominantly in patients with pre-existing bronchospastic disease) dyspnoea, cough

Gastrointestinal disorders: nausea, diarrhoea, dyspepsia

Skin and subcutaneous tissue disorders: alopecia, psoriasiform rash or exacerbation of psoriasis

Musculoskeletal, connective tissue and bone disorders: systemic lupus erythematosus

Renal and urinary disorders: Peyronie's disease

General disorders and administration site conditions: oedema, chest pain

4.9 Overdose

No data are available with regard to overdose with Combigan.

Brimonidine

In cases where brimonidine has been used as part of the medical treatment of congenital glaucoma, symptoms of brimonidine overdose such as hypotension, bradycardia, hypothermia and apnoea have been reported in a few neonates receiving brimonidine.

Oral overdoses of other alpha-2-agonists have been reported to cause symptoms such as hypotension, asthenia, vomiting, lethargy, sedation, bradycardia, arrhythmias, miosis, apnoea, hypotonia, hypothermia, respiratory depression and seizure.

Timolol

Symptoms of systemic timolol overdose are: bradycardia, hypotension, bronchospasm, headache, dizziness and cardiac arrest. A study of patients showed that timolol did not dialyse readily.

If overdose occurs treatment should be symptomatic and supportive.

5. PHARMACOLOGICAL PROPERTIES

5.1 Pharmacodynamic properties

Pharmacotherapeutic group:

Ophthalmological – beta-blocking agents – timolol, combinations

ATC code: SO1ED 51

Mechanism of action:

Combigan consists of two active substances: brimonidine tartrate and timolol maleate. These two components decrease elevated intraocular pressure (IOP) by complementary mechanisms of action and the combined effect results in additional IOP reduction compared to either compound administered alone. Combigan has a rapid onset of action.

Brimonidine tartrate is an alpha-2 adrenergic receptor agonist that is 1000-fold more selective for the alpha-2 adrenoceptor than the alpha-1 adrenoreceptor. This selectivity results in no mydriasis and the absence of vasoconstriction in microvessels associated with human retinal xenografts.

It is thought that brimonidine tartrate lowers IOP by enhancing uveoscleral outflow and reducing aqueous humour formation.

Timolol is a $beta_1$ and $beta_2$ non-selective adrenergic receptor blocking agent that does not have significant intrinsic sympathomimetic, direct myocardial depressant, or local anaesthetic (membrane-stabilising) activity. Timolol lowers IOP by reducing aqueous humour formation. The precise mechanism of action is not clearly established, but inhibition of the increased cyclic AMP synthesis caused by endogenous beta-adrenergic stimulation is probable.

Clinical effects:

In three well-controlled, double-masked clinical studies, Combigan (twice daily) produced significantly greater decreases in mean diurnal IOP compared with timolol (twice daily) and brimonidine (twice daily or three times a day) when administered as monotherapy.

In a study in patients whose IOP was insufficiently controlled following a minimal 3-week run-in on any monotherapy, additional decreases in mean diurnal IOP of 4.5, 3.3 and 3.5 mmHg were observed during 3 months of treatment for Combigan (twice daily), timolol (twice daily) and brimonidine (twice daily), respectively.

In addition, the IOP-lowering effect of Combigan was consistently non-inferior to that achieved by adjunctive therapy of brimonidine and timolol (all twice daily).

The IOP-lowering effect of Combigan has been shown to be maintained in double-masked studies of up to 12 months.

5.2 Pharmacokinetic properties

Combigan:

Plasma brimonidine and timolol concentrations were determined in a crossover study comparing the monotherapy treatments to Combigan treatment in healthy subjects. There were no statistically significant differences in brimonidine or timolol AUC between Combigan and the respective monotherapy treatments. Mean plasma C_{max} values for brimonidine and timolol following dosing with Combigan were 0.0327 and 0.406 ng/ml respectively.

Brimonidine:

After ocular administration of 0.2% eye drops solution in humans, plasma brimonidine concentrations are low. Brimonidine is not extensively metabolised in the human eye and human plasma protein binding is approximately 29%. The mean apparent half-life in the systemic circulation was approximately 3 hours after topical dosing in man.

Following oral administration to man, brimonidine is well absorbed and rapidly eliminated. The major part of the dose (around 74% of the dose) was excreted as metabolites in urine within five days; no unchanged drug was detected in urine. In vitro studies, using animal and human liver, indicate that the metabolism is mediated largely by aldehyde oxidase and cytochrome P450. Hence, the systemic elimination seems to be primarily hepatic metabolism.

Brimonidine binds extensively and reversibly to melanin in ocular tissues without any untoward effects. Accumulation does not occur in the absence of melanin.

Brimonidine is not metabolised to a great extent in human eyes. After instillation of brimonidine tartrate 0.2% eye drops to the rabbit, peak drug concentration was 0.647 mg/ml in the aqueous humour within 1 hour post-dose. Brimonidine concentrations declined subsequently in a biphasic manner with an initial half-life of 1 hour, followed by a slower terminal elimination phase from 6 to 24 hours post dose.

Timolol:

After ocular administration of a 0.5% eye drops solution in humans undergoing cataract surgery, peak timolol concentration was 898 ng/ml in the aqueous humour at one hour post-dose. Part of the dose is absorbed systemically where it is extensively metabolised in the liver. The half-life of timolol in plasma is about 7 hours. Timolol is partially metabolised by the liver with timolol and its metabolites excreted by the kidney. Timolol is not extensively bound to plasma.

5.3 Preclinical safety data

The ocular and systemic safety profile of the individual components is well established. Preclinical data reveal no special hazard for humans based on conventional studies of the individual components of safety pharmacology, repeated dose toxicity, genotoxicity, carcinogenic potential, toxicity to reproduction. Additional repeated dose toxicity studies on Combigan also showed no special hazard for humans.

6. PHARMACEUTICAL PARTICULARS

6.1 List of excipients

Benzalkonium chloride

Sodium phosphate, monobasic

Sodium phosphate, dibasic

Hydrochloric acid or sodium hydroxide to adjust pH

Purified water

6.2 Incompatibilities

None applicable

6.3 Shelf life

21 months.

After first opening: Use within 28 days.

6.4 Special precautions for storage

Keep the bottle in the outer carton.

6.5 Nature and contents of container

Bottles and tips are manufactured from white low density polyethylene (LDPE). Caps are manufactured from high impact polystyrene (HIPS).

The following pack size is available: carton containing 1 bottle of 5ml.

6.6 Instructions for use and handling

No special requirements

7. MARKETING AUTHORISATION HOLDER

Allergan Pharmaceuticals Ireland

Castlebar Road

Westport

Co. Mayo

Ireland

8. MARKETING AUTHORISATION NUMBER(S)

PL 05179/0006

9. DATE OF FIRST AUTHORISATION/RENEWAL OF THE AUTHORISATION

12 April 2005

10. DATE OF REVISION OF THE TEXT

Combivent UDVs

(Boehringer Ingelheim Limited)

1. NAME OF THE MEDICINAL PRODUCT

Combivent® UDVs®

2. QUALITATIVE AND QUANTITATIVE COMPOSITION

Each 2.5 ml single dose unit contains 500 micrograms ipratropium bromide (as 520 micrograms ipratropium bromide monohydrate Ph. Eur.) and 3 mg salbutamol sulphate Ph. Eur. (corresponds to 2.5mg salbutamol base).

3. PHARMACEUTICAL FORM

Nebuliser solution.

4. CLINICAL PARTICULARS

4.1 Therapeutic indications

The management of bronchospasm in patients suffering from chronic obstructive pulmonary disease who require regular treatment with both ipratropium and salbutamol.

4.2 Posology and method of administration

For inhalation.

COMBIVENT UDVs may be administered from a suitable nebuliser or an intermittent positive pressure ventilator. The single dose units should not be taken orally or administered parenterally.

The recommended dose is:

Adults (including elderly patients and children over 12 years): 1 single dose unit three or four times daily.

Children under 12 years: There is no experience of the use of COMBIVENT UDVs in children under 12 years.

4.3 Contraindications

COMBIVENT UDVs are contraindicated in patients with hypertrophic obstructive cardio- myopathy or tachyarrhythmia. COMBIVENT UDVs are also contraindicated in patients with a history of hypersensitivity to ipratropium bromide, salbutamol sulphate or to atropine or its derivatives.

4.4 Special warnings and special precautions for use

Immediate hypersensitivity reactions may occur after administration of COMBIVENT UDVs, as demonstrated by rare cases of urticaria, angioedema, rash, bronchospasm and oropharyngeal oedema.

Ocular complications: There have been rare reports of ocular complications (i.e. mydriasis, blurring of vision, narrow-angle glaucoma and eye pain) when the contents of metered aerosols containing ipratropium bromide have been sprayed inadvertently into the eye.

Patients must be instructed in the correct use of COMBIVENT UDVs and warned not to allow the solution or mist to enter the eyes. This is particularly important in patients who may be pre-disposed to glaucoma. Such patients should be warned specifically to protect their eyes. Eye pain or discomfort, blurred vision, visual halos or coloured images, in association with red eyes from conjunctival congestion and corneal oedema may be signs of acute narrow-angle glaucoma. Should any combination of these symptoms develop, treatment with miotic drops should be initiated and specialist advice sought immediately.

In the following conditions COMBIVENT UDVs should only be used after careful risk/benefit assessment: insufficiently controlled diabetes mellitus, recent myocardial infarction and/or severe organic heart or vascular disorders, hyperthyroidism, pheochromocytoma, prostatic hypertrophy and risk of narrow-angle glaucoma.

Potentially serious hypokalaemia may result from beta$_2$-agonist therapy. Particular caution is advised in severe airway obstruction as this effect may be potentiated by concomitant treatment with xanthine derivatives, steroids and diuretics. Additionally, hypoxia may aggravate the effects of hypokalaemia on cardiac rhythm (especially in patients receiving digoxin). It is recommended that serum potassium levels are monitored in such situations.

Patients with cystic fibrosis may be more prone to gastro-intestinal motility disturbances.

The patient should be instructed to consult a doctor immediately in the event of acute, rapidly worsening dyspnoea. In addition, the patient should be warned to seek medical advice should a reduced response become apparent.

4.5 Interaction with other medicinal products and other forms of Interaction

The use of additional beta-agonists, xanthine derivatives and corticosteroids may enhance the effect of COMBIVENT UDVs. The concurrent administration of other beta-mimetics, systemically absorbed anticholinergics and xanthine derivatives may increase the severity of side effects. A potentially serious reduction in effect may occur during concurrent administration of beta-blockers.

Beta-adrenergic agonists should be administered with caution to patients being treated with monoamine oxidase inhibitors or tricyclic antidepressants, since the action of beta-adrenergic agonists may be enhanced.

Inhalation of halogenated hydrocarbon anaesthetics such as halothane, trichloroethylene and enflurane may increase the susceptibility to the cardiovascular effects of beta-agonists.

4.6 Pregnancy and lactation

Ipratropium bromide has been in general use for several years and there is no definite evidence of ill-consequence during pregnancy; animal studies have shown no hazard.

Salbutamol has been in widespread use for many years without apparent ill-consequence during pregnancy. There is inadequate published evidence of safety in the early stages of human pregnancy but in animal studies there has been evidence of some harmful effects on the foetus at very high dose levels.

As with all medicines, COMBIVENT UDVs should not be used in pregnancy, especially the first trimester, unless the expected benefit is thought to outweigh any possible risk to the foetus. Similarly, COMBIVENT UDVs should not be administered to breast-feeding mothers unless the expected benefit is thought to outweigh any possible risk to the neonate.

4.7 Effects on ability to drive and use machines

None stated.

4.8 Undesirable effects

Nebulisation-induced bronchospasm, dyspnoea and cough have been reported infrequently following the use of COMBIVENT UDVs.

In common with other beta-agonist bronchodilators the undesirable effects of COMBIVENT UDVs include fine tremor of skeletal muscles and nervousness and less frequently, tachycardia, dizziness, palpitations or headache, especially in hypersensitive patients.

Potentially serious hypokalemia may result from beta$_2$-agonist therapy.

As with other beta-mimetics, nausea, vomiting, sweating, weakness and myalgia/muscle cramps may occur. In rare cases decrease in diastolic blood pressure, increase in systolic blood pressure, arrhythmias, particularly after higher doses, may occur.

In individual cases psychological alterations have been reported under inhalational therapy with beta-mimetics.

Dry mouth and dysphonia have occasionally been reported.

Isolated reports of ocular complications (i.e. mydriasis, increased intraocular pressure, angle-closure glaucoma, eye pain) when aerosolised ipratropium bromide either alone or in combination with an adrenergic beta$_2$-agonist, has escaped into the eyes.

Ocular side effects, gastro-intestinal motility disturbances and urinary retention may occur in rare cases and are reversible (see Special Precautions).

4.9 Overdose

Acute effects of overdosage with ipratropium bromide are unlikely due to its poor systemic absorption after either inhalation or oral administration. Any effects of overdosage are therefore likely to be related to the salbutamol component.

Manifestations of overdosage with salbutamol may include anginal pain, hypertension, hypokalaemia and tachycardia. The preferred antidote for overdosage with salbutamol is a cardioselective beta-blocking agent but caution should be used in administering these drugs in patients with a history of bronchospasm.

5. PHARMACOLOGICAL PROPERTIES

5.1 Pharmacodynamic properties

Ipratropium bromide is an anticholinergic agent which inhibits vagally-mediated reflexes by antagonising the action of acetylcholine, the transmitter agent released from the vagus nerve. The bronchodilation following inhalation of ipratropium bromide is primarily local and site specific to the lung and not systemic in nature.

Salbutamol is a beta$_2$-adrenergic agent which acts on airway smooth muscle resulting in relaxation. Salbutamol relaxes all smooth muscle from the trachea to the terminal bronchioles and protects against bronchoconstrictor challenges.

COMBIVENT UDVs provide the simultaneous delivery of ipratropium bromide and salbutamol sulphate allowing effects on both muscarinic and beta$_2$-adrenergic receptors in the lung leading to increased bronchodilation over that provided by each agent singly.

5.2 Pharmacokinetic properties

Ipratropium bromide is not readily absorbed into the systemic circulation either from the surface of the lung or from the gastrointestinal tract as assessed by blood level and renal excretion studies. The elimination half-life of drug and metabolites is about 3 to 4 hours after inhalation or intravenous administration. Ipratropium bromide does not cross the blood-brain barrier.

Salbutamol is rapidly and completely absorbed following oral administration either by the inhaled or the gastric route. Peak plasma salbutamol concentrations are seen within three hours of administration and the drug is excreted unchanged in the urine after 24 hours. The elimination half-life is 4 hours. Salbutamol will cross the blood brain barrier reaching concentrations amounting to about five percent of the plasma concentrations.

It has been shown that co-nebulisation of ipratropium bromide and salbutamol sulphate does not potentiate the systemic absorption of either component and that therefore the additive activity of COMBIVENT UDVs is due to the combined local effect on the lung following inhalation.

5.3 Preclinical safety data

None stated.

6. PHARMACEUTICAL PARTICULARS

6.1 List of excipients

Sodium chloride

1N Hydrochloric acid

Purified water

6.2 Incompatibilities

None stated.

6.3 Shelf life

24 months.

6.4 Special precautions for storage

Store below 25°C. Do not freeze. Keep vials in the outer carton in order to protect from light. Do not use if solution is discoloured.

6.5 Nature and contents of container

Low density polyethylene (Ph.Eur.) vials containing 2.5 ml solution, formed into strips of 10 and packed into cartons containing 10, 20, 40, 60, 80 or 100 vials.

6.6 Instructions for use and handling

i) Prepare the nebuliser by following the manufacturer's instructions and the advice of your doctor.

ii) Carefully separate a new vial from the strip. NEVER use one that has been opened already.

iii) Open the vial by simply twisting off the top, always taking care to hold it in an upright position.

iv) Unless otherwise instructed by your doctor squeeze all the contents of the plastic vial into the nebuliser chamber.

v) Assemble the nebuliser and use it as directed by your doctor.

vi) After nebulisation clean the nebuliser according to the manufacturer's instructions.

Since the single dose units contain no preservatives, it is important that the contents are used soon after opening and a fresh vial is used for each administration to avoid microbial contamination. Partly used, opened or damaged single dose units should be discarded.

It is strongly recommended not to mix COMBIVENT with other drugs in the same nebuliser.

7. MARKETING AUTHORISATION HOLDER

Boehringer Ingelheim Limited

Ellesfield Avenue

Bracknell

Berkshire

RG12 8YS

United Kingdom

8. MARKETING AUTHORISATION NUMBER(S)

PL 00015/0197

9. DATE OF FIRST AUTHORISATION/RENEWAL OF THE AUTHORISATION

7 June 1995

10. DATE OF REVISION OF THE TEXT

March 2004

11. Legal Category

POM

C4b/UK/SPC/6

Combivir Film Coated Tablets

(GlaxoSmithKline UK)

1. NAME OF THE MEDICINAL PRODUCT

Combivir film-coated tablets

2. QUALITATIVE AND QUANTITATIVE COMPOSITION

Each film-coated tablet contains 150 mg lamivudine and 300 mg zidovudine.

For excipients see section 6.1.

3. PHARMACEUTICAL FORM

Film-coated tablet

White to off-white, capsule-shaped film-coated tablets engraved with GXFC3 on one side.

4. CLINICAL PARTICULARS

4.1 Therapeutic indications

Combivir is indicated in antiretroviral combination therapy for the treatment of Human Immunodeficiency Virus (HIV) infected adults and adolescents over 12 years of age.

4.2 Posology and method of administration

Therapy should be initiated by a physician experienced in the management of HIV infection.

Adults and adolescents over the age of 12 years: the recommended dose of Combivir is one tablet twice daily. Combivir may be administered with or without food.

For situations where discontinuation of therapy with one of the active substances of Combivir, or dose reduction is necessary separate preparations of lamivudine and zidovudine are available in tablets/capsules and oral solution.

Renal impairment: Lamivudine and zidovudine concentrations are increased in patients with renal impairment due to decreased clearance. Therefore as dosage adjustment of these may be necessary it is recommended that separate preparations of lamivudine and zidovudine be administered to patients with reduced renal function (creatinine clearance ⩽ 50 ml/min). Physicians should refer to the individual prescribing information for these medicinal products.

Hepatic impairment: Limited data in patients with cirrhosis suggest that accumulation of zidovudine may occur in patients with hepatic impairment because of decreased glucuronidation. Data obtained in patients with moderate to severe hepatic impairment show that lamivudine pharmacokinetics are not significantly affected by hepatic dysfunction. However, as dosage adjustments for zidovudine may be necessary, it is recommended that separate preparations of lamivudine and zidovudine be administered to patients with severe hepatic impairment. Physicians should refer to the individual prescribing information for these medicinal products.

Dosage adjustments in patients with haematological adverse reactions: Dosage adjustment of zidovudine may be necessary if the haemoglobin level falls below 9 g/dl or 5.59 mmol/l or the neutrophil count falls below 1.0×10^9/l (see sections 4.3 and 4.4). As dosage adjustment of Combivir is not possible, separate preparations of zidovudine and lamivudine should be used. Physicians should refer to the individual prescribing information for these medicinal products.

Dosage in the elderly: No specific data are available, however special care is advised in this age group due to age associated changes such as the decrease in renal function and alteration of haematological parameters.

4.3 Contraindications

Hypersensitivity to lamivudine, zidovudine or to any of the excipients.

Zidovudine is contraindicated in patients with abnormally low neutrophil counts ($< 0.75 \times 10^9$/l), or abnormally low haemoglobin levels (< 7.5 g/dl or 4.65 mmol/l). Combivir is therefore contra-indicated in these patients (see section 4.4).

4.4 Special warnings and special precautions for use

The special warnings and precautions relevant to both lamivudine and zidovudine are included in this section. There are no additional precautions and warnings relevant to the combination Combivir.

It is recommended that separate preparations of lamivudine and zidovudine should be administered in cases where dosage adjustment is necessary (see section 4.2). In these cases the physician should refer to the individual prescribing information for these medicinal products.

Patients should be cautioned about the concomitant use of self-administered medications (see section 4.5).

Opportunistic infections: Patients receiving Combivir or any other antiretroviral therapy may continue to develop opportunistic infections and other complications of HIV infection. Therefore patients should remain under close clinical observation by physicians experienced in the treatment of HIV infection.

Transmission of HIV: Patients should be advised that current antiretroviral therapy, including Combivir, has not been proven to prevent the risk of transmission of HIV to others through sexual contact or blood contamination. Appropriate precautions should continue to be taken.

Haematological adverse reactions: Anaemia, neutropenia and leucopenia (usually secondary to neutropenia) can be expected to occur in patients receiving zidovudine. These occurred more frequently at higher zidovudine dosages (1200-1500 mg/day) and in patients with poor bone marrow reserve prior to treatment, particularly with advanced HIV disease. Haematological parameters should therefore be carefully monitored (see section 4.3) in patients receiving Combivir. These haematological effects are not usually observed before four to six weeks therapy. For patients with advanced symptomatic HIV disease, it is generally recommended that blood tests are performed at least every two weeks for the first three months of therapy and at least monthly thereafter.

In patients with early HIV disease haematological adverse reactions are infrequent. Depending on the overall condition of the patient, blood tests may be performed less often, for example every one to three months. Additionally dosage adjustment of zidovudine may be required if severe anaemia or myelosuppression occurs during treatment with Combivir, or in patients with pre-existing bone marrow compromise e.g. haemoglobin <9 g/dl (5.59 mmol/l) or neutrophil count $<1.0 \times 10^9$/l (see section 4.2). As dosage adjustment of Combivir is not possible separate preparations of zidovudine and lamivudine should be used. Physicians should refer to the individual prescribing information for these medicinal products.

Children: Combivir is not indicated for children <12 years old as appropriate dose reduction for the weight of the child cannot be made. Physicians should refer to the individual prescribing information for lamivudine and zidovudine.

Use in pregnancy: As the active substances of Combivir may inhibit cellular DNA replication, any use, especially during the first trimester of pregnancy, presents a potential risk to the foetus. (see section 4.6).

Pancreatitis: Cases of pancreatitis have occurred rarely in patients treated with lamivudine and zidovudine. However it is not clear whether these cases were due to the antiretroviral treatment or to the underlying HIV disease. Treatment with Combivir should be stopped immediately if clinical signs, symptoms or laboratory abnormalities suggestive of pancreatitis occur.

Lactic acidosis: lactic acidosis usually associated with hepatomegaly and hepatic steatosis has been reported with the use of nucleoside analogues. Early symptoms (symptomatic hyperlactatemia) include benign digestive symptoms (nausea, vomiting and abdominal pain) non-specific malaise, loss of appetite, weight loss, respiratory symptoms (rapid and/or deep breathing) or neurological symptoms (including motor weakness).

Lactic acidosis has a high mortality and may be associated with pancreatitis, liver failure, or renal failure.

Lactic acidosis generally occurred after a few or several months of treatment.

Treatment with nucleoside analogues should be discontinued if there is symptomatic hyperlactatemia and metabolic/lactic acidosis, progressive hepatomegaly, or rapidly elevating aminotransferase levels.

Caution should be exercised when administering nucleoside analogues to any patient (particularly obese women) with hepatomegaly, hepatitis or other known risk factors for liver disease and hepatic steatosis (including certain medicinal products and alcohol). Patients co-infected with hepatitis C and treated with alpha interferon and ribavirin may constitute a special risk.

Patients at increased risk should be followed closely.

Mitochondrial dysfunction: Nucleoside and nucleotide analogues have been demonstrated *in vitro* and *in vivo* to cause a variable degree of mitochondrial damage. There have been reports of mitochondrial dysfunction in HIV-negative infants exposed *in utero* and/or post-natally to nucleoside analogues. The main adverse events reported are haematological disorders (anaemia, neutropenia), metabolic disorders (hyperlactatemia, hyperlipasemia). These events are often transitory. Some late-onset neurological disorders have been reported (hypertonia, convulsion, abnormal behaviour). Whether the neurological disorders are transient or permanent is currently unknown. Any child exposed *in utero* to nucleoside and nucleotide analogues, even HIV-negative children, should have clinical and laboratory follow-up and should be fully investigated for possible mitochondrial dysfunction in case of relevant signs or symptoms. These findings do not affect current national recommendations to use antiretroviral therapy in pregnant women to prevent vertical transmission of HIV.

Lipodystrophy: Combination antiretroviral therapy has been associated with the redistribution of body fat (lipodystrophy) in HIV patients. The long-term consequences of these events are currently unknown. Knowledge about the mechanism is incomplete. A connection between visceral lipomatosis and protease inhibitors (PIs) and lipoatrophy and nucleoside reverse transcriptase inhibitors (NRTIs) has been hypothesised. A higher risk of lipodystrophy has been associated with individual factors such as older age, and with drug related factors such as longer duration of antiretroviral treatment and associated metabolic disturbances. Clinical examination should include evaluation for physical signs of fat redistribution. Consideration should be given to the measurement of fasting serum lipids and blood glucose. Lipid disorders should be managed as clinically appropriate (see section 4.8).

Immune Reactivation Syndrome: In HIV-infected patients with severe immune deficiency at the time of institution of combination antiretroviral therapy (CART), an inflammatory reaction to asymptomatic or residual opportunistic pathogens may arise and cause serious clinical conditions, or aggravation of symptoms. Typically, such reactions have been observed within the first few weeks or months of initiation of CART. Relevant examples are cytomegalovirus retinitis, generalised and/or focal mycobacterium infections, and *Pneumocystis carinii* pneumonia. Any inflammatory symptoms should be evaluated and treatment instituted when necessary.

Liver disease: If lamivudine is being used concomitantly for the treatment of HIV and HBV, additional information relating to the use of lamivudine in the treatment of hepatitis B infection is available in the Zeffix SPC.

The safety and efficacy of zidovudine has not been established in patients with significant underlying liver disorders.

Patients with chronic hepatitis B or C and treated with combination antiretroviral therapy are at an increased risk of severe and potentially fatal hepatic adverse events. In case of concomitant antiviral therapy for hepatitis B or C, please refer also to the relevant product information for these medicinal products.

If Combivir is discontinued in patients co-infected with hepatitis B virus, periodic monitoring of both liver function tests and markers of HBV replication is recommended, as withdrawal of lamivudine may result in an acute exacerbation of hepatitis (see Zeffix SPC).

Patients with pre-existing liver dysfunction, including chronic active hepatitis, have an increased frequency of liver function abnormalities during combination antiretroviral therapy, and should be monitored according to standard practice. If there is evidence of worsening liver disease in such patients, interruption or discontinuation of treatment must be considered.

4.5 Interaction with other medicinal products and other forms of Interaction

As Combivir contains lamivudine and zidovudine, any interactions that have been identified with these agents individually may occur with Combivir. The likelihood of metabolic interactions with lamivudine is low due to limited metabolism and plasma protein binding, and almost complete renal clearance. Zidovudine is primarily eliminated by hepatic conjugation to an inactive glucuronidated metabolite. Medicinal products which are primarily eliminated by hepatic metabolism especially via glucuronidation may have the potential to inhibit metabolism of zidovudine. The interactions listed below should not be considered exhaustive but are representative of the classes of medicinal products where caution should be exercised.

Interactions relevant to lamivudine

The possibility of interactions with other medicinal products administered concurrently with Combivir should be considered, particularly when the main route of elimination is active renal secretion, especially via the cationic transport system e.g. trimethoprim. Nucleoside analogues (e.g. zidovudine, didanosine and zalcitabine) and other medicinal products (e.g. ranitidine, cimetidine) are eliminated only in part by this mechanism and were shown not to interact with lamivudine.

Administration of trimethoprim/sulfamethoxazole 160 mg/800 mg results in a 40% increase in lamivudine exposure, because of the trimethoprim component; the sulfamethoxazole component does not interact. However, unless the patient has renal impairment, no dosage adjustment of lamivudine is necessary (see section 4.2). Lamivudine has no effect on the pharmacokinetics of trimethoprim or sulfamethoxazole. When concomitant administration with co-trimoxazole is warranted, patients should be monitored clinically. Co-administration of Combivir with high doses of co-trimoxazole for the treatment of *Pneumocystis carinii* pneumonia (PCP) and toxoplasmosis should be avoided.

Co-administration of lamivudine with intravenous ganciclovir or foscarnet is not recommended until further information is available.

Lamivudine may inhibit the intracellular phosphorylation of zalcitabine when the two medicinal products are used concurrently. Combivir is therefore not recommended to be used in combination with zalcitabine.

Lamivudine metabolism does not involve CYP3A, making interactions with medicinal products metabolised by this system (e.g. PIs) unlikely.

Interactions relevant to zidovudine

Limited data suggest that co-administration of zidovudine and rifampicin decreases the AUC of zidovudine by 48% ± 34%. However the clinical significance of this is unknown.

Limited data suggest that probenecid increases the mean half-life and area under the plasma concentration curve of zidovudine by decreasing glucuronidation. Renal excretion of the glucuronide (and possibly zidovudine itself) is reduced in the presence of probenecid.

A modest increase in C_{max} (28%) was observed for zidovudine when administered with lamivudine, however overall exposure (AUC) was not significantly altered. Zidovudine has no effect on the pharmacokinetics of lamivudine.

Phenytoin blood levels have been reported to be low in some patients receiving zidovudine, while in one patient a high level was noted. These observations suggest that phenytoin concentrations should be carefully monitored in patients receiving Combivir and phenytoin.

In a pharmacokinetic study co-administration of zidovudine and atovaquone showed a decrease in zidovudine oral clearance leading to a 35% ± 23% increase in plasma zidovudine AUC. Given the limited data available the clinical significance of this is unknown.

Valproic acid or methadone when co-administered with zidovudine have been shown to increase the AUC, with a corresponding decrease in its clearance. As only limited data are available the clinical significance is not known.

Other medicinal products, including but not limited to, acetyl salicylic acid, codeine, morphine, indomethacin, ketoprofen, naproxen, oxazepam, lorazepam, cimetidine, clofibrate, dapsone and isoprinosine, may alter the metabolism of zidovudine by competitively inhibiting glucuronidation or directly inhibiting hepatic microsomal metabolism. Careful thought should be given to the possibility of interactions before using such medicinal products in combination with Combivir, particularly for chronic therapy.

Zidovudine in combination with either ribavirin or stavudine are antagonistic *in vitro*. The concomitant use of either ribavirin or stavudine with Combivir should be avoided.

Concomitant treatment, especially acute therapy, with potentially nephrotoxic or myelosuppressive medicinal products (e.g. systemic pentamidine, dapsone, pyrimethamine, co-trimoxazole, amphotericin, flucytosine, ganciclovir, interferon, vincristine, vinblastine and doxorubicin) may also increase the risk of adverse reactions to zidovudine. If concomitant therapy with Combivir and any of these medicinal products is necessary then extra care should be taken in monitoring renal function and haematological parameters and, if required, the dosage of one or more agents should be reduced.

Since some patients receiving Combivir may continue to experience opportunistic infections, concomitant use of prophylactic antimicrobial therapy may have to be considered. Such prophylaxis has included co-trimoxazole, aerosolised pentamidine, pyrimethamine and acyclovir. Limited data from clinical trials do not indicate a significantly increased risk of adverse reactions to zidovudine with these medicinal products.

4.6 Pregnancy and lactation

Pregnancy: The safety of lamivudine in human pregnancy has not been established. No data are available for the treatment with a combination of lamivudine and zidovudine in humans or animals (see also section 5.3). The use in pregnant women of zidovudine alone, with subsequent treatment of the newborn infants, has been shown to reduce the rate of maternal-foetal transmission of HIV. However, no such data are available for lamivudine.

In reproductive toxicity studies in animals both lamivudine and zidovudine were shown to cross the placenta. In humans, consistent with passive transmission of lamivudine across the placenta, lamivudine concentrations in infant serum at birth were similar to those in maternal and cord serum at delivery. Zidovudine was measured in plasma and gave similar results to those observed for lamivudine (see section 5.2).

As the active ingredients of Combivir may inhibit cellular DNA replication, any use, especially during the first trimester of pregnancy, presents a potential risk to the foetus (see section 4.4). Consequently the administration of Combivir during pregnancy should only be considered if expected benefits outweigh any possible risks.

Based on the animal carcinogenicity and mutagenicity findings a carcinogenic risk to humans cannot be excluded. The relevance of these animal data to both infected and uninfected infants exposed to zidovudine is unknown. However, pregnant women considering using Combivir during pregnancy should be made aware of these findings (see section 5.3).

Neither zidovudine nor lamivudine have shown evidence of impairment of fertility in studies in male and female rats. There are no data on their affect on human female fertility. In men zidovudine has not been shown to affect sperm count, morphology or motility.

Lactation: Both lamivudine and zidovudine are excreted in breast milk at similar concentrations to those found in serum. It is recommended that mothers taking Combivir do not breast-feed their infants. It is recommended that HIV infected women do not breast-feed their infants under any circumstances in order to avoid transmission of HIV.

4.7 Effects on ability to drive and use machines
No studies on the effects on the ability to drive and use machines have been performed.

4.8 Undesirable effects
Adverse events have been reported during therapy for HIV disease with lamivudine and zidovudine separately or in combination. For many of these events, it is unclear whether they are related to lamivudine, zidovudine, the wide range of medicinal products used in the management of HIV disease, or as a result of the underlying disease process.

As Combivir contains lamivudine and zidovudine, the type and severity of adverse reactions associated with each of the compounds may be expected. There is no evidence of added toxicity following concurrent administration of the two compounds.

Cases of lactic acidosis, sometimes fatal, usually associated with severe hepatomegaly and hepatic steatosis, have been reported with the use of nucleoside analogues (see section 4.4).

Combination antiretroviral therapy has been associated with redistribution of body fat (lipodystrophy) in HIV patients including the loss of peripheral and facial subcutaneous fat, increased intra-abdominal and visceral fat, breast hypertrophy and dorsocervical fat accumulation (buffalo hump).

Combination antiretroviral therapy has been associated with metabolic abnormalities such as hypertriglyceridaemia, hypercholesterolaemia, insulin resistance, hyperglycaemia and hyperlactataemia (see section 4.4).

In HIV-infected patients with severe immune deficiency at the time of initiation of combination antiretroviral therapy (CART), an inflammatory reaction to asymptomatic or residual opportunistic infections may arise (see section 4.4).

Lamivudine:

The adverse events considered at least possibly related to the treatment are listed below by body system, organ class and absolute frequency. Frequencies are defined as very common >1/10), common >1/100, <1/10), uncommon >1/1000, <1/100), rare >1/10,000, <1/1000), very rare (<1/10,000).

Blood and lymphatic systems disorders

Uncommon: Neutropenia and anaemia (both occasionally severe), thrombocytopenia

Very rare: Pure red cell aplasia

Nervous system disorders

Common: Headache, insomnia.

Very rare: Cases of peripheral neuropathy (or paraesthesiae) have been reported

Respiratory, thoracic and mediastinal disorders

Common: Cough, nasal symptoms

Gastrointestinal disorders

Common: Nausea, vomiting, abdominal pain or cramps, diarrhoea

Rare: Rises in serum amylase. Cases of pancreatitis have been reported.

Hepatobiliary disorders

Uncommon: Transient rises in liver enzymes (AST, ALT).

Rare: Hepatitis

Skin and subcutaneous tissue disorders

Common: Rash, alopecia

Musculoskeletal and connective tissue disorders

Common: Arthralgia, muscle disorders

Rare: Rhabdomyolysis

General disorders and administration site conditions

Common: Fatigue, malaise, fever.

Zidovudine:

The adverse event profile appears similar for adults and adolescents. The most serious adverse reactions include anaemia (which may require transfusions), neutropenia and leucopenia. These occurred more frequently at higher dosages (1200-1500 mg/day) and in patients with advanced HIV disease (especially when there is poor bone marrow reserve prior to treatment), and particularly in patients with CD4 cell counts less than 100/mm^3. Dosage reduction or cessation of therapy may become necessary (see section 4.4).

The incidence of neutropenia was also increased in those patients whose neutrophil counts, haemoglobin levels and serum vitamin B_{12} levels were low at the start of zidovudine therapy.

The adverse events considered at least possibly related to the treatment are listed below by body system, organ class and absolute frequency. Frequencies are defined as very common >1/10), common >1/100, <1/10), uncommon >1/1000, <1/100), rare >1/10,000, <1/1000), very rare (<1/10,000).

Blood and lymphatic system disorders

Common: Anaemia, neutropenia and leucopenia.

Uncommon: Thrombocytopenia and pancytopenia (with marrow hypoplasia)

Rare: Pure red cell aplasia

Very rare: Aplastic anaemia

Metabolism and nutrition disorders

Rare: Lactic acidosis in the absence of hypoxaemia, anorexia

Psychiatric disorders

Rare: Anxiety and depression

Nervous system disorders

Very common: Headache

Common : Dizziness

Rare: Insomnia, paraesthesiae, somnolence, loss of mental acuity, convulsions,

Cardiac disorders

Rare: Cardiomyopathy

Respiratory, thoracic and mediastinal disorders

Uncommon: Dyspnoea

Rare: Cough

Gastrointestinal disorders

Very common: Nausea

Common : Vomiting, abdominal pain and diarrhoea

Uncommon: Flatulence

Rare: Oral mucosa pigmentation, taste perversion and dyspepsia. Pancreatitis

Hepatobiliary disorders

Common: Raised blood levels of liver enzymes and bilirubin

Rare: Liver disorders such as severe hepatomegaly with steatosis

Skin and subcutaneous tissue disorders

Uncommon: Rash and pruritus

Rare: Nail and skin pigmentation, urticaria and sweating

Musculoskeletal and connective tissue disorders

Common: Myalgia

Uncommon: Myopathy

Renal and urinary disorders

Rare: Urinary frequency

Reproductive system and breast disorders

Rare: Gynaecomastia

General disorders and administration site conditions

Common: Malaise

Uncommon: Fever, generalised pain and asthenia

Rare: Chills, chest pain and influenza-like syndrome

The available data from both placebo-controlled and open-label studies indicate that the incidence of nausea and other frequently reported clinical adverse events consistently decreases over time during the first few weeks of therapy with zidovudine.

4.9 Overdose
There is limited experience of overdosage with Combivir. No specific symptoms or signs have been identified following acute overdose with zidovudine or lamivudine apart from those listed as undesirable effects. No fatalities occurred, and all patients recovered.

If overdosage occurs the patient should be monitored for evidence of toxicity (see section 4.8), and standard supportive treatment applied as necessary. Since lamivudine is dialysable, continuous haemodialysis could be used in the treatment of overdosage, although this has not been studied. Haemodialysis and peritoneal dialysis appear to have a limited effect on elimination of zidovudine, but enhance the elimination of the glucuronide metabolite. For more details physicians should refer to the individual prescribing information for lamivudine and zidovudine.

5. PHARMACOLOGICAL PROPERTIES

5.1 Pharmacodynamic properties
Pharmacotherapeutic group: nucleoside analogue, ATC Code: JO5A F30

Lamivudine and zidovudine are nucleoside analogues which have activity against HIV. Additionally, lamivudine has activity against hepatitis B virus (HBV). Both medicinal products are metabolised intracellularly to their active moieties, lamivudine 5'- triphosphate(TP) and zidovudine 5'-triphosphate respectively Their main modes of action are as chain terminators of viral reverse transcription. Lamivudine-TP and zidovudine-TP have selective inhibitory activity against HIV-1 and HIV-2 replication *in vitro*; lamivudine is also active against zidovudine-resistant clinical isolates of HIV. Lamivudine in combination with zidovudine exhibits synergistic anti-HIV activity against clinical isolates in cell culture.

HIV-1 resistance to lamivudine involves the development of a M184V amino acid change close to the active site of the viral reverse transcriptase (RT). This variant arises both *in vitro* and in HIV-1 infected patients treated with lamivudine-containing antiretroviral therapy. M184V mutants display greatly reduced susceptibility to lamivudine and show diminished viral replicative capacity *in vitro*. *In vitro* studies indicate that zidovudine-resistant virus isolates can become zidovudine sensitive when they simultaneously acquire resistance to lamivudine. The clinical relevance of such findings remains, however, not well defined.

Cross-resistance conferred by the M184V RT is limited within the nucleoside inhibitor class of antiretroviral agents. Zidovudine and stavudine maintain their antiretroviral activities against lamivudine-resistant HIV-1. Abacavir maintains its antiretroviral activities against lamivudine-resistant HIV-1 harbouring only the M184V mutation. The M184V RT mutant shows a <4-fold decrease in susceptibility to didanosine and zalcitabine; the clinical significance of these findings is unknown. *In vitro* susceptibility testing has not been standardised and results may vary according to methodological factors.

Lamivudine demonstrates low cytotoxicity to peripheral blood lymphocytes, to established lymphocyte and monocyte-macrophage cell lines, and to a variety of bone marrow progenitor cells *in vitro*. Resistance to thymidine analogues (of which zidovudine is one) is well characterised and is conferred by the stepwise accumulation of up to six specific mutations in the HIV reverse transcriptase at codons 41, 67, 70, 210, 215 and 219. Viruses acquire phenotypic resistance to thymidine analogues through the combination of mutations at codons 41 and 215 or by the accumulation of at least four of the six mutations. These thymidine analogue mutations alone do not cause high-level cross-resistance to any of the other nucleosides, allowing for the subsequent use of any of the other approved reverse transcriptase inhibitors.

Two patterns of multi-drug resistance mutations, the first characterised by mutations in the HIV reverse transcriptase at codons 62, 75, 77, 116 and 151 and the second involving a T69S mutation plus a 6-base pair insert at the same position, result in phenotypic resistance to AZT as well as to the other approved NRTIs. Either of these two patterns of multinucleoside resistance mutations severely limits future therapeutic options.

Clinical Experience

In clinical trials, lamivudine in combination with zidovudine has been shown to reduce HIV-1 viral load and increase CD4 cell count. Clinical end-point data indicate that lamivudine in combination with zidovudine, results in a significant reduction in the risk of disease progression and mortality.

Lamivudine and zidovudine have been widely used as components of antiretroviral combination therapy with other antiretroviral agents of the same class (NRTIs) or different classes (PIs, non-nucleoside reverse transcriptase inhibitors).

Multiple drug antiretroviral therapy containing lamivudine has been shown to be effective in antiretrovirally-naive patients as well as in patients presenting with viruses containing the M184V mutations.

Evidence from clinical studies shows that lamivudine plus zidovudine delays the emergence of zidovudine resistant isolates in individuals with no prior antiretroviral therapy. Subjects receiving lamivudine and zidovudine with or without additional concomitant antiretroviral therapies and who already present with the M184V mutant virus also experience a delay in the onset of mutations that confer resistance to zidovudine and stavudine (Thymidine Analogue Mutations; TAMs).

The relationship between *in vitro* susceptibility of HIV to lamivudine and zidovudine and clinical response to lamivudine/zidovudine containing therapy remains under investigation.

Lamivudine at a dose of 100 mg once daily has also been shown to be effective for the treatment of adult patients with chronic HBV infection (for details of clinical studies, see the prescribing information for Zeffix). However, for the treatment of HIV infection only a 300 mg daily dose of lamivudine (in combination with other antiretroviral agents) has been shown to be efficacious.

Lamivudine has not been specifically investigated in HIV patients co-infected with HBV.

5.2 Pharmacokinetic properties
Absorption: Lamivudine and zidovudine are well absorbed from the gastrointestinal tract. The bioavailability of oral lamivudine in adults is normally between 80 – 85% and for zidovudine 60 – 70%.

A bioequivalence study compared Combivir with lamivudine 150 mg and zidovudine 300 mg tablets taken together. The effect of food on the rate and extent of absorption was also studied. Combivir was shown to be bioequivalent to lamivudine 150 mg and zidovudine 300 mg given as separate tablets, when administered to fasting subjects.

Following single dose Combivir administration in healthy volunteers, mean (CV) lamivudine and zidovudine C_{max} values were 1.6 μg/ml (32 %) and 2.0 μg/ml (40 %), respectively and the corresponding values for AUC were 6.1 μg.h/ml (20 %) and 2.4 μg.h/ml (29 %) respectively. The median (range) lamivudine and zidovudine t_{max} values were 0.75 (0.50 - 2.00) hours and 0.50 (0.25 - 2.00) hours respectively. The extent of lamivudine and zidovudine absorption (AUC_{∞}) and estimates of half-life following administration of Combivir with food were similar when compared to fasting subjects, although the rates of absorption (C_{max}, t_{max}) were slowed. Based on these data Combivir may be administered with or without food.

Distribution: Intravenous studies with lamivudine and zidovudine showed that the mean apparent volume of distribution is 1.3 and 1.6 l/kg respectively. Lamivudine exhibits linear pharmacokinetics over the therapeutic dose range and displays limited binding to the major plasma protein albumin (< 36% serum albumin *in vitro*). Zidovudine plasma protein binding is 34% to 38%. Interactions involving binding site displacement are not anticipated with Combivir.

Data show that lamivudine and zidovudine penetrate the central nervous system (CNS) and reach the cerebrospinal fluid (CSF). The mean ratios of CSF/serum lamivudine and zidovudine concentrations 2 - 4 hours after oral administration were approximately 0.12 and 0.5 respectively. The true extent of CNS penetration of lamivudine and its relationship with any clinical efficacy is unknown.

Metabolism: Metabolism of lamivudine is a minor route of elimination. Lamivudine is predominately cleared unchanged by renal excretion. The likelihood of metabolic drug interactions with lamivudine is low due to the small extent of hepatic metabolism (5 - 10%) and low plasma binding.

The 5'-glucuronide of zidovudine is the major metabolite in both plasma and urine, accounting for approximately 50 – 80% of the administered dose eliminated by renal excretion. 3'-amino-3'-deoxythymidine (AMT) has been identified as a metabolite of zidovudine following intravenous dosing.

Elimination: The observed lamivudine half-life of elimination is 5 to 7 hours. The mean systemic clearance of lamivudine is approximately 0.32 l/h/kg, with predominantly renal clearance > 70%) via the organic cationic transport system. Studies in patients with renal impairment show lamivudine elimination is affected by renal dysfunction. Dose reduction is required for patients with creatinine clearance ≤ 50 ml/min (see section 4.2).

From studies with intravenous zidovudine, the mean terminal plasma half-life was 1.1 hours and the mean systemic clearance was 1.6 l/h/kg. Renal clearance of zidovudine is estimated to be

0.34 l/h/kg, indicating glomerular filtration and active tubular secretion by the kidneys. Zidovudine concentrations are increased in patients with advanced renal failure.

Pharmacokinetics in pregnancy: The pharmacokinetics of lamivudine and zidovudine were similar to that of non-pregnant women.

5.3 Preclinical safety data

The clinically relevant effects of lamivudine and zidovudine in combination are anaemia, neutropenia and leucopenia.

Neither lamivudine nor zidovudine are mutagenic in bacterial tests, but like many nucleoside analogues they show activity in *in vitro* mammalian tests such as the mouse lymphoma assay.

Lamivudine has not shown any genotoxic activity in *in vivo* studies at doses that gave plasma concentrations up to 40-50 times higher than clinical plasma levels. Zidovudine showed clastogenic effects in an oral repeated dose micronucleus test in mice. Peripheral blood lymphocytes from AIDS patients receiving zidovudine treatment have also been observed to contain higher numbers of chromosome breakages.

A pilot study has demonstrated that zidovudine is incorporated into leukocyte nuclear DNA of adults, including pregnant women, taking zidovudine as treatment for HIV-1 infection, or for the prevention of mother to child viral transmission. Zidovudine was also incorporated into DNA from cord blood leukocytes of infants from zidovudine-treated mothers. A transplacental genotoxicity study conducted in monkeys compared zidovudine alone with the combination of zidovudine and lamivudine at human-equivalent exposures. The study demonstrated that foetuses exposed *in utero* to the combination sustained a higher level of nucleoside analogue-DNA incorporation into multiple foetal organs, and showed evidence of more telomere shortening than in those exposed to zidovudine alone. The clinical significance of these findings is unknown.

The carcinogenic potential of a combination of lamivudine and zidovudine has not been tested

In long-term oral carcinogenicity studies in rats and mice, lamivudine did not show any carcinogenic potential.

In oral carcinogenicity studies with zidovudine in mice and rats, late appearing vaginal epithelial tumours were observed. A subsequent intravaginal carcinogenicity study confirmed the hypothesis that the vaginal tumours were the result of long term local exposure of the rodent vaginal epithelium to high concentrations of unmetabolised zidovudine in urine. There were no other zidovudine-related tumours observed in either sex of either species.

In addition, two transplacental carcinogenicity studies have been conducted in mice. In one study, by the US National Cancer Institute, zidovudine was administered at maximum tolerated doses to pregnant mice from day 12 to 18 of gestation. One year post-natally, there was an increase in the incidence of tumours in the lung, liver and female reproductive tract of offspring exposed to the highest dose level (420 mg/kg term body weight).

In a second study, mice were administered zidovudine at doses up to 40 mg/kg for 24 months, with exposure beginning prenatally on gestation day 10. Treatment related findings were limited to late-occurring vaginal epithelial tumours, which were seen with a similar incidence and time of onset as in the standard oral carcinogenicity study. The second study thus provided no evidence that zidovudine acts as a transplacental carcinogen.

It is concluded that as the increase in incidence of tumours in the first transplacental carcinogenicity study represents a hypothetical risk, this should be balanced against the proven therapeutic benefit.

In reproductive toxicity studies lamivudine has demonstrated evidence of causing an increase in early embryonic deaths in the rabbit at relatively low systemic exposures, comparable to those achieved in man, but not in the rat even at very high systemic exposure. Zidovudine had a similar effect in both species, but only at very high systemic exposures. Lamivudine was not teratogenic in animal studies. At maternally toxic doses, zidovudine given to rats during organogenesis resulted in an increased incidence of malformations, but no evidence of foetal abnormalities was observed at lower doses.

6. PHARMACEUTICAL PARTICULARS

6.1 List of excipients

Tablet core:

Microcrystalline cellulose (E460),

sodium starch glycollate,

colloidal silicon dioxide,

magnesium stearate

Tablet film coat:

Hypromellose (E464),

titanium dioxide (E171),

macrogol 400,

polysorbate 80

6.2 Incompatibilities

Not applicable

6.3 Shelf life

2 years

6.4 Special precautions for storage

Do not store above 30°C

6.5 Nature and contents of container

Tamper-evident cartons containing opaque polyvinyl chloride/foil blister packs or white high density polyethylene (HDPE) bottle with a child-resistant closure. Each pack type contains 60 film-coated tablets.

6.6 Instructions for use and handling

No special requirements

Administrative Data

7. MARKETING AUTHORISATION HOLDER

Glaxo Group Ltd

Greenford Road

Greenford

Middlesex UB6 0NN

United Kingdom

8. MARKETING AUTHORISATION NUMBER(S)

EU/1/98/058/001

EU/1/98/058/002

9. DATE OF FIRST AUTHORISATION/RENEWAL OF THE AUTHORISATION

18 March 2003

10. DATE OF REVISION OF THE TEXT

5 January 2005

Compound W

(SSL International plc)

1. NAME OF THE MEDICINAL PRODUCT

Compound W.

2. QUALITATIVE AND QUANTITATIVE COMPOSITION

Salicylic acid Ph Eur 17.0% w/w.

3. PHARMACEUTICAL FORM

Viscous, faintly yellow liquid for topical administration.

4. CLINICAL PARTICULARS

4.1 Therapeutic indications

For the treatment of common warts and verrucae.

4.2 Posology and method of administration

Adults, the elderly and children over 6 years: Gently rub the hard skin from the surface of the wart with a pumice stone or emery board. Apply to wart one drop at a time with dropper-rod until wart is covered. Allow to dry completely. Avoid surrounding skin. Repeat application daily, with regular washing, for up to twelve weeks.

4.3 Contraindications

Do not use Compound W on moles, birth marks, hairy, genital or facial warts.

4.4 Special warnings and special precautions for use

Do not apply to healthy skin or skin which is inflamed or broken. If the wart does not dissolve or gets worse, consult a doctor. If in doubt or have diabetes, ask a doctor.

4.5 Interaction with other medicinal products and other forms of Interaction

None stated.

4.6 Pregnancy and lactation

No contraindications known.

4.7 Effects on ability to drive and use machines

None known.

4.8 Undesirable effects

None known.

4.9 Overdose

None probable.

5. PHARMACOLOGICAL PROPERTIES

5.1 Pharmacodynamic properties

Salicylic acid facilitates desquamation by solubilising the intercellular cement that binds scales in the stratum corneum thereby loosening the keratin.

5.2 Pharmacokinetic properties

Salicylic acid can be absorbed through the skin. It is excreted unchanged in the urine.

5.3 Preclinical safety data

None stated.

6. PHARMACEUTICAL PARTICULARS

6.1 List of excipients

Acetone BP; Industrial Methylated Spirits 99% BP; Pyroxyline (Nitrocellulose DHM 10/25) BP; Castor Oil Ph Eur.

6.2 Incompatibilities

None known.

6.3 Shelf life

48 months.

6.4 Special precautions for storage

No special precautions required.

6.5 Nature and contents of container

Glass bottle with screw threaded plastic cap and plastic rod wad. Pack size: 6.5ml.

6.6 Instructions for use and handling

Not applicable.

7. MARKETING AUTHORISATION HOLDER

Seton Products Limited, Tubiton House, Oldham, OL1 3HS.

8. MARKETING AUTHORISATION NUMBER(S)

PL 11314/0119.

9. DATE OF FIRST AUTHORISATION/RENEWAL OF THE AUTHORISATION

19th May 2004

10. DATE OF REVISION OF THE TEXT

May 2004

Comtess 200 mg film-coated tablets

(Orion Pharma (UK) Limited)

1. NAME OF THE MEDICINAL PRODUCT

COMTESS 200 mg film-coated tablets

2. QUALITATIVE AND QUANTITATIVE COMPOSITION

Each film-coated tablet contains 200 mg entacapone.

For excipients, see 6.1.

3. PHARMACEUTICAL FORM

Film-coated tablet

Brownish-orange, oval, biconvex film-coated tablet with "Comtess" engraved on one side.

4. CLINICAL PARTICULARS

4.1 Therapeutic indications

Entacapone is indicated as an adjunct to standard preparations of levodopa/benserazide or levodopa/carbidopa for use in patients with Parkinson's disease and end-of-dose motor fluctuations, who cannot be stabilised on those combinations.

4.2 Posology and method of administration

Entacapone should only be used in combination with levodopa/bensarazide or levodopa/carbidopa. The prescribing information for these levodopa preparations is applicable to their concomitant use with entacapone.

Method of Administration

Entacapone is administered orally and simultaneously with each levodopa/carbidopa or levodopa/benserazide dose. Entacaponecan be used with standard preparations of levodopa. The efficacy of entacapone as an adjunct to controlled-release levodopa/dopa decarboxylase inhibitor preparations has not been proven.

Entacapone can be taken with or without food (see section 5.2 Pharmacokinetic properties).

Posology

One 200 mg tablet is taken with each levodopa/dopa decarboxylase inhibitor dose. The maximum recommended dose is 200 mg ten times daily, i.e. 2,000 mg of entacapone.

Entacapone enhances the effects of levodopa. Hence, to reduce levodopa-related dopaminergic adverse effects, e.g. dyskinesias, nausea, vomiting and hallucinations, it is often necessary to adjust levodopa dosage within the first days to first weeks after initiating entacapone treatment. The daily dose of levodopa should be reduced by about 10-30% by extending the dosing intervals and/or by reducing the amount of levodopa per dose, according to the clinical condition of the patient.

If entacapone treatment is discontinued, it is necessary to adjust the dosing of other antiparkinsonian treatments, especially levodopa, to achieve a sufficient level of control of the parkinsonian symptoms.

Entacapone increases the bioavailability of levodopa from standard levodopa/benserazide preparations slightly (5-10%) more than from standard levodopa/carbidopa preparations. Hence, patients who are taking standard levodopa/benserazide preparations may need a larger reduction of levodopa dose when entacapone is initiated.

Renal insufficiency does not affect the pharmacokinetics of entacapone and there is no need for dose adjustment. However, for patients who are receiving dialysis therapy, a longer dosing interval may be considered (see section 5.2 Pharmacokinetic properties).

Elderly: No dosage adjustment of entacapone is required for elderly patients.

Children: As entacapone has not been studied in patients under 18 years of age, the use of the medicinal product in patients under this age cannot be recommended.

4.3 Contraindications

Hypersensitivity to the active substance or to any of the excipients.

Liver impairment.

Pheochromocytoma.

Concomitant use of entacapone and non-selective monoamine oxidase (MAO-A and MAO-B) inhibitors (e.g. phenelzine, tranylcypromine) is contraindicated. Concomitant use of a selective MAO-A inhibitor plus a selective MAO-B inhibitor and entacapone is contraindicated (see section 4.5 Interaction with other medicinal products and other forms of interaction).

A previous history of Neuroleptic Malignant Syndrome (NMS) and/or non-traumatic rhabdomyolysis.

4.4 Special warnings and special precautions for use

Rhabdomyolysis secondary to severe dyskinesias or Neuroleptic Malignant Syndrome (NMS) has been observed rarely in patients with Parkinson's disease.

NMS, including rhabdomyolysis and hyperthermia, is characterised by motor symptoms (rigidity, myoclonus, tremor), mental status changes (e.g. agitation, confusion, coma), hyperthermia, autonomic dysfunction (tachycardia, labile blood pressure) and elevated serum creatine phosphokinase. In individual cases, only some of these symptoms and/or findings may be evident.

Neither NMS nor rhabdomyolysis have been reported in association with entacapone treatment from controlled trials in which entacapone was discontinued abruptly. Since the introduction into the market, isolated cases of NMS have been reported, especially following abrupt reduction or discontinuation of entacapone and other concomitant dopaminergic medications. When considered necessary, withdrawal of entacapone and other dopaminergic treatment should proceed slowly, and if signs and/or symptoms occur despite a slow withdrawal of entacapone, an increase in levodopa dosage may be necessary.

Because of its mechanism of action, entacapone may interfere with the metabolism of medicinal products containing a catechol group and potentiate their action. Thus, entacapone should be administered cautiously to patients being treated with medicinal products metabolised by catechol-O-methyl transferase (COMT), e.g. rimiterole, isoprenaline, adrenaline, noradrenaline, dopamine, dobutamine, alpha-methyldopa, and apomorphine (see also section 4.5 Interaction with other medicinal products and other forms of interaction).

Entacapone is always given as an adjunct to levodopa treatment. Hence, the precautions valid for levodopa treatment should also be taken into account for entacapone treatment. Entacapone increases the bioavailability of levodopa from standard levodopa/benserazide preparations 5-10% more than from standard levodopa/carbidopa preparations. Consequently, undesirable dopaminergic effects may be more frequent when entacapone is added to levodopa/benserazide treatment (see also section 4.8 Undesirable effects). To reduce levodopa-related dopaminergic adverse effects, it is often necessary to adjust levodopa dosage within the first days to first weeks after initiating entacapone treatment, according to the clinical condition of the patient (see section 4.2 Posology and method of administration and 4.8 Undesirable effects).

Entacapone may aggravate levodopa-induced orthostatic hypotension. Entacapone should be given cautiously to patients who are taking other medicinal products which may cause orthostatic hypotension.

In clinical studies, undesirable dopaminergic effects, e.g. dyskinesia, were more common in patients who received entacapone and dopamine agonists (such as bromocriptine), selegiline or amantadine compared to those who received placebo with this combination. The doses of other antiparkinsonian medications may need to be adjusted when entacapone treatment is initiated.

Entacapone in association with levodopa has been associated with somnolence and episodes of sudden sleep onset in patients with Parkinson's disease and caution should therefore be exercised when driving or operating machines (see also section 4.7 Effects on ability to drive and use machines).

For patients experiencing diarrhoea, a follow-up of weight is recommended in order to avoid potential excessive weight decrease.

4.5 Interaction with other medicinal products and other forms of Interaction

No interaction of entacapone with carbidopa has been observed with the recommended treatment schedule. Pharmacokinetic interaction with benserazide has not been studied.

In single-dose studies in healthy volunteers, no interactions were observed between entacapone and imipramine or between entacapone and moclobemide. Similarly, no interactions between entacapone and selegiline were observed in repeated-dose studies in parkinsonian patients. However, the experience of the clinical use of entacapone with several drugs, including MAO-A inhibitors, tricyclic antidepressants, noradrenaline reuptake inhibitors such as desipramine, maprotiline and venlafaxine, and medicinal products that are metabolised by COMT (e.g. catechol-structured compounds: rimiterole, isoprenaline, adrenaline, noradrenaline, dopamine, dobutamine, alphamethyldopa, apomorphine, and paroxetine) is still limited. Caution should be exercised when these medicinal products are used concomitantly with entacapone (see also section 4.3 Contraindications and section 4.4 Special warnings and special precautions for use).

Entacapone may be used with selegiline (a selective MAO-B inhibitor), but the daily dose of selegiline should not exceed 10 mg.

Entacapone may form chelates with iron in the gastrointestinal tract. Entacapone and iron preparations should be taken at least 2-3 hours apart (see section 4.8 Undesirable effects).

Entacapone binds to human albumin binding site II which also binds several other medicinal products, including diazepam and ibuprofen. Clinical interaction studies with diazepam and non-steroidal anti-inflammatory drugs have not been carried out. According to *in vitro* studies, significant displacement is not anticipated at therapeutic concentrations of the medicinal products.

Due to its affinity to cytochrome P450 2C9 *in vitro* (see section 5.2 Pharmacokinetic properties), entacapone may potentially interfere with drugs whose metabolism is dependent on this isoenzyme, such as S-warfarin.

However, in an interaction study with healthy volunteers, entacapone did not change the plasma levels of S-warfarin, while the AUC for R-warfarin increased on average by 18% [CI_{90} 11–26%]. The INR values increased on average by 13% [CI_{90} 6–19%]. Thus, control of INR is recommended when entacapone treatment is initiated for patients receiving warfarin.

4.6 Pregnancy and lactation

Pregnancy

No overt teratogenic or primary foetotoxic effects were observed in animal studies in which the exposure levels of entacapone were markedly higher than the therapeutic exposure levels. As there is no experience in pregnant women, entacapone should not be used during pregnancy.

Lactation

In animal studies entacapone was excreted in milk. The safety of entacapone in infants is unknown. Women should not breast-feed during treatment with entacapone.

4.7 Effects on ability to drive and use machines

Entacapone may together with levodopa cause dizziness and symptomatic orthostatism. Therefore, caution should be exercised when driving or using machines.

Patients being treated with entacapone in association with levodopa and presenting with somnolence and/or sudden sleep onset episodes must be instructed to refrain from driving or engaging in activities where impaired alertness may put themselves or others at risk of serious injury or death (e.g. operating machines) until such recurrent episodes have resolved (see also section 4.4 Special warnings and special precautions for use).

4.8 Undesirable effects

The most frequent adverse reactions caused by entacapone relate to the increased dopaminergic activity and occur most commonly at the beginning of the treatment. Reduction of levodopa dosage decreases the severity and frequency of these reactions. The other major class of adverse reactions are gastrointestinal symptoms, including e.g. nausea, vomiting, abdominal pain, constipation and diarrhoea. Urine may be discoloured reddish-brown by entacapone, but this is a harmless phenomenon.

Usually the adverse reactions caused by entacapone are mild to moderate. In clinical studies the most common adverse reactions leading to discontinuation of entacapone treatment have been gastrointestinal symptoms (e.g. diarrhoea, 2.5%) and increased dopaminergic adverse reactions of levodopa (e.g. dyskinesias, 1.7%).

Dyskinesias (27%), nausea (11%), diarrhoea (8%), abdominal pain (7%) and dry mouth (4.2%) were reported significantly more often with entacapone than with placebo in pooled data from clinical studies involving 406 patients taking the medicinal product and 296 patients taking placebo.

Some of the adverse reactions, such as dyskinesia, nausea, and abdominal pain, may be more common with the higher doses (1,400 to 2,000 mg per day) than with the lower doses of entacapone.

The following adverse drug reactions, listed below in Table 1, have been accumulated both from clinical studies with entacapone and since the introduction of entacapone into the market.

Table 1. Adverse drug reactions*

Psychiatric disorders Common: Insomnia, hallucinations, confusion, paroniria Very rare: Agitation
Nervous system disorders Very common: Dyskinesia Common: Parkinsonism aggravated, dizziness, dystonia, hyperkinesia
Gastrointestinal disorders Very common: Nausea Common: Diarrhoea, abdominal pain, mouth dry, constipation, vomiting Very rare: Anorexia
Hepato-biliary disorders Rare: Hepatic function tests abnormal
Skin and subcutaneous tissue disorders Rare: Erythematous or maculopapular rash Very rare: Urticaria
Renal and urinary disorders Very common: Urine discolouration
General disorders and administration site conditions Common: Fatigue, sweating increased, fall Very rare: Weight decrease

* Adverse reactions are ranked under headings of frequency, the most frequent first, using the following convention: Very common $>1/10$); common $>1/100, <1/10$); uncommon $>1/1,000, <1/100$); rare $>1/10,000, <1/1,000$), very rare $<1/10,000$), including isolated reports.

Isolated cases of hepatitis with cholestatic features have been reported.

Entacapone in association with levodopa has been associated with isolated cases of excessive daytime somnolence and sudden sleep onset episodes.

Isolated cases of NMS have been reported following abrupt reduction or discontinuation of entacapone and other dopaminergic medications.

Isolated cases of rhabdomyolysis have been reported.

4.9 Overdose

No cases of overdose have been reported with entacapone. The highest dose of entacapone given to man is 2,400 mg daily. Management of acute overdosing is symptomatic.

5. PHARMACOLOGICAL PROPERTIES

5.1 Pharmacodynamic properties

Pharmacotherapeutic group: catechol-O-methyl transferase inhibitor, ATC code: NO4BX02.

Entacapone belongs to a new therapeutic class, catechol-O-methyl transferase (COMT) inhibitors. It is a reversible, specific, and mainly peripherally acting COMT inhibitor designed for concomitant administration with levodopa preparations. Entacapone decreases the metabolic loss of levodopa to 3-O-methyldopa (3-OMD) by inhibiting the COMT enzyme. This leads to a higher levodopa AUC. The amount of levodopa available to the brain is increased. Entacapone thus prolongs the clinical response to levodopa.

Entacapone inhibits the COMT enzyme mainly in peripheral tissues. COMT inhibition in red blood cells closely follows the plasma concentrations of entacapone, thus clearly indicating the reversible nature of COMT inhibition.

Clinical studies

In two phase III double-blind studies in altogether 376 patients with Parkinson's disease and end-of-dose motor fluctuations, entacapone or placebo was given with each levodopa/dopa decarboxylase inhibitor dose. The results are given in Table 2. In study I, daily ON time (hours) was measured from home diaries and in study II, the proportion of daily ON time.

Table 2. Daily ON time (Mean ±SD)

(see Table 2 on next page)

There were corresponding decreases in OFF time.

Table 2 Daily ON time (Mean ±SD)

Study I: Daily On time (h)			
	Entacapone(n=85)	**Placebo(n=86)**	**Difference**
Baseline	9.3±2.2	9.2±2.5	
Week 8-24	10.7±2.2	9.4±2.6	1h 20 min (8.3%) $CI_{95\%}$ 45 min, 1 h 56 min
Study II: Proportion of daily On time (%)			
	Entacapone(n=103)	**Placebo(n=102)**	**Difference**
Baseline	60.0±15.2	60.8±14.0	
Week 8-24	66.8±14.5	62.8±16.80	4.5% (0 h 35 min) $CI_{95\%}$ 0.93%, 7.97%

The % change from baseline in OFF time was −24% in the entacapone group and 0% in the placebo group in study I. The corresponding figures in study II were −18% and −5%.

5.2 Pharmacokinetic properties

a) General characteristics of the active substance

Absorption

There are large intra- and interindividual variations in the absorption of entacapone.

The peak concentration (C_{max}) in plasma is usually reached about one hour after a 200 mg entacapone tablet. The drug is subject to extensive first-pass metabolism. The bioavailability of entacapone is about 35% after an oral dose. Food does not affect the absorption of entacapone to any significant extent.

Distribution

After absorption from the gastrointestinal tract, entacapone is rapidly distributed to the peripheral tissues with a distribution volume of 20 litres at steady state (Vd_{ss}). Approximately 92 % of the dose is eliminated during β-phase with a short elimination half-life of 30 minutes. The total clearance of entacapone is about 800 ml/min.

Entacapone is extensively bound to plasma proteins, mainly to albumin. In human plasma the unbound fraction is about 2.0% in the therapeutic concentration range. At therapeutic concentrations, entacapone does not displace other extensively bound drugs (e.g. warfarin, salicylic acid, phenylbutazone, or diazepam), nor is it displaced to any significant extent by any of these drugs at therapeutic or higher concentrations.

Metabolism

A small amount of entacapone, the *(E)*-isomer, is converted to its *(Z)*-isomer. The *(E)*-isomer accounts for 95% of the AUC of entacapone. The *(Z)*-isomer and traces of other metabolites account for the remaining 5%.

Data from *in vitro* studies using human liver microsomal preparations indicate that entacapone inhibits cytochrome P450 2C9 (IC_{50} ~4 μM). Entacapone showed little or no inhibition of other types of P450 isoenzymes (CYP1A2, CYP2A6, CYP2D6, CYP2E1, CYP3A and CYP2C19) (see section 4.5 Interaction with other medicinal products and other forms of interaction).

Elimination

The elimination of entacapone occurs mainly by non-renal metabolic routes. It is estimated that 80-90% of the dose is excreted in faeces, although this has not been confirmed in man. Approximately 10-20% is excreted in urine. Only traces of entacapone are found unchanged in urine. The major part (95%) of the product excreted in urine is conjugated with glucuronic acid. Of the metabolites found in urine only about 1% have been formed through oxidation.

b) Characteristics in patients

The pharmacokinetic properties of entacapone are similar in both young and elderly adults. The metabolism of the medicinal product is slowed in patients with mild to moderate liver insufficiency (Child-Pugh Class A and B), which leads to an increased plasma concentration of entacapone both in the absorption and elimination phases (see section 4.3 Contra-indications). Renal impairment does not affect the pharmacokinetics of entacapone. However, a longer dosing interval may be considered for patients who are receiving dialysis therapy.

5.3 Preclinical safety data

Preclinical data revealed no special hazard for humans based on conventional studies of safety pharmacology, repeated dose toxicity, genotoxicity, and carcinogenic potential. In repeated dose toxicity studies, anaemia most likely due to iron chelating properties of entacapone was observed. Regarding reproduction toxicity, decreased foetal weight and a slightly delayed bone development were noticed in rabbits at systemic exposure levels in the therapeutic range.

6. PHARMACEUTICAL PARTICULARS

6.1 List of excipients

Tablet core:

Microcrystalline cellulose
Mannitol
Croscarmellose sodium
Hydrogenated vegetable oil
Magnesium stearate
Film-coating:
Hypromellose
Polysorbate 80
Glycerol 85%
Sucrose
Magnesium stearate
Yellow iron oxide (E 172)
Red iron oxide (E 172)
Titanium dioxide (E 171).

6.2 Incompatibilities

Not applicable

6.3 Shelf life

3 years.

6.4 Special precautions for storage

No special precautions for storage.

6.5 Nature and contents of container

White high-density polyethylene (HDPE) bottles with white tamper proof HD- polyethylene closures containing 30, 60, 100 or 350 tablets.

All pack sizes may not be marketed.

6.6 Instructions for use and handling

No special requirements.

7. MARKETING AUTHORISATION HOLDER

Orion Corporation
Orionintie 1
FIN-02200 Espoo
Finland

8. MARKETING AUTHORISATION NUMBER(S)

EU/1/98/082/001-004

9. DATE OF FIRST AUTHORISATION/RENEWAL OF THE AUTHORISATION

16.09.98

10. DATE OF REVISION OF THE TEXT

07.03.05

Concerta XL 18 mg prolonged-release tablets, CONCERTA XL 36 mg prolonged-release tablets.

(Janssen-Cilag Ltd)

1. NAME OF THE MEDICINAL PRODUCT

CONCERTA XL 18 mg prolonged-release tablets.

CONCERTA XL 36 mg prolonged-release tablets.

2. QUALITATIVE AND QUANTITATIVE COMPOSITION

One tablet contains either 18 mg or 36 mg of methylphenidate hydrochloride.

For excipients, see 6.1.

3. PHARMACEUTICAL FORM

Prolonged-release Tablet.

18 mg Tablet:

Capsule-shaped yellow tablet with "alza 18" printed on one side in black ink.

36 mg Tablet:

Capsule-shaped white tablet with "alza 36" printed on one side in black ink.

4. CLINICAL PARTICULARS

4.1 Therapeutic indications

CONCERTA® XL is indicated as part of a comprehensive treatment programme for Attention Deficit Hyperactivity Disorder (ADHD) in children (over 6 years of age) and adolescents when remedial measures alone prove insufficient. Diagnosis must be made according to DSM-IV criteria or the guidelines in ICD-10 and should be based on a complete history and evaluation of the patient. The specific aetiology of this syndrome is unknown, and there is no single diagnostic test. Adequate diagnosis requires the use of medical and special psychological, educational, and social resources. Learning may or may not be impaired. Drug treatment may not be necessary for all children with this syndrome. Therefore CONCERTA® XL treatment is not indicated in all children with ADHD and the decision to use the drug must be based on a very thorough assessment of the severity and chronicity of the child's symptoms in relation to the child's age.

Use of CONCERTA® XL should be limited to patients requiring a product with effects lasting through the day to the evening when taken in the morning. A comprehensive treatment programme for the treatment of ADHD should include other measures (psychological, educational, social) for patients with this disorder. Stimulants are not intended for use in the patient who exhibits symptoms secondary to environmental factors and/or other primary psychiatric disorders, including psychosis. Appropriate educational placement is essential, and psychosocial intervention is often helpful.

4.2 Posology and method of administration

Adults: Not applicable.

Elderly: Not applicable.

Children (over 6 years of age) and Adolescents: CONCERTA® XL is administered orally once daily in the morning.

CONCERTA® XL must be swallowed whole with the aid of liquids, and must not be chewed, divided, or crushed (see 4.4. Special Warnings and Special Precautions for Use).

CONCERTA® XL may be administered with or without food (see 5.2. Pharmacokinetic Properties).

Treatment must be initiated under the supervision of a specialist conversant with childhood and/or adolescence behavioural disorders.

Dosage should be individualised according to the needs and responses of the patient.

Dosage may be adjusted in 18 mg increments to a maximum of 54 mg/day taken once daily in the morning. In general, dosage adjustment may proceed at approximately weekly intervals.

Patients New to Methylphenidate: Clinical experience with CONCERTA® XL is limited in these patients (see Section 5.1. Pharmacodynamic Properties). CONCERTA® XL may not be indicated in all children with ADHD syndrome. Lower doses of short-acting methylphenidate formulations may be considered sufficient to treat patients new to methylphenidate. Careful dose titration by the physician in charge is required in order to avoid unnecessarily high doses of methylphenidate. The recommended starting dose of CONCERTA® XL for patients who are not currently taking methylphenidate, or for patients who are on stimulants other than methylphenidate, is 18 mg once daily.

Patients Currently Using Methylphenidate: The recommended dose of CONCERTA® XL for patients who are currently taking methylphenidate three times daily at doses of 15 to 45 mg/day is provided in Table 1. Dosing recommendations are based on current dose regimen and clinical judgement.

TABLE 1

Recommended Dose Conversion from

Other Methylphenidate Regimens, where available, to CONCERTA® XL

Previous Methylphenidate Daily Dose	**Recommended CONCERTA® XL Dose**
5 mg Methylphenidate three times daily	18 mg once daily
10 mg Methylphenidate three times daily	36 mg once daily
15 mg Methylphenidate three times daily	54 mg once daily

Daily dosage above 54 mg is not recommended.

If improvement is not observed after appropriate dosage adjustment over a one-month period, the drug should be discontinued.

Maintenance/Extended Treatment: The long-term use of methylphenidate has not been systematically evaluated in controlled trials. The physician who elects to use CONCERTA® XL for extended periods in patients with ADHD should periodically re-evaluate the long-term usefulness of the drug for the individual patient with trial periods off medication to assess the patient's functioning without pharmacotherapy. Improvement may be sustained when the drug is either temporarily or permanently discontinued.

Dose Reduction and Discontinuation: If paradoxical aggravation of symptoms or other adverse events occur, the dosage should be reduced, or, if necessary, the drug should be discontinued. Drug treatment is usually discontinued during or after puberty.

Children (under 6 years): The safety and efficacy of CONCERTA® XL in children under 6 years of age have not been established. Therefore, CONCERTA® XL should not be used in children under 6 years of age.

4.3 Contraindications

CONCERTA® XL is contraindicated:

- in patients known to be hypersensitive to methylphenidate or other components of the product;
- in patients with marked anxiety and tension, since the drug may aggravate these symptoms;
- in patients with glaucoma;
- in patients with a family history or diagnosis of Tourette's syndrome;
- in combination with non-selective, irreversible monoamine oxidase inhibitors (MAO), and also within a minimum of 14 days following discontinuation of a non-selective, irreversible MAO inhibitor (hypertensive crises may result) (see Section 4.5. Interactions with other Medicinal Products and other forms of Interaction);
- in patients with hyperthyroidism;
- in patients with severe angina pectoris;
- in patients with cardiac arrhythmias;
- in patients with severe hypertension;
- in patients who currently exhibit severe depression, anorexia nervosa, psychotic symptoms or suicidal tendency, since the drug might worsen these conditions;
- in patients with known drug dependence or alcoholism;
- in patients during pregnancy (see Sections 4.6. Pregnancy and Lactation and 5.3. Preclinical Safety Data).

4.4 Special warnings and special precautions for use

CONCERTA® XL should not be used in children under 6 years old. The safety and efficacy of CONCERTA® XL in this age group have not been established.

Because the CONCERTA® XL tablet is nondeformable and does not appreciably change in shape in the gastrointestinal (GI) tract, it should not ordinarily be administered to patients with pre-existing severe GI narrowing (pathologic or iatrogenic) or in patients with dysphagia or significant difficulty in swallowing tablets. There have been rare reports of obstructive symptoms in patients with known strictures in association with the ingestion of drugs in nondeformable prolonged-release formulations.

Due to the prolonged-release design of the tablet, CONCERTA® XL should only be used in patients who are able to swallow the tablet whole. Patients should be informed that CONCERTA® XL must be swallowed whole with the aid of liquids. Tablets should not be chewed, divided, or crushed. The medication is contained within a nonabsorbable shell designed to release the drug at a controlled rate. The tablet shell is eliminated from the body; patients should not be concerned if they occasionally notice in their stool something that looks like a tablet.

The choice between treatment with either CONCERTA® XL or an immediate release formulation, containing methylphenidate, will have to be decided by the treating physician on an individual basis and depends on the intended duration of effect.

CNS stimulants, including methylphenidate, have been associated with the onset or exacerbation of motor and verbal tics. Therefore, clinical evaluation for tics in children should precede use of stimulant medication. Family history should be assessed.

It should not be used for the prevention or treatment of normal fatigue states.

Clinical experience suggests that in psychotic patients, administration of methylphenidate may exacerbate symptoms of behaviour disturbance and thought disorder.

CONCERTA® XL should be given cautiously to patients with a history of drug dependence or alcoholism. Chronic abusive use can lead to marked tolerance and psychological dependence with varying degrees of abnormal behaviour. Frank psychotic episodes can occur, especially with parenteral abuse. Careful supervision is required during withdrawal from abusive use since severe depression may occur. Withdrawal following chronic therapeutic use may unmask symptoms of the underlying disorder that may require follow-up.

There is some clinical evidence that methylphenidate may lower the convulsive threshold in patients with prior history of seizures, in patients with prior EEG abnormalities in absence of seizures, and, very rarely, in absence of history of seizures and no prior EEG evidence of seizures. In the presence of seizures, the drug should be discontinued.

Use cautiously in patients with hypertension. Blood pressure should be monitored at appropriate intervals in patients taking CONCERTA® XL, especially patients with hypertension. In the laboratory classroom clinical trials, both CONCERTA® XL and methylphenidate three times daily increased resting pulse by an average of 2 to 6 bpm and produced average increases of systolic and diastolic blood pressure of roughly 1 to 4 mm Hg during the day, relative to placebo. Therefore, caution is indicated in treating patients whose underlying medical conditions might be compromised by increases in blood pressure or heart rate.

Periodic full blood count, differential, and platelet counts are advised during prolonged therapy.

Symptoms of visual disturbances have been encountered in rare cases. Difficulties with accommodation and blurring of vision have been reported.

There is no experience with the use of CONCERTA® XL in patients with renal insufficiency or hepatic insufficiency (see Section 5.2. Pharmacokinetic Properties).

Sufficient data on the safety of long-term use of methylphenidate in children are not yet available. Although a causal relationship has not been established, suppression of growth (ie, weight gain, and/or height) has been reported with the long-term use of stimulants in children. Therefore, patients requiring long-term therapy should be carefully monitored. Patients who are not growing or gaining weight as expected should have their treatment interrupted temporarily.

Sport: This product contains methylphenidate which results in a positive result during drug testing.

Females of child-bearing potential (females post-menarche) should use effective contraception.

4.5 Interaction with other medicinal products and other forms of Interaction

CONCERTA® XL should not be used in patients being treated (currently or within the preceding 2 weeks) with non-selective, irreversible MAO inhibitors.

Because of possible increases in blood pressure, CONCERTA® XL should be used cautiously with vasopressor agents.

Formal drug-drug interaction studies have not been performed with CONCERTA® XL. Hence, the interaction potential is not fully elucidated. It is not known how methylphenidate may affect plasma concentrations of concomitantly administered drugs. Caution is recommended at combination of methylphenidate with other drugs, especially those with a narrow therapeutic window. Case reports have indicated that methylphenidate may inhibit the metabolism of coumarin anticoagulants, anticonvulsants (eg, phenobarbitone, phenytoin, primidone), and some antidepressants (tricyclics and selective serotonin reuptake inhibitors). Downward dose adjustment of these drugs may be required when given concomitantly with methylphenidate. It may be necessary to adjust the dosage and monitor plasma drug concentrations (or, in the case of coumarin, coagulation times), when initiating or discontinuing concomitant methylphenidate.

Halogenated anaesthetics: There is a risk of sudden blood pressure increase during surgery. If surgery is planned, methylphenidate treatment should not be used on the day of surgery.

Alcohol may exacerbate the adverse CNS effect of psychoactive drugs, including CONCERTA® XL. It is therefore advisable for patients to abstain from alcohol during treatment.

4.6 Pregnancy and lactation

There are no adequate data from the use of methylphenidate in pregnant women.

Studies in animals have shown reproductive toxicity (teratogenic effects) of methylphenidate (see Section 5.3. Preclinical Safety Data). The potential risk for humans is unknown.

From observations in humans there are indications that amphetamines could be harmful to the foetus.

CONCERTA® XL is contraindicated during pregnancy (see Section 4.3. Contraindications).

Females of child-bearing potential (females post-menarche) should use effective contraception.

It is not known whether methylphenidate or its metabolites pass into breast milk, but for safety reasons breast-feeding mothers should not use CONCERTA® XL.

4.7 Effects on ability to drive and use machines

No studies have been performed on the effects of CONCERTA® XL on the ability to drive and use machines. However, CONCERTA® XL may cause dizziness. It is therefore advisable to exercise caution when driving, operating machinery, or engaging in other potentially hazardous activities.

4.8 Undesirable effects

Undesirable effects reported with CONCERTA® XL:

In clinical trials with CONCERTA® XL (n=469), approximately 62% of patients experienced at least one adverse reaction. The most commonly reported undesirable effects were headache (26%), loss of appetite (14%), insomnia (14%), and stomach ache (12%).

Frequency estimate: Very common $\geqslant$10%; Common $\geqslant$1% to $<$10%; Uncommon $\geqslant$0.1% to $<$1%; Rare $\geqslant$0.01% to $<$0.1%; Very Rare $<$0.01%.

Body as a whole: Very Common: Headache, stomach ache. Common: ADHD aggravated, asthenia. Uncommon: chest pain, fever, accidental injury, malaise, pain.

Cardiovascular system disorders: Common: hypertension. Uncommon: migraine, tachycardia.

Digestive system disorders: Very Common: loss of appetite. Common: nausea and/or vomiting, dyspepsia. Uncommon: diarrhoea, faecal incontinence, increased appetite.

Metabolic and nutritional system disorders: Common: weight loss.

Musculoskeletal system disorders: Uncommon: leg cramps.

Nervous system disorders: Common: dizziness, somnolence and twitching (tics). Uncommon: hyperkinesia, speech disorder and vertigo.

Psychiatric disorders: Very common: insomnia. Common: anxiety, depression, emotional lability, hostility and nervousness. Uncommon: abnormal dreams, apathy, confusion, hallucinations, sleep disorder, thinking abnormal, suicide attempt.

Respiratory system disorders: Uncommon: cough increased, epistaxis.

Skin system disorders: Common: rash. Uncommon: alopecia, pruritus, urticaria.

Special senses: Uncommon: diplopia.

Urogenital system disorders: Uncommon: urinary frequency, haematuria, urinary urgency.

Frequency of undesirable effects was similar to that seen with immediate release methylphenidate given three times daily.

Post-marketing Experience with CONCERTA® XL:

Blood and lymphatic system disorders: leucopenia, thrombocytopenia.

Cardiac disorders: arrhythmia, palpitations.

Eye disorders: blurred vision, difficulties in visual accommodation.

Gastro-intestinal disorders: dry mouth.

Hepatobiliary disorders: abnormal liver function tests (eg transaminase elevation), hepatitis.

Musculoskeletal and connective tissue disorders: arthralgia.

Nervous system disorders: convulsions.

Psychiatric disorders: agitation, psychosis.

Miscellaneous: growth retardation/weight loss.

Undesirable effects noted with other methylphenidate formulations:

In addition to the above reactions observed with CONCERTA® XL, the following adverse reactions have been noted with the use of other methylphenidate products:

Nervous system disorders: Very rare: hyperactivity, convulsions, muscle cramps, choreo-athetoid movements, exacerbation of existing tics, Tourette's syndrome.

Very rare reports of poorly documented neuroleptic malignant syndrome (NMS) have been noted.

Psychiatric disorders: Very rare:toxic psychosis (sometimes with visual and tactile hallucinations), transient depressed mood.

Vascular disorders: Very rare: cerebral arteritis, and/or occlusion.

Gastro-intestinal disorders: Very rare: hepatic coma.

Cardiovascular system disorders: Rare: angina pectoris.

Skin and appendages: Common: fever. Very rare: thrombocytopaenic purpura, exfoliative dermatitis, erythema multiforme.

Blood: Very rare: anaemia.

Miscellaneous: Rare: slight growth retardation during prolonged use in children.

4.9 Overdose

The prolonged release of methylphenidate from CONCERTA® XL should be considered when treating patients with overdose.

Signs and Symptoms: Signs and symptoms of acute methylphenidate overdosage, resulting principally from overstimulation of the CNS and from excessive sympathomimetic effects, may include the following: vomiting, agitation, tremors, hyperreflexia, muscle twitching, convulsions (may be followed by coma), euphoria, confusion, hallucinations, delirium, sweating, flushing, headache, hyperpyrexia, tachycardia, palpitations, cardiac arrhythmias, hypertension, mydriasis, and dryness of mucous membranes.

Recommended Treatment: Treatment consists of appropriate supportive measures. The patient must be protected against self-injury and against external stimuli that would aggravate overstimulation already present. Gastric contents may be evacuated by gastric lavage as indicated. Before performing gastric lavage, control agitation and seizures if present and protect the airway. Other measures to detoxify the gut include administration of activated charcoal and a cathartic. Intensive care must be provided to maintain adequate circulation and respiratory exchange; external cooling procedures may be required for hyperpyrexia.

Efficacy of peritoneal dialysis or extracorporeal haemodialysis for CONCERTA® XL overdosage has not been established.

5. PHARMACOLOGICAL PROPERTIES

5.1 Pharmacodynamic properties

Pharmacotherapeutic group: psychoanaleptics, psychostimulants and nootropics, centrally acting sympathomimetics: ATC code: N06BA04

Methylphenidate HCl is a mild central nervous system (CNS) stimulant. The mode of therapeutic action in Attention Deficit Hyperactivity Disorder (ADHD) is not known. Methylphenidate is thought to block the reuptake of noradrenaline and dopamine into the presynaptic neurone and increase the release of these monoamines into the extraneuronal space. Methylphenidate is a racemic mixture comprised of the d- and l-isomers. The d-isomer is more pharmacologically active than the l-isomer.

In the pivotal clinical studies, CONCERTA® XL was assessed in 321 patients already stabilised with immediate release preparations (IR) of methylphenidate and in 95 patients not previously treated with IR preparations of methylphenidate.

Clinical studies showed that the effects of CONCERTA® XL were maintained until 12 hours after dosing when the product was taken once daily in the morning.

5.2 Pharmacokinetic properties

Absorption: Methylphenidate is readily absorbed. Following oral administration of CONCERTA® XL to adults the drug overcoat dissolves, providing an initial maximum drug concentration at about 1 to 2 hours. The methylphenidate contained in the two internal drug layers is gradually released over the next several hours. Peak plasma concentrations are achieved at about 6 to 8 hours, after which plasma levels of methylphenidate gradually decrease. CONCERTA® XL taken once daily minimises the fluctuations between peak and trough concentrations associated with immediate-release methylphenidate three times daily. The extent of absorption of CONCERTA® XL once daily is generally comparable to conventional immediate release preparations.

Following the administration of CONCERTA® XL 18 mg once daily in 36 adults, the mean pharmacokinetic parameters were: C_{max} 3.7 ± 1.0 (ng/mL), T_{max} 6.8 ± 1.8 (h), AUC_{inf} 41.8 ± 13.9 (ng.h/mL), and $t_{½}$ 3.5 ± 0.4 (h).

No differences in the pharmacokinetics of CONCERTA® XL were noted following single and repeated once daily dosing, indicating no significant drug accumulation. The AUC and $t_{1/2}$ following repeated once daily dosing are similar to those following the first dose of CONCERTA® XL 18 mg. Following administration of CONCERTA® XL in single doses of 18, 36, and 54 mg/day to adults, C_{max} and $AUC_{(0-inf)}$ of methylphenidate were proportional to dose.

Distribution: Plasma methylphenidate concentrations in adults decline biexponentially following oral administration. The half-life of methylphenidate in adults following oral administration of CONCERTA® XL was approximately 3.5 h. The rate of protein binding of methylphenidate and of its metabolites is approximately 15%. The apparent volume of distribution of methylphenidate is approximately 13 litres/kg.

Metabolism: In humans, methylphenidate is metabolised primarily by de-esterification to alpha-phenyl-piperidine acetic acid (PPA, approximately 50 fold the level of the unchanged substance) which has little or no pharmacologic activity. In adults the metabolism of CONCERTA® XL once daily as evaluated by metabolism to PPA is similar to that of methylphenidate three times daily. The metabolism of single and repeated once daily doses of CONCERTA® XL is similar.

Excretion: The elimination half-life of methylphenidate in adults following administration of CONCERTA® XL was approximately 3.5 hours. After oral administration, about 90% of the dose is excreted in urine and 1 to 3% in faeces, as metabolites within 48 to 96 hours. Small quantities of unchanged methylphenidate are recovered in urine (less than 1%). The main urinary metabolite is alpha-phenyl-piperidine acetic acid (60-90%).

After oral dosing of radiolabelled methylphenidate in humans, about 90% of the radioactivity was recovered in urine. The main urinary metabolite was PPA, accounting for approximately 80% of the dose.

Food Effects: In patients, there were no differences in either the pharmacokinetics or the pharmacodynamic performance of CONCERTA® XL when administered after a high fat breakfast on an empty stomach.

Special PopulationsGender: In healthy adults, the mean dose-adjusted $AUC_{(0-inf)}$ values for CONCERTA® XL were 36.7 ng.h/mL in men and 37.1 ng.h/mL in women, with no differences noted between the two groups.

Race: In healthy adults receiving CONCERTA® XL, dose-adjusted $AUC_{(0-inf)}$ was consistent across ethnic groups; however, the sample size may have been insufficient to detect ethnic variations in pharmacokinetics.

Age: The pharmacokinetics of CONCERTA® XL has not been studied in children younger than 6 years of age. In children 7-12 years of age, the pharmacokinetics of CONCERTA® XL after 18, 36 and 54 mg were (mean±SD): C_{max} 6.0±1.3, 11.3±2.6, and 15.0±3.8 ng/mL, respectively, T_{max} 9.4±0.02, 8.1±1.1, 9.1±2.5 h, respectively, and $AUC_{0-11.5}$ 50.4±7.8, 87.7±18.2, 121.5±37.3 ng.h/mL, respectively.

Renal Insufficiency: There is no experience with the use of CONCERTA® XL in patients with renal insufficiency. After oral administration of radiolabelled methylphenidate in humans, methylphenidate was extensively metabolised and approximately 80% of the radioactivity was excreted in the urine in the form of PPA. Since renal clearance is not an important route of methylphenidate clearance, renal insufficiency is expected to have little effect on the pharmacokinetics of CONCERTA® XL.

Hepatic Insufficiency: There is no experience with the use of CONCERTA® XL in patients with hepatic insufficiency.

5.3 Preclinical safety data

There is evidence that methylphenidate may be a teratogen in two species. Spina bifida and limb malformations have been reported in rabbits whilst in the rat, equivocal evidence of induction of abnormalities of the vertebrae was found.

Methylphenidate did not affect reproductive performance or fertility at low multiples (2-5 times) of the therapeutic human dose.

There was no evidence of carcinogenicity in the rat. In mice, methylphenidate caused an increase in hepatocellular adenomas, in animals of both sexes and, in males only, hepatoblastomas. In the absence of exposure data, the significance of these findings to humans is not known.

The weight of evidence from the genotoxicity studies reveals no special hazard for humans.

6. PHARMACEUTICAL PARTICULARS

6.1 List of excipients

18 mg

Butylhydroxytoluene (E321), cellulose acetate 398-10, hypromellose 3cp, phosphoric acid concentrated, poloxamer 188, polyethylene oxides 200K and 7000K, povidone K29-32, sodium chloride, stearic acid, succinic acid, black iron oxide (E172), and ferric oxide yellow (E172).

Film Coat: ferric oxide yellow (E172), hypromellose 15cp, lactose monohydrate, stearic acid, titanium dioxide (E171), and triacetin.

Clear Coat: carnauba wax, hypromellose 6cp, and macrogol 400.

Printing Ink: black iron oxide (E172), hypromellose 6cp, isopropyl alcohol, propylene glycol, and purified water.

36 mg

Butylhydroxytoluene (E321), cellulose acetate 398-10, hypromellose 3cp, phosphoric acid concentrated, poloxamer 188, polyethylene oxides 200K and 7000K, povidone K29-32, sodium chloride, stearic acid, succinic acid, black iron oxide (E172), and ferric oxide yellow (E172).

Film Coat: hypromellose 15cp, lactose monohydrate, titanium dioxide (E171), and triacetin.

Clear Coat: carnauba wax, hypromellose 6cp, and macrogol 400.

Printing Ink: black iron oxide (E172), hypromellose 6cp, isopropyl alcohol, propylene glycol, and purified water.

6.2 Incompatibilities

Not applicable.

6.3 Shelf life

3 years

6.4 Special precautions for storage

Keep the container tightly closed. Do not store above 30°C.

6.5 Nature and contents of container

High-density polyethylene (HDPE) bottle with a child-resistant polypropylene closure and a desiccant enclosed.

28 or 30 tablets.

Not all pack sizes may be marketed.

6.6 Instructions for use and handling

No special requirements.

7. MARKETING AUTHORISATION HOLDER

Janssen-Cilag Limited
PO Box 79, Saunderton
High Wycombe
Buckinghamshire
HP14 4HJ
United Kingdom

8. MARKETING AUTHORISATION NUMBER(S)

18 mg Tablets: PL 00242/0372

36 mg Tablets: PL 00242/0373

9. DATE OF FIRST AUTHORISATION/RENEWAL OF THE AUTHORISATION

19 February 2002

10. DATE OF REVISION OF THE TEXT

3 March 2004

Conotrane Cream

(Astellas Pharma Limited)

1. NAME OF THE MEDICINAL PRODUCT

Conotrane Cream.

2. QUALITATIVE AND QUANTITATIVE COMPOSITION

A smooth white cream containing benzalkonium chloride 0.1% w/w and Dimeticone 22.0% w/w.

3. PHARMACEUTICAL FORM

Cream for topical administration.

4. CLINICAL PARTICULARS

4.1 Therapeutic indications

Conotrane is used for protection of the skin from moisture, irritants, chafing and contamination with bacteria or yeasts.

It may be used in situations such as in the prevention/treatment of napkin rash, the prevention of pressure sores and in the management of incontinence.

4.2 Posology and method of administration

The cream should be applied to the affected area several times a day, as necessary or after every napkin change.

4.3 Contraindications

Known hypersensitivity to benzalkonium chloride.

4.4 Special warnings and special precautions for use

None stated.

4.5 Interaction with other medicinal products and other forms of Interaction

None stated.

4.6 Pregnancy and lactation

Not applicable.

4.7 Effects on ability to drive and use machines

None stated.

4.8 Undesirable effects

Local hypersensitivity to benzalkonium chloride is rare.

4.9 Overdose

Not applicable.

5. PHARMACOLOGICAL PROPERTIES

5.1 Pharmacodynamic properties

This is a remedy suitable for both prescription and for self medication. It is a cream for topical application containing dimeticone and benzalkonium chloride. The dimeticone is water repellent allowing transpiration of water vapour from the skin. The benzalkonium chloride is a quaternary ammonium compound, active against bacteria and yeasts.

5.2 Pharmacokinetic properties

Not applicable.

5.3 Preclinical safety data

None stated.

6. PHARMACEUTICAL PARTICULARS

6.1 List of excipients

Cetostearyl alcohol
Macrogol cetostearyl ether
White soft paraffin
Light liquid paraffin
Deionised water
Macrogol 300
Potassium dihydrogen orthophosphate
Geranium SC45

6.2 Incompatibilities

None stated.

6.3 Shelf life

3 years.

6.4 Special precautions for storage

Do not store above 25°C.

6.5 Nature and contents of container

(i) 7 g, 15 g, 50 g and 100 g in white LDPE tubes.

(ii) 500 g white polypropylene pot with screw lid.

6.6 Instructions for use and handling

None stated.

Administrative Data

7. MARKETING AUTHORISATION HOLDER

Yamanouchi Pharma Ltd
Yamanouchi House
Pyrford Road
West Byfleet
Surrey
KT14 6RA

8. MARKETING AUTHORISATION NUMBER(S)

PL 0166/0178.

9. DATE OF FIRST AUTHORISATION/RENEWAL OF THE AUTHORISATION

1 July 1998 / 28th February 2002

10. DATE OF REVISION OF THE TEXT

Date of partial revision 8th January 2002

11. Legal category

GSL

Convulex 150 mg Capsules

(Pharmacia Limited)

1. NAME OF THE MEDICINAL PRODUCT
Convulex 150 mg Capsules

2. QUALITATIVE AND QUANTITATIVE COMPOSITION
Valproic Acid 150.00 mg

3. PHARMACEUTICAL FORM
Enteric-coated soft gelatine capsules

4. CLINICAL PARTICULARS

4.1 Therapeutic indications
Treatment of generalised, partial or other epilepsy.

4.2 Posology and method of administration
Convulex capsules are for oral administration.

Daily dosage requirements vary according to age and body weight.

Convulex capsules may be given twice daily.

The capsules should be swallowed and not crushed or chewed.

Monotherapy:

Usual requirements are as follows:

a) Adults

Dosage should start at 600 mg daily, followed by gradual increases (approx. 300 mg) at three day intervals until control is achieved. This is generally within the dosage range 1000 mg to 2000 mg per day, i.e. 20-30 mg/kg body weight. Where adequate control is not achieved within this range, the dose may be further increased up to 2500 mg per day.

b) Elderly Patients

Although the pharmacokinetics of valproate are modified in the elderly, they have limited clinical significance and dosage should be determined by seizure control. The volume of distribution is increased in the elderly and because of decreased binding to serum albumin, the proportion of free drug is increased. This will affect the clinical interpretation of plasma valproic acid levels.

c) Children

Children over 20kg
Initial dosage is usually not more than 400mg/day (irrespective of weight) with spaced increases until control is achieved; this is usually within the range 20-30mg/kg body weight per day. Where adequate control is not achieved within this range the dose may be increased to 35mg/kg body weight per day.

Children under 20kg
20mg/kg of body weight per day; in severe cases this may be increased but only in patients in whom plasma valproic acid levels can be monitored. Above 40mg/kg/day, clinical chemistry and haematological parameters should be monitored.

Splitting the total daily dose into 2-4 intakes is generally recommended.

d) In patients with renal insufficiency

It may be necessary to decrease dosage. Dosage should be adjusted according to clinical monitoring since monitoring of plasma concentrations may be misleading (see section 5.2 Pharmacokinetic Properties).

e) In patients with hepatic insufficiency

Salicylates should not be used concomitantly with valproate since they employ the same metabolic pathway (see also sections 4.4 Special Warnings and Precautions for Use and 4.8 Undesirable Effects).

Liver dysfunction, including hepatic failure resulting in fatalities, has occurred in patients whose treatment included valproic acid (see sections 4.3 Contraindications and 4.4 Special Warnings and Precautions for Use).

Salicylates should not be used in children under 16 years (see aspirin/salicylate product information on Reye's syndrome). In addition in conjunction with Convulex, concomitant use in children under 3 years can increase the risk of liver toxicity (see section 4.4.1 Special warnings).

Substitution:

A one to one dose relationship of Convulex and products containing sodium valproate has been demonstrated in pharmacokinetic trials. In patients previously receiving sodium valproate therapy, Convulex should be initiated at the same total daily dose.

Combined therapy:

When starting Convulex in patients already on other anticonvulsants, these should be tapered slowly; initiation of Convulex therapy should then be gradual, with target dose being reached after about 2 weeks. In certain cases it may be necessary to raise the dose by 5 to 10mg/kg/day when used in combination with anticonvulsants which induce liver enzyme activity, e.g. phenytoin, phenobarbitone and carbamazepine. Once known enzyme inducers have been withdrawn it may be possible to maintain seizure control on a reduced dose of Convulex. When barbiturates are being administered concomitantly and particularly if sedation is observed (particularly in children)
the dosage of barbiturate should be reduced.

NB: In children requiring doses higher than 40mg/kg/day clinical chemistry and haematological parameters should be monitored.

Optimum dosage is mainly determined by seizure control and routine measurement of plasma levels is unnecessary. However, a method for measurement of plasma levels is available and may be helpful where there is poor control or side effects are suspected (see section 5.2 Pharmacokinetic Properties).

4.3 Contraindications
- Active liver disease
- Personal or family history of severe hepatic dysfunction, especially drug related
- Hypersensitivity to valproic acid
- Porphyria

4.4 Special warnings and special precautions for use
4.4.1 Special warnings
Liver dysfunction:

Conditions of occurrence:

Severe liver damage, including hepatic failure sometimes resulting in fatalities, has been very rarely reported. Experience in epilepsy has indicated that patients most at risk, especially in cases of multiple anticonvulsant therapy, are infants and in particular young children under the age of 3 and those with severe seizure disorders, organic brain disease, and (or) congenital metabolic or degenerative disease associated with mental retardation.

After the age of 3, the incidence of occurrence is significantly reduced and progressively decreases with age.

The concomitant use of salicylates should be avoided in children under 3 due to the risk of liver toxicity. Additionally, salicylates should not be used in children under 16 years (see aspirin/salicylate product information on Reye's syndrome).

Monotherapy is recommended in children under the age of 3 years when prescribing Convulex, but the potential benefit of Convulex should be weighed against the risk of liver damage or pancreatitis in such patients prior to initiation of therapy

In most cases, such liver damage occurred during the first 6 months of therapy, the period of maximum risk being 2-12 weeks.

Suggestive signs:

Clinical symptoms are essential for early diagnosis. In particular the following conditions, which may precede jaundice, should be taken into consideration, especially in patients at risk (see above: 'Conditions of occurrence'):

- non specific symptoms, usually of sudden onset, such as asthenia, malaise, anorexia, lethargy, oedema and drowsiness, which are sometimes associated with repeated vomiting and abdominal pain.
- in patients with epilepsy, recurrence of seizures.

These are an indication for immediate withdrawal of the drug.

Patients (or their family for children) should be instructed to report immediately any such signs to a physician should they occur. Investigations including clinical examination and biological assessment of liver function should be undertaken immediately.

Detection:

Liver function should be measured before and then periodically monitored during the first 6 months of therapy, especially in those who seem most at risk, and those with a prior history of liver disease.

Amongst usual investigations, tests which reflect protein synthesis, particularly prothrombin rate, are most relevant.

Confirmation of an abnormally low prothrombin rate, particularly in association with other biological abnormalities (significant decrease in fibrinogen and coagulation factors; increased bilirubin level and raised transaminases) requires cessation of Convulex therapy.

As a matter of precaution and in case they are taken concomitantly salicylates should also be discontinued since they employ the same metabolic pathway.

As with most antiepileptic drugs, increased liver enzymes are common, particularly at the beginning of therapy; they are also transient.

More extensive biological investigations (including prothrombin rate) are recommended in these patients; a reduction in dosage may be considered when appropriate and tests should be repeated as necessary.

Pancreatitis: Pancreatitis, which may be severe and result in fatalities, has been very rarely reported. Patients experiencing nausea, vomiting or acute abdominal pain should have a prompt medical evaluation (including measurement of serum amylase). Young children are at particular risk; this risk decreases with increasing age. Severe seizures and severe neurological impairment with combination anticonvulsant therapy may be risk factors. Hepatic failure with pancreatitis increases the risk of fatal outcome. In case of pancreatitis, valproate should be discontinued.

4.4.2 Precautions

Haematological: Blood tests (blood cell count, including platelet count, bleeding time and coagulation tests) are recommended prior to initiation of therapy or before surgery, and in case of spontaneous bruising or bleeding (see section 4.8 Undesirable Effects). Renal insufficiency: In patients with renal insufficiency, it may be necessary to decrease dosage. As monitoring of plasma concentrations may be misleading, dosage should be adjusted according to clinical monitoring (see sections 4.2 Posology and Method of Administration and 5.2. Pharmacokinetic Properties).

Systemic lupus erythematosus: Although immune disorders have only rarely been noted during the use of Convulex, the potential benefit of Convulex should be weighed against its potential risk in patients with systemic lupus erythematosus (see also section 4.8 Undesirable Effects).

Hyperammonaemia: When a urea cycle enzymatic deficiency is suspected, metabolic investigations should be performed prior to treatment because of the risk of hyperammonaemia with valproate.

Weight gain: Convulex very commonly causes weight gain, which may be marked and progressive. Patients should be warned of the risk of weight gain at the initiation of therapy and appropriate strategies should be adopted to minimise it (see section 4.8 Undesirable Effects).

Pregnancy: Women of childbearing potential should not be started on Convulex without specialist neurological advice. Convulex is the antiepileptic of choice in patients with certain types of epilepsy such as generalised epilepsy ± myoclonus/photosensitivity. For partial epilepsy, Convulex should be used only in patients resistant to other treatment. Women who are likely to get pregnant, should receive specialist advice because of the potential teratogenic risk to the foetus (see also section 4.6 Pregnancy and Lactation).

Diabetic patients: Valproate is eliminated mainly through the kidneys, partly in the form of ketone bodies; this may give false positives in the urine testing of possible diabetics.

4.5 Interaction with other medicinal products and other forms of Interaction
4.5.1 Effects of Valproate on other drugs

- Neuroleptics, MAO inhibitors, antidepressants and benzodiazepines

Valproate may potentiate the effect of other psychotropics such as neuroleptics, MAO inhibitors, antidepressants and benzodiazepines; therefore, clinical monitoring is advised and dosage should be adjusted when appropriate.

- Phenobarbital

Valproate increases phenobarbital plasma concentrations (due to inhibition of hepatic catabolism) and sedation may occur, particularly in children. Therefore, clinical monitoring is recommended throughout the first 15 days of combined treatment with immediate reduction of phenobarbital doses if sedation occurs and determination of phenobarbital plasma levels when appropriate.

- Primidone

Valproate increases primidone plasma levels with exacerbation of its adverse effects (such as sedation); these signs cease with long term treatment. Clinical monitoring is recommended especially at the beginning of combined therapy with dosage adjustment when appropriate.

- Phenytoin

Valproate decreases phenytoin total plasma concentration. Moreover valproate increases phenytoin free form with possible overdosage symptoms (valproic acid displaces phenytoin from its plasma protein binding sites and reduces its hepatic catabolism). Therefore clinical monitoring is recommended; when phenytoin plasma levels are determined, the free form should be evaluated.

- Carbamazepine

Clinical toxicity has been reported when valproate was administered with carbamazepine as valproate may potentiate toxic effects of carbamazepine. Clinical monitoring is recommended especially at the beginning of combined therapy with dosage adjustment when appropriate.

- Lamotrigine

Valproate may reduce lamotrigine metabolism and increase its mean half-life, dosages should be adjusted (lamotrigine dosage decreased) when appropriate. Co-administration of lamotrigine and Convulex might increase the risk of rash.

- Zidovudine

Valproate may raise zidovudine plasma concentration leading to increased zidovudine toxicity.

- Vitamin K-dependent anticoagulants

The anticoagulant effect of warfarin and other coumarin anticoagulants may be increased following displacement from plasma protein binding sites by valproic acid. The prothrombin time should be closely monitored.

- Temozolomide

Co-administration of temozolomide and valproate may cause a small decrease in the clearance of temozolomide that is not thought to be clinically relevant.

4.5.2 Effects of other drugs on Valproate

Antiepileptics with enzyme inducing effect (including *phenytoin, phenobarbital, carbamazepine*) decrease valproic acid plasma concentrations. Dosages should be adjusted according to blood levels in case of combined therapy.

On the other hand, combination of *felbamate* and valproate may increase valproic acid plasma concentration. Valproate dosage should be monitored.

Mefloquine and *chloroquine* increase valproic acid metabolism and may lower the seizure threshold; therefore epileptic seizures may occur in cases of combined therapy. Accordingly, the dosage of Convulex may need adjustment.

In case of concomitant use of valproate and *highly protein bound agents (e.g. aspirin)*, free valproic acid plasma levels may be increased.

Valproic acid plasma levels may be increased (as a result of reduced hepatic metabolism) in case of concomitant use with *cimetidine* or *erythromycin*.

Carbapenem antibiotics such as *imipenem* and *meropenem*: Decrease in valproic acid blood level, sometimes associated with convulsions, has been observed when imipenem or meropenem were combined. If these antibiotics have to be administered, close monitoring of valproic acid blood levels is recommended.

Cholestyramine may decrease the absorption of valproate.

4.5.3 Other Interactions

Caution is advised when using Convulex in combination with newer anti-epileptics whose pharmacodynamics may not be well established.

Valproate usually has no enzyme-inducing effect; as a consequence, valproate does not reduce efficacy of oestroprogestative agents in women receiving hormonal contraception, including the oral contraceptive pill.

4.6 Pregnancy and lactation

4.6.1. Pregnancy

From experience in treating mothers with epilepsy, the risk associated with the use of valproate during pregnancy has been described as follows:

- Risk associated with epilepsy and antiepileptics

In offspring born to mothers with epilepsy receiving anti-epileptic treatment, the overall rate of malformations has been demonstrated to be 2 to 3 times higher than the rate (approximately 3%) reported in the general population. Although an increased number of children with malformations have been reported in cases of multiple drug therapy, the respective role of treatments and disease in causing the malformations has not been formally established. Malformations most frequently encountered are cleft lip and cardio-vascular malformations.

Epidemiological studies have suggested an association between in-utero exposure to sodium valproate and a risk of developmental delay. Many factors including maternal epilepsy may also contribute to this risk but it is difficult to quantify the relative contribution of these or of maternal anti-epileptic treatment. Notwithstanding those potential risks, no sudden discontinuation in the anti-epileptic therapy should be undertaken as this may lead to breakthrough seizures which could have serious consequences for both the mother and the foetus.

- Risk associated with valproate

In animals: teratogenic effects have been demonstrated in the mouse, rat and rabbit.

There is animal experimental evidence that high plasma peak levels and the size of an individual dose are associated with neural tube defects.

In humans: an increased incidence of congenital abnormalities (including cases of facial dysmorphia, hypospadias and multiple malformations, particularly of the limbs) has been demonstrated in offspring born to mothers with epilepsy treated with valproate. Valproate use is associated with neural tube defects such as myelomeningocele and spina bifida. The frequency of this effect is estimated to be 1 to 2%.

- In view of the above data

When a woman is planning pregnancy, this provides an opportunity to review the need for anti-epileptic treatment. Women of childbearing age should be informed of the risks and benefits of continuing anti-epileptic treatment throughout pregnancy.

Folate supplementation **prior** to pregnancy, has been demonstrated to reduce the incidence of neural tube defects in the offspring of women at high risk. Although no direct evidence exists of such effects in women receiving anti-epileptic drugs, women should be advised to start taking folic acid supplementation (5 mg) as soon as contraception is discontinued.

The available evidence suggests that anticonvulsant monotherapy is preferred. Dosage should be reviewed before conception and the lowest effective dose used, in divided doses, as abnormal pregnancy outcome tends to be associated with higher total daily dosage and with the size of an individual dose. The incidence of neural tube defects rises with increasing dosage, particularly above 1000 mg daily. The administration in several divided doses over the day and the use of a prolonged release formulation is preferable in order to avoid high peak plasma levels.

During pregnancy, valproate anti-epileptic treatment should not be discontinued if it has been effective.

Nevertheless, specialised prenatal monitoring should be instituted in order to detect the possible occurrence of a neural tube defect or any other malformation. Pregnancies should be carefully screened by ultrasound, and other techniques if appropriate (see Section 4.4 Special Warnings and Special Precautions for Use).

- Risk in the neonate

Very rare cases of haemorrhagic syndrome have been reported in neonates whose mothers have taken valproate during pregnancy. This haemorrhagic syndrome is related to hypofibrinogenemia; afibrinogenemia has also been reported and may be fatal. These are possibly associated with a decrease of coagulation factors. However, this syndrome has to be distinguished from the decrease of the vitamin-K factors induced by phenobarbitone and other anti-epileptic enzyme inducing drugs.

Therefore, platelet count, fibrinogen plasma level, coagulation tests and coagulation factors should be investigated in neonates.

4.6.2. Lactation

Excretion of valproate in breast milk is low, with a concentration between 1% to 10% of total maternal serum levels; up to now children breast fed that have been monitored during the neonatal period have not experienced clinical effects. There appears to be no contra-indication to breast feeding by patients on valproate.

4.7 Effects on ability to drive and use machines

Use of Convulex may provide seizure control such that the patient may be eligible to hold a driving licence.

Patients should be warned of the risk of transient drowsiness, especially in cases of anticonvulsant polytherapy or association with benzodiazepines (see section 4.5 Interactions with Other Medicaments and Other Forms of Interaction).

4.8 Undesirable effects

Congenital and familial/genetic disorders: (see section 4.6 Pregnancy and Lactation)

Hepato-biliary disorders: rare cases of liver dysfunction (see section 4.4.1 Warnings)

Severe liver damage, including hepatic failure sometimes resulting in death, has been reported (see also sections 4.2, 4.3 and 4.4.1). Increased liver enzymes are common, particularly early in treatment, and may be transient (see section 4.4.1).

Gastrointestinal disorders (nausea, gastralgia, diarrhoea) frequently occur at the start of treatment. These problems can usually be overcome by taking Convulex capsules with or after food.

Very rare cases of pancreatitis, sometimes lethal, have been reported (see section 4.4 Special Warnings and Special Precautions for Use).

Nervous system disorders:

Sedation has been reported occasionally, usually when in combination with other anticonvulsants. In monotherapy it occurred early in treatment on rare occasions and is usually transient. Rare cases of lethargy and confusion occasionally progressing to stupor, sometimes with associated hallucinations or convulsions have been reported. Encephalopathy and coma have very rarely been observed. These cases have often been associated with too high a starting dose or too rapid a dose escalation or concomitant use of other anticonvulsants, notably phenobarbitone. They have usually been reversible on withdrawal of treatment or reduction of dosage.

Very rare cases of reversible extrapyramidal symptoms including parkinsonism, or reversible dementia associated with reversible cerebral atrophy have been reported. Dose-related ataxia and fine postural tremor have occasionally been reported.

An increase in alertness may occur; this is generally beneficial but occasionally aggression, hyperactivity and behavioural deterioration have been reported.

Metabolic disorders:

Cases of isolated and moderate hyperammonaemia without change in liver function tests may occur frequently, are usually transient and should not cause treatment discontinuation. However, they may present clinically as vomiting, ataxia, and increasing clouding of consciousness. Should these symptoms occur Convulex should be discontinued.

Hyperammonaemia associated with neurological symptoms has also been reported (see section 4.4.2 Precautions). In such cases further investigations should be considered.

Blood and lymphatic system disorders:

Frequent occurrence of thrombocytopenia, rare cases of anaemia, leucopenia or pancytopenia. The blood picture returned to normal when the drug was discontinued.

Isolated reduction of fibrinogen or reversible increase in bleeding time have been reported, usually without associated clinical signs and particularly with high doses (valproate has an inhibitory effect on the second phase of platelet aggregation). Spontaneous bruising or bleeding is an indication for withdrawal of medication pending investigations (see also section 4.6 Pregnancy and Lactation).

Skin and subcutaneous tissue disorders:

Cutaneous reactions such as exanthematous rash rarely occur with valproate. In very rare cases toxic epidermal necrolysis, Stevens-Johnson syndrome and erythema multiforme have been reported.

Transient hair loss, which may sometimes be dose-related, has often been reported. Regrowth normally begins within six months, although the hair may become more curly than previously. Hirsutism and acne have been very rarely reported.

Reproductive system and breast disorders:

Amenorrhoea and irregular periods have been reported. Very rarely gynaecomastia has occurred.

Vascular disorders: The occurrence of vasculitis has occasionally been reported.

Ear disorders:

Hearing loss, either reversible or irreversible has been reported rarely; however a cause and effect relationship has not been established.

Renal and urinary disorders:

There have been isolated reports of a reversible Fanconi's syndrome (a defect in proximal renal tubular function giving rise to glycosuria, amino aciduria, phosphaturia, and uricosuria) associated with valproate therapy, but the mode of action is as yet unclear.

Immune system disorders:

Allergic reactions (ranging from rash to hypersensitivity reactions) have been reported.

General disorders:

Very rare cases of non-severe peripheral oedema have been reported.

Increase in weight may also occur. Weight gain being a risk factor for polycystic ovary syndrome, it should be carefully monitored (see section 4.4 Special Warnings and Special Precautions for Use).

4.9 Overdose

Cases of accidental and deliberate valproate overdosage have been reported.

At plasma concentrations of up to 5-6 times the maximum therapeutic levels, there are unlikely to be any symptoms other than nausea, vomiting and dizziness.

Clinical signs of massive overdose, i.e. plasma concentration 10 to 20 times maximum therapeutic levels, usually include CNS depression or coma with muscular hypotonia, hyporeflexia, miosis, impaired respiratory function.

Symptoms may however be variable and seizures have been reported in the presence of very high plasma levels (see also section 5.2 Pharmacokinetic Properties). Cases of intracranial hypertension related to cerebral oedema have been reported.

Hospital management of overdose should be symptomatic, including cardio-respiratory monitoring. Gastric lavage may be useful up to 10 to 12 hours following ingestion.

Haemodialysis and haemoperfusion have been used successfully.

Naloxone has been successfully used in a few isolated cases, sometimes in association with activated charcoal given orally. Deaths have occurred following massive overdose; nevertheless, a favourable outcome is usual.

5. PHARMACOLOGICAL PROPERTIES

5.1 Pharmacodynamic properties

Valproic acid is an anticonvulsant.

The most likely mode of action for valproate is potentiation of the inhibitory action of gamma amino butyric acid (GABA) through an action on the further synthesis or further metabolism of GABA.

In certain in-vitro studies it was reported that sodium valproate could stimulate HIV replication but studies on peripheral blood mononuclear cells from HIV-infected subjects show that sodium valproate does not have a mitogen-like effect on inducing HIV replication. Indeed the effect of sodium valproate on HIV replication ex-vivo is highly variable, modest in quantity, appears to be unrelated to the dose and has not been documented in man.

5.2 Pharmacokinetic properties

The half-life of valproate is usually reported to be within the range of 8-20 hours. It is usually shorter in children.

In patients with severe renal insufficiency it may be necessary to alter dosage in accordance with free plasma valproic acid levels.

The reported effective therapeutic range for plasma valproic acid levels is 40-100mg/litre (278-694 micromol/litre). This reported range may depend on time of sampling and presence of co-medication. The percentage of free (unbound) drug is usually between 6% and 15% of total plasma levels. An increased incidence of adverse effects may occur with plasma levels above the effective therapeutic range.

The pharmacological (or therapeutic) effects of Convulex may not be clearly correlated with the total or free (unbound) plasma valproic acid levels.

5.3 Preclinical safety data

There are no pre-clinical data of relevance to the prescriber which are additional to those already stated in other sections of the SPC.

6. PHARMACEUTICAL PARTICULARS

6.1 List of excipients

Fractionated Coconut Oil

Gelatine

Glycerol 85 %

Dry substance of Karion 83 (70 %)

Sodium ethyl hydroxybenzoate

Sodium propyl hydroxybenzoate

Titanium dioxide

Cochineal red A 62.5 % (E 124)

Sunset yellow S 92 % (E 110)

Hydroxypropylmethylcellulose phthalate

Dibutylphthalate BP 1963

6.2 Incompatibilities

None.

6.3 Shelf life

60 months

6.4 Special precautions for storage

Do not store above 25°C. Protect from light.

6.5 Nature and contents of container

Blister packs:

Upper: PVC-foil

Lower: aluminium foil

Outer box:

carton folding box

Pack size: 100

6.6 Instructions for use and handling

Not applicable.

7. MARKETING AUTHORISATION HOLDER

Gerot Pharmazeutika GmbH

Arnethgasse 3

A – 1160 Vienna

Austria

8. MARKETING AUTHORISATION NUMBER(S)

PL 08298/0004

9. DATE OF FIRST AUTHORISATION/RENEWAL OF THE AUTHORISATION

11 October 1991 / 13 October 1998 / 2 July 2004

10. DATE OF REVISION OF THE TEXT

November 2004

Legal Status

POM

Convulex 300 mg Capsules

(Pharmacia Limited)

1. NAME OF THE MEDICINAL PRODUCT

Convulex 300 mg Capsules

2. QUALITATIVE AND QUANTITATIVE COMPOSITION

Valproic Acid 300.00 mg

3. PHARMACEUTICAL FORM

Enteric-coated soft gelatine capsules

4. CLINICAL PARTICULARS

4.1 Therapeutic indications

Treatment of generalised, partial or other epilepsy.

4.2 Posology and method of administration

Convulex capsules are for oral administration.

Daily dosage requirements vary according to age and body weight.

Convulex capsules may be given twice daily.

The capsules should be swallowed and not crushed or chewed.

Monotherapy:

Usual requirements are as follows:

a) Adults

Dosage should start at 600 mg daily, followed by gradual increases (approx. 300 mg) at three day intervals until control is achieved. This is generally within the dosage range 1000 mg to 2000 mg per day, i.e. 20-30 mg/kg body weight. Where adequate control is not achieved within this range, the dose may be further increased up to 2500 mg per day.

b) Elderly Patients

Although the pharmacokinetics of valproate are modified in the elderly, they have limited clinical significance and dosage should be determined by seizure control. The volume of distribution is increased in the elderly and because of decreased binding to serum albumin, the proportion of free drug is increased. This will affect the clinical interpretation of plasma valproic acid levels.

c) Children

Children over 20kg

Initial dosage is usually not more than 400mg/day (irrespective of weight) with spaced increases until control is achieved; this is usually within the range 20-30mg/kg body weight per day. Where adequate control is not achieved within this range the dose may be increased to 35mg/kg body weight per day.

Children under 20kg

20mg/kg of body weight per day; in severe cases this may be increased but only in patients in whom plasma valproic acid levels can be monitored. Above 40mg/kg/day, clinical chemistry and haematological parameters should be monitored.

Splitting the total daily dose into 2-4 intakes is generally recommended.

d) In patients with renal insufficiency

It may be necessary to decrease dosage. Dosage should be adjusted according to clinical monitoring since monitoring of plasma concentrations may be misleading (see section 5.2 Pharmacokinetic Properties).

e) In patients with hepatic insufficiency

Salicylates should not be used concomitantly with valproate since they employ the same metabolic pathway (see also sections 4.4 Special Warnings and Precautions for Use and 4.8 Undesirable Effects).

Liver dysfunction, including hepatic failure resulting in fatalities, has occurred in patients whose treatment included valproic acid (see sections 4.3 Contraindications and 4.4 Special Warnings and Precautions for Use).

Salicylates should not be used in children under 16 years (see aspirin/salicylate product information on Reye's syndrome). In addition in conjunction with Convulex, concomitant use in children under 3 years can increase the risk of liver toxicity (see section 4.4.1 Special warnings).

Substitution:

A one to one dose relationship of Convulex and products containing sodium valproate has been demonstrated in pharmacokinetic trials. In patients previously receiving sodium valproate therapy, Convulex should be initiated at the same total daily dose.

Combined therapy:

When starting Convulex in patients already on other anticonvulsants, these should be tapered slowly; initiation of Convulex therapy should then be gradual, with target dose being reached after about 2 weeks. In certain cases it may be necessary to raise the dose by 5 to 10mg/kg/day when used in combination with anticonvulsants which induce liver enzyme activity, e.g. phenytoin, phenobarbitone and carbamazepine. Once known enzyme inducers have been withdrawn it may be possible to maintain seizure control on a reduced dose of Convulex. When barbiturates are being administered concomitantly and particularly if sedation is observed (particularly in children) the dosage of barbiturate should be reduced.

NB: In children requiring doses higher than 40mg/kg/day clinical chemistry and haematological parameters should be monitored.

Optimum dosage is mainly determined by seizure control and routine measurement of plasma levels is unnecessary. However, a method for measurement of plasma levels is available and may be helpful where there is poor control or side effects are suspected (see section 5.2 Pharmacokinetic Properties).

4.3 Contraindications

- Active liver disease
- Personal or family history of severe hepatic dysfunction, especially drug related
- Hypersensitivity to valproic acid
- Porphyria

4.4 Special warnings and special precautions for use

4.4.1 Special warnings

Liver dysfunction:

Conditions of occurrence:

Severe liver damage, including hepatic failure sometimes resulting in fatalities, has been very rarely reported. Experience in epilepsy has indicated that patients most at risk, especially in cases of multiple anticonvulsant therapy, are infants and in particular young children under the age of 3 and those with severe seizure disorders, organic brain disease, and (or) congenital metabolic or degenerative disease associated with mental retardation.

After the age of 3, the incidence of occurrence is significantly reduced and progressively decreases with age.

The concomitant use of salicylates should be avoided in children under 3 due to the risk of liver toxicity. Additionally, salicylates should not be used in children under 16 years (see aspirin/salicylate product information on Reye's syndrome).

Monotherapy is recommended in children under the age of 3 years when prescribing Convulex, but the potential benefit of Convulex should be weighed against the risk of liver damage or pancreatitis in such patients prior to initiation of therapy

In most cases, such liver damage occurred during the first 6 months of therapy, the period of maximum risk being 2-12 weeks.

Suggestive signs:

Clinical symptoms are essential for early diagnosis. In particular the following conditions, which may precede jaundice, should be taken into consideration, especially in patients at risk (see above: 'Conditions of occurrence'):

- non specific symptoms, usually of sudden onset, such as asthenia, malaise, anorexia, lethargy, oedema and drowsiness, which are sometimes associated with repeated vomiting and abdominal pain.
- in patients with epilepsy, recurrence of seizures.

These are an indication for immediate withdrawal of the drug.

Patients (or their family for children) should be instructed to report immediately any such signs to a physician should they occur. Investigations including clinical examination and biological assessment of liver function should be undertaken immediately.

Detection:

Liver function should be measured before and then periodically monitored during the first 6 months of therapy, especially in those who seem most at risk, and those with a prior history of liver disease.

Amongst usual investigations, tests which reflect protein synthesis, particularly prothrombin rate, are most relevant.

Confirmation of an abnormally low prothrombin rate, particularly in association with other biological abnormalities (significant decrease in fibrinogen and coagulation factors; increased bilirubin level and raised transaminases) requires cessation of Convulex therapy.

As a matter of precaution and in case they are taken concomitantly salicylates should also be discontinued since they employ the same metabolic pathway.

As with most antiepileptic drugs, increased liver enzymes are common, particularly at the beginning of therapy; they are also transient.

More extensive biological investigations (including prothrombin rate) are recommended in these patients; a reduction in dosage may be considered when appropriate and tests should be repeated as necessary.

Pancreatitis: Pancreatitis, which may be severe and result in fatalities, has been very rarely reported. Patients experiencing nausea, vomiting or acute abdominal pain should have a prompt medical evaluation (including measurement of serum amylase). Young children are at particular risk; this risk decreases with increasing age. Severe seizures and severe neurological impairment with combination anticonvulsant therapy may be risk factors. Hepatic failure with pancreatitis increases the risk of fatal outcome. In case of pancreatitis, valproate should be discontinued.

4.4.2 Precautions

Haematological: Blood tests (blood cell count, including platelet count, bleeding time and coagulation tests) are recommended prior to initiation of therapy or before surgery, and in case of spontaneous bruising or bleeding (see section 4.8 Undesirable Effects). Renal insufficiency: In patients with renal insufficiency, it may be necessary to decrease dosage. As monitoring of plasma concentrations may be misleading, dosage should be adjusted according to clinical monitoring (see sections 4.2 Posology and Method of Administration and 5.2. Pharmacokinetic Properties).

Systemic lupus erythematosus: Although immune disorders have only rarely been noted during the use of Convulex, the potential benefit of Convulex should be weighed against its potential risk in patients with systemic lupus erythematosus (see also section 4.8 Undesirable Effects).

Hyperammonaemia: When a urea cycle enzymatic deficiency is suspected, metabolic investigations should be performed prior to treatment because of the risk of hyperammonaemia with valproate.

Weight gain: Convulex very commonly causes weight gain, which may be marked and progressive. Patients should be warned of the risk of weight gain at the initiation of therapy and appropriate strategies should be adopted to minimise it (see section 4.8 Undesirable Effects).

Pregnancy: Women of childbearing potential should not be started on Convulex without specialist neurological advice. Convulex is the antiepileptic of choice in patients with certain types of epilepsy such as generalised epilepsy ± myoclonus/photosensitivity. For partial epilepsy, Convulex should be used only in patients resistant to other treatment. Women who are likely to get pregnant, should receive specialist advice because of the potential teratogenic risk to the foetus (see also section 4.6 Pregnancy and Lactation).

Diabetic patients: Valproate is eliminated mainly through the kidneys, partly in the form of ketone bodies; this may give false positives in the urine testing of possible diabetics.

4.5 Interaction with other medicinal products and other forms of Interaction

4.5.1 Effects of Valproate on other drugs

- Neuroleptics, MAO inhibitors, antidepressants and benzodiazepines

Valproate may potentiate the effect of other psychotropics such as neuroleptics, MAO inhibitors, antidepressants and benzodiazepines; therefore, clinical monitoring is advised and dosage should be adjusted when appropriate.

- Phenobarbital

Valproate increases phenobarbital plasma concentrations (due to inhibition of hepatic catabolism) and sedation may occur, particularly in children. Therefore, clinical monitoring is recommended throughout the first 15 days of combined treatment with immediate reduction of phenobarbital doses if sedation occurs and determination of phenobarbital plasma levels when appropriate.

- Primidone

Valproate increases primidone plasma levels with exacerbation of its adverse effects (such as sedation); these signs cease with long term treatment. Clinical monitoring is recommended especially at the beginning of combined therapy with dosage adjustment when appropriate.

- Phenytoin

Valproate decreases phenytoin total plasma concentration. Moreover valproate increases phenytoin free form with possible overdosage symptoms (valproic acid displaces phenytoin from its plasma protein binding sites and reduces its hepatic catabolism). Therefore clinical monitoring is recommended; when phenytoin plasma levels are determined, the free form should be evaluated.

- Carbamazepine

Clinical toxicity has been reported when valproate was administered with carbamazepine as valproate may potentiate toxic effects of carbamazepine. Clinical monitoring is recommended especially at the beginning of combined therapy with dosage adjustment when appropriate.

- Lamotrigine

Valproate may reduce lamotrigine metabolism and increase its mean half-life, dosages should be adjusted (lamotrigine dosage decreased) when appropriate. Co-administration of lamotrigine and Convulex might increase the risk of rash.

- Zidovudine

Valproate may raise zidovudine plasma concentration leading to increased zidovudine toxicity.

- Vitamin K-dependent anticoagulants

The anticoagulant effect of warfarin and other coumarin anticoagulants may be increased following displacement from plasma protein binding sites by valproic acid. The prothrombin time should be closely monitored.

- Temozolomide

Co-administration of temozolomide and valproate may cause a small decrease in the clearance of temozolomide that is not thought to be clinically relevant.

4.5.2 Effects of other drugs on Valproate

Antiepileptics with enzyme inducing effect (including *phenytoin, phenobarbital, carbamazepine*) decrease valproic acid plasma concentrations. Dosages should be adjusted according to blood levels in case of combined therapy.

On the other hand, combination of *felbamate* and valproate may increase valproic acid plasma concentration. Valproate dosage should be monitored.

Mefloquine and *chloroquine* increase valproic acid metabolism and may lower the seizure threshold; therefore epileptic seizures may occur in cases of combined therapy. Accordingly, the dosage of Convulex may need adjustment.

In case of concomitant use of valproate and *highly protein bound agents (e.g. aspirin)*, free valproic acid plasma levels may be increased.

Valproic acid plasma levels may be increased (as a result of reduced hepatic metabolism) in case of concomitant use with *cimetidine* or *erythromycin*.

Carbapenem antibiotics such as *imipenem* and *meropenem*: Decrease in valproic acid blood level, sometimes associated with convulsions, has been observed when imipenem or meropenem were combined. If these antibiotics have to be administered, close monitoring of valproic acid blood levels is recommended.

Cholestyramine may decrease the absorption of valproate.

4.5.3 Other Interactions

Caution is advised when using Convulex in combination with newer anti-epileptics whose pharmacodynamics may not be well established.

Valproate usually has no enzyme-inducing effect; as a consequence, valproate does not reduce efficacy of oestroprogestative agents in women receiving hormonal contraception, including the oral contraceptive pill.

4.6 Pregnancy and lactation

4.6.1. Pregnancy

From experience in treating mothers with epilepsy, the risk associated with the use of valproate during pregnancy has been described as follows:

- Risk associated with epilepsy and antiepileptics

In offspring born to mothers with epilepsy receiving anti-epileptic treatment, the overall rate of malformations has been demonstrated to be 2 to 3 times higher than the rate (approximately 3%) reported in the general population. Although an increased number of children with malformations have been reported in cases of multiple drug therapy, the respective role of treatments and disease in causing the malformations has not been formally established. Malformations most frequently encountered are cleft lip and cardio-vascular malformations.

Epidemiological studies have suggested an association between in-utero exposure to sodium valproate and a risk of developmental delay. Many factors including maternal epilepsy may also contribute to this risk but it is difficult to quantify the relative contribution of these or of maternal anti-epileptic treatment. Notwithstanding those potential risks, no sudden discontinuation in the anti-epileptic therapy should be undertaken as this may lead to breakthrough seizures which could have serious consequences for both the mother and the foetus.

- Risk associated with valproate

In animals: teratogenic effects have been demonstrated in the mouse, rat and rabbit.

There is animal experimental evidence that high plasma peak levels and the size of an individual dose are associated with neural tube defects.

In humans: an increased incidence of congenital abnormalities (including cases of facial dysmorphia, hypospadias and multiple malformations, particularly of the limbs) has been demonstrated in offspring born to mothers with epilepsy treated with valproate. Valproate use is associated with neural tube defects such as myelomeningocele and spina bifida. The frequency of this effect is estimated to be 1 to 2%.

- In view of the above data

When a woman is planning pregnancy, this provides an opportunity to review the need for anti-epileptic treatment. Women of childbearing age should be informed of the risks and benefits of continuing anti-epileptic treatment throughout pregnancy.

Folate supplementation **prior** to pregnancy, has been demonstrated to reduce the incidence of neural tube defects in the offspring of women at high risk. Although no direct evidence exists of such effects in women receiving anti-epileptic drugs, women should be advised to start taking folic acid supplementation (5 mg) as soon as contraception is discontinued.

The available evidence suggests that anticonvulsant monotherapy is preferred. Dosage should be reviewed before conception and the lowest effective dose used, in divided doses, as abnormal pregnancy outcome tends to be associated with higher total daily dosage and with the size of an individual dose. The incidence of neural tube defects rises with increasing dosage, particularly above 1000 mg daily. The administration in several divided doses over the day and the use of a prolonged release formulation is preferable in order to avoid high peak plasma levels.

During pregnancy, valproate anti-epileptic treatment should not be discontinued if it has been effective.

Nevertheless, specialised prenatal monitoring should be instituted in order to detect the possible occurrence of a neural tube defect or any other malformation. Pregnancies should be carefully screened by ultrasound, and other techniques if appropriate (see Section 4.4 Special Warnings and Special Precautions for Use).

- Risk in the neonate

Very rare cases of haemorrhagic syndrome have been reported in neonates whose mothers have taken valproate during pregnancy. This haemorrhagic syndrome is related to hypofibrinogenemia; afibrinogenemia has also been reported and may be fatal. These are possibly associated with a decrease of coagulation factors. However, this syndrome has to be distinguished from the decrease of the vitamin-K factors induced by phenobarbitone and other anti-epileptic enzyme inducing drugs.

Therefore, platelet count, fibrinogen plasma level, coagulation tests and coagulation factors should be investigated in neonates.

4.6.2. Lactation

Excretion of valproate in breast milk is low, with a concentration between 1% to 10% of total maternal serum levels; up to now children breast fed that have been monitored during the neonatal period have not experienced clinical effects. There appears to be no contra-indication to breast feeding by patients on valproate.

4.7 Effects on ability to drive and use machines

Use of Convulex may provide seizure control such that the patient may be eligible to hold a driving licence.

Patients should be warned of the risk of transient drowsiness, especially in cases of anticonvulsant polytherapy or association with benzodiazepines (see section 4.5 Interactions with Other Medicaments and Other Forms of Interaction).

4.8 Undesirable effects

Congenital and familial/genetic disorders: (see section 4.6 Pregnancy and Lactation)

Hepato-biliary disorders: rare cases of liver dysfunction (see section 4.4.1 Warnings)

Severe liver damage, including hepatic failure sometimes resulting in death, has been reported (see also sections 4.2, 4.3 and 4.4.1). Increased liver enzymes are common, particularly early in treatment, and may be transient (see section 4.4.1).

Gastrointestinal disorders (nausea, gastralgia, diarrhoea) frequently occur at the start of treatment. These problems can usually be overcome by taking Convulex capsules with or after food.

Very rare cases of pancreatitis, sometimes lethal, have been reported (see section 4.4 Special Warnings and Special Precautions for Use).

Nervous system disorders:

Sedation has been reported occasionally, usually when in combination with other anticonvulsants. In monotherapy it occurred early in treatment on rare occasions and is usually transient. Rare cases of lethargy and confusion occasionally progressing to stupor, sometimes with associated hallucinations or convulsions have been reported. Encephalopathy and coma have very rarely been observed. These cases have often been associated with too high a starting dose or too rapid a dose escalation or concomitant use of other anticonvulsants, notably phenobarbitone. They have usually been reversible on withdrawal of treatment or reduction of dosage.

Very rare cases of reversible extrapyramidal symptoms including parkinsonism, or reversible dementia associated with reversible cerebral atrophy have been reported. Dose-related ataxia and fine postural tremor have occasionally been reported.

An increase in alertness may occur; this is generally beneficial but occasionally aggression, hyperactivity and behavioural deterioration have been reported.

Metabolic disorders:

Cases of isolated and moderate hyperammonaemia without change in liver function tests may occur frequently, are usually transient and should not cause treatment discontinuation. However, they may present clinically as vomiting, ataxia, and increasing clouding of consciousness. Should these symptoms occur Convulex should be discontinued.

Hyperammonaemia associated with neurological symptoms has also been reported (see section 4.4.2 Precautions). In such cases further investigations should be considered.

Blood and lymphatic system disorders:

Frequent occurrence of thrombocytopenia, rare cases of anaemia, leucopenia or pancytopenia. The blood picture returned to normal when the drug was discontinued.

Isolated reduction of fibrinogen or reversible increase in bleeding time have been reported, usually without associated clinical signs and particularly with high doses (valproate has an inhibitory effect on the second phase of platelet aggregation). Spontaneous bruising or bleeding is an indication for withdrawal of medication pending investigations (see also section 4.6 Pregnancy and Lactation).

Skin and subcutaneous tissue disorders:

Cutaneous reactions such as exanthematous rash rarely occur with valproate. In very rare cases toxic epidermal necrolysis, Stevens-Johnson syndrome and erythema multiforme have been reported.

Transient hair loss, which may sometimes be dose-related, has often been reported. Regrowth normally begins within six months, although the hair may become more curly than previously. Hirsutism and acne have been very rarely reported.

Reproductive system and breast disorders:

Amenorrhoea and irregular periods have been reported. Very rarely gynaecomastia has occurred.

Vascular disorders: The occurrence of vasculitis has occasionally been reported.

Ear disorders:

Hearing loss, either reversible or irreversible has been reported rarely; however a cause and effect relationship has not been established.

Renal and urinary disorders:

There have been isolated reports of a reversible Fanconi's syndrome (a defect in proximal renal tubular function giving rise to glycosuria, amino aciduria, phosphaturia, and uricosuria) associated with valproate therapy, but the mode of action is as yet unclear.

Immune system disorders:

Allergic reactions (ranging from rash to hypersensitivity reactions) have been reported.

General disorders:

Very rare cases of non-severe peripheral oedema have been reported.

Increase in weight may also occur. Weight gain being a risk factor for polycystic ovary syndrome, it should be carefully monitored (see section 4.4 Special Warnings and Special Precautions for Use).

4.9 Overdose

Cases of accidental and deliberate valproate overdosage have been reported.

At plasma concentrations of up to 5-6 times the maximum therapeutic levels, there are unlikely to be any symptoms other than nausea, vomiting and dizziness.

Clinical signs of massive overdose, i.e. plasma concentration 10 to 20 times maximum therapeutic levels, usually include CNS depression or coma with muscular hypotonia, hyporeflexia, miosis, impaired respiratory function.

Symptoms may however be variable and seizures have been reported in the presence of very high plasma levels (see also section 5.2 Pharmacokinetic Properties). Cases of intracranial hypertension related to cerebral oedema have been reported.

Hospital management of overdose should be symptomatic, including cardio-respiratory monitoring. Gastric lavage may be useful up to 10 to 12 hours following ingestion.

Haemodialysis and haemoperfusion have been used successfully.

Naloxone has been successfully used in a few isolated cases, sometimes in association with activated charcoal given orally. Deaths have occurred following massive overdose; nevertheless, a favourable outcome is usual.

5. PHARMACOLOGICAL PROPERTIES

5.1 Pharmacodynamic properties

Valproic acid is an anticonvulsant.

The most likely mode of action for valproate is potentiation of the inhibitory action of gamma amino butyric acid (GABA) through an action on the further synthesis or further metabolism of GABA.

In certain in-vitro studies it was reported that sodium valproate could stimulate HIV replication but studies on peripheral blood mononuclear cells from HIV-infected subjects show that sodium valproate does not have a mitogen-like effect on inducing HIV replication. Indeed the effect of sodium valproate on HIV replication ex-vivo is highly variable, modest in quantity, appears to be unrelated to the dose and has not been documented in man.

5.2 Pharmacokinetic properties

The half-life of valproate is usually reported to be within the range of 8-20 hours. It is usually shorter in children.

In patients with severe renal insufficiency it may be necessary to alter dosage in accordance with free plasma valproic acid levels.

The reported effective therapeutic range for plasma valproic acid levels is 40-100mg/litre (278-694 micromol/litre). This reported range may depend on time of sampling and presence of co-medication. The percentage of free (unbound) drug is usually between 6% and 15% of total plasma levels. An increased incidence of adverse effects may occur with plasma levels above the effective therapeutic range.

The pharmacological (or therapeutic) effects of Convulex may not be clearly correlated with the total or free (unbound) plasma valproic acid levels.

5.3 Preclinical safety data

There are no pre-clinical data of relevance to the prescriber which are additional to those already stated in other sections of the SPC.

6. PHARMACEUTICAL PARTICULARS

6.1 List of excipients

Fractionated Coconut Oil

Gelatine

Glycerol 85 %

Dry substance of Karion 83 (70 %)

Sodium ethyl hydroxybenzoate

Sodium propyl hydroxybenzoate

Titanium dioxide

Cochineal red A 62.5 % (E 124)

Sunset yellow S 92 % (E 110)

Hydroxypropylmethylcellulose phthalate

Dibutylphthalate BP 1963

6.2 Incompatibilities

None.

6.3 Shelf life

60 months

6.4 Special precautions for storage

Do not store above 25°C. Protect from light.

6.5 Nature and contents of container

Blister packs:

Upper: PVC-foil

Lower: aluminium foil

Outer box:

carton folding box

Pack size: 100

6.6 Instructions for use and handling

Not applicable.

7. MARKETING AUTHORISATION HOLDER

Gerot Pharmazeutika GmbH

Arnethgasse 3

A – 1160 Vienna

Austria

8. MARKETING AUTHORISATION NUMBER(S)

PL 08298/0002

9. DATE OF FIRST AUTHORISATION/RENEWAL OF THE AUTHORISATION

11 October 1991 / 13 October 1998 / 2 July 2004

10. DATE OF REVISION OF THE TEXT

November 2004

Legal Status

POM

Convulex 500 mg Capsules

(Pharmacia Limited)

1. NAME OF THE MEDICINAL PRODUCT

Convulex 500 mg Capsules

2. QUALITATIVE AND QUANTITATIVE COMPOSITION

Valproic Acid 500.00 mg

3. PHARMACEUTICAL FORM

Enteric-coated soft gelatine capsules

4. CLINICAL PARTICULARS

4.1 Therapeutic indications

Treatment of generalised, partial or other epilepsy.

4.2 Posology and method of administration

Convulex capsules are for oral administration.

Daily dosage requirements vary according to age and body weight.

Convulex capsules may be given twice daily.

The capsules should be swallowed and not crushed or chewed.

Monotherapy:

Usual requirements are as follows:

a) Adults

Dosage should start at 600 mg daily, followed by gradual increases (approx. 300 mg) at three day intervals until control is achieved. This is generally within the dosage range 1000 mg to 2000 mg per day, i.e. 20-30 mg/kg body weight. Where adequate control is not achieved within this range, the dose may be further increased up to 2500 mg per day. For dosage adjustment, Convulex capsules 150 mg and 300 mg are also available.

b) Elderly Patients

Although the pharmacokinetics of valproate are modified in the elderly, they have limited clinical significance and dosage should be determined by seizure control. The volume of distribution is increased in the elderly and because of decreased binding to serum albumin, the proportion of free drug is increased. This will affect the clinical interpretation of plasma valproic acid levels.

c) Children

Children over 20kg

Initial dosage is usually not more than 400mg/day (irrespective of weight) with spaced increases until control is achieved; this is usually within the range 20-30mg/kg body weight per day. Where adequate control is not achieved within this range the dose may be increased to 35mg/kg body weight per day.

Children under 20kg

20mg/kg of body weight per day; in severe cases this may be increased but only in patients in whom plasma valproic acid levels can be monitored. Above 40mg/kg/day, clinical chemistry and haematological parameters should be monitored.

Splitting the total daily dose into 2-4 intakes is generally recommended.

d) In patients with renal insufficiency

It may be necessary to decrease dosage. Dosage should be adjusted according to clinical monitoring since monitoring of plasma concentrations may be misleading (see section 5.2 Pharmacokinetic Properties).

e) In patients with hepatic insufficiency

Salicylates should not be used concomitantly with valproate since they employ the same metabolic pathway (see also sections 4.4 Special Warnings and Precautions for Use and 4.8 Undesirable Effects).

Liver dysfunction, including hepatic failure resulting in fatalities, has occurred in patients whose treatment included valproic acid (see sections 4.3 Contraindications and 4.4 Special Warnings and Precautions for Use).

Salicylates should not be used in children under 16 years (see aspirin/salicylate product information on Reye's syndrome). In addition in conjunction with Convulex, concomitant use in children under 3 years can increase the risk of liver toxicity (see section 4.4.1 Special warnings).

Substitution:

A one to one dose relationship of Convulex and products containing sodium valproate has been demonstrated in pharmacokinetic trials. In patients previously receiving sodium valproate therapy, Convulex should be initiated at the same total daily dose.

Combined therapy:

When starting Convulex in patients already on other anticonvulsants, these should be tapered slowly; initiation of Convulex therapy should then be gradual, with target dose being reached after about 2 weeks. In certain cases it may be necessary to raise the dose by 5 to 10mg/kg/day when used in combination with anticonvulsants which induce liver enzyme activity, e.g. phenytoin, phenobarbitone and carbamazepine. Once known enzyme inducers have been withdrawn it may be possible to maintain seizure control on a reduced dose of Convulex. When barbiturates are being administered concomitantly and particularly if sedation is observed (particularly in children) the dosage of barbiturate should be reduced.

NB: In children requiring doses higher than 40mg/kg/day clinical chemistry and haematological parameters should be monitored.

Optimum dosage is mainly determined by seizure control and routine measurement of plasma levels is unnecessary. However, a method for measurement of plasma levels is available and may be helpful where there is poor control or side effects are suspected (see section 5.2 Pharmacokinetic Properties).

4.3 Contraindications

- Active liver disease
- Personal or family history of severe hepatic dysfunction, especially drug related
- Hypersensitivity to valproic acid
- Porphyria

4.4 Special warnings and special precautions for use

4.4.1 Special warnings

Liver dysfunction:

Conditions of occurrence:

Severe liver damage, including hepatic failure sometimes resulting in fatalities, has been very rarely reported. Experience in epilepsy has indicated that patients most at risk, especially in cases of multiple anticonvulsant therapy, are infants and in particular young children under the age of 3 and those with severe seizure disorders, organic brain disease, and (or) congenital metabolic or degenerative disease associated with mental retardation.

After the age of 3, the incidence of occurrence is significantly reduced and progressively decreases with age.

The concomitant use of salicylates should be avoided in children under 3 due to the risk of liver toxicity. Additionally, salicylates should not be used in children under 16 years (see aspirin/salicylate product information on Reye's syndrome).

Monotherapy is recommended in children under the age of 3 years when prescribing Convulex, but the potential benefit of Convulex should be weighed against the risk of liver damage or pancreatitis in such patients prior to initiation of therapy

In most cases, such liver damage occurred during the first 6 months of therapy, the period of maximum risk being 2-12 weeks.

Suggestive signs:

Clinical symptoms are essential for early diagnosis. In particular the following conditions, which may precede jaundice, should be taken into consideration, especially in patients at risk (see above: 'Conditions of occurrence'):

- non specific symptoms, usually of sudden onset, such as asthenia, malaise, anorexia, lethargy, oedema and drowsiness, which are sometimes associated with repeated vomiting and abdominal pain.
- in patients with epilepsy, recurrence of seizures.

These are an indication for immediate withdrawal of the drug.

Patients (or their family for children) should be instructed to report immediately any such signs to a physician should they occur. Investigations including clinical examination and biological assessment of liver function should be undertaken immediately.

Detection:

Liver function should be measured before and then periodically monitored during the first 6 months of therapy, especially in those who seem most at risk, and those with a prior history of liver disease.

Amongst usual investigations, tests which reflect protein synthesis, particularly prothrombin rate, are most relevant.

Confirmation of an abnormally low prothrombin rate, particularly in association with other biological abnormalities (significant decrease in fibrinogen and coagulation factors; increased bilirubin level and raised transaminases) requires cessation of Convulex therapy.

As a matter of precaution and in case they are taken concomitantly salicylates should also be discontinued since they employ the same metabolic pathway.

As with most antiepileptic drugs, increased liver enzymes are common, particularly at the beginning of therapy; they are also transient.

More extensive biological investigations (including prothrombin rate) are recommended in these patients; a reduction in dosage may be considered when appropriate and tests should be repeated as necessary.

Pancreatitis: Pancreatitis, which may be severe and result in fatalities, has been very rarely reported. Patients experiencing nausea, vomiting or acute abdominal pain should have a prompt medical evaluation (including measurement of serum amylase). Young children are at particular risk; this risk decreases with increasing age. Severe seizures and severe neurological impairment with combination anticonvulsant therapy may be risk factors. Hepatic failure with pancreatitis increases the risk of fatal outcome. In case of pancreatitis, valproate should be discontinued.

4.4.2 Precautions

Haematological: Blood tests (blood cell count, including platelet count, bleeding time and coagulation tests) are recommended prior to initiation of therapy or before surgery, and in case of spontaneous bruising or bleeding (see section 4.8 Undesirable Effects). Renal insufficiency: In patients with renal insufficiency, it may be necessary to decrease dosage. As monitoring of plasma concentrations may be misleading, dosage should be adjusted according to clinical monitoring (see sections 4.2 Posology and Method of Administration and 5.2. Pharmacokinetic Properties).

Systemic lupus erythematosus: Although immune disorders have only rarely been noted during the use of Convulex, the potential benefit of Convulex should be weighed against its potential risk in patients with systemic lupus erythematosus (see also section 4.8 Undesirable Effects).

Hyperammonaemia: When a urea cycle enzymatic deficiency is suspected, metabolic investigations should be performed prior to treatment because of the risk of hyperammonaemia with valproate.

Weight gain: Convulex very commonly causes weight gain, which may be marked and progressive. Patients should be warned of the risk of weight gain at the initiation of therapy and appropriate strategies should be adopted to minimise it (see section 4.8 Undesirable Effects).

Pregnancy: Women of childbearing potential should not be started on Convulex without specialist neurological advice. Convulex is the antiepileptic of choice in patients with certain types of epilepsy such as generalised epilepsy ± myoclonus/photosensitivity. For partial epilepsy, Convulex should be used only in patients resistant to other treatment. Women who are likely to get pregnant, should receive specialist advice because of the potential teratogenic risk to the foetus (see also section 4.6 Pregnancy and Lactation).

Diabetic patients: Valproate is eliminated mainly through the kidneys, partly in the form of ketone bodies; this may give false positives in the urine testing of possible diabetics.

4.5 Interaction with other medicinal products and other forms of Interaction

4.5.1 Effects of Valproate on other drugs

- Neuroleptics, MAO inhibitors, antidepressants and benzodiazepines

Valproate may potentiate the effect of other psychotropics such as neuroleptics, MAO inhibitors, antidepressants and benzodiazepines; therefore, clinical monitoring is advised and dosage should be adjusted when appropriate.

- Phenobarbital

Valproate increases phenobarbital plasma concentrations (due to inhibition of hepatic catabolism) and sedation may occur, particularly in children. Therefore, clinical monitoring is recommended throughout the first 15 days of combined treatment with immediate reduction of phenobarbital doses if sedation occurs and determination of phenobarbital plasma levels when appropriate.

- Primidone

Valproate increases primidone plasma levels with exacerbation of its adverse effects (such as sedation); these signs cease with long term treatment. Clinical monitoring is recommended especially at the beginning of combined therapy with dosage adjustment when appropriate.

- Phenytoin

Valproate decreases phenytoin total plasma concentration. Moreover valproate increases phenytoin free form with possible overdosage symptoms (valproic acid displaces phenytoin from its plasma protein binding sites and reduces its hepatic catabolism). Therefore clinical monitoring is recommended; when phenytoin plasma levels are determined, the free form should be evaluated.

- Carbamazepine

Clinical toxicity has been reported when valproate was administered with carbamazepine as valproate may potentiate toxic effects of carbamazepine. Clinical monitoring is recommended especially at the beginning of combined therapy with dosage adjustment when appropriate.

- Lamotrigine

Valproate may reduce lamotrigine metabolism and increase its mean half-life, dosages should be adjusted (lamotrigine dosage decreased) when appropriate. Co-administration of lamotrigine and Convulex might increase the risk of rash.

- Zidovudine

Valproate may raise zidovudine plasma concentration leading to increased zidovudine toxicity.

- Vitamin K-dependent anticoagulants

The anticoagulant effect of warfarin and other coumarin anticoagulants may be increased following displacement from plasma protein binding sites by valproic acid. The prothrombin time should be closely monitored.

- Temozolomide

Co-administration of temozolomide and valproate may cause a small decrease in the clearance of temozolomide that is not thought to be clinically relevant.

4.5.2 Effects of other drugs on Valproate

Antiepileptics with enzyme inducing effect (including *phenytoin, phenobarbital, carbamazepine*) decrease valproic acid plasma concentrations. Dosages should be adjusted according to blood levels in case of combined therapy.

On the other hand, combination of *felbamate* and valproate may increase valproic acid plasma concentration. Valproate dosage should be monitored.

Mefloquine and *chloroquine* increase valproic acid metabolism and may lower the seizure threshold; therefore epileptic seizures may occur in cases of combined therapy. Accordingly, the dosage of Convulex may need adjustment.

In case of concomitant use of valproate and *highly protein bound agents (e.g. aspirin)*, free valproic acid plasma levels may be increased.

Valproic acid plasma levels may be increased (as a result of reduced hepatic metabolism) in case of concomitant use with *cimetidine* or *erythromycin*.

Carbapenem antibiotics such as *imipenem* and *meropenem*: Decrease in valproic acid blood level, sometimes associated with convulsions, has been observed when imipenem or meropenem were combined. If these antibiotics have to be administered, close monitoring of valproic acid blood levels is recommended.

Cholestyramine may decrease the absorption of valproate.

4.5.3 Other Interactions

Caution is advised when using Convulex in combination with newer anti-epileptics whose pharmacodynamics may not be well established.

Valproate usually has no enzyme-inducing effect; as a consequence, valproate does not reduce efficacy of oestroprogestative agents in women receiving hormonal contraception, including the oral contraceptive pill.

4.6 Pregnancy and lactation

4.6.1. Pregnancy

From experience in treating mothers with epilepsy, the risk associated with the use of valproate during pregnancy has been described as follows:

- Risk associated with epilepsy and antiepileptics

In offspring born to mothers with epilepsy receiving anti-epileptic treatment, the overall rate of malformations has been demonstrated to be 2 to 3 times higher than the rate (approximately 3%) reported in the general population. Although an increased number of children with malformations have been reported in cases of multiple drug therapy, the respective role of treatments and disease in causing the malformations has not been formally established. Malformations most frequently encountered are cleft lip and cardio-vascular malformations.

Epidemiological studies have suggested an association between in-utero exposure to sodium valproate and a risk of developmental delay. Many factors including maternal epilepsy may also contribute to this risk but it is difficult to quantify the relative contribution of these or of maternal anti-epileptic treatment. Notwithstanding those potential risks, no sudden discontinuation in the anti-epileptic therapy should be undertaken as this may lead to breakthrough seizures which could have serious consequences for both the mother and the foetus.

- Risk associated with valproate

In animals: teratogenic effects have been demonstrated in the mouse, rat and rabbit.

There is animal experimental evidence that high plasma peak levels and the size of an individual dose are associated with neural tube defects.

In humans: an increased incidence of congenital abnormalities (including cases of facial dysmorphia, hypospadias and multiple malformations, particularly of the limbs) has been demonstrated in offspring born to mothers with epilepsy treated with valproate. Valproate use is associated with neural tube defects such as myelomeningocele and spina bifida. The frequency of this effect is estimated to be 1 to 2%.

- In view of the above data

When a woman is planning pregnancy, this provides an opportunity to review the need for anti-epileptic treatment. Women of childbearing age should be informed of the risks and benefits of continuing anti-epileptic treatment throughout pregnancy.

Folate supplementation **prior** to pregnancy, has been demonstrated to reduce the incidence of neural tube defects in the offspring of women at high risk. Although no direct evidence exists of such effects in women receiving anti-epileptic drugs, women should be advised to start taking folic acid supplementation (5 mg) as soon as contraception is discontinued.

The available evidence suggests that anticonvulsant monotherapy is preferred. Dosage should be reviewed before conception and the lowest effective dose used, in divided doses, as abnormal pregnancy outcome tends to be associated with higher total daily dosage and with the size of an individual dose. The incidence of neural tube defects rises with increasing dosage, particularly above 1000 mg daily. The administration in several divided doses over the day and the use of a prolonged release formulation is preferable in order to avoid high peak plasma levels.

During pregnancy, valproate anti-epileptic treatment should not be discontinued if it has been effective.

Nevertheless, specialised prenatal monitoring should be instituted in order to detect the possible occurrence of a neural tube defect or any other malformation. Pregnancies should be carefully screened by ultrasound, and other techniques if appropriate (see Section 4.4 Special Warnings and Special Precautions for Use).

- Risk in the neonate

Very rare cases of haemorrhagic syndrome have been reported in neonates whose mothers have taken valproate during pregnancy. This haemorrhagic syndrome is related to hypofibrinogenemia; afibrinogenemia has also been reported and may be fatal. These are possibly associated with a decrease of coagulation factors. However, this syndrome has to be distinguished from the decrease of the vitamin-K factors induced by phenobarbitone and other anti-epileptic enzyme inducing drugs.

Therefore, platelet count, fibrinogen plasma level, coagulation tests and coagulation factors should be investigated in neonates.

4.6.2. Lactation

Excretion of valproate in breast milk is low, with a concentration between 1% to 10% of total maternal serum levels; up to now children breast fed that have been monitored during the neonatal period have not experienced clinical effects. There appears to be no contra-indication to breast feeding by patients on valproate.

4.7 Effects on ability to drive and use machines

Use of Convulex may provide seizure control such that the patient may be eligible to hold a driving licence.

Patients should be warned of the risk of transient drowsiness, especially in cases of anticonvulsant polytherapy or association with benzodiazepines (see section 4.5 Interactions with Other Medicaments and Other Forms of Interaction).

4.8 Undesirable effects

Congenital and familial/genetic disorders: (see section 4.6 Pregnancy and Lactation)

Hepato-biliary disorders: rare cases of liver dysfunction (see section 4.4.1 Warnings)

Severe liver damage, including hepatic failure sometimes resulting in death, has been reported (see also sections 4.2, 4.3 and 4.4.1). Increased liver enzymes are common, particularly early in treatment, and may be transient (see section 4.4.1).

Gastrointestinal disorders (nausea, gastralgia, diarrhoea) frequently occur at the start of treatment. These problems can usually be overcome by taking Convulex capsules with or after food.

Very rare cases of pancreatitis, sometimes lethal, have been reported (see section 4.4 Special Warnings and Special Precautions for Use).

Nervous system disorders:

Sedation has been reported occasionally, usually when in combination with other anticonvulsants. In monotherapy it occurred early in treatment on rare occasions and is usually transient. Rare cases of lethargy and confusion occasionally progressing to stupor, sometimes with associated hallucinations or convulsions have been reported. Encephalopathy and coma have very rarely been observed. These cases have often been associated with too high a starting dose or too rapid a dose escalation or concomitant use of other anticonvulsants, notably phenobarbitone. They have usually been reversible on withdrawal of treatment or reduction of dosage.

Very rare cases of reversible extrapyramidal symptoms including parkinsonism, or reversible dementia associated with reversible cerebral atrophy have been reported. Dose-related ataxia and fine postural tremor have occasionally been reported.

An increase in alertness may occur; this is generally beneficial but occasionally aggression, hyperactivity and behavioural deterioration have been reported.

Metabolic disorders:

Cases of isolated and moderate hyperammonaemia without change in liver function tests may occur frequently, are usually transient and should not cause treatment discontinuation. However, they may present clinically as vomiting, ataxia, and increasing clouding of consciousness. Should these symptoms occur Convulex should be discontinued.

Hyperammonaemia associated with neurological symptoms has also been reported (see section 4.4.2 Precautions). In such cases further investigations should be considered.

Blood and lymphatic system disorders:

Frequent occurrence of thrombocytopenia, rare cases of anaemia, leucopenia or pancytopenia. The blood picture returned to normal when the drug was discontinued.

Isolated reduction of fibrinogen or reversible increase in bleeding time have been reported, usually without associated clinical signs and particularly with high doses (valproate has an inhibitory effect on the second phase of platelet aggregation). Spontaneous bruising or bleeding is an indication for withdrawal of medication pending investigations (see also section 4.6 Pregnancy and Lactation).

Skin and subcutaneous tissue disorders:

Cutaneous reactions such as exanthematous rash rarely occur with valproate. In very rare cases toxic epidermal necrolysis, Stevens-Johnson syndrome and erythema multiforme have been reported.

Transient hair loss, which may sometimes be dose-related, has often been reported. Regrowth normally begins within six months, although the hair may become more curly than previously. Hirsutism and acne have been very rarely reported.

Reproductive system and breast disorders:

Amenorrhoea and irregular periods have been reported. Very rarely gynaecomastia has occurred.

Vascular disorders: The occurrence of vasculitis has occasionally been reported.

Ear disorders:

Hearing loss, either reversible or irreversible has been reported rarely; however a cause and effect relationship has not been established.

Renal and urinary disorders:

There have been isolated reports of a reversible Fanconi's syndrome (a defect in proximal renal tubular function giving rise to glycosuria, amino aciduria, phosphaturia, and uricosuria) associated with valproate therapy, but the mode of action is as yet unclear.

Immune system disorders:

Allergic reactions (ranging from rash to hypersensitivity reactions) have been reported.

General disorders:

Very rare cases of non-severe peripheral oedema have been reported.

Increase in weight may also occur. Weight gain being a risk factor for polycystic ovary syndrome, it should be carefully monitored (see section 4.4 Special Warnings and Special Precautions for Use).

4.9 Overdose

Cases of accidental and deliberate valproate overdosage have been reported.

At plasma concentrations of up to 5-6 times the maximum therapeutic levels, there are unlikely to be any symptoms other than nausea, vomiting and dizziness.

Clinical signs of massive overdose, i.e. plasma concentration 10 to 20 times maximum therapeutic levels, usually include CNS depression or coma with muscular hypotonia, hyporeflexia, miosis, impaired respiratory function.

Symptoms may however be variable and seizures have been reported in the presence of very high plasma levels (see also section 5.2 Pharmacokinetic Properties). Cases of intracranial hypertension related to cerebral oedema have been reported.

Hospital management of overdose should be symptomatic, including cardio-respiratory monitoring. Gastric lavage may be useful up to 10 to 12 hours following ingestion.

Haemodialysis and haemoperfusion have been used successfully.

Naloxone has been successfully used in a few isolated cases, sometimes in association with activated charcoal given orally. Deaths have occurred following massive overdose; nevertheless, a favourable outcome is usual.

5. PHARMACOLOGICAL PROPERTIES

5.1 Pharmacodynamic properties

Valproic acid is an anticonvulsant.

The most likely mode of action for valproate is potentiation of the inhibitory action of gamma amino butyric acid (GABA) through an action on the further synthesis or further metabolism of GABA.

In certain in-vitro studies it was reported that sodium valproate could stimulate HIV replication but studies on peripheral blood mononuclear cells from HIV-infected subjects show that sodium valproate does not have a mitogen-like effect on inducing HIV replication. Indeed the effect of sodium valproate on HIV replication ex-vivo is highly variable, modest in quantity, appears to be unrelated to the dose and has not been documented in man.

5.2 Pharmacokinetic properties

The half-life of valproate is usually reported to be within the range of 8-20 hours. It is usually shorter in children.

In patients with severe renal insufficiency it may be necessary to alter dosage in accordance with free plasma valproic acid levels.

The reported effective therapeutic range for plasma valproic acid levels is 40-100mg/litre (278-694 micromol/litre). This reported range may depend on time of sampling and presence of co-medication. The percentage of free (unbound) drug is usually between 6% and 15% of total plasma levels. An increased incidence of adverse effects may occur with plasma levels above the effective therapeutic range.

The pharmacological (or therapeutic) effects of Convulex may not be clearly correlated with the total or free (unbound) plasma valproic acid levels.

5.3 Preclinical safety data

There are no pre-clinical data of relevance to the prescriber which are additional to those already stated in other sections of the SPC.

6. PHARMACEUTICAL PARTICULARS

6.1 List of excipients

Gelatine

Glycerol 85 %

Dry substance of Karion 83 (70 %)

Sodium ethyl hydroxybenzoate

Sodium propyl hydroxybenzoate

Titanium dioxide

Cochineal red A 62.5 % (E 124)

Sunset yellow S 92 % (E 110)

Hydroxypropylmethylcellulose phthalate

Dibutylphthalate BP 1963

6.2 Incompatibilities

None.

6.3 Shelf life

60 months

6.4 Special precautions for storage

Do not store above 25°C. Protect from light.

6.5 Nature and contents of container

Blister packs:

Upper: PVC-foil

Lower: aluminium foil

Outer box:

carton folding box

Pack size: 100

6.6 Instructions for use and handling

Not applicable.

7. MARKETING AUTHORISATION HOLDER

Gerot Pharmazeutika GmbH

Arnethgasse 3

A – 1160 Vienna

Austria

8. MARKETING AUTHORISATION NUMBER(S)

PL 08298/0003

9. DATE OF FIRST AUTHORISATION/RENEWAL OF THE AUTHORISATION

11 October 1991 / 16 October 1998 / 2 July 2004

10. DATE OF REVISION OF THE TEXT

November 2004

Legal Status

POM

Copegus 200mg

(Roche Products Limited)

1. NAME OF THE MEDICINAL PRODUCT

Copegus® 200 mg film-coated tablet

2. QUALITATIVE AND QUANTITATIVE COMPOSITION

Each film-coated tablet contains 200 milligrams of ribavirin.

For excipients, see section **6.1.**

3. PHARMACEUTICAL FORM

Film-coated tablet

Light pink, oval-shaped film-coated tablets (marked with RIB 200 on one side and ROCHE on the opposite side).

4. CLINICAL PARTICULARS

4.1 Therapeutic indications

Copegus is indicated for the treatment of chronic hepatitis C and must only be used as part of a combination regimen with peginterferon alfa-2a or with interferon alfa-2a. Copegus monotherapy must not be used.

The combination of Copegus with peginterferon alfa-2a or interferon alfa-2a is indicated in adult patients with elevated transaminases and who are positive for serum HCV-RNA, including patients with compensated cirrhosis (See section 4.4). The combination with peginterferon alfa-2a is also indicated in patients co-infected with clinically stable HIV, including patients with compensated cirrhosis (See section 4.3). The combination regimens are indicated in previously untreated patients as well as in patients who have previously responded to interferon alpha therapy and subsequently relapsed after treatment was stopped.

Please refer to the Summary of Product Characteristics (SPC) of peginterferon alfa-2a or interferon alfa-2a for prescribing information particular to either of these products.

4.2 Posology and method of administration

Treatment should be initiated, and monitored, by a physician experienced in the management of chronic hepatitis C.

Method of Administration

Copegus tablets are administered orally in two divided doses with food (morning and evening). The tablets should not be broken or crushed. Since ribavirin is considered a potential teratogen, caution should be observed in handling broken tablets.

Posology

Copegus is used in combination with peginterferon alfa-2a or interferon alfa-2a. The exact dose and duration of treatment depend on the interferon product used.

Please refer to the SPC of peginterferon alfa-2a or interferon alfa-2a for further information on dosage and duration of treatment when Copegus is to be used in combination with either of these products.

Posology in combination with peginterferon alfa-2a:

Dose to be administered

The recommended dose of Copegus in combination with peginterferon alfa-2a solution for injection depends on viral genotype and the patient's body weight (see Table 1).

Duration of treatment

The duration of combination therapy with peginterferon alfa-2a depends on viral genotype. Patients infected with HCV genotype 1 regardless of viral load should receive 48 weeks of therapy. Patients infected with HCV genotype 2/3 regardless of viral load should receive 24 weeks of therapy (see Table 1).

(see Table 1)

In general, patients infected with genotype 4 are considered hard to treat and limited study data (N=66) are compatible with a posology as for genotype 1. When deciding on the duration of therapy, the presence of additional factors should also be considered. For patients infected with genotype 5 or 6, this posology should also be considered.

HIV-HCV Co-infection

The recommended dosage for Copegus in combination with 180 micrograms once weekly of peginterferon alfa-2a is 800 milligrams, daily for 48 weeks, regardless of genotype. The safety and efficacy of combination therapy with ribavirin doses greater than 800 milligrams daily or a duration of therapy less than 48 weeks has not been studied.

Predictability of response and non-response

Early virological response by week 12, defined as a 2 log viral load decrease or undetectable levels of HCV RNA has been shown to be predictive for sustained response (see Table 2).

(see Table 2 on next page)

A similar negative predictive value has been observed in HIV-HCV co-infected patients treated with peginterferon alfa-2a monotherapy or in combination with ribavirin (100% (130/130) or 98% (83/85), respectively). Positive predictive values of 45% (50/110) and 70% (59/84) were observed for genotype 1 and genotype 2/3 HIV-HCV co-infected patients receiving combination therapy.

Posology in combination with interferon alfa-2a:

Dose to be administered

The recommended dose of Copegus in combination with interferon alfa-2a solution for injection depends on the patient's body weight (see Table 3).

Duration of treatment:

Patients should be treated with combination therapy with interferon alfa-2a for at least six months. Patients with HCV genotype 1 infections should receive 48 weeks of combination therapy. In patients infected with HCV of other genotypes, the decision to extend therapy to 48 weeks should be based on other prognostic factors (such as high viral load at baseline, male gender, age > 40 years and evidence of bridging fibrosis).

(see Table 3 on next page)

Dosage modification for adverse reactions

Please refer to the SPC of peginterferon alfa-2a or interferon alfa-2a for further information on dose adjustment and discontinuation of treatment for either of these products.

If severe adverse reactions or laboratory abnormalities develop during therapy with Copegus and peginterferon

Table 1 Copegus Dosing Recommendations in Combination with Peginterferon alfa-2a for HVC patients

Genotype	Daily Copegus Dose	Duration of treatment	Number of 200mg tablets
Genotype 1	<75 kg = 1,000 mg	48 weeks	5 (2 morning, 3 evening)
	≥75 kg = 1,200 mg	48 weeks	6 (3 morning, 3 evening)
Genotype 2/3	800 mg	24 weeks	4 (2 morning, 2 evening)

Table 2 Predictive Value of Week 12 Virological Response at the Recommended Dosing Regimen while receiving Copegus and peginterferon Combination Therapy

Genotype	Negative			Positive		
	No response by week 12	No sustained response	Predictive Value	Response by week 12	Sustained response	Predictive Value
Genotype 1 (N= 569)	102	97	**95%** (97/102)	467	271	**58%** (271/467)
Genotype 2 and 3 (N=96)	3	3	**100%** (3/3)	93	81	**87%** (81/93)

Table 3 Copegus Dosing Recommendations in Combination with Interferon alfa-2a

Patient weight (kg)	Daily Copegus dose	Duration of treatment	Number of 200 mg tablets
<75	1,000 mg	24 or 48 weeks	5 (2 morning, 3 evening)
≥75	1,200 mg	24 or 48 weeks	6 (3 morning, 3 evening)

alfa-2a or interferon alfa-2a, modify the dosages of each product, until the adverse reactions abate. Guidelines were developed in clinical trials for dose modification (see **Dosage Modification Guidelines for Management of Treatment-Emergent Anaemia**, Table 4).

If intolerance persists after dose adjustment, discontinuation of Copegus or both Copegus and peginterferon alfa-2a or interferon alfa-2a may be needed.

Table 4. Dosage Modification Guidelines for Management of Treatment-Emergent Anaemia

Laboratory Values	Reduce only Copegus dose to 600 mg/day* if:	Discontinue Copegus if:**
Haemoglobin in Patients with No Cardiac Disease	<10 g/dl	<8.5 g/dl
Haemoglobin: Patients with History of Stable Cardiac Disease	≥2 g/dl decrease in haemoglobin during any 4 week period during treatment (permanent dose reduction)	<12 g/dl despite 4 weeks at reduced dose

*Patients whose dose of Copegus is reduced to 600 mg daily receive one 200 mg tablet in the morning and two 200 mg tablets in the evening.

**If the abnormality is reversed, Copegus may be restarted at 600 mg daily, and further increased to 800 mg daily at the discretion of the treating physician. However, a return to higher doses is not recommended.

Special populations

Use in renal impairment: The recommended dose regimens (adjusted by the body weight cutoff of 75 kg) of ribavirin give rise to substantial increases in plasma concentrations of ribavirin in patients with renal impairment. There are insufficient data on the safety and efficacy of ribavirin in patients with serum creatinine > 2 mg/dl or creatinine clearance < 50 ml/min, whether or not on haemodialysis, to support recommendations for dose adjustments. Therefore, ribavirin should be used in such patients only when this is considered to be essential. Therapy should be initiated (or continued if renal impairment develops while on therapy) with extreme caution and intensive monitoring of haemoglobin concentrations, with corrective action as may be necessary, should be employed throughout the treatment period. (see **4.4 Special warnings and special precautions for use** and see **5.2 Pharmacokinetic properties**).

Use in hepatic impairment: No pharmacokinetic interaction appears between ribavirin and hepatic function (see **5.2 Pharmacokinetic properties**). Therefore, no dose adjustment of Copegus is required in patients with hepatic impairment. The use of peginterferon alfa-2a and interferon alfa-2a is contraindicated in patients with decompensated cirrhosis and other forms of severe hepatic impairment.

Use in elderly patients over the age of 65: There does not appear to be a significant age-related effect on the pharmacokinetics of ribavirin. However, as in younger patients, renal function must be determined prior to administration of Copegus.

Use in patients under the age of 18 years: Safety and effectiveness of ribavirin in combination with peginterferon alfa-2a and interferon alfa-2a in these patients have not been fully evaluated. Treatment with Copegus is not recommended for use in children and adolescents under the age of 18.

4.3 Contraindications

See peginterferon alfa-2a or interferon alfa-2a prescribing information for contraindications related to either of these products.

- hypersensitivity to ribavirin or to any of the excipients.

- pregnant women (see **4.4 Special warnings and special precautions for use**). Copegus must not be initiated until a report of a negative pregnancy test has been obtained immediately prior to initiation of therapy.

- women who are breast-feeding (see **4.6 Pregnancy and lactation**).

- a history of severe pre-existing cardiac disease, including unstable or uncontrolled cardiac disease, in the previous six months.

- severe hepatic dysfunction or decompensated cirrhosis of the liver.

- haemoglobinopathies (e.g. thalassaemia, sickle-cell anaemia).

- Initiation of peginterferon alfa-2a is contraindicated in HIV-HCV patients with cirrhosis and a Child-Pugh score ≥ 6 (Please refer to the SPC of peginterferon alfa-2a for Child-Pugh assessment).

4.4 Special warnings and special precautions for use

Please refer to the SPC of peginterferon alfa-2a or interferon alfa-2a for futher information on special warnings and precautions for use related to either of these products.

All patients in the chronic hepatitis C studies had a liver biopsy before inclusion, but in certain cases (ie, patients with genotype 2 or 3), treatment may be possible without histological confirmation. Current treatment guidelines should be consulted as to whether a liver biopsy is needed prior to commencing treatment.

In patients with normal ALT, progression of fibrosis occurs on average at a slower rate than in patients with elevated ALT. This should be considered in conjunction with other factors, such as HCV genotype, age, extrahepatic manifestations, risk of transmission, etc. which influence the decision to treat or not.

Based on results of clinical trials, the use of ribavirin as monotherapy is not effective and Copegus must not be used alone.

Teratogenic risk: See **4.6 Pregnancy and lactation.**

Prior to initiation of treatment with ribavirin the physician must comprehensively inform the patient of the teratogenic risk of ribavirin, the necessity of effective and continuous contraception, the possibility that contraceptive methods may fail and the possible consequences of pregnancy should it occur during treatment with ribavirin.

Carcinogenicity: Ribavirin is mutagenic in some *in vivo* and *in vitro* genotoxicity assays. A potential carcinogenic effect of ribavirin cannot be excluded (see **5.3 Preclinical safety data**).

Haemolysis and Cardiovascular system: A decrease in haemoglobin levels to <10 g/dl was observed in up to 15% of patients treated for 48 weeks with Copegus 1000/1200 milligrams in combination with peginterferon alfa-2a and up to 19% of patients in combination with interferon alfa-2a. When Copegus 800 milligram was combined with peginterferon alfa-2a for 24 weeks, 3% of patients had a decrease in haemoglobin levels to <10 g/dl. The risk of developing anaemia is higher in the female population. Although ribavirin has no direct cardiovascular effects, anaemia associated with Copegus may result in deterioration of cardiac function, or exacerbation of the symptoms of coronary disease, or both. Thus, Copegus must be administered with caution to patients with pre-existing cardiac disease. Cardiac status must be assessed before start of therapy and monitored clinically during therapy; if any deterioration occurs, stop therapy (see **4.2 Posology and method of administration**). Patients with a history of congestive heart failure, myocardial infarction, and/or previous or current arrhythmic disorders must be closely monitored. It is recommended that those patients who have pre-existing cardiac abnormalities have electrocardiograms taken prior to and during the course of treatment. Cardiac arrhythmias (primarily supraventricular) usually respond to conventional therapy but may require discontinuation of therapy.

Acute hypersensitivity: If an acute hypersensitivity reaction (e.g. urticaria, angioedema, bronchoconstriction, anaphylaxis) develops, Copegus must be discontinued immediately and appropriate medical therapy instituted. Transient rashes do not necessitate interruption of treatment.

Liver function: In patients who develop evidence of hepatic decompensation during treatment, Copegus in combination with peginterferon alfa-2a or interferon alfa-2a should be discontinued. When the increase in ALT levels is progressive and clinically significant, despite dose reduction, or is accompanied by increased direct bilirubin, therapy should be discontinued.

Psychiatric and Central Nervous System (CNS):

Patients with existence of history of severe psychiatric conditions:

If treatment with ribavirin and peginterferon alfa-2a or interferon alfa-2a is judged necessary in patients with existence or history of severe psychiatric conditions, this should be only initiated after having ensured appropriate individualised diagnostic and therapeutic management of the psychiatric condition.

Severe CNS effects, particularly depression, suicidal ideation and suicide have been observed in some patients during Copegus combination therapy with peginterferon alfa-2a or interferon alfa-2a. Other CNS effects including aggressive behaviour, confusion and alterations of mental status have been observed with interferon alfa-2a. If patients develop psychiatric or CNS problems, including clinical depression, it is recommended that patients be carefully monitored by the prescribing physician. If such symptoms appear, the potential seriousness of these undesirable effects must be borne in mind by the prescribing physician. If symptoms persist or worsen, discontinue both Copegus and peginterferon alfa-2a or interferon alfa-2a.

Renal impairment: The pharmacokinetics of ribavirin are altered in patients with renal dysfunction due to reduction of apparent clearance in these patients (see **5.2 Pharmacokinetic properties**). Therefore, it is recommended that renal function be evaluated in all patients prior to initiation of Copegus, preferably by estimating the patient's creatinine clearance. Substantial increases in ribavirin plasma concentrations are seen at the recommended dosing regimen in patients with serum creatinine >2 mg/dl or with creatinine clearance <50 ml/minute. There are insufficient data on the safety and efficacy of Copegus in such patients to support recommendations for dose adjustments. Copegus therapy should not be initiated (or continued if renal impairment occurs while on treatment) in such patients, whether or not on haemodialysis, unless it is considered to be essential. Extreme caution is required. Haemoglobin concentrations should be monitored intensively during treatment and corrective action taken as necessary (see 4.2. **Posology and method of administration** and see **5.2 Pharmacokinetic properties**).

HIV/HCV Co-infection: Please refer to the respective Summary of Product Characteristics of the antiretroviral medicinal products that are to be taken concurrently with HCV therapy for awareness and management of toxicities specific for each product and the potential for overlapping toxicities with peginterferon alfa-2a with or without ribavirin. In study NR15961, patients concurrently treated with stavudine and interferon therapy with or without ribavirin, the incidence of pancreatitis and/or lactic acidosis was 3% (12/398).

Chronic hepatitis C patients co-infected with HIV and receiving Highly Active Anti-Retroviral Therapy (HAART) may be at increased risk of serious adverse effects (e.g. lactic acidosis; peripheral neuropathy; pancreatitis).

Co-infected patients with advanced cirrhosis receiving HAART may also be at increased risk of hepatic decompensation and possibly death if treated with Copegus in combination with interferons. Baseline variables in co-infected cirrhotic patients that may be associated with hepatic decompensation include: increased serum bilirubin, decreased haemoglobin, increased alkaline phosphatase or decreased platelet count, and treatment with didanosine (ddI). Caution should therefore be exercised when adding peginterferon alfa-2a and Copegus to HAART therapy. (see **4.5 Interaction with other medicinal products and other forms of interaction).**

Co-infected patients should be closely monitored, assessing their Child-Pugh score during treatment, and should be immediately discontinued if they progress to a Child-Pugh score of 7 or greater.

Laboratory tests: Standard haematologic tests and blood chemistries (complete blood count [CBC] and differential, platelet count, electrolytes, serum creatinine, liver function tests, uric acid) must be conducted in all patients prior to initiating therapy. Acceptable baseline values that may be considered as a guideline prior to initiation of Copegus in combination with peginterferon alfa-2a or interferon alfa-2a:

Haemoglobin	⩾12 g/dl (females); ⩾13 g/dl (males)
Platelets	⩾ 90,000/mm³
Neutrophil Count	⩾1,500/mm³

In patients co-infected with HIV-HCV, limited efficacy and safety data (N=51) are available in subjects with CD4 counts less than 200 cells/μL. Caution is therefore warranted in the treatment of patients with low CD4 counts.

Laboratory evaluations are to be conducted at weeks 2 and 4 of therapy, and periodically thereafter as clinically appropriate.

For women of childbearing potential: Female patients must have a routine pregnancy test performed monthly during treatment and for 6 months thereafter. Female partners of male patients must have a routine pregnancy test performed monthly during treatment and for 6 months thereafter.

Uric acid may increase with Copegus due to haemolysis and therefore the potential for development of gout must be carefully monitored in predisposed patients.

4.5 Interaction with other medicinal products and other forms of Interaction

Interaction studies have been conducted with ribavirin in combination with peginterferon alfa-2a, interferon alfa-2b and antacids. Ribavirin concentrations are similar when given alone or concomitantly with interferon alfa-2b or peginterferon alfa-2a.

Any potential for interactions may persist for up to 2 months (5 half lives for ribavirin) after cessation of Copegus therapy due to the long half-life.

Results of *in vitro* studies using both human and rat liver microsome preparations indicated no cytochrome P450 enzyme mediated metabolism of ribavirin. Ribavirin does not inhibit cytochrome P450 enzymes. There is no evidence from toxicity studies that ribavirin induces liver enzymes. Therefore, there is a minimal potential for P450 enzyme-based interactions.

Antacid: The bioavailability of ribavirin 600 milligrams was decreased by co-administration with an antacid containing magnesium, aluminium and methicone; AUC_{tf} decreased 14%. It is possible that the decreased bioavailability in this study was due to delayed transit of ribavirin or modified pH. This interaction is not considered to be clinically relevant.

Nucleoside analogs: Ribavirin was shown *in vitro* to inhibit phosphorylation of zidovudine and stavudine. The clinical significance of these findings is unknown. However, these *in vitro* findings raise the possibility that concurrent use of Copegus with either zidovudine or stavudine might lead to increased HIV plasma viraemia. Therefore, it is recommended that plasma HIV RNA levels be closely monitored in patients treated with Copegus concurrently with either of these two agents. If HIV RNA levels increase, the use of Copegus concomitantly with reverse transcriptase inhibitors must be reviewed.

Didanosine (ddI): Ribavirin potentiated the antiretroviral effect of didanosine (ddI) *in vitro* and in animals by increasing the formation of the active triphosphate anabolite (ddATP). This observation also raised the possibility that concomitant administration of ribavirin and ddI might increase the risk of adverse reactions related to ddI (such as peripheral neuropathy, pancreatitis, and hepatic steatosis with lactic acidosis). While the clinical significance of these findings is unknown, one study of concomitant ribavirin and ddI in patients with HIV disease did not result in further reductions in viraemia or an increase in adverse reactions. Plasma pharmacokinetics of ddI were not significantly affected by concomitant ribavirin in this study, although intracellular ddATP was not measured.

HIV-HCV co-infected patients

No apparent evidence of drug interaction was observed in 47 HIV-HCV co-infected patients who completed a 12 week pharmacokinetic substudy to examine the effect of ribavirin on the intracellular phosphorylation of some nucleoside reverse transcriptase inhibitors (lamivudine and zidovudine or stavudine). However, due to high variability, the confidence intervals were quite wide Plasma exposure of ribavirin did not appear to be affected by concomitant administration of nucleoside reverse transcriptase inhibitors (NRTIs).

Co-administration of ribavirin and didanosine is not recommended. Exposure to didanosine or its active metabolite (dideoxyadenosine 5'-triphosphate) is increased *in vitro* when didanosine is co-administered with ribavirin. Reports of fatal hepatic failure as wells as peripheral neuropathy, pancreatitis, and symptomatic hyperlactataemia/lactic acidosis have been reported with use of ribavirin.

4.6 Pregnancy and lactation

Preclinical data: Significant teratogenic and/or embryocidal potential have been demonstrated for ribavirin in all animal species in which adequate studies have been conducted, occurring at doses well below the recommended human dose. Malformations of the skull, palate, eye, jaw, limbs, skeleton and gastrointestinal tract were noted. The incidence and severity of teratogenic effects increased with escalation of the ribavirin dose. Survival of foetuses and offspring was reduced.

Female patients: Copegus must not be used by women who are pregnant (see **4.3 Contraindications** and see **4.4 Special warnings and special precautions for use**). Extreme care must be taken to avoid pregnancy in female patients. Copegus therapy must not be initiated until a report of a negative pregnancy test has been obtained immediately prior to initiation of therapy. Any birth control method can fail. Therefore, it is critically important that women of childbearing potential and their partners must use 2 forms of effective contraception simultaneously, during treatment and for 6 months after treatment has been concluded; routine monthly pregnancy tests must be performed during this time. If pregnancy does occur during treatment or within 6 months from stopping treatment the patient must be advised of the significant teratogenic risk of ribavirin to the foetus.

Male patients and their female partners: Extreme care must be taken to avoid pregnancy in partners of male patients taking Copegus. Ribavirin accumulates intracellularly and is cleared from the body very slowly. In animal studies, ribavirin produced changes in sperm at doses below the clinical dose. It is unknown whether the ribavirin that is contained in sperm will exert its known teratogenic effects upon fertilisation of the ova. Male patients and their female partners of childbearing age must, therefore, be counselled to use 2 forms of effective contraception simultaneously during treatment with Copegus and for 6 months after treatment has been concluded. Women must have a negative pregnancy test before therapy is started. Men whose partners are pregnant must be instructed to use a condom to minimise delivery of ribavirin to the partner.

Lactation: It is not known whether ribavirin is excreted in human milk. Because of the potential for adverse reactions in nursing infants, nursing must be discontinued prior to initiation of treatment.

4.7 Effects on ability to drive and use machines

Copegus has no or negligible influence; however, peginterferon alfa-2a or interferon alfa-2a used in combination may have an effect. Thus, patients who develop fatigue, somnolence, or confusion during treatment must be cautioned to avoid driving or operating machinery.

4.8 Undesirable effects

See peginterferon alfa-2a or interferon alfa-2a prescribing information for additional undesirable effects for either of these products.

The most frequently reported adverse reactions with Copegus in combination with peginterferon alfa-2a 180 micrograms were mostly mild to moderate in severity and were manageable without the need for modification of doses or discontinuation of therapy.

HIV-HCV co-infected patients

In HIV-HCV co-infected patients, the clinical adverse event profiles reported for peginterferon alfa-2a, alone or in combination with ribavirin, were similar to those observed in HCV mono-infected patients. Peginterferon alfa-2a treatment was associated with decreases in absolute CD4+ cell counts within the first 4 weeks without a reduction in CD4+ cell percentage. The decrease in CD4+ cell counts was reversible upon dose reduction or cessation of therapy. The use of peginterferon alfa-2a had no observable negative impact on the control of HIV viraemia during therapy or follow-up. Limited safety data (N = 31) are available in co-infected patients with CD4+ cell counts < 200/μl. (see peginterferon alfa-2a SPC).

Table 5 summarises the safety overview of different treatment regimens of Copegus in combination with peginterferon alfa-2a for HCV and HIV-HCV patients.

(see Table 5 below)

Table 6 shows the most common undesirable effects reported in ⩾ 10% of patients who have received Copegus and peginterferon alfa-2a or interferon alfa-2a therapy.

Adverse events reported in patients receiving Copegus in combination with interferon alfa-2a are essentially the same as for those reported for Copegus in combination with peginterferon alfa-2a.

(see Table 6 on next page)

Undesirable effects reported in <10% patients on Copegus in combination with peginterferon alfa-2a or Copegus in combination with interferon alfa-2a are reported in table 7.

(see Table 7 on page 578)

Very rarely, alpha interferons including peginterferon alfa-2a, used in combination with Copegus, may be associated with pancytopenia including aplastic anaemia.

For HIV-HCV patients receiving Copegus and peginterferon alfa-2a combination therapy, other undesirable effects have been reported in ⩾ 1% to ⩽ 2% of patients: hyperlactacidaemia/lactic acidosis, influenza, pneumonia, affect lability, apathy, tinnitus, pharyngolaryngeal pain, cheilitis, acquired lipodystrophy and chromaturia.

Laboratory values: In clinical trials of Copegus in combination with peginterferon alfa-2a or interferon alfa-2a, the majority of cases of abnormal laboratory values were managed with dose modifications (see **4.2 Posology and method of administration, Dosage Modification Guidelines**). With peginterferon alfa-2a and Copegus combination treatment, up to 2% of patients experienced increased ALT levels that led to dose modification or discontinuation of treatment.

Haemolysis is the defining toxicity of ribavirin therapy. A decrease in haemoglobin levels to <10 g/dl was observed in up to 15% of patients treated for 48 weeks with Copegus 1000/1200 milligrams in combination with peginterferon alfa-2a and up to 19% of patients in combination with interferon alfa-2a. When Copegus 800 milligram was combined with peginterferon alfa-2a for 24 weeks, 3% of patients had a decrease in haemoglobin levels to <10 g/dl. It is not expected that patients will need to discontinue therapy because of decrease in haemoglobin levels alone. In most cases the decrease in haemoglobin occurred early in the treatment period and stabilised concurrently with a compensatory increase in reticulocytes.

Most cases of anaemia, leukopenia and thrombocytopenia were mild (WHO grade 1). WHO grade 2 laboratory changes was reported for haemoglobin (4% of patients), leucocytes (24% of patients) and thrombocytes (2% of patients). Moderate (absolute neutrophil count (ANC): 0.749-0.5x109/L) and severe (ANC: <0.5x109/L) neutropenia was observed in 24% (216/887) and 5% (41/887) of patients receiving 48 weeks of Copegus 1000/1200 milligrams in combination with peginterferon alfa-2a.

An increase in uric acid and indirect bilirubin values associated with haemolysis were observed in some patients treated with Copegus used in combination with peginterferon alfa-2a or interferon alfa-2a and values returned to baseline levels within 4 weeks after the end of therapy. In rare cases (2/755) this was associated with clinical manifestation (acute gout).

Laboratory values for HIV-HCV co-infected patients

Although haematological toxicities of neutropenia, thrombocytopenia and anaemia occurred more frequently in HIV-HCV patients, the majority could be managed by dose modification and the use of growth factors and infrequently required premature discontinuation of treatment. Decrease in ANC levels below 500 cells/mm³ was observed in 13% and 11% of patients receiving peginterferon alfa-2a monotherapy and combination therapy, respectively. Decrease in platelets below 50,000/mm³ was observed in 10% and 8% of patients receiving peginterferon alfa-2a monotherapy and combination therapy respectively. Anaemia (haemoglobin < 10g/dL) was reported in 7% and 14% of patients treated with peginterferon alfa-2a monotherapy or in combination therapy, respectively.

4.9 Overdose

No cases of overdose of Copegus have been reported in clinical trials. Hypocalcaemia and hypomagnesaemia have been observed in persons administered dosages greater than four times the maximal recommended dosages. In many of these instances ribavirin was administered intra-

Table 5 Safety Overview of Copegus Treatment Regimens in Combination with Pegintefer on alfa-2a for HCV and HIV-HCV patients

	HCV mono-infection Copegus 800 mg 24 weeks & PEG-IFN alfa-2a 180 mcg	HCV mono-infection Copegus 1000/1200 mg 48 weeks & PEG-IFN alfa-2a 180 mcg	HIV-HCV co-Infection Copegus 800 mg 48 weeks & PEG-INF alfa-2a 180 mcg
Serious adverse events	3%	11%	17%
Anaemia (haemoglobin < 10g/dl)	3%	15%	14%
Ribavirin dose modification	19%	39%	37%
Premature withdrawals due to adverse events	4%	10%	12%
Premature withdrawals due to laboratory abnormalities	1%	3%	3%

Table 6 Adverse Reactions (⩾ 10 % Incidence in Any Treatment Group) for HCV and HIV-HCV patients

	HCV Copegus 800 mg & Peginterferon alfa-2a 180 micrograms (NV15942) 24 weeks N=207	**HCV** Copegus 1,000 or 1,200 mg & Peginterferon alfa-2a 180 micrograms (NV15801 + NV15942) 48 weeks N=887	**HIV-HCV** Copegus 800 mg & Peginterferon Alfa-2a 180 micrograms (NR15961) 48 weeks N=288
Body System	%	%	%
Metabolism & Nutrition disorders			
Anorexia	20 %	27 %	23%
Weight Decrease	2%	7%	16%
Psychiatric Disorders			
Insomnia	30 %	32 %	19%
Irritability	28 %	24 %	15%
Depression	17 %	21 %	22%
Concentration Impairment	8 %	10 %	2%
Nervous system disorders			
Headache	48 %	47 %	35%
Dizziness	13 %	15 %	7%
Respiratory, thoracic and mediastinal disorders			
Dyspnoea	11 %	13 %	7%
Cough	8 %	13 %	3%
Gastrointestinal Disorders			
Nausea	29 %	28 %	24%
Diarrhoea	15 %	14 %	16%
Abdominal Pain	9 %	10 %	7%
Skin and subcutaneous tissue disorders			
Alopecia	25 %	24 %	10%
Pruritus	25 %	21 %	5%
Dermatitis	15 %	16 %	1%
Dry skin	13 %	12 %	4%
Musculoskeletal, connective tissue and bone disorders			
Myalgia	42 %	38 %	32%
Arthralgia	20 %	22 %	16%
General disorders and administration site conditions			
Fatigue	45 %	49 %	40%
Pyrexia	37 %	39 %	41%
Rigors	30 %	25 %	16%
Asthenia	18 %	15 %	26%
Pain	9 %	10 %	6%
Injection Site Reaction	28 %	21 %	10%

venously. Ribavirin is not effectively removed by haemodialysis.

5. PHARMACOLOGICAL PROPERTIES

5.1 Pharmacodynamic properties

Pharmacotherapeutic group: Direct acting antivirals, nucleosides and nucleotides (excl. reverse transcriptase inhibitors), ATC code: J05A B04.

Mechanism of Action: Ribavirin is a synthetic nucleoside analog that shows *in vitro* activity against some RNA and DNA viruses. The mechanism by which ribavirin in combination with peginterferon alfa-2a or interferon alfa-2a exerts its effects against HCV is unknown.

HCV RNA levels decline in a biphasic manner in responding patients with hepatitis C who have received treatment with 180 micrograms peginterferon alfa-2a. The first phase of decline occurs 24 to 36 hours after the first dose of peginterferon alfa-2a and is followed by the second phase of decline which continues over the next 4 to 16 weeks in patients who achieve a sustained response. Copegus had no significant effect on the initial viral kinetics over the first 4 to 6 weeks in patients treated with the combination of Copegus and pegylated interferon alfa-2a or interferon alfa.

Oral formulations of ribavirin monotherapy have been investigated as therapy for chronic hepatitis C in several clinical trials. Results of these investigations showed that ribavirin monotherapy had no effect on eliminating hepatitis virus (HCV-RNA) or improving hepatic histology after 6 to 12 months of therapy and 6 months of follow-up.

Clinical Trial Results

Copegus in combination with peginterferon alfa-2a

Predictability of response

Please refer to section **4.2 Posology and method of administration**, in Table 2.

Study results

Efficacy and safety of the combination of Copegus and peginterferon alfa-2a were established in two pivotal studies (NV15801 + NV15942), including a total of 2405 patients. The study population comprised interferon-naïve patients with CHC confirmed by detectable levels of serum HCV RNA, elevated levels of ALT, and a liver biopsy consistent with chronic hepatitis C infection. Only HIV-HCV co-infected patients were included in the study NR15961 (see Table 10). These patients had stable HIV disease and mean CD4 T-cell count was about 500 cells/μl.

Study NV15801 (1121 patients treated) compared the efficacy of 48 weeks of treatment with peginterferon alfa-2a (180 mcg once weekly) and Copegus (1000/1200 mg daily) with either peginterferon alfa-2a monotherapy or combination therapy with interferon-alfa-2b and ribavirin. The combination of peginterferon alfa-2a and Copegus was significantly more efficacious than either the combination of interferon alfa-2b and ribavirin or peginterferon alfa-2a monotherapy.

Study NV15942 (1284 patients treated) compared the efficacy of two durations of treatment (24 weeks with 48 weeks) and two dosages of Copegus (800 mg with 1000/1200 mg).

For HCV monoinfected patients and HIV-HCV co-infected patients, for treatment regimens, duration of therapy and study outcome see tables 8, 9 and 10, respectively. Virological response was defined as undetectable HCV RNA as measured by the COBAS AMPLICOR™ HCV Test, version 2.0 (limit of detection 100 copies/ml equivalent to 50 International Units/ml) and sustained response as one negative sample approximately 6 months after the end of therapy.

(see Table 8 on page 579)

The virological responses of patients treated with Copegus and peginterferon alfa-2a combination therapy in relation to genotype and viral load are summarised in table 9 for HCV monoinfected patients and 10 for HIV-HCV co-infected patients respectively. The results of study NV15942 provide the rationale for recommending treatment regimens based on genotype (see table 1).

The difference between treatment regimens was in general not influenced by viral load or presence/absence of cirrhosis; therefore treatment recommendations for genotype 1, 2 or 3 are independent of these baseline characteristics.

(see Table 9 on page 579)

HCV patients with normal ALT

In study NR16071, HCV patients with normal ALT values were randomised to receive peginterferon alfa-2a 180 micrograms/week with a Copegus dose of 800 milligrams/day for either 24 or 48 weeks followed by a 24 week treatment free follow-up period or an untreated control group for 72 weeks. The SVRs reported in the treatment arms or this study were similar to the corresponding treatment arms from study NV15942.

HIV-HCV co-infected patients

(see Table 10 on page 579)

Ribavirin in combination with interferon alfa-2a

The therapeutic efficacy of interferon alfa-2a alone and in combination with oral ribavirin was compared in clinical trials in naïve (previously untreated) and relapsed patients who had virologically, biochemically and histologically documented chronic hepatitis C. Six months after end of treatment sustained biochemical and virological response as well as histological improvement were assessed.

A statistically significant 10-fold increase (from 4% to 43%; $p < 0.01$) in sustained virological and biochemical response was observed in relapsed patients (M23136; N=99). The favourable profile of the combination therapy was also reflected in the response rates relative to HCV genotype or baseline viral load. In the combination and interferon monotherapy arms, respectively, the sustained response rates in patients with HCV genotype-1 were 28% versus 0% and with genotype non-1 were 58% versus 8%. In addition the histological improvement favoured the combination therapy. Supportive favourable results (monotherapy vs combination; 6% vs 48%, $p<0.04$) from a small published study in naïve patients (N=40) were reported using interferon alfa-2a (3 MIU 3 times per week) with ribavirin.

5.2 Pharmacokinetic properties

Ribavirin is absorbed rapidly following oral administration of a single dose of Copegus (median T_{max} = 1-2 hours). The mean terminal phase half-life of ribavirin following

Table 7 Undesirable Effects (<10% Incidence) Reported for HCV and HIV-HCV patients

Body system	Common	Common	Uncommon to Rare serious adverse events
	<10% - 5%	<5% -1%	<1% - <0.1%
Infections and infestations		herpes simplex, URI infection, bronchitis, oral candidiasis	Skin infection, lower respiratory tract infection, otitis externa, endocarditis
Neoplasms benign and malignant			Hepatic neoplasm
Blood and lymphatic system disorders		Anaemia, lymphadenopathy, thrombocytopenia	
Immune system disorders			ITP, thyroiditis, psoriasis, rheumatoid arthritis, SLE, sarcoidosis, anaphylaxis
Endocrine disorders		Hypothyroidism, hyperthyroidism	Diabetes
Psychiatric disorders	mood alteration, emotional disorders, anxiety	Nervousness, libido decreased, aggression	Suicide ideation, suicide, anger
Nervous system disorders	memory impairment	taste disturbance, weakness, paraesthesia, hypoaesthesia, tremor, migraine, somnolence, hyperaesthesia, nightmares, syncope	Peripheral neuropathy, coma
Eye disorders		vision blurred, eye inflammation, xerophthalmia, eye pain	Corneal ulcer, retinopathy, retinal vascular disorder, retinal haemorrhage, papilloedema, optic neuropathy, vision loss
Ear and labyrinth disorders		vertigo, earache	
Cardiac disorders		Palpitations, oedema peripheral, tachycardia	Arrhythmia, supraventricular tachycardia, atrial fibrillation, CHF, angina, myocardial infarction, pericarditis
Vascular disorders		Flushing	Cerebral haemorrhage, hypertension
Respiratory, thoracic and mediastinal disorders		sore throat, dyspnoea exertional, epistaxis, nasopharyngitis, sinus congestion, rhinitis, nasal congestion	Bronchoconstriction, interstitial pneumonitis with fatal outcome, pulmonary embolism
Gastrointestinal disorders	vomiting, dry mouth, dyspepsia	mouth ulceration, flatulence, gingival bleeding, stomatitis, dysphagia, glossitis	Peptic ulcer, gastrointestinal bleeding, reversible pancreatic reaction (ie, amylase/lipase increase with or without abdominal pain)
Hepato-biliary disorders			Hepatic failure, hepatic dysfunction, fatty liver, cholangitis
Skin and subcutaneous tissue disorders	rash, sweating increased	Eczema, night sweats, psoriasis, photosensitivity reaction, urticaria, skin disorder	Angioedema
Musculoskeletal, connective tissue and bone disorders	back pain	muscle cramps, neck pain, musculoskeletal pain, bone pain, arthritis, muscle weakness	Myositis
Reproductive system and breast disorders		Impotence	
General disorders and administration site conditions		Malaise, lethargy, chest pain, hot flushes, thirst, influenza like illness	
Injury and poisoning			Substance overdose

single doses of Copegus range from 140 to 160 hours. Ribavirin data from the literature demonstrates absorption is extensive with approximately 10% of a radiolabeled dose excreted in the faeces. However, absolute bioavailability is approximately 45%-65%, which appears to be due to first pass metabolism. There is a linear relationship between dose and AUC_{tf} following single doses of 200-1,200 milligrams ribavirin. Mean apparent oral clearance of ribavirin following single 600 milligram doses of Copegus ranges from 22 to 29 litres/hour. Volume of distribution is approximately 4,500 1itres following administration of Copegus. Ribavirin does not bind to plasma proteins.

Ribavirin has been shown to produce high inter- and intra-subject pharmacokinetic variability following single oral doses of Copegus(intra-subject variability of ⩽25% for both AUC and C_{max}), which may be due to extensive first pass metabolism and transfer within and beyond the blood compartment.

Ribavirin transport in non-plasma compartments has been most extensively studied in red cells, and has been identified to be primarily via an e_s-type equilibrative nucleoside transporter. This type of transporter is present on virtually all cell types and may account for the high volume of distribution of ribavirin. The ratio of whole blood: plasma ribavirin concentrations is approximately 60:1; the excess of ribavirin in whole blood exists as ribavirin nucleotides sequestered in erythrocytes.

Ribavirin has two pathways of metabolism: 1) a reversible phosphorylation pathway, 2) a degradative pathway involving deribosylation and amide hydrolysis to yield a triazole carboxyacid metabolite. Ribavirin and both its triazole carboxamide and triazole carboxylic acid metabolites are excreted renally.

Upon multiple dosing, ribavirin accumulates extensively in plasma with a six-fold ratio of multiple-dose to single-dose AUC_{12hr} based on literature data. Following oral dosing with 600 milligrams BID, steady-state was reached by approximately 4 weeks, with mean steady state plasma concentrations of approximately 2,200 ng/ml. Upon discontinuation of dosing the half-life was approximately 300 hours, which probably reflects slow elimination from non-plasma compartments.

Food effect: The bioavailability of a single oral 600 mg dose Copegus was increased by coadministration of a high fat meal. The ribavirin exposure parameters of $AUC_{(0-192h)}$ and C_{max} increased by 42% and 66%, respectively, when Copegus was taken with a high fat breakfast compared to being taken in the fasted state. The clinical relevance of results from this single dose study is unknown. Ribavirin exposure after multiple dosing when taken with food was comparable in patients receiving peginterferon alfa-2a and Copegus and interferon alfa-2b and ribavirin. In order to achieve optimal ribavirin plasma concentrations, it is recommended to take ribavirin with food.

Renal function: Single-dose ribavirin pharmacokinetics were altered (increased AUC_{tf} and C_{max}) in patients with renal dysfunction compared with control subjects whose creatinine clearance was greater than 90 ml/minute. The clearance of ribavirin is substantially reduced in patients with serum creatinine > 2 mg/dl or creatinine clearance < 50 ml/min. There are insufficient data on the safety and efficacy of ribavirin in such patients to support recommendations for dose adjustments. Plasma concentrations of ribavirin are essentially unchanged by haemodialysis.

Hepatic function: Single-dose pharmacokinetics of ribavirin in patients with mild, moderate or severe hepatic dysfunction (Child-Pugh Classification A, B or C) are similar to those of normal controls.

Use in elderly patients over the age of 65: Specific pharmacokinetic evaluations for elderly subjects have not been performed. However, in a published population pharmacokinetic study, age was not a key factor in the kinetics of ribavirin; renal function is the determining factor.

Patients under the age of 18 years: The pharmacokinetic properties of ribavirin have not been fully evaluated in patients under the age of 18 years. Copegus in combination with peginterferon alfa-2 or interferon alfa-2a is indicated for the treatment of chronic hepatitis C only in patients 18 years of age or older.

Population Pharmacokinetics: A population pharmacokinetic analysis was performed using plasma concentration values from five clinical trials. While body weight and race were statistically significant covariates in the clearance model only the effect of body weight was clinically significant. Clearance increased as a function of body weight and was predicted to vary from 17.7 to 24.8 L/h over a weight range of 44 to 155 kg. Creatinine clearance (as low as 34 ml/min) did not affect ribavirin clearance.

5.3 Preclinical safety data

Ribavirin is embryotoxic and/or teratogenic at doses well below the recommended human dose in all animal species in which adequate studies have been conducted. Malformations of the skull, palate, eye, jaw, limbs, skeleton and gastrointestinal tract were noted. The incidence and severity of teratogenic effects increased with escalation of the dose. Survival of foetuses and offspring is reduced.

Erythrocytes are a primary target of toxicity for ribavirin in animal studies, including studies in dogs and monkeys. Anaemia occurs shortly after initiation of dosing, but is rapidly reversible upon cessation of treatment. Hypoplastic anaemia was observed only in rats at the high dose of 160 milligrams/kg/day in the subchronic study.

Reduced leucocyte and/or lymphocyte counts were consistently noted in the repeat-dose rodent and dog toxicity studies with ribavirin and transiently in monkeys administered ribavirin in the subchronic study. Repeat-dose rat toxicity studies showed thymic lymphoid depletion and/or depletion of thymus-dependent areas of the spleen (periarteriolar lymphoid sheaths, white pulp) and mesenteric lymph node. Following repeat-dosing of dogs with ribavirin, increased dilatation/necrosis of the intestinal crypts of the duodenum was noted, as well as chronic inflammation of the small intestine and erosion of the ileum.

In repeat dose studies in mice to investigate ribavirin-induced testicular and sperm effects, abnormalities in sperm occurred at doses in animals well below therapeutic doses. Upon cessation of treatment, essentially total recovery from ribavirin-induced testicular toxicity occurred within one or two spermatogenic cycles.

Genotoxicity studies have demonstrated that ribavirin does exert some genotoxic activity. Ribavirin was active in an *in vitro* Transformation Assay. Genotoxic activity was observed in *in vivo* mouse micronucleus assays. A dominant lethal assay in rats was negative, indicating that if

Table 8 Virological Response in the overall population (including non-cirrhotic and cirrhotic patients)

	Study NV15942	Study NV15801	
	Copegus 1,000/1,200 mg & Peginterferon alfa-2a 180 micrograms (N=436) 48 weeks	Copegus 1,000/1,200 mg & Peginterferon alfa-2a 180 micrograms (N=453) 48 weeks	Ribavirin 1,000/1,200 mg & Interferon alfa-2b 3 MIU (N=444) 48 weeks
Response at End of Treatment	68%	69%	52%
Overall Sustained Response	63%	54%*	45%*

*95% CI for difference: 3% to 16% p-value (stratified Cochran-Mantel-Haenszel test) = 0.003

Table 9 Sustained Virological Response based on Genotype and Viral Load after Copegus Combination Therapy with peginterferon alfa-2a

	Study NV15942				Study NV15801	
	Copegus 800 mg & **PEG-IFN alfa-2a** 180 mcg 24 weeks	**Copegus** 1000/1200 mg & **PEG-IFN alfa-2a** 180 mcg 24 weeks	**Copegus** 800 mg & **PEG-IFN alfa-2a** 180 mcg 48 weeks	**Copegus** 1000/1200 mg & **PEG-IFN alfa-2a** 180 mcg 48 weeks	**Copegus** 1000/1200 mg & **PEG-IFN alfa-2a** 180 mcg 48 weeks	**Ribavirin** 1000/1200 mg & **Interferon alfa-2b** 3 MIU 48 weeks
Genotype 1	29% (29/101)	42% (49/118)†	41% (102/250)*	52% (142/271)*†	45% (134/298)	36% (103/285)
Low viral load	41% (21/51)	52% (37/71)	55% (33/60)	65% (55/85)	53% (61/115)	44% (41/94)
High viral load	16% (8/50)	26% (12/47)	36% (69/190)	47% (87/186)	40% (73/182)	33% (62/189)
Genotype 2/3	84% (81/96)	81% (117/144)	79% (78/99)	80% (123/153)	71% (100/140)	61% (88/145)
Low viral load	85% (29/34)	83% (39/47)	88% (29/33)	77% (37/48)	76% (28/37)	65% (34/52)
High viral load	84% (52/62)	80% (78/97)	74% (49/66)	82% (86/105)	70% (72/103)	58% (54/93)
Genotype 4	0% (0/5)	67% (8/12)	63% (5/8)	82% (9/11)	77% (10/13)	45% (5/11)

*Copegus 1000/1200 mg + peginterferon alfa-2a 180 mcg, 48 w vs. Copegus 800 mg + peginterferon alfa-2a 180 mcg, 48 w: Odds Ratio (95% CI) = 1.52 (1.07 to 2.17) P-value (stratified Cochran-Mantel-Haenszel test) = 0.020

†Copegus 1000/1200 mg + peginterferon alfa-2a 180 mcg, 48 w vs. Copegus 1000/1200 mg + peginterferon alfa-2a 180 mcg, 24 w: Odds Ratio (95% CI) = 2.12 (1.30 to 3.46) P-value (stratified Cochran-Mantel-Haenszel test) = 0.002

Table 10 Sustained Virological Response based on Genotype and Viral Load after Copegus Combination Therapy with peginterferon alfa-2a in HIV-HCV co-infected patients

Study NR15961			
	Interferon alfa-2a 3 MIU & **Copegus 800 mg** 48 weeks	**Peginterferon alfa-2a** 180 mcg & **Placebo** 48 weeks	**Peginterferon alfa-2a** 180 mcg & **Copegus 800 mg** 48 weeks
All patients	12% (33/285)*	20% (58/286)*	40% (116/289)*
Genotype 1	7% (12/171)	14% (24/175)	29% (51/176)
Low viral load	19% (8/42)	38% (17/45)	61% (28/46)
High viral load	3% (4/129)	5% (7/130)	18% (23/130)
Genotype 2-3	20% (18/89)	36% (32/90)	62% (59/95)
Low viral load	27% (8/30)	38% (9/24)	61% (17/28)
High viral load	17% (10/59)	35% (23/66)	63% (42/67)

* peginterferon alfa-2a 180 mcg Copegus 800mg vs. Interferon alfa-2a 3MIU ribavirin 800mg: Odds Ratio (95% CI) = 5.40 (3.42 to 8.54), ….P-value (stratified Cochran-Mantel-Haenszel test) = < 0.0001

* peginterferon alfa-2a 180 mcg Copegus 800mg vs. peginterferon alfa-2a 180μg: Odds Ratio (95% CI) = 2.89 (1.93 to 4.32),…. P-value (stratified Cochran-Mantel-Haenszel test) = < 0.0001

* Interferon alfa-2a 3MIU Copegus 800mg vs. peginterferon alfa-2a 180mcg: Odds Ratio (95% CI) = 0.53 (0.33 to 0.85), … P-value (stratified Cochran-Mantel-Haenszel test) = < 0.0084.

mutations occurred in rats they were not transmitted through male gametes. Ribavirin is a possible human carcinogen.

Administration of ribavirin and peginterferon alfa-2a in combination did not produce any unexpected toxicity in monkeys. The major treatment-related change was reversible mild to moderate anaemia, the severity of which was greater than that produced by either active substance alone.

6. PHARMACEUTICAL PARTICULARS

6.1 List of excipients

Tablet core:

Pregelatinised starch

Sodium starch glycolate

Microcrystalline cellulose

Maize starch

Magnesium stearate

Film-coating:

Hypromellose

Talc

Titanium dioxide (E171)

Yellow iron oxide (E172)

Red iron oxide (E172)

Ethylcellulose aqueous dispersion

Triacetin

6.2 Incompatibilities

Not applicable

6.3 Shelf life

3 years

6.4 Special precautions for storage

No special precautions for storage

6.5 Nature and contents of container

Copegus is supplied in high density polyethylene (HDPE) bottles with a child-resistant polypropylene screw cap containing 28, 42, 112 or 168 tablets. Not all pack sizes may be marketed.

6.6 Instructions for use and handling

No special requirements

7. MARKETING AUTHORISATION HOLDER

Roche Products Limited, 40 Broadwater Road, Welwyn Garden City, Hertfordshire AL7 3AY, England.

8. MARKETING AUTHORISATION NUMBER(S)

PL 0031/0604

PA 50/153/1

9. DATE OF FIRST AUTHORISATION/RENEWAL OF THE AUTHORISATION

UK 13 November 2002

Ireland 4 April 2003

10. DATE OF REVISION OF THE TEXT

September 2005

LEGAL STATUS

POM

Coracten SR Capsules 10mg or 20mg

(UCB Pharma Limited)

1. NAME OF THE MEDICINAL PRODUCT

Coracten SR Capsules 10mg or 20mg

BIDNIF 10 or 20

2. QUALITATIVE AND QUANTITATIVE COMPOSITION

Each capsule contains 10mg or 20mg Nifedipine USP in sustained release form.

For excipients, see 6.1

3. PHARMACEUTICAL FORM

Modified-release capsule, hard

10 mg:

Sustained release capsules with opaque grey body and opaque brownish-pink cap, overprinted in white with 'Coracten' on the body and '10mg' on the cap, and filled with yellow pellets.

20 mg:

Sustained release capsules with opaque brownish-pink body and opaque reddish-brown cap, overprinted in white with 'Coracten' on the body and '20mg' on the cap, and filled with yellow pellets.

4. CLINICAL PARTICULARS

4.1 Therapeutic indications

Coracten SR Capsules are indicated for the prophylaxis of chronic stable angina pectoris and the treatment of hypertension.

They are also indicated for the treatment of Prinzmetal (variant) angina when diagnosed by a cardiologist.

4.2 Posology and method of administration

Adults only: The recommended starting dose of Coracten SR Capsules is 10mg every 12 hours swallowed with water, with subsequent titration of dosage according to response. The dose may be adjusted to 40mg every 12 hours.

Children: Coracten SR Capsules are not recommended for use in children.

Elderly: The pharmacokinetics of nifedipine are altered in the elderly so that lower maintenance doses of nifedipine may be required compared to younger patients.

Hepatic impairment: Caution should be exercised in treating patients with hepatic impairment. In these patients the use of one 10mg Coracten SR Capsule every 12 hours, together with careful monitoring, is suggested when commencing therapy.

Renal impairment: Dosage adjustments are not usually required in patients with renal impairment.

4.3 Contraindications

Coracten SR Capsules are contraindicated in patients with known hypersensitivity to nifedipine or other dihydropyridines because of the theoretical risk of cross reactivity. They should not be used in women who are or who may become pregnant (see section 4.6. Pregnancy and Lactation).

Coracten SR Capsules should not be used in clinically significant aortic stenosis, unstable angina, or during or within one month of a myocardial infarction. They should not be used in patients in cardiogenic shock.

Coracten SR Capsules should not be used for the treatment of acute attacks of angina, or in patients who have had ischaemic pain following its administration previously.

The safety of Coracten SR Capsules in malignant hypertension has not been established.

Coracten SR Capsules should not be used for secondary prevention of myocardial infarction.

Coracten SR Capsules are contraindicated in patients with acute porphyria.

Coracten SR Capsules should not be administered concomitantly with rifampicin since effective plasma levels of nifedipine may not be achieved owing to enzyme induction.

4.4 Special warnings and special precautions for use

The dose of nifedipine should be reduced in patients with hepatic impairment (***see section 4.2. Posology and Method of Administration***). Nifedipine should be used with caution in patients who are hypotensive; in patients with poor cardiac reserve; in patients with heart failure or significantly impaired left ventricular function as their condition may deteriorate; in diabetic patients as they may require adjustment of their diabetic therapy; and in dialysis patients with malignant hypertension and irreversible renal failure with hypovolaemia, since a significant drop in blood pressure may occur due to the vasodilator effects of nifedipine.

Excessive falls in blood pressure may result in transient blindness. If affected the patient should not attempt to drive or use machinery (see section 4.8. Undesirable Effects).

Since nifedipine has no beta-blocking activity, it gives no protection against the dangers of abrupt withdrawal of beta-blocking drugs. Withdrawal of any previously prescribed beta-blockers should be gradual, preferably over 8 to 10 days.

Nifedipine may be used in combination with beta-blockers and other antihypertensive agents, but the possibility of an additive effect resulting in postural hypotension and/or cardiac failure must be borne in mind.

Cardiac ischaemic pain has been reported in a minority of patients within 30 minutes of starting nifedipine treatment; such patients should stop treatment.

4.5 Interaction with other medicinal products and other forms of Interaction

As with other dihydropyridines, nifedipine should not be taken with grapefruit juice because bioavailability is increased.

The simultaneous administration of nifedipine and digoxin may lead to reduced digoxin clearance and hence an increase in the plasma digoxin. Digoxin levels should be monitored and, if necessary, the digoxin dose reduced.

Nifedipine may increase the spectrophotometric values of urinary vanillylmandelic acid falsely. However, HPLC measurements are unaffected.

Coracten SR Capsules should not be administered concomitantly with rifampicin since effective plasma levels of nifedipine may not be achieved owing to enzyme induction (see section 4.3. Contra-indications).

Increased plasma levels of nifedipine have been reported during concomitant use of H_2-receptor antagonists (specifically cimetidine), other calcium channel blockers (specifically diltiazem), alcohol and cyclosporin. Azole antifungals may increase serum concentrations of nifedipine.

Plasma levels of nifedipine are possibly decreased by the concomitant use of antiepileptics.

When used in combination with nifedipine, plasma concentrations of quinidine have been shown to be suppressed regardless of quinidine dosage. The plasma concentrations of phenytoin, theophylline and non-depolarising muscle relaxants (e.g. tubocurarine) are increased when used in combination with nifedipine. Tacrolimus concentrations may be increased by nifedipine.

Enhanced hypotensive effect of nifedipine may occur with: Aldesleukin, Alprostadil, Anaesthetics, Antipsychotics, Diuretics, Phenothiazides, Prazosin and Intravenous ionic X-ray contrast medium. Profound hypotension has been reported with nifedipine and intravenous magnesium sulphate in the treatment of pre-eclampsia.

Ritonavir and quinupristin/dalfopristin may result in increased plasma concentrations of nifedipine.

Effective plasma levels of nifedipine may not be achieved due to enzyme induction with concurrent administration of carbamazepine, erythromycin and phenobarbitone.

There is an increased risk of excessive hypotension, bradycardia and heart failure with β-blockers.

An increased rate of absorption of nifedipine from sustained release preparation may occur if given concurrently with cisapride.

Nifedipine may result in increased levels of mizolastine due to inhibition of cytochrome CYP3A4.

Nifedipine may increase the neuromuscular blocking effects of vecuronium.

4.6 Pregnancy and lactation

Pregnancy

Because animal studies show embryotoxicity and teratogenicity, Coracten SR Capsules are contra-indicated during pregnancy (see also section 4.3. Contra-indications). Embryotoxicity was noted at 6 to 20 times the maximum recommended dose for Coracten SR Capsules given to rats, mice and rabbits, and teratogenicity was noted in rabbits given 20 times the maximum recommended dose for Coracten SR Capsules.

Lactation

Nifedipine is excreted in breast milk, therefore Coracten SR Capsules are not recommended during lactation.

4.7 Effects on ability to drive and use machines

Dizziness and lethargy are potential undesirable effects. If affected do not attempt to drive or use machinery (see also section 4.8. Undesirable Effects).

Excessive falls in blood pressure may result in transient blindness. If affected do not attempt to drive or use machinery (see also section 4.8. Undesirable Effects).

4.8 Undesirable effects

Side-effects are generally transient and mild, and usually occur at the start of treatment only. They include headache, flushing and, usually at higher dosages, nausea, dyspepsia, heartburn, gastrointestinal disturbances such as constipation and diarrhoea, dizziness, lethargy, skin reactions (such as rash, pruritus and urticaria), paraesthesia, hypotension, palpitation, tachycardia, dependent oedema, increased frequency of micturition, eye pain, depression, fever, gingival hyperplasia telangiectasia and erythema multiforme.

Other less frequently reported side-effects include myalgia, tremor, pemphigoid reaction and and visual disturbances. Impotence may occur rarely.

Excessive falls in blood pressure may result in cerebral or myocardial ischaemia or transient blindness.

As with other sustained release dihydropyridines, exacerbation of angina pectoris may occur rarely at the start of treatment with sustained release formulations of nifedipine. The occurrence of myocardial infarction has been described although it is not possible to distinguish such an event from the natural course of ischaemic heart disease.

There are reports in older men on long-term therapy of gynaecomastia which usually regresses upon withdrawal of therapy.

Side-effects which may occur in isolated cases are photosensitivity, exfoliative dermatitis, systemic allergic reactions and purpura. Usually, these regress after discontinuation of the drug.

Rare cases of hypersensitivity-type jaundice have been reported. In addition, disturbances of liver function such as intra-hepatic cholestasis may occur. These regress after discontinuation of therapy.

4.9 Overdose

Human experience:

Reports of nifedipine overdosage are limited and symptoms are not necessarily dose-related. Severe hypotension due to vasodilation, and tachycardia or bradycardia are the most likely manifestations of overdose.

Metabolic disturbances include hyperglycaemia, metabolic acidosis and hypo- or hyperkalaemia.

Cardiac effects may include heart block, AV dissociation and asystole, and cardiogenic shock with pulmonary oedema.

Other toxic effects include nausea, vomiting, drowsiness, dizziness, confusion, lethargy, flushing, hypoxia, unconsciousness and coma.

Management of overdose in man:

Treatment consists of gastric lavage followed by oral activated charcoal together with supportive and symptomatic measures, principally intravenous fluids to maintain circulating blood volume. If the latter is not sufficient, dopamine or dobutamine may be given. Intravenous calcium gluconate may be considered as an antidote.

5. PHARMACOLOGICAL PROPERTIES

5.1 Pharmacodynamic properties

ATC Code: C08C A05

Nifedipine is a potent calcium-channel blocker which, by dilating peripheral arterial smooth muscle, decreases cardiac work and myocardial oxygen requirement. It also dilates coronary arteries, thereby improving myocardial perfusion and reducing coronary artery spasm. In hypertension, it reduces blood pressure but has little or no effect in normotensive subjects. It has no therapeutic antiarrhythmic effect.

5.2 Pharmacokinetic properties

Coracten SR Capsules are a sustained release formulation of nifedipine designed to provide less fluctuation and more prolonged nifedipine blood concentrations than standard immediate release preparations.

Nifedipine is highly protein bound. It undergoes hepatic oxidation to inactive metabolites which are excreted in the urine (80%) and faeces (20%).

5.3 Preclinical safety data

There are no pre-clinical data of relevance to the prescriber which are additional to that already included in other sections of the Summary of Product Characteristics.

6. PHARMACEUTICAL PARTICULARS

6.1 List of excipients

Capsule contents:

Sucrose, Maize Starch, Lactose, Povidone K30, Methacrylic acid copolymer type A (Eudragit L100), Talc, Purified Water.

Capsule shells:

Gelatin, Red iron oxide (E172), Yellow iron oxide (E172), Titanium dioxide (E171), Black iron oxide (E172, 10mg only).

6.2 Incompatibilities

None known.

6.3 Shelf life

36 months.

6.4 Special precautions for storage

Store in original pack at a temperature not exceeding 30°C and protect from light.

6.5 Nature and contents of container

Coracten SR Capsules are presented in blister strips packed in cartons containing 60 capsules. The blister strips are formed from PVC with a coating of PVdC backed with aluminium foil.

(Cartons of 10, 15, 30, 56, 100, 150, 250, 500 and 600 capsules are licensed but not marketed.)

6.6 Instructions for use and handling

None.

7. MARKETING AUTHORISATION HOLDER

UCB Pharma Ltd

208 Bath Road

Slough

Berkshire

SL1 3WE

UK

8. MARKETING AUTHORISATION NUMBER(S)

10 mg:

PL 00039/0365

20 mg:

PL 00039/0367

9. DATE OF FIRST AUTHORISATION/RENEWAL OF THE AUTHORISATION

11 April 1991

10. DATE OF REVISION OF THE TEXT

June 2005

11. Legal Category

POM

Coracten XL Joint SPC 30mg, 60mg

(UCB Pharma Limited)

1. NAME OF THE MEDICINAL PRODUCT

Coracten XL 30 mg

Coracten XL 60 mg.

2. QUALITATIVE AND QUANTITATIVE COMPOSITION

Each capsule contains 30 mg or 60 mg Nifedipine Ph.Eur in sustained release form.

For excipients, see 6.1

3. PHARMACEUTICAL FORM

Prolonged release capsule, hard.

4. CLINICAL PARTICULARS

4.1 Therapeutic indications

Coracten XL capsules are indicated for the treatment of hypertension and the prophylaxis of chronic stable angina pectoris.

4.2 Posology and method of administration

The capsules are for oral administration and should be swallowed whole with a little fluid.

Dosage - Angina Pectoris and Hypertension

Adults only: Normally treatment is initiated with one 30mg Coracten XL capsule every 24 hours. Dosage may be titrated to a higher level as clinically warranted. The dose may be adjusted to 90mg every 24 hours.

Children: Coracten XL capsules are not recommended for use in children.

Elderly: The pharmacokinetics of nifedipine are altered in the elderly so that lower maintenance doses of nifedipine may be required compared to younger patients.

Hepatic impairment: As Coracten XL is a long acting formulation, it should not be administered to patients with hepatic impairment.

Renal impairment: Dosage adjustments are not usually required in patients with renal impairment.

4.3 Contraindications

Coracten XL capsules are contraindicated in patients with known hypersensitivity to nifedipine or other dihydropyridines because of the theoretical risk of cross reactivity. They should not be used in nursing mothers and women who are or who may become pregnant (see section 4.6. Pregnancy and Lactation).

Coracten XL capsules should not be used in clinically significant aortic stenosis, unstable angina, or during or within one month of a myocardial infarction. They should not be used in patients in cardiogenic shock.

Coracten XL capsules should not be used for the treatment of acute attacks of angina, or in patients who have had ischaemic pain following its administration previously.

The safety of Coracten XL capsules in malignant hypertension has not been established.

Coracten XL capsules should not be used for secondary prevention of myocardial infarction.

Coracten XL capsules are contraindicated in patients with acute porphyria.

Coracten XL capsules should not be administered concomitantly with rifampicin since effective plasma levels of nifedipine may not be achieved owing to enzyme induction.

As Coracten XL is a long acting formulation, it should not be administered to patients with hepatic impairment.

4.4 Special warnings and special precautions for use

Nifedipine should be used with caution in patients who are hypotensive; in patients with poor cardiac reserve; in patients with heart failure or significantly impaired left ventricular function as their condition may deteriorate; in diabetic patients as they may require adjustment of their diabetic therapy; and in dialysis patients with malignant hypertension and irreversible renal failure with hypovolaemia, since a significant drop in blood pressure may occur due to the vasodilator effects of nifedipine.

Excessive falls in blood pressure may result in transient blindness. If affected do not attempt to drive or use machinery (see also section 4.8. Undesirable Effects).

Since nifedipine has no beta-blocking activity, it gives no protection against the dangers of abrupt withdrawal of beta-blocking drugs. Withdrawal of any previously prescribed beta-blockers should be gradual, preferably over 8 to 10 days.

The dose of nifedipine should be reduced in patients with hepatic impairment (see section 4.2. Posology and Method of Administration).

Nifedipine may be used in combination with beta-blocking drugs and other antihypertensive agents, but the possibility of an additive effect resulting in postural hypotension should be borne in mind. Nifedipine will not prevent possible rebound effects after cessation of other anti-hypertensive therapy.

4.5 Interaction with other medicinal products and other forms of Interaction

As with other dihydropyridines, nifedipine should not be taken with grapefruit juice because bioavailability is increased.

The simultaneous administration of nifedipine and digoxin may lead to reduced digoxin clearance and hence an increase in the plasma digoxin. Digoxin levels should be monitored and, if necessary, the digoxin dose reduced.

Nifedipine may increase the spectrophotometric values of urinary vanillylmandelic acid falsely. However, HPLC measurements are unaffected.

Coracten XL capsules should not be administered concomitantly with rifampicin since effective plasma levels of nifedipine may not be achieved owing to enzyme induction (see section 4.3. Contra-indications).

Increased plasma levels of nifedipine have been reported during concomitant use of H2-receptor antagonists (specifically cimetidine), other calcium channel blockers (specifically diltiazem), alcohol and cyclosporin. Azole antifungals may increase serum concentrations of nifedipine.

Decreased plasma levels of nifedipine have been reported during concomitant use of antibacterials (specifically rifampicin), and probably also antiepileptics.

When used in combination with nifedipine, plasma concentrations of quinidine have been shown to be suppressed regardless of quinidine dosage. The plasma concentrations of phenytoin, theophylline, non-depolarising muscle relaxants (e.g. tubocurarine) and possibly digoxin are increased when used in combination with nifedipine. Tacrolimus concentrations may be increased by nifedipine.

Enhanced hypotensive effect of nifedipine may occur with: aldesleukin, alprostadil, anaesthetics, antipsychotics, diuretics, phenothiazides, prazosin and intravenous ionic X-ray contrast medium. Profound hypotension has been reported with nifedipine and intravenous magnesium sulphate in the treatment of pre-eclampsia.

Ritonavir and quinupristin/dalfopristin may result in increased plasma concentrations of nifedipine.

Effective plasma levels of nifedipine may not be achieved due to enzyme induction with concurrent administration of carbamazepine, erythromycin and phenobarbitone.

There is an increased risk of excessive hypotension, bradycardia and heart failure with β-blockers.

An increased rate of absorption of nifedipine from sustained release preparation may occur if given concurrently with cisapride.

Nifedipine may result in increased levels of mizolastine due to inhibition of cytochrome CYP3A4.

Nifedipine may increase the neuromuscular blocking effects of vecuronium.

4.6 Pregnancy and lactation

Pregnancy

Because animal studies show embryotoxicity and teratogenicity, nifedipine is contraindicated during pregnancy (see also section 4.3. Contra-indications). Embryotoxicity was noted at 6 to 20 times the maximum recommended dose for nifedipine given to rats, mice and rabbits, and teratogenicity was noted in rabbits given 20 times the maximum recommended dose for nifedipine.

Lactation

Nifedipine is secreted in breast milk, therefore, Coracten XL capsules are not recommended during lactation.

4.7 Effects on ability to drive and use machines

Dizziness and lethargy are potential undesirable effects. If affected do not attempt to drive or use machinery (see also section 4.8. Undesirable Effects).

Excessive falls in blood pressure may result in transient blindness. If affected do not attempt to drive or use machinery (see also section 4.8. Undesirable Effects).

4.8 Undesirable effects

Most side-effects are consequences of the vasodilatory effects of nifedipine. They include headache, flushing and, usually at higher dosages, nausea, dyspepsia, heartburn, constipation, diarrhoea, dizziness, lethargy, skin reactions (rash, urticaria and pruritus), paraesthesia, hypotension, palpitation, tachycardia, dependent oedema, increased frequency of micturition, eye pain, depression, allergic hepatitis, fever, gingival hyperplasia, telangiectasia. and erythema multiforme.

Other less frequently reported side-effects include myalgia,, pemphigoid reaction tremor and visual disturbances. Impotence may occur rarely. Mood changes may occur rarely. Altered bowel habit may occur occasionally.

Excessive falls in blood pressure may result in cerebral or myocardial ischaemia or transient blindness.

As with other sustained release dihydropyridines, exacerbation of angina pectoris may occur rarely at the start of treatment with sustained release formulations of nifedipine. The occurrence of myocardial infarction has been described although it is not possible to distinguish such an event from the natural course of ischaemic heart disease.

Ischaemic pain has been reported in a small proportion of patients following the introduction of nifedipine therapy. Although a 'steal' effect has not been demonstrated, patients experiencing this effect should discontinue nifedipine therapy.

There are reports in older men on long-term therapy of gynaecomastia which usually regresses upon withdrawal of therapy.

Side-effects which may occur in isolated cases are photosensitivity, exfoliative dermatitis, systemic allergic reactions and purpura. Usually, these regress after discontinuation of the drug.

Rare cases of hypersensitivity-type jaundice have been reported. In addition, disturbances of liver function such as intra-hepatic cholestasis may occur. These regress after discontinuation of therapy.

4.9 Overdose

Clinical effects

Reports of nifedipine overdosage are limited and symptoms are not necessarily dose-related. Severe hypotension due to vasodilation, and tachycardia and bradycardia are the most likely manifestations of overdose.

Metabolic disturbances include hyperglycaemia, metabolic acidosis and hypo- or hyperkalaemia.

Cardiac effects may include heart block, AV dissociation and asystole, and cardiogenic shock with pulmonary oedema.

Other toxic effects include nausea, vomiting, drowsiness, dizziness, confusion, lethargy, flushing, hypoxia and unconsciousness to the point of coma.

Treatment

As far as treatment is concerned, elimination of nifedipine and the restoration of stable cardiovascular conditions have priority.

After oral ingestion, gastric lavage is indicated, if necessary in combination with irrigation of the small intestine. Ipecacuanha should be given to children.

Elimination must be as complete as possible, including the small intestine, to prevent the otherwise inevitable subsequent absorption of the active substance.

Activated charcoal should be given in 4-hourly doses of 25g for adults, 10g for children.

Blood pressure, ECG, central arterial pressure, pulmonary wedge pressure, urea and electrolytes should be monitored.

Hypotension as a result of cardiogenic shock and arterial vasodilation should be treated with elevation of the feet and plasma expanders. If these measures are ineffective, hypotension may be treated with 10% calcium gluconate 10-20 ml intravenously over 5-10 minutes. If the effects are inadequate, the treatment can be continued, with ECG monitoring. In addition, beta-sympathomimetics may be given, e.g. isoprenaline 0.2 mg slowly i.v. or as a continuous infusion of 5μg/min. If an insufficient increase in blood pressure is achieved with calcium and isoprenaline, vasoconstricting sympathomimetics such as dopamine or noradrenaline should be administered. The dosage of these drugs should be determined by the patient's response.

Bradycardia may be treated with atropine, beta-sympathomimetics or a temporary cardiac pacemaker, as required.

Additional fluids should be administered with caution to avoid cardiac overload.

5. PHARMACOLOGICAL PROPERTIES

5.1 Pharmacodynamic properties

ATC Code: C08C A05

Nifedipine is a potent calcium-channel blocker which, by dilating peripheral arterial smooth muscle, decreases cardiac work and myocardial oxygen requirement. It also dilates coronary arteries, thereby improving myocardial perfusion and reducing coronary artery spasm. In hypertension, it reduces blood pressure but has little or no effect in normotensive subjects. It has no therapeutic antiarrhythmic effect.

5.2 Pharmacokinetic properties

Coracten XL capsules are a sustained release formulation of nifedipine designed to provide less fluctuation and more prolonged nifedipine blood concentrations than standard immediate release preparations.

Nifedipine is highly protein bound. It undergoes hepatic oxidation to inactive metabolites which are excreted in the urine (80%) and faeces (20%).

5.3 Preclinical safety data

There are no pre-clinical data of relevance to the prescriber which are additional to that already included in other sections of the Summary of Product Characteristics.

6. PHARMACEUTICAL PARTICULARS

6.1 List of excipients

Capsule contents:

Lactose monohydrate

Microcrystalline Cellulose

Hydroxylpropyl methylcellulose K100

Povidone K30

Magnesium Stearate

Hydroxypropylcellulose

Ammonio methacrylate copolymer type B

Polyethylene Glycol 6000

Dibutylphthalate

Titanium dioxide E171

Talc

Coracten XL 30 mg

(Capsule shells (size 3)

Yellow iron oxide E172

Red iron oxide E172

Titanium dioxide E171

Gelatin

Coracten XL 60 mg

Capsule shells (size 1):

Red iron oxide E172

Titanium dioxide E171

Gelatin

The printing ink is made of shellac, purified water, black iron oxide (E172) with 2-ethoxyethanol, soya lecithin, antifoam and IMS or with ethyl alcohol, isopropyl alcohol, n-butyl alcohol, propylene glycol, ammonium hydroxide and potassium hydroxide.

6.2 Incompatibilities

None known.

6.3 Shelf life

36 months.

6.4 Special precautions for storage

Do not store above 25°C. Store in the original package.

6.5 Nature and contents of container

Coracten XL capsules are available in blister strips packed in cartons containing 28, 30, 56 and 60 capsules. The blister strips are formed from PVC with a coating of PVdC backed with aluminium foil.

6.6 Instructions for use and handling

None.

7. MARKETING AUTHORISATION HOLDER

UCB Pharma Limited

208 Bath Road

Slough

Berkshire

SL1 3WE

UK

8. MARKETING AUTHORISATION NUMBER(S)

Coracten XL 30 mg – PL 00039/0506

Coracten XL 60 mg - PL 00039/0507

9. DATE OF FIRST AUTHORISATION/RENEWAL OF THE AUTHORISATION

7 October 1998

10. DATE OF REVISION OF THE TEXT

June 2005

11. Legal Category

POM

Cordarone X 100, Cordarone X 200

(sanofi-aventis)

1. NAME OF THE MEDICINAL PRODUCT

Cordarone X 100.

Cordarone X 200

2. QUALITATIVE AND QUANTITATIVE COMPOSITION

Cordarone X 100 contain 100mg of amiodarone hydrochloride.

Cordarone X 200 contain 200mg of amiodarone hydrochloride.

For excipients, see 6.1

3. PHARMACEUTICAL FORM

Tablet.

Cordarone X 100: Round, white tablet with a breakline on one side, imprinted with 100 on the other.

Cordarone X 200: Round, white tablet with a breakline on one side, imprinted with 200 on the other.

4. CLINICAL PARTICULARS

4.1 Therapeutic indications

Treatment should be initiated and normally monitored only under hospital or specialist supervision. Oral Cordarone X is indicated only for the treatment of severe rhythm disorders not responding to other therapies or when other treatments cannot be used.

Tachyarrhythmias associated with Wolff-Parkinson-White Syndrome.

Atrial flutter and fibrillation when other drugs cannot be used.

All types of tachyarrhythmias of paroxysmal nature including: supraventricular, nodal andventricular tachycardias, ventricular fibrillation: when other drugs cannot be used

4.2 Posology and method of administration

Adults

It is particularly important that the minimum effective dose be used. In all cases the patient's management must be judged on the individual response and well being. The following dosage regimen is generally effective.

Initial Stabilisation

Treatment should be started with 200mg, three times a day and may be continued for 1 week. The dosage should then be reduced to 200mg, twice daily for a further week.

Maintenance

After the initial period the dosage should be reduced to 200mg daily, or less if appropriate. Rarely, the patient may require a higher maintenance dose. The scored 100mg tablet should be used to titrate the minimum dosage required to maintain control of the arrhythmia. The maintenance dose should be regularly reviewed, especially where this exceeds 200mg daily.

General Considerations

Initial dosing

A high dose is needed in order to achieve adequate tissue levels rapidly.

Maintenance

Too high a dose during maintenance therapy can cause side effects which are believed to be related to high tissue levels of amiodarone and its metabolites.

Amiodarone is strongly protein bound and has an average plasma half life of 50 days (reported range 20-100 days). It follows that sufficient time must be allowed for a new distribution equilibrium to be achieved between adjustments of dosage. In patients with potentially lethal arrhythmias the long half life is a valuable safeguard, as omission of occasional doses does not significantly influence the overall therapeutic effect. It is particularly important that the minimum effective dosage is used and the patient is monitored regularly to detect the clinical features of excess amiodarone dosage. Therapy may then be adjusted accordingly.

Dosage reduction/withdrawal

Side effects slowly disappear as tissue levels fall. Following drug withdrawal, residual tissue bound amiodarone may protect the patient for up to a month. However, the likelihood of recurrence of arrhythmia during this period should be considered.

Paediatric population

No controlled paediatric studies have been undertaken. In published uncontrolled studies effective doses for children were:

• Loading dose: 10 to 20mg/kg/day for 7 to 10 days (or 500mg/m^2/day if expressed per square metre)

• Maintenance dose: the minimum effective dosage should be used; according to individual response, it may range between 5 to 10 mg/kg/day (or 250mg/m^2/day if expressed per square metre).

Elderly

As with all patients it is important that the minimum effective dose is used. Whilst there is no evidence that dosage requirements are different for this group of patients they may be more susceptible to bradycardia and conduction defects if too high a dose is employed. Particular attention should be paid to monitoring thyroid function. *(see sections 4.3, 4.4 and 4.8).*

Cordarone X is for oral administration.

4.3 Contraindications

Sinus bradycardia and sino-atrial heart block. In patients with severe conduction disturbances (high grade AV block, bifascicular or trifascicular block) or sinus node disease, Cordarone X should be used only in conjunction with a pacemaker.

Evidence or history of thyroid dysfunction. Thyroid function tests should be performed in all patients prior to therapy.

Known hypersensitivity to iodine or to amiodarone, or to any of the excipients. (One 100mg tablet contains approximately 37.5mg iodine).

The combination of Cordarone X with drugs which may induce torsades de pointes is contra-indicated *(see section 4.5).*

Pregnancy - except in exceptional circumstances *(see section 4.6)*

Lactation *(see section 4.6).*

4.4 Special warnings and special precautions for use

Patients with rare hereditary problems of galactose intolerance, the Lapp lactase deficiency or glucose-galactose malabsorption should not take this medicine.

Amiodarone can cause serious adverse reactions affecting the eyes, heart, lung, liver, thyroid gland, skin and peripheral nervous system *(see section 4.8.)*. Because these reactions may be delayed, patients on long-term treatment should be carefully supervised. As undesirable effects are usually dose-related, the minimum effective maintenance dose should be given.

Before surgery, the anaesthetist should be informed that the patient is taking amiodarone *(see sections 4.5 and 4.8).*

Cardiac disorders *(see section 4.8):*

Too high a dosage may lead to severe bradycardia and to conduction disturbances with the appearance of an idioventricular rhythm, particularly in elderly patients or during digitalis therapy. In these circumstances, Cordarone X treatment should be withdrawn. If necessary beta-adrenostimulants or glucagon may be given. Because of the long half-life of amiodarone, if bradycardia is severe and symptomatic the insertion of a pacemaker should be considered.

Oral Cordarone X is not contra-indicated in patients with latent or manifest heart failure but caution should be exercised as, occasionally, existing heart failure may be worsened. In such cases, Cordarone X may be used with other appropriate therapies.

The pharmacological action of amiodarone induces ECG changes: QT prolongation (related to prolonged repolarisation) with the possible development of U-waves and deformed T-waves; these changes do not reflect toxicity.

In the elderly, heart rate may decrease markedly.

Treatment should be discontinued in case of onset of 2nd or 3rd degree A-V block, sino-atrial block, or bifascicular block.

Amiodarone has a low pro-arrhythmic effect. Onsets of new arrhythmias or worsening of treated arrhythmias, sometimes fatal, have been reported. It is important, but difficult, to differentiate a lack of efficacy of the drug from a proarrhythmic effect, whether or not this is associated with a worsening of the cardiac condition. Proarrhythmic effects generally occur in the context of drug interactions and/or electrolytic disorders *(see sections 4.5. and 4.8).*

Before starting amiodarone, it is recommended to perform an ECG and serum potassium measurement. Monitoring of ECG is recommended during treatment.

Endocrine disorders *(see section 4.8)*

Amiodarone may induce hypothyroidism or hyperthyroidism, particularly in patients with a personal history of thyroid disorders. Clinical and biological [including ultrasensitive TSH (usTSH)] monitoring should be performed prior to therapy in all patients. Monitoring should be carried out during treatment, at six-monthly intervals, and for several months following its discontinuation. This is particularly important in the elderly. In patients whose history indicates an increased risk of thyroid dysfunction, regular assessment is recommended. Serum usTSH level should be measured when thyroid dysfunction is suspected.

Amiodarone contains iodine and thus may interfere with radio-iodine uptake. However, thyroid function tests (free-T_3, free-T_4, usTSH) remain interpretable. Amiodarone inhibits peripheral conversion of levothyroxine (T_4) to triiodothyronine (T_3) and may cause isolated biochemical changes (increase in serum free-T_4, free-T_3 being slightly decreased or even normal) in clinically euthyroid patients. There is no reason in such cases to discontinue amiodarone treatment if there is no clinical or further biological (usTSH) evidence of thyroid disease.

Hypothyroidism

Hypothyroidism should be suspected if the following clinical signs occur: weight gain, cold intolerance, reduced activity, excessive bradycardia. The diagnosis is supported by an increase in serum usTSH and an exaggerated TSH response to TRH. T_3 and T_4 levels may be low. Euthyroidism is usually obtained within 3 months following the discontinuation of treatment. In life-threatening situations, amiodarone therapy can be continued, in combination with levothyroxine. The dose of levothyroxine is adjusted according to TSH levels.

Hyperthyroidism

Hyperthyroidism may occur during amiodarone treatment, or, up to several months after discontinuation. Clinical features, such as weight loss, asthenia, restlessness, increase in heart rate, onset of arrhythmia, angina, congestive heart failure should alert the physician. The diagnosis is supported by a decrease in serum usTSH level, an elevated T_3 and a reduced TSH response to thyrotropin releasing hormone. Elevation of reverse T_3 (rT_3) may also be found.

In the case of hyperthyroidism, therapy should be withdrawn. Clinical recovery usually occurs within a few months, although severe cases, sometimes resulting in fatalities, have been reported. Clinical recovery precedes the normalisation of thyroid function tests.

Courses of anti-thyroid drugs have been used for the treatment of severe thyroid hyperactivity; large doses may be required initially. These may not always be effective and concomitant high dose corticosteroid therapy (e.g. 1mg/kg prednisolone) may be required for several weeks.

Eye disorders *(see section 4.8)*

If blurred or decreased vision occurs, complete ophthalmologic examination including fundoscopy should be promptly performed. Appearance of optic neuropathy and/or optic neuritis requires amiodarone withdrawal due to the potential progression to blindness. Unless blurred or decreased vision occurs, opthamological examination is recommended annually.

Hepato-biliary disorders *(see section 4.8):*

Amiodarone may be associated with a variety of hepatic effects, including cirrhosis, hepatitis, jaundice and hepatic failure. Some fatalities have been reported, mainly following long-term therapy, although rarely they have occurred soon after starting treatment particularly after Cordarone X intravenous. It is advisable to monitor liver function particularly transaminases before treatment and six monthly thereafter.

At the beginning of therapy, elevation of serum transaminases which can be in isolation (1.5 to 3 times normal) may occur. These may return to normal with dose reduction, or sometimes spontaneously.

Isolated cases of acute liver disorders with elevated serum transaminases and/or jaundice may occur; in such cases treatment should be discontinued.

There have been reports of chronic liver disease. Alteration of laboratory tests which may be minimal (transaminases elevated 1.5 to 5 times normal) or clinical signs (possible hepatomegaly) during treatment for longer than 6 months should suggest this diagnosis. Routine monitoring of liver function tests is therefore advised. Abnormal clinical and laboratory test results usually regress upon cessation of treatment, but fatal cases have been reported. Histological findings may resemble pseudo-alcoholic hepatitis, but they can be variable and include cirrhosis.

Although there have been no literature reports on the potentiation of hepatic adverse effects of alcohol, patients should be advised to moderate their alcohol intake while taking Cordarone X.

Nervous system disorders *(see section 4.8):*

Amiodarone may induce peripheral sensorimotor neuropathy and/or myopathy. Both these conditions may be severe, although recovery usually occurs within several months after amiodarone withdrawal, but may sometimes be incomplete.

Respiratory, thoracic and mediastinal disorders *(see section 4.8):*

Onset of dyspnoea or non-productive cough may be related to pulmonary toxicity (hypersensitivity pneumonitis, alveolar/interstitial pneumonitis or fibrosis, pleuritis, bronchiolitis obliterans organising pneumonitis. Presenting features can include dyspnoea (which may be severe and unexplained by the current cardiac status), non-productive cough and deterioration in general health (fatigue, weight loss and fever). The onset is usually slow but may be rapidly progressive. Whilst the majority of cases have been reported with long term therapy, a few have occurred soon after starting treatment.

Patients should be carefully evaluated clinically and consideration given to chest X-rays before starting therapy. During treatment, if pulmonary toxicity is suspected, this should be repeated and associated with lung function testing including, where possible, measurement of transfer factor. Initial radiological changes may be difficult to distinguish from pulmonary venous congestion. Pulmonary toxicity has usually been reversible following early withdrawal of amiodarone therapy, with or without corticosteroid therapy. Clinical symptoms often resolve within a few weeks followed by slower radiological and lung function improvement. Some patients can deteriorate despite discontinuing Cordarone X.

Skin and subcutaneous tissue disorders *(see section 4.8)*

Patients should be instructed to avoid exposure to sun and to use protective measures during therapy as patients taking Cordarone X can become unduly sensitive to sunlight, which may persist after several months of discontinuation of Cordarone X. In most cases symptoms are limited to tingling, burning and erythema of sun-exposed skin but severe phototoxic reactions with blistering may be seen.

Drug interactions (*see section 4.5*)

Concomitant use of amiodarone is not recommended with the following drugs: beta-blockers, heart rate lowering calcium channel inhibitors (verapamil, diltiazem), stimulant laxative agents which may cause hypokalaemia.

Increased plasma levels of flecainide have been reported with co-administration of amiodarone. The flecainide dose should be reduced accordingly and the patient closely monitored.

4.5 Interaction with other medicinal products and other forms of Interaction

Some of the more important drugs that interact with amiodarone include warfarin, digoxin, phenytoin and any drug which prolongs the QT interval.

Amiodarone raises the plasma concentrations of oral anticoagulants (warfarin) and phenytoin by inhibition of CYP 2C9. The dose of warfarin should be reduced accordingly. More frequent monitoring of prothrombin time both during and after amiodarone treatment is recommended. Phenytoin dosage should be reduced if signs of overdosage appear, and plasma levels may be measured.

Administration of Cordarone X to a patient already receiving digoxin will bring about an increase in the plasma digoxin concentration and thus precipitate symptoms and signs associated with high digoxin levels. Clinical, ECG and biological monitoring is recommended and digoxin dosage should be halved. A synergistic effect on heart rate and atrioventricular conduction is also possible.

Combined therapy with the following drugs which prolong the QT interval is contra-indicated (*see section 4.3*) due to the increased risk of torsades de pointes; for example:

- Class Ia anti-arrhythmic drugs e.g. quinidine, procainamide, disopyramide
- Class III anti-arrhythmic drugs e.g. sotalol, bretylium
- intravenous erythromycin, co-trimoxazole or pentamidine injection
- some anti-psychotics e.g. chlorpromazine, thioridazine, fluphenazine, pimozide, haloperidol, amisulpiride and sertindole
- lithium and tricyclic anti-depressants e.g. doxepin, maprotiline, amitriptyline
- certain antihistamines e.g. terfenadine, astemizole, mizolastine
- anti-malarials e.g. quinine, mefloquine, chloroquine, halofantrine.

Combined therapy with the following drugs is not recommended:

- Beta blockers and certain calcium channel inhibitors (diltiazem, verapamil); potentiation of negative chronotropic properties and conduction slowing effects may occur.
- Stimulant laxatives, which may cause hypokalaemia thus increasing the risk of torsades de pointes; other types of laxatives should be used.

Caution should be exercised over combined therapy with the following drugs which may also cause hypokalaemia and/or hypomagnesaemia, e.g. diuretics, systemic corticosteroids, tetracosactide, intravenous amphotericin.

In cases of hypokalaemia, corrective action should be taken and QT interval monitored. In case of torsades de pointes antiarrhythmic agents should not be given; pacing may be instituted and IV magnesium may be used.

Caution is advised in patients undergoing general anaesthesia, or receiving high dose oxygen therapy.

Potentially severe complications have been reported in patients taking amiodarone undergoing general anaesthesia: bradycardia unresponsive to atropine, hypotension, disturbances of conduction, decreased cardiac output.

A few cases of adult respiratory distress syndrome, most often in the period immediately after surgery, have been observed. A possible interaction with a high oxygen concentration may be implicated.

Drugs metabolised by cytochrome P450 3A4

When drugs are co-administered with amiodarone, an inhibitor of CYP 3A4, this may result in a higher level of their plasma concentrations, which may lead to a possible increase in their toxicity:

- Cyclosporin: plasma levels of cyclosporin may increase as much as 2-fold when used in combination. A reduction in the dose of cyclosporin may be necessary to maintain the plasma concentration within the therapeutic range.
- Other drugs metabolised by cytochrome P450 3A4: examples of such drugs are the statins (such as simvastatin), lidocaine, tacrolimus, sildenafil, fentanyl, midazolam and ergotamine.

Flecainide

Given that flecainide is mainly metabolised by CYP 2D6, by inhibiting this isoenzyme, amiodarone may increase flecainide plasma levels; it is advised to reduce the flecainide dose by 50% and to monitor the patient closely for adverse effects. Monitoring of flecainide plasma levels is strongly recommended in such circumstances.

Interaction with substrates of other CYP 450 isoenzymes

In vitro studies show that amiodarone also has the potential to inhibit CYP 1A2, CYP 2C19 and CYP 2D6 through its main metabolite. When co-administered, amiodarone would be expected to increase the plasma concentration of drugs whose metabolism is dependent upon CYP 1A2, CYP 2C19 and CYP 2D6.

4.6 Pregnancy and lactation

Pregnancy

There are insufficient data on the use of amiodarone during pregnancy in humans to judge any possible toxicity. However, in view of its effect on the foetal thyroid gland, amiodarone is contraindicated during pregnancy, except in exceptional circumstances.

If, because of the long half life of amiodarone, discontinuation of the drug is considered prior to planned conception, the real risk of reoccurrence of life threatening arrhythmias should be weighed against the possible hazard for the foetus.

Lactation

Amiodarone is excreted into the breast milk in significant quantities and breast-feeding is contra-indicated.

4.7 Effects on ability to drive and use machines

The ability to drive or to operate machinery may be impaired in patients with clinical symptoms of amiodarone-induced eye disorders.

4.8 Undesirable effects

The following adverse reactions are classified by system organ class and ranked under heading of frequency using the following convention: very common >= 10%), common >= 1% and < 10%); uncommon >= 0.1% and < 1%); rare >= 0.01% and < 0.1%), very rare (< 0.01%).

Blood and lymphatic system disorders:

- Very rare:
- haemolytic anemia
- aplastic anaemia
- thrombocytopenia.

Cardiac disorders:

- Common: bradycardia, generally moderate and dose-related.
- Uncommon:
- onset or worsening of arrhythmia, sometimes followed by cardiac arrest (*see sections 4.4 and 4.5.)*
- conduction disturbances (sinoatrial block, AV block of various degrees) (*see section 4.4*)
- Very rare: marked bradycardia or sinus arrest in patients with sinus node dysfunction and/or in elderly patients.

Endocrine disorders (*see section 4.4*):

- Common:
- hypothyroidism
- hyperthyroidism, sometimes fatal.

Eye disorders:

- Very common: corneal microdeposits usually limited to the area under the pupil, which are usually only discernable by slit-lamp examinations. They may be associated with colored halos in dazzling light or blurred vision. Corneal micro-deposits consist of complex lipid deposits and are reversible following discontinuation of treatment. The deposits are considered essentially benign and do not require discontinuation of amiodarone.
- Very rare: optic neuropathy/neuritis that may progress to blindness (*see section 4.4*).

Gastrointestinal disorders:

- Very common: benign gastrointestinal disorders (nausea, vomiting, dysgeusia) usually occurring with loading dosage and resolving with dose reduction.

Hepato-biliary disorders: (*see section 4.4*).

- Very common: isolated increase in serum transaminases, which is usually moderate (1.5 to 3 times normal range), occurring at the beginning of therapy. It may return to normal with dose reduction or even spontaneously.
- Common: acute liver disorders with high serum transaminases and/or jaundice, including hepatic failure, which are sometimes fatal
- Very rare: chronic liver disease (pseudo alcoholic hepatitis, cirrhosis), sometimes fatal.

Investigations:

- Very rare: increase in blood creatinine.

Nervous system disorders:

- Common:
- extrapyramidal tremor, for which regression usually occurs after reduction of dose or withdrawal
- nightmares
- sleep disorders.
- Uncommon: peripheral sensorimotor neuropathy and/or myopathy, usually reversible on withdrawal of the drug (*see section 4.4*).
- Very rare:
- cerebellar ataxia, for which regression usually occurs after reduction of dose or withdrawal
- benign intracranial hypertension (pseudo- tumor cerebri)
- headache
- vertigo.

Reproductive system and breast disorders:

- Very rare:
- epididymo-orchitis
- impotence.

Respiratory, thoracic and mediastinal disorders:

- Common: pulmonary toxicity [hypersensitivity pneumonitis, alveolar/interstitial pneumonitis or fibrosis, pleuritis, bronchiolitis obliterans organising pneumonia (BOOP)], sometimes fatal (*see section 4.4*).
- Very rare:
- bronchospasm in patients with severe respiratory failure and especially in asthmatic patients
- surgery (possible interaction with a high oxygen concentration) (*see sections 4.4 and 4.5*).

Skin and subcutaneous tissue disorders:

- Very common: photosensitivity (*see section 4.4*).
- Common: slate grey or bluish pigmentations of light-exposed skin, particularly the face, in case of prolonged treatment with high daily dosages; such pigmentations slowly disappear following treatment discontinuation.
- Very rare:
- erythema during the course of radiotherapy
- skin rashes, usually non- specific
- exfoliative dermatitis
- alopecia.

Vascular disorders:

- Very rare: vasculitis.

4.9 Overdose

Little information is available regarding acute overdosage with oral amiodarone. Few cases of sinus bradycardia, heart block, attacks of ventricular tachycardia, torsades de pointes, circulatory failure and hepatic injury have been reported.

In the event of overdose treatment should be symptomatic, gastric lavage may be employed to reduce absorption in addition to general supportive measures. The patient should be monitored and if bradycardia occurs beta-adrenostimulants or glucagon may be given. Spontaneously resolving attacks of ventricular tachycardia may also occur. Due to the pharmacokinetics of amiodarone, adequate and prolonged surveillance of the patient, particularly cardiac status, is recommended. Neither amiodarone nor its metabolites are dialysable.

5. PHARMACOLOGICAL PROPERTIES

5.1 Pharmacodynamic properties

Amiodarone hydrochloride is an antiarrhythmic.

5.2 Pharmacokinetic properties

Amiodarone is strongly protein bound and the plasma half life is usually of the order of 50 days. However there may be considerable inter-patient variation; in individual patients a half life of less than 20 days and a half life of more than 100 days has been reported. High doses of Cordarone X, for example 600mg/day, should be given initially to achieve effective tissue levels as rapidly as possible. Owing to the long half life of the drug, a maintenance dose of only 200mg/day, or less is usually necessary. Sufficient time must be allowed for a new distribution equilibrium to be achieved between adjustments of dose.

The long half life is a valuable safeguard for patients with potentially lethal arrhythmias as omission of occasional doses does not significantly influence the protection afforded by Cordarone X.

5.3 Preclinical safety data

There are no pre-clinical data of relevance to the prescriber which are additional to that already included in other sections of the SPC.

6. PHARMACEUTICAL PARTICULARS

6.1 List of excipients

Lactose monohydrate, Maize starch, Povidone, Colloidal anhydrous silica, Magnesium stearate.

6.2 Incompatibilities

Not applicable.

6.3 Shelf life

60 months.

6.4 Special precautions for storage

The tablets should be protected from light.

6.5 Nature and contents of container

Cordarone X tablets are supplied in blister packs of 28 tablets packed in cardboard cartons.

6.6 Instructions for use and handling

Not applicable.

7. MARKETING AUTHORISATION HOLDER

Sanofi-Synthelabo
PO Box 597
Guildford
Surrey

8. MARKETING AUTHORISATION NUMBER(S)
Cordarone X 100: PL 11723/0012.

Cordarone X 200: PL 11723/0013

9. DATE OF FIRST AUTHORISATION/RENEWAL OF THE AUTHORISATION
Cordarone X 100: 15 January 2001.

Cordarone X 200: 18 June 2003

10. DATE OF REVISION OF THE TEXT
May 2004

Legal category: POM

Cordarone X Intravenous

(sanofi-aventis)

1. NAME OF THE MEDICINAL PRODUCT
Cordarone X Intravenous.

2. QUALITATIVE AND QUANTITATIVE COMPOSITION
Each 3ml ampoule contains 150mg amiodarone hydrochloride.

For excipients, see 6.1

3. PHARMACEUTICAL FORM
Solution for injection.

4. CLINICAL PARTICULARS

4.1 Therapeutic indications
Treatment should be initiated and normally monitored only under hospital or specialist supervision. Cordarone X Intravenous is indicated only for the treatment of severe rhythm disorders not responding to other therapies or when other treatments cannot be used.

Tachyarrhythmias associated with Wolff-Parkinson-White syndrome.

All types of tachyarrhythmias including supraventricular, nodal and ventricular tachycardias; atrial flutter and fibrillation; ventricular fibrillation; when other drugs cannot be used.

Cordarone X Intravenous can be used where a rapid response is required or where oral administration is not possible.

4.2 Posology and method of administration
Cordarone X Intravenous should only be used when facilities exist for cardiac monitoring, defibrillation, and cardiac pacing.

Cordarone X Intravenous may be used prior to DC cardioversion.

The standard recommended dose is 5mg/kg bodyweight given by intravenous infusion over a period of 20 minutes to 2 hours. This should be administered as a dilute solution in 250ml 5% dextrose. This may be followed by repeat infusion up to 1200mg (approximately 15mg/kg bodyweight) in up to 500ml 5% dextrose per 24 hours, the rate of infusion being adjusted on the basis of clinical response. *(see section 4.4)*.

In extreme clinical emergency the drug may, at the discretion of the clinician, be given as a slow injection of 150-300mg in 10-20ml 5% dextrose over a minimum of 3 minutes. This should not be repeated for at least 15 minutes. Patients treated in this way with Cordarone X Intravenous must be closely monitored, e.g. in an intensive care unit.*(see section 4.4)*.

Changeover from Intravenous to Oral Therapy

As soon as an adequate response has been obtained, oral therapy should be initiated concomitantly at the usual loading dose (i.e. 200mg three times a day). Cordarone X Intravenous should then be phased out gradually.

Paediatric population

Due to the presence of benzyl alcohol, intravenous amiodarone is usually contraindicated in neonates and premature babies *(see section 4.3)*.

No controlled paediatric studies have been undertaken. In published uncontrolled studies effective doses for children were *(see section 4.4)*:

• Loading dose: 5mg/kg body weight over 20 minutes to 2 hours

• Maintenance dose: 10 to 15mg/kg/day from a few hours to several days.

If needed, oral therapy may be initiated concomitantly.

Elderly

As with all patients it is important that the minimum effective dose is used. Whilst there is no evidence that dosage requirements are different for this group of patients they may be more susceptible to bradycardia and conduction defects if too high a dose is employed. Particular attention should be paid to monitoring thyroid function *(see sections 4.3, 4.4 and 4.8)*.

See section 6.2 for information on incompatibilities

4.3 Contraindications
Sinus bradycardia and sino-atrial heart block. In patients with severe conduction disturbances (high grade AV block, bifascicular or trifascicular block) or sinus node disease, Cordarone X should be used only in conjunction with a pacemaker.

Evidence or history of thyroid dysfunction. Thyroid function tests should be performed where appropriate prior to therapy in all patients.

Severe respiratory failure, circulatory collapse, or severe arterial hypotension; hypotension, heart failure and cardiomyopathy are also contra-indications when using Cordarone X Intravenous as a bolus injection.

Known hypersensitivity to iodine or to amiodarone, or to any of the excipients. (One ampoule contains approximately 56mg iodine).

The combination of Cordarone X with drugs which may induce torsades de pointes is contra-indicated *(see section 4.5)*.

Cordarone X Intravenous ampoules contain benzyl alcohol. There have been reports of fatal 'gasping syndrome' in neonates (hypotension, bradycardia and cardiovascular collapse) following the administration of intravenous solution containing this preservative. Cordarone X Intravenous should not be given to neonates or premature babies unless the rhythm disturbance is life threatening and either resistant to other medication or alternative therapy is deemed inappropriate.

Pregnancy - except in exceptional circumstances *(see section 4.6)*

Lactation *(see section 4.6)*

4.4 Special warnings and special precautions for use
Benzyl alcohol may cause toxic reactions and allergic reactions in infants and children up to 3 years old.

Cordarone X Intravenous should only be used in a special care unit under continuous monitoring (ECG and blood pressure).

IV infusion is preferred to bolus due to the haemodynamic effects sometimes associated with rapid injection *(see section 4.8)*. Circulatory collapse may be precipitated by too rapid administration or overdosage (atropine has been used successfully in such patients presenting with bradycardia).

Repeated or continuous infusion via peripheral veins may lead to injection site reactions *(see section 4.8)*. When repeated or continuous infusion is anticipated, administration by a central venous catheter is recommended.

When given by infusion Cordarone X may reduce drop size and, if appropriate, adjustments should be made to the rate of infusion.

Anaesthesia *(see section 4.5)*: Before surgery, the anaesthetist should be informed that the patient is taking amiodarone.

Cardiac disorders:

Caution should be exercised in patients with hypotension and decompensated cardiomyopathy and severe heart failure *(also see section 4.3)*.

Amiodarone has a low pro-arrhythmic effect. Onsets of new arrhythmias or worsening of treated arrhythmias, sometimes fatal, have been reported. It is important, but difficult to differentiate a lack of efficacy of the drug from a proarrhythmic effect, whether or not this is associated with a worsening of the cardiac condition. Proarrhythmic effects generally occur in the context of drug interactions and/or electrolytic disorders *(see sections 4.5 and 4.8)*.

Too high a dosage may lead to severe bradycardia and to conduction disturbances with the appearance of an idioventricular rhythm, particularly in elderly patients or during digitalis therapy. In these circumstances, Cordarone X treatment should be withdrawn. If necessary beta-adrenostimulants or glucagon may be given. Because of the long half-life of amiodarone, if bradycardia is severe and symptomatic the insertion of a pacemaker should be considered.

The pharmacological action of amiodarone induces ECG changes: QT prolongation (related to prolonged repolarisation) with the possible development of U-waves and deformed T-waves; these changes do not reflect toxicity.

Respiratory, thoracic and mediastinal disorders *(see section 4.8)*:

Very rare cases of interstitial pneumonitis have been reported with intravenous amiodarone. When the diagnosis is suspected, a chest X-ray should be performed. Amiodarone therapy should be re-evaluated since interstitial pneumonitis is generally reversible following early withdrawal of amiodarone, and corticosteroid therapy should be considered *(see section 4.8)*. Clinical symptoms often resolve within a few weeks followed by slower radiological and lung function improvement. Some patients can deteriorate despite discontinuing Cordarone X. Fatal cases of pulmonary toxicity have been reported.

Very rare cases of severe respiratory complications, sometimes fatal, have been observed usually in the period immediately following surgery (adult acute respiratory distress syndrome); a possible interaction with a high oxygen concentration may be implicated *(see sections 4.5 and 4.8)*.

Hepato-biliary disorders *(see section 4.8)*

Severe hepatocellular insufficiency may occur within the first 24 hours of IV amiodarone, and may sometimes be fatal. Close monitoring of transaminases is therefore recommended as soon as amiodarone is started.

Drug interactions *(see section 4.5)*

Concomitant use of amiodarone with the following drugs is not recommended; beta-blockers, heart rate lowering calcium channel inhibitors (verapamil, diltiazem), stimulant laxative agents which may cause hypokalaemia.

Increased plasma levels of flecainide have been reported with co-administration of amiodarone. The flecainide dose should be reduced accordingly and the patient closely monitored.

4.5 Interaction with other medicinal products and other forms of Interaction
Some of the more important drugs that interact with amiodarone include warfarin, digoxin, phenytoin and any drug which prolongs the QT interval.

Amiodarone raises the plasma concentrations of oral anticoagulants (warfarin) and phenytoin by inhibition of CYP 2C9. The dose of warfarin should be reduced accordingly. More frequent monitoring of prothrombin time both during and after amiodarone treatment is recommended. Phenytoin dosage should be reduced if signs of overdosage appear, and plasma levels may be measured.

Administration of Cordarone X to a patient already receiving digoxin will bring about an increase in the plasma digoxin concentration and thus precipitate symptoms and signs associated with high digoxin levels. Clinical, ECG and biological monitoring is recommended and digoxin dosage should be halved. A synergistic effect on heart rate and atrioventricular conduction is also possible.

Combined therapy with the following drugs which prolong the QT interval is contra-indicated (*see 4.3 Contra-indications*) due to the increased risk of torsades de pointes; for example:

• Class Ia anti-arrhythmic drugs e.g. quinidine, procainamide, disopyramide

• Class III anti-arrhythmic drugs e.g. sotalol, bretylium

• intravenous erythromycin, co-trimoxazole or pentamidine injection

• some anti-psychotics e.g. chlorpromazine, thioridazine, fluphenazine, pimozide, haloperidol, amisulpride and sertindole

• lithium and tricyclic anti-depressants e.g. doxepin, maprotiline, amitriptyline

• certain antihistamines e.g. terfenadine, astemizole, mizolastine

• anti-malarials e.g. quinine, mefloquine, chloroquine, halofantrine.

Combined therapy with the following drugs is not recommended:

• Beta blockers and certain calcium channel inhibitors (diltiazem, verapamil); potentiation of negative chronotropic properties and conduction slowing effects may occur.

• Stimulant laxatives, which may cause hypokalaemia thus increasing the risk of torsades de pointes; other types of laxatives should be used.

Caution should be exercised over combined therapy with the following drugs which may also cause hypokalaemia and/or hypomagnesaemia: e.g. diuretics, systemic corticosteroids, tetracosactide, intravenous amphotericin.

In cases of hypokalaemia, corrective action should be taken and QT interval monitored. In case of torsades de pointes antiarrhythmic agents should not be given; pacing may be instituted and IV magnesium may be used.

Caution is advised in patients undergoing general anaesthesia, or receiving high dose oxygen therapy. Potentially severe complications have been reported in patients taking amiodarone undergoing general anaesthesia: bradycardia unresponsive to atropine, hypotension, disturbances of conduction, decreased cardiac output. A few cases of adult respiratory distress syndrome, most often in the period immediately after surgery, have been observed. A possible interaction with a high oxygen concentration may be implicated.

Drugs metabolised by cytochrome P450 3A4

When such drugs are co-administered with amiodarone, an inhibitor of CYP 3A4, this may result in a higher level of their plasma concentrations, which may lead to a possible increase in their toxicity:

• Cyclosporin: plasma levels of cyclosporin may increase as much as 2-fold when used in combination. A reduction in the dose of cyclosporin may be necessary to maintain the plasma concentration within the therapeutic range.

• Other drugs metabolised by cytochrome P450 3A4: examples of such drugs are the statins (such as simvastatin), lidocaine, tacrolimus, sildenafil, fentanyl, midazolam and ergotamine.

Flecainide

Given that flecainide is mainly metabolised by CYP 2D6, by inhibiting this isoenzyme, amiodarone may increase flecainide plasma levels; it is advised to reduce the flecainide dose by 50% and to monitor the patient closely for adverse effects. Monitoring of flecainide plasma levels is strongly recommended in such circumstances.

Interaction with substrates of other CYP 450 isoenzymes

In vitro studies show that amiodarone also has the potential to inhibit CYP 1A2, CYP 2C19 and CYP 2D6 through its main metabolite. When co-administered, amiodarone would be expected to increase the plasma concentration of drugs whose metabolism is dependent upon CYP 1A2, CYP 2C19 and CYP 2D6.

4.6 Pregnancy and lactation

Pregnancy

There are insufficient data on the use of amiodarone during pregnancy in humans to judge any possible toxicity. However, in view of its effect on the foetal thyroid gland, amiodarone is contraindicated during pregnancy, except in exceptional circumstances.

Lactation

Amiodarone is excreted into the breast milk in significant quantities and breast-feeding is contra-indicated.

4.7 Effects on ability to drive and use machines

Not relevant.

4.8 Undesirable effects

The following adverse reactions are classified by system organ class and ranked under heading of frequency using the following convention: very common > = 10%), common > = 1% and < 10%); uncommon > = 0.1% and < 1%); rare > = 0.01% and < 0.1%), very rare (< 0.01%).

Cardiac disorders:

- Common: bradycardia, generally moderate.
- Very rare:

- marked bradycardia, sinus arrest requiring discontinuation of amiodarone, especially in patients with sinus node dysfunction and/or in elderly patients

- onset of worsening of arrythmia, sometimes followed by cardiac arrest *(see sections 4.4 and 4.5)*.

Gastrointestinal disorders:

- Very rare: nausea.

General disorders and administration site conditions:

- Common: injection site reactions such as pain, erythema, oedema, necrosis, extravasation, infiltration, inflammation, induration, thrombophlebitis, phlebitis, cellulitis, infection, pigmentation changes.

Hepato-biliary disorders:

- Very rare:

- isolated increase in serum transaminases, which is usually moderate (1.5 to 3 times normal range) at the beginning of therapy. They may return to normal with dose reduction or even spontaneously.

- acute liver disorders with high serum transaminases and/or jaundice, including hepatic failure, sometimes fatal *(see section 4.4)*.

Immune system disorders:

- Very rare: anaphylactic shock.

Nervous system disorders:

- Very rare: benign intra-cranial hypertension (pseudo tumor cerebri), headache.

Respiratory, thoracic and mediastinal disorders:

- Very rare:

- interstitial pneumonitis *(see section 4.4)*

- severe respiratory complications (adult acute respiratory distress syndrome), sometimes fatal *(see sections 4.4 and 4.5)*

- bronchospasm and/or apnoea in case of severe respiratory failure, and especially in asthmatic patients.

Skin and subcutaneous tissue disorders:

- Very rare: sweating.

Vascular disorders:

- Common: decrease in blood pressure, usually moderate and transient. Cases of hypotension or collapse have been reported following overdosage or a too rapid injection.
- Very rare: hot flushes.

4.9 Overdose

There is no information regarding overdosage with intravenous amiodarone.

Little information is available regarding acute overdosage with oral amiodarone. Few cases of sinus bradycardia, heart block, attacks of ventricular tachycardia, torsades de pointes, circulatory failure and hepatic injury have been reported.

In the event of overdose, treatment should be symptomatic, in addition to general supportive measures. The patient should be monitored and if bradycardia occurs beta-adrenostimulants or glucagon may be given.

Spontaneously resolving attacks of ventricular tachycardia may also occur. Due to the pharmacokinetics of amiodarone, adequate and prolonged surveillance of the patient, particularly cardiac status, is recommended.

Neither amiodarone nor its metabolites are dialysable.

5. PHARMACOLOGICAL PROPERTIES

5.1 Pharmacodynamic properties

Cordarone is a product for the treatment of tachyarrhythmias and has complex pharmacological actions. Its effects are anti-adrenergic (partial alpha and beta blocker). It has haemodynamic effects (increased blood flow and systemic/coronary vasodilation). The drug reduces myocardial oxygen consumption and has been shown to have a sparing effect of rat myocardial ATP utilisation, with decreased oxidative processes. Amiodarone inhibits the metabolic and biochemical effects of catecholamines on the heart and inhibits Na^+ and K^+ activated ATP-ase.

5.2 Pharmacokinetic properties

Pharmacokinetics of amiodarone are unusual and complex, and have not been completely elucidated. Absorption following oral administration is variable and may be prolonged, with enterohepatic cycling. The major metabolite is desethylamiodarone. Amiodarone is highly protein bound > 95%). Renal excretion is minimal and faecal excretion is the major route. A study in both healthy volunteers and patients after intravenous administration of amiodarone reported that the calculated volumes of distribution and total blood clearance using a two-compartment open model were similar for both groups. Elimination of amiodarone after intravenous injection appeared to be biexponential with a distribution phase lasting about 4 hours. The very high volume of distribution combined with a relatively low apparent volume for the central compartment suggests extensive tissue distribution. A bolus IV injection of 400mg gave a terminal T½ of approximately 11 hours.

5.3 Preclinical safety data

There are no pre-clinical data of relevance to the prescriber which are additional to that already included in other sections of the SPC.

6. PHARMACEUTICAL PARTICULARS

6.1 List of excipients

Benzyl alcohol, Polysorbate and Water for Injections.

6.2 Incompatibilities

Cordarone X Intravenous is incompatible with saline and should be administered solely in 5% dextrose solution. Cordarone X Intravenous, diluted with 5% dextrose solution to a concentration of less than 0.6mg/ml, is unstable. Solutions containing less than 2 ampoules Cordarone X Intravenous in 500ml dextrose 5% are unstable and should not be used.

The use of administration equipment or devices containing plasticizers such as DEHP (di-2-ethylhexylphthalate) in the presence of amiodarone may result in leaching out of DEHP. In order to minimise patient exposure to DEHP, the final amiodarone dilution for infusion should preferably be administered through non DEHP-containing sets.

6.3 Shelf life

24 months.

6.4 Special precautions for storage

Do not store above 25°C. Store in the original container.

6.5 Nature and contents of container

Each carton contains ten glass ampoules.

6.6 Instructions for use and handling

Refer to 4.2 above.

7. MARKETING AUTHORISATION HOLDER

Sanofi-Synthelabo

PO Box 597

Guildford

Surrey

8. MARKETING AUTHORISATION NUMBER(S)

PL 11723/0014.

9. DATE OF FIRST AUTHORISATION/RENEWAL OF THE AUTHORISATION

14th May 1998

10. DATE OF REVISION OF THE TEXT

May 2004

Legal category: POM

Corgard Tablets 80mg

(sanofi-aventis)

1. NAME OF THE MEDICINAL PRODUCT

Corgard Tablets 80mg

2. QUALITATIVE AND QUANTITATIVE COMPOSITION

The tablets contain Nadolol 80.0mg.

3. PHARMACEUTICAL FORM

Tablet.

White, capsule-shaped, biconvex scored tablet.

4. CLINICAL PARTICULARS

4.1 Therapeutic indications

Corgard is indicated in the management of:

Angina Pectoris: For the long-term management of patients with angina pectoris by continuous medication.

Hypertension: For the long-term management of essential hypertension, either alone or in combination with other antihypertensive agents, especially thiazide-type diuretics.

Arrhythmias: For the treatment of cardiac tachyarrhythmias.

Migraine: For the prophylactic management of migraine headache. The efficacy of

Corgard in the treatment of a migraine attack that has already started has not been established, and Corgard is not indicated for such use.

Thyrotoxicosis: For the relief of the symptoms of hyperthyroidism and the pre-operative preparation of patients for surgery. Nadolol may be used in conjunction with conventional antithyroid therapy.

4.2 Posology and method of administration

Adults:

Dosage should be titrated gradually with at least a week between increments to assess response; individuals show considerable variation in their response to beta-adrenergic blockade.

Corgard may be given in a once daily dosage without regard to meals. The dosage interval should be increased when creatinine clearance is below 50ml/min/1.73m².

If Corgard is to be discontinued, reduce dosage over a period of at least two weeks (see warnings).

Angina pectoris: Initially 40mg once daily. This may be increased at weekly intervals until an adequate response is obtained or excessive bradycardia occurs. Most patients respond to 160mg or less daily. The value and safety of daily doses exceeding 240mg have not been established.

Hypertension: Initially 80mg once daily. This may be increased by a weekly increment of 80mg or less until an optimum response is obtained. Many patients respond to 80mg daily, and most patients respond to 240mg or less, daily, but higher doses have been required for a few patients. In some patients it is necessary to administer a diuretic, peripheral vasolidator and/or other antihypertensive agents in conjunction with nadolol in order to achieve satisfactory response.

Treatment of hypertension associated with phaeochromocytoma may require the addition of an alpha-blocking agent.

Cardiac tachyarrhythmias: Initially 40mg once daily. This may be increased if necessary to 160mg once daily. If bradycardia occurs dosage should be reduced to 40mg once daily.

Migraine: The initial dose of nadolol is 40mg once daily. Dosage may be gradually increased in 40mg increments until optimum migraine prophylaxis is achieved. The usual maintenance dose is 80 to 160mg administered once daily. After 4 to 6 weeks at the maximum dose if a satisfactory response is not obtained, therapy with nadolol should be withdrawn gradually.

Thyrotoxicosis: The dosage range is 80-160mg once daily. It has been found that most patients require a dose of 160mg once daily. Nadolol may be used together with conventional anti-thyroid treatment. For the preparation of patients for partial thyroidectomy, nadolol should be administered in conjunction with potassium iodide for a period of 10 days prior to operation. Nadolol should be administered on the morning of operation. Post-operatively, nadolol dosage should be slowly reduced and then withdrawn following clinical stability.

Children:

Safety and effectiveness in children have not been established.

Elderly:

In elderly patients a low initial dose should be used so that sensitivity to side-effects may be assessed.

Renal or hepatic impairment

As with all drugs patients with impaired renal or hepatic function should be monitored.

4.3 Contraindications

- Bronchial asthma or a history of asthma
- Sinus bradycardia
- Greater than first degree atrioventricular conduction block
- Cardiogenic shock
- Right ventricular failure secondary to pulmonary hypertension
- Overt cardiac failure (see 4.4 – Special warnings and special precautions for use)
- Previously demonstrated hypersensitivity to nadolol

4.4 Special warnings and special precautions for use

Warnings

Exacerbation of Ischaemic Heart Disease Following Abrupt Withdrawal

Hypersensitivity to catecholamines has been observed in patients withdrawn from beta-blocker therapy; exacerbation of angina, hypertension, and, in some cases, myocardial infarction have occurred after *abrupt* discontinuation of such therapy. When discontinuing chronically administered nadolol, particularly in patients with ischaemic heart disease, the dosage should be gradually reduced over a period of one to two weeks, and the patient should be carefully monitored. If angina markedly worsens or acute coronary insufficiency develops, nadolol administration should be re-instituted promptly (at least temporarily), and other measures appropriate for the management of unstable angina should be taken. Patients should be warned against interruption or discontinuation of therapy without the physician's advice. Because coronary artery disease is common and may be unrecognised, it may be prudent not to discontinue nadolol therapy abruptly, even in patients under treatment for hypertension alone.

Patients with a History of Cardiac Failure - Sympathetic stimulation may be a vital component supporting circulatory function in patients with congestive heart failure, and beta-blockade may worsen failure.

Although beta-blockers including nadolol should be avoided in overt congestive heart failure, they can be cautiously used, if necessary, in patients with a history of heart failure who are well compensated (usually with digitalis and diuretics). Beta-adrenergic blocking agents do not abolish the inotropic action of digitalis on heart muscle.

Patients Without a History of Heart Failure - Continued depression of the myocardium with beta blockade over a period of time can, in some cases, lead to cardiac failure. At the first sign or symptom of impending heart failure, the patient should be fully digitalised and/or treated with diuretics, and the response observed closely.

If cardiac failure continues despite adequate digitalisation and diuresis, Corgard should be withdrawn (gradually, if possible).

Major Surgery - Beta-blockade impairs the ability of the heart to respond to reflex stimuli and may increase the risks of general anaesthesia and surgical procedures, resulting in protracted hypotension or low cardiac output. It has generally been suggested that beta blocker therapy should be withdrawn several days prior to surgery. Recognition of the increased sensitivity to catecholamines of patients recently withdrawn from beta-blocker therapy, however, has made this recommendation controversial. If possible, beta-blockers including nadolol should be withdrawn well before surgery takes place.

In no circumstances should beta-blockers be discontinued prior to surgery in patients with phaeochromocytoma or thyrotoxicosis.

In the event of emergency surgery, the anaesthesiologist should be informed that the patient is on beta-blocker therapy. The effects of nadolol can be reversed by administration of beta-receptor agonists such as isoprenaline or dobutamine. However, such patients may be subject to protracted severe hypotension. Difficulty in restarting and maintaining the heart beat has also been reported with beta-adrenergic receptor blocking agents.

(An exception to the above paragraph is thyroid surgery—see under 'Thyrotoxicosis' in section 4.1 Indications and section 4.2 Posology and method of administration).

Nonallergic Bronchospasm (e.g. chronic bronchitis, emphysema) - Patients with bronchospastic diseases should not, in general, receive beta-blockers since they may block bronchodilation produced by endogenous or exogenous catecholamine stimulation of beta receptors.

(NOTE: Corgard is contra-indicated in asthmatic patients.)

Diabetes and Hypoglycaemia - Beta-adrenergic blockade may prevent the appearance of warning signs and symptoms (e.g. tachycardia and blood pressure changes) of acute hypoglycaemia. This is especially important with labile diabetics. Beta-blockade also reduces the release of insulin in response to hyperglycaemia; therefore, it may be necessary to adjust the dose of anti-diabetic drugs.

Skin Rashes - There have been reports of skin rashes (including a psoriasiform type) and/or ocular changes (conjunctivitis and 'dry eye') associated with the use of beta-adrenergic blocking drugs. The reported incidence is small and in most cases the symptoms have cleared when the treatment was withdrawn. Discontinuation of the drug should be considered if any such reaction is not otherwise explicable. Cessation of the therapy with a beta-adrenergic blocker should be gradual.

Treatment for Anaphylactic Reaction - While taking beta-blockers, patients with a history of severe anaphylactic reaction may be more reactive to repeated challenge, either accidental, diagnostic, or therapeutic. Such patients may be unresponsive to the usual doses of epinephrine used to treat allergic reaction.

(NOTE: Epinephrine combined with non cardio-selective beta blockers such as nadolol can cause a hypertensive episode followed by bradycardia.)

Thyrotoxicosis - Beta-adrenergic blockade may mask certain clinical signs of hyperthyroidism (e.g. tachycardia). Abrupt withdrawal of nadolol in thyroid patients can precipitate thyroid storm.

Precautions

Occasionally, beta-blockade with drugs such as nadolol may produce hypotension and/or marked bradycardia, resulting in vertigo, syncope or orthostatic hypotension.

Impaired Renal or Hepatic Function - Nadolol should be used with caution in patients with impaired renal or hepatic function (see section 4.2 Posology and method of administration).

Carcinogenesis, Mutagenesis, Impairment of Fertility - In chronic oral toxicologic studies lasting one to two years, nadolol did not produce any significant toxic effects in mice, rats, or dogs. In two-year oral carcinogenic studies in rats and mice, nadolol did not produce any neoplastic, pre-neoplastic, or non-neoplastic pathologic lesions. In fertility and general reproductive performance studies in rats, nadolol caused no adverse effects.

4.5 Interaction with other medicinal products and other forms of Interaction

General anaesthetics - Those which cause myocardial depression such as chloroform, cyclopropane, trichloroethylene and ether should be avoided as the patient may be subject to protracted severe hypotension. (see Major Surgery in section 4.4 Special warnings and special precautions for use).

Myocardial depressants such as lignocaine and procainamide may subject the patient to protracted severe hypotension.

Adrenoceptor Stimulants - Beta-adrenoceptor stimulants such as isoprenaline and verapamil, or alpha-adrenoceptor stimulants such as noradrenaline and adrenaline, will reverse the hypotensive effects and increase vasoconstrictor activity.

Catecholamine Depleting Drugs - - Additive effects may occur with nadolol; monitor closely for evidence of hypotension and/or excessive bradycardia (e.g. vertigo, syncope, postural hypotension).

Antihypertensives (*e.g. neurone-blocking drugs, vasodilators, diuretics*) Additive hypotensive effect.

Clonidine - If Corgard and clonidine are given concurrently, clonidine should not be discontinued until several days after Corgard withdrawal.

Antidiabetic drugs *(oral agents and insulin)* - Hypoglycaemia or hyperglycaemia; adjust dosage of anti-diabetic drug accordingly (see Diabetes and Hypoglycaemia in section 4.4 Special warnings and special precautions for use).

Monoamine oxidase inhibitors (MAOIs) - Isolated cases of bradycardia have occurred during concurrent use of beta blockers and MAOIs.

Antimuscarinic agents - May counteract the bradycardia caused by beta blockers.

Calcium-channel blockers - Calcium channel blockers generally potentiate the pharmacologic effects of beta-blockers. Patients taking both agents should be carefully monitored for adverse cardiovascular events.

Other antiarrhythmic agents - Additive or antagonistic effects may occur with nadolol.

Lidocaine, IV - Significant reduction of lidocaine clearance can occur when a beta blocker is administered concurrently.

Non-steroidal anti-inflammatory agents (NSAIDs) - The antihypertensive effects of beta blockers may be reduced during concurrent administration of indomethacin and possibly other NSAIDs.

Phenothiazines and other antipsychotic agents - Additive antihypertensive effects have occurred with other beta blockers when they were given concurrently with phenothiazines or haloperidol.

Vasoconstrictor Agents - Effects with nadolol can be additive (e.g. with ergot alkaloids).

4.6 Pregnancy and lactation

Pregnancy

There are no adequate and well-controlled studies in pregnant women. In animal reproduction studies with nadolol, evidence of embryo- and foetotoxicity was found in rabbits, but not in rats or hamsters, at doses 5 to 10 times greater (on a mg/kg basis) than the maximum indicated human dose. No teratogenic potential was observed in any of these species.

Nadolol should be used during pregnancy only if the potential benefit justifies the potential risk to the foetus.

Neonates whose mothers are receiving nadolol at parturition have exhibited bradycardia, hypoglycaemia, and associated symptoms.

Lactation

Nadolol is excreted in human milk. Because of the potential for adverse effects in nursing infants, a decision should be made whether to discontinue nursing or to discontinue therapy, taking into account the importance of nadolol to the mother.

4.7 Effects on ability to drive and use machines

There are no studies on the effect of this medicine on the ability to drive. When driving vehicles or operating machines it should be taken into account that occasionally dizziness or fatigue may occur.

4.8 Undesirable effects

Most adverse effects have been mild and transient and have rarely required withdrawal of therapy. The percentages given below were based on a population of 1440 patients taking nadolol in clinical trials.

Cardiovascular:

Bradycardia (heart rate <60 BPM) occurs commonly in nadolol-treated patients; heart rate <40 BPM and/or symptomatic bradycardia occurred in approximately 2% of patients; Symptoms of peripheral vascular insufficiency, usually of the Raynaud type (approximately 2%);

Cardiac failure, hypotension, and rhythm/conduction disturbances (about 1%). Single instances of first-degree and third-degree heart block have been reported; intensification of AV block is a known effect of beta-blockers (see also section 4.3 Contra-indications, and section 4.4 Special warnings and special precautions for use).

Central Nervous System:

Dizziness or fatigue has been reported in approximately 2% of patients; paraesthesias, sedation, and change in behaviour have each been reported in approximately 0.6% of patients. Light-headedness, insomnia and cold extremities have also been reported.

Gastrointestinal:

Nausea, diarrhoea, abdominal discomfort, constipation, vomiting, indigestion, anorexia, bloating and flatulence have been reported in 0.1% to 0.5% of patients.

Respiratory:

Bronchospasm has been reported in approximately 0.1% of patients (see section 4.3 Contraindications and section 4.4 Special warnings and precautions for use).

Miscellaneous:

Each of the following has been reported in 0.1% to 0.5% of patients: rash; pruritus; headache; dry mouth, eyes or skin; impotence or decreased libido; facial swelling; weight gain; slurred speech; cough; nasal stuffiness; sweating; tinnitus; blurred vision. Reversible alopaecia has been reported infrequently.

The events listed below have also occurred with nadolol and/or other beta-adrenergic blocking agents; however, no causal relationship to nadolol was established:

Central Nervous System - Reversible depression progressing to catatonia; visual disturbances; hallucinations; an acute reversible syndrome characterised by disorientation for time and place, short-term memory loss, emotional lability, slightly clouded sensorium, and decreased performance on neuropsychologic tests.

Gastrointestinal - Mesenteric arterial thrombosis; ischaemic colitis; elevated liver enzymes.

Haematologic - Agranulocytosis; thrombocytopaenic or non-thrombocytopaenic purpura.

Allergic - Fever combined with aching, and sore throat; laryngospasm; respiratory distress.

Miscellaneous - Pemphigoid rash; hypertensive reaction in patients with pheochromocytoma; sleep disturbances; Peyronie's disease.

4.9 Overdose

In the event of overdosage, nadolol may cause excessive bradycardia, cardiac failure, hypotension, or bronchospasm.

Transitory increase in BUN has been reported, and serum electrolyte changes may occur, especially in patients with impaired renal function.

Treatment

Nadolol can be removed from the general circulation by haemodialysis. In determining the duration of corrective therapy, note must be taken of the long duration of the effect of nadolol.

In addition to gastric lavage, the following measures should be employed, as appropriate:

Excessive Bradycardia - Administer atropine (0.25 to 1.0 mg). If there is no response to vagal blockade, administer isoprenaline cautiously.

Cardiac Failure - Administer a digitalis glycoside and diuretic. It has been reported that glucagon may also be useful in this situation.

Hypotension - If fluid administration is ineffective, administer vasopressors such as dopamine, dobutamine or adrenaline.

Bronchospasm - Administer a beta-2-agonist agent and/or a theophylline derivative.

Stupor or coma - Supportive therapy as warranted.

Gastrointestinal Effects - Symptomatic treatment as needed.

BUN and/or Serum Electrolyte Abnormalities - Institute supportive measures as required to maintain hydration, electrolyte balance, respiration, and cardiovascular and renal function.

5. PHARMACOLOGICAL PROPERTIES

5.1 Pharmacodynamic properties

Nadolol is a beta-adrenergic receptor blocking agent with a prolonged activity, permitting once-daily dosage in angina, hypertension, cardiac arrhythmias, the prophylaxis of migraine, and the relief of hyperthyroid symptoms.

Nadolol is not metabolised. It has no membrane stabilising or intrinsic sympathomimetic activity, and its only effect on the autonomic nervous system is one of beta-adrenergic blockade. Nadolol is nonselective.

Receptor blockade by nadolol results in protection from excessive inappropriate sympathetic activity. Nadolol reduces the number and severity of attacks of angina pectoris by blocking response to catecholamine stimulation and thus lowers the oxygen requirement of the heart at any given level of effort.

Nadolol reduces both supine and erect blood pressure. Like other beta-blockers nadolol exerts an antiarrhythmic action. Nadolol has been shown to reduce the rapid ventricular response which accompanies atrial fibrillation/flutter by slowing conduction through the A-V node. Beta-blockade is of particular value in arrhythmias caused by increased levels of, or sensitivity of the heart to, circulating catecholamines, e.g. arrhythmias associated with phaeochromocytoma, thyrotoxicosis, or exercise. Nadolol is effective in reducing ventricular premature beats in selected patients.

Nadolol exerts an effect in the prophylaxis of migraine by a mechanism which may involve prevention of vasoconstriction in the area served by the internal carotid artery and prevention of excessive adrenergic vasodilation in the external carotid artery.

Nadolol alleviates the symptoms of thyrotoxicosis and provides symptomatic control before and during thyroid surgery.

Beta-blocking agents have been shown in large scale studies to reduce mortality by preventing reinfarction and sudden death in patients surviving their first myocardial infarction.

5.2 Pharmacokinetic properties

About 30 percent of an oral dose of Corgard is absorbed. Peak serum concentrations usually occur in 3 to 4 hours after drug administration. The presence of food in the gastrointestinal tract does not affect the rate or extent of Corgard absorption. Approximately 30 percent of the Corgard present in serum is reversibly bound to plasma protein. Unlike most available beta-blocking agents, Corgard is not metabolised, and is excreted unchanged principally by the kidneys. The serum half-life of therapeutic doses of Corgard is relatively long, ranging from 20 to 24 hours (permitting once daily dosage). A significant correlation between minimum steady-state serum concentrations of Corgard and total oral daily dose has been demonstrated in hypertensive patients; however, the observed dose-response range is wide and proper dosage requires individual titration.

5.3 Preclinical safety data

None stated.

6. PHARMACEUTICAL PARTICULARS

6.1 List of excipients

The tablets also contain microcrystalline cellulose and magnesium stearate.

6.2 Incompatibilities

Not applicable.

6.3 Shelf life

36 months.

6.4 Special precautions for storage

Do not store above 25°C.

6.5 Nature and contents of container

PVC/aluminium foil blister packs in cartons containing 28 tablets.

6.6 Instructions for use and handling

None stated.

7. MARKETING AUTHORISATION HOLDER

Sanofi-Synthelabo
PO Box 597
Guildford
Surrey

8. MARKETING AUTHORISATION NUMBER(S)

PL 11723/0100

9. DATE OF FIRST AUTHORISATION/RENEWAL OF THE AUTHORISATION

24 November 1995/23 September 2004

10. DATE OF REVISION OF THE TEXT

24 September 2004

Legal Category POM

Corlan Pellets

(UCB Pharma Limited)

1. NAME OF THE MEDICINAL PRODUCT

Corlan Pellets

2. QUALITATIVE AND QUANTITATIVE COMPOSITION

Each pellet contains 2.5mg Hydrocortisone in the form of the ester hydrocortisone sodium succinate

For excipients, see 6.1

3. PHARMACEUTICAL FORM

Muco-adhesive buccal tablet

Small white pellet engraved 'Corlan Evans' on one side

4. CLINICAL PARTICULARS

4.1 Therapeutic indications

Local use in previously diagnosed aphthous ulceration of the mouth, whether simple or occurring as a complication in diseases such as sprue, idiopathic steatorrhoea or ulcerative colitis.

4.2 Posology and method of administration

Adults and elderly:

Corlan Pellets should not be sucked, but kept in the mouth and allowed to dissolve slowly in close proximity to the ulcers. One pellet should be used in this way four times a day. If the ulcers have not healed after 5 days of treatment (completion of one pack), or if they recur quickly after healing, a doctor should be consulted.

Children under 12 years of age:

Children under 12 years old must see a doctor before starting each course of Corlan Pellets.

4.3 Contraindications

Corlan Pellets should not be used in the presence of oral infection unless effective appropriate anti-infective therapy is also employed. Hypersensitivity to any component of the product.

4.4 Special warnings and special precautions for use

If aphthous ulceration is severe or recurring, serious underlying disease should be excluded.

4.5 Interaction with other medicinal products and other forms of Interaction

None known.

4.6 Pregnancy and lactation

There is inadequate evidence of safety in human pregnancy. Topical administration of corticosteroids to pregnant animals can cause abnormalities of foetal development including cleft palate and intra-uterine growth retardation. There may, therefore, be a very small risk of such effects in the human foetus.

4.7 Effects on ability to drive and use machines

None known.

4.8 Undesirable effects

Corticosteroids may worsen diabetes.

Occasionally, topical therapy may result in an exacerbation of local infection.

Hypersensitivity reactions have occurred with corticosteroids, mainly when administered topically.

Most topically applied corticosteroids may, under certain circumstances, be absorbed in sufficient amounts to produce systemic effects.

4.9 Overdose

Treatment is unlikely to be needed in cases of acute overdosage.

5. PHARMACOLOGICAL PROPERTIES

5.1 Pharmacodynamic properties

ATC Code: A01A C03

None stated.

5.2 Pharmacokinetic properties

None stated.

5.3 Preclinical safety data

None stated.

6. PHARMACEUTICAL PARTICULARS

6.1 List of excipients

Lactose

Acacia

Magnesium Stearate

6.2 Incompatibilities

None known.

6.3 Shelf life

3 years.

6.4 Special precautions for storage

Store below 25°C. Replace cap firmly after use.

6.5 Nature and contents of container

Tamper evident polypropylene container with polythene lid containing 20 pellets.

Tubular glass vials with snap-plug closure containing 20 pellets.

6.6 Instructions for use and handling

None.

7. MARKETING AUTHORISATION HOLDER

UCB Pharma Limited
208 Bath Road
Slough
Berkshire
SL1 3WE
UK

8. MARKETING AUTHORISATION NUMBER(S)

PL 00039/0397

9. DATE OF FIRST AUTHORISATION/RENEWAL OF THE AUTHORISATION

20 January 1993

10. DATE OF REVISION OF THE TEXT

June 2005

Cortisone acetate 25mg

(sanofi-aventis)

1. NAME OF THE MEDICINAL PRODUCT

Cortisone Acetate 25mg Tablets

2. QUALITATIVE AND QUANTITATIVE COMPOSITION

Each tablet contains 25mg of Cortisone Acetate BP

3. PHARMACEUTICAL FORM

Tablet

4. CLINICAL PARTICULARS

4.1 Therapeutic indications

Replacement therapy as in Addison's disease or when the adrenals have been removed surgically or damaged as result of haemorrhage or shock.

4.2 Posology and method of administration

Adults

Acute episodes: doses up to 300mg daily for several days may be required.

Maintenance dosage: 12.5 to 37.5mg daily with, if necessary 0.1mg daily of fludrocortisone to supplement the salt retaining properties of cortisone acetate.

Children

The use of cortisone acetate in children would be limited, as in adults to replacement therapy. Dosage should be limited to a single dose on alternate days to lessen retardation of growth and to minimise suppression of the hypothalamo-pituitary axis.

Elderly

Treatment of elderly patients, particularly if long term, should be planned bearing in mind the more serious consequences of the common side effects of corticosteroids in old age, especially osteoporosis, diabetes, hypertension, susceptibility to infection and thinning of the skin.

4.3 Contraindications

This product is intended for use solely as replacement therapy. Corticosteroids are contraindicated in systemic fungal and viral infections, acute bacterial infections unless specific anti-infective therapy is given.

4.4 Special warnings and special precautions for use

Corticosteroids should be given with care to patients with a history of tuberculosis or the characteristic appearance of tuberculous disease on X-ray. The emergence of tuberculosis can however be prevented by the prophylactic use of anti-tuberculosis therapy.

Administration of corticosteroids may impair the ability to resist and counteract infections: in addition, the clinical signs of and symptoms of infection may be suppressed.

Prolonged corticosteroid treatment is likely to reduce the response of the Pituitary-Adrenal Axis to stress, and relative insufficiency may persist for a year after withdrawal of therapy.

Cortisone acetate should be used with care in diabetes, osteoporosis (post-menopausal women are especially at risk), hypertension, patients with a history of severe affective disorders (especially a history of steroid psychosis), glaucoma or a family history of glaucoma, previous steroid myopathy and epilepsy.

In patients who have received more than physiological doses of systemic corticosteroids (approximately 40mg cortisone or equivalent) for greater than 3 weeks, withdrawal should not be abrupt. How dose reduction should be carried out depends largely on whether the disease is likely to relapse as the dose of systemic corticosteroids is reduced. Clinical assessment of disease activity may be needed during withdrawal. If the disease is unlikely to relapse on withdrawal of systemic corticosteroids but there is uncertainty about HPA suppression, the dose of systemic corticosteroid may be reduced rapidly to physiological doses. Once a daily dose equivalent to 40mg of cortisone is reached, dose reduction should be slower to allow the HPA-axis to recover.

Abrupt withdrawal of systemic corticosteroid treatment, which has continued up to 3 weeks, is appropriate if it is considered that the disease is unlikely to relapse. Abrupt withdrawal of doses of up to 200mg daily cortisone, or equivalent for 3 weeks is unlikely to lead to clinically relevant HPA-axis suppression, in the majority of patients. In the following patient groups, gradual withdrawal of systemic corticosteroid therapy should be considered even after courses lasting 3 weeks or less:

* patients who have had repeated courses of systemic corticosteroids, particularly if taken for greater than 3 weeks.

* when a short course has been prescribed within one year of cessation of long term therapy.

* patients who may have reasons for adrenocortical insufficiency other than exogenous corticosteroid therapy.

* patients receiving doses of systemic corticosteroid greater than 40mg daily of prednisolone or equivalent.

* patients repeatedly taking doses in the evening.

4.5 Interaction with other medicinal products and other forms of Interaction

The effectiveness of anti-coagulants may be increased or decreased with concurrent corticosteroid therapy.

Serum levels of salicylates may increase considerably if corticosteroid therapy is withdrawn, possibly causing intoxication. Since both salicylates and corticosteroids are ulcerogenic, it is possible that there will be an increased rate of gastro-intestinal ulceration.

The action of hypoglycaemic drugs is antagonised by the hypoglycaemic action of corticosteroids.

Since both amphotericin and corticosteroids have potassium depleting effects, signs of hypokalaemia should be looked for during their concurrent use.

There is a small amount of evidence that the use of corticosteroids and methotrexate simultaneously, may cause increased methotrexate toxicity and possible death, although the combination of drugs has been used successfully.

Barbiturates, phenytoin and rifampicin are known to reduce the effects of corticosteroids.

Live virus vaccines should not be administered to patients on immunosuppressant doses of corticosteroids. If inactivated vaccines are administered to such individuals the expected serum antibody response may not be obtained.

In patients treated with systemic corticosteroids, use of non-depolarizing muscle relaxants can result in prolonged relaxation and acute myopathy. Risk factors for this include prolonged and high dose corticosteroids treatment and prolonged duration of muscle paralysis. This interaction is more likely to occur following prolonged ventililation (such as in an ITU setting).

Corticosteroid requirements may be reduced in patients taking estrogens (e.g. contraceptive products)

4.6 Pregnancy and lactation

Pregnancy

The ability of corticosteroids to cross the placenta varies between individual drugs, however cortisone readily crosses the placenta. Administration of corticosteroids to pregnant animals can cause abnormalities of foetal development including cleft palate, intra-uterine growth retardation and affects on brain growth and development. There is no evidence that corticosteroids cause an increased incidence of congenital abnormalities, such as cleft palate/lip in man. However, when administered for prolonged periods or repeatedly during pregnancy, corticosteroids may increase the risk of intrauterine growth retardation. Hypoadrenalism may occur in the neonate following prenatal exposure to corticosteroids but usually resolves spontaneously following birth and is rarely clinically important. As with all drugs, corticosteroids should only be prescribed when the benefits to the mother and child outweigh the risks. When corticosteroids are essential, however, patients with abnormal pregnancies may be treated as though they were in the non-gravid state.

Lactation

Corticosteroids are excreted in breast milk. However, doses of up to 200mg daily of cortisone are unlikely to cause systemic effects in the infant. Infants of mothers taking higher doses than this may have a degree of adrenal suppression but the benefits of breast feeding are likely to out-weigh any theoretical risk.

4.7 Effects on ability to drive and use machines

Not applicable.

4.8 Undesirable effects

The following side-effects may be associated with the long-term systemic use of corticosteroids:-

1. *Gastro-intestinal:* perforations and haemorrhage from peptic ulcer may be presenting features. Fatalities have been reported: perforation of the small and large bowel, particularly in patients with inflammatory bowel disease; other gastro-intestinal side effects include dyspepsia, abdominal distension, oesophageal ulceration candidiasis and acute pancreatitis.

2. *Musculo-skeletal:* muscle weakness, wasting and loss of muscle mass, osteoporosis, vertebral compression fractures, avascular necrosis of bone, pathological fractures of the long bones and tendon rupture. Acute myopathy may be precipitated in patients administered non-depolarising muscle relaxants (See section 4.5).

3. *Endocrine and metabolic:* suppression of growth in childhood and adolescence, menstrual irregularities, amenorrhoea, cushingoid face, hirsutism and weight gain, decreased carbohydrate tolerance with development of classical symptoms of diabetes mellitus, increased need for insulin or oral hypoglycaemic agents in diabetics, negative nitrogen balance due to protein catabolism.

4. *Fluid and electrolyte disturbance:* sodium and water retention leading to congestive heart failure in susceptible subjects, hypertension, potassium loss and hypokalaemic alkalosis.

5. *Dermatological:* impaired wound healing, skin atrophy, patechial haemorrhage and ecchymoses, erythema, telangiectasia, skin striae and acne.

6. *Neuropsychiatric:* euphoria may be marked and may lead to dependence. Insomnia, hypomania and depression have all been reported. Schizophrenia may be aggravated. There is an increased risk of increased intracranial pressure and papilloedema in children. Psychological dependence may be marked.

7. *Opthalmic:* increased intra-ocular pressure with the development of glaucoma, papilloedema, posterior subcapsular cataracts, corneal and scleral thinning or perforation after prolonged use. Viral ophthalmic disease may be re-ignited or spread.

8. *Miscellaneous:* opportunistic infections occur more frequently in corticosteroids recipients; hypersensitivity; thromboembolism and increased appetite have also been reported. Clinical reactivation of previously dormant tuberculosis, leukocytosis (sometimes an almost leukaemoid-like reaction) may occur and there may be a suppression of the hypothalamic-pituitary axis on stopping treatment. Withdrawal after prolonged therapy may result in the characteristic withdrawal symptoms including fever, myalgia, arthralgia and malaise. These may occur even without evidence of adrenal insufficiency. The latter arises from too rapid withdrawal of long-term corticosteroids and may be minimised by gradual reduction of dosage.

4.9 Overdose

Treatment is symptomatic but is unlikely to be required. Blood electrolytes should be observed.

5. PHARMACOLOGICAL PROPERTIES

5.1 Pharmacodynamic properties

Cortisone is a glucocorticoid. It has appreciable mineralocorticoid properties and is used mainly for replacement therapy in Addison's disease or chronic adrenocortical insufficiency secondary to hypopituitarism.

5.2 Pharmacokinetic properties

Cortisone acetate is readily absorbed from the gastro-intestinal tract and the cortisone is rapidly converted in the liver to its active metabolite hydrocortisone. The biological half-life of cortisone itself is about 30 minutes.

It is metabolised mainly in the liver, but also in the kidney. It is excreted in the urine.

5.3 Preclinical safety data

Not applicable.

6. PHARMACEUTICAL PARTICULARS

6.1 List of excipients

Lactose

Maize Starch

Povidone

Soluble Starch (Amisol)

Colloidal Silicon Dioxide (Aerosil)

Magnesium Stearate

Purified Talc.

6.2 Incompatibilities

None.

6.3 Shelf life

Blister packs: 3 years

6.4 Special precautions for storage

Protect from light.

Store below 25°C in a dry place.

6.5 Nature and contents of container

Opaque PVC blister sealed with an aluminium foil: packs of 56 tablets.

6.6 Instructions for use and handling

Not applicable.

7. MARKETING AUTHORISATION HOLDER

Aventis Pharma Ltd, 50 Kings Hill Avenue, West Malling, ME19 4AH. UK.

Distributed by: Beacon Pharmaceuticals Ltd, 85 High Street, Tunbridge Wells, Kent. TN1 1YG. UK.

8. MARKETING AUTHORISATION NUMBER(S)

PL 04425/0332

9. DATE OF FIRST AUTHORISATION/RENEWAL OF THE AUTHORISATION

08/03/02

10. DATE OF REVISION OF THE TEXT

11. LEGAL CLASSIFICATION

POM

Cosmegen Lyovac

(Merck Sharp & Dohme Limited)

1. NAME OF THE MEDICINAL PRODUCT

COSMEGEN® Lyovac®

2. QUALITATIVE AND QUANTITATIVE COMPOSITION

When reconstituted the resulting solution will contain approximately 500 mcg dactinomycin (as a yellow-orange lyophilised powder) per ml.

3. PHARMACEUTICAL FORM

Powder for solution for injection.

4. CLINICAL PARTICULARS

4.1 Therapeutic indications

'Cosmegen' is a cytotoxic, antineoplastic antibiotic with immunosuppressant properties.

'Cosmegen', as part of a combination chemotherapy and/ or multi-modality treatment regimen, is indicated for the treatment of Wilms' tumor, childhood rhabdomyosarcoma, Ewing's sarcoma, and metastatic nonseminomatous testicular cancer.

'Cosmegen' is indicated as a single agent, or as part of a combination chemotherapy regimen, for the treatment of gestational trophoblastic neoplasia.

'Cosmegen', as a component of regional perfusion in combination with melphalan, is indicated for the treatment of locally recurrent or locoregionally metastatic melanoma.

4.2 Posology and method of administration

Toxic reactions due to 'Cosmegen' are frequent and may be severe (see 4.8 'Undesirable effects'), thus limiting the amount that may be administered in many cases. However, the severity of toxicity varies markedly and is only partly dependent on the dosage used.

Intravenous use

The dosage of 'Cosmegen' will vary with the tolerance of the patient, the size and location of the neoplasm, and the use of other forms of therapy. It may be necessary to reduce the usual dosage suggested below when additional chemotherapy or radiation therapy is used concurrently or has been employed previously.

The dosage of 'Cosmegen' is calculated in micrograms. The dose intensity per-two-week cycle for adults or children should not exceed 15 micrograms per kg per day or 400-600 micrograms per square meter of body surface daily, intravenously, for five days. Calculation of the dosage for obese or oedematous patients should be on the basis of surface area in an effort to relate dosage to lean body mass.

As there is a greater frequency of toxic effects of 'Cosmegen' in infants, 'Cosmegen' should only be given to infants under the age of 12 months, when the benefit outweighs the risk.

Use in the elderly: The general considerations already outlined also apply to elderly patients.

A wide variety of single agent and combination chemotherapy regimens with 'Cosmegen' may be employed. Because chemotherapeutic regimens are constantly changing, dosing and administration should be performed under the direct supervision of physicians familiar with current oncologic practices and new advances in therapy. The following suggested regimens are based upon a review of current literature concerning therapy with 'Cosmegen' and are on a per-cycle basis.

Wilm's tumor, rhabdomyosarcoma and Ewing's sarcoma

Regimens of 15 mcg/kg intravenously daily for five days administered in various combinations and schedules with other chemotherapeutic agents have been utilised in the treatment of Wilm's tumor, rhabdomyosarcoma and Ewing's sarcoma.

Testicular carcinoma

1,000 mcg/m^2 intravenously on Day 1 as part of a combination regimen with cyclophosphamide, bleomycin, vinblastine, and cisplatin.

Gestational trophoblastic neoplasia

12 mcg/kg intravenously daily for five days as a single agent.

500 mcg intravenously on Days 1 and 2 as part of a combination regimen with etoposide, methotrexate, folinic acid, vincristine, cyclophosphamide and cisplatin.

Regional perfusion in locally recurrent and locoregionally metastatic melanoma

The dosage schedules and the technique itself vary from one investigator to another, and the published literature should, therefore, be consulted for details. In general the following doses are suggested:

For a lower extremity or pelvis - 50 micrograms per kg bodyweight.

For an upper extremity - 35 micrograms per kg bodyweight.

It may be advisable to use lower doses in obese patients, or when previous chemotherapy or radiation therapy has been employed.

When reconstituted, the solution of dactinomycin can be added to an infusion solution of 5% dextrose injection or sodium chloride injection, either directly or into the tubing of a running intravenous infusion.

Although reconstituted 'Cosmegen' is chemically stable, the product does not contain a preservative and accidental microbial contamination might result. Any unused portion of the solution should be discarded.

Partial removal of dactinomycin from intravenous solutions by cellulose ester membrane filters used in some intravenous in-line filters has been reported.

If 'Cosmegen' is to be injected directly into the vein without the use of an infusion, the 'two-needle' technique should be used. The calculated dose should be reconstituted and withdrawn from the vial with one sterile needle; direct injection into the vein should then be performed with another sterile needle.

4.3 Contraindications

Use in patients with varicella or herpes zoster.

If 'Cosmegen' is given at or about the time of infection with chickenpox or herpes zoster, a severe generalised disease, which may be fatal can occur.

4.4 Special warnings and special precautions for use

'Cosmegen' should be administered only under the supervision of a physician who is experienced in the use of a cancer chemotherapeutic agent. Due to the toxic properties of dactinomycin (e.g. corrosivity, carcinogenicity, mutagenicity, teratogenicity). Special handling procedures should be reviewed prior to handling and followed diligently.

'Cosmegen' is HIGHLY TOXIC and both powder and solution must be handled and administered with care. Since 'Cosmegen' is extremely corrosive to soft tissues, it is intended for intravenous use. Inhalation of dust or vapours and contact with skin or mucous membranes, especially those of the eyes, must be avoided. Appropriate protective equipment should be worn when handling 'Cosmegen'. Should accidental eye contact occur, copious irrigation for at least 15 minutes with water, normal saline or a balanced salt ophthalmic irrigating solution should be instituted immediately, followed by prompt ophthalmic consultation. Should accidental skin contact occur, the affected part must be irrigated immediately with copious amounts of water for at least 15 minutes while removing contaminated clothing and shoes. Medical attention should be sought immediately. Contaminated clothing should be destroyed and shoes cleaned thoroughly before reuse (see 6.6 'Instructions for use/handling').

If extravasation occurs during intravenous use, severe damage to soft tissue may occur (see 6.6 'Instructions for use/handling').

'Cosmegen', like all antineoplastic agents, is a toxic drug, and very careful and frequent observation of the patient for adverse reactions is necessary. These reactions may involve any tissue of the body, most commonly the haematopoietic system resulting in myelosuppression. The possibility of an anaphylactic reaction should be borne in mind.

It is extremely important to observe the patient daily for toxic side effects when combined therapy is employed, since a full course of therapy is occasionally not tolerated. If stomatitis, diarrhoea or severe haematopoietic depression appear during therapy, these drugs should be discontinued until the patient has recovered.

'Cosmegen' and radiation therapy

An increased incidence of gastrointestinal toxicity and marrow suppression has been reported with combination therapy incorporating 'Cosmegen' and radiation. Moreover, the normal skin, as well as the buccal and pharyngeal mucosa, may show early erythema. A smaller than usual radiation dose administered in combination with 'Cosmegen' causes erythema and vesiculation, which progress more rapidly through the stages of tanning and desquamation. Healing may occur in four to six weeks rather than two to three months. Erythema from previous radiation therapy may be reactivated by 'Cosmegen' alone, even when radiotherapy was administered many months earlier, and especially when the interval between the two forms of therapy is brief. This potentiation of radiation effect represents a special problem when the radiotherapy involves the mucous membrane. When irradiation is directed toward the nasopharynx, the combination may produce severe oropharyngeal mucositis. Severe reactions may ensue if high doses of both 'Cosmegen' and radiation therapy are used or if the patient is particularly sensitive to such combined therapy.

Particular caution is necessary when administering 'Cosmegen' within two months of irradiation for the treatment of right-sided Wilm's tumor, since hepatomegaly and elevated AST levels have been noted.

In general, 'Cosmegen' should not be concomitantly administered with radiotherapy in the treatment of Wilm's tumor unless the benefit outweighs the risk.

Reports indicate an increased incidence of secondary primary tumours (including leukaemia) following treatment with radiation and antineoplastic agents, such as 'Cosmegen'. Multi-modal therapy creates the need for careful, long-term observation of cancer survivors.

Laboratory tests

A variety of abnormalities of renal, hepatic and bone-marrow function have been reported in patients with neoplastic disease receiving 'Cosmegen'. Renal, hepatic and bone-marrow functions should be assessed frequently.

4.5 Interaction with other medicinal products and other forms of Interaction

Much evidence suggests that 'Cosmegen' potentiates the effects of X-ray therapy. The converse also appears likely: that 'Cosmegen' may be more effective when radiation therapy is given concurrently. See 4.4 ''Cosmegen' and radiation therapy.'

'Cosmegen' may interfere with bio-assay procedures for the determination of antibacterial drug levels.

4.6 Pregnancy and lactation

Dactinomycin has been shown to be teratogenic in animals and should not normally be given to pregnant women.

'Cosmegen', dactinomycin should not be administered to mothers who are breast-feeding.

4.7 Effects on ability to drive and use machines

There are side effects associated with this product such as fatigue and lethargy, that may affect some patients ability to drive or operate machinery (see 4.8 'Undesirable effects').

4.8 Undesirable effects

Toxic effects (except nausea and vomiting) do not usually become apparent until two to four days after a course of therapy is stopped, and may not peak until one to two weeks have elapsed. Deaths have been reported. However, side effects are usually reversible on discontinuing therapy, they include the following:

General: malaise, fatigue, lethargy, fever, myalgia, proctitis, hypocalcaemia, renal abnormalities, growth retardation, infection.

Lung: pneumonitis.

Oral: cheilitis, dysphagia, oesophagitis, ulcerative stomatitis, pharyngitis.

Gastro-intestinal: anorexia, nausea, vomiting, abdominal pain, diarrhoea, gastro-intestinal ulceration, liver toxicity including ascites, hepatomegaly, hepatitis and liver-function test abnormalities. Nausea and vomiting, which occur early during the first few hours after administration, may be alleviated by the administration of anti-emetics.

Hepatic veno-occusive disease has been reported in patients receiving 'Cosmegen' as part of a multidrug chemotherapy regimen. However, relationship to the individual components could not be established.

Haematological: anaemia (even to the point of aplastic anaemia, agranulocytosis, leucopenia, thrombocytopenia, pancytopenia, reticulocytopenia). Platelet and white blood-cell counts should be performed frequently to detect severe haemopoietic depression. If either count shows a marked decrease, dactinomycin should be withheld to allow marrow recovery. This often takes up to three weeks.

Dermatological: alopecia, skin eruptions, acne, flare-up of erythema or increased pigmentation of previously irradiated skin.

Soft tissues: dactinomycin is extremely corrosive to soft tissues. If extravasation occurs during intravenous use, severe damage to soft tissues will occur. In at least one instance this has led to contracture of the arms. Epidermolysis, erythema, and oedema, at times severe, have been reported with regional limb perfusion.

'Cosmegen' and regional-perfusion therapy

Complications of the perfusion technique are related mainly to the amount of drug that escapes into the systemic circulation and may consist of haemopoietic depression, increased susceptibility of infection, absorption of toxic products from massive destruction of neoplastic tissue, impaired wound healing and superficial ulceration of the gastric mucosa. Other side effects may include oedema of the extremity involved, damage to the soft tissues of the perfused area, and potentially venous thrombosis.

4.9 Overdose

In the event of overdosage, dactinomycin therapy should be withdrawn immediately. Limited information is available on overdosage in humans. Manifestations of overdose have included nausea, vomiting, diarrhoea, stomatitis, gastro-intestinal ulceration, severe haemopoietic depression, acute renal failure and death. Treatment should be symptomatic and supportive. There is no known antidote. It is advisable to check renal, hepatic and bone-marrow functions frequently.

5. PHARMACOLOGICAL PROPERTIES

5.1 Pharmacodynamic properties

Mode of action: 'Cosmegen' inhibits the proliferation of cells by forming a stable complex with DNA and interfering with DNA-dependent RNA synthesis.

Generally, the actinomycins exert an inhibitory effect on Gram-positive and Gram-negative bacteria and on some fungi. However, the toxic properties of the actinomycins (including dactinomycin) in relation to antibacterial activity are such as to preclude their use as antibiotics in the treatment of infectious diseases.

Because the actinomycins are cytotoxic, they have an antineoplastic effect which has been demonstrated in experimental animals with various types of tumour implant. This cytotoxic action is the basis for their use in the palliative treatment of certain types of cancer.

5.2 Pharmacokinetic properties

Results of a study in patients with malignant melanoma indicate that dactinomycin (^3H actinomycin D) is minimally metabolised, is concentrated in nucleated cells and does not penetrate the blood brain barrier. Approximately 30% of the dose was recovered in urine and faeces in one week. The terminal plasma half-life for radioactivity was approximately 36 hours.

5.3 Preclinical safety data

The international Agency on Research on Cancer has judged that dactinomycin is a positive carcinogen in animals. Local sarcomas were produced in mice and rats after repeated subcutaneous or intraperitoneal injection. Mesenchymal tumours occurred in male F344 rats given intraperitoneal injections of 50 mcg/kg, two to five times per week for 18 weeks. The first tumour appeared at 23 weeks.

Dactinomycin has been shown to be mutagenic in a number of test systems *in vitro* and *in vivo*, including human fibroblasts and leucocytes, and HELA cells. DNA damage and cytogenetic effects have been demonstrated in the mouse and the rat.

Impairment of fertility

Adequate fertility studies have not been reported, although, an increased incidence of infertility following treatment with other antineoplastic agents has been reported.

Teratogenicity

'Cosmegen' has been shown to cause malformations and embryotoxicity in the rat, rabbit and hamster when given in doses of 50-100 mcg/kg intravenously (three to seven times the maximum recommended human dose).

6. PHARMACEUTICAL PARTICULARS

6.1 List of excipients

Mannitol EP.

6.2 Incompatibilities

Use of water containing preservatives (benzyl alcohol or parabens) to reconstitute 'Cosmegen' for injection results in the formation of a precipitate.

6.3 Shelf life

The shelf-life is 36 months.

6.4 Special precautions for storage

Do not store above 25°C. Store the vial in the outer carton. Do not freeze.

Discard open unused product immediately.

6.5 Nature and contents of container

Amber Type I glass vials with 13 mm red rubber stoppers. The vial contains an aluminium seal with a flip-off cap.

Pack size: single vials containing 500 micrograms dactinomycin.

6.6 Instructions for use and handling

Reconstitution and administration

'Cosmegen' is reconstituted by adding 1.1 ml of water for Injections Ph Eur without preservative to the vial. For injection, 1.0 ml of the reconstituted solution, which will contain 500 micrograms of dactinomycin, is withdrawn into the syringe. Only Water for Injections Ph Eur (which does not contain preservatives) should be used. Other injection fluids may cause precipitation. 'Cosmegen' should be inspected for particulate matter and discoloration, whenever possible. The reconstituted solution is clear and gold-coloured.

Special Handling

Animal studies have shown dactinomycin to be corrosive to skin, irritating to the eyes and mucous membranes of the respiratory tract and highly toxic by the oral route. It has also been shown to be carcinogenic, mutagenic, embryotoxic and teratogenic. Due to the drug's toxic properties, appropriate precautions including the use of appropriate safety equipment are recommended for the preparation of 'Cosmegen' for parenteral administration. Inhalation of dust or vapours and contact with skin or mucous membranes, especially those of the eyes must be avoided. It is recommended that the preparation of injectable antineoplastic drugs should be performed in a Class II laminar flow biological safety cabinet. Personnel preparing drugs of this class should wear chemical resistant, impervious gloves, safety goggles, outer garments, and shoe covers. Additional body garments should be used based upon the task being performed (e.g. sleevelets, apron, gauntlets, disposable suits) to avoid exposed skin surfaces and inhalation of vapours and dust. Appropriate techniques should be used to remove potentially contaminated clothing.

Several guidelines for proper handling and disposal of antineoplastic drugs have been published and should be considered.

Accidental contact measures

Should accidental eye contact occur, copious irrigation for at least 15 minutes with water, normal saline or a balanced salt ophthalmic irrigating solution should be instituted immediately, followed by prompt ophthalmic consultation. Should accidental skin contact occur, the affected part must be irrigated immediately with copious amounts of water for at least 15 minutes while removing contaminated clothing and shoes. Medical attention should be sought immediately. Contaminated clothing should be destroyed and shoes cleaned thoroughly before reuse (see 4.4 'Special warnings and precautions for use').

Care in the administration of 'Cosmegen' will reduce the chance of perivenous infiltration (See 4.4 'Special warnings and precautions for use' and 4.8 'Undesirable effects'). It may also decrease the chance of local reactions such as urticaria and erythematous streaking. On intravenous administration of 'Cosmegen', extravasation may occur with or without an accompanying burning or stinging sensation, even if blood returns well on aspiration of the infusion needle. If any signs or symptoms of extravasation have occurred, the injection or infusion should be terminated and restarted in another vein. If extravasation is suspected, intermittent application of ice to the site for 15 minutes 4 times daily for 3 days may be useful. The benefit of local administration of drugs has not been clearly established. Because of the progressive nature of extravasation reactions, close observation and plastic surgery consultation is recommended. Blistering, ulceration and/or persistent pain are indications for wide excision surgery, followed by split-thickness skin grafting.

7. MARKETING AUTHORISATION HOLDER

Merck Sharp & Dohme Limited

Hertford Road, Hoddesdon, Hertfordshire EN11 9BU, UK

8. MARKETING AUTHORISATION NUMBER(S)
PL 0025/5075R

9. DATE OF FIRST AUTHORISATION/RENEWAL OF THE AUTHORISATION
Date of grant at last renewal:
27 March 1996

10. DATE OF REVISION OF THE TEXT
November 2001.

LEGAL CATEGORY
POM

® denotes registered trademark of Merck & Co., Inc., Whitehouse Station, NJ, USA.

SPC.CMG.98.GB/IRL.0166

Cosopt Ophthalmic Solution

(Merck Sharp & Dohme Limited)

1. NAME OF THE MEDICINAL PRODUCT
COSOPT® eye drops, solution

2. QUALITATIVE AND QUANTITATIVE COMPOSITION
Each millilitre contains 22.26 mg of dorzolamide hydrochloride corresponding to 20 mg dorzolamide and 6.83 mg of timolol maleate corresponding to 5 mg timolol.

For excipients, see 6.1.

3. PHARMACEUTICAL FORM
Eye drops, solution.

'Cosopt' is a clear, colourless to nearly colourless, slightly viscous solution.

4. CLINICAL PARTICULARS

4.1 Therapeutic indications
'Cosopt' is indicated in the treatment of elevated intra-ocular pressure (IOP) in patients with open-angle glaucoma or pseudo-exfoliative glaucoma when topical beta-blocker monotherapy is not sufficient.

4.2 Posology and method of administration
The dose is one drop of 'Cosopt' in the (conjunctival sac of the) affected eye(s) two times daily.

If another topical ophthalmic agent is being used, 'Cosopt' and the other agent should be administered at least ten minutes apart.

Please see section 6.6 'Instructions for use and handling'.

Paediatric use

Safety and effectiveness in children have not been established.

4.3 Contraindications
'Cosopt' is contra-indicated in patients with:

• reactive airway disease, including bronchial asthma or a history of bronchial asthma, or severe chronic obstructive pulmonary disease

• sinus bradycardia, second- or third-degree atrioventricular block, overt cardiac failure, cardiogenic shock

• severe renal impairment (CrCl < 30 ml/min) or hyperchloraemic acidosis

• hypersensitivity to one or both active substances or to any of the excipients.

The above are based on the components and are not unique to the combination.

4.4 Special warnings and special precautions for use
Cardiovascular/respiratory reactions

As with other topically-applied ophthalmic agents, this drug may be absorbed systemically. The timolol component is a beta-blocker. Therefore, the same types of adverse reactions found with systemic administration of beta-blockers may occur with topical administration, including worsening of Prinzmetal's angina, worsening of severe peripheral and central circulatory disorders, and hypotension.

Because of the timolol maleate component, cardiac failure should be adequately controlled before beginning therapy with 'Cosopt'. In patients with a history of severe cardiac disease, signs of cardiac failure should be watched for and pulse rates should be checked.

Respiratory reactions and cardiac reactions, including death due to bronchospasm in patients with asthma and rarely death in association with cardiac failure, have been reported following administration of timolol maleate.

Hepatic impairment

'Cosopt' has not been studied in patients with hepatic impairment and therefore should be used with caution in such patients.

Immunology and hypersensitivity

As with other topically-applied ophthalmic agents, this drug may be absorbed systemically. The dorzolamide component is a sulphonamide. Therefore the same types of adverse reactions found with systemic administration of sulphonamides may occur with topical administration. If signs of serious reactions or hypersensitivity occur, discontinue use of this preparation.

Local ocular adverse effects, similar to those observed with dorzolamide hydrochloride eye drops, have been seen with 'Cosopt'. If such reactions occur, discontinuation of 'Cosopt' should be considered.

While taking β-blockers, patients with a history of atopy or a history of severe anaphylactic reaction to a variety of allergens may be more reactive to accidental, diagnostic, or therapeutic repeated challenge with such allergens. Such patients may be unresponsive to the usual doses of epinephrine used to treat anaphylactic reactions.

Concomitant therapy

The following concomitant medication is not recommended:

– dorzolamide and oral carbonic anhydrase inhibitors

– topical beta-adrenergic blocking agents.

Withdrawal of therapy

As with systemic beta-blockers, if discontinuation of ophthalmic timolol is needed in patients with coronary heart disease, therapy should be withdrawn gradually.

Additional effects of beta-blockade

Therapy with beta-blockers may mask certain symptoms of hypoglycaemia in patients with diabetes mellitus or hypoglycaemia.

Therapy with beta-blockers may mask certain symptoms of hyperthyroidism. Abrupt withdrawal of beta-blocker therapy may precipitate a worsening of symptoms.

Therapy with beta-blockers may aggravate symptoms of myasthenia gravis.

Additional effects of carbonic anhydrase inhibition

Therapy with oral carbonic anhydrase inhibitors has been associated with urolithiasis as a result of acid-base disturbances, especially in patients with a prior history of renal calculi. Although no acid-base disturbances have been observed with 'Cosopt', urolithiasis has been reported infrequently. Because 'Cosopt' contains a topical carbonic anhydrase inhibitor that is absorbed systemically, patients with a prior history of renal calculi may be at increased risk of urolithiasis while using 'Cosopt'.

Other

The management of patients with acute angle-closure glaucoma requires therapeutic interventions in addition to ocular hypotensive agents. 'Cosopt' has not been studied in patients with acute angle-closure glaucoma.

Corneal oedema and irreversible corneal decompensation have been reported in patients with pre-existing chronic corneal defects and/or a history of intra-ocular surgery while using dorzolamide. Topical dorzolamide should be used with caution in such patients.

Choroidal detachment concomitant with ocular hypotony have been reported after filtration procedures with administration of aqueous suppressant therapies.

As with the use of other antiglaucoma drugs, diminished responsiveness to ophthalmic timolol maleate after prolonged therapy has been reported in some patients. However, in clinical studies in which 164 patients have been followed for at least three years, no significant difference in mean intra-ocular pressure has been observed after initial stabilisation.

Contact lens use

'Cosopt' contains the preservative benzalkonium chloride, which may cause eye irritation. Remove contact lenses prior to application and wait at least 15 minutes before reinsertion. Benzalkonium chloride is known to discolour soft contact lenses.

4.5 Interaction with other medicinal products and other forms of Interaction
Specific drug interaction studies have not been performed with 'Cosopt'.

In clinical studies, 'Cosopt' was used concomitantly with the following systemic medications without evidence of adverse interactions: ACE-inhibitors, calcium channel blockers, diuretics, non-steroidal anti-inflammatory drugs including aspirin, and hormones (e.g. oestrogen, insulin, thyroxine).

However, the potential exists for additive effects and production of hypotension and/or marked bradycardia when timolol maleate ophthalmic solution is administered together with oral calcium channel blockers, catecholamine-depleting drugs or beta-adrenergic blocking agents, antiarrhythmics (including amiodarone), digitalis glycosides, parasympathomimetics, narcotics, and monoamine oxidase (MAO) inhibitors.

Potentiated systemic beta-blockade (e.g., decreased heart rate) has been reported during combined treatment with quinidine and timolol, possibly because quinidine inhibits the metabolism of timolol via the P-450 enzyme, CYP2D6.

The dorzolamide component of 'Cosopt' is a carbonic anhydrase inhibitor and although administered topically, is absorbed systemically. In clinical studies, dorzolamide hydrochloride ophthalmic solution was not associated with acid-base disturbances. However, these disturbances have been reported with oral carbonic anhydrase inhibitors and have in some instances, resulted in drug interactions (e.g., toxicity associated with high-dose salicylate therapy). Therefore, the potential for such drug interactions should be considered in patients receiving 'Cosopt'.

Although 'Cosopt' alone has little or no effect on pupil size, mydriasis resulting from concomitant use of ophthalmic timolol maleate and epinephrine has been reported occasionally.

Beta-blockers may increase the hypoglycaemic effect of antidiabetic agents.

Oral beta-adrenergic blocking agents may exacerbate the rebound hypertension which can follow the withdrawal of clonidine.

4.6 Pregnancy and lactation
Use during pregnancy

No studies were performed in pregnant women. In rabbits given maternotoxic doses of dorzolamide associated with metabolic acidosis, malformations of the vertebral bodies were observed. 'Cosopt' should not be used during pregnancy.

Use during lactation

It is not known whether dorzolamide is excreted in human milk. In lactating rats receiving dorzolamide, decreases in the body weight gain of offspring were observed. Timolol does appear in human milk. 'Cosopt' should not be used during lactation.

4.7 Effects on ability to drive and use machines
Possible side effects such as blurred vision may affect some patients' ability to drive and/or operate machinery.

4.8 Undesirable effects
In clinical studies no adverse experiences specific to 'Cosopt' have been observed; adverse experiences have been limited to those that were reported previously with dorzolamide hydrochloride and/or timolol maleate. In general, common adverse experiences were mild and did not cause discontinuation.

During clinical studies, 1,035 patients were treated with 'Cosopt'. Approximately 2.4% of all patients discontinued therapy with 'Cosopt' because of local ocular adverse reactions, approximately 1.2% of all patients discontinued because of local adverse reactions suggestive of allergy or hypersensitivity (such as lid inflammation and conjunctivitis).

The following adverse reactions have been reported with 'Cosopt' or one of its components either during clinical trials or during post-marketing experience:

[Very Common: >1/10), Common: >1/100, <1/10), Uncommon: >1/1000, <1/100), and Rare: >1/10,000, <1/1000)]

Blood and lymphatic system disorders:

Timolol maleate ophthalmic solution:

Rare: systemic lupus erythematosus

Nervous system and psychiatric disorders:

Dorzolamide hydrochloride ophthalmic solution:

Common: headache*

Rare: dizziness*, paresthesia*

Timolol maleate ophthalmic solution:

Common: headache*

Uncommon: dizziness*, depression*

Rare: insomnia*, nightmares*, memory loss, paraesthesia*, increase in signs and symptoms of myasthenia gravis, decreased libido*, cerebrovascular accident*

Eye disorders:

'Cosopt':

Very Common: burning and stinging

Common: conjunctival injection, blurred vision, corneal erosion, ocular itching, tearing

Dorzolamide hydrochloride ophthalmic solution:

Common: eyelid inflammation*, eyelid irritation*

Uncommon: iridocyclitis*

Rare: irritation including redness*, pain*, eyelid crusting*, transient myopia (which resolved upon discontinuation of therapy), corneal oedema*, ocular hypotony*, choroidal detachment (following filtration surgery)*

Timolol maleate ophthalmic solution:

Common: signs and symptoms of ocular irritation including blepharitis*, keratitis*, decreased corneal sensitivity, and dry eyes*

Uncommon: visual disturbances including refractive changes (due to withdrawal of miotic therapy in some cases)*

Rare: ptosis, diplopia, choroidal detachment (following filtration surgery)*

Ear and labyrinth disorders:

Timolol maleate ophthalmic solution:

Rare: tinnitus*

Cardiac and vascular disorders:

Timolol maleate ophthalmic solution:

Uncommon: bradycardia*, syncope*

Rare: hypotension*, chest pain*, palpitation*, oedema*, arrhythmia*, congestive heart failure*, heart block*, cardiac arrest*, cerebral ischaemia, claudication, Raynaud's phenomenon*, cold hands and feet*

Respiratory, thoracic, and mediastinal disorders:

'Cosopt':

Common: sinusitis

Rare: shortness of breath, respiratory failure, rhinitis

Dorzolamide hydrochloride ophthalmic solution:

Rare: epistaxis*

Timolol maleate ophthalmic solution:

Uncommon: dyspnoea*

Rare: bronchospasm (predominantly in patients with pre-existing bronchospastic disease)*, cough*

Gastro-intestinal disorders:

'Cosopt':

Very Common: taste perversion

Dorzolamide hydrochloride ophthalmic solution:

Common: nausea*

Rare: throat irritation, dry mouth*

Timolol maleate ophthalmic solution:

Uncommon: nausea*, dyspepsia*

Rare: diarrhoea, dry mouth*

Skin and subcutaneous tissue disorders:

'Cosopt':

Rare: contact dermatitis

Dorzolamide hydrochloride ophthalmic solution:

Rare: rash*

Timolol maleate ophthalmic solution:

Rare: alopecia*, psoriasiform rash or exacerbation of psoriasis*

Renal disorders:

'Cosopt':

Uncommon: urolithiasis

Reproductive system and breast disorders:

Timolol maleate ophthalmic solution:

Rare: Peyronie's disease*

General disorders and administration site disorders:

'Cosopt':

Rare: signs and symptoms of systemic allergic reactions, including angioedema, urticaria, pruritus, rash, anaphylaxis, rarely bronchospasm

Dorzolamide hydrochloride ophthalmic solution:

Common: asthenia/fatigue*

Timolol maleate ophthalmic solution:

Uncommon: asthenia/fatigue*

*These adverse reactions were also observed with 'Cosopt' during post-marketing experience.

Laboratory findings

'Cosopt' was not associated with clinically meaningful electrolyte disturbances in clinical studies.

4.9 Overdose

No data are available in humans in regard to overdosage by accidental or deliberate ingestion of 'Cosopt'.

There have been reports of inadvertent overdosage with timolol maleate ophthalmic solution resulting in systemic effects similar to those seen with systemic beta-adrenergic blocking agents such as dizziness, headache, shortness of breath, bradycardia, bronchospasm, and cardiac arrest. The most common signs and symptoms to be expected with overdosage of dorzolamide are electrolyte imbalance, development of an acidotic state, and possibly central nervous system effects.

Only limited information is available with regard to human overdosage by accidental or deliberate ingestion of dorzolamide hydrochloride. With oral ingestion, somnolence has been reported. With topical application the following have been reported: nausea, dizziness, headache, fatigue, abnormal dreams, and dysphagia.

Treatment should be symptomatic and supportive. Serum electrolyte levels (particularly potassium) and blood pH levels should be monitored. Studies have shown that timolol does not dialyse readily.

5. PHARMACOLOGICAL PROPERTIES

5.1 Pharmacodynamic properties

Pharmacotherapeutic group: S01E D51

(Ophthalmologicals - Beta-Blocking Agents - Timolol, Combinations)

Mechanism of action

'Cosopt' is comprised of two components: dorzolamide hydrochloride and timolol maleate. Each of these two components decreases elevated intra-ocular pressure by reducing aqueous humor secretion, but does so by a different mechanism of action.

Dorzolamide hydrochloride is a potent inhibitor of human carbonic anhydrase II. Inhibition of carbonic anhydrase in the ciliary processes of the eye decreases aqueous humor secretion, presumably by slowing the formation of bicarbonate ions with subsequent reduction in sodium and fluid transport. Timolol maleate is a non-selective beta-adrenergic receptor blocking agent. The precise mechanism of action of timolol maleate in lowering intra-ocular pressure is not clearly established at this time, although a fluorescein study and tonography studies indicate that the predominant action may be related to reduced aqueous formation. However, in some studies a slight increase in outflow facility was also observed. The combined effect of these two agents results in additional intra-ocular pressure reduction compared to either component administered alone.

Following topical administration, 'Cosopt' reduces elevated intra-ocular pressure, whether or not associated with glaucoma. Elevated intra-ocular pressure is a major risk factor in the pathogenesis of optic nerve damage and glaucomatous visual field loss. 'Cosopt' reduces intra-ocular pressure without the common side effects of miotics such as night blindness, accommodative spasm and pupillary constriction.

Pharmacodynamic effects

Clinical effects:

Clinical studies of up to 15 months duration were conducted to compare the IOP-lowering effect of 'Cosopt' b.i.d. (dosed morning and bedtime) to individually- and concomitantly-administered 0.5% timolol and 2.0% dorzolamide in patients with glaucoma or ocular hypertension for whom concomitant therapy was considered appropriate in the trials. This included both untreated patients and patients inadequately controlled with timolol monotherapy. The majority of patients were treated with topical beta-blocker monotherapy prior to study enrollment. In an analysis of the combined studies, the IOP-lowering effect of 'Cosopt' b.i.d. was greater than that of monotherapy with either 2% dorzolamide t.i.d. or 0.5% timolol b.i.d. The IOP-lowering effect of 'Cosopt' b.i.d. was equivalent to that of concomitant therapy with dorzolamide b.i.d. and timolol b.i.d. The IOP-lowering effect of 'Cosopt' b.i.d. was demonstrated when measured at various time points throughout the day and this effect was maintained during long-term administration.

5.2 Pharmacokinetic properties

Dorzolamide hydrochloride:

Unlike oral carbonic anhydrase inhibitors, topical administration of dorzolamide hydrochloride allows for the drug to exert its effects directly in the eye at substantially lower doses and therefore with less systemic exposure. In clinical trials, this resulted in a reduction in IOP without the acid-base disturbances or alterations in electrolytes characteristic of oral carbonic anhydrase inhibitors.

When topically applied, dorzolamide reaches the systemic circulation. To assess the potential for systemic carbonic anhydrase inhibition following topical administration, drug and metabolite concentrations in red blood cells (RBCs) and plasma and carbonic anhydrase inhibition in RBCs were measured. Dorzolamide accumulates in RBCs during chronic dosing as a result of selective binding to CA-II while extremely low concentrations of free drug in plasma are maintained. The parent drug forms a single N-desethyl metabolite that inhibits CA-II less potently than the parent drug but also inhibits a less active isoenzyme (CA-I). The metabolite also accumulates in RBCs where it binds primarily to CA-I. Dorzolamide binds moderately to plasma proteins (approximately 33%). Dorzolamide is primarily excreted unchanged in the urine; the metabolite is also excreted in urine. After dosing ends, dorzolamide washes out of RBCs non-linearly, resulting in a rapid decline of drug concentration initially, followed by a slower elimination phase with a half-life of about four months.

When dorzolamide was given orally to simulate the maximum systemic exposure after long term topical ocular administration, steady state was reached within 13 weeks. At steady state, there was virtually no free drug or metabolite in plasma; CA inhibition in RBCs was less than that anticipated to be necessary for a pharmacological effect on renal function or respiration. Similar pharmacokinetic results were observed after chronic, topical administration of dorzolamide hydrochloride. However, some elderly patients with renal impairment (estimated CrCl 30-60 millilitre/min) had higher metabolite concentrations in RBCs, but no meaningful differences in carbonic anhydrase inhibition and no clinically significant systemic side effects were directly attributable to this finding.

Timolol maleate:

In a study of plasma drug concentration in six subjects, the systemic exposure to timolol was determined following twice daily topical administration of timolol maleate ophthalmic solution 0.5%. The mean peak plasma concentration following morning dosing was 0.46 ng/millilitre and following afternoon dosing was 0.35 ng/millilitre.

5.3 Preclinical safety data

The ocular and systemic safety profile of the individual components is well established. Furthermore, no adverse ocular effects were seen in animals treated topically with dorzolamide hydrochloride and timolol maleate ophthalmic solution or with concomitantly-administered dorzolamide hydrochloride and timolol maleate. *In vitro* and *in vivo* studies with each of the components did not reveal a mutagenic potential. Therefore, no significant risk for human safety is expected with therapeutic doses of 'Cosopt'.

6. PHARMACEUTICAL PARTICULARS

6.1 List of excipients

Hyetellose, mannitol, sodium citrate, sodium hydroxide, water for injection and benzalkonium chloride.

6.2 Incompatibilities

Not applicable.

6.3 Shelf life

2 years.

'Cosopt' should be used no longer than 4 weeks after first opening the container.

6.4 Special precautions for storage

Keep the bottle in the outer carton, in order to protect from light.

6.5 Nature and contents of container

The OCUMETER Plus Ophthalmic Dispenser consists of a translucent, high-density polyethylene container with a sealed dropper tip, a flexible fluted side area which is depressed to dispense the drops, and a two-piece cap assembly. The two-piece cap mechanism punctures the sealed dropper tip upon initial use, then locks together to provide a single cap during the usage period. Tamper evidence is provided by a safety strip on the container label. The OCUMETER Plus ophthalmic dispenser contains 5 ml of solution.

'Cosopt' is available in the following packaging configurations:

1 × 5 ml (single 5-ml container)

3 × 5 ml (three 5-ml containers)

6 × 5 ml (six 5-ml containers)

Not all pack sizes may be marketed.

6.6 Instructions for use and handling

Patients should be instructed to avoid allowing the tip of the dispensing container to contact the eye or surrounding structures.

Patients should also be instructed that ocular solutions, if handled improperly, can become contaminated by common bacteria known to cause ocular infections. Serious damage to the eye and subsequent loss of vision may result from using contaminated solutions.

Patients should be informed of the correct handling of the OCUMETER PLUS bottles.

Usage instructions:

1. Before using the medication for the first time, be sure the safety strip on the front of the bottle is unbroken. A gap between the bottle and the cap is normal for an unopened bottle.
2. Tear off the safety strip to break the seal.
3. To open the bottle, unscrew the cap by turning as indicated by the arrows.
4. Tilt your head back and pull your lower eyelid down slightly to form a pocket between your eyelid and your eye.
5. Invert the bottle, and press lightly with the thumb or index finger over the "Finger Push Area" until a single drop is dispensed into the eye as directed by your doctor. DO NOT TOUCH YOUR EYE OR EYELID WITH THE DROPPER TIP.
6. Repeat steps 4 and 5 with the other eye if instructed to do so by your doctor.
7. Replace the cap by turning until it is firmly touching the bottle. Do not overtighten the cap.
8. The dispenser tip is designed to provide a pre-measured drop; therefore, do NOT enlarge the hole of the dispenser tip.
9. After you have used all doses, there will be some 'Cosopt' left in the bottle. You should not be concerned since an extra amount of 'Cosopt' has been added and you will get the full amount of 'Cosopt' that your doctor prescribed. Do not attempt to remove the excess medicine from the bottle.

7. MARKETING AUTHORISATION HOLDER

Merck Sharp & Dohme Limited

Hertford Road, Hoddesdon, Hertfordshire EN11 9BU, UK.

8. MARKETING AUTHORISATION NUMBER(S)

PL 0025/0373

9. DATE OF FIRST AUTHORISATION/RENEWAL OF THE AUTHORISATION

4 August 1998.

10. DATE OF REVISION OF THE TEXT

Revision approved March 2003.

LEGAL CATEGORY

POM

® denotes registered trademark of Merck & Co., Inc., Whitehouse Station, NJ, USA.

MSD (logo)

Merck Sharp & Dohme Limited

Hertford Road, Hoddesdon, Hertfordshire EN11 9BU, UK

SPC.CST.03.UK.0930-N01 (UK)

Coversyl

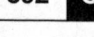

(Servier Laboratories Limited)

1. NAME OF THE MEDICINAL PRODUCT

Coversyl 2 mg

Coversyl 4 mg

Coversyl 8 mg Tablets

2. QUALITATIVE AND QUANTITATIVE COMPOSITION

2 mg perindopril tert-butylamine salt, equivalent to 1.669 mg perindopril

4 mg perindopril tert-butylamine salt, equivalent to 3.338 mg perindopril

8 mg perindopril tert-butylamine salt, equivalent to 6.676 mg perindopril

For excipients, see Section 6.1.

3. PHARMACEUTICAL FORM

Coversyl 2 mg: Tablets, white, biconvex.

Coversyl 4 mg: Tablets, light green, oblong, engraved with on one face and scored on both edges.

Coversyl 8 mg Tablets: Tablets, green, round, biconvex, engraved with on one face and on the other.

4. CLINICAL PARTICULARS

4.1 Therapeutic indications

Hypertension

Treatment of hypertension

Heart Failure

Treatment of symptomatic heart failure

4.2 Posology and method of administration

It is recommended that COVERSYL is taken once daily in the morning before a meal.

The dose should be individualised according to the patient profile (see 4.4 "Special warnings and special precautions for use") and blood pressure response.

Hypertension

COVERSYL may be used in monotherapy or in combination with other classes of antihypertensive therapy.

The recommended starting dose is 4 mg given once daily in the morning.

Patients with a strongly activated renin-angiotensin-aldosterone system (in particular, renovascular hypertension, salt and/or volume depletion, cardiac decompensation or severe hypertension) may experience an excessive drop in blood pressure following the initial dose. A starting dose of 2 mg is recommended in such patients and the initiation of treatment should take place under medical supervision.

The dose may be increased to 8 mg once daily after one month of treatment.

Symptomatic hypotension may occur following initiation of therapy with COVERSYL; this is more likely in patients who are being treated concurrently with diuretics. Caution is therefore recommended since these patients may be volume and/or salt depleted.

If possible, the diuretic should be discontinued 2 to 3 days before beginning therapy with COVERSYL (see section 4.4 "Special warnings and special precautions for use").

In hypertensive patients in whom the diuretic cannot be discontinued, therapy with COVERSYL should be initiated with a 2 mg dose. Renal function and serum potassium should be monitored. The subsequent dosage of COVERSYL should be adjusted according to blood pressure response. If required, diuretic therapy may be resumed.

In elderly patients treatment should be initiated at a dose of 2 mg which may be progressively increased to 4 mg after one month then to 8 mg if necessary depending on renal function (see table below).

Symptomatic heart failure

It is recommended that COVERSYL, generally associated with a non-potassium-sparing diuretic and/or digoxin and/or a beta blocker, be introduced under close medical supervision with a recommended starting dose of 2 mg taken in the morning. This dose may be increased by increments of 2 mg at intervals of no less than 2 weeks to 4 mg once daily if tolerated. The dose adjustment should be based on the clinical response of the individual patient.

In severe heart failure and in other patients considered to be at high risk (patients with impaired renal function and a tendency to have electrolyte disturbances, patients receiving simultaneous treatment with diuretics and/or treatment with vasodilating agents), treatment should be initiated under careful supervision (see 4.4 "Special warnings and special precautions for use").

Patients at high risk of symptomatic hypotension e.g. patients with salt depletion with or without hyponatraemia, patients with hypovolaemia or patients who have been receiving vigorous diuretic therapy should have these conditions corrected, if possible, prior to therapy with COVERSYL. Blood pressure, renal function and serum potassium should be monitored closely, both before and during treatment with COVERSYL (see section 4.4 "Special warnings and special precautions for use").

Dosage adjustment in renal impairment

Dosage in patients with renal impairment should be based on creatinine clearance as outlined in table 1 below:

Table 1: dosage adjustment in renal impairment

Creatinine clearance (ml/min)	Recommended dose
$Cl_{CR} \geqslant 60$	4 mg per day
$30 < Cl_{CR} < 60$	2 mg per day
$15 < Cl_{CR} < 30$	2 mg every other day
Haemodialysed patients *, $Cl_{CR} < 15$	2 mg on the day of dialysis

* Dialysis clearance of perindoprilat is 70 ml/min. For patients on haemodialysis, the dose should be taken after dialysis.

Dosage adjustment in hepatic impairment

No dosage adjustment is necessary in patients with hepatic impairment (see sections 4.4 "Special warnings and special precautions for use" and 5.2 "Pharmacokinetic properties")

Paediatric use

Efficacy and safety of use in children has not been established. Therefore, use in children is not recommended.

4.3 Contraindications

- Hypersensitivity to perindopril, to any of the excipients or to any other ACE inhibitor;
- History of angioedema associated with previous ACE inhibitor therapy;
- Hereditary or idiopathic angioedema;
- Second and third trimesters of pregnancy (see 4.6 "Pregnancy and lactation").

4.4 Special warnings and special precautions for use

Hypotension

ACE inhibitors may cause a fall in blood pressure. Symptomatic hypotension is seen rarely in uncomplicated hypertensive patients and is more likely to occur in patients who have been volume-depleted e.g. by diuretic therapy, dietary salt restriction, dialysis, diarrhoea or vomiting, or who have severe renin-dependent hypertension (see sections 4.5 "Interaction with other medicaments and other forms of interaction" and 4.8 "Undesirable effects"). In patients with symptomatic heart failure, with or without associated renal insufficiency, symptomatic hypotension has been observed. This is most likely to occur in those patients with more severe degrees of heart failure, as reflected by the use of high doses of loop diuretics, hyponatraemia or functional renal impairment. In patients at increased risk of symptomatic hypotension, initiation of therapy and dose adjustment should be closely monitored (see 4.2 "Posology and method of administration" and 4.8 "Undesirable effects"). Similar considerations apply to patients with ischaemic heart or cerebrovascular disease in whom an excessive fall in blood pressure could result in a myocardial infarction or cerebrovascular accident.

If hypotension occurs, the patient should be placed in the supine position and, if necessary, should receive an intravenous infusion of normal saline. A transient hypotensive response is not a contraindication to further doses, which can be given usually without difficulty once the blood pressure has increased after volume expansion.

In some patients with congestive heart failure who have normal or low blood pressure, additional lowering of systemic blood pressure may occur with COVERSYL. This effect is anticipated and is usually not a reason to discontinue treatment. If hypotension becomes symptomatic, a reduction of dose or discontinuation of COVERSYL may be necessary.

Aortic and mitral valve stenosis / hypertrophic cardiomyopathy

As with other ACE inhibitors, COVERSYL should be given with caution to patients with mitral valve stenosis and obstruction in the outflow of the left ventricle such as aortic stenosis or hypertrophic cardiomyopathy.

Renal impairment

In cases of renal impairment (creatinine clearance < 60 ml/min) the initial perindopril dosage should be adjusted according to the patient's creatinine clearance (see 4.2 "Posology and method of administration") and then as a function of the patient's response to treatment. Routine monitoring of potassium and creatinine are part of normal medical practice for these patients (see 4.8 "Undesirable effects").

In patients with symptomatic heart failure, hypotension following the initiation of therapy with ACE inhibitors may lead to some further impairment in renal function. Acute renal failure, usually reversible, has been reported in this situation.

In some patients with bilateral renal artery stenosis or stenosis of the artery to a solitary kidney, who have been treated with ACE inhibitors, increases in blood urea and serum creatinine, usually reversible upon discontinuation of therapy, have been seen. This is especially likely in patients with renal insufficiency. If renovascular hypertension is also present there is an increased risk of severe hypotension and renal insufficiency. In these patients, treatment should be started under close medical supervision with low doses and careful dose titration. Since treatment with diuretics may be a contributory factor to the above, they should be discontinued and renal function should be monitored during the first weeks of COVERSYL therapy.

Some hypertensive patients with no apparent pre-existing renal vascular disease have developed increases in blood urea and serum creatinine, usually minor and transient, especially when COVERSYL has been given concomitantly with a diuretic. This is more likely to occur in patients with pre-existing renal impairment. Dosage reduction and/or discontinuation of the diuretic and/or COVERSYL may be required.

Haemodialysis patients

Anaphylactoid reactions have been reported in patients dialysed with high flux membranes, and treated concomitantly with an ACE inhibitor. In these patients consideration should be given to using a different type of dialysis membrane or different class of antihypertensive agent.

Kidney transplantation

There is no experience regarding the administration of COVERSYL in patients with a recent kidney transplantation.

Hypersensitivity/Angioedema

Angioedema of the face, extremities, lips, mucous membranes, tongue, glottis and/or larynx has been reported rarely in patients treated with ACE inhibitors, including COVERSYL (see 4.8 Undesirable effects). This may occur at any time during therapy. In such cases, COVERSYL should promptly be discontinued and appropriate monitoring should be initiated and continued until complete resolution of symptoms has occurred. In those instances where swelling was confined to the face and lips the condition generally resolved without treatment, although antihistamines have been useful in relieving symptoms.

Angioedema associated with laryngeal oedema may be fatal. Where there is involvement of the tongue, glottis or larynx, likely to cause airway obstruction, emergency therapy should be administered promptly. This may include the administration of adrenaline and/or the maintenance of a patent airway. The patient should be under close medical supervision until complete and sustained resolution of symptoms has occurred.

Angiotensin converting enzyme inhibitors cause a higher rate of angioedema in black patients than in non-black patients.

Patients with a history of angioedema unrelated to ACE inhibitor therapy may be at increased risk of angioedema while receiving an ACE inhibitor (See 4.3 Contraindications).

Anaphylactoid reactions during low-density lipoproteins (LDL) apheresis

Rarely, patients receiving ACE inhibitors during low-density lipoprotein (LDL) apheresis with dextran sulphate have experienced life-threatening anaphylactoid reactions. These reactions were avoided by temporarily withholding ACE inhibitor therapy prior to each apheresis.

Anaphylactic reactions during desensitisation

Patients receiving ACE inhibitors during desensitisation treatment (e.g. hymenoptera venom) have experienced anaphylactoid reactions. In the same patients, these reactions have been avoided when the ACE inhibitors were temporarily withheld, but they reappeared upon inadvertent rechallenge.

Hepatic failure

Rarely, ACE inhibitors have been associated with a syndrome that starts with cholestatic jaundice and progresses to fulminant hepatic necrosis and (sometimes) death. The mechanism of this syndrome is not understood. Patients receiving ACE inhibitors who develop jaundice or marked elevations of hepatic enzymes should discontinue the ACE inhibitor and receive appropriate medical follow-up (4.8 Undesirable effects).

Neutropenia/Agranulocytosis/Thrombocytopenia/Anaemia

Neutropenia/agranulocytosis, thrombocytopenia and anaemia have been reported in patients receiving ACE inhibitors. In patients with normal renal function and no other complicating factors, neutropenia occurs rarely. Perindopril should be used with extreme caution in patients with collagen vascular disease, immunosuppressant therapy, treatment with allopurinol or procainamide, or a combination of these complicating factors, especially if there is pre-existing impaired renal function. Some of these patients developed serious infections, which in a few instances did not respond to intensive antibiotic therapy. If perindopril is used in such patients, periodic monitoring of white blood cell counts is advised and patients should be instructed to report any sign of infection.

Race

ACE inhibitors cause a higher rate of angioedema in black patients than in non-black patients.

As with other ACE inhibitors, perindopril may be less effective in lowering blood pressure in black people than in non-blacks, possibly because of a higher prevalence of low-renin states in the black hypertensive population.

Cough

Cough has been reported with the use of ACE inhibitors. Characteristically, the cough is non-productive, persistent and resolves after discontinuation of therapy. ACE inhibitor-induced cough should be considered as part of the differential diagnosis of cough.

Surgery/Anaesthesia

In patients undergoing major surgery or during anaesthesia with agents that produce hypotension, COVERSYL may block angiotensin II formation secondary to compensatory renin release. The treatment should be discontinued one day prior to the surgery. If hypotension occurs and is considered to be due to this mechanism, it can be corrected by volume expansion.

Hyperkalaemia

Elevations in serum potassium have been observed in some patients treated with ACE inhibitors, including perindopril. Patients at risk for the development of hyperkalaemia include those with renal insufficiency, uncontrolled diabetes mellitus, or those using concomitant potassium-sparing diuretics, potassium supplements or potassium-containing salt substitutes; or those patients taking other drugs associated with increases in serum potassium (e.g. heparin). If concomitant use of the above-mentioned agents is deemed appropriate, regular monitoring of serum potassium is recommended.

Diabetic patients

In diabetic patients treated with oral antidiabetic agents or insulin, glycaemic control should be closely monitored during the first month of treatment with an ACE inhibitor. (See 4.5 Interaction with other medicinal products and other forms of interaction, Antidiabetics.)

Lithium

The combination of lithium and perindopril is generally not recommended (see 4.5 Interaction with other medicinal products and other forms of interaction).

Potassium sparing diuretics, potassium supplements or potassium-containing salt substitutes

The combination of perindopril and potassium sparing diuretics, potassium supplements or potassium-containing salt substitutes is generally not recommended (see 4.5 Interaction with other medicinal products and other forms of interaction).

Pregnancy and lactation

(See section 4.3 "Contraindications" and section 4.6 "Pregnancy and lactation").

4.5 Interaction with other medicinal products and other forms of Interaction

Diuretics

Patients on diuretics, and especially those who are volume and/or salt depleted, may experience excessive reduction in blood pressure after initiation of therapy with an ACE inhibitor. The possibility of hypotensive effects can be reduced by discontinuation of the diuretic, by increasing volume or salt intake prior to initiating therapy with low and progressive doses of perindopril.

Potassium sparing diuretics, potassium supplements or potassium-containing salt substitutes

Although serum potassium usually remains within normal limits, hyperkalaemia may occur in some patients treated with perindopril. Potassium sparing diuretics (e.g. spironolactone, triamterene, or amiloride), potassium supplements, or potassium-containing salt substitutes may lead to significant increases in serum potassium. Therefore the combination of perindopril with the above-mentioned drugs is not recommended (see section 4.4). If concomitant use is indicated because of demonstrated hypokalaemia they should be used with caution and with frequent monitoring of serum potassium.

Lithium

Reversible increases in serum lithium concentrations and toxicity have been reported during concomitant administration of lithium with ACE inhibitors. Concomitant use of thiazide diuretics may increase the risk of lithium toxicity and enhance the already increased risk of lithium toxicity with ACE inhibitors. Use of perindopril with lithium is not recommended, but if the combination proves necessary, careful monitoring of serum lithium levels should be performed (see section 4.4).

Non-steroidal anti-inflammatory drugs (NSAIDs) including aspirin ≥ 3 g/day

The administration of a non-steroidal anti-inflammatory drug may reduce the antihypertensive effect of ACE inhibitors. Additionally, NSAIDs and ACE inhibitors exert an additive effect on the increase in serum potassium and may result in a deterioration of renal function. These effects are usually reversible. Rarely, acute renal failure may occur, especially in patients with compromised renal function such as those who are elderly or dehydrated.

Antihypertensive agents and vasodilators

Concomitant use of these agents may increase the hypotensive effects of perindopril. Concomitant use with nitroglycerin and other nitrates, or other vasodilators, may further reduce blood pressure.

Antidiabetic agents

Epidemiological studies have suggested that concomitant administration of ACE inhibitors and antidiabetic medicines (insulins, oral hypoglycaemic agents) may cause an increased blood-glucose lowering effect with risk of hypoglycaemia. This phenomenon appeared to be more likely to occur during the first weeks of combined treatment and in patients with renal impairment.

Acetylsalicylic acid, thrombolytics, beta-blockers, nitrates

Perindopril may be used concomitantly with acetylsalicylic acid (when used as a thrombolytic), thrombolytics, beta-blockers and/or nitrates.

Tricyclic antidepressants/Antipsychotics/Anaesthetics

Concomitant use of certain anaesthetic medicinal products, tricyclic antidepressants and antipsychotics with ACE inhibitors may result in further reduction of blood pressure (see section 4.4).

Sympathomimetics

Sympathomimetics may reduce the antihypertensive effects of ACE inhibitors.

4.6 Pregnancy and lactation

Pregnancy

COVERSYL should not be used during the first trimester of pregnancy. When a pregnancy is planned or confirmed, the switch to an alternative treatment should be initiated as soon as possible. Controlled studies with ACE inhibitors have not been done in humans, but in a limited number of cases with first trimester exposure there do not appear to have been any malformations consistent with human foetotoxicity as described below.

Perindopril is contraindicated during the second and third trimesters of pregnancy.

Prolonged ACE inhibitor exposure during the second and third trimesters is known to induce human foetotoxicity (decreased renal function, oligohydramnios, skull ossification retardation) and neonatal toxicity (renal failure, hypotension, hyperkalaemia). (see 5.3 "Preclinical safety data")

Should exposure to perindopril have occurred from the second trimester of pregnancy, ultrasound check of renal function and skull is recommended.

Lactation

It is not known whether perindopril is excreted into human breast milk. Therefore the use of COVERSYL is not recommended in women who are breast-feeding.

4.7 Effects on ability to drive and use machines

When driving vehicles or operating machines it should be taken into account that occasionally dizziness or weariness may occur.

4.8 Undesirable effects

The following undesirable effects have been observed during treatment with perindopril and ranked under the following frequency:

Very common (>1/10); common (>1/100, <1/10); uncommon (>1/1000, <1/100); rare (>1/10000, <1/1000); very rare (<1/10000), including isolated reports.

Psychiatric disorders:

Uncommon: mood or sleep disturbances

Nervous system disorders:

Common: headache, dizziness, vertigo, paresthaesia

Very rare: confusion

Eye disorders:

Common: vision disturbance

Ear and labyrinth disorders:

Common: tinnitus

Cardio-vascular disorders:

Common: hypotension and effects related to hypotension

Very rare: arrhythmia, angina pectoris, myocardial infarction and stroke, possibly secondary to excessive hypotension in high risk patients (see 4.4 Special warnings and special precautions for use).

Respiratory, thoracic and mediastinal disorders:

Common: cough, dyspnoea

Uncommon: bronchospasm

Very rare: eosinophilic pneumonia, rhinitis

Gastro-intestinal disorders:

Common: nausea, vomiting, abdominal pain, dysgeusia, dyspepsia, diarrhoea, constipation

Uncommon: dry mouth

Very rare: pancreatitis

Hepato-biliary disorders:

Very rare: hepatitis either cytolytic or cholestatic (see section 4.4 Special warnings and special precautions for use)

Skin and subcutaneous tissue disorders:

Common: rash, pruritus

Uncommon: angioedema of face, extremities, lips, mucous membranes, tongue, glottis and/or larynx, urticaria (see 4.4 Special warnings and special precautions for use).

Very rare: erythema multiforme

Musculoskeletal, connective tissue and bone disorders:

Common: muscle cramps

Renal and urinary disorders:

Uncommon: renal insufficiency

Very rare: acute renal failure

Reproductive system and breast disorders:

Uncommon: impotence

General disorders:

Common: asthenia

Uncommon: sweating

Blood and the lymphatic system disorders:

Decreases in haemoglobin and haematocrit, thrombocytopenia, leucopenia/neutropenia, and cases of agranulocytosis or pancytopenia, have been reported very rarely. In patients with a congenital deficiency of G-6PDH, very rare cases of haemolytic anaemia have been reported (see section 4.4 Special warnings and special precautions for use).

Investigations:

Increases in blood urea and plasma creatinine, hyperkalaemia reversible on discontinuation may occur, especially in the presence of renal insufficiency, severe heart failure and renovascular hypertension. Elevation of liver enzymes and serum bilirubin have been reported rarely.

4.9 Overdose

Limited data are available for overdosage in humans. Symptoms associated with overdosage of ACE inhibitors may include hypotension, circulatory shock, electrolyte disturbances, renal failure, hyperventilation, tachycardia, palpitations, bradycardia, dizziness, anxiety, and cough.

The recommended treatment of overdosage is intravenous infusion of normal saline solution. If hypotension occurs, the patient should be placed in the shock position. If available, treatment with angiotensin II infusion and/or intravenous catecholamines may also be considered. Perindopril may be removed from the general circulation by haemodialysis. (See 4.4 Special warnings and special precautions for use, Haemodialysis Patients.) Pacemaker therapy is indicated for therapy-resistant bradycardia. Vital signs, serum electrolytes and creatinine concentrations should be monitored continuously.

5. PHARMACOLOGICAL PROPERTIES

5.1 Pharmacodynamic properties

ATC code: C09A A04

Perindopril is an inhibitor of the enzyme that converts angiotensin I into angiotensin II (Angiotensin Converting Enzyme ACE). The converting enzyme, or kinase, is an exopeptidase that allows conversion of angiotensin I into the vasoconstrictor angiotensin II as well as causing the degradation of the vasodilator bradykinin into an inactive heptapeptide. Inhibition of ACE results in a reduction of angiotensin II in the plasma, which leads to increased plasma renin activity (by inhibition of the negative feedback of renin release) and reduced secretion of aldosterone. Since ACE inactivates bradykinin, inhibition of ACE also results in an increased activity of circulating and local kallikrein-kinin systems (and thus also activation of the prostaglandin system). It is possible that this mechanism contributes to the blood pressure-lowering action of ACE inhibitors and is partially responsible for certain of their side effects (e.g. cough).

Perindopril acts through its active metabolite, perindoprilat. The other metabolites show no inhibition of ACE activity *in vitro*.

Hypertension

Perindopril is active in all grades of hypertension: mild, moderate, severe; a reduction in systolic and diastolic blood pressures in both supine and standing positions is observed.

Perindopril reduces peripheral vascular resistance, leading to blood pressure reduction. As a consequence, peripheral blood flow increases, with no effect on heart rate.

Renal blood flow increases as a rule, while the glomerular filtration rate (GFR) is usually unchanged.

The antihypertensive activity is maximal between 4 and 6 hours after a single dose and is sustained for at least 24 hours: trough effects are about 87-100 % of peak effects.

The decrease in blood pressure occurs rapidly. In responding patients, normalisation is achieved within a month and persists without the occurrence of tachyphylaxis.

Discontinuation of treatment does not lead to a rebound effect.

Perindopril reduces left ventricular hypertrophy.

In man, perindopril has been confirmed to demonstrate vasodilatory properties. It improves large artery elasticity and decreases the media:lumen ratio of small arteries.

An adjunctive therapy with a thiazide diuretic produces an additive-type of synergy. The combination of an ACE inhibitor and a thiazide also decreases the risk of hypokalaemia induced by the diuretic treatment.

Heart failure

COVERSYL reduces cardiac work by a decrease in preload and after-load.

Studies in patients with heart failure have demonstrated:

- decreased left and right ventricular filling pressures,
- reduced total peripheral vascular resistance,
- increased cardiac output and improved cardiac index.

In comparative studies, the first administration of 2 mg of COVERSYL to patients with mild to moderate heart failure was not associated with any significant reduction of blood pressure as compared to placebo.

5.2 Pharmacokinetic properties
After oral administration, the absorption of perindopril is rapid and the peak concentration complete within 1 hour. Bioavailability is 65 to 70 %.

About 20 % of the total quantity of perindopril absorbed is converted into perindoprilat, the active metabolite. In addition to active perindoprilat, perindopril yields five metabolites, all inactive. The plasma half-life of perindopril is equal to 1 hour. The peak plasma concentration of perindoprilat is achieved within 3 to 4 hours.

As ingestion of food decreases conversion to perindoprilat, hence bioavailability, COVERSYL should be administered orally in a single daily dose in the morning before a meal.

The volume of distribution is approximately 0.2 l/kg for unbound perindoprilat. Protein binding is slight (binding of perindoprilat to angiotensin converting enzyme is less than 30 %), but is concentration-dependent.

Perindoprilat is eliminated in the urine and the half-life of the unbound fraction is approximately 3 to 5 hours. Dissociation of perindoprilat bound to angiotensin converting enzyme leads to an "effective" elimination half-life of 25 hours, resulting in steady-state within 4 days.

After repeated administration, no accumulation of perindopril is observed.

Elimination of perindoprilat is decreased in the elderly, and also in patients with heart or renal failure. Dosage adjustment in renal insufficiency is desirable depending on the degree of impairment (creatinine clearance).

Dialysis clearance of perindoprilat is equal to 70 ml/min.

Perindopril kinetics are modified in patients with cirrhosis: hepatic clearance of the parent molecule is reduced by half. However, the quantity of perindoprilat formed is not reduced and therefore no dosage adjustment is required (see also sections 4.2 "Posology and method of administration" and 4.4 "Special warnings and special precautions for use").

5.3 Preclinical safety data
In the chronic oral toxicity studies (rats and monkeys), the target organ is the kidney, with reversible damage.

No mutagenicity has been observed in *in vitro* or *in vivo* studies.

Reproduction toxicology studies (rats, mice, rabbits and monkeys) showed no sign of embryotoxicity or teratogenicity. However, angiotensin converting enzyme inhibitors, as a class, have been shown to induce adverse effects on late foetal development, resulting in foetal death and congenital effects in rodents and rabbits: renal lesions and an increase in peri- and postnatal mortality have been observed.

No carcinogenicity has been observed in long term studies in rats and mice.

6. PHARMACEUTICAL PARTICULARS

6.1 List of excipients
Microcrystalline cellulose

Lactose monohydrate

Hydrophobic colloidal silica

Magnesium stearate

Aluminium copper complexes of chloryphyllins lake

6.2 Incompatibilities
None

6.3 Shelf life
2 years

6.4 Special precautions for storage
Coversyl 2 mg: Store below 25° C

Coversyl 4 mg: Store below 25° C

Coversyl 8 mg Tablets: Do not store above 30° C

6.5 Nature and contents of container
PVC /aluminium blisters.

7, 14, 28, 30, 56 or 112 tablets per carton.

Not all pack sizes may be marketed.

6.6 Instructions for use and handling
Not applicable

7. MARKETING AUTHORISATION HOLDER
LES LABORATOIRES Servier

22 rue Garnier

92200 Neuilly-sur-Seine - France

8. MARKETING AUTHORISATION NUMBER(S)
Coversyl 2 mg: 05815/0001

Coversyl 4 mg: 05815/0002

Coversyl 8 mg Tablets: 05815/0023

9. DATE OF FIRST AUTHORISATION/RENEWAL OF THE AUTHORISATION
Coversyl 2 mg: 15 December 1989

Coversyl 4 mg: 15 December 1989

Coversyl 8 mg Tablets: 12 June 2002

10. DATE OF REVISION OF THE TEXT
December 2003

Coversyl Plus Tablets

(Servier Laboratories Limited)

1. NAME OF THE MEDICINAL PRODUCT
COVERSYL® PLUS Tablets

2. QUALITATIVE AND QUANTITATIVE COMPOSITION
One tablet contains:

Perindopril tert-butylamine, 4.00 mg, equivalent to 3.338 mg perindopril

Indapamide, 1.25 mg

For excipients, see 6.1

3. PHARMACEUTICAL FORM
Tablet.

White, rod-shaped tablet.

4. CLINICAL PARTICULARS

4.1 Therapeutic indications
Treatment of essential hypertension, Coversyl® Plus Tablets are indicated in patients whose blood pressure is not adequately controlled on perindopril alone.

4.2 Posology and method of administration
Oral route.

One Coversyl® Plus tablet per day as a single dose, preferably to be taken in the morning, and before a meal.

When possible individual dose titration with the components can be recommended. When clinically appropriate, direct change from monotherapy to Coversyl® Plus Tablets may be considered.

Patients with renal insufficiency (see Special warnings and special precautions for use).

In severe renal insufficiency (creatinine clearance below 30 ml/min), treatment is contraindicated.

In patients with creatinine clearance greater than or equal to 30 ml/min and less than 60 ml/min, it is recommended to start treatment with the adequate dosage of the free combination. It is not necessary to change the dose when creatinine clearance is greater than 60 ml/min. Usual medical follow-up will include frequent monitoring of creatinine and potassium.

Children

Coversyl® Plus Tablets should not be used in children as the efficacy and tolerability of perindopril in children, alone or in combination, have not been established.

4.3 Contraindications
-LINKED TO PERINDOPRIL:

- Hypersensitivity to perindopril or any other ACE inhibitor
- History of angioneurotic oedema (Quincke's oedema) associated with previous ACE inhibitor therapy
- Hereditary/idiopathic angioneurotic oedema
- Pregnancy
- Lactation
- The drug is usually not recommended in case of: combinations with potassium-sparing diuretics, potassium salts, lithium (see Interaction with other medicinal products); bilateral renal artery stenosis or single functioning kidney; raised plasma levels of potassium.

- LINKED TO INDAPAMIDE:

- Hypersensitivity to sulphonamides
- Severe renal failure (creatinine clearance below 30 ml/min)
- Hepatic encephalopathy
- Severe impairment of liver function
- Hypokalaemia
- As a general rule, this medicine is inadvisable in combination with non-antiarrhythmic agents causing torsades de pointes (see Interaction with other medicinal products).

LINKED TO COVERSYL® PLUS TABLETS:

- Hypersensitivity to any of the excipients

Due to the lack of sufficient therapeutic experience, Coversyl® Plus Tablets should not be used in:

- dialysis patients
- patients with untreated decompensated heart failure.

4.4 Special warnings and special precautions for use
Special warnings

LINKED TO PERINDOPRIL:

RISK OF NEUTROPENIA/AGRANULOCYTOSIS IN IMMUNO-SUPPRESSED PATIENTS:

The risk of neutropenia appears to be dose- and type-related and is dependent on patient's clinical status. It is rarely seen in uncomplicated patients but may occur in patients with some degree of renal impairment especially when it is associated with collagen vascular disease *e.g.* systemic lupus erythematosus, scleroderma and therapy with immunosuppressive agents. It is reversible after discontinuation of the ACE inhibitor.

Strict compliance with the predetermined dose seems to be the best way to prevent the onset of these events. However, if an angiotensin converting enzyme inhibitor is to be administered to this type of patient, the risk/benefit ratio should be evaluated carefully.

ANGIONEUROTIC OEDEMA (QUINCKE'S OEDEMA):

Angioneurotic oedema of the face, extremities, lips, tongue, glottis and/or larynx has been reported rarely in patients receiving treatment with angiotensin converting enzyme inhibitors, including perindopril. In such cases, treatment with perindopril should be stopped immediately and the patient should be monitored until the oedema has disappeared.

When the oedema only affects the face and the lips, the effect generally recedes without treatment, even though antihistamines may be used to relieve symptoms.

Angioneurotic oedema combined with laryngeal oedema may be fatal. Involvement of the tongue, glottis or larynx may lead to an obstruction of the airways. A subcutaneous injection of adrenaline at 1:1000 (0.3 ml to 0.5 ml) should be administered quickly and other appropriate measures taken.

The prescription of an angiotensin converting enzyme inhibitor should not subsequently be considered in these patients (see Contraindications).

Patients with a previous history of Quincke's oedema which was not linked to taking an angiotensin converting enzyme inhibitor have an increased risk of Quincke's oedema with an angiotensin converting enzyme inhibitor.

ANAPHYLACTIC REACTIONS DURING DESENSITISATION:

There have been isolated reports of patients experiencing sustained, life-threatening anaphylactoid reactions while receiving ACE inhibitors during desensitisation treatment with hymenoptera (bees, wasps) venom. ACE inhibitors should be used with caution in allergic patients treated with desensitisation, and avoided in those undergoing venom immunotherapy. However these reactions could be prevented by temporary withdrawal of ACE inhibitor for at least 24 hours before treatment in patients who require both ACE inhibitors and desensitisation.

ANAPHYLACTIC REACTONS DURING MEMBRANE EXPOSURE:

There have been reports of patients experiencing sustained, life-threatening anaphylactoid reactions while receiving ACE inhibitors during dialysis with high-flux membranes or low-density lipoprotein apheresis with dextran sulphate adsorption. ACE inhibitors should be avoided in patients undergoing dialysis with high-flux membranes or LDL apheresis with dextran sulphate adsorption. However these reactions could be prevented by temporary withdrawal of ACE inhibitor for at least 24 hours before treatment in patients who require both ACE inhibitors and LDL apheresis.

LINKED TO INDAPAMIDE:

When liver function is impaired, thiazide diuretics and thiazide-related diuretics may cause hepatic encephalopathy. Administration of the diuretic should be stopped immediately if this occurs.

Special precautions for use

LINKED TO COVERSYL® PLUS TABLETS:

RENAL INSUFFICIENCY:

In cases of severe renal insufficiency (creatinine clearance < 30 ml/min), treatment is contraindicated.

In certain hypertensive patients without pre-existing apparent renal lesion and for whom renal blood tests show functional renal insufficiency, treatment should be stopped and possibly restarted either at a low dose or with one constituent only.

In these patients usual medical follow-up will include frequent monitoring of potassium and creatinine, after two weeks of treatment and then every two months during therapeutic stability period. Renal failure has been reported mainly in patients with severe heart failure or underlying renal failure including renal artery stenosis.

HYPOTENSION AND WATER AND ELECTROLYTE DEPLETION:

There is a risk of sudden hypotension in the presence of pre-existing sodium depletion (in particular in individuals with renal artery stenosis). Therefore systematic testing should be carried out for clinical signs of water and electrolyte depletion, which may occur with an intercurrent episode of diarrhoea or vomiting. Regular monitoring of plasma electrolytes should be carried out in such patients.

Marked hypotension may require the implementation of an intravenous infusion of isotonic saline.

Transient hypotension is not a contraindication to continuation of treatment. After re-establishment of a satisfactory blood volume and blood pressure, treatment can be started again either at a reduced dose or with only one of the constituents.

POTASSIUM LEVELS:

The combination of perindopril and indapamide does not prevent the onset of hypokalaemia particularly in diabetic patients or in patients with renal failure. As with any antihypertensive agent containing a diuretic, regular monitoring of plasma potassium levels should be carried out.

LINKED TO PERINDOPRIL:

COUGH:

A dry cough has been reported with the use of angiotensin converting enzyme inhibitors. It is characterised by its persistence and by its disappearance when treatment is withdrawn. An iatrogenic aetiology should be considered in the event of this symptom. If the prescription of an angiotensin converting enzyme inhibitor is still preferred, continuation of treatment may be considered.

CHILDREN:

The efficacy and tolerability of perindopril in children, alone or in combination, have not been established.

RISK OF ARTERIAL HYPOTENSION AND/OR RENAL INSUFFICIENCY (IN CASES OF CARDIAC INSUFFICIENCY, WATER AND ELECTROLYTE DEPLETION, ETC...):

Marked stimulation of the renin-angiotensin-aldosterone system has been observed particularly during marked water and electrolyte depletions (strict sodium-free diet or prolonged diuretic treatment), in patients whose blood pressure was initially low, in cases of renal artery stenosis, congestive heart failure or cirrhosis with oedema and ascites.

The blocking of this system with an angiotensin converting enzyme inhibitor may therefore cause, particularly at the time of the first administration and during the first two weeks of treatment, a sudden drop in blood pressure and/or an increase in plasma levels of creatinine, showing a functional renal insufficiency. Occasionally this can be acute in onset, although rare, and with a variable time to onset.

In such cases, the treatment should then be initiated at a lower dose and increased progressively.

ELDERLY:

Renal function and potassium levels should be tested before the start of treatment. The initial dose is subsequently adjusted according to blood pressure response, especially in cases of water and electrolyte depletion, in order to avoid sudden onset of hypotension.

PATIENTS WITH KNOWN ATHEROSCLEROSIS:

The risk of hypotension exists in all patients but particular care should be taken in patients with ischaemic heart disease or cerebral circulatory insufficiency, with treatment being started at a low dose.

RENOVASCULAR HYPERTENSION:

The treatment for renovascular hypertension is revascularisation. Nonetheless, angiotensin converting enzyme inhibitors can be beneficial in patients presenting with renovascular hypertension who are awaiting corrective surgery or when such a surgery is not possible.

Treatment should be started in a hospital setting at a low dose and renal function and potassium levels should be monitored, since some patients have developed a functional renal insufficiency which was reversed when treatment was stopped.

OTHER POPULATIONS AT RISK:

In patients with severe cardiac insufficiency (grade IV) or in patients with insulin dependent diabetes mellitus (spontaneous tendency to increased levels of potassium), treatment should be started under medical supervision with a reduced initial dose. Treatment with beta-blockers in hypertensive patients with coronary insufficiency should not be stopped: the ACE inhibitor should be added to the beta-blocker.

ANAEMIA:

Anaemia has been observed in patients who have had a kidney transplant or have been undergoing dialysis. The reduction in haemoglobin levels is more apparent as initial values were high. This effect does not seem to be dose-dependent but may be linked to the mechanism of action of angiotensin converting enzyme inhibitors.

This reduction in haemoglobin is slight, occurs within 1 to 6 months, and then remains stable. It is reversible when treatment is stopped. Treatment can be continued with regular haematological testing.

SURGERY:

Angiotensin converting enzyme inhibitors can cause hypotension in cases of anaesthesia, especially when the anaesthetic administered is an agent with hypotensive potential. It is therefore recommended that treatment with long-acting angiotensin converting enzyme inhibitors such as perindopril should be discontinued where possible two days before surgery.

AORTIC STENOSIS/HYPERTROPHIC CARDIOMYOPATHY:

ACE inhibitors should be used with caution in patient with an obstruction in the outflow tract of the left ventricle.

LINKED TO INDAPAMIDE:

WATER AND ELECTROLYTE BALANCE:

Sodium levels:

These should be tested before treatment is started, then at regular intervals. All diuretic treatment can cause a reduction in sodium levels, which may have serious consequences. Reduction in sodium levels can be initially asymptomatic and regular testing is therefore essential. Testing should be more frequent in elderly and cirrhotic patients (see Undesirable effects and Overdose).

Potassium levels:

Potassium depletion with hypokalaemia is a major risk with thiazide diuretics and thiazide-related diuretics. The risk of onset of lowered potassium levels (< 3.4 mmol/l) should be prevented in some high risk populations such as elderly and/or malnourished subjects, whether or not they are taking multiple medications, cirrhotic patients with oedema and ascites, coronary patients and patients with heart failure.

In such cases hypokalaemia increases the cardiac toxicity of cardiac glycosides and the risk of rhythm disorders.

Subjects presenting with a long QT interval are also at risk, whether the origin is congenital or iatrogenic. Hypokalaemia, as with bradycardia, acts as a factor which favours the onset of severe rhythm disorders, in particular torsades de pointes, which may be fatal.

In all cases more frequent testing of potassium levels is necessary. The first measurement of plasma potassium levels should be carried out during the first week following the start of treatment.

If low potassium levels are detected, correction is required.

Calcium levels:

Thiazide diuretics and thiazide-related diuretics may reduce urinary excretion of calcium and cause a mild and transient increase in plasma calcium levels. Markedly raised levels of calcium may be related to undiagnosed hyperparathyroidism. In such cases the treatment should be stopped before investigating the parathyroid function.

BLOOD GLUCOSE:

Monitoring of blood glucose is important in diabetic patients, particularly when potassium levels are low.

URIC ACID:

Tendency to gout attacks may be increased in hyperuricaemic patients.

RENAL FUNCTION AND DIURETICS:

Thiazide diuretics and thiazide-related diuretics are only fully effective when renal function is normal or only slightly impaired (creatinine levels lower than approximately 25 mg/l, i.e. 220 μmol/l for an adult).

In the elderly the value of plasma creatinine levels should be adjusted to take account of the age, weight and sex of the patient, according to the Cockroft formula:

cl_{cr} = (140 - age) × body weight / 0.814 × plasma creatinine level

with: age expressed in years, body weight in kg, plasma creatinine level in micromol/l

This formula is suitable for an elderly male and should be adapted for women by multiplying the result by 0.85.

Hypovolaemia, resulting from the loss of water and sodium caused by the diuretic at the start of treatment, causes a reduction in glomerular filtration. It may result in an increase in blood urea and creatinine levels. This transitory functional renal insufficiency is of no adverse consequence in patients with normal renal function but may however worsen a pre-existing renal insufficiency.

ATHLETES:

Athletes should note that this product contains an active substance which may cause a positive reaction in doping tests.

4.5 Interaction with other medicinal products and other forms of Interaction

LINKED TO COVERSYL® PLUS TABLETS:

Combinations which are NOT RECOMMENDED:

- Lithium

An increase in lithium levels may produce signs of overdose, as occurs with a sodium-free diet (reduction in renal excretion of lithium). If the combination of an angiotensin converting enzyme inhibitor and a diuretic is unavoidable, strict monitoring of lithium levels and adjustment of the dose are necessary.

Combinations which require special care:

- Antidiabetic agents (insulin, hypoglycaemic sulphonamides)

Reported with captopril and enalapril: The use of angiotensin converting enzyme inhibitors may increase the hypoglycaemic effect in diabetics receiving treatment with insulin or with hypoglycaemic sulphonamides. The onset of hypoglycaemic episodes is very rare (improvement in glucose tolerance with a resulting reduction in insulin requirements).

- Baclofen

Potentiation of antihypertensive effect: Monitoring of blood pressure and renal function, and dose adaptation of the antihypertensive if necessary.

- N.S.A.I.D (systemic route), high-dose salicylates

Acute renal insufficiency in dehydrated patients (reduction in glomerular filtration). The patient should be well hydrated; renal function should be monitored at the start of treatment.

Combinations which require some care:

- Imipramine-like antidepressants (tricyclics), neuroleptics

Increased antihypertensive effect and increased risk of orthostatic hypotension (additive effect).

- Corticosteroids, tetracosactide

Reduction in antihypertensive effect (salt and water retention due to corticosteroids).

LINKED TO PERINDOPRIL:

Combinations which are NOT RECOMMENDED:

- Potassium-sparing diuretics (spironolactone, triamterene, alone or in combination.), potassium (salts)

Increased levels of potassium (potentially lethal), particularly in cases of renal insufficiency (addition of potassium-sparing effects). Potassium-raising agents should not be combined with angiotensin converting enzyme inhibitors, except when potassium levels are low.

- Anaesthetic drugs

ACE inhibitors may enhance the hypotensive effects of certain anaesthetic drugs.

- Allopurinol, cytostatic or immunosuppressive agents, systemic corticosteroids or procainamide

Concomitant administration with ACE inhibitors may lead to an increased risk for leucopenia.

- Antihypertensive agents

Increase of the hypotensive effect of ACE inhibitors.

LINKED TO INDAPAMIDE:

Combinations which are NOT RECOMMENDED:

- Non antiarrhythmic drugs which prolong the QT interval or cause torsades de pointes (astemizole, bepridil, erythromycin IV, halofantrine, pentamidine, sultopride, terfenadine, vincamine)

Torsades de pointes (low potassium levels is a risk, as are bradycardia and pre-existing long QT interval).

Substances which do not have the unwanted effect of causing torsades de pointes should be used in cases of low potassium levels.

Combinations which require special care:

- N.S.A.I.D (systemic route), high-dose salicylates

Possible reduction in the antihypertensive effect of indapamide.

Acute renal insufficiency in dehydrated patients (reduction in glomerular filtration).

Hydrate the patient; monitor renal function at the start of treatment.

- Potassium-lowering drugs: amphotericin B (IV route), glucocorticoids and mineralocorticoids (systemic route), tetracosactide, stimulant laxatives

Increased risk of low potassium levels (additive effect).

Monitoring of potassium levels, and correction if necessary; particular consideration required in cases of treatment with cardiac glycosides. Non-stimulant laxatives should be used.

- Cardiac glycosides

Low potassium levels favour the toxic effects of cardiac glycosides.

Potassium levels and ECG should be monitored and treatment reconsidered if necessary.

Combinations which require some care:

- Potassium-sparing diuretics (amiloride, spironolactone, triamterene)

The rational combination, which is useful for some patients, does not exclude the onset of low potassium levels or, particularly in patients with renal insufficiency or diabetes, raised potassium levels.

Potassium levels and ECG should be monitored and treatment reconsidered if necessary.

- Antiarrhythmic drugs which produce torsades de pointes: Class IA antiarrhythmic agents (quinidine, hydroquinidine, disopyramide), amiodarone, bretylium, sotalol

Torsades de pointes (low potassium levels is a risk factor, as are bradycardia and a pre-existing long QT interval).

Prevention of low potassium levels and correction if necessary: monitoring of the QT interval. Antiarrythmics should not be administered in cases of torsades de pointes (management by pacemaker).

- Metformin

Lactic acidosis due to metformin caused by possible functional renal insufficiency linked to diuretics and in particular to loop diuretics.

Do not use metformin when plasma creatinine levels exceed 15 mg/l (135 micromol/l) in men and 12 mg/l (110 micromol/l) in women.

- Iodinated contrast media

In cases of dehydration caused by diuretics, there is an increased risk of acute renal insufficiency, particularly when high doses of iodinated contrast media are used.

Rehydration should be carried out before the iodinated compound is administered.

- Imipramine-like antidepressants (tricyclics), neuroleptics

Increased antihypertensive effect and increased risk of orthostatic hypotension (additive effect).

- Calcium (salts)

Risk of increased levels of calcium due to reduced elimination of calcium in the urine.

- Ciclosporin

Risk of increased creatinine levels with no change in circulating levels of ciclosporin, even when there is no salt and water depletion.

- Corticosteroids, tetracosactide (systemic route)

Reduction in antihypertensive effect (salt and water retention due to corticosteroids).

4.6 Pregnancy and lactation

As this combination includes an ACE inhibitor, Coversyl® Plus Tablets are contraindicated during pregnancy and lactation.

LINKED TO PERINDOPRIL:

Pregnancy:

Appropriate and well-controlled studies have not been done in humans. ACE inhibitors cross the placenta and can cause foetal and neonatal morbidity and mortality when administered to pregnant women.

Foetal exposure to ACE inhibitors during the second and third trimesters has been associated with neonatal hypotension, renal failure, face or skull deformities and/or death. Maternal oligohydramnios has also been reported reflecting decreasing renal function in the foetus. Limb contractures, craniofacial deformities, hypoplastic lung development and intrauterine growth retardation have been reported in association with oligohydramnios. Infants exposed in utero to ACE inhibitors should be closely observed for hypotension, oliguria and hyperkalaemia. Oliguria should be treated with support of blood pressure and renal perfusion.

Intrauterine growth retardation, prematurity, patent ductus arteriosus and foetal death have also been reported but it is not clear whether they are related to the ACE inhibition or the underlying maternal disease.

It is not known whether exposure limited to the first trimester can adversely affect foetal outcome. Women who become pregnant while receiving an ACE inhibitor should be informed of the potential hazard to the foetus.

Lactation:

ACE inhibitors may be excreted in breast milk and their effect on the nursing infant has not been determined. It is recommended that lactating mothers should not breast feed while taking ACE inhibitors.

LINKED TO INDAPAMIDE:

Pregnancy:

As a general rule, the administration of diuretics should be avoided in pregnant women and should never be given as treatment for physiological oedema (and therefore do not require treatment) of pregnancy. Diuretics may lead to foeto-placental ischaemia, with a risk of impaired foetal growth.

Nonetheless diuretics remain an essential part of the treatment of oedema from cardiac, hepatic and renal origin arising in pregnant women.

Lactation:

Indapamide is excreted in small quantities in breast milk. Nonetheless, it should not be used in breast-feeding period due to:

- the decrease and even suppression of the milk secretion,

- its undesirable effects in particular biological (potassium levels),

- its belonging to the sulphonamide group with the risks of allergy and nuclear icterus.

4.7 Effects on ability to drive and use machines

LINKED TO PERINDOPRIL, INDAPAMIDE AND COVERSYL® PLUS TABLETS:

Neither the two active substances nor Coversyl® Plus Tablets affect alertness but individual reactions related to low blood pressure may occur in some patients, particularly at the start of treatment or in combination with another antihypertensive medication.

As a result the ability to drive or operate machinery may be impaired.

4.8 Undesirable effects

The administration of perindopril inhibits the renin-angiotensin-aldosterone axis and tends to reduce the potassium loss caused by indapamide. Four percent of the patients on treatment with Coversyl® Plus Tablets experience hypokalaemia (potassium level < 3.4 mmol/l).

GASTRO-INTESTINAL TRACT

- Common (>1/100, <1/10): constipation, dry mouth, nausea, epigastric pain, anorexia, abdominal pains, taste disturbance

- Very rare (<1/10,000): pancreatitis

- In case of hepatic insufficiency, there is a possibility of onset of hepatic encephalopathy (see Contraindications and Special warnings)

RESPIRATORY SYSTEM

Common (>1/100, <1/10):

A dry cough has been reported with the use of angiotensin converting enzyme inhibitors. It is characterised by its persistence and by its disappearance when treatment is withdrawn. An iatrogenic aetiology should be considered in the presence of this symptom.

CARDIO-VASCULAR SYSTEM

Uncommon (>1/1,000, <1/100):

- Hypotension whether orthostatic or not (see Special precautions for use).

SKIN APPENDAGES

Uncommon (>1/1,000, <1/100):

- Hypersensitivity reactions, mainly dermatological, in subjects with a predisposition to allergic and asthmatic reactions

- Maculopapular eruptions, purpura, possible aggravation of pre-existing acute disseminated lupus erythematosus

- Skin rash

Very rare (<1/10,000):

- Angioneurotic oedema (Quincke's oedema) (see Special warnings)

NERVOUS SYSTEM

Uncommon (>1/1,000, <1/100):

- Headache, asthenia, feelings of dizziness, mood disturbances and/or sleep disturbances.

MUSCULAR SYSTEM

Uncommon (>1/1,000, <1/100):

- Cramps, paresthesia.

HAEMIC SYSTEM

Very rare (<1/10,000):

- Thrombocytopenia, leucopenia, agranulocytosis, aplastic anaemia, haemolytic anaemia.

- Anaemia (see Special precautions for use) has been reported with angiotensin converting enzyme inhibitors in specific circumstances (patients who have had kidney transplants, patients undergoing haemodialysis).

LABORATORY PARAMETERS

- Potassium depletion with particularly serious reduction in levels of potassium in some at risk populations (see Special precautions for use).

- Reduced sodium levels with hypovolaemia causing dehydration and orthostatic hypotension.

- Increase in uric acid levels and in blood glucose levels during treatment

- Slight increase in urea and in plasma creatinine levels, reversible when treatment is stopped. This increase is more frequent in cases of renal artery stenosis, arterial hypertension treated with diuretics, renal insufficiency.

- Increased levels of potassium, usually transitory.

Rare (>1/10,000, <1/1,000):

- raised plasma calcium levels.

4.9 Overdose

The most likely adverse event in cases of overdose is hypotension, sometimes associated with nausea, vomiting, cramps, dizziness, sleepiness, mental confusion, oliguria which may progress to anuria (due to hypovolaemia). Salt and water disturbances (low sodium levels, low potassium levels) may occur.

The first measures to be taken consist of rapidly eliminating the product(s) ingested by gastric lavage and/or administration of activated charcoal, then restoring fluid and electrolyte balance in a specialised centre until they return to normal.

If marked hypotension occurs, this can be treated by placing the patient in a supine position with the head lowered. If necessary an IV infusion of isotonic saline may be given, or any other method of volaemic expansion may be used.

Perindoprilat, the active form of perindopril, can be dialysed (see Pharmacokinetic properties).

5. PHARMACOLOGICAL PROPERTIES

5.1 Pharmacodynamic properties

Pharmacotherapeutic group: perindopril and diuretics

ATC code: C09BA04

Coversyl® Plus is a combination of perindopril tert-butylamine salt, an angiotensin converting enzyme inhibitor, and indapamide, a chlorosulphamoyl diuretic. Its pharmacological properties are derived from those of each of the components taken separately, in addition to those due to the additive synergic action of the two products when combined.

PHARMACOLOGICAL MECHANISM OF ACTION

LINKED TO COVERSYL® PLUS TABLETS:

Coversyl® Plus Tablets produce an additive synergy of the antihypertensive effects of the two components.

LINKED TO PERINDOPRIL:

Perindopril is an inhibitor of the angiotensin converting enzyme (ACE inhibitor) which converts angiotensin I to angiotensin II, a vasoconstricting substance; in addition the enzyme stimulates the secretion of aldosterone by the adrenal cortex and stimulates the degradation of bradykinin, a vasodilatory substance, into inactive heptapeptides.

This results in:

- a reduction in aldosterone secretion,

- an increase in plasma renin activity, since aldosterone no longer exercises negative feedback,

- a reduction in total peripheral resistance with a preferential action on the vascular bed in muscle and the kidney, with no accompanying salt and water retention or reflex tachycardia, with chronic treatment.

The antihypertensive action of perindopril also occurs in patients with low or normal renin concentrations.

Perindopril acts through its active metabolite, perindoprilat. The other metabolites are inactive.

Perindopril reduces the work of the heart:

- by a vasodilatory effect on veins, probably caused by changes in the metabolism of prostaglandins: reduction in pre-load,

- by reduction of the total peripheral resistance: reduction in afterload.

Studies carried out on patients with cardiac insufficiency have shown:

- a reduction in left and right ventricular filling pressures,

- a reduction in total peripheral vascular resistance,

- an increase in cardiac output and an improvement in the cardiac index,

- an increase in regional blood flow in muscle.

Exercise test results also showed improvement.

LINKED TO INDAPAMIDE:

Indapamide is a sulphonamide derivative with an indole ring, pharmacologically related to the thiazide group of diuretics. Indapamide inhibits the reabsorption of sodium in the cortical dilution segment. It increases the urinary excretion of sodium and chlorides and, to a lesser extent, the excretion of potassium and magnesium, thereby increasing urine output and having an antihypertensive action.

CHARACTERISTICS OF ANTIHYPERTENSIVE ACTION

LINKED TO COVERSYL® PLUS TABLETS:

In hypertensive patients regardless of age, Coversyl® Plus Tablets exert a dose-dependent antihypertensive effect on diastolic and systolic arterial pressure whilst supine or standing. This antihypertensive effect lasts for 24 hours. The reduction in blood pressure is obtained in less than one month without tachyphylaxis; stopping treatment has no rebound effect. During clinical trials, the concomitant administration of perindopril and indapamide produced antihypertensive effects of a synergic nature in relation to each of the products administered alone.

LINKED TO PERINDOPRIL:

Perindopril is active in all grades of hypertension: mild to moderate or severe. A reduction in systolic and diastolic arterial pressure is observed in the lying and standing position.

The antihypertensive activity after a single dose is maximal at between 4 and 6 hours and is maintained over 24 hours.

There is a high degree of residual blocking of angiotensin converting enzyme at 24 hours, approximately 80%.

In patients who respond, normalised blood pressure is reached after one month and is maintained without tachyphylaxis.

Withdrawal of treatment has no rebound effect on hypertension.

Perindopril has vasodilatory properties and restores elasticity of the main arterial trunks, corrects histomorphometric changes in resistance arteries and produces a reduction in left ventricular hypertrophy.

If necessary, the addition of a thiazide diuretic leads to an additive synergy.

The combination of an angiotensin converting enzyme inhibitor with a thiazide diuretic decreases the hypokalaemia risk associated with the diuretic alone.

LINKED TO INDAPAMIDE:

Indapamide, as monotherapy, has an antihypertensive effect which lasts for 24 hours. This effect occurs at doses at which the diuretic properties are minimal.

Its antihypertensive action is proportional to an improvement in arterial compliance and a reduction in total and arteriolar peripheral vascular resistance.

Indapamide reduces left ventricular hypertrophy.

When a dose of thiazide diuretic and thiazide-related diuretics is exceeded, the antihypertensive effect reaches a plateau, whereas the adverse effects continue to increase. If the treatment is ineffective, the dose should not be increased.

Furthermore, it has been shown that in the short-term, mid-term and long-term in hypertensive patients, indapamide:

- has no effect on lipid metabolism: triglycerides, LDL-cholesterol and HDL-cholesterol,

- has no effect on carbohydrate metabolism, even in diabetic hypertensive patients.

5.2 Pharmacokinetic properties

LINKED TO COVERSYL® PLUS TABLETS:

The co-administration of perindopril and indapamide does not change their pharmacokinetic properties by comparison to separate administration.

LINKED TO PERINDOPRIL:

Perindopril is rapidly absorbed by the oral route. The quantity absorbed is 65 to 70 % of the dose administered.

It is hydrolysed into perindoprilat which is a specific angiotensin converting enzyme inhibitor. The quantity of perindoprilat formed is altered by food intake. The peak plasma concentration of perindoprilat is reached after 3 to 4 hours. Plasma protein binding is less than 30 % but is concentration-dependent.

After repeated administration of perindopril as a single daily dose, steady-state is reached after an average of 4 days. The effective elimination half-life of perindoprilat is approximately 24 hours.

Plasma concentrations of perindoprilat are significantly higher in patients with creatinine clearance below 60 ml/min, whether they are patients with renal insufficiency or elderly. Elimination is also slowed down in patients with cardiac insufficiency.

The clearance of perindopril by dialysis is 70 ml/min.

In cirrhotic patients, the kinetics of perindopril is altered: hepatic clearance of the parent substance is reduced by half. However, the quantity of perindoprilat formed is not reduced and dose adjustment is therefore not necessary.

Angiotensin converting enzyme inhibitors cross the placenta.

LINKED TO INDAPAMIDE:

Indapamide is rapidly and completely absorbed from the digestive tract.

The peak plasma level is reached in humans approximately one hour after oral administration of the product. Plasma protein binding is 79 %.

The elimination half-life is between 14 and 24 hours (average 18 hours). Repeated administration does not produce accumulation. Elimination is mainly in the urine

(70 % of the dose) and faeces (22 %) in the form of inactive metabolites.

The pharmacokinetics are unchanged in patients with renal insufficiency.

5.3 Preclinical safety data
Coversyl® Plus has a slightly increased toxicity than that of its components. Renal manifestations do not seem to be potentiated in the rat. However, the combination produces gastro-intestinal toxicity in the dog and the toxic effects on the mother seem to be increased in the rat (compared to perindopril).

Nonetheless, these adverse effects are shown at dose levels corresponding to a very marked safety margin by comparison to the therapeutic doses used.

6. PHARMACEUTICAL PARTICULARS

6.1 List of excipients
Colloidal hydrophobic silica, lactose monohydrate, magnesium stearate, microcrystalline cellulose.

6.2 Incompatibilities
Not applicable

6.3 Shelf life
2 years.

6.4 Special precautions for storage
Do not store above 30°C.

6.5 Nature and contents of container
14, 20, 28, 30, 50, 56, 60, 90, 100 and 500 tablets in blister (PVC/aluminium).

Not all pack sizes may be marketed.

6.6 Instructions for use and handling
No special requirements.

7. MARKETING AUTHORISATION HOLDER
LES LABORATOIRES SERVIER

22, rue Garnier

92200 Neuilly-sur-Seine – France

8. MARKETING AUTHORISATION NUMBER(S)
PL 05815/0013

9. DATE OF FIRST AUTHORISATION/RENEWAL OF THE AUTHORISATION
23 September 1998/European Renewal: 15 December 2002

10. DATE OF REVISION OF THE TEXT
October 2003

COZAAR 25 mg, 50 mg and 100 mg Tablets

(Merck Sharp & Dohme Limited)

1. NAME OF THE MEDICINAL PRODUCT
COZAAR® 100 mg Film Coated Tablets

COZAAR® 50 mg Film Coated Tablets

COZAAR® 25 mg Film Coated Tablets

2. QUALITATIVE AND QUANTITATIVE COMPOSITION
There are three strengths of 'Cozaar' Tablets available:

Each 'Cozaar' 100 mg Tablet contains 91.6 mg of losartan, present as 100 mg of losartan potassium.

Each 'Cozaar' 50 mg Tablet contains 45.8 mg of losartan, present as 50 mg of losartan potassium.

Each 'Cozaar' 25 mg Tablet contains 22.9 mg of losartan, present as 25 mg of losartan potassium.

For excipients see section 6.1

3. PHARMACEUTICAL FORM
Film-coated tablet

'Cozaar' 100 mg Tablet is supplied as a white, teardrop-shaped, film-coated tablet marked '960' on one side and plain on the other.

'Cozaar' 50 mg Tablet is supplied as a white, oval-shaped, film-coated tablet marked '952' on one side and a single score line on the other.

'Cozaar' 25 mg Tablet is supplied as a white, oval-shaped, film-coated tablet marked '951' on one side and plain on the other.

4. CLINICAL PARTICULARS

4.1 Therapeutic indications
Hypertension

'Cozaar' is indicated for the treatment of hypertension.

Hypertensive patients with left ventricular hypertrophy

In hypertensive patients with left ventricular hypertrophy a reduced risk of stroke was demonstrated. The data do not support the use of 'Cozaar' for this indication in black patients (see section 4.4 Special warnings and Precautions for Use-*Race* and section 5.1 Pharmacodynamic Properties, LIFE study, *Race*).

Renal protection in type 2 diabetic patients with nephropathy (macroalbuminuria)

'Cozaar' is indicated to delay the progression of renal disease as measured by a reduction in the combined incidence of doubling of serum creatinine, end stage renal disease (need for dialysis or renal transplantation) or death; and to reduce proteinuria.

4.2 Posology and method of administration
'Cozaar' may be administered with or without food.

'Cozaar' may be administered with other antihypertensive agents. The concomitant use of 'Cozaar' and ACE inhibitors has not been adequately studied.

Hypertension

The starting and maintenance dose is 50 mg once daily for most patients. The maximal antihypertensive effect is attained 3-6 weeks after initiation of therapy. Some patients may receive an additional benefit by increasing the dose to 100 mg once daily.

Reduction in the risk of stroke in hypertensive patients with left ventricular hypertrophy

The usual starting dose is 50 mg of 'Cozaar' once daily. A low dose of hydrochlorothiazide may be added and/or the dose of 'Cozaar' may be increased to 100 mg once daily based on blood pressure.

Renal protection in type 2 diabetic patients with nephropathy.

The usual starting dose is 50 mg once daily. The dose may be increased to 100 mg once daily according to blood pressure response from one month after initiation of therapy onwards. 'Cozaar' may be administered with other antihypertensive agents (e.g., diuretics, calcium channel blockers, alpha- or beta-blockers, and centrally acting agents) as well as with insulin and other commonly used hypoglycaemic agents (e.g., sulfonylureas, glitazones and glucosidase inhibitors).

'Cozaar' was not studied in type 2 diabetic patients with severe renal impairment.

Use in patients with intravascular volume depletion: For the very small proportion of patients who have intravascular volume depletion (e.g. those treated with high-dose diuretics), a starting dose of 25 mg once daily is recommended (see 4.4 'Special warnings and precautions for use').

Use in renal impairment: No initial dosage adjustment is necessary in patients with mild renal impairment (i.e. creatinine clearance 20-50 ml/min). For patients with moderate to severe renal impairment (i.e. creatinine clearance <20 ml/min) or patients on dialysis, a lower starting dose of 25 mg once daily is recommended.

Use in hepatic impairment: A lower dose should be considered for patients with a history of hepatic impairment (see 4.4 'Special warnings and precautions for use').

Use in the elderly: *Patients up to 75 years*: No initial dosage adjustment is necessary for this group of patients.

Patients over 75 years: Presently there is limited clinical experience in this group; a lower starting dose of 25 mg once daily is recommended.

4.3 Contraindications
'Cozaar' is contraindicated in pregnancy (see 4.6 'Pregnancy and lactation') and in patients who are hypersensitive to any component of this product.

4.4 Special warnings and special precautions for use
Hypersensitivity:

Angioedema. See 4.8 'Undesirable effects'.

The use of 'Cozaar' in patients with haemodynamically significant obstructive valvular disease or cardiomyopathy has not been adequately studied.

Hypotension and electrolyte/fluid imbalance

In patients who are intravascularly volume depleted (e.g. those treated with high-dose diuretics), symptomatic hypotension may occur. These conditions should be corrected prior to administration of 'Cozaar', or a lower starting dose should be used (see 4.2 'Posology and method of administration').

Electrolyte imbalances are common in patients with renal impairment, with or without diabetes, and should be addressed. In a clinical study conducted in type 2 diabetic patients with nephropathy, the incidence of hyperkalaemia was higher in the group treated with 'Cozaar' as compared to the placebo group (see 4.8 'Undesirable effects' and *Laboratory test findings*).

Liver function impairment

Based on pharmacokinetic data which demonstrate significantly increased plasma concentrations of losartan in cirrhotic patients, a lower dose should be considered for patients with a history of hepatic impairment (see 4.2 'Posology and method of administration' and 5.2 'Pharmacokinetic properties').

Renal function impairment

As a consequence of inhibiting the renin-angiotensin-aldosterone system, changes in renal function including renal failure have been reported (in particular, in patients whose renal function is dependent on the renin-angiotensin-aldosterone system such as those with severe cardiac insufficiency or pre-existing renal dysfunction).

As with other drugs that affect the renin-angiotensin-aldosterone system, increases in blood urea and serum creatinine have also been reported in patients with bilateral renal artery stenosis or stenosis of the artery to a solitary kidney; these changes in renal function may be reversible upon discontinuation of therapy.

Caution is required in patients with significant renal disease and renal transplant recipients as there have been reports of anaemia developing in such patients treated with 'Cozaar'.

Race (Black patients):

There is no evidence that Cozaar reduces the risk of stroke in black patients with hypertension and left ventricular hypertrophy (see Section 5.1 Pharmacodynamic properties, LIFE Study, *Race*).

4.5 Interaction with other medicinal products and other forms of Interaction
In clinical pharmacokinetic trials, no drug interactions of clinical significance have been identified with hydrochlorothiazide, digoxin, warfarin, cimetidine, ketoconazole, erythromycin and phenobarbital (phenobarbitone). Rifampicin and fluconazole have been reported to reduce levels of active metabolite. The clinical consequences of these interactions have not been evaluated.

As with other drugs that block angiotensin II or its effects, concomitant use of other drugs which retain potassium or may increase potassium levels (e.g. potassium-sparing diuretics, potassium supplements or salt substitutes containing potassium) may lead to increases in serum potassium. Co-medication is not advisable.

As with other antihypertensive agents, the antihypertensive effect of losartan may be attenuated by non-steroidal anti-inflammatory drugs such as indomethacin.

4.6 Pregnancy and lactation
Use during pregnancy

Although there is no experience with the use of 'Cozaar' in pregnant women, animal studies with losartan potassium have demonstrated foetal and neonatal injury and death, the mechanism of which is believed to be pharmacologically mediated through effects on the renin-angiotensin-aldosterone system.

In humans, foetal renal perfusion, which is dependent upon the development of the renin-angiotensin-aldosterone system, begins in the second trimester; thus, risk to the foetus increases if 'Cozaar' is administered during the second or third trimesters of pregnancy.

When used in pregnancy during the second and third trimesters, drugs that act directly on the renin-angiotensin-aldosterone system can cause injury and even death in the developing foetus. 'Cozaar' should not be used in pregnancy, and if pregnancy is detected 'Cozaar' should be discontinued as soon as possible.

Use during lactation

It is not known whether losartan is excreted in human milk. However, significant levels of losartan and the active metabolite were shown to be present in rat milk. Because of the potential for adverse effects on the nursing infant, a decision should be made whether to discontinue breast-feeding or discontinue the drug, taking into account the importance of the drug to the mother.

4.7 Effects on ability to drive and use machines
There are no data to suggest that 'Cozaar' affects the ability to drive and use machines.

4.8 Undesirable effects
Side effects have usually been mild and transient in nature and have not required discontinuation of therapy. The overall incidence of side effects reported with 'Cozaar' was comparable to placebo.

In controlled clinical trials for essential hypertension, dizziness was the only side effect reported as drug related that occurred with an incidence greater than placebo in 1% or more of patients treated with 'Cozaar'. In addition, dose-related orthostatic effects were seen in less than 1% of patients.

'Cozaar' was generally well tolerated in a controlled clinical trial in hypertensive patients with left ventricular hypertrophy. The most common drug-related side effects were dizziness, asthenia/fatigue and vertigo.

'Cozaar' was generally well tolerated in a controlled clinical trial in type 2 diabetic patients with nephropathy. The most common drug-related side effects were asthenia/fatigue, dizziness, hypotension and hyperkalaemia. In this study, few patients discontinued due to hyperkalaemia (see 4.4 'Special warnings and precautions for use', *Hypotension and electrolyte/fluid imbalance*).

The following adverse reactions have been reported in post-marketing experience:

Hypersensitivity: Anaphylactic reactions, angioedema including swelling of the larynx and glottis causing airway obstruction and/or swelling of the face, lips, pharynx, and/ or tongue have been reported rarely in patients treated with losartan; some of these patients previously experienced angioedema with other drugs including ACE inhibitors. Vasculitis, including Henoch-Schonlein purpura, has been reported rarely.

Gastro-intestinal: Hepatitis (reported rarely), diarrhoea, liver function abnormalities.

Haematologic: Anaemia (see 4.4 'Special warnings and precautions for use').

Musculoskeletal: Myalgia, arthralgia.

Nervous system/Psychiatric: Migraine.

Respiratory: Cough.

Skin: Urticaria, pruritus, rash.

Laboratory test findings

In controlled clinical trials, clinically important changes in standard laboratory parameters were rarely associated with administration of 'Cozaar'. Hyperkalaemia (serum potassium >5.5 mmol/l) occurred in 1.5% of patients in hypertension clinical trials. In a clinical study conducted in type 2 diabetic patients with nephropathy, 9.9% of patients treated with 'Cozaar' and 3.4% of patients treated with placebo developed hyperkalaemia (see 4.4 'Special warnings and precautions for use', *Hypotension and electrolyte/ fluid imbalance*). Serum potassium should be monitored, particularly in the elderly and patients with renal impairment. Elevations of ALT occurred rarely and usually resolved upon discontinuation of therapy.

4.9 Overdose

Significant lethality was observed in mice and rats after oral administration of 1,000 mg/kg (3,000 mg/m^2) and 2,000 mg/kg (11,800 mg/m^2) (500 and 1,000 times the maximum recommended daily human dose), respectively.

Limited data are available in regard to overdosage in humans. The most likely manifestation of overdosage would be hypotension and tachycardia; bradycardia could occur from parasympathetic (vagal) stimulation. If symptomatic hypotension should occur, supportive treatment should be instituted.

Neither losartan nor the active metabolite can be removed by haemodialysis.

*Based on a patient weight of 50 kg.

5. PHARMACOLOGICAL PROPERTIES

5.1 Pharmacodynamic properties

ATC code: CO9C A

Losartan is an oral, specific angiotensin-II receptor (type AT$_1$) antagonist. Angiotensin II binds to the AT$_1$ receptor found in many tissues (e.g. vascular smooth muscle, adrenal gland, kidneys, and the heart) and elicits several important biological actions, including vasoconstriction and the release of aldosterone. Angiotensin II also stimulates smooth-muscle proliferation. Based on binding and pharmacological bioassays, it binds selectively to the AT$_1$ receptor. *In vitro* and *in vivo*, both losartan and its pharmacologically active carboxylic acid metabolite (E-3174) block all physiologically relevant actions of angiotensin II, regardless of the source or route of synthesis.

During losartan administration, removal of angiotensin-II negative feedback on renin secretion leads to increased plasma renin activity. Increases in plasma renin activity lead to increases in angiotensin II in plasma. Even with these increases, antihypertensive activity and suppression of plasma aldosterone concentration are maintained, indicating effective angiotensin-II receptor blockade.

Losartan binds selectively to the AT$_1$ receptor and does not bind to or block other hormone receptors or ion channels important in cardiovascular regulation. Furthermore, losartan does not inhibit ACE (kininase II), the enzyme that degrades bradykinin. Consequently, effects not directly related to blocking the AT$_1$ receptor, such as the potentiation of bradykinin-mediated effects, the generation of oedema (losartan 1.7%, placebo 1.9%) or fatigue (losartan 3.8%, placebo 3.9%), are not associated with losartan.

Losartan has been shown to block responses to angiotensin I and angiotensin II without affecting responses to bradykinin, a finding which is consistent with the specific mechanism of action of losartan. In contrast, ACE inhibitors have been shown to block responses to angiotensin I and enhance responses to bradykinin without altering the response to angiotensin II, thus providing a pharmacodynamic distinction between losartan and ACE inhibitors.

A study was carried out which was specifically designed to assess the incidence of cough in patients treated with 'Cozaar' as compared to patients treated with ACE inhibitors. In this study and in the controlled clinical trials for hypertension, the incidence of cough reported by patients receiving 'Cozaar' or an agent not associated with ACE-inhibitor-induced cough (hydrochlorothiazide or placebo) was similar and was significantly less than in patients treated with an ACE inhibitor. In addition, in an overall analysis of 16 double-blind clinical trials in 4,131 patients, the incidence of spontaneously reported cough in patients treated with 'Cozaar' was similar (3.1%) to that of patients treated with placebo (2.6%) or hydrochlorothiazide (4.1%), whereas the incidence with ACE inhibitors was 8.8%.

In non-diabetic hypertensive patients with proteinuria, the administration of losartan potassium significantly reduces proteinuria, fractional excretion of albumin and IgG. Losartan maintains glomerular filtration rate and reduces filtration fraction. Generally, losartan causes a decrease in serum uric acid (usually <24 micromol) which was persistent in chronic therapy.

Losartan has no effect on autonomic reflexes and no sustained effect on plasma noradrenaline.

Losartan potassium administered in doses of up to 150 mg once daily did not cause clinically important changes in fasting triglycerides, total cholesterol or HDL cholesterol in patients with hypertension. The same doses of losartan had no effect on fasting glucose levels.

Hypertension Studies:

In clinical studies, once-daily administration of 50 mg 'Cozaar' to patients with mild to moderate essential hypertension produced statistically significant reductions in systolic and diastolic blood pressure; the antihypertensive effect was maintained in clinical studies for up to one year. Measurement of blood pressure at trough (24 hours post-dose) relative to peak (5-6 hours post-dose) demonstrated relatively smooth blood pressure reduction over 24 hours. The antihypertensive effect paralleled the natural diurnal rhythms. Blood-pressure reduction at the end of the dosing interval was approximately 70-80% of the effect seen 5-6 hours post-dose. Discontinuation of losartan in hypertensive patients did not result in an abrupt rebound of blood pressure. Despite the significant decrease in blood pressure, administration of 'Cozaar' had no clinically significant effect on heart rate.

The antihypertensive effect of 50 mg of 'Cozaar' is similar to once-daily administration of enalapril 20 mg. The antihypertensive effect of once-daily administration of 50-100 mg of 'Cozaar' is comparable to once-daily administration of atenolol 50-100 mg. The effect of administration of 50-100 mg of 'Cozaar' once daily also is equivalent to felodipine extended-release 5-10 mg in older hypertensives (≥65 years) after 12 weeks of therapy.

Although 'Cozaar' is antihypertensive in all races, as with other drugs that affect the renin-angiotensin-aldosterone system, black hypertensive patients have a smaller average response to losartan monotherapy than non-black patients.

If 'Cozaar' is given together with thiazide-type diuretics, the blood-pressure-lowering effects are approximately additive.

LIFE Study

The Losartan Intervention For Endpoint reduction in hypertension (LIFE) study was a randomised, triple-blind, active-controlled study in 9193 hypertensive patients aged 55 to 80 years with ECG-documented left ventricular hypertrophy. Patients were randomised to once daily Cozaar' 50 mg or atenolol 50 mg. If goal blood pressure (<140/90 mmHg) was not reached, hydrochlorothiazide (12.5 mg) was added first and, if needed, the dose of 'Cozaar' or atenolol was then increased to 100 mg once daily. Other antihypertensives, with the exception of ACE inhibitors, angiotensin II antagonists or beta-blockers were added if necessary to reach the goal blood pressure. The mean length of follow up was 4.8 years.

The primary endpoint was the composite of cardiovascular morbidity and mortality as measured by a reduction in the combined incidence of cardiovascular death, stroke and myocardial infarction. Blood pressure was significantly lowered to similar levels in the two groups. Treatment with 'Cozaar' resulted in a 13.0% risk reduction (p=0.021, 95 % confidence interval 0.77-0.98) compared with atenolol for patients reaching the primary composite endpoint. This was mainly attributable to a reduction of the incidence of stroke. Treatment with 'Cozaar' reduced the risk of stroke by 25% relative to atenolol (p=0.001 95% confidence interval 0.63-0.89). The rates of cardiovascular death and myocardial infarction were not significantly different between the treatment groups.

Race: There were 533 black patients in the study. In this group, treatment with 'Cozaar' resulted in a 67% increase in risk compared with atenolol for the primary composite endpoint (p=0.033, 95% confidence interval 1.04-2.66) and a 118% increase relative to atenolol in the risk of stroke (p=0.030, 95% confidence interval 1.08-4.40).

RENAAL Study

The Reduction of Endpoints in NIDDM with the Angiotensin II Receptor Antagonist Losartan (RENAAL) study was a multicentre, randomised, placebo-controlled, double-blind study 1,513 type 2 diabetic patients with nephropathy (751 treated with 'Cozaar'), with or without hypertension. Patients were recruited with proteinuria as defined by urinary albumin to creatinine ratio >25 mg/mmol or 24-hour urinary protein excretion >500 mg and a serum creatinine of 115-265 micromol/l (a lower limit of 133 micromol/l was used for patients weighing more than 60 kg). The patients were randomised to receive 'Cozaar' 50 mg once daily, titrated if necessary, to achieve blood pressure response, or to placebo, on a background of conventional antihypertensive therapy excluding ACE inhibitors and angiotensin II antagonists. Investigators were instructed to titrate study drug to 100 mg daily as appropriate after one month; 72% of patients were taking the 100 mg daily dose the majority of the time they were on study drug. Patients were followed for 3.4 years on average.

The results showed that treatment with 'Cozaar' (327 events) as compared with placebo (359 events) resulted in a 16.1% risk reduction (p=0.022) in the number of patients reaching the primary composite endpoint, of doubling of serum creatinine, end-stage renal disease (need for dialysis or transplantation), or death. The benefit exceeded that attributable to changes in blood pressure alone. For the following individual and combined components of the primary composite end point, the results also showed significant risk reduction in the group treated with 'Cozaar': 25.3% risk reduction in doubling of serum creatinine (p=0.006); 28.6% risk reduction in end-stage renal disease (p=0.002); 19.9% risk reduction in end-stage renal disease or death (p=0.009); 21.0% risk reduction in doubling of serum creatinine or end-stage renal disease (p=0.010). All-cause mortality alone was not significantly different between the two treatment groups.

For the secondary endpoints, the results showed an average reduction of 34.3% in the level of proteinuria in the group treated with 'Cozaar' (p<0.001) over the mean of 3.4 years. Treatment with 'Cozaar' reduced the rate of decline in renal function during the chronic phase of the study by 13.9%, p=0.003 (median rate of decline of 25.5%, p<0.0001) as measured by the reciprocal of the serum creatinine concentration-time curve. There was no significant difference between the group treated with 'Cozaar' (247 events) and the placebo group (268 events) in the composite endpoint of cardiovascular morbidity and mortality, although the study was not powered to detect such an effect.

5.2 Pharmacokinetic properties

Absorption

Following oral administration, losartan is well absorbed and undergoes first-pass metabolism, forming an active carboxylic acid metabolite and other inactive metabolites. The systemic bioavailability of losartan tablets is approximately 33%. Mean peak concentrations of losartan and its active metabolite are reached in 1 hour and in 3-4 hours, respectively. There was no clinically significant effect on the plasma concentration profile of losartan when the drug was administered with a standardised meal.

Distribution

Both losartan and its active metabolite are ≥99% bound to plasma proteins, primarily albumin. The volume of distribution of losartan is 34 litres. Studies in rats indicate that losartan crosses the blood-brain barrier poorly, if at all.

Biotransformation

About 14% of an intravenously or orally-administered dose of losartan is converted to its active metabolite. Following oral and intravenous administration of ^{14}C-labelled losartan potassium, circulating plasma radioactivity primarily is attributed to losartan and its active metabolite.

In addition to the active metabolite, inactive metabolites are formed, including two major metabolites formed by hydroxylation of the butyl side chain and a minor metabolite, an N-2 tetrazole glucuronide.

Elimination

Plasma clearance of losartan and its active metabolite is about 600 ml/min and 50 ml/min, respectively. Renal clearance of losartan and its active metabolite is about 74 ml/ min and 26 ml/min, respectively. When losartan is administered orally, about 4% of the dose is excreted unchanged in the urine, and about 6% of the dose is excreted in the urine as active metabolite. The pharmacokinetics of losartan and its active metabolite are linear with oral losartan potassium doses up to 200 mg.

Following oral administration, plasma concentrations of losartan and its active metabolite decline polyexponentially with a terminal half-life of about 2 hours and 6-9 hours, respectively. During once-daily dosing with 100 mg, neither losartan nor its active metabolite accumulates significantly in plasma.

Both biliary and urinary excretion contribute to the elimination of losartan and its metabolites. Following an oral dose of ^{14}C-labelled losartan in man, about 35% of radioactivity is recovered in the urine and 58% in the faeces.

Characteristics in patients

Following oral administration in patients with mild to moderate alcoholic cirrhosis of the liver, plasma concentrations of losartan and its active metabolite were, respectively, 5-fold and 1.7-fold greater than those seen in young male volunteers.

Plasma concentrations of losartan are not altered in patients with creatinine clearance above 10 ml/min. Compared to patients with normal renal function, the AUC for losartan is approximately 2-fold greater in haemodialysis patients. Plasma concentrations of the active metabolite are not altered in patients with renal impairment or in haemodialysis patients. Neither losartan nor the active metabolite can be removed by haemodialysis.

5.3 Preclinical safety data
The toxic potential of losartan potassium was evaluated in a series of repeated dose oral toxicity studies of up to three months in monkeys and up to one year in rats and dogs. There were no findings that would preclude administration at the therapeutic dosage level.

Losartan potassium was not carcinogenic when administered at maximum tolerated dosage levels to rats and mice for 105 and 92 weeks, respectively. These maximum tolerated dosage levels provided respective margins of systemic exposure for losartan and its pharmacologically active metabolite over that achieved in humans treated with 50 mg of losartan of approximately 270- and 150-fold in rats and 45- and 27-fold in mice.

There was no evidence of direct genotoxicity in studies conducted with losartan potassium or its primary pharmacologically active metabolite (E-3174).

Fertility and reproductive performance were not affected in studies with male and female rats given oral doses of losartan potassium up to approximately 150 and 300 mg/kg/day, respectively. These dosages provide respective margins of systemic exposure for losartan and its pharmacologically active metabolite of approximately 150/125-fold in male rats and 300/170-fold in female rats over that achieved in man at the recommended daily dose.

Losartan potassium has been shown to produce adverse effects in rat foetuses and neonates. The effects include decreased bodyweight, mortality and/or renal toxicity. In addition, significant levels of losartan and its active metabolite were shown to be present in rat milk. Based on pharmacokinetic assessments, these findings are attributed to drug exposure in late gestation and during lactation.

6. PHARMACEUTICAL PARTICULARS
6.1 List of excipients
'Cozaar' Tablets contain the following excipients:

hydroxypropyl cellulose E463

hypromellose E464

lactose monohydrate

magnesium stearate E572

microcrystalline cellulose E460

pregelatinised starch

titanium dioxide E171

carnauba wax.

'Cozaar' 100 mg also contains 8.48 mg (0.216 mmol) of potassium.

'Cozaar' 50 mg also contains 4.24 mg (0.108 mmol) of potassium.

'Cozaar' 25 mg also contains 2.12 mg (0.054 mmol) of potassium.

6.2 Incompatibilities
None.

6.3 Shelf life
36 months.

6.4 Special precautions for storage
Do not store above 30°C. Store in the original package.

6.5 Nature and contents of container
White, opaque PVC/PE/PVDC blisters with aluminium foil lidding.

100 mg and 50 mg tablets: Packs of 28 tablets

25 mg tablets: Pack of 7 and 28 tablets

6.6 Instructions for use and handling
None.

7. MARKETING AUTHORISATION HOLDER
Merck Sharp & Dohme Limited

Hertford Road, Hoddesdon, Hertfordshire EN11 9BU, UK.

8. MARKETING AUTHORISATION NUMBER(S)
100 mg tablet: PL 0025/0416

50 mg tablet: PL 0025/0324

25 mg tablet: PL 0025/0336

9. DATE OF FIRST AUTHORISATION/RENEWAL OF THE AUTHORISATION
50 mg and 25 mg: Granted 15 December 1994.

100 mg: Granted 28 November 2001.

10. DATE OF REVISION OF THE TEXT
May 2005.

LEGAL CATEGORY:
POM

® denotes registered trademark of E. I. du Pont de Nemours and Company, Wilmington, Delaware, USA.

MSD (logo)

Merck Sharp & Dohme Limited

Hertford Road, Hoddesdon, Hertfordshire EN11 9BU, UK

SPC.CZR.05.UK.2133

COZAAR-Comp 50/12.5 Tablets

(Merck Sharp & Dohme Limited)

1. NAME OF THE MEDICINAL PRODUCT
COZAAR®-Comp 50/12.5 Tablets

2. QUALITATIVE AND QUANTITATIVE COMPOSITION
The active ingredients in 'Cozaar'-Comp are losartan and hydrochlorothiazide. Each 'Cozaar'-Comp Tablet contains 45.8 mg of losartan, present as 50 mg of losartan potassium, and 12.5 mg hydrochlorothiazide.

3. PHARMACEUTICAL FORM
'Cozaar'-Comp is supplied as oval, yellow, film-coated tablets with '717' on one side and plain on the other.

4. CLINICAL PARTICULARS
4.1 Therapeutic indications
For the treatment of hypertension in patients whose blood pressure is not adequately controlled on hydrochlorothiazide or losartan monotherapy.

In hypertensive patients with left ventricular hypertrophy a reduced risk of stroke was demonstrated with losartan administered usually in combination with HCTZ. The data do not support the use of losartan for this indication in black patients (see section 4.4 Special warnings and Precautions for Use-*Race* and section 5.1 Pharmacodynamic Properties, LIFE study, *Race*.

4.2 Posology and method of administration
Where possible titration with the individual components (ie losartan and hydrochlorothiazide) is recommended.

When clinically appropriate direct change from monotherapy to the fixed combinations may be considered in patients whose blood pressure is not adequately controlled.

The usual starting and maintenance dose is 1 tablet once daily for most patients. For patients who do not respond adequately, the dosage may be increased to 2 tablets once daily. The maximum dose is 2 tablets once daily. In general, the antihypertensive effect is attained within three weeks after initiation of therapy.

Reduction in the risk of stroke in hypertensive patients with left ventricular hypertrophy

The usual starting dose is 50 mg of losartan once daily. If goal blood pressure is not reached with losartan 50 mg, therapy should be titrated using a combination of losartan and a low dose of hydrochlorothiazide (12.5 mg) and, if needed the dose should then be increased to losartan 100 mg/hydrochlorothiazide 12.5 mg once daily. If necessary, the dose should be increased to losartan 100 mg/hydrochlorothiazide 25 mg daily.

Use in the elderly: Patients over 75 years: Presently there is limited clinical experience in this group. Any therapy involving the angiotensin II antagonist, losartan, should be initiated with 25 mg losartan in these patients.

Use in renal impairment: No initial dosage adjustment is necessary in patients with mild renal impairment (i.e. creatinine clearance 20-50 ml/min). 'Cozaar'-Comp is not recommended for patients with moderate to severe renal impairment (i.e. creatinine clearance <20 ml/min) or patients on dialysis.

Use in patients with intravascular volume depletion: 'Cozaar'-Comp should not be initiated in patients who are intravascularly volume depleted (e.g. those treated with high-dose diuretics).

Use in hepatic impairment: 'Cozaar'-Comp is not recommended for patients with hepatic impairment.

Concomitant therapy: 'Cozaar'-Comp may be administered with other antihypertensive agents.

'Cozaar'-Comp may be administered with or without food.

Use in children: Safety and efficacy in children have not been established.

4.3 Contraindications
'Cozaar'-Comp is contra-indicated in pregnancy (see 4.6 'Pregnancy and lactation'), in patients who are hypersensitive to any component of this product, in patients with anuria, and in patients who are hypersensitive to other sulphonamide-derived drugs.

4.4 Special warnings and special precautions for use
Losartan and hydrochlorothiazide combination tablet

Hypersensitivity: Angioedema. See 4.8 'Undesirable effects'.

Hepatic and renal impairment: 'Cozaar'-Comp is not recommended for patients with hepatic impairment or moderate to severe renal impairment (creatinine clearance <20 ml/min). (See 4.2 'Posology and method of administration'.)

Losartan

Renal function impairment: As a consequence of inhibiting the renin-angiotensin-aldosterone system, changes in renal function, including renal failure, have been reported (in particular, in patients whose renal function is dependent on the renin-angiotensin-aldosterone system, such as those with severe cardiac insufficiency or pre-existing renal dysfunction).

As with other drugs that affect the renin-angiotensin-aldosterone system, increases in blood urea and serum creatinine have also been reported in patients with bilateral renal artery stenosis or stenosis of the artery to a solitary kidney; these changes in renal function may be reversible upon discontinuation of therapy.

Caution is required in patients with significant renal disease and renal transplant recipients as there have been reports of anaemia developing in such patients treated with 'Cozaar'.

Hydrochlorothiazide

Hypotension and electrolyte/fluid imbalance: As with all antihypertensive therapy, symptomatic hypotension may occur in some patients. This was rarely seen in uncomplicated hypertensive patients, but was more likely in the presence of fluid depletion or electrolyte imbalance. Periodic determination of serum electrolytes should be performed at appropriate intervals, as in any patients receiving diuretics.

Metabolic and endocrine effects

Thiazide therapy may impair glucose tolerance. Dosage adjustment of antidiabetic agents, including insulin, may be required (see 4.5 'Interaction with other medicinal productsand other forms of interaction').

Thiazides may decrease urinary calcium excretion and may cause intermittent and slight elevation of serum calcium. Marked hypercalcaemia may be evidence of hidden hyperparathyroidism. Thiazides should be discontinued before carrying out tests for parathyroid function.

Increases in cholesterol and triglyceride levels may be associated with thiazide diuretic therapy.

Thiazide therapy may precipitate hyperuricaemia and/or gout in certain patients. Because losartan decreases uric acid, losartan in combination with hydrochlorothiazide attenuates the diuretic-induced hyperuricaemia.

Other

In patients receiving thiazides, hypersensitivity reactions may occur with or without a history of allergy or bronchial asthma. Exacerbation or activation of systemic lupus erythematosus has been reported with the use of thiazides.

The use of 'Cozaar' in patients with haemodynamically significant obstructive valvular disease and cardiomyopathy has not been adequately studied.

Race (Black patients):

There is no evidence that losartan reduces the risk of stroke in black hypertensive patients with LVH (see section 5.1 Pharmacodynamic Properties, LIFE Study Race).

4.5 Interaction with other medicinal products and other forms of Interaction
Losartan

In clinical pharmacokinetic trials no drug interactions of clinical significance have been identified with hydrochlorothiazide, digoxin, warfarin, cimetidine, phenobarbital (phenobarbitone), (see ***Hydrochlorothiazide***; *Alcohol, barbiturates, or narcotics* below) ketoconazole and erythromycin. Rifampicin and fluconazole have been reported to reduce levels of active metabolite. The clinical consequences of these interactions have not been evaluated.

As with other drugs that block angiotensin II or its effects, concomitant use of other drugs which retain potassium or may increase potassium levels (e.g. potassium-sparing diuretics, potassium supplements, or salt substitutes containing potassium) may lead to increases in serum potassium. Co-medication is not advisable.

As with other antihypertensive agents, the antihypertensive effect of losartan may be attenuated by non-steroidal anti-inflammatory drugs such as indomethacin.

Hydrochlorothiazide

When given concurrently, the following drugs may interact with thiazide diuretics:

Alcohol, barbiturates, or narcotics—potentiation of orthostatic hypotension may occur.

Antidiabetic drugs (oral agents and insulin)—dosage adjustment of the antidiabetic drug may be required.

Other antihypertensive drugs—there may be an additive effect.

Cholestyramine and colestipol resins—absorption of hydrochlorothiazide is impaired in the presence of anionic exchange resins. Single doses of either cholestyramine or colestipol resins bind the hydrochlorothiazide and reduce its absorption from the gastro-intestinal tract by up to 85% and 43%, respectively.

Corticosteroids, ACTH—there may be intensified electrolyte depletion, particularly hypokalaemia.

Pressor amines (e.g. adrenaline)—possible decreased response to pressor amines, but not sufficient to preclude their use.

Skeletal muscle relaxants, non-depolarising (e.g. tubocurarine)—possible increased responsiveness to the muscle relaxant.

Lithium—diuretic agents reduce the renal clearance of lithium and add a high risk of lithium toxicity. Therefore, concomitant use is not recommended. Refer to the prescribing information for lithium preparations before use of such preparations.

Non-steroidal anti-inflammatory drugs—in some patients, the administration of a non-steroidal anti-inflammatory agent can reduce the diuretic, natriuretic, and antihypertensive effects of diuretics.

Drug/laboratory test interactions

Because of their effects on calcium metabolism, thiazides may interfere with tests for parathyroid function (see 4.4 'Special warnings and precautions for use').

4.6 Pregnancy and lactation

Use during pregnancy

Although there is no experience with the use of 'Cozaar'-Comp in pregnant women, animal studies with losartan potassium have demonstrated foetal and neonatal injury and death, the mechanism of which is believed to be pharmacologically mediated through effects on the renin-angiotensin system.

In humans, foetal renal perfusion, which is dependent upon the development of the renin-angiotensin system, begins in the second trimester; thus, risk to the foetus increases if 'Cozaar'-Comp is administered during the second or third trimesters of pregnancy.

Thiazides cross the placental barrier and appear in cord blood. The routine use of diuretics in otherwise healthy pregnant women is not recommended and exposes mother and foetus to unnecessary hazard, including foetal or neonatal jaundice, thrombocytopenia and possibly other adverse reactions which have occurred in the adult. Diuretics do not prevent development of toxaemia of pregnancy and there is no satisfactory evidence that they are useful in the treatment of toxaemia.

When used in pregnancy during the second and third trimesters, drugs that act directly on the renin-angiotensin system can cause injury and even death to the developing foetus. When pregnancy is detected, 'Cozaar'-Comp should be discontinued as soon as possible.

Use during lactation

It is not known whether losartan is excreted in human milk. Significant levels of losartan and the active metabolite were shown to be present in rat milk. Thiazides appear in human milk. Because of the potential for adverse effects on the breast-feeding infant, a decision should be made whether to discontinue breast-feeding or discontinue the drug, taking into account the importance of the drug to the mother.

4.7 Effects on ability to drive and use machines

There are no data to suggest that 'Cozaar'-Comp affects the ability to drive and use machines.

4.8 Undesirable effects

In clinical trials with the combination tablet of losartan and hydrochlorothiazide, no adverse experiences peculiar to this combination drug have been observed. Adverse experiences have been limited to those that were reported previously with losartan potassium and/or hydrochlorothiazide. The overall incidence of adverse experiences reported with the combination was comparable to placebo. The percentage of discontinuations of therapy was also comparable to placebo. For the most part, adverse experiences have been mild and transient in nature and have not required discontinuation of therapy.

In controlled clinical trials for essential hypertension, dizziness was the only adverse experience reported as drug related that occurred with an incidence greater than placebo in 1% or more of patients treated with losartan potassium-hydrochlorothiazide.

In a controlled trial in hypertensive patients with left ventricular hypertrophy, losartan used usually with hydrochlorothiazide was generally well tolerated. The most common drug-related side effects were dizziness, asthenia/fatigue, and vertigo.

The following adverse reactions have been reported in post-marketing experience:

Hypersensitivity

Anaphylactic reactions, angioedema including swelling of the larynx and glottis causing airway obstruction and/or swelling of the face, lips, pharynx, and/or tongue has been reported rarely in patients treated with losartan; some of these patients previously experienced angioedema with other drugs including ACE inhibitors. Vasculitis including Henoch-Schonlein purpura, has been reported rarely with losartan.

Gastro-intestinal: Hepatitis has been reported rarely in patients treated with losartan, diarrhoea.

Respiratory: Cough has been reported with losartan.

Skin: Urticaria

Additional side effects that have been seen with one of the individual components and may be potential side effects with 'Cozaar'-Comp are the following:

Losartan

Dose-related orthostatic effects, liver function abnormalities, myalgia, migraine, rash, anaemia, pruritus.

Hydrochlorothiazide

Anorexia, gastric irritation, nausea, vomiting, cramping, diarrhoea, constipation, jaundice (intrahepatic cholestatic jaundice), pancreatitis, sialoadenitis, vertigo, paraesthesiae, headache, xanthopsia, leucopenia, agranulocytosis, thrombocytopenia, aplastic anaemia, haemolytic anaemia, purpura, photosensitivity, fever, necrotising angiitis, respiratory distress (including pneumonitis and pulmonary oedema), anaphylactic reactions, toxic epidermal necrolysis, hyperglycaemia, glycosuria, hyperuricaemia, electrolyte imbalance (including hyponatraemia and hypokalaemia), renal dysfunction, interstitial nephritis, renal failure, muscle spasm, weakness, restlessness, transient blurred vision.

Laboratory test findings

In controlled clinical trials, clinically important changes in standard laboratory parameters were rarely associated with administration of losartan potassium-hydrochlorothiazide. Hyperkalaemia (serum potassium >5.5 mmol/l) occurred in 0.7% of patients, but in these trials discontinuation of losartan potassium-hydrochlorothiazide due to hyperkalaemia was not necessary. Serum potassium should be monitored, particularly in the elderly and patients with renal impairment. Elevations of ALT occurred rarely and usually resolved upon discontinuation of therapy.

4.9 Overdose

No specific information is available on the treatment of overdosage with 'Cozaar'-Comp. Treatment is symptomatic and supportive. Therapy with 'Cozaar'-Comp should be discontinued and the patient observed closely. Suggested measures include induction of emesis if ingestion is recent, and correction of dehydration, electrolyte imbalance, hepatic coma, and hypotension by established procedures.

Losartan

Limited data are available in regard to overdosage in humans. The most likely manifestation of overdosage would be hypotension and tachycardia; bradycardia could occur from parasympathetic (vagal) stimulation. If symptomatic hypotension should occur, supportive treatment should be instituted.

Neither losartan nor the active metabolite can be removed by haemodialysis.

Hydrochlorothiazide

The most common signs and symptoms observed are those caused by electrolyte depletion (hypokalaemia, hypochloraemia, hyponatraemia) and dehydration resulting from excessive diuresis. If digitalis has also been administered, hypokalaemia may accentuate cardiac arrhythmias.

The degree to which hydrochlorothiazide is removed by haemodialysis has not been established.

5. PHARMACOLOGICAL PROPERTIES

5.1 Pharmacodynamic properties

Losartan and hydrochlorothiazide combination tablet

The components of 'Cozaar'-Comp have been shown to have an additive effect on blood-pressure reduction, reducing blood pressure to a greater degree than either component alone. This effect is thought to be a result of the complimentary actions of both components. Further, as a result of its diuretic effect, hydrochlorothiazide increases plasma-renin activity, increases aldosterone secretion, decreases serum potassium, and increases the levels of angiotensin II. Administration of losartan blocks all the physiologically relevant actions of angiotensin II and through inhibition of aldosterone could tend to attenuate the potassium loss associated with the diuretic.

Losartan has been shown to have a mild and transient uricosuric effect. Hydrochlorothiazide has been shown to cause modest increases in uric acid; the combination of losartan and hydrochlorothiazide tends to attenuate the diuretic-induced hyperuricaemia.

The antihypertensive effect of 'Cozaar'-Comp is sustained for a 24-hour period. In clinical studies of at least one year's duration, the antihypertensive effect was maintained with continued therapy. Despite the significant decrease in blood pressure, administration of 'Cozaar'-Comp had no clinically significant effect on heart rate. In clinical trials, after 12 weeks of therapy with losartan 50 mg/hydrochlorothiazide 12.5 mg, trough sitting diastolic blood pressure was reduced by an average of up to 13.2 mm Hg.

'Cozaar'-Comp is effective in reducing blood pressure in males and females, blacks and non-blacks, and in younger (<65 years) and older (≥65 years) patients and is effective in all degrees of hypertension.

Losartan

Losartan is an oral, specific angiotensin-II receptor (type AT_1) antagonist. Angiotensin II binds to the AT_1 receptor found in many tissues (e.g. vascular smooth muscle, adrenal gland, kidneys, and the heart) and elicits several important biological actions, including vasoconstriction and the release of aldosterone. Angiotensin II also stimulates smooth-muscle proliferation. Based on binding and pharmacological bioassays, angiotensin II binds selectively to the AT_1 receptor. *In vitro* and *in vivo*, both losartan and its pharmacologically active carboxylic acid metabolite (E-3174) block all physiologically relevant actions of angiotensin II, regardless of the source or route of synthesis.

During losartan administration, removal of angiotensin-II negative feedback on renin secretion leads to increased plasma-renin activity. Increases in plasma-renin activity lead to increases in angiotensin II in plasma. Even with these increases, antihypertensive activity and suppression of plasma-aldosterone concentration are maintained, indicating effective angiotensin-II receptor blockade.

Losartan binds selectively to the AT_1 receptor and does not bind to or block other hormone receptors or ion channels important in cardiovascular regulation. Furthermore, losartan does not inhibit ACE (kininase II), the enzyme that degrades bradykinin. Consequently, effects not directly related to blocking the AT_1 receptor, such as the potentiation of bradykinin-mediated effects or the generation of oedema (losartan 1.7%, placebo 1.9%), are not associated with losartan.

Losartan has been shown to block responses to angiotensin I and angiotensin II without affecting responses to bradykinin, a finding which is consistent with the specific mechanism of action of losartan. In contrast, ACE inhibitors have been shown to block responses to angiotensin I and enhance responses to bradykinin without altering the response to angiotensin II, thus providing a pharmacodynamic distinction between losartan and ACE inhibitors.

A study was carried out which was specifically designed to assess the incidence of cough in patients treated with losartan as compared to patients treated with ACE inhibitors. In this study, the incidence of cough reported by patients receiving losartan or hydrochlorothiazide was similar and was significantly less than in patients treated with an ACE inhibitor. In addition, in an overall analysis of 16 double-blind clinical trials in 4,131 patients, the incidence of spontaneously reported cough in patients treated with losartan was similar (3.1%) to that of patients treated with placebo (2.6%) or hydrochlorothiazide (4.1%), whereas the incidence with ACE inhibitors was 8.8%.

In non-diabetic hypertensive patients with proteinuria, the administration of losartan potassium significantly reduces proteinuria, fractional excretion of albumin and IgG. Losartan maintains glomerular filtration rate and reduces filtration fraction. Generally, losartan causes a decrease in serum uric acid (usually <24 micro mol/l) which was persistent in chronic therapy.

Losartan has no effect on autonomic reflexes and no sustained effect on plasma noradrenaline.

In clinical studies, once-daily administration of losartan to patients with mild to moderate essential hypertension produced statistically significant reductions in systolic and diastolic blood pressure; in clinical studies of up to one year the antihypertensive effect was maintained. Measurement of blood pressure at trough (24 hours post-dose) relative to peak (5-6 hours post-dose) demonstrated relatively smooth blood pressure reduction over 24 hours. The antihypertensive effect paralleled the natural diurnal rhythms. Blood-pressure reduction at the end of the dosing interval was approximately 70-80% of the effect seen 5-6 hours post-dose. Discontinuation of losartan in hypertensive patients did not result in an abrupt rebound of blood pressure. Despite the significant decrease in blood pressure, administration of losartan had no clinically significant effect on heart rate.

In a study comparing losartan 50 mg with the once-daily administration of enalapril 20 mg, the antihypertensive responses were shown to be similar in both treatment groups. The efficacy of once-daily administration of losartan 50-100 mg in hypertension has also been found to be comparable to once-daily administration of atenolol 50-100 mg. In older hypertensives (≥65 years), the effect of administration of losartan 50-100 mg once daily has been reported to be equivalent to felodopine extended-release 5-10 mg after 12 weeks of therapy.

Losartan is equally effective in males and females and in younger (<65 years) and older (≥65 years) hypertensives. Although losartan is antihypertensive in all races, as with other drugs that affect the renin-angiotensin system, black hypertensive patients have a smaller average response to losartan monotherapy than non-black patients.

When given together with thiazide-type diuretics, the blood-pressure lowering effects of losartan are approximately additive.

LIFE Study

The Losartan Intervention For Endpoint reduction in hypertension (LIFE) study was a randomised, triple-blind, active-controlled study in 9193 hypertensive patients aged 55 to 80 years with ECG-documented left ventricular hypertrophy. Patients were randomised to once daily 'Cozaar' 50 mg or atenolol 50 mg. If goal blood pressure (<140/90 mmHg) was not reached, hydrochlorothiazide (12.5 mg) was added first and, if needed, the dose of 'Cozaar' or atenolol was then increased to 100 mg once daily. Other antihypertensives (e.g., increase in dose of hydrochlorothiazide therapy to 25 mg or addition of other diuretic therapy, calcium channel blockers, alpha blockers, or centrally acting agents, but not ACE inhibitors, angiotensin II antagonists or beta-blockers) were added if necessary to reach the goal blood pressure. In efforts to control blood pressure, the patients in both arms of the LIFE study were coadministered hydrochlorothiazide the majority of time they were on study drug (73.9% and 72.4% of days in the losartan and atenolol arms respectively). The mean length of follow up was 4.8 years.

The primary endpoint was the composite of cardiovascular morbidity and mortality as measured by a reduction in the combined incidence of cardiovascular death, stroke and myocardial infarction. Blood pressure was significantly lowered to similar levels in the two groups. Treatment with 'Cozaar' resulted in a 13.0% risk reduction (p=0.021, 95 % confidence interval 0.77-0.98) compared with atenolol for patients reaching the primary composite endpoint. This was mainly attributable to a reduction of the incidence of stroke. Treatment with 'Cozaar' reduced the risk of stroke by 25% relative to atenolol (p=0.001 95% confidence interval 0.63-0.89). The rates of cardiovascular death and myocardial infarction were not significantly different between the treatment groups.

Race: There were 533 black patients in the study. In this group, treatment with 'Cozaar' resulted in a 67% increase in risk compared with atenolol for the primary composite endpoint (p=0.033, 95% confidence interval 1.04-2.66) and a 118% increase relative to atenolol in the risk of stroke (p=0.030, 95% confidence interval 1.08-4.40).

Hydrochlorothiazide

The mechanism of the antihypertensive effect of thiazides is unknown. Thiazides do not usually affect normal blood pressure.

Hydrochlorothiazide is a diuretic and antihypertensive. It affects the distal renal tubular mechanism of electrolyte reabsorption. Hydrochlorothiazide increases excretion of sodium and chloride in approximately equivalent amounts. Natriuresis may be accompanied by some loss of potassium and bicarbonate.

After oral use, diuresis begins within 2 hours, peaks in about 4 hours and lasts about 6 to 12 hours.

5.2 Pharmacokinetic properties

Absorption

Losartan:

Following oral administration, losartan is well absorbed and undergoes first-pass metabolism, forming an active carboxylic acid metabolite and other inactive metabolites. The systemic bioavailability of losartan tablets is approximately 33%. Mean peak concentrations of losartan and its active metabolite are reached in 1 hour and in 3-4 hours, respectively. There was no clinically significant effect on the plasma-concentration profile of losartan when the drug was administered with a standardised meal.

Distribution

Losartan:

Both losartan and its active metabolite are ⩾99% bound to plasma proteins, primarily albumin. The volume of distribution of losartan is 34 litres. Studies in rats indicate that losartan crosses the blood-brain barrier poorly, if at all.

Hydrochlorothiazide:

Hydrochlorothiazide crosses the placental but not the blood-brain barrier and is excreted in breast milk.

Biotransformation

Losartan:

About 14% of an intravenously or orally administered dose of losartan is converted to its active metabolite. Following oral and intravenous administration of ^{14}C-labelled losartan potassium, circulating plasma radioactivity primarily is attributed to losartan and its active metabolite. Minimal conversion of losartan to its active metabolite was seen in about 1% of individuals studied.

In addition to the active metabolite, inactive metabolites are formed, including two major metabolites formed by hydroxylation of the butyl side chain and a minor metabolite, an N-2 tetrazole glucuronide.

Elimination

Losartan:

Plasma clearance of losartan and its active metabolite is about 600 ml/min and 50 ml/min, respectively. Renal clearance of losartan and its active metabolite is about 74 ml/min and 26 ml/min, respectively. When losartan is administered orally, about 4% of the dose is excreted unchanged in the urine, and about 6% of the dose is excreted in the urine as active metabolite. The pharmacokinetics of losartan and its active metabolite are linear with oral losartan potassium doses up to 200 mg.

Following oral administration, plasma concentrations of losartan and its active metabolite decline polyexponentially with a terminal half-life of about 2 hours and 6-9 hours, respectively. During once-daily dosing with 100 mg, neither losartan nor its active metabolite accumulates significantly in plasma.

Both biliary and urinary excretion contribute to the elimination of losartan and its metabolites. Following an oral dose of ^{14}C-labelled losartan in man, about 35% of radioactivity is recovered in the urine and 58% in the faeces.

Hydrochlorothiazide:

Hydrochlorothiazide is not metabolised but is eliminated rapidly by the kidney. When plasma levels have been followed for at least 24 hours, the plasma half-life has been observed to vary between 5.6 and 14.8 hours. At least 61% of the oral dose is eliminated unchanged within 24 hours.

Characteristics in Patients

Losartan and hydrochlorothiazide combination tablet:

The plasma concentrations of losartan and its active metabolite and the absorption of hydrochlorothiazide in elderly hypertensives are not significantly different from those in young hypertensives.

Losartan:

Following oral administration in patients with mild to moderate alcoholic cirrhosis of the liver, plasma concentrations of losartan and its active metabolite were, respectively, 5-fold and 1.7-fold greater than those seen in young male volunteers.

Neither losartan nor the active metabolite can be removed by haemodialysis.

5.3 Preclinical safety data

The toxic potential of losartan potassium and hydrochlorothiazide was evaluated in repeated-dose oral toxicity studies for up to six months in rats and dogs. There were no findings that would preclude administration to man at the therapeutic dosage level.

There was no evidence of direct genotoxicity in studies conducted with the losartan and hydrochlorothiazide combination.

Losartan potassium and hydrochlorothiazide administration had no effect on the reproductive performance or fertility in male rats at dosage levels of up to 135 mg/kg/day losartan in combination with 33.75 mg/kg/day hydrochlorothiazide. These dosage levels provided respective plasma concentrations (AUC) for losartan, the active metabolite and hydrochlorothiazide that were approximately 260-, 120-, and 50-fold greater than those achieved in man with 50 mg losartan potassium in combination with 12.5 mg hydrochlorothiazide. In female rats, however, the coadministration of losartan potassium and hydrochlorothiazide (10/2.5 mg/kg/day) induced a slight but statistically significant decrease in fecundity and fertility indices. Compared to plasma concentrations in man (see above) these dosage levels provided respective increases in plasma concentration (AUC) for losartan, the active metabolite, and hydrochlorothiazide of approximately 15-, 4-, and 5-fold.

There was no evidence of teratogenicity in rats or rabbits treated with losartan potassium and hydrochlorothiazide combination. Foetal toxicity in rats, as evidenced by a slight increase in supernumerary ribs in the F_1 generation, was observed when females were treated prior to and throughout gestation. As observed in studies with losartan alone, adverse foetal and neonatal effects, including decreased bodyweight, mortality and/or renal toxicity, also occurred when pregnant rats were treated with losartan potassium and hydrochlorothiazide combination during late gestation and/or lactation.

6. PHARMACEUTICAL PARTICULARS

6.1 List of excipients

Each 'Cozaar'-Comp Tablet contains the following inactive ingredients:

hydroxypropylcellulose E463

hypromellose E464

lactose monohydrate

magnesium stearate E572

microcrystalline cellulose E460

pregelatinised maize starch

titanium dioxide E171

quinoline yellow aluminum lake E104

carnauba wax

'Cozaar'-Comp also contains 4.24 mg (0.108 mmol) of potassium.

6.2 Incompatibilities

None.

6.3 Shelf life

36 months.

6.4 Special precautions for storage

Store in a dry place at temperatures below 30°C (86°F).

6.5 Nature and contents of container

White, opaque PVC/PE/PVDC blisters with aluminium foil lidding.

Available in blister calendar packs of 28 tablets.

6.6 Instructions for use and handling

None.

7. MARKETING AUTHORISATION HOLDER

Merck Sharp & Dohme Limited

Hertford Road, Hoddesdon, Hertfordshire EN11 9BU, UK.

8. MARKETING AUTHORISATION NUMBER(S)

PL 0025/0338

9. DATE OF FIRST AUTHORISATION/RENEWAL OF THE AUTHORISATION

12 April 1996.

10. DATE OF REVISION OF THE TEXT

November 2004.

LEGAL CATEGORY:

POM

® denotes registered trademark of E. I. du Pont de Nemours and Company, Wilmington, Delaware, USA.

SPC.HYZ.04.UK.1088

Creon 10000 Capsules

(Solvay Healthcare Limited)

1. NAME OF THE MEDICINAL PRODUCT

Creon® 10000 Capsules

2. QUALITATIVE AND QUANTITATIVE COMPOSITION

Each capsule contains:

Lipase	10,000	PhEur units
Amylase	8,000	PhEur units
Protease	600	PhEur units

3. PHARMACEUTICAL FORM

Brown/clear capsules containing gastro-resistant granules.

4. CLINICAL PARTICULARS

4.1 Therapeutic indications

For the treatment of pancreatic exocrine insufficiency.

4.2 Posology and method of administration

Adults (including the elderly) and children:

Initially one to two capsules with each meal. Dose increases, if required, should be added slowly, with careful monitoring of response and symptomatology.

It is important to ensure adequate hydration of patients at all times whilst dosing Creon.

The capsules can be swallowed whole, or for ease of administration they may be opened and the granules taken with fluid or soft food, but without chewing. If the granules are mixed with food it is important that they are taken immediately, otherwise dissolution of the enteric coating may result.

Colonic damage has been reported in patients with cystic fibrosis taking in excess of 10,000 units of lipase/kg/day (see Undesirable effects).

4.3 Contraindications

Patients with known hypersensitivity to porcine proteins.

4.4 Special warnings and special precautions for use

The product is of porcine origin.

Oral medications should not be administered during the early stages of acute pancreatitis.

4.5 Interaction with other medicinal products and other forms of Interaction

None known.

4.6 Pregnancy and lactation

There are no adequate data from the use of Creon in pregnant women. Animal studies are insufficient with respect to effects on pregnancy and embryonal/foetal development, parturition/ and postnatal development. The potential risk for humans is unknown. Creon should not be used during pregnancy or lactation unless clearly necessary but if required should be used in doses providing adequate nutritional status (see warnings about high dose sections 4.2 and 4.8).

4.7 Effects on ability to drive and use machines

None known.

4.8 Undesirable effects

Diarrhoea, constipation, gastric discomfort, nausea and skin reactions have been reported occasionally in patients receiving enzyme replacement therapy.

Rarely cases of hyper-uricosuria and hyper-uricaemia have been reported with very high doses of pancreatin.

Stricture of the ileo-caecum and large bowel and colitis has been reported in children with cystic fibrosis taking high doses of pancreatic enzyme supplements. To date, Creon has not been implicated in the development of colonic damage. However, unusual abdominal symptoms or changes in abdominal symptoms should be reviewed to exclude the possibility of colonic damage - especially if the patient is taking in excess of 10,000 units of lipase/kg/day.

4.9 Overdose

Most cases respond to supportive measures including stopping enzyme therapy, ensuring adequate rehydration.

5. PHARMACOLOGICAL PROPERTIES

5.1 Pharmacodynamic properties

Replacement therapy in pancreatic enzyme deficiency states. The enzymes have hydrolytic activity on fat, carbohydrates and proteins.

5.2 Pharmacokinetic properties

Pharmacokinetic data are not available as the enzymes act locally in the gastro-intestinal tract. After exerting their action, the enzymes are digested themselves in the intestine.

5.3 Preclinical safety data

None stated.

6. PHARMACEUTICAL PARTICULARS

6.1 List of excipients

Granules:	Macrogol 4000, liquid paraffin, hypromellose phthalate, dibutylphthalate, dimeticone.
Capsule shell:	gelatin, red, yellow and black iron oxides (E172), titanium dioxide (E171).

6.2 Incompatibilities
Not applicable.

6.3 Shelf life
2 years.

6.4 Special precautions for storage
Do not store above 30°C.

6.5 Nature and contents of container
HDPE container with LDPE cap. Containers hold 100, 250 or 300 capsules.

6.6 Instructions for use and handling
No special instructions.

Administrative Data

7. MARKETING AUTHORISATION HOLDER
Solvay Healthcare Limited
Mansbridge Road
West End
Southampton
SO18 3JD
United Kingdom

8. MARKETING AUTHORISATION NUMBER(S)
PL 00512/0149

9. DATE OF FIRST AUTHORISATION/RENEWAL OF THE AUTHORISATION
01 January 2001

10. DATE OF REVISION OF THE TEXT
September 2003

Creon 25000 Capsules

(Solvay Healthcare Limited)

1. NAME OF THE MEDICINAL PRODUCT
Creon® 25000 Capsules

2. QUALITATIVE AND QUANTITATIVE COMPOSITION
Each capsule contains pancreatin PhEur 300 mg equivalent to:

Lipase 25,000 PhEur units
Amylase 18,000 PhEur units
Protease 1,000 PhEur units

3. PHARMACEUTICAL FORM
Orange/colourless capsules filled with brownish minimicrospheres.

4. CLINICAL PARTICULARS

4.1 Therapeutic indications
For the treatment of pancreatic exocrine insufficiency.

4.2 Posology and method of administration
Adults (including the elderly) and children:

Initially one capsule with meals. Dose increases, if required, should be added slowly, with careful monitoring of response and symptomatology.

It is important to ensure adequate hydration of patients at all times whilst dosing Creon 25000.

The capsules can be swallowed whole, or for ease of administration they may be opened and the granules taken with fluid or soft food. If the granules are mixed with food, it is important that they are taken immediately, otherwise dissolution of the enteric coating may result. In order to protect the enteric coating, it is important that the granules are not crushed or chewed.

Colonic damage has been reported in patients with cystic fibrosis taking in excess of 10,000 units of lipase/kg/day (see Undesirable Effects).

4.3 Contraindications
Patients with known hypersensitivity to porcine proteins.

4.4 Special warnings and special precautions for use
The product is of porcine origin.

Oral medications should not be administered during the early stages of acute pancreatitis.

4.5 Interaction with other medicinal products and other forms of Interaction
None known.

4.6 Pregnancy and lactation
There are no adequate data from the use of Creon in pregnant women. Animal studies are insufficient with respect to effects on pregnancy and embryonal/foetal development, parturition/ and postnatal development. The potential risk for humans is unknown. Creon should not be used during pregnancy or lactation unless clearly necessary but if required should be used in doses providing adequate nutritional status (see warnings about high dose sections 4.2 & 4.8).

4.7 Effects on ability to drive and use machines
None known.

4.8 Undesirable effects
Diarrhoea, constipation, gastric discomfort, nausea and skin reactions have been reported occasionally in patients receiving enzyme replacement therapy.

Rarely cases of hyper-uricosuria and hyper-uricaemia have been reported with very high doses of Pancreatin

Stricture of the ileo-caecum and large bowel and colitis has been reported in children with cystic fibrosis taking high doses of pancreatic enzyme supplements. To date, Creon 25000 has not been implicated in the development of colonic damage. However, unusual abdominal symptoms or changes in abdominal symptoms should be reviewed to exclude the possibility of colonic damage - especially if the patient is taking in excess of 10,000 units of lipase/kg/day.

4.9 Overdose
Most cases respond to supportive measures including stopping enzyme therapy, ensuring adequate rehydration.

5. PHARMACOLOGICAL PROPERTIES

5.1 Pharmacodynamic properties
Replacement therapy in pancreatic enzyme deficiency states. The enzymes have hydrolytic activity on fat, carbohydrates and proteins.

5.2 Pharmacokinetic properties
Pharmacokinetic data are not available as the enzymes act locally in the gastro-intestinal tract. After exerting their action, the enzymes are digested themselves in the intestine.

5.3 Preclinical safety data
Not applicable.

6. PHARMACEUTICAL PARTICULARS

6.1 List of excipients
Granules: Macrogol 4000, liquid paraffin, hypromellose phthalate, dibutyl phthalate, dimeticone.

Capsules: Gelatin, E171, E172.

6.2 Incompatibilities
None known.

6.3 Shelf life
2 years

6.4 Special precautions for storage
Store below 25°C.

6.5 Nature and contents of container
HDPE tablet container with LDPE closure. Each container contains 100 capsules.

6.6 Instructions for use and handling
No special instructions.

Administrative Data

7. MARKETING AUTHORISATION HOLDER
Solvay Healthcare Limited
Mansbridge Road
West End
Southampton
SO18 3JD
United Kingdom

8. MARKETING AUTHORISATION NUMBER(S)
PL 00512/0150

9. DATE OF FIRST AUTHORISATION/RENEWAL OF THE AUTHORISATION
01 January 2001

10. DATE OF REVISION OF THE TEXT
September 2003

Legal category
POM

Creon 40000 Capsules

(Solvay Healthcare Limited)

1. NAME OF THE MEDICINAL PRODUCT
Creon® 40000 Capsules

2. QUALITATIVE AND QUANTITATIVE COMPOSITION
Each capsule contains pancreatin PhEur 400 mg equivalent to:

Lipase 40,000 PhEur units
Amylase 25,000 PhEur units
Protease 1,600 PhEur units

3. PHARMACEUTICAL FORM
Capsules.

Brown/clear size 00 capsules containing light brown, gastro-resistant granules.

4. CLINICAL PARTICULARS

4.1 Therapeutic indications
For the treatment of pancreatic exocrine insufficiency.

4.2 Posology and method of administration
Adults (including the elderly) and children:

Creon 40000 should only be used if the patient requires equal to or more than 40,000 lipase units per meal or snack. Creon 40000 should only be used in patients in whom the minimum effective dose has already been determined using lower strength pancreatic enzyme products.

Initially one or two capsules with meals. The capsules should be swallowed whole. Dose increases, if required, should be added slowly, with careful monitoring of response and symptomatology.

It is important to ensure adequate hydration of patients at all times whilst dosing Creon 40000.

Colonic damage has been reported in patients with cystic fibrosis taking in excess of 10,000 units of lipase/kg/day (see Undesirable Effects).

4.3 Contraindications
Patients with known hypersensitivity to porcine proteins.

4.4 Special warnings and special precautions for use
The product is of porcine origin.

Oral medications should not be administered during the early stages of acute pancreatitis.

4.5 Interaction with other medicinal products and other forms of Interaction
None known.

4.6 Pregnancy and lactation
There are no adequate data from the use of Creon in pregnant women. Animal studies are insufficient with respect to effects on pregnancy and embryonal/foetal development, parturition/ and postnatal development. The potential risk for humans is unknown. Creon should not be used during pregnancy or lactation unless clearly necessary but if required should be used in doses providing adequate nutritional status (see warnings about high dose sections 4.2 and 4.8).

4.7 Effects on ability to drive and use machines
Creon 40000 has no influence on the ability to drive or use machines.

4.8 Undesirable effects
Diarrhoea, constipation, gastric discomfort, nausea and skin reactions have been reported occasionally in patients receiving enzyme replacement therapy.

Rarely cases of hyper-uricosuria and hyperuricaemia have been reported with very high doses of pancreatin.

Stricture of the ileocaecum and large bowel and colitis has been reported in children with cystic fibrosis taking high doses of pancreatic enzyme supplements. To date, Creon 10000 and 25000 have not been implicated in the development of colonic damage. Experience with Creon 40000 in clinical use is limited. Unusual abdominal symptoms or changes in abdominal symptoms should be reviewed to exclude the possibility of colonic damage - especially if the patient is taking in excess of 10,000 units of lipase/kg/day.

4.9 Overdose
Most cases respond to supportive measures including stopping enzyme therapy, ensuring adequate rehydration.

5. PHARMACOLOGICAL PROPERTIES

5.1 Pharmacodynamic properties
The ATC code is A09A A (Enzyme preparations).

Replacement therapy in pancreatic enzyme deficiency states. The enzymes have hydrolytic activity on fat, carbohydrates and proteins.

5.2 Pharmacokinetic properties
Pharmacokinetic data are not available as the enzymes act locally in the gastro-intestinal tract. After exerting their action, the enzymes are digested themselves in the intestine.

5.3 Preclinical safety data
None stated.

6. PHARMACEUTICAL PARTICULARS

6.1 List of excipients
Granules: Macrogol 4000, light liquid paraffin, hypromellose phthalate, dimeticone, dibutyl phthalate.

Capsules: Gelatin, Iron oxide E172, Titanium dioxide E171.

6.2 Incompatibilities
None known.

6.3 Shelf life
3 years.

6.4 Special precautions for storage
Do not store above 25°C. Keep container tightly closed.

6.5 Nature and contents of container
HDPE tablet container with LDPE closure. Each container contains 100 capsules.

6.6 Instructions for use and handling
No special instructions.

7. MARKETING AUTHORISATION HOLDER
Solvay Healthcare Limited
Mansbridge Road
West End
Southampton
SO18 3JD
United Kingdom

8. MARKETING AUTHORISATION NUMBER(S)
PL 00512/0177

9. DATE OF FIRST AUTHORISATION/RENEWAL OF THE AUTHORISATION
5 July 2002

10. DATE OF REVISION OF THE TEXT
August 2005

Legal Category
POM

Creon Micro

(Solvay Healthcare Limited)

1. NAME OF THE MEDICINAL PRODUCT
Creon® Micro Pancreatin 60.36 mg Gastro-resistant Granules

2. QUALITATIVE AND QUANTITATIVE COMPOSITION
Each 100 mg of gastro-resistant granules (equivalent to one measuring spoonful) contains 60.36mg of pancreatin, containing the following pancreatic enzymes:

Lipase 5,000 PhEur units

Amylase 3,600 PhEur units

Protease 200 PhEur units

For excipients, see 6.1.

3. PHARMACEUTICAL FORM
Gastro-resistant granules.

Round, light brown gastro-resistant granules.

4. CLINICAL PARTICULARS
4.1 Therapeutic indications
For the treatment of pancreatic exocrine insufficiency.

4.2 Posology and method of administration
Initially 100 mg (5000 lipase units) of gastro-resistant granules (one measure). should be taken with each feed or meal. Dose increases, if required, should be added slowly, with careful monitoring of response and symptomatology. The maximum daily dosage should not exceed 10,000 units lipase/kg/day. The required quantity of gastro-resistant granules should be dispensed using the measuring scoop contained in the pack which holds 100 mg.

In young infants,

Creon Micro granules should be mixed with a small amount of apple juice and given from a spoon directly before the feed. In weaned infants, granules should be taken with acidic liquids or soft foods (e.g. mixed with apple juice or apple puree), but without chewing, directly before the meal. When giving Creon Micro to young or weaned infants the apple juice should not be diluted.

It is important to ensure adequate hydration of patients at all times whilst dosing with Creon.

Colonic damage has been reported in patients with cystic fibrosis taking in excess of 10000 units of lipase/kg/day (see Undesirable effects)

4.3 Contraindications
Patients with known hypersensitivity to porcine proteins or to any of the excipients.

4.4 Special warnings and special precautions for use
The product is of porcine origin.

Oral medications should not be administered during the early stages of acute pancreatitis.

4.5 Interaction with other medicinal products and other forms of Interaction
None known.

4.6 Pregnancy and lactation
There are no adequate data from the use of Creon in pregnant women. Animal studies are insufficient with respect to effects on pregnancy and embryonal/foetal development, parturition and postnatal development. The potential risk to humans is unknown. Creon should not be used during pregnancy or lactation unless clearly necessary.

4.7 Effects on ability to drive and use machines
Creon has no influence on the ability to drive or use machines.

4.8 Undesirable effects
In pooled data from clinical trials, the overall incidence of adverse drug events reported with Creon was the same as with placebo. The incidence tended to reflect the general symptomatology of the underlying disease.

Very common (Frequency > 10%):

Gastrointestinal disorders: abdominal pain

Common (Frequency 1-10%):

Gastrointestinal disorders: diarrhoea, constipation, abnormal stool, nausea and vomiting.

Skin and subcutaneous tissue: allergic or hypersensitivity reactions.

Stricture of the ileo-caecum and large bowel an colitis has been reported in children with cystic fibrosis taking high doses of pancreatic enzyme supplements. To date, Creon 10000 and 25000 have not been implicated in the development of colonic damage. Experience with Creon 40000 and Creon Micro in clinical use is limited. Unusual abdominal symptoms or changes in abdominal symptoms should be reviewed to exclude the possibility of colonic damage especially if the patient is taking in excess of 10,000 units lipase/kg/day.

4.9 Overdose
Most cases respond to supportive measures including stopping enzyme therapy, ensuring adequate rehydration. Rarely cases of hyperuricosuria and hyperuricaemia have been reported with very high doses of pancreatin.

5. PHARMACOLOGICAL PROPERTIES
5.1 Pharmacodynamic properties
The ATC code is A09A A (Enzyme preparations).

Replacement therapy in pancreatic enzyme deficiency states. The enzymes have hydrolytic activity on fat, carbohydrates and proteins.

5.2 Pharmacokinetic properties
Pharmacokinetic data are not available as the enzymes act locally in the gastro-intestinal tract. After exerting their action, the enzymes are digested themselves in the intestine.

5.3 Preclinical safety data
None stated.

6. PHARMACEUTICAL PARTICULARS
6.1 List of excipients
Hypromellose phthalate

Macrogol 4000

Liquid paraffin

Dibutylphthalate

Dimeticone

6.2 Incompatibilities
Not applicable.

6.3 Shelf life
2 years. 12 weeks after first opening.

6.4 Special precautions for storage
Do not store above 25°C.

Keep the container tightly closed in order to protect from moisture.

6.5 Nature and contents of container
Glass bottle with LDPE stopper. Containers hold 20 g of gastro-resistant granules.

6.6 Instructions for use and handling
No special requirements.

7. MARKETING AUTHORISATION HOLDER
Solvay Healthcare Limited

Mansbridge Road

West End

Southampton

SO18 3JD

United Kingdom

8. MARKETING AUTHORISATION NUMBER(S)
PL 00512/0179

9. DATE OF FIRST AUTHORISATION/RENEWAL OF THE AUTHORISATION
August 2004

10. DATE OF REVISION OF THE TEXT
June 2004

Legal category
P

Crestor 10 mg, 20 mg and 40 mg film-coated tablets

(AstraZeneca UK Limited)

1. NAME OF THE MEDICINAL PRODUCT
Crestor 10 mg, 20 mg and 40 mg film-coated tablets. ▼

2. QUALITATIVE AND QUANTITATIVE COMPOSITION
Each tablet contains 10 mg rosuvastatin (as rosuvastatin calcium).

Each tablet contains 20 mg rosuvastatin (as rosuvastatin calcium).

Each tablet contains 40 mg rosuvastatin (as rosuvastatin calcium).

For excipients see 6.1.

3. PHARMACEUTICAL FORM
Film-coated tablet.

Crestor 10 mg Tablet

Round, pink coloured, intagliated with 'ZD4522' and '10' on one side and plain on the reverse.

Crestor 20 mg Tablet

Round, pink coloured, intagliated with 'ZD4522' and '20' on one side and plain on the reverse.

Crestor 40 mg Tablet

Oval, pink coloured, intagliated with 'ZD4522' on one side and '40' on the reverse.

4. CLINICAL PARTICULARS
4.1 Therapeutic indications
Primary hypercholesterolaemia (type IIa including heterozygous familial hypercholesterolaemia) or mixed dyslipidaemia (type IIb) as an adjunct to diet when response to diet and other non-pharmacological treatments (e.g. exercise, weight reduction) is inadequate.

Homozygous familial hypercholesterolaemia as an adjunct to diet and other lipid lowering treatments (e.g. LDL apheresis) or if such treatments are not appropriate.

4.2 Posology and method of administration
Before treatment initiation the patient should be placed on a standard cholesterol-lowering diet that should continue during treatment. The dose should be individualised according to the goal of therapy and patient response, using current consensus guidelines.

The recommended start dose is 10 mg orally once daily and the majority of patients are controlled at this dose. Patients who are switched over from another HMG-CoA reductase inhibitor should also start with the 10 mg dose. A dose adjustment to 20 mg can be made after 4 weeks, if necessary (see Section 5.1 Pharmacodynamic properties). In light of the increased reporting rate of adverse reactions with the 40 mg dose compared to lower doses (see Section 4.8 Undesirable effects), a doubling of the dose to 40 mg after an additional 4 weeks should only be considered in patients with severe hypercholesterolaemia at high cardiovascular risk (in particular those with familial hypercholesterolaemia), who do not achieve their treatment goal on 20 mg, and in whom routine follow-up will be performed (see Section 4.4 Special warnings and precautions). Specialist supervision is recommended when the 40 mg dose is initiated.

Crestor may be given at any time of day, with or without food.

Paediatric use
Safety and efficacy have not been established in children. Paediatric experience is limited to a small number of children (aged 8 years or above) with homozygous familial hypercholesterolaemia. Therefore, Crestor is not recommended for paediatric use at this time.

Use in the elderly
No dose adjustment is necessary.

Dosage in patients with renal insufficiency
No dose adjustment is necessary in patients with mild to moderate renal impairment. The use of Crestor in patients with severe renal impairment is contraindicated for all doses. The 40 mg dose is also contraindicated in patients with moderate renal impairment (creatinine clearance < 60 ml/min, see Section 4.3 Contraindications and Section 5.2 Pharmacokinetic properties).

Dosage in patients with hepatic impairment
There was no increase in systemic exposure to rosuvastatin in subjects with Child-Pugh scores of 7 or below. However, increased systemic exposure has been observed in subjects with Child-Pugh scores of 8 and 9 (see Section 5.2 Pharmacokinetic properties). In these patients an assessment of renal function should be considered (see Section 4.4 Special warnings and special precautions for use). There is no experience in subjects with Child-Pugh scores above 9. Crestor is contraindicated in patients with active liver disease (see Section 4.3 Contraindications).

Race
Increased systemic exposure has been seen in Asian subjects (see section 4.4 Special warnings and special precautions for use and section 5.2 Pharmacokinetic properties). This should be considered when making dose decisions for patients of Asian ancestry. The 40 mg dose is contraindicated in these patients.

4.3 Contraindications
Crestor is contraindicated:

- in patients with hypersensitivity to rosuvastatin or to any of the excipients.

- in patients with active liver disease including unexplained, persistent elevations of serum transaminases and any serum transaminase elevation exceeding 3 × the upper limit of normal (ULN).

- in patients with severe renal impairment (creatinine clearance <30 ml/min).

- in patients with myopathy.

- in patients receiving concomitant cyclosporin.

- during pregnancy and lactation and in women of child-bearing potential not using appropriate contraceptive measures.

The 40 mg dose is contraindicated in patients with pre-disposing factors for myopathy/rhabdomyolysis. Such factors include:

– moderate renal impairment (creatinine clearance < 60 ml/min)

– hypothyroidism

– personal or family history of hereditary muscular disorders

– previous history of muscular toxicity with another HMG-CoA reductase inhibitor or fibrate

– alcohol abuse

– situations where an increase in plasma levels may occur

– Asian patients

– concomitant use of fibrates.

(see sections 4.4 Special warnings and special precautions for use, 4.5 Interaction with other medicinal products and other forms of interaction and 5.2 Pharmacokinetic properties)

In patients with secondary hypercholesterolaemia caused by hypothyroidism or nephrotic syndrome, the underlying disease should be treated prior to initiating therapy with Crestor.

Race

Pharmacokinetic studies show an increase in exposure in Asian subjects compared with Caucasians (see section 4.2 Posology and Method of administration and section 5.2 Pharmacokinetic properties)

4.4 Special warnings and special precautions for use

Renal Effects

Proteinuria, detected by dipstick testing and mostly tubular in origin, has been observed in patients treated with higher doses of Crestor, in particular 40 mg, where it was transient or intermittent in most cases. Proteinuria has not been shown to be predictive of acute or progressive renal disease (see Section 4.8 Undesirable effects). An assessment of renal function should be considered during routine follow-up of patients treated with a dose of 40 mg.

Skeletal Muscle Effects

Effects on skeletal muscle e.g. myalgia, myopathy and, rarely, rhabdomyolysis have been reported in Crestor-treated patients with all doses and in particular with doses > 20 mg.

Creatine Kinase Measurement

Creatine Kinase (CK) should not be measured following strenuous exercise or in the presence of a plausible alternative cause of CK increase which may confound interpretation of the result. If CK levels are significantly elevated at baseline >5xULN) a confirmatory test should be carried out within 5 – 7 days. If the repeat test confirms a baseline CK>5xULN, treatment should not be started.

Before Treatment

Crestor, as with other HMG-CoA reductase inhibitors, should be prescribed with caution in patients with predisposing factors for myopathy/rhabdomyolysis. Such factors include:

- renal impairment
- hypothyroidism
- personal or family history of hereditary muscular disorders
- previous history of muscular toxicity with another HMG-CoA reductase inhibitor or fibrate
- alcohol abuse
- age >70 years
- situations where an increase in plasma levels may occur (see section 5.2 Pharmacokinetic properties)
- concomitant use of fibrates.

In such patients the risk of treatment should be considered in relation to possible benefit and clinical monitoring is recommended. If CK levels are significantly elevated at baseline >5xULN) treatment should not be started.

Whilst on Treatment

Patients should be asked to report inexplicable muscle pain, weakness or cramps immediately, particularly if associated with malaise or fever. CK levels should be measured in these patients. Therapy should be discontinued if CK levels are markedly elevated >5xULN) or if muscular symptoms are severe and cause daily discomfort (even if CK levels are ⩽ 5x ULN). If symptoms resolve and CK levels return to normal, then consideration should be given to re-introducing Crestor or an alternative HMG-CoA reductase inhibitor at the lowest dose with close monitoring. Routine monitoring of CK levels in asymptomatic patients is not warranted.

In clinical trials there was no evidence of increased skeletal muscle effects in the small number of patients dosed with Crestor and concomitant therapy. However, an increase in the incidence of myositis and myopathy has been seen in patients receiving other HMG-CoA reductase inhibitors together with fibric acid derivatives including gemfibrozil, cyclosporin, nicotinic acid, azole antifungals, protease inhibitors and macrolide antibiotics. Gemfibrozil increases the risk of myopathy when given concomitantly with some HMG-CoA reductase inhibitors. Therefore, the combination of Crestor and gemfibrozil is not recommended. The benefit of further alterations in lipid levels by the combined use of Crestor with fibrates or niacin should be carefully weighed against the potential risks of such combinations. The 40 mg dose is contraindicated with concomitant use of a fibrate.

(See Section 4.5 Interaction with other medicinal products and other forms of interaction and Section 4.8 Undesirable effects.)

Crestor should not be used in any patient with an acute, serious condition suggestive of myopathy or predisposing to the development of renal failure secondary to rhabdomyolysis (e.g. sepsis, hypotension, major surgery, trauma, severe metabolic, endocrine and electrolyte disorders; or uncontrolled seizures).

Liver Effects

As with other HMG-CoA reductase inhibitors, Crestor should be used with caution in patients who consume excessive quantities of alcohol and/or have a history of liver disease.

It is recommended that liver function tests be carried out prior to, and 3 months following, the initiation of treatment. Crestor should be discontinued or the dose reduced if the level of serum transaminases is greater than 3 times the upper limit of normal.

4.5 Interaction with other medicinal products and other forms of Interaction

Cyclosporin: During concomitant treatment with Crestor and cyclosporin, rosuvastatin AUC values were on average 7 times higher than those observed in healthy volunteers (see Section 4.3 Contraindications).

Concomitant administration did not affect plasma concentrations of cyclosporin.

Vitamin K antagonists: As with other HMG-CoA reductase inhibitors, the initiation of treatment or dosage up-titration of Crestor in patients treated concomitantly with vitamin K antagonists (e.g. warfarin) may result in an increase in International Normalised Ratio (INR). Discontinuation or down-titration of Crestor may result in a decrease in INR. In such situations, appropriate monitoring of INR is desirable.

Gemfibrozil and other lipid-lowering products: Concomitant use of Crestor and gemfibrozil resulted in a 2-fold increase in rosuvastatin C_{max} and AUC (see Section 4.4 Special warnings and special precautions for use).

Based on data from specific interaction studies no pharmacokinetic relevant interaction with fenofibrate is expected, however a pharmacodynamic interaction may occur. Gemfibrozil, fenofibrate, other fibrates and lipid lowering doses > or equal to 1g/day) of niacin (nicotinic acid) increase the risk of myopathy when given concomitantly with HMG-CoA reductase inhibitors, probably because they can produce myopathy when given alone. The 40 mg dose is contraindicated with concomitant use of a fibrate (see Section 4.3 Contraindications and Section 4.4 Special warnings and special precautions for use).

Antacid: The simultaneous dosing of Crestor with an antacid suspension containing aluminium and magnesium hydroxide resulted in a decrease in rosuvastatin plasma concentration of approximately 50%. This effect was mitigated when the antacid was dosed 2 hours after Crestor. The clinical relevance of this interaction has not been studied.

Erythromycin: Concomitant use of Crestor and erythromycin resulted in a 20% decrease in AUC (0-t) and a 30% decrease in C_{max} of rosuvastatin. This interaction may be caused by the increase in gut motility caused by erythromycin.

Oral contraceptive/hormone replacement therapy (HRT): Concomitant use of Crestor and an oral contraceptive resulted in an increase in ethinyl oestradiol and norgestrel AUC of 26% and 34%, respectively. These increased plasma levels should be considered when selecting oral contraceptive doses. There are no pharmacokinetic data available in subjects taking concomitant Crestor and HRT and therefore a similar effect cannot be excluded. However, the combination has been extensively used in women in clinical trials and was well tolerated.

Other medicinal products: Based on data from specific interaction studies no clinically relevant interaction with digoxinis expected.

Cytochrome P450 enzymes: Results from *in vitro* and *in vivo* studies show that rosuvastatin is neither an inhibitor nor an inducer of cytochrome P450 isoenzymes. In addition, rosuvastatin is a poor substrate for these isoenzymes. No clinically relevant interactions have been observed between rosuvastatin and either fluconazole (an inhibitor of CYP2C9 and CYP3A4) or ketoconazole (an inhibitor of CYP2A6 and CYP3A4). Concomitant administration of itraconazole (an inhibitor of CYP3A4) and rosuvastatin resulted in a 28% increase in AUC of rosuvastatin. This small increase is not considered clinically significant. Therefore, drug interactions resulting from cytochrome P450-mediated metabolism are not expected.

4.6 Pregnancy and lactation

Crestor is contraindicated in pregnancy and lactation.

Women of child bearing potential should use appropriate contraceptive measures.

Since cholesterol and other products of cholesterol biosynthesis are essential for the development of the foetus, the potential risk from inhibition of HMG-CoA reductase outweighs the advantage of treatment during pregnancy. Animal studies provide limited evidence of reproductive toxicity (see Section 5.3 Preclinical safety data). If a patient becomes pregnant during use of this product, treatment should be discontinued immediately.

Rosuvastatin is excreted in the milk of rats. There are no data with respect to excretion in milk in humans.

(see Section 4.3 Contraindications).

4.7 Effects on ability to drive and use machines

Studies to determine the effect of Crestor on the ability to drive and use machines have not been conducted. However, based on its pharmacodynamic properties, Crestor is unlikely to affect this ability. When driving vehicles or operating machines, it should be taken into account that dizziness may occur during treatment.

4.8 Undesirable effects

The adverse events seen with Crestor are generally mild and transient. In controlled clinical trials, less than 4% of Crestor-treated patients were withdrawn due to adverse events.

The frequencies of adverse events are ranked according to the following: Common >1/100, <1/10); Uncommon >1/1,000, <1/100); Rare >1/10,000, <1/1000); Very rare (<1/10,000).

Immune system disorders

Rare: hypersensitivity reactions including angioedema

Nervous system disorders

Common: headache, dizziness

Gastrointestinal disorders

Common: constipation, nausea, abdominal pain

Skin and subcutaneous tissue disorders

Uncommon: pruritus, rash and urticaria

Musculoskeletal, connective tissue and bone disorders

Common: myalgia

Rare: myopathy and rhabdomyolysis

General disorders

Common: asthenia

As with other HMG-CoA reductase inhibitors, the incidence of adverse drug reactions tends to be dose dependent.

Renal Effects: Proteinuria, detected by dipstick testing and mostly tubular in origin, has been observed in patients treated with Crestor. Shifts in urine protein from none or trace to ++ or more were seen in <1% of patients at some time during treatment with 10 and 20 mg, and in approximately 3% of patients treated with 40 mg. A minor increase in shift from none or trace to + was observed with the 20 mg dose. In most cases, proteinuria decreases or disappears spontaneously on continued therapy, and has not been shown to be predictive of acute or progressive renal disease.

Skeletal muscle effects: Effects on skeletal muscle e.g.myalgia, myopathy and, rarely, rhabdomyolysishave been reported in Crestor-treated patients with all doses and in particular with doses > 20 mg.

A dose-related increase in CK levels has been observed inpatients taking rosuvastatin; the majority of cases were mild, asymptomatic and transient. If CK levels are elevated (>5xULN), treatment should bediscontinued (see Section 4.4 Special warnings and special precautions for use).

Liver Effects: As with other HMG-CoA reductase inhibitors, a dose-related increase in transaminases has been observed in a small number of patients taking rosuvastatin; the majority of cases were mild, asymptomatic and transient.

Post Marketing Experience:

In addition to the above, the following adverse events have been reported during post marketing experience for CRESTOR:

Hepatobiliary disorders: very rare: jaundice, hepatitis; *rare:* increased hepatic transaminases.

Musculoskeletal disorders:rare: arthralgia

Nervous system disorders: very rare: polyneuropathy

4.9 Overdose

There is no specific treatment in the event of overdose. In the event of overdose, the patient should be treated symptomatically and supportive measures instituted as required. Liver function and CK levels should be monitored. Haemodialysis is unlikely to be of benefit.

5. PHARMACOLOGICAL PROPERTIES

5.1 Pharmacodynamic properties

Pharmacotherapeutic group: HMG-CoA reductase inhibitors

ATC code: C10A A07

Mechanism of action

Rosuvastatin is a selective and competitive inhibitor of HMG-CoA reductase, the rate-limiting enzyme that converts 3-hydroxy-3-methylglutaryl coenzyme A to mevalonate, a precursor for cholesterol. The primary site of action of rosuvastatin is the liver, the target organ for cholesterol lowering.

Rosuvastatin increases the number of hepatic LDL receptors on the cell-surface, enhancing uptake and catabolism of LDL and it inhibits the hepatic synthesis of VLDL, thereby reducing the total number of VLDL and LDL particles.

Pharmacodynamic effects

Crestor reduces elevated LDL-cholesterol, total cholesterol and triglycerides and increases HDL-cholesterol. It also lowers ApoB, nonHDL-C, VLDL-C, VLDL-TG and increases ApoA-I (see Table 1). Crestor also lowers the LDL-C/HDL-C, total C/HDL-C and nonHDL-C/HDL-C and the ApoB/ApoA-I ratios.

Table 1 Dose response in patients with primary hypercholesterolaemia (type IIa and IIb) (adjusted mean percent change from baseline)

(see Table 1 on next page)

Table 1 Dose response in patients with primary hypercholesterolaemia (type IIa and IIb) (adjusted mean percent change from baseline)

Dose	N	LDL-C	Total-C	HDL-C	TG	nonHDL-C	ApoB	ApoA-I
Placebo	13	-7	-5	3	-3	-7	-3	0
10	17	-52	-36	14	-10	-48	-42	4
20	17	-55	-40	8	-23	-51	-46	5
40	18	-63	-46	10	-28	-60	-54	0

A therapeutic effect is obtained within 1 week following treatment initiation and 90% of maximum response is achieved in 2 weeks. The maximum response is usually achieved by 4 weeks and is maintained after that.

Clinical efficacy

Crestor is effective in adults with hypercholesterolaemia, with and without hypertriglyceridaemia, regardless of race, sex, or age and in special populations such as diabetics, or patients with familial hypercholesterolaemia.

From pooled phase III data, Crestor has been shown to be effective at treating the majority of patients with type IIa and IIb hypercholesterolaemia (mean baseline LDL-C about 4.8 mmol/l) to recognised European Atherosclerosis Society (EAS; 1998) guideline targets; about 80% of patients treated with 10 mg reached the EAS targets for LDL-C levels (<3 mmol/l).

In a large study, 435 patients with heterozygous familial hypercholesterolaemia were given Crestor from 20 mg to 80 mg in a force-titration design. All doses showed a beneficial effect on lipid parameters and treatment to target goals. Following titration to a daily dose of 40 mg (12 weeks of treatment), LDL-C was reduced by 53%. 33% of patients reached EAS guidelines for LDL-C levels (<3 mmol/l).

In a force-titration, open label trial, 42 patients with homozygous familial hypercholesterolaemia were evaluated for their response to Crestor 20 - 40 mg. In the overall population, the mean LDL-C reduction was 22%.

In clinical studies with a limited number of patients, Crestor has been shown to have additive efficacy in lowering triglycerides when used in combination with fenofibrate and in increasing HDL-C levels when used in combination with niacin (see Section 4.4 Special warnings and special precautions for use).

Rosuvastatin has not been proven to prevent the associated complications of lipid abnormalities, such as coronary heart disease as mortality and morbidity studies with Crestor have not yet been completed.

5.2 Pharmacokinetic properties

Absorption: Maximum rosuvastatin plasma concentrations are achieved approximately 5 hours after oral administration. The absolute bioavailability is approximately 20%.

Distribution: Rosuvastatin is taken up extensively by the liver which is the primary site of cholesterol synthesis and LDL-C clearance. The volume of distribution of rosuvastatin is approximately 134 L. Approximately 90% of rosuvastatin is bound to plasma proteins, mainly to albumin.

Metabolism: Rosuvastatin undergoes limited metabolism (approximately 10%). *In vitro* metabolism studies using human hepatocytes indicate that rosuvastatin is a poor substrate for cytochrome P450-based metabolism. CYP2C9 was the principal isoenzyme involved, with 2C19, 3A4 and 2D6 involved to a lesser extent. The main metabolites identified are the N-desmethyl and lactone metabolites. The N-desmethyl metabolite is approximately 50% less active than rosuvastatin whereas the lactone form is considered clinically inactive. Rosuvastatin accounts for greater than 90% of the circulating HMG-CoA reductase inhibitor activity.

Excretion: Approximately 90% of the rosuvastatin dose is excreted unchanged in the faeces (consisting of absorbed and non-absorbed active substance) and the remaining part is excreted in urine. Approximately 5% is excreted unchanged in urine. The plasma elimination half-life is approximately 19 hours. The elimination half-life does not increase at higher doses. The geometric mean plasma clearance is approximately 50 litres/hour (coefficient of variation 21.7%). As with other HMG-CoA reductase inhibitors, the hepatic uptake of rosuvastatin involves the membrane transporter OATP-C. This transporter is important in the hepatic elimination of rosuvastatin.

Linearity: Systemic exposure of rosuvastatin increases in proportion to dose. There are no changes in pharmacokinetic parameters following multiple daily doses.

Special populations:

Age and sex: There was no clinically relevant effect of age or sex on the pharmacokinetics of rosuvastatin.

Race: Pharmacokinetic studies show an approximate 2-fold elevation in median AUC and Cmax in Asian subjects in Asia compared with Caucasians living in Asia and Europe. The contribution of environmental and genetic factors to these observed differences has not been determined. A population pharmacokinetic analysis revealed no clinically relevant differences in pharmacokinetics between Caucasian and Black groups.

Renal insufficiency: In a study in subjects with varying degrees of renal impairment, mild to moderate renal disease had no influence on plasma concentration of rosuvastatin or the N-desmethyl metabolite. Subjects with severe impairment (CrCl <30 ml/min) had a 3-fold increase in plasma concentration and a 9-fold increase in the N-desmethyl metabolite concentration compared to healthy volunteers. Steady-state plasma concentrations of rosuvastatin in subjects undergoing haemodialysis were approximately 50% greater compared to healthy volunteers.

Hepatic insufficiency: In a study with subjects with varying degrees of hepatic impairment there was no evidence of increased exposure to rosuvastatin in subjects with Child-Pugh scores of 7 or below. However, two subjects with Child-Pugh scores of 8 and 9 showed an increase in systemic exposure of at least 2-fold compared to subjects with lower Child-Pugh scores. There is no experience in subjects with Child-Pugh scores above 9.

5.3 Preclinical safety data

Preclinical data reveal no special hazard for humans based on conventional studies of safety pharmacology, repeated dose toxicity, genotoxicity and carcinogenicity potential. In a rat pre- and postnatal study, reproductive toxicity was evident from reduced litter sizes, litter weight and pup survival. These effects were observed at maternotoxic doses at systemic exposures several times above the therapeutic exposure level.

6. PHARMACEUTICAL PARTICULARS

6.1 List of excipients

Tablet core

Lactose monohydrate

Microcrystalline cellulose

Calcium phosphate

Crospovidone

Magnesium stearate

Tablet coat

Lactose monohydrate

Hypromellose

Glycerol triacetate

Titanium dioxide (E171)

Ferric oxide, red (E172)

6.2 Incompatibilities

Not applicable.

6.3 Shelf life

3 years.

6.4 Special precautions for storage

Blisters: Do not store above 30°C. Store in the original package.

HDPE bottles: Do not store above 30°C. Keep container tightly closed.

6.5 Nature and contents of container

Blisters of aluminium laminate/aluminium foil of 7, 14, 15, 20, 28, 30, 42, 50, 56, 60, 84, 98 and 100 tablets and HDPE bottles of 30 and 100 tablets.

Not all pack sizes may be marketed.

6.6 Instructions for use and handling

No special requirements.

7. MARKETING AUTHORISATION HOLDER

AstraZeneca UK Ltd

600 Capability Green

Luton

LU1 3LU

United Kingdom

8. MARKETING AUTHORISATION NUMBER(S)

Crestor 10mg - PL 17901/0201

Crestor 20mg - PL 17901/0202

Crestor 40mg - PL 17901/0203

9. DATE OF FIRST AUTHORISATION/RENEWAL OF THE AUTHORISATION

21st March 2003

10. DATE OF REVISION OF THE TEXT

28th February 2005

Crinone 8% Progesterone Vaginal Gel

(Serono Ltd)

1. NAME OF THE MEDICINAL PRODUCT

CRINONE* 8% PROGESTERONE VAGINAL GEL.

2. QUALITATIVE AND QUANTITATIVE COMPOSITION

Active Ingredient

	mg/dose	% w/w
Progesterone	90	8.0

3. PHARMACEUTICAL FORM

Vaginal gel.

4. CLINICAL PARTICULARS

4.1 Therapeutic indications

Treatment of infertility due to inadequate luteal phase.

For use during in-vitro fertilisation, where infertility is mainly due to tubal, idiopathic or endometriosis linked sterility associated with normal ovulatory cycles.

4.2 Posology and method of administration

Intravaginal application.

Treatment of infertility due to inadequate luteal phase: one application (1.125g 8% gel) every day, starting after documented ovulation or arbitrarily on the 18th-21st day of the cycle.

When used during in-vitro fertilisation, daily application of Crinone 8% gel should be continued for 30 days if there is laboratory evidence of pregnancy.

Children: Not applicable.

The Elderly: Not applicable.

4.3 Contraindications

Known allergy to any of the excipients.

Undiagnosed uterine bleeding.

Porphyria

4.4 Special warnings and special precautions for use

Cautious use in severe hepatic insufficiency.

The product should not be used concurrently with other local intravaginal therapy.

4.5 Interaction with other medicinal products and other forms of Interaction

No interaction reported

4.6 Pregnancy and lactation

In case of corpus luteum deficiency, CRINONE can be used during the first month of pregnancy.

Do not use during lactation.

4.7 Effects on ability to drive and use machines

Drivers and users of machines are warned that risk of somnolence may occur.

4.8 Undesirable effects

Rare cases of somnolence.

Occasional spotting.

4.9 Overdose

Not applicable.

5. PHARMACOLOGICAL PROPERTIES

5.1 Pharmacodynamic properties

The pharmacological particulars of the product are those of the naturally occurring progesterone with induction of a full secretory endometrium.

5.2 Pharmacokinetic properties

The progesterone vaginal gel is based on a polycarbophil delivery system which attaches to the vaginal mucosa and provides a prolonged release of progesterone for at least three days.

5.3 Preclinical safety data

In rabbits, Crinone was an eye irritant categorised class IV (minimal effects clearing in less than 24 hours), but not a dermal irritant.

A moderate vaginal irritation was found in rabbits after application of 2.0ml/day of 8% gel for 5 days.

6. PHARMACEUTICAL PARTICULARS

6.1 List of excipients

Glycerin, Light Liquid Paraffin, Hydrogenated Palm Oil Glyceride, Carbopol 974P, Sorbic acid, Polycarbophil, Sodium hydroxide, Purified water.

6.2 Incompatibilities

No incompatibilities were found with the usual contraceptive devices.

6.3 Shelf life

36 months.

6.4 Special precautions for storage

Store below 25°C.

6.5 Nature and contents of container

A single use, one piece, white polyethylene applicator with a twist-off top, designed for intravaginal application.

Each applicator contains 1.45 g of gel and delivers 1.125g of gel. Each one is wrapped up and sealed in a paper/aluminium/polyethylene foil overwrap.

The applicators are packed in cardboard boxes containing 6 or 15 units of Crinone 8% progesterone vaginal gel.

6.6 Instructions for use and handling
Crinone is applied directly from the specially designed sealed applicator into the vagina. Remove the applicator from the sealed wrapper. DO NOT remove the twist-off cap at this time. Grip the applicator firmly by the thick end. Shake down like a thermometer to ensure that the contents are at the thin end. Twist off the tab and discard. The applicator may be inserted while you are in a sitting position or when lying on your back with the knees bent. Gently insert the thin end of applicator well into the vagina. Press the thick end of the applicator firmly to deposit gel. Remove the applicator and discard in a waste container. CRINONE coats the vaginal mucosa to provide long-lasting release of progesterone.

7. MARKETING AUTHORISATION HOLDER
Serono Pharmaceuticals Ltd
Bedfont Cross
Stanwell Road
Feltham
Middlesex TW14 8NX
United Kingdom
Tel: 020 8818 7200

8. MARKETING AUTHORISATION NUMBER(S)
PL 03400/0081

9. DATE OF FIRST AUTHORISATION/RENEWAL OF THE AUTHORISATION
26 January 2000

10. DATE OF REVISION OF THE TEXT
November 2000

CRIXIVAN 200 mg and 400 mg hard capsules

(Merck Sharp & Dohme Limited)

1. NAME OF THE MEDICINAL PRODUCT
CRIXIVAN 200 mg hard capsules
CRIXIVAN 400 mg hard capsules

2. QUALITATIVE AND QUANTITATIVE COMPOSITION
CRIXIVAN 200 mg - Each hard capsule contains 250 mg of indinavir sulphate corresponding to 200 mg of indinavir.

CRIXIVAN 400 mg - Each hard capsule contains 500 mg of indinavir sulphate corresponding to 400 mg of indinavir.

For excipients, see 6.1

3. PHARMACEUTICAL FORM
Hard capsules.

CRIXIVAN 200 mg - The capsules are semi–translucent white and coded CRIXIVAN™ 200 mg in blue.

CRIXIVAN 400 mg - The capsules are semi–translucent white and coded CRIXIVAN™ 400 mg in green.

4. CLINICAL PARTICULARS
4.1 Therapeutic indications
CRIXIVAN is indicated in combination with antiretroviral nucleoside analogues for the treatment of HIV–1 infected adults, adolescents, and children 4 years of age and older. In adolescents and children, the benefit of indinavir therapy versus the increased risk of nephrolithiasis should particularly be considered (see section 4.4).

4.2 Posology and method of administration
CRIXIVAN should be administered by physicians who are experienced in the treatment of HIV infection. On the basis of current pharmacodynamic data, indinavir must be used in combination with other antiretroviral agents. When indinavir is administered as monotherapy resistant viruses rapidly emerge (see section 5.1).

Adults

The recommended dosage of CRIXIVAN is 800 mg orally every 8 hours.

Children and adolescents (4 to 17 years of age)

The recommended dosage of CRIXIVAN for patients 4 to 17 years of age is 500 mg/m^2 (dose adjusted from calculated body surface area [BSA] based on height and weight) orally every 8 hours (see table below). This dose should not exceed the equivalent of the adult dose of 800 mg every 8 hours. CRIXIVAN hard capsules should only be given to children who are able to swallow hard capsules. CRIXIVAN has not been studied in children under the age of 4 years (see section 5.1 and 5.2).

Paediatric dose (500 mg/m^2) to be administered every 8 hours

Body Surface Area (m^2)	CRIXIVAN dose Every 8 hours (mg)
0.50	300
0.75	400
1.00	500
1.25	600
1.50	800

General administration recommendations

The hard capsules should be swallowed whole.

Since CRIXIVAN must be taken at intervals of 8 hours, a schedule convenient for the patient should be developed. For optimal absorption, CRIXIVAN should be administered without food but with water 1 hour before or 2 hours after a meal. Alternatively, CRIXIVAN may be administered with a low–fat, light meal.

To ensure adequate hydration, it is recommended that adults drink at least 1.5 litres of liquids during the course of 24 hours. It is also recommended that children who weigh less than 20 kg drink at least 75 ml/kg/day and that children who weigh 20 to 40 kg drink at least 50 ml/kg/day.

Medical management in patients with one or more episodes of nephrolithiasis must include adequate hydration and may include temporary interruption of therapy (e.g., 1 to 3 days) during the acute episode of nephrolithiasis or discontinuation of therapy (see section 4.4).

Special dosing considerations in adults

Due to an increase in the plasma concentrations of rifabutin and a decrease in the plasma concentrations of indinavir, a dosage reduction of rifabutin to half the standard dose (consult manufacturer's package circular for rifabutin) and a dosage increase of CRIXIVAN to 1,000 – 1,200 mg every 8 hours is suggested when rifabutin is co–administered with CRIXIVAN. For dosages of 1,000 mg, use the 333–mg hard capsules, and for all other dosages, use the 100–mg, 200–mg or 400–mg hard capsules. This dose regimen has not been confirmed in clinical studies and could result in a clinically significant increase in the plasma concentration of rifabutin.

A dosage reduction of CRIXIVAN to 600 mg every 8 hours should be considered when administering itraconazole concurrently (see section 4.5).

In patients with mild–to–moderate hepatic impairment due to cirrhosis, the dosage of CRIXIVAN should be reduced to 600 mg every 8 hours. The recommendation is based on limited pharmacokinetic data (see section 5.2). Patients with severe hepatic impairment have not been studied; therefore, no dosing recommendations can be made (see section 4.4).

Safety in patients with impaired renal function has not been studied; however, less than 20 % of indinavir is excreted in the urine as unchanged drug or metabolites (see section 4.4).

4.3 Contraindications
Hypersensitivity to the active substance or to any excipients of this medicinal product.

Indinavir should not be administered concurrently with medicinal products with narrow therapeutic windows and which are substrates of CYP3A4. CRIXIVAN should not be administered concurrently with terfenadine, cisapride, astemizole, alprazolam, triazolam, midazolam, pimozide, or ergot derivatives. Inhibition of CYP3A4 by CRIXIVAN could result in elevated plasma concentrations of these medicines, potentially causing serious or life–threatening reactions.

Indinavir should not be administered concurrently with rifampicin because co–administration results in 90 % reduction in the plasma concentration of indinavir.

Herbal preparations containing St. John's wort (*Hypericum perforatum)* must not be used while taking CRIXIVAN because co–administration substantially reduces plasma concentrations of indinavir. This may result in reduced clinical effects of CRIXIVAN (see section 4.5).

4.4 Special warnings and special precautions for use
Nephrolithiasis and tubulointerstitial nephritis

Nephrolithiasis has occurred with indinavir therapy in adult and paediatric patients. The frequency of nephrolithiasis is higher in paediatric patients than in adult patients. In some cases, nephrolithiasis has been associated with renal insufficiency or acute renal failure; in the majority of these cases renal insufficiency and acute renal failure were reversible. If signs and symptoms of nephrolithiasis, including flank pain with or without haematuria (including microscopic haematuria) occur, temporary interruption of therapy (e.g. for 1–3 days) during the acute episode of nephrolithiasis or discontinuation of therapy may be considered. Paediatric patients who experience flank pain should be evaluated for the possibility of nephrolithiasis. Evaluation may consist of urinalysis, serum BUN and creatinine, and ultrasound of the bladder and kidneys. The long–term effects of nephrolithiasis in paediatric patients are unknown. Adequate hydration is recommended in all patients on indinavir (see section 4.2 and 4.8).

Cases of interstitial nephritis with medullary calcification and cortical atrophy have been observed in patients with asymptomatic severe leucocyturia > 100 cells/high power field). In patients at increased risk such as children, urinary screening should be considered. If persistent severe leucocyturia is found, further investigation might be warranted.

Drug interactions

Indinavir should be used cautiously with other medicinal products that are potent inducers of CYP3A4. Co–administration may result in decreased plasma concentrations of indinavir and as a consequence an increased risk for suboptimal treatment and facilitation of development of resistance (see section 4.5).

If indinavir is given with ritonavir, the potential drug interaction may be increased. The Drug Interactions section of the SPC for ritonavir should also be consulted for information about potential drug interactions.

Concomitant use of indinavir with lovastatin or simvastatin is not recommended due to an increased risk of myopathy including rhabdomyolysis. Caution must also be exercised if indinavir is used concurrently with atorvastatin (see section 4.5).

Co–administration of CRIXIVAN with sildenafil is expected to substantially increase sildenafil plasma concentrations and may result in an increase in sildenafil–associated adverse events, including hypotension, visual changes, and priapism (see section 4.5).

Acute haemolytic anaemia

Acute haemolytic anaemia has been reported which in some cases was severe and progressed rapidly. Once a diagnosis is apparent, appropriate measures for the treatment of haemolytic anaemia should be instituted which may include discontinuation of indinavir.

Hyperglycaemia

New onset diabetes mellitus, hyperglycaemia or exacerbation of existing diabetes mellitus has been reported in patients receiving protease inhibitors (PIs). In some of these the hyperglycaemia was severe and in some cases also associated with ketoacidosis. Many patients had confounding medical conditions, some of which required therapy with agents that have been associated with the development of diabetes mellitus or hyperglycaemia.

Fat redistribution

Combination antiretroviral therapy has been associated with the redistribution of body fat (lipodystrophy) in HIV patients. The long term-consequences of these events are currently unknown. Knowledge about the mechanism is incomplete. A connection between visceral lipomatosis and PIs and lipoatrophy and nucleoside reverse transcriptase inhibitors (NRTIs) has been hypothesised. A higher risk of lipodystrophy has been associated with individual factors such as older age, and with drug related factors such as longer duration of antiretroviral treatment and associated metabolic disturbances. Clinical examination should include evaluation for physical signs of fat redistribution. Consideration should be given to the measurement of fasting serum lipids and blood glucose. Lipid disorders should be managed as clinically appropriate (see section 4.8).

Liver disease

The safety and efficacy of indinavir has not been established in patients with significant underlying liver disorders. Patients with chronic hepatitis B or C and treated with combination antiretroviral therapy are at an increased risk for severe and potentially fatal hepatic adverse events. In case of concomitant antiviral therapy for hepatitis B or C, please refer also to the relevant product information for these medicinal products.

Patients with pre-existing liver dysfunction including chronic active hepatitis have an increased frequency of liver function abnormalities during combination antiretroviral therapy and should be monitored according to standard practice. If there is evidence of worsening liver disease in such patients, interruption or discontinuation of treatment must be considered.

An increased incidence of nephrolithiasis has been observed in patients with underlying liver disorders when treated with indinavir.

Immune Reactivation Syndrome

In HIV-infected patients with severe immune deficiency at the time of institution of combination antiretroviral (CART), an inflammatory reaction to asymptomatic or residual opportunistic pathogens may arise and cause serious clinical conditions, or aggravation of symptoms. Typically, such reactions have been observed within the first few weeks or months of initiation of CART. Relevant examples are cytomegalovirus retinitis, generalised and/or focal myobacterial infections, and *Pneumocystis carinii* pneumonia. Any inflammatory symptoms should be evaluated and treatment instituted when necessary.

Patients with coexisting conditions

There have been reports of increased bleeding, including spontaneous skin haematomas and haemarthroses, in haemophiliac patients type A and B treated with PIs. In some patients additional factor VIII was given. In more than a half of the reported cases, treatment with PIs was continued or re-introduced if treatment had been discontinued. A causal relationship has been evoked, although the mechanism of action has not been elucidated. Haemophiliac patients should therefore be made aware of the possibility of increased bleeding.

Patients with mild–to–moderate hepatic insufficiency due to cirrhosis will require a dosage reduction of indinavir due to decreased metabolism of indinavir (see section 4.2). Patients with severe hepatic impairment have not been studied. In the absence of such studies, caution should be exercised as increased levels of indinavir may occur.

Safety in patients with impaired renal function has not been studied; however, less than 20 % of indinavir is excreted in the urine as unchanged drug or metabolites (see section 4.2).

Lactose

This medicinal product contains 299.2 mg of lactose in each 800-mg dose (maximum single dose). This quantity is not likely to induce symptoms of lactose intolerance (milk intolerance).

CRIXIVAN 200 mg - Each 200 mg capsule contains 74.8 mg of lactose.

CRIXIVAN 400 mg - Each 400 mg capsule contains 149.6 mg of lactose.

Patients with rare hereditary problems of galactose intolerance, the Lapp lactose deficiency or glucose-galactose malabsorption should not take this medicine.

4.5 Interaction with other medicinal products and other forms of Interaction

All drug interaction studies were performed in adults. The relevance of the results from these studies in paediatric patients is unknown.

The metabolism of indinavir is mediated by the cytochrome P450 enzyme CYP3A4. Therefore, other substances that either share this metabolic pathway or modify CYP3A4 activity may influence the pharmacokinetics of indinavir. Similarly, indinavir might also modify the pharmacokinetics of other substances that share this metabolic pathway.

Refer also to section 4.3 Contra-indications and 4.2 Posology and method of administration.

Specific interaction studies were performed with indinavir and the following medicinal products: zidovudine, zidovudine/lamivudine, stavudine, trimethoprim/sulfamethoxazole, fluconazole, isoniazid, clarithromycin, quinidine, cimetidine, theophylline, methadone and an oral contraceptive (norethindrone/ethinyl estradiol 1/35). No clinically significant interactions were observed with these medicinal products. Clinically significant interactions with other medicinal products are described below.

A formal interaction study has not been performed between indinavir and warfarin. Combined treatment could result in increased levels of warfarin.

Calcium channel blockers

Calcium channel blockers are metabolised by CYP 3A4 which is inhibited by indinavir. Coadministration with CRIXIVAN may result in increased plasma concentrations of the calcium channel blockers which could increase or prolong the therapeutic and adverse effects.

Rifabutin

The co–administration of indinavir 800 mg every 8 hours with rifabutin either 300 mg once daily or 150 mg once daily was evaluated in two separate clinical studies. The results of these studies showed a decrease in indinavir AUC (34 % and 33 %, respectively, versus indinavir 800 mg every 8 hours alone) and an increase in rifabutin AUC (173 % and 55 %, respectively, versus rifabutin 300 mg once daily alone). This increase in rifabutin plasma concentrations is likely to be related to inhibition of CYP3A4–mediated metabolism of rifabutin by indinavir. A dosage increase of indinavir and a dosage reduction of rifabutin are necessary when indinavir and rifabutin are co–administered (see section 4.2).

Ketoconazole

Co–administration of indinavir and ketoconazole could result in somewhat increased indinavir levels. This is not expected to substantially influence the safety profile of indinavir, and hence no general dose reduction is recommended.

Itraconazole

Administration of indinavir 600 mg every 8 hours with itraconazole 200 mg twice daily, an inhibitor of CYP3A4, resulted in an indinavir AUC similar to that observed during administration of indinavir 800 mg every 8 hours alone (see section 4.2).

Nevirapine

Administration of nevirapine 200 mg twice daily, an inducer of CYP3A4, with indinavir 800 mg every 8 hours resulted in a 28 % mean decrease in indinavir AUC. Indinavir had no effect on nevirapine pharmacokinetics. A dose increase of indinavir to 1,000 mg every 8 hours should be considered if given with nevirapine. Relevant safety and efficacy data are not available for this combination.

Delavirdine

Administration of delavirdine 400 mg three times daily, an inhibitor of CYP3A4, with a single 400–mg dose of indinavir resulted in indinavir AUC values 14 % less than those observed following administration of an 800–mg dose of indinavir alone. Co–administration of delavirdine and a 600–mg dose of indinavir resulted in indinavir AUC values approximately 40 % greater than those observed following administration of an 800–mg dose of indinavir alone. Indinavir had no effect on delavirdine pharmacokinetics. A dose reduction of indinavir to 400–600 mg every 8 hours should be considered if given with delavirdine. Relevant safety and efficacy data are not available for this combination.

Efavirenz

When indinavir (800 mg every 8 hours) was given with efavirenz (200 mg once daily) the indinavir AUC and C_{trough} were decreased by approximately 31 % and 40 %, respectively. When indinavir at an increased dose (1,000 mg every 8 hours) was given with efavirenz (600 mg once daily) in uninfected volunteers, the indinavir AUC and C_{trough} were decreased on average by 33-46% and 39-57%, respectively, compared to when indinavir was given alone at the standard dose (800 mg every 8 hours). Similar differences in indinavir AUC and C_{trough} were also observed in HIV-infected patients who received indinavir (1,000 mg every 8 hours) with efavirenz (600 mg once daily) compared to indinavir given alone (800 mg every 8 hours). While the clinical significance of decreased indinavir concentrations has not been established, the magnitude of the observed pharmacokinetic interaction should be taken into consideration when choosing a regimen containing both efavirenz and indinavir. No adjustment of the dose of efavirenz is necessary when given with indinavir.

HMG –CoA reductase inhibitors

HMG-CoA reductase inhibitors which are highly dependent on CYP3A4 metabolism, such as lovastatin and simvastatin, are expected to have markedly increased plasma concentrations when co-administered with indinavir. Since increased concentrations of HMG-CoA reductase inhibitors may cause myopathy, including rhabdomyolysis, the combination of these medicinal products with indinavir is not recommended. Atorvastatin is less dependent on CYP3A4 for metabolism. Clinical data on the combination of indinavir with HMG–CoA reductase inhibitors, not predominantly metabolised by CYP3A4, are not available. The metabolism of pravastatin and fluvastatin is not dependent on CYP3A4, and interactions are not expected with PIs. If treatment with an HMG-CoA reductase inhibitor is indicated, pravastatin or fluvastatin is recommended.

St. John's wort (*Hypericum perforatum*)

Plasma levels of indinavir have been shown to be substantially reduced by the concomitant use of the herbal preparation St. John's wort (*Hypericum perforatum)* to about 20 % of those when indinavir is given alone. This is due to induction of drug metabolising and/or transport proteins by St. John's wort. Herbal preparations containing St. John's wort must not be used concomitantly with CRIXIVAN. If a patient is already taking St. John's wort, stop St. John's wort, check viral levels and if possible indinavir levels. Indinavir levels may increase on stopping St. John's wort, and the dose of CRIXIVAN may need adjusting. The inducing effect may persist up to 2 weeks after cessation of treatment with St. John's wort (see section 4.3).

Pimozide

Pimozide should not be used together with indinavir. Inhibition of CYP3A4 by indinavir could result in elevated plasma concentrations of pimozide which could potentially result in QT prolongation and associated ventricular arrhythmias.

Rifampicin

Rifampicin should not be used together with indinavir. The use of rifampicin in patients receiving indinavir dramatically reduces the plasma levels of indinavir to 1/10 of that when indinavir is given alone. This effect is due to an induction of CYP3A4 by rifampicin (see section 4.3).

Ritonavir

Twice daily co–administration to volunteers of indinavir (800 mg) and ritonavir (100, 200, or 400 mg) with food for 2 weeks resulted in indinavir AUC_{24h} increases of 178 %, 266 %, and 220 %, respectively, compared to historical indinavir AUC_{24h} values in patients who received CRIXIVAN 800 mg every 8 hours alone. In addition, twice daily co–administration of indinavir (400 mg) and ritonavir (400 mg) resulted in indinavir AUC_{24h} increases of 68 %. In the same study, twice daily co–administration of indinavir (800 mg) and ritonavir (100 or 200 mg) resulted in ritonavir AUC_{24h} increases of 72 % and 96 %, respectively, versus the same doses of ritonavir alone. By contrast, twice daily co–administration of indinavir (800 mg or 400 mg) and ritonavir (400 mg) had a negligible effect (7 % and 7 % decrease, respectively) on ritonavir AUC_{24h}. Currently, there are no safety or efficacy data available on the use of this combination in patients. In cases of co-administration of ritonavir and indinavir (dosed at 800 mg twice daily), caution is warranted as the risk of nephrolithiasis can be increased. Appropriate hydration is highly recommended. If the indinavir dose is reduced due to tolerability problems, plasma drug monitoring may be valuable. There is insufficient data available to support a definitive relationship between indinavir plasma levels and efficacy and the occurrence of nephrolithiasis (see section 4.4).

Saquinavir

Co–administration of indinavir with saquinavir (600–mg hard capsules or 800–mg soft capsules or 1,200–mg soft capsules single dose) in healthy subjects resulted in a 500 %, 620 %, and 360 % increase in saquinavir plasma AUC_{24h}, respectively. Relevant safety and efficacy data are not available for this combination. The design of the study does not allow for definitive evaluation of the effect of saquinavir on indinavir, but suggests there is less than a two–fold increase in indinavir AUC_{8h} during co–administration with saquinavir.

Didanosine

A formal interaction study between indinavir and didanosine has not been performed. However, a normal (acidic) gastric pH may be necessary for optimum absorption of indinavir whereas acid rapidly degrades didanosine which is formulated with buffering agents to increase pH. Indinavir and didanosine should be administered at least one hour apart on an empty stomach (consult the manufacturer's prescribing information for didanosine). Antiretroviral activity was unaltered when didanosine was administered 3 hours after treatment with indinavir in one clinical study.

Sildenafil

Because indinavir is a CYP3A4 inhibitor, co–administration of CRIXIVAN with sildenafil is likely to result in an increase of sildenafil plasma concentrations by competitive inhibition of metabolism. In one published study of HIV–infected men chronically treated with 800 mg indinavir, administration of a single dose of 25 mg sildenafil had no significant effect on the AUC of indinavir, but resulted in a 340 % increase in sildenafil AUC compared to historical control data on sildenafil pharmacokinetics dose–normalised to 25 mg. A starting dose of 25 mg of sildenafil should be considered if indinavir and sildenafil are used concomitantly (see the manufacturer's complete prescribing information for sildenafil).

Other

Concomitant use of other medicinal products that are inducers of CYP3A4, such as phenobarbital, phenytoin, dexamethasone and carbamazepine, may reduce indinavir plasma concentrations. For information regarding diet or the effect of food on indinavir absorption (see section 4.2 and 5.2).

4.6 Pregnancy and lactation

Use during pregnancy

There are no adequate and well-controlled studies in pregnant patients. Indinavir should be used during pregnancy only if the potential benefit justifies the potential risk to the foetus. Given that substantially lower antepartum exposures have been observed in a small study of HIV-infected pregnant patients and the limited data in this patient population, indinavir use is not recommended in HIV-infected pregnant patients (see section 5.2).

Hyperbilirubinaemia, reported predominantly as elevated indirect bilirubin, has occurred in 14 % of patients during treatment with indinavir. Because it is unknown whether indinavir will exacerbate physiologic hyperbilirubinaemia in neonates, careful consideration must be given to the use of indinavir in pregnant women at the time of delivery (see section 4.8).

In Rhesus monkeys, administration of indinavir to neonates caused a mild exacerbation of the transient physiologic hyperbilirubinaemia seen in this species after birth. Administration of indinavir to pregnant Rhesus monkeys during the third trimester did not cause a similar exacerbation in neonates; however, only limited placental transfer of indinavir occurred.

Use during lactation

It is recommended that HIV–infected women do not breast–feed their infants under any circumstances in order to avoid transmission of HIV. It is not known whether indinavir is excreted in human milk. Mothers should be instructed to discontinue breast–feeding during treatment.

4.7 Effects on ability to drive and use machines

There are no data to suggest that indinavir affects the ability to drive and use machines. However, patients should be informed that dizziness and blurred vision have been reported during treatment with indinavir.

4.8 Undesirable effects

Clinical experience

In controlled clinical trials conducted world–wide, indinavir was administered alone or in combination with other antiretroviral agents (zidovudine, didanosine, stavudine, and/or lamivudine) to approximately 2,000 patients, the majority of whom were adult Caucasian males (15 % females).

Indinavir did not alter the type, frequency, or severity of known major adverse effects associated with the use of zidovudine, didanosine, or lamivudine.

Clinical adverse experiences reported by the investigators as possibly, probably, or definitely related to CRIXIVAN in $\geqslant$ 5 % of patients treated with CRIXIVAN alone or in combination (n = 309) for 24 weeks are listed below. Many of these adverse experiences were also identified as common pre–existing or frequently occurring medical conditions in this population. These adverse experiences were: nausea (35.3 %), headache (25.2 %), diarrhoea (24.6 %), asthenia/fatigue (24.3 %), rash (19.1 %), taste perversion (19.1 %), dry skin (16.2 %), abdominal pain (14.6 %), vomiting (11.0 %), dizziness (10.7 %). With the exception of dry skin, rash, and taste perversion, the incidence of clinical adverse experiences was similar or higher among patients treated with antiretroviral nucleoside analogue controls than among patients treated with CRIXIVAN alone or in combination. This overall safety profile remained similar for 107 patients treated with CRIXIVAN alone or in combination for up to 48 weeks. Adverse events, including nephrolithiasis, may lead to treatment interruption.

Very Common (> 10 %)

Nervous system disorders: headache; dizziness.

Gastrointestinal disorders: nausea; vomiting; diarrhoea; dyspepsia.

Skin and subcutaneous tissue disorders: rash; dry skin.

Renal and urinary disorders: nephrolithiasis in paediatric patients 3 years of age and older.

General disorders and administration site conditions: asthenia/fatigue; taste perversion; abdominal pain.

Common (5 – 10 %)

Nervous system disorders: insomnia; hypoaesthesia; paraesthesia.

Gastrointestinal disorders: flatulence; dry mouth; acid regurgitation.

Skin and subcutaneous tissue disorders: pruritus.

Musculoskeletal, connective tissue and bone disorders: myalgia.

Renal and urinary disorders: nephrolithiasis in adults; dysuria.

Nephrolithiasis, including flank pain with or without haematuria (including microscopic haematuria), has been reported in approximately 10 % (252/2,577) of patients receiving CRIXIVAN in clinical trials at the recommended dose compared to 2.2 % in the control arms. In general, these events were not associated with renal dysfunction and resolved with hydration and temporary interruption of therapy (e.g., 1–3 days).

In clinical trials in paediatric patients 3 years of age and older, the adverse experience profile was similar to that for adult patients except for a higher frequency of nephrolithiasis of 29 % (20/70) in paediatric patients who were treated with CRIXIVAN at the recommended dose of 500 mg/m^2 every 8 hours.

Laboratory test findings

The laboratory abnormalities reported by the investigators as possibly, probably, or definitely related to CRIXIVAN in ⩾ 10 % of patients treated with CRIXIVAN alone or in combination were:

Very Common (> 10 %)

Blood and lymphatic system disorders: increases in MCV, decreases in neutrophils.

Renal and urinary disorders: haematuria, proteinuria, crystalluria; pyuria in paediatric patients 3 years of age and older.

Hepato-biliary disorders: isolated asymptomatic hyperbilirubinaemia (total bilirubin ⩾ 2.5 mg/dl, 43 mcmol/l), reported predominantly as elevated indirect bilirubin and rarely associated with elevations in ALT, AST, or alkaline phosphatase, has occurred in approximately 14 % of patients treated with CRIXIVAN alone or in combination with other antiretroviral agents. Most patients continued treatment with CRIXIVAN without dosage reduction and bilirubin values gradually declined toward baseline. Hyperbilirubinaemia occurred more frequently at doses exceeding 2.4 g/day compared to doses less than 2.4 g/day. Increased ALT and AST.

In clinical trials with CRIXIVAN in paediatric patients 3 years of age and older, asymptomatic pyuria of unknown etiology was noted in 10.9 % (6/55) of patients who received CRIXIVAN at the recommended dose of 500 mg/m^2 every 8 hours. Some of these events were associated with mild elevation of serum creatinine.

Post–marketing experience

The following additional adverse reactions have been reported during post–marketing experience; they are derived from spontaneous reports for which incidences cannot be determined:

Blood and the lymphatic system disorders: increased spontaneous bleeding in patients with haemophilia; anemia including acute haemolytic anaemia; thrombocytopenia (see section 4.4).

Immune system disorders: anaphylactoid reactions.

Endocrine disorders: new onset diabetes mellitus or hyperglycaemia, or exacerbation of pre-existing diabetes mellitus (see section 4.4).

Nervous system disorders: oral paraesthesia.

Gastrointestinal disorders: hepatitis, including reports of hepatic failure; pancreatitis

Skin and subcutaneous tissue disorders: rash including erythema multiforme and Stevens Johnson syndrome; hypersensitivity vasculitis; alopecia, hyperpigmentation; urticaria; ingrown toenails and/or paronychia

Musculoskeletal, connective tissue and bone disorders: myalgia, myositis; rhabdomyolysis.

Renal and urinary disorders: nephrolithiasis, in some cases with renal insufficiency or acute renal failure; interstitial nephritis, sometimes associated with indinavir crystal deposits. In some patients, resolution of the interstitial nephritis did not occur following discontinuation of indinavir therapy; leucocyturia (see section 4.4).

General disorders and administration site conditions: Combination antiretroviral therapy has been associated with redistribution of body fat (lipodystrophy) in HIV patients, including the loss of peripheral and facial subcutaneous fat, increased intra-abdominal fat and visceral fat, breast hypertrophy and dorsocervical fat accumulation (buffalo hump).

Combination antiretroviral therapy has been associated with metabolic abnormalities such as hypertriglyceridaemia, hypercholesterolaemia, insulin resistance, hyperglycaemia and hyperlactataemia (see section 4.4).

In HIV-infected patients with severe immune deficiency at the time of initiation of combination antiretroviral therapy (CART), an inflammatory reaction to asymptomatic or residual opportunistic infections may arise (see section 4.4).

Laboratory test findings

The following additional laboratory abnormalities have been reported during post-marketing experience; they are derived from spontaneous reports for which precise incidences cannot be determined:

Metabolic and nutritional disorders: increased serum triglycerides, increased serum cholesterol.

Hepato-biliary disorders: liver function abnormalities.

Musculoskeletal and connective tissue and bone disorders: increased CPK.

4.9 Overdose

There have been reports of human overdose with CRIXIVAN. The most commonly reported symptoms were gastro-intestinal (e.g., nausea, vomiting, diarrhoea) and renal (e.g., nephrolithiasis, flank pain, haematuria).

It is not known whether indinavir is dialysable by peritoneal or haemodialysis.

5. PHARMACOLOGICAL PROPERTIES

5.1 Pharmacodynamic properties

Pharmacotherapeutic group: Protease inhibitor, ATC code JO5AE02

Mechanism of action

Indinavir inhibits recombinant HIV-1 and HIV-2 protease with an approximate tenfold selectivity for HIV–1 over HIV–2 proteinase. Indinavir binds reversibly to the protease active site and inhibits competitively the enzyme, thereby preventing cleavage of the viral precursor polyproteins that occurs during maturation of the newly formed viral particle. The resulting immature particles are non–infectious and are incapable of establishing new cycles of infection. Indinavir did not significantly inhibit the eukaryotic proteases human renin, human cathepsin D, human elastase, and human factor Xa.

Microbiology

Indinavir at concentrations of 50 to 100 nM mediated 95 % inhibition (IC_{95}) of viral spread (relative to an untreated virus–infected control) in human T–lymphoid cell cultures and primary human monocytes/macrophages infected with HIV–1 variants LAI, MN, RF, and a macrophage-tropic variant SF–162, respectively. Indinavir at concentrations of 25 to 100 nM mediated 95 % inhibition of viral spread in cultures of mitogen–activated human peripheral blood mononuclear cells infected with diverse, primary clinical isolates of HIV–1, including isolates resistant to zidovudine and non–nucleoside reverse transcriptase inhibitors (NNRTIs). Synergistic antiretroviral activity was observed when human T–lymphoid cells infected with the LAI variant of HIV–1 were incubated with indinavir and either zidovudine, didanosine, or NNRTIs.

Drug resistance

Loss of suppression of viral RNA levels occurred in some patients; however, CD4 cell counts were often sustained above pre–treatment levels. When loss of viral RNA suppression occurred, it was typically associated with replacement of circulating susceptible virus with resistant viral variants. Resistance was correlated with the accumulation of mutations in the viral genome that resulted in the expression of amino acid substitutions in the viral protease.

At least eleven amino acid sites in the protease have been associated with indinavir resistance: L10, K20, L24, M46, I54, L63, I64, A71, V82, I84, and L90. The basis for their contributions to resistance, however, is complex. None of these substitutions was either necessary or sufficient for resistance. For example, no single substitution or pair of substitutions was capable of engendering measurable (⩾ four–fold) resistance to indinavir, and the level of resistance was dependent on the ways in which multiple substitutions were combined. In general, however, higher levels of resistance resulted from the co–expression of greater numbers of substitutions at the eleven identified positions. Among patients experiencing viral RNA rebound during indinavir monotherapy at 800 mg q8h, substitutions at only three of these sites were observed in the majority of patients: V82 (to A or F), M46 (to I or L), and L10 (to I or R). Other substitutions were observed less frequently. The observed amino acid substitutions appeared to accumulate sequentially and in no consistent order, probably as a result of ongoing viral replication.

It should be noted that the decrease in suppression of viral RNA levels was seen more frequently when therapy with indinavir was initiated at doses lower than the recommended oral dose of 2.4 g/day. **Therefore, therapy with indinavir should be initiated at the recommended dose to increase suppression of viral replication and therefore inhibit the emergence of resistant virus.**

The concomitant use of indinavir with nucleoside analogues (to which the patient is naive) may lessen the risk of the development of resistance to both indinavir and the nucleoside analogues. In one comparative trial, combination therapy with nucleoside analogues (triple therapy with zidovudine plus didanosine) conferred protection against the selection of virus expressing at least one resistance–associated amino acid substitution to both indinavir (from 13/24 to 2/20 at therapy week 24) and to the nucleoside analogues (from 10/16 to 0/20 at therapy week 24).

Cross resistance

HIV–1 patient isolates with reduced susceptibility to indinavir expressed varying patterns and degrees of cross–resistance to a series of diverse HIV PIs, including ritonavir and saquinavir. Complete cross–resistance was noted between indinavir and ritonavir; however, cross–resistance to saquinavir varied among isolates. Many of the protease amino acid substitutions reported to be associated with resistance to ritonavir and saquinavir were also associated with resistance to indinavir.

Pharmacodynamic effects

Adults

Treatment with indinavir alone or in combination with other antiretroviral agents (i.e., nucleoside analogues) has so far been documented to reduce viral load and increase CD4 lymphocytes in patients with CD4 cell counts below 500 cells/mm^3.

Indinavir alone or in combination with nucleoside analogues (zidovudine/stavudine and lamivudine) has been shown to delay clinical progression rate compared with nucleoside analogues and to provide a sustained effect on viral load and CD4 count.

In zidovudine experienced patients, indinavir, zidovudine and lamivudine in combination compared with lamivudine added to zidovudine reduced the probability of AIDS defining illness or death (ADID) at 48 weeks from 13 % to 7 %. Similarly, in antiretroviral naive patients, indinavir with and without zidovudine compared with zidovudine alone reduced the probability of ADID at 48 weeks from 15 % with zidovudine alone to approximately 6 % with indinavir alone or in combination with zidovudine.

Effects on viral load were consistently more pronounced in patients treated with indinavir in combination with nucleoside analogues, but the proportion of patients with serum viral RNA below the limit of quantification (500 copies/ml) varied between studies, at week 24 from 40 % to more than 80 %. This proportion tends to remain stable over prolonged periods of follow–up. Similarly, effects on CD4 cell count tend to be more pronounced in patients treated with indinavir in combination with nucleoside analogues compared with indinavir alone. Within studies, this effect is sustained also after prolonged periods of follow–up.

Paediatric patients

Two ongoing clinical trials in 41 paediatric patients (4 to 15 years of age) were designed to characterise the safety, antiretroviral activity, and pharmacokinetics of indinavir in combination with stavudine and lamivudine. In one study, at week 24, the proportion of patients with plasma viral RNA below 400 copies/ml was 60 %; the mean increase in CD4 cell counts was 242 cells/mm^3; and the mean increase in percent CD4 cell counts was 4.2 %. At week 60, the proportion of patients with plasma viral RNA below 400 copies/ml was 59 %. In another study, at week 16, the proportion of patients with plasma viral RNA below 400 copies/ml was 59 %; the mean increase in CD4 cell counts was 73 cells/mm^3; and the mean increase in percent CD4 cell counts was 1.2 %. At week 24, the proportion of patients with plasma viral RNA below 400 copies/ml was 60 %.

5.2 Pharmacokinetic properties

Absorption

Indinavir is rapidly absorbed in the fasted state with a time to peak plasma concentration of 0.8 hours ± 0.3 hours (mean ± S.D.). A greater than dose–proportional increase in indinavir plasma concentrations was observed over the 200 – 800 mg dose range. Between 800–mg and 1,000–mg dose levels, the deviation from dose–proportionality is less pronounced. As a result of the short half–life, 1.8 ± 0.4 hours, only a minimal increase in plasma concentrations occurred after multiple dosing. The bioavailability of a single 800–mg dose of indinavir was approximately 65 % (90 % CI, 58 – 72 %).

Data from a steady state study in healthy volunteers indicate that there is a diurnal variation in the pharmacokinetics of indinavir. Following a dosage regimen of 800 mg every 8 hours, measured peak plasma concentrations (C_{max}) after morning, afternoon and evening doses were 15,550 nM, 8,720 nM and 8,880 nM, respectively. Corresponding plasma concentrations at 8 hours post dose were 220 nM, 210 nM and 370 nM, respectively. The relevance of these findings for ritonavir boosted indinavir is unknown. At steady state following a dosage regimen of 800 mg every 8 hours, HIV–seropositive adult patients in one study achieved geometric means of: AUC_{0-8h} of 27813 nM*h (90% confidence interval = 22185, 34869), peak plasma concentrations 11144 nM (90% confidence interval = 9192, 13512) and plasma concentrations at 8 hours post dose 211 nM (90% confidence interval = 163, 274).

At steady state following a dosage regimen of 800 mg/100 mg of indinavir/ritonavir every 12 hours with a low-fat meal, healthy volunteers in one study achieved geometric means: AUC_{0-12h} 116067 nM*h (90% confidence interval = 101680, 132490), peak plasma concentrations 19001 nM (90% confidence interval = 17538, 20588), and plasma concentrations at 12 hours post dose 2274 nM (90% confidence interval = 1701, 3042). No significant difference in exposure was seen when the regimen was given with a high-fat meal.

In HIV–infected paediatric patients, a dosage regimen of indinavir hard capsules, 500 mg/m^2 every 8 hours, produced AUC_{0-8hr} values of 27,412 nM ˙h, peak plasma concentrations of 12,182 nM, and plasma concentrations at 8 hours post dose of 122 nM. The AUC and peak plasma concentrations were generally similar to those previously observed in HIV–infected adults receiving the recommended dose of 800 mg every 8 hours; it should be observed that the plasma concentrations 8 hours post dose were lower.

During pregnancy, it has been demonstrated that the systemic exposure of indinavir is relevantly decreased (PACTG 358. Crixivan, 800 mg every 8 hours + zidovudine 200 mg every 8 hours and lamivudine 150 mg twice a day). The mean indinavir plasma AUC_{0-8hr} at week 30-32 of gestation (n=11) was 9231 nM*hr, which is 74% (95% CI: 50%, 86%) lower than that observed 6 weeks postpartum. Six of these 11 (55%) patients had mean indinavir plasma concentrations 8 hours post-dose (C_{min}) below assay threshold of reliable quantification. The pharmacokinetics of indinavir in these 11 patients at 6 weeks postpartum were generally similar to those observed in non-pregnant patients in another study (see section 4.6).

Administration of indinavir with a meal high in calories, fat, and protein resulted in a blunted and reduced absorption with an approximate 80 % reduction in AUC and an 86 % reduction in C_{max}. Administration with light meals (e.g., dry toast with jam or fruit conserve, apple juice, and coffee with skimmed or fat–free milk and sugar or corn flakes, skimmed or fat–free milk and sugar) resulted in plasma concentrations comparable to the corresponding fasted values.

The pharmacokinetics of indinavir taken as indinavir sulphate salt (from opened hard capsules) mixed in apple sauce were generally comparable to the pharmacokinetics of indinavir taken as hard capsules, under fasting conditions. In HIV–infected paediatric patients, the pharmacokinetic parameters of indinavir in apple sauce were: AUC_{0-8hr} of 26,980 nM ˙h peak plasma concentration of 13,711 nM; and plasma concentration at 8 hours post dose of 146 nM.

Distribution

Indinavir was not highly bound to human plasma proteins (39 % unbound).

There are no data concerning the penetration of indinavir into the central nervous system in humans.

Biotransformation

Seven major metabolites were identified and the metabolic pathways were identified as glucuronidation at the pyridine nitrogen, pyridine–N–oxidation with and without 3'–hydroxylation on the indane ring, 3'–hydroxylation of indane, p–hydroxylation of phenylmethyl moiety, and N–depyridomethylation with and without the 3'–hydroxylation. *In vitro* studies with human liver microsomes indicated that CYP3A4 is the only P450 isozyme that plays a major role in the oxidative metabolism of indinavir. Analysis of plasma and urine samples from subjects who received indinavir indicated that indinavir metabolites had little proteinase inhibitory activity.

Elimination

Over the 200–1,000–mg dose range administered in both volunteers and HIV infected patients, there was a slightly greater than dose–proportional increase in urinary recovery of indinavir. Renal clearance (116 ml/min) of indinavir is concentration–independent over the clinical dose range. Less than 20 % of indinavir is excreted renally. Mean urinary excretion of unchanged drug following single dose administration in the fasted state was 10.4 % following a 700–mg dose, and 12.0 % following a 1,000–mg dose. Indinavir was rapidly eliminated with a half–life of 1.8 hours.

Characteristics in patients

Pharmacokinetics of indinavir do not appear to be affected by race.

There are no clinically significant differences in the pharmacokinetics of indinavir in HIV seropositive women compared to HIV seropositive men.

Patients with mild–to–moderate hepatic insufficiency and clinical evidence of cirrhosis had evidence of decreased metabolism of indinavir resulting in approximately 60 % higher mean AUC following a

400–mg dose. The mean half–life of indinavir increased to approximately 2.8 hours.

5.3 Preclinical safety data

Crystals have been seen in the urine of rats, one monkey, and one dog. The crystals have not been associated with drug–induced renal injury. An increase in thyroidal weight and thyroidal follicular cell hyperplasia, due to an increase in thyroxine clearance, was seen in rats treated with indinavir at doses ⩾ 160 mg/kg/day. An increase in hepatic weight occurred in rats treated with indinavir at doses ⩾ 40 mg/kg/day and was accompanied by hepatocellular hypertrophy at doses ⩾ 320 mg/kg/day.

The maximum non–lethal oral dose of indinavir was at least 5,000 mg/kg in rats and mice, the highest dose tested in acute toxicity studies.

Studies in rats indicated that uptake into brain tissue was limited, distribution into and out of the lymphatic system was rapid, and excretion into the milk of lactating rats was extensive. Distribution of indinavir across the placental barrier was significant in rats, but limited in rabbits.

Mutagenicity

Indinavir did not have any mutagenic or genotoxic activity in studies with or without metabolic activation.

Carcinogenicity

No carcinogenicity was noted in mice at the maximum tolerated dose, which corresponded to a systemic exposure approximately 2 to 3 times higher than the clinical exposure. In rats, at similar exposure levels, an increased incidence of thyroid adenomas was seen, probably related to an increase in release of thyroid stimulating hormone secondary to an increase in thyroxine clearance. The relevance of the findings to humans is likely limited.

Developmental Toxicity

Developmental toxicity studies were performed in rats, rabbits and dogs (at doses which produced systemic exposures comparable to or slightly greater than human exposure) and revealed no evidence of teratogenicity. No external or visceral changes were observed in rats, however, increases in the incidence of supernumerary ribs and of cervical ribs were seen. No external, visceral, or skeletal changes were observed in rabbits or dogs. In rats and rabbits, no effects on embryonic/foetal survival or foetal weights were observed. In dogs, a slight increase in resorptions was seen; however, all foetuses in medication–treated animals were viable, and the incidence of live foetuses in medication–treated animals was comparable to that in controls.

6. PHARMACEUTICAL PARTICULARS

6.1 List of excipients

- Capsule content

- anhydrous lactose

- magnesium stearate

- Capsule shell:

- gelatin

- titanium dioxide

- silicon dioxide

- sodium lauryl sulphate

CRIXIVAN 200 mg also contains printing ink: titanium dioxide (E 171), and indigo carmine (E 132).

CRIXIVAN 400 mg also contains printing ink: titanium dioxide (E 171), indigo carmine (E 132) and iron oxide (E172).

6.2 Incompatibilities

Not applicable.

6.3 Shelf life

CRIXIVAN 200 mg - 3 years

CRIXIVAN 400 mg – 2 years for HDPE bottles containing 18 hard capsules

3 years for HDPE bottles containing 90 and 180 hard capsules

6.4 Special precautions for storage

Store in the original container. Keep the container tightly closed in order to protect from moisture.

6.5 Nature and contents of container

CRIXIVAN 200 mg hard capsules are supplied in HDPE bottles with a polypropylene cap and a foil induction cap containing 180, 270 or 360 capsules.

CRIXIVAN 400 mg hard capsules are supplied in HDPE bottles with a polypropylene cap and a foil induction cap containing 18, 90 or 180 capsules.

Not all pack sizes may be marketed.

6.6 Instructions for use and handling

The bottles contain desiccant canisters that should remain in the container.

7. MARKETING AUTHORISATION HOLDER

Merck Sharp & Dohme Limited

Hertford Road, Hoddesdon

Hertfordshire EN11 9BU

United Kingdom

8. MARKETING AUTHORISATION NUMBER(S)

CRIXIVAN 200 mg

EU/1/96/024/001

EU/1/96/024/002

EU/1/96/024/003

CRIXIVAN 400 mg

EU/1/96/024/004

EU/1/96/024/005

EU/1/96/024/008

9. DATE OF FIRST AUTHORISATION/RENEWAL OF THE AUTHORISATION

21 November 2001

10. DATE OF REVISION OF THE TEXT

January 2005.

SPC.CRX.05.UK/IRL.2146 (II/66)

Crystapen Injection

(Britannia Pharmaceuticals Limited)

1. NAME OF THE MEDICINAL PRODUCT

Crystapen Injection

2. QUALITATIVE AND QUANTITATIVE COMPOSITION

Benzylpenicillin sodium BP available as 600 mg and 1200 mg vials.

3. PHARMACEUTICAL FORM

White crystalline, water-soluble sterile powder for injection.

4. CLINICAL PARTICULARS

4.1 Therapeutic indications

Crystapen is indicated for most wound infections, pyogenic infections of the skin, soft tissue infections and infections of the nose, throat, nasal sinuses, respiratory tract and middle ear, etc.

It is also indicated for the following infections caused by penicillin-sensitive microorganisms: Generalised infections, septicaemia and pyaemia from susceptible bacteria. Acute and chronic osteomyelitis, sub-acute bacterial endocarditis and meningitis caused by susceptible organisms. Suspected meningococcal disease. Gas gangrene, tetanus, actinomycosis, anthrax, leptospirosis, rat-bite fever, listeriosis, severe Lyme disease, and prevention of neonatal group B streptococcal infections. Complications secondary to gonorrhoea and syphilis (e.g. gonococcal arthritis or endocarditis, congenital syphilis and neurosyphilis). Diphtheria, brain abscesses and pasteurellosis.

Consideration should be given to official local guidance (e.g. national recommendations) on the appropriate use of antibacterial agents.

Susceptibility of the causative organism to the treatment should be tested (if possible), although therapy may be initiated before the results are available.

4.2 Posology and method of administration

Route of administration:

Intramuscular, intravenous.

Preparation of solutions:

Pharmaceutical preparation

Only freshly prepared solutions should be used. Reconstituted solutions of benzylpenicillin sodium BP are intended for immediate administration.

600 mg vial

Intramuscular injection: 600 mg (1 mega unit) is usually dissolved in 1.6 to 2.0 ml of Water for Injections BP.

600 mg and 1200 mg vials

Intravenous Injection: A suitable concentration is 600 mg (1 mega unit) dissolved in 4 to 10 ml of Water for Injections BP or Sodium Chloride Injection BP and 1200 mg (2 mega units) dissolved in at least 8 ml of Sodium Chloride Injection BP or Water for Injections BP.

Intravenous Infusion: It is recommended that 600 mg (1 mega unit) should be dissolved in at least 10 ml of Sodium Chloride Injection BP or Water for Injections BP and 1200 mg (2 mega units) should be dissolved in at least 20 ml of Sodium Chloride Injection BP or Water for Injections BP.

Sodium overload and/or heart failure may occur if benzylpenicillin sodium BP is administered in sodium-containing solvents to patients who suffer from renal failure and/or heart failure. Therefore, for such patients, benzylpenicillin sodium BP should not be reconstituted in sodium-containing liquids such as Sodium Chloride Injection BP or Ringer's solution.

Dosage and administration:

The following dosages apply to both intramuscular and intravenous injection.

Alternate sites should be used for repeated injections.

Adults

600 to 3,600 mg (1 to 6 mega units) daily, divided into 4 to 6 doses, depending on the indication. Higher doses (up to 14.4 g/day (24 mega units) in divided doses) may be given in serious infections such as adult meningitis by the intravenous route.

In bacterial endocarditis, 7.2 to 12 g (12 to 20 mega units) or more may be given daily in divided doses by the intravenous route, often by infusion.

Doses up to 43.2 g (72 mega units) per day may be necessary for patients with rapidly spreading gas gangrene.

High doses should be administered by intravenous injection or infusion, with intravenous doses in excess of 1.2g (2 mega units) being given slowly, taking at least one minute for each 300 mg (0.5 mega unit) to avoid high levels causing irritation of the central nervous system and/or electrolyte imbalance.

High dosage of benzylpenicillin sodium BP may result in hypernatraemia and hypokalaemia unless the sodium content is taken into account.

For the prevention of Group B Streptococcal disease of the newborn, a 3 g (5 mega units) loading dose should be given to the mother initially, followed by 1.5 g (2.5 mega units) every 4 hours until delivery.

Children aged 1 month to 12 years

100 mg/kg/day in 4 divided doses; not exceeding 4 g/day.

Infants 1-4 weeks

75 mg/kg/day in 3 divided doses.

Newborn Infants

50 mg/kg/day in 2 divided doses.

Meningococcal disease

Children 1 month to 12 years: 180-300 mg/kg/day in 4-6 divided doses,

not exceeding 12 g/day.

Infants 1-4 weeks: 150 mg/kg/day in 3 divided doses.

Newborn infants: 100 mg/kg/day in 2 divided doses.

Adults and children over 12 years: 2.4 g every 4 hours

Suspected meningococcal disease

If meningococcal disease is suspected general practitioners should give a single dose of benzylpenicillin sodium BP, before transferring the patient to hospital, as follows:

Adults and children over 10 years: 1,200 mg IV (or IM)

Children 1-9 years: 600 mg IV (or IM)

Children under 1 year: 300 mg IV (or IM)

Premature babies and neonates

Dosing should not be more frequent than every 8 or 12 hours in this age group, since renal clearance is reduced at this age and the mean half-life of benzylpenicillin may be as long as 3 hours.

Since infants have been found to develop severe local reactions to intramuscular injections, intravenous treatment should preferably be used.

Patients with renal insufficiency

For doses of 0.6-1.2 g (1-2 mega units) the dosing interval should be no more frequent than every 8-10 hours.

For high doses e.g. 14.4 g (24 mega units) required for the treatment of serious infections such as meningitis, the dosage and dose interval of benzylpenicillin sodium BP should be adjusted in accordance with the following schedule:

(see Table 1 below)

The dose in the above table should be further reduced to 300 mg (0.5 mega units) 8 hourly if advanced liver disease is associated with severe renal failure.

If haemodialysis is required, an additional dose of 300 mg (0.5 mega units) should be given 6 hourly during the procedure.

Elderly Patients

Elimination may be delayed in elderly patients and dose reduction may be necessary.

4.3 Contraindications

Allergy to penicillins. Hypersensitivity to any ingredient of the preparation.

Cross allergy to other beta-lactams such as cephalosporins should be taken into account.

4.4 Special warnings and special precautions for use

600 mg benzylpenicillin contains 1.68 mmol of sodium. Massive doses of Benzylpenicillin Sodium BP can cause hypokalaemia and sometimes hypernatraemia. Use of a potassium-sparing diuretic may be helpful. In patients undergoing high-dose treatment for more than 5 days, electrolyte balance, blood counts and renal functions should be monitored.

In the presence of impaired renal function, large doses of penicillin can cause cerebral irritation, convulsions and coma.

Skin sensitisation may occur in persons handling the antibiotic and care should be taken to avoid contact with the substance.

It should be recognised that any patient with a history of allergy, especially to drugs, is more likely to develop a hypersensitivity reaction to penicillin. Patients should be observed for 30 minutes after administration and if an allergic reaction occurs the drug should be withdrawn and appropriate treatment given.

Table 2

Organism	S ⩽ (mg/L)	I (mg/L)	R ⩾ (mg/L)
Streptococcus pneumoniae Neisseria gonorrhoeae	0.06	0.12-1.0	2.0
Neisseria meningitides	0.06		0.12
Haemolytic streptococci Staphylococci Moraxella catarrhalis Haemophilus influenzae	0.12		0.25
Rapidly growing anaerobes	1.0		2.0

S = Susceptible, I = Intermediate susceptibility, R = Resistant

Delayed absorption from the intramuscular depot may occur in diabetics.

Prolonged use of benzylpenicillin may occasionally result in an overgrowth of non-susceptible organisms or yeast and patients should be observed carefully for superinfections.

Pseudomembranous colitis should be considered in patients who develop severe and persistent diarrhoea during or after receiving benzylpenicillin. In this situation, even if Clostridium difficile is only suspected, administration of benzylpenicillin should be discontinued and appropriate treatment given.

4.5 Interaction with other medicinal products and other forms of Interaction

The efficacy of oral contraceptives may be impaired under concomitant administration of benzylpenicillin sodium BP, which may result in unwanted pregnancy. Women taking oral contraceptives should be aware of this and should be informed about alternative methods of contraception.

There is reduced excretion of methotrexate (and therefore increased risk of methotrexate toxicity) when used with benzylpenicillin sodium BP.

Probenecid inhibits tubular secretion of benzylpenicillin sodium BP and so may be given to increase the plasma concentrations.

4.6 Pregnancy and lactation

Benzylpenicillin sodium BP has been taken by a large number of pregnant women and women of childbearing age without an increase in malformations or other direct or indirect harmful effects on the foetus having been observed.

Although it is not known if benzylpenicillin sodium BP may be excreted into the breast milk of nursing mothers, it is actively transported from the blood to milk in animals and trace amounts of other penicillins in human milk have been detected.

4.7 Effects on ability to drive and use machines

None

4.8 Undesirable effects

Blood and Lymphatic System Disorders

Rare (0.01% - 0.1%)

Haemolytic anaemia and granulocytopenia (neutropenia), agranulocytosis, leucopenia and thrombocytopenia, have been reported in patients receiving prolonged high doses of benzylpenicillin sodium BP (eg. Subacute bacterial endocarditis).

Immune System Disorders

Very Common >10%)

Patients undergoing treatment for syphilis or neurosyphilis with benzylpenicillin may develop a Jarisch-Herxheimer reaction.

Common (1-10%)

Hypersensitivity to penicillin in the form of rashes (all types), fever, and serum sickness may occur (1-10% treated patients). These may be treated with antihistamine drugs.

Rare (0.01%-0.1%)

More rarely, anaphylactic reactions have been reported (<0.05% treated patients).

Nervous System Disorders

Rare (0.01%-0.1%)

Central nervous system toxicity, including convulsions, has been reported with massive doses over 60 g per day and in patients with severe renal impairment.

Renal and Urinary Disorders

Rare (0.01%-0.1%)

Interstitial nephritis has been reported after intravenous benzylpenicillin sodium BP at doses of more than 12 g per day.

4.9 Overdose

Excessive blood levels of benzylpenicillin sodium BP can be corrected by haemodialysis.

5. PHARMACOLOGICAL PROPERTIES

5.1 Pharmacodynamic properties

Pharmacotherapeutic group: Beta-lactamase sensitive penicillins.

ATC code: J01 CE01.

General Properties:

Benzylpenicillin sodium BP is a beta-lactam antibiotic. It is bacteriocidal by inhibiting bacterial cell wall biosynthesis.

Breakpoints:

The tentative breakpoints (British Society for Antimicrobial Chemotherapy, BSAC) for benzylpenicillin sodium BP are as follows:

(see Table 2 above)

Susceptibility:

The prevalence of resistance may vary geographically and with time for selected species and local information on resistance is desirable, particularly when treating severe infections. The following table gives only approximate guidance on probabilities whether microorganisms will be susceptible to benzylpenicillin sodium BP or not.

Susceptible and intermediately susceptible microorganisms		
Type of Microorganism	Microorganism	Range of acquired resistance
Aerobic Gram-positive microorganisms	• Bacillus anthracis	0%**
	• Corynebacterium diphtheriae	0%*
	• Haemolytic streptococci (including Streptococcus pyogenes)	0%*-3%**
	• Listeria monocytogenes	0%**
	• Streptococcus pneumoniae	4%*-40%**
	• Streptococcus viridans	3-32%*
Aerobic Gram-negative microorganisms	• Neisseria gonorrhoeae	9-10%*
	• Neisseria meningitidis	18%*
	• Pasteurella multocida	0%***
Anaerobic microorganisms	• Actinomyces israelii	8%**

Table 1

Creatinine clearance (ml per minute)	Dose (g)	Dose (mega units)	Dosing interval (hours)
125	1.2 or 1.8	2 or 3	2 3
60	1.2	2	4
40	0.9	1.5	4
20	0.6	1.0	4
10	0.6	1.0	6
Nil	0.3 or 0.6	0.5 or 1.0	6 8

	• Fusobacterium nucleatum and Fusobacterium necrophorum	Usually sensitive
	• Gram-positive sporing bacilli (including Clostridium tetani and Clostridium perfringens (welchii))	14%**
	• Gram-positive cocci (including peptostreptococcus)	7%*
Other microorganisms	• Borrelia bugdorferi	Usually sensitive
	• Capnocytophaga canimorosus	Usually sensitive
	• Leptospirae	Usually sensitive
	• Streptobacillus moniliformis and spirillum minus	Usually sensitive
	• Treponema pallidum	0%***

* UK data; ** European data, ***Global data

Insusceptible microorganisms		
Type of Microorganism	Microorganism	Range of acquired resistance
Aerobic Gram-positive microorganisms	• Coagulase negative Staphylococcus	71-81%*
	• Enterococcus Spp	Resistant
	• Staphylococcus aureus	79-87%*
Aerobic Gram-negative microorganisms	• Acinetobacter	Resistant
	• Bordetella pertussis	Generally resistant
	• Brucella spp.	Resistant
	• Enterobacteriaceae (including Escherichia coli, Salmonella, Shigella, Enterobacter, Klebsiella, Proteus, Citrobacter).	Generally resistant
	• Haemophilus influenzae	Resistant
	• Pseudomonas	Resistant
Anaerobic microorganisms	• Bacteroides fragilis	100%***

* UK data; ** European data, *** Global data

Other Information:

Known Resistance Mechanisms and Cross-resistance

Penicillin resistance can be mediated by alteration of penicillin binding proteins or development of beta-lactamases.

Resistance to penicillin may be associated with cross-resistance to a variety of other beta lactam antibiotics either due to a shared target site that is altered, or due to a beta-lactamase with a broad range of substrate molecules. In addition to this, cross resistance to unrelated antibiotics can develop due to more than one resistance gene being present on a mobile section of DNA (e.g. plasmid, transposon etc) resulting in two or more resistance mechanisms being transferred to a new organism at the same time.

5.2 Pharmacokinetic properties

Benzylpenicillin sodium BP rapidly appears in the blood following intramuscular injection of water-soluble salts and maximum concentrations are usually reached in 15-30 minutes. Peak plasma concentrations of about 12 mcg/ml have been reported after doses of 600 mg with therapeutic plasma concentrations for most susceptible organisms detectable for about 5 hours. Approximately 60% of the dose injected is reversibly bound to plasma protein.

In adults with normal renal function the plasma half-life is about 30 minutes. Most of the dose (60-90%) undergoes renal elimination, 10% by glomerular filtration and 90% by tubular secretion. Tubular secretion is inhibited by probenecid, which is sometimes given to increase plasma penicillin concentrations. Biliary elimination of benzylpenicillin sodium BP accounts for only a minor fraction of the dose.

5.3 Preclinical safety data

There are no pre-clinical data of relevance to the prescriber which are additional to that already included in other sections of the SmPC.

6. PHARMACEUTICAL PARTICULARS

6.1 List of excipients

None

6.2 Incompatibilities

Benzylpenicillin sodium BP and solutions that contain metal ions should be administered separately.

Benzylpenicillin sodium should not be administered in the same syringe / giving set as amphotericin B, cimetidine, cytarabine, flucloxacillin, hydroxyzine, methylprednisolone, or promethazine since it is incompatible with these drugs.

6.3 Shelf life

Unopened 36 months.

Reconstituted product should be used immediately.

6.4 Special precautions for storage

Store below 25°C.

6.5 Nature and contents of container

Tubular type III glass vials sealed with bromobutyl rubber plugs with aluminium overseals or plastic 'flip-top' caps. This product is supplied in vials containing 600 mg and 1.2 g of powder in boxes containing 25 vials and "GP pack" containing 2 vials of 600 mg.

6.6 Instructions for use and handling

After contact with skin, wash immediately with water. In case of contact with eyes, rinse immediately with plenty of water and seek medical advice if discomfort persists.

7. MARKETING AUTHORISATION HOLDER

Britannia Pharmaceuticals Limited

41 Brighton Road

Redhill

Surrey

RH1 6YS

8. MARKETING AUTHORISATION NUMBER(S)

PL 04483/0039

PA 356/8/1

9. DATE OF FIRST AUTHORISATION/RENEWAL OF THE AUTHORISATION

10th March 2003

10. DATE OF REVISION OF THE TEXT

17th June 2004

Cuprofen for Children

(SSL International plc)

1. NAME OF THE MEDICINAL PRODUCT

Cuprofen For Children

2. QUALITATIVE AND QUANTITATIVE COMPOSITION

Ibuprofen 100mg / 5ml

For excipients see 6.1

3. PHARMACEUTICAL FORM

Oral Suspension

A white, opaque smooth suspension

4. CLINICAL PARTICULARS

4.1 Therapeutic indications

For reduction in fever (including post immunization fever) and relief of mild to moderate pain such as headache, sore throat, earache, teething pain and toothache, cold and flu symptoms, minor aches and sprains.

4.2 Posology and method of administration

Children 8 to 12 years: 10ml three to four times daily.

Children 3 to 7 years: 5ml three to four times daily.

Children 1 to 2 years: 2.5ml three to four times daily.

Infants 6 months to 1 year: 2.5ml three times daily.

Not recommended for children under 6 months of age.

For post immunization fever: 2.5ml followed by one further 2.5ml 6 hours later, if necessary. No more than 2 doses in 24 hours. If fever is not reduced, consult your doctor.

4.3 Contraindications

Patients with a known hypersensitivity to Ibuprofen, Aspirin or any of the products constituents.

Patients with a history of bronchospasm, rhinitis or urticaria particularly associated with therapy with aspirin or other anti-inflammatory drugs.

Patients with active peptic ulceration or a history of peptic ulceration.

Children under 6 months.

4.4 Special warnings and special precautions for use

Should be used with care in patients with renal, hepatic or cardiac impairment as the use of non-steroidal anti-inflammatory drugs may result in the deterioration of renal function. The dose should be kept as low as possible and renal function should be monitored.

For short term use only.

In patients suffering from or with a previous history of bronchial asthma or allergic disease, bronchospasm may be precipitated.

Undesirable effects may be minimised by using the minimum effective dose for the shortest possible duration.

The elderly are at increased risk of the serious consequence of adverse reactions.

The label will state:

Do not use if your child has ever had a stomach ulcer or is allergic to ibuprofen or aspirin. If your child is allergic to or is taking any other painkiller or suffers from asthma speak to your doctor before taking ibuprofen. Pregnant women should only take this product on the advice of a doctor. Do not exceed the stated dose. Keep out of the reach of children. If symptoms persist, consult your doctor.

4.5 Interaction with other medicinal products and other forms of Interaction

Concurrent aspirin or other NSAIDs may result in an increased incidence of adverse reactions. May enhance the effects of anti-coagulants. NSAIDs may diminish the effect of anti-hypertensives or diuretics.

Lithium concentrations are increased by Ibuprofen.

4.6 Pregnancy and lactation

Whilst no teratogenic effects have been demonstrated in animal studies, the use of Ibuprofen is best avoided during pregnancy. The onset of labour may be delayed and the duration of labour increased. Ibuprofen has been found in breast milk in very low concentrations and is unlikely to adversely effect for breast fed infant.

4.7 Effects on ability to drive and use machines

None, although not applicable in children under 12 years.

4.8 Undesirable effects

Hypersensitivity reactions have been reported following treatment with ibuprofen. These may consist of

a) non-specific allergic reaction and anaphylaxis,

b) respiratory tract reactivity comprising of asthma, aggravated asthma, bronchospasm or dyspnoea, or

c) associated skin disorders, including skin rashes of various types, pruritis, urticaria, purpura, angiodema and, less commonly, bullous dermatoses (including epidermal necrolysis and erythema multiforme).

Gastrointestinal: abdominal pain, nausea and dyspepsia. Occasionally peptic ulcer and gastrointestinal haemorrhage.

Haematological: thrombocytopenia.

Others: rarely hepatic dysfunction, headache, dizziness, hearing disturbance.

NSAID's have been reported to cause nephrotoxicity in various forms and their use can lead to interstitial nephritis, nephrotic syndrome and renal failure.

4.9 Overdose

Symptoms include headache, vomiting, drowsiness and hypotension.

There is no specific antidote to Ibuprofen. Treatment should consist of gastric lavage and if necessary, correction of serum electrolytes.

5. PHARMACOLOGICAL PROPERTIES

5.1 Pharmacodynamic properties

Ibuprofen has analgesic, anti-inflammatory and antipyretic properties. It is an inhibitor of prostaglandin synthesis.

5.2 Pharmacokinetic properties

Ibuprofen is absorbed from the gastro-intestinal tract and peak plasma concentrations occur about 1-2 hours after ingestion. It is extensively bound to plasma proteins and has a half life of about 2 hours.

Ibuprofen is rapidly excreted in the urine mainly as metabolites and their conjugates. About 1% is excreted in urine as unchanged Ibuprofen, and about 14% as conjugated Ibuprofen.

In limited studies, ibuprofen appears in the breast milk in very low concentrations.

5.3 Preclinical safety data

No relevant information additional to that contained elsewhere in the SPC.

6. PHARMACEUTICAL PARTICULARS

6.1 List of excipients

Sodium Methyl Parahydroxybenzoate; Sodium Propyl Parahydroxybenzoate; Citric Acid Anhydrous; Saccharin Sodium; Sodium Benzoate; Dispersible Cellulose; Orange Juicy Flavour; Polysorbate 80; Maltitol Liquid; Xanthan Gum; Purified Water.

6.2 Incompatibilities

None.

6.3 Shelf life
2 years.

6.4 Special precautions for storage
Do not store above 25°C. Keep container in the outer carton.

6.5 Nature and contents of container
Amber glass or PET bottles with polypropylene child resistant cap, containing 100 or 150ml enclosed in an outer carton. A measuring spoon is provided.

6.6 Instructions for use and handling
Not applicable.

7. MARKETING AUTHORISATION HOLDER
Galpharm Healthcare Limited

Hugh House

Upper Cliffe Road

Dodworth Business Park

Dodworth

Barnsley

South Yorkshire

S75 3SP

8. MARKETING AUTHORISATION NUMBER(S)
PL 16028/0075

9. DATE OF FIRST AUTHORISATION/RENEWAL OF THE AUTHORISATION
15 May 2003

10. DATE OF REVISION OF THE TEXT
October 2003

Cuprofen Gel

(SSL International plc)

1. NAME OF THE MEDICINAL PRODUCT
Cuprofen Gel

2. QUALITATIVE AND QUANTITATIVE COMPOSITION
Ibuprofen BP 5% w/w.

3. PHARMACEUTICAL FORM
Gel containing 5.0%w/w ibuprofen.

4. CLINICAL PARTICULARS

4.1 Therapeutic indications
Symptomatic relief of: rheumatic pain; pain due to non-serious arthritic conditions; and muscular aches, pains and swellings such as strains, sprains and sports injuries.

4.2 Posology and method of administration
Route of administration: Cutaneous. Adults, including the elderly, and children over 12 years: The recommended dose of ibuprofen is 50-125 mg 3-4 times daily. 2.5-6.25 cm of gel is equivalent to about 50-125 mg of ibuprofen. Apply the gel to affected area 3-4 times daily. Approximately 2.5-6.25 cm (1-2.5 inches) of gel should be expressed from the tube and rubbed gently onto the skin. Do not give to children under 12 years of age except on the advice of a doctor. The dose should not be repeated more frequently than every 4 hours and no more than 4 times in any 24-hour period.

4.3 Contraindications
Hypersensitivity to ibuprofen or to any of the other constituents. Hypersensitivity to aspirin or other non-steroidal anti-inflammatory drugs including patients predisposed to asthma, rhinitis or urticaria.

4.4 Special warnings and special precautions for use
Apply with gentle massage, avoid contact with the eyes, mucous membranes and inflamed or broken skin. Discontinue use if a rash develops. Not to be used under an occlusive dressing. Wash hands immediately after use. The label states: Do not exceed the stated dose. Keep out of the reach of children. For external use only. If symptoms persist consult your doctor or pharmacist. Do not use if allergic to ibuprofen or any other ingredients, aspirin or any other painkillers. Consult your doctor before use if you are taking aspirin or any other pain relieving medication or if you are pregnant. Not recommended in children under 12 years.

4.5 Interaction with other medicinal products and other forms of Interaction
If used concurrently with aspirin or other non-steroidal anti-inflammatory drugs, there may be increased incidence of adverse reactions.

4.6 Pregnancy and lactation
Pregnancy: Whilst no teratogenic effects have been observed in animal experiments, ibuprofen should be avoided during pregnancy. The onset of labour may be delayed and the duration of labour increased. Lactation: Ibuprofen appears in breast milk in very low concentrations and is unlikely to affect the breast-fed infant adversely.

4.7 Effects on ability to drive and use machines
No effects are known.

4.8 Undesirable effects
Hypersensitivity reactions have been reported following treatment with ibuprofen. These may consist of (a) non-specific allergic reaction and anaphylaxis, (b) respiratory tract reactivity comprising of asthma, aggravated asthma, bronchospasm or dyspnoea, or (c) assorted skin disorders, including rashes of various types, pruritis, urticaria, purpura, angiodema and, less commonly, bullous dermatoses (including epidermal necrolysis and erythema multiforme). Gastrointestinal effects such as abdominal pain and dyspepsia may occur.

Very rare: renal failure.

4.9 Overdose
Overdosage with topical ibuprofen is unlikely to occur. Symptoms of ibuprofen overdose include headache, vomiting, drowsiness and hypotension. When treating symptoms, correction of severe electrolyte abnormalities should be considered.

5. PHARMACOLOGICAL PROPERTIES

5.1 Pharmacodynamic properties
The active constituent is a phenyl propionic acid derivative possessing analgesic, anti-inflammatory and antipyretic properties.

5.2 Pharmacokinetic properties
Percutaneous absorption amounts to about 5% of that which occurs after oral dosing with ibuprofen.

5.3 Preclinical safety data
There is no relevant information additional to that contained elsewhere in this Summary of Product Characteristics.

6. PHARMACEUTICAL PARTICULARS

6.1 List of excipients
Solketal; Poloxamer 407; Miglyol 812; Purified Water; Isopropyl Alcohol; Lavender Oil; Neroli Oil.

6.2 Incompatibilities
None known.

6.3 Shelf life
36 months unopened.

6.4 Special precautions for storage
Store below 25°C.

6.5 Nature and contents of container
Aluminium tubes with tamper-evident diaphragm and safety caps, containing 30 or 50g of gel. The interior surfaces of the tubes are coated with protected varnish.

6.6 Instructions for use and handling
Not applicable.

7. MARKETING AUTHORISATION HOLDER
Seton Healthcare Group plc, Tubiton House, Oldham, OL1 3HS.

8. MARKETING AUTHORISATION NUMBER(S)
PL 0223/0049.

9. DATE OF FIRST AUTHORISATION/RENEWAL OF THE AUTHORISATION
23rd January 1998/ 7th March 2003.

10. DATE OF REVISION OF THE TEXT
February 2005

Cuprofen Ibuprofen Tablets 200mg BP

(SSL International plc)

1. NAME OF THE MEDICINAL PRODUCT
Cuprofen Ibuprofen Tablets 200mg BP.

2. QUALITATIVE AND QUANTITATIVE COMPOSITION
Ibuprofen BP 200mg.

3. PHARMACEUTICAL FORM
Film-coated tablet.

4. CLINICAL PARTICULARS

4.1 Therapeutic indications
For the relief of rheumatic, muscular, dental and period pains and pain in backache, neuralgia, migraine and headache, and for the symptomatic relief of colds, flu and feverishness.

4.2 Posology and method of administration
For oral administration. Tablets to be taken preferably after food. Adults and children over 12 years: An initial dose of 2 tablets to be taken with water. The initial dose may be followed by further doses of 1 or 2 tablets every four hours. Maximum daily dose of 6 tablets in 24 hours. Children under 12 years: Not suitable.

4.3 Contraindications
Patients with a history of peptic ulceration or bleeding disorders. Bronchospasm may be precipitated in patients suffering from a previous history of bronchial asthma. Cuprofen should not be given to patients in whom aspirin or other non-steroidal anti-inflammatory drug induces the symptoms; rhinitis or urticaria.

4.4 Special warnings and special precautions for use
Bronchospasm may be precipitated in patients suffering from or with a previous history of bronchial asthma or allergic disease. Undesirable effects may be minimised by using the minimum effective dose for the shortest possible duration. The elderly are at an increased risk of the serious consequences of adverse reactions. Caution is required in patients with renal, cardiac or hepatic impairment since renal function may deteriorate. Do not take Cuprofen with any lithium-containing medication.

The label states: Do not exceed the stated dose. Consult a doctor if asthmatic, sensitive to aspirin or other NSAIDs or are pregnant. If symptoms persist, consult your doctor. Do not take if you have a stomach ulcer or other stomach disorders. Keep out of the reach of children. Not suitable for children under 12 years of age.

4.5 Interaction with other medicinal products and other forms of Interaction
NSAIDS may enhance the effects of anticoagulants and diminish the effects of antihypertensives or thiazide diuretics. Concurrent aspirin or other NSAIDS may result in an increased incidence of adverse reaction. Lithium excretion reduced by ibuprofen, risk of toxicity, avoid concomitant use.

4.6 Pregnancy and lactation
Whilst no teratogenic effects have been demonstrated in animal studies, ibuprofen should be avoided during pregnancy. The onset of labour may be delayed and duration of labour increased. Ibuprofen appears in breast milk in very low concentrations and is unlikely to affect the breast-fed infant adversely.

4.7 Effects on ability to drive and use machines
None stated.

4.8 Undesirable effects
The most frequent side effects which may occur are gastrointestinal disturbances, including dyspepsia, abdominal distension or pain, nausea, vomiting, gastrointestinal bleeding or activation of peptic ulcers. Skin: rashes, pruritis, urticaria, rarely exfoliative dermatitis and epidermal necrolysis. Central nervous system related side effects which may occur include dizziness, headache, drowsiness, depression, nervousness, insomnia and tinnitus. More rarely, hypersensitivity reactions may occur, including fever and rashes. Hepatotoxicity and aseptic meningitis rarely may occur may also be hypersensitivity reactions. Renal: papillary necrosis which can lead to renal failure. Other adverse effects include anaemias, thrombocytopenia, neutropenia, eosinophilia, agranulocytosis, abnormalities in liver function tests, blurred vision, changes in visual colour perception, toxic amblyopia, cystitis and haematuria. Non-steroidal anti-inflammatory drugs have been reported to cause nephrotoxicity in various forms and their use can lead to interstitial nephritis, nephrotic syndrome and renal failure.

4.9 Overdose
In case of overdose, supportive measures should be taken, such as gastric lavage and correction of serum electrolytes if necessary.

5. PHARMACOLOGICAL PROPERTIES

5.1 Pharmacodynamic properties
Ibuprofen has analgesic, anti-inflammatory and antipyretic properties, it is an inhibitor prostaglandin synthetase.

5.2 Pharmacokinetic properties
Following oral administration, ibuprofen is rapidly and almost completely absorbed. Peak serum levels are achieved between 1 and 2 hours after dosing. The relationship between the administered dose and the area of the total ibuprofen concentration-time curve appears to be non-linear, though a linear relationship does exist between free ibuprofen plasma concentration and dose. Thus, plasma protein binding of the drug may be non-linear. Total urinary excretion of ibuprofen and its metabolites is a linear function of dosage. The absorption and elimination of ibuprofen are not affected by the dosage regimen. Peak serum levels are lower and later when the drug is taken after food. Ibuprofen is rapidly eliminated from the plasma with a half-life of about 2 hours. Except at very high concentrations, about 99% of ibuprofen is bound to a single site on plasma albumin although a second primary site can be occupied. The high plasma protein binding of ibuprofen results in relatively low volume of distribution, about $0.11kg^{-1}$. Only very small amounts of ibuprofen are excreted in breast milk, not sufficient to have any effect on the infant. It is not known if the drug crosses the placenta. Ibuprofen is extensively metabolised in the liver, with more than 90% of the dose excreted in the urine and the remainder presumably in the faeces. Less than 10% of the dose is excreted unchanged. Excretion is essentially complete within 24 hours. Renal impairment has no effect on the kinetics of the drug, rapid elimination still occurring as a consequence of metabolism. There is no accumulation of ibuprofen or its metabolites in normal subjects on repeated administration of the drug. Old age has no significant effect on the elimination of ibuprofen.

Summary: Oral absorption: >95%.

Plasma half life: 2 hours.

Volume of distribution: $0.11kg^{-1}$.

Plasma protein binding: 99%.

5.3 Preclinical safety data
None stated.

6. PHARMACEUTICAL PARTICULARS

6.1 List of excipients

Core: Lactose BP; Ac-di-Sol; Methyl Cellulose BP (Methocel A4C); Magnesium Stearate BP. *Coating:* Methyl Cellulose (Methocel E15); Polyethylene Glycol 400; Mastercoat Pink FA0430.

6.2 Incompatibilities

None stated.

6.3 Shelf life

Three years.

6.4 Special precautions for storage

In glass bottle – normal storage conditions

In blister pack - store below 25°C in a dry place.

6.5 Nature and contents of container

60ml amber glass universal tablet containing 96 tablets

20μ hard temper aluminium foil blister packs containing 12, 24 and 48 tablets.

6.6 Instructions for use and handling

Not applicable.

7. MARKETING AUTHORISATION HOLDER

Cupal Limited, Tubiton House, Oldham, OL1 3HS.

8. MARKETING AUTHORISATION NUMBER(S)

PL 0338/0055.

9. DATE OF FIRST AUTHORISATION/RENEWAL OF THE AUTHORISATION

24th October 1985 / 12th January 2001

10. DATE OF REVISION OF THE TEXT

January 2001

Cuprofen Maximum Strength Tablets

(SSL International plc)

1. NAME OF THE MEDICINAL PRODUCT

Cuprofen Maximum Strength Tablets.

2. QUALITATIVE AND QUANTITATIVE COMPOSITION

Ibuprofen BP 400mg.

3. PHARMACEUTICAL FORM

Coated tablet.

4. CLINICAL PARTICULARS

4.1 Therapeutic indications

For the relief of rheumatic, muscular, dental and period pains and pain in backache, neuralgia, migraine and headache, and for the symptomatic relief of colds, flu and feverishness.

4.2 Posology and method of administration

Route of administration: Oral. Adults and children over 12 years of age: Initial dose: one tablet to be taken with water. The initial dose may be followed by further doses of one tablet not more frequently than every four hours. Maximum daily dose: three tablets in 24 hours. Not suitable for children under 12 years of age. To be taken preferably after food.

4.3 Contraindications

Hypersensitivity to any of the constituents. Hypersensitivity to aspirin or other NSAIDS including asthma, rhinitis or urticaria. Current or previous peptic ulceration.

4.4 Special warnings and special precautions for use

Caution should be exercised in administering ibuprofen to patients with asthma and especially patients who have developed bronchospasm with other non-steroidal agents. Special care should be taken when using ibuprofen in elderly patients, in whom increased tissue levels may result with an attendant increase in the risk of adverse reactions. Undesirable effects may be minimised by using the minimum effective dose for the shortest possible duration. In patients with renal, cardiac or hepatic impairment caution is required, since the use of non-steroidal anti-inflammatory drugs may result in deterioration of renal function. The dose should be kept as low as possible and renal function should be monitored. Do not take Cuprofen with any lithium-containing medication.

The label will state: Do not exceed the stated dose. Consult your doctor if you are asthmatic, sensitive to aspirin or other NSAIDs or are pregnant. If symptoms persist, consult your doctor. Do not take if you have a stomach ulcer or other stomach disorders. Keep out of the reach of children. Not suitable for children under 12 years of age.

4.5 Interaction with other medicinal products and other forms of Interaction

NSAIDS may enhance the effects of anticoagulants and diminish the effects of antihypertensives or thiazide diuretics. Concurrent aspirin or other NSAIDS may result in an increased incidence of adverse reaction. Lithium excretion reduced by ibuprofen, risk of toxicity, avoid concomitant use.

4.6 Pregnancy and lactation

Whilst no teratogenic effects have been demonstrated in animal studies, ibuprofen should be avoided during pregnancy. The onset of labour may be delayed and duration of labour increased. Ibuprofen appears in breast milk in very low concentrations and is unlikely to affect the breast-fed infant adversely.

4.7 Effects on ability to drive and use machines

None known.

4.8 Undesirable effects

Adverse effects reported include dyspepsia, gastrointestinal intolerance and bleeding, and skin rashes. Less frequently, thrombocytopenia has occurred. Very rarely toxic amblyopia has occurred; on cessation of treatment recovery has occurred. Non-steroidal anti-inflammatory drugs have been reported to cause nephrotoxicity in various forms and their use can lead to interstitial nephritis, nephrotic syndrome and renal failure. Skin rashes, pruritis, urticaria, rarely exfoliative dermatitis and epidermal necrolysis, headache, dizziness, and hearing disturbance.

4.9 Overdose

Symptoms include headache, vomiting, drowsiness and hypotension. Gastric lavage and correction of severe electrolyte abnormalities should be considered.

5. PHARMACOLOGICAL PROPERTIES

5.1 Pharmacodynamic properties

Ibuprofen is a non-steroidal anti-inflammatory agent which exhibits analgesic and antipyretic properties. It is an effective inhibitor of cyclo-oxygenase responsible for the biosynthesis of prostaglandins which forms part of the inflammatory process. It also inhibits the same enzymes in the gastric mucosa. Based on data from clinical trials, which indicate that the time taken for onset for onset of pain relief to be felt is within 30 minutes after dosing with ibuprofen.

5.2 Pharmacokinetic properties

Ibuprofen is rapidly absorbed following oral administration: t_{max}:approximately 2 hours; $t_{0.5}$: 2$\pm$0.5 hours; clearance = 0.75 $\pm$ 0.20 ml/min/kg; Vd: 0.151/kg. The excretion of ibuprofen is rapid and complete. Greater than 90% of an ingested dose is excreted and no ibuprofen per se is found in the urine. The major metabolites are a hydroxylated and a carboxylated compound.

5.3 Preclinical safety data

Not applicable.

6. PHARMACEUTICAL PARTICULARS

6.1 List of excipients

Lactose; Ac-di-Sol; Methyl Cellulose (Methocel A4C); Magnesium Stearate; Water; IMS; Polyethylene Glycol; Methyl Cellulose (Methocel E15); Sepisperse Rose AP5002 or Mastercote Pink FA0430.

6.2 Incompatibilities

None known.

6.3 Shelf life

Three years.

6.4 Special precautions for storage

Store at or below 25°C.

6.5 Nature and contents of container

Blister packs comprised of 250μ plain white rigid uPVC and 20μ hard temper aluminium foil. Packs of 12, 24, 48 and 96 tablets.

6.6 Instructions for use and handling

None.

7. MARKETING AUTHORISATION HOLDER

Cupal Limited, Tubiton House, Oldham, OL1 3HS.

8. MARKETING AUTHORISATION NUMBER(S)

PL0338/0085.

9. DATE OF FIRST AUTHORISATION/RENEWAL OF THE AUTHORISATION

4th July 1994 / 12th January 2001.

10. DATE OF REVISION OF THE TEXT

April 2004

Cuprofen Plus

(SSL International plc)

1. NAME OF THE MEDICINAL PRODUCT

Cuprofen PLUS

2. QUALITATIVE AND QUANTITATIVE COMPOSITION

Ibuprofen Ph Eur 200 mg

Codeine Phosphate Hemihydrate Ph Eur 12.8 mg

3. PHARMACEUTICAL FORM

White film-coated capsule-shaped tablets.

4. CLINICAL PARTICULARS

4.1 Therapeutic indications

Symptomatic relief of mild to moderate pain in such conditions as soft tissue injuries, including sprains, strains and musculo-tendonitis, backache, non-serious arthritic and rheumatic conditions. Also for the relief of mild to moderate pain in neuralgia, migraine, headache, dental pain and dysmenorrhoea.

4.2 Posology and method of administration

Dosage:

Do not take for more than 3 days without consulting a doctor.

Adults:

One or two tablets every four to six hours.

Not more than 6 tablets should be taken in 24 hours.

Children under 12 years:

Not recommended

Elderly:

No specific dosage recommendations are required unless renal or hepatic function is impaired, in which case dosage should be assessed individually.

Route of Administration:

Oral.

4.3 Contraindications

Cuprofen PLUS are contraindicated in individuals with hypersensitivity to the active ingredients or a history of peptic ulceration.

4.4 Special warnings and special precautions for use

Cuprofen PLUS should be used with caution in patients with gastro-intestinal disease. In patients receiving anticoagulant therapy, prothrombin time should be monitored daily for the first few days of combined treatment.

Bronchospasm may be precipitated in patients suffering from, or with a history of, bronchial asthma or allergic disease. The possibility of cross-sensitivity with aspirin and other non-steroidal anti-inflammatory agents should be considered.

Patients should be advised to consult their doctor if their headaches become persistent.

Patient Information Leaflet:

Do not take more than the stated dose and do not take every day for more than 3 days unless told to do so by your doctor. Contains codeine: regular use for long periods of time may result in symptoms such as restlessness and irritability when you stop taking this medicine. If you need to use this product all the time, see you doctor straight away.

4.5 Interaction with other medicinal products and other forms of Interaction

Caution should be exercised in patients taking monoamine oxidase inhibitors, thiazide diuretics or oral anticoagulants.

4.6 Pregnancy and lactation

Based on animal studies and clinical experience there is no evidence to suggest that foetal abnormalities are associated with the use of ibuprofen or codeine. As with all drugs, use should be avoided in pregnancy and lactation unless essential.

4.7 Effects on ability to drive and use machines

Patients should be advised not to drive or operate machinery if affected by dizziness or sedation.

4.8 Undesirable effects

Adverse effects occurring with ibuprofen include gastrointestinal disturbance, peptic ulceration and gastro-intestinal bleeding. Thrombocytopenia is a less frequent adverse effect.

Codeine may cause constipation, nausea, dizziness and drowsiness according to dosage and individual susceptibility.

Hypersensitivity reactions have been reported following treatment with ibuprofen. These may consist of (a) non-specific allergic reactions and anaphylaxis, (b) respiratory tract reactivity comprising of asthma, aggravated asthma, bronchospasm or dyspnoea, or (c) assorted skin disorders, including rashes of various types, pruritis, urticaria, purpura, angiodema and, less commonly, bullous dermatoses (including epidermal necrolysis and erythema multiforme)

4.9 Overdose

Overuse of this product, defined as consumption of quantities in excess of the recommended dose, or consumption for a prolonged period of time may lead to physical or psychological dependency. Symptoms of restlessness and irritability may result when treatment is stopped.

Ibuprofen overdose should be treated with gastric lavage and, if necessary, correction of serum electrolytes. There is no specific antidote to ibuprofen. Nausea and vomiting are prominent symptoms of codeine toxicity and there is evidence of circulatory and respiratory depression. Suggested treatment includes gastric lavage or use of emetics. If CNS depression is severe, artificial respiration, oxygen and parenteral naloxone may be needed.

5. PHARMACOLOGICAL PROPERTIES

5.1 Pharmacodynamic properties

Ibuprofen is an analgesic and anti-inflammatory agent which acts peripherally, inhibiting prostaglandin synthesis and the action of chemical mediators of pain.

Codeine is a centrally-acting opioid analgesic.

5.2 Pharmacokinetic properties

Ibuprofen is rapidly and efficiently absorbed following oral administration and peak concentrations in plasma are observed after 1-2 hours. The half-life in plasma is about 2 hours. Ibuprofen is extensively (99%) bound to plasma proteins. It passes slowly into the synovial spaces and may remain there in higher concentrations for long after concentrations in plasma have declined. About 60 - 90% of an ingested dose is excreted in the urine as metabolites or their conjugates. The major metabolites are a hydroxylated and a carboxylated compound.

Codeine phosphate is absorbed from the gastrointestinal tract, with a relative bioavailability (versus parenteral administration) of about 75%. The half-life in plasma is about 2.5 - 3 hours, whilst its analgesic effect occurs from 15 minutes up to 4 - 6 hours after oral administration. Peak plasma concentrations occur about one hour post-dose. Codeine and its metabolites are excreted almost entirely via the kidneys.

5.3 Preclinical safety data

Both ibuprofen and codeine are well established analgesics with well-documented preclinical safety profiles.

6. PHARMACEUTICAL PARTICULARS

6.1 List of excipients

Microcrystalline cellulose

Hydrogenated vegetable oil

Sodium starch glycollate

Colloidal silicon dioxide

Cellactose 80

Hydroxypropyl methyl cellulose

Polyethylene glycol 400

6.2 Incompatibilities

Not applicable.

6.3 Shelf life

Three years.

6.4 Special precautions for storage

None.

6.5 Nature and contents of container

White opaque polyvinyl chloride (250μm)/aluminium foil (20μm) blister packs containing 4, 6, 12, 24, 48 or 96 tablets.

6.6 Instructions for use and handling

Not applicable.

7. MARKETING AUTHORISATION HOLDER

SmithKline Beecham (SWG) Limited

980 Great West Road

Brentford

Middlesex

TW8 9GS

United Kingdom

Trading as: GlaxoSmithKline Consumer Healthcare, Brentford, TW8 9GS, U.K.

8. MARKETING AUTHORISATION NUMBER(S)

PL 00071/0431

9. DATE OF FIRST AUTHORISATION/RENEWAL OF THE AUTHORISATION

8 February 1996

10. DATE OF REVISION OF THE TEXT

9 September 2003

Cutivate Cream 0.05%

(GlaxoSmithKline UK)

1. NAME OF THE MEDICINAL PRODUCT

Cutivate Cream 0.05%.

2. QUALITATIVE AND QUANTITATIVE COMPOSITION

Fluticasone Propionate (micronised) HSE 0.05% w/w.

3. PHARMACEUTICAL FORM

Cream

4. CLINICAL PARTICULARS

4.1 Therapeutic indications

Adults:

For the relief of the inflammatory and pruritic manifestations of corticosteroid-responsive dermatoses such as: eczema including atopic and discoid eczemas; prurigo nodularis; psoriasis (excluding widespread plaque psoriasis); neurodermatoses including lichen simplex; lichen planus; seborrhoeic dermatitis; contact sensitivity reactions; discoid lupus erythematosus; an adjunct to systemic steroid therapy in generalised erythroderma; insect bite reactions; or prickly heat.

Children:

For children aged one year and over who are unresponsive to lower potency corticosteroids Cutivate Cream is indicated for the relief of the inflammatory and pruritic manifestations of atopic dermatitis under the supervision of a specialist. Expert opinion should be sought prior to the use of Cutivate Cream in other corticosteroid responsive dermatoses in children.

4.2 Posology and method of administration

Eczema/Dermatitis

For adults and children aged one year and over, apply a thin film of Cutivate Cream to the affected skin areas once daily.

Other indications

Apply a thin film of Cutivate Cream to the affected skin areas twice daily

Duration of use:

Daily treatment should be continued until adequate control of the condition is achieved. Frequency of application should thereafter be reduced to the lowest effective dose.

When Cutivate is used in the treatment of children, if there is no improvement within 7 – 14 days, treatment should be withdrawn and the child re-evaluated. Once the condition has been controlled (usually within 7-14 days), frequency of application should be reduced to the lowest effective dose for the shortest possible time. Continuous daily treatment for longer than 4 weeks is not recommended

For topical administration.

4.3 Contraindications

Rosacea, acne vulgaris, perioral dermatitis, primary cutaneous viral infections (e.g. herpes simplex, chickenpox). Hypersensitivity to any of the ingredients. Perianal and genital pruritus. The use of fluticasone propionate skin preparations is not indicated in the treatment of primarily infected skin lesions caused by infection with fungi or bacteria and dermatoses in children under one year of age, including dermatitis and napkin eruptions.

4.4 Special warnings and special precautions for use

Fluticasone propionate has a very low propensity for systemic absorption, nevertheless, prolonged application of high doses to large areas of body surface, especially in infants and small children, might lead to adrenal suppression. Children may absorb proportionally larger amounts of topical corticosteroids and thus be more susceptible to systemic toxicity. Care should be taken when using Cutivate Cream to ensure the amount applied is the minimum that provides therapeutic benefit.

Long-term continuous use should be avoided in children. The safety and efficacy of fluticasone propionate when used continuously for longer than 4 weeks has not been established.

The face, more than other areas of the body may exhibit atrophic changes after prolonged treatment with potent topical corticosteroids. This must be borne in mind when treating such conditions as psoriasis, discoid lupus erythematosus and severe eczema.

If applied to the eyelids, care is needed to ensure that the preparation does not enter the eye so as to avoid the risk of local irritation or glaucoma.

Topical steroids may be hazardous in psoriasis for a number of reasons, including rebound relapses, development of tolerance, risk of generalised pustular psoriasis and development of local or systemic toxicity due to impaired barrier function of the skin. If used in psoriasis careful patient supervision is important and referral to a dermatologist is required before using Cutivate Cream to treat psoriasis in children.

Appropriate antimicrobial therapy should be used whenever treating inflammatory lesions, which have become infected. Any infection requires withdrawal of topical corticosteroid therapy and systemic administration of antimicrobial agents. Bacterial infection is encouraged by the warm, moist conditions induced by occlusive dressing, and so the skin should be cleansed before a fresh dressing is applied.

4.5 Interaction with other medicinal products and other forms of Interaction

None known.

4.6 Pregnancy and lactation

Pregnancy: Topical administration of corticosteroids to pregnant animals can cause abnormalities of foetal development, but in humans there is no convincing evidence that systemic corticosteroids cause an increased incidence of congenital abnormalities. However, administration of fluticasone propionate during pregnancy should only be considered if the expected benefit to the mother is greater than any possible risk to the foetus.

Lactation: The excretion of fluticasone propionate into human breast milk has not been investigated. When measurable, plasma levels were obtained in lactating laboratory rats following subcutaneous administration, there was evidence of fluticasone propionate in the breast milk. However plasma levels in patients following dermal application of fluticasone propionate at recommended doses are likely to be low.

When fluticasone propionate is used in breast feeding mothers, the therapeutic benefits must be weighed against the potential hazards to mother and baby.

4.7 Effects on ability to drive and use machines

None known.

4.8 Undesirable effects

Adverse events are listed below by system organ class and frequency. Frequencies are defined as: very common ($\geqslant$ 1/10), common ($\geqslant$ 1/100 and < 1/10), uncommon ($\geqslant$ 1/1000 and < 1/100), rare ($\geqslant$ 1/10,000 and < 1/1000) and very rare (< 1/10,000) including isolated reports. Very common, common and uncommon events were generally determined from clinical trial data. The background rates in placebo and comparator groups were not taken into account when assigning frequency categories to adverse events derived from clinical trial data, since these rates were generally comparable to those in the active treatment group. Rare and very rare events were generally derived from spontaneous data.

Infections and infestations

Very rare: Secondary infection.

Secondary infections, particularly when occlusive dressings are used or when skin folds are involved have been reported with corticosteroid use.

Immune system disorders

Very rare: Hypersensitivity.

If signs of hypersensitivity appear, application should stop immediately.

Endocrine disorders

Very rare: Features of hypercortisolism.

Prolonged use of large amounts of corticosteroids, or treatment of extensive areas, can result in sufficient systemic absorption to produce the features of hypercortisolism. This effect is more likely to occur in infants and children, and if occlusive dressings are used. In infants, the napkin may act as an occlusive dressing (See 4.4 Special Warnings and Special Precautions for Use).

Vascular disorders

Very rare: Dilation of superficial blood vessels.

Prolonged and intensive treatment with potent corticosteroid preparations may cause dilation of the superficial blood vessels.

Skin and subcutaneous tissue disorders

Common: Pruritus.

Uncommon: Local burning.

Very rare: Allergic contact dermatitis, exacerbation of signs and symptoms of dermatoses, pustular psoriasis. Prolonged and intensive treatment with potent corticosteroid preparations may cause thinning, striae, hypertrichosis and hypopigmentation.

Treatment of psoriasis with a corticosteroid (or its withdrawal) may provoke the pustular form of the disease.

4.9 Overdose

Acute overdosage is very unlikely to occur, however, in the case of chronic overdosage or misuse, the features of hypercortisolism may appear and in this situation, topical steroids should be discontinued gradually. However, because of the risk of acute adrenal suppression this should be done under medical supervision.

5. PHARMACOLOGICAL PROPERTIES

5.1 Pharmacodynamic properties

Fluticasone propionate is a glucocorticoid with high topical anti-inflammatory potency but low HPA-axis suppressive activity after dermal administration. It therefore has a therapeutic index which is greater than most of the commonly available steroids.

It shows high systemic glucocorticoid potency after subcutaneous administration but very weak oral activity, probably due to metabolic inactivation. *In vitro* studies show a strong affinity for, and agonist activity at, human glucocorticoid receptors.

Fluticasone propionate has no unexpected hormonal effects, and no overt, marked effects upon the central and peripheral nervous systems, the gastrointestinal system, or the cardiovascular or respiratory systems.

5.2 Pharmacokinetic properties

Pharmacokinetic data for the rat and dog indicate rapid elimination and extensive metabolic clearance. Bioavailability is very low after topical or oral administration, due to limited absorption through the skin or from the gastrointestinal tract, and because of extensive first-pass metabolism. Distribution studies have shown that only minute traces of orally administered compound reach the systemic circulation, and that any systemically-available radiolabel is rapidly eliminated in the bile and excreted in the faeces.

Fluticasone propionate does not persist in any tissue, and does not bind to melanin. The major route of metabolism is hydrolysis of the S-fluoromethyl carbothioate group, to yield a carboxylic acid (GR36264), which has very weak glucocorticoid or anti-inflammatory activity. In all test animal species, the route of excretion of radioactivity is independent of the route of administration of radiolabelled fluticasone propionate. Excretion is predominantly faecal and is essentially complete within 48 hours.

In man too, metabolic clearance is extensive, and elimination is consequently rapid. Thus drug entering the systemic circulation via the skin, will be rapidly inactivated. Oral bioavailability approaches zero, due to poor absorption and extensive first-pass metabolism. Therefore systemic exposure to any ingestion of the topical formulation will be low.

5.3 Preclinical safety data

Reproductive studies suggest that administration of corticosteroids to pregnant animals can result in abnormalities of foetal development including cleft palate/lip. However, in humans, there is no convincing evidence of congenital abnormalities, such as cleft palate or lip.

Studies of safety pharmacology, repeated dose toxicity, genotoxicity, carcinogenic potential, fertility and general reproductive performance revealed no special hazard for humans, other than that anticipated for a potent steroid.

6. PHARMACEUTICAL PARTICULARS

6.1 List of excipients

Liquid Paraffin

Cetostearyl Alcohol

Isopropyl Myristate

Cetomacrogol 1000

Propylene Glycol

Imidurea

Sodium Phosphate

Citric Acid Monohydrate

Purified Water

6.2 Incompatibilities

None reported.

6.3 Shelf life

24 months.

6.4 Special precautions for storage

Store below 30°C.

6.5 Nature and contents of container

15g, 30g, 50g and 100g collapsible internally-laquered, blind-end aluminium tubes, with latex bands and closed with polypropylene caps.

Not all pack sizes may be marketed

6.6 Instructions for use and handling

No special instructions.

Administrative Data

7. MARKETING AUTHORISATION HOLDER

Glaxo Wellcome UK Ltd T/A Glaxo Laboratories

and / or GlaxoSmithKline UK

Stockley Park West

Uxbridge

Middlesex, UB11 1BT.

8. MARKETING AUTHORISATION NUMBER(S)

PL 10949/0013.

9. DATE OF FIRST AUTHORISATION/RENEWAL OF THE AUTHORISATION

17 February 1993.

10. DATE OF REVISION OF THE TEXT

30 July 2003

11. Legal Status

POM.

Cutivate Ointment 0.005%

(GlaxoSmithKline UK)

1. NAME OF THE MEDICINAL PRODUCT

Cutivate Ointment 0.005%.

2. QUALITATIVE AND QUANTITATIVE COMPOSITION

Fluticasone Propionate (micronised) HSE 0.005% w/w.

3. PHARMACEUTICAL FORM

Ointment.

4. CLINICAL PARTICULARS

4.1 Therapeutic indications

Adults:

For the relief of the inflammatory and pruritic manifestations of corticosteroid-responsive dermatoses such as: eczema including atopic and discoid eczemas; prurigo nodularis; psoriasis (excluding widespread plaque psoriasis); neurodermatoses including lichen simplex; lichen planus; seborrhoeic dermatitis; contact sensitivity reactions; discoid lupus erythematosus; an adjunct to systemic steroid therapy in generalised erythroderma; insect bite reactions; or prickly heat.

Children:

For children aged one year and over who are unresponsive to lower potency corticosteroids Cutivate Ointment is indicated for the relief of the inflammatory and pruritic manifestations of atopic dermatitis under the supervision of a specialist. Expert opinion should be sought prior to the use of Cutivate Ointment in other corticosteroid responsive dermatoses in children.

4.2 Posology and method of administration

For adults and children aged one year and over, apply a thin film of Cutivate Ointment to the affected skin areas twice daily.

Duration of use:

Daily treatment should be continued until adequate control of the condition is achieved. Frequency of application should thereafter be reduced to the lowest effective dose.

When Cutivate is used in the treatment of children, if there is no improvement within 7 - 14 days, treatment should be withdrawn and the child re-evaluated. Once the condition has been controlled (usually within 7 -14 days), frequency of application should be reduced to the lowest effective dose for the shortest possible time. Continuous daily treatment for longer than 4 weeks is not recommended.

For topical administration.

4.3 Contraindications

Rosacea, acne vulgaris, perioral dermatitis, primary cutaneous viral infections (e.g. herpes simplex, chickenpox). Hypersensitivity to any of the ingredients. Perianal and genital pruritus. The use of fluticasone propionate skin preparations is not indicated in the treatment of primarily infected skin lesions caused by infection with fungi or bacteria and dermatoses in children under one year of age, including dermatitis and napkin eruptions.

4.4 Special warnings and special precautions for use

Prolonged applications of high doses to large areas of body surface, especially in infants and small children, might lead to adrenal suppression. Children may absorb proportionally larger amounts of topical corticosteroids and thus be more susceptible to systemic toxicity. Care should be taken when using Cutivate Ointment to ensure the amount applied is the minimum that provides therapeutic benefit.

Long-term continuous use should be avoided in children. The safety and efficacy of fluticasone propionate when used continuously for longer than 4 weeks has not been established.

The face, more than other areas of the body may exhibit atrophic changes after prolonged treatment with potent topical corticosteroids. This must be borne in mind when treating such conditions as psoriasis, discoid lupus erythematosus and severe eczema.

If applied to the eyelids, care is needed to ensure that the preparation does not enter the eye so as to avoid the risk of local irritation or glaucoma.

Topical steroids may be hazardous in psoriasis for a number of reasons, including rebound relapses, development of tolerance, risk of generalised pustular psoriasis and development of local or systemic toxicity due to impaired barrier function of the skin. If used in psoriasis careful patient supervision is important and referral to a dermatologist is required before using Cutivate Ointment to treat psoriasis in children.

Appropriate antimicrobial therapy should be used whenever treating inflammatory lesions, which have become infected. Any infection requires withdrawal of topical corticosteroid therapy and systemic administration of antimicrobial agents. Bacterial infection is encouraged by the warm, moist conditions induced by occlusive dressing, and so the skin should be cleansed before a fresh dressing is applied.

4.5 Interaction with other medicinal products and other forms of Interaction

None known.

4.6 Pregnancy and lactation

Pregnancy: Topical administration of corticosteroids to pregnant animals can cause abnormalities of foetal development, but in humans there is no convincing evidence that systemic corticosteroids cause an increased incidence of congenital abnormalities. However, administration of fluticasone propionate during pregnancy should only be considered if the expected benefit to the mother is greater than any possible risk to the foetus.

Lactation: The excretion of fluticasone propionate into human breast milk has not been investigated. When measurable, plasma levels were obtained in lactating laboratory rats following subcutaneous administration, there was evidence of fluticasone propionate in the breast milk. However plasma levels in patients following dermal application of fluticasone propionate at recommended doses are likely to be low.

When fluticasone propionate is used in breast feeding mothers, the therapeutic benefits must be weighed against the potential hazards to mother and baby.

4.7 Effects on ability to drive and use machines

None known.

4.8 Undesirable effects

Adverse events are listed below by system organ class and frequency. Frequencies are defined as: very common (≥1/10), common (≥1/100 and <1/10), uncommon (≥1/1000 and <1/100), rare (≥1/10,000 and <1/1000) and very rare (<1/10,000) including isolated reports. Very common, common and uncommon events were generally determined from clinical trial data. The background rates in placebo and comparator groups were not taken into account when assigning frequency categories to adverse events derived from clinical trial data, since these rates were generally comparable to those in the active treatment group. Rare and very rare events were generally derived from spontaneous data.

Infections and infestations

Very rare: Secondary infection.

Secondary infections, particularly when occlusive dressings are used or when skin folds are involved have been reported with corticosteroid use.

Immune system disorders

Very rare: Hypersensitivity.

If signs of hypersensitivity appear, application should stop immediately.

Endocrine disorders

Very rare: Features of hypercortisolism.

Prolonged use of large amounts of corticosteroids, or treatment of extensive areas, can result in sufficient systemic absorption to produce the features of hypercortisolism. This effect is more likely to occur in infants and children, and if occlusive dressings are used. In infants, the napkin may act as an occlusive dressing (See 4.4 Special Warnings and Special Precautions for Use).

Vascular disorders

Very rare: Dilation of superficial blood vessels.

Prolonged and intensive treatment with potent corticosteroid preparations may cause dilation of the superficial blood vessels.

Skin and subcutaneous tissue disorders

Common: Pruritus.

Uncommon: Local burning.

Very rare: Allergic contact dermatitis, exacerbation of signs and symptoms of dermatoses, pustular psoriasis. Prolonged and intensive treatment wih potent corticosteroid preparations may cause thinning, striae, hypertrichosis and hypopigmentation.

Treatment of psoriasis with a corticosteroid (or its withdrawal) may provoked the pustular form of the disease.

4.9 Overdose

Acute overdosage is very unlikely to occur, however, in the case of chronic overdosage or misuse, the features of hypercortisolism may appear and in this situation, topical steroids should be discontinued gradually. However, because of the risk of acute adrenal suppression this should be done under medical supervision.

5. PHARMACOLOGICAL PROPERTIES

5.1 Pharmacodynamic properties

Fluticasone propionate is a glucocorticoid with high topical anti-inflammatory potency but low HPA-axis suppressive activity after dermal administration. It therefore has a therapeutic index which is greater than most of the commonly available steroids.

It shows high systemic glucocorticoid potency after subcutaneous administration but very weak oral activity, probably due to metabolic inactivation. *In vitro* studies show a strong affinity for and agonist activity at, human glucocorticoid receptors.

Fluticasone propionate has no unexpected hormonal effects, and no overt, marked effects upon the central and peripheral nervous systems, the gastrointestinal system, or the cardiovascular or respiratory systems.

5.2 Pharmacokinetic properties

Pharmacokinetic data for the rat and dog indicate rapid elimination and extensive metabolic clearance. Bioavailability is very low after topical or oral administration, due to limited absorption through the skin or from the gastrointestinal tract, and because of extensive first-pass metabolism. Distribution studies have shown that only minute traces of orally administered compound reach the systemic circulation, and that any systemically-available radiolabel is rapidly eliminated in the bile and excreted in the faeces.

Fluticasone propionate does not persist in any tissue, and does not bind to melanin. The major route of metabolism is hydrolysis of the S-fluoromethyl carbothioate group, to yield a carboxylic acid (GR36264), which has very weak glucocorticoid or anti-inflammatory activity. In all test animal species, the route of excretion of radioactivity is independent of the route of administration of radiolabelled fluticasone propionate. Excretion is predominantly faecal and is essentially complete within 48 hours.

In man too, metabolic clearance is extensive, and elimination is consequently rapid. Thus drug entering the systemic circulation via the skin, will be rapidly inactivated. Oral bioavailability approaches zero, due to poor absorption and extensive first-pass metabolism. Therefore systemic exposure to any ingestion of the topical formulation will be low.

5.3 Preclinical safety data

Reproductive studies suggest that administration of corticosteroids to pregnant animals can result in abnormalities of foetal development including cleft palate/lip. However, in humans, there is no convincing evidence of congenital abnormalities, such as cleft palate or lip.

Studies of safety pharmacology, repeated dose toxicity, genotoxicity, carcinogenic potential, fertility and general reproductive performance revealed no special hazard for humans, other than that anticipated for a potent steroid.

6. PHARMACEUTICAL PARTICULARS

6.1 List of excipients

Propylene Glycol

Sorbitan Sesquioleate

Microcrystalline Wax

Liquid Paraffin

6.2 Incompatibilities

None reported.

6.3 Shelf life
24 months.

6.4 Special precautions for storage
Store below 30°C.

6.5 Nature and contents of container
15g, 30g, 50g and 100g collapsible blind-end aluminium tubes, with latex bands and closed with polypropylene caps.

Not all pack sizes may be marketed

6.6 Instructions for use and handling
None.

Administrative Data

7. MARKETING AUTHORISATION HOLDER
Glaxo Wellcome UK Ltd T/A Glaxo Laboratories

and / or GlaxoSmithKline UK

Stockley Park West

Uxbridge

Middlesex, UB11 1BT.

8. MARKETING AUTHORISATION NUMBER(S)
PL 10949/0012

9. DATE OF FIRST AUTHORISATION/RENEWAL OF THE AUTHORISATION
17 February 1993.

10. DATE OF REVISION OF THE TEXT
30 July 2003

11. Legal Status
POM

Cyclimorph 10 and 15 Injection

(Amdipharm)

1. NAME OF THE MEDICINAL PRODUCT
Cyclimorph 10 Injection

Cyclimorph 15 Injection

2. QUALITATIVE AND QUANTITATIVE COMPOSITION
Cyclimorph 10 Injection:

Morphine Tartrate 10mg

Cyclizine 39.01mg

Cyclimorph 15 Injection:

Morphine Tartrate 15mg

Cyclizine 39.01mg

For excipients see section 6.1.

3. PHARMACEUTICAL FORM
Injection.

4. CLINICAL PARTICULARS

4.1 Therapeutic indications
Cyclimorph Injection is indicated for the relief of moderate to severe pain in all suitable medical and surgical conditions (see Contraindications and Precautions & Warnings) in which reduction of the nausea and vomiting associated with the administration of morphine is required.

4.2 Posology and method of administration
Route of Administration
By subcutaneous, intramuscular or intravenous injection.

Adults
The usual dose is 10-20 mg morphine tartrate, given subcutaneously, intramuscularly or intravenously.

Additional doses may not be given more frequently than 4 hourly.

Not more than 3 doses (representing 150 mg cyclizine: i.e. 3ml of Cyclimorph 10 Injection or Cyclimorph 15 Injection) should be given in any 24-hour period.

Use in the elderly
Morphine doses should be reduced in elderly patients and titrated to provide optimal pain relief with minimal side effects since:

- Increased duration of pain relief from a standard dose of morphine has been reported in elderly patients.

- A review of pharmacokinetic studies has suggested that morphine clearance decreases and half-life increases in older patients.

- The elderly may be particularly sensitive to the adverse effects of morphine.

Children
Cyclimorph Injection should not be used in children under 12 years of age.

4.3 Contraindications
Cyclimorph Injection is contra-indicated in individuals with known hypersensitivity to morphine, cyclizine or any of the other constituents.

Cyclimorph Injection, like other opioid-containing preparations, is contra-indicated in patients with respiratory depression. Patients with excessive bronchial secretions should not be given Cyclimorph Injection as morphine diminishes the cough response.

Cyclimorph Injection should not be given during an attack of bronchial asthma or in heart failure secondary to chronic lung disease.

Cyclimorph Injection is contra-indicated in patients with head injury or raised intra-cranial pressure.

Renal impairment
Severe and prolonged respiratory depression may occur in patients with renal impairment given morphine; this is attributed to the accumulation of the active metabolite morphine-6-glucuronide. Therefore Cyclimorph Injection should not be administered to patients with moderate or severe renal impairment (glomerular filtration rate <20 ml/min).

Hepatic impairment
As with other opioid analgesic containing preparations Cyclimorph Injection should not be administered to patients with severe hepatic impairment as it may precipitate coma.

Cyclimorph Injection is contra-indicated in the presence of acute alcohol intoxication. The anti-emetic properties of cyclizine may increase the toxicity of alcohol.

Cyclimorph Injection is contra-indicated in individuals receiving monoamine oxidase inhibitors or within 14 days of stopping such treatment.

Cyclimorph Injection, as with other opioid containing preparations, is contra-indicated in patients with ulcerative colitis, since such preparations may precipitate toxic dilation or spasm of the colon.

Cyclimorph Injection is contra-indicated in biliary and renal tract spasm.

4.4 Special warnings and special precautions for use
In common with the other opioid containing preparations, Cyclimorph Injection has the potential to produce tolerance and physical and psychological dependence in susceptible individuals. Abrupt cessation of therapy after prolonged use may result in withdrawal symptoms.

Cyclimorph Injection should be used with caution in the debilitated since they may be more sensitive to the respiratory depressant effects.

Cyclimorph Injection should be used with caution (including consideration of dose administered) in the presence of the following:

hypothyroidism

adrenocortical insufficiency

hypopituitarism

prostatic hypertrophy

shock

diabetes mellitus

Extreme caution should be exercised when administering Cyclimorph Injection to patients with phaeochromocytoma, since aggravated hypertension has been reported in association with diamorphine.

Cyclizine may cause a fall in cardiac output associated with increases in heart rate, mean arterial pressure and pulmonary wedge pressure. Cyclimorph Injection should therefore be used with caution in patients with severe heart failure.

Because cyclizine has anticholinergic activity it may precipitate incipient glaucoma. It should be used with caution and appropriate monitoring in patients with glaucoma and also in obstructive disease of the gastrointestinal tract.

4.5 Interaction with other medicinal products and other forms of Interaction
The central nervous system depressant effects of Cyclimorph Injection may be enhanced by other centrally-acting agents such as phenothiazines, hypnotics, neuroleptics, alcohol and muscle relaxants.

Monoamine oxidase inhibitors (MAOI's) may prolong and enhance the respiratory depressant effects of morphine. Opioids and MAOI's used together may cause fatal hypotension and coma (see Contra-indications).

Because of its anticholinergic activity cyclizine may enhance the side effects of other anticholinergic drugs.

The analgesic effect of opioids tends to be enhanced by co-administration of dexamphetamine, hydroxyzine, and some phenothiazines although respiratory depression may also be enhanced by the latter combination.

Morphine may reduce the efficacy of diuretics by inducing the release of antidiuretic hormone.

Propranolol has been reported to enhance the lethality of toxic doses of opioids in animals, although the significance of this finding is not known for man. Caution should be exercised when these drugs are administered concurrently.

Interference with laboratory tests

Morphine can react with Folin-Ciocalteau reagent in the Lowry method of protein estimation.

Morphine can also interfere with the determination of urinary 17-ketosteroids due to chemical structure effects in the Zimmerman procedure.

4.6 Pregnancy and lactation
Pregnancy
There is no evidence on the safety of the combination in human pregnancy nor is there evidence from animal work that the constituents are free from hazard. However, limited data from epidemiological studies of cyclizine and morphine in human pregnancies have found no evidence of teratogenicity. In the absence of definitive human data with the combination, the use of Cyclimorph Injection in pregnancy is not advised.

Administration of morphine during labour may cause respiratory depression in the newborn infant.

Lactation
Cyclizine is excreted in human milk, however, the amount has not been quantified.

Morphine can significantly suppress lactation. Morphine is excreted in human milk, but the amount is generally considered to be less than 1% of any dose.

4.7 Effects on ability to drive and use machines
In common with other opioids, morphine may produce orthostatic hypotension and drowsiness in ambulatory patients. Sedation of short duration has been reported in patients receiving intravenous cyclizine. The CNS depressant effects of Cyclimorph Injection may be enhanced by combination with other centrally acting agents (see Drug interactions). Patients should therefore be cautioned against activities requiring vigilance including driving vehicles and operating machinery.

4.8 Undesirable effects
As Cyclimorph Injection contains morphine and cyclizine, the type and frequency of adverse effects associated with such compounds may be expected.

Adverse reactions attributable to morphine include respiratory depression, raised intra-cranial pressure, orthostatic hypotension, drowsiness, confusion, dysphoria, restlessness, miosis, constipation, nausea, vomiting, skin reactions (e.g. urticaria) biliary tract and renal spasm, vertigo and difficulty with micturition.

Adverse reactions attributable to cyclizine include urticaria, drug rash, drowsiness/sedation, dryness of the mouth, nose and throat, blurred vision, tachycardia, urinary retention, constipation, restlessness, nervousness, insomnia, auditory and visual hallucination and cholestatic jaundice. Other central nervous system effects which have been reported rarely include dystonia, dyskinesia, extrapyramidal motor disturbances, tremor, twitching, muscle spasms, convulsions, disorientation, dizziness, decreased consciousness and transient speech disorders.

A single case of anaphylaxis has been reported following intravenous administration of cyclizine co-administered in the same syringe as propanidid.

Anaphylactic shock is a rare adverse reaction to morphine.

A case of hyperactivity following intravenous administration of morphine during induction of anaesthesia has been reported.

A case of morphine-induced thrombocytopenia has been reported.

Morphine has a depressant effect on gonadal hormone secretion which can result in a reduction of testosterone leading to regression of secondary sexual characteristics in men on long-term therapy.

Injection site reactions including vein tracking, erythema, pain and thrombophlebitis have been reported rarely.

4.9 Overdose
Signs
The signs of overdosage with Cyclimorph Injection are those pathognomic of opioid poisoning i.e. respiratory depression, pin point pupils, hypotension, circulatory failure and deepening coma. Mydriasis may replace miosis as asphyxia intervenes.

Drowsiness, floppiness, miosis and apnoea are signs of opioid overdosage in children as are convulsions.

Treatment
It is imperative to maintain and support respiration and circulation.

The specific opioid antagonist naloxone is the treatment of choice for the reversal of coma and restoration of spontaneous respiration. The literature should be consulted for details of appropriate dosage.

The use of a specific opioid antagonist in patients tolerant to morphine may produce withdrawal symptoms.

Patients should be monitored closely for at least 48 hours in case of relapse.

5. PHARMACOLOGICAL PROPERTIES

5.1 Pharmacodynamic properties
Cyclizine is a histamine H_1 receptor antagonist of the piperazine class. It possesses anticholinergic and antiemetic properties. The exact mechanism by which cyclizine can prevent or suppress both nausea and vomiting from various causes is unknown. Cyclizine increases lower oesophageal sphincter tone and reduces the sensitivity of the labyrinthine apparatus.

Morphine is a competitive agonist at the μ-opioid receptor and is a potent analgesic. It is thought that activity at the $\mu1$-receptor subtype may mediate the analgesic and euphoric actions of morphine whilst activity at the $\mu2$-receptor subtype may mediate respiratory depression and inhibition of gut motility. An action at the k-opioid receptor may mediate spinal analgesia.

5.2 Pharmacokinetic properties

In a healthy adult volunteer the administration of a single oral dose of 50mg cyclizine resulted in a peak plasma concentration of approximately 70 ng/ml, occurring at about 2 hours after administration. Urine collected over 24 hours contained less than 1% of the total dose administered. In a separate study in one healthy adult volunteer the plasma elimination half-life of cyclizine was approximately 20 hours.

Cyclizine is metabolised to its N-dimethylated derivative norcyclizine, which has little antihistaminic (H_1) activity compared to cyclizine.

The mean elimination half-life for morphine in blood and plasma is 2.7h (range 1.2-4.9h) and 2.95 (range 0.8-5h) respectively.

Morphine is extensively metabolised by hepatic biotransformation. In addition, the kidney has been shown to have the capacity to form morphine glucuronides. The major metabolite is morphine-3-glucuronide (approximately 45% of a dose). Morphine-6-glucuronide is a minor metabolite (approx 5% of the dose) but is highly active. Although renal excretion is a minor route of elimination for unchanged morphine, it constitutes the major mechanism of elimination of conjugated morphine metabolites including the active morphine-6-glucuronide.

Morphine is bound to plasma proteins only to the extent of 25-35% and therefore functions that change the extent of protein binding will have only a minor impact on its pharmacodynamic effects.

5.3 Preclinical safety data

A. Mutagenicity

Cyclizine was not mutagenic in an Ames test (at a dose level of 100 μg/plate), with or without metabolic activation.

No bacterial mutagenicity studies with morphine have been reported. A review of the literature has indicated that morphine was negative in gene mutation assays in *Drosophila melanogaster*, but was positive in a mammalian spermatocyte test. The results of another study by the same authors has indicated that morphine causes chromosomal aberrations, in germ cells of male mice when given at dose levels of 10, 20, 40 or 60mg/kg bodyweight for 3 consecutive days.

B. Carcinogenicity

No long term studies have been conducted in animals to determine whether cyclizine or morphine are potentially carcinogenic.

C. Teratogenicity

Some animal studies indicate that cyclizine may be teratogenic at dose levels up to 25 times the clinical dose level. In another study, cyclizine was negative at oral dose levels up to 65 mg/kg in rats and 75 mg/kg in rabbits.

Morphine was not teratogenic in rats when dosed for up to 15 days at 70 mg/kg/day. Morphine given subcutaneously to mice at very high doses (200, 300 or 400 mg/kg/day) on days 8 or 9 of gestation, resulted in a few cases of exencephaly and axial skeletal fusions. The hypoxic effects of such high doses could account for the defects seen.

Lower doses of morphine (40, 4.0 or 0.4 mg/ml) given to mice as a continuous i.v. infusion (at a dose volume of 0.3 ml/kg) between days 7 and 10 of gestation, caused soft tissue and skeletal malformations as shown in previous studies.

D. Fertility

In a study involving prolonged administration of cyclizine to male and female rats, there was no evidence of impaired fertility after continuous treatment for 90-100 days at dose levels of approximately 15 and 25 mg/kg/day.

Effects of morphine exposure on sexual maturation of male rats, their reproductive capacity and the development of their progeny have been examined. Results indicated that exposure during adolescence led to pronounced inhibition of several indices of sexual maturation (e.g. hormone levels, reduced gonad weights), smaller litters and selective gender specific effects on endocrine function in the offspring.

A disruption in ovulation and amenorrhoea can occur in women given morphine.

6. PHARMACEUTICAL PARTICULARS

6.1 List of excipients

Tartaric Acid

Sodium Metabisulphite

Water for Injections

6.2 Incompatibilities

See Interactions with other medicaments and other forms of interaction and Contraindications.

6.3 Shelf life

3 years.

6.4 Special precautions for storage

Store below 30°C.

Protect from light. Do not freeze.

6.5 Nature and contents of container

Ampoules which comply with the requirements of the European Pharmacopoeia for type 1 neutral glass.

Pack size: 1ml ampoules: Box of five.

6.6 Instructions for use and handling

No special instructions.

7. MARKETING AUTHORISATION HOLDER

Amdipharm PLC

Regency House

Miles Gray Road

Basildon

Essex

SS14 3AF

8. MARKETING AUTHORISATION NUMBER(S)

Cyclimorph 10 Injection: PL 20072/0007

Cyclimorph 15 Injection: PL 20072/0008

9. DATE OF FIRST AUTHORISATION/RENEWAL OF THE AUTHORISATION

3rd November 2003

10. DATE OF REVISION OF THE TEXT

October 2004

Cyclogest 200mg

(Alpharma Limited)

1. NAME OF THE MEDICINAL PRODUCT

CYCLOGEST 200mg

2. QUALITATIVE AND QUANTITATIVE COMPOSITION

Each pessary contains 200mg Progesterone PhEur.

3. PHARMACEUTICAL FORM

Off-white pessaries.

4. CLINICAL PARTICULARS

4.1 Therapeutic indications

1) Treatment of premenstrual syndrome, including premenstrual tension and depression.

2) Treatment of puerperal depression.

4.2 Posology and method of administration

Posology

200mg daily to 400mg twice a day, by vaginal or rectal insertion. For premenstrual syndrome commence treatment on day 14 of menstrual cycle and continue treatment until onset of menstruation. If symptoms are present at ovulation commence treatment on day 12.

Children: Not applicable.

Elderly: Not applicable.

Method of Administration

For rectal or vaginal insertion.

4.3 Contraindications

Undiagnosed vaginal bleeding.

4.4 Special warnings and special precautions for use

Use rectally if barrier methods of contraception are used.

Use vaginally if patients suffer from colitis or faecal incontinence. Use rectally if patients suffer from vaginal infection (especially moniliasis) or recurrent cystitis. Use rectally in patients who have recently given birth.

Progesterone is metabolised in the liver and should be used with caution in patients with hepatic dysfunction.

Cyclogest contains the hormone progesterone which is present in significant concentrations in women during the second half of the menstrual cycle and during pregnancy. This should be borne in mind when treating patients with conditions that may be hormone-sensitive.

4.5 Interaction with other medicinal products and other forms of Interaction

None known.

4.6 Pregnancy and lactation

Due to the indications of the product, it is anticipated that it will not be administered to pregnant women. As progesterone is a natural hormone, it is not expected to have adverse effects, however, no evidence is available to this effect.

4.7 Effects on ability to drive and use machines

None known.

4.8 Undesirable effects

Menstruation may occur earlier than expected, or, more rarely, menstruation may be delayed.

Soreness, diarrhoea and flatulence may occur with rectal administration.

As with other vaginal and rectal preparations, some leakage of the pessary base may occur.

4.9 Overdose

There is a wide margin of safety with Cyclogest pessaries, but overdosage may produce euphoria or dysmenorrhoea.

5. PHARMACOLOGICAL PROPERTIES

5.1 Pharmacodynamic properties

ATC code: G03D A

Progesterone is a progestational steroid.

5.2 Pharmacokinetic properties

Not applicable.

5.3 Preclinical safety data

Not applicable.

6. PHARMACEUTICAL PARTICULARS

6.1 List of excipients

Also contains: vegetable fat.

6.2 Incompatibilities

None known.

6.3 Shelf life

Shelf-life

Three years from the date of manufacture.

Shelf-life after dilution/reconstitution

Not applicable.

Shelf-life after first opening

Not applicable.

6.4 Special precautions for storage

Store below 25°C in a dry place.

6.5 Nature and contents of container

The product may be supplied in strip packs contained in cartons:

Carton: White backed folding box board printed on white.

Strip pack: Aluminium foil lacquer-laminated to 20μm polypropylene foil and coated on the reverse with polythene (20mg/m^2). The alternative is thermoplastic film and laminated PVC to 95μm and polyethylene to 27-30μm.

Pack sizes: 5s, 12s, 15s

6.6 Instructions for use and handling

Not applicable.

Administrative Data

7. MARKETING AUTHORISATION HOLDER

Alpharma Limited (Trading styles: Alpharma, Cox Pharmaceuticals)

Whiddon Valley

Barnstaple

North Devon

EX32 8NS

United Kingdom

8. MARKETING AUTHORISATION NUMBER(S)

PL 00142/0507

9. DATE OF FIRST AUTHORISATION/RENEWAL OF THE AUTHORISATION

23 August 2000

10. DATE OF REVISION OF THE TEXT

April 2001

Cyclogest 400mg

(Alpharma Limited)

1. NAME OF THE MEDICINAL PRODUCT

CYCLOGEST 400mg

2. QUALITATIVE AND QUANTITATIVE COMPOSITION

Each pessary contains 400mg Progesterone PhEur.

3. PHARMACEUTICAL FORM

Off-white pessaries.

4. CLINICAL PARTICULARS

4.1 Therapeutic indications

1) Treatment of premenstrual syndrome, including premenstrual tension and depression.

2) Treatment of puerperal depression.

4.2 Posology and method of administration

Posology

200mg daily to 400mg twice a day, by vaginal or rectal insertion. For premenstrual syndrome commence treatment on day 14 of menstrual cycle and continue treatment until onset of menstruation. If symptoms are present at ovulation commence treatment on day 12.

Children: Not applicable.

Elderly: Not applicable.

Method of Administration

For rectal or vaginal insertion.

4.3 Contraindications

Undiagnosed vaginal bleeding.

4.4 Special warnings and special precautions for use

Use rectally if barrier methods of contraception are used.

Use vaginally if patients suffer from colitis or faecal incontinence. Use rectally if patients suffer from vaginal infection (especially moniliasis) or recurrent cystitis. Use rectally in patients who have recently given birth.

Progesterone is metabolised in the liver and should be used with caution in patients with hepatic dysfunction.

Cyclogest contains the hormone progesterone which is present in significant concentrations in women during the second half of the menstrual cycle and during pregnancy. This should be borne in mind when treating patients with conditions that may be hormone-sensitive.

4.5 Interaction with other medicinal products and other forms of Interaction
None known.

4.6 Pregnancy and lactation
Due to the indications of the product, it is anticipated that it will not be administered to pregnant women. As progesterone is a natural hormone, it is not expected to have adverse effects, however, no evidence is available to this effect.

4.7 Effects on ability to drive and use machines
None known.

4.8 Undesirable effects
Menstruation may occur earlier than expected, or, more rarely, menstruation may be delayed.

Soreness, diarrhoea and flatulence may occur with rectal administration.

As with other vaginal and rectal preparations, some leakage of the pessary base may occur.

4.9 Overdose
There is a wide margin of safety with Cyclogest pessaries, but overdosage may produce euphoria or dysmenorrhoea.

5. PHARMACOLOGICAL PROPERTIES

5.1 Pharmacodynamic properties
ATC code: G03D A

Progesterone is a progestational steroid.

5.2 Pharmacokinetic properties
Not applicable.

5.3 Preclinical safety data
Not applicable.

6. PHARMACEUTICAL PARTICULARS

6.1 List of excipients
Also contains: vegetable fat.

6.2 Incompatibilities
None known.

6.3 Shelf life
Shelf-life

Three years from the date of manufacture.

Shelf-life after dilution/reconstitution

Not applicable.

Shelf-life after first opening

Not applicable.

6.4 Special precautions for storage
Store below 25°C in a dry place.

6.5 Nature and contents of container
The product may be supplied in strip packs contained in cartons:

Carton: White backed folding box board printed on white.

Strip pack: Aluminium foil lacquer-laminated to 20μm polypropylene foil and coated on the reverse with polythene (20mg/m^2). The alternative is thermoplastic film and laminated PVC to 95μm and polyethylene to 27-30μm.

Pack sizes: 5s, 12s, 15s

6.6 Instructions for use and handling
Not applicable.

Administrative Data

7. MARKETING AUTHORISATION HOLDER
Alpharma Limited (Trading styles: Alpharma, Cox Pharmaceuticals)

Whiddon Valley

Barnstaple

North Devon

EX32 8NS

United Kingdom

8. MARKETING AUTHORISATION NUMBER(S)
PL 00142/0508

9. DATE OF FIRST AUTHORISATION/RENEWAL OF THE AUTHORISATION
23 August 2000

10. DATE OF REVISION OF THE TEXT
April 2001

Cyclophosphamide 50 Tablets

(Pharmacia Limited)

1. NAME OF THE MEDICINAL PRODUCT
Cyclophosphamide Tablets.

2. QUALITATIVE AND QUANTITATIVE COMPOSITION
Cyclophosphamide monohydrate BP 53.50 mg equivalent to 50 mg anhydrous cyclophosphamide.

3. PHARMACEUTICAL FORM
Sugar-coated tablets

4. CLINICAL PARTICULARS

4.1 Therapeutic indications
Alkylating, antineoplastic agent. Cyclophosphamide has been used successfully to induce and maintain regressions in a wide range of neoplastic conditions, including leukaemias, lymphomas, soft tissue and osteogenic sarcomas, paediatric malignancies and adult solid tumours; in particular, breast and lung carcinomas.

Cyclophosphamide is frequently used in combination chemotherapy regimens involving other cytotoxic drugs.

4.2 Posology and method of administration
Route of administration: Oral.

Adults and children

The recommended dose for cyclophosphamide tablets is 50-250 mg/m^2 daily (doses towards the upper end of this range should be used only for short courses).

The dose may be amended at the discretion of the physician.

It is recommended that the calculated dose of cyclophosphamide be reduced when it is given in combination with other antineoplastic agents or radiotherapy, and in patients with bone marrow depression.

Cyclophosphamide tablets should be swallowed whole, preferably on an empty stomach, but if gastric irritation is severe, they may be taken with meals.

A minimum output of 100 ml/hour should be maintained during therapy with conventional doses to avoid cystitis. If the larger doses are used, an output of at least this level should be maintained for 24 hours following administration, if necessary by forced diuresis. Alkalinisation of the urine is not recommended.

Cyclophosphamide should be given early in the day and the bladder voided frequently. The patient should be well hydrated and maintained in fluid balance.

Mesna (Uromitexan) can be used concurrently with cyclophosphamide to reduce urotoxic effects (for dosage see Uromitexan data sheet). If Mesna (Uromitexan) is used to reduce uroethelial toxicity, frequent emptying of the bladder should be avoided.

If the leucocyte count is below 4,000/mm^3 or the platelet count is below 100,000/mm^3, treatment with cyclophosphamide should be temporarily withheld until the blood count returns to normal levels.

4.3 Contraindications
Hypersensitivity and haemorrhagic cystitis.

4.4 Special warnings and special precautions for use
Cyclophosphamide should be withheld in the presence of severe bone marrow depression and reduced doses should be used in the presence of lesser degrees of bone marrow depression. Regular blood counts should be performed in patients receiving cyclophosphamide.

It should not normally be given to patients with severe infections and should be withdrawn if such infections become life threatening.

Cyclophosphamide should be used with caution in debilitated patients and those with renal and/or hepatic failure. Cyclophosphamide is not recommended in patients with a plasma creatinine greater than 120 μmol/l (1.5 mg/100 ml) bilirubin greater than 17 μmol/l (1 mg/100 ml); or serum transaminases or alkaline phosphatase more than 2-3 times the upper limit of normal. In all such cases, dosage should be reduced.

Cyclophosphamide should be used only under the directions of physicians experienced in cytotoxic or immunosuppressant therapy.

Further Information:

The dosage regimen for mesna (Uromitexan) varies according to the dose of cyclophosphamide administered. In general i.v. Uromitexan is given as 60% w/w of the dose of i.v. Cyclophosphamide in three equal doses of 20% at 0, 4 and 8 hours. With the higher doses of cyclophosphamide, the dose and frequency of administration may need to be increased. Uromitexan Tablets are also available; full prescribing information for both presentations is available on the appropriate data sheet.

4.5 Interaction with other medicinal products and other forms of Interaction
Oral hypoglycaemic agents may be potentiated by cyclophosphamide.

4.6 Pregnancy and lactation
This product should not normally be administered to patients who are pregnant or to mothers who are breastfeeding. Alkylating agents, including cyclophosphamide, have been shown to possess mutagenic, teratogenic and carcinogenic potential. Pregnancy should therefore be avoided during cyclophosphamide therapy and for three months thereafter.

4.7 Effects on ability to drive and use machines
None known.

4.8 Undesirable effects
Single doses will produce a leucopenia which may be severe but usually returns to normal within 21 days.

Amenorrhoea and azoospermia often occur during treatment with cyclophosphamide but in most cases are reversible.

Haematuria may occur during or after therapy with Cyclophosphamide. Cyclophosphamide is excreted mainly in the urine, largely in the form of active metabolites which may give rise to a chemical cystitis which may be haemorrhagic. Acute sterile haemorrhagic cystitis may occur in up to 10% of patients not given mesna (Uromitexan) in conjunction with Cyclophosphamide. Late sequelae of this cystitis are bladder contracture and fibrosis.

Because of this, a high fluid intake should be maintained with frequent emptying of the bladder. Cyclophosphamide therapy may lead to inappropriate secretion of anti-diuretic hormone, fluid retention and hyponatremia, with subsequent water intoxication. Should this arise, a diuretic may be given. Cyclophosphamide may cause myocardial toxicity, especially at high dosage.

Cyclophosphamide may induce permanent sterility in children.

In addition to those noted above, the following may accompany cyclophosphamide therapy: hair loss, which may be total, although generally reversible; mucosal ulcertation; anorexia, nausea and vomiting; pigmentation, typically affecting the palms and nails of the hands and the soles of the feet, and interstitial pulmonary fibrosis.

Hepatic toxicity has rarely been reported.

4.9 Overdose
Myelosuppression (particularly granulocytopenia) and haemorrhagic cystitis are the most serious consequences of overdosage. Recovery from myelosuppression will occur by the 21st day after the overdosage in the great majority of patients (at doses up to 200 mg/kg i.v.) while granulocytopenia is usually seen by day 6 and lasts for a mean period of 12 days (up to 18 days). A broad spectrum antibiotic may be administered until recovery occurs. Transfusion of whole blood, platelets or white cells and reverse barrier nursing may be necessary.

If the drug has been taken in the form of tablets, early gastric lavage may reduce the amount of drug absorbed.

During the first 24 hours and possibly up to 48 hours after overdosage, i.v. mensa may be beneficial in ameliorating damage to the urinary system. Normal supportive measures such as analgesics and maintenance of fluid balance should be instituted. If the cystitis does not resolve more intensive treatment may be necessary.

No further courses should be given until the patient has fully recovered.

5. PHARMACOLOGICAL PROPERTIES

5.1 Pharmacodynamic properties
Cyclophosphamide is an antineoplastic agent which is converted in the body to an active alkylating metabolite. It also possesses marked immunosuppressant properties. The principal site of cyclophosphamide activation is the liver. The chemotherapeutic and immunosuppressant activity of cyclophosphamide is thought to be mediated by the cytotoxic intermediates produced by activation by mixed function oxidases in hepatic microsomes. Non-enzymatic cleavage, possibly taking place in the tumour cells, results in the formulation of highly cytotoxic forms of the drug.

5.2 Pharmacokinetic properties
Cyclophosphamide may be incompletely absorbed from the gastro-intestinal tract. It rapidly disappears from the plasma and peak concentrations occur about 1 hour after an oral dose.

The metabolites of cyclophosphamide are excreted in the urine and these have an irritant effect on the bladder mucosa. Unchanged drug is also excreted in the urine and accounts for only 5-25% of the administered dose.

Metabolites have been found to be more protein bound than the parent compound.

5.3 Preclinical safety data
No further preclinical data are available.

6. PHARMACEUTICAL PARTICULARS

6.1 List of excipients
Maize starch

Pregelatinised starch

Lactose monohydrate

Gelatin

Microcrystalline cellulose

Sodium stearyl fumarate

Magnesium stearate

Coating

Polyethylene glycol

Sucrose

Maize starch

Calcium carbonate

Povidone

Opalux AS-9486 consisting of

- titanium dioxide
- red iron oxide
- yellow iron oxide
- sucrose
- purified water
- polyvinylpyrrolidone
- sodium benzoate

Carnauba wax

6.2 Incompatibilities
None stated.

6.3 Shelf life
60 months.

6.4 Special precautions for storage
Do not store above 25°C. Store in the original container in order to protect from moisture.

6.5 Nature and contents of container
White polyethylene containers with polyethylene snap-caps, containing a white capsule of desiccant.

6.6 Instructions for use and handling
None stated.

7. MARKETING AUTHORISATION HOLDER
Pharmacia Limited
Davy Avenue
Milton Keynes
MK5 8PH
UK

8. MARKETING AUTHORISATION NUMBER(S)
PL 00032/0335

9. DATE OF FIRST AUTHORISATION/RENEWAL OF THE AUTHORISATION
16 August 2002

10. DATE OF REVISION OF THE TEXT

Legal Category
POM.

CYCLOSERINE

(King Pharmaceuticals Ltd)

1. NAME OF THE MEDICINAL PRODUCT
CYCLOSERINE

2. QUALITATIVE AND QUANTITATIVE COMPOSITION
Each capsule contains as active ingredient 250mg of cycloserine.

3. PHARMACEUTICAL FORM
Capsule

4. CLINICAL PARTICULARS

4.1 Therapeutic indications
Actions: Cycloserine inhibits cell wall synthesis in susceptible strains of Gram-positive and Gram-negative bacteria and in *Mycobacterium tuberculosis.*

Indications: Cycloserine is indicated in the treatment of active pulmonary and extra-pulmonary tuberculosis (including renal disease) when the organisms are susceptible to this drug and after failure of adequate treatment with the primary medications (streptomycin, isoniazid, rifampicin and ethambutol). Like all anti-tuberculous drugs, cycloserine should be administered in conjunction with other effective chemotherapy and not as the sole therapeutic agent.

Cycloserine may be effective in the treatment of acute urinary tract infections caused by susceptible strains of Gram-positive and Gram-negative bacteria, especially *Klebsiella/Enterobacter* species and *Escherichia coli*. It is generally no more and may be less effective than other antimicrobial agents in the treatment of urinary tract infections caused by bacteria other than mycobacteria. Use of cycloserine in these infections should be considered only when the more conventional therapy has failed and when the organism has been demonstrated to be sensitive to the drug.

4.2 Posology and method of administration
Adults: the usual dosage is 500mg to 1g daily in divided doses, monitored by blood level determinations. The initial adult dosage most frequently given is 250mg twice daily at 12-hour intervals for the first two weeks. A daily dosage of 1g should not be exceeded.

Children: the usual starting dose is 10mg/ kg/ day, then adjusted according to blood levels obtained and therapeutic response.

The elderly: as for adults but reduce dosage if renal function is impaired.

4.3 Contraindications
Cycloserine is contra-indicated in the presence of any of the following: hypersensitivity to cycloserine; epilepsy; depression, severe anxiety or psychosis; severe renal insufficiency; alcohol abuse.

4.4 Special warnings and special precautions for use
Administration of cycloserine should be discontinued or the dosage reduced if the patient develops allergic dermatitis or symptoms of central nervous system toxicity such as convulsions, psychosis, somnolence, depression, confusion, hyper-reflexia, headache, tremor, vertigo, paresis or dysarthria.

Toxicity is usually associated with blood levels of greater than 30mg/l, which may be the result of high dosage or inadequate renal clearance. The therapeutic index for this drug is low. The risk of convulsions is increased in chronic alcoholics (see 'Precautions' section).

Patients should be monitored by haematological, renal excretion, blood level and liver function studies.

Before treatment with cycloserine is begun, cultures should be taken and the susceptibility of the organism to the drug should be established. In tuberculous infections, sensitivity to the other anti-tuberculous agents in the regimen should also be demonstrated.

Blood levels should be determined at least weekly for patients having reduced renal function, for individuals receiving a daily dosage of more than 500mg, and for those showing signs and symptoms suggestive of toxicity. The dosage should be adjusted to keep the blood level below 30mg/l.

Anticonvulsant drugs or sedatives may be effective in controlling symptoms of central nervous system toxicity, such as convulsions, anxiety or tremor. Patients receiving more than 500mg of cycloserine daily should be closely observed for such symptoms. The value of pyridoxine in preventing CNS toxicity from cycloserine has not been proven.

Administration of cycloserine and other anti-tuberculous drugs has been associated in a few instances with vitamin B_{12} and/or folic acid deficiency, megaloblastic anaemia and sideroblastic anaemia. If evidence of anaemia develops during treatment, appropriate investigations and treatment should be carried out.

Cycloserine has been associated with clinical exacerbations of porphyria and is not recommended in porphyric patients.

4.5 Interaction with other medicinal products and other forms of Interaction
Drug interactions: Concurrent administration of ethionamide has been reported to potentiate neurotoxic side-effects. Alcohol and cycloserine are incompatible, especially during a regimen calling for large doses of the latter. Alcohol increases the possibility and risk of epileptic episodes. Patients receiving cycloserine and isoniazid should be monitored for signs of CNS toxicity, such as dizziness and drowsiness, as these drugs have a combined toxic action on the CNS. Dosage adjustments may be necessary.

4.6 Pregnancy and lactation
Usage in pregnancy: Concentrations in fetal blood approach those found in the serum. A study in 2 generations of rats given doses up to 100mg/ kg/ day demonstrated no teratogenic effect in offspring. It is not known whether cycloserine can cause fetal harm when administered to a pregnant woman or can affect reproductive capability. Cycloserine should be given to a pregnant woman only if clearly needed.

Usage in nursing mothers: Concentrations in the mother's milk approach those found in the serum. A decision should be made whether to discontinue nursing or to discontinue the drug, taking into account the importance of the drug to the mother.

4.7 Effects on ability to drive and use machines
None known

4.8 Undesirable effects
Most side-effects occurring during treatment with cycloserine involve the nervous system or are manifestations of drug hypersensitivity. The following side-effects have been observed: nervous system manifestations, which appear to be related to higher dosages of drug, i.e. more than 500mg daily, can be convulsions, drowsiness, somnolence, headache, tremor, dysarthria, vertigo, confusion and disorientation with loss of memory, psychosis, possibly with suicidal tendencies, character changes, hyperirritability, aggression, paresis, hyper-reflexia, paraesthesiae, major and minor localised clonic seizures and coma.

Other reported side-effects include allergy, rash, megaloblastic anaemia and elevated serum aminotransferases, especially in patients with pre-existing liver disease.

Sudden development of congestive heart failure, in patients receiving 1 to 1.5g of cycloserine daily, has been reported.

4.9 Overdose
Signs and symptoms: Acute toxicity can occur if more than 1g is ingested by an adult. Chronic toxicity is dose related and can occur if more than 500mg is administered daily. For patients with renal impairment see 'Contra-indications' and 'Warnings'. Toxicity commonly affects the central nervous system. Effects may include headache, vertigo, confusion, drowsiness, hyper-irritability, paraesthesias, dysarthria and psychosis. Following larger ingestions, paresis, convulsions and coma often occur. Ethanol may increase the risk of seizures.

Treatment: Symptomatic and supportive therapy is recommended. Activated charcoal may be more effective in reducing absorption than emesis or lavage. In adults, many neurotoxic effects can be both treated and prevented with 200-300mg of pyridoxine daily. Haemodialysis removes cycloserine from the bloodstream but should be reserved for life-threatening toxicity.

5. PHARMACOLOGICAL PROPERTIES

5.1 Pharmacodynamic properties
Actions: Cycloserine inhibits cell wall synthesis (by competing with D-alanine for incorporation into the cell wall) in susceptible strains of Gram-positive and Gram-negative bacteria and in *Mycobacterium tuberculosis.*

Indications: Cycloserine is indicated in the treatment of active pulmonary and extra-pulmonary tuberculosis (including renal disease) when the organisms are susceptible to this drug and after failure of adequate treatment with the primary medications (streptomycin, isoniazid, rifampicin and ethambutol). Like all anti-tuberculous drugs, cycloserine should be administered in conjunction with other effective chemotherapy and not as the sole therapeutic agent.

Cycloserine may be effective in the treatment of acute urinary tract infections caused by susceptible strains of Gram-positive and Gram-negative bacteria, especially *Klebsiella/Enterobacter* species and *Escherichia coli*. It is generally no more and may be less effective than other antimicrobial agents in the treatment of urinary tract infections caused by bacteria other than mycobacteria. Use of cycloserine in these infections should be considered only when the more conventional therapy has failed and when the organism has been demonstrated to be sensitive to the drug.

5.2 Pharmacokinetic properties
Cycloserine is rapidly and almost completely absorbed from the GI tract after oral administration. Following the administration of a 250mg dose plasma levels are detectable within an hour and peak plasma concentrations of approximately 10mg/l are achieved 3-4 hours after dosage administration. It is widely distributed throughout body fluids and tissues.

There is no appreciable blood-brain barrier, and CSF levels are approximately the same as plasma levels. It is found in the sputum of tuberculous patients and has been detected in pleural and ascitic fluids, bile, amniotic fluid and fetal blood, breast milk, lung and lymph tissues.

Cycloserine is excreted into the urine, levels appearing within half an hour of oral ingestion. Approximately 66 per cent of a dose appears unchanged in the urine in 24 hours. A further 10 per cent is excreted over the next 48 hours. It is not significantly excreted in the faeces. Approximately 35 per cent is metabolised, but the metabolites have not yet been identified.

The half-life of cycloserine is in the range 8-12 hours.

5.3 Preclinical safety data
A study in two generations of rats given doses up to 100mg/ kg/ day demonstrated no teratogenic effect in offspring.

6. PHARMACEUTICAL PARTICULARS

6.1 List of excipients
Talc
Liquid Paraffin
Amaranth
Erthrosine
Sunset Yellow
Titanium Dioxide
Black Iron Oxide
Gelatin

6.2 Incompatibilities
None known

6.3 Shelf life
Eighteen months when stored appropriately.

6.4 Special precautions for storage
Keep tightly closed. Protect from moisture. Store below 25°C.

6.5 Nature and contents of container
HDPE bottles of 100 capsules and HDPE bottles with an extruded polyethylene (PE) / PET / Al foil Liner for Induction Heat Seal also containing 100 capsules.

6.6 Instructions for use and handling
For oral administration

Administrative Data

7. MARKETING AUTHORISATION HOLDER
King Pharmaceuticals Ltd
Donegal Street
Ballybofey
County Donegal
Ireland

8. MARKETING AUTHORISATION NUMBER(S)
PL 14385/0005

9. DATE OF FIRST AUTHORISATION/RENEWAL OF THE AUTHORISATION
October 1996

10. DATE OF REVISION OF THE TEXT
March 2001

Legal Category
POM

Cyklokapron Injection

(Pharmacia Limited)

1. NAME OF THE MEDICINAL PRODUCT
Cyklokapron® Injection

2. QUALITATIVE AND QUANTITATIVE COMPOSITION
Active ingredient: Tranexamic Acid Ph.Eur 500 mg

3. PHARMACEUTICAL FORM
Ampoules containing 5ml colourless solution

4. CLINICAL PARTICULARS

4.1 Therapeutic indications

Local fibrinolysis

For short term use in prophylaxis and treatment in patients at high risk of per - and post-operative haemorrhage following:

a) prostatectomy

b) conisation of the cervix

c) surgical procedures and dental extractions in haemophiliacs

General fibrinolysis

a) haemorrhagic complications in association with thrombolytic therapy.

b) Haemorrhage associated with disseminated intravascular coagulation with predominant activation of the fibrinolytic system.

4.2 Posology and method of administration
Route of administration: by slow intravenous injection.

Local fibrinolysis: the recommended standard dose is 5-10ml (500-1000mg) by slow intravenous injection (1 ml/min), three times daily. If treatment continues for more than three days, consideration should be given to the use of Cyklokapron tablets or syrup. Alternatively, following an initial intravenous injection, subsequent treatment may proceed by intravenous infusion. Following addition to a suitable diluent (see Section 4.5), Cyklokapron may be administered at a rate of 25-50 mg/kg body wt/day.

Children: According to body weight (10mg/kg body wt/ 2-3 times daily)

Elderly patients: No reduction in dosage is necessary unless there is evidence of renal failure.

General fibrinolysis

1 In disseminated intravascular coagulation with predominant activation of the fibrinolytic system, usually a single dose of 10ml (1g) is sufficient to control bleeding.

2 Neutralisation of thrombolytic therapy; 10mg/kg body wt by slow intravenous injection.

4.3 Contraindications
Cyklokapron is contra-indicated in patients with a history of thromboembolic disease.

4.4 Special warnings and special precautions for use
In patients with renal insufficiency, because of the risk of accumulation. The dose should be reduced according to the following table:

Serum Creatinine	Dose iv	Dose Frequency
120-250 mcmol/l	10 mg/kg	Twice daily
250-500 mcmol/l	10 mg/kg	Every 24th hour
> 500 mcmol/l	5 mg/kg	Every 24th hour

In massive haematuria from the upper urinary tract (especially in haemophilia) since, in a few cases, ureteric obstruction has been reported.

In patients with disseminated intravascular coagulation (DIC) treatment must be restricted to those in whom there is predominant activation of the fibrinolytic system with acute severe bleeding. Characteristically, the haematological profile approximates to the following: reduced euglobulin clot lysis time; prolonged prothrombin time; reduced plasma levels of fibrinogen, factors V and VIII, plasminogen and alpha-2 macroglobulin; normal plasma levels of P and P complex; i.e. factors II (prothrombin), VIII and X; increased plasma levels of fibrinogen degradation products; a normal platelet count. The foregoing presumes that the underlying disease state does not of itself modify the various elements in this profile. In such acute cases a single dose of 1g tranexamic acid is frequently sufficient to control bleeding. The fibrinolytic activity in the blood will be reduced for about 4 hours if renal function is normal. Anticoagulation with heparin should be instigated in order to prevent further fibrin deposition. Administration of Cyklokapron in DIC should be considered only when appropriate haematological laboratory facilities and expertise are available. Cyklokapron must not be administered in DIC with predominant activation of the coagulation system.

4.5 Interaction with other medicinal products and other forms of Interaction
The solution for injection may be mixed with the following solutions: isotonic sodium chloride; isotonic glucose; 20% fructose; 10% invertose; dextran 40; dextran 70; ringer's solution.

Cyklokapron solution for injection may be mixed with Heparin.

4.6 Pregnancy and lactation
Although there is no evidence from animal studies of a teratogenic effect, the usual caution with the use of drugs in pregnancy should be observed.

Tranexamic acid passes into breast milk to a concentration of approximately one hundredth of the concentration in the maternal blood. An antifibrinolytic effect in the infant is unlikely.

4.7 Effects on ability to drive and use machines
None known.

4.8 Undesirable effects
Gastro-intestinal disorders (nausea, vomiting, diarrhoea) may occur but disappear when the dosage is reduced. Rapid intravenous injection may cause dizziness and/or hypotension. Rare cases of thromboembolic events have been reported.

4.9 Overdose
No cases of overdosage have been reported. Symptoms may be nausea, vomiting, orthostatic symptoms and/or hypotension. Maintain a high fluid intake to promote renal excretion.

5. PHARMACOLOGICAL PROPERTIES

5.1 Pharmacodynamic properties
Tranexamic acid is an antifibrinolytic agent, which competitively inhibits the activation of plasminogen to plasmin.

5.2 Pharmacokinetic properties
Approximately 90% of an intravenously administered tranexamic acid dose is excreted, largely unchanged, in the urine within 24 hours. The plasma half-life is approximately 2 hours.

5.3 Preclinical safety data
There are no preclinical data of relevance to the prescriber which are additional to that already included in other sections of the Summary of Product Characteristics.

6. PHARMACEUTICAL PARTICULARS

6.1 List of excipients
Water for injections

6.2 Incompatibilities
Cyklokapron solution for injection should not be added to blood for transfusion, or to injections containing penicillin.

6.3 Shelf life
3 years.

6.4 Special precautions for storage
None.

6.5 Nature and contents of container
Type I glass 5ml ampoules packed in outer cardboard carton.

6.6 Instructions for use and handling
See Section 4.2

7. MARKETING AUTHORISATION HOLDER
Pharmacia Limited

Davy Avenue

Milton Keynes

MK5 8PH

UK

8. MARKETING AUTHORISATION NUMBER(S)
PL 00032/0314

9. DATE OF FIRST AUTHORISATION/RENEWAL OF THE AUTHORISATION
9th February 1987

10. DATE OF REVISION OF THE TEXT
20th November 2001

Legal Category
POM.

Cyklokapron Tablets

(Meda Pharmaceuticals)

1. NAME OF THE MEDICINAL PRODUCT
Cyklokapron Tablets

Tranexamic Acid Tablets

2. QUALITATIVE AND QUANTITATIVE COMPOSITION
Each tablet contains Tranexamic acid 500 mg as the active ingredient.

For excipients, see section 6.1.

3. PHARMACEUTICAL FORM
Film-coated tablets.

White, oblong tablets, 8x18 mm, engraved CY with an arc above and below the lettering, for oral use.

4. CLINICAL PARTICULARS

4.1 Therapeutic indications
Short-term use for haemorrhage or risk of haemorrhage in increased fibrinolysis or fibrinogenolysis. Local fibrinolysis as occurs in the following conditions:

Prostatectomy and bladder surgery

Menorrhagia

Epistaxis

Conisation of the cervix

Traumatic hyphaema

Hereditary angioneurotic oedema

Management of dental extraction in haemophiliacs

4.2 Posology and method of administration
Route of administration: Oral.

Local fibrinolysis: The recommended standard dosage is 15-25 mg/kg bodyweight (i.e. 2-3 tablets) two to three times daily. For the indications listed below the following doses may be used:

1a. Prostatectomy: Prophylaxis and treatment of haemorrhage in high risk patients should commence pre- or post-operatively with Cyklokapron Injection; thereafter 2 tablets three to four times daily until macroscopic haematuria is no longer present.

1b. Menorrhagia: Recommended dosage is 2 tablets 3 times daily as long as needed for up to 4 days. If very heavy menstrual bleeding, dosage may be increased. A total dose of 4g daily (8 tablets) should not be exceeded. Treatment with Cyklokapron should not be initiated until menstrual bleeding has started.

1c. Epistaxis: Where recurrent bleeding is anticipated oral therapy (2 tablets three times daily) should be administered for 7 days.

1d. Conisation of the cervix: 3 tablets three times daily.

1e. Traumatic hyphaema: 2-3 tablets three times daily. The dose is based on 25 mg/kg three times a day.

2. Haemophilia: In the management of dental extractions 2-3 tablets every eight hours. The dose is based on 25 mg/kg.

3. Hereditary angioneurotic oedema: Some patients are aware of the onset of the illness; suitable treatment for these patients is intermittently 2-3 tablets two to three times daily for some days. Other patients are treated continuously at this dosage.

Renal insufficiency: By extrapolation from clearance data relating to the intravenous dosage form, the following reduction in the oral dosage is recommended for patients with mild to moderate renal insufficiency.

Serum Creatinine (μmol/l) Dose tranexamic acid

120-249 15 mg/kg body weight twice daily

250-500 15 mg/kg body weight/day

Children's dosage: This should be calculated according to body weight at 25 mg/kg per dose.

Elderly patients: No reduction in dosage is necessary unless there is evidence of renal failure (see guidelines below).

4.3 Contraindications
Severe renal failure because of risk of accumulation,

Hypersensitivity to tranexamic acid or any of the other ingredients,

Active thromboembolic disease.

4.4 Special warnings and special precautions for use
In massive haematuria from the upper urinary tract (especially in haemophilia) since, in a few cases, ureteric obstruction has been reported.

When disseminated intravascular coagulation is in progress.

In the long-term treatment of patients with hereditary angioneurotic oedema, regular eye examinations (e.g. visual acuity, slit lamp, intraocular pressure, visual fields) and liver function tests should be performed.

Patients with irregular menstrual bleeding should not use Cyklokapron until the cause of irregular bleeding has been established. If menstrual bleeding is not adequately reduced by Cyklokapron, an alternative treatment should be considered.

Patients with a previous thromboembolic event and a family history of thromboembolic disease (patients with thrombophilia) should use Cyklokapron only if there is a strong medical indication and under strict medical supervision.

The blood levels are increased in patients with renal insufficiency. Therefore a dose reduction is recommended (see section 4.2).

The use of tranexamic acid in cases of increased fibrinolysis due to disseminated intravascular coagultion is not recommended.

Clinical experience with Cyklokapron in menorrhagic children under 15 years of age is not available.

4.5 Interaction with other medicinal products and other forms of Interaction
Cyklokapron will counteract the thrombolytic effect of fibrinolytic preparations.

4.6 Pregnancy and lactation

Pregnancy

Although there is no evidence from animal studies of a teratogenic effect, the usual caution with use of drugs in pregnancy should be observed.

Tranexamic acid crosses the placenta.

Lactation

Tranexamic acid passes into breast milk to a concentration of approximately one hundredth of the concentration in the maternal blood. An antifibrinolytic effect in the infant is unlikely.

4.7 Effects on ability to drive and use machines

None known.

4.8 Undesirable effects

Gastrointestinal disorders (nausea, vomiting, diarrhoea) may occur but disappear when the dosage is reduced. Rare instances of colour vision disturbances have been reported. Patients who experience disturbance of colour vision should be withdrawn from treatment. Rare cases of thromboembolic events have been reported.

Rare cases of allergic skin reactions have also been reported.

4.9 Overdose

Symptoms may be nausea, vomiting, orthostatic symptoms and/or hypotension. Initiate vomiting, then stomach lavage, and charcoal therapy. Maintain a high fluid intake to promote renal excretion. There is a risk of thrombosis in predisposed individuals. Anticoagulant treatment should be considered.

5. PHARMACOLOGICAL PROPERTIES

5.1 Pharmacodynamic properties

Tranexamic acid is an antifibrinolytic compound which is a potent competitive inhibitor of the activation of plasminogen to plasmin. At much higher concentrations it is a non-competitive inhibitor of plasmin. The inhibitory effect of tranexamic acid in plasminogen activation by urokinase has been reported to be 6-100 times and by streptokinase 6-40 times greater than that of aminocaproic acid. The antifibrinolytic activity of tranexamic acid is approximately ten times greater than that of aminocaproic acid.

5.2 Pharmacokinetic properties

Following oral administration, 1.13% and 39% of the administered dose were recovered after 3 and 24 hours respectively. Tranexamic acid administered parenterally is distributed in a two compartment model. Tranexamic acid crosses the placenta, and may reach one hundredth of the serum peak concentration in the milk of lactating women. Tranexamic acid crosses the blood brain barrier.

Following intravenous administration, the biological half-life of tranexamic acid has been determined to be 1.9 hours and 2.7 hours.

5.3 Preclinical safety data

There are no preclinical data of relevance to the prescriber which are additional to that already included in other sections of the Summary of Product Characteristics.

6. PHARMACEUTICAL PARTICULARS

6.1 List of excipients

Core

Microcrystalline cellulose;

Hydroxypropyl cellulose;

Talc;

Magnesium stearate;

Colloidal anhydrous silica;

Povidone.

Coating

Methacrylate polymers;

Titanium dioxide;

Talc;

Magnesium stearate;

Polyethylene glycol 8000;

Vanillin.

6.2 Incompatibilities

None known.

6.3 Shelf life

Sixty months.

6.4 Special precautions for storage

Do not store above 25°C (blister packs only).

6.5 Nature and contents of container

White, high density polyethylene container with white, medium-density polyethylene screw cap and a polyethylene tamper-proof membrane, containing 50 tablets.

Blister packs of PVC/PVDC with aluminium foil backing containing 1 or 5 blister strips of 12 tablets each.

6.6 Instructions for use and handling

None

7. MARKETING AUTHORISATION HOLDER

Meda Pharmaceuticals Ltd

Regus House

Herald Way

Pegasus Business Park

Castle Donington Derbyshire

DE74 2TZ

United Kingdom

8. MARKETING AUTHORISATION NUMBER(S)

PL 19477/0016

9. DATE OF FIRST AUTHORISATION/RENEWAL OF THE AUTHORISATION

14th February 2005

10. DATE OF REVISION OF THE TEXT

11. LEGAL CATEGORY

POM

Cymbalta 30mg hard gastro-resistant capsules, Cymbalta 60mg hard gastro-resistant capsules

(Eli Lilly and Company Limited)

1. NAME OF THE MEDICINAL PRODUCT

Cymbalta* ▼ 30mg hard gastro-resistant capsules.

Cymbalta ▼60mg hard gastro-resistant capsules.

2. QUALITATIVE AND QUANTITATIVE COMPOSITION

The active ingredient in Cymbalta is duloxetine.

Each capsule contains 30mg of duloxetine as duloxetine hydrochloride.

Each capsule contains 60mg of duloxetine as duloxetine hydrochloride.

For excipients, see section 6.1.

3. PHARMACEUTICAL FORM

Hard gastro-resistant capsule.

The Cymbalta 30mg capsule has an opaque white body, imprinted with '30mg', and an opaque blue cap, imprinted with '9543'.

The Cymbalta 60mg capsule has an opaque green body, imprinted with '60mg', and an opaque blue cap, imprinted with '9542'.

4. CLINICAL PARTICULARS

4.1 Therapeutic indications

Treatment of major depressive episodes.

Treatment of diabetic peripheral neuropathic pain in adults.

4.2 Posology and method of administration

For oral use.

Adults

Major depressive episodes: The starting and recommended maintenance dose is 60mg once daily, with or without food. Dosages above 60mg once daily, up to a maximum dose of 120mg per day administered in evenly divided doses, have been evaluated from a safety perspective in clinical trials. However, there is no clinical evidence suggesting that patients not responding to the initial recommended dose may benefit from dose up-titrations.

Therapeutic response is usually seen after 2-4 weeks of treatment.

After consolidation of the antidepressive response, it is recommended to continue treatment for several months, in order to avoid relapse.

Diabetic peripheral neuropathic pain: The starting and recommended maintenance dose is 60mg daily, with or without food. Dosages above 60mg once daily, up to a maximum dose of 120mg per day administered in evenly divided doses, have been evaluated from a safety perspective in clinical trials. The plasma concentration of duloxetine displays large interindividual variability (see section 5.2). Hence, some patients that respond insufficiently to 60mg may benefit from a higher dose.

The medicinal product response should be evaluated after 2 months of treatment. Additional response after this time is unlikely (see section 5.1).

The therapeutic benefit should regularly (at least every 3 months) be reassessed.

Elderly

Major depressive episodes: No dosage adjustment is recommended for elderly patients solely on the basis of age. However, as with any medicine, caution should be exercised when treating the elderly, especially with Cymbalta 120mg per day for which data are limited (see sections 4.4 and 5.2).

Diabetic peripheral neuropathic pain: No dosage adjustment is recommended for elderly patients solely on the basis of age. However, caution should be exercised when treating the elderly (see section 5.2).

Children and Adolescents

The safety and efficacy of duloxetine in these age groups have not been studied. Therefore, administration of Cymbalta to children and adolescents is not recommended (see section 4.4).

Hepatic Impairment

Cymbalta should not be used in patients with liver disease resulting in hepatic impairment (see sections 4.3 and 5.2).

Renal Insufficiency

No dosage adjustment is necessary for patients with mild or moderate renal dysfunction (creatinine clearance 30 to 80ml/min). See section 4.3 for severe renal impairment.

Discontinuation of Treatment

When discontinuing Cymbalta after more than 1 week of therapy, it is generally recommended that the dose be tapered over no less than 2 weeks before discontinuation in an effort to decrease the risk of discontinuation symptoms. As a general recommendation, the dose should be reduced by half or administered on alternate days during this period. The precise regimen followed should, however, take into account the individual circumstances of the patient, such as duration of treatment, dose at discontinuation, etc.

4.3 Contraindications

Hypersensitivity to the active substance or to any of the excipients.

Concomitant use of Cymbalta with non-selective, irreversible monoamine oxidase inhibitors (MAOIs) is contra-indicated (see section 4.5).

Liver disease resulting in hepatic impairment (see section 5.2).

Cymbalta should not be used in combination with fluvoxamine, ciprofloxacin, or enoxacine (ie, potent CYP1A2 inhibitors), since the combination results in elevated plasma concentrations of duloxetine (see section 4.5).

Severe renal impairment (creatinine clearance <30ml/min).

4.4 Special warnings and special precautions for use

Mania and Seizures

Cymbalta should be used with caution in patients with a history of mania or a diagnosis of bipolar disorder and/or seizures.

Mydriasis

Mydriasis has been reported in association with duloxetine, therefore, caution should be used when prescribing Cymbalta to patients with increased intra-ocular pressure or those at risk of acute narrow-angle glaucoma.

Blood Pressure

In patients with known hypertension and/or other cardiac disease, blood pressure monitoring is recommended as appropriate.

Renal Impairment

Increased plasma concentrations of duloxetine occur in patients with severe renal impairment on haemodialysis (creatinine clearance <30ml/min). For patients with severe renal impairment, see section 4.3. See section 4.2 for information on patients with mild or moderate renal dysfunction.

Use With Antidepressants

Caution should be exercised when using Cymbalta in combination with antidepressants. In particular, the combination with selective, reversible MAOIs is not recommended.

St John's Wort

Undesirable effects may be more common during concomitant use of Cymbalta and herbal preparations containing St John's Wort (*Hypericum perforatum*).

Suicide

Major depressive episodes: Depression is associated with an increased risk of suicidal thoughts, self-harm, and suicide. This risk persists until significant remission occurs. As improvement may not occur during the first few weeks or more of treatment, patients should be closely monitored until such improvement occurs. It is general clinical experience with all antidepressant therapies that the risk of suicide may increase in the early stages of recovery. Cases of suicidal ideation and suicidal behaviours have been reported during duloxetine therapy or early after treatment discontinuation. Close supervision of high-risk patients should accompany drug therapy. Patients (and caregivers of patients) should be alerted about the need to monitor for the emergence of suicidal ideation/behaviour or thoughts of harming themselves and to seek medical advice immediately if these symptoms present.

No clinical trials have been conducted in the depressed paediatric population. Due to lack of clinical experience, duloxetine should not be used in children and adolescents under the age of 18 years for the treatment of major depressive episode. Safety and efficacy from data collected in adults with major depressive episode cannot be extrapolated to the paediatric population. For SSRIs/SNRIs, suicidal behaviour has been reported.

Diabetic peripheral neuropathic pain: As with other medicinal products with similar pharmacological action (antidepressants), isolated cases of suicidal ideation and suicidal behaviours have been reported during duloxetine therapy or early after treatment discontinuation. Physicians should encourage patients to report any distressing thoughts or feelings at any time.

Sucrose

Cymbalta hard gastro-resistant capsules contain sucrose. Patients with rare hereditary problems of fructose intolerance, glucose-galactose malabsorption, or sucrose-isomaltase insufficiency should not take this medicine.

Haemorrhage

There have been reports of cutaneous bleeding abnormalities, such as ecchymoses and purpura, with selective serotonin reuptake inhibitors (SSRIs). Caution is advised in patients taking anticoagulants and/or medicinal products known to affect platelet function, and in patients with known bleeding tendencies.

Hyponatraemia

Hyponatraemia has been reported rarely, predominantly in the elderly, when administering Cymbalta and other drugs of the same pharmacodynamic class.

Discontinuation of Treatment

Some patients may experience symptoms on discontinuation of Cymbalta, particularly if treatment is stopped abruptly (see sections 4.2 and 4.8).

Elderly

Major depressive episodes: Data on the use of Cymbalta 120mg in elderly patients with major depressive disorders are limited. Therefore, caution should be exercised when treating the elderly with the maximum dosage (see sections 4.2 and 5.2).

Medicinal Products Containing Duloxetine

Duloxetine is used under different trademarks in several indications (treatment of diabetic neuropathic pain, major depressive episodes, as well as stress urinary incontinence). The use of more than one of these products concomitantly should be avoided.

4.5 Interaction with other medicinal products and other forms of Interaction

CNS Medicinal Products

The risk of using duloxetine in combination with other CNS-active medicinal products has not been systematically evaluated, except in the cases described in this section. Consequently, caution is advised when Cymbalta is taken in combination with other centrally acting medicinal products and substances including alcohol and sedative medicinal products (eg, benzodiazepines, morphinomimetics, antipsychotics, phenobarbital, sedative antihistamines).

Monoamine Oxidase Inhibitors (MAOIs)

Due to the risk of serotonin syndrome, Cymbalta should not be used in combination with non-selective, irreversible monoamine oxidase inhibitors (MAOIs) or within at least 14 days of discontinuing treatment with an MAOI. Based on the half-life of duloxetine, at least 5 days should be allowed after stopping Cymbalta before starting an MAOI (see section 4.3).

For selective, reversible MAOIs, like moclobemide, the risk of serotonin syndrome is lower. However, the concomitant use of Cymbalta with selective, reversible MAOIs is not recommended (see section 4.4).

Serotonin Syndrome

In rare cases, serotonin syndrome has been reported in patients using SSRIs (eg, paroxetine, fluoxetine) concomitantly with serotonergic medicinal products. Caution is advisable if Cymbalta is used concomitantly with serotonergic antidepressants like SSRIs, tricyclics like clomipramine or amitriptyline, St John's Wort (*Hypericum perforatum*), venlafaxine, or triptans, tramadol, pethidine, and tryptophan.

Effect of Duloxetine on Other Drugs

Medicinal products metabolised by CYP1A2: In a clinical study, the pharmacokinetics of theophylline, a CYP1A2 substrate, were not significantly affected by co-administration with duloxetine (60mg twice daily). The study was performed in males and it cannot be excluded that females having a lower CYP1A2 activity and higher plasma concentrations of duloxetine may experience an interaction with a CYP1A2 substrate.

Medicinal products metabolised by CYP2D6: The co-administration of duloxetine (40mg twice daily) increases steady-state AUC of tolterodine (2mg twice daily) by 71%, but does not affect the pharmacokinetics of its 5-hydroxyl metabolite and no dosage adjustment is recommended. Caution is advised if Cymbalta is co-administered with medicinal products that are predominantly metabolised by CYP2D6 if they have a narrow therapeutic index.

Oral contraceptives and other steroidal agents: Results of *in vitro* studies demonstrate that duloxetine does not induce the catalytic activity of CYP3A. Specific *in vivo* drug interaction studies have not been performed.

Effects of Other Drugs on Duloxetine

Antacids and H_2 antagonists: Co-administration of duloxetine with aluminium- and magnesium-containing antacids or duloxetine with famotidine had no significant effect on the rate or extent of duloxetine absorption after administration of a 40mg oral dose.

Inhibitors of CYP1A2: Because CYP1A2 is involved in duloxetine metabolism, concomitant use of duloxetine with potent inhibitors of CYP1A2 is likely to result in higher concentrations of duloxetine. Fluvoxamine (100mg once daily), a potent inhibitor of CYP1A2, decreased the apparent plasma clearance of duloxetine by about 77% and increased $AUC_{0\text{-}t}$ 6-fold. Therefore, Cymbalta should not be administered in combination with potent inhibitors of CYP1A2 like fluvoxamine (see section 4.3).

Inducers of CYP1A2: Population pharmacokinetic studies have shown that smokers have almost 50% lower plasma concentrations of duloxetine compared with non-smokers.

4.6 Pregnancy and lactation

Pregnancy

There are no data on the use of duloxetine in pregnant women. Studies in animals have shown reproductive toxicity at systemic exposure levels (AUC) of duloxetine lower than the maximum clinical exposure (see section 5.3).

The potential risk for humans is unknown. As with other serotonergic drugs, discontinuation symptoms may occur in the neonate after maternal duloxetine use near term. Cymbalta should be used in pregnancy only if the potential benefit justifies the potential risk to the foetus. Women should be advised to notify their physician if they become pregnant, or intend to become pregnant, during therapy.

Breast-Feeding

Duloxetine and/or its metabolites are excreted into the milk of lactating rats. Adverse behavioural effects were seen in offspring in a perinatal/postnatal toxicity study in rats (see section 5.3). Excretion of duloxetine and/or metabolites into human milk has not been studied. The use of Cymbalta while breast-feeding is not recommended.

4.7 Effects on ability to drive and use machines

Although in controlled studies duloxetine has not been shown to impair psychomotor performance, cognitive function, or memory, it may be associated with sedation. Patients should be cautioned about their ability to drive a car or operate hazardous machinery.

4.8 Undesirable effects

Tables 1 and 2 give the frequency of adverse reactions from placebo-controlled clinical trials in depression and diabetic neuropathic pain. The adverse reactions reported in these tables are those events that occurred in 1% or more of patients treated with duloxetine and were reported significantly more often in patients taking duloxetine than placebo or where the event was considered clinically relevant.

The most commonly reported adverse reactions in patients with depression treated with Cymbalta were nausea, dry mouth, and constipation. However, the majority of common adverse reactions were mild to moderate, they usually started early in therapy, and most tended to subside even as therapy was continued. The most commonly observed adverse reactions in patients with diabetic neuropathic pain treated with Cymbalta were nausea, somnolence, dizziness, constipation, and fatigue.

Table 1. **Very Common Adverse Reactions (⩾10%)**

System Organ Class	Adverse Reaction	Cymbalta n = 1,592 (%)	Placebo n = 1,000 (%)
Psychiatric disorders	Insomnia	10	6
Nervous system disorders	Dizziness Somnolence	11 10	5 3
Gastro-intestinal disorders	Nausea Dry mouth Constipation	22 13 12	7 6 4

Table 2. **Common Adverse Reactions (⩾1%, <10%)**
(see Table 2 below)

Discontinuation symptoms have been reported when stopping Cymbalta. Common symptoms, particularly on abrupt discontinuation, include dizziness, nausea, insomnia, headache, and anxiety (see sections 4.2 and 4.4).

Duloxetine treatment in clinical trials was associated with numerically significant, but not clinically related, increases in ALT, AST, alkaline phosphatase, and creatinine phosphokinase (CPK); transient, abnormal values of these enzymes were infrequently observed in duloxetine-treated patients compared with placebo-treated patients.

Duloxetine is known to affect urethral resistance. In placebo-controlled trials, urinary hesitation was reported rarely (<1%) in male patients. If symptoms of urinary hesitation develop during treatment with duloxetine, consideration should be given that they might be drug-related.

In clinical trials of duloxetine in patients with diabetic neuropathic pain, small but statistically significant increases in fasting blood glucose were observed in duloxetine-treated patients compared to placebo at 12 weeks and routine care at 52 weeks. The increase was similar at both time points and was not considered clinically relevant. Relative to placebo or routine care, mean HbA_{1c} values were stable, there was no mean weight gain, mean lipid concentrations (cholesterol, LDL, HDL, triglycerides) were stable, and there were no differences in incidence of serious and non-serious diabetes-related adverse reactions.

Electrocardiograms were obtained from 1,139 duloxetine-treated patients and 777 placebo-treated patients in 8-week clinical trials in major depressive disorder, and from 528 duloxetine-treated and 205 placebo-treated patients with diabetic neuropathic pain in clinical trials lasting up to 13 weeks. The heart rate-corrected QT interval in duloxetine-treated patients did not differ from that seen in placebo-treated patients. No clinically significant differences

Table 2 Common Adverse Reactions (⩾1%, <10%)

System Organ Class	Adverse Reaction	Cymbalta n = 1,592 (%)	Placebo n = 1,000 (%)
Metabolism and nutrition disorders	Decreased appetite Anorexia	6 2	2 <1
Psychiatric disorders	Decreased libido Anorgasmia Middle insomnia	2 2 1	<1 0 <1
Nervous system disorders	Tremor Sedation Hypersomnia	3 1[a] 1	1 <1[a] <1
Eye disorders	Vision blurred	3	1
Vascular disorders	Hot flush	2	1
Respiratory, thoracic, and mediastinal disorders	Yawning	1	0
Gastro-intestinal disorders	Diarrhoea Vomiting	8 5	6 3
Skin and subcutaneous tissue disorders	Increased sweat Night sweats	7 1	2 <1
Musculoskeletal and connective tissue disorders	Muscle tightness	1	<1
Reproductive system and breast disorders	Erectile dysfunction* Ejaculation disorder*	5 2	1 <1
General disorders and administration site conditions	Fatigue Lethargy Feeling jittery	9 1 1	4 <1 <1
Investigations	Weight decreased	2	1

*Adjusted for gender (n males = duloxetine 660, placebo 375).

[a]Values rounded from a frequency of 1.3% (duloxetine) and 0.6% (placebo).

were observed for QT, PR, QRS, or QTcB measurements between duloxetine-treated and placebo-treated patients.

Cases of suicidal ideation and suicidal behaviours have been reported during duloxetine therapy or early after treatment discontinuation (see section 4.4).

4.9 Overdose

There is limited clinical experience with duloxetine overdose in humans. In pre-marketing clinical trials, no cases of fatal overdose of duloxetine have been reported. Cases of acute ingestions up to 1400mg, alone or in combination with other medicinal products, have been reported.

No specific antidote is known for duloxetine. A free airway should be established. Monitoring of cardiac and vital signs is recommended, along with appropriate symptomatic and supportive measures. Gastric lavage may be indicated if performed soon after ingestion or in symptomatic patients. Activated charcoal may be useful in limiting absorption. Duloxetine has a large volume of distribution and forced diuresis, haemoperfusion, and exchange perfusion are unlikely to be beneficial.

5. PHARMACOLOGICAL PROPERTIES

5.1 Pharmacodynamic properties

Pharmacotherapeutic group: Other antidepressants. *ATC code:* N06AX21.

Duloxetine is a combined serotonin (5-HT) and noradrenaline (NA) reuptake inhibitor. It weakly inhibits dopamine reuptake, with no significant affinity for histaminergic, dopaminergic, cholinergic, and adrenergic receptors. Duloxetine dose-dependently increases extracellular levels of serotonin and noradrenaline in various brain areas of animals.

Duloxetine normalised pain thresholds in several preclinical models of neuropathic and inflammatory pain and attenuated pain behaviour in a model of persistent pain. The pain inhibitory action of duloxetine is believed to be a result of potentiation of descending inhibitory pain pathways within the central nervous system.

Major Depressive Episodes

Cymbalta was studied in a clinical programme involving 3,158 patients (1,285 patient-years of exposure) meeting DSM-IV criteria for major depression. The efficacy of Cymbalta at the recommended dose of 60mg once a day was demonstrated in three out of three randomised, double-blind, placebo-controlled, fixed dose acute studies in adult outpatients with major depressive disorder. Overall, Cymbalta's efficacy has been demonstrated at daily doses between 60 and 120mg in a total of five out of seven randomised, double-blind, placebo-controlled, fixed dose acute studies in adult outpatients with major depressive disorder.

Cymbalta demonstrated statistical superiority over placebo as measured by improvement in the 17-item Hamilton Depression Rating Scale (HAM-D) total score (including both the emotional and somatic symptoms of depression). Response and remission rates were also statistically significantly higher with Cymbalta compared with placebo. Only a small proportion of patients included in pivotal clinical trials had severe depression (baseline HAM-D >25).

In a relapse prevention study, patients responding to 12 weeks of acute treatment with open-label Cymbalta 60mg once daily were randomised to either Cymbalta 60mg once daily or placebo for a further 6 months. Cymbalta 60mg once daily demonstrated a statistically significant superiority compared to placebo ($P = 0.004$) on the primary outcome measure, the prevention of depressive relapse, as measured by time to relapse. The incidence of relapse during the 6 months double-blind follow-up period was 17% and 29% for duloxetine and placebo, respectively.

The effect of Cymbalta 60mg once a day in elderly depressed patients (⩾65 years) was specifically examined in a study that showed a statistically significative difference in the reduction of the $HAM\text{-}D_{17}$ score for duloxetine-treated patients compared to placebo. Tolerability of Cymbalta 60mg once daily in elderly patients was comparable to that seen in the younger adults. However, data on elderly patients exposed to the maximum dose (120mg per day) are limited and thus, caution is recommended when treating this population.

Diabetic Peripheral Neuropathic Pain

The efficacy of duloxetine as a treatment for diabetic neuropathic pain was established in 2 randomised, 12-week, double-blind, placebo-controlled, fixed dose studies in adults (22 to 88 years) having diabetic neuropathic pain for at least 6 months. Patients meeting diagnostic criteria for major depressive disorder were excluded from these trials. The primary outcome measure was the weekly mean of 24-hour average pain, which was collected in a daily diary by patients on an 11-point Likert scale.

In both studies, duloxetine 60mg once daily and 60mg twice daily significantly reduced pain compared with placebo. The effect in some patients was apparent in the first week of treatment. The difference in mean improvement between the two active treatment arms was not significant. At least 30% reported pain reduction was recorded in approximately 65% of duloxetine-treated patients versus 40% for placebo. The corresponding figures for at least 50% pain reduction were 50% and 26%, respectively. Clinical response rates (50% or greater improvement in pain) were analysed according to whether or not the patient experienced somnolence during treatment. For patients not experiencing somnolence, clinical response was observed in 47% of patients receiving duloxetine and 27% patients on placebo. Clinical response rates in patients experiencing somnolence were 60% on duloxetine and 30% on placebo. Patients not demonstrating a pain reduction of 30% within 60 days of treatment were unlikely to reach this level during further treatment.

Although data from a one-year open label study offer some evidence for longer-term efficacy, no conclusive efficacy data for treatments longer than 12 weeks duration are available from placebo-controlled studies.

5.2 Pharmacokinetic properties

Duloxetine is administered as a single enantiomer. Duloxetine is extensively metabolised by oxidative enzymes (CYP1A2 and the polymorphic CYP2D6), followed by conjugation. The pharmacokinetics of duloxetine demonstrate large intersubject variability (generally 50-60%), partly due to gender, age, smoking status, and CYP2D6 metaboliser status.

Duloxetine is well absorbed after oral administration, with a C_{max} occurring 6 hours post-dose. The absolute oral bioavailability of duloxetine ranged from 32% to 80% (mean of 50%). Food delays the time to reach the peak concentration from 6 to 10 hours and it marginally decreases the extent of absorption (approximately 11%). These changes do not have any clinical significance. Duloxetine is approximately 96% bound to human plasma proteins. Duloxetine binds to both albumin and alpha$_1$-acid glycoprotein. Protein binding is not affected by renal or hepatic impairment.

Duloxetine is extensively metabolised and the metabolites are excreted principally in urine. Both cytochromes P450-2D6 and 1A2 catalyse the formation of the two major metabolites, glucuronide conjugate of 4-hydroxy duloxetine and sulphate conjugate of 5-hydroxy,6-methoxy duloxetine. Based upon *in vitro* studies, the circulating metabolites of duloxetine are considered pharmacologically inactive. The pharmacokinetics of duloxetine in patients who are poor metabolisers with respect to CYP2D6 has not been specifically investigated. Limited data suggest that the plasma levels of duloxetine are higher in these patients.

The elimination half-life of duloxetine ranges from 8 to 17 hours (mean of 12 hours). After an intravenous dose the plasma clearance of duloxetine ranges from 22 l/hr to 46 l/hr (mean of 36 l/hr). After an oral dose the apparent plasma clearance of duloxetine ranges from 33 to 261 l/hr (mean 101 l/hr).

Special Populations

Gender: Pharmacokinetic differences have been identified between males and females (apparent plasma clearance is approximately 50% lower in females). Based upon the overlap in the range of clearance, gender-based pharmacokinetic differences do not justify the recommendation for using a lower dose for female patients.

Age: Pharmacokinetic differences have been identified between younger and elderly females (⩾65 years) (AUC increases by about 25% and half-life is about 25% longer in the elderly), although the magnitude of these changes is not sufficient to justify adjustments to the dose. As a general recommendation, caution should be exercised when treating the elderly (see sections 4.2 and 4.4).

Renal impairment: End stage renal disease (ESRD) patients receiving dialysis had 2-fold higher duloxetine C_{max} and AUC values compared with healthy subjects. Pharmacokinetic data on duloxetine is limited in patients with mild or moderate renal impairment.

Hepatic impairment: Moderate liver disease (Child-Pugh class B) affected the pharmacokinetics of duloxetine. Compared with healthy subjects, the apparent plasma clearance of duloxetine was 79% lower, the apparent terminal half-life was 2.3-times longer, and the AUC was 3.7-times higher in patients with moderate liver disease. The pharmacokinetics of duloxetine and its metabolites have not been studied in patients with mild or severe hepatic insufficiency.

5.3 Preclinical safety data

Duloxetine was not genotoxic in a standard battery of tests and was not carcinogenic in rats.

Multinucleated cells were seen in the liver in the absence of other histopathological changes in the rat carcinogenicity study. The underlying mechanism and the clinical relevance are unknown. Female mice receiving duloxetine for 2 years had an increased incidence of hepatocellular adenomas and carcinomas at the high dose only (144mg/kg/day), but these were considered to be secondary to hepatic microsomal enzyme induction. The relevance of this mouse data to humans is unknown. Female rats receiving duloxetine (45mg/kg/day) before and during mating and early pregnancy had a decrease in maternal food consumption and body weight, oestrous cycle disruption, decreased live birth indices and progeny survival, and progeny growth retardation at systemic exposure levels estimated to be at the most at maximum clinical exposure (AUC). In an embryotoxicity study in the rabbit, a higher incidence of cardiovascular and skeletal malformations was observed at systemic exposure levels below the maximum clinical exposure (AUC). No malformations were observed in another study testing a higher dose of a different salt of duloxetine. In prenatal/postnatal toxicity studies in the rat, duloxetine induced adverse behavioural effects in the offspring at exposures below maximum clinical exposure (AUC).

6. PHARMACEUTICAL PARTICULARS

6.1 List of excipients

Capsule Content

Hypromellose

Hydroxypropyl methylcellulose acetate succinate

Sucrose

Sugar spheres

Talc

Titanium dioxide (E171)

Triethyl citrate

Capsule Shell

30 mg:

Gelatin, sodium lauryl sulfate, titanium dioxide (E171), indigo carmine (E132), edible green ink. Edible green ink contains: black iron oxide - synthetic (E172), yellow iron oxide - synthetic (E172), propylene glycol, shellac.

60 mg:

Gelatin, sodium lauryl sulfate, titanium dioxide (E171), indigo carmine (E132), yellow iron oxide (E172), edible white ink. Edible white ink contains: titanium dioxide (E171), propylene glycol, shellac, povidone.

Capsule Shell Cap Colour

30 mg:

Opaque blue.

60 mg:

Opaque blue.

Capsule Shell Body Colour

30 mg:

Opaque white.

60 mg:

Opaque green.

6.2 Incompatibilities

Not applicable.

6.3 Shelf life

3 years.

6.4 Special precautions for storage

Store in the original package. Do not store above 30°C.

6.5 Nature and contents of container

Polyvinylchloride (PVC), polyethylene (PE), and polychlorotrifluoroethylene (PCTFE) blister sealed with an aluminium foil.

Cymbalta 30mg is available in packs of 7 and 28 capsules.

Cymbalta 60mg is available in packs of 28, 56, 84, and 98 capsules.

Not all pack sizes may be marketed.

6.6 Instructions for use and handling

No special requirements.

7. MARKETING AUTHORISATION HOLDER

Eli Lilly Nederland BV, Grootslag 1-5, NL-3991 RA Houten, The Netherlands.

8. MARKETING AUTHORISATION NUMBER(S)

30mg, 7 capsules: EU/1/04/296/006

30mg, 28 capsules: EU/1/04/296/001

60mg, 28 capsules: EU/1/04/296/002

60mg, 56 capsules: EU/1/04/296/005

60mg, 84 capsules: EU/1/04/296/003

60mg, 98 capsules: EU/1/04/296/004

9. DATE OF FIRST AUTHORISATION/RENEWAL OF THE AUTHORISATION

Date of first authorisation: 17 December 2004

10. DATE OF REVISION OF THE TEXT

4 July 2005

LEGAL CATEGORY

POM

*CYMBALTA (duloxetine) is a trademark of Eli Lilly and Company. CYM2M

Cymevene IV

(Roche Products Limited)

1. NAME OF THE MEDICINAL PRODUCT

Cymevene® powder for infusion.

2. QUALITATIVE AND QUANTITATIVE COMPOSITION

Ganciclovir 500mg (as ganciclovir sodium 546mg).

3. PHARMACEUTICAL FORM

Sterile, freeze-dried powder for reconstitution with Water for Injections.

4. CLINICAL PARTICULARS

4.1 Therapeutic indications

Cymevene is indicated for the treatment of life-threatening or sight-threatening cytomegalovirus (CMV) infections in immunocompromised individuals. These states include acquired immunodeficiency syndrome (AIDS), iatrogenic immunosuppression associated with organ transplantation, or chemotherapy for neoplasia.

Cymevene may also be used for the prevention of CMV disease, specifically in those patients receiving immunosuppressive therapy secondary to organ transplantation.

4.2 Posology and method of administration

For intravenous infusion following reconstitution with 10ml Water for Injections BP. Based on patient weight and therapeutic indication the appropriate calculated dose volume should be removed from the vial (ganciclovir concentration 50mg/ml) and added to an acceptable infusion fluid (typically 100ml) for delivery over the course of 1 hour. Infusion concentrations greater than 10mg/ml are not recommended. (See section *6.6 Instructions for use/handling*).

Adults

Treatment of CMV infection

Initial (induction) treatment: 5mg/kg infused at a constant rate over 1 hour every 12 hours (10mg/kg/day) for 14 to 21 days.

Long-term (maintenance) treatment: For immunocompromised patients at risk of relapse of CMV retinitis a course of maintenance therapy may be given. Intravenous infusion of 6mg/kg once daily 5 days per week, or 5mg/kg once daily 7 days per week is recommended.

Treatment of disease progression: Indefinite treatment may be required in patients with AIDS, but even with continued maintenance treatment, patients may have progression of retinitis. Any patient in whom the retinitis progresses, either while on maintenance treatment or because treatment with Cymevene has been withdrawn, may be re-treated using the induction treatment regimen.

Prevention of CMV disease

Induction regimen: 5mg/kg infused every 12 hours (10mg/kg/day) for 7 to 14 days.

Maintenance regimen: Intravenous infusion of 6mg/kg once daily 5 days per week, or 5mg/kg once daily 7 days per week is recommended.

Special dosage instructions

Patients with renal impairment:

Serum creatinine levels or creatinine clearance should be monitored carefully. Dosage adjustment is required according to creatinine clearance as shown in the table below (see section *4.4 Special warnings and precautions for use and section 5.2 Pharmacokinetic properties*).

An estimated creatinine clearance (ml/min) can be related to serum creatinine by the following formulae:

$$\text{For males} = \frac{(140 - \text{age[years]}) \times (\text{body weight [kg]})}{(72 \times (0.011 \times \text{serum creatinine [micromol/L]})}$$

For females = 0.85 × male value

CrCl	Induction dose of ganciclovir
⩾ 70ml/min	5.0mg/kg every 12 hours
50 - 69ml/min	2.5mg/kg every 12 hours
25 - 49ml/min	2.5mg/kg/day
10 - 24ml/min	1.25mg/kg/day
< 10ml/min	1.25mg/kg/day after haemodialysis

Elderly patients

No studies on the efficacy or safety of Cymevene in elderly patients have been conducted. Since elderly individuals often have reduced renal function, Cymevene should be administered to elderly patients with special consideration for their renal status (see above).

Paediatric patients

There has been limited clinical experience in treating patients under the age of 12 years (see section *4.4 Special warnings and precautions for use* and *5.2 Pharmacokinetic properties*). Reported adverse events were similar to those seen in adults. However, the use of Cymevene in children warrants extreme caution due to the potential for long-term carcinogenicity and reproductive toxicity. The benefits of treatment should outweigh the risks. Cymevene is not indicated for the treatment of congenital or neonatal CMV infections.

Dosage reductions

For less severe neutropenia or other cytopenias a reduction in the total daily dose should be considered. Cell counts usually normalise within 3 to 7 days after discontinuing the drug or decreasing the dose. As evidence of marrow recovery becomes apparent gradual increases in dose, with careful monitoring of white blood cell counts, may be appropriate.

Patients with severe leucopenia, neutropenia, anaemia, thrombocytopenia and pancytopenia

See section *4.4 Special warnings and precautions for use* before initiation of therapy.

If there is a significant deterioration of blood cell counts during therapy with Cymevene, treatment with haematopoetic growth factors and/or dose interruption should be considered (see section *4.4 Special warnings and precautions for use* and section *4.8 Undesirable effects*).

Method of administration

Cymevene is a powder for solution for intravenous infusion. For directions on the preparation of the infusion solution, see section *6.6 Instructions for use and handling, and disposal*.

Cymevene must only be given by intravenous infusion, preferably via a plastic cannula, into a vein with adequate blood flow.

Caution - do not administer by rapid or bolus i.v. injection! The toxicity of Cymevene may be increased as a result of excessive plasma levels.

Caution - i.m. or s.c. injection may result in severe tissue irritation due to the high pH (~11) of ganciclovir solutions.

The recommended dosage, frequency, or infusion rates should not be exceeded.

Caution should be exercised in the handling of Cymevene, see section *6.6 Instructions for use and handling, and disposal*.

4.3 Contraindications

Cymevene is contra-indicated in patients with hypersensitivity to ganciclovir or valganciclovir.

Due to the similarity of the chemical structure of Cymevene and that of aciclovir and valaciclovir, a cross-hypersensitivity reaction between these drugs is possible. Therefore, Cymevene is contra-indicated in patients with hypersensitivity to aciclovir and valaciclovir.

Cymevene is contra-indicated during pregnancy and lactation, refer to section *4.6 Pregnancy and lactation*.

4.4 Special warnings and special precautions for use

Prior to initiation of ganciclovir treatment, patients should be advised of the potential risks to the foetus. In animal studies ganciclovir was found to be mutagenic, teratogenic, aspermatogenic and carcinogenic and a suppressor of female fertility. Cymevene should therefore be considered a potential teratogen and carcinogen in humans with the potential to cause birth defects and cancers (see section *5.3 Preclinical safety data*). It is also considered likely that Cymevene causes temporary or permanent inhibition of spermatogenesis. Women of child bearing potential must be advised to use effective contraception during treatment. Men must be advised to practise barrier contraception during treatment, and for at least 90 days thereafter, unless it is certain that the female partner is not at risk of pregnancy (see section *4.6 Pregnancy and lactation*, section *4.8 Undesirable effects* and section *5.3 Preclinical safety data*).

The use of Cymevene in children and adolescents warrants extreme caution due to the potential for long-term carcinogenicity and reproductive toxicity. The benefits of treatment should outweigh the risks.

Severe leucopenia, neutropenia, anaemia, thrombocytopenia, pancytopenia, bone marrow depression and aplastic anaemia have been observed in patients treated with Cymevene. Therapy should not be initiated if the absolute neutrophil count is less than 500 cells/μL, or the platelet count is less than 25000/μL, or the haemoglobin level is less than 8g/dL (see section 4.2 Posology and method of administration, Special dosage instructions and section 4.8 Undesirable effects).

Cymevene should be used with caution in patients with pre-existing haematological cytopenia or a history of drug-related haematological cytopenia and in patients receiving radiotherapy.

It is recommended that complete blood counts and platelet counts be monitored during therapy. Increased haematological monitoring may be warranted in patients with renal impairment. In patients developing severe leucopenia, neutropenia, anaemia and/or thrombocytopenia, it is recommended that treatment with haematopoietic growth factors and/or dose interruption be considered (see section *4.2 Posology and method of administration*, Special dosage instructions and section *4.8 Undesirable effects*).

In patients with impaired renal function, dosage adjustments based on creatinine clearance are required (see section *4.2 Posology and method of administration*, Special dosage instructions and section *5.2 Pharmacokinetic properties, Pharmacokinetics in special populations*).

Convulsions have been reported in patients taking imipenem-cilastatin and ganciclovir. Cymevene should not be used concomitantly with imipenem-cilastatin unless the potential benefits outweigh the potential risks (see section *4.5 Interaction with other medicinal products and other forms of interaction*).

Patients treated with Cymevene and (a) didanosine, (b) drugs that are known to be myelosuppressive (e.g. zidovudine), or (c) substances affecting renal function, should be closely monitored for signs of added toxicity (see section *4.5 Interaction with other medicinal products and other forms of interaction*).

4.5 Interaction with other medicinal products and other forms of Interaction

Imipenem-cilastatin

Convulsions have been reported in patients taking ganciclovir and imipenem-cilastatin concomitantly. These drugs should not be used concomitantly unless the potential benefits outweigh the potential risks (see section *4.4 Special warnings and precautions for use*).

Probenecid

Probenecid given with oral ganciclovir resulted in statistically significantly decreased renal clearance of ganciclovir (20%) leading to statistically significantly increased exposure (40%). These changes were consistent with a mechanism of interaction involving competition for renal tubular secretion. Therefore, patients taking probenecid and Cymevene should be closely monitored for ganciclovir toxicity.

Zidovudine

When zidovudine was given in the presence of oral ganciclovir there was a small (17%), but statistically significant increase in the AUC of zidovudine. There was also a trend towards lower ganciclovir concentrations when administered with zidovudine, although this was not statistically significant. However, since both zidovudine and ganciclovir have the potential to cause neutropenia and anaemia, some patients may not tolerate concomitant therapy at full dosage (see section *4.4 Special warnings and precautions for use*).

Didanosine

Didanosine plasma concentrations were found to be consistently raised when given with ganciclovir (both intravenous and oral). At ganciclovir oral doses of 3 and 6g/day, an increase in the AUC of didanosine ranging from 84 to 124% has been observed, and likewise at intravenous doses of 5 and 10 mg/kg/day, an increase in the AUC of didanosine ranging from 38 to 67% has been observed. There was no clinically significant effect on ganciclovir concentrations. Patients should be closely monitored for didanosine toxicity (see section *4.4 Special warnings and precautions for use*).

Mycophenolate Mofetil

Based on the results of a single dose administration study of recommended doses of oral mycophenolate mofetil (MMF) and intravenous ganciclovir and the known effects of renal impairment on the pharmacokinetics of MMF and ganciclovir, it is anticipated that co-administration of these agents (which have the potential to compete for renal tubular secretion) will result in increases in phenolic glucuronide of mycophenolic acid (MPAG) and ganciclovir concentration. No substantial alteration of mycophenolic acid (MPA) pharmacokinetics is anticipated and MMF dose adjustment is not required. In patients with renal impairment to whom MMF and ganciclovir are co-administered, the dose recommendation of ganciclovir should be observed and the patients monitored carefully.

Zalcitabine

No clinically significant pharmacokinetic changes were observed after concomitant administration of ganciclovir and zalcitabine. Both valganciclovir and zalcitabine have the potential to cause peripheral neuropathy and patients should be monitored for such events.

Stavudine

No clinically significant interactions were observed when stavudine and oral ganciclovir were given in combination.

Trimethoprim

No clinically significant pharmacokinetic interaction was observed when trimethoprim and oral ganciclovir were given in combination. However, there is a potential for toxicity to be enhanced since both drugs are known to be myelosuppressive and therefore both drugs should be used concomitantly only if the potential benefits outweigh the risks.

Other antiretrovirals

At clinically relevant concentrations, there is unlikely to be either a synergistic or antagonistic effect on the inhibition of either HIV in the presence of ganciclovir or CMV in the presence of a variety of antiretroviral drugs. Metabolic interactions with, for example, protease inhibitors and non-nucleoside reverse transcriptase inhibitors (NNRTIs) are unlikely due to the lack of P450 involvement in the metabolism of ganciclovir.

Other potential drug interactions

Toxicity may be enhanced when ganciclovir is co-administered with, or is given immediately before or after, other drugs that inhibit replication of rapidly dividing cell populations such as occur in the bone marrow, testes and germinal layers of the skin and gastrointestinal mucosa. Examples of these types of drugs are dapsone, pentamidine, flucytosine, vincristine, vinblastine, adriamycin, amphotericin B, trimethoprim/sulpha combinations, nucleoside analogues and hydroxyurea.

Since ganciclovir is excreted through the kidney (section *5.2*), toxicity may also be enhanced during co-administration of ganciclovir with drugs that might reduce the renal clearance of ganciclovir and hence increase its exposure. The renal clearance of ganciclovir might be inhibited by two mechanisms: (a) nephrotoxicity, caused by drugs such as cidofovir and foscarnet, and (b) competitive inhibition of active tubular secretion in the kidney by, for example, other nucleoside analogues.

Therefore, all of these drugs should be considered for concomitant use with ganciclovir only if the potential benefits outweigh the potential risks (see section *4.4 Special warnings and precautions for use*).

4.6 Pregnancy and lactation

The safety of Cymevene for use in human pregnancy has not been established. Ganciclovir readily diffuses across the human placenta. Based on its pharmacological mechanism of action and reproductive toxicity observed in animal studies with ganciclovir (see section *5.3 Preclinical safety data*), there is a theoretical risk of teratogenicity in humans. Therefore, Cymevene should not be given to pregnant women as there is a high likelihood of damage to the developing foetus.

Women of childbearing potential must be advised to use effective contraception during treatment. Male patients should be advised to practise barrier contraception during, and for at least 90 days following treatment unless it is certain that the female partner is not at risk of pregnancy (see section *5.3 Preclinical safety data*).

It is unknown if ganciclovir is excreted in breast milk, but the possibility of ganciclovir being excreted in the breast milk and causing serious adverse reactions in the nursing infant cannot be discounted. Therefore, breastfeeding must be discontinued.

4.7 Effects on ability to drive and use machines

No studies on the effects on the ability to drive and use machines have been performed.

Convulsion, sedation, dizziness, ataxia and/or confusion have been reported with the use of Cymevene. If they occur, such effects may affect tasks requiring alertness including the patient's ability to drive and operate machinery.

4.8 Undesirable effects

In patients who were being treated with ganciclovir the most common haematological side effects were neutropenia, anaemia and thrombocytopenia.

Adverse reactions reported with i.v. ganciclovir, oral ganciclovir and valganciclovir are presented in the table below. Valganciclovir is a pro-drug of ganciclovir, and adverse reactions associated with valganciclovir can be expected to occur with ganciclovir. The frequency groupings of these adverse events are based upon the frequency recorded in clinical trials with CMV retinitis patients with AIDS and in clinical trials with solid organ transplant patients.

Infections and infestations:	
Common (⩾ 1/100, < 1/10):	Sepsis (bacteremia, viraemia), cellulitis, urinary tract infection, oral candidiasis.
Blood and lymphatic disorders:	
Very common (⩾ 1/10):	neutropenia, anaemia.
Common (⩾ 1/100, < 1/10):	thrombocytopenia, leucopenia, pancytopenia.
Uncommon (⩾ 1/1000, < 1/100):	bone marrow depression.
Immune system disorders:	
Uncommon (⩾ 1/1000, < 1/100):	anaphylactic reaction.
Metabolic and nutrition disorders:	
Common (⩾ 1/100, < 1/10):	appetite decreased, anorexia.
Psychiatric disorders:	
Common (⩾ 1/100, < 1/10):	depression, anxiety, confusion, abnormal thinking.
Uncommon (⩾ 1/1000, < 1/100):	agitation, psychotic disorder
Nervous system disorders:	
Common (⩾ 1/100, < 1/10):	headache, insomnia, dysgeusia (taste disturbance), hypoaesthesia, paraesthesia, peripheral neuropathy, convulsions, dizziness (excluding vertigo).
Uncommon (⩾ 1/1000, < 1/100):	tremor.
Eye disorders:	
Common (⩾ 1/100, < 1/10):	macular oedema, retinal detachment, vitreous floaters, eye pain.
Uncommon (⩾ 1/1000, < 1/100):	vision abnormal, conjunctivitis.
Ear and labyrinth disorders:	
Common (⩾ 1/100, < 1/10):	ear pain
Uncommon (⩾ 1/1000, < 1/100):	deafness.
Cardiac disorders:	
Uncommon (⩾ 1/1000, < 1/100):	arrhythmias.
Vascular disorders:	
Uncommon (⩾ 1/1000, < 1/100):	hypotension.
Respiratory, thoracic and mediastinal disorders:	
Very common (⩾ 1/10):	dyspnoea.
Common (⩾ 1/100, < 1/10):	cough.
Gastrointestinal disorders:	
Very common (⩾ 1/10):	diarrhoea.
Common (⩾ 1/100, < 1/10):	nausea, vomiting, abdominal pain, abdominal pain upper, constipation, flatulence, dysphagia, dyspepsia.
Uncommon (⩾1/1000, <1/100):	abdominal distention, mouth ulcerations, pancreatitis.
Hepato-biliary disorders:	
Common (⩾ 1/100, < 1/10):	hepatic function abnormal, blood alkaline phosphatase increased, aspartate aminotransferase increased.
Uncommon (⩾ 1/1000, < 1/100):	alanine aminotransferase increased.
Skin and subcutaneous tissues disorders:	
Common (⩾ 1/100, < 1/10):	dermatitis, night sweats, pruritus.
Uncommon (⩾ 1/1000, < 1/100):	alopecia, urticaria, dry skin.
Musculo-skeletal and connective tissue disorders:	
Common (⩾ 1/100, < 1/10):	back pain, myalgia, arthralgia, muscle cramps.
Renal and urinary disorders:	
Common (⩾ 1/100, < 1/10):	creatinine clearance renal decreased, renal impairment.
Uncommon (⩾ 1/1000, < 1/100):	haematuria, renal failure.
Reproductive system and breast disorders:	
Uncommon (⩾ 1/1000, < 1/100):	male infertility.
General disorders and administration site conditions:	
Common (⩾ 1/100, < 1/10):	fatigue, pyrexia, rigors, pain, chest pain, malaise, asthenia, injection site reaction (intravenous ganciclovir only).
Investigations:	
Common (⩾ 1/100, < 1/10):	weight decreased, blood creatinine increased.

4.9 Overdose

Overdose experience with intravenous ganciclovir

Reports of overdoses with intravenous ganciclovir have been received from clinical trials and during post-marketing experience. In some of these cases no adverse events were reported. The majority of patients experienced one or more of the following adverse events:

– *Haematological toxicity* - pancytopenia, bone marrow depression, medullary aplasia, leucopenia, neutropenia, granulocytopenia.

– *Hepatotoxicity* - hepatitis, liver function disorder.

– *Renal toxicity* - worsening of haematuria in a patient with pre-existing renal impairment, acute renal failure, elevated creatinine.

– *Gastrointestinal toxicity* - abdominal pain, diarrhoea, vomiting.

– *Neurotoxicity* - generalised tremor, convulsion.

In addition, one adult received an excessive volume of i.v. ganciclovir solution by intravitreal injection, and experienced temporary loss of vision and central retinal artery occlusion secondary to increased intraocular pressure related to the injected fluid volume.

Haemodialysis and hydration may be of benefit in reducing blood plasma levels in patients who receive an overdose of ganciclovir (see section 5.2 Pharmacokinetic properties, Patients undergoing haemodialysis).

Overdose experience with valganciclovir

One adult developed fatal bone marrow depression (medullary aplasia) after several days of dosing that was at least 10-fold greater than recommended for the patient's degree of renal impairment (decreased creatinine clearance).

5. PHARMACOLOGICAL PROPERTIES

5.1 Pharmacodynamic properties

Pharmacotherapeutic group: ATC code: J 05 A B 06 (anti-infectives for systemic use, antivirals for systemic use, direct acting antivirals, nucleosides and nucleotides excluding reverse transcriptase inhibitors).

Ganciclovir is a synthetic analogue of 2'-deoxyguanosine which inhibits replication of herpes viruses *in vitro* and *in vivo*. Sensitive human viruses include human cytomegalovirus (HCMV), herpes simplex virus-1 and -2 (HSV-1 and HSV-2), human herpes virus-6, 7 and 8 (HHV-6, HHV-7, HHV-8), Epstein-Barr virus (EBV) and varicella zoster virus (VZV) and hepatitis B virus. Clinical studies have been limited to assessment of efficacy in patients with CMV infection.

In CMV infected cells ganciclovir is initially phosphorylated to ganciclovir monophosphate by the viral protein kinase, UL97. Further phosphorylation occurs by several cellular kinases to produce ganciclovir triphosphate, which is then slowly metabolised intracellularly. This has been shown to occur in HSV- and HCMV-infected cells with half-lives of 18 and between 6 and 24 hours respectively after removal of extracellular ganciclovir. As the phosphorylation is largely dependent on the viral kinase, phosphorylation of ganciclovir occurs preferentially in virus-infected cells.

The virustatic activity of ganciclovir is due to the inhibition of viral DNA synthesis by: (1) competitive inhibition of incorporation of deoxyguanosine triphosphate into DNA by DNA polymerase and (2) incorporation of ganciclovir triphosphate into viral DNA causing termination of, or very limited, viral DNA elongation. The *in vitro* anti-viral activity, measured as IC_{50} of ganciclovir against CMV, is in the range of 0.08μM (0.02μg/ml) to 14 μM (3.5μg/ml).

Viral resistance

The possibility of viral resistance should be considered for patients who repeatedly show poor clinical response or experience persistent viral excretion during therapy. CMV resistant to ganciclovir can arise after prolonged treatment or prophylaxis with ganciclovir by selection of mutations in either the viral protein kinase gene (UL97) responsible for ganciclovir monophosphorylation and/or, but less frequently, in the viral polymerase gene (UL54). Virus with mutations in the UL97 gene are resistant to ganciclovir alone, whereas virus with mutations in the UL54 gene may show cross-resistance to other antivirals with a similar mechanism of action and vice versa.

The working definition of CMV resistance to ganciclovir based on *in vitro* antiviral assays is an IC_{50} value $\geqslant$ 12.0μM with values > 6.0μM < 12.0μM being considered as indicating intermediate resistance. By these definitions up to 4% of untreated patients have CMV isolates with IC_{50} values that meet the criteria for either resistance or intermediate resistance.

In a prospective study of 76 previously untreated severely immunocompromised AIDS patients with CMV retinitis starting therapy with ganciclovir (i.v. induction / i.v. maintenance or i.v. induction / oral maintenance), the number of patients carrying resistant virus (IC_{50} > 6.0μM) increased with time of treatment; 3.7%, 5.4%, 11.4% and 27.5% of those still on treatment at baseline, 3, 6 and 12 months respectively. Similarly in another study of AIDS patients with CMV retinitis treated for $\geqslant$ 3 months with i.v. ganciclovir 7.8% of patients carried virus with IC_{50} $\geqslant$ 12.0μM. Combined data from 4 clinical studies of the treatment of CMV retinitis indicated an incidence of resistance (IC_{50} > 6.0μM) of 3.2% (median exposure 75 days) for i.v. ganciclovir and 6.5% (median exposure 165 days) for oral ganciclovir.

5.2 Pharmacokinetic properties

Systemic exposure

The systemic exposure (AUC_{0-24}) reported following dosing with a single 1-hour i.v. infusion of 5mg/kg ganciclovir in HIV+/CMV+ patients ranged from 21.4 ± 3.1 (N=16) to 26.0 ± 6.06 (N=16) μg.h/ml. In this patient population peak plasma concentration (C_{max}) ranged from 8.27 ± 1.02 (N=16) to 9.03 ± 1.42 (N=16)μg/ml.

Distribution

For i.v. ganciclovir, the volume of distribution is correlated with body weight with values for the steady state volume of distribution ranging from 0.536 ± 0.078 (N=15) to 0.870 ± 0.116 (N=16) L/kg. Cerebrospinal fluid concentrations obtained 0.25 - 5.67 hours post-dose in 2 patients who received 2.5mg/kg ganciclovir i.v. every 8 hours or every 12 hours ranged from 0.50 to 0.68μg/ml representing 24 - 67% of the respective plasma concentrations. Binding to plasma proteins was 1 - 2% over ganciclovir concentrations of 0.5 and 51μg/ml.

Intra-ocular concentrations of ganciclovir range from 40 to 200% of those measured simultaneously in plasma following administration of i.v. ganciclovir. Average intravitreal concentrations following induction and maintenance dosing with i.v. ganciclovir were 1.15 and 1.0 μg/ml respectively. Half-life of ganciclovir within the eye is much longer than that in plasma with estimates ranging from 13.3 to 18.8 hours.

Metabolism and elimination

When administered i.v., ganciclovir exhibits linear pharmacokinetics over the range of 1.6 - 5.0mg/kg. Renal excretion of unchanged drug by glomerular filtration and active tubular secretion is the major route of elimination of ganciclovir. In patients with normal renal function, 89.6 ± 5.0% (N=4) of i.v. administered ganciclovir was recovered unmetabolised in the urine. In subjects with normal renal function, systemic clearance ranged from 2.64 ± 0.38ml/min/kg (N=15) to 4.52 ± 2.79ml/min/kg (N=6) and renal clearance ranged from 2.57 ± 0.69ml/min/kg (N=15) to 3.48 ± 0.68ml/min/kg (N=16), corresponding to 90% - 101% of administered ganciclovir. Half-lives in subjects without renal impairment ranged from 2.73 ± 1.29 (N=6) to 3.98 ± 1.78 hours (N=8).

Pharmacokinetics in special populations

Renal impairment

Renal impairment leads to altered kinetics of ganciclovir as indicated below.

	Ganciclovir	
Serum creatinine (micromol/l)	**Systemic plasma clearance (ml/min/kg)**	**Plasma half-life (hours)**
< 124 (n = 22)	3.64	2.9
125 - 225 (n = 9)	2.00	5.3
226 - 398 (n = 3)	1.11	9.7
> 398 (n = 5)	0.33	28.5

Patients undergoing haemodialysis

Haemodialysis reduces plasma concentrations of ganciclovir by about 50% after both i.v. and oral administration (see section *4.9 Overdosage*).

During intermittent haemodialysis, estimates for the clearance of ganciclovir ranged from 42 to 92 ml/min, resulting in intra-dialytic half-lives of 3.3 to 4.5 hours. Estimates of ganciclovir clearance for continuous dialysis were lower (4.0 to 29.6 ml/min) but resulted in greater removal of ganciclovir over a dose interval. For intermittent haemodialysis, the fraction of ganciclovir removed in a single dialysis session varied from 50% to 63%.

Paediatric patients

Ganciclovir pharmacokinetics were also studied in 10 children, aged 9 months to 12 years. The pharmacokinetic characteristics of ganciclovir are similar after single and multiple (every 12 hours) i.v. doses (5mg/kg). After the administration of a 5mg/kg single dose, exposure as measured by mean AUC∞ was 19.4 ± 7.1 μg.h/ml, the steady-state volume of distribution reported was 0.68 ± 0.20 l/kg, C_{max} was 7.59 ± 3.21μg/ml, systemic clearance was 4.66 ± 1.72ml/min/kg, and $t_{1/2}$ was 2.49 ± 0.57 hours. The pharmacokinetics of i.v. ganciclovir in children are similar to those observed in adults.

Elderly patients

No studies have been conducted in adults older than 65 years of age.

5.3 Preclinical safety data

Ganciclovir was mutagenic in mouse lymphoma cells and clastogenic in mammalian cells. Such results are consistent with the positive mouse carcinogenicity study with ganciclovir. Ganciclovir is a potential carcinogen.

Ganciclovir causes impaired fertility and teratogenicity in animals (see section 4.4 *Special warnings and precautions for use*).

Based upon animals studies where aspermatogenesis was induced at ganciclovir systemic exposures below therapeutic levels, it is considered likely that ganciclovir could cause inhibition of human spermatogenesis.

Data obtained using an *ex vivo* human placental model show that ganciclovir crosses the placenta and that simple diffusion is the most likely mechanism of transfer. The transfer was not saturable over a concentration range of 1 to 10 mg/ml and occurred by passive diffusion.

6. PHARMACEUTICAL PARTICULARS

6.1 List of excipients

None.

6.2 Incompatibilities

The dry powder should not be reconstituted with bacteriostatic water containing parabens, since these are incompatible with ganciclovir sterile powder and may cause precipitation.

6.3 Shelf life

36 months.

6.4 Special precautions for storage

Undiluted vials: Do not store above 30°C.

From a microbiological point of view, the product should be used immediately after reconstitution and dilution. If the product is not used immediately, the in-use storage times and conditions prior to use are the responsibility of the user. Following reconstitution and dilution, the following in-use storage times should be followed unless reconstitution and dilution has taken place in controlled and validated aseptic conditions.

In-use storage times for the reconstituted vial should not be longer than 12 hours. Do not refrigerate.

In-use storage time for the infusion solution should not be longer than 24 hours when stored in a refrigerator at 2 - 8°C. Freezing is not recommended.

6.5 Nature and contents of container

10ml multidose vials (type I, clear glass) with a grey butyl siliconised stopper in quantities of 5 or 25 vials.

6.6 Instructions for use and handling

Caution should be exercised in the handling of Cymevene

Since Cymevene is considered a potential teratogen and carcinogen in humans, caution should be exercised in its handling (see section *4.4 Special warnings and precautions for use*). Avoid inhalation or direct contact of the powder contained in the vials or direct contact of the reconstituted solution with the skin or mucous membranes. Cymevene solutions are alkaline (pH approximately 11). If such contact occurs, wash thoroughly with soap and water, rinse eyes thoroughly with sterile water, or plain water if sterile water is unavailable.

Method of preparation of Cymevene solution

1. Lyophilised Cymevene should be reconstituted by injecting 10ml of sterile Water for Injections into the vial. **Do not use bacteriostatic water for injection containing parabens (para-hydroxybenzoates), since these are incompatible with Cymevene sterile powder and may cause precipitation.**

2. The vial should be shaken to dissolve the drug.

3. Reconstituted solution should be inspected for particulate matter prior to proceeding with the admixture preparation.

4. Reconstituted solution in the vial is stable at room temperature for 12 hours. It should not be refrigerated.

Preparation and administration of infusion solution

Based on patient weight the appropriate calculated dose volume should be removed from the Cymevene vial (concentration 50 mg/ml) and added to an acceptable infusion fluid. Normal saline, dextrose 5% in water, Ringer's or lactated Ringer's solution are determined chemically or physically compatible with Cymevene. Infusion concentrations greater than 10mg/ml are not recommended.

Cymevene should not be mixed with other i.v. products.

Because Cymevene is reconstituted with nonbacteriostatic sterile water, the infusion solution should be used as soon as possible and within 24 hours of dilution in order to reduce the risk of bacterial contamination.

The infusion solution should be refrigerated. Freezing is not recommended.

Any unused product or waste material should be disposed of in accordance with local requirements.

7. MARKETING AUTHORISATION HOLDER

Roche Products Limited, 40 Broadwater Road, Welwyn Garden City, Hertfordshire, AL7 3AY.

8. MARKETING AUTHORISATION NUMBER(S)

PL 0031/0465

9. DATE OF FIRST AUTHORISATION/RENEWAL OF THE AUTHORISATION

June 1998

10. DATE OF REVISION OF THE TEXT

April 2004

Cymevene is a registered trade mark

P222172/404

Cyprostat 50mg and 100mg

(Schering Health Care Limited)

1. NAME OF THE MEDICINAL PRODUCT

Cyprostat® 50mg and 100mg

2. QUALITATIVE AND QUANTITATIVE COMPOSITION

Cyprostat 100mg: Each white, scored tablet contains 100mg cyproterone acetate.

Cyprostat 50mg: Each white, scored tablet contains 50mg cyproterone acetate.

3. PHARMACEUTICAL FORM

Tablets

4. CLINICAL PARTICULARS

4.1 Therapeutic indications

Management of patients with prostatic cancer (1) to suppress "flare" with initial LHRH analogue therapy,(2) in long-term palliative treatment where LHRH analogues or surgery are contraindicated, not tolerated, or where oral therapy is preferred, and (3) in the treatment of hot flushes in patients under treatment with LHRH analogues or who have had orchidectomy.

4.2 Posology and method of administration

Adults, including the elderly:

Dosage for suppression of "flare" with initial LHRH analogue therapy is 300 mg/day, which may be reduced to 200 mg if the higher dose is not tolerated. For long-term palliative treatment where LHRH analogues or surgery are contraindicated, not tolerated, or where oral therapy is preferred the dosage is 200-300 mg/day.

For the above two indications the dosage should be divided into 2 - 3 doses per day and taken after meals.

For the treatment of hot flushes in patients under treatment with LHRH analogues or who have had orchidectomy a 50 mg starting dose, with upward titration if necessary within the range 50-150 mg/day, is recommended. For this indication the dosage should be divided into 1 - 3 doses per day and taken after meals.

All doses should be taken orally.

Children: Not recommended.

4.3 Contraindications

Hypersensitivity to any of the components of Cyprostat.

4.4 Special warnings and special precautions for use

Liver: Direct hepatic toxicity, including jaundice, hepatitis and hepatic failure, which has been fatal in some cases, has been reported in patients treated with 200-300 mg cyproterone acetate. Most reported cases are in men with prostatic cancer. Toxicity is dose-related and develops, usually, several months after treatment has begun. Liver function tests should be performed pre-treatment, regularly during treatment and whenever any symptoms or signs suggestive of hepatotoxicity occur. If hepatotoxicity is confirmed, cyproterone acetate should normally be withdrawn, unless the hepatotoxicity can be explained by another cause, e.g. metastatic disease, in which case cyproterone acetate should be continued only if the perceived benefit outweighs the risk.

As with other sex steroids, benign and malignant liver changes have been reported in isolated cases.

In very rare cases, liver tumours may lead to life-threatening intra-abdominal haemorrhage. If severe upper abdominal complaints, liver enlargement or signs of intra-abdominal haemorrhage occur, a liver tumour should be considered in the differential diagnosis.

Thromboembolism: Patients with a history of thrombosis may be at risk of recurrence of the disease during Cyprostat therapy.

In patients with a history of thromboembolic processes or suffering from sickle-cell anaemia or severe diabetes with vascular changes, the risk: benefit ratio must be considered carefully in each individual case before Cyprostat is prescribed.

In extremely rare cases, the occurrence of thromboembolic events has been reported in temporal association with the use of Cyprostat. However a causal relationship seems to be questionable.

Chronic depression: It has been found that some patients with severe chronic depression deteriorate whilst taking Cyprostat therapy.

Breathlessness: Shortness of breath may occur. This may be due to the stimulatory effect of progesterone and synthetic progestogens on breathing, which is accompanied by hypocapnia and compensatory alkalosis, and which is not considered to require treatment.

Adrenocortical function: During treatment adrenocortical function should be checked regularly, since suppression has been observed.

Diabetes: Cyprostat can influence carbohydrate metabolism. Parameters of carbohydrate metabolism should be examined carefully in all diabetics before and regularly during treatment. See also section 4.5.

Haemoglobin: Hypochromic anaemia has been found rarely during long-term treatment, and blood-counts before and at regular intervals during treatment are advisable.

4.5 Interaction with other medicinal products and other forms of Interaction

The requirement for oral antidiabetics or insulin can change. See also section 4.4.

4.6 Pregnancy and lactation

Not applicable

4.7 Effects on ability to drive and use machines

Fatigue and lassitude are common - patients should be warned about this and if affected should not drive or operate machinery.

4.8 Undesirable effects

Thromboembolism: See section 4.4.

Inhibition of sexual drive and potency: Under treatment with Cyprostat, sexual drive and potency are reduced. These changes are reversible after discontinuation of therapy.

Inhibition of spermatogenesis: The sperm count and the volume of ejaculate are reduced. Infertility is usual, and there may be azoospermia after 8 weeks. There is usually slight atrophy of seminiferous tubules. Follow-up examinations have shown these changes to be reversible, spermatogenesis usually reverting to its previous state about 3-5 months after stopping Cyprostat, or in some users, up to 20 months. That spermatogenesis can recover even after very long treatment is not yet known. There is evidence that abnormal sperms which might give rise to malformed embryos are produced during treatment with Cyprostat.

Tiredness: Fatigue and lassitude are common.

Gynaecomastia: Transient, and perhaps in some cases permanent, enlargement of the mammary glands has been reported. In rare cases, galactorrhoea and tender benign nodules have been reported. Symptoms generally subside after discontinuation of treatment or on reduction of dosage, but this should be weighed against the risk from the tumour of using inadequate doses.

Bodyweight: During long-term treatment, changes in bodyweight have been reported. Both increases and decreases have been seen.

Osteoporosis: Rarely cases of osteoporosis have been reported.

Other changes that have been reported include:

- reduction of sebum production leading to dryness of the skin and improvement of existing acne vulgaris;
- transient patchy loss and reduced growth of body hair, increased growth of scalp hair, lightening of hair colour and female type of pubic hair growth;
- occasionally depressive moods can occur;
- breathlessness can occur (see section 4.4);
- in rare cases, hypersensitivity reactions and rashes may occur.

4.9 Overdose

There have been no reports of ill-effects of overdosage, which it is, therefore, generally unnecessary to treat. There are no specific antidotes and if treatment is required it should be symptomatic.

5. PHARMACOLOGICAL PROPERTIES

5.1 Pharmacodynamic properties

Prostatic carcinoma and its metastases are in general androgen-dependent. Cyproterone acetate exerts a direct anti-androgen action on the tumour and its metastases. It also has progestogenic activity, which exerts a negative feedback effect on the hypothalamic receptors, so leading to a reduction in gonadotrophin release, and hence to diminished production of testicular androgens. Sexual drive and potency are reduced and gonadal function is inhibited.

The antigonadotropic effect of cyproterone acetate is also exerted when administered with LHRH analogues. The initial increase of testosterone caused by this class of substances is reduced by cyproterone acetate.

An occasional tendency for the prolactin levels to increase slightly has been observed under higher doses of cyproterone acetate.

5.2 Pharmacokinetic properties

Following oral administration, cyproterone acetate is completely absorbed over a wide dose range.

Cyprostat 100mg:

The ingestion of 100 mg of cyproterone acetate gives maximum serum levels of about 239 ng/ml at about 3 hours. Thereafter, drug serum levels declined during a time interval of typically 24 to 120 h, with a terminal half-life of 42.8 ± 9.7 h. The total clearance of cyproterone acetate from serum is 3.8 ± 2.2 ml/min/kg.

Cyprostat 50mg:

The ingestion of two cyproterone acetate 50 mg tablets gives maximum serum levels of about 285 ng/ml at about 3 hours. Thereafter, drug serum levels declined during a time interval of typically 24 to 120 h, with a terminal half-life of 43.9 ± 12.8 h. The total clearance of cyproterone acetate from serum is 3.5 ± 1.5 ml/min/kg.

Cyproterone acetate is metabolised by various pathways, including hydroxylations and conjugations. The main metabolite in human plasma is the 15β-hydroxy derivative.

Some drug is excreted unchanged with bile fluid. Most of the dose is excreted in the form of metabolites at a urinary to biliary ratio of 3:7. The renal and biliary excretion proceeds with a half-life of 1.9 days. Metabolites from plasma are eliminated at a similar rate (half-life of 1.7 days).

Cyproterone acetate is almost exclusively bound to plasma albumin. About 3.5 - 4 % of total drug levels are present unbound. Because protein binding is non-specific, changes in SHBG (sex hormone binding globulin) levels do not affect the pharmacokinetics of cyproterone acetate.

The absolute bioavailability of cyproterone acetate is almost complete (88 % of dose).

5.3 Preclinical safety data

Experimental investigations produced corticoid-like effects on the adrenal glands in rats and dogs following higher dosages, which could indicate similar effects in humans at the highest given dose (300 mg/day).

Recognised first-line tests of genotoxicity gave negative results when conducted with cyproterone acetate. However, further tests showed that cyproterone acetate was capable of producing adducts with DNA (and an increase in DNA repair activity) in liver cells from rats and monkeys and also in freshly isolated human hepatocytes. This DNA-adduct formation occurred at exposures that might be expected to occur in the recommended dose regimens for cyproterone acetate. *In vivo* consequences of cyproterone acetate treatment were the increased incidence of focal, possibly preneoplastic, liver lesions in which cellular enzymes were altered in female rats, and an increase of mutation frequency in transgenic rats carrying a bacterial gene as target for mutation. The clinical relevance of these findings is presently uncertain. Clinical experience to date would not support an increased incidence of hepatic tumours in man. However, it must be borne in mind that sex steroids can promote the growth of certain hormone dependent tissues and tumours.

6. PHARMACEUTICAL PARTICULARS

6.1 List of excipients

Maize starch

Povidone 25 000

Magnesium stearate (E572)

Lactose

Aerosil (Cyprostat 50mg only)

6.2 Incompatibilities

None known

6.3 Shelf life

5 years

6.4 Special precautions for storage

None

6.5 Nature and contents of container

Cyprostat 100mg:

Cartons containing PVC film and aluminium foil blister packs of 84 tablets.

Cyprostat 50mg:

Original packs containing 168 tablets (14 blister strips of 12 tablets),

6.6 Instructions for use and handling

Keep out of the reach of children.

7. MARKETING AUTHORISATION HOLDER

Schering Health Care Limited

The Brow

Burgess Hill

West Sussex RH15 9NE

8. MARKETING AUTHORISATION NUMBER(S)

Cyprsotat 100mg: PL 0053/0218

Cyprostat 50mg: PL0053/0133

9. DATE OF FIRST AUTHORISATION/RENEWAL OF THE AUTHORISATION

Cyprostat 100mg: 5 November 1998

Cyprostat 50mg: 8 August 2003

10. DATE OF REVISION OF THE TEXT

2 April 2004

LEGAL CATEGORY

POM

Cystrin 3mg Tablets, Cystrin 5mg Tablets

(sanofi-aventis)

1. NAME OF THE MEDICINAL PRODUCT

Cystrin 3mg Tablets

Cystrin 5mg Tablets

2. QUALITATIVE AND QUANTITATIVE COMPOSITION

Oxybutynin hydrochloride 3.00mg

Oxybutynin hydrochloride 5.00mg

3. PHARMACEUTICAL FORM

Tablet

4. CLINICAL PARTICULARS

4.1 Therapeutic indications

Cystrin is indicated for urinary incontinence, urgency and frequency in unstable bladder conditions due either to idiopathic detrusor instability or neurogenic bladder disorders (detrusor hyperreflexia) in conditions such as spina bifida and multiple sclerosis.

In addition, for children over 5 years of age, oxybutynin may be used in nocturnal enuresis in conjunction with non-drug therapy where this alone, or in conjunction with other drug treatment, has failed.

4.2 Posology and method of administration

Children under 5 years of age: Not recommended

Children over 5 years of age:

Neurogenic bladder disorders: The usual dose is 5mg twice a day. This may be increased to a maximum of 5mg three times a day to obtain a clinical response provided that the side effects are tolerated.

Nocturnal enuresis: The usual dose is 5mg two or three times a day. The last dose should be given before bedtime.

In children the maintenance dose may be achieved by upward titration from an initial dose of 3mg twice daily.

Adults: The usual dose is 5mg two or three times a day. This may be increased to a maximum dosage of 5mg four times a day (20mg) to obtain a satisfactory clinical response provided that the side effects are tolerated.

Elderly: The elimination half-life may be increased in some elderly patients, therefore, dosage should be individually titrated commencing at 3mg twice a day. The final dosage will depend on response and tolerance to side-effects. As with other anticholinergic drugs caution should be observed in frail and elderly patients.

4.3 Contraindications

Hypersensitivity to oxybutynin or any component.

Myasthenia gravis.

Narrow-angle glaucoma or shallow anterior chamber.

Gastrointestinal obstruction including paralytic ileus, intestinal atony.

Patients with toxic megacolon, severe ulcerative colitis.

Patients with bladder outflow obstruction where urinary retention may be precipitated.

4.4 Special warnings and special precautions for use

Oxybutynin should be used with caution in the frail elderly and children who may be more sensitive to the effects of the product and in patients with autonomic neuropathy, hepatic or renal impairment and severe gastro-intestinal motility disorders (also see section 4.3).

Oxybutynin may aggravate the symptoms of hyperthyroidism, congestive heart failure, coronary heart disease, cardiac arrhythmia, tachycardia, hypertension and prostatic hypertrophy.

Oxybutynin can cause decreased sweating; in high environmental temperatures this can lead to heat prostration.

The use of oxybutynin in children under 5 years of age is not recommended; it has not been established whether oxybutynin can be safely used in this age group.

Special care should be taken in patients with hiatus hernia associated with reflux oesophagitis, as anticholinergic drugs can aggravate this condition.

4.5 Interaction with other medicinal products and other forms of Interaction

Care should be taken if other anticholinergic agents are administered together with Cystrin, as potentiation of anticholinergic effects could occur.

Occasional cases of interaction between anticholinergics and phenothiazines, amantidine, butyrophenones, L-dopa, digitalis and tricyclic antidepressants have been reported and care should be taken if Cystrin is administered concurrently with such drugs.

By reducing gastric motility, oxybutynin may affect absorption of other drugs.

4.6 Pregnancy and lactation

<u>Pregnancy</u>

There is no experience of the use of oxybutynin during pregnancy in humans, however, in foetal toxicity and fertility studies in animals, effects were seen on reproductive processes at dosages associated with maternal toxicity. Cystrin should, therefore, only be prescribed during pregnancy if considered essential.

Lactation

Small amounts of oxybutynin have been found in mother's milk of lactating animals. Breast feeding while using oxybutynin is therefore not recommended.

4.7 Effects on ability to drive and use machines

As Cystrin may produce drowsiness or blurred vision, the patient should be cautioned regarding activities requiring mental alertness such as driving, operating machinery or performing hazardous work while taking this drug.

4.8 Undesirable effects

Gastro-intestinal disorders

Nausea, diarrhoea, constipation, dry mouth, abdominal discomfort, anorexia, vomiting, gastroesophageal reflux.

CNS and psychiatric disorders

Agitation, headache, dizziness, drowsiness, disorientation, hallucinations, nightmares, convulsions.

Cardiovascular disorders

Tachycardia, cardiac arrythmia.

Vision disorders
Blurred vision, mydriasis, intraocular hypertension, onset of narrow-angle glaucoma, dry eyes.

Renal and urinary disorders
Urinary retention, difficulty in micturition.

Skin and appendages
Facial flushing which may be more marked in children, dry skin, allergic reactions such as rash, urticaria, angioedema, photosensitivity.

4.9 Overdose
The symptoms of overdosage with oxybutynin progress from an intensification of the usual side-effects of CNS disturbances (from restlessness and excitement to psychotic behaviour), circulatory changes (flushing, fall in blood pressure, circulatory failure etc), respiratory failure, paralysis and coma.

Measures to be taken are:

(1) immediate gastric lavage and

(2) physostigmine by slow intravenous injection

Adults: 0.5 to 2.0 mg of physostigmine by slow intravenous administration. Repeat after 5 minutes, if necessary up to a maximum total dose of 5mg

Children: 30 micrograms/kg of physostigmine by slow intravenous administration. Repeat after 5 minutes, if necessary up to a maximum total dose of 2mg.

Fever should be treated symptomatically with tepid sponging or ice packs.

In pronounced restlessness or excitation, diazepam 10mg may be given by intravenous injection. Tachycardia may be treated with intravenous propanolol and urinary retention managed by bladder catheterization.

In the event of progression of the curare-like effect to paralysis of the respiratory muscles, mechanical ventilation will be required.

5. PHARMACOLOGICAL PROPERTIES

5.1 Pharmacodynamic properties
Pharmacotherapeutic group: Urinary Antispasmodics, ATC code: G04B D04

Oxybutynin hydrochloride is an anticholinergic agent which also exerts a direct antispasmodic effect on smooth muscle. It inhibits bladder contraction and relieves spasm induced by various stimuli; it increases bladder volume, diminishes the frequency of contractions and delays the desire to void in the disturbance of neurogenic bladder. The relaxation of smooth muscle results from the papaverin like effect of the antagonism of the processes distal to the neuromuscular junction in addition to the anticholinergic blocking action of the muscarinic type receptors. In addition oxybutynin hydrochloride has local anaesthetic properties.

5.2 Pharmacokinetic properties
Pharmacodynamic reports show oxybutynin to be rapidly absorbed from the gastrointestinal tract following oral administration with maximum plasma concentrations reached in less than 1 hour subsequently falling bioexponentially with a half-life of between 2 and 3 hours.

Maximum effect can be seen within 3-4 hours with some effect still evident after 10 hours.

Repeated oral administration achieved steady state after eight days. Oxybutynin does not appear to accumulate in elderly patients and the pharmacokinetics are similar to those in other adults. Some excretion via the biliary system has been observed in the rabbit and partial first-pass metabolism occurs, the metabolites also appearing to have antimuscarinic properties. The main elimination route is via the kidneys with only 0.3-0.4% of unchanged drug appearing in the urine of the rat after 24 hours and 1% appearing in the urine of the dog after 48 hours. In rats and dogs therefore, oxybutynin appears to be almost completely absorbed.

5.3 Preclinical safety data
No additional data available.

6. PHARMACEUTICAL PARTICULARS

6.1 List of excipients
Lactose anhydrous, microcrystalline cellulose, calcium stearate, indigo carmine aluminium lake (E132).

6.2 Incompatibilities
None known

6.3 Shelf life
3 years

6.4 Special precautions for storage
Do not store above 30°C.

6.5 Nature and contents of container
Cystrin 3mg: 56 tablets in aluminium/PVC blister strips which are contained within a printed

Cardboard carton.

Cystrin 5mg: 84 tablets in aluminium/PVC blister strips which are contained within a printed cardboard carton.

6.6 Instructions for use and handling
No relevance.

7. MARKETING AUTHORISATION HOLDER
Sanofi-Synthelabo Limited

One Onslow Street

Guildford

Surrey

GU1 4YS

8. MARKETING AUTHORISATION NUMBER(S)
Cystrin 3mg: PL 11723/0343

Cystrin 5mg: PL 11723/0344

9. DATE OF FIRST AUTHORISATION/RENEWAL OF THE AUTHORISATION
Cystrin 3mg: 5 September 2000

Cystrin 5mg: 4 September 2003

10. DATE OF REVISION OF THE TEXT
Cystrin 3mg: March 2005

Cystrin 5mg: April 2004

Legal Category: POM

Cytamen Injection 1000mcg

(UCB Pharma Limited)

1. NAME OF THE MEDICINAL PRODUCT
Cytamen Injection 1000mcg

2. QUALITATIVE AND QUANTITATIVE COMPOSITION
Cyanocobalamin 1.0mg

3. PHARMACEUTICAL FORM
Solution for injection.

4. CLINICAL PARTICULARS

4.1 Therapeutic indications
Addisonian pernicious anaemia. Prophylaxis and treatment of other macrocytic anaemias associated with vitamin B_{12} deficiency. Schilling test.

Not indicated for treatment of toxic amblyopias - use Neo-Cytamen.

4.2 Posology and method of administration
Route of administration: intramuscular.

Adults and Children

Addisonian pernicious anaemia and other macrocytic anaemias without neurological involvement:

Initially: 250 to 1000mcg intramuscularly on alternate days for one to two weeks, then 250mcg weekly until the blood count is normal.

Maintenance: 1000mcg monthly.

Addisonian pernicious anaemia and other macrocytic anaemias with neurological complications:

Initially: 1000mcg intramuscularly on alternate days as long as improvement is occurring.

Maintenance: 1000mcg monthly.

Prophylaxis of macrocytic anaemia associated with vitamin B_{12} deficiency resulting from gastrectomy, some malabsorption syndromes and strict vegetarianism:

250mcg - 1000mcg monthly.

Schilling Test:

An intramuscular injection of 1000mcg cyanocobalamin is an essential part of this test.

4.3 Contraindications
Hypersensitivity to cyanocobalamin or any other constitutents.

Cytomen should not be used for the treatment of megaloblastic anaemia of pregnancy unless vitamin B12 deficiency has be demonstrated.

Not indicated for treatment of toxic amblyopias - use Neo-Cytamen.

4.4 Special warnings and special precautions for use
Precautions:

The dosage schemes given above are usually satisfactory, but regular examination of the blood is advisable. If megaloblastic anaemia fails to respond to Cytamen, folate metabolism should be investigated. Doses in excess of 10mcg daily may produce a haematological response in patients with folate deficiency. Indiscriminate administration may mask the true diagnosis. The haematological and neurological state should be monitored regularly to ensure adequacy of therapy. Cardiac arrhythmias secondary to hypokalaemia during initial therapy have been reported. Plasma potassium should therefore be monitored during this period.

4.5 Interaction with other medicinal products and other forms of Interaction
Chloramphenicol-treated patients may respond poorly to Cytamen. Serum concentrations of cyanocobalamin may be lowered by oral contraceptives but this interaction is unlikely to have clinical significance.

Antimetabolites and most antibiotics invalidate vitamin B_{12} assays by microbiological techniques.

4.6 Pregnancy and lactation
Cytamen should not be used for the treatment of megaloblastic anaemia of pregnancy unless vitamin B_{12} deficiency has been demonstrated. Cytamen is secreted into breast milk but this is unlikely to harm the infant, and may be beneficial if the mother and infant are vitamin B_{12} deficient.

4.7 Effects on ability to drive and use machines
None stated.

4.8 Undesirable effects
Hypersensitivity reactions have been reported including skin reactions (e.g. rash, itching) and exceptionally anaphylaxis. Other symptoms reported include fever, chills, hot flushing, dizziness, malaise, nausea, acneiform and bullous eruptions.

4.9 Overdose
Treatment is unlikely to be needed in cases of overdosage.

5. PHARMACOLOGICAL PROPERTIES

5.1 Pharmacodynamic properties
Cyanocobalamin is a form of vitamin B_{12}.

5.2 Pharmacokinetic properties
Cobalamins are absorbed from the gastro-intestinal tract, but may be irregularly absorbed when given in large therapeutic doses. Absorption is impaired in patients with an absence of intrinsic factor, with a malabsorption syndrome or with a disease or abnormality of the gut, or after gastrectomy.

After injection of cyanocobalamin a large proportion is excreted in the urine within 24 hours; the body retains only 55% of a 100-microgram dose and 15% of a 1000-microgram dose. Vitamin B12 is extensively bound to specific plasma proteins called transcobalamins; transcobalamin II appears to be involved in the rapid transport of the cobalamins to tissues. Vitamin B12 is stored in the liver, excreted in the bile, and undergoes extensive enterohepatic recycling; part of an administered dose is excreted in the urine, most of it in the first 8 hours; urinary excretion, however, accounts for only a small fraction in the reduction of total body stores acquired by dietary means. Vitamin B12 diffuses across the placenta and also appears in breast milk.

5.3 Preclinical safety data
None stated.

6. PHARMACEUTICAL PARTICULARS

6.1 List of excipients
Sodium chloride

Acetic acid

Water for injections

6.2 Incompatibilities
None.

6.3 Shelf life
36 months.

6.4 Special precautions for storage
Protect from light. Do not store above 25°C

6.5 Nature and contents of container
1ml glass ampoules in packs of 5.

6.6 Instructions for use and handling
Not applicable.

7. MARKETING AUTHORISATION HOLDER
UCB Pharma Limited

208 Bath Road

Slough

Berkshire

SL1 3WE

UK

8. MARKETING AUTHORISATION NUMBER(S)
PL 00039/0403

9. DATE OF FIRST AUTHORISATION/RENEWAL OF THE AUTHORISATION
17 December 1992 / 17 December 1997

10. DATE OF REVISION OF THE TEXT
June 2005

Cytarabine Injection Solution 100mg/ml (Pharmacia)

(Pharmacia Limited)

1. NAME OF THE MEDICINAL PRODUCT
Cytarabine 100mg/ml

2. QUALITATIVE AND QUANTITATIVE COMPOSITION
Cytarabine Ph Eur 100 mg/ml

3. PHARMACEUTICAL FORM
Solution for infusion or injection.

4. CLINICAL PARTICULARS

4.1 Therapeutic indications
Cytotoxic. For induction of remission in acute myeloid leukaemia in adults and for other acute leukaemias of adults and children.

4.2 Posology and method of administration

By intravenous infusion or injection, or subcutaneous injection.

Dosage recommendations may be converted from those in terms of bodyweight to those related to surface area by means of nomograms, as presented in Documenta Geigy.

1) Remission induction:

a) Continuous treatment:

i) Rapid injection - 2 mg/kg/day is a judicious starting dose. Administer for 10 days. Obtain daily blood counts. If no antileukaemic effect is noted and there is no apparent toxicity, increase to 4 mg/kg/day and maintain until therapeutic response or toxicity is evident. Almost all patients can be carried to toxicity with these doses.

ii) 0.5 - 1.0 mg/kg/day may be given in an infusion of up to 24 hours duration. Results from one-hour infusions have been satisfactory in the majority of patients. After 10 days this initial daily dose may be increased to 2 mg/kg/day subject to toxicity. Continue to toxicity or until remission occurs.

b) Intermittent treatment:

3 - 5 mg/kg/day are administered intravenously on each of five consecutive days. After a two to nine-day rest period, a further course is given. Continue until response or toxicity occurs.

The first evidence of marrow improvement has been reported to occur 7 - 64 days (mean 28 days) after the beginning of therapy.

In general, if a patient shows neither toxicity nor remission after a fair trial, the cautious administration of higher doses is warranted. As a rule, patients have been seen to tolerate higher doses when given by rapid intravenous injection as compared with slow infusion. This difference is due to the rapid metabolism of cytarabine and the consequent short duration of action of the high dose.

2) Maintenance therapy: Remissions which have been induced by cytarabine, or by other drugs, may be maintained by intravenous or subcutaneous injection of 1 mg/kg once or twice weekly.

Children: Children appear to tolerate higher doses than adults and, where dose ranges are quoted, the children should receive the higher dose and the adults the lower.

Elderly Patients: There is no information to suggest that a change in dosage is warranted in the elderly. Nevertheless, the elderly patient does not tolerate drug toxicity as well as the younger patient, and particular attention should thus be given to drug induced leucopenia, thrombocytopenia, and anaemia, with appropriate initiation of supportive therapy when indicated.

4.3 Contraindications

Therapy with Cytarabine should not be considered in patients with pre-existing drug-induced bone marrow suppression, unless the clinician feels that such management offers the most hopeful alternative for the patient. Cytarabine should not be used in the management of non-malignant disease, except for immunosuppression.

4.4 Special warnings and special precautions for use

Warnings: Cytarabine is a potent bone marrow suppressant. Therapy should be started cautiously in patients with pre-existing drug-induced bone marrow suppression. Patients receiving this drug must be under close medical supervision and, during induction therapy, should have leucocyte and platelet counts performed daily. Bone marrow examinations should be performed frequently after blasts have disappeared from the peripheral blood.

Facilities should be available for management of complications, possibly fatal, of bone marrow suppression (infection resulting from granulocytopenia and other impaired body defences, and haemorrhage secondary to thrombocytopenia). One case of anaphylaxis that resulted in acute cardiopulmonary arrest and required resuscitation has been reported. This occurred immediately after the intravenous administration of cytarabine.

Severe and at times fatal CNS, GI and pulmonary toxicity (different from that seen with conventional therapy regimens of cytarabine) has been reported following some experimental cytarabine dose schedules. These reactions include reversible corneal toxicity; cerebral and cerebellar dysfunction, usually reversible; severe gastro-intestinal ulceration, including pneumatosis cystoides intestinalis, leading to peritonitis; sepsis and liver abscess; and pulmonary oedema.

Cytarabine has been shown to be carcinogenic in animals. The possibility of a similar effect should be borne in mind when designing the long-term management of the patient.

Precautions: Patients receiving cytarabine must be monitored closely. Frequent platelet and leucocyte counts are mandatory. Suspend or modify therapy when drug-induced marrow depression has resulted in a platelet count under 50,000 or a polymorphonuclear count under 1,000 per cubic mm. Counts of formed elements in the peripheral blood may continue to fall after the drug is stopped, and reach lowest values after drug-free intervals of five to seven days. If indicated, restart therapy when definite signs of marrow recovery appear (on successive bone marrow studies). Patients whose drug is withheld until 'normal' peripheral blood values are attained may escape from control.

When intravenous doses are given quickly, patients are frequently nauseated and may vomit for several hours afterwards. This problem tends to be less severe when the drug is infused.

The human liver apparently detoxifies a substantial fraction of an administered dose. Use the drug with caution and at reduced dose in patients whose liver function is poor.

Periodic checks of bone marrow, liver and kidney functions should be performed in patients receiving Cytarabine.

The safety of this drug for use in infants is not established.

Like other cytotoxic drugs, cytarabine may induce hyperuricaemia secondary to rapid lysis of neoplastic cells. The clinician should monitor the patient's blood uric acid level and be prepared to use such supportive and pharmacological measures as may be necessary to control this problem.

4.5 Interaction with other medicinal products and other forms of Interaction

5-Fluorocytosine should not be administered with cytarabine as the therapeutic efficacy of 5-fluorocytosine has been shown to be abolished during such therapy.

4.6 Pregnancy and lactation

Cytarabine is known to be teratogenic in some animal species. The use of cytarabine in women who are, or who may become, pregnant should be undertaken only after due consideration of the potential benefits and hazards.

This product should not normally be administered to patients who are pregnant or to mothers who are breast-feeding.

4.7 Effects on ability to drive and use machines

Cytarabine has no effect on intellectual function or psychomotor performance. Nevertheless, patients receiving chemotherapy may have an impaired ability to drive or operate machinery and should be warned of the possibility and advised to avoid such tasks if so affected.

4.8 Undesirable effects

Adverse reactions seen with cytarabine treatment have included those seen with cytotoxic agents having an effect on bone marrow, such as: leucopenia, thrombocytopenia, anaemia, bone marrow suppression and megaloblastosis. Other side-effects have included: nausea, vomiting, diarrhoea, oral ulceration, hepatic dysfunction. Occasional adverse experiences have been reported as follows: renal dysfunction, anorexia, sepsis, gastro-intestinal haemorrhage, irritation or sepsis at site of injection, neuritis or neurotoxicity, rash, freckling, oesophagitis, skin and mucosal bleeding, chest pain, joint pain and reduction in reticulocytes.

A cytarabine syndrome has been described. It is characterised by fever, myalgia, bone pain, occasionally chest pain, maculopapular rash, conjunctivitis and malaise. It usually occurs 6 - 12 hours following drug administration. Corticosteroids have been shown to be beneficial in treating or preventing this syndrome. If the symptoms of the syndrome are serious enough to warrant treatment, corticosteroids should be contemplated as well as continuation of therapy with cytarabine.

Cases of pancreatitis have been observed with the induction of cytarabine.

Cytarabine is not recommended for intrathecal use; however, the following side-effects have been reported with such use. Expected systemic reactions: bone marrow depression, nausea, vomiting. Occasionally, severe spinal cord toxicity even leading to quadriplegia and paralysis, necrotising encephalopathy, blindness and other isolated neurotoxicities have been reported.

4.9 Overdose

Cessation of therapy, followed by management of ensuing bone marrow depression including whole blood or platelet transfusion and antibiotics as required.

5. PHARMACOLOGICAL PROPERTIES

5.1 Pharmacodynamic properties

Cytarabine, a pyrimidine nucleoside analogue, is an antineoplastic agent which inhibits the synthesis of deoxyribonucleic acid. It also has antiviral and immunosuppressant properties. Detailed studies on the mechanism of cytotoxicity in vitro suggests that the primary action of cytarabine is inhibition of deoxycytidine synthesis, although inhibition of cytidylic kinases and incorporation of the compound into nucleic acids may also play a role in its cytostatic and cytocidal actions.

5.2 Pharmacokinetic properties

Cytarabine is deaminated to arabinofuranosyl uracil in the liver and kidneys. After intravenous administration to humans, only 5.8% of the administered doses is excreted unaltered in urine within 12-24 hours, 90% of the dose is excreted as the deaminated product. Cytarabine appears to be metabolised rapidly, primarily by the liver and perhaps by the kidney. After single high intravenous doses, blood levels fall to unmeasurable levels witching 15 minutes in most patients. Some patients have in demonstrable circulating drug as early as 5 minutes after injection.

5.3 Preclinical safety data

There are no preclinical data of relevance to the prescriber which are additional to that already included in other sections of the Summary of Product Characteristics.

6. PHARMACEUTICAL PARTICULARS

6.1 List of excipients

Hydrochloric Acid

Sodium Hydroxide

Nitrogen

Water for injections

6.2 Incompatibilities

Not applicable.

6.3 Shelf life

18 months

6.4 Special precautions for storage

Store at 15°C - 25°C. Keep container in outer carton.

Cytarabine should not be stored at refrigerated temperatures (2-8°C).

6.5 Nature and contents of container

Polypropylene vials, closed with either a West S63/1704 Grey EPDM rubber stopper or a West 4110/40 Grey FlurоTec® Plus-faced rubber stopper, and sealed with an aluminium crimp with a plastic flip-off top.

Cytarabine is supplied as single vials containing 100 mg/ml cytarabine in 10 ml (1g) or 20ml (2g)

6.6 Instructions for use and handling

Prior to use, vials of cytarabine 100mg/ml must be warmed to 55°C, for 30 minutes, with adequate shaking, and allowed to cool to room temperature.

Once opened, the contents of each vial must be used immediately and not stored. Discard any unused portion.

Water for injections, 0.9% saline or 5% dextrose are commonly used infusion fluids for cytarabine. Compatibility must be assured before mixing with any other substance.

Infusion fluids containing cytarabine must be used immediately.

Disposal and Spills: To destroy, place in a high risk (for cytotoxics) waste disposal bag and incinerate at 1100°C. If spills occur, restrict access to the affected area and adequate protection including gloves and safety spectacles should be worn. Limit the spread and clean the area with absorbent paper/material. Spills may also be treated with 5% sodium hypochlorite. The spill area should be cleaned with copious amounts of water. Place the contaminated material in a leak proof disposal bag for cytotoxics and incinerate at 1100°C.

7. MARKETING AUTHORISATION HOLDER

Pharmacia Limited

Davy Avenue

Milton Keynes

MK5 8PH

UK

8. MARKETING AUTHORISATION NUMBER(S)

PL 0032/0198

9. DATE OF FIRST AUTHORISATION/RENEWAL OF THE AUTHORISATION

3 June 1999

10. DATE OF REVISION OF THE TEXT

March 2003

Cytarabine Injection Solution 20mg/ml (Pharmacia)

(Pharmacia Limited)

1. NAME OF THE MEDICINAL PRODUCT

Cytarabine 20mg/ml

2. QUALITATIVE AND QUANTITATIVE COMPOSITION

Cytarabine Ph. Eur. 20 mg/ml

3. PHARMACEUTICAL FORM

Solution for infusion or injection.

4. CLINICAL PARTICULARS

4.1 Therapeutic indications

Cytotoxic. For induction of remission in acute myeloid leukaemia in adults and for other acute leukaemias of adults and children.

4.2 Posology and method of administration

By intravenous infusion or injection, or subcutaneous injection.

Dosage recommendations may be converted from those in terms of bodyweight to those related to surface area by means of nomograms, as presented in Documenta Geigy.

1) Remission induction:

a) Continuous treatment:

i) Rapid injection - 2 mg/kg/day is a judicious starting dose. Administer for 10 days. Obtain daily blood counts. If no antileukaemic effect is noted and there is no apparent toxicity, increase to 4 mg/kg/day and maintain until therapeutic response or toxicity is evident. Almost all patients can be carried to toxicity with these doses.

ii) 0.5 - 1.0 mg/kg/day may be given in an infusion of up to 24 hours duration. Results from one-hour infusions have been satisfactory in the majority of patients. After 10 days this initial daily dose may be increased to 2 mg/kg/day subject to toxicity. Continue to toxicity or until remission occurs.

b) Intermittent treatment:

3 - 5 mg/kg/day are administered intravenously on each of five consecutive days. After a two to nine-day rest period, a further course is given. Continue until response or toxicity occurs.

The first evidence of marrow improvement has been reported to occur 7 - 64 days (mean 28 days) after the beginning of therapy.

In general, if a patient shows neither toxicity nor remission after a fair trial, the cautious administration of higher doses is warranted. As a rule, patients have been seen to tolerate higher doses when given by rapid intravenous injection as compared with slow infusion. This difference is due to the rapid metabolism of cytarabine and the consequent short duration of action of the high dose.

2) Maintenance therapy: Remissions which have been induced by cytarabine, or by other drugs, may be maintained by intravenous or subcutaneous injection of 1 mg/kg once or twice weekly.

Children: Children appear to tolerate higher doses than adults and, where dose ranges are quoted, the children should receive the higher dose and the adults the lower.

Elderly Patients: There is no information to suggest that a change in dosage is warranted in the elderly. Nevertheless, the elderly patient does not tolerate drug toxicity as well as the younger patient, and particular attention should thus be given to drug induced leucopenia, thrombocytopenia, and anaemia, with appropriate initiation of supportive therapy when indicated.

4.3 Contraindications

Therapy with Cytarabine should not be considered in patients with pre-existing drug-induced bone marrow suppression, unless the clinician feels that such management offers the most hopeful alternative for the patient. Cytarabine should not be used in the management of non-malignant disease, except for immunosuppression.

4.4 Special warnings and special precautions for use

Warnings: Cytarabine is a potent bone marrow suppressant. Therapy should be started cautiously in patients with pre-existing drug-induced bone marrow suppression. Patients receiving this drug must be under close medical supervision and, during induction therapy, should have leucocyte and platelet counts performed daily. Bone marrow examinations should be performed frequently after blasts have disappeared from the peripheral blood.

Facilities should be available for management of complications, possibly fatal, of bone marrow suppression (infection resulting from granulocytopenia and other impaired body defences, and haemorrhage secondary to thrombocytopenia). One case of anaphylaxis that resulted in acute cardiopulmonary arrest and required resuscitation has been reported. This occurred immediately after the intravenous administration of cytarabine.

Severe and at times fatal CNS, GI and pulmonary toxicity (different from that seen with conventional therapy regimens of cytarabine) has been reported following some experimental cytarabine dose schedules. These reactions include reversible corneal toxicity; cerebral and cerebellar dysfunction, usually reversible; severe gastro-intestinal ulceration, including pneumatosis cystoides intestinalis, leading to peritonitis; sepsis and liver abscess; and pulmonary oedema.

Cytarabine has been shown to be carcinogenic in animals. The possibility of a similar effect should be borne in mind when designing the long-term management of the patient.

Precautions: Patients receiving cytarabine must be monitored closely. Frequent platelet and leucocyte counts are mandatory. Suspend or modify therapy when drug-induced marrow depression has resulted in a platelet count under 50,000 or a polymorphonuclear count under 1,000 per cubic mm. Counts of formed elements in the peripheral blood may continue to fall after the drug is stopped, and reach lowest values after drug-free intervals of five to seven days. If indicated, restart therapy when definite signs of marrow recovery appear (on successive bone marrow studies). Patients whose drug is withheld until 'normal' peripheral blood values are attained may escape from control.

When intravenous doses are given quickly, patients are frequently nauseated and may vomit for several hours afterwards. This problem tends to be less severe when the drug is infused.

The human liver apparently detoxifies a substantial fraction of an administered dose. Use the drug with caution and at reduced dose in patients whose liver function is poor.

Periodic checks of bone marrow, liver and kidney functions should be performed in patients receiving Cytarabine.

The safety of this drug for use in infants is not established.

Like other cytotoxic drugs, cytarabine may induce hyperuricaemia secondary to rapid lysis of neoplastic cells. The clinician should monitor the patient's blood uric acid level and be prepared to use such supportive and pharmacological measures as may be necessary to control this problem.

4.5 Interaction with other medicinal products and other forms of Interaction

5-Fluorocytosine should not be administered with cytarabine as the therapeutic efficacy of 5-fluorocytosine has been shown to be abolished during such therapy.

4.6 Pregnancy and lactation

Cytarabine is known to be teratogenic in some animal species. The use of cytarabine in women who are, or who may become, pregnant should be undertaken only after due consideration of the potential benefits and hazards.

This product should not normally be administered to patients who are pregnant or to mothers who are breast-feeding.

4.7 Effects on ability to drive and use machines

Cytarabine has no effect on intellectual function or psychomotor performance. Nevertheless, patients receiving chemotherapy may have an impaired ability to drive or operate machinery and should be warned of the possibility and advised to avoid such tasks if so affected.

4.8 Undesirable effects

Adverse reactions seen with cytarabine treatment have included those seen with cytotoxic agents having an effect on bone marrow, such as: leucopenia, thrombocytopenia, anaemia, bone marrow suppression and megaloblastosis. Other side-effects have included: nausea, vomiting, diarrhoea, oral ulceration, hepatic dysfunction. Occasional adverse experiences have been reported as follows: renal dysfunction, anorexia, sepsis, gastro-intestinal haemorrhage, irritation or sepsis at site of injection, neuritis or neurotoxicity, rash, freckling, oesophagitis, skin and mucosal bleeding, chest pain, joint pain and reduction in reticulocytes.

A cytarabine syndrome has been described. It is characterised by fever, myalgia, bone pain, occasionally chest pain, maculopapular rash, conjunctivitis and malaise. It usually occurs 6 - 12 hours following drug administration. Corticosteroids have been shown to be beneficial in treating or preventing this syndrome. If the symptoms of the syndrome are serious enough to warrant treatment, corticosteroids should be contemplated as well as continuation of therapy with cytarabine.

Cases of pancreatitis have been observed with the induction of cytarabine.

Cytarabine is not recommended for intrathecal use; however, the following side-effects have been reported with such use. Expected systemic reactions: bone marrow depression, nausea, vomiting. Occasionally, severe spinal cord toxicity even leading to quadriplegia and paralysis, necrotising encephalopathy, blindness and other isolated neurotoxicities have been reported.

4.9 Overdose

Cessation of therapy, followed by management of ensuing bone marrow depression including whole blood or platelet transfusion and antibiotics as required.

5. PHARMACOLOGICAL PROPERTIES

5.1 Pharmacodynamic properties

Cytarabine, a pyrimidine nucleoside analogue, is an antineoplastic agent which inhibits the synthesis of deoxyribonucleic acid. It also has antiviral and immunosuppressant properties. Detailed studies on the mechanism of cytotoxicity in vitro suggests that the primary action of cytarabine is inhibition of deoxycytidine synthesis, although inhibition of cytidylic kinases and incorporation of the compound into nucleic acids may also play a role in its cytostatic and cytocidal actions.

5.2 Pharmacokinetic properties

Cytarabine is deaminated to arabinofuranosyl uracil in the liver and kidneys. After intravenous administration to humans, only 5.8% of the administered doses is excreted unaltered in urine within 12-24 hours, 90% of the dose is excreted as the deaminated product. Cytarabine appears to be metabolised rapidly, primarily by the liver and perhaps by the kidney. After single high intravenous doses, blood levels fall to unmeasurable levels within 15 minutes in most patients. Some patients have in demonstrable circulating drug as early as 5 minutes after injection.

5.3 Preclinical safety data

There are no preclinical data of relevance to the prescriber which are additional to that already included in other sections of the Summary of Product Characteristics.

6. PHARMACEUTICAL PARTICULARS

6.1 List of excipients

Hydrochloric Acid

Sodium Hydroxide

Nitrogen

Water for injections

Sodium Chloride

6.2 Incompatibilities

Not applicable.

6.3 Shelf life

12 months

6.4 Special precautions for storage

Store at 15°C - 25°C. Keep container in outer carton.

Cytarabine should not be stored at refrigerated temperatures (2-8°C).

6.5 Nature and contents of container

Polypropylene vials, closed with either a West S63/1704 Grey EPDM rubber stopper or a West 4110/40 Grey FluroTec® Plus-faced rubber stopper, and sealed with an aluminium crimp with a plastic flip-off top.

Cytarabine is supplied as vials containing 20 mg/ml cytarabine in 5 ml (100mg) in packs of 5, or 25ml (500mg) as single vials

6.6 Instructions for use and handling

Once opened, the contents of each vial must be used immediately and not stored. Discard any unused portion.

Water for injections, 0.9% saline or 5% dextrose are commonly used infusion fluids for cytarabine. Compatibility must be assured before mixing with any other substance.

Infusion fluids containing cytarabine should be used immediately.

Disposal and Spills: To destroy, place in a high risk (for cytotoxics) waste disposal bag and incinerate at 1100°C. If spills occur, restrict access to the affected area and adequate protection including gloves and safety spectacles should be worn. Limit the spread and clean the area with absorbent paper/material. Spills may also be treated with 5% sodium hypochlorite. The spill area should be cleaned with copious amounts of water. Place the contaminated material in a leak proof disposal bag for cytotoxics and incinerate at 1100°C.

7. MARKETING AUTHORISATION HOLDER

Pharmacia Limited

Davy Avenue

Milton Keynes

MK5 8PH

UK

8. MARKETING AUTHORISATION NUMBER(S)

PL 0032/0197

9. DATE OF FIRST AUTHORISATION/RENEWAL OF THE AUTHORISATION

3 June 1999

10. DATE OF REVISION OF THE TEXT

March 2003

LEGAL CATEGORY

POM

Cytotec Tablets

(Pharmacia Limited)

1. NAME OF THE MEDICINAL PRODUCT

Cytotec 200mcg tablets.

2. QUALITATIVE AND QUANTITATIVE COMPOSITION

Each tablet contains 200 micrograms misoprostol.

For excipients, see 6.1.

3. PHARMACEUTICAL FORM

White to off-white hexagonal tablets scored both sides, engraved SEARLE 1461 on one side for oral administration.

4. CLINICAL PARTICULARS

4.1 Therapeutic indications

Cytotec is indicated for the healing of duodenal ulcer and gastric ulcer including those induced by nonsteroidal anti-inflammatory drugs (NSAID) in arthritic patients at risk, whilst continuing their NSAID therapy. In addition, Cytotec can be used for the prophylaxis of NSAID-induced ulcers.

4.2 Posology and method of administration

Adults

Healing of duodenal ulcer, gastric ulcer and NSAID-induced peptic ulcer: 800 micrograms daily in two or four divided doses taken with breakfast and / or each main meal and at bedtime.

Treatment should be given initially for at least 4 weeks even if symptomatic relief has been achieved sooner. In most patients ulcers will be healed in 4 weeks but treatment may be continued for up to 8 weeks if required. If the ulcer relapses further treatment courses may be given.

Prophylaxis of NSAID-induced peptic ulcer: 200 micrograms twice daily, three times daily or four times daily. Treatment can be continued as required. Dosage should be individualised according to the clinical condition of each patient.

Elderly

The usual dosage may be used.

Renal impairment: Available evidence indicates that no adjustment of dosage is necessary in patients with renal impairment.

Hepatic impairment: Cytotec is metabolised by fatty acid oxidising systems present in organs throughout the body. Its metabolism and plasma levels are therefore unlikely to be affected markedly in patients with hepatic impairment.

Children

Use of Cytotec in children has not yet been evaluated in the treatment of peptic ulceration or NSAID-induced peptic ulcer disease.

4.3 Contraindications

Use in pregnancy and lactation:

Cytotec is contraindicated in pregnant women and in women planning a pregnancy as it increases uterine tone and contractions in pregnancy which may cause partial or complete expulsion of the products of conception. Use in pregnancy has been associated with birth defects.

It is also contraindicated in patients with a known allergy to prostaglandins.

4.4 Special warnings and special precautions for use

Warnings

Use in pre-menopausal women (see also Contraindications): Cytotec should not be used in pre-menopausal women unless the patient requires nonsteroidal anti-inflammatory (NSAID) therapy and is at high risk of complications from NSAID-induced ulceration.

In such patients it is advised that Cytotec should only be used if the patient:

- takes effective contraceptive measures
- has been advised of the risks of taking Cytotec if pregnant (see Contraindications)

If pregnancy is suspected the product should be discontinued.

Precautions

The results of clinical studies indicate that Cytotec does not produce hypotension at dosages effective in promoting the healing of gastric and duodenal ulcers. Nevertheless, Cytotec should be used with caution in the presence of disease states where hypotension might precipitate severe complications, e.g., cerebrovascular disease, coronary artery disease or severe peripheral vascular disease including hypertension.

There is no evidence that Cytotec has adverse effects on glucose metabolism in human volunteers or patients with diabetes mellitus.

4.5 Interaction with other medicinal products and other forms of Interaction

Cytotec is predominantly metabolised via fatty acid oxidising systems and has shown no adverse effect on the hepatic microsomal mixed function oxidase (P450) enzyme system. In specific studies no clinically significant pharmacokinetic interaction has been demonstrated with antipyrine, diazepam and propranolol. In extensive clinical studies no drug interactions have been attributed to Cytotec. Additional evidence shows no clinically important pharmacokinetic or pharmacodynamic interaction with nonsteroidal anti-inflammatory drugs including aspirin, diclofenac and ibuprofen.

4.6 Pregnancy and lactation

Pregnancy

See Contraindications.

Lactation

It is not known if the active metabolite of Cytotec is excreted in breast milk; therefore Cytotec should not be administered during breast feeding.

4.7 Effects on ability to drive and use machines

Not applicable.

4.8 Undesirable effects

Gastrointestinal system: Diarrhoea has been reported and is occasionally severe and prolonged and may require withdrawal of the drug. It can be minimised by using single doses not exceeding 200 micrograms with food and by avoiding the use of predominantly magnesium containing antacids when an antacid is required.

Abdominal pain with or without associated dyspepsia or diarrhoea can follow misoprostol therapy.

Other gastrointestinal adverse effects reported include dyspepsia, flatulence, nausea and vomiting.

Female reproductive system: Menorrhagia, vaginal bleeding and intermenstrual bleeding have been reported in pre-and post-menopausal women.

Other adverse events: Skin rashes have been reported. Dizziness has been infrequently reported.

The pattern of adverse events associated with Cytotec is similar when an NSAID is given concomitantly.

A number of side effects have been reported in clinical studies or in the literature following use of misoprostol for non-approved indications. These include abnormal uterine contractions, uterine haemorrhage, retained placenta, amniotic fluid embolism, incomplete abortion and premature birth.

4.9 Overdose

Intensification of pharmacological effects may occur with overdose. In the event of overdosage symptomatic and supportive therapy should be given as appropriate. In clinical trials patients have tolerated 1200 micrograms daily for three months without significant adverse effects.

5. PHARMACOLOGICAL PROPERTIES

5.1 Pharmacodynamic properties

Cytotec is an analogue of naturally occurring prostaglandin E_1 which promotes peptic ulcer healing and symptomatic relief.

Cytotec protects the gastroduodenal mucosa by inhibiting basal, stimulated and nocturnal acid secretion and by reducing the volume of gastric secretions, the proteolytic activity of the gastric fluid, and increasing bicarbonate and mucus secretion.

5.2 Pharmacokinetic properties

Cytotec is rapidly absorbed following oral administration, with peak plasma levels of the active metabolite (misoprostol acid) occurring after about 30 minutes. The plasma elimination half-life of misoprostol acid is 20-40 minutes. No accumulation of misoprostol acid in plasma occurs after repeated dosing of 400 micrograms twice daily.

5.3 Preclinical safety data

In single and repeat-dose studies in dogs, rats and mice at multiples of the human dose, toxicological findings were consistent with the known pharmacological effects of the E-type prostaglandins, the main symptoms being diarrhoea, vomiting, mydriasis, tremors and hyperpyrexia. Gastric mucosal hyperplasia was also observed in the mouse, rat and the dog. In the rat and the dog the hyperplasia was reversible on discontinuation of misoprostol following one year of dosing. Histological examination of gastric biopsies in humans has shown no adverse tissue response after up to one year's treatment. In studies of fertility, teratogenicity and peri/post-natal toxicity in rats and rabbits there were no major findings. A decrease in implantations and some pup growth retardation was observed at doses greater than 100 times the human dose. It was concluded that misoprostol does not significantly affect fertility, is not teratogenic or embryotoxic and does not affect rat pups in the peri/post-natal period.

Misoprostol was negative in a battery of 6 in vitro assays and one in vivo test to assess mutagenic potential. In carcinogenicity studies in the rat and mouse it was concluded that there was no risk of carcinogenic hazard.

6. PHARMACEUTICAL PARTICULARS

6.1 List of excipients

Microcrystalline cellulose,

Sodium starch glycolate (Type A),

Hydrogenated castor oil,

Hypromellose.

6.2 Incompatibilities

Not applicable.

6.3 Shelf life

3 Years.

6.4 Special precautions for storage

Do not store above 30°C. Store in the original package.

6.5 Nature and contents of container

Cold-formed aluminium blister packs of 56, 60, 112, 120 or 140 tablets.

Not all pack sizes may be marketed.

6.6 Instructions for use and handling

No Special Requirements.

7. MARKETING AUTHORISATION HOLDER

Pharmacia Limited

Davy Avenue

Milton Keynes

Buckinghamshire

MK5 8PH

United Kingdom

8. MARKETING AUTHORISATION NUMBER(S)

PL 00032/0404

9. DATE OF FIRST AUTHORISATION/RENEWAL OF THE AUTHORISATION

First authorised: 10 May 2002

10. DATE OF REVISION OF THE TEXT

July 2004.

Dacarbazine 100mg, 200mg, 500mg, 1000mg

(medac GmbH)

1. NAME OF THE MEDICINAL PRODUCT

Dacarbazine medac 100 mg, Powder for solution for injection or infusion

Dacarbazine medac 200 mg, Powder for solution for injection or infusion

Dacarbazine medac 500 mg, Powder for solution for infusion

Dacarbazine medac 1000 mg, Powder for solution for infusion

2. QUALITATIVE AND QUANTITATIVE COMPOSITION

Each single-dose vial of Dacarbazine medac 100 mg (-200 mg, -500 mg, -1000 mg) contains 100 mg (200 mg, 500 mg, 1000 mg) dacarbazine (as dacarbazine citrate, formed in situ).

After reconstitution, Dacarbazine medac 100 mg (-200 mg) contains 10 mg/ml dacarbazine (see 6.6 a).

After reconstitution and final dilution, Dacarbazine medac 500 mg (-1000 mg) contains 1.4 – 2.0 mg/ml (2.8 – 4.0 mg/ml) dacarbazine (see 6.6 b).

For excipients, see section 6.1.

3. PHARMACEUTICAL FORM

Dacarbazine medac 100 mg (-200 mg-):

Powder for solution for injection or infusion.

Dacarbazine medac 500 mg (-1000 mg-):

Powder for solution for infusion.

Dacarbazine medac is a white or pale yellow powder.

4. CLINICAL PARTICULARS

4.1 Therapeutic indications

Dacarbazine is indicated for the treatment of patients with metastasized malignant melanoma.

Further indications for dacarbazine as part of a combination chemotherapy are:

advanced Hodgkin's disease, advanced adult soft tissue sarcomas (except mesotheliomas, Kaposi sarcoma).

4.2 Posology and method of administration

The use of dacarbazine should be confined to physicians experienced in oncology or hematology respectively.

Dacarbazine is sensitive to light exposure. All reconstituted solutions should be suitably protected from light also during administration (light-resistant infusion set).

Care should be taken of administration of the injection to avoid extravasation into tissues since this will cause local pain and tissue damage. If extravasation occurs, the injection should be discontinued immediately and any remaining portion of the dose should be introduced into another vein.

The following regimes can be used. For further details cf. current scientific literature.

<u>Malignant Melanoma</u>

Dacarbazine can be administered as single agent in doses of 200 to 250 mg/m^2 body surface area/day as an i.v. injection for 5 days every 3 weeks.

As an alternative to an intravenous bolus injection dacarbazine can be administered as a short-term infusion (over 15 - 30 minutes).

It is also possible to give 850 mg/m^2 body surface area on day 1 and then once every 3 weeks as intravenous infusion.

<u>Hodgkin's disease</u>

Dacarbazine is administered in a daily dose of 375 mg/m^2 body surface area i.v. every 15 days in combination with doxorubicin, bleomycin and vinblastine (ABVD regimen).

<u>Adult soft tissue sarcomas</u>

For adult soft tissue sarcomas dacarbazine is given in daily doses of 250 mg/m^2 body surface area i.v. (days 1 - 5) in combination with doxorubicin every 3 weeks (ADIC regimen).

During dacarbazine treatment frequent monitoring of blood counts should be conducted as well as monitoring of hepatic and renal function. Since severe gastrointestinal reactions frequently occur, antiemetic and supportive measures are advisable.

Because severe gastrointestinal and hematological disturbances can occur, an extremely careful benefit-risk analysis has to be made before every course of therapy with dacarbazine.

Duration of therapy

The treating physician should individually decide about the duration of therapy taking into account the type and stage of the underlying disease, the combination therapy administered and the response to and adverse effects of dacarbazine. In advanced Hodgkin's disease, a usual recommendation is to administer 6 cycles of ABVD combination therapy. In metastasized malignant melanoma and in advanced tissue sarcoma, the duration of treatment depends on the efficacy and tolerability in the individual patient.

Rate of administration

Doses up to 200 mg/m^2 may be given as a slow intravenous injection. Larger doses (ranging from 200 to 850 mg/m^2) should be administered as an i.v. infusion over 15 - 30 minutes.

It is recommended to test the patency of the vein first with a 5 to 10-ml flush of sodium chloride infusion solution or glucose 5 %. The same solutions should be used after infusion to flush any remaining drug from the tubing.

After reconstitution with water for injections without further dilution with sodium chloride infusion solution or glucose 5 %, dacarbazine 100 mg and 200 mg preparations are hypoosmolar (ca. 100 mOsmol/kg) and should therefore be given by slow intravenous injection e.g. over 1 minute rather than rapid intravenous bolus injection over a few seconds.

Special populations

Patients with kidney/liver insufficiency:

If there is mild to moderate renal or hepatic insufficiency alone, a dose reduction is not usually required. In patients with combined renal and hepatic impairment elimination of dacarbazine is prolonged. However, no validated recommendations on dose reductions can be given currently.

Elderly patients:

As limited experience in elderly patients is available no special instructions for the use in elderly patients can be given.

Children:

No special recommendations for the use of dacarbazine in the pediatric age group can be given until further data become available.

4.3 Contraindications

Dacarbazine is contraindicated in patients

- who have a history of hypersensitivity reactions to dacarbazine or to any of the excipients,
- in pregnant or breast-feeding women,
- in patients with leucopenia and/or thrombocytopenia,
- in patients with severe liver or kidney diseases.

4.4 Special warnings and special precautions for use

It is recommended that dacarbazine should only be administered under the supervision of a physician specialized in oncology, having the facilities for regular monitoring of clinical, biochemical and hematological effects, during and after therapy.

If symptoms of a liver or kidney functional disorder or symptoms of a hypersensitivity reaction are observed, immediate cessation of therapy is required. If veno-occlusive disease of the liver occurs, further therapy with dacarbazine is contraindicated.

Note: The responsible physician should be aware of a rarely observed severe complication during therapy resulting from liver necrosis due to occlusion of intrahepatic veins. Therefore, frequent monitoring of liver size, function and blood counts (especially eosinophils) is required (see 4.8).

Long-term therapy can cause cumulative bone marrow toxicity.

The possible bone marrow depression requires careful monitoring of white blood cells, red blood cells and platelet levels. Hemopoetic toxicity may warrant temporary suspension or cessation of therapy.

Extravasation of the drug during i.v. administration may result in tissue damage and severe pain.

Furthermore, dacarbazine is a moderate immunosuppressive agent.

Hepatotoxic drugs and alcohol should be avoided during chemotherapy.

Contraceptive measures:

Men are advised to take contraceptive measures during and for 6 months after cessation of therapy.

Administration of dacarbazine in the pediatric age group:

Dacarbazine is not recommended for use in the pediatric age group until further data become available.

Handling of dacarbazine:

Dacarbazine should be handled according to standard procedures for cytostatics that have mutagenic, carcinogenic and teratogenic effects.

4.5 Interaction with other medicinal products and other forms of Interaction

In case of previous or concomitant treatment having adverse effects on the bone marrow (particularly cytostatic agents, irradiation) myelotoxic interactions are possible.

Studies to investigate the presence of phenotypic metabolism have not been undertaken but hydroxylation of the parent compound to metabolites with anti-tumour activity has been identified.

Dacarbazine is metabolised by cytochrome P450 (CYP1A1, CYP1A2, and CYP2E1). This has to be taken into account if other drugs are co-administered which are metabolised by the same hepatic enzymes.

Dacarbazine can enhance the effects of methoxypsoralen because of photosensitization.

4.6 Pregnancy and lactation

Dacarbazine has been shown to be mutagenic, teratogenic and carcinogenic in animals. It must be assumed that an increased risk for teratogenic effects exists in humans. Therefore, dacarbazine must not be used during pregnancy and during breast-feeding (see: 4.3 und 4.4).

Women of child-bearing potential:

Women of child-bearing age must avoid pregnancy during dacarbazine treatment.

4.7 Effects on ability to drive and use machines

Dacarbazine may influence the ability to drive or operate machines because of its central nervous side effects or because of nausea and vomiting.

4.8 Undesirable effects

Frequencies

Very common (>1/10)

Common (>1/100, <1/10)

Uncommon (>1/1,000, <1/100)

Rare (>1/10,000, <1/1,000)

Very rare (<1/10,000), including isolated reports

The most commonly reported ADRs are gastrointestinal disorders (anorexia, nausea and vomiting) and blood and lymphatic system disorders as anemia, leukopenia and thrombocytopenia. The latter are dose-dependant and delayed, with the nadirs often only occurring after 3 to 4 weeks.

Blood and lymphatic system disorders	<u>Common (≥ 1/100, ≤ 1/10)</u> Anemia, leukopenia, thrombocytopenia <u>Rare (≥ 1/10,000, ≤ 1/1,000)</u> Pancytopenia, agranulocytosis
Immune system disorders	<u>Rare (≥ 1/10,000, ≤ 1/1,000)</u> Anaphylactic reactions
Nervous system disorders	<u>Rare (≥ 1/10,000, ≤ 1/1,000)</u> Headaches, impaired vision, confusion, lethargy, convulsions, facial paraesthesia
Vascular disorders	<u>Rare (≥ 1/10,000, ≤ 1/1,000)</u> Facial flushing
Gastrointestinal disorders	<u>Common (≥ 1/100, ≤ 1/10)</u> Anorexia, nausea, vomiting <u>Rare (≥ 1/10,000, ≤ 1/1,000)</u> Diarrhoea
Hepatobiliary disorders	<u>Very rare (≤ 1/10,000), including isolated reports</u> Hepatic necrosis due to veno-occlusive disease (VOD) of the liver
Renal and urinary disorders	<u>Rare (≥ 1/10,000, ≤ 1/1,000)</u> Impaired renal function
Skin and subcutaneous tissue disorders	<u>Uncommon (≥ 1/1,000, ≤ 1/100)</u> Alopecia, hyperpigmentation, photosensitivity <u>Rare (≥ 1/10,000, ≤ 1/1,000)</u> Erythema, maculopapular exanthema, urticaria
General disorders and administration site conditions	<u>Uncommon (≥ 1/1,000, ≤ 1/100)</u> Flu-like symptoms <u>Rare (≥ 1/10,000, ≤ 1/1,000)</u> Application site irritation
Investigations	<u>Rare (≥ 1/10,000, ≤ 1/1,000)</u> Elevation of liver enzymes

Disturbances of the digestive tract such as anorexia, nausea and vomiting are common and severe. In rare cases diarrhoea has been observed.

Changes in blood counts often observed (anemia, leukopenia, thrombocytopenia) are dose-dependent and delayed, with the nadirs often only occurring after 3 to 4 weeks. In rare cases pancytopenia and agranulocytosis have been described.

Flu-like symptoms with exhaustion, chills, fever and muscular pain are occasionally observed during or often only days after dacarbazine administration. These disturbances may recur with the next infusion.

Elevation of liver enzymes (e.g. alkaline phosphatase) is observed in rare cases.

In isolated cases liver necrosis due to occlusion of intrahepatic veins (veno-occlusive disease of the liver) has been observed after administration of dacarbazine in monotherapy or in combined treatment modalities. In general the syndrome occurred during the second cycle of therapy. Symptoms included fever, eosinophilia, abdominal pain, enlarged liver, jaundice and shock which worsened rapidly over a few hours or days. As fatal outcome has been described special care has to be taken of frequently monitoring of liver size, function and blood counts (especially eosinophils) (see 4.2 and 4.4).

Application site irritations and some of the systemic adverse reactions are thought to result from formation of photodegradation products.

Impaired renal function with increased blood levels of substances obligatory excreted by urine is rare.

Central nervous side effects such as headaches, impaired vision, confusion, lethargy and convulsions rarely may occur. Facial paraesthesia and flushing may occur shortly after injection.

Allergic reactions of the skin in the form of erythema, maculopapular exanthema or urticaria are observed rarely. Infrequently alopecia, hyperpigmentation and photosensitivity of the skin may occur. In rare cases anaphylactic reactions have been described.

Inadvertent paravenous injection is expected to cause local pain and necrosis.

4.9 Overdose

The primary anticipated complications of overdose are severe bone marrow suppression, eventually bone marrow aplasia which may be delayed by up to two weeks.

Time to occurrence of nadirs of leucocytes and thrombocytes can be 4 weeks. Even if overdosage is only suspected, long-term careful hematologic monitoring is essential. There is no known antidote for dacarbazine overdose. Therefore, special care has to be taken to avoid overdose of this drug.

5. PHARMACOLOGICAL PROPERTIES

5.1 Pharmacodynamic properties

Pharmacotherapeutic group: Alkylating agents, ATC code: L01AX04

Dacarbazine is a cytostatic agent. The antineoplastic effect is due to an inhibition of cell growth which is independent of the cell cycle and due to an inhibition of DNA synthesis. An alkylating effect has also been shown and other cytostatic mechanisms may also be influenced by dacarbazine.

Dacarbazine is considered not to show an antineoplastic effect by itself. However, by microsomal N-demethylation it is quickly converted to 5-amino-imidazole-4-carboxamide and a methyl cation which is responsible for the alkylating effect of the drug.

5.2 Pharmacokinetic properties

After intravenous administration, dacarbazine is quickly distributed into tissue. Plasma protein binding is 5 %. Kinetics in plasma are biphasic; the initial (distribution) half-life is only 20 minutes, terminal half-life is 0.5 - 3.5 hours.

Dacarbazine is inactive until metabolised in the liver by cytochromes P450 to form the reactive N-demethylated species HMMTIC and MTIC. This is catalysed by CYP1A1, CYP1A2, and CYP2E1. MTIC is further metabolised to 5-aminoimidazole-4-carboxamide (AIC).

Dacarbazine is metabolised mainly in the liver by both hydroxylation and demethylation, approx. 20 - 50% of the drug is excreted unmodified by the kidney via renal tubular secretion.

5.3 Preclinical safety data

Because of its pharmacodynamic properties dacarbazine shows mutagenic, carcinogenic and teratogenic effects which are detectable in experimental test systems.

6. PHARMACEUTICAL PARTICULARS

6.1 List of excipients

Citric acid, anhydrous, and mannitol.

6.2 Incompatibilities

Dacarbazine solution is chemically incompatible with heparin, hydrocortisone, L-cysteine and sodium hydrogen carbonate.

6.3 Shelf life

The shelf-life is 3 years.

<u>Shelf life of the reconstituted solution of Dacarbazine medac 100 mg (-200 mg):</u>

A chemical and physical in-use stability has been demonstrated for 24 hours at 20°C protected from light.

From a microbiological point of view, the product should be used immediately. If not used immediately, in-use storage times and conditions prior to use are the responsibility of the user and would normally be no longer than 24 hours at 2 to 8°C, unless reconstitution has taken place in controlled and validated aseptic conditions.

<u>Shelf life of the reconstituted and further diluted solution of Dacarbazine medac 100 mg (-200 mg):</u>

The reconstituted and further diluted solution must be used immediately.

<u>Shelf life of the reconstituted and further diluted solution of Dacarbazine medac 500 mg (-1000 mg):</u>

The reconstituted and further diluted solution must be used immediately.

6.4 Special precautions for storage

Do not store above 25 °C, keep the vial in outer carton in order to protect from light. Reconstituted solutions should also be protected from light.

For storage of the reconstituted product, see 6.3.

6.5 Nature and contents of container

Dacarbazine medac 100 mg (-200 mg-) is supplied as a sterile powder for solution for injection or infusion in single-dose vials made of amber glass (Type I, Ph.Eur.) and closed with butyl rubber stoppers. Each carton of Dacarbazine medac 100 mg (-200 mg-) contains 10 vials.

Dacarbazine medac 500 mg (-1000 mg-) is supplied as a sterile powder for solution for infusion in single-dose vials made of amber glass (Type I, Ph.Eur.) and closed with butyl rubber stoppers. Each carton of Dacarbazine medac 500 mg (-1000 mg-) contains one vial.

6.6 Instructions for use and handling

Recommendations for the safe handling:

Dacarbazine is an antineoplastic agent. Before commencing, local cytotoxic guidelines should be referred to.

Dacarbazine should only be opened by trained staff and as with all cytotoxic agents, precautions should be taken to avoid exposing staff. Handling of cytotoxic drugs should be generally avoided during pregnancy. Preparation of solution for administration should be carried out in a designated handling area and working over a washable tray or disposable plastic-backed absorbent paper.

Suitable eye protection, disposable gloves, face mask and disposable apron should be worn. Syringes and infusion sets should be assembled carefully to avoid leakage (use of Luer lock fittings is recommended).

On completion, any exposed surface should be thoroughly cleaned and hands and face washed.

In the event of spillage, operators should put on gloves, face masks, eye-protection and disposable apron and mop up the spilled material with an absorbent material tapped in the area for that purpose. The area should then be cleaned and all contaminated material transferred to a cytotoxic spillage bag or bin or sealed for incineration.

Preparation for the intravenous administration:

Dacarbazine solutions are prepared immediately before use.

Dacarbazine is sensitive to light exposure. During administration, the infusion container and administration set should be protected from exposure to daylight, e.g. by using light-resistant PVC infusion sets. Normal infusion sets should be wrapped up in e.g. UV-resistant foils.

a) Preparation of Dacarbazine medac 100 mg (-200 mg-):

Aseptically transfer the required amount of water for injections (Dacarbazine medac 100 mg: 10 ml; Dacarbazine medac 200 mg: 20 ml) into the vial and shake until a solution is obtained. This freshly prepared solution (dacarbazine: 10 mg/ml*) is administered as a slow injection.

For preparation of Dacarbazine medac 100 mg (-200 mg-) for i.v. infusion the freshly prepared solution is further diluted with 200 - 300 ml sodium chloride infusion solution or glucose 5 %. This solution is given as a short-term infusion over a period between 15 - 30 minutes.

b) Preparation of Dacarbazine medac 500 mg (-1000 mg):

Aseptically transfer the required amount of 50 ml water for injections into the Dacarbazine medac 500 mg (-1000 mg-) vial and shake until a solution is obtained⁺. The resulting solution has to be further diluted with 200 - 300 ml sodium chloride infusion solution or glucose 5 %. The obtained infusion solution is ready for i.v. administration (Dacarbazine medac 500 mg: 1.4 - 2.0 mg/ml; Dacarbazine medac 1000 mg: 2.8 - 4.0 mg/ml) and should be given within 20 - 30 minutes.

Dacarbazine medac 100 mg (-200 mg, -500 mg, -1000 mg) is for single use only.

The diluted solution for infusion should be visually inspected and only clear solutions practically free from particles should be used. Do not use the solution if particles are present.

Any portion of the contents remaining after use should be discarded, as well as solutions where the visual appearance of the product has changed.

Disposal: All materials that have been utilized for dilution and administration should be disposed of according to standard procedures (incineration).

* Density of the solution:

1.007 mg/ml

⁺ Density of the solution:

1.007 mg/ml (Dacarbazine medac 500 mg)

1.015 mg/ml (Dacarbazine medac 1000 mg)

7. MARKETING AUTHORISATION HOLDER

medac

Gesellschaft fur klinische Spezialpraparate mbH

Fehlandtstrasse 3

D-20354 Hamburg

8. MARKETING AUTHORISATION NUMBER(S)

Dacarbazine medac 100 mg

MA-no.: PL 11587/0008

Dacarbazine medac 200 mg

MA-no.: PL 11587/0009

Dacarbazine medac 500 mg

MA-no.: PL 11587/0010

Dacarbazine medac 1000 mg

MA-no.: PL 11587/0011

9. DATE OF FIRST AUTHORISATION/RENEWAL OF THE AUTHORISATION

November 28, 1997 / April 24, 2005

10. DATE OF REVISION OF THE TEXT

May 11, 2005

Full information is available on request from

medac UK

Scion House

Stirling University Innovation Park

Stirling FK9 4NF

Tel: 01786 458 086

Daktacort Cream & Ointment

(Janssen-Cilag Ltd)

1. NAME OF THE MEDICINAL PRODUCT

Daktacort® Cream

Daktacort® Ointment

2. QUALITATIVE AND QUANTITATIVE COMPOSITION

Miconazole nitrate 2% w/w and hydrocortisone 1% w/w.

3. PHARMACEUTICAL FORM

Cream: White, homogenous cream.

Ointment: White, odourless, fatty ointment.

4. CLINICAL PARTICULARS

4.1 Therapeutic indications

For the topical treatment of inflamed dermatoses where infection by susceptible organisms and inflammation co-exist, eg intertrigo and infected eczema.

Moist or dry eczema or dermatitis including atopic eczema, primary irritant or contact allergic eczema or seborrhoeic eczema including that associated with acne.

Intertriginous eczema including inframammary intertrigo, perianal and genital dermatitis.

Organisms which are susceptible to miconazole are dermatophytes and pathogenic yeasts (eg *Candida* spp.). Also many Gram-positive bacteria including most strains of *Streptococcus* and *Staphylococcus*.

The properties of Daktacort indicate it particularly for the initial stages of treatment. Once the inflammatory symptoms have disappeared (after about 7 days), treatment can be continued where necessary with Daktarin® Cream or Daktarin® Powder.

4.2 Posology and method of administration

For topical administration.

Cream:

Apply the cream two or three times a day to the affected area, rubbing in gently until the cream has been absorbed by the skin.

Ointment:

Daktacort Ointment should be applied topically two or three times daily.

The same dosage applies to both adults and children.

<u>*Use in elderly*</u>:

Natural thinning of the skin occurs in the elderly, hence corticosteroids should be used sparingly and for short periods of time.

In infants, long term continuous topical corticosteroid therapy should be avoided.

If after about 7 days' application, no improvement has occurred, cultural isolation of the offending organism should be followed by appropriate local or systemic antimicrobial therapy.

4.3 Contraindications
True hypersensitivity to any of the ingredients. Tubercular or viral infections of the skin or those caused by Gram-negative bacteria.

4.4 Special warnings and special precautions for use
As with any topical corticosteroid, care is advised with infants and children when Daktacort is to be applied to extensive surface areas or under occlusive dressings including baby napkins; similarly, application to the face should be avoided.

In infants, long term continuous topical corticosteroid therapy should be avoided. Adrenal suppression can occur even without occlusion.

4.5 Interaction with other medicinal products and other forms of Interaction
Miconazole administered systemically is known to inhibit CYP3A4/2C9. Due to the limited systemic availability after topical application, clinically relevant interactions are rare. However, in patients on oral anticoagulants, such as warfarin, caution should be exercised and anticoagulant effect should be monitored.

4.6 Pregnancy and lactation
In animals, miconazole nitrate has shown no teratogenic effects but is foetotoxic at high oral doses and administration of corticosteroids to pregnant animals can cause abnormalities of foetal development. The relevance of these findings to humans has not been established. However, combinations of topical steroids with imidazoles should be used in pregnant women only if the practitioner considers it to be necessary.

4.7 Effects on ability to drive and use machines
None known.

4.8 Undesirable effects
Rarely, local sensitivity may occur requiring discontinuation of treatment.

4.9 Overdose
Topically applied corticosteroids can be absorbed in sufficient amounts to produce systemic effects. If accidental ingestion of large quantities of the product occurs, an appropriate method of gastric emptying may be used if considered necessary.

5. PHARMACOLOGICAL PROPERTIES

5.1 Pharmacodynamic properties
Miconazole nitrate is a potent broad-spectrum antifungal and antibacterial agent with marked activity against dermatophytes, pathogenic yeasts (eg *Candida* spp) and many Gram-positive bacteria including most strains of *Streptococcus* and *Staphylococcus*.

Hydrocortisone is a widely used topical anti-inflammatory of value in the treatment of inflammatory skin conditions including atrophic and infantile eczema, contact sensitivity reactions and intertrigo.

5.2 Pharmacokinetic properties
Following topical administration of 100 mg miconazole nitrate cream, plasma concentrations of 0.01 μg/ml were never exceeded. Allowing for a 100 fold increase due to the occlusive effects of the ointment base, if the whole of a 30 g tube (containing 600 mg miconazole) was applied at once, maximum plasma levels would be of the order of 6 μg/ml. This would correspond approximately to an iv dose of 5 mg/kg.

Similar plasma levels are achieved in rabbits after an oral dose of 40 mg/kg and in rats and rabbits after an intravenous dose of 20 mg/kg (extrapolated value).

Reproduction studies showed that there were no effects at these doses.

5.3 Preclinical safety data
Not applicable.

6. PHARMACEUTICAL PARTICULARS

6.1 List of excipients
Cream:
PEG-6, PEG-32 and glycol stearate
Polyoxyethylene glycol glycerides
Mineral oil
Benzoic acid
Disodium edetate
Butylated hydroxyanisole
Purified water
Ointment:
Polyethylene 5.5% liquid paraffin gel

6.2 Incompatibilities
None known.

6.3 Shelf life
36 months.

6.4 Special precautions for storage
Cream: Store in a refrigerator (2-8°C).
Ointment: Store at or below 25°C.

6.5 Nature and contents of container
Aluminium tube with polypropylene cap.
Cream: Each tube contains 30 g cream.
Ointment: Each tube contains 30 g ointment.

6.6 Instructions for use and handling
None.

7. MARKETING AUTHORISATION HOLDER
Janssen-Cilag Ltd
Saunderton
High Wycombe
Buckinghamshire
HP14 4HJ

8. MARKETING AUTHORISATION NUMBER(S)
Cream: PL 00242/0042
Ointment: PL 00242/0130

9. DATE OF FIRST AUTHORISATION/RENEWAL OF THE AUTHORISATION
Date of First Authorisation:
Cream: 04/02/77
Ointment: 05/03/87
Renewal of Authorisation:
Cream: 16/04/97
Ointment: 28/02/97

10. DATE OF REVISION OF THE TEXT
Cream: 12/07/04
Ointment: 12/07/04

Legal category POM.

Daktacort Hydrocortisone Cream
(Janssen-Cilag Ltd)

1. NAME OF THE MEDICINAL PRODUCT
Daktacort Hydrocortisone Cream

2. QUALITATIVE AND QUANTITATIVE COMPOSITION
Miconazole nitrate 2%w/w; Hydrocortisone acetate equivalent to hydrocortisone 1%w/w.

For excipients, see 6.1.

3. PHARMACEUTICAL FORM
Cream.

White, homogeneous, odourless cream

4. CLINICAL PARTICULARS

4.1 Therapeutic indications
Athlete's foot and candidal intertrigo where there are co-existing symptoms of inflammation.

Organisms which are susceptible to miconazole are dermatophytes and pathogenic yeasts (eg, *Candida* spp.). Also many Gram-positive bacteria including most strains of *Streptococcus* and *Staphylococcus*.

The properties of Daktacort HC indicate it particularly for the initial stages of treatment. Once the inflammatory symptoms have disappeared, treatment can be continued with Daktarin cream or Daktarin powder.

4.2 Posology and method of administration
For topical administration

Apply the cream twice a day to the affected area, rubbing in gently until the cream has been absorbed by the skin.

The maximum period of treatment is 7 days.

4.3 Contraindications
Hypersensitivity to any of the ingredients. Tubercular or viral infections of the skin or those caused by Gram-negative bacteria.

Daktacort HC should not be used in the following conditions:

- If the skin is broken
- On large areas of skin
- Used for longer than 7 days
- To treat cold sores and acne
- Use on the face, eyes and mucous membranes
- Children under 10 years of age, unless prescribed by a doctor
- On the ano-genital region unless prescribed by a doctor
- To treat ringworm unless prescribed by a doctor
- To treat secondary infected conditions unless prescribed by a doctor

4.4 Special warnings and special precautions for use
As with any topical corticosteroid, care is advised when Daktacort HC is to be applied to extensive surface areas or under occlusive dressings including baby napkins; similarly application to the face should be avoided.

Long term continuous topical corticosteroid therapy should be avoided. Adrenal suppression can occur even without occlusion.

4.5 Interaction with other medicinal products and other forms of Interaction
Miconazole administered systemically is known to inhibit CYP3A4/2C9. Due to the limited systemic availability after topical application, clinically relevant interactions are rare. However, in patients on oral anticoagulants, such as warfarin, caution should be exercised and anticoagulant effect should be monitored.

4.6 Pregnancy and lactation
In animals, miconazole nitrate has shown no teratogenic effects but is foetotoxic at high oral doses and administration of corticosteroids to pregnant animals can cause abnormalities of foetal development. The relevance of these findings to humans has not been established. However, combinations of topical steroids with imidazoles should be used in pregnant women only if the practitioner considers it to be necessary.

4.7 Effects on ability to drive and use machines
None known.

4.8 Undesirable effects
Rarely, local sensitivity may occur requiring discontinuation of treatment.

4.9 Overdose
Topically applied corticosteroids can be absorbed in sufficient amounts to produce systemic effects. If accidental ingestion of large quantities of the product occurs, an appropriate method of gastric emptying may be used if considered necessary.

5. PHARMACOLOGICAL PROPERTIES

5.1 Pharmacodynamic properties
Miconazole nitrate is active against dermatophytes and pathogenic yeasts and many Gram-positive bacteria. Hydrocortisone has anti-inflammatory activity.

5.2 Pharmacokinetic properties
Not applicable.

5.3 Preclinical safety data
Not applicable.

6. PHARMACEUTICAL PARTICULARS

6.1 List of excipients
Macrogol 6-32 stearate and glycol stearate
Oleyl macrogolglycerides
Liquid paraffin
Butylhydroxyanisole
Benzoic acid
Disodium edetate
Sodium hydroxide solution
Purified water

6.2 Incompatibilities
None known

6.3 Shelf life
24 months

6.4 Special precautions for storage
None

6.5 Nature and contents of container
Aluminium tubes with internal epoxyphenolic resin lacquer and polypropylene screw cap or tubes made of a multi-laminate aluminium/low density polyethylene foil with a polypropylene screw cap.

Each tube contains 5g, 10g or 15g cream.

6.6 Instructions for use and handling
None.

7. MARKETING AUTHORISATION HOLDER
Janssen-Cilag Limited
Saunderton
High Wycombe
Buckinghamshire
HP14 4HJ

8. MARKETING AUTHORISATION NUMBER(S)
PL 00242/0367

9. DATE OF FIRST AUTHORISATION/RENEWAL OF THE AUTHORISATION
24 August 2001

10. DATE OF REVISION OF THE TEXT
16/02/05

LEGAL STATUS: P

Daktarin Cream
(Janssen-Cilag Ltd)

1. NAME OF THE MEDICINAL PRODUCT
Daktarin® Cream.

2. QUALITATIVE AND QUANTITATIVE COMPOSITION
Miconazole nitrate 2% w/w.

3. PHARMACEUTICAL FORM
White homogeneous cream.

4. CLINICAL PARTICULARS

4.1 Therapeutic indications
For the treatment of mycotic infections of the skin and nails and superinfections due to Gram-positive bacteria.

4.2 Posology and method of administration

Route of administration:

Cutaneous use.

Recommended dosage: For all ages:

Skin infections: Apply the cream twice daily to the lesions. Treatment should be prolonged for 10 days after all lesions have disappeared to prevent relapse.

Nail infections: Apply the cream once or twice daily to the lesions. Treatment should be prolonged for 10 days after all lesions have disappeared to prevent relapse.

4.3 Contraindications

None known.

4.4 Special warnings and special precautions for use

None.

4.5 Interaction with other medicinal products and other forms of Interaction

Miconazole administered systemically is known to inhibit CYP3A4/2C9. Due to the limited systemic availability after topical application, clinically relevant interactions are rare. However, in patients on oral anticoagulants, such as warfarin, caution should be exercised and anticoagulant effect should be monitored.

4.6 Pregnancy and lactation

In animals miconazole nitrate has shown no teratogenic effects but is foetotoxic at high oral doses. Only small amounts of miconazole nitrate are absorbed following topical administration. However, as with other imidazoles, miconazole nitrate should be used with caution during pregnancy.

4.7 Effects on ability to drive and use machines

None known.

4.8 Undesirable effects

Occasionally irritation has been reported. Rarely, local sensitisation may occur in which case administration of the product should be discontinued.

4.9 Overdose

Daktarin cream is intended for topical use. If accidental ingestion of the product occurs, an appropriate method of gastric emptying may be used if considered advisable.

5. PHARMACOLOGICAL PROPERTIES

5.1 Pharmacodynamic properties

Miconazole nitrate is an imidazole antifungal agent and may act by interfering with the permeability of the fungal cell membrane. It possesses a wide antifungal spectrum and has some antibacterial activity.

5.2 Pharmacokinetic properties

There is little absorption through skin or mucous membranes when miconazole nitrate is applied topically.

When administered orally, miconazole is incompletely absorbed from the gastro-intestinal tract. Peak plasma concentrations occur at about 4 hours after administration. Miconazole disappears from the plasma in a triphasic manner with a biological half-life of about 24 hours. Over 90% are reported to be bound to plasma proteins.

5.3 Preclinical safety data

No relevant information additional to that contained elsewhere in the Summary of Product Characteristics.

6. PHARMACEUTICAL PARTICULARS

6.1 List of excipients

Macrogol 6-32 stearate and glycol stearate

Unsaturated polyglycolysed glycerides

Liquid paraffin

Benzoic acid (E210)

Butylated hydroxyanisole (E320)

Purified water

6.2 Incompatibilities

None known.

6.3 Shelf life

24months.

6.4 Special precautions for storage

Do not store above 25°C.

6.5 Nature and contents of container

Aluminium tube inner lined with heat polymerised epoxyphenol resin with a white polypropylene cap containing 15 g, 30 g or 70 g of cream, or aluminium tube inner lined with heat polymerised epoxy-phenol resin with a high density polyethylene cap containing 5 g of cream.

6.6 Instructions for use and handling

Not applicable.

7. MARKETING AUTHORISATION HOLDER

Janssen-Cilag Ltd,

PO Box 79

Saunderton,

High Wycombe

HP14 4HJ

8. MARKETING AUTHORISATION NUMBER(S)

PL 00242/0016

9. DATE OF FIRST AUTHORISATION/RENEWAL OF THE AUTHORISATION

13 May 1974 / 11 August 2000

10. DATE OF REVISION OF THE TEXT

12/07/04

Legal Category: P

Daktarin Dual Action Cream

(Janssen-Cilag Ltd)

1. NAME OF THE MEDICINAL PRODUCT

Daktarin Dual Action Cream

2. QUALITATIVE AND QUANTITATIVE COMPOSITION

Miconazole Nitrate Ph.Eur 2.0% w/w

3. PHARMACEUTICAL FORM

Cream

4. CLINICAL PARTICULARS

4.1 Therapeutic indications

For the treatment of athlete's foot.

4.2 Posology and method of administration

For all ages.

Apply the cream twice daily to the lesions. Treatment should be prolonged for 10 days after all lesions have disappeared to prevent relapse.

Method of administration: Cutaneous application.

4.3 Contraindications

None known.

4.4 Special warnings and special precautions for use

None.

4.5 Interaction with other medicinal products and other forms of Interaction

Miconazole administered systemically is known to inhibit CYP3A4/2C9. Due to the limited systemic availability after topical application, clinically relevant interactions are rare. However, in patients on oral anticoagulants, such as warfarin, caution should be exercised and anticoagulant effect should be monitored.

4.6 Pregnancy and lactation

In animals, miconazole nitrate has shown no teratogenic effects but is foetotoxic at high oral doses. Only small amounts of miconazole nitrate are absorbed following topical administration. However, as with other imidazoles, miconazole nitrate should be used with caution during pregnancy.

4.7 Effects on ability to drive and use machines

None known.

4.8 Undesirable effects

Occasionally irritation has been reported. Rarely local sensitisation or hypersensitivity may occur in which case administration of the product should be discontinued.

4.9 Overdose

Daktarin Dual Action Cream is intended for topical use. If accidental ingestion of the product occurs, an appropriate method of gastric emptying may be used if considered advisable.

5. PHARMACOLOGICAL PROPERTIES

5.1 Pharmacodynamic properties

Miconazole is an imidazole antifungal agent and may act by interfering with the permeability of the fungal cell membrane. It possesses a wide antifungal spectrum and has some antibacterial activity.

5.2 Pharmacokinetic properties

There is little absorption through skin or mucous membranes when miconazole nitrate is applied topically.

When administered orally miconazole is incompletely absorbed from the gastro-intestinal tract. Peak plasma concentrations occur at about 4 hours after administration. Miconazole disappears from the plasma in a triphasic manner with a biological half life of about 24 hours. Over 90% is reported to be bound to plasma proteins.

5.3 Preclinical safety data

No relevant information additional to that contained elsewhere in the Summary of Product Characteristics.

6. PHARMACEUTICAL PARTICULARS

6.1 List of excipients

Macrogol 6-32 stearate and glycol stearate

Unsaturated polyglycolysed glycerides

Liquid paraffin

Benzoic acid (E210)

Butylated hydroxyanisole (E320)

Purified water

6.2 Incompatibilities

None known.

6.3 Shelf life

24 months.

6.4 Special precautions for storage

Do not store above 25°C.

6.5 Nature and contents of container

Aluminium tube lined with epoxyphenol resin. Cap made of white polypropylene for the 15, 30 and 70g sizes. Cap for 5g size made of high density polyethylene.

Daktarin Dual Action Cream may be supplied in packs of 5, 15, 30 and 70g.

6.6 Instructions for use and handling

Not applicable.

7. MARKETING AUTHORISATION HOLDER

Janssen-Cilag Ltd.

Saunderton,

High Wycombe,

Bucks HP14 4HJ,

UK

8. MARKETING AUTHORISATION NUMBER(S)

PL 00242/0324

9. DATE OF FIRST AUTHORISATION/RENEWAL OF THE AUTHORISATION

17 November 1997/16 November 2002

10. DATE OF REVISION OF THE TEXT

12/07/04

Legal category GSL

Daktarin Dual Action Powder

(Janssen-Cilag Ltd)

1. NAME OF THE MEDICINAL PRODUCT

Daktarin Dual Action Powder

2. QUALITATIVE AND QUANTITATIVE COMPOSITION

Miconazole nitrate 2.0% w/w

3. PHARMACEUTICAL FORM

Cutaneous powder

4. CLINICAL PARTICULARS

4.1 Therapeutic indications

For the treatment of athlete's foot.

4.2 Posology and method of administration

Adults

Twice daily application of the powder to the lesions, treatment being prolonged for some 10 days after all lesions have disappeared to prevent relapse.

Elderly

As for adults

Children

As for adults

Method of administration: Cutaneous use

4.3 Contraindications

Known hypersensitivity to miconazole or any other component of this product.

The powder should not be recommended for treatment of infections of the hair and nails

4.4 Special warnings and special precautions for use

If a reaction suggesting sensitivity or irritation should occur, the treatment should be discontinued.

4.5 Interaction with other medicinal products and other forms of Interaction

Miconazole administered systemically is known to inhibit CYP3A4/2C9. Due to the limited systemic availability after topical application, clinically relevant interactions are rare. However, in patients on oral anticoagulants, such as warfarin, caution should be exercised and anticoagulant effect should be monitored.

4.6 Pregnancy and lactation

In animals, miconazole nitrate has shown no teratogenic effects but is foetotoxic at high oral doses. Only small amounts of miconazole nitrate are absorbed following topical administration. However, as with other imidazoles, miconazole nitrate should be used with caution during pregnancy.

4.7 Effects on ability to drive and use machines

None known

4.8 Undesirable effects

Hypersensitivity has rarely been recorded, if it should occur the treatment should be discontinued.

4.9 Overdose

Daktarin Dual Action Powder is intended for topical use. If accidental ingestion of large quantities of the product occur, an appropriate method of gastric emptying may be used if considered desirable.

5. PHARMACOLOGICAL PROPERTIES

5.1 Pharmacodynamic properties

Miconazole is an imidazole antifungal agent and may act by interfering with the permeability of the fungal cell membrane. It possesses a wide antifungal spectrum and has some antibacterial activity.

5.2 Pharmacokinetic properties

There is little absorption through skin or mucous membranes when miconazole nitrate is applied topically.

When administered orally miconazole is incompletely absorbed from the gastro-intestinal tract. Peak plasma concentrations occur at about 4 hours after administration. Miconazole disappears from the plasma in a triphasic manner with a biological half life of about 24 hours. Over 90% is reported to be bound to plasma proteins.

5.3 Preclinical safety data
No relevant information additional to that contained elsewhere in the Summary of Product Characteristics.

6. PHARMACEUTICAL PARTICULARS
6.1 List of excipients
Talc

Zinc oxide

Colloidal anhydrous silica

6.2 Incompatibilities
Not applicable.

6.3 Shelf life
60 months

6.4 Special precautions for storage
Store at room temperature.

6.5 Nature and contents of container
High density polyethylene bottle with polypropylene dredger cap and screw cap containing 20 grams or 30 grams of powder.

6.6 Instructions for use and handling
No special instructions.

Administrative Data
7. MARKETING AUTHORISATION HOLDER
Janssen-Cilag Ltd.

Saunderton, High Wycombe

Bucks HP14 4HJ,

UK

8. MARKETING AUTHORISATION NUMBER(S)
PL 00242/0325

9. DATE OF FIRST AUTHORISATION/RENEWAL OF THE AUTHORISATION
20 January 1998/16 November 2002

10. DATE OF REVISION OF THE TEXT
12/07/04

Legal category GSL.

Daktarin Dual Action Spray Powder

(Janssen-Cilag Ltd)

1. NAME OF THE MEDICINAL PRODUCT
Daktarin Dual Action Spray Powder

2. QUALITATIVE AND QUANTITATIVE COMPOSITION
Miconazole nitrate Ph.Eur 0.16% w/w

3. PHARMACEUTICAL FORM
Cutaneous spray powder

4. CLINICAL PARTICULARS
4.1 Therapeutic indications
Cutaneous administration for the treatment and prevention of athlete's foot.

4.2 Posology and method of administration
Apply to infected area twice daily until the lesions are healed.

Method of administration: Cutaneous use

4.3 Contraindications
Known hypersensitivity to miconazole or any other component of this product.

Not to be used on hair infections, nail infections or broken skin.

4.4 Special warnings and special precautions for use
The spray should be kept away from the eyes and mucous membranes.

If a reaction suggesting sensitivity or irritation should occur, the treatment should be discontinued.

4.5 Interaction with other medicinal products and other forms of Interaction
Miconazole administered systemically is known to inhibit CYP3A4/2C9. Due to the limited systemic availability after topical application, clinically relevant interactions are rare. However, in patients on oral anticoagulants, such as warfarin, caution should be exercised and anticoagulant effect should be monitored.

4.6 Pregnancy and lactation
In animals, miconazole nitrate has shown no teratogenic effects but is foetotoxic at high oral doses. Only small amounts of miconazole nitrate are absorbed following topical administration. However, as with other imidazoles, miconazole nitrate should be used with caution during pregnancy.

4.7 Effects on ability to drive and use machines
None known

4.8 Undesirable effects
Hypersensitivity has rarely been recorded, if it should occur the treatment should be discontinued.

4.9 Overdose
Daktarin Dual Action Spray Powder is intended for topical use. If accidental ingestion of large quantities of the product occur, an appropriate method of gastric emptying may be used if considered desirable.

5. PHARMACOLOGICAL PROPERTIES
5.1 Pharmacodynamic properties
Miconazole is an imidazole antifungal agent and may act by interfering with the permeability of the fungal cell membrane. It possesses a wide antifungal spectrum and has some antibacterial activity.

5.2 Pharmacokinetic properties
There is little absorption through skin or mucous membranes when miconazole nitrate is applied topically.

When administered orally miconazole is incompletely absorbed from the gastro-intestinal tract. Peak plasma concentrations occur at about 4 hours after administration. Miconazole disappears from the plasma in a triphasic manner with a biological half life of about 24 hours. Over 90% is reported to be bound to plasma proteins.

5.3 Preclinical safety data
No relevant information additional to that contained elsewhere in the Summary of Product Characteristics.

6. PHARMACEUTICAL PARTICULARS
6.1 List of excipients
Stearalkonuim hectorite

Denatured alcohol

Hydrocarbon propellant

Sorbitan sesquioleate

Talc

6.2 Incompatibilities
Not applicable.

6.3 Shelf life
24 months

6.4 Special precautions for storage
Store in a cool dry place away from direct heat and sunlight.

Keep out of reach and sight of children.

6.5 Nature and contents of container
Three piece aerosol container with epoxy lining and welded side seam with protective epoxy side strip. 1 inch opening to accommodate a standard aerosol valve.

The aerosol container contains 100g of product.

6.6 Instructions for use and handling
Shake well. Hold can 3 inches from skin, then generously spray affected area.

7. MARKETING AUTHORISATION HOLDER
Janssen-Cilag Ltd.

Saunderton, High Wycombe

Bucks HP14 4HJ

UK

8. MARKETING AUTHORISATION NUMBER(S)
PL 00242/0326

9. DATE OF FIRST AUTHORISATION/RENEWAL OF THE AUTHORISATION
20 January 1998

10. DATE OF REVISION OF THE TEXT
12 /07/04

Legal status GSL

Daktarin Gold (Nizoral Cream)

(Janssen-Cilag Ltd)

1. NAME OF THE MEDICINAL PRODUCT
POM: Nizoral Cream

P: Daktarin Gold

2. QUALITATIVE AND QUANTITATIVE COMPOSITION
Ketoconazole Ph.Eur 2% w/w.

3. PHARMACEUTICAL FORM
Cream

4. CLINICAL PARTICULARS
4.1 Therapeutic indications
POM

For topical application in the treatment of dermatophyte infections of the skin such as tinea corporis, tinea cruris, tinea manus and tinea pedis infections due to Trichophyton spp, Microsporon spp and Epidermophyton spp. Nizoral cream is also indicated for the treatment of cutaneous candidosis (including vulvitis), pityriasis versicolor and seborrhoeic dermatitis caused by Pityrosporum spp.

P

For the treatment of the following mycotic infections of the skin: tinea pedis, tinea cruris and candidal intertrigo.

4.2 Posology and method of administration
POM

Tinea pedis:

Nizoral cream should be applied to the affected areas twice daily. The usual duration of treatment for mild infections is 1 week. For more severe or extensive infections (eg involving the sole or sides of the feet) treatment should be continued until a few days after all signs and symptoms have disappeared in order to prevent relapse.

For other infections:

Nizoral cream should be applied to the affected areas once or twice daily, depending on the severity of the infection.

The treatment should be continued until a few days after the disappearance of all signs and symptoms. The usual duration of treatment is: pityriasis versicolor 2–3 weeks, tinea corporis 3–4 weeks.

The diagnosis should be reconsidered if no clinical improvement is noted after 4 weeks. General measures in regard to hygiene should be observed to control sources of infection or reinfection.

Seborrhoeic dermatitis is a chronic condition and relapse is highly likely.

If a potent topical corticosteroid has been used previously in the treatment of seborrhoeic dermatitis, a recovery period of 2 weeks should be allowed before using Nizoral cream, as an increased incidence of steroid induced skin sensitisation has been reported when no recovery period is allowed.

P

For the treatment of tinea pedis (athlete's foot) and tinea cruris (dhobie itch) and candidal intertrigo (sweat rash).

For tinea pedis, Daktarin Gold cream should be applied to the affected areas twice daily. The usual duration of treatment for mild infections is 1 week. For more severe or extensive infections (eg involving the sole or sides of the feet) treatment should be continued for 2–3 days after all signs of infection have disappeared to prevent relapse.

For tinea cruris and candidal intertrigo, apply cream to the affected areas once or twice daily until 2-3 days after all signs of infection have disappeared to prevent relapse. Treatment for up to 6 weeks may be necessary. If no improvement in symptoms is experienced after 4 weeks treatment, a doctor should be consulted.

Method of administration: Topical administration.

4.3 Contraindications
Ketoconazole cream is contra-indicated in patients who have shown hypersensitivity to any of the ingredients or to ketoconazole itself.

4.4 Special warnings and special precautions for use
Not for ophthalmic use.

4.5 Interaction with other medicinal products and other forms of Interaction
None known except possible corticosteroid interaction (see POM dosage section).

4.6 Pregnancy and lactation
After topical application, ketoconazole cream is not systematically absorbed and does not produce detectable plasma concentrations. However, as with any medication, ketoconazole cream should only be used in pregnant women if its use is considered essential by a doctor. Since no ketoconazole is detected in plasma following topical administration, use of ketoconazole cream is not contra-indicated for breast feeding women.

4.7 Effects on ability to drive and use machines
None.

4.8 Undesirable effects
A few instances of irritation, dermatitis and burning sensation have been observed during treatment with ketoconazole cream.

4.9 Overdose
If accidental ingestion of ketoconazole cream occurs, an appropriate method of gastric emptying may be used if considered appropriate.

5. PHARMACOLOGICAL PROPERTIES
5.1 Pharmacodynamic properties
Ketoconazole has a potent antimycotic action against dermatophytes and yeasts. Ketoconazole cream acts rapidly on the pruritus, which is commonly seen in dermatophyte and yeast infections. This symptomatic improvement often occurs before the first signs of healing are observed.

5.2 Pharmacokinetic properties
After topical application, ketoconazole is not systematically absorbed and does not produce detectable plasma concentrations.

5.3 Preclinical safety data
Since ketoconazole administered topically as a cream is not systemically absorbed and does not produce detectable plasma concentrations, there is no specific relevant information. However, oral administration of high doses >80mg/kg) of ketoconazole to pregnant rats has been shown to cause abnormalities of foetal development. The relevance of this finding to humans has not been established and it is not of practical relevance to ketoconazole cream which is for external use only.

6. PHARMACEUTICAL PARTICULARS

6.1 List of excipients

Propylene Glycol

Stearyl Alcohol

Cetyl Alcohol

Sorbitan Stearate

Polysorbate 60

Isopropyl Myristate

Sodium Sulphite Anhydrous

Polysorbate 80

Purified Water

6.2 Incompatibilities

Not applicable.

6.3 Shelf life

60 months.

6.4 Special precautions for storage

Do not store above 25°C.

6.5 Nature and contents of container

Tube made of 99.7% aluminum, lined on inner side with heat polymerised epoxyphenol resin with a latex coldseal ring at the end of the tube. The cap is made of 60% polypropylene, 30% calcium carbonate and 10% glyceryl monostearate.

Tubes of 5, 15 and 30g.

6.6 Instructions for use and handling

Not applicable.

7. MARKETING AUTHORISATION HOLDER

Janssen-Cilag Ltd

Saunderton

High Wycombe

Bucks

HP14 4HJ

UK

8. MARKETING AUTHORISATION NUMBER(S)

PL 00242/0107

9. DATE OF FIRST AUTHORISATION/RENEWAL OF THE AUTHORISATION

Renewed 25 April 1996

10. DATE OF REVISION OF THE TEXT

December 2002

Legal Category

POM: Nizoral Cream

P: Daktarin Gold

Daktarin Oral Gel

(Janssen-Cilag Ltd)

1. NAME OF THE MEDICINAL PRODUCT

DAKTARIN® Oral Gel

2. QUALITATIVE AND QUANTITATIVE COMPOSITION

Each gram of Daktarin Oral Gel contains 20 mg of miconazole.

3. PHARMACEUTICAL FORM

White gel with orange taste.

4. CLINICAL PARTICULARS

4.1 Therapeutic indications

POM

Oral treatment and prevention of fungal infections of the oropharynx and gastrointestinal tract, and of super infections due to Gram-positive bacteria.

P

Oral treatment and prevention of fungal infections of the oropharynx and of superinfections due to Gram-positive bacteria.

4.2 Posology and method of administration

POM only

For oral administration.

Dosage is based on 15 mg/kg/day (0.625 ml/kg/day).

Adults:

1-2 spoonfuls (5-10 ml) of gel four times per day.

Elderly:

As for adults.

Children aged 6 years and over:

One spoonful (5 ml) of gel four times per day.

Children aged 2-6 years:

One spoonful (5 ml) of gel twice per day.

Infants under 2 years:

Half a spoonful (2.5 ml) of gel twice per day.

POM and P

For localised lesions of the mouth, a small amount of gel may be applied directly to the affected area with a clean finger.

For topical treatment of the oropharynx, the gel should be kept in the mouth for as long as possible.

Treatment should be continued for up to 2 days after the symptoms have cleared.

For oral candidosis, dental prostheses should be removed at night and brushed with the gel.

4.3 Contraindications

Known hypersensitivity to miconazole or to any of the excipients.

Liver dysfunction.

Daktarin Oral Gel should not be given concurrently with the drugs terfenadine, astemizole, mizolastine, cisapride, triazolam, oral midazolam, dofetilide, quinidine, pimozide, CYP3A4 metabolised HMG-CoA reductase inhibitors such as simvastatin and lovastatin. (See also section 4.5 Interactions with other medicaments and other forms of interaction).

4.4 Special warnings and special precautions for use

If the concomitant use of Daktarin and anticoagulants is envisaged, the anti-coagulant effect should be carefully monitored and titrated. It is advisable to monitor miconazole and phenytoin levels, if they are used concomitantly.

Particularly in infants and young children, caution is required to ensure that the gel does not obstruct the throat. Hence, the gel should not be applied to the back of the throat and the full dose should be divided into smaller portions. Observe the patient for possible choking.

4.5 Interaction with other medicinal products and other forms of Interaction

Miconazole can inhibit the metabolism of drugs metabolised by the Cytochrome P450-3A and -2C9 families. This can result in an increase and/or prolongation of their effects, including side effects. Examples are:

Daktarin Oral Gel should not be used during treatment with the following drugs:

- terfenadine, astemizole, mizolastine, cisapride, triazolam, oral midazolam, dofetilide, quinidine, pimozide, CYP3A4 metabolised HMG-CoA reductase inhibitors such as simvastatin and lovastatin.

Drugs whose plasma levels effects or side effects should be monitored. Their dosage, if co-administered with miconazole, should be reduced if necessary.

- oral anticoagulants,
- HIV Protease Inhibitors such as saquinavir;
- Certain antineoplastic agents such as vinca alkaloids, busulfan and docetaxel;
- CYPA4 metabolised calcium channel blockers such as dihydropyridines and probably verapamil;
- Certain immunosuppressive agents: cyclosporin, tacrolimus, sirolimus (= rapamycin)
- Others: phenytoin, oral hypoglycaemics, carbamazepine, buspirone, alfentanil, sildenafil, alprazolam, brotizolam, midazolam IV, rifabutin, methylprednisolone, trimetrexate, ebastine and reboxetine.

4.6 Pregnancy and lactation

In animals, miconazole has shown no teratogenic effects but is foetotoxic at high oral doses. The significance of this to man is unknown. However, as with other imidazoles, Daktarin Oral Gel should be avoided in pregnant women if possible. The potential hazards should be balanced against the possible benefits.

It is not known whether miconazole is excreted in human milk. Caution should be exercised when prescribing Daktarin Oral Gel to nursing mothers.

4.7 Effects on ability to drive and use machines

Daktarin should not affect alertness or driving ability.

4.8 Undesirable effects

Occasionally, nausea and vomiting have been reported, and with long term treatment, diarrhoea. In rare instances, allergic reactions have been reported. There are isolated reports of hepatitis, for which the causal relationship with Daktarin has not been established.

4.9 Overdose

Symptoms:

In general, miconazole is not highly toxic. In the event of accidental overdosage, vomiting and diarrhoea may occur.

Treatment:

Treatment is symptomatic and supportive. A specific antidote is not available.

5. PHARMACOLOGICAL PROPERTIES

5.1 Pharmacodynamic properties

The active ingredient, miconazole, is a synthetic imidazole anti-fungal agent with a broad spectrum of activity against pathogenic fungi (including yeast and dermatophytes) and gram-positive bacteria (*Staphylococcus* and *Streptococcus* spp). It may act by interfering with the permeability of the fungal cell membranes.

5.2 Pharmacokinetic properties

When administered orally, miconazole is incompletely absorbed from the gastrointestinal tract, peak plasma levels of about 1 μg per ml have been achieved after a dose of 1 g per day.

Miconazole is inactivated in the body and 10-20% of an oral dose is excreted in the urine, mainly as metabolites, within 6 days. About 50% of an oral dose may be excreted unchanged in the faeces.

5.3 Preclinical safety data

No relevant information additional to that contained elsewhere in the Summary of Product Characteristics.

6. PHARMACEUTICAL PARTICULARS

6.1 List of excipients

Purified water

Pregelatinised potato starch

Alcohol

Polysorbate 20

Sodium saccharin

Cocoa flavour

Orange flavour

Glycerol

6.2 Incompatibilities

None known.

6.3 Shelf life

5 years.

6.4 Special precautions for storage

Do not Store above 30°C.

6.5 Nature and contents of container

Aluminium tubes containing 15 g, or 80 g gel.

A 5 ml plastic spoon, marked with a 2.5 ml graduation is provided.

6.6 Instructions for use and handling

Not applicable.

Administrative Data

7. MARKETING AUTHORISATION HOLDER

Janssen-Cilag Limited

Saunderton

High Wycombe

Buckinghamshire

HP14 4HJ

UK

8. MARKETING AUTHORISATION NUMBER(S)

PL 0242/0048

9. DATE OF FIRST AUTHORISATION/RENEWAL OF THE AUTHORISATION

Date of First Authorisation: 19 July 1977

Date of Renewal of Authorisation: 22 September 1997

10. DATE OF REVISION OF THE TEXT

19/09/03

Legal category POM/P.

External use: Pharmacy Medicine Only.

Other: Prescription Only Medicine.

Daktarin Powder

(Janssen-Cilag Ltd)

1. NAME OF THE MEDICINAL PRODUCT

Daktarin powder

2. QUALITATIVE AND QUANTITATIVE COMPOSITION

Daktarin powder contains miconazole nitrate Ph Eur 2.0% w/w.

3. PHARMACEUTICAL FORM

Cutaneous powder.

4. CLINICAL PARTICULARS

4.1 Therapeutic indications

For the treatment of mycotic infections of the skin and superinfections due to Gram positive bacteria.

4.2 Posology and method of administration

Daktarin powder is for cutaneous administration.

Adults

Twice daily application of powder to the lesions, treatment being prolonged for some 10 days after all lesions have disappeared to prevent relapse.

Elderly and children

As for adults.

4.3 Contraindications

Known hypersensitivity to miconazole or any other component of this product.

The powder should not be recommended for the treatment of infections of the hair and nails.

4.4 Special warnings and special precautions for use

If a reaction suggesting sensitivity or irritation should occur, the treatment should be discontinued.

4.5 Interaction with other medicinal products and other forms of Interaction

Miconazole administered systemically is known to inhibit CYP3A4/2C9. Due to the limited systemic availability after topical application, clinically relevant interactions are rare. However, in patients on oral anticoagulants, such as warfarin, caution should be exercised and anticoagulant effect should be monitored

4.6 Pregnancy and lactation

In animals, miconazole nitrate has shown no teratogenic effects but is foetotoxic at high oral doses. Only small amounts of miconazole nitrate are absorbed following topical administration. However, as with other imidazoles, miconazole nitrate should be used with caution during pregnancy.

4.7 Effects on ability to drive and use machines

None known.

4.8 Undesirable effects

Hypersensitivity has rarely been recorded, if it should occur the treatment should be discontinued.

4.9 Overdose

Daktarin powder is intended for topical use. If accidental ingestion of large quantities of product occurs, an appropriate method of gastric emptying may be used if considered desirable.

5. PHARMACOLOGICAL PROPERTIES

5.1 Pharmacodynamic properties

Miconazole is an imidazole antifungal agent and may act by interfering with the permeability of the fungal cell membrane. It possesses a wide antifungal spectrum and has some antifungal activity.

5.2 Pharmacokinetic properties

There is little absorption through skin or mucous membranes when miconazole nitrate is applied topically.

When administered orally miconazole is incompletely absorbed from the gastrointestinal tract. Peak plasma concentrations occur at about 4 hours after administration. Miconazole disappears from the plasma in a triphasic manner with a biological half-life of about 24 hours. Over 90% is reported to be bound to plasma proteins.

5.3 Preclinical safety data

No relevant information additional to that contained elsewhere in the Summary of Product Characteristics.

6. PHARMACEUTICAL PARTICULARS

6.1 List of excipients

Talc

Zinc oxide

Colloidal anhydrous silica

6.2 Incompatibilities

Not applicable.

6.3 Shelf life

Five years.

6.4 Special precautions for storage

Do not store above 25°C.

6.5 Nature and contents of container

High-density polyethylene bottle with a polypropylene dredger-cap and screw-cap containing 20 gram or 30 gram of powder.

6.6 Instructions for use and handling

Not applicable.

7. MARKETING AUTHORISATION HOLDER

Janssen-Cilag Limited

Saunderton

High Wycombe

Bucks

HP14 4HJ

England

8. MARKETING AUTHORISATION NUMBER(S)

PL 00242/0017

9. DATE OF FIRST AUTHORISATION/RENEWAL OF THE AUTHORISATION

Date of first Authorisation: 15/09/1975

Date of Renewal of Authorisation: 27/3/01

10. DATE OF REVISION OF THE TEXT

12/07/04

Legal status P

Dalacin C Capsules 150mg

(Pharmacia Limited)

1. NAME OF THE MEDICINAL PRODUCT

Dalacin C Capsules 150 mg or Clindamycin Hydrochloride Capsules 150mg

2. QUALITATIVE AND QUANTITATIVE COMPOSITION

One Dalacin C capsule contains 150mg clindamycin hydrochloride

For excipients, see section 6.1 ('List of Excipients')

3. PHARMACEUTICAL FORM

Hard gelatin capsule

Capsule (maroon/lavender) with markings 'P & U 225' on cap and body.

4. CLINICAL PARTICULARS

4.1 Therapeutic indications

Antibacterial. Serious infections caused by susceptible Gram-positive organisms, staphylococci (both penicillinase- and non-penicillinase-producing), streptococci (except *Streptococcus faecalis*) and pneumococci. It is also indicated in serious infections caused by susceptible anaerobic pathogens.

Clindamycin does not penetrate the blood/brain barrier in therapeutically effective quantities.

4.2 Posology and method of administration

Oral. Dalacin C Capsules should always be taken with a glass of water. Absorption of Dalacin C is not appreciably modified by the presence of food.

Adults: Moderately severe infection, 150 - 300 mg every six hours; severe infection, 300 - 450 mg every six hours.

Elderly patients: The half-life, volume of distribution and clearance, and extent of absorption after administration of clindamycin hydrochloride are not altered by increased age. Analysis of data from clinical studies has not revealed any age-related increase in toxicity. Dosage requirements in elderly patients, therefore, should not be influenced by age alone. See *Precautions* for other factors which should be taken into consideration.

Children: 3 - 6 mg/kg every six hours depending on the severity of the infection

Note: In cases of beta-haemolytic streptococcal infection, treatment with Dalacin C should continue for at least 10 days to diminish the likelihood of subsequent rheumatic fever or glomerulonephritis.

4.3 Contraindications

Dalacin C is contra-indicated in patients previously found to be sensitive to clindamycin, lincomycin or to any component of the formulation.

4.4 Special warnings and special precautions for use

Warnings: Dalacin C should only be used in the treatment of serious infections. In considering the use of the product, the practitioner should bear in mind the type of infection and the potential hazard of the diarrhoea which may develop, since cases of colitis have been reported during, or even two or three weeks following, the administration of clindamycin.

Studies indicate a toxin(s) produced by clostridia (especially *Clostridium difficile*) is the principal direct cause of antibiotic-associated colitis. These studies also indicate that this toxigenic clostridium is usually sensitive *in vitro* to vancomycin. When 125 mg to 500 mg of vancomycin are administered orally four times a day for 7 - 10 days, there is a rapid observed disappearance of the toxin from faecal samples and a coincident clinical recovery from the diarrhoea. (Where the patient is receiving cholestyramine in addition to vancomycin, consideration should be given to separating the times of administration).

Colitis is a disease which has a clinical spectrum from mild, watery diarrhoea to severe, persistent diarrhoea, leucocytosis, fever, severe abdominal cramps, which may be associated with the passage of blood and mucus. If allowed to progress, it may produce peritonitis, shock and toxic megacolon. This may be fatal.

The appearance of marked diarrhoea should be regarded as an indication that the product should be discontinued immediately. The disease is likely to follow a more severe course in older patients or patients who are debilitated. Diagnosis is usually made by the recognition of the clinical symptoms, but can be substantiated by endoscopic demonstration of pseudomembranous colitis. The presence of the disease may be further confirmed by culture of the stool for *Clostridium difficile* on selective media and assay of the stool specimen for the toxin(s) of *C. difficile.*

Precautions: Caution should be used when prescribing Dalacin C to individuals with a history of gastro-intestinal disease, especially colitis.

Periodic liver and kidney function tests should be carried out during prolonged therapy. Such monitoring is also recommended in neonates and infants.

The dosage of Dalacin C may require reduction in patients with renal or hepatic impairment due to prolongation of the serum half-life.

Prolonged administration of Dalacin C, as with any anti-infective, may result in super-infection due to organisms resistant to clindamycin.

Care should be observed in the use of Dalacin C in atopic individuals.

4.5 Interaction with other medicinal products and other forms of Interaction

Clindamycin has been shown to have neuromuscular blocking properties that may enhance the action of other neuromuscular blocking agents. It should be used with caution, therefore, in patients receiving such agents.

Antagonism has been demonstrated between clindamycin and erythromycin *in vitro*. Because of possible clinical significance the two drugs should not be administered concurrently.

4.6 Pregnancy and lactation

Safety for use in pregnancy has not yet been established.

Clindamycin is excreted in human milk. Caution should be exercised when Dalacin C is administered to a nursing mother. It is unlikely that a nursing infant can absorb a significant amount of clindamycin from its gastro-intestinal tract.

4.7 Effects on ability to drive and use machines

Not applicable

4.8 Undesirable effects

Gastro-intestinal tract: Nausea, vomiting, abdominal pain, diarrhoea and oesophagitis (see *Warnings*)

Haematopoietic: Transient neutropenia (leucopenia), eosinophilia, agranulocytosis and thrombocytopenia have been reported. No direct aetiologic relationship to concurrent clindamycin therapy could be made in any of the foregoing.

Skin and mucous membranes: Pruritus, vaginitis and rare instances of exfoliative and vesiculobullous dermatitis have been reported.

Hypersensitivity reactions: Maculopapular rash and urticaria have been observed during drug therapy. Generalised mild to moderate morbilliform-like skin rashes are the most frequently reported reactions. Rare instances of erythema multiforme and Stevens-Johnson syndrome, have been associated with clindamycin. A few cases of anaphylactoid reactions have been reported.

Liver: Jaundice and abnormalities in liver function tests have been observed during clindamycin therapy.

4.9 Overdose

In cases of overdosage no specific treatment is indicated.

The serum biological half-life of clindamycin is 2.4 hours. Clindamycin cannot readily be removed from the blood by dialysis or peritoneal dialysis.

If an allergic adverse reaction occurs, therapy should be with the usual emergency treatments, including corticosteroids, adrenaline and antihistamines.

5. PHARMACOLOGICAL PROPERTIES

Antibacterials for Systemic Use ATC Code: J01 F F

5.1 Pharmacodynamic properties

Clindamycin is a lincosamide antibiotic with a primarily bacteriostatic action against Gram-positive aerobes and a wide range of anaerobic bacteria. Most Gram-negative aerobic bacteria, including the Enterobacteriaceae, are resistant to clindamycin. Lincosamides such as clindamycin bind to the 50S subunit of the bacterial ribosome similarly to macrolides such as erythromycin and inhibit the early stages of protein synthesis. The action of clindamycin is predominantly bacteriostatic although high concentrations may be slowly bactericidal against sensitive strains.

5.2 Pharmacokinetic properties

General characteristics of active substance

About 90% of a dose of clindamycin hydrochloride is absorbed from the gastro-intestinal tract; concentrations of 2 to 3 micrograms per ml occur within one hour after a 150 mg dose of clindamycin, with average concentrations of about 0.7 micrograms per ml after 6 hours. After doses of 300 and 600 mg peak plasma concentrations of 4 and 8 micrograms per ml, respectively, have been reported. Absorption is not significantly diminished by food in the stomach but the rate of absorption may be reduced.

Clindamycin is widely distributed in body fluids and tissues including bone, but it does not reach the csf in significant concentrations. It diffuses across the placenta into the fetal circulation and has been reported to appear in breast milk. High concentrations occur in bile. It accumulates in leucocytes and macrophages. Over 90% of clindamycin in the circulation is bound to plasma proteins. The half-life is 2 to 3 hours, although this may be prolonged in pre-term neonates and patients with severe renal impairment.

Clindamycin undergoes metabolism, presumably in the liver, to the active *N*-demethyl and sulphoxide metabolites, and also some inactive metabolites. About 10% of a dose is excreted in the urine as active drug or metabolites and about 4% in the faeces; the remainder is excreted as inactive metabolites. Excretion is slow, and takes place over several days. It is not effectively removed from the blood by dialysis.

Characteristics in patients

No special characteristics. See section 4.4 "Special warnings and special precautions for use" for further information.

6. PHARMACEUTICAL PARTICULARS

6.1 List of excipients

Lactose

Maize starch

Talc

Magnesium stearate

Capsule shell:

Gelatin

Capsule cap:

Indigo carmine (E132)

Erythrosine (E127)

Titanium dioxide

Capsule body:

Indigo carmine (E132)

Erythrosine (E127

Printing ink:

Shellac

Soya lecithin

Dimeticone (Antifoam DC 1510)

Titanium dioxide (E171)

6.2 Incompatibilities

Not applicable.

6.3 Shelf life

Bottle: 60 months

Blister: 60 months

6.4 Special precautions for storage

Do not store above 25°C.

6.5 Nature and contents of container

Dalacin C Capsules 150 mg are available in blister packs (aluminium foil/PVC) of 24 capsules and bottle packs (high density polyethylene or amber glass) of 24, 100 or 500 capsules.

Not all pack sizes may be marketed.

6.6 Instructions for use and handling

None stated

7. MARKETING AUTHORISATION HOLDER

Pharmacia Limited

Davy Avenue

Milton Keynes

MK5 8PH

UK

8. MARKETING AUTHORISATION NUMBER(S)

PL 0032/5007R

9. DATE OF FIRST AUTHORISATION/RENEWAL OF THE AUTHORISATION

20 February 1989/22nd May 2001

10. DATE OF REVISION OF THE TEXT

February 2004

Legal category: POM

Dalacin C Capsules 75mg

(Pharmacia Limited)

1. NAME OF THE MEDICINAL PRODUCT

Dalacin C Capsules 75 mg or Clindamycin Hydrochloride Capsules 75mg

2. QUALITATIVE AND QUANTITATIVE COMPOSITION

One Dalacin C capsule contains 75mg clindamycin hydrochloride

For excipients, see section 6.1 ('List of Excipients')

3. PHARMACEUTICAL FORM

Hard gelatin capsule

Capsule (lavender/lavender) with markings of 'P & U 331'.

4. CLINICAL PARTICULARS

4.1 Therapeutic indications

Antibacterial. Serious infections caused by susceptible Gram-positive organisms, staphylococci (both penicillinase- and non-penicillinase-producing), streptococci (except *Streptococcus faecalis*) and pneumococci. It is also indicated in serious infections caused by susceptible anaerobic pathogens.

Clindamycin does not penetrate the blood/brain barrier in therapeutically effective quantities.

4.2 Posology and method of administration

Oral. Dalacin C Capsules should always be taken with a glass of water. Absorption of Dalacin C is not appreciably modified by the presence of food.

Adults: Moderately severe infection, 150 - 300 mg every six hours; severe infection, 300 - 450 mg every six hours.

Elderly patients: The half-life, volume of distribution and clearance, and extent of absorption after administration of clindamycin hydrochloride are not altered by increased age. Analysis of data from clinical studies has not revealed any age-related increase in toxicity. Dosage requirements in elderly patients, therefore, should not be influenced by age alone. See *Precautions* for other factors which should be taken into consideration.

Children: 3 - 6 mg/kg every six hours depending on the severity of the infection

Note: In cases of beta-haemolytic streptococcal infection, treatment with Dalacin C should continue for at least 10 days to diminish the likelihood of subsequent rheumatic fever or glomerulonephritis.

4.3 Contraindications

Dalacin C is contra-indicated in patients previously found to be sensitive to clindamycin, lincomycin or to any component of the formulation.

4.4 Special warnings and special precautions for use

Warnings: Dalacin C should only be used in the treatment of serious infections. In considering the use of the product, the practitioner should bear in mind the type of infection and the potential hazard of the diarrhoea which may develop, since cases of colitis have been reported during, or even two or three weeks following, the administration of clindamycin.

Studies indicate a toxin(s) produced by clostridia (especially *Clostridium difficile*) is the principal direct cause of antibiotic-associated colitis. These studies also indicate that this toxigenic clostridium is usually sensitive *in vitro* to vancomycin. When 125 mg to 500 mg of vancomycin are administered orally four times a day for 7 - 10 days, there is a rapid observed disappearance of the toxin from faecal samples and a coincident clinical recovery from the diarrhoea. (Where the patient is receiving cholestyramine in addition to vancomycin, consideration should be given to separating the times of administration).

Colitis is a disease which has a clinical spectrum from mild, watery diarrhoea to severe, persistent diarrhoea, leucocytosis, fever, severe abdominal cramps, which may be associated with the passage of blood and mucus. If allowed to progress, it may produce peritonitis, shock and toxic megacolon. This may be fatal.

The appearance of marked diarrhoea should be regarded as an indication that the product should be discontinued immediately. The disease is likely to follow a more severe course in older patients or patients who are debilitated. Diagnosis is usually made by the recognition of the clinical symptoms, but can be substantiated by endoscopic demonstration of pseudomembranous colitis. The presence of the disease may be further confirmed by culture of the stool for *Clostridium difficile* on selective media and assay of the stool specimen for the toxin(s) of *C. difficile*.

Precautions: Caution should be used when prescribing Dalacin C to individuals with a history of gastro-intestinal disease, especially colitis.

Periodic liver and kidney function tests should be carried out during prolonged therapy. Such monitoring is also recommended in neonates and infants.

The dosage of Dalacin C may require reduction in patients with renal or hepatic impairment due to prolongation of the serum half-life.

Prolonged administration of Dalacin C, as with any anti-infective, may result in super-infection due to organisms resistant to clindamycin.

Care should be observed in the use of Dalacin C in atopic individuals.

4.5 Interaction with other medicinal products and other forms of Interaction

Clindamycin has been shown to have neuromuscular blocking properties that may enhance the action of other neuromuscular blocking agents. It should be used with caution, therefore, in patients receiving such agents.

Antagonism has been demonstrated between clindamycin and erythromycin *in vitro*. Because of possible clinical significance the two drugs should not be administered concurrently.

4.6 Pregnancy and lactation

Safety for use in pregnancy has not yet been established.

Clindamycin is excreted in human milk. Caution should be exercised when Dalacin C is administered to a nursing mother. It is unlikely that a nursing infant can absorb a significant amount of clindamycin from its gastro-intestinal tract.

4.7 Effects on ability to drive and use machines

Not applicable

4.8 Undesirable effects

Gastro-intestinal tract: Nausea, vomiting, abdominal pain, diarrhoea and oesophagitis (see *Warnings*)

Haematopoietic: Transient neutropenia (leucopenia), eosinophilia, agranulocytosis and thrombocytopenia have been reported. No direct aetiologic relationship to concurrent clindamycin therapy could be made in any of the foregoing.

Skin and mucous membranes: Pruritus, vaginitis and rare instances of exfoliative and vesiculobullous dermatitis have been reported.

Hypersensitivity reactions: Maculopapular rash and urticaria have been observed during drug therapy. Generalised mild to moderate morbilliform-like skin rashes are the most frequently reported reactions. Rare instances of erythema multiforme and Stevens-Johnson syndrome, have been associated with clindamycin. A few cases of anaphylactoid reactions have been reported.

Liver: Jaundice and abnormalities in liver function tests have been observed during clindamycin therapy.

4.9 Overdose

In cases of overdosage no specific treatment is indicated.

The serum biological half-life of clindamycin is 2.4 hours. Clindamycin cannot readily be removed from the blood by dialysis or peritoneal dialysis.

If an allergic adverse reaction occurs, therapy should be with the usual emergency treatments, including corticosteroids, adrenaline and antihistamines.

5. PHARMACOLOGICAL PROPERTIES

Antibacterials for Systemic Use ATC Code: J01 F F

5.1 Pharmacodynamic properties

Clindamycin is a lincosamide antibiotic with a primarily bacteriostatic action against Gram-positive aerobes and a wide range of anaerobic bacteria. Most Gram-negative aerobic bacteria, including the Enterobacteriaceae, are resistant to clindamycin. Lincosamides such as clindamycin bind to the 50S subunit of the bacterial ribosome similarly to macrolides such as erythromycin and inhibit the early stages of protein synthesis. The action of clindamycin is predominantly bacteriostatic although high concentrations may be slowly bactericidal against sensitive strains.

5.2 Pharmacokinetic properties

General characteristics of active substance

About 90% of a dose of clindamycin hydrochloride is absorbed from the gastro-intestinal tract; concentrations of 2 to 3 micrograms per ml occur within one hour after a 150 mg dose of clindamycin, with average concentrations of about 0.7 micrograms per ml after 6 hours. After doses of 300 and 600 mg peak plasma concentrations of 4 and 8 micrograms per ml, respectively, have been reported. Absorption is not significantly diminished by food in the stomach but the rate of absorption may be reduced.

Clindamycin is widely distributed in body fluids and tissues including bone, but it does not reach the csf in significant concentrations. It diffuses across the placenta into the fetal circulation and has been reported to appear in breast milk. High concentrations occur in bile. It accumulates in leucocytes and macrophages. Over 90% of clindamycin in the circulation is bound to plasma proteins. The half-life is 2 to 3 hours, although this may be prolonged in pre-term neonates and patients with severe renal impairment.

Clindamycin undergoes metabolism, presumably in the liver, to the active *N*-demethyl and sulphoxide metabolites, and also some inactive metabolites. About 10% of a dose is excreted in the urine as active drug or metabolites and about 4% in the faeces; the remainder is excreted as inactive metabolites. Excretion is slow, and takes place over several days. It is not effectively removed from the blood by dialysis.

Characteristics in patients

No special characteristics. See section 4.4 "Special warnings and special precautions for use" for further information.

6. PHARMACEUTICAL PARTICULARS

6.1 List of excipients

Lactose

Maize starch

Talc

Magnesium stearate

Capsule shell:

Gelatin

Indigo carmine (E132)

Erythrosine (E127)

Printing ink:

Shellac

Soya lecithin

Dimeticone (antifoam DC 1510)

Titanium dioxide (E171)

6.2 Incompatibilities

Not applicable.

6.3 Shelf life

Bottles: 60 months

Blisters: 60 months

6.4 Special precautions for storage

Do not store above 25°C.

6.5 Nature and contents of container

Dalacin C Capsules 75 mg are available in blister packs (aluminium foil/PVC) of 24 capsules and bottle packs (high density polyethylene or amber glass) of 24, 100 or 500 capsules.

Not all pack sizes may be marketed.

6.6 Instructions for use and handling

None stated

7. MARKETING AUTHORISATION HOLDER

Pharmacia Limited

Davy Avenue

Milton Keynes

MK5 8PH

UK

8. MARKETING AUTHORISATION NUMBER(S)

PL 0032/5006R

9. DATE OF FIRST AUTHORISATION/RENEWAL OF THE AUTHORISATION

20 February 1989/22nd May 2001

10. DATE OF REVISION OF THE TEXT

February 2004

Legal category: POM

Dalacin C Phosphate

(Pharmacia Limited)

1. NAME OF THE MEDICINAL PRODUCT
Dalacin C Phosphate Sterile Solution

2. QUALITATIVE AND QUANTITATIVE COMPOSITION
Each ml of solution contains clindamycin phosphate equivalent to 150 mg clindamycin.

For excipients, see section 6.1.

3. PHARMACEUTICAL FORM
Solution for Injection

Clear, colourless, sterile solution.

4. CLINICAL PARTICULARS

4.1 Therapeutic indications
Antibacterial. Serious infections caused by susceptible Gram-positive organisms, staphylococci (both penicillinase- and non-penicillinase-producing), streptococci (except *Streptococcus faecalis*) and pneumococci. It is also indicated in serious infections caused by susceptible anaerobic pathogens such as *Bacteroides* spp, *Fusobacterium* spp, *Propionibacterium* spp, *Peptostreptococcus* spp. and microaerophilic streptococci.

Clindamycin does not penetrate the blood/brain barrier in therapeutically effective quantities.

4.2 Posology and method of administration
Parenteral (i.m. or IV. administration). Dalacin C Phosphate **must** be diluted prior to IV. administration and should be infused over at least 10-60 minutes.

Adults: Serious infections: 600 mg - 1.2 g/day in two, three or four equal doses.

More severe infections: l.2-2.7 g/day in two, three or four equal doses.

Single i.m. injections of greater than 600 mg are not recommended nor is administration of more than 1.2 g in a single one-hour infusion.

For more serious infections, these doses may have to be increased. In life-threatening situations, doses as high as 4.8 g daily have been given intravenously to adults.

Alternatively, the drug may be administered in the form of a single rapid infusion of the first dose followed by continuous IV. infusion.

Children (over 1 month of age): Serious infections: 15-25 mg/kg/day in three or four equal doses.

More severe infections: 25-40 mg/kg/day in three or four equal doses. In severe infections it is recommended that children be given no less than 300 mg/day regardless of body weight.

Elderly patients: The half-life, volume of distribution and clearance, and extent of absorption after administration of clindamycin phosphate are not altered by increased age. Analysis of data from clinical studies has not revealed any age-related increase in toxicity. Dosage requirements in elderly patients should not be influenced, therefore, by age alone. See *Precautions* for other factors which should be taken into consideration.

Treatment for infections caused by beta-haemolytic streptococci should be continued for at least 10 days to guard against subsequent rheumatic fever or glomerulonephritis.

The concentration of clindamycin in diluent for infusion should not exceed 18 mg per mL and INFUSION RATES SHOULD NOT EXCEED 30 MG PER MINUTE. The usual infusion rates are as follows:

Dose	Diluent	Time
300 mg	50 mL	10 min
600 mg	50 mL	20 min
900 mg	50-100 mL	30 min
1200 mg	100 mL	40 min

4.3 Contraindications
Dalacin C Phosphate is contra-indicated in patients previously found to be sensitive to clindamycin, lincomycin or to any component of the formulation.

4.4 Special warnings and special precautions for use
Warnings

This product contains benzyl alcohol. Benzyl alcohol has been reported to be associated with a fatal "Gasping syndrome" in premature infants.

Dalacin C Phosphate should only be used in the treatment of serious infections. In considering the use of the product, the practitioner should bear in mind the type of infection and the potential hazard of the diarrhoea which may develop, since cases of colitis have been reported during, or even two or three weeks following, the administration of clindamycin.

Studies indicate a toxin(s) produced by clostridia (especially *Clostridium difficile*) is the principal direct cause of antibiotic-associated colitis. These studies also indicate that this toxigenic clostridium is usually sensitive *in vitro* to vancomycin. When 125 mg to 500 mg of vancomycin are administered orally four times a day for 7 - 10 days, there is a rapid observed disappearance of the toxin from faecal samples and a coincident clinical recovery from the diarrhoea. (Where the patient is receiving cholestyramine in addition to vancomycin, consideration should be given to separating the times of administration).

Colitis is a disease which has a clinical spectrum from mild, watery diarrhoea to severe, persistent diarrhoea, leucocytosis, fever, severe abdominal cramps, which may be associated with the passage of blood and mucus. If allowed to progress, it may produce peritonitis, shock and toxic megacolon. This may be fatal. The appearance of marked diarrhoea should be regarded as an indication that the product should be discontinued immediately. The disease is likely to follow a more severe course in older patients or patients who are debilitated. Diagnosis is usually made by the recognition of the clinical symptoms, but can be substantiated by endoscopic demonstration of pseudomembranous colitis. The presence of the disease may be further confirmed by culture of the stool for *C. difficile* on selective media and assay of the stool specimen for the toxin(s) of *C. difficile*.

Precautions

Caution should be used when prescribing Dalacin C Phosphate to individuals with a history of gastro-intestinal disease, especially colitis.

Periodic liver and kidney function tests should be carried out during prolonged therapy. Such monitoring is also recommended in neonates and infants. Safety and appropriate dosage in infants less than one month old have not been established.

The dosage of Dalacin C Phosphate may require reduction in patients with renal or hepatic impairment due to prolongation of the serum half-life.

Prolonged administration of Dalacin C Phosphate, as with any anti-infective, may result in super-infection due to organisms resistant to clindamycin.

Care should be observed in the use of Dalacin C Phosphate in atopic individuals.

4.5 Interaction with other medicinal products and other forms of Interaction
Clindamycin has been shown to have neuromuscular blocking properties that may enhance the action of other neuromuscular blocking agents. It should be used with caution, therefore, in patients receiving such agents.

Antagonism has been demonstrated between clindamycin and erythromycin *in vitro*. Because of possible clinical significance, the two drugs should not be administered concurrently.

4.6 Pregnancy and lactation
Safety for use in pregnancy has not been established.

Clindamycin is excreted in human milk. Caution should be exercised when Dalacin C Phosphate is administered to a nursing mother. It is unlikely that a nursing infant can absorb a significant amount of clindamycin from its gastro-intestinal tract.

4.7 Effects on ability to drive and use machines
None known

4.8 Undesirable effects
Gastro-intestinal tract: Nausea, vomiting, abdominal pain and diarrhoea (See *Warnings*).

Haematopoietic: Transient neutropenia (leucopenia), eosinophilia, agranulocytosis and thrombocytopenia have been reported. No direct aetiologic relationship to concurrent clindamycin therapy could be made in any of the foregoing.

Skin and mucous membranes: Pruritus, vaginitis and rare instances of exfoliative and vesiculobullous dermatitis have been reported.

Hypersensitivity reactions: Maculopapular rash and urticaria have been observed during drug therapy. Generalised mild to moderate morbilliform-like skin rashes are the most frequently reported reactions. Rare instances of erythema multiforme and Stevens-Johnson syndrome, have been associated with clindamycin. A few cases of anaphylactoid reactions have been reported.

Liver: Jaundice and abnormalities in liver function tests have been observed during clindamycin therapy.

Cardiovascular: Rare instances of cardiopulmonary arrest and hypotension have been reported following too rapid intravenous administration. (See **Dosage and administration** section)

Local reactions: Local irritation, pain, abscess formation have been seen with i.m. injection. Thrombophlebitis has been reported with IV. injection. These reactions can be minimized by deep i.m. injection and avoiding the use of an indwelling catheter.

4.9 Overdose
In cases of overdosage no specific treatment is indicated.

The serum biological half-life of lincomycin is 2.4 hours. Clindamycin cannot readily be removed from the blood by dialysis or peritoneal dialysis.

If an allergic adverse reaction occurs, therapy should be with the usual emergency treatments, including corticosteroids, adrenaline and antihistamines.

5. PHARMACOLOGICAL PROPERTIES

5.1 Pharmacodynamic properties
Clindamycin is a lincosamide antibiotic with a primarily bacteriostatic action against Gram-positive aerobes and a wide range of anaerobic bacteria. Lincosamides such as clindamycin bind to the 50S subunit of the bacterial ribosome similarly to macrolides such as erythromycin and inhibit the early stages of protein synthesis. The action of clindamycin is predominantly bacteriostatic although high concentrations may be slowly bactericidal against sensitive strains.

Most Gram-negative aerobic bacteria, including the Enterobacteriaceae, are resistant to clindamycin. Clindamycin demonstrates cross-resistance with lincomycin. When tested by *in vitro* methods, some staphylococcal strains originally resistant to erythromycin rapidly developed resistance to clindamycin. The mechanisms for resistance are the same as for erythromycin, namely methylation of the ribosomal binding site, chromosomal mutation of the ribosomal protein and in a few staphylococcal isolates enzymic inactivation by a plasmid-mediated adenyltransferase.

5.2 Pharmacokinetic properties
General characteristics of active substance

Following parenteral administration, the biologically inactive clindamycin phosphate is hydrolysed to clindamycin. When the equivalent of 300 mg of clindamycin is injected intramuscularly, a mean peak plasma concentration of 6 microgram/ml is achieved within three hours; 600 mg gives a peak concentration of 9 microgram/ml. In children, peak concentration may be reached within one hour. When the same doses are infused intravenously, peak concentrations of 7 and 10 micrograms per ml respectively are achieved by the end of infusion.

Clindamycin is widely distributed in body fluids and tissues including bone, but it does not reach the cerebrospinal fluid in significant concentrations. It diffuses across the placenta into the fetal circulation and appears in breast milk. High concentrations occur in bile. It accumulates in leucocytes and macrophages. Over 90% of clindamycin in the circulation is bound to plasma proteins. The half-life is 2 to 3 hours, although this may be prolonged in pre-term neonates and patients with severe renal impairment.

Clindamycin undergoes metabolism, to the active *N*-demethyl and sulphoxide metabolites and also some inactive metabolites. About 10% of the drug is excreted in the urine as active drug or metabolites and about 4% in the faeces; the remainder is excreted as inactive metabolites. Excretion is slow and takes place over several days, It is not effectively removed from the blood by dialysis.

Characteristics in patients

No special characteristics. See section 4.4 "**Special warnings and special precautions for use**" for further information.

6. PHARMACEUTICAL PARTICULARS

6.1 List of excipients
Benzyl alcohol

Disodium edetate

Sterilised water for injections

6.2 Incompatibilities
Solutions of clindamycin salts have a low pH and incompatibilities may reasonably be expected with alkaline preparations or drugs unstable at low pH. Incompatibility has been reported with: ampicillin sodium, aminophylline, barbiturates, calcium gluconate, ceftriaxone sodium, ciprofloxacin, diphenylhydantoin, idarubicin hydrochloride, magnesium sulphate, phenytoin sodium and ranitidine hydrochloride.

6.3 Shelf life
24 months

6.4 Special precautions for storage
Do not store above 25°C. Do not refrigerate or freeze.

6.5 Nature and contents of container
Type 1 flint glass ampoule containing 2 ml or 4 ml sterile, aqueous solution, packed in cardboard carton, together with a leaflet.

6.6 Instructions for use and handling
Dalacin C Phosphate has been shown to be physically and chemically compatible for at least 24 hours in dextrose 5% water and sodium chloride injection solutions containing the following antibiotics in usually administered concentrations: Amikacin sulphate, aztreonam, cefamandole nafate, cephazolin sodium, cefotaxime sodium, cefoxitin sodium, ceftazidime sodium, ceftizoxime sodium, gentamicin sulphate, netilmicin sulphate, piperacillin and tobramycin.

The compatibility and duration of stability of drug admixtures will vary depending upon concentration and other conditions.

7. MARKETING AUTHORISATION HOLDER
Pharmacia Limited

Davy Avenue

Milton Keynes

MK5 8PH

UK

8. MARKETING AUTHORISATION NUMBER(S)
PL 0032/0042R

9. DATE OF FIRST AUTHORISATION/RENEWAL OF THE AUTHORISATION
27th December 1997 / 22nd May 2002

10. DATE OF REVISION OF THE TEXT
December 2002

11. LEGAL CATEGORY
POM

Ref: DAB 1_0

Dalacin Cream 2%

(Pharmacia Limited)

1. NAME OF THE MEDICINAL PRODUCT
Dalacin Cream 2%.

2. QUALITATIVE AND QUANTITATIVE COMPOSITION
Each gram of cream contains clindamycin phosphate equivalent to 20 mg or 2.0% w/w clindamycin.

For Excipients, see section 6.1

3. PHARMACEUTICAL FORM
Cream
White, semi-solid.

4. CLINICAL PARTICULARS

4.1 Therapeutic indications
Antibiotic for the treatment of bacterial vaginosis.

4.2 Posology and method of administration
One applicator full (approximately 5 grams) intravaginally at bedtime for 7 consecutive days.

In patients in whom a shorter treatment course is desirable, a 3 day regimen has been shown to be effective.

Children and the elderly: No clinical studies have been conducted in populations younger than 15 or older than 60. Dalacin Cream is not recommended in children under 12 years of age.

4.3 Contraindications
Dalacin Cream is contra-indicated in patients previously found to be hypersensitive to preparations containing clindamycin or any of the components of the cream base (see "Presentation"). Although cross-sensitisation to lincomycin has not been demonstrated, it is recommended that Dalacin Cream should not be used in patients who have demonstrated lincomycin sensitivity.

4.4 Special warnings and special precautions for use
As there are no data available on the use of Dalacin Cream in patients younger than 12 years of age, it should not be used in this population. The use of clindamycin may result in the overgrowth of non-susceptible organisms, particularly yeasts.

Virtually all antibiotics have been associated with diarrhoea and in some cases pseudomembranous colitis. Therefore, even though only a minimal amount of drug is absorbed, if significant diarrhoea occurs, the drug should be discontinued and appropriate diagnostic procedures and treatment provided as necessary.

Dalacin Cream contains oil-based components. Some of these have been shown to weaken the rubber of condoms and diaphragms and make them less effective as a barrier method of contraception or as protection from sexually transmitted disease, including AIDS. Do not rely on condoms and diaphragms when using Dalacin Cream.

4.5 Interaction with other medicinal products and other forms of Interaction
Cross resistance has been demonstrated between clindamycin and lincomycin, and erythromycin and clindamycin. Antagonism has been demonstrated between clindamycin and erythromycin *in vitro.*

No information is available on concomitant use with other intravaginal products, which is not recommended.

4.6 Pregnancy and lactation
Pregnancy
Reproduction studies have been performed in rats and mice using subcutaneous and oral doses of clindamycin ranging from 20 to 600 mg/kg/day and have revealed no evidence of impaired fertility or harm to the foetus due to clindamycin. In one mouse strain, cleft palates were observed in treated foetuses; this response was not produced in other mouse strains or in other species, and is therefore considered to be a strain specific effect.

There are no adequate and well-controlled studies in pregnant women during their first trimester, and because animal reproduction studies are not always predictive of human response, this drug should be used during the first trimester of pregnancy only if clearly needed. In a clinical trial in pregnant women during the second trimester, Dalacin Cream was effective in treating bacterial vaginosis, and no drug-related medical events were reported in the neonates. However, as with any drug used during pregnancy, a careful risk-benefit assessment should take place beforehand.

Lactation
It is not known if clindamycin is excreted in breast milk following the use of vaginally administered clindamycin phosphate. However, orally and parenterally administered clindamycin has been reported to appear in breast milk. Therefore, a full assessment of benefit-risk should be made when consideration is given to using vaginal clindamycin phosphate in a nursing mother.

4.7 Effects on ability to drive and use machines
Not applicable.

4.8 Undesirable effects
In clinical trials medical events judged to be related, probably related, or possibly related to vaginally administered clindamycin phosphate cream were reported for (24%) of patients as indicated below:

Genital tract: cervicitis/vaginitis (14%); vulvo-vaginal irritation (6%).

Central nervous system: dizziness, headache, vertigo.

Gastro-intestinal: heartburn, nausea, vomiting, diarrhoea, constipation, abdominal pain.

Dermatological: rash, exanthema.

Hypersensitivity: urticaria.

(Events without percentages were reported by less than 1% of the patients.)

4.9 Overdose
Intravaginal overdose is not possible. Accidental ingestion of the product could be accompanied by effects related to therapeutic levels of oral clindamycin.

5. PHARMACOLOGICAL PROPERTIES

5.1 Pharmacodynamic properties
Clindamycin is an antimicrobial agent which has been shown to be effective in the treatment of infection caused by susceptible anaerobic bacteria or susceptible strains of Gram positive aerobic bacteria. It has been shown to have *in-vitro* activity against the following organisms which are associated with bacterial vaginosis.:

Gardnerella vaginalis;

Mobiluncus spp;

Bacteroides spp;

Mycoplasma hominis;

Peptostreptococcus spp.

5.2 Pharmacokinetic properties
Following once a day dosing of 100 mg of vaginally administered clindamycin phosphate, at a concentration equivalent to 20 mg of clindamycin per gram of cream, peak serum clindamycin levels average 20 nanograms/ml (range 3-93 nanograms/ml in normal volunteers. Approximately 3% (range 0.1-7%) of the administered dose is absorbed systematically.

In women with bacterial vaginosis, the amount of clindamycin absorbed following vaginal administration of 100 mg of Dalacin Cream (20 mg/g) is 4% (range 0.8-8%), which is approximately the same as in normal women.

Characteristics in patients

No special characteristics. See section 4.4 "**Special warnings and special precautions for use**" for further information.

6. PHARMACEUTICAL PARTICULARS

6.1 List of excipients
Sorbitan stearate

polysorbate 60

propylene glycol

stearic acid

cetostearyl alcohol

cetyl palmitate

liquid paraffin

benzyl alcohol

water.

6.2 Incompatibilities
Not applicable.

6.3 Shelf life
2 years

6.4 Special precautions for storage
Do not store above 25°C. Do not freeze.

6.5 Nature and contents of container
Laminate tube (consisting of LMDPE and aluminium foil) with polypropylene cap containing 7.8 g, 20 g or 40 g cream, packed in cardboard carton, together with a leaflet.

Not all pack sizes may be marketed.

6.6 Instructions for use and handling
None.

Administrative Data

7. MARKETING AUTHORISATION HOLDER
Pharmacia Limited

Davy Avenue

Milton Keynes

MK5 8PH

UK

8. MARKETING AUTHORISATION NUMBER(S)
PL 0032/0176

9. DATE OF FIRST AUTHORISATION/RENEWAL OF THE AUTHORISATION
Date of first authorisation: 27 April 1993 / Renewal 21st May 2001

10. DATE OF REVISION OF THE TEXT
July 2003

Legal category: POM

Dalacin T Topical Lotion or Clindamycin Phosphate Topical Lotion

(Pharmacia Limited)

1. NAME OF THE MEDICINAL PRODUCT
Dalacin T Topical Lotion

Clindamycin Phosphate Topical Lotion

2. QUALITATIVE AND QUANTITATIVE COMPOSITION
One ml of Dalacin T Topical Lotion contains the equivalent of 10mg clindamycin.

For excipients see Section 6.1 ('List of excipients').

3. PHARMACEUTICAL FORM
Topical Emulsion.

White to off-white aqueous emulsion.

4. CLINICAL PARTICULARS

4.1 Therapeutic indications
Dalacin T Topical is indicated for the treatment of acne vulgaris.

4.2 Posology and method of administration
Apply a thin film of Dalacin T Topical Lotion twice daily to the affected area.

4.3 Contraindications
Dalacin T is contra-indicated in patients previously found to be hypersensitive to preparations containing clindamycin or any of the excipients. Although cross- sensitisation to lincomycin has not been demonstrated, it is recommended that Dalacin T is not used in patients who have demonstrated lincomycin sensitivity.

4.4 Special warnings and special precautions for use
Oral and parenteral clindamycin, as well as most other antibiotics, have been associated with severe pseudomembranous colitis. However, post-marketing studies have indicated a very low incidence of colitis with Dalacin T Solution. The physician should, nonetheless, be alert to the development of antibiotic-associated diarrhoea or colitis. If diarrhoea occurs, the product should be discontinued immediately.

Studies indicate a toxin(s) produced by *Clostridium difficile* is the major cause of antibiotic-associated colitis. Colitis is usually characterized by persistent, severe diarrhoea and abdominal cramps. Endoscopic examination may reveal pseudomembranous colitis. Stool culture for *C. difficile* andlor assay for *C. difficile* toxin may be helpful to diagnosis.

Vancomycin is effective in the treatment of antibiotic-associated colitis produced by *C. difficile.* The usual dose is 125 - 500 mg orally every 6 hours for 7 - 10 days. Additional supportive medical care may be necessary.

Mild cases of colitis may respond to discontinuance of clindamycin alone. Cholestyramine and colestipol resins have been shown to bind *C. difficile* toxin *in vitro,* and cholestyramine has been effective in the treatment of some mild cases of antibiotic-associated colitis. Cholestyramine resins have been shown to bind vancomycin; therefore, when both cholestyramine and vancomycin are used concurrently, their administration should be separated by at least two hours.

The lotion has an unpleasant taste and caution should be exercised when applying medication around the mouth.

4.5 Interaction with other medicinal products and other forms of Interaction
None.

4.6 Pregnancy and lactation
Safety for use in pregnancy has not been established.

Reproduction studies have been performed in rats and mice using subcutaneous and oral doses of clindamycin ranging from 100 to 600 mg/kg/day and have revealed no evidence of impaired fertility or harm to the foetus due to clindamycin. There are, however, no adequate and well-controlled studies in pregnant women. Because animal reproduction studies are not always predictive of human response, this drug should be used during pregnancy only if clearly needed.

It is not known whether clindamycin is excreted in human milk following use of Dalacin T Topical Lotion. However, orally and parenterally administered clindamycin has been reported to appear in breast milk. As a general rule, breast-feeding should not be undertaken while a patient is on a drug since many drugs are excreted in human milk.

4.7 Effects on ability to drive and use machines
None.

4.8 Undesirable effects
Side-effects: Adverse reactions reported in clinical trials have been minor and of a similar incidence to placebo.

4.9 Overdose
Improbable given route of application.

5. PHARMACOLOGICAL PROPERTIES
Anti-infectives for treatment of acne. D10A F

5.1 Pharmacodynamic properties
The active constituent, clindamycin, is a known antibiotic. When applied topically it is found in comedone samples at sufficient levels to be active against most strains of *P. acnes*.

5.2 Pharmacokinetic properties
When applied topically in an alcoholic solution, clindamycin has been shown to be absorbed from the skin in small amounts. Very low levels, more than 1,000 times lower than those from normal systemic doses of clindamycin, have been found in the plasma. Using a sensitive RIA method, clindamycin has been detected in the urine at levels of < 1 to 53 ng/ml, 0.15-0.25% of the cumulative dose being recovered from the urine. No clindamycin has been detected in the serum following topical application.

5.3 Preclinical safety data
None stated.

6. PHARMACEUTICAL PARTICULARS

6.1 List of excipients
Glycerol,
sodium lauroyl sarcosinate,
stearic acid,
tegin,
cetostearyl alcohol,
isostearyl alcohol,
methylparaben,
purified water.

6.2 Incompatibilities
None.

6.3 Shelf life
36 months.

6.4 Special precautions for storage
Do not store above 25°C.

6.5 Nature and contents of container
HDPE/LDPE bottles and polypropylene cap containing, 15 ml, 30 ml and 60 ml of Dalacin T Topical lotion and HDPE bottle, polypropylene roller-ball and cap containing 15 ml, 30 ml and 50 ml of Dalacin Topical Lotion.

Only the 30 ml and 50 ml packs are marketed in the UK.

6.6 Instructions for use and handling
None.

7. MARKETING AUTHORISATION HOLDER
Pharmacia Limited
Davy Avenue
Milton Keynes
MK5 8PH
UK

8. MARKETING AUTHORISATION NUMBER(S)
PL 00032/0156

9. DATE OF FIRST AUTHORISATION/RENEWAL OF THE AUTHORISATION
18th September 1990/21st May 2001

10. DATE OF REVISION OF THE TEXT
April 2003

11. LEGAL CATEGORY
POM

DAD 1_0

Dalacin T Topical Solution

(Pharmacia Limited)

1. NAME OF THE MEDICINAL PRODUCT
Dalacin® T Topical Solution
Clindamycin Phosphate Topical Solution.

2. QUALITATIVE AND QUANTITATIVE COMPOSITION
One ml of Dalacin T Topical Solution contains the equivalent of 10 mg Clindamycin.

For excipients see Section 6.1 ('List of excipients').

3. PHARMACEUTICAL FORM
Topical solution.

Clear colourless aqueous solution.

4. CLINICAL PARTICULARS

4.1 Therapeutic indications
Dalacin T Topical Solution is indicated in the treatment of acne vulgaris

4.2 Posology and method of administration
Apply a thin film of Dalacin T Topical Solution twice daily to the affected area.

4.3 Contraindications
Dalacin T is contra-indicated in patients previously found to be hypersensitive to preparations containing clindamycin or any of the excipients. Although cross-sensitisation to lincomycin has not been demonstrated, it is recommended that Dalacin T is not used in patients who have demonstrated lincomycin sensitivity.

4.4 Special warnings and special precautions for use
Products containing benzoyl peroxide should not be used concurrently with Dalacin T Topical Solution.

Oral and parenteral clindamycin, as well as most other antibiotics, have been associated with severe pseudomembranous colitis. Post-marketing studies, however, have indicated a very low incidence of colitis with Dalacin T Topical Solution. The physician should, nonetheless, be alert to the development of antibiotic associated diarrhoea or colitis. If significant or prolonged diarrhoea occurs, the product should be discontinued immediately.

Studies indicate a toxin(s) produced by *Clostridium difficile* is the major cause of antibiotic associated colitis. Colitis is usually characterised by persistent, severe diarrhoea and abdominal cramps. Endoscopic examination may reveal pseudomembranous colitis. Stool culture for *C. difficile* and/or assay for *C. difficile* toxin may be helpful to diagnosis.

Vancomycin is effective in the treatment of antibiotic-associated colitis produced by *C. difficile*. The usual dose is 125-500 mg orally every 6 hours for 7-10 days. Additional supportive medical care may be necessary.

Mild cases of colitis may respond to discontinuance of clindamycin alone. Cholestyramine and colestipol resins have been shown to bind *C. difficile* toxin *in vitro*, and cholestyramine has been effective in the treatment of some mild cases of antibiotic-associated colitis. Cholestyramine resins have been shown to bind vancomycin; therefore, when both cholestyramine and vancomycin are used concurrently, their administration should be separated by at least two hours.

Dalacin T Topical Solution contains an alcohol base which can cause burning and irritation of the eye. In the event of accidental contact with sensitive surfaces (eye, abraded skin, mucous membranes), bathe with copious amounts of cool tap water. The solution has an unpleasant taste and caution should be exercised when applying medication around the mouth.

4.5 Interaction with other medicinal products and other forms of Interaction
Not known.

4.6 Pregnancy and lactation
Safety for use in pregnancy has not been established.

It is not known if clindamycin is excreted in breast milk following the use of Dalacin T Topical Solution.

4.7 Effects on ability to drive and use machines
Not applicable.

4.8 Undesirable effects
Skin dryness is the most common side-effect reported. Other side-effects include skin irritation, contact dermatitis, oily skin, stinging of the eye, Gram-negative folliculitis, gastro-intestinal disturbances and abdominal pain.

4.9 Overdose
Not applicable.

5. PHARMACOLOGICAL PROPERTIES
Anti-infectives for treatment of acne. D10A F

5.1 Pharmacodynamic properties
The active constituent, clindamycin, is a known antibiotic. When applied topically it is found in comedone samples at sufficient levels to be active against most strains of *Propionibacterium acnes*.

5.2 Pharmacokinetic properties
When applied topically, clindamycin has been shown to be absorbed from the skin in small amounts.

Very low levels, more than 1000 times lower than those from normal systemic doses of clindamycin, have been found in the plasma. Using a sensitive RIA method clindamycin has been detected in the urine at levels of < 1 to 53 nanograms/ml, 0.15 - 0.25% of the cumulative dose being recovered from the urine. No clindamycin has been detected in the serum following topical applications.

5.3 Preclinical safety data
No further pre-clinical safety data are available.

6. PHARMACEUTICAL PARTICULARS

6.1 List of excipients
Isopropyl alcohol
Propylene glycol
Purified water
Hydrochloric acid (10%)
Sodium hydroxide (10%)

6.2 Incompatibilities
Not applicable.

6.3 Shelf life
24 months.

6.4 Special precautions for storage
None.

6.5 Nature and contents of container
Dab-O-Matic bottle containing 30 ml, 50 ml or 60 ml.

Novonette wipe (1 g)

Webril wipe (2 g)

6.6 Instructions for use and handling
None.

7. MARKETING AUTHORISATION HOLDER
Pharmacia Limited
Davy Avenue
Milton Keynes
MK5 8PH
UK

8. MARKETING AUTHORISATION NUMBER(S)
PL 0032/0135

9. DATE OF FIRST AUTHORISATION/RENEWAL OF THE AUTHORISATION
Date of first authorisation: 18 January 1988

Date of renewal of authorisation: 22nd May 2001

10. DATE OF REVISION OF THE TEXT
April 2003

LEGAL CATEGORY: POM

DAC 1_0

DALMANE CAPSULES 15MG

(Valeant Pharmaceuticals Ltd)

1. NAME OF THE MEDICINAL PRODUCT
Dalmane 15 mg Capsules

2. QUALITATIVE AND QUANTITATIVE COMPOSITION
Capsules with opaque grey cap and opaque yellow body with ICN/15 printed in red on both cap

And body, containing 16.4 mg flurazepam monohydrochloride (equivalent to 15 mg flurazepam).

3. PHARMACEUTICAL FORM
Dalmane capsules 15 mg.

4. CLINICAL PARTICULARS

4.1 Therapeutic indications
Short-term treatment of insomnia when it is severe, disabling or subjecting the individual to extreme distress. Dalmane is helpful in overcoming difficulties in getting to sleep and also in the problem of frequent nocturnal awakenings. Its properties make it particularly indicated where the total duration of sleep is less than adequate.

An underlying cause for insomnia should be sought before deciding upon the use of benzodiazepines for symptomatic relief.

Benzodiazepines are not recommended for the primary treatment of psychotic illness.

4.2 Posology and method of administration

Adults
The dosage of Dalmane should be determined on an individual basis taking into account the severity of the insomnia and the patient's response to treatment. Dosage is important in determining the duration of effect and the occurrence of residual effects. For most patients the optimum dose if 15 mg – this will ensure a full night's sleep with minimal residual effects on wakening. Patients with severe insomnia may require 30 mg but residual effects on awakening, associated with an anxiolytic effect, are more frequent at this dose.

Elderly
Elderly or debilitated patients: the elderly or patients with impaired renal and/or hepatic function will be particularly susceptible to the adverse effects of Dalmane. The initial dose should not exceed 15 mg. If organic brain changes are present, the dosage of Dalmane should not exceed 15 mg in these patients.

In patients with chronic pulmonary insufficiency and in patients which chronic renal or hepatic disease, dosage may need to be reduced.

Children
Dalmane is contra-indicated for use in children.

Treatment should, if possible, be on an intermittent basis.

Treatment should be as short as possible and should be started with the lowest recommended dose. The maximum dose should not be exceeded. Generally the duration of treatment varies from a few days to two weeks with a maximum of four weeks, including the tapering off process. Patients who have taken benzodiazepines for a prolonged time may require a longer period during which doses are reduced. Specialist help may be appropriate. Little is known regarding the efficacy or safety of benzodiazepines in long-term use.

In certain cases, extension beyond the maximum treatment period may be necessary; if so, it should not take place without re-evaluation of the patient's status. Long-term chronic use is not recommended.

The product should be taken just before going to bed.

Dalmane capsules are for oral administration.

4.3 Contraindications
Patients with known sensitivity to benzodiazepines; acute pulmonary insufficiency; respiratory depression; phobic or obsessional states; chronic psychosis; myasthenia gravis;

sleep apnoea syndrome; severe hepatic insufficiency; use in children.

Use of this drug is contra-indicated in patients with a known hypersensitivity to benzodiazepines and any of the excipients. Hypersensitivity reactions with the benzodiazepines including rash, angioedema and hypotension have been reported on rare occasions in susceptible patients.

4.4 Special warnings and special precautions for use
In patients with chronic pulmonary insufficiency, and in patients with chronic renal or hepatic disease, dosage may need to be reduced.

Dalmane should not be used alone to treat depression or anxiety associated with depression, since suicide may be precipitated in such patients.

In cases of loss or bereavement, psychological adjustment may be inhibited by benzodiazepines.

If the patient is awoken during the period of maximum drug activity, recall may be impaired.

Use of benzodiazepines may lead to the development of physical and psychological dependence. The dependence potential of the benzodiazepines is low, particularly when limited to short-term use, but this increases when high doses are used, especially when given over long periods. This is particularly so in patients with a history of alcoholism or drug abuse or in patients with marked personality disorders. Regular monitoring in such patients is essential, routine repeat prescriptions should be avoided and treatment should be withdrawn gradually. Symptoms such as depression, nervousness, extreme anxiety, tension, restlessness, confusion, mood changes, rebound insomnia, irritability, sweating, diarrhoea, headaches and muscle pain have been reported following abrupt cessation of treatment in patients receiving even normal therapeutic doses for short periods of time.

In severe cases the following symptoms may occur: derealisation, depersonalisation, hyperacusis, numbness and tingling of the extremities, hypersensitivity to light, noise and physical contact and hallucinations or epileptic seizures. In rare instances, withdrawal following excessive dosages may produce confusional states, psychotic manifestations and convulsions. Abuse of the benzodiazepines has been reported.

Some loss of efficacy to the hypnotic effects of short-acting benzodiazepines may develop after repeated use for a few weeks.

Abnormal psychological reactions to benzodiazepines have been reported. Rare behavioural effects include paradoxical aggressive outbursts, excitement, confusion, restlessness, agitation, irritability, delusion, rages, nightmares, hallucinations, psychoses, inappropriate behaviour and the uncovering of depression with suicidal tendencies. Extreme caution should therefore be used in prescribing benzodiazepines to patients with personality disorders. If any of these reactions occur, use of the drug should be discontinued. These reactions may be quite severe and are more likely to occur in children and the elderly.

Benzodiazepines may induce anterograde amnesia. The condition usually occurs 1-2 hours after ingesting the product and may last up to several hours. Therefore, to reduce the risk, patients should ensure that they will be able to have an uninterrupted sleep of 7 to 8 hours.

4.5 Interaction with other medicinal products and other forms of Interaction
Enhancement of the central depressive effect may occur if benzodiazepines are combined with centrally-acting drugs such as neuroleptics, tranquilisers, antidepressants, hypnotics, analgesics, enhancement of the euphoria may also occur leading to an increase in psychological dependence. The elderly require special supervision.

When Dalmane is used in conjunction with anti-epileptic drugs, side-effects and toxicity may be more evident, particularly with hydantoins or barbiturates or combinations including them. This requires extra care in adjusting dosage in the initial stages of treatment.

Known inhibitors of hepatic enzymes, eg cimetidine, have been shown to reduce the clearance of benzodiazepines and may potentiate their action and known inducers of hepatic enzymes, eg rifampicin, may increase the clearance of benzodiazepines.

Concomitant intake with alcohol should be avoided. The sedative effect may be enhanced when the product is used in combination with alcohol. This adversely affects the ability to drive or use machines.

4.6 Pregnancy and lactation
There is no evidence as to drug safety in human pregnancy, nor is there evidence from animal work that it is free from hazard. Do not use during pregnancy, especially during the first and last trimesters, unless there are compelling reasons.

If the product is prescribed to a woman of childbearing potential, she should be warned to contact her physician regarding discontinuance of the product if she intends to become or suspects that she is pregnant.

Administration of benzodiazepines in the last trimester of pregnancy or during labour has been reported to produce irregularities in the foetal heart rate, and hypotonia, poor sucking and hypothermia and moderate respiratory depression in the neonate.

Infants born to mothers who took benzodiazepines chronically during the latter stages of pregnancy may have developed physical dependence and may be at some risk of developing withdrawal symptoms in the postnatal period.

No data regarding the passage of flurazepam into breast milk are available. However, in common with other benzodiazepines, its passage into breast milk might be expected. If possible, the use of Dalmane in mothers who are breast-feeding should be avoided.

4.7 Effects on ability to drive and use machines
Patients should be advised that, like all medicaments of this type, Dalmane might modify patients' performance at skilled tasks (driving, operating machinery, etc) to a varying degree depending upon dosage, administration, and sleep pattern and individual susceptibility. Patients should further be advised that alcohol may intensify any impairment, and should therefore be avoided during treatment.

4.8 Undesirable effects
Common adverse effects include drowsiness during the day, numbed emotions, reduced alertness, confusion, fatigue, headache, dizziness, muscle weakness, ataxia and double vision. These phenomena are dose-related and are likely to be uncommon with the recommended dosage; they occur predominantly at the start of therapy and usually disappear with repeated administration. The elderly are particularly sensitive to the effects of centrally depressant drugs.

Other adverse effects are rare and include vertigo, hypotension, gastro-intestinal upsets, skin rashes, visual disturbances, changes in libido, and urinary retention. Isolated cases of blood dyscrasias and jaundice have also been reported.

Occasionally patients treated with Dalmane experience a bitter after-taste.

4.9 Overdose
When taken alone in overdosage Dalmane presents few problems in management and should not present a threat to life unless combined with other CNS depressants (including alcohol).

In the management of overdose with any medicinal product, it should be borne in mind that multiple agents might have been taken.

Following overdose with oral benzodiazepines, vomiting should be induced if the patient is conscious or gastric lavage undertaken with the airway protected if the patient is unconscious. If there is no advantage in emptying the stomach, activated charcoal should be given to reduce absorption.

Special attention should be paid to respiratory and cardiovascular functions in intensive care. Overdose of benzodiazepines is usually manifested by degrees of central nervous system depression ranging from drowsiness to coma. In mild cases, symptoms include drowsiness, mental confusion, dysarthria and lethargy; in more serious cases, symptoms may include ataxia, hypotonia, hypotension, respiratory depression, rarely coma and very rarely death.

The value of dialysis has not been determined. Anexate is a specific IV antidote for use in emergency situations. Patients requiring such intervention should be monitored closely in hospital (see separate prescribing information).

If excitation occurs, barbiturates should not be used.

5. PHARMACOLOGICAL PROPERTIES

5.1 Pharmacodynamic properties
Dalmane is a benzodiazepine drug with hypnotic properties.

5.2 Pharmacokinetic properties
The pharmacokinetic properties of Dalmane make it particularly indicated for patients whose total duration of sleep is less than adequate. The dosage of the drug is important in balancing the duration of effect with the occurrence of residual effects. On repeated dosing there is accumulation of an active metabolite, desalkylflurazepam, with steady state levels being reached within 2 to 3 weeks. Psychomotor studies have demonstrated, however, that a dose of 15 mg given for 7 consecutive nights did not significantly affect performance on the morning after final administration. However, impairment of performance was recorded on the morning after final administration of 30 mg for 7 consecutive nights. This latter dose is associated with daytime anxiolytic effects.

5.3 Preclinical safety data
Not applicable.

6. PHARMACEUTICAL PARTICULARS

6.1 List of excipients
15 mg capsules contain the following excipients: lactose, talc purified, magnesium stearate, black iron oxide E172, titanium dioxide E171 and yellow iron oxide E172.

6.2 Incompatibilities
Not applicable.

6.3 Shelf life
Amber glass bottles and plastic adept containers - 5 years.

PVDC blister packs - 3 years.

Polythene bags in tins and small HDPE bottles - 2 years.

White securitainers - 1 year.

6.4 Special precautions for storage
Dalmane capsules should be stored in a dry place with a recommended maximum storage temperature of 25°C.

6.5 Nature and contents of container
PVDC blister packs, amber glass bottles, polythene bags in tins, plastic adept containers, white securitainers and small HDPE bottles, containing 30 capsules.

6.6 Instructions for use and handling
None.

7. MARKETING AUTHORISATION HOLDER
ValeantPharmaceuticals Limited, Cedarwood, Chineham Business Park, Crockford Lane, Basingstoke, Hants, RG24 8WD.

8. MARKETING AUTHORISATION NUMBER(S)
PL 15142/0016

9. DATE OF FIRST AUTHORISATION/RENEWAL OF THE AUTHORISATION
3rd May 1999

10. DATE OF REVISION OF THE TEXT
December 2004

DALMANE CAPSULES 30MG

(Valeant Pharmaceuticals Ltd)

1. NAME OF THE MEDICINAL PRODUCT
Dalmane 30 mg Capsules

2. QUALITATIVE AND QUANTITATIVE COMPOSITION
Capsules with black cap and opaque grey body with ICN 30 printed in red on both cap and body, containing 32.8 mg flurazepam monohydrochloride (equivalent to 30 mg flurazepam).

3. PHARMACEUTICAL FORM
Dalmane capsules 30 mg.

4. CLINICAL PARTICULARS

4.1 Therapeutic indications
Short-term treatment of insomnia when it is severe, disabling or subjecting the individual to extreme distress. Dalmane is helpful in overcoming difficulties in getting to sleep and also in the problem of frequent nocturnal awakenings. Its properties make it particularly indicated where the total duration of sleep is less than adequate.

An underlying cause for insomnia should be sought before deciding upon the use of benzodiazepines for symptomatic relief.

Benzodiazepines are not recommended for the primary treatment of psychotic illness.

4.2 Posology and method of administration
Adults
The dosage of Dalmane should be determined on an individual basis taking into account the severity of the insomnia and the patient's response to treatment. Dosage is important in determining the duration of effect and the occurrence of residual effects. For most patients the optimum dose is 15 mg – this will ensure a full night's sleep with minimal residual effects on wakening. Patients with severe insomnia may require 30 mg but residual effects on awakening, associated with an anxiolytic effect, are more frequent at this dose.

Elderly
Elderly or debilitated patients: the elderly or patients with impaired renal and/or hepatic function will be particularly susceptible to the adverse effects of Dalmane. The initial dose should not exceed 15 mg. If organic brain changes are present, the dosage of Dalmane should not exceed 15 mg in these patients.

In patients with chronic pulmonary insufficiency and in patients which chronic renal or hepatic disease, dosage may need to be reduced.

Children
Dalmane is contra-indicated for use in children.

Treatment should, if possible, be on an intermittent basis.

Treatment should be as short as possible and should be started with the lowest recommended dose. The maximum dose should not be exceeded. Generally the duration of treatment varies from a few days to two weeks with a maximum of four weeks, including the tapering off process. Patients who have taken benzodiazepines for a prolonged time may require a longer period during which doses are reduced. Specialist help may be appropriate. Little is known regarding the efficacy or safety of benzodiazepines in long-term use.

In certain cases, extension beyond the maximum treatment period may be necessary; if so, it should not take place without re-evaluation of the patient's status. Long-term chronic use is not recommended.

The product should be taken just before going to bed.

Dalmane capsules are for oral administration.

4.3 Contraindications
Patients with known sensitivity to benzodiazepines; acute pulmonary insufficiency; respiratory depression; phobic or obsessional states; chronic psychosis; myasthenia gravis; sleep apnoea syndrome; severe hepatic insufficiency; use in children.

Use of this drug is contra-indicated in patients with a known hypersensitivity to benzodiazepines and any of the excipients. Hypersensitivity reactions with the benzodiazepines including rash, angioedema and hypotension have been reported on rare occasions in susceptible patients.

4.4 Special warnings and special precautions for use
In patients with chronic pulmonary insufficiency, and in patients with chronic renal or hepatic disease, dosage may need to be reduced.

Dalmane should not be used alone to treat depression or anxiety associated with depression, since suicide may be precipitated in such patients.

In cases of loss or bereavement, psychological adjustment may be inhibited by benzodiazepines.

If the patient is awoken during the period of maximum drug activity, recall may be impaired.

Use of benzodiazepines may lead to the development of physical and psychological dependence. The dependence potential of the benzodiazepines is low, particularly when limited to short-term use, but this increases when high doses are used, especially when given over long periods. This is particularly so in patients with a history of alcoholism or drug abuse or in patients with marked personality disorders. Regular monitoring in such patients is essential, routine repeat prescriptions should be avoided and treatment should be withdrawn gradually. Symptoms such as depression, nervousness, extreme anxiety, tension, restlessness, confusion, mood changes, rebound insomnia, irritability, sweating, diarrhoea, headaches and muscle pain have been reported following abrupt cessation of treatment in patients receiving even normal therapeutic doses for short periods of time.

In severe cases the following symptoms may occur: derealisation, depersonalisation, hyperacusis, numbness and tingling of the extremities, hypersensitivity to light, noise and physical contact and hallucinations or epileptic seizures. In rare instances, withdrawal following excessive dosages may produce confusional states, psychotic manifestations and convulsions. Abuse of the benzodiazepines has been reported.

Some loss of efficacy to the hypnotic effects of short-acting benzodiazepines may develop after repeated use for a few weeks.

Abnormal psychological reactions to benzodiazepines have been reported. Rare behavioural effects include paradoxical aggressive outbursts, excitement, confusion, restlessness, agitation, irritability, delusion, rages, nightmares, hallucinations, psychoses, inappropriate behaviour and the uncovering of depression with suicidal tendencies. Extreme caution should therefore be used in prescribing benzodiazepines to patients with personality disorders. If any of these reactions occur, use of the drug should be discontinued. These reactions may be quite severe and are more likely to occur in children and the elderly.

Benzodiazepines may induce anterograde amnesia. The condition usually occurs 1-2 hours after ingesting the product and may last up to several hours. Therefore, to reduce the risk, patients should ensure that they will be able to have an uninterrupted sleep of 7 to 8 hours.

4.5 Interaction with other medicinal products and other forms of Interaction
Enhancement of the central depressive effect may occur if benzodiazepines are combined with centrally-acting drugs such as neuroleptics, tranquilisers, antidepressants, hypnotics, analgesics, enhancement of the euphoria may also occur leading to an increase in psychological dependence. The elderly require special supervision.

When Dalmane is used in conjunction with anti-epileptic drugs, side-effects and toxicity may be more evident, particularly with hydantoins or barbiturates or combinations including them. This requires extra care in adjusting dosage in the initial stages of treatment.

Known inhibitors of hepatic enzymes, eg cimetidine, have been shown to reduce the clearance of benzodiazepines and may potentiate their action and known inducers of hepatic enzymes, eg rifampicin, may increase the clearance of benzodiazepines.

Concommitant intake with alcohol should be avoided. The sedative effect may be enhanced when the product is used in combination with alcohol. This adversely affects the ability to drive or use machines.

4.6 Pregnancy and lactation
There is no evidence as to drug safety in human pregnancy, nor is there evidence from animal work that it is free from hazard. Do not use during pregnancy, especially during the first and last trimesters, unless there are compelling reasons.

If the product is prescribed to a woman of childbearing potential, she should be warned to contact her physician regarding discontinuance of the product if she intends to become or suspects that she is pregnant.

Administration of benzodiazepines in the last trimester of pregnancy or during labour has been reported to produce irregularities in the foetal heart rate, and hypotonia, poor sucking and hypothermia and moderate respiratory depression in the neonate.

Infants born to mothers who took benzodiazepines chronically during the latter stages of pregnancy may have developed physical dependence and may be at some risk of developing withdrawal symptoms in the postnatal period.

No data regarding the passage of flurazepam into breast milk are available. However, in common with other benzodiazepines, its passage into breast milk might be expected. If possible, the use of Dalmane in mothers who are breast-feeding should be avoided.

4.7 Effects on ability to drive and use machines
Patients should be advised that, like all medicaments of this type, Dalmane might modify patients' performance at skilled tasks (driving, operating machinery, etc) to a varying degree depending upon dosage, administration, and sleep pattern and individual susceptibility. Patients should further be advised that alcohol may intensify any impairment, and should, therefore, be avoided during treatment.

4.8 Undesirable effects
Common adverse effects include drowsiness during the day, numbed emotions, reduced alertness, confusion, fatigue, headache, dizziness, muscle weakness, ataxia and double vision. These phenomena are dose-related and are likely to be uncommon with the recommended dosage; they occur predominantly at the start of therapy and usually disappear with repeated administration. The elderly are particularly sensitive to the effects of centrally-depressant drugs.

Other adverse effects are rare and include vertigo, hypotension, gastro-intestinal upsets, skin rashes, visual disturbances, changes in libido, and urinary retention. Isolated cases of blood dyscrasias and jaundice have also been reported.

Occasionally patients treated with Dalmane experience a bitter after-taste.

4.9 Overdose
When taken alone in overdosage Dalmane presents few problems in management and should not present a threat to life unless combined with other CNS depressants (including alcohol).

In the management of overdose with any medicinal product, it should be borne in mind that multiple agents might have been taken.

Following overdose with oral benzodiazepines, vomiting should be induced if the patient is conscious or gastric lavage undertaken with the airway protected if the patient is unconscious. If there is no advantage in emptying the stomach, activated charcoal should be given to reduce absorption.

Special attention should be paid to respiratory and cardiovascular functions in intensive care. Overdose of benzodiazepines is usually manifested by degrees of central nervous system depression ranging from drowsiness to coma. In mild cases, symptoms include drowsiness, mental confusion, dysarthria and lethargy; in more serious cases, symptoms may include ataxia, hypotonia, hypotension, respiratory depression, rarely coma and very rarely death.

The value of dialysis has not been determined. Anexate is a specific IV antidote for use in emergency situations. Patients requiring such intervention should be monitored closely in hospital (see separate prescribing information).

If excitation occurs, barbiturates should not be used.

5. PHARMACOLOGICAL PROPERTIES

5.1 Pharmacodynamic properties
Dalmane is a benzodiazepine drug with hypnotic properties.

5.2 Pharmacokinetic properties
The pharmacokinetic properties of Dalmane make it particularly indicated for patients whose total duration of sleep is less than adequate. The dosage of the drug is important in balancing the duration of effect with the occurrence of residual effects. On repeated dosing there is accumulation of an active metabolite, desalkylflurazepam, with steady state levels being reached within 2 to 3 weeks. Psychomotor studies have demonstrated, however, that a dose of 15 mg given for 7 consecutive nights did not significantly affect performance on the morning after final administration. However, impairment of performance was recorded on the morning after final administration of 30 mg for 7 consecutive nights. This latter dose is associated with daytime anxiolytic effects.

5.3 Preclinical safety data
Not applicable.

6. PHARMACEUTICAL PARTICULARS

6.1 List of excipients
30 mg capsules contain the following excipients: lactose, talc purified, magnesium stearate, black iron oxide E172, titanium dioxide E171 and yellow iron oxide E172.

6.2 Incompatibilities
Not applicable.

6.3 Shelf life
Amber glass bottles and plastic adept containers - 5 years.

PVDC blister packs - 3 years.

Polythene bags in tins and small HDPE bottles - 2 years.

White securitainers - 1 year.

6.4 Special precautions for storage
Dalmane capsules should be stored in a dry place with a recommended maximum storage temperature of 25°C.

6.5 Nature and contents of container
PVDC blister packs, amber glass bottles, polythene bags in tins, plastic adept containers, white securitainers and small HDPE bottles, containing 30 capsules.

6.6 Instructions for use and handling
None.

7. MARKETING AUTHORISATION HOLDER
ValeantPharmaceuticals Limited, Cedarwood, Chineham Business Park, Crockford Lane, Basingstoke, Hants, RG24 8WD.

8. MARKETING AUTHORISATION NUMBER(S)
PL 15142/0017

9. DATE OF FIRST AUTHORISATION/RENEWAL OF THE AUTHORISATION
3rd May 1999

10. DATE OF REVISION OF THE TEXT
December 2004

Danol 100mg Capsules, Danol 200mg Capsules

(sanofi-aventis)

1. NAME OF THE MEDICINAL PRODUCT
Danol 100mg Capsules

Danol 200mg Capsules

2. QUALITATIVE AND QUANTITATIVE COMPOSITION
Danol 100mg Capsules: danazol 100mg

Danol 200mg Capsules: danazol 200mg

3. PHARMACEUTICAL FORM
Danol 100mg: Capsule

Danol 200mg: Capsule with white body and orange cap.

4. CLINICAL PARTICULARS

4.1 Therapeutic indications
Danol capsules are recommended for the treatment of:

Endometriosis: treatment of endometriosis-associated symptoms or/and to reduce the extent of endometriosis foci. Danazol may be used either in conjunction with surgery or, as sole hormonal therapy, in patients not responding to other treatments.

Benign fibrocystic breast disease: symptomatic relief of severe pain and tenderness. Danazol should be used only in patients not responsive to other therapeutic measures or for whom such measures are inadvisable.

4.2 Posology and method of administration
Adults:

Danol capsules should be given as a continuous course, dosage being adjusted according to the severity of the condition and the patient's response. A reduction in dosage once a satisfactory response has been achieved may prove possible. In fertile females, Danol capsules should be started during menstruation, preferably on the first day, to avoid exposing a pregnancy to its possible effects. Where doubt exists, appropriate checks should be made to exclude pregnancy before starting medication. Females of child-bearing age should employ non-hormonal contraception throughout the course of treatment.

In endometriosis the recommended dosage is 200mg to 800mg daily in a course of treatment lasting normally three to six months. Dosage should be increased if normal cyclical bleeding still persists after two months therapy, a higher dosage (not exceeding 800mg per day) may also be needed for severe disease.

In benign fibrocystic breast disease, treatment should commence at a dose of 300mg daily, a course of treatment normally lasting 3 to 6 months.

Elderly: Danol is not recommended.

Children: Danol is not recommended.

The capsules are for oral administration.

4.3 Contraindications
1. Pregnancy
2. Breast feeding
3. Markedly impaired hepatic, renal or cardiac function
4. Porphyria
5. Active thrombosis or thromboembolic disease and a history of such events
6. Androgen dependent tumour
7. Undiagnosed abnormal genital bleeding.

4.4 Special warnings and special precautions for use
4.4.1

Special Warnings

In the event of virilisation, Danol should be withdrawn. Androgenic reactions generally prove reversible, but continued use of Danol after evidence of androgenic virilisation increases the risk of irreversible androgenic effects.

Danol should be stopped if any clinically significant adverse event arises, and particularly if there is evidence of papilloedema, headache, visual disturbances or other signs or symptoms of raised intracranial pressure, jaundice or other indication of significant hepatic disturbance, thrombosis or thromboembolism.

Whilst a course of therapy may need to be repeated, care should be observed as no safety data are available in relation to repeated courses of treatment over time. The long-term risk of 17-alkylated steroids (including benign hepatic adenomata, peliosis hepatis and hepatic carcinoma), should be considered when danazol, which is chemically related to those compounds, is used.

Data, from two case-control epidemiological studies, were pooled to examine the relationship between endometriosis, endometriosis treatments and ovarian cancer. These preliminary results suggest that the use of danazol might increase the baseline risk of ovarian cancer in - patients treated for endometriosis.

4.4.2

Precautions

In view of its pharmacology, known interactions and side effects, particular care should be observed when using Danol in patients with hepatic or renal disease, hypertension or other cardiovascular disease and in any state which may be exacerbated by fluid retention as well as in diabetes mellitus, polycythaemia, epilepsy, lipoprotein disorder, and in those who have shown marked or persistent androgenic reaction to previous gonadal steroid therapy.

Caution is advised in patients with migraine.

Until more is known, caution is advised in the use of Danol in the presence of known or suspected malignant disease (see also contra-indications). Before treatment initiation, the presence of hormone–dependent carcinoma should be excluded at least by careful clinical examination, as well as if breast nodules persist or enlarge during danazol treatment.

In addition to clinical monitoring in all patients, appropriate laboratory monitoring should be considered which may include periodic measurement of hepatic function and haematological state. For long-term treatment > 6 months) or repeated courses of treatment, biannual hepatic ultrasonography is recommended.

Danazol should be initiated during menstruation. An effective, non-hormonal method of contraception should be employed (see Section 4.2 and 4.6 Pregnancy and Lactation).

The lowest effective dose of Danol should always be sought.

4.5 Interaction with other medicinal products and other forms of Interaction

Anti-convulsant therapy: Danol may affect the plasma level of carbamazepine and possibly the patient's response to this agent and to phenytoin. With phenobarbitone it is likely that similar interaction would occur.

Anti-diabetic therapy: Danol can cause insulin resistance.

Oral anti-coagulant therapy: Danol can potentiate the action of warfarin.

Anti-hypertensive therapy: Possibly through promotion of fluid retention, Danol can oppose the action of anti-hypertensive agents.

Cyclosporin and tacrolimus: Danol can increase the plasma level of cyclosporin and tacrolimus, leading to an increase of the renal toxicity of these drugs.

Concomitant steroids: Although specific instances have not been described, it is likely that interactions will occur between Danol and gonadal steroid therapy.

Migraine therapy: Danol may itself provoke migraine and possibly reduce the effectiveness of medication to prevent that condition.

Ethyl alcohol: Subjective intolerance in the form of nausea and shortness of breath has been reported.

Alpha calcidol: Danol may increase the calcaemic response in primary hypoparathyroidism necessitating a reduction in dosage of this agent.

Interactions with laboratory function tests: Danazol treatment may interfere with laboratory determination of testosterone or plasma proteins (See also section4.8 Undesirable effects)

4.6 Pregnancy and lactation

There is epidemiological and toxicological evidence of hazard in human pregnancy. Danazol is known to be associated with the risk of virilisation to the female foetus if administered during human pregnancy. Danazol should not be used during pregnancy. Women of childbearing age should be advised to use an effective, non-hormonal, method of contraception. If the patient conceives during therapy, danazol should be stopped. Danazol has the theoretical potential for androgenic effects in breast-fed infants and therefore either danazol therapy or breast-feeding should be discontinued.

4.7 Effects on ability to drive and use machines

No special warning is felt necessary.

4.8 Undesirable effects

Androgenic effects include weight gain, increased appetite, acne and seborrhoea. Hirsutism, hair loss, voice change, which may take the form of hoarseness, sore throat or of instability or deepening of pitch may occur. Hypertrophy of the clitoris as well as fluid retention are rare.

Other possible endocrine effects include menstrual disturbances in the form of spotting, alteration of the timing of the cycle and amenorrhoea. Although cyclical bleeding and ovulation usually return within 60-90 days after Danol, persistent amenorrhoea has occasionally been reported. Flushing, vaginal dryness, changes in libido, irritation and reduction in breast size may reflect a lowering of oestrogen. In the male a modest reduction in spermatogenesis may be evident during treatment.

Insulin resistance may be increased in diabetes mellitus but symptomatic hypoglycaemia in non-diabetic patients has also been reported as has an increase in plasma glucagon level. Coupled with elevated plasma insulin levels, danazol can also cause a mild impairment of glucose tolerance.

Danol may aggravate epilepsy and expose the condition in those so predisposed.

Cutaneous reactions include rashes, which may be maculopapular, petechial or purpuric or may take an urticarial form and may be accompanied by facial oedema. Associated fever has also been reported. Rarely, sun-sensitive rash has been noted. Inflammatory erythematous nodules, changes in skin pigmentation, exfoliative dermatitis and erythema multiforme have also been reported.

Musculo-skeletal reactions include backache and muscle cramps which can be severe, creatine phosphokinase levels may also rise. Muscle tremors, fasciculation, limb pain, joint pain and joint swelling have also been reported.

Cardiovascular reactions may include hypertension, palpitations and tachycardia.

Thrombotic events have also been observed. Sagittal sinus and cerebrovascular thrombosis as well as arterial thrombosis have been observed. Cases of myocardial infarction have been reported.

Benign intracranial hypertension, visual disturbances such as blurring of vision, difficulty in focusing, difficulty in wearing contact lenses and refraction disorders requiring correction have been noted.

Haematological responses include an increase in red cell and platelet count. Reversible polycythaemia may be provoked. Eosinophilia, leucopenia thrombocytopenia and splenic peliosis have also been noted.

Hepatic-pancreatic reactions include isolated increases in serum transaminase levels and rarely cholestatic jaundice and benign hepatic adenomata and pancreatitis. Very rarely peliosis hepatitis as well as malignant hepatic tumour have been observed with long term use.

Fluid retention may explain the occasional reports of carpal tunnel syndrome. Danol capsules may also provoke migraine.

Possible psychical reactions include emotional lability, anxiety, depressed mood and nervousness. Dizziness, vertigo, nausea, headache, fatigue and epigastric and pleuritic pain have also been noted.

A temporary alteration of lipoproteins in the form of an increase in LDL cholesterol, a decrease in HDL cholesterol, affecting all subfractions, and a decrease in apolipoproteins AI and AII have been reported with Danol in the female.

Other metabolic events have been reported, including induction of aminolevulinic acid (ALA) synthetase, and reduction in thyroid binding globulin, T4, with increased uptake of T3 but without disturbance of thyroid stimulating hormone or free thyroxine index, is also likely during therapy.

Haematuria has rarely been reported with prolonged use in patients with hereditary angioedema. Cases of interstitial pneumonitis have been reported

4.9 Overdose

Available evidence suggests that acute overdosage would be unlikely to give rise to immediate serious reaction.

In the case of acute overdose, consideration should be given to reducing the absorption of the drug with activated charcoal and the patient should be kept under observation in case of any delayed reactions.

5. PHARMACOLOGICAL PROPERTIES

5.1 Pharmacodynamic properties

Danazol, 17a-pregna-2,4-dien-20-yno(2,3-d)-isoxazol-17-ol, is a synthetic steroid derived from ethisterone. Its pharmacological properties include:

1. Relatively marked affinity for androgen receptors, less marked affinity for progesterone receptors and least affinity for oestrogen receptors. Danazol is a weak androgen but in addition antiandrogenic, progestogenic, antiprogestogenic, oestrogenic and antioestrogenic actions have been observed.

2. Interference with the synthesis of gonadal steroids, possibly by inhibition of the enzymes of steroidogenesis, including 3β hydroxysteroid dehydrogenase,17β hydroxysteroid dehydrogenase, 17 hydroxylase, 17, 20 lyase, 11β hydroxylase, 21 hydroxylase and cholesterol side chain cleavage enzymes, or alternatively by inhibition of the cyclic AMP accumulation usually induced by gonadotrophic hormones in granulosa and luteal cells.

3. Inhibition of the mid-cycle surge of FSH and LH as well as alterations in the pulsatility of LH. Danazol can also reduce the mean plasma levels of these gonadotrophins after the menopause.

4. A wide range of actions on plasma proteins, including increasing prothrombin, plasminogen, antithrombin III, alpha-2 macroglobulin, C1 esterase inhibitor, and erythropoietin and reducing fibrinogen, thyroid binding and sex hormone binding globulins. Danazol increases the proportion and concentration of testosterone carried unbound in plasma.

5 The suppressive effects of danazol on the hypothalmic-pituitary-gonadal axis are reversible, cyclical activity reappearing normally within 60-90 days after therapy.

5.2 Pharmacokinetic properties

Danazol is absorbed from the gastrointestinal tract, peak plasma concentrations of 50-80ng/ml being reached approximately 2-3 hours after dosing. Compared to the fasting state, the bioavailability has been shown to increase 3 fold when the drug is taken with a meal with a high fat content. It is thought that food stimulates bile flow which facilitates the dissolution and absorption of danazol, a highly lipophilic compound.

The apparent plasma elimination half life of danazol in a single dose is approximately 3-6 hours. With multiple doses this may increase to approximately 26 hours.

None of the metabolites of danazol, which have been isolated, exhibits pituitary inhibiting activity comparable to that of danazol.

Few data on excretion routes and rates exist. In the monkey 36% of a radioactive dose was recoverable in the urine and 48% in the faeces within 96 hours.

5.3 Preclinical safety data

There are no pre-clinical data of relevance to the prescriber which are additional to that already included in other sections of the SPC.

6. PHARMACEUTICAL PARTICULARS

6.1 List of excipients

Maize starch, Lactose, Purified talc, Magnesium stearate, Gelatin, Titanium dioxide, Red iron oxide, Yellow iron oxide, Shellac, Soya Lecithin, 2-ethoxyethanol, Dimethylpolysiloxane, Black iron oxide.

6.2 Incompatibilities

None.

6.3 Shelf life

60 months.

6.4 Special precautions for storage

None.

6.5 Nature and contents of container

PVC blister pack compound of polyvinyl chloride (thickness 250μm) sealed to aluminium foil (thickness 20μm). The blisters are then packed in a cardboard carton.

Pack size: 60 capsules.

6.6 Instructions for use and handling

Not applicable.

7. MARKETING AUTHORISATION HOLDER

Sanofi-Synthelabo

PO Box 597

Guildford

Surrey

8. MARKETING AUTHORISATION NUMBER(S)

Danol 100mg: PL 11723/0015

Danol 200mg: PL 11723/0016

9. DATE OF FIRST AUTHORISATION/RENEWAL OF THE AUTHORISATION

28th October 1993

10. DATE OF REVISION OF THE TEXT

Danol 100mg: July 2003

Danol 200mg: August 2004

Legal Category: POM

Dantrium 100mg Capsules

(Procter & Gamble Pharmaceuticals UK Limited)

1. NAME OF THE MEDICINAL PRODUCT

Dantrium 100mg capsules.

2. QUALITATIVE AND QUANTITATIVE COMPOSITION

Dantrium 100mg capsules contain 100mg dantrolene sodium per capsule.

3. PHARMACEUTICAL FORM

Dantrium capsules are presented in orange/light brown capsules. The 100mg capsule carries the monogram Dantrium 100mg on the cap and 0149, 0033 and triple coding bars on the body.

4. CLINICAL PARTICULARS

4.1 Therapeutic indications

For the treatment of chronic, severe spasticity of skeletal muscle in adults.

4.2 Posology and method of administration

Adults

For the individual patient, the lowest dose compatible with optimal response is recommended.

A recommended dosage increment scale is shown below:-

Week	*Recommended dosage*
First	One 25mg capsule daily
Second	One 25mg capsule twice daily
Third	Two 25mg capsules twice daily
Fourth	Two 25mg capsules three times daily
Fifth	Three 25mg capsules three times daily
Sixth	Three 25mg capsules four times daily
Seventh	One 100mg capsule four times daily

Each dosage level should be maintained for seven days in order to determine the patient's response. Therapy with a dose four times daily may offer maximum benefit to some patients. The maximum daily dose should not exceed 400mg. In view of the potential for hepatoxicity in long term use, if no observable benefit is derived from the administration of Dantrium after a total of 45 days, therapy should be discontinued.

Elderly

A similar dosage scheme should be used with the elderly.

Children

Dantrium is not recommended for use in children.

4.3 Contraindications

Dantrium is contraindicated where spasticity is utilised to sustain upright posture and balance in locomotion or whenever spasticity is utilised to obtain or maintain increased function. Dantrium is contraindicated in patients with evidence of hepatic dysfunction. Dantrium is not indicated for the treatment of acute skeletal muscle spasm. Dantrium should not be administered to children.

4.4 Special warnings and special precautions for use

Fatal and non-fatal liver disorders of an idiosyncratic or hypersensitivity type may occur with Dantrium therapy.

Patients should be instructed to contact their physician should signs or symptoms of hepatotoxicity (e.g., discolored feces, generalized pruritus, jaundice, anorexia, nausea, vomiting) occur during therapy.

Factors that may increase the risk of developing hepatotoxicity include:

- Higher daily doses (doses exceeding 400 mg daily)
- Duration of therapy (most frequently reported between 2 and 12 months of treatment)
- Female gender
- Age greater than 30 years
- Prior history of liver disease/dysfunction
- Receiving other hepatotoxic therapies concomitantly.

Spontaneous reports also suggest a higher proportion of hepatic events with fatal outcome in elderly patients.

At the start of Dantrium therapy, it is desirable to do liver function studies (SGOT/ALT, SGPT/AST, alkaline phosphatase, total bilirubin) for a baseline or to establish whether there is pre-existing liver disease. If baseline liver abnormalities exist and are confirmed, there is a clear possibility that the potential for Dantrium hepatotoxicity could be enhanced, although such a possibility has not yet been established.

Liver functions studies (e.g. serum, SGOT/AST, SGPT/ALT) should be performed at appropriate intervals during Dantrium therapy. If such studies reveal abnormal values, therapy should generally be discontinued. Only where benefits of the drug have been of major importance to the patient, should re-introduction or continuation of therapy be considered. Some patients have revealed a return to normal laboratory values in the face of continued therapy while others have not.

If symptoms compatible with hepatitis, accompanied by abnormalities in liver function tests or jaundice appear, Dantrium should be discontinued. If caused by Dantrium and detected early, the abnormalities in liver function have reverted to normal when the drug was discontinued.

Dantrium has been re-introduced in a few patients who have developed clinical signs, or elevated serum enzymes, of hepatocellular injury.

Re-introduction of Dantrium therapy should only be contemplated in patients who clearly need the drug, and only after complete reversal of the signs of hepatotoxicity and liver function tests. Patients being re-challenged with Dantrium should be hospital in-patients, and small, gradually increasing doses should be used. Laboratory test monitoring should be frequent, and the drug should be withdrawn immediately if there is any indication of recurrent liver abnormality. Some patients have reacted with unmistakable signs of liver abnormality upon administration of a challenge dose, whilst others have not.

The use of Dantrium with other potentially hepatotoxic drugs should be avoided.

There are isolated cases of possibly significant effects of Dantrium on the cardiovascular and respiratory systems. These cases also have other features suggesting a predisposition to cardiovascular disease, and impaired respiratory function, particularly obstructive pulmonary disease. Dantrium should be used with caution in such patients.

Dantrolene sodium showed some evidence of tumourgenicity at high dose levels in Sprague-Dawley female rats. However, these effects were not seen in other studies in Fischer 344 rats or HaM/ICR mice. There is no clinical evidence of carcinogenicity in humans, however, this possibility cannot be absolutely excluded.

Caution should be exercised in the simultaneous administration of tranquillising agents and alcohol.

4.5 Interaction with other medicinal products and other forms of Interaction

An idiosyncratic interaction between verapamil and intravenous Dantrium, involving hypotension, hyperkalaemia, and myocardial depression, has been reported as a single case. This interaction has been replicated in dogs and pigs.

4.6 Pregnancy and lactation

Although teratological studies in animals have proved satisfactory, the use of Dantrium is not advised in pregnant or nursing mothers.

4.7 Effects on ability to drive and use machines

Patients should be advised not to drive a motor vehicle or to undertake potentially dangerous work until Dantrium therapy has been stabilised, because some patients experience drowsiness and dizziness.

4.8 Undesirable effects

The most frequently reported unwanted effects associated with the use of Dantrium have been drowsiness, dizziness, weakness, general malaise, fatigue and diarrhoea. These effects are generally transient, occur early in treatment, and can often be obviated by careful determination and regulation of the dosage. Diarrhoea may be severe, and may necessitate temporary withdrawal of Dantrium. If diarrhoea recurs upon re-introduction of Dantrium, then Dantrium therapy should probably be withdrawn permanently. Other frequent side effects include anorexia, nausea, headache and skin rash. Less frequent side effects include constipation, dysphagia, speech disturbance, visual disturbance, confusion, nervousness, depression, seizures, increased urinary frequency, and insomnia. Rare reports include tachycardia, erratic blood pressure, dyspnoea, haematuria, crystalluria (unconfirmed reports), urinary incontinence, and urinary retention. Pleural effusion and/or pericarditis in patients using Dantrium have been rarely reported. Chills and fever have occasionally been reported.

Dantrium has a potential for hepatotoxicity. Symptomatic hepatitis (fatal and non-fatal) has been reported at various dose levels although the incidence is greater in patients taking more than 400 mg/day. Liver dysfunction as evidenced by blood chemical abnormalities alone (liver enzyme elevation) has been observed in patients exposed to Dantrium for varying periods of time.

Overt hepatitis has occurred at varying intervals after initiation of therapy, but has most frequently been observed between the second and twelfth month of treatment. The risk of hepatic injury appears to be greater in females, in patients over 30 years old and in patients taking concomitant medication. There is some evidence that hepatic injury is more likely in patients using concomitant oral oestrogen.

4.9 Overdose

For acute overdosage, general supportive measures and gastric lavage should be employed as well as measures to reduce the absorption of Dantrium. The theoretical possibility of crystalluria in overdose has not been reported for Dantrium, but would be treated according to general principles, including administration of fluids.

5. PHARMACOLOGICAL PROPERTIES

5.1 Pharmacodynamic properties

<u>Molecular Pharmacology</u>

The receptor molecule for dantrolene has not been identified. Radiolabelled dantrolene sodium binds to specific components of the striated muscle cell, namely the t-tubules and the sarcoplastic reticulum; however the kinetics of binding varies between these two organelles. The binding of ryanodine is thought to compete with the binding of calcium in these organelles; further evidence for the specificity of binding is that dantrolene inhibits the binding of the insecticide ryanodine to heavy sarcoplastic reticulum vesicles from rabbit skeletal muscle. Under some conditions, dantrolene will lower intra-sarcoplasmic calcium concentrations in the resting state. This may be more important in diseased muscle (e.g. in malignant hyperthermia in humans and swine stress syndrome) than in muscle with normal function.

Dantrolene does not bind to the same sites as calcium channel blocking drugs such as nitrendipine or calmodulin. There is no electrophysiological evidence that dantrolene interferes with the influx of calcium from outside the cell. This may be one reason why paralysis by dantrolene has never been reported in animals or man; the muscle cell has alternative sources of calcium which are not influenced by dantrolene.

<u>Biochemical Pharmacology</u>

Whatever the molecular mechanism, the cardinal property of dantrolene sodium is that it lowers intracellular calcium concentration in skeletal muscle. Calcium concentrations may be lower in both the quiescent state, and as a result of a reduction in the release of calcium form the sarcoplasmic reticulum in response to a standard stimulus. This effect has been observed in striated muscle fibres from several species, and is not seen in myocardium. Fast fibres may be more sensitive than slow fibres to the action of dantrolene sodium.

Diverse other properties of dantrolene sodium have been observed <u>in-vitro</u>, and in animal studies. Dantrolene sodium may inhibit the release of calcium from the smooth endoplasmic reticulum of smooth muscle, but the significance of this observation is questionable; for example, dantrolene sodium has no effect on isolated human urinary bladder smooth muscle. Calcium dependent, pre-synaptic neurotransmitter release may also be inhibited by dantrolene sodium. Again, the clinical significance of this has not been demonstrated.

<u>Studies on Isolated, Functional Muscle</u>

Elevation of intracellular, free calcium ion concentration is an obligatory step in excitation-contraction coupling of skeletal muscle. Dantrolene sodium, therefore, acts as a muscle relaxant by a peripheral mechanism which is quite different, and easily distinguishable from neuromuscular junction blocking drugs. In contrast with compounds that relax skeletal muscle by acting principally on the central nervous system, dantrolene sodium acts directly on skeletal muscle cells. In rabbit atria, dantrolene sodium has no effect alone, but it may antagonise inotropic agents which act by increasing intramyocardial cell calcium e.g. the experimental drug anthopleurin-A.

5.2 Pharmacokinetic properties

<u>Absorption</u>

Dantrium is easily and almost completely absorbed from the gastrointestinal tract. After dosing on an empty stomach, plasma dantrolene levels peak within three hours in most subjects.

<u>Distribution</u>

Dantrolene sodium is a highly lipophobic drug. In addition it lacks hydrophilicity. Dantrolene sodium binds to human serum albumin (HSA) with a molar ratio of 0.95 to 1.68 <u>in-vitro</u>. The association constant <u>in-vitro</u> is higher (2.3 to 5.4×10^{-5} per mol). <u>In-vitro</u> dantrolene sodium can be displaced from HSA by warfarin, clofibrate and tolbutamide but these interactions have not been confirmed in humans (re. manufacturer's database). Single intravenous dose studies suggest that the primary volume of distribution is about 15 litres. Single oral doses achieve peak plasma concentration of about a quarter of that for a similarly sized intravenous dose.

<u>Metabolism and Excretion</u>

The biological half life in plasma in most human subjects is between 5 and 9 hours, although half-lives as long as 12.1 ± 1.9 hours have been reported after a single intravenous dose. Inactivation is by hepatic metabolism in the first instance. There are two alternative pathways. Most of the drug is hydroxylated to 5-hydroxy-dantrolene. The minor pathway involves nitro-reduction to amino-dantrolene which is then acetylated (compound F-490). The 5-hydroxy metabolite is a muscle relaxant with nearly the same potency as the parent molecule, and may have a longer half life than the parent compound. Compound F-490 is much less potent and is probably inactive at the concentrations achieved in clinical samples. Metabolites are subsequently excreted in the urine in the ratio of 79 5-hydroxy-dantrolene:17 compound F-490: 4 unaltered dantrolene (salt or free acid). The proportion of drug excreted in the faeces depends upon dose size.

5.3 Preclinical safety data

Sprague-Dawley female rats fed dantrolene sodium for 18 months at dosage levels of 15, 30 and 60 mg/kg/day showed an increased incidence of benign and malignant mammary tumors compared with concurrent controls. At the highest dose level, there was an increase in the incidence of benign hepatic lymphatic neoplasms. In a 30-month study at the same dose levels also in Sprague-Dawley rats, dantrolene sodium produced a decrease in the time of onset of mammary neoplasms. Female rats at the highest dose level showed an increased incidence of hepatic lymphangiomas and hepatic angiosarcomas.

The only drug-related effect seen in a 30-month study in Fischer-344 rats was a dose-related reduction in the time of onset of mammary and testicular tumors. A 24-month study in HaM/ICR mice revealed no evidence of carcinogenic activity.

The significance of carcinogenicity data relative to use of dantrolene sodium in humans is unknown.

Dantrolene sodium has produced positive results in the Ames S. Typhimurium bacterial mutagenesis assay in the presence and absence of a liver activating system.

Dantrolene sodium administered to male and female rats at dose levels up to 45 mg/kg/day showed no adverse effects on fertility or general reproductive performance.

6. PHARMACEUTICAL PARTICULARS

6.1 List of excipients

Gelatin, starch, talc, magnesium stearate, lactose, E110, E171 and E172.

6.2 Incompatibilities

None.

6.3 Shelf life

Three years.

6.4 Special precautions for storage

Store below 30°C.

6.5 Nature and contents of container

Dantrium 100mg capsules are supplied in polypropylene containers of 100 capsules.

6.6 Instructions for use and handling

A patient leaflet is provided for details of use and handling of the product.

7. MARKETING AUTHORISATION HOLDER

Procter & Gamble Pharmaceuticals UK Limited
Rusham Park
Whitehall Lane
Egham
Surrey
TW20 9NW, UK

8. MARKETING AUTHORISATION NUMBER(S)

PL 0364/0016R

9. DATE OF FIRST AUTHORISATION/RENEWAL OF THE AUTHORISATION

25 October 1989

10. DATE OF REVISION OF THE TEXT

October 2002

Dantrium 25mg Capsules

(Procter & Gamble Pharmaceuticals UK Limited)

1. NAME OF THE MEDICINAL PRODUCT

Dantrium 25mg capsules.

2. QUALITATIVE AND QUANTITATIVE COMPOSITION

Dantrium 25mg capsules contain 25mg dantrolene sodium per capsule.

3. PHARMACEUTICAL FORM

Dantrium capsules are presented in orange/light brown capsules. The 25mg capsule carries the monogram Dantrium 25mg on the cap and 0149, 0030 and a single coding bar on the body.

4. CLINICAL PARTICULARS

4.1 Therapeutic indications

For the treatment of chronic, severe spasticity of skeletal muscle in adults.

4.2 Posology and method of administration

Adults

For the individual patient, the lowest dose compatible with optimal response is recommended.

A recommended dosage increment scale is shown below:-

Week	*Recommended dosage*
First	One 25mg capsule daily
Second	One 25mg capsule twice daily
Third	Two 25mg capsules twice daily
Fourth	Two 25mg capsules three times daily
Fifth	Three 25mg capsules three times daily
Sixth	Three 25mg capsules four times daily
Seventh	One 100mg capsule four times daily

Each dosage level should be maintained for seven days in order to determine the patient's response. Therapy with a dose four times daily may offer maximum benefit to some patients. The maximum daily dose should not exceed 400mg. In view of the potential for hepatoxicity in long term use, if no observable benefit is derived from the administration of Dantrium after a total of 45 days, therapy should be discontinued.

Elderly

A similar dosage scheme should be used with the elderly.

Children

Dantrium is not recommended for use in children.

4.3 Contraindications

Dantrium is contraindicated where spasticity is utilised to sustain upright posture and balance in locomotion or whenever spasticity is utilised to obtain or maintain increased function. Dantrium is contraindicated in patients with evidence of hepatic dysfunction. Dantrium is not indicated for the treatment of acute skeletal muscle spasm. Dantrium should not be administered to children.

4.4 Special warnings and special precautions for use

Fatal and non-fatal liver disorders of an idiosyncratic or hypersensitivity type may occur with Dantrium therapy.

Patients should be instructed to contact their physician should signs or symptoms of hepatotoxicity (e.g., discolored feces, generalized pruritus, jaundice, anorexia, nausea, vomiting) occur during therapy.

Factors that may increase the risk of developing hepatotoxicity include:

- Higher daily doses (doses exceeding 400 mg daily)
- Duration of therapy (most frequently reported between 2 and 12 months of treatment)
- Female gender
- Age greater than 30 years
- Prior history of liver disease/dysfunction
- Receiving other hepatotoxic therapies concomitantly.

Spontaneous reports also suggest a higher proportion of hepatic events with fatal outcome in elderly patients.

At the start of Dantrium therapy, it is desirable to do liver function studies (SGOT/ALT, SGPT/AST, alkaline phosphatase, total bilirubin) for a baseline or to establish whether there is pre-existing liver disease. If baseline liver abnormalities exist and are confirmed, there is a clear possibility that the potential for Dantrium hepatotoxicity could be enhanced, although such a possibility has not yet been established.

Liver functions studies (e.g. serum, SGOT/AST, SGPT/ALT) should be performed at appropriate intervals during Dantrium therapy. If such studies reveal abnormal values, therapy should generally be discontinued. Only where benefits of the drug have been of major importance to the patient, should re-introduction or continuation of therapy be considered. Some patients have revealed a return to normal laboratory values in the face of continued therapy while others have not.

If symptoms compatible with hepatitis, accompanied by abnormalities in liver function tests or jaundice appear, Dantrium should be discontinued. If caused by Dantrium and detected early, the abnormalities in liver function have reverted to normal when the drug was discontinued.

Dantrium has been re-introduced in a few patients who have developed clinical signs, or elevated serum enzymes, of hepatocellular injury.

Re-introduction of Dantrium therapy should only be contemplated in patients who clearly need the drug, and only after complete reversal of the signs of hepatotoxicity and liver function tests. Patients being re-challenged with Dantrium should be hospital in-patients, and small, gradually increasing doses should be used. Laboratory test monitoring should be frequent, and the drug should be withdrawn immediately if there is any indication of recurrent liver abnormality. Some patients have reacted with unmistakable signs of liver abnormality upon administration of a challenge dose, whilst others have not.

The use of Dantrium with other potentially hepatotoxic drugs should be avoided.

There are isolated cases of possibly significant effects of Dantrium on the cardiovascular and respiratory systems. These cases also have other features suggesting a predisposition to cardiovascular disease, and impaired respiratory function, particularly obstructive pulmonary disease. Dantrium should be used with caution in such patients.

Dantrolene sodium showed some evidence of tumourgenicity at high dose levels in Sprague-Dawley female rats. However, these effects were not seen in other studies in Fischer 344 rats or HaM/ICR mice. There is no clinical evidence of carcinogenicity in humans, however, this possibility cannot be absolutely excluded.

Caution should be exercised in the simultaneous administration of tranquillising agents and alcohol.

4.5 Interaction with other medicinal products and other forms of Interaction

An idiosyncratic interaction between verapamil and intravenous Dantrium, involving hypotension, hyperkalaemia, and myocardial depression, has been reported as a single case. This interaction has been replicated in dogs and pigs.

4.6 Pregnancy and lactation

Although teratological studies in animals have proved satisfactory, the use of Dantrium is not advised in pregnant or nursing mothers.

4.7 Effects on ability to drive and use machines

Patients should be advised not to drive a motor vehicle or to undertake potentially dangerous work until Dantrium therapy has been stabilised, because some patients experience drowsiness and dizziness.

4.8 Undesirable effects

The most frequently reported unwanted effects associated with the use of Dantrium have been drowsiness, dizziness, weakness, general malaise, fatigue and diarrhoea. These effects are generally transient, occur early in treatment, and can often be obviated by careful determination and regulation of the dosage. Diarrhoea may be severe, and may necessitate temporary withdrawal of Dantrium. If diarrhoea recurs upon re-introduction of Dantrium, then Dantrium therapy should probably be withdrawn permanently. Other frequent side effects include anorexia, nausea, headache and skin rash. Less frequent side effects include constipation, dysphagia, speech disturbance, visual disturbance, confusion, nervousness, depression, seizures, increased urinary frequency, and insomnia. Rare reports include tachycardia, erratic blood pressure, dyspnoea, haematuria, crystalluria (unconfirmed reports), urinary incontinence, and urinary retention. Pleural effusion and/or pericarditis in patients using Dantrium have been rarely reported. Chills and fever have occasionally been reported.

Dantrium has a potential for hepatotoxicity. Symptomatic hepatitis (fatal and non-fatal) has been reported at various dose levels although the incidence is greater in patients taking more than 400 mg/day. Liver dysfunction as evidenced by blood chemical abnormalities alone (liver enzyme elevation) has been observed in patients exposed to Dantrium for varying periods of time.

Overt hepatitis has occurred at varying intervals after initiation of therapy, but has most frequently been observed between the second and twelfth month of treatment. The risk of hepatic injury appears to be greater in females, in patients over 30 years old and in patients taking concomitant medication. There is some evidence that hepatic injury is more likely in patients using concomitant oral oestrogen.

4.9 Overdose

For acute overdosage, general supportive measures and gastric lavage should be employed as well as measures to reduce the absorption of Dantrium. The theoretical possibility of crystalluria in overdose has not been reported for Dantrium, but would be treated according to general principles, including administration of fluids.

5. PHARMACOLOGICAL PROPERTIES

5.1 Pharmacodynamic properties

Molecular Pharmacology

The receptor molecule for dantrolene has not been identified. Radiolabelled dantrolene sodium binds to specific components of the striated muscle cell, namely the t-tubules and the sarcoplastic reticulum; however the kinetics of binding varies between these two organelles. The binding of ryanodine is thought to compete with the binding of calcium in these organelles; further evidence for the specificity of binding is that dantrolene inhibits the binding of the insecticide ryanodine to heavy sarcoplastic reticulum vesicles from rabbit skeletal muscle. Under some conditions, dantrolene will lower intra-sarcoplasmic calcium concentrations in the resting state. This may be more important in diseased muscle (e.g. in malignant hyperthermia in humans and swine stress syndrome) than in muscle with normal function.

Dantrolene does not bind to the same sites as calcium channel blocking drugs such as nitrendipine or calmodulin. There is no electrophysiological evidence that dantrolene interferes with the influx of calcium from outside the cell. This may be one reason why paralysis by dantrolene has never been reported in animals or man; the muscle cell has alternative sources of calcium which are not influenced by dantrolene.

Biochemical Pharmacology

Whatever the molecular mechanism, the cardinal property of dantrolene sodium is that it lowers intracellular calcium concentration in skeletal muscle. Calcium concentrations may be lower in both the quiescent state, and as a result of a reduction in the release of calcium form the sarcoplasmic reticulum in response to a standard stimulus. This effect has been observed in striated muscle fibres from several species, and is not seen in myocardium. Fast fibres may be more sensitive than slow fibres to the action of dantrolene sodium.

Diverse other properties of dantrolene sodium have been observed in-vitro, and in animal studies. Dantrolene sodium may inhibit the release of calcium from the smooth endoplasmic reticulum of smooth muscle, but the significance of this observation is questionable; for example, dantrolene sodium has no effect on isolated human urinary bladder smooth muscle. Calcium dependent, pre-synaptic neurotransmitter release may also be inhibited by dantrolene sodium. Again, the clinical significance of this has not been demonstrated.

Studies on Isolated, Functional Muscle

Elevation of intracellular, free calcium ion concentration is an obligatory step in excitation-contraction coupling of skeletal muscle. Dantrolene sodium, therefore, acts as a muscle relaxant by a peripheral mechanism which is quite different, and easily distinguishable from neuromuscular junction blocking drugs. In contrast with compounds that relax skeletal muscle by acting principally on the central nervous system, dantrolene sodium acts directly on skeletal muscle cells. In rabbit atria, dantrolene sodium has no effect alone, but it may antagonise inotropic agents which act by increasing intramyocardial cell calcium e.g. the experimental drug anthopleurin-A.

5.2 Pharmacokinetic properties

Absorption

Dantrium is easily and almost completely absorbed from the gastrointestinal tract. After dosing on an empty stomach, plasma dantrolene levels peak within three hours in most subjects.

Distribution

Dantrolene sodium is a highly lipophobic drug. In addition it lacks hydrophilicity. Dantrolene sodium binds to human serum albumin (HSA) with a molar ratio of 0.95 to 1.68 in-vitro. The association constant in-vitro is higher (2.3 to 5.4 × 10^{-5} per mol). In-vitro dantrolene sodium can be displaced from HSA by warfarin, clofibrate and tolbutamide but these interactions have not been confirmed in humans (re. manufacturer's database). Single intravenous dose studies suggest that the primary volume of distribution is about 15 litres. Single oral doses achieve peak plasma concentration of about a quarter of that for a similarly sized intravenous dose.

Metabolism and Excretion

The biological half life in plasma in most human subjects is between 5 and 9 hours, although half-lives as long as 12.1 ± 1.9 hours have been reported after a single intravenous dose. Inactivation is by hepatic metabolism in the first instance. There are two alternative pathways. Most of the drug is hydroxylated to 5-hydroxy-dantrolene. The minor pathway involves nitro-reduction to amino-dantrolene which is then acetylated (compound F-490). The 5-hydroxy metabolite is a muscle relaxant with nearly the same potency as the parent molecule, and may have a longer half life than the parent compound. Compound F-490 is much less potent and is probably inactive at the concentrations achieved in clinical samples. Metabolites are subsequently excreted in the urine in the ratio of 79 5-hydroxy-dantrolene:17 compound F-490: 4 unaltered dantrolene (salt or free acid). The proportion of drug excreted in the faeces depends upon dose size.

5.3 Preclinical safety data

Sprague-Dawley female rats fed dantrolene sodium for 18 months at dosage levels of 15, 30 and 60 mg/kg/day showed an increased incidence of benign and malignant mammary tumors compared with concurrent controls. At the highest dose level, there was an increase in the incidence of benign hepatic lymphatic neoplasms. In a 30-month study at the same dose levels also in Sprague-Dawley rats, dantrolene sodium produced a decrease in the time of onset of mammary neoplasms. Female rats at the highest dose level showed an increased incidence of hepatic lymphangiomas and hepatic angiosarcomas.

The only drug-related effect seen in a 30-month study in Fischer-344 rats was a dose-related reduction in the time of onset of mammary and testicular tumors. A 24-month study in HaM/ICR mice revealed no evidence of carcinogenic activity.

The significance of carcinogenicity data relative to use of dantrolene sodium in humans is unknown.

Dantrolene sodium has produced positive results in the Ames S. Typhimurium bacterial mutagenesis assay in the presence and absence of a liver activating system.

Dantrolene sodium administered to male and female rats at dose levels up to 45 mg/kg/day showed no adverse effects on fertility or general reproductive performance.

6. PHARMACEUTICAL PARTICULARS

6.1 List of excipients

Gelatin, starch, talc, magnesium stearate, lactose, E110, E171 and E172.

6.2 Incompatibilities

None.

6.3 Shelf life

Three years.

6.4 Special precautions for storage

Store below 30°C.

6.5 Nature and contents of container

Dantrium 25mg capsules are supplied in polypropylene containers of 100 capsules.

6.6 Instructions for use and handling

A patient leaflet is provided for details of use and handling of the product.

7. MARKETING AUTHORISATION HOLDER

Procter & Gamble Pharmaceuticals UK Limited
Rusham Park
Whitehall Lane
Egham
Surrey
TW20 9NW, UK

8. MARKETING AUTHORISATION NUMBER(S)

PL 0364/0015R

9. DATE OF FIRST AUTHORISATION/RENEWAL OF THE AUTHORISATION

25 October 1989

10. DATE OF REVISION OF THE TEXT

October 2002

Dantrium Intravenous

(Procter & Gamble Pharmaceuticals UK Limited)

1. NAME OF THE MEDICINAL PRODUCT

Dantrium Intravenous

2. QUALITATIVE AND QUANTITATIVE COMPOSITION

Each vial contains 20 mg dantrolene sodium. For excipients, see 6.1

3. PHARMACEUTICAL FORM

Powder for solution for injection.

4. CLINICAL PARTICULARS

4.1 Therapeutic indications

For the treatment of malignant hyperthermia.

4.2 Posology and method of administration

As soon as the malignant hyperthermia syndrome is recognised all anaesthetic agents should be discontinued. An initial Dantrium intravenous dose of 1 mg/kg should be given rapidly into the vein. If the physiological and metabolic abnormalities persist or reappear, this dose may be repeated up to a cumulative dose of 10 mg/kg. Clinical experience to date has shown that the average dose of Dantrium intravenous required to reverse the manifestations of malignant hyperthermia has been 2.5 mg/kg. If a relapse or recurrence occurs, Dantrium intravenous should be readministered at the last effect dose.

4.3 Contraindications

None stated.

4.4 Special warnings and special precautions for use

In some subjects as much as 10 mg/kg of Dantrium intravenous has been needed to reverse the crisis. In a 70 kg man this dose would require approximately 36 vials. Such a volume has been administered in approximately one and a half hours.

Because of the high pH of the intravenous formulation of Dantrium, care must be taken to prevent extravasation of the intravenous solution into the surrounding tissues.

The use of Dantrium intravenous in the management of malignant hyperthermia is not a substitute for previously known supportive measures. It will be necessary to discontinue the suspect triggering agents, attend to increased oxygen requirements and manage the metabolic acidosis. When necessary institute cooling, attend to urinary output and monitor for electrolyte imbalance.

4.5 Interaction with other medicinal products and other forms of Interaction

The combination of therapeutic doses of intravenous dantrolene sodium and verapamil in halothane/alpha-chloralose anaesthetised swine has resulted in ventricular fibrillation and cardiovascular collapse in association with marked hyperkalaemia. It is recommended that the combination of intravenous dantrolene sodium and calcium channel blockers, such as verapamil, is not used during the reversal of a malignant hyperthermia crisis until the relevance of these findings to humans is established.

4.6 Pregnancy and lactation

The safety of Dantrium intravenous in pregnant women has not been established; it should be given only when the potential benefits have been weighed against the possible risk to mother and child.

4.7 Effects on ability to drive and use machines

A decrease in grip strength and weakness of leg muscles, especially walking down stairs, can be expected post-operatively. In addition, symptoms such as "lightheadedness" may be noted. Since some of these symptoms may persist for up to 48 hours, patients must not operate an automobile or engage in other hazardous activity during this time.

4.8 Undesirable effects

There have been occasional reports of death following malignant hyperthermia crisis even when treated with intravenous dantrolene sodium; incidence figures are not available (the pre-dantrolene mortality of malignant hyperthermia crisis was approximately 50%). Most of these deaths can be accounted for by late recognition, delayed treatment, inadequate dosage, lack of supportive therapy, intercurrent disease and/or the development of delayed complications such as renal failure or disseminated intravascular coagulopathy. In some cases there are insufficient data to completely rule out therapeutic failure of dantrolene sodium.

The administration of intravenous dantrolene sodium to human volunteers is associated with loss of grip strength and weakness in the legs, as well as subjective central nervous system complaints.

There are rare reports of pulmonary oedema developing during the treatment of malignant hyperthermia crisis in which the diluent volume and mannitol needed to deliver i.v. dantrolene sodium possibly contributed.

There have been reports of thrombophlebitis following administration of intravenous dantrolene sodium.

Hepatotoxic reactions have been noted in a small number of subjects given long-term oral dantrolene therapy.

4.9 Overdose

None stated.

5. PHARMACOLOGICAL PROPERTIES

5.1 Pharmacodynamic properties

Molecular Pharmacology

The receptor molecule for dantrolene has not been identified. Radiolabelled dantrolene sodium binds to specific components of the striated muscle cell, namely the t-tubules and the sarcoplasmic reticulum. However, the kinetics of binding vary between these two organelles. The binding of ryanodine is thought to compete with the binding of calcium in these organelles; further evidence for the specificity of binding is that dantrolene inhibits the binding of ryanodine to heavy sarcoplasmic reticulum vesicles from rabbit skeletal muscle. Under some conditions, dantrolene will lower intra-sarcoplasmic calcium concentrations in the resting state. This may be more important in diseased muscle [e.g. in malignant hyperthermia in humans and swine stress syndrome] than in muscle with normal function.

Dantrolene does not bind to the same sites as calcium channel blocking drugs such as nitrendipine or calmodulin. There is no electrophysiological evidence that dantrolene interferes with the influx of calcium from outside the cell. This may be one reason why paralysis by dantrolene has never been reported in animals or man; the muscle cell has alternative sources of calcium which are not influenced by dantrolene.

Biochemical Pharmacology

Whatever the molecular mechanism, the cardinal property of dantrolene sodium is that it lowers intracellular calcium concentration in skeletal muscle. Calcium concentrations may be lower in both the quiescent state, and as a result of a reduction in the release of calcium from the sarcoplasmic reticulum in response to a standard stimulus. This effect has been observed in striated muscle fibres from several species, and is not seen in myocardium. Fast fibres may be more sensitive than slow fibres to the action of dantrolene sodium.

Diverse other properties of dantrolene sodium have been observed *in vitro*, and in animal studies. Dantrolene sodium may inhibit the release of calcium from the smooth endoplasmic reticulum of smooth muscle, but the significance of this observation is questionable; for example, dantrolene sodium has no effect on isolated human urinary bladder smooth muscle. Calcium dependent, pre-synaptic neurotransmitter release may also be inhibited by dantrolene sodium. Again, the clinical significance of this has not been demonstrated.

Studies on Isolated, Functional Muscle

Elevation of intracellular, free calcium ion concentration is an obligatory step in excitation-contraction coupling of skeletal muscle. Dantrolene sodium, therefore, acts as a muscle relaxant by a peripheral mechanism which is quite different, and easily distinguishable from neuromuscular junction blocking drugs. In contrast with compounds that relax skeletal muscle by acting principally on the central nervous system, dantrolene sodium acts directly on skeletal muscle cells. In rabbit atria, dantrolene sodium has no effect alone, but it may antagonise inotropic agents which act by increasing intramyocardial cell calcium e.g. anthopleurin-a.

5.2 Pharmacokinetic properties

Distribution

Dantrolene sodium is a highly lipophobic drug. In addition, it lacks hydrophilicity. Dantrolene sodium binds to human serum albumin (HSA) with a molar ratio of 0.95 to 1.68 *in vitro*. The association constant *in vitro* is 2.3 to 5.4 × 10^{-5} per mol. *In vitro* dantrolene sodium can be displaced from HSA by warfarin, clofibrate and tolbutamide but these interactions have not been confirmed in humans (re. manufacturer's database). Single intravenous dose studies suggest that the primary volume of distribution is about 15 litres.

Metabolism and Excretion

The biological half life in plasma in most human subjects is between 5 and 9 hours, although half-lives as long as 12.1 ± 1.9 hours have been reported after a single intravenous dose. Inactivation is by hepatic metabolism in the first instance. There are two alternative pathways. Most of the drug is hydroxylated to 5-hydroxy-dantrolene. The minor pathway involves nitro-reduction to amino-dantrolene which is then acetylated (compound F-490). The 5-hydroxy metabolite is a muscle relaxant with nearly the same potency as the parent molecule, and may have a longer half life than the parent compound. Compound F-490 is much less potent and is probably inactive at the concentrations achieved in clinical samples. Metabolites are subsequently excreted in the urine in the ratio of 79 5-hydroxy dantrolene: 17 compound F-490: 4 unaltered dantrolene (salt or free acid). The proportion of drug excreted in the faeces depends upon dose size.

5.3 Preclinical safety data

Whilst there is no clinical evidence of carcinogenicity in humans, this possibility cannot be absolutely excluded. Dantrolene sodium has shown some evidence of tumourgenicity at high dose levels in Sprague-Dawley female rats, but these effects have not been seen in other studies in Fischer 344 rats or HaM/ICR mice.

6. PHARMACEUTICAL PARTICULARS

6.1 List of excipients

Mannitol and sodium hydroxide.

6.2 Incompatibilities

Dantrium intravenous should not be mixed with other intravenous infusions.

6.3 Shelf life

Three years. The reconstituted solution should be used within six hours.

6.4 Special precautions for storage
Unopened product: Do not store above 30°C. Reconstituted solution: Do not store above 30°C. Do not refrigerate or freeze. Protect from direct light.

Because of the nature of the freeze-drying process used in the manufacture of Dantrium intravenous, the freeze-dried cake of Dantrium intravenous may have a mottled orange/ white appearance or be in the form of loose aggregates. This is an entirely normal artefact and in no way compromises the stability of the product.

6.5 Nature and contents of container
Type I glass vial with butyl rubber stopper and aluminium seal. Twelve vials per carton.

6.6 Instructions for use and handling
Each vial of Dantrium IV should be reconstituted by adding 60ml of water for injection PhEur, and shaken until the solution is clear. Any unused portion of the reconstituted solution should be discarded. There are no special requirements relating to the disposal of the container or contents.

7. MARKETING AUTHORISATION HOLDER
Procter & Gamble Pharmaceuticals UK Limited

Rusham Park

Whitehall Lane

Egham

Surrey

TW20 9NW, UK

8. MARKETING AUTHORISATION NUMBER(S)
PL 0364/0030

9. DATE OF FIRST AUTHORISATION/RENEWAL OF THE AUTHORISATION
14 February 1980

10. DATE OF REVISION OF THE TEXT
October 2002

Daonil Tablets, Semi-Daonil Tablets

(sanofi-aventis)

1. NAME OF THE MEDICINAL PRODUCT
Daonil™ 5mg Tablets

Semi-Daonil™ 2.5mg Tablets

2. QUALITATIVE AND QUANTITATIVE COMPOSITION
Daonil: Glibenclamide BP 5mg.

Semi Daonil: Glibenclamide BP 2.5mg.

3. PHARMACEUTICAL FORM
Tablet.

4. CLINICAL PARTICULARS

4.1 Therapeutic indications
Daonil is a hypoglycaemic agent, indicated for the oral treatment of patients with non-insulin dependent diabetes who respond inadequately to dietary measures alone.

4.2 Posology and method of administration
1. TREATMENT OF PREVIOUSLY UNTREATED DIABETICS:Stabilisation can be started with one 5 mg tablet of Daonil daily. The dose should be taken by mouth, with or immediately after breakfast or the first main meal. Where control is satisfactory, 1 tablet is continued as the maintenance dose. If control is unsatisfactory, the dose can be adjusted by increments of 2.5 or 5 mg at weekly intervals. The total daily dosage rarely exceeds 15 mg and increasing the daily dosage above this does not generally produce any additional effect. The total daily requirement should normally be administered as a single dose at breakfast, or with the first main meal; due consideration should be given to the patient's dietary habits and daily activity in apportioning the dosage.

ELDERLY: In debilitated or aged patients, who may be more liable to hypoglycaemia, treatment should be initiated with one Semi-Daonil tablet daily.

2. CHANGE-OVER FROM OTHER ORAL ANTI-DIABETICS:The change over to Daonil from other drugs with a similar mode of action can be carried out without any break in therapy. Daonil treatment should be started with one 5 mg tablet daily and adjusted by increments of 2.5 - 5 mg to achieve control. For patients not adequately controlled on other oral agents, treatment is commenced with the equivalent dose of Daonil, without exceeding an initial dose of 10 mg. If response is inadequate, the dose can be raised in a stepwise fashion to 15 mg daily. One 5 mg tablet of Daonil is approximately equivalent to 1 g tolbutamide or glymidine, 250 mg chlorpropamide or tolazamide, 500 mg acetohexamide, 25 mg glibornuride or 5 mg glipizide.

3. CHANGE-OVER FROM BIGUANIDES:Daonil treatment should be started with 1 tablet of Semi-Daonil (2.5 mg) and the biguanide withdrawn. The dosage should then be adjusted by increments of 2.5 mg to achieve control.

COMBINATION WITH BIGUANIDES: If adequate control is not possible with diet and 15 mg of Daonil, control can often be re-established by combined administration of Daonil and a biguanide derivative.

4. CHANGE-OVER FROM INSULIN:While it is appreciated that most patients who are on insulin therapy will continue to need it, there may be a few patients, particularly those on low daily doses, who will remain stabilised if transferred from insulin to Daonil.

The tablets should always be taken with, or immediately after, the first main meal.

CHILDREN:As non-insulin dependent diabetes is not usually a disease of childhood, Daonil is not recommended for use in children.

4.3 Contraindications
Daonil should not be used in patients who have or have ever had diabetic ketoacidosis or diabetic coma/precoma or in patients who have insulin-dependent diabetes mellitus, serious impairment of renal, hepatic or adrenocortical function, in patients who are hypersensitive to glibenclamide, or in circumstances of unusual stress, e.g. surgical operations or during pregnancy, when dietary measures and insulin are essential.

4.4 Special warnings and special precautions for use
The hypoglycaemic effect of glibenclamide may be enhanced by ACE inhibitors, anabolic steroids, beta-adrenergic blocking agents, benzafibrate, chloramphenicol, clofibrate, coumarin derivatives, cyclophosphamide, disopyramide, fenfluramine, fluoxetine, guanethidine, monoamine oxidase inhibitors, miconazole, phenylbutazone, probenecid, quinolone antibacterials, salicylates, sulphinpyrazone, sulphonamides and tetracycline compounds or diminished by clonidine, corticosteroids, diazoxide, diuretics, glucagon, laxative abuse, nicotinic acid (high dose), oral contraceptives, phenothiazine derivatives, phenytoin, sympathomimetic agents and thyroid hormones.

Both a potentiation and a reduction in blood sugar lowering have been reported in patients treated concomitantly with clonidine or H_2 receptor antagonists.

The warning symptoms of a hypoglycaemic attack may be masked during concomitant treatment with beta-adrenergic blocking agents, clonidine or guanethidine.

4.5 Interaction with other medicinal products and other forms of Interaction
See "Special Warnings and Special Precautions for Use".

4.6 Pregnancy and lactation
There is no information on the use of Daonil in human pregnancy but it has been in wide, general use for many years without apparent ill consequence. Animal studies have shown no hazard.

NURSING MOTHERS: It has not yet been established whether glibenclamide is transferred to human milk. However, other sulphonylureas have been found in milk and there is no evidence to suggest that glibenclamide differs from the group in this respect.

4.7 Effects on ability to drive and use machines
Not applicable.

4.8 Undesirable effects
Adverse reactions serious enough to warrant discontinuation of treatment are uncommon, but mild gastro-intestinal or allergic skin reactions have occurred. Cross-sensitivity to sulphonamides or their derivatives may occur. Transient visual disturbances may occur at the start of treatment. Reversible leucopenia and thrombocytopenia have been reported but are rare. Agranulocytosis, pancytopenia and haemolytic anaemia have been reported very rarely. Treatment with sulphonylureas has been associated with occasional disturbances of liver function and cholestatic jaundice. If hepatitis or cholestatic jaundice occurs, glibenclamide should be discontinued. Hypoglycaemic symptoms have occasionally been reported when the dose has been administered without due regard to the patient's dietary habits.

4.9 Overdose
Hypoglycaemia may be treated in the conscious patient by the administration of glucose, or three to four lumps of table sugar with water. This may be repeated as necessary.

If the patient is comatose, glucose should be administered as an intravenous infusion and the patient monitored. Bolus glucose injections are not recommended because of the possibility of rebound hypoglycaemia which may be delayed. Alternatively, glucagon may be administered in a dose of 1 mg subcutaneously or intramuscularly to restore consciousness.

5. PHARMACOLOGICAL PROPERTIES

5.1 Pharmacodynamic properties
The pharmacodynamic effect of glibenclamide is to lower blood glucose levels. Mechanisms proposed for this effect include:

- stimulation of insulin release from pancreatic beta-cells
- increasing insulin-releasing response to beta-cells
- formation of new alpha- and beta-cells
- increasing insulin binding and receptor density in peripheral tissues.

Plasma glucose levels affect the insulin-releasing response to glibenclamide, (a high glucose level increases the response). The minimum active concentration for effect is considered to be 30 - 50 nanograms/ml glibenclamide.

Investigations of the relationship between insulin, glucose levels and glibenclamide in the hypoglycaemic effect continue.

5.2 Pharmacokinetic properties
Orally administered Daonil is rapidly absorbed and substantially metabolised. 50% of the administered dose is excreted in the urine and 50% in the bile.

The major (hydroxylated) metabolite in man has no significant hypoglycaemic activity. After absorption, the plasma half-life of the drug follows a 2-compartment model.

1st phase: 2.1 hours

2nd phase: 8 - 10 hours

The second phase has been reported to affect insulin levels for longer, owing to the existence of a "deep compartment".

97% binds to serum protein.

5.3 Preclinical safety data
None of clinical relevance.

6. PHARMACEUTICAL PARTICULARS

6.1 List of excipients
Lactose, maize starch, pregelatinised maize starch, talc, anhydrous silica, magnesium stearate.

6.2 Incompatibilities
None known.

6.3 Shelf life
3 years.

6.4 Special precautions for storage
Do not store above 25°C. Store in the original packaging, keep container in the outer carton.

6.5 Nature and contents of container
Blister packs of 28 tablets.

6.6 Instructions for use and handling
None.

7. MARKETING AUTHORISATION HOLDER
Hoechst Marion Roussel Limited

Broadwater Park

Denham

Uxbridge

Middlesex UB9 5HP

8. MARKETING AUTHORISATION NUMBER(S)
Daonil™ 5mg Tablets: PL 13402/0027

Semi-Daonil™ 2.5mg Tablets: PL 13402/0028

9. DATE OF FIRST AUTHORISATION/RENEWAL OF THE AUTHORISATION
Daonil™ 5mg Tablets: 19 November 1998

Semi-Daonil™ 2.5mg Tablets: 23 June 2005

10. DATE OF REVISION OF THE TEXT
June 2005

11. LEGAL CATEGORY
POM

Daraprim Tablets

(GlaxoSmithKline UK)

1. NAME OF THE MEDICINAL PRODUCT
Daraprim 25mg Tablets

2. QUALITATIVE AND QUANTITATIVE COMPOSITION
Pyrimethamine 25.0 mg

For excipients see 6.1.

3. PHARMACEUTICAL FORM
Tablet

Each tablet is white and round with the markingGS A3A.

4. CLINICAL PARTICULARS

4.1 Therapeutic indications
Malaria prophylaxis

Daraprim is indicated for chemoprophylaxis of malaria due to susceptible strains of Plasmodia. However, since resistance to pyrimethamine is increasing worldwide, Daraprim can only be considered suitable for use in individuals who are resident in areas where pyrimethamine is acknowledged to be effective. It is not suitable as a prophylactic for travellers.

Toxoplasmosis

Treatment is not normally required for asymtomatic or mild toxoplasma infection. Daraprim, in conjunction with a sulphonamide, is effective in the treatment of the following conditions associated with toxoplasma infections:

Toxoplasmic encephalitis and other manifestations in immune deficient individuals including those with AIDS.

Ocular infections where there is considered to be a risk of visual damage.

Proven foetal infection following maternal infection during pregnancy.

For the treatment of toxoplasmosis, Daraprim should not be used as monotherapy. It must be combined with a synergistic agent, normally an orally administered sulphonamide as recommended in section 4.2, Posology and Method of Administration.

4.2 Posology and method of administration

Malaria Prophylaxis:

Adults: 1 tablet regularly each week.

Children: Over 10 years: 1 tablet regularly each week.

5 to 10 years: ½ tablet regularly each week.

Under 5 years: Formulation not applicable.

Daraprim is rapidly absorbed and therefore prophylactic cover can be expected shortly after the first dose. Prophylaxis should commence before arrival in an endemic area and be continued once weekly. On returning to a non-malarious area dosage should be maintained for a further four weeks.

Toxoplasmosis treatment:

Daraprim should be given concurrently with sulphadiazine or another appropriate sulphonamide. Data on the extent to which other combinations might be better than pyrimethamine alone are limited. For patients who are intolerant of sulphonamides however, consideration should be given to substituting the sulphonamide for another agent such as clindamycin.

In the treatment of toxoplasmosis, all patients receiving Daraprim should be given a folate supplement to reduce the risk of bone marrow depression. Whenever possible calcium folinate should be administered. Folic acid is likely to be less effective than calcium folinate.

Daraprim treatment should generally be given for 3 to 6 weeks and not less than three weeks in immunosuppressed patients. If further therapy is indicated, a period of two weeks should elapse between treatments.

There have been no dose response studies of pyrimethamine in the treatment of toxoplasmosis. The following recommendations are therefore for guidance only.

Dosage for Toxoplasmic encephalitis and other manifestations in immune-deficient patients (adults and children over 5 years)

Daraprim

A loading dose of 100 mg – 200 mg daily should be given for the first 2 - 3 days of treatment.

The optimal dose subsequently for the treatment of toxoplasmic encephalitis in AIDS patients is not fully established but is generally in the range 25mg-75mg/day. Doses up to 100mg/day have been used successfully. The duration of treatment of the acute infection will depend on the clinical response and tolerability, but should normally be not less than three to six weeks.

Maintenance treatment is required indefinitely in immunocompromised patients if relapses are to be avoided. There is insufficient evidence to establish the optimal dose regimen, but doses of 25-100mg daily have been employed successfully.

Sulphadiazine 2 - 6 g per day in divided doses.

Dosage for treatment of ocular infections (adults and children over 5 years)

Daraprim

A loading dose of 100mg for 1-2 days followed by maintenance doses of 25-50mg daily. The optimal maintenance dose has not been clearly established.

Sulphadiazine 2-4g daily in divided doses.

• Dosage for treatment of foetal toxoplasmosis during pregnancy

See Section 4.4 Special Warnings and Precautions for Use and Section 4.6 Pregnancy and Lactation

Daraprim: ***25 - 50 mg daily***

Sulphadiazine ***2 - 4 g daily in divided doses***

Children under 5 years

There is insufficient data to provide specific dose recommendations in children. This formulation is not suitable for children under 5 years.

Use in the elderly

There is no definitive information on the effect of Daraprim on elderly individuals. It is theoretically possible that elderly patients might be more susceptible to folate depression associated with the daily administration of Daraprim in the treatment of toxoplasmosis, and folate supplements are therefore essential (See Special Warnings and Precautions for Use).

4.3 Contraindications

Daraprim should not be given to patients with a history of pyrimethamine sensitivity.

Daraprim should not be used during the first trimester of pregnancy. (See Section 4.6 Pregnancy and Lactation).

Breast-feeding should be avoided during toxoplasmosis treatment. (See Section 4.6 Pregnancy and Lactation).

4.4 Special warnings and special precautions for use

During pregnancy and in other conditions predisposing to folate deficiency, a folate supplement should be given. The co-administration of a folate supplement is necessary for treatment of toxoplasmosis (see Dosage & Method of Administration). Full blood counts should be carried out weekly during therapy and for a further two weeks after treatment is stopped. In immunosuppressed patients, full blood counts should be carried out twice weekly. Should signs of folate deficiency develop, treatment must be discontinued and high doses of calcium folinate administered. Calcium folinate should be used because folic acid does not correct folate deficiency due to dihydrofolate reductase inhibitors.

Daraprim may exacerbate folate deficiency in subjects predisposed to this condition through disease or malnutrition. Accordingly, a calcium folinate supplement should be given to such individuals. In patients with megaloblastic anaemia due to folate deficiency the risks versus benefits of administering Daraprim require careful consideration.

Caution should be exercised in administering Daraprim to patients with a history of seizures; large loading doses should be avoided in such patients (see Undesirable Effects).

When a sulphonamide is given an adequate fluid intake should be ensured to minimise the risk of crystalluria.

Since pyrimethamine is administered with a sulphonamide for the conditions indicated the general precautions applicable to sulphonamides should be observed.

Occasional reports suggest that individuals taking pyrimethamine as malarial prophylaxis at doses in excess of 25 mg weekly may develop megaloblastic anaemia if co-trimoxazole is prescribed concurrently.

Use in renal impairment

The kidney is not the major route of excretion of pyrimethamine and excretion is not significantly altered in patients with renal failure. There are, however, no substantial data on the use of Daraprim in renally impaired subjects. Due to lack of data on the theoretical possibility of active metabolites with prolonged treatment, caution should be exercised in renally impaired patients. It is not known if Daraprim is dialyzable. Since Daraprim is co-administered with a sulphonamide, care should be taken to avoid accumulation of the sulphonamide in renally impaired patients.

Use in hepatic impairment

The liver is the main route for metabolism of pyrimethamine. Data on the use of pyrimethamine in patients with liver disease are limited. Daraprim in combination with sulphonamides has been used effectively to treat toxoplasmosis in a patient with mild hepatic disease. There are no general recommendations for dosage reductions for liver-impaired states but consideration should be given to dose adjustment for individual cases.

4.5 Interaction with other medicinal products and other forms of Interaction

Daraprim, by its mode of action, may further depress folate metabolism in patients receiving treatment with other folate inhibitors, or agents associated with myelosuppression, including co-trimoxazole, trimethoprim, proguanil, zidovudine, or cytostatic agents (eg. methotrexate). Cases of fatal bone marrow aplasia have been associated with the administration of daunorubicin, cytosine arabinoside and pyrimethamine to individuals suffering from acute myeloid leukaemia. Megaloblastic anaemia has been reported occasionally in individuals who took pyrimethamine in excess of 25 mg weekly concurrently with a trimethoprim/sulphonamide combination.

Convulsions have occurred after concurrent administration of methotrexate and pyrimethamine to children with central nervous system leukaemia. Also, seizures have occasionally been reported when pyrimethamine was used in combination with other antimalarial drugs.

The concurrent administration of lorazepam and Daraprim may induce hepatotoxicity.

In vitro data suggest that antacid salts and the anti-diarrhoeal agent kaolin reduce the absorption of pyrimethamine.

The high protein binding exhibited by pyrimethamine may prevent protein binding by other compounds (eg. quinine or warfarin). This could affect the efficacy or toxicity of the concomitant drug depending on the levels of unbound drug.

4.6 Pregnancy and lactation

Pregnancy

Pyrimethamine in combination with sulphonamide has been used for many years in the treatment of toxoplasmosis during pregnancy. This infection carries a high risk to the foetus. Pyrimethamine crosses the placenta and, although there is a theoretical risk of foetal abnormalities from all folate inhibitors given during pregnancy, there have been no reports that have shown with any certainty that pyrimethamine is associated with human teratogenicity. Nevertheless, caution should be exercised in the administration of pyrimethamine. A folate supplement should be given to pregnant women receiving Daraprim.

Consideration should be given to the treatment of all suspected cases of acquired toxoplasmosis in pregnancy. The risks associated with the administration of Daraprim must be balanced against the dangers of abortion or foetal malformation due to the infection.

Treatment with pyrimethamine and sulfadiazine during pregnancy is indicated in the presence of confirmed placental or foetal infection or when the mother is at risk of serious sequelae. However, in view of the theoretical risk of foetal abnormality arising from the use of Daraprim in early pregnancy, its use in combination therapy should be restricted to the second and third trimesters. Alternative therapy is therefore advised in the first trimester of pregnancy and until diagnosis has been confirmed.

Lactation

Pyrimethamine enters human breast milk. It has been estimated that over a 9-day period an average weight infant would receive about 45% of the dose ingested by the mother. In view of the high doses of pyrimethamine and concurrent sulphonamides needed in toxoplasmosis treatment, breast feeding should be avoided for the duration of treatment.

4.7 Effects on ability to drive and use machines

Not known.

4.8 Undesirable effects

At the recommended dose for malaria prophylaxis, side-effects are rare. Occasionally, rashes have been observed. At the doses required for treatment of toxoplasmosis, pyrimethamine may produce myleosuppression with anaemia, leucopenia and thrombocytopenia.

Precipitation of a grand mal attack in one patient predisposed to epilepsy has been reported but the clinical significance has not been defined.

Since a concurrent sulphonamide is to be taken with pyrimethamine for the indications listed the relevant sulphonamide data sheet/SPC or published literature should be consulted for sulphonamide associated adverse events.

4.9 Overdose

Symptoms and signs:-

Vomiting and convulsions occur in cases of severe, acute overdoses. Ataxia, tremor and respiratory depression can also occur. There have been isolated cases with fatal outcomes following acute overdose of pyrimethamine.

Chronic excess doses can result in bone marrow depression (eg. megaloblastic anaemia, leucopenia, thrombocytopenia) resulting from folic acid deficiency.

Management:-

Routine supportive treatment, including maintenance of a clear airway and control of convulsions.

Adequate fluids should be given to ensure optimal diuresis.

Gastric lavage may be of value only if instituted within two hours of ingestion in view of the rapid absorption of Daraprim.

To counteract possible folate deficiency, calcium folinate should be given until signs of toxicity have subsided. There may a delay of 7 to 10 days before the full leucopenic side effects become evident, therefore calcium folinate therapy should be continued for the period at risk.

5. PHARMACOLOGICAL PROPERTIES

5.1 Pharmacodynamic properties

Pyrimethamine is an antiparasitic agent.

Group: diaminopyrimidines

ATC code:- P01B D01

Mode of Action:-

The antiparasitic action of pyrimethamine is due to its specific activity on folic acid metabolism in the Plasmodium and Toxoplasma parasites. In this respect it competitively inhibits the dihydrofolate reductase enzyme with an affinity far greater for the protozoal than for the human enzyme.

5.2 Pharmacokinetic properties

Absorption:-

Pyrimethamine is rapidly absorbed from the gastrointestinal tract after administration. Time to peak plasma concentration is 2 to 4 hours in healthy volunteers. Peak plasma concentrations vary widely between individuals and can range from 260 to 1411ng/ml after daily doses of 25mg. A similar degree of inter-patient variability in serum levels has been noted in patients with AIDS.

Distribution:-

The volume of distribution for pyrimethamine is approximately 2L/kg. In patients with HIV infection, population pharmacokinetic analysis has indicated that the mean volume of distribution (corrected for bioavailability) is 246+/-64L.

About 87% of the drug is bound to plasma proteins. Pyrimethamine has been shown to reach the cerebrospinal fluid of patients with AIDS given daily doses, achieving concentrations approximately one fifth of those in serum.

Metabolism and elimination:-

Pyrimethamine is predominantly eliminated by metabolism, with up to 30% recovered in the urine as parent compound over a period of several weeks. The mean elimination half-life is 85 hours (ranging from 35 to 175 hours). In AIDS patients, the total clearance is 1.28+/-0.41L/h resulting in an elimination half life of 139+/-34h. Data are lacking on the nature of the metabolites of pyrimethamine, their route/rate of formation and elimination in man and any pharmacological activity, particularly after prolonged daily dosing.

Multiple dose studies indicate that steady state is achieved in 12 to 20 days with daily dosing. It is theoretically possible that metabolic pathways might be saturable, leading to excessive accumulation of the drug in some patients. However, it has been demonstrated that plasma levels are approximately proportional to dose at steady state so this appears unlikely. Genetic variation in the exposure to pyrimethamine has been reported but these data are unsubstantiated.

Some studies in patients with AIDS have indicated shorter half lives than those noted above: these are very likely to be a consequence of inappropriate sampling and analytical techniques. However, if there are patients in whom the half-life is particularly short, steady state therapeutic levels might be inadequate.

5.3 Preclinical safety data

Mutagenicity:-

In microbial tests, pyrimethamine was found to be non-mutagenic in the Ames Salmonella assay whereas DNA damage was seen in the Escherichia coli repair assay.

Further in vitro data indicate that pyrimethamine induces mutagenic activity in mouse lymphoma cells in the absence, but not in the presence of metabolic activation.

Pyrimethamine also showed clastogenic activity in mammalian lymphocytes in the absence of metabolic activation.

Following intraperitoneal administration, pyrimethamine has been shown to induce chromosomal damage in male rodent germ cells although studies in somatic cells (micronucleus tests) are either negative or inconclusive. Studies following oral administration of pyrimethamine in rodents showed negative results in female germ cells and in male and female bone marrow/peripheral blood cells.

Carcinogenicity

A study in mice (dosed with either 500 or 1000 ppm pyrimethamine in the diet for 5 days per week, for 78 weeks) showed no evidence of carcinogenicity in females. Survival in the male mice did not allow for an assessment of carcinogenicity in this sex.

A similar study in rats dosed at 200 or 400 ppm pyrimethamine showed no evidence of carcinogenicity.

Teratogenicity

No changes in early development were seen in embryos from 15 mice given a single intra-gastric dose of pyrimethamine (50mg/kg bodyweight) on the first day of gestation. However development of mouse and rat embryos in culture was severely hindered by pyrimethamine in a dose-dependent manner.

Pyrimethamine was teratogenic in rodents and in the Gottingen minipig in a dose-dependent manner.

Other studies in rats dosed at either 1mg/kg or 10mg/kg bodyweight showed some inhibition of developmental processes but no teratological effects.

Pyrimethamine was not teratogenic in rabbits at dose levels up to 100mg/kg bodyweight/day administered on days 6 to 18 of pregnancy. Pyrimethamine markedly reduced early stage cell division in rabbit embryos but implantation and foetal development were normal.

Fertility

A study in rats dosed with 5mg/kg bodyweight/day for 6 weeks resulted in reduced sperm concentrations and testis weights, but there were no effects on fertility. Reversible arrest of spermatogenesis was shown in a study on mice dosed with 200mg/kg/day for 50 days. However, this dose is far in excess of human therapeutic doses.

6. PHARMACEUTICAL PARTICULARS

6.1 List of excipients

Lactose Monohydrate

Maize Starch

Hydrolysed Starch

Docusate sodium

Magnesium stearate

6.2 Incompatibilities

Not applicable

6.3 Shelf life

5 years

6.4 Special precautions for storage

Do not store above 30°C.

Store in the original container.

6.5 Nature and contents of container

Vinyl - lacquered aluminium foil strip-packs.

Pack size: 30 tablets

6.6 Instructions for use and handling

Not applicable

Administrative Data

7. MARKETING AUTHORISATION HOLDER

The Wellcome Foundation Ltd	t/a GlaxoSmithKline UK
Glaxo Wellcome House	Stockley Park West,
Berkeley Avenue	Uxbridge
Greenford	Middlesex, UB11 1BT
Middlesex	
UB6 ONN	

8. MARKETING AUTHORISATION NUMBER(S)

PL 00003/5026R

9. DATE OF FIRST AUTHORISATION/RENEWAL OF THE AUTHORISATION

26th November 1998

10. DATE OF REVISION OF THE TEXT

18/07/03

Daunorubicin

(sanofi-aventis)

1. NAME OF THE MEDICINAL PRODUCT

DAUNORUBICIN

2. QUALITATIVE AND QUANTITATIVE COMPOSITION

The active ingredient in Daunorubicin is daunorubicin hydrochloride Eur. Ph. Each vial contains 21.4 mg daunorubicin hydrochloride (equivalent to 20 mg as base).

3. PHARMACEUTICAL FORM

Vial containing a red lyophilised powder for intravenous administration following reconstitution in Water for Injections and dilution with saline.

4. CLINICAL PARTICULARS

4.1 Therapeutic indications

Daunorubicin is indicated for the following:

Inducing remissions of acute myelogenous and lymphocytic leukaemias.

4.2 Posology and method of administration

ADULTS: 40 - 60 mg/m^2 on alternate days for a course of up to three injections for the induction of remissions.

Acute myelogenous leukaemia: The recommended dose is 45 mg/m^2

Acute lymphocytic leukaemia: The recommended dose is 45 mg/m^2

CHILDREN: Over 2 years - Same as for adults

Under 2 years or if less than 0.5 m^2 surface area: 1 mg/kg/day.

ELDERLY: Daunorubicin should be used with care in patients with inadequate bone marrow reserves due to old age. A reduction of up to 50% in dosage is recommended.

The number of injections required varies widely from patient to patient and must be determined in each case according to response and tolerance.

The dosage should be reduced in patients with impaired hepatic or renal function. A 25% reduction is recommended in patients with serum bilirubin concentrations of 20 - 50 μmol/l or creatinine of 105 - 265 μmol/l. A 50% reduction is recommended in cases with serum bilirubin concentrations of above 50 μmol/l or creatinine of above 265 μmol/l.

Daunorubicin is extremely irritating to tissues and may only be administered intravenously after dilution. Daunorubicin should be administered through a large vein and the infusion should be kept free flowing. When second or subsequent injections are given, the doses and time intervals depend on the effect of the previous doses and must be the subject of careful deliberation, examination of the peripheral blood and, under some circumstances, of the bone marrow.

The effect of Daunorubicin on the disease process and on normal blood precursors cannot be exactly predicted for any particular case. The difference between incomplete treatment, a satisfactory remission and overdosage with possible irreversible aplasia of the bone marrow depends on the correct choice of dosage, time intervals and total number of doses.

4.3 Contraindications

Daunorubicin should not be used in patients recently exposed to, or with existing chicken pox or herpes zoster.

Do not administer by the intramuscular route.

4.4 Special warnings and special precautions for use

Daunorubicin should be used under the direction of a clinician conversant with the management of acute leukaemia and cytotoxic chemotherapy. The haematological status of patients should be monitored regularly.

Daunorubicin should be used with care in patients at risk of hyperuricaemia (eg in the presence of gout, urate and renal calculi), tumour cell infiltration of the bone marrow and in patients with inadequate bone marrow reserves due to previous cytotoxic drug or radiation therapy. The cumulative dose of Daunorubicin should be limited to 400 mg/m^2 when radiation therapy to the mediastinum has been previously administered. The dose of Daunorubicin should not be repeated in the presence of bone marrow depression or buccal ulceration.

Care should be taken to avoid extravasation during intravenous administration. All steps should be taken to avoid tissuing and bandages should be avoided. Facial flushing or erythematous streaking along veins indicates too rapid injection. If tissue necrosis is suspected, the infusion should be stopped immediately and resumed in another vein. Where extravasation has occurred, an attempt should be made to aspirate the fluid back through the needle. The affected area may be injected with hydrocortisone. Sodium bicarbonate (5 ml of 8.4% w/v solution) may also be injected in the hope that through pH change the drug will hydrolyse. The opinion of a plastic surgeon should be sought as skin grafting may be required.

Application of ice packs may help decrease local discomfort and also prevent extension. Liberal application of corticosteroid cream and dressing the area with sterile gauze should then be carried out.

Each patient should be given a clinical and bacteriological examination to determine whether infection is present; any infection should be adequately eliminated before treatment with Daunorubicin which might depress the bone marrow to the point where anti-infective agents would no longer be effective. If facilities are available, patients should be treated in a germ-free environment or, where it is not possible, reverse barrier nursing and aseptic precautions should be employed.

Anti-infective therapy should be employed in the presence of suspected or confirmed infection and during a phase of aplasia. It should be continued for some time after the marrow has regenerated. Care should also be used in patients at risk of infection.

4.5 Interaction with other medicinal products and other forms of Interaction

None.

4.6 Pregnancy and lactation

Daunorubicin crosses the placenta and experiments in animals have shown it to be mutagenic, carcinogenic and teratogenic.

There is also the possibility that treatment during pregnancy may produce delayed effects in the offspring. If appropriate, the mother should be offered the opportunity of a therapeutic abortion.

Owing to potential toxic risk to the infant, breastfeeding should be discontinued during treatment.

4.7 Effects on ability to drive and use machines

Not applicable

4.8 Undesirable effects

Bone marrow depression: In every patient bone marrow function will be depressed by treatment with Daunorubicin and in a variable proportion of cases, severe aplasia will develop.

Leucopenia is usually more significant than thrombocytopenia. The nadir for leucopenia usually occurs between 10 - 14 days and recovery occurs gradually over the next 1 - 2 weeks. Bone marrow depression must be anticipated in every case by eliminating infection before treatment, by isolating the patient from infection during treatment and by means of supportive therapy. This includes the continuous administration of anti-infective agents, the administration of platelet-rich plasma or fresh whole blood transfusion and, under some circumstances, the transfusion of white cell concentrates.

Other less serious reactions have been reported (in order of reducing frequency) are: stomatitis, alopecia, phlebitis, fever, anaemia, nausea, vomiting, mucositis, diarrhoea and rash. The urine may be temporarily coloured red after treatment.

Rapid destruction of a large number of leukaemia cells may cause a rise in blood uric acid or urea and so it is a wise precaution to check these concentrations three or four times a week during the first week of treatment. Fluids should be administered and allopurinol used in severe cases to prevent the development of hyperuricaemia.

Patients with heart disease should not be treated with this potentially cardiotoxic drug. Cardiotoxicity if it occurs is likely to be heralded by either a persistent tachycardia, shortness of breath, swelling of feet and lower limbs or by minor changes in the electrocardiogram and for this reason an electrocardiographic examination should be made at regular intervals during the treatment. Cardiotoxicity usually appears within 1 to 6 months after initiation of therapy. It may develop suddenly and not be detected by routine ECG. It may be irreversible and fatal but responds to treatment if detected early.

The risk of congestive heart failure increases significantly when the total cumulative dosage exceeds 600 mg/m^2 in adults, 300 mg/m^2 in children over 2 years or 10 mg/kg in children under 2 years. Cardiotoxicity may be more frequent in children and the elderly. The dosage should be modified if previous or concomitant cardiotoxic drug therapy is used.

4.9 Overdose

Although no cases have been reported to our knowledge, overdosage may result in drastic myelosupression and severe cardiotoxicity with or without transient reversible ECG changes leading to congestive heart failure. Treatment should be supportive and symptomatic.

5. PHARMACOLOGICAL PROPERTIES

5.1 Pharmacodynamic properties

Daunorubicin is an anthracycline glycoside antibiotic and is a potent antileukaemic agent. It also has immunosuppressant effects.

The exact mechanism of antineoplastic action is uncertain but may involve binding to DNA by intercalation between base pairs and inhibition of DNA and RNA synthesis by template disordering and steric obstruction. Daunorubicin is most active in the S-phase of cell division but is not cycle phase specific. Tumour cell cross-resistance has been observed between daunorubicin and doxorubicin.

5.2 Pharmacokinetic properties
Daunorubicin is rapidly taken up by tissues, especially by the kidneys, spleen, liver and heart. It does not cross the blood-brain barrier, subsequent release of drug and its metabolites from the tissues is slow ($t½ = 55$ hours). Daunorubicin is rapidly metabolised in the liver. The major metabolite daunorubicinol is also active. Daunorubicin is excrete slowly in the urine, mainly as metabolites with 25% excreted in the first 5 days. Biliary excretion also makes a significant (40%) contribution to elimination.

5.3 Preclinical safety data
No further information available.

6. PHARMACEUTICAL PARTICULARS

6.1 List of excipients
Mannitol.

6.2 Incompatibilities
The reconstituted solution is incompatible with heparin sodium injection and dexamethasone sodium phosphate.

6.3 Shelf life
The shelf-life of Daunorubicin is 3 years. After reconstitution Daunorubicin should be used within 24 hours.

6.4 Special precautions for storage
Daunorubicin vials should be stored below 25°C, protected from light. After reconstitution Daunorubicin should be stored at 2 - 8°C, protected from light.

6.5 Nature and contents of container
Glass vial with rubber cap containing 21.4 mg of daunorubicin hydrochloride (equivalent to
20 mg as base).

6.6 Instructions for use and handling
The contents of a vial should be reconstituted with 4ml of Water for Injection giving a concentration of 5 mg per ml. The calculated dose of Daunorubicin should be further diluted with normal saline to give a final concentration of 1 mg per ml. The solution should be injected over a 20 minute period into the tubing, or side arm, of a well placed, rapidly flowing i.v. infusion of normal saline (to minimise extravasation and possible tissue necrosis). Alternatively, the Daunorubicin may be added to a minibag of sodium chloride injection 0.9% and this solution infused into the side arm of a rapidly flowing infusion of normal saline.

7. MARKETING AUTHORISATION HOLDER
May & Baker Ltd. 50 Kings Hill Avenue, West Malling ME19 4AH

8. MARKETING AUTHORISATION NUMBER(S)
PL0012/0220

9. DATE OF FIRST AUTHORISATION/RENEWAL OF THE AUTHORISATION
8 June 1994

10. DATE OF REVISION OF THE TEXT
July 2000

Daunorubicin is distributed by:

Beacon Pharmaceuticals Ltd

85 High Street, Tunbridge Wells TN1 1YG

Daunoxome

(Gilead Sciences International Limited)

1. NAME OF THE MEDICINAL PRODUCT
DaunoXome Injection (liposomal daunorubicin)

2. QUALITATIVE AND QUANTITATIVE COMPOSITION
Daunorubicin hydrochloride, Ph.Eur., present as citrate salt, equivalent to daunorubicin 2.0mg/ml, (50mg) encapsulated in liposomes. The liposomes are small unilamellar vesicles with mean diameter of about 45 nm. The active ingredient is daunorubicin, an anthracycline antibiotic with antineoplastic activity originally obtained from *Streptomyces peucetius*. Daunorubicin has a four-ring anthracycline moiety linked by a glycosidic bond to daunosamin, an amino sugar. Daunorubicin is currently isolated from *Streptomyces coeruleorubidus* and is described by the following chemical name:

(8S,10S)-8-acetyl-10-[(3-amino-2,3,6-trideoxy- α -L-lyxo-hexopyranosyl)oxy]-6,8,11-trihydroxy-1-methoxy-7,8,9,10-tetrahydronaphthacene-5,12-dione.

Daunorubicin has a molecular weight of 527.5 and is represented by the formula

$C_{27}H_{29}NO_{10}$.

3. PHARMACEUTICAL FORM
Each vial contains a sterile, pyrogen-free, preservative-free liposomal emulsion. This emulsion is red and clear to slightly opalescent in appearance. The product is an injectable intended to be administered by intravenous infusion.

4. CLINICAL PARTICULARS

4.1 Therapeutic indications
DaunoXome is indicated for the treatment of advanced HIV-related Kaposi's Sarcoma.

4.2 Posology and method of administration
Dosage of DaunoXome must be adjusted for each patient. Therapy should be instituted at 40 mg/m^2 every two weeks. Therapy should be continued as long as disease control can be maintained.

DaunoXome should be diluted with 5% Dextrose Injection before administration. The recommended concentration after dilution is between 0.2 mg and 1 mg daunorubicin/ml of solution. DaunoXome should be administered intravenously over a 30-60 minute period and within six hours of dilution with dextrose. (See also Section 6.2, 6.3 and 6.6)

Myelosuppression is a known reaction to DaunoXome therapy. The colony stimulating factor G-CSF has been used to manage patients whose absolute neutrophil count (ANC) fell below 1000/mm^3.

Safety and effectiveness in children and the elderly has not been established.

4.3 Contraindications
DaunoXome is a bone marrow suppressant. Suppression may occur in patients given therapeutic doses of this drug. Combination of DaunoXome with other cancer chemotherapeutic agents which suppress blood counts is contraindicated. Therapy with DaunoXome is contraindicated in patients who have had a serious hypersensitivity reaction to previous doses of DaunoXome or to any of its constituents unless the benefit from such treatment warrants the risk.

4.4 Special warnings and special precautions for use
Myelosuppression is a known reaction to DaunoXome and frequent monitoring of the bone marrow function is recommended. The colony stimulating factor G-CSF has been used to manage patients with neutropenia.

A small number of cardiac events were reported in patients treated with DaunoXome during clinical trials. All patients receiving DaunoXome should routinely undergo frequent ECG monitoring. Transient ECG changes such as T-wave flattening, S-T segment depression and benign arrhythmias are not considered mandatory indications for the withdrawal of DaunoXome therapy. However, reduction of the QRS complex is considered indicative of cardiac toxicity.

A more specific method for the evaluation and monitoring of cardiac function is a measurement of left ventricular ejection fraction by echocardiography or preferably by MUGA (Multiple Gated Acquisition). These methods should be applied in patients with an increased risk of cardiomyopathy (those who have received prior anthracycline therapy or who have pre-existing cardiac disease) before the initiation of DaunoXome therapy and should be repeated periodically during treatment.

Infrequently, clinically significant, but asymptomatic, drops in the left ventricular ejection fraction (LVEF) have been seen, in patients treated with cumulative doses of 320 mg/m^2 DaunoXome. Out of a group of 979 Kaposi's Sarcoma patients, 1 patient developed congestive heart failure and 8 patients experienced a drop in LVEF without clinical symptoms. Determination of LVEF is recommended at cumulative doses of 320 mg/m^2 and every 160 mg/m^2 thereafter, in order to identify at an early stage any changes in LVEF that may be a precursor to cardiomyopathy if DaunoXome therapy is continued.

Whenever cardiomyopathy is suspected, i.e. LVEF has decreased as compared to pre-treatment values and/or LVEF is lower than a prognostically relevant value (e.g. $<45\%$), the benefit of continued therapy must be carefully evaluated against the risk of producing irreversible cardiac damage.

Congestive heart failure due to cardiomyopathy may occur suddenly, without prior ECG changes and may also occur several weeks after discontinuation of therapy.

Patients with a history of cardiovascular disease should receive DaunoXome only when the benefit outweighs the risk to the patient. Caution should be exercised in patients with impaired cardiac function.

Caution should also be observed in patients who have received other anthracycline therapy as this may increase the risk of cardiac events. The total dose of daunorubicin HCl should take into account any previous (or concomitant) therapy with cardiotoxic compounds such as other anthracyclines/- cenedions or 5-FU.

Conventional daunorubicin has also been associated with local tissue necrosis at the site of drug infiltrations. No such local necrosis has been observed with DaunoXome. Nonetheless, care should be taken to ensure that there is no extravasation of drug when DaunoXome is administered.

4.5 Interaction with other medicinal products and other forms of Interaction
No interactions between DaunoXome and other drugs have been observed to date. DaunoXome has been safely administered during antiretroviral therapy with zidovudine (AZT), dideoxycytidene (ddC, zalcitabine), and dideoxyinosine (ddI, didanosine) and with the colony stimulating factor G-CSF. Although interaction of DaunoXome with other drugs has not been observed, patients requiring concomitant drug therapy should be monitored closely. During preparation and administration DaunoXome should not be mixed with saline; aggregation of the liposomes may result.

So far no safety information is available on the combination of DaunoXome with other cancer chemotherapeutic agents which suppress blood counts. Concomitant use of DaunoXome and parenteral nutritional lipid solutions or other liposomal products should be avoided.

4.6 Pregnancy and lactation
Safety for use of DaunoXome in pregnant and lactating women has not been established. Since it is not known if the administration of DaunoXome during pregnancy can cause fetal harm, DaunoXome should only be used during pregnancy if the possible benefits to be derived outweigh the potential risks involved. Breast feeding should be discontinued during treatment.

Daunorubicin, the active component of DaunoXome, has been shown to impair fertility and to have teratogenic effects in experimental animals, and there is also positive evidence of human fetal risk. Daunorubicin is also mutagenic both *in vitro* and *in vivo*, and carcinogenic *in vivo.* A high incidence of mammary tumours was observed in rats treated with daunorubicin. Although no such studies have been conducted with DaunoXome, it is most likely that DaunoXome will have a similar profile for carcinogenesis, teratogenesis, mutagenesis, and impairment of fertility as that of daunorubicin.

4.7 Effects on ability to drive and use machines
Since DaunoXome is being administered to sick patients and may induce delayed nausea and vomiting, administration prior to driving or the use of heavy machinery is contraindicated.

4.8 Undesirable effects
The primary toxicity of DaunoXome is myelosuppression and, as such, close patient observation and frequent monitoring of the blood cell counts is mandated. In patients with malignancies or with HIV infection, the immune system is already compromised, and the use of a cytotoxic agent decreasing the white blood cell count may cause further immunosuppression and make the patient more susceptible to febrile neutropenia, intercurrent or opportunistic infections.

Back pain, flushing, and chest tightness were occasionally reported during the clinical trials. This syndrome may occur during a patient's initial infusion and may also occur in patients who have previously been exposed to DaunoXome without incident. This combination of symptoms does not always appear to be dose related, and generally occurs during the first ten minutes of the infusion. The etiology is unclear. The symptoms usually subside when the infusion is slowed or halted, and acetaminophen (paracetamol) may be used for analgesia. Other allergic or immune reactions may also be seen, and have been reported to be associated with hypotension. Anaphylactic reactions have been reported in rare cases.

Conventional daunorubicin has been associated with cardiomyopathy and congestive heart failure. Cardiac side effects typical for anthracyclines/ anthracenedions appear to occur at a lower frequency with DaunoXome than with conventional anthracyclin preparations. In clinical studies in patients with Kaposi's Sarcoma treated at a dose level of 40 mg/m^2 administered every two weeks, congestive heart failure is infrequent (1 case in 979 patients treated). Although this includes patients who have been treated with cumulative doses over 2,000mg/m^2, due to the relatively small numbers a safe upper limit for the cumulative dose cannot be defined.

From clinical trials using higher doses (60 to 180 mg/m^2 every three weeks), there appears to be a trend towards a higher incidence of congestive heart failure.

Thus the possibility of anthracyclin/- cenedion induced cardiomyopathy should be considered during and after treatment with DaunoXome. See Section 4.4

Various other minor reactions, such as headache, fatigue, chills, mucositis, lightheadedness, nausea, and vomiting, have also been reported.

4.9 Overdose
No experience exists for an overdose with this medication. The primary anticipated toxicity from such an overdose would be myelosuppression, and under these circumstances bone marrow function should be carefully monitored with appropriate therapy for any severe side-effects.

5. PHARMACOLOGICAL PROPERTIES

5.1 Pharmacodynamic properties
DaunoXome is a liposomal preparation of daunorubicin formulated to maximise the selectivity of daunorubicin for solid tumours *in situ*. This tumour selectivity has been demonstrated for transplanted tumours in animal models. While in the circulation, the DaunoXome formulation protects the entrapped daunorubicin from chemical and enzymatic degradation, minimises protein binding, and generally decreases uptake by normal tissues, as well as by the non-reticuloendothelial system. The specific mechanism by which DaunoXome is able to deliver daunorubicin to solid tumours *in situ* is not known. However, it is believed to be a function of increased permeability of the tumour neovasculature to some particulates in the size range of DaunoXome. Thus, by a decrease in distribution and uptake of normal tissues and binding to plasma

Table 1

Diluent	Dilution Ratio mL to mL	Final Concentration Daunorubicin mg/mL	Duration of Chemical Stability at 25°C	Duration of Chemical Stability at 2° - 8°C
5% Dextrose	1:2	1.0	24 hours	24 hours
	1:4	0.5	24 hours	24 hours
	1:8	0.25	24 hours	24 hours
	1:10	0.2	24 hours	24 hours

proteins and by selective extravasation in tumour neovasculature, the pharmacokinetics of daunorubicin are favourably shifted towards an accumulation of DaunoXome in tumour tissue. Once within the tumour environment, DaunoXome vesicles enter the tumour cells intact. Daunorubicin is then released over time in the cytoplasm, where it is able to exert its anti-neoplastic activity over a longer period.

5.2 Pharmacokinetic properties

DaunoXome has a pharmacokinetic profile significantly different from that of conventional daunorubicin. DaunoXome was administered intravenously over approximately 30 minutes as a single dose of 10, 20, 40, 60, or 80 mg/m^2. Plasma pharmacokinetic profiles for most patients demonstrated monoexponential declines, although biexponential or Michaelis-Menton (saturation) kinetics occurred in some instances. Peak plasma levels at 40 mg/m^2 ranged from 14.8 to 22.0 μg/ml with a mean peak plasma level of 18.0 μg/ml. The mean terminal half-life at this dose was 4.0 hours and mean total body clearance was 10.5 ml/minute. This resulted in a mean area under the plasma curve of 120 μg·hr/ml. Metabolism of DaunoXome appeared not to be significant at lower doses. At 60 mg/m^2 and above, three metabolites were observed, although they have not yet been identified.

DaunoXome pharmacokinetic parameters were also compared to published values for conventional daunorubicin. At 80 mg/m^2, peak plasma levels ranged from 33.4 to 52.3 μg/ml for DaunoXome compared to 0.40 μg/ml for conventional drug. At this dose, DaunoXome plasma levels decline monoexponentially with a terminal half-life of 5.2 hours versus an initial half-life of 0.77 hours and a final half-life of 55.4 hours for conventional daunorubicin. Mean clearance for DaunoXome is 6.6 ml/min versus 223 ml/minute for daunorubicin. When combined, these parameters indicate that DaunoXome produces a 36-fold increase in mean area under the plasma curve compared to conventional drug (375.3 versus 10.33 μg·hr/ml).

5.3 Preclinical safety data

Animal studies with tumour models in mice have demonstrated that DaunoXome can increase daunorubicin tumour exposure ten-fold (in terms of area under the tumour concentration vs. time curve, AUC) when compared with equivalent doses of conventional (free) drug. The rate of drug accumulation in tumour tissues, however, appears to be slower for DaunoXome than for conventional daunorubicin. This difference is thought to be due to a slow diffusion process by which DaunoXome extravasates through the tumour neovasculature into the extracellular space while free drug, in contrast, is able to rapidly equilibrate from the circulation to both normal and neoplastic tissues. Since tumour accumulation of DaunoXome-delivered daunorubicin is a gradual process, it is important that DaunoXome remains in the circulation at high levels for prolonged periods. This has been shown to occur in animal studies where plasma AUC values for daunorubicin were approximately 200-fold greater for DaunoXome than for conventional drug. In contrast to tumour tissue, however, AUC values for normal tissues were only moderately elevated in DaunoXome-treated animals, relative to conventional daunorubicin. Exclusive of reticuloendothelial tissues (liver and spleen, AUC values increased by 110% and 60%, respectively) and brain tissue (AUC value increased by 3.5 fold) AUC increases ranged from 10% for heart and lungs to 30% for kidney and small intestines.

6. PHARMACEUTICAL PARTICULARS

6.1 List of excipients

Liposome

Distearoylphosphatidylcholine

Cholesterol, USNF

Citric acid, Ph.Eur.

Buffer

Sucrose, Ph.Eur.

Glycine, B.P.

Calcium chloride, Ph.Eur.

q.s. to approximately 25 ml with Water for Injection, Ph.Eur.

6.2 Incompatibilities

To date, no incompatibilities of DaunoXome with other drugs have been reported. However, it is known that the active component daunorubicin is physically incompatible with heparin sodium and with dexamethasone phosphate when directly admixed. A precipitate is produced with either drug. Additionally, because of the chemical instability of the glycosidic bond of daunorubicin, admixture into a highly alkaline media (pH> 8.0) is not recommended. DaunoXome should not be mixed with saline; aggregation of the liposomes may result.

Admixtures containing bacteriostatic agents such as benzyl alcohol or other detergent-like molecules should be avoided because such compounds can rupture the bilayer wall of the liposomes causing premature leakage of the active drug.

6.3 Shelf life

The shelf-life is 52 weeks when stored at 2°-8°C.

Chemical and physical in-use stability has been demonstrated for DaunoXome diluted with 5% dextrose, see table below for details.

From a microbial point of view, diluted DaunoXome should be used immediately. If not used immediately, in-use storage times and conditions prior to use are the responsibility of the user and should not be longer than 24 hours at 2-8°C for the 5% dextrose dilutions. This recommendation is made on the assumption that dilution has taken place in controlled and validated aseptic conditions.

(see Table 1 above)

6.4 Special precautions for storage

Store at 2° - 8°C. Do not freeze. Protect against exposure to light. Do not store partially used vials for future patient use. Vials are for single use only.

6.5 Nature and contents of container

DaunoXome is presented in 50-ml, sterile, Type I glass vials. The closure consists of a butyl rubber stopper and aluminium ring seal fitted with a removable plastic cap. Each single-dose vial is packed in a white chipboard carton. Included in each carton are directions for use.

6.6 Instructions for use and handling

Use Aseptic Technique. Aseptic technique must be strictly observed in all handling, since no preservative or bacteriostatic agent is present in DaunoXome or in the materials recommended for dilution.

Withdraw the calculated volume of DaunoXome into a sterile syringe. Instill the DaunoXome preparation into a sterile container with the correct amount of 5% Dextrose Injection. The recommended concentration after dilution is between 0.2 mg and 1 mg daunorubicin/ml of solution. Infuse over a 30-60 minute period. As with all parenteral drug products, inspect the solution visually for particulate matter prior to administration.

Caution: The only fluid which may be mixed with DaunoXome is 5% Dextrose Injection; DaunoXome should not be mixed with saline, bacteriostatic agents such as benzyl alcohol, or any other solution.

An in-line filter is not recommended for the intravenous infusion of DaunoXome. However, if such a filter is used, the mean pore diameter of the filter should not be less than 5 μm.

Procedures for proper handling and disposal of anticancer drugs should be followed.

7. MARKETING AUTHORISATION HOLDER

Gilead Sciences International Limited

Granta Park

Abington

Cambridge

CB1 6GT

United Kingdom

8. MARKETING AUTHORISATION NUMBER(S)

PL 16807/0002

9. DATE OF FIRST AUTHORISATION/RENEWAL OF THE AUTHORISATION

12 October 1995

10. DATE OF REVISION OF THE TEXT

18 December 2000

DDAVP Tablets 0.1mg

(Ferring Pharmaceuticals Ltd)

1. NAME OF THE MEDICINAL PRODUCT

DDAVP® Tablets 0.1mg.

2. QUALITATIVE AND QUANTITATIVE COMPOSITION

Each tablet contains 0.1mg Desmopressin acetate

For excipients, see 6.1

3. PHARMACEUTICAL FORM

Tablet

Uncoated, white, oval, convex tablets scored on one side and engraved '0.1' on the other side.

4. CLINICAL PARTICULARS

4.1 Therapeutic indications

DDAVP® Tablets are indicated for the treatment of vasopressin-sensitive cranial diabetes insipidus or in the treatment of post-hypophysectomy polyuria/polydipsia.

4.2 Posology and method of administration

Treatment of Diabetes Insipidus:

Dosage is individual in diabetes insipidus but clinical experience has shown that the total daily dose normally lies in the range of 0.2 to 1.2mg. A suitable starting dose in adults and children is 0.1mg three times daily. This dosage regimen should then be adjusted in accordance with the patient's response. For the majority of patients, the maintenance dose is 0.1mg to 0.2mg three times daily.

Post-hypophysectomy polyuria/polydipsia:

The dose of DDAVP® Tablets should be controlled by measurement of urine osmolality.

4.3 Contraindications

DDAVP® Tablets are contraindicated in cases of cardiac insufficiency and other conditions requiring treatment with diuretic agents.

Before prescribing DDAVP® Tablets the diagnoses of psychogenic polydipsia and alcohol abuse should be excluded.

4.4 Special warnings and special precautions for use

Care should be taken with patients who have reduced renal function and/or cardiovascular disease. In chronic renal disease the antidiuretic effect of DDAVP® Tablets would be less than normal.

Precautions to prevent fluid overload must be taken in:

- conditions characterised by fluid and/or electrolyte imbalance

- patients at risk for increased intracranial pressure

4.5 Interaction with other medicinal products and other forms of Interaction

Substances which are known to induce SIADH e.g. tricyclic antidepressants, selective serotonin re-uptake inhibitors, chlorpromazine and carbamazepine, may cause an additive antidiuretic effect leading to an increased risk of water retention and/or hyponatraemia.

NSAIDs may induce water retention and/or hyponatraemia.

Concomitant treatment with loperamide may result in a 3-fold increase of desmopressin plasma concentrations, which may lead to an increased risk of water retention and/or hyponatraemia. Although not investigated, other drugs slowing transport might have the same effect.

A standardised 27% fat meal significantly decreased the absorption (rate and extent) of a 0.4mg dose of oral desmopressin. Although it did not significantly affect the pharmacodynamic effect (urine production and osmolality), there is the potential for this to occur at lower doses. If a diminution of effect is noted, then the effect of food should be considered before increasing the dose.

4.6 Pregnancy and lactation

Pregnancy:

Data on a limited number (n=53) of exposed pregnancies in women with diabetes insipidus indicate rare cases of malformations in children treated during pregnancy. To date, no other relevant epidemiological data are available. Animal studies do not indicate direct or indirect harmful effects with respect to pregnancy, embryonal/fetal development, parturition or postnatal development.

Caution should be exercised when prescribing to pregnant women. Blood pressure monitoring is recommended due to the increased risk of pre-eclampsia.

Lactation:

Results from analyses of milk from nursing mothers receiving high dose desmopressin (300 micrograms intranasally) indicate that the amounts of desmopressin that may be transferred to the child are considerably less than the amounts required to influence diuresis.

4.7 Effects on ability to drive and use machines

None

4.8 Undesirable effects

Side-effects include headache, stomach pain and nausea. Isolated cases of allergic skin reactions and more severe general allergic reactions have been reported. Very rare cases of emotional disturbances in children have been reported. Treatment with desmopressin without concomitant reduction of fluid intake may lead to water retention/hyponatraemia with accompanying symptoms of headache, nausea, vomiting, weight gain, decreased serum sodium and in serious cases, convulsions.

4.9 Overdose
An overdose of DDAVP® Tablets leads to a prolonged duration of action with an increased risk of water retention and/or hyponatraemia.

Treatment:

Although the treatment of hyponatraemia should be individualised, the following general recommendations can be given. Hyponatraemia is treated by discontinuing the desmopressin treatment, fluid restriction and symptomatic treatment if needed.

5. PHARMACOLOGICAL PROPERTIES

5.1 Pharmacodynamic properties
In its main biological effects, DDAVP® does not differ qualitatively from vasopressin. However, DDAVP® is characterised by a high antidiuretic activity whereas the uterotonic and vasopressor actions are extremely low.

5.2 Pharmacokinetic properties
The absolute bioavailability of orally administered desmopressin varies between 0.08% and 0.16%. Mean maximum plasma concentration is reached within 2 hours. The distribution volume is 0.2 – 0.32 l/kg. Desmopressin does not cross the blood-brain barrier. The oral terminal half-life varies between 2.0 and 3.11 hours.

In vitro, in human liver microsome preparations, it has been shown that no significant amount of desmopressin is metabolised in the liver and thus human liver metabolism *in vivo* is not likely to occur.

About 65% of the amount of desmopressin absorbed after oral administration could be recovered in the urine within 24 hours.

It is unlikely that desmopressin will interact with drugs affecting hepatic metabolism, since desmopressin has been shown not to undergo significant liver metabolism in *in vitro* studies with human microsomes. However, formal *in vivo* interaction studies have not been performed.

5.3 Preclinical safety data
There are no pre-clinical data of relevance to the prescriber which are additional to that already included in other sections of the SPC.

6. PHARMACEUTICAL PARTICULARS

6.1 List of excipients
Lactose monohydrate

Potato starch

Povidone

Magnesium stearate

6.2 Incompatibilities
Not applicable

6.3 Shelf life
24 months

6.4 Special precautions for storage
Do not store above 25°C. Keep the container tightly closed.

6.5 Nature and contents of container
30ml High Density Polyethylene (HDPE) bottle with a tamper-proof, twist-off polypropylene (PP) closure with a silica gel desiccant insert. Each bottle contains either 30 or 90 tablets.

Not all pack sizes may be marketed.

6.6 Instructions for use and handling
None

7. MARKETING AUTHORISATION HOLDER
Ferring Pharmaceuticals Limited, The Courtyard, Waterside Drive, Langley, Berkshire SL3 6EZ

8. MARKETING AUTHORISATION NUMBER(S)
PL 3194/0040

9. DATE OF FIRST AUTHORISATION/RENEWAL OF THE AUTHORISATION
12th January 2003

10. DATE OF REVISION OF THE TEXT
May 2003

11. Legal Category
POM

DDAVP Tablets 0.2mg

(Ferring Pharmaceuticals Ltd)

1. NAME OF THE MEDICINAL PRODUCT
DDAVP® Tablets 0.2mg.

2. QUALITATIVE AND QUANTITATIVE COMPOSITION
Each tablet contains 0.2mg Desmopressin acetate

For excipients, see 6.1

3. PHARMACEUTICAL FORM
Tablet

Uncoated, white, round, convex tablets scored on one side and engraved '0.2' on the other side.

4. CLINICAL PARTICULARS

4.1 Therapeutic indications
DDAVP® Tablets are indicated for the treatment of vasopressin-sensitive cranial diabetes insipidus or in the treatment of post-hypophysectomy polyuria/polydipsia.

4.2 Posology and method of administration
Treatment of Diabetes Insipidus:

Dosage is individual in diabetes insipidus but clinical experience has shown that the total daily dose normally lies in the range of 0.2 to 1.2mg. A suitable starting dose in adults and children is 0.1mg three times daily. This dosage regimen should then be adjusted in accordance with the patient's response. For the majority of patients, the maintenance dose is 0.1mg to 0.2mg three times daily.

Post-hypophysectomy polyuria/polydipsia:

The dose of DDAVP® Tablets should be controlled by measurement of urine osmolality.

4.3 Contraindications
DDAVP® Tablets are contraindicated in cases of cardiac insufficiency and other conditions requiring treatment with diuretic agents.

Before prescribing DDAVP® Tablets the diagnoses of psychogenic polydipsia and alcohol abuse should be excluded.

4.4 Special warnings and special precautions for use
Care should be taken with patients who have reduced renal function and/or cardiovascular disease. In chronic renal disease the antidiuretic effect of DDAVP® Tablets would be less than normal.

Precautions to prevent fluid overload must be taken in:

- conditions characterised by fluid and/or electrolyte imbalance

- patients at risk for increased intracranial pressure

4.5 Interaction with other medicinal products and other forms of Interaction
Substances which are known to induce SIADH e.g. tricyclic antidepressants, selective serotonin re-uptake inhibitors, chlorpromazine and carbamazepine, may cause an additive antidiuretic effect leading to an increased risk of water retention and/or hyponatraemia.

NSAIDs may induce water retention and/or hyponatraemia.

Concomitant treatment with loperamide may result in a 3-fold increase of desmopressin plasma concentrations, which may lead to an increased risk of water retention and/or hyponatraemia. Although not investigated, other drugs slowing transport might have the same effect.

A standardised 27% fat meal significantly decreased the absorption (rate and extent) of a 0.4mg dose of oral desmopressin. Although it did not significantly affect the pharmacodynamic effect (urine production and osmolality), there is the potential for this to occur at lower doses. If a diminution of effect is noted, then the effect of food should be considered before increasing the dose.

4.6 Pregnancy and lactation
Pregnancy:

Data on a limited number (n=53) of exposed pregnancies in women with diabetes insipidus indicate rare cases of malformations in children treated during pregnancy. To date, no other relevant epidemiological data are available. Animal studies do not indicate direct or indirect harmful effects with respect to pregnancy, embryonal/fetal development, parturition or postnatal development.

Caution should be exercised when prescribing to pregnant women. Blood pressure monitoring is recommended due to the increased risk of pre-eclampsia.

Lactation:

Results from analyses of milk from nursing mothers receiving high dose desmopressin (300 micrograms intranasally) indicate that the amounts of desmopressin that may be transferred to the child are considerably less than the amounts required to influence diuresis.

4.7 Effects on ability to drive and use machines
None

4.8 Undesirable effects
Side-effects include headache, stomach pain and nausea. Isolated cases of allergic skin reactions and more severe general allergic reactions have been reported. Very rare cases of emotional disturbances in children have been reported. Treatment with desmopressin without concomitant reduction of fluid intake may lead to water retention/hyponatraemia with accompanying symptoms of headache, nausea, vomiting, weight gain, decreased serum sodium and in serious cases, convulsions.

4.9 Overdose
An overdose of DDAVP® Tablets leads to a prolonged duration of action with an increased risk of water retention and/or hyponatraemia.

Treatment:

Although the treatment of hyponatraemia should be individualised, the following general recommendations can be given. Hyponatraemia is treated by discontinuing the desmopressin treatment, fluid restriction and symptomatic treatment if needed.

5. PHARMACOLOGICAL PROPERTIES

5.1 Pharmacodynamic properties
In its main biological effects, DDAVP® does not differ qualitatively from vasopressin. However, DDAVP® is characterised by a high antidiuretic activity whereas the uterotonic and vasopressor actions are extremely low.

5.2 Pharmacokinetic properties
The absolute bioavailability of orally administered desmopressin varies between 0.08% and 0.16%. Mean maximum plasma concentration is reached within 2 hours. The distribution volume is 0.2 – 0.32 l/kg. Desmopressin does not cross the blood-brain barrier. The oral terminal half-life varies between 2.0 and 3.11 hours.

In vitro, in human liver microsome preparations, it has been shown that no significant amount of desmopressin is metabolised in the liver and thus human liver metabolism *in vivo* is not likely to occur.

About 65% of the amount of desmopressin absorbed after oral administration could be recovered in the urine within 24 hours.

It is unlikely that desmopressin will interact with drugs affecting hepatic metabolism, since desmopressin has been shown not to undergo significant liver metabolism in *in vitro* studies with human microsomes. However, formal *in vivo* interaction studies have not been performed.

5.3 Preclinical safety data
There are no pre-clinical data of relevance to the prescriber which are additional to that already included in other sections of the SPC.

6. PHARMACEUTICAL PARTICULARS

6.1 List of excipients
Lactose monohydrate

Potato starch

Povidone

Magnesium stearate

6.2 Incompatibilities
Not applicable

6.3 Shelf life
24 months.

6.4 Special precautions for storage
Do not store above 25°C. Keep the container tightly closed.

6.5 Nature and contents of container
30ml High Density Polyethylene (HDPE) bottle with a tamper-proof, twist-off polypropylene (PP) closure with a silica gel desiccant insert. Each bottle contains either 30 or 90 tablets.

Not all pack sizes may be marketed.

6.6 Instructions for use and handling
None

7. MARKETING AUTHORISATION HOLDER
Ferring Pharmaceuticals Limited, The Courtyard, Waterside Drive, Langley, Berkshire SL3 6EZ

8. MARKETING AUTHORISATION NUMBER(S)
PL 3194/0041

9. DATE OF FIRST AUTHORISATION/RENEWAL OF THE AUTHORISATION
12th January 2003

10. DATE OF REVISION OF THE TEXT
May 2003

11. Legal Category
POM

DDAVP/Desmopressin Injection

(Ferring Pharmaceuticals Ltd)

1. NAME OF THE MEDICINAL PRODUCT
DDAVP®/Desmopressin Injection.

2. QUALITATIVE AND QUANTITATIVE COMPOSITION
Each 1ml ampoule contains Desmopressin acetate 4 micrograms per ml.

3. PHARMACEUTICAL FORM
Solution for injection.

4. CLINICAL PARTICULARS

4.1 Therapeutic indications
DDAVP®/Desmopressin Injection is indicated as follows:

1) Diagnosis and treatment of cranial diabetes insipidus.

2) To increase Factor VIII:C and Factor VIII:Ag in patients with mild to moderate haemophilia or von Willebrand's disease undergoing surgery or following trauma.

3) To establish renal concentration capacity.

4) To treat headache resulting from a lumbar puncture.

5) To test for fibrinolytic response.

4.2 Posology and method of administration
Treatment of cranial Diabetes Insipidus:

By subcutaneous, intramuscular or intravenous injection.

Adults:

The usual dose is 1 to 4 micrograms given once daily.

Children and infants:

Doses from 0.4 micrograms (0.1ml) may be used.

Diagnosis of cranial Diabetes Insipidus:

The diagnostic dose in adults and children is 2 micrograms given by subcutaneous or intramuscular injection. Failure to elaborate a concentrated urine after water deprivation, followed by the ability to do so after the administration of Desmopressin confirms a diagnosis of cranial diabetes insipidus. Failure to concentrate after the administration suggests nephrogenic diabetes insipidus.

Mild to moderate haemophilia and von Willebrand's disease:

By intravenous administration.

The dose for adults, children and infants is 0.4 micrograms per kilogram body weight administered by intravenous infusion. Further doses may be administered at 12 hourly intervals so long as cover is required. As some patients have shown a diminishing response to successive doses, it is recommended that monitoring of Factor VIII levels should continue. The dose should be diluted in 50ml of 0.9% sodium chloride for injection and given over 20 minutes. This dose should be given immediately prior to surgery or following trauma. During administration of intravenous Desmopressin, vasodilation may occur resulting in decreased blood pressure and tachycardia with facial flushing in some patients.

Increase of Factor VIII levels are dependent on basal levels and are normally between 2 and 5 times the pre-treatment levels. If results from a previous administration of Desmopressin are not available then blood should be taken pre-dose and 20 minutes post-dose for assay of Factor VIII levels in order to monitor response.

Unless contraindicated, when surgery is undertaken, tranexamic acid may be given orally at the recommended dose from 24 hours beforehand until healing is complete.

Renal Function Testing:

By subcutaneous or intramuscular injection.

Adults and children can be expected to achieve urine concentrations above 700mOsm/kg in the period of 5 to 9 hours following a dose of 2 micrograms DDAVP®/Desmopressin Injection. It is recommended that the bladder should be emptied at the time of administration.

In normal infants, a urine concentration of 600mOsm/kg should be achieved in the five hour period following a dose of 0.4 micrograms DDAVP®/Desmopressin Injection. The fluid intake at the two meals following the administration should be restricted to 50% of the ordinary intake to avoid water overload.

Post Lumbar Puncture Headache:

By subcutaneous or intramuscular injection.

Where a headache is thought to be due to a lumbar puncture, an adult patient can be given a dose of 4 micrograms DDAVP®/Desmopressin Injection which may be repeated 24 hours later if necessary. Alternatively, a prophylactic dose of 4 micrograms can be given immediately prior to the lumbar puncture and repeated 24 hours later.

Fibrinolytic Response Testing:

By intravenous administration.

The dose for adults and children is 0.4 micrograms per kilogram body weight administered by intravenous infusion. The dose should be diluted in 50ml of 0.9% sodium chloride for injection and given over 20 minutes.

A sample of venous blood should be taken 20 minutes after the infusion. In patients with a normal response the sample should show fibrinolytic activity of euglobulin clot precipitate on fibrin plates of at least 240mm^2.

4.3 Contraindications

DDAVP®/Desmopressin Injection is contraindicated in cases of:

GENERAL:

- habitual and psychogenic polydipsia

RENAL FUNCTION TESTING, TREATMENT OF LUMBAR PUNCTURE HEADACHE OR FIBRINOLYTIC RESPONSE TESTING:

- should not be carried out in patients with hypertension, heart disease, cardiac insufficiency and other conditions requiring treatment with diuretic agents

FOR HAEMOSTATIC USE

- unstable angina pectoris
- decompensated cardiac insufficiency
- von Willebrand's Disease Type IIB where the administration of Desmopressin may result in pseudothrombocytopenia due to the release of clotting factors which cause platelet aggregation.

4.4 Special warnings and special precautions for use

GENERAL

Precautions to prevent fluid overload must be taken in:

- conditions characterised by fluid and/or electrolyte imbalance
- patients at risk for increased intracranial pressure

Care should be taken with patients who have reduced renal function and/or cardiovascular disease.

When DDAVP®/Desmopressin Injection is used for diagnostic purposes, fluid intake must be limited and not exceed 0.5 litres from 1 hour before until 8 hours after administration.

Renal concentration capacity testing in children below the age of 1 year should only be performed under carefully supervised conditions in hospital.

FOR HAEMOSTATIC USE

When repeated doses are used to control bleeding in haemophilia or von Willebrand's disease, care should be taken to prevent fluid overload. Fluid should not be forced, orally or parenterally, and patients should only take as much fluid as they require to satisfy thirst. Intravenous infusions should not be left up as a routine after surgery. Fluid accumulation can be readily monitored by weighing the patient or by determining plasma sodium or osmolality.

Measures to prevent fluid overload must be taken in patients with conditions requiring treatment with diuretic agents.

Special attention must be paid to the risk of water retention. The fluid intake should be restricted to the least possible and the body weight should be checked regularly.

If there is a gradual increase of the body weight, decrease of serum sodium to below 130mmol/l or plasma osmolality to below 270mOsm/kg, the fluid intake must be reduced drastically and the administration of DDAVP®/Desmopressin Injection interrupted.

During infusion of DDAVP®/Desmopressin Injection for haemostatic use, it is recommended that the patient's blood pressure is monitored continuously.

DDAVP®/Desmopressin Injection does not reduce prolonged bleeding time in thrombocytopenia.

4.5 Interaction with other medicinal products and other forms of Interaction

Substances which are known to induce SIADH e.g. tricyclic antidepressants, selective serotonin re-uptake inhibitors, chlorpromazine and carbamazepine, may cause an additive antidiuretic effect leading to an increased risk of water retention and/or hyponatraemia.

NSAIDs may induce water retention and/or hyponatraemia.

4.6 Pregnancy and lactation

Pregnancy:

Data on a limited number (n=53) of exposed pregnancies in women with diabetes insipidus indicate rare cases of malformations in children treated during pregnancy. To date, no other relevant epidemiological data are available. Animal studies do not indicate direct or indirect harmful effects with respect to pregnancy, embryonal/fetal development, parturition or postnatal development.

Caution should be exercised when prescribing to pregnant women. Blood pressure monitoring is recommended due to the increased risk of pre-eclampsia.

Lactation:

Results from analyses of milk from nursing mothers receiving high dose Desmopressin (300 micrograms intranasally) indicate that the amounts of Desmopressin that may be transferred to the child are considerably less than the amounts required to influence diuresis or haemostasis.

4.7 Effects on ability to drive and use machines

None

4.8 Undesirable effects

Side-effects include headache, stomach pain and nausea. Isolated cases of allergic skin reactions and more severe general allergic reactions have been reported. Treatment with Desmopressin without concomitant reduction of fluid intake may lead to water retention/hyponatraemia with accompanying symptoms of headache, nausea, vomiting, weight gain, decreased serum sodium and in serious cases, convulsions.

4.9 Overdose

An overdose of DDAVP®/Desmopressin injection leads to a prolonged duration of action with an increased risk of water retention and/or hyponatraemia.

Treatment:

Although the treatment of hyponatraemia should be individualised, the following general recommendations can be given. Hyponatraemia is treated by discontinuing the desmopressin treatment, fluid restriction and symptomatic treatment if needed.

5. PHARMACOLOGICAL PROPERTIES

5.1 Pharmacodynamic properties

Desmopressin is a structural analogue of vasopressin in which the antidiuretic activity has been enhanced by the order of 10, while the vasopressor effect has been reduced by the order of 1500. The clinical advantage of this highly changed ratio of antidiuretic to vasopressor effect is that clinically active antidiuretic doses are far below the threshold for a vasopressor effect.

Like vasopressin, Desmopressin also increases concentrations of Factor VIII:C, Factor VIII:Ag and Plasminogen Activator.

5.2 Pharmacokinetic properties

Following intravenous injection, plasma concentrations of Desmopressin follow a biexponential curve. The initial fast phase of a few minutes duration and with a half life of less than 10 minutes is thought mainly to represent the diffusion of Desmopressin from plasma to its volume of distribution. The second phase with a half life of 51-158 minutes represents the elimination rate of Desmopressin from the body.

As a comparison, the half life of vasopressin is less than 10 minutes.

In vitro, in human liver microsome preparations, it has been shown that no significant amount of desmopressin is metabolised in the liver and thus human liver metabolism *in vivo* is not likely to occur.

It is unlikely that desmopressin will interact with drugs affecting hepatic metabolism, since desmopressin has been shown not to undergo significant liver metabolism in *in vitro* studies with human microsomes. However, formal *in vivo* interaction studies have not been performed.

5.3 Preclinical safety data

There are no pre-clinical data of relevance to the prescriber which are additional to those already included in other sections of the SPC.

6. PHARMACEUTICAL PARTICULARS

6.1 List of excipients

Sodium Chloride Ph. Eur.

Hydrochloric Acid Ph. Eur.

Water for Injection Ph. Eur.

6.2 Incompatibilities

None known

6.3 Shelf life

Shelf life of unopened ampoule: 24 months.

6.4 Special precautions for storage

To be stored in a refrigerator at 4°C to 8°C.

6.5 Nature and contents of container

Carton containing 10 × 1ml clear Type I glass ampoules. Each ampoule contains 1ml of a sterile, clear, colourless solution for injection.

6.6 Instructions for use and handling

As indicated under the posology and method of administration section.

7. MARKETING AUTHORISATION HOLDER

Ferring Pharmaceuticals Limited, The Courtyard, Waterside Drive, Langley, Berkshire SL3 6EZ

8. MARKETING AUTHORISATION NUMBER(S)

PL 3194/0002

9. DATE OF FIRST AUTHORISATION/RENEWAL OF THE AUTHORISATION

10th September 1998

10. DATE OF REVISION OF THE TEXT

September 2002

11. Legal Category

POM

DDAVP/Desmopressin Intranasal Solution

(Ferring Pharmaceuticals Ltd)

1. NAME OF THE MEDICINAL PRODUCT

DDAVP®/Desmopressin Intranasal Solution

2. QUALITATIVE AND QUANTITATIVE COMPOSITION

Desmopressin acetate 0.01% w/v

3. PHARMACEUTICAL FORM

Aqueous solution for intranasal administration

4. CLINICAL PARTICULARS

4.1 Therapeutic indications

DDAVP®/Desmopressin Intranasal Solution is indicated for:

1) The diagnosis and treatment of vasopressin-sensitive cranial diabetes insipidus

2) The treatment of nocturia associated with multiple sclerosis where other treatments have failed.

3) Establishing renal concentration capacity.

4.2 Posology and method of administration

Treatment of Diabetes Insipidus:

Dosage is individual but clinical experience has shown that the average maintenance doses are as follows:

Adults: 10 to 20 micrograms once or twice daily.

Elderly: 10 to 20 micrograms once or twice daily.

Children: 5 to 20 micrograms daily, (a lower dose may be required for infants).

Diagnosis of Diabetes Insipidus:

The diagnostic dose in adults and children is 20 micrograms. Failure to elaborate a concentrated urine after water deprivation, followed by the ability to do so after the administration of Desmopressin confirms the diagnosis of cranial diabetes insipidus. Failure to concentrate after the administration suggests nephrogenic diabetes insipidus.

Treatment of Nocturia:

For multiple sclerosis patients up to 65 years of age with normal renal function suffering from nocturia the dose is 10 to 20 micrograms at bed time. Not more than one dose should be used in any 24 hour period.

Renal Function Testing:

To establish renal concentration capacity, the following single doses are recommended:

Adults: 40 micrograms

Elderly: 40 micrograms

Children (1 - 15 years): 20 micrograms

Infants (to 1 year): 10 micrograms

Adults and children with normal renal function can be expected to achieve concentrations above 700mOsm/kg in the period of 5-9 hours following administration of DDAVP®/Desmopressin Intranasal Solution. It is recommended that the bladder should be emptied at the time of administration.

In normal infants a urine concentration of 600mOsm/kg should be achieved in the 5 hour period following the administration of DDAVP®/Desmopressin Intranasal Solution. The fluid intake at the two meals following the administration should be restricted to 50% of the ordinary intake in order to avoid water overload.

4.3 Contraindications

DDAVP®/Desmopressin Intranasal Solution is contraindicated in cases of:

- cardiac insufficiency and other conditions requiring treatment with diuretic agents
- hypersensitivity to the preservative

Before prescribing DDAVP®/Desmopressin Intranasal the diagnoses of psychogenic polydipsia and alcohol abuse should be excluded.

When used to control nocturia in patients with multiple sclerosis, Desmopressin should not be used in patients with hypertension or cardiovascular disease.

Desmopressin should not be prescribed to patients over the age of 65 for the treatment of nocturia associated with multiple sclerosis.

4.4 Special warnings and special precautions for use

Care should be taken with patients who have reduced renal function and/or cardiovascular disease or cystic fibrosis.

When DDAVP®/Desmopressin Intranasal Solution is used for the treatment of nocturia associated with multiple sclerosis, fluid intake must be limited from 1 hour before until 8 hours after administration. Periodic assessments should be made of blood pressure and weight to monitor the possibility of fluid overload.

When used for diagnostic purposes, fluid intake must be limited and not exceed 0.5 litres from 1 hour before until 8 hours after administration.

Following diagnostic testing for diabetes insipidus or renal concentration, care should be taken to prevent fluid overload. Fluid should not be forced, orally or parenterally, and patients should only take as much fluid as they require to satisfy thirst.

Precautions to prevent fluid overload must be taken in:

- conditions characterised by fluid and/or electrolyte imbalance
- patients at risk for increased intracranial pressure

Renal concentration capacity testing in children below the age of 1 year should only be performed under carefully supervised conditions in hospital.

4.5 Interaction with other medicinal products and other forms of Interaction

Substances which are known to induce SIADH e.g. tricyclic antidepressants, selective serotonin re-uptake inhibitors, chlorpromazine and carbamazepine, may cause an additive antidiuretic effect leading to an increased risk of water retention and/or hyponatraemia.

NSAIDs may induce water retention and/or hyponatraemia.

4.6 Pregnancy and lactation

Pregnancy:

Data on a limited number (n=53) of exposed pregnancies in women with diabetes insipidus indicate rare cases of malformations in children treated during pregnancy. To date, no other relevant epidemiological data are available. Animal studies do not indicate direct or indirect harmful effects with respect to pregnancy, embryonal/fetal development, parturition or postnatal development.

Caution should be exercised when prescribing to pregnant women. Blood pressure monitoring is recommended due to the increased risk of pre-eclampsia.

Lactation:

Results from analyses of milk from nursing mothers receiving high dose Desmopressin (300 micrograms intranasally) indicate that the amounts of Desmopressin that may be transferred to the child are considerably less than the amounts required to influence diuresis.

4.7 Effects on ability to drive and use machines

None

4.8 Undesirable effects

Side-effects include headache, stomach pain, nausea, nasal congestion, rhinitis and epistaxis. Isolated cases of allergic skin reactions and more severe general allergic reactions have been reported. Very rare cases of emotional disturbances in children have been reported. Treatment with Desmopressin without concomitant reduction of fluid intake may lead to water retention/hyponatraemia with accompanying symptoms of headache, nausea, vomiting, weight gain, decreased serum sodium and in serious cases, convulsions.

4.9 Overdose

An overdose of DDAVP®/Desmopressin Intranasal Solution leads to a prolonged duration of action with an increased risk of water retention and/or hyponatraemia.

Treatment:

Although the treatment of hyponatraemia should be individualised, the following general recommendations can be given. Hyponatraemia is treated by discontinuing the desmopressin treatment, fluid restriction and symptomatic treatment if needed.

5. PHARMACOLOGICAL PROPERTIES

5.1 Pharmacodynamic properties

Desmopressin is a structural analogue of vasopressin, with two chemical changes namely desamination of the N-terminal and replacement of the 8-L-Arginine by 8-D-Arginine. These changes have increased the antidiuretic activity and prolonged the duration of action. The pressor activity is reduced to less than 0.01% of the natural peptide as a result of which side-effects are rarely seen.

5.2 Pharmacokinetic properties

Following intranasal administration, the bioavailability of Desmopressin is of the order of 10%.

Pharmacokinetic parameters following intravenous administration were reported as follows:

Total clearance: 2.6ml/min/kg body weight.

T½: 55 mins

Plasma kinetics of DDAVP in man

H.Vilhardt, S. Lundin, J. Falch.

Acta Pharmacol. et. Toxicol. 1986, 58, 379-381

In vitro, in human liver microsome preparations, it has been shown that no significant amount of desmopressin is metabolised in the liver and thus human liver metabolism *in vivo* is not likely to occur.

It is unlikely that desmopressin will interact with drugs affecting hepatic metabolism, since desmopressin has been shown not to undergo significant liver metabolism in *in vitro* studies with human microsomes. However, formal *in vivo* interaction studies have not been performed.

5.3 Preclinical safety data

There are no pre-clinical data of relevance to the prescriber which are additional to those already included in other sections of the SPC.

6. PHARMACEUTICAL PARTICULARS

6.1 List of excipients

Sodium Chloride BP

Chlorobutanol Ph. Eur.

Hydrochloric Acid Ph. Eur.

Purified Water Ph. Eur.

6.2 Incompatibilities

None.

6.3 Shelf life

36 months.

6.4 Special precautions for storage

Store in a refrigerator at a temperature of 2°C to 8°C. Protect from light.

6.5 Nature and contents of container

Brown glass vial, 1st hydrolytic glass. Fitted with a dropper set composed of poly-propylene and a cap of polyethylene.

6.6 Instructions for use and handling

None.

7. MARKETING AUTHORISATION HOLDER

Ferring Pharmaceuticals Limited, The Courtyard, Waterside Drive, Langley, Berkshire SL3 6EZ

8. MARKETING AUTHORISATION NUMBER(S)

PL 03194/0001R

9. DATE OF FIRST AUTHORISATION/RENEWAL OF THE AUTHORISATION

28th April 2002

10. DATE OF REVISION OF THE TEXT

May 2003

11. Legal Category

POM

Decadron Tablets

(Merck Sharp & Dohme Limited)

1. NAME OF THE MEDICINAL PRODUCT

DECADRON® Tablets

2. QUALITATIVE AND QUANTITATIVE COMPOSITION

Each tablet of 'Decadron' contains 500 micrograms dexamethasone Ph Eur.

3. PHARMACEUTICAL FORM

'Decadron' is supplied as a round, white, half-scored tablet, marked 'MSD 41'.

4. CLINICAL PARTICULARS

4.1 Therapeutic indications

'Decadron' is indicated as a treatment for certain endocrine and non-endocrine disorders, in certain cases of cerebral oedema, and for diagnostic testing of adrenocortical hyperfunction.

Endocrine disorders: Primary or secondary adrenocortical insufficiency, congenital adrenal hyperplasia.

Non-endocrine disorders: Dexamethasone may be used in the treatment of non-endocrine corticosteroid responsive conditions, including:

Allergy and anaphylaxis: Angioneurotic oedema, anaphylaxis.

Arteritis collagenosis: Polymyalgia rheumatica, polyarteritis nodosa.

Blood disorders: Haemolytic anaemia, leukaemia, myeloma.

Cardiovascular disorders: Post-myocardial infarction syndrome.

Gastro-intestinal: Crohn's disease, ulcerative colitis.

Hypercalcaemia: Sarcoidosis.

Infections (with appropriate chemotherapy): Miliary tuberculosis.

Muscular disorders: Polymyositis.

Neurological disorders: Raised intra-cranial pressure secondary to cerebral tumours.

Ocular disorders: Anterior and posterior uveitis, optic neuritis.

Renal disorders: Lupus nephritis.

Respiratory disease: Bronchial asthma, aspiration pneumonitis.

Rheumatic disorders: Rheumatoid arthritis.

Skin disorders: Pemphigus vulgaris.

4.2 Posology and method of administration

General considerations: Dosage must be individualised on the basis of the disease and the response of the patient. In order to minimise side effects, the lowest possible dosage adequate to control the disease process should be used (see 'Undesirable effects').

The initial dosage varies from 0.5 mg to 9 mg a day depending on the disease being treated. In more severe diseases, doses higher than 9 mg may be required. The initial dosage should be maintained or adjusted until the patient's response is satisfactory. Both the dose in the evening, which is useful in alleviating morning stiffness, and the divided dosage regimen are associated with greater suppression of the hypothalamo-pituitary-adrenal axis. If satisfactory clinical response does not occur after a reasonable period of time, discontinue 'Decadron' Tablets and transfer the patient to other therapy.

After a favourable initial response, the proper maintenance dosage should be determined by decreasing the initial dosage in small amounts to the lowest dosage that maintains an adequate clinical response. Chronic dosage should preferably not exceed 1.5 mg dexamethasone daily.

Patients should be monitored for signs that might require dosage adjustment, including changes in clinical status resulting from remissions or exacerbations of the disease, individual drug responsiveness, and the effect of stress (e.g. surgery, infection, trauma). During stress it may be necessary to increase dosage temporarily.

To avoid hypoadrenalism and/or a relapse of the underlying disease, it may be necessary to withdraw the drug gradually (see 'Special warnings and special precautions for use').

The following equivalents facilitate changing to 'Decadron' from other glucocorticoids.

Milligram for milligram, dexamethasone is approximately equivalent to betamethasone, 4 to 6 times more potent than methylprednisolone and triamcinolone, 6 to 8 times more potent than prednisone and prednisolone, 25 to 30 times more potent than hydrocortisone, and about 35 times more potent than cortisone.

In acute, self-limiting allergic disorders or acute exacerbations of chronic allergic disorders, the following dosage schedule combining parenteral and oral therapy is suggested.

First day 'Decadron' Injection, 4 mg or 8 mg (1 ml or 2 ml) intramuscularly

Second day Two 500 microgram 'Decadron' Tablets twice a day

Third day Two 500 microgram 'Decadron' Tablets twice a day

Fourth day One 500 microgram 'Decadron' Tablet twice a day

Fifth day One 500 microgram 'Decadron' Tablet twice a day

Sixth day One 500 microgram 'Decadron' Tablet

Seventh day One 500 microgram 'Decadron' Tablet

Eighth day Reassessment day

This schedule is designed to ensure adequate therapy during acute episodes while minimising the risk of overdosage in chronic cases.

Dexamethasone suppression tests:

1. *Tests for Cushing's syndrome*: 2 milligram 'Decadron' is given orally at 11 p.m., then blood is drawn for plasma cortisol determination at 8 a.m. the following morning.

For greater accuracy, 500 microgram 'Decadron' is given orally every 6 hours for 48 hours. Plasma cortisol is measured at 8 a.m. on the third morning. Twenty-four-hour urine collections are made for determination of 17-hydroxycorticosteroid excretion.

2. *Test to distinguish Cushing's syndrome caused by pituitary ACTH excess from the syndrome induced by other causes*: 2 milligram 'Decadron' is given orally every 6 hours for 48 hours. Plasma cortisol is measured at 8 a.m. on the morning following the last dose. Twenty-four-hour urine collections are made for determination of 17-hydroxycorticosteroid excretion.

Use in children: Dosage should be limited to a single dose on alternate days to lessen retardation of growth and minimise suppression of hypothalamo-pituitary-adrenal axis.

Use in the elderly: Treatment of elderly patients, particularly if long term, should be planned bearing in mind the more serious consequences of the common side effects of corticosteroids in old age, especially osteoporosis, diabetes, hypertension, hypokalaemia, susceptibility to infection and thinning of the skin. Close clinical supervision is required to avoid life-threatening reactions (see 'Undesirable effects').

4.3 Contraindications

Systemic fungal infections; systemic infection unless specific anti-infective therapy is employed; hypersensitivity to any component of the drug. Administration of live virus vaccines (see 'Special warnings and special precautions for use').

4.4 Special warnings and special precautions for use

Undesirable effects may be minimised by using the lowest effective dose for the minimum period and when appropriate by administering the daily requirement as a single morning dose or whenever possible as a single morning dose on alternative days. Frequent patient review is required to appropriately titrate the dose against disease activity. When reduction in dosage is possible, the reduction should be gradual (see 'Posology and method of administration').

Corticosteroids may exacerbate systemic fungal infections and should not be used in the presence of such infections unless they are needed to control life-threatening drug reactions due to amphotericin. Moreover, there have been cases reported in which concomitant use of amphotericin and hydrocortisone was followed by cardiac enlargement and heart failure.

Reports in the literature suggest an apparent association between use of corticosteroids and left-ventricular free-wall rupture after a recent myocardial infarction; therefore, corticosteroids should be used with great caution in these patients.

A report shows that the use of corticosteroids in cerebral malaria is associated with a prolonged coma and an increased incidence of pneumonia and gastro-intestinal bleeding.

Average and large doses of hydrocortisone or cortisone can cause elevation of blood pressure, retention of salt and water, and increased excretion of potassium, but these effects are less likely to occur with synthetic derivatives, except when used in large doses. Dietary salt restriction and potassium supplementation may be necessary. All corticosteroids increase calcium excretion.

In patients on corticosteroid therapy subjected to unusual stress (e.g. intercurrent illness, trauma, or surgical procedure), dosage should be increased before, during and after the stressful situation. Drug-induced secondary adrenocortical insufficiency may result from too rapid withdrawal of corticosteroids and may be minimised by gradual dosage reduction, being tapered off over weeks and months, depending on the dose and duration of treatment, but may persist for up to a year after discontinuation of therapy. In any stressful situation during that period, therefore, corticosteroid therapy should be reinstated. If the patient is already receiving corticosteroids, the current dosage may have to be temporarily increased. Salt and/or a mineralocorticoid should be given concurrently, since mineralocorticoid secretion may be impaired.

Stopping corticosteroids after prolonged therapy may cause withdrawal symptoms including fever, myalgia, arthralgia, and malaise. This may occur in patients even without evidence of adrenal insufficiency.

In patients who have received more than physiological doses of systemic corticosteroids (approximately 1 mg dexamethasone) for greater than three weeks, withdrawal should not be abrupt. How dose reduction should be carried out depends largely on whether the disease is likely to relapse as the dose of systemic corticosteroids is reduced. Clinical assessment of disease activity may be needed during withdrawal. If the disease is unlikely to relapse on withdrawal of systemic corticosteroids but there is uncertainty about hypothalamic-pituitary adrenal (HPA) suppression, the dose of systemic corticosteroids ***may*** be reduced rapidly to physiological doses. Once a daily dose of 1 mg dexamethasone is reached, dose reduction should be slower to allow the HPA-axis to recover.

Abrupt withdrawal of systemic corticosteroid treatment, which has continued up to three weeks is appropriate if it is considered that the disease is unlikely to relapse. Abrupt withdrawal of doses of up to 6 mg daily of dexamethasone for three weeks is unlikely to lead to clinically relevant HPA-axis suppression, in the majority of patients. In the following patient groups, gradual withdrawal of systemic corticosteroid therapy should be ***considered*** even after courses lasting three weeks or less:

- Patients who have had repeated courses of systemic corticosteroids, particularly if taken for greater than three weeks.
- When a short course has been prescribed within one year of cessation of long-term therapy (months or years).
- Patients who may have reasons for adrenocortical insufficiency other than exogenous corticosteroid therapy.
- Patients receiving doses of systemic corticosteroid greater than 6 mg daily of dexamethasone.
- Patients repeatedly taking doses in the evening.

Patients should carry 'steroid treatment' cards, which give clear guidance on the precautions to be taken to minimise risk, and which provide details of prescriber, drug, dosage, and the duration of treatment.

Administration of live virus vaccines is contra-indicated in individuals receiving immunosuppressive doses of corticosteroids. If inactivated viral or bacterial vaccines are administered to individuals receiving immunosuppressive doses of corticosteroids, the expected serum antibody response may not be obtained. However, immunisation procedures may be undertaken in patients who are receiving corticosteroids as replacement therapy, e.g. for Addison's disease.

The use of 'Decadron' Tablets in active tuberculosis should be restricted to those cases of fulminating or disseminated tuberculosis in which the corticosteroid is used for the management of the disease in conjunction with an appropriate antituberculous regimen. If corticosteroids are indicated in patients with latent tuberculosis or tuberculin reactivity, close observation of the disease is necessary as reactivation may occur. During prolonged corticosteroid therapy, these patients should receive prophylactic chemotherapy.

There is an enhanced effect of corticosteroids in patients with hypothyroidism and in those with cirrhosis.

Corticosteroids may mask some signs of infection, and new infections may appear during their use. Suppression of the inflammatory response and immune function increases the susceptibility to infections and their severity. The clinical presentation may often be atypical, and serious infections such as septicaemia and tuberculosis may be masked and reach an advanced stage before being recognised. There may be decreased resistance and inability to localise infection in patients on corticosteroids.

Chickenpox is of particular concern, since this normally minor illness may be fatal in immunosuppressed patients. Patients (or parents of children) without a definite history of chickenpox should be advised to avoid close personal contact with chickenpox or herpes zoster, and if exposed they should seek urgent medical attention. Passive immunisation with varicella/zoster immunoglobulin (VZIG) is needed by exposed non-immune patients who are receiving systemic corticosteroids or who have used them within the previous three months; this should be given within ten days of exposure to chickenpox. **If a diagnosis of chickenpox is confirmed, the illness warrants specialist care and urgent treatment. Corticosteroids should not be stopped and the dose may need to be increased.**

Measles can have a more serious or even fatal course in immunosuppressed patients. In such children or adults particular care should be taken to avoid exposure to measles. If exposed, prophylaxis with intramuscular pooled immunoglobulin (IG) may be indicated. Exposed patients should be advised to seek medical advice without delay.

Corticosteroids may activate latent amoebiasis or strongyloidiasis or exacerbate active disease. Therefore, it is recommended that latent or active amoebiasis and strongyloidiasis be ruled out before initiating corticosteroid therapy in any patient at risk of or with symptoms suggestive of either condition.

Prolonged use of corticosteroids may produce subcapsular cataracts, glaucoma with possible damage to the optic nerves, and may enhance the establishment of secondary ocular infections due to fungi or viruses. Steroids may increase or decrease the motility and number of spermatozoa.

Special precautions: Particular care is required when considering the use of systemic corticosteroids in patients with the following conditions, and frequent patient monitoring is necessary: renal insufficiency, hypertension, diabetes or in those with a family history of diabetes, congestive heart failure, osteoporosis, previous steroid myopathy, glaucoma (or family history of glaucoma), myasthenia gravis, non-specific ulcerative colitis, diverticulitis, fresh intestinal anastomosis, active or latent peptic ulcer, existing or previous history of severe affective disorders (especially previous steroid psychosis), liver failure, and epilepsy. Signs of peritoneal irritation following gastro-intestinal perforation in patients receiving large doses of corticosteroids may be minimal or absent. Fat embolism has been reported as a possible complication of hypercortisonism.

Corticosteroids should be used cautiously in patients with ocular herpes simplex, because of possible corneal perforation.

Children: Corticosteroids cause growth retardation in infancy, childhood and adolescence, which may be irreversible. Treatment should be limited to the minimum dosage for the shortest possible time. In order to minimise suppression of the hypothalamo-pituitary-adrenal axis and growth retardation, treatment should be limited, where possible, to a single dose on alternate days.

Growth and development of infants and children on prolonged corticosteroid therapy should be carefully monitored.

4.5 Interaction with other medicinal products and other forms of Interaction

'Decadron' should be used with caution with thalidomide, as toxic epidermal necrolysis has been reported with concomitant administration of these two drugs.

Aspirin should be used cautiously in conjunction with corticosteroids in hypoprothrombinaemia.

The renal clearance of salicylates is increased by corticosteroids and, therefore, salicylate dosage should be reduced along with steroid withdrawal.

Dexamethasone is metabolised by cytochrome P450 3A4 (CYP 3A4). Concomitant administration of dexamethasone with cytochrome P450 3A4 enzyme inducers (e.g. phenytoin, barbiturates,, rifabutin, carbamazepine, and rifampicin), may enhance the metabolic clearance of corticosteroids, resulting in decreased blood levels and reduced physiological activity. This may necessitate adjustment of the dosage of 'Decadron'. In addition, the concomitant administration of dexamethasone with known inhibitors of CYP 3A4 (e.g ketoconazole, macrolide antibiotics such as erythromycin) has the potential to result in increased plasma concentrations of dexamethasone. Effects of other drugs on the metabolism of dexamethasone may interfere with dexamethasone suppression tests, which should be interpreted with caution during administration of such drugs.

Dexamethasone is a moderate inducer of CYP 3A4. Co-administration with other drugs that are metabolised by CYP 3A4 (e.g. erythromycin and anti-HIV drugs such as indinavir, ritonavir, lopinavir, saquinavir) may increase their clearance, resulting in decreased plasma concentrations.

In post-marketing experience, there have been reports of both increases and decreases in phenytoin levels with dexamethasone co-administration, leading to alterations in seizure control.

Although ketoconazole may increase dexamethasone plasma concentrations through inhibition of CYP 3A4, ketoconazole alone can inhibit adrenal corticosteroid synthesis and may cause adrenal insufficiency during corticosteroid withdrawal.

Aminoglutethimide and ephedrine may enhance metabolic clearance of corticosteroids and an increase in corticosteroid dosage may be necessary.

False-negative results in the dexamethasone suppression test in patients being treated with indomethacin have been reported.

The prothrombin time should be checked frequently in patients who are receiving corticosteroids and coumarin anticoagulants at the same time as there have been reports that corticosteroids have altered the response to these anticoagulants. Studies have shown that the usual effect produced by adding corticosteroids is inhibition of response to coumarins, although there have been some conflicting reports of potentiation not substantiated by studies.

The desired effects of hypoglycaemic agents (including insulin) are antagonised by corticosteroids.

When corticosteroids are administered concomitantly with potassium-depleting diuretics, patients should be observed closely for development of hypokalaemia.

Corticosteroids may affect the nitrobluetetrazolium test for bacterial infection and produce false-negative results.

4.6 Pregnancy and lactation

The ability of corticosteroids to cross the placenta varies between individual drugs, however, dexamethasone readily crosses the placenta.

Administration of corticosteroids to pregnant animals can cause abnormalities of foetal development including cleft palate, intra-uterine growth retardation and effects on brain growth and development. There is no evidence that corticosteroids result in an increased incidence of congenital abnormalities, such as cleft palate/lip in man. However, when administered for prolonged periods or repeatedly during pregnancy, corticosteroids may increase the risk of intra-uterine growth retardation. Hypoadrenalism may, in theory, occur in the neonate following prenatal exposure to corticosteroids but usually resolves spontaneously following birth and is rarely clinically important. As with all drugs, corticosteroids should only be prescribed when the benefits to the mother and child outweigh the risks. When corticosteroids are essential however, patients with normal pregnancies may be treated as though they were in the non-gravid state.

Corticosteroids may pass into breast milk, although no data are available for dexamethasone. Infants of mothers taking high doses of systemic corticosteroids for prolonged periods may have a degree of adrenal suppression.

4.7 Effects on ability to drive and use machines
None reported.

4.8 Undesirable effects
The incidence of predictable undesirable effects, including hypothalamic-pituitary-adrenal suppression, correlates with the relative potency of the drug, dosage, timing of administration and the duration of treatment (see 'Special warnings and special precautions for use').

Fluid and electrolyte disturbances: Sodium retention, fluid retention, congestive heart failure in susceptible patients, potassium loss, hypokalaemic alkalosis, hypertension, increased calcium excretion (see 'Special warnings and special precautions for use').

Musculoskeletal effects: Muscle weakness, steroid myopathy, loss of muscle mass, osteoporosis (especially in post-menopausal females), vertebral compression fractures, aseptic necrosis of femoral and humeral heads, pathological fracture of long bones, tendon rupture.

Gastro-intestinal: Peptic ulcer with possible perforation and haemorrhage, perforation of the small and large bowel particularly in patients with inflammatory bowel disease, pancreatitis, abdominal distension, ulcerative oesophagitis, dyspepsia, oesophageal candidiasis.

Dermatological: Impaired wound healing, thin fragile skin, petechiae and ecchymoses, erythema, striae, telangiectasia, acne, increased sweating, suppressed reaction to skin tests, other cutaneous reactions such as allergic dermatitis, urticaria, angioneurotic oedema.

Neurological: Convulsions, vertigo, headache. Increased intracranial pressure with papilloedema (pseudotumour cerebri) may occur usually after treatment, psychic disturbances (e.g. euphoria, psychological dependence, depression, insomnia).

Endocrine: Menstrual irregularities, amenorrhoea, development of Cushingoid state, suppression of growth in children and adolescents, secondary adrenocortical and pituitary unresponsiveness (particularly in times of stress as in trauma, surgery or illness), decreased carbohydrate tolerance, manifestations of latent diabetes mellitus, hyperglycemia, increased requirements for insulin or oral hypoglycaemic agents in diabetics, hirsutism.

Anti-inflammatory and immunosuppressive effects: Increased susceptibility and severity of infections with suppression of clinical symptoms and signs. Opportunistic infections, recurrence of dormant tuberculosis (see 'Special warnings and special precautions for use').

Ophthalmic: Posterior subcapsular cataracts, increased intra-ocular pressure, papilloedema, corneal or scleral thinning, exacerbation of ophthalmic viral disease, glaucoma, exophthalmos.

Metabolic: Negative nitrogen balance due to protein catabolism. Negative calcium balance.

Cardiovascular: Myocardial rupture following recent myocardial infarction (see 'Special warnings and special precautions for use').

Other: Hypersensitivity, including anaphylaxis has been reported, leucocytosis, thrombo-embolism, weight gain, increased appetite, nausea, malaise, hiccups.

Withdrawal symptoms and signs

Too rapid a reduction of corticosteroid dosage following prolonged treatment can lead to acute adrenal insufficiency, hypotension, and death (see 'Special warnings and special precautions for use').

In some instances, withdrawal symptoms may simulate a clinical relapse of the disease for which the patient has been undergoing treatment.

4.9 Overdose
Reports of acute toxicity and/or deaths following overdosage with glucocorticoids are rare. No antidote is available. Treatment is probably not indicated for reactions due to chronic poisoning unless the patient has a condition that would render him unusually susceptible to ill effects from corticosteroids. In this case, the stomach should be emptied and symptomatic treatment should be instituted as necessary.

Anaphylactic and hypersensitivity reactions may be treated with epinephrine (adrenaline), positive-pressure artificial respiration and aminophylline. The patient should be kept warm and quiet.

The biological half-life of dexamethasone in plasma is about 190 minutes.

5. PHARMACOLOGICAL PROPERTIES

5.1 Pharmacodynamic properties
Dexamethasone is a glucocorticoid. It possesses the actions and effects of other basic glucocorticoids, and is among the most active members. Glucocorticoids are adrenocortical steroids, both naturally occurring and synthetic, which are readily absorbed from the gastro-intestinal tract. They cause profound and varied metabolic effects and in addition they modify the body's immune responses to diverse stimuli.

Naturally occurring glucocorticoids (hydrocortisone and cortisone), which also have salt-retaining properties, are used as replacement therapy in adrenocortical deficiency states. Their synthetic analogs, including dexamethasone, are used primarily for their potent anti-inflammatory effects in disorders of many organ systems.

5.2 Pharmacokinetic properties
Dexamethasone is readily absorbed from the gastro-intestinal tract.

Its biological half-life in plasma is about 190 minutes.

Binding of dexamethasone to plasma proteins is less than for most other corticosteroids and is estimated to be about 77%.

Up to 65% of a dose is excreted in the urine in 24 hours, the rate of excretion being increased following concomitant administration of phenytoin.

The more potent halogenated corticosteroids such as dexamethasone, appear to cross the placental barrier with minimal inactivation.

Dexamethasone has predominant glucocorticoid activity with little propensity to promote renal retention of sodium and water. Therefore, it does not offer complete replacement therapy, and must be supplemented with salt and/or deoxycorticosterone. Cortisone and hydrocortisone also act predominately as glucocorticoids, although their mineralocorticoid action is greater than that of dexamethasone. Their use in patients with total adrenocortical insufficiency also may require supplemental salt, deoxycortisone, or both.

5.3 Preclinical safety data
No relevant information.

6. PHARMACEUTICAL PARTICULARS

6.1 List of excipients
Calcium hydrogen phosphate E341, lactose Ph Eur, magnesium stearate E572, maize starch Ph Eur, purified water Ph Eur

6.2 Incompatibilities
None reported.

6.3 Shelf life
Three years.

6.4 Special precautions for storage
Store in a dry place below 25°C.

6.5 Nature and contents of container
Opaque PVC blister lidded with aluminium foil, containing 30 tablets.

6.6 Instructions for use and handling
None.

7. MARKETING AUTHORISATION HOLDER
Merck Sharp & Dohme Limited
Hertford Road, Hoddesdon, Hertfordshire EN11 9BU

8. MARKETING AUTHORISATION NUMBER(S)
PL 0025/5046R.

9. DATE OF FIRST AUTHORISATION/RENEWAL OF THE AUTHORISATION
11 February 1987/9 June 1997.

10. DATE OF REVISION OF THE TEXT
October 2003

LEGAL CATEGORY
POM.

® denotes registered trademark of Merck & Co., Inc., Whitehouse Station, NJ, USA.

MSD (logo)

Merck Sharp & Dohme Limited

Hertford Road, Hoddesdon, Hertfordshire EN11 9BU

SPC.DRNT.03.UK.0900

Decapeptyl SR 11.25mg

(Ipsen Ltd)

1. NAME OF THE MEDICINAL PRODUCT
DECAPEPTYL SR 11.25 mg, powder for suspension for injection.

2. QUALITATIVE AND QUANTITATIVE COMPOSITION
Triptorelin (I.N.N.) 15 mg, as triptorelin acetate.

The vial contains an overage to ensure that a dose of 11.25 mg is administered to the patient.

For excipients, see 6.1.

3. PHARMACEUTICAL FORM
Powder for suspension for injection, sustained release formulation.

4. CLINICAL PARTICULARS

4.1 Therapeutic indications
Treatment of advanced prostate cancer.

Treatment of endometriosis.

4.2 Posology and method of administration

__Prostate cancer__

One intramuscular injection should be administered every 3 months.

No dosage adjustment is necessary in the elderly.

__Endometriosis__

One intramuscular injection should be administered every 3 months. The treatment must be initiated in the first five days of the menstrual cycle. Treatment duration depends on the initial severity of the endometriosis and the changes observed in the clinical features (functional and anatomical) during treatment. The maximum duration of treatment should be 6 months (two injections).

A second course of treatment with DECAPEPTYL SR 11.25 mg or with other GnRH analogues should not be undertaken due to concerns about bone density losses.

4.3 Contraindications
Hypersensitivity to GnRH analogues or to any of the excipients.

In prostate cancer, DECAPEPTYL SR 11.25 mg is contraindicated in patients presenting with spinal cord compression or evidence of spinal metastases.

In endometriosis, confirm that the patient is not pregnant before beginning treatment.

4.4 Special warnings and special precautions for use
In adults the prolonged use of GnRH analogues may lead to bone loss which enhances the risk of osteoporosis.

__Prostate cancer__

Initially, DECAPEPTYL SR 11.25 mg like other GnRH analogues causes a transient increase in serum testosterone and consequent worsening of symptoms including increase in bone pain (and serum acid phosphatase levels). Continued treatment with DECAPEPTYL SR 11.25 mg leads to suppression of testosterone (and dihydrotestosterone) and consequent improvement in the disease.

During the first month of treatment, patients presenting with, or at particular risk of developing, urinary tract obstruction should be carefully monitored, as should those at risk of developing spinal cord compression. Consideration should be given to the use of an anti-androgen for three days prior to DECAPEPTYL SR 11.25 mg treatment, to counteract this initial rise in serum testosterone levels.

__Endometriosis__

At the recommended dose, DECAPEPTYL SR 11.25 mg causes a persistent hypogonadotrophic amenorrhoea. A supervening metrorrhagia in the course of treatment, other than in the first month, should lead to measurement of plasma oestradiol levels. Should this level be less than 50 pg/ml, possible associated organic lesions should be sought. After withdrawal of treatment, ovarian function resumes, with ovulation expected to occur approximately 5 months after the last injection.

A non-hormonal method of contraception should be used throughout treatment including for 3 months after the last injection.

Due to concerns about bone density losses, DECAPEPTYL SR 11.25 mg should be used with caution in women with known metabolic bone disease.

4.5 Interaction with other medicinal products and other forms of Interaction
Drugs which raise prolactin levels should not be prescribed concomitantly as they reduce the level of LHRH receptors in the pituitary.

4.6 Pregnancy and lactation
Animal studies have not revealed any teratogenic effects. During post-marketing surveillance and in a limited number of pregnant women who were exposed inadvertently to triptorelin, there were no reports of malformation or foetotoxicity attributable to the product. However, as the number of patients is too small to draw conclusions regarding the risk of foetal malformations or foetotoxicity, if a patient becomes pregnant while receiving triptorelin, therapy should be discontinued.

Triptorelin is not recommended for use during lactation.

4.7 Effects on ability to drive and use machines
No effects on ability to drive and use machines have been observed.

4.8 Undesirable effects

__Prostate cancer__

The most frequently occurring side-effects of treatment with triptorelin are hot flushes, decreased libido and impotence, each reported by > 10 % of patients in clinical trials using DECAPEPTYL SR 11.25 mg.

At the beginning of treatment increased bone pain, worsening of genito-urinary obstruction symptoms (haematuria, urinary disorders) and/or worsening of neurological signs of vertebral metastases (back pain, weakness or paresthesia of the lower limbs) are commonly observed, resulting from the initial and transient increase in plasma testosterone. These symptoms disappear in one or two weeks.

The following uncommon adverse reactions have been observed during clinical trials with other triptorelin formulations: hypertension, gynaecomastia, insomnia, mood disorders, emergence of psychiatric disorders, vertigo, dizziness.

Additional rare adverse reactions reported among patients treated with other marketed triptorelin formulations are: allergic reactions (rash, pruritus, urticaria, and very occasionally Quincke's oedema), phlebitis, dry mouth or excessive salivation, headaches, recurrence of asthma, fever, sweating, weight increase, pain/erythema/induration at injection site, gastralgia, gastric disturbance, nausea, vomiting, slight hair loss, visual disturbances.

Endometriosis

At the beginning of treatment the symptoms of endometriosis (pelvic pain, dysmenorrhoea) may be exacerbated during the initial and transient increase in plasma oestradiol levels. These symptoms should disappear in one or two weeks. Genital haemorrhage including menorrhagia, metrorrhagia or spotting may occur in the month following the first injection.

During clinical trials the adverse reactions showed a general pattern of hypo-oestrogenic events related to pituitary-ovarian blockade such as hot flushes, sweating, sleep disturbances, headache, mood changes, vaginal dryness, dyspareunia, and decreased libido.

Transient pain, redness or local inflammation at the injection site may occur.

The following adverse reactions have been observed during clinical trials with other triptorelin formulations: breast pain, muscle cramps, joint pain, weight gain, nausea, abdominal pain or discomfort, asthenia, increased blood pressure, episodes of blurred or abnormal vision, cutaneous rash, oedema, hair loss.

As with any GnRH analogue, a small loss in bone density, specifically trabecular bone density, occurs during six months of DECAPEPTYL SR 11.25 mg treatment. Clinical data suggests that this loss is reversible.

4.9 Overdose

No case of overdose has been reported. Animal data do not predict any effects other than those on sex hormone concentration and consequent effect on the reproductive tract. If overdose occurs, symptomatic management is indicated.

5. PHARMACOLOGICAL PROPERTIES

5.1 Pharmacodynamic properties

Pharmacotherapeutic group:

Gonadotrophin-Releasing Hormone analogue

L 02 A E 04: Antineoplastic and immunomodulator

Triptorelin is a synthetic decapeptide analogue of natural GnRH.

The first administration of DECAPEPTYL SR 11.25 mg stimulates the release of pituitary gonadotrophins with a transient increase in testosterone levels ("flare-up") in men and in oestradiol levels in women. Prolonged administration leads to a suppression of gonadotrophins and a fall in plasma testosterone or oestradiol to castrate levels after approximately 20 days, which is maintained for as long as the product is administered.

Continued administration of DECAPEPTYL SR 11.25 mg induces suppression of oestrogen secretion and thus enables resting of ectopic endometrial tissue.

5.2 Pharmacokinetic properties

Following intramuscular injection of DECAPEPTYL SR 11.25 mg in patients (men and women), a peak of plasma triptorelin is observed in the first 3 hours after injection. After a phase of decrease, the circulating triptorelin levels remain stable at around 0.04-0.05 ng/ml in endometriosis patients and around 0.1ng/ml in prostate cancer patients until day 90.

5.3 Preclinical safety data

The compound did not demonstrate any specific toxicity in animal toxicological studies. The effects observed are related to the pharmacological properties of triptorelin on the endocrine system.

6. PHARMACEUTICAL PARTICULARS

6.1 List of excipients

D,L lactide-glycolide copolymer

Mannitol

Carmellose sodium

Polysorbate 80.

6.2 Incompatibilities

This medicinal product must not be mixed with other medicinal products except the one mentioned in 6.6.

6.3 Shelf life

2 years.

The product should be used immediately after reconstitution.

6.4 Special precautions for storage

Do not store above 25°C. Keep container in the outer carton.

6.5 Nature and contents of container

A type I, 4 ml capacity glass vial with an elastomer stopper and an aluminium cap containing the powder.

A type I, 3 ml capacity glass ampoule containing 2 ml of the suspension vehicle.

One syringe and 2 needles.

6.6 Instructions for use and handling

The suspension for injection must be reconstituted following the aseptic technique and using exclusively the provided ampoule of mannitol solution 0.8% for injection, suspension vehicle for DECAPEPTYL SR 11.25mg.

The suspension vehicle should be drawn into the syringe provided using the pink needle and transferred to the vial containing the powder for injection. The vial should be gently shaken and the mixture then drawn back into the syringe without inverting the vial. The needle should then be changed and the green needle used to administer the injection immediately. The vial is intended for single use only and any remaining product should be discarded.

7. MARKETING AUTHORISATION HOLDER

Ipsen Limited

190 Bath Road

Slough

Berkshire

SL1 3XE

United Kingdom

8. MARKETING AUTHORISATION NUMBER(S)

06958/0016

9. DATE OF FIRST AUTHORISATION/RENEWAL OF THE AUTHORISATION

10. DATE OF REVISION OF THE TEXT

09 September 2004

Decapeptyl SR 3mg

(Ipsen Ltd)

1. NAME OF THE MEDICINAL PRODUCT

DECAPEPTYL SR 3 mg, powder for suspension for injection.

2. QUALITATIVE AND QUANTITATIVE COMPOSITION

Triptorelin (I.N.N.) 4.2 mg, as triptorelin acetate.

The vial contains an overage to ensure that a dose of 3 mg is administered to the patient.

For excipients, see 6.1.

3. PHARMACEUTICAL FORM

Powder for suspension for injection, sustained release formulation.

4. CLINICAL PARTICULARS

4.1 Therapeutic indications

Treatment of advanced prostate cancer.

Treatment of endometriosis.

Treatment of uterine fibroids prior to surgery or when surgery is not appropriate.

4.2 Posology and method of administration

Advanced prostate cancer

One intramuscular injection should be administered every 4 weeks (28 days). No dosage adjustment is necessary in the elderly.

Endometriosis and uterine fibroids

One intramuscular injection every 28 days. For the treatment of endometriosis and uterine fibroids the treatment must be initiated in the first five days of the cycle. The maximum duration of treatment should be 6 months. For patients with uterine fibroids DECAPEPTYL SR 3 mg should be administered for a minimum of 3 months.

A second course of treatment by DECAPEPTYL SR 3 mg or by other GnRH analogues should not be undertaken due to concerns about bone density losses.

4.3 Contraindications

Hypersensitivity to GnRH analogues or to any of the excipients.

In prostate cancer, DECAPEPTYL SR 3 mg should not be prescribed in patients presenting with spinal cord compression or evidence of spinal metastases.

In endometriosis and uterine fibroid treatment, confirm that the patient is not pregnant before beginning treatment.

4.4 Special warnings and special precautions for use

Advanced prostate cancer

Initially, DECAPEPTYL SR 3 mg causes a transient increase in serum testosterone and consequent worsening of symptoms including increase in bone pain (and acid phosphatase levels). Consideration should be given to the use of an anti-androgen for three days prior to DECAPEPTYL SR 3 mg treatment, to counteract this initial rise in serum testosterone levels. During the first month of treatment, patients presenting with, or at particular risk of developing, ureteric obstruction should be carefully monitored, as should those at risk of developing spinal cord compression. Continued treatment with DECAPEPTYL SR 3 mg leads to suppression of testosterone (and dihydrotestosterone) and consequent improvement in the disease.

Endometriosis and uterine fibroids

Regular administration, every 28 days of one vial of DECAPEPTYL SR 3 mg causes a persistent hypogonadotrophic amenorrhoea. During the first month of treatment, a non-hormonal contraception should be given. A supervening metrorrhagia in the course of treatment, other than in the first month, should lead to measurement of plasma oestradiol levels. Should this level be less than 50 pg/ml, possible associated organic lesions should be sought. After withdrawal of treatment, ovarian function resumes and ovulation occurs on average 58 days after the last injection, with first menses occurring on average 70 days after the last injection. Contraception may therefore be required. Due to concerns about bone density losses, DECAPEPTYL SR 3 mg should be used with caution in women with known metabolic bone disease.

4.5 Interaction with other medicinal products and other forms of Interaction

Drugs which raise prolactin levels should not be prescribed concomitantly as they reduce the level of LHRH receptors in the pituitary.

4.6 Pregnancy and lactation

Reproductive studies in primates have shown no maternal toxicity or embryotoxicity, and there was no effect on parturition. Inadvertent administration of triptorelin during human pregnancy has not demonstrated a teratogenic or other foetal risk. However, it is recommended that DECAPEPTYL SR 3 mg should not be used during pregnancy or lactation.

4.7 Effects on ability to drive and use machines

There is no evidence that DECAPEPTYL SR 3 mg has any effect on the ability to drive or operate machinery.

4.8 Undesirable effects

Prostate cancer

In prostate cancer patients, the most frequent side-effects of hot flushes, decreased libido, and impotence are a result of the decrease in testosterone levels. Bone pain, as a result of "disease flare", occurs occasionally. Pain and erythema at injection site, phlebitis and moderate and transient hypertension have been reported. On rare occasions the following have been reported: gynaecomastia, gastralgia, dry mouth, headaches, recurrence of asthma, increased dysuria, fever, pruritus, sweating, paresthesias, dizziness, insomnia, excessive salivation, gastric disturbance, nausea, vertigo, slight hair loss, induration at injection site.

Endometriosis and uterine fibroid patients

In endometriosis and uterine fibroid patients, adverse effects such as hot flushes, menorrhagia and vaginal dryness, reflect the efficacy of pituitary-ovarian blockade. Cutaneous rash, hair loss, asthenia, headache, weight gain, oedema, arthralgia, myalgia, transient sight disturbances and temporary hypertension may occur. As with any GnRH analogue, a small loss in bone density, specifically trabecular bone density, occurs during six months of DECAPEPTYL SR 3 mg treatment. Clinical data suggests that this loss is reversible.

In the studies of uterine fibroids, surgical intervention as a result of an increase in vaginal haemorrhage was a rare complication of GnRH therapy.

With uterine fibroid patients it is important to monitor the early response to GnRH analogues and if there is no change or even an increase in uterine volume then the possibility of uterine leiomyosarcoma should be considered.

4.9 Overdose

There is no human experience of overdosage. Animal data do not predict any effects other than those on sex hormone concentration and consequent effect on the reproductive tract. If overdosage occurs, symptomatic management is indicated.

5. PHARMACOLOGICAL PROPERTIES

5.1 Pharmacodynamic properties

Pharmacotherapeutic group: Gonadotrophin-Releasing Hormone analogue

L 02 A E 04: Antineoplastic and immunomodulator

Triptorelin is a decapeptide analogue of GnRH which initially stimulates release of pituitary gonadotrophins.

Prostate cancer patients

This results in an increase in peripheral circulating levels of testosterone and dihydrotestosterone. Continued administration (over 7 days) however, leads to suppression of gonadotrophins and a consequent fall in plasma testosterone. In prostate cancer patients, plasma testosterone levels fall to castrate levels after 2-3 weeks of treatment, frequently resulting in an improvement of function and objective symptoms.

Endometriosis and Uterine fibroid patients

Continued administration of DECAPEPTYL SR 3 mg induces suppression of oestrogen secretion and thus enables resting of ectopic endometrial tissue. In pre-operative therapy for uterine fibroids there appears to be a beneficial effect on the blood loss at surgery. Studies have demonstrated a consistent and marked reduction in uterine and/or fibroid volume becoming maximal in a three to six month treatment period. Clinical studies have shown that 90-100% of fibroid patients become amenorrhoeic within two months of treatment and triptorelin provides relief from the symptoms of abdominal pain, dysmenorrhoea and menorrhagia associated with uterine fibroids.

5.2 Pharmacokinetic properties
SUBCUTANEOUS FORM
In healthy volunteers
Subcutaneously administered triptorelin (100 μg) is rapidly absorbed (Tmax = 0.63 ± 0.26 hr for peak plasma concentration = 1.85 ± 0.23 ng/ml). Elimination is effected with a biological half-life of 7.6 ± 1.6 hr, after a 3 to 4 hr distribution phase. Total plasma clearance is: 161 ± 28 ml/min. Distribution volume is 104.1 ± 11.7 litres.
In prostate cancer patients
With subcutaneous administration (100 μg), triptorelin blood levels oscillate between maximum values of 1.28 ± 0.24 ng/ml (Cmax) obtained in general one hour after injection (Tmax) and minimum values of 0.28 ± 0.15 ng/ml (Cmin) obtained 24 hrs after injection.

The biological half-life is on average 11.7 ± 3.4 hr but varies according to patients. Plasma clearance (118 ± 32 ml/min) reflects slower elimination in patients, whilst distribution volumes are close to those of healthy volunteers (113.4 ± 21.6 litres).

SUSTAINED RELEASE FORM
Prostate cancer patients
Following intramuscular injection of the sustained release form, an initial phase of release of the active principle present on the surface of the microspheres is observed, followed by further fairly regular release (Cmax = 0.32 ± 0.12 ng/ml), with a mean rate of release of triptorelin of 46.6 ± 7.1 μg/day. The bioavailability of the microparticles is approximately 53% at one month.
Endometriosis and uterine fibroid patients
After intramuscular injection of DECAPEPTYL SR 3 mg in endometriosis and uterine fibroid patients the maximum blood level of triptorelin is obtained between 2 to 6 hours after injection, the peak value reached is 11 ng/ml. There was no evidence of accumulation of the product following monthly injections over six months. The minimum blood level oscillates between 0.1 and 0.2 ng/ml. The bioavailability of the sustained release product is approximately 50%.

5.3 Preclinical safety data
Preclinical findings were only those related to the expected pharmacological activity of triptorelin, namely down-regulation of the hypothalamic-pituitary-gonadal axis. These included atrophy of the testes and genital tract, with resultant suppression of spermatogenesis, together with decreased weight of the prostate gland. These findings were largely reversible within the recovery period. In a small number of rats, in a 24 months oncogenicity study, a low incidence of benign histological changes were seen in the non-glandular part of the fore stomach. Erosions, ulcers, necrosis and inflammation were seen at varying degrees of severity. The clinical relevance of these findings is unknown. The increased incidence of adenomatous tumours in the rat pituitary observed with DECAPEPTYL following long-term repeated dosing is thought to be a class specific action of GnRH analogues due to an hormonally-mediated mechanism and has not been found in the mouse nor has it been described in man.

Standard mutagenicity testing revealed no mutagenic activity of triptorelin.

6. PHARMACEUTICAL PARTICULARS
6.1 List of excipients
D,L-lactide/glycolide copolymer

Mannitol

Carmellose sodium

Polysorbate 80

6.2 Incompatibilities
This medicinal product must not be mixed with other medicinal products except those mentioned in 6.6.

6.3 Shelf life
18 months.

The product should be used immediately after reconstitution.

6.4 Special precautions for storage
Do not store above 25°C. Keep the container in the outer carton.

6.5 Nature and contents of container
A type I, 5 ml capacity glass vial with an elastomer stopper and an aluminium cap containing the powder.

A type I, 3 ml capacity glass ampoule containing 2 ml of the suspension vehicle.

One syringe and two needles.

6.6 Instructions for use and handling
The suspension for injection must be reconstituted following the aseptic technique and using exclusively the provided ampoule of mannitol solution 0.8% for injection, suspension vehicle for DECAPEPTYL SR 3 mg.

The vehicle should be drawn into the syringe provided using the pink needle and transferred to the vial containing the powder for injection. The vial should be gently shaken and the mixture then drawn back into the syringe without inverting the vial. The needle should then be changed and the green needle used to administer the injection immediately.

7. MARKETING AUTHORISATION HOLDER
Ipsen Limited

190 Bath Road

Slough

Berkshire

SL1 3XE

United Kingdom

8. MARKETING AUTHORISATION NUMBER(S)
PL 06958/0017

9. DATE OF FIRST AUTHORISATION/RENEWAL OF THE AUTHORISATION
10 January 2002

10. DATE OF REVISION OF THE TEXT
September 2003

Decubal Clinic

(Alpharma Limited)

1. NAME OF THE MEDICINAL PRODUCT
DECUBAL® CLINIC

2. QUALITATIVE AND QUANTITATIVE COMPOSITION
Dimeticone 50mg/g

Wool fat 60mg/g

Glycerol (85%) 100mg/g

Isopropyl myristate 170mg/g

3. PHARMACEUTICAL FORM
Cream.

4. CLINICAL PARTICULARS
4.1 Therapeutic indications
Treatment and prophylactic care of dry and sensitive skin, for example in Ichthyosis, Psoriasis, Dermatitis and Hyperkeratosis.

4.2 Posology and method of administration
Posology
A thin layer of the cream should be gently massaged into the skin three times daily or at appropriate intervals.

4.3 Contraindications
Known hypersensitivity to the ingredients.

4.4 Special warnings and special precautions for use
Should not be used on open wounds but can be used on cracked skin associated with dry skin conditions. Avoid contact with the eyes.

4.5 Interaction with other medicinal products and other forms of Interaction
None known.

4.6 Pregnancy and lactation
No restrictions for use.

4.7 Effects on ability to drive and use machines
None.

4.8 Undesirable effects
No serious adverse reactions have been reported.

4.9 Overdose
Not applicable.

5. PHARMACOLOGICAL PROPERTIES
5.1 Pharmacodynamic properties
Decubal Clinic cream is a cream base consisting of well-known excipients commonly used in medicinal products for topical use. Decubal Clinic is an oil-in-water emulsion and therefore suitable for use on dry and moist skin. The cream has emollient, moisturising, and protective properties.

5.2 Pharmacokinetic properties
Not applicable.

5.3 Preclinical safety data
None.

6. PHARMACEUTICAL PARTICULARS
6.1 List of excipients
Also contains: Sorbic acid, cetyl alcohol, polysorbate 60, sorbitan monostearate, purified water

6.2 Incompatibilities
None known.

6.3 Shelf life
Shelf-life
3 years

Shelf-life after dilution/reconstitution
Not applicable.

Shelf-life after first opening
Not applicable.

6.4 Special precautions for storage
Store below 25°C.

6.5 Nature and contents of container
Aluminium polyethylene laminate tubes, with screwcap closure. Packaged in cartons.

Package sizes: 50g, 100g, and 250g.

6.6 Instructions for use and handling
None

Administrative Data
7. MARKETING AUTHORISATION HOLDER
Dumex Ltd

Whiddon Valley

BARNSTAPLE

N Devon

EX32 8NS

8. MARKETING AUTHORISATION NUMBER(S)
PL 10183/0002

9. DATE OF FIRST AUTHORISATION/RENEWAL OF THE AUTHORISATION
November 1991

November 1996

10. DATE OF REVISION OF THE TEXT
September 1999

Deltacortril Enteric

(Pfizer Limited)

1. NAME OF THE MEDICINAL PRODUCT
DELTACORTRIL ® ENTERIC

2. QUALITATIVE AND QUANTITATIVE COMPOSITION
Prednisolone 2.5mg

Prednisolone 5mg

3. PHARMACEUTICAL FORM
Tablets 2.5 mg, uniformly brown in colour and coded 'Pfizer'.

Tablets 5mg, uniformly maroon in colour and coded 'Pfizer'.

4. CLINICAL PARTICULARS
4.1 Therapeutic indications
Allergy and anaphylaxis: bronchial asthma, drug hypersensitivity reactions, serum sickness, angioneurotic oedema, anaphylaxis.

Arteritis/collagenosis: giant cell arteritis/polymyalgia rheumatica, mixed connective tissue disease, polyarteritis nodosa, polymyositis.

Blood disorders: haemolytic anaemia (auto-immune), leukaemia (acute and chronic lymphocytic), lymphoma, multiple myeloma, idiopathic thrombocytopenic purpura.

Cardiovascular disorders: post-myocardial infarction syndrome, rheumatic fever with severe carditis.

Endocrine disorders: primary and secondary adrenal insufficiency, congenital adrenal hyperplasia.

Gastro-intestinal disorders: Crohn's disease, ulcerative colitis, persistent coeliac syndrome (coeliac disease unresponsive to gluten withdrawal), auto-immune chronic active hepatitis, multisystem disease affecting liver, biliary peritonitis.

Hypercalcaemia: sarcoidosis, vitamin D excess.

Infections (with appropriate chemotherapy): helminthic infestations, Herxheimer reaction, infectious mononucleosis, miliary tuberculosis, mumps orchitis (adult), tuberculous meningitis, rickettsial disease.

Muscular disorders: polymyositis, dermatomyositis.

Neurological disorders: infantile spasms, Shy-Drager syndrome, sub-acute demyelinating polyneuropathy.

Ocular disease: scleritis, posterior uveitis, retinal vasculitis, pseudo-tumours of the orbit, giant cell arteritis, malignant ophthalmic Graves disease.

Renal disorders: lupus nephritis, acute interstitial nephritis, minimal change glomerulonephritis.

Respiratory disease: allergic pneumonitis, asthma, occupational asthma, pulmonary aspergillosis, pulmonary fibrosis, pulmonary alveolitis, aspiration of foreign body, aspiration of stomach contents, pulmonary sarcoid, drug induced lung disease, adult respiratory distress syndrome, spasmodic croup.

Rheumatic disorders: rheumatoid arthritis, polymyalgia rheumatica, juvenile chronic arthritis, systemic lupus erythematosus, dermatomyositis, mixed connective tissue disease.

Skin disorders: pemphigus vulgaris, bullous pemphigoid, systemic lupus erythematosus, pyoderma gangrenosum.

Miscellaneous: sarcoidosis, hyperpyrexia, Behçets disease, immunosuppression in organ transplantation.

4.2 Posology and method of administration
The initial dosage of Deltacortril Enteric may vary from 5mg to 60mg daily depending on the disorder being treated. Divided daily dosage is usually used.

The following therapeutic guidelines should be kept in mind for all therapy with corticosteroids:

Corticosteroids are palliative symptomatic treatment by virtue of their anti-inflammatory effects; they are never curative.

The appropriate individual dose must be determined by trial and error and must be re-evaluated regularly according to activity of the disease.

As corticosteroid therapy becomes prolonged and as the dose is increased, the incidence of disabling side-effects increases.

In general, initial dosage shall be maintained or adjusted until the anticipated response is observed. The dose should be gradually reduced until the lowest dose which will maintain an adequate clinical response is reached. Use of the lowest effective dose may also minimise side-effects (see 'Special warnings and special precautions for use').

In patients who have received more than physiological dose for systemic corticosteroids (approximately 7.5mg prednisolone or equivalent) for greater than 3 weeks, withdrawal should not be abrupt. How dose reduction should be carried out depends largely on whether the disease is likely to relapse as the dose of systemic corticosteroids is reduced. Clinical assessment of disease activity may be needed during withdrawal. If the disease is unlikely to relapse on withdrawal of systemic corticosteroids but there is uncertainty about hypothalamic-pituitary-adrenal (HPA) suppression, the dose of corticosteroid may be reduced rapidly to physiological doses. Once a daily dose equivalent to 7.5mg of prednisolone is reached, dose reduction should be slower to allow the HPA-axis to recover.

Abrupt withdrawal of systemic corticosteroid treatment, which has continued up to 3 weeks is appropriate if it is considered that the disease is unlikely to relapse. Abrupt withdrawal of doses of up to 40mg daily of prednisolone, or equivalent for 3 weeks is unlikely to lead to clinically relevant HPA-axis suppression, in the majority of patients. In the following patient groups, gradual withdrawal of systemic corticosteroid therapy should be considered even after courses lasting 3 weeks or less:

- patients who have had repeated courses of systemic corticosteroids, particularly if taken for greater than 3 weeks.
- when a short course has been prescribed within one year of cessation of long-term therapy (months or years).
- patients who may have reasons for adrenocortical insufficiency other than exogenous corticosteroid therapy.
- patients receiving doses of systemic corticosteroid greater than 40mg daily of prednisolone (or equivalent).
- patients repeatedly taking doses in the evening.

(See 'Special warnings and special precautions for use' and 'Undesirable effects')

During prolonged therapy, dosage may need to be temporarily increased during periods of stress or during exacerbations of the disease (see 'Special warnings and special precautions for use')

If there is lack of a satisfactory clinical response to Deltacortril Enteric, the drug should be gradually discontinued and the patient transferred to alternative therapy.

Intermittent dosage regimen A single dose of Deltacortril Enteric in the morning on alternate days or at longer intervals is acceptable therapy for some patients. When this regimen is practical, the degree of pituitary-adrenal suppression can be minimised.

Specific dosage guidelines The following recommendations for some corticosteroid-responsive disorders are for guidance only. Acute or severe disease may require initial high dose therapy with reduction to the lowest effective maintenance dose as soon as possible. Dosage reductions should not exceed 5-7.5mg daily during chronic treatment.

Allergic and skin disorders Initial doses of 5-15mg daily are commonly adequate.

Collagenosis Initial doses of 20-30mg daily are frequently effective. Those with more severe symptoms may require higher doses.

Rheumatoid arthritis The usual initial dose is 10-15mg daily. The lowest daily maintenance dose compatible with tolerable symptomatic relief is recommended.

Blood disorders and lymphoma An initial daily dose of 15-60mg is often necessary with reduction after an adequate clinical or haematological response. Higher doses may be necessary to induce remission in acute leukaemia.

Use in childrenAlthough appropriate fractions of the actual dose may be used, dosage will usually be determined by clinical response as in adults (see also 'Special warnings and special precautions for use'). Alternate day dosage is preferable where possible.

Use in elderlyTreatment of elderly patients, particularly if long-term, should be planned bearing in mind the more serious consequences of the common side-effects of corticosteroids in old age (see also 'Special warnings and special precautions for use').

4.3 Contraindications

Systemic infections unless specific anti-infective therapy is employed. Hypersensitivity to any ingredient. Ocular herpes simplex because of possible perforation.

4.4 Special warnings and special precautions for use

Caution is necessary when oral corticosteroids, including Deltacortril Enteric, are prescribed in patients with the following conditions, and frequent patient monitoring is necessary.

- Tuberculosis: Those with a previous history of, or X-ray changes characteristic of, tuberculosis. The emergence of active tuberculosis can, however, be prevented by the prophylactic use of anti-tuberculosis therapy.

- Hypertension.

- Congestive heart failure.

- Liver failure.

- Renal insufficiency.

- Diabetes mellitus or in those with a family history of diabetes.

- Osteoporosis: This is of special importance in post-menopausal females who are at particular risk.

- Patients with a history of severe affective disorders and particularly those with a previous history of steroid-induced psychoses.

- Also, existing emotional instability or psychotic tendencies may be aggravated by corticosteroids including prednisolone

- Epilepsy,. and/or seizure disorders

- Peptic ulceration.

- Previous steroid myopathy.

- Glucocorticoids should be used cautiously in patients with myasthenia gravis receiving anticholinesterase therapy.

- Because cortisone has been reported rarely to increase blood coagulability and to precipitate intravascular thrombosis, thromboembolism, and thrombophlebitis, corticosteroids should be used with caution in patients with thromboembolic disorders.

A Patient Information Leaflet is supplied with this product.

Undesirable effects may be minimised by using the lowest effective dose for the minimum period and by administering the daily requirement as a single morning dose on alternate days. Frequent patient review is required to titrate the dose appropriately against disease activity (see 'Posology and method of administration').

Adrenocortical Insufficiency Pharmacologic doses of corticosteroids administered for prolonged periods may result in hypothalamic-pituitary-adrenal (HPA) suppression (secondary adrenocortical insufficiency). The degree and duration of adrenocortical insufficiency produced is variable among patients and depends on the dose, frequency, time of administration, and duration of glucocorticoid therapy.

In addition, acute adrenal insufficiency leading to a fatal outcome may occur if glucocorticoids are withdrawn abruptly. Drug-induced secondary adrenocortical insufficiency may therefore be minimized by gradual reduction of dosage. This type of relative insufficiency may persist for months after discontinuation of therapy; therefore, in any situation of stress occurring during that period, hormone therapy should be reinstituted. Since mineralocorticoid secretion may be impaired, salt and/or a mineralocorticoid should be administered concurrently. During prolonged therapy any intercurrent illness, trauma, or surgical procedure will require a temporary increase in dosage; if corticosteroids have been stopped following prolonged therapy they may need to be temporarily re-introduced.

Patients should carry "Steroid treatment" cards which give clear guidance on the precautions to be taken to minimise risk and which provide details of prescriber, drug, dosage and the duration of treatment.

Anti-inflammatory/Immunosuppressive effects and Infection Suppression of the inflammatory response and immune function increases the susceptibility to infections and their severity. The clinical presentation may often be atypical and serious infection such as septicaemia and tuberculosis may be masked and may reach an advanced stage before being recognised when corticosteroids including prednisolone are used. The immunosuppressive effects of glucocorticoids may result in activation of latent infection or exacerbation of intercurrent infections.

Chickenpox Chickenpox is of particular concern since this normally minor illness may be fatal in immunosuppressed patients. Patients (or parents of children) without a definite history of chickenpox should be advised to avoid close personal contact with chickenpox or herpes zoster and if exposed they should seek urgent medical attention. Passive immunisation with varicella-zoster immunoglobulin (VZIG) is needed by exposed non-immune patients who are receiving systemic corticosteroids or who have used them within the previous 3 months; this should be given within 10 days of exposure to chickenpox. If a diagnosis of chickenpox is confirmed, the illness warrants specialist care and urgent treatment. Corticosteroids should not be stopped and the dose may need to be increased. The effect of corticosteroids may be enhanced in patients with hypothyroidism and in those with chronic liver disease with impaired hepatic function.

Measles Patients should be advised to take particular care to avoid exposure to measles, and to seek immediate medical advice if exposure occurs. Prophylaxis with intramuscular normal immunoglobulin may be needed.

Administration of Live Vaccines Live vaccines should not be given to individuals on high doses of corticosteroids, due to impaired immune response. Live vaccines should be postponed until at least 3 months after stopping corticosteroid therapy. (See also section 4.5 Interactions.)

Ocular EffectsProlonged use of corticosteroids may produce posterior subcapsular cataracts and nuclear cataracts (particularly in children), exophthalmos, or increased intraocular pressure, which may result in glaucoma with possible damage to the optic nerves. Establishment of secondary fungal and viral infections of the eye may also be enhanced in patients receiving glucocorticoids.

Corticosteroids should be used cautiously in patients with ocular herpes simplex because of possible perforation.

Cushing's disease Because glucocorticoids can produce or aggravate *Cushing's syndrome*, glucocorticoids should be avoided in patients with Cushing's disease

There is an enhanced effect of corticosteroids in patients with hypothyroidism and in those with cirrhosis.

Psychic derangements may appear when corticosteroids, including prednisolone, are used, ranging from euphoria, insomnia, mood swings, personality changes, and severe depression, to frank psychotic manifestations.

Use in children Corticosteroids cause growth retardation in infancy, childhood and adolescence, which may be irreversible, and therefore long-term administration of pharmacological doses should be avoided. If prolonged therapy is necessary, treatment should be limited to the minimum suppression of the hypothalamo-pituitary adrenal axis and growth retardation. The growth and development of infants and children should be closely monitored. Treatment should be administered where possible as a single dose on alternate days

Use in the elderly Treatment of elderly patients, particularly if long term, should be planned bearing in mind the more serious consequences of the common side-effects of corticosteroids in old age, especially osteoporosis, diabetes, hypertension, hypokalaemia, susceptibility to infection and thinning of the skin. Close clinical supervision is required to avoid life threatening reactions.

4.5 Interaction with other medicinal products and other forms of Interaction

Hepatic microsomal enzyme inducers Drugs that induce hepatic enzyme cytochrome P-450 (CYP) isoenzyme 3A4 such as phenobarbital, phenytoin, rifampicin, rifabutin, carbamazepine, primidone and aminoglutethimide may reduce the therapeutic efficacy of corticosteroids by increasing the rate of metabolism. Lack of expected response may be observed and dosage of Deltacortril Enteric may need to be increased.

Hepatic microsomal enzyme inhibitors Drugs that inhibit hepatic enzyme cytochrome P-450 (CYP) isoenzyme 3A4 (e.g. ketoconazole, troleandomycin) may decrease glucocorticoid clearance. Dosages of glucocorticoids given in combination with such drugs may need to be decreased to avoid potential adverse effects.

Antidiabetic agents Glucocorticoids may increase blood glucose levels. Patients with diabetes mellitus receiving concurrent insulin and/or oral hypoglycemic agents may require dosage adjustments of such therapy.

Non-steroidal anti-inflammatory drugs Concomitant administration of ulcerogenic drugs such as indomethacin during corticosteroid therapy may increase the risk of GI ulceration. Aspirin should be used cautiously in conjunction with glucocorticoids in patients with hypoprothrombinaemia. Although concomitant therapy with salicylate and corticosteroids does not appear to increase the incidence or severity of GI ulceration, the possibility of this effect should be considered.

Serum salicylate concentrations may decrease when corticosteroids are administered concomitantly. The renal clearance of salicylates is increased by corticosteroids and steroid withdrawal may result in salicylate intoxication. Salicylates and corticosteroids should be used concurrently with caution. Patients receiving both drugs should be observed closely for adverse effects of either drug.

Antibacterials Rifamycins accelerate metabolism of corticosteroids and thus may reduce their effect. Erythromycin inhibits metabolism of methylprednisolone and possibly other corticosteroids.

Anticoagulants Response to anticoagulants may be reduced or, less often, enhanced by corticosteroids. Close monitoring of the INR or prothrombin time is required to avoid spontaneous bleeding.

Antiepileptics Carbamazepine, phenobarbital, phenytoin, and primidone accelerate metabolism of corticosteroids and may reduce their effect.

AntifungalsRisk of hypokalaemia may be increased with amphotericin, therefore concomitant use with corticosteroids should be avoided unless corticosteroids are required to control reactions; ketoconazole inhibits metabolism of methylprednisolone and possibly other corticosteroids.

Antivirals Ritonavir possibly increases plasma concentrations of prednisolone and other corticosteroids.

Cardiac Glycosides Increased toxicity if hypokalaemia occurs with corticosteroids.

Ciclosporin Concomitant administration of prednisolone and ciclosporin may result in decreased plasma clearance of prednisolone (i.e. increased plasma concentration of prednisolone). The need for appropriate dosage adjustment should be considered when these drugs are administered concomitantly.

Cytotoxics Increased risk of haematological toxicity with methotrexate.

Mifepristone Effect of corticosteroids may be reduced for 3-4 days after mifepristone.

Vaccines Live vaccines should not be given to individuals with impaired immune responsiveness. The antibody response to other vaccines may be diminished.

Oestrogens Oestrogens may potentiate the effects of glucocorticoids and dosage adjustments may be required if oestrogens are added to or withdrawn from a stable dosage regimen.

Somatropin Growth promoting effect may be inhibited.

Sympathomimetics Increased risk of hypokalaemia if high doses of corticosteroids given with high doses of bambuterol, fenoteral, formoterol, ritodrine, salbutamol, salmeterol and terbutaline.

Other The desired effects of hypoglycaemic agents (including insulin), antihypertensives and diuretics are antagonised by corticosteroids; and the hypokalaemic effect of acetazolamide, loop diuretics, thiazide diuretics, carbenoxolone and theophylline are enhanced.

4.6 Pregnancy and lactation

Use in pregnancy The ability of corticosteroids to cross the placenta varies between individual drugs, however, 88% of prednisolone is inactivated as it crosses the placenta. Administration of corticosteroids to pregnant animals can cause abnormalities of foetal development including cleft palate, intra-uterine growth retardation and effects on brain growth and development. There is no evidence that corticosteroids result in an increased incidence of congenital abnormalities, such as cleft palate/lip in man. However, when administered for prolonged periods or repeatedly during pregnancy, corticosteroids may increase the risk of intra-uterine growth retardation. Hypoadrenalism may, in theory, occur in the neonate following prenatal exposure to corticosteroids but usually resolves spontaneously following birth and is rarely clinically important. Cataracts have been observed in infants born to mothers treated with long-term prednisolone during pregnancy. As with all drugs, corticosteroids should only be prescribed when the benefits to the mother and child outweigh the risks. When corticosteroids are essential however, patients with normal pregnancies may be treated as though they were in the non-gravid state.

Patients with pre-eclampsia or fluid retention require close monitoring.

Use in lactation Corticosteroids are excreted in small amounts in breast milk. Corticosteroids distributed into breast milk may suppress growth and interfere with endogenous glucocorticoid production in nursing infants. Since adequate reproductive studies have not been performed in humans with glucocorticoids, these drugs should be administered to nursing mothers only if the benefits of therapy are judged to outweigh the potential risks to the infant.

4.7 Effects on ability to drive and use machines

The effect of Deltacortril Enteric on the ability to drive or use machinery has not been evaluated. There is no evidence to suggest that prednisolone may affect these abilities.

4.8 Undesirable effects

The incidence of predictable undesirable effects, including hypothalamic-pituitary adrenal suppression correlates with the relative potency of the drug, dosage, timing of administration and the duration of treatment (see 'Special warnings and special precautions for use').

Body as a WholeLeucocytosis, hypersensitivity including anaphylaxis, thromboembolism, fatigue, malaise.

Cardiovascular congestive heart failure in susceptible patients, hypertension

Gastro-intestinal Dyspepsia, nausea, peptic ulceration with perforation and haemorrhage, abdominal distension, abdominal pain, increased appetite which may result in weight gain, diarrhoea, oesophageal ulceration, oesophageal candidiasis, acute pancreatitis.

Musculo-skeletal Proximal myopathy, osteoporosis, vertebral and long bone fractures, avascular osteonecrosis, tendon rupture, myalgia.

Metabolic/Nutritional Sodium and water retention, hypokalaemic alkalosis, potassium loss, negative nitrogen and calcium balance.

Skin/Appendages Impaired healing, hirsutism, skin atrophy, bruising, striae, telangiectasia, acne, increased sweating, may suppress reactions to skin tests, pruritis, rash, urticaria.

Endocrine Suppression of the hypothalamo-pituitary adrenal axis particularly in times of stress, as in trauma, surgery or illness, growth suppression in infancy, childhood and adolescence, menstrual irregularity and amenorrhoea. Cushingoid facies, weight gain, impaired carbohydrate tolerance with increased requirement for antidiabetic therapy, manifestation of latent diabetes mellitus, Increased appetite.

Central and Peripheral Nervous System Euphoria, psychological dependence, depression, insomnia, dizziness, headache, vertigo. Raised intracranial pressure with papilloedema (pseudotumor cerebri) in children, usually after treatment withdrawal. Aggravation of schizophrenia. Aggravation of epilepsy.

VisionIncreased intra-ocular pressure, glaucoma, papilloedema, posterior subcapsular cataracts, exophthalmos, corneal or scleral thinning, exacerbation of ophthalmic viral or fungal disease.

Anti-inflammatory and immunosuppressive effects Increases susceptibility to, and severity of infections with suppression of clinical symptoms and signs, opportunistic infections, recurrence of dormant tuberculosis (see 'Special warnings and special precautions for use').

Withdrawal symptoms Too rapid a reduction of corticosteroid dosage following prolonged treatment can lead to acute adrenal insufficiency, hypotension and death (see 'Special warnings and special precautions for use' and 'Posology and method of administration'). A steroid "withdrawal syndrome" seemingly unrelated to adrenocortical insufficiency may also occur following abrupt discontinuance of glucocorticoids. This syndrome includes symptoms such as: anorexia, nausea, vomiting, lethargy, headache, fever, joint pain, desquamation, myalgia, arthralgia, rhinitis, conjunctivitis, painful itchy skin nodules weight loss, and/or hypotension. These effects are thought to be due to the sudden change in glucocorticoid concentration rather than to low corticosteroid levels.

4.9 Overdose

Reports of acute toxicity and/or death following overdosage of glucocorticoids are rare. No specific antidote is available; treatment is supportive and symptomatic. Serum electrolytes should be monitored.

5. PHARMACOLOGICAL PROPERTIES

5.1 Pharmacodynamic properties

Naturally occurring glucocorticoids (hydrocortisone and cortisone), which also have salt- retaining properties, are used as replacement therapy in adrenocortical deficiency states. Their synthetic analogs are primarily used for their potent anti-inflammatory effects in disorders of many organ systems.

Glucocorticoids cause profound and varied metabolic effects. In addition, they modify the body's immune responses to diverse stimuli.

5.2 Pharmacokinetic properties

Prednisolone is rapidly and apparently almost completely absorbed after oral administration; it reaches peak plasma concentrations after 1-3 hours. There is however wide inter-subject variation suggesting impaired absorption in some individuals. Plasma half-life is about 3 hours in adults and somewhat less in children. Its initial absorption, but not its overall bioavailability, is affected by food. Prednisolone has a biological half-life lasting several hours, making it suitable for alternate-day administration regimens.

Although peak plasma prednisolone levels are somewhat lower after administration of Deltacortril Enteric and absorption is delayed, total absorption and bioavailability are the same as after plain prednisolone. Prednisolone shows dose dependent pharmacokinetics, with an increase in dose leading to an increase in volume of distribution and plasma clearance. The degree of plasma protein binding determines the distribution and clearance of free, pharmacologically active drug. Reduced doses are necessary in patients with hypoalbuminaemia.

Prednisolone is metabolised primarily in the liver to a biologically inactive compound. Liver disease prolongs the half-life of prednisolone and, if the patient has hypoalbuminaemia, also increases the proportion of unbound drug and may thereby increase adverse effects.

Prednisolone is excreted in the urine as free and conjugated metabolites, together with small amounts of unchanged prednisolone.

6. PHARMACEUTICAL PARTICULARS

6.1 List of excipients

Core: calcium carbonate, lactose, magnesium stearate, maize starch

2.5 mg Coating:

polyvinyl alcohol, titanium dioxide (E171), purified talc, lecithin, xanthan gum (E415), polyvinyl acetate phthalate, polyethylene glycol, sodium hydrogen carbonate, triethyl citrate, purified stearic acid, sodium alginate (E401), colloidal silicon dioxide, lactose, methylcellulose (E461), sodium carboxymethyl cellulose, iron oxide (E172), beeswax (E901), carnauba wax (E903), polysorbate 20 (E432) and sorbic acid (E200).

5 mg Coating:

polyvinyl alcohol, titanium dioxide (E171), purified talc, lecithin, xanthan gum (E415), polyvinyl acetate phthalate, polyethylene glycol, sodium hydrogen carbonate, triethyl citrate, purified stearic acid, sodium alginate (E401), colloidal silicon dioxide, lactose monohydrate, methylcellulose (E461), sodium carboxymethyl cellulose, carmine (E120), indigo carmine aluminium lake (E132), beeswax (E901), carnauba wax (E903), polysorbate 20 (E432) and sorbic acid (E200).

Printing ink: titanium dioxide (E171), shellac, propylene glycol, indigo carmine aluminium lake (E132).

6.2 Incompatibilities

None.

6.3 Shelf life

24 months.

6.4 Special precautions for storage

Store below 25°C.

6.5 Nature and contents of container

Polypropylene container with HDPE Child-Resistant screw cap containing 30 or 100 tablets. Supplied with a patient information leaflet.

6.6 Instructions for use and handling

None.

7. MARKETING AUTHORISATION HOLDER

Pfizer Limited

Ramsgate Road

Sandwich

CT13 9NJ

United Kingdom

8. MARKETING AUTHORISATION NUMBER(S)

PL0057/5012R

PL0057/0128

9. DATE OF FIRST AUTHORISATION/RENEWAL OF THE AUTHORISATION

18 September 2002

10. DATE OF REVISION OF THE TEXT

January 2004

LEGAL CATEGORY

POM

Company Ref: DE 6_2

Deltastab Injection

(Sovereign Medical)

1. NAME OF THE MEDICINAL PRODUCT

Deltastab Injection

2. QUALITATIVE AND QUANTITATIVE COMPOSITION

Prednisolone Acetate BP 25 mg/ml

3. PHARMACEUTICAL FORM

A white or almost white suspension.

4. CLINICAL PARTICULARS

4.1 Therapeutic indications

Deltastab Injection is indicated for the local treatment, by intra-articular or periarticular injection, of the following conditions: rheumatoid arthritis; osteoarthritis; synovitis not associated with infection; tennis elbow; golfer's elbow, and bursitis.

Deltastab Injection is also suitable for administration by the intramuscular route in conditions requiring systemic corticosteroids, e.g. suppression of inflammatory and allergic disorders such as bronchial asthma, anaphylaxis, ulcerative colitis and Crohn's disease.

4.2 Posology and method of administration

For intra-articular, periarticular or intramuscular injection.

Adults

For articular use: 5-25 mg depending upon the size of the joint. The injections may be repeated when relapse occurs. No more than three joints should be treated in one day.

For intramuscular use: Dosage will depend upon the clinical circumstances and the judgement of the physician. The suggested dose is 25-100 mg once or twice weekly.

Elderly

Steroids should be used cautiously in the elderly since adverse effects are enhanced by old age (see section 4.4, 'Special Warnings and Precautions for Use').

Undesirable effects may be minimised by using the lowest effective dose for the minimum period, and by administering the daily requirement as a single morning dose or whenever possible, as a single morning dose on alternate days. Frequent patient review is required to titrate the dose against disease activity.

4.3 Contraindications

Deltastab Injection is contra-indicated in patients with known hypersensitivity to any of the ingredients. It is also contra-indicated in patients with systemic infections (unless specific anti-infective therapy is employed) and in patients vaccinated with live vaccines (see section 4.4, 'Special Warnings and Precautions for Use').

Intra-articular and periarticular injections of Deltastab Injection are contra-indicated when the joint or surrounding tissues are infected. The presence of infection also precludes injection into tendon sheaths and bursae. Deltastab Injection must not be injected directly into tendons, nor should it be injected into spinal or other non-diarthrodial joints.

4.4 Special warnings and special precautions for use

A patient information leaflet should be supplied with this product.

Intra-articular corticosteroids are associated with a substantially increased risk of inflammatory response in the joint, particularly bacterial infection introduced with the injection. Great care is required that all intra-articular steroid injections should be undertaken under aseptic conditions.

Adrenal suppression

Adrenal cortical atrophy develops during prolonged therapy and may persist for years after stopping treatment. Withdrawal of corticosteroids after prolonged therapy must therefore always be gradual to avoid acute adrenal insufficiency, being tapered off over weeks or months according to the dose and duration of treatment. During prolonged therapy, any intercurrent illness, trauma or surgical procedure will require a temporary increase in dosage. If corticosteroids have been stopped following prolonged therapy, they may need to be temporarily re-introduced.

Patients should carry 'Steroid Treatment' cards which give clear guidance on the precautions to be taken to minimise risk and which provide details of prescriber, drug, dosage and the duration of treatment.

Anti-inflammatory/immunosuppressive effects and infection

Suppression of inflammatory response and immune function increases the susceptibility to infections and their severity. The clinical presentation may often be atypical and serious infections such as septicaemia and tuberculosis may be masked and may reach an advanced stage before being recognised. New infections may appear during their use.

Chickenpox is of particular concern since this normally minor illness may be fatal in immunosuppressed patients. Patients (or parents of children) without a definite history of chickenpox should be advised to avoid close personal contact with chickenpox or herpes zoster and if exposed they should seek urgent medical attention. Passive immunisation with varicella zoster immunoglobin (VZIG) is needed by exposed, non-immune patients who are receiving systemic corticosteroids or who have used them within the previous 3 months; this should be given within 10 days of exposure to chickenpox. If a diagnosis of chickenpox is confirmed, the illness warrants specialist care and urgent treatment. Corticosteroids should not be stopped and the dose may need to be increased.

Live vaccines should not be given to individuals with impaired immune responsiveness. Killed vaccines or toxoids may be given though their effects may be attenuated.

Particular care is required when prescribing systemic corticosteroids in patients with the following conditions and frequent patient monitoring is necessary:

(a) Osteoporosis (postmenopausal females are particularly at risk).

(b) Hypertension or congestive heart failure.

(c) Existing or previous history of severe affective disorders (especially previous history of steroid psychosis).

(d) Diabetes mellitus (or a family history of diabetes).

(e) Previous history of tuberculosis or characteristic appearance on chest X-ray. The emergence of active tuberculosis can, however, be prevented by the prophylactic use of antituberculous therapy.

(f) Glaucoma (or a family history of glaucoma).

(g) Previous corticosteroid-induced myopathy.

(h) Liver failure.

(i) Renal insufficiency.

(j) Epilepsy.

(k) Peptic ulceration.

During treatment, the patient should be observed for psychotic reactions, muscular weakness, electrocardiographic changes, hypertension and untoward hormonal effects.

Corticosteroids should be used with caution in patients with hypothyroidism.

Use in children

Corticosteroids cause growth retardation in infancy, childhood and adolescence; this may be irreversible. Treatment should be limited to the minimum dosage for the shortest possible time, in order to minimise suppression of the hypothalamo-pituitary-adrenal (HPA) axis and growth retardation (see section 4.2, 'Posology and Method of Administration').

Use in the elderly

The common adverse effects of systemic corticosteroids may be associated with more serious consequences in old age, especially osteoporosis, hypertension, hypokalaemia, diabetes, susceptibility to infection and thinning of the skin. Close clinical supervision is required to avoid life-threatening reactions (see section 4.2, 'Posology and Method of Administration').

4.5 Interaction with other medicinal products and other forms of Interaction

The effectiveness of anticoagulants may be increased or decreased with concurrent corticosteroid therapy, and close monitoring of the INR or prothrombin time is required to avoid spontaneous bleeding.

Serum levels of salicylates may increase considerably if corticosteroid therapy is withdrawn, possible causing intoxication. Since both salicylates and corticosteroids are ulcerogenic, it is possible that there will be an increased rate of gastrointestinal ulceration.

The desired actions of hypoglycaemic drugs (including insulin), antihypertensives and diuretics will be antagonised by corticosteroids.

The potassium-depleting effects of amphotericin, carbenoxolone and diuretics (acetazolamide, loop diuretics and thiazides) are enhanced by corticosteroids and signs of hypokalaemia should be looked for during their concurrent use.

There is a small amount of evidence that the simultaneous use of corticosteroids and methotrexate may cause increased methotrexate toxicity and possibly death, although this combination of drugs has been used very successfully.

The metabolism of corticosteroids may be enhanced and the therapeutic effects reduced by certain barbiturates (e.g. phenobarbitone), and by phenytoin, rifampicin, rifabutin, primidone, carbamazepine and aminoglutethimide.

4.6 Pregnancy and lactation

Pregnancy

The ability of corticosteroids to cross the placenta varies between individual drugs. However, 88% of prednisolone is inactivated as it crosses the placenta.

Administration of corticosteroids to pregnant animals can cause abnormalities of foetal development including cleft palate, intra-uterine growth retardation and effects on brain growth and development. There is no evidence that corticosteroids result in an increased incidence of congenital abnormalities such as cleft palate/lip in man. However, when administered for prolonged periods or repeatedly during pregnancy, corticosteroids may increase the risk of intra-uterine growth retardation. Hypoadrenalism may, in theory, occur in the neonate following pre-natal exposure to corticosteroids but usually resolves spontaneously following birth and is rarely clinically important. As with all drugs, corticosteroids should only be prescribed when the benefits to the mother and child outweigh the risks. When corticosteroids are essential, however, patients with normal pregnancies may be treated as though they were in the non-gravid state.

Lactation

Corticosteroids are excreted in small amounts in breast milk. However, doses of up to 40 mg daily of prednisolone are unlikely to cause systemic effects in the infant. Infants of mothers taking higher doses than this may have a degree of adrenal suppression but the benefits of breast feeding are likely to outweigh any theoretical risk.

4.7 Effects on ability to drive and use machines

No adverse effects known.

4.8 Undesirable effects

With intra-articular or other local injections, the principal side effect encountered is a temporary local exacerbation with increased pain and swelling. This normally subsides after a few hours.

The incidence of predictable undesirable effects, including hypothalamo-pituitary-adrenal suppression, correlates with the relative potency of the drug, dosage, timing of administration and the duration of treatment (see section 4.4, 'Special Warnings and Precautions for Use').

The following side effects may be associated with the long-term systemic use of corticosteroids.

Anti-inflammatory and immunosuppressive effects

Increased susceptibility and severity of infections with suppression of clinical symptoms and signs, opportunistic infections, recurrence of dormant tuberculosis (see section 4.4, 'Special Warnings and Precautions for Use').

Gastrointestinal

Dyspepsia, peptic ulceration with perforation and haemorrhage, abdominal distension, oesophageal ulceration, candidiasis, acute pancreatitis.

Musculoskeletal

Proximal myopathy, osteoporosis, vertebral and long bone fractures, avascular osteonecrosis, tendon rupture.

Fluid and electrolyte disturbance

Sodium and water retention, hypertension, potassium loss, hypokalaemic alkalosis.

Dermatological

Impaired healing, skin atrophy, bruising, striae, acne, telangiectasia.

Endocrine/Metabolic

Suppression of the HPA axis, growth suppression in infancy, childhood and adolescence, menstrual irregularity and amenorrhoea. Cushingoid facies, hirsutism, weight gain, impaired carbohydrate tolerance with increased requirement for antidiabetic therapy, negative protein and calcium balance, increased appetite.

Neuropsychiatric

Euphoria, psychological dependence, depression, insomnia and aggravation of schizophrenia. Increased intracranial pressure with papilloedema in children (pseudotumour cerebri), usually after treatment withdrawal. Aggravation of epilepsy.

Ophthalmic

Increased intra-ocular pressure, glaucoma, papilloedema, posterior subcapsular cataracts, corneal or scleral thinning, exacerbation of ophthalmic viral or fungal diseases.

General

Hypersensitivity, including anaphylaxis, has been reported. Nausea, malaise, leucocytosis, thromboembolism.

Withdrawal

In patients who have received more than physiological doses of systemic corticosteroids (approximately 7.5 mg prednisolone or equivalent) for greater than 3 weeks, withdrawal should not be abrupt. How dose reduction should be carried out depends largely on whether the disease is likely to relapse as the dose of systemic corticosteroids is reduced. Clinical assessment of disease activity may be needed during withdrawal. If the disease is unlikely to relapse on withdrawal of systemic corticosteroids but there is uncertainty about HPA suppression, the dose of systemic corticosteriod may be reduced rapidly to physiological doses. Once a daily dose equivalent to 7.5 mg of prednisolone is reached, dose reduction should be slower to allow the HPA-axis to recover.

Abrupt withdrawal of systemic corticosteriod treatment which has continued up to 3 weeks is appropriate if it is considered that the disease is unlikely to relapse. Abrupt withdrawal of doses of up to 40 mg daily of prednisolone (or equivalent) for 3 weeks is unlikely to lead to clinically relevant HPA-axis suppression in the majority of patients. In the following patient groups, gradual withdrawal of systemic coticosteroid therapy should be *considered* even after courses lasting 3 weeks or less:

- Patients who have had repeated courses of systemic corticosteroids, particularly if taken for greater than 3 weeks,
- When a short course has been prescribed within one year of cessation of long-term therapy (months or years),
- Patients who may have reasons for adrenocortical insufficiency other than exogenous corticosteriod therapy,
- Patients receiving doses of systemic corticosteriod greater than 40 mg daily of prednisolone (or equivalent),
- Patients repeatedly taking doses in the evening.

4.9 Overdose

Overdosage is unlikely with Deltastab Injection but there is no specific antidote available. Treatment should be symptomatic.

5. PHARMACOLOGICAL PROPERTIES

5.1 Pharmacodynamic properties

Prednisolone is a glucocorticoid which has anti-inflammatory activity.

5.2 Pharmacokinetic properties

Absorption following intramuscular injection is relatively slow. Systemic absorption occurs slowly after local, intra-articular injection. Prednisolone is extensively bound to plasma proteins. Excretion takes place via the urine as free and conjugated metabolites, together with an appreciable proportion of unchanged prednisolone.

5.3 Preclinical safety data

There is no pre-clinical data of relevance to a prescriber which is additional to that already included in other sections of the SmPC.

6. PHARMACEUTICAL PARTICULARS

6.1 List of excipients

Water for injections, sodium chloride for injections, benzyl alcohol, sodium carboxymethylcellulose, polysorbate 80 (Tween 80), with sodium hydroxide and/or sterile sodium hydroxide and/or hydrochloric acid as pH adjusters.

6.2 Incompatibilities

Not applicable.

6.3 Shelf life

36 months.

6.4 Special precautions for storage

Store at 15-25°C and protect from light.

6.5 Nature and contents of container

1 ml flint neutral glass ampoules. 10 ampoules are packed in a polystyrene pack within a cardboard sleeve.

6.6 Instructions for use and handling

Shake the ampoule well before use.

Administrative Data

7. MARKETING AUTHORISATION HOLDER

Waymade PLC

T/A Sovereign Medical

Sovereign House

Miles Gray Road

Basildon

Essex

SS14 3FR

8. MARKETING AUTHORISATION NUMBER(S)

PL 06464/0703

9. DATE OF FIRST AUTHORISATION/RENEWAL OF THE AUTHORISATION
11/01/1999

10. DATE OF REVISION OF THE TEXT
18 June 2002

Legal Category
POM

De-Noltab
(Astellas Pharma Limited)

1. NAME OF THE MEDICINAL PRODUCT
DE-NOLTAB

2. QUALITATIVE AND QUANTITATIVE COMPOSITION
Tri-potassium di-citrato bismuthate equivalent to 120mg Bi_2O_3

3. PHARMACEUTICAL FORM
Film-coated tablet

4. CLINICAL PARTICULARS

4.1 Therapeutic indications
For the treatment of gastric and duodenal ulcers.

4.2 Posology and method of administration
For Adults, and the Elderly:

One tablet to be taken four times a day, half an hour before each of the three main meals and two hours after the last meal of the day, or

Two tablets to be taken twice daily, half an hour before breakfast and half an hour before the evening meal, or

As directed by the physician

The maximum duration for one course of treatment is two months; De-Noltab should not be used for maintenance therapy.

For children:

Not recommended.

4.3 Contraindications
In cases of severe renal insufficiency.

Harmful to people on a low potassium diet.

4.4 Special warnings and special precautions for use
None stated.

4.5 Interaction with other medicinal products and other forms of interaction
The efficacy of oral tetracyclines may be inhibited.

4.6 Pregnancy and lactation
On theoretical grounds De-Noltab is contraindicated in pregnancy. No information is available on excretion in breast milk.

4.7 Effects on ability to drive and use machines
None reported.

4.8 Undesirable effects
Blackening of the stool usually occurs; nausea and vomiting have been reported.

4.9 Overdose
Extremely few cases of overdosage have been reported; contact the company for further information.

5. PHARMACOLOGICAL PROPERTIES

5.1 Pharmacodynamic properties
The active constituent exerts a local healing effect at the ulcer site, and by eradication or reduction of *Helicobacter pylori* defers relapse.

5.2 Pharmacokinetic properties
The action is local in the gastro-intestinal tract.

5.3 Preclinical safety data
No relevant pre-clinical safety data has been generated.

6. PHARMACEUTICAL PARTICULARS

6.1 List of excipients
Povidone K 30

Polacrillin potassium

Macrogol 6000

Magnesium stearate

Maize starch

Hypromellose

6.2 Incompatibilities
None

6.3 Shelf life
Four years

6.4 Special precautions for storage
Do not store above 25°C

6.5 Nature and contents of container
Amber glass bottles and/or aluminium foil strips, containing 112 tablets

6.6 Instructions for use and handling
None

7. MARKETING AUTHORISATION HOLDER
Yamanouchi Pharma Ltd

Yamanouchi House

Pyrford Road

West Byfleet

Surrey

KT14 6RA

8. MARKETING AUTHORISATION NUMBER(S)
0166/0124

9. DATE OF FIRST AUTHORISATION/RENEWAL OF THE AUTHORISATION
1 December 1986; 15th July 2002.

10. DATE OF REVISION OF THE TEXT
Date of revision = 8th March 2004

11. LEGAL CATEGORY
P

Depakote tablets
(sanofi-aventis)

1. NAME OF THE MEDICINAL PRODUCT
Depakote 250mg Tablets.

Depakote 500mg Tablets

2. QUALITATIVE AND QUANTITATIVE COMPOSITION
Depakote 250mg Tablets: Containing 269.10mg of valproate semisodium* per tablet (equivalent to 250mg of valproic acid).

Depakote 500mg Tablets: Containing 538.20mg of valproate semisodium* per tablet (equivalent to 500mg of valproic acid).

*Valproate semisodium is a stable coordination compound comprised of sodium valproate and valproic acid in a 1:1 molar relationship. It is also known as divalproex sodium (USAN).

3. PHARMACEUTICAL FORM
Gastro-resistant tablets.

4. CLINICAL PARTICULARS

4.1 Therapeutic indications
Depakote is indicated for the acute treatment of a manic episode associated with bipolar disorder.

4.2 Posology and method of administration
For oral administration. The tablets should be swallowed whole with a drink of water, and not chewed.

The daily dosage should be established according to age and body weight. The wide individual sensitivity to valproate semisodium should also be considered.

There is no clear correlation between daily dose, plasma concentration and therapeutic effect. Optimum dosage should be determined mainly by clinical response. Measurement of valproate plasma levels may be considered in addition to clinical monitoring when adequate therapeutic effect is not achieved or adverse effects are suspected.

In mania it is generally agreed that plasma levels around 45 to 50μg/ml are needed to allow efficacy; most patients receiving Depakote during controlled clinical trials achieved a maximum plasma concentration of greater than 75μg/ml.

Dosage

Adults

The recommended initial dose is 750mg daily in 2 to 3 divided doses. The dose should be increased as rapidly as possible to achieve the lowest therapeutic dose which produces the desired clinical effect. Daily doses usually range between 1000 and 2000mg.

Patients receiving daily doses higher than 45mg/kg should be carefully monitored.

Elderly

Although the pharmacokinetics of Depakote are modified in the elderly, they have limited clinical significance and dosage should be determined on the basis of clinical response.

Children and adolescents

The safety and effectiveness of Depakote for the treatment of manic episodes have not been studied in individuals below the age of 18 years.

In patients with renal insufficiency

It may be necessary to decrease dosage. Dosage should be adjusted according to clinical monitoring since monitoring of plasma concentrations may be misleading (see section 5.2 Pharmacokinetic Properties).

In patients with hepatic insufficiency

Salicylates should not be used concomitantly with valproate since they employ the same metabolic pathway (see also sections 4.4 Special Warnings and Precautions for Use and 4.8 Undesirable Effects).

Liver dysfunction, including hepatic failure resulting in fatalities, has occurred in patients whose treatment included valproic acid (see sections 4.3 Contraindications and 4.4 Special Warnings and Precautions for Use).

Salicylates should not be used in children under 16 years (see aspirin/salicylate product information on Reye's syndrome). In addition in conjunction with Depakote, concomitant use in children under 3 years can increase the risk of liver toxicity (see section 4.4.1 Special warnings).

4.3 Contraindications
Active liver disease

Personal or family history of severe hepatic dysfunction, drug related

Hypersensitivity to valproate semisodium or any other ingredient of the preparation.

Porphyria

4.4 Special warnings and special precautions for use
To ensure the correct medication is prescribed for the patient's condition, care must be taken not to confuse Depakote with Epilim or sodium valproate. Patients with bipolar disorder and epilepsy are distinct populations. These differences are reflected in the patient information leaflets which clearly indicate specific indications for these differing medications.

4.4.1 Special Warnings
Liver dysfunction:

Conditions of occurrence:

Severe liver damage, including hepatic failure sometimes resulting in fatalities, has been very rarely reported. Experience in epilepsy has indicated that patients most at risk are infants and in particular young children under the age of 3 and those with severe seizure disorders, organic brain disease, and (or) congenital metabolic or degenerative disease associated with mental retardation.

After the age of 3, the incidence of occurrence is significantly reduced and progressively decreases with age.

The concomitant use of salicylates should be avoided in children under 3 due to the risk of liver toxicity. Additionally, salicylates should not be used in children under 16 years (see aspirin/salicylate product information on Reye's syndrome).

In most cases, such liver damage occurred during the first 6 months of therapy, the period of maximum risk being 2-12 weeks.

Suggestive signs:

Clinical symptoms are essential for early diagnosis. In particular, the following conditions which may precede jaundice should be taken into consideration, especially in patients at risk (see above: 'Conditions of occurrence'):

- non specific symptoms, usually of sudden onset, such as asthenia, malaise, anorexia, lethargy, oedema and drowsiness, which are sometimes associated with repeated vomiting and abdominal pain.

- in patients with epilepsy, recurrence of seizures,

These are an indication for immediate withdrawal of the drug. Patients (or their family for children) should be instructed to report immediately any such signs to a physician should they occur. Investigations including clinical examination and biological assessment of liver function should be undertaken immediately.

Detection:

Liver function should be measured before and then periodically monitored during the first 6 months of therapy, especially in those who seem most at risk, and those with a prior history of liver disease. Amongst usual investigations, tests which reflect protein synthesis, particularly prothrombin rate, are most relevant. Confirmation of an abnormally low prothrombin rate, particularly in association with other biological abnormalities (significant decrease in fibrinogen and coagulation factors; increased bilirubin level and raised transaminases) requires cessation of treatment. As a matter of precaution and in case they are taken concomitantly salicylates should also be discontinued since they employ the same metabolic pathway.

Increased liver enzymes are common, particularly at the beginning of therapy; they are also transient.

More extensive biological investigations (including prothrombin rate) are recommended in these patients; a reduction in dosage may be considered when appropriate and tests should be repeated as necessary.

Pancreatitis: Pancreatitis, which may be severe and result in fatalities, has been very rarely reported. Patients experiencing nausea, vomiting or acute abdominal pain should have a prompt medical evaluation (including measurement of serum amylase). Young children are at particular risk; this risk decreases with increasing age. Hepatic failure with pancreatitis increases the risk of fatal outcome. In case of pancreatitis, valproate should be discontinued.

4.4.2 Precautions
Haematological: Blood tests (blood cell count, including platelet count, bleeding time and coagulation tests) are recommended prior to initiation of therapy or before surgery, and in case of spontaneous bruising or bleeding (see section 4.8. Undesirable Effects)

Renal insufficiency: In patients with renal insufficiency, it may be necessary to decrease dosage. As monitoring of plasma concentrations may be misleading, dosage should be adjusted according to clinical monitoring (see sections 4.2 Posology and Method of Administration and 5.2. Pharmacokinetic Properties).

Systemic lupus erythematosus: Although immune disorders have only rarely been noted during the use of valproate, the potential benefit of Depakote should be weighed against its potential risk in patients with systemic lupus erythematosus (see also section 4.8 Undesirable Effects).

Hyperammonaemia: When a urea cycle enzymatic deficiency is suspected, metabolic investigations should be performed prior to treatment because of the risk of hyperammonaemia with Depakote.

Weight gain: Depakote very commonly causes weight gain, which may be marked and progressive.

Patients should be warned of the risk of weight gain at the initiation of therapy and appropriate strategies should be adopted to minimise it (see section 4.8 Undesirable Effects).

Pregnancy: Women of child-bearing potential, should receive specialist psychiatric advice prior to starting Depakote and if planning a pregnancy whilst taking Depakote because of the potential teratogenic risk to the foetus (see also section 4.6 Pregnancy and Lactation).

Diabetic patients: Valproate is eliminated mainly through the kidneys, partly in the form of ketone bodies; this may give false positives in the urine testing of possible diabetics.

4.5 Interaction with other medicinal products and other forms of Interaction

4.5.1 Effects of Depakote on other drugs

- Clozapine, haloperidol, lithium

No significant interaction was observed when clozapine and haloperidol were administered concurrently with Depakote. Co-administration of Depakote and lithium does not appear to affect the steady state kinetics of lithium.

- Neuroleptics, MAO inhibitors, antidepressants and benzodiazepines

Valproate may potentiate the effect of antipsychotics, MAO inhibitors, antidepressants and benzodiazepines; therefore, clinical monitoring is advised and dosage should be adjusted when appropriate.

- Phenobarbital

Valproate increases phenobarbital plasma concentrations (due to inhibition of hepatic catabolism) and sedation may occur. Therefore, clinical monitoring is recommended throughout the first 15 days of combined treatment with immediate reduction of phenobarbital doses if sedation occurs and determination of phenobarbital plasma levels when appropriate.

- Primidone

Valproate increases primidone plasma levels with exacerbation of its adverse effects (such as sedation); these signs cease with long term treatment. Clinical monitoring is recommended especially at the beginning of combined therapy with dosage adjustment when appropriate.

- Phenytoin

Valproate decreases phenytoin total plasma concentration. Moreover valproate increases phenytoin free form with possible overdosage symptoms (valproic acid displaces phenytoin from its plasma protein binding sites and reduces its hepatic catabolism). Therefore clinical monitoring is recommended; when phenytoin plasma levels are determined, the free form should be evaluated.

- Carbamazepine

Clinical toxicity has been reported when valproate was administered with carbamazepine as valproate may potentiate toxic effects of carbamazepine. Clinical monitoring is recommended especially at the beginning of combined therapy with dosage adjustment when appropriate.

- Lamotrigine

Depakote may reduce the metabolism of lamotrigine and increase the mean half-life. Dose should be adjusted (lamotrigine dosage decreased) when appropriate. Co-administration of lamotrigine and Depakote might increase the risk of rash.

- Zidovudine

Valproate may raise zidovudine plasma concentration leading to increased zidovudine toxicity.

- Vitamin K-dependent anticoagulants

The anticoagulant effect of warfarin and other coumarin anticoagulants may be increased following displacement from plasma protein binding sites by valproic acid. The prothrombin time should be closely monitored.

4.5.2 Effects of other drugs on Depakote

Anticonvulsants with enzyme inducing effects (including *phenytoin, phenobarbital, carbamazepine*) decrease valproic acid plasma concentrations. Dosages should be adjusted according to blood levels in case of combined therapy.

On the other hand, combination of *felbamate* and valproate may increase valproic acid plasma concentration. Valproate dosage should be monitored.

Mefloquine and *Chloroquine* increase valproic acid metabolism. Accordingly, the dosage of Depakote may need adjustment.

In case of concomitant use of valproate and *highly protein bound agents (e.g. aspirin)*, free valproic acid plasma levels may be increased.

Valproic acid plasma levels may be increased (as a result of reduced hepatic metabolism) in case of concomitant use with *cimetidine* or *erythromycin*

Carbapenem antibiotics such as *imipenem* and *meropenem*: Decrease in valproic acid blood level, sometimes associated with convulsions, has been observed when imipenem or meropenem were combined. If these antibiotics have to be administered, close monitoring of valproic acid blood level is recommended.

Cholestyramine may decrease the absorption of valproate.

4.5.3 Other Interactions

Valproate usually has no enzyme inducing effect; as a consequence, valproate does not reduce efficacy of oestroprogestative agents in women receiving horminal contraception, including the oral contraceptive pill.

4.6 Pregnancy and lactation

4.6.1 Pregnancy

From experience in treating mothers with epilepsy, the risk associated with the use of valproate during pregnancy has been described as follows:

- Risk associated with valproate

In animals: teratogenic effects have been demonstrated in the mouse, rat and rabbit.

There is animal experimental evidence that high plasma peak levels and the size of an individual dose are associated with neural tube defects.

In humans: an increased incidence of congenital abnormalities (including cases of facial dysmorphia, hypospadias and multiple malformations, particularly of the limbs) has been demonstrated in offspring born to mothers treated with valproate.

Valproate use is associated with neural tube defects such as myelomeningocele and spina bifida. The frequency of this effect is estimated to be 1 to 2%.

Epidemiological studies, of women with epilepsy, have suggested an association between in-utero exposure to sodium valproate and a risk of developmental delay. Many factors including maternal epilepsy may also contribute to this risk but it is difficult to quantify the relative contributions of these or of maternal anti-epileptic treatment.

- In view of the above data

Women of childbearing age should be informed of the risks and benefits of continuing Depakote treatment throughout pregnancy.

Folate supplementation, **prior** to pregnancy, has been demonstrated to reduce the incidence of neural tube defects in the offspring of women at high risk. Although no direct evidence exists of such effects in women receiving Depakote, women should be advised to start taking folic acid supplementation (5mg) as soon as contraception is discontinued.

Dosage should be reviewed before conception and the lowest effective dose used, in divided doses, as abnormal pregnancy outcome tends to be associated with higher total daily dosage and with the size of an individual dose. The incidence of neural tube defects rises with increasing dosage, particularly above 1000mg daily. The administration in several divided doses over the day is preferable in order to avoid high peak plasma levels.

Nevertheless, specialised prenatal monitoring should be instituted in order to detect the possible occurrence of a neural tube defect or any other malformation. Pregnancies should be carefully screened by ultrasound, and other techniques if appropriate (see Section 4.4 Special Warnings and Precautions for Use).

- Risk in the neonate

Very rare cases of haemorrhagic syndrome have been reported in neonates whose mothers have taken valproate during pregnancy. This haemorrhagic syndrome is related to hypofibrinogenemia; afibrinogenemia has also been reported and may be fatal. These are possibly associated with a decrease of coagulation factors. However, this syndrome has to be distinguished from the decrease of the vitamin-K factors induced by phenobarbitone and other enzyme inducing drugs.

Therefore, platelet count, fibrinogen plasma level, coagulation tests and coagulation factors should be investigated in neonates.

4.6.2 Lactation

Excretion of valproate in breast milk is low, with a concentration between 1 % to 10 % of total maternal serum levels; up to now children breast fed that have been monitored during the neonatal period have not experienced clinical effects. There appears to be no contra-indication to breast feeding by patients on valproate.

4.7 Effects on ability to drive and use machines

Patients should be warned of the risk of transient drowsiness, especially in cases of polytherapy or association with benzodiazepines (see section 4.5 Interactions with Other Medicaments and Other Forms of Interaction).

4.8 Undesirable effects

The following adverse events have been described from experience of sodium valproate in epilepsy; no other adverse event that could be specifically associated with the use of Depakote in the treatment of manic episodes have been identified.

Congenital and familial/genetic disorders: (see section 4.6. Pregnancy and Lactation)

Hepato-biliary disorders: rare cases of liver dysfunction (see section 4.4.1 Special Warnings)

Severe liver damage, including hepatic failure sometimes resulting in death, has been reported (see also sections 4.2, 4.3 and 4.4.1). Increased liver enzymes are common, particularly early in treatment, and may be transient (see section 4.4.1 Special Warnings).

Gastrointestinal disorders: (nausea, gastralgia, diarrhoea) frequently occur at the start of treatment, but they usually disappear after a few days without discontinuing treatment. These problems can usually be overcome by taking Depakote Tablets with or after food.

Very rare cases of pancreatitis, sometimes lethal, have been reported (see section 4.4 Special Warnings and Precautions for Use).

Nervous system disorders: Sedation has been reported occasionally. In monotherapy it occurred early in treatment on rare occasions and is usually transient. Rare cases of lethargy and confusion occasionally progressing to stupor, sometimes with associated hallucinations or convulsions have been reported. Encephalopathy and coma have very rarely been observed. These cases have often been associated with too high a starting dose or too rapid a dose escalation or concomitant use of anticonvulsants, notably phenobarbitone. They have usually been reversible on withdrawal of treatment or reduction of dosage.

Very rare cases of reversible extrapyramidal symptoms including parkinsonism, or reversible dementia associated with reversible cerebral atrophy have been reported. Dose-related ataxia and fine postural tremor have occasionally been reported.

An increase in alertness may occur; this is generally beneficial but occasionally aggression, hyperactivity and behavioural deterioration have been reported.

Metabolic disorders: Cases of isolated and moderate hyperammonaemia without change in liver function tests may occur frequently, are usually transient and should not cause treatment discontinuation. However, they may present clinically as vomiting, ataxia, and increasing clouding of consciousness. Should these symptoms occur Depakote should be discontinued.

Hyperammonaemia associated with neurological symptoms has also been reported (see section 4.4.2. Precautions). In such cases further investigations should be considered

Blood and lymphatic system disorders: frequent occurrence of thrombocytopenia, rare cases of anaemia, leucopenia or pancytopenia. The blood picture returned to normal when the drug was discontinued.

Isolated reduction of fibrinogen or reversible increase in bleeding time have been reported, usually without associated clinical signs and particularly with high doses (sodium valproate has an inhibitory effect on the second phase of platelet aggregation). Spontaneous bruising or bleeding is an indication for withdrawal of medication pending investigations (see also section 4.6 Pregnancy and Lactation).

Skin and subcutaneous tissue disorders: cutaneous reactions such as exanthematous rash rarely occur with valproate. In very rare cases, toxic epidermal necrolysis, Stevens-Johnson syndrome and erythema multiforme have been reported.

Transient hair loss, which may sometimes be dose-related, has often been reported. Regrowth normally begins within six months, although the hair may become more curly than previously. Hirsutism and acne have been very rarely reported.

Reproductive system and breast disorders: Amenorrhea and irregular periods have been reported. Very rarely gynaecomastia has occurred.

Vascular disorders: the occurrence of vasculitis has occasionally been reported.

Ear disorders: hearing loss, either reversible or irreversible, has been reported rarely; however a cause and effect relationship has not been established.

Renal and urinary disorders: there have been isolated reports of a reversible Fanconi's syndrome (a defect in proximal renal tubular function giving rise to glycosuria, amino aciduria, phosphaturia, and uricosuria) associated with valproate therapy, but the mode of action is as yet unclear.

Immune system disorders: allergic reactions (ranging from rash to hypersensitivity reactions) have been reported

General disorders: very rare cases of non severe peripheral oedema have been reported.

Increase in weight may also occur. Weight gain being a risk factor for polycystic ovary syndrome, it should be carefully monitored (see section 4.4 Special Warnings and Precautions for Use).

4.9 Overdose
Clinical signs of acute massive overdose, i.e. plasma concentration 10 to 20 times maximum therapeutic levels, usually include CNS depression, or coma with muscular hypotonia, hyporeflexia, miosis, impaired respiratory functions.

Symptoms may however be variable and seizures have been reported in the presence of very high plasma levels in epileptic patients. Cases of intracranial hypertension related to cerebral oedema have been reported.

Hospital management of overdose should be symptomatic, including cardio-respiratotgastric monitoring. Gastric lavage may be useful up to 10 to 12 hours following ingestion.

Haemodialysis and haemoperfusion have been used successfully.

Naloxone has been successfully used in a few isolated cases, sometimes in association with activated charcoal given orally.

Deaths have occurred following massive overdose; nevertheless, a favourable outcome is usual.

5. PHARMACOLOGICAL PROPERTIES

5.1 Pharmacodynamic properties
Depakote exerts its effects mainly on the central nervous system.

The most likely mode of action for Depakote is potentiation of the inhibitory action of gamma amino butyric acid (GABA) through an action on the further synthesis or further metabolism of GABA.

The effectiveness of Depakote in acute mania was demonstrated in two 3-week, double-blind, placebo-controlled trials conducted in bipolar patients. Depakote was initiated at a dose of 250mg tid and subsequently titrated up to a maximum daily dose not exceeding 2500mg; the concomitant use of a benzodiazepine was allowed during the first 10 days of treatment to manage associated symptoms such as severe agitation.

Pharmacological studies have demonstrated activity in experimental models of animal behaviour in mania.

5.2 Pharmacokinetic properties
Following oral administration of Depakote the absolute bioavailability of valproic acid approaches 100%. Mean terminal half life is about 14 hours, steady state conditions usually being achieved within 3 to 4 days. Peak plasma concentrations are achieved within 3 to 5 hours. Administration with food increases T_{max} by about 4 hours but does not modify the extent of absorption.

Depakote is extensively metabolised in the liver with less than 3% of an administered dose excreted unchanged in the urine. Principal metabolites found in urine are those originating from β-oxidation (up to 45% of the dose) and glucuronidation (up to 60% of the dose). Plasma clearance ranges from 0.4 to 0.6L/h and is independent of hepatic blood flow.

Plasma protein binding of Depakote ranges from 85 to 94% over plasma drug concentrations of 40 to 100 mcg/ml. It is concentration-dependent and the free fraction increases non-linearly with plasma drug concentration.

In elderly patients and those with liver cirrhosis (including alcoholic), acute hepatitis or renal failure the elimination of valproic acid is reduced. Reduction in intrinsic clearance and protein binding are reported. Thus, monitoring of total concentrations may be misleading and dosage adjustment may need to be considered according to clinical response.

Haemodialysis reduces serum valproic acid concentrations by about 20%.

5.3 Preclinical safety data
There are no pre-clinical data of relevance to the prescriber which are additional to that already included in other sections of the SPC.

6. PHARMACEUTICAL PARTICULARS

6.1 List of excipients
Depakote 250mg Tablets: Colloidal silica, hydrated; Starch pregelatinised; Povidone; Titanium dioxide (E171); Talc; Hypromellose phthalate; Diacetylated monoglycerides; Sunset yellow aluminium lake (E110); Vanillin.

Depakote 500mg Tablets: Colloidal silica, hydrated; Starch pregelatinised; Povidone; Titanium dioxide (E171); Talc; Hypromellose phthalate; Diacetylated monoglycerides; Ponceau 4R aluminium lake (E124); Indigo carmine aluminium lake (E132); Vanillin.

6.2 Incompatibilities
Not relevant.

6.3 Shelf life
3 years.

6.4 Special precautions for storage
None.

6.5 Nature and contents of container
Aluminium/aluminium blister packs containing 90 tablets.

6.6 Instructions for use and handling
None.

7. MARKETING AUTHORISATION HOLDER
Sanofi-Synthelabo Limited
One Onslow Street
Guildford
Surrey
GU1 4YS
Trading as:
Sanofi-Synthelabo
PO Box 597
Guildford
Surrey

8. MARKETING AUTHORISATION NUMBER(S)
Depakote 250mg Tablets: 11723/0251
Depakote 500mg Tablets: 11723/0252

9. DATE OF FIRST AUTHORISATION/RENEWAL OF THE AUTHORISATION
21 December 2000

10. DATE OF REVISION OF THE TEXT
May 2004

Legal Status: POM

Depixol Injection, Conc. Injection

(Lundbeck Limited)

1. NAME OF THE MEDICINAL PRODUCT
Depixol® Injection, Conc. Injection

2. QUALITATIVE AND QUANTITATIVE COMPOSITION
Depixol Injection
20 mg/mL (2% w/v) cis(Z)-flupentixol decanoate in thin vegetable oil. Ampoules 1mL and 2 mL, Syringes 1 mL and 2 mL and Vial 10 mL.

Depixol Conc Injection
100 mg/mL (10%w/v) cis (Z)-flupentixol decanoate in thin vegetable oil. Ampoules 0.5 mL and 1 mL and Vial 5 mL.

3. PHARMACEUTICAL FORM
Oily solution for deep intramuscular injection.

4. CLINICAL PARTICULARS

4.1 Therapeutic indications
The treatment of schizophrenia and other psychoses.

4.2 Posology and method of administration
Route of administration: Deep intramuscular injection into the upper outer buttock or lateral thigh. Dosage and dosage interval should be adjusted according to the patients' symptoms and response to treatment.

Note: As with all oil based injections it is important to ensure, by aspiration before injection, that inadvertent intravascular entry does not occur.

Adults: The usual dosage of flupentixol decanoate lies between 50 mg every 4 weeks and 300 mg every 2 weeks, but some patients may require up to 400 mg weekly. Other patients may be adequately maintained on dosages of 20-40 mg flupentixol decanoate every 2-4 weeks. In patients who have not previously received depot antipsychotic, treatment is usually started with a small dose (e.g. 20 mg) to assess tolerability. An interval of at least one week should be allowed before the second injection is given at a dose consistent with the patients' condition.

Adequate control of severe psychotic symptoms may take up to 4 to 6 months at high enough dosage. Once stabilised lower maintenance doses may be considered, but must be sufficient to prevent relapse.

The appropriate presentation of Depixol should be selected to achieve an injection volume which does not exceed 2 mL. Volumes greater than 2 mL should be distributed between two injection sites.

Elderly: In accordance with standard medical practice, initial dosage may need to be reduced to a quarter or half the normal starting dose in the frail or elderly.

Children: Depixol Injection and Depixol Conc Injection are not indicated for children.

4.3 Contraindications
Comatose states, including alcohol, barbiturates, or opiate poisoning. Not recommended for excitable or agitated patients.

4.4 Special warnings and special precautions for use
Caution should be exercised in patients having: liver disease; cardiac disease or arrhythmias; severe respiratory disease; renal failure; epilepsy (and conditions predisposing to epilepsy e.g. alcohol withdrawal or brain damage); Parkinson's disease; narrow angle glaucoma; prostatic hypertrophy; hypothyroidism; hyperthyroidism; myasthenia gravis; phaeochromocytoma and patients who have shown hypersensitivity to thioxanthenes or other antipsychotics.

The elderly require close supervision because they are specially prone to experience such adverse effects as sedation, hypotension, confusion and temperature changes.

Acute withdrawal symptoms, including nausea, vomiting, sweating and insomnia have been described after abrupt cessation of antipsychotic drugs. Recurrence of psychotic symptoms may also occur, and the emergence of involuntary movement disorders (such as akathisia, dystonia and dyskinesia) has been reported. Therefore gradual withdrawal is usually advisable. The plasma concentrations of Depixol Injection and Depixol Conc Injection gradually decrease over several weeks which makes gradual dose tapering unnecessary.

When transferring patients from oral to depot antipsychotics treatment, the oral medication should not be discontinued immediately, but gradually withdrawn over a period of several days after administering the first injection.

4.5 Interaction with other medicinal products and other forms of Interaction
In common with other antipsychotics, flupentixol enhances the response to alcohol, the effects of barbiturates and other CNS depressants. Flupentixol may potentiate the effects of general anaesthetics and anticoagulants and prolong the action of neuromuscular blocking agents.

The anticholinergic effects of atropine or other drugs with anticholinergic properties may be increased. Concomitant use of drugs such as metoclopramide, piperazine or anti-parkinson drugs may increase the risk of extrapyramidal effects such as tardive dyskinesia. Combined use of antipsychotics and lithium or sibutramine has been associated with an increased risk of neurotoxicity.

Antipsychotics may enhance the cardiac depressant effects of quinidine, the absorption of corticosteroids and digoxin. The hypotensive effect of vasodilator antihypertensive agents such as hydralazine and α-blockers (e.g. doxazosin), or methyl-dopa may be enhanced. Concomitant use of flupentixol and drugs known to cause QT prolongation or cardiac arrhythmias, such as tricyclic antidepressants, other antipsychotics or terfenadine should be avoided.

Antipsychotics may antagonise the effects of adrenaline and other sympathomimetic agents, and reverse the antihypertensive effects of guanethidine and similar adrenergic-blocking agents. Antipsychotics may also impair the effect of levodopa, adrenergic drugs and anticonvulsants.

The metabolism of tricyclic antidepressants may be inhibited and the control of diabetes may be impaired.

4.6 Pregnancy and lactation
As the safety of this drug during pregnancy has not been established, use during pregnancy, especially the first and last trimesters, should be avoided, unless the expected benefit to the patient outweighs the potential risk to the foetus.

Flupentixol is excreted into the breast milk. If the use of Depixol is considered essential, nursing mothers should be advised to stop breast feeding.

The newborn of mothers treated with antipsychotics in late pregnancy, or labour, may show signs of intoxication such as lethargy, tremor and hyperexcitability, and have a low apgar score.

4.7 Effects on ability to drive and use machines
Alertness may be impaired, especially at the start of treatment, or following the consumption of alcohol; patients should be warned of this risk and advised not to drive or operate machinery until their susceptibility is known. Patients should not drive if they have blurred vision.

4.8 Undesirable effects
Drowsiness and sedation are unusual. Sedation, if it occurs, is more often seen with high dosage and at the start of treatment, particularly in the elderly. Other adverse effects include blurring of vision, tachycardia and urinary incontinence and frequency. Dose-related postural hypotension may occur, particularly in the elderly.

Because Depixol may impair alertness, especially at the start of treatment or following the consumption of alcohol, patients should be warned of the risk and advised not to drive or operate machinery, until their susceptibility is known.

Extrapyramidal reactions in the form of acute dystonias (including oculogyric crisis), parkinsonian rigidity, tremor, akinesia and akathisia have been reported and may occur even at lower dosage in susceptible patients. Such effects would usually be encountered early in treatment, but delayed reactions may also occur. Antiparkinson agents should not be prescribed routinely because of the possible risk of precipitating toxic-confusional states, impairing therapeutic efficacy or causing anticholinergic side-effects. They should only be given if required and their requirement reassessed at regular intervals.

Tardive dyskinesia can occur with antipsychotic treatment. It is more common at high doses for prolonged periods but has been reported at lower dosages for short periods. The risk seems to be greater in the elderly, especially females. It has been reported that fine vermicular movements of the tongue are an early sign. It has been observed occasionally in patients receiving Depixol. The concurrent use of anticholinergic antiparkinson drugs may exacerbate this effect. The potential irreversibility and seriousness, as well as the unpredictability of the syndrome, requires especially careful assessment of the risk versus benefit, and the lowest possible dosage and duration of treatment consistent with therapeutic efficacy. Short-lived dyskinesia may occur after abrupt withdrawal of the drug (see section 4.4).

The neuroleptic malignant syndrome has rarely been reported in patients receiving antipsychotics, including flupentixol. This potentially fatal syndrome is characterised by hyperthermia, a fluctuating level of consciousness, muscular rigidity and autonomic dysfunction with pallor, tachycardia, labile blood pressure, sweating and urinary incontinence. Antipsychotic therapy should be discontinued immediately and vigorous symptomatic treatment implemented.

Epileptic fits have occasionally been reported. Confusional states can occur.

The hormonal effects of antipsychotic drugs include hyperprolactinaemia, which may be associated with galactorrhoea, gynaecomastia, oligomenorrhoea or amenorrhoea. Sexual function, including erection and ejaculation may be impaired; but increased libido has also been reported.

ECG changes with prolongation of the QT interval and T-wave changes may occur with moderate to high doses; they are reversible on reducing the dose.

Flupentixol may impair body temperature control, and cases of hyperthermia have occurred rarely. The possible development of hypothermia, particularly in the elderly and hypothyroid, should be borne in mind.

Blood dyscrasias, including thrombocytopenia, have occasionally been reported. Blood counts should be carried out if a patient develops signs of persistent infection. Jaundice and other liver abnormalities have been reported rarely.

Weight gain and less commonly weight loss have been reported; oedema has occasionally been reported and has been considered to be allergic in origin. Rashes have occurred rarely. Although less likely than with phenothiazines, flupentixol can rarely cause increased susceptibility to sunburn.

Occasional local reactions, such as erythema, swelling or tender fibrous nodules have been reported.

Flupentixol, even in low doses, in susceptible (especially non-psychotic) individuals may unusually cause nausea, dizziness or headache, excitement, agitation, insomnia, or unpleasant subjective feelings of being mentally dulled or slowed down.

4.9 Overdose

Overdosage may cause somnolence, or even coma, extrapyramidal symptoms, convulsions, hypotension, shock, hyper-or hypothermia. Treatment is symptomatic and supportive, with measures aimed at supporting the respiratory and cardiovascular systems. The following specific measures may be employed if required.

- anticholinergic antiparkinson drugs if extrapyramidal symptoms occur.
- sedation (with benzodiazepines) in the unlikely event of agitation or excitement or convulsions.
- noradrenaline in saline intravenous drip if the patient is in shock. Adrenaline must not be given.

5. PHARMACOLOGICAL PROPERTIES

5.1 Pharmacodynamic properties

Flupentixol is a non-sedating antipsychotic drug of the thioxanthene group. Its primary pharmacological action is dopamine blockade. Flupentixol has a high affinity for D_1 and D_2 receptors.

5.2 Pharmacokinetic properties

After intramuscular injection, the ester is slowly released from the oil depot and is rapidly hydrolysed to release flupentixol. Flupentixol is widely distributed in the body and extensively metabolized in the liver. Peak circulating levels occur around 7 days after administration.

5.3 Preclinical safety data

Nil of relevance

6. PHARMACEUTICAL PARTICULARS

6.1 List of excipients

Thin vegetable oil "Viscoleo" (fractionated coconut oil).

6.2 Incompatibilities

This product may be mixed in the same syringe with other products in the Depixol Injection range. It should not be mixed with any other injection fluids.

6.3 Shelf life

Depixol Injection

Ampoules 1 mL and 2 mL: 4 years

Syringes 1 mL and 2 mL: 2 years

Depixol Conc Injection

Ampoule 0.5 mL: 2 years

Ampoule 1 mL: 4 years

Vial 5 mL: 3 years

6.4 Special precautions for storage

Store at or below 25°C. Protect from light.

6.5 Nature and contents of container

Depixol Injection

Ampoules containing 1 mL and 2 mL of 20 mg/mL (2% w/v) cis (Z)-flupentixol decanoate in thin vegetable oil. Pack size = 10 ampoules per box.

Syringes containing 1 mL and 2 mL of 20 mg/mL (2%w/v) cis (Z)-flupentixol decanoate in thin vegetable oil. Pack size = 5 syringes per box.

Vial containing 10 mL of 20 mg/mL (2%w/v) cis (Z)-flupentixol decanoate in thin vegetable oil. Pack size = 1 vial per box.

Depixol Conc Injection

Ampoules containing 0.5 mL and 1 mL of 100 mg/ml (10% w/v) cis (Z)-flupentixol decanoate in thin vegetable oil. Pack size = 10 ampoules per box.

Vial containing 5 mL of 100 mg/ml (10%) cis(Z)- flupentixol decanoate in thin vegetable oil. Pack size = 1 vial per box.

6.6 Instructions for use and handling

Nil.

7. MARKETING AUTHORISATION HOLDER

Lundbeck Limited

Lundbeck House

Caldecotte Lake Business Park

Caldecotte

Milton Keynes

MK7 8LF

8. MARKETING AUTHORISATION NUMBER(S)

Depixol Injection	PL 0458/0007R
Depixol Conc Injection	PL 0458/0015R

9. DATE OF FIRST AUTHORISATION/RENEWAL OF THE AUTHORISATION

First Authorisation	28 January 1987
Renewal of Authorisation	17 March 2002

10. DATE OF REVISION OF THE TEXT

17 September 2004

® Registered trademark

Depixol Low Volume Injection

(Lundbeck Limited)

1. NAME OF THE MEDICINAL PRODUCT

Depixol® Low Volume Injection

2. QUALITATIVE AND QUANTITATIVE COMPOSITION

200mg/mL (20% w/v) cis (Z)-flupentixol decanoate in thin vegetable oil.

Ampoules 1 mL and 2 mL and Glass Vial 5 mL.

3. PHARMACEUTICAL FORM

Oily solution for deep intramuscular injection.

4. CLINICAL PARTICULARS

4.1 Therapeutic indications

The treatment of schizophrenia and other psychoses.

4.2 Posology and method of administration

Route of administration: Deep intramuscular injection into the upper outer buttock or lateral thigh. Dosage and dosage interval should be adjusted according to the patients' symptoms and response to treatment.

Note: As with all oil based injections it is important to ensure, by aspiration before injection, that inadvertent intravascular entry does not occur.

Adults: The usual dosage of flupentixol decanoate lies between 50 mg every 4 weeks and 300 mg every 2 weeks, but some patients may require up to 400 mg weekly. Other patients may be adequately maintained on dosages of 20-40 mg flupentixol decanoate every 2-4 weeks. In patients who have not previously received depot antipsychotic, treatment is usually started with a small dose (e.g. 20 mg) to assess tolerability. An interval of at least one week should be allowed before the second injection is given at a dose consistent with the patients' condition.

Adequate control of severe psychotic symptoms may take up to 4 to 6 months at high enough dosage. Once stabilised lower maintenance doses may be considered, but must be sufficient to prevent relapse.

The appropriate presentation of Depixol should be selected to achieve an injection volume which does not exceed 2 mL. Volumes greater than 2 mL should be distributed between two injection sites.

Elderly: In accordance with standard medical practice, initial dosage may need to be reduced to a quarter or half the normal starting dose in the frail or elderly.

Children: Depixol Low Volume Injection is not indicated for children.

4.3 Contraindications

Comatose states, including alcohol, barbiturates, or opiate poisoning. Not recommended for excitable or agitated patients.

4.4 Special warnings and special precautions for use

Caution should be exercised in patients having: liver disease; cardiac disease or arrhythmias; severe respiratory disease; renal failure; epilepsy (and conditions predisposing to epilepsy e.g. alcohol withdrawal or brain damage); Parkinson's disease; narrow angle glaucoma; prostatic hypertrophy; hypothyroidism; hyperthyroidism; myasthenia gravis; phaeochromocytoma and patients who have shown hypersensitivity to thioxanthenes or other antipsychotics.

The elderly require close supervision because they are specially prone to experience such adverse effects as sedation, hypotension, confusion and temperature changes.

Acute withdrawal symptoms, including nausea, vomiting, sweating and insomnia have been described after abrupt cessation of antipsychotic drugs. Recurrence of psychotic symptoms may also occur, and the emergence of involuntary movement disorders (such as akathisia, dystonia and dyskinesia) has been reported. Therefore gradual withdrawal is usually advisable. The plasma concentrations of Depixol Low Volume Injection gradually decrease over several weeks which makes gradual dose tapering unnecessary.

When transferring patients from oral to depot antipsychotics treatment, the oral medication should not be discontinued immediately, but gradually withdrawn over a period of several days after administering the first injection.

4.5 Interaction with other medicinal products and other forms of Interaction

In common with other antipsychotics, flupentixol enhances the response to alcohol, the effects of barbiturates and other CNS depressants. Flupentixol may potentiate the effects of general anaesthetics and anticoagulants and prolong the action of neuromuscular blocking agents.

The anticholinergic effects of atropine or other drugs with anticholinergic properties may be increased. Concomitant use of drugs such as metoclopramide, piperazine or antiparkinson drugs may increase the risk of extrapyramidal effects such as tardive dyskinesia. Combined use of antipsychotics and lithium or sibutramine has been associated with an increased risk of neurotoxicity.

Antipsychotics may enhance the cardiac depressant effects of quinidine; the absorption of corticosteroids and digoxin. The hypotensive effect of vasodilator antihypertensive agents such as hydralazine and α-blockers (e.g. doxazosin), or methyl-dopa may be enhanced. Concomitant use of flupentixol and drugs known to cause QT prolongation or cardiac arrhythmias, such as tricyclic antidepressants, other antipsychotics or terfenadine should be avoided.

Antipsychotics may antagonise the effects of adrenaline and other sympathomimetic agents, and reverse the antihypertensive effects of guanethidine and similar adrenergic-blocking agents. Antipsychotics may also impair the effect of levodopa, adrenergic drugs and anticonvulsants.

The metabolism of tricyclic antidepressants may be inhibited and the control of diabetes may be impaired.

4.6 Pregnancy and lactation

As the safety of this drug during pregnancy has not been established, use during pregnancy, especially the first and last trimesters, should be avoided, unless the expected benefit to the patient outweighs the potential risk to the foetus.

Flupentixol is excreted into the breast milk. If the use of Depixol is considered essential, nursing mothers should be advised to stop breast feeding.

The newborn of mothers treated with antipsychotics in late pregnancy, or labour, may show signs of intoxication such as lethargy, tremor and hyperexcitability, and have a low apgar score.

4.7 Effects on ability to drive and use machines

Alertness may be impaired, especially at the start of treatment, or following the consumption of alcohol; patients should be warned of this risk and advised not to drive or operate machinery until their susceptibility is known. Patients should not drive if they have blurred vision.

4.8 Undesirable effects

Drowsiness and sedation are unusual. Sedation, if it occurs, is more often seen with high dosage and at the start of treatment, particularly in the elderly. Other adverse effects include blurring of vision, tachycardia and urinary incontinence and frequency. Dose-related postural hypotension may occur, particularly in the elderly.

Because Depixol may impair alertness, especially at the start of treatment or following the consumption of alcohol, patients should be warned of the risk and advised not to drive or operate machinery, until their susceptibility is known.

Extrapyramidal reactions in the form of acute dystonias (including oculogyric crisis), parkinsonian rigidity, tremor, akinesia and akathisia have been reported and may occur even at lower dosage in susceptible patients. Such effects would usually be encountered early in treatment, but delayed reactions may also occur. Antiparkinson agents should not be prescribed routinely because of the possible risk of precipitating toxic-confusional states, impairing therapeutic efficacy or causing anticholinergic side-effects.

They should only be given if required and their requirement reassessed at regular intervals.

Tardive dyskinesia can occur with antipsychotic treatment. It is more common at high doses for prolonged periods but has been reported at lower dosage for short periods. The risk seems to be greater in the elderly, especially females. It has been reported that fine vermicular movements of the tongue are an early sign. It has been observed occasionally in patients receiving Depixol. The concurrent use of anticholinergic antiparkinson drugs may exacerbate this effect. The potential irreversibility and seriousness, as well as the unpredictability of the syndrome, requires especially careful assessment of the risk versus benefit, and the lowest possible dosage and duration of treatment consistent with therapeutic efficacy. Short-lived dyskinesia may occur after abrupt withdrawal of the drug (see section 4.4).

The neuroleptic malignant syndrome has rarely been reported in patients receiving antipsychotics, including flupentixol. This potentially fatal syndrome is characterised by hyperthermia, a fluctuating level of consciousness, muscular rigidity and autonomic dysfunction with pallor, tachycardia, labile blood pressure, sweating and urinary incontinence. Antipsychotic therapy should be discontinued immediately and vigorous symptomatic treatment implemented.

Epileptic fits have occasionally been reported. Confusional states can occur.

The hormonal effects of antipsychotic drugs include hyperprolactinaemia, which may be associated with galactorrhoea, gynaecomastia, oligomenorrhoea or amenorrhoea. Sexual function, including erection and ejaculation may be impaired; but increased libido has also been reported.

ECG changes with prolongation of the QT interval and T-wave changes may occur with moderate to high doses; they are reversible on reducing the dose.

Flupentixol may impair body temperature control, and cases of hyperthermia have occurred rarely. The possible development of hypothermia, particularly in the elderly and hypothyroid, should be borne in mind.

Blood dyscrasias, including thrombocytopenia, have occasionally been reported. Blood counts should be carried out if a patient develops signs of persistent infection. Jaundice and other liver abnormalities have been reported rarely.

Weight gain and less commonly weight loss have been reported; oedema has occasionally been reported and has been considered to be allergic in origin. Rashes have occurred rarely. Although less likely than with phenothiazines, flupentixol can rarely cause increased susceptibility to sunburn.

Occasional local reactions, such as erythema, swelling or tender fibrous nodules have been reported.

Flupentixol, even in low doses, in susceptible (especially non-psychotic) individuals may unusually cause nausea, dizziness or headache, excitement, agitation, insomnia, or unpleasant subjective feelings of being mentally dulled or slowed down.

4.9 Overdose

Overdosage may cause somnolence, or even coma, extrapyramidal symptoms, convulsions, hypotension, shock, hyper-or hypothermia. Treatment is symptomatic and supportive, with measures aimed at supporting the respiratory and cardiovascular systems. The following specific measures may be employed if required.

- anticholinergic antiparkinson drugs if extrapyramidal symptoms occur.
- sedation (with benzodiazepines) in the unlikely event of agitation or excitement or convulsions.
- noradrenaline in saline intravenous drip if the patient is in shock. Adrenaline must not be given.

5. PHARMACOLOGICAL PROPERTIES

5.1 Pharmacodynamic properties

Cis(Z)-flupentixol is a antipsychotic of the thioxanthene series.

The antipsychotic effect antipsychotics is related to their dopamine receptor blocking effect. The thioxanthenes have high affinity for both the adenylate cyclase coupled dopamine D_1 receptors and for the dopamine D_2 receptors; in the phenothiazine group the affinity for D_1 receptors is much lower than that for D_2 receptors, whereas butyrophenones, diphenylbutylpiperidines and benzamides only have affinity for D_2 receptors.

In the traditional tests for antipsychotic effect, eg antagonism of stereotypic behaviour induced by dopamine agonists, the chemical groups of antipsychotics mentioned reveal equal but dosage-dependent activity. However, the antistereotypic effects of phenothiazines, butyrophenones, diphenylbutylpiperidines, and benzamides is strongly counteracted by the anticholinergic drug scopolamine, while the antistereotypic effect of thioxanthenes, eg cis(Z)-flupentixol is not, or only very slightly, influenced by concomitant treatment with anticholinergics.

5.2 Pharmacokinetic properties

By esterification of cis(Z)-flupentixol with decanoic acid cis(Z)-flupentixol has been converted to a highly lipophilic substance, cis(Z)-flupentixol decanoate. When dissolved in oil and injected intramuscularly this substance diffuses slowly into the surrounding body water, where enzymatic breakdown occurs releasing the active component cis(Z)-flupentixol. The duration of action is 2-4 weeks with maximum serum levels being reached by the end of the first week after injection.

Cis(Z)-flupentixol is distributed in the body in a similar way to other antipsychotics; with the highest concentrations of drug and metabolites in liver lungs, intestines and kidneys and lower concentrations in heart, spleen, brain and blood. The apparent volume of distribution is about 14 L/kg and the protein binding >95%.

Cis(Z)-flupentixol crosses the placental barrier in small amounts; it is also excreted in breast milk in very small amounts.

The metabolism of cis(Z)-flupentixol proceeds via three main routes - sulphoxidation, side chain N-dealkylation and glucuronic acid conjugation. The metabolites are devoid of psychopharmacological activity. The excretion proceeds mainly with the faeces but also to some degree with the urine. Systemic clearance is about 0.4-0.5 L/min.

5.3 Preclinical safety data

Nil of relevance

6. PHARMACEUTICAL PARTICULARS

6.1 List of excipients

Thin vegetable oil "Viscoleo" (fractionated coconut oil).

6.2 Incompatibilities

This product may be mixed in the same syringe with other products in the Depixol Injection range. It should not be mixed with any other injection fluids.

6.3 Shelf life

Ampoules 1 mL and 2 mL:	2 years
Vial 5 mL	2 years

6.4 Special precautions for storage

Store below 25°C. Protect from light.

6.5 Nature and contents of container

Ampoules containing 1 mL and 2 mL of 200 mg/mL (20%w/v) cis(Z)-flupentixol decanoate in thin vegetable oil. Pack size = 5 ampoules per box.

Vial containing 5 mL of 200 mg/mL (20%w/v) cis(Z)-flupentixol decanoate in thin vegetable oil. Pack size = 1 vial per box.

6.6 Instructions for use and handling

Nil.

7. MARKETING AUTHORISATION HOLDER

Lundbeck Limited

Lundbeck House

Caldecotte Lake Business Park

Caldecotte

Milton Keynes

MK7 8LF

8. MARKETING AUTHORISATION NUMBER(S)

PL 0458/0065

9. DATE OF FIRST AUTHORISATION/RENEWAL OF THE AUTHORISATION

First Authorisation	October 1991
Renewal of Authorisation	January 2002

10. DATE OF REVISION OF THE TEXT

17 September 2004

® Registered trademark

Depixol Tablets 3mg

(Lundbeck Limited)

1. NAME OF THE MEDICINAL PRODUCT

Depixol® Tablets 3 mg

2. QUALITATIVE AND QUANTITATIVE COMPOSITION

3.504 mg flupentixol dihydrochloride corresponding to 3 mg flupentixol base.

3. PHARMACEUTICAL FORM

Round, biconvex, yellow, sugar-coated tablets.

4. CLINICAL PARTICULARS

4.1 Therapeutic indications

The treatment of schizophrenia and other psychoses.

4.2 Posology and method of administration

Route of administration: Oral.

Adults: 1 - 3 tablets twice daily to a maximum of 18 mg (6 tablets) per day. It is recommended that commencement of treatment and increase in dosage should be carried out under close supervision. As with all antipsychotic drugs, the dose of Depixol should be titrated to the needs of each patient.

When transferring patients from oral to depot antipsychotic treatment, the oral medication should not be discontinued immediately, but gradually withdrawn over a period of several days after administering the first injection.

Elderly: In accordance with standard medical practice, initial dosage may need to be reduced to a quarter or half the normal starting dose in the frail or elderly.

Children: Not indicated for children.

4.3 Contraindications

Comatose states, including alcohol, barbiturate, or opiate poisoning. Not recommended for excitable or agitated patients.

4.4 Special warnings and special precautions for use

Caution should be exercised in patients having: liver disease; cardiac disease or arrhythmias; severe respiratory disease; renal failure; epilepsy (and conditions predisposing to epilepsy e.g. alcohol withdrawal or brain damage); Parkinson's disease; narrow angle glaucoma; prostatic hypertrophy; hypothyroidism; hyperthyroidism; myasthenia gravis; phaeochromocytoma and patients who have shown hypersensitivity to thioxanthenes or other antipsychotics.

The elderly require close supervision because they are specially prone to experience such adverse effects as sedation, hypotension, confusion and temperature changes.

Acute withdrawal symptoms, including nausea, vomiting, sweating and insomnia have been described after abrupt cessation of antipsychotic drugs. Recurrence of psychotic symptoms may also occur, and the emergence of involuntary movement disorders (such as akathisia, dystonia and dyskinesia) has been reported. Therefore, gradual withdrawal is advisable.

4.5 Interaction with other medicinal products and other forms of Interaction

In common with other antipsychotics, flupentixol enhances the response to alcohol, the effects of barbiturates and other CNS depressants. Flupentixol may potentiate the effects of general anaesthetics and anticoagulants and prolong the action of neuromuscular blocking agents.

The anticholinergic effects of atropine or other drugs with anticholinergic properties may be increased. Concomitant use of drugs such as metoclopramide, piperazine or antiparkinson drugs may increase the risk of extrapyramidal effects such as tardive dyskinesia. Combined use of antipsychotics and lithium or sibutramine has been associated with an increased risk of neurotoxicity.

Antipsychotics may enhance the cardiac depressant effects of quinidine; the absorption of corticosteroids and digoxin. The hypotensive effect of vasodilator antihypertensive agents such as hydralazine and α-blockers (e.g. doxazosin), or methyl-dopa may be enhanced. Concomitant use of flupentixol and drugs known to cause QT prolongation or cardiac arrhythmias, such as tricyclic antidepressants, other antipsychotics or terfenadine should be avoided.

Antipsychotics may antagonise the effects of adrenaline and other sympathomimetic agents, and reverse the antihypertensive effects of guanethidine and similar adrenergic-blocking agents. Antipsychotics may also impair the effect of levodopa, adrenergic drugs and anticonvulsants.

The metabolism of tricyclic antidepressants may be inhibited and the control of diabetes may be impaired.

Antacids may impair absorption, as may tea or coffee.

4.6 Pregnancy and lactation

As the safety of this drug during pregnancy has not been established, use during pregnancy, especially the first and last trimesters, should be avoided, unless the expected benefit to the patient outweighs the potential risk to the foetus.

Flupentixol is excreted into the breast milk. If the use of Depixol is considered essential, nursing mothers should be advised to stop breast feeding.

The newborn of mothers treated with antipsychotics in late pregnancy, or labour, may show signs of intoxication such as lethargy, tremor and hyperexcitability, and have a low apgar score.

4.7 Effects on ability to drive and use machines

Alertness may be impaired, especially at the start of treatment, or following the consumption of alcohol; patients should be warned of this risk and advised not to drive or operate machinery until their susceptibility is known. Patients should not drive if they have blurred vision.

4.8 Undesirable effects

Drowsiness and sedation are unusual. Sedation, if it occurs, is more often seen with high dosage and at the start of treatment, particularly in the elderly. Other adverse effects include blurring of vision, tachycardia and urinary incontinence and frequency. Dose-related postural hypotension may occur, particularly in the elderly.

Because Depixol may impair alertness, especially at the start of treatment or following the consumption of alcohol, patients should be warned of the risk and advised not to drive or operate machinery, until their susceptibility is known.

Extrapyramidal reactions in the form of acute dystonias (including oculogyric crisis), parkinsonian rigidity, tremor, akinesia and akathisia have been reported and may occur even at lower dosage in susceptible patients. Such effects would usually be encountered early in treatment, but delayed reactions may also occur. Antiparkinson agents should not be prescribed routinely because of the possible risk of precipitating toxic-confusional states, impairing therapeutic efficacy or causing anticholinergic side-effects. They should only be given if required and their requirement reassessed at regular intervals.

Tardive dyskinesia can occur with antipsychotic treatment. It is more common at high doses for prolonged periods but has been reported at lower dosage for short periods. The risk seems to be greater in the elderly, especially females. It has been reported that fine vermicular movements of the tongue are an early sign. It has been observed occasionally in patients receiving Depixol. The concurrent use of anticholinergic antiparkinson drugs may exacerbate this effect. The potential irreversibility and seriousness, as well as the unpredictability of the syndrome, requires especially careful assessment of the risk versus benefit, and the lowest possible dosage and duration of treatment consistent with therapeutic efficacy. Short-lived dyskinesia may occur after abrupt withdrawal of the drug (see section 4.4).

The neuroleptic malignant syndrome has rarely been reported in patients receiving antipsychotics, including flupentixol. This potentially fatal syndrome is characterised by hyperthermia, a fluctuating level of consciousness, muscular rigidity and autonomic dysfunction with pallor, tachycardia, labile blood pressure, sweating and urinary incontinence. Antipsychotic therapy should be discontinued immediately and vigorous symptomatic treatment implemented.

Epileptic fits have occasionally been reported. Confusional states can occur.

The hormonal effects of antipsychotic drugs include hyperprolactinaemia, which may be associated with galactorrhoea, gynaecomastia, oligomenorrhoea or amenorrhoea. Sexual function, including erection and ejaculation may be impaired; but increased libido has also been reported.

ECG changes with prolongation of the QT interval and T-wave changes may occur with moderate to high doses; they are reversible on reducing the dose.

Flupentixol may impair body temperature control, and cases of hyperthermia have occurred rarely. The possible development of hypothermia, particularly in the elderly and hypothyroid, should be borne in mind.

Blood dyscrasias, including thrombocytopenia, have occasionally been reported. Blood counts should be carried out if a patient develops signs of persistent infection. Jaundice and other liver abnormalities have been reported rarely.

Weight gain and less commonly weight loss have been reported; oedema has occasionally been reported and has been considered to be allergic in origin. Rashes have occurred rarely. Although less likely than with phenothiazines, flupentixol can rarely cause increased susceptibility to sunburn.

Flupentixol, even in low doses, in susceptible (especially non-psychotic) individuals may unusually cause nausea, dizziness or headache, excitement, agitation, insomnia, or unpleasant subjective feelings of being mentally dulled or slowed down.

4.9 Overdose

Overdosage may cause somnolence, or even coma, extrapyramidal symptoms, convulsions, hypotension, shock, hyper-or hypothermia. Treatment is symptomatic and supportive, with measures aimed at supporting the respiratory and cardiovascular systems. The following specific measures may be employed if required.

- anticholinergic antiparkinson drugs if extrapyramidal symptoms occur.
- sedation (with benzodiazepines) in the unlikely event of agitation or excitement or convulsions.
- noradrenaline in saline intravenous drip if the patient is in shock. Adrenaline must not be given.
- gastric lavage should be considered.

5. PHARMACOLOGICAL PROPERTIES

5.1 Pharmacodynamic properties

Flupentixol is a antipsychotic of the thioxanthene series.

The antipsychotic effect of antipsychotic is believed to be related to their dopamine receptor blocking effect. The thioxanthenes have high affinity for D_1 and D_2 receptors.

5.2 Pharmacokinetic properties

Oral administration to volunteers (8 mg single dose and 1.5 mg/day) and patients (5-60 mg/d) resulted in serum drug concentration curves with a maximum around four hours after administration. Mean biological half-life was about 35 hours in patients. No difference was seen in patients between half-lives estimated after single-dose administration and those estimated after repeated administration. Mean oral bioavailability of flupentixol varied between 40% and 55%.

5.3 Preclinical safety data

Nil of relevance

6. PHARMACEUTICAL PARTICULARS

6.1 List of excipients

Potato starch, lactose, gelatin, talc, magnesium stearate, sucrose and yellow iron oxide (E172).

6.2 Incompatibilities

Not applicable.

6.3 Shelf life

Depixol tablets are stable for 3 years.

6.4 Special precautions for storage

Store in original container, protected from light and moisture. Do not store above 30°C.

6.5 Nature and contents of container

Grey polypropylene container with screw cap or glass bottles with white plastic stoppers. Contents 100 tablets.

6.6 Instructions for use and handling

Nil.

7. MARKETING AUTHORISATION HOLDER

Lundbeck Limited

Lundbeck House

Caldecotte Lake Business Park

Caldecotte

Milton Keynes

MK7 8LF

8. MARKETING AUTHORISATION NUMBER(S)

PL 0458/0013R

9. DATE OF FIRST AUTHORISATION/RENEWAL OF THE AUTHORISATION

First Authorisation 29 January 1987

Renewal of Authorisation 17 March 2002

10. DATE OF REVISION OF THE TEXT

17 September 2004

® Registered trademark

DepoCyte 50 mg suspension for injection

(Napp Pharmaceuticals Limited)

1. NAME OF THE MEDICINAL PRODUCT

DepoCyte® 50 mg suspension for injection ▼

2. QUALITATIVE AND QUANTITATIVE COMPOSITION

Each vial contains 50 mg cytarabine.

For excipients, see Section 6.1.

3. PHARMACEUTICAL FORM

Suspension for injection.

4. CLINICAL PARTICULARS

4.1 Therapeutic indications

Intrathecal treatment of lymphomatous meningitis. In the majority of patients such treatment will be part of symptomatic palliation of the disease.

4.2 Posology and method of administration

Adults and the elderly

DepoCyte should be administered only under the supervision of a physician experienced in the use of cancer chemotherapeutic agents.

For the treatment of lymphomatous meningitis, the dose for adults is 50 mg (one vial) administered intrathecally (lumbar puncture or intraventricularly via an Ommaya reservoir). The following regimen of induction, consolidation and maintenance therapy is recommended:

Induction therapy: 50 mg administered every 14 days for 2 doses (weeks 1 and 3).

Consolidation therapy: 50 mg administered every 14 days for 3 doses (weeks 5, 7 and 9) followed by an additional dose of 50 mg at week 13.

Maintenance therapy: 50 mg administered every 28 days for 4 doses (weeks 17, 21, 25 and 29).

Method of administration: ***DepoCyte*** is to be administered by slow injection over a period of 1-5 minutes directly into the CSF via either an intraventricular reservoir or by direct injection into the lumbar sac. Following administration by lumbar puncture, it is recommended that the patient should be instructed to lie flat for one hour. Patients should be started on dexamethasone 4 mg twice daily orally or intravenously for 5 days beginning on the day of injection of ***DepoCyte.***

DepoCyte must not be administered by any other route of administration.

DepoCyte must be used as supplied; do not dilute (see also Section 6.2).

Patients should be observed by the physician for immediate toxic reactions.

If neurotoxicity develops the dose should be reduced to 25 mg. If it persists, treatment with ***DepoCyte*** should be discontinued.

Children

Safety and efficacy in children have not been demonstrated.

4.3 Contraindications

Hypersensitivity to cytarabine or any of the excipients.

Patients with active meningeal infection.

4.4 Special warnings and special precautions for use

Patients receiving ***DepoCyte*** should be concurrently treated with corticosteroids (e.g. dexamethasone) to mitigate the symptoms of arachnoiditis (see Undesirable Effects) which is a common adverse event.

Arachnoiditis is a syndrome manifested primarily by nausea, vomiting, headache and fever.

Patients should be informed about the expected adverse events of headache, nausea, vomiting and fever, and about the early signs and symptoms of neurotoxicity. The importance of concurrent dexamethasone administration should be emphasised at the initiation of each cycle of ***DepoCyte*** treatment. Patients should be instructed to seek medical attention if signs or symptoms of neurotoxicity develop, or if oral dexamethasone is not well tolerated.

Cytarabine, when administered intrathecally, has been associated with nausea, vomiting and serious central nervous system toxicity including blindness, myelopathy and other neurological toxicity sometimes leading to a permanent neurological deficit.

Administration of ***DepoCyte*** in combination with other neurotoxic chemotherapeutic agents or with cranial/spinal irradiation may increase the risk of neurotoxicity.

Blockage of CSF flow may result in increased free cytarabine concentrations in the CSF with increased risk of neurotoxicity.

Although significant systemic exposure to free cytarabine is not expected following intrathecal treatment, some effects on bone marrow function cannot be excluded. Systemic toxicity due to intravenous administration of cytarabine consists primarily of bone marrow suppression with leucopenia, thrombocytopenia and anaemia. Therefore monitoring of the haemopoietic system is advised.

Anaphylactic reactions following intravenous administration of free cytarabine have been rarely reported.

Since ***DepoCyte's*** particles are similar in size and appearance to white blood cells, care must be taken in interpreting CSF examination following ***DepoCyte*** administration.

4.5 Interaction with other medicinal products and other forms of Interaction

No definite interactions between ***DepoCyte*** delivered intrathecally and other drugs have been established.

Concomitant administration of ***DepoCyte*** with other antineoplastic agents administered by the intrathecal route has not been studied.

Intrathecal co-administration of cytarabine with other cytotoxic agents may increase the risk of neurotoxicity.

4.6 Pregnancy and lactation

Teratology studies in animals have not been conducted with ***DepoCyte*** and there are no adequate and well controlled studies in pregnant women; however cytarabine can cause foetal harm when administered during pregnancy. Therefore, women of childbearing potential should not receive the treatment until pregnancy is excluded and should be advised to use a reliable contraceptive method.

Given that cytarabine has a mutagenic potential which could induce chromosomal damage in the human spermatozoa, males undergoing ***DepoCyte*** treatment and their partner should be advised to use a reliable contraceptive method.

It is not known whether cytarabine is excreted in human milk following intrathecal administration. The systemic exposure to free cytarabine following intrathecal treatment with ***DepoCyte*** was negligible. Because of possible excretion in human milk and because of the potential for serious adverse reactions in nursing infants, the use of ***DepoCyte*** is not recommended in nursing women.

4.7 Effects on ability to drive and use machines

There have been no reports explicitly relating to effects of ***DepoCyte*** treatment on the ability to drive or use machines. However, on the basis of reported adverse reactions, patients should be advised against driving or using machines during treatment.

4.8 Undesirable effects

DepoCyte has the potential of producing serious toxicity.

All patients receiving ***DepoCyte*** should be treated concurrently with corticosteroids (e.g., dexamethasone) to mitigate the symptoms of arachnoiditis. Toxic effects may be related to a single dose or to cumulative doses. Because toxic effects can occur at any time during therapy (although they are most likely within 5 days of administration), patients receiving ***DepoCyte*** therapy should be monitored continuously for the development of neurotoxicity. If patients develop neurotoxicity, subsequent doses of ***DepoCyte*** should be reduced, and ***DepoCyte*** should be discontinued if toxicity persists.

Arachnoiditis, a syndrome manifested primarily by headache, nausea, vomiting, fever, neck rigidity, neck or back pain, meningism, CSF pleocytosis, with or without altered state of consciousness, is a common adverse event. Arachnoiditis can be fatal if left untreated.

The incidence of adverse events determined from all the patients treated in the Phase II-IV clinical trials is given in the table below:

(see Table 1 on next page)

Transient elevations in CSF protein and white blood cells have also been observed in patients following ***DepoCyte***

Table 1 Adverse events possibly reflecting meningeal irritation in Phase II, III, and IV patients (n [%] of cycles* of therapy)

	DepoCyte (n = 689 cycles)	Methotrexate (n = 69.5 cycles)	Cytarabine (n = 56.25 cycles)
Headache	25%	22%	12%
Nausea	19%	17%	16%
Vomiting	17%	24%	16%
Fever	13%	12%	21%
Back pain	11%	14%	9%
Convulsions	7%	9%	1%
Neck pain	5%	3%	3%
Neck rigidity	3%	0%	4%
Hydrocephalus	2%	3%	0%
Meningism	1%	0%	1%

*Cycle length was 2 weeks during which the patient received either 1 dose of ***DepoCyte*** or 4 doses of cytarabine or methotrexate. Cytarabine and methotrexate patients not completing all 4 doses are counted as a fraction of a cycle.

administration and also been noted after intrathecal treatment with methotrexate or cytarabine.

4.9 Overdose

No overdosages with ***DepoCyte*** have been reported. An overdose with ***DepoCyte*** may be associated with severe arachnoiditis including encephalopathy.

In an early uncontrolled study without dexamethasone prophylaxis, single doses up to 125 mg were administered. One patient at the 125 mg dose level died of encephalopathy 36 hours after receiving ***DepoCyte*** intraventricularly. This patient, however, was also receiving concomitant whole brain irradiation and had previously received intraventricular methotrexate.

There is no antidote for intrathecal ***DepoCyte*** or unencapsulated cytarabine released from ***DepoCyte***. Exchange of cerebrospinal fluid with isotonic saline has been carried out in a case of intrathecal overdose of free cytarabine and such a procedure may be considered in the case of ***DepoCyte*** overdose. Management of overdose should be directed at maintaining vital functions.

5. PHARMACOLOGICAL PROPERTIES

5.1 Pharmacodynamic properties

Pharmacotherapeutic group: Antimetabolite (pyrimidine analogue). ATC code L01B C01

DepoCyte is a sustained-release formulation of cytarabine, designed for direct administration into the cerebrospinal fluid (CSF).

Cytarabine is a cell-cycle phase specific antineoplastic agent, affecting cells only during the S-phase of cell division. Intracellularly, cytarabine is converted into cytarabine-5'-triphosphate (ara-CTP), which is the active metabolite. The mechanism of action is not completely understood, but it appears that ara-CTP acts primarily through inhibition of DNA synthesis. Incorporation into DNA and RNA may also contribute to cytarabine cytotoxicity. Cytarabine is cytotoxic to a wide variety of proliferating mammalian cells in culture.

For cell-cycle phase specific antimetabolites the duration of exposure of neoplastic cells to cytotoxic concentrations is an important determination of drug efficacy.

In vitro studies, examining more than 60 cell lines, demonstrated that the median cytarabine concentration resulting in 50% growth inhibition (IC_{50}) was approximately 10 μM (2.4 μg/ml) for two days of exposure and 0.1 μM (0.024 μg/ml) for 6 days of exposure. The studies also demonstrated susceptibility of many solid tumour cell lines to cytarabine, particularly after longer periods of exposure to cytarabine.

In an open-label, active-controlled, multicentre clinical study, 35 patients with lymphomatous meningitis (with malignant cells found on CSF cytology) were randomised to intrathecal therapy with either ***DepoCyte*** (n=18) or unencapsulated cytarabine (n=17). During the 1 month Induction phase of treatment, ***DepoCyte*** was administered intrathecally as 50 mg every 2 weeks, and unencapsulated cytarabine as 50 mg twice a week. Patients who did not respond discontinued protocol treatment after 4 weeks. Patients who achieved a response (defined as clearing of the CSF of malignant cells in the absence of progression of neurological symptoms) went on to receive Consolidation and Maintenance therapy for up to 29 weeks.

Responses were observed in 13/18 (72%, 95% confidence intervals: 47, 90) of ***DepoCyte*** patients versus 3/17 (18% patients, 95% confidence intervals: 4, 43) in the unencapsulated cytarabine arm. A statistically significant association between treatment and response was observed (Fisher's exact test p-value = 0.002). The majority of ***DepoCyte*** patients went on beyond Induction to receive additional therapy. ***DepoCyte*** patients received a median of 5 cycles (doses) per patient (range 1 to 10 doses) with a median time on therapy of 90 days (range 1 to 207 days).

No statistically significant differences were noted in secondary endpoints such as duration of response, progression-free survival, neurological signs and symptoms, Karnofsky performance status, quality of life and overall survival. Median progression-free survival (defined as time to neurological progression or death) for all treated patients was 77 versus 48 days for ***DepoCyte*** versus unencapsulated cytarabine, respectively. The proportion of patients alive at 12 months was 24% for ***DepoCyte*** versus 19% for unencapsulated cytarabine.

5.2 Pharmacokinetic properties

Analysis of the available pharmacokinetic data shows that following intrathecal ***DepoCyte*** administration in patients, either via the lumbar sac or by intraventricular reservoir, peaks of free cytarabine were observed within 5 hours in both the ventricle and lumbar sac. These peaks were followed by a biphasic elimination profile consisting of an initial sharp decline and subsequent slow decline with a terminal phase half-life of 100 to 263 hours over a dose-range of 12.5 mg to 75 mg. In contrast, intrathecal administration of 30 mg free cytarabine has shown a biphasic CSF concentration profile with a terminal phase half-life of about 3.4 hours.

Pharmacokinetic parameters of ***DepoCyte*** (75 mg) in neoplastic meningitis patients in whom the drug was administered either intraventricularly or by lumbar puncture suggest that exposure to the drug in the ventricular or lumbar spaces is similar regardless of the route of administration. In addition, compared with free cytarabine, the formulation increases the biological half-life by a factor of 27 to 71 depending upon the route of administration and the compartment sampled. Encapsulated cytarabine concentrations and the counts of the lipid particles in which the cytarabine is encapsulated in ***DepoCyte*** followed a similar distribution pattern. AUCs of free and encapsulated cytarabine after ventricular injection of ***DepoCyte*** appeared to increase linearly with increasing dose, indicating that the release of cytarabine from ***DepoCyte*** and the pharmacokinetics of cytarabine are linear in human CSF.

The transfer rate of cytarabine from CSF to plasma is slow and the conversion to uracil arabinoside (ara-U), the inactive metabolite, in the plasma is fast. Systemic exposure to cytarabine was determined to be negligible following intrathecal administration of 50 mg and 75 mg of ***DepoCyte***.

Metabolism and Elimination

The primary route of elimination of cytarabine is metabolism to the inactive compound ara-U, (1-β-D-arabinofuranosyluracil or uracil arabinoside) followed by urinary excretion of ara-U. In contrast with systemically administered cytarabine which is rapidly metabolised to ara-U, conversion to ara-U in the CSF is negligible after intrathecal administration because of the significantly lower cytidine deaminase activity in the CNS tissues and CSF. The CSF clearance rate of cytarabine is similar to the CSF bulk flow rate of 0.24 ml/min.

The distribution and clearance of cytarabine and of the predominant phospholipid component of the lipid particle (DOPC) following intrathecal administration of ***DepoCyte*** was evaluated in rodents. Radiolabels for cytarabine and DOPC were distributed rapidly throughout the neuraxis. More than 90% of cytarabine was excreted by day 4 and an additional 2.7% by 21 days. The results suggest that the lipid components undergo hydrolysis and are largely incorporated in the tissues following breakdown in the intrathecal space.

5.3 Preclinical safety data

A review of the toxicological data available for the constituent lipids (DOPC and DPPG) or similar phospholipids to those in ***DepoCyte*** indicates that such lipids are well tolerated in various animal species even when administered for prolonged periods at doses in the g/kg range.

The results of acute and subacute toxicity studies performed in monkeys suggested that intrathecal ***DepoCyte*** was tolerated up to a dose of 10 mg (comparable to a human dose of 100 mg). Slight to moderate inflammation of the meninges in the spinal cord and brain and/or astrocytic activation were observed in animals receiving intrathecal ***DepoCyte***. These changes were believed to be consistent with the toxic effects of other intrathecal agents such as unencapsulated cytarabine. Similar changes (generally described as minimal to slight) were also observed in some animals receiving DepoFoam alone (***DepoCyte*** vesicles without cytarabine) but not in saline control animals. Mouse, rat and dog studies have shown that free cytarabine is highly toxic for the haemopoietic system.

No carcinogenicity, mutagenicity or impairment of fertility studies have been conducted with ***DepoCyte***. The active ingredient of ***DepoCyte***, cytarabine, was mutagenic in *in vitro* tests and was clastogenic *in vitro* (chromosome aberrations and sister chromatid exchange in human leukocytes) and *in vivo* (chromosome aberrations and sister chromatid exchange assay in rodent bone marrow, mouse micronucleus assay). Cytarabine caused the transformation of hamster embryo cells and rat H43 cells *in vitro*. Cytarabine was clastogenic to meiotic cells; a dose-dependent increase in sperm-head abnormalities and chromosomal aberrations occurred in mice given i.p. cytarabine. No studies assessing the impact of cytarabine on fertility are available in the literature. Because the systemic exposure to free cytarabine following intrathecal treatment with ***DepoCyte*** was negligible, the risk of impaired fertility is likely to be low.

6. PHARMACEUTICAL PARTICULARS

6.1 List of excipients

Cholesterol, triolein, dioleylphosphatidylcholine (DOPC), dipalmitoylphosphatidylglycerol (DPPG), sodium chloride, water for injections.

6.2 Incompatibilities

No formal assessments of pharmacokinetic drug-drug interactions between ***DepoCyte*** and other agents have been conducted. ***DepoCyte*** should not be diluted or mixed with any other medicinal products, as any change in concentration or pH may affect the stability of the microparticles.

6.3 Shelf life

2 years

6.4 Special precautions for storage

Store at 2°C - 8°C (in a refrigerator). Do not freeze.

6.5 Nature and contents of container

DepoCyte is supplied in individual cartons each containing one single-dose glass vial (Ph.Eur. type I glass), closed with a fluororesin faced butyl rubber stopper and sealed with an aluminium flip-off seal.

6.6 Instructions for use and handling

Preparation of ***DepoCyte***

Given its toxic nature, special precautions should be taken in handling ***DepoCyte***. See 'Precautions for the handling and disposal of ***DepoCyte***' below.

Vials of ***DepoCyte*** should be allowed to warm to room temperature (18°C -22°C) for a minimum of 30 minutes and be gently inverted to resuspend the particles immediately prior to withdrawal from the vial. Avoid vigorous shaking. No further reconstitution or dilution is required.

DepoCyte administration

DepoCyte should be withdrawn from the vial immediately before administration. Since ***DepoCyte*** is a single use vial and does not contain any preservative, the drug should be used within 4 hours of withdrawal from the vial. Unused drug must be discarded and not used subsequently. Do not mix ***DepoCyte*** with any other medicinal products (see Section 6.2).

In-line filters must not be used when administering ***DepoCyte. DepoCyte*** is administered directly into the CSF via an intraventricular reservoir or by direct injection into the lumbar sac. ***DepoCyte*** should be injected slowly over a period of 1-5 minutes. Following drug administration by lumbar puncture, the patient should be instructed to lie flat for one hour. Patients should be observed by the physician for immediate toxic reactions.

Patients should be started on corticosteroids (e.g. dexamethasone 4 mg twice daily either orally or intravenously) for 5 days beginning on the day of ***DepoCyte*** injection.

DepoCyte must only be administered by the intrathecal route.

Do not dilute ***DepoCyte*** suspension.

Precautions for the handling and disposal of ***DepoCyte***

The following protective recommendations are given due to the toxic nature of this substance:

- personnel should be trained in good technique for handling anticancer agents

• male and female staff who are trying to conceive and female staff who are pregnant should be excluded from working with the substance

• personnel must wear protective clothing: goggles, gowns, disposable gloves and masks

• a designated area should be defined for preparation (preferably under a laminar flow system). The work surface should be protected by disposable, plastic backed, absorbent paper

• all items used during administration or cleaning, should be placed in high risk, waste-disposal bags for high temperature incineration

• in the event of accidental contact with the skin, exposed areas should be washed immediately with soap and water

• in the event of accidental contact with the mucous membranes, exposed areas should be treated immediately by copious lavage with water; medical attention should be sought.

7. MARKETING AUTHORISATION HOLDER

SkyePharma PLC
105 Piccadilly
London
W1V 9FN
UK

8. MARKETING AUTHORISATION NUMBER(S)

EU/1/01/187/001

9. DATE OF FIRST AUTHORISATION/RENEWAL OF THE AUTHORISATION

11 July 2001

10. DATE OF REVISION OF THE TEXT

11. LEGAL CATEGORY

POM

® The Napp device and ***DepoCyte*** are Registered Trade Marks.

Depo-Medrone 40mg/ml

(Pharmacia Limited)

1. NAME OF THE MEDICINAL PRODUCT

Depo-Medrone 40 mg/ml.

2. QUALITATIVE AND QUANTITATIVE COMPOSITION

Methylprednisolone Acetate BP 40 mg/ml.

3. PHARMACEUTICAL FORM

Sterile, aqueous suspension.

4. CLINICAL PARTICULARS

4.1 Therapeutic indications

Depo-Medrone may be used locally or systemically, particularly where oral therapy is not feasible.

Depo-Medrone may be used by any of the following routes: intramuscular, intra-articular, periarticular, intrabursal, intralesional or into the tendon sheath. It must not be used by the intrathecal or intravenous routes (see Contra-indications and Undesirable effects).

Intramuscular administration:

1. Rheumatic disorders
Rheumatoid arthritis

2. Collagen diseases/arteritis
Systemic lupus erythematosus

3. Dermatological diseases
Severe erythema multiforme (Stevens-Johnson syndrome)

4. Allergic states
Bronchial asthma
Severe seasonal and perennial allergic rhinitis
Drug hypersensitivity reactions
Angioneurotic oedema

5. Gastro-intestinal diseases
Ulcerative colitis
Crohn's disease

6. Respiratory diseases
Fulminating or disseminated tuberculosis (with appropriate antituberculous chemotherapy)
Aspiration of gastric contents

7. Miscellaneous
TB meningitis (with appropriate antituberculous chemotherapy)

Intra-articular administration:

Rheumatoid arthritis
Osteo-arthritis with an inflammatory component

Soft tissue administration (intrabursal, periarticular, into tendon sheath):

Synovitis not associated with infection
Epicondylitis
Tenosynovitis
Plantar fasciitis
Bursitis

Intralesional:

Keloids
Localized lichen planus
Localized lichen simplex
Granuloma annulare
Discoid lupus erythematosus
Alopecia areata

4.2 Posology and method of administration

Depo-Medrone should not be mixed with any other suspending agent or solution. Parenteral drug products should be inspected visually for particulate matter and discoloration prior to administration, whenever suspension and container permit. Depo-Medrone may be used by any of the following routes: intramuscular, intra-articular, periarticular, intrabursal, intralesional and into the tendon sheath. It must not be used by the intrathecal or intravenous routes (see Contra-indications and Undesirable effects).

Undesirable effects may be minimised by using the lowest effective dose for the minimum period (see Special warnings and special precautions for use).

Depo-Medrone vials are intended for single dose use only.

Intramuscular - for sustained systemic effect: Allergic conditions (severe seasonal and perennial allergic rhinitis, asthma, drug reactions), 80 - 120 mg (2 - 3 ml).

Dermatological conditions, 40 - 120 mg (1 - 3 ml).

Rheumatic disorders and collagen diseases (rheumatoid arthritis, SLE), 40 - 120 mg (1 - 3 ml) per week.

Dosage must be individualized and depends on the condition being treated and its severity.

Note: Depo-Medrone is not intended for the prophylaxis of severe seasonal and perennial allergic rhinitis or other seasonal allergies and should be administered only when symptoms are present.

The frequency of intramuscular injections should be determined by the duration of clinical response.

In the case of seasonal allergic rhinitis a single injection is frequently sufficient. If necessary, however, a second injection may be given after two to three weeks.

On average the effect of a single 2 ml (80 mg) injection may be expected to last approximately two weeks.

Intra-articular: Rheumatoid arthritis, osteo-arthritis. The dose of Depo-Medrone depends upon the size of the joint and the severity of the condition. Repeated injections, if needed, may be given at intervals of one to five or more weeks depending upon the degree of relief obtained from the initial injection. A suggested dosage guide is: large joint (knee, ankle, shoulder), 20 - 80 mg (0.5 - 2 ml); medium joint (elbow, wrist), 10 - 40 mg (0.25 - 1 ml); small joint (metacarpophalangeal, interphalangeal, sternoclavicular, acromioclavicular), 4 - 10 mg (0.1 - 0.25 ml).

Intrabursal: Subdeltoid bursitis, prepatellar bursitis, olecranon bursitis. For administration directly into bursae, 4 - 30 mg (0.1 - 0.75 ml). In most cases, repeat injections are not needed.

Intralesional: Keloids, localised lichen planus, localized lichen simplex, granuloma annulare, alopecia areata, and discoid lupus erythematosus. For administration directly into the lesion for local effect in dermatological conditions, 20 - 60 mg (0.5 - 1.5 ml). For large lesions, the dose may be distributed by repeated local injections of 20 - 40 mg (0.5 - 1 ml). One to four injections are usually employed. Care should be taken to avoid injection of sufficient material to cause blanching, since this may be followed by a small slough.

Peri-articular: Epicondylitis. Infiltrate 4 - 30 mg (0.1 - 0.75 ml) into the affected area.

Into the tendon sheath: Tenosynovitis, epicondylitis. For administration directly into the tendon sheath, 4 - 30 mg (0.1 - 0.75 ml). In recurrent or chronic conditions, repeat injections may be necessary.

Special precautions should be observed when administering Depo-Medrone. Intramuscular injections should be made deeply into the gluteal muscles. The usual technique of aspirating prior to injection should be employed to avoid intravascular administration. Doses recommended for intramuscular injection must not be administered superficially or subcutaneously.

Intra-articular injections should be made using precise, anatomical localisation into the synovial space of the joint involved. The injection site for each joint is determined by that location where the synovial cavity is most superficial and most free of large vessels and nerves. Suitable sites for intra-articular injection are the knee, ankle, wrist, elbow, shoulder, phalangeal and hip joints. The spinal joints, unstable joints and those devoid of synovial space are not suitable. Treatment failures are most frequently the result of failure to enter the joint space. Intra-articular injections should be made with care as follows: ensure correct positioning of the needle into the synovial space and aspirate a few drops of joint fluid. The aspirating syringe should then be replaced by another containing Depo-Medrone. To ensure position of the needle, synovial fluid should be aspirated and the injection made. After injection the joint is moved slightly to aid mixing of the synovial fluid and the suspension. Subsequent to therapy care should be taken for the patient not to overuse the joint in which benefit has been obtained. Negligence in this matter may permit an increase in joint deterioration that will more than offset the beneficial effects of the steroid.

Intrabursal injections should be made as follows: the area around the injection site is prepared in a sterile way and a wheal at the site made with 1 per cent procaine hydrochloride solution. A 20 to 24 gauge needle attached to a dry syringe is inserted into the bursa and the fluid aspirated. The needle is left in place and the aspirating syringe changed for a small syringe containing the desired dose. After injection, the needle is withdrawn and a small dressing applied. In the treatment of tenosynovitis care should be taken to inject Depo-Medrone into the tendon sheath rather than into the substance of the tendon. Due to the absence of a true tendon sheath, the Achilles tendon should not be injected with Depo-Medrone.

Children: Dosage may be reduced for infants and children but should be governed more by the severity of the condition and response of the patient, than by age or size.

Elderly patients: When used according to instructions, there is no information to suggest that a change in dosage is warranted in the elderly. However, treatment of elderly patients, particularly if long-term, should be planned bearing in mind the more serious consequences of the common side-effects of corticosteroids in old age and close clinical supervision is required (see Special warnings and special precautions for use).

4.3 Contraindications

Depo-medrone is contra-indicated where there is known hypersensitivity to components and in systemic infection unless specific anti-infective therapy is employed.

Due to its potential for neurotoxicity, Depo-Medrone must not be given by the intrathecal route. In addition, as the product is a suspension it must not be given by the intravenous route (see Undesirable effects).

4.4 Special warnings and special precautions for use

Warnings and Precautions:

1. A Patient Information Leaflet is provided in the pack by the manufacturer.

2. Undesirable effects may be minimised by using the lowest effective dose for the minimum period. Frequent patient review is required to appropriately titrate the dose against disease activity (see Posology and method of administration).

3. Patients should carry 'Steroid Treatment' cards which give clear guidance on the precautions to be taken to minimise risk and which provide details of prescriber, drug, dosage and the duration of treatment.

4. Depo-Medrone vials are intended for single dose use only. Any multidose use of the product may lead to contamination.

5. Depo-Medrone is not recommended for epidural, intranasal, intra-ocular, or any other unapproved route of administration. See Undesirable effects section for details of side-effects reported from some non-recommended routes of administration.

6. Due to the absence of a true tendon sheath, the Achilles tendon should not be injected with Depo-Medrone.

7. While crystals of adrenal steroids in the dermis suppress inflammatory reactions, their presence may cause disintegration of the cellular elements and physiochemical changes in the ground substance of the connective tissue. The resultant infrequently occurring dermal and/or subdermal changes may form depressions in the skin at the injection site. The degree to which this reaction occurs will vary with the amount of adrenal steroid injected. Regeneration is usually complete within a few months or after all crystals of the adrenal steroid have been absorbed. In order to minimize the incidence of dermal and subdermal atrophy, care must be exercised not to exceed recommended doses in injections. Multiple small injections into the area of the lesion should be made whenever possible. The technique of intra-articular and intramuscular injection should include precautions against injection or leakage into the dermis. Injection into the deltoid muscle should be avoided because of a high incidence of subcutaneous atrophy.

8. Intralesional doses should not be placed too superficially, particularly in easily visible sites in patients with deeply pigmented skins, since there have been rare reports of subcutaneous atrophy and depigmentation.

9. Systemic absorption of methylprednisolone occurs following intra-articular injection of Depo-Medrone. Systemic as well as local effects can therefore be expected.

10. Intra-articular corticosteroids are associated with a substantially increased risk of inflammatory response in the joint, particularly bacterial infection introduced with the injection. Charcot-like arthropathies have been reported particularly after repeated injections. Appropriate examination of any joint fluid present is necessary to exclude any bacterial infection, prior to injection.

11. Following a single dose of Depo-Medrone, plasma cortisol levels are reduced and there is evidence of hypothalamic-pituitary-adrenal (HPA) axis suppression. This suppression lasts for a variable period of up to 4 weeks. The usual dynamic tests of HPA axis function can be used to diagnose evidence of impaired activity (e.g. Synacthen test).

12. Adrenal cortical atrophy develops during prolonged therapy and may persist for months after stopping treatment. In patients who have received more than physiological doses of systemic corticosteroids (approximately 6 mg methylprednisolone) for greater than 3 weeks, withdrawal should not be abrupt. How dose reduction should be carried out depends largely on whether the disease is likely to relapse as the dose of systemic corticosteroids is reduced. Clinical assessment of disease activity may be needed during withdrawal. If the disease is unlikely to relapse on withdrawal of systemic corticosteroids, but there is uncertainty about HPA suppression, the dose of systemic corticosteroid may be reduced rapidly to physiological doses. Once a daily dose of 6 mg methylprednisolone is reached, dose reduction should be slower to allow the HPA-axis to recover.

Abrupt withdrawal of systemic corticosteroid treatment, which has continued up to 3 weeks is appropriate if it considered that the disease is unlikely to relapse. Abrupt withdrawal of doses up to 32 mg daily of methylprednisolone for 3 weeks is unlikely to lead to clinically relevant HPA-axis suppression, in the majority of patients. In the following patient groups, gradual withdrawal of systemic corticosteroid therapy should be *considered* even after courses lasting 3 weeks or less:

- Patients who have had repeated courses of systemic corticosteroids, particularly if taken for greater than 3 weeks.
- When a short course has been prescribed within one year of cessation of long-term therapy (months or years).
- Patients who may have reasons for adrenocortical insufficiency other than exogenous corticosteroid therapy.
- Patients receiving doses of systemic corticosteroid greater than 32 mg daily of methylprednisolone.
- Patients repeatedly taking doses in the evening.

13. Since mineralocorticoid secretion may be impaired, salt and/or a mineralocorticoid should be administered concurrently.

14. Because rare instances of anaphylactic reactions have occurred in patients receiving parenteral corticosteroid therapy, appropriate precautionary measures should be taken prior to administration, especially when the patient has a history of drug allergy.

15. Corticosteroids may mask some signs of infection, and new infections may appear during their use. Suppression of the inflammatory response and immune function increases the susceptibility to fungal, viral and bacterial infections and their severity. The clinical presentation may often be atypical and may reach an advanced stage before being recognised.

16. Chickenpox is of serious concern since this normally minor illness may be fatal in immunosuppressed patients. Patients (or parents of children) without a definite history of chickenpox should be advised to avoid close personal contact with chickenpox or herpes zoster and if exposed they should seek urgent medical attention. Passive immunization with varicella/zoster immunoglobin (VZIG) is needed by exposed non-immune patients who are receiving systemic corticosteroids or who have used them within the previous 3 months; this should be given within 10 days of exposure to chickenpox. If a diagnosis of chickenpox is confirmed, the illness warrants specialist care and urgent treatment. Corticosteroids should not be stopped and the dose may need to be increased.

17. Live vaccines should not be given to individuals with impaired immune responsiveness. The antibody response to other vaccines may be diminished.

18. The use of Depo-Medrone in active tuberculosis should be restricted to those cases of fulminating or disseminated tuberculosis in which the corticosteroid is used for the management of the disease in conjunction with an appropriate antituberculous regimen. If corticosteroids are indicated in patients with latent tuberculosis or tuberculin reactivity, close observation is necessary as reactivation of the disease may occur. During prolonged corticosteroid therapy, these patients should receive chemoprophylaxis.

19. Care should be taken for patients receiving cardioactive drugs such as digoxin because of steroid induced electrolyte disturbance/potassium loss (see Undesirable effects).

20. *The following precautions apply for parenteral corticosteroids:* Following intra-articular injection, the occurrence of a marked increase in pain accompanied by local swelling, further restriction of joint motion, fever, and malaise are suggestive of septic arthritis. If this complication occurs and the diagnosis of sepsis is confirmed, appropriate antimicrobial therapy should be instituted.

Local injection of a steroid into a previously infected joint is to be avoided.

Corticosteroids should not be injected into unstable joints.

Sterile technique is necessary to prevent infections or contamination.

The slower rate of absorption by intramuscular administration should be recognised.

Special precautions:

Particular care is required when considering the use of systemic corticosteroids in patients with the following conditions and frequent patient monitoring is necessary.

1. Osteoporosis (post-menopausal females are particularly at risk).
2. Hypertension or congestive heart failure.
3. Existing or previous history of severe affective disorders (especially previous steroid psychosis).
4. Diabetes mellitus (or a family history of diabetes).
5. History of tuberculosis.
6. Glaucoma (or a family history of glaucoma).
7. Previous corticosteroid-induced myopathy.
8. Liver failure or cirrhosis.
9. Renal insufficiency.
10. Epilepsy.
11. Peptic ulceration.
12. Fresh intestinal anastomoses.
13. Predisposition to thrombophlebitis.
14. Abscess or other pyogenic infections.
15. Ulcerative colitis.
16. Diverticulitis.
17. Myasthenia gravis.
18. Ocular herpes simplex, for fear of corneal perforation.
19. Hypothyroidism.

Use in Children: Corticosteroids cause growth retardation in infancy, childhood and adolescence which may be irreversible. Treatment should be limited to the minimum dosage for the shortest possible time.

Use in the elderly: The common adverse effects of systemic corticosteroids may be associated with more serious consequences in old age, especially osteoporosis, hypertension, hypokalaemia, diabetes, susceptibility to infection and thinning of the skin. Close clinical supervision is required to avoid life-threatening reactions.

4.5 Interaction with other medicinal products and other forms of Interaction

1. Convulsions have been reported with concurrent use of methylprednisolone and cyclosporin. Since concurrent administration of these agents results in a mutual inhibition of metabolism, it is possible that convulsions and other adverse effects associated with the individual use of either drug may be more apt to occur.

2. Drugs that induce hepatic enzymes, such as rifampicin, rifabutin, carbamazepine, phenobarbitone, phenytoin, primidone, and aminoglutethimide enhance the metabolism of corticosteroids and its therapeutic effects may be reduced.

3. Drugs such as erythromycin and ketoconazole may inhibit the metabolism of corticosteroids and thus decrease their clearance.

4. Steroids may reduce the effects of anticholinesterases in myasthenia gravis. The desired effects of hypoglycaemic agents (including insulin), anti-hypertensives and diuretics are antagonised by corticosteroids, and the hypokalaemic effects of acetazolamide, loop diuretics, thiazide diuretics and carbenoxolone are enhanced.

5. The efficacy of coumarin anticoagulants may be enhanced by concurrent corticosteroid therapy and close monitoring of the INR or prothrombin time is required to avoid spontaneous bleeding.

6. The renal clearance of salicylates is increased by corticosteroids and steroid withdrawal may result in salicylate intoxication. Salicylates and non-steroidal anti-inflammatory agents should be used cautiously in conjunction with corticosteroids in hypothrombinaemia.

7. Steroids have been reported to interact with neuromuscular blocking agents such as pancuronium with partial reversal of the neuromuscular block.

4.6 Pregnancy and lactation

Pregnancy

The ability of corticosteroids to cross the placenta varies between individual drugs, however, methylprednisolone does cross the placenta.

Administration of corticosteroids to pregnant animals can cause abnormalities of foetal development including cleft palate, intra-uterine growth retardation and affects on brain growth and development. There is no evidence that corticosteroids result in an increased incidence of congenital abnormalities, such as cleft palate in man, however, when administered for long periods or repeatedly during pregnancy, corticosteroids may increase the risk of intra-uterine growth retardation. Hypoadrenalism may, in theory, occur in the neonate following prenatal exposure to corticosteroids but usually resolves spontaneously following birth and is rarely clinically important. As with all drugs, corticosteroids should only be prescribed when the benefits to the mother and child outweigh the risks. When corticosteroids are essential, however, patients with normal pregnancies may be treated as though they were in the non-gravid state.

Lactation

Corticosteroids are excreted in small amounts in breast milk, however, doses of up to 40 mg daily of methylprednisolone are unlikely to cause systemic effects in the infant. Infants of mothers taking higher doses than this may have a degree of adrenal suppression, but the benefits of breast-feeding are likely to outweigh any theoretical risk.

4.7 Effects on ability to drive and use machines

None stated.

4.8 Undesirable effects

The incidence of predictable undesirable side-effects associated with the use of corticosteroids, including hypothalamic-pituitary-adrenal suppression correlates with the relative potency of the drug, dosage, timing of administration and duration of treatment (see Special warnings and special precautions for use).

PARENTERAL CORTICOSTEROID THERAPY - Anaphylactic reaction or allergic reactions, hypopigmentation or hyperpigmentation, subcutaneous and cutaneous atrophy, sterile abscess, post injection flare (following intra-articular use), Charcot-like arthropathy, rare instances of blindness associated with intralesional therapy around the face and head.

GASTRO-INTESTINAL - Dyspepsia, peptic ulceration with perforation and haemorrhage, abdominal distension, oesophageal ulceration, oesophageal candidiasis, acute pancreatitis, perforation of bowel.

Increases in alanine transaminase (ALT, SGPT) aspartate transaminase (AST, SGOT) and alkaline phosphatase have been observed following corticosteroid treatment. These changes are usually small, not associated with any clinical syndrome and are reversible upon discontinuation.

ANTI-INFLAMMATORY AND IMMUNOSUPPRESSIVE EFFECTS - Increased susceptibility and severity of infections with suppression of clinical symptoms and signs, opportunistic infections, may suppress reactions to skin tests, recurrence of dormant tuberculosis (see Special warnings and special precautions for use).

MUSCULOSKELETAL - Proximal myopathy, osteoporosis, vertebral and long bone fractures, avascular osteonecrosis, tendon rupture, aseptic necrosis, muscle weakness.

FLUID AND ELECTROLYTE DISTURBANCE - Sodium and water retention, potassium loss, hypertension, hypokalaemic alkalosis, congestive heart failure in susceptible patients.

DERMATOLOGICAL - Impaired healing, petechiae and ecchymosis, thin fragile skin, skin atrophy, bruising, striae, telangiectasia, acne.

ENDOCRINE/METABOLIC - Suppression of the hypothalamo-pituitary-adrenal axis, growth suppression in infancy, childhood and adolescence, menstrual irregularity and amenorrhoea. Cushingoid facies, hirsutism, weight gain, impaired carbohydrate tolerance with increased requirement for antidiabetic therapy, negative nitrogen and calcium balance. Increased appetite.

NEUROPSYCHIATRIC - Euphoria, psychological dependence, mood swings, depression, personality changes, insomnia. Increased intra-cranial pressure with papilloedema in children (pseudotumour cerebri), usually after treatment withdrawal. Psychosis, aggravation of schizophrenia, seizures.

OPHTHALMIC - Increased intra-ocular pressure, glaucoma, papilloedema, cataracts with possible damage to the optic nerve, corneal or scleral thinning, exacerbation of ophthalmic viral or fungal disease, exophthalmos.

GENERAL - Leucocytosis, hypersensitivity including anaphylaxis, thrombo-embolism, nausea, vertigo.

WITHDRAWAL SYMPTOMS - Too rapid a reduction of corticosteroid dosage following prolonged treatment can lead to acute adrenal insufficiency, hypotension and death. However, this is more applicable to corticosteroids with an indication where continuous therapy is given (see Special warnings and special precautions for use).

A 'withdrawal syndrome' may also occur including, fever, myalgia, arthralgia, rhinitis, conjunctivitis, painful itchy skin nodules and loss of weight.

CERTAIN SIDE-EFFECTS REPORTED WITH SOME NON-RECOMMENDED ROUTES OF ADMINISTRATION.

Intrathecal: Usual systemic corticoid adverse reactions, headache, meningismus, meningitis, paraplegia, spinal fluid abnormalities, nausea, vomiting, sweating, arachnoiditis, convulsions.

Extradural: Wound dehiscence, loss of sphincter control.

Intranasal: Permanent/temporary blindness, rhinitis.

Ophthalmic: (Subconjunctival) - Redness and itching, abscess, slough at injection site, residue at injection site, increased intra-ocular pressure, decreased vision - blindness, infection.

Miscellaneous injection sites - Scalp, tonsillar fauces, sphenopalatine ganglion: blindness.

4.9 Overdose

There is no clinical syndrome of acute overdosage with Depo-Medrone. Following overdosage the possibility of adrenal suppression should be guarded against by gradual diminution of dose levels over a period of time. In such event the patient may require to be supported during any further traumatic episode.

5. PHARMACOLOGICAL PROPERTIES

5.1 Pharmacodynamic properties

Methylprednisolone acetate is a synthetic glucocorticoid. An aqueous suspension may be injected directly into joints and soft tissues in the treatment of rheumatoid arthritis, osteoarthritis, bursitis and similar inflammatory conditions.

For prolonged systemic effect it may be administered intramuscularly.

5.2 Pharmacokinetic properties
Methylprednisolone acetate is absorbed from joints in a few days, with peak serum levels being reached 2-12 hours after injection.

It is more slowly absorbed following deep intramuscular injection with plasma levels detected up to 17 days afterwards.

Methylprednisolone acetate is less soluble than methylprednisolone.

6. PHARMACEUTICAL PARTICULARS

6.1 List of excipients
Polyethylene glycol, sodium chloride, myristyl-gamma-picolinium chloride and sterile water for injections.

6.2 Incompatibilities
None stated.

6.3 Shelf life
Shelf-life of the medicinal product as packaged for sale: 60 months.

Depo-Medrone should not be mixed with any other fluid. Discard any remaining suspension after use.

6.4 Special precautions for storage
Depo-Medrone should be protected from freezing.

6.5 Nature and contents of container
Type I flint glass vial with a butyl rubber plug and metal seal. Each vial contains 1 ml, 2ml, or 3 ml of Depo-Medrone 40 mg/ml.

6.6 Instructions for use and handling
No special requirements.

7. MARKETING AUTHORISATION HOLDER
Pharmacia Ltd

Davy Avenue

Milton Keynes

MK5 8PH

UK

8. MARKETING AUTHORISATION NUMBER(S)
PL 0032/5038

9. DATE OF FIRST AUTHORISATION/RENEWAL OF THE AUTHORISATION
Date of first authorisation: 7 March 1989.

Last renewal date: 5 September 1996

10. DATE OF REVISION OF THE TEXT
April 2001

Depo-Medrone with Lidocaine

(Pharmacia Limited)

1. NAME OF THE MEDICINAL PRODUCT
Depo-Medrone with Lidocaine

2. QUALITATIVE AND QUANTITATIVE COMPOSITION
Methylprednisolone BP 4%, Lidocaine Hydrochloride BP 1%

3. PHARMACEUTICAL FORM
White, sterile aqueous suspension for injection

4. CLINICAL PARTICULARS

4.1 Therapeutic indications
Corticosteroid (glucocorticoid). Depo-Medrone with Lidocaine is indicated in conditions requiring a glucocorticoid effect: e.g. anti-inflammatory or anti-rheumatic. It is recommended for local use where the added anaesthetic effect would be considered advantageous.

Depo-Medrone with Lidocaine may be used as follows:

Intra-articular administration

Rheumatoid arthritis

Osteo-arthritis with an inflammatory component

Periarticular administration

Epicondylitis

Intrabursal administration

Subacromial bursitis

Prepatellar bursitis

Olecranon bursitis

Tendon sheath administration

Tendinitis

Tenosynovitis

Epicondylitis

Therapy with Depo-Medrone with Lidocaine does not obviate the need for the conventional measures usually employed. Although this method of treatment will ameliorate symptoms, it is in no sense a cure and the hormone has no effect on the cause of the inflammation.

4.2 Posology and method of administration
Depo-Medrone with Lidocaine should not be mixed with any other preparation as flocculation of the product may occur. Parenteral drug products should be inspected visually for particulate matter and discoloration prior to administration whenever suspension and container permit. Depo-Medrone with Lidocaine may be used by any of the following routes: intra-articular, periarticular, intrabursal, and into the tendon sheath. It must not be used by the intrathecal or intravenous routes (see Contra-indications and Side-effects)

Adults

Intra-articular: Rheumatoid arthritis, osteo-arthritis. The dose of Depo-Medrone with Lidocaine depends on the size of the joint and the severity of the condition. Repeated injections, if needed, may be given at intervals of one to five or more weeks depending upon the degree of relief obtained from the initial injection. A suggested dosage guide is: large joint (knee, ankle, shoulder), 0.5 - 2 ml (20 - 80 mg of steroid); medium joint (elbow, wrist), 0.25 - 1 ml (10 - 40 mg of steroid); small joint (metacarpophalangeal, interphalangeal, sternoclavicular, acromioclavicular), 0.1 - 0.25 ml (4 - 10 mg of steroid).

Periarticular: Epicondylitis. Infiltrate 0.1 - 0.75 ml (4 - 30 mg of steroid) into the affected area.

Intrabursal: Subdeltoid bursitis, prepatellar bursitis, olecranon bursitis. For administration directly into bursae, 0.1 - 0.75 ml (4 - 30 mg of steroid). In most acute cases, repeat injections are not needed.

Into the tendon sheath: Tendinitis, tenosynovitis, epicondylitis. For administration directly into the tendon sheath, 0.1 - 0.75 ml (4 - 30 mg of steroid). In recurrent or chronic conditions, repeat injections may be necessary.

Children:

For infants and children, the recommended dosage should be reduced, but dosage should be governed by the severity of the condition rather than by strict adherence to the ratio indicated by age or body weight.

Elderly:

When used according to instructions, there is no information to suggest that a change in dosage is warranted in the elderly. However, treatment of elderly patients, particularly if long-term, should be planned bearing in mind the more serious consequences of the common side-effects of corticosteroids in old age and close clinical supervision is required (see Other special warnings and precautions).

Special precautions should be observed when administering Depo-Medrone with Lidocaine:

Intra-articular injections should be made using precise, anatomical localisation into the synovial space of the joint involved. The injection site for each joint is determined by that location where the synovial cavity is most superficial and most free of large vessels and nerves. Suitable sites for intra-articular injection are the knee, ankle, wrist, elbow, shoulder, phalangeal and hip joints. The spinal joints, unstable joints and those devoid of synovial space are not suitable. Treatment failures are most frequently the result of failure to enter the joint space. Intra-articular injections should be made with care as follows: ensure correct positioning of the needle into the synovial space and aspirate a few drops of joint fluid. The aspirating syringe should then be replaced by another containing Depo-Medrone with Lidocaine. To ensure position of the needle synovial fluid should be aspirated and the injection made.

After injection the joint is moved slightly to aid mixing of the synovial fluid and the suspension. Subsequent to therapy care should be taken for the patient not to overuse the joint in which benefit has been obtained. Negligence in this matter may permit an increase in joint deterioration that will more than offset the beneficial effects of the steroid.

Intrabursal injections should be made as follows: the area around the injection site is prepared in a sterile way and a wheal at the site made with 1 percent procaine hydrochloride solution. A 20 to 24 gauge needle attached to a dry syringe is inserted into the bursa and the fluid aspirated. The needle is left in place and the aspirating syringe changed for a small syringe containing the desired dose. After injection, the needle is withdrawn and a small dressing applied. In the treatment of tenosynovitis and tendinitis, care should be taken to inject Depo-Medrone with Lidocaine into the tendon sheath rather than into the substance of the tendon. Due to the absence of a true tendon sheath, the Achilles tendon should not be injected with Depo-Medrone with Lidocaine.

4.3 Contraindications
Depo-Medrone with Lidocaine is contra-indicated where there is known hypersensitivity to components or to any local anaesthetics of the amide type and in systemic infection unless anti-infective therapy is employed.

Due to its potential for neurotoxicity, Depo-Medrone with Lidocaine must not be given by the intrathecal route. In addition, as the product is a suspension it must not be given by the intravenous route (see Side-effects).

4.4 Special warnings and special precautions for use
1. Undesirable effects may be minimised by using the lowest effective dose for the minimum period. Frequent patient review is required to appropriately titrate the dose against disease activity (see Dosage and administration).

2. Patients should carry 'Steroid Treatment' cards which give clear guidance on the precautions to be taken to minimise risk and which provide details of prescriber, drug, dosage and the duration of treatment.

3. Depo-Medrone with Lidocaine vials are intended for single dose use only. Any multidose use of the product may lead to contamination.

4. Depo-Medrone with Lidocaine is not recommended for epidural, intranasal, intra-ocular, or any other unapproved route of administration. See Side-effects section for details of side-effects reported from some non-recommended routes of administration.

5. Due to the absence of a true tendon sheath, the Achilles tendon should not be injected with Depo-Medrone with Lidocaine.

6. While crystals of adrenal steroids in the dermis suppress inflammatory reactions, their presence may cause disintegration of the cellular elements and physiochemical changes in the ground substance of the connective tissue. The resultant infrequently occurring dermal and/or subdermal changes may form depressions in the skin at the injection site and the possibility of depigmentation. The degree to which this reaction occurs will vary with the amount of adrenal steroid injected. Regeneration is usually complete within a few months or after all crystals of the adrenal steroid have been absorbed. In order to minimize the incidence of dermal and subdermal atrophy, care must be exercised not to exceed recommended doses in injections. Multiple small injections into the area of the lesion should be made whenever possible. The technique of intra-articular injection should include precautions against injection or leakage into the dermis.

7. Systemic absorption of methylprednisolone occurs following intra-articular injection of Depo-Medrone with Lidocaine. Systemic as well as local effects can therefore be expected.

8. Intra-articular corticosteroids are associated with a substantially increased risk of inflammatory response in the joint, particularly bacterial infection introduced with the injection. Charcot-like arthropathies have been reported particularly after repeated injections. Appropriate examination of any joint fluid present is necessary to exclude any bacterial infection, prior to injection.

9 Following a single dose of Depo-Medrone with Lidocaine, plasma cortisol levels are reduced and there is evidence of hypothalamic-pituitary-adrenal axis (HPA) suppression. This suppression lasts for a variable period of up to 4 weeks. The usual dynamic tests of HPA axis function can be used to diagnose evidence of impaired activity (e.g. Synacthen test).

10. Adrenal cortical atrophy develops during prolonged therapy and may persist for months after stopping treatment. In patients who have received more than physiological doses of systemic corticosteroids (approximately 6 mg methylprednisolone) for greater than 3 weeks, withdrawal should not be abrupt. How dose reduction should be carried out depends largely on whether the disease is likely to relapse as the dose of systemic corticosteroids is reduced. Clinical assessment of disease activity may be needed during withdrawal. If the disease is unlikely to relapse on withdrawal of systemic corticosteroids, but there is uncertainty about HPA suppression, the dose of systemic corticosteroid may be reduced rapidly to physiological doses. Once a daily dose of 6 mg methylprednisolone is reached, dose reduction should be slower to allow the HPA-axis to recover.

Abrupt withdrawal of systemic corticosteroid treatment, which has continued up to 3 weeks is appropriate if it considered that the disease is unlikely to relapse. Abrupt withdrawal of doses up to 32 mg daily of methylprednisolone for 3 weeks is unlikely to lead to clinically relevant HPA-axis suppression, in the majority of patients. In the following patient groups, gradual withdrawal of systemic corticosteroid therapy should be *considered* even after courses lasting 3 weeks or less:

• Patients who have had repeated courses of systemic corticosteroids, particularly if taken for greater than 3 weeks.

• When a short course has been prescribed within one year of cessation of long-term therapy (months or years).

• Patients who may have reasons for adrenocortical insufficiency other than exogenous corticosteroid therapy.

• Patients receiving doses of systemic corticosteroid greater than 32 mg daily of methylprednisolone.

• Patients repeatedly taking doses in the evening.

11. Since mineralocorticoid secretion may be impaired, salt and/or a mineralocorticoid should be administered concurrently.

12. Because rare instances of anaphylactic reactions have occurred in patients receiving parenteral corticosteroid therapy, appropriate precautionary measures should be taken prior to administration, especially when the patient has a history of drug allergy.

13. Corticosteroids may mask some signs of infection, and new infections may appear during their use. Suppression of the inflammatory response and immune function increases the susceptibility to fungal, viral and bacterial infections and their severity. The clinical presentation may often be atypical and may reach an advanced stage before being recognised.

14. Chickenpox is of serious concern since this normally minor illness may be fatal in immunosuppressed patients. Patients (or parents of children) without a definite history of

chickenpox should be advised to avoid close personal contact with chickenpox or herpes zoster and if exposed they should seek urgent medical attention. Passive immunization with varicella/zoster immunoglobin (VZIG) is needed by exposed non-immune patients who are receiving systemic corticosteroids or who have used them within the previous 3 months; this should be given within 10 days of exposure to chickenpox. If a diagnosis of chickenpox is confirmed, the illness warrants specialist care and urgent treatment. Corticosteroids should not be stopped and the dose may need to be increased.

15. Live vaccines should not be given to individuals with impaired immune responsiveness. The antibody response to other vaccines may be diminished.

16. If corticosteroids are indicated in patients with latent tuberculosis or tuberculin reactivity, close observation is necessary as reactivation of the disease may occur. During prolonged corticosteroid therapy, these patients should receive chemoprophylaxis.

17. This product contains benzyl alcohol. Benzyl alcohol has been reported to be associated with a fatal "Gasping Syndrome" in premature infants.

18. Care should be taken for patients receiving cardioactive drugs such as digoxin because of steroid induced electrolyte disturbance/potassium loss (see Side-effects).

19. *The following precautions apply for parenteral corticosteroids:* Following intra-articular injection, a marked increase in pain accompanied by local swelling, further restriction of joint motion, fever, and malaise are suggestive of septic arthritis. If this complication occurs and the diagnosis of sepsis is confirmed, appropriate antimicrobial therapy should be instituted.

No additional benefit derives from the intramuscular administration of Depo-Medrone with Lidocaine. Where parenteral corticosteroid therapy for sustained systemic effect is desired, plain Depo-Medrone should be used.

Local injection of a steroid into a previously infected joint is to be avoided.

Corticosteroids should not be injected into unstable joints.

Sterile technique is necessary to prevent infections or contamination.

Special precautions:

Particular care is required when considering the use of systemic corticosteroids in patients with the following conditions and frequent patient monitoring is necessary.

1. Osteoporosis (post-menopausal females are particularly at risk).
2. Hypertension or congestive heart failure.
3. Existing or previous history of severe affective disorders (especially previous steroid psychosis).
4. Diabetes mellitus (or a family history of diabetes).
5. History of tuberculosis.
6. Glaucoma (or a family history of glaucoma).
7. Previous corticosteroid-induced myopathy.
8. Liver failure or cirrhosis.
9. Renal insufficiency.
10. Epilepsy.
11. Peptic ulceration.
12. Fresh intestinal anastomoses.
13. Predisposition to thrombophlebitis.
14. Abscess or other pyogenic infections.
15. Ulcerative colitis.
16. Diverticulitis.
17. Myasthenia gravis.
18. Ocular herpes simplex, for fear of corneal perforation.
19. Hypothyroidism.

Use in children: Corticosteroids cause growth retardation in infancy, childhood and adolescence which may be irreversible. Treatment should be limited to the minimum dosage for the shortest possible time.

Use in the elderly: The common adverse effects of systemic corticosteroids may be associated with more serious consequences in old age, especially osteoporosis, hypertension, hypokalaemia, diabetes, susceptibility to infection and thinning of the skin. Close clinical supervision is required to avoid life-threatening reactions.

4.5 Interaction with other medicinal products and other forms of Interaction

1. Convulsions have been reported with concurrent use of methylprednisolone and cyclosporin. Since concurrent administration of these agents results in a mutual inhibition of metabolism, it is possible that convulsions and other adverse effects associated with the individual use of either drug may be more apt to occur.

2. Drugs that induce hepatic enzymes, such as rifampicin, rifabutin, carbamazepine, phenobarbitone, phenytoin, primidone, and aminoglutethimide enhance the metabolism of corticosteroids and its therapeutic effects may be reduced.

3. Drugs such as erythromycin and ketoconazole may inhibit the metabolism of corticosteroids and thus decrease their clearance.

4. Steroids may reduce the effects of anticholinesterases in myasthenia gravis. The desired effects of hypoglycaemic agents (including insulin), anti-hypertensives and diuretics are antagonised by corticosteroids, and the hypokalaemic effects of acetazolamide, loop diuretics, thiazide diuretics and carbenoxolone are enhanced.

5. The efficacy of coumarin anticoagulants may be enhanced by concurrent corticosteroid therapy and close monitoring of the INR or prothrombin time is required to avoid spontaneous bleeding.

6. The renal clearance of salicylates is increased by corticosteroids and steroid withdrawal may result in salicylate intoxication. Salicylates and non-steroidal anti-inflammatory agents should be used cautiously in conjunction with corticosteroids in hypothrombinaemia.

7. Steroids have been reported to interact with neuromuscular blocking agents such as pancuronium with partial reversal of the neuromuscular block.

4.6 Pregnancy and lactation

Pregnancy

The ability of corticosteroids to cross the placenta varies between individual drugs, however, methylprednisolone does cross the placenta.

Administration of corticosteroids to pregnant animals can cause abnormalities of foetal development including cleft palate, intra-uterine growth retardation and affects on brain growth and development. There is no evidence that corticosteroids result in an increased incidence of congenital abnormalities, such as cleft palate in man, however, when administered for long periods or repeatedly during pregnancy, corticosteroids may increase the risk of intra-uterine growth retardation. Hypoadrenalism may, in theory, occur in the neonate following prenatal exposure to corticosteroids but usually resolves spontaneously following birth and is rarely clinically important. As with all drugs, corticosteroids should only be prescribed when the benefits to the mother and child outweigh the risks. When corticosteroids are essential, however, patients with normal pregnancies may be treated as though they were in the non-gravid state.

The use of local anaesthetics such as lidocaine during labour and delivery may be associated with adverse effects on mother and foetus. Lidocaine readily crosses the placenta.

Lactation

Corticosteroids are excreted in small amounts in breast milk, however, doses of up to 40 mg daily of methylprednisolone are unlikely to cause systemic effects in the infant. Infants of mothers taking higher doses than this may have a degree of adrenal suppression, but the benefits of breastfeeding are likely to outweigh any theoretical risk.

It is not known whether lidocaine is excreted in human breast milk.

4.7 Effects on ability to drive and use machines

None stated.

4.8 Undesirable effects

The incidence of predictable undesirable side-effects associated with the use of corticosteroids, including hypothalamic-pituitary-adrenal suppression correlates with the relative potency of the drug, dosage, timing of administration and duration of treatment (See other special warnings and precautions).

Side-effects for the Depo-Medrone component may be observed including:

PARENTERAL CORTICOSTEROID THERAPY - Anaphylactic reaction or allergic reactions, hypopigmentation or hyperpigmentation, subcutaneous and cutaneous atrophy, sterile abscess, post injection flare (following intra-articular use), charcot-like arthropathy.

GASTRO-INTESTINAL - Dyspepsia, peptic ulceration with perforation and haemorrhage, abdominal distension, oesophageal ulceration, oesophageal candidiasis, acute pancreatitis, perforation of bowel.

Increases in alanine transaminase (ALT, SGPT) aspartate transaminase (AST, SGOT) and alkaline phosphatase have been observed following corticosteroid treatment. These changes are usually small, not associated with any clinical syndrome and are reversible upon discontinuation.

ANTI-INFLAMMATORY AND IMMUNOSUPPRESSIVE EFFECTS - Increased susceptibility and severity of infections with suppression of clinical symptoms and signs, opportunistic infections, may suppress reactions to skin tests, recurrence of dormant tuberculosis (see Other special warnings and precautions).

MUSCULOSKELETAL - Proximal myopathy, osteoporosis, vertebral and long bone fractures, avascular osteonecrosis, tendon rupture, aseptic necrosis, muscle weakness.

FLUID AND ELECTROLYTE DISTURBANCE - Sodium and water retention, potassium loss, hypertension, hypokalaemic alkalosis, congestive heart failure in susceptible patients.

DERMATOLOGICAL - Impaired healing, petechiae and ecchymosis, thin fragile skin, skin atrophy, bruising, striae, telangiectasia, acne.

ENDOCRINE/METABOLIC - Suppression of the hypothalamo-pituitary-adrenal axis; growth suppression in infancy, childhood and adolescence; menstrual irregularity and amenorrhoea. Cushingoid facies, hirsutism, weight gain, impaired carbohydrate tolerance with increased requirement for antidiabetic therapy, negative nitrogen and calcium balance. Increased appetite.

NEUROPSYCHIATRIC - Euphoria, psychological dependence, mood swings, depression, personality changes, insomnia. Increased intra-cranial pressure with papilloedema in children (pseudotumour cerebri), usually after treatment withdrawal. Psychosis, aggravation of schizophrenia, seizures.

OPHTHALMIC - Increased intra-ocular pressure, glaucoma, papilloedema, cataracts with possible damage to the optic nerve, corneal or scleral thinning, exacerbation of ophthalmic viral or fungal disease, exophthalmos.

GENERAL - Leucocytosis, hypersensitivity including anaphylaxis, thrombo-embolism, nausea, vertigo.

WITHDRAWAL SYMPTOMS - Too rapid a reduction of corticosteroid dosage following prolonged treatment can lead to acute adrenal insufficiency, hypotension and death. However, this is more applicable to corticosteroids with an indication where continuous therapy is given (see Other special warnings and precautions).

A 'withdrawal syndrome' may also occur including, fever, myalgia, arthralgia, rhinitis, conjunctivitis, painful itchy skin nodules and loss of weight.

Side-effects for the Lidocaine component include:

CENTRAL NERVOUS SYSTEM - Lightheadedness, nervousness, apprehension, euphoria, confusion, dizziness, drowsiness, tinnitus, blurred or double vision, vomiting, sensation of heat, cold, numbness, twitching, tremors, convulsions, loss of consciousness, respiratory depression, respiratory arrest.

CARDIOVASCULAR SYSTEM - Bradycardia, hypotension, cardiovascular collapse, cardiac arrest.

ALLERGIC REACTIONS - Cutaneous lesions, urticaria, oedema, anaphylactic reactions.

CERTAIN SIDE-EFFECTS REPORTED WITH SOME NON RECOMMENDED ROUTES OF ADMINISTRATION:

Intrathecal: Usual systemic corticoid adverse reactions, headache, meningismus, meningitis, paraplegia, spinal fluid abnormalities, nausea, vomiting, sweating, arachnoiditis, convulsions.

Extradural: Wound dehiscence, loss of sphincter control.

Intranasal: Permanent/temporary blindness, allergic reactions, rhinitis.

Ophthalmic (Subconjunctival): Redness and itching, abscess, slough at injection site, residue at injection site, increased intra-ocular pressure, decreased vision - blindness, infection.

Miscellaneous: Scalp, tonsillar fauces, sphenopalatine ganglion: blindness.

4.9 Overdose

There is no clinical syndrome of acute overdosage with Depo-Medrone with Lidocaine. Following overdosage the possibility of adrenal suppression should be guarded against by gradual diminution of dose levels over a period of time. In such event the patient may require to be supported during any further traumatic episode.

5. PHARMACOLOGICAL PROPERTIES

5.1 Pharmacodynamic properties

Methylprednisolone acetate is a synthetic glucocorticoid with the actions and use of natural corticosteroids. However the slower metabolism of the synthetic corticosteroid with their lower protein-binding affinity may account for their increased potency compared with the natural corticosteroids.

Lidocaine has the actions of a local anaesthetic.

5.2 Pharmacokinetic properties

Administration of methylprednisolone acetate 40 mg intramuscularly produced measurable plasma concentrations of methylprednisolone for 11-17 days. The average peak plasma concentration was 14.8 ng per ml and occurred after 6-8 hours.

Plasma concentrations of lidocaine decline rapidly after an intravenous dose with an initial half life of less than 30 minutes; the elimination half life is 1-2 hours.

5.3 Preclinical safety data

Due to the age and well established safety nature of this product, preclinical data has not been included.

6. PHARMACEUTICAL PARTICULARS

6.1 List of excipients

Sodium chloride, myristyl-gamma-picolinium chloride, benzyl alcohol, ***macrogol***, sodium hydroxide, hydrochloric acid and water for injection.

6.2 Incompatibilities

None

6.3 Shelf life

24 months

6.4 Special precautions for storage

Store at room temperature. Protect from freezing.

6.5 Nature and contents of container

Glass vials with rubber cap containing 1 or 2 ml of suspension.

6.6 Instructions for use and handling

None

7. MARKETING AUTHORISATION HOLDER
Pharmacia Limited,
Davy Avenue,
Milton Keynes,
MK5 8PH
U.K.

8. MARKETING AUTHORISATION NUMBER(S)
PL 0032/0076

9. DATE OF FIRST AUTHORISATION/RENEWAL OF THE AUTHORISATION
MA granted: 03 March 1981
MA renewed: 25 November 1991

10. DATE OF REVISION OF THE TEXT
April 2001

Legal category
POM

Deponit 10

(SCHWARZ PHARMA Limited)

1. NAME OF THE MEDICINAL PRODUCT
DEPONIT 10

2. QUALITATIVE AND QUANTITATIVE COMPOSITION
One patch contains glyceryl trinitrate 37.4 mg

The average amount of glyceryl trinitrate absorbed from each patch in 24 hours is 10mg.

3. PHARMACEUTICAL FORM
Transdermal patch

White to translucent square patch with convex round corners with "Deponit® 10" marked on the outer face.

4. CLINICAL PARTICULARS

4.1 Therapeutic indications
Prophylaxis of angina pectoris alone or in combination with other anti-anginal therapy.

4.2 Posology and method of administration
Dermal

Adults: Treatment should be initiated with one patch daily. If necessary the dosage may be increased to two patches.

It is recommended that the patch is applied to healthy, undamaged, relatively crease free and hairless skin. The best places to apply Deponit patches are the easily reached, fairly static areas at the front or side of the chest. However, Deponit patches may also be applied to the upper arm, thigh, abdomen or shoulder. Skin care products should not be used before applying the patch. The replacement patch should be applied to a new area of skin. Allow several days to elapse before applying a fresh patch to the same area of skin.

Tolerance may occur during chronic nitrate therapy. Tolerance is likely to be avoided by allowing a patch-free period of 8-12 hours each day, usually at night. Additional anti-anginal therapy with drugs not containing nitro compounds should be considered for the nitrate-free interval if required.

As with any nitrate therapy, treatment with these patches should not be stopped abruptly. If the patient is being changed to another type of treatment, the two should overlap.

Elderly: No specific information on use in the elderly is available, however there is no evidence to suggest that an alteration in dose is required.

Children: The safety and efficacy of this patch in children has yet to be established

4.3 Contraindications
- Known hypersensitivity to nitrates or to the adhesives used in the patch
- Raised intracranial pressure including that caused by head trauma or cerebral haemorrhage
- Marked anaemia
- Closed angle glaucoma
- Hypotensive conditions and hypovolaemia
- Hypertrophic obstructive cardiomyopathy
- Aortic stenosis and mitral stenosis
- Constrictive pericarditis
- Cardiac tamponade
- Concomitant use of phosphodiesterase type-5 inhibitors. Phosphodiesterase type-5 inhibitors (eg sildenafil, tadalafil, vardenafil) have been shown to potentiate the hypotensive effects of nitrates, and their co-administration with nitrates or nitric oxide donors is therefore contra-indicated.

4.4 Special warnings and special precautions for use
This patch should be used with caution in patients with
- Severe hepatic or renal impairment
- Hypothyroidism
- Hypothermia
- Malnutrition
- A recent history of myocardial infarction
- Hypoxaemia or a ventilation/perfusion imbalance due to lung disease or ischaemic heart failure.

The patch is not indicated for use in acute angina attacks. In the event of an acute angina attack, sublingual treatment such as a spray or tablet should be used. As with all nitrate preparations withdrawal of long-term treatment should be gradual by replacement with decreasing doses of long acting oral nitrates.

If the patches are not used as indicated (see Section 4.2) tolerance to the medication could develop.

4.5 Interaction with other medicinal products and other forms of Interaction
Concomitant treatment with other vasodilators, calcium antagonists, ACE inhibitors, beta-blockers, diuretics, antihypertensives, tricyclic antidepressants and major tranquillisers, as well as the consumption of alcohol, may potentiate the hypotensive effect of the preparation.

The blood pressure lowering effect of these patches will be increased if used together with phosphodiesterase inhibitors (e.g. sildenafil) which are used for erectile dysfunction (see Section 4.3). This might lead to life threatening cardiovascular complications. Patients who are on nitrate therapy must not use phosphodiesterase inhibitors (e.g. sildenafil).

If administered concurrently, these patches may increase the blood level of dihydroergotamine and lead to coronary vasoconstriction.

The possibility that ingestion of acetylsalicylic acid and non-steroidal anti-inflammatory drugs might diminish the therapeutic response to the patch cannot be excluded.

4.6 Pregnancy and lactation
These patches should not be used during pregnancy or lactation unless considered absolutely essential by the physician.

It is not known whether the active substance passes into the breast milk. Benefits to the mother must be weighed against risk to the child.

4.7 Effects on ability to drive and use machines
Glyceryl trinitrate can cause postural hypotension and dizziness. Patients should not drive or operate machinery if they feel affected.

4.8 Undesirable effects
A very common (>10% of patients) adverse reaction to the patch is headache. The incidence of headache diminishes gradually with time and continued use.

At start of therapy or when the dosage is increased, hypotension and/or light-headedness on standing are observed commonly (i.e. in 1-10% of patients). These symptoms may be associated with dizziness, drowsiness, reflex tachycardia, and a feeling of weakness.

Infrequently (i.e. in less than 1% of patients), nausea, vomiting, flushing and allergic skin reaction (e.g. rash), which may be severe can occur. Exfoliative dermatitis has been reported

Severe hypotensive responses have been reported for organic nitrates and include nausea, vomiting, restlessness, pallor and excessive perspiration. Uncommonly collapse may occur (sometimes accompanied by bradyarrhythmia and syncope). Uncommonly severe hypotension may lead to enhanced angina symptoms.

A few reports of heartburn, most likely due to a nitrate-induced sphincter relaxation, have been recorded.

Allergic skin reactions to glyceryl trinitrate and ingredients can occur, but they are uncommon (i.e. > 0.1% but < 1 %). Patients may commonly experience slight itching or burning at the site of application. Slight reddening usually disappears without therapeutic measures after the patch has been removed. Allergic contact dermatitis is uncommon.

During the treatment with these patches, a temporary hypoxaemia may occur due to a relative redistribution of the blood flow in hypoventilated alveolar areas. Particularly in patients with coronary artery disease this may lead to a myocardial hypoxia.

4.9 Overdose
In view of the transdermal mode of delivery, an overdose of glyceryl trinitrate is unlikely to occur. However, in the unlikely event of an overdose, the symptoms could include the following:
- Fall in blood pressure ≤ 90 mmHg
- Paleness
- Sweating
- Weak pulse
- Tachycardia
- Flushing
- Light-headedness on standing
- Headache
- Weakness
- Dizziness
- Nausea
- Vomiting
- Methaemoglobinaemia has been reported in patients receiving other organic nitrates. During glyceryl trinitrate biotransformation nitrite ions are released, which may induce methaemoglobinaemia and cyanosis with subsequent tachypnoea, anxiety, loss of consciousness and cardiac arrest. It can not be excluded that an overdose of glyceryl trinitrate may cause this adverse reaction
- In very high doses the intracranial pressure may be increased. This might lead to cerebral symptoms

General procedure:
- Stop delivery of the drug. Since these patches are applied to the skin, removing the patch immediately stops delivery of the drug.
- General procedures in the event of nitrate-related hypotension

- Patient should be kept horizontal with the head lowered and legs raised
- Supply oxygen
- Expand plasma volume
- For specific shock treatment admit patient to intensive care unit

Special procedure:
- Raising the blood pressure if the blood pressure is very low
- Treatment of methaemoglobinaemia

-Treatment with intravenous methylene blue
- Initially 1 to 2 mg/kg, not exceed 4 mg/kg of a 1% solution over 5 minutes.
- Repeat dose in 60 minutes if there is no response.
- Administer oxygen (if necessary)
- Initiate artificial ventilation

Treatment with methylene blue is contraindicated in patients with glucose-6-phosphate dehydrogenase (G-6-PD) deficiency or methaemaglobin reductase deficiency.

Where treatment with methylene blue is contraindicated or is not effective, exchange transfusion and / or transfusion of packed red blood cells is recommended.

Resuscitation measures:

In case of signs of respiratory and circulatory arrest, initiate resuscitation measures immediately.

5. PHARMACOLOGICAL PROPERTIES

5.1 Pharmacodynamic properties
The main pharmacological activity of organic nitrates is the relaxation of smooth vascular muscles. The systemic vasodilation induces an increase of venous capacitance. Venous return is reduced. Ventricular volume, filling pressures and diastolic wall tension are diminished (preload reduction).

A diminished ventricular radius and reduced wall tension, lower myocardial energy and oxygen consumption, respectively.

The dilation of the large arteries near the heart leads to a decrease in both the systemic (reduction of afterload) and the pulmonary vascular resistance. In addition, this relieves the myocardium and lowers oxygen demands.

By dilating the large epicardial coronary arteries, glyceryl trinitrate enhances blood supply to the myocardium, improving its pump function and increasing the oxygen supply.

At molecular level, nitrates form nitric oxide (NO), which corresponds to the physical EDRF (endothelium derived relaxing factor). EDRF mediated production of cyclic guanosine monophosphate (cGMP) leads to relaxation of smooth muscle cells.

5.2 Pharmacokinetic properties
(a) *General characteristics of the active substance*

The transdermal absorption of glyceryl trinitrate circumvents the extensive hepatic first pass metabolism so the bioavailability is about 70% of that achieved after i.v. administration.

The steady-state concentration in the plasma depends on the patch dosage and the corresponding rate of absorption. At a rate of absorption of 0.4 mg/h, the steady-state concentration is about 0.2 μg/h on average. Plasma protein binding is about 60%. Glyceryl trinitrate is metabolized to 1,2- and 1,3-dinitroglycerols. The dinitrates exert less vasodilatory activity than glyceryl trinitrate. The contribution to the overall effect is not known. The dinitrates are further metabolized to inactive mononitrates, glyceryl and carbon dioxide.

The elimination half-life of glyceryl trinitrate is 2-4 min. The metabolism of glyceryl trinitrate, which is effected in the liver, but also in many other cells, e.g. the red blood cells, includes the separation of one or more nitrate groups. In addition to the metabolism of glyceryl trinitrate, there is a renal excretion of the catabolites.

(b) *Characteristics in patients*

There is no evidence that a dosage adjustment is required in the elderly or in diseases such as renal failure or hepatic insufficiency.

5.3 Preclinical safety data
Glyceryl trinitrate is a well-known active substance, established for more than a hundred years. Thus new preclinical studies have not been carried out with Deponit 10.

6. PHARMACEUTICAL PARTICULARS

6.1 List of excipients

Acrylate/vinyl acetate copolymer (adhesive matrix)

Polypropylene (backing foil)

Polyethylene (siliconised release liner)

6.2 Incompatibilities

No incompatibilities have so far been demonstrated.

6.3 Shelf life

Shelf life of the product as packaged for sale: 36 months.

6.4 Special precautions for storage

Do not store above 25°C

6.5 Nature and contents of container

Multilaminate film/foil pouch with heat-sealed edges.

28 patches per carton.

6.6 Instructions for use and handling

The patch should be removed from the package just before application. After removal of the protective foil, the patch should be applied to unbroken, clean and dry skin that is smooth and with few hairs. The same area of skin should not be used again for some days.

7. MARKETING AUTHORISATION HOLDER

SCHWARZ PHARMA Limited

East Street

Chesham

Bucks

HP5 1DG

England

8. MARKETING AUTHORISATION NUMBER(S)

PL 4438/0037

9. DATE OF FIRST AUTHORISATION/RENEWAL OF THE AUTHORISATION

26 October 2000

10. DATE OF REVISION OF THE TEXT

February 2005

Deponit 5

(SCHWARZ PHARMA Limited)

1. NAME OF THE MEDICINAL PRODUCT

DEPONIT 5

2. QUALITATIVE AND QUANTITATIVE COMPOSITION

One patch contains glyceryl trinitrate 18.7 mg

The average amount of glyceryl trinitrate absorbed from each patch in 24 hours is 5mg.

3. PHARMACEUTICAL FORM

Transdermal patch

White to translucent square patch with convex round corners with "Deponit® 5" marked on the outer face.

4. CLINICAL PARTICULARS

4.1 Therapeutic indications

Prophylaxis of angina pectoris alone or in combination with other anti-anginal therapy.

4.2 Posology and method of administration

Dermal

Adults: Treatment should be initiated with one patch daily. If necessary the dosage may be increased to two patches.

It is recommended that the patch is applied to healthy, undamaged, relatively crease free and hairless skin. The best places to apply Deponit patches are the easily reached, fairly static areas at the front or side of the chest. However, Deponit patches may also be applied to the upper arm, thigh, abdomen or shoulder. Skin care products should not be used before applying the patch. The replacement patch should be applied to a new area of skin. Allow several days to elapse before applying a fresh patch to the same area of skin.

Tolerance may occur during chronic nitrate therapy. Tolerance is likely to be avoided by allowing a patch-free period of 8-12 hours each day, usually at night. Additional anti-anginal therapy with drugs not containing nitro compounds should be considered for the nitrate-free interval if required.

As with any nitrate therapy, treatment with these patches should not be stopped abruptly. If the patient is being changed to another type of treatment, the two should overlap.

Elderly: No specific information on use in the elderly is available, however there is no evidence to suggest that an alteration in dose is required.

Children: The safety and efficacy of this patch in children has yet to be established.

4.3 Contraindications

- Known hypersensitivity to nitrates or to the adhesives used in the patch
- Raised intracranial pressure including that caused by head trauma or cerebral haemorrhage
- Marked anaemia
- Closed angle glaucoma
- Hypotensive conditions and hypovolaemia
- Hypertrophic obstructive cardiomyopathy
- Aortic stenosis and mitral stenosis
- Constrictive pericarditis
- Cardiac tamponade
- Concomitant use of phosphodiesterase type-5 inhibitors.

Phosphodiesterase type-5 inhibitors (eg sildenafil, tadalafil, vardenafil) have been shown to potentiate the hypotensive effects of nitrates, and their co-administration with nitrates or nitric oxide donors is therefore contra-indicated.

4.4 Special warnings and special precautions for use

This patch should be used with caution in patients with

- Severe hepatic or renal impairment
- Hypothyroidism
- Hypothermia
- Malnutrition
- A recent history of myocardial infarction
- Hypoxaemia or a ventilation/perfusion imbalance due to lung disease or ischaemic heart failure.

The patch is not indicated for use in acute angina attacks. In the event of an acute angina attack, sublingual treatment such as a spray or tablet should be used. As with all nitrate preparations withdrawal of long-term treatment should be gradual by replacement with decreasing doses of long acting oral nitrates.

If the patches are not used as indicated (see Section 4.2) tolerance to the medication could develop.

4.5 Interaction with other medicinal products and other forms of interaction

Concomitant treatment with other vasodilators, calcium antagonists, ACE inhibitors, beta-blockers, diuretics, antihypertensives, tricyclic antidepressants and major tranquillisers, as well as the consumption of alcohol, may potentiate the hypotensive effect of the preparation.

The blood pressure lowering effect of these patches will be increased if used together with phosphodiesterase inhibitors (e.g. sildenafil) which are used for erectile dysfunction (see Section 4.3). This might lead to life threatening cardiovascular complications. Patients who are on nitrate therapy must not use phosphodiesterase inhibitors (e.g. sildenafil).

If administered concurrently, these patches may increase the blood level of dihydroergotamine and lead to coronary vasoconstriction.

The possibility that ingestion of acetylsalicylic acid and non-steroidal anti-inflammatory drugs might diminish the therapeutic response to the patch cannot be excluded.

4.6 Pregnancy and lactation

These patches should not be used during pregnancy or lactation unless considered absolutely essential by the physician.

It is not known whether the active substance passes into the breast milk. Benefits to the mother must be weighed against risk to the child.

4.7 Effects on ability to drive and use machines

Glyceryl trinitrate can cause postural hypotension and dizziness. Patients should not drive or operate machinery if they feel affected.

4.8 Undesirable effects

A very common (> 10% of patients) adverse reaction to the patch is headache. The incidence of headache diminishes gradually with time and continued use.

At start of therapy or when the dosage is increased, hypotension and/or light-headedness on standing are observed commonly (i.e. in 1-10% of patients). These symptoms may be associated with dizziness, drowsiness, reflex tachycardia, and a feeling of weakness.

Infrequently (i.e. in less than 1% of patients), nausea, vomiting, flushing and allergic skin reaction (e.g. rash), which may be severe can occur. Exfoliative dermatitis has been reported.

Severe hypotensive responses have been reported for organic nitrates and include nausea, vomiting, restlessness, pallor and excessive perspiration. Uncommonly collapse may occur (sometimes accompanied by bradyarrhythmia and syncope). Uncommonly severe hypotension may lead to enhanced angina symptoms.

A few reports of heartburn, most likely due to a nitrate-induced sphincter relaxation, have been recorded.

Allergic skin reactions to glyceryl trinitrate and ingredients can occur, but they are uncommon (i.e. > 0.1% but < 1 %). Patients may commonly experience slight itching or burning at the site of application. Slight reddening usually disappears without therapeutic measures after the patch has been removed. Allergic contact dermatitis is uncommon.

During the treatment with these patches, a temporary hypoxaemia may occur due to a relative redistribution of the blood flow in hypoventilated alveolar areas. Particularly in patients with coronary artery disease this may lead to a myocardial hypoxia.

4.9 Overdose

In view of the transdermal mode of delivery, an overdose of glyceryl trinitrate is unlikely to occur. However, in the unlikely event of an overdose, the symptoms could include the following:

- Fall in blood pressure ≤ 90 mmHg
- Paleness
- Sweating
- Weak pulse
- Tachycardia
- Flushing
- Light-headedness on standing
- Headache
- Weakness
- Dizziness
- Nausea
- Vomiting
- Methaemoglobinaemia has been reported in patients receiving other organic nitrates. During glyceryl trinitrate biotransformation nitrite ions are released, which may induce methaemoglobinaemia and cyanosis with subsequent tachypnoea, anxiety, loss of consciousness and cardiac arrest. It can not be excluded that an overdose of glyceryl trinitrate may cause this adverse reaction
- In very high doses the intracranial pressure may be increased. This might lead to cerebral symptoms

General procedure:

- Stop delivery of the drug. Since these patches are applied to the skin, removing the patch immediately stops delivery of the drug.
- General procedures in the event of nitrate-related hypotension

- Patient should be kept horizontal with the head lowered and legs raised
- Supply oxygen
- Expand plasma volume
- For specific shock treatment admit patient to intensive care unit

Special procedure:

- Raising the blood pressure if the blood pressure is very low
- Treatment of methaemoglobinaemia

-Treatment with intravenous methylene blue

- Initially 1 to 2 mg/kg, not exceed 4 mg/kg of a 1% solution over 5 minutes.
- Repeat dose in 60 minutes if there is no response.
- Administer oxygen (if necessary)
- Initiate artificial ventilation

Treatment with methylene blue is contraindicated in patients with glucose-6-phosphate dehydrogenase (G-6-PD) deficiency or methaemaglobin reductase deficiency.

Where treatment with methylene blue is contraindicated or is not effective, exchange transfusion and / or transfusion of packed red blood cells is recommended.

Resuscitation measures:

In case of signs of respiratory and circulatory arrest, initiate resuscitation measures immediately.

5. PHARMACOLOGICAL PROPERTIES

5.1 Pharmacodynamic properties

The main pharmacological activity of organic nitrates is the relaxation of smooth vascular muscles. The systemic vasodilation induces an increase of venous capacitance. Venous return is reduced. Ventricular volume, filling pressures and diastolic wall tension are diminished (preload reduction).

A diminished ventricular radius and reduced wall tension, lower myocardial energy and oxygen consumption, respectively.

The dilation of the large arteries near the heart leads to a decrease in both the systemic (reduction of afterload) and the pulmonary vascular resistance. In addition, this relieves the myocardium and lowers oxygen demands.

By dilating the large epicardial coronary arteries, glyceryl trinitrate enhances blood supply to the myocardium, improving its pump function and increasing the oxygen supply.

At molecular level, nitrates form nitric oxide (NO), which corresponds to the physical EDRF (endothelium derived relaxing factor). EDRF mediated production of cyclic guanosine monophosphate (cGMP) leads to relaxation of smooth muscle cells.

5.2 Pharmacokinetic properties

(a) *General characteristics of the active substance*

The transdermal absorption of glyceryl trinitrate circumvents the extensive hepatic first pass metabolism so the bioavailability is about 70% of that achieved after i.v. administration.

The steady-state concentration in the plasma depends on the patch dosage and the corresponding rate of absorption. At a rate of absorption of 0.4 mg/h, the steady-state concentration is about 0.2 μg/h on average. Plasma protein binding is about 60%. Glyceryl trinitrate is metabolized to 1,2- and 1,3-dinitroglycerols. The dinitrates exert less vasodilatory activity than glyceryl trinitrate. The contribution to the overall effect is not known. The dinitrates are further metabolized to inactive mononitrates, glyceryl and carbon dioxide.

The elimination half-life of glyceryl trinitrate is 2-4 min. The metabolism of glyceryl trinitrate, which is effected in the liver, but also in many other cells, e.g. the red blood cells, includes the separation of one or more nitrate groups. In addition to the metabolism of glyceryl trinitrate, there is a renal excretion of the catabolites.

(b) *Characteristics in patients*

There is no evidence that a dosage adjustment is required in the elderly or in diseases such as renal failure or hepatic insufficiency.

5.3 Preclinical safety data

Glyceryl trinitrate is a well-known active substance, established for more than a hundred years. Thus new preclinical studies have not been carried out with Deponit 5.

6. PHARMACEUTICAL PARTICULARS

6.1 List of excipients

Acrylate/vinyl acetate copolymer (adhesive matrix)

Polypropylene (backing foil)

Polyethylene (siliconised release liner)

6.2 Incompatibilities

No incompatibilities have so far been demonstrated.

6.3 Shelf life

Shelf life of the product as packaged for sale: 36 months.

6.4 Special precautions for storage

Do not store above 25°C.

6.5 Nature and contents of container

Multi-laminate film/foil pouch with heat-sealed edges.

28 patches per carton.

6.6 Instructions for use and handling

Each patch should be removed from the package just before application. After removal of the protective foil, the patch should be applied to unbroken, clean and dry skin that is smooth and with few hairs. The same area of skin should not be used again for some days.

7. MARKETING AUTHORISATION HOLDER

SCHWARZ PHARMA Limited

East Street

Chesham

Bucks

HP5 1DG

England

8. MARKETING AUTHORISATION NUMBER(S)

PL 4438/0036

9. DATE OF FIRST AUTHORISATION/RENEWAL OF THE AUTHORISATION

26 October 2000

10. DATE OF REVISION OF THE TEXT

February 2005

Depo-Provera 150mg/ml Injection

(Pharmacia Limited)

1. NAME OF THE MEDICINAL PRODUCT

Depo-Provera 150 mg/ml

2. QUALITATIVE AND QUANTITATIVE COMPOSITION

Each ml of suspension contains 150 mg medroxyprogesterone acetate Ph. Eur.

For excipients, see section 6.1

3. PHARMACEUTICAL FORM

Sterile suspension for injection.

4. CLINICAL PARTICULARS

4.1 Therapeutic indications

Progestogen: for contraception.

Depo-Provera is a long-term contraceptive agent suitable for use in women who have been appropriately counselled concerning the likelihood of menstrual disturbance and the potential for a delay in return to full fertility.

Depo-Provera may also be used for short-term contraception in the following circumstances:

(i) For partners of men undergoing vasectomy, for protection until the vasectomy becomes effective.

(ii) In women who are being immunised against rubella, to prevent pregnancy during the period of activity of the virus.

(iii) In women awaiting sterilisation.

Since loss of bone mineral density (BMD) may occur in females of all ages who use Depo-Provera injection long-term (see section 4.4 Special Warnings and Special Precautions for Use), a risk/benefit assessment, which also takes into consideration the decrease in BMD that occurs during pregnancy and/or lactation, should be considered.

Use in Adolescents (12-18 years)

In adolescents, Depo-Provera may be used, but <u>**only**</u> after other methods of contraception have been discussed with the patient and considered unsuitable or unacceptable.

It is of the greatest importance that adequate explanations of the long-term nature of the product, of its possible side-effects and of the impossibility of immediately reversing the effects of each injection are given to potential users and that every effort is made to ensure that each patient receives such counselling as to enable her to fully understand these explanations. Patient information leaflets are supplied by the manufacturer. It is recommended that the doctor uses these leaflets to aid counselling of the patient.

Consistent with good clinical practice a general medical as well as gynaecological examination should be undertaken before administration of Depo-Provera and at appropriate intervals thereafter.

4.2 Posology and method of administration

The sterile aqueous suspension of Depo-Provera should be vigorously shaken just before use to ensure that the dose being given represents a uniform suspension of Depo-Provera.

Doses should be given by deep intramuscular injection. Care should be taken to ensure that the depot injection is given into the muscle tissue, preferably the gluteus maximus, but other muscle issue such as the deltoid may be used.

The site of injection should be cleansed using standard methods prior to administration of the injection.

Adults:

First injection: To provide contraceptive cover in the first cycle of use, an injection of 150 mg i.m. should be given during the first five days of a normal menstrual cycle. If the injection is carried out according to these instructions, no additional contraceptive cover is required.

Post Partum: To increase assurance that the patient is not pregnant at the time of first administration, this injection should be given within 5 days post partum if not breast-feeding.

There is evidence that women prescribed Depo-Provera in the immediate puerperium can experience prolonged and heavy bleeding. Because of this, the drug should be used with caution in the puerperium. Women who are considering use of the product immediately following delivery or termination should be advised that the risk of heavy or prolonged bleeding may be increased. Doctors are reminded that in the non breast-feeding, post partum patient, ovulation may occur as early as week 4.

If the puerperal woman will be breast-feeding, the initial injection should be given no sooner than six weeks post partum, when the infant's enzyme system is more fully developed. Further injections should be given at 12 week intervals.

Further doses: These should be given at 12 week intervals, however, as long as the injection is given no later than five days after this time, no additional contraceptive measures (e.g. barrier) are required. (N.B. For partners of men undergoing vasectomy a second injection of 150 mg i.m. 12 weeks after the first may be necessary in a small proportion of patients where the partner's sperm count has not fallen to zero.) If the interval from the preceding injection is greater than 89 days (12 weeks and five days) for any reason, then pregnancy should be excluded before the next injection is given and the patient should use additional contraceptive measures (e.g. barrier) for fourteen days after this subsequent injection.

Elderly: Not appropriate.

Children: . Depo-Provera is not indicated before menarche (see Section 4.1 Therapeutic Indications).

Data in adolescent females (12-18 years) is available (see section 4.4 Special Warnings and Special Precautions for Use and Section 5.1 Pharmacodynamic properties). Other than concerns about loss of BMD, the safety and effectiveness of Depo-Provera is expected to be the same for adolescents after menarche and adult females

4.3 Contraindications

Depo-Provera is contra-indicated in patients with a known sensitivity to medroxyprogesterone acetate or any ingredient of the vehicle.

Depo-Provera should not be used during pregnancy, either for diagnosis or therapy.

Depo-Provera is contra-indicated as a contraceptive at the above dosage in known or suspected hormone-dependent malignancy of breast or genital organs.

Whether administered alone or in combination with oestrogen, Depo-Provera should not be employed in patients with abnormal uterine bleeding until a definite diagnosis has been established and the possibility of genital tract malignancy eliminated.

4.4 Special warnings and special precautions for use

Warnings:

Loss of Bone Mineral Density: Use of Depo-Provera injection reduces serum oestrogen levels and is associated with significant loss of BMD due to the known effect of oestrogen deficiency on the bone remodelling system. Bone loss is greater with increasing duration of use and appears to be at least partially reversible after Depo-Provera injection is discontinued and ovarian oestrogen production increases.

This loss of BMD is of particular concern during adolescence and early adulthood, a critical period of bone accretion (see section 4.1, Therapeutic Indications). It is unknown if use of Depo-Provera injection by adolescent women will reduce peak bone mass and increase the risk for osteoporotic fracture in later life.

A study to assess the reversibility of loss of BMD in adolescent females is ongoing. In adolescents, Depo-Provera may be used, but only after other methods of contraception have been discussed with the patients and considered to be unsuitable or unacceptable. In women of all ages, careful re-evaluation of the risks and benefits of treatment should be carried out in those who wish to continue use for more than 2 years. In women with significant lifestyle and/or medical risk factors for osteoporosis, other methods of contraception should be considered prior to use of Depo-Provera.

Menstrual Irregularity: The administration of Depo-Provera usually causes disruption of the normal menstrual cycle. Bleeding patterns include amenorrhoea (present in up to 30% of women during the first 3 months and increasing to 55% by month 12 and 68% by month 24); irregular bleeding and spotting; prolonged >10 days) episodes of bleeding (up to 33% of women in the first 3 months of use decreasing to 12% by month 12). Rarely, heavy prolonged bleeding may occur. Evidence suggests that prolonged or heavy bleeding requiring treatment may occur in 0.5-4 occasions per 100 women years of use. If abnormal bleeding persists or is severe, appropriate investigation should take place to rule out the possibility of organic pathology and appropriate treatment should be instituted when necessary. Excessive or prolonged bleeding can be controlled by the co-administration of oestrogen. This may be delivered either in the form of a low dose (30 micrograms oestrogen) combined oral contraceptive pill or in the form of oestrogen replacement therapy such as conjugated equine oestrogen (0.625-1.25 mg daily). Oestrogen therapy may need to be repeated for 1-2 cycles. Long-term co-administration of oestrogen is not recommended.

Return to Fertility: There is no evidence that Depo-Provera causes permanent infertility. Pregnancies have occurred as early as 14 weeks after a preceding injection, however, in clinical trials, the mean time to return of ovulation was 5.3 months following the preceding injection. Women should be counselled that there is a potential for delay in return to full fertility following use of the method, regardless of the duration of use, however, 83% of women may be expected to conceive within 12 months of the first "missed" injection (i.e. 15 months after the last injection administered). The median time to conception was 10 months (range 4-31) after the last injection.

Cancer Risks: Long-term case-controlled surveillance of Depo-Provera users found no overall increased risk of ovarian, liver, or cervical cancer and a prolonged, protective effect of reducing the risk of endometrial cancer in the population of users. A meta-analysis in 1996 from 54 epidemiological studies[1] reported that there is a slight increased relative risk of having breast cancer diagnosed in women who are currently using hormonal contraceptives. The observed pattern of increased risk may be due to an earlier diagnosis of breast cancer in hormonal contraceptive users, biological effects or a combination of both. The additional breast cancers diagnosed in current users of hormonal contraceptives or in women who have used them in the last ten years are more likely to be localised to the breast than those in women who never used hormonal contraceptives.

Breast cancer is rare among women under 40 years of age whether or not they use hormonal contraceptives. In the meta-analysis the results for injectable progestogens (1.5% of the data) and progestogen only pills (0.8% of the data) did not reach significance although there was no evidence that they differed from other hormonal contraceptives. Whilst the background risk of breast cancer increases with age, the excess number of breast cancer diagnoses in current and recent injectable progestogen (IP) users is small in relation to the overall risk of breast cancer, possibly of similar magnitude to that associated with combined oral contraceptives. However, for IPs, the evidence is based on much smaller populations of users (less than 1.5% of the data) and is less conclusive than for combined oral contraceptives. It is not possible to infer from these data whether it is due to an earlier diagnosis of breast cancer in ever-users, the biological effects of hormonal contraceptives, or a combination of reasons.

The most important risk factor for breast cancer in IP users is the age women discontinue the IP; the older the age at stopping, the more breast cancers are diagnosed. Duration of use is less important and the excess risk gradually disappears during the course of the 10 years after stopping IP use, such that by 10 years there appears to be no excess.

The evidence suggests that compared with never-users, among 10,000 women who use IPs for up to 5 years but stop by age 20, there would be much less than 1 extra case of breast cancer diagnosed up to 10 years afterwards. For those stopping by age 30 after 5 years use of the IP, there would be an estimated 2-3 extra cases (additional to the 44 cases of breast cancer per 10,000 women in this age group never exposed to oral contraceptives). For those stopping by age 40 after 5 years use, there would be an estimated 10 extra cases diagnosed up to 10 years afterwards (additional to the 160 cases of breast cancer per 10,000 never-exposed women in this age group).

It is important to inform patients that users of all hormonal contraceptives appear to have a small increase in the risk of being diagnosed with breast cancer, compared with non-users of hormonal contraceptives, but that this has to be weighed against the known benefits.

Weight Gain: There is a tendency for women to gain weight while on Depo-Provera therapy. Studies indicate that over the first 1-2 years of use, average weight gain was 5-8 lbs. Women completing 4-6 years of therapy gained an average of 14-16.5 lbs. There is evidence that weight is gained as a result of increased fat and is not secondary to an anabolic effect or fluid retention.

Anaphylaxis: Very few reports of anaphylactoid reactions have been received.

Thrombo-embolic Disorders: Should the patient experience pulmonary embolism, cerebrovascular disease or retinal thrombosis while receiving Depo-Provera, the drug should not be readministered.

Psychiatric Disorders: Patients with a history of endogenous depression should be carefully monitored. Some patients may complain of premenstrual-type depression while on Depo-Provera therapy.

Abscess formation: As with any intramuscular injection, especially if not administered correctly, there is a risk of abscess formation at the site of injection, which may require medical and/or surgical intervention.

Precautions:

History or emergence of the following conditions require careful consideration and appropriate investigation: migraine or unusually severe headaches, acute visual disturbances of any kind, pathological changes in liver function and hormone levels. Patients with thromboembolic or coronary vascular disease should be carefully evaluated before using Depo-Provera.

A decrease in glucose tolerance has been observed in some patients treated with progestogens. The mechanism for this decrease is obscure. For this reason, diabetic patients should be carefully monitored while receiving progestogen therapy.

Rare cases of thrombo-embolism have been reported with use of Depo-Provera, but causality has not been established.

The effects of medroxyprogesterone acetate on lipid metabolism have been studied with no clear impact demonstrated. Both increases and decreases in total cholesterol, triglycerides and low-density lipoprotein (LDL) cholesterol have been observed in studies. The use of Depo-Provera appears to be associated with a 15-20% reduction in serum high density lipoprotein (HDL) cholesterol levels which may protect women from cardiovascular disease. The clinical consequences of this observation are unknown. The potential for an increased risk of coronary disease should be considered prior to use.

Doctors should carefully consider the use of Depo-Provera in patients with recent trophoblastic disease before levels of human chorionic gonadotrophin have returned to normal.

Physicians should be aware that pathologists should be informed of the patient's use of Depo-Provera if endometrial or endocervical tissue is submitted for examination.

The results of certain laboratory tests may be affected by the use of Depo-Provera. These include gonadotrophin levels (decreased), plasma progesterone levels (decreased), urinary pregnanediol levels (decreased), plasma oestrogen levels (decreased), plasma cortisol levels (decreased), glucose tolerance test, metyrapone test, liver function tests (may increase), thyroid function tests (protein bound iodine levels may increase and T3 uptake levels may decrease). Coagulation test values for prothrombin (Factor II), and Factors VII, VIII, IX and X may increase.

4.5 Interaction with other medicinal products and other forms of Interaction

Aminoglutethimide administered concurrently with Depo-Provera may significantly depress the bioavailability of Depo-Provera.

Interactions with other medicinal treatments (including oral anticoagulants) have rarely been reported, but causality has not been determined. The possibility of interaction should be borne in mind in patients receiving concurrent treatment with other drugs.

The clearance of medroxyprogesterone acetate is approximately equal to the rate of hepatic blood flow. Because of this fact, it is unlikely that drugs which induce hepatic enzymes will significantly affect the kinetics of medroxyprogesterone acetate. Therefore, no dose adjustment is recommended in patients receiving drugs known to affect hepatic metabolising enzymes.

Table 1 Mean Percent Change from Baseline in BMD in Adults by Skeletal Site and Cohort after 5 Years of Therapy with Depo-Provera 150 mg IM and after 2 Years Post-Therapy or 7 Years of Observation (Control)

Time in Study	Spine		Total Hip		Femoral Neck	
	Depo-Provera	Control	Depo-Provera	Control	Depo-Provera	Control
5 years*	n=33 -5.38%	n=105 0.43%	n=21 -5.16%	n=65 0.19%	n=34 -6.12%	n=106 -0.27%
7 years**	n=12 -3.13%	n=60 0.53%	n=7 -1.34%	n=39 0.94%	n=13 -5.38%	n=63 -0.11%

*The treatment group consisted of women who received Depo-Provera Contraceptive Injection for 5 years and the control group consisted of women who did not use hormonal contraception for this time period.

** The treatment group consisted of women who received Depo-Provera Contraceptive Injection for 5 years and were then followed up for 2 years post-use and the control group consisted of women who did not use hormonal contraceptive for 7 years.

4.6 Pregnancy and lactation

Doctors should check that patients are not pregnant before initial injection of Depo-Provera, and also if administration of any subsequent injection is delayed beyond 89 days (12 weeks and five days).

Infants from accidental pregnancies that occur 1-2 months after injection of Depo-Provera may be at an increased risk of low birth weight, which in turn is associated with an increased risk of neonatal death. The attributable risk is low because such pregnancies are uncommon.

Children exposed to medroxyprogesterone acetate *in utero* and followed to adolescence, showed no evidence of any adverse effects on their health including their physical, intellectual, sexual or social development.

Medroxyprogesterone acetate and/or its metabolites are secreted in breast milk, but there is no evidence to suggest that this presents any hazard to the child. Infants exposed to medroxyprogesterone via breast milk have been studied for developmental and behavioural effects to puberty. No adverse effects have been noted.

4.7 Effects on ability to drive and use machines

None

4.8 Undesirable effects

In a large clinical trial of over 3900 women, who were treated with Depo-Provera for up to 7 years, the following adverse events were reported.

The following adverse events were commonly (by more than 5% of subjects) reported: menstrual irregularities (bleeding and/or amenorrhoea), weight changes, headache, nervousness, abdominal pain or discomfort, dizziness, asthenia (weakness or fatigue).

Adverse events reported by 1% to 5% of subjects using Depo-Provera were: decreased libido or anorgasmia, backache, leg cramps, depression, nausea, insomnia, leucorrhoea, acne, vaginitis, pelvic pain, breast pain, no hair growth or alopecia, bloating, rash, oedema, hot flushes.

Other events were reported infrequently (by fewer than 1 % of subjects), and included: galactorrhoea, melasma, chloasma, convulsions, changes in appetite, gastrointestinal disturbances, jaundice, genitourinary infections, vaginal cysts, dyspareunia, paraesthesia, chest pain, pulmonary embolus, allergic reactions, anaemia, syncope, dyspnoea, thirst, hoarseness, somnolence, decreased glucose tolerance, hirsutism, pruritus, arthralgia, pyrexia, pain at injection site, injection site abscess, blood dyscrasia, rectal bleeding, changes in breast size, breast lumps or nipple bleeding, axillary swelling, prevention of lactation, sensation of pregnancy, lack of return to fertility, paralysis, facial palsy, scleroderma, osteoporosis, uterine hyperplasia, varicose veins, dysmenorrhoea, thrombophlebitis, deep vein thrombosis.

In postmarketing experience, there have been rare cases of osteoporosis including osteoporotic fractures reported in patients taking Depo-Provera.

4.9 Overdose

No positive action is required other than cessation of therapy.

5. PHARMACOLOGICAL PROPERTIES

5.1 Pharmacodynamic properties

Medroxyprogesterone acetate exerts anti-oestrogenic, anti-androgenic and antigonadotrophic effects.

BMD Changes in Adult Women

In a controlled, clinical study adult women using Depo-Provera injection (150 mg IM) for up to 5 years showed spine and hip mean BMD decreases of 5-6%, compared to no significant change in BMD in the control group. The decline in BMD was more pronounced during the first two years of use, with smaller declines in subsequent years. Mean changes in lumbar spine BMD of –2.86%, -4.11%, -4.89%, -4.93% and –5.38% after 1, 2, 3, 4 and 5 years, respectively, were observed. Mean decreases in BMD of the total hip and femoral neck were similar. Please refer to Table 1 below for further details.

After stopping use of Depo-Provera injection (150 mg IM), there was partial recovery of BMD toward baseline values during the 2-year post-therapy period. A longer duration of treatment was associated with a slower rate of BMD recovery.

Table 1. Mean Percent Change from Baseline in BMD in Adults by Skeletal Site and Cohort after 5 Years of Therapy with Depo-Provera 150 mg IM and after 2 Years Post-Therapy or 7 Years of Observation (Control)

(see Table 1)

BMD Changes in Adolescent Females (12-18 years)

Preliminary results from an ongoing, open-label clinical study of Depo-Provera injectable (150 mg IM every 12 weeks for up to 5 years) in adolescent females (12-18 years) also showed that Depo-Provera IM use was associated with a significant decline in BMD from baseline. The mean decrease in lumbar spine BMD was 4.2% after 5 years; mean decreases for the total hip and femoral neck were 6.9% and 6.1%, respectively. In contrast, most adolescent girls will significantly increase bone density during this period of growth following menarche. Preliminary data from a small number of adolescents have shown partial recovery of BMD during the 2-year follow-up period.

5.2 Pharmacokinetic properties

Parenteral medroxyprogesterone acetate (MPA) is a long acting progestational steroid. The long duration of action results from its slow absorption from the injection site. Immediately after injection of 150 mg/ml MPA, plasma levels were 1.7 ± 0.3 nmol/l. Two weeks later, levels were 6.8 ± 0.8 nmol/l. Concentrations fell to the initial levels by the end of 12 weeks. At lower doses, plasma levels of MPA appear directly related to the dose administered. Serum accumulation over time was not demonstrated. MPA is eliminated via faecal and urinary excretion. Plasma half-life is about six weeks after a single intramuscular injection. At least 11 metabolites have been reported. All are excreted in the urine, some, but not all, conjugated.

6. PHARMACEUTICAL PARTICULARS

6.1 List of excipients

Excipients are methylparaben, macrogol 3350, polysorbate 80, propylparaben, sodium chloride, hydrochloric acid, sodium hydroxide and water for injections.

6.2 Incompatibilities

None known.

6.3 Shelf life

Syringe: 36 months.

Vial: 18 months

6.4 Special precautions for storage

Do not store above 25 C.

Do not freeze.

6.5 Nature and contents of container

1 ml disposable syringe with plunger stopper and tip cap.

1 ml vial with stopper and tip cap.

6.6 Instructions for use and handling

No special instructions are applicable.

Administrative Data

7. MARKETING AUTHORISATION HOLDER

Pharmacia Limited
Davy Avenue
Milton Keynes
MK5 8PH
UK

8. MARKETING AUTHORISATION NUMBER(S)

PL 0032/0082

9. DATE OF FIRST AUTHORISATION/RENEWAL OF THE AUTHORISATION

Date of Grant: 27 August 1991

Date of Renewal: 6 February 1997

10. DATE OF REVISION OF THE TEXT

November 2004

LEGAL CATEGORY: POM

Company Reference: DPB1_5

Derbac-M Liquid

(SSL International plc)

1. NAME OF THE MEDICINAL PRODUCT
Derbac-M Liquid.

2. QUALITATIVE AND QUANTITATIVE COMPOSITION
Malathion 0.5% w/w.

3. PHARMACEUTICAL FORM
Liquid emulsion.

4. CLINICAL PARTICULARS

4.1 Therapeutic indications
For the eradication of head lice, pubic lice and their eggs. Treatment of scabies.

4.2 Posology and method of administration
For topical external use only. Adults, the elderly and children aged 6 months and over: As this product does not contain alcohol, it may be more suitable for those with asthma or eczema. *Treatment of head lice:* Rub the liquid into the scalp until all the hair and scalp is thoroughly moistened. Leave the hair to dry naturally in a warm but well ventilated room. After 12 hours, or the next day if preferred, shampoo the hair in the normal way. Rinse the hair and comb whilst wet to remove the dead lice and eggs (nits) using a fine toothed metal nit comb. *Treatment of crab (pubic) lice:* Apply Derbac-M Liquid to the entire skin surface. Pay particular attention to all hairy areas including beards and moustaches. Avoid any other areas above the neck. Leave on for at least one hour before washing but preferably Derbac-M Liquid should be left on overnight. Wash off in the usual manner. *Treatment of scabies:* Apply Derbac-M Liquid to the entire skin surface. In adults it may not be necessary to apply above the neck but children under the age of two years should have a thin film of Derbac-M Liquid applied to the scalp, face and ears, avoiding the eyes and mouth. Do not wash off or bathe for 24 hours. If hands or any other parts must be washed during this period, the treatment must be reapplied to those areas immediately. No special sterilisation of clothing is necessary: ordinary laundering or dry cleaning with hot iron pressing are sufficient. The infestation is cleared by the treatment. However, the itching and rash may persist for up to 7 days. An anti-irritant cream can be applied if necessary. Family members and close contacts should also be treated simultaneously. Children aged 6 months and under: On medical advice only.

4.3 Contraindications
Known sensitivity to malathion. Not to be used on infants less than 6 months except on medical advice.

4.4 Special warnings and special precautions for use
Avoid contact with the eyes. For external use only. Keep out of the reach of children. If inadvertently swallowed, a doctor or casualty department should be contacted at once. When Derbac-M Liquid is used by a school nurse or other health officer in the mass treatment of large numbers of children, it is advisable that protective plastic or rubber gloves be worn. Continued prolonged treatment with this product should be avoided. It should be used not more than once a week and for not more than 3 consecutive weeks.

4.5 Interaction with other medicinal products and other forms of Interaction
None stated.

4.6 Pregnancy and lactation
No known effects in pregnancy and lactation. However, as with all medicines, use with caution.

4.7 Effects on ability to drive and use machines
None stated.

4.8 Undesirable effects
Very rarely, skin irritation has been reported.

4.9 Overdose
It is most unlikely that a toxic dose of malathion will be ingested. Treatment consists of gastric lavage, assisted respiration and, if necessary in the event of massive ingestion, administration of atropine together with pralidoxime.

5. PHARMACOLOGICAL PROPERTIES

5.1 Pharmacodynamic properties
Derbac-M Liquid contains malathion, a widely used organophosphorus insecticide which is active by cholinesterase inhibition. It is effective against a wide range of insects, but is one of the least toxic organophosphorus insecticides since it is rapidly detoxified by plasma carboxylesterases.

5.2 Pharmacokinetic properties
None stated. Derbac-M Liquid is applied topically to the affected area.

5.3 Preclinical safety data
None stated.

6. PHARMACEUTICAL PARTICULARS

6.1 List of excipients
Methylhydroxybenzoate; Propylhydroxybenzoate; Lanette Wax SX; Potassium Citrate; Citric Acid; Perfume HT 52; Water.

6.2 Incompatibilities
None stated.

6.3 Shelf life
Two and a half years.

6.4 Special precautions for storage
Store at or below 25°C. Protect from light.

6.5 Nature and contents of container
Cartoned, clear or amber glass bottles with polyethylene caps and polypropylene faced wads containing 50 or 200 ml of product.

6.6 Instructions for use and handling
None stated.

7. MARKETING AUTHORISATION HOLDER
Seton Products Limited, Tubiton House, Oldham, OL1 3HS.

8. MARKETING AUTHORISATION NUMBER(S)
PL 11314/0046.

9. DATE OF FIRST AUTHORISATION/RENEWAL OF THE AUTHORISATION
13th October 1995/11th September 2000.

10. DATE OF REVISION OF THE TEXT
September 2000.

Dermalo Bath Emollient

(Dermal Laboratories Limited)

1. NAME OF THE MEDICINAL PRODUCT
DERMALO® BATH EMOLLIENT

2. QUALITATIVE AND QUANTITATIVE COMPOSITION
Liquid Paraffin 65.0% w/w; Acetylated Wool Alcohols 5.0% w/w.

3. PHARMACEUTICAL FORM
Bath additive - dye- and fragrance-free colourless to straw coloured clear oily liquid.

4. CLINICAL PARTICULARS

4.1 Therapeutic indications
For the symptomatic relief of contact dermatitis, atopic dermatitis, senile pruritus, ichthyosis and related dry skin disorders.

4.2 Posology and method of administration
Adults, including the elderly: Add 15 to 20 ml (1½ to 2 capfuls) to a standard bath of water (8 inch depth). Immerse and cover the affected areas with the bath water and soak for 10 to 20 minutes. Pat dry with a towel. Alternatively, use a similar amount smoothed onto wet skin following a shower. Rinse off thoroughly and pat dry with a towel.

Infants and children: Add 5 to 10 ml (½ to 1 capful) to a small bath or wash basin of water. Immerse and cover the affected areas with the bath water and soak for 10 to 20 minutes. Alternatively, repeatedly gently sponge over the affected areas. Pat dry with a towel.

There is no differentiation between the dosage quantities for the symptomatic relief of the conditions listed.

4.3 Contraindications
Sensitivity to any of the ingredients.

4.4 Special warnings and special precautions for use
Take care not to slip in the bath or shower. Surfaces that have been in contact with the product should be cleaned with a proprietary detergent. For external use only.

4.5 Interaction with other medicinal products and other forms of Interaction
None known.

4.6 Pregnancy and lactation
The constituents are not percutaneously absorbed or toxic if ingested. There is no evidence of safety of the drug used in pregnancy or lactation, but the active constituents have been in widespread use and in similar preparations for many years without apparent ill consequence.

4.7 Effects on ability to drive and use machines
None known.

4.8 Undesirable effects
Contact sensitivity reactions or mild irritant reactions may occur occasionally. In either case, treatment should be discontinued.

4.9 Overdose
Accidental ingestion may result in a purgative action due to the liquid paraffin and the oily nature of the product. Treat symptomatically. Fluid and electrolyte replacement may be necessary.

5. PHARMACOLOGICAL PROPERTIES

5.1 Pharmacodynamic properties
For dry skin conditions it is important to use an emollient while bathing. Dermalo Bath Emollient contains 65% Liquid Paraffin and 5% Acetylated Wool Alcohols for their moisturising and skin softening properties, and is specially formulated to facilitate dispersion in bath water or for ease of application after a shower.

5.2 Pharmacokinetic properties
The active constituents are not absorbed percutaneously. Pharmacokinetic particulars are thus not relevant.

5.3 Preclinical safety data
No relevant information additional to that contained elsewhere in the SPC.

6. PHARMACEUTICAL PARTICULARS

6.1 List of excipients
Isopropyl Myristate; Macrogol 3 Lauryl Ether.

6.2 Incompatibilities
None known.

6.3 Shelf life
36 months.

6.4 Special precautions for storage
Do not store above 25°C.

6.5 Nature and contents of container
500 ml white plastic bottle fitted with a dispensing plug and screw cap. Supplied in original packs (OP).

6.6 Instructions for use and handling
Not applicable.

7. MARKETING AUTHORISATION HOLDER
Dermal Laboratories

Tatmore Place, Gosmore

Hitchin, Herts SG4 7QR, UK.

8. MARKETING AUTHORISATION NUMBER(S)
0173/0182.

9. DATE OF FIRST AUTHORISATION/RENEWAL OF THE AUTHORISATION
24 February 2002.

10. DATE OF REVISION OF THE TEXT
October 2001.

Dermamist

(Astellas Pharma Limited)

1. NAME OF THE MEDICINAL PRODUCT
Dermamist

2. QUALITATIVE AND QUANTITATIVE COMPOSITION
White Soft Paraffin BP 10.0% w/w.

3. PHARMACEUTICAL FORM
Pressurised aerosol

4. CLINICAL PARTICULARS

4.1 Therapeutic indications
Treatment of dry skin conditions including eczema, ichthyosis and pruritus of the elderly.

4.2 Posology and method of administration
Adults, children and the elderly: Shake before use. Bathe or shower for not more than ten minutes. Pat dry and apply spray without delay. Do not spray on face. Spray from a distance of approximately 8 inches. Spray away from the face and move the can while spraying to achieve a very light coverage of the body. Spray sparingly; over application may cause the skin to feel oily.

4.3 Contraindications
Hypersensitivity to any of the ingredients.

4.4 Special warnings and special precautions for use
For external use only. Keep out of reach of children. Do not spray on face. Use in a ventilated area. Avoid inhalation. Guard against slipping. Discontinue use if the condition is made worse. Do not apply to broken skin.

4.5 Interaction with other medicinal products and other forms of Interaction
None.

4.6 Pregnancy and lactation
Can be used.

4.7 Effects on ability to drive and use machines
Not relevant.

4.8 Undesirable effects
Not relevant

4.9 Overdose
None

5. PHARMACOLOGICAL PROPERTIES

5.1 Pharmacodynamic properties
Emollients are fats or oils used for their local action on the skin and, occasionally, the mucous membranes. These oleaginous substances, also known as occlusive agents and humectants, are employed as protectives and as agents for softening the skin and rendering it more pliable. White soft paraffin forms an effective occlusive lipid film. The mechanism of action is by occluding water loss from the outer layer of skin.

5.2 Pharmacokinetic properties
White soft paraffin exerts its physiological effects by forming an occlusive layer on the surface of the skin. It is effective because it is not subject to absorption or subsequent distribution in the body, excretion or metabolism. Pharmacokinetic particulars are not appropriate in these circumstances.

5.3 Preclinical safety data
No relevant pre-clinical data has been generated.

6. PHARMACEUTICAL PARTICULARS

6.1 List of excipients
Liquid paraffin BP

Fractionated coconut oil BP

Butane 40 (butane: isobutane: propane) HSE

6.2 Incompatibilities
None

6.3 Shelf life
60 months.

6.4 Special precautions for storage
Store below 25°C. Pressurised container. Highly flammable, protect from sunlight and do not puncture, burn or expose to temperatures over 50°C even when empty. Do not spray on a naked flame or any incandescent material.

6.5 Nature and contents of container
Pressurised aerosol. Pack sizes 50 ml, 250 ml, 75 ml, 150 ml, 200 ml, 300 ml, 400 ml, and 500 ml. (75 ml, 150 ml, 200 ml, 300 ml, 400 ml, and 500 ml are currently not marketed.)

6.6 Instructions for use and handling
No special instructions for use or handling.

Administrative Data

7. MARKETING AUTHORISATION HOLDER
Caraderm Ltd

6 Pine Valley

Rostrevor

Co Down, BT34 3DE.

8. MARKETING AUTHORISATION NUMBER(S)
PL 13147/0001

9. DATE OF FIRST AUTHORISATION/RENEWAL OF THE AUTHORISATION
15/03/94

10. DATE OF REVISION OF THE TEXT
8th December 1998

Dermol 200 Shower Emollient

(Dermal Laboratories Limited)

1. NAME OF THE MEDICINAL PRODUCT
DERMOL™ 200 SHOWER EMOLLIENT

2. QUALITATIVE AND QUANTITATIVE COMPOSITION
Liquid Paraffin 2.5% w/w; Isopropyl Myristate 2.5% w/w; Benzalkonium Chloride 0.1% w/w; Chlorhexidine Dihydrochloride 0.1% w/w.

3. PHARMACEUTICAL FORM
White, non-greasy cutaneous emulsion.

4. CLINICAL PARTICULARS

4.1 Therapeutic indications
An antimicrobial shower emollient for the management of dry and pruritic skin conditions, especially eczema and dermatitis. Dermol 200 Shower Emollient is for direct application onto the skin and is suitable for use as a soap substitute.

4.2 Posology and method of administration
For adults, children and the elderly: For application to the skin (eg after showering): Apply to the affected areas as required. Massage into the skin, until absorbed. For use as a soap substitute in the shower: As required, use the shower emollient instead of an ordinary shower gel or soap. Pat dry.

4.3 Contraindications
Do not use in cases of known sensitivity to any of the ingredients.

4.4 Special warnings and special precautions for use
Avoid contact with the eyes, especially when used on the face. Take care to avoid slipping in the shower or bath.

4.5 Interaction with other medicinal products and other forms of Interaction
None known.

4.6 Pregnancy and lactation
No special precautions.

4.7 Effects on ability to drive and use machines
None known.

4.8 Undesirable effects
Although the shower emollient has been specially formulated for use on dry or problem skin, in the unlikely event of a reaction, discontinue treatment.

4.9 Overdose
Not applicable.

5. PHARMACOLOGICAL PROPERTIES

5.1 Pharmacodynamic properties
Bacteria (especially *Staphylococcus aureus*) are implicated in the pathogenesis of inflammatory dry skin conditions such as atopic eczema and dermatitis.

Dermol 200 Shower Emollient contains 5% of emollient oils in a non-greasy aqueous system which also contains the well-known and effective antiseptics benzalkonium chloride and chlorhexidine dihydrochloride. Its antimicrobial properties assist in overcoming infection, whether from *Staph aureus*, the pathogen which often complicates eczema and associated pruritus, or secondary infection caused by scratching.

The emollients, liquid paraffin and isopropyl myristate, permit rehydration of dry skin by forming an occlusive barrier within the skin surface, thus reducing drying from evaporation of water that diffuses from the underlying layers.

Patients with dry skin conditions have a deficiency of the natural oils which assist in the retention of moisture.

A non-ionic emollient soap substitute such as Dermol 200 Shower Emollient, will cleanse the skin, helping to remove surface debris without removing the skin's natural oils.

5.2 Pharmacokinetic properties
The active ingredients are presented in an aqueous emulsion system and so are readily absorbed into the stratum corneum when the product is gently massaged over the areas of dry skin. The antiseptic ingredients are in intimate contact with the skin, and as they are in solution, their availability is optimal.

5.3 Preclinical safety data
No special information.

6. PHARMACEUTICAL PARTICULARS

6.1 List of excipients
Cetostearyl Alcohol; Cetomacrogol 1000; Phenoxyethanol; Purified Water.

6.2 Incompatibilities
None known.

6.3 Shelf life
30 months.

6.4 Special precautions for storage
Do not store above 25°C.

6.5 Nature and contents of container
Plastic 200 ml bottle with a hooked overcap. This is supplied as an original pack (OP).

6.6 Instructions for use and handling
Not applicable.

7. MARKETING AUTHORISATION HOLDER
Dermal Laboratories

Tatmore Place, Gosmore

Hitchin, Herts SG4 7QR, UK.

8. MARKETING AUTHORISATION NUMBER(S)
0173/0156.

9. DATE OF FIRST AUTHORISATION/RENEWAL OF THE AUTHORISATION
22 February 2004.

10. DATE OF REVISION OF THE TEXT
October 2003.

Dermol 500 Lotion

(Dermal Laboratories Limited)

1. NAME OF THE MEDICINAL PRODUCT
DERMOL™ 500 LOTION

2. QUALITATIVE AND QUANTITATIVE COMPOSITION
Benzalkonium Chloride 0.1% w/w; Chlorhexidine Hydrochloride 0.1% w/w; Liquid Paraffin 2.5% w/w; Isopropyl Myristate 2.5% w/w.

3. PHARMACEUTICAL FORM
White, non-greasy cutaneous emulsion.

4. CLINICAL PARTICULARS

4.1 Therapeutic indications
An antimicrobial emollient for the management of dry and pruritic skin conditions, especially eczema and dermatitis. The lotion is suitable for direct application, and for use as a soap substitute.

4.2 Posology and method of administration
For adults, children and the elderly: For application to the skin: apply the lotion to the affected areas as required. Massage into the skin, until absorbed. For use as a soap substitute: use as a cleanser in the bath or shower, or for other toiletry purposes, instead of ordinary soap or shower gel.

4.3 Contraindications
Do not use in cases of known sensitivity to any of the ingredients.

4.4 Special warnings and special precautions for use
Avoid contact with the eyes.

4.5 Interaction with other medicinal products and other forms of Interaction
None known.

4.6 Pregnancy and lactation
No special precautions.

4.7 Effects on ability to drive and use machines
None known.

4.8 Undesirable effects
Although the lotion has been specially formulated for use on dry or problem skin, in the unlikely event of a reaction discontinue treatment.

4.9 Overdose
Not applicable.

5. PHARMACOLOGICAL PROPERTIES

5.1 Pharmacodynamic properties
Bacteria (especially *Staphylococcus aureus*) are implicated in the pathogenesis of inflammatory dry skin conditions such as atopic eczema or dermatitis. Dermol 500 Lotion contains 5% of emollient oils in a non-greasy aqueous lotion which also contains the well-known and effective antiseptics benzalkonium chloride and chlorhexidine hydrochloride. Its antimicrobial properties assist in overcoming infection, whether from *Staph. aureus*, the pathogen which often complicates eczema and associated pruritus, or secondary infection caused by scratching.

Massaged into the skin, the emollients, liquid paraffin and isopropyl myristate, permit rehydration of dry skin by forming an occlusive barrier within the skin surface, thus reducing drying from evaporation of water that diffuses from the underlying layers.

5.2 Pharmacokinetic properties
The active ingredients are presented in an aqueous lotion and so are readily absorbed into the stratum corneum when the product is gently massaged over the areas of dry skin. The antiseptic ingredients are in intimate contact with the skin, and as they are in solution, their availability is optimal.

5.3 Preclinical safety data
No special information.

6. PHARMACEUTICAL PARTICULARS

6.1 List of excipients
Cetostearyl Alcohol; Cetomacrogol 1000; Phenoxyethanol; Purified Water.

6.2 Incompatibilities
None known.

6.3 Shelf life
30 months.

6.4 Special precautions for storage
Do not store above 25°C.

6.5 Nature and contents of container
Plastic 500 ml bottle with a white pump dispenser. Supplied as an original pack (OP).

6.6 Instructions for use and handling
Not applicable.

7. MARKETING AUTHORISATION HOLDER
Dermal Laboratories

Tatmore Place, Gosmore

Hitchin, Herts SG4 7QR, UK.

8. MARKETING AUTHORISATION NUMBER(S)
0173/0051.

9. DATE OF FIRST AUTHORISATION/RENEWAL OF THE AUTHORISATION
2 October 2002.

10. DATE OF REVISION OF THE TEXT
July 2001.

Dermol 600 Bath Emollient

(Dermal Laboratories Limited)

1. NAME OF THE MEDICINAL PRODUCT
DERMOL™ 600 BATH EMOLLIENT

2. QUALITATIVE AND QUANTITATIVE COMPOSITION
Liquid Paraffin 25.0% w/w; Isopropyl Myristate 25.0% w/w; Benzalkonium Chloride 0.5% w/w.

3. PHARMACEUTICAL FORM
White bath additive.

4. CLINICAL PARTICULARS

4.1 Therapeutic indications
An antimicrobial bath emollient for use as an aid in the treatment of dry and pruritic skin conditions, especially eczema, dermatitis, ichthyosis or xeroderma. It permits the rehydration of the keratin by replacing lost lipids, and its antiseptic properties assist in overcoming secondary infection.

4.2 Posology and method of administration
For use in the bath: For adults, children and the elderly: Add up to 30 ml to a bath of warm water (more or less according to the size of the bath and individual patient requirements). For infants: Add up to 15ml to a bath of warm water (more or less according to the size of the bath and individual patient requirements). Soak for 5 to 10 minutes. Pat dry.

4.3 Contraindications
Sensitivity to any of the ingredients.

4.4 Special warnings and special precautions for use
Keep away from the eyes. For external use only. Take care to avoid slipping in the bath.

4.5 Interaction with other medicinal products and other forms of Interaction
None known.

4.6 Pregnancy and lactation
No special precautions.

4.7 Effects on ability to drive and use machines
None known.

4.8 Undesirable effects
None known.

4.9 Overdose
Not applicable.

5. PHARMACOLOGICAL PROPERTIES

5.1 Pharmacodynamic properties
For dry skin conditions it is important to add an emollient to the bath water. Dermol 600 Bath Emollient contains 50% of oils emulsified in water as well as the well-known antiseptic, benzalkonium chloride which assists in overcoming secondary infection.

5.2 Pharmacokinetic properties
Dermol 600 Bath Emollient contains 0.5% of the quaternary ammonium antiseptic, benzalkonium chloride. The large positively charged cation is readily adsorbed from the formulation onto negatively charged bacterial cell surfaces, thereby conferring substantial antimicrobial activity. Even at extended dilution, it is particularly effective against *Staphylococcus aureus*, a bacterium which is known to colonise the skin in large numbers in patients with eczema, especially atopic eczema. Apart from its emollient properties, Dermol 600 Bath Emollient therefore also helps to prevent and overcome secondary infection which may exacerbate the eczematous condition.

5.3 Preclinical safety data
The safety and efficacy of the emollients (liquid paraffin and isopropyl myristate) and the antiseptic (benzalkonium chloride) in topical dosage forms have been well established over many years of widespread clinical usage.

6. PHARMACEUTICAL PARTICULARS

6.1 List of excipients
Sorbitan Stearate; Polysorbate 60; IMS 95%; Purified Water.

6.2 Incompatibilities
None known.

6.3 Shelf life
36 months.

6.4 Special precautions for storage
Do not store above 25°C. Always replace the cap after use.

6.5 Nature and contents of container
600 ml plastic bottle with a measuring cap, supplied as an original pack.

6.6 Instructions for use and handling
Not applicable.

7. MARKETING AUTHORISATION HOLDER
Dermal Laboratories

Tatmore Place, Gosmore

Hitchin, Herts SG4 7QR, UK.

8. MARKETING AUTHORISATION NUMBER(S)
0173/0155.

9. DATE OF FIRST AUTHORISATION/RENEWAL OF THE AUTHORISATION
21 February 2004.

10. DATE OF REVISION OF THE TEXT
October 2003.

Dermol Cream

(Dermal Laboratories Limited)

1. NAME OF THE MEDICINAL PRODUCT
DERMOL™ CREAM

2. QUALITATIVE AND QUANTITATIVE COMPOSITION
Liquid Paraffin 10.0% w/w; Isopropyl Myristate 10.0% w/w; Benzalkonium Chloride 0.1% w/w; Chlorhexidine Dihydrochloride 0.1% w/w.

3. PHARMACEUTICAL FORM
Cream.

White non-greasy topical emulsion.

4. CLINICAL PARTICULARS

4.1 Therapeutic indications
An antimicrobial emollient cream for the management of dry and pruritic skin conditions, especially eczema and dermatitis. The cream is suitable for direct application, and for use as a soap substitute.

4.2 Posology and method of administration
For external use only.

Before using the 500g pump bottle, turn the top of the pump dispenser anti-clockwise to unlock it.

For adults, the elderly, infants and children.

For application to the skin

Apply Dermol Cream to the affected areas as often as necessary.

For use as a soap substitute

Dermol Cream may also be used as a cleanser in the bath or shower, or for other toiletry purposes, instead of ordinary soap or shower gel.

4.3 Contraindications
Do not use in cases of known sensitivity to any of the ingredients.

4.4 Special warnings and special precautions for use
Avoid contact with the eyes.

4.5 Interaction with other medicinal products and other forms of Interaction
None known.

4.6 Pregnancy and lactation
No special precautions.

4.7 Effects on ability to drive and use machines
None known.

4.8 Undesirable effects
Although the cream has been specially formulated for use on dry or problem skin, in the unlikely event of a reaction discontinue treatment.

4.9 Overdose
Excessive topical use is very unlikely to cause any untoward effects other than making the skin feel greasy.

In the event of a significant quantity being accidentally swallowed, nausea and vomiting may occur but serious effects are unlikely. Unless there are signs that give cause for concern, treatment should be conservative.

5. PHARMACOLOGICAL PROPERTIES

5.1 Pharmacodynamic properties
ATC Code: D02AX - Dermatologicals, other emollients and protectives.

Bacteria (especially *Staphylococcus aureus*) are implicated in the pathogenesis of inflammatory dry skin conditions such as atopic eczema or dermatitis.

Dermol Cream contains 20% of emollient oils in a non-greasy aqueous cream which also contains the well-known and effective antiseptics benzalkonium chloride and chlorhexidine dihydrochloride. Its antimicrobial properties assist in overcoming infection, whether from *Staph aureus*, the pathogen which often complicates eczema and associated pruritus, or secondary infection caused by scratching.

Massaged into the skin, the emollients, liquid paraffin and isopropyl myristate, permit rehydration of dry skin by forming an occlusive barrier within the skin surface, thus reducing drying from evaporation of water that diffuses from the underlying layers.

5.2 Pharmacokinetic properties
The active ingredients are presented in an aqueous cream and so are readily absorbed into the stratum corneum when the product is gently massaged over the areas of dry skin. The antiseptic ingredients are in intimate contact with the skin, and as they are in solution, their availability is optimal.

5.3 Preclinical safety data
No special information.

6. PHARMACEUTICAL PARTICULARS

6.1 List of excipients
Cetostearyl Alcohol; Glycerol; Cetomacrogol 1000; Phenoxyethanol; Disodium Phosphate Dodecahydrate; Sodium Dihydrogen Phosphate Dihydrate; Purified Water.

6.2 Incompatibilities
None known.

6.3 Shelf life
30 months - for 500g pack.

24 months - for 100g pack.

6.4 Special precautions for storage
Do not store above 30°C. Replace cap after use.

6.5 Nature and contents of container
High density polyethylene squeezable **Bottle** (500g) with a polypropylene flip top cap.

High density polyethylene **Tube** (100g) with a polypropylene screw cap.

6.6 Instructions for use and handling
Not applicable.

7. MARKETING AUTHORISATION HOLDER
Dermal Laboratories

Tatmore Place, Gosmore

Hitchin, Herts SG4 7QR, UK.

8. MARKETING AUTHORISATION NUMBER(S)
0173/0171.

9. DATE OF FIRST AUTHORISATION/RENEWAL OF THE AUTHORISATION
17 May 2004.

10. DATE OF REVISION OF THE TEXT
May 2004.

Dermovate Cream

(GlaxoSmithKline UK)

1. NAME OF THE MEDICINAL PRODUCT
Dermovate Cream

2. QUALITATIVE AND QUANTITATIVE COMPOSITION
Clobetasol propionate 0.0525% w/w

3. PHARMACEUTICAL FORM
Cream

4. CLINICAL PARTICULARS

4.1 Therapeutic indications
Clobetasol propionate is a very active topical corticosteroid which is of particular value when used in short courses for the treatment of more resistant dermatoses such as psoriasis (excluding widespread plaque psoriasis), recalcitrant eczemas, lichen planus, discoid lupus erythematosus, and other skin conditions which do not respond satisfactorily to less active steroids.

4.2 Posology and method of administration
Apply sparingly to the affected area once or twice daily until improvement occurs. As with other highly active topical steroid preparations, therapy should be discontinued when control is achieved. In the more responsive conditions this may be within a few days.

If no improvement is seen within two to four weeks, reassessment of the diagnosis, or referral, may be necessary.

Repeated short courses of Dermovate may be used to control exacerbations. If continuous steroid treatment is necessary, a less potent preparation should be used.

In very resistant lesions, especially where there is hyperkeratosis, the anti-inflammatory effect of Dermovate can be enhanced, if necessary, by occluding the treatment area with polythene film. Overnight occlusion only is usually adequate to bring about a satisfactory response. Thereafter improvement can usually be maintained by application without occlusion.

For topical administration.

4.3 Contraindications
Rosacea.

Acne vulgaris.

Perioral dermatitis.

Perianal and genital pruritus.

Primary cutaneous viral infections (e.g. herpes simplex, chickenpox).

Hypersensitivity to the preparation.

The use of Dermovate skin preparations is not indicated in the treatment of primary infected skin lesions caused by infection with fungi (e.g. candidiasis, tinea) or bacteria (e.g. impetigo); or dermatoses in children under one year of age, including dermatitis and napkin eruptions.

4.4 Special warnings and special precautions for use
Long-term continuous therapy should be avoided where possible, particularly in infants and children, as adrenal suppression can occur even without occlusion. If Dermovate is required for use in children, it is recommended that the treatment should be reviewed weekly. It should be noted that the infant's napkin may act as an occlusive dressing.

If used in childhood or on the face, courses should be limited if possible to five days and occlusion should not be used.

The face, more than other areas of the body, may exhibit atrophic changes after prolonged treatment with potent topical corticosteroids. This must be borne in mind when treating such conditions as psoriasis, discoid lupus erythematosus and severe eczema.

If applied to the eyelids, care is needed to ensure that the preparation does not enter the eye, as glaucoma might result. If Dermovate Cream does enter the eye, the affected eye should be bathed in copious amounts of water.

Topical steroids may be hazardous in psoriasis for a number of reasons including rebound relapses, development of tolerance, risk of generalised pustular psoriasis and development of local or systemic toxicity due to impaired barrier function of the skin. If used in psoriasis careful patient supervision is important.

Appropriate antimicrobial therapy should be used whenever treating inflammatory lesions which have become infected. Any spread of infection requires withdrawal of topical corticosteroid therapy and systemic administration of antimicrobial agents. Bacterial infection is encouraged by the warm, moist conditions induced by occlusive dressings, and so the skin should be cleansed before a fresh dressing is applied.

4.5 Interaction with other medicinal products and other forms of Interaction
None reported.

4.6 Pregnancy and lactation
There is inadequate evidence of safety in human pregnancy. Topical administration of corticosteroids to pregnant animals can cause abnormalities of foetal development including cleft palate and intrauterine growth retardation. The relevance of this finding to humans has not

been established, therefore, topical steroids should not be used extensively in pregnancy, i.e. in large amounts or for prolonged periods.

The safe use of clobetasol propionate during lactation has not been established.

4.7 Effects on ability to drive and use machines
Clobetasol propionate is not expected to have any effects.

4.8 Undesirable effects
As with other topical corticosteroids, prolonged use of large amounts, or treatment of extensive areas can result in sufficient systemic absorption to produce the features of hypercortisolism. This effect is more likely to occur in infants and children, and if occlusive dressings are used. In infants, the napkin may act as an occlusive dressing.

Provided the weekly dosage is less than 50g in adults, any suppression of the HPA axis is likely to be transient with a rapid return to normal values once the short course of steroid therapy has ceased. The same applies to children given proportionate dosage.

Prolonged and intensive treatment with highly active corticosteroid preparations may cause local atrophic changes, such as thinning, striae, and dilatation of the superficial blood vessels, particularly when occlusive dressings are used or when skin folds are involved.

There are reports of pigmentation changes and hypertrichosis with topical steroids.

In rare instances, treatment of psoriasis with corticosteroids (or its withdrawal) is thought to have provoked the pustular form of the disease (see Special warnings and special precautions for use).

Dermovate is usually well tolerated, but if signs of hypersensitivity appear, application should be stopped immediately.

Exacerbation of symptoms may occur.

4.9 Overdose
Acute overdosage is very unlikely to occur, however, in the case of chronic overdosage or misuse, the features of hypercortisolism may appear and in this situation topical steroids should be discontinued gradually. However, because of the risk of acute adrenal suppression this should be done under medical supervision.

5. PHARMACOLOGICAL PROPERTIES

5.1 Pharmacodynamic properties
Clobetasol propionate is a highly active corticosteroid with topical anti-inflammatory activity. The major effect of clobetasol propionate on skin is a non-specific anti-inflammatory response, partially due to vasoconstriction and decrease in collagen synthesis.

5.2 Pharmacokinetic properties
Percutaneous penetration of clobetasol propionate varies among individuals and can be increased by the use of occlusive dressings, or when the skin is inflamed or diseased.

Mean peak plasma clobetasol propionate concentrations of 0.63 ng/ml occurred in one study eight hours after the second application (13 hours after an initial application) of 30 g clobetasol propionate 0.05% ointment to normal individuals with healthy skin. Following the application of a second dose of 30 g clobetasol propionate cream 0.05% mean peak plasma concentrations were slightly higher than the ointment and occurred 10 hours after application.

In a separate study, mean peak plasma concentrations of approximately 2.3 ng/ml and 4.6 ng/ml occurred respectively in patients with psoriasis and eczema three hours after a single application of 25 g clobetasol propionate 0.05% ointment.

Following percutaneous absorption of clobetasol propionate, the drug probably follows the metabolic pathway of systemically administered corticosteroids, i.e. metabolised primarily by the liver and then excreted by the kidneys. However, systemic metabolism of clobetasol has never been fully characterised or quantified.

5.3 Preclinical safety data
There are no preclinical data of relevance to the prescriber which are additional to that in other sections of the SmPC.

6. PHARMACEUTICAL PARTICULARS

6.1 List of excipients
Cetostearyl alcohol
Glyceryl monostearate
Arlacel 165
Beeswax substitute 6621
Propylene glycol
Chlorocresol
Sodium citrate
Citric acid monohydrate
Purified water

6.2 Incompatibilities
None reported.

6.3 Shelf life
24 months.

6.4 Special precautions for storage
Store below 25°C.

6.5 Nature and contents of container
Collapsible latex banded aluminium tube internally coated with epoxy resin based lacquer, with polypropylene cap.

Pack sizes: 25 g, 30 g or 100 g.

Not all pack sizes may be marketed.

6.6 Instructions for use and handling
No special instructions.

Administrative Data

7. MARKETING AUTHORISATION HOLDER
Glaxo Wellcome UK Ltd
trading as Glaxo Laboratories
Stockley Park West
Uxbridge
Middlesex
UB11 1BT

8. MARKETING AUTHORISATION NUMBER(S)
PL 10949/0025

9. DATE OF FIRST AUTHORISATION/RENEWAL OF THE AUTHORISATION
August 04

10. DATE OF REVISION OF THE TEXT
August 04

Dermovate -NN Cream

(GlaxoSmithKline UK)

1. NAME OF THE MEDICINAL PRODUCT
Dermovate-NN Cream

2. QUALITATIVE AND QUANTITATIVE COMPOSITION
Dermovate-NN skin preparations contain clobetasol propionate 0.05% w/w, neomycin sulphate 0.5% and nystatin 100,000 units per gram.

3. PHARMACEUTICAL FORM
Cream.

4. CLINICAL PARTICULARS

4.1 Therapeutic indications
Clobetasol propionate is a highly active topical corticosteroid which is of particular value when used in short courses for the treatment of recalcitrant eczemas, neurodermatoses, and other conditions which do not respond satisfactorily to less active steroids.

Dermovate-NN is indicated in more resistant dermatoses such as recalcitrant eczemas and psoriasis (excluding widespread plaque psoriasis) where secondary bacterial or candidal infection is present, suspected or likely to occur, as when using occlusive dressings.

4.2 Posology and method of administration
Adults and children over 2 years:

Apply sparingly to the affected area once or twice daily until improvement occurs. As with other highly-active topical steroid preparations therapy should be discontinued when control is achieved. In the more responsive conditions this may be within a few days.

In very resistant lesions, especially where there is hyperkeratosis, the anti-inflammatory effect of Dermovate-NN can be enhanced, if necessary, by occluding the treatment area with polythene. Overnight occlusion only is usually adequate to bring about a satisfactory response, thereafter improvement can be usually maintained by application without occlusion.

Treatment should not be continued for more than 7 days without medical supervision. If a longer course is necessary, it is recommended that treatment should not be continued for more than 4 weeks without the patient's condition being reviewed.

Repeated short courses of Dermovate-NN may be used to control exacerbations. If continuous steroid treatment is necessary, a less potent preparation should be used.

Dosage in Renal Impairment: Dosage should be reduced in patients with reduced renal function (see Special Warnings and Special Precautions for Use).

Elderly:

Dermovate-NN is suitable for use in the elderly. Caution should be exercised in cases where a decrease in renal function exists and significant systemic absorption of neomycin sulphate may occur. (See Special Warnings and Special Precautions for Use.)

Children:

Dermovate-NN is suitable for use in children (2 years and over) at the same dose as adults. A possibility of increased absorption exists in very young children, thus Dermovate-NN is not recommended for use in neonates and infants (younger than 2 years) (see Contra-indications and Special Warnings and Special Precautions for Use).

For topical administration.

4.3 Contraindications
Rosacea, acne vulgaris and perioral dermatitis.

Primary cutaneous viral infections (eg. herpes simplex, chickenpox).

Hypersensitivity to the preparations.

Use of Dermovate-NN skin preparations is not indicated in the treatment of primary infected skin lesions caused by infection with fungi (eg. candidiasis, tinea), bacteria (eg. impetigo), or yeast; secondary infections due to Pseudomonas or Proteus species; perianal and genital pruritus, dermatoses in children under 2 years of age, including dermatitis and napkin eruptions.

Preparations containing neomycin should not be used for the treatment of otitis externa when the ear drum is perforated, because of the risk of ototoxicity.

Due to the known ototoxic and nephrotoxic potential of neomycin sulphate the use of Dermovate-NN in large quantities or on large areas for prolonged periods is not recommended in circumstances where significant systemic absorption may occur.

A possibility of increased absorption exists in very young children, therefore Dermovate-NN is not recommended for use in neonates and infants (up to 2 years). In neonates and infants, absorption by immature skin may be enhanced, and renal function may be immature.

4.4 Special warnings and special precautions for use
Long-term continuous topical therapy should be avoided where possible, particularly in infants and children, as adrenal suppression can occur readily even without occlusion.

If used in childhood, or on the face, courses should be limited to 5 days and occlusion should not be used. It should be noted that the child's napkin may act as an occlusive dressing.

The face, more than other areas of the body, may exhibit atrophic changes after prolonged treatment with potent topical corticosteroids. This must be borne in mind when treating such conditions as psoriasis and severe eczema.

If applied to the eyelids, care is needed to ensure that the preparation does not enter the eye, as glaucoma might result. If Dermovate-NN Cream does enter the eye, the affected eye should be bathed in copious amounts of water.

Topical corticosteroids may be hazardous in psoriasis for a number of reasons, including rebound relapses, development of tolerance, risk of generalized pustular psoriasis and development of local or systemic toxicity due to impaired barrier function of the skin. If used in psoriasis careful patient supervision is important.

Extension of the infection may occur due to the masking effect of the steroid.

If infection persists, systemic chemotherapy is required. Any spread of infection requires withdrawal of topical corticosteroid therapy.

Bacterial infection is encouraged by the warm, moist conditions induced by occlusive dressings, and the skin should be cleansed before a fresh dressing is applied.

Following significant systemic absorption, aminoglycosides such as neomycin can cause irreversible ototoxicity; and neomycin has nephrotoxic potential.

In renal impairment, the plasma clearance of neomycin is reduced (see Dosage in Renal Impairment).

Extended or recurrent application may increase the risk of contact sensitization.

Products which contain antimicrobial agents should not be diluted.

Dermovate NN Cream contains arachis oil (peanut oil) and should not be taken/applied by patients known to be allergic to peanut. As there is a possible relationship between allergy to peanut and allergy to Soya, patients with Soya allergy should also avoid Dermovate NN Cream.

4.5 Interaction with other medicinal products and other forms of Interaction
Neomycin sulphate can intensify and prolong the respiratory depressant effects of neuromuscular blocking agents following significant systemic absorption. However, if used in accordance with the recommendations systemic exposure to neomycin sulphate is expected to be minimal and drug interactions are unlikely to be significant. No hazardous interactions have been reported with use of clobetasol propionate or nystatin.

4.6 Pregnancy and lactation
There is little information to demonstrate the possible effect of topically applied neomycin in pregnancy and lactation. However, neomycin present in maternal blood can cross the placenta and may give rise to a theoretical risk of foetal toxicity, thus the use of Dermovate-NN is not recommended in pregnancy and lactation.

The safe use of clobetasol propionate during lactation has not been established.

4.7 Effects on ability to drive and use machines
Dermovate-NN Cream is not expected to have any effect.

4.8 Undesirable effects
As with other topical corticosteroids prolonged use of large amounts or treatment of extensive areas can result in sufficient systemic absorption to produce the features of hypercortisolism. This effect is more likely to occur in infants and children and if occlusive dressings are used. In infants, the napkin may act as an occlusive dressing. Provided the weekly dosage is less than 50g in adults, any

suppression of the HPA axis is likely to be transient with a rapid return to normal values once the short course of steroid therapy has ceased. The same applies to children given a proportionate dosage.

Prolonged and intensive treatment with highly active corticosteroid preparations may cause local atrophic changes in the skin such as thinning, striae, and dilatation of the superficial blood vessels, particularly when occlusive dressings are used, or when skin folds are involved.

In rare instances, treatment of psoriasis with corticosteroids (or its withdrawal) is thought to have provoked the pustular form of the disease (see Special Warnings and Special Precautions for Use).

There are reports of pigmentation changes and hypertrichosis with topical steroids.

Dermovate-NN is usually well tolerated, but if signs of hypersensitivity appear, application should be stopped immediately.

Exacerbation of symptoms may occur.

4.9 Overdose
Acute overdosage is very unlikely to occur, however, in the case of chronic overdosage or misuse the features of hypercortisolism may appear and in this situation topical steroids should be discontinued gradually. However, because of the risk of acute adrenal suppression this should be done under medical supervision.

Also, consideration should be given to significant systemic absorption of neomycin sulphate (see Special Warnings and Special Precautions for Use). If this is suspected, use of the product should be stopped and the patient's general status, hearing acuity, renal and neuromuscular functions should be monitored.

Blood levels of neomycin sulphate should also be determined. Haemodialysis may reduce the serum level of neomycin sulphate.

5. PHARMACOLOGICAL PROPERTIES

5.1 Pharmacodynamic properties
Clobetasol propionate is a highly active corticosteroid with topical anti-inflammatory activity. The major effect of clobetasol propionate on skin is a non-specific anti-inflammatory response, partially due to vasoconstriction and decrease in collagen synthesis.

The use of nystatin in the local treatment of candidal infections of the skin and of neomycin as a broad spectrum antibiotic is well known.

The principle action of the preparation is based on the anti-inflammatory activity of the corticosteroid. The broad spectrum antibacterial and anti-candidal activity provided by the combination of neomycin and nystatin allow this effect to be utilized in the treatment of conditions which are or are likely to become infected.

5.2 Pharmacokinetic properties
Percutaneous penetration of clobetasol propionate varies among individuals and can be increased by the use of occlusive dressings, or when the skin is inflamed or diseased.

Mean peak plasma clobetasol propionate concentrations of 0.63ng/ml occurred in one study 8 hours after the second application (13 hours after an initial application) of 30g clobetasol propionate 0.05% ointment to normal individuals with healthy skin. Following the application of a second dose of 30g clobetasol propionate cream 0.05% mean peak plasma concentrations were slightly higher than the ointment and occurred 10 hours after application.

In a separate study, mean peak plasma concentrations of approximately 2.3ng/ml and 4.6ng/ml occurred respectively in patients with psoriasis and eczema 3 hours after a single application of 25g clobetasol propionate 0.05% ointment. However, systemic metabolism of clobetasol has never been fully characterised or quantified. Following percutaneous absorption of clobetasol propionate the drug probably follows the metabolic pathway of systemically administered corticosteroids, i.e. metabolised primarily by the liver and then excreted by the kidneys.

5.3 Preclinical safety data
There are no preclinical data of relevance to the prescriber which are in addition to that in other sections of the SmPC.

6. PHARMACEUTICAL PARTICULARS

6.1 List of excipients
Microcrystalline wax, arachis oil (peanut oil), polyoxyethylene cetyl ether, white beeswax or beeswax substitute 6621, titanium dioxide (E171), propyl gallate and ultra light liquid paraffin.

6.2 Incompatibilities
None known.

6.3 Shelf life
18 months.

6.4 Special precautions for storage
Store below 25°C.

6.5 Nature and contents of container
Collapsible aluminium tube, with a polypropylene cap.

Pack sizes: 25g or 30g.

6.6 Instructions for use and handling
Do not dilute.

Administrative Data

7. MARKETING AUTHORISATION HOLDER
Glaxo Wellcome UK Ltd

trading style GlaxoSmithKline UK

Stockley Park West

Uxbridge

Middlesex UB11 1BT

8. MARKETING AUTHORISATION NUMBER(S)
PL 10949/0026

9. DATE OF FIRST AUTHORISATION/RENEWAL OF THE AUTHORISATION
14 June 2002

10. DATE OF REVISION OF THE TEXT
10 September 2003

Dermovate -NN Ointment

(GlaxoSmithKline UK)

1. NAME OF THE MEDICINAL PRODUCT
Dermovate-NN Ointment

2. QUALITATIVE AND QUANTITATIVE COMPOSITION
Dermovate-NN skin preparations contain clobetasol propionate 0.05% w/w, neomycin sulphate 0.5% and nystatin 100,000 units per gram.

3. PHARMACEUTICAL FORM
Ointment.

4. CLINICAL PARTICULARS

4.1 Therapeutic indications
Clobetasol propionate is a highly active topical corticosteroid which is of particular value when used in short courses for the treatment of recalcitrant eczemas, neurodermatoses, and other conditions which do not respond satisfactorily to less active steroids.

Dermovate-NN is indicated in more resistant dermatoses such as recalcitrant eczemas and psoriasis (excluding widespread plaque psoriasis) where secondary bacterial or candidal infection is present, suspected or likely to occur, as when using occlusive dressings.

4.2 Posology and method of administration
Adults and children over 2 years:

Apply sparingly to the affected area once or twice daily until improvement occurs. As with other highly-active topical steroid preparations therapy should be discontinued when control is achieved. In the more responsive conditions this may be within a few days.

In very resistant lesions, especially where there is hyperkeratosis, the anti-inflammatory effect of Dermovate-NN can be enhanced, if necessary, by occluding the treatment area with polythene. Overnight occlusion only is usually adequate to bring about a satisfactory response, thereafter improvement can be usually maintained by application without occlusion.

Treatment should not be continued for more than 7 days without medical supervision. If a longer course is necessary, it is recommended that treatment should not be continued for more than 4 weeks without the patient's condition being reviewed.

Repeated short courses of Dermovate-NN may be used to control exacerbations. If continuous steroid treatment is necessary, a less potent preparation should be used.

Dosage in Renal Impairment: Dosage should be reduced in patients with reduced renal function (see Special Warnings and Special Precautions for use).

Elderly:

Dermovate-NN is suitable for use in the elderly. Caution should be exercised in cases where a decrease in renal function exists and significant systemic absorption of neomycin sulphate may occur. (See Special Warnings and Special Precautions for Use.)

Children:

Dermovate-NN is suitable for use in children (2 years and over) at the same dose as adults. A possibility of increased absorption exists in very young children, thus Dermovate-NN is not recommended for use in neonates and infants (younger than 2 years) (see Contra-indications and Special Warnings and Special Precautions for Use).

For topical administration.

4.3 Contraindications
Rosacea, acne vulgaris and perioral dermatitis.

Primary cutaneous viral infections (eg. herpes simplex, chickenpox).

Hypersensitivity to the preparations.

Use of Dermovate-NN skin preparations is not indicated in the treatment of primary infected skin lesions caused by infection with fungi (eg. candidiasis, tinea), bacteria (eg. impetigo), or yeast; secondary infections due to Pseudomonas or Proteus species; perianal and genital pruritus, dermatoses in children under 2 years of age, including dermatitis and napkin eruptions.

Preparations containing neomycin should not be used for the treatment of otitis externa when the ear drum is perforated, because of the risk of ototoxicity.

Due to the known ototoxic and nephrotoxic potential of neomycin sulphate the use of Dermovate-NN in large quantities or on large areas for prolonged periods is not recommended in circumstances where significant systemic absorption may occur.

A possibility of increased absorption exists in very young children, therefore Dermovate-NN is not recommended for use in neonates and infants (up to 2 years). In neonates and infants, absorption by immature skin may be enhanced, and renal function may be immature.

4.4 Special warnings and special precautions for use
Long-term continuous topical therapy should be avoided where possible, particularly in infants and children, as adrenal suppression can occur readily even without occlusion.

If used in childhood, or on the face, courses should be limited to 5 days and occlusion should not be used. It should be noted that the child's napkin may act as an occlusive dressing.

The face, more than other areas of the body, may exhibit atrophic changes after prolonged treatment with potent topical corticosteroids. This must be borne in mind when treating such conditions as psoriasis and severe eczema.

If applied to the eyelids, care is needed to ensure that the preparation does not enter the eye, as glaucoma might result. If Dermovate-NN Ointment does enter the eye, the affected eye should be bathed in copious amounts of water.

Topical corticosteroids may be hazardous in psoriasis for a number of reasons, including rebound relapses, development of tolerance, risk of generalized pustular psoriasis and development of local or systemic toxicity due to impaired barrier function of the skin. If used in psoriasis careful patient supervision is important.

Extension of the infection may occur due to the masking effect of the steroid.

If infection persists, systemic chemotherapy is required. Any spread of infection requires withdrawal of topical corticosteroid therapy.

Bacterial infection is encouraged by the warm, moist conditions induced by occlusive dressings, and the skin should be cleansed before a fresh dressing is applied.

Following significant systemic absorption, aminoglycosides such as neomycin can cause irreversible ototoxicity; and neomycin has nephrotoxic potential.

In renal impairment, the plasma clearance of neomycin is reduced (see Dosage in Renal Impairment).

Extended or recurrent application may increase the risk of contact sensitization.

Products which contain antimicrobial agents should not be diluted.

4.5 Interaction with other medicinal products and other forms of Interaction
Neomycin sulphate can intensify and prolong the respiratory depressant effects of neuromuscular blocking agents following systemic absorption. However, if used in accordance with the recommendations systemic exposure to neomycin sulphate is expected to be minimal and drug interactions are unlikely to be significant. No hazardous interactions have been reported with use of clobetasol propionate or nystatin.

4.6 Pregnancy and lactation
There is little information to demonstrate the possible effect of topically applied neomycin in pregnancy and lactation. However, neomycin present in maternal blood can cross the placenta and may give rise to a theoretical risk of foetal toxicity, thus the use of Dermovate-NN is not recommended in pregnancy and lactation.

The safe use of clobetasol propionate during lactation has not been established.

4.7 Effects on ability to drive and use machines
Dermovate-NN Ointment is not expected to have any effect.

4.8 Undesirable effects
As with other topical corticosteroids prolonged use of large amounts or treatment of extensive areas can result in sufficient systemic absorption to produce the features of hypercortisolism. This effect is more likely to occur in infants and children if occlusive dressings are used. Provided the weekly dosage is less than 50g in adults, any suppression of the HPA axis is likely to be transient with a rapid return to normal values once the short course of steroid therapy has ceased. The same applies to children given a proportionate dosage.

Prolonged and intensive treatment with highly active corticosteroid preparations may cause local atrophic changes in the skin such as thinning, striae, and dilatation of the superficial blood vessels, particularly when occlusive dressings are used, or when skin folds are involved.

In rare instances, treatment of psoriasis with corticosteroids (or its withdrawal) is thought to have provoked the pustular form of the disease (see Special Warnings and Special Precautions for Use).

There are reports of pigmentation changes and hypertrichosis with topical steroids.

Dermovate-NN is usually well tolerated, but if signs of hypersensitivity appear, application should be stopped immediately.

Exacerbation of symptoms may occur.

4.9 Overdose

Acute overdosage is very unlikely to occur, however, in the case of chronic overdosage or misuse the features of hypercortisolism may appear and in this situation topical steroids should be discontinued gradually. However, because of the risk of acute adrenal suppression this should be done under medical supervision.

Also, consideration should be given to significant systemic absorption of neomycin sulphate (see Special Warnings and Special Precautions for Use). If this is suspected, use of the product should be stopped and the patient's general status, hearing acuity, renal and neuromuscular functions should be monitored.

Blood levels of neomycin sulphate should also be determined. Haemodialysis may reduce the serum level of neomycin sulphate.

5. PHARMACOLOGICAL PROPERTIES

5.1 Pharmacodynamic properties

Clobetasol propionate is a highly active corticosteroid with topical anti-inflammatory activity. The major effect of clobetasol propionate on skin is a non-specific anti-inflammatory response, partially due to vasoconstriction and decrease in collagen synthesis.

The use of nystatin in the local treatment of candidial infections of the skin and of neomycin as a broad spectrum antibiotic is well known.

The principle action of the preparation is based on the anti-inflammatory activity of the corticosteroid. The broad spectrum antibacterial and anti-candidal activity provided by the combination of neomycin and nystatin allow this effect to be utilized in the treatment of conditions which are or are likely to become infected.

5.2 Pharmacokinetic properties

Percutaneous penetration of clobetasol propionate varies among individuals and can be increased by the use of occlusive dressings, or when the skin is inflamed or diseased.

Mean peak plasma clobetasol propionate concentrations of 0.63ng/ml occurred in one study 8 hours after the second application (13 hours after an initial application) of 30g clobetasol propionate 0.05% ointment to normal individuals with healthy skin. Following the application of a second dose of 30g of clobetasol propionate cream 0.05% mean peak plasma concentrations were slightly higher than the ointment and occurred 10 hours after application.

In a separate study, mean peak plasma concentrations of approximately 2.3ng/ml and 4.6ng/ml occurred respectively in patients with psoriasis and eczema 3 hours after a single application of 25g clobetasol propionate 0.05% ointment. However, systemic metabolism of clobetasol has never been fully characterised or quantified. Following percutaneous absorption of clobetasol propionate the drug probably follows the metabolic pathway of systemically administered corticosteroids, i.e. metabolised primarily by the liver and then excreted by the kidneys.

5.3 Preclinical safety data

There are no preclinical data of relevance to the prescriber which are additional to that in other sections of the SmPC.

6. PHARMACEUTICAL PARTICULARS

6.1 List of excipients

Titanium dioxide (E171)

Liquid paraffin

Soft white paraffin

6.2 Incompatibilities

None known.

6.3 Shelf life

36 months.

6.4 Special precautions for storage

Store below 25°C.

6.5 Nature and contents of container

Collapsible aluminum tube, with a polypropylene cap.

Pack sizes: 25g or 30g.

6.6 Instructions for use and handling

Do not dilute.

Administrative Data

7. MARKETING AUTHORISATION HOLDER

Glaxo Wellcome UK Ltd

trading style GlaxoSmithKline UK

Stockley Park West

Uxbridge

Middlesex

UB11 1BT

8. MARKETING AUTHORISATION NUMBER(S)

PL 10949/0027

9. DATE OF FIRST AUTHORISATION/RENEWAL OF THE AUTHORISATION

31 August 1994/19 November 1999

10. DATE OF REVISION OF THE TEXT

29 January 2003

11. Legal Status

POM

Dermovate Ointment

(GlaxoSmithKline UK)

1. NAME OF THE MEDICINAL PRODUCT

Dermovate Ointment

2. QUALITATIVE AND QUANTITATIVE COMPOSITION

Clobetasol 17-propionate 0.05375% w/w

3. PHARMACEUTICAL FORM

Ointment

4. CLINICAL PARTICULARS

4.1 Therapeutic indications

Clobetasol propionate is a very active topical corticosteroid which is of particular value when used in short courses for the treatment of more resistant dermatoses such as psoriasis (excluding widespread plaque psoriasis), recalcitrant eczemas, lichen planus, discoid lupus erythematosus, and other conditions which do not respond satisfactorily to less active steroids.

4.2 Posology and method of administration

Apply sparingly to the affected area once or twice daily until improvement occurs. As with other highly active topical steroid preparations, therapy should be discontinued when control is achieved. In the more responsive conditions this may be within a few days.

If no improvement is seen within two to four weeks, reassessment of the diagnosis, or referral, may be necessary.

Repeated short courses of Dermovate may be used to control exacerbations. If continuous steroid treatment is necessary, a less potent preparation should be used.

In very resistant lesions, especially where there is hyperkeratosis, the anti-inflammatory effect of Dermovate can be enhanced, if necessary, by occluding the treatment area with polythene film. Overnight occlusion only is usually adequate to bring about a satisfactory response. Thereafter improvement can usually be maintained by application without occlusion.

For topical administration.

4.3 Contraindications

Rosacea.

Acne vulgaris.

Perioral dermatitis.

Perianal and genital pruritus.

Primary cutaneous viral infections (e.g. herpes simplex, chickenpox).

Hypersensitivity to the preparation.

The use of Dermovate skin preparations is not indicated in the treatment of primary infected skin lesions caused by infection with fungi (e.g. candidiasis, tinea), or bacteria (e.g. impetigo); or dermatoses in children under one year of age, including dermatitis and napkin eruptions.

4.4 Special warnings and special precautions for use

Long term continuous topical therapy should be avoided where possible, particularly in infants and children, as adrenal suppression can occur readily even without occlusion. If Dermovate is required for use in children, it is recommended that the treatment should be reviewed weekly. It should be noted that the infant's napkin may act as an occlusive dressing.

If used in childhood or on the face, courses should be limited if possible to five days and occlusion should not be used.

The face, more than other areas of the body, may exhibit atrophic changes after prolonged treatment with potent topical corticosteroids. This must be borne in mind when treating such conditions as psoriasis, discoid lupus erythematosus and severe eczema.

If applied to the eyelids, care is needed to ensure that the preparation does not enter the eye, as glaucoma might result. If Dermovate Ointment does enter the eye, the affected eye should be bathed in copious amounts of water.

Topical corticosteroids may be hazardous in psoriasis for a number of reasons including rebound relapses, development of tolerance, risk of generalised pustular psoriasis and development of local or systemic toxicity due to impaired barrier function of the skin. If used in psoriasis careful patient supervision is important.

Appropriate antimicrobial therapy should be used whenever treating inflammatory lesions which have become infected. Any spread of infection requires withdrawal of topical corticosteroid therapy and systemic administration of antimicrobial agents. Bacterial infection is encouraged by the warm, moist conditions induced by occlusive dressings, and so the skin should be cleansed before a fresh dressing is applied.

4.5 Interaction with other medicinal products and other forms of Interaction

None reported.

4.6 Pregnancy and lactation

There is inadequate evidence of safety in human pregnancy. Topical administration of corticosteroids to pregnant animals can cause abnormalities of fetal development including cleft palate and intrauterine growth retardation. The relevance of this finding to humans has not been established, therefore, topical steroids should not be used extensively in pregnancy, i.e. in large amounts or for prolonged periods.

The safe use of clobetasol propionate during lactation has not been established.

4.7 Effects on ability to drive and use machines

Clobetasol propionate is not expected to have any effects.

4.8 Undesirable effects

As with other topical corticosteroids, prolonged use of large amounts, or treatment of extensive areas can result in sufficient systemic absorption to produce the features of hypercortisolism. This effect is more likely to occur in infants and children, and if occlusive dressings are used. In infants, the napkin may act as an occlusive dressing.

Provided the weekly dosage is less than 50g in adults, any suppression of the HPA axis is likely to be transient with a rapid return to normal values once the short course of steroid therapy has ceased. The same applies to children given proportionate dosage.

Prolonged and intensive treatment with a highly active corticosteroid preparation may cause local atrophic changes in the skin such as thinning, striae, and dilatation of the superficial blood vessels, particularly when occlusive dressings are used or when skin folds are involved.

There are reports of pigmentation changes and hypertrichosis with topical steroids.

In rare instances, treatment of psoriasis with corticosteroids (or its withdrawal) is thought to have provoked the pustular form of the disease (see Special warnings and special precautions for use).

Dermovate is usually well tolerated, but if signs of hypersensitivity appear, application should be stopped immediately.

Exacerbation of symptoms may occur.

4.9 Overdose

Acute overdosage is very unlikely to occur, however, in the case of chronic overdosage or misuse, the features of hypercortisolism may appear and in this situation topical steroids should be discontinued gradually. However, because of the risk of acute adrenal suppression this should be done under medical supervision.

5. PHARMACOLOGICAL PROPERTIES

5.1 Pharmacodynamic properties

Clobetasol propionate is a highly active corticosteroid with topical anti-inflammatory activity. The major effect of clobetasol propionate on skin is a non-specific anti-inflammatory response, partially due to vasoconstriction and decrease in collagen synthesis.

5.2 Pharmacokinetic properties

Percutaneous penetration of clobetasol propionate varies among individuals and can be increased by the use of occlusive dressings, or when the skin is inflamed or diseased.

Mean peak plasma clobetasol propionate concentrations of 0.63 ng/ml occurred in one study eight hours after the second application (13 hours after an initial application) of 30 g clobetasol propionate 0.05% ointment to normal individuals with healthy skin. Following the application of a second dose of 30 g clobetasol propionate cream 0.05% mean peak plasma concentrations were slightly higher than the ointment and occurred 10 hours after application.

In a separate study, mean peak plasma concentrations of approximately 2.3 ng/ml and 4.6 ng/ml occurred respectively in patients with psoriasis and eczema three hours after a single application of 25 g clobetasol propionate 0.05% ointment.

Following percutaneous absorption of clobetasol propionate, the drug probably follows the metabolic pathway of systemically administered corticosteroids, i.e. metabolised primarily by the liver and then excreted by the kidneys. However, systemic metabolism of clobetasol has never been fully characterised or quantified.

5.3 Preclinical safety data

There are no preclinical data of relevance to the prescriber which are additional to that in other sections of the SmPC.

6. PHARMACEUTICAL PARTICULARS

6.1 List of excipients

Propylene glycol

Sorbitan sesquioleate

White soft paraffin

6.2 Incompatibilities

None known.

6.3 Shelf life
24 months.

6.4 Special precautions for storage
Store below 30°C.

6.5 Nature and contents of container
Collapsible tubes either internally coated with epoxy resin based lacquer or uncoated with wadless polypropylene caps.

Pack sizes: 25 g, 30 g or 100 g.

Not all pack sizes may be marketed

6.6 Instructions for use and handling
No special instructions.

Administrative Data

7. MARKETING AUTHORISATION HOLDER
Glaxo Wellcome UK Ltd
trading as Glaxo Laboratories
Stockley Park West
Uxbridge
Middlesex
UB11 1BT

8. MARKETING AUTHORISATION NUMBER(S)
PL 10949/0028

9. DATE OF FIRST AUTHORISATION/RENEWAL OF THE AUTHORISATION
August 04

10. DATE OF REVISION OF THE TEXT
August 04

Dermovate Scalp Application

(GlaxoSmithKline UK)

1. NAME OF THE MEDICINAL PRODUCT
Dermovate Scalp Application

2. QUALITATIVE AND QUANTITATIVE COMPOSITION
Clobetasol propionate 0.05 % w/w

3. PHARMACEUTICAL FORM
Scalp application

4. CLINICAL PARTICULARS

4.1 Therapeutic indications
Psoriasis and recalcitrant eczemas of the scalp.

Clobetasol propionate is a highly active topical corticosteroid which is indicated for use in short courses for conditions which do not respond satisfactorily to less active steroids.

4.2 Posology and method of administration
Route of administration: Topical, on the scalp.

Apply sparingly to the scalp night and morning until improvement occurs. As with other highly active topical steroid preparations, therapy should be discontinued when control is achieved. Repeated short courses of Dermovate Scalp Application may be used to control exacerbations. If continuous steroid treatment is necessary, a less potent preparation should be used.

These recommendations apply to both children and adults, including the elderly.

4.3 Contraindications
Infections of the scalp.

Hypersensitivity to the preparation.

Dermatoses in children under one year of age, including dermatitis.

4.4 Special warnings and special precautions for use
Care must be taken to keep the preparation away from the eyes. Do not use near a naked flame.

Long-term continuous topical therapy should be avoided, particularly in infants and children, as adrenal suppression can occur readily even without occlusion.

Development of secondary infection requires withdrawal of topical corticosteroid therapy and commencement of appropriate systemic antimicrobial therapy.

Topical corticosteroids may be hazardous in psoriasis for a number of reasons, including rebound relapses, development of tolerance, risk of generalised pustular psoriasis and development of local or systemic toxicity due to impaired barrier function of the skin. If used in psoriasis careful patient supervision is important.

The least potent corticosteroid which will control the disease should be selected. The viscosity of the scalp application has been adjusted so that the preparation spreads easily without being too fluid. The specially designed bottle and nozzle allow easy application direct to the scalp through the hair.

4.5 Interaction with other medicinal products and other forms of Interaction
None known.

4.6 Pregnancy and lactation
There is inadequate evidence of safety in human pregnancy. Topical administration of corticosteroids to pregnant animals can cause abnormalities of foetal development, including cleft palate and intrauterine growth retardation. The relevance of this finding to human beings has not been established; therefore, topical steroids should not be used extensively in pregnancy, i.e. in large amounts or for prolonged periods.

The safe use of clobetasol propionate during lactation has not been established.

4.7 Effects on ability to drive and use machines
None known.

4.8 Undesirable effects
Dermovate preparations are usually well tolerated, but if signs of hypersensitivity appear, application should be stopped immediately.

As with other topical corticosteroids, prolonged use of large amounts or treatment of extensive areas can result in sufficient systemic absorption to produce the features of hypercortisolism and suppression of the HPA axis. These effects are more likely to occur in infants and children, and if occlusive dressings are used. Local atrophy may occur after prolonged treatment.

In rare instances, treatment of psoriasis with corticosteroids (or its withdrawal) is thought to have provoked the pustular form of the disease. See *Special Warnings and Precautions for Use.*

4.9 Overdose
Acute overdosage is very unlikely to occur, however, in the case of chronic overdosage or misuse, the features of hypercortisolism may appear and in this situation topical steroids should be discontinued gradually. However, because of the risk of acute adrenal suppression this should be done under medical supervision.

5. PHARMACOLOGICAL PROPERTIES

5.1 Pharmacodynamic properties
Clobetasol propionate is a highly active corticosteroid with topical anti-inflammatory activity. The major effect of clobetasol propionate on skin is a non-specific anti-inflammatory response partially due to vasoconstriction and decrease in collagen synthesis.

5.2 Pharmacokinetic properties
Percutaneous penetration of clobetasol propionate varies among individuals and can be increased by the use of occlusive dressings, or when the skin is inflamed or diseased.

Following percutaneous absorption of clobetasol propionate the drug follows the metabolic pathway of systemically administered corticosteroids, i.e. metabolised primarily by the liver and then excreted by the kidneys. However, systemic metabolism of clobetasol has never been fully characterised or quantified.

5.3 Preclinical safety data
There are no preclinical data of relevance to the prescriber which are additional to that in other sections of the SmPC.

6. PHARMACEUTICAL PARTICULARS

6.1 List of excipients
Carbomer
Isopropyl Alcohol
Sodium Hydroxide
Purified Water

6.2 Incompatibilities
None known.

6.3 Shelf life
24 months

6.4 Special precautions for storage
None.

6.5 Nature and contents of container
White opaque low density polyethylene squeeze bottle with a polyethylene nozzle and either a polystyrene or high density polyethylene cap

or

White High Density Polyethylene (HDPE) Hostalen GF4750 and Remafin white CEG 020 container with a polyethylene nozzle and either a polystyrene or polyethylene cap.

Pack size: 25ml, 30ml, 100ml.

6.6 Instructions for use and handling
For detailed instructions for use refer to the Patient Information Leaflet in every pack.

Do not use near a naked flame.

Administrative Data

7. MARKETING AUTHORISATION HOLDER
Glaxo Wellcome UK Ltd
trading as
GlaxoSmithKline UK
Stockley Park West
Uxbridge
Middlesex
UB11 1BT

8. MARKETING AUTHORISATION NUMBER(S)
PL 10949/0046

9. DATE OF FIRST AUTHORISATION/RENEWAL OF THE AUTHORISATION
1 April 1993/31 August 1994/10 November 1999

10. DATE OF REVISION OF THE TEXT
29 January 2003

11. Legal Status
POM

Deseril Tablets 1mg

(Alliance Pharmaceuticals)

1. NAME OF THE MEDICINAL PRODUCT
Deseril® tablets 1mg

2. QUALITATIVE AND QUANTITATIVE COMPOSITION
Methysergide maleate BP 1.33 mg.

3. PHARMACEUTICAL FORM
White, biconvex, sugar-coated tablet, branded DSL on one side.

4. CLINICAL PARTICULARS

4.1 Therapeutic indications
Prophylactic treatment of migraine with or without aura, and cluster headache and other vascular headaches in patients who, despite attempts at control, experience headaches of such severity or regularity that social or economic life is seriously disrupted. (Note: Deseril is not recommended for treatment of the acute attack).

Diarrhoea caused by carcinoid disease.

4.2 Posology and method of administration
Prophylactic treatment of headache: 1 or 2 tablets three times a day with meals. Treatment should start with one tablet at bedtime and dosage should then be increased gradually over about two weeks until effective levels are reached. The minimum effective dose should be used, often that which will prevent 75% of attacks rather than all headaches.

From the outset, patients should understand that regular clinical supervision and periodic withdrawal of treatment are essential so that adverse effects can be recognised and minimised (see Section 4.4 Special warnings and precautions for use).

Carcinoid Syndrome: High doses are usually necessary. In most reported cases, dosage ranged between 12 and 20 tablets daily.

Children: Not recommended.

Elderly: No evidence exists that elderly patients require different dosage from younger patients.

4.3 Contraindications
Hypersensitivity to methysergide or any of the excipients of Deseril, pregnancy, lactation, peripheral vascular disorders, progressive arteriosclerosis, severe hypertension, coronary heart disease, valvular heart disease, phlebitis or cellulitis of the lower extremities, history of drug – induced fibrotic disorders (e.g. retroperitoneal fibrosis), pulmonary disease, collagen disease, impaired kidney or liver function, disease of the urinary tract, cachectic or septic conditions.

4.4 Special warnings and special precautions for use
Continuous Deseril administration should not exceed six months without a drug-free interval of at least one month for re-assessment; dosage should be reduced gradually over two to three weeks to avoid rebound headaches. In patients undergoing treatment with Deseril the dose of ergotamine required to control acute attacks may have to be reduced.

Regular clinical supervision of patients treated with Deseril is essential. Particular attention should be paid to complaints of urinary dysfunction, pain in the loin, flank or chest, and pain, coldness or numbness in the limbs. Patients should be regularly examined for the presence of cardiac murmurs, vascular bruits, pleural or pericardial friction rubs and abdominal or flank masses or tenderness. Treatment with Deseril should be stopped should any of these symptoms or signs occur. Caution is also advised during drug administration to patients with a past history of peptic ulceration.

In carcinoid syndrome the risk of adverse reactions due to the higher dosage must be weighed against the therapeutic benefit.

4.5 Interaction with other medicinal products and other forms of Interaction
Concomitant use of Deseril and vasoconstrictors or vasopressors may result in enhanced vasoconstriction. Methysergide should not be administered within six hours of therapy with 5-HT_1 receptor agonists. In addition, use of 5-HT_1 receptor agonists should be avoided for at least 24 hours after the last methysergide dose.

The concomitant use of cytochrome P450 3A (CYP3A) inhibitors such as macrolide antibiotics (e.g. troleandomycin, erythromycin, clarithromycin), HIV protease or reverse transcriptase inhibitors (e.g. ritonavir, indinavir, nelfinavir, delavirdine), azole antifungals (e.g. ketoconazole, itraconazole) or cimetidine and Deseril must be avoided, since this can result in an elevated exposure to methysergide and ergot toxicity (vasospasm and ischemia of the extremities and other tissues). Ergot alkaloids have also been shown to be inhibitors of CYP3A. No pharmacokinetic interactions involving other cytochrome P450 isoenzymes are known.

4.6 Pregnancy and lactation
Deseril is contra-indicated during pregnancy. It is likely that methysergide is excreted in breast milk. Deseril is therefore contra-indicated for nursing mothers.

4.7 Effects on ability to drive and use machines
Patients should be warned of the potential hazards of driving or operating machinery if they experience side effects such as dizziness, drowsiness or disturbances in vision.

4.8 Undesirable effects
General: The most commonly reported side-effects are nausea, heartburn, abdominal discomfort, vomiting, dizziness, lassitude and drowsiness. These side-effects can often be minimised by taking Deseril with food. Tissue oedema, insomnia, leg cramps and weight gain have occurred, and skin eruptions or loss of scalp hair have occasionally been reported. Mental and behavioural disturbances have occurred in isolated instances.

Inflammatory fibrosis: Retroperitoneal fibrosis: Continuous long-term Deseril administration has been associated with the development of retroperitoneal fibrosis. This is very rare when continuous treatment has not exceeded 6 months. Retroperitoneal fibrosis usually presents with symptoms of urinary tract obstruction such as persistent loin or flank pain, oliguria, dysuria, increased blood nitrogen and vascular insufficiency of the lower limbs. Deseril must be withdrawn if retroperitoneal fibrosis develops; drug withdrawal is often associated with clinical improvement over a few days to several weeks.

Fibrosis in other areas: fibrotic processes involving lungs, pleura, heart valves and major vessels have been reported in a small number of patients. Presenting symptoms include chest pain, dyspnoea or pleural friction rub and pleural effusion. Cardiac murmurs or vascular bruits have also been reported. Appearance of these symptoms demands immediate withdrawal of Deseril. These fibrotic manifestations are often reversible although less readily so than retroperitoneal fibrosis.

Vascular: Vascular reactions, including arterial spasm, have been seen in some patients. The following have all been described; arterial spasm in a limb causing coldness, numbness, pain or intermittent claudication; renal artery spasm giving rise to transitory hypertension; mesenteric artery spasm causing abdominal pain; retinal artery spasm causing reversible loss of vision; coronary artery spasm causing angina and questionably resulting in myocardial infarction. Arterial spasm is rapidly reversible following drug withdrawal.

4.9 Overdose
Experience with cases of overdoses with Deseril is limited. Symptoms: headache, agitation, hyperactivity, nausea, vomiting, abdominal pain, mydriasis, tachycardia, cyanosis, peripheral vasospasm with diminished pulses and coldness of extremities.

Treatment: Treatment is essentially symptomatic and supportive. Administration of activated charcoal is recommended; in case of very recent intake, gastric lavage may be considered. For controlling hyperactivity, conventional sedative measures may be used. In the event of severe vasospastic reactions, i.v. administration of a peripheral vasodilator such as nitroprusside or phentolamine, local administration of warmth to the affected area and nursing care to prevent tissue damage are recommended. In the case of coronary constriction, appropriate treatment should be initiated.

5. PHARMACOLOGICAL PROPERTIES

5.1 Pharmacodynamic properties
Deseril is effective in the prevention of migraine chiefly on account of its marked 5–HT receptor antagonism, probably by inhibition of 5-HT_{2B} receptors (inhibition of pain-facilitating and permeability-increasing actions of 5-HT).

5.2 Pharmacokinetic properties
Methysergide is rapidly and well absorbed. The parent drug is metabolised in the liver mainly to methylergometrine. Unchanged parent drug and metabolites are excreted predominantly via the kidney; the elimination is biphasic, with a half-life of 2.7 hours for the α-phase and 10 hours for the β-phase. Protein binding is moderate (66%).

5.3 Preclinical safety data
There are no findings of relevance to the prescriber which are additional to those already included in other sections of the SmPC.

6. PHARMACEUTICAL PARTICULARS

6.1 List of excipients
Maleic acid, gelatin, stearic acid, talc, maize starch, lactose. The coating constituents are gum acacia, sugar, talc, titanium dioxide, silica, carnauba wax and printing ink (consisting of Shellac, black iron oxide, ethanol and isopropanol).

6.2 Incompatibilities
None.

6.3 Shelf life
5 years.

6.4 Special precautions for storage
None.

6.5 Nature and contents of container
Aluminium/PVdC blister strips of 60 tablets.

6.6 Instructions for use and handling
None.

Administrative Data

7. MARKETING AUTHORISATION HOLDER
Alliance Pharmaceuticals Ltd
Avonbridge House
Bath Road
Chippenham
Wiltshire
SN15 2BB

8. MARKETING AUTHORISATION NUMBER(S)
PL16853/0006

9. DATE OF FIRST AUTHORISATION/RENEWAL OF THE AUTHORISATION
25 June 1998

10. DATE OF REVISION OF THE TEXT
February 2003

11. Legal status
POM

Alliance, Alliance Pharmaceuticals and associated devices are registered Trademarks of Alliance Pharmaceuticals Ltd.

Desferal Vials, 500mg or 2g

(Novartis Pharmaceuticals UK Ltd)

1. NAME OF THE MEDICINAL PRODUCT
Desferal® Vials, 500mg or 2g.

2. QUALITATIVE AND QUANTITATIVE COMPOSITION
Each vial contains desferrioxamine mesilate 500mg or 2g.

3. PHARMACEUTICAL FORM
A sterile, lyophilised powder available in vials containing 500mg or 2g of desferrioxamine mesilate.

4. CLINICAL PARTICULARS

4.1 Therapeutic indications
Treatment for chronic iron overload, e.g.

- transfusional haemosiderosis in patients receiving regular transfusions e.g. thalassaemia major
- primary and secondary haemochromatosis in patients in whom concomitant disorders (e.g. severe anaemia, hypoproteinaemia, renal or cardiac failure) preclude phlebotomy.

Treatment for acute iron poisoning.

For the diagnosis of iron storage disease and certain anaemias.

Aluminium overload - In patients on maintenance dialysis for end stage renal failure where preventative measures (e.g. reverse osmosis) have failed and with proven aluminium-related bone disease and/or anaemia, dialysis encephalopathy; and for diagnosis of aluminium overload.

4.2 Posology and method of administration
Desferal may be administered parenterally.

For parenteral administration:

The drug should preferably be employed in the form of a 10% solution, e.g. 500 mg: by dissolving the contents of one 500mg vial in 5ml of water for injection or 2 g: by dissolving the contents of one 2 g vial in 20 ml of water for injection. When administered subcutaneously the needle should not be inserted too close to the dermis. The 10% Desferal solution can be diluted with routinely employed infusion solutions (saline, glucose, dextrose or dextrose-saline), although these should not be used as solvent for the dry substance. Dissolved Desferal can also be added to dialysis fluid and given intraperitoneally to patients on continuous ambulatory peritoneal dialysis (CAPD) or continuous cyclic peritoneal dialysis (CCPD).

Only clear pale yellow Desferal solutions should be used. Opaque, cloudy or discoloured solutions should be discarded. Heparin is pharmaceutically incompatible with Desferal solutions.

Treatment of acute iron poisoning

Adults and children:

Desferal may be administered parenterally. Desferal is an adjunct to standard measures generally used in treating acute iron poisoning. It is important to initiate treatment as soon as possible.

Parenteral Desferal treatment should be considered in any of the following situations:

- all symptomatic patients exhibiting more than transient minor symptoms (e.g. more than one episode of emesis or passage of one soft stool),
- patients with evidence of lethargy, significant abdominal pain, hypovolaemia, or acidosis,
- patients with positive abdominal radiograph results demonstrating multiple radio-opacities (the great majority of these patients will go on to develop symptomatic iron poisoning),
- any symptomatic patient with a serum iron level greater than 300 to 350 micro g/dL regardless of the total iron binding capacity (TIBC). It has also been suggested that a conservative approach without Desferal therapy or challenge should be considered when serum iron levels are in the 300 to 500 micro g/dL range in asymptomatic patients, as well as in those with self-limited, non-bloody emesis or diarrhoea without other symptoms.

The dosage and route of administration should be adapted to the severity of the poisoning.

Dosage:

The continuous intravenous administration of Desferal is the preferred route and the recommended rate for infusion is 15 mg/kg per hour and should be reduced as soon as the situation permits, usually after 4 to 6 hours so that the total intravenous dose does not exceed a recommended 80 mg/kg in any 24 hour period.

However, if the option to infuse intravenously is not available and if the intramuscular route is used the normal dosage is 2 g for an adult and 1g for a child, administered as a single intramuscular dose.

The decision to discontinue Desferal therapy must be a clinical decision; however, the following suggested criteria are believed to represent appropriate requirements for the cessation of Desferal. Chelation therapy should be continued until all of the following criteria are satisfied:

- the patient must be free of signs and symptoms of systemic iron poisoning (e.g. no acidosis, no worsening hepatoxicity),
- ideally, a corrected serum iron level should be normal or low (when iron level falls below 100 micro g/dL). Given that laboratories cannot measure serum iron concentrations accurately in the presence of Desferal, it is acceptable to discontinue Desferal when all other criteria are met if the measured serum iron concentration is not elevated.
- Repeat abdominal radiograph test should be obtained in patients who initially demonstrated multiple radio-opacities to ensure they have disappeared before Desferal is discontinued because they serve as a marker for continued iron absorption,
- If the patient initially developed vin-rose coloured urine with Desferal therapy, it seems reasonable that urine colour should return to normal before halting Desferal (absence of vin-rose urine is not sufficient by itself to indicate discontinuation of Desferal).

The effectiveness of treatment is dependent on an adequate urine output in order that the iron complex (ferrioxamine) is excreted from the body. Therefore if oliguria or anuria develop, peritoneal dialysis or haemodialysis may become necessary to remove ferrioxamine.

It should be noted that the serum iron level may rise sharply when the iron is released from the tissues.

Theoretically 100 mg Desferal can chelate 8.5 mg of ferric iron.

Chronic Iron Overload.

The main aim of therapy in younger patients is to achieve an iron balance and prevent haemosiderosis, whilst in the older patient a negative iron balance is desirable in order to slowly deplete the increased iron stores and to prevent the toxic effects of iron.

Adults and children:

Desferal therapy should be commenced after the first 10-20 blood transfusions, or when serum ferritin levels reach 1000 ng/mL, indicating saturation of the transferrin. The dose and mode of administration should be individually adapted according to the degree of iron overload.

Growth retardation may result from iron overload or excessive Desferal doses. If chelation is started before 3 years of age growth must be monitored carefully and the mean daily dose should not exceed 40mg/kg. (see section 4.4 **Special warnings and precautions for use**).

Dose:

The lowest effective dose should be used. The average daily dose will probably lie between 20 and 60 mg/kg/day. Patients with serum ferritin levels of < 2000 ng/mL should require about 25 mg/kg/day, and those with levels between 2000 and 3000 ng/mL about 35 mg/kg/day. Higher doses should only be employed if the benefit for the patient outweighs the risk of unwanted effects.

Patients with higher serum ferritin may require up to 55 mg/kg/day. It is inadvisable regularly to exceed an average daily dose of 50 mg/kg/day except when very intensive chelation is needed in patients who have completed growth. If ferritin values fall below 1000 ng/mL, the risk of Desferal toxicity increases; it is important to monitor these patients particularly carefully and perhaps to consider lowering the total weekly dose.

To assess the chelation therapy, 24 hour urinary iron excretion should initially be monitored daily. Starting with a dose of 500 mg daily the dose should be raised until a plateau of iron excretion is reached. Once the appropriate dose has been established, urinary iron excretion rates can be assessed at intervals of a few weeks.

Alternatively the mean daily dose may be adjusted according to the ferritin value to keep the therapeutic index less than 0.025 (i.e. mean daily dose (mg/kg) of Desferal divided by the serum ferritin level (micro g/L) below 0.025).

Mode of administration:

Slow subcutaneous infusion by means of a portable, lightweight, infusion pump over a period of 8-12 hours is effective and particularly convenient for ambulant patients. It may be possible to achieve a further increase in iron excretion by infusing the same daily dose over a 24 hour period. Patients should be treated 5-7 times a week depending on the degree of iron overload.

Since the subcutaneous infusions are more effective, intramuscular injections are given only when subcutaneous infusions are not feasible.

Desferal can be administered by intravenous infusion during blood transfusion.

The Desferal solution should not be put directly into the blood bag but may be added to the blood line by means of a "Y" adaptor located near to the venous site of injection. The patient's pump should be used to administer Desferal as usual. Patients and nurses should be warned against accelerating the infusion, as an intravenous bolus of Desferal may lead to flushing, hypotension and acute collapse (see section 4.4 **Special warnings and special precautions for use**).

Continuous intravenous infusion is recommended for patients incapable of continuing subcutaneous infusions and in those who have cardiac problems secondary to iron overload. 24 hour urinary iron excretion should be measured regularly where intensive chelation (i.v.) is required, and the dose adjusted accordingly. Implanted intravenous systems can be used when intensive chelation is carried out.

Care should be taken when flushing the line to avoid the sudden infusion of residual Desferal which may be present in the dead space of the line, as this may lead to flushing; hypotension and acute collapse (see section 4.4 **Special warnings and special precautions for use**).

Diagnosis of iron storage disease and certain anaemias

The Desferal test for iron overload is based on the principle that normal subjects do not excrete more than a fraction of a milligram of iron in their urine daily, and that a standard intramuscular injection of 500 mg of Desferal will not increase this above 1 mg (18 micro mol). In iron storage diseases, however, the increase may be well over 1.5 mg (27 micro mol). It should be borne in mind that the test only yields reliable results when renal function is normal.

Desferal is administered as 500 mg intramuscular injection. Urine is then collected for a period of 6 hours and its iron content determined.

Excretion of 1-1.5 mg (18-27 micro mol) of iron during this 6-hour period is suggestive of iron overload; values greater than 1.5 mg (27 micro mol) can be regarded as pathological.

Treatment for aluminium overload in patients with end stage renal failure

Patients should receive Desferal if:

- they have symptoms or evidence of organ impairment due to aluminium overload

- they are asymptomatic but their serum aluminium levels are consistently above 60 ng/mL and associated with a positive Desferal test (see below), particularly if a bone biopsy provides evidence of aluminium related bone disease.

The iron and aluminium complexes of Desferal are dialysable. In patients with renal failure their elimination will be increased by dialysis.

Adults and children:

Patients on maintenance haemodialysis or haemofiltration: 5 mg/kg once a week. Patients with post-desferrioxamine test serum aluminium levels up to 300 ng/mL: Desferal should be given as a slow i.v. infusion during the last 60 minutes of a dialysis session (to reduce loss of free drug in the dialysate). Patients with a post-desferrioxamine test serum aluminium value above 300 ng/ml: Desferal should be administered by slow i.v. infusion 5 hours prior to the dialysis session.

Four weeks after the completion of a three month course of Desferal treatment a Desferal infusion test should be performed, followed by a second test 1 month later. Serum aluminium increases of less than 50ng/mL above baseline measured in 2 successive infusion tests indicate that further Desferal treatment is not necessary.

Patients on CAPD or CCPD:

5 mg/kg once a week prior to the final exchange of the day. It is recommended that the intraperitoneal route be used in these patients. However, Desferal can also be given i.m., by slow infusion i.v. or s.c.

Diagnosis of aluminium overload in patients with end stage renal failure

A Desferal infusion test is recommended in patients with serum aluminium levels > 60ng/mL associated with serum ferritin levels >100 ng/mL.

Just before starting the haemodialysis session, a blood sample is taken to determine the baseline level serum aluminium level.

During the last 60 minutes of the haemodialysis session a 5mg/kg dose is given as a slow intravenous infusion.

At the start of the next haemodialysis session (i.e. 44 hours after the aforementioned Desferal infusion) the second blood sample is taken to determine the serum aluminium level once more.

An increase in serum aluminium above baseline of more than 150 ng/mL is suggestive of aluminium overload. It should be noted that a negative test does not completely exclude the possibility of aluminium overload.

Theoretically 100 mg Desferal can bind 4.1 mg Al^{+++}.

Use in the elderly

No special dosage regime is necessary but concurrent renal insufficiency should be taken into account.

4.3 Contraindications

Hypersensitivity to desferrioxamine mesilate unless the patients can be desensitised.

4.4 Special warnings and special precautions for use

Desferal should be used with caution in patients with renal impairment since the metal complexes are excreted via the kidneys. In these patients, dialysis will increase the elimination of chelated iron and aluminium.

Used alone Desferal may exacerbate neurological impairment in patients with aluminium-related encelphalopathy. This deterioration (manifest as seizures) is probably related to an acute increase in brain aluminium secondary to elevated circulating levels. Pretreatment with clonazepam has been shown to afford protection against such impairment. Also, treatment of aluminium overload may result in decreased serum calcium and aggravation of hyperparathyroidism.

Treatment with Desferal by the intravenous route should only be administered in the form of slow infusions. Rapid intravenous infusion may lead to hypotension and shock (e.g. flushing, tachycardia, collapse and urticaria).

Desferal should not be administered s.c. in concentrations and/or doses higher than those recommended as local irritation at the site of administration may occur more frequently.

Patients suffering from iron overload are particularly susceptible to infection. There have been reports of Desferal promoting some infections such as *Yersinia enterocolitica* and *Y. pseudotuberculosis*. If patients develop fever with pharyngitis, diffuse abdominal pain or enteritis/enterocolitis, Desferal therapy should be stopped, and appropriate treatment with antibiotics should be instituted. Desferal therapy may be resumed once the infection has cleared.

In patients, receiving Desferal for aluminium and/or iron overload there have been rare reports of mucormycosis (a severe fungal infection), some with fatal outcome. If any characteristic signs or symptoms occur Desferal treatment should be discontinued, mycological tests carried out and appropriate treatment immediately instituted. Mucormycosis has been reported to occur in dialysis patients not receiving Desferal, thus no causal link with the use of the drug has been established.

Disturbances of vision and hearing have been reported during prolonged Desferal therapy. In particular, this has occurred in patients on higher than recommended therapy or in patients with low serum ferritin levels. Patients with renal failure who are receiving maintenance dialysis and have low ferritin levels may be particularly prone to adverse reactions, visual symptoms having been reported after single doses of Desferal. Therefore, ophthalmological and audiological tests should be carried out both prior to the institution of long-term therapy with Desferal and at 3-monthly intervals during treatment. By keeping the ratio of the mean daily dose (mg/kg of Desferal) divided by the serum ferritin (micro g/L) below 0.025 the risk of audiometric abnormalities may be reduced in thalassaemia patients. A detailed ophthalmological assessment is recommended (visual field measurements, fundoscopy, and colour vision testing using pseudoisochromatic plates and the Farnsworth D-15 colour test, slit lamp investigation, visual evoked potential studies).

If disturbances of vision or hearing do occur, treatment with Desferal should be stopped. Such disturbances are usually reversible. If Desferal therapy is re-instituted later at a lower dosage, close monitoring of ophthalmological/auditory function should be carried out with due regard to the risk-benefit ratio.

The use of inappropriately high doses of Desferal in patients with low ferritin levels or young children (<3 years at commencement of treatment) has also been associated with growth retardation; dose reduction has been found to restore the growth rate to pretreatment levels in some cases. Three monthly checks on body weight and height are recommended in children.

Growth retardation if associated with excessive doses of Desferal must be distinguished from growth retardation from iron overload. Growth retardation from Desferal use is rare if the dose is kept below 40 mg/kg; if growth retardation has been associated with doses above this value, then reduction of the dose may result in return in growth velocity, however, predicted adult height is not attained.

Acute respiratory distress syndrome has been described following treatment with excessively high i.v. doses of Desferal in patients with acute iron intoxication, and also in thalassaemic patients (see section 4.8 Undesirable effects). The recommended daily doses should therefore not be exceeded.

It should be noted that desferrioxamine will affect aluminium levels and may necessitate some dosage adjustment of erythropoietin if co-prescribed.

4.5 Interaction with other medicinal products and other forms of Interaction

Oral administration of vitamin C (up to a maximum of 200 mg daily, given in divided doses) may serve to enhance excretion of the iron complex in response to Desferal; larger doses of vitamin C fail to produce an additional effect. Monitoring of cardiac function is indicated during such combined therapy. Vitamin C should be given only if the patient is receiving Desferal regularly and should not be administered within the first month of Desferal therapy. In patients with severe chronic iron-storage disease undergoing combined treatment with Desferal and high doses of vitamin C (more than 500 mg daily) impairment of cardiac function has been encountered; this proved reversible when the vitamin C was withdrawn. Vitamin C supplements should not, therefore, be given to patients with cardiac failure.

Desferal should not be used in combination with prochlorperazine (a phenothiazine derivative) since prolonged unconsciousness may result.

Gallium^{67} imaging results may be distorted because of the rapid urinary excretion of Desferal-bound radiolabel. Discontinuation of Desferal 48 hours prior to scintigraphy is advised.

4.6 Pregnancy and lactation

Desferal has caused teratogenic effects in animals when given during pregnancy, particularly in the first trimester.

In rabbits, desferrioxamine caused skeletal malformations. However, these teratogenic effects in the foetuses were observed at doses which were toxic to the mother. In mice and rats desferrioxamine appears to be free of teratogenic activity.

Malformations have not occurred in children born to patients reported to have received Desferal during pregnancy.

It is not known whether Desferal is excreted into the breast milk.

Desferal should not be given to pregnant or lactating women, unless, in the judgement of the physician, the expected benefits to the mother outweigh the potential risk to the child. This particularly applies to the first trimester.

4.7 Effects on ability to drive and use machines

Patients experiencing CNS effects such as dizziness or impaired vision or hearing should be warned against driving or operating machinery.

4.8 Undesirable effects

Frequency estimate: very common ⩾ 10%, common ⩾ 1% to < 10%; uncommon ⩾ 0.1% to < 1%; rare ⩾ 0.01% to < 0.1%; very rare < 0.01%.

Some signs and symptoms reported as adverse effects may also be manifestations of the underlying disease (iron and/or aluminium overload).

Local reactions/associated systemic reactions

At the injection site pain, swelling, induration, erythema, pruritus and eschar/crust are very common; vesicles, local oedema and burning are uncommon reactions. The local manifestations may be accompanied by systemic reactions like arthralgia/myalgia (very common), headache (common), urticaria (common), nausea (common), fever (common), vomiting (uncommon), or abdominal pain (uncommon) or asthma (uncommon).

Allergy

Very rare: analphylactic/anaphylactoid reactions with or without shock, angioedema.

Special senses:

High frequency sensorineural hearing loss and tinnitus are uncommon if doses are kept within guidelines and if doses are reduced when ferritin levels fall (ratio of the mean daily dose of Desferal divided by the serum ferritin should be below 0.025): blurred vision, decreased visual acuity, loss of vision, impairment of colour vision (dyschromatopsia), night blindness (nyctalopia), visual field defects, scotoma, retinopathy (pigmentary degeneration of the retina), optic neuritis, cataracts (lens opacities), corneal opacities are rare, except if high doses are given (see 4.4 **Special warnings and precautions** for use).

Skin

Very rare: generalised rash.

Musco-Skeletal system

Growth retardation and bone changes (e.g. metaphyseal dysplasia) are common in chelated patients given doses of 60 mg/kg, especially those who begin iron chelation in the first three years of life. If doses are kept to 40 mg/kg or below, the risk is considerably reduced.

Pulmonary system

Very rare: acute respiratory distress syndrome (with dyspnoea, cyanosis, and interstitial pulmonary infiltrates) (see 4.4 Special warnings and special precautions for use).

Central nervous system

Very rare: neurological disturbances, dizziness, precipitation or exacerbation of aluminium-related dialysis encephalopathy, peripheral sensory, motor or mixed neuropathy, paraesthesia (see 4.4 **Special warnings and precautions** for use).

Gastrointestinal system

Very rare: Diarrhoea.

Renal system

Very rare: impaired renal function (see 4.4 **Special warnings and precautions** for use).

Cardiovascular system

Hypotension may occur if the recommended precautions for the administration of Desferal are not followed (see 4.2 **Posology and method of administration** and 4.4 **Special warnings and precautions** for use).

Haematological system

Very rare: blood dyscrasias (e.g. thrombocytopenia).

Susceptibility to infections

In very rare cases *Yersinia* and *Mucormycosis* infections have been reported in association with Desferal treatment (see 4.4 **Special warnings and precautions** for use).

4.9 Overdose

Desferal is usually administered parenterally and acute poisoning is unlikely to occur.

Signs and symptoms: tachycardia, hypotension and gastro-intestinal symptoms have occasionally occurred in patients who received an overdose of Desferal. Accidental administration of Desferal by the i.v. route may be associated with acute but transient loss of vision, aphasia, agitation, headache, nausea, bradycardia, hypotension and acute renal failure.

Treatment: there is no specific antidote to Desferal but signs and symptoms may be eliminated by reducing the dosage and Desferal is dialysable. Appropriate supportive therapy should be instituted.

5. PHARMACOLOGICAL PROPERTIES

5.1 Pharmacodynamic properties

Chelating agent (ATC code: V03AC01)

Desferal is a chelating agent for trivalent iron and aluminium ions; the resulting chelates (ferrioxamine and aluminoxamine) are stable and non-toxic. Neither chelate undergoes intestinal absorption, and any formed systemically as a result of parenteral administration is rapidly excreted via the kidneys without deleterious effects. Desferal takes up iron either free or bound to ferritin and haemosiderin. Similarly it mobilises and chelates tissue bound aluminium. It does not remove iron from haemin containing substances including haemoglobin and transferrin. Since both ferrioxamine and aluminoxamine are completely excreted, Desferal promotes the excretion of iron and aluminium in urine and faeces, thus reducing pathological iron or aluminium deposits in the organs and tissues.

5.2 Pharmacokinetic properties

Absorption

Desferrioxamine is rapidly absorbed after intramuscular bolus injection or slow subcutaneous infusion, but only poorly absorbed from the gastrointestinal tract in the presence of intact mucosa.

During peritoneal dialysis desferrioxamine is absorbed if administered in the dialysis fluid.

Distribution

In healthy volunteers peak plasma concentrations of desferrioxamine (15.5 micro mol/L (87 micro g/mL)) were measured 30 minutes after an intramuscular injection of 10 mg/kg desferrioxamine. One hour after injection the peak concentration of ferrioxamine was 3.7 micro mol/L (2.3 micro g/mL). Less than 10% of desferrioxamine is bound to serum proteins in vitro.

Biotransformation

Four metabolites of desferrioxamine were isolated from urine of patients with iron overload. The following biotransformation reactions were found to occur with desferrioxamine: transamination and oxidation yielding an acid metabolite, beta-oxidation also yielding an acid metabolite, decarboxylation and N-hydroxylation yielding neutral metabolites.

Elimination

Both desferrioxamine and ferrioxamine a biphasic elimination after intramuscular injection in healthy volunteers; for desferrioxamine the apparent distribution half-life is 1 hour, and for ferrioxamine 2.4 hours. The apparent terminal half-life is 6 hours for both. Within six hours of injection, 22% of the dose appears in the urine as desferrioxamine and 1% as ferrioxamine.

Characteristics in patients

In patients with haemochromatosis peak plasma levels of 7.0 micro mol/L (3.9 micro g/mL) were measured for desferrioxamine, and 15.7 micro mol/L (9.6 micro g/mL) for ferrioxamine, 1 hour after an intramuscular injection of 10 mg/kg desferrioxamine. These patients eliminated desferrioxamine and ferrioxamine with half-lives of 5.6 and 4.6 hours respectively. Six hours after the injection 17% of the dose was excreted in the urine as desferrioxamine and 12% as ferrioxamine.

In patients dialysed for renal failure who received 40 mg/kg desferrioxamine infused i.v. within 1 hour, the plasma concentration at the end of the infusion was 152 micro mol/L (85.2 micro g/mL) when the infusion was given between dialysis sessions. Plasma concentrations of desferrioxamine were between 13% and 27% lower when the infusion was administered during dialysis. Concentrations of ferrioxamine were in all cases approximately 7.0 micro mol/L (4.3 micro g/mL) with concomitant aluminoxamine levels of 2-3 micro mol/litre (1.2-1.8 micro g/mL). After the infusion was discontinued, the plasma concentrations of desferrioxamine decreased rapidly with a half-life of 20 minutes. A smaller fraction of the dose was eliminated with a longer half-life of 14 hours. Plasma concentrations of aluminoxamine continued to increase for up to 48 hours post-infusion and reached values of approximately 7 micro mol/L (4 micro g/mL). Following dialysis the plasma concentration of aluminoxamine fell to 2.2 micro mol/L (1.3 micro g/mL), indicating that the aluminoxamine complex is dialysable.

In patients with thalassaemia continuous intravenous infusion of 50mg/kg/24h of desferrioxamine resulted in plasma steady state levels of desferrioxamine of 7.4 micro mol/L. Elimination of desferrioxamine from plasma was biphasic with a mean distribution half-life of 0.28 hours and an apparent terminal half-life of 3.0 hours. The total plasma clearance was 0.5 L/h/kg and the volume of distribution at steady state was estimated at 1.35 L/kg. Exposure to the main iron binding metabolite was around 54% of that of desferrioxamine in terms of AUC. The apparent monoexponential elimination half-life of the metabolite was 1.3 hours.

5.3 Preclinical safety data

There are no preclinical data of relevance to the prescriber which are additional to that already included in other sections of the Summary of Product Characteristics.

6. PHARMACEUTICAL PARTICULARS

6.1 List of excipients

None present.

6.2 Incompatibilities

None known.

6.3 Shelf life

48 months.

6.4 Special precautions for storage

Vial: Store below 25°C.

Reconstituted solution: Single use only.

From a microbiological point of view, the product should be used immediately after reconstitution (commencement of treatment within 3 hours). When the reconstitution is carried out under validated aseptic conditions the reconstituted solution may be stored for a maximum of 24 hours at room temperature (25°C or below) before administration. If not used immediately, in-use storage times and conditions prior to administration are the responsibility of the user. Unused solution should be discarded.

6.5 Nature and contents of container

Each vial contains a white to practically white lyophilisate supplied in a clear glass vial in a pack size of 10 (500 mg) or 1 (2 g).

6.6 Instructions for use and handling

None stated.

7. MARKETING AUTHORISATION HOLDER

Novartis Pharmaceuticals UK Limited
Trading as Ciba Laboratories
Frimley Business Park
Frimley
Camberley
Surrey
GU16 7SR

8. MARKETING AUTHORISATION NUMBER(S)

PL 00101/0523.

9. DATE OF FIRST AUTHORISATION/RENEWAL OF THE AUTHORISATION

31 October 1997 / 12 December 2000

10. DATE OF REVISION OF THE TEXT

25 February 2004

LEGAL CATEGORY:

POM

Desmospray, Desmopressin Nasal Spray

(Ferring Pharmaceuticals Ltd)

1. NAME OF THE MEDICINAL PRODUCT

DESMOSPRAY®, Desmopressin Nasal Spray.

2. QUALITATIVE AND QUANTITATIVE COMPOSITION

Desmospray® contains 10 micrograms of Desmopressin acetate per actuation.

3. PHARMACEUTICAL FORM

Nasal spray.

4. CLINICAL PARTICULARS

4.1 Therapeutic indications

Desmospray® is indicated for:

i) The treatment of primary nocturnal enuresis

ii) The treatment of nocturia associated with multiple sclerosis where other treatments have failed.

iii) The diagnosis and treatment of vasopressin-sensitive cranial diabetes insipidus.

iv) Establishing renal concentration capacity.

4.2 Posology and method of administration

Primary Nocturnal Enuresis:

The starting dose for children (from 5 years of age) and adults (up to 65 years of age) with normal urine concentrating ability who have primary nocturnal enuresis is one spray (10 micrograms) into each nostril (a total of 20 micrograms) at bedtime and only if needed should the dose be increased up to two sprays (20 micrograms) into each nostril (a total of 40 micrograms).

The need for continued treatment should be reassessed after 3 months by means of a period of at least 1 week without Desmospray®.

Treatment of Nocturia:

For multiple sclerosis patients up to 65 years of age with normal renal function suffering from nocturia the dose is one or two sprays intranasally (10 to 20 micrograms) at bedtime. Not more than one dose should be used in any 24 hour period. If a dose of two sprays is required, this should be as one spray into each nostril.

Treatment of Diabetes Insipidus:

Dosage is individual but clinical experience has shown that the average maintenance dose in adults and children is one or two sprays (10 to 20 micrograms) once or twice daily. If a dose of two sprays is required, this should be as one spray into each nostril.

Diagnosis of Diabetes Insipidus:

The diagnostic dose in adults and children is two sprays (20 micrograms). Failure to elaborate a concentrated urine after water deprivation, followed by the ability to do so after the administration of Desmospray® confirms the diagnosis of cranial diabetes insipidus. Failure to concentrate after the administration suggests nephrogenic diabetes insipidus.

Renal Function Testing:

Recommended doses for the renal concentration capacity test:

Adults: Two sprays into each nostril (a total of 40 micrograms)

Children: (1-15 years): One spray into each nostril (a total of 20 micrograms).

Infants (to 1 year): One spray (10 micrograms).

Adults and children with normal renal function can be expected to achieve concentrations above 700mOsm/kg in the period of 5-9 hours following administration of Desmospray®. It is recommended that the bladder should be emptied at the time of administration.

In normal infants a urine concentration of 600mOsm/kg should be achieved in the 5 hour period following the administration of Desmospray®. The fluid intake at the two meals following the administration should be restricted to 50% of the ordinary intake in order to avoid water overload.

4.3 Contraindications

Desmospray® is contraindicated in cases of:

- cardiac insufficiency and other conditions requiring treatment with diuretic agents

- hypersensitivity to the preservative

When used to control primary nocturnal enuresis Desmospray® should only be used in patients with normal blood pressure.

Before prescribing Desmospray® the diagnoses of psychogenic polydipsia and alcohol abuse should be excluded.

When used to control nocturia in patients with multiple sclerosis, Desmopressin should not be used in patients with hypertension or cardiovascular disease.

Desmopressin should not be prescribed to patients over the age of 65 for the treatment of primary nocturnal enuresis or nocturia associated with multiple sclerosis.

4.4 Special warnings and special precautions for use

Care should be taken with patients who have reduced renal function and/or cardiovascular disease or cystic fibrosis.

Patients being treated for primary nocturnal enuresis should be warned to avoid ingesting water while swimming and to discontinue Desmospray® during an episode of vomiting and/or diarrhoea until their fluid balance is once again normal.

When Desmospray® is used for the treatment of enuresis or nocturia associated with multiple sclerosis, fluid intake must be limited from 1 hour before until 8 hours after administration.

When Desmospray® is used in the treatment of nocturia, periodic assessments should be made of blood pressure and weight to monitor the possibility of fluid overload.

When used for diagnostic purposes, fluid intake must be limited and not exceed 0.5 litres from 1 hour before until 8 hours after administration.

Following diagnostic testing for diabetes insipidus or renal concentration capacity, care should be taken to prevent fluid overload. Fluid should not be forced, orally or parenterally, and patients should only take as much fluid as they require to satisfy thirst.

Precautions to prevent fluid overload must be taken in:

- conditions characterised by fluid and/or electrolyte imbalance

- patients at risk for increased intracranial pressure

Renal concentration capacity testing in children below the age of 1 year should only be performed under carefully supervised conditions in hospital.

4.5 Interaction with other medicinal products and other forms of Interaction

Substances which are known to induce SIADH e.g. tricyclic antidepressants, selective serotonin re-uptake inhibitors, chlorpromazine and carbamazepine, may cause an additive antidiuretic effect leading to an increased risk of water retention and/or hyponatraemia.

NSAIDs may induce water retention and/or hyponatraemia.

4.6 Pregnancy and lactation

Pregnancy:

Data on a limited number (n=53) of exposed pregnancies in women with diabetes insipidus indicate rare cases of malformations in children treated during pregnancy. To date, no other relevant epidemiological data are available. Animal studies do not indicate direct or indirect harmful effects with respect to pregnancy, embryonal/fetal development, parturition or postnatal development.

Caution should be exercised when prescribing to pregnant women. Blood pressure monitoring is recommended due to the increased risk of pre-eclampsia.

Lactation:

Results from analyses of milk from nursing mothers receiving high dose Desmopressin (300 micrograms intranasally) indicate that the amounts of Desmopressin that may be transferred to the child are considerably less than the amounts required to influence diuresis.

4.7 Effects on ability to drive and use machines

None

4.8 Undesirable effects

Side-effects include headache, stomach pain, nausea, nasal congestion, rhinitis and epistaxis. Isolated cases of allergic skin reactions and more severe general allergic reactions have been reported. Very rare cases of emotional disturbances in children have been reported. Treatment with Desmopressin without concomitant reduction of fluid intake may lead to water retention/hyponatraemia with accompanying symptoms of headache, nausea, vomiting, weight gain, decreased serum sodium and in serious cases, convulsions.

4.9 Overdose

An overdose of Desmospray® leads to a prolonged duration of action with an increased risk of water retention and/or hyponatraemia.

Treatment:

Although the treatment of hyponatraemia should be individualised, the following general recommendations can be given. Hyponatraemia is treated by discontinuing the Desmopressin treatment, fluid restriction and symptomatic treatment if needed.

5. PHARMACOLOGICAL PROPERTIES

5.1 Pharmacodynamic properties

Desmopressin is a structural analogue of vasopressin, with two chemical changes, namely desamination of the N-terminal and replacement of the 8-L-Arginine by D-8-Arginine. These changes have increased the antidiuretic activity and prolonged the duration of action. The pressor activity is reduced to less than 0.01% of the natural peptide as a result of which side-effects are rarely seen.

5.2 Pharmacokinetic properties

Following intranasal administration, the bioavailability of Desmopressin is of the order of 10%.

Pharmacokinetic parameters following intravenous administration have been reported as follows:

Total clearance: 2.6 ml / min / kg body wt.

T ½: 55mins

Plasma kinetics of DDAVP in man

H Vilhardt, S Lundin, J Falch

Acta Pharmacol et Toxicol, 1986, 58, 379-381

In vitro, in human liver microsome preparations, it has been shown that no significant amount of Desmopressin is metabolised in the liver and thus human liver metabolism *in vivo* is not likely to occur.

It is unlikely that Desmopressin will interact with drugs affecting hepatic metabolism, since Desmopressin has been shown not to undergo significant liver metabolism in *in vitro* studies with human microsomes. However, formal *in vivo* interaction studies have not been performed.

5.3 Preclinical safety data

There are no pre-clinical data of relevance to the prescriber which are additional to that already included in other sections of the SPC.

6. PHARMACEUTICAL PARTICULARS

6.1 List of excipients

Sodium Chloride Ph. Eur.

Citric Acid Monohydrate Ph. Eur.

Disodium Phosphate Dihydrate Ph. Eur.

Benzalkonium Chloride Solution 50% Ph. Eur.

Purified Water Ph. Eur.

6.2 Incompatibilities

None known.

6.3 Shelf life

2 years.

6.4 Special precautions for storage

Store at room temperature (up to 25°C). Protect from light.

6.5 Nature and contents of container

The spray pack comprises of a 10ml amber glass injection vial fitted with a snap-on tamper-proof pre-compression pump spray device, to which a 20mm nasal adaptor is attached. It contains a clear, colourless solution of Desmopressin acetate 0.1mg/ml. The fill volume is 7.1ml including overage to allow delivery of 60 doses of 0.1 ml.

6.6 Instructions for use and handling

None

7. MARKETING AUTHORISATION HOLDER

Ferring Pharmaceuticals Limited, The Courtyard, Waterside Drive, Langley, Berkshire SL3 6EZ

8. MARKETING AUTHORISATION NUMBER(S)

PL 3194/0024

9. DATE OF FIRST AUTHORISATION/RENEWAL OF THE AUTHORISATION

30th April 1997

10. DATE OF REVISION OF THE TEXT

September 2002

11. Legal Category

POM

Desmotabs 0.2mg

(Ferring Pharmaceuticals Ltd)

1. NAME OF THE MEDICINAL PRODUCT

Desmotabs® 0.2mg

2. QUALITATIVE AND QUANTITATIVE COMPOSITION

Each tablet contains 0.2mg Desmopressin acetate

For excipients, see 6.1.

3. PHARMACEUTICAL FORM

Tablet

Uncoated, white, round, convex tablets scored on one side and engraved '0.2' on the other side.

4. CLINICAL PARTICULARS

4.1 Therapeutic indications

Desmotabs® are indicated for the treatment of primary nocturnal enuresis.

4.2 Posology and method of administration

Children (from 5 years of age) and adults (up to 65 years of age) with normal urine concentrating ability who have primary nocturnal enuresis should take 0.2mg at bedtime and only if needed should the dose be increased to 0.4mg.

The need for continued treatment should be reassessed after 3 months by means of a period of at least 1 week without Desmotabs®.

4.3 Contraindications

Desmotabs® are contraindicated in cases of cardiac insufficiency and other conditions requiring treatment with diuretic agents. Desmotabs® should only be used in patients with normal blood pressure.

Before prescribing Desmotabs® the diagnoses of psychogenic polydipsia and alcohol abuse should be excluded.

Desmopressin should not be prescribed to patients over the age of 65 for the treatment of primary nocturnal enuresis.

4.4 Special warnings and special precautions for use

Care should be taken with patients who have reduced renal function and/or cardiovascular disease or cystic fibrosis. In chronic renal disease the antidiuretic effect of Desmotabs® would be less than normal.

When Desmotabs® are used for the treatment of enuresis, fluid intake must be limited from 1 hour before until 8 hours after administration.

Patients being treated for primary nocturnal enuresis should be warned to avoid ingesting water while swimming and to discontinue Desmotabs® during an episode of vomiting and/or diarrhoea until their fluid balance is once again normal.

Precautions to prevent fluid overload must be taken in:

- conditions characterised by fluid and/or electrolyte imbalance

- patients at risk for increased intracranial pressure

4.5 Interaction with other medicinal products and other forms of Interaction

Substances which are known to induce SIADH e.g. tricyclic antidepressants, selective serotonin re-uptake inhibitors, chlorpromazine and carbamazepine, may cause an additive antidiuretic effect leading to an increased risk of water retention and/or hyponatraemia.

NSAIDs may induce water retention and/or hyponatraemia.

Concomitant treatment with loperamide may result in a 3-fold increase of desmopressin plasma concentrations, which may lead to an increased risk of water retention and/or hyponatraemia. Although not investigated, other drugs slowing transport might have the same effect.

A standardised 27% fat meal significantly decreased the absorption (rate and extent) of a 0.4mg dose of oral desmopressin. Although it did not significantly affect the pharmacodynamic effect (urine production and osmolality), there is the potential for this to occur at lower doses. If a diminution of effect is noted, then the effect of food should be considered before increasing the dose.

4.6 Pregnancy and lactation

Pregnancy:

Data on a limited number (n=53) of exposed pregnancies in women with diabetes insipidus indicate rare cases of malformations in children treated during pregnancy. To date, no other relevant epidemiological data are available. Animal studies do not indicate direct or indirect harmful effects with respect to pregnancy, embryonal/fetal development, parturition or postnatal development.

Caution should be exercised when prescribing to pregnant women. Blood pressure monitoring is recommended due to the increased risk of pre-eclampsia.

Lactation:

Results from analyses of milk from nursing mothers receiving high dose Desmopressin (300 micrograms intranasally) indicate that the amounts of Desmopressin that may be transferred to the child are considerably less than the amounts required to influence diuresis.

4.7 Effects on ability to drive and use machines

None

4.8 Undesirable effects

Side-effects include headache, stomach pain and nausea. Isolated cases of allergic skin reactions and more severe general allergic reactions have been reported. Very rare cases of emotional disturbances in children have been reported. Treatment with Desmopressin without concomitant reduction of fluid intake may lead to water retention/hyponatraemia with accompanying symptoms of headache, nausea, vomiting, weight gain, decreased serum sodium and in serious cases, convulsions.

4.9 Overdose

An overdose of Desmotabs® leads to a prolonged duration of action with an increased risk of water retention and/or hyponatraemia.

Treatment:

Although the treatment of hyponatraemia should be individualised, the following general recommendations can be given. Hyponatraemia is treated by discontinuing the desmopressin treatment, fluid restriction and symptomatic treatment if needed.

5. PHARMACOLOGICAL PROPERTIES

5.1 Pharmacodynamic properties

In its main biological effects, Desmopressin does not differ qualitatively from vasopressin. However, Desmopressin is characterised by a high antidiuretic activity whereas the uterotonic and vasopressor actions are extremely low.

5.2 Pharmacokinetic properties

The absolute bioavailability of orally administered desmopressin varies between 0.08% and 0.16%. Mean maximum plasma concentration is reached within 2 hours. The distribution volume is 0.2 – 0.32 l/kg. Desmopressin does not cross the blood-brain barrier. The oral terminal half-life varies between 2.0 and 3.11 hours.

In vitro, in human liver microsome preparations, it has been shown that no significant amount of desmopressin is metabolised in the liver and thus human liver metabolism *in vivo* is not likely to occur.

About 65% of the amount of desmopressin absorbed after oral administration could be recovered in the urine within 24 hours.

It is unlikely that desmopressin will interact with drugs affecting hepatic metabolism, since desmopressin has been shown not to undergo significant liver metabolism in *in vitro* studies with human microsomes. However, formal *in vivo* interaction studies have not been performed.

5.3 Preclinical safety data

There are no pre-clinical data of relevance to the prescriber which are additional to that already included in other sections of the SPC.

6. PHARMACEUTICAL PARTICULARS

6.1 List of excipients

Lactose monohydrate

Potato starch

Povidone

Magnesium stearate

6.2 Incompatibilities

Not applicable

6.3 Shelf life

24 months.

6.4 Special precautions for storage

Do not store above 25°C. Keep the container tightly closed.

6.5 Nature and contents of container

30ml High Density Polyethylene (HDPE) bottle with a tamper-proof, twist-off polypropylene (PP) closure with a silica gel desiccant insert. Each bottle contains 7, 30 or 90 tablets.

Not all pack sizes may be marketed.

6.6 Instructions for use and handling

None.

7. MARKETING AUTHORISATION HOLDER

Ferring Pharmaceuticals Limited, The Courtyard, Waterside Drive, Langley, Berkshire SL3 6EZ

8. MARKETING AUTHORISATION NUMBER(S)

PL 3194/0046

9. DATE OF FIRST AUTHORISATION/RENEWAL OF THE AUTHORISATION

19th April 1999.

10. DATE OF REVISION OF THE TEXT

September 2002

11. Legal Category

POM

Destolit

(Norgine Limited)

1. NAME OF THE MEDICINAL PRODUCT

Destolit 150 mg tablets

2. QUALITATIVE AND QUANTITATIVE COMPOSITION

Each tablet contains 150 mg ursodeoxycholic acid (UDCA)

3. PHARMACEUTICAL FORM

Tablet

4. CLINICAL PARTICULARS

4.1 Therapeutic indications

The dissolution of radiolucent (i.e. non-radio opaque) cholesterol gallstones in patients with a functioning gallbladder

4.2 Posology and method of administration

Adults and the elderly

Dissolution of gallstones:

A daily dose of 8 to 12mg/kg UDCA will produce cholesterol desaturation in the majority of cases. The measurement of the lithogenic index on bile-rich duodenal drainage fluid after 4-6 weeks of therapy may be useful for determining the minimum effective dose. The lowest effective dose has been found to be 4 mg/kg. The daily dose for most patients is 3 or 4 tablets, according to body weight. The dose should be divided into two administrations after meals, with one administration always after the evening meal.

The duration of treatment needed to achieve dissolution will not usually exceed 2 years, and should be monitored with regular cholecystograms. Treatment should be continued for 3-4 months after the radiological disappearance of gallstones.

Any temporary discontinuation of treatment, if prolonged for 3-4 weeks, will allow the bile to return to a state of supersaturation, and will extend the total time taken for litholysis. In some cases stones may recur after successful treatment.

For oral administration.

4.3 Contraindications

Active gastric or duodenal ulcers, a non-functioning gall bladder, radio-opaque gall stones and inflammatory bowel disease are contraindicated, as are hepatic and intestinal conditions interfering with the enterohepatic circulation of bile acids (ileal resection and stoma, regional ileitis, extra and intra-hepatic cholestasis, severe, acute, and chronic liver diseases).

4.4 Special warnings and special precautions for use

Excessive dietary intake of calories and cholesterol should be avoided; a low cholesterol diet will probably improve the effectiveness of Destolit tablets.

4.5 Interaction with other medicinal products and other forms of Interaction

Drugs such as cholestyramine and some antacids bind bile acids *in vitro*, and may inhibit the absorption of UDCA.

There is a possibility of increased serum ciclosporin levels in some patients taking ursodeoxycholic acid and ciclosporin simultaneously.

It is recommended that drugs known to increase cholesterol elimination in bile, such as oestrogenic hormones, oral contraceptive agents and certain blood cholesterol lowering agents, such as clofibrate, should also not be prescribed concomitantly.

4.6 Pregnancy and lactation

It is advised that women of child bearing age should use adequate non-hormonal or low oestrogen oral contraceptive measures during treatment with UDCA, and that the drug should not be given during the first trimester of pregnancy unless, in the opinion of the physician, the benefit outweighs the risk.

There are no clinical data available on the safety of UDCA in women who are breast-feeding. Therefore, Destolit is not recommended in this patient group.

4.7 Effects on ability to drive and use machines

None known

4.8 Undesirable effects

Destolit is normally well tolerated. Diarrhoea has been found to occur only occasionally. No significant alterations have so far been observed in liver function. Nausea, vomiting, pruritus and gallstone calcification may occur.

4.9 Overdose

It is unlikely that overdosage will cause serious adverse effects. Diarrhoea may occur and it is recommended that liver function tests be monitored. Ion-exchange resins may be useful to bind bile acids in the intestine.

5. PHARMACOLOGICAL PROPERTIES

5.1 Pharmacodynamic properties

Ursodeoxycholic acid is a gallstone dissolving agent which acts by reducing the content of cholesterol in bile. This may be due either to a reduction in hepatic cholesterol synthesis or reduced absorption of cholesterol or both.

5.2 Pharmacokinetic properties

Intestinal absorption after an oral dose of UDCA is high, with a first-pass clearance of about 50 to 60%. Studies show that passive diffusion occurs, whereupon the drug enters the enterohepatic circulation and is subject to an efficient hepatic extraction mechanism. The 'spillover' into the systemic blood supply is therefore minimal. Plasma levels are not clinically important but may be useful in estimating patient compliance; they reach maximum concentrations at about 60 minutes after ingestion with another peak recorded at 3 hours.

Ursodeoxycholic acid is rapidly conjugated with glycine and taurine in the liver. Microbial biotransformation of the drug and its metabolites occurs when they leave the enterohepatic circulation and is responsible for high levels of faecal lithocholic and 7-ketolithocholic acids during ursodeoxycholic acid therapy. Intestinal flora also hydrolyse conjugated drug back to the parent compound and interconvert ursodeoxycholic and chenodeoxycholic acids.

5.3 Preclinical safety data

UDCA has not shown teratogenic potential in rats and rabbits; embryotoxicity seen in the rat at high doses appears to occur early in gestation.

UDCA was not genotoxic in bacterial mutation tests. It has shown genotoxic potential in vitro in a mammalian chromosome aberration study and in a gene mutation study using yeast, however, the relevance of this is questionable since UDCA was not carcinogenic in long term studies in mice and rats.

Bile acids act as tumour promoters in colon carcinogenesis, but there is no evidence that they are direct carcinogens. In two year carcinogenicity studies UDCA was not tumourigenic in mice. In rats an increase in adrenal phaeochromocytomas was observed which is not considered to be clinically significant

6. PHARMACEUTICAL PARTICULARS

6.1 List of excipients

Lactose, pregelatinised maize starch, acacia gum, talc, magnesium stearate, purified water.

6.2 Incompatibilities

None known

6.3 Shelf life

3 years

6.4 Special precautions for storage

None

6.5 Nature and contents of container

Blister pack of 60 tablets

6.6 Instructions for use and handling

None

7. MARKETING AUTHORISATION HOLDER

Norgine Ltd

Chaplin House

Widewater Place

Moorhall Road

Harefield

Uxbridge

Middlesex

UB9 5NS

8. MARKETING AUTHORISATION NUMBER(S)

PL 00322/0076

9. DATE OF FIRST AUTHORISATION/RENEWAL OF THE AUTHORISATION

22 August 2002

10. DATE OF REVISION OF THE TEXT

11th June 2005

Legal category POM

Deteclo Tablets

(Wyeth Pharmaceuticals)

1. NAME OF THE MEDICINAL PRODUCT

DETECLO tablets 300mg.

2. QUALITATIVE AND QUANTITATIVE COMPOSITION

Active Constituent	Quantity/ Dose	Specification Reference
Tetracycline hydrochloride	115.4mg	BP
Demeclocyline hydrochloride	69.2mg	BP
Chlortetracycline hydrochloride	115.4mg	BP

For excipients, see Section 6.1.

3. PHARMACEUTICAL FORM

Tablet.

Round, convex, blue film-coated tablets, embossed LL on one side and 5422 on the reverse side.

4. CLINICAL PARTICULARS

4.1 Therapeutic indications

The treatment of infections caused by tetracycline-sensitive organisms. For example, DETECLO is highly effective in the treatment of infections caused by Borrellia recurrentis (relapsing fever), Calymmatobacterium granulomatis (granuloma inguinale), Chlamydia species (psittacosis, lymphogranuloma venereum, trachoma, inclusion conjunctivitis), Francisella tularensis (tularaemia), Haemophilus ducreyi (chancroid), Leptospira (meningitis, jaundice), Mycoplasma pneumoniae (non-gonococcal urethritis), Pseudomonas mallei and pseudomallei (glanders and melioidosis), Rickettsiae (typhus fever, Q fever, rocky mountain spotted fever), Vibrio species (cholera). It is also highly effective, alone or in combination with streptomycin, in the treatment of infections due to Brucella species (brucellosis), and Yersina pestis (bubonic plague). Severe acne vulgaris.

Other sensitive organisms include: Actinomyces israelii, Bacillus anthracis (pneumonia), Clostridium species (gas gangrene, tetanus), Entamoeba histolytica (dysentery), Neisseria gonorrhoeae, and anaerobic species, Treponema pallidum and pertenue (syphilis and yaws).

4.2 Posology and method of administration

For oral administration

Adults: One tablet every 12 hours. This may be increased to 3 or 4 tablets daily for short periods in more severe infections.

Gonorrhoea: 1,200mg (4 tablets) followed by a similar dose six hours later.

Non-gonococcal urethritis: One tablet twice daily for 10-21 days.

Children: Not recommended for children under 12 years of age.

Elderly: DETECLO should be used with caution in the treatment of elderly patients where accumulation is a possibility.

In patients with renal and/or liver impairment: Tetracyclines should be used cautiously in patients with impaired liver function. Total dosage should be decreased by reduction of recommended individual doses and/or by extending the time intervals between doses. See Section 4.4 Special Warnings and Special Precautions for Use.

Administration: DETECLO should be swallowed whole with plenty of fluid while sitting or standing to reduce the risk of oesophageal irritation and ulceration. DETECLO should be taken at least an hour before or two hours after meals. It should be noted that absorption of tetracyclines is impaired by foods and some dairy products, antacids containing aluminium, calcium or magnesium, and by iron-containing preparations. Therapy should be continued for up to three days after characteristic symptoms of the infection have subsided.

4.3 Contraindications
i) A history of hypersensitivity to tetracyclines or any of the components of the product formulation.

ii) Overt renal insufficiency.

iii) Children under 12 years of age.

iv) Use during pregnancy or during lactation in women breast feeding infants is contraindicated (see also Section 4.6 Pregnancy and Lactation)

4.4 Special warnings and special precautions for use
The use of tetracyclines during tooth development in children under the age of 12 years may cause permanent discolouration. Enamel hypoplasia has also been reported.

DETECLO should be used with caution in patients with renal or hepatic dysfunction or in conjunction with other potentially hepatotoxic or nephrotoxic drugs.

Concurrent use with the anaesthetic methoxyflurane increases the risk of kidney failure and has been reported to result in fatal kidney failure. The anti-anabolic action of the tetracyclines may cause an increase in BUN.

Lower doses are indicated in cases of renal impairment to avoid excessive systemic accumulation, and if therapy is prolonged, serum level determinations are advisable. Patients who have known liver disease should not receive more than 1g daily. In long-term therapy, periodic laboratory evaluation of organ systems, including haematopoietic, renal and hepatic studies should be performed.

Photosensitivity manifested by an exaggerated sunburn reaction has been observed in some individuals taking tetracyclines. Patients apt to be exposed to direct sunlight or ultraviolet light should be advised that this reaction can occur with tetracycline drugs, be warned to avoid direct exposure to natural or artificial sunlight and that treatment should be discontinued at the first evidence of skin erythema or skin discomfort.

Cross-resistance between tetracyclines may develop in micro-organisms and cross-sensitisation in patients. DETECLO should be discontinued if there are signs/symptoms of overgrowth of resistant organisms including candida, enteritis, glossitis, stomatitis, vaginitis, pruritus ani or staphylococcal enterocolitis.

Patients taking oral contraceptives should be warned that if diarrhoea or breakthrough bleeding occur there is a possibility of contraceptive failure.

All patients with gonorrhoea should have a serologic test for syphilis at the time of diagnosis. Patients treated with demeclocycline hydrochloride should have a follow-up serologic test for syphilis after 3 months.

4.5 Interaction with other medicinal products and other forms of Interaction
DETECLO should not be used with penicillins.

Tetracyclines depress plasma prothrombin activity and reduced doses of concomitant anti-coagulants may be required.

Absorption of DETECLO is impaired by the concomitant administration of iron, calcium, zinc, magnesium and particularly aluminium salts, commonly used as antacids. Absorption of tetracyclines is also impaired by food and some dairy products.

The concomitant use of tetracyclines may reduce the efficacy of oral contraceptives; an increased incidence of breakthrough bleeding may also be experienced (see Special Warnings and Precautions for Use).

The concurrent use of tetracyclines and methoxyflurane has been reported to result in fatal renal toxicity.

4.6 Pregnancy and lactation
Use in pregnancy

Contraindicated in pregnancy. Demeclocycline hydrochloride, like other tetracycline-class antibiotics, can cause foetal harm when administered to a pregnant woman. If either drug is used during pregnancy or if the patient becomes pregnant while taking these drugs, the patient should be informed of the potential hazard to the foetus.

Results of animal studies indicate that tetracyclines cross the placenta, are found in foetal tissues and can have toxic effects on the developing foetus (often related to retardation of skeletal development). Evidence of embryotoxicity has also been noted in animals treated early in pregnancy. DETECLO therefore, should not be used in pregnancy unless considered essential, in which case the maximum daily dose should be 1g.

The use of tetracyclines during tooth development (last half of pregnancy) may cause permanent discolouration of the teeth (yellow-grey-brown). This adverse reaction is more common during long-term use of the drugs but has been observed following repeated short-term courses. Enamel hypoplasia has also been reported.

Use in lactation
Contraindicated during lactation.

Tetracyclines have been found in the milk of lactating women who are taking a drug in this class. Permanent tooth discolouration may occur in the developing infant and enamel hypoplasia has been reported. Therefore, DETECLO should not be administered to lactating women.

4.7 Effects on ability to drive and use machines
Headache, dizziness, visual disturbances and, rarely, impaired hearing have been reported with tetracyclines and patients should be warned about the possible hazards of driving or operating machinery during treatment.

4.8 Undesirable effects
Blood and Lymphatic System Disorders:

Haemolytic anaemia, thrombocytopenia, neutropenia, eosinophilia, agranulocytosis, aplastic anaemia.

Ear and Labyrinth Disorders:

Tinnitus.

Eye Disorders:

Visual disturbances.

Gastrointestinal Disorders:

Nausea, vomiting, diarrhoea, glossitis, dysphagia, enterocolitis, pancreatitis, increases in liver enzymes, hepatitis and liver failure. Instances of oesophagitis and oesophageal ulcerations have been reported in patients receiving particularly the capsule and also the tablet forms of tetracyclines. Most of these patients were reported to have taken the medication immediately before going to bed.

Tooth discolouration in paediatric patients less than 12 years of age and also, rarely, in adults.

Immune System Disorders:

Anaphylaxis, anaphylactoid purpura, serum sickness-like reactions.

Infections and Infestations:

Candidal overgrowth in the anogenital region.

Metabolism and Nutrition Disorders:

Anorexia.

Nervous System Disorders:

Pseudomotor cerebri (benign intracranial hypertension) in adults, bulging fontanels in infants, dizziness, headache.

Renal and Urinary Disorders:

Elevations in BUN are often dose-related. Acute renal failure.

Skin and Subcutaneous Tissue Disorders:

Urticaria, angioneurotic oedema, maculopapular and erythematous rashes, exfoliative dermatitis, fixed drug eruptions including balanitis, erythema multiforme, Stevens-Johnson syndrome, photosensitivity.

4.9 Overdose
No specific antidote. In case of overdosage, discontinue medication, treat symptomatically and institute supportive measures (gastric lavage plus oral administration of milk or antacids. Maintain fluid and electrolyte balance). Tetracyclines are not removed in significant quantities by haemodialysis or peritoneal dialysis.

5. PHARMACOLOGICAL PROPERTIES
5.1 Pharmacodynamic properties
Pharmacotherapeutic Group: Antibacterials for systemic use – tetracyclines

ATC Code: J01A A20.

Tetracyclines are bacteriostatic at the concentrations usually achieved in the body and interfere with protein synthesis in susceptible organisms.

Tetracyclines are active against a wide range of Gram-negative and Gram-positive bacteria, including some which are resistant to penicillin.

5.2 Pharmacokinetic properties
DETECLO tablets contain a mixture of tetracycline hydrochloride, chlortetracycline hydrochloride and demeclocycline hydrochloride. This combination is designed to take advantage of the different pharmacokinetic properties of the individual components and to produce high plasma antibiotic levels of long duration with a twice daily dosage.

Tetracyclines are incompletely and irregularly absorbed from the gastro-intestinal tract. Absorption is affected by the soluble salts of divalent and trivalent metals, milk and food.

Doses of 300mg of DETECLO every 12 hours produce plasma concentrations in the range of 5-9μg/ml expressed in tetracycline-equivalent units.

24-65% of circulating tetracycline, 47% chlortetracycline and 41-90% demeclocycline are bound to plasma proteins. Tetracyclines are widely distributed throughout the body tissues and are retained at sites of new bone formation and recent calcification. Biological half-lives: tetracycline - 8.5 hours, chlortetracycline - 5.5 hours, demeclocycline - 12 hours.

Tetracyclines are excreted in the urine and faeces.

5.3 Preclinical safety data
Carcinogenesis, Mutagenesis, Impairment of Fertility:

Long-term studies in animals to evaluate carcinogenic potential of demeclocycline hydrochloride have not been conducted. Dietary administration of tetracycline hydrochloride at levels of 0, 12, 500, or 25000ppm to rats and mice in long-term carcinogenesis studies produced no evidence of carcinogenic activity of tetracycline hydrochloride. However, there has been evidence of oncogenic activity in rats in studies with the related antibiotics oxytetracycline (adrenal and pituitary tumours) and minocycline (thyroid tumours).

Although mutagenicity studies of demeclocycline hydrochloride have not been conducted, positive results in *in vitro* mammalian cell assays (i.e. mouse lymphoma and Chinese hamster lung cells) have been reported for related antibiotics (tetracycline hydrochloride and oxytetracycline).

Demeclocycline hydrochloride and tetracycline hydrochloride had no effect on fertility when administered in the diet to male and female rats at a daily intake of 45 and 25 times respectively the human dose.

6. PHARMACEUTICAL PARTICULARS
6.1 List of excipients
Tablet core:

Corn starch

Alginic acid

Ethyl cellulose

Magnesium stearate

Film coating:

Opadry OY 6531

Purified water

Talc

Opaspray K-IF-4336

Liquid paraffin

IMS

Chloroform

Hydroxypropylmethyl cellulose

6.2 Incompatibilities
None.

6.3 Shelf life
3 years.

6.4 Special precautions for storage
Do not store above 25°C.

Store in the original pack or in containers which prevent access of light and moisture.

6.5 Nature and contents of container
Tamper-evident, white polypropylene bottle with plastic screw-on cap or amber glass bottle with metal screw-on cap.

Pack size: 10 or 14 tablets.

White polypropylene bottle with plastic screw-on cap or amber glass bottle with metal screw-on cap.

Pack size: 100 or 500 tablets.

PVC or ACLAR blister pack.

Pack size: 2 tablets.

6.6 Instructions for use and handling
Not applicable.

7. MARKETING AUTHORISATION HOLDER
Cyanamid of Great Britain Ltd

Fareham Road

Gosport

Hants

PO13 0AS

8. MARKETING AUTHORISATION NUMBER(S)
PL 0095/5070R.

9. DATE OF FIRST AUTHORISATION/RENEWAL OF THE AUTHORISATION
First Authorisation: 4 July 1991 (Review Licence). Renewed 26 January 1999. Renewed 26 January 2004.

10. DATE OF REVISION OF THE TEXT
Approved: 19 July 2004

Detrunorm 15 mg Tablets

(Amdipharm)

1. NAME OF THE MEDICINAL PRODUCT
Detrunorm® 15 mg Coated Tablets

2. QUALITATIVE AND QUANTITATIVE COMPOSITION
Each coated tablet contains 15 mg propiverine hydrochloride equivalent to 13.64 mg propiverine.

For excipients, see section 6.1.

3. PHARMACEUTICAL FORM
Coated tablets.

Rose-coloured, lenticular glazing coated tablets.

4. CLINICAL PARTICULARS
4.1 Therapeutic indications
The treatment of urinary incontinence, as well as urgency and frequency in patients who have either idiopathic detrusor overactivity (overactive bladder) or neurogenic detrusor overactivity (detrusor hyperreflexia) from spinal cord injuries, e.g. transverse lesion paraplegia.

4.2 Posology and method of administration
Coated tablets for oral application.

The recommended daily doses are as follows:

Adults: As a standard dose one coated tablet (= 15 mg propiverine hydrochloride) twice a day is recommended, this may be increased to three times a day. Some patients may already respond to a dosage of 15 mg a day.

For neurogenic detrusor overactivity a dose of one coated tablet three times a day is recommended. This may be increased to four times a day if necessary and tolerated (maximum recommended daily dose).

Elderly: Generally there is no special dosage regimen for the elderly (see 5.2).

There is no clinically relevant effect of food on the pharmacokinetics of propiverine (see 5.2). Accordingly, there is no particular recommendation for the intake of propiverine in relation to food.

This medicinal product contains 0.61 mg of glucose. Accordingly, a daily dose of 2 coated tablets supplies 1.22 mg of glucose.

4.3 Contraindications

The drug is contraindicated in patients who have demonstrated hypersensitivity to the active substance or to any of the excipients and in patients suffering from one of the following disorders:

- obstruction of the bowel
- significant degree of bladder outflow obstruction where urinary retention may be anticipated
- myasthenia gravis
- intestinal atony
- severe ulcerative colitis
- toxic megacolon
- uncontrolled angle closure glaucoma
- moderate or severe hepatic impairment
- tachyarrhythmias.

4.4 Special warnings and special precautions for use

The drug should be used with caution in patients suffering from:

- autonomic neuropathy.

Symptoms of the following diseases may be aggravated following administration of the drug:

- severe congestive heart failure (NYHA IV)
- prostatic hypertrophy
- hiatus hernia with reflux oesophagitis
- cardiac arrhythmia
- tachycardia.

Propiverine, like other anticholinergics, induces mydriasis. Therefore, the risk to induce acute angle-closure glaucoma in individuals predisposed with narrow angles of the anterior chamber may be increased.

Drugs of this class have been reported to induce or precipitate acute angle-closure glaucoma.

Pollakiuria and nocturia due to renal disease or congestive heart failure as well as organic bladder diseases (e.g. urinary tract infections, malignancy) should be ruled out prior to treatment.

Cochineal red A (E124, lake) may cause allergic reactions.

Due to a lack of data Detrunorm® 15 mg Coated Tablets should not be used in children.

4.5 Interaction with other medicinal products and other forms of Interaction

Increased effects due to concomitant medication with tricyclic antidepressants (e.g. imipramine), tranquillisers (e.g. benzodiazepines), anticholinergics, amantadine, neuroleptics (e.g. phenothiazines) and beta-adrenoceptor agonists (beta-sympathomimetics). Decreased effects due to concomitant medication with cholinergic drugs. Reduced blood pressure in patients treated with isoniazid. The effect of prokinetics such as metoclopramide may be decreased.

Pharmacokinetic interactions are possible with other drugs metabolised by cytochrome P450 3A4 (CYP 3A4). However, a very pronounced increase of concentrations for such drugs is not expected as the effects of propiverine are small compared to classical enzyme inhibitors (e.g. ketoconazole or grapefruit juice). Propiverine may be considered as weak inhibitor of cytochrome P450 3A4. Pharmacokinetic studies with patients concomitantly receiving potent CYP 3A4 inhibitors such as azole antifungals (e.g. ketoconazole, itraconazole) or macrolide antibiotics (e.g. erythromycin, clarithromycin) have not been performed.

4.6 Pregnancy and lactation

There are no adequate data from the use of propiverine hydrochloride in pregnant women. Studies in animals have shown reproductive toxicity (see section 5.3). The potential risk for humans is unknown.

The drug is secreted into the milk of lactating mammals.

Propiverine hydrochloride should not be used during pregnancy and should not be administered to nursing women.

4.7 Effects on ability to drive and use machines

Propiverine hydrochloride may produce drowsiness and blurred vision. This may impair the patient's ability to exert activities that require mental alertness such as operating a motor vehicle or other machinery, or to exert hazardous work while taking this drug.

Sedative drugs may enhance the drowsiness caused by propiverine hydrochloride.

4.8 Undesirable effects

Adverse reactions	System organ class (Disorders according to MedDRA)
Very common (>1/10)	
- dry mouth	Gastrointestinal
Common (>1/100, <1/10)	
- accommodation abnormal, accommodation disturbances, vision abnormal	Eye
- constipation	Gastrointestinal
Uncommon (>1/1,000, <1/100)	
- fatigue	General disorders and administration site conditions
- nausea/vomiting	Gastrointestinal
- dizziness	Nervous system
- tremor	Nervous system
- urinary retention	Urinary system
- flushing	Vascular
- decreased blood pressure with drowsiness	Vascular
Rare (>1/10,000, <1/1,000)	
- rash due to idiosyncrasy (propiverine hydrochloride) or hypersensitivity (excipients, e.g. colorant)	Skin and subcutaneous tissue
Very rare (<1/10,000, including isolated reports)	
- palpitation	Cardiac
- restlessness, confusion	Psychiatric

All undesirable effects are transient and recede after a dose reduction or termination of the therapy after maximum 1 - 4 days.

During long-term therapy hepatic enzymes should be monitored, because reversible changes of liver enzymes might occur in rare cases. Monitoring of intraocular pressure is recommended in patients at risk of developing glaucoma.

Particular attention should be paid to the residual urine volume in cases of urinary tract infection.

4.9 Overdose

Overdose with the muscarinic receptor antagonist propiverine hydrochloride can potentially result in central anticholinergic effects, e.g. restlessness, dizziness, vertigo, disorders in speech and vision and muscular weakness. Moreover, severe dryness of mucosa, tachycardia and urinary retention may occur.

Treatment should be symptomatic and supportive. Management of overdose may include initiation of vomiting or gastric lavage using an oiled tube (attention: dryness of mucosa!), followed by symptomatic and supportive treatment as for atropine overdose (e.g. physostigmine) with a dosage of 1.0 to 2.0 mg in adults by slow intravenous injection (may be repeated as necessary to a total of 5 mg).

A 14-year old girl who ingested 450 mg propiverine hydrochloride presented with confabulation. The adolescent fully recovered.

5. PHARMACOLOGICAL PROPERTIES

5.1 Pharmacodynamic properties

ATC code: G04B D06

Pharmacotherapeutic group: spasmolytic, anticholinergic.

Mechanism of action

Inhibition of calcium influx and modulation of intracellular calcium in urinary bladder smooth muscle cells causing musculotropic spasmolysis.

Inhibition of the efferent connection of the nervus pelvicus due to anticholinergic action.

- Pharmacodynamic effects

In animal models propiverine hydrochloride causes a dose-dependent decrease of the intravesical pressure and an increase in bladder capacity.

The effect is based on the sum of the pharmacological properties of propiverine and three active urinary metabolites as shown in isolated detrusor strips of human and animal origin.

5.2 Pharmacokinetic properties

General characteristics of the active substance

Propiverine is nearly completely absorbed from the gastrointestinal tract. It undergoes extensive first pass metabolism. Effects on urinary bladder smooth muscle cells are due to the parent compound and three active metabolites as well, which are rapidly excreted into the urine.

Absorption

After oral administration of Detrunorm® 15 mg Coated Tablets propiverine is rapidly absorbed from the gastrointestinal tract with maximal plasma concentrations reached after 2.3 hours. The mean absolute bioavailability of Detrunorm® 15 mg Coated Tablets is 40.5% (arithmetic mean value for $AUC_{0-\infty\ (p.o.)}$ / $AUC_{0-\infty\ (i.v.)}$).

Food intake increases the bioavailability of propiverine (mean increase 1.3 fold), but does not significantly affect the maximum plasma concentrations of propiverine or of its main metabolite, propiverine-N-oxide. This difference in bioavailability is unlikely to be of clinical significance and adjustment of dose in relation to food intake is not required.

Distribution

After administration of Detrunorm® 15 mg Coated Tablets t.i.d., steady state is reached after four to five days at a higher concentration level than after single dose application ($C_{average}$ = 61 ng/ml). The volume of distribution was estimated in 21 healthy volunteers after intravenous administration of propiverine hydrochloride to range from 125 to 473 l (mean 279 l) indicating that a large amount of available propiverine is distributed to peripheral compartments. The binding to plasma proteins is 90 - 95% for the parent compound and about 60% for the main metabolite.

Plasma concentrations of propiverine in 16 healthy volunteers after single and repeated administration of Detrunorm® 15 mg Coated Tablets (t.i.d. for 6 days):

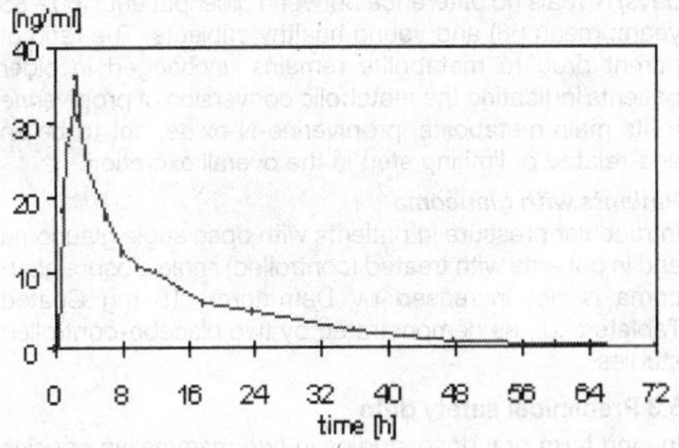

single dose

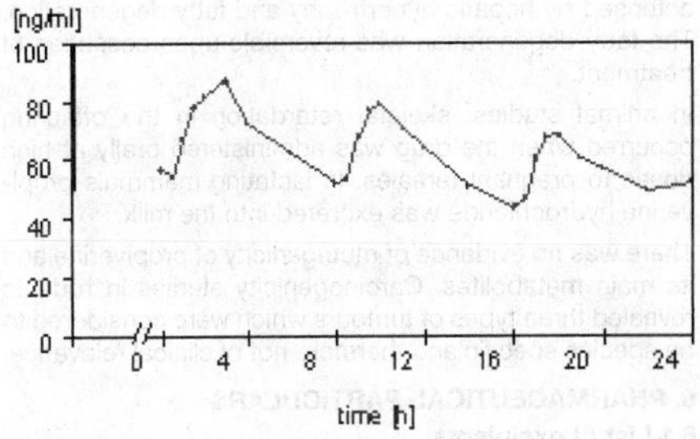

multiple dose

Steady state characteristics of propiverine following multiple-dose administration to 16 healthy volunteers of Detrunorm® 15 mg Coated Tablets (t.i.d. for 6 days):

(see Table 1 below)

Table 1

Dose interval [h]	$AUC_{0-\tau}$ [ng>/>h/ml]	CV [%]	PTF [%]	CV [%]	$C_{average}$ [ng/ml]	CV [%]
0 - 8	515	35	57	16	64	36
8 - 16	460	33	70	25	57	33
16 - 24	421	36	52	39	52	36

CV: coefficient of variation

PTF: peak-trough fluctuation

Biotransformation

Propiverine is extensively metabolised by intestinal and hepatic enzymes. The primary metabolic route involves the oxidation of the Piperidyl-N and is mediated by CYP 3A4 and Flavin-monoxygenases (FMO) 1 and 3 and leads to the formation of the much less active N-oxide, the plasma concentration of which greatly exceeds that of the parent substance. Four metabolites were identified in urine; two of them are pharmacologically active and may contribute to the therapeutic efficacy of Detrunorm® 15 mg Coated Tablets.

In vitro there is a slight inhibition of CYP 3A4 and CYP 2D6 detectable which occurs at concentrations exceeding therapeutic plasma concentrations 10- to 100-fold (see section 4.5).

Elimination

Following administration of 30 mg oral dose of ^{14}C-propiverine hydrochloride to healthy volunteers, 60% of radioactivity was recovered in urine and 21% was recovered in faeces within 12 days. Less than 1% of an oral dose is excreted unchanged in the urine. Mean total clearance after single dose administration of 30 mg is 371 ml/min (191 – 870 ml/min). In three studies including a total of 37 healthy volunteers the mean elimination half-life was 14.1, 20.1, and 22.1 hours, respectively.

Linearity/non-linearity

Pharmacokinetic parameters of propiverine and propiverine-N-oxide following oral administration of 10 - 30 mg of propiverine hydrochloride are linearly related to dose. There are no changes of pharmacokinetics during steady state compared to single dose administration.

Characteristics in patients

Renal impairment

Severe renal impairment does not significantly alter the disposition of propiverine and its main metabolite, propiverine-N-oxide, as deduced from a single dose study in 12 patients with creatinine clearance < 30 ml/min. No dose adjustment is to be recommended as long as the total daily dose does not exceed 30 mg (i.e. Detrunorm® 15 mg Coated Tablets given b.i.d.). In case that higher dose (i.e. 45 mg) shall be administered a careful titration of dose is recommended considering anticholinergic effects as a marker for tolerability.

Hepatic insufficiency

There were similar steady state pharmacokinetics in 12 patients with mild to moderate impairment of liver function due to fatty liver disease as compared to 12 healthy controls. No data are available for severe hepatic impairment.

Age

The comparison of trough plasma concentrations during steady state (Detrunorm® 15 mg Coated Tablets t.i.d. for 28 days) reveals no difference between older patients (60 – 85 years; mean 68) and young healthy subjects. The ratio of parent drug to metabolite remains unchanged in older patients indicating the metabolic conversion of propiverine to its main metabolite, propiverine-N-oxide, not to be an age-related or limiting step in the overall excretion.

Patients with glaucoma

Intraocular pressure in patients with open angle glaucoma and in patients with treated (controlled) angle closure glaucoma is not increased by Detrunorm® 15 mg Coated Tablets t.i.d., as demonstrated by two placebo-controlled studies.

5.3 Preclinical safety data

In long term oral dose studies in two mammalian species the main treatment related effects were changes in the liver (including elevation of hepatic enzymes). These were characterised by hepatic hypertrophy and fatty degeneration. The fatty degeneration was reversible upon cessation of treatment.

In animal studies, skeletal retardation in the offspring occurred when the drug was administered orally at high doses to pregnant females. In lactating mammals propiverine hydrochloride was excreted into the milk.

There was no evidence of mutagenicity of propiverine and its main metabolites. Carcinogenicity studies in rodents revealed three types of tumours which were considered to be species specific and therefore not of clinical relevance.

6. PHARMACEUTICAL PARTICULARS

6.1 List of excipients

Lactose monohydrate, powdered cellulose, magnesium stearate, sucrose, talc, heavy kaolin, calcium carbonate, titanium dioxide (E171), acacia gum, colloidal anhydrous silica, Macrogol 6000, glucose monohydrate, Cochineal red A (E124, lake), montan wax.

6.2 Incompatibilities

Not applicable.

6.3 Shelf life

3 years.

6.4 Special precautions for storage

No special precautions for storage.

6.5 Nature and contents of container

PVC/aluminium blisters in carton with 56 coated tablets per carton.

6.6 Instructions for use and handling

Not applicable.

7. MARKETING AUTHORISATION HOLDER

Amdipharm Plc
Regency House
Miles Gray Road
Basildon
Essex
SS14 3AF

8. MARKETING AUTHORISATION NUMBER(S)

PL 20072/0015

9. DATE OF FIRST AUTHORISATION/RENEWAL OF THE AUTHORISATION

15 July 2004

10. DATE OF REVISION OF THE TEXT

Detrusitol 1mg & 2mg tablets

(Pharmacia Limited)

1. NAME OF THE MEDICINAL PRODUCT

Detrusitol 1 mg filmcoated tablets

Detrusitol 2 mg filmcoated tablets

2. QUALITATIVE AND QUANTITATIVE COMPOSITION

Each filmcoated tablet contains tolterodine tartrate 1 mg or 2 mg corresponding to 0.68 mg and 1.37 mg tolterodine, respectively

For excipients, see 6.1

3. PHARMACEUTICAL FORM

Filmcoated tablets

The filmcoated tablets are white, round and biconvex. The 1 mg tablet is engraved with arcs above and below the letters TO and the 2 mg tablet is engraved with arcs above and below the letters DT.

4. CLINICAL PARTICULARS

4.1 Therapeutic indications

Symptomatic treatment of urge incontinence and/or increased urinary frequency and urgency as may occur in patients with overactive bladder syndrome.

4.2 Posology and method of administration

Adults (including elderly):

The recommended dose is 2 mg twice daily except in patients with impaired liver function or severely impaired renal function (GFR≤30 ml/min) for whom the recommended dose is 1 mg twice daily (see section 4.4). In case of troublesome side effects the dose may be reduced from 2 mg to 1 mg twice daily.

The effect of treatment should be re-evaluated after 2-3 months (see section 5.1).

Children:

Safety and effectiveness in children have not yet been established. Therefore Detrusitol is not recommended for children, until more information is available

4.3 Contraindications

Tolterodine is contraindicated in patients with

- Urinary retention
- Uncontrolled narrow angle glaucoma
- Myasthenia gravis
- Known hypersensitivity to tolterodine or excipients
- Severe ulcerative colitis
- Toxic megacolon

4.4 Special warnings and special precautions for use

Tolterodine shall be used with caution in patients with

- Significant bladder outlet obstruction at risk of urinary retention
- Gastrointestinal obstructive disorders, e.g. pyloric stenosis
- Renal impairement (see section 4.2)
- Hepatic disease. (see section 4.2 and 5.2)
- Autonomic neuropathy
- Hiatus hernia
- Risk for decreased gastrointestinal motility

Caution should be used in patients with known risk factors for QT-prolongation (i.e. hypokalaemia, bradycardia, and concurrent administration of drugs known to prolong QT-interval) and relevant pre-existing cardiac diseases (i.e. myocardial ischaemia, arrhythmia, congestive heart failure) (see section 5.3).

As with all treatments for symptoms of urgency and urge incontinence, organic reasons for urge and frequency should be considered before treatment.

The combination of tolterodine with strong inhibitors of CYP3A4 is not recommended (see Section 4.5 Interactions).

4.5 Interaction with other medicinal products and other forms of Interaction

Concomitant systemic medication with potent CYP3A4 inhibitors such as macrolide antibiotics (e.g. erythromycin and clarithromycin), antifungal agents (e.g. ketoconazole and itraconazole) and antiproteases is not recommended due to increased serum concentrations of tolterodine in poor CYP2D6 metabolisers with (subsequent) risk of overdosage (see section 4.4).

Concomitant medication with other drugs that possess antimuscarinic properties may result in more pronounced therapeutic effect and side-effects. Conversely, the therapeutic effect of tolterodine may be reduced by concomitant administration of muscarinic cholinergic receptor agonists.

The effect of prokinetics like metoclopramide and cisapride may be decreased by tolterodine.

Concomitant treatment with fluoxetine (a potent CYP2D6 inhibitor) does not result in a clinically significant interaction since tolterodine and its CYP2D6-dependent metabolite, 5-hydroxymethyl tolterodine are equipotent.

Drug interaction studies have shown no interactions with warfarin or combined oral contraceptives (ethinyl estradiol/levonorgestrel).

A clinical study has indicated that tolterodine is not a metabolic inhibitor of CYP2D6, 2C19, 3A4 or 1A2. Therefore an increase of plasma levels of drugs metabolised by the isoenzyme systems is not expected when dosed in combination with tolterodine.

4.6 Pregnancy and lactation

Pregnancy

There are no adequate data from the use of tolterodine in pregnant women.

Studies in animals have shown reproductive toxicity (see section 5.3). The potential risk for humans is unknown.

Consequently, Detrusitol is not recommended during pregnancy.

Lactation

No data concerning the excretion of tolterodine into human milk are available. Tolterodine should be avoided during lactation.

4.7 Effects on ability to drive and use machines

Since this drug may cause accommodation disturbances and influence reaction time, the ability to drive and use machines may be negatively affected.

4.8 Undesirable effects

Due to the pharmacological effect of tolterodine it may cause mild to moderate antimuscarinic effects, like dryness of the mouth, dyspepsia and dry eyes.

The table below reflects the data obtained with Detrusitol in clinical trials and from postmarketing experience. The most commonly reported adverse reaction was dry mouth, which occurred in 35% of patients treated with Detrusitol tablets and in 10% of placebo treated patients.

(see Table 1 on next page)

Other adverse effects reported with the use of tolterodine are anaphylactoid reactions including angioedema (very rare) and cardiac failure (very rare).

Palpitations and arrhythmia (rare) are known adverse effects for this drug class.

4.9 Overdose

The highest dose given to human volunteers of tolterodine L-tartrate is 12.8 mg as single dose. The most severe adverse events observed were accommodation disturbances and micturition difficulties.

In the event of tolterodine overdose, treat with gastric lavage and give activated charcoal. Treat symptoms as follows:

- Severe central anticholinergic effects (e.g. hallucinations, severe excitation): treat with physostigmine
- Convulsions or pronounced excitation: treat with benzodiazepines
- Respiratory insufficiency: treat with artificial respiration
- Tachycardia: treat with beta-blockers
- Urinary retention: treat with catheterization
- Mydriasis: treat with pilocarpine eye drops and/or place patient in dark room

5. PHARMACOLOGICAL PROPERTIES

5.1 Pharmacodynamic properties

Pharmacotherapeutic group: Urinary antispasmodics

ATC code: G04B D07

Tolterodine is a competitive, specific muscarinic receptor antagonist with a selectivity for the urinary bladder over salivary glands in vivo. One of the tolterodine metabolites (5-hydroxymethyl derivative) exhibits a pharmacological profile similar to that of the parent compound. In extensive metabolisers this metabolite contributes significantly to the therapeutic effect (see 5.2).

Effect of the treatment can be expected within 4 weeks.

Effect of treatment with Detrusitol 2 mg twice daily after 4 and 12 weeks, respectively, compared with placebo (pooled data). Absolute change and percentage change relative to baseline.

(see Table 2 on next page)

The effect of tolterodine was evaluated in patients, examined with urodynamic assessment at baseline and, depending on the urodynamic result, they were allocated to a urodynamic positive (motor urgency) or a urodynamic negative (sensory urgency) group. Within each group, the

Table 1

	Common > 1/100, < 1/10	Uncommon > 1/1000, < 1/100	Rare > 1/10000, < 1/1000
Immune system disorders		Hypersensitivity not otherwise specified	
Psychiatric disorders	Nervousness	Confusion	Hallucinations
Nervous system disorders	Dizziness, somnolence, paresthesia		
Eye disorders	Dry eyes, abnormal vision including abnormal accommodation		
Cardiac disorders			Tachycardia
Gastrointestinal disorders	Dyspepsia, constipation, abdominal pain, flatulence, vomiting		
Skin and subcutaneous tissue disorders	Dry skin		
Renal and urinary disorders		Urinary retention	
General disorders	Fatigue, headache, chest pain	Peripheral oedema	

Table 2

Variable	4-week studies			12-week studies		
	Detrusitol 2 mg b.i.d.	Placebo	Statistical significance vs. placebo	Detrusitol 2 mg b.i.d.	Placebo	Statistical significance vs. placebo
Number of micturitions per 24 hours	-1.6 (-14%) n=392	-0.9 (-8%) n=189	*	-2.3 (-20%) n=354	-1.4 (-12%) n=176	**
Number of incontinence episodes per 24 hours	-1.3 (-38%) n=288	-1.0 (-26%) n=151	n.s.	-1.6 (-47%) n=299	-1.1 (-32%) n=145	*
Mean volume voided per micturition (ml)	+25 (+17%) n=385	+12 (+8%) n=185	***	+35 (+22%) n=354	+10 (+6%) n=176	***
Number of patients with no or minimal bladder problems after treatment (%)	16% n=394	7% n=190	**	19% n=356	15% n=177	n.s.

n.s. = not significant; * = $p \leq 0.05$; ** = $p \leq 0.01$; *** = $p \leq 0.001$

patients were randomised to receive either tolterodine or placebo. The study could not provide convincing evidence that tolterodine had effects over placebo in patients with sensory urgency.

Clinical effects of tolterodine on QT interval were investigated in a variety of clinical studies. The clinical trial information is based on ECGs that were obtained from over 600 treated patients, and which included the elderly and patients with pre-existing cardiovascular disease. The changes in QT intervals did not significantly differ between placebo and treatment groups. Overall, there does not appear to be a significant change in QT interval.

5.2 Pharmacokinetic properties

Pharmacokinetic characteristics specific for this formulation: Tolterodine is rapidly absorbed. Both tolterodine and the 5-hydroxymethyl metabolite reach maximal serum concentrations 1-3 hours after dose. The half-life for tolterodine given as the tablet is 2-3 hours in extensive and about 10 hours in poor metabolisers (devoid of CYP2D6). Steady state concentrations are reached within 2 days after administration of the tablets.

Food does not influence the exposure to the unbound tolterodine and the active 5-hydroxymethyl metabolite in extensive metabolisers, although the tolterodine levels increase when taken with food. Clinically relevant changes are likewise not expected in poor metabolisers.

Absorption: After oral administration tolterodine is subject to CYP2D6 catalysed first-pass metabolism in the liver, resulting in the formation of the 5-hydroxymethyl derivative, a major pharmacologically equipotent metabolite.

The absolute bioavailability of tolterodine is 17 % in extensive metabolisers, the majority of the patients, and 65% in poor metabolisers (devoid of CYP2D6).

Distribution: Tolterodine and the 5-hydroxymethyl metabolite bind primarily to orosomucoid. The unbound fractions are 3.7% and 36%, respectively. The volume of distribution of tolterodine is 113 l.

Elimination: Tolterodine is extensively metabolised by the liver following oral dosing. The primary metabolic route is mediated by the polymorphic enzyme CYP2D6 and leads to the formation of the 5-hydroxymethyl metabolite. Further metabolism leads to formation of the 5-carboxylic acid and N-dealkylated 5-carboxylic acid metabolites, which account for 51 % and 29 % of the metabolites recovered in the urine, respectively. A subset (about 7%) of the population is devoid of CYP2D6 activity. The identified pathway of metabolism for these individuals (poor metabolisers) is dealkylation via CYP3A4 to N-dealkylated tolterodine, which does not contribute to the clinical effect. The remainder of the population is referred to as extensive metabolisers. The systemic clearance of tolterodine in extensive metabolisers is about 30 L/h. In poor metabolisers the reduced clearance leads to significantly higher serum concentrations of tolterodine (about 7-fold) and negligible concentrations of the 5-hydroxymethyl metabolite are observed.

The 5-hydroxymethyl metabolite is pharmacologically active and equipotent with tolterodine. Because of the differences in the protein-binding characteristics of tolterodine and the 5-hydroxymethyl metabolite, the exposure (AUC) of unbound tolterodine in poor metabolisers is similar to the combined exposure of unbound tolterodine and the 5-hydroxymethyl metabolite in patients with CYP2D6 activity given the same dosage regimen. The safety, tolerability and clinical response are similar irrespective of phenotype.

The excretion of radioactivity after administration of [^{14}C]-tolterodine is about 77% in urine and 17% in faeces. Less than 1% of the dose is recovered as unchanged drug, and about 4% as the 5-hydroxymethyl metabolite. The carboxylated metabolite and the corresponding dealkylated metabolite account for about 51% and 29% of the urinary recovery, respectively.

The pharmacokinetics is linear in the therapeutic dosage range.

Specific patient groups:

Impaired liver function: About 2-fold higher exposure of unbound tolterodine and the 5-hydroxymethyl metabolite is found in subjects with liver cirrhosis (see section 4.2 and 4.4).

Impaired renal function: The mean exposure of unbound tolterodine and its 5-hydroxymethyl metabolite is doubled in patients with severe renal impairment (inulin clearance GFR ≤ 30 ml/min). The plasma levels of other metabolites were markedly (up to 12-fold) increased in these patients. The clinical relevance of the increased exposure of these metabolites is unknown. There is no data in mild to moderate renal impairment (see section 4.2 and 4.4).

5.3 Preclinical safety data

In toxicity, genotoxicity, carcinogenicity and safety pharmacology studies no clinically relevant effects have been observed, except those related to the pharmacological effect of the drug.

Reproduction studies have been performed in mice and rabbits.

In mice, there was no effect of tolterodine on fertility or reproductive function. Tolterodine produced embryo death and malformations at plasma exposures (C_{max} or AUC) 20 or 7 times higher than those seen in treated humans.

In rabbits, no malformative effect was seen, but the studies were conducted at 20 or 3 times higher plasma exposure (C_{max} or AUC) than those expected in treated humans.

Tolterodine, as well as its active human metabolites prolong action potential duration (90% repolarisation) in canine purkinje fibres (14 - 75 times therapeutic levels) and block the K+-current in cloned human ether-a-go-go-related gene (hERG) channels (0.5 – 26.1 times therapeutic levels). In dogs prolongation of the QT interval has been observed after application of tolterodine and its human metabolites (3.1 – 61.0 times therapeutic levels). The clinical relevance of these findings is unknown.

In clinical trials, overall there does not appear to be a significant change in QT interval (see 5.1).

6. PHARMACEUTICAL PARTICULARS

6.1 List of excipients

Core:

Cellulose, microcrystalline

Calcium hydrogen phosphate dihydrate

Sodium starch glycollate (Type B)

Magnesium stearate

Colloidal anhydrous silica

Film coating:

Coating granules containing

Hypromellose

Cellulose, microcrystalline

Stearic acid

Titanium dioxide

6.2 Incompatibilities

Not applicable.

6.3 Shelf life

3 years.

6.4 Special precautions for storage

No special precautions for storage

6.5 Nature and contents of container

Tablets are packed in either blister package made of PVC/PVDC and aluminium foil with a heat seal coating of PVDC or plastic containers made of polyethylene provided with screw caps of polypropylene.

Pack sizes:

Detrusitol tablets are available in blisters of 2x10, 3x10, 5x10 and 10x10 tablets, 1x14, 2x14 and 4x14 tablets, 280 and 560 tablets and in bottles of 60 and 500 tablets.

Not all pack sizes may be marketed.

6.6 Instructions for use and handling

No special requirements.

7. MARKETING AUTHORISATION HOLDER

Pharmacia Ltd

Ramsgate Road

Sandwich

Kent

CT 13 9NJ

UK

8. MARKETING AUTHORISATION NUMBER(S)

PL 00032/0222

PL 00032/0223

9. DATE OF FIRST AUTHORISATION/RENEWAL OF THE AUTHORISATION

3rd February 1998

10. DATE OF REVISION OF THE TEXT

28th October 2004

POM

Ref: DT 3_0

Detrusitol XL 4mg

(Pharmacia Limited)

1. NAME OF THE MEDICINAL PRODUCT

Detrusitol XL 4 mg, prolonged-release capsules, hard

2. QUALITATIVE AND QUANTITATIVE COMPOSITION

Each prolonged-release capsule contains tolterodine tartrate 4 mg corresponding to 2.74 mg tolterodine.

For excipients see 6.1

3. PHARMACEUTICAL FORM

Prolonged-release capsule, hard

The 4 mg prolonged-release capsule is blue with white printing (symbol and 4).

4. CLINICAL PARTICULARS

4.1 Therapeutic indications

Symptomatic treatment of urge incontinence and/or increased urinary frequency and urgency as may occur in patients with overactive bladder syndrome.

4.2 Posology and method of administration

Adults (including the elderly):

The recommended dose is 4 mg once daily except in patients with impaired liver function or severely impaired renal function (GFR ≤ 30 ml/min) for whom the recommended dose is 2 mg once daily (see sections 4.4 and 5.2). In case of troublesomeside-effects the dose may be reduced from 4 mg to 2 mg once daily.

The prolonged-release capsules can be taken with or without food and must be swallowed whole.

The effect of treatment should be re-evaluated after 2-3 months (see section 5.1).

Children:

Safety and effectiveness in children have not yet been established. Therefore Detrusitol XL prolonged-release capsules are not recommended for children, until more information is available.

4.3 Contraindications

Tolterodine is contraindicated in patients with

- Urinary retention
- Uncontrolled narrow angle glaucoma
- Myasthenia gravis
- Known hypersensitivity to tolterodine or excipients
- Severe ulcerative colitis
- Toxic megacolon

4.4 Special warnings and special precautions for use

Tolterodine shall be used with caution in patients with

- Significant bladder outlet obstruction at risk ofurinary retention
- Gastrointestinal obstructive disorders, e.g. pyloric stenosis
- Renal impairment (see sections 4.2 and 5.2)
- Hepatic disease (see sections 4.2 and 5.2)
- Autonomic neuropathy
- Hiatus hernia
- Risk of decreased gastrointestinal motility

Caution should be used in patients with known risk factors for QT-prolongation (i.e. hypokalaemia, bradycardia, and concurrent administration of drugs known to prolong QT-interval) and relevant pre-existing cardiac diseases (i.e. myocardial ischaemia, arrhythmia, congestive heart failure). (See Section 5.3)

As with all treatments for symptoms of urgency and urge incontinence, organic reasons for urge and frequency should be considered before treatment.

The combination of tolterodine with strong inhibitors of CYP3A4 is not recommended (see Section 4.5. Interactions).

Patients with rare hereditary problems of fructose intolerance, glucose-galactose malabsorption or sucrase-isomaltase insufficiency should not take this medicine.

4.5 Interaction with other medicinal products and other forms of Interaction

Concomitant systemic medication with potent CYP3A4 inhibitors such as macrolide antibiotics (erythromycin and clarithromycin), antifungal agents (e.g. ketoconazole and itraconazole) and antiproteases is not recommended due to increased serumconcentrations of tolterodine in poor CYP2D6 metabolisers with (subsequent) risk of overdosage (see section 4.4).

Concomitant medication with other drugs that possess antimuscarinic properties may result in more pronounced therapeutic effect and side-effects. Conversely, the therapeutic effect of tolterodine may be reduced by concomitant administration of muscarinic cholinergic receptor agonists.

The effect of prokinetics like metoclopramide and cisapride may be decreased by tolterodine.

Concomitant treatment with fluoxetine (a potent CYP2D6 inhibitor) does not result in a clinically significant interaction since tolterodine and its CYP2D6-dependent metabolite, 5-hydroxymethyl tolterodine are equipotent.

Drug interaction studies have shown no interactions with warfarin or combined oral contraceptives (ethinyl estradiol/levonorgestrel).

A clinical study has indicated that tolterodine is not a metabolic inhibitor of CYP2D6, 2C19, 3A4 or 1A2. Therefore an increase of plasma levels of drugs metabolised by the isoenzyme systems is not expected when dosed in combination with tolterodine.

4.6 Pregnancy and lactation

Pregnancy

There are no adequate data from the use of tolterodine in pregnant women.

Studies in animals have shown reproductive toxicity (see section 5.3). The potential risk for humans is unknown.

Consequently, Detrusitol XL is not recommended during pregnancy.

Lactation

No data concerning the excretion of tolterodine into human milk are available. Tolterodine should be avoided during lactation.

4.7 Effects on ability to drive and use machines

Since this drug may cause accommodation disturbances and influence reaction time, the ability to drive and use machines may be negatively affected.

4.8 Undesirable effects

Due to the pharmacological effect of tolterodine it may cause mild to moderate antimuscarinic effects, like dryness of the mouth, dyspepsia and dry eyes.

The table below reflects the data obtained with Detrusitol in clinical trials and from post marketing experience. The most commonly reported adverse reaction was dry mouth, which occurred in 23.4 % of patients treated with Detrusitol XL and in 7.7 % of placebo-treated patients.

(see Table 1)

Other adverse effects reported with the use of tolterodine are anaphylactoid reactions including angioedema (very rare) and cardiac failure (very rare).

Palpitations and arrhythmia (rare) are known adverse effects for this drug class

4.9 Overdose

The highest dose given to human volunteers of tolterodine tartrate is 12.8 mg as single dose of the immediate release formulation. The most severe adverse events observed were accommodation disturbances and micturition difficulties.

In the event of tolterodine overdose, treat with gastric lavage and give activated charcoal. Treat symptoms as follows:

- Severe central anticholinergic effects (e.g. hallucinations, severe excitation): treat with physostigmine
- Convulsions or pronounced excitation: treat with benzodiazepines
- Respiratory insufficiency: treat with artificial respiration
- Tachycardia: treat with beta-blockers
- Urinary retention: treat with catheterisation
- Mydriasis: treat with pilocarpine eye drops and/or place patient in dark room

5. PHARMACOLOGICAL PROPERTIES

5.1 Pharmacodynamic properties

Pharmacotherapeutic group: Urinary antispasmodics

ATC code: G04B D07

Tolterodine is a competitive, specific muscarinic receptor antagonist with a selectivity for the urinary bladder over salivary glands in vivo. One of the tolterodine metabolites (5-hydroxymethyl derivative) exhibits a pharmacological profile similar to that of the parent compound. In extensive metabolisers this metabolite contributes significantly to the therapeutic effect (see 5.2).

Effect of the treatment can be expected within 4 weeks.

In the Phase III program, the primary endpoint was reduction of incontinence episodes per week and the secondary endpoints were reduction of micturitions per 24 hours and increase of mean volume voided per micturition. These parameters are presented in the following table.

Effect of treatment with Detrusitol XL 4 mg once daily after 12 weeks, compared with placebo. Absolute change and percentage change relative to baseline. Treatment difference Detrusitol vs. placebo: Least Squares estimated mean change and 95% confidence interval.

(see Table 2 on next page)

After 12 weeks of treatment 23.8% (121/507) in the Detrusitol XL group and 15.7% (80/508) in the placebo group reported that they subjectively had no or minimal bladder problems.

The effect of tolterodine was evaluated in patients, examined with urodynamic assessment at baseline and, depending on the urodynamic result, they were allocated to a urodynamic positive (motor urgency) or a urodynamic negative (sensory urgency) group. Within each group, the patients were randomised to receive either tolterodine or placebo. The study could not provide convincing evidence that tolterodine had effects over placebo in patients with sensory urgency.

Clinical effects of tolterodine on QT interval were investigated in a variety of clinical studies. The clinical trial information is based on ECGs that were obtained from over 600 treated patients, and which included the elderly and patients with pre-existing cardiovascular disease. The changes in QT intervals did not significantly differ between placebo and treatment groups. Overall, there does not appear to be a significant change in QT interval.

5.2 Pharmacokinetic properties

Pharmacokinetic characteristics specific for this formulation: Tolterodine prolonged-release capsules give a slower absorption of tolterodine than the immediate-release tablets do. As a result, the maximum serum concentrations are observed 4 (2-6) hours after administration of the capsules. The apparent half-life for tolterodine given as the capsule is about 6 hours in extensive and about 10 hours in poor metabolisers (devoid of CYP2D6). Steady state concentrations are reached within 4 days after administration of the capsules.

There is no effect of food on the bioavailability of the capsules.

Absorption: After oral administration tolterodine is subject to CYP2D6 catalysed first-pass metabolism in the liver, resulting in the formation of the 5-hydroxymethyl derivative, a major pharmacologically equipotent metabolite.

The absolute bioavailability of tolterodine is 17 % in extensive metabolisers, the majority of the patients, and 65% in poor metabolisers (devoid of CYP2D6).

Distribution: Tolterodine and the 5-hydroxymethyl metabolite bind primarily to orosomucoid. The unbound fractions are 3.7% and 36%, respectively. The volume of distribution of tolterodine is 113 l.

Elimination: Tolterodine is extensively metabolised by the liver following oral dosing. The primary metabolic route is

Table 1

	Common >1/100, <1/10	Uncommon >1/1000, <1/100)	Rare >1/10.000, <1/1000)
Immune system disorders		Hypersensitivity not otherwise specified	
Psychiatric disorders	Nervousness	Confusion	Hallucinations
Nervous system disorders	Dizziness, somnolence, paresthesia		
Eye disorders	Dry eyes, abnormal vision (including abnormal accomodation)		
Cardiac disorders			Tachycardia
Gastrointestinal disorders	Dyspepsia, constipation, abdominal pain, flatulence, vomiting		
Skin and subcutaneous tissue disorders	Dry skin		
Renal and urinary disorders		Urinary retention	
General disorders	Fatigue, headache, chest pain	Peripheral oedema	

Table 2

	Detrusitol XL 4 mg once daily (n=507)	Placebo (n=508)	Treatment difference vs. placebo: Mean change and 95% CI	Statistical significance vs. placebo (p-value)
Number of incontinence episodes per week	-11.8 (-54%)	-6.9 (-28%)	-4.8 (-7.2; -2.5)*	<0.001
Number of micturitions per 24 hours	-1.8 (-13%)	-1.2 (-8%)	-0.6 (-1.0; -0.2)	0.005
Mean volume voided per micturition (ml)	+34 (+27%)	+14 (+12%)	+20 (14; 26)	<0.001

) 97.5% confidence interval according to Bonferroni

mediated by the polymorphic enzyme CYP2D6 and leads to the formation of the 5-hydroxymethyl metabolite. Further metabolism leads to formation of the 5-carboxylic acid and N-dealkylated 5-carboxylic acid metabolites, which account for 51 % and 29 % of the metabolites recovered in the urine, respectively. A subset (about 7%) of the population is devoid of CYP2D6 activity. The identified pathway of metabolism for these individuals (poor metabolisers) is dealkylation via CYP3A4 to N-dealkylated tolterodine, which does not contribute to the clinical effect. The remainder of the population is referred to as extensive metabolisers. The systemic clearance of tolterodine in extensive metabolisers is about 30 L/h. In poor metabolisers the reduced clearance leads to significantly higher serum concentrations of tolterodine (about 7-fold) and negligible concentrations of the 5-hydroxymethyl metabolite are observed.

The 5-hydroxymethyl metabolite is pharmacologically active and equipotent with tolterodine. Because of the differences in the protein-binding characteristics of tolterodine and the 5-hydroxymethyl metabolite, the exposure (AUC) of unbound tolterodine in poor metabolisers is similar to the combined exposure of unbound tolterodine and the 5-hydroxymethyl metabolite in patients with CYP2D6 activity given the same dosage regimen. The safety, tolerability and clinical response are similar irrespective of phenotype.

The excretion of radioactivity after administration of [^{14}C]-tolterodine is about 77% in urine and 17% in faeces. Less than 1% of the dose is recovered as unchanged drug, and about 4% as the 5-hydroxymethyl metabolite. The carboxylated metabolite and the corresponding dealkylated metabolite account for about 51% and 29% of the urinary recovery, respectively.

The pharmacokinetics is linear in the therapeutic dosage range.

Specific patient groups:

Impaired liver function: About 2-fold higher exposure of unbound tolterodine and the 5-hydroxymethyl metabolite is found in subjects with liver cirrhosis (see section 4.2 and 4.4).

Impaired renal function: The mean exposure of unbound tolterodine and its 5-hydroxymethyl metabolite is doubled in patients with severe renal impairment (inulin clearance GFR $\leqslant$ 30 ml/min). The plasma levels of other metabolites were markedly (up to 12-fold) increased in these patients. The clinical relevance of the increased exposure of these metabolites is unknown. There is no data in mild to moderate renal impairment (see section 4.2 and 4.4).

5.3 Preclinical safety data

In toxicity, genotoxicity, carcinogenicity and safety pharmacology studies no clinically relevant effects have been observed except those related to the pharmacological effect of the drug.

Reproduction studies have been performed in mice and rabbits.

In mice, there was no effect of tolterodine on fertility or reproductive function. Tolterodine produced embryo death and malformations at plasma exposures (C_{max} or AUC) 20 or 7 times higher than those seen in treated humans.

In rabbits, no malformative effect was seen, but the studies were conducted at 20 or 3 times higher plasma exposure (C_{max} or AUC) than those expected in treated humans.

Tolterodine, as well as its active human metabolites prolong action potential duration (90% repolarisation) in canine purkinje fibres (14 - 75 times therapeutic levels) and block the K+-current in cloned human ether-a-go-go-related gene (hERG) channels (0.5 – 26.1 times therapeutic levels). In dogs prolongation of the QT interval has been observed after application of tolterodine and its human metabolites (3.1 – 61.0 times therapeutic levels). The clinical relevance of these findings is unknown.

In clinical trials, overall there does not appear to be a significant change in QT interval (see 5.1)

6. PHARMACEUTICAL PARTICULARS

6.1 List of excipients

Prolonged release capsule contents:

Sugar spheres (containing sucrose and maize starch)

Hypromellose

Surelease E-7-9010 clear:

Ethylcellulose

Medium Chain Triglycerides

Oleic acid

Prolonged release capsule shell contents:

Gelatin

Printing ink:

Shellac glaze

Titanium dioxide, E 171

Propylene glycol

Simeticone

Colorants in the blue 4 mg prolonged release capsule:

Indigo carmine, E132

Titanium dioxide, E 171

6.2 Incompatibilities

Not applicable.

6.3 Shelf life

2 years

6.4 Special precautions for storage

Do not store above 30 °C

Bottles: Store in the original container.

Blisters: Keep container in the outer carton.

6.5 Nature and contents of container

Detrusitol XL prolonged-release capsules are packed in either blisters made of PVC/PVDC and aluminium foil with a heat seal coating of PVDC or HDPE bottles with screw caps of polypropylene.

Pack sizes:

Detrusitol XL prolonged release capsules of 4 mg are available in blisters of 1 × 7, 2 × 7, 4 × 7, 7 × 7, 12 × 7, 14 × 7, 40 × 7 capsules and in bottles of 30, 90 and 100. Hospital packs are available in blisters of 10 × 2 × 4, 20 × 2 × 4 and 40 × 2 × 4 capsules.

Not all pack sizes may be marketed.

6.6 Instructions for use and handling

No special requirements.

7. MARKETING AUTHORISATION HOLDER

Pharmacia Limited

Ramsgate Road

Sandwich

Kent

CT13 9NJ

UK

8. MARKETING AUTHORISATION NUMBER(S)

PL 00032/ 0287

9. DATE OF FIRST AUTHORISATION/RENEWAL OF THE AUTHORISATION

14th August 2001

10. DATE OF REVISION OF THE TEXT

28th October 2004

11 LEGAL CATEGORY

POM

DT3_0

Dexa-Rhinaspray Duo

(Boehringer Ingelheim Limited)

1. NAME OF THE MEDICINAL PRODUCT

Dexa-Rhinaspray® Duo

2. QUALITATIVE AND QUANTITATIVE COMPOSITION

Tramazoline hydrochloride (INN) 120 micrograms/metered dose (as monohydrate) and dexamethasone isonicotinate 20 micrograms/metered dose.

For excipients, see 6.1

3. PHARMACEUTICAL FORM

Nasal spray, suspension.

4. CLINICAL PARTICULARS

4.1 Therapeutic indications

Treatment of allergic rhinitis.

4.2 Posology and method of administration

Adults (including the elderly): 1 metered dose into each nostril up to six times in 24 hours, although 2 or 3 applications a day are usually sufficient.

Children 5-12 years: 1 metered dose into each nostril up to twice daily.

Children under 5 years: Not recommended.

The dose should be titrated to the lowest dose at which effective control of symptoms is maintained.

Each course of treatment should not exceed 14 days.

No specific information on the use of this product in the elderly is available. No adverse reactions specific to this age group have been reported with tramazoline and dexamethasone.

4.3 Contraindications

The use of Dexa-Rhinaspray Duo is contraindicated in patients hypersensitive to any of the components and in infants and nursing mothers.

4.4 Special warnings and special precautions for use

Care should be used to avoid contact with the eyes as conjunctival irritation may occur. The use of Dexa-Rhinaspray Duo for prolonged periods is not recommended. The possibility of side-effects from the systemic absorption of dexamethasone should be borne in mind.

Systemic effects of nasal corticosteroids may occur, particularly at high doses prescribed for prolonged periods. Growth retardation has been reported in children receiving nasal corticosteroids at licensed doses.

It is recommended that the height of children receiving prolonged treatment with nasal corticosteroids is regularly monitored. If growth is slowed, therapy should be reviewed with the aim of reducing the dose of nasal corticosteroid if possible, to the lowest dose at which effective control of symptoms is maintained. In addition, consideration should be given to referring the patient to a paediatric specialist.

Treatment with higher than recommended doses of nasal corticosteroids may result in clinically significant adrenal suppression. If there is evidence of higher than recommended doses being used then additional systemic corticosteroid cover should be considered during periods of stress or elective surgery.

4.5 Interaction with other medicinal products and other forms of Interaction

None stated.

4.6 Pregnancy and lactation

There is inadequate evidence of safety in human pregnancy. Topical administration of corticosteroids to pregnant animals can cause abnormalities of foetal development including cleft palate and intra-uterine growth retardation. There may therefore be a very small risk of such effects in the human foetus. Dexa-Rhinaspray Duo should not be used by nursing mothers.

4.7 Effects on ability to drive and use machines

None stated.

4.8 Undesirable effects

A slight burning sensation in the nose, with sneezing, has been reported when using tramazoline hydrochloride alone. Rebound congestion of the nasal mucosa has been reported following prolonged use of nasal decongestants.

Systemic effects of nasal corticosteroids may occur, particularly when prescribed at high doses for prolonged periods.

4.9 Overdose

Absorption of tramazoline may produce pallor, sweating, tachycardia and anxiety. These should be treated symptomatically if necessary.

5. PHARMACOLOGICAL PROPERTIES

5.1 Pharmacodynamic properties

Tramazoline hydrochloride is a sympathomimetic with local vasoconstrictor activity. It has a quick-acting, long lasting decongestant effect on the nasal mucosa.

Dexamethasone 21-isonicotinate is a corticosteroid with marked anti-inflammatory and anti-allergic properties.

5.2 Pharmacokinetic properties

Although Dexa-Rhinaspray Duo is intended for topical administration, the possibility of systemic absorption, particularly of the steroid component, should be borne in mind.

5.3 Preclinical safety data

None stated.

6. PHARMACEUTICAL PARTICULARS

6.1 List of excipients

Benzalkonium chloride

Sodium chloride

Polyoxyethylene-sorbitan monooleate (Polysorbate 80)

Glycerol 85%

Purified water

0.1N Sodium hydroxide is used for pH adjustment.

6.2 Incompatibilities
Not applicable.

6.3 Shelf life
36 months.

After opening use within 6 months after which discard any remaining product.

6.4 Special precautions for storage
Do not store above 25°C.

6.5 Nature and contents of container
Amber-coloured glass (Type I) bottle fitted with 0.07 ml metering pump and white nasal adaptor and a protective cap. Nominal contents 10 ml equivalent to not less than 110 doses.

6.6 Instructions for use and handling
1. Shake the bottle each time before use.
2. Remove the dust cap. (Diagram)
3. Blow your nose to clear your nostrils, if necessary.
4. The nasal pump spray must be primed before Dexa-Rhinaspray Duo is used for the first time. To prime the pump, hold the bottle with your thumb at the base and your index and middle fingers on the white shoulder area. Make sure the bottle points upwards and away from your eyes. Press your thumb firmly and quickly against the bottle seven times. The pump is now primed and can be used. Your pump should be be reprimed if you have not used the medication for more than 24 hours; repriming the pump will only require one or two sprays. (Diagram)
5. Close one nostril by gently placing your finger against the side of your nose. Tilt your head slightly forward and, keeping the bottle upright, insert the nasal tip into the other nostril. Point the tip toward the back and outer side of the nose. (Diagram)

Press firmly and quickly upwards with the thumb at the base while holding the white shoulder portion of the pump between your index and middle fingers. Following each spray, sniff and breathe out through your mouth.

After spraying the nostril and removing the unit, tilt your head backwards for a few seconds to let the spray spread over the back of the nose.
6. Repeat step 5 in the other nostril.
7. Replace the cap.

Avoid spraying Dexa-Rhinaspray Duo in or around your eye. Should this occur, immediately flush your eye with cold tap water for several minutes.

If the nasal tip becomes clogged, remove the clear plastic dust cap. Hold the nasal tip under running warm tap water for about a minute. Dry the nasal tip, reprime the nasal pump spray and replace the plastic dust cap.

7. MARKETING AUTHORISATION HOLDER
Boehringer Ingelheim Limited
Ellesfield Avenue
Bracknell
Berkshire RG12 8YS
United Kingdom

8. MARKETING AUTHORISATION NUMBER(S)
PL 00015/0213

9. DATE OF FIRST AUTHORISATION/RENEWAL OF THE AUTHORISATION
22 December 1997

10. DATE OF REVISION OF THE TEXT
June 2003

11. Legal Category
Prescription only medicine.

D1/UK/SPC/7

Dexedrine Tablets 5mg

(UCB Pharma Limited)

1. NAME OF THE MEDICINAL PRODUCT
Dexedrine Tablets 5mg

2. QUALITATIVE AND QUANTITATIVE COMPOSITION
Dexamfetamine Sulphate 5mg

3. PHARMACEUTICAL FORM
Tablets for oral administration

4. CLINICAL PARTICULARS

4.1 Therapeutic indications
Dexedrine is a symphathomimetic amine with central stimulant and anorectic activity. It is indicated in narcolepsy. It is also indicated for children with refractory hyperkinetic states under the supervision of a physician specialising in child psychiatry.

4.2 Posology and method of administration
Adults: In narcolepsy, the usual starting dose is 10mg Dexedrine a day, given in divided doses. Dosage may be increased if necessary by 10mg a day at weekly intervals to a suggested maximum of 60mg a day.

Elderly: Start with 5mg a day, and increase by increments of 5mg at weekly intervals.

Children: In hyperkinetic states, the usual starting dosage for children aged 3-5 years is 2.5mg a day, increased if necessary by 2.5mg a day at weekly intervals; for children aged 6 years and over, the usual starting dose is 5-10mg a day increasing if necessary by 5mg at weekly intervals.

The usual upper limit is 20mg a day though some older children have needed 40mg or more for optimal response.

4.3 Contraindications
Do not use in patients known to be intolerant of sympathomimetic amines; during, or for 14 days after treatment with an MAO inhibitor; in those with a history of drug abuse; with symptomatic cardiovascular disease and/or moderate or severe hypertensive disease; in those suffering from hyperthyroidism or hyperexcitability or in those with glaucoma; Gilles de la Tourette syndrome or similar dystonias; porphyria.

Do not use in patients with a history of alcohol abuse.

4.4 Special warnings and special precautions for use
Use with caution in patients on guanethidine and patients with mild hypertension or a family history of dystonias. If tics develop, discontinue treatment with dexedrine. Dexamfetamine is likely to reduce the convulsant threshold therefore caution is advised in patients with epilepsy. Height and weight should be carefully monitored in children as growth retardation may occur.

Caution should be used when administering dexamfetamine to patients with impaired kidney function or unstable personality.

4.5 Interaction with other medicinal products and other forms of Interaction
Adrenoreceptor blocking agents (e.g. propanolol), lithium and α methyltyrosine may antagonise the effects of dexamfetamine. Disulfiram may inhibit metabolism and excretion.

The concurrent use of tricyclic antidepressants may increase the risk of cardiovascular side effects.

Concurrent use of MAOI's or use within the preceding 14 days may precipitate a hypertensive crisis.

Concurrent use of beta-blockers may result in severe hypertension and dexamfetamine may result in diminished effect of other anti-hypertensives such as guanethidine.

Phenothiazines may inhibit the actions of dexamfetamine.

Amfetamines may delay the absorption of ethosuximide, phenobarbital and phenytoin.

Acute dystonia has been noted with concurrent administration of haloperidol.

The analgesic effect of morphine may be increased and its respiratory depressant effects decreased with concurrent use of morphine and dexamfetamine.

4.6 Pregnancy and lactation
Dexamfetamine has been thought to produce embryotoxic effects in rodents and retrospective evidence of certain significance in man has suggested a similar possibility. Dexedrine should therefore be avoided in pregnancy, especially during the first trimester.

Dexedrine passes into breast milk.

4.7 Effects on ability to drive and use machines
Dexedrine may affect ability to drive or operate machinery.

4.8 Undesirable effects
Insomnia, restlessness, irritability, euphoria, tremor, dizziness, headache and other symptoms of over-stimulation have been reported. Also dry mouth, unwanted anorexia and other gastro-intestinal symptoms, sweating, convulsions and cardiovascular effects such as tachycardia, palpitations and minor increases in blood pressure. There have been isolated reports of cardiomyopathy associated with chronic amphetamine use.

Drug dependence, with consumption of increasing doses to levels many times those recommended, may occur as tolerance develops. At such levels, a psychosis which may be clinically indistinguishable from schizophrenia can occur.

Treatment should be stopped gradually since abrupt cessation may produce extreme fatigue and mental depression.

Intracranial haemorrhages have been reported, presumably precipitated by the hypertensive effect and possibly associated with pre-existing vascular malformation.

A toxic hypermetabolic state, characterised by transient hyperactivity, hyperpyrexia, acidosis and death due to cardiovascular collapse have been reported.

Rhabdomyolysis and renal damage.

The following adverse effects have been noted: psychosis/psychotic reactions, night terrors, nervousness, abdominal cramps, decreased blood pressure, altered libido and impotence, growth retardation, hyperpyrexia, mydriasis, hyperflexia, chest pain, confusion, panic states, aggressive behaviour, delirium, visual disturbance, choreoathetoid movements, tics and Tourettes syndrome in predisposed individuals.

4.9 Overdose
Symptoms of overdosage include excitement, hallucinations, convulsions leading to coma; tachycardia and cardiac arrhythmias; and respiratory depression.

Treatment consists of the induction of vomiting and/or gastric lavage together with supportive and symptomatic measures. Excessive stimulation or convulsions may be treated with diazepam. Excretion of dexamfetamine may be increased by forced acid diuresis.

5. PHARMACOLOGICAL PROPERTIES

5.1 Pharmacodynamic properties
Dexedrine is a sympathomimetic amine with a central stimulant and anorectic activity.

5.2 Pharmacokinetic properties
Dexamfetamine is readily absorbed from the gastrointestinal tract. It is resistant to metabolism by monoamine oxidase. It is excreted in the urine as unchanged parent drug together with some hydroxylated metabolites. Elimination is increased in acidic urine. After high doses, elimination in the urine may take several days.

5.3 Preclinical safety data
Dexamfetamine has been thought to produce embryotoxic effects in rodents, and retrospective evidence of uncertain significance in man has suggested a similar possibility. 'Dexedrine' should therefore be avoided in pregnancy, especially during the first trimester 'Dexedrine' passes into breast milk.

6. PHARMACEUTICAL PARTICULARS

6.1 List of excipients
Stearic acid
Acacia powder
Lactose
Paraffin, Light Liquid
Maize starch
Sucrose
Purified talc
Purified water

6.2 Incompatibilities
None stated

6.3 Shelf life
5 years

6.4 Special precautions for storage
No special storage precautions are necessary.

6.5 Nature and contents of container
Polypropylene securitainers, amber glass bottles or polythene vials containing 1000 and 100 tablets. Blister packs containing 100 and 28 tablets

6.6 Instructions for use and handling
None.

7. MARKETING AUTHORISATION HOLDER
UCB Pharma Ltd.
208 Bath Road
Slough
Berkshire
SL1 3WE
UK.

8. MARKETING AUTHORISATION NUMBER(S)
PL 0039/0385

9. DATE OF FIRST AUTHORISATION/RENEWAL OF THE AUTHORISATION
13 October 1992

10. DATE OF REVISION OF THE TEXT
June 2005

11. LEGAL CATEGORY
CD (Sch 2), POM

Dexsol 2mg/5ml Oral Solution

(Rosemont Pharmaceuticals Limited)

1. NAME OF THE MEDICINAL PRODUCT
Dexsol 2mg/5ml Oral Solution, Dexamethasone

2. QUALITATIVE AND QUANTITATIVE COMPOSITION
Dexamethasone 2mg/5ml (as dexamethasone sodium phosphate)

3. PHARMACEUTICAL FORM
Oral Solution

4. CLINICAL PARTICULARS

4.1 Therapeutic indications
Dexamethasone is a corticosteroid. It is designed for use in certain endocrine and non-endocrine disorders, in certain cases of cerebral oedema and for diagnostic testing of adrenocortical hyperfunction.

Endocrine disorders:

Primary or secondary adrenocortical insufficiency (the first choice is hydrocortisone or cortisone, but synthetic analogues may be used with mineralocorticoids where applicable; in infancy, mineralocorticoid supplementation is particularly important) and congenital adrenal hyperplasia.

Non-endocrine disorders:

Dexamethasone may be used in the treatment of non-endocrine corticosteroid responsive conditions including:

Allergy and anaphylaxis: Angioneurotic oedema, anaphylaxis.

Arteritis collagenosis: Polymyalgia rheumatica, polyarteritis nodosa.

Blood disorders: Haemolytic anaemia, leukaemia, myeloma.

Cardiovascular disorders: Post-myocardial infarction syndrome.

Gastro-intestinal: Crohn's disease, ulcerative colitis.

Hypercalcaemia: Sarcoidosis.

Infections (with appropriate chemotherapy): Miliary tuberculosis.

Muscular disorders: Polymyositis.

Neurological disorders: Raised intra-cranial pressure secondary to cerebral tumours.

Ocular disorders: Anterior and posterior uveitis, optic neuritis.

Renal disorders: Lupus nephritis.

Respiratory disease: Bronchial asthma, aspiration pneumonitis.

Rheumatic disorders: Rheumatoid arthritis.

Skin disorders: Pemphigus vulgaris.

4.2 Posology and method of administration

Adults

General considerations:

The dosage should be titrated to the individual response and the nature of the disease. In order to minimise side effects, the lowest effective possible dosage should be used (see 'Side effects').

The initial dosage varies from 0.5 – 9mg a day depending on the disease being treated. In more severe diseases, doses higher than 9mg may be required. The initial dosage should be maintained or adjusted until the patient's response is satisfactory. Both the dose in the evening, which is useful in alleviating morning stiffness, and the divided dosage regimen are associated with greater suppression of the hypothalamo-pituitary-adrenal axis. If satisfactory clinical response does not occur after a reasonable period of time, discontinue treatment with dexamethasone and transfer the patient to another therapy.

If the initial response is favourable, the maintenance dosage should be determined by lowering the dose gradually to the lowest dose required to maintain an adequate clinical response. Chronic dosage should preferably not exceed 1.5mg dexamethasone daily.

Patients should be monitored for signs that may require dosage adjustment. These may be changes in clinical status resulting from remissions or exacerbations of the disease, individual drug responsiveness and the effect of stress (e.g. surgery, infection, trauma). During stress it may be necessary to increase dosage temporarily.

If the drug is to be stopped after more than a few days of treatment, it should be withdrawn gradually.

The following equivalents facilitate changing to dexamethasone from other glucocorticoids:

Milligram for milligram, dexamethasone is approximately equivalent to betamethasone, 4 to 6 times more potent than methylprednisolone and triamcinolone, 6 to 8 times more potent than prednisone and prednisolone, 25 to 30 times more potent than hydrocortisone, and about 35 times more potent than cortisone.

Acute, self-limiting allergic disorders or acute exacerbations of chronic allergic disorders. The following dosage schedule combining parenteral and oral therapy is suggested:

First day: Dexamethasone sodium phosphate injection 4mg or 8mg (1ml or 2ml) intramuscularly.

Second day: 1mg (2.5ml) Dexamethasone Oral Solution twice a day.

Third day: 1mg (2.5ml) Dexamethasone Oral Solution twice a day.

Fourth day: 500micrograms (1.25ml) Dexamethasone Oral Solution twice a day.

Fifth day: 500micrograms (1.25ml) Dexamethasone Oral Solution twice a day.

Sixth day: 500micrograms (1.25ml) Dexamethasone Oral Solution.

Seventh day: 500micrograms (1.25ml) Dexamethasone Oral Solution.

Eighth day: Re-assessment.

If a dose of less than 5ml is required, an oral dosing device should be employed.

This schedule is designed to ensure adequate therapy during acute episodes whilst minimising the risk of overdosage in chronic cases.

Dexamethasone suppression tests:

1. *Tests for Cushing's syndrome*:

2mg (5ml) Dexamethasone Oral Solution should be administered at 11pm. Blood samples are then taken at 8am the next morning for plasma cortisol determination.

If greater accuracy is required, 500 micrograms (1.25ml) Dexamethasone Oral Solution should be administered every 6 hours for 48 hours. Blood should be drawn at 8am for plasma cortisol determination on the third morning.

24-hour urine collection should be employed for 17-hydroxycorticosteroid excretion determination.

2. *Test to distinguish Cushing's syndrome caused by pituitary ACTH excess from the syndrome induced by other causes*:

2mg (5ml) Dexamethasone Oral Solution should be administered every 6 hours for 48 hours. Blood should be drawn at 8am for plasma cortisol determination on the third morning.

24-hour urine collection should be employed for 17-hydroxycorticosteroid excretion determination.

Children:

Dosage should be limited to a single dose on alternate days to lessen retardation of growth and minimize suppression of hypothalamo-pituitary-adrenal axis.

Elderly:

Treatment of elderly patients, particularly if long term, should be planned bearing in mind the more serious consequences of the common side effects of corticosteroids in old age.

4.3 Contraindications

Hypersensitivity to dexamethasone or any of the excipients listed. Systemic infection unless specific anti-infective therapy is employed. Systemic fungal infections. Administration of live vaccines (see 'Precautions').

4.4 Special warnings and special precautions for use

Patients should carry 'steroid treatment' cards, which give clear guidance on the precautions to be taken to minimise risk, and which provides details of prescriber, drug, dosage and the duration of treatment.

Undesirable effects may be minimised by using the lowest effective dose for the minimum period. Dexamethasone Oral Solution may be given in divided doses as appropriate. Frequent patient review is required to appropriately titrate the dose against disease activity. When reduction in dosage is possible, the reduction should be gradual (Refer to 'Posology and Administration).

Anti-inflammatory/Immunosuppressive effects/Infection

Corticosteroids may exacerbate systemic fungal infections and should not be used unless they are needed to control drug reactions due to amphotericin. There have also been reports in which concomitant use of amphotericin and hydrocortisone was followed by cardiac enlargement and heart failure.

Live vaccines should not be given to individuals with impaired immune response. The antibody response to other vaccines may be diminished.

Suppression of the inflammatory response and immune function increases the susceptibility to infections and their severity. The clinical presentation may be atypical, and serious infections such as septicaemia and tuberculosis may be masked and may reach an advanced stage before being recognised.

Appropriate anti-microbial therapy should accompany glucocorticoid therapy when necessary e.g. in tuberculosis and viral and fungal infections of the eye.

There may be decreased resistance and inability to localise infection in patients on corticosteroids.

Chickenpox is of particular concern, since this normally minor illness may be fatal in immunosuppressed patients. Patients (or parents of children) without a definite history of chickenpox should be advised to avoid close personal contact with chickenpox or herpes zoster, and if exposed they should seek urgent medical attention. Passive immunisation with varicella/zoster immunoglobulin (VZIG) is needed by exposed non-immune patients who are receiving systemic corticosteroids or who have used them within the previous three months; this should be given within ten days of exposure to chickenpox. *If a diagnosis of chickenpox is confirmed, the illness warrants specialist care and urgent treatment. Corticosteroids should not be stopped and the dose may need to be increased.*

Measles can have a more serious or even fatal course in immunosuppressed patients. In such children or adults particular care should be taken to avoid exposure to measles. If exposed, prophylaxis with intramuscular pooled immunoglobulin (IG) may be indicated. Exposed patients should be advised to seek medical advice without delay.

Corticosteroids may activate latent amoebiasis or strongyloidiasis or exacerbate active disease. It is recommended that these are ruled out before initiating corticosteroid therapy.

General

A report shows that the use of corticosteroids in cerebral malaria is associated with a prolonged coma and an increased incidence of pneumonia and gastro-intestinal bleeding.

Dietary salt restriction and potassium supplementation may be necessary with corticosteroid therapy.

Adrenal Suppression:

Adrenal cortical atrophy develops during prolonged therapy and may persist for years after stopping treatment. Withdrawal of corticosteroids after prolonged therapy must therefore always be gradual to avoid acute adrenal insufficiency, being tapered off over weeks or months according to the dose and duration of treatment.

During prolonged therapy, any intercurrent illness, trauma or surgical procedure will require a temporary increase in dosage; if corticosteroids have been stopped following prolonged therapy they may need to be temporarily reintroduced.

Stopping corticosteroids after prolonged therapy may cause withdrawal symptoms including fever, myalgia, arthralgia and malaise. This may occur in patients even without evidence of adrenal insufficiency.

There is an enhanced effect of corticosteroids in patients with hypothyroidism and in those with cirrhosis.

Particular care is required when considering the use of systemic corticosteroids in patients with the following conditions and frequent patient monitoring is necessary:

- renal insufficiency
- hypertension or congestive heart failure
- diabetes mellitus (or a family history of diabetes)
- osteoporosis (especially post-menopausal females)
- previous corticosteroid-induced myopathy
- glaucoma (or family history of glaucoma)
- myasthenia gravis
- non-specific ulcerative colitis, diverticulitis or fresh intestinal anastomosis
- peptic ulceration
- existing or previous history of severe affective disorders (especially previous steroid psychosis)
- liver failure
- epilepsy
- migraine
- history of allergy to corticosteroids.

Large doses of corticosteroids may mask the symptoms of gastro-intestinal perforation.

Use in Children

Corticosteroids cause growth retardation. Treatment should be limited to the minimum dose for the shortest period.

Children on prolonged therapy should be carefully monitored.

Excipient Warnings

The medicine contains benzoic acid which is a mild irritant to the skin, eyes and mucous membrane. It may also increase the risk of jaundice in newborn babies.

It also contains 0.7g sorbitol in each 5ml. When given according to the recommended dosage instructions, each dose will provide up to 3.1g of sorbitol. It is unsuitable in hereditary fructose intolerance and can cause stomach upset and diarrhoea.

It also contains liquid maltitol which may cause diarrhoea.

4.5 Interaction with other medicinal products and other forms of Interaction

The efficacy of coumarin anticoagulants may be changed by concurrent corticosteroid treatment. The prothrombin time should be monitored frequently to avoid spontaneous bleeding.

The renal clearance of salicylates is increased by corticosteroids and therefore, salicylate dosage should be reduced along with steroidal withdrawal.

The desired effects of hypoglycaemic agents (including insulin), anti-hypertensives and diuretics are antagonised by corticosteroids and the hypokalaemic effects of acetazolamide, loop diuretics, thiazide diuretics and carbenoxolone are enhanced.

As phenytoin, barbiturates, ephedrine, rifabutin, carbamazepine, rifampicin, primidone and aminoglutethimide may enhance the metabolic clearance of corticosteroids, resulting in decreased blood levels and reduced physiological activity, the dosage of Dexamethasone Oral Solution may require adjustment. These interactions may interfere with dexamethasone suppression tests and these should be interpreted with caution during administration of these drugs.

Patients taking NSAID's should be monitored since the incidence and/or severity of gastro-ulceration may increase. Aspirin should also be used cautiously in conjunction with corticosteroids in hypoprothrombinaemia.

False-negative results in the dexamethasone suppression test in patients being treated with indometacin have been reported.

Antacids, particularly those containing magnesium trisilicate have been reported to impair the gastro-intestinal absorption of glucocorticoid steroids. Therefore doses of one reagent should be spaced as far as possible from the other.

Corticosteroids may affect the nitrobuletetrazolium test for bacterial infection and produce false-negative results.

4.6 Pregnancy and lactation

There is evidence of harmful effects on pregnancy in animals. Intra-uterine growth retardation in the foetus and a small increased risk of cleft palate have been reported. Infants born of mothers who have received substantial doses of corticosteroids during pregnancy should be carefully observed for signs of hypoadrenalism.

When corticosteroids are essential however, patients with normal pregnancies may be treated as though they were in the non-gravid state. Patients with pre-eclampsia or fluid retention require close monitoring.

Corticosteroids are excreted in small amounts in breast milk and may suppress growth, interfere with endogenous corticosteroid production or cause other unwanted effects.

Mothers taking pharmacological doses of glucocorticoids should be advised not to breast feed.

4.7 Effects on ability to drive and use machines

None known

4.8 Undesirable effects

The incidence of predictable undesirable effects, including hypothalamic-pituitary-adrenal suppression correlates with the relative potency of the drug, dosage, timing of administration and the duration of treatment (refer to Special Warnings and Precautions).

Reports in the literature suggest an apparent association between use of corticosteroids and left ventricular free wall rupture after a recent myocardial infarction; therefore corticosteroids should be used with great caution in these patients.

Fluid and electrolyte disturbances

Sodium retention, fluid retention, congestive heart failure in susceptible patients, potassium loss, hypokalaemic alkalosis, hypertension, increased calcium excretion.

Musculoskeletal

Osteoporosis, vertebral and long bone fractures, avascular necrosis, tendon rupture. Proximal myopathy.

Gastro-intestinal

Dyspepsia, peptic ulceration with perforation and haemorrhage, acute pancreatitis, candidiasis. Abdominal distension and vomiting. Ulcerative oesophagitis.

Dermatological

Impaired wound healing, thin fragile skin, petechiae and ecchymoses, erythema, striae, telangiectasia, acne, increased sweating, suppressed reaction to skin tests, other cutaneous reactions such as allergic dermatitis, urticaria, angioneurotic oedema.

Ophthalmic

Posterior subcapsular cataracts, increased intra-ocular pressure, glaucoma, papilloedema, corneal or scleral thinning, exacerbation of ophthalmic viral or fungal diseases, exopthalmos.

Cardiovascular

Myocardial rupture following recent myocardial infarction.

Anti-inflammatory and immunosuppressive effects

Increased susceptibility and severity of infections with suppression of clinical symptoms and signs, opportunistic infections, recurrence of dormant tuberculosis.

Endocrine/metabolic

Menstrual irregularities and amenorrhoea, suppression of the hypothalamic-pituitary-adrenal axis, growth suppression in children and adolescents, premature epiphyseal closure, development of Cushingoid state, hirsutism, weight gain, impaired carbohydrate tolerance with increased requirement for anti-diabetic therapy. Negative protein and calcium balance.

Neurological

Convulsions and aggravation of epilepsy, vertigo, headache, increased intra-cranial pressure with papilloedema in children (Pseudotumour cerebri), usually after treatment withdrawal, psychological dependence, depression, insomnia, aggravation of schizophrenia and psychic disturbances ranging from euphoria to frank psychotic manifestations.

General

Hypersensitivity including anaphylaxis has been reported. Leucocytosis, thromboembolism, increased appetite, nausea, malaise, hiccups.

Withdrawal symptoms and signs

Too rapid a reduction of corticosteroid dosage following prolonged treatment can lead to acute adrenal insufficiency, hypotension and death (See 'Special Warnings and Precautions').

A 'withdrawal syndrome' may also occur including fever, myalgia, arthralgia, rhinitis, conjunctivitis, painful itchy skin nodules and loss of weight.

4.9 Overdose

Reports of acute toxicity and/or deaths following overdosage with glucocorticoids are rare. No antidote is available. Treatment is probably not indicated for reactions due to chronic poisoning unless the patient has a condition that would render him unusually susceptible to ill effects from corticosteroids. In this case, the stomach should be emptied and symptomatic treatment should be instituted as necessary. Anaphylactic and hypersensitivity reactions may be treated with epinephrine (adrenaline), positive-pressure artificial respiration and aminophylline. The patient should be kept warm and quiet. The biological half life of dexamethasone in plasma is about 190 minutes.

5. PHARMACOLOGICAL PROPERTIES

5.1 Pharmacodynamic properties

Dexamethasone is a highly potent and long-acting glucocorticoid with negligible sodium retaining properties and is therefore, particularly suitable for the use in patients with cardiac failure and hypertension. It's anti-inflammatory potency is 7 times greater than prednisolone and like other glucocorticoids, dexamethasone also has anti-allergic, antipyretic and immunosuppressive properties.

Dexamethasone has a biological half life of 36 - 54 hours and therefore is suitable in conditions where continuous glucocorticoid action is required.

5.2 Pharmacokinetic properties

Dexamethasone is well absorbed when given by mouth; peak plasma levels are reached between 1 and 2 hours after ingestion and show wide interindividual variations. The mean plasma half life is 3.6 ± 0.9h. Dexamethasone is bound (up to 77%) to plasma proteins. Percentage protein binding of dexamethasone, unlike that of cortisol, remains practically unchanged with increasing steroid concentrations. Corticosteroids are rapidly distributed to all body tissues. They cross the placenta and may be excreted in small amounts in breast milk. Corticosteroids are metabolised mainly in the liver but also in the kidney and are excreted in the urine.

5.3 Preclinical safety data

Dexamethasone is a glucocorticoid which has been used clinically over 30 years and its clinical efficacy and safety are well published.

6. PHARMACEUTICAL PARTICULARS

6.1 List of excipients

Benzoic acid, propylene glycol, citric acid monohydrate, liquid maltitol, garden mint flavour (containing isopropanol and propylene glycol), sorbitol 70%, sodium citrate and purified water.

6.2 Incompatibilities

Not applicable.

6.3 Shelf life

24 months

3 months once open.

6.4 Special precautions for storage

Do not store above 25°C. Do not refrigerate.

6.5 Nature and contents of container

Bottles: Amber (Type III) glass.

Closures:

a) Aluminium, EPE wadded, roll-on pilfer-proof (ROPP) screw cap.

b) HDPE, EPE wadded, tamper evident screw cap.

c) HDPE, EPE wadded, tamper evident, child resistant closure.

6.6 Instructions for use and handling

Not applicable.

Administrative Data

7. MARKETING AUTHORISATION HOLDER

Rosemont Pharmaceuticals Ltd., Rosemont House, Yorkdale Industrial Park, Braithwaite Street, Leeds, LS11 9XE, UK.

8. MARKETING AUTHORISATION NUMBER(S)

PL 00427/0125

9. DATE OF FIRST AUTHORISATION/RENEWAL OF THE AUTHORISATION

14th April 2000.

10. DATE OF REVISION OF THE TEXT

June 2004

11. Legal Category

POM

Dextrose Injection BP 50%

(UCB Pharma Limited)

1. NAME OF THE MEDICINAL PRODUCT

Dextrose Injection BP 50%

2. QUALITATIVE AND QUANTITATIVE COMPOSITION

Anhydrous Glucose 50%w/v

3. PHARMACEUTICAL FORM

Sterile solution intended for parenteral use

4. CLINICAL PARTICULARS

4.1 Therapeutic indications

1. Treatment of carbohydrate and fluid depletion

2. Treatment of hypoglycaemia

4.2 Posology and method of administration

By the intravenous route only. Dextrose should be administered via a central venous vein, preferably using a catheter.

Treatment of Carbohydrate and Fluid Depletion

Non-diabetic adults (including the elderly) and children:

1 to 3 litres daily of 50% dextrose solution, administered at a rate not exceeding 3ml/minute.

Treatment of Hypoglycaemia

Adults (including the elderly):

20-50ml of 50% dextrose solution by slow injection. Repeated doses may be required in severe cases.

4.3 Contraindications

Dextrose 50% solution is contra-indicated in patients with anuria, intra-cranial or intra-spinal haemorrhage an in delirium tremens where there is dehydration.

4.4 Special warnings and special precautions for use

Changes in fluid balance, electrolyte concentrations and acid-base balance should be evaluated during prolonged therapy.

Dextrose injections or infusions should be used with caution in patients with overt or sub-clinical diabetes mellitus, carbohydrate intolerance, severe under-nutrition, thiamine deficiency, hypophosphataemia, haemodilution, sepsis, trauma, shock, metabolic acidosis and severe dehydration. Monitor blood glucose levels in diabetic patients.

4.5 Interaction with other medicinal products and other forms of Interaction

None known.

4.6 Pregnancy and lactation

Intravenous dextrose infusion to the mother may result in foetal insulin production and a risk of rebound hypoglycaemia in the neonate. Infusions of dextrose administered during Caesarian Section and labour should not exceed 5-10mg dextrose/hour.

4.7 Effects on ability to drive and use machines

None known.

4.8 Undesirable effects

Fever, phlebitis, extravasation, thrombosis, pain at site of injection.

A too rapid administration of dextrose injection may result in hyperglycaemia and glycosuria.

Sodium retention, oedema and heart failure may be induced in patients with severe under-nutrition. Wernicke's Encephalopathy may be induced in patients with thiamine deficiency unless thiamine is administered concurrently with the dextrose.

Fluid and electrolyte imbalances including oedema, hypokalaemia, hypomagnesaemia and hypophosphataemia.

4.9 Overdose

Accidental overdose will result in hyperglycaemia, fluid and electrolyte imbalances. Following overdose, administration of dextrose should be reduced or discontinued and electrolyte balance restored. Further dextrose administration should be undertaken with careful monitoring of blood glucose.

5. PHARMACOLOGICAL PROPERTIES

5.1 Pharmacodynamic properties

Dextrose is a natural sugar, whose presence in the blood is essential to life. It is transported into all living cells by facilitated diffusion.

5.2 Pharmacokinetic properties

After intravenous administration glucose goes through fast (approximately 20 minutes) and slow phases of equilibration. The mean volume of distribution has been shown to be 18.4 ±3.39L in healthy adults and 18 ±4.36 in diabetic adults. Dextrose is metabolised to carbon dioxide and water with the release of energy.

5.3 Preclinical safety data

Not applicable.

6. PHARMACEUTICAL PARTICULARS

6.1 List of excipients

Sodium hydroxide BP

Acetic acid BP

Water for Injections HSE

6.2 Incompatibilities

Dextrose solutions have been reported to be incompatible with the following drugs: cyanocobalamin, kanamycin sulphate, novobiocin sodium and warfarin sodium.

Dextrose solution should not be combined with blood transfusion as clumping of the red blood cells may occur.

6.3 Shelf life

36 months

6.4 Special precautions for storage

Store below 25°C.

6.5 Nature and contents of container

25mL × 10 Type I neutral glass ampoules.

50mL × 10 Type I neutral glass ampoules

Not all pack sizes may be marketed.

6.6 Instructions for use and handling

The product should be stored below 25°C. Do not use the product after the expiry date on the label. Keep out of the reach of children.

Administrative Data

7. MARKETING AUTHORISATION HOLDER

Celltech Pharmaceuticals Limited

208 Bath Road

Slough

Berkshire

SL1 3 WE

UK

8. MARKETING AUTHORISATION NUMBER(S)

PL 00039/5661R

9. DATE OF FIRST AUTHORISATION/RENEWAL OF THE AUTHORISATION

16 August 1993

10. DATE OF REVISION OF THE TEXT

March 2001

POM

DHC Continus prolonged release tablets 60mg, 90mg, and 120mg

(Napp Pharmaceuticals Limited)

1. NAME OF THE MEDICINAL PRODUCT

DHC® CONTINUS® prolonged release tablets 60 mg, 90 mg, 120 mg.

2. QUALITATIVE AND QUANTITATIVE COMPOSITION

Dihydrocodeine tartrate 60 mg, 90 mg, 120 mg.

3. PHARMACEUTICAL FORM

Prolonged release tablet.

White capsule shaped tablets, 60 mg are marked DHC 60, 90 mg are marked DHC 90 and 120 mg are marked DHC 120.

4. CLINICAL PARTICULARS

4.1 Therapeutic indications

For the relief of severe pain in cancer and other chronic conditions.

4.2 Posology and method of administration

Adults and children over 12 years: 60 mg - 120 mg every 12 hours.

Elderly: Dosage should be reduced.

Children 12 years or under: Not recommended.

Method of administration

Oral

4.3 Contraindications

Hypersensitivity to dihydrocodeine or any of the tablet constituents; respiratory depression; obstructive airways disease; paralytic ileus; head injury; raised intracranial pressure; acute alcoholism. As dihydrocodeine may cause the release of histamine, it should not be given during an asthma attack and should be given with caution to asthmatics.

Patients with rare hereditary problems of galactose intolerance, the Lapp lactase deficiency or glucose-galactose malabsorption should not take this medicine.

4.4 Special warnings and special precautions for use

Dosage should be reduced in the elderly, in hypothyroidism, chronic hepatic disease and renal insufficiency.

Dihydrocodeine should be administered with caution to patients with a history of opioid abuse, biliary tract disorders, prostatic hypertrophy, pancreatitis and severe cor pulmonale.

Dihydrocodeine has a recognised abuse and addiction profile similar to other opioids. Tolerance to analgesic effects may develop upon repeated administration.

DHC CONTINUS tablets must be swallowed whole, and not broken, chewed or crushed. The administration of broken, chewed or crushed tablets may lead to a rapid release and absorption of a potential overdose of dihydrocodeine (see Section 4.9).

4.5 Interaction with other medicinal products and other forms of Interaction

Other central nervous system depressants, including sedatives or hypnotics, phenothiazines, other tranquillisers and alcohol, may result in respiratory depression or sedation. Dihydrocodeine should be used with caution in patients taking monoamine oxidase inhibitors or within two weeks of such therapy.

4.6 Pregnancy and lactation

There is little published evidence on safety in human pregnancy but dihydrocodeine has been used for many years without apparent ill effects. Dihydrocodeine has not been reported to be excreted in breast milk. However, it is advisable that dihydrocodeine only be administered to breast-feeding mothers if considered essential.

4.7 Effects on ability to drive and use machines

Dihydrocodeine may cause drowsiness and, if affected, patients should not drive or operate machinery.

4.8 Undesirable effects

Common adverse drug reactions seen during therapy are constipation, nausea, vomiting, headache, somnolence, pruritus and rash. Uncommon adverse reactions are urinary retention, ureteric or biliary spasm, dry mouth, mood changes, blurred vision, sweating, decreased libido, flushing, abdominal pain, hypotension, paraesthesia, confusion, dizziness, hallucinations, urticaria, paralytic ileus and respiratory depression. Tolerance and dependence may occur.

4.9 Overdose

Acute overdosage with dihydrocodeine can be manifested by somnolence progressing to stupor or coma, miotic pupils, rhabdomyolysis, non-cardiac pulmonary oedema, bradycardia, hypotension and respiratory depression or apnoea.

Primary attention should be given to the establishment of a patent airway and institution of assisted or controlled ventilation.

In the case of massive overdosage, administer naloxone intravenously (0.4 to 2 mg for an adult and 0.01 mg/kg body weight for children) if the patient is in a coma or respiratory depression is present. Repeat the dose at 2 minute intervals if there is no response, or by an infusion. An infusion of 60% of the initial dose per hour is a useful starting point. A solution of 10 mg made up in 50 ml dextrose will produce 200 micrograms/ml for infusion using an IV pump (dose adjusted to the clinical response). Infusions are not a substitute for frequent review of the patient's clinical state. Intramuscular naloxone is an alternative in the event that IV access is not possible.

As the duration of action of naloxone is relatively short, the patient must be carefully monitored until spontaneous respiration is reliably re-established. Naloxone is a competitive antagonist and large doses (4 mg) may be required in seriously poisoned patients. For less severe overdosage, administer naloxone 0.2 mg intravenously followed by increments of 0.1 mg every 2 minutes if required.

Naloxone should not be administered in the absence of clinically significant respiratory or circulatory depression secondary to dihydrocodeine overdosage. Naloxone should be administered cautiously to persons who are known, or suspected, to be physically dependent on dihydrocodeine. In such cases, an abrupt or complete reversal of opioid effects may precipitate pain and an acute withdrawal syndrome.

Additional/other considerations:

- Consider activated charcoal (50 g for adults, 10-15 g for children), if a substantial amount has been ingested within 1 hour, provided the airway can be protected. It may be reasonable to assume that late administration of activated charcoal may be beneficial for prolonged release preparations but there is no evidence to support this.
- DHC CONTINUS tablets will continue to release and add to the dihydrocodeine load for up to 12 hours after administration and the management of overdosage should be modified accordingly. Gastric contents may therefore need to be emptied, as this can be useful in removing unabsorbed drug, particularly when a prolonged release formulation has been taken.

5. PHARMACOLOGICAL PROPERTIES

5.1 Pharmacodynamic properties

Dihydrocodeine is a semisynthetic narcotic analgesic with a potency between morphine and codeine. It acts on opioid receptors in the brain to reduce the patient's perception of pain and improve the psychological reaction to pain by reducing the associated anxiety.

5.2 Pharmacokinetic properties

Dihydrocodeine is well absorbed from the gastrointestinal tract following administration of DHC CONTINUS tablets and plasma levels are maintained throughout the twelve hour dosing interval.

Like other phenanthrene derivatives, dihydrocodeine is mainly metabolised in the liver with the resultant metabolites being excreted mainly in the urine. Metabolism of dihydrocodeine includes o-demethylation, n-demethylation and 6-keto reduction.

5.3 Preclinical safety data

There are no pre-clinical data of relevance to the prescriber which are additional to that already included in other sections of the SPC.

6. PHARMACEUTICAL PARTICULARS

6.1 List of excipients

Lactose (anhydrous)

Hydroxyethylcellulose

Cetostearyl Alcohol

Magnesium Stearate

Purified Talc

Purified Water

6.2 Incompatibilities

None known.

6.3 Shelf life

Three years.

6.4 Special precautions for storage

Do not store above 25°C.

6.5 Nature and contents of container

Polypropylene containers with polyethylene lids containing 56 tablets.

6.6 Instructions for use and handling

None stated.

Administrative Data

7. MARKETING AUTHORISATION HOLDER

Napp Pharmaceuticals Limited

Cambridge Science Park

Milton Road

Cambridge CB4 0GW

8. MARKETING AUTHORISATION NUMBER(S)

PL 16950/0019-0021

9. DATE OF FIRST AUTHORISATION/RENEWAL OF THE AUTHORISATION

60 mg -5.11.86/5.3.2001

90 mg and 120 mg -12.7.90/5.3.2001

10. DATE OF REVISION OF THE TEXT

April 2005

Legal Category

POM

® The Napp device, DHC and DHC CONTINUS are Registered Trade Marks

Diamicron

(Servier Laboratories Limited)

1. NAME OF THE MEDICINAL PRODUCT

DIAMICRON®

2. QUALITATIVE AND QUANTITATIVE COMPOSITION

Gliclazide 80 mg

3. PHARMACEUTICAL FORM

Tablets.

4. CLINICAL PARTICULARS

4.1 Therapeutic indications

Non insulin dependent diabetes mellitus.

4.2 Posology and method of administration

Oral administration.

Adults: The total daily dose may vary from 40 to 320 mg taken orally. The dose should be adjusted according to the individual patient's response, commencing with 40-80 mg daily (1/2 - 1 tablet) and increasing until adequate control is achieved. A single dose should not exceed 160 mg (2 tablets). When higher doses are required, DIAMICRON® should be taken twice daily and according to the main meals of the day.

In obese patients or those not showing adequate response to DIAMICRON® alone, additional therapy may be required.

Elderly: Plasma clearance of gliclazide is not altered in the elderly and steady state plasma levels can therefore be expected to be similar to those in adults under 65 years. Clinical experience in the elderly to date shows that DIAMICRON® is effective and well tolerated. Care should be exercised, however, when prescribing sulphonylureas in the elderly due to a possible age-related increased risk of hypoglycaemia.

Children: DIAMICRON® as with other sulphonylureas, is not indicated for the treatment of juvenile onset diabetes mellitus.

4.3 Contraindications

DIAMICRON® should not be used in:

- Juvenile onset diabetes.
- Diabetes complicated by ketosis and acidosis.
- Pregnancy.
- Diabetics undergoing surgery, after severe trauma or during infections.
- Patients known to have hypersensitivity to other sulphonylureas and related drugs.
- Diabetic pre-coma and coma.
- Severe renal or hepatic insufficiency.

4.4 Special warnings and special precautions for use

Hypoglycaemia: all sulphonylurea drugs are capable of producing moderate or severe hypoglycaemia, particularly in the following conditions:

- in patients controlled by diet alone,
- in cases of accidental overdose,
- when calorie or glucose intake is deficient,
- in patients with hepatic and/or renal impairment; however, in long-term clinical trials, patients with renal insufficiency have been treated satisfactorily, using DIAMICRON® at reduced doses.

In order to reduce the risk of hypoglycaemia it is therefore recommended:

- to initiate treatment for non-insulin dependent diabetics by diet alone, if this is possible,

- to take into account the age of the patient: blood sugar levels not strictly controlled by diet alone might be acceptable in the elderly,

- to adjust the dose of DIAMICRON® according to the blood glucose response and to the 24 hour urinary glucose during the first days of treatment.

Dosage adjustments may be necessary:

- on the occurrence of mild symptoms of hypoglycaemia (sweating, pallor, hunger pangs, tachycardia, sensation of malaise). Such findings should be treated with oral glucose and adjustments made in drug dosage and/or meal patterns,

- on the occurrence of severe hypoglycaemic reactions (coma or neurological impairment, see overdose),

- loss of control of blood glucose (hyperglycaemia). When a patient stabilised on any diabetic regimen is exposed to stress such as fever, trauma, infection or surgery, a loss of control may occur. At such times, it may be necessary to increase progressively the dosage of DIAMICRON® and if this is insufficient, to discontinue the treatment with DIAMICRON® and to administer insulin. As with other sulphonylureas, hypoglycaemia will occur if the patients' dietary intake is reduced or if they are receiving a larger dose of DIAMICRON® than required.

Care should be exercised in patients with hepatic and/or renal impairment and a small starting dose should be used with careful patient monitoring.

4.5 Interaction with other medicinal products and other forms of Interaction

Care should be taken when giving DIAMICRON® with drugs which are known to alter the diabetic state or potentiate the drug's action.

The hypoglycaemic effect of DIAMICRON® may be potentiated by phenylbutazone, salicylates, sulphonamides, coumarin derivatives, MAOIs, beta adrenergic blocking agents, tetracycline compounds, chloramphenicol, clofibrate, disopyramide, miconazole (oral forms) and cimetidine.

It may be diminished by corticosteroids, oral contraceptives, thiazide diuretics, phenothiazine derivatives, thyroid hormones and abuse of laxatives.

4.6 Pregnancy and lactation

Pregnancy: See "Contra-indications".

Lactation: It has not been established whether gliclazide is transferred to human milk. However, other sulphonylureas have been found in milk and there is no evidence to suggest that gliclazide differs from the group in this respect.

4.7 Effects on ability to drive and use machines

Patients should be informed that their concentration may be affected if their diabetes is not satisfactorily controlled, especially at the beginning of treatment (see special warnings and precautions).

4.8 Undesirable effects

- Hypoglycaemia (see special warnings and precautions).

- Abnormalities of hepatic function are not uncommon during DIAMICRON® therapy. There are rare reports of hepatic failure, hepatitis and jaundice following treatment with DIAMICRON®.

- Mild gastro-intestinal disturbances including nausea, dyspepsia, diarrhoea, constipation have been reported but this type of adverse reaction can be avoided if DIAMICRON® is taken during a meal.

- Skin reactions including rash, pruritus, erythema, bullous eruption; blood dyscrasia including anaemia, leukopenia, thrombocytopenia and granulocytopenia have been observed during treatment with DIAMICRON® but are not known to be directly attributable to the drug.

4.9 Overdose

The symptom to be expected of overdose would be hypoglycaemia. The treatment is gastric lavage and correction of the hypoglycaemia by appropriate means with continual monitoring of the patient's blood sugar until the effect of the drug has ceased.

5. PHARMACOLOGICAL PROPERTIES

5.1 Pharmacodynamic properties

Gliclazide is a hypoglycaemic sulphonylurea differing from other related compounds by the addition of an azabicyclo-octane ring.

In man, apart from having similar hypoglycaemic effect to the other sulphonylureas, gliclazide has been shown to reduce platelet adhesiveness and aggregation and increase fibrinolytic activity. These factors are thought to be implicated in the pathogenesis of long-term complications of diabetes mellitus.

Gliclazide primarily enhances the first phase of insulin secretion, but also to a lesser degree its second phase. Both phases are diminished in non-insulin dependent diabetes mellitus.

5.2 Pharmacokinetic properties

The drug is well absorbed and its half-life in man is approximately 10-12 hours. Gliclazide is metabolised in the liver; less than 5% of the dose is excreted unchanged in the urine.

5.3 Preclinical safety data

No findings in the preclinical testing which could be of relevance for the prescriber.

6. PHARMACEUTICAL PARTICULARS

6.1 List of excipients

Lactose monohydrate, maize starch, pregelatinised maize starch, talc, magnesium stearate.

6.2 Incompatibilities

None

6.3 Shelf life

5 years

6.4 Special precautions for storage

None

6.5 Nature and contents of container

Blister strip (PVC/Aluminium) of 20 tablets. 3 strips per carton.

Blister strip (PVC/Aluminium) of 28 tablets. 1 strip per carton.

Blister strip (PVC/Aluminium) of 28 tablets. 2 strips per carton.

Blister strip (PVC/Aluminium) of 28 tablets. 4 strips per carton.

6.6 Instructions for use and handling

Not applicable.

7. MARKETING AUTHORISATION HOLDER

Servier Laboratories Limited
Gallions, Wexham Springs,
Framewood Road, Wexham
Slough
SL3 6RJ

8. MARKETING AUTHORISATION NUMBER(S)

PL 0093/0024

9. DATE OF FIRST AUTHORISATION/RENEWAL OF THE AUTHORISATION

21 December 1979

10. DATE OF REVISION OF THE TEXT

5 July 2005

Diamicron 30 mg MR

(Servier Laboratories Limited)

1. NAME OF THE MEDICINAL PRODUCT

DIAMICRON 30 mg MR

2. QUALITATIVE AND QUANTITATIVE COMPOSITION

One tablet contains gliclazide 30 mg.

3. PHARMACEUTICAL FORM

Modified release tablet.

White, oblong tablet engraved on both faces, 'DIA 30' on one face and on the other.

4. CLINICAL PARTICULARS

4.1 Therapeutic indications

Non insulin-dependent diabetes (type 2) in adults when dietary measures, physical exercise and weight loss alone are not sufficient to control blood glucose.

4.2 Posology and method of administration

Oral use.

For adult use only.

The daily dose may vary between 1 and 4 tablets per day, *i.e.* from 30 to 120 mg taken orally, once daily.

It is recommended that the tablet(s) be taken at breakfast time.

If a dose is forgotten, there must be no increase in the dose taken the next day.

As with any hypoglycaemic agent, the dose should be adjusted according to the individual patient's metabolic response (blood glucose, HbA_{1C}).

Initial dose

The recommended starting dose is 30 mg daily.

If blood glucose is effectively controlled, this dose may be used for maintenance treatment.

If blood glucose is not adequately controlled, the dose may be increased to 60, 90 or 120 mg daily, in successive steps. The interval between each dose increment should be at least 1 month except in patients whose blood glucose has not reduced after two weeks of treatment. In such cases, the dose may be increased at the end of the second week of treatment.

The maximum recommended daily dose is 120 mg.

Switching from Diamicron 80 mg tablets to Diamicron 30 mg modified release tablets:

1 tablet of Diamicron 80 mg is comparable to 1 tablet of Diamicron 30 mg MR. Consequently the switch can be performed provided a careful blood monitoring is carried out.

Switching from another oral antidiabetic agent to Diamicron 30 mg MR:

Diamicron 30 mg MR can be used to replace other oral antidiabetic agents.

The dosage and the half-life of the previous antidiabetic agent should be taken into account when switching to Diamicron 30 mg MR.

A transitional period is not generally necessary. A starting dose of 30 mg should be used and this should be adjusted to suit the patient's blood glucose response, as described above.

When switching from a hypoglycaemic sulphonylurea with a prolonged half-life, a treatment free period of a few days may be necessary to avoid an additive effect of the two products, which might cause hypoglycaemia. The procedure described for initiating treatment should also be used when switching to treatment with Diamicron 30 mg MR, *i.e.* a starting dose of 30 mg/day, followed by a stepwise increase in dose, depending on the metabolic response.

Combination treatment with other antidiabetic agents:

Diamicron 30 mg MR can be given in combination with biguanides, alpha glucosidase inhibitors or insulin.

In patients not adequately controlled with Diamicron 30 mg MR, concomitant insulin therapy can be initiated under close medical supervision.

In the elderly (over 65).

Diamicron 30 mg MR should be prescribed using the same dosing regimen recommended for patients under 65 years of age. In patients with mild to moderate renal insufficiency the same dosing regimen can be used as in patients with normal renal function with careful patient monitoring. These data have been confirmed in clinical trials.

- In patients at risk of hypoglycaemia:

- undernourished or malnourished,

- severe or poorly compensated endocrine disorders (hypopituitarism, hypothyroidism, adrenocorticotrophic insufficiency),

- withdrawal of prolonged and/or high dose corticosteroid therapy,

- severe vascular disease (severe coronary heart disease, severe carotid impairment, diffuse vascular disease);

It is recommended that the minimum daily starting dose of 30 mg is used.

There are no data and clinical studies available in children.

4.3 Contraindications

- known hypersensitivity to gliclazide or to any of the excipients, other sulphonylureas, sulphonamides,
- type 1 diabetes,
- diabetic pre-coma and coma, diabetic keto-acidosis,
- severe renal or hepatic insufficiency: in these cases the use of insulin is recommended,
- treatment with miconazole (see Section "Interactions with other medicinal products and other forms of interaction"),
- lactation (see Section "Pregnancy and lactation").

4.4 Special warnings and special precautions for use

HYPOGLYCAEMIA

This treatment should be prescribed only if the patient is likely to have a regular food intake (including breakfast). It is important to have a regular carbohydrate intake due to the increased risk of hypoglycaemia if a meal is taken late, if an inadequate amount of food is consumed or if the food is low in carbohydrate. Hypoglycaemia is more likely to occur during low-calorie diets, following prolonged or strenuous exercise, alcohol intake or if a combination of hypoglycaemic agents is being used.

Hypoglycaemia may occur following administration of sulphonylureas (see 4.8. Undesirable effects). Some cases may be severe and prolonged. Hospitalisation may be necessary and glucose administration may need to be continued for several days.

Careful selection of patients, of the dose used, and clear patient directions are necessary to reduce the risk of hypoglycaemic episodes.

Factors which increase the risk of hypoglycaemia:

- patient refuses or (particularly in elderly subjects) is unable to co-operate,
- malnutrition, irregular mealtimes, skipping meals, periods of fasting or dietary changes,
- imbalance between physical exercise and carbohydrate intake,
- renal insufficiency,
- severe hepatic insufficiency,
- overdose of Diamicron 30 mg MR,
- certain endocrine disorders: thyroid disorders, hypopituitarism and adrenal insufficiency,
- concomitant administration of certain other medicines (see Interactions).

Renal and hepatic insufficiency: the pharmacokinetics and/or pharmacodynamics of gliclazide may be altered in patients with hepatic insufficiency or severe renal failure. A hypoglycaemic episode occurring in these patients may be prolonged, so appropriate management should be initiated.

Patient information:

The risks of hypoglycaemia, together with its symptoms, treatment, and conditions that predispose to its development, should be explained to the patient and to family members.

The patient should be informed of the importance of following dietary advice, of taking regular exercise, and of regular monitoring of blood glucose levels.

Poor blood glucose control:

Blood glucose control in a patient receiving antidiabetic treatment may be affected by any of the following: fever, trauma, infection or surgical intervention. In some cases, it may be necessary to administer insulin.

The hypoglycaemic efficacy of any oral antidiabetic agent, including gliclazide, is attenuated over time in many patients: this may be due to progression in the severity of the diabetes, or to a reduced response to treatment. This phenomenon is known as secondary failure which is distinct from primary failure, when an active substance is ineffective as first-line treatment. Adequate dose adjustment and dietary compliance should be considered before classifying the patient as secondary failure.

Laboratory tests: Measurement of glycated haemoglobin levels (or fasting venous plasma glucose) is recommended in assessing blood glucose control. Blood glucose self-monitoring may also be useful.

4.5 Interaction with other medicinal products and other forms of Interaction

The following products are likely to increase the risk of hypoglycaemia:

Contra-indicated combination

• Miconazole (systemic route, oromucosal gel): increases the hypoglycaemic effect with possible onset of hypoglycaemic symptoms, or even coma.

Combinations which are not recommended

• Phenylbutazone (systemic route): increases the hypoglycaemic effect of sulphonylureas (displaces their binding to plasma proteins and/or reduces their elimination).

It is preferable to use a different anti-inflammatory agent, or else to warn the patient and emphasise the importance of self-monitoring. Where necessary, adjust the dose during and after treatment with the anti-inflammatory agent.

• Alcohol: increases the hypoglycaemic reaction (by inhibiting compensatory reactions) that can lead to the onset of hypoglycaemic coma.

Avoid alcohol or medicines containing alcohol.

Combinations requiring precautions for use

Potentiation of the blood glucose lowering effect and thus, in some instances, hypoglycaemia may occur when one of the following drugs is taken, for example:

Other antidiabetic agents (insulins, acarbose, biguanides), beta-blockers, fluconazole, angiotensin converting enzyme inhibitors (captopril, enalapril), H2-receptor antagonists, MAOIs, sulphonamides, and nonsteroidal anti-inflammatory agents.

The following products may cause an increase in blood glucose levels:

Combination which is not recommended

• Danazol: diabetogenic effect of danazol.

If the use of this active substance cannot be avoided, warn the patient and emphasise the importance of urine and blood glucose monitoring. It may be necessary to adjust the dose of the antidiabetic agent during and after treatment with danazol.

Combinations requiring precautions during use

• Chlorpromazine (neuroleptic agent): high doses >100 mg per day of chlorpromazine) increase blood glucose levels (reduced insulin release).

Warn the patient and emphasise the importance of blood glucose monitoring. It may be necessary to adjust the dose of the antidiabetic active substance during and after treatment with the neuroleptic agent.

• Glucocorticoids (systemic and local route: intra-articular, cutaneous and rectal preparations) and tetracosactrin: increase in blood glucose levels with possible ketosis (reduced tolerance to carbohydrates due to glucocorticoids).

Warn the patient and emphasise the importance of blood glucose monitoring, particularly at the start of treatment. It may be necessary to adjust the dose of the antidiabetic active substance during and after treatment with glucocorticoids.

• Ritodrine, salbutamol, terbutaline: (I.V.)

Increased blood glucose levels due to beta-2 agonist effects.

Emphasise the importance of monitoring blood glucose levels. If necessary, switch to insulin.

Combination which must be taken into account

• Anticoagulant therapy (Warfarin.):

Sulphonylureas may lead to potentiation of anticoagulation during concurrent treatment.

Adjustment of the anticoagulant may be necessary.

4.6 Pregnancy and lactation

Pregnancy

There is no experience with the use of gliclazide during pregnancy in humans, even though there are few data with other sulphonylureas.

In animal studies, gliclazide is not teratogenic.

Control of diabetes should be obtained before the time of conception to reduce the risk of congenital abnormalities linked to uncontrolled diabetes.

Oral hypoglycaemic agents are not suitable, insulin is the drug of first choice for treatment of diabetes during pregnancy. It is recommended that oral hypoglycaemic therapy is changed to insulin before a pregnancy is attempted, or as soon as pregnancy is discovered.

Lactation

It is not known whether gliclazide or its metabolites are excreted in breast milk. Given the risk of neonatal hypoglycaemia, the product is contra-indicated in breastfeeding mothers.

4.7 Effects on ability to drive and use machines

Patients should be made aware of the symptoms of hypoglycaemia and should be careful if driving or operating machinery, especially at the beginning of treatment.

4.8 Undesirable effects

Hypoglycaemia

As for other sulphonylureas, treatment with Diamicron 30 mg MR can cause hypoglycaemia, if mealtimes are irregular and, in particular, if meals are skipped. Possible symptoms of hypoglycaemia are: headache, intense hunger, nausea, vomiting, lassitude, drowsiness, sleep disorders, agitation, aggression, poor concentration, reduced awareness and slowed reactions, depression, confusion, visual and speech disorders, aphasia, tremor, paresis, sensory disorders, dizziness, feeling of powerlessness, loss of self-control, delirium, convulsions, shallow respiration, bradycardia, drowsiness and loss of consciousness, possibly resulting in coma and lethal outcome.

In addition, signs of adrenergic counter-regulation may be observed: sweating, clammy skin, anxiety, tachycardia, hypertension, palpitations, angina pectoris and cardiac arrhythmia.

Usually, symptoms disappear after intake of carbohydrates (sugar). However, artificial sweeteners have no effect. Experience with other sulphonylureas shows that hypoglycaemia can recur even when measures prove effective initially.

If a hypoglycaemic episode is severe or prolonged, and even if it is temporarily controlled by intake of sugar, immediate medical treatment or even hospitalisation are required.

Gastrointestinal disturbances, including abdominal pain, nausea, vomiting, dyspepsia, diarrhoea, and constipation have been reported: if these should occur they can be avoided or minimised if gliclazide is taken with breakfast.

The following **undesirable effects** have been more rarely reported:

• Skin and subcutaneous tissue disorders: rash, pruritus, urticaria, erythema, maculopapular rashes, bullous reactions.

Allergic vasculitis has been reported in very rare cases for other sulphonylureas.

• Blood and lymphatic system disorders: Changes in haematology are rare. They may include anaemia, leucopenia, thrombocytopenia, granulocytopenia. These are in general reversible upon discontinuation of medication.

Rare cases of erythrocytopenia, agranulocytosis, haemolytic anaemia and pancytopenia have been described for other sulphonylureas.

• Hepato-biliary disorders: raised hepatic enzyme levels (AST, ALT, alkaline phosphatase), hepatitis (isolated reports). Discontinue treatment if cholestatic jaundice appears.

With other sulphonylureas rare cases were observed of elevated liver enzyme levels and even impairment of liver function (e.g. with cholestasis and jaundice) and hepatitis which regressed after withdrawal of the sulphonylurea or led to life-threatening liver failure in isolated cases.

These symptoms usually disappear after discontinuation of treatment.

• Eye disorders

Transient visual disturbances may occur especially on initiation of treatment, due to changes in blood glucose levels.

4.9 Overdose

An overdose of sulphonylureas may cause hypoglycaemia.

Moderate symptoms of hypoglycaemia, without any loss of consciousness or neurological signs, must be corrected by carbohydrate intake, dose adjustment and/or change of diet. Strict monitoring should be continued until the doctor is sure that the patient is out of danger.

Severe hypoglycaemic reactions, with coma, convulsions or other neurological disorders are possible and must be treated as a medical emergency, requiring immediate hospitalisation.

If hypoglycaemic coma is diagnosed or suspected, the patient should be given a rapid I.V. injection of 50 mL of concentrated glucose solution (20 to 30 %). This should be followed by continuous infusion of a more dilute glucose solution (10 %) at a rate that will maintain blood glucose levels above 1g/L. Patients should be monitored closely and, depending on the patient's condition after this time, the doctor will decide if further monitoring is necessary.

Dialysis is of no benefit to patients due to the strong binding of gliclazide to proteins.

5. PHARMACOLOGICAL PROPERTIES

5.1 Pharmacodynamic properties

HYPOGLYCAEMIC SULPHONYLUREA - ORAL BLOOD GLUCOSE LOWERING DRUG

(A10BB09: Alimentary tract and metabolism)

Gliclazide is a hypoglycaemic sulphonylurea oral antidiabetic active substance differing from other related compounds by an N-containing heterocyclic ring with an endocyclic bond.

Gliclazide reduces blood glucose levels by stimulating insulin secretion from the β-cells of the islets of Langerhans. Increase in postprandial insulin and C-peptide secretion persists after two years of treatment.

In addition to these metabolic properties, gliclazide has haemovascular properties.

Effects on insulin release

In type 2 diabetics, gliclazide restores the first peak of insulin secretion in response to glucose and increases the second phase of insulin secretion. A significant increase in insulin response is seen in response to stimulation induced by a meal or glucose.

Haemovascular properties:

Gliclazide decreases microthrombosis by two mechanisms which may be involved in complications of diabetes:

• a partial inhibition of platelet aggregation and adhesion, with a decrease in the markers of platelet activation (beta thromboglobulin, thromboxane B_2).

• an action on the vascular endothelium fibrinolytic activity with an increase in tPA activity.

5.2 Pharmacokinetic properties

Plasma levels increase progressively during the first 6 hours, reaching a plateau which is maintained from the sixth to the twelfth hour after administration.

Intra-individual variability is low.

Gliclazide is completely absorbed. Food intake does not affect the rate or degree of absorption.

The relationship between the dose administered ranging up to 120 mg and the area under the concentration time curve is linear.

Plasma protein binding is approximately 95%.

Gliclazide is mainly metabolised in the liver and excreted in the urine: less than 1% of the unchanged form is found in the urine. No active metabolites have been detected in plasma.

The elimination half-life of gliclazide varies between 12 and 20 hours.

The volume of distribution is around 30 litres.

No clinically significant changes in pharmacokinetic parameters have been observed in elderly patients.

A single daily dose of Diamicron 30 mg MR maintains effective gliclazide plasma concentrations over 24 hours.

5.3 Preclinical safety data

Preclinical data reveal no special hazards for humans based on conventional studies of repeated dose toxicity and genotoxicity. Long term carcinogenicity studies have not been done. No teratogenic changes have been shown in animal studies, but lower foetal body weight was observed in animals receiving doses 25 fold higher than the maximum recommended dose in humans.

6. PHARMACEUTICAL PARTICULARS

6.1 List of excipients

Calcium hydrogen phosphate dihydrate, maltodextrin, hypromellose, magnesium stearate, anhydrous colloidal silica.

6.2 Incompatibilities

Not applicable.

6.3 Shelf life

3 years.

6.4 Special precautions for storage

Store in the original package.

6.5 Nature and contents of container

7, 10, 14, 20, 28, 30, 56, 60, 84, 90, 100, 112, 120, 180, or 500 tablets in blisters (PVC/Aluminium).

6.6 Instructions for use and handling

No special requirements.

7. MARKETING AUTHORISATION HOLDER

Les Laboratoires Servier

22 rue Garnier

92200 Neuilly-sur-Seine

France

8. MARKETING AUTHORISATION NUMBER(S)

PL 05815/0019

9. DATE OF FIRST AUTHORISATION/RENEWAL OF THE AUTHORISATION

7 December 2000

10. DATE OF REVISION OF THE TEXT

July 2002

Diamorphine Injection BP 100mg

(Wockhardt UK Ltd)

1. NAME OF THE MEDICINAL PRODUCT
Diamorphine Hydrochloride 100mg for Injection BP

2. QUALITATIVE AND QUANTITATIVE COMPOSITION
Each ampoule contains 100mg of Diamorphine Hydrochloride BP.

3. PHARMACEUTICAL FORM
A white to off-white, sterile, freeze dried powder of Diamorphine Hydrochloride BP for reconstitution for injection.

4. CLINICAL PARTICULARS
4.1 Therapeutic indications
Diamorphine may be used in the treatment of severe pain associated with surgical procedures, myocardial infarction or pain in the terminally ill and for the relief of dyspnoea in acute pulmonary oedema.

4.2 Posology and method of administration
Diamorphine may be given by the intramuscular, intravenous or subcutaneous routes. Glucose intravenous infusion is the preferred diluent, particularly when the drug is administered by a continuous infusion pump over 24 to 48 hours, although it is also compatible with sodium chloride intravenous infusion.

The dose should be suited to the individual patient.

Adults:

Acute pain, 5mg repeated every four hours if necessary (up to 10mg for heavier, well muscled patients) by subcutaneous or intramuscular injection. By slow intravenous injection, one quarter to one half the corresponding intramuscular dose.

Chronic pain, 5-10mg regularly every four hours by subcutaneous or intramuscular injection. The dose may be increased according to individual needs.

Myocardial infarction, 5mg by slow intravenous injection (1mg/minute) followed by a further 2.5mg to 5mg if necessary.

Acute pulmonary oedema, 2.5mg to 5mg by slow intravenous injection (1mg/minute).

Children and Elderly:

As diamorphine has a respiratory depressant effect, care should be taken when giving the drug to the very young and the elderly and a lower starting dose than normal is recommended.

4.3 Contraindications
Respiratory depression and obstructive airways disease.

Phaeochromocytoma (endogenous release of histamine may stimulate catecholamine release).

Raised intracranial pressure.

Concurrent use of monoamine oxidase inhibitors or within two weeks of their discontinuation.

4.4 Special warnings and special precautions for use
Diamorphine should be administered with care to patients with head injuries as there is an increased risk of respiratory depression which may lead to elevation of CSF pressure. The sedation and pupillary changes produced may interfere with accurate monitoring of the patient.

Repeated administration of diamorphine may lead to dependence and tolerance developing. Abrupt withdrawal in patients who have developed dependence may precipitate a withdrawal syndrome. Great caution should be exercised in patients with a known tendency or history of drug abuse.

Use with caution in patients with toxic psychosis, CNS depression, myxoedema, prostatic hypertrophy or urethral stricture, kyphoscoliosis, acute alcoholism, delirium tremens, severe inflammatory or obstructive bowel disorders, adrenal insufficiency or severe diarrhoea. Care should be exercised in treating the elderly or debilitated patients and those with hepatic or renal impairment.

4.5 Interaction with other medicinal products and other forms of Interaction
The depressant effects of diamorphine may be exaggerated and prolonged by phenothiazines, monoamine oxidase inhibitors, tricyclic antidepressants, anxiolytics and hypnotics. There may be antagonism of the gastrointestinal effects of cisapride, domperidone and metoclopramide. The risk of severe constipation and/or urinary retention is increased by administration of antimuscarinic drugs (e.g. atropine). There may be increased risk of toxicity with 4-quinolone antibacterials.

Alcohol may enhance the sedative and hypotensive effects of diamorphine.

Cimetidine inhibits metabolism of opioid analgesics.

Hyperpyrexia and CNS toxicity have been reported when opioid analgesics are used with selegiline.

4.6 Pregnancy and lactation
Safety has not been established in pregnancy.

Administration during labour may cause respiratory depression in the neonate and gastric stasis during labour, increasing the risk of inhalation pneumonia.

Diamorphine should not be given to women who are breast-feeding as there is limited information available on diamorphine in breast milk.

4.7 Effects on ability to drive and use machines
Diamorphine causes drowsiness and mental clouding. If affected patients should not drive or use machines.

4.8 Undesirable effects
The most serious hazard of therapy is respiratory depression although circulatory depression is also possible. The most common side effects are sedation, nausea and vomiting, constipation and sweating. Other side effects include dizziness, miosis, confusion, urinary retention, biliary spasm, orthostatic hypotension, facial flushing, vertigo, palpitations, mood changes, dry mouth, dependence, urticaria, pruritus and raised intracranial pressure.

4.9 Overdose
a) Symptoms

Respiratory depression, pulmonary oedema, muscle flaccidity, coma or stupor, constricted pupils, cold, clammy skin and occasionally bradycardia and hypotension.

b) Treatment

Respiration and circulation should be maintained and naloxone is indicated if coma or bradypnoea are present. A dose of 0.4 to 2mg repeated at intervals of two to three minutes (up to 10mg) may be given by subcutaneous, intramuscular or intravenous injection. The usual initial dosage for children is 10 micrograms per kg body weight. Naloxone may also be given by continuous intravenous infusion, 2mg diluted in 500ml, at a rate adjusted to the patient's response. Oxygen and assisted ventilation should be administered if necessary.

5. PHARMACOLOGICAL PROPERTIES
5.1 Pharmacodynamic properties
Diamorphine is a narcotic analgesic which acts primarily on the central nervous system and smooth muscle. It is predominantly a central nervous system depressant but it has stimulant actions resulting in nausea, vomiting and miosis.

5.2 Pharmacokinetic properties
Diamorphine is a potent opiate analgesic which has a more rapid onset of activity than morphine as the first metabolite, monoacetylmorphine, more readily crosses the blood brain barrier. In man, diamorphine has a half life of two to three minutes. Its first metabolite, monoacetylmorphine, is more slowly hydrolysed in the blood to be concentrated mainly in skeletal muscle, kidney, lung, liver and spleen. Monoacetylmorphine is metabolised to morphine. Morphine forms conjugates with glucuronic acid. The majority of the drug is excreted via the kidney as glucuronides and to a much lesser extent as morphine. About 7-10% is eliminated via the biliary system into the faeces.

Diamorphine does not bind to protein. However, morphine is about 35% bound to human plasma proteins, mainly to albumin. The analgesic effect lasts approximately three to four hours.

5.3 Preclinical safety data
There are no additional pre-clinical data of relevance to the prescriber.

6. PHARMACEUTICAL PARTICULARS
6.1 List of excipients
Water for Injections BP*

Not detectable in the finished product.

6.2 Incompatibilities
Physical incompatibility has been reported with mineral acids and alkalis.

6.3 Shelf life
Three years from date of manufacture.

6.4 Special precautions for storage
Do not store above 25°C.

Keep container in the outer carton.

6.5 Nature and contents of container
5ml Neutral glass ampoules, PhEur. Type 1. Ampoules are packed into cartons of 5, 10 or 50.

6.6 Instructions for use and handling
The solution should be used immediately after preparation.

Administrative Data
7. MARKETING AUTHORISATION HOLDER
CP Pharmaceuticals Ltd
Ash Road North
Wrexham
LL13 9UF

8. MARKETING AUTHORISATION NUMBER(S)
4543/0306

9. DATE OF FIRST AUTHORISATION/RENEWAL OF THE AUTHORISATION
22/3/93

10. DATE OF REVISION OF THE TEXT
January 2001

Diamorphine Injection BP 10mg

(Wockhardt UK Ltd)

1. NAME OF THE MEDICINAL PRODUCT
Diamorphine Hydrochloride 10mg for Injection BP.

2. QUALITATIVE AND QUANTITATIVE COMPOSITION
Each ampoule contains 10mg of Diamorphine Hydrochloride BP.

3. PHARMACEUTICAL FORM
A white to off-white, sterile, freeze dried powder of Diamorphine Hydrochloride BP for reconstitution for injection.

4. CLINICAL PARTICULARS
4.1 Therapeutic indications
Diamorphine may be used in the treatment of severe pain associated with surgical procedures, myocardial infarction or pain in the terminally ill and for the relief of dyspnoea in acute pulmonary oedema.

4.2 Posology and method of administration
Diamorphine may be given by the intramuscular, intravenous or subcutaneous routes. Glucose intravenous infusion is the preferred diluent, particularly when the drug is administered by a continuous infusion pump over 24 to 48 hours, although it is also compatible with sodium chloride intravenous infusion.

The dose should be suited to the individual patient.

Adults:

Acute pain, 5mg repeated every four hours if necessary (up to 10mg for heavier, well muscled patients) by subcutaneous or intramuscular injection. By slow intravenous injection, one quarter to one half the corresponding intramuscular dose.

Chronic pain, 5-10mg regularly every four hours by subcutaneous or intramuscular injection. The dose may be increased according to individual needs.

Myocardial infarction, 5mg by slow intravenous injection (1mg/minute) followed by a further 2.5mg to 5mg if necessary.

Acute pulmonary oedema, 2.5mg to 5mg by slow intravenous injection (1mg/minute).

Children and Elderly:

As diamorphine has a respiratory depressant effect, care should be taken when giving the drug to the very young and the elderly and a lower starting dose than normal is recommended.

4.3 Contraindications
Respiratory depression and obstructive airways disease.

Phaeochromocytoma (endogenous release of histamine may stimulate catecholamine release).

Raised intracranial pressure.

Concurrent use of monoamine oxidase inhibitors or within two weeks of their discontinuation.

4.4 Special warnings and special precautions for use
Diamorphine should be administered with care to patients with head injuries as there is an increased risk of respiratory depression which may lead to elevation of CSF pressure. The sedation and pupillary changes produced may interfere with accurate monitoring of the patient.

Repeated administration of diamorphine may lead to dependence and tolerance developing. Abrupt withdrawal in patients who have developed dependence may precipitate a withdrawal syndrome. Great caution should be exercised in patients with a known tendency or history of drug abuse.

Use with caution in patients with toxic psychosis, CNS depression, myxoedema, prostatic hypertrophy or urethral stricture, kyphoscoliosis, acute alcoholism, delirium tremens, severe inflammatory or obstructive bowel disorders, adrenal insufficiency or severe diarrhoea. Care should be exercised in treating the elderly or debilitated patients and those with hepatic or renal impairment.

4.5 Interaction with other medicinal products and other forms of Interaction
The depressant effects of diamorphine may be exaggerated and prolonged by phenothiazines, monoamine oxidase inhibitors, tricyclic antidepressants, anxiolytics and hypnotics. There may be antagonism of the gastrointestinal effects of cisapride, domperidone and metoclopramide. The risk of severe constipation and/or urinary retention is increased by administration of antimuscarinic drugs (e.g. atropine). There may be increased risk of toxicity with 4-quinolone antibacterials.

Alcohol may enhance the sedative and hypotensive effects of diamorphine.

Cimetidine inhibits metabolism of opioid analgesics.

Hyperpyrexia and CNS toxicity have been reported when opioid analgesics are used with selegiline.

4.6 Pregnancy and lactation
Safety has not been established in pregnancy.

Administration during labour may cause respiratory depression in the neonate and gastric stasis during labour, increasing the risk of inhalation pneumonia.

Diamorphine should not be given to women who are breast-feeding as there is limited information available on diamorphine in breast milk.

4.7 Effects on ability to drive and use machines
Diamorphine causes drowsiness and mental clouding. If affected patients should not drive or use machines.

4.8 Undesirable effects
The most serious hazard of therapy is respiratory depression although circulatory depression is also possible. The most common side effects are sedation, nausea and vomiting, constipation and sweating. Other side effects include dizziness, miosis, confusion, urinary retention, biliary spasm, orthostatic hypotension, facial flushing, vertigo, palpitations, mood changes, dry mouth, dependence, urticaria, pruritus and raised intracranial pressure.

4.9 Overdose
a) Symptoms

Respiratory depression, pulmonary oedema, muscle flaccidity, coma or stupor, constricted pupils, cold, clammy skin and occasionally bradycardia and hypotension.

b) Treatment

Respiration and circulation should be maintained and naloxone is indicated if coma or bradypnoea are present. A dose of 0.4 to 2mg repeated at intervals of two to three minutes (up to 10mg) may be given by subcutaneous, intramuscular or intravenous injection. The usual initial dosage for children is 10 micrograms per kg body weight. Naloxone may also be given by continuous intravenous infusion, 2mg diluted in 500ml, at a rate adjusted to the patient's response. Oxygen and assisted ventilation should be administered if necessary.

5. PHARMACOLOGICAL PROPERTIES
5.1 Pharmacodynamic properties
Diamorphine is a narcotic analgesic which acts primarily on the central nervous system and smooth muscle. It is predominantly a central nervous system depressant but it has stimulant actions resulting in nausea, vomiting and miosis.

5.2 Pharmacokinetic properties
Diamorphine is a potent opiate analgesic which has a more rapid onset of activity than morphine as the first metabolite, monoacetylmorphine, more readily crosses the blood brain barrier. In man, diamorphine has a half life of two to three minutes. Its first metabolite, monoacetylmorphine, is more slowly hydrolysed in the blood to be concentrated mainly in skeletal muscle, kidney, lung, liver and spleen. Monoacetylmorphine is metabolised to morphine. Morphine forms conjugates with glucuronic acid. The majority of the drug is excreted via the kidney as glucuronides and to a much lesser extent as morphine. About 7-10% is eliminated via the biliary system into the faeces.

Diamorphine does not bind to protein. However, morphine is about 35% bound to human plasma proteins, mainly to albumin. The analgesic effect lasts approximately three to four hours.

5.3 Preclinical safety data
There are no additional pre-clinical data of relevance to the prescriber.

6. PHARMACEUTICAL PARTICULARS
6.1 List of excipients
Water for Injections BP*

Not detectable in the finished product.

6.2 Incompatibilities
Physical incompatibility has been reported with mineral acids and alkalis.

6.3 Shelf life
Three years from date of manufacture

6.4 Special precautions for storage
Do not store above 25°C.

Keep container in the outer carton.

6.5 Nature and contents of container
2ml Neutral glass ampoules, PhEur. Type 1. Ampoules are packed into cartons of 5, 10 or 50.

6.6 Instructions for use and handling
The solution should be used immediately after preparation.

Administrative Data
7. MARKETING AUTHORISATION HOLDER
CP Pharmaceuticals Ltd

Ash Road North

Wrexham

LL13 9UF

8. MARKETING AUTHORISATION NUMBER(S)
4543/0304

9. DATE OF FIRST AUTHORISATION/RENEWAL OF THE AUTHORISATION
22/3/93

10. DATE OF REVISION OF THE TEXT
January 2001

Diamorphine Injection BP 30mg

(Wockhardt UK Ltd)

1. NAME OF THE MEDICINAL PRODUCT
Diamorphine Hydrochloride 30mg for Injection BP.

2. QUALITATIVE AND QUANTITATIVE COMPOSITION
Each ampoule contains 30mg of Diamorphine Hydrochloride BP.

3. PHARMACEUTICAL FORM
A white to off-white, sterile, freeze dried powder of Diamorphine Hydrochloride BP for reconstitution for injection.

4. CLINICAL PARTICULARS
4.1 Therapeutic indications
Diamorphine may be used in the treatment of severe pain associated with surgical procedures, myocardial infarction or pain in the terminally ill and for the relief of dyspnoea in acute pulmonary oedema.

4.2 Posology and method of administration
Diamorphine may be given by the intramuscular, intravenous or subcutaneous routes. Glucose intravenous infusion is the preferred diluent, particularly when the drug is administered by a continuous infusion pump over 24 to 48 hours, although it is also compatible with sodium chloride intravenous infusion.

The dose should be suited to the individual patient.

Adults:

Acute pain, 5mg repeated every four hours if necessary (up to 10mg for heavier, well muscled patients) by subcutaneous or intramuscular injection. By slow intravenous injection, one quarter to one half the corresponding intramuscular dose.

Chronic pain, 5-10mg regularly every four hours by subcutaneous or intramuscular injection. The dose may be increased according to individual needs.

Myocardial infarction, 5mg by slow intravenous injection (1mg/minute) followed by a further 2.5mg to 5mg if necessary.

Acute pulmonary oedema, 2.5mg to 5mg by slow intravenous injection (1mg/minute).

Children and Elderly:

As diamorphine has a respiratory depressant effect, care should be taken when giving the drug to the very young and the elderly and a lower starting dose than normal is recommended.

4.3 Contraindications
Respiratory depression and obstructive airways disease.

Phaeochromocytoma (endogenous release of histamine may stimulate catecholamine release).

Raised intracranial pressure.

Concurrent use of monoamine oxidase inhibitors or within two weeks of their discontinuation.

4.4 Special warnings and special precautions for use
Diamorphine should be administered with care to patients with head injuries as there is an increased risk of respiratory depression which may lead to elevation of CSF pressure. The sedation and pupillary changes produced may interfere with accurate monitoring of the patient.

Repeated administration of diamorphine may lead to dependence and tolerance developing. Abrupt withdrawal in patients who have developed dependence may precipitate a withdrawal syndrome. Great caution should be exercised in patients with a known tendency or history of drug abuse.

Use with caution in patients with toxic psychosis, CNS depression, myxoedema, prostatic hypertrophy or urethral stricture, kyphoscoliosis, acute alcoholism, delirium tremens, severe inflammatory or obstructive bowel disorders, adrenal insufficiency or severe diarrhoea. Care should be exercised in treating the elderly or debilitated patients and those with hepatic or renal impairment.

4.5 Interaction with other medicinal products and other forms of Interaction
The depressant effects of diamorphine may be exaggerated and prolonged by phenothiazines, monoamine oxidase inhibitors, tricyclic antidepressants, anxiolytics and hypnotics. There may be antagonism of the gastrointestinal effects of cisapride, domperidone and metoclopramide. The risk of severe constipation and/or urinary retention is increased by administration of antimuscarinic drugs (e.g. atropine). There may be increased risk of toxicity with 4-quinolone antibacterials.

Alcohol may enhance the sedative and hypotensive effects of diamorphine.

Cimetidine inhibits metabolism of opioid analgesics.

Hyperpyrexia and CNS toxicity has been reported when opioid analgesics are used with selegiline.

4.6 Pregnancy and lactation
Safety has not been established in pregnancy.

Administration during labour may cause respiratory depression in the neonate and gastric stasis during labour, increasing the risk of inhalation pneumonia.

Diamorphine should not be given to women who are breast-feeding as there is limited information available on diamorphine in breast milk.

4.7 Effects on ability to drive and use machines
Diamorphine causes drowsiness and mental clouding. If affected patients should not drive or use machines.

4.8 Undesirable effects
The most serious hazard of therapy is respiratory depression although circulatory depression is also possible. The most common side effects are sedation, nausea and vomiting, constipation and sweating. Other side effects include dizziness, miosis, confusion, urinary retention, biliary spasm, orthostatic hypotension, facial flushing, vertigo, palpitations, mood changes, dry mouth, dependence, urticaria, pruritus and raised intracranial pressure.

4.9 Overdose
a) Symptoms

Respiratory depression, pulmonary oedema, muscle flaccidity, coma or stupor, constricted pupils, cold, clammy skin and occasionally bradycardia and hypotension.

b) Treatment

Respiration and circulation should be maintained and naloxone is indicated if coma or bradypnoea are present. A dose of 0.4 to 2mg repeated at intervals of two to three minutes (up to 10mg) may be given by subcutaneous, intramuscular or intravenous injection. The usual initial dosage for children is 10 micrograms per kg body weight. Naloxone may also be given by continuous intravenous infusion, 2mg diluted in 500ml, at a rate adjusted to the patient's response. Oxygen and assisted ventilation should be administered if necessary.

5. PHARMACOLOGICAL PROPERTIES
5.1 Pharmacodynamic properties
Diamorphine is a narcotic analgesic which acts primarily on the central nervous system and smooth muscle. It is predominantly a central nervous system depressant but it has stimulant actions resulting in nausea, vomiting and miosis.

5.2 Pharmacokinetic properties
Diamorphine is a potent opiate analgesic which has a more rapid onset of activity than morphine as the first metabolite, monoacetylmorphine, more readily crosses the blood brain barrier. In man, diamorphine has a half life of two to three minutes. Its first metabolite, monoacetylmorphine, is more slowly hydrolysed in the blood to be concentrated mainly in skeletal muscle, kidney, lung, liver and spleen. Monoacetylmorphine is metabolised to morphine. Morphine forms conjugates with glucuronic acid. The majority of the drug is excreted via the kidney as glucuronides and to a much lesser extent as morphine. About 7-10% is eliminated via the biliary system into the faeces.

Diamorphine does not bind to protein. However, morphine is about 35% bound to human plasma proteins, mainly to albumin. The analgesic effect lasts approximately three to four hours.

5.3 Preclinical safety data
There are no additional pre-clinical data of relevance to the prescriber.

6. PHARMACEUTICAL PARTICULARS
6.1 List of excipients
Water for Injections BP*

Not detectable in the finished product.

6.2 Incompatibilities
Physical incompatibility has been reported with mineral acids and alkalis.

6.3 Shelf life
Three years from date of manufacture

6.4 Special precautions for storage
Do not store above 25°C.

Keep container in the outer container.

6.5 Nature and contents of container
2ml Neutral glass ampoules, PhEur. Type 1. Ampoules are packed into cartons of 5, 10 or 50.

6.6 Instructions for use and handling
The solution should be used immediately after preparation.

Administrative Data
7. MARKETING AUTHORISATION HOLDER
CP Pharmaceuticals Ltd

Ash Road North

Wrexham

LL13 9UF

8. MARKETING AUTHORISATION NUMBER(S)
4543/0305

9. DATE OF FIRST AUTHORISATION/RENEWAL OF THE AUTHORISATION
22/3/93

10. DATE OF REVISION OF THE TEXT
January 2001

Diamorphine Injection BP 500mg

(Wockhardt UK Ltd)

1. NAME OF THE MEDICINAL PRODUCT
Diamorphine Hydrochloride 500mg for Injection BP.

2. QUALITATIVE AND QUANTITATIVE COMPOSITION
Each ampoule contains 500mg of Diamorphine Hydrochloride BP.

3. PHARMACEUTICAL FORM
A white to off-white, sterile, freeze dried powder of Diamorphine Hydrochloride BP for reconstitution for injection.

4. CLINICAL PARTICULARS

4.1 Therapeutic indications
Diamorphine may be used in the treatment of severe pain associated with surgical procedures, myocardial infarction or pain in the terminally ill and for the relief of dyspnoea in acute pulmonary oedema.

4.2 Posology and method of administration
Diamorphine may be given by the intramuscular, intravenous or subcutaneous routes. Glucose intravenous infusion is the preferred diluent, particularly when the drug is administered by a continuous infusion pump over 24 to 48 hours, although it is also compatible with sodium chloride intravenous infusion.

The dose should be suited to the individual patient.

Adults:

Acute pain, 5mg repeated every four hours if necessary (up to 10mg for heavier, well muscled patients) by subcutaneous or intramuscular injection. By slow intravenous injection, one quarter to one half the corresponding intramuscular dose.

Chronic pain, 5-10mg regularly every four hours by subcutaneous or intramuscular injection. The dose may be increased according to individual needs.

Myocardial infarction, 5mg by slow intravenous injection (1mg/minute) followed by a further 2.5mg to 5mg if necessary.

Acute pulmonary oedema, 2.5mg to 5mg by slow intravenous injection (1mg/minute).

Children and Elderly:

As diamorphine has a respiratory depressant effect, care should be taken when giving the drug to the very young and the elderly and a lower starting dose than normal is recommended.

4.3 Contraindications
Respiratory depression and obstructive airways disease.

Phaeochromocytoma (endogenous release of histamine may stimulate catecholamine release).

Raised intracranial pressure.

Concurrent use of monoamine oxidase inhibitors or within two weeks of their discontinuation.

4.4 Special warnings and special precautions for use
Diamorphine should be administered with care to patients with head injuries as there is an increased risk of respiratory depression which may lead to elevation of CSF pressure. The sedation and pupillary changes produced may interfere with accurate monitoring of the patient.

Repeated administration of diamorphine may lead to dependence and tolerance developing. Abrupt withdrawal in patients who have developed dependence may precipitate a withdrawal syndrome. Great caution should be exercised in patients with a known tendency or history of drug abuse.

Use with caution in patients with toxic psychosis, CNS depression, myxoedema, prostatic hypertrophy or urethral stricture, kyphoscoliosis, acute alcoholism, delirium tremens, severe inflammatory or obstructive bowel disorders, adrenal insufficiency or severe diarrhoea. Care should be exercised in treating the elderly or debilitated patients and those with hepatic or renal impairment.

4.5 Interaction with other medicinal products and other forms of Interaction
The depressant effects of diamorphine may be exaggerated and prolonged by phenothiazines, monoamine oxidase inhibitors, tricyclic antidepressants, anxiolytics and hypnotics. There may be antagonism of the gastrointestinal effects of cisapride, domperidone and metoclopramide. The risk of severe constipation and/or urinary retention is increased by administration of antimuscarinic drugs (e.g. atropine). There may be increased risk of toxicity with 4-quinolone antibacterials.

Alcohol may enhance the sedative and hypotensive effects of diamorphine.

Cimetidine inhibits metabolism of opioid analgesics.

Hyperpyrexia and CNS toxicity have been reported when opioid analgesics are used with selegiline.

4.6 Pregnancy and lactation
Safety has not been established in pregnancy.

Administration during labour may cause respiratory depression in the neonate and gastric stasis during labour, increasing the risk of inhalation pneumonia.

Diamorphine should not be given to women who are breast-feeding as there is limited information available on diamorphine in breast milk.

4.7 Effects on ability to drive and use machines
Diamorphine causes drowsiness and mental clouding. If affected patients should not drive or use machines.

4.8 Undesirable effects
The most serious hazard of therapy is respiratory depression although circulatory depression is also possible. The most common side effects are sedation, nausea and vomiting, constipation and sweating. Other side effects include dizziness, miosis, confusion, urinary retention, biliary spasm, orthostatic hypotension, facial flushing, vertigo, palpitations, mood changes, dry mouth, dependence, urticaria, pruritus and raised intracranial pressure.

4.9 Overdose
a) Symptoms

Respiratory depression, pulmonary oedema, muscle flaccidity, coma or stupor, constricted pupils, cold, clammy skin and occasionally bradycardia and hypotension.

b) Treatment

Respiration and circulation should be maintained and naloxone is indicated if coma or bradypnoea are present. A dose of 0.4 to 2mg repeated at intervals of two to three minutes (up to 10mg) may be given by subcutaneous, intramuscular or intravenous injection. The usual initial dosage for children is 10 micrograms per kg body weight. Naloxone may also be given by continuous intravenous infusion, 2mg diluted in 500ml, at a rate adjusted to the patient's response. Oxygen and assisted ventilation should be administered if necessary.

5. PHARMACOLOGICAL PROPERTIES

5.1 Pharmacodynamic properties
Diamorphine is a narcotic analgesic which acts primarily on the central nervous system and smooth muscle. It is predominantly a central nervous system depressant but it has stimulant actions resulting in nausea, vomiting and miosis.

5.2 Pharmacokinetic properties
Diamorphine is a potent opiate analgesic which has a more rapid onset of activity than morphine as the first metabolite, monoacetylmorphine, more readily crosses the blood brain barrier. In man, diamorphine has a half life of two to three minutes. Its first metabolite, monoacetylmorphine, is more slowly hydrolysed in the blood to be concentrated mainly in skeletal muscle, kidney, lung, liver and spleen. Monoacetylmorphine is metabolised to morphine. Morphine forms conjugates with glucuronic acid. The majority of the drug is excreted via the kidney as glucuronides and to a much lesser extent as morphine. About 7-10% is eliminated via the biliary system into the faeces.

Diamorphine does not bind to protein. However, morphine is about 35% bound to human plasma proteins, mainly to albumin. The analgesic effect lasts approximately three to four hours.

5.3 Preclinical safety data
There are no additional pre-clinical data of relevance to the prescriber.

6. PHARMACEUTICAL PARTICULARS

6.1 List of excipients
Water for Injections BP*

Not detectable in the finished product.

6.2 Incompatibilities
Physical incompatibility has been reported with mineral acids and alkalis.

6.3 Shelf life
Three years from date of manufacture

6.4 Special precautions for storage
Do not store above 25°C.

Keep container in the outer carton.

6.5 Nature and contents of container
5ml Neutral glass ampoules, PhEur. Type 1. Ampoules are packed into cartons of 5, 10 or 50.

6.6 Instructions for use and handling
The solution should be used immediately after preparation.

Administrative Data

7. MARKETING AUTHORISATION HOLDER
CP Pharmaceuticals Ltd

Ash Road North

Wrexham

LL13 9UF

8. MARKETING AUTHORISATION NUMBER(S)
4543/0308

9. DATE OF FIRST AUTHORISATION/RENEWAL OF THE AUTHORISATION
22/3/93

10. DATE OF REVISION OF THE TEXT
January 2001

Diamorphine Injection BP 5mg

(Wockhardt UK Ltd)

1. NAME OF THE MEDICINAL PRODUCT
Diamorphine Hydrochloride 5mg for Injection BP

2. QUALITATIVE AND QUANTITATIVE COMPOSITION
Each ampoule contains 5mg of Diamorphine Hydrochloride BP.

3. PHARMACEUTICAL FORM
A white to off-white, sterile, freeze dried powder of Diamorphine Hydrochloride BP for reconstitution for injection.

4. CLINICAL PARTICULARS

4.1 Therapeutic indications
Diamorphine may be used in the treatment of severe pain associated with surgical procedures, myocardial infarction or pain in the terminally ill and for the relief of dyspnoea in acute pulmonary oedema.

4.2 Posology and method of administration
Diamorphine may be given by the intramuscular, intravenous or subcutaneous routes. Glucose intravenous infusion is the preferred diluent, particularly when the drug is administered by a continuous infusion pump over 24 to 48 hours, although it is also compatible with sodium chloride intravenous infusion.

The dose should be suited to the individual patient.

Adults:

Acute pain, 5mg repeated every four hours if necessary (up to 10mg for heavier, well muscled patients) by subcutaneous or intramuscular injection. By slow intravenous injection, one quarter to one half the corresponding intramuscular dose.

Chronic pain, 5-10mg regularly every four hours by subcutaneous or intramuscular injection. The dose may be increased according to individual needs.

Myocardial infarction, 5mg by slow intravenous injection (1mg/minute) followed by a further 2.5mg to 5mg if necessary.

Acute pulmonary oedema, 2.5mg to 5mg by slow intravenous injection (1mg/minute).

Children and Elderly:

As diamorphine has a respiratory depressant effect, care should be taken when giving the drug to the very young and the elderly and a lower starting dose than normal is recommended.

4.3 Contraindications
Respiratory depression and obstructive airways disease.

Phaeochromocytoma (endogenous release of histamine may stimulate catecholamine release).

Raised intracranial pressure.

Concurrent use of monoamine oxidase inhibitors or within two weeks of their discontinuation.

4.4 Special warnings and special precautions for use
Diamorphine should be administered with care to patients with head injuries as there is an increased risk of respiratory depression which may lead to elevation of CSF pressure. The sedation and pupillary changes produced may interfere with accurate monitoring of the patient.

Repeated administration of diamorphine may lead to dependence and tolerance developing. Abrupt withdrawal in patients who have developed dependence may precipitate a withdrawal syndrome. Great caution should be exercised in patients with a known tendency or history of drug abuse.

Use with caution in patients with toxic psychosis, CNS depression, myxoedema, prostatic hypertrophy or urethral stricture, kyphoscoliosis, acute alcoholism, delirium tremens, severe inflammatory or obstructive bowel disorders, adrenal insufficiency or severe diarrhoea. Care should be exercised in treating the elderly or debilitated patients and those with hepatic or renal impairment.

4.5 Interaction with other medicinal products and other forms of Interaction
The depressant effects of diamorphine may be exaggerated and prolonged by phenothiazines, monoamine oxidase inhibitors, tricyclic antidepressants, anxiolytics and hypnotics. There may be antagonism of the gastrointestinal effects of cisapride, domperidone and metoclopramide. The risk of severe constipation and/or urinary retention is increased by administration of antimuscarinic drugs (e.g. atropine). There may be increased risk of toxicity with 4-quinolone antibacterials.

Alcohol may enhance the sedative and hypotensive effects of diamorphine.

Cimetidine inhibits metabolism of opioid analgesics.

Hyperpyrexia and CNS toxicity have been reported when opioid analgesics are used with selegiline.

4.6 Pregnancy and lactation
Safety has not been established in pregnancy.

Administration during labour may cause respiratory depression in the neonate and gastric stasis during labour, increasing the risk of inhalation pneumonia.

Diamorphine should not be given to women who are breast-feeding as there is limited information available on diamorphine in breast milk.

4.7 Effects on ability to drive and use machines
Diamorphine causes drowsiness and mental clouding. If affected patients should not drive or use machines.

4.8 Undesirable effects
The most serious hazard of therapy is respiratory depression although circulatory depression is also possible. The most common side effects are sedation, nausea and vomiting, constipation and sweating. Other side effects include dizziness, miosis, confusion, urinary retention, biliary spasm, orthostatic hypotension, facial flushing, vertigo, palpitations, mood changes, dry mouth, dependence, urticaria, pruritus and raised intracranial pressure.

4.9 Overdose
a) Symptoms

Respiratory depression, pulmonary oedema, muscle flaccidity, coma or stupor, constricted pupils, cold, clammy skin and occasionally bradycardia and hypotension.

b) Treatment

Respiration and circulation should be maintained and naloxone is indicated if coma or bradypnoea are present. A dose of 0.4 to 2mg repeated at intervals of two to three minutes (up to 10mg) may be given by subcutaneous, intramuscular or intravenous injection. The usual initial dosage for children is 10 micrograms per kg body weight. Naloxone may also be given by continuous intravenous infusion, 2mg diluted in 500ml, at a rate adjusted to the patient's response. Oxygen and assisted ventilation should be administered if necessary.

5. PHARMACOLOGICAL PROPERTIES
5.1 Pharmacodynamic properties
Diamorphine is a narcotic analgesic which acts primarily on the central nervous system and smooth muscle. It is predominantly a central nervous system depressant but it has stimulant actions resulting in nausea, vomiting and miosis.

5.2 Pharmacokinetic properties
Diamorphine is a potent opiate analgesic which has a more rapid onset of activity than morphine as the first metabolite, monoacetylmorphine, more readily crosses the blood brain barrier. In man, diamorphine has a half life of two to three minutes. Its first metabolite, monoacetylmorphine, is more slowly hydrolysed in the blood to be concentrated mainly in skeletal muscle, kidney, lung, liver and spleen. Monoacetylmorphine is metabolised to morphine. Morphine forms conjugates with glucuronic acid. The majority of the drug is excreted via the kidney as glucuronides and to a much lesser extent as morphine. About 7-10% is eliminated via the biliary system into the faeces.

Diamorphine does not bind to protein. However, morphine is about 35% bound to human plasma proteins, mainly to albumin. The analgesic effect lasts approximately three to four hours.

5.3 Preclinical safety data
There are no additional pre-clinical data of relevance to the prescriber.

6. PHARMACEUTICAL PARTICULARS
6.1 List of excipients
Water for Injections BP*

Not detectable in the finished product.

6.2 Incompatibilities
Physical incompatibility has been reported with mineral acids and alkalis.

6.3 Shelf life
Three years from date of manufacture

6.4 Special precautions for storage
Do not store above 25°C.

Keep container in the outer carton.

6.5 Nature and contents of container
2ml Neutral glass ampoules, PhEur. Type 1. Ampoules are packed into cartons of 5, 10 or 50.

6.6 Instructions for use and handling
The solution should be used immediately after preparation.

Administrative Data
7. MARKETING AUTHORISATION HOLDER
CP Pharmaceuticals Ltd

Ash Road North

Wrexham

LL13 9UF

8. MARKETING AUTHORISATION NUMBER(S)
4543/0303

9. DATE OF FIRST AUTHORISATION/RENEWAL OF THE AUTHORISATION
22/3/93

10. DATE OF REVISION OF THE TEXT
January 2001

Dianette

(Schering Health Care Limited)

1. NAME OF THE MEDICINAL PRODUCT
Dianette ®

2. QUALITATIVE AND QUANTITATIVE COMPOSITION
Each beige tablet contains 2 milligrams of the anti-androgen, cyproterone acetate and 35 micrograms of the oestrogen, ethinylestradiol.

3. PHARMACEUTICAL FORM
Sugar-coated tablets.

4. CLINICAL PARTICULARS
4.1 Therapeutic indications
Dianette is recommended for use in women only for the treatment of (a) severe acne, refractory to prolonged oral antibiotic therapy; (b) moderately severe hirsutism.

Although Dianette also acts as an oral contraceptive, it should not be used in women solely for contraception, but should be reserved for those women requiring treatment for the androgen-dependent conditions described.

Complete remission of acne is to be expected in nearly all cases, often within a few months, but in particularly severe cases treatment for longer may be necessary before the full benefit is seen. It is recommended that treatment be withdrawn 3 to 4 cycles after the indicated condition(s) has/have completely resolved and that Dianette is not continued solely to provide oral contraception. Repeat courses of Dianette may be given if the androgen-dependent condition(s) recur.

4.2 Posology and method of administration
Dianette inhibits ovulation and thereby prevents conception. Patients who are using Dianette should not therefore use an additional hormonal contraceptive, as this will expose the patient to an excessive dose of hormones and is not necessary for effective contraception.

First treatment course: One tablet daily for 21 days, starting on the first day of the menstrual cycle (the first day of menstruation counting as Day 1).

Subsequent courses: Each subsequent course is started after 7 tablet-free days have followed the preceding course.

When the contraceptive action of Dianette is also to be employed, it is essential that the above instructions be rigidly adhered to. Should bleeding fail to occur during the tablet-free interval, the possibility of pregnancy must be excluded before the next pack is started.

When changing from an oral contraceptive and relying on the contraceptive action of Dianette, follow the instructions given below:

Changing from 21-day combined oral contraceptives: The first tablet of Dianette should be taken on the first day immediately after the end of the previous oral contraceptive course. Additional contraceptive precautions are not required.

Changing from a combined Every Day pill (28 day tablets):

Dianette should be started after taking the last active tablet from the Every Day Pill pack. The first Dianette tablet is taken the next day. Additional contraceptive precautions are not then required.

Changing from a progestogen-only pill (POP):

The first tablet of Dianette should be taken on the first day of bleeding, even if a POP has already been taken on that day. Additional contraceptive precautions are not then required. The remaining progestogen-only pills should be discarded.

Post-partum and post-abortum use:

After pregnancy, Dianette can be started 21 days after a vaginal delivery, provided that the patient is fully ambulant and there are no puerperal complications. Additional contraceptive precautions will be required for the first 7 days of pill taking. Since the first post-partum ovulation may precede the first bleeding, another method of contraception should be used in the interval between childbirth and the first course of tablets. Lactation is contra-indicated with Dianette. After a first-trimester abortion, Dianette may be started immediately in which case no additional contraceptive precautions are required.

Special circumstances requiring additional contraception

Incorrect administration: A single delayed tablet should be taken as soon as possible, and if this can be done within 12 hours of the correct time, contraceptive protection is maintained. With longer delays, additional contraception is needed. Only the most recently delayed tablet should be taken, earlier missed tablets being omitted, and additional non-hormonal methods of contraception (except the rhythm or temperature methods) should be used for the next 7 days, while the next 7 tablets are being taken. Additionally, therefore, if tablet(s) have been missed during the last 7 days of a pack, there should be no break before the next pack is started. In this situation, a withdrawal bleed should not be expected until the end of the second pack. Some breakthrough bleeding may occur on tablet taking days but this is not clinically significant. If the patient does not have a withdrawal bleed during the tablet-free interval following the end of the second pack, the possibility of pregnancy must be ruled out before starting the next pack.

Gastro-intestinal upset: Vomiting or diarrhoea may reduce the efficacy of oral contraceptives by preventing full absorption. Tablet-taking from the current pack should be continued. Additional non-hormonal methods of contraception (except the rhythm or temperature methods) should be used during the gastro-intestinal upset and for 7 days following the upset. If these 7 days overrun the end of a pack, the next pack should be started without a break. In this situation, a withdrawal bleed should not be expected until the end of the second pack. If the patient does not have a withdrawal bleed during the tablet-free interval following the end of the second pack, the possibility of pregnancy must be ruled out before starting the next pack. Other methods of contraception should be considered if the gastro-intestinal disorder is likely to be prolonged.

4.3 Contraindications
1. Pregnancy or lactation

2. Severe disturbances of liver function, jaundice or persistent itching during a previous pregnancy, Dubin-Johnson syndrome, Rotor syndrome, previous or existing liver tumours.

3. Personal or family history of confirmed, idiopathic venous thromboembolism (VTE) (where a family history refers to VTE in a sibling or parent at a relatively early age).

4. Current venous thrombotic or embolic processes.

5. Existing or previous arterial thrombotic or embolic processes.

6. The presence of a severe or multiple risk factor(s) for venous or arterial thrombosis may also constitute a contra-indication (see section 4.4).

7. Sickle-cell anaemia.

8. Mammary or endometrial carcinoma, or a history of these conditions.

9. Severe diabetes mellitus with vascular changes.

10. Disorders of lipid metabolism.

11. History of herpes gestationis.

12. Deterioration of otosclerosis during pregnancy.

13. Undiagnosed abnormal vaginal bleeding.

14. Hypersensitivity to any of the components of Dianette.

4.4 Special warnings and special precautions for use
Warnings: Like many other steroids, Dianette, when given in very high doses and for the majority of the animal's life-span, has been found to cause an increase in the incidence of tumours, including carcinoma, in the liver of rats. The relevance of this finding to humans is unknown.

In rare cases benign and in even rarer cases malignant liver tumours leading in isolated cases to life-threatening intra-abdominal haemorrhage have been observed after the use of hormonal substances such as those contained in Dianette. If severe upper abdominal complaints, liver enlargement or signs of intra-abdominal haemorrhage occur, a liver tumour should be included in the differential diagnosis.

Animal studies have revealed that feminisation of male foetuses may occur if cyproterone acetate is administered during the phase of embryogenesis at which differentiation of the external genitalia occurs. Although the results of these tests are not necessarily relevant to man, the possibility must be considered that administration of Dianette to women after the 45th day of pregnancy could cause feminisation of male foetuses. It follows from this that pregnancy is an absolute contra-indication for treatment with Dianette, and must be excluded before such treatment is begun.

Dianette is composed of the progestogen cyproterone acetate and the oestrogen ethinylestradiol and is administered for 21 days of a monthly cycle. It therefore has a similar composition to that of a combined oral contraceptive (COC). The use of any COC or Dianette carries an increased risk for venous thromboembolism (VTE), including deep venous thrombosis and pulmonary embolism, compared with no use. The excess risk of VTE is highest during the first year a woman ever uses a COC. This increased risk is less than the risk of VTE associated with pregnancy, which is estimated as 60 per 100,000 pregnancies.

Full recovery from such disorders does not always occur; VTE is fatal in 1-2% of cases.

Epidemiological studies have shown that the incidence of VTE in users of oral contraceptives with low oestrogen content ($< 50\ \mu g$ ethinylestradiol) is up to 40 cases per 100,000 women-years. This compares with 5-10 cases per 100,000 women-years for non-users.

Certain factors may increase the risk of venous thrombosis e.g. severe obesity (body mass index $> 30kg/m^2$), increasing age, a genetic predisposition to clotting or a personal or family history of confirmed, idiopathic VTE (where family history refers to VTE in a sibling or parent at a relatively early age, see contraindications section 4.3). In addition, the risk of VTE may be temporarily increased by prolonged immobilisation, major surgery, any surgery to the legs, or major trauma (see "Reasons for stopping Dianette immediately").

Figure 1 Estimated cumulative numbers of breast cancers per 10,000 women diagnosed in 5 years of use and up to 10 years after stopping COCs, compared with numbers of breast cancers diagnosed in 10,000 women who had never used COCs

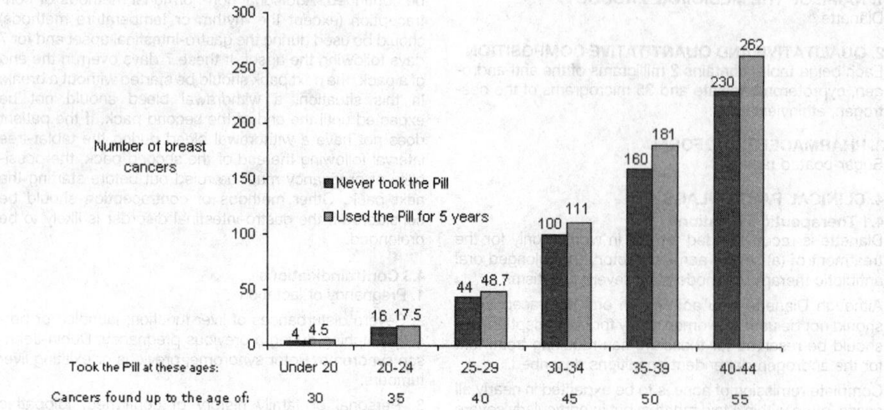

There is some epidemiological evidence that the incidence of VTE is higher in users of Dianette when compared to users of COCs with low oestrogen content (< 50μg).

The user group of Dianette as a treatment for severe acne or moderately severe hirsutism is likely to include patients that may have an inherently increased cardiovascular risk such as that associated with polycystic ovarian syndrome.

Epidemiological studies have also associated the use of COCs with an increased risk for arterial (myocardial infarction, transient ischaemic attack) thromboembolism. Certain factors such as smoking, obesity, cardiovascular disease, hypertension, diabetes and migraine may increase the risk of arterial thromboembolism. The risk of arterial thrombosis associated with oral contraceptives increases with age, and this risk is aggravated by cigarette smoking.

Numerous epidemiological studies have been reported on the risks of ovarian, endometrial, cervical and breast cancer in women using combined oral contraceptives. The evidence is clear that combined oral contraceptives offer substantial protection against both ovarian and endometrial cancer.

An increased risk of cervical cancer in long-term users of combined oral contraceptives has been reported in some studies, but there continues to be controversy about the extent to which this is attributable to the confounding effects of sexual behaviour and other factors.

A meta-analysis from 54 epidemiological studies reported that there is a slightly increased relative risk (RR = 1.24) of having breast cancer diagnosed in women who are currently using combined oral contraceptives (COCs). The observed pattern of increased risk may be due to an earlier diagnosis of breast cancer in COC users, the biological effects of COCs or a combination of both. The additional breast cancers diagnosed in current users of COCs or in women who have used COCs in the last ten years are more likely to be localised to the breast than those in women who never used COCs.

Breast cancer is rare among women under 40 years of age whether or not they take COCs. Whilst this background risk increases with age, the excess number of breast cancer diagnoses in current and recent COC users is small in relation to the overall risk of breast cancer (see bar chart).

The most important risk factor for breast cancer in COC users is the age women discontinue the COC; the older the age at stopping, the more breast cancers are diagnosed. Duration of use is less important and the excess risk gradually disappears during the course of the 10 years after stopping COC use such that by 10 years there appears to be no excess.

The possible increase in risk of breast cancer should be discussed with the user and weighed against the benefits of COCs taking into account the evidence that they offer substantial protection against the risk of developing certain other cancers (e.g. ovarian and endometrial cancer).

Estimated cumulative numbers of breast cancers per 10,000 women diagnosed in 5 years of use and up to 10 years after stopping COCs, compared with numbers of breast cancers diagnosed in 10,000 women who had never used COCs

(see Figure 1 above)

The possibility cannot be ruled out that certain chronic diseases may occasionally deteriorate during the use of Dianette (see *Precautions*)

Reasons for stopping Dianette immediately:

1. Occurrence for the first time, or exacerbation, of migrainous headaches or unusually frequent or unusually severe headaches.

2. Sudden disturbances of vision or hearing or other perceptual disorders.

3. First signs of thrombophlebitis or thromboembolic symptoms (e.g. unusual pains in or swelling of the leg(s), stabbing pains on breathing or coughing for no apparent reason). Feeling of pain and tightness in the chest.

4. Six weeks before an elective major operation (e.g. abdominal, orthopaedic), any surgery to the legs, medical treatment for varicose veins or prolonged immobilisation, e.g. after accidents or surgery. Do not restart until 2 weeks after full ambulation. In case of emergency surgery, thrombotic prophylaxis is usually indicated e.g. subcutaneous heparin.

5. Onset of jaundice, hepatitis, itching of the whole body.

6. Increase in epileptic seizures.

7. Significant rise in blood pressure.

8. Onset of severe depression.

9. Severe upper abdominal pain or liver enlargement.

10. Clear worsening of conditions known to deteriorate during use of hormonal contraception or during pregnancy.

11. Pregnancy is a reason for stopping immediately because it has been suggested by some investigations that oral contraceptives taken in early pregnancy may slightly increase the risk of foetal malformations. Other investigations have failed to support these findings. The possibility therefore cannot be excluded, but it is certain that if a risk exists at all, it is small.

Precautions:

Assessment of women prior to starting oral contraceptives (and at regular intervals thereafter) should include a personal and family medical history of each woman. Physical examination should be guided by this and by the contra-indications (section 4.3) and warnings (section 4.4) for this product. The frequency and nature of these assessments should be based upon relevant guidelines and should be adapted to the individual woman, but should include measurement of blood pressure and, if judged appropriate by the clinician, breast, abdominal and pelvic examination including cervical cytology.

The following conditions require strict medical supervision during medication with oral contraceptives. Deterioration or first appearance of any of these conditions may indicate that Dianette should be discontinued:

Diabetes mellitus, or a tendency towards diabetes mellitus (e.g. unexplained glycosuria), hypertension, varicose veins, a history of phlebitis, otosclerosis, multiple sclerosis, epilepsy, porphyria, tetany, disturbed liver function, Sydenham's chorea, renal dysfunction, family history of clotting disorders, obesity, family history of breast cancer and patient history of benign breast disease, history of clinical depression, systemic lupus erythematosus, uterine fibroids, an intolerance to contact lenses, migraine, gallstones, cardiovascular diseases, chloasma, asthma, or any disease that is prone to worsen during pregnancy.

It should be borne in mind that the use of ultraviolet lamps, for the treatment of acne, or prolonged exposure to sunlight, increases the risk of the deterioration of chloasma.

Some women may experience amenorrhoea or oligomenorrhoea after discontinuation of Dianette, especially when these conditions existed prior to use. Women should be informed of this possibility.

4.5 Interaction with other medicinal products and other forms of Interaction

Hepatic enzyme inducers such as barbiturates, primidone, phenobarbitone, phenytoin, phenylbutazone, rifampicin, carbamazepine and griseofulvin can impair the contraceptive efficacy of Dianette. For women receiving long-term therapy with hepatic enzyme inducers, another method of contraception should be used. The use of antibiotics may also reduce the contraceptive efficacy of Dianette, possibly by altering the intestinal flora.

Women receiving short courses of enzyme inducers and broad spectrum antibiotics should take additional, non-hormonal (except rhythm or temperature method) contraceptive precautions during the time of concurrent medication and for 7 days afterwards. If these 7 days overrun the end of a pack, the next pack should be started without a break. In this situation, a withdrawal bleed should not be expected until the end of the second pack. If the patient does not have a withdrawal bleed during the tablet-free interval following the end of the second pack, the possibility of pregnancy must be ruled out before resuming with the next pack.

The possibility cannot be ruled out that oral tetracyclines, if used in conjunction with Dianette may reduce its contraceptive efficacy, although it has not been shown. When drugs of these classes are being taken it is, therefore, advisable to use additional non-hormonal methods of contraception (except the rhythm or temperature methods) since an extremely high degree of protection must be provided when Dianette is being taken. With rifampicin, additional contraceptive precautions should be continued for 4 weeks after treatment stops, even if only a short course was administered.

The requirement for oral antidiabetics or insulin can change as a result of the effect on glucose tolerance.

The herbal remedy St John's wort (Hypericum perforatum) should not be taken concomitantly with Dianette as this could potentially lead to a loss of contraceptive effect.

4.6 Pregnancy and lactation

Contra-indicated.

Animal studies have revealed that feminisation of male foetuses may occur if cyproterone acetate is administered during the phase of embryogenesis at which differentiation of the external genitalia occurs. Although the results of these tests are not necessarily relevant to man, the possibility must be considered that administration of Dianette to women after the 45th day of pregnancy could cause feminisation of male foetuses. It follows from this that pregnancy is an absolute contra-indication for treatment with Dianette, and must be excluded before such treatment is begun.

4.7 Effects on ability to drive and use machines

None known.

4.8 Undesirable effects

There is an increased risk of venous thromboembolism for all women who use Dianette. For more information see section 4.4

In rare cases, headaches, gastric upsets, nausea, vomiting, breast tenderness, changes in body weight, changes in libido, depressive moods can occur.

In predisposed women, use of Dianette can sometimes cause chloasma which is exacerbated by exposure to sunlight. Such women should avoid prolonged exposure to sunlight.

Individual cases of poor tolerance of contact lenses have been reported with use of oral contraceptives. Contact lens wearers who develop changes in lens tolerance should be assessed by an ophthalmologist.

Menstrual changes:

1. Reduction of menstrual flow:

This is not abnormal and it is to be expected in some patients. Indeed, it may be beneficial where heavy periods were previously experienced.

2. Missed menstruation:

Occasionally, withdrawal bleeding may not occur at all. If the tablets have been taken correctly, pregnancy is unlikely. Should bleeding fail to occur during the tablet-free interval the possibility of pregnancy must be excluded before the next pack is started.

Intermenstrual bleeding: "Spotting" or heavier "breakthrough bleeding" sometimes occur during tablet taking, especially in the first few cycles, and normally cease spontaneously. Dianette should therefore, be continued even if irregular bleeding occurs. If irregular bleeding is persistent, appropriate diagnostic measures to exclude an organic cause are indicated and may include curettage. This also applies in the case of spotting which occurs at regular intervals in several consecutive cycles or which occurs for the first time after long use of Dianette.

Effect on blood chemistry: The use of oral contraceptives may influence the results of certain laboratory tests including biochemical parameters of liver, thyroid, adrenal and renal function, plasma levels of carrier proteins and lipid/lipoprotein fractions, parameters of carbohydrate metabolism and parameters of coagulation and fibrinolysis. Laboratory staff should therefore be informed about oral contraceptive use when laboratory tests are requested.

Refer to Section 4.4. "Special warnings and special precautions for use" for additional information.

4.9 Overdose

Overdose may cause nausea, vomiting and, in females, withdrawal bleeding.

There are no specific antidotes and further treatment should be symptomatic.

5. PHARMACOLOGICAL PROPERTIES

5.1 Pharmacodynamic properties

Dianette blocks androgen-receptors. It also reduces androgen synthesis both by negative feedback effect on the hypothalamo-pituitiary-ovarian systems and by the inhibition of androgen-synthesising enzymes.

Although Dianette also acts as an oral contraceptive, it is not recommended in women solely for contraception, but should be reserved for those women requiring treatment for the androgen-dependent skin conditions described.

5.2 Pharmacokinetic properties

Cyproterone acetate: Following oral administration cyproterone acetate is completely absorbed in a wide dose range. The ingestion of Dianette effects a maximum serum level of 15ng cyproterone acetate/ml at 1.6 hours. Thereafter drug serum levels decrease in two disposition phases characterised by half-lives of 0.8 hours and 2.3 days. The total clearance of cyproterone acetate from serum was determined to be 3.6 ml/min/kg. Cyproterone acetate is metabolised by various pathways including hydroxylations and conjugations. The main metabolite in human plasma is the 15β-hydroxy derivative.

Some dose parts are excreted unchanged with the bile fluid. Most of the dose is excreted in form of metabolites at a urinary to biliary ratio of 3:7. The renal and biliary excretion was determined to proceed with half-life of 1.9 days. Metabolites from plasma were eliminated at a similar rate (half-life of 1.7 days). Cyproterone acetate is almost exclusively bound to plasma albumin. About 3.5 - 4.0% of total drug levels are present unbound. Because protein binding is non-specific changes in sex hormone binding globulin (SHBG) levels do not affect cyproterone acetate pharmacokinetics.

According to the long half-life of the terminal disposition phase from plasma (serum) and the daily intake cyproterone acetate accumulates during one treatment cycle. Mean maximum drug serum levels increased from 15ng/ml (day 1) to 21ng/ml and 24ng/ml at the end of the treatment cycles 1 and 3 respectively. The area under the concentration versus time profile increased 2.2 fold (end of cycle 1) and 2.4 fold (end of cycle 3). Steady state conditions were reached after about 16 days. During long term treatment cyproterone acetate accumulates over treatment cycles by a factor of 2.

The absolute bioavailability of cyproterone acetate is almost complete (88% of dose). The relative bioavailability of cyproterone acetate from Dianette was 109% when compared to an aqueous microcrystalline suspension.

Ethinylestradiol: Orally administered ethinylestradiol is rapidly and completely absorbed. Following ingestion of Dianette maximum drug serum levels of about 80pg/ml are reached at 1.7 hours. Thereafter ethinylestradiol plasma levels decrease in two phases characterised by half-lives of 1 - 2 hours and about 20 hours. For analytical reasons these parameters can only be calculated for higher dosages.

For ethinylestradiol an apparent volume of distribution of about 5 l/kg and a metabolic clearance rate from plasma of about 5 ml/min/kg were determined.

Ethinylestradiol is highly but non-specifically bound to serum albumin. 2% of the drug levels are present unbound. During absorption and first liver passage ethinylestradiol is metabolised resulting in a reduced absolute and variable oral bioavailability. Unchanged drug is not excreted. Ethinylestradiol metabolites are excreted at a urinary to biliary ratio of 4:6 with a half-life of about 1 day.

According to the half-life of the terminal disposition phase from plasma and the daily ingestion steady state plasma levels are reached after 3 - 4 days and are higher by 30 - 40% as compared to a single dose. The relative bioavailability (reference: aqueous microcrystalline suspension) of ethinylestradiol was almost complete.

The systemic bioavailability of ethinylestradiol might be influenced in both directions by other drugs. There is, however, no interaction with high doses of vitamin C.

Ethinylestradiol induces the hepatic synthesis of SHBG and corticosteroid binding globulin (CBG) during continuous use. The extent of SHBG induction, however, is dependent upon the chemical structure and dose of the co-administered progestin. During treatment with Dianette SHBG concentrations in serum increased from about 100nmol/l to 300nmol/l and the serum concentrations of CBG were increased from about 50μg/ml to 95μg/ml.

5.3 Preclinical safety data

There are no preclinical safety data which could be of relevance to the prescriber and which are not already included in other relevant sections of the SPC.

6. PHARMACEUTICAL PARTICULARS

6.1 List of excipients

Lactose, maize starch, povidone, talc, magnesium stearate (E 572), sucrose, polyethylene glycol 6,000, calcium carbonate (E 170), titanium dioxide (E 171), glycerol 85%, montan glycol wax, yellow ferric oxide pigment (E 172).

6.2 Incompatibilities

None known.

6.3 Shelf life

5 years

6.4 Special precautions for storage

Not applicable.

6.5 Nature and contents of container

Outer carton contains aluminium foil and PVC blister memo packs each containing 21 tablets. Each carton contains either 1 or 3 blister memo packs.

6.6 Instructions for use and handling

Keep out of the reach of children.

7. MARKETING AUTHORISATION HOLDER

Schering Health Care Limited

The Brow

Burgess Hill

West Sussex

RH15 9NE

8. MARKETING AUTHORISATION NUMBER(S)

0053/0190

9. DATE OF FIRST AUTHORISATION/RENEWAL OF THE AUTHORISATION

1st August 2003

10. DATE OF REVISION OF THE TEXT

15 July 2004

LEGAL CATEGORY

POM

Diazemuls

(Alpharma Limited)

1. NAME OF THE MEDICINAL PRODUCT

Diazemuls

2. QUALITATIVE AND QUANTITATIVE COMPOSITION

Each emulsion contains Diazepam 0.5w/v

3. PHARMACEUTICAL FORM

Sterile, milky white emulsion

4. CLINICAL PARTICULARS

4.1 Therapeutic indications

1. Sedation prior to procedures such as endoscopy, dentistry, cardiac catheterisation and cardioversion.

2. Premedication prior to general anaesthesia.

3. Control of acute muscle spasm due to tetanus or poisoning.

4. Control of convulsions; status epilepticus.

5. Management of severe acute anxiety or agitation including delirium tremens.

4.2 Posology and method of administration

Diazemuls may be ad-ministered by slow intravenous injection (1ml per min), or by continuous infusion. Diazemuls should be drawn into the syringe immediately prior to administration.

1. *Sedation:* 0.1-0.2mg diazepam/kg body weight by iv injection. The normal adult dose is 10-20 mg, but dosage should be titrated to the patient's response.

2. *Premedication:* 0.1-0.2mg diazepam/kg body weight by iv injection. Dosage should be titrated to the patient's response. In this indication, prior treat-ment with diazepam leads to a reduction in fascicula-tions and postoperative myalgia associated with the use of suxamethonium.

3. *Tetanus:* 0.1-0.3mg diazepam/kg body weight by iv injection repeated every 1-4 hours as required. Alternatively, continuous infusion of 3-10mg/kg body weight over 24 hours may be infused.

4. *Status epilepticus:* An initial dose 0.15-0.25mg/kg body weight by iv injection repeated in 30 to 60 minutes if required, and followed if necessary by infusion (see below) of up to 3mg/kg body weight over 24 hours.

5. *Anxiety and tension, acute muscle spasm, acute states of excitation, delirium tremens:* The usual dose is 10mg repeated at intervals of 4 hours, or as required.

Elderly or debilitated patients: Elderly and debilitated patients are particularly sensitive to benzodiazepines. Dosage should initially be reduced to one half of the normal recommendations.

If a continuous infusion is required, Diazemuls can be added to dextrose solution 5% or 10% to achieve a final diazepam concentration within the range 0.1-0.4mg/ml (i.e. 2-8ml Diazemuls per 100ml dextrose solution). A dextrose solution containing Diazemuls should be used within 6 hours of the admixture. Diazemuls can be mixed in all proportions with intralipid 10% or 20% but not with saline solutions. It can be injected into the infusion tube during an ongoing infusion of isotonic saline or dextrose solution 5% or 10%. As with other diazepam injections, adsorption may occur to plastic infusion equipment. This adsorption may occur to a lesser degree with Diazemuls than with aqueous diazepam injection preparations when mixed with dextrose solutions.

4.3 Contraindications

1. Should not be used in phobic or obsessional states since there is inadequate evidence of efficacy and safety.

2. Should not be used in the treatment of chronic psychosis.

3. Hypersensitivity to diazepam or any of the excipients. Hypersensitivity to egg or soybean as egg phospholipid and soybean oil are included in the preparation.

4. Acute porphyria.

4.4 Special warnings and special precautions for use

Use with caution in patients with impairment of renal or hepatic function and in patients with pulmonary insufficiency or myasthenia gravis.

Should not be used alone to treat depression or anxiety associated with depression.

Amnesia may occur. In cases of loss or bereavement psychological adjustment may be inhibited by benzodiazepines.

Disinhibiting effects may be manifested in various ways. Suicide may be precipitated in patients who are depressed and aggressive behaviour toward self and others may be precipitated. Extreme caution should therefore be used in prescribing benzodiazepines in patients with personality disorders.

Physiological and psychological symptoms of withdrawal including depression may be associated with discontinuation of benzodiazepines even after normal therapeutic doses for short periods of time.

4.5 Interaction with other medicinal products and other forms of Interaction

Not recommended: Concomitant intake with alcohol.

The sedative effects may be enhanced when the product is used in combination with alcohol. This affects the ability to drive or use machines. Concomitant use of neuroleptics (antipsychotics), hypnotics, sedative antihistamines, and central nervous system depressants, e.g. general anaesthetics, narcotic analgesics, or antidepressants, including MAOI's will result in accentuation of their sedative effects. When Diazemuls is combined with centrally depressant drugs administered parenterally, severe respiratory and cardiovascular depression may occur. It is recommended that Diazemuls is administered following the analgesic, and that the dose should be carefully titrated to the patient's response. Diazepam clearance is increased by concomitant administration of phenobarbitone, and is decreased by administration of cimetidine. Omeprazole and Isoniazid inhibit diazepam metabolism. Concurrent use of zidovudine with benzodiazepines may decrease zidovudine clearance.

4.6 Pregnancy and lactation

If Diazemuls is prescribed to a woman of childbearing potential, she should be warned to contact her physician regarding discontinuance of Diazemuls if she intends to become, or suspects that she is pregnant.

If, for compelling medical reasons, Diazemuls is administered during the late phase of pregnancy, or during labour at high doses, effects on neonate, such as hypothermia, hypotonia and moderate respiratory depression; can be expected, due to the pharmacological action of Diazemuls.

Moreover, infants borne to mothers who took benzodiazepines chronically during the latter stages of pregnancy may have developed physical dependence and may be at some risk for developing withdrawal symptoms in the postnatal period.

Since benzodiazepines are found in the breast milk, benzodiazepines should not be given to breast feeding mothers.

4.7 Effects on ability to drive and use machines

Sedation, amnesia, impaired concentration, and impaired muscular function may adversely affect the ability to drive or use machines. If insufficient sleep duration occurs, the likelihood of impaired alertness may be increased (see also Interactions).

4.8 Undesirable effects

This formulation may rarely cause local pain of thrombophlebitis in the vein used for administration.

Rare instances have been reported of a local painless erythematous rash round the site of injection, which has resolved in 1-2 days. Urticaria and, rarely anaphylaxis have been reported following the injection of Diazemuls.

Dose related adverse effects which occur commonly with diazepam and which may persist into the following day, even after a single dose include sedation, drowsiness, unsteadiness and ataxia.

The elderly are particularly sensitive to the effects of centrally-depressant drugs and may experience confusion, especially if organic brain changes are present.

Less commonly, headache, vertigo, hypotension, gastrointestinal disturbances, visual disturbances, changes in libido and urinary retention have been reported. Isolated cases of blood dyscrasias and jaundice have been reported.

Abnormal psychological reactions have been reported and are more likely to occur in children and the elderly.

4.9 Overdose

Symptoms of diazepam overdosage are mainly an intensification of its therapeutic effects - sedation, muscle weakness, profound sleep or paradoxical excitation. In more severe cases, symptoms may include ataxia, hypotonia, hypotension, respiratory depression, and rarely, coma and death. When combined with other CNS depressants, including alcohol, the effects of overdosage are likely to be severe and may prove fatal.

Treatment is symptomatic.

Respiratory and cardiovascular functions should be carefully monitored in intensive care. If excitation occurs, barbiturates should not be used. Flumazenil, a specific competitive inhibitor of the central effects of benzodiazepines, may be useful as an antidote. Benzodiazepines are not significantly removed from the body by dialysis.

5. PHARMACOLOGICAL PROPERTIES

5.1 Pharmacodynamic properties

Diazepam is a potent anxiolytic, anticonvulsant and central muscle relaxant mediating its effects mainly via the limbic system as well as the postsynaptic spinal reflexes. Diazemuls contains diazepam dissolved in the oil phase of an oil-in-water emulsion. Release of the diazepam from the lipid particles of the emulsion has been demonstrated by clinical studies showing comparable efficacy with injectable diazepam preparations.

5.2 Pharmacokinetic properties

Diazepam is metabolised to two active metabolites, one of which, desmethyldiazepam, has an extended half-life. Diazepam is therefore a long acting benzodiazepine and repeated doses may lead to accumulation.

Diazepam is metabolised in the liver and excreted via the kidney. Impaired hepatic or renal function may prolong the duration of action of diazepam. It is recommended that elderly and debilitated patients receive initially one half the normal recommended dose.

During prolonged administration, for example in the treatment of tetanus, the dosage should generally be reduced after 6-7 days, to reduce the likelihood of accumulation and prolonged CNS depression.

5.3 Preclinical safety data

Not applicable.

6. PHARMACEUTICAL PARTICULARS

6.1 List of excipients

Fractionated soy bean oil, diacetylated monoglycerides, fractionated egg phospholipids, glycerol (anhydrous), sodium hydroxide (to pH8), water for injections (to 2ml).

6.2 Incompatibilities

Diazemuls should only be mixed in the same container or syringe with dextrose solution 5% or 10% or intralipid 10% or 20%. The contents of the ampoule should not be mixed with any drugs other than the infusion solutions mentioned above. Store at room temperature. Do not freeze.

6.3 Shelf life

24 months.

6.4 Special precautions for storage

Store below 25°C. Do not freeze.

6.5 Nature and contents of container

2ml glass type 1 ampoules in cartons of 10.

6.6 Instructions for use and handling

Not applicable.

Administrative Data

7. MARKETING AUTHORISATION HOLDER

Dumex Limited

Whiddon Valley

Barnstaple

Devon EX32 8NS

8. MARKETING AUTHORISATION NUMBER(S)

PL 10183/0001

9. DATE OF FIRST AUTHORISATION/RENEWAL OF THE AUTHORISATION

15.3.89

Renewed: 10.2.97; 10.2.02

10. DATE OF REVISION OF THE TEXT

January 2004

Diazepam Injection BP

(Wockhardt UK Ltd)

1. NAME OF THE MEDICINAL PRODUCT

Diazepam 5.0mg/ml Injection BP

2. QUALITATIVE AND QUANTITATIVE COMPOSITION

Diazepam 5.0mg/ml

For excipients, see section 6.1.

3. PHARMACEUTICAL FORM

Solution for Injection.

Clear, colourless to yellow liquid.

4. CLINICAL PARTICULARS

4.1 Therapeutic indications

Diazepam injection may be used in severe or disabling anxiety and agitation; for the control of status epilepticus, epileptic and febrile convulsions; to relieve muscle spasm; as a sedative in minor surgical and dental procedures; or other circumstances in which a rapid effect is required.

4.2 Posology and method of administration

Dosage depends on individual response, age and weight.

Adults:

In severe anxiety or acute muscle spasm, diazepam 10mg may be given intravenously or intramuscularly and repeated after 4 hours.

In tetanus, 0.1 to 0.3mg per kg bodyweight may be given intravenously and repeated every 1-4 hours; alternatively, a continuous infusion of 3 to 10mg per kg every 24 hours may be used or similar doses may be given by nasoduodenal tube.

In status epilepticus or epileptic convulsions, 0.15-0.25mg per kg (usually 10-20mg) is given by intravenous injection. If no effect is seen after 5 minutes, the dose can be repeated, up to a maximum of 30mg. Once the patient is controlled, recurrence of seizures may be prevented by a slow infusion (maximum total dose 3mg per kg over 24 hours).

In minor surgical procedures and dentistry, 0.1-0.2mg per kg by injection (usually 10-20mg) adjusted to the patient's requirements.

Elderly:

Elderly or debilitated patients should be given not more than half of the usual dose.

Hepatic/renal impairment

Dosage reduction may also be required in patients with liver or kidney dysfunction.

Children:

In status epilepticus, epileptic or febrile convulsions: 0.2-0.3mg per kg (or 1mg per year of life) is given by intravenous injection. If no effect is seen after 5 minutes, the dose can be repeated.

Sedation or muscle relaxation: up to 0.2mg per kg may be given parenterally.

Neonates:

Not recommended; dosage has not been established and Diazepam Injection BP contains benzyl alcohol which should be avoided in injections to neonates.

IMPORTANT: In order to reduce the likelihood of adverse effects during intravenous administration the injection should be given slowly (1.0ml solution per minute). It is advisable to keep the patient supine for at least an hour after administration. Except in emergencies, a second person should always be present during intravenous use and facilities for resuscitation should always be available.

It is recommended that patients should remain under medical supervision until at least one hour has elapsed from the time of injection. They should always be accompanied home by a responsible adult, with a warning not to drive or operate machinery for 24 hours.

Intravenous injection may be associated with local reactions and thrombophlebitis and venous thrombosis may occur. In order to minimise the likelihood of these effects, intravenous injections of diazepam should be given into a large vein of the antecubital fossa.

Where continuous intravenous infusion is necessary it is suggested that 2ml Diazepam Injection is mixed with at least 200ml of infusion fluid such as Sodium Chloride Injection or Dextrose Injection and that such solutions should be used immediately. There is evidence that diazepam is adsorbed onto plastic infusion bags and giving sets. It is therefore recommended that glass bottles should be used for the administration of diazepam by intravenous infusion.

4.3 Contraindications

Known sensitivity to benzodiazepines or any of the ingredients

Myasthenia gravis

Severe respiratory insufficiency

Sleep apnoea syndrome

Avoid injection in neonates (contains benzyl alcohol)

Diazepam injection should not be used in phobic or obsessional states nor be used alone in the treatment of depression or anxiety associated with depression due to the risk of suicide being precipitated in this patient group. Diazepam Injection should not be used in the treatment of chronic psychosis. In common with other benzodiazepines the use of diazepam may be associated with amnesia and Diazepam Injection should not be used in cases of loss or bereavement as psychological adjustment may be inhibited.

4.4 Special warnings and special precautions for use

Diazepam injection should be used with caution in patients with renal or hepatic dysfunction (see 4.2 Posology and Method of Administration), chronic pulmonary insufficiency, porphyria, a known history of drug or alcohol abuseor organic brain changes, particularly arteriosclerosis.

Diazepam may enhance the effects of other CNS depressants; their concurrent use should be avoided.

The dependence potential of diazepam increases with dose and duration of treatment and is greater in patients with a history of alcohol or drug abuse (see 4.8 Undesirable Effects). It is low when limited to short term use. Withdrawal symptoms may occur with benzodiazepines following normal use of therapeutic doses for only short periods and may be associated with physiological and psychological sequelae, including depression. This should be considered when treating patients for more than a few days; abrupt discontinuation should be avoided and the dose reduced gradually As with other benzodiazepines extreme caution should be used if prescribing diazepam for patients with personality disorders. The disinhibiting effects of benzodiazepines may be manifested as the precipitation of suicide in patients who are depressed or show aggressive behaviour towards self and others.

There is a risk of benzyl alcohol poisoning with prolonged use of high-dose intravenous infusions of diazepam injection containing benzyl alcohol.

4.5 Interaction with other medicinal products and other forms of Interaction

Alcohol

Alcohol increases the sedative effect of diazepam and should therefore be avoided.

CNS depressants

Enhanced sedation or respiratory and cardiovascular depression may occur if diazepam is given with other drugs that have CNS depressant properties, e.g. antipsychotics (enhanced sedative effect, increased plasma concentrations of zotepine), other anxiolytics, sedatives, antidepressants, hypnotics, narcotic analgesics, lofexidine, nabilone, anaesthetics, antiepileptics, sedative antihistamines and antihypertensives (enhanced hypotensive effect, enhanced sedative effect with alpha blockers and possibly moxonidine.).

If such centrally acting depressant drugs are given parenterally in conjunction with intravenous diazepam, severe respiratory and cardiovascular depression may occur. When intravenous diazepam is to be administered concurrently with a narcotic analgesic agent (e.g. in dentistry), it is recommended that diazepam be given after the analgesic and that the dose be carefully titrated to meet the patient's needs.

Hepatic enzyme inducers and inhibitors

Agents that interfere with metabolism by hepatic enzymes (e.g. isoniazid, disulfiram, cimetidine, omeprazole, oral contraceptives, amprenavir and ritonavir) have been shown to reduce the clearance of benzodiazepines and may potentiate their actions., whilst kKnown inducers of hepatic enzymes, for example, rifampicin and phenytoin, may increase the clearance of benzodiazepines.

Diazepam metabolism is accelerated by theophylline and smoking.

Diazepam may interact with other hepatically metabolised drugs, causing inhibition (levodopa) or potentiation (muscle relaxants – enhanced sedative effect with baclofen and tizanidine). Serum phenytoin levels may rise, fall or remain unaltered. In addition, phenytoin may cause diazepam serum levels to fall.

4.6 Pregnancy and lactation

There is no evidence regarding the safety of diazepam in pregnancy. It should not be used, especially in the first and third trimesters, unless the benefit is considered to outweigh the risk.

If the product is prescribed to a woman of childbearing potential she should be warned to contact her physician regarding the discontinuance of the product if she intends to become or suspects that she is pregnant.

There may be a small increase in the risk of congenital malformation, particularly oral cleft, with the use of benzodiazepines in the first trimester.

In labour, high single doses or repeated low doses have been reported to produce hypothermia, hypotonia, respiratory depression and poor suckling (floppy infant syndrome) in the neonate and irregularities in the foetal heart.

Infants born to mothers who take benzodiazepines chronically during the latter stages of pregnancy may develop physical dependence and may be at some risk for developing withdrawal symptoms in the postnatal period A small number of children exposed in utero to benzodiazepines have shown slow development in the early years but by four years of age had developed normally.

Since benzodiazepines are found in the breast milk, benzodiazepines should not be given to breast feeding mothers.

4.7 Effects on ability to drive and use machines

Patients treated with Diazepam Injection should not drive or use machinery.

4.8 Undesirable effects

High dosage or parenteral administration can produce respiratory depression and hypotension.

The side effects of diazepam are usually mild and infrequent. The most common side effects are sedation, drowsiness, headaches, muscle weakness, dizziness (with risk of falls in the elderly), ataxia, confusion, slurred speech, tremor, numbed emotions, reduced alertness, fatigue, double vision, anterograde amnesia and a hangover effect. Elderly or debilitated patients are particularly susceptible to side effects and may require lower doses (see 4.2 Posology and method of administration).

Development of dependence is common after regular use, even in therapeutic doses for short periods, particularly in patients with a history of drug or alcohol abuse or marked personality disorders. Discontinuation may be associated with withdrawal symptoms (see 4.4 Special Warnings and Precautions for Use).

Diazepam injection may be associated with pain and thrombophlebitis.

Other effects which may occur rarely are dry mouth, increased appetite, gastrointestinal and visual disturbances, raised liver enzymes, jaundice, urinary retention, incontinence, hypotension, bradycardia, changes in libido, menstrual disturbances, skin reactions, hypersensitivity, blood dyscrasias, laryngeal spasm, chest pain, respiratory depression and apnoea.

In susceptible patients, an unnoticed depression may become evident. Paradoxical reactions (restlessness, agitation, instability, rages, hallucinations) are known to occur with benzodiazepines and are more likely in children and the elderly.

4.9 Overdose

a) Symptoms

The symptoms of mild overdose may include confusion, somnolence, ataxia, dysarthria, hypotension, muscular weakness. In severe overdose, depression of vital functions may occur, particularly the respiratory centre. As drug levels fall severe agitation may develop.

b) Treatment

Treatment is symptomatic. Respiration, heart rate, blood pressure and body temperature should be monitored and supportive measures taken to maintain cardiovascular and respiratory function. Flumazenil is indicated to counteract the central depressive effect of benzodiazepines but expert advice is essential since adverse effects may occur (e.g. convulsions in patients dependent on benzodiazepines).

5. PHARMACOLOGICAL PROPERTIES

5.1 Pharmacodynamic properties

Diazepam is a psychotropic substance from the class of 1,4-benzodiazepines with marked properties of suppression of tension, agitation and anxiety as well as sedative and hypnotic effects. In addition, diazepam demonstrates muscle relaxant and anticonvulsive properties. It is used in the short-term treatment of anxiety and tension states, as a sedative and premedicant, in the control of muscle spasm and in the management of alcohol withdrawal symptoms.

Diazepam binds to specific receptors in the central nervous system and particular peripheral organs. The benzodiazepine receptors in the CNS have a close functional connection with receptors of the GABA-ergic transmitter system. After binding to the benzodiazepine receptor, diazepam augments the inhibitory effect of GABA-ergic transmission.

5.2 Pharmacokinetic properties

Diazepam is highly lipid soluble and crosses the blood brain barrier. These properties qualify it for intravenous use in short term anaesthetic procedures since it acts promptly on the brain, and its initial effects decrease rapidly as it is distributed into fat deposits and tissues. Following the administration of an adequate intravenous dose of diazepam, effective plasma concentrations are usually reached within 5 minutes (ca. 150-400 ng/ml).

Absorption is erratic following intramuscular administration and lower peak plasma concentrations may be obtained than those following oral administration.

Diazepam is extensively protein bound (95-99%). The volume of distribution is between 0.95 and 2 l/kg depending on age. Diazepam and its main metabolite, N-desmethyldiazepam, cross the placenta and are secreted in breast milk.

Diazepam is metabolised predominantly in the liver. Its metabolites, N-desmethyldiazepam (nordiazepam), temazepam and oxazepam, which appear in the urine as glucuronides, are also pharmacologically active substances. Only 20% of the metabolites are detected in the urine in the first 72 hours.

Diazepam has a biphasic half life with an initial rapid distribution phase followed by a prolonged terminal elimination phase of 1-2 days. For the active metabolites N-desmethyldiazepam, temazepam and oxazepam, the half lives are 30-100 hours, 10-20 hours and 5-15 hours, respectively.

Excretion is mainly renal and also partly biliary. It is dependent on age as well as hepatic and renal function.

Metabolism and elimination in the neonate are markedly slower than in children and adults. In the elderly, elimination is prolonged by a factor of 2 to 4. In patients with impaired renal function, elimination is also prolonged. In patients with hepatic disorders (liver cirrhosis, hepatitis), elimination is prolonged by a factor of 2.

5.3 Preclinical safety data

Chronic toxicity studies have demonstrated no evidence of drug induced changes. There are no long term animal studies to investigate the carcinogenic potential of diazepam. Several investigations pointed to a weakly mutagenic potential at doses far above the human therapeutic dose.

Local tolerability has been studied following single and repeat dose applications into the conjunctival sac of rabbits and the rectum of dogs. Only minimal irritation was observed. There were no systemic changes.

In humans it would appear that the risk of congenital abnormalities from the ingestion of therapeutic doses of benzodiazepines is slight, although a few epidemiological studies have pointed to an increased risk of cleft palate. There are case reports of congenital abnormalities and mental retardation in prenatally exposed children following overdosage and intoxication with benzodiazepines.

6. PHARMACEUTICAL PARTICULARS

6.1 List of excipients

Benzoic acid

Ethanol

Propylene glycol

Sodium benzoate

Benzyl alcohol

Water for Injections

6.2 Incompatibilities

Diazepam Injection should not be mixed with other drugs in the same infusion solution or the same syringe.

6.3 Shelf life

Three years

6.4 Special precautions for storage

Store in the original packaging in order to protect from light.

Do not store above 25°C

6.5 Nature and contents of container

Amber glass ampoules (2ml or 4ml) packed in 10s in an outer printed carton.

6.6 Instructions for use and handling

None

Administrative Data

7. MARKETING AUTHORISATION HOLDER

CP Pharmaceuticals Ltd

Ash Road North

Wrexham

LL13 9UF

8. MARKETING AUTHORISATION NUMBER(S)

4543/0179

9. DATE OF FIRST AUTHORISATION/RENEWAL OF THE AUTHORISATION

Date of last renewal – 31 May 1996

10. DATE OF REVISION OF THE TEXT

May 2003

Diazepam RecTubes 10mg

(Wockhardt UK Ltd)

1. NAME OF THE MEDICINAL PRODUCT

Diazepam RecTubes 10mg

2. QUALITATIVE AND QUANTITATIVE COMPOSITION

Diazepam Ph Eur 10mg in 2.5ml (4mg/ml)

For excipients, see 6.1

3. PHARMACEUTICAL FORM

Rectal solution

A clear, colourless or almost yellow solution

4. CLINICAL PARTICULARS

4.1 Therapeutic indications

Diazepam rectal tubes may be used in severe or disabling anxiety and agitation; epileptic and febrile convulsions; to relieve muscle spasm caused by tetanus; as a sedative in minor surgical and dental procedures, or other circumstances in which a rapid effect is required but where intravenous injection is impracticable or undesirable.

Diazepam rectal tubes may be of particular value for the immediate treatment of convulsions in children.

4.2 Posology and method of administration

Dosage depends on age and weight.

Children: 0.5mg/kg

(not recommended for use in children less than one year old)

Adults: 0.5mg/kg

If convulsions are not controlled other anticonvulsive measures should be instituted.

The dose can be repeated every 12 hours.

Elderly and debilitated patients should be given not more than one half the appropriate adult dose.

Dosage reduction may also be required in patients with liver or kidney dysfunction.

The solution is administered rectally. Adults should be in the lateral position; children should be in the prone or lateral position.

a) Tear open the foil pack. Remove the cap.

b) Insert the tube nozzle completely into the rectum. For children under 15kg, insert only half way. Hold the tube with the spout downwards. The contents of the tube should be completely emptied by using firm pressure with the index finger and thumb.

c) To avoid suction, maintain pressure on the tube until it is withdrawn from the rectum. Press together the patients buttocks for a short time.

In anxiety, the duration of treatment should be as short as possible and generally not more than 8-12 weeks, including a tapering off process (see 4.4 Special Warnings and Special Precautions for Use).

Patients requiring chronic dosing should be checked regularly at the start of treatment in order to decrease, if necessary, the dose or frequency of administration, to prevent overdose due to accumulation.

4.3 Contraindications

Known hypersensitivity to benzodiazepines or any of the ingredients.

Myasthenia gravis.

Severe respiratory insufficiency.

Sleep apnoea syndrome

Severe hepatic insufficiency

Diazepam should not be used in phobic or obsessional states, nor be used alone in the treatment of depression or anxiety associated with depression due to the risk of suicide being precipitated in this patient group. Diazepam should not be used for the primary treatment of psychotic illness. In common with other benzodiazepines the use of diazepam may be associated with amnesia and diazepam should not be used in cases of loss or bereavement as psychological adjustments may be inhibited.

4.4 Special warnings and special precautions for use

Use in patients with concomitant physical illness

Diazepam should be used with caution in patients with renal or hepatic dysfunction, chronic pulmonary insufficiency, closed angle glaucoma or organic brain changes, particularly arteriosclerosis.

Dependence and withdrawal symptoms

Use of benzodiazepines may lead to the development of physical and psychological dependence upon these products. This should be considered when treating patients for more than a few days. The dependence potential of diazepam is low when limited to short-term use but increases with the dose and duration of treatment; it is also greater in patients with a history of alcohol or drug abuse.

Once physical dependence has developed, abrupt termination of treatment will be accompanied by withdrawal symptoms. These may consist of headaches, muscle pain, extreme anxiety, tension, restlessness, confusion and irritability. In severe cases the following symptoms may occur: derealisation, depersonalisation, hyperacusis, numbness and tingling of the extremities, hypersensitivity to light, noise and physical contact, hallucinations or epileptic seizures.

Since the risk of withdrawal phenomena/rebound phenomena is greater after abrupt discontinuation of treatment, it is recommended that dose is decreased gradually.

When benzodiazepines with a long duration of action, such as diazepam, are being used, it is important to warn against changing to a benzodiazepine with a short duration of action, as withdrawal symptoms may develop.

Treatment of anxiety (see 4.2 Posology and Method of Administration)

It may be useful to inform the patient when treatment is started that it will be of limited duration and to explain precisely how the dosage will be progressively decreased. In certain cases, extension beyond the maximum treatment period may be necessary; if so, it should not take place without re-evaluation of the patient's status with special expertise.

Rebound anxiety, a transient syndrome whereby the symptoms that led to treatment with a benzodiazepine recur in an enhanced form, may occur on withdrawal of treatment. It may be accompanied by other reactions including mood changes or sleep disturbances and restlessness. It is important that the patient should be aware of the possibility of rebound phenomena, thereby minimising anxiety over such symptoms should they occur while the medicinal product is being discontinued.

Benzodiazepines should not be given to children for anxiety without careful assessment of the need to do so.

Amnesia

Benzodiazepines may induce anterograde amnesia (see 4.8 Undesirable Effects). The condition occurs most often several hours after administration. To reduce the risk, where appropriate and possible, patients should be able to have an uninterrupted sleep of 7-8 hours after administration.

Psychiatric and paradoxical reactions

Reactions like restlessness, agitation, irritability, aggressiveness, delusion, rages, nightmares, hallucinations, psychoses, inappropriate behaviour and other adverse behavioural effects are known to occur when using benzodiazepines (See 4.8 Undesirable Effects). Should they occur, use of diazepam should be discontinued.

Use in patients with concomitant mental illness or addiction

Benzodiazepines should be used with extreme caution in patients with a history of alcohol or drug abuse. As with other benzodiazepines, extreme caution should be used if prescribing diazepam for patients with personality disorders. The disinhibiting effects of benzodiazepines may be manifested as the precipitation of suicide in patients who show aggressive behaviour towards self and others.

4.5 Interaction with other medicinal products and other forms of Interaction

Alcohol

Concomitant intake of alcohol is not recommended. The sedative effect of diazepam may be enhanced. This affects the ability to drive or use machines (see 4.7 Effects on ability to drive and use machines).

CNS depressants

The effects of concurrent CNS depressants should be taken into account. Enhanced sedation or respiratory and cardiovascular depression may occur if diazepam is given with other drugs that have CNS depressant properties (e.g. antipsychotics [neuroleptics], anxiolytics, sedatives, antidepressants, hypnotics, narcotic analgesics, anaesthetics, antiepileptics and sedative antihistamines). In the case of narcotic analgesics, enhancement of euphoria may also occur leading to an increase in psychological dependence.

Hepatic enzyme inducers and inhibitors

Agents that interfere with their metabolism by hepatic enzymes (particularly cytochrome P450), e.g. isoniazid, disulfiram, cimetidine, omeprazole, oral contraceptives, amprenavir may reduce the clearance of benzodiazepines and potentiate their action. Known inducers of hepatic enzymes e.g. rifampicin, may increase the clearance of benzodiazepines.

Diazepam metabolism is accelerated by theophylline and smoking.

Diazepam may interact with other hepatically metabolised drugs, causing inhibition (levodopa) or potentiation (phenytoin, muscle relaxants).

4.6 Pregnancy and lactation

There is no evidence regarding the safety of diazepam in pregnancy. It should not be used, especially in the first and third trimesters, unless the benefit is considered to outweigh the risk.

If diazepam is prescribed to a woman of childbearing potential, she should be warned to contact her physician regarding discontinuation of the product if she intends to become, or suspects that she is, pregnant.

If, for compelling medical reasons, diazepam is administered during the late phase of pregnancy or in labour as high single doses or repeated low doses, effects on the neonate, such as hypothermia, hypotonia, moderate respiratory depression and poor suckling (floppy infant syndrome) and irregularities in the foetal heart can be expected.

Moreover, infants born to mothers who take benzodiazepines chronically during the latter stages of pregnancy may develop physical dependence and may be at some risk for developing withdrawal symptoms in the postnatal period.

Diazepam is excreted in the breast milk and therefore its use during lactation should be avoided.

4.7 Effects on ability to drive and use machines

Patients treated with Diazepam Rectal Tubes should not drive or operate machines as sedation, amnesia, impaired concentration and impaired muscular function may adversely affect their ability (see 4.5 Interaction with Other Medicaments). If insufficient sleep duration occurs, the likelihood of impaired alertness may be increased.

4.8 Undesirable effects

The side effects of diazepam are usually mild and infrequent, occur predominantly at the start of therapy and usually disappear with repeated administration. The most common side effects are sedation, drowsiness, headaches, muscle weakness, dizziness (with risk of falls in the elderly), ataxia, confusion, slurred speech, tremor, numbed emotions, reduced alertness, fatigue, double vision, anterograde amnesia and a hangover effect. Elderly or debilitated patients are particularly susceptible to side effects and may require lower doses. Gastrointestinal disturbances, changes in libido or skin reactions have been reported occasionally. Other effects which may occur rarely are dry mouth, increased appetite, visual disturbances, jaundice, urinary retention, hypotension, bradycardia, menstrual disturbances, blood dyscrasias, laryngeal spasm, chest pain, respiratory depression and apnoea.

Anterograde amnesia may occur using therapeutic doses, the risk increasing at higher doses (see 4.4 Special Warnings and Special Precautions for Use). Amnestic effects may be associated with inappropriate behaviour.

In susceptible patients, an unnoticed pre-existingdepression may become evident. Paradoxical reactions (restlessness, agitation, instability, rages, hallucinations, irritability, aggressiveness, delusion, nightmares, psychoses, inappropriate behaviour and other adverse behavioural effects) are known to occur with benzodiazepines and may be quite severe with diazepam (see 4.4 Special Warnings and Special Precautions for Use). They are more likely to occur in children and the elderly.

Use (even at therapeutic doses) may lead to the development of physical dependence; discontinuation of diazepam may result in withdrawal or rebound phenomena (see 4.4 Special Warnings and Special Precautions for Use). Psychological dependence may occur. Abuse of benzodiazepines has been reported.

4.9 Overdose

a) Symptoms

Overdose of benzodiazepines is usually manifest by degrees of central nervous system depression ranging from drowsiness to coma. The symptoms of mild overdose may include confusion, somnolence, lethargy, ataxia, dysarthria, muscular weakness. In severe overdose, symptoms may include hypotonia, hypotension, respiratory depression, rarely coma and, very rarely, death. As drug levels fall severe agitation may develop.

As with other benzodiazepines, overdose should not present a threat to life unless combined with other CNS depressants (including alcohol).

b) Treatment

In the management of overdose with any medicinal product, it should be borne in mind that multiple agents may have been taken.

Treatment is symptomatic. Respiration, heart rate, blood pressure and body temperature should be monitored in intensive care and supportive measures taken to maintain cardiovascular and respiratory function. Flumazenil may be indicated to counteract the central depressive effect of benzodiazepines.

5. PHARMACOLOGICAL PROPERTIES

5.1 Pharmacodynamic properties

Diazepam is a psychotropic substance from the class of 1,4-benzodiazepines with marked properties of suppression of tension, agitation and anxiety as well as sedative and hypnotic effects. In addition, diazepam demonstrates muscle relaxant and anticonvulsive properties. It is used in the short-term treatment of anxiety and tension states, as a sedative and premedicant, in the control of muscle spasm and in the management of alcohol withdrawal symptoms.

Diazepam binds to specific receptors in the central nervous system and particular peripheral organs. The benzodiazepine receptors in the CNS have a close functional connection with receptors of the GABA-ergic transmitter system. After binding to the benzodiazepine receptor, diazepam augments the inhibitory effect of GABA-ergic transmission.

5.2 Pharmacokinetic properties

After rectal administration of the solution, diazepam is absorbed rapidly and almost completely from the rectum.

The onset of the therapeutic effect occurs within a few minutes of rectal administration. The rapidity of the rise in the serum level following rectal administration corresponds approximately to that following an intravenous dose but peak plasma concentrations are lower after rectal tubes than after intravenous administration. In adults maximal plasma concentrations following the administration of 10 mg diazepam in rectal solution are reached after about 10 - 30 minutes (ca. 150 - 400 ng/ml).

Diazepam is extensively protein bound (95-99%). The volume of distribution is between 0.95 and 2 l/kg depending on age. Diazepam is lipophilic and rapidly enters the cerebrospinal fluid. Diazepam and its main metabolite, N-desmethyldiazepam, cross the placenta and are secreted in breast milk.

Diazepam is metabolised predominantly in the liver. Its metabolites, N-desmethyldiazepam (nordiazepam), temazepam and oxazepam, which appear in the urine as glucuronides, are also pharmacologically active substances. Only 20% of the metabolites are detected in the urine in the first 72 hours.

Diazepam has a biphasic half life with an initial rapid distribution phase followed by a prolonged terminal elimination phase of 1-2 days. The time to reach steady state plasma levels is therefore 4-10 days. For the active metabolites N-desmethyldiazepam, temazepam and oxazepam, the half lives are 30-100 hours, 10-20 hours and 5-15 hours, respectively.

Excretion is mainly renal and also partly biliary. It is dependent on age as well as hepatic and renal function.

Metabolism and elimination in the neonate are markedly slower than in children and adults. In the elderly, elimination is prolonged by a factor of 2 to 4. In patients with impaired renal function, elimination is also prolonged. In patients with hepatic disorders (liver cirrhosis, hepatitis), elimination is prolonged by a factor of 2.

5.3 Preclinical safety data

Chronic toxicity studies in animals have demonstrated no evidence of drug-induced changes. There are no long-term animal studies to investigate the carcinogenic potential of diazepam. Several investigations pointed to a weakly mutagenic potential at doses far above the human therapeutic dose.

Local tolerability has been studied following single and repeat dose applications into the conjunctival sac of rabbits and the rectum of dogs. Only minimal irritation was observed. There were no systemic changes.

In humans it would appear that the risk of congenital abnormalities from the ingestion of therapeutic doses of benzodiazepines is slight, although a few epidemiological studies have pointed to an increased risk of cleft palate. There are case reports of congenital abnormalities and mental retardation in prenatally exposed children following overdosage and intoxication with benzodiazepines.

6. PHARMACEUTICAL PARTICULARS

6.1 List of excipients

Benzyl alcohol

Ethanol 96%

Propylene glycol

Benzoic acid

Sodium benzoate

Purified Water

6.2 Incompatibilities

None known.

6.3 Shelf life

Three years.

6.4 Special precautions for storage

Do not store above 25°C.

6.5 Nature and contents of container

Packs of 2 or 5 rectal tubes each containing 2.5ml of solution

The tubes are made of low-density polyethylene.

6.6 Instructions for use and handling

No special requirements.

Administrative Data

7. MARKETING AUTHORISATION HOLDER

CP Pharmaceuticals Ltd

Wrexham Industrial Estate

Wrexham

LL13 9UF

UK

8. MARKETING AUTHORISATION NUMBER(S)

PL 04543/0341

9. DATE OF FIRST AUTHORISATION/RENEWAL OF THE AUTHORISATION

14th June 1994

10. DATE OF REVISION OF THE TEXT

February 2002

Diazepam RecTubes 2.5mg

(Wockhardt UK Ltd)

1. NAME OF THE MEDICINAL PRODUCT

Diazepam RecTubes 2.5mg

2. QUALITATIVE AND QUANTITATIVE COMPOSITION

Diazepam 2.5mg in 1.25ml (2mg/ml)

For excipients, see 6.1

3. PHARMACEUTICAL FORM

Rectal solution

A clear, colourless or almost yellow solution

4. CLINICAL PARTICULARS

4.1 Therapeutic indications

Diazepam rectal tubes may be used in severe or disabling anxiety and agitation; epileptic and febrile convulsions; to relieve muscle spasm caused by tetanus; as a sedative in minor surgical and dental procedures, or other circumstances in which a rapid effect is required but where intravenous injection is impracticable or undesirable.

Diazepam rectal tubes may be of particular value for the immediate treatment of convulsions in children.

4.2 Posology and method of administration

Dosage depends on age and weight.

Children: 0.5mg/kg

(not recommended for use in children less than one year old)

Adults: 0.5mg/kg

If convulsions are not controlled other anticonvulsive measures should be instituted.

The dose can be repeated every 12 hours.

Elderly and debilitated patients should be given not more than one half the appropriate adult dose.

Dosage reduction may also be required in patients with liver or kidney dysfunction.

The solution is administered rectally. Adults should be in the lateral position; children should be in the prone or lateral position.

a) Tear open the foil pack. Remove the cap.

b) Insert the tube nozzle completely into the rectum. For children under 15kg, insert only half way. Hold the tube with the spout downwards. The contents of the tube should be completely emptied by using firm pressure with the index finger and thumb.

c) To avoid suction, maintain pressure on the tube until it is withdrawn from the rectum. Press together the patient's buttocks for a short time.

In anxiety, the duration of treatment should be as short as possible and generally not more than 8-12 weeks, including a tapering off process (see 4.4 Special Warnings and Special Precautions for Use).

Patients requiring chronic dosing should be checked regularly at the start of treatment in order to decrease, if necessary, the dose or frequency of administration, to prevent overdose due to accumulation.

4.3 Contraindications

Known hypersensitivity to benzodiazepines or any of the ingredients.

Myasthenia gravis.

Severe respiratory insufficiency.

Sleep apnoea syndrome

Severe hepatic insufficiency

Diazepam should not be used in phobic or obsessional states, nor be used alone in the treatment of depression or anxiety associated with depression due to the risk of suicide being precipitated in this patient group. Diazepam should not be used for the primary treatment of psychotic illness. In common with other benzodiazepines the use of diazepam may be associated with amnesia and diazepam should not be used in cases of loss or bereavement as psychological adjustments may be inhibited.

4.4 Special warnings and special precautions for use

Use in patients with concomitant physical illness

Diazepam should be used with caution in patients with renal or hepatic dysfunction, chronic pulmonary insufficiency, closed angle glaucoma or organic brain changes, particularly arteriosclerosis.

Dependence and withdrawal symptoms

Use of benzodiazepines may lead to the development of physical and psychological dependence upon these products. This should be considered when treating patients for more than a few days. The dependence potential of diazepam is low when limited to short-term use but increases with the dose and duration of treatment; it is also greater in patients with a history of alcohol or drug abuse.

Once physical dependence has developed, abrupt termination of treatment will be accompanied by withdrawal symptoms. These may consist of headaches, muscle pain, extreme anxiety, tension, restlessness, confusion and irritability. In severe cases the following symptoms may occur: derealisation, depersonalisation, hyperacusis, numbness and tingling of the extremities, hypersensitivity to light, noise and physical contact, hallucinations or epileptic seizures.

Since the risk of withdrawal phenomena/rebound phenomena is greater after abrupt discontinuation of treatment, it is recommended that dose is decreased gradually.

When benzodiazepines with a long duration of action, such as diazepam, are being used, it is important to warn against changing to a benzodiazepine with a short duration of action, as withdrawal symptoms may develop.

Treatment of anxiety (see 4.2 Posology and Method of Administration)

It may be useful to inform the patient when treatment is started that it will be of limited duration and to explain precisely how the dosage will be progressively decreased. In certain cases, extension beyond the maximum treatment period may be necessary; if so, it should not take place without re-evaluation of the patient's status with special expertise.

Rebound anxiety, a transient syndrome whereby the symptoms that led to treatment with a benzodiazepine recur in an enhanced form, may occur on withdrawal of treatment. It may be accompanied by other reactions including mood changes or sleep disturbances and restlessness. It is important that the patient should be aware of the possibility of rebound phenomena, thereby minimising anxiety over such symptoms should they occur while the medicinal product is being discontinued.

Benzodiazepines should not be given to children for anxiety without careful assessment of the need to do so.

Amnesia

Benzodiazepines may induce anterograde amnesia (see 4.8 Undesirable Effects). The condition occurs most often several hours after administration. To reduce the risk, where appropriate and possible, patients should be able to have an uninterrupted sleep of 7-8 hours after administration.

Psychiatric and paradoxical reactions

Reactions like restlessness, agitation, irritability, aggressiveness, delusion, rages, nightmares, hallucinations, psychoses, inappropriate behaviour and other adverse behavioural effects are known to occur when using benzodiazepines (See 4.8 Undesirable Effects). Should they occur, use of diazepam should be discontinued.

Use in patients with concomitant mental illness or addiction

Benzodiazepines should be used with extreme caution in patients with a history of alcohol or drug abuse. As with other benzodiazepines, extreme caution should be used if prescribing diazepam for patients with personality disorders. The disinhibiting effects of benzodiazepines may be manifested as the precipitation of suicide in patients who show aggressive behaviour towards self and others.

4.5 Interaction with other medicinal products and other forms of Interaction

Alcohol

Concomitant intake of alcohol is not recommended. The sedative effect of diazepam may be enhanced. This affects the ability to drive or use machines (see 4.7 Effects on ability to drive and use machines).

CNS depressants

The effects of concurrent CNS depressants should be taken into account. Enhanced sedation or respiratory and cardiovascular depression may occur if diazepam is given with other drugs that have CNS depressant properties (e.g. antipsychotics [neuroleptics], anxiolytics, sedatives, antidepressants, hypnotics, narcotic analgesics, anaesthetics, antiepileptics and sedative antihistamines). In the case of narcotic analgesics, enhancement of euphoria may also occur leading to an increase in psychological dependence.

Hepatic enzyme inducers and inhibitors

Agents that interfere with their metabolism by hepatic enzymes (particularly cytochrome P450), e.g. isoniazid, disulfiram, cimetidine, omeprazole, oral contraceptives, amprenavir may reduce the clearance of benzodiazepines and potentiate their action. Known inducers of hepatic enzymes e.g. rifampicin, may increase the clearance of benzodiazepines.

Diazepam metabolism is accelerated by theophylline and smoking.

Diazepam may interact with other hepatically metabolised drugs, causing inhibition (levodopa) or potentiation (phenytoin, muscle relaxants).

4.6 Pregnancy and lactation

There is no evidence regarding the safety of diazepam in pregnancy. It should not be used, especially in the first and third trimesters, unless the benefit is considered to outweigh the risk.

If diazepam is prescribed to a woman of childbearing potential, she should be warned to contact her physician regarding discontinuation of the product if she intends to become, or suspects that she is, pregnant.

If, for compelling medical reasons, diazepam is administered during the late phase of pregnancy or in labour as high single doses or repeated low doses, effects on the neonate, such as hypothermia, hypotonia, moderate respiratory depression and poor suckling (floppy infant syndrome) and irregularities in the foetal heart can be expected.

Moreover, infants born to mothers who take benzodiazepines chronically during the latter stages of pregnancy may develop physical dependence and may be at some risk for developing withdrawal symptoms in the postnatal period.

Diazepam is excreted in the breast milk and therefore its use during lactation should be avoided.

4.7 Effects on ability to drive and use machines

Patients treated with Diazepam Rectal Tubes should not drive or operate machines as sedation, amnesia, impaired concentration and impaired muscular function may adversely affect their ability (see 4.5 Interaction with Other Medicaments). If insufficient sleep duration occurs, the likelihood of impaired alertness may be increased.

4.8 Undesirable effects

The side effects of diazepam are usually mild and infrequent, occur predominantly at the start of therapy and usually disappear with repeated administration. The most common side effects are sedation, drowsiness, headaches, muscle weakness, dizziness (with risk of falls in the elderly), ataxia, confusion, slurred speech, tremor, numbed emotions, reduced alertness, fatigue, double vision, anterograde amnesia and a hangover effect. Elderly or debilitated patients are particularly susceptible to side effects and may require lower doses. Gastrointestinal disturbances, changes in libido or skin reactions have been reported occasionally. Other effects which may occur rarely are dry mouth, increased appetite, visual disturbances, jaundice, urinary retention, hypotension, bradycardia, menstrual disturbances, blood dyscrasias, laryngeal spasm, chest pain, respiratory depression and apnoea.

Anterograde amnesia may occur using therapeutic doses, the risk increasing at higher doses (see 4.4 Special Warnings and Special Precautions for Use). Amnestic effects may be associated with inappropriate behaviour.

In susceptible patients, an unnoticed pre-existing depression may become evident. Paradoxical reactions (restlessness, agitation, instability, rages, hallucinations, irritability, aggressiveness, delusion, nightmares, psychoses, inappropriate behaviour and other adverse behavioural effects) are known to occur with benzodiazepines and may be quite severe with diazepam (see 4.4 Special Warnings and Special Precautions for Use). They are more likely to occur in children and the elderly.

Use (even at therapeutic doses) may lead to the development of physical dependence; discontinuation of diazepam may result in withdrawal or rebound phenomena (see 4.4 Special Warnings and Special Precautions for Use). Psychological dependence may occur. Abuse of benzodiazepines has been reported.

4.9 Overdose

a) Symptoms

Overdose of benzodiazepines is usually manifest by degrees of central nervous system depression ranging from drowsiness to coma. The symptoms of mild overdose may include confusion, somnolence, lethargy, ataxia, dysarthria, muscular weakness. In severe overdose, symptoms may include hypotonia, hypotension, respiratory depression, rarely coma and, very rarely, death. As drug levels fall severe agitation may develop.

As with other benzodiazepines, overdose should not present a threat to life unless combined with other CNS depressants (including alcohol).

b) Treatment

In the management of overdose with any medicinal product, it should be borne in mind that multiple agents may have been taken.

Treatment is symptomatic. Respiration, heart rate, blood pressure and body temperature should be monitored in intensive care and supportive measures taken to maintain cardiovascular and respiratory function. Flumazenil may be indicated to counteract the central depressive effect of benzodiazepines.

5. PHARMACOLOGICAL PROPERTIES

5.1 Pharmacodynamic properties

Diazepam is a psychotropic substance from the class of 1,4-benzodiazepines with marked properties of suppression of tension, agitation and anxiety as well as sedative and hypnotic effects. In addition, diazepam demonstrates muscle relaxant and anticonvulsive properties. It is used in the short-term treatment of anxiety and tension states, as a sedative and premedicant, in the control of muscle spasm and in the management of alcohol withdrawal symptoms.

Diazepam binds to specific receptors in the central nervous system and particular peripheral organs. The benzodiazepine receptors in the CNS have a close functional connection with receptors of the GABA-ergic transmitter system. After binding to the benzodiazepine receptor, diazepam augments the inhibitory effect of GABA-ergic transmission.

5.2 Pharmacokinetic properties

After rectal administration of the solution, diazepam is absorbed rapidly and almost completely from the rectum.

The onset of the therapeutic effect occurs within a few minutes of rectal administration. The rapidity of the rise in the serum level following rectal administration corresponds approximately to that following an intravenous dose but peak plasma concentrations are lower after rectal tubes than after intravenous administration. In adults maximal plasma concentrations following the administration of 10 mg diazepam in rectal solution are reached after about 10 - 30 minutes (ca. 150 - 400 ng/ml).

Diazepam is extensively protein bound (95-99%). The volume of distribution is between 0.95 and 2 l/kg depending on age. Diazepam is lipophilic and rapidly enters the cerebrospinal fluid. Diazepam and its main metabolite, N-desmethyldiazepam, cross the placenta and are secreted in breast milk.

Diazepam is metabolised predominantly in the liver. Its metabolites, N-desmethyldiazepam (nordiazepam), temazepam and oxazepam, which appear in the urine as glucuronides, are also pharmacologically active substances. Only 20% of the metabolites are detected in the urine in the first 72 hours.

Diazepam has a biphasic half life with an initial rapid distribution phase followed by a prolonged terminal elimination phase of 1-2 days. The time to reach steady state plasma levels is therefore 4-10 days. For the active metabolites N-desmethyldiazepam, temazepam and oxazepam, the half lives are 30-100 hours, 10-20 hours and 5-15 hours, respectively.

Excretion is mainly renal and also partly biliary. It is dependent on age as well as hepatic and renal function.

Metabolism and elimination in the neonate are markedly slower than in children and adults. In the elderly, elimination is prolonged by a factor of 2 to 4. In patients with impaired renal function, elimination is also prolonged. In patients with hepatic disorders (liver cirrhosis, hepatitis), elimination is prolonged by a factor of 2.

5.3 Preclinical safety data

Chronic toxicity studies in animals have demonstrated no evidence of drug-induced changes. There are no long-term animal studies to investigate the carcinogenic potential of diazepam. Several investigations pointed to a weakly mutagenic potential at doses far above the human therapeutic dose.

Local tolerability has been studied following single and repeat dose applications into the conjunctival sac of rabbits and the rectum of dogs. Only minimal irritation was observed. There were no systemic changes.

In humans it would appear that the risk of congenital abnormalities from the ingestion of therapeutic doses of benzodiazepines is slight, although a few epidemiological studies have pointed to an increased risk of cleft palate. There are case reports of congenital abnormalities and mental retardation in prenatally exposed children following overdosage and intoxication with benzodiazepines.

6. PHARMACEUTICAL PARTICULARS

6.1 List of excipients
Benzyl alcohol
Ethanol 96%
Propylene glycol
Benzoic acid
Sodium benzoate
Purified Water

6.2 Incompatibilities
None known.

6.3 Shelf life
Three years

6.4 Special precautions for storage
Do not store above 25°C.

6.5 Nature and contents of container
Packs of 2 or 5 rectal tubes each containing 1.25ml of solution

The tubes are made of low density polyethylene.

6.6 Instructions for use and handling
No special requirements.

Administrative Data

7. MARKETING AUTHORISATION HOLDER
CP Pharmaceuticals Ltd
Wrexham Industrial Estate
Wrexham
LL13 9UF
UK

8. MARKETING AUTHORISATION NUMBER(S)
PL 04543/0364

9. DATE OF FIRST AUTHORISATION/RENEWAL OF THE AUTHORISATION
14 August 1996

10. DATE OF REVISION OF THE TEXT
February 2002

Diazepam RecTubes 5mg

(Wockhardt UK Ltd)

1. NAME OF THE MEDICINAL PRODUCT
Diazepam RecTubes 5mg

2. QUALITATIVE AND QUANTITATIVE COMPOSITION
Diazepam 5mg in 2.5ml (2mg/ml)

For excipients, see 6.1

3. PHARMACEUTICAL FORM
Rectal solution

A clear, colourless or almost yellow solution

4. CLINICAL PARTICULARS

4.1 Therapeutic indications
Diazepam rectal tubes may be used in severe or disabling anxiety and agitation; epileptic and febrile convulsions; to relieve muscle spasm caused by tetanus; as a sedative in minor surgical and dental procedures, or other circumstances in which a rapid effect is required but where intravenous injection is impracticable or undesirable.

Diazepam rectal tubes may be of particular value for the immediate treatment of convulsions in children.

4.2 Posology and method of administration
Dosage depends on age and weight.

Children: 0.5mg/kg

(not recommended for use in children less than one year old)

Adults: 0.5mg/kg

If convulsions are not controlled other anticonvulsive measures should be instituted.

The dose can be repeated every 12 hours.

Elderly and debilitated patients should be given not more than one half the appropriate adult dose.

Dosage reduction may also be required in patients with liver or kidney dysfunction.

The solution is administered rectally. Adults should be in the lateral position; children should be in the prone or lateral position.

a) Tear open the foil pack. Remove the cap.

b) Insert the tube nozzle completely into the rectum. For children under 15kg, insert only half way. Hold the tube with the spout downwards. The contents of the tube should be completely emptied by using firm pressure with the index finger and thumb.

c) To avoid suction, maintain pressure on the tube until it is withdrawn from the rectum. Press together the patients buttocks for a short time.

In anxiety, the duration of treatment should be as short as possible and generally not more than 8-12 weeks, including a tapering off process (see 4.4 Special Warnings and Special Precautions for Use).

Patients requiring chronic dosing should be checked regularly at the start of treatment in order to decrease, if necessary, the dose or frequency of administration, to prevent overdose due to accumulation.

4.3 Contraindications
Known hypersensitivity to benzodiazepines or any of the ingredients.

Myasthenia gravis.

Severe respiratory insufficiency.

Sleep apnoea syndrome

Severe hepatic insufficiency

Diazepam should not be used in phobic or obsessional states, nor be used alone in the treatment of depression or anxiety associated with depression due to the risk of suicide being precipitated in this patient group. Diazepam should not be used for the primary treatment of psychotic illness. In common with other benzodiazepines the use of diazepam may be associated with amnesia and diazepam should not be used in cases of loss or bereavement as psychological adjustments may be inhibited.

4.4 Special warnings and special precautions for use
Use in patients with concomitant physical illness

Diazepam should be used with caution in patients with renal or hepatic dysfunction, chronic pulmonary insufficiency, closed angle glaucoma or organic brain changes, particularly arteriosclerosis.

Dependence and withdrawal symptoms

Use of benzodiazepines may lead to the development of physical and psychological dependence upon these products. This should be considered when treating patients for more than a few days. The dependence potential of diazepam is low when limited to short-term use but increases with the dose and duration of treatment; it is also greater in patients with a history of alcohol or drug abuse.

Once physical dependence has developed, abrupt termination of treatment will be accompanied by withdrawal symptoms. These may consist of headaches, muscle pain, extreme anxiety, tension, restlessness, confusion and irritability. In severe cases the following symptoms may occur: derealisation, depersonalisation, hyperacusis, numbness and tingling of the extremities, hypersensitivity to light, noise and physical contact, hallucinations or epileptic seizures.

Since the risk of withdrawal phenomena/rebound phenomena is greater after abrupt discontinuation of treatment, it is recommended that dose is decreased gradually.

When benzodiazepines with a long duration of action, such as diazepam, are being used, it is important to warn against changing to a benzodiazepine with a short duration of action, as withdrawal symptoms may develop.

Treatment of anxiety (see 4.2 Posology and Method of Administration)

It may be useful to inform the patient when treatment is started that it will be of limited duration and to explain precisely how the dosage will be progressively decreased. In certain cases, extension beyond the maximum treatment period may be necessary; if so, it should not take place without re-evaluation of the patient's status with special expertise.

Rebound anxiety, a transient syndrome whereby the symptoms that led to treatment with a benzodiazepine recur in an enhanced form, may occur on withdrawal of treatment. It may be accompanied by other reactions including mood changes or sleep disturbances and restlessness. It is important that the patient should be aware of the possibility of rebound phenomena, thereby minimising anxiety over such symptoms should they occur while the medicinal product is being discontinued.

Benzodiazepines should not be given to children for anxiety without careful assessment of the need to do so.

Amnesia

Benzodiazepines may induce anterograde amnesia (see 4.8 Undesirable Effects). The condition occurs most often several hours after administration. To reduce the risk, where appropriate and possible, patients should be able to have an uninterrupted sleep of 7-8 hours after administration.

Psychiatric and paradoxical reactions

Reactions like restlessness, agitation, irritability, aggressiveness, delusion, rages, nightmares, hallucinations, psychoses, inappropriate behaviour and other adverse behavioural effects are known to occur when using benzodiazepines (See 4.8 Undesirable Effects). Should they occur, use of diazepam should be discontinued.

Use in patients with concomitant mental illness or addiction

Benzodiazepines should be used with extreme caution in patients with a history of alcohol or drug abuse. As with other benzodiazepines, extreme caution should be used if prescribing diazepam for patients with personality disorders. The disinhibiting effects of benzodiazepines may be manifested as the precipitation of suicide in patients who show aggressive behaviour towards self and others.

4.5 Interaction with other medicinal products and other forms of Interaction
Alcohol

Concomitant intake of alcohol is not recommended. The sedative effect of diazepam may be enhanced. This affects the ability to drive or use machines (see 4.7 Effects on ability to drive and use machines).

CNS depressants

The effects of concurrent CNS depressants should be taken into account. Enhanced sedation or respiratory and cardiovascular depression may occur if diazepam is given with other drugs that have CNS depressant properties (e.g. antipsychotics [neuroleptics], anxiolytics, sedatives, antidepressants, hypnotics, narcotic analgesics, anaesthetics, antiepileptics and sedative antihistamines). In the case of narcotic analgesics, enhancement of euphoria may also occur leading to an increase in psychological dependence.

Hepatic enzyme inducers and inhibitors

Agents that interfere with their metabolism by hepatic enzymes (particularly cytochrome P450), e.g. isoniazid, disulfiram, cimetidine, omeprazole, oral contraceptives, amprenavir, may reduce the clearance of benzodiazepines and potentiate their action. Known inducers of hepatic enzymes e.g. rifampicin, may increase the clearance of benzodiazepines.

Diazepam metabolism is accelerated by theophylline and smoking.

Diazepam may interact with other hepatically metabolised drugs, causing inhibition (levodopa) or potentiation (phenytoin, muscle relaxants).

4.6 Pregnancy and lactation
There is no evidence regarding the safety of diazepam in pregnancy. It should not be used, especially in the first and third trimesters, unless the benefit is considered to outweigh the risk.

If diazepam is prescribed to a woman of childbearing potential, she should be warned to contact her physician regarding discontinuation of the product if she intends to become, or suspects that she is, pregnant.

If, for compelling medical reasons, diazepam is administered during the late phase of pregnancy or in labour as high single doses or repeated low doses, effects on the neonate, such as hypothermia, hypotonia, moderate respiratory depression and poor suckling (floppy infant syndrome) and irregularities in the foetal heart can be expected.

Moreover, infants born to mothers who take benzodiazepines chronically during the latter stages of pregnancy may develop physical dependence and may be at some risk for developing withdrawal symptoms in the postnatal period.

Diazepam is excreted in the breast milk and therefore its use during lactation should be avoided.

4.7 Effects on ability to drive and use machines
Patients treated with Diazepam Rectal Tubes should not drive or operate machines as sedation, amnesia, impaired concentration and impaired muscular function may adversely affect their ability (see 4.5 Interaction with Other Medicaments). If insufficient sleep duration occurs, the likelihood of impaired alertness may be increased.

4.8 Undesirable effects
The side effects of diazepam are usually mild and infrequent, occur predominantly at the start of therapy and usually disappear with repeated administration. The most common side effects are sedation, drowsiness, headaches, muscle weakness, dizziness (with risk of falls in the elderly), ataxia, confusion, slurred speech, tremor, numbed emotions, reduced alertness, fatigue, double vision, anterograde amnesia and a hangover effect. Elderly or debilitated patients are particularly susceptible to side effects and may require lower doses. Gastrointestinal disturbances, changes in libido or skin reactions have been reported occasionally. Other effects which may occur rarely are dry mouth, increased appetite, visual disturbances, jaundice, urinary retention, hypotension, bradycardia, menstrual disturbances, blood dyscrasias, laryngeal spasm, chest pain, respiratory depression and apnoea.

Anterograde amnesia may occur using therapeutic doses, the risk increasing at higher doses (see 4.4 Special Warnings and Special Precautions for Use). Amnestic effects may be associated with inappropriate behaviour.

In susceptible patients, an unnoticed pre-existingdepression may become evident. Paradoxical reactions (restlessness, agitation, instability, rages, hallucinations, irritability, aggressiveness, delusion, nightmares, psychoses, inappropriate behaviour and other adverse behavioural effects) are known to occur with benzodiazepines and may be quite severe with diazepam (see 4.4 Special Warnings and Special Precautions for Use). They are more likely to occur in children and the elderly.

Use (even at therapeutic doses) may lead to the development of physical dependence; discontinuation of diazepam may result in withdrawal or rebound phenomena (see 4.4 Special Warnings and Special Precautions for Use). Psychological dependence may occur. Abuse of benzodiazepines has been reported.

4.9 Overdose

a) Symptoms

Overdose of benzodiazepines is usually manifest by degrees of central nervous system depression ranging from drowsiness to coma. The symptoms of mild overdose may include confusion, somnolence, lethargy, ataxia, dysarthria, muscular weakness. In severe overdose, symptoms may include hypotonia, hypotension, respiratory depression, rarely coma and, very rarely, death. As drug levels fall severe agitation may develop.

As with other benzodiazepines, overdose should not present a threat to life unless combined with other CNS depressants (including alcohol).

b) Treatment

In the management of overdose with any medicinal product, it should be borne in mind that multiple agents may have been taken.

Treatment is symptomatic. Respiration, heart rate, blood pressure and body temperature should be monitored in intensive care and supportive measures taken to maintain cardiovascular and respiratory function. Flumazenil may be indicated to counteract the central depressive effect of benzodiazepines.

5. PHARMACOLOGICAL PROPERTIES

5.1 Pharmacodynamic properties

Diazepam is a psychotropic substance from the class of 1,4-benzodiazepines with marked properties of suppression of tension, agitation and anxiety as well as sedative and hypnotic effects. In addition, diazepam demonstrates muscle relaxant and anticonvulsive properties. It is used in the short-term treatment of anxiety and tension states, as a sedative and premedicant, in the control of muscle spasm and in the management of alcohol withdrawal symptoms.

Diazepam binds to specific receptors in the central nervous system and particular peripheral organs. The benzodiazepine receptors in the CNS have a close functional connection with receptors of the GABA-ergic transmitter system. After binding to the benzodiazepine receptor, diazepam augments the inhibitory effect of GABA-ergic transmission.

5.2 Pharmacokinetic properties

After rectal administration of the solution, diazepam is absorbed rapidly and almost completely from the rectum.

The onset of the therapeutic effect occurs within a few minutes of rectal administration. The rapidity of the rise in the serum level following rectal administration corresponds approximately to that following an intravenous dose but peak plasma concentrations are lower after rectal tubes than after intravenous administration. In adults maximal plasma concentrations following the administration of 10 mg diazepam in rectal solution are reached after about 10 - 30 minutes (ca. 150 - 400 ng/ml).

Diazepam is extensively protein bound (95-99%). The volume of distribution is between 0.95 and 2 l/kg depending on age. Diazepam is lipophilic and rapidly enters the cerebrospinal fluid. Diazepam and its main metabolite, N-desmethyldiazepam, cross the placenta and are secreted in breast milk.

Diazepam is metabolised predominantly in the liver. Its metabolites, N-desmethyldiazepam (nordiazepam), temazepam and oxazepam, which appear in the urine as glucuronides, are also pharmacologically active substances. Only 20% of the metabolites are detected in the urine in the first 72 hours.

Diazepam has a biphasic half life with an initial rapid distribution phase followed by a prolonged terminal elimination phase of 1-2 days. The time to reach steady state plasma levels is therefore 4-10 days. For the active metabolites N-desmethyldiazepam, temazepam and oxazepam, the half lives are 30-100 hours, 10-20 hours and 5-15 hours, respectively.

Excretion is mainly renal and also partly biliary. It is dependent on age as well as hepatic and renal function.

Metabolism and elimination in the neonate are markedly slower than in children and adults. In the elderly, elimination is prolonged by a factor of 2 to 4. In patients with impaired renal function, elimination is also prolonged. In patients with hepatic disorders (liver cirrhosis, hepatitis), elimination is prolonged by a factor of 2.

5.3 Preclinical safety data

Chronic toxicity studies in animals have demonstrated no evidence of drug-induced changes. There are no long-term animal studies to investigate the carcinogenic potential of diazepam. Several investigations pointed to a weakly mutagenic potential at doses far above the human therapeutic dose.

Local tolerability has been studied following single and repeat dose applications into the conjunctival sac of rabbits and the rectum of dogs. Only minimal irritation was observed. There were no systemic changes.

In humans it would appear that the risk of congenital abnormalities from the ingestion of therapeutic doses of benzodiazepines is slight, although a few epidemiological studies have pointed to an increased risk of cleft palate. There are case reports of congenital abnormalities and mental retardation in prenatally exposed children following overdosage and intoxication with benzodiazepines.

6. PHARMACEUTICAL PARTICULARS

6.1 List of excipients

Benzyl alcohol

Ethanol 96%

Propylene glycol

Benzoic acid

Sodium benzoate

Purified Water

6.2 Incompatibilities

None known.

6.3 Shelf life

Three years

6.4 Special precautions for storage

Do not store above 25°C.

6.5 Nature and contents of container

Packs of 2 or 5 rectal tubes each containing 2.5ml of solution

The tubes are made of low-density polyethylene.

6.6 Instructions for use and handling

No special requirements.

Administrative Data

7. MARKETING AUTHORISATION HOLDER

CP Pharmaceuticals Ltd

Wrexham Industrial Estate

Wrexham

LL13 9UF

UK

8. MARKETING AUTHORISATION NUMBER(S)

PL 04543/0340

9. DATE OF FIRST AUTHORISATION/RENEWAL OF THE AUTHORISATION

14th June 1994

10. DATE OF REVISION OF THE TEXT

February 2002

Diclomax SR / Diclomax Retard

(Provalis Healthcare)

1. NAME OF THE MEDICINAL PRODUCT

Diclomax Retard® and Diclomax SR®

2. QUALITATIVE AND QUANTITATIVE COMPOSITION

Each Diclomax Retard® capsule contains diclofenac sodium 100mg.

Each Diclomax SR® capsule contains diclofenac sodium 75mg.

For excipients, see 6.1.

3. PHARMACEUTICAL FORM

Modified release capsules for oral use.

4. CLINICAL PARTICULARS

4.1 Therapeutic indications

For rheumatoid arthritis; osteoarthritis; low back pain; acute musculo-skeletal disorders and trauma such as periarthritis (especially frozen shoulder), tendinitis, tenosynovitis, bursitis, sprains, strains and dislocations; relief of pain in fractures; ankylosing spondylitis; acute gout; control of pain and inflammation in orthopaedic, dental and other minor surgery.

4.2 Posology and method of administration

For oral use.

Adults

Diclomax Retard®: One 100 mg capsule taken whole daily preferably with food or after food.

Diclomax SR®: One or two 75mg capsules taken whole daily in single or divided doses preferably with or after food.

Children

Not recommended.

Elderly

The elderly are at an increased risk of serious consequences of adverse reactions. Studies indicate the pharmacokinetics of diclofenac sodium are not impaired to any clinical extent in the elderly, however, as with all nonsteroidal anti-inflammatory drugs, Diclomax should be used with caution in elderly patients and the lowest effective dose used for the shortest possible duration. These patients should be monitored regularly for GI bleeding during NSAID therapy.

4.3 Contraindications

Diclomax is contra-indicated in patients with a known sensitivity to diclofenac sodium or to any of its constituents, patients with a history of/or active peptic ulcer, history of/or upper gastrointestinal bleeding or perforation related to previous NSAID therapy. NSAIDs are contraindicated in patients who have previously shown hypersensitivity reactions (e.g. asthma, rhinitis, angioedema or urticaria) in response to ibuprofen, aspirin, or other nonsteroidal anti-inflammatory drugs.

Diclomax should not be used in patients with severe hepatic, renal or cardiac failure (see section 4.4) or during the last trimester of pregnancy (see section 4.6)

Diclomax should not be used concomitantly with other NSAIDs including the cyclooxygenase 2 specific inhibitors (see section 4.5).

As Diclomax contains lactose and sucrose, patients with rare hereditary problems of fructose / galactose intolerance, Lapp lactase deficiency, glucose-galactose malabsorption or sucrase-isomaltase insufficiency should not take this medicine.

4.4 Special warnings and special precautions for use

As with all non-steroidal anti-inflammatory drugs (NSAIDs), Diclomax should only be given to the elderly after other forms of treatment have been carefully considered, as the elderly have an increased frequency of adverse reactions to NSAIDs especially gastrointestinal bleeding and perforation which may be fatal (see section 4.2).

Undesirable effects may be minimised in all patients by using the minimum effective dose for the shortest possible duration.

Cardiovascular, Renal and Hepatic impairment:

The administration of an NSAID may cause a dose dependent reduction in prostaglandin formation and precipitate renal failure. Patients at greatest risk of this reaction are those with impaired renal function, cardiac impairment, liver dysfunction, those taking diuretics and the elderly. Renal function should be monitored in these patients (see section 4.3).

NSAIDs should be given with care to patients with a history of heart failure and/or hypertension since fluid retention and oedema has been reported in association with NSAID administration.

All patients who are receiving long-term treatment with NSAIDs should be monitored as a precautionary measure, e.g. renal, hepatic function (elevation of liver enzymes may occur) and blood counts.

If abnormal liver function tests persist or worsen, clinical signs or symptoms consistent with liver disease develop or if other manifestations occur (eosinophilia, rash), Diclomax should be discontinued.

Respiratory disorders:

Caution is required if administered to patients suffering from, or with a previous history of, bronchial asthma since NSAIDs have been reported to cause bronchospasm in such patients.

Gastrointestinal bleeding, ulceration and perforation:

Diclomax should be used with caution in patients with gastro-intestinal disorders or haematological abnormalities, as GI bleeding, ulceration or perforation, which can be fatal, has been reported with NSAID therapy at any time during treatment, with or without warning symptoms or a previous history of serious GI events.

Patients with a history of GI toxicity, particularly the elderly, should report any unusual abdominal symptoms (especially GI bleeding) particularly in the initial stages of treatment.

Caution is advised in patients receiving concomitant medications which could increase the risk of gastrotoxicity or bleeding, such as corticosteroids, or anticoagulants such as warfarin or anti-platelet agents such as aspirin (see section 4.5).

When GI bleeding or ulceration occurs in patients receiving Diclomax, the treatment should be withdrawn.

NSAIDs should be given with care to patients with a history of gastrointestinal disease (ulcerative colitis, Crohns disease) as these conditions may be exacerbated (see section 4.8).

Haematological:

Diclomax, in common with other NSAIDs, can reversibly inhibit platelet aggregation.

SLE and mixed connective tissue disease:

In patients with systemic lupus erythematosus (SLE) and mixed connective tissue disorders there may be an increased risk of aseptic meningitis (see section 4.8).

Female fertility:

The use of Diclomax may impair female fertility and is not recommended in women attempting to conceive. In women who have difficulties conceiving or who are undergoing investigation of infertility, withdrawal of Diclomax should be considered.

4.5 Interaction with other medicinal products and other forms of Interaction

Lithium:

Diclomax may increase plasma concentrations and decrease elimination of lithium.

Cardiac glycosides:

NSAIDs may exacerbate cardiac failure, reduce GFR and increase plasma glycoside levels.

Anticoagulants:

NSAIDs may enhance the effects of anti-coagulants, such as warfarin (see section 4.4).

Antidiabetic agents:

Clinical studies have shown that Diclomax can be given together with oral hypoglycaemic agents without influencing their clinical effect.

However there have been isolated reports of hyperglycaemic and hypoglycaemic effects, which have required adjustments to the dosage of hypoglycaemic agents.

Ciclosporin:

Ciclosporin nephrotoxicity may be increased by the effect of NSAIDs on renal prostaglandins.

Mifepristone:

NSAIDs should not be used for 8-12 days after mifepristone administration as NSAIDs can reduce the effect of mifepristone.

Methotrexate:

Caution should be exercised if NSAIDs and methotrexate are administered within 24 hours of each other, since NSAIDs may increase methotrexate plasma levels with decreased elimination, resulting in increased toxicity.

Quinolone antibiotics:

Animal data indicate that NSAIDs can increase the risk of convulsions associated with quinolone antibiotics.

Patients taking NSAIDs and quinolones may have an increased risk of developing convulsions.

Other analgesics:

Concomitant therapy with other systemic NSAIDs (including aspirin) may increase the frequency of side effects (see section 4.3).

Corticosteroids:

Corticosteroids can increase the risk of gastrointestinal bleeding (see section 4.4).

Diuretics:

Various NSAIDs are liable to inhibit the activity of diuretics. Diuretics can increase the risk of nephrotoxicity of NSAIDs. Concomitant treatment with potassium-sparing diuretics may be associated with increased serum potassium levels, hence serum potassium should be monitored.

Anti-hypertensives:

Reduced anti-hypertensive effect.

Tacrolimus:

Possible increased risk of nephrotoxicity when NSAIDS are given with tacrolimus.

4.6 Pregnancy and lactation

Congenital abnormalities have been reported in association with NSAID administration in man; however, these are low in frequency and do not appear to follow any discernible pattern. In view of the known effects of NSAIDS on the foetal cardiovascular system (risk of closure of the ductus arteriosus), use in the last trimester of pregnancy is contra-indicated. The onset of labour may be delayed and the duration increased with increased bleeding tendency in both mother and child (see section 4.3). NSAIDs should not be used during the first two trimesters of pregnancy or labour unless the potential benefit to the patient outweighs the potential risk to the foetus.

In limited studies so far available, NSAIDs can appear in breast milk in very low concentrations with traces of diclofenac sodium found in breast milk following oral doses of 50mg every 8 hours. NSAIDs should, if possible, be avoided when breastfeeding (see section 4.4 regarding female fertility).

4.7 Effects on ability to drive and use machines

Undesirable effects such as dizziness, drowsiness, fatigue and visual disturbances are possible after taking NSAIDs. If affected, patients should not drive or operate machinery.

4.8 Undesirable effects

The following adverse events have been reported with NSAIDs:

Gastrointestinal:

The most commonly observed adverse events are gastrointestinal in nature. Peptic ulcers, perforation or GI bleeding, sometimes fatal, particularly in the elderly, may occur (see section 4.4). Nausea, vomiting, diarrhoea, flatulence, constipation, dyspepsia, abdominal pain, melaena, haematemesis, ulcerative stomatitis, exacerbation of colitis and Crohns disease (see section 4.4) have been reported following administration. Less frequently, gastritis, has been observed.

Hypersensitivity:

Hypersensitivity reactions have been reported following treatment with NSAIDs. These may consist of a) non-specific allergic reactions and anaphylaxis b) respiratory tract reactivity comprising asthma, aggravated asthma, bronchospasm or dyspnoea, or c) assorted skin disorders, including rashes of various types, pruritus, urticaria, purpura, angioedema and, more rarely exfoliative and bullous dermatoses (including epidermal necrolysis and erythema multiforme).

Cardiovascular:

Oedema has been reported in association with NSAID treatment.

Other adverse events reported less commonly include:

Renal:

Nephrotoxicity in various forms, including interstitial nephritis, nephrotic syndrome and renal failure.

Hepatic

Abnormal liver function, hepatitis and jaundice.

Neurological & special senses:

Visual disturbances, optic neuritis, headaches, paraesthesia, reports of aseptic meningitis (especially in patients with existing auto-immune disorders, such as systemic lupus erythematosus, mixed connective tissue disease), with symptoms such as stiff neck, headache, nausea, vomiting, fever or disorientation (see section 4.4), depression, confusion, hallucinations, tinnitus, vertigo, dizziness, malaise, fatigue and drowsiness.

Haematological:

Thrombocytopenia, neutropenia, agranulocytosis, aplastic anaemia and haemolytic anaemia.

Dermatological:

Photosensitivity.

4.9 Overdose

a) Symptoms

Symptoms include headache, nausea, vomiting, epigastric pain, gastrointestinal bleeding, rarely diarrhoea, disorientation, excitation, coma, drowsiness, dizziness, tinnitus, fainting, occasionally convulsions. In cases of significant poisoning, acute renal failure and liver damage are possible.

b) Therapeutic measures

Patients should be treated symptomatically as required.

Within one hour of ingestion of a potentially toxic amount, activated charcoal should be considered. Alternatively, in adults, gastric lavage should be considered within one hour of ingestion of a potentially life-threatening overdose.

Good urine output should be ensured.

Renal and liver function should be closely monitored.

Patients should be observed for at least four hours after ingestion of potentially toxic amounts.

Frequent or prolonged convulsions should be treated with intravenous diazepam.

Other measures may be indicated by the patient's clinical condition.

5. PHARMACOLOGICAL PROPERTIES

5.1 Pharmacodynamic properties

Diclofenac Sodium is a non-steroidal agent with marked analgesic/anti-inflammatory and anti-pyretic properties. It is an inhibitor of prostaglandin synthetase (cyclo-oxygenase).

5.2 Pharmacokinetic properties

Diclofenac Sodium is rapidly absorbed from the gut and is subject to first-pass metabolism. Capsules give peak plasma concentrations after approximately 2.5 hours. The active substance is 99.7% protein bound and plasma half-life for the terminal elimination phase is 1-2 hours. Approximately 60% of the administered dose is excreted via the kidneys in the form of metabolites and less than 1% in unchanged form. About 30% of the dose is excreted via the bile in metabolised form.

The Diclomax slow release preparation:

- Increases the duration of action of the drug
- Maintains relatively constant rate of absorption in the gastrointestinal tract over a longer period of time
- Increases the fraction of the ingested dose absorbed in the G.I.tract
- Regulates the rate at which the drug is made available for absorption, thereby reducing the possibility of malabsorption and occurrence of side-effects.

5.3 Preclinical safety data

The results of the preclinical tests do not add anything of further significance to the prescriber.

6. PHARMACEUTICAL PARTICULARS

6.1 List of excipients

Diclomax Retard® capsules contain the following excipients:

Sucrose, maize starch, polyethylene glycol 6000, ammonio methacrylate copolymer type A, talc, lactose, polysorbate 80, purified water, ethanol 96%, acetone, gelatin, titanium dioxide E171 and imprinting ink – Opacode S-1-8100 Black HV 1007 (shellac, iron oxide black, 2-ethoxyethanol, soya lecithin and simeticone).

Diclomax SR® capsules contain the following excipients:

Sucrose, maize starch, polyethylene glycol 6000, ammonio methacrylate copolymer type A, talc, lactose, polysorbate 80, purified water, ethanol 96%, acetone, gelatin, E172, E171 and imprinting ink - opacode S-1-8100 black HV 1007 (shellac, iron oxide black, 2-ethoxyethanol, soya lecithin and simeticone).

6.2 Incompatibilities

None known.

6.3 Shelf life

Diclomax Retard®: 24 months – PVC/PE/PVDC blister packs.

18 months – PVC blister packs.

Diclomax SR®: 24 months – PVC/PE/PVDC blister packs

18 months – PVC blister packs

6.4 Special precautions for storage

Store between 10°C and 25°C. Protect from moisture. Do not refrigerate.

6.5 Nature and contents of container

Diclomax Retard®: White opaque PVC/Al blister strips or white opaque PVC/PE/PVDC/Al blister strips in packs of 4 or 28 capsules.

Diclomax SR®: White opaque PVC blister pack with hard tempered foil or white opaque PVC/PE/PVDC/hard tempered foil blister strips in packs of 4 and 56 capsules.

6.6 Instructions for use and handling

No special instructions needed.

Administrative Data

7. MARKETING AUTHORISATION HOLDER

Provalis Healthcare Ltd

Newtech Square

Deeside Industrial Park

Deeside

Flintshire

CH5 2NT

8. MARKETING AUTHORISATION NUMBER(S)

Diclomax Retard®: PL 14658/0010

Diclomax SR®: PL 14658/0011

9. DATE OF FIRST AUTHORISATION/RENEWAL OF THE AUTHORISATION

1st March 2002

10. DATE OF REVISION OF THE TEXT

May 2005

Dicobalt Edetate Injection 300mg

(Cambridge Laboratories)

1. NAME OF THE MEDICINAL PRODUCT

Dicobalt Edetate Injection 300mg

2. QUALITATIVE AND QUANTITATIVE COMPOSITION

Each ampoule contains 300mg Dicobalt Edetate INN (15mg/ml)

3. PHARMACEUTICAL FORM

Solution for Injection

4. CLINICAL PARTICULARS

4.1 Therapeutic indications

Dicobalt Edetate Injection is a specific antidote for acute cyanide poisoning. In view of the difficulty of certain diagnosis in emergency situations, it is recommended that Dicobalt Edetate Injection only be given when the patient is tending to lose or has lost consciousness. The product should not be used as a precautionary measure.

4.2 Posology and method of administration

Cyanide poisoning must be treated as quickly as possible and intensive supportive measures must be instituted: clear airways and adequate ventilation are essential. 100% oxygen should be administered concurrently with Dicobalt Edetate.

Expert advice on the treatment of poisoning is available at the local poisons centre.

Adults

One 300mg ampoule intravenously over approximately one minute. If the patient shows inadequate response, a second ampoule may be given. If there is no response after a further five minutes, a third ampoule maybe administered.

Each ampoule of Dicobalt Edetate Injection may be followed immediately by 50ml Glucose Intravenous Infusion BP 500g/l.

When the patient's condition is less severe but in the physician's judgement still warrants the use of Dicobalt Edetate Injection, the period over which the injection is given should be extended to 5 minutes.

Children

There is no clinical experience of the use of Dicobalt Edetate Injection in children. As with adults the dose required will be related to the quantity of cyanide ingested.

The elderly

There is no clinical evidence of the use of Dicobalt Edetate Injection in the elderly, but there is no reason to believe that the dosage schedule should be different from that for adults.

4.3 Contraindications

None.

4.4 Special warnings and special precautions for use

There is a reciprocal antidote action between cyanide and cobalt. Thus in the absence of cyanide, Dicobalt Edetate Injection itself is toxic. It is therefore essential that the product only be used in cases of cyanide poisoning. When the patient is fully conscious, it is likely that the extent of poisoning warrants the use of Dicobalt Edetate Injection.

4.5 Interaction with other medicinal products and other forms of Interaction

No information is available.

4.6 Pregnancy and lactation

No information is available.

4.7 Effects on ability to drive and use machines
Not applicable.

4.8 Undesirable effects
The initial effects of Dicobalt Edetate Injection are vomiting, a fall in blood pressure and compensatory tachycardia. After this the patient should recover.

4.9 Overdose
Signs and symptoms – these may be due to cobalt toxicity or to an anaphylactic type reaction, which may be dramatic. Oedema (particularly of the face and neck), vomiting, chest pain, sweating, hypotension, cardiac irregularities and rashes may occur.

Treatment – intensive supportive therapy is required.

5. PHARMACOLOGICAL PROPERTIES
5.1 Pharmacodynamic properties
Cyanide blocks intracellular respiration by binding to cytochrome oxidase. Dicobalt Edetate Injection forms a stable complex with the cyanide thereby acting as an antidote.

5.2 Pharmacokinetic properties
Only very limited data are available. Intravenous infusion of Dicobalt Edetate Injection is likely to result in rapid distribution in the extracellular fluid compartment. Excretion is entirely via the kidneys within 24 hours and it is not metabolised.

5.3 Preclinical safety data
There are no pre-clinical data of relevance to the prescriber which are additional to that already included in other sections of the SPC.

6. PHARMACEUTICAL PARTICULARS
6.1 List of excipients
Dextrose Monohydrate

Water for Injections

6.2 Incompatibilities
Not applicable.

6.3 Shelf life
Three years.

6.4 Special precautions for storage
Store below 25°C away from light.

6.5 Nature and contents of container
Packs of six Ph.Eur Type 1 glass ampoules each containing 20ml of rose-violet coloured sterile pyrogen free solution.

6.6 Instructions for use and handling
None.

7. MARKETING AUTHORISATION HOLDER
L'Arguenon Limited

The Cricketers

Turgis Green

Nr Basingstoke

RG27 0AH

8. MARKETING AUTHORISATION NUMBER(S)
PL: 14945/0001

9. DATE OF FIRST AUTHORISATION/RENEWAL OF THE AUTHORISATION
31st May 1996

10. DATE OF REVISION OF THE TEXT
March 2000

Diconal Tablets

(Amdipharm)

1. NAME OF THE MEDICINAL PRODUCT
Diconal Tablets.

2. QUALITATIVE AND QUANTITATIVE COMPOSITION
Each tablet contains 10 mg of Dipipanone Hydrochloride BP and 30 mg of Cyclizine Hydrochloride BP, coloured deep pink, scored and coded 'F3A'.

3. PHARMACEUTICAL FORM
Tablet.

4. CLINICAL PARTICULARS
4.1 Therapeutic indications
Diconal Tablets are indicated for the management of moderate to severe pain in medical and surgical conditions in which morphine may be indicated.

Cyclizine is effective in preventing nausea and vomiting associated with the administration of narcotic analgesics.

4.2 Posology and method of administration
Adults: The initial dose in all conditions is one tablet every 6 hours. It is unwise to exceed this dose in view of the difficulty in accurately predicting the initial central effects of dipipanone.

Should this dose fail to prove adequate analgesia, as in severe intractable pain or when other potent opioids have been used, it may be increased by half a tablet every six hours.

It is seldom necessary to exceed a dose of 30 mg dipipanone given 6-hourly (i.e. 12 tablets in 24 hours).

Children: There is no specific information on the use of Diconal in children. Diconal is very rarely indicated in children and dosage guidelines cannot be stated.

Use in the elderly: There is no specific information on the use of Diconal in elderly patients. In common with opioid drugs, Diconal may be expected to cause confusion in this age group, and careful monitoring is advised (see *Precautions*).

4.3 Contraindications
Diconal is contra-indicated in individuals who are hypersensitive to dipipanone or cyclizine.

Diconal is generally contra-indicated in patients with respiratory depression, especially in the presence of cyanosis and excessive bronchial secretions.

Diconal should not be given during an attack of bronchial asthma.

Diconal is generally contra-indicated in the presence of acute alcoholism, head injury and raised intracranial pressure.

Diconal is contra-indicated in individuals receiving monoamine oxidase inhibitors, or within 14 days of stopping such treatment.

Diconal is contra-indicated in patients with ulcerative colitis since in common with other narcotic analgesics it may precipitate toxic dilatation or spasm of the colon.

As with all narcotic analgesics Diconal should not be administered to patients with severe hepatic impairment as it may precipitate hepatic encephalopathy.

In severe renal impairment Diconal, in common with all narcotic analgesics, may precipitate coma and should not be administered.

Diconal, in common with morphine and most other narcotics, may cause spasm of the biliary and renal tracts; it is contra-indicated in these conditions.

4.4 Special warnings and special precautions for use
The repeated use of Diconal may lead to tolerance and physical dependence as well as to psychological dependence on the product.

Misuse of Diconal has been reported, particularly by young addicts who have previously been dependent on, or have misused other agents both opiate and non-opiate. Extreme caution is warranted when prescribing Diconal to this group of patients.

Diconal should be used with extreme caution in the presence of the following: hypothyroidism; adrenocortical insufficiency; prostatic hypertrophy; hypotension secondary to hypovolaemic shock; diabetes mellitus.

Diconal is metabolised in the liver and excreted along with its metabolites in the urine. Where not contra-indicated in patients with impaired hepatic and/or renal function, Diconal should be given at less than the usual recommended dose, and the patient's response used as a guide to further dosage requirements.

Extreme caution should be exercised when administering Diconal to patients with phaeochromocytoma, since hypertension has been reported in association with other potent opioids.

No data are available as to whether or not dipipanone has carcinogenic, mutagenic or teratogenic potential. It is not known whether cyclizine has carcinogenic or mutagenic potential. Some animal studies are interpreted as indicating that cyclizine may be teratogenic, but relevance to the human situation is not known.

In a study involving prolonged administration of cyclizine to male and female rats, there was no evidence of impaired fertility after continuous treatment for 90-100 days. There are no similar data for dipipanone. There is no information on the effect of Diconal on human fertility.

4.5 Interaction with other medicinal products and other forms of Interaction
The central nervous system depressant effects of Diconal may be increased by phenothiazine drugs, alcohol, sedatives and tricyclic antidepressants. Concurrent administration of some phenothiazines increases the respiratory depressant effects of narcotic analgesics and also produces hypotension.

Because of its anticholinergic activity, cyclizine may enhance the side effects of other anticholinergic agents.

Analgesic effects of opioid drugs tend to be enhanced by co-administration of dexamphetamine, however their use in combination is not recommended.

4.6 Pregnancy and lactation
The use of Diconal during pregnancy is not recommended. No data are available on the therapeutic use of Diconal in human pregnancy. It may be anticipated that if given in the last trimester, Diconal would cause withdrawal symptoms in the neonate.

Diconal is not recommended for use in labour because of its potential to cause respiratory depression in the neonate.

No data are available on the excretion of dipipanone, cyclizine or their metabolites in human milk.

4.7 Effects on ability to drive and use machines
Ambulatory patients receiving Diconal should be cautioned against driving cars or operating machinery in view of its tendency to cause drowsiness.

4.8 Undesirable effects
The adverse effects of dipipanone are common to all opioid agents, and may include:- respiratory depression; mental clouding, drowsiness and sedation, confusion, mood changes, euphoria, dysphoria, psychosis, restlessness, miosis and raised intracranial pressure; constipation, nausea and vomiting; sweating, facial flushing and hypotension; urticaria and rashes; difficulty with micturition; biliary and renal tract spasm; vertigo.

In addition, cyclizine may cause urticaria, drug rash, drowsiness, dryness of the mouth, nose and throat, blurred vision, tachycardia, urinary retention, constipation, restlessness, nervousness, insomnia and auditory and visual hallucinations, particularly when dosage recommendations have been exceeded. Other central nervous system effects which have been reported rarely include dystonia, dyskenesia, extrapyramidal motor disturbances, tremor, twitching, muscle spasms, convulsions, disorientation, dizziness, decreased consciousness and transient speech disorders. Cholestatic jaundice has occurred in association with cyclizine. Single case reports have been documented of fixed drug eruption; generalised chorea; hypersensitivity hepatitis and agranulocytosis.

4.9 Overdose
The signs of overdosage with Diconal are typically those of opioid poisoning i.e. respiratory depression, pin-point pupils, hypotension, circulatory failure and deepening coma. Mydriasis may replace miosis as asphyxia intervenes. Drowsiness, floppiness, miosis and apnoea have been reported in children, as have convulsions.

General supportive measures should be employed as required. Gastric lavage should be performed if indicated. The specific opioid antagonist naloxone is the treatment of choice for the reversal of coma and the restoration of spontaneous respiration; the literature should be consulted for details of appropriate dosage. Patients should be monitored closely for at least 48 hours after recovery in case of relapse, since the duration of action of the antagonist may be substantially shorter than that of dipipanone.

5. PHARMACOLOGICAL PROPERTIES
5.1 Pharmacodynamic properties
The onset of analgesic action of dipipanone is approximately one hour and lasts for 4 to 6 hours. Cyclizine produces its anti-emetic effect within 2 hours and lasts for approximately 4 hours.

5.2 Pharmacokinetic properties
Dipipanone is absorbed from the gastro-intestinal tract. It is metabolised in the liver and excreted in the urine and faeces, although data on the proportions of parent compound and metabolites so excreted are lacking.

In healthy adult volunteers, the administration of a single oral dose of 50 mg cyclizine resulted in a peak plasma concentration of approximately 70 nanogram/ml occurring approximately 2 hours after drug administration. The plasma elimination half-life was approximately 20 hours.

The N-demethylated derivative, norcyclizine, has been identified as a metabolite of cyclizine. Norcyclizine has little antihistaminic (H_1) activity compared with cyclizine and has a plasma elimination half life of approximately 20 hours. After a single oral dose of 50 mg cyclizine given to a single adult male volunteer, urine collected over the following 24 hours contained less than 1% of the total dose administered.

5.3 Preclinical safety data
No additional data of relevance.

6. PHARMACEUTICAL PARTICULARS
6.1 List of excipients
Lactose, starches, dye (FD and C Red No. 3), gelatin, magnesium stearate.

6.2 Incompatibilities
None stated.

6.3 Shelf life
60 months.

6.4 Special precautions for storage
Store below 25°C. Protect from light. Keep dry.

6.5 Nature and contents of container
PVC/aluminium foil blister packs containing 50 tablets.

6.6 Instructions for use and handling
None stated.

7. MARKETING AUTHORISATION HOLDER
Amdipharm PLC

Trading as Amdipharm

Regency House

Miles Gray Road

Basildon

Essex

SS14 3AF

8. MARKETING AUTHORISATION NUMBER(S)
PL 20072/0009

9. DATE OF FIRST AUTHORISATION/RENEWAL OF THE AUTHORISATION
15th September 2003

10. DATE OF REVISION OF THE TEXT

Dicynene 500 Tablets

(sanofi-aventis)

1. NAME OF THE MEDICINAL PRODUCT

Dicynene 500 Tablets

2. QUALITATIVE AND QUANTITATIVE COMPOSITION

Each tablet contains 500mg etamsylate as the active ingredient.

For excipients, see 6.1.

3. PHARMACEUTICAL FORM

White capsule-shaped tablet imprinted "D500" on one face, with a break-mark on the other.

4. CLINICAL PARTICULARS

4.1 Therapeutic indications

Dicynene is used clinically for the short term treatment of blood loss in primary and IUCD-induced menorrhagia.

4.2 Posology and method of administration

Adults only

The usual dosage is 500mg four times daily from the start of bleeding until menstruation ceases.

Route of administration: oral

4.3 Contraindications

Treatment should only be undertaken following exclusion of other pelvic pathology, in particular the presence of fibroids. Use in patients with a known hypersensitivity to etamsylate or to any of the excipients. Use in patients with porphyria.

4.4 Special warnings and special precautions for use

The drug contains:

- Sulfites which may cause anaphylactic reactions (see 4.8 Undesirable effects).
- Wheat starch which may be harmful to people with coeliac disease.

If the patient develops a fever then treatment should be discontinued.

In patients receiving Dicynene for menorrhagia the use of the product before onset of bleeding is not recommended.

4.5 Interaction with other medicinal products and other forms of Interaction

None stated.

4.6 Pregnancy and lactation

Clinical use in pregnancy is not relevant for this indication. Studies in animals have revealed no teratogenic effect of etamsylate however there is inadequate evidence of safety in human pregnancy.

Etamsylate is secreted in breast milk and administration to nursing mothers is not recommended.

4.7 Effects on ability to drive and use machines

None stated.

4.8 Undesirable effects

Fever may occur.

Occasional headaches or skin rashes may also occur but usually disappear on reduced dosage. A few patients may experience gastrointestinal disturbances such as nausea, vomiting or diarrhoea; however this may be overcome by administering the dose after food.

Due to the presence of sulfites, allergic reactions may occur including anaphylactic symptoms ranging from rash to anaphylactic shock (see 4.4 Special warnings and precautions for use).

4.9 Overdose

There is no experience of overdosage with Dicynene 500 tablets.

5. PHARMACOLOGICAL PROPERTIES

5.1 Pharmacodynamic properties

Dicynene is a non-hormonal agent which reduces capillary exudation and blood loss. Dicynene does not affect the normal coagulation mechanism since administration is without effect on prothrombin times, fibrinolysis, platelet count or function.

Dicynene is thought to act by increasing capillary vascular wall resistance and platelet adhesiveness; in the presence of a vascular lesion, it inhibits the biosynthesis and action of those prostaglandins which cause platelet disaggregation, vasodilation and increased capillary permeability. Dicynene does not have a vasoconstricting action.

5.2 Pharmacokinetic properties

Dicynene is fully absorbed when given orally and is excreted unchanged, largely by the urinary route.

5.3 Preclinical safety data

No further information is available.

6. PHARMACEUTICAL PARTICULARS

6.1 List of excipients

Sodium sulphite anhydrous, sodium dihydrogen citrate, microcrystalline cellulose, povidone, wheat starch and stearic acid.

6.2 Incompatibilities

None known.

6.3 Shelf life

3 years.

6.4 Special precautions for storage

Do not store above 25°C. Store in the original packaging. Dispense in airtight containers.

6.5 Nature and contents of container

Securitainer with lid and foam wad or moulded pack insert (jayfilla) containing 100 tablets.

6.6 Instructions for use and handling

Not applicable.

7. MARKETING AUTHORISATION HOLDER

Sanofi-Synthelabo
PO Box 597
Guildford
Surrey

8. MARKETING AUTHORISATION NUMBER(S)

PL 11723/0319

9. DATE OF FIRST AUTHORISATION/RENEWAL OF THE AUTHORISATION

15th August 2001

10. DATE OF REVISION OF THE TEXT

February 2004

Legal Category POM

Didronel 200mg Tablets

(Procter & Gamble Pharmaceuticals UK Limited)

1. NAME OF THE MEDICINAL PRODUCT

Didronel 200mg Tablets.

2. QUALITATIVE AND QUANTITATIVE COMPOSITION

Each tablet contains 200mg of Etidronate Disodium, USP.

3. PHARMACEUTICAL FORM

White rectangular tablets marked with 'P&G' on one face and '402' on the other.

4. CLINICAL PARTICULARS

4.1 Therapeutic indications

Paget's disease of bone:

Effectiveness has been demonstrated primarily in patients with polyostotic Paget's disease with symptoms of pain and with clinically significant elevations of urinary hydroxyproline and serum alkaline phosphatase. In other circumstances in which there is extensive involvement of the skull or the spine with the prospect of irreversible neurological damage, or when a weight-bearing bone may be involved, the use of Didronel may also be considered.

4.2 Posology and method of administration

5mg/kg/day to 20mg/kg/day as detailed below.

Didronel should be given on an empty stomach. It is recommended that patients take the therapy with water, at the mid point of a four hour fast (ie. two hours before and two after food).

Adults and Elderly:

The recommended initial dose of Didronel for most patients is 5mg/kg body weight/day, for a period not exceeding six months. Doses above 10mg/kg should be reserved for use when there is an overriding requirement for suppression of increased bone turnover associated with Paget's disease or when the patient requires more prompt reduction of elevated cardiac output. Treatment with doses above 10mg/kg/day should be approached cautiously and should not exceed three months duration. Doses in excess of 20mg/kg/day are not recommended.

Re-treatment should be undertaken only after a drug-free period of at least three months and after it is evident that reactivation of the disease has occurred and biochemical indices of the disease have become substantially re-elevated or approach pretreatment values (approximately twice the upper limit of normal or 75% of pre-treatment value). In no case should duration of treatment exceed the maximum duration of the initial treatment. Premature re-treatment should be avoided. In clinical trials the biochemical improvements obtained during drug therapy have generally persisted for a period of three months to 2 years after drug withdrawal.

Daily Dosage Guide

(see Table 1 below)

Children:

Disorders of bone in children, referred to as juvenile Paget's disease, have been reported rarely. The relationship to adult Paget's disease has not been established. Didronel has not been studied in children for Paget's disease.

4.3 Contraindications

Known hypersensitivity to the drug. Clinically overt osteomalacia.

4.4 Special warnings and special precautions for use

In Pagetic patients the physician should adhere to the recommended dose regimen in order to avoid over-treatment with Didronel. The response to therapy may be of slow onset and may continue even for months after treatment with the drug has been discontinued. Dosage should not be increased prematurely nor should treatment be resumed before there is clear evidence of reactivation of the disease process. Re-treatment should not be initiated until the patient has had at least a three-month drug-free interval.

Didronel is not metabolised but excreted unchanged via the kidney; therefore, a reduced dose should be used in patients with mild renal impairment and treatment of patients with moderate to severe renal impairment should be avoided. Caution should be taken in patients with a history of renal stone formation. In patients with impaired renal function or a history of renal stone formation, serum and urinary calcium should be monitored regularly.

It is recommended that serum phosphate, serum alkaline phosphatase and if possible urinary hydroxyproline be measured before commencing medication and at three month intervals during treatment. If after three months of medication the pre-treatment levels have not been reduced by at least 25%, the patient may be relatively resistant to therapy. If the serum phosphate level is unchanged in the "resistant" patient, consideration should be given to increasing the dose since the absorption of pharmacologically active amounts of Didronel is typically accompanied by a rise in serum phosphate. This rise usually correlates with reductions in the biochemical indices of disease activity. If after three or more months of medication elevations of serum phosphate above the upper limit of normal are not accompanied by clinical or biochemical evidence of reduced activity, resistance of the disease to the action of Didronel is probable and termination of Didronel medication should be considered. Etidronate disodium suppresses bone turnover and may retard mineralisation of osteoid laid down during the bone accretion process. These effects are dose and time dependent. Osteoid, which may accumulate noticeably at doses of 10-20 mg/kg/day, mineralises normally post-therapy. Patients in whom serum phosphate elevations are high and reductions of disease activity are low may be particularly prone to retarded mineralisation of new osteoid. In those cases where 200mg per day (a single tablet) may be excessive, doses may be administered less frequently.

Patients with Paget's disease of bone should maintain an adequate intake of calcium and vitamin D. Patients with low vitamin D and calcium intake may be particularly sensitive to drugs that affect calcium homeostasis and should be closely monitored during Didronel therapy.

Etidronate disodium does not adversely affect serum levels of parathyroid hormone or calcium.

Hyperphosphataemia has been observed in patients receiving etidronate disodium, usually in association with doses of 10-20mg/kg/day. No adverse effects have been traced to this, and it does not constitute grounds for discontinuing therapy. It is apparently due to a drug-related increase in renal tubular reabsorption of phosphate. Serum phosphate levels generally return to normal 2-4 weeks post therapy.

Patients with significant chronic diarrhoeal disease may experience increased frequency of bowel movements and diarrhoea, particularly at higher doses.

Table 1 Daily Dosage Guide

Body Weight		Required Daily Regimen of 200mg Tablets		
Kilogrames	Stones	5mg/kg*	10mg/kg*	20mg/kg+
50	8	1	3	5
60	9.5	2	3	6
70	11	2	4	7
80	12.5	2	4	8
90	14	2	5	9

*Course of therapy - 6 months
+Course of therapy - 3 months

Increased or recurrent bone pain at existing Pagetic sites and/or the appearance of pain at sites previously asymptomatic have been reported at a dose of 5mg/kg/day.

Fractures are recognised as a common feature in patients with Paget's disease. There has been no evidence of increased risk of fractures at the recommended dose of 5mg/kg/day for six months. At doses of 20mg/kg/day in excess of three months' duration, mineralisation of newly formed osteoid may be impaired and the risk of fracture may be increased. The risk of fracture may also be greater in patients with extensive and severe disease, a history of multiple fractures, and/or rapidly advancing osteolytic lesions. It is therefore recommended that the drug is discontinued when fractures occur and therapy not reinstated until the fracture healing is complete.

Patients with predominantly lytic lesions should be monitored radiographically and biochemically to permit termination of etidronate disodium in those patients unresponsive to treatment. The incidence of osteogenic sarcoma is known to be increased in Paget's disease. Pagetic lesions, with or without therapy, may appear by X-ray to progress markedly, possibly with some loss of definition of periosteal margins. Such lesions should be evaluated carefully to differentiate these from osteogenic sarcoma.

4.5 Interaction with other medicinal products and other forms of Interaction

Food in the stomach or upper portions of the small intestine, particularly materials with a high calcium content such as milk, may reduce absorption of etidronate disodium. Vitamins with mineral supplements such as iron, calcium supplements, laxatives containing magnesium, or antacids containing calcium or aluminium should not be taken within two hours of dosing etidronate disodium.

There have been isolated reports of patients experiencing changes in their prothrombin times when etidronate was added to warfarin therapy. The majority of these reports concerned variable elevations in prothrombin times without clinically significant sequelae. Although the relevance of these reports and any mechanism of coagulation alterations is unclear, patients on warfarin should have their prothrombin time monitored.

4.6 Pregnancy and lactation

The safety of this medicinal product for use in human pregnancy has not been established. Reproductive studies have shown skeletal abnormalities in rats. It is therefore recommended that Didronel should not be used in women of childbearing potential unless adequate contraceptive measures are taken.

It is not known whether this drug is excreted in human milk, and therefore caution should be exercised when Didronel is administered to a nursing woman.

4.7 Effects on ability to drive and use machines

Etidronate disodium does not interfere with the ability to drive or use machines.

4.8 Undesirable effects

Gastro-intestinal

The most common effects reported are diarrhoea and nausea. Reports of exacerbation of peptic ulcer with complications in a few patients.

Dermatological/hypersensitivity

Hypersensitivity reactions, including angio-oedema/urticaria, rash and/or pruritus, have been reported rarely.

Nervous System

Paresthesia, confusion, have been reported rarely.

Haematological

In patients receiving etidronate disodium, there have been rare reports of leucopenia, agranulocytosis and pancytopenia.

Other

Less common effects believed to be related to therapy include arthropathies (arthralgia and arthritis), and rarely burning of the tongue, alopecia, erythema multiforme and exacerbation of asthma.

4.9 Overdose

Overdose would manifest as the signs and symptoms of hypocalcaemia. Treatment should involve cessation of therapy and correction of hypocalcaemia with administration of Ca^{2+} intravenously.

5. PHARMACOLOGICAL PROPERTIES

5.1 Pharmacodynamic properties

Etidronate acts primarily on bone. It can inhibit the formation, growth and dissolution of hydroxyapatite crystals and amorphous precursors by chemisorption to calcium phosphate surfaces. Inhibition of crystal resorption occurs at lower doses than are required for the inhibition of crystal growth. Both effects increase as dose increases.

5.2 Pharmacokinetic properties

Etidronate is not metabolised. Absorption averages about 1% of an oral dose of 5mg/kg body weight/day. This increases to about 1.5% at 10mg/kg/day and 6% at 20mg/kg/day. Most of the drug is cleared from the blood within 6 hours. Within 24 hours about half of the absorbed dose is excreted in the urine. The remainder is chemically absorbed to bone, especially to areas of elevated osteogenesis, and is slowly eliminated. Unabsorbed drug is excreted in the faeces.

5.3 Preclinical safety data

In long term studies in mice and rats, there was no evidence of carcinogenicity with etidronate disodium. All *in vitro* and *in vivo* assays conducted to assess the mutagenic potential of etidronate disodium have been negative.

6. PHARMACEUTICAL PARTICULARS

6.1 List of excipients

Starch, magnesium stearate and microcrystalline cellulose.

6.2 Incompatibilities

See section 4.5 Interactions with other medicaments and other forms of interaction.

6.3 Shelf life

Four years.

6.4 Special precautions for storage

None.

6.5 Nature and contents of container

Supplied in high density polypropylene bottles or blister packs of 60 tablets.

6.6 Instructions for use and handling

None.

7. MARKETING AUTHORISATION HOLDER

Procter & Gamble Pharmaceuticals UK Limited

Rusham Park

Whitehall Lane

Egham

Surrey

TW20 9NW

UK

8. MARKETING AUTHORISATION NUMBER(S)

PL 0364/0039

9. DATE OF FIRST AUTHORISATION/RENEWAL OF THE AUTHORISATION

26th November 1987

10. DATE OF REVISION OF THE TEXT

October 2002

Didronel PMO

(Procter & Gamble Pharmaceuticals UK Limited)

1. NAME OF THE MEDICINAL PRODUCT

Didronel PMO.

2. QUALITATIVE AND QUANTITATIVE COMPOSITION

A two component therapy consisting of 14 Didronel 400mg tablets and 76 Cacit 500mg effervescent tablets (equivalent to 500mg elemental calcium). Each Didronel tablet contains 400mg of etidronate disodium, USP. Each Cacit 500mg effervescent tablet contains 1250mg of calcium carbonate, Ph.Eur, which when dispersed in water provides 500mg of elemental calcium as calcium citrate.

3. PHARMACEUTICAL FORM

Each Didronel 400mg tablet is white, capsule-shaped and marked with "NE" on one face and "406" on the other. The Cacit 500mg effervescent tablet is round, flat, white with pink speckles and has a distinctive orange flavour.

4. CLINICAL PARTICULARS

4.1 Therapeutic indications

Treatment of osteoporosis, and prevention of bone loss in postmenopausal women considered at risk of developing osteoporosis. Didronel PMO is particularly indicated in patients who are unable or unwilling to take oestrogen replacement therapy. Didronel PMO is also indicated for the prevention and treatment of corticosteroid - induced osteoporosis.

4.2 Posology and method of administration

Didronel PMO therapy is a long-term cyclical regimen administered in 90-day cycles. Each cycle consists of Didronel 400mg tablets for the first 14 days, followed by Cacit 500mg tablets for the remaining 76 days.

The majority of patients have been treated for 3 years, with a small number of patients treated for up to 7 years, with no clinical safety concerns. The optimum duration of treatment has not been established.

***Didronel 400mg component:**

One tablet should be taken each day for 14 consecutive days on an empty stomach. It is recommended that patients take the tablet with water at the midpoint of a four hour fast (ie. two hours before and two hours after food).

***Cacit 500mg component:**

Following 14 days treatment with Didronel 400mg tablets, one Cacit tablet should be taken on a daily basis. The Cacit tablet should be dissolved in water and drunk immediately after complete dissolution.

Adults and Elderly

The patient should adhere to the prescribed regimen above. Modification of the dosage for the elderly is not required.

Children

No data exists in the use of this therapy in juvenile osteoporosis.

4.3 Contraindications

Known hypersensitivity to any of the ingredients. Treatment of patients with severe renal impairment. Patients with hypercalcaemia or hypercalciuria. Clinically overt osteomalacia. Use in pregnancy and lactation.

4.4 Special warnings and special precautions for use

Clinicians should advise patients to adhere to the recommended treatment regimen, and compliance pack.

In long-term trials no clinical osteomalacia was observed in patients receiving cyclical etidronate. Following long-term therapy in excess of 4 years, analysis of bone biopsies showed an increased prevalence of peritrabecular fibrosis and histologically defined atypical and focal osteomalacia (not to be confused with the syndrome associated with "clinical osteomalacia" due to vitamin D deficiency). In addition, these laboratory findings were not associated with any clinical consequences. Osteoid, which may accumulate at high doses of continuous etidronate therapy (10-20mg/kg/day) mineralises normally after discontinuation of therapy. Continuous administration of etidronate should be avoided.

Patients with significant chronic diarrhoeal disease may experience increased frequency of bowel movements and diarrhoea. Therapy should be withheld from patients with enterocolitis because of increased frequency of bowel movements.

Caution should be taken in patients with impaired renal function, or a history of renal stone formation. In these patients, serum and urinary calcium should be monitored regularly.

Etidronate disodium does not adversely effect serum levels of parathyroid hormone or calcium.

Hyperphosphataemia has been observed in patients receiving etidronate disodium, usually in association with doses of 10-20mg/kg/day. No adverse effects have been traced to this, and it does not constitute grounds for discontinuing therapy. It is apparently due to a drug-related increase in renal tubular re absorption of phosphate. Serum phosphate levels generally return to normal 2-4 weeks post therapy.

4.5 Interaction with other medicinal products and other forms of Interaction

Food in the stomach or upper gastrointestinal tract, particularly materials with a high calcium content such as milk, may reduce absorption of etidronate disodium. Vitamins with mineral supplements such as iron, calcium supplements, laxatives containing magnesium, or antacids containing calcium or aluminium should not be taken within two hours of dosing etidronate disodium.

A small number of patients in clinical trials (involving more than 600 patients) received either thiazide diuretics or intravaginal oestrogen while on this treatment. The concomitant use of either of these agents did not interfere with the positive effects of the therapy on vertebral bone mass or fracture rates.

Calcium salts may reduce the absorption of some drugs, eg. tetracyclines. It is therefore suggested that administration of Cacit tablets be separated from these products by at least three hours.

Vitamin D causes an increase in calcium absorption and plasma calcium levels may continue to rise after stopping vitamin D therapy. Concomitant administration of Cacit tablets and vitamin D should therefore be carried out with caution.

The effects of digoxin and other cardiac glycosides may be accentuated by calcium and toxicity may be produced, especially in combination with vitamin D therapy.

There have been isolated reports of patients experiencing changes in their prothrombin times when etidronate was added to warfarin therapy. The majority of these reports concerned variable elevations in prothrombin times without clinically significant sequelae. Although the relevance of these reports and any mechanism of coagulation alterations is unclear, patients on warfarin should have their prothrombin time monitored.

4.6 Pregnancy and lactation

Contra-indicated.

4.7 Effects on ability to drive and use machines

Etidronate disodium does not interfere with the ability to drive or use machines.

4.8 Undesirable effects

Gastro-intestinal

In clinical studies of 2-3 years duration, the incidence of these events were comparable to placebo. The most common effects reported in order of incidence were diarrhoea, nausea, flatulence, dyspepsia, abdominal pain, gastritis, constipation and vomiting. Reports of exacerbation of peptic ulcer with complications in a few patients.

Dermatological/hypersensitivity

Hypersensitivity reactions including angio-oedema, urticaria, rash and/or pruritus have been reported rarely. The colouring agent E110 can cause allergic-type reactions including asthma. Allergy is more common in those people who are allergic to aspirin.

Nervous System

Headache, and rarely paresthesia, peripheral neuropathy and confusion.

Haematological

There have been rare reports of leucopenia, agranulocytosis and pancytopenia

Other

Less common effects believed to be related to therapy include arthropathies (arthralgia and arthritis), and rarely burning of the tongue, alopecia, erythema multiforme and exacerbation of asthma.

Occasional mild leg cramps have been reported in less than 5% of patients on the Didronel PMO regimen. These cramps were transient, often nocturnal and generally associated with other underlying conditions.

4.9 Overdose

Clinical experience of acute overdosage with etidronate is limited and unlikely with this compliance kit. Theoretically it would be manifested as the signs and symptoms of hypocalcaemia and possibly paresthesia of the fingers. Treatment would consist of gastric lavage to remove unabsorbed drug along with correction of hypocalcaemia with administration of Ca^{2+} intravenously.

Prolonged continuous treatment (chronic overdose) has been reported to cause nephrotic syndrome and fractures.

5. PHARMACOLOGICAL PROPERTIES

5.1 Pharmacodynamic properties

Etidronate in an intermittent cyclical regimen, works indirectly to increase bone mass. By timing delivery and withdrawal, the etidronate disodium component acts to modulate osteoclasts and reduce the mean resorption depth of the affected basic multicellular units (BMU). Calcium is an essential element which has been shown to help prevent bone loss.

Epidemiological studies have suggested that there are a number of risk factors associated with postmenopausal osteoporosis, such as early menopause, a family history of osteoporosis, prolonged exposure to corticosteroid therapy, small and thin skeletal frame and excessive cigarette smoking.

5.2 Pharmacokinetic properties

Within 24 hours, about one half of the absorbed dose of etidronate is excreted in the urine. The remainder is chemically absorbed on bone and is slowly eliminated. Unabsorbed drug is excreted in the faeces. Etidronate disodium is not metabolised. After oral doses of up to 1600mg of the disodium salt, the amount of drug absorbed is approximately 3-4%. In normal subjects, plasma half life ($t_{1/2}$) of etidronate, based on non-compartmental pharmacokinetics is 1-6 hours.

Calcium carbonate is converted into soluble calcium salts in the stomach under the influence of hydrochloric acid. 30-80% of orally ingested calcium is absorbed both by active transport (primarily in the upper small intestine) and by passive diffusion. The distribution of calcium in the body is subject to the mechanism of physiological regulation controlled by parathyroid hormone, calcitonin, calciferol and other hormones.

When calcium effervescent tablets are added to water, insoluble calcium carbonate is converted into calcium citrate.

5.3 Preclinical safety data

In long-term studies in mice and rats, there was no evidence of carcinogenicity with etidronate disodium. All *in vitro* and *in vivo* assays conducted to assess the mutagenic potential of etidronate disodium have been negative.

6. PHARMACEUTICAL PARTICULARS

6.1 List of excipients

Etidronate disodium tablets contain microcrystalline cellulose, pregelatinised starch and magnesium stearate. Cacit tablets contain citric acid, sodium saccharin, sodium cyclamate, sunset yellow (E110) and orange flavouring.

6.2 Incompatibilities

None.

6.3 Shelf life

The expiry date for the compliance pack should not exceed 3 years from the date of its manufacture.

6.4 Special precautions for storage

Store in a dry place below 30°C. Since Cacit 500mg tablets are hygroscopic, the stopper should be carefully replaced after use.

6.5 Nature and contents of container

14 Didronel 400mg tablets in a blister plus four polypropylene tubes, each containing 19 Cacit 500mg tablets, all packaged in a compliance kit.

6.6 Instructions for use and handling

None.

7. MARKETING AUTHORISATION HOLDER

Procter & Gamble Pharmaceuticals UK Limited
Rusham Park
Whitehall Lane
Egham
Surrey
TW209NW
UK

8. MARKETING AUTHORISATION NUMBER(S)

PL 0364/0051

9. DATE OF FIRST AUTHORISATION/RENEWAL OF THE AUTHORISATION

1 November 1991

10. DATE OF REVISION OF THE TEXT

October 2002

Differin Cream

(Galderma (U.K.) Ltd)

1. NAME OF THE MEDICINAL PRODUCT

Differin Cream 0.1% w/w

2. QUALITATIVE AND QUANTITATIVE COMPOSITION

Adapalene 0.1% w/w.

For excipients, see 6.1

3. PHARMACEUTICAL FORM

Cream

White shiny cream

4. CLINICAL PARTICULARS

4.1 Therapeutic indications

Differin Cream is proposed for the cutaneous treatment of mild to moderate acne vulgaris where comedones, papules and pustules predominate. Differin Cream is best suited for use on dry and fair skin. Acne of the face, chest or back is appropriate for treatment.

4.2 Posology and method of administration

Differin Cream should be applied to the acne affected areas once a day before retiring and after washing. A thin film of cream should be applied, with the fingertips, avoiding the eyes and lips (see 4.4 *Special warnings and special precautions for use*, below). Ensure that the affected areas are dry before application.

Since it is customary to alternate therapies in the treatment of acne, it is recommended that the physician assess the continued improvement of the patient after three months of treatment with Differin Cream.

With patients for whom it is necessary to reduce the frequency of application or to temporarily discontinue treatment, frequency of application may be restored or therapy resumed once it is judged that the patient can again tolerate the treatment.

If patients use cosmetics, these should be non-comedogenic and non-astringent.

The safety and effectiveness of Differin Cream have not been studied in neonates and young children.

4.3 Contraindications

Hypersensitivity to any ingredient of the product.

4.4 Special warnings and special precautions for use

If a reaction suggesting sensitivity or severe irritation occurs, use of the medication should be discontinued. If the degree of local irritation warrants, patients should be directed to use the medication less frequently, to discontinue use temporarily, or to discontinue use altogether. Differin Cream should not come into contact with the eyes, mouth, angles of the nose or mucous membranes.

If product enters the eye, wash immediately with warm water. The product should not be applied to either broken (cuts and abrasions), sunburnt or eczematous skin, nor should it be used in patients with severe acne, or acne involving large areas of the body, especially in women of child bearing age who are not on effective contraception.

Exposure to sunlight and artificial UV irradiation, including sunlamps, should be minimised during use of adapalene. Patients who normally experience high levels of sun exposure and those with inherent sensitivity to sun, should be warned to exercise caution. Use of sunscreen products and protective clothing over treated areas is recommended when exposure cannot be avoided.

Methyl parahydroxybenzoate (E218) and propyl parahydroxybenzoate (E216) may cause allergic reactions which can possibly be delayed.

4.5 Interaction with other medicinal products and other forms of Interaction

There are no known interactions with other medications which might be used cutaneously and concurrently with Differin Cream; however, other retinoids or drugs with a similar mode of action should not be used concurrently with adapalene.

Adapalene is essentially stable to oxygen and light and is chemically non-reactive. Whilst extensive studies in animals and man have shown neither phototoxic nor photoallergic potential for adapalene, the safety of using adapalene during repeated exposure to sunlight or UV irradiation has not been established in either animals or man. Exposure to excessive sunlight or UV irradiation should be avoided.

Absorption of adapalene through human skin is low (see Pharmacokinetic Properties) and therefore interaction with systemic medications is unlikely. There is no evidence that the efficacy of oral drugs such as contraceptives and antibiotics is influenced by the cutaneous use of Differin Cream.

Differin Cream has a potential for mild local irritation, and therefore it is possible that concomitant use of peeling agents, astringents or irritant products may produce additive irritant effects. However, cutaneous antiacne treatment e.g. erythromycin (up to 4%) or clindamycin phosphate (1% as the base) solutions or benzoyl peroxide water based gels up to 10% may be used in the morning when Differin Cream is used at night as there is no mutual degradation or cumulative irritation.

4.6 Pregnancy and lactation

No information on the effects of Adapalene in pregnant women is available and therefore this product should not be used during pregnancy, unless considered essential by the physician. Because of the risk of teratogenicity shown in animal studies and since there is no information on the use of adapalene in pregnant women, it should not be used in women of child bearing age unless they are using an effective means of contraception.

Adapalene produces teratogenic effects by the oral route in rats and rabbits. At cutaneous doses up to 200-fold the therapeutic dose, producing circulating plasma levels of adapalene at least 35 to 120 times higher than plasma levels demonstrated in therapeutic use, adapalene increased the incidence of additional ribs in rats and rabbits, without increasing the incidence of major malformations.

It is not known whether adapalene is secreted in animal or human milk. In animal studies, infant rats suckled by mother with circulating levels of adapalene at least 300 times those demonstrated in clinical use developed normally.

Its use in women breast feeding infants should be avoided but when it is used in breast feeding women, to avoid contact exposure of the infant, application of adapalene to the chest should be avoided.

4.7 Effects on ability to drive and use machines

Based upon the pharmacodynamic profile and clinical experience, performance related to driving and using machines should not be affected.

4.8 Undesirable effects

Side effects include skin irritation (erythema, dryness, scaling, burning) and stinging at the site of application which is reversible when treatment is reduced in frequency or discontinued. Eyelid oedema as well as eye irritation when the product comes into contact with the eyes have been reported rarely.

4.9 Overdose

Differin Cream is not to be taken orally and is for cutaneous use only. If the medication is applied excessively, no more rapid or better results will be obtained and marked redness, peeling or discomfort may occur.

The acute oral dose of Differin Cream required to produce toxic effects in mice is greater than 10 g/kg. Nevertheless, unless the amount accidentally ingested is small, an appropriate method of gastric emptying should be considered.

5. PHARMACOLOGICAL PROPERTIES

5.1 Pharmacodynamic properties

Adapalene is a retinoid-like compound which in, in vivo and in vitro models of inflammation, has been demonstrated to possess anti-inflammatory properties. Adapalene is essentially stable to oxygen and light and is chemically non-reactive. Mechanically, adapalene binds like tretinoin to specific retinoic acid nuclear receptors but, unlike tretinoin not to cytosolic receptor binding proteins.

Adapalene applied cutaneously is comedolytic in the rhino mouse model and also has effects on the abnormal processes of epidermal keratinisation and differentiation, both of which are present in the pathogenesis of acne vulgaris. The mode of action of adapalene is suggested to be a normalisation of differentiation of follicular epithelial cells resulting in decreased microcomedone formation.

Adapalene is superior to reference retinoids in standard anti-inflammatory assays, both in vivo and in vitro. Mechanistically, it inhibits chemotactic and chemokinetic responses of human polymorphonuclear leucocytes and also the metabolism by lipoxidation of arachidonic acid to pro-inflammatory mediators. This profile suggests that the cell mediated inflammatory component of acne may be modified by adapalene. Studies in human patients provide clinical evidence that cutaneous adapalene is effective in reducing the inflammatory components of acne (papules and pustules).

5.2 Pharmacokinetic properties

Absorption of adapalene through human skin is low, in clinical trials measurable plasma adapalene levels were not found following chronic cutaneous application to large areas of acneic skin with an analytical sensitivity of 0.15 ng/ml.

After administration of [^{14}C]-adapalene in rats (IV, IP, oral and cutaneous), rabbits (IV, oral and cutaneous) and dogs (IV and oral), radioactivity was distributed in several tissues, the highest levels being found in liver, spleen, adrenals and ovaries. Metabolism in animals has been tentatively identified as being mainly by O-demethylation, hydroxylation and conjugation, and excretion is primarily by the biliary route.

5.3 Preclinical safety data
In animal studies, adapalene was well tolerated on cutaneous application for periods of up to six months in rabbits and for up to two years in mice. The major symptoms of toxicity found in all animal species by the oral route were related to an hypervitaminosis A syndrome, and included bone dissolution, elevated alkaline phosphatase and a slight anaemia. Large oral doses of adapalene produced no adverse neurological, cardiovascular or respiratory effects in animals. Adapalene is not mutagenic. Lifetime studies with adapalene have been completed in mice at cutaneous doses of 0.6, 2 and 6 mg/kg/day and in rats at oral doses of 0.15, 0.5 and 1.5 mg/kg/day. The only significant finding was a statistically significant increase of benign phaeochromocytomas of the adrenal medulla among male rats receiving adapalene at 1.5 mg/kg/day. These changes are unlikely to be of relevance to the cutaneous use of adapalene.

6. PHARMACEUTICAL PARTICULARS
6.1 List of excipients
Carbomer 934P
Macrogol -20 methyl glucose sesquistearate
Glycerol (E422)
Natural squalane
Methyl parahydroxybenzoate (E218)
Propyl parahydroxybenzoate (E216)
Disodium edetate
Methyl glucose sesquistearate
Phenoxyethanol
Cyclomethicone
Sodium hydroxide
Purified water

6.2 Incompatibilities
None known.

6.3 Shelf life
The shelf life expiry date for this product shall not exceed three years from the date of its manufacture.

6.4 Special precautions for storage
Do not store above 25°C.
Do not freeze.
Keep out of the reach and sight of children.

6.5 Nature and contents of container
Collapsible Aluminium tube coated internally with an epoxy-phenolic resin and fitted with a white Polypropylene screw cap. Pack sizes: 30g and 45g.

6.6 Instructions for use and handling
A thin film of the cream should be applied, avoiding eyes, lips and mucous membranes.

7. MARKETING AUTHORISATION HOLDER
Galderma (UK) Limited
Galderma House
Church Lane
Kings Langley
Hertfordshire, WD4 8JP
England

8. MARKETING AUTHORISATION NUMBER(S)
PL 10590/0029

9. DATE OF FIRST AUTHORISATION/RENEWAL OF THE AUTHORISATION
9 January 1998

10. DATE OF REVISION OF THE TEXT
April 2005

11. Legal Category
POM

Differin Gel

(Galderma (U.K.) Ltd)

1. NAME OF THE MEDICINAL PRODUCT
Differin Gel 0.1% w/w

2. QUALITATIVE AND QUANTITATIVE COMPOSITION
Adapalene 0.1% w/w
For excipients, see 6.1

3. PHARMACEUTICAL FORM
Topical Gel
A smooth white gel

4. CLINICAL PARTICULARS
4.1 Therapeutic indications
Differin Gel is proposed for the cutaneous treatment of mild to moderate acne where comedones, papules and pustules predominate. Acne of the face, chest or back is appropriate for treatment.

4.2 Posology and method of administration
Differin Gel should be applied to the acne affected areas once a day before retiring and after washing. A thin film of gel should be applied, with the fingertips, avoiding the eyes and lips (see 4.4 Special Warnings and Special Precautions for Use, below). Ensure that the affected areas are dry before application.

Since it is customary to alternate therapies in the treatment of acne, it is recommended that the physician assess the continued improvement of the patient after three months of treatment with Differin Gel.

With patients for whom it is necessary to reduce the frequency of application or to temporarily discontinue treatment, frequency of application may be restored or therapy resumed once it is judged that the patient can again tolerate the treatment.

If patients use cosmetics, these should be non-comedogenic and non-astringent.

The safety and effectiveness of Differin Gel have not been studied in neonates and young children. Differin gel should not be used in patients with severe acne.

4.3 Contraindications
Hypersensitivity to any ingredient of the product.

4.4 Special warnings and special precautions for use
If a reaction suggesting sensitivity or severe irritation occurs, use of the medication should be discontinued. If the degree of local irritation warrants, patients should be directed to use the medication less frequently, to discontinue use temporarily, or to discontinue use altogether. Differin Gel should not come into contact with the eyes, mouth, nostrils or mucous membranes.

If product enters the eye, wash immediately with warm water. The product should not be applied to either broken (cut and abrasions) or eczematous skin, nor should it be used in patients with severe acne involving large areas of the body, especially in women of child bearing age who are not on effective contraception.

The excipient propylene glycol (E1520) may cause skin irritation and methyl parahydroxybenzoate (E218) may cause allergic reactions which can possibly be delayed.

4.5 Interaction with other medicinal products and other forms of Interaction
There are no known interactions with other medications which might be used cutaneously and concurrently with Differin Gel, however, other retinoids or drugs with a similar mode of action should not be used concurrently with adapalene.

Adapalene is essentially stable to oxygen and light and is chemically non-reactive. Whilst extensive studies in animals and man have shown neither phototoxic nor photo-allergic potential for adapalene, the safety of using adapalene during repeated exposure to sunlight or UV irradiation has not been established in either animals or man. Exposure to excessive sunlight or UV irradiation should be avoided.

Absorption of adapalene through human skin is low (see 5.2 Pharmacokinetic Properties) and therefore interaction with systemic medications is unlikely. There is no evidence that the efficacy of oral drugs such as contraceptives and antibiotics is influenced by the cutaneous use of Differin Gel.

Differin Gel has a potential for mild local irritation, and therefore it is possible that concomitant use of peeling agents, abrasive cleansers, strong drying agents, astringents or irritant products (aromatic and alcoholic agents) may produce additive irritant effects. However, cutaneous antiacne treatment (eg erythromycin up to 4%) or clindamycin phosphate (1% as the base) solutions or benzoyl peroxide water based gels up to 10% may be used in the morning when Differin Gel is used at night as there is no mutual degradation or cumulative irritation.

4.6 Pregnancy and lactation
No information on the effects of Adapalene in pregnant women is available and therefore this product should not be used during pregnancy, unless considered essential by the physician. Because of the risk of teratogenicity shown in animal studies and since there is no information on the use of adapalene in pregnant women, it should not be used in women of child bearing age unless they are using an effective means of contraception.

Adapalene produces teratogenic effects by the oral route in rats and rabbits. At cutaneous doses up to 200-fold the therapeutic dose, producing circulating plasma levels of adapalene at least 35 to 120 times higher than plasma levels demonstrated in therapeutic use, adapalene increased the incidence of additional ribs in rats and rabbits, without increasing the incidence of major malformations.

It is not known whether adapalene is secreted in animal or human milk. In animal studies, infant rats suckled by mother with circulating levels of adapalene at least 300 times those demonstrated in clinical use developed normally.

Its use in women breast feeding infants should be avoided but when it is used in breast feeding women, to avoid contact exposure of the infant, application of adapalene to the chest should be avoided.

4.7 Effects on ability to drive and use machines
Based upon the pharmodynamic profile and clinical experience, performance related to driving and using machines should not be affected.

4.8 Undesirable effects
Local reactions include burning, erythema, stinging, pruritus, dry or peeling skin. Eye irritation and oedema, and blistering or crusting of skin have been reported rarely.

The major undesirable effect which may occur is irritation of the skin which is reversible when treatment is reduced in frequency or discontinued.

4.9 Overdose
Differin Gel is not to be taken orally and is for cutaneous use only. If the medication is applied excessively, no more rapid or better results will be obtained and marked redness, peeling or discomfort may occur.

The acute oral dose of Differin Gel required to produce toxic effects in mice is greater that 10 mg/kg. Nevertheless, unless the amount accidentally ingested is small, an appropriate method of gastric emptying should be considered.

5. PHARMACOLOGICAL PROPERTIES
5.1 Pharmacodynamic properties
Adapalene is a retinoid-like compound which in, in vivo and in vitro models of inflammation, has been demonstrated to possess anti-inflammatory properties. Adapalene is essentially stable to oxygen and light and is chemically non-reactive. Mechanically, adapalene binds like tretinoin to specific retinoic acid nuclear receptors but, unlike tretinoin not to cytosolic receptor binding proteins.

Adapalene applied cutaneously is comedolytic in the rhino mouse model and also has effects on the abnormal processes of epidermal keratinization and differentiation, both of which are present in the pathogenesis of acne vulgaris. The mode of action of adapalene is suggested to be a normalisation of differentiation of follicular epithelial cells resulting in decreased microcomedone formation.

Adapalene is superior to reference retinoids in standard anti-inflammatory assays, both in vivo and in vitro. Mechanistically, it inhibits chemotactic and chemokinetic responses of human polymorphonuclear leucocytes and also the metabolism by lipoxidation of arachidonic acid to pro-inflammatory mediators. This profile suggests that the cell mediated inflammatory component of acne may be modified by adapalene.

5.2 Pharmacokinetic properties
Absorption of adapalene through human skin is low, in clinical trial measurable plasma adapalene levels where not found following chronic cutaneous application to large areas of acneic skin with an analytical sensitivity of 0.15 ng/ml.

After administration of [^{14}C] adapalene in rats (IV, IP, oral and cutaneous), rabbits (IV, oral and cutaneous) and dogs (IV and oral), radioactivity was distributed in several tissues, the highest levels being found in liver, spleen, adrenals and ovaries. Metabolism in animals has been tentatively identified as being mainly by O-demethylation, hydroxylation and conjugation, and excretion is primarily by the biliary route.

5.3 Preclinical safety data
In animal studies, adapalene was well tolerated on cutaneous application for periods of up to six months in rabbits and for up to two years in mice. The major symptom of toxicity found in all animal species by the oral route were related to a hypervitaminosis A syndrome, and included bone dissolution, elevated alkaline phosphatase and a slight anaemia. Large oral doses of adapalene produced no adverse neurological, caridovascular or respiratory effects in animals. Adapalene is not mutagenic. Lifetime studies with adapalene have been completed in mice at cutaneous doses of 0.6,2 and 6 mg/kg/day and in rats at oral doses of 0.15, 0.5 and 1.5 mg/kg/day. The only significant finding was a statistically significant increase of benign phaeochromocytomas of the adrenal medulla among male rats receiving adapalene at 1.5 mg/kg/day. These changes are unlikely to be of relevance to the cutaneous use of adapalene.

6. PHARMACEUTICAL PARTICULARS
6.1 List of excipients
Carbomer 940
Propylene Glycol (E1520)
Poloxamer 182
Disodium Edetate
Methyl Parahydroxybenzoate (E218)
Phenoxyethanol
Sodium Hydroxide
Purified Water

6.2 Incompatibilities
None Known

6.3 Shelf life
The shelf life expiry date for this product shall not exceed three years from the date of its manufacture.

6.4 Special precautions for storage
Do not store above 25°C.

Do not freeze.

Keep out of the reach and sight of children

6.5 Nature and contents of container
White LDPE tube with white PP screw cap. Pack size 30g and 45g.

6.6 Instructions for use and handling
A thin film of the gel should be applied, avoiding eyes, lips and mucous membranes

7. MARKETING AUTHORISATION HOLDER
Galderma (UK) Limited

Galderma House

Church Lane

Kings Langley

Hertfordshire WD4 8JP

England

8. MARKETING AUTHORISATION NUMBER(S)
PL 10590/0015

9. DATE OF FIRST AUTHORISATION/RENEWAL OF THE AUTHORISATION

10. DATE OF REVISION OF THE TEXT
April 2005

Difflam Cream

(3M Health Care Limited)

1. NAME OF THE MEDICINAL PRODUCT
Difflam Cream

or

Difflam-P Cream

2. QUALITATIVE AND QUANTITATIVE COMPOSITION
Each tube of Difflam Cream/ Difflam-P Cream contains Benzydamine Hydrochloride 3% w/w.

3. PHARMACEUTICAL FORM
Cream.

4. CLINICAL PARTICULARS

4.1 Therapeutic indications
Difflam Cream/ Difflam-P Cream is a topical analgesic and non-steroidal anti-inflammatory agent.

It is recommended as a short-term treatment for the relief of symptoms associated with painful inflammatory conditions of the musculo-skeletal system, including:

Acute inflammatory disorders such as myalgia and bursitis.

Traumatic conditions such as sprains, strains, contusions and the after-effects of fractures.

Difflam Cream/ Difflam-P Cream is well absorbed through the skin and has been shown to have anti-inflammatory and local anaesthetic actions.

4.2 Posology and method of administration
Difflam Cream/ Difflam-P Cream should be massaged lightly into the affected area. Depending on the size of the site to be treated, 35 - 85 mm (1 - 2 g) should be applied three times daily and at the discretion of the doctor, up to six times daily in more severe conditions. It is recommended that treatment be limited to not more than ten days.

<u>ELDERLY</u>:

No special dosage recommendations are made for elderly patients.

4.3 Contraindications
Difflam Cream is contraindicated in patients with known hypersensitivity to any of the ingredients.

4.4 Special warnings and special precautions for use
To avoid possible irritation, Difflam Cream/ Difflam-P Cream should be kept away from eyes and mucosal surfaces.

4.5 Interaction with other medicinal products and other forms of Interaction
None.

4.6 Pregnancy and lactation
There is inadequate evidence of safety of the drug in human pregnancy, but it has been in wide use for many years without apparent ill consequence.

4.7 Effects on ability to drive and use machines
None.

4.8 Undesirable effects
Photosensitivity reactions have been reported and local skin reactions which have varied from erythema to papular eruption. The skin returned to normal on stopping treatment.

4.9 Overdose
Difflam is unlikely to cause adverse systemic effects, even if accidental ingestion should occur. No special measures are required.

5. PHARMACOLOGICAL PROPERTIES

5.1 Pharmacodynamic properties
Benzydamine exerts an anti-inflammatory and analgesic action by stabilising the cellular membrane and inhibiting prostaglandin synthesis.

5.2 Pharmacokinetic properties
Following topical administration, benzydamine is absorbed through intact skin and reaches peak levels between 24 - 32 hours, amounting to about 20 - 25% of the plasma levels obtained after the oral administration of the same dose.

About half of the benzydamine is excreted unchanged via the kidney at a rate of 10% of the dose within the first 24 hours. The remainder is metabolised, mostly to N-oxide.

5.3 Preclinical safety data
Not applicable.

6. PHARMACEUTICAL PARTICULARS

6.1 List of excipients
'Cutina' MD

Cetyl Alcohol USNF

'Cetiol' V

'Eumulgin' B1

Propylene Glycol Ph Eur

Perfume, 'Crematest' 0/064060

Methyl Hydroxybenzoate Ph Eur

Propyl Hydroxybenzoate Ph Eur

Purified Water Ph Eur

6.2 Incompatibilities
None known.

6.3 Shelf life
3 years.

6.4 Special precautions for storage
Store between 5 - 30°C. Do not freeze.

6.5 Nature and contents of container
Collapsible Aluminium tube closed with plastic screwcap

<u>or</u>

Laminate tube closed with plastic screwcap.

Contents: 35 g, 50 g or 100 g

6.6 Instructions for use and handling
Not applicable.

7. MARKETING AUTHORISATION HOLDER
3M Health Care Limited

3M House

Morley Street

Loughborough

Leicestershire

LE11 1EP

8. MARKETING AUTHORISATION NUMBER(S)
0068/0088

9. DATE OF FIRST AUTHORISATION/RENEWAL OF THE AUTHORISATION
6 March 1980.

10. DATE OF REVISION OF THE TEXT
April 2003

Difflam Oral Rinse

(3M Health Care Limited)

1. NAME OF THE MEDICINAL PRODUCT
Difflam Oral Rinse

2. QUALITATIVE AND QUANTITATIVE COMPOSITION
A pleasant tasting, clear, green solution, containing benzydamine hydrochloride 0.15% w/v.

3. PHARMACEUTICAL FORM
Liquid for use as mouthwash/gargle.

4. CLINICAL PARTICULARS

4.1 Therapeutic indications
Difflam Oral Rinse is a locally acting analgesic and anti-inflammatory treatment for the relief of painful inflammatory conditions of the mouth and throat including:

Traumatic conditions: Pharyngitis following tonsillectomy or the use of a naso-gastric tube.

Inflammatory conditions: Pharyngitis, aphthous ulcers and oral ulceration due to radiation therapy.

Dentistry: For use after dental operations.

4.2 Posology and method of administration
Adults: Rinse or gargle with 15 ml (approximately 1 tablespoonful) every 1½ to 3 hours as required for pain relief.

The solution should be expelled from the mouth after use.

Children: Not suitable for children aged 12 years or under.

Elderly: No special dosage recommendations are made for elderly patients.

Difflam Oral Rinse should generally be used undiluted, but if 'stinging' occurs the rinse may be diluted with water.

Uninterrupted treatment should not exceed seven days, except under medical supervision.

4.3 Contraindications
Difflam Oral Rinse is contra-indicated in patients with known hypersensitivity to any of the ingredients.

4.4 Special warnings and special precautions for use
Difflam Oral Rinse should generally be used undiluted, but if 'stinging' occurs the rinse may be diluted with water.

Avoid contact with eyes.

4.5 Interaction with other medicinal products and other forms of Interaction
None known.

4.6 Pregnancy and lactation
There is inadequate evidence of safety of the drug in human pregnancy, but it has been in wide use for many years without apparent ill consequence.

4.7 Effects on ability to drive and use machines
Not applicable.

4.8 Undesirable effects
Side-effects are minor. Occasionally, oral tissue numbness or 'stinging' sensations may occur. Hypersensitivity reactions occur very rarely but may be associated with pruritus rash, urticaria, photodermatitis and occasionally laryngospasm or bronchospasm.

4.9 Overdose
Difflam is unlikely to cause adverse systemic effects, even if accidental ingestion should occur. No special measures are required.

5. PHARMACOLOGICAL PROPERTIES

5.1 Pharmacodynamic properties
Benzydamine exerts an anti-inflammatory and analgesic effect by stabilising the cellular membrane and inhibiting prostaglandin synthesis.

5.2 Pharmacokinetic properties
Oral doses of benzydamine are well absorbed and plasma drug concentrations reach a peak fairly rapidly and then decline with a half-life of about 13 hours. Less than 20% of the drug is bound to plasma proteins.

Although local drug concentrations are relatively large, the systemic absorption of mouthwash-gargle doses of benzydamine is relatively low compared to oral doses. This low absorption should greatly diminish the potential for any systemic drug side-effects when benzydamine is administered by this route. Benzydamine is metabolized primarily by oxidation, conjugation and dealkylation.

5.3 Preclinical safety data
Not applicable.

6. PHARMACEUTICAL PARTICULARS

6.1 List of excipients
Ethanol (96% v/v) BP

Glycerol Ph Eur

Saccharin Sodium BP

Mouthwash flavour, 52 503/T

Polysorbate 20 Ph Eur

Methyl Hydroxybenzoate Ph Eur

Quinoline Yellow (E104)

Patent Blue V (E131)

Purified Water Ph Eur

6.2 Incompatibilities
None known.

6.3 Shelf life
3 years

6.4 Special precautions for storage
Do not leave the uncartonned bottle in direct sunlight. Store between 5°C and 30°C. Do not freeze.

6.5 Nature and contents of container
Clear glass bottle with screwcap containing 300 ml.

6.6 Instructions for use and handling
The solution should be expelled from the mouth after use.

7. MARKETING AUTHORISATION HOLDER
3M Health Care Limited, 3M House, Morley Street, Loughborough, Leics, LE11 1EP

8. MARKETING AUTHORISATION NUMBER(S)
0068/0096

9. DATE OF FIRST AUTHORISATION/RENEWAL OF THE AUTHORISATION
Date of first authorisation 11 June 1981

Date of last renewal 14 May 1997

10. DATE OF REVISION OF THE TEXT
February 2001

Difflam Spray

(3M Health Care Limited)

1. NAME OF THE MEDICINAL PRODUCT
Difflam Spray.

2. QUALITATIVE AND QUANTITATIVE COMPOSITION
Each metered dose pump spray delivers Benzydamine Hydrochloride
0.15% w/v, approximately 175 microlitres per puff.

3. PHARMACEUTICAL FORM
Difflam Spray is a metered dose pump throat spray.

4. CLINICAL PARTICULARS

4.1 Therapeutic indications
Difflam Spray is a locally acting analgesic and anti-inflammatory treatment for the throat and mouth.

It is especially useful for the relief of pain in traumatic conditions such as following tonsillectomy or the use of a naso-gastric tube; dental surgery.

4.2 Posology and method of administration
For oral administration.

ADULTS AND ELDERLY: 4 to 8 puffs, 1½-3 hourly.

CHILDREN (6-12): 4 puffs, 1½-3 hourly.

CHILDREN UNDER 6: One puff to be administered per 4 kg body weight, up to a maximum of 4 puffs, 1½-3 hourly.

Because of the small amount of drug applied, elderly patients can receive the same dose as adults.

4.3 Contraindications
Difflam Spray is contra-indicated in patients with known hypersensitivity to any of the ingredients.

4.4 Special warnings and special precautions for use
Avoid contact with the eyes.

4.5 Interaction with other medicinal products and other forms of Interaction
None known.

4.6 Pregnancy and lactation
There is inadequate evidence of safety of the drug in human pregnancy, but it has been in wide use for many years without apparent ill consequence.

4.7 Effects on ability to drive and use machines
None.

4.8 Undesirable effects
Side-effects are minor. Occasionally, oral tissue numbness or 'stinging' sensations may occur. The stinging has been reported to disappear upon continuation of the treatment, however if it persists it is recommended that treatment be discontinued. Hypersensitivity reactions occur very rarely but may be associated with pruritus rash, urticaria, photodermatitis and occasionally laryngospasm or bronchospasm.

4.9 Overdose
Difflam is unlikely to cause adverse systemic effects, even if accidental ingestion should occur. No special measures are required.

5. PHARMACOLOGICAL PROPERTIES

5.1 Pharmacodynamic properties
Benzydamine exerts an anti-inflammatory and analgesic action by stabilising the cellular membrane and inhibiting prostaglandin synthesis.

5.2 Pharmacokinetic properties
Following oral administration, Benzydamine is rapidly absorbed from the gastrointestinal tract and maximum plasma levels reached after 2-4 hours. The most important aspect of the tissue distribution of Benzydamine is its tendency to concentrate at the site of inflammation.

About half of the Benzydamine is excreted unchanged via the kidney at a rate of 10% of the dose within the first 24 hours. The remainder is metabolised, mostly to N-Oxide.

5.3 Preclinical safety data
Not applicable.

6. PHARMACEUTICAL PARTICULARS

6.1 List of excipients
The excipients in Difflam Spray include:-

Glycerol Ph Eur, Saccharin FU, Sodium Bicarbonate Ph Eur. Ethanol FU, Methylhydroxybenzoate Ph Eur, Mouthwash Flavour, Polysorbate 20

Ph Eur, Purified Water Ph Eur.

6.2 Incompatibilities
None.

6.3 Shelf life
The shelf life expiry date for this product shall not exceed 3 years from the date of its manufacture.

6.4 Special precautions for storage
Do not store above 30°C, do not refrigerate or freeze. Keep out of the reach of children.

6.5 Nature and contents of container
Difflam Spray is presented in a 30 ml HDPE bottle with 170 μl valve pump spray.

6.6 Instructions for use and handling
The patient should read the instruction leaflet before use.

7. MARKETING AUTHORISATION HOLDER
3M Health Care Limited
3M House
Morley Street
Loughborough
Leicestershire
LE11 1EP

8. MARKETING AUTHORISATION NUMBER(S)
PL0068/0112.

9. DATE OF FIRST AUTHORISATION/RENEWAL OF THE AUTHORISATION
Date of first authorisation 30 November 1984

Date of last renewal 22 August 1996

10. DATE OF REVISION OF THE TEXT
December 2003

Diflucan 150 Capsules

(Pfizer Limited)

1. NAME OF THE MEDICINAL PRODUCT
DIFLUCAN® 150 CAPSULE.

2. QUALITATIVE AND QUANTITATIVE COMPOSITION
Diflucan 150 capsule contains as its active ingredient fluconazole 150mg.

3. PHARMACEUTICAL FORM
Diflucan 150 capsules are light turquoise blue, coded 'FLU 150' and 'PFIZER'.

4. CLINICAL PARTICULARS

4.1 Therapeutic indications
Diflucan 150 is indicated for the treatment of the following conditions:

Genital candidiasis. Vaginal candidiasis, acute or recurrent. Candidal balanitis. The treatment of partners who present with symptomatic genital candidiasis should be considered.

4.2 Posology and method of administration
In adults Vaginal candidiasis or candidal balanitis - 150mg single oral dose.

In children Despite extensive data supporting the use of Diflucan in children there are limited data available on the use of Diflucan for genital candidiasis in children below 16 years. Use at present is not recommended unless antifungal treatment is imperative and no suitable alternative agent exists.

Use in elderly The normal adult dose should be used.

Use in renal impairment Fluconazole is excreted predominantly in the urine as unchanged drug. No adjustments in single dose therapy are required.

4.3 Contraindications
Diflucan 150 should not be used in patients with known hypersensitivity to fluconazole or to related azole compounds or any other ingredient in the formulation.

Fluconazole should not be co-adminstered with cisapride or terfenadine which are known to both prolong the QT –interval and are metabolised by CYP3A4 (See "Interactions with other medicinal products and other forms of interaction".)

4.4 Special warnings and special precautions for use
In some patients, particularly those with serious underlying diseases such as AIDS and cancer, abnormalities in haematological, hepatic, renal and other biochemical function test results have been observed during treatment with Diflucan but the clinical significance and relationship to treatment is uncertain.

Very rarely, patients who died with severe underlying disease and who had received multiple doses of Diflucan had post-mortem findings which included hepatic necrosis. These patients were receiving multiple concomitant medications, some known to be potentially hepatotoxic, and/or had underlying diseases which could have caused the hepatic necrosis.

In cases of hepatotoxicity, no obvious relationship to total daily dose of Diflucan, duration of therapy, sex or age of the patient has been observed; the abnormalities have usually been reversible on discontinuation of Diflucan therapy.

As a causal relationship with Diflucan cannot be excluded, patients who develop abnormal liver function tests during Diflucan therapy should be monitored for the development of more serious hepatic injury. Diflucan should be discontinued if clinical signs or symptoms consistent with liver disease develop during treatment with Diflucan.

Patients have rarely developed exfoliative cutaneous reactions, such as Stevens-Johnson Syndrome and toxic epidermal necrolysis, during treatment with fluconazole. AIDS patients are more prone to the development of severe cutaneous reactions to many drugs.

If a rash develops in a patient which is considered attributable to Diflucan 150, further therapy with this agent is not recommended.

In rare cases, as with other azoles, anaphylaxis has been reported.

Some azoles, including fluconazole, have been associated with prolongation of the QT interval on the electrocardiogram. During post-marketing surveillance, there have been very rare cases of QT prolongation and torsade de pointes in patients taking fluconazole. Although the association of fluconazole and QT-prolongation has not been fully established, fluconazole should be used with caution in patients with potentially proarrythmic conditions such as:

Congenital or documented acquired QT prolongation

Cardiomyopathy, in particular when heart failure is present

Sinus bradycardia

Existing symptomatic arrythmias

Concomitant medication not metabolized by CY34A but known to prolong QT interval

Electrolyte disturbances such as hypokalaemia, hypomagnesaemia and hypocalaemia

(See Section 4.5 Interactions with other medicinal products and other forms of interaction)

4.5 Interaction with other medicinal products and other forms of Interaction
The following drug interactions relate to the use of multiple-dose fluconazole, and the relevance to single-dose Diflucan 150 has not yet been established:

Rifampicin Concomitant administration of Diflucan and rifampicin resulted in a 25% decrease in the AUC and 20% shorter half-life of fluconazole. In patients receiving concomitant rifampicin, an increase in the Diflucan dose should be considered.

Hydrochlorothiazide In a kinetic interaction study, co-administration of multiple-dose hydrochlorothiazide to healthy volunteers receiving Diflucan increased plasma concentrations of fluconazole by 40%. An effect of this magnitude should not necessitate a change in the Diflucan dose regimen in subjects receiving concomitant diuretics, although the prescriber should bear it in mind.

Anticoagulants In an interaction study, fluconazole increased the prothrombin time (12%) after warfarin administration in healthy males. In post-marketing experience, as with other azole antifungals, bleeding events (bruising, epistaxis, gastrointestinal bleeding, hematuria and melena) have been reported in association with increases in prothrombin time in patients receiving fluconazole concurrently with warfarin. Prothrombin time in patients receiving coumarin-type anticoagulants should be carefully monitored. ***Benzodiazepines*** (Short Acting) Following oral administration of midazolam, fluconazole resulted in substantial increases in midazolam concentrations and psychomotor effects. This effect on midazolam appears to be more pronounced following oral administration of fluconazole than with fluconazole administered intravenously. If concomitant benzodiazepine therapy is necessary in patients being treated with fluconazole, consideration should be given to decreasing the benzodiazepine dosage and the patients should be appropriately monitored.

Sulphonylureas Fluconazole has been shown to prolong the serum half-life of concomitantly administered oral sulphonylureas (chlorpropamide, glibenclamide, glipizide and tolbutamide) in healthy volunteers. Fluconazole and oral sulphonylureas may be co-administered to diabetic patients, but the possibility of a hypoglycaemic episode should be borne in mind.

Phenytoin Concomitant administration of fluconazole and phenytoin may increase the levels of phenytoin to a clinically significant degree. If it is necessary to administer both drugs concomitantly, phenytoin levels should be monitored and the phenytoin dose adjusted to maintain therapeutic levels.

Oral contraceptives Two kinetic studies with combined oral contraceptives have been performed using multiple doses of fluconazole. There were no relevant effects on either hormone level in the 50mg fluconazole study, while at 200mg daily the AUCs of ethinyloestradiol and levonorgestrel were increased 40% and 24% respectively Thus multiple dose use of fluconazole at these doses is unlikely to have an effect on the efficacy of the combined oral contraceptive.

In a 300 mg once weekly fluconazole study, the AUCs of ethinyl estradiol and norethindrone were increased by 24% and 13%, respectively.

Endogenous steroid Fluconazole 50mg daily does not affect endogenous steroid levels in females: 200-400mg daily has no clinically significant effect on endogenous steroid levels or on ACTH stimulated response in healthy male volunteers.

Cyclosporin A kinetic study in renal transplant patients found fluconazole 200mg daily to slowly increase cyclosporin concentrations. However, in another multiple dose study with 100mg daily, fluconazole did not affect cyclosporin levels in patients with bone marrow transplants. Cyclosporin plasma concentration monitoring in patients receiving fluconazole is recommended.

Theophylline In a placebo controlled interaction study, the administration of fluconazole 200mg for 14 days resulted in an 18% decrease in the mean plasma clearance of theophylline. Patients who are receiving high doses of theophylline or who are otherwise at increased risk for theophylline toxicity should be observed for signs of theophylline toxicity while receiving fluconazole, and the therapy modified appropriately if signs of toxicity develop.

Terfenadine Because of the occurrence of serious dysrhythmias secondary to prolongation of the QTc interval in patients receiving other azole antifungals in conjunction with terfenadine, interactions studies have been performed. One study at a 200mg daily dose of fluconazole failed to demonstrate a prolongation in QTc interval. Another study at a 400mg and 800mg daily dose of fluconazole demonstrated that fluconazole taken in multiple doses of 400mg per day or greater significantly increased plasma levels of terfenadine when taken concomitantly. There have been spontaneously reported cases of palpitations, tachycardia, dizziness, and chest pain in patients taking concomitant fluconazole and terfenadine where the relationship of the reported adverse events to drug therapy or underlying medical conditions was not clear. Because of the potential seriousness of such an interaction, it is recommended that terfenadine not be taken in combination with fluconazole. (See "Contra-indications".)

Cisapride There have been reports of cardiac events including torsades de pointes in patients to whom fluconazole and cisapride were co-administered. A controlled study found that concomitant fluconazole 200 mg once daily and cisapride 20 mg four times a day yielded a significant increase in cisapride plasma levels and prolongation of QTc interval. In most of these cases, the patients appear to have been predisposed to arrhythmias or had serious underlying illnesses, and the relationship of the reported events to a possible fluconazole-cisapride drug interaction is unclear. Because of the potential seriousness of such an interaction, co-administration of cisapride is contra-indicated in patients receiving fluconazole. (See "Contra-indications".)

Zidovudine Two kinetic studies resulted in increased levels of zidovudine most likely caused by the decreased conversion of zidovudine to its major metabolite. One study determined zidovudine levels in AIDS or ARC patients before and following fluconazole 200mg daily for 15 days. There was a significant increase in zidovudine AUC (20%). A second randomised, two-period, two-treatment cross-over study examined zidovudine levels in HIV infected patients. On two occasions, 21 days apart, patients received zidovudine 200mg every eight hours either with or without fluconazole 400mg daily for seven days. The AUC of zidovudine significantly increased (74%) during co-administration with fluconazole. Patients receiving this combination should be monitored for the development of zidovudine-related adverse reactions.

Rifabutin There have been reports that an interaction exists when fluconazole is administered concomitantly with rifabutin, leading to increased serum levels of rifabutin. There have been reports of uveitis in patients to whom fluconazole and rifabutin were co-administered. Patients receiving rifabutin and fluconazole concomitantly should be carefully monitored.

Tacrolimus There have been reports that an interaction exists when fluconazole is administered concomitantly with tacrolimus, leading to increased serum levels of tacrolimus. There have been reports of nephrotoxicity in patients to whom fluconazole and tacrolimus were co-administered. Patients receiving tacrolimus and fluconazole concomitantly should be carefully monitored.

The use of fluconazole in patients concurrently taking astemizole or other drugs metabolised by the cytochrome P450 system may be associated with elevations in serum levels of these drugs. In the absence of definitive information, caution should be used when co-administering fluconazole. This is particularly important for drugs known to prolong QT interval. Patients should be carefully monitored.

Interaction studies have shown that when oral fluconazole is co-administered with food, cimetidine, antacids or following total body irradiation for bone marrow transplantation, no clinically significant impairment of fluconazole absorption occurs.

Physicians should be aware that drug-drug interaction studies with other medications have not been conducted, but that such interactions may occur.

4.6 Pregnancy and lactation

Use during pregnancy There are no adequate and well controlled studies in pregnant women. There have been reports of multiple congenital abnormalities in infants whose mothers were being treated for 3 or more months with high dose (400-800 mg/day) fluconazole therapy for coccidioidomycosis. The relationship between fluconazole and these events is unclear. Accordingly, Diflucan 150 should not be used in pregnancy, or in women of child-bearing potential unless adequate contraception is employed.

Use during lactation Fluconazole is found in human breast milk at concentrations similar to plasma, hence its use in nursing mothers is not recommended.

4.7 Effects on ability to drive and use machines

Experience with Diflucan indicates that therapy is unlikely to impair a patient's ability to drive or use machinery.

4.8 Undesirable effects

Fluconazole is generally well tolerated. The most common undesirable effects observed during clinical trials and associated with fluconazole are:

__Nervous SystemDisorders:__ Headache.

__Skinand Subcutaneous Tissue Disorders:__ Rash.

__GastrointestinalDisorders:__ Abdominal pain, diarrhoea, flatulence, nausea.

In some patients, particularly those with serious underlying diseases such as AIDS and cancer, changes in renal and haematological function test results and hepatic abnormalities have been observed during treatment with fluconazole and comparative agents, but the clinical significance and relationship to treatment is uncertain (see Section 4.4 "Special warnings and special precautions for use").

__Hepatobiliary Disorders:__ Hepatic toxicity including rare cases of fatalities, elevated alkaline phosphatase, elevated bilirubin, elevated SGOT, elevated SGPT.

In addition, the following undesirable effects have occurred during post-marketing:

__Nervous SystemDisorders:__ Dizziness, seizures, taste perversion.

__Skinand Subcutaneous Tissue Disorders:__ Alopecia, exfoliative skin disorders including Stevens-Johnson syndrome and toxic epidermal necrosis.

__GastrointestinalDisorders:__Dyspepsia, vomiting.

__Blood and Lymphatic System Disorders:__ Leukopenia including neutropenia and agranulocytosis, thrombocytopenia.

__Immune System Disorders:__

Allergic reaction:Anaphylaxis(including angioedema, face oedema, pruritus), urticaria.

__Hepatobiliary Disorders:__ Hepatic failure, hepatitis, hepatocellular necrosis, jaundice.

__Metabolism and Nutrition Disorders:__ Hypercholesterolaemia, hypertriglyceridaemia, hypokalaemia.

__Cardiac Disorders:__ QT prolongation, torsade de pointes (see section 4.4 **Special Warnings and Special Precautions for Use**).

4.9 Overdose

There have been reports of overdosage with fluconazole and in one case, a 42 year-old patient infected with human immunodeficiency virus developed hallucinations and exhibited paranoid behaviour after reportedly ingesting 8200mg of fluconazole, unverified by his physician. The patient was admitted to the hospital and his condition resolved within 48 hours.

In the event of overdosage, supportive measures and symptomatic treatment, with gastric lavage if necessary, may be adequate.

As fluconazole is largely excreted in the urine, forced volume diuresis would probably increase the elimination rate. A three hour haemodialysis session decreases plasma levels by approximately 50%.

5. PHARMACOLOGICAL PROPERTIES

5.1 Pharmacodynamic properties

Pharmacotherapeutic group: Triazole derivatives, ATC code J02AC.

Fluconazole, a member of the triazole class of antifungal agents, is a potent and selective inhibitor of fungal enzymes necessary for the synthesis of ergosterol.

Fluconazole shows little pharmacological activity in a wide range of animal studies. Some prolongation of pentobarbitone sleeping times in mice (p.o.), increased mean arterial and left ventricular blood pressure and increased heart rate in anaesthetised cats (i.v.) occurred. Inhibition of rat ovarian aromatase was observed at high concentrations.

Both orally and intravenously administered fluconazole was active in a variety of animal fungal infection models. Activity has been demonstrated against opportunistic mycoses, such as infections with *Candida* spp. Including systemic candidiasis in immunocompromised animals; with *Cryptococcus neoformans,* including intracranial infections; with *Microsporum* spp. and with *Trichophyton* spp. Fluconazole has also been shown to be active in animal models of endemic mycoses, including infections with *Blastomyces dermatitides;* with *Coccidoides immitis,* including intracranial infection and with *Histoplasma capsulatum* in normal and immunosuppressed animals.

There have been reports of cases of superinfection with *Candida* species other than *C. albicans*, which are often inherently not susceptible to fluconazole (e.g. *Candida krusei).* Such cases may require alternative antifungal therapy.

Fluconazole is highly specific for fungal cytochrome P-450 dependent enzymes. Fluconazole 50mg daily given up to 28 days has been shown not to affect testosterone plasma concentrations in males or steroid concentrations in females of child-bearing age. Fluconazole 200-400mg daily has no clinically significant effect on endogenous steroid levels or on ACTH stimulated response in healthy male volunteers. Interaction studies with antipyrine indicate that single or multiple doses of fluconazole 50mg do not affect its metabolism.

5.2 Pharmacokinetic properties

The pharmacokinetic properties of fluconazole are similar following administration by the intravenous or oral route. After oral administration fluconazole is well absorbed and plasma levels (and systemic bioavailability) are over 90% of the levels achieved after intravenous administration. Oral absorption is not affected by concomitant food intake. Peak plasma concentrations in the fasting state occur between 0.5 and 1.5 hours post-dose with a plasma elimination half-life of approximately 30 hours. Plasma concentrations are proportional to dose. Ninety percent steady-state levels are reached by day 4 -5 with multiple once daily dosing.

Administration of loading dose (on day 1) of twice the usual daily dose enables plasma levels to approximate to 90% steady-state levels by day 2. The apparent volume of distribution approximates to total body water. Plasma protein binding is low (11-12%).

Fluconazole achieves good penetration in all body fluids studied. The levels of fluconazole in saliva and sputum are similar to plasma levels. In patients with fungal meningitis, fluconazole levels in the CSF are approximately 80% of the corresponding plasma levels.

High skin concentrations of fluconazole, above serum concentrations, are achieved in the stratum corneum, epidemis-dermis and eccrine sweat. Fluconazole accumulates in the stratum corneum. At a dose of 50mg once daily, the concentration of fluconazole after 12 days was 73 microgram/g and 7 days after cessation of treatment the concentration was still 5.8 microgram/g.

The major route of excretion is renal, with approximately 80% of the administered dose appearing in the urine as unchanged drug. Fluconazole clearance is proportional to creatinine clearance. There is no evidence of circulating metabolites.

The long plasma elimination half-life provides the basis for single dose therapy for genital candidiasis.

A study compared the saliva and plasma concentrations of a single fluconazole 100mg dose administration in a capsule or in an oral suspension by rinsing and retaining in mouth for 2 minutes and swallowing. The maximum concentration of fluconazole in saliva after the suspension was observed 5 minutes after ingestion, and was 182 times higher than the maximum saliva concentration after the capsule which occurred 4 hours after ingestion. After about 4 hours, the saliva concentrations of fluconazole were similar. The mean AUC (0-96) in saliva was significantly greater after the suspension compared to the capsule. There was no significant difference in the elimination rate from saliva or the plasma pharmacokinetic parameters for the two formulations.

Pharmacokinetics in Children

In children, the following pharmacokinetics data have been reported:

(see Table 1 on next page)

In premature new-borns (gestational age around 28 weeks), intravenous administration of fluconazole of 6mg/kg was given every third day for a maximum of five doses while the premature new-borns remained in the intensive care unit. The mean half-life (hours) was 74 (range 44-185) on day 1 which decreased with time to a mean of 53 (range 30-131) on day 7 and 47 (range 27-68) on day 13.

The area under the curve (microgram.h/ml) was 271 (range 173-385) on day 1 and increased with a mean of 490 (range 292-734) on day 7 and decreased with a mean of 360 (range 167-566) on day 13.

The volume of distribution (ml/kg) was 1183 (range 1070-1470) on day 1 and which increased with time to a mean of 1184 (range 510-2130) on day 7 and 1328 (range 1040-1680) on day 13.

5.3 Preclinical safety data

Reproductive toxicity Increases in fetal anatomical variants (supernumerary ribs, renal pelvis dilation) and delays in ossification were observed at 25 and 50mg/kg and higher doses. At doses ranging from 80mg/kg (approximately 20-60x the recommended human dose) to 320mg/kg embryolethality in rats was increased and fetal abnormalities included wavy ribs, cleft palate and abnormal craniofacial ossification. These effects are consistent with the inhibition of oestrogen synthesis in rats and may be a result of known effects of lowered oestrogen on pregnancy, organogenesis and parturition.

Carcinogenesis Fluconazole showed no evidence of carcinogenic potential in mice and rats treated orally for 24 months at doses of 2.5, 5 or 10mg/kg/day. Male rats treated with 5 and 10mg/ kg/day had an increased incidence of hepatocellular adenomas.

Mutagenesis Fluconazole, with or without metabolic activation, was negative in tests for mutagenicity in 4 strains of S.typhimurium and in the mouse lymphoma L5178Y system. Cytogenetic studies in vivo (murine bone marrow cells, following oral administration of fluconazole) and in vitro (human lymphocytes exposed to fluconazole at 1000μg/ml) showed no evidence of chromosomal mutations.

Table 1

Age Studied	Dose (mg/kg)	Half-life (hours)	AUC (microgram.h/ml)
11 days- 11 months	Single-IV 3mg/kg	23	110.1
9 months- 13 years	Single-Oral 2mg/kg	25.0	94.7
9 months- 13 years	Single-Oral 8mg/kg	19.5	362.5
5 years- 15 years	Multiple-IV 2mg/kg	17.4*	67.4
5 years- 15 years	Multiple-IV 4mg/kg	15.2*	139.1
5 years- 15 years	Multiple-IV 8mg/kg	17.6*	196.7
Mean age 7 years	Multiple-Oral 3mg/kg	15.5	41.6

* Denotes final day

Impairment of fertility Fluconazole did not affect the fertility of male or female rats treated orally with daily doses of 5, 10 or 20mg/kg or with parenteral doses of 5, 25 or 75mg/kg, although the onset of parturition was slightly delayed at 20mg/kg p.o. In an intravenous perinatal study in rats at 5, 20 and 40mg/kg, dystocia and prolongation of parturition were observed in a few dams at 20mg/kg and 40mg/kg, but not at 5mg/kg. The disturbances in parturition were reflected by a slight increase in the number of still-born pups and decrease of neonatal survival at these dose levels. The effects on parturition in rats are consistent with the species specific oestrogen-lowering property produced by high doses of fluconazole. Such a hormone change has not been observed in women treated with Diflucan.

6. PHARMACEUTICAL PARTICULARS

6.1 List of excipients

Diflucan 150 capsules contain lactose, maize starch, colloidal silicon dioxide, magnesium stearate and sodium lauryl sulphate as excipients.

In addition, capsule shells contain: patent blue V (E131), titanium dioxide (E171) and gelatin.

6.2 Incompatibilities

No specific incompatibilities have been noted.

6.3 Shelf life

Current stability data support a shelf life of 5 years.

6.4 Special precautions for storage

Store below 30°C.

6.5 Nature and contents of container

Diflucan 150 capsules will be supplied as a pack containing one capsule in clear or opaque PVC blister packs with aluminium foil backing.

6.6 Instructions for use and handling

Diflucan 150 capsules should be swallowed whole.

7. MARKETING AUTHORISATION HOLDER

Pfizer Limited

Sandwich

Kent CT13 9NJ

United Kingdom

8. MARKETING AUTHORISATION NUMBER(S)

PL 00057/0290

9. DATE OF FIRST AUTHORISATION/RENEWAL OF THE AUTHORISATION

11 January 2000

10. DATE OF REVISION OF THE TEXT

November 2004

Legal Category

POM

Diflucan Capsules 50mg and 200mg, Powder for Oral Suspension 50mg/ml and 200mg/ml, Intravenous Infusion 2mg/ml

(Pfizer Limited)

1. NAME OF THE MEDICINAL PRODUCT

DIFLUCAN® CAPSULES 50MG

DIFLUCAN® CAPSULES 200MG

DIFLUCAN® POWDER FOR ORAL SUSPENSION 50MG/5ML

DIFLUCAN® POWDER FOR ORAL SUSPENSION 200MG/5ML

DIFLUCAN® INTRAVENOUS INFUSION 2MG/ML

2. QUALITATIVE AND QUANTITATIVE COMPOSITION

Diflucan contains as its active ingredient fluconazole 50mg and 200mg as capsules, 50mg or 200mg per 5ml as powder for oral suspension on reconstitution with water, and as 2mg/ml in a saline solution for intravenous infusion.

3. PHARMACEUTICAL FORM

Diflucan Capsules 50mg are light turquoise blue and white, coded 'FLU 50' and 'PFIZER'.

Diflucan Capsules 200mg are purple and white, coded 'FLU 200' and 'PFIZER'.

Diflucan Powder for Oral Suspension is a dry white to off-white powder which yields, on reconstitution with water (24ml), an orange flavoured suspension containing the equivalent of 50mg or 200mg fluconazole per 5ml.

Diflucan Intravenous Infusion 2mg/ml is available in a 0.9% aqueous sodium chloride solution, presented in glass infusion vials (25 or 100ml).

4. CLINICAL PARTICULARS

4.1 Therapeutic indications

Therapy may be instituted before the results of the cultures and other laboratory studies are known; however, once these results become available, anti-infective therapy should be adjusted accordingly.

Diflucan is indicated for the treatment of the following conditions:

1. Genital candidiasis. Vaginal candidiasis, acute or recurrent. Candidal balanitis. The treatment of partners who present with symptomatic genital candidiasis should be considered.

2. Mucosal candidiasis. These include oropharyngeal, oesophageal, non-invasive bronchopulmonary infections, candiduria, mucocutaneous and chronic oral atrophic candidiasis (denture sore mouth). Normal hosts and patients with compromised immune function may be treated.

3. Tinea pedis, tinea corporis, tinea cruris, tinea versicolor and dermal *Candida* infections. Diflucan is not indicated for nail infections and tinea capitis.

4. Systemic candidiasis including candidaemia, disseminated candidiasis and other forms of invasive candidal infection. These include infections of the peritoneum, endocardium and pulmonary and urinary tracts. Candidal infections in patients with malignancy, in intensive care units or those receiving cytotoxic or immunosuppressive therapy may be treated.

5. Cryptococcosis, including cryptococcal meningitis and infections of other sites (e.g. pulmonary, cutaneous). Normal hosts, and patients with AIDS, organ transplants or other causes of immunosuppression may be treated. Diflucan can be used as maintenance therapy to prevent relapse of cryptococcal disease in patients with AIDS.

6. For the prevention of fungal infections in immunocompromised patients considered at risk as a consequence of neutropenia following cytotoxic chemotherapy or radiotherapy, including bone marrow transplant patients.

4.2 Posology and method of administration

Diflucan may be administered either orally or by intravenous infusion at a rate of approximately 5-10ml/min, the route being dependent on the clinical state of the patient. On transferring from the intravenous route to the oral route or vice versa, there is no need to change the daily dose. Diflucan intravenous infusion is formulated in 0.9% sodium chloride solution, each 200mg (100ml bottle) containing 15mmol each of Na^+ and Cl^-.

The daily dose of Diflucan should be based on the nature and severity of the fungal infection. Most cases of vaginal candidiasis respond to single dose therapy. Therapy for those types of infections requiring multiple dose treatment should be continued until clinical parameters or laboratory tests indicate that active fungal infection has subsided. An inadequate period of treatment may lead to recurrence of active infection. Patients with AIDS and cryptococcal meningitis usually require maintenance therapy to prevent relapse.

Use in adults

1. Candidal vaginitis or balanitis - 150mg single oral dose.

2. Mucosal Candidiasis

Oropharyngeal candidiasis - the usual dose is 50mg once daily for 7 - 14 days. Treatment should not normally exceed 14 days except in severely immunocompromised patients.

For atrophic oral candidiasis associated with dentures - the usual dose is 50mg once daily for 14 days administered concurrently with local antiseptic measures to the denture.

For other candidal infections of mucosa except genital candidiasis (see above), e.g. oesophagitis, non-invasive bronchopulmonary infections, candiduria, mucocutaneous candidiasis etc., the usual effective dose is 50mg daily, given for 14 - 30 days.

In unusually difficult cases of mucosal candidal infections the dose may be increased to 100mg daily.

3. For tinea pedis, corporis, cruris, versicolor and dermal *Candida* infections the recommended dosage is 50mg once daily. Duration of treatment is normally 2 to 4 weeks but tinea pedis may require treatment for up to 6 weeks. Duration of treatment should not exceed 6 weeks.

4. For candidaemia, disseminated candidiasis and other invasive candidal infections the usual dose is 400mg on the first day followed by 200mg daily. Depending on the clinical response the dose may be increased to 400mg daily. Duration of treatment is based upon the clinical response.

5a. For cryptococcal meningitis and cryptococcal infections at other sites, the usual dose is 400mg on the first day followed by 200mg - 400mg once daily. Duration of treatment for cryptococcal infections will depend on the clinical and mycological response, but is usually at least 6-8 weeks for cryptococcal meningitis.

5b. For the prevention of relapse of cryptococcal meningitis in patients with AIDS, after the patient receives a full course of primary therapy, Diflucan may be administered indefinitely at a daily dose of 100 - 200mg.

6. For the prevention of fungal infections in immunocompromised patients considered at risk as a consequence of neutropenia following cytotoxic chemotherapy or radiotherapy, the dose should be 50 to 400mg once daily, based on the patient's risk for developing fungal infection. For patients at high risk of systemic infection, e.g. patients who are anticipated to have profound or prolonged neutropenia such as during bone marrow transplantation, the recommended dose is 400mg once daily. Diflucan administration should start several days before the anticipated onset of neutropenia, and continue for 7 days after the neutrophil count rises above 1000 cells per mm^3.

Use in children

As with similar infections in adults, the duration of treatment is based on the clinical and mycological response. Diflucan is administered as a single daily dose each day.

For children with impaired renal function, see dosing in "Use in patients with impaired renal function".

Children over four weeks of age The recommended dose of Diflucan for mucosal candidiasis is 3mg/kg daily. A loading dose of 6mg/kg may be used on the first day to achieve steady state levels more rapidly.

For the treatment of systemic candidiasis and cryptococcal infections, the recommended dosage is 6-12mg/kg daily, depending on the severity of the disease.

For the prevention of fungal infections in immunocompromised patients considered at risk as a consequence of neutropenia following cytotoxic chemotherapy or radiotherapy, the dose should be 3-12mg/kg daily, depending on the extent and duration of the induced neutropenia (see adult dosing).

A maximum dosage of 400mg daily should not be exceeded in children.

Despite extensive data supporting the use of Diflucan in children there are limited data available on the use of Diflucan for genital candidiasis in children below 16 years. Use at present is not recommended unless antifungal treatment is imperative and no suitable alternative agent exists.

Children four weeks of age and younger Neonates excrete fluconazole slowly. In the first two weeks of life, the same mg/kg dosing as in older children should be used but administered every 72 hours. During weeks 3 and 4 of life, the same dose should be given every 48 hours.

A maximum dosage of 12mg/kg every 72 hours should not be exceeded in children in the first two weeks of life. For children between 3 and 4 weeks of life, 12mg/kg every 48 hours should not be exceeded.

To facilitate accurate measurement of doses less than 10mg, Diflucan should only be administered to children in hospital using the 50mg/5ml suspension orally or the intravenous infusion, depending on the clinical condition of the child. A suitable measuring device should be used for administration of the suspension. Once reconstituted the suspension should not be further diluted.

Use in the elderly The normal dose should be used if there is no evidence of renal impairment. In patients with renal impairment (creatinine clearance less than 50ml/min) the dosage schedule should be adjusted as described below.

Use in patients with impaired renal function Fluconazole is excreted predominantly in the urine as unchanged drug. No adjustments in single dose therapy are required. In patients (including children) with impaired renal function who will receive multiple doses of Diflucan, the normal recommended dose (according to indication) should be given on day 1, followed by a daily dose based on the following table:

Creatinine clearance (ml/min)	*Percent of recommended dose*
>50	100%
⩽50 (no dialysis)	50%
Regular dialysis	100% after each dialysis

Compatibility of intravenous infusion

Although further dilution is unnecessary Diflucan Intravenous Infusion is compatible with the following administration fluids:

a) Dextrose 20%

b) Ringer's solution

c) Hartmann's solution

d) Potassium chloride in dextrose

e) Sodium bicarbonate 4.2%

f) Normal saline (0.9%)

Diflucan may be infused through an existing line with one of the above listed fluids. No specific incompatibilities have been noted, although mixing with any other drug prior to infusion is not recommended.

4.3 Contraindications

Diflucan should not be used in patients with known hypersensitivity to fluconazole or to related azole compounds or any other ingredient in the formulation.

Fluconazole should not be co-adminstered with cisapride or terfenadine which are known to both prolong the QT – interval and are metabolised by CYP3A4 (See "Interactions with other medicinal products and other forms of interaction").

4.4 Special warnings and special precautions for use

In some patients, particularly those with serious underlying diseases such as AIDS and cancer, abnormalities in haematological, hepatic, renal and other biochemical function test results have been observed during treatment with Diflucan but the clinical significance and relationship to treatment is uncertain.

Very rarely, patients who died with severe underlying disease and who had received multiple doses of Diflucan had post-mortem findings which included hepatic necrosis. These patients were receiving multiple concomitant medications, some known to be potentially hepatotoxic, and/or had underlying diseases which could have caused the hepatic necrosis.

In cases of hepatotoxicity, no obvious relationship to total daily dose of Diflucan, duration of therapy, sex or age of the patient has been observed; the abnormalities have usually been reversible on discontinuation of Diflucan therapy.

As a causal relationship with Diflucan cannot be excluded, patients who develop abnormal liver function tests during Diflucan therapy should be monitored for the development of more serious hepatic injury. Diflucan should be discontinued if clinical signs or symptoms consistent with liver disease develop during treatment with Diflucan.

Patients have rarely developed exfoliative cutaneous reactions, such as Stevens-Johnson Syndrome and toxic epidermal necrolysis, during treatment with fluconazole. AIDS patients are more prone to the development of severe cutaneous reactions to many drugs. If a rash develops in a patient treated for a superficial fungal infection which is considered attributable to Diflucan, further therapy with this agent should be discontinued. If patients with invasive/systemic fungal infections develop rashes, they should be monitored closely and Diflucan discontinued if bullous lesions or erythema multiforme develop.

In rare cases, as with other azoles, anaphylaxis has been reported.

Some azoles, including fluconazole, have been associated with prolongation of the QT interval on the electrocardiogram. During post-marketing surveillance, there have been very rare cases of QT prolongation and torsade de pointes in patients taking fluconazole. Although the association of fluconazole and QT-prolongation has not been fully established, fluconazole should be used with caution in patients with potentially proarrythmic conditions such as:

- Congenital or documented acquired QT prolongation
- Cardiomyopathy, in particular when heart failure is present
- Sinus bradycardia
- Existing symptomatic arrythmias
- Concomitant medication not metabolized by CY34A but known to prolong QT interval
- Electrolyte disturbances such as hypokalaemia, hypomagnesaemia and hypocalaemia

(See Section 4.5 Interactions with other medical products and other forms of interaction)

4.5 Interaction with other medicinal products and other forms of Interaction

The following drug interactions relate to the use of multiple-dose fluconazole, and the relevance to single-dose 150mg fluconazole has not yet been established.

Rifampicin Concomitant administration of fluconazole and rifampicin resulted in a 25% decrease in the AUC and 20% shorter half-life of fluconazole. In patients receiving concomitant rifampicin, an increase in the fluconazole dose should be considered.

Hydrochlorothiazide In a kinetic interaction study, co-administration of multiple-dose hydrochlorothiazide to healthy volunteers receiving fluconazole increased plasma concentrations of fluconazole by 40%. An effect of this magnitude should not necessitate a change in the fluconazole dose regimen in subjects receiving concomitant diuretics, although the prescriber should bear it in mind.

Anticoagulants In an interaction study, fluconazole increased the prothrombin time (12%) after warfarin administration in healthy males. In post-marketing experience, as with other azole antifungals, bleeding events (bruising, epistaxis, gastrointestinal bleeding, hematuria and melaena) have been reported in association with increases in prothrombin time in patients receiving fluconazole concurrently with warfarin. Prothrombin time in patients receiving coumarin-type anticoagulants should be carefully monitored.

Benzodiazepines (Short Acting) Following oral administration of midazolam, fluconazole resulted in substantial increases in midazolam concentrations and psychomotor effects. This effect on midazolam appears to be more pronounced following oral administration of fluconazole than with fluconazole administered intravenously. If concomitant benzodiazepine therapy is necessary in patients being treated with fluconazole, consideration should be given to decreasing the benzodiazepine dosage and the patients should be appropriately monitored.

Sulphonylureas Fluconazole has been shown to prolong the serum half-life of concomitantly administered oral sulphonylureas (chlorpropamide, glibenclamide, glipizide and tolbutamide) in healthy volunteers. Fluconazole and oral sulphonylureas may be co-administered to diabetic patients, but the possibility of a hypoglycaemic episode should be borne in mind.

Phenytoin Concomitant administration of fluconazole and phenytoin may increase the levels of phenytoin to a clinically significant degree. If it is necessary to administer both drugs concomitantly, phenytoin levels should be monitored and the phenytoin dose adjusted to maintain therapeutic levels.

Oral contraceptives Two kinetic studies with combined oral contraceptives have been performed using multiple doses of fluconazole. There were no relevant effects on either hormone level in the 50mg fluconazole study, while at 200mg daily the AUCs of ethinyloestradiol and levonorgestrel were increased 40% and 24% respectively. Thus multiple dose use of fluconazole at these doses is unlikely to have an effect on the efficacy of the combined oral contraceptive.

In a 300 mg once weekly fluconazole study, the AUCs of ethinyl estradiol and norethindrone were increased by 24% and 13%, respectively.

Endogenous steroid Fluconazole 50mg daily does not affect endogenous steroid levels in females: 200-400mg daily has no clinically significant effect on endogenous steroid levels or on ACTH stimulated response in healthy male volunteers.

Cyclosporin A kinetic study in renal transplant patients found fluconazole 200mg daily to slowly increase cyclosporin concentrations. However, in another multiple dose study with 100mg daily, fluconazole did not affect cyclosporin levels in patients with bone marrow transplants. Cyclosporin plasma concentration monitoring in patients receiving fluconazole is recommended.

Theophylline In a placebo controlled interaction study, the administration of fluconazole 200mg for 14 days resulted in an 18% decrease in the mean plasma clearance of theophylline. Patients who are receiving high doses of theophylline or who are otherwise at increased risk for theophylline toxicity should be observed for signs of theophylline toxicity while receiving fluconazole, and the therapy modified appropriately if signs of toxicity develop.

Terfenadine Because of the occurrence of serious dysrhythmias secondary to prolongation of the QTc interval in patients receiving other azole antifungals in conjunction with terfenadine, interactions studies have been performed. One study at a 200mg daily dose of fluconazole failed to demonstrate a prolongation in QTc interval. Another study at a 400mg and 800mg daily dose of fluconazole demonstrated that fluconazole taken in multiple doses of 400mg per day or greater significantly increased plasma levels of terfenadine when taken concomitantly. There have been spontaneously reported cases of palpitations, tachycardia, dizziness, and chest pain in patients taking concomitant fluconazole and terfenadine where the relationship of the reported adverse events to drug therapy or underlying medical conditions was not clear. Because of the potential seriousness of such an interaction, it is recommended that terfenadine not be taken in combination with fluconazole. (See "Contra-indications".)

Cisapride There have been reports of cardiac events including torsades de pointes in patients to whom fluconazole and cisapride were co-administered. A controlled study found that concomitant fluconazole 200 mg once daily and cisapride 20 mg four times a day yielded a significant increase in cisapride plasma levels and prolongation of QTc interval. In most of these cases, the patients appear to have been predisposed to arrhythmias or had serious underlying illnesses, and the relationship of the reported events to a possible fluconazole-cisapride drug interaction is unclear. Because of the potential seriousness of such an interaction, co-administration of cisapride is contra-indicated in patients receiving fluconazole. (See "Contra-indications".)

Zidovudine Two kinetic studies resulted in increased levels of zidovudine most likely caused by the decreased conversion of zidovudine to its major metabolite. One study determined zidovudine levels in AIDS or ARC patients before and following fluconazole 200mg daily for 15 days. There was a significant increase in zidovudine AUC (20%). A second randomised, two-period, two-treatment cross-over study examined zidovudine levels in HIV infected patients. On two occasions, 21 days apart, patients received zidovudine 200mg every eight hours either with or without fluconazole 400mg daily for seven days. The AUC of zidovudine significantly increased (74%) during co-administration with fluconazole. Patients receiving this combination should be monitored for the development of zidovudine-related adverse reactions.

Rifabutin There have been reports that an interaction exists when fluconazole is administered concomitantly with rifabutin, leading to increased serum levels of rifabutin. There have been reports of uveitis in patients to whom fluconazole and rifabutin were co-administered. Patients receiving rifabutin and fluconazole concomitantly should be carefully monitored.

Tacrolimus There have been reports that an interaction exists when fluconazole is administered concomitantly with tacrolimus, leading to increased serum levels of tacrolimus. There have been reports of nephrotoxicity in patients to whom fluconazole and tacrolimus were co-administered. Patients receiving tacrolimus and fluconazole concomitantly should be carefully monitored.

The use of fluconazole in patients concurrently taking astemizole or other drugs metabolised by the cytochrome P450 system may be associated with elevations in serum levels of these drugs. In the absence of definitive information, caution should be used when co-administering fluconazole. This is particularly important for drugs known to prolong QT interval. Patients should be carefully monitored.

Interaction studies have shown that when oral fluconazole is co-administered with food, cimetidine, antacids or following total body irradiation for bone marrow transplantation, no clinically significant impairment of fluconazole absorption occurs.

Physicians should be aware that drug-drug interaction studies with other medications have not been conducted, but that such interactions may occur.

4.6 Pregnancy and lactation

Use during pregnancy There are no adequate and well controlled studies in pregnant women. There have been reports of multiple congenital abnormalities in infants whose mothers were being treated for 3 or more months with high dose (400-800 mg/day) fluconazole therapy for coccidioidomycosis. The relationship between fluconazole and these events is unclear.

Accordingly, Diflucan should not be used in pregnancy, or in women of childbearing potential unless adequate contraception is employed.

Use during lactation Fluconazole is found in human breast milk at concentrations similar to plasma, hence its use in nursing mothers is not recommended.

4.7 Effects on ability to drive and use machines

Experience with Diflucan indicates that therapy is unlikely to impair a patient's ability to drive or use machinery.

4.8 Undesirable effects

Fluconazole is generally well tolerated. The most common undesirable effects observed during clinical trials and associated with fluconazole are:

Nervous System Disorders: Headache.

Skin and Subcutaneous Tissue Disorders: Rash.

Gastrointestinal Disorders: Abdominal pain, diarrhoea, flatulence, nausea.

In some patients, particularly those with serious underlying diseases such as AIDS and cancer, changes in renal and haematological function test results and hepatic abnormalities have been observed during treatment with fluconazole and comparative agents, but the clinical significance and relationship to treatment is uncertain (see Section 4.4 "Special warnings and special precautions for use").

Hepatobiliary Disorders: Hepatic toxicity including rare cases of fatalities, elevated alkaline phosphatase, elevated bilirubin, elevated SGOT, elevated SGPT.

In addition, the following undesirable effects have occurred during post-marketing:

Nervous SystemDisorders: Dizziness, seizures, taste perversion.

Skinand Subcutaneous Tissue Disorders: Alopecia, exfoliative skin disorders including Stevens-Johnson syndrome and toxic epidermal necrolysis.

Gastrointestinal Disorders: Dyspepsia, vomiting.

Blood and Lymphatic System Disorders: Leukopenia including neutropenia and agranulocytosis, thrombocytopenia.

Immune System Disorders:

Allegic reaction:Anaphylaxis(including angioedema, face oedema, pruritus), urticaria.

Hepatobiliary Disorders: Hepatic failure, hepatitis, hepatocellular necrosis, jaundice.

Metabolism and Nutrition Disorders: Hypercholesterolaemia, hypertriglyceridaemia, hypokalaemia.

Cardiac Disorders: QT prolongation, torsade de pointes (see section 4.4 **Special Warnings and Special Precautions for Use**).

4.9 Overdose

There have been reports of overdosage with fluconazole and in one case, a 42 year-old patient infected with human immunodeficiency virus developed hallucinations and exhibited paranoid behaviour after reportedly ingesting 8200mg of fluconazole, unverified by his physician. The patient was admitted to the hospital and his condition resolved within 48 hours.

In the event of overdosage, supportive measures and symptomatic treatment, with gastric lavage if necessary, may be adequate.

As fluconazole is largely excreted in the urine, forced volume diuresis would probably increase the elimination rate. A three hour haemodialysis session decreases plasma levels by approximately 50%.

5. PHARMACOLOGICAL PROPERTIES

5.1 Pharmacodynamic properties

Pharmacotherapeutic group: Triazole derivatives, ATC code J02AC.

Fluconazole, a member of the triazole class of antifungal agents, is a potent and selective inhibitor of fungal enzymes necessary for the synthesis of ergosterol.

Fluconazole shows little pharmacological activity in a wide range of animal studies. Some prolongation of pentobarbitone sleeping times in mice (p.o.), increased mean arterial and left ventricular blood pressure and increased heart rate in anaesthetised cats (i.v.) occurred. Inhibition of rat ovarian aromatase was observed at high concentrations.

Both orally and intravenously administered fluconazole was active in a variety of animal fungal infection models. Activity has been demonstrated against opportunistic mycoses, such as infections with *Candida* spp. including systemic candidiasis in immunocompromised animals; with *Cryptococcus neoformans,* including intracranial infections; with *Microsporum* spp. and with *Trichophyton* spp. Fluconazole has also been shown to be active in animal models of endemic mycoses, including infections with *Blastomyces dermatitides;* with *Coccidoides immitis,* including intracranial infection and with *Histoplasma capsulatum* in normal and immunosuppressed animals.

There have been reports of cases of superinfection with *Candida* species other than *C. albicans*, which are often inherently not susceptible to fluconazole (e.g. *Candida krusei*). Such cases may require alternative antifungal therapy.

Fluconazole is highly specific for fungal cytochrome P-450 dependent enzymes. Fluconazole 50mg daily given up to 28 days has been shown not to affect testosterone plasma concentrations in males or steroid concentrations in females of child-bearing age. Fluconazole 200-400mg daily has no clinically significant effect on endogenous steroid levels or on ACTH stimulated response in healthy male volunteers. Interaction studies with antipyrine indicate that single or multiple doses of fluconazole 50mg do not affect its metabolism.

The efficacy of fluconazole in tinea capitis has been studied in 2 randomised controlled trials in a total of 878 patients comparing fluconazole with griseofulvin. Fluconazole at 6 mg/kg/day for 6 weeks was not superior to griseofulvin administered at 11 mg/kg/day for 6 weeks. The overall success rate at week 6 was low (fluconazole 6 weeks: 18.3%; fluconazole 3 weeks: 14.7%; griseofulvin: 17.7%) across all treatment groups. These findings are not inconsistent with the natural history of tinea capitis without therapy.

5.2 Pharmacokinetic properties

The pharmacokinetic properties of fluconazole are similar following administration by the intravenous or oral route. After oral administration fluconazole is well absorbed and plasma levels (and systemic bioavailability) are over 90% of the levels achieved after intravenous administration. Oral absorption is not affected by concomitant food intake. Peak plasma concentrations in the fasting state occur between 0.5 and 1.5 hours post-dose with a plasma elimination half-life of approximately 30 hours. Plasma concentrations are proportional to dose. Ninety percent steady-state levels are reached by day 4 -5 with multiple once daily dosing.

Administration of a loading dose (on day 1) of twice the usual daily dose enables plasma levels to approximate to 90% steady-state levels by day 2. The apparent volume of distribution approximates to total body water. Plasma protein binding is low (11-12%).

Fluconazole achieves good penetration in all body fluids studied. The levels of fluconazole in saliva and sputum are similar to plasma levels. In patients with fungal meningitis, fluconazole levels in the CSF are approximately 80% of the corresponding plasma levels.

High skin concentrations of fluconazole, above serum concentrations, are achieved in the stratum corneum, epidermis-dermis and eccrine sweat. Fluconazole accumulates in the stratum corneum. At a dose of 50mg once daily, the concentration of fluconazole after 12 days was 73 microgram/g and 7 days after cessation of treatment the concentration was still 5.8 microgram/g.

The major route of excretion is renal, with approximately 80% of the administered dose appearing in the urine as unchanged drug. Fluconazole clearance is proportional to creatinine clearance. There is no evidence of circulating metabolites.

The long plasma elimination half-life provides the basis for single dose therapy for genital candidiasis and once daily dosing for other indications.

A study compared the saliva and plasma concentrations of a single fluconazole 100mg dose administration in a capsule or in an oral suspension by rinsing and retaining in mouth for 2 minutes and swallowing. The maximum concentration of fluconazole in saliva after the suspension was observed 5 minutes after ingestion, and was 182 times higher than the maximum saliva concentration after the capsule which occurred 4 hours after ingestion. After about 4 hours, the saliva concentrations of fluconazole were similar. The mean AUC (0-96) in saliva was significantly greater after the suspension compared to the capsule. There was no significant difference in the elimination rate from saliva or the plasma pharmacokinetic parameters for the two formulations.

Pharmacokinetics in Children

In children, the following pharmacokinetic data have been reported:

(see Table 1)

In premature new-borns (gestational age around 28 weeks), intravenous administration of fluconazole of 6mg/kg was given every third day for a maximum of five doses while the premature new-borns remained in the intensive care unit. The mean half-life (hours) was 74 (range 44-185) on day 1 which decreased with time to a mean of 53 (range 30-131) on day 7 and 47 (range 27-68) on day 13.

The area under the curve (microgram.h/ml) was 271 (range 173-385) on day 1 and increased with a mean of 490 (range 292-734) on day 7 and decreased with a mean of 360 (range 167-566) on day 13.

The volume of distribution (ml/kg) was 1183 (range 1070-1470) on day 1 and increased with time to a mean of 1184 (range 510-2130) on day 7 and 1328 (range 1040-1680) on day 13.

5.3 Preclinical safety data

Reproductive Toxicity Increases in fetal anatomical variants (supernumerary ribs, renal pelvis dilation) and delays in ossification were observed at 25 and 50mg/kg and higher doses. At doses ranging from 80mg/kg (approximately 20-60x the recommended human dose) to 320mg/kg embryolethality in rats was increased and fetal abnormalities included wavy ribs, cleft palate and abnormal craniofacial ossification. These effects are consistent with the inhibition of oestrogen synthesis in rats and may be a result of known effects of lowered oestrogen on pregnancy, organogenesis and parturition.

Carcinogenesis Fluconazole showed no evidence of carcinogenic potential in mice and rats treated orally for 24 months at doses of 2.5, 5 or 10mg/kg/day. Male rats treated with 5 and 10mg/kg/day had an increased incidence of hepatocellular adenomas.

Mutagenesis Fluconazole, with or without metabolic activation, was negative in tests for mutagenicity in 4 strains of S.typhimurium and in the mouse lymphoma L5178Y system. Cytogenetic studies in vivo (murine bone marrow cells, following oral administration of fluconazole) and in vitro (human lymphocytes exposed to fluconazole at 1000μg/ml) showed no evidence of chromosomal mutations.

Impairment of fertility Fluconazole did not affect the fertility of male or female rats treated orally with daily doses of 5, 10 or 20mg/kg or with parenteral doses of 5, 25 or 75mg/kg, although the onset of parturition was slightly delayed at 20mg/kg p.o. In an intravenous perinatal study in rats at 5, 20 and 40mg/kg, dystocia and prolongation of parturition were observed in a few dams at 20mg/kg and 40mg/kg, but not at 5mg/kg. The disturbances in parturition were reflected by a slight increase in the number of still-born pups and decrease of neonatal survival at these dose levels. The effects on parturition in rats are consistent with the species specific oestrogen-lowering property produced by high doses of fluconazole. Such a hormone change has not been observed in women treated with fluconazole.

6. PHARMACEUTICAL PARTICULARS

6.1 List of excipients

Diflucan Capsules (all strengths) contain lactose, maize starch, colloidal silicon dioxide, magnesium stearate and sodium lauryl sulphate as excipients.

In addition, capsule shells contain:

50mg - patent blue V (E131), titanium dioxide (E171) and gelatin.

200mg - titanium dioxide (E171), erythrosine (E127), indigotine (E132) and gelatin.

Diflucan Intravenous Infusion is a sterile aqueous solution which is made iso-osmotic with sodium chloride.

Diflucan Powder for Oral Suspension contains sucrose (2.88g per 50mg dose; 2.73g per 200mg dose), colloidal silicon dioxide, titanium dioxide, xanthan gum, sodium citrate dihydrate, citric acid anhydrous, sodium benzoate and natural orange flavour.

6.2 Incompatibilities

No specific incompatibilities have been noted.

6.3 Shelf life

Current stability data support a shelf life of 5 years for the capsules, 5 years for the intravenous infusion and 2 years for the dry powder for oral suspension. There is a use period of 14 days for the reconstituted suspension.

6.4 Special precautions for storage

Store below 30°C.

Reconstituted suspension should be stored at 5°C - 30°C.

Do not freeze reconstituted suspension or intravenous infusion.

6.5 Nature and contents of container

Diflucan Capsules will be supplied in clear or opaque PVC blister packs with aluminium foil backing, as follows:

7 × 50mg or 200mg Diflucan capsules for multiple dose therapy.

Diflucan Intravenous Infusion will be supplied in clear Type I glass infusion vials (25 or 100ml) sealed with rubber bungs on crimping with aluminium over-caps.

Table 1

Age Studied	Dose (mg/kg)	Half-life (hours)	AUC (microgram.h/ml)
11 days- 11 months	Single-IV 3mg/kg	23	110.1
9 months- 13 years	Single-Oral 2mg/kg	25.0	94.7
9 months- 13 years	Single-Oral 8mg/kg	19.5	362.5
5 years- 15 years	Multiple IV 2mg/kg	17.4*	67.4
5 years- 15 years	Multiple IV 4mg/kg	15.2*	139.1
5 years- 15 years	Multiple IV 8mg/kg	17.6*	196.7
Mean Age 7 Years	Multiple Oral 3mg/kg	15.5	41.6

* Denotes final day

Diflucan Powder for Oral Suspension will be supplied in high density polyethylene bottles with child resistant closures, containing 35ml of suspension (50mg/5ml or 200mg/5ml)on reconstitution with 24ml of water.

6.6 Instructions for use and handling

Diflucan Capsules should be swallowed whole.

Diflucan Intravenous Infusion Do not freeze. The infusion does not contain any preservative. It is for single use only. Discard any remaining solution.

To reconstitute the ***Diflucan Powder for Oral Suspension***: Tap the bottle to loosen powder. Add 24ml of water. Shake well. Shake immediately prior to use. Where doses of less than 5ml are required, a suitable measuring device should be used. Dilution is not appropriate.

7. MARKETING AUTHORISATION HOLDER

Pfizer Limited
Sandwich
Kent CT13 9NJ
United Kingdom

8. MARKETING AUTHORISATION NUMBER(S)

Diflucan Capsules 50mg PL 00057/0289

Diflucan Capsules 200mg PL 00057/0317

Diflucan Intravenous Infusion 2mg/ml PL 00057/0315

Diflucan Powder for Oral Suspension 50mg/5ml PL 00057/0343

Diflucan Powder for Oral Suspension 200mg/5ml PL 00057/0344

9. DATE OF FIRST AUTHORISATION/RENEWAL OF THE AUTHORISATION

Diflucan Capsules 50mg	11 January 2000
Diflucan Capsules 200mg	30 May 1996
Diflucan IV Infusion	24 November 1994
Diflucan POS	18 December 1996

10. DATE OF REVISION OF THE TEXT

March 2005

Legal Category

POM

Company Reference: DF11_0

Diflucan One

(Pfizer Consumer Healthcare)

1. NAME OF THE MEDICINAL PRODUCT

DIFLUCAN ONE (150 mg)

2. QUALITATIVE AND QUANTITATIVE COMPOSITION

Diflucan One contains as its active ingredient fluconazole, 150 mg.

3. PHARMACEUTICAL FORM

Diflucan One capsules are available for oral administration, as follows:

150 mg: No 1 hard gelatin capsules, blue opaque cap and body: marked with Pfizer logo and code FLU-150.

4. CLINICAL PARTICULARS

4.1 Therapeutic indications

Diflucan One is indicated for the treatment of the following conditions:

Vaginal candidiasis, acute or recurrent; or candidal balanitis associated with vaginal candidiasis.

4.2 Posology and method of administration

In adults aged 16 - 60 years

Vaginal candidiasis or candidal balanitis – 150 mg single oral dose.

In Children - Not recommended in children aged under 16 years.

Use in Elderly - not recommended in patients aged over 60 years.

Use in Renal Impairment

Fluconazole is excreted predominantly in the urine as unchanged drug. No adjustments in single dose therapy are required.

4.3 Contraindications

Diflucan One should not be used in patients with known hypersensitivity to the drug or to related azole compounds or any other ingredient in the formulation.

Fluconazole should not be co-administered with cisapride or terfenadine, which are known both to prolong the QT interval and be metabolised by CYP3A4 (See section 4.5 Interactions with other medicinal products and other forms of interaction.)

4.4 Special warnings and special precautions for use

Fluconazole has been associated with rare cases of serious hepatic toxicity including fatalities, primarily in patients with serious underlying medical conditions. In cases of fluconazole-associated hepatotoxicity, no obvious relationship to total daily dose, duration of therapy, sex or age of patients has been observed. Fluconazole hepatotoxicity has usually been reversible on discontinuation of therapy. Fluconazole should not be used again if clinical signs or symptoms consistent with liver disease develop that may be attributable to fluconazole.

Rarely patients have developed exfoliative cutaneous reactions, such as Stevens-Johnson syndrome and toxic epidermal necrolysis, during treatment with fluconazole. AIDS patients are more prone to the development of severe cutaneous reactions to many drugs. Fluconazole should not be used again, if a rash develops, which is considered attributable to fluconazole.

In rare cases, as with other azoles, anaphylaxis has been reported.

Some azoles, including fluconazole, have been associated with prolongation of the QT interval on the electrocardiogram. During post-marketing surveillance, there have been very rare cases of QT prolongation and torsade de pointes in patients taking fluconazole. Although the association of fluconazole and QT-prolongation has not been fully established, fluconazole should be administered with caution to patients with potential proarrhythmic conditions such as:

- Congenital or documented acquired QT prolongation
- Cardiomyopathy, in particular when heart failure is present
- Sinus bradycardia
- Existing symptomatic arrhythmias
- Concomitant medication known to prolong QT interval
- Electrolyte disturbances such as hypokalaemia, hypomagnesaemia and hypocalcaemia

(See Section 4.5 Interactions with other medicinal products and other forms of interaction.)

Patients with rare hereditary problems of galactose intolerance, the Lapp lactase deficiency or glucose-galactose malabsorption should not take this medicine.

The product intended for pharmacy availability without prescription will carry a leaflet which will advise the patient:

<u>Do not use Diflucan One without first consulting your doctor:</u>

If you are under 16 or over 60 years of age.

If you are allergic to any of the ingredients in Diflucan One or other antifungals and other thrush treatments, or have previously had a rash after taking fluconazole (see section "After taking Diflucan One").

If you have an intolerance to lactose.

If you are taking any medicine other than the Pill.

If you are taking the antihistamines terfenadine or astemizole
Cisapride (for indigestion)

If you have had thrush more than twice in the last six months.

If you suffer from heart disease including heart rhythm problems.

If you have low potassium, magnesium or calcium in your blood (ask your doctor if you are not sure).

If you have any disease or illness affecting your liver or have had unexplained jaundice.

If you suffer from any other chronic disease or illness.

If you or your partner have had exposure to a sexually transmitted disease.

If you are unsure about the cause of your symptoms.

Women Only:

If you are pregnant, suspect you might be pregnant or are breast-feeding.

If you have any abnormal or irregular vaginal bleeding or a blood-stained discharge.

If you have vulval or vaginal sores, ulcers or blisters.

If you are experiencing lower abdominal pain or burning on passing urine.

Men Only:

If your sexual partner does <u>not</u> have vaginal thrush

If you have penile sores, ulcers or blisters

If you have an abnormal penile discharge (leakage)

If your penis has started to smell

If you have pain on passing urine.

The product should never be used again if the patient experiences a rash or anaphylaxis follows the use of the drug.

Recurrent use (men and women): Patients should be advised to consult their physician if the symptoms have not been relieved within one week of taking Diflucan One. Diflucan One can be used if the candidal infection returns after 7 days. However, if the candidal infection recurs more than twice within six months, patients should be advised to consult their physician.

4.5 Interaction with other medicinal products and other forms of Interaction

The following drug interactions relate to the use of multiple-dose fluconazole, and the relevance to single-dose Diflucan One has not yet been established. Patients on other medications should consult their doctor or pharmacist before starting fluconazole.

Rifampicin: Concomitant administration of fluconazole and rifampicin resulted in a 25% decrease in the AUC and 20% shorter half-life of fluconazole. In patients receiving concomitant rifampicin, an increase in the fluconazole dose should be considered.

Hydrochlorothiazide: In a kinetic interaction study, co-administration of multiple-dose hydrochlorothiazide to healthy volunteers receiving fluconazole increased plasma concentrations of fluconazole by 40%. An effect of this magnitude should not necessitate a change in the fluconazole dose regimen in subjects receiving concomitant diuretics, although the prescriber should bear it in mind.

Anticoagulants: In an interaction study, fluconazole increased the prothrombin time (12%) after warfarin administration in healthy males. In post-marketing experience, as with other azole antifungals, bleeding events (bruising, epistaxis, gastrointestinal bleeding, haematuria and melaena) have been reported in association with increases in prothrombin time in patients receiving fluconazole concurrently with warfarin. Prothrombin times in patients receiving coumarin-type anticoagulants should be carefully monitored.

Benzodiazepines (short acting)

Following oral administration of midazolam, fluconazole resulted in substantial increases in midazolam concentrations and psychomotor effects. If concomitant benzodiazepine therapy is necessary in patients being treated with fluconazole, consideration should be given to decreasing the benzodiazepine dosage, and the patients should be appropriately monitored.

Sulfonylureas: Fluconazole has been shown to prolong the serum half life of concomitantly administered oral sulfonylureas (chlorpropamide, glibenclamide, glipizide and tolbutamide) in healthy volunteers. Fluconazole and oral sulfonylureas may be co-administered to diabetic patients, but the possibility of a hypoglycaemic episode should be borne in mind.

Phenytoin: Concomitant administration of fluconazole and phenytoin may increase the levels of phenytoin to a clinically significant degree. If it is necessary to administer both drugs concomitantly, phenytoin levels should be monitored and the phenytoin dose adjusted to maintain therapeutic levels.

Oral contraceptives: Three kinetic studies with combined oral contraceptives have been performed using multiple doses of fluconazole. There were no relevant effects on either hormone level in the 50 mg fluconazole study, while at 200 mg daily the AUCs of ethinylestradiol and levonorgestrel were increased 40% and 24% respectively. In a 300 mg once weekly fluconazole study, the AUCs of ethinyl estradiol and norethindrone were increased by 24% and 13%, respectively. Thus single dose use of fluconazole at these doses is unlikely to have an effect on the efficacy of the combined oral contraceptive.

Ciclosporin: A kinetic study in renal transplant patients found fluconazole 200 mg daily to slowly increase ciclosporin concentrations. However, in another multiple dose study with 100 mg daily, fluconazole did not affect ciclosporin levels in patients with bone marrow transplants. Ciclosporin plasma concentration monitoring in patients receiving fluconazole is recommended.

Theophylline: In a placebo-controlled interaction study, the administration of fluconazole 200 mg for 14 days resulted in an 18% decrease in the mean plasma clearance of theophylline. Patients who are receiving high doses of theophylline or who are otherwise at increased risk for theophylline toxicity should be observed for signs of theophylline toxicity while receiving fluconazole, and the therapy modified appropriately if signs of toxicity develop.

Terfenadine: Interaction studies have been performed because of the occurrence of serious dysrhythmias secondary to prolongation of the QTc interval in patients receiving azole antifungals and terfenadine concomitantly. One study at a 200 mg daily dose of fluconazole failed to demonstrate a prolongation in QTc interval. Another study at a 400 mg and 800 mg daily dose of fluconazole demonstrated that fluconazole, taken in doses of 400 mg per day or greater, significantly increased plasma levels of terfenadine when taken concomitantly. There have been spontaneously reported cases of palpitations, tachycardia, dizziness, and chest pain in patients taking concomitant fluconazole and terfenadine where the relationship of the reported adverse events to drug therapy or underlying medical conditions was not clear. Because of the potential seriousness of such an interaction, it is recommended that terfenadine should not be taken in combination with fluconazole. (See section 4.3 Contraindications.)

Cisapride: There have been reports of cardiac events including *torsade de pointes* in patients to whom fluconazole and cisapride were co-administered. A controlled study found that concomitant fluconazole 200 mg once daily and cisapride 20 mg four times a day yielded a significant increase in cisapride plasma levels and prolongation of QTc interval. Co-administration of cisapride is contraindicated in patients receiving fluconazole. (See section 4.3 Contraindications.)

Zidovudine: The AUC of zidovudine can be significantly increased during co-administration with fluconazole. Patients receiving this combination should be monitored for the development of zidovudine-related adverse reactions.

Rifabutin: There have been reports that an interaction exists when fluconazole is administered concomitantly with rifabutin, leading to increased serum levels of rifabutin. There have been reports of uveitis in patients to whom fluconazole and rifabutin were co-administered. Patients receiving rifabutin and fluconazole concomitantly should be carefully monitored.

Tacrolimus: There have been reports that an interaction exists when fluconazole is administered concomitantly with tacrolimus, leading to increased serum levels of tacrolimus. There have been reports of nephrotoxicity in patients to whom fluconazole and tacrolimus were co-administered. Patients receiving tacrolimus and fluconazole concomitantly should be carefully monitored.

The use of fluconazole in patients concurrently taking astemizole or other drugs metabolised by the cytochrome P450 system may be associated with elevations in serum levels of these drugs. In the absence of definitive information, caution should be used when co-administering fluconazole. This is particularly important for drugs that are also known to prolong QT interval. Patients should be carefully monitored.

Interaction studies have shown that when oral fluconazole is co-administered with food, cimetidine, antacids or following total body irradiation for bone marrow transplantation, no clinically significant impairment of fluconazole absorption occurs.

Physicians should be aware that drug-drug interaction studies with other medications have not been conducted, but that such interactions may occur.

4.6 Pregnancy and lactation

Use during pregnancy

There are no adequate and well controlled studies in pregnant women. There have been reports of multiple congenital abnormalities in infants whose mothers were being treated for 3 months with high dose (400-800 mg/day) fluconazole therapy for coccidioidomycosis. The relationship between fluconazole use and these events is unclear (see section 5.3 Preclinical safety data). Accordingly, Diflucan One should not be used in pregnancy, or in women of childbearing potential unless adequate contraception is employed.

Use during lactation

Fluconazole is found in human breast milk at concentrations similar to plasma, hence its use in nursing mothers is not recommended.

4.7 Effects on ability to drive and use machines

Experience with fluconazole indicates that therapy is unlikely to impair a patient's ability to drive or use machinery.

4.8 Undesirable effects

Diflucan One is generally well tolerated.

Nervous System Disorders: Headache, dizziness, seizures, taste perversion

Gastrointestinal Disorders: Abdominal pain, diarrhoea, flatulence, nausea, dyspepsia, vomiting

Hepatobiliary Disorders: Hepatic failure, hepatitis, hepatocellular necrosis, jaundice (see section 4.4 Special warnings and precautions for use).

Skin and Subcutaneous Tissue Disorders: Rash, alopecia, exfoliative skin disorders including Stevens-Johnson syndrome and toxic epidermal necrolysis.

Blood and Lymphatic System Disorders: Leukopenia including neutropenia and agranulocytosis, thrombocytopenia.

Immune System Disorders: Anaphylaxis (including angiooedema, face oedema, pruritus, urticaria).

Metabolism and Nutritional Disorders: Hypercholesterolaemia, hypertriglyceridaemia, hypokalaemia.

Cardiac Disorders: QT prolongation, torsade de pointes (see section 4.4 Special warnings and precautions for use)

4.9 Overdose

There have been reports of overdosage with fluconazole and in one case a 42 year-old patient infected with human immunodeficiency virus developed hallucinations and exhibited paranoid behaviour after reportedly ingesting 8200 mg of fluconazole. The patient was admitted to hospital and his condition resolved within 48 hours.

In the event of overdosage, symptomatic treatment (with supportive measures and gastric lavage if necessary) may be adequate.

As fluconazole is largely excreted in the urine, forced volume diuresis would probably increase the elimination rate. A three hour haemodialysis session decreases plasma levels by approximately 50%.

5. PHARMACOLOGICAL PROPERTIES

5.1 Pharmacodynamic properties

Pharmacotherapeutic Group: Triazole derivatives, ATC code J02AC.

Fluconazole, a member of the triazole class of antifungal agents, is a potent and selective inhibitor of fungal enzymes necessary for the synthesis of ergosterol.

Fluconazole is highly specific for fungal cytochrome P-450 dependent enzymes.

Fluconazole 50 mg daily given for up to 28 days has been shown not to affect testosterone plasma concentrations in males or steroid concentrations in females of child-bearing age. Fluconazole 200-400 mg daily has no clinically significant effect on endogenous steroid levels or on ACTH stimulated response in healthy male volunteers.

There have been reports of cases of superinfection with *Candida* species other than *C. albicans*, which are often inherently not susceptible to fluconazole (e.g. *Candida krusei*). Such cases may require alternative antifungal therapy.

5.2 Pharmacokinetic properties

After oral administration fluconazole is well absorbed, and plasma levels (and systemic bioavailability) are over 90% of the levels achieved after intravenous administration. Oral absorption is not affected by concomitant food intake. Peak plasma concentrations in the fasting state occur between 0.5 and 1.5 hours post dose with a plasma elimination half-life of approximately 30 hours. Plasma concentrations are proportional to dose. The apparent volume of distribution approximates to total body water. Plasma protein binding is low (11-12%).

Fluconazole achieves good penetration in all body fluids studied. The levels of fluconazole in saliva and sputum are similar to plasma levels.

The major route of excretion is renal with approximately 80% of the administered dose appearing in the urine as unchanged drug. Fluconazole clearance is proportional to creatinine clearance. There is no evidence of circulating metabolites.

The long plasma elimination half-life provides the basis for single dose therapy for vaginal candidiasis.

5.3 Preclinical safety data

Reproductive Toxicity

Adverse foetal effects have been seen in animals only at high dose levels associated with maternal toxicity. There were no foetal effects at 5 or 10 mg/kg; increases in foetal anatomical variants (supernumerary ribs, renal pelvis dilation) and delays in ossification were observed at 25 and 50 mg/kg and higher doses. At doses ranging from 80 mg/kg (approximately 20-60 times the recommended human dose) to 320 mg/kg embryolethality in rats was increased and foetal abnormalities included wavy ribs, cleft palate and abnormal cranio-facial ossification. These effects are consistent with the inhibition of estrogen synthesis in rats and may be a result of known effects of lowered estrogen in pregnancy, organogenesis and parturition.

Carcinogenesis

Fluconazole showed no evidence of carcinogenic potential in mice and rats treated orally for 24 months at doses of 2.5, 5 or 10 mg/kg/day (approximately 2-7 times the recommended human dose). Male rats treated with 5 and 10 mg/kg/day had an increased incidence of hepatocellular adenomas.

Mutagenesis

Fluconazole, with or without metabolic activation, was negative in tests for mutagenicity in 4 strains of *S. typhimurium* and in the mouse lymphoma L5178Y system. Cytogenetic studies *in vivo* (murine bone marrow cells, following oral administration of fluconazole) and *in vitro* (human lymphocytes exposed to fluconazole at 1000 μg/ml) showed no evidence of chromosomal mutations.

Impairment of Fertility

Fluconazole did not affect the fertility of male or female rats treated orally with daily doses of 5, 10 or 20 mg/kg or with parenteral doses of 5, 25 or 75 mg/kg, although the onset of parturition was slightly delayed at 20mg/kg orally. In an intravenous perinatal study in rats at 5, 20 and 40 mg/kg, dystocia and prolongation of parturition were observed in a few dams at 20 mg/kg (approximately 5-15 times the recommended human dose) and 40 mg/kg, but not at 5 mg/kg. The disturbances in parturition were reflected by a slight increase in the number of still-born pups and decrease of neonatal survival at these dose levels. The effects on parturition in rats are consistent with the species specific estrogen-lowering property produced by high doses of fluconazole. Such a hormone change has not been observed in women treated with fluconazole (see section 5.1 Pharmacodynamic properties).

6. PHARMACEUTICAL PARTICULARS

6.1 List of excipients

Diflucan One capsules contain lactose, maize starch, colloidal silicon dioxide, magnesium stearate and sodium lauryl sulphate as excipients. The capsule shells contain gelatin and the colours Patent Blue V (E131) and titanium dioxide (E171).

6.2 Incompatibilities

No specific incompatibilities have been noted.

6.3 Shelf life

Current stability data support a shelf life of 5 years.

6.4 Special precautions for storage

Store below 30°C.

6.5 Nature and contents of container

Diflucan One capsules are supplied as a pack containing one capsule in aluminium/PVC laminate blister packs with aluminium foil backing.

6.6 Instructions for use and handling

Diflucan One capsules should be swallowed whole.

Administrative Data

7. MARKETING AUTHORISATION HOLDER

Pfizer Consumer Healthcare,

Walton Oaks,

Dorking Road

Walton-on-the-Hill

Surrey, KT20 7NS

United Kingdom

8. MARKETING AUTHORISATION NUMBER(S)

PL 15513/0099.

9. DATE OF FIRST AUTHORISATION/RENEWAL OF THE AUTHORISATION

17 December 2001

10. DATE OF REVISION OF THE TEXT

17 January 2005

DIGIBIND*

(GlaxoSmithKline UK)

DIGOXIN-SPECIFIC ANTIBODY FRAGMENTS (FAB)

Presentation Each vial of Digibind contains a sterile, lyophilised, crystalline off-white powder, comprising 38 mg of antigen-binding fragments (Fab) derived from specific anti-digoxin antibodies raised in sheep, approximately 75 mg Sorbitol BP and approximately 28 mg Sodium Chloride BP.

Uses Digibind is indicated for the treatment of known or strongly suspected digoxin or digitoxin toxicity, where measures beyond the withdrawal of the digitalis glycoside and correction of any serum electrolyte abnormality are felt to be necessary.

Dosage and administration

Dosage: The dosage of Digibind varies according to the amount of digoxin (or digitoxin) to be neutralised. The average dose used during clinical testing was 10 vials. When determining the dose for Digibind, the following guidelines should be considered:

- Dosage estimates are based on a steady-state volume of distribution of 5 l/kg for digoxin (0.5 l/kg for digitoxin) to convert serum digitalis concentration to the amount of digitalis in the body. These volumes are population averages and vary widely among individuals. Many patients may require higher doses for complete neutralisation. Doses should ordinarily be rounded up to the next whole vial.
- Erroneous calculations may result from inaccurate estimates of the amount of digitalis ingested or absorbed or from non steady-state serum digitalis concentrations. Inaccurate serum digitalis concentration measurements are a possible source of error; this is especially so for very high values, since most digoxin assay kits are not designed to measure values above 5 nanogram/ml.
- If after several hours toxicity has not adequately reversed or appears to recur, re-administration of Digibind at a dose guided by clinical judgement may be required.

Acute ingestion of unknown amount of glycoside: Adults and children over 20 kg: If a patient presents with potentially life-threatening digitalis toxicity after acute ingestion of an unknown amount of digoxin or digitoxin, and neither a serum digoxin concentration nor an estimate of the ingested amount of glycoside is available, 20 vials of Digibind can be administered. This amount will be adequate to treat most life-threatening ingestions in adults and large children.

As an alternative, the physician may consider administering 10 vials of Digibind, observing the patient's response, and following with an additional 10 vials if clinically indicated.

Infants and children ⩽ 20 kg: In infants and small children (⩽ 20 kg) with potentially life- threatening digitalis toxicity after acute ingestion of an unknown amount of digoxin or digitoxin, when neither a serum concentration nor an estimate of the ingested amount is available, clinical judgement must be exercised to estimate an appropriate number of vials of Digibind to administer.

This estimate should be based on the maximum likely total body load of glycoside and the neutralising capacity of Digibind (one vial of Digibind per 0.5 mg of digoxin or digitoxin). It is important to monitor for volume overload during administration of Digibind.

Acute ingestion of known amount of glycoside: Each vial of Digibind contains 38 mg of purified digoxin-specific Fab fragments which will bind approximately 0.5 mg of digoxin or digitoxin. Thus one can calculate the total number of vials required by dividing the total digitalis body load in mg by 0.5 (see formula 1).

Formula 1

$$\text{Dose (in number of vials)} = \frac{\text{Total body load (mg)}}{0.5}$$

For toxicity from an acute ingestion, total body load in milligrams will be approximately equal to the amount ingested in milligrams for digitoxin, or the amount ingested in milligrams multiplied by 0.80 (to account for incomplete absorption) for digoxin. Table 1 gives Digibind doses based on an estimate of the number of digoxin tablets (0.25 mg) ingested as a single dose and is applicable to children or adults.

TABLE 1: Approximate Digibind Dose for Reversal of a Single Large Digoxin Overdose

Number of Digoxin Tablets*	Digibind dose number of vials
25	10
50	20
75	30
100	40
150	60
200	80

* 0.25 mg tablets with 80% bioavailability.

Toxicity during chronic therapy: Adults and children over 20 kg: In adults and children over 20 kg with digitalis toxicity resulting from chronic digoxin or digitoxin therapy and for whom a steady-state serum concentration is not available, a dose of 6 vials of Digibind will usually be adequate to reverse toxicity.

Table 2 gives dosage estimates in number of vials for adult patients for whom a steady-state serum digoxin concentration is known. The Digibind dose (in number of vials) represented in Table 2 can be approximated using the following formula:

(see Formula 2 below)

(see Table 2 below)

In patients for whom a steady-state serum digitoxin concentration is known the Digibind dose (in number of vials) can be approximated using the following formula:

(see Formula 3 below)

Infants and children ⩽ 20kg: In infants and small children with toxicity resulting from chronic digoxin or digitoxin therapy and for whom a steady-state serum concentration is not available, a dose of one vial of Digibind will usually suffice.

Clinical experience in children has indicated that the calculation of dose of Digibind from steady-state serum digoxin concentration may be carried out as for adults.

Table 3 (see next page) gives dosage estimates in milligrams for infants and small children based on the steady-state serum digoxin concentration. The Digibind dose represented in Table 3 can be estimated by multiplying the dose (in number of vials) calculated from Formula 2, by the amount of Digibind contained in a vial (38 mg/vial).

Formula 4

Dose (in mg) = 38 x dose (in number of vials)

(see Table 3 below)

For very small doses, it may be necessary to dilute the reconstituted vial with sterile isotonic saline to achieve a concentration of 1 mg/ml, and to administer the dose with a tuberculin syringe.

Use in the elderly: Clinical experience has indicated that Digibind is effective and that calculation of dose may be carried out as for adults.

Use in renal impairment: See *Precautions.*

Administration: The contents of each vial to be used should be dissolved in 4 ml of sterile Water for Injections BP, by gentle mixing, thus producing an approximately isosmotic solution with a protein concentration of between 8.5 and 10.5mg/ml. This may be diluted further to any convenient volume with sterile saline suitable for infusion.

The final solution of Digibind should be infused intravenously over a 30 minute period. Infusion through a 0.22 micron membrane filter is recommended to remove any incompletely dissolved aggregates of Digibind. If cardiac arrest seems imminent, Digibind can be given as a bolus intravenous injection.

Pharmacology: The affinity constant (K_D) of Fab for digoxin is high ($10^{11} M^{-1}$) and greater than that of digoxin for its receptor (Na-K ATPase). The affinity constant of Fab for digitoxin is also high (fifteen fold lower than for digoxin). Digoxin and digitoxin are therefore attracted away from the receptor on heart tissue (and presumably other tissues as well, though this has not been studied) and their rate of elimination is changed from that governed by the kinetics of receptor binding to that governed by the kinetics of access and elimination of Fab.

In dogs, anti-digoxin Fab reverses arrhythmic manifestations of digoxin toxicity much more quickly than does IgG. There is a suggestion that reversal of inotropy with Fab lags behind reversal of cardiac electrophysiological effects.

The plasma elimination (β) half-life of ovine digoxin-specific Fab in the baboon is 9 to l3h and that of the parent IgG antibody is 61h. The total volume of distribution of Digibind in the baboon appears to be about 9 times greater than that of IgG and more ready diffusion of the smaller moiety sufficiently accounts for this.

About 93% of radioactively labelled Fab, injected into baboons, was recovered in the urine within 24h and the corresponding amount of recoverable digoxin-specific IgG was less than 1%. Much of the urinary Fab was not intact; after glomerular filtration, low molecular weight proteins are taken into proximal renal tubular cells and catabolised.

Corresponding information on human patients is sparse, but the close relationship of therapeutic performance to predictions suggest that the animal data will be helpful. The human plasma elimination half-life after intravenous administration of Digibind is about l6 to 20h with good renal function.

Ordinarily, following administration of Digibind, improvements in signs and symptoms of digitalis intoxication begins within 30 minutes.

Contra-indications, warnings, etc

Contra-indications: None known.

Precautions: Failure to respond to Digibind raises the possibility that the clinical problem is not caused by digitalis intoxication. If there is no response to an adequate dose of Digibind, the diagnosis of digitalis toxicity should be questioned.

Although allergic reactions have been reported rarely, the possibility of anaphylactic, hypersensitive or febrile reactions should be borne in mind. The likelihood of an allergic reaction is distinctly greater where there is a history of allergy to antibiotics or asthma. Since papain is used to cleave the whole antibody into Fab and Fc fragments, and traces of papain or inactivated papain residues may be present in Digibind, patients with known allergies to papain, chymopapain or other papaya extracts would be at particular risk, as would those allergic to ovine proteins. However, as the Fab fragment of the antibody lacks the antigenic determinants of the Fc fragment it should present less of an immunogenic threat to patients than does an intact immunoglobulin molecule.

Many patients with mild or moderate renal dysfunction and some with severe renal dysfunction have been treated successfully with Digibind. There has been no evidence that administration of Digibind to patients with renal dysfunction will exacerbate that dysfunction; the dominant pattern of serial serum creatinine measurements has been one of stable or improved renal function after Digibind administration. The time course and general pattern of therapeutic effect have not been different in patients with severe renal dysfunction, although excretion of the Fab-digoxin complexes from the body is slowed in this situation. A theoretical possibility exists that digoxin could be released after some days from Fab-digoxin complexes which remained in the circulation because their excretion was prevented by renal failure. However, this phenomenon has proved to be rare.

Patients previously dependent on the inotropism of digoxin may develop signs of heart failure when treated with Digibind. After successful management of poisoning, digoxin has had to be reinstituted in some cases. If deemed absolutely necessary, additional inotropic support can be obtained from a non-glycoside inotropic drug such as dopamine or dobutamine, but caution is required as catecholamines and catecholamine analogues can aggravate arrhythmias caused by cardiac glycosides.

Parenteral drug products should be inspected visually for particulate matter and discoloration prior to administration, whenever solution and container permit.

Monitoring and laboratory tests: Patients should have continuous electrocardiographic monitoring during and for at least 24 hours after administration of Digibind.

Presence of the exogenous antibody fragments will interfere with radioimmunoassay measurements of digoxin.

The total serum digoxin concentration may rise precipitously following administration of Digibind, but this will be almost entirely bound to the Fab fragment and therefore not able to react with receptors in the body.

Serum potassium concentrations should be followed carefully, since severe digitalis intoxication can cause life-threatening elevation in serum potassium concentration by shifting it from within the cells. When the effect of digitalis is reversed by Digibind, potassium returns to the cell causing the serum potassium concentrations to fall. It is possible for there to be a total body deficit of potassium in the presence of digitalis toxicity-induced hyperkalaemia and Digibind treatment could result in a significant hypokalaemia.

Side- and adverse effects: Allergic responses of possible or probable attribution to Digibind have been reported rarely. The development of a pruritic rash (either with or without facial flushing and swelling) or shaking or chills without fever, have occurred on the day of treatment. Urticaria and thrombocytopenia have occurred up to 16 days post treatment. There are no reports of any allergic reactions to re-administration of Digibind in the same patient, but there are few instances on which information is available.

Use in pregnancy and lactation: To date there is no evidence that Digibind administered during human pregnancy causes foetal abnormalities; however, the use of Digibind should be considered only if the expected clinical benefit of treatment to the mother outweighs any possible risk to the developing foetus.

Formula 2

$$\text{Dose (in number of vials)} = \frac{\text{serum digoxin concentration in ng/ml} \times \text{weight in kg}}{100}$$

Formula 3

$$\text{Dose (in number of vials)} = \frac{\text{serum digitoxin concentration in ng/ml} \times \text{weight in kg}}{1000}$$

Table 2 Adult Dose Estimate of Digibind (in number of vials) from Steady-State Serum Digoxin Concentration

Patient Weight	Serum Digoxin Concentration (ng/ml)						
(kg)	1	2	4	8	12	16	20
40	0.5v	1v	2v	3v	5v	7v	8v
60	0.5v	1v	3v	5v	7v	10v	12v
70	1v	2v	3v	6v	9v	11v	14v
80	1v	2v	3v	7v	10v	13v	16v
100	1v	2v	4v	8v	12v	16v	20v

v = vials

Table 3 Infants and Small Children Dose Estimates of Digibind (in mg) from Steady-State Serum Digoxin Concentration

Patient	Serum Digoxin Concentration (ng/ml)						
Weight (kg)	1	2	4	8	12	16	20
1	0.4mg*	1mg*	1.5mg*	3mg	5mg	6mg	8mg
3	1mg*	2mg*	5mg	9mg	14mg	18mg	23mg
5	2mg*	4mg	8mg	15mg	23mg	30mg	38mg
10	4mg	8mg	15mg	30mg	46mg	61mg	76mg
20	8mg	15mg	30mg	61mg	91mg	122mg	152mg

* Dilution of reconstituted vial to 1 mg/ml may be desirable.

Carcinogenesis, mutagenesis, impairment of fertility: There have been no long-term studies performed in animals to evaluate carcinogenic or mutagenic potential or effects on fertility.

Drug interactions: No drug interactions have been identified.

Toxicity and treatment of overdosage: Not relevant.

Pharmaceutical precautions Store between 2 & 8°C. Protect from light. After reconstitution store between 2 and 8°C for up to 4 hours.

Reconstituted product should be used promptly. If it is not used immediately, it may be stored under refrigeration between 2 and 8°C for up to 4 hours. The reconstituted product may be diluted with sterile isotonic saline to a convenient volume.

Legal category POM.

Package quantities Single vial of lyophilised powder containing 38 mg of antigen-binding fragments (Fab).

Further information Digoxin-specific antibody Fab fragments have been used successfully to treat a case of lanatoside C intoxication. Reversal of ß-methyl digoxin and ß-acetyl digoxin-induced arrhythmias by Digibind has been verified in guinea-pigs.

Product licence number 00003/0207

Product licence holder

The Wellcome Foundation Limited

Glaxo Wellcome

House Berkeley Avenue

Greenford

Middlesex

UB6 0NN

Trading as GlaxoSmithKline UK, Stockley Park West, Uxbridge, Middlesex UB11 1BT

Date of preparation April 1997.

Digitoxin Tablets BP 100mcg

(Celltech Manufacturing Services Limited)

1. NAME OF THE MEDICINAL PRODUCT
Digitoxin Tablets BP 100 micrograms.

2. QUALITATIVE AND QUANTITATIVE COMPOSITION
Digitoxin BP 0.10 mg.

3. PHARMACEUTICAL FORM
White, biconvex uncoated tablets, engraved EVANS 128 on one side and plain on the obverse.

4. CLINICAL PARTICULARS

4.1 Therapeutic indications
Digitoxin tablets are indicated in the treatment of heart failure and supraventricular arrhythmias particularly atrial fibrillation.

Digitoxin is metabolised in the liver and is therefore preferable to digoxin in patients with impaired renal function.

4.2 Posology and method of administration
Adults and the elderly

Initial dose:

a) Rapid digitalisation (titrated to individual patients needs)

1 to 1.5 mg in divided doses over 24 hours.

b) Slow digitalisation

200 micrograms twice daily for 4 days.

Maintenance dose: 50 to 200 micrograms once a day (usually 10% of loading dose).

Renal Disease

These patients may be maintained at lower serum digitoxin concentrations than other patients.

Children

There is no dosage recommendation in children.

Route of administration:

Oral

4.3 Contraindications
Supraventricular arrhythmias caused by Wolff-Parkinson-White syndrome.

Ventricular fibrillation; ventricular tachycardia, unless congestive failure supervenes after a protracted episode not due to digitalis; presence of digitalis toxicity; Beri Beri, heart disease and some instances of hypersensitive carotid sinus syndrome. There may be cross-sensitivity between different formulations of cardiac glycosides.

4.4 Special warnings and special precautions for use
Digitoxin should be used with caution in patients with abnormalities of thyroid function or impaired hepatic function. Digitoxin should also be used with caution in heart block; complete heart block may be induced if cardiac glycosides are used in partial heart block. Almost any deterioration in the conditions of the heart or circulation may increase the sensitivity to digitoxin.

4.5 Interaction with other medicinal products and other forms of Interaction
Concomitant administration of some drugs may increase serum levels of digitoxin or the risk of toxicity:

There is a risk of increased toxicity with digitoxin if hypokalaemia occurs. This is likely with loop diuretics, thiazides, acetazolamide, carbenoxolone, antifungals and corticosteroids.

NSAIDs may exacerbate heart failure, reduce GFR and increase cardiac glycoside concentrations.

Macrolide antibiotics (such as azithromycin, erythromycin and clarithromycin) may cause digitoxin toxicity.

Quinidine, amiodarone and propafenone appear to increase digitoxin serum levels by reducing its non-renal clearance.

Calcium channel blockers (eg verapamil or diltiazem) may lead to increased digitoxin serum levels.

Beta blockers can cause increased AV block and bradycardia.

Edrophonium and other anticholinesterase drugs (eg neostigmine and pyridostigmine) may cause excessive bradycardia and AV-block in patients on digitalis glycosides.

The use of suxamethonium or pancuronium in digitalised patients may cause arrhythmias.

Intravenous calcium should be avoided in patients on cardiac glycosides as arrhythmias may be precipitated.

Anti-malarial drugs such as quinine, hydroxychloroquine and possibly chloroquine can increase the plasma concentration of digoxin. Mefloquine may increase the risk of bradycardia.

Other drugs may reduce serum levels of digitoxin:

The absorption of digitoxin may be reduced by concomitant administration of cholestyramine and colestipol.

Rifampicin, phenytoin, barbiturates and aminoglutethimide accelerate the metabolism of digitoxin, thus lowering its serum level.

4.6 Pregnancy and lactation
Safety for use in pregnancy and lactation has not been established hence digitoxin should not be given to pregnant or lactating women.

4.7 Effects on ability to drive and use machines
Digitoxin can cause fatigue, dizziness and drowsiness and patients should be advised not to drive or to use machines.

4.8 Undesirable effects
Cardiac glycosides commonly produce side effects because the margin between the therapeutic and toxic doses is small.

The most serious adverse effects are those on the heart. Toxic doses may cause or aggravate heart failure. Atrial or ventricular arrhythmias and defects of conduction are common and may be an early indication of excessive dosage.

In general, the incidence and severity of arrhythmias is related to the severity of the underlying heart disease. Almost any arrhythmia may ensue, but particular note should be made of supraventricular tachycardia, especially atrioventricular (AV) junctional tachycardia and atrial tachycardia and block.

Nausea, vomiting, anorexia, abdominal pain, diarrhoea, headache, fatigue, weakness, dizziness, drowsiness, disorientation, mental confusion, chorea, hypersensitivity reactions (skin desquamation, urticaria, angioneurotic oedema, eosiniphilia and fever), facial pain and rarely delirium. Acute psychoses, bad dreams and hallucinations may also occur.

Disturbances of vision have been reported, as have occasional reports of convulsions, gynaecomastia or thrombocytopenia.

4.9 Overdose
The main effects of overdose are cardiac and consist of arrhythmias (usually ventricular) in combination with heart block. Hyperkalaemia may develop because of Na^+K^+-ATPase inhibition.

Perform gastric lavage or induce emesis immediately following ingestion of a single toxic dose. Oral administration of activated charcoal or an insoluble stero-binding resin such as colestipol or cholestyramine has also been advocated. Monitor ECG continuously and potassium regularly. Specific antidigitoxin antibody fragments may be appropriate.

5. PHARMACOLOGICAL PROPERTIES

5.1 Pharmacodynamic properties
Digitoxin is a cardiac glycoside. Cardiac glycosides have a positive inotropic effect on myocardial cells, increasing the force and velocity of myocardial systolic contraction. In patients with congestive cardiac failure this results in increased cardiac output, more complete systolic emptying and a decreased diastolic heart size. Cardiac glycosides reduce the conductivity of the heart, particularly by reducing conduction through the atrioventricular node. At the cellular level, cardiac glycosides inhibit the activity of the enzyme Na^+K^+-ATPase, thus increasing plasma K^+.

5.2 Pharmacokinetic properties
Digitoxin is well absorbed orally with a bioavailability of more than 90%. Peak plasma concentrations occur 1.5 - 2.5 hours after an oral dose.

Digitoxin is more than 90% bound to plasma protein. Digitoxin is not removed by haemodialysis.

Digitoxin is widely distributed to all body tissues except fat. High concentrations are found in the kidney, liver, skeletal muscle and ventricular myocardium. It is not known if digitoxin is distributed into milk.

Steady-state plasma concentrations of digitoxin range from 10 to 35 nanograms per mL.

Digitoxin is extensively metabolised in the liver and undergoes some enterohepatic recirculation. The intermediate metabolites of digitoxin have pharmacological activity. At steady-state about 25% of a dose is excreted unchanged. The clearance of digitoxin is prolonged in hypothyroid patients and decreased in hyperthyroid patients. The excretion of digitoxin appears unaltered by renal impairment. The plasma half-life of digitoxin averages about 7.5 days.

5.3 Preclinical safety data
Not applicable since Digitoxin Tablets have been used in clinical practice for many years and its effects in man are well known.

6. PHARMACEUTICAL PARTICULARS

6.1 List of excipients
Maize Starch BP

Lactose BP

Magnesium Stearate BP

Purified Water BP

6.2 Incompatibilities
None.

6.3 Shelf life
36 months.

6.4 Special precautions for storage
Store below 25°C.

6.5 Nature and contents of container
Pigmented polypropylene containers fitted with a tamper evident closure of low density polyethylene containing 28 or 250 tablets.

6.6 Instructions for use and handling
No special precautions are required.

Administrative Data

7. MARKETING AUTHORISATION HOLDER
Celltech Manufacturing Services Limited

Vale of Bardsley

Ashton-under-Lyne

Lancashire

OL7 9RR

United Kingdom

8. MARKETING AUTHORISATION NUMBER(S)
18816/0005

9. DATE OF FIRST AUTHORISATION/RENEWAL OF THE AUTHORISATION
18 July 2001

10. DATE OF REVISION OF THE TEXT

Diloxanide Tablets 500mg

(Sovereign Medical)

1. NAME OF THE MEDICINAL PRODUCT
Diloxanide Tablets 500mg

2. QUALITATIVE AND QUANTITATIVE COMPOSITION

Active ingredient	Quantity
Diloxanide Furoate	500 mg

3. PHARMACEUTICAL FORM
A flat, white tablet, scored and with a characteristic engraving E/F on one face.

4. CLINICAL PARTICULARS

4.1 Therapeutic indications
For the treatment of acute and chronic intestinal amoebiasis.

4.2 Posology and method of administration
Adults: One tablet three times daily for ten days.

Children: 20 mg/kg bodyweight daily in divided doses for ten days. Furamide is not suitable for use in children weighing less than 25 kg.

Elderly: There is no need for dosage reduction in the elderly.

If required, a second course of treatment may be prescribed.

4.3 Contraindications
Hypersensitivity to diloxanide furoate.

4.4 Special warnings and special precautions for use
Keep all medicines out of the reach of children.

4.5 Interaction with other medicinal products and other forms of Interaction
No clinically-significant drug interactions known.

4.6 Pregnancy and lactation
The safety of Furamide during pregnancy and lactation has not been established and use during these periods should therefore be avoided.

4.7 Effects on ability to drive and use machines
No adverse effects known.

4.8 Undesirable effects
No serious side effects have been reported and the bacterial flora of the gut is not upset. Flatulence sometimes occurs but may usually be disregarded. Occasionally, vomiting, pruritus and urticaria may occur.

4.9 Overdose
Furamide tablets are unlikely to constitute a hazard in overdosage. In severe overdosage, early gastric lavage is recommended. There is no specific antidote. Treatment should be symptomatic and supportive.

5. PHARMACOLOGICAL PROPERTIES

5.1 Pharmacodynamic properties
Diloxanide furoate is a luminal amoebicide acting principally in the bowel lumen, although its mode of action is not known.

5.2 Pharmacokinetic properties
In the gut, diloxanide furoate is largely, if not wholly, hydrolysed into diloxanide and furoic acid under the combined action of bacterial and gut esterases. After absorption, diloxanide is very rapidly conjugated to form a glucuronide. In circulating blood, it is present to about 99% as a glucuronide and 1% as free diloxanide. Diloxanide is predominantly excreted in the urine. It is believed that the unabsorbed diloxanide is the active anti-amoebic substance, up to 10% remaining in the gut which is subsequently excreted as diloxanide in the faeces.

5.3 Preclinical safety data
Not applicable.

6. PHARMACEUTICAL PARTICULARS

6.1 List of excipients
Maize starch, pregelatinized maize starch, dried maize starch, magnesium stearate, purified water.

6.2 Incompatibilities
None known.

6.3 Shelf life
36 months.

6.4 Special precautions for storage
None.

6.5 Nature and contents of container
A white aluminium tube with a polythene foam disc and a white aluminium screw cap with flowed-in PVC. Pack size: 15 tablets.

A white polythene cylindrical bottle and white polypropylene screw cap fitted with a waxed aluminium-faced pulpboard liner. Pack size: 30 tablets.

A rectangular amber-glass bottle with a white tin-plate screw cap fitted with a waxed aluminium-faced pulpboard liner. Pack size: 250 tablets.

A white polythene cylindrical bottle and white polypropylene screw cap fitted with a waxed aluminium-faced pulpboard liner. Pack size: 250 tablets.

6.6 Instructions for use and handling
Not applicable.

Administrative Data

7. MARKETING AUTHORISATION HOLDER
Waymade PLC
Sovereign House
Miles Gray Road
Basildon, Essex, SS14 3FR
United Kingdom

8. MARKETING AUTHORISATION NUMBER(S)
PL 06464/0900

9. DATE OF FIRST AUTHORISATION/RENEWAL OF THE AUTHORISATION
17 November 1999

10. DATE OF REVISION OF THE TEXT
29 February 2000

Legal Category
POM

Dilzem SR 120mg

(Zeneus Pharma Ltd)

1. NAME OF THE MEDICINAL PRODUCT
Dilzem SR 120mg Prolonged-release Hard Capsules

2. QUALITATIVE AND QUANTITATIVE COMPOSITION
Each Dilzem SR 120mg capsule contains diltiazem hydrochloride 120mg.
For excipients, see 6.1.

3. PHARMACEUTICAL FORM
Prolonged-release capsule, hard.

Buff coloured, hard gelatin capsules, printed with 120mg and containing roughly spherical white to off-white beads.

4. CLINICAL PARTICULARS

4.1 Therapeutic indications
Treatment of angina pectoris including Prinzmetal's angina.

Treatment of mild to moderate hypertension.

4.2 Posology and method of administration
Oral use only.

Adults:

Hypertension: The usual initial dose is 90 mg twice daily (corresponding to 180 mg of diltiazem hydrochloride). Depending upon clinical response the patient's dosage may be increased to 180 mg twice daily if required.

Angina Pectoris: The usual initial dose is 90 mg twice daily (corresponding to 180 mg of diltiazem hydrochloride). Depending upon clinical response the patient's dosage may be increased to 180 mg twice daily if required.

Elderly patients and those with renal or hepatic impairment:

Dosage should commence at the lower level of 60 mg twice daily and be increased slowly. Do not increase the dose if the heart rate falls below 50 beats per minute.

Children:

This product is not recommended for use in children.

4.3 Contraindications
- Use in women of child-bearing potential
- Concomitant administration of dantrolene infusion due to the risk of ventricular fibrillation
- Shock
- Acute cardiac infarct with complications (bradycardia, severe hypotension, left heart insufficiency)
- Bradycardia (pulse rate, at rest, of less than 50 bpm), hypotension (less than 90 mm Hg systole), second or third degree heart block or sick sinus syndrome, except in the presence of a functioning ventricular pacemaker
- Atrial fibrillation/flutter and simultaneous presence of a WPW (Wolff-Parkinson-White) syndrome (increased risk of triggering a ventricular tachycardia)
- Manifest myocardial insufficiency
- Left ventricular failure with stasis
- Hypersensitivity to diltiazem or any of the excipients

4.4 Special warnings and special precautions for use
- Capsules should not be sucked or chewed.
- The use of diltiazem hydrochloride in diabetic patients may require adjustment of their control.
- The product should be used with caution in patients with hepatic dysfunction. Abnormalities of liver function may occur during therapy. Very occasional reports of abnormal liver function have been received, these reactions have been reversible upon discontinuation of therapy.
- First degree AV block or prolonged PR interval. Diltelan prolongs AV node refractory periods without significantly prolonging sinus node recovery time, except in patients with sick sinus syndrome. This effect may rarely result in abnormally slow heart rates (particularly in patients with sick sinus syndrome) or second or third degree AV block (see interactions section for information concerning beta-blockers and digitalis).
- Mild bradycardia.
- Patients with reduced left ventricular function.
- Renally impaired patients.
- Owing to the presence of sucrose, patients with rare hereditary problems of fructose intolerance, glucose-galactose malabsorption or sucrase-isomaltase insufficiency should not take this medicine.

As with any drug given over prolonged periods, laboratory parameters should be monitored at regular intervals.

4.5 Interaction with other medicinal products and other forms of Interaction
Diltiazem undergoes biotransformation by cytochrome P-450 mixed function oxidase. Coadministration with other agents which follow the same route of biotransformation may result in competitive inhibition of metabolism.

Diltiazem hydrochloride should only be administered with great care to patients receiving concurrent treatment with antihypertensives or other hypotensive agents including halogenated anaesthetics or drugs with moderate protein binding.

Diltiazem hydrochloride will not protect against effects of withdrawal of β-adrenoceptor blocking agents, nor the rebound effects seen with various antihypertensives. Combination with β-adrenoceptor blockers having a significant "first pass" loss, e.g. propranolol may require a decrease in their dose and may lead to bradycardia. There may be an additive effect when used with drugs which may induce bradycardia or with other antihypertensives. Concomitant H_2 antagonist therapy may increase diltiazem blood levels.

Diltiazem may affect the blood levels of concomitant carbamazepine, theophylline, ciclosporin and digoxin. Careful attention should therefore be given to signs of overdosage. The levels should be determined and the dose of carbamazepine, theophylline, ciclosporin, or digoxin reduced if necessary. Patients receiving β-blockers, diuretics, ACE inhibitors or other antihypertensive agents should be regularly monitored. Use with alpha blockers should be strictly monitored.

The simultaneous administration of diltiazem with drugs such as β-blockers, antiarrhythmics or heart glycosides may cause a greater degree of AV blocking, reduce the heart rate or induce a hypotensive effect. Intravenous administration of β-blockers should be discontinued during therapy with diltiazem.

Anaesthetists should be warned that a patient is on a calcium antagonist. The depression of cardiac contractility, conductivity, and automaticity as well as the vascular dilation associated with anaesthetics may be potentiated by calcium channel blockers. When used concomitantly, anaesthetics and calcium channel blockers should be titrated carefully.

There have been reports in the literature of diltiazem interactions with warfarin, rifampicin, and lithium.

4.6 Pregnancy and lactation
Diltiazem must not be taken during pregnancy as experimental studies have shown indications of teratogenicity. There is no experience of its effects in humans. As diltiazem is known to enter the breast milk and there is no experience of possible effects in infants, infants should be weaned if treatment of the mother with diltiazem is necessary.

4.7 Effects on ability to drive and use machines
Not applicable.

4.8 Undesirable effects
In studies carried out to date, serious adverse reactions with diltiazem have been rare; however, it should be recognised that patients with impaired ventricular function and cardiac conduction abnormalities have usually been excluded from these studies.

In 900 patients with hypertension, the most common adverse events were oedema (9%), headache (8%), dizziness (6%), asthenia (5%), sinus bradycardia (3%), flushing (3%), and first degree AV block (3%). Only oedema and perhaps bradycardia were dose related. The most common adverse events (>1%) observed in clinical studies of over 2100 angina and hypertensive patients receiving diltiazem were: oedema (5.4%), headache (4.5%), dizziness (3.4%), asthenia (2.8%), first-degree AV block (1.8%), flushing (1.7%), nausea (1.6%), bradycardia (1.5%) and rash (1.5%).

Less common adverse events have included the following:

Cardiovascular: angina, arrhythmia, AV block (second or third degree), congestive heart failure, hypotension, palpitations, syncope.

Nervous system: amnesia, depression, gait abnormality, hallucinations, insomnia, nervousness, paraesthesia, personality change, somnolence, tinnitus, tremor.

Gastrointestinal: anorexia, constipation, diarrhoea, dyspepsia, mild elevations of alkaline phosphatase, SGOT, SGPT and LDH (see Special Warnings and Precautions), vomiting, weight increase, gingivitis.

Dermatologic: petechiae, pruritus, photosensitivity, urticaria. Allergic skin reactions including erythema multiforme, vasculitis, lymphadenopathy and eosinophilia have been observed in isolated cases. Dermatological events may be transient and may disappear despite continued use of diltiazem. Should a dermatologic reaction persist, the drug should be discontinued.

Other: amblyopia, CK elevation, dyspnoea, epistaxis, eye irritation, hyperglycaemia, nasal congestion, nocturia, osteoarticular pain, polyuria, sexual difficulties.

4.9 Overdose
Experience of overdosage in man is limited but cases of spontaneous recovery have been reported. However, it is recommended that patients with suspected overdose should be placed under observation in a coronary care unit with facilities available for treatment of any possible hypotension and conduction disturbances that may occur. Most patients suffering from overdosage of diltiazem become hypotensive within 8 hours of ingestion. With bradycardia and first to third degree atrioventricular block also developing cardiac arrest may ensue. Hyperglycaemia is also a recognised complication. The elimination half-life of diltiazem after overdosage is estimated to be about 5.5 - 10.2 hours. If a patient presents early after overdose, gastric lavage should be performed and activated charcoal administered to reduce diltiazem absorption.

Hypotension should be corrected with plasma expanders, intravenous calcium gluconate and inotropic agents (dopamine, dobutamine or isoprenaline). Symptomatic bradycardia and high grade AV block may respond to atropine, isoprenaline or occasionally cardiac pacing which may be useful if cardiac standstill occurs.

5. PHARMACOLOGICAL PROPERTIES

5.1 Pharmacodynamic properties
Diltiazem has pharmacologic actions similar to those of other calcium channel blocking agents such as nifedipine or verapamil. The principal physiologic action of diltiazem is to inhibit the transmembrane influx of extracellular

calcium ions across the membranes of myocardial cells and vascular smooth muscle cells.

Calcium plays important roles in the excitation-contraction coupling processes of the heart and vascular smooth muscle cells and in the electrical discharge of the specialised conduction cells of the heart. The membranes of these cells contain numerous channels that carry a slow inward current and that are selective for calcium.

By inhibiting calcium influx, diltiazem inhibits the contractile processes of cardiac and vascular smooth muscle, thereby dilating the main coronary and systemic arteries. Dilation of systemic arteries by diltiazem results in a decrease in total peripheral resistance, a decrease in systemic blood pressure and a decrease in the afterload of the heart. The reduction in afterload, seen at rest and with exercise, and its resultant decrease in myocardial oxygen consumption are thought to be responsible for the beneficial effects of diltiazem in patients with chronic stable angina pectoris. In patients with prinzmetal variant angina, inhibition of spontaneous and ergonovine-induced coronary artery spasm by diltiazem results in increased myocardial oxygen delivery.

5.2 Pharmacokinetic properties

a) General Characteristics

Absorption: Capsules seem to have a similar bioavailability to tablets (30-40%), with peak concentrations for the prolonged release product after 8-11 hours compared with 1-2 hours after the conventional release product. The relatively low bioavailability is due to first pass metabolism in the liver to an active metabolite.

Distribution: Diltiazem hydrochloride is lipophilic and has a high volume of distribution. Typical study results are in the range of 3-8 litres/kg. Protein binding is about 80% and is not concentration-dependent at levels likely to be found clinically. Protein binding does not appear to be influenced by phenylbutazone, warfarin, propranolol, salicylic acid or digoxin.

Metabolism: Diltiazem hydrochloride is extensively metabolised in the liver. N-monodesmethyl diltiazem is the predominant metabolite followed quantitatively by the desacetyl metabolite, which has some pharmacological activity. The efficacy of the metabolites, desacetyl diltiazem and N-monodesmethyl diltiazem is 25-50% and about 20% respectively of that of diltiazem. In liver function disorders delayed metabolism in the liver is likely. These metabolites are converted to conjugates, generally the glucuronide or the sulphate.

Elimination: Diltiazem is excreted in the form of its metabolites (about 35%) and in the non-metabolised form (about 2-4%) via the kidneys while about 60% is excreted via the faeces. The average elimination half life period for diltiazem is 6-8 hours but may vary between 2 and 11 hours. Although the elimination half life is not changed after repeated oral administration, diltiazem and also the desacetyl metabolite show a slight accumulation in the plasma.

b) Characteristics in Patients

Decreased first-pass metabolism in the elderly tends to result in increased plasma concentrations of calcium antagonists but no major changes have been found with diltiazem. Renal impairment did not cause significant changes in diltiazem pharmacokinetics. Plasma concentrations of diltiazem also tend to be higher in hepatic cirrhosis due to impaired oxidative metabolism.

5.3 Preclinical safety data

Chronic toxicity studies in rats revealed no remarkable changes at oral doses up to 125 mg/kg/day although there was a 60% mortality at this dose. In dogs chronically treated with oral doses of 20 mg/kg/day, transient rises in SGPT were observed. Embryotoxicity has been reported in mice, rats and rabbits following i.p. administration of diltiazem. Main types of malformations included limb and tail defects with a small number of vertebral and rib deformities also noted.

6. PHARMACEUTICAL PARTICULARS

6.1 List of excipients

Fumaric acid

Talc

Povidone

Sugar spheres (containing sucrose and maize starch)

Ammonio methacrylate copolymer Type B

Ammonio methacrylate copolymer Type A

The capsule shell contains:

Yellow iron oxide (E172)

Erythrosine (E127)

Titanium dioxide (E171)

Gelatin

The printing ink contains:

Shellac

Soya lecithin

Black iron oxide (E172)

Dimethylpolysiloxane

6.2 Incompatibilities

Not applicable.

6.3 Shelf life

Three years from date of manufacture for all presentations.

6.4 Special precautions for storage

Do not store above 25°C. Store in the original package

6.5 Nature and contents of container

Securitainer containing 30 or 100 capsules.

Clear PVC blister pack containing 60 capsules.

Opaque PVC/PVDC blister pack containing 56 or 60 capsules.

6.6 Instructions for use and handling

Not applicable.

7. MARKETING AUTHORISATION HOLDER

Elan Pharma Limited,

Monksland,

Athlone,

Co. Westmeath,

Ireland

Trading as:

Elan Pharma,

Abel Smith House,

Gunnels Wood Road,

Stevenage,

Hertfordshire SG1 2FG

8. MARKETING AUTHORISATION NUMBER(S)

PL 10038/0026

9. DATE OF FIRST AUTHORISATION/RENEWAL OF THE AUTHORISATION

30 April 1998

10. DATE OF REVISION OF THE TEXT

December 2003

11. LEGAL CATEGORY

POM

Dilzem SR 60mg

(Zeneus Pharma Ltd)

1. NAME OF THE MEDICINAL PRODUCT

Dilzem SR 60mg Prolonged-release Hard Capsules

2. QUALITATIVE AND QUANTITATIVE COMPOSITION

Each Dilzem SR 60mg capsule contains diltiazem hydrochloride 60mg.

For excipients, see 6.1.

3. PHARMACEUTICAL FORM

Prolonged-release capsule, hard.

Buff coloured, hard gelatin capsules, printed with 60mg and containing roughly spherical white to off-white beads.

4. CLINICAL PARTICULARS

4.1 Therapeutic indications

Treatment of angina pectoris including Prinzmetal's angina.

Treatment of mild to moderate hypertension.

4.2 Posology and method of administration

Oral use only.

Adults:

Hypertension: The usual initial dose is 90mg twice daily (corresponding to 180mg of diltiazem hydrochloride). Depending upon clinical response the patient's dosage may be increased to 180mg twice daily if required.

Angina Pectoris: The usual initial dose is 90mg twice daily (corresponding to 180mg of diltiazem hydrochloride). Depending upon clinical response the patient's dosage may be increased to 180mg twice daily if required.

Elderly patients and those with renal or hepatic impairment:

Dosage should commence at the lower level of 60mg twice daily and be increased slowly. Do not increase the dose if the heart rate falls below 50 beats per minute.

Children:

This product is not recommended for use in children.

4.3 Contraindications

- Use in women of child-bearing potential
- Concomitant administration of dantrolene infusion due to the risk of ventricular fibrillation
- Shock
- Acute cardiac infarct with complications (bradycardia, severe hypotension, left heart insufficiency)
- Bradycardia (pulse rate, at rest, of less than 50 bpm), hypotension (less than 90 mm Hg systole), second or third degree heart block or sick sinus syndrome, except in the presence of a functioning ventricular pacemaker
- Atrial fibrillation/flutter and simultaneous presence of a WPW (Wolff-Parkinson-White) syndrome (increased risk of triggering a ventricular tachycardia)
- Manifest myocardial insufficiency
- Left ventricular failure with stasis
- Hypersensitivity to diltiazem or any of the excipients

4.4 Special warnings and special precautions for use

- Capsules should not be sucked or chewed.
- The use of diltiazem hydrochloride in diabetic patients may require adjustment of their control.
- The product should be used with caution in patients with hepatic dysfunction. Abnormalities of liver function may occur during therapy. Very occasional reports of abnormal liver function have been received, these reactions have been reversible upon discontinuation of therapy.
- First degree AV block or prolonged PR interval. Diltelan prolongs AV node refractory periods without significantly prolonging sinus node recovery time, except in patients with sick sinus syndrome. This effect may rarely result in abnormally slow heart rates (particularly in patients with sick sinus syndrome) or second or third degree AV block (see interactions section for information concerning beta-blockers and digitalis).
- Mild bradycardia.
- Patients with reduced left ventricular function.
- Renally impaired patients.
- Owing to the presence of sucrose, patients with rare hereditary problems of fructose intolerance, glucose-galactose malabsorption or sucrase-isomaltase insufficiency should not take this medicine.

As with any drug given over prolonged periods, laboratory parameters should be monitored at regular intervals.

4.5 Interaction with other medicinal products and other forms of Interaction

Diltiazem undergoes biotransformation by cytochrome P-450 mixed function oxidase. Coadministration with other agents which follow the same route of biotransformation may result in competitive inhibition of metabolism.

Diltiazem hydrochloride should only be administered with great care to patients receiving concurrent treatment with antihypertensives or other hypotensive agents including halogenated anaesthetics or drugs with moderate protein binding.

Diltiazem hydrochloride will not protect against effects of withdrawal of β-adrenoceptor blocking agents, nor the rebound effects seen with various antihypertensives. Combination with β-adrenoceptor blockers having a significant "first pass" loss, e.g. propranolol may require a decrease in their dose and may lead to bradycardia. There may be an additive effect when used with drugs which may induce bradycardia or with other antihypertensives. Concomitant H_2 antagonist therapy may increase diltiazem blood levels. Diltiazem may affect the blood levels of concomitant carbamazepine, theophylline, ciclosporin and digoxin. Careful attention should therefore be given to signs of overdosage. The levels should be determined and the dose of carbamazepine, theophylline, ciclosporin, or digoxin reduced if necessary. Patients receiving β-blockers, diuretics, ACE inhibitors or other antihypertensive agents should be regularly monitored. Use with alpha blockers should be strictly monitored.

The simultaneous administration of diltiazem with drugs such as β-blockers, antiarrhythmics or heart glycosides may cause a greater degree of AV blocking, reduce the heart rate or induce a hypotensive effect. Intravenous administration of β-blockers should be discontinued during therapy with diltiazem.

Anaesthetists should be warned that a patient is on a calcium antagonist. The depression of cardiac contractility, conductivity, and automaticity as well as the vascular dilation associated with anaesthetics may be potentiated by calcium channel blockers. When used concomitantly, anaesthetics and calcium channel blockers should be titrated carefully.

There have been reports in the literature of diltiazem interactions with warfarin, rifampicin, and lithium.

4.6 Pregnancy and lactation

Diltiazem must not be taken during pregnancy as experimental studies have shown indications of teratogenicity. There is no experience of its effects in humans. As diltiazem is known to enter the breast milk and there is no experience of possible effects in infants, infants should be weaned if treatment of the mother with diltiazem is necessary.

4.7 Effects on ability to drive and use machines

Not applicable.

4.8 Undesirable effects

In studies carried out to date, serious adverse reactions with diltiazem have been rare; however, it should be recognised that patients with impaired ventricular function and cardiac conduction abnormalities have usually been excluded from these studies.

In 900 patients with hypertension, the most common adverse events were oedema (9%), headache (8%), dizziness (6%), asthenia (5%), sinus bradycardia (3%), flushing (3%), and first degree AV block (3%). Only oedema and perhaps bradycardia were dose related. The most common adverse events (> 1%) observed in clinical studies of over 2100 angina and hypertensive patients receiving diltiazem were: oedema (5.4%), headache (4.5%), dizziness (3.4%), asthenia (2.8%), first-degree AV block (1.8%), flushing (1,7%), nausea (1.6%), bradycardia (1.5%) and rash (1.5%).

Less common adverse events have included the following:

Cardiovascular: angina, arrhythmia, AV block (second or third degree), congestive heart failure, hypotension, palpitations, syncope.

Nervous system: amnesia, depression, gait abnormality, hallucinations, insomnia, nervousness, paraesthesia, personality change, somnolence, tinnitus, tremor.

Gastrointestinal: anorexia, constipation, diarrhoea, dyspepsia, mild elevations of alkaline phosphatase, SGOT, SGPT and LDH (see Special Warnings and Precautions), vomiting, weight increase, gingivitis.

Dermatologic: petechiae, pruritus, photosensitivity, urticaria. Allergic skin reactions including erythema multiforme, vasculitis, lymphadenopathy and eosinophilia have been observed in isolated cases. Dermatological events may be transient and may disappear despite continued use of diltiazem. Should a dermatologic reaction persist, the drug should be discontinued.

Other: amblyopia, CK elevation, dyspnoea, epistaxis, eye irritation, hyperglycaemia, nasal congestion, nocturia, osteoarticular pain, polyuria, sexual difficulties.

4.9 Overdose

Experience of overdosage in man is limited but cases of spontaneous recovery have been reported. However, it is recommended that patients with suspected overdose should be placed under observation in a coronary care unit with facilities available for treatment of any possible hypotension and conduction disturbances that may occur. Most patients suffering from overdosage of diltiazem become hypotensive within 8 hours of ingestion. With bradycardia and first to third degree atrioventricular block also developing cardiac arrest may ensue. Hyperglycaemia is also a recognised complication. The elimination half-life of diltiazem after overdosage is estimated to be about 5.5 - 10.2 hours. If a patient presents early after overdose, gastric lavage should be performed and activated charcoal administered to reduce diltiazem absorption.

Hypotension should be corrected with plasma expanders, intravenous calcium gluconate and inotropic agents (dopamine, dobutamine or isoprenaline). Symptomatic bradycardia and high grade AV block may respond to atropine, isoprenaline or occasionally cardiac pacing which may be useful if cardiac standstill occurs.

5. PHARMACOLOGICAL PROPERTIES

5.1 Pharmacodynamic properties

Diltiazem has pharmacologic actions similar to those of other calcium channel blocking agents such as nifedipine or verapamil. The principal physiologic action of diltiazem is to inhibit the transmembrane influx of extracellular calcium ions across the membranes of myocardial cells and vascular smooth muscle cells.

Calcium plays important roles in the excitation-contraction coupling processes of the heart and vascular smooth muscle cells and in the electrical discharge of the specialised conduction cells of the heart. The membranes of these cells contain numerous channels that carry a slow inward current and that are selective for calcium.

By inhibiting calcium influx, diltiazem inhibits the contractile processes of cardiac and vascular smooth muscle, thereby dilating the main coronary and systemic arteries. Dilation of systemic arteries by diltiazem results in a decrease in total peripheral resistance, a decrease in systemic blood pressure and a decrease in the afterload of the heart. The reduction in afterload, seen at rest and with exercise, and its resultant decrease in myocardial oxygen consumption are thought to be responsible for the beneficial effects of diltiazem in patients with chronic stable angina pectoris. In patients with prinzmetal variant angina, inhibition of spontaneous and ergonovine-induced coronary artery spasm by diltiazem results in increased myocardial oxygen delivery.

5.2 Pharmacokinetic properties

a) General Characteristics

Absorption: Capsules seem to have a similar bioavailability to tablets (30-40%), with peak concentrations for the prolonged release product after 8-11 hours compared with 1-2 hours after the conventional release product. The relatively low bioavailability is due to first pass metabolism in the liver to an active metabolite.

Distribution: Diltiazem hydrochloride is lipophilic and has a high volume of distribution. Typical study results are in the range of 3-8 litres/kg. Protein binding is about 80% and is not concentration-dependent at levels likely to be found clinically. Protein binding does not appear to be influenced by phenylbutazone, warfarin, propranolol, salicylic acid or digoxin.

Metabolism: Diltiazem hydrochloride is extensively metabolised in the liver. N-monodesmethyl diltiazem is the predominant metabolite followed quantitatively by the desacetyl metabolite, which has some pharmacological activity. The efficacy of the metabolites, desacetyl diltiazem and N-monodesmethyl diltiazem is 25-50% and about 20% respectively of that of diltiazem. In liver function disorders delayed metabolism in the liver is likely. These metabolites are converted to conjugates, generally the glucuronide or the sulphate.

Elimination: Diltiazem is excreted in the form of its metabolites (about 35%) and in the non-metabolised form (about 2-4%) via the kidneys while about 60% is excreted via the faeces. The average elimination half life period for diltiazem is 6-8 hours but may vary between 2 and 11 hours. Although the elimination half life is not changed after repeated oral administration, diltiazem and also the desacetyl metabolite show a slight accumulation in the plasma.

b) Characteristics in Patients

Decreased first-pass metabolism in the elderly tends to result in increased plasma concentrations of calcium antagonists but no major changes have been found with diltiazem. Renal impairment did not cause significant changes in diltiazem pharmacokinetics. Plasma concentrations of diltiazem also tend to be higher in hepatic cirrhosis due to impaired oxidative metabolism.

5.3 Preclinical safety data

Chronic toxicity studies in rats revealed no remarkable changes at oral doses up to 125 mg/kg/day although there was a 60% mortality at this dose. In dogs chronically treated with oral doses of 20 mg/kg/day, transient rises in SGPT were observed. Embryotoxicity has been reported in mice, rats and rabbits following i.p. administration of diltiazem. Main types of malformations included limb and tail defects with a small number of vertebral and rib deformities also noted.

6. PHARMACEUTICAL PARTICULARS

6.1 List of excipients

Fumaric acid

Talc

Povidone

Sugar spheres (containing sucrose and maize starch)

Ammonio methacrylate copolymer Type B

Ammonio methacrylate copolymer Type A

The capsule shell contains:

Yellow iron oxide (E172)

Erythrosine (E127)

Titanium dioxide (E171)

Gelatin

The printing ink contains:

Shellac

Soya lecithin

Black iron oxide (E172)

Dimethylpolysiloxane

6.2 Incompatibilities

Not applicable.

6.3 Shelf life

Three years from date of manufacture for all presentations.

6.4 Special precautions for storage

Do not store above 25°C. Store in the original package.

6.5 Nature and contents of container

Securitainer containing 30 or 100 capsules.

Clear PVC blister pack containing 100 capsules.

Opaque PVC/PVDC blister pack containing 56 or 100 capsules.

6.6 Instructions for use and handling

Not applicable.

7. MARKETING AUTHORISATION HOLDER

Elan Pharma Limited

Monksland

Athlone

Co. Westmeath

Ireland

Trading as:

Elan Pharma

Abel Smith House

Gunnels Wood Road

Stevenage

Hertfordshire SG1 2FG

8. MARKETING AUTHORISATION NUMBER(S)

PL 10038/0024

9. DATE OF FIRST AUTHORISATION/RENEWAL OF THE AUTHORISATION

30 April 1998

10. DATE OF REVISION OF THE TEXT

December 2003

11. LEGAL CATEGORY

POM

Dilzem SR 90mg

(Zeneus Pharma Ltd)

1. NAME OF THE MEDICINAL PRODUCT

Dilzem SR 90mg Prolonged-release Hard Capsules

2. QUALITATIVE AND QUANTITATIVE COMPOSITION

Each Dilzem SR 90mg capsule contains diltiazem hydrochloride 90mg.

For excipients, see 6.1.

3. PHARMACEUTICAL FORM

Prolonged-release capsule, hard.

Buff coloured, hard gelatin capsules, printed with 90mg and containing roughly spherical white to off-white beads.

4. CLINICAL PARTICULARS

4.1 Therapeutic indications

Treatment of angina pectoris including Prinzmetal's angina.

Treatment of mild to moderate hypertension.

4.2 Posology and method of administration

Oral use only.

Adults:

Hypertension: The usual initial dose is 90 mg twice daily (corresponding to 180 mg of diltiazem hydrochloride). Depending upon clinical response the patient's dosage may be increased to 180 mg twice daily if required.

Angina Pectoris: The usual initial dose is 90 mg twice daily (corresponding to 180 mg of diltiazem hydrochloride). Depending upon clinical response the patient's dosage may be increased to 180 mg twice daily if required.

Elderly patients and those with renal or hepatic impairment:

Dosage should commence at the lower level of 60 mg twice daily and be increased slowly. Do not increase the dose if the heart rate falls below 50 beats per minute.

Children:

This product is not recommended for use in children.

4.3 Contraindications

- Use in women of child-bearing potential
- Concomitant administration of dantrolene infusion due to the risk of ventricular fibrillation
- Shock
- Acute cardiac infarct with complications (bradycardia, severe hypotension, left heart insufficiency)
- Bradycardia (pulse rate, at rest, of less than 50 bpm), hypotension (less than 90 mm Hg systole), second or third degree heart block or sick sinus syndrome, except in the presence of a functioning ventricular pacemaker
- Atrial fibrillation/flutter and simultaneous presence of a WPW (Wolff-Parkinson-White) syndrome (increased risk of triggering a ventricular tachycardia)
- Manifest myocardial insufficiency
- Left ventricular failure with stasis
- Hypersensitivity to diltiazem or any of the excipients

4.4 Special warnings and special precautions for use

- Capsules should not be sucked or chewed.
- The use of diltiazem hydrochloride in diabetic patients may require adjustment of their control.
- The product should be used with caution in patients with hepatic dysfunction. Abnormalities of liver function may occur during therapy. Very occasional reports of abnormal liver function have been received, these reactions have been reversible upon discontinuation of therapy.
- First degree AV block or prolonged PR interval. Diltelan prolongs AV node refractory periods without significantly prolonging sinus node recovery time, except in patients with sick sinus syndrome. This effect may rarely result in abnormally slow heart rates (particularly in patients with sick sinus syndrome) or second or third degree AV block (see interactions section for information concerning beta-blockers and digitalis).
- Mild bradycardia.
- Patients with reduced left ventricular function.
- Renally impaired patients.
- Owing to the presence of sucrose, patients with rare hereditary problems of fructose intolerance, glucose-galactose malabsorption or sucrase-isomaltase insufficiency should not take this medicine.

As with any drug given over prolonged periods, laboratory parameters should be monitored at regular intervals.

4.5 Interaction with other medicinal products and other forms of Interaction

Diltiazem undergoes biotransformation by cytochrome P-450 mixed function oxidase. Coadministration with other agents which follow the same route of biotransformation may result in competitive inhibition of metabolism.

Diltiazem hydrochloride should only be administered with great care to patients receiving concurrent treatment with antihypertensives or other hypotensive agents including halogenated anaesthetics or drugs with moderate protein binding.

Diltiazem hydrochloride will not protect against effects of withdrawal of β-adrenoceptor blocking agents, nor the rebound effects seen with various antihypertensives. Combination with β-adrenoceptor blockers having a significant "first pass" loss, e.g. propranolol may require a decrease in their dose and may lead to bradycardia. There may be an additive effect when used with drugs which may induce bradycardia or with other antihypertensives. Concomitant H_2 antagonist therapy may increase diltiazem blood levels.

Diltiazem may affect the blood levels of concomitant carbamazepine, theophylline, ciclosporin and digoxin. Careful attention should therefore be given to signs of overdosage. The levels should be determined and the dose of carbamazepine, theophylline, ciclosporin, or digoxin reduced if necessary. Patients receiving β-blockers, diuretics, ACE inhibitors or other antihypertensive agents should be regularly monitored. Use with alpha blockers should be strictly monitored.

The simultaneous administration of diltiazem with drugs such as β-blockers, antiarrhythmics or heart glycosides may cause a greater degree of AV blocking, reduce the heart rate or induce a hypotensive effect. Intravenous administration of β-blockers should be discontinued during therapy with diltiazem.

Anaesthetists should be warned that a patient is on a calcium antagonist. The depression of cardiac contractility, conductivity, and automaticity as well as the vascular dilation associated with anaesthetics may be potentiated by calcium channel blockers. When used concomitantly, anaesthetics and calcium channel blockers should be titrated carefully.

There have been reports in the literature of diltiazem interactions with warfarin, rifampicin, and lithium.

4.6 Pregnancy and lactation

Diltiazem must not be taken during pregnancy as experimental studies have shown indications of teratogenicity. There is no experience of its effects in humans. As diltiazem is known to enter the breast milk and there is no experience of possible effects in infants, infants should be weaned if treatment of the mother with diltiazem is necessary.

4.7 Effects on ability to drive and use machines

Not applicable.

4.8 Undesirable effects

In studies carried out to date, serious adverse reactions with diltiazem have been rare; however, it should be recognised that patients with impaired ventricular function and cardiac conduction abnormalities have usually been excluded from these studies.

In 900 patients with hypertension, the most common adverse events were oedema (9%), headache (8%), dizziness (6%), asthenia (5%), sinus bradycardia (3%), flushing (3%), and first degree AV block (3%). Only oedema and perhaps bradycardia were dose related. The most common adverse events (>1%) observed in clinical studies of over 2100 angina and hypertensive patients receiving diltiazem were: oedema (5.4%), headache (4.5%), dizziness (3.4%), asthenia (2.8%), first-degree AV block (1.8%), flushing (1.7%), nausea (1.6%), bradycardia (1.5%) and rash (1.5%).

Less common adverse events have included the following:

Cardiovascular: angina, arrhythmia, AV block (second or third degree), congestive heart failure, hypotension, palpitations, syncope.

Nervous system: amnesia, depression, gait abnormality, hallucinations, insomnia, nervousness, paraesthesia, personality change, somnolence, tinnitus, tremor.

Gastrointestinal: anorexia, constipation, diarrhoea, dyspepsia, mild elevations of alkaline phosphatase, SGOT, SGPT and LDH (see Special Warnings and Precautions), vomiting, weight increase, gingivitis.

Dermatologic: petechiae, pruritus, photosensitivity, urticaria. Allergic skin reactions including erythema multiforme, vasculitis, lymphadenopathy and eosinophilia have been observed in isolated cases. Dermatological events may be transient and may disappear despite continued use of diltiazem. Should a dermatologic reaction persist, the drug should be discontinued.

Other: amblyopia, CK elevation, dyspnoea, epistaxis, eye irritation, hyperglycaemia, nasal congestion, nocturia, osteoarticular pain, polyuria, sexual difficulties.

4.9 Overdose

Experience of overdosage in man is limited but cases of spontaneous recovery have been reported. However, it is recommended that patients with suspected overdose should be placed under observation in a coronary care unit with facilities available for treatment of any possible hypotension and conduction disturbances that may occur. Most patients suffering from overdosage of diltiazem become hypotensive within 8 hours of ingestion. With bradycardia and first to third degree atrioventricular block also developing cardiac arrest may ensue. Hyperglycaemia is also a recognised complication. The elimination half-life of diltiazem after overdosage is estimated to be about 5.5 - 10.2 hours. If a patient presents early after overdose, gastric lavage should be performed and activated charcoal administered to reduce diltiazem absorption.

Hypotension should be corrected with plasma expanders, intravenous calcium gluconate and inotropic agents (dopamine, dobutamine or isoprenaline). Symptomatic bradycardia and high grade AV block may respond to atropine, isoprenaline or occasionally cardiac pacing which may be useful if cardiac standstill occurs.

5. PHARMACOLOGICAL PROPERTIES

5.1 Pharmacodynamic properties

Diltiazem has pharmacologic actions similar to those of other calcium channel blocking agents such as nifedipine or verapamil. The principal physiologic action of diltiazem is to inhibit the transmembrane influx of extracellular calcium ions across the membranes of myocardial cells and vascular smooth muscle cells.

Calcium plays important roles in the excitation-contraction coupling processes of the heart and vascular smooth muscle cells and in the electrical discharge of the specialised conduction cells of the heart. The membranes of these cells contain numerous channels that carry a slow inward current and that are selective for calcium.

By inhibiting calcium influx, diltiazem inhibits the contractile processes of cardiac and vascular smooth muscle, thereby dilating the main coronary and systemic arteries. Dilation of systemic arteries by diltiazem results in a decrease in total peripheral resistance, a decrease in systemic blood pressure and a decrease in the afterload of the heart. The reduction in afterload, seen at rest and with exercise, and its resultant decrease in myocardial oxygen consumption are thought to be responsible for the beneficial effects of diltiazem in patients with chronic stable angina pectoris. In patients with prinzmetal variant angina, inhibition of spontaneous and ergonovine-induced coronary artery spasm by diltiazem results in increased myocardial oxygen delivery.

5.2 Pharmacokinetic properties

a) General Characteristics

Absorption: Capsules seem to have a similar bioavailability to tablets (30-40%), with peak concentrations for the prolonged release product after 8-11 hours compared with 1-2 hours after the conventional release product. The relatively low bioavailability is due to first pass metabolism in the liver to an active metabolite.

Distribution: Diltiazem hydrochloride is lipophilic and has a high volume of distribution. Typical study results are in the range of 3-8 litres/kg. Protein binding is about 80% and is not concentration-dependent at levels likely to be found clinically. Protein binding does not appear to be influenced by phenylbutazone, warfarin, propranolol, salicylic acid or digoxin.

Metabolism: Diltiazem hydrochloride is extensively metabolised in the liver. N-monodesmethyl diltiazem is the predominant metabolite followed quantitatively by the desacetyl metabolite, which has some pharmacological activity. The efficacy of the metabolites, desacetyl diltiazem and N-monodesmethyl diltiazem is 25-50% and about 20% respectively of that of diltiazem. In liver function disorders delayed metabolism in the liver is likely. These metabolites are converted to conjugates, generally the glucuronide or the sulphate.

Elimination: Diltiazem is excreted in the form of its metabolites (about 35%) and in the non-metabolised form (about 2-4%) via the kidneys while about 60% is excreted via the faeces. The average elimination half life period for diltiazem is 6-8 hours but may vary between 2 and 11 hours. Although the elimination half life is not changed after repeated oral administration, diltiazem and also the desacetyl metabolite show a slight accumulation in the plasma.

b) Characteristics in Patients

Decreased first-pass metabolism in the elderly tends to result in increased plasma concentrations of calcium antagonists but no major changes have been found with diltiazem. Renal impairment did not cause significant changes in diltiazem pharmacokinetics. Plasma concentrations of diltiazem also tend to be higher in hepatic cirrhosis due to impaired oxidative metabolism.

5.3 Preclinical safety data

Chronic toxicity studies in rats revealed no remarkable changes at oral doses up to 125 mg/kg/day although there was a 60% mortality at this dose. In dogs chronically treated with oral doses of 20 mg/kg/day, transient rises in SGPT were observed. Embryotoxicity has been reported in mice, rats and rabbits following i.p. administration of diltiazem. Main types of malformations included limb and tail defects with a small number of vertebral and rib deformities also noted.

6. PHARMACEUTICAL PARTICULARS

6.1 List of excipients

Fumaric acid

Talc

Povidone

Sugar spheres (containing sucrose and maize starch)

Ammonio methacrylate copolymer Type B

Ammonio methacrylate copolymer Type A

The capsule shell contains:

Yellow iron oxide (E172)

Erythrosine (E127)

Titanium dioxide (E171)

Gelatin

The printing ink contains:

Shellac

Soya lecithin

Black iron oxide (E172)

Dimethylpolysiloxane

6.2 Incompatibilities

Not applicable.

6.3 Shelf life

Three years from date of manufacture for all presentations.

6.4 Special precautions for storage

Do not store above 25°C. Store in the original package.

6.5 Nature and contents of container

Securitainer containing 30 or 100 capsules.

Clear PVC blister pack containing 4 or 60 capsules.

Opaque PVC/PVDC blister pack containing 56 or 60 capsules.

6.6 Instructions for use and handling

Not applicable.

7. MARKETING AUTHORISATION HOLDER

Elan Pharma Limited

Monksland

Athlone

Co. Westmeath

Ireland

Trading as:

Elan Pharma

Abel Smith House

Gunnels Wood Road

Stevenage

Hertfordshire SG1 2FG

8. MARKETING AUTHORISATION NUMBER(S)

PL 10038/0025

9. DATE OF FIRST AUTHORISATION/RENEWAL OF THE AUTHORISATION

30 April 1998

10. DATE OF REVISION OF THE TEXT

December 2003

11. LEGAL CATEGORY

POM

Dilzem XL 120mg

(Zeneus Pharma Ltd)

1. NAME OF THE MEDICINAL PRODUCT

Dilzem XL 120mg Prolonged-release Hard Capsules

2. QUALITATIVE AND QUANTITATIVE COMPOSITION

Each Dilzem XL 120mg capsule contains diltiazem hydrochloride 120mg.

For excipients, see 6.1.

3. PHARMACEUTICAL FORM

Prolonged-release capsule, hard.

White, hard gelatin capsules, printed with e120 and containing roughly spherical white to off-white beads.

4. CLINICAL PARTICULARS

4.1 Therapeutic indications

Prophylaxis and treatment of angina pectoris.

Treatment of mild to moderate hypertension.

4.2 Posology and method of administration

Oral use only.

Adults:

Hypertension: The usual initial dose is one 180mg capsule per day (corresponding to 180mg of diltiazem hydrochloride once daily). Depending upon the clinical response the dosage may be increased stepwise to 360mg/day if required.

Angina Pectoris: The usual initial dose is one 180mg capsule per day (corresponding to 180mg of diltiazem hydrochloride once daily). Depending upon the clinical response the dosage may be increased stepwise to 360mg/day if required.

Elderly patients and those with renal or hepatic impairment:

Dosage should commence at the lower level of 120mg once daily and be increased slowly. Do not increase the dose if the heart rate falls below 50 beats per minute.

Children:

This product is not recommended for use in children.

4.3 Contraindications

- Use in women of child-bearing potential
- Concomitant administration of dantrolene infusion due to the risk of ventricular fibrillation
- Shock
- Acute cardiac infarct with complications (bradycardia, severe hypotension, left heart insufficiency)
- Bradycardia (pulse rate, at rest, of less than 50 bpm), hypotension (less than 90 mm Hg systole), second or third degree heart block or sick sinus syndrome, except in the presence of a functioning ventricular pacemaker
- Atrial fibrillation/flutter and simultaneous presence of a WPW (Wolff-Parkinson-White) syndrome (increased risk of triggering a ventricular tachycardia)
- Manifest myocardial insufficiency
- Left ventricular failure with stasis
- Hypersensitivity to diltiazem or any of the excipients

4.4 Special warnings and special precautions for use

- Capsules should not be sucked or chewed.
- The use of diltiazem hydrochloride in diabetic patients may require adjustment of their control.
- The product should be used with caution in patients with hepatic dysfunction. Abnormalities of liver function may occur during therapy. Very occasional reports of abnormal liver function have been received, these reactions have been reversible upon discontinuation of therapy.
- First degree AV block or prolonged PR interval. Diltelan prolongs AV node refractory periods without significantly prolonging sinus node recovery time, except in patients with sick sinus syndrome. This effect may rarely result in abnormally slow heart rates (particularly in patients with sick sinus syndrome) or second or third degree AV block (see interactions section for information concerning beta-blockers and digitalis).
- Mild bradycardia.
- Patients with reduced left ventricular function.
- Renally impaired patients.
- Owing to the presence of sucrose, patients with rare hereditary problems of fructose intolerance, glucose-galactose malabsorption or sucrase-isomaltase insufficiency should not take this medicine.

As with any drug given over prolonged periods, laboratory parameters should be monitored at regular intervals.

4.5 Interaction with other medicinal products and other forms of Interaction

Diltiazem undergoes biotransformation by cytochrome P-450 mixed function oxidase. Coadministration with other agents which follow the same route of biotransformation may result in competitive inhibition of metabolism.

Diltiazem hydrochloride should only be administered with great care to patients receiving concurrent treatment with antihypertensives or other hypotensive agents including halogenated anaesthetics or drugs with moderate protein binding.

Diltiazem hydrochloride will not protect against effects of withdrawal of β-adrenoceptor blocking agents, nor the rebound effects seen with various antihypertensives. Combination with β-adrenoceptor blockers having a significant "first pass" loss, e.g. propranolol may require a decrease in their dose and may lead to bradycardia. There may be an additive effect when used with drugs which may induce bradycardia or with other antihypertensives. Concomitant H_2 antagonist therapy may increase diltiazem blood levels.

Diltiazem may affect the blood levels of concomitant carbamazepine, theophylline, ciclosporin and digoxin. Careful attention should therefore be given to signs of overdosage. The levels should be determined and the dose of carbamazepine, theophylline, ciclosporin, or digoxin reduced if necessary. Patients receiving β-blockers, diuretics, ACE inhibitors or other antihypertensive agents should be regularly monitored. Use with alpha blockers should be strictly monitored.

The simultaneous administration of diltiazem with drugs such as β-blockers, antiarrhythmics or heart glycosides may cause a greater degree of AV blocking, reduce the heart rate or induce a hypotensive effect. Intravenous administration of β-blockers should be discontinued during therapy with diltiazem.

Anaesthetists should be warned that a patient is on a calcium antagonist. The depression of cardiac contractility, conductivity, and automaticity as well as the vascular dilation associated with anaesthetics may be potentiated by calcium channel blockers. When used concomitantly, anaesthetics and calcium channel blockers should be titrated carefully.

There have been reports in the literature of diltiazem interactions with warfarin, rifampicin, and lithium.

4.6 Pregnancy and lactation

Diltiazem must not be taken during pregnancy as experimental studies have shown indications of teratogenicity. There is no experience of its effects in humans. As diltiazem is known to enter the breast milk and there is no experience of possible effects in infants, infants should be weaned if treatment of the mother with diltiazem is necessary.

4.7 Effects on ability to drive and use machines

Not applicable.

4.8 Undesirable effects

In studies carried out to date, serious adverse reactions with diltiazem have been rare; however, it should be recognised that patients with impaired ventricular function and cardiac conduction abnormalities have usually been excluded from these studies.

In 900 patients with hypertension, the most common adverse events were oedema (9%), headache (8%), dizziness (6%), asthenia (5%), sinus bradycardia (3%), flushing (3%), and first degree AV block (3%). Only oedema and perhaps bradycardia were dose related. The most common adverse events (>1%) observed in clinical studies of over 2100 angina and hypertensive patients receiving diltiazem were: oedema (5.4%), headache (4.5%), dizziness (3.4%), asthenia (2.8%), first-degree AV block (1.8%), flushing (1.7%), nausea (1.6%), bradycardia (1.5%) and rash (1.5%).

Less common adverse events have included the following:

Cardiovascular: angina, arrhythmia, AV block (second or third degree), congestive heart failure, hypotension, palpitations, syncope.

Nervous system: amnesia, depression, gait abnormality, hallucinations, insomnia, nervousness, paraesthesia, personality change, somnolence, tinnitus, tremor.

Gastrointestinal: anorexia, constipation, diarrhoea, dyspepsia, mild elevations of alkaline phosphatase, SGOT, SGPT and LDH (see Special Warnings and Precautions), vomiting, weight increase, gingivitis.

Dermatologic: petechiae, pruritus, photosensitivity, urticaria. Allergic skin reactions including erythema multiforme, vasculitis, lymphadenopathy and eosinophilia have been observed in isolated cases. Dermatological events may be transient and may disappear despite continued use of diltiazem. Should a dermatologic reaction persist, the drug should be discontinued.

Other: amblyopia, CK elevation, dyspnoea, epistaxis, eye irritation, hyperglycaemia, nasal congestion, nocturia, osteoarticular pain, polyuria, sexual difficulties.

4.9 Overdose

Experience of overdosage in man is limited but cases of spontaneous recovery have been reported. However, it is recommended that patients with suspected overdose should be placed under observation in a coronary care unit with facilities available for treatment of any possible hypotension and conduction disturbances that may occur. Most patients suffering from overdosage of diltiazem become hypotensive within 8 hours of ingestion. With bradycardia and first to third degree atrioventricular block also developing cardiac arrest may ensue. Hyperglycaemia is also a recognised complication. The elimination half-life of diltiazem after overdosage is estimated to be about 5.5 - 10.2 hours. If a patient presents early after overdose, gastric lavage should be performed and activated charcoal administered to reduce diltiazem absorption.

Hypotension should be corrected with plasma expanders, intravenous calcium gluconate and inotropic agents (dopamine, dobutamine or isoprenaline). Symptomatic bradycardia and high grade AV block may respond to atropine, isoprenaline or occasionally cardiac pacing which may be useful if cardiac standstill occurs.

5. PHARMACOLOGICAL PROPERTIES

5.1 Pharmacodynamic properties

Diltiazem has pharmacologic actions similar to those of other calcium channel blocking agents such as nifedipine or verapamil. The principal physiologic action of diltiazem is to inhibit the transmembrane influx of extracellular calcium ions across the membranes of myocardial cells and vascular smooth muscle cells.

Calcium plays important roles in the excitation-contraction coupling processes of the heart and vascular smooth muscle cells and in the electrical discharge of the specialised conduction cells of the heart. The membranes of these cells contain numerous channels that carry a slow inward current and that are selective for calcium.

By inhibiting calcium influx, diltiazem inhibits the contractile processes of cardiac and vascular smooth muscle, thereby dilating the main coronary and systemic arteries. Dilation of systemic arteries by diltiazem results in a decrease in total peripheral resistance, a decrease in systemic blood pressure and a decrease in the afterload of the heart. The reduction in afterload, seen at rest and with exercise, and its resultant decrease in myocardial oxygen consumption are thought to be responsible for the beneficial effects of diltiazem in patients with chronic stable angina pectoris. In patients with prinzmetal variant angina, inhibition of spontaneous and ergonovine-induced coronary artery spasm by diltiazem results in increased myocardial oxygen delivery.

5.2 Pharmacokinetic properties

a) General Characteristics

Absorption: Capsules seem to have a similar bioavailability to tablets (30-40%), with peak concentrations for the prolonged release product after 8-11 hours compared with 1-2 hours after the conventional release product. The relatively low bioavailability is due to first pass metabolism in the liver to an active metabolite.

Distribution: Diltiazem hydrochloride is lipophilic and has a high volume of distribution. Typical study results are in the range of 3-8 litres/kg. Protein binding is about 80% and is not concentration-dependent at levels likely to be found clinically. Protein binding does not appear to be influenced by phenylbutazone, warfarin, propranolol, salicylic acid or digoxin.

Metabolism: Diltiazem hydrochloride is extensively metabolised in the liver. N-monodesmethyl diltiazem is the predominant metabolite followed quantitatively by the desacetyl metabolite, which has some pharmacological activity. The efficacy of the metabolites, desacetyl diltiazem and N-monodesmethyl diltiazem is 25-50% and about 20% respectively of that of diltiazem. In liver function disorders delayed metabolism in the liver is likely. These metabolites are converted to conjugates, generally the glucuronide or the sulphate.

Elimination: Diltiazem is excreted in the form of its metabolites (about 35%) and in the non-metabolised form (about 2-4%) via the kidneys while about 60% is excreted via the faeces. The average elimination half life period for diltiazem is 6-8 hours but may vary between 2 and 11 hours. Although the elimination half life is not changed after repeated oral administration, diltiazem and also the desacetyl metabolite show a slight accumulation in the plasma.

b) Characteristics in Patients

Decreased first-pass metabolism in the elderly tends to result in increased plasma concentrations of calcium antagonists but no major changes have been found with diltiazem. Renal impairment did not cause significant changes in diltiazem pharmacokinetics. Plasma concentrations of diltiazem also tend to be higher in hepatic cirrhosis due to impaired oxidative metabolism.

5.3 Preclinical safety data

Chronic toxicity studies in rats revealed no remarkable changes at oral doses up to 125 mg/kg/day although there was a 60% mortality at this dose. In dogs chronically treated with oral doses of 20 mg/kg/day, transient rises in SGPT were observed. Embryotoxicity has been reported in mice, rats and rabbits following i.p. administration of diltiazem. Main types of malformations included limb and tail defects with a small number of vertebral and rib deformities also noted.

6. PHARMACEUTICAL PARTICULARS

6.1 List of excipients

Fumaric acid

Talc

Povidone

Sugar spheres (containing sucrose and maize starch)

Ammonio methacrylate copolymer Type B

Ammonio methacrylate copolymer Type A

The capsule shell contains:

Gelatin

Titanium dioxide (E171)

The printing ink contains:

Shellac

Soya lecithin

Black iron oxide (E172)

Dimethylpolysiloxane

6.2 Incompatibilities

Not applicable.

6.3 Shelf life

Two years from the date of manufacture.

6.4 Special precautions for storage

Do not store above 25°C. Store in the original package.

6.5 Nature and contents of container

Jaysquare container, containing 7, 20, 30, 50, 60 or 100 capsules.

PVC/PVDC blister pack, containing 4, 28 or 30 capsules.

6.6 Instructions for use and handling

Not applicable.

7. MARKETING AUTHORISATION HOLDER

Elan Pharma Limited

Monksland

Athlone

Co. Westmeath

Ireland

Trading as:

Elan Pharma

Abel Smith House

Gunnels Wood Road

Stevenage

Hertfordshire SG1 2FG

8. MARKETING AUTHORISATION NUMBER(S)

PL 10038/0027

9. DATE OF FIRST AUTHORISATION/RENEWAL OF THE AUTHORISATION

30 April 1998

10. DATE OF REVISION OF THE TEXT

December 2003

11. LEGAL CATEGORY

POM

Dilzem XL 180mg

(Zeneus Pharma Ltd)

1. NAME OF THE MEDICINAL PRODUCT

Dilzem XL 180mg Prolonged-release Hard Capsules

2. QUALITATIVE AND QUANTITATIVE COMPOSITION

Each Dilzem XL 180mg capsule contains diltiazem hydrochloride 180mg.

For excipients, see 6.1.

3. PHARMACEUTICAL FORM

Prolonged-release capsule, hard.

White, hard gelatin capsules, printed with e180 and containing roughly spherical white to off-white beads.

4. CLINICAL PARTICULARS

4.1 Therapeutic indications

Prophylaxis and treatment of angina pectoris.

Treatment of mild to moderate hypertension.

4.2 Posology and method of administration

Oral use only.

Adults:

Hypertension: The usual initial dose is one 180mg capsule per day (corresponding to 180mg of diltiazem hydrochloride once daily). Depending upon the clinical response the dosage may be increased stepwise to 360mg/day if required.

Angina Pectoris: The usual initial dose is one 180mg capsule per day (corresponding to 180mg of diltiazem hydrochloride once daily). Depending upon the clinical response the dosage may be increased stepwise to 360mg/day if required.

Elderly patients and those with renal or hepatic impairment:

Dosage should commence at the lower level of 120mg once daily and be increased slowly. Do not increase the dose if the heart rate falls below 50 beats per minute.

Children:

This product is not recommended for use in children.

4.3 Contraindications

- Use in women of child-bearing potential
- Concomitant administration of dantrolene infusion due to the risk of ventricular fibrillation
- Shock
- Acute cardiac infarct with complications (bradycardia, severe hypotension, left heart insufficiency)
- Bradycardia (pulse rate, at rest, of less than 50 bpm), hypotension (less than 90 mm Hg systole), second or third degree heart block or sick sinus syndrome, except in the presence of a functioning ventricular pacemaker
- Atrial fibrillation/flutter and simultaneous presence of a WPW (Wolff-Parkinson-White) syndrome (increased risk of triggering a ventricular tachycardia)
- Manifest myocardial insufficiency
- Left ventricular failure with stasis
- Hypersensitivity to diltiazem or any of the excipients

4.4 Special warnings and special precautions for use

- Capsules should not be sucked or chewed.
- The use of diltiazem hydrochloride in diabetic patients may require adjustment of their control.
- The product should be used with caution in patients with hepatic dysfunction. Abnormalities of liver function may occur during therapy. Very occasional reports of abnormal liver function have been received, these reactions have been reversible upon discontinuation of therapy.
- First degree AV block or prolonged PR interval. Diltelan prolongs AV node refractory periods without significantly prolonging sinus node recovery time, except in patients with sick sinus syndrome. This effect may rarely result in abnormally slow heart rates (particularly in patients with sick sinus syndrome) or second or third degree AV block (see interactions section for information concerning beta-blockers and digitalis).
- Mild bradycardia.
- Patients with reduced left ventricular function.
- Renally impaired patients.
- Owing to the presence of sucrose, patients with rare hereditary problems of fructose intolerance, glucose-galactose malabsorption or sucrase-isomaltase insufficiency should not take this medicine.

As with any drug given over prolonged periods, laboratory parameters should be monitored at regular intervals.

4.5 Interaction with other medicinal products and other forms of Interaction

Diltiazem undergoes biotransformation by cytochrome P-450 mixed function oxidase. Coadministration with other agents which follow the same route of biotransformation may result in competitive inhibition of metabolism.

Diltiazem hydrochloride should only be administered with great care to patients receiving concurrent treatment with antihypertensives or other hypotensive agents including halogenated anaesthetics or drugs with moderate protein binding.

Diltiazem hydrochloride will not protect against effects of withdrawal of β-adrenoceptor blocking agents, nor the rebound effects seen with various antihypertensives. Combination with β-adrenoceptor blockers having a significant "first pass" loss, e.g. propranolol may require a decrease in their dose and may lead to bradycardia. There may be an additive effect when used with drugs which may induce bradycardia or with other antihypertensives. Concomitant H_2 antagonist therapy may increase diltiazem blood levels.

Diltiazem may affect the blood levels of concomitant carbamazepine, theophylline, ciclosporin and digoxin. Careful attention should therefore be given to signs of overdosage. The levels should be determined and the dose of carbamazepine, theophylline, ciclosporin, or digoxin reduced if necessary. Patients receiving β-blockers, diuretics, ACE inhibitors or other antihypertensive agents should be regularly monitored. Use with alpha blockers should be strictly monitored.

The simultaneous administration of diltiazem with drugs such as β-blockers, antiarrhythmics or heart glycosides may cause a greater degree of AV blocking, reduce the heart rate or induce a hypotensive effect. Intravenous administration of β-blockers should be discontinued during therapy with diltiazem.

Anaesthetists should be warned that a patient is on a calcium antagonist. The depression of cardiac contractility, conductivity, and automaticity as well as the vascular dilation associated with anaesthetics may be potentiated by calcium channel blockers. When used concomitantly, anaesthetics and calcium channel blockers should be titrated carefully.

There have been reports in the literature of diltiazem interactions with warfarin, rifampicin, and lithium.

4.6 Pregnancy and lactation

Diltiazem must not be taken during pregnancy as experimental studies have shown indications of teratogenicity. There is no experience of its effects in humans. As diltiazem is known to enter the breast milk and there is no experience of possible effects in infants, infants should be weaned if treatment of the mother with diltiazem is necessary.

4.7 Effects on ability to drive and use machines

Not applicable.

4.8 Undesirable effects

In studies carried out to date, serious adverse reactions with diltiazem have been rare; however, it should be recognised that patients with impaired ventricular function and cardiac conduction abnormalities have usually been excluded from these studies.

In 900 patients with hypertension, the most common adverse events were oedema (9%), headache (8%), dizziness (6%), asthenia (5%), sinus bradycardia (3%), flushing (3%), and first degree AV block (3%). Only oedema and perhaps bradycardia were dose related. The most common adverse events (>1%) observed in clinical studies of over 2100 angina and hypertensive patients receiving diltiazem were: oedema (5.4%), headache (4.5%), dizziness (3.4%), asthenia (2.8%), first-degree AV block (1.8%), flushing (1.7%), nausea (1.6%), bradycardia (1.5%) and rash (1.5%).

Less common adverse events have included the following:

Cardiovascular: angina, arrhythmia, AV block (second or third degree), congestive heart failure, hypotension, palpitations, syncope.

Nervous system: amnesia, depression, gait abnormality, hallucinations, insomnia, nervousness, paraesthesia, personality change, somnolence, tinnitus, tremor.

Gastrointestinal: anorexia, constipation, diarrhoea, dyspepsia, mild elevations of alkaline phosphatase, SGOT, SGPT and LDH (see Special Warnings and Precautions), vomiting, weight increase, gingivitis.

Dermatologic: petechiae, pruritus, photosensitivity, urticaria. Allergic skin reactions including erythema multiforme, vasculitis, lymphadenopathy and eosinophilia have been observed in isolated cases. Dermatological events may be transient and may disappear despite continued use of diltiazem. Should a dermatologic reaction persist, the drug should be discontinued.

Other: amblyopia, CK elevation, dyspnoea, epistaxis, eye irritation, hyperglycaemia, nasal congestion, nocturia, osteoarticular pain, polyuria, sexual difficulties.

4.9 Overdose

Experience of overdosage in man is limited but cases of spontaneous recovery have been reported. However, it is recommended that patients with suspected overdose should be placed under observation in a coronary care unit with facilities available for treatment of any possible hypotension and conduction disturbances that may occur. Most patients suffering from overdosage of diltiazem become hypotensive within 8 hours of ingestion. With bradycardia and first to third degree atrioventricular block also developing cardiac arrest may ensue. Hyperglycaemia is also a recognised complication. The elimination half-life of diltiazem after overdosage is estimated to be about 5.5 - 10.2 hours. If a patient presents early after overdose, gastric lavage should be performed and activated charcoal administered to reduce diltiazem absorption.

Hypotension should be corrected with plasma expanders, intravenous calcium gluconate and inotropic agents (dopamine, dobutamine or isoprenaline). Symptomatic bradycardia and high grade AV block may respond to atropine, isoprenaline or occasionally cardiac pacing which may be useful if cardiac standstill occurs.

5. PHARMACOLOGICAL PROPERTIES

5.1 Pharmacodynamic properties

Diltiazem has pharmacologic actions similar to those of other calcium channel blocking agents such as nifedipine or verapamil. The principal physiologic action of diltiazem is to inhibit the transmembrane influx of extracellular calcium ions across the membranes of myocardial cells and vascular smooth muscle cells.

Calcium plays important roles in the excitation-contraction coupling processes of the heart and vascular smooth muscle cells and in the electrical discharge of the specialised conduction cells of the heart. The membranes of these cells contain numerous channels that carry a slow inward current and that are selective for calcium.

By inhibiting calcium influx, diltiazem inhibits the contractile processes of cardiac and vascular smooth muscle, thereby dilating the main coronary and systemic arteries. Dilation of systemic arteries by diltiazem results in a decrease in total peripheral resistance, a decrease in systemic blood pressure and a decrease in the afterload of the heart. The reduction in afterload, seen at rest and with exercise, and its resultant decrease in myocardial oxygen consumption are thought to be responsible for the beneficial effects of diltiazem in patients with chronic stable angina pectoris. In patients with prinzmetal variant angina, inhibition of spontaneous and ergonovine-induced coronary artery spasm by diltiazem results in increased myocardial oxygen delivery.

5.2 Pharmacokinetic properties

a) General Characteristics

Absorption: Capsules seem to have a similar bioavailability to tablets (30-40%), with peak concentrations for the prolonged release product after 8-11 hours compared with 1-2 hours after the conventional release product. The relatively low bioavailability is due to first pass metabolism in the liver to an active metabolite.

Distribution: Diltiazem hydrochloride is lipophilic and has a high volume of distribution. Typical study results are in the range of 3-8 litres/kg. Protein binding is about 80% and is not concentration-dependent at levels likely to be found clinically. Protein binding does not appear to be influenced by phenylbutazone, warfarin, propranolol, salicylic acid or digoxin.

Metabolism: Diltiazem hydrochloride is extensively metabolised in the liver. N-monodesmethyl diltiazem is the predominant metabolite followed quantitatively by the desacetyl metabolite, which has some pharmacological activity. The efficacy of the metabolites, desacetyl diltiazem and N-monodesmethyl diltiazem is 25-50% and about 20% respectively of that of diltiazem. In liver function disorders delayed metabolism in the liver is likely. These metabolites are converted to conjugates, generally the glucuronide or the sulphate.

Elimination: Diltiazem is excreted in the form of its metabolites (about 35%) and in the non-metabolised form (about 2-4%) via the kidneys while about 60% is excreted via the faeces. The average elimination half life period for diltiazem is 6-8 hours but may vary between 2 and 11 hours. Although the elimination half life is not changed after repeated oral administration, diltiazem and also the desacetyl metabolite show a slight accumulation in the plasma.

b) Characteristics in Patients

Decreased first-pass metabolism in the elderly tends to result in increased plasma concentrations of calcium antagonists but no major changes have been found with diltiazem. Renal impairment did not cause significant changes in diltiazem pharmacokinetics. Plasma concentrations of diltiazem also tend to be higher in hepatic cirrhosis due to impaired oxidative metabolism.

5.3 Preclinical safety data

Chronic toxicity studies in rats revealed no remarkable changes at oral doses up to 125 mg/kg/day although there was a 60% mortality at this dose. In dogs chronically treated with oral doses of 20mg/kg/day, transient rises in SGPT were observed. Embryotoxicity has been reported in mice, rats and rabbits following i.p. administration of diltiazem. Main types of malformations included limb and tail defects with a small number of vertebral and rib deformities also noted.

6. PHARMACEUTICAL PARTICULARS

6.1 List of excipients

Fumaric acid

Talc

Povidone

Sugar spheres (containing sucrose and maize starch)

Ammonio methacrylate copolymer Type B

Ammonio methacrylate copolymer Type A

The capsule shell contains:

Gelatin

Titanium dioxide (E171)

The printing ink contains:

Shellac

Soya lecithin

Black iron oxide (E172)

Dimethylpolysiloxane

6.2 Incompatibilities

Not applicable.

6.3 Shelf life

Two years from the date of manufacture.

6.4 Special precautions for storage

Do not store above 25°C. Store in the original package.

6.5 Nature and contents of container
Jaysquare container, containing 7, 20, 30, 50, 60 or 100 capsules.

PVC/PVDC blister pack, containing 4, 28 or 30 capsules.

6.6 Instructions for use and handling
Not applicable.

7. MARKETING AUTHORISATION HOLDER
Elan Pharma Limited
Monksland
Athlone
Co. Westmeath
Ireland
Trading as:
Elan Pharma
Abel Smith House
Gunnels Wood Road
Stevenage
Hertfordshire SG1 2FG

8. MARKETING AUTHORISATION NUMBER(S)
PL 10038/0028

9. DATE OF FIRST AUTHORISATION/RENEWAL OF THE AUTHORISATION
30 April 1998

10. DATE OF REVISION OF THE TEXT
December 2003

11. LEGAL CATEGORY
POM

Dilzem XL 240mg

(Zeneus Pharma Ltd)

1. NAME OF THE MEDICINAL PRODUCT
Dilzem XL 240mg Prolonged-release Hard Capsules

2. QUALITATIVE AND QUANTITATIVE COMPOSITION
Each Dilzem XL 240mg capsule contains diltiazem hydrochloride 240mg.

For excipients, see 6.1.

3. PHARMACEUTICAL FORM
Prolonged-release capsule, hard.

White, hard gelatin capsules, printed with e240 and containing roughly spherical white to off-white beads.

4. CLINICAL PARTICULARS

4.1 Therapeutic indications
Prophylaxis and treatment of angina pectoris.

Treatment of mild to moderate hypertension.

4.2 Posology and method of administration
Oral use only.

Adults:

Hypertension: The usual initial dose is one 180mg capsule per day (corresponding to 180mg of diltiazem hydrochloride once daily). Depending upon the clinical response the dosage may be increased stepwise to 360mg/day if required.

Angina Pectoris: The usual initial dose is one 180mg capsule per day (corresponding to 180mg of diltiazem hydrochloride once daily). Depending upon the clinical response the dosage may be increased stepwise to 360mg/day if required.

Elderly patients and those with renal or hepatic impairment:

Dosage should commence at the lower level of 120mg once daily and be increased slowly. Do not increase the dose if the heart rate falls below 50 beats per minute.

Children:

This product is not recommended for use in children.

4.3 Contraindications
- Use in women of child-bearing potential
- Concomitant administration of dantrolene infusion due to the risk of ventricular fibrillation
- Shock
- Acute cardiac infarct with complications (bradycardia, severe hypotension, left heart insufficiency)
- Bradycardia (pulse rate, at rest, of less than 50 bpm), hypotension (less than 90 mm Hg systole), second or third degree heart block or sick sinus syndrome, except in the presence of a functioning ventricular pacemaker
- Atrial fibrillation/flutter and simultaneous presence of a WPW (Wolff-Parkinson-White) syndrome (increased risk of triggering a ventricular tachycardia)
- Manifest myocardial insufficiency
- Left ventricular failure with stasis
- Hypersensitivity to diltiazem or any of the excipients

4.4 Special warnings and special precautions for use
- Capsules should not be sucked or chewed.
- The use of diltiazem hydrochloride in diabetic patients may require adjustment of their control.
- The product should be used with caution in patients with hepatic dysfunction. Abnormalities of liver function may occur during therapy. Very occasional reports of abnormal liver function have been received, these reactions have been reversible upon discontinuation of therapy.
- First degree AV block or prolonged PR interval. Diltelan prolongs AV node refractory periods without significantly prolonging sinus node recovery time, except in patients with sick sinus syndrome. This effect may rarely result in abnormally slow heart rates (particularly in patients with sick sinus syndrome) or second or third degree AV block (see interactions section for information concerning beta-blockers and digitalis).
- Mild bradycardia.
- Patients with reduced left ventricular function.
- Renally impaired patients.
- Owing to the presence of sucrose, patients with rare hereditary problems of fructose intolerance, glucose-galactose malabsorption or sucrase-isomaltase insufficiency should not take this medicine.

As with any drug given over prolonged periods, laboratory parameters should be monitored at regular intervals.

4.5 Interaction with other medicinal products and other forms of Interaction
Diltiazem undergoes biotransformation by cytochrome P-450 mixed function oxidase. Coadministration with other agents which follow the same route of biotransformation may result in competitive inhibition of metabolism.

Diltiazem hydrochloride should only be administered with great care to patients receiving concurrent treatment with antihypertensives or other hypotensive agents including halogenated anaesthetics or drugs with moderate protein binding.

Diltiazem hydrochloride will not protect against effects of withdrawal of β-adrenoceptor blocking agents, nor the rebound effects seen with various antihypertensives. Combination with β-adrenoceptor blockers having a significant "first pass" loss, e.g. propranolol may require a decrease in their dose and may lead to bradycardia. There may be an additive effect when used with drugs which may induce bradycardia or with other antihypertensives. Concomitant H_2 antagonist therapy may increase diltiazem blood levels.

Diltiazem may affect the blood levels of concomitant carbamazepine, theophylline, ciclosporin and digoxin. Careful attention should therefore be given to signs of overdosage. The levels should be determined and the dose of carbamazepine, theophylline, ciclosporin, or digoxin reduced if necessary. Patients receiving β-blockers, diuretics, ACE inhibitors or other antihypertensive agents should be regularly monitored. Use with alpha blockers should be strictly monitored.

The simultaneous administration of diltiazem with drugs such as β-blockers, antiarrhythmics or heart glycosides may cause a greater degree of AV blocking, reduce the heart rate or induce a hypotensive effect. Intravenous administration of β-blockers should be discontinued during therapy with diltiazem.

Anaesthetists should be warned that a patient is on a calcium antagonist. The depression of cardiac contractility, conductivity, and automaticity as well as the vascular dilation associated with anaesthetics may be potentiated by calcium channel blockers. When used concomitantly, anaesthetics and calcium channel blockers should be titrated carefully.

There have been reports in the literature of diltiazem interactions with warfarin, rifampicin, and lithium.

4.6 Pregnancy and lactation
Diltiazem must not be taken during pregnancy as experimental studies have shown indications of teratogenicity. There is no experience of its effects in humans. As diltiazem is known to enter the breast milk and there is no experience of possible effects in infants, infants should be weaned if treatment of the mother with diltiazem is necessary.

4.7 Effects on ability to drive and use machines
Not applicable.

4.8 Undesirable effects
In studies carried out to date, serious adverse reactions with diltiazem have been rare; however, it should be recognised that patients with impaired ventricular function and cardiac conduction abnormalities have usually been excluded from these studies.

In 900 patients with hypertension, the most common adverse events were oedema (9%), headache (8%), dizziness (6%), asthenia (5%), sinus bradycardia (3%), flushing (3%), and first degree AV block (3%). Only oedema and perhaps bradycardia were dose related. The most common adverse events (>1%) observed in clinical studies of over 2100 angina and hypertensive patients receiving diltiazem were: oedema (5.4%), headache (4.5%), dizziness (3.4%), asthenia (2.8%), first-degree AV block (1.8%), flushing (1.7%), nausea (1.6%), bradycardia (1.5%) and rash (1.5%).

Less common adverse events have included the following:

Cardiovascular: angina, arrhythmia, AV block (second or third degree), congestive heart failure, hypotension, palpitations, syncope.

Nervous system: amnesia, depression, gait abnormality, hallucinations, insomnia, nervousness, paraesthesia, personality change, somnolence, tinnitus, tremor.

Gastrointestinal: anorexia, constipation, diarrhoea, dyspepsia, mild elevations of alkaline phosphatase, SGOT, SGPT and LDH (see Special Warnings and Precautions), vomiting, weight increase, gingivitis.

Dermatologic: petechiae, pruritus, photosensitivity, urticaria. Allergic skin reactions including erythema multiforme, vasculitis, lymphadenopathy and eosinophilia have been observed in isolated cases. Dermatological events may be transient and may disappear despite continued use of diltiazem. Should a dermatologic reaction persist, the drug should be discontinued.

Other: amblyopia, CK elevation, dyspnoea, epistaxis, eye irritation, hyperglycaemia, nasal congestion, nocturia, osteoarticular pain, polyuria, sexual difficulties.

4.9 Overdose
Experience of overdosage in man is limited but cases of spontaneous recovery have been reported. However, it is recommended that patients with suspected overdose should be placed under observation in a coronary care unit with facilities available for treatment of any possible hypotension and conduction disturbances that may occur. Most patients suffering from overdosage of diltiazem become hypotensive within 8 hours of ingestion. With bradycardia and first to third degree atrioventricular block also developing cardiac arrest may ensue. Hyperglycaemia is also a recognised complication. The elimination half-life of diltiazem after overdosage is estimated to be about 5.5 - 10.2 hours. If a patient presents early after overdose, gastric lavage should be performed and activated charcoal administered to reduce diltiazem absorption.

Hypotension should be corrected with plasma expanders, intravenous calcium gluconate and inotropic agents (dopamine, dobutamine or isoprenaline). Symptomatic bradycardia and high grade AV block may respond to atropine, isoprenaline or occasionally cardiac pacing which may be useful if cardiac standstill occurs.

5. PHARMACOLOGICAL PROPERTIES

5.1 Pharmacodynamic properties
Diltiazem has pharmacologic actions similar to those of other calcium channel blocking agents such as nifedipine or verapamil. The principal physiologic action of diltiazem is to inhibit the transmembrane influx of extracellular calcium ions across the membranes of myocardial cells and vascular smooth muscle cells.

Calcium plays important roles in the excitation-contraction coupling processes of the heart and vascular smooth muscle cells and in the electrical discharge of the specialised conduction cells of the heart. The membranes of these cells contain numerous channels that carry a slow inward current and that are selective for calcium.

By inhibiting calcium influx, diltiazem inhibits the contractile processes of cardiac and vascular smooth muscle, thereby dilating the main coronary and systemic arteries. Dilation of systemic arteries by diltiazem results in a decrease in total peripheral resistance, a decrease in systemic blood pressure and a decrease in the afterload of the heart. The reduction in afterload, seen at rest and with exercise, and its resultant decrease in myocardial oxygen consumption are thought to be responsible for the beneficial effects of diltiazem in patients with chronic stable angina pectoris. In patients with prinzmetal variant angina, inhibition of spontaneous and ergonovine-induced coronary artery spasm by diltiazem results in increased myocardial oxygen delivery.

5.2 Pharmacokinetic properties
a) General Characteristics

Absorption: Capsules seem to have a similar bioavailability to tablets (30-40%), with peak concentrations for the prolonged release product after 8-11 hours compared with 1-2 hours after the conventional release product. The relatively low bioavailability is due to first pass metabolism in the liver to an active metabolite.

Distribution: Diltiazem hydrochloride is lipophilic and has a high volume of distribution. Typical study results are in the range of 3-8 litres/kg. Protein binding is about 80% and is not concentration-dependent at levels likely to be found clinically. Protein binding does not appear to be influenced by phenylbutazone, warfarin, propranolol, salicylic acid or digoxin.

Metabolism: Diltiazem hydrochloride is extensively metabolised in the liver. N-monodesmethyl diltiazem is the predominant metabolite followed quantitatively by the desacetyl metabolite, which has some pharmacological activity. The efficacy of the metabolites, desacetyl diltiazem and N-monodesmethyl diltiazem is 25-50% and about 20% respectively of that of diltiazem. In liver function disorders delayed metabolism in the liver is likely. These metabolites are converted to conjugates, generally the glucuronide or the sulphate.

Elimination: Diltiazem is excreted in the form of its metabolites (about 35%) and in the non-metabolised form (about 2-4%) via the kidneys while about 60% is excreted

GSL Classification: Patients suffering Irritable Bowel Syndrome should not use this product. The first line of treatment in acute diarrhoea is the prevention or treatment of fluid and electrolyte depletion; this is of particular importance to frail and elderly patients.

The following will appear on the product labeling (P or GSL): Warning: do not exceed the stated dose. Keep out of reach of children. If symptoms persist for more than 24 hours consult your doctor. If you are pregnant, consult your doctor before use. This medicine is for the relief of the symptoms of diarrhoea and is not a substitute for oral rehydration therapy.

4.5 Interaction with other medicinal products and other forms of Interaction
None stated.

4.6 Pregnancy and lactation
No teratogenic effects have been shown in animals. However safety in humans has not been established and the product should only be taken under medical supervision. Caution is advised during lactation.

4.7 Effects on ability to drive and use machines
None stated.

4.8 Undesirable effects
Rarely, skin rashes, including urticaria, have been reported.

4.9 Overdose
The following effects may be observed in cases of overdose: constipation, ileus and neurological symptoms. Treatment would be symptomatic. In severe overdose, naloxone can be given as an antidote if required.

5. PHARMACOLOGICAL PROPERTIES
5.1 Pharmacodynamic properties
By binding to opiate receptors in the gut wall, loperamide hydrochloride reduces propulsive peristalsis, increases intestinal transit time and enhances resorption of water and electrolytes.

5.2 Pharmacokinetic properties
Following partial absorption in the gastrointestinal tract, loperamide undergoes first-pass metabolism in the liver and is excreted predominantly in the faeces. The elimination half-life is reported as about ten hours.

5.3 Preclinical safety data
Not applicable.

6. PHARMACEUTICAL PARTICULARS
6.1 List of excipients
Lactose (DMV), Maize Starch (Dried), Microcrystalline Cellulose (Avicel PH101), Pregelatinised Starch (Dried), Croscarmellose Sodium, Dimeticone. *Shell cap:* Yellow Iron Oxide (E172), Black Iron Oxide (E172), Indigo Carmine (E132), Titanium Dioxide (E171), Gelatin. *Shell body:* Titanium Dioxide (E171), Gelatin.

6.2 Incompatibilities
None stated.

6.3 Shelf life
36 months unopened.

6.4 Special precautions for storage
None.

6.5 Nature and contents of container
Clear blisters of hard polyvinylchloride $250\mu m$ thick backed with aluminium foil 0.02 hard silver, smooth shiny-sided hot sealable against PVC and PVdC dull sided unprinted. 6 or 12 capsules per strip are packed in a cardboard carton.

6.6 Instructions for use and handling
Not applicable.

7. MARKETING AUTHORISATION HOLDER
Seton Products Limited, Tubiton House, Oldham, OL1 3HS.

8. MARKETING AUTHORISATION NUMBER(S)
PL 11314/0068.

9. DATE OF FIRST AUTHORISATION/RENEWAL OF THE AUTHORISATION
19th August 1996 / 6th June 2001.

10. DATE OF REVISION OF THE TEXT
June 2001.

Dioctyl Capsules

(SCHWARZ PHARMA Limited)

1. NAME OF THE MEDICINAL PRODUCT
Dioctyl Capsules

2. QUALITATIVE AND QUANTITATIVE COMPOSITION
Docusate sodium 100 mg.

For excipients, see Section 6.1.

3. PHARMACEUTICAL FORM
Capsules

A two colour (opaque white and opaque yellow) soft, oval, gelatin capsule with a clear, colourless liquid fill.

4. CLINICAL PARTICULARS
4.1 Therapeutic indications
a) To prevent and treat chronic constipation.

(i) to soften hard, dry stools in order to ease defaecation and reduce straining at stool; and

(ii) in the presence of haemorrhoids and anal fissure, to prevent hard, dry stools and reduce straining.

b) As an adjunct in abdominal radiological procedures.

4.2 Posology and method of administration
Route of administration: Oral

Adults and elderly:

Up to 500 mg should be taken daily in divided doses. Treatment should be commenced with large doses, which should be decreased as the condition of the patient improves.

For use with barium meals:

400 mg to be taken with the meal.

Children under 12 years:

Not recommended.

4.3 Contraindications
These capsules should not be administered when abdominal pain, nausea, vomiting or intestinal obstruction is present.

This product should not be given to patients with a known hypersensitivity to Dioctyl capsules or any of the components.

Patients with rare hereditary problems of fructose intolerance should not take this medicine.

4.4 Special warnings and special precautions for use
Organic disorders should be excluded prior to the administration of any laxative.

The treatment of constipation with any medicinal product is only adjuvant to a healthy lifestyle and diet, for example:

- Increased intake of fluids and dietary fibre.
- Advice on appropriate physical activity

If laxatives are needed every day, or if there is persistent abdominal pain, consult your doctor.

Contains sorbitol: do not use this medicine if you are intolerant to small quantities of sugar (sorbitol, fructose).

Contains colouring E110 which may cause allergic reactions.

4.5 Interaction with other medicinal products and other forms of Interaction
These capsules should not be taken concurrently with mineral oil.

4.6 Pregnancy and lactation
There are no adequate data from the use of the drug in pregnant women. Animal studies are insufficient with respect to effects on pregnancy and embryonic foetal development. The potential risk for humans is unknown. During wide use, no adverse consequences have been reported.

Use in pregnancy only if the benefits outweigh the risks.

Docusate sodium is excreted in breast milk and should therefore, be used with caution in lactating mothers.

4.7 Effects on ability to drive and use machines
None known.

4.8 Undesirable effects
Rarely, these capsules can cause diarrhoea, nausea, abdominal cramps or skin rash.

4.9 Overdose
In rare cases of overdose, excessive loss of water and electrolytes should be treated by encouraging the patient to drink plenty of fluid.

Electrolyte loss should be replenished where appropriate.

5. PHARMACOLOGICAL PROPERTIES
5.1 Pharmacodynamic properties
ATC code: A06A02 Laxatives, softeners, emollients

Docusate sodium is an anionic wetting agent, which acts as a faecal softener by lowering the surface tension and allowing penetration of accumulated hard dry faeces by water and salts.

Docusate Sodium also possesses stimulant activity.

5.2 Pharmacokinetic properties
Docusate sodium exerts its clinical effect in the gastrointestinal tract. There is some evidence that docusate sodium is absorbed and is excreted in the bile. There is also evidence that docusate sodium is capable of enhancing absorption of certain compounds administered concomitantly

5.3 Preclinical safety data
None stated.

6. PHARMACEUTICAL PARTICULARS
6.1 List of excipients
Macrogol 400

Propylene glycol

Gelatin 195 bloom

Purified water

Sorbitol special

Glycerol

Titanium dioxide E171

Quinoline yellow E104

Sunset yellow E110

6.2 Incompatibilities
None.

6.3 Shelf life
3 years

6.4 Special precautions for storage
Do not store above 25°C.

6.5 Nature and contents of container
PVC/PVdC blister packs with aluminium foil containing 30 capsules.

Polyethylene / polypropylene containers, e.g.: securitainers / tampertainers containing 100 capsules.

6.6 Instructions for use and handling
None

7. MARKETING AUTHORISATION HOLDER
SCHWARZ PHARMA Limited

Schwarz House

East Street

Chesham

Bucks HP5 1DG

England

8. MARKETING AUTHORISATION NUMBER(S)
PL 04438/0032

9. DATE OF FIRST AUTHORISATION/RENEWAL OF THE AUTHORISATION
September 2003

10. DATE OF REVISION OF THE TEXT
August 2005

Dioderm

(Dermal Laboratories Limited)

1. NAME OF THE MEDICINAL PRODUCT
DIODERM®

2. QUALITATIVE AND QUANTITATIVE COMPOSITION
Hydrocortisone 0.1% w/w.

3. PHARMACEUTICAL FORM
Smooth white aqueous cream.

4. CLINICAL PARTICULARS
4.1 Therapeutic indications
For the topical treatment of eczema and dermatitis.

4.2 Posology and method of administration
For adults, children and the elderly: Apply to the affected areas twice daily. For infants, the treatment period should not normally exceed 7 days.

4.3 Contraindications
As with all topical steroids, Dioderm is not to be used where there is bacterial, viral or fungal infection.

Not to be used on open wounds, ulcers or broken skin.

Not to be used in cases of sensitivity to any of the ingredients.

4.4 Special warnings and special precautions for use
Although generally regarded as safe, even for long-term administration in adults, there is a potential for overdosage in infancy. Extreme caution is required in dermatoses in infancy, including napkin eruption. In such patients, courses of treatment should not normally exceed 7 days.

Prolonged or extensive uninterrupted application should be avoided, particularly if used on the face or with occlusive dressings.

Keep away from the eyes.

For external use only.

4.5 Interaction with other medicinal products and other forms of Interaction
None known.

4.6 Pregnancy and lactation
There is inadequate evidence of safety in human pregnancy. Topical administration of corticosteroids to pregnant animals can cause abnormalities of foetal development including cleft palate and intra-uterine

growth retardation. There may therefore be a very small risk of such effects in the human foetus.

4.7 Effects on ability to drive and use machines
None known.

4.8 Undesirable effects
Reported side effects of corticosteroids include skin thinning and striae. Although rare, these could occur even with hydrocortisone, especially when used under occlusion or in the folds of the skin.

Dioderm is usually well tolerated but in the event of a hypersensitivity reaction (allergic contact dermatitis) treatment should be discontinued.

4.9 Overdose
Under exceptional circumstances, if Dioderm is used excessively, particularly in young children, it is theoretically possible that adrenal suppression and skin thinning may occur. The symptoms are normally reversible on cessation of treatment.

5. PHARMACOLOGICAL PROPERTIES
5.1 Pharmacodynamic properties
Corticosteroids are used in pharmacological doses for their anti-inflammatory and immunosuppressive glucocorticoid properties which suppress the clinical manifestations of a wide range of diseases. Although many synthetic derivatives have been developed, hydrocortisone is still used widely in topical formulations for inflammatory dermatoses. It has the advantage over its synthetic derivatives that it is metabolised in the skin and therefore cannot accumulate to form a depot which may result in local side effects.

5.2 Pharmacokinetic properties
The cream formulation of Dioderm was developed in order to optimise the release and partition of its active ingredient, hydrocortisone, into the skin. The hydrocortisone is presented as a saturated or near saturated solution in aqueous propylene glycol, which represents the continuous phase of the emulsion system. It has been shown, by the vasoconstrictor assay on normal skin, that, in this environment, a 0.1% concentration of the hydrocortisone is equivalent to the 1.0% concentration of the official cream formulations appearing in the British Pharmacopoeia where the drug substance is in suspension. Clinical studies have confirmed that 0.1% Dioderm is equivalent to 1.0% Hydrocortisone Cream BP whilst the reduced strength of Dioderm increases the margin of safety.

5.3 Preclinical safety data
No special information.

6. PHARMACEUTICAL PARTICULARS
6.1 List of excipients
Citric Acid; Emulsifying Ointment; Propylene Glycol; Purified Water.

6.2 Incompatibilities
None known.

6.3 Shelf life
30 months.

6.4 Special precautions for storage
Do not store above 25°C. Replace cap tightly after use.

6.5 Nature and contents of container
30 g collapsible tube. This is supplied as an original pack (OP).

6.6 Instructions for use and handling
Not applicable.

7. MARKETING AUTHORISATION HOLDER
Dermal Laboratories
Tatmore Place, Gosmore
Hitchin, Herts SG4 7QR, UK.

8. MARKETING AUTHORISATION NUMBER(S)
0173/0047.

9. DATE OF FIRST AUTHORISATION/RENEWAL OF THE AUTHORISATION
23 February 2003.

10. DATE OF REVISION OF THE TEXT
June 2003.

Diovan

(Novartis Pharmaceuticals UK Ltd)

1. NAME OF THE MEDICINAL PRODUCT
Diovan 40 mg Capsules.
Diovan 80 mg Capsules.
Diovan 160 mg Capsules.
Diovan 40 mg Tablets.

2. QUALITATIVE AND QUANTITATIVE COMPOSITION
Active substance: (S)-N-valeryl-N-{[2'-(1H-tetrazol-5-yl)biphenyl-4-yl]methyl}-valine
(INN = valsartan).

Diovan 40mg Capsules: One capsule contains 40 mg valsartan.

Diovan 80mg Capsules: One capsule contains 80 mg valsartan.

Diovan 160mg Capsules: One capsule contains 160 mg valsartan.

Diovan 40mg Tablets: One tablet contains 40 mg valsartan.

For excipients, see 6.1

3. PHARMACEUTICAL FORM
Capsules:
Diovan 40mg Capsules: Appearance: Light grey cap and body, marked CG HBH in black ink on the cap.

Diovan 80mg Capsules: Appearance: Light grey cap and flesh opaque body, marked CG FZF in black ink on the cap.

Diovan 160mg Capsules: Appearance: Dark grey cap and flesh opaque body, marked CG GOG in white ink on the cap.

Film Coated Tablets:
Diovan 40mg Tablets: Yellow, ovaloid, scored on one side, slightly convex, bevelled edges, debossed on one side with DO and NVR on the other side.

4. CLINICAL PARTICULARS
4.1 Therapeutic indications
Hypertension
Treatment of hypertension

Post-myocardial infarction
Diovan is indicated to improve survival following myocardial infarction in clinically stable patients with signs, symptoms or radiological evidence of left ventricular failure and/ or with left ventricular systolic dysfunction (see Section 5.1 "**Pharmacodynamic properties**").

4.2 Posology and method of administration
Hypertension
The recommended dose of Diovan is 80 mg once daily for most patients. The antihypertensive effect is substantially present within 2 weeks and maximal effects are seen after 4 weeks. In some patients whose blood pressure is not adequately controlled, the dose can either be increased to 160 mg, or a greater decrease in BP may be achieved by adding in a thiazide diuretic.

Diovan may also be administered with other antihypertensive agents.

Use in patients over 75 years:
A lower starting dose of 40 mg once daily is recommended.

Use in renal impairment:
No initial dose adjustment is required in patients with mild renal impairment (i.e. creatinine clearance 20-50 ml/min). For patients with moderate to severe renal impairment (i.e. creatinine less than 20 ml/min) or patients on dialysis, a lower starting dose of 40 mg once daily is recommended.

Use in patients with intravascular volume depletion:
For those patients who have intravascular volume depletion (e.g. those treated with high dose diuretics who are unable to have their dose of diuretic reduced) a starting dose of 40 mg is recommended.

Use in patients with mild to moderate hepatic impairment:
Treatment should commence at a dose of 40 mg once daily. A daily dose of 80 mg should not be exceeded. Patients with severe hepatic impairment, cirrhosis or biliary obstruction should not use Diovan (see Section 4.3 "**Contraindications**").

Use in children:
The safety and efficacy of Diovan have not been established in children.

Post-myocardial infarction
Therapy may be initiated as early as 12 hours after a myocardial infarction. After an initial dose of 20 mg twice daily, valsartan therapy should be titrated to 40 mg, 80 mg, and 160 mg twice daily over the next few weeks. The starting dose is provided by the 40 mg divisible tablet.

Achievement of the target dose of 160 mg twice daily should be based on the patient's tolerability to valsartan during titration. If symptomatic hypotension or renal dysfunction occur, consideration should be given to a dosage reduction.

Valsartan may be used in patients treated with other post-myocardial infarction therapies, e.g. thrombolytics, acetylsalicylic acid, beta blockers, and statins.

Use in renal impairment:
In the indication of post myocardial infarction no dosage adjustment is required for patients with mild to moderate renal impairment. There are currently no data available in post myocardial patients with severe renal impairment (serum creatinine ⩾ 221 μmol/l). Diovan should therefore be used with caution in such patients, with appropriate assessment of renal function (see Section 4.4 "**Special Warnings and Precautions**").

Use in patients with mild to moderate hepatic impairment:
Doses higher than 80mg twice daily should only be considered if the clinical benefit is likely to outweigh the possible risk associated with increased exposure of valsartan. Patients with severe hepatic impairment, cirrhosis or biliary obstruction should not use Diovan (see Section 4.3 " **Contraindications** ").

Use in children:
The safety and efficacy of Diovan have not been established in children.

4.3 Contraindications
Hypersensitivity to any of the components of Diovan.

Pregnancy (see Section 4.6. "**Pregnancy and lactation**").

Severe hepatic impairment, cirrhosis, biliary obstruction.

4.4 Special warnings and special precautions for use
Hypertension
Sodium and/or volume depleted patients:
In severely sodium-depleted and/or volume-depleted patients, such as those receiving high doses of diuretics, symptomatic hypotension may occur in rare cases after initiation of therapy with Diovan. For those patients whose diuretic dose cannot be reduced in order to correct their sodium and/or volume depletion a starting dose of 40 mg is recommended.

Renal artery stenosis:
Short-term administration of Diovan to twelve patients with renovascular hypertension secondary to unilateral renal artery stenosis did not induce any significant changes in renal haemodynamics, serum creatinine, or blood urea nitrogen (BUN). However, since other drugs that affect the renin-angiotensin-aldosterone system may increase blood urea and serum creatinine in patients with bilateral or unilateral renal artery stenosis, monitoring is recommended as a safety measure.

Hepatic impairment:
Based on pharmacokinetic data which demonstrate significantly increased plasma concentrations of valsartan in mild to moderately hepatically impaired patients, a lower dose is recommended in patients with hypertension (see Section 4.2 "**Posology and method of administration**"). In these patients the dose of 80 mg should not be exceeded. Patients with severe hepatic hepatic impairment, cirrhosis, biliary obstruction are contra-indicated from using Diovan (see Section 4.3 "**Contraindications**").

Renal function impairment:
As a consequence of inhibiting the renin-aldosterone-angiotensin system, increases of blood urea and serum creatinine and changes in renal function including renal failure (very rarely) have been reported particularly in patients with pre-existing renal dysfunction or those with severe cardiac insufficiency.

Post-myocardial infarction
Use of Diovan in patients with post-myocardial infarction commonly results in some reduction in blood pressure, but discontinuation of Diovan therapy because of continuing symptomatic hypotension is not usually necessary if the dosing instructions are followed.

Caution should be observed when initiating therapy in patients with post-myocardial infarction (see Section 4.2 "**Posology and method of administration**").

As a consequence of inhibiting the renin-angiotensin-aldosterone system, changes in renal function may be anticipated in susceptible individuals. Evaluation of patients with post-myocardial infarction should always include assessment of renal function.

Use in hepatic impairment:
Based on pharmacokinetic data which demonstrate approximately 2-fold increases in plasma concentrations of valsartan in mild to moderately hepatically impaired patients, doses higher than 80mg twice daily should only be considered if the clinical benefit is likely to outweigh the possible risk associated with increased exposure of valsartan (see Section 4.2 "**Posology and method of administration**"). Patients with severe hepatic impairment, cirrhosis, biliary obstruction are contra-indicated from using Diovan (see Section 4.3 " **Contraindications** ").

4.5 Interaction with other medicinal products and other forms of Interaction
Compounds which have been studied in clinical trials include cimetidine, warfarin, furosemide, digoxin, atenolol, indometacin, hydrochlorothiazide, amlodipine, glibenclamide. Used together with cimetidine, the systemic exposure of valsartan may be marginally increased. A combination with glibenclamide may cause a decrease in the systemic exposure to valsartan.

As Diovan is not metabolised to a significant extent, clinically relevant drug-drug interactions in the form of metabolic induction or inhibition of the cytochrome P450 system are not expected with valsartan. Although valsartan is highly bound to plasma proteins, *in vitro* studies have not shown any interaction at this level with a range of molecules which are also highly protein-bound, such as diclofenac, furosemide, and warfarin.

Concomitant use of potassium-sparing diuretics (e.g. spironolactone, triamterene, amiloride), potassium supplements, or salt substitutes containing potassium may lead to increases in serum potassium. Comedication is not advisable.

4.6 Pregnancy and lactation

Due to the mechanism of action of angiotensin II antagonists, a risk factor for the fetus cannot be excluded. In utero exposure to angiotensin converting enzyme (ACE) inhibitors given to pregnant women during the second and third trimesters has been reported to cause injury and death to the developing fetus. As for any drug that also acts directly on the renin-angiotensin-aldosterone system (RAAS), Diovan should not be used during pregnancy. If pregnancy is detected during therapy, Diovan should be discontinued as soon as possible.

It is not known whether valsartan is excreted in human milk. Valsartan was excreted in the milk of lactating rats. Thus, it is not advisable to use Diovan in lactating mothers.

4.7 Effects on ability to drive and use machines

There are no data to suggest that Diovan affects the ability to drive or use machines. When driving vehicles or operating machines, it should be recognised that occasionally dizziness or weariness may occur during treatment with any antihypertensive agent.

4.8 Undesirable effects

Hypertension

In general in clinical trials, Diovan had a side-effect profile comparable to placebo; adverse experiences have been mild and transient in nature.

In controlled clinical trials, clinically significant changes in laboratory parameters were rarely seen in patients taking Diovan. In rare cases, Diovan was associated with decreases in haemoglobin and haematocrit; neutropenia was observed occasionally.

Occasional elevation of serum potassium was seen but rarely was this of clinical significance and no patient discontinued for hyperkalaemia. Serum potassium should be monitored in renally impaired or elderly patients if they are also taking potassium supplements.

Adverse events reported during post marketing experience have, in general, been mild and transient in nature. The following have been reported very rarely since licensing:

Body as a whole: Fatigue

Cardiovascular: Syncope

Gastrointestinal: Diarrhoea, liver function abnormalities

Haematological: thrombocytopenia

Musculoskeletal: Arthralgia, myalgia

Nervous system: Dizziness, headache, mild and transient taste disturbance

Renal: Renal dysfunction and isolated cases of renal impairment

Respiratory: Cough, epistaxis

Hypersensitivity: Angioedema, rash, pruritis and isolated cases of other hypersensitivity/allergic reactions including serum sickness and vasculitis.

Post-myocardial infarction

In the double-blind, randomized, active-controlled, parallel-group VALIANT trial comparing the efficacy and safety of long-term treatment with valsartan, captopril and their combination in high-risk patients after myocardial infarction, the safety profile of valsartan was consistent with the pharmacology of the drug and the background diseases, cardiovascular risk factors, and clinical course of patients treated in the post-myocardial infarction setting.

Serious adverse events (SAEs) were primarily cardiovascular and generally related to the underlying disease as reflected in the primary efficacy endpoint of all-cause mortality. Non-fatal SAEs with suspected study drug relationship observed with an incidence of $\geqslant$0.1% and more frequent in valsartan-treated patients than in captopril-treated patients were hypotension and events related to renal dysfunction.

The percentage of permanent discontinuations due to adverse events was 5.8% in valsartan-treated patients and 7.7% in captopril-treated patients.

In post-mycocardial infarction patients, doubling of serum creatinine was observed in 4.2% of valsartan-treated patients, 4.8% of valsartan + captopril-treated patients, and 3.4 % of captopril-treated patients.

4.9 Overdose

Although there is no experience of overdosage with Diovan, the major sign that might be expected is marked hypotension. If the ingestion is recent, vomiting should be induced. Otherwise, the usual treatment would be intravenous infusion of normal saline solution.

Valsartan is unlikely to be removed by haemodialysis.

5. PHARMACOLOGICAL PROPERTIES

5.1 Pharmacodynamic properties

Pharmacotherapeutic groups: angiotensin II antagonists (valsartan) (ATC code: C09C A03).

The active hormone of the RAAS is angiotensin II, which is formed from angiotensin I through ACE. Angiotensin II binds to specific receptors located in the cell membranes of various tissues. It has a wide variety of physiological effects, including in particular both direct and indirect involvement in the regulation of blood pressure. As a potent vasoconstrictor, angiotensin II exerts a direct pressor response. In addition it promotes sodium retention and stimulation of aldosterone secretion.

Diovan (valsartan) is an orally active, potent, and specific angiotensin II (Ang II) receptor antagonist. It acts selectively on the AT_1 receptor subtype, which is responsible for the known actions of angiotensin II. The AT_2 subtype is unrelated to cardiovascular effects. Valsartan does not exhibit any partial agonist activity at the AT_1 receptor and has much (about 20,000 fold) greater affinity for the AT_1 receptor than for the AT_2 receptor.

Valsartan does not inhibit ACE, also known as kininase II, which converts Ang I to Ang II and degrades bradykinin. Since there is no effect on ACE and no potentiation of bradykinin or substance P, angiotensin II antagonists are unlikely to be associated with cough. In clinical trials where valsartan was compared with an ACE inhibitor, the incidence of dry cough was significantly ($P < 0.05$) less in patients treated with valsartan than in those treated with an ACE inhibitor (2.6 % versus 7.9 % respectively). In a clinical trial of patients with a history of dry cough during ACE inhibitor therapy, 19.5 % of trial subjects receiving valsartan and 19.0 % of those receiving a thiazide diuretic experienced cough compared to 68.5 % of those treated with an ACE inhibitor ($P < 0.05$). Valsartan does not bind to or block other hormone receptors or ion channels known to be important in cardiovascular regulation.

Hypertension

Administration of Diovan to patients with hypertension results in reduction of blood pressure without affecting pulse rate.

In most patients, after administration of a single oral dose, onset of antihypertensive activity occurs within 2 hours, and the peak reduction of blood pressure is achieved within 4-6 hours. The antihypertensive effect persists over 24 hours after dosing. During repeated dosing, the maximum reduction in blood pressure with any dose is generally attained within 2-4 weeks and is sustained during long-term therapy. Combined with hydrochlorothiazide, a significant additional reduction in blood pressure is achieved.

Abrupt withdrawal of Diovan has not been associated with rebound hypertension or other adverse clinical events.

In multiple dose studies in hypertensive patients valsartan had no notable effects on total cholesterol, fasting triglycerides, fasting serum glucose, or uric acid.

Post-myocardial infarction

The VALsartan In Acute myocardial iNfarcTion trial (VALIANT) was a randomized, controlled, multinational, double-blind study in 14,703 patients with acute myocardial infarction and evidence of congestive heart failure and/or left ventricular systolic dysfunction (manifested as an ejection fraction $\leqslant$ 40% by radionuclide ventriculography or $\leqslant$ 35% by echocardiography or ventricular contrast angiography). Patients were randomized within 12 hours to 10 days after the onset of myocardial infarction symptoms to one of three treatment groups, for a mean treatment duration of two years: valsartan, captopril, or the combination of valsartan plus captopril. Baseline therapy included acetylsalicylic acid, beta-blockers, ACE inhibitors, thrombolytics, and statins. The population studied was 69 % male, 94 % Caucasian, and 53 % were 65 years of age or older. The primary endpoint was time to all-cause mortality.

Valsartan was as effective as captopril in reducing all-cause mortality after myocardial infarction. All-cause mortality was similar in the valsartan (19.9 %), captopril (19.5 %), and valsartan + captopril (19.3 %) groups. Valsartan was also effective in prolonging the time to and reducing cardiovascular mortality, hospitilization for heart failure, and recurrent myocardial infarction.

Since this was a trial with an active control (captopril), an additional analysis of all-cause mortality was performed to estimate how valsartan would have performed versus placebo. Using the results of the previous reference myocardial infarction trials - SAVE, AIRE, and TRACE – the estimated effect of valsartan preserved 99.6 % of the effect of captopril (97.5 % CI = 60-139 %). Combining valsartan with captopril did not add further benefit over captopril alone, therefore this combination is not recommended. There was no difference in all-cause mortality based on age, gender, race, baseline therapies or underlying disease.

There was no difference in all-cause mortality or cardiovascular mortality or morbidity when beta-blockers were administered together with the combination of valsartan + captopril, valsartan alone, or captopril alone. In addition, the treatment benefits of the combination of valsartan + captopril, valsartan monotherapy, and captopril monotherapy were maintained in patients treated with beta-blockers.

5.2 Pharmacokinetic properties

Absorption of valsartan after oral administration is rapid, although the amount absorbed varies widely. Mean absolute bioavailability for Diovan is 23%. Valsartan shows multi-exponential decay kinetics ($t_{1/2}\ \alpha < 1$h and $t_{1/2}\ \beta$ about 9 h).

The pharmacokinetics of valsartan are linear in the dose range tested. There is no change in the kinetics of valsartan on repeated administration, and little accumulation when dosed once daily. Plasma concentrations were observed to be similar in males and females.

Valsartan is highly bound to serum protein (94-97 %), mainly serum albumin. Steady-state volume of distribution is low (about 17 L). Plasma clearance is relatively slow (about 2 L/h) when compared with hepatic blood flow (about 30 L/h). After oral dosing, 83% is excreted in the faeces and 13% in the urine, mainly as unchanged compound.

Diovan may be given with or without food.

Special populations

Elderly:

A somewhat higher systemic exposure to valsartan was observed in some elderly subjects compared with young subjects; and a lower starting dose (40 mg) is recommended for the elderly.

Impaired renal function:

As expected for a compound where renal clearance accounts for only 30% of total plasma clearance, no correlation was seen between renal function and systemic exposure to valsartan. Dose adjustment is therefore not required in patients with mild renal impairment (creatinine clearance 20-50 ml/min). Limited data are available in patients with moderate-severe impairment of renal function and a starting dose of 40 mg is recommended for these patients. No studies have been performed in patients undergoing dialysis. However, valsartan is highly bound to plasma protein and is unlikely to be removed by dialysis.

Hepatic impairment:

In a pharmacokinetics trial in patients with mild to moderate hepatic dysfunction, exposure to valsartan was increased approximately 2-fold compared with healthy volunteers.

5.3 Preclinical safety data

In a variety of preclinical safety studies conducted in several animal species, there was no evidence of systemic or target organ toxicity, apart from fetotoxicity. Offspring from rats given 600 mg/kg during the last trimester and during lactation showed a slightly reduced survival rate and a slight developmental delay (see Section 4.6. "**Pregnancy and lactation**"). The main preclinical safety findings are attributed to the pharmacological action of the compound, and have not been demonstrated to have any clinical significance.

There was no evidence of mutagenicity, clastogenicity or carcinogenicity.

6. PHARMACEUTICAL PARTICULARS

6.1 List of excipients

Diovan Capsules:

Microcrystalline cellulose, polyvidone, sodium lauryl sulfate, crospovidone, magnesium stearate.

Diovan Tablets:

Core

Microcrystalline cellulose

Crospovidone

Colloidal anhydrous silica

Magnesium stearate

Film-coat

Hypromellose

Titanium dioxide (E171)

Macrogol 8000

Red iron oxide (E172)

Yellow iron oxide (E172)

Black iron oxide (E172)

6.2 Incompatibilities

None known.

6.3 Shelf life

Diovan Capsules and Tablets: 3 years.

6.4 Special precautions for storage

Diovan Capsules:

Protect from moisture and heat. Store below 30°C.

Diovan Tablets:

Do not store above 30°C. Store in the original package.

6.5 Nature and contents of container

Diovan Capsules:

PVC/PE/PVDC blister packs.

Diovan 40 mg capsules are supplied in packs of 7 capsules.

Diovan 80mg and 160 mg capsules are supplied in packs 28 capsules.

Diovan Tablets:

Blisters strips of laminated plastic film of polyvinylchloride / polyethylene / poly-vinyldichloride (PVC/PE/PVDC) with a heat-sealable lacquered aluminium foil backing closure.

Diovan 40mg tablets are supplied in packs of 7 tablets.

6.6 Instructions for use and handling

No specific instructions for use/handling.

7. MARKETING AUTHORISATION HOLDER
Novartis Pharmaceuticals UK Limited
Trading as Ciba Laboratories
Frimley Business Park
Frimley
Camberley
Surrey GU16 7SR
United Kingdom

8. MARKETING AUTHORISATION NUMBER(S)
Diovan 40mg Capsules: PL 00101/0524
Diovan 80mg Capsules: PL 00101/0525
Diovan 160mg Capsules: PL 00101/0526
Diovn 40mg Tablets: PL 00101/0599

9. DATE OF FIRST AUTHORISATION/RENEWAL OF THE AUTHORISATION
Diovan Capsules: 31 October 1997/16 October 2001
Diovan Tablets: 22 March 2002

10. DATE OF REVISION OF THE TEXT
Diovan Capsules: 28 September 2004
Diovan Tablets: 28 September 2004

LEGAL CATEGORY
POM

Dipentum Capsules 250 mg, Dipentum Tablets 500 mg

(UCB Pharma Limited)

1. NAME OF THE MEDICINAL PRODUCT
Dipentum Capsules 250 mg
Dipentum Tablets 500 mg

2. QUALITATIVE AND QUANTITATIVE COMPOSITION
Each capsule contains Olsalazine sodium, 250 mg
Each tablet contains Olsalazine sodium, 500 mg

3. PHARMACEUTICAL FORM
Capsule
Tablet

4. CLINICAL PARTICULARS
4.1 Therapeutic indications
Oral treatment of mild active ulcerative colitis and maintenance of remission.

4.2 Posology and method of administration
Oral

General

Olsalazine taken on an empty stomach may sometimes lead to loose stools or diarrhoea. By taking the drug at the end of a meal, this may be avoided.

Acute mild disease
Adults including elderly: Commence on 1 g daily in divided doses and depending upon the patient response, titrate the dose upwards to a maximum of 3 g daily over one week.

A single dose should not exceed 1 g.

Olsalazine should be taken with food.

Remission
Adults including the elderly: A dose of 0.5g twice daily, taken with food.

Olsalazine has been used concomitantly with gluco-corticosteroids.

4.3 Contraindications
Hypersensitivity to salicylates. There is no experience of the use of olsalazine in patients with significant renal impairment. Olsalazine is contra-indicated in patients with significant renal impairment.

4.4 Special warnings and special precautions for use
Serious blood dyscrasias have been reported very rarely with olsalazine. Haematological investigations should be performed if the patient develops unexplained bleeding, bruising, purpura, anaemia, fever or sore throat. Treatment should be stopped if there is a suspicion or evidence of a blood dyscrasia.

4.5 Interaction with other medicinal products and other forms of Interaction
Those characteristic of salicylates are a theoretical possibility, although with the low blood levels of salicylate during therapy such effects have not been seen.

4.6 Pregnancy and lactation
Reproduction studies performed in mice, rats and rabbits have revealed no evidence of impaired fertility, harm to the foetus or teratogenic effects due to olsalazine administration. However, the experience of use in pregnant women is limited.

Dipentum should not be used during pregnancy unless the clinician considers that the potential benefit outweighs the possible risk to the foetus.

4.7 Effects on ability to drive and use machines
Such effects are not theoretically likely and have not been found in practice.

4.8 Undesirable effects
As with sulphasalazine and mesalazine gastrointestinal side effects are the most common. The most frequently reported adverse reactions are diarrhoea, abdominal cramps, headache, nausea, dyspepsia, arthralgia and rash.

Diarrhoea is often transient, clearing in a few days. Where it does not, taking the drug at the end of a more substantial meal, dose titration or dose reduction are usually effective. Withdrawal in clinical studies when the drug was taken at the end of meals was around 3%. Where diarrhoea persists, the drug should be stopped.

Blood dyscrasias have been reported in a few patients: leucopenia, neutropenia, plastic anaemia, pancytopenia, thrombocytopenia, anaemia and haemolytic anaemia.

4.9 Overdose
There is no specific antidote to olsalazine. Treatment should be supportive. As a salicylate, interference in biochemical and other tests characteristic of salicylates may occur.

5. PHARMACOLOGICAL PROPERTIES
5.1 Pharmacodynamic properties
Olsalazine is itself a relatively inert compound. Absorption in the small intestine is slight. On entering the colon it is split by bacteria into two molecules of 5-amino salicylate (5-ASA, mesalazine). 5-ASA is believed to be principal active fragment of sulphasalazine, which has been in use for 40 years in the treatment of ulcerative colitis. 5-ASA is believed to be the active form of Dipentum as olsalazine has little effect in in-vitro tests or on experimental animals. The clinical benefits of sulphasalazine, 5-ASA and olsalazine are evident in ulcerative colitis, but the pharmacological mechanism is not established.

5.2 Pharmacokinetic properties
Studies in man and animals indicate a low uptake of olsalazine and its metabolites, which is in keeping with the desired aim to deliver a high local concentration of 5-ASA to the colon.

In man an oral dose of olsalazine is negligibly absorbed in the gut. Bacteria split olsalazine in the colon into two molecules of 5-ASA. Local concentrations of 5-ASA in the colon can be 1000 times the plasma levels. Uptake by colonic mucosal cells leads to acetyl 5-ASA generation (the principle metabolite), traces of 5-ASA and olsalazine-O-SO_4 also being found in plasma. 500 mg b.d. in 6 volunteers gave a steady state level of amino salicylate of 0.8-2.9 mcg/ml after 6-9 days. In ileostomised patients almost all the olsalazine could be recovered in ileal fluid. Intravenous administration of olsalazine showed bilary excretion and traces of Ac-5-ASA in the urine and a half life of 56 minutes. Olsalazine given with or without food was taken up to the extent of 1.3 or 1.6% respectively. After a 1 g dose p.o. a maximum plasma level of 12.2 mcg/ml was noted at 1 hour of olsalazine. 22-33% of an oral dose appears in the urine almost all as Ac-5-ASA. The metabolite olsalazine-O-SO_4 is 99% plasma bound and has a half life of 6-10 days. Olsalazine does not penetrate red cells nor displace warfarin, naproxen, diazepam or digitoxin from plasma binding.

Autoradiography in rats showed no activity in the brain, testes, placenta or foetus, some activity in the bile duct and kidney and high activity in the gut.

5.3 Preclinical safety data
None stated.

6. PHARMACEUTICAL PARTICULARS
6.1 List of excipients
Dipentum Capsules 250 mg
Magnesum stearate
Gelatin
Dipentum Tablets 500 mg
Magnesium stearate Ph. Eur.
Colloidal silicon dioxide Ph. Eur.
Polyvidone 30 Ph. Eur.
Crospovidone NF
Ethanol 99.5% BP

6.2 Incompatibilities
As a salicylate, interference in biochemical and other tests characteristics of salicylates may occur.

6.3 Shelf life
Capsules - 60 month, unopened
Tablets - 48 months, unopened.

6.4 Special precautions for storage
Capsules – Store at room temperature in a dry place.
Tablets - Store in a dry place.

6.5 Nature and contents of container
Capsules:
White, square, polyethylene bottles with knurled tamper-evident cap containing 112 capsules, with a label incorporating a pull-out leaflet.

Tablets:
HD polyethylene securitainers with cap,
or
HD polyethylene square section pots with child and tamper resistant cap.

Packs of 60 tablets
Packs of 100 tablets (not marketed)

6.6 Instructions for use and handling
None stated.

7. MARKETING AUTHORISATION HOLDER
UCB Pharma Limited
208 Bath Road
Slough
Berkshire
SL1 3WE
United Kingdom

8. MARKETING AUTHORISATION NUMBER(S)
Dipentum Capsules 250 mg - PL 00039/0526
Dipentum Tablets 500 mg - PL 00039/0527

9. DATE OF FIRST AUTHORISATION/RENEWAL OF THE AUTHORISATION
31st October 2002

10. DATE OF REVISION OF THE TEXT
June 2005

11. Legal Category
POM

Diprivan 1%

(AstraZeneca UK Limited)

1. NAME OF THE MEDICINAL PRODUCT
'Diprivan' 1%.

2. QUALITATIVE AND QUANTITATIVE COMPOSITION
10 mg propofol per 1 ml.

3. PHARMACEUTICAL FORM
Oil-in-water emulsion for intravenous injection.

4. CLINICAL PARTICULARS
4.1 Therapeutic indications
'Diprivan' 1% is a short-acting intravenous anaesthetic agent suitable for induction and maintenance of general anaesthesia.

'Diprivan' 1% may also be used for sedation of ventilated patients receiving intensive care.

'Diprivan' 1% may also be used for sedation for surgical and diagnostic procedures.

4.2 Posology and method of administration
For specific guidance relating to the administration of 'Diprivan' 1% with a target controlled infusion (TCI) device, which incorporates 'Diprifusor' TCI Software, see Section 4.2.5. Such use is restricted to induction and maintenance of anaesthesia in adults. The 'Diprifusor' TCI system is not recommended for use in ICU sedation or sedation for surgical and diagnostic procedures, or in children.

4.2.1 Induction of General Anaesthesia
Adults
In unpremedicated and premedicated patients, it is recommended that 'Diprivan' 1% should be titrated (approximately 4 ml [40 mg] every 10 seconds in an average healthy adult by bolus injection or infusion) against the response of the patient until the clinical signs show the onset of anaesthesia. Most adult patients aged less than 55 years are likely to require 1.5 to 2.5 mg/kg of 'Diprivan' 1%. The total dose required can be reduced by lower rates of administration (2 to 5 ml/min [20 to 50 mg/min]). Over this age, the requirement will generally be less. In patients of ASA Grades 3 and 4, lower rates of administration should be used (approximately 2 ml [20 mg] every 10 seconds).

Elderly Patients
In elderly patients the dose requirement for induction of anaesthesia with 'Diprivan' 1% is reduced. The reduction should take into account of the physical status and age of the patient. The reduced dose should be given at a slower rate and titrated against the response.

Children
'Diprivan' 1% is not recommended for induction of anaesthesia in children aged less than 1 month.

When used to induce anaesthesia in children, it is recommended that 'Diprivan' 1% be given slowly until the clinical signs show the onset of anaesthesia. The dose should be adjusted for age and/or weight. Most patients over 8 years of age are likely to require approximately 2.5 mg/kg of 'Diprivan' 1% for induction of anaesthesia. Under this age the requirement may be more. Lower dosage is recommended for children of ASA grades 3 and 4.

Administration of 'Diprivan' 1% by a 'Diprifusor' TCI system is not recommended for induction of general anaesthesia in children.

4.2.2 Maintenance Of General Anaesthesia
Adults
Anaesthesia can be maintained by administering 'Diprivan' 1% either by continuous infusion or by repeat bolus injections to prevent the clinical signs of light anaesthesia. Recovery from anaesthesia is typically rapid and it is therefore important to maintain 'Diprivan' 1% administration until the end of the procedure.

Continuous Infusion

The required rate of administration varies considerably between patients, but rates in the region of 4 to 12 mg/kg/h usually maintain satisfactory anaesthesia.

Repeat Bolus Injections

If a technique involving repeat bolus injections is used, increments of 25 mg (2.5 ml) to 50 mg (5.0 ml) may be given according to clinical need.

Elderly Patients

When 'Diprivan' 1% is used for maintenance of anaesthesia the rate of infusion or 'target concentration' should also be reduced. Patients of ASA grades 3 and 4 will require further reductions in dose and dose rate. Rapid bolus administration (single or repeated) should not be used in the elderly as this may lead to cardiorespiratory depression.

Children

'Diprivan' 1% is not recommended for maintenance of anaesthesia in children less than 3 years of age.

Anaesthesia can be maintained by administering 'Diprivan' 1% by infusion or repeat bolus injection to prevent the clinical signs of light anaesthesia. The required rate of administration varies considerably between patients, but rates in the region of 9 to 15 mg/kg/h usually achieve satisfactory anaesthesia.

Administration of 'Diprivan' 1% by a 'Diprifusor' TCI system is not recommended for maintenance of general anaesthesia in children.

4.2.3 Sedation During Intensive Care

Adults

For sedation during intensive care it is advised that Diprivan 1% should be administered by continuous infusion. The infusion rate should be determined by the desired depth of sedation. In most patients sufficient sedation can be obtained with a dosage of 0.3 - 4 mg/kg/h of Diprivan 1% (See 4.4 Special warnings and precautions for use). Diprivan 1% is not indicated for sedation in intensive care of patients of 16 years of age or younger (see 4.3 Contraindications). Administration of Diprivan 1% by Diprifusor TCI system is not advised for sedation in the intensive care unit.

Diprivan' 1% may be diluted with 5% Dextrose (see "Dilution and Co-administration" table below).

It is recommended that blood lipid levels be monitored should 'Diprivan' 1% be administered to patients thought to be at particular risk of fat overload. Administration of 'Diprivan' 1% should be adjusted appropriately if the monitoring indicates that fat is being inadequately cleared from the body. If the patient is receiving other intravenous lipid concurrently, a reduction in quantity should be made in order to take account of the amount of lipid infused as part of the 'Diprivan' 1% formulation; 1.0 ml of 'Diprivan' 1% contains approximately 0.1g of fat.

If the duration of sedation is in excess of 3 days, lipids should be monitored in all patients.

Elderly Patients

When 'Diprivan' 1% is used for sedation the rate of infusion should also be reduced. Patients of ASA grades 3 and 4 will require further reductions in dose and dose rate. Rapid bolus administration (single or repeated) should not be used in the elderly as this may lead to cardiorespiratory depression.

Children

'Diprivan' 1% is contra-indicated for the sedation of ventilated children aged 16 years or younger receiving intensive care.

4.2.4 Sedation For Surgical And Diagnostic Procedures

Adults

To provide sedation for surgical and diagnostic procedures, rates of administration should be individualised and titrated to clinical response.

Most patients will require 0.5 to 1 mg/kg over 1 to 5 minutes for onset of sedation.

Maintenance of sedation may be accomplished by titrating 'Diprivan' 1% infusion to the desired level of sedation - most patients will require 1.5 to 4.5 mg/kg/h. In addition to the infusion, bolus administration of 10 to 20 mg may be used if a rapid increase in the depth of sedation is required. In patients of ASA Grades 3 and 4 the rate of administration and dosage may need to be reduced.

Administration of 'Diprivan' 1% by a 'Diprifusor' TCI system is not recommended for sedation for surgical and diagnostic procedures.

Elderly Patients

When 'Diprivan' 1% is used for sedation the rate of infusion or 'target concentration' should also be reduced. Patients of ASA grades 3 and 4 will require further reductions in dose and dose rate. Rapid bolus administration (single or repeated) should not be used in the elderly as this may lead to cardiorespiratory depression.

Children

'Diprivan' 1% is not recommended for sedation in children as safety and efficacy have not been demonstrated.

4.2.5 Administration

'Diprivan' 1% has no analgesic properties and therefore supplementary analgesic agents are generally required in addition to 'Diprivan' 1%.

'Diprivan' 1% can be used for infusion undiluted from glass containers, plastic syringes or 'Diprivan' 1% pre-filled syringes or diluted with 5% Dextrose (Intravenous Infusion BP) only, in PVC infusion bags or glass infusion bottles. Dilutions, which must not exceed 1 in 5 (2 mg propofol per ml) should be prepared aseptically immediately before administration and must be used within 6 hours of preparation.

It is recommended that, when using diluted 'Diprivan' 1%, the volume of 5% Dextrose removed from the infusion bag during the dilution process is totally replaced in volume by 'Diprivan' 1% emulsion. (see "Dilution and Co-administration" table below).

The dilution may be used with a variety of infusion control techniques, but a giving set used alone will not avoid the risk of accidental uncontrolled infusion of large volumes of diluted 'Diprivan' 1%. A burette, drop counter or volumetric pump must be included in the infusion line. The risk of uncontrolled infusion must be taken into account when deciding the maximum amount of 'Diprivan' 1% in the burette.

When 'Diprivan' 1% is used undiluted to maintain anaesthesia, it is recommended that equipment such as syringe pumps or volumetric infusion pumps should always be used to control infusion rates.

'Diprivan' 1% may be administered via a Y-piece close to the injection site into infusions of the following:

- Dextrose 5% Intravenous Infusion B.P.
- Sodium Chloride 0.9% Intravenous Infusion B.P.
- Dextrose 4% with Sodium Chloride 0.18% Intravenous Infusion B.P.

The glass pre-filled syringe (PFS) has a lower frictional resistance than plastic disposable syringes and operates more easily. Therefore, if 'Diprivan' 1% is administered using a hand held pre-filled syringe, the line between the syringe and the patient must not be left open if unattended.

When the pre-filled syringe presentation is used in a syringe pump appropriate compatibility should be ensured. In particular, the pump should be designed to prevent syphoning and should have an occlusion alarm set no greater than 1000 mm Hg. If using a programmable or equivalent pump that offers options for use of different syringes then choose only the 'B-D' 50/60 ml 'PLASTIPAK' setting when using the 'Diprivan' 1% pre-filled syringe.

'Diprivan' 1% may be premixed with alfentanil injection containing 500 micrograms/ml alfentanil in the ratio of 20:1 to 50:1 v/v. Mixtures should be prepared using sterile technique and used within 6 hours of preparation.

In order to reduce pain on initial injection, 'Diprivan' 1% may be mixed with preservative-free Lignocaine Injection 0.5% or 1%; (see "Dilution and Co-administration" table below).

Target Controlled Infusion - Administration of 'Diprivan' 1% by a 'Diprifusor' TCI System in Adults

Administration of 'Diprivan' 1% by a 'Diprifusor' TCI system is restricted to induction and maintenance of general anaesthesia in adults. It is not recommended for use in ICU sedation or sedation for surgical and diagnostic procedures, or in children.

'Diprivan' 1% may be administered by TCI only with a 'Diprifusor' TCI system incorporating 'Diprifusor' TCI software. Such systems will operate only on recognition of electronically tagged pre-filled syringes containing 'Diprivan' 1% or 2% Injection. The 'Diprifusor' TCI system will automatically adjust the infusion rate for the concentration of 'Diprivan' recognised. Users must be familiar with the infusion pump users' manual, and with the administration of 'Diprivan' 1% by TCI and with the correct use of the syringe identification system.

The system allows the anaesthetist or intensivist to achieve and control a desired speed of induction and depth of anaesthesia by setting and adjusting target (predicted) blood concentrations of propofol.

The 'Diprifusor' TCI system assumes that the initial blood propofol concentration in the patient is zero. Therefore, in patients who have received prior propofol, there may be a need to select a lower initial target concentration when commencing 'Diprifusor' TCI. Similarly, the immediate recommencement of 'Diprifusor' TCI is not recommended if the pump has been switched off.

Guidance on propofol target concentrations is given below. In view of interpatient variability in propofol pharmacokinetics and pharmacodynamics, in both premedicated and unpremedicated patients the target propofol concentration should be titrated against the response of the patient in order to achieve the depth of anaesthesia required.

Induction and Maintenance of General Anaesthesia

In adult patients under 55 years of age anaesthesia can usually be induced with target propofol concentrations in the region of 4 to 8 microgram/ml. An initial target of 4 microgram/ml is recommended in premedicated patients and in unpremedicated patients an initial target of 6 microgram/ml is advised. Induction time with these targets is generally within the range of 60 to 120 seconds. Higher targets will allow more rapid induction of anaesthesia but may be associated with more pronounced haemodynamic and respiratory depression.

A lower initial target concentration should be used in patients over the age of about 55 years and in patients of ASA grades 3 and 4. The target concentration can then be increased in steps of 0.5 to 1.0 microgram/ml at intervals of 1 minute to achieve a gradual induction of anaesthesia.

Supplementary analgesia will generally be required and the extent to which target concentrations for maintenance of anaesthesia can be reduced will be influenced by the amount of concomitant analgesia administered. Target propofol concentrations in the region of 3 to 6 microgram/ml usually maintain satisfactory anaesthesia.

The predicted propofol concentration on waking is generally in the region of 1.0 to 2.0 microgram/ml and will be influenced by the amount of analgesia given during maintenance.

Sedation during intensive care

Target blood propofol concentration settings in the range of 0.2 to 2.0 μg/ml will generally be required. Administration should begin at low target setting which should be titrated against the response of the patient to achieve the depth of sedation desired.

DILUTION AND CO-ADMINISTRATION OF 'DIPRIVAN' 1% WITH OTHER DRUGS OR INFUSION FLUIDS (see also 'Additional Precautions' Section)

(see Table 1)

4.3 Contraindications

Known hypersensitivity for any of the components of Diprivan 1% or Diprivan 2%.

Diprivan 1% is contraindicated for sedation in intensive care of patients of 16 years of age or younger (See 4.4 Special warnings and precautions for use).

4.4 Special warnings and special precautions for use

'Diprivan' 1% should be given by those trained in anaesthesia or, where appropriate, doctors trained in the care of patients in Intensive Care. Patients should be constantly monitored and facilities for maintenance of a patient

Table 1

Co-administration Technique	Additive or Diluent	Preparation	Precautions
Pre-mixing.	Dextrose 5% Intravenous Infusion	Mix 1 part of 'Diprivan' 1% with up to 4 parts of Dextrose 5% Intravenous Infusion B.P in either PVC infusion bags or glass infusion bottles. When diluted in PVC bags it is recommended that the bag should be full and that the dilution be prepared by withdrawing a volume of infusion fluid and replacing it with an equal volume of 'Diprivan' 1%.	Prepare aseptically immediately before administration. The mixture is stable for up to 6 hours.
	Lignocaine hydrochloride injection (0.5% or 1% without preservatives).	Mix 20 parts of 'Diprivan' 1% with up to 1 part of either 0.5% or 1% lignocaine hydrochloride injection.	Prepare mixture aseptically immediately prior to administration. Use for Induction only.
	Alfentanil injection (500 microgram/ml).	Mix 'Diprivan' 1% with alfentanil injection in a ratio of 20:1 to 50:1 v/v.	Prepare mixture aseptically; use within 6 hours of preparation.
Co-administration via a Y-piece connector.	Dextrose 5% intravenous infusion	Co-administer via a Y-piece connector.	Place the Y-piece connector close to the injection site.
	Sodium chloride 0.9% intravenous infusion	As above	As above
	Dextrose 4% with sodium chloride 0.18% intravenous infusion	As above	As above

airway, artificial ventilation, oxygen enrichment and other resuscitative facilities should be readily available at all times. 'Diprivan' 1% should not be administered by the person conducting the diagnostic or surgical procedure.

When 'Diprivan' 1% is administered for sedation for surgical and diagnostic procedures patients should be continually monitored for early signs of hypotension, airway obstruction and oxygen desaturation.

As with other sedative agents, when Diprivan is used for sedation during operative procedures, involuntary patient movements may occur. During procedures requiring immobility these movements may be hazardous to the operative site.

As with other intravenous anaesthetic and sedative agents, patients should be instructed to avoid alcohol before and for at least 8 hours after administration of 'Diprivan' 1%.

'Diprivan' 1% should be used with caution when used to sedate patients undergoing some procedures where spontaneous movements are particularly undesirable, such as ophthalmic surgery.

As with other intravenous sedative agents, when 'Diprivan' 1% is given along with central nervous system depressants, such as potent analgesics, the sedative effect may be intensified and the possibility of severe respiratory or cardiovascular depression should be considered.

During bolus administration for operative procedures, extreme caution should be exercised in patients with acute pulmonary insufficiency or respiratory depression.

Concomitant use of central nervous system depressants e.g., alcohol, general anaesthetics, narcotic analgesics will result in accentuation of their sedative effects. When 'Diprivan' 1% is combined with centrally depressant drugs administered parenterally, severe respiratory and cardiovascular depression may occur. It is recommended that 'Diprivan' 1% is administered following the analgesic and the dose should be carefully titrated to the patient's response (see Section 4.5).

During induction of anaesthesia, hypotension and transient apnoea may occur depending on the dose and use of premedicants and other agents.

Occasionally, hypotension may require use of intravenous fluids and reduction of the rate of administration of 'Diprivan' 1% during the period of anaesthetic maintenance.

An adequate period is needed prior to discharge of the patient to ensure full recovery after general anaesthesia. Very rarely the use of 'Diprivan' may be associated with the development of a period of post-operative unconsciousness, which may be accompanied by an increase in muscle tone. This may or may not be preceded by a period of wakefulness. Although recovery is spontaneous, appropriate care of an unconscious patient should be administered.

When 'Diprivan' 1% is administered to an epileptic patient, there may be a risk of convulsion.

As with other intravenous anaesthetic agents, caution should be applied in patients with cardiac, respiratory, renal or hepatic impairment or in hypovolaemic, elderly or debilitated patients.

The risk of relative vagal overactivity may be increased because 'Diprivan' 1% lacks vagolytic activity; it has been associated with reports of bradycardia (occasionally profound) and also asystole. The intravenous administration of an anticholinergic agent before induction, or during maintenance of anaesthesia should be considered, especially in situations where vagal tone is likely to predominate, or when 'Diprivan' 1% is used in conjunction with other agents likely to cause a bradycardia.

Appropriate care should be applied in patients with disorders of fat metabolism and in other conditions where lipid emulsions must be used cautiously.

Use is not recommended with electroconvulsive treatment.

As with other anaesthetics, sexual disinhibition may occur during recovery.

Diprivan 1% is not advised for general anaesthesia in children younger than 1 month of age. The safety and efficacy of Diprivan 1% for (background) sedation in children younger than 16 years of age have not been demonstrated. Although no causal relationship has been established, serious undesirable effects with (background) sedation in patients younger than 16 years of age (including cases with fatal outcome) have been reported during unlicensed use. In particular these effects concerned occurrence of metabolic acidosis, hyperlipidemia, rhabdomyolysis and/or cardiac failure. These effects were most frequently seen in children with respiratory tract infections who received dosages in excess of those advised in adults for sedation in the intensive care unit.

Similarly very rare reports have been received of occurrence of metabolic acidosis, rhabdomyolysis, hyperkalaemia and/or rapidly progressive cardiac failure (in some cases with fatal outcome) in adults who were treated for more than 58 hours with dosages in excess of 5 mg/kg/h. This exceeds the maximum dosage of 4 mg/kg/h currently advised for sedation in the intensive care unit. The patients affected were mainly (but not only) seriously head-injured patients with raised ICP. The cardiac failure in such cases was usually unresponsive to inotropic supportive treatment. Treating physicians are reminded if possible not to exceed the dosage of 4 mg/kg/h. Prescribers should be alert to these possible undesirable effects and consider decreasing the Diprivan 1% dosage or switching to an alternative sedative at the first sign of occurrence of symptoms. Patients with raised ICP should be given appropriate treatment to support the cerebral perfusion pressure during these treatment modifications.

Additional Precautions

'Diprivan' 1% contains no antimicrobial preservatives and supports growth of micro-organisms. When 'Diprivan' 1% is to be aspirated, it must be drawn aseptically into a sterile syringe or giving set immediately after opening the ampoule or breaking the vial seal. Administration must commence without delay. Asepsis must be maintained for both 'Diprivan' 1% and infusion equipment throughout the infusion period. Any drugs or fluids added to the 'Diprivan' 1% line must be administered close to the cannula site. 'Diprivan' 1% must not be administered via a microbiological filter.

'Diprivan' 1% and any syringe containing 'Diprivan' 1% are for single use in an individual patient. For use in long term maintenance of anaesthesia or sedation in intensive care it is recommended that the infusion line and reservoir of 'Diprivan' 1% be discarded and replaced at regular intervals.

4.5 Interaction with other medicinal products and other forms of Interaction

'Diprivan' 1% has been used in association with spinal and epidural anaesthesia and with commonly used premedicants, neuromuscular blocking drugs, inhalational agents and analgesic agents; no pharmacological incompatibility has been encountered. Lower doses of 'Diprivan' 1% may be required where general anaesthesia is used as an adjunct to regional anaesthetic techniques.

The concurrent administration of other CNS depressants such as pre-medication drugs, inhalation agents, analgesic agents may add to the sedative, anaesthetic and cardiorespiratory depressant effects of propofol (see Section 4.4).

4.6 Pregnancy and lactation

Pregnancy The safety of Diprivan during pregnancy has not been established. Therefore Diprivan should not be used in pregnancy unless clearly necessary. Diprivan has been used, however, during termination of pregnancy in the first trimester.

Obstetrics 'Diprivan' 1% crosses the placenta and may be associated with neonatal depression. It should not be used for obstetric anaesthesia unless clearly necessary.

Lactation Safety to the neonate has not been established following the use of 'Diprivan' 1% in mothers who are breast feeding.

4.7 Effects on ability to drive and use machines

Patients should be advised that performance at skilled tasks, such as driving and operating machinery, may be impaired for some time after general anaesthesia.

4.8 Undesirable effects

General

Induction of anaesthesia is generally smooth with minimal evidence of excitation. The most commonly reported ADRs are pharmacologically predictable side effects of an anaesthetic agent, such as hypotension. Given the nature of anaesthesia and those patients receiving intensive care, events reported in association with anaesthesia and intensive care may also be related to the procedures being undertaken or the recipient's condition.

Very common (>1/10)	*General disorders and administration site conditions:*	Local pain on induction (1)
Common (>1/100, <1/10)	*Vascular disorder:*	Hypotension (2)
	Cardiac disorders:	Bradycardia (3)
	Respiratory, thoracic and mediastinal disorders:	Transient apnoea during induction
	Gastrointestinal disorders:	Nausea and vomiting during recovery phase
	Nervous system disorders:	Headache during recovery phase
	General disorders and administration site conditions:	Withdrawal symptoms in children (4)
	Vascular disorders:	Flushing in children (4)
Uncommon (>1/1000, <1/100)	*Vascular disorders:*	Thrombosis and phlebitis
Rare (>1/10 000, <1/1000)	*Nervous system:*	Epileptiform movements, including convulsions and opisthotonus during induction, maintenance and recovery
Very rare (<1/10 000)	*Musculoskeletal and connective tissue disorders:*	Rhabdomyolysis (5)
	Gastrointestinal disorders:	Pancreatitis
	Injury, poisoning and procedural complications:	Post-operative fever
	Renal and urinary disorders:	Discolouration of urine following prolonged administration
	Immune system disorders:	Anaphylaxis – may include angioedema, bronchospasm, erythema and hypotension
	Reproductive system and breast:	Sexual disinhibition
	Cardiac disorders:	Pulmonary oedema
	Nervous system disorders:	Postoperative unconsciousness

(1) May be minimised by using the larger veins of the forearm and antecubital fossa. With Diprivan 1% local pain can also be minimised by the co-administration of lignocaine.

(2) Occasionally, hypotension may require use of intravenous fluids and reduction of the administration rate of Diprivan.

(3) Serious bradycardias are rare. There have been isolated reports of progression to asystole.

(4) Following abrupt discontinuation of Diprivan during intensive care.

(5) Very rare reports of rhabdomyolysis have been received where Diprivan has been given at doses greater than 4 mg/kg/hr for ICU sedation.

Pulmonary oedema, hypotension, asystole, bradycardia, and convulsions, have been reported. In very rare cases rhabdomyolysis, metabolic acidosis, hyperkalaemia or cardiac failure, sometimes with fatal outcome, have been observed when propofol was administered at dosages in excess of 4 mg/kg/h for sedation in the intensive care unit (see 4.4 Special warnings and precautions for use).

Reports from off-label use of Diprivan for induction of anaesthesia in neonates indicates that cardio-respiratory depression may occur if the paediatric dose regimen is applied.

Local

The local pain which may occur during the induction phase of 'Diprivan' 1% anaesthesia can be minimised by the co-administration of lignocaine (see "Dosage and Administration") and by the use of the larger veins of the forearm and antecubital fossa. Thrombosis and phlebitis are rare. Accidental clinical extravasation and animal studies showed minimal tissue reaction. Intra-arterial injection in animals did not induce local tissue effects.

4.9 Overdose

Accidental overdosage is likely to cause cardiorespiratory depression. Respiratory depression should be treated by artificial ventilation with oxygen. Cardiovascular depression would require lowering of the patient's head and, if severe, use of plasma expanders and pressor agents.

5. PHARMACOLOGICAL PROPERTIES

5.1 Pharmacodynamic properties

Propofol (2, 6-diisopropylphenol) is a short-acting general anaesthetic agent with a rapid onset of action of approximately 30 seconds. Recovery from anaesthesia is usually rapid. The mechanism of action, like all general anaesthetics, is poorly understood.

In general, falls in mean arterial blood pressure and slight changes in heart rate are observed when 'Diprivan' 1% is administered for induction and maintenance of anaesthesia. However, the haemodynamic parameters normally remain relatively stable during maintenance and the incidence of untoward haemodynamic changes is low.

Although ventilatory depression can occur following administration of 'Diprivan' 1%, any effects are qualitatively similar to those of other intravenous anaesthetic agents and are readily manageable in clinical practice.

'Diprivan' 1% reduces cerebral blood flow, intracranial pressure and cerebral metabolism. The reduction in intracranial pressure is greater in patients with an elevated baseline intracranial pressure.

Recovery from anaesthesia is usually rapid and clear headed with a low incidence of headache and post-operative nausea and vomiting.

In general, there is less post-operative nausea and vomiting following anaesthesia with 'Diprivan' 1% than following anaesthesia with inhalational agents. There is evidence that this may be related to a reduced emetic potential of propofol.

'Diprivan' 1%, at the concentrations likely to occur clinically, does not inhibit the synthesis of adrenocortical hormones.

5.2 Pharmacokinetic properties

The decline in propofol concentrations following a bolus dose or following the termination of an infusion can be described by a three compartment open model with very rapid distribution (half-life 2 to 4 minutes), rapid elimination (half-life 30 to 60 minutes), and a slower final phase, representative of redistribution of propofol from poorly perfused tissue.

Propofol is extensively distributed and rapidly cleared from the body (total body clearance 1.5 to 2 litres/minute). Clearance occurs by metabolic processes, mainly in the liver, to form inactive conjugates of propofol and its corresponding quinol, which are excreted in urine.

When 'Diprivan' 1% is used to maintain anaesthesia, blood concentrations asymptotically approach the steady-state value for the given administration rate. The pharmacokinetics are linear over the recommended range of infusion rates of 'Diprivan' 1%.

5.3 Preclinical safety data

Propofol is a drug on which extensive clinical experience has been obtained. All relevant information for the prescriber is provided elsewhere in the Summary of Product Characteristics.

6. PHARMACEUTICAL PARTICULARS

6.1 List of excipients

Glycerol Ph Eur

Purified Egg Phosphatide

Sodium Hydroxide Ph Eur

Soya-bean Oil Ph Eur

Water for Injections Ph Eur

Nitrogen Ph Eur

6.2 Incompatibilities

The neuromuscular blocking agents, atracurium and mivacurium should not be given through the same intravenous line as 'Diprivan' 1% without prior flushing.

6.3 Shelf life

6.3.1 Shelf life of the product as packaged for sale

Ampoules - 3 years

Vials - 3 years

Pre-filled syringe - 2 years.

6.3.2 Shelf life after dilution

When diluted, 'Diprivan' 1% must be used within 6 hours of preparation.

6.4 Special precautions for storage

Store between 2°C and 25°C.

Do not freeze.

6.5 Nature and contents of container

a) Clear neutral glass ampoules of 20 ml in boxes of 5

b) Clear neutral glass vials of 50 ml and 100 ml

c) Type 1 glass pre-filled syringe of 50 ml

6.6 Instructions for use and handling

In-use precautions Containers should be shaken before use.

Any portion of the contents remaining after use should be discarded.

'Diprivan' 1% should not be mixed prior to administration with injections or infusion fluids other than 5% Dextrose or Lignocaine Injection (see Section 4.2.5).

7. MARKETING AUTHORISATION HOLDER

AstraZeneca UK Limited,

600 Capability Green,

Luton, LU1 3LU, UK.

8. MARKETING AUTHORISATION NUMBER(S)

PL 17901/0007.

9. DATE OF FIRST AUTHORISATION/RENEWAL OF THE AUTHORISATION

8th July 2000 / 24th September 2004

10. DATE OF REVISION OF THE TEXT

24th September 2004

Diprivan 2%

(AstraZeneca UK Limited)

1. NAME OF THE MEDICINAL PRODUCT

Diprivan 2%.

2. QUALITATIVE AND QUANTITATIVE COMPOSITION

White, aqueous and isotonic emulsion for intravenous injection containing 20 mg propofol per 1 ml.

3. PHARMACEUTICAL FORM

Oil-in-water emulsion for intravenous injection.

4. CLINICAL PARTICULARS

4.1 Therapeutic indications

Diprivan 2% is a short-acting intravenous anaesthetic agent suitable for induction and maintenance of general anaesthesia.

Diprivan 2% may also be used for sedation of ventilated patients receiving intensive care.

4.2 Posology and method of administration

For specific guidance relating to the administration of Diprivan 2% with a target controlled infusion (TCI) device, which incorporates 'Diprifusor' TCI Software, see Section 4.2.4. Such use is restricted to induction and maintenance of anaesthesia in adults. The 'Diprifusor' TCI system is not recommended for use in ICU sedation or in children.

4.2.1 Induction of General Anaesthesia

Adults

Diprivan 2% may be used to induce anaesthesia by infusion.

Administration of Diprivan 2% by bolus injection is not recommended.

Diprivan 2% may be used to induce anaesthesia by infusion but only in those patients who will receive Diprivan 2% for maintenance of anaesthesia.

In unpremedicated and premedicated patients, it is recommended that Diprivan 2% should be titrated (approximately 2 ml [40 mg] every 10 seconds in an average healthy adult by infusion) against the response of the patient until the clinical signs show the onset of anaesthesia. Most adult patients aged less than 55 years are likely to require 1.5 to 2.5 mg/kg of Diprivan 2%. The total dose required can be reduced by lower rates of administration (1 to 2.5 ml/min [20 to 50 mg/min]). Over this age, the requirement will generally be less. In patients of ASA Grades 3 and 4, lower rates of administration should be used (approximately 1 ml [20 mg] every 10 seconds).

Elderly Patients

In elderly patients the dose requirement for induction of anaesthesia with Diprivan 2% is reduced. The reduction should take into account of the physical status and age of the patient. The reduced dose should be given at a slower rate and titrated against the response.

Children

Diprivan 2% is not recommended for induction of anaesthesia in children less than 3 years of age.

When used to induce anaesthesia in children, it is recommended that Diprivan 2% be given by slow infusion until the clinical signs show the onset of anaesthesia. The dose should be adjusted for age and/or weight. Most patients over 8 years of age are likely to require approximately 2.5 mg/kg of Diprivan 2% for induction of anaesthesia. Under this age the requirement may be more. Lower dosage is recommended for children of ASA grades 3 and 4.

Administration of Diprivan 2% by a 'Diprifusor' TCI system is not recommended for induction of general anaesthesia in children.

4.2.2 Maintenance Of General Anaesthesia

Anaesthesia can be maintained by administering Diprivan 2% by continuous infusion to prevent the clinical signs of light anaesthesia. Administration of Diprivan 2% by bolus injection is not recommended. Recovery from anaesthesia is typically rapid and it is therefore important to maintain Diprivan 2% administration until the end of the procedure.

Adults

The required rate of administration varies considerably between patients, but rates in the region of 4 to 12 mg/kg/h usually maintain satisfactory anaesthesia.

Elderly Patients

When Diprivan 2% is used for maintenance of anaesthesia the rate of infusion or 'target concentration' should also be reduced. Patients of ASA grades 3 and 4 will require further reductions in dose and dose rate. Rapid bolus administration (single or repeated) should not be used in the elderly as this may lead to cardiorespiratory depression.

Children

Diprivan 2% is not recommended for maintenance of anaesthesia in children less than 3 years of age.

The required rate of administration varies considerably between patients but rates in the region of 9 to 15 mg/kg/h usually achieve satisfactory anaesthesia.

Administration of Diprivan 2% by a 'Diprifusor' TCI System is not recommended for maintenance of general anaesthesia in children.

4.2.3 Sedation During Intensive Care

Adults

For sedation during intensive care it is advised that Diprivan 2% should be administered by continuous infusion. The infusion rate should be determined by the desired depth of sedation. In most patients sufficient sedation can be obtained with a dosage of 0.3 - 4 mg/kg/h of Diprivan 2% (See 4.4 Special warnings and precautions for use). Diprivan 2% is not indicated for sedation in intensive care of patients of 16 years of age or younger (see 4.3 Contraindications). Administration of Diprivan 2% by Diprifusor TCI system is not advised for sedation in the intensive care unit.

It is recommended that blood lipid levels be monitored should Diprivan 2% be administered to patients thought to be at particular risk of fat overload.

Administration of Diprivan 2% should be adjusted appropriately if the monitoring indicates that fat is being inadequately cleared from the body. If the patient is receiving other intravenous lipid concurrently, a reduction in quantity should be made in order to take account of the amount of lipid infused as part of the Diprivan 2% formulation: 1.0 ml of Diprivan 2% contains approximately 0.1 g of fat.

If the duration of sedation is in excess of 3 days, lipids should be monitored in all patients.

Elderly Patients

When Diprivan 2% is used for sedation of anaesthesia the rate of infusion should also be reduced. Patients of ASA grades 3 and 4 will require further reductions in dose and dose rate. Rapid bolus administration (single or repeated) should not be used in the elderly as this may lead to cardiorespiratory depression.

Children

Diprivan 2% is contra-indicated for the sedation of ventilated children aged 16 years or younger receiving intensive care.

4.2.4 Administration

Diprivan 2% has no analgesic properties and therefore supplementary analgesic agents are generally required in addition to Diprivan 2%.

Diprivan has been used in association with spinal and epidural anaesthesia and with commonly used premedicants, neuromuscular blocking drugs, inhalational agents and analgesic agents; no pharmacological incompatibility has been encountered. Lower doses of Diprivan 2% may be required where general anaesthesia is used as an adjunct to regional anaesthetic techniques.

Diprivan 2% should not be diluted. Diprivan 2% can be used for infusion undiluted from glass containers, plastic syringes or Diprivan 2% pre-filled syringes.

When Diprivan 2% is used to maintain anaesthesia, it is recommended that equipment such as syringe pumps or volumetric infusion pumps should always be used to control infusion rates.

Diprivan 2% should not be mixed prior to administration with injections or infusion fluids. However, Diprivan 2% may be co-administered via a Y-piece connector close to the injection site into infusions of the following:

- Dextrose 5% Intravenous Infusion B.P.
- Sodium Chloride 0.9% Intravenous Infusion B.P.
- Dextrose 4% with Sodium Chloride 0.18% Intravenous Infusion B.P.

The glass pre-filled syringe (PFS) has a lower frictional resistance than plastic disposable syringes and operates more easily. Therefore, if 'Diprivan 2% is administered using a hand held pre-filled syringe, the line between the syringe and the patient must not be left open if unattended.

When the pre-filled syringe presentation is used in a syringe pump appropriate compatibility should be ensured. In particular, the pump should be designed to prevent siphoning and should have an occlusion alarm set no greater than 1000 mm Hg. If using a programmable or equivalent pump that offers options for use of different syringes then choose only the 'B-D' 50/60 ml 'PLASTIPAK' setting when using the Diprivan 2% pre-filled syringe.

Target Controlled Infusion - Administration of Diprivan 2% by a 'Diprifusor' TCI System in Adults

Administration of Diprivan 2% by a 'Diprifusor' TCI system is restricted to induction and maintenance of general anaesthesia in adults. It is not recommended for use in ICU sedation or in children.

Diprivan may be administered by TCI only with a Diprifusor TCI system incorporating Diprifusor TCI software

Such systems will operate only on recognition of electronically tagged prefilled syringes containing Diprivan 1% or 2% Injection. The 'Diprifusor' TCI system will automatically adjust the infusion rate for the concentration of Diprivan recognised. Users must be familiar with the infusion pump users manual, and with the administration of Diprivan 2% by TCI and with the correct use of the syringe identification system.

The system allow the anaesthetist or intensivist to achieve and control a desired speed of induction and depth of anaesthesia by setting and adjusting target (predicted) blood concentrations of propofol.

The 'Diprifusor' TCI system assumes that the initial blood propofol concentration in the patient is zero. Therefore, in patients who have received prior propofol, there may be a need to select a lower initial target concentration when commencing 'Diprifusor' TCI. Similarly, the immediate recommencement of 'Diprifusor' TCI is not recommended if the pump has been switched off.

Guidance on propofol target concentrations is given below. In view of interpatient variability in propofol pharmacokinetics and pharmacodynamics, in both premedicated and unpremedicated patients the target propofol concentration should be titrated against the response of the patient in order to achieve the depth of anaesthesia required.

In adult patients under 55 years of age anaesthesia can usually be induced with target propofol concentrations in the region of 4 to 8 microgram/ml. An initial target of 4 microgram/ml is recommended in premedicated patients and in unpremedicated patients an initial target of 6 microgram/ml is advised. Induction time with these targets is generally within the range of 60 to 120 seconds. Higher targets will allow more rapid induction of anaesthesia but may be associated with more pronounced haemodynamic and respiratory depression.

A lower initial target concentration should be used in patients over the age of about 55 years and in patients of ASA Grades 3 and 4. The target concentration can then be increased in steps of 0.5 to 1.0 microgram/ml at intervals of 1 minute to achieve a gradual induction of anaesthesia.

Supplementary analgesia will generally be required and the extent to which target concentrations for maintenance of anaesthesia can be reduced will be influenced by the amount of concomitant analgesia administered. Target propofol concentrations in the region of 3 to 6 microgram/ml usually maintain satisfactory anaesthesia.

The predicted propofol concentration on waking is generally in the region of 1.0 to 2.0 microgram/ml and will be influenced by the amount of analgesia given during maintenance.

Sedation during intensive care

Target blood propofol concentration settings in the range of 0.2 to 2.0 μg/ml will generally be required. Administration should begin at a low target setting which should be titrated against the response of the patient to achieve the depth of sedation desired.

4.3 Contraindications

Known hypersensitivity for any of the components of Diprivan 1% or Diprivan 2%.

Diprivan 2% is contraindicated for sedation in intensive care of patients of 16 years of age or younger (See 4.4 Special warnings and precautions for use).

4.4 Special warnings and special precautions for use

Diprivan 2% should be given by those trained in anaesthesia, or where appropriate, doctors trained in the care of patients in Intensive Care. Facilities for maintenance of a patient airway, artificial ventilation and oxygen enrichment should be available.

During induction of anaesthesia, hypotension and transient apnoea may occur depending on the dose and use of premedicants and other agents.

Occasionally, hypotension may require use of intravenous fluids and reduction of the rate of administration of Diprivan 2% during the period of anaesthetic maintenance.

As with other sedative agents, when Diprivan is used for sedation during operative procedures, involuntary patient movements may occur. During procedures requiring immobility these movements may be hazardous to the operative site.

An adequate period is needed prior to discharge of the patient to ensure full recovery after general anaesthesia. Very rarely the use of Diprivan may be associated with the development of a period of post-operative unconsciousness, which may be accompanied by an increase in muscle tone. This may or may not be preceded by a period of wakefulness. Although recovery is spontaneous, appropriate care of an unconscious patient should be administered.

When Diprivan 2% is administered to an epileptic patient, there may be a risk of convulsion.

As with other intravenous anaesthetic agents, caution should be applied in patients, with cardiac, respiratory, renal or hepatic impairment or in hypovolaemic or debilitated patients.

The risk of relative vagal overactivity may be increased because Diprivan 2% lacks vagolytic activity. Diprivan has been associated with reports of bradycardia (occasionally profound) and also asystole. The intravenous administration of an anticholinergic agent before induction, or during maintenance of anaesthesia should be considered, especially in situations where vagal tone is likely to predominate or when Diprivan 2% is used in conjunction with other agents likely to cause a bradycardia.

Appropriate care should be applied in patients with disorders of fat metabolism and in other conditions where lipid emulsions must be used cautiously.

Use is not recommended with electroconvulsive treatment.

As with other anaesthetics sexual disinhibition may occur during recovery.

Diprivan 2% is not advised for general anaesthesia in children younger than 1 month of age. The safety and efficacy of Diprivan 2% for (background) sedation in children younger than 16 years of age have not been demonstrated. Although no causal relationship has been established, serious undesirable effects with (background) sedation in patients younger than 16 years of age (including cases with fatal outcome) have been reported during unlicensed use. In particular these effects concerned occurrence of metabolic acidosis, hyperlipidemia, rhabdomyolysis and/or cardiac failure. These effects were most frequently seen in children with respiratory tract infections who received dosages in excess of those advised in adults for sedation in the intensive care unit.

Similarly very rare reports have been received of occurrence of metabolic acidosis, rhabdomyolysis, hyperkalaemia and/or rapidly progressive cardiac failure (in some cases with fatal outcome) in adults who were treated for more than 58 hours with dosages in excess of 5 mg/kg/h. This exceeds the maximum dosage of 4 mg/kg/h currently advised for sedation in the intensive care unit. The patients affected were mainly (but not only) seriously head-injured patients with raised ICP. The cardiac failure in such cases was usually unresponsive to inotropic supportive treatment. Treating physicians are reminded if possible not to exceed the dosage of 4 mg/kg/h. Prescribers should be alert to these possible undesirable effects and consider decreasing the Diprivan 2% dosage or switching to an alternative sedative at the first sign of occurrence of symptoms. Patients with raised ICP should be given appropriate treatment to support the cerebral perfusion pressure during these treatment modifications.

Additional Precautions

Diprivan 2% contains no antimicrobial preservatives and supports growth of micro-organisms. Asepsis must be maintained for both Diprivan 2% and infusion equipment throughout the infusion period. Any drugs or fluids added to the Diprivan 2% infusion line must be administered close to the cannula site. Diprivan 2% must not be administered via a microbiological filter.

Diprivan 2% and any syringe containing Diprivan 2% are for single use in an individual patient. For use in long-term maintenance of anaesthesia or sedation in intensive care it is recommended that the infusion line and reservoir of Diprivan 2% be discarded and replaced at regular intervals.

4.5 Interaction with other medicinal products and other forms of Interaction

See Section 4.2.4 Administration.

4.6 Pregnancy and lactation

Pregnancy Teratology studies in rats and rabbits showed no teratogenic effects. Diprivan has been used during termination of pregnancy in the first trimester. Diprivan 2% should not be used in pregnancy.

Obstetrics Diprivan crosses the placenta and may be associated with neonatal depression. It should not be used for obstetric anaesthesia.

Lactation Safety to the neonate has not been established following the use of Diprivan 2% in mothers who are breast feeding. Diprivan 2% should be avoided, or mothers should stop breast feeding.

4.7 Effects on ability to drive and use machines

Patients should be advised that performance at skilled tasks, such as driving and operating machinery, may be impaired for some time after general anaesthesia.

4.8 Undesirable effects

General

Induction of anaesthesia is generally smooth with minimal evidence of excitation. The most commonly reported ADRs are pharmacologically predictable side effects of an anaesthetic agent, such as hypotension. Given the nature of anaesthesia and those patients receiving intensive care, events reported in association with anaesthesia and intensive care may also be related to the procedures being undertaken or the recipient's condition.

(see Table 1)

Pulmonary edema, hypotension, asystole, bradycardia, and convulsions, have been reported. In very rare cases rhabdomyolysis, metabolic acidosis, hyperkalaemia or cardiac failure, sometimes with fatal outcome, have been observed when propofol was administered at dosages in excess of 4 mg/kg/h for sedation in the intensive care unit (see 4.4 Special warnings and precautions for use).

Reports from off-label use of Diprivan for induction of anaesthesia in neonates indicates that cardio-respiratory depression may occur if the paediatric dose regimen is applied.

Local

The local pain which may occur during the induction phase can be minimised by the use of the larger veins of the forearm and antecubital fossa. Thrombosis and phlebitis are rare. Accidental clinical extravasation and animal studies showed minimal tissue reaction. Intra-arterial injection in animals did not induce local tissue effects.

Table 1

Very common (>1/10)	*General disorders and administration site conditions:*	Local pain on induction [1]
Common (>1/100, <1/10)	*Vascular disorder:*	Hypotension [2]
	Cardiac disorders:	Bracdycardia [3]
	Respiratory, thoracic and mediastinal disorders:	Transient aponea during induction
	Gastrointestinal disorders:	Nausea and vomiting during recovery phase
	Nervous system disorders:	Headache during recovery phase
	General disorders and administration site conditions:	Withdrawal symptoms in children [4]
	Vascular disorders:	Flushing in children [4]
Uncommon (>1/1000, <1/100)	*Vascular disorders:*	Thrombosis and phlebitis
Rare (>1/10 000, <1/1000)	*Nervous system:*	Epileptiform movements, including convulsions and opisthotonus during induction, maintenance and recovery
Very rare (<1/10 000)	*Musculoskeletal and connective tissue disorders:*	Rhabdomyolysis [5]
	Gastrointestinal disorders:	Pancreatitis
	Injury, poisoning and procedural complications:	Post-operative fever
	Renal and urinary disorders:	Discolouration of urine Following prolonged administration
	Immune system disorders:	Anaphylaxis – may include angioedema, bronchospasm, erythema and hypotension
	Reproductive system and breast:	Sexual disinhibition
	Cardiac disorders:	Pulmonary oedema
	Nervous system disorders:	Postoperative unconsciousness

(1) May be minimised by using the larger veins of the forearm and antecubital fossa. With Diprivan 1% local pain can also be minimised by the co-administration of lignocaine.

(2) Occasionally, hypotension may require use of intravenous fluids and reduction of the administration rate of Diprivan.

(3) Serious bradycardias are rare. There have been isolated reports of progression to asystole.

(4) Following abrupt discontinuation of Diprivan during intensive care.

(5) Very rare reports of rhabdomyolysis have been received where Diprivan has been given at doses greater than 4 mg/kg/hr for ICU sedation.

4.9 Overdose
Accidental overdosage is likely to cause cardiorespiratory depression. Respiratory depression should be treated by artificial ventilation with oxygen. Cardiovascular depression would require lowering of the patient's head and, if severe, use of plasma expanders and pressor agents.

5. PHARMACOLOGICAL PROPERTIES

5.1 Pharmacodynamic properties
Propofol (2, 6-diisopropylphenol) is a short-acting general anaesthetic agent with a rapid onset of action of approximately 30 seconds. Recovery from anaesthesia is usually rapid. The mechanism of action, like all general anaesthetics, is poorly understood.

In general, falls in mean arterial blood pressure and slight changes in heart rate are observed when Diprivan 2% is administered for induction and maintenance of anaesthesia. However, the haemodynamic parameters normally remain relatively stable during maintenance and the incidence of untoward haemodynamic changes is low.

Although ventilatory depression can occur following administration of Diprivan 2%, any effects are qualitatively similar to those of other intravenous anaesthetic agents and are readily manageable in clinical practice.

Diprivan 2% reduces cerebral blood flow, intracranial pressure and cerebral metabolism. The reduction in intracranial pressure is greater in patients with an elevated baseline intracranial pressure.

Recovery from anaesthesia is usually rapid and clear headed with a low incidence of headache and post-operative nausea and vomiting.

In general, there is less post-operative nausea and vomiting following anaesthesia with Diprivan 2% than following anaesthesia with inhalational agents. There is evidence that this may be related to a reduced emetic potential of propofol.

Diprivan 2%, at the concentrations likely to occur clinically, does not inhibit the synthesis of adrenocortical hormones.

5.2 Pharmacokinetic properties
The decline in propofol concentrations following a bolus dose or following the termination of an infusion can be described by a three compartment open model with very rapid distribution (half-life 2 to 4 minutes), rapid elimination (half-life 30 to 60 minutes), and a slower final phase, representative of redistribution of propofol from poorly perfused tissue.

Propofol is extensively distributed and rapidly cleared from the body (total body clearance 1.5 to 2 litres/minute). Clearance occurs by metabolic processes, mainly in the liver, to form inactive conjugates of propofol and its corresponding quinol, which are excreted in urine.

When Diprivan 2% is used to maintain anaesthesia, blood concentrations asymptotically approach the steady-state value for the given administration rate. The pharmacokinetics are linear over the recommended range of infusion rates of Diprivan 2%.

5.3 Preclinical safety data
Propofol is a drug on which extensive clinical experience has been obtained. All relevant information for the prescriber is provided elsewhere in this document.

6. PHARMACEUTICAL PARTICULARS

6.1 List of excipients
Glycerol Ph Eur

Purified Egg Phosphatide

Sodium Hydroxide Ph Eur

Soya-Bean Oil Ph Eur

Water for Injections Ph Eur

Nitrogen Ph Eur

6.2 Incompatibilities
Diprivan 2% should not be mixed prior to administration with injections or infusion fluids. However, Diprivan 2% may be co-administered via a Y-piece connector close to the injection site into infusions of the following:

- Dextrose 5% Intravenous Infusion B.P.
- Sodium Chloride 0.9% B.P.
- Dextrose 4% with Sodium Chloride 0.18% Intravenous Infusion B.P.

The neuromuscular blocking agents, atracurium and mivacurium should not be given through the same intravenous line as Diprivan 2% without prior flushing.

6.3 Shelf life

6.3.1 Shelf life of the product as packaged for sale
2 years.

6.3.2 Shelf life after dilution:
Diprivan 2% should not be diluted.

6.4 Special precautions for storage
Store between 2°C and 25°C. Do not freeze.

6.5 Nature and contents of container
Emulsion for injection:

a) 10 ml pre-filled syringe containing propofol 20 mg/ml

b) 50 ml pre-filled syringe containing propofol 20 mg/ml.

6.6 Instructions for use and handling

In use precautions:
Containers should be shaken before use. Any portion of the contents remaining after use should be discarded.

Diprivan 2% should not be mixed prior to administration with injections or infusion fluids. However, Diprivan 2% may be co-administered via a Y-piece connector close to the injection site into infusions of the following:

- Dextrose 5% Intravenous Infusion B.P.
- Sodium Chloride 0.9% Intravenous Infusion B.P.
- Dextrose 4% with Sodium Chloride 0.18% Intravenous Infusion B.P.

When the pre-filled syringe presentation is used in a syringe pump, appropriate compatibility should be ensured. In particular, the pump should be designed to prevent siphoning and should have an occlusion arm set no greater than 1000 mm Hg. If using a programmable or equivalent pump that offers options for use of different syringes then choose only the "B - D" 50/60 ml "PLASTIPAK" setting when using the Diprivan pre-filled syringe.

Additional precautions:
Diprivan 2% contains no antimicrobial preservatives and supports growth of micro-organisms. Asepsis must be maintained for both Diprivan 2% and infusion equipment throughout the infusion period. Any drugs or fluids added to the Diprivan 2% infusion line must be administered close to the cannula site. Diprivan 2% must not be administered via a microbiological filter.

Diprivan 2% and any syringe containing Diprivan 2% are for single use in an individual patient. For use in long-term maintenance of anaesthesia or sedation in intensive care it is recommended that the infusion line and reservoir of Diprivan 2% be discarded and replaced at regular intervals.

7. MARKETING AUTHORISATION HOLDER
AstraZeneca UK Limited,

600 Capability Green,

Luton, LU1 3LU, UK.

8. MARKETING AUTHORISATION NUMBER(S)
PL 17901/0008

9. DATE OF FIRST AUTHORISATION/RENEWAL OF THE AUTHORISATION
8 July 2000 / 26 February 2002

10. DATE OF REVISION OF THE TEXT
17 February 2004

Diprivan 2% (vials)

(AstraZeneca UK Limited)

1. NAME OF THE MEDICINAL PRODUCT
Diprivan 2% (vials).

2. QUALITATIVE AND QUANTITATIVE COMPOSITION
White, aqueous and isotonic emulsion for intravenous injection containing 20 mg propofol per 1 ml.

3. PHARMACEUTICAL FORM
Oil-in-water emulsion for intravenous injection.

4. CLINICAL PARTICULARS

4.1 Therapeutic indications
Diprivan 2% is a short-acting intravenous anaesthetic agent suitable for induction and maintenance of general anaesthesia.

Diprivan 2% may also be used for sedation of ventilated patients receiving intensive care.

4.2 Posology and method of administration

4.2.1 Induction of General Anaesthesia Adults
Diprivan 2% may be used to induce anaesthesia by infusion.

Administration of Diprivan 2% by bolus injection is not recommended.

Diprivan 2% may be used to induce anaesthesia by infusion but only in those patients who will receive Diprivan 2% for maintenance of anaesthesia.

In unpremedicated and premedicated patients, it is recommended that

Diprivan 2% should be titrated (approximately 2 ml [40 mg] every 10 seconds in an average healthy adult by infusion) against the response of the patient until the clinical signs show the onset of anaesthesia. Most adult patients aged less than 55 years are likely to require 1.5 to 2.5 mg/kg of Diprivan 2%. The total dose required can be reduced by lower rates of administration (1 to 2.5 ml/min [20 to 50 mg/min]). Over this age, the requirement will generally be less. In patients of ASA Grades 3 and 4, lower rates of administration should be used (approximately 1 ml [20 mg] every 10 seconds).

Elderly Patients
In elderly patients the dose requirement for induction of anaesthesia with Diprivan 2% is reduced. The reduction should take into account of the physical status and age of the patient. The reduced dose should be given at a slower rate and titrated against the response.

Children
Diprivan 2% is not recommended for induction of anaesthesia in children less than 3 years of age.

When used to induce anaesthesia in children, it is recommended that Diprivan 2% be given by slow infusion until the clinical signs show the onset of anaesthesia. The dose should be adjusted for age and/or weight. Most patients over 8 years of age are likely to require approximately 2.5 mg/kg of Diprivan 2% for induction of anaesthesia. Under this age the requirement may be more. Lower dosage is recommended for children of ASA grades 3 and 4.

4.2.2 Maintenance of General Anaesthesia
Anaesthesia can be maintained by administering Diprivan 2% by continuous infusion to prevent the clinical signs of light anaesthesia. Administration of Diprivan 2% by bolus injection is not recommended. Recovery from anaesthesia is typically rapid and it is therefore important to maintain Diprivan 2% administration until the end of the procedure.

Adults
The required rate of administration varies considerably between patients, but rates in the region of 4 to 12 mg/kg/h usually maintain satisfactory anaesthesia.

Elderly Patients
When Diprivan 2% is used for maintenance of anaesthesia the rate of infusion should also be reduced. Patients of ASA grades 3 and 4 will require further reductions in dose and dose rate. Rapid bolus administration (single or repeated) should not be used in the elderly as this may lead to cardiorespiratory depression.

Children
Diprivan 2% is not recommended for maintenance of anaesthesia in children less than 3 years of age.

The required rate of administration varies considerably between patients but rates in the region of 9 to 15 mg/kg/h usually achieve satisfactory anaesthesia.

4.2.3 Sedation During Intensive Care Adults
For sedation during intensive care it is advised that Diprivan 2% should be administered by continuous infusion. The infusion rate should be determined by the desired depth of sedation. In most patients sufficient sedation can be obtained with a dosage of 0.3 - 4 mg/kg/h of Diprivan 2% (See 4.4 Special warnings and precautions for use). Diprivan 2% is not indicated for sedation in intensive care of patients of 16 years of age or younger (see 4.3 Contraindications).

It is recommended that blood lipid levels be monitored should Diprivan 2% be administered to patients thought to be at particular risk of fat overload.

Administration of Diprivan 2% should be adjusted appropriately if the monitoring indicates that fat is being inadequately cleared from the body. If the patient is receiving other intravenous lipid concurrently, a reduction in quantity should be made in order to take account of the amount of lipid infused as part of the Diprivan 2% formulation: 1.0 ml of Diprivan 2% contains approximately 0.1 g of fat.

If the duration of sedation is in excess of 3 days, lipids should be monitored in all patients.

Elderly Patients
When Diprivan 2% is used for sedation of anaesthesia the rate of infusion should also be reduced. Patients of ASA grades 3 and 4 will require further reductions in dose and dose rate. Rapid bolus administration (single or repeated) should not be used in the elderly as this may lead to cardiorespiratory depression.

Children
Diprivan 2% is contra-indicated for the sedation of ventilated children aged 16 years or younger receiving intensive care.

4.2.4 Administration
Diprivan 2% has no analgesic properties and therefore supplementary analgesic agents are generally required in addition to Diprivan 2%.

Diprivan has been used in association with spinal and epidural anaesthesia and with commonly used premedicants, neuromuscular blocking drugs, inhalational agents and analgesic agents; no pharmacological incompatibility has been encountered. Lower doses of Diprivan 2% may be required where general anaesthesia is used as an adjunct to regional anaesthetic techniques.

Diprivan 2% should not be diluted.

When Diprivan 2% is used to maintain anaesthesia, it is recommended that equipment such as syringe pumps or volumetric infusion pumps should always be used to control infusion rates.

Diprivan 2% should not be mixed prior to administration with injections or infusion fluids. However, Diprivan 2% may be co-administered via a Y-piece connector close to the injection site with the following:

- Dextrose 5% Intravenous Infusion B.P.
- Sodium Chloride 0.9% Intravenous Infusion B.P.
- Dextrose 4% with Sodium Chloride 0.18% Intravenous Infusion B.P.

4.3 Contraindications
Known hypersensitivity for any of the components of Diprivan 1% or Diprivan 2%.

Diprivan 2% is contraindicated for sedation in intensive care of patients of 16 years of age or younger (See 4.4 Special warnings and precautions for use).

4.4 Special warnings and special precautions for use

Diprivan 2% should be given by those trained in anaesthesia, or where appropriate, doctors trained in the care of patients in Intensive Care. Facilities for maintenance of a patient airway, artificial ventilation and oxygen enrichment should be available.

During induction of anaesthesia, hypotension and transient apnoea may occur depending on the dose and use of premedicants and other agents.

Occasionally, hypotension may require use of intravenous fluids and reduction of the rate of administration of Diprivan 2% during the period of anaesthetic maintenance.

An adequate period is needed prior to discharge of the patient to ensure full recovery after general anaesthesia. Very rarely, the use of Diprivan may be associated with the development of a period of post-operative unconsciousness, which may be accompanied by an increase in muscle tone. This may or may not be preceded by a period of wakefulness. Although recovery is spontaneous, appropriate care of an unconscious patient should be administered.

When Diprivan 2% is administered to an epileptic patient, there may be a risk of convulsion.

As with other sedative agents, when Diprivan is used for sedation during operative procedures, involuntary patient movements may occur. During procedures requiring immobility these movements may be hazardous to the operative site.

As with other intravenous anaesthetic agents, caution should be applied in patients, with cardiac, respiratory, renal or hepatic impairment or in hypovolaemic or debilitated patients.

The risk of relative vagal overactivity may be increased because Diprivan 2% lacks vagolytic activity. Diprivan has been associated with reports of bradycardia (occasionally profound) and also asystole. The intravenous administration of an anticholinergic agent before induction, or during maintenance of anaesthesia should be considered, especially in situations where vagal tone is likely to predominate or when Diprivan 2% is used in conjunction with other agents likely to cause a bradycardia.

Appropriate care should be applied in patients with disorders of fat metabolism and in other conditions where lipid emulsions must be used cautiously.

Use is not recommended with electroconvulsive treatment.

As with other anaesthetics sexual disinhibition may occur during recovery.

Diprivan 2% is not advised for general anaesthesia in children younger than 1 month of age. The safety and efficacy of Diprivan 2% for (background) sedation in children younger than 16 years of age have not been demonstrated. Although no causal relationship has been established, serious undesirable effects with (background) sedation in patients younger than 16 years of age (including cases with fatal outcome) have been reported during unlicensed use. In particular these effects concerned occurrence of metabolic acidosis, hyperlipidemia, rhabdomyolysis and/or cardiac failure. These effects were most frequently seen in children with respiratory tract infections who received dosages in excess of those advised in adults for sedation in the intensive care unit.

Similarly very rare reports have been received of occurrence of metabolic acidosis, rhabdomyolysis, hyperkalaemia and/or rapidly progressive cardiac failure (in some cases with fatal outcome) in adults who were treated for more than 58 hours with dosages in excess of 5 mg/kg/h. This exceeds the maximum dosage of 4 mg/kg/h currently advised for sedation in the intensive care unit. The patients affected were mainly (but not only) seriously head-injured patients with raised ICP. The cardiac failure in such cases was usually unresponsive to inotropic supportive treatment. Treating physicians are reminded if possible not to exceed the dosage of 4 mg/kg/h. Prescribers should be alert to these possible undesirable effects and consider decreasing the Diprivan 2% dosage or switching to an alternative sedative at the first sign of occurrence of symptoms. Patients with raised ICP should be given appropriate treatment to support the cerebral perfusion pressure during these treatment modifications.

Additional Precautions

Diprivan 2% contains no antimicrobial preservatives and supports growth of micro-organisms. Asepsis must be maintained for both Diprivan 2% and infusion equipment throughout the infusion period. Any drugs or fluids added to the Diprivan 2% infusion line must be administered close to the cannula site. Diprivan 2% must not be administered via a microbiological filter.

Diprivan 2% and any syringe containing Diprivan 2% are for single use in an individual patient. For use in long-term maintenance of anaesthesia or sedation in intensive care it is recommended that the infusion line and reservoir of Diprivan 2% be discarded and replaced at regular intervals.

4.5 Interaction with other medicinal products and other forms of Interaction

See Section 4.2.4 Administration.

4.6 Pregnancy and lactation

Pregnancy Teratology studies in rats and rabbits showed no teratogenic effects. Diprivan has been used during termination of pregnancy in the first trimester. Diprivan 2% should not be used in pregnancy.

Obstetrics Diprivan crosses the placenta and may be associated with neonatal depression. It should not be used for obstetric anaesthesia.

Lactation Safety to the neonate has not been established following the use of Diprivan 2% in mothers who are breast feeding. Diprivan 2% should be avoided, or mothers should stop breast feeding.

4.7 Effects on ability to drive and use machines

Patients should be advised that performance at skilled tasks, such as driving and operating machinery, may be impaired for some time after general anaesthesia.

4.8 Undesirable effects

General

Induction of anaesthesia is generally smooth with minimal evidence of excitation.

Side effects during induction, maintenance and recovery occur uncommonly.

The most commonly reported ADRs are pharmacologically predictable side effects of an anaesthetic agent, such as hypotension. Given the nature of anaesthesia and those patients receiving intensive care, events reported in association with anaesthesia and intensive care may also be related to the procedures being undertaken or the recipient's condition.

(see Table 1)

Pulmonary edema, hypotension, asystole, bradycardia, and convulsions, have been reported. In very rare cases rhabdomyolysis, metabolic acidosis, hyperkalaemia or cardiac failure, sometimes with fatal outcome, have been observed when propofol was administered at dosages in excess of 4 mg/kg/h for sedation in the intensive care unit (see 4.4 Special warnings and precautions for use).

Reports from off-label use of Diprivan for induction of anaesthesia in neonates indicates that cardio-respiratory depression may occur if the paediatric dose regimen is applied.

Local

The local pain which may occur during the induction phase can be minimised by the use of the larger veins of the forearm and antecubital fossa. Thrombosis and phlebitis are rare. Accidental clinical extravasation and animal studies showed minimal tissue reaction. Intra-arterial injection in animals did not induce local tissue effects.

4.9 Overdose

Accidental overdosage is likely to cause cardiorespiratory depression. Respiratory depression should be treated by artificial ventilation with oxygen. Cardiovascular depression would require lowering of the patient's head and, if severe, use of plasma expanders and pressor agents.

5. PHARMACOLOGICAL PROPERTIES

5.1 Pharmacodynamic properties

Propofol (2, 6-diisopropylphenol) is a short-acting general anaesthetic agent with a rapid onset of action of approximately 30 seconds. Recovery from anaesthesia is usually rapid. The mechanism of action, like all general anaesthetics, is poorly understood.

In general, falls in mean arterial blood pressure and slight changes in heart rate are observed when Diprivan 2% is administered for induction and maintenance of anaesthesia. However, the haemodynamic parameters normally remain relatively stable during maintenance and the incidence of untoward haemodynamic changes is low.

Although ventilatory depression can occur following administration of Diprivan 2%, any effects are qualitatively similar to those of other intravenous anaesthetic agents and are readily manageable in clinical practice.

Diprivan 2% reduces cerebral blood flow, intracranial pressure and cerebral metabolism. The reduction in intracranial pressure is greater in patients with an elevated baseline intracranial pressure.

Recovery from anaesthesia is usually rapid and clear headed with a low incidence of headache and post-operative nausea and vomiting.

In general, there is less post-operative nausea and vomiting following anaesthesia with Diprivan 2% than following anaesthesia with inhalational agents. There is evidence that this may be related to a reduced emetic potential of propofol.

Diprivan 2%, at the concentrations likely to occur clinically, does not inhibit the synthesis of adrenocortical hormones.

5.2 Pharmacokinetic properties

The decline in propofol concentrations following a bolus dose or following the termination of an infusion can be described by a three compartment open model with very rapid distribution (half-life 2 to 4 minutes), rapid elimination (half-life 30 to 60 minutes), and a slower final phase, representative of redistribution of propofol from poorly perfused tissue.

Table 1

Very common (>1/10)	*General disorders and administration site conditions:*	Local pain on induction (1)
Common (>1/100, <1/10)	*Vascular disorder:*	Hypotension (2)
	Cardiac disorders:	Bradycardia (3)
	Respiratory, thoracic and mediastinal disorders:	Transient apnoea during induction
	Gastrointestinal disorders:	Nausea and vomiting during recovery phase
	Nervous system disorders:	Headache during recovery phase
	General disorders and administration site conditions:	Withdrawal symptoms in children (4)
	Vascular disorders:	Flushing in children (4)
Uncommon (>1/1000, <1/100)	*Vascular disorders:*	Thrombosis and phlebitis
Rare (>1/10 000, <1/1000)	*Nervous system:*	Epileptiform movements, including convulsions and opisthotonus during induction, maintanence and recovery
Very rare (<1/10 000)	*Musculoskeletal and connective tissue disorders:*	Rhabdomyolysis (5)
	Gastrointestinal disorders:	Pancreatitis
	Injury, poisoning and procedural complications:	Post-operative fever
	Renal and urinary disorders:	Discolouration of urine Following prolonged administration
	Immune system disorders:	Anaphylaxis – may include angioedema, bronchospasm, erythema and hypotension
	Reproductive system and breast:	Sexual disinhibition
	Cardiac disorders:	Pulmonary oedema
	Nervous system disorders:	Postoperative unconsciousness

(1) May be minimised by using the larger veins of the forearm and antecubital fossa. With Diprivan 1% local pain can also be minimised by the co-administration of lignocaine.

(2) Occasionally, hypotension may require use of intravenous fluids and reduction of the administration rate of Diprivan.

(3) Serious bradycardias are rare. There have been isolated reports of progression to asystole.

(4) Following abrupt discontinuation of Diprivan during intensive care.

(5) Very rare reports of rhadbomyolysis have been received where Diprivan has been given at doses greater than 4 mg/kg/hr for ICU sedation.

Propofol is extensively distributed and rapidly cleared from the body (total body clearance 1.5 to 2 litres/minute). Clearance occurs by metabolic processes, mainly in the liver, to form inactive conjugates of propofol and its corresponding quinol, which are excreted in urine.

When Diprivan 2% is used to maintain anaesthesia, blood concentrations asymptotically approach the steady-state value for the given administration rate. The pharmacokinetics are linear over the recommended range of infusion rates of Diprivan 2%.

5.3 Preclinical safety data
Propofol is a drug on which extensive clinical experience has been obtained. All relevant information for the prescriber is provided elsewhere in the Summary of Product Characteristics.

6. PHARMACEUTICAL PARTICULARS
6.1 List of excipients
Glycerol Ph Eur
Nitrogen Ph Eur
Purified Egg Phosphatide
Sodium Hydroxide Ph Eur
Soya-Bean Oil Ph Eur
Water for Injections Ph Eur

6.2 Incompatibilities
Diprivan' 2% should not be mixed prior to administration with injections or infusion fluids. However, Diprivan 2% may be co-administered via a Y-piece connector close to the injection site into infusions of the following:
- Dextrose 5% Intravenous Infusion B.P.
- Sodium Chloride 0.9% Intravenous Infusion B.P.
- Dextrose 4% with Sodium Chloride 0.18% Intravenous Infusion B.P.

The neuromuscular blocking agents, atracurium and mivacurium should not be given through the same intravenous line as Diprivan 2% without prior flushing.

6.3 Shelf life
6.3.1 Shelf life of the product as packaged for sale
2 years.
6.3.2 Shelf life after dilution
Diprivan 2% should not be diluted.

6.4 Special precautions for storage
Store between 2°C and 25°C. Do not freeze.

6.5 Nature and contents of container
Emulsion for injection:
50 ml vial containing propofol 20 mg/ml.

6.6 Instructions for use and handling
In-use precautions:
Containers should be shaken before use. Any portion of the contents remaining after use should be discarded.
Diprivan 2% should not be mixed prior to administration with injections or infusion fluids. However, Diprivan 2% may be co-administered via a Y-piece connector close to the injection site into infusions of the following:
- Dextrose 5% Intravenous Infusion B.P.
- Sodium Chloride 0.9% Intravenous Infusion B.P.
- Dextrose 4% with Sodium Chloride 0.18% Intravenous Infusion B.P.

7. MARKETING AUTHORISATION HOLDER
AstraZeneca UK Limited,
600 Capability Green,
Luton, LU1 3LU, UK.

8. MARKETING AUTHORISATION NUMBER(S)
PL 17901/0009

9. DATE OF FIRST AUTHORISATION/RENEWAL OF THE AUTHORISATION
8 July 2000 / 26 February 2002

10. DATE OF REVISION OF THE TEXT
17 February 2004

Diprobase Cream

(Schering-Plough Ltd)

1. NAME OF THE MEDICINAL PRODUCT
Diprobase Cream

2. QUALITATIVE AND QUANTITATIVE COMPOSITION
No pharmacologically active components.

3. PHARMACEUTICAL FORM
Cream

4. CLINICAL PARTICULARS
4.1 Therapeutic indications
Diprobase Cream is an emollient, moisturising and protective cream for the follow-up treatment with topical steroids or in spacing such treatment. It may also be used as diluent for topical steroids. Diprobase Cream is recommended for the symptomatic treatment of red inflamed, damaged, dry or chapped skin, the protection of raw skin areas and as a pre-bathing emollient for dry/eczematous skin to alleviate drying areas.

4.2 Posology and method of administration
Adults and Children:
The cream should be applied to the dry skin areas as often as is required and rubbed well into the skin.

4.3 Contraindications
There are no absolute contraindications to the use of the cream other than hypersensitivity to any of the ingredients.

4.4 Special warnings and special precautions for use
None stated.

4.5 Interaction with other medicinal products and other forms of Interaction
None stated

4.6 Pregnancy and lactation
None stated.

4.7 Effects on ability to drive and use machines
None stated.

4.8 Undesirable effects
Rarely, mild skin reactions have been observed.

4.9 Overdose
None stated.

5. PHARMACOLOGICAL PROPERTIES
5.1 Pharmacodynamic properties
Diprobase Cream contains no active ingredients and has no pharmacological action. The ingredients provide emollient, moisturising action on dry or chapped skin.

5.2 Pharmacokinetic properties
Not applicable due to topical administration and direct action on the skin.

5.3 Preclinical safety data
There are no pre-clinical data of relevance to the prescriber which are additional to that already included in other sections of the SmPC.

6. PHARMACEUTICAL PARTICULARS
6.1 List of excipients
Chlorocresol; Cetomacrogol; Cetostearyl alcohol; Liquid paraffin; White soft paraffin; Phosphoric acid; Sodium dihydrogen phosphate; Purified water.

6.2 Incompatibilities
None Known

6.3 Shelf life
60 months

6.4 Special precautions for storage
Store below 25°C.

6.5 Nature and contents of container
50gm aluminium epoxy lined tubes with plastic caps.
500gm polypropylene piston pack with polyethylene cap and daplen pump, disc and tube or PVC cap, polypropylene pump, polyolefin disc and HDPE tube.

6.6 Instructions for use and handling
Not applicable

7. MARKETING AUTHORISATION HOLDER
Schering-Plough Ltd
Shire Park
Welwyn Garden City
Hertfordshire AL7 1TW
England

8. MARKETING AUTHORISATION NUMBER(S)
PL 0201/0076

9. DATE OF FIRST AUTHORISATION/RENEWAL OF THE AUTHORISATION
12 April 1996

10. DATE OF REVISION OF THE TEXT
29 April 1996

Legal Category
GSL

DipCrm/UK/3-01/2

Diprobase Ointment

(Schering-Plough Ltd)

1. NAME OF THE MEDICINAL PRODUCT
Diprobase Ointment

2. QUALITATIVE AND QUANTITATIVE COMPOSITION
No pharmacologically active components

3. PHARMACEUTICAL FORM
Ointment

4. CLINICAL PARTICULARS
4.1 Therapeutic indications
Diprobase Ointment is an emollient, moisturising and protective ointment for the follow-up treatment with topical steroids or in spacing such treatment. It may also be used as diluent for topical steroids. Diprobase Ointment is recommended for the symptomatic treatment of red inflamed, damaged, dry or chapped skin, the protection of raw skin areas and as a pre-bathing emollient for dry/eczematous skin to alleviate drying areas.

4.2 Posology and method of administration
Adults and Children:
The ointment should be thinly applied to cover the affected area completely, massaging gently and thoroughly into the skin. Frequency of application should be established by the physician. Generally, Diprobase Ointment can be used as often as required.

4.3 Contraindications
Hypersensitivity to any of the components of the ointment is a contraindication to its use.

4.4 Special warnings and special precautions for use
None stated.

4.5 Interaction with other medicinal products and other forms of Interaction
None stated

4.6 Pregnancy and lactation
None stated.

4.7 Effects on ability to drive and use machines
None stated.

4.8 Undesirable effects
Rarely, mild skin reactions have been observed.

4.9 Overdose
None stated.

5. PHARMACOLOGICAL PROPERTIES
5.1 Pharmacodynamic properties
Diprobase Ointment contains no active ingredients and has no pharmacological action. The ingredients have an emollient action on dry or chapped skin.

5.2 Pharmacokinetic properties
Not applicable due to topical administration and direct action on the skin.

5.3 Preclinical safety data
There are no pre-clinical data of relevance to the prescriber which are additional to that already included in other sections of the SmPC.

6. PHARMACEUTICAL PARTICULARS
6.1 List of excipients
White soft paraffin and liquid paraffin.

6.2 Incompatibilities
None Known

6.3 Shelf life
60 months (tube presentations)
24 months (460gm pump dispenser pack)

6.4 Special precautions for storage
Store below 25°C.

6.5 Nature and contents of container
5, 50, 100 and 500gm:Epoxy lined aluminium tubes with plastic caps or polypropylene tubes.
460gm: Polypropylene piston pack with polyethylene cap, polypropylene pump and tube and polyester disc.

6.6 Instructions for use and handling
Not applicable

Administrative Data
7. MARKETING AUTHORISATION HOLDER
Schering-Plough Ltd
Shire Park
Welwyn Garden City
Hertfordshire AL7 1TW
England

8. MARKETING AUTHORISATION NUMBER(S)
PL 0201/0075

9. DATE OF FIRST AUTHORISATION/RENEWAL OF THE AUTHORISATION
12 April 1996

10. DATE OF REVISION OF THE TEXT
January 2002

Legal Category
GSL

Diprobath

(Schering-Plough Ltd)

1. NAME OF THE MEDICINAL PRODUCT
Diprobath

2. QUALITATIVE AND QUANTITATIVE COMPOSITION
Light Liquid Paraffin 46.0% w/w
Isopropyl Myristate 39.0% w/w

3. PHARMACEUTICAL FORM
Liquid bath emollient

4. CLINICAL PARTICULARS
4.1 Therapeutic indications
Treatment of dry skin conditions and other hyperkeratoses, including those associated with dermatitis and eczema.

To be diluted in bath water for external application.

4.2 Posology and method of administration
Adults including elderly patients:

25ml or approximately 2.5 capsful to be diluted in a bath of water (100 L approximately). For particularly dry skin the quantity of oil emollient may be doubled.

Children:

10ml or one capful is sufficient for children's baths.

Frequency and duration of bathing will depend on the type and severity of the conditions, but generally 2 to 3 baths should be taken weekly.

4.3 Contraindications
Known hypersensitivity to any of the ingredients.

4.4 Special warnings and special precautions for use
As Diprobath deposits a film of oil over the skin, care should be taken to avoid slipping in the bath.

The following warning will appear on the label:

'Take care when entering or leaving the bath which may be more slippery than usual'.

4.5 Interaction with other medicinal products and other forms of Interaction
None known.

4.6 Pregnancy and lactation
No special precautions.

4.7 Effects on ability to drive and use machines
None known.

4.8 Undesirable effects
None known.

4.9 Overdose
Not applicable.

5. PHARMACOLOGICAL PROPERTIES
5.1 Pharmacodynamic properties
Both active ingredients have established emollient properties which are of relevance to use as a bathing emollient.

5.2 Pharmacokinetic properties
Pharmacokinetic principles are not involved due to direct topical application.

5.3 Preclinical safety data
There are no pre-clinical data of relevance to the prescriber which are additional to that already included in other sections of the SPC.

6. PHARMACEUTICAL PARTICULARS
6.1 List of excipients
Laureth-4

6.2 Incompatibilities
None Known

6.3 Shelf life
24 months

6.4 Special precautions for storage
Store upright at a temperature below 30°C.

6.5 Nature and contents of container
50ml and 500ml natural opaque HDPE single neck container with polypropylene or urea/formaldehyde, steran or expanded polyethylene wadded screw cap.

6.6 Instructions for use and handling
Not applicable

Administrative Data
7. MARKETING AUTHORISATION HOLDER
Schering-Plough Ltd

Shire Park

Welwyn Garden City

Hertfordshire AL7 1TW

UK

8. MARKETING AUTHORISATION NUMBER(S)
PL 0201/0174

9. DATE OF FIRST AUTHORISATION/RENEWAL OF THE AUTHORISATION
11 November 1991 / 02 January 2001

10. DATE OF REVISION OF THE TEXT
June 2001

Legal Category
P

Diprobath/UK/1-02/2

Diprosalic Ointment

(Schering-Plough Ltd)

1. NAME OF THE MEDICINAL PRODUCT
Diprosalic Ointment

2. QUALITATIVE AND QUANTITATIVE COMPOSITION
Betamethasone Dipropionate 0.064% w/w*
(* equivalent to 0.05% Betamethasone)
Salicylic Acid 3.00% w/w

3. PHARMACEUTICAL FORM
Ointment

4. CLINICAL PARTICULARS
4.1 Therapeutic indications
Betamethasone Dipropionate is a synthetic fluorinated corticosteroid. It is active topically and produces a rapid and sustained response in those inflammatory dermatoses that are normally responsive to topical corticosteroid therapy, and it is also effective in the less responsive conditions, such as psoriasis of the scalp, chronic plaque psoriasis of the hands and feet, but excluding widespread plaque psoriasis.

Topical salicylic acid softens keratin, loosens cornified epithelium and desquamates the epidermis.

Diprosalic presentations are therefore indicated for the treatment of hyperkeratotic and dry corticosteroid-responsive dermatoses where the cornified epithelium may resist penetration of the steroid. The salicylic acid constituent of Diprosalic preparations, as a result of its descaling action, allows access of the dermis more rapidly than by applying steroid alone.

4.2 Posology and method of administration
Adults :

Once to twice daily. In most cases a thin film should be applied to cover the affected area twice daily.

For some patients adequate maintenance therapy may be achieved with less frequent application.

It is recommended that Diprosalic preparations are prescribed for two weeks, and that treatment is reviewed at that time. The maximum weekly dose should not exceed 60g.

Children:

Dosage in children should be limited to 5 days.

4.3 Contraindications
Rosacea, acne, perioral dermatitis, perianal and genital pruritus. Hypersensitivity to any of the ingredients of the Diprosalic presentations contra-indicates their use as does tuberculous and most viral lesions of the skin, particularly herpes simplex, vacinia, varicella. Diprosalic should not be used in napkin eruptions, fungal or bacterial skin infections without suitable concomitant anti-infective therapy.

4.4 Special warnings and special precautions for use
Occlusion must not be used, since under these circumstances the keratolytic action of salicylic acid may lead to enhanced absorption of the steroid.

Local and systemic toxicity is common, especially following long continuous use on large areas of damaged skin, in flexures or with polythene occlusion. If used in children or on the face courses should be limited to 5 days. Long term continuous therapy should be avoided in all patients irrespective of age.

Topical corticosteroids may be hazardous in psoriasis for a number of reasons, including rebound relapses following development of tolerance, risk of generalised pustular psoriasis and local systemic toxicity due to impaired barrier function of the skin. Careful patient supervision is important.

It is dangerous if Diprosalic presentations come into contact with the eyes. Avoid contact with the eyes and mucous membranes.

The systemic absorption of betamethasone dipropionate and salicylic acid may be increased if extensive body surface areas or skin folds are treated for prolonged periods or with excessive amounts of steroids. Suitable precautions should be taken in these circumstances, particularly with infants and children.

4.5 Interaction with other medicinal products and other forms of Interaction
None stated

4.6 Pregnancy and lactation
There is inadequate evidence of safety in human pregnancy. Topical administration of corticosteroids to pregnant animals can cause abnormalities of foetal development, including cleft palate and intrauterine growth retardation. There may therefore, be a very small risk of such effects in the human foetus.

4.7 Effects on ability to drive and use machines
None stated.

4.8 Undesirable effects
Diprosalic skin preparations are generally well tolerated and side-effects are rare.

Continuous application without interruption may result in local atrophy of the skin, striae and superficial vascular dilation, particularly on the face.

In addition, prolonged use of salicylic acid preparations may cause dermatitis.

4.9 Overdose
Excessive prolonged use of topical corticosteroids can suppress pituitary-adrenal functions resulting in secondary adrenal insufficiency which is usually reversible. In such cases appropriate symptomatic treatment is indicated.

With topical preparations containing salicylic acid excessive prolonged use may result in symptoms of salicyclism. Treatment is symptomatic.

The steroid content of each tube is so low as to have little or no toxic effect in the unlikely event of accidental oral ingestion.

5. PHARMACOLOGICAL PROPERTIES
5.1 Pharmacodynamic properties
Diprosalic preparations contain the dipropionate ester of betamethasone which is a glucocorticoid exhibiting the general properties of corticosteroids, and salicylic acid which has keratolytic properties.

Salicylic acid is applied topically in the treatment of hyperkeratotic and scaling conditions where its keratolytic action facilitates penetration of the corticosteroid.

In pharmacological doses, corticosteroids are used primarily for their anti-inflammatory and/or immune suppressive effects.

Topical corticosteroids such as betamethasone dipropionate are effective in the treatment of a range of dermatoses because of their anti-inflammatory, anti-pruritic and vasoconstrictive actions. However, while the physiologic, pharmacologic and clinical effects of the corticosteroids are well known, the exact mechanisms of their action in each disease are uncertain.

5.2 Pharmacokinetic properties
Salicylic acid exerts only local action after topical application.

The extent of percutaneous absorption of topical corticosteroids is determined by many factors including vehicle, integrity of the epidermal barrier and the use of occlusive dressings.

Topical corticosteroids can be absorbed through intact, normal skin. Inflammation and/or other disease processes in the skin may increase percutaneous absorption.

Occlusive dressings substantially increase the percutaneous absorption of topical corticosteroids.

Once absorbed through the skin, topical corticosteroids enter pharmacokinetic pathways similar to systemically administered corticosteroids. Corticosteroids are bound to plasma proteins in varying degrees, are metabolised primarily in the liver and excreted by the kidneys. Some of the topical corticosteroids and their metabolites are also excreted in the bile.

5.3 Preclinical safety data
There are no pre-clinical data of relevance to the prescriber which are additional to that already included in other sections of the SPC.

6. PHARMACEUTICAL PARTICULARS
6.1 List of excipients
Liquid Paraffin

White Soft Paraffin

6.2 Incompatibilities
None Stated.

6.3 Shelf life
60 months

6.4 Special precautions for storage
Do not store above 25°C.

6.5 Nature and contents of container
15, 30 or 100gm expoxy-lined aluminium tubes with plastic caps.

6.6 Instructions for use and handling
Not applicable

Administrative Data
7. MARKETING AUTHORISATION HOLDER
Schering-Plough Ltd

Shire Park

Welwyn Garden City

Hertfordshire AL7 1TW

England

8. MARKETING AUTHORISATION NUMBER(S)
PL 0201/0070

9. DATE OF FIRST AUTHORISATION/RENEWAL OF THE AUTHORISATION
10th June 1986 / 25th July 1997

10. DATE OF REVISION OF THE TEXT
July 2004

Legal Category
POM

Diprosalic-O/UK/10-04/4

Diprosalic Scalp Application

(Schering-Plough Ltd)

1. NAME OF THE MEDICINAL PRODUCT

Diprosalic Scalp Application

2. QUALITATIVE AND QUANTITATIVE COMPOSITION

Betamethasone Dipropionate 0.064% w/w*

(* equivalent to 0.05% Betamethasone)

Salicylic Acid 2.00% w/w

3. PHARMACEUTICAL FORM

Lotion

4. CLINICAL PARTICULARS

4.1 Therapeutic indications

Betamethasone Dipropionate is a synthetic fluorinated corticosteroid. It is active topically and produces a rapid and sustained response in those inflammatory dermatoses that are normally responsive to topical corticosteroid therapy, and it is also effective in the less responsive conditions, such as psoriasis of the scalp.

Topical salicylic acid softens keratin, loosens cornified epithelium and desquamates the epidermis.

Diprosalic presentations are therefore indicated for the treatment of hyperkeratotic and dry corticosteroid-responsive dermatoses where the cornified epithelium may resist penetration of the steroid. The salicylic acid constituent of Diprosalic preparations, as a result of its descaling action, allows access of the dermis more rapidly than by applying steroid alone.

4.2 Posology and method of administration

Adults:

Once to twice daily. In most cases a thin film should be applied to the affected areas twice daily and massaged gently and thoroughly into the skin.

For some patients adequate maintenance therapy may be achieved with less frequent application.

It is recommended that Diprosalic preparations are prescribed for two weeks, and that treatment is reviewed at that time. The maximum weekly dose should not exceed 60g.

Children:

Dosage in children should be limited to 5 days.

4.3 Contraindications

Rosacea, acne, perioral dermatitis, perianal and genital pruritus. Hypersensitivity to any of the ingredients of the Diprosalic presentations contra-indicates their use as does tuberculous and most viral lesions of the skin, particularly herpes simplex, vacinia, varicella. Diprosalic should not be used in napkin eruptions, fungal or bacterial skin infections without suitable concomitant anti-infective therapy.

4.4 Special warnings and special precautions for use

Occlusion must not be used, since under these circumstances the keratolytic action of salicylic acid may lead to enhanced absorption of the steroid.

Local and systemic toxicity is common, especially following long continuous use on large areas of damaged skin, in flexures or with polythene occlusion. If used in children or on the face courses should be limited to 5 days. Long term continuous therapy should be avoided in all patients irrespective of age.

Topical corticosteroids may be hazardous in psoriasis for a number of reasons, including rebound relapses following development of tolerance, risk of generalised pustular psoriasis and local systemic toxicity due to impaired barrier function of the skin. Careful patient supervision is important.

It is dangerous if Diprosalic presentations come into contact with the eyes. Avoid contact with the eyes and mucous membranes.

The systemic absorption of betamethasone dipropionate and salicylic acid may be increased if extensive body surface areas or skin folds are treated for prolonged periods or with excessive amounts of steroids. Suitable precautions should be taken in these circumstances, particularly with infants and children.

4.5 Interaction with other medicinal products and other forms of Interaction

None stated

4.6 Pregnancy and lactation

There is inadequate evidence of safety in human pregnancy. Topical administration of corticosteroids to pregnant animals can cause abnormalities of foetal development, including cleft palate and intrauterine growth retardation. There may therefore, be a very small risk of such effects in the human foetus.

4.7 Effects on ability to drive and use machines

None stated.

4.8 Undesirable effects

Diprosalic skin preparations are generally well tolerated and side-effects are rare.

Continuous application without interruption may result in local atrophy of the skin, striae and superficial vascular dilation, particularly on the face.

In addition, prolonged use of salicylic acid preparations may cause dermatitis.

4.9 Overdose

Excessive prolonged use of topical corticosteroids can suppress pituitary-adrenal functions resulting in secondary adrenal insufficiency which is usually reversible. In such cases appropriate symptomatic treatment is indicated.

With topical preparations containing salicylic acid excessive prolonged use may result in symptoms of salicyclism. Treatment is symptomatic.

The steroid content of each tube is so low as to have little or no toxic effect in the unlikely event of accidental oral ingestion.

5. PHARMACOLOGICAL PROPERTIES

5.1 Pharmacodynamic properties

Diprosalic preparations contain the dipropionate ester of betamethasone which is a glucocorticoid exhibiting the general properties of corticosteroids, and salicylic acid which has keratolytic properties.

Salicylic acid is applied topically in the treatment of hyperkeratotic and scaling conditions where its keratolytic action facilitates penetration of the corticosteroid.

In pharmacological doses, corticosteroids are used primarily for their anti-inflammatory and/or immune suppressive effects.

Topical corticosteroids such as betamethasone dipropionate are effective in the treatment of a range of dermatoses because of their anti-inflammatory, anti-pruritic and vasoconstrictive actions. However, while the physiologic, pharmacologic and clinical effects of the corticosteroids are well known, the exact mechanisms of their action in each disease are uncertain.

5.2 Pharmacokinetic properties

Salicylic acid exerts only local action after topical application.

The extent of percutaneous absorption of topical corticosteroids is determined by many factors including vehicle, integrity of the epidermal barrier and the use of occlusive dressings.

Topical corticosteroids can be absorbed through intact, normal skin. Inflammation and/or other disease processes in the skin may increase percutaneous absorption.

Occlusive dressings substantially increase the percutaneous absorption of topical corticosteroids.

Once absorbed through the skin, topical corticosteroids enter pharmacokinetic pathways similar to systemically administered corticosteroids. Corticosteroids are bound to plasma proteins in varying degrees, are metabolised primarily in the liver and excreted by the kidneys. Some of the topical corticosteroids and their metabolites are also excreted in the bile.

5.3 Preclinical safety data

There are no pre-clinical data of relevance to the prescriber which are additional to that already included in other sections of the SPC.

6. PHARMACEUTICAL PARTICULARS

6.1 List of excipients

Disodium edetate

Hydroxypropyl methylcellulose

Sodium hydroxide

Isopropyl alcohol

Purified water

6.2 Incompatibilities

None Stated.

6.3 Shelf life

24 months

6.4 Special precautions for storage

Do not store above 25°C.

6.5 Nature and contents of container

30ml or 100ml polyethylene containers with polypropylene closures

6.6 Instructions for use and handling

Not applicable

Administrative Data

7. MARKETING AUTHORISATION HOLDER

Schering-Plough Ltd

Shire Park

Welwyn Garden City

Hertfordshire AL7 1TW

England

8. MARKETING AUTHORISATION NUMBER(S)

0201/0069

9. DATE OF FIRST AUTHORISATION/RENEWAL OF THE AUTHORISATION

30 July 1997

10. DATE OF REVISION OF THE TEXT

July 2004

Legal Category

POM

Diprosalic-SA/UK/10-04/5

Diprosone Cream & Ointment

(Schering-Plough Ltd)

1. NAME OF THE MEDICINAL PRODUCT

Diprosone Cream and Ointment

2. QUALITATIVE AND QUANTITATIVE COMPOSITION

Betamethasone Dipropionate 0.064% w/w*

(* equivalent to 0.05% Betamethasone)

3. PHARMACEUTICAL FORM

Cream

Ointment

4. CLINICAL PARTICULARS

4.1 Therapeutic indications

Betamethasone Dipropionate is a synthetic fluorinated corticosteroid. It is active topically and produces a rapid and sustained response in eczema and dermatitis of all types, including atopic eczema, photodermatitis., lichen planus, lichen simplex, prurigo nodularis, discoid lupus erythematosus, necrobiosis lipoidica, pretibial myxodemea and erythroderma. It is also effective in the less responsive conditions such as psoriasis of the scalp and chronic plaque psoriasis of the hands and feet, but excluding widespread plaque psoriasis.

4.2 Posology and method of administration

Adults and Children:

Once to twice daily. In most cases a thin film of Diprosone Cream or Ointment should be applied to cover the affected area twice daily. For some patients adequate maintenance therapy may be achieved with less frequent application.

Diprosone Cream is especially appropriate for moist or weeping surfaces and the ointment for dry, lichenifield or scaly lesions but this is not invariably so.

Control over the dosage regimen may be achieved during intermittent and maintenance therapy by using Diprobase Cream or Ointment, (PL 0201/0076 and 0201/0075), the base vehicles of Diprosone Cream and Ointment. Such control may be necessary in mild and improving dry skin conditions requiring low dose steroid treatment.

4.3 Contraindications

Rosacea, acne, perioral dermatitis, perianal and genital pruritus. Hypersensitivity to any of the ingredients of the Diprosone presentations contra-indicates their use as does tuberculous and most viral lesions of the skin, particularly herpes simplex, vacinia, varicella. Diprosone should not be used in napkin eruptions, fungal or bacterial skin infections without suitable concomitant anti-infective therapy.

4.4 Special warnings and special precautions for use

Local and systemic toxicity is common, especially following long continuous use on large areas of damaged skin, in flexures or with polythene occlusion. If used in children or on the face courses should be limited to 5 days. Long term continuous therapy should be avoided in all patients irrespective of age.

Occlusion must not be used.

Topical corticosteroids may be hazardous in psoriasis for a number of reasons, including rebound relapses following development of tolerance, risk of generalised pustular psoriasis and local systemic toxicity due to impaired barrier function of the skin. Careful patient supervision is important.

4.5 Interaction with other medicinal products and other forms of Interaction

None stated

4.6 Pregnancy and lactation

There is inadequate evidence of safety in human pregnancy. Topical administration of corticosteroids to pregnant animals can cause abnormalities of foetal development, including cleft palate and intrauterine growth retardation. There may therefore, be a very small risk of such effects in the human foetus.

4.7 Effects on ability to drive and use machines

None stated.

4.8 Undesirable effects

Diprosone skin preparations are generally well tolerated and side-effects are rare. The systemic absorption of betamethasone dipropionate may be increased if extensive body surface areas or skin folds are treated for prolonged periods or with excessive amounts of steroids. Suitable precautions should be taken in these circumstances, particularly with infants and children.

Continuous application without interruption may result in local atrophy of the skin, striae and superficial vascular dilation, particularly on the face.

4.9 Overdose

Excessive prolonged use of topical corticosteroids can suppress pituitary-adrenal functions resulting in secondary adrenal insufficiency which is usually reversible. In such cases appropriate symptomatic treatment is indicated.

The steroid content of each tube is so low as to have little or no toxic effect in the unlikely event of accidental oral ingestion.

5. PHARMACOLOGICAL PROPERTIES

5.1 Pharmacodynamic properties

Diprosone preparations contain the dipropionate ester of betamethasone which is a glucocorticoid exhibiting the general properties of corticosteroids.

In pharmacological doses, corticosteroids are used primarily for their anti-inflammatory and/or immune suppressive effects.

Topical corticosteroids such as betamethasone dipropionate are effective in the treatment of a range of dermatoses because of their anti-inflammatory, anti-pruritic and vasoconstrictive actions. However, while the physiologic, pharmacologic and clinical effects of the corticosteroids are well known, the exact mechanisms of their action in each disease are uncertain.

5.2 Pharmacokinetic properties

The extent of percutaneous absorption of topical corticosteroids is determined by many factors including vehicle, integrity of the epidermal barrier and the use of occlusive dressings.

Topical corticosteroids can be absorbed through intact, normal skin. Inflammation and/or other disease processes in the skin may increase percutaneous absorption.

Occlusive dressings substantially increase the percutaneous absorption of topical corticosteroids.

Once absorbed through the skin, topical corticosteroids enter pharmacokinetic pathways similar to systemically administered corticosteroids. Corticosteroids are bound to plasma proteins in varying degrees, are metabolised primarily in the liver and excreted by the kidneys. Some of the topical corticosteroids and their metabolites are also excreted in the bile.

5.3 Preclinical safety data

There are no pre-clinical data of relevance to the prescriber which are additional to that already included in other sections of the SPC.

6. PHARMACEUTICAL PARTICULARS

6.1 List of excipients

Diprosone Cream: Chlorocresol, Sodium dihydrogen phosphate, Phosphoric Acid, White Soft Paraffin, Liquid Paraffin, Cetomacrogol 1000, Cetostearyl Alcohol and Purified Water

Diprosone Ointment: Liquid Paraffin and White Soft Paraffin.

6.2 Incompatibilities

None Known

6.3 Shelf life

60 months

6.4 Special precautions for storage

Do not store above 25°C.

6.5 Nature and contents of container

30 or 100g expoxy-lined aluminium tubes with polypropylene caps.

6.6 Instructions for use and handling

Not applicable

7. MARKETING AUTHORISATION HOLDER

Schering-Plough Ltd

Shire Park

Welwyn Garden City

Hertfordshire AL7 1TW

England

8. MARKETING AUTHORISATION NUMBER(S)

Cream: PL 0201/0072

Ointment: PL 0201/0074

9. DATE OF FIRST AUTHORISATION/RENEWAL OF THE AUTHORISATION

10. DATE OF REVISION OF THE TEXT

May 1999

Legal Category

POM

DipsoC&O/UK/7-77/3

Diprosone Lotion

(Schering-Plough Ltd)

1. NAME OF THE MEDICINAL PRODUCT

Diprosone Lotion

2. QUALITATIVE AND QUANTITATIVE COMPOSITION

Betamethasone Dipropionate 0.064% w/w*

(* equivalent to 0.05% Betamethasone)

3. PHARMACEUTICAL FORM

Lotion

4. CLINICAL PARTICULARS

4.1 Therapeutic indications

Diprosone Lotion is indicated for eczema and dermatitis of all types effecting the scalp including atopic eczema, photodermatitis, primary irritant and allergic dermatitis, lichen planus, lichen simplex, discoid lupus erythematosus, erythroderma.

It is also indicated for psoriasis of the scalp.

4.2 Posology and method of administration

Adults and Children:

A few drops of Diprosone Lotion should be applied to the affected areas twice daily and massaged gently and thoroughly into the affected area. For some patients adequate maintenance therapy may be achieved with less frequent application.

4.3 Contraindications

Rosacea, acne, perioral dermatitis, perianal and genital pruritus. Hypersensitivity to any of the ingredients of the Diprosone presentations contraindicates their use as does tuberculous and most viral lesions of the skin, particularly herpes simplex, vacinia, varicella. Diprosone should not be used in napkin eruptions, fungal or bacterial skin infections without suitable concomitant anti-infective therapy.

4.4 Special warnings and special precautions for use

Local and systemic toxicity is common, especially following long continuous use on large areas of damaged skin, in flexures or with polythene occlusion. If used in children or on the face courses should be limited to 5 days. Long term continuous therapy should be avoided in all patients irrespective of age.

Occlusion must not be used.

Topical corticosteroids may be hazardous in psoriasis for a number of reasons, including rebound relapses following development of tolerance, risk of generalised pustular psoriasis and local systemic toxicity due to impaired barrier function of the skin. Careful patient supervision is important.

4.5 Interaction with other medicinal products and other forms of Interaction

None stated

4.6 Pregnancy and lactation

There is inadequate evidence of safety in human pregnancy. Topical administration of corticosteroids to pregnant animals can cause abnormalities of foetal development, including cleft palate and intrauterine growth retardation. There may therefore, be a very small risk of such effects in the human foetus.

4.7 Effects on ability to drive and use machines

None stated.

4.8 Undesirable effects

Diprosone skin preparations are generally well tolerated and side-effects are rare. The systemic absorption of betamethasone dipropionate may be increased if extensive body surface areas or skin folds are treated for prolonged periods or with excessive amounts of steroids. Suitable precautions should be taken in these circumstances, particularly with infants and children.

Continuous application without interruption may result in local atrophy of the skin, striae and superficial vascular dilation, particularly on the face.

4.9 Overdose

Excessive prolonged use of topical corticosteroids can suppress pituitary-adrenal functions resulting in secondary adrenal insufficiency which is usually reversible. In such cases appropriate symptomatic treatment is indicated.

The steroid content of each tube is so low as to have little or no toxic effect in the unlikely event of accidental oral ingestion.

5. PHARMACOLOGICAL PROPERTIES

5.1 Pharmacodynamic properties

Diprosone preparations contain the dipropionate ester of betamethasone which is a glucocorticoid exhibiting the general properties of corticosteroids.

In pharmacological doses, corticosteroids are used primarily for their anti-inflammatory and/or immune suppressive effects.

Topical corticosteroids such as betamethasone dipropionate are effective in the treatment of a range of dermatoses because of their anti-inflammatory, anti-pruritic and vasoconstrictive actions. However, while the physiologic, pharmacologic and clinical effects of the corticosteroids are well known, the exact mechanisms of their action in each disease are uncertain.

5.2 Pharmacokinetic properties

The extent of percutaneous absorption of topical corticosteroids is determined by many factors including vehicle, integrity of the epidermal barrier and the use of occlusive dressings.

Topical corticosteroids can be absorbed through intact, normal skin. Inflammation and/or other disease processes in the skin may increase percutaneous absorption.

Occlusive dressings substantially increase the percutaneous absorption of topical corticosteroids.

Once absorbed through the skin, topical corticosteroids enter pharmacokinetic pathways similar to systemically administered corticosteroids. Corticosteroids are bound to plasma proteins in varying degrees, are metabolised primarily in the liver and excreted by the kidneys. Some of the topical corticosteroids and their metabolites are also excreted in the bile.

5.3 Preclinical safety data

There are no pre-clinical data of relevance to the prescriber which are additional to that already included in other sections of the SPC.

6. PHARMACEUTICAL PARTICULARS

6.1 List of excipients

Carbomer, Isopropyl Alcohol, Sodium Hydroxide and Purified Water.

6.2 Incompatibilities

None Known

6.3 Shelf life

36 months

6.4 Special precautions for storage

Store in a cool place.

6.5 Nature and contents of container

Polyethylene containers of 5, 30 or 100ml with polyethylene closures.

6.6 Instructions for use and handling

Not applicable

Administrative Data

7. MARKETING AUTHORISATION HOLDER

Schering-Plough Ltd

Shire Park

Welwyn Garden City

Hertfordshire AL7 1TW

England

8. MARKETING AUTHORISATION NUMBER(S)

PL 0201/0073

9. DATE OF FIRST AUTHORISATION/RENEWAL OF THE AUTHORISATION

30 July 1997

10. DATE OF REVISION OF THE TEXT

March 2002

Legal Category

POM

Dip-O/UK/8-03/2

Dipyridamole 50mg/5ml Oral Suspension

(Rosemont Pharmaceuticals Limited)

1. NAME OF THE MEDICINAL PRODUCT

Dipyridamole 50mg/5ml Oral Suspension

2. QUALITATIVE AND QUANTITATIVE COMPOSITION

Dipyridamole 50mg/5ml

For excipients see section 6.1

3. PHARMACEUTICAL FORM

Oral Suspension

Bright yellow suspension with odour of almond

4. CLINICAL PARTICULARS

4.1 Therapeutic indications

An adjunct to oral anticoagulation for prophylaxis of thromboembolism associated with prosthetic heart valves.

4.2 Posology and method of administration

Administration:

For oral use only.

Dipyridamole suspension should usually be taken before meals.

Adults: 300mg to a maximum of 600mg daily in three or four doses.

Children: Dipyridamole is not recommended for children.

4.3 Contraindications

Hypersensitivity to any of the ingredients in the product.

4.4 Special warnings and special precautions for use

Among other properties, dipyridamole acts as a vasodilator. It should be used with caution in patients with severe coronary artery disease, including unstable angina and/or recent myocardial infarction, left ventricular outflow obstruction or haemodynamic instability (e.g. decompensated heart failure).

Dipyridamole should be used with caution in patients with coagulation disorders.

In patients with myasthenia gravis, readjustment of therapy may be necessary after changes in dipyridamole dosage (see Drug Interactions).

Patients treated with regular oral doses of dipyridamole should not receive additional intravenous dipyridamole. If pharmacological stress testing with intravenous dipyridamole for coronary artery disease is considered necessary, then oral dipyridamole should be discontinued 24 hours prior to testing.

Excipients in the formulation

Dipyridamole suspension contains liquid maltitol. Patients with a rare hereditary problems of fructose intolerance should not take this medicine.

The medicine also contains parahydroxybenzoates which are known to cause urticaria, generally delayed type reactions such as contact dermatitis and rarely, immediate reaction with urticaria and bronchospasm.

4.5 Interaction with other medicinal products and other forms of Interaction

Adenosine:

Dipyridamole increases plasma levels and cardiovascular effects of adenosine. Adjustment of adenosine dosage should be considered if use with dipyridamole is unavoidable.

Aspirin:

There is evidence that the effects of aspirin and dipyridamole on platelet behaviour are additive.

Antacids:

The administration of antacids may reduce the efficacy of dipyridamole.

Anticoagulants:

It is possible that dipyridamole may enhance the effects of oral anticoagulants. When dipyridamole is used in combination with anticoagulants and acetylsalicylic acid, the statements on intolerance and risks for these preparations must be observed. Addition of dipyridamole to acetylsalicylic acid does not increase the incidence of bleeding events. When dipyridamole was administered concomitantly with warfarin, bleeding was no greater in frequency or severity than that observed when warfarin was administered alone.

Anti-Hypertensives:

Dipyridamole may increase the hypotensive effect of drugs which reduce blood pressure.

Anti-cholinesterases:

Dipyridamole may counteract the anticholinesterase effect of cholinesterase inhibitors thereby potentially aggravating myasthenia gravis.

4.6 Pregnancy and lactation

There is inadequate evidence of safety in human pregnancy but dipyridamole has been used for many years without apparent ill consequence. Animal studies have shown no hazard. Medicines should not be used in pregnancy, especially in the first trimester, unless the expected benefit is thought to outweigh the possible risk to the foetus.

Dipyridamole is excreted in breast milk at levels approximately 6% of the plasma concentration. Therefore, dipyridamole should only be used during lactation if considered essential by the physician.

4.7 Effects on ability to drive and use machines

None stated.

4.8 Undesirable effects

If side effects do occur, it is usually during the early part of treatment.

Blood and the lymphatic system disorders

Isolated cases of thrombocytopenia have been reported in conjunction with treatment of dipyridamole.

Cardiac Disorders

In rare cases, worsening of symptoms of coronary heart disease has been observed.

Vascular Disorders

The vasodilating properties may occasionally produce a vascular headache which normally disappears with long-term use.

As a result of its vasodilator properties, dipyridamole may cause hypotension, hot flushes and tachycardia.

Hepato-biliary disorders

Dipyridamole has been shown to be incorporated into gallstones.

General Disorders

Vomiting, diarrhoea and symptoms such as dizziness, faintness, nausea, dyspepsia, and myalgia have been observed.

Hypersensitivity reactions such as rash, urticaria, severe bronchospasm and angio-oedema have been reported.

Surgical and medical procedures

In very rare cases, increased bleeding during or after surgery has been observed.

4.9 Overdose

Due to the low number of observations, experience with dipyridamole overdose is limited. Symptoms such as a warm feeling, flushes, sweating, restlessness, feeling of weakness, dizziness and anginal complaints can be expected. A drop in blood pressure and tachycardia might be observed.

Symptomatic therapy is recommended. Administration of xanthine derivatives (e.g. aminophylline) may reverse the haemodynamic effects of dipyridamole overdose. Due to its wide distribution to tissues and its predominantly hepatic elimination, dipyridamole is not likely to be accessible to enhanced removal procedures.

5. PHARMACOLOGICAL PROPERTIES

5.1 Pharmacodynamic properties

Dipyridamole has an antithrombotic action based on its ability to modify various aspects of platelet function, such as platelet aggregation, adhesion and survival, which have been shown to be factors associated with the initiation of thrombus formation. Dipyridamole also has coronary vasodilator properties.

5.2 Pharmacokinetic properties

Oral administration of dipyridamole gives a peak plasma level 0.5 - 2 hours after dosing. The drug has an apparent bioavailability of 37-66%. These figures were obtained with other oral immediate release forms of dipyridamole.

The volume of distribution is 2.43 ± 1.1l/kg. When given orally the elimination half life is 9 –12 hours. The major route of excretion of dipyridamole is in the bile.

5.3 Preclinical safety data

There are no preclinical data of relevance to the prescriber additional to those already included in other sections of the SPC.

6. PHARMACEUTICAL PARTICULARS

6.1 List of excipients

Methyl hydroxybenzoate (E218), propyl hydroxybenzoate (E216), propylene glycol (E1520), xanthan gum (E415), ammonium glycyrrhizinate, almond flavour (including propylene glycol and ethanol), levomenthol, liquid maltitol (E965), polysorbate 80 (E433), simethicone emulsion, aluminium magnesium silicate, disodium hydrogen phosphate (E339), citric acid monohydrate (E330) and purified water.

6.2 Incompatibilities

Not applicable.

6.3 Shelf life

24 months

1 month- once open

6.4 Special precautions for storage

Do not store above 25°C.

6.5 Nature and contents of container

Bottle: Amber (Type III) glass

Closure: HDPE, EPE wadded, tamper evident screw cap

HDPE, EPE wadded, tamper evident, child resistant closure.

Capacity: 150ml

6.6 Instructions for use and handling

This product may settle during storage. Please shake the bottle thoroughly before use.

7. MARKETING AUTHORISATION HOLDER

Rosemont Pharmaceuticals Ltd, Rosemont House, Yorkdale Industrial Park, Braithwaite Street, Leeds, LS11 9XE, UK

8. MARKETING AUTHORISATION NUMBER(S)

PL 00427/0133

9. DATE OF FIRST AUTHORISATION/RENEWAL OF THE AUTHORISATION

8/8/02

10. DATE OF REVISION OF THE TEXT

9/02

Disipal Tablets

(Astellas Pharma Limited)

1. NAME OF THE MEDICINAL PRODUCT

DISIPAL TABLETS

2. QUALITATIVE AND QUANTITATIVE COMPOSITION

Orphenadrine hydrochloride BP 50 mg

3. PHARMACEUTICAL FORM

Tablet

4. CLINICAL PARTICULARS

4.1 Therapeutic indications

Anti-cholinergic, for the treatment of all forms of Parkinsonism, including drug-induced extra-pyramidal symptoms (neuroleptic syndrome).

4.2 Posology and method of administration

For Adults, and the Elderly:

Initially 150 mg daily in divided doses, increasing by 50 mg every two or three days until maximum benefit is obtained. Optimal dosage is usually 250 - 300 mg daily in divided doses in idiopathic and post-encephalitic Parkinsonism, 100 - 300 mg daily in divided doses in the neuroleptic syndrome. Maximal dosage, 400 mg daily in divided doses. The elderly may be more susceptible to side-effects at doses which are clinically optimal.

For children:

A dosage for children has not been established.

4.3 Contraindications

Contraindicated in patients with tardive dyskinesia, glaucoma, or prostatic hypertrophy, untreated urinary retention, gastro-intestinal obstruction, porphyria.

4.4 Special warnings and special precautions for use

Use with caution in patients with micturition difficulties, in pregnancy and breast feeding, and in the presence of cardiovascular disease and hepatic or renal impairment. Use in caution in the elderly (see 4.2). Avoid abrupt discontinuation of treatment. For some patients, orphenadrine may be a drug of abuse.

The sodium benzoate E211 used in the sugar coat can be mildly irritating to the skin, eyes and mucous membranes.

4.5 Interaction with other medicinal products and other forms of Interaction

Concomitant use of other antimuscarinic drugs can lead to an increase in side effects such as dry mouth and urine retention.

4.6 Pregnancy and lactation

No recommendations; if considered necessary, it should be used with caution, see 4.4.

4.7 Effects on ability to drive and use machines

Patients must be advised to exercise caution while driving or operating machinery or whilst carrying out other skilled tasks.

4.8 Undesirable effects

Occasionally dry mouth, disturbances of visual accommodation, gastro-intestinal disturbances, dizziness and micturition difficulties may occur; these usually disappear spontaneously or may be controlled by a slight reduction in dosage. Less commonly, tachycardia, hypersensitivity, nervousness, euphoria and insomnia may be seen.

4.9 Overdose

Toxic effects are anti-cholinergic in nature and the treatment is gastric lavage, cholinergics such as carbachol, anticholinesterases such as physostigmine, and general non-specific treatment.

5. PHARMACOLOGICAL PROPERTIES

5.1 Pharmacodynamic properties

Orphenadrine, which is a congener of diphenhydramine without sharing its soporific effect, is an antimuscarinic agent. It also has weak antihistaminic and local anaesthetic properties.

Orphenadrine is used as the hydrochloride in the symptomatic treatment of Parkinsonism. It is also used to alleviate the extrapyramidal syndrome induced by drugs such as the phenothiazine derivatives, but is of no value in tardive dyskinesia, which may be exacerbated.

5.2 Pharmacokinetic properties

Orphenadrine is readily absorbed from the gastro-intestinal tract, and very readily absorbed following intramuscular injection. It is rapidly distributed in tissues and most of a dose is metabolised and excreted in the urine along with a small proportion of unchanged drug. A half life of 14 hours has been reported.

5.3 Preclinical safety data

No relevant pre-clinical safety data has been generated

6. PHARMACEUTICAL PARTICULARS

6.1 List of excipients

Lactose

Sucrose

Acacia

Maize starch

Tribasic calcium phosphate

Stearic acid

Magnesium stearate

Opaseal P-17-0200 (containing IMS, polyvinylacetate phthalate and stearic acid)

Calcium carbonate

Talc

Kaolin

Titanium dioxide

Gelatin

Opalux yellow AS 3026 (containing sucrose, titanium dioxide, tartrazine E102, sunset yellow E110, povidone, amaranth E123 and sodium benzoate E211)

Opaglos 6000 (containing ethanol, shellac, beeswax and yellow carnuba wax)

Black printing ink

6.2 Incompatibilities

None

6.3 Shelf life

Three years

6.4 Special precautions for storage

Store at room temperature (15°C - 25°C)

6.5 Nature and contents of container

Amber glass click-lock bottles and/or securitainers and/or plastic lid-seal containers, containing 100, 250, 1,000, or 10,000 tablets.

6.6 Instructions for use and handling

None

Administrative Data

7. MARKETING AUTHORISATION HOLDER

Yamanouchi Pharma Ltd
Yamanouchi House
Pyrford Road
West Byfleet
Surrey
KT14 6RA

8. MARKETING AUTHORISATION NUMBER(S)

PL 0166/5001R

9. DATE OF FIRST AUTHORISATION/RENEWAL OF THE AUTHORISATION

6 May 1987; renewed March 2003.

10. DATE OF REVISION OF THE TEXT

17 March 2004.

11. Legal Category

POM

Distaclor MR Tablets

(Flynn Pharma Ltd)

1. NAME OF THE MEDICINAL PRODUCT

Distaclor MR* tablets.

2. QUALITATIVE AND QUANTITATIVE COMPOSITION

Each extended release tablet contains cefaclor monohydrate equivalent to 375mg of cefaclor as active ingredient.

3. PHARMACEUTICAL FORM

Extended release tablets of cefaclor 'Modified Release' are blue and engraved with 'Distaclor MR 375' or 'Lilly TA4220'.

4. CLINICAL PARTICULARS

4.1 Therapeutic indications

Distaclor MR is indicated in the treatment of the following infections when caused by susceptible strains of the designated organisms:

Acute bronchitis and acute exacerbations of chronic bronchitis caused by *Streptococcus pneumoniae, Haemophilus influenzae* (including beta-lactamase producing strains), *Haemophilus parainfluenzae, Moraxella catarrhalis* (including beta-lactamase producing strains) and *Staphylococcus aureus.*

Pharyngitis and tonsillitis caused by *Streptococcus pyogenes* (group A streptococci).

Pneumonia caused by *S. pneumoniae, H. influenzae* (including beta-lactamase producing strains) and *M. catarrhalis* (including beta-lactamase producing strains).

Uncomplicated lower urinary tract infections, including cystitis and asymptomatic bacteriuria, caused by *Escherichia coli, Klebsiella pneumoniae, Proteus mirabilis* and *Staphylococcus saprophyticus.*

Skin and skin structure infections caused by *S. pyogenes* (group A streptococci), *S. aureus* (including beta-lactamase producing strains) and *Staphylococcus epidermidis* (including beta-lactamase producing strains).

Bacteriological studies, to determine the causative organism and its susceptibility to cefaclor, should be performed. Therapy may be started while awaiting the results of these studies. Once these results become available, antimicrobial therapy should be adjusted accordingly.

Note: Distaclor MR is generally effective in the eradication of streptococci from the oropharynx. However, data establishing the efficacy of this antibiotic in the subsequent prevention of rheumatic fever are not available.

4.2 Posology and method of administration

Distaclor MR is administered orally.

Adults and the elderly:

Pharyngitis, bronchitis, tonsillitis, skin and skin structure infections: 375mg twice daily.

Lower urinary tract infections: 375mg twice daily.

Pneumonia: 750mg twice daily.

In clinical trials, doses of 1.5g/day of Distaclor MR have been administered safely for 14 days. Doses of 4g/day of cefaclor have been administered safely, to normal subjects, for 28 days.

Elderly subjects with normal renal function do not require dosage adjustment.

Children: The safety and effectiveness of Distaclor MR have not been established. Cefaclor suspensions are available (see Distaclor Summary of Product Characteristics for dosages).

In the treatment of infections caused by *S. pyogenes* (group A streptococci), a therapeutic dosage should be administered for at least 10 days.

Distaclor MR is well absorbed from the gastro-intestinal tract. Since absorption is enhanced by administration with food, Distaclor MR should be taken with meals.

The tablets should not be cut, crushed or chewed.

There is no evidence of metabolism in humans.

4.3 Contraindications

Hypersensitivity to cefaclor and other cephalosporins.

4.4 Special warnings and special precautions for use

Warnings

Before instituting therapy with cefaclor, every effort should be made to determine whether the patient has had previous hypersensitivity reactions to the cephalosporins, penicillins or other drugs. Cefaclor should be given cautiously to penicillin-sensitive patients and to any patient who has demonstrated some form of allergy, particularly to drugs.

If an allergic reaction to cefaclor occurs, the drug should be discontinued and the patient treated with the appropriate agents.

Pseudomembranous colitis has been reported with virtually all broad-spectrum antibiotics, including macrolides, semi-synthetic penicillins and cephalosporins. It is important, therefore, to consider its diagnosis in patients who develop diarrhoea in association with the use of antibiotics. Such colitis may range in severity from mild to life-threatening. Mild cases usually respond to drug discontinuance alone. In moderate to severe cases, appropriate measures should be taken.

Precautions

Prolonged use of cefaclor may result in the overgrowth of non-susceptible organisms. If superinfection occurs during therapy, appropriate measures should be taken.

A false-positive reaction for glucose in the urine may occur with Benedict's or Fehling's solutions or with copper sulphate test tablets.

4.5 Interaction with other medicinal products and other forms of Interaction

The extent of absorption of Distaclor MR is diminished if magnesium hydroxide or aluminium hydroxide containing antacids are taken within 1 hour of administration. H_2-blockers do not alter either the rate or extent of absorption.

The renal excretion of cefaclor is inhibited by probenecid.

4.6 Pregnancy and lactation

Usage in pregnancy: Although animal studies have shown no evidence of impaired fertility or harm to the foetus due to cefaclor, there are no adequate and well-controlled studies in pregnant women. Distaclor MR should be used during pregnancy only if clearly needed.

Usage in nursing mothers: Small amounts of cefaclor have been detected in breast milk following administration of single 500mg doses. Average levels of about 0.2 micrograms/ml or less were detected up to 5 hours later. Trace amounts were detected at one hour. As the effect on nursing infants is not known, caution should be exercised when cefaclor is administered to a nursing woman. No studies have been done with Distaclor MR.

Usage during labour and delivery: Treatment should be given only if clearly needed.

4.7 Effects on ability to drive and use machines

None known.

4.8 Undesirable effects

The majority of adverse reactions observed in clinical trials of Distaclor MR were mild and transient. Drug-related adverse reactions requiring discontinuation of therapy occurred in 1.7% of patients. The following adverse reactions were reported in clinical trials. Incidence rates were less than 1 in 100 (less than 1%), except as stated:

Gastro-intestinal: Diarrhoea (3.4%), nausea (2.5%), vomiting and dyspepsia.

Hypersensitivity: Rash, urticaria or pruritus occurred in approximately 1.7% of patients. One serum sickness-like reaction (0.03%) was reported among the 3,272 patients treated with Distaclor MR during the controlled clinical trials.

Serum sickness-like reactions (erythema multiforme minor, rashes or other skin manifestations accompanied by arthritis/arthralgia, with or without fever) have been reported with cefaclor. Lymphadenopathy and proteinuria are infrequent; there are no circulating immune complexes and no evidence of sequelae. Occasionally, solitary symptoms may occur but do not represent a serum sickness-like reaction. Serum sickness-like reactions are apparently due to hypersensitivity and have usually occurred during or following a second (or subsequent) course of therapy with cefaclor. Such reactions have been reported more frequently in children than in adults. Signs and symptoms usually occur a few days after initiation of therapy and usually subside within a few days of cessation of therapy. Antihistamines and corticosteroids appear to enhance resolution of the syndrome. No serious sequelae have been reported.

Haematological and lymphatic systems: Eosinophilia.

Genitourinary: Vaginal moniliasis (2.5%) and vaginitis (1.7%).

The following adverse effects have been reported, but causal relationship is uncertain:

Central nervous system: Headache, dizziness and somnolence.

Hepatic: Transient elevations in AST, ALT and alkaline phosphatase.

Renal: Transient increase in BUN or creatinine.

Laboratory tests: Transient thrombocytopenia, leucopenia, lymphocytosis, neutropenia and abnormal urinalysis.

In addition to the adverse reactions listed above that have been observed in patients taking Distaclor MR, the following have been reported in patients treated with cefaclor:

Erythema multiforme, fever, anaphylaxis (may be more common in patients with a history of penicillin allergy), Stevens-Johnson syndrome, positive direct Coombs' test and genital pruritus. Symptoms of pseudomembranous colitis may appear either during or after antibiotic treatment. Anaphylactoid events may present as solitary symptoms, including angioedema, asthenia, oedema (including face and limbs), dyspnoea, paraesthesias, syncope, or vasodilatation.

Rarely, hypersensitivity symptoms may persist for several months.

The following reactions have been reported rarely in patients treated with cefaclor:

Toxic epidermal necrolysis, reversible interstitial nephritis, hepatic dysfunction, including cholestasis, increased prothrombin time in patients receiving cefaclor and warfarin concomitantly, reversible hyperactivity, agitation, nervousness, insomnia, confusion, hallucinations, hypertonia, aplastic anaemia, agranulocytosis and haemolytic anaemia.

The following adverse reactions have been reported in patients treated with other beta-lactam antibiotics:

Colitis, renal dysfunction and toxic nephropathy.

Several beta-lactam antibiotics have been implicated in triggering seizures, particularly in patients with renal impairment when the dosage was not reduced. If seizures associated with drug therapy should occur, the drug should be discontinued. Anticonvulsant therapy can be given if clinically indicated.

4.9 Overdose

Symptoms of nausea, vomiting, epigastric distress and diarrhoea would be anticipated.

General management consists of supportive therapy. Consider activated charcoal instead of, or in addition to, gastric emptying.

Forced diuresis, peritoneal dialysis, haemodialysis or charcoal haemoperfusion have not been established as beneficial.

5. PHARMACOLOGICAL PROPERTIES

5.1 Pharmacodynamic properties

Distaclor MR has been shown to be active *in vitro* against most strains of the following organisms, although clinical efficacy has not been established:

Gram-negative organisms:

Citrobacter diversus

Neisseria gonorrhoeae

Anaerobic organisms:

Propionibacterium acnes

Bacteroides species (excluding *Bacteroides fragilis*)

Peptococci

Peptostreptococci

Note: *Pseudomonas* sp, *Acinetobacter calcoaceticus*, most strains of enterococci, *Enterobacter* sp, indole-positive *Proteus* and *Serratia* sp are resistant to cefaclor. Cefaclor is inactive against methicillin-resistant staphylococci.

Using the NCCLS recommended methods for sensitivity testing, the criteria for dilution methods are:

MIC ≤8 micrograms/ml: susceptible

MIC = 16 micrograms/ml: moderately susceptible

MIC ≥32 micrograms/ml: resistant and for the standard disc test, using a 30 microgram cefaclor disc (zone diameters):

MIC ≥18 mm: susceptible

MIC = 15-17 mm: moderately susceptible

MIC ≤14 mm: resistant

Cefaclor is a semi-synthetic cephalosporin antibiotic.

5.2 Pharmacokinetic properties

Following administration of 375mg, 500mg and 750mg tablets to fed subjects, average peak serum concentrations of 4, 8 and 11 micrograms/ml, respectively, were obtained within 2.5 to 3 hours. No drug accumulation was noted when this was given twice daily.

Plasma half-life in healthy subjects is independent of dosage form and averages 1 hour. Elderly subjects with normal, mildly diminished renal function do not require dosage adjustment, since higher peak plasma concentrations and AUC had no apparent clinical significance.

There is no evidence of metabolism in humans.

5.3 Preclinical safety data

There are no preclinical data of relevance to the prescriber which are additional to that already included in other sections of the SPC.

6. PHARMACEUTICAL PARTICULARS

6.1 List of excipients

Mannitol

Methylhydroxypropylcellulose

Hydroxypropylcellulose

Methacrylic acid copolymer

Stearic acid

Magnesium stearate

Titanium dioxide (E171)

Polyethylene glycol

Propylene glycol

Indigo carmine aluminium lake (E132)

Talc

6.2 Incompatibilities

Not applicable.

6.3 Shelf life

Two years.

6.4 Special precautions for storage

Store at room temperature (15°-25°C). Protect from light.

6.5 Nature and contents of container

Blister packs consisting of clear PVC with aluminium foil backing containing either 2 or 14 tablets.

6.6 Instructions for use and handling

Take by mouth.

7. MARKETING AUTHORISATION HOLDER

Eli Lilly and Company Limited
Kingsclere Road
Basingstoke
Hampshire
RG21 6XA
England

8. MARKETING AUTHORISATION NUMBER(S)

PL 0006/0274

9. DATE OF FIRST AUTHORISATION/RENEWAL OF THE AUTHORISATION

Date of first authorisation: 27 November 1992

Date of last renewal of authorisation: 18 September 1998

10. DATE OF REVISION OF THE TEXT

February 2002

LEGAL CATEGORY

POM

*DISTACLOR MR (cefaclor MR) is a trademark of Eli Lilly and Company. DCR26M

Distaclor/cefaclor 500mg capsules. Distaclor/cefaclor 125mg/5ml. Distaclor/ cefaclor 250mg/5ml.

(Flynn Pharma Ltd)

1. NAME OF THE MEDICINAL PRODUCT

Distaclor/cefaclor 500mg capsules.

Distaclor/cefaclor 125mg/5ml.

Distaclor/cefaclor 250mg/5ml.

2. QUALITATIVE AND QUANTITATIVE COMPOSITION

Each capsule contains, as the active ingredient, cefaclor monohydrate PhEur, equivalent to 500mg of cefaclor base.

Each 5ml of reconstituted 125mg/5ml suspension contains, as the active ingredient, cefaclor monohydrate PhEur, equivalent to 125mg of cefaclor base.

Each 5ml of reconstituted 250mg/5ml suspension contains, as the active ingredient, cefaclor monohydrate PhEur, equivalent to 250mg of cefaclor base.

3. PHARMACEUTICAL FORM

500mg capsule, size 0, with opaque purple cap and opaque grey body, printed with 'Lilly' and '3062'.

Granules for oral suspension.

4. CLINICAL PARTICULARS

4.1 Therapeutic indications

Distaclor is indicated for the treatment of the following infections due to susceptible micro-organisms:

Respiratory tract infections, including pneumonia, bronchitis, exacerbations of chronic bronchitis, pharyngitis and tonsillitis, and as part of the management of sinusitis

Otitis media

Skin and soft tissue infections

Urinary tract infections, including pyelonephritis and cystitis

Distaclor has been found to be effective in both acute and chronic urinary tract infections.

Cefaclor is generally effective in the eradication of streptococci from the nasopharynx, however, data establishing efficacy in the subsequent prevention of either rheumatic fever or bacterial endocarditis are not available.

4.2 Posology and method of administration

Distaclor is administered orally.

Adults: The usual adult dosage is 250mg every eight hours. For more severe infections or those caused by less susceptible organisms, doses may be doubled. Doses of 4g per day have been administered safely to normal subjects for 28 days, but the total daily dosage should not exceed this amount.

Distaclor may be administered in the presence of impaired renal function. Under such conditions, dosage is usually unchanged (see 'Special warning and special precautions for use').

Patients undergoing haemodialysis: Haemodialysis shortens serum half-life by 25-30%. In patients undergoing regular haemodialysis, a loading dose of 250mg-1g administered prior to dialysis and a therapeutic dose of 250-500mg every six to eight hours maintained during interdialytic periods is recommended.

The elderly: As for adults.

Children: The usual recommended daily dosage for children is 20mg/kg/day in divided doses, every eight hours, as indicated. For bronchitis and pneumonia, the dosage is 20mg/kg/day in divided doses, administered 3 times daily. For otitis media and pharyngitis, the total daily dosage may be divided and administered every 12 hours. Safety and efficacy have not been established for use in infants aged less than one month.

Distaclor Suspension

	125mg/5ml	250mg/5ml
<1 year (9kg)	2.5ml tid	
1-5 years (9-18kg)	5.0ml tid	
Over 5 years		5.0ml tid

In more serious infections, otitis media, sinusitis and infections caused by less susceptible organisms, 40mg/kg/day in divided doses is recommended, up to a daily maximum of 1g.

In the treatment of beta-haemolytic streptococcal infections, therapy should be continued for at least 10 days.

4.3 Contraindications

Hypersensitivity to cephalosporins.

4.4 Special warnings and special precautions for use

Warnings

Before instituting therapy with cefaclor, every effort should be made to determine whether the patient has had previous hypersensitivity reactions to cefaclor, cephalosporins, penicillins or other drugs. Cefaclor should be given cautiously to penicillin-sensitive patients, because cross-hypersensitivity, including anaphylaxis, among beta-lactam antibiotics has been clearly documented.

If an allergic reaction to cefaclor occurs, the drug should be discontinued and the patient treated with the appropriate agents.

Pseudomembranous colitis has been reported with virtually all broad-spectrum antibiotics, including macrolides, semi-synthetic penicillins and cephalosporins. It is important, therefore, to consider its diagnosis in patients who develop diarrhoea in association with the use of antibiotics. Such colitis may range in severity from mild to life-threatening. Mild cases usually respond to drug discontinuance alone. In moderate to severe cases, appropriate measures should be taken.

Precautions

Cefaclor should be administered with caution in the presence of markedly impaired renal function. Since the half-life of cefaclor in anuric patients is 2.3 to 2.8 hours (compared to 0.6-0.9 hours in normal subjects), dosage adjustments for patients with moderate or severe renal impairment are not usually required. Clinical experience with cefaclor under such conditions is limited; therefore, careful clinical observation and laboratory studies should be made.

Broad-spectrum antibiotics should be prescribed with caution in individuals with a history of gastro-intestinal disease, particularly colitis.

Prolonged use of cefaclor may result in the overgrowth of non-susceptible organisms. If superinfection occurs during therapy, appropriate measures should be taken.

Positive direct Coombs' tests have been reported during treatment with the cephalosporin antibiotics. In haematological studies or in transfusion cross-matching procedures, when anti-globulin tests are performed on the minor side, or in Coombs' testing of newborns whose mothers have received cephalosporin antibiotics before parturition, it should be recognised that a positive Coombs' test may be due to the drug.

A false-positive reaction for glucose in the urine may occur with Benedict's or Fehling's solutions or with copper sulphate test tablets.

4.5 Interaction with other medicinal products and other forms of Interaction

There have been rare reports of increased prothrombin time, with or without clinical bleeding, in patients receiving cefaclor and warfarin concomitantly. It is recommended that in such patients, regular monitoring of prothrombin time should be considered, with adjustment of dosage if necessary.

The renal excretion of cefaclor is inhibited by probenecid.

4.6 Pregnancy and lactation

Usage in pregnancy: Animal studies have shown no evidence of impaired fertility or teratogenicity. However, since there are no adequate or well-controlled studies in pregnant women, caution should be exercised when prescribing for the pregnant patient.

Usage in nursing mothers: Small amounts of cefaclor have been detected in breast milk following administration of single 500mg doses. Average levels of about 0.2 micrograms/ml or less were detected up to 5 hours later. Trace amounts were detected at one hour. As the effect on nursing infants is not known, caution should be exercised when cefaclor is administered to a nursing woman.

4.7 Effects on ability to drive and use machines

Not applicable.

4.8 Undesirable effects

Gastro-intestinal: The most frequent side-effect has been diarrhoea. It is rarely severe enough to warrant cessation of therapy. Colitis, including rare instances of pseudomembranous colitis, has been reported. Nausea and vomiting have also occurred.

Hypersensitivity: Allergic reactions such as morbilliform eruptions, pruritus and urticaria have been observed. These reactions usually subside upon discontinuation of therapy. Serum sickness-like reactions (erythema multiforme minor, rashes or other skin manifestations accompanied by arthritis/arthralgia, with or without fever) have been reported. Lymphadenopathy and proteinuria are infrequent; there are no circulating immune complexes and no evidence of sequelae. Occasionally, solitary symptoms may occur, but do not represent a serum sickness-like reaction. Serum sickness-like reactions are apparently due to hypersensitivity and have usually occurred during or following a second (or subsequent) course of therapy with cefaclor. Such reactions have been reported more frequently in children than in adults. Signs and symptoms usually occur a few days after initiation of therapy and usually subside within a few days of cessation of therapy. Antihistamines and corticosteroids appear to enhance resolution of the syndrome. No serious sequelae have been reported.

There are rare reports of erythema multiforme major (Stevens-Johnson syndrome), toxic epidermal necrolysis, and anaphylaxis. Anaphylaxis may be more common in patients with a history of penicillin allergy. Anaphylactoid events may present as solitary symptoms, including angioedema, asthenia, oedema (including face and limbs), dyspnoea, paraesthesias, syncope, or vasodilatation.

Rarely, hypersensitivity symptoms may persist for several months.

Haematological: Eosinophilia, positive Coombs' tests and, rarely, thrombocytopenia. Transient lymphocytosis, leucopenia and, rarely, haemolytic anaemia, aplastic anaemia, agranulocytosis and reversible neutropenia of possible clinical significance. See 'Interactions with other medicaments and other forms of interaction'.

Hepatic: Transient hepatitis and cholestatic jaundice have been reported rarely, slight elevations in AST, ALT or alkaline phosphatase values.

Renal: Reversible interstitial nephritis has occurred rarely, also slight elevations in blood urea or serum creatinine or abnormal urinalysis.

Central nervous system: Reversible hyperactivity, agitation, nervousness, insomnia, confusion, hypertonia, dizziness, hallucinations and somnolence have been reported rarely.

Miscellaneous: Genital pruritus, vaginitis and vaginal moniliasis.

4.9 Overdose

Symptoms of nausea, vomiting, epigastric distress and diarrhoea would be anticipated.

Treatment: Unless 5 times the normal total daily dose has been ingested, gastro-intestinal decontamination will not be necessary.

General management may consist of supportive therapy.

5. PHARMACOLOGICAL PROPERTIES

5.1 Pharmacodynamic properties

Cefaclor is active against the following organisms *in vitro:*

Alpha- and beta-haemolytic streptococci

Staphylococci; including coagulase-positive, coagulase-negative and penicillinase-producing strains

Streptococcus pneumoniae

Streptococcus pyogenes (group A beta-haemolytic streptococci)

Branhamella catarrhalis

Escherichia coli

Proteus mirabilis

Klebsiella species

Haemophilus influenzae, including ampicillin-resistant strains.

Cefaclor has no activity against *Pseudomonas* species or *Acinetobacter* species. Methicillin-resistant staphylococci and most strains of enterococci (eg, *Str. faecalis*) are resistant to cefaclor. Cefaclor is not active against most strains of *Enterobacter* spp, *Serratia* spp, *Morganella morganii, Proteus vulgaris* and *Providencia rettgeri.*

5.2 Pharmacokinetic properties

Cefaclor is well absorbed after oral administration to fasting subjects. Total absorption is the same whether the drug is given with or without food; however, when it is taken with food, the peak concentration achieved is 50-75% of that observed when the drug is administered to fasting subjects and generally appears from ¾ to one hour later. Following administration of 250mg, 500mg and 1g doses to fasting subjects, average peak serum levels of approximately 7, 13 and 23 mg/l, respectively, were obtained within 30–60 minutes. Approximately 60–85% of the drug is excreted unchanged in the urine within eight hours, the greater portion being excreted within the first two hours. During the eight hour period, peak urine concentrations following the 250mg, 500mg and 1g doses were approximately 600, 900 and 1,900 mg/l, respectively. The serum half-life in normal subjects is 0.6–0.9 hours. In patients with reduced renal function, the serum half-life of cefaclor is slightly prolonged. In those with complete absence of renal function, the plasma half-life of the intact molecule is 2.3–2.8 hours. Excretion pathways in patients with markedly impaired renal function have not been determined. Haemodialysis shortens the half-life by 25-30%.

5.3 Preclinical safety data

There are no pre-clinical data of relevance to the prescriber which are additional to that already included in other sections of the SPC.

6. PHARMACEUTICAL PARTICULARS

6.1 List of excipients

500 mg capsule

Magnesium Stearate

Dimeticone

Starch Flowable

Erythrosine

Patent Blue V

Black Iron Oxide

Titanium Dioxide

Gelatin

Pharmaceutical Grade Edible Printing Ink

125 mg/5ml and 250mg/5ml suspensions

Sucrose

Erythrosine Aluminium Lake

Methylcellulose 15

Sodium Lauryl Sulphate

Artificial Strawberry Flavour

Dimeticone

Xanthan Gum F

Starch Modified

6.2 Incompatibilities

None Known.

6.3 Shelf life

Capsule: 3 years.

Suspensions: 24 months.

6.4 Special precautions for storage

Capsule: Store below 25°C. Keep containers tightly closed and protect from light.

Suspensions: Store at room temperature (15-25°C). Keep containers tightly closed and protect from light. After reconstitution, the suspension should be stored in a refrigerator (2-8°C) and be used within 14 days.

6.5 Nature and contents of container

Capsule: High-density polyethylene bottles with screw caps containing 50 capsules.

Suspensions: The product is filled into high-density polyethylene bottles with screw caps containing 100ml of cefaclor.

6.6 Instructions for use and handling

Capsule: None.

Suspensions: When dilution is unavoidable, syrup BP should be used after the suspension has been prepared according to the manufacturer's instruction.

7. MARKETING AUTHORISATION HOLDER

Eli Lilly and Company Limited

Kingsclere Road

Basingstoke

Hampshire

RG21 6XA

England

Trading as:

Greenfield Pharmaceuticals

Lilly Industries Limited

Dista Products Limited

8. MARKETING AUTHORISATION NUMBER(S)

500 mg capsule: PL 0006/0119

125mg/5ml suspension: PL 0006/0120

250mg/5ml suspension: PL 0006/0121

9. DATE OF FIRST AUTHORISATION/RENEWAL OF THE AUTHORISATION

Date of first authorisation: 21 August 1978

Date of last renewal of authorisation: *Capsule:* 4 October 1994

Suspensions: 29 July 1994

10. DATE OF REVISION OF THE TEXT

Capsule: May 1999

Suspensions: April 1999

'Distaclor' is an Eli Lilly and Company Limited trademark DCR.22M

DISTALGESIC CO-PROXAMOL Tablets

(Meda Pharmaceuticals)

1. NAME OF THE MEDICINAL PRODUCT

'DISTALGESIC' CO-PROXAMOL Tablets

2. QUALITATIVE AND QUANTITATIVE COMPOSITION

Each tablet contains 32.5mg dextropropoxyphene Hydrochloride BP (equivalent to approximately 30mg dextropropoxyphene base) with 325mg Paracetamol Ph. Eur.

3. PHARMACEUTICAL FORM

White, pillow-shaped, film-coated tablets

4. CLINICAL PARTICULARS

4.1 Therapeutic indications

Actions: Dextropropoxyphene is a mild narcotic analgesic structurally related to methadone.

Indication: For the management of mild to moderate pain.

4.2 Posology and method of administration

For oral administration to adults only. The usual dose is 2 tablets three or four times daily and should not normally be exceeded. Take every 6-8 hours, as required.

Consideration should be given to a reduced total daily dosage in patients with hepatic or renal impairment.

The elderly: There is evidence of prolonged half-life in the elderly, so reduction in dosage should be considered.

Children: Distalgesic is not recommended for use in children.

4.3 Contraindications

Hypersensitivity to dextropropoxyphene or paracetamol and/or any other constituents.

Use in patients who are suicidal or addiction-prone.

4.4 Special warnings and special precautions for use

Warnings

PATIENTS SHOULD BE ADVISED NOT TO EXCEED THE RECOMMENDED DOSE AND TO AVOID ALCOHOL.

Dextropropoxyphene products in excessive doses, either alone or in combination with other CNS depressants, including alcohol, are a major cause of drug-related deaths. Fatalities within the first hour of overdosage are not uncommon and can occur within 15 minutes. Some deaths have occurred as a consequence of the accidental ingestion of excessive quantities of Distalgesic alone, or in combination with other drugs.

Distalgesic should not be taken with any other paracetamol-containing products.

Overdosage may damage the liver, due predominantly to the accumulation of intermediate metabolites of paracetamol which cause hepatic necrosis. Immediate medical advice should be sought in the event of an overdose, even if the patient feels well, because of the risk of delayed, serious liver damage. Compared to the general population, the hazards of overdose are greater in those with non-cirrhotic alcoholic liver disease.

Distalgesic should be prescribed with caution for those patients whose medical condition requires the concomitant administration of sedatives, tranquillisers, muscle relaxants, antidepressants or other CNS-depressant drugs; patients should be advised of the additive depressant effects of these combinations. Distalgesic should also be prescribed with caution in patients who use alcohol in excess.

Drug dependence: Dextropropoxyphene, when taken in higher than recommended doses over long periods of time, can produce drug dependence.

Precautions

Distalgesic should be administered with caution to patients with hepatic or renal impairment since higher serum concentrations or delayed elimination may occur.

4.5 Interaction with other medicinal products and other forms of Interaction

Drug interactions: The CNS-depressant effect of dextropropoxyphene is additive with that of other CNS depressants, including alcohol.

Dextropropoxyphene may interfere with the metabolism of antidepressants, anticonvulsants and warfarin-like drugs. Severe neurological signs, including coma, have occurred with concomitant use of carbamazepine.

Speed and/or extent of absorption may be altered by other agents with substantial gastrointestinal effects; for example, metoclopramide or domperidone may speed passage from the stomach to the intestines; and cholestyramine may reduce absorption.

4.6 Pregnancy and lactation

Pregnancy: Safety in pregnancy has not been established relative to possible adverse effects on fetal development. Withdrawal symptoms in neonates have been reported following use during pregnancy. Therefore, Distalgesic should not be used in pregnant women unless, in the judgement of the physician, the potential benefits outweigh the possible hazards.

Nursing mothers: Low levels of dextropropoxyphene have been detected in human milk. In postpartum studies involving nursing mothers who were given dextropropoxyphene, no adverse effects were noted in the infants. Paracetamol is excreted in breast milk but not in a clinically significant amount. Available published data do not contra-indicate breast feeding.

4.7 Effects on ability to drive and use machines

Ambulatory patients: Dextropropoxyphene may impair abilities required for tasks such as driving a car or operating machinery. The patient should be cautioned accordingly.

4.8 Undesirable effects

The most frequently reported have been dizziness, sedation, nausea and vomiting. Some of these side-effects may be alleviated if the patient lies down.

Other side-effects include constipation, abdominal pain, rashes, light-headedness, headache, weakness, euphoria, dysphoria, hallucinations and minor visual disturbances.

Adverse effects of paracetamol are rare but hypersensitivity including skin rash may occur. There have been reports of blood dyscrasias including thrombocytopenia and agranulocytosis, but these were not necessarily causally related to paracetamol.

Dextropropoxyphene therapy has been associated with abnormal liver function tests and, more rarely, with instances of reversible jaundice (including cholestatic jaundice).

Hepatic necrosis may result from acute overdose of paracetamol. In chronic alcohol abusers, this has been reported rarely with short-term use of paracetamol dosages of 2.5 to 10g/day. Fatalities have occurred.

Renal papillary necrosis may result from chronic paracetamol use, particularly when the dosage is greater than recommended and when combined with aspirin.

Subacute painful myopathy has occurred following chronic dextropropoxyphene overdosage.

Chronic ingestion of dextropropoxyphene in doses exceeding 720mg per day has caused toxic psychoses and convulsions.

4.9 Overdose

Initial consideration should be given to the management of the CNS effects of dextropropoxyphene overdosage. Resuscitative measures should be initiated promptly.

Dextropropoxyphene: In the acute phase dextropropoxyphene produces symptoms typical of narcosis, with somnolence or coma and respiratory depression, sometimes with convulsions. Blood pressure falls and cardiac performance deteriorates. Cardiac arrhythmias and conduction delay may be present. A combined respiratory-metabolic acidosis occurs, which may be severe if large amounts of salicylates have also been ingested. Death may occur.

Naloxone will reduce the respiratory depression and 0.4-2mg iv should be administered promptly. (This may be repeated at 2-3 minute intervals, but if there is no response after 10mg of naloxone the diagnosis should be questioned.) The duration of antagonism may be brief and need repeating for up to 24 hours. Mechanical ventilation, with oxygen may be required, and PEEP ventilation is desirable if pulmonary oedema is present.

Blood gases, pH and electrolytes should be monitored and electrocardiographic monitoring is essential. Ventricular fibrillation or cardiac arrest may occur. Respiratory acidosis rapidly subsides as ventilation is restored and hypercapnoea eliminated, but lactic acidosis may require iv bicarbonate for prompt correction. In addition to the use of a narcotic antagonist, the patient may require titration with an anti-convulsant to control convulsions. Gastric lavage may be useful and activated charcoal can absorb a significant amount of ingested dextropropoxyphene.

Treatment of dextropropoxyphene overdose in children: See general comments above. Naloxone at 0.01mg/kg body weight iv should be administered promptly. If there is no response a dose of 0.1mg/kg iv may be used.

Paracetamol: Overdose symptoms may not become apparent until later but early measurement of paracetamol levels is essential. Oral methionine or intravenous N-acetylcysteine given as early as possible is effective in reducing the toxic effects of paracetamol and may have a beneficial effect up to at least 48 hours after the overdose. Treatment should be instituted within 16 hours of ingestion. Symptoms in the first 24 hours are pallor, anorexia, nausea, vomiting, profuse sweating, malaise and abdominal pain. However, the patient may have no symptoms. Abnormalities of glucose metabolism and metabolic acidosis may occur.

Subsequent evidence of liver dysfunction may be apparent up to 72 hours after ingestion, and if severe lead to irreversible hepatic necrosis and death within 3-7 days. Hepatic toxicity has rarely been reported with acute overdoses of less than 10g. However, liver damage is possible in adults who have taken 10g or more of paracetamol. In severe poisoning, with greater than 15g, hepatic failure may progress to encephalopathy, coma and death.

Cardiac arrhythmias and pancreatitis have been reported.

Acute renal failure may accompany the hepatic dysfunction and can occur without signs of fulminant hepatic failure. Typically renal impairment is more apparent 6-9 days after overdose.

5. PHARMACOLOGICAL PROPERTIES

5.1 Pharmacodynamic properties

The product is a compound analgesic containing the non-narcotic drug (paracetamol) for the relief of pain of musculoskeletal conditions and a narcotic drug (dextropropoxyphene) for the relief of pain of visceral origin.

5.2 Pharmacokinetic properties

Single dose studies have shown peak plasma levels of 0.06mg/l two hours after administration of 65mg of dextropropoxyphene HCl. Variation of plasma levels between subjects may be due to individual differences in drug absorption and metabolism.

Multiple dose studies have shown that differences in plasma levels obtained with the hydrochloride salt or the napsylate salt have little therapeutic significance and that a 65mg dextropropoxyphene HCl dose administered six hourly will achieve steady state plasma levels in the 0.13 - 0.19 mg/l range after 48 hours. The minimum lethal dose of dextropropoxyphene has been reported to be 500-800 mg and could result in blood concentrations of 0.45 - 0.74 mg/l. Mean half lives of 11.8 hours for dextropropoxyphene and 36.6 hours for norpropoxyphene have been demonstrated.

5.3 Preclinical safety data

There are no preclinical data of relevance to the prescriber in addition to that summarised in other sections of the Summary of Product Characteristics.

6. PHARMACEUTICAL PARTICULARS

6.1 List of excipients

Maize Starch

Pregelatinised Maize Starch

Magnesium Stearate

Methylhydroxypropylcellulose 15

Glycerol

Titanium Dioxide.

6.2 Incompatibilities

Not applicable.

6.3 Shelf life

3 years.

6.4 Special precautions for storage

None.

6.5 Nature and contents of container

Blister packs containing 100 white, pillow-shaped, film coated tablets, 14 mm in length and marked 'DG' (10 strips of 10 tablets).

6.6 Instructions for use and handling

None.

7. MARKETING AUTHORISATION HOLDER

Meda Pharmaceuticals Ltd
Sherwood House
7 Gregory Boulevard
Nottingham
NG7 6LB
UK
Trading as:
Meda Pharmaceuticals
Regus House
Herald Way
Pegasus Business Park
Castle Donington
DE74 2TZ
UK

8. MARKETING AUTHORISATION NUMBER(S)

PL19477/0011

9. DATE OF FIRST AUTHORISATION/RENEWAL OF THE AUTHORISATION

Date of first authorisation: 24th May 1973

Date of last renewal of authorisation: 18th March 2003

10. DATE OF REVISION OF THE TEXT

30th September 2003.

Distamine 125mg

(Alliance Pharmaceuticals)

1. NAME OF THE MEDICINAL PRODUCT

Distamine 125mg tablets.

2. QUALITATIVE AND QUANTITATIVE COMPOSITION

Each tablet contains 125mg D-penicillamine base.

3. PHARMACEUTICAL FORM

Tablet.

White, film-coated tablet with a diameter of 8mm, marked "DS" on one face and "125" on the other.

4. CLINICAL PARTICULARS

4.1 Therapeutic indications

a) Severe active rheumatoid arthritis, including juvenile forms

b) Wilson's disease (hepatolenticular degeneration)

c) Cystinuria – dissolution and prevention of cystine stones

d) Lead poisoning

e) Chronic active hepatitis

4.2 Posology and method of administration

For oral administration.

Distamine should be taken on an empty stomach at least half an hour before meals, or on retiring.

a) Rheumatoid arthritis

Adults: 125 to 250mg daily for the first month. Increase by the same amount every four to 12 weeks until remission occurs. The minimum maintenance dose to achieve suppression of symptoms should be used and treatment should be discontinued if no benefit is obtained within 12 months. Improvement may not occur for some months.

The usual maintenance dose is 500 to 750mg daily. Up to 1500mg daily may be required.

If remission is established and has been sustained for six months, gradual reduction by 125 to 250mg amounts every 12 weeks may be attempted.

The elderly: Initial dose should not exceed 125mg daily for the first month, increasing by similar increments every four to 12 weeks until the minimum maintenance dose to suppress symptoms is reached. Daily dosage should not exceed 1000mg (see Section 4.4, "Special Warnings and Special Precautions for Use").

Children: The usual maintenance dose is 15 to 20mg/kg/day. The initial dose should be lower (2.5 to 5mg/kg/day) and increased every four weeks over a period of three to six months. Please note that as the smallest available tablet is 125mg, this may not be suitable for children under eight years (or less than 26kg in weight).

Renal insufficiency: Distamine therapy should be initiated at a low dose with intervals between dose increase of at least twelve weeks. Fortnightly monitoring for toxicity is mandatory throughout treatment for rheumatoid arthritis.

b) Wilson's disease

Patients must be maintained in negative copper balance and the minimum dose of Distamine required to achieve this should be given.

Adults: 1500 to 2000mg daily in divided doses. Dose may be reduced to 750 to 1000mg daily when control of the disease is achieved. It is advisable that a dose of 2000mg/day should not be continued for more than a year.

The elderly: 20mg/kg/day in divided doses adjusting the dose to minimal level necessary to control disease.

Children: Up to 20mg/kg/day in divided doses. Minimum dose 500mg/day.

Renal insufficiency: Extra precautions should be taken to monitor for adverse effects in patients with Wilson's disease and renal insufficiency.

c) Cystinuria

Ideally, establish the lowest effective dose by quantitative amino acid chromatography of urine.

(i) Dissolution of cystine stones:

Adults: 1000 to 3000mg daily in divided doses.

Urine cystine levels of not more than 200mg/l should be maintained.

(ii) Prevention of cystine stones:

Adults: 500 to 1000mg on retiring. Fluid intake should be not less than 3 litres/day. Urine cystine levels of not more than 300mg/l should be maintained.

The elderly: Use the minimum dose to maintain urinary cystine levels below 200mg/l.

Children: No dose range established, but urinary cystine levels must be kept below 200mg/l. The minimum dose of Distamine required to achieve this should be given.

Renal insufficiency: If renal insufficiency is present at the onset of therapy, the starting dose should be lower, but it will be necessary to give sufficient Distamine to achieve urine cystine levels of not more than 300mg/l. The maintenance dose should be reviewed at intervals of not more than four weeks.

d) Lead poisoning

Adults: 1000 to 1500mg daily in divided doses until urinary lead is stabilised at less than 0.5mg/day.

The elderly: 20mg/kg/day in divided doses until urinary lead is stabilised at less than 0.5mg/day.

Children: 20mg/kg/day.

e) Chronic active hepatitis

Adults: For maintenance treatment after the disease process has been brought under control with corticosteroids. The initial dose of 500mg daily, in divided doses, should be increased gradually over three months to a maintenance dose of 1250mg daily. During this period, the dose of corticosteroids should be phased out. Throughout therapy, liver function tests should be carried out periodically to assess the disease status.

The elderly: Not recommended.

4.3 Contraindications

Hypersensitivity to penicillamine or any of the ingredients.

Agranulocytosis or severe thrombocytopenia due to penicillamine.

Lupus erythematosus.

Moderate or severe renal impairment.

4.4 Special warnings and special precautions for use

Full blood and platelet counts should be performed and renal function should be assessed prior to treatment with penicillamine.

During the first eight weeks of therapy full blood counts should be carried out weekly or fortnightly and also in the week after any increase in dose, otherwise monthly thereafter. In cystinuria or Wilson's disease, longer intervals may be adequate.

Withdrawal of treatment should be considered if platelets fall below 120,000/mm^3 or white blood cells below 2,500/mm^3, or if three successive falls are noted within the normal range. Treatment may be restarted at a reduced dose when counts return to normal, but should be permanently withdrawn on recurrence of leucopenia or thrombocytopenia.

In patients with normal renal function, urinalysis for detection of haematuria and proteinuria should be carried out weekly at first, and following each increase in dose, then monthly, although longer intervals may be adequate for cystinuria and Wilson's disease. Increasing or persistent proteinuria may necessitate withdrawal of therapy.

Care should be exercised in patients with renal insufficiency; modification of dosage may be necessary (see Section 4.2, "Posology and Method of Administration").

Especially careful monitoring is necessary in the elderly since increased toxicity has been observed in this patient population regardless of renal function.

Concomitant use of NSAIDs and other nephrotoxic drugs may increase the risk of renal damage.

Penicillamine should be used with caution in patients who have had adverse reactions to gold.

Concomitant or previous treatment with gold may increase the risk of side effects with penicillamine treatment. Therefore penicillamine should be used with caution in patients who have previously had adverse reactions to gold and concomitant treatment with gold should be avoided.

If concomitant oral iron therapy is indicated, this should not be given within two hours of taking penicillamine.

Antihistamines, steroid cover, or temporary reduction of dose will control urticarial reactions.

Reversible loss of taste may occur. Mineral supplements to overcome this are not recommended.

Haematuria is rare, but if it occurs in the absence of renal stones or other known cause, treatment should be stopped immediately.

A late rash, described as acquired epidermolysis bullosa and penicillamine dermopathy, may occur after several months or years of therapy. This may necessitate a reduction in dosage.

Breast enlargement has been reported as a rare complication of penicillamine therapy in both women and men. Danazol has been used successfully to treat breast enlargement which does not regress on drug discontinuation.

4.5 Interaction with other medicinal products and other forms of Interaction

Concomitant iron and penicillamine treatment: oral absorption of penicillamine may be reduced by concomitant administration of iron (see Section 4.4 "Special Warnings and Special Precautions for Use").

Concomitant use of NSAIDs and other nephrotoxic drugs may increase the risk of renal damage (see Section 4.4 "Special Warnings and Special Precautions for Use").

Concomitant gold and penicillamine treatment: concomitant use not recommended (see Section 4.4 "Special Warnings and Special Precautions for Use").

4.6 Pregnancy and lactation

Usage in pregnancy: The safety of penicillamine for use during pregnancy has not been established (see Section 5.3, "Preclinical Safety Data").

Wilson's disease: There has been one case reported of reversible cutis laxa in an infant born to a mother taking 1500mg penicillamine daily throughout pregnancy. Although there have been no controlled studies on the use of penicillamine during pregnancy, two retrospective studies have reported the successful delivery of 43 normal infants to 28 women receiving between 500 and 2000mg of penicillamine daily.

Cystinuria: Whilst normal infants have been delivered, there is one report of a severe connective tissue abnormality in the infant of a mother who received 2000mg penicillamine daily throughout pregnancy. Whenever possible, penicillamine should be withheld during pregnancy, but if stones continue to form, the benefit of resuming treatment must be weighed against the possible risk to the foetus.

Rheumatoid arthritis or chronic active hepatitis: Penicillamine should not be administered to patients who are pregnant, and therapy should be stopped when pregnancy is diagnosed or suspected, unless considered to be absolutely essential by the physician.

Usage in lactation: Due to the lack of data on use in breast feeding patients and the possibility that penicillamine may be transmitted to newborns through breast milk, Distamine should only be used in breast feeding patients when it is considered absolutely essential by the physician.

4.7 Effects on ability to drive and use machines
None known.

4.8 Undesirable effects
NB: The incidence and severity of some of the adverse reactions, noted below, varies according to the dosage and nature of the disease under treatment.

Nausea, anorexia, fever and rash may occur early in therapy, especially when full doses are given from the start.

Urticarial reactions have been reported (see Section 4.4, "Special Warnings and Special Precautions for Use").

Reversible loss of taste may occur (see Section 4.4, "Special Warnings and Special Precautions for Use").

Rarely, mouth ulceration/stomatitis has occurred.

Thrombocytopenia occurs commonly and leucopenia less often. These reactions may occur at any time during treatment and are usually reversible (see Section 4.4, "Special Warnings and Special Precautions for Use").

Deaths from agranulocytosis and aplastic anaemia have occurred.

Proteinuria occurs in up to 30% of patients and is partially dose-related (see Section 4.4, "Special Warnings and Special Precautions for Use").

Haematuria may occur rarely (see Section 4.4, "Special Warnings and Special Precautions for Use").

Other rare adverse reactions are as follows: alopecia and inflammatory conditions of the respiratory system, such as bronchiolitis and pneumonitis.

Other complications have included haemolytic anaemia, nephrotic syndrome, pancreatitis, cholestatic jaundice (including raised liver function tests), drug induced lupus erythematosus, and conditions closely resembling myasthenia gravis, polymyositis (with rare cardiac involvement), dermatomyositis, pemphigus, Goodpasture's syndrome, Stevens-Johnson syndrome and rheumatoid arthritis.

A late rash, described as acquired epidermolysis bullosa and penicillamine dermopathy, may occur after several months or years of therapy (see Section 4.4, "Special Warnings and Special Precautions for Use").

Pseudoxanthoma elasticum and skin laxity have been reported rarely. Breast enlargement has been reported as a rare complication of penicillamine therapy in both women and men. In some patients breast enlargement was considerable and/or prolonged with poor resolution and others required surgery (see Section 4.4, "Special Warnings and Special Precautions for Use").

4.9 Overdose
No instances of adverse reactions to an overdose of penicillamine have been recorded and no specific measures are indicated.

5. PHARMACOLOGICAL PROPERTIES

5.1 Pharmacodynamic properties
Pharmacotherapeutic group: M01C C

1. Penicillamine is used to treat severe active rheumatoid arthritis not adequately controlled by NSAID therapy.

2. Penicillamine is a chelating agent which aids the elimination from the body of certain heavy metal ions, including copper, lead and mercury, by forming stable soluble complexes with them that are readily excreted by the kidney.

3. It is used in the treatment of Wilson's disease (hepatolenticular degeneration), in conjunction with a low copper diet, to promote the excretion of copper.

4. It may be used to treat asymptomatic lead intoxication.

5. Penicillamine is used as an adjunct to diet and urinary alkalinisation in the management of cystinuria. By reducing urinary concentrations of cystine, penicillamine prevents the formation of calculi and promotes the gradual dissolution of existing calculi.

6. Desensitisation. Should the physician deem it necessary to attempt to desensitise a patient to penicillamine, it should be noted that this formulation is not suitable for this purpose.

5.2 Pharmacokinetic properties
Penicillamine is a thiol-group containing chelating agent, variably absorbed from the gastrointestinal tract. The drug undergoes a rapid distribution phase, followed by a slower elimination phase.

Penicillamine is strongly plasma-protein bound. Most penicillamine is bound to albumin but some is bound to α-globulins or ceruloplasmin.

Penicillamine is not extensively metabolised in man.

About 80% of the absorbed dose is excreted rapidly in the urine, mostly as mixed disulphides. Some of the dose is excreted as a penicillamine copper complex and some as the S-methyl derivative.

5.3 Preclinical safety data
Penicillamine has been shown to be teratogenic in rats when given in doses several times higher than those recommended for human use.

There is no known LD50 value for penicillamine. In studies some rats died after oral administration of 10,000mg/kg, but intra-peritoneal injections of a dose of 660mg/kg caused no deaths.

6. PHARMACEUTICAL PARTICULARS

6.1 List of excipients
Tablet Core

Microcrystalline cellulose

Sodium starch glycolate

Povidone

Stearic acid

Tablet coating

Glycerol

Titanium dioxide

Hydroxypropylmethyl cellulose

6.2 Incompatibilities
None known.

6.3 Shelf life
3 years

6.4 Special precautions for storage
Do not store above 25°C. Keep the container tightly closed.

6.5 Nature and contents of container
HDPE bottle with screw cap, containing 100 tablets.

6.6 Instructions for use and handling
None.

7. MARKETING AUTHORISATION HOLDER
Alliance Pharmaceuticals Ltd

Avonbridge House

Bath Road

Chippenham

Wiltshire

SN15 2BB

United Kingdom

8. MARKETING AUTHORISATION NUMBER(S)
PL 16853/0057

9. DATE OF FIRST AUTHORISATION/RENEWAL OF THE AUTHORISATION
28th September 2001

10. DATE OF REVISION OF THE TEXT
September 2003

Distamine 250 mg

(Alliance Pharmaceuticals)

1. NAME OF THE MEDICINAL PRODUCT
Distamine 250mg tablets.

2. QUALITATIVE AND QUANTITATIVE COMPOSITION
Each tablet contains 250mg D-penicillamine base.

3. PHARMACEUTICAL FORM
Tablet.

White, film-coated tablet with a diameter of 10mm, marked "DM" on one face and "250" on the other.

4. CLINICAL PARTICULARS

4.1 Therapeutic indications
a) Severe active rheumatoid arthritis, including juvenile forms

b) Wilson's disease (hepatolenticular degeneration)

c) Cystinuria – dissolution and prevention of cystine stones

d) Lead poisoning

e) Chronic active hepatitis

4.2 Posology and method of administration
For oral administration.

Distamine should be taken on an empty stomach at least half an hour before meals, or on retiring.

a) Rheumatoid arthritis

Adults: 125 to 250mg daily for the first month. Increase by the same amount every four to 12 weeks until remission occurs. The minimum maintenance dose to achieve suppression of symptoms should be used and treatment should be discontinued if no benefit is obtained within 12 months. Improvement may not occur for some months.

The usual maintenance dose is 500 to 750mg daily. Up to 1500mg daily may be required.

If remission is established and has been sustained for six months, gradual reduction by 125 to 250mg amounts every 12 weeks may be attempted.

The elderly: Initial dose should not exceed 125mg daily for the first month, increasing by similar increments every four to 12 weeks until the minimum maintenance dose to suppress symptoms is reached. Daily dosage should not exceed 1000mg (see Section 4.4, "Special Warnings and Special Precautions for Use").

Children: The usual maintenance dose is 15 to 20mg/kg/day. The initial dose should be lower (2.5 to 5mg/kg/day) and increased every four weeks over a period of three to six months. Please note that as the smallest available tablet is 125mg, this may not be suitable for children under eight years (or less than 26kg in weight).

Renal insufficiency: Distamine therapy should be initiated at a low dose with intervals between dose increase of at least twelve weeks. Fortnightly monitoring for toxicity is mandatory throughout treatment for rheumatoid arthritis.

b) Wilson's disease

Patients must be maintained in negative copper balance and the minimum dose of Distamine required to achieve this should be given.

Adults: 1500 to 2000mg daily in divided doses. Dose may be reduced to 750 to 1000mg daily when control of the disease is achieved. It is advisable that a dose of 2000mg/day should not be continued for more than a year.

The elderly: 20mg/kg/day in divided doses adjusting the dose to minimal level necessary to control disease.

Children: Up to 20mg/kg/day in divided doses. Minimum dose 500mg/day.

Renal insufficiency: Extra precautions should be taken to monitor for adverse effects in patients with Wilson's disease and renal insufficiency.

c) Cystinuria

Ideally, establish the lowest effective dose by quantitative amino acid chromatography of urine.

(i) Dissolution of cystine stones:

Adults: 1000 to 3000mg daily in divided doses.

Urine cystine levels of not more than 200mg/l should be maintained.

(ii) Prevention of cystine stones:

Adults: 500 to 1000mg on retiring. Fluid intake should be not less than 3 litres/day. Urine cystine levels of not more than 300mg/l should be maintained.

The elderly: Use the minimum dose to maintain urinary cystine levels below 200mg/l.

Children: No dose range established, but urinary cystine levels must be kept below 200mg/l. The minimum dose of Distamine required to achieve this should be given.

Renal insufficiency: If renal insufficiency is present at the onset of therapy, the starting dose should be lower, but it will be necessary to give sufficient Distamine to achieve urine cystine levels of not more than 300mg/l. The maintenance dose should be reviewed at intervals of not more than four weeks.

d) Lead poisoning

Adults: 1000 to 1500mg daily in divided doses until urinary lead is stabilised at less than 0.5mg/day.

The elderly: 20mg/kg/day in divided doses until urinary lead is stabilised at less than 0.5mg/day.

Children: 20mg/kg/day.

e) Chronic active hepatitis

Adults: For maintenance treatment after the disease process has been brought under control with corticosteroids. The initial dose of 500mg daily, in divided doses, should be increased gradually over three months to a maintenance dose of 1250mg daily. During this period, the dose of corticosteroids should be phased out. Throughout therapy, liver function tests should be carried out periodically to assess the disease status.

The elderly: Not recommended.

4.3 Contraindications
Hypersensitivity to penicillamine or any of the ingredients.

Agranulocytosis or severe thrombocytopenia due to penicillamine.

Lupus erythematosus.

Moderate or severe renal impairment.

4.4 Special warnings and special precautions for use
Full blood and platelet counts should be performed and renal function should be assessed prior to treatment with penicillamine.

During the first eight weeks of therapy full blood counts should be carried out weekly or fortnightly and also in the week after any increase in dose, otherwise monthly thereafter. In cystinuria or Wilson's disease, longer intervals may be adequate.

Withdrawal of treatment should be considered if platelets fall below 120,000/mm^3 or white blood cells below 2,500/mm^3, or if three successive falls are noted within the normal range. Treatment may be restarted at a reduced dose when counts return to normal, but should be permanently withdrawn on recurrence of leucopenia or thrombocytopenia.

In patients with normal renal function, urinalysis for detection of haematuria and proteinuria should be carried out weekly at first, and following each increase in dose, then monthly, although longer intervals may be adequate for cystinuria and Wilson's disease. Increasing or persistent proteinuria may necessitate withdrawal of therapy.

Care should be exercised in patients with renal insufficiency; modification of dosage may be necessary (see Section 4.2, "Posology and Method of Administration").

Especially careful monitoring is necessary in the elderly since increased toxicity has been observed in this patient population regardless of renal function.

Concomitant use of NSAIDs and other nephrotoxic drugs may increase the risk of renal damage.

Penicillamine should be used with caution in patients who have had adverse reactions to gold.

Concomitant or previous treatment with gold may increase the risk of side effects with penicillamine treatment. Therefore penicillamine should be used with caution in patients who have previously had adverse reactions to gold and concomitant treatment with gold should be avoided.

If concomitant oral iron therapy is indicated, this should not be given within two hours of taking penicillamine.

Antihistamines, steroid cover, or temporary reduction of dose will control urticarial reactions.

Reversible loss of taste may occur. Mineral supplements to overcome this are not recommended.

Haematuria is rare, but if it occurs in the absence of renal stones or other known cause, treatment should be stopped immediately.

A late rash, described as acquired epidermolysis bullosa and penicillamine dermopathy, may occur after several months or years of therapy. This may necessitate a reduction in dosage.

Breast enlargement has been reported as a rare complication of penicillamine therapy in both women and men. Danazol has been used successfully to treat breast enlargement which does not regress on drug discontinuation.

4.5 Interaction with other medicinal products and other forms of Interaction

Concomitant iron and penicillamine treatment: oral absorption of penicillamine may be reduced by concomitant administration of iron (see Section 4.4 "Special Warnings and Special Precautions for Use").

Concomitant use of NSAIDs and other nephrotoxic drugs may increase the risk of renal damage (see Section 4.4 "Special Warnings and Special Precautions for Use").

Concomitant gold and penicillamine treatment: concomitant use not recommended (see Section 4.4 "Special Warnings and Special Precautions for Use").

4.6 Pregnancy and lactation

Usage in pregnancy: The safety of penicillamine for use during pregnancy has not been established (see Section 5.3, "Preclinical Safety Data").

Wilson's disease: There has been one case reported of reversible cutis laxa in an infant born to a mother taking 1500mg penicillamine daily throughout pregnancy. Although there have been no controlled studies on the use of penicillamine during pregnancy, two retrospective studies have reported the successful delivery of 43 normal infants to 28 women receiving between 500 and 2000mg of penicillamine daily.

Cystinuria: Whilst normal infants have been delivered, there is one report of a severe connective tissue abnormality in the infant of a mother who received 2000mg penicillamine daily throughout pregnancy. Whenever possible, penicillamine should be withheld during pregnancy, but if stones continue to form, the benefit of resuming treatment must be weighed against the possible risk to the foetus.

Rheumatoid arthritis or chronic active hepatitis: Penicillamine should not be administered to patients who are pregnant, and therapy should be stopped when pregnancy is diagnosed or suspected, unless considered to be absolutely essential by the physician.

Usage in lactation: Due to the lack of data on use in breast feeding patients and the possibility that penicillamine may be transmitted to newborns through breast milk, Distamine should only be used in breast feeding patients when it is considered absolutely essential by the physician.

4.7 Effects on ability to drive and use machines

None known.

4.8 Undesirable effects

NB: The incidence and severity of some of the adverse reactions, noted below, varies according to the dosage and nature of the disease under treatment.

Nausea, anorexia, fever and rash may occur early in therapy, especially when full doses are given from the start.

Urticarial reactions have been reported (see Section 4.4, "Special Warnings and Special Precautions for Use").

Reversible loss of taste may occur (see Section 4.4, "Special Warnings and Special Precautions for Use").

Rarely, mouth ulceration/stomatitis has occurred.

Thrombocytopenia occurs commonly and leucopenia less often. These reactions may occur at any time during treatment and are usually reversible (see Section 4.4, "Special Warnings and Special Precautions for Use").

Deaths from agranulocytosis and aplastic anaemia have occurred.

Proteinuria occurs in up to 30% of patients and is partially dose-related (see Section 4.4, "Special Warnings and Special Precautions for Use").

Haematuria may occur rarely (see Section 4.4, "Special Warnings and Special Precautions for Use").

Other rare adverse reactions are as follows: alopecia and inflammatory conditions of the respiratory system, such as bronchiolitis and pneumonitis.

Other complications have included haemolytic anaemia, nephrotic syndrome, pancreatitis, cholestatic jaundice (including raised liver function tests), drug induced lupus erythematosus, and conditions closely resembling myasthenia gravis, polymyositis (with rare cardiac involvement), dermatomyositis, pemphigus, Goodpasture's syndrome, Stevens-Johnson syndrome and rheumatoid arthritis.

A late rash, described as acquired epidermolysis bullosa and penicillamine dermopathy, may occur after several months or years of therapy (see Section 4.4, "Special Warnings and Special Precautions for Use").

Pseudoxanthoma elasticum and skin laxity have been reported rarely. Breast enlargement has been reported as a rare complication of penicillamine therapy in both women and men. In some patients breast enlargement was considerable and/or prolonged with poor resolution and others required surgery (see Section 4.4, "Special Warnings and Special Precautions for Use").

4.9 Overdose

No instances of adverse reactions to an overdose of penicillamine have been recorded and no specific measures are indicated.

5. PHARMACOLOGICAL PROPERTIES

5.1 Pharmacodynamic properties

Pharmacotherapeutic group: M01C C

1. Penicillamine is used to treat severe active rheumatoid arthritis not adequately controlled by NSAID therapy.

2. Penicillamine is a chelating agent which aids the elimination from the body of certain heavy metal ions, including copper, lead and mercury, by forming stable soluble complexes with them that are readily excreted by the kidney.

3. It is used in the treatment of Wilson's disease (hepatolenticular degeneration), in conjunction with a low copper diet, to promote the excretion of copper.

4. It may be used to treat asymptomatic lead intoxication.

5. Penicillamine is used as an adjunct to diet and urinary alkalinisation in the management of cystinuria. By reducing urinary concentrations of cystine, penicillamine prevents the formation of calculi and promotes the gradual dissolution of existing calculi.

6. Desensitisation. Should the physician deem it necessary to attempt to desensitise a patient to penicillamine, it should be noted that this formulation is not suitable for this purpose.

5.2 Pharmacokinetic properties

Penicillamine is a thiol-group containing chelating agent, variably absorbed from the gastrointestinal tract. The drug undergoes a rapid distribution phase, followed by a slower elimination phase.

Penicillamine is strongly plasma-protein bound. Most penicillamine is bound to albumin but some is bound to α-globulins or ceruloplasmin.

Penicillamine is not extensively metabolised in man.

About 80% of the absorbed dose is excreted rapidly in the urine, mostly as mixed disulphides. Some of the dose is excreted as a penicillamine copper complex and some as the S-methyl derivative.

5.3 Preclinical safety data

Penicillamine has been shown to be teratogenic in rats when given in doses several times higher than those recommended for human use.

There is no known LD50 value for penicillamine. In studies some rats died after oral administration of 10,000mg/kg, but intra-peritoneal injections of a dose of 660mg/kg caused no deaths.

6. PHARMACEUTICAL PARTICULARS

6.1 List of excipients

Tablet Core

Microcrystalline cellulose

Sodium starch glycolate

Povidone

Stearic acid

Tablet coating

Glycerol

Titanium dioxide

Hydroxypropylmethyl cellulose

6.2 Incompatibilities

None known.

6.3 Shelf life

3 years

6.4 Special precautions for storage

Do not store above 25°C. Keep the container tightly closed.

6.5 Nature and contents of container

HDPE bottle with screw cap, containing 100 tablets.

6.6 Instructions for use and handling

None.

7. MARKETING AUTHORISATION HOLDER

Alliance Pharmaceuticals Ltd
Avonbridge House
Bath Road
Chippenham
Wiltshire
SN15 2BB
United Kingdom

8. MARKETING AUTHORISATION NUMBER(S)

PL 16853/0058

9. DATE OF FIRST AUTHORISATION/RENEWAL OF THE AUTHORISATION

28th September 2001

10. DATE OF REVISION OF THE TEXT

September 2003

Dithrocream

(Dermal Laboratories Limited)

1. NAME OF THE MEDICINAL PRODUCT

DITHROCREAM®

2. QUALITATIVE AND QUANTITATIVE COMPOSITION

Dithranol 0.1%, 0.25%, 0.5%, 1.0% or 2.0% w/w.

3. PHARMACEUTICAL FORM

Yellow aqueous cream.

4. CLINICAL PARTICULARS

4.1 Therapeutic indications

For the topical treatment of subacute and chronic psoriasis including psoriasis of the scalp.

4.2 Posology and method of administration

Dithranol therapy customarily involves titrating the concentration applied to skin to suit individual patient's circumstances. Dithrocream is, therefore, available in five strengths. The different packs are colour coded as follows:

0.1%	pale blue
0.25%	red
0.5%	purple
1.0%	brown
2.0%	yellow

For adults and the elderly: It is important to determine each patient's optimal treatment strength, as too high a strength may induce a burning sensation. Where the response to Dithrocream has not previously been established, always commence with Dithrocream 0.1%, continuing for at least one week and then, if necessary, increase to the 0.25% followed by the 0.5%, the 1.0% and finally the 2.0% strength. The aim should be to build up gradually over approximately 4 weeks to the highest tolerated strength to produce the optimum therapeutic effect. This optimum concentration will depend upon such factors as the thickness and location of the psoriatic plaques, as well as the variation between individual patients in their reaction to dithranol.

Dithrocream should be applied sparingly, and only to the affected areas, once every 24 hours, at any convenient time of the day or evening. Rub the cream gently and carefully into the skin until completely absorbed. For use on the scalp, first comb the hair to remove scalar debris and, after suitably parting, rub the cream well into the affected areas. Remove by washing off the skin or scalp, usually no more than one hour after application (Short Contact Therapy). Alternatively, it may be applied at night before retiring and washed off in the morning.

Treatment should be continued until the skin is entirely clear, i.e. when there is nothing to feel with the fingers and the texture is normal. By gradually increasing the strength of cream applied, it should be possible to clear psoriasis patches within 4 to 6 weeks.

For children No additional special precautions necessary. However, use cautiously as described above for adults and the elderly, with regular supervision.

4.3 Contraindications

Not to be used on the face, or for acute or pustular psoriasis.

Not to be used in cases of sensitivity to any of the ingredients.

4.4 Special warnings and special precautions for use

Dithrocream 0.5%, Dithrocream 1.0% and Dithrocream 2.0% should only be used for those patients who have failed to respond to lower strengths of dithranol.

Dithrocream 1.0% and 2.0% should normally only be applied for 'short contact' periods.

Dithrocream 0.5%, Dithrocream 1.0% and Dithrocream 2.0% should always be used under medical supervision.

It is most important to avoid applying an excessive amount of the cream, which may cause unnecessary soiling and staining of the clothing and/or bed linen. After each period of treatment, a bath/shower should be taken to remove any residual cream. To prevent the possibility of discolouration, particularly where Dithrocream 1.0% or 2.0% has been used, always rinse the bath/shower with hot water immediately after washing/showering and then use a suitable cleanser to remove any deposit on the surface of the bath/shower.

After use on the scalp, a shampoo may be used to remove the Dithrocream residue. Great care must be taken when washing out the shampoo (which may contain some Dithrocream residue), to ensure that it does not get into the eyes or on the face. This is particularly important when the higher strengths of Dithrocream have been used.

Although a feeling of warmth at the application site is normal, if this amounts to a burning sensation, or if the lesions spread, treatment should be stopped at once, and the dosage re-evaluated by a doctor.

Dithrocream is not normally recommended for use on areas of folded skin such as the groin and beneath the breasts. Do not use high strengths on these sites.

Keep away from the eyes and mucous membranes.

Always wash the hands after use.

As long term use of topical corticosteroids is known to destabilise psoriasis, and withdrawal may give rise to a rebound phenomenon, an interval of at least one week should be allowed between the discontinuance of such steroids and the commencement of Dithrocream therapy. A suitably bland emollient may usefully be applied in the intervening period.

Contact with fabrics, plastics and other materials may cause permanent staining and should be avoided.

4.5 Interaction with other medicinal products and other forms of Interaction
None known.

4.6 Pregnancy and lactation
Although there is no experimental evidence to support the safety of the drug in pregnancy or during lactation, no adverse effects have been reported.

4.7 Effects on ability to drive and use machines
None known.

4.8 Undesirable effects
Some skin irritation and/or a feeling of warmth at the site of application is normally associated with dithranol therapy. Dithrocream applied at too high a strength or left in contact with the skin for too long may induce a burning sensation.

Dithrocream may cause temporary staining of the skin and/or hair.

4.9 Overdose
Dithranol is a cathartic (laxative) and if accidentally swallowed, it should be removed by gastric lavage.

5. PHARMACOLOGICAL PROPERTIES

5.1 Pharmacodynamic properties
Dithranol has been used in the treatment of sub-acute and chronic psoriasis for over 70 years and, during that time, it has become established as a safe and effective form of therapy. Its precise mode of action is still to be confirmed, although it has been shown to inhibit DNA replication, cellular respiration and key cellular enzymes eg glucose-6-phosphate dehydrogenase.

Because dithranol causes staining and irritation, it is now widely used in short contact therapy where the preparation is washed off the skin after periods of one hour or less. For this purpose, Dithrocream is particularly suitable, as it is convenient to apply and washes off easily with ordinary soap and warm water in a bath or shower.

5.2 Pharmacokinetic properties
The traditional formulations of dithranol are based on soft paraffin from which it is effectively released into the skin. In Dithrocream, during manufacture, the oily paraffin phase of the cream is heated until the dithranol entirely dissolves so that, on cooling, it is retained solely within the paraffin phase and does not spread into the aqueous phase. After application of Dithrocream to the skin, the water is lost through absorption and evaporation, leaving the oily phase which then acts in the same way as a dithranol ointment. However, since the cream may be rubbed into the skin more effectively than the ointment, it is convenient to apply and, owing to the presence of the emulsifying components, is easier to wash off.

The availability of the dithranol has now been confirmed in numerous publications detailing the results of clinical trials.

5.3 Preclinical safety data
No special information.

6. PHARMACEUTICAL PARTICULARS

6.1 List of excipients
White Soft Paraffin; Cetostearyl Alcohol; Salicylic Acid; Ascorbic Acid; Sodium Lauryl Sulphate; Chlorocresol; Purified Water.

Dithrocream 2.0% also contains Liquid Paraffin.

6.2 Incompatibilities
None known.

6.3 Shelf life
48 months.

6.4 Special precautions for storage
Do not store above 25°C. Replace cap tightly after use.

6.5 Nature and contents of container
All strengths of Dithrocream are supplied in collapsible tubes containing 50 g. These are supplied as original packs (OP).

6.6 Instructions for use and handling
Not applicable.

7. MARKETING AUTHORISATION HOLDER
Dermal Laboratories
Tatmore Place, Gosmore
Hitchin, Herts SG4 7QR, UK.

8. MARKETING AUTHORISATION NUMBER(S)

Dithrocream 0.1%	0173/0029
Dithrocream 0.25%	0173/0028
Dithrocream 0.5%	0173/0027
Dithrocream 1.0%	0173/0039
Dithrocream 2.0%	0173/0045

9. DATE OF FIRST AUTHORISATION/RENEWAL OF THE AUTHORISATION
19 July 2005.

10. DATE OF REVISION OF THE TEXT
November 2004.

Ditropan Elixir 2.5mg/5ml

(sanofi-aventis)

1. NAME OF THE MEDICINAL PRODUCT
Ditropan elixir 2.5mg/5ml

2. QUALITATIVE AND QUANTITATIVE COMPOSITION
Ditropan elixir contains 2.5mg oxybutynin hydrochloride per 5ml.

3. PHARMACEUTICAL FORM
Ditropan elixir is a clear and colourless elixir.

4. CLINICAL PARTICULARS

4.1 Therapeutic indications
For use in urinary incontinence, urgency and frequency in the unstable bladder; whether due to neurogenic bladder disorders (detrusor hyperreflexia) in conditions such as multiple sclerosis and spina bifida or to idiopathic detrusor instability (motor urge incontinence).

Children over 5 years of age: In addition to neurogenic bladder disorders, Ditropan may also be used in nocturnal enuresis in conjunction with non-drug therapy where this alone, or in conjunction with other drug treatment, has failed.

4.2 Posology and method of administration
Dosage and administration
Adults: The usual dose is 5mg (10ml) two or three times a day. This may be increased to a maximum of 5 mg four times a day to obtain a clinical response provided that the side effects are tolerated.

Elderly: The elimination half-life is increased in the elderly, therefore, a dose of 2.5mg (5ml) twice a day, particularly if the patient is frail, is likely to be adequate. This dose may be titrated upwards to 5mg two times a day to obtain a clinical response provided the side effects are tolerated.

Children (under 5 years of age): Not recommended

Children (over 5 years of age): Neurogenic bladder: the usual dose is 2.5mg (5ml) twice a day. This dose may be titrated upwards to 5mg (10ml) two or three times a day to obtain a clinical response provided that the side effects are tolerated. Nocturnal enuresis: the usual dose is 2.5mg (5ml) twice a day. This dose may be titrated upwards to 5mg (10ml) two or three times a day to obtain a clinical response provided that the side effects are tolerated. The last dose should be given before bedtime.

4.3 Contraindications
Hypersensitivity to oxybutynin or any component.

Myasthenia gravis.

Narrow-angle glaucoma or shallow anterior chamber.

Gastrointestinal obstruction including paralytic ileus, intestinal atony.

Patients with toxic megacolon, severe ulcerative colitis.

Patients with bladder outflow obstruction where urinary retention may be precipitated.

4.4 Special warnings and special precautions for use
Oxybutynin should be used with caution in the frail elderly and children who may be more sensitive to the effects of the product and in patients with autonomic neuropathy, hepatic or renal impairment and severe gastro-intestinal motility disorders (also see section 4.3).

Oxybutynin may aggravate the symptoms of hyperthyroidism, congestive heart failure, coronary heart disease, cardiac arrhythmias, tachycardia, hypertension and prostatic hypertrophy.

Oxybutynin can cause decreased sweating; in high environmental temperatures this can lead to heat prostration.

The use of oxybutynin in children under 5 years of age is not recommended; it has not been established whether oxybutynin can be safely used in this age group.

Special care should be taken in patients with hiatus hernia associated with reflux oesophagitis, as anticholinergic drugs can aggravate this condition.

4.5 Interaction with other medicinal products and other forms of Interaction
Care should be taken if other anticholinergic agents are administered together with Ditropan as potentiation of anticholinergic effects could occur.

Occasional cases of interaction between anticholinergics and phenothiazines, amantidine, butyrophenones, L-dopa, digitalis and tricyclic antidepressants have been reported and care should be taken if Ditropan is administered concurrently with such drugs.

By reducing gastric motility, oxybutynin may affect the absorption of other drugs.

4.6 Pregnancy and lactation
Pregnancy
There is no evidence as to the safety of Ditropan in human pregnancy nor is there evidence from animal work that it is totally free from hazard. Avoid in pregnancy unless there is no safer alternative.

Lactation
Small amounts of oxybutynin have been found in mother's milk of lactating animals. Breast feeding while using oxybutynin is therefore not recommended.

4.7 Effects on ability to drive and use machines
As Ditropan may produce drowsiness or blurred vision, the patient should be cautioned regarding activities requiring mental alertness such as driving, operating machinery or performing hazardous work while taking this drug.

4.8 Undesirable effects
Gastro-intestinal disorders
Nausea, diarrhoea, constipation, dry mouth, abdominal discomfort, anorexia, vomiting, gastroesophageal reflux.

CNS and psychiatric disorders
Agitation, headache, dizziness, drowsiness, disorientation, hallucinations, nightmares, convulsions.

Cardiovascular disorders
Tachycardia, cardiac arrythmia.

Vision disorders
Blurred vision, mydriasis, intraocular hypertension, onset of narrow-angle glaucoma, dry eyes.

Renal and urinary disorders
Urinary retention, difficulty in micturition.

Skin and appendages
Facial flushing which may be more marked in children, dry skin, allergic reactions such as rash, urticaria, angioedema, photosensitivity.

4.9 Overdose
The symptoms of overdosage with oxybutynin progress from an intensification of the usual side effects of CNS disturbances (from restlessness and excitement to psychotic behaviour), circulatory changes (flushing, fall in blood pressure, circulatory failure etc), respiratory failure, paralysis and coma.

Measures to be taken are:

1) immediate gastric lavage

2) physostigmine by slow intravenous injection

Adults: 0.5 to 2.0 mg of physostigmine by slow intravenous administration. Repeat after 5 minutes, if necessary up to a maximum total dose of 5mg.

Children: 30 micrograms/kg of physostigmine by slow intravenous administration. Repeat after 5 minutes, if necessary up to a maximum total dose of 2mg.

Fever should be treated symptomatically with tepid sponging or ice packs.

In pronounced restlessness or excitation, diazepam 10mg may be given by intravenous injection, tachycardia may be treated by intravenous injection of propranolol and urinary retention can be managed by catheterisation.

In the event of progression of the curare like effect to the paralysis of the respiratory muscles, mechanical ventilation will be required.

5. PHARMACOLOGICAL PROPERTIES

5.1 Pharmacodynamic properties
Oxybutynin hydrochloride has both direct antispasmodic action on the smooth muscle of the bladder detrusor muscle as well as an anticholinergic action in blocking the muscarinic effects of acetylcholine on smooth muscle. These properties cause relaxation of the detrusor muscle of the bladder in patients with an unstable bladder. Ditropan increases bladder capacity and reduces the incidence of spontaneous contractions of the detrusor muscle.

5.2 Pharmacokinetic properties
Oxybutynin is poorly absorbed from the gastrointestinal tract. It is highly bound to plasma proteins, the peak plasma level is reached between 0.5 to 1 hour after administration. The half life is biexponential, the first phase being about 40 minutes and the second about 2-3 hours. The elimination half life may be increased in the elderly, particularly if they are frail.

Oxybutynin and its metabolites are excreted in the faeces and urine. There is no evidence of accumulation.

5.3 Preclinical safety data
No data of therapeutic relevance.

6. PHARMACEUTICAL PARTICULARS
6.1 List of excipients
itropan elixir contains citric acid, sodium citrate, sucrose (1.3g per 5ml dose), sorbitol, glycerol, sodium methyl-*p*-hydroxybenzoate (E219), purified water.

6.2 Incompatibilities
None known.

6.3 Shelf life
Ditropan Elixir 2.5mg/5ml has a 30 month shelf life.

6.4 Special precautions for storage
Ditropan Elixir 2.5mg/5ml: Store below 25°C. Protect from light

Discard any medicine remaining 28 days after opening the bottle

6.5 Nature and contents of container
Ditropan Elixir 2.5mg/5ml: 150ml amber glass bottle with a child resistant screw cap.

6.6 Instructions for use and handling
No special requirements.

7. MARKETING AUTHORISATION HOLDER
Sanofi-Synthelabo
PO Box 597
Guildford
Surrey

8. MARKETING AUTHORISATION NUMBER(S)
PL 11723/0316

9. DATE OF FIRST AUTHORISATION/RENEWAL OF THE AUTHORISATION
24 January 2001

10. DATE OF REVISION OF THE TEXT
March 2005

Legal Category POM

Ditropan Tablets 2.5mg, Ditropan Tablets 5mg

(sanofi-aventis)

1. NAME OF THE MEDICINAL PRODUCT
Ditropan tablets 2.5mg
Ditropan tablets 5mg

2. QUALITATIVE AND QUANTITATIVE COMPOSITION
Each tablet contains 2.5mg or 5mg oxybutynin hydrochloride as the active ingredient.

3. PHARMACEUTICAL FORM
Ditropan tablets 2.5mg are pale blue oval bi-convex tablets 8 mm × 5.5 mm, marked OXB2.5 on one side.

Ditropan tablets 5mg are pale blue circular tablets with a 8.0 mm nominal diameter, with a centre breakline on one side, and marked OXB5 on the reverse.

4. CLINICAL PARTICULARS
4.1 Therapeutic indications
Urinary incontinence, urgency and frequency in the unstable bladder, whether due to neurogenic bladder disorders (detrusor hyperreflexia) in conditions such as multiple sclerosis and spina bifida, or to idiopathic detrusor instability (motor urge incontinence).

Children over 5 years of age: In addition to neurogenic bladder disorders, Ditropan may also be used in nocturnal enuresis in conjunction with non-drug therapy where this alone, or in conjunction with other drug treatment, has failed.

4.2 Posology and method of administration
Dosage and administration
Adults: The usual dose is 5mg two or three times a day. This may be increased to a maximum of 5 mg four times a day to obtain a clinical response provided that the side effects are tolerated.

Elderly (including frail elderly): The elimination half-life is increased in the elderly. Therefore, a dose of 2.5mg twice a day, particularly if the patient is frail, is likely to be adequate. This dose may be titrated upwards to 5mg two times a day to obtain a clinical response provided the side effects are well tolerated.

Children (under 5 years of age): Not recommended

Children (over 5 years of age): Neurogenic bladder instability: the usual dose is 2.5mg twice a day. This dose may be titrated upwards to 5mg two or three times a day to obtain a clinical response provided the side effects are well tolerated. Nocturnal enuresis: the usual dose is 2.5mg twice a day. This dose may be titrated upwards to 5mg two or three times a day to obtain a clinical response provided the side effects are tolerated. The last dose should be given before bedtime.

4.3 Contraindications
Hypersensitivity to oxybutynin or any component.

Myasthenia gravis.

Narrow-angle glaucoma or shallow anterior chamber.

Gastrointestinal obstruction including paralytic ileus, intestinal atony.

Patients with toxic megacolon, severe ulcerative colitis.

Patients with bladder outflow obstruction where urinary retention may be precipitated.

4.4 Special warnings and special precautions for use
Oxybutynin should be used with caution in the frail elderly and children who may be more sensitive to the effects of the product and in patients with autonomic neuropathy, hepatic or renal impairment and severe gastro-intestinal motility disorders (also see section 4.3).

Oxybutynin may aggravate the symptoms of hyperthyroidism, congestive heart failure, coronary heart disease, cardiac arrhythmias, tachycardia, hypertension and prostatic hypertrophy.

Oxybutynin can cause decreased sweating; in high environmental temperatures this can lead to heat prostration.

The use of oxybutynin in children under 5 years of age is not recommended; it has not been established whether oxybutynin can be safely used in this age group.

Special care should be taken in patients with hiatus hernia associated with reflux oesophagitis, as anticholinergic drugs can aggravate this condition.

4.5 Interaction with other medicinal products and other forms of Interaction
Care should be taken if other anticholinergic agents are administered together with Ditropan, as potentiation of anticholinergic effects could occur.

Occasional cases of interaction between anticholinergics and phenothiazines, amantidine, butyrophenones, L-dopa, digitalis and tricyclic antidepressants have been reported and care should be taken if Ditropan is administered concurrently with such drugs.

By reducing gastric motility, oxybutynin may affect the absorption of other drugs.

4.6 Pregnancy and lactation
Pregnancy
There is no evidence as to the safety of Ditropan in human pregnancy nor is there evidence from animal work that it is totally free from hazard. Avoid in pregnancy unless there is no safer alternative.

Lactation
Small amounts of oxybutynin have been found in mother's milk of lactating animals. Breast feeding while using oxybutynin is therefore not recommended.

4.7 Effects on ability to drive and use machines
As Ditropan may produce drowsiness or blurred vision, the patient should be cautioned regarding activities requiring mental alertness such as driving, operating machinery or performing hazardous work while taking this drug.

4.8 Undesirable effects
Gastro-intestinal disorders
Nausea, diarrhoea, constipation, dry mouth, abdominal discomfort, anorexia, vomiting, gastroesophageal reflux.

CNS and psychiatric disorders
Agitation, headache, dizziness, drowsiness, disorientation, hallucinations, nightmares, convulsions.

Cardiovascular disorders
Tachycardia, cardiac arrythmia.

Vision disorders
Blurred vision, mydriasis, intraocular hypertension, onset of narrow-angle glaucoma, dry eyes.

Renal and urinary disorders
Urinary retention, difficulty in micturition.

Skin and appendages
Facial flushing which may be more marked in children, dry skin, allergic reactions such as rash, urticaria, angioedema, photosensitivity.

4.9 Overdose
The symptoms of overdose with oxybutynin progress from an intensification of the usual side effects of CNS disturbances (from restlessness and excitement to psychotic behaviour), circulation changes (flushing, fall in blood pressure, circulatory failure etc), respiratory failure, paralysis and coma.

Measures to be taken are:

1) Immediate gastric lavage

2) physostigmine by slow intravenous injection

Adults: 0.5 to 2.0 mg of physostigmine by slow intravenous administration. Repeat after 5 minutes, if necessary up to a maximum total dose of 5mg.

Children: 30 micrograms/kg of physostigmine by slow intravenous administration. Repeat after 5 minutes, if necessary up to a maximum total dose of 2mg.

Fever should be treated symptomatically with tepid sponging or ice packs.

In pronounced restlessness or excitation, diazepam 10mg may be given by intravenous injection, tachycardia may be treated by intravenous injection of propranolol and urinary retention can be managed by catheterisation.

In the event of progression of the curare- like effect to the paralysis of the respiratory muscles, mechanical ventilation will be required.

5. PHARMACOLOGICAL PROPERTIES
5.1 Pharmacodynamic properties
Oxybutynin has both direct antispasmodic action on the smooth muscle of the bladder detrusor muscle as well as an anticholinergic action in blocking the muscarinic effects of acetylcholine on smooth muscle. These properties cause relaxation of the detrusor muscle of the bladder in patients with an unstable bladder. Ditropan increases bladder capacity and reduces the incidence of spontaneous contractions of the detrusor muscle.

5.2 Pharmacokinetic properties
Oxybutynin is poorly absorbed from the gastrointestinal tract. It is highly bound to plasma proteins, the peak plasma level is reached between 0.5 to 1 hour after administration. The half life is biexponential, the first phase being about 40 minutes and the second about 2-3 hours. The elimination half life may be increased in the elderly, particularly if they are frail.

Oxybutynin and its metabolites are excreted in the faeces and urine. There is no evidence of accumulation.

5.3 Preclinical safety data
No data of therapeutic relevance.

6. PHARMACEUTICAL PARTICULARS
6.1 List of excipients
Ditropan tablets contain lactose, cellulose, calcium stearate and indigo carmine (E132).

6.2 Incompatibilities
None known.

6.3 Shelf life
4 years

6.4 Special precautions for storage
Store at or below 30°C.

6.5 Nature and contents of container
Cartons containing 21 or 84 tablets in blister strips.

6.6 Instructions for use and handling
No special requirements.

7. MARKETING AUTHORISATION HOLDER
Sanofi-Synthelabo
PO Box 597
Guildford
Surrey

8. MARKETING AUTHORISATION NUMBER(S)
Ditropan 2.5mg tablets: PL 11723/0314
Ditropan 5mg tablets: PL 11723/0315

9. DATE OF FIRST AUTHORISATION/RENEWAL OF THE AUTHORISATION
12th December 2000

10. DATE OF REVISION OF THE TEXT
March 2005

Legal category POM

Dolmatil Tablets 200mg, Dolmatil 400mg Tablets

(sanofi-aventis)

1. NAME OF THE MEDICINAL PRODUCT
Dolmatil Tablets 200mg.
Dolmatil 400mg Tablets.

2. QUALITATIVE AND QUANTITATIVE COMPOSITION
Dolmatil Tablets 200mg: active ingredient is sulpiride 200mg.

Dolmatil 400mg Tablets: active ingredient is sulpiride 400mg.

Sulpiride is a benzamide derivative.

3. PHARMACEUTICAL FORM
Dolmatil Tablets 200mg: Plain white round tablet with a transverse breakline on one side and D200 on the other.

Dolmatil 400mg Tablets: White film coated stick shaped tablet with break bar engraved SLP 400 on one side

4. CLINICAL PARTICULARS
4.1 Therapeutic indications
Acute and chronic schizophrenia.

4.2 Posology and method of administration

Adults

A starting dose of 400mg to 800mg daily, given as one or two tablets twice daily (morning and early evening) is recommended.

Predominantly positive symptoms (formal thought disorder, hallucinations, delusions, incongruity of affect) respond to higher doses, and a starting dose of at least 400mg twice daily is recommended, increasing if necessary up to a suggested maximum of 1200mg twice daily. Increasing the dose beyond this level has not been shown to produce further improvement.

Predominantly negative symptoms (flattening of affect, poverty of speech, anergia, apathy, as well as depression), respond to doses below 800mg daily; therefore, a starting dose of 400mg twice daily is recommended. Reducing this dose towards 200mg twice daily will normally increase the alerting effect of Dolmatil.

Patients with mixed positive and negative symptoms, with neither predominating, will normally respond to dosage of 400-600mg twice daily.

Children

Clinical experience in children under 14 years of age is insufficient to permit specific recommendations.

Elderly

The same dose ranges are applicable in the elderly, but should be reduced if there is evidence of renal impairment.

4.3 Contraindications

Phaeochromocytoma and acute porphyria.

Hypersensitivity to the active ingredient or to other ingredients of the drug.

Concomitant prolactin-dependent tumours e.g. pituitary gland prolactinomas and breast cancer (See 4.8 Undesirable effects).

Association with levodopa (See 4.5 Interactions with other medicinal products and other forms of interaction).

4.4 Special warnings and special precautions for use

Increased motor agitation has been reported at high dosage in a small number of patients: in aggressive, agitated or excited phases of the disease process, low doses of Dolmatil may aggravate symptoms. Care should be exercised where hypomania is present.

Extrapyramidal reactions, principally akathisia have been reported in a small number of cases. If warranted, reduction in dosage or anti-parkinsonian medication may be necessary.

As with other neuroleptics, rare cases of neuroleptic malignant syndrome, characterised by hyperthermia, muscle rigidity, autonomic instability, altered consciousness and elevated CPK levels, have been reported. In such an event, all antipsychotic drugs, including Dolmatil, should be discontinued.

Elderly patients are more susceptible to postural hypotension, sedation and extrapyramidal effects.

Acute withdrawal symptoms, including nausea, vomiting, sweating and insomnia have been described after abrupt cessation of antipsychotic drugs. Recurrence of psychotic symptoms may also occur, and the emergence of involuntary movement disorders (such as akathisia, dystonia and dyskinesia) have been reported. Therefore, gradual withdrawal is advisable.

Precautions:

In elderly patients, as with other neuroleptics, sulpiride should be used with particular caution (see 4.2 Posology and method of administration).

In children, sulpiride has not been thoroughly investigated. Therefore, caution should be exercised when prescribing to children (see 4.2 Posology and method of administration).

When neuroleptic treatment is absolutely necessary in a patient with Parkinson's disease, sulpiride can be used, although caution is in order.

Dolmatil induces slight EEG modifications only, and whilst neuroleptics may lower the epileptogenic threshold, this has not been evaluated with sulpiride. Caution is advised in prescribing it for patients with unstable epilepsy, and patients with a history of epilepsy should be closely monitored during therapy with sulpiride.

In patients requiring Dolmatil who are receiving anti-convulsant therapy, the dose of the anti-convulsant should not be changed.

Cases of convulsions, sometimes in patients with no previous history, have been reported.

Dolmatil has no significant anticholinergic effect. As with all drugs for which the kidney is the major elimination pathway, the dose should be reduced and titrated in small steps in cases of renal insufficiency.

Prolongation of the QT interval

Sulpiride may induce a prolongation of the QT interval. This effect, known to potentiate the risk of serious ventricular arrhythmias such as torsade de pointes is enhanced by the pre-existence of bradycardia, hypokalaemia, congenital or acquired long QT interval.

Before any administration, and if possible according to the patient's clinical status, it is recommended to monitor factors which could favour the occurrence of this rhythm disorder

- bradycardia less than 55 bpm,
- hypokalaemia (which should be corrected),
- congenital prolongation of the QT interval.
- on-going treatment with a medication likely to produce pronounced bradycardia (< 55 bpm), hypokalaemia, decreased intracardiac conduction, or prolongation of the QTc interval (see § 4.5 Interaction with other medicinal products and other forms of interactions).

4.5 Interaction with other medicinal products and other forms of Interaction

4.5.1 Associations contra-indicated

Levodopa: reciprocal antagonism of effects between levopoda and neuroleptics.

4.5.2 Associations not recommended.

Alcohol: alcohol enhances the sedative effects of neuroleptics.

Avoid the consumption of alcoholic beverages and drugs containing alcohol.

Combination with the following medications which could induce torsades de pointes:

– Bradycardia-inducing medications such as beta-blockers, bradycardia-inducing calcium channel blockers such as diltiazem and verapamil, clonidine; digitalics.

– Medications which induce hypokalaemia: hypokalaemic diuretics, stimulant laxatives, IV amphotericin B, glucocorticoids, tetracosactides.

– Class Ia antiarrhythmic agents such as quinidine, disopyramide.

– Class III antiarrhythmic agents such as amiodarone, sotalol.

– Other medications such as pimozide, haloperidol; imipramine antidepressants; cisapride, thioridazine, IV erythromycin, pentamidine.

4.5.3 Associations to be taken into account.

Antihypertensive agents: antihypertensive effect and possibility of enhanced postural hypotension (additive effect).

CNS depressants including narcotics, analgesics, sedative H1 antihistamines, barbiturates, benzodiazepines and other anxiolytics, clonidine and derivatives.

Antacids or sucralfate: The absorption of sulpiride is decreased after co-administration. Therefore, sulpiride should be administered two hours before these drugs

Lithium increases the risk of extrapyramidal side effects.

Sulpiride may reduce the effectiveness of ropinorole.

4.6 Pregnancy and lactation

Pregnancy:

Animal studies do not indicate direct or indirect harmful effects with respect to embryonal/foetal development, parturition or postnatal development.

In humans, no increase in the risk of birth defects was seen in a small sample of women given low-dose sulpiride (approximately 200 mg/d). No data are available on the effects of higher dosages.

There are no data on the potential effects on the foetal brain of neuroleptic agents given throughout pregnancy.

These data suggest that sulpiride has little or no potential for inducing congenital defects. However, it seems reasonable to reduce the duration of the treatment during pregnancy if possible.

A few cases of extrapyramidal syndrome have been reported in neonates born to mothers under long-term, high-dose neuroleptic therapy.

It seems warranted to monitor neurological function for some time after birth.

A decrease in fertility linked to the pharmacological effects of the drug (prolactin mediated effect) was observed in treated animals. This effect was reversible upon discontinuation.

Lactation: Sulpiride has been found in the breast milk of treated women. Therefore breast-feeding is not recommended during treatment.

4.7 Effects on ability to drive and use machines

Even used as recommended, sulpiride may affect reaction time so that the ability to drive vehicles or operate machinery can be impaired.

4.8 Undesirable effects

Neuroleptic malignant syndrome:

As with other neuroleptics, rare cases of neuroleptic malignant syndrome, characterised by hyperthermia, muscle rigidity, autonomic instability, altered consciousness and elevated CPK levels, have been reported. In such an event, all antipsychotic drugs, including Dolmatil, should be discontinued (See 4.4 Special Warnings and Precautions for Use).

Neurological events: Sedation or drowsiness. Insomnia has been reported.

Very rare cases of convulsions have been reported, in particular in epileptic patients (See 4.4 Special warnings and special precautions for use).

Extrapyramidal symptoms and related disorders:

- parkinsonism and related symptoms: tremor, hypertonia, hypokinesia, hypersalivation,
- acute dyskinesia and dystonia (spasm torticollis, oculogyric crisis, trismus),
- akathisia.

These symptoms are generally reversible upon administration of antiparkinsonian medication.

- tardive dyskinesia (characterised by rhythmic, involuntary movements primarily of the tongue and/or the face) have been reported, as with all neuroleptics, after a neuroleptic administration of more than 3 months. Antiparkinsonian medication is ineffective or may induce aggravation of the symptoms.

Autonomic events: postural hypotension.

Very rare cases of QT prolongation and very rare cases of torsades de pointes have been reported.

Hyperprolactinaemia and related disorders: galactorrhoea, amenorrhoea, gynaecomastia, breast enlargement and breast pain, orgasmic dysfunction and impotence.

Hepatic reactions have been reported.

Bodyweight gain, potentially significant in very rare cases.

Very rare cases of hypersensitivity reactions such as skin reactions have been reported.

4.9 Overdose

Experience with sulpiride in overdosage is limited

The range of single toxic doses is 1 to 16g but no death has occurred even at the 16g dose.

The clinical manifestations of poisoning vary depending upon the size of the dose taken. After single doses of 1 to 3g restlessness and clouding of consciousness have been reported and (rarely) extrapyramidal symptoms. Doses of 3 to 7g may produce a degree of agitation, confusion and extrapyramidal symptoms; more than 7g can cause, in addition, coma and low blood pressure.

The duration of intoxication is generally short, the symptoms disappearing within a few hours. Comas which have occurred after large doses have lasted up to four days.

No haematological or hepatic toxicity has been reported.

Overdose may be treated with alkaline osmotic diuresis and, if necessary, anti-parkinsonian drugs. Coma needs appropriate nursing, and cardiac monitoring is recommended until the patient recovers. Emetic drugs are unlikely to be effective in Dolmatil overdosage.

5. PHARMACOLOGICAL PROPERTIES

5.1 Pharmacodynamic properties

Dolmatil is a member of the group of substituted benzamides, which are structurally distinct from the phenothiazines, butyrophenones and thioxanthenes. Current evidence suggests that the actions of Dolmatil hint at an important distinction between different types of dopamine receptors or receptor mechanisms in the brain.

Behaviourally and biochemically, Dolmatil shares with these classical neuroleptics a number of properties indicative of cerebral dopamine receptor antagonism. Essential and intriguing differences include lack of catalepsy at doses active in other behavioural tests, lack of effect in the dopamine sensitive adenylate cyclase systems, lack of effect upon noradrenaline or 5HT turnover, negligible anticholinesterase activity, no effect on muscarinic or GABA receptor binding, and a radical difference in the binding of tritiated sulpiride to striatal preparations in-vitro, compared to ^{3}H-spiperone or ^{3}H-haloperidol. These findings indicate a major differentiation between Dolmatil and classical neuroleptics which lack such specificity.

One of the characteristics of Dolmatil is its bimodal activity, as it has both antidepressant and neuroleptic properties. Schizophrenia characterised by a lack of social contact can benefit strikingly. Mood elevation is observed after a few days treatment, followed by disappearance of the florid schizophrenic symptoms. The sedation and lack of affect characteristically associated with classical neuroleptics of the phenothiazine or butyrophenone type are not features of Dolmatil therapy.

5.2 Pharmacokinetic properties

Peak sulpiride serum levels are reached 3 - 6 hours after an oral dose. The plasma half-life in man is approximately 8 hours. Approximately 40% sulpiride is bound to plasma proteins. 95% of the compound is excreted in the urine and faeces as unchanged sulpiride.

5.3 Preclinical safety data

In long-term animal studies with neuroleptic drugs, including sulpiride, an increased incidence of various endocrine tumours (some of which have occasionally been malignant) has been seen in some but not all strains of rats and mice studied. The significance of these findings to man is not known; there is no current evidence of an association between neuroleptic use and tumour risk in man.

6. PHARMACEUTICAL PARTICULARS

6.1 List of excipients

Dolmatil Tablets 200mg: Starch, lactose, methylcellulose, magnesium stearate, talc, silica.

Dolmatil 400mg Tablets: Lactose, sodium starch glycollate, microcrystalline cellulose, hydroxypropylmethyl-cellulose and magnesium stearate.

6.2 Incompatibilities
None known.

6.3 Shelf life
5 years.

6.4 Special precautions for storage
Store at or below 25°C.

6.5 Nature and contents of container
Cartons containing 100 tablets in blister strips.

Dolmatil 400mg Tablets: Strip-wrapped in a moulded bubble blister pack in 200μg PVC, heat sealed with 0.02mm printed laminated aluminium foil. Contains 100 tablets.

6.6 Instructions for use and handling
Not applicable.

7. MARKETING AUTHORISATION HOLDER
Sanofi-Synthelabo

PO Box 597

Guildford

Surrey

8. MARKETING AUTHORISATION NUMBER(S)
Dolmatil Tablets 200mg: PL 11723/0339

Dolmatil 400mg Tablets: PL 11723/0340

9. DATE OF FIRST AUTHORISATION/RENEWAL OF THE AUTHORISATION
Dolmatil Tablets 200mg: 15 October 2002

Dolmatil 400mg Tablets: 15 October 2002

10. DATE OF REVISION OF THE TEXT
Dolmatil Tablets 200mg: 15 October 2002

Dolmatil 400mg Tablets: 15 October 2002

Legal Category: POM

Dolobid 250mg, 500mg Tablets

(Merck Sharp & Dohme Limited)

1. NAME OF THE MEDICINAL PRODUCT
DOLOBID® 250 mg Tablets
DOLOBID® 500 mg Tablets

2. QUALITATIVE AND QUANTITATIVE COMPOSITION
'Dolobid' 250 mg contains 250 mg of the active ingredient, diflunisal.

'Dolobid' 500 mg contains 500 mg of the active ingredient, diflunisal.

3. PHARMACEUTICAL FORM
'Dolobid' 250 mg Tablets are supplied as peach-coloured, capsule-shaped, film-coated tablets, marked 'MSD 675'.

'Dolobid' 500 mg Tablets are supplied as orange-coloured, film-coated tablets, marked 'MSD 697'.

4. CLINICAL PARTICULARS

4.1 Therapeutic indications
'Dolobid' is indicated in the relief of pain.

'Dolobid' is also indicated in the relief of pain and inflammation associated with osteoarthritis and rheumatoid arthritis.

'Dolobid' is also indicated in the relief of pain and associated symptoms of primary dysmenorrhoea.

4.2 Posology and method of administration
Tablets should be swallowed whole, not crushed or chewed.

It is prudent to start at the bottom end of the dose range. In certain cases, it will be necessary to start with a high initial dose, as described in the dosage recommendations below.

For relief of pain

An initial dose of 1,000 mg, followed by 500 mg every 12 hours, is recommended for most patients. Following the initial dose, some patients may require 500 mg every eight hours.

Maintenance doses higher than 1,500 mg a day are not recommended.

For osteoarthritis and rheumatoid arthritis

The recommended dosage range is 500 mg to 1,000 mg per day. 'Dolobid' may be administered once or twice a day.

Dosage should be adjusted to the nature and intensity of the pain being treated.

For dysmenorrhoea

The recommended dosage is 1,000 mg at the onset of cramps or bleeding, followed by 500 mg every 12 hours for as long as symptoms last, usually a maximum of five days.

Use in children: 'Dolobid' is not recommended for children.

Use in the elderly: The dosage does not require modification for elderly patients.

4.3 Contraindications
Hypersensitivity to any component of this product.

In patients who have previously experienced acute asthmatic attacks, urticaria, or rhinitis precipitated by aspirin or non-steroidal anti-inflammatory drugs (NSAIDs).

The drug should not be administered to patients with active gastro-intestinal bleeding.

NSAIDs, including 'Dolobid', should not be given to patients with active peptic ulceration.

'Dolobid' is contra-indicated in pregnancy and lactation (see 4.6 'Pregnancy and lactation').

4.4 Special warnings and special precautions for use

Infections

NSAIDs, including 'Dolobid', may mask the usual signs and symptoms of infection. Therefore, the physician must be continually on the alert for this and should use the drug with extra care in the presence of existing infection.

Platelet aggregation

Although 'Dolobid' has less effect on platelet function and bleeding time than aspirin, at higher doses it is an inhibitor of platelet function; therefore, patients who may be adversely affected should be carefully observed when 'Dolobid' is administered.

Ocular effects

Because of reports of adverse eye findings with agents of this class, it is recommended that patients who develop eye complaints during treatment with 'Dolobid' have ophthalmological evaluations.

Gastro-intestinal effects

'Dolobid' should be used with caution in patients having a history of gastro-intestinal haemorrhage or ulcers. Fatalities have occurred, rarely.

In patients with a history of peptic-ulcer disease and in the elderly, NSAIDs should be given only after other forms of treatment have been carefully considered.

'Dolobid' should be used with caution in patients suffering from, or with a previous history of bronchial asthma.

Reye's syndrome

Although there have been no known reports associated with the use of 'Dolobid' to date, acetylsalicylic acid has been associated with Reye's syndrome. Because diflunisal is a compound related to salicylic acid, the possibility of an association with Reye's syndrome cannot be excluded.

Renal effects

As with other NSAIDs, there have been reports of acute interstitial nephritis with haematuria, proteinuria, and occasionally nephrotic syndrome in patients receiving diflunisal.

In patients with reduced renal blood flow where renal prostaglandins play a major role in maintaining renal perfusion, administration of a NSAID may precipitate overt renal decompensation. Patients at greatest risk of this reaction are those with renal or hepatic dysfunction, diabetes mellitus, advanced age, extracellular volume depletion, congestive heart failure, sepsis, or concomitant use of any nephrotoxic drug. An NSAID should be given with caution and renal function should be monitored in any patient who may have reduced renal reserve. Discontinuation of NSAID therapy is usually followed by recovery to the pretreatment state.

Since 'Dolobid' is eliminated primarily by the kidneys, patients with significantly impaired renal function should be closely monitored; a lower daily dosage should be used to avoid excessive drug accumulation. In patients with severe renal impairment, the drug should not be used.

In rats and dogs, high oral doses of diflunisal (50 to 200 mg/kg/day), as with aspirin, produced similar pathological changes (gastro-intestinal ulceration and renal papillary oedema). These dosages are approximately 3 to 12 times the maximum dosages recommended in man.

Cardiovascular effects

Peripheral oedema has been observed in some patients taking 'Dolobid'. Therefore, as with other drugs in this class, 'Dolobid' should be used with caution in patients with compromised cardiac function, hypertension, or other conditions predisposing to fluid retention.

Hypersensitivity syndrome

A potentially life-threatening, apparent hypersensitivity syndrome has been reported. In cases where this syndrome is suspected, therapy should be discontinued immediately and not reinstituted. This multisystem syndrome includes constitutional symptoms (fever, chills), and cutaneous findings (see 4.8 'Undesirable effects', *Dermatological*). It may also include involvement of major organs (changes in liver function), jaundice, leucopenia, thrombocytopenia, eosinophilia, disseminated intravascular coagulation, renal impairment (including renal failure), and less specific findings (adenitis, arthralgia, myalgia, arthritis, malaise, anorexia, disorientation).

Laboratory tests

AST (SGOT) and ALT (SGPT) levels rose significantly by three times the upper limit of normal in less than 1% of patients in controlled clinical trials of NSAIDs.

A patient on 'Dolobid' with signs or symptoms suggesting liver disease, or in whom abnormal liver-function tests have occurred, should be evaluated for evidence of a more severe hepatic reaction. If abnormal liver tests persist or worsen, if signs or symptoms of liver disease develop, or if systemic manifestations such as eosinophilia or rash occur, 'Dolobid' should be discontinued.

4.5 Interaction with other medicinal products and other forms of Interaction

Indomethacin: The combined use of indomethacin and 'Dolobid' has been associated with fatal gastro-intestinal haemorrhage. The combination should not be used. Co-administration of 'Dolobid' with indomethacin increases the plasma level of indomethacin by about 30 to 35% with a concomitant decrease in renal clearance of indomethacin and its conjugate.

Other NSAIDs: The concomitant use of 'Dolobid' and other NSAIDs is not recommended owing to the increased possibility of gastro-intestinal toxicity, with little or no increase in efficacy.

Aspirin: Co-administration of aspirin causes approximately a 15% decrease in plasma levels of 'Dolobid'.

Naproxen: Normal volunteers given naproxen and 'Dolobid' showed no changes in plasma levels of either drug, but a significant decrease in urinary excretion of naproxen and its glucuronide metabolite.

Sulindac: Normal volunteers given sulindac and 'Dolobid' showed substantial but not statistically significant lower levels of the active sulphide metabolite of sulindac.

Paracetamol: Co-administration significantly increased the plasma levels of paracetamol by approximately 50% but the plasma levels of 'Dolobid' were unaffected. Since paracetamol in high doses has been associated with hepatotoxicity, administration of 'Dolobid' and paracetamol should be used cautiously, with careful monitoring of patients.

Gold salts: In clinical studies of patients with rheumatoid arthritis, 'Dolobid' added to the regimen of gold salts usually resulted in additional symptomatic relief.

Codeine: Co-administration with 'Dolobid' improves the analgesic efficacy of either drug taken alone.

Methotrexate: Caution should be used if 'Dolobid' is administered concomitantly with methotrexate. NSAIDs have been reported to decrease the tubular secretion of methotrexate and potentiate the toxicity.

Cyclosporin: Administration of NSAIDs concomitantly with cyclosporin has been associated with an increase in cyclosporin-induced toxicity, possibly due to decreased synthesis of renal prostacyclin. NSAIDs should be used with caution in patients taking cyclosporin, and renal function should be monitored carefully.

Oralanticoagulant drugs: The concomitant administration of 'Dolobid' and warfarin or nicoumalone resulted in prolongation of prothrombin time in normal volunteers. This may occur because diflunisal competitively displaces coumarins from protein binding sites. Accordingly, prothrombin time should be monitored during, and for several days after, the concomitant drug administration of 'Dolobid' and oral anticoagulants. The dosage of oral anticoagulants may require adjustment.

Antihypertensives: the antihypertensive effects of some antihypertensive agents including ACE inhibitors, beta-blocking agents and diuretics, may be reduced when used concomitantly with NSAIDs. Caution should therefore be exercised when considering the addition of NSAID therapy to the regimen of a patient taking antihypertensives therapy.

Cardiac glycosides: an increase in serum-digoxin concentration has been reported with concomitant use of aspirin, indomethacin and other NSAIDs. Therefore when concomitant digoxin and NSAID therapy is initiated or discontinued, serum-digoxin levels should be closely monitored.

Lithium: concomitant use of indomethacin with lithium, produced a clinically relevant elevation of plasma lithium and reduction in renal lithium clearance in psychiatric patients and normal subjects with steady-state plasma lithium concentrations. This effect has been attributed to inhibition of prostaglandin synthesis and the potential exists for a similar effect with other NSAIDs.

As a consequence, when an NSAID and lithium are given concomitantly, the patient should be observed carefully for signs of lithium toxicity. In addition the frequency of monitoring serum lithium concentrations should be increased at the outset of such combination therapy.

Corticosteroids: the risk of gastro-intestinal bleeding and ulceration associated with NSAIDs is increased when used with corticosteroids.

Mifepristone: NSAIDs and aspirin should be avoided until at least 8 to 12 days after administration of mifepristone.

Quinolone antibiotics: there have been reports that 4-quinolones may induce convulsions, in patients with or without a history of convulsions. Taking NSAIDs at the same time may also induce them.

Tolbutamide: No significant changes occurred in the plasma levels of tolbutamide or in the fasting blood sugar levels of diabetic patients who also took 'Dolobid'.

Hydrochlorothiazide: Co-administration increases the plasma levels of hydrochlorothiazide by 25 to 35% with a concomitant decrease in renal clearance of the diuretic. This change is not clinically important. 'Dolobid' counteracts the hyperuricaemic effect of hydrochlorothiazide.

Frusemide: Co-administration did not affect the diuretic activity of frusemide in normal volunteers, but its hyperuricaemic activity was decreased by 'Dolobid'.

Antacids: The clinical effect of occasional doses of antacid is insignificant, but this becomes significant when antacids are used continuously. Co-administration of aluminium hydroxide suspension significantly decreases the absorption of 'Dolobid' by approximately 40%.

Drug/laboratory test interactions: Serum salicylate assays: Caution should be used in interpreting the results of serum salicylate assays when diflunisal is present. Because of the cross-reactivity between the two compounds, salicylate levels have been found to be falsely elevated with some assay methods.

4.6 Pregnancy and lactation

There are no data relating to the safe use of 'Dolobid' during the first two trimesters of pregnancy. Use of 'Dolobid' during the third trimester of pregnancy is not recommended. The known effects of drugs of this class on the human foetus during the third trimester of pregnancy include: constriction of the ductus arteriosus prenatally, tricuspid incompetence, and pulmonary hypertension; non-closure of the ductus arteriosus post-natally which may be resistant to medical management; myocardial degenerative changes; platelet dysfunction with resultant bleeding; intracranial bleeding, renal dysfunction or failure; renal injury/dysgenesis which may result in prolonged or permanent renal failure; oligohydramnios; gastro-intestinal bleeding or perforation; and increased risk of necrotising enterocolitis.

Breast-feeding mothers should not take 'Dolobid', or should stop breast-feeding.

4.7 Effects on ability to drive and use machines

There are no data to suggest that 'Dolobid' affects the ability to drive and use machines. 'Dolobid' may cause dizziness in some patients. If patients experience dizziness, they should be instructed not to drive, and to avoid operating machinery or performing other hazardous activities requiring alertness.

4.8 Undesirable effects

3 % to 9% incidence

Gastro-intestinal: gastro-intestinal pain, dyspepsia, diarrhoea, nausea.

Dermatological: rash.

Central nervous system: headache.

1 % to 3% incidence

Gastro-intestinal: vomiting, constipation, flatulence.

Centralnervous system/psychiatric: dizziness, somnolence, insomnia.

Special senses: tinnitus.

Miscellaneous: fatigue.

Less than 1% incidence

Gastro-intestinal: peptic ulcer, gastro-intestinal perforation and bleeding, anorexia, jaundice, cholestasis, liver-function abnormality, hepatitis, gastritis.

Dermatological: pruritus, sweating, dry mucous membranes, stomatitis, photosensitivity, urticaria, erythema multiforme and Stevens-Johnson syndrome, toxic epidermal necrolysis, exfoliative dermatitis.

Genito-urinary: dysuria, renal impairment including renal failure, interstitial nephritis, haematuria.

Central nervous system/psychiatric: vertigo, light-headedness, paraesthesiae, nervousness, depression, hallucinations, confusion.

Haematological: thrombocytopenia, agranulocytosis, haemolytic anaemia.

Special senses: transient visual disturbances including blurred vision.

Miscellaneous: asthenia, oedema.

Hypersensitivity reactions: acute anaphylactic reaction with bronchospasm, angioedema, hypersensitivity vasculitis, hypersensitivity syndrome (see 4.4 'Special warnings and special precautions for use').

Causal relationship unknown

Other reactions have been reported in clinical trials or since the drug was marketed, but occurred under circumstances where a causal relationship could not be established. However, in these rarely reported events, that possibility cannot be excluded. Therefore, the following observations are listed to serve as alerting information to physicians.

Respiratory: dyspnoea.

Cardiovascular: palpitations, syncope.

Musculoskeletal: muscle cramps.

Genito-urinary: nephrotic syndrome.

Miscellaneous: chest pain, fulminant necrotising fasciitis, particularly in association with Group A β-haemolytic streptococcus (see 4.4 'Special warnings and special precautions for use').

4.9 Overdose

Cases of overdosage have occurred and fatalities have been reported. The most common signs and symptoms observed with overdosage were drowsiness, vomiting, nausea, diarrhoea, hyperventilation, tachycardia, sweating, tinnitus, disorientation, stupor and coma. Diminished urine output and cardiorespiratory arrest have also been reported. The lowest dose of 'Dolobid' alone at which death was reported was 15 g; death has been reported from a mixed drug overdose that included 7.5 g 'Dolobid'.

In the event of recent overdosage, the stomach should be emptied by inducing vomiting or by gastric lavage. The patient should be observed carefully and given symptomatic and supportive treatment.

To facilitate urinary elimination of the drug, attempt to maintain renal function. Because of the high degree of protein binding, haemodialysis is not recommended.

The initial plasma half-life following single oral doses of diflunisal seems to be dose dependent, ranging from approximately 7.5 hours for a 250 mg dose to 11 hours for a 500 mg dose.

5. PHARMACOLOGICAL PROPERTIES

5.1 Pharmacodynamic properties

'Dolobid' in man has been shown to possess analgesic activity lasting up to 12 hours or more. In clinical trials, 'Dolobid' produced highly effective levels of analgesia when administered twice a day.

As an inhibitor of prostaglandin synthetase, 'Dolobid' has a dose-related effect on platelet function. In normal volunteers given 'Dolobid' twice a day for eight days at doses within the recommended range 500-1,000 mg daily, 500 mg daily had no effect on platelet function and 1,000 mg daily had a slight effect. However, at 2,000 mg daily, which exceeds the maximum recommended dosage, 'Dolobid' inhibited platelet function. In contrast to aspirin, these effects of 'Dolobid' were reversible.

A loading dose of 1,000 mg provides faster onset of pain relief, shorter time to peak analgesic effect, and greater peak analgesic effects than an initial 500 mg dose.

'Dolobid' at 1,000 mg twice daily (NOTE: exceeds the recommended dosage) causes a statistically significant increase in faecal blood loss, but this increase was only one-half as large as that associated with aspirin 1,300 mg twice daily.

5.2 Pharmacokinetic properties

'Dolobid' is rapidly and completely absorbed following oral administration with peak plasma concentrations occurring between two and three hours. The drug is excreted in the urine as two soluble glucuronide conjugates accounting for about 90% of the administered dose. Little or no diflunisal is excreted in the faeces. As diflunisal is excreted primarily by the kidney, the greater the degree of renal impairment, the slower the plasma disappearance rate of the drug and its glucuronides. Diflunisal appears in human milk in concentrations of 2 to 7% of those in plasma. More than 99% of diflunisal in plasma is bound to proteins.

The plasma half-life of diflunisal is 8 to 12 hours. Because of this long half-life and non-linear pharmacokinetics, several days are required for diflunisal plasma levels to reach steady state following multiple doses. For this reason, an initial loading dose is necessary to shorten the time to reach steady-state levels, and two to three days of observation are necessary for evaluating changes in treatment regimens if a loading dose is not used.

5.3 Preclinical safety data

There are no pre-clinical data of relevance which are additional to that already included in other sections of the SPC.

6. PHARMACEUTICAL PARTICULARS

6.1 List of excipients

'Dolobid' 250 mg and 500 mg Tablets contain the following inactive ingredients:

Cellulose, microcrystalline E460

Hydroxypropylcellulose E463

Magnesium stearate E572

Pregelatinised maize starch

Sunset yellow aluminum lake E110

Talc

Titanium dioxide E171

Methylhydroxypropylcellulose E464

'Dolobid' 250 mg Tablets also contain carnauba wax E903.

6.2 Incompatibilities

None.

6.3 Shelf life

HDPE bottles: 60 months.

PVC blister packs of 60 tablets: 36 months.

6.4 Special precautions for storage

Store below 25°C, protected from light.

6.5 Nature and contents of container

'Dolobid' 250 mg tablets are available in:

Packs of 50 tablets containing five PVC blister strips of 10 tablets, to give a total of 50 tablets.

Packs of 60 tablets containing six PVC blister strips of 10 tablets, to give a total of 60 tablets.

HDPE bottles with tamper-evident closures containing 100 tablets.

HDPE bottles with securitainer containing 1000 tablets.

'Dolobid' 500 mg tablets are available in:

Packs of 60 tablets containing six PVC blister strips of 10 tablets, to give a total of 60 tablets.

PVC/aluminium blister packs containing 2 tablets (sample packs only).

HDPE bottles with Jay-caps containing 100 tablets.

6.6 Instructions for use and handling

None.

7. MARKETING AUTHORISATION HOLDER

Merck Sharp & Dohme Limited

Hertford Road, Hoddesdon, Hertfordshire EN11 9BU, UK

8. MARKETING AUTHORISATION NUMBER(S)

250 mg tablets: 0025/0128

500 mg tablets: 0025/0146

9. DATE OF FIRST AUTHORISATION/RENEWAL OF THE AUTHORISATION

PL 0025/0128 (250 mg): granted 29 September 1977, renewed 15 May 1998.

PL 0025/0146 (500 mg): granted 23 April 1980, renewed 21 May 1998.

10. DATE OF REVISION OF THE TEXT

8 March 2000.

LEGAL CATEGORY

POM

® denotes registered trademark of Merck & Co., Inc., Whitehouse Station, NJ, USA.

SPC.DLB.96.GB.0072.B. DLB-002a.

7 July 1999

Dopacard

(Zeneus Pharma Ltd)

1. NAME OF THE MEDICINAL PRODUCT

Dopacard 50mg/5ml Concentrate for Solution for Infusion

2. QUALITATIVE AND QUANTITATIVE COMPOSITION

Dopexamine hydrochloride as a 1% solution (w/v). Each 5 ml ampoule contains 50 mg of dopexamine hydrochloride.

3. PHARMACEUTICAL FORM

Concentrate for solution for infusion.

4. CLINICAL PARTICULARS

4.1 Therapeutic indications

Dopacard is indicated for short-term intravenous administration to patients in whom afterload reduction, (through peripheral vasodilatation, and/or renal and mesenteric vasodilatation), combined with a mild positive inotropic effect is required for the treatment of exacerbations of chronic heart failure, or heart failure associated with cardiac surgery.

4.2 Posology and method of administration

For intravenous use only.

Dopacard must be diluted before use.

Dosage

Adults and the elderly:

Infusion should begin at a dose of 0.5 microgram/kg/min and may be increased to 1 microgram/kg/min and then in increments (0.5-1 microgram/kg/min) up to 6 micrograms/kg/min at not less than 15 minute intervals according to the patient's haemodynamic and clinical response. Smaller increments (0.5 microgram/kg/min) may be justified in certain patients according to haemodynamic and clinical response.

Children:

The safety and efficacy of Dopacard for use in children have not been established.

Administration

Dopacard should only be administered intravenously by infusion through a cannula or catheter in a central or large peripheral vein. Contact with metal parts in infusion apparatus should be minimised. A device which provides accurate control of the rate of flow is essential.

Central administration: Dopacard can be administered via a cannula or catheter sited in a central vein. The concentration of the infusion solution for administration via this route must not exceed 4mg/ml.

Peripheral administration: Dopacard can be administered via a cannula in a large peripheral vein. The concentration of the infusion solution for administration via this route must not exceed 1mg/ml. Thrombophlebitis has been reported with peripheral administration using concentrations of Dopacard exceeding 1mg/ml.

During the administration of Dopacard, as with any parenteral catecholamine, the rate of administration and duration of therapy should be adjusted according to the patient's response as determined by heart rate and rhythm (ECG), blood pressure, urine flow and, whenever possible, measurement of cardiac output.

It is recommended that the infusion of Dopacard is reduced gradually rather than withdrawn abruptly.

The duration of therapy is dependent upon the patient's overall response to treatment. Extended therapy beyond 48 hours has not been fully evaluated.

4.3 Contraindications
Known hypersensitivity to dopexamine hydrochloride or excipients (disodium edetate).

Patients who are receiving monoamine oxidase inhibitors (MAOIs).

Phaeochromocytoma.

Thrombocytopenia.

Patients with left ventricular outlet obstruction such as hypertrophic obstructive cardiomyopathy or aortic stenosis. In such patients, positive inotropic activity may increase left ventricular outflow obstruction and sudden vasodilatation may cause hypotension.

4.4 Special warnings and special precautions for use
Correction of hypovolaemia must be achieved prior to administration of Dopacard. Hypovolaemia should also be corrected during therapy as vasodilatation occurs due to treatment.

Care should be exercised so as to restrict the sodium and fluid load during administration of Dopacard.

Dopacard should not be administered to patients with severe hypotension or a markedly reduced systemic vascular resistance until specific resuscitative measures have been taken to restore blood pressure to a clinically acceptable level.

In patients with a marked reduction in systemic vascular resistance, Dopacard should not be used as a direct substitute for pressor agents or other inotropes.

As with other catecholamines, Dopacard should be administered with caution to patients with a clinical history of ischaemic heart disease especially following acute myocardial infarction or recent episodes of angina pectoris as a tachycardia may increase myocardial oxygen demand and further exacerbate myocardial ischaemia.

As has been observed with other β_2-adrenergic agonists, a small reversible fall in circulating platelet numbers has been observed in some patients. No adverse effects attributable to alterations in platelet count have been seen in clinical studies.

Care must be exercised when administering Dopacard in the presence of hypokalaemia or hyperglycaemia. In common with other β_2-agonists, Dopacard depresses plasma potassium and raises plasma glucose. These effects are minor and reversible.

Monitoring of potassium and glucose is advisable in patients likely to be at risk from such changes, e.g. diabetics, patients with myocardial infarction or patients being treated with diuretics or cardiac glycosides.

Benign arrhythmias such as ventricular premature beats and, more rarely, serious arrhythmias have been reported in some patients. If excessive tachycardia occurs during Dopacard administration, then a reduction or temporary discontinuation of the infusion should be considered.

As with other parenteral catecholamines, there have been occasional reports of partial tolerance, with some attenuation of the haemodynamic response developing during long-term infusions of Dopacard.

The risk of thrombophlebitis and local necrosis may be increased if the concentration of Dopacard administered via a peripheral vein exceeds 1 mg/ml. Thrombophlebitis is rare when the concentration of drug used for peripheral administration is less than 1 mg/ml.

4.5 Interaction with other medicinal products and other forms of Interaction
As Dopacard inhibits the Uptake-1 mechanism, it may potentiate the effects of exogenous catecholamines such as noradrenaline. Caution is recommended when these agents are administered concomitantly with Dopacard or soon after its discontinuation.

There is no evidence of an interaction with dopamine, other than possible attenuation of the indirect sympathomimetic inotropic effects of higher doses of dopamine due to Uptake-1 blockade by Dopacard.

Concomitant use with β_2-adrenergic and dopamine receptor antagonists requires caution since possible attenuation of the pharmacological effects of Dopacard may occur.

4.6 Pregnancy and lactation
There is no experience of the use of Dopacard in pregnant or lactating women and therefore its safety in these situations has not been established. There is insufficient evidence from animal studies to indicate it is free from hazard. Dopacard is not therefore currently recommended for use in pregnant or lactating women.

4.7 Effects on ability to drive and use machines
Not applicable.

4.8 Undesirable effects
The most common undesirable effect reported with Dopacard administration in studies of use in heart failure is tachycardia (11.8% in studies of exacerbations of chronic heart failure; 19.4% in studies of use in cardiac surgery). The increases in heart rate are dose-related and, in most cases, not clinically significant.

Hypertension and transient hypotension have been reported after cardiac surgery (at an incidence of 8.8% and 7.0% respectively). These events, however, are not uncommon as compensatory mechanisms following cardiac surgery. Transient hypotension was reported in studies of exacerbations of chronic heart failure at an incidence of 6.3%.

Other undesirable effects reported in clinical trials in both exacerbations of chronic heart failure and cardiac surgery at an incidence of 1% or more include:

Cardiovascular: A number of tachyarrhythmias such as premature ventricular contractions (PVCs) and atrial fibrillation, bradycardia, both sinus and nodal, worsening heart failure leading to asystole and cardiac arrest, angina, myocardial infarction, cardiac enzyme changes and non-specific ECG changes have occurred.

Non-cardiovascular: Nausea and vomiting, tremor, headache, diaphoresis and dyspnoea.

Careful titration of the dose may minimise the incidence of adverse events.

More rarely a number of serious adverse events have been reported in patients undergoing cardiac surgery: renal failure, respiratory failure, acute respiratory distress syndrome (ARDS), pulmonary oedema, pulmonary hypertension, bleeding and septicaemia. However, such events may also be due to the condition of the patients in such populations.

4.9 Overdose
The half-life of Dopacard in blood is short. Consequently, the effects of overdosage are likely to be short-lived provided that administration is discontinued. However, in some cases, it may be necessary to initiate prompt supportive measures.

Effects of overdosage are likely to be related to the pharmacological actions and include tachycardia, tremulousness and tremor, nausea and vomiting, and anginal pain. Treatment should be supportive and directed to these symptoms.

5. PHARMACOLOGICAL PROPERTIES
5.1 Pharmacodynamic properties
The primary actions of Dopacard (dopexamine hydrochloride) are the stimulation of adrenergic β2-receptors and peripheral dopamine receptors of DA_1 and DA_2 subtypes. In addition, Dopacard is an inhibitor of neuronal re-uptake of noradrenaline (Uptake-1). These pharmacological actions result in an increase in cardiac output mediated by afterload reduction (β_2, DA_1) and mild positive inotropism (β_2, Uptake-1 inhibition) together with an increase in blood flow to vascular beds (DA_1) such as the renal and mesenteric beds. Dopacard therefore provides an increase in systemic and regional oxygen delivery. Dopacard is not an α-adrenergic agonist and does not cause vasoconstriction and is not a pressor agent.

5.2 Pharmacokinetic properties
Dopacard is rapidly eliminated from blood with a half-life of approximately 6-7 minutes in healthy volunteers and around 11 minutes in patients with cardiac failure. Subsequent elimination of the metabolites is by urinary and biliary excretion. The response to Dopacard is rapid in onset and effects subside rapidly on discontinuation of the infusion.

5.3 Preclinical safety data
There is no information relevant to the prescriber, which has not been included in other sections of this Summary of Product Characteristics.

6. PHARMACEUTICAL PARTICULARS
6.1 List of excipients
Disodium edetate, Hydrochloric acid, Water for Injections.

6.2 Incompatibilities
Dopacard should only be diluted with 0.9% Sodium Chloride Injection, 5% Dextrose Injection, Hartmann's Solution (Compound Sodium Lactate Intravenous Infusion) or Dextrose 4%/Saline 0.18% Injection, and should not be added to sodium bicarbonate or any other strongly alkaline solutions as inactivation will occur.

Dopacard should not be mixed with any other drugs before administration.

Contact with metal parts, in infusion apparatus for example, should be minimised.

6.3 Shelf life
The shelf life of unopened ampoules is 3 years.

Prepared intravenous solutions in 0.9% Sodium Chloride Injection or 5% Dextrose Injection are stable for 24 hours at room temperature.

6.4 Special precautions for storage
Do not store above 25°C, protect from light.

6.5 Nature and contents of container
Box of 10 clear glass ampoules each containing 5ml of 1% (w/v) solution of dopexamine hydrochloride (50mg per ampoule).

6.6 Instructions for use and handling
The contents of four ampoules (20ml) should be injected aseptically into one of the following:

0.9% Sodium Chloride Injection 500 or 250 ml

5% Dextrose Injection 500 or 250 ml

These dilutions give a concentration for administration as follows:-

4 ampoules of Dopacard diluted to 500ml = 400 micrograms/ml

4 ampoules of Dopacard diluted to 250ml = 800 micrograms/ml

Dopacard, in common with other catecholamines, may turn slightly pink in prepared solutions. There is no significant loss of potency associated with this change.

7. MARKETING AUTHORISATION HOLDER
Zeneus Pharma Limited
The Magdalen Centre
Oxford Science Park
Oxford
OX4 4GA
UK

8. MARKETING AUTHORISATION NUMBER(S)
PL 21799/0009

9. DATE OF FIRST AUTHORISATION/RENEWAL OF THE AUTHORISATION
5 July, 1999

10. DATE OF REVISION OF THE TEXT
October 2005

11. LEGAL CATEGORY
POM

Doralese Tiltab Tablets
(GlaxoSmithKline UK)

1. NAME OF THE MEDICINAL PRODUCT
Doralese® Tiltab® Tablets

2. QUALITATIVE AND QUANTITATIVE COMPOSITION
Indoramin hydrochloride 20 mg

3. PHARMACEUTICAL FORM
Coated tablets

4. CLINICAL PARTICULARS
4.1 Therapeutic indications
Conditions for which alpha blockade is indicated.

Management of urinary outflow obstruction due to benign prostatic hyperplasia.

4.2 Posology and method of administration
Hyperplasia

Adults:

20 mg twice daily

Dosage may be increased in 20 mg increments at two-weekly intervals up to max. 100 mg per day if required.

Elderly:

20 mg at night may be adequate.

Children:

Not recommended.

Route of administration

Oral.

4.3 Contraindications
Patients with established heart failure.

Patients already under treatment with a monoamine oxidase inhibitor.

4.4 Special warnings and special precautions for use
Incipient cardiac failure should be controlled before treatment with Doralese.

Caution should be observed in prescribing Doralese for patients with hepatic or renal insufficiency.

A few cases of extrapyramidal disorders have been reported in patients treated with Doralese. Caution should be observed in prescribing Doralese in patients with Parkinson's disease.

In animals and in the one reported case of overdose in humans, convulsions have occurred. Due consideration should be given and great caution exercised in the use of Doralese in patients with epilepsy.

Caution should be observed in prescribing Doralese for patients with a history of depression.

Clearance of Doralese may be affected in the elderly. A reduced dose, and/or reduced frequency of dosing may be sufficient in some elderly patients.

4.5 Interaction with other medicinal products and other forms of Interaction
Do not use Doralese in patients being treated with a monoamine oxidase (MAO) inhibitor.

Concomitant use of Doralese with antihypertensive drugs or drugs with hypotensive properties e.g. antidepressants, anxiolytics, hypnotics and moxisylyte, may enhance their hypotensive action. Titration of dosage of the latter may therefore be needed.

Alcohol can increase both the rate and extent of absorption of Doralese, but no untoward effects have been reported at recommended doses.

4.6 Pregnancy and lactation

Animal experiments indicate no teratogenic effects but Doralese tablets should not be prescribed for pregnant women unless considered essential by the physician.

There are no data available on the excretion of Doralese in human milk but the drug should not be administered during lactation unless in the judgement of the physician such administration is clinically justifiable.

4.7 Effects on ability to drive and use machines

Drowsiness is sometimes seen in the initial stages of treatment with Doralese or when dosage is increased too rapidly. If drowsiness occurs, patients should be warned not to drive or operate machinery and to avoid CNS depressants including alcohol.

4.8 Undesirable effects

Drowsiness or sedation can occur on starting treatment with Doralese, and also if dosage is increased too rapidly. Less commonly, dry mouth, nasal congestion, weight gain, dizziness, failure of ejaculation, depression, fatigue, headache and hypotension (including postural hypotension) with or without syncope may occur.

Rarely, Parkinson's disease could be exacerbated.

Rarely, hypersensitivity reactions including rash and pruritus may occur.

4.9 Overdose

Information available at present of the effects of acute overdosage in human beings with Doralese is limited. Effects seen have included deep sedation leading to coma, hypotension and fits. Results of animal work suggest that hypothermia may also occur.

Suggested therapy is along the following lines:

1. Recent ingestion of large numbers of tablets would require gastric lavage or a dose of ipecacuanha to remove any of the product still in the stomach of the conscious patient.

2. Ventilation should be monitored and assisted if necessary.

3. Circulation support and control of hypotension should be maintained.

4. If convulsions occur diazepam may be tried.

Temperature should be closely monitored. If hypothermia occurs, rewarming should be carried out very slowly to avoid possible convulsions.

5. PHARMACOLOGICAL PROPERTIES

5.1 Pharmacodynamic properties

Doralese is an alpha adrenoceptor blocking agent. It acts selectively and competitively on post-synaptic alpha-1 receptors, causing a decrease in peripheral resistance. It also produces relaxation of hyperplastic muscle in the prostate.

5.2 Pharmacokinetic properties

Doralese is rapidly absorbed from Doralese tablets and has a half-life of about five hours. There is little accumulation during long-term treatment. When three volunteers and four hypertensive patients were treated with radiolabelled Doralese at doses of 40-60 mg daily for up to three days, plasma concentrations reached a peak one to two hours after administration of single doses. Over 90% of plasma Doralese was protein bound. After two or three days 35% of the radioactivity was excreted in the urine and 46% in the faeces. Extensive first pass metabolism was suggested.

Clearance of Doralese may be affected in the elderly. A reduced dose or reduced frequency of dosing may be sufficient in some elderly patients.

5.3 Preclinical safety data

Not applicable.

6. PHARMACEUTICAL PARTICULARS

6.1 List of excipients

Lactose

Microcrystalline Cellulose

Amberlite IRP

Magnesium Stearate

Film-coating:

Opadry OY-3736

Purified Water

6.2 Incompatibilities

Not applicable.

6.3 Shelf life

Three years.

6.4 Special precautions for storage

Store below 25°C.

6.5 Nature and contents of container

Blister packs - packs of 60, stored below 25°C.

6.6 Instructions for use and handling

Not applicable.

Administrative Data

7. MARKETING AUTHORISATION HOLDER

Smith Kline & French Laboratories Limited

Great West Road, Brentford,

Middlesex TW8 9GS

Trading as:

GlaxoSmithKline UK,

Stockley Park West,

Uxbridge,

Middlesex UB11 1BT

8. MARKETING AUTHORISATION NUMBER(S)

PL 0002/0168

9. DATE OF FIRST AUTHORISATION/RENEWAL OF THE AUTHORISATION

25 February 98

10. DATE OF REVISION OF THE TEXT

22 December 2003

11. Legal Status

POM

Dostinex Tablets

(Pharmacia Limited)

1. NAME OF THE MEDICINAL PRODUCT

DOSTINEX

2. QUALITATIVE AND QUANTITATIVE COMPOSITION

One DOSTINEX tablet contains 0.5 mg cabergoline.

For excipients see Section 6.1 ('List of Excipients').

3. PHARMACEUTICAL FORM

Tablet.

Flat, capsule-shaped, 4 × 8 mm, scored, white tablets.

4. CLINICAL PARTICULARS

4.1 Therapeutic indications

Inhibition/suppression of physiological lactation

DOSTINEX is indicated for the inhibition of physiological lactation soon after delivery and for suppression of already established lactation:

1. After parturition, when the mother elects not to breast feed the infant or when breast feeding is contraindicated due to medical reasons related to the mother or the newborn.

2. After stillbirth or abortion.

DOSTINEX prevents/suppresses physiological lactation by inhibiting prolactin secretion.

In controlled clinical trials, DOSTINEX given as a single 1 mg administration during the first day post-partum, was effective in inhibiting milk secretion, as well as breast engorgement and pain in 70 - 90% of the women. Less than 5% of women experienced rebound breast symptomatology during the third post-partum week (which was usually mild in severity).

Suppression of milk secretion and relief of breast engorgement and pain are obtained in approximately 85% of nursing women treated with a total dose of 1 mg DOSTINEX given in four divided doses over two days. Rebound breast symptomatology after day 10 is uncommon (approximately 2% of cases).

Treatment of hyperprolactinaemic disorders

DOSTINEX is indicated for the treatment of dysfunctions associated with hyperprolactinaemia, including amenorrhoea, oligomenorrhoea, anovulation and galactorrhoea. DOSTINEX is indicated in patients with prolactin-secreting pituitary adenomas (micro- and macroprolactinomas), idiopathic hyperprolactinaemia, or empty sella syndrome with associated hyperprolactinaemia, which represent the basic underlying pathologies contributing to the above clinical manifestations.

On chronic therapy, DOSTINEX at doses ranging between 1 and 2 mg per week, was effective in normalising serum prolactin levels in approximately 84% of hyperprolactinaemic patients. Regular cycles were resumed in 83% of previously amenorrhoeic women. Restoration of ovulation was documented in 89% of women with progesterone levels monitored during the luteal phase. Galactorrhoea disappeared in 90% of cases showing this symptom before therapy. Reduction in tumour size was obtained in 50 - 90% of female and male patients with micro- or macroprolactinoma.

4.2 Posology and method of administration

DOSTINEX is to be administered by the oral route. Since in clinical studies DOSTINEX has been mainly administered with food and since the tolerability of this class of compounds is improved with food, it is recommended that DOSTINEX be preferably taken with meals for all the therapeutic indications.

Inhibition/suppression of physiological lactation

For inhibition of lactation DOSTINEX should be administered during the first day post-partum. The recommended therapeutic dose is 1 mg (two 0.5 mg tablets) given as a single dose.

For suppression of established lactation the recommended therapeutic dosage regimen is 0.25 mg (one-half 0.5 mg tablet) every 12 hours for two days (1 mg total dose). This dosage regimen has been demonstrated to be better tolerated than the single dose regimen in women electing to suppress lactation having a lower incidence of adverse events, in particular of hypotensive symptoms.

Treatment of hyperprolactinaemic disorders

The recommended initial dosage of DOSTINEX is 0.5 mg per week given in one or two (one-half of one 0.5 mg tablet) doses (e.g. on Monday and Thursday) per week. The weekly dose should be increased gradually, preferably by adding 0.5 mg per week at monthly intervals until an optimal therapeutic response is achieved. The therapeutic dosage is usually 1 mg per week and ranges from 0.25 mg to 2 mg per week. Doses of DOSTINEX up to 4.5 mg per week have been used in hyperprolactinaemic patients.

The weekly dose may be given as a single administration or divided into two or more doses per week according to patient tolerability. Division of the weekly dose into multiple administrations is advised when doses higher than 1 mg per week are to be given since the tolerability of doses greater than 1 mg taken as a single weekly dose has been evaluated only in a few patients.

Patients should be evaluated during dose escalation to determine the lowest dosage that produces the therapeutic response. Monitoring of serum prolactin levels at monthly intervals is advised since, once the effective therapeutic dosage regimen has been reached, serum prolactin normalisation is usually observed within two to four weeks.

After DOSTINEX withdrawal, recurrence of hyperprolactinaemia is usually observed. However, persistent suppression of prolactin levels has been observed for several months in some patients. Of the group of women followed up, 23/29 had ovulatory cycles which continued for greater than 6 months after DOSTINEX discontinuation.

Use in children

The safety and efficacy of DOSTINEX has not been established in subjects less than 16 years of age.

Use in the elderly

As a consequence of the indications for which DOSTINEX is presently proposed, the experience in elderly is very limited. Available data do not indicate a special risk.

4.3 Contraindications

Hypersensitivity to any ergot alkaloid.

DOSTINEX is contraindicated in patients with hepatic insufficiency and with toxaemia of pregnancy. DOSTINEX should not be co-administered with anti-psychotic medications or administered to women with a history of puerperal psychosis.

4.4 Special warnings and special precautions for use

General

The safety and efficacy of DOSTINEX have not yet been established in patients with renal and hepatic disease. DOSTINEX should be given with caution to subjects with cardiovascular disease, Raynaud's syndrome, renal insufficiency, peptic ulcer, gastrointestinal bleeding, or a history of serious, particularly psychotic, mental disease. Particular care should be taken when patients are taking concomitant psychoactive medication.

Symptomatic hypotension can occur with DOSTINEX administration for any indication. Care should be exercised when administering DOSTINEX concomitantly with other drugs known to lower blood pressure.

The effects of alcohol on overall tolerability of DOSTINEX are currently unknown.

Before DOSTINEX administration, pregnancy should be excluded and after treatment pregnancy should be prevented for at least one month.

Cabergoline has been associated with somnolence and episodes of sudden sleep onset, particularly in patients with Parkinson's disease. Sudden onset of sleep during daily activities, in some cases without awareness or warning signs, has been reported uncommonly. Patients must be informed of this and advised to exercise caution while driving or operating machines during treatment with cabergoline. Patients who have experienced somnolence and/or an episode of sudden sleep onset must refrain from driving or operating machines. Furthermore a reduction of dosage or termination of therapy may be considered.

Inhibition/suppression of physiological lactation

By analogy with other ergot alkaloids, DOSTINEX should not be used in women with pre-eclampsia and should be used with caution in patients with post-partum hypertension.

In post-partum studies with DOSTINEX, blood pressure decreases were mostly asymptomatic and were frequently observed on a single occasion 2 to 4 days after treatment. Since decreases in blood pressure are frequently noted during the puerperium, independently of drug therapy, it is likely that many of the observed decreases in blood pressure after DOSTINEX administration were not drug-induced. However, periodic monitoring of blood pressure, particularly during the first few days after DOSTINEX administration, is advised.

DOSTINEX should not be administered as a single dose greater than 0.25 mg in nursing women treated for suppression of established lactation since a clinical study exploring the efficacy and tolerability of 0.5 mg of DOSTINEX given as a single dose for suppression of lactation has shown that the risk of side effects is approximately doubled in this indication if the drug is administered as a single dose of 0.5 mg.

In rats DOSTINEX and/or its metabolites are excreted in milk. Therefore, while no information on the excretion of DOSTINEX in maternal milk in humans is available, puerperal women should be advised not to breast-feed in case of failed lactation inhibition/suppression by DOSTINEX.

Treatment of hyperprolactinaemic disorders

Since hyperprolactinaemia with amenorrhoea/galactorrhoea and infertility may be associated with pituitary tumours, a complete evaluation of the pituitary is indicated before treatment with DOSTINEX is initiated.

DOSTINEX restores ovulation and fertility in women with hyperprolactinaemic hypogonadism: since pregnancy might occur prior to reinitiation of menses, a pregnancy test is recommended at least every four weeks during the amenorrhoeic period and, once menses are reinitiated, every time a menstrual period is delayed by more than three days. Women not seeking pregnancy should be advised to use mechanical contraception during treatment and after DOSTINEX withdrawal until recurrence of anovulation. Because of the still limited experience on the safety of foetal exposure to DOSTINEX, until further data become available it is advisable that women seeking pregnancy conceive at least one month after DOSTINEX discontinuation given that ovulatory cycles persist in some patients for 6 months after drug withdrawal. Should pregnancy occur during treatment, DOSTINEX is to be discontinued. As a precautionary measure, women who become pregnant should be monitored to detect signs of pituitary enlargement since expansion of pre-existing pituitary tumours may occur during gestation.

Regular gynaecological assessment, including cervical and endometrial cytology, is recommended for patients taking DOSTINEX for extensive periods.

4.5 Interaction with other medicinal products and other forms of Interaction

The concomitant use of other drugs during early puerperium, particularly of ergot alkaloids, was not associated with detectable interactions modifying the efficacy and safety of DOSTINEX.

Although there is no conclusive evidence of an interaction between DOSTINEX and other ergot alkaloids the concomitant use of these medications during long term treatment with DOSTINEX is not recommended.

Since DOSTINEX exerts its therapeutic effect by direct stimulation of dopamine receptors, it should not be concurrently administered with drugs which have dopamine antagonist activity (such as phenothiazines, butyrophenones, thioxanthenes, metoclopramide) since these might reduce the prolactin-lowering effect of DOSTINEX.

By analogy with other ergot derivatives, DOSTINEX should not be used in association with macrolide antibiotics (e.g. erythromycin) since the systemic bioavailability and also adverse effects could increase.

4.6 Pregnancy and lactation

Pregnancy

DOSTINEX crossed the placenta in rats: it is unknown whether this occurs in humans. Studies in animal models have not demonstrated any teratogenic effect or effects on overall reproductive performance. However, there are no adequate and well-controlled studies in pregnant women. DOSTINEX should be used during pregnancy only if clearly needed.

In clinical studies there have been over 100 pregnancies in women treated for hyperprolactinaemic disorders. DOSTINEX was generally taken during the first 8 weeks after conception. Among the pregnancies evaluable so far, there were approximately 85% live births and about 10% spontaneous abortions. Three cases of congenital abnormalities (Down's Syndrome, hydrocephalus, malformation of lower limbs) which led to therapeutic abortion and three cases of minor abnormalities in live births were observed. These incidence rates are comparable with those quoted for normal populations and for women exposed to other ovulation-inducing drugs. Based on the above data, the use of DOSTINEX does not appear to be associated with an increased risk of abortion, premature delivery, multiple pregnancy, or congenital abnormalities.

Because clinical experience is still limited and the drug has a long half-life, as a precautionary measure it is recommended that once regular ovulatory cycles have been achieved women seeking pregnancy discontinue DOSTINEX one month before intended conception.

This will prevent possible foetal exposure to the drug and will not interfere with the possibility of conception since ovulatory cycles persist in some cases for six months after drug withdrawal. If conception occurs during therapy, treatment is to be discontinued as soon as pregnancy is confirmed to limit foetal exposure to the drug.

Before DOSTINEX administration, pregnancy should be excluded and after treatment pregnancy should be prevented for at least one month.

Lactation

DOSTINEX should not be administered to mothers who elect to breast-feed their infants since it prevents lactation and no information is available on excretion of the drug in maternal milk.

4.7 Effects on ability to drive and use machines

During the first days of DOSTINEX administration, patients should be cautioned about re-engaging in activities requiring rapid and precise responses such as driving an automobile or operating machinery.

Patients being treated with cabergoline and presenting with somnolence and/or sudden sleep episodes must be informed to refrain from driving or engaging in activities where impaired alertness may put themselves and others at risk of serious injury or death (e.g. operating machines) until such recurrent episodes and somnolence have resolved see also section 4.4 ('Special Warnings and Special Precautions for Use').

4.8 Undesirable effects

Adverse events are generally dose-related. In patients known to be intolerant to dopaminergic drugs, the likelihood of adverse events may be lessened by starting therapy with DOSTINEX at reduced doses, e.g. 0.25mg once a week, with subsequent gradual increase until the therapeutic dosage is reached. If persistent or severe adverse events occur, temporary reduction of dosage followed by a more gradual increase, e.g. increments of 0.25mg/week every two weeks, may increase tolerability.

Inhibition/Suppression of lactation:

Approximately 14% of women treated with a single 1 mg dose of DOSTINEX for inhibition of physiological lactation complained of at least one side effect. All side effects were mild to moderate in severity and of a transient nature.

Hyperprolactinaemic disorders:

Data obtained in a controlled clinical trial of 6 months therapy with doses ranging between 1 and 2 mg per week given in two weekly administrations, indicate a 68% incidence of adverse events during DOSTINEX therapy; this was significantly lower than the incidence observed for the reference standard compound. Moreover, the symptoms were generally mild to moderate in degree, mainly appearing during the first two weeks of therapy, and mostly disappearing despite continued therapy. Severe adverse events were reported at least once during therapy by 14% of patients, but therapy was discontinued because of adverse events in only approximately 3% of patients. DOSTINEX withdrawal results in reversal of side effects, usually within a few days after discontinuation.

Cardiovascular system disorders:

Uncommon (< 1 %): decrease in haemoglobin in amenorrhoeic women after menses resumption. Asymptomatic decreases in blood pressure may occur usually once during the first 3-4 days post-partum.

Rare (< 0.1%): cardiovascular regulation (hypotension) in chronic treatment, palpitations, epistaxis.

Central and peripheral nervous system disorders:

Common (1-10 %): headache, dizziness/vertigo, syncope, breast pain.

rare (< 0.1 %): paraesthesia, digital vasospasm, leg cramps.

Psychiatric disorders:

Very common > 10 %): somnolence.

uncommon (< 1 %): excessive daytime somnolence and episodes of sudden sleep onset.

Common (1-10 %): depression.

rare (< 0.1 %): hot flushes.

Vision disorders:

rare (< 0.1%): transient hemianopia.

Gastrointestinal disorders:

Very common > 10 %): nausea.

Common (1-10%): abdominal pain/dyspepsia/gastritis, constipation.

rare (< 0.1%): vomiting.

Skin and appendages disorders:

Common (1-10 %):

uncommon (< 1 %): dermal reactions, e.g. alopecia, pruritus, rash.

Musculo-Skeletal system disorders:

rare (< 0.1%): muscle weakness/fatigue.

Body as a whole:

rare (< 0.1 %): allergic skin reactions.

4.9 Overdose

There is no experience in humans of overdosage with DOSTINEX in the proposed indications: it is likely to lead to symptoms due to overstimulation of dopamine receptors. These might include nausea, vomiting, gastric complaints, hypotension, confusion/psychosis or hallucinations.

General supportive measures should be undertaken to remove any unabsorbed drug and maintain blood pressure if necessary. In addition, the administration of dopamine antagonist drugs may be advisable.

5. PHARMACOLOGICAL PROPERTIES

5.1 Pharmacodynamic properties

DOSTINEX is a dopaminergic ergoline derivative endowed with a potent and long-lasting PRL-lowering activity. It acts by direct stimulation of the D_2-dopamine receptors on pituitary lactotrophs, thus inhibiting PRL secretion. In rats the compound decreases PRL secretion at oral doses of 3-25 mcg/kg, and *in-vitro* at a concentration of 45 pg/ml. In addition, DOSTINEX exerts a central dopaminergic effect via D_2 receptor stimulation at oral doses higher than those effective in lowering serum PRL levels. The long lasting PRL-lowering effect of DOSTINEX is probably due to its long persistence in the target organ as suggested by the slow elimination of total radioactivity from the pituitary after single oral dose in rats ($t_{1/2}$ of approximately 60 hours).

The pharmacodynamic effects of DOSTINEX have been studied in healthy volunteers, puerperal women and hyperprolactinaemic patients. After a single oral administration of DOSTINEX (0.3 - 1.5 mg), a significant decrease in serum PRL levels was observed in each of the populations studied. The effect is prompt (within 3 hours from administration) and persistent (up to 7 - 28 days in healthy volunteers and hyperprolactinaemic patients, and up to 14 - 21 days in puerperal women). The PRL-lowering effect is dose-related both in terms of degree of effect and duration of action.

With regard to the endocrine effects of DOSTINEX not related to the antiprolactinaemic effect, available data from humans confirm the experimental findings in animals indicating that the test compound is endowed with a very selective action with no effect on basal secretion of other pituitary hormones or cortisol. The pharmacodynamic actions of DOSTINEX not correlated with the therapeutic effect only relate to blood pressure decrease. The maximal hypotensive effect of DOSTINEX as single dose usually occurs during the first 6 hours after drug intake and is dose-dependent both in terms of maximal decrease and frequency.

5.2 Pharmacokinetic properties

The pharmacokinetic and metabolic profiles of DOSTINEX have been studied in healthy volunteers of both sexes and in female hyperprolactinaemic patients.

After oral administration of the labelled compound, radioactivity was rapidly absorbed from the gastrointestinal tract as the peak of radioactivity in plasma was between 0.5 and 4 hours.

Ten days after administration about 18% and 72% of the radioactive dose was recovered in urine and faeces, respectively. Unchanged drug in urine accounted for 2-3% of the dose.

In urine, the main metabolite identified was 6-allyl-8β-carboxy-ergoline, which accounted for 4-6% of the dose. Three additional metabolites were identified in urine, which accounted overall for less than 3% of the dose. The metabolites have been found to be much less potent than DOSTINEX in inhibiting prolactin secretion *in vitro*. DOSTINEX biotransformation was also studied in plasma of healthy male volunteers treated with [^{14}C]-cabergoline: a rapid and extensive biotransformation of cabergoline was shown.

The low urinary excretion of unchanged DOSTINEX has been confirmed also in studies with non-radioactive product. The elimination half-life of DOSTINEX, estimated from urinary excretion rates, is long (63-68 hours in healthy volunteers (using a radio-immuno assay), 79-115 hours in hyperprolactinaemic patients (using a HPLC method).

On the basis of the elimination half-life, steady state conditions should be achieved after 4 weeks, as confirmed by the mean peak plasma levels of DOSTINEX obtained after a single dose (37 ± 8 pg/ml) and after a 4 week multiple regimen (101 ± 43 pg/ml).

In vitro experiments showed that the drug at concentrations of 0.1-10 ng/ml is 41-42% bound to plasma proteins. Food does not appear to affect absorption and disposition of DOSTINEX.

5.3 Preclinical safety data

Almost all the findings noted throughout the series of preclinical safety studies are a consequence of the central dopaminergic effects or the long-lasting inhibition of PRL in species (rodents) with a specific hormonal physiology different to man. Preclinical safety studies of DOSTINEX indicate a large safety margin for this compound in rodents and in monkeys, as well as a lack of teratogenic, mutagenic or carcinogenic potential.

6. PHARMACEUTICAL PARTICULARS

6.1 List of excipients

Lactose

Leucine

6.2 Incompatibilities

Not applicable.

6.3 Shelf life

24 months.

6.4 Special precautions for storage

Do not store above 25°C.

6.5 Nature and contents of container

The tablets are contained in type I amber glass bottles with tamper resistant screw caps and containing silica gel desiccant.

Each bottle contains 2, 4 or 8 tablets and is enclosed in an outer cardboard carton.

6.6 Instructions for use and handling
Bottles of DOSTINEX are supplied with desiccant in caps. This desiccant must not be removed.

7. MARKETING AUTHORISATION HOLDER
Pharmacia Limited

Davy Avenue

Knowlhill

Milton Keynes

MK5 8PH

United Kingdom

8. MARKETING AUTHORISATION NUMBER(S)
PL 00032/0372

9. DATE OF FIRST AUTHORISATION/RENEWAL OF THE AUTHORISATION
24 June 2002

10. DATE OF REVISION OF THE TEXT
February 2004

Doublebase Gel

(Dermal Laboratories Limited)

1. NAME OF THE MEDICINAL PRODUCT
DOUBLEBASE® GEL

2. QUALITATIVE AND QUANTITATIVE COMPOSITION
Isopropyl Myristate 15% w/w; Liquid Paraffin 15% w/w.

For excipients see List of Excipients.

3. PHARMACEUTICAL FORM
White opaque gel.

4. CLINICAL PARTICULARS

4.1 Therapeutic indications
A highly emollient and protective hydrating base for regular first-line treatment and prophylaxis of dry or chapped skin conditions which may also be pruritic (itchy) or inflamed. Doublebase may also be used as an adjunct to other topical treatments.

4.2 Posology and method of administration
For external use only. Before using the 500 g bottle, turn the top of the pump dispenser anti-clockwise to unlock it.

For adults, the elderly, infants and children:

• Apply Doublebase to the affected areas as often as necessary. For best results use a few gentle strokes to smooth Doublebase across the skin in the same direction as hair growth. If necessary, allow time for any excess to soak in. Do not rub vigorously.

• Doublebase may also be applied before washing, showering or having a bath to prevent further drying of the skin.

If additional topical treatments are being used on the same skin areas, Doublebase should be applied between these applications.

4.3 Contraindications
Do not use in cases of known sensitivity to any of the ingredients.

4.4 Special warnings and special precautions for use
None.

4.5 Interaction with other medicinal products and other forms of Interaction
None known.

4.6 Pregnancy and lactation
No special precautions.

4.7 Effects on ability to drive and use machines
No special precautions.

4.8 Undesirable effects
Although Doublebase has been specially formulated for use on dry, problem or sensitive skin, local skin reactions can occur in rare cases. In this event, treatment should be discontinued.

4.9 Overdose
Not applicable.

5. PHARMACOLOGICAL PROPERTIES

5.1 Pharmacodynamic properties
The oily ingredients, isopropyl myristate and liquid paraffin, encourage rehydration and softening of dry skin by forming an occlusive barrier within the skin surface, thus reducing drying from evaporation of water that diffuses from the underlying layers.

5.2 Pharmacokinetic properties
Because Doublebase is designed to deliver the emollient ingredients into the stratum corneum when gently applied to areas of dry skin, it is relatively non-greasy despite its high oil content.

5.3 Preclinical safety data
No relevant information additional to that contained elsewhere in this SPC.

6. PHARMACEUTICAL PARTICULARS

6.1 List of excipients
Glycerol; Carbomer; Sorbitan Laurate; Triethanolamine; Phenoxyethanol; Purified Water.

6.2 Incompatibilities
None known.

6.3 Shelf life
30 months.

6.4 Special precautions for storage
Do not store above 25°C. Do not freeze.

6.5 Nature and contents of container
500 g plastic bottle with pump dispenser or 100 g plastic laminate tube with screw cap. These are supplied as original packs (OP).

6.6 Instructions for use and handling
Not applicable.

7. MARKETING AUTHORISATION HOLDER
Dermal Laboratories

Tatmore Place, Gosmore

Hitchin, Herts SG4 7QR, UK.

8. MARKETING AUTHORISATION NUMBER(S)
0173/0183.

9. DATE OF FIRST AUTHORISATION/RENEWAL OF THE AUTHORISATION
21 March 2001.

10. DATE OF REVISION OF THE TEXT
January 2003.

Dovobet Ointment

(Leo Laboratories Limited)

1. NAME OF THE MEDICINAL PRODUCT
Dovobet® 50 microgram/g + 0.5 mg/g ointment

2. QUALITATIVE AND QUANTITATIVE COMPOSITION
Calcipotriol 50 microgram/g (as hydrate), betamethasone 0.5 mg/g (as dipropionate).

For excipients, see section 6.1.

3. PHARMACEUTICAL FORM
Ointment.

Off-white to yellow.

4. CLINICAL PARTICULARS

4.1 Therapeutic indications
Initial topical treatment of stable plaque psoriasis vulgaris amenable to topical therapy.

4.2 Posology and method of administration
Dovobet should be applied to the affected area once daily. The recommended duration of treatment should not exceed 4 weeks.

The maximum daily dose should not exceed 15 g, the maximum weekly dose should not exceed 100 g, and the treated area should not be more than 30% of the body surface.

There is no experience of repeated use.

There is no recommendation for the use of this product in children and adolescents below the age of 18 years.

4.3 Contraindications
Known hypersensitivity to the active substances or to any of the excipients.

Due to the content of calcipotriol Dovobet is contra-indicated in patients with known disorders of calcium metabolism.

Due to the content of corticosteroid Dovobet is contra-indicated in the following conditions: Viral (e.g. herpes or varicella) lesions of the skin, fungal or bacterial skin infections, parasitic infections, skin manifestations in relation to tuberculosis or syphilis, rosacea, perioral dermatitis, acne vulgaris, atrophic skin, striae atrophicae, fragility of skin veins, ichthyosis, acne rosacea, ulcers, wounds, perianal and genital pruritus.

Dovobet is contraindicated in guttate, erythrodermic, exfoliative and pustular psoriasis.

Dovobet is contraindicated in patients with severe renal insufficiency or severe hepatic disorders.

4.4 Special warnings and special precautions for use
The patient must be instructed in correct use of the product to avoid application and accidental transfer to the scalp, face, mouth and eyes. Hands must be washed after each application.

Treatment of more than 30% of the body surface should be avoided.

The risk of hypercalcaemia is minimal when the recommendations relevant to calcipotriol are fulfilled. Due to the content of calcipotriol hypercalcaemia may occur if the maximum weekly dose (100 g) is exceeded. Serum calcium is quickly normalised, however, when treatment is discontinued.

Dovobet contains a group III-steroid (strong) and concurrent treatment with other steroids must be avoided. Adverse effects found in connection with systemic corticosteroid treatment such as adrenocortical suppression or impact on the metabolic control of diabetes mellitus may occur also during topical corticosteroid treatment due to systemic absorption.

Application on large areas of damaged skin and under occlusive dressings or on mucous membranes or in skin folds should be avoided since it increases the systemic absorption of corticosteroids. Skin of the face and genitals are very sensitive to corticosteroids. Long-term treatment of these parts of the body should be avoided. These areas should only be treated with the weaker corticosteroids. When lesions become secondarily infected, they should be treated with antimicrobiological therapy. However, when infection worsens, treatment with corticosteroids should be stopped.

When treating psoriasis with topical corticosteroids there may be a risk of generalised pustular psoriasis.

There is no experience for the use of this product on the scalp. There is no experience with concurrent use of other anti-psoriatic products administered locally or systemically or phototherapy.

4.5 Interaction with other medicinal products and other forms of Interaction
None known.

4.6 Pregnancy and lactation
Pregnancy

There are no adequate data from the use of Dovobet in pregnant women. Studies in animals with glucocorticoids have shown reproductive toxicity (see section 5.3), but a number of epidemiological studies have not revealed congenital anomalies among infants born to women treated with corticosteroids during pregnancy. The potential risk for humans is uncertain. Therefore, during pregnancy, Dovobet should only be used when the potential benefit justifies the potential risk.

Lactation

Betamethasone passes into breast milk but risk of an adverse effect on the infant seems unlikely with therapeutic doses. There are no data on the excretion of calcipotriol in breast milk. Caution should be exercised when prescribing Dovobet to women who breast feed. The patient should be instructed not to use Dovobet on the breast when breast feeding.

4.7 Effects on ability to drive and use machines
Dovobet has no or negligible influence on the ability to drive and to use machines.

4.8 Undesirable effects
Very common >1/10

Common >1/100 and <1/10

Uncommon >1/1,000 and <1/100

Rare >1/10,000 and <1/1000

Very rare <1/10,000

The trial programme for Dovobet ointment has so far included more than 2,500 patients and has shown that approximately 10% of patients can be expected to experience a non-serious undesirable effect.

Based on data from clinical trials and postmarket use the common undesirable effects are pruritus, rash and burning sensation of skin. Uncommon undesirable effects are skin pain or irritation, dermatitis, erythema, exacerbation of psoriasis, folliculitis and application site pigmentation changes. Pustular psoriasis is a rare undesirable effect.

The undesirable effects are listed by MedDRA SOC and the individual undesirable effects are listed starting with the most frequently reported.

• Skin and subcutaneous tissue disorders

Common: Pruritus

Common: Rash

Common: Burning sensation of skin

Uncommon: Skin pain or irritation

Uncommon: Dermatitis

Uncommon: Erythema

Uncommon: Exacerbation of psoriasis

Uncommon: Folliculitis

Uncommon: Application site pigmentation changes

Rare: Pustular psoriasis

Undesirable effects observed for calcipotriol and betamethasone, respectively:

Calcipotriol

Undesirable effects include application site reactions, pruritus, skin irritation, burning and stinging sensation, dry skin, erythema, rash, dermatitis, eczema, psoriasis aggravated, photosensitivity and hypersensitivity reactions including very rare cases of angioedema and facial oedema.

Systemic effects after topical use may appear very rarely causing hypercalcaemia or hypercalciuria, cf. section 4.4.

Betamethasone (as dipropionate)

Local reactions can occur after topical use, especially during prolonged application, including skin atrophy, telangiectasia, striae, folliculitis, hypertrichosis, perioral dermatitis, allergic contact dermatitis, depigmentation and colloid milia. When treating psoriasis there may be a risk of generalised pustular psoriasis.

Systemic effects due to topical use of corticosteroids are rare in adults, however they can be severe. Adrenocortical suppression, cataract and increase of intra-ocular pressure can occur, especially after long term treatment. Systemic effects occur more frequently when applied under occlusion (plastic, skin folds), when applied on large areas and during long term treatment, cf. section 4.4.

4.9 Overdose
Use above the recommended dose may cause elevated serum calcium which should rapidly subside when treatment is discontinued.

Excessive prolonged use of topical corticosteroids may suppress the pituitary-adrenal functions resulting in secondary adrenal insufficiency which is usually reversible. In such cases symptomatic treatment is indicated.

In case of chronic toxicity the corticosteroid treatment must be discontinued gradually.

It has been reported that due to misuse one patient with extensive erythrodermic psoriasis treated with 240g of Dovobet ointment weekly (maximum dose 100 g weekly, cf. section 4.2 and 4.4) for 5 months (recommended treatment period up to 4 weeks, cf. section 4.2) developed Cushing's syndrome and pustular psoriasis after abrupt stopping treatment.

5. PHARMACOLOGICAL PROPERTIES
5.1 Pharmacodynamic properties
DO5AX52 Calcipotriol, combinations.

Calcipotriol is a vitamin D analogue. In vitro data suggests that calcipotriol induces differentiation and suppresses proliferation of keratinocytes. This is the proposed basis for its effect in psoriasis.

Like other topical corticosteroids, betamethasone dipropionate has anti-inflammatory, antipruritic, vasoconstrictive and immunosuppresive properties, however, without curing the underlying condition. Through occlusion the effect can be enhanced due to increased penetration of the stratum corneum (approximately by a factor of 10). The incidence of adverse events will increase because of this. The mechanism of the anti-inflammatory activity of the topical steroids, in general, is unclear.

5.2 Pharmacokinetic properties
Clinical studies with radiolabelled ointment indicate that the systemic absorption of calcipotriol and betamethasone from Dovobet is less than 1% of the dose (2.5 g) when applied to normal skin (625 cm^2) for 12 hours. Application to psoriasis plaques and under occlusive dressings may increase the absorption of topical corticosteroids.

Absorption through damaged skin is approx 24%. Protein binding is approx 64%. Plasma elimination half-life after intravenous application is 5-6 hours. Due to the formation of a depot in the skin elimination after dermal application is in order of days. Betamethasone is metabolised especially in the liver, but also in the kidneys to glucuronide and sulphate esters. Excretion takes place by urine and faeces.

5.3 Preclinical safety data
Studies of corticosteroids in animals have shown reproductive toxicity (cleft palate, skeletal malformations). In reproduction toxicity studies with long-term oral administration of corticosteroids to rats prolonged gestation and prolonged and difficult labour was detected. Moreover reduction in offspring survival, in body weight and body weight gain was observed. There was no impairment of fertility. The relevance for humans is unknown.

For calcipotriol there are no preclinical data of relevance to the prescriber which are additional to the data already included in other sections of the SmPC.

6. PHARMACEUTICAL PARTICULARS
6.1 List of excipients
Liquid paraffin

Polyoxypropylene-15-stearyl ether

α-tocopherol

White soft paraffin

6.2 Incompatibilities
Not to be mixed with other medicinal products.

6.3 Shelf life
Unopened container: 2 years.

After first opening of container: 12 months.

6.4 Special precautions for storage
Do not store above 25°C.

6.5 Nature and contents of container
Aluminium/epoxyphenol tubes with polyethylene screw cap.

Tube sizes: 3 (sample), 15, 30, 60, 100 and 120 g.

Not all pack sizes may be marketed.

6.6 Instructions for use and handling
No special requirements.

7. MARKETING AUTHORISATION HOLDER
LEO Pharmaceutical Products

Industriparken 55

DK-2750 Ballerup

Denmark

8. MARKETING AUTHORISATION NUMBER(S)
PL 05293/0003

9. DATE OF FIRST AUTHORISATION/RENEWAL OF THE AUTHORISATION
18 December 2001

10. DATE OF REVISION OF THE TEXT
28 October 2004

Dovonex Cream

(Leo Laboratories Limited)

1. NAME OF THE MEDICINAL PRODUCT
Dovonex Cream

2. QUALITATIVE AND QUANTITATIVE COMPOSITION
Calcipotriol 50 micrograms per g (as the hydrate)

3. PHARMACEUTICAL FORM
Cream

4. CLINICAL PARTICULARS
4.1 Therapeutic indications
Dovonex Cream is indicated for the topical treatment of plaque psoriasis (psoriasis vulgaris) amenable to topical therapy.

4.2 Posology and method of administration
Adults: Dovonex Cream should be applied to the affected area once or twice daily. For maximum benefit use the cream twice daily. Maximum weekly dose should not exceed 100g.

Children over 12 years: Dovonex Cream should be applied to the affected area twice daily. Maximum weekly dose should not exceed 75g.

Children aged 6 to 12 years: Dovonex Cream should be applied to the affected area twice daily. Maximum weekly dose should not exceed 50g.

Children under 6 years: There is limited experience of the use of Dovonex in this age group. A maximum safe dose has not been established.

These dose recommendations are based on extensive experience in adults. In respect of children, clinical experience in children has shown Dovonex to be safe and effective over eight weeks at a mean dose of 15g per week but with wide variability in dose among patients. Individual dose requirement depends on the extent of psoriasis but should not exceed the above recommendations. There is no experience of use of Dovonex in combination with other therapies in children.

4.3 Contraindications
Dovonex Cream is contra-indicated in patients with known disorders of calcium metabolism. As with other topical preparations, Dovonex Cream is contra-indicated in patients with hypersensitivity to any of the ingredients.

4.4 Special warnings and special precautions for use
Dovonex Cream should not be used on the face. Patients should be advised to wash their hands after applying the cream and to avoid inadvertent transfer to other body areas, especially the face. Care should be exercised in patients with other types of psoriasis, since hypercalcaemia, which rapidly reversed on cessation of treatment, has been reported in patients with generalized pustular or erythrodermic exfoliative psoriasis.

4.5 Interaction with other medicinal products and other forms of Interaction
There is no experience of concomitant therapy with other antipsoriatic products applied to the same skin area at the same time.

Dovonex Cream will not increase the overall effectiveness of UVB treatment. However, Dovonex has a light-saving effect when used in combination with UVB in adults and response is achieved at a lower dose of UVB. Dovonex Cream should be applied at least 2 hours before UVB therapy. Dovonex should not be initiated where patients may already be receiving an erythemogenic or sub-erythemogenic dose of UVB.

4.6 Pregnancy and lactation
Safety for use during human pregnancy has not yet been established, although studies in experimental animals have not shown teratogenic effects. Avoid use in pregnancy unless there is no safer alternative. It is not known whether calcipotriol is excreted in breast milk.

4.7 Effects on ability to drive and use machines
Not applicable.

4.8 Undesirable effects
The most common side effect is transient local irritation which seldom requires discontinuation of treatment. Other local reactions may occur including dermatitis, pruritus, erythema, aggravation of psoriasis, photosensitivity. Facial or perioral dermatitis may occur rarely.

4.9 Overdose
Hypercalcaemia should not occur at the recommended dose of Dovonex Cream.

Excessive use may cause elevated serum calcium which rapidly subsides when the treatment is discontinued.

5. PHARMACOLOGICAL PROPERTIES
5.1 Pharmacodynamic properties
Calcipotriol is a vitamin D derivative. *In vitro* data suggest that calcipotriol induces differentiation and suppresses proliferation of keratinocytes. This is the proposed basis for its effect in psoriasis.

5.2 Pharmacokinetic properties
Not applicable.

5.3 Preclinical safety data
The effect on calcium metabolism is approximately 100 times less than that of the hormonally active form of vitamin D_3.

6. PHARMACEUTICAL PARTICULARS
6.1 List of excipients
Macrogol cetostearyl ether, cetostearyl alcohol, chloroallylhexaminium chloride, disodium edetate, disodium phosphate dihydrate, glycerol 85%, liquid paraffin, purified water, white soft paraffin.

6.2 Incompatibilities
None known.

6.3 Shelf life
2 years.

6.4 Special precautions for storage
Store below 25°C

6.5 Nature and contents of container
Aluminium tubes of 60g (OP) and 120g (OP).

6.6 Instructions for use and handling
None

7. MARKETING AUTHORISATION HOLDER
LEO Laboratories Limited

Longwick Road

Princes Risborough

Bucks

HP27 9RR

8. MARKETING AUTHORISATION NUMBER(S)
PL 0043/0188

9. DATE OF FIRST AUTHORISATION/RENEWAL OF THE AUTHORISATION
10 August 1993

10. DATE OF REVISION OF THE TEXT
May 2005

11. LEGAL CATEGORY
POM

Dovonex Ointment

(Leo Laboratories Limited)

1. NAME OF THE MEDICINAL PRODUCT
Dovonex® Ointment

2. QUALITATIVE AND QUANTITATIVE COMPOSITION
Calcipotriol 50 micrograms/g

3. PHARMACEUTICAL FORM
Ointment

4. CLINICAL PARTICULARS
4.1 Therapeutic indications
Dovonex Ointment is indicated for the topical treatment of plaque psoriasis (psoriasis vulgaris) amenable to topical therapy.

4.2 Posology and method of administration
Adults: Dovonex Ointment should be applied to the affected area once or twice daily. For maximum benefit use the ointment twice daily. Maximum weekly dose should not exceed 100g.

Children over 12 years: Dovonex Ointment should be applied to the affected area twice daily. Maximum weekly dose should not exceed 75g.

Children aged 6 to 12 years: Dovonex Ointment should be applied to the affected area twice daily. Maximum weekly dose should not exceed 50g.

Children under 6 years: There is limited experience of the use of Dovonex Ointment in this age group. A maximum safe dose has not been established.

These dose recommendations are based on extensive experience in adults. In respect of children, clinical experience in children has shown Dovonex to be safe and effective over eight weeks at a mean dose of 15g per week but with wide variability in dose among patients. Individual dose requirement depends on the extent of psoriasis but should not exceed the above recommendations. There is no experience of use of Dovonex in combination with other therapies in children.

4.3 Contraindications
Dovonex Ointment is contra-indicated in patients with known disorders of calcium metabolism. As with other topical preparations, Dovonex Ointment is contra-indicated in patients with hypersensitivity to any of its constituents.

4.4 Special warnings and special precautions for use
Dovonex Ointment should not be used on the face. Patients should be advised to wash their hands after applying the ointment and to avoid inadvertent transfer to other body areas, especially the face. Patients should be advised to use no more than the recommended dose (see section 4.2) since hypercalcaemia, which rapidly reverses on cessation of treatment, may occur.

4.5 Interaction with other medicinal products and other forms of Interaction
There is no experience of concomitant therapy with other antipsoriatic products applied to the same skin area at the same time.

Dovonex Ointment will not increase the overall effectiveness of UVB treatment. However, Dovonex has a light-saving effect when used in combination with UVB in adults and response is achieved at a lower dose of UVB. Dovonex Ointment should be applied at least 2 hours before UVB therapy. Dovonex should not be initiated where patients may already be receiving an erythemogenic or sub-erythemogenic dose of UVB.

4.6 Pregnancy and lactation
Safety for use during human pregnancy has not yet been established, although studies in experimental animals have not shown teratogenic effects. Avoid use in pregnancy unless there is no safer alternative. It is not known whether calcipotriol is excreted in breast milk.

4.7 Effects on ability to drive and use machines
Not applicable.

4.8 Undesirable effects
The most common side effect is transient local irritation which seldom requires discontinuation of treatment. Other local reactions may occur including dermatitis, pruritus, erythema, aggravation of psoriasis, photosensitivity. Facial or perioral dermatitis may occur rarely.

4.9 Overdose
Hypercalcaemia may occur in patients with plaque psoriasis who use more than the recommended dose of Dovonex Ointment weekly and has been reported at lower doses in patients with generalized pustular or erythrodermic exfoliative psoriasis.

5. PHARMACOLOGICAL PROPERTIES

5.1 Pharmacodynamic properties
Calcipotriol is a vitamin D derivative. *In vitro* data suggest that calcipotriol induces differentiation and suppresses proliferation of keratinocytes. This is the proposed basis for its effect in psoriasis.

5.2 Pharmacokinetic properties
Data from a single study containing 5 evaluable patients with psoriasis treated with 0.3 - 1.7g of a 50 micrograms/g tritium labelled calcipotriol ointment suggested that less than 1% of the dose was absorbed.

However, total recovery of the tritium label over a 96 hour period ranged from 6.7 to only 32.6%, figures maximised by uncorrected chemiluminescence. There were no data on ^3H tissue distribution or excretion from the lungs.

5.3 Preclinical safety data
The effect on calcium metabolism is approximately 100 times less than that of the hormonally active form of vitamin D_3.

6. PHARMACEUTICAL PARTICULARS

6.1 List of excipients
Disodium edetate, disodium phosphate dihydrate, DL-α-tocopherol, liquid paraffin, macrogol (2) stearyl ether, propylene glycol, purified water and white soft paraffin.

6.2 Incompatibilities
Not applicable.

6.3 Shelf life
2 years.

6.4 Special precautions for storage
Do not store above 25°C.

6.5 Nature and contents of container
Lacquered aluminium tube with polypropylene screw cap.

Pack sizes: 60g and 120g.

6.6 Instructions for use and handling
None

7. MARKETING AUTHORISATION HOLDER
LEO Laboratories Limited
Longwick Road
Princes Risborough
Bucks
HP27 9RR

8. MARKETING AUTHORISATION NUMBER(S)
PL 0043/0177

9. DATE OF FIRST AUTHORISATION/RENEWAL OF THE AUTHORISATION
10 January 1991

10. DATE OF REVISION OF THE TEXT
February 2003

11. LEGAL CATEGORY
POM

Dovonex Scalp Solution

(Leo Laboratories Limited)

1. NAME OF THE MEDICINAL PRODUCT
Dovonex® Scalp Solution

2. QUALITATIVE AND QUANTITATIVE COMPOSITION
Calcipotriol 50 micrograms per ml (as the hydrate)

3. PHARMACEUTICAL FORM
Solution.

4. CLINICAL PARTICULARS

4.1 Therapeutic indications
Dovonex Scalp Solution is indicated for the topical treatment of scalp psoriasis.

4.2 Posology and method of administration
Adults:Dovonex Scalp Solution should be applied twice daily (morning and evening) to the affected areas. Maximum weekly dose should not exceed 60 ml.

When used together with Dovonex Cream or Ointment, the total dose of calcipotriol should not exceed 5mg in any week, e.g. 60 ml of Scalp Solution plus 30g of Cream or Ointment, or 30ml of Scalp Solution plus 60g of Cream or Ointment.

Children: Not recommended as there is no experience of the use of Dovonex Scalp Solution in children.

4.3 Contraindications
Dovonex Scalp Solution is contraindicated in patients with known disorders of calcium metabolism. As with other topical preparations, Dovonex Scalp Solution is contraindicated in patients with hypersensitivity to any of its constituents.

4.4 Special warnings and special precautions for use
Application of Dovonex to the face may cause local irritation. Dovonex Scalp Solution should not therefore be applied directly to the face. Patients should be advised to wash their hands after applying the scalp solution and to avoid inadvertent transfer to the face. Patients should be advised to use no more than the maximum weekly dose since hypercalcaemia, which rapidly reverses on cessation of treatment, may occur.

4.5 Interaction with other medicinal products and other forms of Interaction
There is no interaction between calcipotriol and UV light. There is no experience of concomitant therapy with other antipsoriatic products applied to the same area.

4.6 Pregnancy and lactation
Safety for use during human pregnancy has not yet been established, although studies in experimental animals have not shown teratogenic effects. Avoid use in pregnancy unless there is no safer alternative. It is not known whether calcipotriol is excreted in breast milk.

4.7 Effects on ability to drive and use machines
Not applicable

4.8 Undesirable effects
The most common side-effect is local irritation on the scalp or face. Facial or perioral dermatitis may occur. Other local reactions which have been reported with Dovonex Ointment include dermatitis, pruritus, erythema, aggravation of psoriasis, photosensitivity, and rarely hypercalcaemia or hypercalciuria.

4.9 Overdose
Hypercalcaemia may occur in patients with plaque psoriasis who use more than 100g of Dovonex Ointment weekly and has been reported at lower doses in patients with generalised pustular or erythrodermic exfoliative psoriasis.

5. PHARMACOLOGICAL PROPERTIES

5.1 Pharmacodynamic properties
Calcipotriol is a vitamin D derivative. *In vitro* data suggest that calcipotriol induces differentiation and suppresses proliferation of keratinocytes. This effect is the proposed basis for its effect in psoriasis.

5.2 Pharmacokinetic properties
Not applicable.

5.3 Preclinical safety data
The effect on the calcium metabolism is approximately 100 times less than that of the hormonally active form of vitamin D_3.

6. PHARMACEUTICAL PARTICULARS

6.1 List of excipients
Hydroxypropyl cellulose, isopropanol, levomenthol, sodium citrate, propylene glycol, purified water.

6.2 Incompatibilities
None known.

6.3 Shelf life
2 years.

6.4 Special precautions for storage
Store below 25°C.

The alcohol base is flammable.

6.5 Nature and contents of container
60ml and 120ml polyethylene bottles with nozzle.

6.6 Instructions for use and handling
None.

7. MARKETING AUTHORISATION HOLDER
LEO Laboratories Limited,
Longwick Road,
Princes Risborough,
Buckinghamshire HP27 9RR,
United Kingdom.

8. MARKETING AUTHORISATION NUMBER(S)
0043/0190

9. DATE OF FIRST AUTHORISATION/RENEWAL OF THE AUTHORISATION
8.6.94

10. DATE OF REVISION OF THE TEXT
August 2001

11. Legal Category
POM

Doxorubicin Rapid Dissolution

(Pharmacia Limited)

1. NAME OF THE MEDICINAL PRODUCT
Doxorubicin Rapid Dissolution 10 mg, 20 mg, 50 mg and 150 mg.

2. QUALITATIVE AND QUANTITATIVE COMPOSITION
Doxorubicin Hydrochloride HSE 10.0 mg

Doxorubicin Hydrochloride HSE 20.0 mg

Doxorubicin Hydrochloride HSE 50.0 mg

Doxorubicin Hydrochloride HSE 150.0 mg

3. PHARMACEUTICAL FORM
Freeze-dried powder for injection.

4. CLINICAL PARTICULARS

4.1 Therapeutic indications
The treatment of a wide range of neoplastic diseases including acute leukaemia, lymphoma, paediatric malignancies and adult solid tumours, in particular, breast and lung carcinomas.

4.2 Posology and method of administration
Route of administration: The proposed routes of administration are intravenous and intra-arterial injection and intravesical instillation. Doxorubicin cannot be used as an antibacterial agent.

Adults and Children:

Intravenous Administration:

The reconstituted solution is given via the tubing of a freely-running intravenous infusion, taking 2-3 minutes over the injection. Commonly used acceptable solutions are sodium chloride injection, dextrose injection 5% or sodium chloride and dextrose injection.

Dosage is usually calculated on the basis of body surface area. On this basis, 60-70 mg/m^2 may be given every three weeks when doxorubicin is used alone. If it is used in combination with other antitumour agents having overlapping toxicity, the dosage for doxorubicin may need to be reduced to 30-40 mg/m^2 every three weeks. If dosage is to be calculated on the basis of body weight, 1.2-2.4 mg/kg should be given as a single dose every three weeks.

It has been shown that giving doxorubicin as a single dose every three weeks greatly reduces the distressing toxic effect, mucositis; however there are still some who believe that dividing the dose over three successive days (0.4-0.8 mg/kg or 20-25 mg/m^2 on each day) gives greater effectiveness even though at the cost of high toxicity.

Administration of doxorubicin in a weekly regimen has been shown to be as effective as the 3-weekly regimen. The recommended dosage is 20 mg/m^2 weekly although objective responses have been seen at 6-12 mg/m^2. Weekly administration leads to a reduction in cardiotoxicity.

Dosage may need to be reduced for patients who have had prior treatment with other cytotoxic agents. Dosage may also need to be reduced in children and the elderly.

If hepatic function is impaired, doxorubicin should be reduced according to the following table:

Serum bilirubin levels	BSP retention	Recommended dose
1.2-3.0 mg/100 ml	9 - 15%	50% normal dose
> 3.0 mg/100 ml	> 15%	25% normal dose

Intra-arterial Administration:

Intra-arterial injection has been used in attempts to produce intense local activity while keeping the total dose low and therefore reducing general toxicity. It should be emphasised that this technique is potentially extremely hazardous and can lead to widespread necrosis of the perfuse tissue unless due precautions are taken.

Intra-arterial injection should only be attempted by those fully conversant with this technique.

Intravesical Administration:

Doxorubicin is being increasingly used by intravesical administration for the treatment of transitional cell carcinoma, papillary bladder tumours and carcinoma-in-situ. It should not be employed in this way for the treatment of invasive tumours which have penetrated the bladder wall. It has also been found useful to instil doxorubicin into the bladder at intervals after transurethral resection of a tumour in order to reduce the probability of recurrence.

While at present many regimens are in use, making interpretation difficult, the following may be helpful guides:

The concentration of doxorubicin in the bladder should be 50 mg per 50 ml.

To avoid undue dilution with urine, the patient should be instructed not to drink any fluid in the 12 hours prior to instillation.

This should limit urine production to approximately 50 ml per hour. The patient should be rotated a quarter turn every 15 minutes while the drug is in situ.

Exposure to the drug solution for one hour is generally adequate and the patient should be instructed to void at the end of this time.

4.3 Contraindications

Hypersensitivity to hydroxybenzoates is a contra-indication. Dosage should not be repeated in the presence of bone-marrow depression or buccal ulceration. The latter may be preceded by premonitory buccal burning sensations and repetition in the presence of this symptom is not advised.

4.4 Special warnings and special precautions for use

A cumulative dose of 450-550 mg/m^2 should only be exceeded with extreme caution. Above this level, the risk of irreversible congestive cardiac failure increases greatly. The total dose of doxorubicin administered to the individual patient should also take account of any previous or concomitant therapy with other potentially cardiotoxic agents such as high-dose i.v. cyclophosphamide, mediastinal irradiation or related anthracycline compounds such as daunorubicin. Administration of doxorubicin weekly has been shown to be associated with reduced cardiotoxicity compared with a 3-weekly schedule allowing patients to be treated to a higher cumulative dose. It should be noted that cardiac failure may also occur several weeks after administration and may not respond to treatment.

Baseline and follow-up ECGs during and immediately after drug administration are advisable. Transient ECG changes, such as T-wave flattening, S-T segment depression and arrhythmias, are not considered indications for the suspension of doxorubicin therapy. A reduction of the QRS wave is considered more indicative of cardiac toxicity. If this change occurs, the benefit of continued therapy must be carefully evaluated against the risk of producing irreversible cardiac damage.

Accidental contact with the skin or eyes should be treated immediately by copious lavage with water or soap and water or if available sodium bicarbonate solution.

4.5 Interaction with other medicinal products and other forms of Interaction

High dose ciclosporin increases the serum levels and myelotoxicity of doxorubicin.

4.6 Pregnancy and lactation

There is no conclusive evidence as to whether doxorubicin may adversely affect human fertility or cause teratogenesis. Experimental data, however, suggest that doxorubicin may harm the foetus and should, therefore, not be administered to pregnant women or to mothers who are breast-feeding.

4.7 Effects on ability to drive and use machines

None stated.

4.8 Undesirable effects

Haematological monitoring should be undertaken regularly in both haematological and non-haematological conditions, because of the possibility of bone-marrow depression which may become evident around ten days from the time of administration. Clinical consequences of doxorubicin bone marrow/haematological toxicity may be fever, infections, sepsis/septicaemia, septic shock, haemorrhages, tissue hypoxia or death.

The occurrence of secondary acute myeloid leukaemia with or without a pre-leukaemic phase has been reported rarely in patients concurrently treated with doxorubicin in association with DNA-damaging antineoplastic agents. Such cases could have a short (1-3 year) latency period.

Cardiotoxicity may be manifested in tachycardia including supraventricular tachycardia and ECG changes. Routine ECG monitoring is recommended and caution should be exercised in patients with impaired cardiac function.

Severe cardiac failure may occur suddenly, without premonitory ECG changes.

Doxorubicin Rapid Dissolution may impart a red colour to the urine, particularly to the first specimen passed after the injection, and patients should be advised that this is no cause for alarm.

Alopecia occurs frequently, including the interruption of beard growth, but all hair growth normally resumes after treatment is stopped. Nausea, vomiting and diarrhoea may also occur.

The risk of thrombophlebitis at the injection site may be minimised by following the procedure for administration recommended above. A stinging or burning sensation at the site of administration signifies a small degree of extravasation and the infusion should be stopped and re-started in another vein.

Other side effects include mucositis, skin rashes, fever, hyperuricaemia, amenorrhoea, anaphylaxis, bronchospasm and dyspnoea.

Following intravesical administration: symptoms of bladder irritation, haematuria, haemorrhagic cystitis, necrosis of the bladder wall.

4.9 Overdose

Single doses of 250 mg and 500 mg of doxorubicin have proved fatal. Such doses may cause acute myocardial degeneration within 24 hours and severe myelosuppression, the effects of which are greatest between 10 and 15 days after administration. Treatment should aim to support the patient during this period and should utilise such measures as blood transfusions and reverse barrier nursing. Delayed cardiac failure may occur up to six months after the overdose. Patients should be observed carefully and should signs of cardiac failure arise, be treated along conventional lines.

5. PHARMACOLOGICAL PROPERTIES

5.1 Pharmacodynamic properties

Doxorubicin is an antitumour agent. Tumour cells are probably killed through drug-induced alterations of nucleic acid synthesis although the exact mechanism of action have not yet been clearly elucidated.

Proposed mechanism of action include:

DNA intercalation (leading to an inhibition of synthesis of DNA, RNA and proteins), formation of highly reactive free-radicals and superoxides, chelation of divalent cations, the inhibition of Na-K ATPase and the binding of doxorubicin to certain constituents of cell membranes (particularly to the membrane lipids, spectrin and cardiolipin). Highest drug concentrations are attained in the lung, liver, spleen, kidney, heart, small intestine and bone-marrow. Doxorubicin does not cross the blood-brain barrier.

5.2 Pharmacokinetic properties

After i.v. administration, the plasma disappearance curve of doxorubicin is triphasic with half-lives of 12 minutes, 3.3 hours and 30 hours. The relatively long terminal elimination half-life reflects doxorubicin's distribution into a deep tissue compartment. Only about 33 to 50% of fluorescent or tritiated drug (or degradation products), respectively, can be accounted for in urine, bile and faeces for up to 5 days after i.v. administration. The remainder of the doxorubicin and degradation products appear to be retained for long periods of time in body tissues.

In cancer patients, doxorubicin is reduced to adriamycinol, which is an active cytotoxic agent. This reduction appears to be catalysed by cytoplasmic nadph-dependent aldo-keto reductases that are found in all tissues and play an important role in determining the overall pharmacokinetics of doxorubicin.

Microsomal glycosidases present in most tissues split doxorubicin and adriamycinol into inactive aglycones. The aglycones may then undergo 0-demethylation, followed by conjugation to sulphate or glucuronide esters, and excretion in the bile.

5.3 Preclinical safety data

No further preclinical safety data available.

6. PHARMACEUTICAL PARTICULARS

6.1 List of excipients

Lactose	Ph. Eur.
Methyl hydroxybenzoate	Ph. Eur.
Water for Injections	Ph. Eur.

6.2 Incompatibilities

Doxorubicin Rapid Dissolution should not be mixed with heparin as a precipitate may form and it is not recommended that Doxorubicin Rapid Dissolution be mixed with other drugs. Prolonged contact with any solution of an alkaline pH should be avoided as it will result in hydrolysis of the drug

6.3 Shelf life

The shelf-life for Doxorubicin Rapid Dissolution is 48 months. Once reconstituted, the solution should be used straight away. If not it may be stored for up to 24 hours.

6.4 Special precautions for storage

None.

6.5 Nature and contents of container

Glass vial, type III, with white or grey rubber stopper, aluminium seal and snap cap (10, 20, 50 and 150 mg vials).

6.6 Instructions for use and handling

The vial contents are under a negative pressure to minimise aerosol formation during reconstitution, particular care should be taken when the needle is inserted. Inhalation of any aerosol produced during reconstitution must be avoided.

The following protective recommendations are given due to the toxic nature of this substance:

- Personnel should be trained in good technique for reconstitution and handling.
- Pregnant staff should be excluded from working with this drug.
- Personnel handling Doxorubicin should wear protective clothing: goggles, gowns and disposable gloves and masks.
- A designated area should be defined for reconstitution (preferably under a laminar flow system). The work surface should be protected by disposable plastic-backed absorbent paper.
- All items used for reconstitution, administration or cleaning, including gloves, should be placed in high-risk waste-disposal bags for high temperature incineration.

The vial contents must be reconstituted before use with water for injections or normal saline. For reconstitution the contents of the 10mg vial may be dissolved in 5ml Water for injections or Sodium Chloride Injection and those of the 20mg vial in 10ml of the same solvents; 50mg vial in 25ml of the same solvents and 150mg vial in 75ml of the same solvents.

After adding the diluent, the vial contents will dissolve with gentle shaking, without inversion, within 30 seconds. The approximate displacement value of the contents of a 50mg vial, after 25ml of solvent has been added is 0.15ml.

The reconstituted solution contains 0.02% methylhydroxybenzoate. This is not a preservative solution. Discard any unused solution.

Accidental contact with the skin or eyes should be treated immediately by copious lavage with water, or soap and water, or sodium bicarbonate solution: medical attention should be sought.

Spillage or leakage should be treated with dilute sodium hypochlorite (1% available chlorine) solution, preferably soaking overnight and then water. All cleaning materials should be disposed of as indicated previously.

Administrative Data

7. MARKETING AUTHORISATION HOLDER

Farmitalia Carlo Erba Limited

Davy Avenue

Milton Keynes

MK5 8PH

UK

8. MARKETING AUTHORISATION NUMBER(S)

PL 3433/0110

9. DATE OF FIRST AUTHORISATION/RENEWAL OF THE AUTHORISATION

25 June 1987/29 April 1998

10. DATE OF REVISION OF THE TEXT

07 March 2002

Legal Category

POM

Doxorubicin Solution for Injection

(Pharmacia Limited)

1. NAME OF THE MEDICINAL PRODUCT

Doxorubicin Solution for Injection

2. QUALITATIVE AND QUANTITATIVE COMPOSITION

Doxorubicin Hydrochloride 2mg/ml

3. PHARMACEUTICAL FORM

Solution for intravenous use.

4. CLINICAL PARTICULARS

4.1 Therapeutic indications

Antimitotic and cytotoxic. Doxorubicin has been used successfully to produce regression in a wide range of neoplastic conditions including acute leukaemia, lymphomas, soft-tissue and osteogenic sarcomas, paediatric malignancies and adult solid tumours; in particular breast and lung carcinomas.

Doxorubicin is frequently used in combination chemotherapy regimens with other cytotoxic drugs. Doxorubicin cannot be used as an antibacterial agent.

4.2 Posology and method of administration

The solution is given via the tubing of a freely running intravenous infusion, taking 2 to 3 minutes over the injection. This technique minimises the risk of thrombosis or perivenous extravasation which can lead to severe cellulitis and vesication.

Dosage is usually calculated on the basis of body surface area. On this basis, 60-75 mg/m^2 may be given every three weeks when doxorubicin is used alone. If it used in combination with other antitumour agents having overlapping toxicity, the dosage of doxorubicin may need to be reduced to 30-40mg/m^2 every three weeks.

If dosage is calculated on the basis of body weight, it has been shown that giving doxorubicin as a single dose every three weeks greatly reduces the distressing toxic effect, mucositis; however, there are still some who believe that dividing the dose over three successive days (0.4-0.8mg/kg or 20-25mg/m^2 on each day) gives greater effectiveness though at the cost of higher toxicity. If dosage is to be calculated on the basis of body weight, 1.2-2.4 mg/kg should be given as a single dose every three weeks.

Administration of doxorubicin in a weekly regimen has been shown to be as effective as the 3-weekly regimen. The recommended dosage is 20mg/m^2 weekly, although, objective responses have been seen at 16mg/m^2. Weekly administration leads to a reduction in cardiotoxicity.

Dosage may also need to be reduced in children and the elderly.

If hepatic function is impaired, doxorubicin dosage should be reduced according to the following table:

Serum Bilirubin Levels	BSP Retention	Recommended Dose
1.2 – 3.0 mg/100ml	9 - 15%	50% Normal dose
> 3.0 mg/100ml	>15%	25% Normal Dose

4.3 Contraindications

Dosage should not be repeated in the presence of bone marrow depression or buccal ulceration. The latter may be preceded by premonitory buccal burning sensations and repetition in the presence of this symptom is not advised.

4.4 Special warnings and special precautions for use

A cumulative dose of 450-500 mg/m^2 should only be exceeded with extreme caution. Above this level, the risk of irreversible congestive cardiac failure increases greatly. The total dose of doxorubicin administered to the individual patient should also take into account any previous or concomitant therapy with other potentially cardiotoxic agents such as high-dose i.v. cyclophosphamide, mediastinal irradiation or related anthracycline compounds such as daunorubicin.

Administration weekly has been shown to be associated with reduced cardiotoxicity compared with a 3-weekly schedule, allowing patients to be treated with a higher cumulative dose.

It should be noted that cardiac failure may also occur several weeks after administration and may not respond to treatment. Baseline and follow-up ECGs during and immediately after drug administration are advisable. Transient ECG changes, such as T-wave flattening, S-T segment depression and arrhythmias are not considered indications for suspension of doxorubicin therapy. A reduction of the QRS wave is considered more indicative of cardiac toxicity. If this change occurs, the benefit of continued therapy must be carefully evaluated against the risk of producing irreversible cardiac damage.

4.5 Interaction with other medicinal products and other forms of Interaction

High dose ciclosporin increases the serum levels and myelotoxicity of doxorubicin.

4.6 Pregnancy and lactation

There is no conclusive evidence as to whether doxorubicin may adversely affect human fertility or cause teratogenesis. Experimental data however suggest that doxorubicin may harm the foetus and should not therefore be administered to pregnant women or those who are breast feeding.

4.7 Effects on ability to drive and use machines

None stated

4.8 Undesirable effects

Haematological monitoring should be undertaken regularly in both haematological and non haematological conditions, because of the possibility of bone-marrow depression which may become evident around ten days from the time of administration. Clinical consequences of doxorubicin bone marrow/haematological toxicity may be fever, infections, sepsis/septicaemia, septic shock, haemorrhages, tissue hypoxia or death.

The occurrence of secondary acute myeloid leukaemia with or without a pre-leukaemic phase has been reported rarely in patients concurrently treated with doxorubicin in association with DNA damaging anti-neoplastic agents. Such cases could have a short (1-3 year) latency period.

Cardiotoxicity may be manifested in tachycardia including supraventricular tachycardia and ECG changes. Routine ECG monitoring is recommended and caution should be exercised in patients with impaired cardiac function. Severe cardiac failure may occur suddenly, without premonitory ECG changes.

Doxorubicin solution for injection may impart a red colour to the urine particularly to the first specimen passed after the injection, and patients should be advised that there is no cause for alarm.

Alopecia occurs frequently, including the interruption of beard growth, but all hair growth normally returns after treatment is stopped. Nausea, vomiting and diarrhoea may also occur.

The risk of thrombophlebitis at the injection site may be minimised by following the procedure for administration recommended above. A stinging or burning sensation signifies a small degree of extravasation and the infusion should be stopped and restarted in another vein.

Other side effects include mucositis, skin rashes, fever, hyperuricaemia, amenorrhoea, anaphylaxis, bronchospasm and dyspnoea.

4.9 Overdose

Single doses of 250mg and 500mg of doxorubicin have proved fatal. Such doses may cause acute myocardial degeneration within 24 hours and severe myelosupression, the effects of which are greatest between 10 and 15 days after administration. Treatment should aim to support the patient during this period and should utilise such measures as blood transfusions and reverse barrier nursing.

Delayed cardiac failure may occur up to six months after the overdosage. Patients should be observed carefully and should signs of cardiac failure arise, be treated along conventional lines.

5. PHARMACODYNAMIC PROPERTIES

5.1 Pharmacodynamic properties

Doxorubicin is an antitumour agent. Tumour cells are probably killed through drug-induced alterations of nucleic acid synthesis although the exact mechanism of action have not yet been clearly elucidated.

Proposed mechanism of action include:

DNA intercalation (leading to an inhibition of synthesis of DNA, RNA and proteins), formation of highly reactive free-radicals and superoxides, chelation of divalent cations, the inhibition of Na-K ATPase and the binding of doxorubicin to certain constituents of cell membranes (particularly to the membrane lipids, spectrin and cardiolipin). Highest drug concentrations are attained in the lung, liver, spleen, kidney, heart, small intestine and bone-marrow. Doxorubicin does not cross the blood-brain barrier.

5.2 Pharmacokinetic properties

After i.v. administration, the plasma disappearance curve of doxorubicin is triphasic with half-lives of 12 minutes, 3.3 hours and 30 hours. The relatively long terminal elimination half-life reflects doxorubicin's distribution into a deep tissue compartment. Only about 33 to 50% of fluorescent or tritiated drug (or degradation products), respectively, can be accounted for in urine, bile and faeces for up to 5 days after i.v. administration. The remainder of the doxorubicin and degradation products appear to be retained for long periods of time in body tissues.

In cancer patients, doxorubicin is reduced to adriamycinol, which is an active cytotoxic agent. This reduction appears to be catalysed by cytoplasmic nadph-dependent aldo-keto reductases that are found in all tissues and play an important role in determining the overall pharmacokinetics of doxorubicin.

Microsomal glycosidases present in most tissues split doxorubicin and adriamycinol into inactive aglycones. The aglycones may then undergo 0-demethylation, followed by conjugation to sulphate or glucuronide esters, and excretion in the bile.

5.3 Preclinical safety data

No information in addition to that presented elsewhere in this Summary of Product Characteristics is available.

6. PHARMACEUTICAL PARTICULARS

6.1 List of excipients

Water for Injections Ph Eur

Sodium chloride Ph Eur

Hydrochloric acid Ph Eur

6.2 Incompatibilities

Doxorubicin should not be mixed with heparin as a precipitate may form and it is not recommended that doxorubicin be mixed with other drugs. Prolonged contact with any solution of an alkaline pH should be avoided as it will result in hydrolysis of the drug.

6.3 Shelf life

2 years

6.4 Special precautions for storage

Store refrigerated between 2- 8°C

6.5 Nature and contents of container

Single glass vials of 5ml (10mg), 10ml (20mg), 25ml (50mg) and 100ml (200mg)

Single Cytosafe® polypropylene vials of 5ml (10mg), 10ml (20mg), 25ml (50mg) and 100ml (200mg)

6.6 Instructions for use and handling

For use only under the direction of those experienced in cytotoxic therapy.

Unused solution should be discarded after use

Accidental contact with the skin or eyes should be treated immediately by copious lavage with water, or soap and water, or sodium bicarbonate solution: medical attention should be sought.

Spillage or leakage should be treated with dilute sodium hypochlorite (1% available chlorine) solution, preferably soaking overnight and then water. All cleaning materials should be disposed of as indicated previously.

7. MARKETING AUTHORISATION HOLDER

Farmitalia Carlo Erba Limited

Davy Avenue

Milton Keynes

MK5 8PH

United Kingdom

8. MARKETING AUTHORISATION NUMBER(S)

PL 3433/0127

9. DATE OF FIRST AUTHORISATION/RENEWAL OF THE AUTHORISATION

Renewed 25 January 1995

10. DATE OF REVISION OF THE TEXT

07 March 2002

Legal Category

POM

Doxorubin 0.2%

(medac GmbH)

1. NAME OF THE MEDICINAL PRODUCT

Doxorubin 0.2%

2. QUALITATIVE AND QUANTITATIVE COMPOSITION

Doxorubin 0.2% injection contains doxorubicin hydrochloride 2 mg/ml.

3. PHARMACEUTICAL FORM

Solution for Injection.

4. CLINICAL PARTICULARS

4.1 Therapeutic indications

In combination with other antineoplastic drugs, doxorubicin is intended for the treatment of acute lymphocytic leukaemia, except acute lymphatic leukaemia of low risk in children, acute myeloid leukaemia (Hodgkin- and non-Hodgkin lymphomas) osteosarcoma, Ewing sarcoma, adult soft tissue sarcoma, metastatic breastcarcinoma, gastric carcinoma, small-cell lung cancer, neuroblastoma, Wilms tumour and bladder carcinoma.

Doxorubicin may be used intravesically as single agent for treatment and prophylaxis of superficial bladder carcinoma.

4.2 Posology and method of administration

Dosage depends on tumour type, hepatic function, and concurrent chemo-therapy.

The commonly recommended dosage schedule as a single agent is 60-75 mg/m^2 by intravenous injection, once every 3 weeks. An alternative dose schedule is 20 mg/m^2 intravenously, on 3 consecutive days, once every 3 weeks.

In combination with other cytotoxic agents doses of 50-75 mg/m^2 are administered. Myelosuppresion may be more pronounced because of the additive effects of the drugs.

The risk of development of cardiomyopathy gradually increases with the dosage. A cumulative dose of 550 mg/m^2 should not be exceeded. The administration of doxorubicin should be monitored by electrocardiography, echocardiography and carotid pulse curve: when the voltage of the QRS wave decreases by 30% or at a fractional shortening of 5% it is recommended that treatment is stopped.

If a patient received mediastinal irradiation, has concomitant heart disease, or is also treated with other cardiotoxic, non-anthracyclinecytotoxic agents, a maximal cumulative dose of 400 mg/m^2 is recommended. Doxorubicin dosage should be reduced if the bilirubin is elevated as follows: serum bilirubin 12 to 30 mg/l - give $^1/_2$ of the normal dose, biliru-bin > 30 mg/l - give $^1/_4$ of the normal dose.

In general, impaired renal function does not require dose reduction.

Doxorubicin may be given by intravenous bolus injection, or as continuous infusion. Bolus injection causes higher peak plasma concentrations and therefore is probably more cardiotoxic.

Doxorubicin should not be administered intramuscularly or subcutaneously.

Intravenous administration occurs preferably through a running intravenous infusion, over 3 to 5 minutes.

Patients at increased risk for cardiotoxicity should be considered for treatment with a 24 hours continuous infusion, rather than bolus injection. In this way, cardiotoxicity may be less frequent, without a reduction in therapeutic efficacy. In these patients, the ejection fraction should be measured before each course.

Dosage in children:

Dosage in children may be lowered, since they have an increased risk for late cardiotoxicity. Myelotoxicity should be anticipated, with nadirs at 10 to 12 days after start of treatment, but is usually followed by a rapid recovery due to the large bone marrow reserve of children as compared to adults.

Superficial bladder carcinoma and bladder carcinoma in situ:

The recommended dosage is 50 mg in 50 ml normal saline, administered via a sterile catheter. Initially, this dose is given weekly, later on, monthly. The optimal duration of treatment has not yet been determined; it ranges from 6 to 12 months.

Restrictions regarding the maximal cumulative dose, as with intravenous administration, do not apply to intravesical administration, because systemic absorption of doxorubicin is negligible.

4.3 Contraindications
Myelosuppression, pre-existing heart disease, previous treatment with complete cumulative doses of doxorubicin or other anthracyclines.

Doxorubicin should not be used intravesically for the treatment of bladder carcinoma in patients with urethral stenosis who can not be catheterised.

4.4 Special warnings and special precautions for use
Nausea, vomiting and mucositis are often severe and should be treated appropriately.

Doxorubicin should not be administered intramuscularly or subcutaneously.

Extravasation results in a severe and progressive tissue necrosis. If extravasation occurs, the injection should be terminated immediately and restarted in another vein. Flooding with normal saline, local infiltration with corticosteroids, or sodium hydrogen carbonate solution (8.4%), and application of dimethylsulphoxide have been reported with varying success. The advice of the plastic surgery consultant should be asked for, and wide excision of the involved area should be considered.

Exceeding the maximum cumulative dose of 550 mg/m^2 increases the risk of severe, irreversible and therapy-resistant cardiomyopathy and resulting congestive heart failure. Age over 70 or below 15 years should be considered a risk factor, as well as concomitant heart disease. In addition, ECG changes may occur including a reduction in the voltage of the QRS wave, and a prolongation of the systolic time interval, and the ejection fraction may be reduced.

In patients previously treated with other anthracyclines or cyclophos-phamide, mitomycin C or dacarbazine and patients who received radiotherapy to the mediastinal area, cardiotoxicity may occur at doses lower than the recommended cumulative limit.

Acute severe arrhythmias have been reported to occur during or within a few hours after doxorubicin administration.

Heart function should be assessed before, during and after doxorubicin therapy, e.g., by ECG, echocardiography or determination of the ejection fraction.

The high incidence of bone marrow depression requires careful haematologic monitoring. Doxorubicin therapy should not be started or continued when polynuclear granulocyte counts are below 2000/mm^3, except in the treatment of acute leukaemia, where lower limits may be applied.

Careful haematologic monitoring is also required because of the risk of secondary leukaemias after treatment with cytotoxic agents (see section 4.8 "Undesirable effects"). These leukaemias can be cured when detected at an early stage.

Hepatic function should be evaluated before and during therapy.

Doxorubicin may induce hyperuricemia. The blood uric acid level should be monitored; sufficient fluid intake should be ascertained (with a daily minimum of 3 l/m^2). If necessary, a xanthine-oxidase inhibitor (allopurinol) may be administered.

Men as well as woment should take effective contraceptive measures during and for at least 3 months after doxorubicin therapy.

Doxorubicin may impart a red coloration to the urine.

4.5 Interaction with other medicinal products and other forms of Interaction
Doxorubicin cardiotoxicity is enhanced by previous or concurrent use of other anthracyclines, mitomycin C, dacarbazine, dactinomycin and, possibly, cyclophosphamide.

Doxorubicin may cause exacerbations of haemorragic cystitis caused by previous cyclophosphamide therapy.

The effects of radiation may be enhanced, and recall of these reactions may occur with doxorubicin therapy, even some time after termination of radiotherapy.

Inducers of the enzyme cytochrome P-450 (e.g. rifampicin and barbiturates) may stimulate the metabolism of doxorubicin, with a possible decrease in efficacy.

Inhibitors of cytochrome P-450 (e.g. cimetidine) may decrease the metabolism of doxorubicin, with a possible increase in toxic effects.

4.6 Pregnancy and lactation
Clinical evidence suggests a possible adverse effect on the foetus. In animals doxorubicin has embryotoxic and teratogenic effects.

Doxorubicin is excreted in breast milk. Usage during pregnancy and lactation is therefore not recommended.

4.7 Effects on ability to drive and use machines
Due to the frequent occurrence of nausea and vomiting, driving and operation of machinery should be discouraged.

4.8 Undesirable effects
Dose limiting toxicities of therapy are myelosuppression and cardio-toxicity. Myelosuppression includes a transient leukopenia, anemia and thrombocytopenia, reaching its nadir at 10 to 14 days after treatment.

Cardiotoxicity may occur as arrhythmia directly following drug administration; ECG changes, including T-wave flattening and S-T depression, may last up to 2 weeks after administration.

The risk of cardiomyopathy increases at cumulative doses higher than 550 mg/m^2. Age over 70 or below 15 years should be regarded as a risk factor. Also, concomitant or previous treatment with mitomycin C, cyclophosphamide or dacarbazine has been reported to potentiate doxorubicin induced cardiomyopathy.

Cardiotoxicity may be encountered several weeks or months after discontinuation of doxorubicin therapy.

Other adverse reactions reported are: a generally reversible alopecia; gastrointestinal disturbances, including nausea, vomiting and diarrhea. Mucositis (stomatitis or esophagitis) may occur 5 to 10 days after administration.

Hypersensitivity reactions, such as fever, urticaria and anaphylaxis have been occasionally reported. Doxorubicin influences and potentiates normal tissue reactions to radiation. Also, late ("recall") reactions may occur when doxorubicin is administered some time after irradiation.

Facial flushing may occur if the injection is given too rapidly.

Thrombophlebitis and conjunctivitis have been reported.

Slight transient increases of liver enzymes have been reported. Concomitant irradiation of the liver may cause severe hepatotoxicity, sometimes progressing to cirrhosis

As with other cytotoxic agents, myelodysplastic syndrome and acute myeloid leukaemia have been observed after treatment with combination therapy including doxorubicin. With topoisomerase II inhibitors, secondary leukaemias have been reported more frequently than expected in the form of acute myeloid leukaemia classification 2, 3, and 4. These forms of leukaemia can have a short period of latency (1 to 3 years). They can be cured when detected at an early stage and with an appropriate curative treatment (see section 4.4 "Special warnings and special precautions for use").

Intravesical administration may cause the following adverse reactions: haematuria, vesical and urethral irritation, stranguria and pollakisuria. These reactions are usually of moderate severity and of short duration.

Intravesical administration of doxorubicin may cause a sometimes hemorrhagic cystitis; this may cause a decrease in bladder capacity.

Doxorubicin may impart a red colouration to the urine.

4.9 Overdose
Acute overdosage of doxorubicin enhances the toxic effects of mucositis, leukopenia and thrombocytopenia. Overdosage at intravesical administration may cause severe cystitis. Treatment of acute overdosage consists of treatment of the severely myelosuppressed patient with hospitalization, antibiotics and transfusions after consultation with an oncologist.

Chronic overdosage with cumulative doses exceeding 550 mg/m^2 increases the risk of cardiomyopathy and resultant congestive heart failure. Treatment consists of vigorous management of congestive heart failure with digitalis preparations and diuretics.

Administration of a very high single dose may cause myocardial degeneration within 24 hours.

5. PHARMACOLOGICAL PROPERTIES

5.1 Pharmacodynamic properties
Doxorubicin is a cytotoxic anthracycline antibiotic isolated from cultures of *Streptomyces peucetius var. caesius*. Animal studies have shown a cytotoxic action in several solid and haematologic tumours. The mechanism of action is not completely elucidated. A major mechanism is probably inhibition of topoisomerase II, resulting in DNA breakage. Intercalation and free-radical formation is probably of minor importance. Drug resistance, due to increased expression of the MDR-1 gene encoding for a multidrug efflux pump, has been reported regularly.

5.2 Pharmacokinetic properties
The intravenous administration of doxorubicin is followed by a rapid plasma clearance (t½ approx. 10 min.) and significant tissue binding. The terminal half-life is approximately 30 hours.

Doxorubicin is partly metabolised, mainly to doxorubicinol and to a lesser extent, to the aglycon, and is conjugated to the glucuronide and sulfate. Biliary and fecal excretion represents the major excretion route. About 5% of the dose is eliminated by renal excretion. Plasma protein binding of doxorubicin ranges from 50-85%. The volume of distribution is 800-3500 l/m^2.

Doxorubicin is not absorbed after oral administration; it does not cross the blood-brain barrier.

Impairment of liver function may decrease the clearance of doxorubicin and its metabolites.

5.3 Preclinical safety data
Non stated.

6. PHARMACEUTICAL PARTICULARS

6.1 List of excipients
Sodium chloride, hydrochloric acid/sodium hydroxide, water for injections.

6.2 Incompatibilities
Doxorubicin should not be mixed with 5-fluorouracil or heparin. Contact with aluminium should be avoided.

6.3 Shelf life
Following the special precautions for storage (see section 6.4) the shelf-life of the 5 ml, 10 ml, and 25 ml vials is 36 months and the shelf life of the 100 ml vial is 24 months as printed on the label.

The injection may be diluted with 0.9% sodium chloride solution or 5% glucose solution.

Chemical and physical in-use stability has been demonstrated for 7 days at room temperature (15-25°C) and protected from light.

From a microbiological point of view, the product should be used immediately. If not used immediately, in-use storage times and conditions prior to use are the responsibility of the user and would normally not be longer than 24 hours at 2 to 8°C, unless dilution has taken place in controlled and validated aseptic conditions.

6.4 Special precautions for storage
Doxorubin 0.2%, injection should be stored at 2-8°C, protected from light.

6.5 Nature and contents of container
Doxorubin 0.2%, injection is supplied as a red-orange, sterile solution in injection vials containing 5 ml (10 mg), 10 ml (20 mg), 25 ml (50 mg), or 100 ml (200 mg), respectively, of doxorubicin hydrochloride 2 mg/ml.

6.6 Instructions for use and handling
Any contact with the solution should be avoided. During preparation and reconstitution a strictly aseptic working technique should be used; protective measures should include the use of gloves, mask, safety goggles and protective clothing. Use of a vertical laminair airflow (LAF) hood is recommended.

Gloves should be worn during administration. Waste-disposal procedures should take into account the cytotoxic nature of this substance.

If doxorubicin solution contacts skin, mucosae, or eyes, immediately wash thoroughly with water. Soap may be used for skin cleansing.

7. MARKETING AUTHORISATION HOLDER
Pharmachemie B.V.

Postbus 552

2003 RN Haarlem

The Netherlands.

8. MARKETING AUTHORISATION NUMBER(S)
PL 4946/0016.

9. DATE OF FIRST AUTHORISATION/RENEWAL OF THE AUTHORISATION
4 January 1996

10. DATE OF REVISION OF THE TEXT
January 2001

Doxorubin 10 mg, 50 mg

(medac GmbH)

1. NAME OF THE MEDICINAL PRODUCT
Doxorubin 10 mg.

Doxorubin 50 mg.

2. QUALITATIVE AND QUANTITATIVE COMPOSITION
Doxorubin 10 mg:

Doxorubin, powder for solution for injection contains 10 mg of doxorubicin hydrochloride E.P.

Doxorubin 50 mg:

Doxorubin, powder for solution for injection contains 50 mg of doxorubicin hydrochloride E.P.

3. PHARMACEUTICAL FORM
Powder for solution for injection.

4. CLINICAL PARTICULARS

4.1 Therapeutic indications
In combination with other antineoplastic drugs, doxorubicin is intended for the treatment of acute lymphocytic leukaemia, (except acute lymphatic leukaemia of low risk in children), acute myeloid leukaemia, Hodgkin- and non-Hodgkin lymphomas, osteosarcoma, Ewing sarcoma, adult soft tissue sarcoma, metastatic breast carcinoma, gastric carcinoma, small-cell lung cancer, neuroblastoma, Wilms tumour and bladder carcinoma.

Doxorubicin may be used intravesically as single agent for treatment and prophylaxis of superficial bladder carcinoma.

4.2 Posology and method of administration
The route of administration is by intravenous injection.

The vial contents must be reconstituted before use with water for injection or normal saline (see Section 6.6 Instructions for Use/Handling).

Doxorubicin should **not** be administered intramuscularly or subcutaneously.

INTRAVENOUS ADMINISTRATION

Doxorubicin may be given by intravenous bolus injection, or as continuous infusion. Bolus injection causes higher peak plasma concentration and therefore is probably more cardiotoxic. Intravenous administration occurs preferably through a running, recently applied intravenous infusion, of sodium chloride injection, dextrose injection 5% or sodium chloride and dextrose injection over 3 to 5 minutes.

Patients with an increased risk for cardiotoxicity (see section 4.4 Special warnings and precautions for use) should be considered for treatment with a 24 hours continuous infusion, rather than bolus injection. In this way, cardiotoxicity may be less frequent, without a reduction in therapeutic efficacy. In these patients, the ejection fraction should be measured before each course.

ADULTS

Dosage depends on tumour type, hepatic function, and concurrent chemotherapy.

The commonly recommended dosage schedule as single agent is 60-75 mg/m^2 by intravenous injection, once every 3 weeks. An alternative dose schedule is 20 mg/m^2 intravenously, during 3 consecutive days, once every 3 weeks.

Lower doses may be required in patients with inadequate marrow reserves and in patients who have had prior treatment with other cytotoxic agents. When used in combination with other chemotherapeutic agents the dosage of 30-60 mg/m^2 are administered. Myelosuppression may be more pronounced because of the additive effect of the drugs.

The risk of development of cardiomyopathy gradually increases with the dosage. The maximum cumulative dose of 450 mg/m^2 should not be exceeded. The administration of doxorubicin should be monitored by electrocardiography, echocardiography and carotid pulse curve: When the voltage of the QRS wave decreases by 30% or at a fractional shortening of 5% it is recommended to stop treatment.

If a patient receives mediastinal irradiation, has concomitant heart disease, or is also treated with other cardiotoxic, non-anthracycline oncolytics, a maximal cumulative dose of 400 mg/m^2 is recommended.

Doxorubicin dosage should be reduced if the bilirubin is elevated. When bilirubin is 12 to 30 mg/l - half the dosage should be given; when bilirubin concentrations > 30 mg/l, one quarter of the dosage should be given.

In general, impaired renal function does not require dose reduction.

CHILDREN

Dosage for children may be lowered, since they have an increased risk for late cardiotoxicity. Myelotoxicity should be anticipated, with nadirs at 10 to 14 days after start of treatment, but is usually followed by a rapid recovery due to the large bone marrow reserve of children as compared to adults.

SUPERFICIAL BLADDER CARCINOMA AND BLADDER CARCINOMA IN SITU:

The recommended dosage is 50 mg in 50 ml normal saline, administered via a sterile catheter. Initially, this dose is given weekly, later on monthly. The optimal duration of treatment has not yet been determined; it ranges from 6 to 12 months.

Restrictions regarding the maximal cumulative dose, as with intravenous administration, do not apply to intravesical administration, because systemic absorption of doxorubicin is negligible.

4.3 Contraindications

Doxorubicin therapy should not be started in the following cases:

1. Marked myelosuppression induced by previous chemotherapy or by radiotherapy.
2. Pre-existing heart disease.
3. Previous treatment with complete cumulative doses of doxorubicin or other anthracyclines.
4. Doxorubicin should not be used intravesically for the treatment of bladder carcinoma in patients with urethral stenosis who can not be catheterised.

4.4 Special warnings and special precautions for use

General precautions

Doxorubicin should only be used under supervision of a physician who is experienced in cytotoxic therapy. Nausea, vomiting and mucositis are often severe and should be treated appropriately.

Doxorubicin should **not** be administered intramuscularly or subcutaneously.

The total dose of doxorubicin administered to the individual patient should take into account any previous or concomitant therapy with related compounds such as daunorubicin.

Extravasation

Extravasation results in a severe and progressive tissue necrosis. If extravasation occurs, the injection should be terminated immediately and restarted in another vein. Flooding with normal saline, local infiltration with corticosteroids with or without sodium hydrogen carbonate solution (8.4%), and application of dimethylsulfoxide have been reported with varying success. The advice of a plastic surgeon should be sought, and wide excision of the involved area should be considered.

Cardiotoxicity

Congestive heart failure and/or cardiomyopathy may be encountered several weeks after discontinuation of doxorubicin therapy. Severe cardiac failure may occur precipitously without antecedent ECG change.

The risk of severe, irreversible and therapy-resistant cardiomyopathy and resulting congestive heart failure gradually increases with increasing dosages. A cumulative dose of 450 mg/m^2 should not be exceeded.

Age over 70 or below 15 years and female gender in children should be considered a risk factor, as well as concomitant heart disease. In addition, ECG changes may occur including a reduction in the voltage of the QRS wave, and a prolongation of the systolic time interval, and the ejection fraction may be reduced.

In patients previously treated with other anthracyclines or cyclophosphamide, mitomycin C or dacarbazine, and patients who received radiotherapy to the mediastinal area, cardiotoxicity may occur at doses lower than the recommended cumulative limit. The concurrent use of trastuzumab and anthracyclines (like doxorubicin) is not recommended (see section 4.5).

Acute severe arrhythmias have been reported to occur during or within a few hours after doxorubicin administration.

Heart function should be assessed before, during and after doxorubicin therapy, e.g., by ECG, echocardiography or determination of the ejection fraction. If test results indicate change in cardiac function associated with doxorubicin the benefit of continued therapy must be carefully evaluated against the risk of producing irreversible cardiac damage.

Myelosuppression

The high incidence of bone marrow depression requires careful haematologic monitoring. The nadir is reached between 10-14 days after administration. Blood values usually return to normal within 21 days after administration. Doxorubicin therapy should not be started or continued when polynuclear granulocyte counts are below 2000/mm^3, except in the treatment of acute leukaemia, where lower limits may be applied, depending on the circumstances.

Careful haematologic monitoring is also required because of the risk of secondary leukaemias after treatment with cytotoxic agents (see section 4.8 Undesirable effects). A remission of acute leukaemia can be achieved when detected at an early stage.

Hepatic impairment

Hepatic function (SGOT, SGPT, alkaline phosphatase and bilirubin) should be evaluated before and during therapy.

Hyperuricaemia

Doxorubicin may induce hyperuricemia. The blood uric acid level should be monitored. Sufficient fluid intake should be ascertained (with a daily minimum of 3 l/m^2). If necessary, a xanthine-oxidase inhibitor (allopurinol) may be administered.

Discoloration of urine

Doxorubicin may impart a red coloration to the urine.

4.5 Interaction with other medicinal products and other forms of Interaction

Doxorubicin cardiotoxicity is enhanced by previous or concurrent use of other anthracyclines, mitomycin C, dacarbazine, dactinomycin and, possibly, cyclophosphamide. Also the risk of cardiotoxicity is increased if trastuzumab is given with or after doxorubicin. Trastuzumab and anthracyclines should not be used concurrently in combination except in a well-controlled clinical trial setting with cardiac monitoring. Furthermore, paclitaxel decreases the elimination of doxorubicin. Care should be taken in case of co- administration of both drugs, because of an increased risk of cardiotoxic effects of doxorubicin. The severity of neutropenia or stomatitis may also be increased.

Doxorubicin may cause exacerbations of haemorrhagic cystitis caused by previous cyclophosphamide therapy.

Doxorubicin may enhance the hepatotoxicity of 6-mercaptopurine.

The effects of radiation may be enhanced, and recall of these reactions may occur with doxorubicin therapy, even some time after termination of radiotherapy.

Inducers of the enzyme cytochrome P-450 (e.g. rifampicin and barbiturates) may stimulate the metabolism of doxorubicin, with a possible decrease in efficacy.

Inhibitors of cytochrome P-450 (e.g. cimetidine) may decrease the metabolism of doxorubicin, with a possible increase in toxic effects.

4.6 Pregnancy and lactation

Clinical evidence suggests a possible adverse effect on the foetus. In animals doxorubicin has embryotoxic and teratogenic effects.

Doxorubicin is excreted into breast milk. Usage during pregnancy and lactation is therefore not recommended.

Men as well as women should take effective contraceptive measures during and for at least three months after doxorubicin therapy.

4.7 Effects on ability to drive and use machines

Due to the frequent occurrence of nausea and vomiting, driving cars and operation of machinery should be discouraged.

4.8 Undesirable effects

Dose limiting toxicities of therapy are myelosuppression and cardiotoxicity.

Blood and Lymphatic System Disorder

Myelosuppression includes a transient leucopenia very commonly. Anaemia and thrombocytopenia are less common. Myelosuppression reaches its nadir at 10 to 14 days after treatment. Blood levels usually return to normal within 21 days after administration.

Myelodysplastic syndrome and acute myeloid leukaemia have been observed after treatment with combination therapy including doxorubicin. With topoisomerase II inhibitors, secondary leukaemias have been reported more frequently than expected in the form of acute myeloid leukaemia classification 2, 3, and 4. These forms of leukaemia can have a short period of latency (1 to 3 years) but much longer periods have been reported. They can be cured when detected at an early stage and with an appropriate curative treatment (see section 4.4 Special warnings and special precautions for use).

Immune Disorder

Hypersensitivity reactions, such as fever, urticaria and anaphylaxis occur rarely. Doxorubicin influences and potentiates normal tissue reactions to radiation. Also, late (recall) reactions may occur when doxorubicin is administered some time after irradiation. Facial flushing may occur if the injection is given too rapidly.

Cardiac Disorder

Cardiotoxicity may occur as arrhythmia directly following drug administration; ECG changes, including T-wave flattening and S-T depression, may last up to 2 weeks after administration.

The risk of cardiomyopathy increases with an increasing dosage. Severe cardiotoxicity is more likely after high cumulative doses of doxorubicin (see section 4.4 Special Warnings and Precautions for Use) and may occur months or years after administration.

Gastrointestinal Disorder

Nausea and vomiting are very common and diarrhoea occurs occasionally.

Mucositis (stomatitis or oesophagitis) may occur 5 to 10 days after administration.

Hepato-biliary Disorder

Slight transient increases of liver enzymes have been reported. Concomitant irradiation of the liver may cause severe hepatotoxicity, sometimes progressing to cirrhosis.

Other adverse reactions:

A generally reversible alopecia is very common.

A red colouration of the urine, imparted by doxorubicin, is very common.

Thrombophlebitis and conjunctivitis have been reported.

Doxorubicin may induce hyperuricemia.

Intravesical Administration

Intravesical administration may cause the following adverse reactions: haematuria, vesical and urethral irritation, dysuria, stranguria and pollakisuria. These reactions are usually of moderate severity and of short duration. Intravesical administration of doxorubicin may sometimes cause a haemorrhagic cystitis; this may cause a decrease in bladder capacity.

4.9 Overdose

Acute overdose of doxorubicin enhances the toxic effects, particularly-mucositis, leucopenia and thrombocytopenia. Overdose of intravesical administration may result in more severe cystitis. Treatment of acute overdose consists of treatment of the severely myelosuppressed patient with hospitalisation, antibiotics and transfusions after consultation of an oncologist.

Chronic overdosage with cumulative doses exceeding 450 mg/m^2 increases the risk of cardiomyopathy and resultant congestive heart failure. Treatment consists of vigorous management of congestive heart failure with digitalis preparations and diuretics. Single doses of 250 mg and 500 mg of doxorubicin have proved fatal. Such doses may cause acute myocardial degeneration within 24 hours and severe myelosuppression, the effects of which are greatest between 10 and 15 days after administration. Treatment should be symptomatic and supportive. Delayed cardiac failure may occur up to six months after the overdose.

5. PHARMACOLOGICAL PROPERTIES

5.1 Pharmacodynamic properties

Doxorubicin is an oncolytic drug of the anthracycline group. It is isolated from cultures of Streptomyces peucetius var. caesius. Animal studies have shown an oncolytic action in several solid and haematologic tumours. The mechanism of action is not completely elucidated. A major mechanism is probably inhibition of topoisomerase II, resulting in DNA breakage. Intercalation and free-radical formation is probably of minor importance. Drug resistance, due to increased expression of the MDR-1 gene encoding for a multidrug efflux pump, has been reported regularly.

5.2 Pharmacokinetic properties

The intravenous administration of doxorubicin is followed by a rapid plasma clearance (t1/2 ~ 10 min.) and significant tissue binding. The terminal half-life is approximately 30 hours.

Doxorubicin is partly metabolised, mainly to doxorubicinol and to a lesser extent, to the aglycone, and is conjugated to the glucuronide and sulphate. Biliary and faecal excretion represents the major excretion route. About 10% of the dose is eliminated by renal excretion. Plasma protein binding of doxorubicin ranges from 50-85%. The volume of distribution is 800-3500 $1/m^2$.

Doxorubicin is not absorbed after oral administration; it does not cross the blood-brain barrier.

Impairment of liver function may decrease the clearance of doxorubicin and its metabolites.

5.3 Preclinical safety data

There are no preclinical safety data of relevance to the prescriber which are additional to those already stated in other sections of the SPC.

6. PHARMACEUTICAL PARTICULARS

6.1 List of excipients

Lactose

6.2 Incompatibilities

Doxorubicin should not be mixed with other drugs. Alkaline solutions may hydrolyse doxorubicin. Doxorubicin should not be mixed with heparin or 5-fluorouracil. Contact with aluminium should be avoided.

6.3 Shelf life

Following the special precautions for storage (see below) the shelf life for the powder for solution for injection is 5 years. The expiration date is printed on the label.

Chemical and physical in-use stability of the reconstituted solution in 0.9% sodium chloride solution has been demonstrated for 7 days at 15-25 C and for 14 days under refrigeration (2-8 C).

Chemical and physical in-use stability of a 0.5 mg/ml solution in water for injections has been demonstrated for 24 hours at temperatures below 25 C.

Chemical and physical in-use stability of solutions in the range 0.05 mg/ml to 5 mg/ml in 0.9% sodium chloride solution has been demonstrated for 7 days at room temperature (15-25 C).

From a microbiological point of view, the product should be used immediately. If not used immediately, in-use storage times and conditions prior to use are the responsibility of the user and would normally not be longer than 24 hours at 2 to 8 C, unless reconstitution has taken place in controlled and validated aseptic conditions.

6.4 Special precautions for storage

Doxorubin, powder for solution for injection, 10 mg (50 mg) should be stored at 15-25 C, protected from light.

6.5 Nature and contents of container

Doxorubin, powder for solution for injection, 10 mg (50 mg) is supplied as a red-orange, sterile, lyophilized powder, in glass injection vials with aluminium seal. The package size is 1 or 10 vials.

6.6 Instructions for use and handling

Instructions for reconstitution:

For intravenous injection, Doxorubicin powder for solution for injection should be reconstituted to a concentration of 2 mg/ml in water for injections immediately before use. Alternatively, sodium chloride for injections may be used as a solvent, however, the product may take longer to dissolve.

In order to reconstitute the product, ensure the powder, solutions and equipment are at room temperature, add 5 (25) ml to the 10 (50) mg vial and shake for at least 60 seconds and leave to stand at room temperature for at least 5 minutes before administration to get a clear red mobile liquid. If gelatinous fragments are seen, leave the solution to stand for 5 minutes and shake again. Should the fragments still be visible, discard the solution.

When water for injections is used, immediate dilution to a concentration of less than 0.4mg/ml doxorubicin with 0.9% sodium chloride solution or 5% glucose solution is needed in order to obtain an isotonic solution.

Due to the toxic nature of doxorubicin it is recommended that the following protective measures be taken:

-General instructions for safe use of cytotoxics:

- Training in good techniques for reconstitution and handling should be given to relevant personnel.

- Pregnant staff should be excluded from working with this drug

- Protective clothing should be worn while administering, handling or reconstituting doxorubicin

- Contact with skin or eyes should be avoided. If it occurs, the affected area should be washed immediately with water, soap and water or sodium bicarbonate solution.

- Any spillages should be cleaned with dilute sodium hypochlorite solution.

- All equipment used for the handling, preparation and administration of doxorubicin should be incinerated.

Unused products should be disposed of in a suitable labelled container, marked as hazardous waste.

7. MARKETING AUTHORISATION HOLDER

Pharmachemie B.V.

Swensweg 5

PO Box 552

2003 RN Haarlem

The Netherlands.

8. MARKETING AUTHORISATION NUMBER(S)

Doxorubin 10 mg: PL 4946/0001

Doxorubin 50 mg: PL 4946/0002

9. DATE OF FIRST AUTHORISATION/RENEWAL OF THE AUTHORISATION

12-July-1993

10. DATE OF REVISION OF THE TEXT

April 2005

Driclor

(Stiefel Laboratories (UK) Limited)

1. NAME OF THE MEDICINAL PRODUCT

Driclor

2. QUALITATIVE AND QUANTITATIVE COMPOSITION

Aluminium Chloride Hexahydrate USP 20% w/w

3. PHARMACEUTICAL FORM

Solution for topical application

4. CLINICAL PARTICULARS

4.1 Therapeutic indications

Driclor is indicated for the treatment of hyperhidrosis.

4.2 Posology and method of administration

Apply Driclor last thing at night after drying the affected areas carefully. Wash off in the morning. Do not re-apply the product during the day.

Initially the product may be applied each night until sweating stops during the day. The frequency of application may then be reduced to twice a week or less.

4.3 Contraindications

None known.

4.4 Special warnings and special precautions for use

Ensure that the affected areas to be treated are completely dry before application.

Do not apply Driclor to broken, irritated or recently shaven skin. Avoid contact with eyes.

Avoid direct contact with clothing and polished metal surfaces.

4.5 Interaction with other medicinal products and other forms of Interaction

None known

4.6 Pregnancy and lactation

There are no restrictions on the use of Driclor during pregnancy or lactation.

4.7 Effects on ability to drive and use machines

None

4.8 Undesirable effects

Driclor may cause irritation which may be alleviated by use of a weak corticosteroid cream.

4.9 Overdose

Not applicable.

5. PHARMACOLOGICAL PROPERTIES

5.1 Pharmacodynamic properties

Aluminium chloride hexahydrate acts locally, in the stratum corneum and in the terminal duct, to relieve hyperhidrosis.

5.2 Pharmacokinetic properties

Not applicable

5.3 Preclinical safety data

Not applicable.

6. PHARMACEUTICAL PARTICULARS

6.1 List of excipients

Ethanol

Purified water

6.2 Incompatibilities

None

6.3 Shelf life

a) For the product as packaged for sale

3 years

b) After first opening the container

Comply with expiry date

6.4 Special precautions for storage

Store in a cool place. Keep away from naked flame. Store upright.

6.5 Nature and contents of container

High density polyethylene bottle with roll-on applicator.

Pack size: 60ml

6.6 Instructions for use and handling

There are no special instructions for use or handling of Driclor.

Administrative Data

7. MARKETING AUTHORISATION HOLDER

Stiefel Laboratories (UK) Ltd

Holtspur Lane,

Wooburn Green,

High Wycombe,

Bucks HP10 0AU

8. MARKETING AUTHORISATION NUMBER(S)

PL 0174/0044

9. DATE OF FIRST AUTHORISATION/RENEWAL OF THE AUTHORISATION

7th January 2005

10. DATE OF REVISION OF THE TEXT

September 2005

Legal Category

Pharmacy

DTIC-DOME

(Bayer plc)

1. NAME OF THE MEDICINAL PRODUCT

DTIC-DOME 200mg

2. QUALITATIVE AND QUANTITATIVE COMPOSITION

Each vial contains 200mg dacarbazine citrate equivalent to 200mg of dacarbazine USP.

3. PHARMACEUTICAL FORM

DTIC-DOME is a sterile, colourless to ivory-coloured solid to be reconstituted with Water for Injections BP for intravenous administration.

4. CLINICAL PARTICULARS

4.1 Therapeutic indications

The treatment of metastatic malignant melanoma, sarcoma and Hodgkin's disease. In addition, dacarbazine has been shown, when used in combination with other cytotoxic agents, to be of value in treatment of other malignant diseases, including: carcinoma of the colon, ovary, breast, lung, testicular teratoma, and solid tumours in children.

4.2 Posology and method of administration

4.2.1 Dosage

Adults:

The following standard dosage schedules are recommended:

1. 2.0 to 4.5mg/kg/day for 10 days, which may be repeated at four week intervals.

2. 250mg/m²/day for five days, which may be repeated at three week intervals.

3. A further alternative is to administer the total schedule on the first day.

Other schedules may be used at the discretion of the physician.

Children:

The dosage for children is calculated on a mg/kg or mg/m^2 basis as per the standard adult dose.

Special Populations:

Patients with kidney/liver insufficiency: If there is mild to moderate renal or hepatic insufficiency alone, a dose reduction is not usually required. In patients with combined renal and hepatic impairment elimination of dacarbazine is prolonged. However, no validated recommendations on dose reductions can be given currently.

4.2.2 Administration

DTIC-DOME 200mg vials are reconstituted with 19.7ml of Water for Injections BP. The resulting solution contains dacarbazine 10mg/ml, citric acid and mannitol, at pH 3.0 to 4.0. After the solution has been prepared, the calculated dose is drawn into a syringe and injected intravenously. Injection may be completed in approximately one minute.

If desired, the reconstituted solution may be diluted further with 125 to 250ml of Dextrose Injection BP 5% or Sodium Chloride Injection BP 0.9% and administered by intravenous infusion over a period of 15 to 30 minutes.

4.3 Contraindications

Patients who are hypersensitive to dacarbazine.

Patients with severe liver or kidney diseases.

4.4 Special warnings and special precautions for use

DTIC-DOME should be administered preferably to patients who are hospitalised and who can be observed carefully and frequently during and after therapy, with particular reference to the haemopoietic system.

Care must be taken to avoid extravasation of the drug subcutaneously during intravenous administration as this may result in tissue damage and severe pain.

It is recommended that DTIC-DOME be administered under the supervision of a physician experienced in the use of cancer chemotherapeutic agents. Since facilities for necessary laboratory studies must be available, hospitalisation is recommended.

4.5 Interaction with other medicinal products and other forms of Interaction
None known.

4.6 Pregnancy and lactation
DTIC-Dome is teratogenic. DTIC-DOME should not normally be administered to patients who are pregnant or to mothers who are breast feeding.

4.7 Effects on ability to drive and use machines
None known.

4.8 Undesirable effects
Haemopoietic depression is the most common toxic side-effect of dacarbazine and involves primarily the leucocytes and platelets, although mild anaemia may sometimes occur. Leucopenia and thrombocytopenia may be severe enough to cause death. The possible bone marrow depression requires careful monitoring of white blood cell, red blood cell and platelet levels. Haemopoietic toxicity may warrant temporary suspension or cessation of dacarbazine therapy.

Symptoms of anorexia, nausea and vomiting are the most frequently noticed side-effects. Over 90% of patients are affected with the first few doses. The vomiting lasts for one to 12 hours and may be completely but unpredictably palliated byprochlorperazine. Rarely, dacarbazine causes diarrhoea in which case restricting the patient's oral intake of fluids and food four to six hours prior to treatment may be helpful. The rapid toleration of these symptoms suggests a central nervous system mechanism, and usually these symptoms subside after the first one or two days.

Infrequently, some patients have experienced an influenza-like syndrome of fever to 39°C, myalgias and malaise. This syndrome occurs usually after large single doses and approximately seven days after treatment with dacarbazine and lasts seven to 21 days, and may recur with successive treatments.

Alopecia has been noted, as has facial flushing and facial paraesthesia.

There have been a few cases of significant liver or renal function test abnormalities.

Hepatic toxicity, accompanied by hepatic vein thrombosis and hepatocellular necrosis resulting in death, has been reported. The incidence of such reactions has been low; approximately 0.01% of patients treated. This toxicity has been observed mostly when dacarbazine has been administered concomitantly with other anti-neoplastic drugs; however, it has also been reported in some patients treated with dacarbazine alone.

Anaphylaxis can occur very rarely following administration of dacarbazine.

Erythematous and urticarial rashes have been observed infrequently after administration of dacarbazine.

Rarely, photosensitivity reactions may occur.

4.9 Overdose
Give supportive treatment and monitor blood cell counts.

5. PHARMACOLOGICAL PROPERTIES

5.1 Pharmacodynamic properties
Dacarbazine is a cell cycle non-specific antineoplastic agent.

Although the exact mechanism of action of dacarbazine is unknown, three hypotheses have been proposed:

1. Inhibition of DNA synthesis by acting as a purine analogue.
2. Action as an alkylating agent.
3. Interaction with sulphydryl groups.

5.2 Pharmacokinetic properties
A pharmacokinetic study in 6 patients at a dose range of 4.8–9mg/kg body weight (single intravenous injection) showed an average plasma half-life of 38 minutes. A further study in 6 patients at a dose of 4.5mg/kg body weight by single intravenous administration resulted in a mean plasma half-life of 75 minutes, and after an oral dose of 4.5mg/kg body weight to four patients the plasma half-life was 66 minutes. Dacarbazine is not significantly protein bound (approximately 5%).

5.3 Preclinical safety data
The drug has been shown to be teratogenic and carcinogenic in animals.

6. PHARMACEUTICAL PARTICULARS

6.1 List of excipients
Citric acid

Mannitol

6.2 Incompatibilities
None known.

6.3 Shelf life
DTIC-DOME can be stored for up to 48 months under refrigeration (2°C to 8°C) and protected from light.

After reconstitution with Water for Injections BP, the solution may be stored, suitably protected from light, at 4°C for 72 hours or at normal room temperature (20°C) for up to 8 hours.

Following reconstitution, if the solution is diluted further in Dextrose Injection BP 5% or Sodium Chloride Injection BP 0.9%, the resulting solution may be stored at 4°C for up to 24 hours.

6.4 Special precautions for storage
The product should be protected from light and stored in the manufacturer's original container in a refrigerator between 2°C and 8°C.

The reconstituted solution should also be protected from light.

6.5 Nature and contents of container
20ml amber glass vial with butyl rubber stopper and aluminium seal containing 200mg DTIC-DOME as sterile dacarbazine.

6.6 Instructions for use and handling
Users should avoid contact of DTIC-DOME with the skin and eyes when reconstituting or administering.

7. MARKETING AUTHORISATION HOLDER
Bayer plc
Bayer House
Strawberry Hill
Newbury, Berkshire
RG14 1JA
Trading as Pharmaceutical Division, Baypharm or Baymet.

8. MARKETING AUTHORISATION NUMBER(S)
PL 0010/0128

9. DATE OF FIRST AUTHORISATION/RENEWAL OF THE AUTHORISATION
Date of first authorisation: 12 March 1984

Date of last renewal: 30 January 2003

10. DATE OF REVISION OF THE TEXT
September 2004

LEGAL CATEGORY
POM

Duac Once Daily Gel

(Stiefel Laboratories (UK) Limited)

1. NAME OF THE MEDICINAL PRODUCT
Duac Once Daily Gel

2. QUALITATIVE AND QUANTITATIVE COMPOSITION
Clindamycin Phosphate 1.28% w/w equivalent to clindamycin 1% w/w (10mg/g)

Hydrous Benzoyl Peroxide 6.67% w/w equivalent to anhydrous benzoyl peroxide 5% w/w (50mg/g)

For excipients, see 6.1.

3. PHARMACEUTICAL FORM
Gel

Description: White to slightly yellow homogeneous gel

4. CLINICAL PARTICULARS

4.1 Therapeutic indications
Mild to moderate acne vulgaris.

4.2 Posology and method of administration
Adults

Duac Once Daily Gel should be applied once daily in the evening, to affected areas after the skin has been thoroughly washed, rinsed with warm water and gently patted dry.

Use in Children

The safety and efficacy of Duac Once Daily Gel has not been established in prepubescent children (under 12 years of age), since acne vulgaris rarely presents in this age group.

Use in the Elderly

No specific recommendations.

4.3 Contraindications
Duac Once Daily Gel should not be used in patients with known hypersensitivity to clindamycin, benzoyl peroxide or any of the excipients in the formulation. Duac Once Daily Gel should not be used in patients with a history of regional enteritis or ulcerative colitis, or a history of antibiotic-associated colitis.

4.4 Special warnings and special precautions for use
Contact with the mouth, eyes and mucous membranes and with abraded or eczematous skin should be avoided. Application to sensitive areas of skin should be made with caution.

The product may bleach hair or coloured fabrics.

Patients should be advised that, in some cases, 4-6 weeks of treatment may be required before the full therapeutic effect is observed.

4.5 Interaction with other medicinal products and other forms of Interaction
Concomitant topical antibiotics, medicated or abrasive soaps and cleansers, soaps and cosmetics that have a strong drying effect, and products with high concentrations of alcohol and/or astringents, should be used with caution as a cumulative irritant effect may occur.

4.6 Pregnancy and lactation
The safety of benzoyl peroxide is established.

With regard to clindamycin animal studies do not indicate direct or indirect harmful effects with respect to pregnancy. Reproduction studies in rats and mice, using subcutaneous and oral doses of clindamycin ranging from 100 to 600 mg/kg/day, revealed no evidence of impaired fertility or harm to the foetus due to clindamycin.

The safety of Duac Once Daily Gel in human pregnancy is not established. Therefore, caution should be exercised when prescribing to pregnant women.

Women of child-bearing potential
There are no contraindications in women of child-bearing potential who are practising adequate contraception. However, due to the lack of clinical studies in pregnant women, Duac Once Daily Gel should be used with caution when adequate contraception is not being practised.

Use during lactation
There is no restriction on the use of benzoyl peroxide during lactation.

It is not known whether clindamycin is excreted in human milk following the use of Duac Once Daily Gel, but oral and parenteral administration of clindamycin has been reported to result in the appearance of clindamycin in breast milk. For this reason, treatment of nursing mothers with Duac Once Daily Gel should be restricted to essential cases.

4.7 Effects on ability to drive and use machines
Not relevant

4.8 Undesirable effects
Duac Once Daily Gel may rarely cause pruritus, paraesthesia, erythema and skin dryness at the site of application. Local skin reactions are infrequent, modest and usually resolved with continued use.

4.9 Overdose
No case of overdose has been reported.

5. PHARMACOLOGICAL PROPERTIES

5.1 Pharmacodynamic properties
Pharmacotherapeutic group: Anti-acne preparations for topical use

ATC Code: D10A X30

Clindamycin is a lincosamide antibiotic with bacteriostatic action against Gram-positive aerobes and a wide range of anaerobic bacteria. Lincosamides such as clindamycin bind to the 23S subunit of the bacterial ribosome and inhibit the early stages of protein synthesis. The action of clindamycin is predominantly bacteriostatic although high concentrations may be slowly bactericidal against sensitive strains.

Although clindamycin phosphate is inactive *in-vitro*, rapid *in-vivo* hydrolysis converts this compound to the antibacterial active clindamycin. Clindamycin activity has been demonstrated clinically in comedones from acne patients at sufficient levels to be active against most strains of *Propionibacterium acnes*. Clindamycin *in-vitro* inhibits all *Propionibacterium acnes* cultures tested (MIC 0.4mcg/ml). Free fatty acids on the skin surface have been decreased from approximately 14% to 2% following application of clindamycin.

Benzoyl peroxide is keratolytic acting against comedones at all stages of their development. It is an oxidising agent with bactericidal activity against *Propionibacterium acnes*, the organism implicated in acne vulgaris. Furthermore it is sebostatic, counteracting the excessive sebum production associated with acne.

Duac Once Daily Gel has a combination of keratolytic and antibacterial properties providing activity against all the inflamed and non-inflamed lesions of mild to moderate acne vulgaris.

The inclusion of benzoyl peroxide reduces the potential for the emergence of organisms resistant to Clindamycin.

The presentation of both active ingredients in one product is more convenient and ensures patient compliance.

5.2 Pharmacokinetic properties
In a maximised percutaneous absorption study the mean plasma clindamycin levels during a four week dosing period for Duac Once Daily Gel were negligible (0.043% of applied dose).

The presence of benzoyl peroxide in the formulation did not have an effect on the percutaneous absorption of clindamycin.

Radio-labelled studies have shown that absorption of benzoyl peroxide through the skin can only occur following its conversion to benzoic acid. Benzoic acid is mostly conjugated to form hippuric acid which is excreted via the kidneys.

5.3 Preclinical safety data
Benzoyl peroxide
Animal toxicity studies of benzoyl peroxide have shown that the compound is non-toxic when applied topically.

Benzoic acid, to which benzoyl peroxide is converted prior to absorption, has a wide margin of safety. Benzoic acid is an approved food additive.

Benzoyl peroxide is a free radical generating compound. The release of oxygen during its conversion to benzoic acid may be implicated in a tumour promoting effect seen in mouse skin.

Benzoyl peroxide at high doses (>20 times the normal human dose) has been shown to increase tumour growth initiated by dimethyl benzanthracene (DMBA) in mice. DMBA is a powerful chemical carcinogen to which patients are unlikely to be exposed. The relevance of these results to man is limited. Studies in mice have also shown that benzoyl peroxide does not increase the growth of tumours initiated by ultra violet light.

Clindamycin

The main safety concern highlighted in preclinical studies is a pseudomembranous colitis suffered by hamsters. Hamsters have been shown to be particularly susceptible to this reaction when administered low doses of Clindamycin by all routes, even topical application (dose equivalent to 1mg/kg), and is considered unlikely to be predictive of the occurrence of pseudomembranous colitis in man.

In addition, the absorption of Clindamycin following topical application in man is very limited and the results of specific studies to investigate its percutaneous absorption have confirmed it to be 0.82% of dose in normal human cadaver skin in vitro and 0.33% in vivo. Hence systemic exposure to clindamycin after treatment with Duac Once Daily Gel is likely to be clinically insignificant.

Otherwise, preclinical data reveal no special hazard for humans based on conventional studies of single and repeat-dose toxicity and toxicity to reproduction. Results of local tolerance studies have revealed no significant effects. No mutagenicity or carcinogenicity data are available, but clindamycin is not structurally related to any known carcinogens.

6. PHARMACEUTICAL PARTICULARS

6.1 List of excipients

Carbomer

Dimeticone

Disodium Lauryl Sulfosuccinate

Edetate Disodium

Glycerol

Colloidal Hydrated Silica

Poloxamer

Purified Water

Sodium Hydroxide

6.2 Incompatibilities

None known.

6.3 Shelf life

Unopened: 18 months

In-use: Two months

6.4 Special precautions for storage

Store at 2°C-8°C. Do not freeze.

The patient may store the product at temperatures up to 25°C.

6.5 Nature and contents of container

Internally lacquered membrane-sealed aluminium tubes fitted with a polyethylene screw-cap, packed into a carton.

Pack sizes: 25 and 50 grams.

6.6 Instructions for use and handling

None

7. MARKETING AUTHORISATION HOLDER

Stiefel Laboratories (UK) Ltd

Holtspur Lane

Wooburn Green

High Wycombe

Bucks, HP10 0AU

8. MARKETING AUTHORISATION NUMBER(S)

PL 0174/0217

9. DATE OF FIRST AUTHORISATION/RENEWAL OF THE AUTHORISATION

17th September 2003

10. DATE OF REVISION OF THE TEXT

29th March 2005

DULCO-LAX Perles

(Boehringer Ingelheim Limited Self-Medication Division)

1. NAME OF THE MEDICINAL PRODUCT

Dulco-lax® Perles®

2. QUALITATIVE AND QUANTITATIVE COMPOSITION

Each capsule contains 2.5 mg sodium picosulfate as Sodium Picosulfate Monohydrate.

For excipients, see 6.1

3. PHARMACEUTICAL FORM

Small, pearl-shaped, soft gelatin capsules.

4. CLINICAL PARTICULARS

4.1 Therapeutic indications

Short term relief of constipation.

For the management of constipation of any aetiology.

For bowel clearance before surgery, childbirth or radiological investigations.

4.2 Posology and method of administration

For oral administration.

Unless otherwise prescribed by the doctor, the following dosages are recommended:

Adults and children over 10 years:

Two to four capsules (5 - 10 mg) at night

Children under 10 years:

Not to be taken by children under 10 years without medical advice.

Children (4 - 10 years):

One to two capsules (2.5 - 5 mg) at night.

Children under 4 years:

Not recommended for children under 4 years of age.

Once regularity has restarted dosage should be reduced and can usually be stopped.

The capsules should be swallowed with adequate fluid.

4.3 Contraindications

DULCO-LAX PERLES are contra-indicated in patients with ileus, intestinal obstruction, acute surgical abdominal conditions like acute appendicitis, acute inflammatory bowel diseases, and in severe dehydration.

Not to be used in patients with a known hypersensitivity to sodium picosulfate or any other component of the product.

4.4 Special warnings and special precautions for use

As with all laxatives, DULCO-LAX PERLES should not be taken on a continuous daily basis for long periods.

If laxatives are needed every day, the cause of constipation should be investigated.

Prolonged excessive use may lead to fluid and electrolyte imbalance and hypokalaemia, and may precipitate onset of rebound constipation.

DULCO-LAX PERLES should not to be taken by children under 10 years without medical advice.

4.5 Interaction with other medicinal products and other forms of Interaction

The concomitant use of diuretics or adreno-corticosteroids may increase the risk of electrolyte imbalance. However, this situation only arises if excessive doses are taken (See Overdose Section).

Concurrent administration of broad spectrum antibiotics may reduce the laxative action of DULCO-LAX PERLES.

4.6 Pregnancy and lactation

There are no reports of undesirable or damaging effects during pregnancy or to the foetus attributable to the use of DULCO-LAX PERLES. Nevertheless, medicines should not be used in pregnancy, especially the first trimester, unless the expected benefit is thought to outweigh any possible risk to the foetus.

Although the active ingredient is not known to be excreted in breast milk, use of DULCO-LAX PERLES during breast feeding is not recommended.

4.7 Effects on ability to drive and use machines

None stated.

4.8 Undesirable effects

Adverse events have been ranked under headings of frequency using the following convention:

Very common ($\geqslant$ 1/10); common ($\geqslant$ 1/100, < 1/10); uncommon ($\geqslant$ 1/1000, <1/100); rare ($\geqslant$ 1/10000, <1/1000); very rare (<1/10000).

Immune system disorders

Rare: Allergic reactions, including skin reactions and angio-oedema.

Gastrointestinal disorders

Common: Abdominal discomfort, abdominal pain, abdominal cramps and diarrhoea.

Abdominal discomfort (including abdominal pain and cramps) and diarrhoea may occasionally occur.

4.9 Overdose

Symptoms: If high doses are taken diarrhoea, abdominal cramps and a clinically significant loss of potassium and other electrolytes can occur. This may also lead to increased sensitivity to cardiac glycosides.

Furthermore, cases of colonic mucosal ischaemia have been reported in association with doses of Dulco-lax considerably higher than those recommended for the routine management of constipation.

Laxatives in chronic overdosage are known to cause chronic diarrhoea, abdominal pain, hypokalaemia, secondary hyperaldosteronism and renal calculi. Renal tubular damage, metabolic alkalosis and muscle weakness secondary to hypokalaemia have also been described in association with chronic laxative abuse.

Therapy: Within a short time of ingestion, absorption can be minimised or prevented by inducing vomiting or by gastric lavage. Replacement of fluids and correction of electrolyte imbalance may be required. This is especially important in the elderly and the young. Administration of antispasmodics may be of some value.

5. PHARMACOLOGICAL PROPERTIES

5.1 Pharmacodynamic properties

Sodium picosulfate, the active ingredient of DULCO-LAX PERLESis a locally acting laxative from the triarylmethane group, which after bacterial cleavage in the colon, has the dual-action of stimulating the mucosa of both the large intestine causing peristalsis and of the rectum causing increased motility and a feeling of rectal fullness. The rectal effect may help to restore the "call to stool" although its clinical relevance remains to be established.

5.2 Pharmacokinetic properties

After oral ingestion, sodium picosulfate reaches the colon without any appreciable absorption. Therefore, enterohepatic circulation is avoided. By bacterial cleavage the active form, the free diphenol, is formed in the colon. Consequently, there is an onset of action between 6 - 12 hours, which is determined by the release of the active substance from the preparation.

After administration, only small amounts of the drug are systemically available. Urinary excretion reflects low systemic burden after oral administration.

There is no relationship between the laxative effect and plasma levels of the active diphenol.

5.3 Preclinical safety data

There are no pre-clinical data of relevance to the prescriber which are additional to that already included in other sections of the SPC.

6. PHARMACEUTICAL PARTICULARS

6.1 List of excipients

Propylene glycol

Polyethylene glycol 400

Gelatin

Glycerol

Purified water

6.2 Incompatibilities

None stated.

6.3 Shelf life

36 months

6.4 Special precautions for storage

Do not store above 25°C

Keep the bottle within the outer carton

6.5 Nature and contents of container

Type III colourless glass bottles with polypropylene screw caps or child resistant polypropylene screw caps, each containing 20, 24 or 50 capsules

6.6 Instructions for use and handling

Not applicable.

7. MARKETING AUTHORISATION HOLDER

Boehringer Ingelheim Ltd

Self Medication Division

Ellesfield Avenue

Bracknell

Berkshire

RG12 8YS

United Kingdom

8. MARKETING AUTHORISATION NUMBER(S)

PL 00015/0254

9. DATE OF FIRST AUTHORISATION/RENEWAL OF THE AUTHORISATION

14 July 2000

10. DATE OF REVISION OF THE TEXT

March 2004

11. Legal Category

Pharmacy only, unless General Sale List: packs up to 24 capsules, with child resistant caps

D5a-UK-SPC-10

DULCO-LAX Tablets, 5 mg

(Boehringer Ingelheim Limited Self-Medication Division)

1. NAME OF THE MEDICINAL PRODUCT

DULCO-LAX Tablets, 5 mg

2. QUALITATIVE AND QUANTITATIVE COMPOSITION

Each tablet contains Bisacodyl 5mg.

For excipients, see 6.1

3. PHARMACEUTICAL FORM

Gastro-resistant tablet for oral administration.

Circular, biconvex, yellow, sugar-coated and enteric-coated tablet.

4. CLINICAL PARTICULARS

4.1 Therapeutic indications

Short term relief of constipation.

4.2 Posology and method of administration
Adults and children over 10 years: one to two tablets, swallowed whole at night.

4.3 Contraindications
DULCO-LAX must not be used in patients with ileus, intestinal obstruction, acute surgical abdominal conditions such as acute appendicitis, acute inflammatory bowel diseases, and in severe dehydration. DULCO-LAX is also contraindicated in patients with a known hypersensitivity to bisacodyl or any other ingredient in the product.

4.4 Special warnings and special precautions for use
As with all laxatives, DULCO-LAX should not be taken on a continuous basis for more than five days.

If laxatives are needed every day, the cause of constipation should be investigated. Prolonged excessive use may lead to fluid and electrolyte imbalance and hypokalaemia, and may precipitate the onset of rebound constipation.

Dizziness and / or syncope have been reported in patients during defecation, consistent with defecation syncope (or syncope attributable to straining at stool), or with a vasovagal response to abdominal pain which may be related to the constipation that prompted these patients to resort to the use of laxatives.

Children under 10 years should not take DULCO-LAX without medical advice.

4.5 Interaction with other medicinal products and other forms of Interaction
The concomitant use of antacids and milk products may reduce the resistance of the coating of the tablets and result in dyspepsia and gastric irritation.

The concomitant use of diuretics or adreno-corticosteroids may increase the risk of electrolyte imbalance. However, this situation only arises if excessive doses of DULCO-LAX are taken (See Overdose Section).

4.6 Pregnancy and lactation
There are no reports of undesirable or damaging effects during pregnancy or to the foetus attributable to the use of DULCO-LAX. Nevertheless, medicines should not be used in pregnancy, especially the first trimester, unless the expected benefit is thought to outweigh any possible risk to the foetus.

Although the active ingredient of DULCO-LAX is not known to be excreted in breast milk, its use during breast feeding is not recommended.

4.7 Effects on ability to drive and use machines
DULCO-LAX has no effect on ability to drive and use machinery.

4.8 Undesirable effects
Abdominal discomfort (including cramps and abdominal pain) and diarrhoea may occasionally occur.

Very rarely allergic reactions, including isolated cases of angio-oedema and anaphylactoid reactions have been reported.

4.9 Overdose
Symptoms: If high doses are taken diarrhoea, abdominal cramps and a clinically significant loss of potassium and other electrolytes can occur. This may also lead to increased sensitivity to cardiac glycosides.

Chronic overdose with laxatives may cause chronic diarrhoea, abdominal pain, hypokalaemia, secondary hyperaldosteronism and renal calculi.

Renal tubular damage, metabolic alkalosis and muscle weakness secondary to hypokalaemia have also been described in association with chronic laxative abuse.

Therapy: Within a short time after ingestion of oral forms of DULCO-LAX, absorption can be minimised or prevented by inducing vomiting. Otherwise, gastric lavage should be performed. Replacement of fluids and correction of electrolyte imbalance (particularly hypokalaemia) may be required. This is especially important in the elderly and the young. Administration of antispasmodics may be of some value.

5. PHARMACOLOGICAL PROPERTIES

5.1 Pharmacodynamic properties
Bisacodyl is a locally acting laxative from the triarylmethane group, which after bacterial cleavage in the colon, has the dual-action of stimulating the mucosa of both the large intestine causing peristalsis and of the rectum causing increased motility and a feeling of rectal fullness. The rectal effect may help to restore the "call to stool" although its clinical relevance remains to be established.

5.2 Pharmacokinetic properties
Hydrolysis of bisacodyl by enzymes of the enteric mucosa forms desacetylbisacodyl which is absorbed and excreted partly via urine and bile as glucuronide. By bacterial cleavage the active form, the free diphenol, is formed in the colon. DULCO-LAX Tablets are resistant to gastric and small intestinal juice, reaching the colon without any appreciable absorption and thereby avoiding enterohepatic circulation. Consequently, DULCO-LAX Tablets have an onset of action between 6 - 12 hours after administration.

After administration, only small amounts of the drug are systemically available. Urinary excretion reflects the low systemic burden after oral and rectal administration.

There is no relationship between the laxative effect and plasma levels of the active diphenol.

5.3 Preclinical safety data
There are no pre-clinical data of relevance to the prescriber which are additional to that already included in other sections of the SPC.

6. PHARMACEUTICAL PARTICULARS

6.1 List of excipients
Lactose, maize starch (dried), soluble maize starch, glycerol (85%), magnesium stearate, sucrose, talc, acacia (powdered), titanium dioxide, eudragit L, eudragit S, dibutyl phthalate, macrogol 6000, yellow iron oxide, white beeswax, carnauba wax and shellac.

6.2 Incompatibilities
None stated.

6.3 Shelf life
5 years

6.4 Special precautions for storage
Do not store above 25°C.

Keep container in the outer carton.

6.5 Nature and contents of container
Blister packs consisting of opaque white PVC/PVDC blister foil and aluminium foil (covering foil).

Blister packs consisting of colourless PVC blister foil and aluminium foil (covering foil).

Packs of 6, 8, 10, 20, 30, and 40.

Not all pack sizes may be marketed.

6.6 Instructions for use and handling
None stated.

7. MARKETING AUTHORISATION HOLDER
Boehringer Ingelheim Limited,

Ellesfield Avenue,

Bracknell,

Berkshire,

RG12 8YS,

United Kingdom.

Trading as Boehringer Ingelheim Self-Medication Division

8. MARKETING AUTHORISATION NUMBER(S)
PL 00015/0240

9. DATE OF FIRST AUTHORISATION/RENEWAL OF THE AUTHORISATION
1 April 1999

10. DATE OF REVISION OF THE TEXT
March 2005

11. Legal category
GSL

D5c/GSL/UK/SPC/12

Duofilm

(Stiefel Laboratories (UK) Limited)

1. NAME OF THE MEDICINAL PRODUCT
Duofilm

2. QUALITATIVE AND QUANTITATIVE COMPOSITION
Salicylic acid BP 16.7% w/w

Lactic acid BP 16.7% w/w

3. PHARMACEUTICAL FORM
Solution for topical administration.

4. CLINICAL PARTICULARS

4.1 Therapeutic indications
Duofilm is indicated for the treatment of warts.

4.2 Posology and method of administration
Adults and the elderly:

Apply daily to the affected areas only.

Children:

Children under the age of 12 years should be treated under supervision. Treatment of infants under the age of 2 years is not recommended.

4.3 Contraindications
Duofilm should not be used on the face or anogenital regions. Avoid applying to normal skin.

4.4 Special warnings and special precautions for use
None.

4.5 Interaction with other medicinal products and other forms of Interaction
None known.

4.6 Pregnancy and lactation
There are no restrictions on the use of Duofilm during pregnancy or lactation.

4.7 Effects on ability to drive and use machines
None.

4.8 Undesirable effects
None.

4.9 Overdose
Not Applicable.

5. PHARMACOLOGICAL PROPERTIES

5.1 Pharmacodynamic properties
Lactic acid affects the keratinisation process, reducing the hyperkeratosis which is characteristic of warts. It is caustic, leading to the destruction of the keratotic tissue of the wart and of the causative virus.

Salicylic acid is keratolytic, producing desquamation by solubilising the intercellular cement in the stratum corneum.

5.2 Pharmacokinetic properties
Not applicable.

5.3 Preclinical safety data
Not applicable.

6. PHARMACEUTICAL PARTICULARS

6.1 List of excipients
Flexible Collodion.

6.2 Incompatibilities
None.

6.3 Shelf life
a) For the product as packaged for sale

3 years.

b) After first opening the container

Comply with expiry date.

6.4 Special precautions for storage
Do not store above 25°C. Keep away from naked flame.

6.5 Nature and contents of container
Amber screw capped applicator bottle containing 15ml.

6.6 Instructions for use and handling
There are no special instructions for use or handling of Duofilm.

7. MARKETING AUTHORISATION HOLDER
Stiefel Laboratories (UK) Ltd

Holtspur Lane

Wooburn Green

High Wycombe

Bucks HP10 0AU

8. MARKETING AUTHORISATION NUMBER(S)
PL 0174/0025R

9. DATE OF FIRST AUTHORISATION/RENEWAL OF THE AUTHORISATION
14th February 1990

10. DATE OF REVISION OF THE TEXT
September 2005

Duovent UDVs

(Boehringer Ingelheim Limited)

1. NAME OF THE MEDICINAL PRODUCT
Duovent UDVs

2. QUALITATIVE AND QUANTITATIVE COMPOSITION
Each single dose unit contains Fenoterol Hydrobromide Ph.Eur. 1.25 mg and Ipratropium Bromide Ph.Eur. 0.5 mg.

For excipients, see Section 6.1.

3. PHARMACEUTICAL FORM
Nebuliser solution.

4. CLINICAL PARTICULARS

4.1 Therapeutic indications
The management of acute severe asthma or acute exacerbation of chronic asthma presenting as an emergency requiring treatment by nebuliser.

4.2 Posology and method of administration
DUOVENT UDVs may be administered from an intermittent positive pressure ventilator or from a properly maintained and functioning nebuliser.

The recommended dose for adults and children over 14 years is one vial (4 ml) to be nebulised immediately upon presentation. Each dose should be inhaled to dryness from the nebuliser. Repeat dosing may be given at the discretion of the treating physician, up to a maximum of 4 vials in 24 hours.

In acute severe asthma additional doses may be necessary depending on clinical response. Nebuliser treatment of acute severe asthma should be replaced by standard inhaler devices 24 - 48 hours before discharge unless the patient requires a nebuliser at home.

Clinical trials have included patients over 65 years. No adverse reactions specific to this age group have been reported.

Administration

DUOVENT UDVs should only be used in a nebuliser approved by your doctor.

1. The nebuliser or ventilator unit should be prepared by following the manufacturer's instructions and /or the advice of the physician.

2. A new single dose unit should be carefully separated from the strip. NEVER use one which has been previously opened.

3. Open the single dose unit by simply twisting off the top, always taking care to hold it in an upright position.

4. Unless otherwise instructed, all the contents of the single dose unit should be squeezed into the nebuliser chamber. If dilution of the single dose unit contents is necessary this should be done using ONLY sterile sodium chloride 0.9% solution as directed by the physician.

5. Use your nebuliser as directed by your doctor.

6. After nebulisation has finished, throw away any remaining solution from the single dose unit or nebuliser chamber.

7. Follow the manufacturer's instructions for cleaning the nebuliser. It is important that the nebuliser is kept clean.

4.3 Contraindications
Hypertrophic obstructive cardiomyopathy, tachyarrhythmia. Hypersensitivity to fenoterol hydrobromide or atropine-like substances.

4.4 Special warnings and special precautions for use
Patients must be instructed in the correct use of a nebuliser and warned not to exceed the prescribed dose. The patient must be instructed to seek medical advice in the event of DUOVENT failing to provide relief of bronchospasm. In the case of acute, rapidly worsening dyspnoea (difficulty in breathing) a doctor should be consulted immediately.

For prolonged use, on demand (symptom-oriented) treatment may be preferable to regular use. Patients should be evaluated for the addition or the increase of anti-inflammatory therapy (e.g. inhaled corticosteroids) to control airway inflammation and to prevent deterioration of disease control.

The use of increasing amounts of beta$_2$-agonist containing products such as DUOVENT on a regular basis to control symptoms of bronchial obstruction may suggest declining disease control. If bronchial obstruction deteriorates it is inappropriate and possibly hazardous to simply increase the use of beta$_2$-agonist containing products such as DUOVENT, beyond the recommended dose over extended periods of time. In this situation, the patient's therapy plan, and in particular the adequacy of anti-inflammatory therapy with inhaled corticosteroids should be reviewed to prevent potentially life threatening deterioration of disease control.

Other sympathomimetic bronchodilators should only be used with DUOVENT under medical supervision.

In the following conditions DUOVENT should only be used after careful risk/benefit assessment, especially when doses higher than recommended are used:

Insufficiently controlled diabetes mellitus, myocardial insufficiency, angina, cardiac dysrhythmias, hypertension, recent myocardial infarction, hypertrophic subvalvular aortic stenosis, severe organic heart or vascular disorders, hyperthyroidism, pheochromocytoma.

The administration of nebuliser solutions has occasionally been associated with cases of paradoxical bronchoconstriction.

Potentially serious hypokalemia may result from beta$_2$-agonist therapy. Caution is advocated in the use of anticholinergic agents in patients with narrow-angle glaucoma, or with prostatic hypertrophy.

Patients must be instructed in the correct administration of DUOVENT UDVs. Care should be taken to prevent the solution or mist from entering the eyes. It is recommended that the nebulised solution be administered via a mouth piece. If this is not available and a nebuliser mask is used, it must fit properly. Patients who may be predisposed to glaucoma should be warned specifically to protect their eyes.

There have been isolated reports of ocular complications (i.e. mydriasis, increased intra-ocular pressure, narrow-angle glaucoma, eye pain) when aerosolised ipratropium bromide either alone or in combination with an adrenergic beta$_2$-agonist was sprayed into the eyes.

Inhaled doses of ipratropium bromide nebuliser solution up to 1 mg have not been associated with elevation of intra-ocular pressure.

Eye pain or discomfort, blurred vision, visual halos or coloured images in association with red eyes from conjunctival and corneal congestion may be signs of acute narrow-angle glaucoma.

Should any combination of these symptoms develop, treatment with miotic eye drops should be initiated and specialist advice sought immediately.

As patients with cystic fibrosis may be more prone to gastro-intestinal motility disturbances, DUOVENT as with other anticholinergics should be used with caution in these patients.

4.5 Interaction with other medicinal products and other forms of Interaction
In view of a possible interaction between sympathomimetic amines and monoamine oxidase inhibitors or tricyclic antidepressants, care should be exercised if it is proposed to administer these compounds concurrently with DUOVENT UDVs.

DUOVENT UDVs should be used with caution in patients already receiving other sympathomimetic agents as cardiovascular effects may be additive.

Other beta-adrenergics and anticholinergics and xanthine derivatives (such as theophylline) may enhance the bronchodilatory effect. The concurrent administration of other beta-mimetics, systemically available anticholinergics and xanthine derivatives (e.g. theophylline) may increase the side effects.

Beta-adrenergic blocking agents may antagonise fenoterol hydrobromide and potentially seriously reduce its bronchodilator effect if administered concurrently.

Beta-agonist induced hypokalemia may be increased by concomitant treatment with xanthine derivatives, steroids and diuretics. This should be taken into account particularly in patients with severe airway obstruction.

Hypokalemia may result in an increased susceptibility to arrhythmias in patients receiving digoxin. Additionally, hypoxia may aggravate the effect of hypokalemia on cardiac rhythm. It is recommended that serum potassium levels are monitored in such situations.

Inhalation of halogenated hydrocarbon anaesthetics such as halothane, trichloroethylene and enflurane may increase the susceptibility to the cardiovascular effects of beta-agonists.

4.6 Pregnancy and lactation
Although both fenoterol hydrobromide and ipratropium bromide have been in general use for several years, there is no definite evidence of ill-consequence during human pregnancy; animal studies have shown no hazard. Medicines should, however, not be used in pregnancy, especially during the first trimester, unless the expected benefit is thought to outweigh any possible risk to the foetus.

Beta-adrenergic agents have been shown to prolong pregnancy and inhibit labour although the amount in the recommended dose of DUOVENT UDVs is probably insufficient to do so.

Preclinical studies have shown that fenoterol hydrobromide is secreted in breast milk. Safety in breast fed infants has not been established.

4.7 Effects on ability to drive and use machines
None stated.

4.8 Undesirable effects
Frequent undesirable effects of DUOVENT are fine tremor of skeletal muscles, nervousness and dryness of the mouth; less frequent are headache, dizziness, tachycardia and palpitations, especially in susceptible patients.

Potentially serious hypokalemia may result from beta$_2$-agonist therapy.

As with use of other inhalation therapy, cough, local irritation and less common, inhalation induced bronchospasm have been reported.

As with other beta-agonist containing products, nausea, vomiting, sweating, weakness and myalgia/muscle cramps may occur. In rare cases decrease in diastolic blood pressure, increase in systolic blood pressure, arrhythmias, particularly after higher doses, may occur.

In individual cases psychological alterations have been reported under inhalational therapy with beta-agonist containing products.

Ocular accommodation disturbances, gastrointestinal motility disturbances and urinary retention are rare and reversible.

Ocular side effects have been reported (see: Special warnings and special precautions for use).

In rare cases skin reactions or allergic-type reactions such as skin rash, angioedema of the tongue, lips and face and urticaria may occur.

As with all β_2-agonists hyperactivity in children is possible.

4.9 Overdose
Symptoms
The effects of overdosage are expected to be primarily related to fenoterol. The expected symptoms of overdosage are those of excessive beta-adrenergic-stimulation, the most prominent being tachycardia, palpitation, hypertension, hypotension, widening of the pulse pressure, anginal pain, arrhythmias, flushing, nausea, restlessness, dizziness, headache and tremor.

Hypokalaemia may occur following overdose with fenoterol. Serum potassium levels should be monitored.

Inhaled doses of 5 mg ipratropium produce an increase in heart rate and palpitation but single doses of 2 mg have been given to adults and 1 mg to children without causing side-effects. Single doses of ipratropium bromide 30 mg by mouth cause anticholinergic side-effects but these are not severe and do not require specific reversal.

Therapy
It is suggested that the patient should be treated symptomatically. Beta$_1$-selective beta-adrenergic blocking agents should be chosen and blood pressure should be monitored. Should the administration of a beta-adrenergic blocking agent be considered necessary to counteract the effects of overdosage, its use in a patient liable to bronchospasm should be carefully monitored.

5. PHARMACOLOGICAL PROPERTIES

5.1 Pharmacodynamic properties
Fenoterol hydrobromide is a direct acting sympathomimetic agent where the catechol nucleus of isoprenaline has been replaced by a resorcinol nucleus, and the substituent moiety on the amino group is larger. This substitution has the effect of depressing the affinity of the molecule to the beta-$_1$ (cardiac and lipolytic) adrenergic receptors and enhancing the affinity towards the beta-$_2$ (bronchial, vascular and intestinal) adrenergic receptors.

Ipratropium bromide affects airway function primarily through its neural effect on the parasympathetic nervous system. Ipratropium bromide blocks the acetylcholine receptors on smooth muscle in the lung. Stimulation of these receptors normally produces contraction and, depending on the degree of actuation, bronchoconstriction. Thus, even in normal subjects, ipratropium bromide will cause bronchodilatation.

5.2 Pharmacokinetic properties
Fenoterol hydrobromide: In man fenoterol is very rapidly distributed through the tissues following intravenous administration. The kidneys excrete up to 65% mainly in the form of acidic conjugates. Following oral administration, the plasma levels reach their maximum 2 hours after ingestion and then drop exponentially. Renal excretion is 39% following peroral administration and over 98% of the renal excretory products consist of acidic conjugates. The half life for total excretion is 7.2 hours and absorption was calculated to be 60%.

The duration of action following use of a metered dose aerosol is considerably larger and can be explained by the dose independent absorption in the upper bronchial tree. The concentration-independent absorption at this site, from the depot produced by the metered dose aerosol is maintained for several hours.

Ipratropium bromide: It is a quaternary ammonium compound which is poorly absorbed from the gastro-intestinal tract and is slow to cross mucous membranes and the blood brain barrier. Following inhalation, uptake into the plasma is minimal, a peak blood concentration is attained 1 ½ to 3 hours after inhalation (and similarly for oral administration). Excretion is chiefly via the kidneys.

5.3 Preclinical safety data
None stated.

6. PHARMACEUTICAL PARTICULARS

6.1 List of excipients
Sodium chloride

Hydrochloric acid

Purified water

6.2 Incompatibilities
Not applicable.

6.3 Shelf life
3 years.

As the product contains no preservative, a fresh vial should be used for each dose and the vial should be opened immediately before administration. Any solution left in the vial should be discarded.

6.4 Special precautions for storage
Do not store above 25°C. Protect from heat. Keep vials in the outer carton.

6.5 Nature and contents of container
Low density polyethylene (LDPE) vials formed in strips of 10 packed into cartons containing 10, 20, 30, 50, 60, 80, 100, 120, 150, 200, 500 and 1000 vials. Each vial contains 4 ml of solution.

Not all pack sizes may be marketed.

6.6 Instructions for use and handling
None

7. MARKETING AUTHORISATION HOLDER
Boehringer Ingelheim Limited,

Ellesfield Avenue,

Bracknell,

Berkshire,

RG12 8YS,

United Kingdom.

8. MARKETING AUTHORISATION NUMBER(S)
PL 00015/0164

9. DATE OF FIRST AUTHORISATION/RENEWAL OF THE AUTHORISATION
09/06/93

10. DATE OF REVISION OF THE TEXT
March 2005

11. Legal Category
POM

D6c/UK/SPC/7

Duphaston, Duphaston HRT

(Solvay Healthcare Limited)

1. NAME OF THE MEDICINAL PRODUCT

Duphaston® and Duphaston®-HRT

2. QUALITATIVE AND QUANTITATIVE COMPOSITION

Each tablet contains 10 mg dydrogesterone B.P.

3. PHARMACEUTICAL FORM

Round, white tablet, scored on one side with the imprint '155' on each half of the tablet and imprinted '§' on the reverse.

4. CLINICAL PARTICULARS

4.1 Therapeutic indications

To counteract the effects of unopposed oestrogen in hormone replacement therapy, pre-menstrual syndrome, endometriosis, dysmenorrhoea, infertility, irregular cycles, dysfunctional bleeding (with added oestrogen), secondary amenorrhoea (with added oestrogen), threatened and habitual abortion (associated with proven progesterone deficiency).

4.2 Posology and method of administration

Adults

Hormone replacement therapy

The standard dose is 10 mg Duphaston daily for the last 14 days of each 28-day oestrogen treatment cycle. The dose may be increased to 10 mg twice daily if either early withdrawal bleeding occurs or if endometrial biopsy reveals inadequate progestational response.

Pre-menstrual syndrome

10 mg twice daily from day 12 to 26 of the cycle. The dosage may be increased if necessary.

Endometriosis

10 mg two to three times daily from day 5 to 25 of the cycle, or continuously.

Dysmenorrhoea

10 mg twice daily from day 5 to 25 of the cycle.

Infertility or Irregular cycles

10 mg twice daily from day 11 to 25 of the cycle. Treatment should be maintained for at least six consecutive cycles. If the patient conceives, it is advisable to continue treatment for the first few months of pregnancy as described under 'habitual abortion'.

Dysfunctional bleeding - to arrest bleeding

10 mg twice daily together with an oestrogen once daily for five to seven days.

Dysfunctional bleeding - to prevent bleeding

10 mg twice daily together with an oestrogen once daily from day 11 to day 25 of the cycle.

Amenorrhoea

An oestrogen once daily from day 1 to 25 of the cycle, and Duphaston 10 mg twice daily from day 11 to 25 of the cycle.

Threatened abortion

40 mg at once then 10 mg every eight hours until symptoms remit. If symptoms persist or return during treatment the dose can be increased by one tablet every eight hours. The effective dose must be maintained for a week after symptoms have ceased and can then be gradually decreased unless symptoms return.

Habitual abortion

Treatment should be started as early as possible, preferably before conception: 10 mg should be given twice daily from day 11 to 25 of the cycle until conception and then continuously (10 mg twice daily) until the twentieth week of pregnancy, then dosage may be gradually reduced.

Elderly

Hormone replacement therapy: Standard adult dosage is recommended.

Children

Primary dysmenorrhoea: 10 mg twice daily at the discretion of the physician.

4.3 Contraindications

Duphaston: None known.

Duphaston-HRT: Known or suspected carcinoma of the breast.

4.4 Special warnings and special precautions for use

Duphaston: None known.

Duphaston-HRT: Assessment of each woman prior to taking hormone replacement therapy (and at regular intervals thereafter) should include a personal and family medical history. Physical examination should be guided by this and by the contraindications (section 4.3) and warnings (section 4.4) for this product. During assessment of each individual woman clinical examination of the breasts and pelvic examination should be performed where clinically indicated rather than as a routine procedure. Women should be encouraged to participate in the national breast cancer screening programme (mammography) and the national cervical cancer screening programme (cervical cytology) as appropriate for their age). Breast awareness should also be encouraged and women advised to report any changes in their breasts to their doctor or nurse.

A reanalysis of original data from 51 epidemiological studies reported a small or moderate increase in the probability of having breast cancer *diagnosed* in women currently or recently using HRT. The findings may be due to biological effects of HRT, earlier diagnosis, or a combination of both. The relative risk increased with duration of treatment (by 2.3% per year of use) and returned to normal in the course of five years after cessation of HRT use. This is comparable to the increase in relative risk when natural menopause is delayed in the absence of HRT. Breast cancers diagnosed in current or recent users of HRT are more likely to be localised to the breast than those found in non-users. HRT use may not be associated with increased mortality from breast cancer.

Between the ages of 50 and 70, about 45 women in every 1000 not using HRT will have breast cancer diagnosed. It is estimated that among those who use HRT for 5 years starting at age 50, 2 extra cases of breast cancer will be detected by age 70 in every 1000 women. For those who use HRT for 10 years there will be 6 extra cases of breast cancer, and for 15 years use, 12 extra cases of breast cancer in every 1000 women during the 20 year period until age 70.

It is important that the increased risk of being diagnosed with breast cancer is discussed with the patient and weighed against the known benefits of HRT.

4.5 Interaction with other medicinal products and other forms of Interaction

None known.

4.6 Pregnancy and lactation

Pregnancy: There is no known risk in pregnancy. Duphaston is indicated for threatened or habitual abortion, until the twentieth week of pregnancy.

Lactation: Small amounts are expected to be excreted, but exact amounts are unknown. There have been no reports of adverse experiences.

4.7 Effects on ability to drive and use machines

None known.

4.8 Undesirable effects

Serious side effects are not expected. Breakthrough bleeding may occur in a few patients. It can, however, be prevented by increasing the dosage. Nausea, breast tenderness, headache, bloated feeling, transient dizziness and skin reactions have occasionally been reported.

4.9 Overdose

Symptoms

No reports of ill-effects from overdosage have been reported and remedial action is generally unnecessary.

Treatment

If a large overdosage is discovered within 2-3 hours and treatment seems desirable, gastric lavage is recommended. There are no special antidotes and treatment should be symptomatic.

5. PHARMACOLOGICAL PROPERTIES

5.1 Pharmacodynamic properties

Dydrogesterone is an orally-active progestogen, which produces a complete secretory endometrium in an oestrogen-primed uterus, thereby providing protection for oestrogen-induced increased risk of endometrial hyperplasia and/or carcinogenesis. It is indicated in all cases of endogenous progesterone deficiency. Duphaston is non-androgenic, non-oestrogenic, non-thermogenic, non-corticoid and non-anabolic.

5.2 Pharmacokinetic properties

After oral administration of labelled dydrogesterone, on average 63% of the dose is excreted into the urine. Within 72 hours, excretion is complete. Dydrogesterone is completely metabolised.

The main metabolite of dydrogesterone is 20α-dihydrodydrogesterone (DHD) and is present in the urine predominantly as the glucuronic acid conjugate. A common feature of all metabolites characterised is the retention of the 4,6 diene-3-one configuration of the parent compound and the absence of 17α-hydroxylation. This explains the lack of oestrogenic and androgenic effects of dydrogesterone.

After oral administration of dydrogesterone, plasma concentrations of DHD are substantially higher as compared to the parent drug. The AUC and C_{max} ratios of DHD to dydrogesterone are in the order of 40 and 25, respectively.

Dydrogesterone is rapidly absorbed. The T_{max} values of dydrogesterone and DHD vary between 0.5 and 2.5 hours.

Mean terminal half lives of dydrogesterone and DHD vary between 5 to 7 and 14 to 17 hours, respectively.

Unlike progesterone, dydrogesterone is not excreted in the urine as pregnanediol. It is therefore possible to analyse production of endogenous progesterone even in the presence of dydrogesterone.

5.3 Preclinical safety data

Dydrogesterone has been used in several animal models and has been proven to be an entity with low toxicity, not having mutagenic or carcinogenic properties.

No effects were seen in reproduction experiments.

6. PHARMACEUTICAL PARTICULARS

6.1 List of excipients

Lactose, maize starch, methylhydroxypropylcellulose, polyethylene glycol 400, silica, magnesium stearate, titanium dioxide (E171).

6.2 Incompatibilities

Not applicable.

6.3 Shelf life

Five years.

6.4 Special precautions for storage

Do not store above 30°C. Store in the original package.

6.5 Nature and contents of container

Cartons containing 42 (Duphaston-HRT) or 60 (Duphaston) tablets in blister strips.

6.6 Instructions for use and handling

None.

7. MARKETING AUTHORISATION HOLDER

Solvay Healthcare Limited

Mansbridge Road

West End

Southampton

SO18 3JD

8. MARKETING AUTHORISATION NUMBER(S)

PL 00512/5004R

9. DATE OF FIRST AUTHORISATION/RENEWAL OF THE AUTHORISATION

17 October 1995

10. DATE OF REVISION OF THE TEXT

May 2001

Legal category

POM

Durogesic DTrans 25/50/75/100 Transdermal Patch

(Janssen-Cilag Ltd)

1. NAME OF THE MEDICINAL PRODUCT

Durogesic® DTrans® 25/50/75/100 Transdermal Patch

2. QUALITATIVE AND QUANTITATIVE COMPOSITION

Each Durogesic DTrans 25/50/75/100 patch contains fentanyl 4.2/8.4/12.6/16.8 mg.

Release rate approximately 25/50/75/100 μg/h; active surface area 10.5/21.0/31.5/42.0 cm^2.

For excipients, see 6.1

3. PHARMACEUTICAL FORM

Transdermal patch.

4. CLINICAL PARTICULARS

4.1 Therapeutic indications

Durogesic DTrans is indicated

- in the management of chronic intractable pain due to cancer
- in the management of chronic intractable pain

4.2 Posology and method of administration

For transdermal use.

Durogesic DTrans should be applied to non-irritated and non-irradiated skin on a flat surface of the torso or upper arm. A non-hairy area should be selected. If the site of Durogesic DTrans application requires to be cleansed prior to application of the patch, this should be done with water. Soaps, oils, lotions or any other agent that might irritate the skin or alter its characteristics should not be used. The skin should be completely dry before the patch is applied.

The Durogesic DTrans patch should be removed from the protective pouch by first folding the notch (located close to the tip of the arrow on the pouch label) and then carefully tearing the pouch material. If scissors are used to open the pouch, this should be done close to the sealed edge so as not to damage the patch inside.

Durogesic DTrans should be applied immediately after removal from the sealed pouch. Following removal of both parts of the protective liner, the transdermal patch should be pressed firmly in place with the palm of the hand for approximately 30 seconds, making sure the contact is complete, especially around the edges.

Durogesic DTrans should be worn continuously for 72 hours. A new patch should then be applied to a different skin site after removal of the previous transdermal patch. Several days should elapse before a new patch is applied to the same area of skin.

The need for continued treatment should be assessed at regular intervals.

Adults:

Initial dose selection

The initial Durogesic DTrans dose should be based on the patient's opioid history, including the degree of opioid tolerance, if any, as well as on the current general condition and medical status of the patient.

In strong opioid-naive patients, the lowest Durogesic DTrans dose 25 μg/h, should be used as the initial dose.

In opioid-tolerant patients, the initial dose of Durogesic DTrans should be based on the previous 24 hour opioid analgesic requirement. A recommended conversion scheme from oral morphine to Durogesic DTrans is given below:

Oral 24-Hour Morphine (mg/day)	Durogesic DTrans (μ g/h)
<135	25
135 - 224	50
225 - 314	75
315 - 404	100
405 - 494	125
495 - 584	150
585 - 674	175
675 - 764	200
765 - 854	225
855 - 944	250
945 - 1034	275
1035 - 1124	300

Previous analgesic therapy should be phased out gradually from the time of the first patch application until analgesic efficacy with Durogesic DTrans is attained. For both strong opioid-naive and opioid tolerant patients, the initial evaluation of the analgesic effect of Durogesic DTrans should not be made before the patch has been worn for 24 hours due to the gradual increase in serum fentanyl concentrations up to this time.

Dose titration and maintenance therapy

The Durogesic DTrans patch should be replaced every 72 hours. The dose should be titrated individually until analgesic efficacy is attained. If analgesia is insufficient at the end of the initial application period, the dose may be increased. Dose adjustment, when necessary, should normally be performed in 25 μg/h increments, although the supplementary analgesic requirements (oral morphine 90 mg/day ≈ Durogesic DTrans 25 μg/h) and pain status of the patient should be taken into account. More than one Durogesic DTrans patch may be used for doses greater than 100 μg/h. Patients may require periodic supplemental doses of a short-acting analgesic for 'breakthrough' pain. Additional or alternative methods of analgesia should be considered when the Durogesic DTrans dose exceeds 300 μg/h.

Discontinuation of Durogesic DTrans

If discontinuation of Durogesic DTrans is necessary, any replacement with other opioids should be gradual, starting at a low dose and increasing slowly. This is because fentanyl levels fall gradually after Durogesic DTrans is removed; it may take 17 hours or more for the fentanyl serum concentration to decrease by 50%. As a general rule, the discontinuation of opioid analgesia should be gradual, in order to prevent withdrawal symptoms.

Use in elderly patients

Data from intravenous studies with fentanyl suggest that elderly patients may have reduced clearance, a prolonged half-life and they may be more sensitive to the drug than younger patients. Studies of Durogesic DTrans in elderly patients demonstrated fentanyl pharmacokinetics which did not differ significantly from young patients although serum concentrations tended to be higher. Elderly, cachectic, or debilitated patients should be observed carefully for signs of fentanyl toxicity and the dose reduced if necessary.

Use in Children

The safety and efficacy of Durogesic DTrans in children has not been established and is therefore not recommended.

4.3 Contraindications

Durogesic DTrans is contra-indicated in patients with known hypersensitivity to fentanyl or to the adhesive in the patch.

Durogesic DTrans is a sustained-release preparation indicated for the treatment of chronic intractable pain and is contra-indicated in acute pain because of the lack of opportunity for dosage titration in the short term and the resultant possibility of significant respiratory depression.

4.4 Special warnings and special precautions for use

Patients who have experienced serious adverse events should be monitored for up to 24 hours after Durogesic DTrans removal since serum fentanyl concentrations decline gradually and are reduced by about 50% in approximately 17 (range 13-22) hours.

Durogesic DTrans should be kept out of reach and sight of children at all times before and after use.

Durogesic DTrans patches should not be cut. No data are available on cut or divided patches.

When Durogesic DTrans is administered for chronic intractable pain that will require prolonged treatment, it is strongly recommended that the physician defines treatment outcomes with regards to pain relief and functional improvement in accordance with locally defined pain management guidelines. Physician and patient should agree to discontinue treatment if these objectives are not met.

Respiratory depression

As with all potent opioids, some patients may experience significant respiratory depression with Durogesic DTrans; patients must be observed for these effects. Respiratory depression may persist beyond the removal of the Durogesic DTrans patch. The incidence of respiratory depression increases as the Durogesic DTrans dose is increased. See also 'overdosage' concerning respiratory depression. CNS active drugs may increase the respiratory depression (see 'interactions').

Chronic pulmonary disease

Fentanyl, like other opioids, may have more severe adverse effects in patients with chronic obstructive or other pulmonary disease. In such patients, they may decrease respiratory drive and increase airway resistance.

Drug dependence

Tolerance and physical and psychological dependence may develop upon repeated administration of opioids such as fentanyl. Iatrogenic addiction following opioid administration is rare.

Increased intracranial pressure

Durogesic DTrans should be used with caution in patients who may be particularly susceptible to the intracranial effects of CO_2 retention such as those with evidence of increased intracranial pressure, impaired consciousness or coma. Durogesic DTrans should be used with caution in patients with brain tumours.

Cardiac disease

Fentanyl may produce bradycardia and Durogesic DTrans should therefore be administered with caution to patients with bradyarrhythmias.

Hepatic disease

Because fentanyl is metabolised to inactive metabolites in the liver, hepatic disease might delay its elimination. In patients with hepatic cirrhosis, the pharmacokinetics of a single application of Durogesic DTrans were not altered although serum concentrations tended to be higher in these patients. Patients with hepatic impairment should be observed carefully for signs of fentanyl toxicity and the dose of Durogesic DTrans reduced if necessary.

Renal disease

Less than 10% of fentanyl is excreted unchanged by the kidney and, unlike morphine, there are no known active metabolites eliminated by the kidney. Data obtained with intravenous fentanyl in patients with renal failure suggest that the volume of distribution of fentanyl may be changed by dialysis. This may affect serum concentrations. If patients with renal impairment receive Durogesic DTrans, they should be observed carefully for signs of fentanyl toxicity and the dose reduced if necessary.

Patients with fever/external heat

Patients who develop fever should be monitored for opioid side effects since significant increases in body temperature can potentially increase fentanyl delivery rate.

Patients should also be advised to avoid exposing the Durogesic DTrans application site to direct external heat sources such as heating pads, hot water bottles, electric blankets, heat lamps, saunas or hot whirlpool spa baths while wearing the patch, since there is potential for temperature dependent increases in release of fentanyl from the patch.

Patch disposal

Used patches may contain significant residues of active substance. After removal, therefore, used patches should be folded firmly in half, adhesive side inwards, so that the adhesive membrane is not exposed, and then discarded safely and out of the reach of children according to the instructions in the pack.

4.5 Interaction with other medicinal products and other forms of Interaction

The concomitant use of other CNS depressants, including opioids, anxiolytics, hypnotics, general anaesthetics, antipsychotics, skeletal muscle relaxants, sedating antihistamines and alcoholic beverages may produce additive depressant effects; hypoventilation, hypotension and profound sedation or coma may occur. Therefore, the use of any of the above mentioned concomitant drugs requires special care and observation.

Fentanyl, a high clearance drug, is rapidly and extensively metabolised mainly by CYP3A4.

Itraconazole (a potent CYP3A4 inhibitor) at 200 mg/day given orally for four days had no significant effect on the pharmacokinetics of IV fentanyl. Oral ritonavir (one of the most potent CYP3A4 inhibitors) reduced the clearance of IV fentanyl by two thirds.

The concomitant use of potent CYP3A4 inhibitors such as ritonavir with transdermal fentanyl may result in an increase in fentanyl plasma concentrations, which could increase or prolong both the therapeutic and adverse effects, and may cause serious respiratory depression. In this situation, special patient care and observation are appropriate. The concomitant use of ritonavir and transdermal fentanyl is not recommended, unless the patient is closely monitored.

4.6 Pregnancy and lactation

The safety of fentanyl in pregnancy has not been established. Durogesic DTrans should not be used in women of child-bearing potential without adequate contraception unless in the judgement of the doctor the potential benefits outweigh the possible hazards.

Fentanyl is excreted into breast milk hence Durogesic DTrans should not be used by women who are breast feeding.

4.7 Effects on ability to drive and use machines

Durogesic DTrans may impair the mental or physical ability required to perform potentially hazardous tasks such as driving or operating machinery.

4.8 Undesirable effects

The most serious adverse reaction, as with all potent opioids, is hypoventilation. Other opioid-related adverse reactions include: nausea; vomiting; constipation; hypotension; bradycardia; somnolence; headache; confusion; hallucinations; euphoria; pruritus; sweating and urinary retention.

Skin reactions such as rash, erythema and itching have occasionally been reported. These reactions usually resolve within 24 hours of removal of the patch.

Opioid withdrawal symptoms (such as nausea, vomiting, diarrhoea, anxiety and shivering) are possible in some patients after conversion from their previous analgesic to Durogesic DTrans.

4.9 Overdose

Symptoms

The symptoms of fentanyl overdosage are an extension of its pharmacological actions, the most serious effect being respiratory depression.

Treatment

For management of respiratory depression, immediate countermeasures include removing Durogesic DTrans and physically or verbally stimulating the patient. These actions can be followed by administration of a specific opioid antagonist such as naloxone. The interval between IV antagonist doses should be carefully chosen and repeated administration or a continuous infusion of naloxone may be necessary because of continued absorption of fentanyl from the skin after patch removal, which may result in prolonged respiratory depression. Reversal of the narcotic effect may result in acute onset of pain and release of catecholamines.

A patent airway should be established and maintained. An oropharyngeal airway or endotracheal tube and oxygen should be administered and respiration assisted or controlled, as appropriate. Adequate body temperature and fluid intake should be maintained.

If severe or persistent hypotension occurs, hypovolaemia should be considered, and the condition should be managed with appropriate parenteral fluid therapy.

5. PHARMACOLOGICAL PROPERTIES

5.1 Pharmacodynamic properties

Fentanyl is an opioid analgesic with a high affinity for the μ-opioid receptor.

5.2 Pharmacokinetic properties

Durogesic DTrans provides continuous systemic delivery of fentanyl over the 72 hour administration period. After the first Durogesic DTrans application, serum fentanyl concentrations increase gradually, generally levelling off between 12 and 24 hours, and remaining relatively constant for the remainder of the 72-hour application period. The serum fentanyl concentrations attained are proportional to the Durogesic DTrans patch size. For all practical purposes by the second 72-hour application, a steady state serum concentration is reached and is maintained during subsequent applications of a patch of the same size.

After Durogesic DTrans is removed, serum fentanyl concentrations decline gradually, falling approximately 50% in 17 (range 13-22) hours. Continued absorption of fentanyl from the skin accounts for a slower disappearance of the drug from the serum than is seen after an IV infusion. Fentanyl is metabolised primarily in the liver. Around 75% of fentanyl is excreted into the urine, mostly as metabolites, with less than 10% as unchanged drug. About 9% of the dose is recovered in the faeces, primarily as metabolites. The major metabolite, norfentanyl, is inactive. Mean values for unbound fractions of fentanyl in plasma are estimated to be between 13 and 21%.

5.3 Preclinical safety data

No relevant information other than that contained elsewhere in the Summary of Product Characteristics.

6. PHARMACEUTICAL PARTICULARS

6.1 List of excipients

Polyacrylate adhesive

Polyethylene terephthalate/ethyl vinyl acetate film

Red/Green/Blue/Grey printing ink

Siliconised polyester film

6.2 Incompatibilities

To prevent interference with the adhesive properties of Durogesic DTrans, no creams, oils, lotions or powder should be applied to the skin area when the Durogesic DTrans transdermal patch is applied.

6.3 Shelf life
2 years.

6.4 Special precautions for storage
This medicinal product does not require any special storage precautions.

6.5 Nature and contents of container
Each patch is packed in a heat-sealed pouch made acrylonitrate film, polyethylene terephthalate (PET), low density polyethylene/aluminium foil and adhesive (Adcote 548)

Pouches are packed into cardboard cartons (five pouches per carton).

6.6 Instructions for use and handling
Please refer to section 4.2 for instructions on how to apply the patch.

After removal, the used patch should be folded in half, adhesive side inwards so that the adhesive is not exposed, placed in the original sachet and then discarded safely out of reach of children.

Wash hands after applying or removing the patch.

Administrative Data

7. MARKETING AUTHORISATION HOLDER
Janssen-Cilag Limited
Saunderton
High Wycombe
Buckinghamshire
HP14 4HJ
UK

8. MARKETING AUTHORISATION NUMBER(S)
PL 0242/0192-5

9. DATE OF FIRST AUTHORISATION/RENEWAL OF THE AUTHORISATION
10 December 1999

10. DATE OF REVISION OF THE TEXT
February 2005

Legal category POM/CD2

Dynastat 40 mg Injection

(Pharmacia Limited)

1. NAME OF THE MEDICINAL PRODUCT
Dynastat▼ 40 mg powder for solution for injection

Dynastat▼ 40 mg powder and solvent for solution for injection

2. QUALITATIVE AND QUANTITATIVE COMPOSITION
40 mg vial: Each vial contains 40 mg parecoxib (present as 42.36 mg parecoxib sodium) for reconstitution. After reconstitution, the final concentration of parecoxib is 20 mg/ml.

For excipients, see section 6.1.

3. PHARMACEUTICAL FORM
Powder for solution for injection

Powder and solvent for solution for injection

White to off-white powder

Solvent: clear, colourless solution

4. CLINICAL PARTICULARS

4.1 Therapeutic indications
For the short-term treatment of postoperative pain.

The decision to prescribe a selective COX-2 inhibitor should be based on an assessment of the individual patient's overall risks (see sections 4.3, 4.4).

4.2 Posology and method of administration
The recommended dose is 40 mg administered intravenously (IV) or intramuscularly (IM), followed every 6 to 12 hours by 20 mg or 40 mg as required, not to exceed 80 mg/day. The IV bolus injection may be given rapidly and directly into a vein or into an existing IV line. The IM injection should be given slowly and deeply into the muscle (see section 6.6 for instructions for reconstitution).

Elderly: No dosage adjustment is generally necessary in elderly patients (⩾ 65 years). However, for elderly patients weighing less than 50 kg, initiate treatment with half the usual recommended dose of Dynastat and reduce the maximum daily dose to 40 mg (see section 5.2).

Hepatic Impairment: No dosage adjustment is generally necessary in patients with mild hepatic impairment (Child-Pugh score 5-6). Introduce Dynastat with caution and at half the usual recommended dose in patients with moderate hepatic impairment (Child-Pugh score 7-9) and reduce the maximum daily dose to 40 mg. There is no clinical experience in patients with severe hepatic impairment (Child-Pugh score ⩾10), therefore its use is contraindicated in these patients (see sections 4.3 and 5.2).

Renal Impairment: On the basis of pharmacokinetics, no dosage adjustment is necessary in patients with mild to moderate (creatinine clearance of 30-80 ml/min.) or severe (creatinine clearance < 30 ml/min.) renal impairment. However, caution should be observed in patients with renal impairment or patients who may be predisposed to fluid retention (see sections 4.4 and 5.2).

Children and adolescents: Dynastat has not been studied in patients under 18 years. Therefore, its use is not recommended in these patients.

4.3 Contraindications
History of hypersensitivity to the active substance or to any of the excipients (see section 6.1).

Known hypersensitivity to sulphonamides (see sections 4.4 & 4.8).

Active peptic ulceration or gastrointestinal (GI) bleeding.

Patients who have experienced bronchospasm, acute rhinitis, nasal polyps, angioneurotic oedema, urticaria or other allergic-type reactions after taking acetylsalicylic acid or NSAIDs including COX-2 (cyclooxygenase-2) inhibitors.

The third trimester of pregnancy and breast-feeding (see sections 4.6 and 5.3).

Severe hepatic dysfunction (serum albumin <25 g/l or Child-Pugh score ⩾ 10).

Inflammatory bowel disease.

Congestive heart failure (NYHA II-IV).

Treatment of post-operative pain following coronary artery bypass graft (CABG) surgery (see section 4.8 and 5.1).

Established ischaemic heart disease and/or cerebrovascular disease

4.4 Special warnings and special precautions for use
There is limited clinical experience with Dynastat treatment beyond three days.

Because of the possibility for increased adverse reactions at higher doses parecoxib, other COX-2 inhibitors and NSAIDs, patients treated with parecoxib should be reviewed following dose increase and, in the absence of an increase in efficacy, other therapeutic options should be considered (see section 4.2).

Patients with significant risk factors for cardiovascular events (e.g. hypertension, hyperlipidaemia, diabetes mellitus, smoking), or peripheral arterial disease should only be treated with parecoxib sodium after careful consideration (see 5.1).

Appropriate measures should be taken and discontinuation of parecoxib therapy should be considered if there is clinical evidence of deterioration in the condition of specific clinical symptoms in these patients (see section 5.1). Dynastat has not been studied in cardiovascular revascularization procedures other than coronary artery bypass graft procedures. Studies in other surgeries than CABG procedures included patients with ASA (American Society of Anaesthesiology) Physical Status Class I-III only.

COX-2 inhibitors are not a substitute for acetylsalicylic acid for prophylaxis of cardiovascular thrombo-embolic diseases because of their lack of antiplatelet effects. Therefore, antiplatelet therapies should not be discontinued (see section 5.1).

Upper gastrointestinal complications [perforations, ulcers or bleedings (PUBs)], some of them resulting in fatal outcome, have occurred in patients treated with parecoxib. Caution is advised in the treatment of patients most at risk of developing a gastrointestinal complication with NSAIDs; the elderly, patients using any other NSAID or acetylsalicylic acid concomitantly or patients with a prior history of gastrointestinal disease, such as ulceration and GI bleeding. There is further increase in the risk of gastrointestinal adverse effects (gastrointestinal ulceration or other gastrointestinal complications), when parecoxib sodium istaken concomitantly with acetylsalicylic acid (even at low doses).

Dynastat has been studied in dental, orthopaedic, gynaecologic (principally hysterectomy) and coronary artery bypass graft surgery. There is little experience in other types of surgery, for example gastrointestinal or urological surgery.

Serious skin reactions, some of them fatal, including erythema multiforme, exfoliative dermatitis, Stevens-Johnson syndrome, and toxic epidermal necrolysis, have been reported through post marketing surveillance in patients receiving valdecoxib. These serious cutaneous reactions cannot be ruled out for parecoxib (the prodrug of valdecoxib) (see section 4.8). Patients appear to be at highest risk for these events early in the course of therapy; the onset of the event occurring in the majority of cases within the first 2 weeks of treatment.

Parecoxib should be discontinued at the first appearance of skin rash, mucosal lesions, or any other sign of hypersensitivity. The reported rate of serious skin events appears to be greater for valdecoxib as compared to other COX-2 selective inhibitors. Patients with a history of sulphonamide allergy may be at greater risk of skin reactions (see section 4.3). Patients without a history of sulphonamide allergy may also be at risk for serious skin reactions.

Hypersensitivity reactions (anaphylaxis and angioedema) have been reported in post-marketing experience with valdecoxib, and cannot be ruled out for parecoxib (see section 4.8). Some of these reactions have occurred in patients with a history of allergic-type reactions to sulphonamides (see section 4.3). Parecoxib should be discontinued at the first sign of hypersensitivity.

Acute renal failure has been reported through post-marketing surveillance in patients receiving parecoxib (see section 4.8). Since prostaglandin synthesis inhibition may result in deterioration of renal function and fluid retention, caution should be observed when administering Dynastat in patients with impaired renal function (see section 4.2) or hypertension, or in patients with compromised cardiac or hepatic function or other conditions predisposing to fluid retention.

Caution should be used when initiating treatment with Dynastat in patients with dehydration. In this case, it is advisable to rehydrate patients first and then start therapy with Dynastat.

Dynastat should be used with caution in patients with moderate hepatic dysfunction (Child-Pugh score 7-9) (see section 4.2).

If during treatment, patients deteriorate with repect to any of the events described above, appropriate measures should be taken and discontinuation of parecoxib sodium therapy should be considered.

Dynastat may mask fever and other signs of inflammation (see section 5.1). In isolated cases, an aggravation of soft tissue infections has been described in connection with the use of NSAIDs and in nonclinical studies with Dynastat (see section 5.3). Caution should be exercised with respect to monitoring the incision for signs of infection in surgical patients receiving Dynastat.

Caution should be exercised when co-administering Dynastat with warfarin and other oral anticoagulants (see section 4.5).

The use of Dynastat, as with any medicinal product known to inhibit cyclooxygenase/prostaglandin synthesis, is not recommended in women attempting to conceive. (see sections 4.6 and 5.1)

4.5 Interaction with other medicinal products and other forms of Interaction

Pharmacodynamic interactions

Anticoagulant therapy should be monitored, particularly during the first few days after initiating Dynastat therapy in patients receiving warfarin or other anticoagulants, since these patients have an increased risk of bleeding complications. Therefore, patients receiving oral anticoagulants should be closely monitored for their prothrombin time INR, particularly in the first few days when therapy with parecoxib is initiated or the dose of parecoxib is changed (see section 4.4).

Dynastat had no effect on acetylsalicylic acid-mediated inhibition of platelet aggregation or bleeding times. Clinical trials indicate that Dynastat can be given with low dose acetylsalicylic acid (⩽ 325 mg). In the submitted studies, as with other NSAIDs, an increased risk of gastrointestinal ulceration or other gastrointestinal complications compared to use of parecoxib alone was shown for concomitant administration of low-dose acetylsalicylic acid (see section 5.1).

Co-administration of parecoxib sodium and heparin did not affect the pharmacodynamics of heparin (activated partial thromboplastin time) compared to heparin alone.

NSAIDs may reduce the effect of diuretics and antihypertensive medicinal products. As for NSAIDs, the risk of acute renal insufficiency may be increased when ACE inhibitors or diuretics are co-administered with parecoxib sodium.

Co-administration of NSAIDs and cyclosporin or tacrolimus has been suggested to increase the nephrotoxic effect of cyclosporin and tacrolimus. Renal function should be monitored when parecoxib sodium and any of these medicinal products are co-administered.

Dynastat may be co-administered with opioid analgesics. When Dynastat was co-administered with morphine, a smaller dose (by 28-36%) of morphine could be used to achieve the same clinical level of analgesia.

Effects of other medicinal products on the pharmacokinetics of parecoxib (or its active metabolite valdecoxib)

Parecoxib is rapidly hydrolysed to the active metabolite valdecoxib. In humans, studies demonstrated that valdecoxib metabolism is predominantly mediated via CYP3A4 and 2C9 isozymes.

Plasma exposure (AUC and C_{max}) to valdecoxib was increased (62% and 19%, respectively) when co-administered with fluconazole (predominantly a CYP2C9 inhibitor), indicating that the dose of parecoxib sodium should be reduced in those patients who are receiving fluconazole therapy.

Plasma exposure (AUC and C_{max}) to valdecoxib was increased (38% and 24%, respectively) when co-administered with ketoconazole (CYP3A4 inhibitor), however, a dosage adjustment should not generally be necessary for patients receiving ketoconazole.

The effect of enzyme induction has not been studied. The metabolism of valdecoxib may increase when co-administered with enzyme inducers such as rifampicin, phenytoin, carbamazepine or dexamethasone.

Effect of parecoxib (or its active metabolite valdecoxib) on the pharmacokinetics of other medicinal products

Treatment with valdecoxib (40 mg twice daily for 7 days) produced a 3-fold increase in plasma concentrations of dextromethorphan (CYP2D6 substrate). Therefore, caution should be observed when co-administering Dynastat and medicinal products that are predominantly metabolised by

CYP2D6 and which have narrow therapeutic margins (e.g. flecainide, propafenone, metoprolol).

Plasma exposure of omeprazole (CYP 2C19 substrate) 40 mg once daily was increased by 46% following administration of valdecoxib 40 mg twice daily for 7 days, while the plasma exposure to valdecoxib was unaffected. These results indicate that although valdecoxib is not metabolised by CYP2C19, it may be an inhibitor of this isoenzyme. Therefore, caution should be observed when administering Dynastat with medicinal products known to be substrates of CYP2C19 (e.g. phenytoin, diazepam, or imipramine).

In interaction studies in rheumatoid arthritis patients receiving weekly methotrexate intramuscularly, orally administered valdecoxib (40 mg twice daily) did not have a clinically significant effect on the plasma concentrations of methotrexate. However, adequate monitoring of methotrexate-related toxicity should be considered when co-administering these two medicinal products.

Co-administration of valdecoxib and lithium produced significant decreases in lithium serum clearance (25%) and renal clearance (30%) with a 34% higher serum exposure compared to lithium alone. Lithium serum concentration should be monitored closely when initiating or changing parecoxib sodium therapy in patients receiving lithium.

Co-administration of valdecoxib with glibenclamide (CYP3A4 substrate) did not affect either the pharmacokinetics (exposure) or the pharmacodynamics (blood glucose and insulin levels) of glibenclamide.

Injectable anaesthetics: Coadministration of IV parecoxib sodium 40 mg with propofol (CYP2C9 substrate) or midazolam (CYP3A4 substrate) did not affect either the pharmacokinetics (metabolism and exposure) or the pharmacodynamics (EEG effects, psychomotor tests and waking from sedation) of IV propofol or IV midazolam. Additionally, coadministration of valdecoxib had no clinically significant effect on the hepatic or intestinal CYP 3A4-mediated metabolism of orally administered midazolam. Administration of IV parecoxib sodium 40 mg had no significant effect on the pharmacokinetics of either IV fentanyl or IV alfentanil (CYP3A4 substrates).

Inhalation anaesthetics: No formal interaction studies have been done. In surgery studies in which parecoxib sodium was administered pre-operatively, no evidence of pharmacodynamic interaction was observed in patients receiving parecoxib sodium and the inhalation anaesthetic agents nitrous oxide and isoflurane. (see section 5.1)

4.6 Pregnancy and lactation

Pregnancy:

The use of Dynastat is contraindicated in the last trimester of pregnancy because as with other medicinal products known to inhibit prostaglandin synthesis, it may cause premature closure of the ductus arteriosus or uterine inertia. (see sections 4.3, 5.1 and 5.3)

Like other medicinal products that inhibit COX-2, Dynastat is not recommended in women attempting to conceive. (see sections 4.4, 5.1 and 5.3)

There are no adequate data from the use of parecoxib sodium in pregnant women or during labour. Studies in animals have shown reproductive effects (see sections 5.1 and 5.3). The potential risk for humans is unknown. Dynastat should not be used during the first two trimesters of pregnancy or labour unless the potential benefit to the patient outweighs the potential risk to the foetus.

Lactation:

Parecoxib, valdecoxib (its active metabolite) and a valdecoxib active metabolite are excreted in the milk of rats. It is not known whether valdecoxib is excreted in human milk. Dynastat should not be administered to women who breast-feed. (see sections 4.3 and 5.3)

4.7 Effects on ability to drive and use machines

No studies on the effect of Dynastat on the ability to drive or use machines have been performed. However, patients who experience dizziness, vertigo or somnolence after receiving Dynastat should refrain from driving or operating machines.

4.8 Undesirable effects

Of the Dynastat treated patients in controlled trials, 1962 were patients with post-surgical pain.

The following undesirable effects had a rate greater than placebo and have been reported among 1543 patients administered Dynastat 20 or 40 mg as a single or multiple dose (up to 80 mg/day) in 12 placebo controlled studies, including dental, gynaecologic, orthopaedic surgery or coronary artery bypass graft surgery as well as pre-operative administration in dental and orthopaedic surgeries. The discontinuation rate due to adverse events in these studies was 5.0 % for patients receiving Dynastat and 4.3% for patients receiving placebo.

[Very Common >1/10), Common (≥1/100, <1/10) Uncommon (≥1/1000, <1/100) Rare (≥1/10,000, <1/1000) Very rare (<1/10,000 including isolated cases)]

<u>Infections and infestations</u>

Uncommon: abnormal sternal serous wound drainage, wound infection.

<u>Blood and lymphatic system disorders</u>

Common: post-operative anaemia

Uncommon: thrombocytopenia

<u>Metabolism and nutrition disorders</u>

Common: hypokalaemia

<u>Pyschiatric disorders:</u>

Common: agitation, insomnia

<u>Nervous system disorders</u>

Common: hypoaesthesia

Uncommon: cerebrovascular disorder

<u>Cardiac disorders</u>

Uncommon: bradycardia

<u>Vascular disorders</u>

Common: hypertension, hypotension

Uncommon: aggravated hypertension

<u>Respiratory, thoracic and mediastinal disorders</u>

Common: pharyngitis, respiratory insufficiency

<u>Gastrointestinal disorders</u>

Common: alveolar osteitis (dry socket), dyspepsia, flatulence

Uncommon: gastroduodenal ulceration

<u>Skin and subcutaneous tissue disorders</u>

Common: pruritus

Uncommon: ecchymosis

<u>Musculoskeletal and connective tissue disorders</u>

Common: back pain

<u>Renal and urinary disorders</u>

Common: oliguria

<u>General disorders and administration site conditions</u>

Common: peripheral oedema

<u>Investigations</u>

Common: blood creatinine increased

Uncommon: SGOT increased, SGPT increased, blood urea nitrogen increased

The following rare, serious adverse events have been reported in association with the use of NSAIDs and cannot be ruled out for Dynastat: bronchospasm, hepatitis.

Following coronary artery bypass graft surgery, patients administered Dynastat have a higher risk of adverse events, such as cardiovascular/ thromboembolic events, deep surgical infections and sternal wound healing complications. Cardiovascular/thromboembolic events include myocardial infarction, stroke/TIA, pulmonary embolus and deep vein thrombosis (see section 4.3 and 5.1).

In post-marketing experience, the following rare, serious adverse events have been reported in association with the use of parecoxib: acute renal failure, congestive heart failure, erythema multiforme and hypersensitivity reactions including anaphylaxis and angioedema (see section 4.4).

In post marketing experience, the following reactions have been reported in association with the use of valdecoxib, and cannot be ruled out for parecoxib: myocardial infarction (very rare), exfoliative dermatitis, Stevens-Johnson syndrome and toxic epidermal necrolysis (see section 4.4).

4.9 Overdose

No case of parecoxib overdose has been reported.

In case of overdose, patients should be managed by symptomatic and supportive care. Valdecoxib is not removed by haemodialysis. Diuresis or alkalisation of urine may not be useful due to high protein binding of valdecoxib.

5. PHARMACOLOGICAL PROPERTIES

5.1 Pharmacodynamic properties

Pharmacotherapeutic group: Coxib, ATC code: M01AH04

Parecoxib is a prodrug of valdecoxib. Valdecoxib is a selective cyclooxygenase-2 (COX-2) inhibitor within the clinical dose range. Cyclooxygenase is responsible for generation of prostaglandins. Two isoforms, COX-1 and COX-2, have been identified. COX-2 is the isoform of the enzyme that has been shown to be induced by pro-inflammatory stimuli and has been postulated to be primarily responsible for the synthesis of prostanoid mediators of pain, inflammation, and fever. COX-2 is also involved in ovulation, implantation and closure of the ductus arteriosus, regulation of renal function, and central nervous system functions (fever induction, pain perception and cognitive function). It may also play a role in ulcer healing. COX-2 has been identified in tissue around gastric ulcers in man but its relevance to ulcer healing has not been established.

The difference in antiplatelet activity between some COX-1 inhibiting NSAIDs and COX-2 selective inhibitors may be of clinical significance in patients at risk of thrombo-embolic reactions. COX-2 selective inhibitors reduce the formation of systemic (and therefore possibly endothelial) prostacyclin without affecting platelet thromboxane. The clinical relevance of these observations has not been established.

The efficacy of Dynastat was established in studies of dental, gynaecologic (hysterectomy), orthopaedic (knee and hip replacement), and coronary artery bypass graft surgical pain. The first perceptible analgesic effect occurred in 7 -13 minutes, with clinically meaningful analgesia demonstrated in 23-39 minutes and a peak effect within 2 hours following administration of single doses of 40 mg IV or IM Dynastat. The magnitude of analgesic effect of the 40 mg dose was comparable with that of ketorolac 60 mg IM or ketorolac 30 mg IV. After a single dose, the duration of analgesia was dose and clinical pain model dependent, and ranged from 6 to greater than 12 hours.

Gastrointestinal studies: In short-term studies (7 days), the incidence of endoscopically observed gastroduodenal ulcers or erosions in healthy young and elderly (≥ 65 years) subjects administered Dynastat (5-21%), although higher than placebo (5-12%), was statistically significantly lower than the incidence observed with NSAIDs (66-90%).

CABG post-operative Safety Studies: In addition to routine adverse event reporting, pre-specified event categories, adjudicated by an independent expert committee, were examined in two placebo-controlled safety studies in which patients received parecoxib sodium for at least 3 days and then were transitioned to oral valdecoxib for a total duration of 10-14 days. All patients received standard of care analgesia during treatment.

Patients received low-dose acetylsalicylic acid prior to randomization and throughout the two CABG surgery studies.

The first CABG surgery study evaluated patients treated with IV parecoxib sodium 40 mg bid for a minimum of 3 days, followed by treatment with valdecoxib 40 mg bid (parecoxib sodium/valdecoxib group) (n=311) or placebo/placebo (n=151) in a 14-day, double-blind placebo-controlled study. Nine pre-specified adverse event categories were evaluated (cardiovascular thromboembolic events, pericarditis, new onset or exacerbation of congestive heart failure, renal failure/dysfunction, upper GI ulcer complications, major non-GI bleeds, infections, non-infectious pulmonary complications, and death). There was a significantly ($p < 0.05$) greater incidence of cardiovascular/thromboembolic events (myocardial infarction, ischemia, cerebrovascular accident, deep vein thrombosis and pulmonary embolism) detected in the parecoxib/valdecoxib treatment group compared to the placebo/placebo treatment group for the IV dosing period (2.2% and 0.0% respectively) and over the entire study period (4.8% and 1.3% respectively). Surgical wound complications (most involving the sternal wound) were observed at an increased rate with parecoxib/valdecoxib treatment.

In the second CABG surgery study, four pre-specified event categories were evaluated (cardiovascular/thromboembolic; renal dysfunction/renal failure; upper GI ulcer/bleeding; surgical wound complication). Patients were randomized within 24-hours post-CABG surgery to: parecoxib initial dose of 40 mg IV, then 20 mg IV Q12H for a minimum of 3 days followed by valdecoxib PO (20 mg Q12H) (n=544) for the remainder of a 10 day treatment period; placebo IV followed by valdecoxib PO (n=544); or placebo IV followed by placebo PO (n=548). A significantly ($p=0.033$) greater incidence of events in the cardiovascular/thromboembolic category was detected in the parecoxib /valdecoxib treatment group (2.0%) compared to the placebo/placebo treatment group (0.5%). Placebo/valdecoxib treatment was also associated with a higher incidence of CV thromboembolic events versus placebo treatment, but this difference did not reach statistical significance. Three of the six cardiovascular thromboembolic events in the placebo/valdecoxib treatment group occurred during the placebo treatment period; these patients did not receive valdecoxib. Pre-specified events that occurred with the highest incidence in all three treatment groups involved the category of surgical wound complications, including deep surgical infections and sternal wound healing events.

There were no significant differences between active treatments and placebo for any of the other pre-specified event categories (renal dysfunction/failure, upper GI ulcer complications or surgical wound complications).

General Surgery: In a large (N=1050) major orthopedic/general surgery trial, patients received an initial dose of parecoxib 40 mg IV, then 20 mg IV Q12H for a minimum of 3 days followed by valdecoxib PO (20 mg Q12H) (n=525) for the remainder of a 10 day treatment period, or placebo IV followed by placebo PO (n=525). There were no significant differences in the overall safety profile, including the four pre-specified event categories described above for the second CABG surgery study, for parecoxib sodium/valdecoxib compared to placebo treatment in these post-surgical patients.

Platelet studies: In a series of small, multiple dose studies in healthy young and elderly subjects, Dynastat 20 mg or 40 mg twice daily had no effect on platelet aggregation or bleeding compared to placebo. In young subjects, Dynastat 40 mg twice daily had no clinically significant effect on acetylsalicylic acid -mediated inhibition of platelet function. (see section 4.5)

5.2 Pharmacokinetic properties

Following IV or IM injection, parecoxib is rapidly converted to valdecoxib, the pharmacologically active substance, by enzymatic hydrolysis in the liver.

Absorption

Exposure of valdecoxib following single doses of Dynastat, as measured by both the area under the plasma concentration vs. time curve (AUC) and peak concentration (C_{max}), is approximately linear in the range of clinical doses. AUC and C_{max} following twice daily administration is linear up to 50 mg IV and 20 mg IM. Steady state plasma concentrations of valdecoxib were reached within 4 days with twice daily dosing.

Following single IV and IM doses of parecoxib sodium 20 mg, C_{max} of valdecoxib is achieved in approximately 30 minutes and approximately 1 hour, respectively. Exposure to valdecoxib was similar in terms of AUC and C_{max} following IV and IM administration. Exposure to parecoxib was similar after IV or IM administration in terms of AUC. Average C_{max} of parecoxib after IM dosing was lower compared to bolus IV dosing, which is attributed to slower extravascular absorption after IM administration. These decreases were not considered clinically important since C_{max} of valdecoxib is comparable after IM and IV parecoxib sodium administration.

Distribution

The volume of distribution of valdecoxib after its IV administration is approximately 55 litres. Plasma protein binding is approximately 98% over the concentration range achieved with the highest recommended dose, 80 mg/ day. Valdecoxib, but not parecoxib, is extensively partitioned into erythrocytes.

Metabolism

Parecoxib is rapidly and almost completely converted to valdecoxib and propionic acid in vivo with a plasma half-life of approximately 22 minutes. Elimination of valdecoxib is by extensive hepatic metabolism involving multiple pathways, including cytochrome P 450 (CYP) 3A4 and CYP2C9 isoenzymes and glucuronidation (about 20%) of the sulphonamide moiety. A hydroxylated metabolite of valdecoxib (via the CYP pathway) has been identified in human plasma that is active as a COX-2 inhibitor. It represents approximately 10% of the concentration of valdecoxib; because of this metabolite's low concentration, it is not expected to contribute a significant clinical effect after administration of therapeutic doses of parecoxib sodium.

Elimination

Valdecoxib is eliminated via hepatic metabolism with less than 5% unchanged valdecoxib recovered in the urine. No unchanged parecoxib is detected in urine and only trace amounts in the faeces. About 70% of the dose is excreted in the urine as inactive metabolites. Plasma clearance (CL) for valdecoxib is about 6 l/hr. After IV or IM dosing of parecoxib sodium, the elimination half-life ($t_{1/2}$) of valdecoxib is about 8 hours.

Elderly Subjects: Dynastat has been administered to 335 elderly patients (65-96 years of age) in pharmacokinetic and therapeutic trials. In healthy elderly subjects, the apparent oral clearance of valdecoxib was reduced, resulting in an approximately 40% higher plasma exposure of valdecoxib compared to healthy young subjects. When adjusted for body weight, steady state plasma exposure of valdecoxib was 16% higher in elderly females compared to elderly males. (see section 4.2)

Renal Impairment: In patients with varying degrees of renal impairment administered 20 mg IVDynastat, parecoxib was rapidly cleared from plasma. Because renal elimination of valdecoxib is not important to its disposition, no changes in valdecoxib clearance were found even in patients with severe renal impairment or in patients undergoing dialysis. (see section 4.2)

Hepatic Impairment: Moderate hepatic impairment did not result in a reduced rate or extent of parecoxib conversion to valdecoxib. In patients with moderate hepatic impairment (Child-Pugh score 7-9), treatment should be initiated with half the usual recommended dose of Dynastat and the maximum daily dose should be reduced to 40 mg since valdecoxib exposures were more than doubled (130%) in these patients. Patients with severe hepatic impairment have not been studied and therefore the use of Dynastat in patients with severe hepatic impairment is not recommended. (see sections 4.2 and 4.3)

5.3 Preclinical safety data

Preclinical data reveal no special hazard for humans based on conventional studies of safety pharmacology or repeated dose toxicity at 2-fold the maximum human exposure to parecoxib. However, in the repeated dose toxicity studies in dogs and rats, the systemic exposures to valdecoxib (the active metabolite of parecoxib) were approximately 0.8-fold the systemic exposure in elderly human subjects at the maximum recommended therapeutic dose of 80 mg daily. Higher doses were associated with aggravation and delayed healing of skin infections, an effect probably associated with COX-2 inhibition.

In reproduction toxicity tests, the incidence of post-implantation losses, resorptions and foetal body weight retardation occurred at doses not producing maternal toxicity in the rabbit studies. No effects of parecoxib on male or female fertilities were found in rats.

The effects of parecoxib have not been evaluated in late pregnancy or in the pre- and postnatal period. Parecoxib sodium administered intravenously to lactating rats as a single dose showed concentrations of parecoxib, valdecoxib and a valdecoxib active metabolite in milk similar to that of maternal plasma.

The carcinogenic potential of parecoxib sodium has not been evaluated.

6. PHARMACEUTICAL PARTICULARS

6.1 List of excipients

Powder

Dibasic sodium phosphate, heptahydrate

Phosphoric acid and/or sodium hydroxide (for pH adjustment).

Solvent

Sodium chloride

Hydrochloric acid or sodium hydroxide (for pH adjustment)

Water for injections.

40 mg vial: When reconstituted in sodium chloride 9 mg/ml (0.9%) solution, Dynastat contains approximately 0.44 mEq of sodium per vial.

6.2 Incompatibilities

This medicinal product must **not** be mixed with other medicinal products other than those mentioned in 6.6.

Dynastat and opioids should not be administered together in the same syringe.

Use of Ringer-Lactate solution for injection or glucose 50 g/l (5%) in Ringer Lactate solution for injection for reconstitution will cause the parecoxib to precipitate from solution and therefore is **not** recommended.

Use of Sterile Water for Injection is **not** recommended, as the resulting solution is not isotonic.

Injection into an IV line delivering glucose 50 g/l (5%) in Ringer-Lactate solution for injection, or other IV fluids not listed in 6.6, is **not** recommended as this may cause precipitation from solution.

6.3 Shelf life

3 years.

Chemical and physical in-use stability of the reconstituted solution has been demonstrated for 24 hours at 25°C. From a microbiological point of view, the aseptically prepared product should be used immediately. If not used immediately, in-use storage times and conditions prior to use are the responsibility of the user and would not normally be longer than 12 hours at 25°C, unless reconstitution has taken place in controlled and validated aseptic conditions.

6.4 Special precautions for storage

No special precautions for storage prior to reconstitution.

Do not refrigerate or freeze reconstituted solutions.

6.5 Nature and contents of container

Parecoxib sodium vials

40 mg vials: Type I colourless glass vials (5 ml) with a laminated stopper, sealed with a purple flip-off cap on the aluminium overseal.

Dynastat is available in packs containing 10 vials.

Solvent ampoules

2 ml ampoule: colourless neutral glass, Type I.

Dynastat is supplied as a sterile, single unit-of-use vial that is packaged with a 2 ml ampoule with a fill volume of 2 ml sodium chloride 9 mg/ml (0.9%) solution (see below for various pack sizes and configurations).

Pack Sizes

1 × 1 pack: contains 1 vial with parecoxib 40 mg and 1 ampoule with 2 ml sodium chloride 9 mg/ml (0.9%) solution.

3 × 3 pack: contains 3 vials with parecoxib 40 mg and 3 ampoule with 2 ml sodium chloride 9 mg/ml (0.9%) solution.

5 × 5 pack: contains 5 vials with parecoxib 40 mg and 5 ampoule with 2 ml sodium chloride 9 mg/ml (0.9%) solution.

Not all pack sizes may be marketed.

6.6 Instructions for use and handling

Reconstitute Dynastat 40 mg with 2 ml sodium chloride 9 mg/ml (0.9%) solution using aseptic technique. The **only** other acceptable solvents for reconstitution are:

glucose 50 g/l (5%) solution for infusion

sodium chloride 4.5 mg/ml (0.45%) and glucose 50 g/l (5%) solution for injection

Use aseptic technique to reconstitute lyophilised parecoxib (as parecoxib sodium).

Remove the purple flip-off cap to expose the central portion of the rubber stopper of the 40 mg parecoxib vial. Withdraw, with a sterile needle and syringe, 2 ml of an acceptable solvent and insert the needle through the central portion of the rubber stopper transferring the solvent into the 40 mg vial. Dissolve the powder completely using a gentle swirling motion and inspect the reconstituted product before use. The entire contents of the vial should be withdrawn for a single administration.

The reconstituted solution is clear and colourless. It should be inspected visually for particulate matter and discoloration prior to administration. The solution should not be used if discoloured or cloudy or if particulate matter is observed.

The reconstituted product is isotonic.

After reconstitution with acceptable solvents, Dynastat may **only** be injected IV or IM, or into IV lines delivering:

sodium chloride 9 mg/ml (0.9%) solution

glucose 50 g/l (5%) solution for infusion

sodium chloride 4.5 mg/ml (0.45%) and glucose 50 g/l (5%) solution for injection

Ringer-Lactate solution for injection

For single use only. Any unused solution, solvent or waste material should be disposed of according to local requirements.

7. MARKETING AUTHORISATION HOLDER

Pharmacia Europe EEIG
Sandwich
Kent CT13 9NJ
United Kingdom

8. MARKETING AUTHORISATION NUMBER(S)

EU/1/02/209/001-008

9. DATE OF FIRST AUTHORISATION/RENEWAL OF THE AUTHORISATION

22nd March 2002

10. DATE OF REVISION OF THE TEXT

17th February 2005

Company Ref: DY 3_0

Dysport

(Ipsen Ltd)

1. NAME OF THE MEDICINAL PRODUCT

Dysport

2. QUALITATIVE AND QUANTITATIVE COMPOSITION

Active Constituent	**Per Vial**
Clostridium botulinum type A toxin-haemagglutinin complex	500U*
Other Constituents	
Albumin solution Lactose	125 MCG 2.5 MG

* One unit (U) is defined as the median lethal intraperitoneal dose in mice.

3. PHARMACEUTICAL FORM

Injection.

4. CLINICAL PARTICULARS

4.1 Therapeutic indications

Dysport is indicated for focal spasticity, including the treatment of:

arm symptoms associated with focal spasticity in conjunction with physiotherapy;

and

dynamic equinus foot deformity due to spasticity in ambulant paediatric cerebral palsy patients, two years of age or older, only in hospital specialist centres with appropriately trained personnel.

Dysport is also indicated for the following treatments:

Spasmodic torticollis in adults

Blepharospasm in adults

Hemifacial spasm in adults

4.2 Posology and method of administration

The units of Dysport are specific to the preparation and are not interchangeable with other preparations of botulinum toxin.

Training: Dysport should only be administered by appropriately trained physicians.

Ipsen can facilitate training in administration of Dysport injections.

The exposed central portion of the rubber stopper should be cleaned with alcohol immediately prior to piercing the septum. A sterile 23 or 25 gauge needle should be used.

Arm spasticity:

Posology

The recommended dose is 1000 units in total, distributed amongst the following five muscles:

(see Table 1 on next page)

The sites of injection should be guided by standard locations used for electromyography, although actual location of the injection site will be determined by palpation. All muscles except the biceps brachii (BB) should be injected at one site, whilst the biceps should be injected at two sites.

The dose should be lowered if there is evidence to suggest that this dose may result in excessive weakness of the target muscles, such as for patients whose target muscles are small, where the BB muscle is not to be injected or patients who are to be administered multi-level injections. Clinical improvement may be expected within two weeks after injection. Data on repeated and long term treatment are limited.

Children: The safety and effectiveness of Dysport in the treatment of arm spasticity in children have not been demonstrated.

Method of administration

The exposed central portion of the rubber stopper should be cleaned with alcohol immediately prior to piercing the septum. A sterile 23 or 25 gauge needle should be used.

Table 1

Biceps brachii (BB)	Flexor digitorum profundus (FDP)	Flexor digitorum superficialis (FDS)	Flexor carpi ulnaris (FCU)	Flexor carpi radialis FCR)	Total Dose
300 - 400 units (0.6 - 0.8 ml)	150 units (0.3 ml)	150 - 250 units (0.3 - 0.5 ml)	150 units (0.3 ml)	150 units (0.3 ml)	1,000 units (2.0 ml)

Dysport is reconstituted with 1.0 ml of sodium chloride injection B.P. (0.9%) to yield a solution containing 500 units per ml of Dysport. Dysport is administered by intramuscular injection into the five muscles detailed above when treating arm spasticity.

***Paediatric cerebral palsy spasticity*:**

Posology

The initial recommended dose is 20 units/kg body weight given as a divided dose between both calf muscles. If only one calf is affected, a dose of 10 units/kg bodyweight should be used. Consideration should be given to lowering this starting dose if there is evidence to suggest that this dose may result in excessive weakness of the target muscles, such as for patients whose target muscles are small or patients who require concomitant injections to other muscle groups. Following evaluation of response to the starting dose subsequent treatment may be titrated within the range 10 units/kg and 30 units/kg divided between both legs. The maximum dose administered must not exceed 1000 units/patient.

Administration should primarily be targeted to the gastrocnemius, although injections of the soleus and injection of the tibialis posterior should also be considered.

The use of electromyography (EMG) is not routine clinical practice but may assist in identifying the most active muscles.

Clinical improvement may be expected within two weeks after injection. Injections may be repeated approximately every 16 weeks or as required to maintain response, but not more frequently than every 12 weeks.

Method of administration

When treating paediatric cerebral palsy spasticity, Dysport is reconstituted with 1.0 ml of sodium chloride injection B.P. (0.9%) to yield a solution containing 500 units per ml of Dysport. Dysport is administered by intramuscular injection into the calf muscles when treating spasticity.

Spasmodic torticollis:

Posology

Adults and elderly: The doses recommended for torticollis are applicable to adults of all ages providing the adults are of normal weight with no evidence of low neck muscle mass. A reduced dose may be appropriate if the patient is markedly underweight or in the elderly, where reduced muscle mass may exist.

The initial recommended dose for the treatment of spasmodic torticollis is 500 units per patient given as a divided dose and administered to the two or three most active neck muscles.

For rotational torticollis distribute the 500 units by administering 350 units into the splenius capitis muscle, ipsilateral to the direction of the chin/head rotation and 150 units into the sternomastoid muscle, contralateral to the rotation.

For laterocollis, distribute the 500 units by administering 350 units into the ipsilateral splenius capitis muscle and 150 units into the ipsilateral sternomastoid muscle. In cases associated with shoulder elevation the ipsilateral trapezoid or levator scapulae muscles may also require treatment, according to visible hypertrophy of the muscle or electromyographic (EMG) findings. Where injections of three muscles are required, distribute the 500 units as follows, 300 units splenius capitis, 100 units sternomastoid and 100 units to the third muscle.

For retrocollis distribute the 500 units by administering 250 units into each of the splenius capitis muscles. This may be followed by bilateral trapezius injections (up to 250 units per muscle) after 6 weeks, if there is insufficient response. Bilateral splenii injections may increase the risk of neck muscle weakness.

All other forms of torticollis are highly dependent on specialist knowledge and EMG to identify and treat the most active muscles. EMG should be used diagnostically for all complex forms of torticollis, for reassessment after unsuccessful injections in non complex cases, and for guiding injections into deep muscles or in overweight patients with poorly palpable neck muscles.

On subsequent administration, the doses may be adjusted according to the clinical response and side effects observed. Doses within the range of 250-1000 units are recommended, although the higher doses may be accompanied by an increase in side effects, particularly dysphagia. Doses above 1000 units are not recommended.

The relief of symptoms of torticollis may be expected within a week after the injection. Injections should be repeated approximately every 12 weeks or as required to prevent recurrence of symptoms.

Children: The safety and effectiveness of Dysport in the treatment of spasmodic torticollis in children have not been demonstrated.

Method of administration

When treating spasmodic torticollis Dysport is reconstituted with 1.0 ml of sodium chloride injection B.P. (0.9%) to yield a solution containing 500 units per ml of Dysport. Dysport is administered by intramuscular injection as above when treating spasmodic torticollis.

Blepharospasm and hemifacial spasm:

Posology

Adults and elderly: In the treatment of bilateral blepharospasm the recommended initial dose is 120 units per eye.

Injection of 0.1 ml (20 units) should be made medially and of 0.2.ml (40 units) should be made laterally into the junction between the preseptal and orbital parts of both the upper and lower orbicularis oculi muscles of each eye.

For injections into the upper lid the needle should be directed away from its centre to avoid the levator muscle. A diagram to aid placement of these injections is provided. The relief of symptoms may be expected to begin within two to four days with maximal effect within two weeks.

Injections should be repeated approximately every 12 weeks or as required to prevent recurrence of symptoms. On such subsequent administrations the dose may need to be reduced to 80 units per eye - viz -: 0.1 ml (20 units) medially and 0.1 ml (20 units) laterally above and below each eye in the manner previously described. The dose may be further reduced to 60 units per eye by omitting the medial lower lid injection.

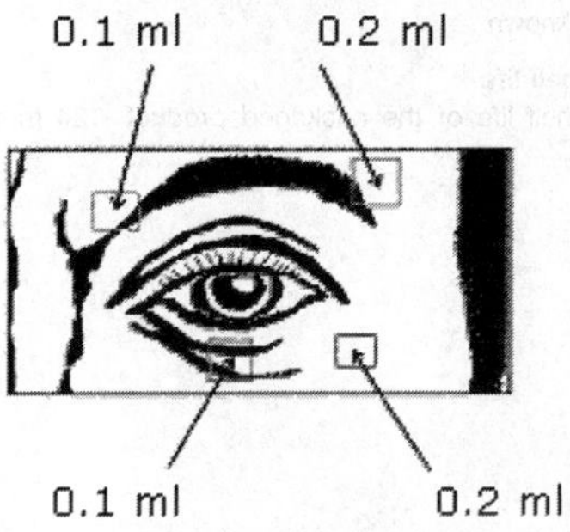

In cases of unilateral blepharospasm the injections should be confined to the affected eye. Patients with hemifacial spasm should be treated as for unilateral blepharospasm. The doses recommended are applicable to adults of all ages including the elderly.

Children: The safety and effectiveness of Dysport in the treatment of blepharospasm and hemifacial spasm in children have not been demonstrated.

Method of administration

When treating blepharospasm and hemifacial spasm Dysport is reconstituted with 2.5 ml of sodium chloride injection BP (0.9%) to yield a solution containing 200 units per ml of Dysport. Dysport is administered by subcutaneous injection medially and laterally into the junction between the preseptal and orbital parts of both the upper and lower orbicularis oculi muscles of the eyes.

4.3 Contraindications

Dysport is contraindicated in individuals with known hypersensitivity to any components of Dysport.

4.4 Special warnings and special precautions for use

Dysport should be administered with caution to patients with existing problems in swallowing or breathing as these problems can worsen if toxin spreads to the relevant muscles. Aspiration has occurred in rare cases, and is a risk when treating patients with spasmodic torticollis who have a chronic respiratory disorder.

Careful consideration should be given before the injection of patients who have experienced a previous allergic reaction to a product containing botulinum toxin type A. The risk of a further allergic reaction must be considered in relation to the benefit of treatment.

Dysport should only be used with caution under close supervision in patients with subclinical or clinical evidence of marked defective neuro-muscular transmission (eg myasthenia gravis). Such patients may have an increased sensitivity to agents such as Dysport which may result in excessive muscle weakness.

There are no reports of any immune response after the local administration of *Clostridium botulinum* type A toxin-haemagglutinin complex in accordance with the doses recommended when treating hemifacial spasm. Antibody formation to botulinum toxin has been noted rarely in patients (approximately 1 in 10, 000 cases) receiving Dysport.

Clinically, neutralizing antibodies have been detected by substantial deterioration in response to therapy or a need for consistently increasing doses.

For the treatment of cerebral palsy in children, Dysport should only be used in children over 2 years of age.

As with any intramuscular injection, Dysport should be used only where strictly necessary in patients with prolonged bleeding times, infection or inflammation at the proposed injection site.

This product contains a small amount of human albumin. The risk of transmission of viral infection cannot be excluded with absolute certainty following the use of human blood or blood products.

4.5 Interaction with other medicinal products and other forms of Interaction

Drugs which affect neuromuscular transmission, such as aminoglycoside antibiotics, should be used with caution.

4.6 Pregnancy and lactation

Teratological and other reproductive studies have not been performed with Dysport. The safety of its use in pregnant or lactating women has not been demonstrated.

Dysport should not be used in pregnant or lactating women, unless clearly necessary.

4.7 Effects on ability to drive and use machines

None known.

4.8 Undesirable effects

Very common >1/10: Common >1/100, <1/10: Uncommon >1/1000, <1/100:

Rare >1/10 000, < 1/1000: Very rare <1/10 000.

General:

A total of approximately 7500 patients were treated with Dysport during a series of clinical trials in patients suffering blepharospasm, hemifacial spasm, torticollis or spasticity associated with cerebral palsy or stroke.

Approximately 2200 patients included in these trials experienced an adverse event.

Nervous system disorders

Rare: Neuralgic amyotrophy

Skin and subcutaneous tissue disorders

Uncommon: Itching

Rare: Skin rashes

General disorders and administration site conditions

Common: Generalised weakness, fatigue, flu-like syndrome, pain / bruising at injection site.

Arm spasticity:

In 5 clinical trials involving 141 patients treated with Dysport the following adverse reactions were reported.

Gastrointestinal disorders

Common: Dysphagia

Musculoskeletal and connective tissue disorders

Common: Arm muscle weakness

Injury, poisoning and procedural complications

Common: Accidental injury/falls

Paediatric cerebral palsy spasticity:

In 14 clinical trials involving approximately 900 patients treated with Dysport, the following adverse reactions were reported:

Gastrointestinal disorders

Common: Diarrhoea, vomiting

Musculoskeletal and connective tissue disorders

Common: Leg muscle weakness

Renal and urinary disorders

Common: Urinary incontinence

General disorders and administration site conditions

Common: Abnormal gait

Injury, poisoning and procedural complications

Common: Accidental injury due to falling

Accidental injury due to falling and abnormal gait may have been due to the over-weakening of the target muscle and / or the local spread of Dysport to other muscles involved in ambulation and balance.

Spasmodic torticollis:

In 21 clinical trials involving approximately 4100 patients the following adverse reactions were reported:

Nervous system disorders

Common: Dysphonia

Uncommon: Headache

Eye disorders

Uncommon: Diplopia, blurred vision

Respiratory, thoracic and mediastinal disorders

Rare: Respiratory disorders

Gastrointestinal disorders

Very common: Dysphagia

Uncommon: Dry mouth

Musculoskeletal and connective tissue disorders

Common: Neck muscle weakness

Dysphagia appeared to be dose related and occurred most frequently following injection into the sternomastoid muscle. A soft diet may be required until symptoms resolve.

These side effects may be expected to resolve within two to four weeks.

Blepharospasm and hemifacial spasm:

In 13 clinical trials involving approximately 1400 patients treated with Dysport, the following adverse reactions were reported:

Nervous system disorders

Common: Facial muscle weakness

Uncommon: Facial nerve paresis

Eye disorders

Very common: Ptosis

Common: Diplopia, dry eyes, tearing

Rare: Ophthalmoplegia

Skin and subcutaneous tissue disorders

Common: Eyelid oedema

Rare: Entropion

Side effects may occur due to deep or misplaced injections of Dysport temporarily paralysing other nearby muscle groups.

The profile of adverse reactions reported to the company during post-marketing use reflects the pharmacology of the product and those seen during clinical trials.

4.9 Overdose

Excessive doses may produce distant and profound neuromuscular paralysis. Respiratory support may be required where excessive doses cause paralysis of respiratory muscles. There is no specific antidote; antitoxin should not be expected to be beneficial and general supportive care is advised. Overdose could lead to an increased risk of the neurotoxin entering the bloodstream and may cause complications associated with the effects of oral botulinum poisoning (e.g deglutition and phonation).

5. PHARMACOLOGICAL PROPERTIES

5.1 Pharmacodynamic properties

Clostridium botulinum type A toxin-haemagglutinin complex blocks peripheral cholinergic transmission at the neuromuscular junction by a presynaptic action at a site proximal to the release of acetylcholine. The toxin acts within the nerve ending to antagonise those events that are triggered by Ca2+ which culminate in transmitter release. It does not affect postganglionic cholinergic transmission or postganglionic sympathetic transmission.

The action of toxin involves an initial binding step whereby the toxin attaches rapidly and avidly to the presynaptic nerve membrane. Secondly, there is an internalisation step in which toxin crosses the presynaptic membrane, without causing onset of paralysis. Finally the toxin inhibits the release of acetylcholine by disrupting the Ca2+ mediated acetylcholine release mechanism, thereby diminishing the endplate potential and causing paralysis.

Recovery of impulse transmission occurs gradually as new nerve terminals sprout and contact is made with the post synaptic motor endplate, a process which takes 6 - 8 weeks in the experimental animal.

5.2 Pharmacokinetic properties

Pharmacokinetic studies with botulinum toxin pose problems in animals because of the high potency, the minute doses involved, the large molecular weight of the compound and the difficulty of labelling toxin to produce sufficiently high specific activity. Studies using I125 labelled toxin have shown that the receptor binding is specific and saturable, and the high density of toxin receptors is a contributory factor to the high potency. Dose and time responses in monkeys showed that at low doses there was a delay of 2 - 3 days with peak effect seen 5 - 6 days after injection. The duration of action, measured by changes of ocular alignment and muscle paralysis varied between 2 weeks and 8 months. This pattern is also seen in man, and is attributed to the process of binding, internalisation and changes at the neuromuscular junction.

5.3 Preclinical safety data

There is no further pre-clinical information relevant to the prescribing physician that has not been included in other sections of the Summary of Product Characteristics.

6. PHARMACEUTICAL PARTICULARS

6.1 List of excipients

Albumin and Lactose.

6.2 Incompatibilities

None known.

6.3 Shelf life

The shelf life of the packaged product - 24 months at 2 - 8°C.

The product may be stored for up to 8 hours at 2 - 8°C following reconstitution.

Since the product does not contain an anti-microbial agent, from a microbiological point of view, it is recommended that the product should be used immediately following reconstitution.

6.4 Special precautions for storage

Unopened vials must be maintained at temperatures between 2°C and 8°C. Dysport must be stored in a refrigerator at the hospital where the injections are to be carried out and should not be given to the patient to store.

Reconstituted Dysport may be stored in a refrigerator (2 - 8°C) for up to 8 hours prior to use.

Dysport should not be frozen.

6.5 Nature and contents of container

Nature of container/closure:

Type 1 glass vials 3 ml capacity. 13 mm chlorbutyl freeze-drying closures oversealed by 13 mm aluminium overseals with centre hole, crimped over.

Contents of container:

A white lyophilised powder for reconstitution.

6.6 Instructions for use and handling

Immediately after treatment of the patient, any residual Dysport which may be present in either vial or syringe should be inactivated with dilute hypochlorite solution (1% available chlorine). Thereafter, all items should be disposed of in accordance with standard hospital practice.

Spillage of Dysport should be wiped up with an absorbent cloth soaked in dilute hypochlorite solution.

7. MARKETING AUTHORISATION HOLDER

Ipsen Limited

190 Bath Road, Slough

Berkshire, SL1 3XE

8. MARKETING AUTHORISATION NUMBER(S)

PL 6958/0005

9. DATE OF FIRST AUTHORISATION/RENEWAL OF THE AUTHORISATION

9th December 1990

10. DATE OF REVISION OF THE TEXT

February 2005

DYSPORT is a registered trademark.

Earex Plus Ear Drops

(SSL International plc)

1. NAME OF THE MEDICINAL PRODUCT

Earex Plus Ear Drops.

2. QUALITATIVE AND QUANTITATIVE COMPOSITION

Choline Salicylate Solution BP 43.22% w/v; and Glycerol BP 12.62% w/v.

3. PHARMACEUTICAL FORM

Solution for topical administration to the ear.

4. CLINICAL PARTICULARS

4.1 Therapeutic indications

For the symptomatic relief of ear pain in acute and chronic otitis media and externa. Patients with ear pain should always seek medical advice. Softening of ear wax as an aid to ear wax removal.

4.2 Posology and method of administration

Auricular Use. Adults, the elderly and children: *For pain relief:* With the head tilted to one side, the external ear canal is filled completely with Earex Plus Ear Drops using the dropper provided. The ear should be plugged with cotton wool soaked with the ear drops. A wick may be inserted, if preferred, using the ear drops to keep it moist. Earex Plus Ear Drops should be instilled every three to four hours. For the softening of ear wax: Apply as described above, twice daily, for four days.

4.3 Contraindications

Not to be used in children under one year of age without medical advice being sought. Salicylate sensitivity. Perforated ear drum. Hypersensitivity to any of the ingredients.

4.4 Special warnings and special precautions for use

None stated.

4.5 Interaction with other medicinal products and other forms of Interaction

None stated.

4.6 Pregnancy and lactation

There is no known hazard with the use of this product during pregnancy and lactation.

4.7 Effects on ability to drive and use machines

None stated.

4.8 Undesirable effects

None stated.

4.9 Overdose

Each bottle of Earex Plus Ear Drops contains 1.6g of choline salicylate, equivalent to 1.2g of aspirin. Accidental or deliberate ingestion of the contents of a bottle of Earex Plus Ear Drops is therefore only of concern in small infants. In such cases, signs of intoxication may include dizziness, tinnitus, sweating, vomiting, confusion and hyperventilation. Gross overdosage may lead to central nervous system depression. Management should include, as appropriate, induced vomiting, correction of fluid and electrolyte balance and measurement of plasma salicylate levels. At concentrations in excess of 300mg/litre measures such as forced alkaline diuresis and haemodialysis to enhance clearance may be appropriate.

5. PHARMACOLOGICAL PROPERTIES

5.1 Pharmacodynamic properties

Choline salicylate has actions similar to those of aspirin, that is analgesic, anti-inflammatory and antipyretic actions considered to be due to inhibition of the biosynthesis of prostaglandins. Glycerol softens ear wax due to its water-retaining and emollient properties.

5.2 Pharmacokinetic properties

Not applicable as Earex Plus Ear Drops are applied topically.

5.3 Preclinical safety data

None stated.

6. PHARMACEUTICAL PARTICULARS

6.1 List of excipients

Ethylene Oxide Polyoxypropylene Glycol; Chlorbutol (Hemihydrate) BP; Hydrochloric Acid; Propylene Glycol BP.

6.2 Incompatibilities

None stated.

6.3 Shelf life

Three years unopened.

6.4 Special precautions for storage

Store at or below 25°C.

6.5 Nature and contents of container

Cartoned amber glass bottle with screw cap and integral dropper containing 10ml of product.

6.6 Instructions for use and handling

Not applicable.

7. MARKETING AUTHORISATION HOLDER

Seton Healthcare Group plc, Tubiton House, Oldham, OL1 3HS.

8. MARKETING AUTHORISATION NUMBER(S)

PL 00223/0047.

9. DATE OF FIRST AUTHORISATION/RENEWAL OF THE AUTHORISATION

11th January 1996 / 22nd May 2001.

10. DATE OF REVISION OF THE TEXT

May 2001.

Ebixa 10 mg Film-Coated Tablets

(Lundbeck Limited)

1. NAME OF THE MEDICINAL PRODUCT

Ebixa▼ 10 mg film-coated tablets.

2. QUALITATIVE AND QUANTITATIVE COMPOSITION

Each tablet contains 10 mg of memantine hydrochloride (equivalent to 8.31 mg memantine).

For excipients, see section 6.1.

3. PHARMACEUTICAL FORM

Film-coated tablets.

The film-coated tablets are white to off-white, centrally tapered oblong, biconvex, with a single breakline on both sides.

4. CLINICAL PARTICULARS

4.1 Therapeutic indications

Treatment of patients with moderately severe to severe Alzheimer's disease.

4.2 Posology and method of administration

Treatment should be initiated and supervised by a physician experienced in the diagnosis and treatment of Alzheimer's dementia. Therapy should only be started if a caregiver is available who will regularly monitor drug intake by the patient. Diagnosis should be made according to current guidelines.

Adults: The maximum daily dose is 20 mg per day. In order to reduce the risk of side effects the maintenance dose is achieved by upward titration 5 mg per week over the first 3 weeks as follows: Treatment should be started with 5 mg daily (half a tablet in the morning) during the 1st week. In the 2nd week 10 mg per day (half a tablet twice a day) and in the 3rd week 15 mg per day is recommended (one tablet in the morning and half a tablet in the afternoon). From the 4th week on, treatment can be continued with the recommended maintenance dose of 20 mg per day (one tablet twice a day).

The tablets can be taken with or without food.

Elderly: On the basis of the clinical studies the recommended dose for patients over the age of 65 years is 20 mg per day (10 mg twice a day) as described above.

Children and adolescents under the age of 18 years: The safety and efficacy of memantine in children and adolescents have not been established.

Renal impairment: In patients with normal to mildly impaired renal function (serum creatinine levels of up to 130 μmol/l) no dose reduction is needed. In patients with moderate renal impairment (creatinine clearance 40 - 60 ml/min/1.73 m^2) daily dose should be reduced to 10 mg per day. No data are available for patients with severely reduced kidney function (see sections 4.4 and 5.2).

Hepatic impairment: There are no data on the use of memantine in patients with hepatic impairment (see section 5.2).

4.3 Contraindications

Hypersensitivity to the active substance or to any of the excipients.

4.4 Special warnings and special precautions for use

As no data are available for patients with severe renal impairment (creatinine clearance less than 9 ml/min/1.73 m^2) therapy is not recommended (see section 4.2).

Caution is recommended in patients with epilepsy, former history of convulsions or patients with predisposing factors for epilepsy.

Concomitant use of N-methyl-D-aspartate(NMDA)-antagonists such as amantadine, ketamine or dextromethorphan should be avoided. These compounds act at the same receptor system as memantine, and therefore adverse drug reactions (mainly CNS-related) may be more frequent or more pronounced (see also section 4.5).

Some factors that may raise urine pH (see section 5.2 "Elimination") may necessitate careful monitoring of the patient. These factors include drastic changes in diet, e.g. from a carnivore to a vegetarian diet, or a massive ingestion of alkalising gastric buffers. Also, urine pH may be elevated by states of renal tubular acidosis (RTA) or severe infections of the urinary tract with *Proteus bacteria*.

In most clinical trials, patients with recent myocardial infarction, uncompensated congestive heart failure (NYHA III-IV), and uncontrolled hypertension were excluded. As a consequence, only limited data are available and patients with these conditions should be closely supervised.

4.5 Interaction with other medicinal products and other forms of Interaction

Due to the pharmacological effects and the mechanism of action of memantine the following interactions may occur:

- The mode of action suggests that the effects of L-dopa, dopaminergic agonists, and anticholinergics may be enhanced by concomitant treatment with NMDA-antagonists such as memantine. The effects of barbiturates and neuroleptics may be reduced. Concomitant administration of memantine with the antispasmodic agents, dantrolene or baclofen, can modify their effects and a dosage adjustment may be necessary.
- Concomitant use of memantine and amantadine should be avoided, owing to the risk of pharmacotoxic psychosis. Both compounds are chemically related NMDA-antagonists. The same may be true for ketamine and dextromethorphan (see also section 4.4). There is one published case report on a possible risk also for the combination of memantine and phenytoin.
- Other drugs such as cimetidine, ranitidine, procainamide, quinidine, quinine and nicotine that use the same renal cationic transport system as amantadine may also possibly interact with memantine leading to a potential risk of increased plasma levels.
- There may be a possibility of reduced serum level of hydrochlorothiazide (HCT) when memantine is co-administered with HCT or any combination with HCT.

Memantine did not inhibit CYP 1A2, 2A6, 2C9, 2D6, 2E1, 3A, flavin containing monoxygenase, epoxide hydrolase and sulphation *in vitro*.

4.6 Pregnancy and lactation

Pregnancy: For memantine, no clinical data on exposed pregnancies are available. Animal studies indicate a potential for reducing intrauterine growth at exposure levels which are identical or slightly higher than at human exposure (see section 5.3). The potential risk for humans is unknown. Memantine should not be used during pregnancy unless clearly necessary.

Lactation: It is not known whether memantine is excreted in humans breast milk but, taking into consideration the lipophilicity of the substance, this probably occurs. Women taking memantine should not breast-feed.

4.7 Effects on ability to drive and use machines

Moderately severe to severe Alzheimer's disease usually causes impairment of driving performance and compromises the ability to use machinery. Furthermore, memantine may change reactivity such that outpatients should be warned to take special care when driving a vehicle or operating machinery.

4.8 Undesirable effects

In clinical trials in moderately severe to severe dementia, overall incidence rates for adverse events did not differ from placebo treatment and adverse events were usually mild to moderate in severity.

The following table gives an overview of the most frequent (>4% for memantine) adverse events (irrespective of causal relationship) that were observed in the trial population of patients with moderately severe to severe dementia.

Preferred term (WHO ART)	Memantine n=299	Placebo n=288
Agitation	27 (9.0%)	50 (17.4%)
Inflicted Injury	20 (6.7%)	20 (6.9%)
Urinary Incontinence	17 (5.7%)	21 (7.3%)
Diarrhoea	16 (5.4%)	14 (4.9%)
Insomnia	16 (5.4%)	14 (4.9%)
Dizziness	15 (5.0%)	8 (2.8%)
Headache	15 (5.0%)	9 (3.1%)
Hallucination	15 (5.0%)	6 (2.1%)
Fall	14 (4.7%)	14 (4.9%)
Constipation	12 (4.0%)	13 (4.5%)
Coughing	12 (4.0%)	17 (5.9%)

Common adverse reactions (1 - 10% and more frequent than with placebo) for memantine and placebo patients respectively were: hallucinations (2.0 vs. 0.7%), confusion (1.3 vs. 0.3%), dizziness (1.7 vs. 1.0%), headache (1.7 vs. 1.4%) and tiredness (1.0 vs. 0.3%).

Uncommon adverse reactions (0.1 - 1% and more frequent than with placebo) were anxiety, hypertonia (increased muscle tone), vomiting, cystitis and increased libido.

Based on spontaneous reports, seizures have been reported, mostly in patients with a history of convulsions.

4.9 Overdose

In one case of suicidal overdosage the patient survived the oral intake of up to 400 mg memantine with effects on the central nervous system (e. g. restlessness, psychosis, visual hallucinations, proconvulsiveness, somnolence, stupor and unconsciousness) which resolved without permanent sequelae.

Treatment of overdosage should be symptomatic.

5. PHARMACOLOGICAL PROPERTIES

5.1 Pharmacodynamic properties

Pharmacotherapeutic group: Anti-dementia drugs, ATC code: N06DX01.

There is increasing evidence that malfunctioning of glutamatergic neurotransmission, in particular at NMDA-receptors, contributes to both expression of symptoms and disease progression in neurodegenerative dementia.

Memantine is a voltage-dependent, moderate-affinity uncompetitive NMDA-receptor antagonist. It blocks the effects of pathologically elevated tonic levels of glutamate that may lead to neuronal dysfunction.

Clinical studies: A clinical trial in a population of patients suffering from moderately severe to severe Alzheimer's disease (MMSE total scores at baseline of 3 - 14) showed beneficial effects of memantine treatment in comparison to placebo over a treatment period of 6 months.

In this multicenter, double-blind, randomised, placebo-controlled study, a total of 252 outpatients (33% male, 67% female, mean age 76 years) were included. The dosing was 10 mg memantine twice a day. Primary outcome parameters included assessment of the global domain (using the Clinicians Interview-Based Impression of Change (CIBIC-Plus)) and the functional domain (using the Activities of Daily Living Inventory (ADCS-ADLsev)). Cognition was assessed as a secondary endpoint with the Severe Impairment Battery (SIB). The results in these domains favoured memantine over placebo (Observed Cases Analysis for CIBIC-Plus: $p=0.025$; ADCS-ADLsev: $p=0.003$; SIB: $p=0.002$).

After 6 months, the rate of individual responders (response prospectively defined as stabilisation or improvement in two independent domains) was 29% for the memantine group versus 10% for placebo ($p=0.0004$). With a triple criterion (response defined as stabilisation or improvement in all three domains: cognition, functional and global domain), there were 11% responders for memantine versus 6% for placebo ($p=0.17$).

5.2 Pharmacokinetic properties

Absorption: Memantine has an absolute bioavailability of approximately 100%. t_{max} is between 3 and 8 hours. There is no indication that food influences the absorption of memantine.

Linearity: Studies in volunteers have demonstrated linear pharmacokinetics in the dose range of 10 to 40 mg.

Distribution: Daily doses of 20 mg lead to steady-state plasma concentrations of memantine ranging from 70 to 150 ng/ml (0.5 - 1 μmol) with large interindividual variations. When daily doses of 5 to 30 mg were administered, a mean CSF/serum ratio of 0.52 was calculated. The volume of distribution is around 10 l/kg. About 45% of memantine is bound to plasma-proteins.

Biotransformation: In man, about 80% of the circulating memantine-related material is present as the parent compound. Main human metabolites are N-3,5-dimethyl-gludantan, the isomeric mixture of 4- and 6-hydroxy-memantine, and 1-nitroso-3,5-dimethyl-adamantane. None of these metabolites exhibit NMDA-antagonistic activity. No cytochrome P 450 catalysed metabolism has been detected *in vitro*.

In a study using orally administered ^{14}C-memantine, a mean of 84% of the dose was recovered within 20 days, more than 99% being excreted renally.

Elimination: Memantine is eliminated in a monoexponential manner with a terminal $t_{½}$ of 60 to 100 hours. In volunteers with normal kidney function, total clearance (Cl_{tot}) amounts to 170 ml/min/1.73 m^2 and part of total renal clearance is achieved by tubular secretion.

Renal handling also involves tubular reabsorption, probably mediated by cation transport proteins. The renal elimination rate of memantine under alkaline urine conditions may be reduced by a factor of 7 to 9 (see section 4.4). Alkalisation of urine may result from drastic changes in diet, e.g. from a carnivore to a vegetarian diet, or from the massive ingestion of alkalising gastric buffers.

Specific patient population: In elderly volunteers with normal and reduced renal function (creatinine clearance of 50 - 100 ml/min/1.73 m^2), a significant correlation was observed between creatinine clearance and total renal clearance of memantine (see section 4.2).

The effect of liver disease on the pharmacokinetics of memantine has not been studied. As memantine is metabolised to a minor extent only, and into metabolites with no NMDA-antagonistic activity, clinically relevant changes in the pharmacokinetics are not expected in mild to moderate liver impairment.

Pharmacokinetic/pharmacodynamic relationship: At a dose of memantine of 20 mg per day the cerebrospinal fluid (CSF) levels match the k_i-value (k_i = inhibition constant) of memantine, which is 0.5 μmol in human frontal cortex.

5.3 Preclinical safety data

In short term studies in rats memantine like other NMDA-antagonists have induced neuronal vacuolisation and necrosis (Olney lesions) only after doses leading to very high peak serum concentrations. Ataxia and other preclinical signs have preceded the vacuolisation and necrosis. As the effects have neither been observed in long term studies in rodents nor in non-rodents, the clinical relevance of these findings is unknown.

Ocular changes were inconsistently observed in repeat dose toxicity studies in rodents and dogs, but not in monkeys. Specific ophthalmoscopic examinations in clinical studies with memantine did not disclose any ocular changes.

Phospholipidosis in pulmonary macrophages due to accumulation of memantine in lysosomes was observed in rodents. This effect is known from other drugs with cationic amphiphilic properties. There is a possible relationship between this accumulation and the vacuolisation observed in lungs. This effect was only observed at high doses in rodents. The clinical relevance of these findings is unknown.

No genotoxicity has been observed following testing of memantine in standard assays. There was no evidence of any carcinogenicity in life long studies in mice and rats. Memantine was not teratogenic in rats and rabbits, even at maternally toxic doses, and no adverse effects of memantine were noted on fertility. In rats, foetal growth reduction was noted at exposure levels which are identical or slightly higher than at human exposure.

6. PHARMACEUTICAL PARTICULARS

6.1 List of excipients

Tablet core:

Lactose monohydrate

Microcrystalline cellulose

Colloidal anhydrous silica

Talc

Magnesium stearate

Tablet coat:

Methacrylic acid - ethyl acrylate copolymer (1:1)

Sodium lauryl sulphate

Polysorbate 80

Talc

Triacetin

Simethicone emulsion

6.2 Incompatibilities

Not applicable.

6.3 Shelf life

4 years.

6.4 Special precautions for storage

No special precautions for storage.

6.5 Nature and contents of container

Blister packs containing either 7, 10, 14 or 20 tablets per blister strip (Alu/PP). Pack sizes of 28, 30, 49 × 1, 50, 56, 100, 100 × 1, 112 or 1000 (20 × 50) tablets are presented. The pack sizes 49 × 1 film-coated tablets and 100 × 1 film-coated tablets are presented in perforated unit dose blister.

Not all pack sizes may be marketed.

6.6 Instructions for use and handling

No special requirements.

7. MARKETING AUTHORISATION HOLDER

H. Lundbeck A/S

Ottiliavej 9,

DK-2500 Valby

Denmark

8. MARKETING AUTHORISATION NUMBER(S)

EU/1/02/219/001-3

EU/1/02/219/007-012

9. DATE OF FIRST AUTHORISATION/RENEWAL OF THE AUTHORISATION

17/05/2002

10. DATE OF REVISION OF THE TEXT

24 March 2004

Ebixa 10 mg/g Oral Drops, Solution

(Lundbeck Limited)

1. NAME OF THE MEDICINAL PRODUCT

Ebixa 10 mg/g oral drops, solution ▼.

2. QUALITATIVE AND QUANTITATIVE COMPOSITION

1 g of solution contains 10 mg of memantine hydrochloride (equivalent to 8.31 mg memantine).

For excipients, see section 6.1.

3. PHARMACEUTICAL FORM

Oral drops, solution.

The solution is clear and colourless to light yellowish.

4. CLINICAL PARTICULARS

4.1 Therapeutic indications

Treatment of patients with moderately severe to severe Alzheimer's disease.

4.2 Posology and method of administration

Treatment should be initiated and supervised by a physician experienced in the diagnosis and treatment of Alzheimer's dementia. Therapy should only be started if a caregiver is available who will regularly monitor drug intake by the patient. Diagnosis should be made according to current guidelines.

Adults: The maximum daily dose is 20 mg per day. In order to reduce the risk of side effects the maintenance dose is achieved by upward titration 5 mg per week over the first 3 weeks as follows: Treatment should be started with 5 mg daily (10 drops in the morning) during the 1st week. In the 2nd week 10 mg per day (10 drops twice a day) and in the 3rd week 15 mg per day is recommended (20 drops in the morning and 10 drops in the afternoon). From the 4th week on, treatment can be continued with the recommended maintenance dose of 20 mg per day (20 drops twice a day).

The drops can be taken with or without food.

Elderly: On the basis of the clinical studies the recommended dose for patients over the age of 65 years is 20 mg per day (10 mg twice a day) as described above.

Children and adolescents under the age of 18 years: The safety and efficacy of memantine in children and adolescents have not been established.

Renal impairment: In patients with normal to mildly impaired renal function (serum creatinine levels of up to 130 μmol/l) no dose reduction is needed. In patients with moderate renal impairment (creatinine clearance 40 - 60 ml/min/1.73 m^2) daily dose should be reduced to 10 mg per day. No data are available for patients with severely reduced kidney function (see sections 4.4 and 5.2).

Hepatic impairment: There are no data on the use of memantine in patients with hepatic impairment (see section 5.2).

4.3 Contraindications

Hypersensitivity to the active substance or to any of the excipients.

4.4 Special warnings and special precautions for use

As no data are available for patients with severe renal impairment (creatinine clearance less than 9 ml/min/1.73 m^2) therapy is not recommended (see section 4.2).

Caution is recommended in patients with epilepsy, former history of convulsions or patients with predisposing factors for epilepsy.

Concomitant use of N-methyl-D-aspartate(NMDA)-antagonists such as amantadine, ketamine or dextromethorphan should be avoided. These compounds act at the same receptor system as memantine, and therefore adverse drug reactions (mainly CNS-related) may be more frequent or more pronounced (see also section 4.5).

Some factors that may raise urine pH (see section 5.2 "Elimination") may necessitate careful monitoring of the patient. These factors include drastic changes in diet, e.g. from a carnivore to a vegetarian diet, or a massive ingestion of alkalising gastric buffers. Also, urine pH may be elevated by states of renal tubulary acidosis (RTA) or severe infections of the urinary tract with *Proteus bacteria*.

In most clinical trials, patients with recent myocardial infarction, uncompensated congestive heart failure (NYHA III-IV), and uncontrolled hypertension were excluded. As a consequence, only limited data are available and patients with these conditions should be closely supervised.

4.5 Interaction with other medicinal products and other forms of Interaction

Due to the pharmacological effects and the mechanism of action of memantine the following interactions may occur:

- The mode of action suggests that the effects of L-dopa, dopaminergic agonists, and anticholinergics may be enhanced by concomitant treatment with NMDA-antagonists such as memantine. The effects of barbiturates and neuroleptics may be reduced. Concomitant administration of memantine with the antispasmodic agents, dantrolene or baclofen, can modify their effects and a dosage adjustment may be necessary.

- Concomitant use of memantine and amantadine should be avoided, owing to the risk of pharmacotoxic psychosis. Both compounds are chemically related NMDA-antagonists. The same may be true for ketamine and dextromethorphan (see also section 4.4). There is one published case report on a possible risk also for the combination of memantine and phenytoin.
- Other drugs such as cimetidine, ranitidine, procainamide, quinidine, quinine and nicotine that use the same renal cationic transport system as amantadine may also possibly interact with memantine leading to a potential risk of increased plasma levels.
- There may be a possibility of reduced serum level of hydrochlorothiazide (HCT) when memantine is co-administered with HCT or any combination with HCT

Memantine did not inhibit CYP 1A2, 2A6, 2C9, 2D6, 2E1, 3A, flavin containing monoxygenase, epoxide hydrolase and sulphation *in vitro*.

4.6 Pregnancy and lactation

Pregnancy: For memantine, no clinical data on exposed pregnancies are available. Animal studies indicate a potential for reducing intrauterine growth at exposure levels which are identical or slightly higher than at human exposure (see section 5.3). The potential risk for humans is unknown. Memantine should not be used during pregnancy unless clearly necessary.

Lactation: It is not known whether memantine is excreted in humans breast milk but, taking into consideration the lipophilicity of the substance, this probably occurs. Women taking memantine should not breast-feed.

4.7 Effects on ability to drive and use machines

Moderately severe to severe Alzheimer's disease usually causes impairment of driving performance and compromises the ability to use machinery. Furthermore, memantine may change reactivity such that outpatients should be warned to take special care when driving a vehicle or operating machinery.

4.8 Undesirable effects

In clinical trials in moderately severe to severe dementia, overall incidence rates for adverse events did not differ from placebo treatment and adverse events were usually mild to moderate in severity.

The following table gives an overview of the most frequent (>4% for memantine) adverse events (irrespective of causal relationship) that were observed in the trial population of patients with moderately severe to severe dementia.

Preferred term (WHO ART)	Memantine n=299	Placebo n=288
Agitation	27 (9.0%)	50 (17.4%)
Inflicted Injury	20 (6.7%)	20 (6.9%)
Urinary Incontinence	17 (5.7%)	21 (7.3%)
Diarrhoea	16 (5.4%)	14 (4.9%)
Insomnia	16 (5.4%)	14 (4.9%)
Dizziness	15 (5.0%)	8 (2.8%)
Headache	15 (5.0%)	9 (3.1%)
Hallucination	15 (5.0%)	6 (2.1%)
Fall	14 (4.7%)	14 (4.9%)
Constipation	12 (4.0%)	13 (4.5%)
Coughing	12 (4.0%)	17 (5.9%)

Common adverse reactions (1 - 10% and more frequent than with placebo) for memantine and placebo patients respectively were: hallucinations (2.0 vs. 0.7%), confusion (1.3 vs. 0.3%), dizziness (1.7 vs. 1.0%), headache (1.7 vs. 1.4%) and tiredness (1.0 vs. 0.3%).

Uncommon adverse reactions (0.1 - 1% and more frequent than with placebo) were anxiety, hypertonia (increased muscle tone), vomiting, cystitis and increased libido.

Based on spontaneous reports, seizures have been reported, mostly in patients with a history of convulsions.

4.9 Overdose

In one case of suicidal overdosage the patient survived the oral intake of up to 400 mg memantine with effects on the central nervous system (e. g. restlessness, psychosis, visual hallucinations, proconvulsiveness, somnolence, stupor and unconsciousness) which resolved without permanent sequelae.

Treatment of overdosage should be symptomatic.

5. PHARMACOLOGICAL PROPERTIES

5.1 Pharmacodynamic properties

Pharmacotherapeutic group: Anti-dementia drugs, ATC code: N06DX01.

There is increasing evidence that malfunctioning of glutamatergic neurotransmission, in particular at NMDA-receptors, contributes to both expression of symptoms and disease progression in neurodegenerative dementia.

Memantine is a voltage-dependent, moderate-affinity uncompetitive NMDA-receptor antagonist. It blocks the effects of pathologically elevated tonic levels of glutamate that may lead to neuronal dysfunction.

Clinical studies: A clinical trial in a population of patients suffering from moderately severe to severe Alzheimer's disease (MMSE total scores at baseline of 3 - 14) showed beneficial effects of memantine treatment in comparison to placebo over a treatment period of 6 months.

In this multicenter, double-blind, randomised, placebo-controlled study, a total of 252 outpatients (33% male, 67% female, mean age 76 years) were included. The dosing was 10 mg memantine twice a day. Primary outcome parameters included assessment of the global domain (using the Clinicians Interview-Based Impression of Change (CIBIC-Plus)) and the functional domain (using the Activities of Daily Living Inventory (ADCS-ADLsev)). Cognition was assessed as a secondary endpoint with the Severe Impairment Battery (SIB). The results in these domains favoured memantine over placebo (Observed Cases Analysis for CIBIC-Plus: p=0.025; ADCS-ADLsev: p=0.003; SIB: p=0.002).

After 6 months, the rate of individual responders (response prospectively defined as stabilisation or improvement in two independent domains) was 29% for the memantine group versus 10% for placebo (p=0.0004). With a triple criterion (response defined as stabilisation or improvement in all three domains: cognition, functional and global domain), there were 11% responders for memantine versus 6% for placebo (p=0.17).

5.2 Pharmacokinetic properties

Absorption: Memantine has an absolute bioavailability of approximately 100%. t_{max} is between 3 and 8 hours. There is no indication that food influences the absorption of memantine.

Linearity: Studies in volunteers have demonstrated linear pharmacokinetics in the dose range of 10 to 40 mg.

Distribution: Daily doses of 20 mg lead to steady-state plasma concentrations of memantine ranging from 70 to 150 ng/ml (0.5 - 1 μmol) with large interindividual variations. When daily doses of 5 to 30 mg were administered, a mean CSF/serum ratio of 0.52 was calculated. The volume of distribution is around 10 l/kg. About 45% of memantine is bound to plasma-proteins.

Biotransformation: In man, about 80% of the circulating memantine-related material is present as the parent compound. Main human metabolites are N-3,5-dimethyl-gludantan, the isomeric mixture of 4- and 6-hydroxy-memantine, and 1-nitroso-3,5-dimethyl-adamantane. None of these metabolites exhibit NMDA-antagonistic activity. No cytochrome P 450 catalysed metabolism has been detected *in vitro*.

In a study using orally administered ^{14}C-memantine, a mean of 84% of the dose was recovered within 20 days, more than 99% being excreted renally.

Elimination: Memantine is eliminated in a monoexponential manner with a terminal $t_{½}$ of 60 to 100 hours. In volunteers with normal kidney function, total clearance (Cl_{tot}) amounts to 170 ml/min/1.73 m^2 and part of total renal clearance is achieved by tubular secretion.

Renal handling also involves tubular reabsorption, probably mediated by cation transport proteins. The renal elimination rate of memantine under alkaline urine conditions may be reduced by a factor of 7 to 9 (see section 4.4). Alkalisation of urine may result from drastic changes in diet, e.g. from a carnivore to a vegetarian diet, or from the massive ingestion of alkalising gastric buffers.

Specific patient population: In elderly volunteers with normal and reduced renal function (creatinine clearance of 50 - 100 ml/min/1.73 m^2), a significant correlation was observed between creatinine clearance and total renal clearance of memantine (see section 4.2).

The effect of liver disease on the pharmacokinetics of memantine has not been studied. As memantine is metabolised to a minor extent only, and into metabolites with no NMDA-antagonistic activity, clinically relevant changes in the pharmacokinetics are not expected in mild to moderate liver impairment.

Pharmacokinetic/pharmacodynamic relationship: At a dose of memantine of 20 mg per day the cerebrospinal fluid (CSF) levels match the k_i-value (k_i = inhibition constant) of memantine, which is 0.5 μmol in human frontal cortex.

5.3 Preclinical safety data

In short term studies in rats memantine like other NMDA-antagonists have induced neuronal vacuolisation and necrosis (Olney lesions) only after doses leading to very high peak serum concentrations. Ataxia and other preclinical signs have preceded the vacuolisation and necrosis. As the effects have neither been observed in long term studies in rodents nor in non-rodents, the clinical relevance of these findings is unknown.

Ocular changes were inconsistently observed in repeat dose toxicity studies in rodents and dogs, but not in monkeys. Specific ophthalmoscopic examinations in clinical studies with memantine did not disclose any ocular changes.

Phospholipidosis in pulmonary macrophages due to accumulation of memantine in lysosomes was observed in rodents. This effect is known from other drugs with cationic amphiphilic properties. There is a possible relationship between this accumulation and the vacuolisation observed in lungs. This effect was only observed at high doses in rodents. The clinical relevance of these findings is unknown.

No genotoxicity has been observed following testing of memantine in standard assays. There was no evidence of any carcinogenicity in life long studies in mice and rats. Memantine was not teratogenic in rats and rabbits, even at maternally toxic doses, and no adverse effects of memantine were noted on fertility. In rats, foetal growth reduction was noted at exposure levels which are identical or slightly higher than at human exposure.

6. PHARMACEUTICAL PARTICULARS

6.1 List of excipients

Potassium sorbate

Sorbitol

Purified water

6.2 Incompatibilities

Not applicable.

6.3 Shelf life

4 years.

Once opened, the contents of the bottle should be used within 3 months.

6.4 Special precautions for storage

Do not store above 30°C.

6.5 Nature and contents of container

Brown glass bottles (Hydrolytic Class III) with dropper containing either 20, 50, 100 or 10 × 50 g solution.

Not all pack sizes may be marketed.

6.6 Instructions for use and handling

No special requirements.

7. MARKETING AUTHORISATION HOLDER

H. Lundbeck A/S

Ottiliavej 9,

DK-2500 Valby

Denmark

8. MARKETING AUTHORISATION NUMBER(S)

EU/1/02/219/004-6

EU/1/02/219/013

9. DATE OF FIRST AUTHORISATION/RENEWAL OF THE AUTHORISATION

15/05/2002

10. DATE OF REVISION OF THE TEXT

24 March 2004

Eccoxolac

(Viatris Pharmaceuticals Ltd)

1. NAME OF THE MEDICINAL PRODUCT

Eccoxolac

Etodolac Capsules 300 mg

2. QUALITATIVE AND QUANTITATIVE COMPOSITION

Each capsule contains Etodolac 300 mg.

For excipients see section 6.1.

3. PHARMACEUTICAL FORM

Hard capsules

4. CLINICAL PARTICULARS

4.1 Therapeutic indications

Etodolac is indicated for acute or long term use in:

i) Osteoarthritis

ii) Rheumatoid arthritis.

4.2 Posology and method of administration

Usual adult dose:

400-600 mg daily in two divided doses or as a single daily dose.

Children: It is not recommended for use in children.

Elderly: No dosage adjustment in initial dosage is generally required in the elderly (see precautions).

4.3 Contraindications

Etodolac is contraindicated in patients who have a previous history of hypersensitivity to etodolac. It should not be administered to patients with a history of acute asthma, rhinitis, urticaria or other allergic reactions with aspirin or non-steroidal anti-inflammatory drugs due to possible cross-reactivity. The drug is also contra-indicated in patients with active peptic ulceration or with a history of peptic ulcer disease (including gastrointestinal haemorrhage).

4.4 Special warnings and special precautions for use

• As with other NSAIDs, in renal, cardiac or hepatic impairment caution is generally required since the use may result in deterioration of renal function. The dose should be low and renal function should be monitored.

• Hepatic and renal function, haematological parameters of patients on long-term use of Etodolac should be regularly reviewed.

• Caution is required if Etodolac is administered to patients suffering from or with a previous history of bronchial asthma since NSAIDs have been reported to cause bronchospasm is such patients.

• Etodolac should be used with caution in patients with fluid retention, hypertension or heart failure.

• The patients with long-term use of etodolac, especially the elderly should be monitored for the potential side effects and the dose adjusted or discontinued as required.

• All such drugs, which inhibit the biosynthesis of prostaglandins, may interfere with platelet function. Patients who may be adversely affected due to inhibition of platelet function should be carefully observed.

Geriatrics

No dosage adjustment is generally necessary in the elderly. However, caution should be exercised in treating the elderly, and when individualising their dosage, extra care should be taken while increasing the dose because the elderly seem to tolerate NSAID side effects less well than younger patients.

Paediatrics

Safety and efficacy in children have not been established and therefore etodolac is not recommended in children.

WARNING

Serious gastrointestinal toxicity such as bleeding, ulceration and perforation can occur at any time in patients treated chronically with NSAIDs. If any sign of gastrointestinal bleeding occurs, etodolac should be stopped immediately.

4.5 Interaction with other medicinal products and other forms of Interaction

Warfarin – Prothrombin time may be prolonged when etodolac and other NSAIDs are given along with warfarin thus leading to increased risk of bleeding.

Cyclosporin, Digoxin, Lithium, Methotrexate – Serum levels of these drugs may be increased. Nephrotoxicity associated with cyclosporin may be enhanced.

Since etodolac is extensively protein-bound, it may be necessary to modify the dosage of other highly protein-bound drugs.

Bilirubin tests can give a false positive result due to the presence of phenolic metabolites of etodolac in the urine.

Care should be taken in patients treated with any of the following drugs as interactions have been reported:

Antihypertensives: reduced anti-hypertensive effect.

Mifepristone: NSAIDs should not be used for 8-12 days after mifepristone administration as NSAIDs can reduce the effect of mifepristone.

Other analgesics: avoid the concomitant use of two or more NSAIDs.

Corticosteroids: increased risk of gastrointestinal bleeding.

Quinolone antibiotics: animal data indicate that NSAIDs can increase the risk of convulsions associated with quinolone antibiotics. Patients taking NSAIDs and quinolones may have an increased risk of developing convulsions.

4.6 Pregnancy and lactation

Etodolac should not be used in pregnancy since there are no adequate or well controlled studies in pregnant women. However, in teratogenic studies in animals, drugs which inhibit prostaglandin synthesis have been reported to cause dystocia, delayed parturition and interfere with closure of ductus arteriosus. Etodolac should not be used during pregnancy.

Safety of etodolac during lactation has not been established. Use of etodolac should be avoided in nursing mothers.

4.7 Effects on ability to drive and use machines

Etodolac can cause dizziness, drowsiness or abnormal vision. Patients need to be aware of how they react to this medicine before driving or operating machines.

4.8 Undesirable effects

Gastrointestinal system – Nausea, vomiting, dyspepsia, epigastric pain, stomatitis, gastritis, colitis, abdominal pain, constipation, flatulence, haematemesis, malaena, gastrointestinal ulceration, diarrhoea, indigestion, heartburn, hepatic function abnormalities, rectal bleeding.

Nervous system – Depression, headache, dizziness, insomnia, confusion, paraesthesia, tremor, weakness, nervousness, dyspnoea.

Urogenital system – Dysuria, urinary frequency (<1%), interstitial nephritis, nephritic syndrome, renal failure.

Other – Rash, pruritus, urticaria, vasculitis, Stevens-Johnson syndrome, chills and fever, abnormal vision, tinnitus (1-3%), asthenia, fatigue, bilirubinuria, angioedema, thrombocytopenia, neutropenia, agranulocytosis, anaemia, jaundice, oedema, palpitation, drowsiness, anaphylactoid reaction, photosensitivity.

4.9 Overdose

The standard practice of gastric evacuation, activated charcoal administration and general supportive therapy should be undertaken.

5. PHARMACOLOGICAL PROPERTIES

5.1 Pharmacodynamic properties

Pharmacotherapeutic classification

M01A B (Anti-inflammatory and Anti-rheumatic agents)

Mode of Action

Etodolac is a non-steroidal anti-inflammatory drug (NSAID) with anti-inflammatory, analgesic and antipyretic actions. The mode of action is thought to be through inhibition of the cyclo-oxygenase enzyme involved in prostaglandin synthesis.

5.2 Pharmacokinetic properties

Etodolac is well absorbed when taken orally. Following oral administration of 200 mg or 300 mg of etodolac, the peak plasma concentration of 10-18μg/ml and 36 μg/ml respectively is achieved in about 1-2 hours. Etodolac plasma concentrations, after multiple dose administration within therapeutic range, are only slightly higher than after single dose. Etodolac may be given with food or co-administered with antacids, as the extent of absorption of etodolac is not affected when administered after a meal or with an antacid. Etodolac is more than 99% bound to plasma proteins.

Etodolac penetrates readily into synovial fluid following oral administration in patients with arthritis. Consistent with the lower levels of total protein and albumin in synovial fluid compared to serum, the synovial fluid free Etodolac AUC (0-24h) is 72% higher than the value for serum. In the post-distributive phase, total and free Etodolac concentration in synovial fluid consistently exceeds those in serum, with mean synovial fluid: serum ratios of 1.18 and 3.25, between 8 and 32 hours post dose respectively.

Etodolac is extensively metabolised in the liver. Approximately 72% of the administered dose is recovered in the urine as inactive metabolites. 16% of the dose is excreted through faeces. The plasma half-life of dose is 6-7.4 hours.

Studies in the elderly have shown similar Pharmacokinetics as in younger individuals. No dosage adjustment is needed in the elderly. Since etodolac clearance is dependent on hepatic function, patients with severe hepatic failure may have reduced clearance. No change in Pharmacokinetics has been noticed in patients of mild to moderate renal impairment compared to normal. In usual therapeutic doses etodolac decreases serum uric acid levels by 1-2 mg% after four weeks of administration.

5.3 Preclinical safety data

The pharmacological and toxicological properties of etodolac are well established. Etodolac has no carcinogenic or mutagenic potential. It has shown no embryogenic or teratogenic effects. However, an isolated alteration of limb development has occurred in rats receiving 2-14 mg/kg/day.

6. PHARMACEUTICAL PARTICULARS

6.1 List of excipients

Lactose, sodium starch glycollate (type A), povidone, sodium lauryl sulphate, magnesium Stearate, microcrystalline cellulose and talc. The hard gelatin capsules are coloured with E110, E129, E171 and E172. The black ink contains shellac, iron oxide black (E172), IMS 74 OP, n-butyl alcohol, soya lecithin MC thin and antifoam DC 1510.

6.2 Incompatibilities

No incompatibilities have been reported with etodolac.

6.3 Shelf life

3 Years

6.4 Special precautions for storage

Store in the original package.

6.5 Nature and contents of container

Strip comprising clear transparent PVC film 0.3 mm thick (coated uniformly with PVdC on the inner side) with a backing of aluminium foil 0.025 mm thick (coated with heat seal lacquer).

Pack containing four strips of 15 capsules each or six strips of 10 capsules each.

6.6 Instructions for use and handling

None

7. MARKETING AUTHORISATION HOLDER

Ranbaxy (UK) Limited

95 Park Lane, Mayfair,

London W1Y 3TA

8. MARKETING AUTHORISATION NUMBER(S)

14894/0019

9. DATE OF FIRST AUTHORISATION/RENEWAL OF THE AUTHORISATION

23rd February 2000

10. DATE OF REVISION OF THE TEXT

February 2004

LEGAL CATEGORY

POM

Econacort Cream

(E. R. Squibb & Sons Limited)

1. NAME OF THE MEDICINAL PRODUCT

Econacort Cream

2. QUALITATIVE AND QUANTITATIVE COMPOSITION

Each gram of topical cream contains: Econazole Nitrate EP 10mg and Hydrocortisone EP 10 mg

3. PHARMACEUTICAL FORM

Topical Cream.

4. CLINICAL PARTICULARS

4.1 Therapeutic indications

Econacort is indicated for the topical treatment of inflammatory dermatoses where infection by susceptible organisms co-exist.

4.2 Posology and method of administration

Adults and children:

To be massaged gently into the affected and surrounding skin area morning and evening. The cream is particularly suitable for moist or weeping lesions.

Elderly:

Natural thinning of the skin occurs in the elderly, hence corticosteroids should be used sparingly and for short periods of time.

4.3 Contraindications

Hypersensitivity to either of the active ingredients.

In tuberculous and most viral lesions of the skin, particularly herpes simplex, vaccinia and varicella.

Should not be used for facial rosacea, acne vulgaris or perioral dermatitis.

4.4 Special warnings and special precautions for use

Econacort cream should not be used in or near the eyes.

If used in infants and children, or on the face, courses should be limited to 5 days and occlusion should not be used.

4.5 Interaction with other medicinal products and other forms of Interaction

None stated.

4.6 Pregnancy and lactation

Topical administration of corticosteroids to pregnant animals can cause abnormalities of foetal development including cleft palate and intra-uterine growth retardation. There may, therefore, be a very small risk of such effects in the human foetus.

4.7 Effects on ability to drive and use machines

None stated.

4.8 Undesirable effects

Econazole nitrate and hydrocortisone are well tolerated. Where adverse reactions occur they are usually reversible on cessation of therapy.

Side effects of econazole nitrate are limited to occasional local irritation manifested by erythema, burning or stinging sensation, and pruritus, but these may be minimised by the hydrocortisone component.

The possibility of the systemic effects which are associated with all steroid therapy should be considered. These effects may be enhanced with occlusive dressings.

4.9 Overdose

Topically applied corticosteroids can be absorbed in sufficient amounts to produce systemic effects.

In the event of accidental ingestion, the patient should be observed and treated symptomatically.

5. PHARMACOLOGICAL PROPERTIES

5.1 Pharmacodynamic properties

Econazole nitrate is a broad spectrum antifungal and antibiotic agent, active against dermatophytes (*Trichophyton rubrum, Trichophyton mentagrophytes, Epidermophyton floccosum* and *Malassezia furfur*); pathogenic yeasts; *Candida albicans* and other *Candida* species. It is also active against Gram-positive bacteria.

Hydrocortisone is a widely used topical anti-inflammatory agent of value in the treatment of inflammatory skin conditions including atopic and infantile eczema, contact sensitivity reactions and intertrigo.

5.2 Pharmacokinetic properties

Not applicable.

5.3 Preclinical safety data

No further relevant data available.

6. PHARMACEUTICAL PARTICULARS

6.1 List of excipients

Benzoic acid, butylated hydroxyanisole, liquid paraffin, ethoxylated oleic acid

glycerides, stearate esters of ethylene glycol and polyoxyethylene glycol, and water.

6.2 Incompatibilities

None stated.

6.3 Shelf life
18 months.

6.4 Special precautions for storage
Do not store above 25°C.

Avoid Freezing.

6.5 Nature and contents of container
Aluminium tubes of 30g.

6.6 Instructions for use and handling
Not applicable.

7. MARKETING AUTHORISATION HOLDER
E. R. Squibb & Sons Limited
Uxbridge Business Park,
Sanderson Road,
Uxbridge,
Middlesex UB8 1DH

8. MARKETING AUTHORISATION NUMBER(S)
PL 0034/0249

9. DATE OF FIRST AUTHORISATION/RENEWAL OF THE AUTHORISATION
9 May 1984 / 19 July 2001

10. DATE OF REVISION OF THE TEXT
24th June 2005

Ecostatin -1 Pessary

(E. R. Squibb & Sons Limited)

1. NAME OF THE MEDICINAL PRODUCT
Ecostatin-1 Pessary

2. QUALITATIVE AND QUANTITATIVE COMPOSITION
Ecostatin-1 Pessary contains Econazole Nitrate 150mg.

3. PHARMACEUTICAL FORM
Pessary

4. CLINICAL PARTICULARS

4.1 Therapeutic indications
The treatment of vaginitis due to *Candida albicans* and other yeasts.

4.2 Posology and method of administration
Adults:
The recommended dose is one pessary inserted at bedtime. The pessary should be inserted as high as possible into the vagina, using the applicator, with the patient in the supine position.

Although one course of therapy usually suffices, it may be necessary to institute a second course of therapy.

Elderly:
No specific dosage recommendations or precautions apply.

Children:
Vulvovaginal candidosis is not normally a problem in children, therefore there are no specific dosage recommendations.

4.3 Contraindications
Patients with a known history of sensitivity to any of the components of the preparation.

4.4 Special warnings and special precautions for use
Avoid contact between this product and contraceptive diaphragms and condoms since the rubber may be damaged by the preparation. To prevent re-infection with *Candida*, the male consort should be treated concurrently with Ecostatin Cream. Although one course of therapy usually suffices, it may be necessary to institute a second course of therapy.

4.5 Interaction with other medicinal products and other forms of Interaction
None known.

4.6 Pregnancy and lactation
Ecostatin-1 Pessaries are effective in the candidal vaginitis associated with pregnancy. Safety of systemic econazole has not been established but percutaneous absorption following topical application is likely to be low. However, as with other agents, Ecostatin should not be used during the first trimester of pregnancy unless the physician deems its use essential for the welfare of the patient. In pregnancy, extra care should be taken in using an applicator, to prevent the possibility of mechanical trauma.

4.7 Effects on ability to drive and use machines
None known.

4.8 Undesirable effects
Patients may rarely complain of transitory discomfort.

4.9 Overdose
There have been no recorded cases of overdose.

5. PHARMACOLOGICAL PROPERTIES

5.1 Pharmacodynamic properties
Econazole nitrate has a broad spectrum of antifungal activity. It is highly active against *Candida albicans* and other *Candida* species and is effective in controlling infections of the vagina and vulva caused by such organisms (thrush).

5.2 Pharmacokinetic properties
Not applicable.

5.3 Preclinical safety data
No further relevant information.

6. PHARMACEUTICAL PARTICULARS

6.1 List of excipients
Colloidal silicon dioxide, hard fat, natural polysaccharides, stearyl heptanoate.

6.2 Incompatibilities
None known.

6.3 Shelf life
60 months.

6.4 Special precautions for storage
Do not store above 25°C.

6.5 Nature and contents of container
Pre-formed PVC mould packed in a cardboard carton. The carton includes an applicator with directions for use.

6.6 Instructions for use and handling
No special instructions apply.

7. MARKETING AUTHORISATION HOLDER
E.R. Squibb & Sons Ltd
Uxbridge Business Park,
Sanderson Road,
Uxbridge,
Middlesex UB8 1DH

8. MARKETING AUTHORISATION NUMBER(S)
PL 0034/0266

9. DATE OF FIRST AUTHORISATION/RENEWAL OF THE AUTHORISATION
29 April 1987 / 19 May 1997 / 29 October 2002

10. DATE OF REVISION OF THE TEXT
24th June 2005

Ecostatin Cream

(E. R. Squibb & Sons Limited)

1. NAME OF THE MEDICINAL PRODUCT
Ecostatin Cream

2. QUALITATIVE AND QUANTITATIVE COMPOSITION
Ecostatin Cream contains Econazole Nitrate 1% w/w.

3. PHARMACEUTICAL FORM
Cream

4. CLINICAL PARTICULARS

4.1 Therapeutic indications
All fungal skin infections due to dermatophytes (e.g. trichophyton species), yeasts (e.g. *Candida* species), moulds and other fungi. These include ringworm (*Tinea*) infections, athlete's foot, paronychia, pityriasis versicolor, erythrasma, intertrigo, fungal nappy rash, candidal vulvitis and candidal balanitis. Bacterial skin infections due to gram-positive organisms.

4.2 Posology and method of administration
Adults and Children:
To be massaged gently into the affected and surrounding skin area morning and evening. The cream is particularly suitable for moist or weeping lesions.

Clinical improvement usually occurs promptly; however, complete disappearance of the symptoms of the disease may require prolonged treatment. Therapy should continue for several days following both clinical and mycological cure in order to prevent relapse.

Elderly:
No specific dosage recommendations.

4.3 Contraindications
Patients with a history of sensitivity to any of the components of the preparation.

4.4 Special warnings and special precautions for use
Ecostatin Cream should not be used in or near the eyes. Avoid contact with diaphragms and condoms.

4.5 Interaction with other medicinal products and other forms of Interaction
None.

4.6 Pregnancy and lactation
No specific precautions apply; systemic absorption is likely to be negligible.

4.7 Effects on ability to drive and use machines
Not applicable.

4.8 Undesirable effects
Ecostatin is well tolerated. Side-effects are limited to occasional local irritation manifested by erythema, burning or stinging sensations and pruritus.

4.9 Overdose
Not applicable.

5. PHARMACOLOGICAL PROPERTIES

5.1 Pharmacodynamic properties
Econazole nitrate is a broad spectrum antifungal agent, active against dermatophytes (trichophyton rubrum, trichophyton mentagrophytes; epidermophyton floccosum and malassezia furfur); pathogenic yeasts; *Candida albicans* and other *Candida* species. Also active against some gram-positive bacteria, e.g. *Staphylococci* and *Streptococci*.

5.2 Pharmacokinetic properties
Not applicable.

5.3 Preclinical safety data
Not applicable.

6. PHARMACEUTICAL PARTICULARS

6.1 List of excipients
Benzoic acid, butylated hydroxyanisole, ethoxylated oleic acid glycerides, liquid paraffin, stearate esters of ethylene glycol and polyoxyethylene glycol, perfume, water.

6.2 Incompatibilities
None known.

6.3 Shelf life
60 months.

6.4 Special precautions for storage
Store below 25°C. Avoid freezing.

6.5 Nature and contents of container
Blind end epoxy resin lined aluminium 15g or 30g tube packed in a carton.

The twin pack includes 3 pessaries and a 15g tube of cream.

6.6 Instructions for use and handling
No special instructions apply.

7. MARKETING AUTHORISATION HOLDER
E.R. Squibb & Sons Ltd
Uxbridge Business Park,
Sanderson Road,
Uxbridge,
Middlesex UB8 1DH

8. MARKETING AUTHORISATION NUMBER(S)
PL 0034/0231

9. DATE OF FIRST AUTHORISATION/RENEWAL OF THE AUTHORISATION
7 November 1983 / 15 June 1999

10. DATE OF REVISION OF THE TEXT
24th June 2005

Ecostatin Twin Pack

(E. R. Squibb & Sons Limited)

1. NAME OF THE MEDICINAL PRODUCT
Ecostatin Pessaries

2. QUALITATIVE AND QUANTITATIVE COMPOSITION
Each Ecostatin Pessary contains Econazole Nitrate 150mg.

3. PHARMACEUTICAL FORM
Vaginal pessary

4. CLINICAL PARTICULARS

4.1 Therapeutic indications
Vulvovaginal candidosis. In addition to vaginal treatment, the twin pack contains cream for topical application to the anogenital area.

4.2 Posology and method of administration
Adults:
One pessary to be inserted at bedtime for three consecutive nights. Administration should be continued even if menstruation occurs and despite the disappearance of signs and symptoms of the infection.

The pessary should be inserted high into the vagina while the patient is supine.

Although a three day course of therapy usually suffices, it may be necessary to institute a second course of therapy.

Note: To prevent reinfection with *Candida*, the male consort should be treated concurrently with Ecostatin Cream, applied twice daily to the external genital area during the treatment period.

Elderly:
No specific dosage recommendations or precautions apply.

Children:
Vulvovaginal candidosis is not normally a problem in children, therefore there are no specific dosage recommendations.

4.3 Contraindications
Patients with a history of sensitivity to any of the components of the preparation.

4.4 Special warnings and special precautions for use
Avoid contact between this product and contraceptive diaphragms and condoms since the rubber may be damaged by the preparation.

4.5 Interaction with other medicinal products and other forms of Interaction
None, except see Special Warnings and Special Precautions for Use, above.

4.6 Pregnancy and lactation
Ecostatin Pessaries are effective in the candidal vaginitis associated with pregnancy. Safety of systemic econazole has not been established but percutaneous absorption following topical application is likely to be low. However, as with other agents, Ecostatin should not be used during the first trimester of pregnancy unless the physician deems its use essential for the welfare of the patient. In pregnancy, extra care should be taken in using an applicator, to prevent the possibility of mechanical trauma.

4.7 Effects on ability to drive and use machines
Not applicable.

4.8 Undesirable effects
Patients may rarely complain of discomfort; this is usually transitory and disappears with continued treatment. Seldom is it necessary to discontinue treatment with econazole pessaries.

4.9 Overdose
Not applicable.

5. PHARMACOLOGICAL PROPERTIES

5.1 Pharmacodynamic properties
Econazole nitrate has a broad spectrum of antifungal activity. It is highly active against *Candida albicans* and other *Candida* species and is effective in controlling infections of the vagina and vulva caused by such organisms (thrush).

5.2 Pharmacokinetic properties
Not applicable.

5.3 Preclinical safety data
None.

6. PHARMACEUTICAL PARTICULARS

6.1 List of excipients
Hard vegetable fat.

6.2 Incompatibilities
None known.

6.3 Shelf life
60 months.

6.4 Special precautions for storage
Store below 25°C.

6.5 Nature and contents of container
3 pessaries in plastic foil lined polyvinyl chloride containers, packed in cardboard cartons, with applicator and directions for use.

The twin pack includes a 15g tube of cream.

6.6 Instructions for use and handling
No special instructions apply.

7. MARKETING AUTHORISATION HOLDER
E.R. Squibb & Sons Ltd
Uxbridge Business Park,
Sanderson Road,
Uxbridge,
Middlesex UB8 1DH

8. MARKETING AUTHORISATION NUMBER(S)
PL 0034/0233

9. DATE OF FIRST AUTHORISATION/RENEWAL OF THE AUTHORISATION
Date of first grant: 06.06.83

Date of last renewal: 15.06.99

10. DATE OF REVISION OF THE TEXT
24th June 2005

Edronax 4mg Tablets

(Pharmacia Limited)

1. NAME OF THE MEDICINAL PRODUCT
EDRONAX® 4 mg Tablets

2. QUALITATIVE AND QUANTITATIVE COMPOSITION
One tablet contains 4mg of reboxetine (as methanesulphonate)

For excipients see 6.1.

3. PHARMACEUTICAL FORM
Tablet

White, round, convex, 8 mm diameter tablet with a breakline on one side. A 'P' is marked on the left side of the breakline. A 'U' is marked on the right side of the breakline. The side opposite the breakline is marked '7671'.

4. CLINICAL PARTICULARS

4.1 Therapeutic indications
Reboxetine is indicated for the acute treatment of depressive illness/major depression and for maintaining the clinical improvement in patients initially responding to treatment.

4.2 Posology and method of administration
Edronax tablets are for oral administration.

Use in adults

The recommended therapeutic dose is 4 mg b.i.d. (8 mg/day) administered orally. The full therapeutic dose can be given upon starting treatment. After 3-4 weeks, this dose can be increased to 10 mg/day in case of incomplete clinical response. The maximum daily dose should not exceed 12 mg. The minimum effective dose has not yet been established.

Use in the elderly

Elderly patients have been studied in clinical trials at doses of 2 mg b.i.d. However, safety and efficacy have not been evaluated in placebo-controlled conditions. Therefore, as for other antidepressants that have not been studied in placebo-controlled conditions, reboxetine cannot be recommended.

Use in children

The use of reboxetine in children is not recommended since safety and efficacy have not been evaluated in this population.

Use in patients with renal or hepatic insufficiency

The starting dose in patients with renal or hepatic insufficiency should be 2 mg b.i.d which can be increased based on patient tolerance.

4.3 Contraindications
Known hypersensitivity to reboxetine or any of the components of the product.

Reboxetine is contra-indicated in pregnancy and lactation.

4.4 Special warnings and special precautions for use
As reboxetine has not been tested in patients with convulsive disorders in clinical studies and since rare cases of seizures have been reported in clinical studies, it should be given under close supervision to subjects with a history of convulsive disorders and it must be discontinued if the patient develops seizures.

Concomitant use of MAO-inhibitors and reboxetine should be avoided in view of the potential risk (tyramine-like effect) based on their mechanisms of action.

Concomitant use of reboxetine with other antidepressants (tricyclics, MAO inhibitors, SSRIs and lithium) has not been evaluated during clinical trials.

As with all antidepressants, switches to mania/hypomania have occurred during the clinical studies. Close supervision of bipolar patients is, therefore, recommended.

The risk of a suicidal attempt is inherent in depression and may persist until significant remission occurs: close patient supervision during initial drug therapy is, therefore, recommended.

Clinical experience with reboxetine in patients affected by serious concomitant systemic illnesses is limited. Close supervision should be applied in patients with current evidence of urinary retention, prostatic hypertrophy, glaucoma and history of cardiac disease.

At doses higher than the maximum recommended, orthostatic hypotension has been observed with greater frequency than that observed at recommended doses. Particular attention should be paid when administering reboxetine with other drugs known to lower blood pressure.

Clinical experience with reboxetine in the long-term treatment of elderly patients is, at present, limited. In this population, lowering of mean potassium levels was found starting from week 14; the magnitude of this reduction did not exceed 0.8 mmol/litre and potassium levels never dropped below normal limits.

4.5 Interaction with other medicinal products and other forms of Interaction
In vitro metabolism studies indicate that reboxetine is primarily metabolised by the CYP3A4 isozyme of cytochrome P450; reboxetine is not metabolized by CYP2D6. Therefore potent inhibitors of CYP3A4 (ketoconazole, nefazodone, erythromycin and fluvoxamine), would be expected to increase plasma concentrations of reboxetine. In a study in healthy volunteers, ketoconazole, a potent inhibitor of CYP3A4, was found to increase plasma concentrations of the reboxetine enantiomers by approximately 50%. Because of reboxetine's narrow therapeutic margin, inhibition of elimination is a major concern. Reboxetine, therefore should not be given together with drugs known to inhibit CYP3A4 such as azole antifungal agents, macrolide antibiotics such as erythromycin, or fluvoxamine

In vitro studies have shown that reboxetine does not inhibit the activity of the following P450 isoenzymes: CYP1A2, CYP2C9, CYP2C19 and CYP2E1. Pharmacokinetic interactions would not be expected with compounds metabolised by these enzymes. At concentrations which exceed those in clinical use, reboxetine inhibits CYP2D6 and CYP3A4, however, the results of in vivo studies suggest that interactions with other drugs metabolised by these enzymes are unlikely.

No significant reciprocal pharmacokinetic interaction has been found between reboxetine and lorazepam. During their co-administration in healthy volunteers, mild to moderate drowsiness and short lasting orthostatic acceleration of heart rate have been observed.

Reboxetine does not appear to potentiate the effect of alcohol on cognitive functions in healthy volunteers.

Concomitant use of MAO-inhibitors and reboxetine should be avoided in view of the potential risk (tyramine-like effect) based on their mechanisms of action.

Concomitant use of reboxetine with other antidepressants (tricyclics, MAO inhibitors, SSRIs and lithium) has not been evaluated during clinical trials.

Concomitant use of ergot derivatives and reboxetine might result in increased blood pressure.

Food intake delayed the absorption of reboxetine, but did not significantly influence the extent of absorption.

Although data are not available from clinical studies, the possibility of hypokalaemia with concomitant use of potassium losing diuretics should be considered.

4.6 Pregnancy and lactation
PREGNANCY

In humans experience is very limited. Therefore, administration during pregnancy should be avoided.**WOMEN OF CHILD-BEARING POTENTIAL** If conception occurs during therapy, treatment is to be discontinued as soon as pregnancy is confirmed to limit foetal exposure to the drug.**LACTATION**No information on the excretion of reboxetine in maternal milk in humans is available, reboxetine administration is not recommended in breast feeding women.

4.7 Effects on ability to drive and use machines
Reboxetine is not sedative per se. No cognitive or psychomotor impairment has been observed with reboxetine in clinical studies, also when the compound was co-administered with alcohol. However, as with all psychoactive drugs, patients should be cautioned about operating machinery and driving.

4.8 Undesirable effects
Over 2100 patients received reboxetine in clinical studies, approximately 250 of which received reboxetine for at least 1 year.

Common adverse events causing withdrawal at least twice as often on reboxetine than placebo include insomnia, dizziness, dry mouth, nausea, sweating, sensation of incomplete bladder emptying (males only), urinary hesitancy (males only) and headache.

The information below refers to short-term controlled studies. Very common or common adverse events that are at least two times higher on reboxetine than placebo are listed below.

[Very common (⩾ 1/10, Common (⩾ 1/100, < 1/10)]

Nervous system disorders:

Very common: insomnia, Common: vertigo

Cardiac disorders:

Common: tachycardia, palpitation, vasodilation, postural hypotension

Eye disorders:

Common: abnormality of accommodation

Gastrointestinal disorders:

Very common: dry mouth, constipation

Common: lack or loss of appetite

Skin and subcutaneous disorders:

Very common: sweating

Renal and urinary disorders:

Common: urinary hesitancy, sensation of incomplete bladder emptying, urinary tract infection

Reproductive system and breast disorders:

Common: erectile dysfunction (males only), ejaculatory pain (males only), ejaculatory delay (males only), testicular disorder-primarily pain (males only)

General disorders and administrative site conditions:

Common: chills

In addition there have been spontaneous reports of aggressive behaviour, cold extremities, nausea, vomiting and allergic dermatitis/rash.

As for long-term tolerability, 143 reboxetine-treated and 140 placebo-treated adult patients participated in a long term placebo controlled study. Adverse events newly emerged on long term treatment in 28% of the reboxetine treated patients and 23% of the placebo-treated patients and caused discontinuation in 4% and 1% of the cases respectively. There was a similar risk of the development of individual events with reboxetine and placebo. In the long term studies, no individual events were seen which have not been seen on short term treatment.

In short-term controlled studies of patients with depression, no clinically significant between-gender differences were noted in the frequency of treatment emergent symptoms, with the exception of urologic events (such as the sensation of incomplete bladder emptying, urinary hesitancy and urinary frequency), which were reported in a higher percentage of reboxetine-treated male patients (31.4% [143/456]) than reboxetine-treated female patients (7.0% [59/847]). In contrast, the frequency of urologic-related events was similar among male (5.0% [15/302]) and female (8.4% [37/440]) placebo-treated patients.

In the elderly population, frequency of total adverse events, as well as of individual events, was no higher than that reported above.

Signs and symptoms newly reported on abrupt discontinuation were infrequent and less frequent in patients treated with reboxetine (4%) than in those treated with placebo (6%).

In those short-term studies in depression where heart rate was assessed with ECG, reboxetine was associated with mean increases in heart rate, compared to placebo, of 6 to 12 beats per minute.

In all short-term controlled studies in depression, the mean change in pulse (in beats per minute) for reboxetine-treated patients was 3.0, 6.4 and 2.9 in the standing, sitting and supine positions respectively, compared with 0, 0, and −0.5 for placebo-treated patients in the corresponding positions. In these same studies, 0.8% of reboxetine-treated patients discontinued the drug because of tachycardia compared with 0.1% of placebo-treated patients.

4.9 Overdose

The acute toxicity studies carried out in animals indicate a very low toxicity, with a wide safety margin with respect to the pharmacologically active doses. Clinical signs and cause of death were related to CNS stimulation (mainly convulsive symptoms).

In a few cases doses higher than those recommended were administered to patients (12 mg to 20 mg/day) for a period ranging from a few days to some weeks during clinical studies: newly reported complaints include postural hypotension, anxiety and hypertension. Elderly might be particularly vulnerable to overdose.

In premarketing clinical studies, there were 5 reports of reboxetine overdose alone or in combination with other pharmacologic agents. The amount of reboxetine ingested was 52 mg as the sole agent by 1 patient and 20 mg in combination with other agents by another patient. The remaining 3 patients ingested unknown quantities of reboxetine. All 5 patients recovered fully. There were no reports of ECG abnormalities, coma, or convulsions following overdose with reboxetine alone.

In postmarketing experience, there have been few reports of overdose in patients taking reboxetine alone; none of these have proved fatal. Non-fatal overdoses in patients have been reported for patients taking up to 240 mg of reboxetine. One fatal overdose was reported in a patient who ingested reboxetine in combination with amitriptyline (doses unknown).

In case of overdose, monitoring of cardiac function and vital signs is recommended. General symptomatic supportive and/or emetic measures might be required.

5. PHARMACOLOGICAL PROPERTIES

5.1 Pharmacodynamic properties

Pharmacotherapeutic group: Antidepressants

ATC code: NO6A X18

Reboxetine is a highly selective and potent inhibitor of noradrenaline reuptake. It has only a weak effect on the 5-HT reuptake and does not affect the uptake of dopamine.

Noradrenaline reuptake inhibition and the consequent increase of noradrenaline availability in the synaptic cleft and modification of noradrenergic transmission, reportedly is among the most relevant mechanisms of action of known antidepressant drugs.

In vitro, studies have shown that reboxetine has no significant affinity for adrenergic (α_1, α_2, β) and muscarinic receptors; antagonism of such receptors has been described to be associated with cardiovascular, anticholinergic and sedative side effects of other antidepressant drugs. Reboxetine is devoid of in-vitro binding affinity for either α_1 or α_2 adrenoceptors, however, a functional interference with α-adrenoceptors at high doses in-vivo cannot be excluded.

5.2 Pharmacokinetic properties

After oral administration of a single 4 mg reboxetine dose to healthy volunteers, peak levels of about 130 ng/ml are achieved within 2 h post-dosing. Data indicate that absolute bioavailability is at least 60%.

Reboxetine plasma levels decreased monoexponentially with a half-life of about 13 h. Steady-state conditions are observed within 5 days. Linearity of the pharmacokinetics was shown in the range of single oral doses in the clinically recommended dose-ranges.

The drug appears to be distributed into total body water. Reboxetine is 97 % bound to human plasma proteins in young and 92% in elderly(with affinity markedly higher for α_1 acid glycoprotein than albumin), with no significant dependence of the concentration of drug.

Reboxetine is predominantly metabolised in vitro via cytochrome P4503A (CYP3A4). In vitro studies have shown that reboxetine does not inhibit the activity of the following isozymes of cytochrome P450: CYP1A2, CYP2C9, CYP2C19, and CYP2E1. Reboxetine inhibits both CYP2D6 and CYP3A4 with low binding affinities, but has shown no effect on the in vivo clearance of drugs metabolized by these enzymes. Reboxetine should be co-prescribed with caution with potent inhibitors of CYP3A4.

The amount of radioactivity excreted in urine accounts for 78 % of the dose. Even though unchanged drug is predominant in the systemic circulation (70% of total radioactivity, in terms of AUC), only 10% of the dose is excreted as unchanged drug in urine. These findings suggest that biotransformation rules the overall elimination of reboxetine and that metabolites excretion is limited by their formation. The main metabolic pathways identified are 2-O-dealkylation, hydroxylation of the ethoxyphenoxy ring and oxidation of the morpholine ring, followed by partial or complete glucuro- or sulpho-conjugation.

The drug is available as a racemic mixture (with both enantiomers being active in the experimental models): no chiral inversion, nor reciprocal pharmacokinetic interferences between enantiomers have been observed. Plasma levels of the more potent SS enantiomer are about two times lower and urinary excretion two times higher than those of the enantiomeric counterpart. No significant differences were observed in the terminal half-lives of the two enantiomers.

Increases in systemic exposure and half-life of approximately two-fold are observed in patients with renal insufficiency and hepatic insufficiency. Similar or somewhat greater (3-fold) increases in systemic exposure also occur in elderly patients relative to young healthy volunteers.

5.3 Preclinical safety data

Reboxetine did not induce gene mutations in bacterial or mammalian cells in vitro but induced chromosomal aberrations in human lymphocytes in vitro. Reboxetine did not cause DNA damage in yeast cells or rat hepatocytes in vitro. Reboxetine did not cause chromosomal damage in an in vivo mouse micronucleus test, and did not increase tumor incidence in carcinogenecity studies in mice and rats.

Haemosiderosis was reported in toxicity studies in rats only.

Studies in animals have not demonstrated any teratogenic effect or any effect of the compound on global reproductive performance. Dosages that produced plasma concentrations within the therapeutic range for humans induced an impairment of growth and development and long term behavioural changes in offspring of rats.

In rats reboxetine is excreted in milk.

6. PHARMACEUTICAL PARTICULARS

6.1 List of excipients

Cellulose microcrystalline

Calcium hydrogen phosphate dihydrate

Crospovidone

Silica, colloidal hydrated

Magnesium stearate

6.2 Incompatibilities

None known.

6.3 Shelf life

36 months

6.4 Special precautions for storage

Do not store above 25° C.

6.5 Nature and contents of container

The tablets are contained either in amber glass, type III, bottle, closed with an aluminium pilfer-proof screw cap equipped with a polyethylene undercap or in aluminium-PVDC / PVC-PVDC opaque blisters.

Each pack contains: 10, 20, 50, 60, 100, 120, and 180 tablets in blisters;

and 60 tablets in glass bottles.

Not all pack sizes may be marketed.

6.6 Instructions for use and handling

There are no special instructions for handling.

7. MARKETING AUTHORISATION HOLDER

Pharmacia Limited

Ramsgate Road

Sandwich

Kent

CT13 9NJ

United Kingdom

8. MARKETING AUTHORISATION NUMBER(S)

PL 0032/0216

9. DATE OF FIRST AUTHORISATION/RENEWAL OF THE AUTHORISATION

10 April 1997

10. DATE OF REVISION OF THE TEXT

2 September 2004

Edrophonium Injection BP 10mg/1ml

(Cambridge Laboratories)

1. NAME OF THE MEDICINAL PRODUCT

Edrophonium Injection BP 10mg/1ml.

2. QUALITATIVE AND QUANTITATIVE COMPOSITION

Each ampoule contains 10mg Edrophonium Chloride BP in 1ml of solution.

3. PHARMACEUTICAL FORM

Ampoules

4. CLINICAL PARTICULARS

4.1 Therapeutic indications

Myasthenia gravis, as a diagnostic test; to distinguish between overdosage and underdosage of cholinergic drugs in myasthenic patients; diagnosis of suspected 'dual block'; antagonist to non-depolarising neuromuscular blockade.

4.2 Posology and method of administration

Edrophonium Injection BP is for intramuscular or intravenous injection. In view of the possibility of provoking a cholinergic crisis it is recommended that facilities for resuscitation should be available whenever Edrophonium Injection BP is administered.

Adults - Test for myasthenia gravis:

A syringe is filled with the contents of 1 ampoule (10mg) and 2mg is given intravenously, the needle and syringe being left in situ. If no response occurs within 30 seconds, the remaining 8mg is injected. In adults with unsuitable veins, 10mg is given by intramuscular injection.

To differentiate between 'myasthenic' and 'cholinergic' crises:

In a myasthenic patient who is suffering from marked muscle weakness, in spite of taking large doses of Mestinon or Prostigmin, a test dose of 2mg Edrophonium Injection BP is given intravenously one hour after the last dose of the cholinergic compound. If therapy has been inadequate, there is a rapid, transient increase in muscle strength; if the patient has been overtreated, Edrophonium Injection BP causes a transient increase of muscle weakness.

Diagnosis of suspected 'dual block':

Edrophonium Injection BP 10mg intravenously. If the block is due to depolarisation, it is briefly potentiated, whereas in a 'dual block', it is reversed.

Children: Diagnostic tests:

A total dose of 100micrograms/kg body-weight may be given intravenously. One fifth of this dose should be injected initially; if no reaction occurs, the remainder of the dose is administered 30 seconds later.

Antagonist to non-depolarising neuromuscular blockade:

Generally, reversal of neuromuscular block with Edrophonium Injection BP should not be attempted until there is evidence of spontaneous recovery from paralysis. It is recommended that the patient be well ventilated and a patent airway maintained until complete recovery of normal respiration is assured.

Adults and children:

Edrophonium Injection BP 500 - 700micrograms/kg body-weight and atropine 7micrograms/kg body-weight, by slow intravenous injection over several minutes, is usually adequate for reversal of non-depolarising muscle relaxants within 5 - 15 minutes. The two drugs are usually given simultaneously, but in patients who show bradycardia the pulse rate should be increased to about 80/minute with atropine before administering Edrophonium Injection BP.

The speed of recovery from neuromuscular blockade is primarily determined by the intensity of the block at the time of antagonism but it is also subject to other factors, including the presence of drugs (eg. anaesthetic agents, antibiotics, antiarrhythmic drugs) and physiological changes (electrolyte and acid-base imbalance, renal impairment). These factors may prevent successful reversal with Edrophonium Injection BP or lead to recurarisation after apparently successful reversal. Therefore it is imperative that patients should not be left unattended until these possibilities have been excluded.

Elderly:

There are no specific dosage recommendations for Edrophonium Injection BP in elderly patients.

4.3 Contraindications

Edrophonium Injection BP should not be given to patients with mechanical intestinal or urinary obstruction.

Edrophonium Injection BP is contra-indicated in patients with known hypersensitivity to the drug.

4.4 Special warnings and special precautions for use

Extreme caution is required when administering Edrophonium Injection BP to patients with bronchial asthma.

Care should also be taken in patients with bradycardia, recent coronary occlusion, vagotonia, hypotension, peptic ulcer, epilepsy or Parkinsonism.

In diagnostic uses of Edrophonium Injection BP, a syringe containing 1mg of atropine should be kept at hand to counteract severe cholinergic reactions, should they occur. In view of the possibility of provoking a cholinergic crisis it is recommended that facilities for resuscitation should always be available.

When Edrophonium Injection BP is used as an antagonist to neuromuscular blockade bradycardia may occur, to a possibly dangerous level, unless atropine is given simultaneously. In this indication, Edrophonium Injection BP should not be given during cyclopropane or halothane anaesthesia; however, it may be used after withdrawal of these agents.

There is no evidence to suggest that Edrophonium Injection BP has any special effects in the elderly. However, elderly patients may be more susceptible to dysrhythmias than younger adults.

4.5 Interaction with other medicinal products and other forms of Interaction

With doses above 10mg, especially the higher dosage employed to antagonise neuromuscular blockade, Edrophonium Injection BP should not be used in conjunction with depolarising muscle relaxants such as suxamethonium as neuromuscular blockade may be potentiated and prolonged apnoea may result.

4.6 Pregnancy and lactation

The safety of Edrophonium Injection BP during pregnancy or lactation has not been established. Although the possible hazards to mother and child must be weighed against the potential benefits in every case, experience with Edrophonium Injection BP in pregnant patients with myasthenia gravis has revealed no untoward effect of the drug on the course of pregnancy.

There is no information on the excretion of Edrophonium Injection BP into breast milk. Although only negligible amounts would be expected to be present, due regard should be paid to possible effects on the breast-feeding infant.

4.7 Effects on ability to drive and use machines

None.

4.8 Undesirable effects

These may include nausea and vomiting, increased salivation, diarrhoea and abdominal cramps.

4.9 Overdose

Edrophonium Injection BP overdosage may give rise to bradycardia, arrhythmias, hypotension and bronchiolar spasm. Perspiration, gastro-intestinal hypermotility and visual disturbances may also occur.

Artificial ventilation should be instituted if respiration is severely depressed. Atropine sulphate 1 - 2mg intravenously is an antidote to the muscarinic effects.

5. PHARMACOLOGICAL PROPERTIES

5.1 Pharmacodynamic properties

Edrophonium Injection BP is an antagonist to cholinesterase, the enzyme which normally destroys acetylcholine. The action of Edrophonium Injection BP can briefly be described, therefore, as the potentiation of naturally occurring acetylcholine. It differs from Prostigmin (neostigmine) and Mestinon (pyridostigmine) in the rapidity and brevity of its action.

5.2 Pharmacokinetic properties

Following intravenous injection of Edrophonium Injection BP an initial rapid phase of elimination (0.5 - 2 minutes) precedes a much slower decline (24 - 45 minutes). It is suggested that the rapid fall in plasma concentration of edrophonium is not primarily due to metabolism and excretion but to the rapid uptake of the drug by other tissues.

5.3 Preclinical safety data

There are no pre-clinical data of relevance to the prescriber which are additional to that already included in other sections of the SPC.

6. PHARMACEUTICAL PARTICULARS

6.1 List of excipients

Sodium Sulphite anhydrous

Sodium Citrate BP

Citric Acid BP

Water for Injections BP

6.2 Incompatibilities

None known.

6.3 Shelf life

Five years.

6.4 Special precautions for storage

Protect from light.

6.5 Nature and contents of container

Colourless glass ampoules each containing 1ml of solution, in packs of 10 ampoules.

The ampoule solution is almost colourless.

6.6 Instructions for use and handling

None.

7. MARKETING AUTHORISATION HOLDER

Cambridge Laboratories Limited

Deltic House

Kingfisher Way

Silverlink Business Park

Wallsend

Tyne & Wear

NE28 9NX

8. MARKETING AUTHORISATION NUMBER(S)

PL 12070/0008

9. DATE OF FIRST AUTHORISATION/RENEWAL OF THE AUTHORISATION

24 April 1992

10. DATE OF REVISION OF THE TEXT

March 2000

Efcortelan Cream 0.5%

(GlaxoSmithKline UK)

1. NAME OF THE MEDICINAL PRODUCT

Efcortelan Cream 0.5%

2. QUALITATIVE AND QUANTITATIVE COMPOSITION

Hydrocortisone BP 0.5% $^{W}/_{W}$

3. PHARMACEUTICAL FORM

Aqueous Cream

4. CLINICAL PARTICULARS

4.1 Therapeutic indications

Hydrocortisone has topical anti-inflammatory activities of value in the treatment of a wide variety of dermatological conditions, including the following: eczema, including atopic, infantile, discoid and stasis eczemas; prurigo nodularis, neurodermatoses, seborrhoeic dermatitis, intertrigo and contact sensitivity reactions.

Efcortelan preparations can also be used in the management of insect bites and otitis externa.

Efcortelan 0.5% preparations can be used as continuation therapy in mild cases of seborrhoeic or atopic eczema once the acute inflammatory phase has passed.

4.2 Posology and method of administration

<u>Adults, children and elderly</u>

A small quantity should be applied to the affected area two or three times daily.

Efcortelan Cream is often appropriate for moist or weeping surfaces, and Efcortelan Ointment for dry-lichenified or scaly lesions, but this is not invariably so.

For topical application.

4.3 Contraindications

Skin lesions caused by infection with viruses (e.g. herpes simplex, chicken pox), fungi (e.g. candidiasis, tinea) or bacteria (e.g. impetigo).

Hypersensitivity to the preparation.

4.4 Special warnings and special precautions for use

In infants and children, long-term continuous topical therapy should be avoided where possible, as adrenal suppression can occur even without occlusion. In infants, the napkin may act as an occlusive dressing, and increase absorption. Treatment should therefore be limited, if possible, to a maximum of 7 days.

Appropriate antimicrobial therapy should be used whenever treating inflammatory lesions which have become infected. Any spread of infection requires withdrawal of topical corticosteroid therapy, and systemic administration of antimicrobial agents.

As with all corticosteroids, prolonged application to the face is undesirable.

4.5 Interaction with other medicinal products and other forms of Interaction

None.

4.6 Pregnancy and lactation

There is inadequate evidence of safety in human pregnancy. Topical application of corticosteroids to pregnant animals can cause abnormalities of fetal development including cleft palate and intrauterine growth retardation. There may therefore be a very small risk of such effects in the human fetus.

4.7 Effects on ability to drive and use machines

None.

4.8 Undesirable effects

Efcortelan preparations are usually well tolerated but if signs of hypersensitivity appear, application should be stopped immediately.

Local atrophic changes may occur where skin folds are involved, or in areas such as the nappy area in small children, where constant moist conditions favour the absorption of hydrocortisone. Sufficient systemic absorption may also occur in such sites to produce the features of hypercorticism and suppression of the HPA axis after prolonged treatment.

The effect is more likely to occur in infants and children, and if occlusive dressings are used.

There are reports of pigmentation changes and hypertrichosis with topical steroids.

Exacerbation of symptoms may occur.

4.9 Overdose

Acute overdosage is very unlikely to occur, however, in the case of chronic overdosage or misuse the features of hypercorticism may appear and in this situation topical steroids should be discontinued.

5. PHARMACOLOGICAL PROPERTIES

5.1 Pharmacodynamic properties

Hydrocortisone is the main glucocorticoid secreted by the adrenal cortex. It is used topically for its anti-inflammatory effects which suppress the clinical manifestations of the disease in a wide range of disorders where inflammation is a prominent feature.

5.2 Pharmacokinetic properties

Hydrocortisone is absorbed through the skin particularly in denuded areas. Hydrocortisone is metabolised in the liver and most body tissues to hydrogenated and degraded forms such as tetrahydrocortisone and tetrahydrocortisol. These are excreted in the urine, mainly conjugated as glucuronides, together with a very small proportion of unchanged hydrocortisone.

5.3 Preclinical safety data

There are no preclinical data of relevance to the prescriber which are additional to that in other sections of the SmPC.

6. PHARMACEUTICAL PARTICULARS

6.1 List of excipients

Chlorocresol	BP
Cetomacrogol 1000	BP
Cetostearyl alcohol	BP
White Soft Paraffin	BP
Liquid Paraffin	BP
Sodium Acid Phosphate	BP
Phosphoric Acid	BP
Sodium Hydroxide	BP
Purified Water	BP

6.2 Incompatibilities

None known.

6.3 Shelf life

24 months

6.4 Special precautions for storage

Store below 25°C.

6.5 Nature and contents of container

15gm and 30gm collapsible aluminum tubes internally coated with an epoxy resin based lacquer and closed with a wadless polypropylene cap.

6.6 Instructions for use and handling

No special instructions.

Administrative Data

7. MARKETING AUTHORISATION HOLDER

Glaxo Wellcome UK Limited,

Trading as GlaxoSmithKline UK,

Stockley Park West,

Uxbridge,

Middlesex UB11 1BT.

8. MARKETING AUTHORISATION NUMBER(S)

PL10949/0029

9. DATE OF FIRST AUTHORISATION/RENEWAL OF THE AUTHORISATION

9/12/97 / October 04

10. DATE OF REVISION OF THE TEXT

October 04

Efcortelan Cream 1%

(GlaxoSmithKline UK)

1. NAME OF THE MEDICINAL PRODUCT

Efcortelan Cream 1%

2. QUALITATIVE AND QUANTITATIVE COMPOSITION

Hydrocortisone BP 1%$^{W}/_{W}$

3. PHARMACEUTICAL FORM

Aqueous Cream

4. CLINICAL PARTICULARS

4.1 Therapeutic indications

Hydrocortisone has topical anti-inflammatory activities of value in the treatment of a wide variety of dermatological conditions, including the following: eczema, including atopic, infantile, discoid and stasis eczemas; prurigo nodularis, neurodermatoses, seborrhoeic dermatitis, intertrigo and contact sensitivity reactions.

Efcortelan preparations can also be used in the management of insect bites and otitis externa.

Efcortelan 0.5% preparations can be used as continuation therapy in mild cases of seborrhoeic or atopic eczema once the acute inflammatory phase has passed.

4.2 Posology and method of administration

<u>Adults, children and elderly</u>

A small quantity should be applied to the affected area two or three times daily.

Efcortelan Cream is often appropriate for moist or weeping surfaces, and Efcortelan Ointment for dry-lichenified or scaly lesions, but this is not invariably so.

For topical application.

4.3 Contraindications

Skin lesions caused by infection with viruses (e.g. herpes simplex, chicken pox), fungi (e.g. candidiasis, tinea) or bacteria (e.g. impetigo).

Hypersensitivity to the preparation.

4.4 Special warnings and special precautions for use
In infants and children, long-term continuous topical therapy should be avoided where possible, as adrenal suppression can occur even without occlusion. In infants, the napkin may act as an occlusive dressing, and increase absorption. Treatment should therefore be limited, if possible, to a maximum of 7 days.

Appropriate antimicrobial therapy should be used whenever treating inflammatory lesions which have become infected. Any spread of infection requires withdrawal of topical corticosteroid therapy, and systemic administration of antimicrobial agents.

As with all corticosteroids, prolonged application to the face is undesirable.

4.5 Interaction with other medicinal products and other forms of Interaction
None.

4.6 Pregnancy and lactation
There is inadequate evidence of safety in human pregnancy. Topical application of corticosteroids to pregnant animals can cause abnormalities of fetal development including cleft palate and intrauterine growth retardation. There may therefore be a very small risk of such effects in the human fetus.

4.7 Effects on ability to drive and use machines
None.

4.8 Undesirable effects
Efcortelan preparations are usually well tolerated but if signs of hypersensitivity appear, application should be stopped immediately.

Local atrophic changes may occur where skin folds are involved, or in areas such as the nappy area in small children, where constant moist conditions favour the absorption of hydrocortisone. Sufficient systemic absorption may also occur in such sites to produce the features of hypercorticism and suppression of the HPA axis after prolonged treatment.

The effect is more likely to occur in infants and children, and if occlusive dressings are used.

There are reports of pigmentation changes and hypertrichosis with topical steroids.

Exacerbation of symptoms may occur.

4.9 Overdose
Acute overdosage is very unlikely to occur, however, in the case of chronic overdosage or misuse the features of hypercorticism may appear and in this situation topical steroids should be discontinued.

5. PHARMACOLOGICAL PROPERTIES

5.1 Pharmacodynamic properties
Hydrocortisone is the main glucocorticoid secreted by the adrenal cortex. It is used topically for its anti-inflammatory effects which suppress the clinical manifestations of the disease in a wide range of disorders where inflammation is a prominent feature.

5.2 Pharmacokinetic properties
Hydrocortisone is absorbed through the skin particularly in denuded areas. Hydrocortisone is metabolised in the liver and most body tissues to hydrogenated and degraded forms such as tetrahydrocortisone and tetrahydrocortisol. These are excreted in the urine, mainly conjugated as glucuronides, together with a very small proportion of unchanged hydrocortisone.

5.3 Preclinical safety data
There are no preclinical data of relevance to the prescriber which are additional to that in other sections of the SmPC.

6. PHARMACEUTICAL PARTICULARS

6.1 List of excipients

Chlorocresol	BP
Cetomacrogol 1000	BP
Cetostearyl alcohol	BP
White Soft Paraffin	BP
Liquid Paraffin	BP
Sodium Acid Phosphate	BP
Phosphoric Acid	BP
Sodium Hydroxide	BP
Purified Water	BP

6.2 Incompatibilities
None known.

6.3 Shelf life
24 months

6.4 Special precautions for storage
Store below 25°C.

6.5 Nature and contents of container
15gm, 30gm and 50gm collapsible aluminum tubes internally coated with an epoxy resin based lacquer and closed with a wadless polypropylene cap.

6.6 Instructions for use and handling
No special instructions.

Administrative Data

7. MARKETING AUTHORISATION HOLDER
Glaxo Wellcome UK Limited,

Trading as GlaxoSmithKline UK

Stockley Park West,

Uxbridge,

Middlesex UB11 1BT.

8. MARKETING AUTHORISATION NUMBER(S)
PL10949/0030

9. DATE OF FIRST AUTHORISATION/RENEWAL OF THE AUTHORISATION
18 December 1997 / October 04

10. DATE OF REVISION OF THE TEXT
October 04

Efcortelan Cream 2.5%

(GlaxoSmithKline UK)

1. NAME OF THE MEDICINAL PRODUCT
Efcortelan Cream 2.5%

2. QUALITATIVE AND QUANTITATIVE COMPOSITION
Hydrocortisone BP 2.5%$^{W}/_{W}$

3. PHARMACEUTICAL FORM
Aqueous Cream

4. CLINICAL PARTICULARS

4.1 Therapeutic indications
Hydrocortisone has topical anti-inflammatory activities of value in the treatment of a wide variety of dermatological conditions, including the following: eczema, including atopic, infantile, discoid and stasis eczemas; prurigo nodularis, neurodermatoses, seborrhoeic dermatitis, intertrigo and contact sensitivity reactions.

Efcortelan preparations can also be used in the management of insect bites and otitis externa.

Efcortelan 0.5% preparations can be used as continuation therapy in mild cases of seborrhoeic or atopic eczema once the acute inflammatory phase has passed.

4.2 Posology and method of administration
Adults, children and elderly

A small quantity should be applied to the affected area two or three times daily.

Efcortelan Cream is often appropriate for moist or weeping surfaces, and Efcortelan Ointment for dry-lichenified or scaly lesions, but this is not invariably so.

For topical application.

4.3 Contraindications
Skin lesions caused by infection with viruses (e.g. herpes simplex, chicken pox), fungi (e.g. candidiasis, tinea) or bacteria (e.g. impetigo).

Hypersensitivity to the preparation.

4.4 Special warnings and special precautions for use
In infants and children, long-term continuous topical therapy should be avoided where possible, as adrenal suppression can occur even without occlusion. In infants, the napkin may act as an occlusive dressing, and increase absorption. Treatment should therefore be limited, if possible, to a maximum of 7 days.

Appropriate antimicrobial therapy should be used whenever treating inflammatory lesions which have become infected. Any spread of infection requires withdrawal of topical corticosteroid therapy, and systemic administration of antimicrobial agents.

As with all corticosteroids, prolonged application to the face is undesirable.

4.5 Interaction with other medicinal products and other forms of Interaction
None.

4.6 Pregnancy and lactation
There is inadequate evidence of safety in human pregnancy. Topical application of corticosteroids to pregnant animals can cause abnormalities of fetal development including cleft palate and intrauterine growth retardation. There may therefore be a very small risk of such effects in the human fetus.

4.7 Effects on ability to drive and use machines
None.

4.8 Undesirable effects
Efcortelan preparations are usually well tolerated but if signs of hypersensitivity appear, application should be stopped immediately.

Local atrophic changes may occur where skin folds are involved, or in areas such as the nappy area in small children, where constant moist conditions favour the absorption of hydrocortisone. Sufficient systemic absorption may also occur in such sites to produce the features of hypercorticism and suppression of the HPA axis after prolonged treatment.

The effect is more likely to occur in infants and children, and if occlusive dressings are used.

There are reports of pigmentation changes and hypertrichosis with topical steroids.

Exacerbation of symptoms may occur.

4.9 Overdose
Acute overdosage is very unlikely to occur, however, in the case of chronic overdosage or misuse the features of hypercorticism may appear and in this situation topical steroids should be discontinued.

5. PHARMACOLOGICAL PROPERTIES

5.1 Pharmacodynamic properties
Hydrocortisone is the main glucocorticoid secreted by the adrenal cortex. It is used topically for its anti-inflammatory effects which suppress the clinical manifestations of the disease in a wide range of disorders where inflammation is a prominent feature.

5.2 Pharmacokinetic properties
Hydrocortisone is absorbed through the skin particularly in denuded areas. Hydrocortisone is metabolised in the liver and most body tissues to hydrogenated and degraded forms such as tetrahydrocortisone and tetrahydrocortisol. These are excreted in the urine, mainly conjugated as glucuronides, together with a very small proportion of unchanged hydrocortisone.

5.3 Preclinical safety data
There are no preclinical data of relevance to the prescriber which are additional to that in other sections of the SmPC.

6. PHARMACEUTICAL PARTICULARS

6.1 List of excipients

Chlorocresol	BP
Cetomacrogol 1000	BP
Cetostearyl alcohol	BP
White Soft Paraffin	BP
Liquid Paraffin	BP
Sodium Acid Phosphate	BP
Phosphoric Acid	BP
Sodium Hydroxide	BP
Purified Water	BP

6.2 Incompatibilities
None known.

6.3 Shelf life
24 months

6.4 Special precautions for storage
Store below 25°C.

6.5 Nature and contents of container
15gm and 30gm collapsible aluminum tubes internally coated with an epoxy resin based lacquer and closed with a wadless polypropylene cap.

6.6 Instructions for use and handling
No special instructions.

Administrative Data

7. MARKETING AUTHORISATION HOLDER
Glaxo Wellcome UK Limited,

Trading as GlaxoSmithKline UK

Stockley Park West,

Uxbridge,

Middlesex UB11 1BT.

8. MARKETING AUTHORISATION NUMBER(S)
PL10949/0031

9. DATE OF FIRST AUTHORISATION/RENEWAL OF THE AUTHORISATION
18 December 1997 / October 04

10. DATE OF REVISION OF THE TEXT
October 04

Efcortelan Ointment 0.5%

(GlaxoSmithKline UK)

1. NAME OF THE MEDICINAL PRODUCT
Efcortelan Ointment 0.5%

2. QUALITATIVE AND QUANTITATIVE COMPOSITION
Hydrocortisone BP 0.5% w/w

3. PHARMACEUTICAL FORM
Ointment

4. CLINICAL PARTICULARS

4.1 Therapeutic indications
Hydrocortisone has topical anti-inflammatory activities of value in the treatment of a wide variety of dermatological conditions, including the following: eczema, including atopic, infantile, discoid and stasis eczemas: prurigo nodularis, neurodermatoses, seborrhoeic dermatitis, intertrigo and contact sensitivity reactions.

Efcortelan preparations can also be used in the management of insect bites and otitis externa.

Efcortelan 0.5% preparations can be used as continuation therapy in mild cases of seborrhoeic or atopic eczema once the acute inflammatory phase has passed.

4.2 Posology and method of administration

Adults, Children and Elderly

A small quantity should be applied to the affected area two or three times daily.

Efcortelan cream is often appropriate for moist or weeping surfaces, and Efcortelan Ointment for dry-lichenified or scaly lesions, but this is not invariably so. Efcortelan lotion is particularly suitable when a minimal application to a large area is required.

Route of Administration

For topical application.

4.3 Contraindications

Skin lesions, caused by infection with viruses (e.g. herpes simplex, chickenpox), fungi (e.g. candidiasis, tinea) or bacteria (e.g. impetigo). Hypersensitivity to the preparations.

4.4 Special warnings and special precautions for use

In infants and children, long-term continuous topical therapy should be avoided where possible, as adrenal suppression can occur even without occlusion. In infants, the napkin may act as an occlusive dressing, and increase absorption. Treatment should therefore be limited if possible, to a maximum of seven days.

Appropriate antimicrobial therapy should be used whenever treating inflammatory lesions which have become infected. Any spread of infection requires withdrawal of topical corticosteroid therapy, and systemic administration of antimicrobial agents.

As with all corticosteroids, prolonged application to the face is undesirable.

4.5 Interaction with other medicinal products and other forms of Interaction

None known.

4.6 Pregnancy and lactation

There is inadequate evidence of safety in human pregnancy. Topical application of corticosteroids to pregnant animals can cause abnormalities of fetal development including cleft palate and intra-uterine growth retardation. There may, therefore, be a very small risk of such effects in the human fetus.

4.7 Effects on ability to drive and use machines

None known.

4.8 Undesirable effects

Efcortelan preparations are usually well tolerated, but if signs of hypersensitivity appear, application should stop immediately.

Exacerbation of symptoms may occur.

Local atrophic changes may occur where skin folds are involved, or in areas such as the nappy area in small children, where constant moist conditions favour the absorption of hydrocortisone. Sufficient systemic absorption may also occur in such sites to produce the features of hypercorticism and suppression of the HPA axis after prolonged treatment. This effect is more likely to occur in infants and children, and if occlusive dressings are used.

There are reports of pigmentation changes and hypertrichosis with topical steroids.

4.9 Overdose

Acute overdosage is very unlikely to occur, however, in the case of chronic overdosage or misuse the features of hypercorticism may appear and in this situation topical steroids should be discontinued.

5. PHARMACOLOGICAL PROPERTIES

5.1 Pharmacodynamic properties

Hydrocortisone is the main glucocorticoid secreted by the adrenal cortex. It is used topically for its anti-inflammatory effects which suppress the clinical manifestations of the disease in a wide range of disorders where inflammation is a prominent feature.

5.2 Pharmacokinetic properties

Hydrocortisone is absorbed through the skin particularly in denuded areas. Hydrocortisone is metabolised in the liver and most body tissues to hydrogenated and degraded forms such as tetrahydrocortisone and tetrahydrocortisol. These are excreted in the urine, mainly conjugated as glucuronides, together with a very small proportion of unchanged hydrocortisone.

5.3 Preclinical safety data

There are no preclinical data of relevance to the prescriber which are additional to that in other sections of the SPC.

6. PHARMACEUTICAL PARTICULARS

6.1 List of excipients

White soft paraffin BP

Liquid paraffin BP

6.2 Incompatibilities

None known.

6.3 Shelf life

36 months

6.4 Special precautions for storage

Store below 25°C.

6.5 Nature and contents of container

15gm and 30gm collapsible aluminium tubes internally uncoated or coated with an epoxy resin based lacquer and closed with a wadless polypropylene cap.

6.6 Instructions for use and handling

No special instructions.

Administrative Data

7. MARKETING AUTHORISATION HOLDER

Glaxo Wellcome UK Limited

Trading as GlaxoSmithKline UK

Stockley Park West

Uxbridge

Middlesex

UB11 1BT

8. MARKETING AUTHORISATION NUMBER(S)

PL 10949/0032

9. DATE OF FIRST AUTHORISATION/RENEWAL OF THE AUTHORISATION

1 Mrach 1993 / October 04

10. DATE OF REVISION OF THE TEXT

October 04

Efcortelan Ointment 1.0%

(GlaxoSmithKline UK)

1. NAME OF THE MEDICINAL PRODUCT

Efcortelan Ointment 1.0%

2. QUALITATIVE AND QUANTITATIVE COMPOSITION

Hydrocortisone BP 1.0% w/w

3. PHARMACEUTICAL FORM

Ointment

4. CLINICAL PARTICULARS

4.1 Therapeutic indications

Hydrocortisone has topical anti-inflammatory activities of value in the treatment of a wide variety of dermatological conditions, including the following: eczema, including atopic, infantile, discoid and stasis eczemas: prurigo nodularis, neurodermatoses, seborrhoeic dermatitis, intertrigo and contact sensitivity reactions.

Efcortelan preparations can also be used in the management of insect bites and otitis externa.

Efcortelan 0.5% preparations can be used as continuation therapy in mild cases of seborrhoeic or atopic eczema once the acute inflammatory phase has passed.

4.2 Posology and method of administration

Adults, Children and Elderly

A small quantity should be applied to the affected area two or three times daily.

Efcortelan cream is often appropriate for moist or weeping surfaces, and Efcortelan Ointment for dry-lichenified or scaly lesions, but this is not invariably so. Efcortelan lotion is particularly suitable when a minimal application to a large area is required.

Route of Administration

For topical application.

4.3 Contraindications

Skin lesions, caused by infection with viruses (e.g. herpes simplex, chickenpox), fungi (e.g. candidiasis, tinea) or bacteria (e.g. impetigo). Hypersensitivity to the preparations.

4.4 Special warnings and special precautions for use

In infants and children, long-term continuous topical therapy should be avoided where possible, as adrenal suppression can occur even without occlusion. In infants, the napkin may act as an occlusive dressing, and increase absorption. Treatment should therefore be limited if possible, to a maximum of seven days.

Appropriate antimicrobial therapy should be used whenever treating inflammatory lesions which have become infected. Any spread of infection requires withdrawal of topical corticosteroid therapy, and systemic administration of antimicrobial agents.

As with all corticosteroids, prolonged application to the face is undesirable.

4.5 Interaction with other medicinal products and other forms of Interaction

None known.

4.6 Pregnancy and lactation

There is inadequate evidence of safety in human pregnancy. Topical application of corticosteroids to pregnant animals can cause abnormalities of fetal development including cleft palate and intra-uterine growth retardation. There may, therefore, be a very small risk of such effects in the human fetus.

4.7 Effects on ability to drive and use machines

None known.

4.8 Undesirable effects

Efcortelan preparations are usually well tolerated, but if signs of hypersensitivity appear, application should stop immediately.

Exacerbation of symptoms may occur.

Local atrophic changes may occur where skin folds are involved, or in areas such as the nappy area in small children, where constant moist conditions favour the absorption of hydrocortisone. Sufficient systemic absorption may also occur in such sites to produce the features of hypercorticism and suppression of the HPA axis after prolonged treatment. This effect is more likely to occur in infants and children, and if occlusive dressings are used.

There are reports of pigmentation changes and hypertrichosis with topical steroids.

4.9 Overdose

Acute overdosage is very unlikely to occur, however, in the case of chronic overdosage or misuse the features of hypercorticism may appear and in this situation topical steroids should be discontinued.

5. PHARMACOLOGICAL PROPERTIES

5.1 Pharmacodynamic properties

Hydrocortisone is the main glucocorticoid secreted by the adrenal cortex. It is used topically for its anti-inflammatory effects which suppress the clinical manifestations of the disease in a wide range of disorders where inflammation is a prominent feature.

5.2 Pharmacokinetic properties

Hydrocortisone is absorbed through the skin particularly in denuded areas. Hydrocortisone is metabolised in the liver and most body tissues to hydrogenated and degraded forms such as tetrahydrocortisone and tetrahydrocortisol. These are excreted in the urine, mainly conjugated as glucuronides, together with a very small proportion of unchanged hydrocortisone.

5.3 Preclinical safety data

There are no preclinical data of relevance to the prescriber which are additional to that in other sections of the SPC.

6. PHARMACEUTICAL PARTICULARS

6.1 List of excipients

White soft paraffin	BP
Liquid paraffin	BP

6.2 Incompatibilities

None known.

6.3 Shelf life

36 months

6.4 Special precautions for storage

Store below 25°C.

6.5 Nature and contents of container

15gm, 30gm and 50gm collapsible aluminium tubes internally uncoated or coated with an epoxy resin based lacquer and closed with a wadless polypropylene cap.

6.6 Instructions for use and handling

No special instructions.

Administrative Data

7. MARKETING AUTHORISATION HOLDER

Glaxo Wellcome UK Limited

Trading as GlaxoSmithKline UK

Stockley Park West

Uxbridge

Middlesex

UB11 1BT

8. MARKETING AUTHORISATION NUMBER(S)

PL 10949/0033

9. DATE OF FIRST AUTHORISATION/RENEWAL OF THE AUTHORISATION

1 March 1993 / October 04

10. DATE OF REVISION OF THE TEXT

October 04

Efcortelan Ointment 2.5%

(GlaxoSmithKline UK)

1. NAME OF THE MEDICINAL PRODUCT

Efcortelan Ointment 2.5%

2. QUALITATIVE AND QUANTITATIVE COMPOSITION

Hydrocortisone BP 2.5% w/w

3. PHARMACEUTICAL FORM

Ointment

4. CLINICAL PARTICULARS

4.1 Therapeutic indications

Hydrocortisone has topical anti-inflammatory activities of value in the treatment of a wide variety of dermatological conditions, including the following: eczema, including atopic, infantile, discoid and stasis eczemas: prurigo nodularis, neurodermatoses, seborrhoeic dermatitis, intertrigo and contact sensitivity reactions.

Efcortelan preparations can also be used in the management of insect bites and otitis externa.

Efcortelan 0.5% preparations can be used as continuation therapy in mild cases of seborrhoeic or atopic eczema once the acute inflammatory phase has passed.

4.2 Posology and method of administration

Adults, Children and Elderly

A small quantity should be applied to the affected area two or three times daily.

Efcortelan cream is often appropriate for moist or weeping surfaces, and Efcortelan Ointment for dry-lichenified or scaly lesions, but this is not invariably so. Efcortelan lotion is particularly suitable when a minimal application to a large area is required.

Route of Administration

For topical application.

4.3 Contraindications

Skin lesions, caused by infection with viruses (e.g. herpes simplex, chickenpox), fungi (e.g. candidiasis, tinea) or bacteria (e.g. impetigo). Hypersensitivity to the preparations.

4.4 Special warnings and special precautions for use

In infants and children, long-term continuous topical therapy should be avoided where possible, as adrenal suppression can occur even without occlusion. In infants, the napkin may act as an occlusive dressing, and increase absorption. Treatment should therefore be limited if possible, to a maximum of seven days.

Appropriate antimicrobial therapy should be used whenever treating inflammatory lesions which have become infected. Any spread of infection requires withdrawal of topical corticosteroid therapy, and systemic administration of antimicrobial agents.

As with all corticosteroids, prolonged application to the face is undesirable.

4.5 Interaction with other medicinal products and other forms of Interaction

None known.

4.6 Pregnancy and lactation

There is inadequate evidence of safety in human pregnancy. Topical application of corticosteroids to pregnant animals can cause abnormalities of fetal development including cleft palate and intra-uterine growth retardation. There may, therefore, be a very small risk of such effects in the human fetus.

4.7 Effects on ability to drive and use machines

None known.

4.8 Undesirable effects

Efcortelan preparations are usually well tolerated, but if signs of hypersensitivity appear, application should stop immediately.

Exacerbation of symptoms may occur.

Local atrophic changes may occur where skin folds are involved, or in areas such as the nappy area in small children, where constant moist conditions favour the absorption of hydrocortisone. Sufficient systemic absorption may also occur in such sites to produce the features of hypercorticism and suppression of the HPA axis after prolonged treatment. This effect is more likely to occur in infants and children, and if occlusive dressings are used.

There are reports of pigmentation changes and hypertrichosis with topical steroids.

4.9 Overdose

Acute overdosage is very unlikely to occur, however, in the case of chronic overdosage or misuse the features of hypercorticism may appear and in this situation topical steroids should be discontinued.

5. PHARMACOLOGICAL PROPERTIES

5.1 Pharmacodynamic properties

Hydrocortisone is the main glucocorticoid secreted by the adrenal cortex. It is used topically for its anti-inflammatory effects which suppress the clinical manifestations of the disease in a wide range of disorders where inflammation is a prominent feature.

5.2 Pharmacokinetic properties

Hydrocortisone is absorbed through the skin particularly in denuded areas. Hydrocortisone is metabolised in the liver and most body tissues to hydrogenated and degraded forms such as tetrahydrocortisone and tetrahydrocortisol. These are excreted in the urine, mainly conjugated as glucuronides, together with a very small proportion of unchanged hydrocortisone.

5.3 Preclinical safety data

There are no preclinical data of relevance to the prescriber which are additional to that in other sections of the SPC.

6. PHARMACEUTICAL PARTICULARS

6.1 List of excipients

White soft paraffin BP

Liquid paraffin BP

6.2 Incompatibilities

None known.

6.3 Shelf life

36 months

6.4 Special precautions for storage

Store below 25°C.

6.5 Nature and contents of container

15gm and 30gm collapsible aluminium tubes internally uncoated or coated with an epoxy resin based lacquer and closed with a wadless polypropylene cap.

6.6 Instructions for use and handling

No special instructions.

7. MARKETING AUTHORISATION HOLDER

Glaxo Wellcome UK Limited

Trading as GlaxoSmithKline UK

Stockley Park West

Uxbridge

Middlesex

UB11 1BT

8. MARKETING AUTHORISATION NUMBER(S)

PL 10949/0034

9. DATE OF FIRST AUTHORISATION/RENEWAL OF THE AUTHORISATION

1 March 1993 / October 04

10. DATE OF REVISION OF THE TEXT

October 04

Efcortesol Injection

(Sovereign Medical)

1. NAME OF THE MEDICINAL PRODUCT

Efcortesol Injection.

2. QUALITATIVE AND QUANTITATIVE COMPOSITION

Hydrocortisone Sodium Phosphate BP 13.39% $^{w}/_{v}$.

3. PHARMACEUTICAL FORM

Sterile aqueous solution.

4. CLINICAL PARTICULARS

4.1 Therapeutic indications

This presentation permits rapid use in emergency situations involving the following conditions:

Status asthmaticus and acute allergic reactions, including anaphylactic reaction to drugs. Efcortesol supplements the action of adrenaline.

Severe shock arising from surgical or accidental trauma or overwhelming infection.

Acute adrenal insufficiency caused by abnormal stress in Addison's disease, hypopituitarism, following adrenalectomy, and when adrenocortical function has been suppressed by prolonged corticosteroid therapy.

Soft tissue lesions such as tennis elbow, tenosynovitis, or bursitis.

Note: Efcortesol does not replace other forms of therapy for the treatment of shock and status asthmaticus.

4.2 Posology and method of administration

Undesirable effects may be minimised by using the lowest effective dose for the minimum period. Frequent patient review is required to titrate appropriately the dose against disease activity (see Section 4.4).

Systemic therapy in adults: 100 to 500mg hydrocortisone (1 to 5ml) administered by slow intravenous injection, taking at least half to one minute. This dose can be repeated three or four times in 24 hours, depending upon the condition being treated and the patient's response. Alternatively, Efcortesol Injection may be given as an intravenous infusion. A clinical effect is seen in two to four hours, and it persists for up to eight hours after intravenous injection. The same dose can be given by intramuscular injection, but the response is likely to be less rapid, especially in shock.

Systemic therapy in children: As a guide, infants up to 1 year may be given 25mg hydrocortisone intravenously; children 1 to 5 years, 50mg; 6 to 12 years, 100mg (1ml). This dose can be repeated three or four times in 24 hours depending upon the condition being treated and the patient's response.

Other uses: Local treatment of soft-tissue lesions - 100 to 200mg. This daily dose may be repeated on two or three occasions depending upon the patient's response.

Efcortesol Injection is not recommended for intrathecal use.

Route(s) of administration

Intravenous or intramuscular injection, or injection into soft tissues.

4.3 Contraindications

Systemic infections, unless specific anti-infective therapy is employed. Live virus immunisation. Hypersensitivity to any component.

Efcortesol Injection should not be injected directly into tendons.

4.4 Special warnings and special precautions for use

In patients who have received more than physiological doses of systemic corticosteroids (approximately 30mg hydrocortisone) for greater than three weeks, withdrawal should not be abrupt. How dose reduction should be carried out depends largely on whether the disease is likely to relapse as the dose of systemic corticosteroids is reduced. Clinical assessment of disease activity may be needed during withdrawal. If the disease is unlikely to relapse on withdrawal of systemic corticosteroids but there is uncertainty about hypothalamic-pituitary-adrenal (HPA)-axis suppression, the dose of systemic corticosteroid may be reduced rapidly to physiological doses. Once a daily dose of 30mg hydrocortisone is reached, dose reduction should be slower to allow the HPA-axis to recover.

Abrupt withdrawal of systemic corticosteroid treatment, which has continued for up to three weeks is appropriate if it is considered that the disease is unlikely to relapse. Abrupt withdrawal of doses of up to 160mg hydrocortisone for three weeks is unlikely to lead to clinically relevant HPA-axis suppression, in the majority of patients. In the following patient groups, gradual withdrawal of systemic corticosteroid therapy should be *considered* even after courses lasting three weeks or less:

- Patients who have had repeated courses of systemic corticosteroids, particularly if taken for greater than three weeks.
- When a short course has been prescribed within one year of cessation of long-term therapy (months or years).
- Patients who may have reasons for adrenocortical insufficiency other than exogenous corticosteroid therapy.
- Patients receiving doses of systemic corticosteroid greater than 160mg hydrocortisone.
- Patients repeatedly taking doses in the evening.

Suppression of the HPA-axis and other undesirable effects may be minimised by using the lowest effective dose for the minimum period (see Section 4.2). The pronounced hormonal effects associated with prolonged corticosteroid therapy will probably not be seen when this injection is used for short term adjunctive therapy in shock. Frequent patient review is required to titrate appropriately the dose against disease activity.

Patients should carry a 'steroid treatment' card which gives clear guidance on the precautions to be taken to minimise risk and which provides details of prescriber, drug, dosage and the duration of treatment.

Suppression of the inflammatory response and immune function increases the susceptibility to infections and their severity. The clinical presentation may often be atypical and serious infections such as septicaemia and tuberculosis may be masked and may reach an advanced stage before recognised.

Chickenpox is of particular concern since this normally minor illness may be fatal in immunosuppressed patients. Patients without a definite history of chickenpox should be advised to avoid close personal contact with chickenpox or herpes zoster and if exposed they should seek urgent medical attention. If the patient is a child, parents must be given the above advice. Passive immunisation with varicella zoster immunoglobulin (VZIG) is needed by exposed non-immune patients who are receiving systemic corticosteroids or who have used them within the previous three months; this should be given within 10 days of exposure to chickenpox. If a diagnosis of chickenpox is confirmed, the illness warrants specialist care and urgent treatment. Corticosteroids should not be stopped and the dose may need to be increased.

Patients should be advised to take particular care to avoid exposure to measles and to seek immediate medical advice if exposure occurs. Prophylaxis with intramuscular normal immunoglobulins may be needed.

Live vaccines should not be given to individuals with impaired immune responsiveness. The antibody response to other vaccines may be diminished.

Adrenal cortical atrophy develops during prolonged therapy and may persist for years after stopping treatment. Withdrawal of corticosteroids after prolonged therapy must therefore always be gradual to avoid acute adrenal insufficiency, being tapered off over weeks or months according to the dose and duration of treatment. During prolonged therapy any intercurrent illness, trauma or surgical procedure will require a temporary increase in dosage; if corticosteroids have been stopped following prolonged therapy they may need to be temporarily re-introduced.

Because of the possibility of fluid retention, care must be taken when corticosteroids are administered to patients with renal insufficiency or congestive heart failure.

Corticosteroids may worsen diabetes mellitus, osteoporosis, hypertension, glaucoma and epilepsy and therefore patients with these conditions or a family history should be monitored frequently.

Care is required and frequent patient monitoring necessary where there is a history of severe affective disorders (especially a previous history of steroid psychosis), previous steroid myopathy, peptic ulceration or patients with a history of tuberculosis.

In patients with liver failure, blood levels of corticosteroid may be increased, as with other drugs which are metabolised in the liver and therefore patients should be monitored frequently. Care and monitoring is also required in patients with renal insufficiency.

4.5 Interaction with other medicinal products and other forms of Interaction

Drug interactions: rifampicin, rifabutin, carbamazepine, phenobarbitone, phenytoin, primidone, ephedrine and aminoglutethimide enhance the metabolism of corticosteroids and its therapeutic effects may be reduced.

The desired effects of hypoglycaemic agents (including insulin), anti-hypertensives and diuretics are antagonised by corticosteroids, and the hypokalaemic effects of acetazolamide, loop diuretics, thiazide diuretics and carbenoxolone are enhanced. The efficacy of coumarin anticoagulants may be enhanced by concurrent corticosteroid therapy and close monitoring of the INR or prothrombin time is required to avoid spontaneous bleeding.

The renal clearance of salicylates is increased by corticosteroids and steroid withdrawal may result in salicylate intoxication.

Steroids may reduce the effects of anticholinesterases in myasthenia gravis and cholecystographic x-ray media.

Oestrogens may potentiate the effects of glucocorticoids.

4.6 Pregnancy and lactation

Pregnancy: The ability of corticosteroids to cross placenta varies between individual drugs, however, hydrocortisone readily crosses the placenta.

Administration of corticosteroids to pregnant animals can cause abnormalities of foetal development including cleft palate, intra-uterine growth retardation and effects on brain growth and development. There is no evidence that corticosteroids result in an increased incidence of congenital abnormalities, such as cleft palate/lip in man. However, when administered for prolonged periods or repeatedly during pregnancy, corticosteroids may increase the risk of intra-uterine growth retardation. Hypoadrenalism may, in theory, occur in the neonate following prenatal exposure to corticosteroids but usually resolves spontaneously following birth and is rarely clinically important. As with all drugs, corticosteroids should only be prescribed when the benefits to the mother and child outweigh the risks. When corticosteroids are essential however, patients with normal pregnancies may be treated as though they were in the non-gravid state.

Patients with pre-eclampsia or fluid retention require close monitoring.

Depression of hormone levels has been described in pregnancy but the significance of this finding is not clear.

Lactation:

Corticosteroids are excreted in breast milk, although no data are available for hydrocortisone. Doses of up to 160mg daily of hydrocortisone are unlikely to cause systemic effects in the infant. Infants of mothers taking higher doses than this may have a degree of adrenal suppression but the benefits of breast feeding are likely to outweigh any theoretical risk.

4.7 Effects on ability to drive and use machines

None stated.

4.8 Undesirable effects

Side effects: Paraesthesia may occur following intravenous administration and is probably related to the rate of injection. It is often localised to the genital area but in some cases may radiate over the entire body. The unpleasant and sometimes painful sensation usually passes off within a few minutes and no sequelae have been reported. The effect seems to be related to the sodium phosphate salt of hydrocortisone.

The incidence of predictable undesirable effects, including hypothalamic-pituitary-adrenal suppression correlates with the relative potency of the drug, dosage, timing of administration and the duration of treatment. (see Section 4.4).

Endocrine/metabolic

Suppression of the hypothalamic-pituitary-adrenal axis, growth suppression in infancy, childhood and adolescence, menstrual irregularity and amenorrhoea, cushingoid faces, hirsutism, weight gain, impaired carbohydrate tolerance with increased requirement for anti-diabetic therapy. Negative protein and calcium balance. Increased appetite.

Anti-inflammatory and immunosuppressive effects

Increased susceptibility and severity of infections with suppression of clinical symptoms and signs, opportunistic infections, recurrence of dormant tuberculosis (see Section 4.4).

Musculoskeletal

Osteoporosis, vertebral and long bone fractures, avascular osteonecrosis, tendon rupture. Proximal myopathy.

Fluid and electrolyte disturbance

Sodium and water retention, hypertension, potassium loss, hypokalaemic alkalosis.

Neuropsychiatric

Euphoria, psychological dependence, depression, insomnia and aggravation of schizophrenia, increased intra-cranial pressure with papilloedema in children (pseudotumour cerebri), usually after treatment withdrawal. Aggravation of epilepsy.

Ophthalmic

Increased intra-ocular pressure, glaucoma, papilloedema, posterior subcapsular cataracts, corneal or scleral thinning, exacerbation of ophthalmic viral or fungal diseases.

Gastrointestinal

Dyspepsia, peptic ulceration with perforation and haemorrhage, acute pancreatitis, candidiasis.

Dermatological

Impaired healing, skin atrophy, bruising, telangiectasia, striae, acne.

General

Hypersensitivity including anaphylaxis, has been reported. Leucocytosis. Thrombo-embolism. Flushing and pruritis.

Withdrawal symptoms and signs

Too rapid a reduction of corticosteroid dosage following prolonged treatment can lead to acute adrenal insufficiency, hypotension and death. (see Section 4.4)

A 'withdrawal syndrome' may also occur including, fever, myalgia, arthralgia, rhinitis, conjunctivitis, painful itchy skin nodules and loss of weight.

Use in children: Corticosteroids cause dose-related growth retardation in infancy, childhood and adolescence, which may be irreversible.

Use in the elderly: The common adverse effects of systemic corticosteroids may be associated with more serious consequences in old age, especially osteoporosis, hypertension, hypokalaemia, diabetes, susceptibility to infections and thinning of the skin. Close clinical supervision is required to avoid life-threatening reactions.

4.9 Overdose

None stated.

5. PHARMACOLOGICAL PROPERTIES

5.1 Pharmacodynamic properties

Hydrocortisone is a glucocorticoid with anti-inflammatory properties.

5.2 Pharmacokinetic properties

Hydrocortisone is readily absorbed from the gastrointestinal tract and peak blood concentrations are attained in about an hour. It is more than 90% bound to plasma proteins.

Hydrocortisone is metabolised in the liver and most body tissues to hydrogenated and degradated forms such as tetrahydrocortisone and tetrahydrocortisol.

These are then excreted in the urine, mainly conjugated as glucuronides, together with a very small proportion of unchanged hydrocortisone.

5.3 Preclinical safety data

There are no preclinical data of relevance to the prescriber which are additional to that in other sections of the SPC.

6. PHARMACEUTICAL PARTICULARS

6.1 List of excipients

Disodium Edetate

Disodium Hydrogen Phosphate, Anhydrous

Sodium Acid Phosphate

Sodium Formaldehyde Bisulphite Monohydrate

Phosphoric Acid (10% solution)

Water for injections

6.2 Incompatibilities

None known.

6.3 Shelf life

24 months

6.4 Special precautions for storage

Store below 25°C. Keep the ampoules in the outer carton.

6.5 Nature and contents of container

1ml and 5ml neutral glass ampoules.

6.6 Instructions for use and handling

No special instructions

7. MARKETING AUTHORISATION HOLDER

Waymade PLC *Trading as* Sovereign Medical

Sovereign House

Miles Gray Road

Basildon

Essex

SS14 3FR

8. MARKETING AUTHORISATION NUMBER(S)

PL 06464/0915

9. DATE OF FIRST AUTHORISATION/RENEWAL OF THE AUTHORISATION

16 December 1999

10. DATE OF REVISION OF THE TEXT

February 2004

Efexor

(Wyeth Pharmaceuticals)

1. NAME OF THE MEDICINAL PRODUCT

Efexor*

2. QUALITATIVE AND QUANTITATIVE COMPOSITION

Efexor tablets contain 37.5mg, 50mg or 75mg of venlafaxine as hydrochloride.

3. PHARMACEUTICAL FORM

Tablet

Efexor are peach coloured, shield-shaped tablets impressed with the tablet strength and embossed with a "W" on one side, and plain on the other.

4. CLINICAL PARTICULARS

4.1 Therapeutic indications

Moderate to severe major depressive disorder

Initiation of treatment with venlafaxine should be restricted to specialist care and treatment should be managed under specialist supervision or shared care arrangements.

Efexor is indicated for the treatment of moderate to severe major depressive disorder including depression accompanied by anxiety. All patients should be evaluated for the risk of suicidality and monitored for clinical worsening (see section 4.4).

Following an initial response Efexor is indicated for the prevention of relapses of the initial episode of depression or for the prevention of the recurrence of new episodes.

4.2 Posology and method of administration

Treatment with Efexor should not be started until 14 days after discontinuing a monoamine oxidase inhibitor (MAOI).

Depression:

The recommended dose is 75mg per day given in two divided doses (37.5mg twice daily). Most patients respond to this dose.

If, after an adequate trial and evaluation, further clinical improvement is required, the dose may be increased to 150mg per day given in two divided doses (75mg twice daily). There may be an increased risk of side effects at higher doses and dose increments should be made only after a clinical evaluation and after at least 3-4 weeks of therapy (see section 4.4). The lowest effective dose should be maintained.

In more severely depressed or hospitalised patients, and under close supervision of a physician, the daily dose may then be increased by up to 75mg every two or three days until the desired response is achieved. The maximum recommended dose is 375mg per day. The dose should then be gradually reduced, to the minimum effective dose consistent with patient response and tolerance. A limited number of tablets should be provided to reduce the risk from overdose (see section 4.4).

Usually, the dosage for prevention of relapse or for prevention of recurrence of a new episode is similar to that used during the index episode. Patients should be re-assessed regularly in order to evaluate the benefit of long-term therapy.

It is recommended that Efexor be taken with food.

Patients with Renal or Hepatic Impairment:

For patients with mild renal impairment (GFR > 30ml/minute) or mild hepatic impairment (PT < 14 seconds), no change in dosage is necessary.

For patients with moderate renal impairment (GFR 10-30ml/minute) or moderate hepatic impairment (PT 14-18 seconds), the dose should be reduced by 50%. This dose may be given once daily due to the longer half-lives of venlafaxine and O-desmethylvenlafaxine (ODV) in these patients.

Insufficient data are available to support the use of Efexor in patients with severe renal impairment (GFR < 10ml/minute) or severe hepatic impairment (PT > 18 seconds).

Elderly Patients:

No adjustment in the usual dosage is recommended for elderly patients. However, as with any therapy, caution should be exercised in treating the elderly (e.g. due to the possibility of renal impairment. See also dosage recommendations for renal impairment). The lowest effective dose should always be used and patients should be carefully monitored when an increase in the dose is required.

Children/Adolescents:

Controlled clinical studies in children and adolescents with Major Depressive Disorder failed to demonstrate efficacy and do not support the use of Efexor in these patients *(see sections 4.3 Contra-indications and 4.8 Undesirable Effects).*

The efficacy and safety of Efexor for other indications in children and adolescents under the age of 18 have not yet been established.

Maintenance/Continuation/Extended Treatment:

The physician should periodically re-evaluate the usefulness of long-term treatment with Efexor for the individual patient. It is generally agreed that acute episodes of major depression require several months or longer of sustained therapy. Efexor has been shown to be efficacious during long-term (up to 12 months) treatment.

In clinical trials venlafaxine was demonstrated to be effective for preventing relapse, or recurrence of new episodes, in patients responding to venlafaxine treatment during the index episode.

Withdrawal symptoms seen on discontinuation of venlafaxine

Abrupt discontinuation should be avoided (see section 4.4 Special Warnings and Special Precautions for Use and section 4.8 Undesirable Effects). Following treatment with daily doses of venlafaxine greater than 75mg for more than one week, it is recommended that when discontinuing treatment the dose should be gradually reduced over at least a further week. If high doses have been used for more than 6 weeks tapering over at least a 2 week period is recommended. If intolerable symptoms occur following a decrease in the dose or upon discontinuation of treatment, then resuming the previously prescribed dose may be considered. Subsequently, the physician may continue decreasing the dose, but at a more gradual rate.

4.3 Contraindications

1. Known hypersensitivity to venlafaxine or any other component of the product.

2. Concomitant use of venlafaxine with monoamine oxidase inhibitors *(See Interactions with other Medicaments and Other Forms of Interactions)*.

3. Efexor should not be used in children and adolescents under the age of 18 years with Major Depressive Disorder *(see section 4.8 Undesirable Effects)*.

4. Venlafaxine should not be used in patients with heart disease, e.g. cardiac failure, coronary artery disease, ECG abnormalities including pre-existing QT interval prolongation, patients with electrolyte imbalance or in patients who are hypertensive (see section 4.4).

4.4 Special warnings and special precautions for use

1. Suicide/suicidal thoughts

Depression is associated with an increased risk of suicidal thoughts, self harm and suicide (suicide-related events). This risk persists until significant remission occurs. As improvement may not occur during the first few weeks or more of treatment, patients should be closely monitored until such improvement occurs. It is general clinical experience that the risk of self harm is highest shortly after presentation and the risk of suicide may increase again in the early stages of recovery. Furthermore, there is evidence that in a small group of people, antidepressants may increase the risk of suicidal thoughts and self-harm.

Other psychiatric conditions for which venlafaxine is prescribed can also be associated with an increased risk of suicide-related events. In addition, these conditions may be co-morbid with major depressive disorder. The same precautions observed when treating patients with major depressive disorder should therefore be observed when treating patients with other psychiatric disorders.

Patients with a history of suicide-related events, those exhibiting a significant degree of suicidal ideation prior to commencement of treatment, and young adults, are at a greater risk of suicidal thoughts or suicide attempts, and should receive careful monitoring during treatment.

Patients, (and caregivers of patients) should be alerted about the need to monitor for the emergence of suicidal thoughts and to seek medical advice immediately if these symptoms present.

2. Withdrawal symptoms seen on discontinuation of venlafaxine treatment

Withdrawal symptoms when treatment is discontinued are common, particularly if discontinuation is abrupt (see section 4.8 Undesirable effects). In clinical trials adverse events seen on treatment discontinuation occurred in approximately 31% of patients treated with venlafaxine and in approximately 17% of placebo patients. The risk of withdrawal symptoms may be dependent on several factors including the duration and dose of therapy and the rate of dose reduction.

Dizziness, sensory disturbances (including paraesthesia and electric shock sensations), sleep disturbances (including insomnia and abnormal dreams), agitation or anxiety, nausea and/or vomiting, tremor, sweating, headache, diarrhoea, palpitations and emotional instability are the most commonly reported withdrawal reactions. Generally these symptoms are mild to moderate, however, in some patients they may be severe in intensity. They usually occur within the first few days of discontinuing treatment, but there have been very rare reports of such symptoms in patients who have inadvertently missed a dose. Generally these symptoms are self-limiting and usually resolve within 2 weeks, though in some individuals they may be prolonged (2-3 months or more). It is therefore advised that venlafaxine should be gradually tapered when discontinuing treatment over a period of several weeks or months, according to the patient's needs (see "Withdrawal Symptoms Seen on Discontinuation of Venlafaxine", Section 4.2 Posology and Method of Administration).

3. Activation of mania or hypomania has been reported rarely in patients who have received antidepressants, including venlafaxine. As with all antidepressants, Efexor should be used with caution in patients with a history of mania.

4. Treatment with venlafaxine (especially starting and discontinuing treatment) has been associated with reports of aggression.

5. **Psychomotor restlessness**: The use of venlafaxine has been associated with the development of psychomotor restlessness, which clinically may be very similar to akathisia, characterised by a subjectively unpleasant or distressing restlessness and need to move often accompanied by an inability to sit or stand still. This is most likely to occur within the first few weeks of treatment. In patients who develop these symptoms, increasing the dose may be detrimental and it may be necessary to review the use of venlafaxine.

6. There have been reports of cardiotoxicity associated with therapeutic doses of venlafaxine. Before starting treatment with venlafaxine, a baseline ECG and blood pressure measurement should be performed and blood pressure should be monitored at regular intervals.

7. Significant electrocardiogram findings were observed in 0.8% of venlafaxine-treated patients compared with 0.7% of placebo-treated patients. Significant changes in PR, QRS or QTc intervals were rarely observed in patients treated with venlafaxine during clinical trials.

8. Seizures are a potential risk with antidepressant drugs, especially in overdose. Efexor should be introduced with caution in patients with a history of seizure and should be discontinued in any patient developing a seizure or if there is an increase in seizure frequency. Efexor should be avoided in patients with unstable epilepsy and patients with controlled epilepsy should be carefully monitored (see section 4.8).

9. Due to the possibility of drug abuse with CNS-active drugs, physicians should evaluate patients for a history of drug abuse, and follow such patients closely. Clinical studies have shown no evidence of drug-seeking behaviour, development of tolerance, or dose escalation over time among patients taking venlafaxine.

10. Increases in heart rate can occur, particularly at high doses. In clinical trials the mean heart rate was increased by approximately 4 beats/minute in patients treated with venlafaxine. Caution should be exercised in patients whose underlying conditions might be compromised by increases in heart rate.

11. Dosage should be reduced in patients with moderate-severe renal impairment or hepatic cirrhosis (see sections 4.2 and 4.5).

12. Postural hypotension has been observed occasionally during venlafaxine treatment. Patients, especially the elderly, should be alerted to the possibility of dizziness or unsteadiness.

13. Hyponatraemia (usually in the elderly and possibly due to inappropriate secretion of antidiuretic hormone) has been associated with all types of antidepressants and should be considered in all patients who develop drowsiness, confusion or convulsions while taking an antidepressant.

14. Mydriasis has been reported in association with venlafaxine; therefore patients with raised intra-ocular pressure or at a risk of narrow angle glaucoma should be monitored closely.

15. There have been reports of cutaneous bleeding abnormalities, such as ecchymosis and purpura, with serotonin-reuptake inhibitors (SSRIs). Other bleeding manifestations (e.g. gastrointestinal bleeding and mucous membrane bleeding) have been reported. Caution is advised in patients predisposed to bleeding due to factors such as age, underlying medical conditions or concomitant medications.

16. Clinically relevant increases in serum cholesterol were recorded in 5.3% of venlafaxine-treated patients and 0.0% of placebo-treated patients treated for at least 3 months in placebo-controlled trials. Measurement of serum cholesterol levels should be considered during long-term treatment.

17. The safety and efficacy of venlafaxine therapy in combination with weight loss agents, including phentermine, have not been established. Co-administration of venlafaxine and weight loss agents is not recommended. Venlafaxine is not indicated for weight loss alone or in combination with other products.

18. As with SSRIs, venlafaxine should be used with caution in patients already receiving neuroleptics, since symptoms suggestive of Neuroleptic Malignant Syndrome cases have been reported with this combination.

4.5 Interaction with other medicinal products and other forms of Interaction

MAOIs: Adverse reactions, some serious, have been reported when venlafaxine therapy is initiated soon after discontinuation of an MAOI, and when an MAOI is initiated soon after discontinuation of venlafaxine. These reactions have included tremor, myoclonus, diaphoresis, nausea, vomiting, flushing, dizziness, andhyperthermia with features resembling neuroleptic malignant syndrome, seizures and death. Do not use Efexor in combination with an MAOI, or within at least 14 days of discontinuing MAOI treatment. Allow at least 7 days after stopping Efexor before starting an MAOI (see also Contra-indications).

Serotonergic drugs: Based on the known mechanism of action of venlafaxine and the potential for serotonergic syndrome, caution is advised when venlafaxine is co-administered with drugs that may affect the serotonergic neurotransmitter systems (such as triptans, SSRIs or lithium).

Lithium: Reports have been received of an interaction between lithium and venlafaxine leading to increased lithium levels.

Imipramine/desipramine: The metabolism of imipramine and its metabolite 2-OH-imipramine were unaffected by venlafaxine although the total renal clearance of 2-hydroxydesipramine was reduced and desipramine AUC and C_{max} were increased by approximately 35%.

Haloperidol: In a pharmacokinetic study co-administration of venlafaxine with a single 2mg oral dose of haloperidol resulted in a 42% decrease in renal clearance, a 70% increase in AUC and an 88% increase in C_{max} for haloperidol. The elimination half-life remained unchanged.

Diazepam: The pharmacokinetic profiles of venlafaxine and ODV were not significantly altered by the administration of diazepam. Venlafaxine has no effect on the pharmacokinetic profile of diazepam or on the psychomotor or psychometric effects induced by diazepam.

Clozapine: Increased levels of clozapine, that were temporally associated with adverse events, including seizures, have been reported following the addition of venlafaxine.

Alcohol: Venlafaxine has been shown not to increase the impairment of mental or motor skills caused by ethanol. However, as with all CNS-active drugs, patients should be advised to avoid alcohol consumption while taking Efexor.

ECT: There is little clinical experience of the concurrent use of venlafaxine with ECT. As prolonged seizure activity has been reported with concomitant SSRI antidepressants, caution is advised.

Drugs metabolised by Cytochrome P450 isoenzymes: The major elimination pathways for venlafaxine are through CYP2D6 and CYP3A4. Venlafaxine is primarily metabolised to its active metabolite, ODV, by the cytochrome P450 enzyme CYP2D6. Co-administration of ketoconazole suggests that inhibition of CYP3A4 may result in increased venlafaxine plasma levels in poor CYP2D6 metabolisers. Caution should be used with concomitant intake of drugs which inhibit either CYP2D6 or CYP3A4.

Studies indicate that venlafaxine is a relatively weak inhibitor of CYP2D6. Venlafaxine did not inhibit CYP1A2, CYP2C9 or CYP3A4. This was confirmed by *in vivo* studies with the following drugs: alprazolam (CYP3A4), caffeine (CYP1A2), carbamazepine (CYP3A4) and diazepam (CYP3A4 and CYP2C19).

Cimetidine: Cimetidine inhibited the first-pass metabolism of venlafaxine but had no significant effect on the formation or elimination of ODV, which is present in much greater quantities in the systemic circulation. No dosage adjustment therefore seems necessary when Efexor is co-administered with cimetidine. For elderly patients, or patients with hepatic dysfunction the interaction could potentially be more pronounced, and for such patients clinical monitoring is indicated when Efexor is administered with cimetidine.

Warfarin: Potentiation of anticoagulant effects including increases in PT or INR have been reported in patients taking warfarin following the addition of venlafaxine.

Indinavir: A pharmacokinetic study with indinavir has shown a 28% decrease in AUC and a 36% decrease in C_{max} for indinavir. Indinavir did not affect the pharmacokinetics of venlafaxine and ODV. The clinical significance of this interaction is not known.

4.6 Pregnancy and lactation

There are no adequate data from the use of venlafaxine in pregnant women. Animal studies are insufficient with respect to effects on pregnancy. The potential risk for humans is unknown. Efexor should not be used during pregnancy unless clearly necessary. If venlafaxine is used until or shortly before birth, discontinuation effects in the newborn should be considered.

There is evidence to suggest that venlafaxine and its metabolite, ODV, transfers into breast milk. Therefore, a decision should be made whether or not to breast-feed or to discontinue venlafaxine.

4.7 Effects on ability to drive and use machines

Although venlafaxine has been shown not to affect psychomotor, cognitive, or complex behaviour performance in healthy volunteers, any psychoactive drug may impair judgement, thinking or motor skills. Therefore patients should be cautioned about their ability to drive or operate hazardous machinery.

4.8 Undesirable effects

See also Special Warnings and Special Precautions for Use.

The most commonly observed adverse events associated with the use of venlafaxine in clinical trials, and which occurred more frequently than those which were associated with placebo were: nausea, insomnia, dry mouth, somnolence, dizziness, constipation, sweating, nervousness, asthenia and abnormal ejaculation/orgasm.

The occurrence of most of these adverse events was dose-related, and the majority of them decreased in intensity and frequency over time. They generally did not lead to cessation of treatment.

Adverse events observed with venlafaxine, from both spontaneous and clinical trials reports, are classified in body systems and listed below as very common >1/10); common (<1/10 and >1/100); uncommon (<1/100 and >1/1000); rare (<1/1000);very rare (<1/10,000):

Blood and lymphatic system disorders - Uncommon: ecchymosis, mucous membrane bleeding; Rare: prolonged bleeding time, haemorrhage, thrombocytopenia; Very rare: blood dyscrasias (including agranulocytosis, aplastic anaemia, neutropenia and pancytopenia).

Cardiovascular and vascular disorders(*see Special Warnings and Special Precautions for Use*) - Common:hypertension, palpitation, vasodilatation; Uncommon: hypotension/ postural hypotension, syncope, arrhythmias (including tachycardia); Very rare: Torsade de Pointes, QT prolongation, ventricular tachycardia, ventricular fibrillation.

Gastrointestinal disorders - Very common: constipation, nausea (see below); Common: anorexia, appetite decreased, diarrhoea, dyspepsia, vomiting; Uncommon: bruxism; Rare: gastrointestinal bleeding; Very rare: pancreatitis.

General disorders - Very common: asthenia, headache; Common: abdominal pain, chills, pyrexia; Rare: anaphylaxis

Metabolic and nutritional disorders - Common: serum cholesterol increased (particularly with prolonged administration and possibly with higher doses *(seeSpecial Warnings and Special Precautions for Use)*, weight gain or loss; Uncommon: hyponatraemia including SIADH *(see Special Warnings and Special Precautions for Use)*, increased liver enzymes *(see below)*; Rare: hepatitis; Very rare: prolactin increased.

Musculo-skeletal disorders - Common: arthralgia, myalgia; Uncommon: muscle spasm; Very rare: rhabdomyolysis.

Neurological disorders - Very common: dizziness, dry mouth, insomnia, nervousness, somnolence; Common: abnormal dreams, agitation, anxiety, confusion, hypertonia, paraesthesia, tremor; Uncommon: apathy, hallucinations, myoclonus; Rare: ataxia anddisorders of balance and co-ordination, speech disorders including dysarthria, mania or hypomania *(see Special Warnings and Special Precautions for Use)*, neuroleptic malignant syndrome-like effects, seizures *(see below and Special Warnings and Special Precautions for Use)*, serotonergic syndrome; Very rare: delirium, extrapyramidal disorders including dyskinesia and dystonia, tardive dyskinesia, psychomotor restlessness/akathisia (see section 4.4 Special Warnings and Special Precautions for Use).

Renal and urinary disorders - Common: urinary frequency; Uncommon: urinary retention.

Reproductive and breast disorders - Very common: anorgasmia, erectile dysfunction, abnormal ejaculation/ orgasm; Common: decreased libido, impotence, menstrual cycle disorders; Uncommon: menorrhagia; Rare: galactorrhoea.

Respiratory system disorders - Common: dyspnoea, yawning; Very rare: pulmonary eosinophilia.

Skin and subcutaneous tissue disorders -Very common: sweating (including night sweats); Common: pruritus, rash; Uncommon: angioedema, maculopapular eruptions, urticaria, photosensitivity reactions, alopecia; Rare: erythema multiforme, Stevens Johnson syndrome.

Special senses - Common: abnormal vision/ accommodation, mydriasis, tinnitus; Uncommon: altered taste sensation.

Adverse events from paediatric clinical trials

In paediatric MDD clinical trials the following adverse events were reported at a frequency of at least 2% of patients and occurred at a rate of at least twice that of placebo: abdominal pain, chest pain, tachycardia, anorexia, weight loss, constipation, dyspepsia, nausea, ecchymosis, epistaxis, mydriasis, myalgia, dizziness, emotional lability, tremor, hostility and suicidal ideation.

Withdrawal symptoms seen on discontinuation of venlafaxine treatment

Discontinuation of venlafaxine (particularly when abrupt) commonly leads to withdrawal symptoms. Dizziness, sensory disturbances (including paraesthesia and electric shock sensations), sleep disturbances (including insomnia and abnormal dreams), agitation or anxiety, nausea and/or vomiting, tremor, sweating, headache, diarrhoea, palpitations and emotional instability are the most commonly reported withdrawal reactions. Additional withdrawal reactions include hypomania, nervousness, confusion, fatigue, somnolence, convulsion, vertigo, tinnitus, dry mouth and anorexia. Generally these events are mild to moderate and are self-limiting, however, in some patients they may be severe and/or prolonged. It is therefore advised that when venlafaxine treatment is no longer required, gradual discontinuation by dose tapering should be carried out (see section 4.2 Posology and Method of Administration and section 4.4 Special Warnings and Special Precautions for use).

Special Notes:

In all premarketing depression trials with venlafaxine tablets, seizures were reported in 0.3% of all venlafaxine-treated patients. All patients recovered. No seizures occurred in Efexor XL-treated patients in clinical trials for depression and GAD. No seizures occurred in placebo-treated patients in depression studies. Seizures were reported in 0.2% of placebo-treated patients in GAD studies (see section 4.4).

Nausea is most common at the start of treatment with the incidence decreasing over the first few weeks. The nausea experienced with Efexor is usually mild to moderate, and infrequently results in vomiting or withdrawal. The incidence increases with higher doses particularly when the dose is increased rapidly.

Reversible increases in liver enzymes are seen in a small number of patients treated with venlafaxine. These generally resolve on discontinuation of therapy.

4.9 Overdose

Electrocardiogram changes (e.g. prolongation of QT interval, bundle branch block, QRS prolongation), sinus and ventricular tachycardia, bradycardia and seizures, hypotension, vertigo, serotonin syndrome and changes in level of consciousness have been reported in association with overdosage of venlafaxine usually when in combination with alcohol and/or other CNS drugs.

There have been some reports of fatalities in patients taking overdoses of Efexor, predominantly in combination with alcohol and/or other CNS drugs.

Management of Overdosage - Ensure an adequate airway, oxygenation and ventilation. Monitoring of cardiac rhythm and vital signs is recommended, as are general supportive and symptomatic measures. Use of activated charcoal or gastric lavage should be considered. Induction of emesis is not recommended. No specific antidotes for venlafaxine are known. In managing overdose, consider the possibility of multiple drug involvement.

The haemodialysis clearance of venlafaxine and its main active metabolite, are low. Therefore, they are not considered dialysable.

5. PHARMACOLOGICAL PROPERTIES

5.1 Pharmacodynamic properties

Efexor is a structurally novel antidepressant which is chemically unrelated to tricyclic, tetracyclic, or other available antidepressant agents. It is a racemate with two active enantiomers.

The mechanism of Efexor's antidepressant action in humans is believed to be associated with its potentiation of neurotransmitter activity in the central nervous system. Preclinical studies have shown that venlafaxine and its major metabolite, O-desmethylvenlafaxine, are potent neuronal serotonin and noradrenaline re-uptake inhibitors (SNRI) and weak inhibitors of dopamine reuptake. In addition, venlafaxine and O-desmethylvenlafaxine reduce β-adrenergic responsiveness in animals after both acute (single dose) and chronic administration. Venlafaxine and its major metabolite appear to be equipotent with respect to their overall action on neurotransmitter re-uptake.

Venlafaxine has virtually no affinity for rat brain muscarinic, histaminergic or adrenergic receptors *in vitro*. Pharmacologic activity at these receptors may be related to various side effects seen with other antidepressant drugs, such as anticholinergic, sedative and cardiovascular effects.

5.2 Pharmacokinetic properties

Venlafaxine is well absorbed and undergoes extensive first-pass metabolism. Mean peak plasma concentrations of venlafaxine range from approximately 33 to 172ng/ml after 25 to 150mg single doses, and are reached in approximately 2.4 hours. Venlafaxine is extensively metabolised in the liver. O-desmethylvenlafaxine is the major active metabolite of venlafaxine. The mean disposition half-life of venlafaxine and O-desmethylvenlafaxine is approximately 5 and 11 hours, respectively. Mean peak O-desmethylvenlafaxine plasma concentrations range from approximately 61 to 325ng/ml and are reached in approximately 4.3 hours. Plasma concentrations of venlafaxine and O-desmethylvenlafaxine generally correlated well with dose levels. Venlafaxine and O-desmethylvenlafaxine are 27% and 30% bound to plasma proteins respectively. O-desmethylvenlafaxine, other minor venlafaxine metabolites, and non-metabolised venlafaxine are excreted primarily through the kidneys.

5.3 Preclinical safety data

Studies with venlafaxine in rats and mice revealed no evidence of carcinogenesis. Venlafaxine was not mutagenic in a wide range of *in vitro* and *in vivo* tests.

Reduced fertility was observed in a study in which both male and female rats were exposed to the major metabolite of venlafaxine (ODV). This exposure was approximately 2 to 3 times that of a human dose of 225mg/day.

6. PHARMACEUTICAL PARTICULARS

6.1 List of excipients

The active constituent is venlafaxine as hydrochloride. Other constituents are microcrystalline cellulose, lactose, sodium starch glycollate, magnesium stearate, yellow and brown iron oxide.

6.2 Incompatibilities

Not applicable

6.3 Shelf life

Three years

6.4 Special precautions for storage

Store in a dry place at room temperature (at or below 30°C)

6.5 Nature and contents of container

PVC/aluminium foil blisters of 56 tablets

6.6 Instructions for use and handling

None

7. MARKETING AUTHORISATION HOLDER

John Wyeth and Brother Limited

Huntercombe Lane South

Taplow, Maidenhead, Berks SL6 0PH

UK

8. MARKETING AUTHORISATION NUMBER(S)

Efexor 37.5mg: 00011/0199

Efexor 75mg: 00011/0201

9. DATE OF FIRST AUTHORISATION/RENEWAL OF THE AUTHORISATION

22 November 1994

10. DATE OF REVISION OF THE TEXT

6 December 2004

* Trade Mark

Efexor XL

(Wyeth Pharmaceuticals)

1. NAME OF THE MEDICINAL PRODUCT

Efexor* XL

2. QUALITATIVE AND QUANTITATIVE COMPOSITION

Efexor XL 75mg capsules contain 84.8mg of venlafaxine hydrochloride, equivalent to 75mg of venlafaxine free base, in an extended release formulation.

Efexor XL 150mg capsules contain 169.7mg of venlafaxine hydrochloride, equivalent to 150mg of venlafaxine free base, in an extended release formulation.

Venlafaxine is chemically defined as (R/S)-1-[(2-dimethylamino)-1-(4-methoxy phenyl)ethyl]cyclohexanol hydrochloride.

3. PHARMACEUTICAL FORM

Efexor XL 75mg capsules are opaque peach modified release capsules printed in red with "W" and "75".

Efexor XL 150mg capsules are opaque dark orange modified release capsules printed in white with "W" and "150".

4. CLINICAL PARTICULARS

4.1 Therapeutic indications

Moderate to severe major depressive disorder

Initiation of treatment with venlafaxine should be restricted to specialist care and treatment should be managed under specialist supervision or shared care arrangements.

Efexor XL is indicated for the treatment of moderate to severe major depressive disorder including depression accompanied by anxiety. All patients should be evaluated for the risk of suicidality and monitored for clinical worsening (see section 4.4).

Following an initial response Efexor XL is indicated for the prevention of relapses of the initial episode of depression or for the prevention of the recurrence of new episodes.

Moderate to severe Generalised Anxiety Disorder

Initiation of treatment with venlafaxine should be restricted to specialist care and treatment should be managed under specialist supervision or shared care arrangements.

Efexor XL is also indicated for the treatment of moderate to severe Generalised Anxiety Disorder (GAD). This is primarily characterised by chronic and excessive worry and anxiety, sufficient to cause impairment in everyday functioning, for at least 6 months.

4.2 Posology and method of administration

Treatment with Efexor XL should not be started until 14 days after discontinuing a monoamine oxidase inhibitor (MAOI).

Depression:

The recommended dose is 75mg per day given once daily. Most patients respond to this dose.

If, after an adequate trial and evaluation, further clinical improvement is required, the dose may be increased to 150mg per day given once daily. There may be an increased risk of side effects at higher doses and dose increments should be made only after a clinical evaluation and after at least 3-4 weeks of therapy (see section 4.4). The lowest effective dose should be maintained.

In more severely depressed or hospitalised patients, and under close supervision of a physician, the daily dose may then be increased to 225mg given once daily. The dose should then be gradually reduced, to the minimum effective dose consistent with patient response and tolerance. A limited number of tablets should be provided to reduce the risk from overdose (see section 4.4).

Usually, the dosage for prevention of relapse or for prevention of recurrence of a new episode is similar to that used during the index episode. Patients should be reassessed regularly in order to evaluate the benefit of long-term therapy.

Generalised Anxiety Disorder (GAD):

The recommended dose for GAD for Efexor XL is 75mg, given once daily.

Patients should be reviewed at regular intervals and treatment should be discontinued after 8 weeks if there is no evidence of clinical response.

Efexor XL should be taken with food. Each capsule should be swallowed whole with fluid. Do not divide, crush, chew, or place the capsule in water. Efexor XL should be taken once daily, at approximately the same time, either in the morning or in the evening.

Depressed patients who are currently being treated with Efexor Tablets may be switched to Efexor XL. For example, a patient receiving Efexor Tablets 37.5mg b.d. would receive Efexor XL 75mg o.d. When switching, individual dosage adjustments may be necessary.

It is recommended that Efexor XL be taken with food.

Patients with Renal or Hepatic Impairment:

For patients with mild renal impairment (GFR >30ml/minute) or mild hepatic impairment (PT <14 seconds), no change in dosage is necessary.

For patients with moderate renal impairment (GFR 10-30ml/minute) or moderate hepatic impairment (PT 14-18 seconds), the dose should be reduced by 50%. This dose may be given once daily due to the longer half-lives of venlafaxine and O-desmethylvenlafaxine (ODV) in these patients.

Insufficient data are available to support the use of Efexor XL in patients with severe renal impairment (GFR <10ml/minute) or severe hepatic impairment (PT>18 seconds).

Elderly Patients:

No adjustment in the usual dosage is recommended for elderly patients. However, as with any therapy, caution should be exercised in treating the elderly (e.g. due to the possibility of renal impairment. See also dosage recommendations for renal impairment). The lowest effective dose should always be used and patients should be carefully monitored when an increase in the dose is required.

Children/Adolescents:

Controlled clinical studies in children and adolescents with Major Depressive Disorder failed to demonstrate efficacy and do not support the use of Efexor XL in these patients *(see sections 4.3 Contra-indications and 4.8 Undesirable Effects).*

The efficacy and safety of Efexor XL for other indications in children and adolescents under the age of 18 have not yet been established.

Maintenance/Continuation/Extended Treatment:

The physician should periodically re-evaluate the usefulness of long-term treatment with Efexor XL for the individual patient. It is generally agreed that acute episodes of major depression require several months or longer of sustained therapy. Efexor XL has been shown to be efficacious during long-term (up to 12 months) treatment.

In clinical trials venlafaxine was demonstrated to be effective for preventing relapse, or recurrence of new episodes, in patients responding to venlafaxine treatment during the index episode.

Withdrawal symptoms seen on discontinuation of venlafaxine

Abrupt discontinuation should be avoided (see section 4.4 Special Warnings and Special Precautions for Use and section 4.8 Undesirable Effects). Following treatment with daily doses of venlafaxine greater than 75mg for more than one week, it is recommended that when discontinuing treatment the dose should be gradually reduced over at least a further week. If high doses have been used for more than 6 weeks tapering over at least a 2 week period is recommended. If intolerable symptoms occur following a decrease in the dose or upon discontinuation of treatment, then resuming the previously prescribed dose may be considered. Subsequently, the physician may continue decreasing the dose, but at a more gradual rate.

4.3 Contraindications

1. Known hypersensitivity to venlafaxine or any other component of the product.

2. Concomitant use of venlafaxine with monoamine oxidase inhibitors *(See Interactions with other Medicaments and Other Forms of Interactions).*

3. Efexor XL should not be used in children and adolescents under the age of 18 years with Major Depressive Disorder *(see section 4.8 Undesirable Effects).*

4. Venlafaxine should not be used in patients with heart disease, e.g. cardiac failure, coronary artery disease, ECG abnormalities including pre-existing QT interval prolongation, patients with electrolyte imbalance or in patients who are hypertensive (see section 4.4).

4.4 Special warnings and special precautions for use

1. Suicide/suicidal thoughts

Depression is associated with an increased risk of suicidal thoughts, self-harm and suicide (suicide-related events). This risk persists until significant remission occurs. As improvement may not occur during the first few weeks or more of treatment, patients should be closely monitored until such improvement occurs. It is general clinical experience that the risk of self-harm is highest shortly after presentation and the risk of suicide may increase again in the early stages of recovery. Furthermore, there is evidence that in a small group of people, antidepressants may increase the risk of suicidal thoughts and self-harm.

Other psychiatric conditions for which venlafaxine is prescribed can also be associated with an increased risk of suicide-related events. In addition, these conditions may be co-morbid with major depressive disorder. The same precautions observed when treating patients with major depressive disorder should therefore be observed when treating patients with other psychiatric disorders.

Patients with a history of suicide-related events, those exhibiting a significant degree of suicidal ideation prior to commencement of treatment, and young adults, are at a greater risk of suicidal thoughts or suicide attempts, and should receive careful monitoring during treatment.

Patients, (and caregivers of patients) should be alerted about the need to monitor for the emergence of suicidal thoughts and to seek medical advice immediately if these symptoms present.

2. Withdrawal symptoms seen on discontinuation of venlafaxine treatment

Withdrawal symptoms when treatment is discontinued are common, particularly if discontinuation is abrupt (see section 4.8 Undesirable effects). In clinical trials adverse events seen on treatment discontinuation occurred in approximately 31% of patients treated with venlafaxine and in approximately 17% of placebo patients. The risk of withdrawal symptoms may be dependent on several factors including the duration and dose of therapy and the rate of dose reduction.

Dizziness, sensory disturbances (including paraesthesia and electric shock sensations), sleep disturbances (including insomnia and abnormal dreams), agitation or anxiety, nausea and/or vomiting, tremor, sweating, headache, diarrhoea, palpitations and emotional instability are the most commonly reported withdrawal reactions. Generally these symptoms are mild to moderate, however, in some patients they may be severe in intensity. They usually occur within the first few days of discontinuing treatment, but there have been very rare reports of such symptoms in patients who have inadvertently missed a dose. Generally these symptoms are self-limiting and usually resolve within 2 weeks, though in some individuals they may be prolonged (2-3 months or more). It is therefore advised that venlafaxine should be gradually tapered when discontinuing treatment over a period of several weeks or months, according to the patient's needs (see "Withdrawal Symptoms Seen on Discontinuation of Venlafaxine", Section 4.2 Posology and Method of Administration).

3. Activation of mania or hypomania has been reported rarely in patients who have received antidepressants, including venlafaxine. As with all antidepressants, Efexor XL should be used with caution in patients with a history of mania.

4. Treatment with venlafaxine (especially starting and discontinuing treatment) has been associated with reports of aggression.

5. Psychomotor restlessness:

The use of venlafaxine has been associated with the development of psychomotor restlessness, which clinically may be very similar to akathisia, characterised by a subjectively unpleasant or distressing restlessness and need to move often accompanied by an inability to sit or stand still. This is most likely to occur within the first few weeks of treatment. In patients who develop these symptoms, increasing the dose may be detrimental and it may be necessary to review the use of venlafaxine.

6. There have been reports of cardiotoxicity associated with therapeutic doses of venlafaxine. Before starting treatment with venlafaxine, a baseline ECG and blood pressure measurement should be performed and blood pressure should be monitored at regular intervals.

7. Significant electrocardiogram findings were observed in 0.8% of venlafaxine-treated patients compared with 0.7% of placebo-treated patients. Significant changes in PR, QRS or QTc intervals were rarely observed in patients treated with venlafaxine during clinical trials.

8. Seizures are a potential risk with antidepressant drugs, especially in overdose. Efexor XL should be introduced with caution in patients with a history of seizure and should be discontinued in any patient developing a seizure or if there is an increase in seizure frequency. Efexor XL should be avoided in patients with unstable epilepsy and patients with controlled epilepsy should be carefully monitored (see section 4.8).

9. Due to the possibility of drug abuse with CNS-active drugs, physicians should evaluate patients for a history of drug abuse, and follow such patients closely. Clinical studies have shown no evidence of drug-seeking behaviour, development of tolerance, or dose escalation over time among patients taking venlafaxine.

10. Increases in heart rate can occur, particularly at high doses. In clinical trials the mean heart rate was increased by approximately 4 beats/minute in patients treated with venlafaxine. Caution should be exercised in patients whose underlying conditions might be compromised by increases in heart rate.

11. Dosage should be reduced in patients with moderate-severe renal impairment or hepatic cirrhosis (see sections 4.2 and 4.5).

12. Postural hypotension has been observed occasionally during venlafaxine treatment. Patients, especially the elderly, should be alerted to the possibility of dizziness or unsteadiness.

13. Hyponatraemia (usually in the elderly and possibly due to inappropriate secretion of antidiuretic hormone) has been associated with all types of antidepressants and should be considered in all patients who develop drowsiness, confusion or convulsions while taking an antidepressant.

14. Mydriasis has been reported in association with venlafaxine; therefore patients with raised intra-ocular pressure or at a risk of narrow angle glaucoma should be monitored closely.

15. There have been reports of cutaneous bleeding abnormalities, such as ecchymosis and purpura, with serotonin-reuptake inhibitors (SSRIs). Other bleeding manifestations (e.g. gastrointestinal bleeding and mucous membrane bleeding) have been reported. Caution is advised in patients predisposed to bleeding due to factors such as age, underlying medical conditions or concomitant medications.

16. Clinically relevant increases in serum cholesterol were recorded in 5.3% of venlafaxine-treated patients and 0.0% of placebo-treated patients treated for at least 3 months in placebo-controlled trials. Measurement of serum cholesterol levels should be considered during long-term treatment.

17. The safety and efficacy of venlafaxine therapy in combination with weight loss agents, including phentermine, have not been established. Co-administration of venlafaxine and weight loss agents is not recommended. Venlafaxine is not indicated for weight loss alone or in combination with other products.

18. As with SSRIs, venlafaxine should be used with caution in patients already receiving neuroleptics, since symptoms suggestive of Neuroleptic Malignant Syndrome cases have been reported with this combination.

4.5 Interaction with other medicinal products and other forms of Interaction

MAOIs: Adverse reactions, some serious, have been reported when venlafaxine therapy is initiated soon after discontinuation of an MAOI, and when an MAOI is initiated soon after discontinuation of venlafaxine. These reactions have included tremor, myoclonus, diaphoresis, nausea, vomiting, flushing, dizziness, and hyperthermia with features resembling neuroleptic malignant syndrome, seizures and death. Do not use Efexor XL in combination with an MAOI, or within at least 14 days of discontinuing MAOI treatment. Allow at least 7 days after stopping Efexor XL before starting an MAOI (see also Contra-indications).

Serotonergic drugs: Based on the known mechanism of action of venlafaxine and the potential for serotonergic syndrome, caution is advised when venlafaxine is co-administered with drugs that may affect the serotonergic neurotransmitter systems (such as triptans, SSRIs or lithium).

Lithium: Reports have been received of an interaction between lithium and venlafaxine leading to increased lithium levels.

Imipramine/desipramine: The metabolism of imipramine and its metabolite 2-OH-imipramine were unaffected by venlafaxine although the total renal clearance of 2-hydroxydesipramine was reduced and desipramine AUC and C_{max} were increased by approximately 35%.

Haloperidol: In a pharmacokinetic study co-administration of venlafaxine with a single 2mg oral dose of haloperidol resulted in a 42% decrease in renal clearance, a 70% increase in AUC and an 88% increase in C_{max} for haloperidol. The elimination half-life remained unchanged.

Diazepam: The pharmacokinetic profiles of venlafaxine and ODV were not significantly altered by the administration of diazepam. Venlafaxine has no effect on the pharmacokinetic profile of diazepam or on the psychomotor or psychometric effects induced by diazepam.

Clozapine: Increased levels of clozapine, that were temporally associated with adverse events, including seizures, have been reported following the addition of venlafaxine.

Alcohol: Venlafaxine has been shown not to increase the impairment of mental or motor skills caused by ethanol. However, as with all CNS-active drugs, patients should be advised to avoid alcohol consumption while taking Efexor XL.

ECT: There is little clinical experience of the concurrent use of venlafaxine with ECT. As prolonged seizure activity has been reported with concomitant SSRI antidepressants, caution is advised.

Drugs metabolised by Cytochrome P450 isoenzymes: The major elimination pathways for venlafaxine are through CYP2D6 and CYP3A4. Venlafaxine is primarily metabolised to its active metabolite, ODV, by the cytochrome P450 enzyme CYP2D6. Co-administration of ketoconazole suggests that inhibition of CYP3A4 may result in increased venlafaxine plasma levels in poor CYP2D6 metabolisers. Caution should be used with concomitant intake of drugs which inhibit either CYP2D6 or CYP3A4.

Studies indicate that venlafaxine is a relatively weak inhibitor of CYP2D6. Venlafaxine did not inhibit CYP1A2, CYP2C9 or CYP3A4. This was confirmed by *in vivo* studies with the following drugs: alprazolam (CYP3A4), caffeine (CYP1A2), carbamazepine (CYP3A4) and diazepam (CYP3A4 and CYP2C19).

Cimetidine: Cimetidine inhibited the first-pass metabolism of venlafaxine but had no significant effect on the formation or elimination of ODV, which is present in much greater quantities in the systemic circulation. No dosage adjustment therefore seems necessary when Efexor XL is co-administered with cimetidine. For elderly patients, or patients with hepatic dysfunction the interaction could potentially be more pronounced, and for such patients clinical monitoring is indicated when Efexor XL is administered with cimetidine.

Warfarin: Potentiation of anticoagulant effects including increases in PT or INR have been reported in patients taking warfarin following the addition of venlafaxine.

Indinavir: A pharmacokinetic study with indinavir has shown a 28% decrease in AUC and a 36% decrease in C_{max} for indinavir. Indinavir did not affect the pharmacokinetics of venlafaxine and ODV. The clinical significance of this interaction is not known.

4.6 Pregnancy and lactation

There are no adequate data from the use of venlafaxine in pregnant women. Animal studies are insufficient with respect to effects on pregnancy. The potential risk for humans is unknown. Efexor XL should not be used during pregnancy unless clearly necessary. If venlafaxine is used until or shortly before birth, discontinuation effects in the newborn should be considered.

There is evidence to suggest that venlafaxine and its metabolite, ODV, transfers into breast milk. Therefore, a decision should be made whether or not to breast-feed or to discontinue venlafaxine.

4.7 Effects on ability to drive and use machines

Although venlafaxine has been shown not to affect psychomotor, cognitive, or complex behaviour performance in healthy volunteers, any psychoactive drug may impair judgement, thinking or motor skills. Therefore patients should be cautioned about their ability to drive or operate hazardous machinery.

4.8 Undesirable effects

See also Special Warnings and Special Precautions for Use.

The most commonly observed adverse events associated with the use of venlafaxine in clinical trials, and which occurred more frequently than those which were associated with placebo were: nausea, insomnia, dry mouth, somnolence, dizziness, constipation, sweating, nervousness, asthenia and abnormal ejaculation/orgasm.

The occurrence of most of these adverse events was dose-related, and the majority of them decreased in intensity and frequency over time. They generally did not lead to cessation of treatment.

Adverse events observed with venlafaxine, from both spontaneous and clinical trials reports, are classified in body systems and listed below as very common $>1/10$); common ($<1/10$ and $>1/100$); uncommon ($<1/100$ and $>1/1000$); rare ($<1/1000$);very rare ($<1/10,000$):

Blood and lymphatic system disorders - Uncommon: ecchymosis, mucous membrane bleeding; Rare: prolonged bleeding time, haemorrhage, thrombocytopenia; Very rare: blood dyscrasias (including agranulocytosis, aplastic anaemia, neutropenia and pancytopenia).

Cardiovascular and vascular disorders(*see Special Warnings and Special Precautions for Use*) - Common:hypertension, palpitation, vasodilatation; Uncommon: hypotension/postural hypotension, syncope, arrhythmias (including tachycardia); Very rare: Torsade de Pointes, QT prolongation, ventricular tachycardia, ventricular fibrillation.

Gastrointestinal disorders - Very common: constipation, nausea (see below); Common: anorexia, appetite decreased, diarrhoea, dyspepsia, vomiting; Uncommon: bruxism; Rare: gastrointestinal bleeding; Very rare: pancreatitis.

General disorders - Very common: asthenia, headache; Common: abdominal pain, chills, pyrexia; Rare: anaphylaxis

Metabolic and nutritional disorders - Common: serum cholesterol increased (particularly with prolonged administration and possibly with higher doses (*seeSpecial Warnings and Special Precautions for Use*), weight gain or loss; Uncommon: hyponatraemia including SIADH (*see Special Warnings and Special Precautions for Use*), increased liver enzymes (*see below*); Rare: hepatitis; Very rare: prolactin increased.

Musculo-skeletal disorders - Common: arthralgia, myalgia; Uncommon: muscle spasm; Very rare: rhabdomyolysis.

Neurological disorders - Very common: dizziness, dry mouth, insomnia, nervousness, somnolence; Common: abnormal dreams, agitation, anxiety, confusion, hypertonia, paraesthesia, tremor; Uncommon: apathy, hallucinations, myoclonus; Rare: ataxia and disorders of balance and co-ordination, speech disorders including dysarthria, mania or hypomania (*see Special Warnings and Special Precautions for Use*), neuroleptic malignant syndrome-like effects, seizures (*see below and Special Warnings and Special Precautions for Use*), serotonergic syndrome; Very rare: delirium, extrapyramidal disorders including dyskinesia and dystonia, tardive dyskinesia, psychomotor restlessness/akathisia (see section 4.4 Special Warnings and Special Precautions for Use).

Renal and urinary disorders - Common: urinary frequency; Uncommon: urinary retention.

Reproductive and breast disorders - Very common: anorgasmia, erectiledysfunction, abnormal ejaculation/orgasm; Common: decreased libido, impotence, menstrual cycle disorders; Uncommon: menorrhagia; Rare: galactorrhoea.

Respiratory system disorders - Common: dyspnoea, yawning; Very rare: pulmonary eosinophilia.

Skin and subcutaneous tissue disorders -Very common: sweating (including night sweats); Common: pruritus, rash; Uncommon: angioedema, maculopapular eruptions, urticaria, photosensitivity reactions, alopecia; Rare: erythema multiforme, Stevens Johnson syndrome.

Special senses - Common: abnormal vision/accommodation, mydriasis, tinnitus; Uncommon: altered taste sensation.

Adverse events from paediatric clinical trials

In paediatric MDD clinical trials the following adverse events were reported at a frequency of at least 2% of patients and occurred at a rate of at least twice that of placebo: abdominal pain, chest pain, tachycardia, anorexia, weight loss, constipation, dyspepsia, nausea, ecchymosis, epistaxis, mydriasis, myalgia, dizziness, emotional lability, tremor, hostility and suicidal ideation.

Withdrawal symptoms seen on discontinuation of venlafaxine treatment

Discontinuation of venlafaxine (particularly when abrupt) commonly leads to withdrawal symptoms. Dizziness, sensory disturbances (including paraesthesia and electric shock sensations), sleep disturbances (including insomnia and abnormal dreams), agitation or anxiety, nausea and/or vomiting, tremor, sweating, headache, diarrhoea, palpitations and emotional instability are the most commonly reported withdrawal reactions. Additional withdrawal reactions include hypomania, nervousness, confusion, fatigue, somnolence, convulsion, vertigo, tinnitus, dry mouth and anorexia. Generally these events are mild to moderate and are self-limiting, however, in some patients they may be severe and/or prolonged. It is therefore advised that when venlafaxine treatment is no longer required, gradual discontinuation by dose tapering should be carried out (see section 4.2 Posology and Method of Administration and section 4.4 Special Warnings and Special Precautions for use).

Special Notes:

In all premarketing depression trials with venlafaxine tablets, seizures were reported in 0.3% of all venlafaxine-treated patients. All patients recovered. No seizures occurred in Efexor XL-treated patients in clinical trials for depression and GAD. No seizures occurred in placebo-treated patients in depression studies. Seizures were reported in 0.2% of placebo-treated patients in GAD studies (see section 4.4).

Nausea is most common at the start of treatment with the incidence decreasing over the first few weeks. The nausea experienced with Efexor XL is usually mild to moderate, and infrequently results in vomiting or withdrawal. The incidence increases with higher doses particularly when the dose is increased rapidly.

Reversible increases in liver enzymes are seen in a small number of patients treated with venlafaxine. These generally resolve on discontinuation of therapy.

4.9 Overdose

Electrocardiogram changes (e.g. prolongation of QT interval, bundle branch block, QRS prolongation), sinus and ventricular tachycardia, bradycardia and seizures, hypotension, vertigo, serotonin syndrome and changes in level of consciousness have been reported in association with overdosage of venlafaxine usually when in combination with alcohol and/or other CNS drugs.

There have been some reports of fatalities in patients taking overdoses of Efexor XL, predominantly in combination with alcohol and/or other CNS drugs.

Management of Overdosage - Ensure an adequate airway, oxygenation and ventilation. Monitoring of cardiac rhythm and vital signs is recommended, as are general supportive and symptomatic measures. Use of activated charcoal or gastric lavage should be considered. Induction of emesis is not recommended. No specific antidotes for venlafaxine are known. In managing overdose, consider the possibility of multiple drug involvement.

The haemodialysis clearance of venlafaxine and its main active metabolite, are low. Therefore, they are not considered dialysable.

5. PHARMACOLOGICAL PROPERTIES

Venlafaxine is a structurally novel antidepressant that is chemically unrelated to tricyclic, tetracyclic, or other available antidepressants. It is a racemate with two active enantiomers.

5.1 Pharmacodynamic properties

The mechanism of venlafaxine's antidepressant action in humans is believed to be associated with its potentiation of neurotransmitter activity in the central nervous system. Preclinical studies have shown that venlafaxine and its major metabolite, O-desmethylvenlafaxine (ODV), are potent inhibitors of serotonin and noradrenaline reuptake. Venlafaxine also weakly inhibits dopamine uptake. Studies in animals show that tricyclic antidepressants may reduce β-adrenergic responsiveness following chronic administration. In contrast, venlafaxine and its active metabolite reduced β-adrenergic responsiveness after both acute (single dose) and chronic administration. Venlafaxine and ODV are very similar with respect to their overall action on neurotransmitter reuptake.

Venlafaxine has virtually no affinity for rat brain muscarinic cholinergic, H_1-histaminergic or α_1-adrenergic receptors *in vitro*. Pharmacological activity at these receptors may be related to various side effects seen with other antidepressant drugs, such as anticholinergic, sedative and cardiovascular side effects.

Venlafaxine does not possess monoamine oxidase (MAO) inhibitory activity.

In vitro studies revealed that venlafaxine has virtually no affinity for opiate, benzodiazepine, phencyclidine (PCP), or N-methyl-d-aspartic acid (NMDA) receptors. It has no significant central nervous system (CNS) stimulant activity in rodents. In primate drug discrimination studies, venlafaxine showed no significant or depressant abuse liability.

5.2 Pharmacokinetic properties

At least 92% of a single oral dose of venlafaxine is absorbed. After administration of Efexor XL, the peak plasma concentrations of venlafaxine and ODV are attained within 6.0±1.5 and 8.8±2.2 hours, respectively. The rate of absorption of venlafaxine from the Efexor XL capsule is slower than its rate of elimination. Therefore, the apparent elimination half-life of venlafaxine following administration of Efexor XL (15±6 hours) is actually the absorption half-life instead of the true disposition half-life (5±2 hours) observed following administration of an immediate release tablet.

When equal daily doses of venlafaxine were administered as either the immediate release tablet, or the extended release capsule, the exposure (AUC, area under the concentration curve) to both venlafaxine and ODV was similar for the two treatments, and the fluctuation in plasma concentrations was slightly lower following treatment with the Efexor XL capsule. Therefore, the Efexor XL capsule provides a slower rate of absorption, but the same extent of absorption (i.e. AUC), as the Efexor immediate release tablet.

Venlafaxine undergoes extensive first-pass metabolism in the liver, primarily by CYP2D6, to the major metabolite ODV. Venlafaxine is also metabolised to N-desmethylvenlafaxine, catalysed by CYP3A3/4, and to other minor metabolites.

Venlafaxine and its metabolites are excreted primarily through the kidneys. Approximately 87% of a venlafaxine dose is recovered in the urine within 48 hours as either unchanged venlafaxine, unconjugated ODV, conjugated ODV, or other minor metabolites.

The half-lives of venlafaxine and its active metabolite O-desmethylvenlafaxine (ODV) are increased in patients with renal and hepatic impairment.

Administration of Efexor XL with food has no effect on the absorption of venlafaxine, or on the subsequent formation of ODV.

Subject age and sex do not significantly affect the pharmacokinetics of venlafaxine. No accumulation of venlafaxine or ODV has been observed during chronic administration in healthy subjects.

The extended release formulation of venlafaxine contains spheroids which release the drug slowly into the digestive tract. The insoluble portion of these spheroids is eliminated and may be seen in the stools.

5.3 Preclinical safety data

Studies with venlafaxine in rats and mice revealed no evidence of carcinogenesis. Venlafaxine was not mutagenic in a wide range of *in vitro* and *in vivo* tests.

6. PHARMACEUTICAL PARTICULARS

6.1 List of excipients

Microcrystalline cellulose, ethylcellulose, hydroxypropyl methylcellulose, gelatin, red and yellow iron oxides (E172), titanium dioxide (E171) and printing ink.

6.2 Incompatibilities

Not applicable.

6.3 Shelf life

Three years.

6.4 Special precautions for storage

Store in a dry place at room temperature (at or below 25°C).

6.5 Nature and contents of container

PVC/aluminium foil blister packs of 28 capsules.

6.6 Instructions for use and handling

Not applicable

7. MARKETING AUTHORISATION HOLDER

John Wyeth and Brother Limited

trading as: Wyeth Laboratories

Huntercombe Lane South, Taplow, Maidenhead,

Berks SL6 0PH

8. MARKETING AUTHORISATION NUMBER(S)
Efexor XL 75mg: PL 00011/0223

Efexor XL 150mg: PL 00011/0224

9. DATE OF FIRST AUTHORISATION/RENEWAL OF THE AUTHORISATION
5 August 1997

10. DATE OF REVISION OF THE TEXT
6 December 2004

* Trade mark

Effico Tonic

(Forest Laboratories UK Limited)

1. NAME OF THE MEDICINAL PRODUCT
EFFICO TONIC

2. QUALITATIVE AND QUANTITATIVE COMPOSITION
Each 5ml oral liquid contains:

Vitamin B_1 (Thiamine Hydrochloride Ph.Eur.) 0.18mg

Nicotinamide Ph.Eur. 2.10mg

Caffeine Ph.Eur. 20.20mg

3. PHARMACEUTICAL FORM
Clear orange/red slightly viscous liquid

4. CLINICAL PARTICULARS

4.1 Therapeutic indications
A gentle pick-me-up and appetite promoter to combat the depressing effects that occur when tired, listless, run down, after a weakening illness or hospitalisation and due to too little nicotinamide and B_1.

4.2 Posology and method of administration
Adults and elderly:

10ml immediately before meals, three times a day.

Children (over 6 years):

2.5 to 5 ml taken as for adults.

Method of administration - oral use

4.3 Contraindications
Use in patients with known hypersensitivity to the product.

4.4 Special warnings and special precautions for use
None stated

4.5 Interaction with other medicinal products and other forms of Interaction
None stated

4.6 Pregnancy and lactation
Contra-indicated in pregnancy and lactation unless considered essential by the physician.

4.7 Effects on ability to drive and use machines
None stated

4.8 Undesirable effects
None stated

4.9 Overdose
None stated.

5. PHARMACOLOGICAL PROPERTIES

5.1 Pharmacodynamic properties
Caffeine is a mild CNS stimulant and its inclusion in the formulation helps counteract symptoms of tiredness and listlessness after a weakening illness or hospitalisation.

Thiamine and nicotinamide are present as vitamin supplements. Deficiencies of these two vitamins produce symptoms including fatigue and lethargy with anorexia or loss of appetite.

5.2 Pharmacokinetic properties
Nicotinamide is readily absorbed from the gastrointestinal tract. It has a short half-life and after low doses, the principle metabolites are the N-methyl, 2- and 4- pyridone derivatives.

Thiamine is absorbed from the gastrointestinal tract and widely distributed to most body tissues. It is not stored in the body and amounts in excess of the body's requirements are excreted in the urine as unchanged thiamine or as metabolites.

Caffeine is absorbed readily after oral administration. The average half-life is reported to be 3.5 hours. Peak plasma concentrations of 1.5 to 1.8 mg/litre have been measured after a 100mg oral dose.

5.3 Preclinical safety data
There are no preclinical data of relevance to the prescriber which are additional to that already included in other sections of the SPC.

6. PHARMACEUTICAL PARTICULARS

6.1 List of excipients
Ethanol 96%

Sodium Benzoate

Citric acid

Concentrated Hydrochloric Acid

Sucrose

Compound Gentian Infusion

Ponceau 4R (E124)

Quinoline Yellow (E104)

H & R Summer Fruit flavour 288234

Purified Water

6.2 Incompatibilities
None stated.

6.3 Shelf life
Clear colourless glass bottles – 3 years

Clear colourless polyethene terephthalate (PET) bottles – 2 years

6.4 Special precautions for storage
Store away from direct sunlight below 25°C

6.5 Nature and contents of container
Clear colourless glass bottle or clear colourless polyethene terephthalate (PET) bottle with food grade polypropylene tamper-evident caps pigmented with titanium dioxide containing 300ml or 500ml.

6.6 Instructions for use and handling
None stated.

7. MARKETING AUTHORISATION HOLDER
Forest Laboratories UK Limited

Bourne Road

Bexley

Kent DA5 1NX

8. MARKETING AUTHORISATION NUMBER(S)
PL 0108/5013

9. DATE OF FIRST AUTHORISATION/RENEWAL OF THE AUTHORISATION
24th November 1988 / 24 November 1998

10. DATE OF REVISION OF THE TEXT
October 1998

11. Legal Category
GSL

Efudix Cream

(Valeant Pharmaceuticals Ltd)

1. NAME OF THE MEDICINAL PRODUCT
Efudix cream.

2. QUALITATIVE AND QUANTITATIVE COMPOSITION
Efudix cream contains 5% w/w fluorouracil.

3. PHARMACEUTICAL FORM
White, opaque cream.

4. CLINICAL PARTICULARS

4.1 Therapeutic indications
Efudix is used for the topical treatment of superficial premalignant and malignant skin lesions; keratoses including senile, actinic and arsenical forms; keratoacanthoma; Bowen's disease; superficial basal-cell carcinoma. Deep, penetrating or nodular basal cell and squamous cell carcinomas do not usually respond to Efudix therapy. It should be used only as a palliative therapy in such cases where no other form of treatment is possible.

4.2 Posology and method of administration
Efudix cream is for topical application.

Pre-malignant conditions
The cream should be applied thinly to the affected area once or twice daily; an occlusive dressing is not essential.

Malignant conditions
The cream should be applied once or twice daily under an occlusive dressing where this is practicable.

The cream should not harm healthy skin. Treatment should be continued until there is marked inflammatory response from the treated area, preferably with some erosion in the case of pre-malignant conditions. Severe discomfort may be alleviated by the use of topical steroid cream. The usual duration of treatment for an initial course of therapy is three to four weeks, but this may be prolonged. Lesions on the face usually respond more quickly than those on the trunk or lower limbs whilst lesions on the hands and forearms respond more slowly. Healing may not be complete until one or two months after therapy is stopped.

Elderly
Many of the conditions for which Efudix is indicated are common in the elderly. No special precautions are necessary.

Children
In view of the lack of clinical data available, Efudix is not recommended for use in children.

4.3 Contraindications
Efudix is contra-indicated in patients with known hypersensitivity to Efudix or parabens.

4.4 Special warnings and special precautions for use
Efudix is for topical use only and care should be taken to avoid contact with mucous membranes or the eyes. The hands should be washed carefully after applying the cream.

The total area of skin being treated with Efudix at any one time should not exceed $500cm^2$ (approx. 23 × 23cm). Larger areas should be treated a section at a time.

4.5 Interaction with other medicinal products and other forms of Interaction
No significant drug interactions with Efudix have been reported.

4.6 Pregnancy and lactation
There is evidence from animal work that fluorouracil is teratogenic and there is no evidence as to drug safety in human pregnancy. Therefore the use of Efudix is contra-indicated during pregnancy. It should also be regarded as contra-indicated in mothers who are breast-feeding.

4.7 Effects on ability to drive and use machines
None known.

4.8 Undesirable effects
Efudix is well tolerated. Transient erythema may occur in healthy skin surrounding the area being treated. Pre-existing subclinical lesions may become apparent. Exposure to sunlight may increase the intensity of the reaction. Dermatitis, allergic skin reactions and, rarely, erythema multiforme have been reported.

Percutaneous absorption of fluorouracil should not lead to clinically significant systemic toxicity when Efudix is administered as directed. However, this possibility should be borne in mind if the product is used excessively, especially on ulcerated or broken skin.

4.9 Overdose
If Efudix is accidentally ingested, signs of fluorouracil overdosage may include nausea, vomiting and diarrhoea. Stomatitis and blood dyscrasias may occur in severe cases. Appropriate measures should be taken for the prevention of systemic infection and daily white cell counts should be performed.

5. PHARMACOLOGICAL PROPERTIES

5.1 Pharmacodynamic properties
Efudix is a topical cytostatic preparation which exerts a beneficial therapeutic effect on neoplastic and pre-neoplastic skin lesions without damaging normal skin. The pattern of response follows this sequence: erythema, vesiculation, erosion, ulceration, necrosis and epithelisation.

5.2 Pharmacokinetic properties
Animal studies have shown that after topical application of fluorouracil, less than 10% is systemically absorbed. This may be metabolised by catabolic or anabolic routes which are similar to that of endogenous uracil.

5.3 Preclinical safety data
None stated.

6. PHARMACEUTICAL PARTICULARS

6.1 List of excipients
Stearyl Alcohol HSE

White Soft Paraffin BP

Polysorbate 60 EP

Propylene Glycol EP

Methyl Parahydroxybenzoate EP

Propyl Parahydroxybenzoate EP

Purified Water EP

6.2 Incompatibilities
None known.

6.3 Shelf life
The recommended shelf life of Efudix cream is 60 months.

6.4 Special precautions for storage

Storage
The recommended maximum storage temperature for Efudix cream is 30°C.

Dilution
Efudix cream should not be diluted.

6.5 Nature and contents of container
Efudix cream is supplied in a 20g aluminium tube with a plastic screw cap.

6.6 Instructions for use and handling
Efudix is for topical use only and care should be taken to avoid contact with mucous membranes or the eyes. The hands should be washed carefully after applying the cream.

7. MARKETING AUTHORISATION HOLDER
Valeant Pharmaceuticals Limited

Cedarwood

Chineham Business Park

Crockford Lane

Basingstoke

Hampshire RG24 8WD

8. MARKETING AUTHORISATION NUMBER(S)
PL 15142/0003

9. DATE OF FIRST AUTHORISATION/RENEWAL OF THE AUTHORISATION
1 March 1998

10. DATE OF REVISION OF THE TEXT
April 2005

Elantan 10

(SCHWARZ PHARMA Limited)

1. NAME OF THE MEDICINAL PRODUCT
Elantan 10

2. QUALITATIVE AND QUANTITATIVE COMPOSITION
Isosorbide-5-mononitrate-lactose trituration 90%, 11.10mg equivalent to isosorbide-5-mononitrate, 10.00mg.

(The lactose complies with PhEur).

For excipients see 6.1.

3. PHARMACEUTICAL FORM
Tablets

White, upperside flat with bevelled edge and score engraving (E/10), underside rounded.

4. CLINICAL PARTICULARS

4.1 Therapeutic indications
For the prophylaxis of angina pectoris

4.2 Posology and method of administration
For oral administration

Adults

One tablet to be taken asymmetrically (to allow a nitrate low period) two or three times a day.

For patients not already receiving prophylactic nitrate therapy it is recommended that the initial dose be one tablet of Elantan 10 twice a day.

The dosage may be increased up to 120mg per day.

Elderly

There is no evidence to suggest that an adjustment of the dosage is necessary.

Children

The safety and efficacy of Elantan 10 has yet to be established in children.

4.3 Contraindications
Elantan 10 should not be used in cases of acute myocardial infarction with low filling pressure, acute circulatory failure (shock, vascular collapse), or very low blood pressure.

This product should not be given to patients with a known sensitivity to nitrates.

Elantan 10 should not be used in patients with marked anaemia, head trauma, cerebral haemorrhage, severe hypotension or hypovolaemia.

Phosphodiesterase inhibitors (eg sildenafil) have been shown to potentiate the hypotensive effects of nitrates, and their co-administration with nitrates or nitric oxide donors is therefore contraindicated.

4.4 Special warnings and special precautions for use
Elantan 10 should be used with caution in patients who are suffering from hypothyroidism, hypothermia, malnutrition and severe liver or renal disease.

This product may give rise to postural hypotension and syncope in some patients.

Symptoms of circulatory collapse may arise after first dose, particularly in patients with labile circulation.

Elantan 10 should be used with particular caution and under medical supervision in the following:

Hypertrophic obstructive cardiomyopathy (HOCM), constrictive pericarditis, cardiac tamponade, low cardiac filling pressures, aortic/mitral valve stenosis, and diseases associated with a raised intra-cranial pressure.

In the event of an acute angina attack, a sublingual treatment such as a GTN spray or tablet should be used instead of Elantan tablets.

If the tablets are not taken as indicated (see section 4.2.) tolerance to the medication could develop.

4.5 Interaction with other medicinal products and other forms of Interaction
Concurrent administration of drugs with blood pressure lowering properties, e.g. beta-blockers, calcium channel blockers, vasodilators etc and/or alcohol may potentiate the hypotensive effect of Elantan. This may also occur with neuroleptics and tricyclic antidepressants.

Any blood pressure lowering effect of Elantan will be increased if used together with phosphodiesterase inhibitors (eg sildenafil) which are used for erectile dysfunction (see special warnings and contraindications). This might lead to life threatening cardiovascular complications. Patients who are on Elantan therapy therefore must not use phosphodiesterase inhibitors (eg sildenafil)

Reports suggest that concomitant administration of Elantan may increase the blood level of dihydroergotamine and its hypertensive effect.

4.6 Pregnancy and lactation
This product should not be used during pregnancy or by women breast-feeding infants unless considered essential by the physician.

4.7 Effects on ability to drive and use machines
Dizziness and tiredness might occur at the start of treatment. The patient should therefore be advised that if affected, they should not drive or operate machinery. This effect may be increased by alcohol.

4.8 Undesirable effects
A very common (>10% of patients) adverse reaction to Elantan is headache. The incidence of headache diminishes gradually with time and continued use.

At the start of therapy or when the dosage is increased, hypotension and/or light headedness in the upright position are commonly observed (i.e. in 1 – 10% of patients). These symptoms may be associated with dizziness, drowsiness, reflex tachychardia and a feeling of weakness.

Infrequently (i.e. in less than 1% of patients) nausea, vomiting, flushing and allergic skin reaction (e.g. rash) may occur sometimes severely. In single cases exfoliative dermatitis may occur.

Severe hypotensive responses have been reported for organic nitrates and include nausea, vomiting, restlessness, pallor and excessive perspiration. Uncommonly collapse may occur (sometimes accompanied by bradyarrhythmia and syncope). Uncommonly severe hypotension may lead to enhanced angina symptoms.

A few reports of heartburn most likely due to a nitrate induced sphincter relaxation have been recorded.

4.9 Overdose
Symptoms and signs:

Headache, hypotension, nausea, vomiting, sweating, tachycardia, vertigo and syncope. Methaemoglobinaemia (cyanosis, hypoxaemia, restlessness, respiratory depression, convulsions, cardiac arrhythmias, circulatory failure, raised intracranial pressure) occurs rarely.

Treatment:

Symptomatic and supportive measures maintaining airway, breathing and circulation. If ingestion within last 1 hour, administration of activated charcoal. Gastric lavage may also be useful if ingestion within last 1 hour.

Place patient in recumbent position, raise foot of bed to encourage venous return and give IV volume expansion. Also, to maintain adequate blood pressure, the use of inotropes (dopamine/dobutamine) is recommended.

If methaemoglobinaemia (symptoms or > 30% methaemoglobin), IV administration of methylene blue 1-2 mg/kg body weight. If therapy fails with second dose after 1 hour or contraindicated, consider red blood cell concentrates or exchange transfusion. In case of cerebral convulsions, diazepam or clonazepam IV, or if therapy fails, phenobarbital, phenytoin or propofol anaesthesia.

5. PHARMACOLOGICAL PROPERTIES

5.1 Pharmacodynamic properties
ATC Code: C01D A14 Vasodilator used in cardiac diseases

Isosorbide mononitrate is an organic nitrate which, in common with other cardioactive nitrates, is a vasodilator. It produces decreased left and right ventricular end-diastolic pressures to a greater extent than the decrease in systemic arterial pressure, thereby reducing afterload and especially the preload of the heart.

Isosorbide mononitrate influences the oxygen supply to ischaemic myocardium by causing the redistribution of blood flow along collateral channels and from epicardial to endocardial regions by selective dilation of large epicardial vessels.

It reduces the requirement of the myocardium for oxygen by increasing venous capacitance, causing a pooling of blood in peripheral veins, thereby reducing ventricular volume and heart wall distension.

5.2 Pharmacokinetic properties
Isosorbide-5-mononitrate is rapidly absorbed and peak plasma levels occur approx. 1 hour following oral dosing.

Isosorbide-5-mononitrate is completely bioavailable after oral doses and is not subject to pre-systemic elimination processes.

Isosorbide-5-mononitrate is eliminated from the plasma with a half-life of about 5.1 hours. It is metabolised to Isosorbide-5-MN-2-glucoronide, which has a half-life of approximately 2.5 hours. As well as being excreted unchanged in the urine.

After multiple oral dosing plasma concentrations are similar to those that can be predicted from single dose kinetic parameters.

5.3 Preclinical safety data
Preclinical data reveal no special hazard for humans based on conventional studies of single and repeated dose toxicity, genotoxicity, oncogenicity and toxicity to reproduction.

6. PHARMACEUTICAL PARTICULARS

6.1 List of excipients
Lactose monohydrate

Microcrystalline cellulose

Potato starch

Purified talc

Colloidal silicon dioxide

Aluminium stearate.

6.2 Incompatibilities
None Known

6.3 Shelf life
5 years

6.4 Special precautions for storage
None

6.5 Nature and contents of container
Cartons of blister strips of PP/aluminium or of PP/PP.

Aluminium foil thickness 16μm or 20μm.

Pack sizes: 56 and 84 tablets.

6.6 Instructions for use and handling
None

7. MARKETING AUTHORISATION HOLDER
SCHWARZ PHARMA Limited

Schwarz House

East Street

Chesham

Bucks HP5 1DG

England

8. MARKETING AUTHORISATION NUMBER(S)
PL 04438/0018

9. DATE OF FIRST AUTHORISATION/RENEWAL OF THE AUTHORISATION
20 April 1999

10. DATE OF REVISION OF THE TEXT
August 2003

Elantan 20

(SCHWARZ PHARMA Limited)

1. NAME OF THE MEDICINAL PRODUCT
Elantan 20

2. QUALITATIVE AND QUANTITATIVE COMPOSITION
Isosorbide-5-mononitrate-lactose trituration 90%, 22.20mg equivalent to Isosorbide-5-mononitrate, 20.00mg.

(The lactose complies with PhEur).

For excipients see 6.1.

3. PHARMACEUTICAL FORM
Tablets

White tablets with breakscore and marked 'E20'.

4. CLINICAL PARTICULARS

4.1 Therapeutic indications
For the prophylaxis of angina pectoris

As adjunctive therapy in congestive heart failure not responding to cardiac glycosides or diuretics.

4.2 Posology and method of administration
For oral administration

Adults

One tablet to be taken asymmetrically (to allow a nitrate low period) two or three times a day.

For patients not already receiving prophylactic nitrate therapy it is recommended that the initial dose be one tablet of Elantan 20 twice a day.

The dosage may be increased up to 120mg per day.

Elderly

There is no evidence to suggest that an adjustment of the dosage is necessary.

Children

The safety and efficacy of Elantan 20 has yet to be established in children.

4.3 Contraindications
Elantan 20 should not be used in cases of acute myocardial infarction with low filling pressure, acute circulatory failure (shock, vascular collapse), or very low blood pressure.

This product should not be given to patients with a known sensitivity to nitrates.

Elantan 20 should not be used in patients with marked anaemia, head trauma, cerebral haemorrhage, severe hypotension or hypovolaemia.

Phosphodiesterase inhibitors (e.g. sildenafil) have been shown to potentiate the hypotensive effects of nitrates, and their co-administration with nitrates or nitric oxide donors is therefore contraindicated.

4.4 Special warnings and special precautions for use
Elantan 20 should be used with caution in patients who are suffering from hypothyroidism, hypothermia, malnutrition and severe liver or renal disease.

Symptoms of circulatory collapse may arise after first dose, particularly in patients with labile circulation.

This product may give rise to postural hypotension and syncope in some patients.

Elantan 20 should be used with particular caution and under medical supervision in the following:

Hypertrophic obstructive cardiomyopathy (HOCM), constrictive pericarditis, cardiac tamponade, low cardiac filling pressures, aortic/mitral valve stenosis, and diseases associated with a raised intra-cranial pressure.

In the event of an acute angina attack, a sublingual treatment such as a GTN spray or tablet should be used instead of Elantan tablets.

If the tablets are not taken as indicated (see section 4.2.) tolerance to the medication could develop.

4.5 Interaction with other medicinal products and other forms of Interaction

Concurrent administration of drugs with blood pressure lowering properties, e.g. beta-blockers, calcium channel blockers, vasodilators etc and/or alcohol may potentiate the hypotensive effect of Elantan. This may also occur with neuroleptics and tricyclic antidepressants.

Any blood pressure lowering effect of Elantan will be increased if used together with phosphodiesterase inhibitors (e.g. sildenafil) which are used for erectile dysfunction (see special warnings and contraindications). This might lead to life threatening cardiovascular complications. Patients who are on Elantan therapy therefore must not use phosphodiesterase inhibitors (e.g. sildenafil)

Reports suggest that concomitant administration of Elantan may increase the blood level of dihydroergotamine and its hypertensive effect.

4.6 Pregnancy and lactation

This product should not be used during pregnancy or by women breast-feeding infants unless considered essential by the physician.

4.7 Effects on ability to drive and use machines

Dizziness and tiredness may occur at the start of treatment. The patient should therefore be advised that if affected, they should not drive or operate machinery. This effect may be increased by alcohol.

4.8 Undesirable effects

A very common (>10% of patients) adverse reaction to Elantan is headache. The incidence of headache diminishes gradually with time and continued use.

At the start of therapy or when the dosage is increased, hypotension and/or light headedness in the upright position are commonly observed (i.e. in 1 – 10% of patients).

These symptoms may be associated with dizziness, drowsiness, reflex tachychardia and a feeling of weakness.

Uncommonly (i.e. in less than 1% of patients) nausea, vomiting, flushing and allergic skin reaction (e.g. rash) may occur sometimes severely. In single cases exfoliative dermatitis may occur.

Severe hypotensive responses have been reported for organic nitrates and include nausea, vomiting, restlessness, pallor and excessive perspiration. Uncommonly collapse may occur (sometimes accompanied by bradyarrhythmia and syncope). Uncommonly severe hypotension may lead to enhanced angina symptoms.

A few reports of heartburn most likely due to a nitrate induced sphincter relaxation have been reported.

4.9 Overdose

Symptoms and signs:

Headache, hypotension, nausea, vomiting, sweating, tachycardia, vertigo and syncope.

Methaemoglobinaemia (cyanosis, hypoxaemia, restlessness, respiratory depression, convulsions, cardiac arrhythmias, circulatory failure, raised intracranial pressure) occurs rarely.

Treatment:

Symptomatic and supportive measures maintaining airway, breathing and circulation. If ingestion is within the last hour, administration of activated charcoal. Gastric lavage may also be useful if ingestion is within the last hour.

Place patient in recumbent position, raise foot of bed to encourage venous return and give IV volume expansion. Also, to maintain adequate blood pressure, the use of inotropes (dopamine/dobutamine) is recommended.

If methaemoglobinaemia (symptoms or > 30% methaemoglobin), IV administration of methylene blue 1-2 mg/kg body weight. If therapy fails with second dose after 1 hour or contraindicated, consider red blood cell concentrates or exchange transfusion. In case of cerebral convulsions, diazepam or clonazepam IV, or if therapy fails, phenobarbital, phenytoin or propofol anaesthesia.

5. PHARMACOLOGICAL PROPERTIES

5.1 Pharmacodynamic properties

ATC Code: C01D A14 Vasodilator used in cardiac diseases

Isosorbide mononitrate is an organic nitrate which, in common with other cardioactive nitrates, is a vasodilator. It produces decreased left and right ventricular end-diastolic pressures to a greater extent than the decrease in systemic arterial pressure, thereby reducing afterload and especially the preload of the heart.

Isosorbide mononitrate influences the oxygen supply to ischaemic myocardium by causing the redistribution of blood flow along collateral channels and from epicardial to endocardial regions by selective dilation of large epicardial vessels.

It reduces the requirement of the myocardium for oxygen by increasing venous capacitance, causing a pooling of blood in peripheral veins, thereby reducing ventricular volume and heart wall distension.

5.2 Pharmacokinetic properties

Isosorbide-5-mononitrate is rapidly absorbed and peak plasma levels occur approx. 1 hour following oral dosing.

Isosorbide-5-mononitrate is completely bioavailable after oral doses and is not subject to pre-systemic elimination processes.

Isosorbide-5-mononitrate is eliminated from the plasma with a half-life of about 5.1 hours. It is metabolised to Isosorbide-5-MN-2-glucoronide, which has a half-life of approximately 2.5 hours. As well as being excreted unchanged in the urine.

After multiple oral dosing plasma concentrations are similar to those that can be predicted from single dose kinetic parameters.

5.3 Preclinical safety data

Preclinical data reveal no special hazard for humans based on conventional studies of single and repeated dose toxicity, genotoxicity, oncogenicity and toxicity to reproduction.

6. PHARMACEUTICAL PARTICULARS

6.1 List of excipients

Lactose monohydrate

Purified talc

Colloidal silicon dioxide

Potato starch

Microcrystalline cellulose

Aluminium stearate

6.2 Incompatibilities

None Known

6.3 Shelf life

5 years

6.4 Special precautions for storage

None

6.5 Nature and contents of container

Cartons of blister strips of PP/aluminium or of PP/PP.

Aluminium foil thickness 16μm or 20μm.

Pack sizes: 56 and 84 tablets.

6.6 Instructions for use and handling

None

7. MARKETING AUTHORISATION HOLDER

SCHWARZ PHARMA Limited

Schwarz House

East Street

Chesham

Bucks HP5 1DG

England

8. MARKETING AUTHORISATION NUMBER(S)

PL 04438/0005

9. DATE OF FIRST AUTHORISATION/RENEWAL OF THE AUTHORISATION

12th June 2003

10. DATE OF REVISION OF THE TEXT

August 2003

Elantan 40

(SCHWARZ PHARMA Limited)

1. NAME OF THE MEDICINAL PRODUCT

Elantan 40

2. QUALITATIVE AND QUANTITATIVE COMPOSITION

Isosorbide-5-mononitrate-lactose trituration 90%, 44.40mg equivalent to Isosorbide-5-mononitrate, 40.00mg. (The lactose complies with PhEur).

For excipients see 6.1.

3. PHARMACEUTICAL FORM

Tablets

White tablets upperside flat with facet and breakscore; underside arc-shaped marked 'E40'.

4. CLINICAL PARTICULARS

4.1 Therapeutic indications

For the prophylaxis of angina pectoris

As adjunctive therapy in congestive heart failure not responding to cardiac glycosides or diuretics.

4.2 Posology and method of administration

For oral administration

Adults

One tablet to be taken asymmetrically (to allow a nitrate low period) two or three times a day.

For patients not already receiving prophylactic nitrate therapy it is recommended that the initial dose be one tablet of Elantan 40 twice a day.

The dosage may be increased up to 120mg per day.

Elderly

There is no evidence to suggest that an adjustment of the dosage is necessary.

Children

The safety and efficacy of Elantan 40 has yet to be established in children.

4.3 Contraindications

Elantan 40 should not be used in cases of acute myocardial infarction with low filling pressure, acute circulatory failure (shock, vascular collapse), or very low blood pressure.

This product should not be given to patients with a known sensitivity to nitrates.

Elantan 40 should not be used in patients with marked anaemia, head trauma, cerebral haemorrhage, severe hypotension or hypovolaemia.

Phosphodiesterase inhibitors (e.g. sildenafil) have been shown to potentiate the hypotensive effects of nitrates, and their co-administration with nitrates or nitric oxide donors is therefore contraindicated.

4.4 Special warnings and special precautions for use

Elantan 40 should be used with caution in patients who are suffering from hypothyroidism, hypothermia, malnutrition and severe liver or renal disease.

Symptoms of circulatory collapse may arise after first dose, particularly in patients with labile circulation.

This product may give rise to postural hypotension and syncope in some patients.

Elantan 40 should be used with particular caution and under medical supervision in the following:

Hypertrophic obstructive cardiomyopathy (HOCM), constrictive pericarditis, cardiac tamponade, low cardiac filling pressures, aortic/mitral valve stenosis, and diseases associated with a raised intra-cranial pressure.

In the event of an acute angina attack, a sublingual treatment such as a GTN spray or tablet should be used instead of Elantan tablets.

If the tablets are not taken as indicated (see section 4.2.) tolerance to the medication could develop.

4.5 Interaction with other medicinal products and other forms of Interaction

Concurrent administration of drugs with blood pressure lowering properties, e.g. beta-blockers, calcium channel blockers, vasodilators etc and/or alcohol may potentiate the hypotensive effect of Elantan. This may also occur with neuroleptics and tricyclic antidepressants.

The blood pressure lowering effect of Elantan will be increased if used together with phosphodiesterase inhibitors (e.g. sildenafil) which are used for erectile dysfunction (see special warnings and contraindications). This might lead to life threatening cardiovascular complications. Patients who are on Elantan therapy therefore must not use phosphodiesterase inhibitors (e.g. sildenafil)

Reports suggest that concomitant administration of Elantan may increase the blood level of dihydroergotamine and its hypertensive effect.

4.6 Pregnancy and lactation

This product should not be used during pregnancy or by women breast-feeding infants unless considered essential by the physician.

4.7 Effects on ability to drive and use machines

Dizziness and tiredness might occur at the start of treatment. The patient should therefore be advised that if affected, they should not drive or operate machinery. This effect may be increased by alcohol.

4.8 Undesirable effects

A very common (>10% of patients) adverse reaction to Elantan is headache. The incidence of headache diminishes gradually with time and continued use.

At the start of therapy or when the dosage is increased, hypotension and/or light headedness in the upright position are commonly observed (i.e. in 1 – 10% of patients).

These symptoms may be associated with dizziness, drowsiness, reflex tachychardia and a feeling of weakness.

Uncommonly (i.e. in less than 1% of patients) nausea, vomiting, flushing and allergic skin reaction (e.g. rash) may occur sometimes severely. In single cases exfoliative dermatitis may occur.

Severe hypotensive responses have been reported for organic nitrates and include nausea, vomiting, restlessness, pallor and excessive perspiration. Uncommonly collapse may occur (sometimes accompanied by bradyarrhythmia and syncope). Uncommonly severe hypotension may lead to enhanced angina symptoms.

A few reports of heartburn most likely due to a nitrate induced sphincter relaxation have been reported.

4.9 Overdose

Symptoms and signs:

Headache, hypotension, nausea, vomiting, sweating, tachycardia, vertigo and syncope.

Methaemoglobinaemia (cyanosis, hypoxaemia, restlessness, respiratory depression, convulsions, cardiac arrhythmias, circulatory failure, and raised intracranial pressure) occurs rarely.

Treatment:

Symptomatic and supportive measures maintaining airway, breathing and circulation. If ingestion is within the last hour, administration of activated charcoal. Gastric lavage may also be useful if ingestion is within the last hour.

Place patient in recumbent position, raise foot of bed to encourage venous return and give IV volume expansion. Also, to maintain adequate blood pressure, the use of inotropes (dopamine/dobutamine) is recommended.

If methaemoglobinaemia (symptoms or > 30% methaemoglobin), IV administration of methylene blue 1-2 mg/kg body weight. If therapy fails with second dose after 1 hour or contraindicated, consider red blood cell concentrates or exchange transfusion. In case of cerebral convulsions, diazepam or clonazepam IV, or if therapy fails, phenobarbital, phenytoin or propofol anaesthesia.

5. PHARMACOLOGICAL PROPERTIES

5.1 Pharmacodynamic properties

ATC Code: C01D A14 Vasodilator used in cardiac diseases

Isosorbide mononitrate is an organic nitrate which, in common with other cardioactive nitrates, is a vasodilator. It produces decreased left and right ventricular end-diastolic pressures to a greater extent than the decrease in systemic arterial pressure, thereby reducing afterload and especially the preload of the heart.

Isosorbide mononitrate influences the oxygen supply to ischaemic myocardium by causing the redistribution of blood flow along collateral channels and from epicardial to endocardial regions by selective dilation of large epicardial vessels.

It reduces the requirement of the myocardium for oxygen by increasing venous capacitance, causing a pooling of blood in peripheral veins, thereby reducing ventricular volume and heart wall distension.

5.2 Pharmacokinetic properties

Isosorbide-5-mononitrate is rapidly absorbed and peak plasma levels occur approx. 1 hour following oral dosing.

Isosorbide-5-mononitrate is completely bioavailable after oral doses and is not subject to pre-systemic elimination processes.

Isosorbide-5-mononitrate is eliminated from the plasma with a half-life of about 5.1 hours. It is metabolised to Isosorbide-5-mn-2-glucoronide which has a half-life of approximately 2.5 hours. As well as being excreted unchanged in the urine.

After multiple oral dosing plasma concentrations are similar to those that can be predicted from single dose kinetic parameters.

5.3 Preclinical safety data

Preclinical data reveal no special hazard for humans based on conventional studies of single and repeated dose toxicity, genotoxicity, oncogenicity and toxicity to reproduction.

6. PHARMACEUTICAL PARTICULARS

6.1 List of excipients

Lactose monohydrate

Purified talc

Colloidal silicon dioxide

Potato starch

Microcrystalline cellulose

Aluminium stearate

6.2 Incompatibilities

None Known

6.3 Shelf life

5 years

6.4 Special precautions for storage

None

6.5 Nature and contents of container

Cartons of blister strips of PP/aluminium or of PP/PP.

Aluminium foil thickness 16μm or 20μm.

Pack sizes: 56 and 84 tablets.

6.6 Instructions for use and handling

None

7. MARKETING AUTHORISATION HOLDER

SCHWARZ PHARMA Limited

Schwarz House

East Street

Chesham

Bucks HP5 1DG

England

8. MARKETING AUTHORISATION NUMBER(S)

PL 04438/0008

9. DATE OF FIRST AUTHORISATION/RENEWAL OF THE AUTHORISATION

25th May 2004

10. DATE OF REVISION OF THE TEXT

August 2003

Elantan LA 25

(SCHWARZ PHARMA Limited)

1. NAME OF THE MEDICINAL PRODUCT

Elantan LA 25

2. QUALITATIVE AND QUANTITATIVE COMPOSITION

Isosorbide mononitrate 25mg

For excipients see 6.1.

3. PHARMACEUTICAL FORM

Prolonged release capsules

4. CLINICAL PARTICULARS

4.1 Therapeutic indications

For the prophylaxis of angina pectoris

4.2 Posology and method of administration

For oral administration

Adults

One capsule to be taken in the morning.

For patients with higher nitrate requirements the dose may be increased to two capsules taken simultaneously.

Children

The safety and efficacy of these capsules has yet to be established in children.

4.3 Contraindications

The capsules should not be used in cases of acute myocardial infarction with low filling pressure, acute circulatory failure, shock, vascular collapse, or very low blood pressure.

This product should not be given to patients with a known sensitivity to nitrates, marked anaemia, head trauma, cerebral haemorrhage, severe hypotension or hypovolaemia.

Phosphodiesterase inhibitors (e.g. sildenafil) have been shown to potentiate the hypotensive effects of nitrates, and their co-administration with nitrates or nitric oxide donors is therefore contraindicated.

4.4 Special warnings and special precautions for use

The capsules should be used with caution in patients who are suffering from hypothyroidism, hypothermia, malnutrition, severe liver disease or severe renal disease.

Symptoms of circulatory collapse may arise after first dose, particularly in patients with labile circulation.

This product may give rise to postural hypotension and syncope in some patients.

These capsules should be used with particular caution and under medical supervision in the following:

Hypertrophic obstructive cardiomyopathy (HOCM), constrictive pericarditis, cardiac tamponade, low cardiac filling pressures, aortic/mitral valve stenosis, and diseases associated with a raised intra-cranial pressure.

In the event of an acute angina attack, a sublingual treatment such as a GTN spray or tablet should be used instead of these capsules.

If these capsules are not taken as indicated (see section 4.2.) tolerance to the medication could develop.

4.5 Interaction with other medicinal products and other forms of Interaction

Concurrent administration of drugs with blood pressure lowering properties, e.g. beta-blockers, calcium channel blockers, vasodilators etc and/or alcohol may potentiate the hypotensive effect of these capsules. This may also occur with neuroleptics and tricyclic antidepressants.

Any blood pressure lowering effect of these capsules will be increased if used together with phosphodiesterase inhibitors (eg sildenafil) which are used for erectile dysfunction (see special warnings and contraindications). This might lead to life threatening cardiovascular complications. Patients who are on these capsules therefore must not use phosphodiesterase inhibitors (eg sildenafil)

Reports suggest that concomitant administration of these capsules may increase the blood level of dihydroergotamine and its hypertensive effect.

4.6 Pregnancy and lactation

There is inadequate evidence of safety of the drug in human pregnancy but nitrates have been used widely in the treatment of angina for many years without apparent ill consequence; animal studies having shown no hazard. Nevertheless it is not advisable to use this drug during pregnancy and lactation.

4.7 Effects on ability to drive and use machines

Dizziness and tiredness may occur at the start of treatment. The patient should therefore be advised that if affected, they should not drive or operate machinery. This effect may be increased by alcohol.

4.8 Undesirable effects

A very common (>10% of patients) adverse reaction to these capsules is headache. The incidence of headache diminishes gradually with time and continued use.

At the start of therapy or when the dosage is increased, hypotension and/or light headedness in the upright position are commonly observed (i.e. in 1 – 10% of patients). These symptoms may be associated with dizziness, drowsiness, reflex tachychardia and a feeling of weakness.

Infrequently (i.e. in less than 1% of patients) nausea, vomiting, flushing and allergic skin reaction (e.g. rash) may occur sometimes severely. In single cases exfoliative dermatitis may occur.

Severe hypotensive responses have been reported for organic nitrates and include nausea, vomiting, restlessness, pallor and excessive perspiration. Uncommonly collapse may occur (sometimes accompanied by bradyarrhythmia and syncope). Uncommonly severe hypotension may lead to enhanced angina symptoms.

A few reports of heartburn most likely due to a nitrate induced sphincter relaxation have been recorded.

4.9 Overdose

Symptoms and signs:

Headache, hypotension, nausea, vomiting, sweating, tachycardia, vertigo and syncope. Methaemoglobinaemia (cyanosis, hypoxaemia, restlessness, respiratory depression, convulsions, cardiac arrhythmias, circulatory failure, raised intracranial pressure) occurs rarely.

Treatment:

Symptomatic and supportive measures maintaining airway, breathing and circulation. If ingestion within last 1 hour, administration of activated charcoal. Gastric lavage may also be useful if ingestion within last 1 hour.

Place patient in recumbent position, raise foot of bed to encourage venous return and give IV volume expansion. Also, to maintain adequate blood pressure, the use of inotropes (dopamine/dobutamine) is recommended.

If methaemoglobinaemia (symptoms or > 30% methaemoglobin), IV administration of methylene blue 1-2 mg/kg body weight. If therapy fails with second dose after 1 hour or contraindicated, consider red blood cell concentrates or exchange transfusion. In case of cerebral convulsions, diazepam or clonazepam IV, or if therapy fails, phenobarbital, phenytoin or propofol anaesthesia.

5. PHARMACOLOGICAL PROPERTIES

5.1 Pharmacodynamic properties

ATC Code: C01D A14 Vasodilator used in cardiac diseases.

Isosorbide mononitrate is an organic nitrate which, in common with other cardioactive nitrates, is a vasodilator. It produces decreased left and right ventricular end-diastolic pressures to a greater extent than the decrease in systemic arterial pressure, thereby reducing afterload and especially preload of the heart.

Isosorbide mononitrate influences the oxygen supply to the ischaemic myocardium by causing the redistribution of blood flow along collateral channels and from epicardial to endocardial regions by selective dilation of large epicardial vessels.

It reduces the requirement of the myocardium for oxygen by increasing venous capacitance, causing a pooling of blood in peripheral veins, thereby reducing ventricular volume and heart wall distension.

5.2 Pharmacokinetic properties

Isosorbide mononitrate is a vasodilator, which is rapidly absorbed following oral administration. These capsules have a bioavailability of 84 (±7)% when compared to the immediate release isosorbide mononitrate tablets. There is no effect of food on bioavailability.

The capsules contain pellets which are formulated to release 30% of the dose immediately whilst 70% of the dose is released slowly.

Time to peak plasma levels (T_{max}) is 5.0 (±3) hrs; with a half life ($T_{½}$) of 5.02 (±0.68) hrs.

Isosorbide mononitrate is extensively metabolised to nitric oxide (NO-which is the active ingredient) and isosorbide (inactive). In patients with cirrhotic disease or cardiac failure or renal failure, parameters were similar to those obtained in healthy volunteers.

5.3 Preclinical safety data

Preclinical data reveal no special hazard for humans based on conventional studies of single and repeated dose toxicity, genotoxicity, oncogenicity and toxicity to reproduction.

6. PHARMACEUTICAL PARTICULARS

6.1 List of excipients

Lactose monohydrate

Talc

Ethyl cellulose

Polyethylene glycol

Macrogol 20000

Hydroxypropyl cellulose

Sucrose

Starch

Gelatin

Titanium dioxide

Iron oxide red

Iron oxide black

6.2 Incompatibilities

None Known

6.3 Shelf life
3 years

6.4 Special precautions for storage
None

6.5 Nature and contents of container
Cartons of blister strips of PVC and aluminium or of PP and aluminium.

Aluminium foil thickness 20μm or 16μm.

Pack size: 28 capsules.

6.6 Instructions for use and handling
None

7. MARKETING AUTHORISATION HOLDER
SCHWARZ PHARMA Limited
Schwarz House
East Street
Chesham
Bucks HP5 1DG
England

8. MARKETING AUTHORISATION NUMBER(S)
PL 04438/0028

9. DATE OF FIRST AUTHORISATION/RENEWAL OF THE AUTHORISATION
18 March 2003

10. DATE OF REVISION OF THE TEXT
August 2003

Elantan LA50

(SCHWARZ PHARMA Limited)

1. NAME OF THE MEDICINAL PRODUCT
Elantan LA50

2. QUALITATIVE AND QUANTITATIVE COMPOSITION
Isosorbide mononitrate 50mg

For excipients see 6.1.

3. PHARMACEUTICAL FORM
Prolonged release capsules, hard.

Hard capsule, upper half brown opaque and lower half flesh opaque. Contains white to off-white pellets.

4. CLINICAL PARTICULARS
4.1 Therapeutic indications
For the prophylaxis of angina pectoris

4.2 Posology and method of administration
For oral administration. Capsules should be swallowed whole, with water

Adults
One capsule to be taken in the morning.

This may be increased to two capsules if required.

Elderly
There is no evidence to suggest an adjustment of the dosage is necessary.

Children
The safety and efficacy of these capsules has yet to be established in children.

4.3 Contraindications
The capsules should not be used in cases of acute myocardial infarction with low filling pressure, acute circulatory failure, shock, vascular collapse, or very low blood pressure.

This product should not be given to patients with a known sensitivity to nitrates, marked anaemia, head trauma, cerebral haemorrhage, severe hypotension or hypovolaemia. Sildenafil (Viagra®) has been shown to potentiate the hypotensive effects of nitrates, and its co-administration with nitrates or nitric oxide donors is therefore contraindicated. The use of sildenafil (Viagra®) must be stopped at least 24 hours prior to starting treatment with these capsules. Treatment with these capsules must not be interrupted or stopped to take sildenafil-containing products due to the increased risk of inducing an attack of angina pectoris.

4.4 Special warnings and special precautions for use
The capsules should be used with caution in patients who are suffering from hypothyroidism, hypothermia, malnutrition, severe liver disease or severe renal disease.

Symptoms of circulatory collapse may arise after first dose, particularly in patients with labile circulation.

This product may give rise to symptoms of postural hypotension and syncope at high doses.

These capsules should be used with particular caution and under medical supervision in the following:

Hypertrophic obstructive cardiomyopathy (HOCM), constrictive pericarditis, cardiac tamponade, low cardiac filling pressures, aortic/mitral valve stenosis, and diseases associated with a raised intra-cranial pressure.

The onset of action of these capsules is not sufficiently rapid and therefore makes them unsuitable for treatment of acute angina attacks.

If these capsules are not taken as indicated (see section 4.2.) tolerance to the medication could develop.

4.5 Interaction with other medicinal products and other forms of Interaction
Concurrent intake of drugs with blood pressure lowering properties e.g. beta- blockers, calcium antagonists, vasodilators etc. and/or alcohol may potentiate the hypotensive effect of the capsules. Symptoms of circulatory collapse can arise in patients already taking ACE inhibitors.

The hypotensive effect of nitrates is potentiated by concurrent administration of sildenafil (Viagra®). This might also occur with neuroleptics and tricyclic antidepressants.

4.6 Pregnancy and lactation
There is inadequate evidence of safety of the drug in human pregnancy but nitrates have been used widely in the treatment of angina for many years without apparent ill consequence; animal studies having shown no hazard. Nevertheless it is not advisable to use this drug during pregnancy and lactation.

4.7 Effects on ability to drive and use machines
Dizziness and tiredness may occur at the start of treatment. The patient should therefore be advised that if affected, they should not drive or operate machinery. This effect may be increased by alcohol.

4.8 Undesirable effects
A headache may occur at the start of treatment, but this usually disappears after a few days. If headache persists, dosage should be decreased.

Symptoms of circulatory collapse may arise after the first dose in patients with labile circulation. Symptoms of postural hypotension and syncope may result in some patients.

Infrequently (<1% of patients) cases of nausea, vomiting, flushing and allergic rashes can occur.

4.9 Overdose
Symptoms and signs:

Headache, hypotension, nausea, vomiting, sweating, tachycardia, vertigo and syncope. Methaemoglobinaemia (cyanosis, hypoxaemia, restlessness, respiratory depression, convulsions, cardiac arrhythmias, circulatory failure, raised intracranial pressure) occurs rarely.

Treatment:

Symptomatic and supportive measures maintaining airway, breathing and circulation. If ingestion within last 1 hour, administration of activated charcoal. Gastric lavage may also be useful if ingestion within last 1 hour.

Place patient in recumbent position, raise foot of bed to encourage venous return and give IV volume expansion. Also, to maintain adequate blood pressure, the use of inotropes (dopamine/dobutamine) is recommended.

If methaemoglobinaemia (symptoms or >30% methaemoglobin), IV administration of methylene blue 1-2 mg/kg body weight. If therapy fails with second dose after 1 hour or contraindicated, consider red blood cell concentrates or exchange transfusion. In case of cerebral convulsions, diazepam or clonazepam IV, or if therapy fails, phenobarbital, phenytoin or propofol anaesthesia.

5. PHARMACOLOGICAL PROPERTIES
5.1 Pharmacodynamic properties
ATC Code: C01D A14 Vasodilator used in cardiac diseases.

Isosorbide mononitrate is an organic nitrate which, in common with other cardioactive nitrates, is a vasodilator. It produces decreased left and right ventricular end-diastolic pressures to a greater extent than the decrease in systemic arterial pressure, thereby reducing afterload and especially preload of the heart.

Isosorbide mononitrate influences the oxygen supply to the ischaemic myocardium by causing the redistribution of blood flow along collateral channels and from epicardial to endocardial regions by selective dilation of large epicardial vessels.

It reduces the requirement of the myocardium for oxygen by increasing venous capacitance, causing a pooling of blood in peripheral veins, thereby reducing ventricular volume and heart wall distension.

5.2 Pharmacokinetic properties
Isosorbide mononitrate is a vasodilator, which is rapidly absorbed following oral administration. These capsules have a bioavailability of 84 (±7)% when compared to the immediate release isosorbide mononitrate tablets. There is no effect of food on bioavailability.

The capsules contain pellets which are formulated to release 30% of the dose immediately whilst 70% of the dose is released slowly.

Time to peak plasma levels (T_{max}) is 5.0 (±3) hrs; with a half life ($T_{½}$) of 5.02 (±0.68) hrs.

Isosorbide mononitrate is extensively metabolised to nitric oxide (NO-which is the active ingredient) and isosorbide (inactive). In patients with cirrhotic disease or cardiac failure or renal failure, parameters were similar to those obtained in healthy volunteers.

5.3 Preclinical safety data
Preclinical data reveal no special hazard for humans based on conventional studies of single and repeated dose toxicity, genotoxicity, oncogenicity and toxicity to reproduction.

6. PHARMACEUTICAL PARTICULARS
6.1 List of excipients
Lactose monohydrate
Purified talc
Ethyl cellulose
Macrogol 20,000
Hydroxypropyl cellulose
Sucrose
Corn starch
Gelatin
Titanium dioxide (E171)
Iron oxide red (E172)
Iron oxide black (E172)

6.2 Incompatibilities
None Known

6.3 Shelf life
3 years

6.4 Special precautions for storage
None

6.5 Nature and contents of container
Cartons of blister strips of PVC and aluminium or of PP and aluminium.

Aluminium foil thickness 20μm or 16μm.

Pack size: 28 capsules.

6.6 Instructions for use and handling
None

7. MARKETING AUTHORISATION HOLDER
Schwarz Pharma Ltd
Schwarz House
East Street
Chesham
Bucks HP5 1DG
England

8. MARKETING AUTHORISATION NUMBER(S)
PL 04438/0015

9. DATE OF FIRST AUTHORISATION/RENEWAL OF THE AUTHORISATION
17 June 1998

10. DATE OF REVISION OF THE TEXT
May 2004

Eldepryl

(Orion Pharma (UK) Limited)

1. NAME OF THE MEDICINAL PRODUCT
Eldepryl Tablets 5 mg
Eldepryl Tablets 10 mg
Eldepryl syrup 10 mg / 5ml

2. QUALITATIVE AND QUANTITATIVE COMPOSITION
Eldepryl Tablets 5 mg; Selegiline hydrochloride Ph.Eur. 5 mg, Constit. q.s.

Eldepryl Tablets 10 mg; Selegiline hydrochloride Ph.Eur. 10 mg, Constit. q.s.

Eldepryl syrup 10 mg / 5ml; Selegiline hydrochloride Ph.Eur. 2 mg/ml, Constit. q.s.

3. PHARMACEUTICAL FORM
Tablet for peroral administration.

Syrup for peroral administration.

4. CLINICAL PARTICULARS
4.1 Therapeutic indications
Selegiline is indicated for the treatment of Parkinson's disease, or symptomatic parkinsonism. It may be used alone to delay the need for levodopa (with or without decarboxylase inhibitor) or as an adjunct to levodopa (with or without decarboxylase inhibitor).

4.2 Posology and method of administration
10 mg daily either alone or as an adjunct to levodopa or levodopa/peripheral decarboxylase inhibitor. Selegiline may be administered either as a single dose in the morning or in two divided doses of 5 mg, taken at breakfast and lunch. When selegiline is added to a levodopa regimen it is possible to reduce the levodopa dosage by an average of 30%.

4.3 Contraindications
Known hypersensitivity to selegiline or other components of the formulation.

4.4 Special warnings and special precautions for use
Selegiline should be administered cautiously to patients with peptic or duodenal ulcer, labile hypertension, cardiac arrhythmias, severe angina pectoris, severe liver or kidney dysfunction or psychosis. In higher doses (more than 30 mg daily) the selectivity of selegiline begins to diminish resulting in increased inhibition of MAO-A. Thus in higher

doses there is a risk of hypertension after ingestion of food rich in tyramine.

4.5 Interaction with other medicinal products and other forms of Interaction
Foods containing tyramine have not been reported to induce hypertensive reactions during selegiline treatment at doses used in the treatment of Parkinson's disease.

A concomitant use of nonselective MAO-inhibitors may cause severe hypotension.

No tolerability problems have been reported when a combination of selegiline and moclobemide, an inhibitor of MAO-A, has been used. However, when they are used together, the tyramine sensitivity factor may increase up to 8-9 (being 1 for selegiline alone and 2-3 for moclobemide alone). Although tyramine induced hypertensive reactions are unlikely when selegiline and moclobemide are used together, dietary restrictions (excluding foods with large amounts of tyramine such as aged cheese and yeast products) are recommended when using this combination.

Interactions between nonselective MAO-inhibitors and pethidine, as well as selegiline and pethidine have been described. The mechanism of this interaction is not fully understood and therefore, use of pethidine concomitantly with selegiline should be avoided. Tramadol may also potentially interact with Selegiline.

Dopamine should be used with caution in patients receiving Selegiline.

Serious reactions with signs and symptoms that may include diaphoresis, flushing, ataxia, tremor, hyperthermia, hyper/hypotension, seizures, palpitation, dizziness and mental changes that include agitation, confusion and hallucinations progressing to delirium and coma have been reported in some patients receiving a combination of selegiline and fluoxetine. Similar experience has been reported in patients receiving selegiline and four serotonin reuptake inhibitors, fluvoxamine, sertraline, paroxetine or venlafaxine. Since the mechanisms of these reactions are not fully understood, it is recommended to avoid the combination of selegiline with fluoxetine, sertraline, paroxetine or venlafaxine. A minimum period of five weeks should be allowed between discontinuation of fluoxetine and initiation of selegiline treatment, due to the long half-lives of fluoxetine and its active metabolite. As the half-lives of selegiline and its metabolites are short, a wash-out period of 14 days after selegiline treatment would be sufficient before starting fluoxetine. The concomitant use of selegiline and citalopram has been investigated in healthy volunteers. No signs of clinically relevant pharmacokinetic or pharmacodynamic interactions between the two drugs were observed.

Severe CNS toxicity has been reported in patients with the combination of tricyclic antidepressants and selegiline. In one patient receiving amitriptyline and selegiline this included hyperpyrexia and death, and another patient receiving protriptyline and selegiline experienced tremor, agitation, and restlessness followed by unresponsiveness and death two weeks after selegiline was added. Other adverse reactions occasionally reported in patients receiving a combination of selegiline with various tricyclic antidepressants include hyper/hypotension, dizziness, diaphoresis, tremor, seizures, and changes in behavioural and mental status. Since the mechanisms of these reactions are not fully understood, it is recommended to be cautious when using selegiline together with tricyclic antidepressants.

Concomitant use of oral contraceptives (tablets containing the combination of gestodene/ethinyl estradiol or levonorgestrel/ethinyl estradiol) and selegiline may cause an increase in the oral bioavailability of selegiline. Thus appropriate caution during the concomitant administration of selegiline and oral contraceptives should be applied.

4.6 Pregnancy and lactation
The available safety data concerning the use during pregnancy and lactation is insufficient to justify the use of selegiline in these patient groups.

4.7 Effects on ability to drive and use machines
No effects on ability to drive or operate machines.

4.8 Undesirable effects
In monotherapy, selegiline has been found to be well tolerated. Dry mouth, transient rise of serum alanine aminotransferase (ALAT) values and sleeping disorders have been reported more frequently than in patients receiving placebo. Because selegiline potentiates the effects of levodopa, the adverse reactions of levodopa, e.g. abnormal movements (such as dyskinesias), nausea, agitation, confusion, hallucinations, headache, postural hypotension, cardiac arrhythmias and vertigo, may be emphasised, particularly if the dose of levodopa is too high. Such adverse reactions usually disappear when the levodopa dosage is decreased. Levodopa dosage can be reduced by an average of 30% when selegiline is added to the treatment. Micturition difficulties and skin reactions have also been reported during selegiline treatment. Follow-up of these possible adverse reactions is important.

A summary of the undesirable effects in terms of frequency of occurrence is shown below.

(see Table 1)

4.9 Overdose
No overdosage cases are known. However, experience gained during selegiline's development reveals that some individuals exposed to doses of 600 mg/day selegiline suffered severe hypotension and psychomotor agitation.

Theoretically, overdosage causes significant inhibition of both MAO-A and MAO-B and thus, symptoms of overdosage may resemble those observed with non-selective MAO-inhibitors, such as different central nervous and cardiovascular system disorders (e.g. drowsiness, dizziness, faintness, irritability, hyperactivity, agitation, severe headache, hallucination, hypertension, hypotension, vascular collapse, rapid and irregular pulse, precordial pain, respiratory depression and failure, hyperpyrexia, diaphoresis). There is no specific antidote and the treatment is symptomatic.

5. PHARMACOLOGICAL PROPERTIES

5.1 Pharmacodynamic properties
Selegiline is a selective MAO-B-inhibitor which prevents dopamine breakdown in the brain. It also inhibits the reuptake of dopamine at the presynaptic dopamine receptor. These effects potentiate dopaminergic function in the brain and help to even out and prolong the effect of exogenous and endogenous dopamine. Thus, selegiline potentiates and prolongs the effect of levodopa in the treatment of parkinsonism.

Double-blind studies on early phase Parkinsonian patients showed that patients receiving selegiline monotherapy manage significantly longer without levodopa therapy than controls receiving placebo. These patients could also maintain their ability to work longer.

The addition of selegiline to levodopa (with or without decarboxylase inhibitor) therapy helps to alleviate dose related fluctuations and end of dose deterioration.

When selegiline is added to such a regimen it is possible to reduce the levodopa dosage by an average of 30%. Unlike conventional MAO-inhibitors, which inhibit both the MAO-A and MAO-B enzyme, selegiline is a specific MAO-B inhibitor and can be given safely with levodopa.

Selegiline HCl does not cause the so called "cheese effect" either when used alone as monotherapy, or when used with other drugs, except for moclobemide or nonselective MAO-inhibitors.

5.2 Pharmacokinetic properties
Selegiline HCl is readily absorbed from the gastrointestinal tract. The maximal concentrations are reached in half an hour after oral administration. The bioavailability is low; 10% (on the average; interindividual variation is large) of unchanged selegiline can reach the systemic circulation.

Selegiline is a lipophilic, slightly basic compound which quickly penetrates into tissues, also into brain. Selegiline HCl inhibits MAO irreversibly and enzyme activity only increases again after new enzyme is synthesised. The inhibitory effect of a single 10 mg dose lasts for 24 hours. Selegiline is rapidly distributed throughout the body, the apparent volume of distribution being 500 litres after an intravenous 10 mg dose. 75-85 % of selegiline is bound to plasma proteins at therapeutic concentrations.

Selegiline is rapidly metabolised, mainly in the liver, into desmethylselegiline, l-methamphetamine and to l-amphetamine. In humans, the three metabolites have been identified in plasma and urine after single and multiple doses of selegiline. The mean elimination half-life is 1.6 hours for selegiline. The total body clearance of selegiline is about 240 L/hour. Metabolites of selegiline are excreted mainly via the urine with about 15% occurring in the faeces.

5.3 Preclinical safety data
No mutagenicity or carcinogenicity due to selegiline have emerged in routine studies.

6. PHARMACEUTICAL PARTICULARS

6.1 List of excipients
Tablets: Mannitol, maize starch, microcrystalline cellulose, povidone, and magnesium stearate.

Syrup: Methyl parahydroxybenzoate, propyl parahydroxybenzoate, butyl parahydroxybenzoate, sucrose, xanthan gum T, saccharin sodium, flavour mango, purified water.

6.2 Incompatibilities
No other incompatibilities noted.

6.3 Shelf life
36 months

6.4 Special precautions for storage

Tablets

HDPE bottle; Do not store above 25 °C. Keep the container tightly closed.

Al/Al blister; Do not store above 25 °C. Store in the original package.

Syrup

No special precautions.

6.5 Nature and contents of container

5 mg Tablets

White polyethylene bottle with polyethylene closure; 100 tablets

Al/Al blister; 30, 50, 60, 100 tablets

10 mg Tablets

White polyethylene bottle with polyethylene closure; 50, 100 tablets

Al/Al blister; 30, 50, 60, 100 tablets

Syrup

Amber glass bottle (200 ml) sealed with a pilfer-proof type EPE/Aluminium Melinex screw cap. The container is packed in a cardboard box with a graduated dose dispenser.

6.6 Instructions for use and handling
None.

7. MARKETING AUTHORISATION HOLDER
Orion Corporation, Orionintie 1, FIN-02200 Espoo, Finland

8. MARKETING AUTHORISATION NUMBER(S)
5 mg Tablets: PL 06043/0011

10 mg Tablets: PL 06043/0012

Syrup: PL 06043/0013

9. DATE OF FIRST AUTHORISATION/RENEWAL OF THE AUTHORISATION
5 mg Tablets: 1.7.1993 / Renewed 28.7.1997

10 mg Tablets: 1.7.1993 / Renewed 28.7.1997

Syrup: 1.7.1993 / Renewed 27.7.1997

10. DATE OF REVISION OF THE TEXT
5 mg Tablets, 10 mg Tablets and syrup: 20th October 2003

Table 1

Psychiatric disorders	Common (>1/100, <1/10)	Sleeping disorders, confusion, hallucinations
Nervous system disorders	Common (>1/100, <1/10)	Dry mouth, abnormal movements (such as dyskinesias), vertigo
	Rare (>1/10,000, <1/1,000)	Agitation, headache
Cardiac disorders	Rare (>1/10,000, <1/1,000)	Cardiac arrhythmias
Vascular disorders	Common (>1/100, <1/10)	Postural hypotension
Gastrointestinal disorders	Common (>1/100, <1/10)	Nausea
Hepato-biliary disorders	Common (> 1/100, <1/10)	Transient rise of serum alanine aminotransferase (ALAT)
Skin and subcutaneous tissue	Rare (>1/10,000, <1/1,000)	Skin reactions
Renal and urinary disorders	Rare (>1/10,000, <1/1,000)	Micturition difficulties

Elidel 1% Cream

(Novartis Pharmaceuticals UK Ltd)

1. NAME OF THE MEDICINAL PRODUCT
▼ Elidel® 1% cream

2. QUALITATIVE AND QUANTITATIVE COMPOSITION
1 g of cream contains 10 mg of pimecrolimus.

For excipients, see 6.1.

3. PHARMACEUTICAL FORM

Cream.

Whitish and homogeneous.

4. CLINICAL PARTICULARS

4.1 Therapeutic indications

Elidel is indicated in patients with mild to moderate atopic dermatitis (eczema) aged 2 years and over for:

- short-term treatment of signs and symptoms
- intermittent long-term treatment for prevention of progression to flares

4.2 Posology and method of administration

Elidel should be prescribed by physicians with experience in the topical treatment of atopic dermatitis.

Data from clinical studies support intermittent treatment with Elidel for up to 12 months.

If no improvement occurs after 6 weeks, or in case of disease exacerbation, Elidel should be stopped and further therapeutic options considered.

Adults

Apply a thin layer of Elidel to the affected skin twice daily and rub in gently and completely. Each affected region of the skin should be treated with Elidel until clearance occurs and then treatment should be discontinued.

Elidel may be used on all skin areas, including the head and face, neck and intertriginous areas, except on mucous membranes. Elidel should not be applied under occlusion (see Section 4.4 "Special warnings and precautions for use").

In the long-term management of atopic dermatitis (eczema), Elidel treatment should begin at first appearance of signs and symptoms of atopic dermatitis to prevent flares of the disease. Elidel should be used twice daily for as long as signs and symptoms persist. If discontinued, treatment should be resumed upon first recurrence of signs and symptoms to prevent flares of the disease.

Emollients can be applied immediately after using Elidel.

Due to the low level of systemic absorption, there is no restriction either in the total daily dose applied or in the extent of the body surface area treated or in the duration of treatment.

Paediatric patients

For children (2-11 years) and adolescents (12-17 years) the posology and method of administration are the same as for adults.

The use of Elidel in patients under 2 years of age is not recommended until further data become available.

Elderly patients

Atopic dermatitis (eczema) is rarely observed in patients aged 65 and over. Clinical studies with Elidel did not include a sufficient number of patients in this age range to determine whether they respond differently from younger patients.

4.3 Contraindications

Hypersensitivity to pimecrolimus, other macrolactams or to any of the excipients. For excipients, see 6.1.

4.4 Special warnings and special precautions for use

Elidel should not be applied to areas affected by acute cutaneous viral infections (herpes simplex, chicken pox).

Elidel has not been evaluated for its efficacy and safety in the treatment of clinically infected atopic dermatitis. Before commencing treatment with Elidel, clinical infections at treatment sites should be cleared.

While patients with atopic dermatitis are predisposed to superficial skin infections including eczema herpeticum (Kaposi's varicelliform eruption), treatment with Elidel may be associated with an increased risk of skin herpes simplex virus infection, or eczema herpeticum (manifesting as rapid spread of vesicular and erosive lesions).

In the presence of herpes simplex skin infection, Elidel treatment at the site of infection should be discontinued until the viral infection has cleared.

Although patients treated with Elidel experienced overall a lower incidence of bacterial skin infections as compared to patients treated with the vehicle, patients with severe atopic dermatitis may have an increased risk of skin bacterial infections (impetigo) during treatment with Elidel.

Use of Elidel may cause mild and transient reactions at the site of application, such as a feeling of warmth and/or burning sensation. If the application site reaction is severe, the risk-benefit of treatment should be re-evaluated.

Care should be taken to avoid contact with eyes and mucous membranes. If accidentally applied to these areas, the cream should be thoroughly wiped off and/or rinsed off with water.

The use of Elidel under occlusion has not been studied in patients. Occlusive dressings are not recommended.

As the safety of Elidel has not been established in erythrodermic patients, the use of the product in this patient population cannot be recommended.

Elidel has not been studied in patients with Netherton's syndrome. Due to the potential for increased systemic absorption of pimecrolimus, Elidel is not recommended in patients with Netherton's syndrome.

Physicians should advise patients on appropriate sun protection measures, such as minimisation of the time in the sun, use of sunscreen product and covering the skin with appropriate clothing (see Section 4.5 "Interaction with other medicinal products and other forms of interaction").

Elidel has not been studied in immunocompromised patients and in patients with evidence of skin malignancies and there is no data to support its use in these patients.

Long-term effect on the local skin immune response and on the incidence of skin malignancies is unknown.

Elidel contains cetyl alcohol and stearyl alcohol which may cause local skin reactions. Elidel also contains propylene glycol, which may cause skin irritation.

4.5 Interaction with other medicinal products and other forms of Interaction

Potential interactions between Elidel and other medicinal products have not been systematically evaluated. Pimecrolimus is exclusively metabolised by CYP 450 3A4. Based on its minimal extent of absorption, interactions of Elidel with systemically administered medicinal products are unlikely to occur (see Section 5.2 "Pharmacokinetic properties").

The present data indicate that Elidel can be used simultaneously with antibiotics, antihistamines and corticosteroids (oral/nasal/inhaled).

Based on the minimal extent of absorption, a potential systemic interaction with vaccination is unlikely to occur. However, this interaction has not been studied. Therefore, in patients with extensive disease, it is recommended to administer vaccinations during treatment-free intervals.

Concomitant use of other topical anti-inflammatory preparations including corticosteroids has not been investigated, therefore Elidel should not be used concomitantly with topical corticosteroids and other topical anti-inflammatory products. There is no experience with concomitant use of immunosuppressive therapies given for atopic eczema such as UVB, UVA, PUVA, azathioprine and cyclosporin A.

Elidel has no photocarcinogenic potential in animals (see section 5.3. "Preclinical Safety Data"). However, since the relevance to man is unknown excessive exposure of the skin to ultraviolet light including light from a solarium, or therapy with PUVA, UVA or UVB should be avoided during treatment with Elidel.

4.6 Pregnancy and lactation

Pregnancy

There are no adequate data from the use of Elidel in pregnant women. Animal studies using dermal application do not indicate direct or indirect harmful effects with respect to embryonal/fetal development. Studies in animals after oral application have shown reproductive toxicity (see Section 5.3 "Preclinical safety data"). Based on the minimal extent of pimecrolimus absorption after topical application of Elidel (see Section 5.2 "Pharmacokinetic properties"), the potential risk for humans is considered limited. However, Elidel should not be used during pregnancy.

Lactation

Animal studies on milk excretion after topical application were not conducted and the use of pimecrolimus in breast-feeding women has not been studied. It is not known whether pimecrolimus is excreted in the milk after topical application.

However, based on the minimal extent of pimecrolimus absorption after topical application of Elidel, (see Section 5.2 "Pharmacokinetic properties"), the potential risk for humans is considered limited. Caution should be exercised when Elidel is administered to breastfeeding women.

Breastfeeding mothers may use Elidel but should not apply Elidel to the breast in order to avoid unintentional oral uptake by the newborn.

4.7 Effects on ability to drive and use machines

Elidel has no known effect on the ability to drive and use machines.

4.8 Undesirable effects

The most common adverse events were application site reactions which were reported by approximately 19% of the patients treated with Elidel and 16% of patients in the control groups. These reactions generally occurred early in treatment, were mild/moderate and were of short duration.

Frequency estimates: very common ($\geqslant$ 1/10); common ($\geqslant$ 1/100, < 1/10); uncommon ($\geqslant$ 1/1,000, < 1/100); rare ($\geqslant$ 1/10,000, < 1/1,000); very rare (< 1/10,000, including isolated reports)

very common: application site burning.

common: application site reactions (irritation, pruritus and erythema), skin infections (folliculitis).

uncommon: furuncle, impetigo, herpes simplex, herpes zoster, herpes simplex dermatitis (eczema herpeticum), molluscum contagiosum, skin papilloma, application site disorders such as rash, pain, paraesthesia, desquamation, dryness, oedema, and condition aggravated.

rare: alcohol intolerance (in most cases, flushing, rash, burning, itching or swelling occurred shortly after the intake of alcohol), allergic skin reactions (e.g. dermatitis, urticaria).

4.9 Overdose

There has been no experience of overdose with Elidel.

No incidents of accidental ingestion have been reported.

5. PHARMACOLOGICAL PROPERTIES

5.1 Pharmacodynamic properties

Pharmacotherapeutic group: Other dermatologicals, ATC code: D11AX15.

Non-clinical pharmacology

Pimecrolimus is a lipophilic anti-inflammatory ascomycin macrolactam derivative and a cell selective inhibitor of the production and release of pro-inflammatory cytokines.

Pimecrolimus binds with high affinity to macrophilin-12 and inhibits the calcium-dependent phosphatase calcineurin. As a consequence, it blocks the synthesis of inflammatory cytokines in T cells.

Pimecrolimus exhibits high anti-inflammatory activity in animal models of skin inflammation after topical and systemic application. In the pig model of allergic contact dermatitis, topical pimecrolimus is as effective as potent corticosteroids. Unlike corticosteroids, pimecrolimus does not cause skin atrophy in pigs and does not affect Langerhanścells in murine skin.

Pimecrolimus has only a low potential to affect systemic immune responses, as shown in standard models of systemic immunosuppression. Furthermore, pimecrolimus neither impairs the primary immune response nor affects lymph nodes in murine allergic contact dermatitis. Topical pimecrolimus penetrates similarly into, but permeates much less through human skin than corticosteroids, indicating a very low potential of pimecrolimus for systemic absorption.

In conclusion, pimecrolimus has a skin-selective pharmacological profile different from corticosteroids. It combines high anti-inflammatory activity in the skin with a low potential to impair local and systemic immunosurveillance.

Clinical data

The efficacy and safety profile of Elidel has been evaluated in more than 2000 patients including infants ($\geqslant$ 3 months), children, adolescents, and adults enrolled in phase II and III studies. Over 1500 of these patients were treated with Elidel and over 500 were treated with control treatment i.e. either Elidel vehicle and/or topical corticosteroids.

Short-term (acute) treatment

Children and adolescents: Two 6-week, vehicle-controlled trials were conducted including a total of 403 paediatric patients aged 2 to 17 years. Patients were treated twice daily with Elidel. The data of both studies were pooled.

Infants: A similar 6-week study was conducted in 186 patients aged 3-23 months.

In these three 6-week studies, the efficacy results at end-point were as follows:

(see Table 1 on next page)

A significant improvement in pruritus was observed within the first week of treatment in 44% of children and adolescents and in 70% of infants.

Adults: Elidel was less effective than 0.1% betamethasone-17-valerate in the short-term treatment (3 weeks) of adults with moderate to severe atopic dermatitis.

Long-term treatment:

Two double-blind studies of long-term management of atopic dermatitis were undertaken in 713 children and adolescents (2-17 years) and 251 infants (3-23 months). Elidel was evaluated as foundation therapy.

Elidel was used at first signs of itching and redness to prevent progression to flares of atopic dermatitis. Only in case of a flare of severe disease not controlled by Elidel, treatment with medium potency topical corticosteroids was initiated.

When corticosteroid therapy was initiated for the treatment of flares, Elidel therapy was discontinued. The control group received Elidel vehicle in order to maintain blinding.

Both studies showed a significant reduction in the incidence of flares ($p<0.001$) in favour of Elidel treatment; Elidel treatment showed better efficacy in all secondary assessments (Eczema Area Severity Index, Investigators Global Assessment, subject assessment); pruritus was controlled within a week with Elidel.

More patients treated with Elidel completed 6 months [children (61% Elidel vs 34% control), infants (70% Elidel vs 33% control)] and 12 months with no flare [children (51% Elidel vs 28% control), infants (57% Elidel vs 28% control)].

Elidel had a sparing effect on the use of topical corticosteroids: more patients treated with Elidel did not use corticosteroids in 12 months [children (57% Elidel vs 32% control), infants (64% Elidel vs 35% control)]. The efficacy of Elidel was maintained over time.

A 6-month randomized, double-blind, parallel group, vehicle-controlled study of similar design was performed in 192 adults with moderate to severe atopic dermatitis. Topical corticosteroid medication was used on 14.2 ± 24.2% of the days of the 24-week treatment period in Elidel group and on 37.2 ± 34.6% of the days in the control group ($p<0.001$). A total of 50.0% of the patients treated with Elidel did not experience any flare compared with 24.0% of the patients randomized to the control group.

A one year double-blind study in adults with moderate to severe atopic dermatitis was conducted to compare Elidel to 0.1% triamcinolone acetonide cream (for trunk and extremities) plus 1% hydrocortisone acetate cream (for

Table 1

Endpoint	Criteria	Children and adolescents Elidel 1% (N=267)	Vehicle (N=136)	p-value	Infants Elidel 1% (N=123)	Vehicle (N=63)	p-value
IGA*:	Clear or almost clear [1]	34.8%	18.4%	< 0.001	54.5%	23.8%	<0.001
IGA*	Improvement [2]	59.9%	33%	not done	68%	40%	Not done
Pruritus:	Absent or mild	56.6%	33.8%	< 0.001	72.4%	33.3%	<0.001
EASI°:	Overall (mean % change)[3]	-43.6	-0.7	< 0.001	-61.8	+7.35	<0.001
EASI°:	Head/Neck (mean % change)[3]	-61.1	+0.6	< 0.001	-74.0	+31.48	<0.001

* Investigators Global Assessment

° Eczema Area Severity Index (EASI): mean % change in clinical signs (erythema, infiltration, excoriation, lichenification) and body surface area involved

[1]: p-value based on CMH test stratified by centre

[2]Improvement=lower IGA than at baseline

[3]: p-value based on ANCOVA model of EASI at Day 43 endpoint, with centre and treatment as factors and baseline (Day 1) EASI a covariate;

face, neck and intertriginous areas). Both Elidel and topical corticosteroids were used without restrictions. Half of the patients in the control group received topical corticosteroids for more than 95% of study days. Elidel was less effective than 0.1% triamcinolone acetonide cream (for trunk and extremities) plus 1% hydrocortisone acetate cream (for face, neck and intertriginous areas) in the long-term treatment (52 weeks) of adults with moderate to severe atopic dermatitis.

Long-term clinical trials were 1 year in duration. There is no clinical data beyond 1 year of treatment.

Frequency of application greater than twice daily has not been studied.

Special studies:

Tolerability studies demonstrated that Elidel has not shown contact sensitising, phototoxic or photosensitising potential, nor did they show any cumulative irritation.

The atrophogenic potential of Elidel in humans was tested in comparison to medium and highly potent topical steroids (betamethasone-17-valerate 0.1% cream, triamcinolone acetonide 0.1% cream) and vehicle in sixteen healthy volunteers treated for 4 weeks. Both topical corticosteroids induced a significant reduction in skin thickness measured by echography, as compared to Elidel and vehicle, which did not induce a reduction of skin thickness.

5.2 Pharmacokinetic properties

Data in animals

The bioavailability of pimecrolimus in mini-pigs following a single dermal dose (applied for 22h under semi-occlusion) was 0.03%.

The amount of active substance-related material in the skin at the application site (almost exclusively unchanged pimecrolimus) remained practically constant for 10 days.

Data in humans

Absorption in adults

Systemic exposure to pimecrolimus was investigated in 12 adults with atopic dermatitis who were treated with Elidel twice daily for 3 weeks. The affected body surface area (BSA) ranged from 15-59%. 77.5% of pimecrolimus blood concentrations were below 0.5ng/ml and 99.8% of the total samples were below 1 ng/ml. The highest pimecrolimus blood concentration was 1.4 ng/ml in one patient.

In 40 adult patients treated for up to 1 year with Elidel, having 14-62% of their BSA affected at baseline, 98% of pimecrolimus blood concentrations were below 0.5 ng/ml. A maximum blood concentration of 0.8 ng/ml was measured in only 2 patients in week 6 of treatment. There was no increase in blood concentration over time in any patient during the 12 months of treatment. In 8 adult atopic dermatitis patients, in which AUC levels could be quantified, the $AUC_{(0\text{-}12h)}$ values ranged from 2.5 to 11.4 ng·h/ml.

Absorption in children

Systemic exposure to pimecrolimus was investigated in 58 paediatric patients aged 3 months to 14 years. The affected BSA ranged from 10-92%. These children were treated with Elidel twice daily for 3 weeks and five out of them were treated for up to 1 year on a "as needed" basis.

Pimecrolimus blood concentrations were consistently low regardless of the extent of lesions treated or duration of therapy. They were in a range similar to that measured in adult patients. Around 60% of pimecrolimus blood concentrations were below 0.5 ng/ml and 97% of all samples were below 2 ng/ml. The highest blood concentrations measured in 2 paediatric patients aged 8 months to 14 years were 2.0 ng/ml.

In infants (aged 3 to 23 months), the highest blood concentration measured in one patient was 2.6 ng/ml. In the 5 children treated for 1 year, blood concentrations were consistently low (maximum blood concentration was 1.94 ng/ml in 1 patient). There was no increase in blood concentration over time in any patient during the 12 months of treatment.

In 8 paediatric patients aged 2-14 years, $AUC_{(0\text{-}12h)}$ ranged from 5.4 to 18.8 ng·h/ml. AUC ranges observed in patients with <40% BSA affected at baseline were comparable to those in patients with ⩾40% BSA.

The maximum body surface area treated was 92% in clinical pharmacology studies and up to 100% in Phase III trials.

Distribution, Metabolism, and Excretion

Consistent with its skin selectivity, after topical application, pimecrolimus blood levels are very low. Therefore pimecrolimus metabolism could not be determined after topical administration.

After single oral administration of radiolabeled pimecrolimus in healthy subjects, unchanged pimecrolimus was the major active substance-related component in blood and there were numerous minor metabolites of moderate polarity that appeared to be products of O-demethylations and oxygenation.

Active substance-related radioactivity was excreted principally via the faeces (78.4%) and only a small fraction (2.5%) was recovered in urine. Total mean recovery of radioactivity was 80.9%. Parent compound was not detected in urine and less than 1% of radioactivity in faeces was accounted for by unchanged pimecrolimus.

No metabolism of pimecrolimus was observed in human skin *in vitro*.

5.3 Preclinical safety data

Conventional studies of repeated dose toxicity, reproductive toxicity and carcinogenicity using oral administration produced effects at exposures sufficiently in excess of those in man to be of negligible clinical significance. Pimecrolimus had no genotoxic, antigenic, phototoxic, photoallergenic or photocarcinogenic potential. Dermal application in embryo/fetal developmental studies in rats and rabbits and in carcinogenicity studies in mice and rats were negative.

Effects on reproductive organs and altered sex hormone functions were seen in male and female rats in repeated dose toxicity studies after oral administration of 10 or 40 mg/kg/day (= 20 to 60 times the maximum human exposure after dermal application). This is reflected by the findings from the fertility study. The No Observed Adverse Effect Level (NOAEL) for female fertility was 10 mg/kg/day (= 20 times the maximum human exposure after dermal application). In the oral embryotoxicity study in rabbits, a higher resorption rate associated with maternal toxicity was observed at 20 mg/kg/day (= 7 times the maximum human exposure after dermal application); the mean number of live fetuses was not affected.

6. PHARMACEUTICAL PARTICULARS

6.1 List of excipients

Medium chain triglycerides
oleyl alcohol
propylene glycol
stearyl alcohol
cetyl alcohol
mono-and di-glycerides
sodium cetostearyl sulphate
benzyl alcohol
citric acid anhydrous
sodium hydroxide
purified water

6.2 Incompatibilities

Not applicable

6.3 Shelf life

2 years. After first opening of the container: 12 months

6.4 Special precautions for storage

Do not store above 25°C. Do not freeze.

6.5 Nature and contents of container

Aluminium tube with a phenol-epoxy protective inner lacquer and polypropylene screw cap.

Tubes of 30, 60 and 100 grams.

6.6 Instructions for use and handling

Emollients can be applied together with Elidel (see Section 4.2 "Posology and method of administration").

7. MARKETING AUTHORISATION HOLDER

Novartis Pharmaceuticals UK Limited
Frimley Business Park
Frimley
Camberley
Surrey
GU16 7SR

8. MARKETING AUTHORISATION NUMBER(S)

PL 00101/0659

9. DATE OF FIRST AUTHORISATION/RENEWAL OF THE AUTHORISATION

3 October 2002

10. DATE OF REVISION OF THE TEXT

10 May 2005

Legal Category

POM

Elleste Duet 1mg

(Pharmacia Limited)

1. NAME OF THE MEDICINAL PRODUCT

Elleste Duet 1mg

2. QUALITATIVE AND QUANTITATIVE COMPOSITION

One white tablet contains 1mg estradiol (as estradiol hemihydrate)

One green tablet contains 1mg estradiol (as estradiol hemihydrate) and 1mg norethisterone acetate.

For excipients, see 6.1

3. PHARMACEUTICAL FORM

Film coated tablets.

4. CLINICAL PARTICULARS

4.1 Therapeutic indications

Hormone replacement therapy (HRT) for estrogen deficiency symptoms in post- and peri-menopausal women. (See also Section 4.4)

The experience of treating women older than 65 years is limited.

4.2 Posology and method of administration

This product is a continuous sequential HRT. One white tablet to be taken daily for the first 16 days, followed by one pale green tablet for the next 12 days. A new cycle should then begin without any break. Therapy may start at any time in patients with established amenorrhoea or who are experiencing long intervals between spontaneous menses. In patients who are menstruating, it is advised that therapy starts on the first day of bleeding. Patients changing from another cyclical or continuous sequential preparation should complete the cycle and may then change to Elleste Duet 1mg without a break in therapy. Patients changing from a continuous combined preparation may start therapy at any time if amenorrhoea is established, or otherwise start on the first day of bleeding.

Elderly

There are no special dosage requirements in elderly patients.

Children

Not to be used in children.

Elleste Duet tablets are available in two strengths: Elleste Duet 1 mg (containing 1 mg estradiol and 1 mg norethisterone acetate) and Elleste Duet 2 mg (containing 2 mg estradiol and 1 mg norethisterone acetate). For initiation and continuation of treatment of post- and peri-menopausal symptoms, the lowest effective dose for the shortest duration (see also Section 4.4) should be used. Elleste Duet 2 mg is additionally indicated for prevention of osteoporosis in postmenopausal women at high risk of future fractures and who are intolerant of, or contraindicated for, other medicinal products approved for the prevention of osteoporosis.

Missed Tablet: If a tablet is missed it should be taken within 12 hours of when normally taken; otherwise the tablet should be discarded, and the usual tablet should be taken the following day. If a tablet is missed there is an increased likelihood of breakthrough bleeding or spotting.

4.3 Contraindications

Known, past or suspected breast cancer;

Known or suspected estrogen-dependent malignant tumours (e.g. endometrial cancer);

Undiagnosed genital bleeding;

Untreated endometrial hyperplasia;

Previous idiopathic or current venous thromboembolism (deep venous thrombosis, pulmonary embolism);

Active or recent arterial thromboembolic disease (e.g. angina, myocardial infarction);

Acute liver disease, or a history of liver disease as long as liver function tests have failed to return to normal;

Known hypersensitivity to the active substances or to any of the excipients;

Porphyria.

4.4 Special warnings and special precautions for use

For the treatment of postmenopausal symptoms, HRT should only be initiated for symptoms that adversely affect quality of life. In all cases a careful appraisal of the risks and benefits should be undertaken at least annually and HRT should only be continued as long as the benefit outweighs the risk.

Medical Examination/Follow Up

Before initiating or reinstituting HRT, a complete personal and family medical history should be taken. Physical (including pelvic and breast) examination should be guided by this and by the contraindications and warnings for use. During treatment, periodic check-ups are recommended of a frequency and nature adapted to the individual woman. Women should be advised what changes in their breasts should be reported to their doctor or nurse (see 'Breast cancer' below). Investigations, including mammography, should be carried out in accordance with currently accepted screening practices, modified to the clinical needs of the individual.

Conditions Which Need Supervision

If any of the following conditions are present, have occurred previously, and/or have been aggravated during pregnancy or previous hormone treatment, the patient should be closely supervised. It should be taken into account that these conditions may recur or be aggravated during treatment with Elleste Duet 1 mg, in particular:

- Leiomyoma (uterine fibroids) or endometriosis
- A history of, or risk factors for, thromboembolic disorders (see below)
- Risk factors for estrogen dependent tumours, e.g. 1st degree heredity for breast cancer
- Hypertension
- Liver disorders (e.g. liver adenoma)
- Diabetes mellitus with or without vascular involvement
- Cholelithiasis
- Migraine or (severe) headache
- Systemic lupus erythematosus
- A history of endometrial hyperplasia (see below)
- Epilepsy
- Asthma
- Otosclerosis

Reasons for Immediate Withdrawal of Therapy:

Therapy should be discontinued if a contra-indication is discovered and in the following situations:

- Jaundice or deterioration in liver function
- Significant increase in blood pressure
- New onset of migraine-type headache
- Pregnancy

Endometrial Hyperplasia

The risk of endometrial hyperplasia and carcinoma is increased when estrogens are administered alone for prolonged periods (see Section 4.8). The addition of a progestogen for at least 12 days per cycle in non-hysterectomised women greatly reduces this risk.

Break-through bleeding and spotting may occur during the first months of treatment. If break-through bleeding or spotting appears after some time on therapy, or continues after treatment has been discontinued, the reason should be investigated, which may include endometrial biopsy to exclude endometrial malignancy.

Breast Cancer

A randomised placebo-controlled trial, the Women's Health Initiative Study (WHI), and epidemiological studies, including the Million Women Study (MWS), have reported an increased risk of breast cancer in women taking estrogens, estrogen-progesterone combinations or tibolone for HRT for several years (see Section 4.8).

For all HRT, an excess risk becomes apparent within a few years of use and increases with duration of intake but returns to baseline within a few (at most five) years after stopping treatment.

In the MWS, the relative risk of breast cancer with conjugated equine estrogens (CEE) or estradiol (E2) was greater when a progestogen was added, either sequentially or continuously, and regardless of type of progestogen. There was no evidence of a difference in risk between the different routes of administration.

In the WHI study, the continuous combined conjugated equine estrogen and medroxyprogesterone acetate (CEE + MPA) product used was associated with breast cancers that were slightly larger in size and more frequently had local lymph node metastases compared to placebo.

HRT, especially estrogen-progestogen combined treatment, increases the density of mammographic images which may adversely affect the radiological detection of breast cancer.

Venous Thromboembolism

HRT is associated with a higher relative risk of developing venous thromboembolism (VTE), i.e. deep vein thrombosis or pulmonary embolism. One randomised controlled trial and epidemiological studies found a two- to threefold higher risk for users compared with non-users. For non-users it is estimated that the number of cases of VTE that will occur over a 5 year period is about 3 per 1000 women aged 50-59 years and 8 per 1000 women aged 60-69 years. It is estimated that in healthy women who use HRT for 5 years, the number of additional cases of VTE over a 5 year period will be between 2 and 6 (best estimate = 4) per 1000 women aged 50-59 years and between 5 and 15 (best estimate = 9) per 1000 women aged 60-69 years. The occurrence of such an event is more likely in the first year of HRT than later.

Generally recognised risk factors for VTE include a personal history or family history, severe obesity (BM > 30 kg/m^2) and systemic lupus erythematosus (SLE). There is no consensus about the possible role of varicose veins in VTE.

Patients with a history of VTE or known thrombophilic states have an increased risk of VTE. HRT may add to this risk. Personal or strong family history of thromboembolism or recurrent spontaneous abortion should be investigated in order to exclude a thrombophilic predisposition. Until a thorough evaluation of thrombophilic factors has been made or anticoagulant treatment initiated, use of HRT in such patients should be viewed as contraindicated. Those women already on anticoagulant treatment require careful consideration of the benefit-risk of use of HRT.

The risk of VTE may be temporarily increased with prolonged immobilisation, major trauma or major surgery. As in all postoperative patients, scrupulous attention should be given to prophylactic measures to prevent VTE following surgery. Where prolonged immobilisation is liable to follow elective surgery, particularly abdominal or orthopaedic surgery to the lower limbs, consideration should be given to temporarily stopping HRT 4 to 6 weeks earlier, if possible. Treatment should not be restarted until the woman is completely mobilised.

If VTE develops after initiating therapy, the drug should be discontinued. Patients should be told to contact their doctors immediately when they are aware of a potential thromboembolic symptom (e.g., painful swelling of a leg, sudden pain in the chest, dyspnea).

Coronary Artery Disease

There is no evidence from randomised controlled trials of cardiovascular benefit with continuous combined conjugated estrogens and medroxyprogesterone acetate (MPA). Two large clinical trials (WHI and HERS i.e. Heart and Estrogen/progestin Replacement Study) showed a possible increased risk of cardiovascular morbidity in the first year of use and no overall benefit. For other HRT products there are only limited data from randomised controlled trials examining effects in cardiovascular morbidity or mortality. Therefore, it is uncertain whether these findings also extend to other HRT products.

Stroke

One large randomised clinical trial (WHI-trial) found, as a secondary outcome, an increased risk of ischaemic stroke in healthy women during treatment with continuous combined conjugated estrogens and MPA. For women who do not use HRT, it is estimated that the number of cases of stroke that will occur over a 5 year period is about 3 per 1000 women aged 50-59 years and 11 per 1000 women aged 60-69 years. It is estimated that for women who use conjugated estrogen and MPA for 5 years, the number of additional cases will be between 0 and 3 (best estimate = 1) per 1000 users aged 50-59 years and between 1 and 9 (best estimate = 4) per 1000 users aged 60-69 years. It is unknown whether the increased risk also extends to other HRT products.

Ovarian Cancer

Long-term (at least 5 to 10 years) use of estrogen-only HRT products in hysterectomised women has been associated with an increased risk of ovarian cancer in some epidemiological studies. It is uncertain whether long-term use of combined HRT confers a different risk than estrogen-only products.

Other Conditions

Estrogens may cause fluid retention, and therefore patients with cardiac or renal dysfunction should be carefully observed. Patients with terminal renal insufficiency should be closely observed, since it is expected that the level of circulating active ingredients in Elleste Duet 1 mg is increased.

Women with pre-existing hypertriglyceridaemia should be followed closely during estrogen replacement or hormone replacement therapy, since rare cases of large increases of plasma triglycerides leading to pancreatitis have been reported with estrogen therapy in this condition.

Estrogens increase thyroid binding globulin (TBG), leading to increased circulating total thyroid hormone, as measured by protein-bound iodine (PBI), T4 levels (by column or by radio-immunoassay) or T3 levels (by radio-immunoassay). T3 resin uptake is decreased, reflecting the elevated TBG. Free T4 and free T3 concentrations are unaltered. Other binding proteins may be elevated in serum, i.e. corticoid binding globulin (CBG), sex-hormone-binding globulin (SHBG) leading to increased circulating corticosteroids and sex steroids, respectively. Free or biological active hormone concentrations are unchanged. Other plasma proteins may be increased (angiotensinogen/renin substrate, alpha-1-antitrypsin, ceruloplasmin).

There is no conclusive evidence for improvement of cognitive function. There is some evidence from the WHI trial of increased risk of probable dementia in women who start using continuous combined CEE and MPA after the age of 65. It is unknown whether the findings apply to younger post-menopausal women or other HRT products.

There is an increased risk of gall bladder disease in women receiving post-menopausal estrogens.

In rare cases benign, and in even rarer cases malignant liver tumours leading in isolated cases to life-threatening intra-abdominal haemorrhage have been observed after the use of hormonal substances such as those contained in Elleste Duet 1mg. If severe upper abdominal complaints, enlarged liver or signs of intra-abdominal haemorrhage occur, a liver tumour should be considered in the differential diagnosis.

4.5 Interaction with other medicinal products and other forms of Interaction

The metabolism of estrogens and progestogens may be increased by concomitant use of substances known to induce drug-metabolising enzymes, specifically cytochrome P450 enzymes, such as anticonvulsants (e.g. phenobarbital, phenytoin, carbamazepine) and anti-infectives (e.g. rifampicin, rifabutin, nevirapine, efavirenz).

Ritonavir and nelfinavir, although known as strong inhibitors, by contrast exhibit inducing properties when used concomitantly with steroid hormones. Herbal preparations containing St John's Wort (Hypericum Perforatum) may induce the metabolism of estrogens and progestogens.

Clinically, an increased metabolism of estrogens and progestogens may lead to decreased effect and changes in the uterine bleeding profile.

The requirement for oral anti-diabetics or insulin can change as a result of the effect on glucose tolerance. Some laboratory tests can be influenced by estrogens such as tests for thyroid function (see Section 4.4) or glucose tolerance.

4.6 Pregnancy and lactation

Pregnancy:

Elleste Duet 1 mg is not indicated during pregnancy. If pregnancy occurs during medication with Elleste Duet 1 mg treatment should be withdrawn immediately.

Data on a limited number of exposed pregnancies indicate adverse effects of norethisterone on the foetus. At doses higher than normally used in OC and HRT formulations masculinisation of female foetuses was observed.

The results of most epidemiological studies to date relevant to inadvertent foetal exposure to combinations of estrogens + progestogens indicate no teratogenic or foetotoxic effect.

Lactation:

Elleste Duet 1 mg is not indicated during lactation.

4.7 Effects on ability to drive and use machines

No adverse effects on the ability to drive or operate machines have been reported.

4.8 Undesirable effects

Undesirable effects observed with estrogens and progestogens are detailed in the following table. The effects are grouped according to system organ class.

(see Table 1 on next page)

Breast Cancer

According to evidence from a large number of epidemiological studies and one randomised placebo-controlled trial, the Women's Health Initiative (WHI), the overall risk of breast cancer increases with increasing duration of HRT use in current or recent HRT users.

For *estrogen-only* HRT, estimates of relative risk (RR) from a reanalysis of original data from 51 epidemiological studies (in which > 80% of HRT use was estrogen-only HRT) and from the epidemiological Million Women Study (MWS) are similar at 1.35 (95%CI 1.21 – 1.49) and 1.30 (95%CI 1.21 – 1.40), respectively.

For *estrogen plus progestogen* combined HRT, several epidemiological studies have reported an overall higher risk for breast cancer than with estrogens alone.

The MWS reported that, compared to never users, the use of various types of estrogen-progestogen combined HRT was associated with a higher risk of breast cancer (RR = 2.00, 95%CI: 1.88 – 2.12) than use of estrogens alone (RR = 1.30, 95%CI: 1.21 – 1.40) or use of tibolone (RR=1.45; 95%CI 1.25-1.68).

The WHI trial reported a risk estimate of 1.24 (95%CI 1.01 – 1.54) after 5.6 years of use of estrogen-progestogen combined HRT (CEE + MPA) in all users compared with placebo.

Table 1

Organ group	Common >1/100)	Uncommon >1/1,000, <1/100)	Rare >1/10,000, <1/1,000)
Gastrointestinal	Nausea, abdominal pain	Dyspepsia, vomiting, flatulence, gallbladder disease, gallstones	
Skin			Alopecia, hirsutism, rash, itching
CNS	Headache	Dizziness, migraine	
Urogenital	Uterine bleeding, increase in size of uterine fibroids	Vaginal candidiasis	
Cardiovascular		Increase in blood pressure	Venous thromboembolism* Thrombophlebitis
Miscellaneous	Weight increase/decrease, oedema, breast tenderness, breast enlargement, change in mood including anxiety and depressive mood, change in libido	Leg cramps	

* see Sections 4.3 Contraindications and 4.4 Special warnings and precautions for use

The absolute risks calculated from the MWS and the WHI trial are presented below:

The MWS has estimated, from the known average incidence of breast cancer in developed countries, that:

Ø For women not using HRT, about 32 in every 1000 are expected to have breast cancer diagnosed between the ages of 50 and 64 years.

Ø For 1000 current or recent users of HRT, the number of *additional* cases during the corresponding period will be

Ø For users of *estrogen-only* replacement therapy

- between 0 and 3 (best estimate = 1.5) for 5 years' use
- between 3 and 7 (best estimate = 5) for 10 years' use.

Ø For users of *estrogen plus progestogen* combined HRT,

- between 5 and 7 (best estimate = 6) for 5 years' use
- between 18 and 20 (best estimate = 19) for 10 years' use.

The WHI trial estimated that after 5.6 years of follow-up of women between the ages of 50 and 79 years, an *additional* 8 cases of invasive breast cancer would be due to *estrogen-progestogen combined* HRT (CEE + MPA) per 10,000 women years.

According to calculations from the trial data, it is estimated that:

Ø For 1000 women in the placebo group,

- about 16 cases of invasive breast cancer would be diagnosed in 5 years.

Ø For 1000 women who used estrogen + progestogen combined HRT (CEE + MPA), the number of *additional* cases would be

- between 0 and 9 (best estimate = 4) for 5 years' use.

The number of additional cases of breast cancer in women who use HRT is broadly similar for women who start HRT irrespective of age at start of use (between the ages of 45-65) (see Section 4.4).

Endometrial cancer

In women with an intact uterus, the risk of endometrial hyperplasia and endometrial cancer increases with increasing duration of use of unopposed estrogens. According to data from epidemiological studies, the best estimate of the risk is that for women not using HRT, about 5 in every 1000 are expected to have endometrial cancer diagnosed between the ages of 50 and 65. Depending on the duration of treatment and estrogen dose, the reported increase in endometrial cancer risk among unopposed estrogen users varies from 2-to 12-fold greater compared with non-users. Adding a progestogen to estrogen-only therapy greatly reduces, this increased risk.

Very rare cases of myocardial infarction, stroke, chloasma, erythema multiforme, erythema nodosum, vascular purpura, haemorrhagic eruption and probable dementia (see Section 4.4) have been reported in women using HRT.

4.9 Overdose

Overdosage may be manifested by nausea and vomiting. If overdosage is discovered within two or three hours and is so large that treatment seems desirable, gastric lavage can be considered. There are no specific antidotes for overdosage and further treatment should be symptomatic.

5. PHARMACOLOGICAL PROPERTIES

Pharmacotherapeutic group: Progestogens and estrogens, sequential preparations, norethisterone and estrogen.

ATC Code: G03FB05

5.1 Pharmacodynamic properties

Estradiol

The active ingredient, synthetic 17β-estradiol, is chemically and biologically identical to endogenous human estradiol. It substitutes for the loss of estrogen production in menopausal women, and alleviates menopausal symptoms.

Norethisterone acetate

As estrogens promote the growth of the endometrium, unopposed estrogens increase the risk of endometrial hyperplasia and cancer. The addition of a progestogen reduces but does not eliminate the estrogen-induced risk of endometrial hyperplasia in non-hysterectomised women.

5.2 Pharmacokinetic properties

No pharmacokinetic parameters are available for Elleste Duet 1 mg. Pharmacokinetic parameters for Elleste Duet 2 mg (2 mg estradiol + 1 mg norethisterone tablets) are provided in the table below. The data were obtained from an open label, two way crossover pharmacokinetic study in which treatment was admnistered for 7 days to achieve steady state (n=24). Pharmacokinetic data were collected over 24 hours.

(see Table 2 below)

Estradiol

Readily and fully absorbed from the GI tract when given orally, peak levels are generally observed 3-6 hours after ingestion, but by 24 hours concentrations have returned to baseline.

Estradiol is converted to estrone and estriol primarily in the liver. These are excreted into the bile and undergo enterohepatic recirculation and further degradation before being excreted in the urine (90-95%) as biologically inactive glucuronide and sulphate conjugates or in the faeces (5-10%), mostly unconjugated.

Norethisterone acetate

Norethisterone acetate is absorbed from the GI tract and its effects last for at least 24 hours. Maximum blood concentrations are generally reached 1-4 hours after administration. Norethisterone acetate undergoes first pass effect, being transformed to norethisterone which is then metabolised and excreted mainly in the urine as glucuronide and sulphate conjugates.

5.3 Preclinical safety data

Both estradiol and norethisterone acetate have been shown to induce adverse effects in preclinical reproductive toxicity studies. Chiefly, estradiol showed embryotoxic effects and induced anomalies in urogenital tract development, e.g. feminisation of male foetuses in high doses. Norethisterone acetate showed embryotoxic effects and induced anomalies in urogenital tract development. In mice, additional anomalies in non-urogenital foetal development, including hydrocephalus and clubfoot, have been detected.

Table 2

	Serum unconjuated estradiol mean (SD)	Serum unconjugated estrone mean (SD)	Norethisterone mean (SD)
$AUC_{0\text{-}24h}$	967.8 (0.5) pg.h/ml	8366 (1.7) pg.h/ml	43.2 (0.4) ng.h/ml
C_{max}	61.6 (0.4) pg/ml	648.5 (1.5) pg/ml	11.8 (0.4) ng/ml
C_{min}	19.3 (0.6) pg/ml	131.1 (2.5) pg/ml	0.5 (0.5) ng/ml
T_{max}	3.4 (2.1) h	5.07 (1.8) h	0.9 (0.3) h

6. PHARMACEUTICAL PARTICULARS

6.1 List of excipients

Tablet core:

Lactose monohydrate, maize starch, povidone 25, talc (purified) and magnesium stearate.

Film-coating material:

Estradiol only (white) tablets:

Hydroxypropylmethyl cellulose (E464), titanium dioxide (E171) and macrogol 400

Estradiol and Norethisterone Acetate only (green) tablets:

Hydroxypropylmethyl cellulose (E464), titanium dioxide (E171), macrogol 400, quinoline yellow (E104) and indigo carmine (E132)

6.2 Incompatibilities

Not applicable.

6.3 Shelf life

3 years.

6.4 Special precautions for storage

Do not store above 30°C. Store in the original package.

6.5 Nature and contents of container

Aluminium foil and UPVC blister packed in a cardboard carton.

Pack sizes: 28 tablets and 84 (3 × 28) tablets.

6.6 Instructions for use and handling

There are no special instructions for handling.

7. MARKETING AUTHORISATION HOLDER

Shire Pharmaceutical Contracts Limited

Hampshire International Business Park

Chineham

Basingstoke

Hampshire

RG24 8EP

United Kingdom

8. MARKETING AUTHORISATION NUMBER(S)

PL 08081/0028

9. DATE OF FIRST AUTHORISATION/RENEWAL OF THE AUTHORISATION

24th March 1997.

10. DATE OF REVISION OF THE TEXT

June 2004

Elleste Duet 2mg

(Pharmacia Limited)

1. NAME OF THE MEDICINAL PRODUCT

Elleste Duet 2 mg

2. QUALITATIVE AND QUANTITATIVE COMPOSITION

One orange tablet contains 2 mg estradiol (as estradiol hemihydrate).

One grey tablet contains 2 mg estradiol (as estradiol hemihydrate) and 1 mg norethisterone acetate.

For excipients, see 6.1.

3. PHARMACEUTICAL FORM

Film coated tablets.

4. CLINICAL PARTICULARS

4.1 Therapeutic indications

Hormone Replacement Therapy (HRT) for estrogen deficiency symptoms in post- and peri- menopausal women. Prevention of osteoporosis in postmenopausal women at high risk of future fractures who are intolerant of, or contraindicated for, other medicinal products approved for the prevention of osteoporosis. (See also section 4.4)

The experience of treating women older than 65 years is limited.

4.2 Posology and method of administration

This product is a continuous sequential HRT. One orange tablet to be taken daily for the first 16 days, followed by one grey tablet for the next 12 days. A new cycle should then begin without any break. Therapy may start at any time in patients with established amenorrhoea or who are experiencing long intervals between spontaneous menses. In patients who are menstruating it is advised that therapy starts on the first day of bleeding. Patients changing from another cyclical or continuous sequential preparation should complete the cycle and may then change to Elleste Duet 2 mg without a break in therapy. Patients changing from a continuous combined preparation may start therapy at any time if amenorrhoea is established, or otherwise start on the first day of bleeding.

Elderly

There are no special dosage requirements in elderly patients.

Children

Not to be used in children.

Elleste Duet tablets are available in two strengths: Elleste Duet 1 mg (containing 1 mg estradiol and 1 mg norethisterone acetate) and Elleste Duet 2 mg (containing 2 mg estradiol and 1 mg norethisterone acetate). For initiation and continuation of treatment of post- and peri-menopausal symptoms, the lowest effective dose for the shortest duration (see also Section 4.4) should be used.

Missed Tablet: If a tablet is missed it should be taken within 12 hours of when normally taken; otherwise the tablet should be discarded, and the usual tablet should be taken the following day. If a tablet is missed there is an increased likelihood of breakthrough bleeding or spotting.

4.3 Contraindications

Known, past or suspected breast cancer;

Known or suspected estrogen-dependent malignant tumours (e.g. endometrial cancer);

Undiagnosed genital bleeding;

Untreated endometrial hyperplasia;

Previous idiopathic or current venous thromboembolism (deep venous thrombosis, pulmonary embolism);

Active or recent arterial thromboembolic disease (e.g. angina, myocardial infarction);

Acute liver disease, or a history of liver disease as long as liver function tests have failed to return to normal;

Known hypersensitivity to the active substances or to any of the excipients;

Porphyria.

4.4 Special warnings and special precautions for use

For the treatment of postmenopausal symptoms, HRT should only be initiated for symptoms that adversely affect quality of life. In all cases, a careful appraisal of the risks and benefits should be undertaken at least annually and HRT should only be continued as long as the benefit outweighs the risk.

Medical Examination/Follow Up

Before initiating or reinstituting HRT, a complete personal and family medical history should be taken. Physical (including pelvic and breast) examination should be guided by this and by the contraindications and warnings for use. During treatment, periodic check-ups are recommended of a frequency and nature adapted to the individual woman. Women should be advised what changes in their breasts should be reported to their doctor or nurse (see 'Breast Cancer' below). Investigations, including mammography, should be carried out in accordance with currently accepted screening practices, modified to the clinical needs of the individual.

Conditions Which Need Supervision

If any of the following conditions are present, have occurred previously, and/or have been aggravated during pregnancy or previous hormone treatment, the patient should be closely supervised. It should be taken into account that these conditions may recur or be aggravated during treatment wth Elleste Duet 2 mg, in particular:

- Leiomyoma (uterine fibroids) or endometriosis
- A history of, or risk factors for, thromboembolic disorders (see below)
- Risk factors for estrogen dependent tumours, e.g. 1st degree heredity for breast cancer
- Hypertension
- Liver disorders (e.g. liver adenoma)
- Diabetes mellitus with or without vascular involvement
- Cholelithiasis
- Migraine or (severe) headache
- Systemic lupus erythematosus
- A history of endometrial hyperplasia (see below)
- Epilepsy
- Asthma
- Otosclerosis

Reasons for Immediate Withdrawal of Therapy:

Therapy should be discontinued if a contra-indication is discovered and in the following situations:

- Jaundice or deterioration in liver function
- Significant increase in blood pressure
- New onset of migraine-type headache
- Pregnancy

Endometrial Hyperplasia

The risk of endometrial hyperplasia and carcinoma is increased when estrogens are administered alone for prolonged periods (see section 4.8). The addition of a progestogen for at least 12 days per cycle in non-hysterectomised women greatly reduces this risk.

Break-through bleeding and spotting may occur during the first months of treatment. If break-through bleeding or spotting appears after some time on therapy, or continues after treatment has been discontinued, the reason should be investigated, which may include endometrial biopsy to exclude endometrial malignancy.

Breast Cancer

A randomised placebo-controlled trial, the Women's Health Initiative Study (WHI), and epidemiological studies, including the Million Women Study (MWS), have reported an increased risk of breast cancer in women taking estrogens, estrogen-progestogen combinations or tibolone for HRT for several years (see Section 4.8). For all HRT, an excess risk becomes apparent within a few years of use and increases with duration of intake but returns to baseline within a few (at most five) years after stopping treatment.

In the MWS, the relative risk of breast cancer with conjugated equine estrogens (CEE) or estradiol (E2) was greater when a progestogen was added, either sequentially or continuously, and regardless of type of progestogen. There was no evidence of a difference in risk between the different routes of administration.

In the WHI study, the continuous combined conjugated equine estrogen and medroxyprogesterone acetate (CEE + MPA) product used was associated with breast cancers that were slightly larger in size and more frequently had local lymph node metastases compared to placebo.

HRT, especially estrogen-progestogen combined treatment, increases the density of mammographic images which may adversely affect the radiological detection of breast cancer.

Venous Thromboembolism

HRT is associated with a higher relative risk of developing venous thromboembolism (VTE), i.e. deep vein thrombosis or pulmonary embolism. One randomised controlled trial and epidemiological studies found a two to threefold higher risk for users compared with non-users. For non-users, it is estimated that the number of cases of VTE that will occur over a 5 year period is about 3 per 1000 women aged 50-59 years and 8 per 1000 women aged 60-69 years. It is estimated that in healthy women who use HRT for 5 years, the number of additional cases of VTE over a 5 year period will be between 2 and 6 (best estimate = 4) per 1000 women aged 50-59 years and between 5 and 15 (best estimate = 9) per 1000 women aged 60-69 years. The occurrence of such an event is more likely in the first year of HRT than later.

Generally recognised risk factors for VTE include a personal history or family history, severe obesity (BM > 30 kg/m^2) and systemic lupus erythematosus (SLE). There is no consensus about the possible role of varicose veins in VTE.

Patients with a history of VTE or known thrombophilic states have an increased risk of VTE. HRT may add to this risk. Personal or strong family history of thromboembolism or recurrent spontaneous abortion should be investigated in order to exclude a thrombophilic predisposition. Until a thorough evaluation of thrombophilic factors has been made or anticoagulant treatment initiated, use of HRT in such patients should be viewed as contraindicated. Those women already on anticoagulant treatment require careful consideration of the benefit-risk of use of HRT.

The risk of VTE may be temporarily increased with prolonged immobilisation, major trauma or major surgery. As in all postoperative patients, scrupulous attention should be given to prophylactic measures to prevent VTE following surgery. Where prolonged immobilisation is liable to follow elective surgery, particularly abdominal or orthopaedic surgery to the lower limbs, consideration should be given to temporarily stopping HRT 4 to 6 weeks earlier, if possible. Treatment should not be restarted until the woman is completely mobilised.

If VTE develops after initiating therapy, the drug should be discontinued. Patients should be told to contact their doctors immediately when they are aware of a potential thromboembolic symptom (e.g., painful swelling of a leg, sudden pain in the chest, dyspnea).

Coronary Artery Disease

There is no evidence from randomised controlled trials of cardiovascular benefit with continuous combined conjugated estrogens and medroxyprogesterone acetate (MPA). Two large clinical trials (WHI and HERS i.e. Heart and Estrogen/progestin Replacement Study) showed a possible increased risk of cardiovascular morbidity in the first year of use and no overall benefit. For other HRT products there are only limited data from randomised controlled trials examining effects in cardiovascular morbidity or mortality. Therefore, it is uncertain whether these findings also extend to other HRT products.

Stroke

One large randomised clinical trial (WHI-trial) found, as a secondary outcome, an increased risk of ischaemic stroke in healthy women during treatment with continuous combined conjugated estrogens and MPA. For women who do not use HRT, it is estimated that the number of cases of stroke that will occur over a 5 year period is about 3 per 1000 women aged 50-59 years and 11 per 1000 women aged 60-69 years. It is estimated that for women who use conjugated estrogens and MPA for 5 years, the number of additional cases will be between 0 and 3 (best estimate = 1) per 1000 users aged 50-59 years and between 1 and 9 (best estimate = 4) per 1000 users aged 60-69 years. It is unknown whether the increased risk also extends to other HRT products.

Ovarian Cancer

Long-term (at least 5 to 10 years) use of estrogen-only HRT products in hysterectomised women has been associated with an increased risk of ovarian cancer in some epidemiological studies. It is uncertain whether long-term use of combined HRT confers a different risk than estrogen-only products.

Other conditions

Estrogens may cause fluid retention and therefore patients with cardiac or renal dysfunction should be carefully observed. Patients with terminal renal insufficiency should be closely observed, since it is expected that the level of circulating active ingredients in Elleste Duet 2 mg is increased.

Women with pre-existing hypertriglyceridaemia should be followed closely during estrogen replacement or hormone replacement therapy, since rare cases of large increases of plasma triglycerides leading to pancreatitis have been reported with estrogen therapy in this condition.

Estrogens increase thyroid binding globulin (TBG) levels, leading to increased circulating total thyroid hormone, as measured by protein-bound iodine (PBI), T4 levels (by column or by radio-immunoassay) or T3 levels (by radio-immunoassay). T3 resin uptake is decreased, reflecting the elevated TBG. Free T4 and free T3 concentrations are unaltered. Other binding proteins may be elevated in serum, i.e. corticoid binding globulin (CBG), sex-hormone-binding globulin (SHBG) leading to increased circulating corticosteroids and sex steroids, respectively. Free or biological active hormone concentrations are unchanged. Other plasma proteins may be increased (angiotensinogen/renin substrate, alpha-1-antitrypsin, ceruloplasmin).

There is no conclusive evidence for improvement of cognitive function. There is some evidence from the WHI trial of increased risk of probable dementia in women who start using continuous combined CEE and MPA after the age of 65. It is unknown whether the findings apply to younger post-menopausal women or other HRT products.

There is an increased risk of gall bladder disease in women receiving post-menopausal estrogens.

In rare cases benign, and in even rarer cases malignant liver tumours leading in isolated cases to life-threatening intra-abdominal haemorrhage have been observed after the use of hormonal substances such as those contained in Elleste Duet 2mg. If severe upper abdominal complaints, enlarged liver or signs of intra-abdominal haemorrhage occur, a liver tumour should be considered in the differential diagnosis.

4.5 Interaction with other medicinal products and other forms of Interaction

The metabolism of estrogens and progestogens may be increased by concomitant use of substances known to induce drug-metabolising enzymes, specifically cytochrome P450 enzymes, such as anticonvulsants (e.g. phenobarbital, phenytoin, carbamazepine) and anti-infectives (e.g. rifampicin, rifabutin, nevirapine, efavirenz).

Ritonavir and nelfinavir, although known as strong inhibitors, by contrast exhibit inducing properties when used concomitantly with steroid hormones. Herbal preparations containing St John's Wort (Hypericum Perforatum) may induce the metabolism of estrogens and progestogens.

Clinically, an increased metabolism of estrogens and progestogens may lead to decreased effect and changes in the uterine bleeding profile.

The requirement for oral anti-diabetics or insulin can change as a result of the effect on glucose tolerance. Some laboratory tests can be influenced by estrogens such as tests for thyroid function (see section 4.4) or glucose tolerance.

4.6 Pregnancy and lactation

Pregnancy:

Elleste Duet 2 mg is not indicated during pregnancy. If pregnancy occurs during medication with Elleste Duet 2 mg treatment should be withdrawn immediately.

Data on a limited number of exposed pregnancies indicate adverse effects of norethisterone on the foetus. At doses higher than normally used in OC and HRT formulations masculinisation of female foetuses was observed.

The results of most epidemiological studies to date relevant to inadvertent foetal exposure to combinations of estrogens + progestogens indicate no teratogenic or foetotoxic effect.

Lactation:

Elleste Duet 2 mg is not indicated during lactation.

4.7 Effects on ability to drive and use machines

No adverse effects on the ability to drive or operate machines have been reported.

4.8 Undesirable effects

Undesirable effects observed with estrogens and progestogens are detailed in the following table. The effects are grouped according to system organ class.

(see Table 1 on next page)

Breast Cancer

According to evidence from a large number of epidemiological studies and one randomised placebo-controlled trial, the Women's Health Initiative (WHI), the overall risk of breast cancer increases with increasing duration of HRT use in current or recent HRT users.

For *estrogen-only* HRT, estimates of relative risk (RR) from a reanalysis of original data from 51 epidemiological studies (in which > 80% of HRT use was estrogen-only HRT) and from the epidemiological Million Women Study (MWS)

Table 1

Organ group	Common >1/100)	Uncommon >1/1,000, <1/100)	Rare >1/10,000, <1/1,000)
Gastrointestinal	Nausea, abdominal pain	Dyspepsia, vomiting, flatulence, gallbladder disease, gallstones	
Skin			Alopecia, hirsutism, rash, itching.
CNS	Headache	Dizziness, migraine	
Urogenital	Uterine bleeding, increase in size of uterine fibroids	Vaginal candidiasis	
Cardiovascular		Increase in blood pressure	Venous thromboembolism* Thrombophlebitis
Miscellaneous	Weight increase/decrease, oedema, breast tenderness, breast enlargement, change in mood including anxiety and depressive mood, change in libido	Leg cramps	

* see sections 4.3 Contraindications and 4.4 Special warnings and precautions for use

are similar at 1.35 (95%CI 1.21 – 1.49) and 1.30 (95%CI 1.21 – 1.40), respectively.

For *estrogen plus progestogen* combined HRT, several epidemiological studies have reported an overall higher risk for breast cancer than with estrogens alone.

The MWS reported that, compared to never users, the use of various types of estrogen-progestogen combined HRT was associated with a higher risk of breast cancer (RR = 2.00, 95%CI: 1.88 – 2.12) than use of estrogens alone (RR = 1.30, 95%CI: 1.21 – 1.40) or use of tibolone (RR=1.45; 95%CI 1.25-1.68).

The WHI trial reported a risk estimate of 1.24 (95%CI 1.01 – 1.54) after 5.6 years of use of estrogen-progestogen combined HRT (CEE + MPA) in all users compared with placebo.

The absolute risks calculated from the MWS and the WHI trial are presented below:

The MWS has estimated, from the known average incidence of breast cancer in developed countries, that:

- For women not using HRT, about 32 in every 1000 are expected to have breast cancer diagnosed between the ages of 50 and 64 years.

For 1000 current or recent users of HRT, the number of *additional* cases during the corresponding period will be

- For users of *estrogen-only* replacement therapy
- between 0 and 3 (best estimate = 1.5) for 5 years' use
- between 3 and 7 (best estimate = 5) for 10 years' use.
- For users of *estrogen plus progestogen* combined HRT,
- between 5 and 7 (best estimate = 6) for 5 years' use
- between 18 and 20 (best estimate = 19) for 10 years' use.

The WHI trial estimated that after 5.6 years of follow-up of women between the ages of 50 and 79 years, an *additional* 8 cases of invasive breast cancer would be due to *estrogen-progestogen combined* HRT (CEE + MPA) per 10,000 women years.

According to calculations from the trial data, it is estimated that:

- For 1000 women in the placebo group,
- about 16 cases of invasive breast cancer would be diagnosed in 5 years.
- For 1000 women who used estrogen + progestogen combined HRT (CEE + MPA), the number of *additional* cases would be
- between 0 and 9 (best estimate = 4) for 5 years' use.

The number of additional cases of breast cancer in women who use HRT is broadly similar for women who start HRT irrespective of age at start of use (between the ages of 45-65) (see section 4.4).

Endometrial cancer

In women with an intact uterus, the risk of endometrial hyperplasia and endometrial cancer increases with increasing duration of use of unopposed estrogens. According to data from epidemiological studies, the best estimate of the risk is that for women not using HRT, about 5 in every 1000 are expected to have endometrial cancer diagnosed between the ages of 50 and 65. Depending on the duration of treatment and estrogen dose, the reported increase in endometrial cancer risk among unopposed estrogen users varies from 2-to 12-fold greater compared with non-users. Adding a progestogen to estrogen-only therapy greatly reduces this increased risk.

Very rare cases of myocardial infarction, stroke, chloasma, erythema multiforme, erythema nodosum, vascular purpura, haemorrhagic eruption and probable dementia (see section 4.4) have been reported in women using HRT.

4.9 Overdose

Overdosage may be manifested by nausea and vomiting. If overdosage is discovered within two or three hours and is so large that treatment seems desirable, gastric lavage can be considered. There are no specific antidotes for overdosage and further treatment should be symptomatic.

5. PHARMACOLOGICAL PROPERTIES

Pharmacotherapeutic group: Progestogens and estrogens, sequential preparations, norethisterone and estrogen.

ATC Code: G03FB05

5.1 Pharmacodynamic properties

Estradiol

The active ingredient, synthetic 17β-estradiol, is chemically and biologically identical to endogenous human estradiol. It substitutes for the loss of estrogen production in menopausal women, and alleviates menopausal symptoms.

Estrogens prevent bone loss following menopause or ovariectomy. Estrogen deficiency at menopause is associated with an increasing bone turnover and decline in bone mass. The effect of estrogens on the bone mineral density is dose-dependent. Protection appears to be effective for as long as treatment is continued. After discontinuation of HRT, bone mass is lost at a rate similar to that in untreated women.

Evidence from the WHI trial and meta-analysed trials shows that current use of HRT, alone or in combination with a progestogen – given to predominantly healthy women – reduces the risk of hip, vertebral, and other osteoporotic fractures. HRT may also prevent fractures in women with low bone density and/or established osteoporosis, but the evidence for that is limited.

Norethisterone acetate

As estrogens promote the growth of the endometrium, unopposed estrogens increase the risk of endometrial hyperplasia and cancer. The addition of a progestogen reduces but does not eliminate the estrogen-induced risk of endometrial hyperplasia in non-hysterectomised women.

5.2 Pharmacokinetic properties

Pharmacokinetic parameters for Elleste Duet 2 mg (2 mg estradiol + 1 mg norethisterone tablets) are provided in the table below. The data were obtained from an open label, two way crossover pharmacokinetic study in which treatment was administered for 7 days to achieve steady state (n=24). Pharmacokinetic data were collected over 24 hours.

(see Table 2 below)

Table 2

	Serum unconjuated estradiol mean (SD)	Serum unconjugated estrone mean (SD)	Norethisterone mean (SD)
$AUC_{0\text{-}24h}$	967.8 (0.5) pg.h/ml	8366 (1.7) pg.h/ml	43.2 (0.4) ng.h/ml
C_{max}	61.6 (0.4) pg/ml	648.5 (1.5) pg/ml	11.8 (0.4) ng/ml
C_{min}	19.3 (0.6) pg/ml	131.1 (2.5) pg/ml	0.5 (0.5) ng/ml
T_{max}	3.4 (2.1) h	5.07 (1.8) h	0.9 (0.3) h

Estradiol

Readily and fully absorbed from the GI tract when given orally, peak levels are generally observed 3-6 hours after ingestion, but by 24 hours concentrations have returned to baseline.

Estradiol is converted to estrone and estriol primarily in the liver. These are excreted into the bile and undergo enterohepatic recirculation and further degradation before being excreted in the urine (90-95%) as biologically inactive glucuronide and sulphate conjugates or in the faeces (5-10%), mostly unconjugated.

Norethisterone acetate

Norethisterone acetate is absorbed from GI tract and its effects last for at least 24 hours. Maximum blood concentrations are generally reached 1-4 hours after administration. Norethisterone acetate undergoes first pass effect, being transformed to norethisterone which is then metabolised and excreted mainly in the urine as glucuronide and sulphate conjugates.

5.3 Preclinical safety data

Both estradiol and norethisterone acetate have been shown to induce adverse effects in preclinical reproductive toxicity studies. Chiefly, estradiol showed embryotoxic effects and induced anomalies in urogenital tract development, e.g. feminisation of male foetuses in high doses. Norethisterone acetate showed embryotoxic effects and induced anomalies in urogenital tract development. In mice, additional anomalies in non-urogenital foetal development, including hydrocephalus and clubfoot, have been detected.

6. PHARMACEUTICAL PARTICULARS

6.1 List of excipients

Tablet core:

Lactose monohydrate, maize starch, povidone 25, talc (purified) and magnesium stearate.

Film-coating material:

Estradiol only (orange) tablets

Hydroxypropylmethyl cellulose (E464), titanium dioxide (E171), macrogol 400 and sunset yellow (E110).

Estradiol and Norethisterone Acetate (grey) tablets

Hydroxypropylmethyl cellulose (E464), titanium dioxide (E171), macrogol 400, black iron oxide (E172)

6.2 Incompatibilities

Not applicable

6.3 Shelf life

3 years

6.4 Special precautions for storage

Do not store above 25°C. Store in the original package.

6.5 Nature and contents of container

Aluminium foil and UPVC blister packed in a cardboard carton.

Pack sizes: 28 tablets and 84 (3 × 28) tablets.

6.6 Instructions for use and handling

There are no special instructions for handling.

7. MARKETING AUTHORISATION HOLDER

Shire Pharmaceutical Contracts Limited

Hampshire International Business Park

Chineham

Basingstoke

Hampshire

RG24 8EP

United Kingdom

8. MARKETING AUTHORISATION NUMBER(S)

PL 08081/0024

9. DATE OF FIRST AUTHORISATION/RENEWAL OF THE AUTHORISATION

23 February 1995

10. DATE OF REVISION OF THE TEXT

March 2004

Elleste Duet Conti Tablet

(Pharmacia Limited)

1. NAME OF THE MEDICINAL PRODUCT

Elleste Duet Conti Tablets

2. QUALITATIVE AND QUANTITATIVE COMPOSITION

One film-coated tablet contains 2mg estradiol (as estradiol hemihydrate) and 1mg norethisterone acetate

For excipients, see 6.1.

3. PHARMACEUTICAL FORM

Film coated tablets.

4. CLINICAL PARTICULARS

4.1 Therapeutic indications

Hormone Replacement Therapy (HRT) for estrogen deficiency symptoms. in women with an intact uterus who are at least one year post menopause. Prevention of osteoporosis in postmenopausal women at high risk of future fractures who are intolerant of, or contraindicated for, other medicinal products approved for the prevention of osteoporosis. (See also Section 4.4).

The experience of treating women older than 65 years is limited.

4.2 Posology and method of administration

For initiation and continuation of treatment of post-menopausal symptoms the lowest effective dose for the shortest duration (see also Section 4.4) should be used.

The product is a continuous combined HRT. One grey tablet is taken daily continuously without a break thus running one packet into the next.

Therapy may start at any time in patients without prior hormone replacement therapy. Patients changing from another cyclical or continuous sequential preparation should complete the cycle and may then change to Elleste Duet Conti Tablets without a break in therapy. Patients changing from a continuous combined preparation may start therapy at any time if amenorrhoea is established, or otherwise start on the first day of bleeding.

Elderly

There are no special dosage requirements in elderly patients

Children

Not to be used in children.

Missed Tablet: If a tablet is missed it should be taken within 12 hours of when normally taken; otherwise the tablet should be discarded, and the usual tablet should be taken the following day. If a tablet is missed there is an increased likelihood of breakthrough bleeding or spotting.

4.3 Contraindications

Known, past or suspected breast cancer;

Known or suspected estrogen-dependent malignant tumours (e.g. endometrial cancer);

Undiagnosed genital bleeding;

Untreated endometrial hyperplasia;

Previous idiopathic or current venous thromboembolism (deep venous thrombosis, pulmonary embolism);

Active or recent arterial thromboembolic disease (e.g. angina, myocardial infarction).

Acute liver disease, or a history of liver disease as long as liver function tests have failed to return to normal;

Known hypersensitivity to the active substances or to any of the excipients;

Porphyria.

4.4 Special warnings and special precautions for use

For the treatment of postmenopausal symptoms, HRT should only be initiated for symptoms that adversely affect quality of life. In all cases a careful appraisal of the risks and benefits should be undertaken at least annually and HRT should only be continued as long as the benefit outweighs the risk.

Medical Examination and Follow Up

Before initiating or reinstituting HRT, a complete personal and family medical history should be taken. Physical (including pelvic and breast) examination should be guided by this and by the contraindications and warnings for use. During treatment, periodic check-ups are recommended of a frequency and nature adapted to the individual woman. Women should be advised what changes in their breasts should be reported to their doctor or nurse (see 'Breast cancer' below). Investigations, including mammography, should be carried out in accordance with currently accepted screening practices, modified to the clinical needs of the individual.

Conditions Which Need Supervision

If any of the following conditions are present, have occurred previously, and/or have been aggravated during pregnancy or previous hormone treatment, the patient should be closely supervised. It should be taken into account that these conditions may recur or be aggravated during treatment with Elleste Duet Conti Tablets, in particular:

- Leiomyoma (uterine fibroids) or endometriosis
- A history of, or risk factors for, thromboembolic disorders (see below)
- Risk factors for estrogen dependent tumours, e.g. 1st degree heredity for breast cancer
- Hypertension
- Liver disorders (eg, liver adenoma)
- Diabetes mellitus with or without vascular involvement
- Cholelithiasis
- Migraine or (severe) headache
- Systemic lupus erythematosus
- A history of endometrial hyperplasia (see below)
- Epilepsy
- Asthma
- Otosclerosis

Reasons for Immediate Withdrawal of Therapy:

Therapy should be discontinued if a contra-indication is discovered and in the following situations:

- Jaundice or deterioration in liver function
- Significant increase in blood pressure
- New onset of migraine-type headache
- Pregnancy

Endometrial Hyperplasia

The risk of endometrial hyperplasia and carcinoma is increased when estrogens are administered alone for prolonged periods (see Section 4.8). The addition of a progestogen for at least 12 days per cycle in non-hysterectomised women greatly reduces this risk.

Breakthrough bleeding and spotting may occur during the first months of treatment. If breakthrough bleeding or spotting appears after some time on therapy, or continues after treatment has been discontinued, the reason should be investigated, which may include endometrial biopsy to exclude endometrial malignancy.

Breast Cancer

A randomised placebo-controlled trial, the Women's Health Initiative Study (WHI), and epidemiological studies, including the Million Women Study (MWS), have reported an increased risk of breast cancer in women taking estrogens, estrogen-progestogen combinations or tibolone for HRT for several years (see Section 4.8).

For all HRT, an excess risk becomes apparent within a few years of use and increases with duration of intake but returns to baseline within a few (at most five) years after stopping treatment.

In the MWS, the relative risk of breast cancer with conjugated equine estrogens (CEE) or estradiol (E2) was greater when a progestogen was added, either sequentially or continuously, and regardless of type of progestogen. There was no evidence of a difference in risk between the different routes of administration.

In the WHI study, the continuous combined conjugated equine estrogen and medroxyprogesterone acetate (CEE + MPA) product was associated with breast cancers that were slightly larger in size and more frequently had local lymph node metastases compared to placebo.

HRT, especially estrogen-progestogen combined treatment, increases the density of mammographic images which may adversely affect the radiological detection of breast cancer.

Venous Thromboembolism

HRT is associated with a higher relative risk of developing venous thromboembolism (VTE), i.e. deep vein thrombosis or pulmonary embolism. One randomised controlled trial and epidemiological studies found a two- to threefold higher risk for users compared with non-users. For non-users, it is estimated that the number of cases of VTE that will occur over a 5 year period is about 3 per 1000 women aged 50-59 years and 8 per 1000 women aged 60-69 years. It is estimated that in healthy women who use HRT for 5 years, the number of additional cases of VTE over a 5 year period will be between 2 and 6 (best estimate = 4) per 1000 women aged 50-59 years and between 5 and 15 (best estimate = 9) per 1000 women aged 60-69 years. The occurrence of such an event is more likely in the first year of HRT than later.

Generally recognised risk factors for VTE include a personal history or family history, severe obesity (BM > 30kg/m^2) and systemic lupus erythematosus (SLE). There is no consensus about the possible role of varicose veins in VTE.

Patients with a history of VTE or known thrombophilic states have an increased risk of VTE. HRT may add to this risk. Personal or strong family history of thromboembolism or recurrent spontaneous abortion should be investigated in order to exclude a thrombophilic predisposition. Until a thorough evaluation of thrombophilic factors has been made or anticoagulant treatment initiated, use of HRT in such patients should be viewed as contraindicated. Those women already on anticoagulant treatment require careful consideration of the benefit-risk of use of HRT.

The risk of VTE may be temporarily increased with prolonged immobilisation, major trauma or major surgery. As in all postoperative patients, scrupulous attention should be given to prophylactic measures to prevent VTE following surgery. Where prolonged immobilisation is liable to follow elective surgery, particularly abdominal or orthopaedic surgery to the lower limbs, consideration should be given to temporarily stopping HRT 4 to 6 weeks earlier, if possible. Treatment should not be restarted until the woman is completely mobilised.

If VTE develops after initiating therapy, the drug should be discontinued. Patients should be told to contact their doctors immediately when they are aware of a potential thromboembolic symptom (e.g., painful swelling of a leg, sudden pain in the chest, dyspnea).

Coronary Artery Disease

There is no evidence from randomised controlled trials of cardiovasular benefit with continuous combined conjugated estrogens and medroxyprogesterone acetate (MPA). Two large clinical trials (WHI and HERS i.e. Heart and Estrogen/progestin Replacement Study) showed a possible increased risk of cardiovascular morbidity in the first year of use and no overall benefit. For other HRT products there are only limited data from randomised controlled trials examining effects in cardiovascular morbidity or mortality. Therefore, it is uncertain whether these findings also extend to other HRT products.

Stroke

One large randomised clinical trial (WHI-trial) found, as a secondary outcome, an increased risk of ischaemic stroke in healthy women during treatment with continuous combined conjugated estrogens and MPA. For women who do not use HRT, it is estimated that the number of cases of stroke that will occur over a 5 year period is about 3 per 1000 women aged 50-59 years and 11 per 1000 women aged 60-69 years. It is estimated that for women who use conjugated estrogens and MPA for 5 years, the number of additional cases will be between 0 and 3 (best estimate = 1) per 1000 users aged 50-59 years and between 1 and 9 (best estimate = 4) per 1000 users aged 60-69 years. It is unknown whether the increased risk also extends to other HRT products.

Ovarian Cancer

Long-term (at least 5 to 10 years) use of estrogen-only HRT products in hysterectomised women has been associated with an increased risk of ovarian cancer in some epidemiological studies. It is uncertain whether long-term use of combined HRT confers a different risk than estrogen-only products.

Other conditions

Estrogens may cause fluid retention and therefore patients with cardiac or renal dysfunction should be carefully observed. Patients with terminal renal insufficiency should be closely observed, since it is expected that the level of circulating active ingredients in Elleste Duet Conti Tablets are increased.

Women with pre-existing hypertriglyceridemia should be followed closely during estrogen replacement or hormone replacement therapy, since rare cases of large increases of plasma triglycerides leading to pancreatitis have been reported with estrogen therapy in this condition.

Estrogens increase thyroid binding globulin (TBG) levels, leading to increased circulating total thyroid hormone, as measured by protein-bound iodine (PBI), T4 levels (by column or by radio-immunoassay) or T3 levels (by radio-immunoassay). T3 resin uptake is decreased, reflecting the elevated TBG. Free T4 and free T3 concentrations are unaltered. Other binding proteins may be elevated in serum, i.e. corticoid binding globulin (CBG), sex-hormone-binding globulin (SHBG) leading to increased circulating corticosteroids and sex steroids, respectively. Free or biological active hormone concentrations are unchanged. Other plasma proteins may be increased (angiotensinogen/renin substrate, alpha-1-antitrypsin, ceruloplasmin).

There is no conclusive evidence for improvement of cognitive function. There is some evidence from the WHI trial of increased risk of probable dementia in women who start using continuous combined CEE and MPA after the age of 65. It is unknown whether the findings apply to younger post-menopausal women or other HRT products.

There is an increased risk of gall bladder disease in women receiving post-menopausal estrogens.

In rare cases benign and in even rarer cases malignant liver tumours leading in isolated cases to life-threatening intra-abdominal haemorrhage have been observed after the use of hormonal substances such as those contained in Elleste Duet Conti Tablets. If severe upper abdominal complaints, enlarged liver or signs of intra-abdominal haemorrhage occur, a liver tumour should be considered in the differential diagnosis.

4.5 Interaction with other medicinal products and other forms of Interaction

The metabolism of estrogens and progestogens may be increased by concomitant use of substances known to induce drug-metabolising enzymes, specifically cytochrome P450 enzymes, such as anticonvulsants (e.g. phenobarbital, phenytoin, carbamazepine) and anti-infectives (e.g. rifampicin, rifabutin, nevirapine, efavirenz).

Ritonavir and nelfinavir, although known as strong inhibitors by contrast exhibit inducing properties when used concomitantly with steroid hormones. Herbal preparations containing St John's Wort (Hypericum Perforatum) may induce the metabolism of estrogens and progestogens.

Clinically, an increased metabolism of estrogens and progestogens may lead to decreased effect and changes in the uterine bleeding profile.

The requirement for oral anti-diabetics or insulin can change as a result of the effect on glucose tolerance. Some laboratory tests can be influenced by estrogens such as tests for thyroid function (see section 4.4) or glucose tolerance.

4.6 Pregnancy and lactation

Pregnancy:

Elleste Duet Conti Tablets are not indicated during pregnancy. If pregnancy occurs during medication with Elleste Duet Conti Tablets, treatment should be withdrawn immediately.

Data on a limited number of exposed pregnancies indicate adverse effects of norethisterone on the foetus. At doses higher than normally used in OC and HRT formulations masculinisation of female foetuses was observed. The results of most epidemiological studies to date relevant to inadvertent foetal exposure to combinations of estrogens + progestogens indicate no teratogenic or foetotoxic effect.

Lactation:

Elleste Duet Conti Tablets are not indicated during lactation.

4.7 Effects on ability to drive and use machines

No adverse effects on the ability to drive or operate machines have been reported.

4.8 Undesirable effects

Undesirable effects observed with estrogens and progestogens are detailed in the following table. The effects are grouped according to system organ class.

(see Table 1 below)

Breast Cancer

According to evidence from a large number of epidemiological studies and one randomised placebo-controlled trial, the Women's Health Initiative (WHI), the overall risk of breast cancer increases with increasing duration of HRT use in current or recent HRT users.

For *estrogen-only* HRT, estimates of relative risk (RR) from a reanalysis of original data from 51 epidemiological studies (in which >80% of HRT use was estrogen-only HRT) and from the epidemiological Million Women Study (MWS) are similar at 1.35 (95%CI 1.21 – 1.49) and 1.30 (95%CI 1.21 – 1.40), respectively.

For *estrogen plus progestogen* combined HRT, several epidemiological studies have reported an overall higher risk for breast cancer than with estrogens alone.

The MWS reported that, compared to never users, the use of various types of estrogen-progestogen combined HRT was associated with a higher risk of breast cancer (RR = 2.00, 95%CI: 1.88 – 2.12) than use of oestrogens alone (RR = 1.30, 95%CI: 1.21 – 1.40) or use of tibolone (RR=1.45; 95%CI 1.25-1.68).

The WHI trial reported a risk estimate of 1.24 (95%CI 1.01 – 1.54) after 5.6 years of use of estrogen-progestogen combined HRT (CEE + MPA) in all users compared with placebo.

The absolute risks calculated from the MWS and the WHI trial are presented below:

The MWS has estimated, from the known average incidence of breast cancer in developed countries, that:

- For women not using HRT, about 32 in every 1000 are expected to have breast cancer diagnosed between the ages of 50 and 64 years.
- For 1000 current or recent users of HRT, the number of *additional* cases during the corresponding period will be
- For users of *estrogen-only* replacement therapy
- between 0 and 3 (best estimate = 1.5) for 5 years' use
- between 3 and 7 (best estimate = 5) for 10 years' use.
- For users of *estrogen plus progestogen* combined HRT,
- between 5 and 7 (best estimate = 6) for 5 years' use
- between 18 and 20 (best estimate = 19) for 10 years' use.

The WHI trial estimated that after 5.6 years of follow-up of women between the ages of 50 and 79 years, an *additional* 8 cases of invasive breast cancer would be due to *estrogen-progestogen combined* HRT (CEE + MPA) per 10,000 women years.

According to calculations from the trial data, it is estimated that:

- For 1000 women in the placebo group,
- about 16 cases of invasive breast cancer would be diagnosed in 5 years.
- For 1000 women who used oestrogen + progestagen combined HRT (CEE + MPA), the number of *additional* cases would be
- between 0 and 9 (best estimate = 4) for 5 years' use.

The number of additional cases of breast cancer in women who use HRT is broadly similar for women who start HRT irrespective of age at start of use (between the ages of 45-65) (see section 4.4).

Endometrial cancer

In women with an intact uterus, the risk of endometrial hyperplasia and endometrial cancer increases with increasing duration of use of unopposed estrogens. According to data from epidemiological studies, the best estimate of the risk is that for women not using HRT, about 5 in every 1000 are expected to have endometrial cancer diagnosed between the ages of 50 and 65. Depending on the duration of treatment and oestrogen dose, the reported increase in endometrial cancer risk among unopposed oestrogen users varies from 2-to 12-fold greater compared with non-users. Adding a progestogen to estrogen-only therapy greatly reduces, but may not eliminate, this increased risk.

Very rare cases of myocardial infarction, stroke, chloasma, erythema multiforme, erythema nodosum, vascular purpura, haemorrhagic eruption and probable dementia (see section 4.4) have been reported in women using HRT.

4.9 Overdose

Overdose may be manifested by nausea and vomiting. If overdosage is discovered within two or three hours and is so large that treatment seems desirable, gastric lavage can be considered. There are no specific antidotes for overdosage and further treatment should be symptomatic.

5. PHARMACOLOGICAL PROPERTIES

Pharmacotherapeutic group: Progestogens and estrogens, combinations

ATC code: G03F A01

5.1 Pharmacodynamic properties

Estradiol

The active ingredient, synthetic 17β-estradiol, is chemically and biologically identical to endogenous human estradiol. It substitutes for the loss of estrogen production in menopausal women, and alleviates menopausal symptoms.

Estrogens prevent bone loss following menopause or ovariectomy. Estrogen deficiency at menopause is associated with an increasing bone turnover and decline in bone mass. The effect of estrogens on the bone mineral density is dose-dependent. Protection appears to be effective for as long as treatment is continued. After discontinuation of HRT, bone mass is lost at a rate similar to that in untreated women.

Evidence from the WHI trial and meta-analysed trials shows that current use of HRT, alone or in combination with a progestogen – given to predominantly healthy women – reduces the risk of hip, vertebral, and other osteoporotic fractures. HRT may also prevent fractures in women with low bone density and/or established osteoporosis, but the evidence for that is limited.

Norethisterone acetate

As estrogens promote the growth of the endometrium, unopposed estrogens increase the risk of endometrial hyperplasia and cancer. The addition of a progestogen reduces but does not eliminate the estrogen-induced risk of endometrial hyperplasia in non-hysterectomised women.

5.2 Pharmacokinetic properties

Pharmacokinetic parameters for Elleste Duet Conti Tablets (2 mg estradiol + 1 mg norethisterone tablets) are provided in the table below. The data were obtained from an open label, two way crossover pharmacokinetic study in which treatment was administered for 7 days to achieve steady state (n=24). Pharmacokinetic data were collected over 24 hours.

(see Table 2 above)

Table 2

	Serum unconjuated estradiol mean (SD)	Serum unconjugated estrone mean (SD)	Norethisterone mean (SD)
AUC_{0-24}	967.8 (0.5) pg.h/ml	8366 (1.7) pg.h/ml	43.2 (0.4) ng.h/ml
C_{max}	61.6 (0.4) pg/ml	648.5 (1.5) pg/ml	11.8 (0.4) ng/ml
C_{min}	19.3 (0.6) pg/ml	131.1 (2.5) pg/ml	0.5 (0.5) ng/ml
T_{max}	3.4 (2.1) h	5.07 (1.8) h	0.9 (0.3) h

Estradiol

Readily and fully absorbed from the GI tract when given orally, peak levels are generally observed 3-6 hours after ingestion, but by 24 hours concentrations have returned to baseline.

Estradiol is converted to estrone and estriol primarily in the liver. These are excreted into the bile and undergo enterohepatic recirculation and further degradation before being excreted in the urine (90-95%) as biologically inactive glucuronide and sulphate conjugates or in the faeces (5-10%), mostly unconjugated.

Norethisterone acetate

Norethisterone acetate is absorbed from the GI tract and its effects last for at least 24 hours. Maximum blood concentrations are generally reached 1-4 hours after administration. Norethisterone acetate undergoes first pass effect, being transformed to norethisterone which is then metabolised and excreted mainly in the urine as glucuronide and sulphate conjugates.

5.3 Preclinical safety data

Both estradiol and norethisterone acetate have been shown to induce adverse effects in preclinical reproductive toxicity studies. Chiefly, estradiol showed embryotoxic effects and induced anomalies in urogenital tract development, e.g. feminisation of male foetuses in high doses. Norethisterone acetate showed embryotoxic effects and induced anomalies in urogenital tract development. In mice, additional anomalies in non-urogenital foetal development, including hydrocephalus and clubfoot, have been detected.

6. PHARMACEUTICAL PARTICULARS

6.1 List of excipients

Tablet core:

Lactose monohydrate, maize starch, povidone 25, talc (purified) and magnesium stearate.

Film-coating material:

Hydroxypropylmethyl cellulose E464, titanium dioxide (E171), macrogol 400 and black iron oxide (E172).

6.2 Incompatibilities

Not applicable.

6.3 Shelf life

3 years

6.4 Special precautions for storage

Do not store above 25°C. Store in the original package.

6.5 Nature and contents of container

Aluminium foil and UPVC blister packed in a cardboard carton.

Pack sizes: 28 tablets and 84 (3 × 28) tablets.

6.6 Instructions for use and handling

There are no special instructions for handling.

7. MARKETING AUTHORISATION HOLDER

Shire Pharmaceutical Contracts Ltd
Hampshire International Business Park
Chineham
Basingstoke
Hampshire
RG24 8EP
United Kingdom

8. MARKETING AUTHORISATION NUMBER(S)

PL 08081/0030

9. DATE OF FIRST AUTHORISATION/RENEWAL OF THE AUTHORISATION

27 November 1997

10. DATE OF REVISION OF THE TEXT

March 2004

Table 1

Organ group	*Common >1/100)*	*Uncommon >1/1,000, <1/100)*	*Rare >1/10,000, <1/1,000)*
Gastrointestinal	Nausea, abdominal pain	Dyspepsia, vomiting, flatulence, gallbladder disease, gallstones	
Skin			Alopecia, hirsutism, rash, itching.
CNS	Headache	Dizziness, migraine	
Urogenital	Uterine bleeding, increase in size of uterine fibroids	Vaginal candidiasis	
Cardiovascular		Increase in blood pressure	Venous thromboembolism* Thrombophlebitis
Miscellaneous	Weight increase/decrease, oedema, breast tenderness, breast enlargement, change in mood including anxiety and depressive mood, change in libido	Leg cramps	

*see sections 4.3 Contra-indications and 4.4 Special warnings and precautions for use

Elleste Solo 1mg

(Pharmacia Limited)

1. NAME OF THE MEDICINAL PRODUCT

Elleste Solo 1 mg

2. QUALITATIVE AND QUANTITATIVE COMPOSITION

Each tablet contains 1 mg estradiol (as estradiol hemihydrate)

For excipients, see 6.1.

3. PHARMACEUTICAL FORM

Film coated tablets.

4. CLINICAL PARTICULARS

4.1 Therapeutic indications

Hormone Replacement Therapy (HRT) for estrogen deficiency symptoms in post- and peri-menopausal women. (See also Section 4.4)

The experience of treating women older than 65 years is limited.

4.2 Posology and method of administration

One tablet daily to be taken orally. Elleste Solo 1 mg may be taken continuously in hysterectomised women. In women with a uterus, a progestogen should be added for 12 - 14 days each cycle to oppose the production of an estrogen-stimulated hyperplasia of the endometrium. Unless there is a previous diagnosis of endometriosis, it is not recommended to add a progestogen in hysterectomised women.

Therapy may start at any time in women with established amenorrhoea or who are experiencing long intervals between spontaneous menses. In patients who are menstruating, it is advised that therapy starts on the first day of bleeding. Patients changing from a cyclical or continuous sequential preparation should complete the cycle and may then change to Elleste Solo 1 mg without a break in therapy. Patients changing from a continuous combined preparation may start therapy at any time if amenorrhoea is established, or otherwise start on the first day of bleeding.

Elderly

There are no special dosage requirements for elderly patients.

Children

Not to be used in children.

Elleste Solo tablets are available in two strengths: Elleste Solo 1 mg (containing 1 mg estradiol) and Elleste Solo 2 mg (containing 2 mg estradiol). For initiation and continuation of treatment of post-and peri-menopausal symptoms, the lowest effective dose for the shortest duration (see also Section 4.4) should be used. Elleste Solo 2 mg is additionally indicated for prevention of osteoporosis in postmenopausal women at high risk of future fractures and who are intolerant of, or contraindicated for, other medicinal products approved for the prevention of osteoporosis.

Missed or Extra Tablet: If a tablet is missed it should be taken within 12 hours of when normally taken; otherwise the tablet should be discarded, and the usual tablet should be taken the following day. A missed dose may lead to break-through bleeding or spotting in non-hysterectomised women. If one extra tablet is taken inadvertently, the usual tablet should be taken the following day.

4.3 Contraindications

Known, past or suspected breast cancer;

Known or suspected estrogen-dependent malignant tumours (e.g. endometrial cancer);

Undiagnosed genital bleeding;

Untreated endometrial hyperplasia;

Previous idiopathic or current venous thromboembolism (deep venous thrombosis, pulmonary embolism);

Active or recent arterial thromboembolic disease (e.g. angina, myocardial infarction);

Acute liver disease, or a history of liver disease as long as liver function tests have failed to return to normal;

Known hypersensitivity to the active substances or to any of the excipients;

Porphyria.

4.4 Special warnings and special precautions for use

For the treatment of postmenopausal symptoms, HRT should only be initiated for symptoms that adversely affect quality of life. In all cases a careful appraisal of the risks and benefits should be undertaken at least annually and HRT should only be continued as long as the benefit outweighs the risk.

Medical Examination/Follow Up

Before initiating or reinstituting HRT, a complete personal and family medical history should be taken. Physical (including pelvic and breast) examination should be guided by this and by the contraindications and warnings for use. During treatment, periodic check-ups are recommended of a frequency and nature adapted to the individual woman. Women should be advised what changes in their breasts should be reported to their doctor or nurse (see 'Breast Cancer' below). Investigations, including mammography, should be carried out in accordance with currently accepted screening practices, modified to the clinical needs of the individual.

Conditions Which Need Supervision

If any of the following conditions are present, have occurred previously, and/or have been aggravated during pregnancy or previous hormone treatment, the patient should be closely supervised. It should be taken into account that these conditions may recur or be aggravated during treatment with Elleste Solo 1 mg, in particular:

- Leiomyoma (uterine fibroids) or endometriosis
- A history of, or risk factors for, thromboembolic disorders (see below)
- Risk factors for estrogen dependent tumours, e.g. 1st degree heredity for breast cancer
- Hypertension
- Liver disorders (e.g. liver adenoma)
- Diabetes mellitus with or without vascular involvement
- Cholelithiasis
- Migraine or (severe) headache
- Systemic lupus erythematosus
- A history of endometrial hyperplasia (see below)
- Epilepsy
- Asthma
- Otosclerosis

Reasons for Immediate Withdrawal of Therapy:

Therapy should be discontinued if a contraindication is discovered and in the following situations:

- Jaundice or deterioration in liver function
- Significant increase in blood pressure
- New onset of migraine-type headache
- Pregnancy

Endometrial Hyperplasia

The risk of endometrial hyperplasia and carcinoma is increased when estrogens are administered alone for prolonged periods (see Section 4.8). The addition of a progestogen for at least 12 days per cycle in non-hysterectomised women greatly reduces this risk.

Break-through bleeding and spotting may occur during the first months of treatment. If break-through bleeding or spotting appears after some time on therapy, or continues after treatment has been discontinued, the reason should be investigated, which may include endometrial biospy to exclude endometrial malignancy.

Unopposed estrogen stimulation may lead to premalignant or malignant transformation in the residual foci of endometriosis. Therefore, the addition of progestogens to estrogen replacement therapy should be considered in women who have undergone hysterectomy because of endometriosis, if they are known to have residual endometriosis.

Breast Cancer

A randomised placebo-controlled trial, the Women's Health Initiative study (WHI), and epidemiological studies, including the Million Women Study (MWS), have reported an increased risk of breast cancer in women taking estrogens, or estrogen-progestogen combinations or tibolone for HRT for several years (see Section 4.8).

For all HRT, an excess risk becomes apparent within a few years of use and increases with duration of intake but returns to baseline within a few (at most five) years after stopping treatment.

In the MWS, the relative risk of breast cancer with conjugated equine estrogens (CEE) or estradiol (E2) was greater when a progestogen was added, either sequentially or continuously, and regardless of type of progestogen. There was no evidence of a difference in risk between the different routes of administration.

In the WHI study, the continuous combined conjugated equine estrogen and medroxyprogesterone acetate (CEE + MPA)_product used was associated with breast cancers that were slightly larger in size and more frequently had local lymph node metastases compared to placebo.

HRT, especially estrogen-progestogen combined treatment, increases the density of mammographic images which may adversely affect the radiological detection of breast cancer.

Venous Thromboembolism

HRT is associated with a higher relative risk of developing venous thromboembolism (VTE), i.e. deep vein thrombosis or pulmonary embolism. One randomised controlled trial and epidemiological studies found a two- to threefold higher risk for users compared with non-users. For non-users, it is estimated that the number of cases of VTE that will occur over a 5 year period is about 3 per 1000 women aged 50-59 years and 8 per 1000 women aged between 60-69 years. It is estimated that in healthy women who use HRT for 5 years, the number of additional cases of VTE over a 5 year period will be between 2 and 6 (best estimate = 4) per 1000 women aged 50-59 years and between 5 and 15 (best estimate = 9) per 1000 women aged 60-69 years. The occurrence of such an event is more likely in the first year of HRT than later.

Generally recognised risk factors for VTE include a personal history or family history, severe obesity (BM > 30 kg/m^2) and systemic lupus erythematosus (SLE). There is no consensus about the possible role of varicose veins in VTE.

Patients with a history of VTE or known thrombophilic states have an increased risk of VTE. HRT may add to this risk. Personal or strong family history of thromboembolism or recurrent spontaneous abortion should be investigated in order to exclude a thrombophilic predisposition. Until a thorough evaluation of thrombophilic factors has been made or anticoagulant treatment initiated, use of HRT in such patients should be viewed as contraindicated. Those women already on anticoagulant treatment require careful consideration of the benefit-risk of use of HRT.

The risk of VTE may be temporarily increased with prolonged immobilisation, major trauma or major surgery. As in all postoperative patients, scrupulous attention should be given to prophylactic measures to prevent VTE following surgery. Where prolonged immobilisation is liable to follow elective surgery, particularly abdominal or orthopaedic surgery to the lower limbs, consideration should be given to temporarily stopping HRT 4 to 6 weeks earlier, if possible. Treatment should not be restarted until the woman is completely mobilised.

If VTE develops after initiating therapy, the drug should be discontinued. Patients should be told to contact their doctors immediately when they are aware of a potential thromboembolic symptom (e.g., painful swelling of a leg, sudden pain in the chest, dyspnea).

Coronary Artery Disease

There is no evidence from randomised controlled trials of cardiovasular benefit with continuous combined conjugated estrogens and medroxyprogesterone acetate (MPA). Two large clinical trials (WHI and HERS i.e. Heart and Estrogen/progestin Replacement Study) showed a possible increased risk of cardiovascular morbidity in the first year of use and no overall benefit. For other HRT products there are only limited data from randomised controlled trials examining effectsin cardiovascular morbidity or mortality. Therefore, it is uncertain whether these findings also extend to other HRT products.

Stroke

One large randomised clinical trial (WHI-trial) found, as a secondary outcome, an increased risk of ischaemic stroke in healthy women during treatment with continuous combined conjugated estrogens and MPA. For women who do not use HRT, it is estimated that the number of cases of stroke that will occur over a 5 year period is about 3 per 1000 women aged 50-59 years and 11 per 1000 women aged 60-69 years. It is estimated that for women who use conjugated estrogens and MPA for 5 years, the number of additional cases will be between 0 and 3 (best estimate = 1) per 1000 users aged 50-59 years and between 1 and 9 (best estimate = 4) per 1000 users aged 60-69 years. It is unknown whether the increased risk also extends to other HRT products.

Ovarian Cancer

Long-term (at least 5 to 10 years) use of estrogen-only HRT products in hysterectomised women has been associated with an increased risk of ovarian cancer in some epidemiological studies. It is uncertain whether long-term use of combined HRT confers a different risk than estrogen-only products.

Other Conditions

Estrogens may cause fluid retention and therefore patients with cardiac or renal dysfunction should be carefully observed. Patients with terminal renal insufficiency should be closely observed, since it is expected that the level of circulating active ingredients in Elleste Solo 1 mg is increased.

Women with pre-existing hypertriglyceridaemia should be followed closely during estrogen replacement or hormone replacement therapy, since rare cases of large increases of plasma triglycerides leading to pancreatitis have been reported with estrogen therapy in this condition.

Estrogens increase thyroid binding globulin (TBG), leading to increased circulating total thyroid hormone, as measured by protein-bound iodine (PBI), T4 levels (by column or by radio-immunoassay) or T3 levels (by radio-immunoassay). T3 resin uptake is decreased, reflecting the elevated TBG. Free T4 and free T3 concentrations are unaltered. Other binding proteins may be elevated in serum, i.e. corticoid binding globulin (CBG), sex-hormone-binding globulin (SHBG) leading to increased circulating corticosteroids and sex steroids, respectively. Free or biological active hormone concentrations are unchanged. Other plasma proteins may be increased (angiotensinogen/renin substrate, alpha-1-antitrypsin, ceruloplasmin).

There is no conclusive evidence for improvement of cognitive function. There is some evidence from the WHI trial of increased risk of probable dementia in women who start using continuous combined CEE and MPA after the age of 65. It is unknown whether the findings apply to younger post-menopausal women or other HRT products.

There is an increased risk of gall bladder disease in women receiving post-menopausal estrogens.

In rare cases benign, and in even rarer cases malignant liver tumours leading in isolated cases to life-threatening intra-abdominal haemorrhage have been observed after the use of hormonal substances such as those contained in Elleste Solo 1 mg. If severe upper abdominal complaints, enlarged liver or signs of intra-abdominal haemorrhage occur, a liver tumour should be considered in the differential diagnosis.

4.5 Interaction with other medicinal products and other forms of Interaction

The metabolism of estrogens may be increased by concomitant use of substances known to induce drug-metabolising enzymes, specifically cytochrome P450 enzymes, such as anticonvulsants (e.g. phenobarbital, phenytoin, carbamazepine) and anti-infectives (e.g. rifampicin, rifabutin, nevirapine, efavirenz).

Ritonavir and nelfinavir, although known as strong inhibitors, by contrast exhibit inducing properties when used concomitantly with steroid hormones. Herbal preparations containing St John's Wort (Hypericum Perforatum) may induce the metabolism of estrogens.

Clinically, an increased metabolism of estrogens may lead to decreased effect and changes in the uterine bleeding profile.

The requirement for oral anti-diabetics or insulin can change as a result of the effect on glucose tolerance. Some laboratory tests can be influenced by estrogens, such as tests for thyroid function (see Section 4.4) or glucose tolerance.

4.6 Pregnancy and lactation

Pregnancy:

Elleste Solo 1 mg is not indicated during pregnancy. If pregnancy occurs during medication with Elleste Solo 1 mg treatment should be withdrawn immediately. The results of most epidemiological studies to date relevant to inadvertent foetal exposure to estrogens indicate no teratogenic or foetotoxic effects.

Lactation:

Elleste Solo 1 mg is not indicated during lactation.

4.7 Effects on ability to drive and use machines

No adverse effects on the ability to drive or operate machines have been recorded.

4.8 Undesirable effects

Undesirable effects observed with estrogens are detailed in the following table. The effects are grouped according to system organ class.

(see Table 1 below)

Breast Cancer

According to evidence from a large number of epidemiological studies and one randomised placebo-controlled trial, the Women's Health Initiative (WHI), the overall risk of breast cancer increases with increasing duration of HRT use in current or recent HRT users.

For *estrogen-only* HRT, estimates of relative risk (RR) from a reanalysis of original data from 51 epidemiological studies (in which >80% of HRT use was estrogen-only HRT) and from the epidemiological Million Women Study (MWS) are similar at 1.35 (95%CI 1.21 – 1.49) and 1.30 (95%CI 1.21 – 1.40), respectively.

For *estrogen plus progestogen* combined HRT, several epidemiological studies have reported an overall higher risk for breast cancer than with estrogens alone.

The MWS reported that, compared to never users, the use of various types of estrogen-progestogen combined HRT was associated with a higher risk of breast cancer (RR = 2.00, 95%CI: 1.88 – 2.12) than use of estrogens alone (RR = 1.30, 95%CI: 1.21 - 1.40) or use of tibolone (RR=1.45; 95%CI 1.25-1.68).

The WHI trial reported a risk estimate of 1.24 (95%CI 1.01 – 1.54) after 5.6 years of use of estrogen-progestogen combined HRT (CEE + MPA) in all users compared with placebo.

The absolute risks calculated from the MWS and the WHI trial are presented below:

The MWS has estimated, from the known average incidence of breast cancer in developed countries, that:

- For women not using HRT, about 32 in every 1000 are expected to have breast cancer diagnosed between the ages of 50 and 64 years.
- For 1000 current or recent users of HRT, the number of *additional* cases during the corresponding period will be
- For users of *estrogen-only* replacement therapy
- between 0 and 3 (best estimate = 1.5) for 5 years' use
- between 3 and 7 (best estimate = 5) for 10 years' use.
- For users of *estrogen plus progestogen* combined HRT,
- between 5 and 7 (best estimate = 6) for 5 years' use
- between 18 and 20 (best estimate = 19) for 10 years' use.

The WHI trial estimated that after 5.6 years of follow-up of women between the ages of 50 and 79 years, an *additional* 8 cases of invasive breast cancer would be due to *estrogen-progestogen combined* HRT (CEE + MPA) per 10,000 women years.

According to calculations from the trial data, it is estimated that:

- For 1000 women in the placebo group,
- about 16 cases of invasive breast cancer would be diagnosed in 5 years.
- For 1000 women who used estrogen + progestogen combined HRT (CEE + MPA), the number of *additional* cases would be
- between 0 and 9 (best estimate = 4) for 5 years' use.

The number of additional cases of breast cancer in women who use HRT is broadly similar for women who start HRT irrespective of age at start of use (between the ages of 45-65) (see Section 4.4).

Endometrial cancer

In women with an intact uterus, the risk of endometrial hyperplasia and endometrial cancer increases with increasing duration of use of unopposed estrogens. According to data from epidemiological studies, the best estimate of the risk is that for women not using HRT, about 5 in every 1000 are expected to have endometrial cancer diagnosed between the ages of 50 and 65. Depending on the duration of treatment and estrogen dose, the reported increase in endometrial cancer risk among unopposed estrogen users varies from 2-to 12-fold greater compared with non-users. Adding a progestogen to estrogen-only therapy greatly reduces this increased risk.

Very rare cases of myocardial infarction, stroke, chloasma, erythema multiforme, erythema nodosum, vascular purpura, haemorrhagic eruption and probable dementia (see Section 4.4) have been reported in women using HRT.

4.9 Overdose

Overdosage may be manifested by nausea and vomiting. If overdosage is discovered within two or three hours and is so large that treatment seems desirable, gastric lavage can be considered. There are no specific antidotes for overdosage, and further treatment should be symptomatic.

5. PHARMACOLOGICAL PROPERTIES

Pharmacotherapeutic group: Natural and semisynthetic estrogens, plain

ATC Code: G03CA03.

5.1 Pharmacodynamic properties

The active ingredient, synthetic 17β-estradiol, is chemically and biologically identical to endogenous human estradiol. It substitutes for the loss of estrogen production in menopausal women, and alleviates menopausal symptoms.

5.2 Pharmacokinetic properties

No pharmacokinetic parameters are available for Elleste Solo 1 mg. Pharmacokinetic parameters for Elleste Solo 2 mg, are provided in the following table. Elleste Solo 2 mg contains 2 mg estradiol (as hemihydrate). The data were obtained from an open label, single dose, two way cross-over pharmacokinetic study (n=16). Pharmacokinetic data were collected over 48 hours.

	Plasma Unconjugated Estradiol (mean)	**Plasma Unconjugated Estrone (mean)**
AUC_{0-48h}	950 pg.h/ml	2700 pg.h/ml
C_{max}	45 pg/ml	140 pg/ml
T_{max}	5.0 h	4.0 h

Estradiol

Readily and fully absorbed from the GI tract when given orally, peak levels are generally observed 3-6 hours after ingestion, but by 24 hours concentrations have returned to baseline.

Estradiol is converted to estrone and estriol primarily in the liver. These are excreted into the bile and undergo enterohepatic recirculation and further degradation before being excreted in the urine (90-95%) as biologically inactive glucuronide and sulphate conjugates or in the faeces (5-10%), mostly unconjugated.

5.3 Preclinical safety data

Estradiol has been shown to induce adverse effects in preclinical reproductive toxicity studies. Chiefly estradiol showed embryotoxic effects and induced anomalies in urogenital tract development e.g. feminisation of male foetuses in high doses.

6. PHARMACEUTICAL PARTICULARS

6.1 List of excipients

Tablet core:

Lactose monohydrate, maize starch, povidone 25, talc (purified), magnesium stearate.

Film-coating material:

Hydroxypropylmethyl cellulose (E464), titanium dioxide (E171), macrogol 400.

6.2 Incompatibilities

Not applicable

6.3 Shelf life

3 years

6.4 Special precautions for storage

Do not store above 25°C. Store in the original package.

6.5 Nature and contents of container

Aluminium foil and UPVC blister packed in a cardboard carton.

Pack sizes: 20*, 28, 60*, 84 or 100* tablets.

Packs marked with a * are not marketed in the UK.

6.6 Instructions for use and handling

There are no special instructions for handling.

7. MARKETING AUTHORISATION HOLDER

Shire Pharmaceutical Contracts Limited

Hampshire International Business Park

Chineham

Basingstoke

Hampshire

RG24 8EP

United Kingdom

8. MARKETING AUTHORISATION NUMBER(S)

PL 08081/0020

9. DATE OF FIRST AUTHORISATION/RENEWAL OF THE AUTHORISATION

30 September 1994

10. DATE OF REVISION OF THE TEXT

April 2004

Table 1

Organ group	*Common >1/100)*	*Uncommon >1/1,000, <1/100)*	*Rare >1/10,000, <1/1,000)*
Gastrointestinal	Nausea, abdominal pain	Dyspepsia, vomiting, flatulence, gallbladder disease, gallstones	
Skin			Alopecia, hirsutism, rash, itching
CNS	Headache	Dizziness, migraine	
Urogenital	Uterine bleeding, increase in size of uterine fibroids	Vaginal candidiasis	
Cardiovascular		Increase in blood pressure	Venous thromboembolism* Thrombophlebitis
Miscellaneous	Weight increase/decrease, oedema, breast tenderness, breast enlargement, change in mood including anxiety and depressive mood, change in libido	Leg cramps	

* see Sections 4.3 Contraindications and 4.4 Special warnings and precautions for use

Elleste Solo 2mg

(Pharmacia Limited)

1. NAME OF THE MEDICINAL PRODUCT

Elleste Solo 2 mg

2. QUALITATIVE AND QUANTITATIVE COMPOSITION

Each tablet contains 2 mg estradiol (as estradiol hemihydrate)

For excipients, see 6.1.

3. PHARMACEUTICAL FORM

Film coated tablets.

4. CLINICAL PARTICULARS

4.1 Therapeutic indications

Hormone Replacement Therapy (HRT) for estrogen deficiency symptoms in post- and peri-menopausal women.

Prevention of osteoporosis in postmenopausal women at high risk of future fractures who are intolerant of, or contra-indicated for, other medicinal products approved for the prevention of osteoporosis. (See also Section 4.4).

The experience of treating women older than 65 years is limited.

4.2 Posology and method of administration

One tablet daily to be taken orally. Elleste Solo 2 mg may be taken continuously in hysterectomised women. In women with a uterus, a progestogen should be added for 12 - 14 days each cycle to oppose the production of an estrogen-stimulated hyperplasia of the endometrium. Unless there is a previous diagnosis of endometriosis, it is not recommended to add a progestogen in hysterectomised women.

Therapy may start at any time in women with established amenorrhoea or who are experiencing long intervals between spontaneous menses. In patients who are menstruating, it is advised that therapy starts on the first day of bleeding. Patients changing from a cyclical or continuous sequential preparation should complete the cycle and may then change to Elleste Solo 2 mg without a break in therapy. Patients changing from a continuous combined preparation may start therapy at any time if amenorrhoea is established, or otherwise start on the first day of bleeding.

Elderly

There are no special dosage requirements for elderly patients.

Children

Not to be used in children.

Elleste Solo Tablets are available in two strengths: Elleste Solo 1 mg (containing 1 mg estradiol) and Elleste Solo 2 mg (containing 2 mg estradiol). For initiation and continuation of treatment of post- and peri-menopausal symptoms, the lowest effective dose for the shortest duration (see also Section 4.4) should be used. Elleste Solo 1 mg is not indicated for prophylaxis of osteoporosis.

Missed or Extra Tablet: If a tablet is missed it should be taken within 12 hours of when normally taken; otherwise the tablet should be discarded, and the usual tablet should be taken the following day. A missed dose may lead to break-through bleeding or spotting in non-hysterectomised women. If one extra tablet is taken inadvertently, the usual tablet should be taken the following day.

4.3 Contraindications

Known, past or suspected breast cancer;

Known or suspected estrogen-dependent malignant tumours (e.g. endometrial cancer);

Undiagnosed genital bleeding;

Untreated endometrial hyperplasia;

Previous idiopathic or current venous thromboembolism (deep venous thrombosis, pulmonary embolism);

Active or recent arterial thromboembolic disease (e.g. angina, myocardial infarction);

Acute liver disease, or a history of liver disease as long as liver function tests have failed to return to normal;

Known hypersensitivity to the active substances or to any of the excipients;

Porphyria.

4.4 Special warnings and special precautions for use

For the treatment of postmenopausal symptoms, HRT should only be initiated for symptoms that adversely affect quality of life. In all cases, a careful appraisal of the risks and benefits should be undertaken at least annually and HRT should only be continued as long as the benefit outweighs the risk.

Medical Examination/Follow Up

Before initiating or reinstituting HRT, a complete personal and family medical history should be taken. Physical (including pelvic and breast) examination should be guided by this and by the contraindications and warnings for use. During treatment, periodic check-ups are recommended of a frequency and nature adapted to the individual woman. Women should be advised what changes in their breasts should be reported to their doctor or nurse (see "Breast cancer" below). Investigations, including mammography, should be carried out in accordance with currently accepted screening practices, modified to the clinical needs of the individual.

Conditions Which Need Supervision

If any of the following conditions are present, have occurred previously, and/or have been aggravated during pregnancy or previous hormone treatment, the patient should be closely supervised. It should be taken into account that these conditions may recur or be aggravated during treatment with Elleste Solo 2 mg, in particular:

- Leiomyoma (uterine fibroids) or endometriosis
- A history of, or risk factors for, thromboembolic disorders (see below)
- Risk factors for estrogen dependent tumours, e.g. 1st degree heredity for breast cancer
- Hypertension
- Liver disorders (e.g. liver adenoma)
- Diabetes mellitus with or without vascular involvement
- Cholelithiasis
- Migraine or (severe) headache
- Systemic lupus erythematosus
- A history of endometrial hyperplasia (see below)
- Epilepsy
- Asthma
- Otosclerosis

Reasons for Immediate Withdrawal of Therapy

Therapy should be discontinued if a contraindication is discovered and in the following situations:

- Jaundice or deterioration in liver function
- Significant increase in blood pressure
- New onset of migraine-type headache
- Pregnancy

Endometrial Hyperplasia

The risk of endometrial hyperplasia and carcinoma is increased when estrogens are administered alone for prolonged periods (see Section 4.8). The addition of a progestogen for at least 12 days per cycle in non-hysterectomised women greatly reduces this risk.

Break-through bleeding and spotting may occur during the first months of treatment. If break-through bleeding or spotting appears after some time on therapy, or continues after treatment has been discontinued, the reason should be investigated, which may include endometrial biopsy to exclude endometrial malignancy.

Unopposed estrogen stimulation may lead to premalignant or malignant transformation in the residual foci of endometriosis. Therefore, the addition of progestogens to estrogen replacement therapy should be considered in women who have undergone hysterectomy because of endometriosis, if they are known to have residual endometriosis.

Breast Cancer

A randomised placebo-controlled trial, the Women's Health Initiative Study (WHI), and epidemiological studies, including the Million Women Study (MWS), have reported an increased risk of breast cancer in women taking estrogens, estrogen-progestogen combinations or tibolone for HRT for several years (see Section 4.8). For all HRT, an excess risk becomes apparent within a few years of use and increases with duration of intake but returns to baseline within a few (at most five) years after stopping treatment.

In the MWS, the relative risk of breast cancer with conjugated equine estrogens (CEE) or estradiol (E2) was greater when a progestogen was added, either sequentially or continuously, and regardless of type of progestogen. There was no evidence of a difference in risk between the different routes of administration.

In the WHI study, the continuous combined conjugated equine estrogen and medroxyprogesterone acetate (CEE + MPA) product used was associated with breast cancers that were slightly larger in size and more frequently had local lymph node metastases compared to placebo.

HRT, especially estrogen-progestogen combined treatment, increases the density of mammographic images, which may adversely affect the radiological detection of breast cancer.

Venous Thromboembolism

HRT is associated with a higher relative risk of developing venous thromboembolism (VTE), i.e. deep vein thrombosis or pulmonary embolism. One randomised controlled trial and epidemiological studies found a two- to threefold higher risk for users compared with non-users. For non-users, it is estimated that the number of cases of VTE that will occur over a 5 year period is about 3 per 1000 women aged 50-59 years and 8 per 1000 women aged 60-69 years. It is estimated that in healthy women who use HRT for 5 years, the number of additional cases of VTE over a 5 year period will be between 2 and 6 (best estimate = 4) per 1000 women aged 50-59 years and between 5 and 15 (best estimate = 9) per 1000 women aged 60-69 years. The occurrence of such an event is more likely in the first year of HRT than later.

Generally recognised risk factors for VTE include a personal history or family history, severe obesity (BM > 30 kg/m^2) and systemic lupus erythematosus (SLE). There is no consensus about the possible role of varicose veins in VTE.

Patients with a history of VTE or known thrombophilic states have an increased risk of VTE. HRT may add to this risk. Personal or strong family history of thromboembolism or recurrent spontaneous abortion should be investigated in order to exclude a thrombophilic predisposition. Until a thorough evaluation of thrombophilic factors has been made or anticoagulant treatment initiated, use of HRT in such patients should be viewed as contraindicated. Those women already on anticoagulant treatment require careful consideration of the benefit-risk of use of HRT.

The risk of VTE may be temporarily increased with prolonged immobilisation, major trauma or major surgery. As in all postoperative patients, scrupulous attention should be given to prophylactic measures to prevent VTE following surgery. Where prolonged immobilisation is liable to follow elective surgery, particularly abdominal or orthopaedic surgery to the lower limbs, consideration should be given to temporarily stopping HRT 4 to 6 weeks earlier, if possible. Treatment should not be restarted until the woman is completely mobilised.

If VTE develops after initiating therapy, the drug should be discontinued. Patients should be told to contact their doctors immediately when they are aware of a potential thromboembolic symptom (eg, painful swelling of a leg, sudden pain in the chest, dyspnea).

Coronary Artery Disease

There is no evidence from randomised controlled trials of cardiovascular benefit with continuous combined conjugated estrogens and medroxyprogesterone acetate (MPA). Two large clinical trials (WHI and HERS i.e. Heart and Estrogen/progestin Replacement Study) showed a possible increased risk of cardiovascular morbidity in the first year of use and no overall benefit. For other HRT products there are only limited data from randomised controlled trials examining effects in cardiovascular morbidity or mortality. Therefore, it is uncertain whether these findings also extend to other HRT products.

Stroke

One large randomised clinical trial (WHI-trial) found, as a secondary outcome, an increased risk of ischaemic stroke in healthy women during treatment with continuous combined conjugated estrogens and MPA. For women who do not use HRT, it is estimated that the number of cases of stroke that will occur over a 5 year period is about 3 per 1000 women aged 50-59 years and 11 per 1000 women aged 60-69 years. It is estimated that for women who use conjugated estrogens and MPA for 5 years, the number of additional cases will be between 0 and 3 (best estimate = 1) per 1000 users aged 50-59 years and between 1 and 9 (best estimate = 4) per 1000 users aged 60-69 years. It is unknown whether the increased risk also extends to other HRT products.

Ovarian Cancer

Long-term (at least 5 to 10 years) use of estrogen-only HRT products in hysterectomised women has been associated with an increased risk of ovarian cancer in some epidemiological studies. It is uncertain whether long-term use of combined HRT confers a different risk than estrogen-only products.

Other Conditions

Estrogens may cause fluid retention and therefore patients with cardiac or renal dysfunction should be carefully observed. Patients with terminal renal insufficiency should be closely observed, since it is expected that the level of circulating active ingredients in Elleste Solo 2 mg is increased.

Women with pre-existing hypertriglyceridaemia should be followed closely during estrogen replacement or hormone replacement therapy, since rare cases of large increases of plasma triglycerides leading to pancreatitis have been reported with estrogen therapy in this condition.

Estrogens increase thyroid binding globulin (TBG), leading to increased circulating total thyroid hormone, as measured by protein-bound iodine (PBI), T4 levels (by column or by radio-immunoassay) or T3 levels (by radio-immunoassay). T3 resin uptake is decreased, reflecting the elevated TBG. Free T4 and free T3 concentrations are unaltered. Other binding proteins may be elevated in serum i.e. corticoid binding globulin (CBG), sex-hormone-binding globulin (SHBG) leading to increased circulating corticosteroids and sex steroids, respectively. Free or biological active hormone concentrations are unchanged. Other plasma proteins may be increased (angiotensinogen/renin substrate, alpha-1-antitrypsin, ceruloplasmin).

There is no conclusive evidence for improvement of cognitive function. There is some evidence from the WHI trial of increased risk of probable dementia in women who start using continuous combined CEE and MPA after the age of 65. It is unknown whether the findings apply to younger post-menopausal women or other HRT products.

There is an increased risk of gall bladder disease in women receiving post-menopausal estrogens.

In rare cases benign, and in even rarer cases malignant liver tumours leading in isolated cases to life-threatening intra-abdominal haemorrhage have been observed after the use of hormonal substances such as those contained in Elleste Solo 2 mg. If severe upper abdominal complaints, enlarged liver or signs of intra-abdominal haemorrhage occur, a liver tumour should be considered in the differential diagnosis.

4.5 Interaction with other medicinal products and other forms of Interaction

The metabolism of estrogens may be increased by concomitant use of substances known to induce drug-metabolising enzymes, specifically cytochrome P450 enzymes, such as anticonvulsants (e.g. phenobarbital, phenytoin, carbamazepine) and anti-infectives (e.g. rifampicin, rifabutin, nevirapine, efavirenz).

Ritonavir and nelfinavir, although known as strong inhibitors, by contrast exhibit inducing properties when used concomitantly with steroid hormones. Herbal preparations containing St John's Wort (*Hypericum Perforatum*) may induce the metabolism of estrogens.

Clinically, an increased metabolism of estrogens may lead to decreased effect and changes in the uterine bleeding profile.

The requirement for oral anti-diabetics or insulin can change as a result of the effect on glucose tolerance. Some laboratory tests can be influenced by estrogens, such as tests for thyroid function (see section 4.4) or glucose tolerance.

4.6 Pregnancy and lactation

Pregnancy:

Elleste Solo 2 mg is not indicated during pregnancy. If pregnancy occurs during medication with Elleste Solo 2 mg treatment should be withdrawn immediately. The results of most epidemiological studies to date relevant to inadvertent foetal exposure to estrogens indicate no teratogenic or foetotoxic effects.

Lactation:

Elleste Solo 2 mg is not indicated during lactation.

4.7 Effects on ability to drive and use machines

No adverse effects on the ability to drive or operate machines have been recorded.

4.8 Undesirable effects

Undesirable effects observed with estrogens are detailed in the following table. The effects are grouped according to system organ class.

(see Table 1 below)

Breast Cancer

According to evidence from a large number of epidemiological studies and one randomised placebo-controlled trial, the Women's Health Initiative (WHI), the overall risk of breast cancer increases with increasing duration of HRT use in current or recent HRT users.

For *estrogen-only* HRT, estimates of relative risk (RR) from a reanalysis of original data from 51 epidemiological studies (in which >80% of HRT use was estrogen-only HRT) and from the epidemiological Million Women Study (MWS) are similar at 1.35 (95%CI 1.21 – 1.49) and 1.30 (95%CI 1.21 – 1.40), respectively.

For *estrogen plus progestogen* combined HRT, several epidemiological studies have reported an overall higher risk for breast cancer than with estrogens alone.

The MWS reported that, compared to never users, the use of various types of estrogen-progestogen combined HRT was associated with a higher risk of breast cancer (RR = 2.00, 95%CI: 1.88 – 2.12) than use of estrogens alone (RR = 1.30, 95%CI: 1.21 – 1.40) or use of tibolone (RR=1.45; 95%CI 1.25-1.68).

The WHI trial reported a risk estimate of 1.24 (95%CI 1.01 – 1.54) after 5.6 years of use of estrogen-progestogen combined HRT (CEE + MPA) in all users compared with placebo.

The absolute risks calculated from the MWS and the WHI trial are presented below:

The MWS has estimated, from the known average incidence of breast cancer in developed countries, that:

- For women not using HRT, about 32 in every 1000 are expected to have breast cancer diagnosed between the ages of 50 and 64 years.
- For 1000 current or recent users of HRT, the number of *additional* cases during the corresponding period will be
- For users of *estrogen-only* replacement therapy
- between 0 and 3 (best estimate = 1.5) for 5 years' use
- between 3 and 7 (best estimate = 5) for 10 years' use.
- For users of *estrogen plus progestogen* combined HRT,
- between 5 and 7 (best estimate = 6) for 5 years' use
- between 18 and 20 (best estimate = 19) for 10 years' use.

The WHI trial estimated that after 5.6 years of follow-up of women between the ages of 50 and 79 years, an *additional* 8 cases of invasive breast cancer would be due to *estrogen-progestogen combined* HRT (CEE + MPA) per 10,000 women years.

According to calculations from the trial data, it is estimated that:

- For 1000 women in the placebo group,
- about 16 cases of invasive breast cancer would be diagnosed in 5 years.
- For 1000 women who used estrogen + progestogen combined HRT (CEE + MPA), the number of *additional* cases would be
- between 0 and 9 (best estimate = 4) for 5 years' use.

The number of additional cases of breast cancer in women who use HRT is broadly similar for women who start HRT irrespective of age at start of use (between the ages of 45-65) (see section 4.4).

Endometrial cancer

In women with an intact uterus, the risk of endometrial hyperplasia and endometrial cancer increases with increasing duration of use of unopposed estrogens. According to data from epidemiological studies, the best estimate of the risk is that for women not using HRT, about 5 in every 1000 are expected to have endometrial cancer diagnosed between the ages of 50 and 65. Depending on the duration of treatment and estrogen dose, the reported increase in endometrial cancer risk among unopposed estrogen users varies from 2-to 12-fold greater compared with non-users. Adding a progestogen to estrogen-only therapy greatly reduces this increased risk.

Very rare cases of myocardial infarction, stroke, chloasma, erythema multiforme, erythema nodosum, vascular purpura, haemorrhagic eruption and probable dementia (see section 4.4) have been reported in women using HRT.

4.9 Overdose

Overdosage may be manifested by nausea and vomiting. If overdosage is discovered within two or three hours and is so large that treatment seems desirable, gastric lavage can be considered. There are no specific antidotes for overdosage, and further treatment should be symptomatic.

5. PHARMACOLOGICAL PROPERTIES

Pharmacotherapeutic group: Natural and semisynthetic estrogens, plain

ATC Code: G03CA03

5.1 Pharmacodynamic properties

The active ingredient, synthetic 17β-estradiol, is chemically and biologically identical to endogenous human estradiol. It substitutes for the loss of estrogen production in menopausal women, and alleviates menopausal symptoms.

Estrogens prevent bone loss following menopause or ovariectomy. Estrogen deficiency at menopause is associated with an increasing bone turnover and decline in bone mass. The effect of estrogens on the bone mineral density is dose-dependent. Protection appears to be effective for as long as treatment is continued. After discontinuation of HRT, bone mass is lost at a rate similar to that in untreated women.

Evidence from the WHI trial and meta-analysed trials shows that current use of HRT, alone or in combination with a progestogen – given to predominantly healthy women – reduces the risk of hip, vertebral, and other osteoporotic fractures. HRT may also prevent fractures in women with low bone density and/or established osteoporosis, but the evidence for that is limited.

5.2 Pharmacokinetic properties

Pharmacokinetic parameters for Elleste Solo 2 mg, are provided in the following table. The data were obtained from an open label, single dose, two way crossover pharmacokinetic study (n=16). Pharmacokinetic data were collected over 48 hours.

	Plasma Unconjugated Estradiol **(mean)**	**Plasma Unconjugated Estrone (mean)**
AUC_{0-48h}	950 pg.h/ml	2700 pg.h/ml
C_{max}	45 pg/ml	140 pg/ml
T_{max}	5.0 h	4.0 h

Estradiol

Readily and fully absorbed from the GI tract when given orally, peak levels are generally observed 3-6 hours after ingestion, but by 24 hours concentrations have returned to baseline.

Estradiol is converted to estrone and estriol primarily in the liver. These are excreted into the bile and undergo enterohepatic recirculation and further degradation before being excreted in the urine (90-95%) as biologically inactive glucuronide and sulphate conjugates or in the faeces (5-10%), mostly unconjugated.

5.3 Preclinical safety data

Estradiol has been shown to induce adverse effects in preclinical reproductive toxicity studies. Chiefly estradiol showed embryotoxic effects and induced anomalies in urogenital tract development e.g. feminisation of male foetuses in high doses.

6. PHARMACEUTICAL PARTICULARS

6.1 List of excipients

Tablet core:

Lactose monohydrate, maize starch, povidone 25, talc (purified), magnesium stearate.

Film-coating material:

Hydroxypropylmethyl cellulose (E464), titanium dioxide (E171), macrogol 400, sunset yellow (E110).

6.2 Incompatibilities

Not applicable

6.3 Shelf life

3 years

6.4 Special precautions for storage

Do not store above 25°C. Store in the original package.

6.5 Nature and contents of container

Aluminium foil and UPVC blister packed in a cardboard carton.

Pack sizes: 20*, 28, 60*, 84 or 100* tablets.

Packs marked with a * are not marketed in the UK.

6.6 Instructions for use and handling

There are no special instructions for handling.

7. MARKETING AUTHORISATION HOLDER

Shire Pharmaceutical Contracts Limited

Hampshire International Business Park

Chineham

Basingstoke

RG24 8EP

United Kingdom

8. MARKETING AUTHORISATION NUMBER(S)

PL 08081/0017

9. DATE OF FIRST AUTHORISATION/RENEWAL OF THE AUTHORISATION

30 September 1994

10. DATE OF REVISION OF THE TEXT

March 2004

Table 1

Organ group	*Common >1/100)*	*Uncommon >1/1,000, <1/100)*	*Rare >1/10,000, <1/1,000)*
Gastrointestinal	Nausea, abdominal pain	Dyspepsia, vomiting, flatulence, gallbladder disease, gallstones	
Skin			Alopecia, hirsutism, rash, itching
CNS	Headache	Dizziness, migraine	
Urogenital	Uterine bleeding, increase in size of uterine fibroids	Vaginal candidiasis	
Cardiovascular		Increase in blood pressure	Venous thromboembolism* Thrombophlebitis
Miscellaneous	Weight increase/decrease, oedema, breast tenderness, breast enlargement, change in mood including anxiety and depressive mood, change in libido	Leg cramps	

* see sections 4.3 Contraindications and 4.4 Special warnings and precautions for use

Elleste Solo MX40 mcg Transdermal Patch

(Pharmacia Limited)

1. NAME OF THE MEDICINAL PRODUCT

Elleste Solo MX 40 micrograms Transdermal Patch.

2. QUALITATIVE AND QUANTITATIVE COMPOSITION

Elleste Solo MX 40 contains 1.25 mg of estradiol (as hemihydrate) and each patch delivers approximately 40 micrograms of estradiol per 24 hours.

For excipients, see 6.1.

3. PHARMACEUTICAL FORM

Transdermal patch.

Elleste Solo MX 40 is a self-adhesive, flexible transdermal patch comprising a layer of clear adhesive sandwiched between a translucent patch and a metallised polyester backing. Elleste Solo MX 40 is a rectangular shape with rounded corners and has an active surface area of 14.25 cm^2.

4. CLINICAL PARTICULARS

4.1 Therapeutic indications

Hormone replacement therapy (HRT) for estrogen deficiency symptoms in peri-menopausal and post-menopausal women.

4.2 Posology and method of administration

Elleste Solo MX 40 Transdermal Patch is an estrogen-only product for transdermal use.

Adults

Climacteric Symptoms:

For initiation and continuation of treatment of peri- and postmenopausal symptoms, the lowest effective dose for the shortest duration (see also Section 4.4) should be used. Therapy should be initiated with Elleste Solo MX 40 in women who have menopausal symptoms. The dosage may be increased if required by using Elleste Solo MX 80.

Dosage Schedule:

Therapy may start at any time in women with established amenorrhoea or who are experiencing long intervals between spontaneous menses. In women who are menstruating, it is advised that therapy starts within five days of the start of bleeding. Patients changing from a cyclical or continuous sequential preparation should complete the cycle, and after a withdrawal bleed, may then change to Elleste Solo MX 40. Patients changing from a continuous combined preparation may start therapy at any time if amenorrhoea is established, or otherwise start within five days of the start of bleeding.

One Elleste Solo MX 40 transdermal patch should be applied twice weekly on a continuous basis. Each patch should be removed after 3 to 4 days and replaced with a new patch applied to a slightly different site. Patches should be applied to clean, dry and intact areas of skin below the waist on the lower back or buttocks. Elleste Solo MX 40 should not be applied on or near the breasts.

Elleste Solo MX 40 should be given continuously and, in women with an intact uterus, a progestogen is recommended and should be added for at least 12-14 days each cycle. The benefits of the lower risk of endometrial hyperplasia and endometrial cancer, due to adding progestogen, should be weighed against the increased risk of Breast cancer, (See Sections 4.4 and 4.8). Unless there is a previous diagnosis of endometriosis, it is not recommended to add a progestogen in hysterectomised women.

If the patch is not replaced at the normal time, it should be changed as soon as practical.

There is an increased likelihood of break-through bleeding and spotting when a patch is not replaced at the normal time.

Children

Elleste Solo MX 40 is not indicated in children.

4.3 Contraindications

Known, past or suspected breast cancer;

Known or suspected estrogen-dependent malignant tumours, (e.g. endometrial cancer);

Undiagnosed genital bleeding;

Untreated endometrial hyperplasia;

Previous idiopathic or current venous thromboembolism (deep vein thrombosis, pulmonary embolism);

Active or recent arterial thromboembolic disease (e.g. angina, myocardial infarction);

Acute liver disease, or a history of liver disease as long as liver function tests have failed to return to normal;

Known hypersensitivity to the active substances or to any of the excipients;

Porphyria.

4.4 Special warnings and special precautions for use

For the treatment of postmenopausal symptoms, HRT should only be initiated for symptoms that adversely affect quality of life. In all cases, a careful appraisal of the risks and benefits should be undertaken at least annually and HRT should only be continued as long as the benefit outweighs the risk.

Assessment of each woman prior to taking hormone replacement therapy (and at regular intervals thereafter) should include a personal and family medical history. Physical examination should be guided by this and by the contraindications (see Section 4.3) and warnings (see Section 4.4) for this product. During assessment of each individual woman, clinical examination of the breasts and pelvic examination should be performed where clinically indicated rather than as a routine procedure. Women should be encouraged to participate in the national breast screening programme (mammography) and the national cervical screening programme (cervical cytology) as appropriate for their age. Breast awareness should also be encouraged and women advised to report any changes in their breasts to their doctor or nurse, (see "Breast Cancer" below).

Conditions which need supervision:

If any of the following conditions are present, have occurred previously, and/or have been aggravated during pregnancy or previous hormone treatment, the patient should be closely supervised. It should be taken into account that these conditions may recur or be aggravated during treatment with Elleste Solo MX 40, in particular:

- Risk factors for estrogen dependent tumours, e.g. 1st degree heredity for breast cancer (see below);
- Diabetes mellitus with or without vascular involvement;
- Migraine or (severe) headache;
- Epilepsy;
- A history of, or risk of factors for, thromboembolic disorders (see below);
- Systemic lupus erythematosus, SLE;
- Liver disorders (e.g. liver adenoma);
- Leiomyoma (uterine fibroids) or endometriosis;
- Otosclerosis;
- Cholelithiasis;
- A history of endometrial hyperplasia (see below);
- Hypertension;
- Asthma.

Reasons for immediate withdrawal of therapy:

Therapy should be discontinued in case a contra-indication is discovered and in the following situations:

- Jaundice or deterioration in liver function
- ***Significant increase in blood pressure***
- New onset of migraine-type headache
- Pregnancy

Endometrial Hyperplasia

The risk of endometrial hyperplasia and carcinoma is increased when estrogens are administered alone for prolonged periods, (see Section 4.8). The addition of a progestogen for at least 12 days per cycle in non-hysterectomised women greatly reduces this risk (See Section 4.8).

The endometrial safety of added progestogen has not been studied for Elleste Solo MX 40.

The reduction in risk to the endometrium should be weighed against the increase in the risk of breast cancer of added progestogen (See 'Breast cancer' below, and in Section 4.8).

Breakthrough bleeding and spotting may occur during the first months of treatment. If breakthrough bleeding or spotting appears after some time on therapy or continues after treatment has been discontinued, the reason should be investigated which may include endometrial biopsy to exclude endometrial malignancy.

Unopposed estrogen stimulation may lead to premalignant transformation in the residual foci of endometriosis. Therefore, the addition of progestogens to estrogen replacement therapy should be considered in women who have undergone hysterectomy because of endometriosis, if they are known to have residual endometriosis, (but see above).

Breast Cancer

A randomised placebo-controlled trial, the Women's Health Initiative study (WHI), and epidemiological studies, including the Million Women Study (MWS), have reported an increased risk of breast cancer in women taking estrogens, estrogen-progestogen combinations or tibolone for HRT for several years (see Section 4.8). For all HRT, an excess risk becomes apparent within a few years of use and increases with duration of intake but returns to baseline within a few (at most five) years after stopping treatment.

In the MWS, the relative risk of breast cancer with conjugated equine estrogens (CEE) or estradiol (E2) was greater when a progestogen was added, either sequentially or continuously, and regardless of type of progestogen. There was no evidence of a difference in risk between the different routes of administration.

In the WHI study, the continuous combined conjugated equine estrogen and medroxyprogesterone acetate (CEE + MPA) product used was associated with breast cancers that were slightly larger in size and more frequently had local lymph node metastases compared to placebo.

HRT, especially estrogen-progestogen combined treatment, increases the density of mammographic images which may adversely affect the radiological detection of breast cancer.

Venous Thromboembolism

HRT is associated with a higher relative risk of developing venous thromboembolism (VTE), i.e. deep vein thrombosis or pulmonary embolism. One randomised controlled trial and epidemiological studies found a two to threefold higher risk for users compared with non-users. For non-users, it is estimated that the number of cases of VTE that will occur over a 5 year period is about 3 per 1000 women aged 50-59 years and 8 per 1000 women aged between 60-69 years. It is estimated that in healthy women who use HRT for 5 years, the number of additional cases of VTE over a 5 year period will be between 2 and 6 (best estimate = 4) per 1000 women aged 50-59 years and between 5 and 15 (best estimate = 9) per 1000 women aged 60-69 years. The occurrence of such an event is more likely in the first year of HRT than later.

Generally recognised risk factors for VTE include a personal history or family history, severe obesity (BM > 30 kg/m^2) and systemic lupus erythematosus (SLE). There is no consensus about the possible role of varicose veins in VTE.

Patients with a history of VTE or known thrombophilic states have an increased risk of VTE. HRT may add to this risk. Personal or strong family history of thromboembolism or recurrent spontaneous abortion should be investigated in order to exclude a thrombophilic predisposition. Until a thorough evaluation of thrombophilic factors has been made or anticoagulant treatment initiated, use of HRT in such patients should be viewed as contraindicated. Those women already on anticoagulant treatment require careful consideration of the benefit-risk of use of HRT.

The risk of VTE may be temporarily increased with prolonged immobilisation, major trauma or major surgery. As in all postoperative patients, scrupulous attention should be given to prophylactic measures to prevent VTE following surgery. Where prolonged immobilisation is liable to follow elective surgery, particularly abdominal or orthopaedic surgery to the lower limbs, consideration should be given to temporarily stopping HRT 4 to 6 weeks earlier, if possible. Treatment should not be restarted until the woman is completely mobilised.

If VTE develops after initiating therapy, the drug should be discontinued. Patients should be told to contact their doctor immediately when they are aware of a potential thromboembolic symptom (e.g. painful swelling of a leg, sudden pain in the chest, dyspnea).

Coronary Artery Disease

There is no evidence from randomised controlled trials of cardiovascular benefit with continuous combined conjugated estrogens and medroxyprogesterone acetate, (MPA). Two large clinical trials (WHI and HERS, i.e. Heart and Estrogen/progestin Replacement Study) showed a possible increased risk of cardiovascular morbidity in the first year of use and no overall benefit. For other HRT products there are only limited data from randomised controlled trials examining effects in cardiovascular morbidity or mortality. Therefore, it is uncertain whether these findings also extend to other HRT products.

Stroke

One large randomised clinical trial (WHI-trial) found, as a secondary outcome, an increased risk of ischaemic stroke in healthy women during treatment with continuous combined conjugated estrogens and medroxyprogesterone acetate. For women who do not use HRT, it is estimated that the number of cases of stroke that will occur over a 5 year period is about 3 per 1000 women aged 50-59 years and 11 per 1000 women aged 60-69 years. It is estimated that for women who use conjugated estrogens and medroxyprogesterone acetate for 5 years, the number of additional cases will be between 0 and 3 (best estimate = 1) per 1000 users aged 50-59 years and between 1 and 9 (best estimate = 4) per 1000 users aged 60-69 years. It is unknown whether the increased risk also extends to other HRT products.

Ovarian Cancer

Long-term (at least 5 to 10 years) use of estrogen-only HRT products in hysterectomised women has been associated with an increased risk of ovarian cancer in some epidemiological studies. It is uncertain whether long-term use of combined HRT confers a different risk than estrogen-only products.

Other Conditions

Estrogens may cause fluid retention and therefore patients with cardiac or renal dysfunction should be carefully observed. Patients with terminal renal insufficiency should be closely observed, since it is expected that the level of circulating active ingredients in Elleste Solo MX 40 is increased.

Women with pre-existing hypertriglyceridaemia should be followed closely during estrogen replacement or hormone replacement therapy, since rare cases of large increases of plasma triglycerides leading to pancreatitis have been reported with estrogen therapy in this condition.

Estrogens increase thyroid binding globulin (TBG), leading to increased circulating total thyroid hormone, as measured by protein-bound iodine (PBI), T4 levels (by column or by radio-immunoassay) or T3 levels (by radio-immunoassay). T3 resin uptake is decreased, reflecting the elevated TBG. Free T4 and free T3 concentrations are unaltered. Other binding proteins may be elevated in serum, i.e. corticoid binding globulin (CBG), sex-hormone-binding globulin (SHBG) leading to increased circulating corticosteroids and sex steroids, respectively. Free or biologically active hormone concentrations are unchanged. Other plasma proteins may be increased (angiotensinogen/renin substrate, alpha-1-antitrypsin, ceruloplasmin).

There is no conclusive evidence for improvement of cognitive function. There is some evidence from the WHI trial of increased risk of probable dementia in women who start using continuous combined CEE and MPA after the age of 65. It is unknown whether the findings apply to younger post-menopausal women or other HRT products.

In rare cases benign, and in even rarer cases malignant liver tumours leading in isolated cases to life-threatening intra-abdominal haemorrhage have been observed after the use of hormonal substances such as those contained in Elleste Solo MX 40. If severe upper abdominal complaints, enlarged liver or signs of intra-abdominal haemorrhage occur, a liver tumour should be considered in the differential diagnosis.

Women who may be at risk of pregnancy should be advised to adhere to non-hormonal contraceptive methods.

The requirement for oral anti-diabetics or insulin can change as a result of the effect on glucose tolerance.

4.5 Interaction with other medicinal products and other forms of Interaction

The metabolism of estrogens may be increased by concomitant use of substances known to induce drug-metabolising enzymes, specifically cytochrome P450 enzymes, such as anticonvulsants, (e.g. phenobarbitol, phenytoin and carbamezapine) and anti-infectives, (e.g. rifampicin, rifabutin, nevirapine or efavirenz).

Ritonavir and nelfinavir, although known strong inhibitors, by contrast exhibit inducing properties when used concomitantly with steroid hormones. Herbal preparations containing St John's wort (Hypericum Perforatum) may induce the metabolism of estrogens.

At transdermal administration, the first-pass effect in the liver is avoided and, thus, transdermally applied estrogens might be less affected than oral hormones by enzyme inducers.

Clinically, an increased metabolism of estrogens may lead to decreased effect and changes in the uterine bleeding profile.

Some laboratory tests can be influenced by estrogens such as tests for thyroid function or glucose tolerance, (see Section 4.4).

4.6 Pregnancy and lactation

Pregnancy

Elleste Solo MX 40 is not indicated during pregnancy. If pregnancy occurs during medication with Elleste Solo MX 40, treatment should be withdrawn immediately. The results of most epidemiological studies to date relevant to inadvertent foetal exposure to estrogens indicate no teratogenic or foetotoxic effects

Lactation

Elleste Solo MX 40 is not indicated during lactation.

4.7 Effects on ability to drive and use machines

None.

4.8 Undesirable effects

Elleste Solo MX 40 is generally well tolerated. The most frequent side effects, (reported in 10 to 20 % of patients, on at least one occasion, in clinical trials with Elleste Solo MX 40) which do not normally prevent continued treatment include: breast tenderness, headaches and breakthrough bleeding. Some patients experience mild and transient local erythema at the site of application with or without itching; this usually disappears rapidly on removal of the patch. The overall incidence of general patch irritation in clinical studies is less than 5 %. In a clinical study 3 % of 102 patients showed well defined erythema (Draize scale) 30 minutes after patch removal. No instances of permanent skin damage have been reported. If unacceptable topical side effects do occur discontinuation of treatment should be considered.

The following adverse reactions have been reported with Elleste Solo MX 40 and/or estrogen therapy:

1. *Genito-urinary tract:* Endometrial neoplasia*, dysmenorrhoea, intermenstrual bleeding, increase in the size of uterine fibromyomata, endometrial proliferation or aggravation of endometriosis, vaginal haemorrhagic eruptions, changes in cervical eversion and excessive production of cervical mucus, cervical erosion, cystitis-like syndrome, candidal infections, thrush;

2. *Breast:* Tenderness, pain, enlargement or secretion, breast cancer*;

3. *Gastro-intestinal tract*: Nausea, vomiting, abdominal cramp, bloating;

4. *Cardiovascular system*: Hypertension, thrombosis, thrombophlebitis, venous thromboembolism*, myocardial infarction* and stroke*;

5. *Liver/biliary system:* In rare cases benign, and in even rarer cases malignant liver tumours, cholelithiasis, cholestatic jaundice, gall bladder disease;

6. *Skin:* Chloasma which may persist when the drug is discontinued, erythema multiforme, erythema nodosum, muscle cramps, vascular purpura, rash, loss of scalp hair, hirsutism;

7. *Eyes*: Steepening of corneal curvature, visual disturbances, intolerance to contact lenses;

8. *CNS*: Headache, migraine, dizziness, mood changes (elation or depression), chorea, probable dementia (see Section 4.4);

9. *Miscellaneous:* Sodium and water retention, reduced glucose tolerance, leg cramps, oedema, change in body weight, aggravation of porphyria, changes in libido.

* See sections 4.3, Contraindications and Section 4.4 Special Warnings and Special Precautions for Use.

Breast Cancer

According to evidence from a large number of epidemiological studies and one randomised placebo-controlled trial, the Women's Health Initiative (WHI), the overall risk of breast cancer increases with increasing duration of HRT use in current or recent HRT users.

For *estrogen-only* HRT, estimates of relative risk (RR) from a reanalysis of original data from 51 epidemiological studies (in which >80% of HRT use was estrogen-only HRT) and from the epidemiological Million Women Study (MWS) are similar at 1.35 (95% CI 1.21 – 1.49) and 1.30 (95% CI 1.21 – 1.40), respectively.

For *estrogen plus progestogen* combined HRT, several epidemiological studies have reported an overall higher risk for breast cancer than with estrogens alone.

The MWS reported that, compared to never users, the use of various types of estrogen-progestogen combined HRT was associated with a higher risk of breast cancer (RR = 2.00, 95% CI: 1.88 – 2.12) than use of estrogens alone (RR = 1.30, 95% CI: 1.21 – 1.40) or use of tibolone (RR=1.45; 95%CI 1.25-1.68).

The WHI trial reported a risk estimate of 1.24 (95% CI 1.01 – 1.54) after 5.6 years of use of estrogen-progestogen combined HRT (CEE + MPA) in all users compared with placebo.

The absolute risks calculated from the MWS and the WHI trial are presented below:

The MWS has estimated, from the known average incidence of breast cancer in developed countries, that:

Ø *For women not using HRT, about 32 in every 1000 are expected to have breast cancer diagnosed between the ages of 50 and 64 years.*

Ø For 1000 current or recent users of HRT, the number of *additional* cases during the corresponding period will be

Ø For users of *estrogen-only* replacement therapy

- between 0 and 3 (best estimate = 1.5) for 5 years' use
- between 3 and 7 (best estimate = 5) for 10 years' use.

Ø For users of *estrogen plus progestogen* combined HRT,

- between 5 and 7 (best estimate = 6) for 5 years' use
- between 18 and 20 (best estimate = 19) for 10 years' use.

The WHI trial estimated that after 5.6 years of follow-up of women between the ages of 50 and 79 years, an *additional* 8 cases of invasive breast cancer would be due to *estrogen-progestogen combined* HRT (CEE + MPA) per 10,000 women years.

According to calculations from the trial data, it is estimated that:

Ø For 1000 women in the placebo group, about 16 cases of invasive breast cancer would be diagnosed in 5 years.

Ø For 1000 women who used estrogen + progestogen combined HRT (CEE + MPA), the number of *additional* cases would be between 0 and 9 (best estimate = 4) for 5 years' use.

The number of additional cases of breast cancer in women who use HRT is broadly similar for women who start HRT irrespective of age at start of use (between the ages of 45-65) (see Section 4.4).

Endometrial cancer

In women with an intact uterus, the risk of endometrial hyperplasia and endometrial cancer increases with increasing duration of use of unopposed estrogens. According to data from epidemiological studies, the best estimate of the risk is that for women not using HRT, about 5 in every 1000 are expected to have endometrial cancer diagnosed between the ages of 50 and 65. Depending on the duration of treatment and estrogen dose, the reported increase in endometrial cancer risk among unopposed estrogen users varies from 2-to 12-fold greater compared with non-users. Adding a progestogen to estrogen-only therapy greatly reduces this increased risk.

4.9 Overdose

This is not likely due to the mode of administration. If it is necessary to stop delivery then the patch can be removed and plasma estradiol levels will fall rapidly.

5. PHARMACOLOGICAL PROPERTIES

5.1 Pharmacodynamic properties

Pharmacotherapeutic group:

Natural and semisynthetic estrogens, plain.

ATC Code G03C A

The active ingredient, synthetic 17β-estradiol, is chemically and biologically identical to endogenous human estradiol. It substitutes for the loss of estrogen production in menopausal women, and alleviates menopausal symptoms.

5.2 Pharmacokinetic properties

Estradiol is absorbed from the patch across the stratum corneum and is delivered systemically at a low but constant rate throughout the period of application (3 to 4 days). The estimated delivery of estradiol is approximately 40 μg/day for Elleste Solo MX 40.

Steady state plasma estradiol concentrations have been demonstrated in the range of 26 pg/ml to 34 pg/ml for the Elleste Solo MX 40 patch (including baseline levels) and these are maintained throughout the dose interval (for up to four days). Absorption rate may vary between individual patients. After removal of the last patch plasma estradiol and estrone concentrations return to baseline values in less than 24 hours.

Estradiol is mainly metabolized in the liver. Its main metabolites are estriol, estrone, and their conjugates. The plasma half life of estradiol is 1-2 hours. Metabolic plasma clearance varies between 450-625 ml/min/m^2. The metabolites are mainly excreted via the kidneys as glucuronides and sulphates. Estrogens also undergo enterohepatic circulation.

5.3 Preclinical safety data

No additional information is available.

6. PHARMACEUTICAL PARTICULARS

6.1 List of excipients

Diethyltoluamide

Acrylic adhesive (Dow Corning MG-0560)

Acrylic emulsion (Acrysol 33)

Backing: Polyester film (Scotchpak 9733)

Release liner: Siliconised aluminised polyester

6.2 Incompatibilities

Not applicable.

6.3 Shelf life

3 years.

6.4 Special precautions for storage

Do not store above 25 °C. Store in the original package.

6.5 Nature and contents of container

PVC/PVDC blister tray with paper/polythene/aluminium foil lid containing one transdermal patch. Each carton contains eight patches, sufficient for one 28 day cycle and a patient leaflet. An additional pack containing two patches may also be available.

6.6 Instructions for use and handling

Detailed instructions for use are provided in the patient leaflet.

7. MARKETING AUTHORISATION HOLDER

Pharmacia Limited
Davy Avenue
Milton Keynes
MK5 8PH
UK

8. MARKETING AUTHORISATION NUMBER(S)

PL 00032/0303

9. DATE OF FIRST AUTHORISATION/RENEWAL OF THE AUTHORISATION

26 February 2002

10. DATE OF REVISION OF THE TEXT

March 2005

Ref ELA 2_0

(Previously ELB 1_3)

Elleste Solo MX80 mcg Transdermal Patch

(Pharmacia Limited)

1. NAME OF THE MEDICINAL PRODUCT

Elleste Solo MX 80 micrograms Transdermal Patch.

2. QUALITATIVE AND QUANTITATIVE COMPOSITION

Elleste Solo MX 80 contains 2.50 mg of estradiol (as hemihydrate) and each patch delivers approximately 80 micrograms of estradiol per 24 hours.

For excipients, see 6.1.

3. PHARMACEUTICAL FORM

Transdermal patch.

Elleste Solo MX 80 is a self-adhesive, flexible transdermal patch comprising a layer of clear adhesive sandwiched between a translucent patch and a metallised polyester backing. Elleste Solo MX 80 is a rectangular shape with rounded corners and has an active surface area of 28.5 cm^2.

4. CLINICAL PARTICULARS

4.1 Therapeutic indications

Hormone replacement therapy (HRT) for estrogen deficiency symptoms in peri-menopausal and post-menopausal women.

Prevention of osteoporosis in postmenopausal women at high risk of future fractures who are intolerant of, or contra-indicated for, other medicinal products approved for the prevention of osteoporosis (see also Section 4.4).

4.2 Posology and method of administration

Elleste Solo MX 80 Transdermal Patch is an estrogen-only product for transdermal use.

Adults

Climacteric Symptoms:

For initiation and continuation of treatment of peri- and postmenopausal symptoms, the lowest effective dose for the shortest duration (see also Section 4.4) should be used. Therapy should be initiated with Elleste Solo MX 40 in women who have menopausal symptoms. The dosage may be increased if required by using Elleste Solo MX 80.

Prevention of Osteoporosis

Treatment should be with Elleste Solo MX 80.

Dosage Schedule (for both indications)

Therapy may start at any time in women with established amenorrhoea or who are experiencing long intervals between spontaneous menses. In women who are menstruating, it is advised that therapy starts within five days of the start of bleeding. Patients changing from a cyclical or continuous sequential preparation should complete the cycle, and after a withdrawal bleed, may then change to Elleste Solo MX 80. Patients changing from a continuous combined preparation may start therapy at any time if amenorrhoea is established, or otherwise start within five days of the start of bleeding.

One Elleste Solo MX 80 transdermal patch should be applied twice weekly on a continuous basis. Each patch should be removed after 3 to 4 days and replaced with a new patch applied to a slightly different site. Patches should be applied to clean, dry and intact areas of skin below the waist on the lower back or buttocks. Elleste Solo MX 80 should not be applied on or near the breasts.

Elleste Solo MX 80 should be given continuously and, in women with an intact uterus, a progestogen is recommended and should be added for at least 12-14 days each cycle. The benefits of the lower risk of endometrial hyperplasia and endometrial cancer, due to adding progestogen, should be weighed against the increased risk of Breast cancer, (See Sections 4.4 and 4.8). Unless there is a previous diagnosis of endometriosis, it is not recommended to add a progestogen in hysterectomised women.

If the patch is not replaced at the normal time, it should be changed as soon as practical.

There is an increased likelihood of break-through bleeding and spotting when a patch is not replaced at the normal time.

Children

Elleste Solo MX 80 is not indicated in children.

4.3 Contraindications

Known, past or suspected breast cancer;

Known or suspected estrogen-dependent malignant tumours, (e.g. endometrial cancer);

Undiagnosed genital bleeding;

Untreated endometrial hyperplasia;

Previous idiopathic or current venous thromboembolism (deep vein thrombosis, pulmonary embolism);

Active or recent arterial thromboembolic disease (e.g. angina, myocardial infarction);

Acute liver disease, or a history of liver disease as long as liver function tests have failed to return to normal;

Known hypersensitivity to the active substances or to any of the excipients;

Porphyria.

4.4 Special warnings and special precautions for use

For the treatment of postmenopausal symptoms, HRT should only be initiated for symptoms that adversely affect quality of life. In all cases, a careful appraisal of the risks and benefits should be undertaken at least annually and HRT should only be continued as long as the benefit outweighs the risk.

Assessment of each woman prior to taking hormone replacement therapy (and at regular intervals thereafter) should include a personal and family medical history. Physical examination should be guided by this and by the contraindications (see Section 4.3) and warnings (see Section 4.4) for this product. During assessment of each individual woman, clinical examination of the breasts and pelvic examination should be performed where clinically indicated rather than as a routine procedure. Women should be encouraged to participate in the national breast screening programme (mammography) and the national cervical screening programme (cervical cytology) as appropriate for their age. Breast awareness should also be encouraged and women advised to report any changes in their breasts to their doctor or nurse, (see "Breast Cancer" below).

Conditions which need supervision:

If any of the following conditions are present, have occurred previously, and/or have been aggravated during pregnancy or previous hormone treatment, the patient should be closely supervised. It should be taken into account that these conditions may recur or be aggravated during treatment with Elleste Solo MX 80, in particular:

- Risk factors for estrogen dependent tumours, e.g. 1st degree heredity for breast cancer (see below);
- Diabetes mellitus with or without vascular involvement;
- Migraine or (severe) headache;
- Epilepsy;
- A history of, or risk of factors for, thromboembolic disorders (see below);
- Systemic lupus erythematosus, SLE;
- Liver disorders (e.g. liver adenoma);
- Leiomyoma (uterine fibroids) or endometriosis;
- Otosclerosis;
- Cholelithiasis;
- A history of endometrial hyperplasia (see below);
- Hypertension;
- Asthma.

Reasons for immediate withdrawal of therapy:

Therapy should be discontinued in case a contra-indication is discovered and in the following situations:

- Jaundice or deterioration in liver function
- ***Significant increase in blood pressure***
- New onset of migraine-type headache
- Pregnancy

Endometrial Hyperplasia

The risk of endometrial hyperplasia and carcinoma is increased when estrogens are administered alone for prolonged periods, (see Section 4.8). The addition of a progestogen for at least 12 days per cycle in non-hysterectomised women greatly reduces this risk (See Section 4.8).

The endometrial safety of added progestogen has not been studied for Elleste Solo MX 80.

The reduction in risk to the endometrium should be weighed against the increase in the risk of breast cancer of added progestogen (See 'Breast cancer' below, and in Section 4.8)

Breakthrough bleeding and spotting may occur during the first months of treatment. If breakthrough bleeding or spotting appears after some time on therapy or continues after treatment has been discontinued, the reason should be investigated which may include endometrial biopsy to exclude endometrial malignancy.

Unopposed estrogen stimulation may lead to premalignant transformation in the residual foci of endometriosis. Therefore, the addition of progestogens to estrogen replacement therapy should be considered in women who have undergone hysterectomy because of endometriosis, if they are known to have residual endometriosis (but see above).

Breast Cancer

A randomised placebo-controlled trial, the Women's Health Initiative study (WHI), and epidemiological studies, including the Million Women Study (MWS), have reported an increased risk of breast cancer in women taking estrogens, estrogen-progestogen combinations or tibolone for HRT for several years (see Section 4.8). For all HRT, an excess risk becomes apparent within a few years of use and increases with duration of intake but returns to baseline within a few (at most five) years after stopping treatment.

In the MWS, the relative risk of breast cancer with conjugated equine estrogens (CEE) or estradiol (E2) was greater when a progestogen was added, either sequentially or continuously, and regardless of type of progestogen. There was no evidence of a difference in risk between the different routes of administration.

In the WHI study, the continuous combined conjugated equine estrogen and medroxyprogesterone acetate (CEE + MPA) product used was associated with breast cancers that were slightly larger in size and more frequently had local lymph node metastases compared to placebo.

HRT, especially estrogen-progestogen combined treatment, increases the density of mammographic images which may adversely affect the radiological detection of breast cancer.

Venous Thromboembolism

HRT is associated with a higher relative risk of developing venous thromboembolism (VTE), i.e. deep vein thrombosis or pulmonary embolism. One randomised controlled trial and epidemiological studies found a two to threefold higher risk for users compared with non-users. For non-users, it is estimated that the number of cases of VTE that will occur over a 5 year period is about 3 per 1000 women aged 50-59 years and 8 per 1000 women aged between 60-69 years. It is estimated that in healthy women who use HRT for 5 years, the number of additional cases of VTE over a 5 year period will be between 2 and 6 (best estimate = 4) per 1000 women aged 50-59 years and between 5 and 15 (best estimate = 9) per 1000 women aged 60-69 years. The occurrence of such an event is more likely in the first year of HRT than later.

Generally recognised risk factors for VTE include a personal history or family history, severe obesity (BM > 30 kg/m^2) and systemic lupus erythematosus (SLE). There is no consensus about the possible role of varicose veins in VTE.

Patients with a history of VTE or known thrombophilic states have an increased risk of VTE. HRT may add to this risk. Personal or strong family history of thromboembolism or recurrent spontaneous abortion should be investigated in order to exclude a thrombophilic predisposition. Until a thorough evaluation of thrombophilic factors has been made or anticoagulant treatment initiated, use of HRT in such patients should be viewed as contraindicated. Those women already on anticoagulant treatment require careful consideration of the benefit-risk of use of HRT.

The risk of VTE may be temporarily increased with prolonged immobilisation, major trauma or major surgery. As in all postoperative patients, scrupulous attention should be given to prophylactic measures to prevent VTE following surgery. Where prolonged immobilisation is liable to follow elective surgery, particularly abdominal or orthopaedic surgery to the lower limbs, consideration should be given to temporarily stopping HRT 4 to 6 weeks earlier, if possible. Treatment should not be restarted until the woman is completely mobilised.

If VTE develops after initiating therapy, the drug should be discontinued. Patients should be told to contact their doctor immediately when they are aware of a potential thromboembolic symptom (e.g. painful swelling of a leg, sudden pain in the chest, dyspnea).

Coronary Artery Disease

There is no evidence from randomised controlled trials of cardiovascular benefit with continuous combined conjugated estrogens and medroxyprogesterone acetate, (MPA). Two large clinical trials (WHI and HERS, i.e. Heart and Estrogen/progestin Replacement Study) showed a possible increased risk of cardiovascular morbidity in the first year of use and no overall benefit. For other HRT products there are only limited data from randomised controlled trials examining effects in cardiovascular morbidity or mortality. Therefore, it is uncertain whether these findings also extend to other HRT products.

Stroke

One large randomised clinical trial (WHI-trial) found, as a secondary outcome, an increased risk of ischaemic stroke in healthy women during treatment with continuous combined conjugated estrogens and medroxyprogesterone acetate. For women who do not use HRT, it is estimated that the number of cases of stroke that will occur over a 5 year period is about 3 per 1000 women aged 50-59 years and 11 per 1000 women aged 60-69 years. It is estimated that for women who use conjugated estrogens and medroxyprogesterone acetate for 5 years, the number of additional cases will be between 0 and 3 (best estimate = 1) per 1000 users aged 50-59 years and between 1 and 9 (best estimate = 4) per 1000 users aged 60-69 years. It is unknown whether the increased risk also extends to other HRT products.

Ovarian Cancer

Long-term (at least 5 to 10 years) use of estrogen-only HRT products in hysterectomised women has been associated with an increased risk of ovarian cancer in some epidemiological studies. It is uncertain whether long-term use of combined HRT confers a different risk than estrogen-only products.

Other Conditions

Estrogens may cause fluid retention and therefore patients with cardiac or renal dysfunction should be carefully observed. Patients with terminal renal insufficiency should be closely observed, since it is expected that the level of circulating active ingredients in Elleste Solo MX 80 is increased.

Women with pre-existing hypertriglyceridaemia should be followed closely during estrogen replacement or hormone replacement therapy, since rare cases of large increases of plasma triglycerides leading to pancreatitis have been reported with estrogen therapy in this condition.

Estrogens increase thyroid binding globulin (TBG), leading to increased circulating total thyroid hormone, as measured by protein-bound iodine (PBI), T4 levels (by column or by radio-immunoassay) or T3 levels (by radio-immunoassay). T3 resin uptake is decreased, reflecting the elevated TBG. Free T4 and free T3 concentrations are unaltered. Other binding proteins may be elevated in serum, i.e. corticoid binding globulin (CBG), sex-hormone-binding globulin (SHBG) leading to increased circulating corticosteroids and sex steroids, respectively. Free or biologically active hormone concentrations are unchanged. Other plasma proteins may be increased (angiotensinogen/renin substrate, alpha-1-antitrypsin, ceruloplasmin).

There is no conclusive evidence for improvement of cognitive function. There is some evidence from the WHI trial of increased risk of probable dementia in women who start using continuous combined CEE and MPA after the age of 65. It is unknown whether the findings apply to younger post-menopausal women or other HRT products.

In rare cases benign, and in even rarer cases malignant liver tumours leading in isolated cases to life-threatening intra-abdominal haemorrhage have been observed after the use of hormonal substances such as those contained in Elleste Solo MX 80. If severe upper abdominal complaints, enlarged liver or signs of intra-abdominal haemorrhage occur, a liver tumour should be considered in the differential diagnosis.

Women who may be at risk of pregnancy should be advised to adhere to non-hormonal contraceptive methods.

The requirement for oral anti-diabetics or insulin can change as a result of the effect on glucose tolerance.

4.5 Interaction with other medicinal products and other forms of Interaction

The metabolism of estrogens may be increased by concomitant use of substances known to induce drug-metabolising enzymes, specifically cytochrome P450 enzymes, such as anticonvulsants, (e.g. phenobarbitol, phenytoin and carbamezapine) and anti-infectives, (e.g. rifampicin, rifabutin, nevirapine or efavirenz).

Ritonavir and nelfinavir, although known strong inhibitors, by contrast exhibit inducing properties when used concomitantly with steroid hormones. Herbal preparations containing St John's wort (Hypericum Perforatum) may induce the metabolism of estrogens.

At transdermal administration, the first-pass effect in the liver is avoided and, thus, transdermally applied estrogens might be less affected than oral hormones by enzyme inducers.

Clinically, an increased metabolism of estrogens may lead to decreased effect and changes in the uterine bleeding profile.

Some laboratory tests can be influenced by estrogens such as tests for thyroid function or glucose tolerance, (see Section 4.4).

4.6 Pregnancy and lactation

Pregnancy

Elleste Solo MX 80 is not indicated during pregnancy. If pregnancy occurs during medication with Elleste Solo MX

80, treatment should be withdrawn immediately. The results of most epidemiological studies to date relevant to inadvertent foetal exposure to estrogens indicate no teratogenic or foetotoxic effects

Lactation

Elleste Solo MX 80 is not indicated during lactation.

4.7 Effects on ability to drive and use machines

None.

4.8 Undesirable effects

Elleste Solo MX 80 is generally well tolerated. The most frequent side effects, (reported in 10 to 20 % of patients, on at least one occasion, in clinical trials with Elleste Solo MX 80) which do not normally prevent continued treatment include: breast tenderness, headaches and breakthrough bleeding. Some patients experience mild and transient local erythema at the site of application with or without itching; this usually disappears rapidly on removal of the patch. The overall incidence of general patch irritation in clinical studies is less than 5 %. In a clinical study 3 % of 102 patients showed well defined erythema (Draize scale) 30 minutes after patch removal. No instances of permanent skin damage have been reported.

If unacceptable topical side effects do occur discontinuation of treatment should be considered.

The following adverse reactions have been reported with Elleste Solo MX 80 and/or estrogen therapy:

1. *Genito-urinary tract:* Endometrial neoplasia*, dysmenorrhoea, intermenstrual bleeding, increase in the size of uterine fibromyomata, endometrial proliferation or aggravation of endometriosis, vaginal haemorrhagic eruptions, changes in cervical eversion and excessive production of cervical mucus, cervical erosion, cystitis-like syndrome, candidal infections, thrush;

2. *Breast:* Tenderness, pain, enlargement or secretion, breast cancer*

3. *Gastro-intestinal tract*: Nausea, vomiting, abdominal cramp, bloating;

4. *Cardiovascular system*: Hypertension, thrombosis, thrombophlebitis, venous thromboembolism*, myocardial infarction* and stroke*;

5. *Liver/biliary system*: In rare cases benign, and in even rarer cases malignant liver tumours, cholelithiasis, cholestatic jaundice, gall bladder disease;

6. *Skin*: Chloasma which may persist when the drug is discontinued, erythema multiforme, erythema nodosum, muscle cramps, vascular purpura, rash, loss of scalp hair, hirsutism;

7. *Eyes*: Steepening of corneal curvature, visual disturbances, intolerance to contact lenses;

8. *CNS*: Headache, migraine, dizziness, mood changes (elation or depression), chorea, probable dementia (see Section 4.4);

9. Miscellaneous: Sodium and water retention, reduced glucose tolerance, leg cramps, oedema, change in body weight, aggravation of porphyria, changes in libido.

* See sections 4.3, Contraindications and Section 4.4 Special Warnings and Special Precautions for Use.

Breast Cancer

According to evidence from a large number of epidemiological studies and one randomised placebo-controlled trial, the Women's Health Initiative (WHI), the overall risk of breast cancer increases with increasing duration of HRT use in current or recent HRT users.

For *estrogen-only* HRT, estimates of relative risk (RR) from a reanalysis of original data from 51 epidemiological studies (in which >80% of HRT use was estrogen-only HRT) and from the epidemiological Million Women Study (MWS) are similar at 1.35 (95% CI 1.21 – 1.49) and 1.30 (95% CI 1.21 – 1.40), respectively.

For *estrogen plus progestogen* combined HRT, several epidemiological studies have reported an overall higher risk for breast cancer than with estrogens alone.

The MWS reported that, compared to never users, the use of various types of estrogen-progestogen combined HRT was associated with a higher risk of breast cancer (RR = 2.00, 95% CI: 1.88 – 2.12) than use of estrogens alone (RR = 1.30, 95% CI: 1.21 – 1.40) or use of tibolone (RR=1.45; 95%CI 1.25-1.68).

The WHI trial reported a risk estimate of 1.24 (95% CI 1.01 – 1.54) after 5.6 years of use of estrogen-progestogen combined HRT (CEE + MPA) in all users compared with placebo.

The absolute risks calculated from the MWS and the WHI trial are presented below:

The MWS has estimated, from the known average incidence of breast cancer in developed countries, that:

Ø *For women not using HRT, about 32 in every 1000 are expected to have breast cancer diagnosed between the ages of 50 and 64 years.*

Ø For 1000 current or recent users of HRT, the number of *additional* cases during the corresponding period will be

Ø For users of *estrogen-only* replacement therapy

- between 0 and 3 (best estimate = 1.5) for 5 years' use
- between 3 and 7 (best estimate = 5) for 10 years' use.

Ø For users of *estrogen plus progestogen* combined HRT,

- between 5 and 7 (best estimate = 6) for 5 years' use
- between 18 and 20 (best estimate = 19) for 10 years' use.

The WHI trial estimated that after 5.6 years of follow-up of women between the ages of 50 and 79 years, an *additional* 8 cases of invasive breast cancer would be due to *estrogen-progestogen combined* HRT (CEE + MPA) per 10,000 women years.

According to calculations from the trial data, it is estimated that:

Ø For 1000 women in the placebo group, about 16 cases of invasive breast cancer would be diagnosed in 5 years.

Ø For 1000 women who used estrogen + progestogen combined HRT (CEE + MPA), the number of *additional* cases would be between 0 and 9 (best estimate = 4) for 5 years' use.

The number of additional cases of breast cancer in women who use HRT is broadly similar for women who start HRT irrespective of age at start of use (between the ages of 45-65) (see Section 4.4).

Endometrial cancer

In women with an intact uterus, the risk of endometrial hyperplasia and endometrial cancer increases with increasing duration of use of unopposed estrogens. According to data from epidemiological studies, the best estimate of the risk is that for women not using HRT, about 5 in every 1000 are expected to have endometrial cancer diagnosed between the ages of 50 and 65. Depending on the duration of treatment and estrogen dose, the reported increase in endometrial cancer risk among unopposed estrogen users varies from 2-to 12-fold greater compared with non-users. Adding a progestogen to estrogen-only therapy greatly reduces this increased risk.

4.9 Overdose

This is not likely due to the mode of administration. If it is necessary to stop delivery then the patch can be removed and plasma estradiol levels will fall rapidly.

5. PHARMACOLOGICAL PROPERTIES

5.1 Pharmacodynamic properties

Pharmacotherapeutic group:

Natural and semisynthetic estrogens, plain.

ATC Code G03C A

The active ingredient, synthetic 17β-estradiol, is chemically and biologically identical to endogenous human estradiol. It substitutes for the loss of estrogen production in menopausal women, and alleviates menopausal symptoms. Estrogens prevent bone loss following menopause or ovariectomy.

Estrogen deficiency at menopause is associated with an increasing bone turnover and decline in bone mass. The effect of estrogens on the bone mineral density is dose-dependent. Protection appears to be effective for as long as treatment is continued.

After discontinuation of HRT, bone mass is lost at a rate similar to that in untreated women.

Evidence from the WHI trial and meta-analysed trials shows that current use of HRT, alone or in combination with a progestagen – given to predominantly healthy women – reduces the risk of hip, vertebral, and other osteoporotic fractures. HRT may also prevent fractures in women with low bone density and/or established osteoporosis, but the evidence for that is limited.

5.2 Pharmacokinetic properties

Estradiol is absorbed from the patch across the stratum corneum and is delivered systemically at a low but constant rate throughout the period of application (3 to 4 days). The estimated delivery of estradiol is approximately 80 μg/day for Elleste Solo MX 80.

Steady state plasma estradiol concentrations have been demonstrated in the range of 34 pg/ml to 62 pg/ml for the Elleste Solo MX 80 patch (including baseline levels) and these are maintained throughout the dose interval (for up to four days). Absorption rate may vary between individual patients. After removal of the last patch plasma estradiol and estrone concentrations return to baseline values in less than 24 hours.

Estradiol is mainly metabolized in the liver. Its main metabolites are estriol, estrone, and their conjugates. The plasma half life of estradiol is 1-2 hours. Metabolic plasma clearance varies between 450-625 ml/min/m^2. The metabolites are mainly excreted via the kidneys as glucuronides and sulphates. Estrogens also undergo enterohepatic circulation.

5.3 Preclinical safety data

No additional information is available.

6. PHARMACEUTICAL PARTICULARS

6.1 List of excipients

Diethyltoluamide

Acrylic adhesive (Dow Corning MG-0560)

Acrylic emulsion (Acrysol 33)

Backing: Polyester film (Scotchpak 9733)

Release liner: Siliconised aluminised polyester

6.2 Incompatibilities

Not applicable.

6.3 Shelf life

3 years.

6.4 Special precautions for storage

Do not store above 25 °C. Store in the original package.

6.5 Nature and contents of container

PVC/PVDC blister tray with paper/polythene/aluminium foil lid containing one transdermal patch. Each carton contains eight patches, sufficient for one 28 day cycle and a patient leaflet. An additional pack containing two patches may also be available.

6.6 Instructions for use and handling

Detailed instructions for use are provided in the patient leaflet.

7. MARKETING AUTHORISATION HOLDER

Pharmacia Limited

Davy Avenue

Milton Keynes

MK5 8PH

UK

8. MARKETING AUTHORISATION NUMBER(S)

PL 00032/0304

9. DATE OF FIRST AUTHORISATION/RENEWAL OF THE AUTHORISATION

26 February 2002

10. DATE OF REVISION OF THE TEXT

March 2005

Ref ELB 4_0

(Previously EL 3_3)

Elocon Cream

(Schering-Plough Ltd)

1. NAME OF THE MEDICINAL PRODUCT

Elocon Cream

2. QUALITATIVE AND QUANTITATIVE COMPOSITION

Mometasone Furoate 0.1% w/w

3. PHARMACEUTICAL FORM

Cream

4. CLINICAL PARTICULARS

4.1 Therapeutic indications

Elocon Cream is indicated for the treatment of inflammatory and pruritic manifestations of psoriasis (excluding widespread plaque psoriasis) and atopic dermatitis.

4.2 Posology and method of administration

Adults, including elderly patients and Children: A thin film of Elocon Cream should be applied to the affected areas of skin once daily.

Use of topical corticosteroids in children or on the face should be limited to the least amount compatible with an effective therapeutic regimen and duration of treatment should be no more than 5 days.

4.3 Contraindications

Elocon is contraindicated in facial rosacea, acne vulgaris, perioral dermatitis, perianal and genital pruritis, napkin eruptions, bacterial (e.g. impetigo), viral (e.g. herpes simplex, herpes zoster and chickenpox) and fungal (e.g. candida or dermatophyte) infections, varicella, tuberculosis, syphilis or post-vaccine reactions. Elocon should not be used in patients who are sensitive to mometasone furoate or to other corticosteroids.

4.4 Special warnings and special precautions for use

If irritation or sensitisation develop with the use of Elocon, treatment should be withdrawn and appropriate therapy instituted.

Should an infection develop, use of an appropriate antifungal or antibacterial agent should be instituted. If a favourable response does not occur promptly, the corticosteroid should be discontinued until the infection is adequately controlled.

Local and systemic toxicity is common especially following long continued use on large areas of damaged skin, in flexures and with polythene occlusion. If used in childhood, or on the face, courses should be limited to 5 days and occlusion should not be used. Long term continuous therapy should be avoided in all patients irrespective of age.

Topical steroids may be hazardous in psoriasis for a number of reasons including rebound relapses following development of tolerance, risk of centralised pustular psoriasis and development of local or systemic toxicity due to impaired barrier function of the skin. If used in psoriasis careful patient supervision is important.

Elocon topical preparations are not for ophthalmic use.

4.5 Interaction with other medicinal products and other forms of Interaction

None stated

4.6 Pregnancy and lactation

There is inadequate evidence of safety in human pregnancy. Topical administration of corticosteroids to pregnant animals can cause abnormalities of foetal development including cleft palate and intra-uterine growth retardation. There may therefore be a very small risk of such effects in the human foetus.

It is not known whether topical administration of corticosteroids could result in sufficient systemic absorption to produce detectable quantities in breast milk. Elocon should be administered to nursing mothers only after careful consideration of the benefit/risk relationship.

4.7 Effects on ability to drive and use machines
None stated.

4.8 Undesirable effects
Local adverse reactions occasionally reported with Elocon include paresthesia, folliculitis, burning, pruritis, tingling, stinging, allergic contact dermatitis, hypopigmentation, hypertrichosis, secondary infection, striae, acneiform reactions and signs of skin atrophy.

Local adverse reactions reported infrequently with other topical corticosteroids include: irritation, perioral dermatitis, maceration of the skin and miliaria.

Paediatric patients may demonstrate greater susceptibility to topical corticosteroid-induced hypothalamic-pituitary-adrenal axis suppression and Cushing's syndrome than mature patients because of a larger skin surface area to body weight ratio.

Chronic corticosteroids therapy may interfere with the growth and development of children.

4.9 Overdose
None stated.

5. PHARMACOLOGICAL PROPERTIES
5.1 Pharmacodynamic properties
Mometasone furoate exhibits marked anti-inflammatory activity and marked anti-psoriatic activity in standard animal predictive models.

In the croton oil assay in mice, mometasone was equipotent to betamethasone valerate after single application and about 8 times as potent after five applications.

In guinea pigs, mometasone was approximately twice as potent as betamethasone valerate in reducing m.ovalis-induced epidermal acanthosis (i.e. anti-psoriatic activity) after 14 applications.

5.2 Pharmacokinetic properties
Pharmacokinetic studies have indicated that systemic absorption following topical application of mometasone furoate cream 0.1% is minimal, approximately 0.4% of the applied dose in man, the majority of which is excreted within 72 hours following application. Characterisation of metabolites was not feasible owing to the small amounts present in plasma and excreta.

5.3 Preclinical safety data
There are no pre-clinical data of relevance to the prescriber which are additional to that already included in other sections of the SPC.

6. PHARMACEUTICAL PARTICULARS
6.1 List of excipients
Hexylene glycol
phosphoric acid
propylene glycolstearate
stearyl alcohol and ceteareth-20
titanium dioxide
aluminium starch octenylsuccinate
white wax
white petrolatum
purified water

6.2 Incompatibilities
None Known

6.3 Shelf life
36 months

6.4 Special precautions for storage
Store between 2 and 30°C.

6.5 Nature and contents of container
5, 15, 30, 45 and 100gm aluminium tubes with low density polyethylene cap or laminated tubes with high density polyethylene head and polypropylene cap.

6.6 Instructions for use and handling
Not applicable

Administrative Data
7. MARKETING AUTHORISATION HOLDER
Schering-Plough Ltd
Shire Park
Welwyn Garden City
Hertfordshire AL7 1TW
England

8. MARKETING AUTHORISATION NUMBER(S)
PL 0201/0117

9. DATE OF FIRST AUTHORISATION/RENEWAL OF THE AUTHORISATION
19 November 1991

10. DATE OF REVISION OF THE TEXT
September 2001

Elocon Ointment

(Schering-Plough Ltd)

1. NAME OF THE MEDICINAL PRODUCT
Elocon Ointment

2. QUALITATIVE AND QUANTITATIVE COMPOSITION
Mometasone Furoate 0.1% w/w

3. PHARMACEUTICAL FORM
Ointment

4. CLINICAL PARTICULARS
4.1 Therapeutic indications
Elocon Ointment is indicated for the treatment of inflammatory and pruritic manifestations of psoriasis (excluding widespread plaque psoriasis) and atopic dermatitis.

4.2 Posology and method of administration
Adults, including elderly patients and children: A thin film of Elocon Ointment should be applied to the affected areas of skin once daily.

Use of topical corticosteroids in children or on the face should be limited to the least amount compatible with an effective therapeutic regimen and duration of treatment should be no more than 5 days.

4.3 Contraindications
Elocon is contraindicated in facial rosacea, acne vulgaris, perioral dermatitis, perianal and genital pruritis, napkin eruptions, bacterial (e.g. impetigo), viral (e.g. herpes simplex, herpes zoster and chickenpox) and fungal (e.g. candida or dermatophyte) infections, varicella, tuberculosis, syphilis or post-vaccine reactions. Elocon should not be used in patients who are sensitive to mometasone furoate or to other corticosteroids.

4.4 Special warnings and special precautions for use
If irritation or sensitisation develop with the use of Elocon, treatment should be withdrawn and appropriate therapy instituted.

Should an infection develop, use of an appropriate antifungal or antibacterial agent should be instituted. If a favourable response does not occur promptly, the corticosteroid should be discontinued until the infection is adequately controlled.

Local and systemic toxicity is common especially following long continued use on large areas of damaged skin, in flexures and with polythene occlusion. If used in childhood, or on the face, courses should be limited to 5 days and occlusion should not be used. Long term continuous therapy should be avoided in all patients irrespective of age.

Topical steroids may be hazardous in psoriasis for a number of reasons including rebound relapses following development of tolerance, risk of centralised pustular psoriasis and development of local or systemic toxicity due to impaired barrier function of the skin. If used in psoriasis careful patient supervision is important.

Elocon topical preparations are not for ophthalmic use.

4.5 Interaction with other medicinal products and other forms of Interaction
None stated

4.6 Pregnancy and lactation
There is inadequate evidence of safety in human pregnancy. Topical administration of corticosteroids to pregnant animals can cause abnormalities of foetal development including cleft palate and intra-uterine growth retardation. There may therefore be a very small risk of such effects in the human foetus.

It is not known whether topical administration of corticosteroids could result in sufficient systemic absorption to produce detectable quantities in breast milk. Elocon should be administered to nursing mothers only after careful consideration of the benefit/risk relationship.

4.7 Effects on ability to drive and use machines
None stated.

4.8 Undesirable effects
Local adverse reactions occasionally reported with Elocon include paresthesia, folliculitis, burning, pruritis, tingling, stinging, allergic contact dermatitis, hypopigmentation, hypertrichosis, secondary infection, striae, acneiform reactions and signs of skin atrophy.

Local adverse reactions reported infrequently with other topical corticosteroids include: irritation, perioral dermatitis, maceration of the skin and miliaria.

Paediatric patients may demonstrate greater susceptibility to topical corticosteroid-induced hypothalamic-pituitary-adrenal axis suppression and Cushing's syndrome than mature patients because of a larger skin surface area to body weight ratio. Chronic corticosteroids therapy may interfere with the growth and development of children.

4.9 Overdose
None stated.

5. PHARMACOLOGICAL PROPERTIES
5.1 Pharmacodynamic properties
Mometasone furoate exhibits marked anti-inflammatory activity and marked anti-psoriatic activity in standard animal predictive models.

In the croton oil assay in mice, mometasone was equipotent to betamethasone valerate after single application and about 8 times as potent after five applications.

In guinea pigs, mometasone was approximately twice as potent as betamethasone valerate in reducing m.ovalis-induced epidermal acanthosis (i.e. anti-psoriatic activity) after 14 applications.

5.2 Pharmacokinetic properties
Pharmacokinetic studies have indicated that systemic absorption following topical application of mometasone furoate ointment 0.1% is minimal, approximately 0.4% of the applied dose in man, the majority of which is excreted within 72 hours following application. Characterisation of metabolites was not feasible owing to the small amounts present in plasma and excreta.

5.3 Preclinical safety data
There are no pre-clinical data of relevance to the prescriber which are additional to that already included in other sections of the SPC.

6. PHARMACEUTICAL PARTICULARS
6.1 List of excipients
Hexylene glycol
Phosphoric acid
Propylene glycol stearate
White wax
White petrolatum
Purified water.

6.2 Incompatibilities
None known

6.3 Shelf life
36 months

6.4 Special precautions for storage
Store between 2 and 30°C.

6.5 Nature and contents of container
5, 15, 30, 45 and 100gm aluminium tube with low density polyethylene cap or laminated tubes with high density polyethylene head and polypropylene cap.

6.6 Instructions for use and handling
Not applicable

Administrative Data
7. MARKETING AUTHORISATION HOLDER
Schering-Plough Ltd
Shire Park
Welwyn Garden City
Hertfordshire AL7 1TW
England

8. MARKETING AUTHORISATION NUMBER(S)
PL 0201/0118

9. DATE OF FIRST AUTHORISATION/RENEWAL OF THE AUTHORISATION
19 November 1991 / 15 April 2002

10. DATE OF REVISION OF THE TEXT
January 1996

Legal Category
POM

Elocon Scalp Lotion

(Schering-Plough Ltd)

1. NAME OF THE MEDICINAL PRODUCT
Elocon Scalp Lotion

2. QUALITATIVE AND QUANTITATIVE COMPOSITION
Mometasone Furoate 0.1% w/w

3. PHARMACEUTICAL FORM
Lotion

4. CLINICAL PARTICULARS
4.1 Therapeutic indications
Elocon Scalp Lotion is indicated for the treatment of inflammatory and pruritic manifestations of psoriasis and seborrhoeic dermatitis of the scalp.

4.2 Posology and method of administration
Adults, including elderly patients and Children: A few drops of Elocon Scalp Lotion should be applied to affected scalp sites, once daily; massage gently and thoroughly until the medication disappears.

Use of topical corticosteroids in children should be limited to the least amount compatible with an effective therapeutic regimen and duration of treatment should be no more than 5 days.

4.3 Contraindications
Elocon Scalp Lotion is contraindicated in bacterial (e.g. impetigo), viral (e.g. herpes simplex, herpes zoster and chickenpox) and fungal (e.g. candida or dermatophyte) infections of the scalp. Elocon Scalp Lotion should not be used in patients who are sensitive to mometasone furoate or to other corticosteroids.

4.4 Special warnings and special precautions for use
If irritation or sensitisation develop with the use of Elocon, treatment should be withdrawn and appropriate therapy instituted.

Should an infection develop, use of an appropriate anti-fungal or antibacterial agent should be instituted. If a favourable response does not occur promptly, the corticosteroid should be discontinued until the infection is adequately controlled.

Local and systemic toxicity is common especially following long continued use on large areas of damaged skin. If used in childhood, courses should be limited to 5 days. Long term continuous therapy should be avoided in all patients irrespective of age.

Topical steroids may be hazardous in psoriasis for a number of reasons including rebound relapses following development of tolerance, risk of centralised pustular psoriasis and development of local or systemic toxicity due to impaired barrier function of the skin. If used in psoriasis careful patient supervision is important.

Care must be taken to keep the preparation away from the eyes.

4.5 Interaction with other medicinal products and other forms of Interaction
None known.

4.6 Pregnancy and lactation
There is inadequate evidence of safety in human pregnancy. Topical administration of corticosteroids to pregnant animals can cause abnormalities of foetal development including cleft palate and intra-uterine growth retardation. There may therefore be a very small risk of such effects in the human foetus.

It is not known whether topical administration of corticosteroids could result in sufficient systemic absorption to produce detectable quantities in breast milk. Elocon should be administered to nursing mothers only after careful consideration of the benefit/risk relationship.

4.7 Effects on ability to drive and use machines
None known.

4.8 Undesirable effects
Local adverse reactions occasionally reported with Elocon include paresthesia, folliculitis, burning, pruritis, tingling, stinging, allergic contact dermatitis, hypopigmentation, hypertrichosis, secondary infection, striae, acneiform reactions and signs of skin atrophy.

Local adverse reactions reported infrequently with other topical corticosteroids include: irritation, perioral dermatitis, maceration of the skin and miliaria.

Paediatric patients may demonstrate greater susceptibility to topical corticosteroid-induced hypothalamic-pituitary-adrenal axis suppression and Cushing's syndrome than mature patients because of a larger skin surface area to body weight ratio. Chronic corticosteroids therapy may interfere with the growth and development of children.

4.9 Overdose
Excessive prolonged use of topical corticosteroids can suppress pituitary-adrenal function resulting in secondary adrenal insufficiency which is usually reversible. In such cases appropriate symptomatic treatment is indicated.

The steroid content of each container is so low as to have little or no toxic effect in the unlikely event of accidental oral ingestion.

5. PHARMACOLOGICAL PROPERTIES

5.1 Pharmacodynamic properties
Mometasone furoate exhibits marked anti-inflammatory activity and marked anti-psoriatic activity in standard animal predictive models.

In the croton oil assay in mice, mometasone was equipotent to betamethasone valerate after single application and about 8 times as potent after five applications.

In guinea pigs, mometasone was approximately twice as potent as betamethasone valerate in reducing m.ovalis-induced epidermal acanthosis (i.e. anti-psoriatic activity) after 14 applications.

5.2 Pharmacokinetic properties
Pharmacokinetic studies have indicated that systemic absorption following topical application of mometasone furoate 0.1% is minimal, approximately 0.4% of the applied dose in man, the majority of which is excreted within 72 hours following application. Characterisation of metabolites was not feasible owing to the small amounts present in plasma and excreta.

5.3 Preclinical safety data
There are no pre-clinical data of relevance to the prescriber which are additional to that already included in other sections of this SmPC.

6. PHARMACEUTICAL PARTICULARS

6.1 List of excipients
Isopropyl alcohol; propylene glycol; hydroxypropyl cellulose; sodium phosphate monobasic monohydrate; phosphoric acid; purified water.

6.2 Incompatibilities
None Known

6.3 Shelf life
36 months

6.4 Special precautions for storage
Store below 25°C.

6.5 Nature and contents of container
30ml white HDPE bottle with LDPE dropper and white HDPE cap.

6.6 Instructions for use and handling
Not applicable

7. MARKETING AUTHORISATION HOLDER
Schering-Plough Ltd
Shire Park
Welwyn Garden City
Hertfordshire AL7 1TW
England

8. MARKETING AUTHORISATION NUMBER(S)
0201/0156

9. DATE OF FIRST AUTHORISATION/RENEWAL OF THE AUTHORISATION

10. DATE OF REVISION OF THE TEXT
June 1997

Legal Category
POM

EloSL/UK/12-97/1

Eloxatin

(sanofi-aventis)

1. NAME OF THE MEDICINAL PRODUCT
Eloxatin 5 mg/ml powder for solution for infusion

2. QUALITATIVE AND QUANTITATIVE COMPOSITION
Oxaliplatin 50 mg in a 36 ml glass vial

Oxaliplatin 100 mg in a 50 ml glass vial

One ml of reconstituted solution contains oxaliplatin 5 mg.

For excipients, see section 6.1 " List of excipients".

3. PHARMACEUTICAL FORM
White to off-white cake or powder for solution for infusion.

4. CLINICAL PARTICULARS

4.1 Therapeutic indications
Oxaliplatin in combination with 5-fluorouracil (5-FU) and folinic acid (FA) is indicated for:

- Adjuvant treatment of stage III (Duke's C) colon cancer after complete resection of primary tumor
- Treatment of metastatic colorectal cancer.

4.2 Posology and method of administration
Posology

FOR ADULTS ONLY

The recommended dose for oxaliplatin in adjuvant setting is 85 mg/m^2 intravenously repeated every two weeks for 12 cycles (6 months).

The recommended dose for oxaliplatin in treatment of metastatic colorectal cancer is 85 mg/m^2 intravenously repeated every 2 weeks.

Dosage given should be adjusted according to tolerability (see 4.4 "Special warnings and precautions for use").

Oxaliplatin should always be administered before fluoropyrimidines.

Oxaliplatin is administered as a 2- to 6-hour intravenous infusion in 250 to 500 ml of 5% glucose solution.

Oxaliplatin was mainly used in combination with continuous infusion 5-fluorouracil based regimens. For the two-weekly treatment schedule 5-fluorouracil regimens combining bolus and continuous infusion were used.

- Special Populations

- Renal impairment:

Oxaliplatin has not been studied in patients with severe renal impairment(See 4.3 " Contra-indications").

In patients with moderate renal impairment, treatment may be initiated at the normally recommended dose (see 4.4 "Special warnings and precautions for use"). There is no need for dose adjustment in patients with mild renal dysfunction.

- Hepatic insufficiency:

Oxaliplatin has not been studied in patients with severe hepatic impairment. No increase in oxaliplatin acute toxicities was observed in the subset of patients with abnormal liver function tests at baseline. No specific dose adjustment for patients with abnormal liver function tests was performed during clinical development.

- Elderly patients:

No increase in severe toxicities was observed when oxaliplatin was used as a single agent or in combination with 5-fluorouracil in patients over the age of 65. In consequence no specific dose adaptation is required for elderly patients.

Method of administration

Oxaliplatin is administered by intravenous infusion.

The administration of oxaliplatin does not require hyperhydration.

Oxaliplatin diluted in 250 to 500 ml of 5% glucose solution to give a concentration not less than 0.2 mg/ml must be infused via a central venous line or peripheral vein over 2 to 6 hours. Oxaliplatin infusion should always precede that of 5-fluorouracil.

In the event of extravasation, administration must be discontinued immediately.

Instructions for use:

Oxaliplatin must be reconstituted and further diluted before use. Only the recommended diluents should be used to reconstitute and then dilute the freeze-dried product. (See section 6.6 "Instructions for use / handling and disposal").

4.3 Contraindications
Oxaliplatin is contra-indicated in patients who

- have a known history of hypersensitivityto oxaliplatin.

- are breast feeding.

- have myelosuppression prior to starting first course, as evidenced by baseline neutrophils $<2x10^9$/l and/or platelet count of $<100x10^9$/l.

- have a peripheral sensitive neuropathy with functional impairment prior to first course.

- have a severely impaired renal function (creatinine clearance less than 30 ml/min).

4.4 Special warnings and special precautions for use

Oxaliplatin should only be used in specialised departments of oncology and should be administered under the supervision of an experienced oncologist.

For use in pregnant women see section 4.6.

Due to limited information on safety in patients with moderatelyimpaired renal function, administration should only be considered after suitable appraisal of the benefit/risk for the patient.

In this situation, renal function should be closely monitored and dose adjusted according to toxicity.

Patients with a history of allergic reaction to platinum compounds should be monitored for allergic symptoms. In case of an anaphylactic-like reaction to oxaliplatin, the infusion should be immediately discontinued and appropriate symptomatic treatment initiated. Oxaliplatin rechallenge is contra-indicated.

In case of oxaliplatin extravasation, the infusion must be stopped immediately and usual local symptomatic treatment initiated.

Neurological toxicity of oxaliplatin should be carefully monitored, especially if co-administered with other medications with specific neurological toxicity. A neurological examination should be performed before each administration and periodically thereafter.

For patients who develop acute laryngopharyngeal dysaesthesia (see 4.8 "Undesirable effects"), during or within the hours following the 2-hour infusion, the next oxaliplatin infusion should be administered over 6 hours.

If neurological symptoms (paraesthesia, dysaesthesia) occur, the following recommended oxaliplatin dosage adjustment should be based on the duration and severity of these symptoms:

- If symptoms last longer than seven days and are troublesome, the subsequent oxaliplatin dose should be reduced from 85 to 65 mg/m^2 (metastatic setting) or 75 mg/m^2 (adjuvant setting).

- If paraesthesia without functional impairment persists until the next cycle, the subsequent oxaliplatin dose should be reduced from 85 to 65 mg/m^2 (metastatic setting) or 75 mg/m^2 (adjuvant setting).

- If paraesthesia with functional impairment persists until the next cycle, oxaliplatin should be discontinued.

- If these symptoms improve following discontinuation of oxaliplatin therapy, resumption of therapy may be considered.

Patients should be informed of the possibility of persistent symptoms of peripheral sensory neuropathy after the end of the treatment. Localized moderate paraesthesias or paraesthesias that may interfere with functional activities can persist after up to 3 years following treatment cessation in the adjuvant setting.

Gastrointestinal toxicity, which manifests as nausea and vomiting, warrants prophylactic and/or therapeutic anti-emetic therapy (see 4.8. "Undesirable effects").

Dehydration, paralytic ileus, intestinal obstruction, hypokalemia, metabolic acidosis and renal impairment may be caused by severe diarrhoea/emesis particularly when combining oxaliplatin with 5-fluorouracil.

If haematological toxicity occurs (neutrophils $< 1.5x10^9$/l or platelets $< 50x10^9$/l), administration of the next course of therapy should be postponed until haematological values return to acceptable levels. A full blood count with white cell differential should be performed prior to start of therapy and before each subsequent course.

Patients must be adequately informed of the risk of diarrhoea/emesis, mucositis/stomatitis and neutropenia after oxaliplatin and 5-fluorouracil administration so that they can urgently contact their treating physician for appropriate management.

If mucositis/stomatitis occurs with or without neutropenia, the next treatment should be delayed until recovery from mucositis/stomatitis to grade 1 or less and/or until the neutrophil count is $\geqslant 1.5 \times 10^9$/l.

For oxaliplatin combined with 5-fluorouracil (with or without folinic acid), the usual dose adjustments for 5-fluorouracil associated toxicities should apply.

If grade 4 diarrhoea, grade 3-4 neutropenia (neutrophils $< 1.0 \times 10^9$/l), grade 3-4 thrombocytopenia (platelets $< 50 \times 10^9$/l) occur, the dose of oxaliplatin should be reduced from 85 to 65 mg/m^2 (metastatic setting) or 75 mg/m^2 (adjuvant setting), in addition to any 5-fluorouracil dose reductions required.

In the case of unexplained respiratory symptoms such as non-productive cough, dyspnoea, crackles or radiological pulmonary infiltrates, oxaliplatin should be discontinued until further pulmonary investigations exclude an interstitial lung disease (see section 4.8 " Undesirable effects ").

4.5 Interaction with other medicinal products and other forms of Interaction

In patients who have received a single dose of 85 mg/m^2 of oxaliplatin, immediately before administration of 5-fluorouracil, no change in the level of exposure to 5-fluorouracil has been observed.

In vitro, no significant displacement of oxaliplatin binding to plasma proteins has been observed with the following agents: erythromycin, salicylates, granisetron, paclitaxel, and sodium valproate.

4.6 Pregnancy and lactation

To date there is no available information on safety of use in pregnant women. Based on pre-clinical findings, oxaliplatin is likely to be lethal and/or teratogenic to the human foetus at the recommended therapeutic dose, and is consequently not recommended during pregnancy and should only be considered after suitably appraising the patient of the risk to the foetus and with the patient's consent.

Excretion in breast milk has not been studied. Breast-feeding is contra-indicated during oxaliplatin therapy.

4.7 Effects on ability to drive and use machines

No data available.

4.8 Undesirable effects

The most frequent adverse events of oxaliplatin in combination with 5-fluorouracil/folinic acid (5-FU/FA) were gastrointestinal (diarrhea, nausea, vomiting and mucositis), haematological (neutropenia, thrombocytopenia) and neurological (acute and dose cumulative peripheral sensory neurophathy). Overall, these adverse events were more frequent and severe with oxaliplatin and 5-FU/FA combination than with 5-FU/FA alone.

The frequencies reported in the table below are derived from clinical trials in the metastatic and adjuvant settings (having included 416 and 1108 patients respectively in the oxaliplatin + 5-FU/FA treatment arms) and from post marketing experience.

Frequencies in this table are defined using the following convention: very common (>1/10) common (>1/100, ⩽1/10), uncommon (>1/1000, ⩽1/100), rare (>1/10000, ⩽1/1000), very rare (⩽1/10000) including isolated report.

Further details are given after the table.

(see Table 1 below)

(see Table 2 on next page)

Haematological toxicity

Incidence by patient (%), by grade

(see Table 3 on next page)

Digestive toxicity:

Incidence by patient (%), by grade

(see Table 4 on next page)

Prophylaxis and/or treatment with potent antiemetic agents is indicated.

Dehydration, paralytic ileus, intestinal obstruction, hypokalemia, metabolic acidosis and renal impairment may be caused by severe diarrhoea/emesis particularly when combining oxaliplatin with 5-fluorouracil (see 4.4 " Special warnings and precautions for use ").

Nervous system:

The dose limiting toxicity of oxaliplatin is neurological. It involves a sensory peripheral neuropathy characterised by dysaesthesia and/or paraesthesia of the extremities with or without cramps, often triggered by the cold. These symptoms occur in up to 95% of patients treated. The duration of these symptoms, which usually regress between courses of treatment, increases with the number of treatment cycles.

The onset of pain and/or a functional disorder are indications, depending on the duration of the symptoms, for dose adjustment, or even treatment discontinuation (see 4.4 "Special warnings and precautions for use").

This functional disorder includes difficulties in executing delicate movements and is a possible consequence of sensory impairment. The risk of occurrence of persistent symptoms for a cumulative dose of 850 mg/m^2 (10 cycles) is approximately 10% and 20% for a cumulative dose of 1020 mg/m^2 (12 cycles).

In the majority of the cases, the neurological signs and symptoms improve or totally recover when treatment is discontinued. In the adjuvant setting of colon cancer, 6 months after treatment cessation, 87 % of patients had no or mild symptoms. After up to 3 years of follow up, about 3 % of patients presented either with persisting localized paraesthesias of moderate intensity (2.3%) or with paraesthesias that may interfere with functional activities (0.5%).

Acute neurosensory manifestations (see 5.3. "Preclinical safety data") have been reported. They start within hours of administration and often occur on exposure to cold. They may present as transient paraesthesia, dysaesthesia and hypoesthesia or as an acute syndrome of pharyngolaryngeal dysaesthesia. This acute syndrome of pharyngolaryngeal dysaesthesia, with an incidence estimated between 1% and 2%, is characterised by subjective sensations of dysphagia or dyspnoea, without any objective evidence of respiratory distress (no cyanosis or hypoxia) or of laryngospasm or bronchospasm (no stridor or wheezing); jaw spasm, abnormal tongue sensation, dysarthria and a feeling of chest pressure have also been observed. Although antihistamines and bronchodilators have been administered in such cases, the symptoms are rapidly reversible even in the absence of treatment. Prolongation of the infusion helps to reduce the incidence of this syndrome (see 4.4 "Special warnings and precautions for use").

Other neurological symptoms such as dysarthria, loss of deep tendon reflex and Lhermitte's sign were reported during treatment with oxaliplatin. Isolated cases of optic neuritis have been reported.

Allergic reactions:

Incidence by patient (%), by grade

(see Table 5 on next page)

Table 1

Adverse Events by System Organ Class			
Very common	**Common**	**Uncommon**	**Rare**
Application site disorders			
Injection site reaction+			
+ Extravasation may result in local pain and inflammation which may be severe and lead to complications, especially when oxaliplatin is infused through a peripheral vein (see 4.4 "Special Warnings and Precautions for Use").			
Autonomic nervous system disorders			
	Flushing		
Body as a whole – general disorders*			
Fever+++, Fatigue, Allergy/ allergic reaction++ Asthenia, Pain Weight increase (adjuvant setting)	Chest pain Weight decrease (metastatic setting)		Immunoallergic thrombocytopenia, Haemolytic anemia
++ Common allergic reactions such as skin rash (particularly urticaria), conjunctivitis, rhinitis. Common anaphylactic reactions, including bronchospasm, angioedema, hypotension and anaphylactic shock +++ Very common fever, either from infection (with or without febrile neutropenia) or isolated fever from immunological mechanism.			
Central and peripheral nervous system disorders*			
Peripheral sensory neuropathy, Headache Sensory disturbance	Dizziness, Neuritis motor, Meningism		Dysarthria
Gastrointestinal system disorders*			
Diarrhea, Nausea, Vomiting, Stomatitis/mucositis, Abdominal pain, Constipation, Anorexia	Dyspepsia, Gastroesophageal reflux, Hiccup	Ileus, Intestinal obstruction	Colitis including *Clostridium difficile* diarrhea
Metabolic and nutritional disorders			
	Dehydration	Metabolic acidosis	
Musculo-skeletal system disorders			
Back pain	Arthralgia Skeletal pain		

* See detailed section below

4.9 Overdose

There is no known antidote to oxaliplatin. In cases of overdose, exacerbation of adverse events can be expected. Monitoring of haematological parameters should be initiated and symptomatic treatment given.

5. PHARMACOLOGICAL PROPERTIES

5.1 Pharmacodynamic properties

CYTOSTATIC AGENT

(L: anticancer drugs - immunosuppressive agents - platinum)

ATC code: L01XA 03

Oxaliplatin is an antineoplastic drug belonging to a new class of platinum-based compounds in which the platinum atom is complexed with 1,2-diaminocyclohexane ("DACH") and an oxalate group.

Oxaliplatin is a single enantiomer, the Cis -[oxalato (trans-l-1,2- DACH) platinum].

Oxaliplatin exhibits a wide spectrum of both *in vitro* cytotoxicity and *in vivo* antitumour activity in a variety of tumour model systems including human colorectal cancer models. Oxaliplatin also demonstrates *in vitro* and *in vivo* activity in various cisplatin resistant models.

A synergistic cytotoxic action has been observed in combination with 5-fluorouracil both *in vitro* and *in vivo*.

Studies on the mechanism of action of oxaliplatin, although not completely elucidated, show that the aqua-derivatives resulting from the biotransformation of oxaliplatin, interact with DNA to form both inter and intra-strand cross-links, resulting in the disruption of DNA synthesis leading to cytotoxic and antitumour effects.

In patients with metastatic colorectal cancer, the efficacy of oxaliplatin (85mg/m^2 repeated every two weeks) combined with 5-fluorouracil/folinic acid (5-FU/FA) is reported in three clinical studies:

- In front-line treatment, the 2-arm comparative phase III EFC2962 study randomised 420 patients either to 5-FU/FA alone (LV5FU2, N=210) or the combination of oxaliplatin with 5-FU/FA (FOLFOX4, N=210)

- In pretreated patients, the comparative three arms phase III study EFC4584 randomised 821 patients refractory to an irinotecan (CPT-11) + 5-FU/FA combination either to 5-FU/FA alone (LV5FU2, N=275), oxaliplatin single agent (N=275), or combination of oxaliplatin with 5-FU/FA (FOLFOX4, N=271).

- Finally, the uncontrolled phase II EFC2964 study included patients refractory to 5-FU/FA alone, that were treated with the oxaliplatin and 5-FU/FA combination (FOLFOX4, N=57)

The two randomised clinical trials, EFC2962 in front-line therapy and EFC4584 in pretreated patients, demonstrated a significantly higher response rate and a prolonged progression free survival (PFS)/time to

Table 2

Adverse Events by System Organ Class (cont'd)

Very common	Common	Uncommon	Rare
Platelets, bleeding and clotting disorders			
Epistaxis	Haemorrhage nos, Haematuria, Thrombophlebitis deep, Embolism pulmonary, Haemorrhage rectum		
Psychiatric disorders			
	Depression, Insomnia	Nervousness	
Resistance mechanism disorders			
Infection			
Respiratory system disorders			
Dyspnoea, Coughing	Rhinitis, Upper respiratory tract infection		Interstitial lung disease, pulmonary fibrosis**
Skin and appendage disorders			
Skin disorder, Alopecia	Skin exfoliation (i.e.Hand and Foot syndrome), Rash erythematous, Rash, Sweating increased, Nail disorder		
Special senses, other disorders			
Taste perversion		ototoxicity	Deafness
Urinary system disorders			
	Dysuria, Micturition frequency abnormal		
Vision disorders			
	Conjunctivitis, Vision abnormal		Transient fall in visual acuity, Visual field disturbances, Optic neuritis
Laboratory Abnormalities			
Hematological* Anemia, Neutropenia, Thrombocytopenia Leukopenia, Lymphopenia, **Chemistry** Alkaline phosphatase increase, Bilirubin increase, Glycemia abnormalities, LDH increase, Hypokalaemia, Hepatic enzymes (SGPT/ALAT, SGOT/ASAT) increase, *Phosphatase alkaline increase* Natremia abnormalities,	**Hematological*** Febrile neutropenia /Neutropenic sepsis (i.e. neutropenia grade 3,4 and documented infections) **Chemistry** Creatinine increase		

* See detailed section below

** See section 4.4 "Special warning and precaution for use"

Table 3 Incidence by patient (%), by grade

Oxaliplatin and 5-FU/FA 85 mg/m² every 2 weeks	Metastatic Setting			Adjuvant Setting		
	All grades	Gr 3	Gr 4	All grades	Gr 3	Gr 4
Anemia	82.2	3	<1	75.6	0.7	0.1
Neutropenia	71.4	28	14	78.9	28.8	12.3
Thrombocytopenia	71.6	4	<1	77.4	1.5	0.2
Febrile neutropenia	5.0	3.6	1.4	0.7	0.7	0.0
Neutropenic sepsis	1.1	0.7	0.4	1.1	0.6	0.4

Table 4 Incidence by patient (%), by grade

Oxaliplatin and 5-FU/FA 85 mg/m²	Metastatic Setting			Adjuvant Setting		
Every 2 weeks	**All grades**	**Gr 3**	**Gr 4**	**All grades**	**Gr 3**	**Gr 4**
Nausea	69.9	8	<1	73.7	4.8	0.3
Diarrhoea	60.8	9	2	56.3	8.3	2.5
Vomiting	49.0	6	1	47.2	5.3	0.5
Mucositis/Stomatitis	39.9	4	<1	42.1	2.8	0.1

Table 5 Incidence by patient (%), by grade

Oxaliplatin and 5-FU/FA 85 mg/m² every 2 weeks	Metastatic Setting			Adjuvant Setting		
	All grades	Gr 3	Gr 4	All grades	Gr 3	Gr 4
Allergic reactions / Allergy	9.1	1	<1	10.3	2.3	0.6

progression (TTP) as compared to treatment with 5-FU/FA alone. In EFC4584 performed in refractory pretreated patients, the difference in median overall survival (OS) between the combination of oxaliplatin and 5-FU/FA did not reach statistical significance.

Response rate under FOLFOX4 versus LV5FU2

(see Table 6 on next page)

Median Progression Free Survival (PFS) / Median Time to Progression (TTP)

FOLFOX4 versus LV5FU2

(see Table 7 on next page)

Median Overall Survival (OS) under FOLFOX4 versus LV5FU2

(see Table 8 on next page)

In pretreated patients (EFC4584), who were symptomatic at baseline, a higher proportion of those treated with oxaliplatin and 5-FU/FA experienced a significant improvement of their disease-related symptoms compared to those treated with 5-FU/FA alone (27.7% vs 14.6% p = 0.0033).

In non pretreated patients (EFC2962), no statistically significant difference between the two treatment groups was found for any of the quality of life dimensions. However, the quality of life scores were generally better in the control arm for measurement of global health status and pain and worse in the oxaliplatin arm for nausea and vomiting.

In the adjuvant setting, the MOSAIC comparative phase III study (EFC3313) randomised 2246 patients (899 stage II/Duke's B2 and 1347 stage III/Duke's C) further to complete resection of the primary tumor of colon cancer either to 5-FU/FA alone (LV5FU2, N=1123 (B2/C = 448/675) or to combination of oxaliplatin and 5-FU/FA (FOLFOX4, N=1123 (B2/C) = 451/672).

EFC 3313 3-year disease free survival (ITT analysis)* for the overall population.

Treatment arm	LV5FU2	FOLFOX4
Percent 3-year disease free survival (95% CI)	73.3 (70.6-75.9)	78.7 (76.2-81.1)
Hazard ratio (95% CI)	0.76 (0.64-0.89)	
Stratified log rank test	P=0.0008	

* median follow up 44.2 months (all patients followed for at least 3 years)

The study demonstrated an overall significant advantage in 3-year disease free survival for the oxaliplatin and 5-FU/FA combination (FOLFOX4) over 5-FU/FA alone (LV5FU2).

EFC 3313 3-year Disease Free Survival (ITT analysis)* according to Stage of disease

(see Table 9 on next page)

Overall Survival (ITT analysis):

At time of the analysis of the 3-year disease free survival, which was the primary endpoint of the MOSAIC trial, 85.1% of the patients were still alive in the FOLFOX4 arm versus 83.8% in the LV5FU2 arm. This translated into an overall reduction in mortality risk of 10% in favour of FOLFOX4 not reaching statistical significance (hazard ratio = 0.90). The figures were 92.2% versus 92.4% in the stage II (Duke's B2) sub-population (hazard ratio = 1.01) and 80.4% versus 78.1% in the stage III (Duke's C) sub-population (hazard ratio = 0.87), for FOLFOX4 and LV5FU2, respectively.

5.2 Pharmacokinetic properties

The pharmacokinetics of individual active compounds have not been determined. The pharmacokinetics of ultrafiltrable platinum, representing a mixture of all unbound, active and inactive platinum species, following a two-hour infusion of oxaliplatin at 130 mg/m² every three weeks for 1 to 5 cycles and oxaliplatin at 85 mg/m² every two weeks for 1 to 3 cycles are as follows:

Summary of Platinum Pharmacokinetic Parameter Estimates in Ultrafiltrate

Following Multiple Doses of Oxaliplatin at 85 mg/m² Every Two Weeks or at 130 mg/m² Every Three Weeks

(see Table 10 on page 832)

Mean AUC_{0-48}, and C_{max} values were determined on Cycle 3 (85 mg/m²) or cycle 5 (130 mg/m_2).

Mean AUC, V_{ss}, CL, and CL_{R0-48} values were determined on Cycle 1.

C_{end}, C_{max}, AUC, AUC_{0-48}, V_{ss} and CL values were determined by non-compartmental analysis.

$t_{1/2\alpha}$, $t_{1/2\beta}$, and $t_{1/2\gamma}$, were determined by compartmental analysis (Cycles 1-3 combined).

At the end of a 2-hour infusion, 15% of the administered platinum is present in the systemic circulation, the remaining 85% being rapidly distributed into tissues or eliminated in the urine. Irreversible binding to red blood cells and plasma, results in half-lives in these matrices that are close to the natural turnover of red blood cells and serum albumin. No accumulation was observed in plasma ultrafiltrate following 85 mg/m² every two weeks or 130 mg/m²

Table 6 Response rate under FOLFOX4 versus LV5FU2

Response rate, % (95% CI) independent radiological review ITT analysis	LV5FU2	FOLFOX4	Oxaliplatin Single agent
Front-line treatment EFC2962	22 (16-27)	49 (42-46)	NA*
Response assessment every 8weeks	P value = 0.0001		
Pretreated patients EFC4584 (refractory to CPT-11 + 5-FU/FA)	0.7 (0.0-2.7)	11.1 (7.6-15.5)	1.1 (0.2-3.2)
Response assessment every 6 weeks	P value < 0.0001		
Pretreated patients EFC2964 (refractory to 5-FU/FA) Response assessment every 12weeks	NA*	23 (13-36)	NA*

* NA: Not Applicable

Table 7 Median Progression Free Survival (PFS) / Median Time to Progression (TTP) FOLFOX4 versus LV5FU2

Median PFS/TTP, Months (95% CI) independent radiological review ITT analysis	LV5FU2	FOLFOX4	Oxaliplatin Single agent
Front-line treatment EFC2962 (PFS)	6.0 (5.5-6.5)	8.2 (7.2-8.8)	NA*
	Log-rank P value = 0.0003		
Pretreated patients EFC4584 (TTP) (refractory to CPT-11 + 5-FU/FA)	2.6 (1.8-2.9)	5.3 (4.7-6.1)	2.1 (1.6-2.7)
	Log-rank P value <0.0001		
Pretreated patients EFC2964 (refractory to 5-FU/FA)	NA*	5.1 (3.1-5.7)	NA*

* NA: Not Applicable

Table 8 Median Overall Survival (OS) under FOLFOX4 versus LV5FU2

Median OS, months (95% CI) ITT analysis	LV5FU2	FOLFOX4	Oxaliplatin Single agent
Front-line treatment EFC2962	14.7 (13.0-18.2)	16.2 (14.7-18.2)	NA*
	Log-rank P value = 0.12		
Pretreated patients EFC4584 (refractory to CPT-11 + 5-FU/FA)	8.8 (7.3 - 9.3)	9.9 (9.1-10.5)	8.1 (7.2-8.7)
	Log-rank P value = 0.09		
Pretreated patients EFC2964 (refractory to 5-FU/FA)	NA*	10.8 (9.3-12.8)	NA*

*NA: Not Applicable

Table 9 EFC 3313 3-year Disease Free Survival (ITT analysis)* according to Stage of disease

Patient stage	Stage II (Duke's B2)		Stage III (Duke's C)	
Treatment arm	LV5FU2	FOLFOX4	LV5FU2	FOLFOX4
Percent 3-year disease free survival (95% CI)	84.3 (80.9-87.7)	87.4 (84.3-90.5)	65.8 (62.2-69.5)	72.8 (69.4-76.2)
Hazard ratio (95% CI)	0.79 (0.57-1.09)		0.75 (0.62-0.90)	
Log-rank test	P=0.151		P=0.002	

* median follow up 44.2 months (all patients followed for at least 3 years)

every three weeks and steady state was attained by cycle one in this matrix. Inter- and intra-subject variability is generally low.

Biotransformation *in vitro* is considered to be the result of non-enzymatic degradation and there is no evidence of cytochrome P450-mediated metabolism of the diaminocyclohexane (DACH) ring.

Oxaliplatin undergoes extensive biotransformation in patients, and no intact drug was detectable in plasma ultrafiltrate at the end of a 2h-infusion. Several cytotoxic biotransformation products including the monochloro-, dichloro- and diaquo-DACH platinum species have been identified in the systemic circulation together with a number of inactive conjugates at later time points.

Platinum is predominantly excreted in urine, with clearance mainly in the 48 hours following administration.

By day 5, approximately 54% of the total dose was recovered in the urine and < 3% in the faeces.

A significant decrease in clearance from 17.6 ± 2.18 l/h to 9.95 ± 1.91 l/h in renal impairment was observed together with a statistically significant decrease in distribution volume from 330 ± 40.9 to 241 ± 36.1 l. The effect of severe renal impairment on platinum clearance has not been evaluated.

5.3 Preclinical safety data

The target organs identified in preclinical species (mice, rats, dogs, and/or monkeys) in single- and multiple-dose studies included the bone marrow, the gastrointestinal system, the kidney, the testes, the nervous system, and the heart. The target organ toxicities observed in animals are consistent with those produced by other platinum-containing drugs and DNA-damaging, cytotoxic drugs used in the treatment of human cancers with the exception of the effects produced on the heart. Effects on the heart were observed only in the dog and included electrophysiological disturbances with lethal ventricular fibrillation. Cardiotoxicity is considered specific to the dog not only because it was observed in the dog alone but also because doses similar to those producing lethal cardiotoxicity in dogs (150 mg/m^2) were well-tolerated by humans. Preclinical studies using rat sensory neurons suggest that the acute neurosensory symptoms related to Oxaliplatin may involve an interaction with voltage-gated Na^+ channels.

Oxaliplatin was mutagenic and clastogenic in mammalian test systems and produced embryo-fetal toxicity in rats. Oxaliplatin is considered a probable carcinogen, although carcinogenic studies have not been conducted.

6. PHARMACEUTICAL PARTICULARS

6.1 List of excipients

Lactose monohydrate.

6.2 Incompatibilities

- DO NOT use in association with alkaline drugs or solutions (in particular 5-fluorouracil, basic solutions, trometamol and folinic acid products containing trometamol as an excipient).

- DO NOT reconstitute or dilute for infusion with saline solution.

- DO NOT mix with other drugs in the same infusion bag or infusion line (see Section 6.6 for instructions concerning simultaneous administration with folinic acid).

- DO NOT use injection equipment containing aluminium.

6.3 Shelf life

Medicinal product as packaged for sale: 3 years

Reconstituted solution in the original vial:

From a microbiological and chemical point of view, the reconstituted solution should be diluted immediately.

Infusion preparation:

Chemical and physical in-use stability has been demonstrated for 24 hours at 2°C to 8°C.

From a microbiological point of view, the infusion preparation should be used immediately.

If not used immediately, in-use storage times and conditions prior to use are the responsibility of the user and would normally not be longer than 24 hours at 2°C to 8°C unless dilution has taken place in controlled and validated aseptic conditions.

6.4 Special precautions for storage

Medicinal product as packaged for sale: no special storage conditions are required

Reconstituted solution: should be diluted immediately.

Infusion preparation: store at 2°C to 8°C for not longer than 24 hours.

Inspect visually prior to use. Only clear solutions without particles should be used.

The medicinal product is for single use only. Any unused solution should be discarded.

6.5 Nature and contents of container

36 ml glass vial with stopper of chlorobutyl elastomer, containing 50 mg of oxaliplatin.

50 ml glass vial with stopper of chlorobutyl elastomer, containing 100 mg of oxaliplatin.

Not all pack sizes may be marketed.

6.6 Instructions for use and handling

As with other potentially toxic compounds, caution should be exercised when handling and preparing oxaliplatin solutions.

Instructions for Handling

The handling of this cytotoxic agent by nursing or medical personnel requires every precaution to guarantee the protection of the handler and his surroundings.

The preparation of injectable solutions of cytotoxic agents must be carried out by trained specialist personnel with knowledge of the medicines used, in conditions that guarantee the protection of the environment and in particular the protection of the personnel handling the medicines. It requires a preparation area reserved for this purpose. It is forbidden to smoke, eat or drink in this area.

Personnel must be provided with appropriate handling materials, notably long sleeved gowns, protection masks, caps, protective goggles, sterile single-use gloves, protective covers for the work area, containers and collection bags for waste.

Excreta and vomit must be handled with care.

Pregnant women must be warned to avoid handling cytotoxic agents.

Any broken container must be treated with the same precautions and considered as contaminated waste. Contaminated waste should be incinerated in suitably labelled rigid containers. See below section "Disposal".

If oxaliplatin concentrate, reconstituted solution or infusion solution, should come into contact with skin, wash immediately and thoroughly with water.

If oxaliplatin concentrate, premix solution or infusion solution, should come into contact with mucous membranes, wash immediately and thoroughly with water.

Table 10 Summary of Platinum Pharmacokinetic Parameter Estimates in Ultrafiltrate Following Multiple Doses of Oxaliplatin at 85 mg/m^2 Every Two Weeks or at 130 mg/m^2 Every Three Weeks

Dose	C_{max}	AUC_{0-48}	AUC	$t_{1/2}\alpha$	$t_{1/2}\beta$	$t_{1/2}\gamma$	V_{ss}	CL
	μ g/mL	μ g.h/mL	μ g.h/mL	h	h	h	L	L/h
85 mg/m^2 Mean	0.814	4.19	4.68	0.43	16.8	391	440	17.4
SD	0.193	0.647	1.40	0.35	5.74	406	199	6.35
130 mg/m^2 Mean	1.21	8.20	11.9	0.28	16.3	273	582	10.1
SD	0.10	2.40	4.60	0.06	2.90	19.0	261	3.07

-Special precautions for administration

- DO NOT use injection material containing aluminium.

- DO NOT administer undiluted.

- DO NOT reconstitute or dilute for infusion with saline solution.

- DO NOT mix with any other medication in the same infusion bag or administer simultaneously by the same infusion line (in particular 5-fluorouracil, basic solutions, trometamol and folinic acid products containing trometamol as an excipient)

Oxaliplatin can be co-administered with folinic acid infusion using a Y-line placed immediately before the site of injection. The drugs should not be combined in the same infusion bag. Folinic acid must be diluted using isotonic infusion solutions such as 5% glucose solution but NOT sodium chloride solutions or alkaline solutions.

Flush the line after oxaliplatin administration.

- USE ONLY the recommended solvents (see below).

- Any reconstituted solution that shows evidence of precipitation should not be used and should be destroyed with due regard to legal requirements for disposal of hazardous waste (see below).

Reconstitution of the solution

– Water for injections or 5% glucose solution should be used to reconstitute the solution.

– For a vial of 50 mg: add 10 ml of solvent to obtain a concentration of 5 mg oxaliplatin/ml.

– For a vial of 100 mg: add 20 ml of solvent to obtain a concentration of 5 mg oxaliplatin/ml.

From a microbiological and chemical point of view, the reconstituted solution should be diluted immediately with 5% glucose solution.

Inspect visually prior to use. Only clear solutions without particles should be used.

The medicinal product is for single use only. Any unused solution should be discarded.

Dilution before infusion

Withdraw the required amount of reconstituted solution from the vial(s) and then dilute with 250 ml to 500 ml of a 5% glucose solution to give an oxaliplatin concentration not less than 0.2 mg/ml.

Administer by IV infusion.

Chemical and physical in-use stability has been demonstrated for 24 hours at 2°C to 8°C.

From a microbiological point of view, this infusion preparation should be used immediately.

If not used immediately, in-use storage times and conditions prior to use are the responsibility of the user and would normally not be longer than 24 hours at 2°C to 8°C unless dilution has taken place in controlled and validated aseptic conditions.

Inspect visually prior to use. Only clear solutions without particles should be used.

The medicinal product is for single use only. Any unused solution should be discarded.

NEVER use sodium chloride solution for either reconstitution or dilution.

Infusion

The administration of oxaliplatin does not require prehydration.

Oxaliplatin diluted in 250 to 500 ml of a 5% glucose solution to give a concentration not less than 0.2 mg/ml must be infused either by peripheral vein or central venous line over 2 to 6 hours. When oxaliplatin is administered with 5-fluorouracil, the oxaliplatin infusion should precede that of 5-fluorouracil.

Disposal

Remnants of the medicinal product as well as all materials that have been used for reconstitution, for dilution and administration must be destroyed according to hospital standard procedures applicable to cytotoxic agentswith due regard to current laws related to the disposal of hazardous waste.

7. MARKETING AUTHORISATION HOLDER

Sanofi-Synthelabo
PO Box 597
Guildford
Surrey

8. MARKETING AUTHORISATION NUMBER(S)

PL 11723/0288

9. DATE OF FIRST AUTHORISATION/RENEWAL OF THE AUTHORISATION

12 April 2001

10. DATE OF REVISION OF THE TEXT

September 2004

Legal Category:

POM

Emcor, Emcor LS

(Merck Pharmaceuticals)

1. NAME OF THE MEDICINAL PRODUCT

Emcor LS, Emcor

2. QUALITATIVE AND QUANTITATIVE COMPOSITION

Each Emcor LS tablet contains 5 mg bisoprolol fumarate (2:1)

Each Emcor tablet contains 10mg bisoprolol fumarate (2:1)

3. PHARMACEUTICAL FORM

Tablets

4. CLINICAL PARTICULARS

4.1 Therapeutic indications

(i) Management of hypertension

(ii) Management of angina pectoris

4.2 Posology and method of administration

Adults: The usual dose is 10 mg once daily with a maximum recommended dose of 20 mg per day. In some patients 5 mg per day may be adequate. In patients with final stage impairment of renal function (creatinine clearance < 20 ml/min) or liver function, the dose should not exceed 10 mg bisoprolol once daily.

Elderly: No dosage adjustment is normally required, but 5 mg per day may be adequate in some patients; as for other adults, dosage may have to be reduced in cases of severe renal or hepatic dysfunction.

Children: There is no paediatric experience with bisoprolol, therefore its use cannot be recommended for children.

Route of administration: Oral

4.3 Contraindications

Bisoprolol is contra-indicated in patients with:

- acute heart failure or during episodes of heart failure decompensation requiring i.v. inotropic therapy
- cardiogenic shock
- second or third degree AV block (without a pacemaker)
- sick sinus syndrome
- sinoatrial block
- bradycardia (heart rate less than 60 beats/min prior to start of therapy)
- hypotension (systolic blood pressure < 100mmHg)
- severe bronchial asthma or severe chronic obstructive pulmonary disease
- late stages of peripheral arterial occlusive disease and Raynaud's syndrome
- untreated phaeochromocytoma (see Special Warnings and Precautions)
- metabolic acidosis
- hypersensitivity to bisoprolol or to any of the excipients

4.4 Special warnings and special precautions for use

Bisoprolol must be used with caution in:

- heart failure (the treatment of stable chronic heart failure with bisoprolol has to be initiated with a special titration phase [for details, see SPC for bisoprolol indicated for the treatment of stable chronic heart failure])
- bronchospasm (bronchial asthma, obstructive airways diseases)
- concomitant treatment with inhalation anaesthetics (see Interactions section)
- diabetes mellitus with large fluctuations in blood glucose values; symptoms of hypoglycaemia can be masked
- strict fasting
- ongoing desensitisation therapy
- AV block of first degree
- Prinzmetal's angina
- peripheral arterial occlusive disease (intensification of complaints may occur particularly during the start of therapy)

In bronchial asthma or other chronic obstructive lung diseases, which may cause symptoms, bronchodilating therapy should be given concomitantly. Occasionally an increase of the airway resistance may occur in patients with asthma, therefore the dose of β_2-stimulants may have to be increased.

As with other β-blockers, bisoprolol may increase both the sensitivity towards allergens and the severity of anaphylactic reactions. Adrenaline treatment does not always give the expected therapeutic effect.

Patients with psoriasis or with a history of psoriasis should only be given β-blockers (e.g. bisoprolol) after carefully balancing the benefits against the risks.

In patients with phaeochromocytoma bisoprolol must not be administered until after alpha-receptor blockade.

Under treatment with bisoprolol the symptoms of a thyrotoxicosis may be masked.

In patients with ischaemic heart disease, treatment should not be withdrawn abruptly.

Combination with calcium antagonists, clonidine or monoamine oxidase inhibitors (except MAO-B inhibitors) is not recommended. See 'Interactions' section.

4.5 Interaction with other medicinal products and other forms of Interaction

Combinations not recommended

Calcium antagonists such as verapamil and to a lesser extent diltiazem: Negative influence on contractility, atrio-ventricular conduction and blood pressure. Intravenous administration of verapamil in patients on beta-blocker treatment may lead to profound hypotension and atrioventricular block.

Clonidine: Increased risk of "rebound hypertension" as well as exaggerated decrease in heart rate and cardiac conduction.

Monoamineoxidase inhibitors (except MAO-B inhibitors): Enhanced hypotensive effect of β-blockers but also risk of hypertensive crisis.

Combinations to be used with caution

Calcium antagonists such as dihydropyridine derivatives (eg, nifedipine): increased risk of hypotension. In patients with latent cardiac insufficiency, concomitant treatment with beta-blocking agents may lead to cardiac failure.

Class-I antiarrhythmic drugs (e.g. disopyramide, quinidine): Effect on atrial conduction time may be potentiated and negative inotropic effect may be increased.

Class-III antiarrhythmic drugs (e.g. amiodarone): Effect on atrial conduction time may be potentiated.

Parasympathomimetic drugs: Atrio-ventricular conduction time may be increased.

Other β-blockers, including eye drops, have additive effects.

Insulin and oral antidiabetic drugs: Intensification of blood sugar lowering effect. Blockade of β-adrenoceptors may mask symptoms of hypoglycaemia.

Anaesthetic agents: Attenuation of the reflex tachycardia and increase of the risk of hypotension. Continuation of β-blockade reduces the risk of arrhythmia during induction and intubation. The anaesthesiologist should be informed when the patient is receiving bisoprolol.

Digitalis glycosides: Reduction of heart rate, increase of atrio-ventricular conduction time.

Prostaglandin synthetase inhibiting drugs: Decreased hypotensive effects.

Ergotamine derivatives: Exacerbation of peripheral circulatory disturbances.

Sympathomimetic agents: Combination with bisoprolol may reduce the effect of both agents. Higher doses of epinephrine may be necessary for treatment of allergic reactions.

Tricyclic antidepressants, barbiturates, phenothiazines as well as other antihypertensive agents: Increased blood pressure lowering effect.

Rifampicin: Slight reduction of the half-life of bisoprolol possible due to the induction of hepatic drug-metabolising enzymes. Normally no dosage adjustment is necessary.

Moxisylyte: Possibly causes severe postural hypertension.

Combinations to be considered

Mefloquine: increased risk of bradycardia

4.6 Pregnancy and lactation

Pregnancy

Bisoprolol has pharmacological effects that may cause harmful effects on pregnancy and/or the foetus/newborn. In general, β-adrenoceptor blockers reduce placental perfusion, which has been associated with growth retardation, intrauterine death, abortion or early labour. Adverse effects (e.g. hypoglycaemia and bradycardia) may occur in the foetus and newborn infant. If treatment with β-adrenoceptor blockers is necessary, β_1-selective adrenoceptor blockers are preferable.

Bisoprolol should not be used during pregnancy unless clearly necessary. If treatment with bisoprolol is considered necessary, the uteroplacental blood flow and the foetal growth should be monitored. In case of harmful effects on pregnancy or the foetus alternative treatment should be considered. The newborn infant must be closely monitored. Symptoms of hypoglycaemia and bradycardia are generally to be expected within the first 3 days.

Lactation

It is not known whether this drug is excreted in human milk. Therefore, breastfeeding is not recommended during administration of bisoprolol.

4.7 Effects on ability to drive and use machines

In a study of coronary heart disease patients, bisoprolol did not impair driving performance. However, due to individual variations in reactions to the drug, the ability to drive a vehicle or to operate machinery may be impaired. This should be considered particularly at the start of treatment and upon change of medication as well as in conjunction with alcohol.

4.8 Undesirable effects

Common ($\geq$1% and <10%)	*Circ:* Feeling of coldness or numbness in the extremities *CNS:* Tiredness*, exhaustion*, dizziness*, headache* *GI:* Nausea, vomiting, diarrhoea, constipation
Uncommon ($\geq$0.1% and <1%)	*General:* Muscular weakness and cramps *Circ:* Bradycardia, disturbance of AV conduction, worsening of heart failure, orthostatic hypotension *CNS:* Sleep disturbances, depression *Airways:* Bronchospasm in patients with bronchial asthma or a history of obstructive airways disease.
Rare ($\geq$0.01% and <0.1%)	*CNS:* Nightmares, hallucinations *Skin:* hypersensitivity reactions (itching, flush, rash) *Liver:* increased liver enzymes (ALAT, ASAT), hepatitis *Metabolism:* Increased triglycerides *Urogenital:* Potency disorders *Ear-nose-throat:* hearing impairment, allergic rhinitis *Eyes:* reduced tear flow (to be considered if the patient uses lenses)
Very rare (< 0.01%)	*Eyes:* conjunctivitis, visual disturbances *Skin:* β-blockers may provoke or worsen psoriasis or induce psoriasis-like rash, alopecia *Circ:* chest pain

* These symptoms especially occur at the beginning of the therapy. They are generally mild and often disappear within 1-2 weeks.

4.9 Overdose

The most common signs expected with overdosage of a β-blocker are bradycardia, hypotension, bronchospasm, acute cardiac insufficiency and hypoglycaemia. To date a few cases of overdose (maximum: 2000 mg) with bisoprolol have been reported. Bradycardia and/or hypotension were noted. All patients recovered. There is a wide interindividual variation in sensitivity to one single high dose of bisoprolol.

In general, if overdose occurs, bisoprolol treatment should be stopped and supportive and symptomatic treatment should be provided. Limited data suggest that bisoprolol is hardly dialysable. Based on the expected pharmacological actions and recommendations for other β-blockers, the following general measures should be considered when clinically warranted.

Bradycardia: Administer intravenous atropine. If the response is inadequate, isoprenaline or another agent with positive chronotropic properties may be given cautiously. Under some circumstances, transvenous pacemaker insertion may be necessary.

Hypotension: Intravenous fluids and vasopressors should be administered. Intravenous glucagon may be useful.

AV block (second or third degree): Patients should be carefully monitored and treated with isoprenaline infusion or transvenous cardiac pacemaker insertion.

Acute worsening of heart failure: Administer i.v. diuretics, inotropic agents, vasodilating agents.

Bronchospasm: Administer bronchodilator therapy such as isoprenaline, β_2-sympathomimetic drugs and/or aminophylline.

Hypoglycaemia: Administer i.v. glucose.

5. PHARMACOLOGICAL PROPERTIES

5.1 Pharmacodynamic properties

Bisoprolol is a potent, highly β1-selective adrenoreceptor blocking agent devoid of intrinsic sympathomimetic activity and without relevant membrane stabilising activity.

As with other β1-blocking agents, the mode of action in hypertension is not clear but it is known that bisoprolol markedly depresses plasma renin levels.

In patients with angina, the blockade of β1-receptors reduces heart action and thus reduces oxygen demand. Hence bisoprolol is effective in eliminating or reducing the symptoms.

5.2 Pharmacokinetic properties

Bisoprolol is absorbed almost completely from the gastrointestinal tract. Together with the very small first pass effect in the liver, this results in a high bioavailability of approximately 90%. The drug is cleared equally by the liver and kidney.

The plasma elimination half-life (10-12 hours) provides 24 hours efficacy following a once daily dosage. About 95% of the drug substance is excreted through the kidney, half of this is as unchanged bisoprolol. There are no active metabolites in man.

5.3 Preclinical safety data

-

6. PHARMACEUTICAL PARTICULARS

6.1 List of excipients

Tablet core: Silica, colloidal anhydrous; magnesium stearate, crospovidone, microcrystalline cellulose, maize starch, calcium hydrogen phosphate, anhydrous.

Film coating: Iron oxide yellow (E172), Iron oxide red (E172) (10mg only), dimeticone, macrogol 400, titanium dioxide (E171), hypromellose.

6.2 Incompatibilities

None

6.3 Shelf life

4 years

6.4 Special precautions for storage

No special requirement.

6.5 Nature and contents of container

Cartons containing blister packs of 28 tablets.

6.6 Instructions for use and handling

None

7. MARKETING AUTHORISATION HOLDER

E. Merck Ltd

t/a Merck Pharmaceuticals (A Division of Merck Ltd)

Harrier House

High Street

West Drayton

Middlesex

UB7 7QG

8. MARKETING AUTHORISATION NUMBER(S)

Emcor LS PL 0493/0126

Emcor PL 0493/0127

9. DATE OF FIRST AUTHORISATION/RENEWAL OF THE AUTHORISATION

11 February 1988 / 11 February 1993

10. DATE OF REVISION OF THE TEXT

20 December 2002

Legal category

POM

EMEND 80 mg, 125 mg hard capsules

(Merck Sharp & Dohme Limited)

1. NAME OF THE MEDICINAL PRODUCT

EMEND 125 mg hard capsule▼

EMEND 80 mg hard capsules▼

2. QUALITATIVE AND QUANTITATIVE COMPOSITION

Each 125 mg capsule contains 125 mg of aprepitant. Each 80 mg capsule contains 80 mg of aprepitant.

For excipients, see section 6.1.

3. PHARMACEUTICAL FORM

Hard capsule

The 125 mg capsule is opaque with a white body and pink cap with "462" and "125 mg" printed radially in black ink on the body. The 80 mg capsules are opaque with a white body and cap with "461" and "80 mg" printed radially in black ink on the body.

4. CLINICAL PARTICULARS

4.1 Therapeutic indications

Prevention of acute and delayed nausea and vomiting associated with highly emetogenic cisplatin-based cancer chemotherapy.

Prevention of nausea and vomiting associated with moderately emetogenic cancer chemotherapy.

EMEND is given as part of combination therapy (see section 4.2).

4.2 Posology and method of administration

EMEND is available as an 80 mg and a 125 mg hard capsule.

EMEND is given for 3 days as part of a regimen that includes a corticosteroid and a 5-HT_3 antagonist. The recommended dose of EMEND is 125 mg orally Day 1 and 80 mg once daily Days 2 and 3.

In clinical studies, the following regimens were used for the prevention of nausea and vomiting associated with emetogenic cancer chemotherapy:

Highly Emetogenic Chemotherapy Regimen

(see Table 1 below)

EMEND was administered orally 1 hour prior to chemotherapy treatment on Day 1 and in the morning on Days 2 and 3. Dexamethasone was administered 30 minutes prior to chemotherapy treatment on Day 1 and in the morning on Days 2 to 4. The dose of dexamethasone was chosen to account for medicinal product interactions.

Ondansetron was administered intravenously 30 minutes prior to chemotherapy treatment on Day 1.

Moderately Emetogenic Chemotherapy Regimen

(see Table 2 below)

EMEND was administered orally 1 hour prior to chemotherapy treatment on Day 1 and in the morning on Days 2 and 3. Dexamethasone was administered 30 minutes prior to chemotherapy treatment on Day 1. The dose of dexamethasone was chosen to account for medicinal product interactions.

One 8 mg capsule of Ondansetron was administered 30 to 60 minutes prior to chemotherapy treatment and one 8 mg capsule was administered 8 hours after first dose on Day 1.

Efficacy data on combination with other corticosteroids and 5-HT_3 antagonists are limited. For additional information on the administration of EMEND with corticosteroids, see section 4.5.

Table 1 Highly Emetogenic Chemotherapy Regimen

	Day 1	Day 2	Day 3	Day 4
EMEND	125 mg	80 mg	80 mg	none
Dexamethasone	12 mg orally	8 mg orally	8 mg orally	8 mg orally
Ondansetron	32 mg IV	none	none	none

Table 2 Moderately Emetogenic Chemotherapy Regimen

	Day 1	Day 2	Day 3
EMEND	125 mg	80 mg	80 mg
Dexamethasone	12 mg orally	none	none
Ondansetron	2 × 8 mg orally	none	none

Refer to the full product information for coadministered antiemetic agents.

EMEND may be taken with or without food.

The hard capsule should be swallowed whole.

Elderly

No dosage adjustment is necessary for the elderly.

Renal Impairment

No dosage adjustment is necessary for patients with renal insufficiency or for patients with end stage renal disease undergoing haemodialysis (see section 5.2).

Hepatic Impairment

No dosage adjustment is necessary for patients with mild hepatic insufficiency. There are limited data in patients with moderate hepatic insufficiency and no data in patients with severe hepatic insufficiency (see sections 4.4 and 5.2).

Children and adolescents

Safety and efficacy have not been established in children and adolescents. Therefore, use in patients under 18 years of age is not recommended.

4.3 Contraindications

Hypersensitivity to the active substance or to any of the excipients.

EMEND must not be administered concurrently with pimozide, terfenadine, astemizole or cisapride. Inhibition of cytochrome P450 isoenzyme 3A4 (CYP3A4) by aprepitant could result in elevated plasma concentrations of these medicinal products, potentially causing serious or life-threatening reactions (see section 4.5).

4.4 Special warnings and special precautions for use

There are limited data in patients with moderate hepatic insufficiency and no data in patients with severe hepatic insufficiency. Aprepitant should be used with caution in these patients (see section 5.2).

EMEND should be used with caution in patients receiving concomitant medicinal products that are metabolised primarily through CYP3A4 (see section 4.5). Caution is advised both during and up to 2 weeks after the end of treatment with EMEND due to the inhibitory and inductive effects of aprepitant on CYP3A4 substrates (see section 4.5). Consequently, chemotherapeutic agents metabolised via CYP3A4 should be used with caution (see section 4.5). Additionally, concomitant administration with irinotecan should be approached with particular caution as the combination might result in increased toxicity. Furthermore, the extent of induction following concomitant administration of EMEND and dexamethasone, an inducer of CYP3A4 by itself, has not been investigated.

Coadministration of EMEND with ergot alkaloid derivatives, which are CYP3A4 substrates, may result in elevated plasma concentrations of these medicinal products. Therefore, caution is advised due to the potential risk of ergot-related toxicity.

Coadministration of EMEND with warfarin results in decreased prothrombin time, reported as International Normalised Ratio (INR). In patients on chronic warfarin therapy, the INR should be monitored closely during 2 weeks following initiation of each 3-day course of EMEND (see section 4.5).

The efficacy of hormonal contraceptives may be reduced during and for 28 days after administration of EMEND. Alternative or back-up methods of contraception should be used during treatment with EMEND and for 2 months following the last dose of EMEND (see section 4.5).

Concomitant administration of EMEND with medicinal products that strongly induce CYP3A4 activity (e.g. rifampicin, phenytoin, carbamazepine, phenobarbital) should be avoided as the combination results in reductions of the plasma concentrations of aprepitant (see section 4.5). Concomitant administration of EMEND with St. John's wort is not recommended.

Concomitant administration of EMEND with medicinal products that inhibit CYP3A4 activity (e.g. ritonavir, ketoconazole, clarithromycin, telithromycin) should be approached cautiously as the combination results in increased plasma concentrations of aprepitant (see section 4.5).

Patients with rare hereditary problems of fructose intolerance, glucose-galactose malabsorption or sucrase-isomaltase insufficiency should not take this medicine.

4.5 Interaction with other medicinal products and other forms of Interaction

Aprepitant is a substrate, a moderate inhibitor, and an inducer of CYP3A4. Aprepitant is also an inducer of CYP2C9.

Effect of aprepitant on the pharmacokinetics of other agents

As a moderate inhibitor of CYP3A4, aprepitant can increase plasma concentrations of coadministered medicinal products that are metabolised through CYP3A4. The AUC of orally administered CYP3A4 substrates may increase up to approximately 3-fold; the effect of aprepitant on the plasma concentrations of intravenously administered CYP3A4 substrates is expected to be smaller. Caution is advised during concomitant administration with CYP3A4 substrates.

EMEND must not be used concurrently with pimozide, terfenadine, astemizole, or cisapride. Inhibition of CYP3A4 by aprepitant could result in elevated plasma concentrations of these medicinal products, potentially causing serious or life-threatening reactions.

As an inducer of CYP3A4, aprepitant can decrease plasma concentrations of intravenously administered CYP3A4 substrates within 2 weeks following initiation of dosing with EMEND. This effect may become apparent only after the end of treatment with EMEND. The inductive effect of aprepitant on orally administered CYP3A4 substrates has not been studied, but is expected to be larger. Caution is advised when oral medicinal products metabolised by CYP3A4 are administered during this time period.

Aprepitant has been shown to induce the metabolism of S(-) warfarin and tolbutamide, which are metabolised through CYP2C9. Coadministration of EMEND with these medicinal products or other medicinal products that are known to be metabolised by CYP2C9, such as phenytoin, may result in lower plasma concentrations of these medicinal products; therefore caution is advised.

EMEND does not seem to interact with the P-glycoprotein transporter, as demonstrated by the lack of interaction of EMEND with digoxin.

Corticosteroids:

Dexamethasone: The usual oral dexamethasone dose should be reduced by approximately 50 % when coadministered with EMEND. The dose of dexamethasone in clinical trials was chosen to account for medicinal product interactions (see section 4.2). EMEND, when given as a regimen of 125 mg with dexamethasone coadministered orally as 20 mg on Day 1, and EMEND when given as 80 mg/day with dexamethasone coadministered orally as 8 mg on Days 2 through 5, increased the AUC of dexamethasone, a CYP3A4 substrate, 2.2-fold on Days 1 and 5.

Methylprednisolone: The usual intravenously administered methylprednisolone dose should be reduced approximately 25 %, and the usual oral methylprednisolone dose should be reduced approximately 50 % when coadministered with EMEND. EMEND, when given as a regimen of 125 mg on Day 1 and 80 mg/day on Days 2 and 3, increased the AUC of methylprednisolone, a CYP3A4 substrate, by 1.3-fold on Day 1 and by 2.5-fold on Day 3, when methylprednisolone was coadministered intravenously as 125 mg on Day 1 and orally as 40 mg on Days 2 and 3.

During continuous treatment with methylprednisolone, the AUC of methylprednisolone may decrease at later time points within 2 weeks following initiation of dosing with EMEND, due to the inducing effect of aprepitant on CYP3A4. This effect may be expected to be more pronounced for orally administered methylprednisolone.

Chemotherapeutic agents: In clinical studies, EMEND was administered with the following chemotherapeutic agents metabolised primarily or in part by CYP3A4: etoposide, vinorelbine, docetaxel, and paclitaxel. The doses of these agents were not adjusted to account for potential medicinal product interactions. Caution is advised and additional monitoring may be appropriate in patients receiving such agents (see section 4.4).

Docetaxel: In a clinical study, EMEND, when given as a regimen of 125 mg on Day 1 and 80 mg/day on days 2 and 3, did not influence the pharmacokinetics of docetaxel administered intravenously on Day 1.

Midazolam:The potential effects of increased plasma concentrations of midazolam or other benzodiazepines metabolised via CYP3A4 (alprazolam, triazolam) should be considered when coadministering these agents with EMEND.

EMEND increased the AUC of midazolam, a sensitive CYP3A4 substrate, 2.3-fold on Day 1 and 3.3-fold on Day 5, when a single oral dose of midazolam 2 mg was coadministered on Days 1 and 5 of a regimen of EMEND 125 mg on Day 1 and 80 mg/day on Days 2 to 5.

In another study with intravenous administration of midazolam, EMEND was given as 125 mg on Day 1 and 80 mg/day on Days 2 and 3, and midazolam 2 mg was given intravenously prior to the administration of the 3-day regimen of EMEND and on Days 4, 8, and 15. EMEND increased the AUC of midazolam 25 % on Day 4 and decreased the AUC of midazolam 19 % on Day 8 and 4 % on Day 15. These effects were not considered clinically important.

Warfarin: In patients on chronic warfarin therapy, the prothrombin time (INR) should be monitored closely for 2 weeks following initiation of each 3-day course of EMEND (see section 4.4). When a single 125-mg dose of EMEND was administered on Day 1 and 80 mg/day on Days 2 and 3 to healthy subjects who were stabilised on chronic warfarin therapy, there was no effect of EMEND on the plasma AUC of R(+) or S(-) warfarin determined on Day 3; however, there was a 34 % decrease in

S(-) warfarin (a CYP2C9 substrate) trough concentration accompanied by a 14 % decrease in INR 5 days after completion of dosing with EMEND.

Tolbutamide: EMEND, when given as 125 mg on Day 1 and 80 mg/day on Days 2 and 3, decreased the AUC of tolbutamide (a CYP2C9 substrate) by 23 % on Day 4, 28 % on Day 8, and 15 % on Day 15, when a single dose of tolbutamide 500 mg was administered orally prior to the administration of the 3-day regimen of EMEND and on Days 4, 8, and 15.

Oral contraceptives:The efficacy of hormonal contraceptives may be reduced during and for 28 days after administration of EMEND. Alternative or back-up methods of contraception should be used during treatment with EMEND and for 2 months following the last dose of EMEND. Aprepitant, when given once daily for 14 days as a 100-mg capsule with an oral contraceptive containing 35 mcg of ethinyl estradiol and 1 mg of norethindrone, decreased the AUC of ethinyl estradiol by 43 %, and decreased the AUC of norethindrone by 8 %.

In another study, single doses of an oral contraceptive containing ethinyl estradiol and norethindrone were administered on Days 1 through 21 with EMEND, given as a regimen of 125 mg on Day 8 and 80 mg/day on Days 9 and 10 with ondansetron 32 mg IV on Day 8 and oral dexamethasone given as 12 mg on Day 8 and 8 mg/day on Days 9, 10, and 11. During days 9 through 21 in this study, there was as much as a 64% decrease in ethinyl estradiol trough concentrations and as much as a 60% decrease in norethindrone trough concentrations.

*$5\text{-}HT_3$ antagonists*In clinical interaction studies, aprepitant did not have clinically important effects on the pharmacokinetics of ondansetron, granisetron or hydrodolasetron (the active metabolite of dolasetron).

Effect of other agents on the pharmacokinetics of aprepitant

Concomitant administration of EMEND with medicinal products that inhibit CYP3A4 activity (e.g., ritonavir, ketoconazole, clarithromycin, telithromycin) should be approached cautiously, as the combination results in increased plasma concentrations of aprepitant.

Concomitant administration of EMEND with medicinal products that strongly induce CYP3A4 activity (e.g. rifampicin, phenytoin, carbamazepine, phenobarbital) should be avoided as the combination results in reductions of the plasma concentrations of aprepitant that may result in decreased efficacy of EMEND. Concomitant administration of EMEND with St. John's wort is not recommended.

Ketoconazole: When a single 125-mg dose of EMEND was administered on Day 5 of a 10-day regimen of 400 mg/day of ketoconazole, a strong CYP3A4 inhibitor, the AUC of aprepitant increased approximately 5-fold and the mean terminal half-life of aprepitant increased approximately 3-fold.

Rifampicin: When a single 375-mg dose of EMEND was administered on Day 9 of a 14-day regimen of 600 mg/day of rifampicin, a strong CYP3A4 inducer, the AUC of aprepitant decreased 91 % and the mean terminal half-life decreased 68 %.

4.6 Pregnancy and lactation

EMEND should not be used during pregnancy unless clearly necessary. The potential for reproductive toxicity of aprepitant has not been fully characterized, since exposure levels above human exposure were not attained in animal studies. These studies did not indicate direct or indirect harmful effects with respect to pregnancy, embryonal/foetal development, parturition or postnatal development. The potential effects on reproduction of alterations in neurokinin regulation are unknown.

Aprepitant is excreted in the milk of lactating rats. It is not known whether aprepitant is excreted in human milk; therefore, breast-feeding is not recommended during treatment with EMEND.

4.7 Effects on ability to drive and use machines

There is no information to indicate that EMEND affects a patient's ability to drive or operate machinery; however, no studies have been performed.

4.8 Undesirable effects

The safety profile of aprepitant was evaluated in approximately 3,800 individuals.

Clinical adverse reactions defined as events considered to be drug related by the investigator were reported in approximately 17 % of patients treated with the aprepitant regimen compared with approximately 13 % of patients treated with standard therapy in patients receiving highly emetogenic chemotherapy. Aprepitant was discontinued due to adverse reactions in 0.6 % of patients treated with the aprepitant regimen compared with 0.4 % of patients treated with standard therapy. In a clinical study of patients receiving moderately emetogenic chemotherapy, clinical adverse reactions were reported in approximately 21% of patients treated with the aprepitant regimen compared with approximately 20% of patients treated with standard therapy. Aprepitant was discontinued due to adverse reactions in 1.1% of patients treated with the aprepitant regimen compared with 0.5% of patients treated with standard therapy.

The most common adverse reactions reported at a greater incidence in patients treated with the aprepitant regimen than with standard therapy in patients receiving highly emetogenic chemotherapy were: hiccups (4.6 %), asthenia/fatigue (2.9 %), ALT increased (2.8 %), constipation (2.2 %), headache (2.2 %), and anorexia (2.0 %). The most common adverse reaction reported at a greater incidence in patients treated with the aprepitant regimen than with standard therapy in patients receiving moderately emetogenic chemotherapy was fatigue (2.5 %).

The following adverse reactions were observed in patients treated with the aprepitant regimen and at a greater incidence than with standard therapy:

[Very common (> 1/10) Common (> 1/100, < 1/10) Uncommon (> 1/1,000, < 1/100) Rare (> 1/10,000, < 1/1,000) Very rare (< 1/10,000), including isolated reports]

Infection and infestations:

Uncommon: candidiasis, staphylococcal infection.

Blood and the lymphatic system disorders:

Uncommon: anaemia, febrile neutropenia.

Metabolism and nutrition disorders:

Common: anorexia

Uncommon: weight gain, polydipsia.

Psychiatric disorders:

Uncommon: disorientation, euphoria, anxiety.

Nervous system disorders:

Common: headache, dizziness

Uncommon: dream abnormality, cognitive disorder.

Eye disorders:

Uncommon: conjunctivitis.

Ear and labyrinth disorders:

Uncommon: tinnitus.

Cardiac disorders:

Uncommon: bradycardia.

Vascular disorders:

Uncommon: hot flush.

Respiratory, thoracic and mediastinal disorders:

Common: hiccups

Uncommon: pharyngitis, sneezing, cough, postnasal drip, throat irritation.

Gastrointestinal disorders:

Common: constipation, diarrhoea, dyspepsia, eructation

Uncommon: nausea*, vomiting*, acid reflux, dysgeusia, epigastric discomfort, obstipation, gastroesophageal reflux disease, perforating duodenal ulcer abdominal pain, dry mouth, enterocolitis, flatulence, stomatitis.

Skin and subcutaneous tissue disorders:

Uncommon: rash, acne, photosensitivity hyperhidrosis, oily skin, pruritus, skin lesion.

Musculoskeletal and connective tissue disorders:

Uncommon: muscle cramp, myalgia.

Renal and urinary disorders:

Uncommon: polyuria, dysuria, pollakiuria.

General disorders and administration site conditions:

Common: asthaenia/fatigue

Uncommon: abdominal pain, oedema, flushing, chest discomfort, lethargy, thirst.

Investigations:

Common: ALT increased, AST increased

Uncommon: alkaline phosphatase increased, hyperglycaemia, microscopic haematuria, hyponatraemia, weight decreased.

*Nausea and vomiting were efficacy parameters in the first 5 days post-chemotherapy treatment and were reported as adverse experiences only thereafter.

The adverse reactions profile in the Multiple-Cycle extension for up to 5 additional cycles of chemotherapy were generally similar to those observed in Cycle 1.

One case of Stevens-Johnson syndrome was reported as a serious adverse event in a patient receiving aprepitant with cancer chemotherapy. One case of angioedema and urticaria was reported as a serious adverse event in a patient receiving aprepitant in a non-CINV study.

4.9 Overdose

No specific information is available on the treatment of overdosage with EMEND.

Drowsiness and headache were reported in one patient who ingested 1,440 mg of aprepitant.

In the event of overdose, EMEND should be discontinued and general supportive treatment and monitoring should be provided. Because of the antiemetic activity of aprepitant, drug-induced emesis may not be effective.

Aprepitant cannot be removed by haemodialysis.

5. PHARMACOLOGICAL PROPERTIES

5.1 Pharmacodynamic properties

Pharmacotherapeutic group: Antiemetics and Antinauseants, ATC code: A04A D12

Aprepitant is a selective high-affinity antagonist at human substance P neurokinin 1 (NK_1) receptors.

In two randomised, double-blind studies encompassing a total of 1,094 patients receiving chemotherapy that included cisplatin $\geqslant$70 mg/m^2, aprepitant in combination with an ondansetron/dexamethasone regimen (see section 4.2) was compared with a standard regimen (placebo plus ondansetron 32 mg intravenously administered on Day 1 plus dexamethasone 20 mg orally on Day 1 and 8 mg orally twice daily on Days 2 to 4).

Efficacy was based on evaluation of the following composite measure: complete response (defined as no emetic episodes and no use of rescue therapy) primarily during Cycle 1. The results were evaluated for each individual study and for the 2 studies combined.

A summary of the key study results from the combined analysis is shown in Table 3.

Table 3 Percent of Patients Receiving Highly Emetogenic Chemotherapy Responding by Treatment Group and Phase —Cycle 1

(see Table 3)

The estimated time to first emesis in the combined analysis is depicted by the Kaplan-Meier plot in Figure 1.

Figure 1 Percent of Patients Receiving Highly Emetogenic Chemotherapy Who Remain Emesis Free Over Time - Cycle 1

(see Figure 1)

Statistically significant differences in efficacy were also observed in each of the 2 individual studies.

In the same 2 clinical studies, 851 patients continued into the Multiple-Cycle extension for up to 5 additional cycles of chemotherapy. The efficacy of the aprepitant regimen was apparently maintained during all cycles.

In a randomised, double-blind study in a total of 866 patients (864 females, 2 males) receiving chemotherapy that included cyclophosphamide 750-1500 mg/m^2; or cyclophosphamide 500-1500 mg/m^2 and doxorubicin ($\leqslant$60 mg/m^2) or epirubicin ($\leqslant$100 mg/m^2), aprepitant in combination with an ondansetron/dexamethasone regimen (see section 4.2) was compared with standard therapy (placebo plus ondansetron 8 mg orally (twice on Day 1, and every 12 hours on Days 2 and 3) plus dexamethasone 20 mg orally on Day 1).

Efficacy was based on evaluation of the composite measure: complete response (defined as no emetic episodes and no use of rescue therapy) primarily during Cycle 1.

A summary of the key study results is shown in Table 4.

Table 4 Percent of Patients Responding by Treatment Group and Phase —Cycle 1 Moderately Emetogenic Chemotherapy

(see Table 4 on next page)

The estimated time to first emesis in the study is depicted by the Kaplan-Meier plot in Figure 2.

Figure 2 Percent of Patients Receiving Moderately Emetogenic Chemotherapy Who Remain Emesis Free Over Time - Cycle 1

(see Figure 2 on next page)

In the same clinical study, 744 patients continued into the Multiple-Cycle extension for up to 3 additional cycles of chemotherapy. The efficacy of the aprepitant regimen was apparently maintained during all cycles.

5.2 Pharmacokinetic properties

Aprepitant displays non-linear pharmacokinetics. Both clearance and absolute bioavailability decrease with increasing dose.

Absorption

The mean absolute oral bioavailability of aprepitant is 67 % for the 80-mg capsule and 59 % for the 125-mg capsule. The mean peak plasma concentration (C_{max}) of aprepitant occurred at approximately 4 hours (T_{max}). Oral administration of the capsule with an approximately 800 Kcal standard breakfast resulted in an up to 40 % increase in AUC of aprepitant. This increase is not considered clinically relevant.

The pharmacokinetics of aprepitant is non-linear across the clinical dose range. In healthy young adults, the increase in $AUC_{0-\infty}$ was 26 % greater than dose proportional between 80-mg and 125-mg single doses administered in the fed state.

Following oral administration of a single 125 mg dose of EMEND on Day 1 and 80 mg once daily on Days 2 and 3, the AUC_{0-24hr} (mean±SD) was 19.6±2.5 microgram × hr/ml and 21.2±6.3 microgram × hr/ml on Days 1 and 3, respectively. C_{max} was 1.6±0.36 microgram/ml and 1.4±0.22 microgram/ml on Days 1 and 3, respectively.

Distribution

Aprepitant is highly protein bound, with a mean of 97 %. The geometric mean apparent volume of distribution at steady state (Vd_{ss}) is approximately 66 l in humans.

Table 3 Percent of Patients Receiving Highly Emetogenic Chemotherapy Responding by Treatment Group and Phase —Cycle 1

COMPOSITE MEASURES	Aprepitant Regimen (N= 521) %	Standard Therapy (N= 524) %	Differences*	
			%	(95 % CI)
Complete Response (no emesis and no rescue therapy)				
Overall (0-120 hours) 0-24 hours 25-120 hours	67.7 86.0 71.5	47.8 73.2 51.2	19.9 12.7 20.3	(14.0, 25.8) (7.9, 17.6) (14.5, 26.1)
INDIVIDUAL MEASURES				
No Emesis (no emetic episodes regardless of use of rescue therapy)				
Overall (0-120 hours) 0-24 hours 25-120 hours	71.9 86.8 76.2	49.7 74.0 53.5	22.2 12.7 22.6	(16.4, 28.0) (8.0, 17.5) (17.0, 28.2)
No Significant Nausea (maximum VAS < 25 mm on a scale of 0-100 mm)				
Overall (0-120 hours) 25-120 hours	72.1 74.0	64.9 66.9	7.2 7.1	(1.6, 12.8) (1.5, 12.6)

* The confidence intervals were calculated with no adjustment for gender and concomitant chemotherapy, which were included in the primary analysis of odds ratios and logistic models.

Figure 1 Percent of Patients Receiving Highly Emetogenic Chemotherapy Who Remain Emesis Free Over Time - Cycle 1

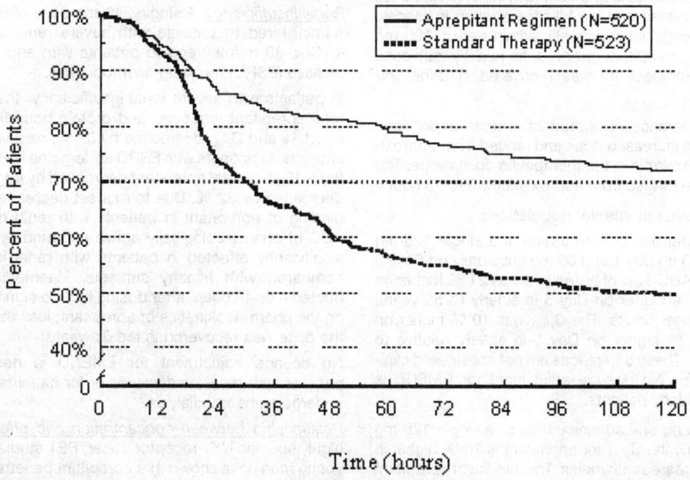

Table 4 Percent of Patients Responding by Treatment Group and Phase —Cycle 1 Moderately Emetogenic Chemotherapy

COMPOSITE MEASURES	Aprepitant Regimen (N= 433) %	Standard Therapy (N= 424) %	Differences* % (95 % CI)	
Complete Response (no emesis and no rescue therapy)				
Overall (0-120 hours)	50.8	42.5	8.3	(1.6, 15.0)
0-24 hours	75.7	69.0	6.7	(0.7, 12.7)
25-120 hours	55.4	49.1	6.3	(-0.4, 13.0)
INDIVIDUAL MEASURES				
No Emesis (no emetic episodes regardless of use of rescue therapy)				
Overall (0-120 hours)	75.7	58.7	17.0	(10.8, 23.2)
0-24 hours	87.5	77.3	10.2	(5.1, 15.3)
25-120 hours	80.8	69.1	11.7	(5.9, 17.5)
No Significant Nausea (maximum VAS < 25 mm on a scale of 0-100 mm)				
Overall (0-120 hours)	60.9	55.7	5.3	(-1.3, 11.9)
0-24 hours	79.5	78.3	1.3	(-4.2, 6.8)
25-120 hours	65.3	61.5	3.9	(-2.6, 10.3)

* The confidence intervals were calculated with no adjustment for age category (<55 years, ⩾55 years) and investigator group, which were included in the primary analysis of odds ratios and logistic models.

Figure 2 Percent of Patients Receiving Moderately Emetogenic Chemotherapy Who Remain Emesis Free Over Time - Cycle 1

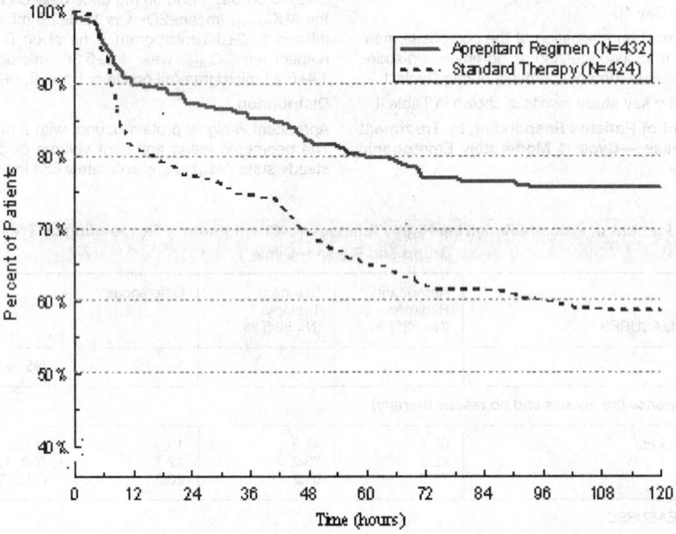

Metabolism

Aprepitant undergoes extensive metabolism. In healthy young adults, aprepitant accounts for approximately 19 % of the radioactivity in plasma over 72 hours following a single intravenous administration 100-mg dose of [^{14}C]-aprepitant prodrug, indicating a substantial presence of metabolites in the plasma. Twelve metabolites of aprepitant have been identified in human plasma. The metabolism of aprepitant occurs largely via oxidation at the morpholine ring and its side chains and the resultant metabolites were only weakly active. *In vitro* studies using human liver microsomes indicate that aprepitant is metabolised primarily by CYP3A4 and potentially with minor contribution by CYP1A2 and CYP2C19.

Elimination

Aprepitant is not excreted unchanged in urine. Metabolites are excreted in urine and via biliary excretion in faeces. Following a single intravenously administered 100-mg dose of [^{14}C]- aprepitant prodrug to healthy subjects, 57 % of the radioactivity was recovered in urine and 45 % in faeces.

The plasma clearance of aprepitant is dose-dependent, decreasing with increased dose and ranged from approximately 60 to 72 ml/min in the therapeutic dose range. The terminal half-life ranged from approximately 9 to 13 hours.

Pharmacokinetics in special populations

Elderly: Following oral administration of a single 125-mg dose of EMEND on Day 1 and 80 mg once daily on Days 2 through 5, the AUC_{0-24hr} of aprepitant was 21 % higher on Day 1 and 36 % higher on Day 5 in elderly (⩾65 years) relative to younger adults. The C_{max} was 10 % higher on Day 1 and 24 % higher on Day 5 in elderly relative to younger adults. These differences are not considered clinically meaningful. No dosage adjustment for EMEND is necessary in elderly patients.

Gender: Following oral administration of a single 125-mg dose of EMEND, the C_{max} for aprepitant is 16 % higher in females as compared with males. The half-life of aprepitant is 25 % lower in females as compared with males and its T_{max} occurs at approximately the same time. These differences are not considered clinically meaningful. No dosage adjustment for EMEND is necessary based on gender.

Paediatric patients: The pharmacokinetics of EMEND have not been evaluated in patients below 18 years of age.

Hepatic insufficiency: Mild hepatic insufficiency (Child-Pugh score 5 to 6) does not affect the pharmacokinetics of aprepitant to a clinically relevant extent. No dosage adjustment is necessary for patients with mild hepatic insufficiency. Conclusions regarding the influence of moderate hepatic insufficiency (Child-Pugh score 7 to 8) on aprepitant pharmacokinetics cannot be drawn from available data. There are no clinical or pharmacokinetic data in patients with severe hepatic insufficiency (Child-Pugh score > 9).

Renal Insufficiency: A single 240-mg dose of EMEND was administered to patients with severe renal insufficiency (CrCl< 30 ml/min) and to patients with end stage renal disease (ESRD) requiring haemodialysis.

In patients with severe renal insufficiency, the $AUC_{0-\infty}$ of total aprepitant (unbound and protein bound) decreased by 21 % and C_{max} decreased by 32 %, relative to healthy subjects. In patients with ESRD undergoing haemodialysis, the $AUC_{0-\infty}$ of total aprepitant decreased by 42 % and C_{max} decreased by 32 %. Due to modest decreases in protein binding of aprepitant in patients with renal disease, the AUC of pharmacologically active unbound drug was not significantly affected in patients with renal insufficiency compared with healthy subjects. Haemodialysis conducted 4 or 48 hours after dosing had no significant effect on the pharmacokinetics of aprepitant; less than 0.2 % of the dose was recovered in the dialysate.

No dosage adjustment for EMEND is necessary for patients with renal insufficiency or for patients with ESRD undergoing haemodialysis.

Relationship between concentration and effect: Using a highly specific NK_1-receptor tracer, PET studies in healthy young men have shown that aprepitant penetrates into the brain and occupies NK_1 receptors in a dose- and plasma-concentration-dependent manner. Aprepitant plasma concentrations achieved with the 3-day regimen of EMEND are predicted to provide greater than 95 % occupancy of brain NK_1 receptors.

5.3 Preclinical safety data

Pre-clinical data reveal no special hazard for humans based on conventional studies of single and repeated dose toxicity, genotoxicity, carcinogenic potential, and toxicity to reproduction. However, it should be noted that systemic exposure in rodents was similar or even lower than therapeutic exposure in humans. In particular, although no adverse effects were noted in reproduction studies at human exposure levels, the animal exposures are not sufficient to make an adequate risk assessment in man.

6. PHARMACEUTICAL PARTICULARS

6.1 List of excipients

Capsule content

sucrose

microcrystalline cellulose (E 460)

hydroxypropyl cellulose (E 463)

sodium lauryl sulfate

Capsule shell (125 mg)

gelatin

titanium dioxide (E 171)

red iron oxide (E 172)

yellow iron oxide (E 172)

Capsule shell (80 mg)

gelatin

titanium dioxide (E 171)

Printing ink

shellac

potassium hydroxide

black iron oxide (E 172)

6.2 Incompatibilities

Not applicable.

6.3 Shelf life

4 years

6.4 Special precautions for storage

No special precautions for storage.

6.5 Nature and contents of container

Different pack sizes including different strengths are available.

Alminium blister containing one 125 mg capsule.

5 aluminium blisters each containing one 125 mg capsule.

Aluminium blister containing one 80 mg capsule.

Aluminium blister containing two 80 mg capsules.

5 aluminium blisters each containing one 80 mg capsule.

Aluminium blister containing one 125 mg capsule and two 80 mg capsules.

Not all pack sizes may be marketed.

6.6 Instructions for use and handling

No special requirements.

7. MARKETING AUTHORISATION HOLDER

Merck Sharp & Dohme Ltd.
Hertford Road, Hoddesdon
Hertfordshire EN 11 9BU
United Kingdom

8. MARKETING AUTHORISATION NUMBER(S)

125 mg x1:	EU/1/03/262/004
125 mg × 5:	EU/1/03/262/005
80 mg x1:	EU/1/03/262/001
80 mg x2:	EU/1/03/262/002
80 mg x5:	EU/1/03/262/003
80 mg x2 and 125 mg x1:	EU/1/03/262/006

9. DATE OF FIRST AUTHORISATION/RENEWAL OF THE AUTHORISATION

11th November 2003

10. DATE OF REVISION OF THE TEXT

28th April 2005.

SPC.EMD.05.UK/IRL.2213 (II-009-010)

Emeside Capsules

(Laboratories for Applied Biology Limited)

1. NAME OF THE MEDICINAL PRODUCT

Emeside Capsules

2. QUALITATIVE AND QUANTITATIVE COMPOSITION

Ethosuximide 250 mg/Capsule

3. PHARMACEUTICAL FORM

Capsule for oral use

4. CLINICAL PARTICULARS

4.1 Therapeutic indications

Emeside gives selective control of absence seizures (petit mal) even when complicated by grand-mal. It is also indicated for myoclonic seizures.

4.2 Posology and method of administration

Adults, the Elderly and Children over 6 Years: Start with a small dose - 500mg daily with increments of 250mg every five to seven days until control is achieved with 1000 - 1500 mg daily. Occasionally 2000 mg in divided doses may be necessary.

Children and Infants under 6 years: Ethosuximide syrup is recommended for infants and children under six years.

Effective plasma levels of ethosuximide normally lie between 40 and 100 mcg per ml, but the clinical response should be the criteria for the regulation of the dosage. The half-life of ethosuximide in the plasma is more than 24 hours but the daily dose if large is more comfortably divided between morning and evening.

4.3 Contraindications

Known hypersensitivity to succinimides. Porphyrias.

4.4 Special warnings and special precautions for use

Use with caution in hepatic or renal impairment. Monitor liver/renal function and ethosuximide concentrations.

If Emeside is being substituted for another anti-epileptic drug the latter must not be withdrawn abruptly but the replacement made gradually with overlap of the preparations otherwise petit mal may break through.

Emeside should always be withdrawn slowly.

4.5 Interaction with other medicinal products and other forms of Interaction

The plasma concentrations of ethosuximide may be reduced by carbamazepine, primidone, phenobarbitone and lamotrigine and increased by isoniazide. No consistent changes in levels of ethosuximide occur when used in combination with phenytoin or sodium valproate.

Phenytoin levels however are increased by concomitant ethosuximide.

4.6 Pregnancy and lactation

Ethosuximide may be excreted into breast milk. Mothers receiving the drug should not breast feed. There is a recognised small increase in the incidence of congenital malformations in children born to mothers receiving anti-convulsants. For women planning pregnancy or who are already pregnant the risk should be weighed carefully against the benefit of treatment.

4.7 Effects on ability to drive and use machines

Patients should be cautioned that ethosuximide may cause drowsiness and if this occurs should avoid driving or operating machinery.

4.8 Undesirable effects

Blood dyscrasias (leucopoenia, agranulocytosis, aplastic anaemia, and pancytopaenia) have been reported, some with fatal outcome. In most cases of leucopoenia the blood picture has returned to normal on reduction of dose or discontinuation. In some instances, patients who become leucopenic on other anticonvulsant therapy have been satisfactorily treated with ethosuximide alone. Elevated neutrophil, monocyte and eosinophil counts have also been noted. Patients should be advised to seek immediate medical attention, for full blood count tests, if symptoms such as fever, sore throat, mouth ulcers, bruising or bleeding develop.

Ethosuximide when used alone in mixed types of epilepsy may increase the frequency of generalised tonic-clonic (grand mal) seizures in some patients.

Other adverse reactions reported include: weight loss, diarrhoea, abdominal pain, gum hypertrophy, swelling of the tongue, hiccoughs, irritability, hyperactivity, sleep disturbances, night terrors, inability to concentrate, aggressiveness, paranoid psychosis, increased libido, myopia, and vaginal bleeding.

Mild side effects, common at first but generally transient, include apathy, euphoria, fatigue, drowsiness, dizziness, headache, ataxia, dyskinesia, photophobia, depression and nausea, vomiting, anorexia, and gastric upset.

Psychotic states thought to be induced or exacerbated by anticonvulsant therapy have been reported.

Rarely cases of skin rash and isolated cases of erythema nodosum have been reported. Lupus-like reactions have occasionally been reported in children given ethosuximide, varying from severe systemic immunological disorders, eg the nephrotic syndrome generally with complete recovery on drug withdrawal, to the detection of antinuclear antibodies without clinical features. Stevens Johnson syndrome has also been reported.

4.9 Overdose

Where more than 2g has been thought to be ingested gastric lavage may be employed, if the time lapse is less than four hours. Routine observation of respiration and circulation will indicate the need for supportive measures.

5. PHARMACOLOGICAL PROPERTIES

5.1 Pharmacodynamic properties

Ethosuximide gives selective control of absence seizures (petit-mal) even when complicated by grand-mal. It is also indicated for myoclonic seizures. Compared to other anti-convulsants, ethosuximide is more specific for pure petit-mal.

The reduction of seizure frequency is thought to be achieved by depression of the motor cortex and elevation of the threshold to convulsive stimuli as seen by the suppression of the characteristic spike and wave EEG pattern.

5.2 Pharmacokinetic properties

Ethosuximide is readily absorbed from the gastro-intestinal tract and extensively metabolised in the liver. It is excreted in the urine mainly in the form of its metabolites. It is widely distributed throughout the body but is not significantly bound to plasma proteins so saliva concentrations may be useful for monitoring. Peak serum levels occur 1 to 7 hours after single oral dose. Therapeutic levels are between 40 and 100 mcg/ml. It has a long elimination half-life: adults: 40 – 60 hours; children 30 hours.

5.3 Preclinical safety data

None stated.

6. PHARMACEUTICAL PARTICULARS

6.1 List of excipients

Polyethylene Glycol 400	160 mg
Gelatine	147.8 mg
Glycerine	70.35 mg
Ethyl p-hydroxybenzoate	0.634 mg
Propyl p-hydroxybenzoate	0.315 mg
Titanium Dioxide	0.708 mg
Sunset Yellow E 110	0.158 mg
Miglycol 812	Trace

6.2 Incompatibilities

Carbamazepine, phenytoin, sodium valproate, or isoniazid.

6.3 Shelf life

5 years.

6.4 Special precautions for storage

Store at 15 - 25° C away from moisture.

6.5 Nature and contents of container

Plastic vial containing capsules and Patient Information Leaflet.

6.6 Instructions for use and handling

No special instructions.

7. MARKETING AUTHORISATION HOLDER

Laboratories for Applied Biology Ltd

91, Amhurst Park

London

N 16 5 DR ML (UK) 0118/01

8. MARKETING AUTHORISATION NUMBER(S)

UK PL 0118/5002R

9. DATE OF FIRST AUTHORISATION/RENEWAL OF THE AUTHORISATION

Granted 01.11.90.

Renewed until 25.02.06

10. DATE OF REVISION OF THE TEXT

05.10 99 Changes to 5.6 Interactions

19.09.00 Rearranged to current format

06.02.2001 Corrected and expanded: 4. Clinical Particulars and 5.2 Pharmacokinetics.

14.06.2001 Changes to 4.2 and 4.8.

11. Legal Category

Prescription only medicine.

Emeside Syrup (Blackcurrant)

(Laboratories for Applied Biology Limited)

1. NAME OF THE MEDICINAL PRODUCT

Emeside Syrup (Blackcurrant)

2. QUALITATIVE AND QUANTITATIVE COMPOSITION

Ethosuximide 5% (250 mg/5 mL)

3. PHARMACEUTICAL FORM

Elixir for oral use.

4. CLINICAL PARTICULARS

4.1 Therapeutic indications

Emeside gives selective control of absence seizures (petit mal) even when complicated by grand-mal. It is also indicated for myoclonic seizures.

4.2 Posology and method of administration

Adults, the Elderly and Children over 6 Years: Start with a small dose - 500mg daily with increments of 250mg every five to seven days until control is achieved with 1000 - 1500 mg daily. Occasionally 2000 mg in divided doses may be necessary.

Children and Infants under 6 years: Begin with a daily dose of 250 mg (5 ml) and increase the dose gradually by small increments every few days until control is achieved. The optimal dose in most children is 20mg/Kg/day. The maximum dose should be 1000 mg.

Effective plasma levels of ethosuximide normally lie between 40 and 100 mcg per ml, but the clinical response should be the criteria for the regulation of the dosage. The half-life of ethosuximide in the plasma is more than 24 hours but the daily dose if large is more comfortably divided between morning and evening.

Larger children and adults will normally take Emeside in capsule form.

4.3 Contraindications

Known hypersensitivity to succinimides. Porphyrias.

4.4 Special warnings and special precautions for use

Use with caution in hepatic or renal impairment. Monitor liver/renal function and ethosuximide concentrations.

If Emeside is being substituted for another anti-epileptic drug the latter must not be withdrawn abruptly but the replacement made gradually with overlap of the preparations otherwise petit mal may break through.

Emeside should always be withdrawn slowly.

It is advisable to brush the teeth or rinse the mouth after taking Emeside syrup.

4.5 Interaction with other medicinal products and other forms of Interaction

The plasma concentrations of ethosuximide may be reduced by carbamazepine, primidone, phenobarbitone and lamotrigine and increased by isoniazide. No consistent changes in levels of ethosuximide occur when used in combination with phenytoin or sodium valproate.

Phenytoin levels however are increased by concomitant ethosuximide.

4.6 Pregnancy and lactation

Ethosuximide may be excreted into breast milk. Mothers receiving the drug should not breast feed. There is a recognised small increase in the incidence of congenital malformations in children born to mothers receiving anti-convulsants. For women planning pregnancy or who are already pregnant the risk should be weighed carefully against the benefit of treatment.

4.7 Effects on ability to drive and use machines

Patients should be cautioned that ethosuximide may cause drowsiness and if this occurs should avoid driving or operating machinery.

4.8 Undesirable effects

Blood dyscrasias (leucopoenia, agranulocytosis, aplastic anaemia, and pancytopaenia) have been reported, some with fatal outcome. In most cases of leucopoenia the blood picture has returned to normal on reduction of dose or discontinuation. In some instances, patients who become leucopenic on other anticonvulsant therapy have been satisfactorily treated with ethosuximide alone. Elevated neutrophil, monocyte and eosinophil counts have also been noted. Patients should be advised to seek immediate medical attention, for full blood count tests, if symptoms such as fever, sore throat, mouth ulcers, bruising or bleeding develop.

Ethosuximide when used alone in mixed types of epilepsy may increase the frequency of generalised tonic-clonic (grand mal) seizures in some patients.

Other adverse reactions reported include: weight loss, diarrhoea, abdominal pain, gum hypertrophy, swelling of the tongue, hiccoughs, irritability, hyperactivity, sleep disturbances, night terrors, inability to concentrate, aggressiveness, paranoid psychosis, increased libido, myopia, and vaginal bleeding.

Mild side effects, common at first but generally transient, include apathy, euphoria, fatigue, drowsiness, dizziness, headache, ataxia, dyskinesia, photophobia, depression and nausea, vomiting, anorexia, and gastric upset.

Psychotic states thought to be induced or exacerbated by anticonvulsant therapy have been reported.

Rarely cases of skin rash and isolated cases of erythema nodosum have been reported. Lupus-like reactions have occasionally been reported in children given ethosuximide, varying from severe systemic immunological disorders, eg the nephrotic syndrome generally with complete recovery on drug withdrawal, to the detection of antinuclear antibodies without clinical features. Stevens Johnson syndrome has also been reported.

4.9 Overdose

Where more than 2g has been thought to be ingested gastric lavage may be employed, if the time lapse is less than four hours. Routine observation of respiration and circulation will indicate the need for supportive measures.

5. PHARMACOLOGICAL PROPERTIES

5.1 Pharmacodynamic properties

Ethosuximide gives selective control of absence seizures (petit-mal) even when complicated by grand-mal. It is also indicated for myoclonic seizures. Compared to other anti-convulsants, ethosuximide is more specific for pure petit-mal.

The reduction of seizure frequency is thought to be achieved by depression of the motor cortex and elevation of the threshold to convulsive stimuli as seen by the suppression of the characteristic spike and wave EEG pattern.

5.2 Pharmacokinetic properties

Ethosuximide is readily absorbed from the gastro-intestinal tract and extensively metabolised in the liver. It is excreted in the urine mainly in the form of its metabolites. It is widely distributed throughout the body but is not significantly bound to plasma proteins so saliva concentrations may be useful for monitoring. Peak serum levels occur 1 to 7 hours after single oral dose. Therapeutic levels are between 40 and 100 mcg/ml. It has a long elimination half-life: adults: 40 – 60 hours; children 30 hours.

5.3 Preclinical safety data

None stated.

6. PHARMACEUTICAL PARTICULARS

6.1 List of excipients

Other Substances

Sucrose	61 % w/v
Saccharine sodium	0.044 % w/v
Water	to 100 %

Colouring, Flavouring and Perfume Compounds

Blackcurrant Juice	7.8 % v/v

6.2 Incompatibilities

Carbamazepine, phenytoin, sodium valproate, or isoniazid.

6.3 Shelf life

5 years.

6.4 Special precautions for storage

Store at ambient temperature.

6.5 Nature and contents of container

200 ml amber glass bottle with plastic cap with polycone liner.

6.6 Instructions for use and handling

No special instructions

7. MARKETING AUTHORISATION HOLDER

Laboratories for Applied Biology Ltd

91, Amhurst Park

London

N 16 5 DR ML (UK) 0118/01

8. MARKETING AUTHORISATION NUMBER(S)

UK PL 0118/5004R

9. DATE OF FIRST AUTHORISATION/RENEWAL OF THE AUTHORISATION

Granted 01.11.90.

Renewed until 26.02.06

10. DATE OF REVISION OF THE TEXT

05.10 99 Changes to 5.6 Interactions

19.09.00 Rearranged to current format

06.02.2001 Corrected and expanded: 4. Clinical Particulars and 5.2 Pharmacokinetics.

14.06.2001 Changes to 4.2 and 4.8.

11. Legal Category

Prescription only medicine.

Emflex Capsules

(Merck Pharmaceuticals)

1. NAME OF THE MEDICINAL PRODUCT

Emflex Capsules

2. QUALITATIVE AND QUANTITATIVE COMPOSITION

Each capsule contains Acemetacin 60mg

3. PHARMACEUTICAL FORM

Gelatine capsule

4. CLINICAL PARTICULARS

4.1 Therapeutic indications

Rheumatoid arthritis, osteoarthritis, low back pain, and post-operative pain and inflammation.

4.2 Posology and method of administration

The recommended starting dose is 120mg/day in divided doses, increasing to 180mg/day in divided doses, depending on patient response.

For the treatment of elderly patients, adjustment of dosage is not normally required. However, non-steroidal anti-inflammatory drugs should be used with particular care in older patients who may be more prone to adverse reactions.

Emflex should be taken with food, milk or an antacid to reduce the possibility of gastro-intestinal disturbance.

4.3 Contraindications

Active peptic ulcer; history of recurrent ulceration; known hypersensitivity to acemetacin or indomethacin. Patients who have experienced asthma attacks, urticaria or acute rhinitis resulting from treatment with aspirin or non-steroidal anti-inflammatory drugs. Patients with nasal polyps associated with angioneurotic oedema. Safety in children is not established.

4.4 Special warnings and special precautions for use

As rare instances of peptic ulceration have been reported administration should be closely supervised in patients with a history of upper gastrointestinal disease. Treatment should be discontinued if peptic ulceration or gastrointestinal bleeding occurs.

Inhibition of platelet aggregation may occur.

Aggravation of psychiatric disorders, epilepsy or parkinsonism may occur.

Signs and symptoms of infection may be masked.

Emflex should be used with caution in patients with reduced renal blood flow where renal perfusion may be maintained by prostaglandins. In patients at particular risk - renal or hepatic dysfunction, congestive heart failure, electrolyte or fluid imbalance, sepsis, concomitant use of nephrotoxic drugs, the dose should be kept as low as possible and renal function should be monitored.

Patients receiving long-term treatment should be periodically screened for renal and hepatic function and blood counts. Borderline elevation of renal and hepatic function test parameters may occur. If this persists or worsens, treatment should be stopped.

Eye changes may occur in chronic rheumatoid disease and patients should receive periodic ophthalmological examinations and therapy discontinued if changes occur.

Hyperkalaemia has been reported with use of indomethacin and this should be considered when administration with potassium sparing diuretics is proposed.

4.5 Interaction with other medicinal products and other forms of Interaction

Emflex is highly protein bound and it may therefore be necessary to modify the dosage of other highly protein bound drugs e.g. anti-coagulants. As there is a possibility of either a pharmacokinetic or pharmacodynamic interaction with aspirin or other salicylates, diflusinal, probenecid, lithium, triamterene, ACE inhibitors, haloperidol and methotrexate, patients receiving such combinations should be carefully monitored and dosages adjusted as necessary. Non-steroidal anti-inflammatory drugs may reduce the anti-hypertensive effects of beta-blockers, although clinical studies showed no propensity for Emflex to antagonise the effects of propranolol. Likewise the reduction of diuretic effects of thiazides and frusemide may occur with non-steroidal anti-inflammatory drugs and this should be borne in mind when treating patients with compromised cardiac function or hypertension.

4.6 Pregnancy and lactation

The safety of this product for use in human pregnancy and lactation has not been established. Animal reproduction studies do not provide reassurance regarding the lack of reproductive toxicity/ teratogenicity. Due to maternal toxicity, the studies were conducted at doses below the therapeutic dose or a very low multiple of the therapeutic dose. It should not therefore be used in pregnancy or lactation in women of childbearing age unless they are taking adequate contraceptive precautions.

4.7 Effects on ability to drive and use machines

The ability to drive a car or operate machinery may be affected.

4.8 Undesirable effects

The following side effects have been either reported with Emflex or could possibly occur as they are common to a number of NSAIDs:

Gastro-intestinal: Gastro-intestinal discomfort/pain, anorexia, nausea, vomiting, indigestion, diarrhoea and constipation, peptic ulceration, gastrointestinal perforation and haemorrhage.

Central Nervous System: Symptoms most frequently encountered are headache, dizziness, vertigo and insomnia. Rarely, confusion, depressed mood, irritability.

Hepatic: Occasional elevation of liver function test parameters without overt clinical symptomatology. Very rarely, symptoms of cholestasis.

Cardiovascular/renal: Rarely, oedema, chest pain, palpitations, blood urea elevation. NSAIDs have been reported to cause nephrotoxicity in various forms and their use can lead to interstitial nephritis, nephrotic syndrome and renal failure.

Dermatological/hypersensitivity: Pruritus, urticaria, erythema, skin rash, alopecia, angio-neurotic oedema and excessive sweating have been reported.

Haematological: Rarely, thrombocytopenia, leucopenia and reduced haemoglobin levels. Very rarely, reversible agranulocytosis, bone marrow depression.

Ocular/auditory: Infrequently, tinnitus, blurred vision and rarely, eye pain.

4.9 Overdose

Symptomatic and supportive therapy is indicated. If ingestion is recent, vomiting should be induced or gastric lavage should be performed. Progress should be followed for several days as gastrointestinal ulceration and haemorrhage have been reported with overdosage of other NSAIDs. Antacids may be helpful.

5. PHARMACOLOGICAL PROPERTIES

5.1 Pharmacodynamic properties

Acemetacin is a glycolic acid ester of indomethacin and the pharmacological activity resulting from acemetacin administration in man is derived from the presence of both acemetacin and indomethacin. The precise pharmacological mode of action of acemetacin is not known. However, unlike other NSAIDs, acemetacin is only a relatively weak inhibitor of prostaglandin synthetase.

Prostaglandins are known to have an antisecretory and cytoprotective effect on the gastric mucosa. Acemetacin shows activity in many of the established in vitro tests of anti-inflammatory activity, including inhibition of the release of a number of mediators of inflammation.

5.2 Pharmacokinetic properties

Acemetacin is well absorbed after oral administration. Its major metabolite is indomethacin which, after repeated administration, is present at levels in excess of those of acemetacin. Acemetacin is bound to plasma protein to a slightly lesser extent than indomethacin and has a relatively short plasma elimination half-life. It is eliminated by both hepatic and renal mechanisms. The pharmacokinetics appear to be linear at recommended therapeutic doses, unaffected by moderate renal or hepatic impairment, and unchanged in the elderly.

5.3 Preclinical safety data

Emflex Capsules show similar toxicity to other non-steroidal anti-inflammatory drugs.

6. PHARMACEUTICAL PARTICULARS

6.1 List of excipients

Gelatine capsule (colourings: Ferric oxide red E172, Ferric oxide yellow E172 and titanium dioxide E171), lactose, magnesium stearate, silicon dioxide, talc and sodium dodecylsulphate.

6.2 Incompatibilities

None known.

6.3 Shelf life

Five years

6.4 Special precautions for storage

Store below 25 degree C.

6.5 Nature and contents of container

White polypropylene bottles with polypropylene screw caps.

Pack sizes: 90, 56, 60 and 30 capsules.

PVC/PVDC foil blister packs in cartons:

Pack sizes: 90, 60, 56, 30, 10, and 6 capsules

6.6 Instructions for use and handling

To be taken with food.

7. MARKETING AUTHORISATION HOLDER

E. Merck Ltd. T/A Merck Pharmaceuticals (A division of Merck Ltd), Harrier House, High Street, West Drayton, Middlesex, UB7 7QG, UK.

8. MARKETING AUTHORISATION NUMBER(S)

PL 0493/0141

9. DATE OF FIRST AUTHORISATION/RENEWAL OF THE AUTHORISATION

26 November 1990/25 March 1996

10. DATE OF REVISION OF THE TEXT

22 December 1998

LEGAL CATEGORY

POM

EMLA Cream 5%

(AstraZeneca UK Limited)

1. NAME OF THE MEDICINAL PRODUCT

EMLA™ Cream 5%

2. QUALITATIVE AND QUANTITATIVE COMPOSITION

Lidocaine 2.5% w/w (25 mg/g)

Prilocaine 2.5% w/w (25 mg/g)

For excipients, see 6.1

3. PHARMACEUTICAL FORM

White soft cream.

4. CLINICAL PARTICULARS

4.1 Therapeutic indications

Local anaesthetic for topical use to produce surface anaesthesia of the skin.

For topical use on the genital mucosa to facilitate the removal of warts in adults.

4.2 Posology and method of administration
Adults (including elderly) and children > 1 year:

Surface	Procedure	Application
Skin (apply a thick layer of cream under an occlusive dressing).	Minor dermatological procedures e.g. needle insertion and surgical treatment of localised lesions.	Approximately 2 g EMLA applied for a minimum of 60 minutes, maximum 5 hours.
	Dermal procedures on larger areas e.g. split skin grafting.	Approximately 1.5-2 g/10 cm^2 EMLA applied for a minimum of 2 hours, maximum 5 hours.
Genital mucosa (adults) (no occlusive dressing required).	Surgical treatment of localised lesions.	Apply up to 10 g EMLA for 5-10 minutes. Commence procedure immediately thereafter.

Analgesic efficacy may decline if the skin application time is more than 5 hours. Procedures on intact skin should begin soon after the occlusive dressing is removed.

On the genital mucosa analgesic efficacy declines after 10-15 minutes and therefore the procedure should be commenced immediately.

Not recommended in infants.

4.3 Contraindications
Known hypersensitivity to anaesthetics of the amide type or to any other component of the product.

4.4 Special warnings and special precautions for use
Patients with glucose-6-phosphate dehydrogenase deficiency or congential or idiopathic methaemoglobinaemia are more susceptible to drug induced methaemoglobinaemia.

Until further clinical experience is available, EMLA Cream should not be applied to wounds, mucous membranes or in areas of atopic dermatitis.

Clinical studies have been unable to demonstrate the efficacy of EMLA during the heal lancing of neonates.

EMLA Cream should not be applied to genital mucosa in children.

Care should be taken not to allow EMLA to come in contact with the eyes as it may cause eye irritation. Also the loss of protective reflexes may allow corneal irritation and potential abrasion. If contact with the eye occurs, immediately rinse the eye with water or sodium chloride solution and protect it until sensation returns.

EMLA, like other local anaesthetics may be ototoxic and should not be instilled in the middle ear nor should it be used for procedures which might allow penetration into the middle ear.

Although the systemic availability of prilocaine by percutaneous absorption of EMLA is low, caution should be exercised in patients with anaemia, congenital or acquired methaemoglobinaemia or patients on concomitant therapy known to produce such conditions.

Lidocaine and prilocaine have bacteriocidal and antiviral properties in concentrations above 0.5 – 2%. For this reason, although one clinical study suggests that the immunization response is not affected when EMLA Cream is used prior to BCG vaccination, the results of intracutaneous injections of live vaccines should be monitored.

4.5 Interaction with other medicinal products and other forms of Interaction
Methaemoglobinaemia may be accentuated in patients already taking drugs known to induce the condition, e.g. Sulphonamides.

The risk of additional systemic toxicity should be considered when large doses of EMLA are applied to patients already using other local anaesthetics or structurally related drugs e.g. tocainide.

4.6 Pregnancy and lactation
Lidocaine and prilocaine cross the placental barrier. However, both drugs have been in widespread clinical use for many years and a large number of women of childbearing age have been exposed to them. No specific effects on the reproductive process have been reported. However, caution should be exercised when used in pregnant women.

Lidocaine and prilocaine are excreted in breast milk in small amounts.

4.7 Effects on ability to drive and use machines
None known.

4.8 Undesirable effects
Transient paleness, redness and oedema have been reported.

Prilocaine has been known to cause methaemoglobinaemia in children when given parenterally.

In rare cases local anaesthetics have been associated with allergic reactions including anaphylactic shock.

Rare cases of discrete local lesions at the application site, described as purpuric or petechial, have been reported, especially after longer application times in children with atopic dermatitis or mollusca contagiosa.

Corneal irritation after accidental eye exposure.

4.9 Overdose
Overdosage with EMLA is unlikely but signs of systemic toxicity will be similar in nature to those observed after administration of other local anaesthetics.

5. PHARMACOLOGICAL PROPERTIES
5.1 Pharmacodynamic properties
Pharmacotherapeutic group: Local anaesthetics

ATC Code: N01B B20

EMLA Cream provides dermal analgesia. The depth of analgesia depends upon the application time and the dose. EMLA causes transient local peripheral vasoconstriction or vasodilation at the treated area.

The use of EMLA prior to measles-mumps-rubella or intramuscular diptheria-pertussis-tetanus-inactivated poliovirus-*Haemophilus influenzae b* or Hepatitis B vaccines does not affect mean antibody titres, rate of seroconversion, or the proportion of patients achieving protective or positive antibody titres post immunization, as compared to placebo treated patients.

5.2 Pharmacokinetic properties
Systemic absorption of lidocaine and prilocaine from EMLA Cream is dependent upon the dose, application time, and the thickness of the skin, which varies between different areas of the body.

Intact skin: in order to provide reliable dermal analgesia, EMLA Cream should be applied under an occlusive dressing for at least 1 hour. The duration of analgesia after an application time of 1-2 hours is at least 2 hours after removal of the dressing.

After application to the thigh in adults (60 g cream/400 cm^2 for 3 hours) the extent of absorption was approximately 5% of lidocaine and prilocaine. Maximum plasma concentrations (mean 0.12 and 0.07 μg/ml) were reached approximately 2-6 hours after the application.

The extent of systemic absorption was approximately 10% following application to the face (10 g/100 cm^2 for 2 hours). Maximum plasma levels (mean 0.16 and 0.06 μg/ml) were reached after approximately 1.5-3 hours.

Genital mucosa: Absorption from the genital mucosa is more rapid than after application to the skin. After the application of 10 g EMLA Cream for 10 minutes to vaginal mucosa maximum plasma concentrations of lidocaine and prilocaine (mean 0.18 μg/ml and 0.15 μg/ml respectively) were reached after 20-45 minutes.

5.3 Preclinical safety data
Lidocaine and prilocaine are well established active ingredients.

6. PHARMACEUTICAL PARTICULARS
6.1 List of excipients
Polyoxyethylene hydrogenated castor oil, Carbomer 974P, sodium hydroxide and water purified.

6.2 Incompatibilities
None known.

6.3 Shelf life
3 years.

6.4 Special precautions for storage
Do not store above 30°C, do not freeze.

6.5 Nature and contents of container
"Pre-medication pack" containing 5 × 5 g tubes EMLA and 12 occlusive dressings.

Pack containing 10 × 5 g tubes of EMLA

1 × 30 g tube

1 × 5 g tube

6.6 Instructions for use and handling
Not applicable.

7. MARKETING AUTHORISATION HOLDER
AstraZeneca UK Limited

600 Capability Green

Luton

LU1 3LU, UK

8. MARKETING AUTHORISATION NUMBER(S)
PL 17901/0120

9. DATE OF FIRST AUTHORISATION/RENEWAL OF THE AUTHORISATION
16th May 1996

10. DATE OF REVISION OF THE TEXT
14th April 2005

Emtriva 10 mg/ml oral solution

(Gilead Sciences International Limited)

1. NAME OF THE MEDICINAL PRODUCT
Emtriva 10 mg/ml oral solution▼

2. QUALITATIVE AND QUANTITATIVE COMPOSITION
Each ml of Emtriva oral solution contains 10 mg emtricitabine.

For excipients, see 6.1.

3. PHARMACEUTICAL FORM
Oral solution.

The clear solution is orange to dark orange in colour.

4. CLINICAL PARTICULARS
4.1 Therapeutic indications
Emtriva is indicated for the treatment of HIV-1 infected adults and children in combination with other antiretroviral agents.

This indication is based on studies in treatment-naïve patients and treatment-experienced patients with stable virological control. There is no experience of the use of Emtriva in patients who are failing their current regimen or who have failed multiple regimens (see 5.1).

When deciding on a new regimen for patients who have failed an antiretroviral regimen, careful consideration should be given to the patterns of mutations associated with different medicinal products and the treatment history of the individual patient. Where available, resistance testing may be appropriate.

4.2 Posology and method of administration
Therapy should be initiated by a physician experienced in the management of HIV infection.

Emtriva 10 mg/ml oral solution may be taken with or without food. A measuring cup is provided (see 6.5).

Adults: The recommended dose of Emtriva 10 mg/ml oral solution is 240 mg (24 ml) once daily.

Infants, children and adolescents up to 18 years of age: The recommended dose of Emtriva 10 mg/ml oral solution is 6 mg/kg up to a maximum of 240 mg (24 ml) once daily.

Children who weigh at least 33 kg may either take one 200 mg hard capsule daily or may take emtricitabine as the oral solution up to a maximum of 240 mg once daily.

There are no data on the safety and efficacy of emtricitabine in infants less than 4 months of age.

Emtriva 200 mg hard capsules are available for adults, adolescents and children who weigh at least 33 kg and can swallow hard capsules. Please refer to the Summary of Product Characteristics for Emtriva 200 mg hard capsules. Due to a difference in the bioavailability of emtricitabine between the hard capsule and oral solution presentations, 240 mg emtricitabine administered as the oral solution (24 ml) should provide similar plasma levels to those observed after administration of one 200 mg emtricitabine hard capsule (see 5.2).

Elderly: There are no safety and efficacy data available in patients over the age of 65 years. However, no adjustment in the recommended daily dose for adults should be required unless there is evidence of renal insufficiency.

Renal insufficiency: Emtricitabine is eliminated by renal excretion and exposure to emtricitabine was significantly increased in patients with renal insufficiency (see 5.2). Dose or dose interval adjustment is required in all patients with creatinine clearance < 50 ml/min (see 4.4).

The table below provides daily doses of Emtriva 10 mg/ml oral solution according to the degree of renal insufficiency. The safety and efficacy of these doses have not been clinically evaluated. Therefore, clinical response to treatment and renal function should be closely monitored in these patients (see 4.4).

Patients with renal insufficiency can also be managed by administration of Emtriva 200 mg hard capsules at modified dose intervals. Please refer to the Summary of Product Characteristics for Emtriva 200 mg hard capsules.

(see Table 1 on next page)

Patients with end-stage renal disease (ESRD) managed with other forms of dialysis such as ambulatory peritoneal dialysis have not been studied and no dose recommendation can be made.

No data are available on which to make a dosage recommendation in paediatric patients with renal insufficiency.

Hepatic insufficiency: No data are available on which to make a dose recommendation for patients with hepatic insufficiency. However, based on the minimal metabolism of emtricitabine and the renal route of elimination it is unlikely that a dose adjustment would be required in patients with hepatic insufficiency (see 5.2).

4.3 Contraindications
Hypersensitivity to emtricitabine or to any of the excipients.

4.4 Special warnings and special precautions for use
General: Emtricitabine is not recommended as monotherapy for the treatment of HIV infection. It must be used in combination with other antiretrovirals. Please also refer to the Summaries of Product Characteristics of the other

Table 1

	Creatinine Clearance (CL_{cr}) (ml/min)			
	⩾ 50	**30-49**	**15-29**	**< 15 (functionally anephric, requiring intermittent haemodialysis)***
Recommended dose of Emtriva 10 mg/ml oral solution every 24 hours	240 mg (24 ml)	120 mg (12 ml)	80 mg (8 ml)	60 mg (6 ml)

* Assumes a 3h haemodialysis session three times a week commencing at least 12h after administration of the last dose of emtricitabine.

antiretroviral medicinal products used in the combination regimen.

Patients receiving emtricitabine or any other antiretroviral therapy may continue to develop opportunistic infections and other complications of HIV infection, and therefore should remain under close clinical observation by physicians experienced in the treatment of patients with HIV associated diseases.

Patients should be advised that antiretroviral therapies, including emtricitabine have not been proven to prevent the risk of transmission of HIV to others through sexual contact or blood contamination. Appropriate precautions should continue to be used. Patients should also be informed that emtricitabine is not a cure for HIV infection.

Renal function: Emtricitabine is principally eliminated by the kidney via glomerular filtration and active tubular secretion. Emtricitabine exposure may be markedly increased in patients with moderate or severe renal insufficiency (creatinine clearance < 50 ml/min) receiving daily doses of 200 mg emtricitabine as hard capsules or 240 mg as the oral solution. Consequently, either a dose interval adjustment (using Emtriva 200 mg hard capsules) or a reduction in the daily dose of emtricitabine (using Emtriva 10 mg/ml oral solution) is required in all patients with creatinine clearance < 50 ml/min. The safety and efficacy of the reduced doses provided in section 4.2 are based on single dose pharmacokinetic data and modelling and have not been clinically evaluated. Therefore, clinical response to treatment and renal function should be closely monitored in patients treated with a reduced dose of emtricitabine (see 4.2 and 5.2).

Caution should be exercised when emtricitabine is co-administered with medicinal products that are eliminated by active tubular secretion as such co-administration may lead to an increase in serum concentrations of either emtricitabine or a co-administered medicinal product, due to competition for this elimination pathway (see 4.5).

Lactic acidosis: Lactic acidosis, usually associated with hepatic steatosis, has been reported with the use of nucleoside analogues. Early symptoms (symptomatic hyperlactataemia) include benign digestive symptoms (nausea, vomiting and abdominal pain), non-specific malaise, loss of appetite, weight loss, respiratory symptoms (rapid and/or deep breathing) or neurological symptoms (including motor weakness). Lactic acidosis has a high mortality and may be associated with pancreatitis, liver failure or renal failure. Lactic acidosis generally occurred after a few or several months of treatment.

Treatment with nucleoside analogues should be discontinued in the setting of symptomatic hyperlactataemia and metabolic/lactic acidosis, progressive hepatomegaly, or rapidly elevating aminotransferase levels.

Caution should be exercised when administering nucleoside analogues to any patient (particularly obese women) with hepatomegaly, hepatitis or other known risk factors for liver disease and hepatic steatosis (including certain medicinal products and alcohol). Patients co-infected with hepatitis C and treated with alpha interferon and ribavirin may constitute a special risk.

Patients at increased risk should be followed closely.

Lipodystrophy: Combination antiretroviral therapy has been associated with the redistribution of body fat (lipodystrophy) in HIV patients. The long-term consequences of these events are currently unknown. Knowledge about the mechanism is incomplete. A connection between visceral lipomatosis and protease inhibitors, and lipoatrophy and nucleoside reverse transcriptase inhibitors has been hypothesised. A higher risk of lipodystrophy has been associated with individual factors such as older age, and with drug related factors such as longer duration of antiretroviral treatment and associated metabolic disturbances. Clinical examination should include evaluation for physical signs of fat redistribution. Consideration should be given to the measurement of fasting serum lipids and blood glucose. Lipid disorders should be managed as clinically appropriate.

Liver function: Patients with pre-existing liver dysfunction including chronic active hepatitis have an increased frequency of liver function abnormalities during combination antiretroviral therapy and should be monitored according to standard practice. Patients with chronic hepatitis B or C infection treated with combination antiretroviral therapy are at increased risk of experiencing severe, and potentially fatal, hepatic adverse events. In case of concomitant antiviral therapy for hepatitis B or C, please also refer to the relevant Summary of Product Characteristics for these medicinal products.

If there is evidence of exacerbations of liver disease in such patients, interruption or discontinuation of treatment must be considered.

Patients co-infected with hepatitis B virus (HBV): Emtricitabine is active *in vitro* against HBV. However, limited data are available on the efficacy and safety of emtricitabine (as a 200 mg hard capsule once daily) in patients who are co-infected with HIV and HBV. The use of emtricitabine in patient with chronic HBV induces the same mutation pattern in the YMDD motif observed with lamivudine therapy. The YMDD mutation confers resistance to both emtricitabine and lamivudine.

Patients co-infected with HIV and HBV should be closely monitored with both clinical and laboratory follow-up for at least several months after stopping treatment with emtricitabine for evidence of exacerbations of hepatitis. Such exacerbations have been seen following discontinuation of emtricitabine treatment in HBV infected patients without concomitant HIV infection and have been detected primarily by serum alanine aminotransferase (ALT) elevations in addition to re-emergence of HBV DNA.

Mitochondrial dysfunction: Nucleoside and nucleotide analogues have been demonstrated *in vitro* and *in vivo* to cause a variable degree of mitochondrial damage. There have been reports of mitochondrial dysfunction in HIV negative infants exposed *in utero* and/or postnatally to nucleoside analogues. The main adverse events reported are haematological disorders (anaemia, neutropenia), metabolic disorders (hyperlactataemia, hyperlipasaemia). These events are often transitory. Some late-onset neurological disorders have been reported (hypertonia, convulsion, abnormal behaviour). Whether the neurological disorders are transient or permanent is currently unknown. Any child exposed *in utero* to nucleoside and nucleotide analogues, even HIV negative children, should have clinical and laboratory follow-up and should be fully investigated for possible mitochondrial dysfunction in case of relevant signs or symptoms. These findings do not affect current national recommendations to use antiretroviral therapy in pregnant women to prevent vertical transmission of HIV.

Immune Reactivation Syndrome: In HIV infected patients with severe immune deficiency at the time of institution of combination antiretroviral therapy (CART), an inflammatory reaction to asymptomatic or residual opportunistic pathogens may arise and cause serious clinical conditions, or aggravation of symptoms. Typically, such reactions have been observed within the first few weeks or months of initiation of CART. Relevant examples are cytomegalovirus retinitis, generalised and/or focal mycobacterium infections, and *Pneumocystis carinii* pneumonia. Any inflammatory symptoms should be evaluated and treatment instituted when necessary.

Sunset yellow (E110), a component of Emtriva oral solution, may cause allergic reactions, including asthma. The methyl parahydroxybenzoate (E218) and propyl parahydroxybenzoate (E216) in the oral solution may cause allergic reactions (possibly delayed).

4.5 Interaction with other medicinal products and other forms of Interaction

In vitro, emtricitabine did not inhibit metabolism mediated by any of the following human CYP450 isoforms: 1A2, 2A6, 2B6, 2C9, 2C19, 2D6 and 3A4. Emtricitabine did not inhibit the enzyme responsible for glucuronidation. Based on the results of these *in vitro* experiments and the known elimination pathways of emtricitabine, the potential for CYP450 mediated interactions involving emtricitabine with other medicinal products is low.

There are no clinically significant interactions when emtricitabine is co-administered with indinavir, zidovudine, stavudine, famciclovir or tenofovir disoproxil fumarate.

Emtricitabine is primarily excreted via glomerular filtration and active tubular secretion. With the exception of famciclovir and tenofovir disoproxil fumarate, the effect of co-administration of emtricitabine with medicinal products that are excreted by the renal route, or other medicinal products known to affect renal function, has not been evaluated. Co-administration of emtricitabine with medicinal products that are eliminated by active tubular secretion may lead to an increase in serum concentrations of either emtricitabine or a co-administered medicinal product due to competition for this elimination pathway.

There is no clinical experience as yet on the co-administration of cytidine analogues. Consequently, the use of emtricitabine in combination with lamivudine or zalcitabine for the treatment of HIV infection cannot be recommended at this time.

4.6 Pregnancy and lactation

The safety of emtricitabine in human pregnancy has not been established.

Animal studies do not indicate direct or indirect harmful effects of emtricitabine with respect to pregnancy, foetal development, parturition or postnatal development (see 5.3).

Emtricitabine should be used during pregnancy only if necessary.

Given that the potential risks to developing human foetuses are unknown, the use of emtricitabine in women of child-bearing potential must be accompanied by the use of effective contraception.

It is not known if emtricitabine is excreted in human milk.

It is recommended that HIV infected women do not breast-feed their infants under any circumstances in order to avoid transmission of HIV.

4.7 Effects on ability to drive and use machines

No studies on the effects of emtricitabine on the ability to drive and use machines have been performed. However, patients should be informed that dizziness has been reported during treatment with emtricitabine.

4.8 Undesirable effects

Assessment of adverse reactions is based on data from three studies in adults (n=1479) and two paediatric studies (n=114). In the adult studies, 1039 treatment-naïve and 440 treatment-experienced patients received emtricitabine (n=814) or comparator medicinal product (n=665) for 48 weeks in combination with other antiretroviral medicinal products. In the paediatric studies, treatment-naïve (n=83) and treatment-experienced (n=31) paediatric patients aged 4 months to 18 years were treated with emtricitabine in combination with other antiretroviral agents.

The adverse reactions with suspected (at least possible) relationship to treatment are listed below by body system organ class and absolute frequency. Frequencies are defined as very common (> 1/10) or common (> 1/100, < 1/10).

Blood and the lymphatic system disorders:

Common: neutropenia, anaemia

Metabolism and nutrition disorders:

Common: hypertriglyceridaemia, hyperglycaemia

Lactic acidosis, usually associated with hepatic steatosis, has been reported with the use of nucleoside analogues (see 4.4).

Nervous system disorders:

Very common: headache

Common: dizziness, asthenia, insomnia, abnormal dreams

Gastrointestinal disorders:

Very common: diarrhoea, nausea

Common: vomiting, dyspepsia, abdominal pain, elevated serum lipase, elevated amylase including elevated pancreatic amylase

Hepato-biliary disorders:

Common: elevated serum aspartate aminotransferase (AST) and/or elevated serum alanine aminotransferase (ALT), hyperbilirubinaemia

Skin and subcutaneous tissue disorders:

Common: rash, pruritus, maculopapular rash, urticaria, vesiculobullous rash, pustular rash, and allergic reaction, skin discolouration (hyper-pigmentation)

Musculoskeletal, connective tissue and bone disorders:

Very common: elevated creatine kinase

General disorders and administration site conditions:

Common: pain

The adverse reaction profile in patients co-infected with HBV is similar to that observed in patients infected with HIV without co-infection with HBV. However, as would be expected in this patient population, elevations in AST and ALT occurred more frequently than in the general HIV infected population.

Combination antiretroviral therapy has been associated with metabolic abnormalities such as hypertriglyceridaemia, hypercholesterolaemia, insulin resistance, hyperglycaemia and hyperlactataemia (see 4.4).

Combination antiretroviral therapy has been associated with redistribution of body fat (lipodystrophy) in HIV patients including the loss of peripheral and facial subcutaneous fat, increased intra-abdominal and visceral fat, breast hypertrophy and dorsocervical fat accumulation (buffalo hump) (see 4.4).

In HIV infected patients with severe immune deficiency at the time of initiation of combination antiretroviral therapy (CART), an inflammatory reaction to asymptomatic or residual opportunistic infections may arise (see section 4.4).

4.9 Overdose

Administration of up to 1200 mg emtricitabine has been associated with the adverse reactions listed above (see 4.8).

If overdose occurs, the patient should be monitored for signs of toxicity and standard supportive treatment applied as necessary.

Up to 30% of the emtricitabine dose can be removed by haemodialysis. It is not known whether emtricitabine can be removed by peritoneal dialysis.

5. PHARMACOLOGICAL PROPERTIES

5.1 Pharmacodynamic properties

Pharmacotherapeutic group: Antiviral for systemic use: Nucleoside and nucleotide reverse transcriptase inhibitors, ATC Code: J05AF09.

Mechanism of action: Emtricitabine is a synthetic nucleoside analogue of cytosine with activity that is specific to human immunodeficiency virus (HIV-1 and HIV-2) and hepatitis B virus (HBV).

Emtricitabine is phosphorylated by cellular enzymes to form emtricitabine 5'-triphosphate, which competitively inhibits HIV-1 reverse transcriptase, resulting in DNA chain termination. Emtricitabine is a weak inhibitor of mammalian DNA polymerase α, β and ε and mitochondrial DNA polymerase γ.

Emtricitabine did not exhibit cytotoxicity to peripheral blood mononuclear cells (PBMCs), established lymphocyte and monocyte-macrophage cell lines or bone marrow progenitor cells *in vitro*. There was no evidence of toxicity to mitochondria *in vitro* or *in vivo*.

Antiviral activity in vitro: The 50% inhibitory concentration (IC_{50}) value for emtricitabine against laboratory and clinical isolates of HIV-1 was in the range of 0.0013 to 0.5 μmol/l. In combination studies of emtricitabine with protease inhibitors, nucleoside, nucleotide and non-nucleoside analogue inhibitors of HIV reverse transcriptase, additive to synergistic effects were observed. Most of these combinations have not been studied in humans.

When tested for activity against laboratory strains of HBV, the 50% inhibitory concentration (IC_{50}) value for emtricitabine was in the range of 0.01 to 0.04 μmol/l.

Resistance: HIV-1 resistance to emtricitabine develops as the result of changes at codon 184 causing the methionine to be changed to a valine (an isoleucine intermediate has also been observed) of the HIV reverse transcriptase. This HIV-1 mutation was observed *in vitro* and in HIV-1 infected patients.

Emtricitabine-resistant viruses were cross-resistant to lamivudine, but retained sensitivity to other nucleoside reverse transcriptase inhibitors (NRTIs) (zidovudine, stavudine, tenofovir, abacavir, didanosine and zalcitabine), all non-nucleoside reverse transcriptase inhibitors (NNRTIs) and all protease inhibitors (PIs). Viruses resistant to zidovudine, zalcitabine, didanosine and NNRTIs retained their sensitivity to emtricitabine (IC_{50}=0.002 μmol/l to 0.08 μmol/l).

Clinical experience: Emtricitabine in combination with other antiretroviral agents, including nucleoside analogues, non-nucleoside analogues and protease inhibitors, has been shown to be effective in the treatment of HIV infection in treatment-naïve patients and treatment-experienced patients with stable virological control. There is no experience of the use of emtricitabine in patients who are failing their current regimen or who have failed multiple regimens. There is no clinical experience of the use of emtricitabine in infants less than 4 months of age.

In antiretroviral treatment-naïve adults, emtricitabine was significantly superior to stavudine when both medicinal products were taken in combination with didanosine and efavirenz through 48 weeks of treatment. Phenotypic analysis showed no significant changes in emtricitabine susceptibility unless the M184V/I mutation had developed.

In virologically stable treatment-experienced adults, emtricitabine, in combination with an NRTI (either stavudine or zidovudine) and a protease inhibitor (PI) or an NNRTI was shown to be non-inferior to lamivudine with respect to the proportion of responders (< 400 copies/ml) through 48 weeks (77% emtricitabine, 82% lamivudine). Additionally, in a second study, treatment-experienced adults on a stable PI based highly active antiretroviral therapy (HAART) regimen were randomised to a once daily regimen containing emtricitabine or to continue with their PI-HAART regimen. At 48 weeks of treatment the emtricitabine-containing regimen demonstrated an equivalent proportion of patients with HIV RNA < 400 copies/ml (94% emtricitabine *versus* 92%) and a greater proportion of patients with HIV RNA < 50 copies/ml (95% emtricitabine *versus* 87%) compared with the patients continuing with their PI-HAART regimen.

In thirty-one virologically stable treatment-experienced and 83 treatment-naïve infants and children ranging in age from 4 months to 18 years old, the majority of patients achieved or maintained complete suppression of plasma HIV-1 RNA through 24 weeks (89% achieved $\leqslant$ 400 copies/ml and 70% achieved $\leqslant$ 50 copies/ml).

5.2 Pharmacokinetic properties

Absorption: Emtricitabine is rapidly and extensively absorbed following oral administration with peak plasma concentrations occurring at 1 to 2 hours post-dose. In 20 HIV infected subjects receiving 200 mg emtricitabine daily as hard capsules, steady-state plasma emtricitabine peak concentrations (C_{max}), trough concentrations (C_{min}) and area under the plasma concentration time curve over a 24-hour dosing interval (AUC) were 1.8±0.7 μg/ml, 0.09±0.07 μg/ml and 10.0±3.1 μg·h/ml, respectively. Steady-state trough plasma concentrations reached levels approximately 4-fold above the *in vitro* IC_{90} values for anti-HIV activity.

The absolute bioavailability of emtricitabine from Emtriva 200 mg hard capsules was estimated to be 93% and the absolute bioavailability from Emtriva 10 mg/ml oral solution was estimated to be 75%.

In a pilot study in children and a definitive bioequivalence study in adults, the Emtriva 10 mg/ml oral solution was shown to have approximately 80% of the bioavailability of the Emtriva 200 mg hard capsules. The reason for this difference is unknown. Due to this difference in bioavailability, 240 mg emtricitabine administered as the oral solution should provide similar plasma levels to those observed after administration of one 200 mg emtricitabine hard capsule. Therefore, children who weigh at least 33 kg may take either one 200 mg hard capsule daily or the oral solution up to a maximum dose of 240 mg (24 ml), once daily.

Administration of Emtriva 200 mg hard capsules with a high-fat meal or administration of Emtriva 10 mg/ml oral solution with a low-fat or high-fat meal did not affect systemic exposure ($AUC_{0-\infty}$) of emtricitabine; therefore Emtriva 200 mg hard capsules and Emtriva 10 mg/ml oral solution may be administered with or without food.

Distribution: In vitro binding of emtricitabine to human plasma proteins was < 4% and independent of concentration over the range of 0.02-200 μg/ml. The mean plasma to blood concentration ratio was approximately 1.0 and the mean semen to plasma concentration ratio was approximately 4.0.

The apparent volume of distribution after intravenous administration of emtricitabine was 1.4±0.3 l/kg, indicating that emtricitabine is widely distributed throughout the body to both intracellular and extracellular fluid spaces.

Biotransformation: There is limited metabolism of emtricitabine. The biotransformation of emtricitabine includes oxidation of the thiol moiety to form the 3'-sulphoxide diastereomers (approximately 9% of dose) and conjugation with glucuronic acid to form 2'-O-glucuronide (approximately 4% of dose).

Emtricitabine did not inhibit *in vitro* drug metabolism mediated by the following human CYP450 isoenzymes: 1A2, 2A6, 2B6, 2C9, 2C19, 2D6 and 3A4.

Also, emtricitabine did not inhibit uridine-5'-diphosphoglucuronyl transferase, the enzyme responsible for glucuronidation.

Elimination: Emtricitabine is primarily excreted by the kidneys with complete recovery of the dose achieved in urine (approximately 86%) and faeces (approximately 14%). Thirteen percent of the emtricitabine dose was recovered in urine as three metabolites. The systemic clearance of emtricitabine averaged 307 ml/min (4.03 ml/min/kg). Following oral administration, the elimination half-life of emtricitabine is approximately 10 hours.

Linearity/non-linearity: The pharmacokinetics of emtricitabine are proportional to dose over the dose range of 25-200 mg following single or repeated administration.

Intracellular pharmacokinetics: In a clinical study, the intracellular half-life of emtricitabine-triphosphate in peripheral blood mononuclear cells was 39 hours. Intracellular triphosphate levels increased with dose, but reached a plateau at doses of 200 mg or greater.

Adults with renal insufficiency: Pharmacokinetic parameters were determined following administration of a single dose of 200 mg emtricitabine hard capsules to 30 non-HIV infected subjects with varying degrees of renal insufficiency. Subjects were grouped according to baseline creatinine clearance > 80 ml/min as normal function; 50-80 ml/min as mild impairment; 30-49 ml/min as moderate impairment; < 30 ml/min as severe impairment; < 15 ml/min as functionally anephric requiring haemodialysis).

The systemic emtricitabine exposure (mean ± standard deviation) increased from 11.8±2.9 μg·h/ml in subjects with normal renal function to 19.9±1.1, 25.0±5.7 and 34.0±2.1 μg·h/ml, in patients with mild, moderate and severe renal impairment, respectively.

In patients with ESRD on haemodialysis, approximately 30% of the emtricitabine dose was recovered in dialysate over a 3 hour dialysis period which had been started within 1.5 hours of emtricitabine dosing (blood flow rate of 400 ml/min and dialysate flow rate of approximately 600 ml/min).

Hepatic insufficiency: The pharmacokinetics of emtricitabine have not been studied in non-HBV infected subjects with varying degrees of hepatic insufficiency. In general, emtricitabine pharmacokinetics in HBV infected subjects were similar to those in healthy subjects and in HIV infected subjects.

Age, gender and ethnicity: In general, the pharmacokinetics of emtricitabine in infants and children (aged 4 months up to 18 years) are similar to those seen in adults.

The mean AUC in 36 infants and children (aged 4 months to 12 years) receiving 6 mg/kg emtricitabine once daily as oral solution and in 12 adolescents (aged 13-18 years) receiving 200 mg emtricitabine as hard capsules once daily were 9.4 μg·h/ml and 10.7 μg·h/ml, respectively. This compares to the mean AUC of 10.0 μg·h/ml in 20 adults receiving 200 mg hard capsules once daily.

Pharmacokinetic data are not available in the elderly.

Although the mean C_{max} and C_{min} were approximately 20% higher and mean AUC was 16% higher in females compared to males, this difference was not considered clinically significant. No clinically important pharmacokinetic difference due to race has been identified.

5.3 Preclinical safety data

Non-clinical data reveal no special hazard for humans based on conventional studies of safety pharmacology, repeated dose toxicity, genotoxicity and reproductive/developmental toxicity. Emtricitabine did not show any carcinogenic potential in long-term oral carcinogenicity studies in mice and rats.

6. PHARMACEUTICAL PARTICULARS

6.1 List of excipients

Cotton candy flavouring

Disodium edetate

Hydrochloric acid

Methyl parahydroxybenzoate (E218)

Propylene glycol

Propyl parahydroxybenzoate (E216)

Sodium hydroxide

Sodium phosphate monobasic hydrate

Sunset yellow (E110)

Purified water

Xylitol (E967)

6.2 Incompatibilities

Not applicable.

6.3 Shelf life

3 years.

After first opening: 45 days.

6.4 Special precautions for storage

Store in a refrigerator (2°C – 8°C).

After opening: Do not store above 25°C.

6.5 Nature and contents of container

Amber-coloured polyethylene terephthalate (PET) bottle with a child-resistant closure. The pack also contains a 30 ml polypropylene measuring cup with 1.0 ml graduations. The bottle contains 170 ml of solution.

6.6 Instructions for use and handling

Patients should be instructed that any solution left in the bottle 45 days after opening should be discarded according to local requirements or returned to the pharmacy.

7. MARKETING AUTHORISATION HOLDER

Gilead Sciences International Limited

Cambridge

CB1 6GT

United Kingdom

8. MARKETING AUTHORISATION NUMBER(S)

EU/1/03/261/003

9. DATE OF FIRST AUTHORISATION/RENEWAL OF THE AUTHORISATION

24 October 2003

10. DATE OF REVISION OF THE TEXT

08/09/05

Emtriva 200 mg hard capsules

(Gilead Sciences International Limited)

1. NAME OF THE MEDICINAL PRODUCT

Emtriva 200 mg hard capsules▼

2. QUALITATIVE AND QUANTITATIVE COMPOSITION

Each hard capsule contains 200 mg emtricitabine.

For excipients, see 6.1.

3. PHARMACEUTICAL FORM

Hard capsule.

Each capsule has a white opaque body with a light blue opaque cap. Each capsule is printed with "200 mg" on the cap and "GILEAD" and [Gilead logo] on the body in black ink.

4. CLINICAL PARTICULARS

4.1 Therapeutic indications

Emtriva is indicated for the treatment of HIV-1 infected adults and children in combination with other antiretroviral agents.

This indication is based on studies in treatment-naïve patients and treatment-experienced patients with stable virological control. There is no experience of the use of Emtriva in patients who are failing their current regimen or who have failed multiple regimens (see 5.1).

When deciding on a new regimen for patients who have failed an antiretroviral regimen, careful consideration should be given to the patterns of mutations associated with different medicinal products and the treatment history of the individual patient. Where available, resistance testing may be appropriate.

4.2 Posology and method of administration

Therapy should be initiated by a physician experienced in the management of HIV infection.

Emtriva 200 mg hard capsules may be taken with or without food.

Adults: The recommended dose of Emtriva is one 200 mg hard capsule, taken orally, once daily.

Children and adolescents up to 18 years of age: The recommended dose of Emtriva for children and adolescents weighing at least 33 kg who are able to swallow hard capsules is one 200 mg hard capsule, taken orally, once daily.

There are no data on the safety and efficacy of emtricitabine in infants less than 4 months of age.

Emtriva is also available as a 10 mg/ml oral solution for use in infants older than 4 months of age, children and patients who are unable to swallow hard capsules and patients with renal insufficiency. Please refer to the Summary of Product Characteristics for Emtriva 10 mg/ml oral solution. Due to a difference in the bioavailability of emtricitabine between the hard capsule and oral solution presentations, 240 mg emtricitabine administered as the oral solution should provide similar plasma levels to those observed after administration of one 200 mg emtricitabine hard capsule (see 5.2).

Elderly: There are no safety and efficacy data available in patients over the age of 65 years. However, no adjustment in the recommended daily dose for adults should be required unless there is evidence of renal insufficiency.

Renal insufficiency: Emtricitabine is eliminated by renal excretion and exposure to emtricitabine was significantly increased in patients with renal insufficiency (see 5.2). Dose or dose interval adjustment is required in all patients with creatinine clearance < 50 ml/min (see 4.4).

The table below provides dose interval adjustment guidelines for the 200 mg hard capsules according to the degree of renal insufficiency. The safety and efficacy of these dose interval adjustment guidelines have not been clinically evaluated. Therefore, clinical response to treatment and renal function should be closely monitored in these patients (see 4.4).

Patients with renal insufficiency can also be managed by administration of Emtriva 10 mg/ml oral solution to provide a reduced daily dose of emtricitabine. Please refer to the Summary of Product Characteristics for Emtriva 10 mg/ml oral solution.

(see Table 1)

Patients with end-stage renal disease (ESRD) managed with other forms of dialysis such as ambulatory peritoneal dialysis have not been studied and no dose recommendations can be made.

No data are available on which to make a dosage recommendation in paediatric patients with renal insufficiency.

Hepatic insufficiency: No data are available on which to make a dose recommendation for patients with hepatic insufficiency. However, based on the minimal metabolism of emtricitabine and the renal route of elimination it is unlikely that a dose adjustment would be required in patients with hepatic insufficiency (see 5.2).

4.3 Contraindications

Hypersensitivity to emtricitabine or to any of the excipients.

4.4 Special warnings and special precautions for use

General: Emtricitabine is not recommended as monotherapy for the treatment of HIV infection. It must be used in combination with other antiretrovirals. Please also refer to the Summaries of Product Characteristics of the other antiretroviral medicinal products used in the combination regimen.

Patients receiving emtricitabine or any other antiretroviral therapy may continue to develop opportunistic infections and other complications of HIV infection, and therefore should remain under close clinical observation by physicians experienced in the treatment of patients with HIV associated diseases.

Patients should be advised that antiretroviral therapies, including emtricitabine, have not been proven to prevent the risk of transmission of HIV to others through sexual contact or blood contamination. Appropriate precautions should continue to be used. Patients should also be informed that emtricitabine is not a cure for HIV infection.

Renal function: Emtricitabine is principally eliminated by the kidney via glomerular filtration and active tubular secretion. Emtricitabine exposure may be markedly increased in patients with moderate or severe renal insufficiency (creatinine clearance < 50 ml/min) receiving daily doses of 200 mg emtricitabine as hard capsules or 240 mg as the oral solution. Consequently, either a dose interval adjustment (using Emtriva 200 mg hard capsules) or a reduction in the daily dose of emtricitabine (using Emtriva 10 mg/ml oral solution) is required in all patients with creatinine clearance < 50 ml/min. The safety and efficacy of the dose interval adjustment guidelines provided in section 4.2 are based on single dose pharmacokinetic data and modelling and have not been clinically evaluated. Therefore, clinical response to treatment and renal function should be closely monitored in patients treated with emtricitabine at prolonged dosing intervals (see 4.2 and 5.2).

Caution should be exercised when emtricitabine is co-administered with medicinal products that are eliminated by active tubular secretion as such co-administration may lead to an increase in serum concentrations of either emtricitabine or a co-administered medicinal product, due to competition for this elimination pathway (see 4.5).

Lactic acidosis: Lactic acidosis, usually associated with hepatic steatosis, has been reported with the use of nucleoside analogues. Early symptoms (symptomatic hyperlactataemia) include benign digestive symptoms (nausea, vomiting and abdominal pain), non-specific malaise, loss of appetite, weight loss, respiratory symptoms (rapid and/or deep breathing) or neurological symptoms (including motor weakness). Lactic acidosis has a high mortality and may be associated with pancreatitis, liver failure or renal failure. Lactic acidosis generally occurred after a few or several months of treatment.

Treatment with nucleoside analogues should be discontinued in the setting of symptomatic hyperlactataemia and metabolic/lactic acidosis, progressive hepatomegaly, or rapidly elevating aminotransferase levels.

Caution should be exercised when administering nucleoside analogues to any patient (particularly obese women) with hepatomegaly, hepatitis or other known risk factors for liver disease and hepatic steatosis (including certain medicinal products and alcohol). Patients co-infected with hepatitis C and treated with alpha interferon and ribavirin may constitute a special risk.

Patients at increased risk should be followed closely.

Lipodystrophy: Combination antiretroviral therapy has been associated with the redistribution of body fat (lipodystrophy) in HIV patients. The long-term consequences of these events are currently unknown. Knowledge about the mechanism is incomplete. A connection between visceral lipomatosis and protease inhibitors, and lipoatrophy and nucleoside reverse transcriptase inhibitors has been hypothesised. A higher risk of lipodystrophy has been associated with individual factors such as older age, and with drug related factors such as longer duration of antiretroviral treatment and associated metabolic disturbances. Clinical examination should include evaluation for physical signs of fat redistribution. Consideration should be given to the measurement of fasting serum lipids and blood glucose. Lipid disorders should be managed as clinically appropriate.

Liver function: Patients with pre-existing liver dysfunction including chronic active hepatitis have an increased frequency of liver function abnormalities during combination antiretroviral therapy and should be monitored according to standard practice. Patients with chronic hepatitis B or C infection treated with combination antiretroviral therapy are at increased risk of experiencing severe, and potentially fatal, hepatic adverse events. In case of concomitant antiviral therapy for hepatitis B or C, please also refer to the relevant Summary of Product Characteristics for these medicinal products.

If there is evidence of exacerbations of liver disease in such patients, interruption or discontinuation of treatment must be considered.

Patients co-infected with hepatitis B virus (HBV): Emtricitabine is active *in vitro* against HBV. However, limited data are available on the efficacy and safety of emtricitabine (as a 200 mg hard capsule once daily) in patients who are co-infected with HIV and HBV. The use of emtricitabine in patient with chronic HBV induces the same mutation pattern in the YMDD motif observed with lamivudine therapy. The YMDD mutation confers resistance to both emtricitabine and lamivudine.

Patients co-infected with HIV and HBV should be closely monitored with both clinical and laboratory follow-up for at least several months after stopping treatment with emtricitabine for evidence of exacerbations of hepatitis. Such exacerbations have been seen following discontinuation of emtricitabine treatment in HBV infected patients without concomitant HIV infection and have been detected primarily by serum alanine aminotransferase (ALT) elevations in addition to re-emergence of HBV DNA.

Mitochondrial dysfunction: Nucleoside and nucleotide analogues have been demonstrated *in vitro* and *in vivo* to cause a variable degree of mitochondrial damage. There have been reports of mitochondrial dysfunction in HIV negative infants exposed *in utero* and/or postnatally to nucleoside analogues. The main adverse events reported are haematological disorders (anaemia, neutropenia), metabolic disorders (hyperlactataemia, hyperlipasaemia). These events are often transitory. Some late-onset neurological disorders have been reported (hypertonia, convulsion, abnormal behaviour). Whether the neurological disorders are transient or permanent is currently unknown. Any child exposed *in utero* to nucleoside and nucleotide analogues, even HIV negative children, should have clinical and laboratory follow-up and should be fully investigated for possible mitochondrial dysfunction in case of relevant signs or symptoms. These findings do not affect current national recommendations to use antiretroviral therapy in pregnant women to prevent vertical transmission of HIV.

Immune Reactivation Syndrome: In HIV infected patients with severe immune deficiency at the time of institution of combination antiretroviral therapy (CART), an inflammatory reaction to asymptomatic or residual opportunistic pathogens may arise and cause serious clinical conditions, or aggravation of symptoms. Typically, such reactions have been observed within the first few weeks or months of initiation of CART. Relevant examples are cytomegalovirus retinitis, generalised and/or focal mycobacterium infections, and *Pneumocystis carinii* pneumonia. Any inflammatory symptoms should be evaluated and treatment instituted when necessary.

4.5 Interaction with other medicinal products and other forms of Interaction

In vitro, emtricitabine did not inhibit metabolism mediated by any of the following human CYP450 isoforms: 1A2, 2A6, 2B6, 2C9, 2C19, 2D6 and 3A4. Emtricitabine did not inhibit the enzyme responsible for glucuronidation. Based on the results of these *in vitro* experiments and the known elimination pathways of emtricitabine, the potential for CYP450 mediated interactions involving emtricitabine with other medicinal products is low.

There are no clinically significant interactions when emtricitabine is co-administered with indinavir, zidovudine, stavudine, famciclovir or tenofovir disoproxil fumarate.

Emtricitabine is primarily excreted via glomerular filtration and active tubular secretion. With the exception of famciclovir and tenofovir disoproxil fumarate, the effect of co-administration of emtricitabine with medicinal products that are excreted by the renal route, or other medicinal products known to affect renal function, has not been evaluated. Co-administration of emtricitabine with medicinal products that are eliminated by active tubular secretion may lead to an increase in serum concentrations of either emtricitabine or a co-administered medicinal product due to competition for this elimination pathway.

There is no clinical experience as yet on the co-administration of cytidine analogues. Consequently, the use of emtricitabine in combination with lamivudine or zalcitabine for the treatment of HIV infection cannot be recommended at this time.

4.6 Pregnancy and lactation

The safety of emtricitabine in human pregnancy has not been established.

Animal studies do not indicate direct or indirect harmful effects of emtricitabine with respect to pregnancy, foetal development, parturition or postnatal development (see 5.3).

Emtricitabine should be used during pregnancy only if necessary.

Given that the potential risks to developing human foetuses are unknown, the use of emtricitabine in women of child-bearing potential must be accompanied by the use of effective contraception.

It is not known if emtricitabine is excreted in human milk.

It is recommended that HIV infected women do not breast-feed their infants under any circumstances in order to avoid transmission of HIV.

4.7 Effects on ability to drive and use machines

No studies on the effects of emtricitabine on the ability to drive and use machines have been performed. However, patients should be informed that dizziness has been reported during treatment with emtricitabine.

Table 1

	Creatinine Clearance (CL_{cr}) (ml/min)			
	≥ 50	30-49	15-29	< 15 (functionally anephric, requiring intermittent haemodialysis)*
Recommended dose interval for 200 mg hard capsules	One 200 mg hard capsule every 24 hours	One 200 mg hard capsule every 48 hours	One 200 mg hard capsule every 72 hours	One 200 mg hard capsule every 96 hours

* Assumes a 3h haemodialysis session three times a week commencing at least 12h after administration of the last dose of emtricitabine.

4.8 Undesirable effects

Assessment of adverse reactions is based on data from three studies in adults (n=1479) and two paediatric studies (n=114). In the adult studies, 1039 treatment-naïve and 440 treatment-experienced patients received emtricitabine (n=814) or comparator medicinal product (n=665) for 48 weeks in combination with other antiretroviral medicinal products. In the paediatric studies, treatment-naïve (n=83) and treatment-experienced (n=31) paediatric patients aged 4 months to 18 years were treated with emtricitabine in combination with other antiretroviral agents.

The adverse reactions with suspected (at least possible) relationship to treatment are listed below by body system organ class and absolute frequency. Frequencies are defined as very common (> 1/10) or common (> 1/100, < 1/10).

Blood and the lymphatic system disorders:

Common: neutropenia, anaemia

Metabolism and nutrition disorders:

Common: hypertriglyceridaemia, hyperglycaemia

Lactic acidosis, usually associated with hepatic steatosis, has been reported with the use of nucleoside analogues (see 4.4).

Nervous system disorders:

Very common: headache

Common: dizziness, asthenia, insomnia, abnormal dreams

Gastrointestinal disorders:

Very common: diarrhoea, nausea

Common: vomiting, dyspepsia, abdominal pain, elevated serum lipase, elevated amylase including elevated pancreatic amylase

Hepato-biliary disorders:

Common: elevated serum aspartate aminotransferase (AST) and/or elevated serum alanine aminotransferase (ALT), hyperbilirubinaemia

Skin and subcutaneous tissue disorders:

Common: rash, pruritus, maculopapular rash, urticaria, vesiculobullous rash, pustular rash, and allergic reaction, skin discolouration (hyper-pigmentation)

Musculoskeletal, connective tissue and bone disorders:

Very common: elevated creatine kinase

General disorders and administration site conditions:

Common: pain

The adverse reaction profile in patients co-infected with HBV is similar to that observed in patients infected with HIV without co-infection with HBV. However, as would be expected in this patient population, elevations in AST and ALT occurred more frequently than in the general HIV infected population.

Combination antiretroviral therapy has been associated with metabolic abnormalities such as hypertriglyceridaemia, hypercholesterolaemia, insulin resistance, hyperglycaemia and hyperlactataemia (see 4.4).

Combination antiretroviral therapy has been associated with redistribution of body fat (lipodystrophy) in HIV patients including the loss of peripheral and facial subcutaneous fat, increased intra-abdominal and visceral fat, breast hypertrophy and dorsocervical fat accumulation (buffalo hump) (see 4.4).

In HIV infected patients with severe immune deficiency at the time of initiation of combination antiretroviral therapy (CART), an inflammatory reaction to asymptomatic or residual opportunistic infections may arise (see section 4.4).

4.9 Overdose

Administration of up to 1200 mg emtricitabine has been associated with the adverse reactions listed above (see 4.8).

If overdose occurs, the patient should be monitored for signs of toxicity and standard supportive treatment applied as necessary.

Up to 30% of the emtricitabine dose can be removed by haemodialysis. It is not known whether emtricitabine can be removed by peritoneal dialysis.

5. PHARMACOLOGICAL PROPERTIES

5.1 Pharmacodynamic properties

Pharmacotherapeutic group: Antiviral for systemic use: Nucleoside and nucleotide reverse transcriptase inhibitors, ATC Code: J05AF09.

Mechanism of action: Emtricitabine is a synthetic nucleoside analogue of cytosine with activity that is specific to human immunodeficiency virus (HIV-1 and HIV-2) and hepatitis B virus (HBV).

Emtricitabine is phosphorylated by cellular enzymes to form emtricitabine 5'-triphosphate, which competitively inhibits HIV-1 reverse transcriptase, resulting in DNA chain termination. Emtricitabine is a weak inhibitor of mammalian DNA polymerase α, β and ε and mitochondrial DNA polymerase γ.

Emtricitabine did not exhibit cytotoxicity to peripheral blood mononuclear cells (PBMCs), established lymphocyte and monocyte-macrophage cell lines or bone marrow progenitor cells *in vitro*. There was no evidence of toxicity to mitochondria *in vitro or in vivo*.

Antiviral activity in vitro: The 50% inhibitory concentration (IC_{50}) value for emtricitabine against laboratory and clinical isolates of HIV-1 was in the range of 0.0013 to 0.5 μmol/l. In combination studies of emtricitabine with protease inhibitors, nucleoside, nucleotide and non-nucleoside analogue inhibitors of HIV reverse transcriptase, additive to synergistic effects were observed. Most of these combinations have not been studied in humans.

When tested for activity against laboratory strains of HBV, the 50% inhibitory concentration (IC_{50}) value for emtricitabine was in the range of 0.01 to 0.04 μmol/l.

Resistance: HIV-1 resistance to emtricitabine develops as the result of changes at codon 184 causing the methionine to be changed to a valine (an isoleucine intermediate has also been observed) of the HIV reverse transcriptase. This HIV-1 mutation was observed *in vitro* and in HIV-1 infected patients.

Emtricitabine-resistant viruses were cross-resistant to lamivudine, but retained sensitivity to other nucleoside reverse transcriptase inhibitors (NRTIs) (zidovudine, stavudine, tenofovir, abacavir, didanosine and zalcitabine), all non-nucleoside reverse transcriptase inhibitors (NNRTIs) and all protease inhibitors (PIs). Viruses resistant to zidovudine, zalcitabine, didanosine and NNRTIs retained their sensitivity to emtricitabine (IC_{50}=0.002 μmol/l to 0.08 μmol/l).

Clinical experience: Emtricitabine in combination with other antiretroviral agents, including nucleoside analogues, non-nucleoside analogues and protease inhibitors, has been shown to be effective in the treatment of HIV infection in treatment-naïve patients and treatment-experienced patients with stable virological control. There is no experience of the use of emtricitabine in patients who are failing their current regimen or who have failed multiple regimens. There is no clinical experience of the use of emtricitabine in infants less than 4 months of age.

In antiretroviral treatment-naïve adults, emtricitabine was significantly superior to stavudine when both medicinal products were taken in combination with didanosine and efavirenz through 48 weeks of treatment. Phenotypic analysis showed no significant changes in emtricitabine susceptibility unless the M184V/I mutation had developed.

In virologically stable treatment-experienced adults, emtricitabine, in combination with an NRTI (either stavudine or zidovudine) and a protease inhibitor (PI) or an NNRTI was shown to be non-inferior to lamivudine with respect to the proportion of responders (< 400 copies/ml) through 48 weeks (77% emtricitabine, 82% lamivudine). Additionally, in a second study, treatment-experienced adults on a stable PI based highly active antiretroviral therapy (HAART) regimen were randomised to a once daily regimen containing emtricitabine or to continue with their PI-HAART regimen. At 48 weeks of treatment the emtricitabine-containing regimen demonstrated an equivalent proportion of patients with HIV RNA < 400 copies/ml (94% emtricitabine *versus* 92%) and a greater proportion of patients with HIV RNA < 50 copies/ml (95% emtricitabine *versus* 87%) compared with the patients continuing with their PI-HAART regimen.

In thirty-one virologically stable treatment-experienced and 83 treatment-naïve infants and children ranging in age from 4 months to 18 years old, the majority of patients achieved or maintained complete suppression of plasma HIV-1 RNA through 24 weeks (89% achieved ⩽ 400 copies/ml and 70% achieved ⩽ 50 copies/ml).

5.2 Pharmacokinetic properties

Absorption: Emtricitabine is rapidly and extensively absorbed following oral administration with peak plasma concentrations occurring at 1 to 2 hours post-dose. In 20 HIV infected subjects receiving 200 mg emtricitabine daily as hard capsules, steady-state plasma emtricitabine peak concentrations (C_{max}), trough concentrations (C_{min}) and area under the plasma concentration time curve over a 24-hour dosing interval (AUC) were 1.8±0.7 μg/ml, 0.09±0.07 μg/ml and 10.0±3.1 μg·h/ml, respectively. Steady-state trough plasma concentrations reached levels approximately 4-fold above the *in vitro* IC_{90} values for anti-HIV activity.

The absolute bioavailability of emtricitabine from Emtriva 200 mg hard capsules was estimated to be 93% and the absolute bioavailability from Emtriva 10 mg/ml oral solution was estimated to be 75%.

In a pilot study in children and a definitive bioequivalence study in adults, the Emtriva 10 mg/ml oral solution was shown to have approximately 80% of the bioavailability of the Emtriva 200 mg hard capsules. The reason for this difference is unknown. Due to this difference in bioavailability, 240 mg emtricitabine administered as the oral solution should provide similar plasma levels to those observed after administration of one 200 mg emtricitabine hard capsule. Therefore, children who weigh at least 33 kg may take either one 200 mg hard capsule daily or the oral solution up to a maximum dose of 240 mg (24 ml), once daily.

Administration of Emtriva 200 mg hard capsules with a high-fat meal or administration of Emtriva 10 mg/ml oral solution with a low-fat or high-fat meal did not affect systemic exposure ($AUC_{0-\infty}$) of emtricitabine; therefore Emtriva 200 mg hard capsules and Emtriva 10 mg/ml oral solution may be administered with or without food.

Distribution: In vitro binding of emtricitabine to human plasma proteins was < 4% and independent of concentration over the range of 0.02-200 μg/ml. The mean plasma to blood concentration ratio was approximately 1.0 and the mean semen to plasma concentration ratio was approximately 4.0.

The apparent volume of distribution after intravenous administration of emtricitabine was 1.4±0.3 l/kg, indicating that emtricitabine is widely distributed throughout the body to both intracellular and extracellular fluid spaces.

Biotransformation: There is limited metabolism of emtricitabine. The biotransformation of emtricitabine includes oxidation of the thiol moiety to form the 3'-sulphoxide diastereomers (approximately 9% of dose) and conjugation with glucuronic acid to form 2'-O-glucuronide (approximately 4% of dose).

Emtricitabine did not inhibit *in vitro* drug metabolism mediated by the following human CYP450 isoenzymes: 1A2, 2A6, 2B6, 2C9, 2C19, 2D6 and 3A4.

Also, emtricitabine did not inhibit uridine-5'-diphosphoglucuronyl transferase, the enzyme responsible for glucuronidation.

Elimination: Emtricitabine is primarily excreted by the kidneys with complete recovery of the dose achieved in urine (approximately 86%) and faeces (approximately 14%). Thirteen percent of the emtricitabine dose was recovered in urine as three metabolites. The systemic clearance of emtricitabine averaged 307 ml/min (4.03 ml/min/kg). Following oral administration, the elimination half-life of emtricitabine is approximately 10 hours.

Linearity/non-linearity: The pharmacokinetics of emtricitabine are proportional to dose over the dose range of 25-200 mg following single or repeated administration.

Intracellular pharmacokinetics: In a clinical study, the intracellular half-life of emtricitabine-triphosphate in peripheral blood mononuclear cells was 39 hours. Intracellular triphosphate levels increased with dose, but reached a plateau at doses of 200 mg or greater.

Adults with renal insufficiency: Pharmacokinetic parameters were determined following administration of a single dose of 200 mg emtricitabine hard capsules to 30 non-HIV infected subjects with varying degrees of renal insufficiency. Subjects were grouped according to baseline creatinine clearance > 80 ml/min as normal function; 50-80 ml/min as mild impairment; 30-49 ml/min as moderate impairment; < 30 ml/min as severe impairment; < 15 ml/min as functionally anephric requiring haemodialysis).

The systemic emtricitabine exposure (mean ± standard deviation) increased from 11.8±2.9 μg·h/ml in subjects with normal renal function to 19.9±1.1, 25.0±5.7 and 34.0±2.1 μg·h/ml, in patients with mild, moderate and severe renal impairment, respectively.

In patients with ESRD on haemodialysis, approximately 30% of the emtricitabine dose was recovered in dialysate over a 3 hour dialysis period which had been started within 1.5 hours of emtricitabine dosing (blood flow rate of 400 ml/min and dialysate flow rate of approximately 600ml/min).

Hepatic insufficiency: The pharmacokinetics of emtricitabine have not been studied in non-HBV infected subjects with varying degrees of hepatic insufficiency. In general, emtricitabine pharmacokinetics in HBV infected subjects were similar to those in healthy subjects and in HIV infected subjects.

Age, gender and ethnicity: In general, the pharmacokinetics of emtricitabine in infants and children (aged 4 months up to 18 years) are similar to those seen in adults.

The mean AUC in 36 infants and children (aged 4 months to 12 years) receiving 6 mg/kg emtricitabine once daily as oral solution and in 12 adolescents (aged 13-18 years) receiving 200 mg emtricitabine as hard capsules once daily were 9.4 μg·h/ml and 10.7 μg·h/ml, respectively. This compares to the mean AUC of 10.0 μg·h/ml in 20 adults receiving 200 mg hard capsules once daily.

Pharmacokinetic data are not available in the elderly.

Although the mean C_{max} and C_{min} were approximately 20% higher and mean AUC was 16% higher in females compared to males, this difference was not considered clinically significant. No clinically important pharmacokinetic difference due to race has been identified.

5.3 Preclinical safety data

Non-clinical data reveal no special hazard for humans based on conventional studies of safety pharmacology, repeated dose toxicity, genotoxicity and reproductive/developmental toxicity. Emtricitabine did not show any carcinogenic potential in long-term oral carcinogenicity studies in mice and rats.

6. PHARMACEUTICAL PARTICULARS

6.1 List of excipients

Capsule contents:

Cellulose, microcrystalline (E460)

Crospovidone

Magnesium stearate (E572)

Povidone (E1201)

Capsule shell:

Gelatin

Indigotine (E132)

Titanium dioxide (E171)

Printing ink containing:

Black iron oxide (E172)

Shellac (E904)

6.2 Incompatibilities
Not applicable.

6.3 Shelf life
2 years.

6.4 Special precautions for storage
This medicinal product does not require any special storage conditions.

6.5 Nature and contents of container
White high-density polyethylene (HDPE) bottle fitted with a child-resistant closure, containing 30 hard capsules.

Blisters made of polychlorotrifluorethylene (PCTFE) / polyethylene (PE) / polyvinylchloride (PVC) / aluminium. Each blister pack contains 30 hard capsules.

Pack size: 30 hard capsules.

6.6 Instructions for use and handling
No special requirements.

7. MARKETING AUTHORISATION HOLDER
Gilead Sciences International Limited

Cambridge

CB1 6GT

United Kingdom

8. MARKETING AUTHORISATION NUMBER(S)
EU/1/03/261/001

EU/1/03/261/002

9. DATE OF FIRST AUTHORISATION/RENEWAL OF THE AUTHORISATION
24 October 2003

10. DATE OF REVISION OF THE TEXT
08/09/05

Emulsiderm Emollient

(Dermal Laboratories Limited)

1. NAME OF THE MEDICINAL PRODUCT
EMULSIDERM® EMOLLIENT

2. QUALITATIVE AND QUANTITATIVE COMPOSITION
Liquid Paraffin 25.0% w/w; Isopropyl Myristate 25.0% w/w; Benzalkonium Chloride 0.5% w/w.

3. PHARMACEUTICAL FORM
Pale blue bath additive and cutaneous emulsion.

4. CLINICAL PARTICULARS

4.1 Therapeutic indications
An antimicrobial bath emollient for use as an aid in the treatment of dry and pruritic skin conditions, especially eczema, dermatitis, ichthyosis or xeroderma. It permits the rehydration of the keratin by replacing lost lipids, and its antiseptic properties assist in overcoming secondary infection.

4.2 Posology and method of administration
For adults, children and the elderly:

For use in the bath Add 7 - 30 ml Emulsiderm to a bath of warm water (more or less according to the size of the bath and individual patient requirements). 1 litre bottle - use graduated measuring cup provided; 300 ml bottle - use ½ to 2 capfuls. Soak for 5 - 10 minutes. Pat dry.

For application to the skin Rub a small amount of undiluted emollient into the dry areas of skin until absorbed.

4.3 Contraindications
Sensitivity to any of the ingredients.

4.4 Special warnings and special precautions for use
Keep away from the eyes. For external use only. Take care to avoid slipping in the bath.

4.5 Interaction with other medicinal products and other forms of Interaction
None known.

4.6 Pregnancy and lactation
No known side effects.

4.7 Effects on ability to drive and use machines
None known.

4.8 Undesirable effects
None known.

4.9 Overdose
Not applicable.

5. PHARMACOLOGICAL PROPERTIES

5.1 Pharmacodynamic properties
For dry skin conditions it is important to add an emollient to the bath water. Emulsiderm contains 50% of oils emulsified in water as well as the well-known antiseptic, benzalkonium chloride which assists in overcoming secondary infection.

5.2 Pharmacokinetic properties
Emulsiderm contains 0.5% of the quaternary ammonium antiseptic, benzalkonium chloride. The large positively charged cation is readily adsorbed from the formulation onto negatively charged bacterial cell surfaces, thereby conferring substantial antimicrobial activity. Even at extended dilution, it is particularly effective against *Staphylococcus aureus*, a bacterium which is known to colonise the skin in large numbers in patients with eczema, especially atopic eczema. Apart from its emollient properties, Emulsiderm therefore also helps to prevent and overcome secondary infection which may exacerbate the eczematous condition.

5.3 Preclinical safety data
The safety and efficacy of the emollients (liquid paraffin and isopropyl myristate) and the antiseptic (benzalkonium chloride) in topical dosage forms have been well established over many years of widespread clinical usage.

6. PHARMACEUTICAL PARTICULARS

6.1 List of excipients
Sorbitan Stearate; Polysorbate 60; Industrial Methylated Spirit 95%; Methylthioninium Chloride; Purified Water.

6.2 Incompatibilities
None known.

6.3 Shelf life
36 months.

6.4 Special precautions for storage
Do not store above 25°C. Always replace the cap after use.

6.5 Nature and contents of container
Supplied in plastic bottles; a 300 ml bottle with a measuring cap, and a 1 litre bottle with a measuring cup. These are supplied as original packs (OP).

6.6 Instructions for use and handling
Not applicable.

7. MARKETING AUTHORISATION HOLDER
Dermal Laboratories

Tatmore Place, Gosmore

Hitchin, Herts SG4 7QR, UK.

8. MARKETING AUTHORISATION NUMBER(S)
0173/0036.

9. DATE OF FIRST AUTHORISATION/RENEWAL OF THE AUTHORISATION
22 February 2004.

10. DATE OF REVISION OF THE TEXT
October 2003.

Enbrel

(Wyeth Pharmaceuticals)

1. NAME OF THE MEDICINAL PRODUCT
Enbrel▼ 25 mg powder and solvent for solution for injection.

2. QUALITATIVE AND QUANTITATIVE COMPOSITION
Each vial contains 25 mg of etanercept.

Etanercept is a human tumour necrosis factor receptor p75 Fc fusion protein produced by recombinant DNA technology in a Chinese hamster ovary (CHO) mammalian expression system. Etanercept is a dimer of a chimeric protein genetically engineered by fusing the extracellular ligand binding domain of human tumour necrosis factor receptor-2 (TNFR2/p75) to the Fc domain of human IgG1. This Fc component contains the hinge, CH_2 and CH_3 regions but not the CH_1 region of IgG1. Etanercept contains 934 amino acids and has an apparent molecular weight of approximately 150 kilodaltons. The potency is determined by measuring the ability of etanercept to neutralise the TNFα-mediated growth inhibition of A375 cells. The specific activity of etanercept is 1.7×10^6 units/mg.

For excipients, see section 6.1.

3. PHARMACEUTICAL FORM
Powder and solvent for solution for injection.

The white powder is supplied in a clear glass vial with rubber stopper, aluminium seal and pink plastic cap. The solvent is a clear, colourless liquid supplied in a pre-filled glass syringe (see section 6.5).

4. CLINICAL PARTICULARS

4.1 Therapeutic indications
Enbrel can be used alone or in combination with methotrexate for the treatment of active rheumatoid arthritis in adults when the response to disease-modifying antirheumatic drugs, including methotrexate (unless contraindicated), has been inadequate.

Enbrel is also indicated in the treatment of severe, active and progressive rheumatoid arthritis in adults not previously treated with methotrexate.

In patients with rheumatoid arthritis, Enbrel used alone or in combination with methotrexate has been shown to slow the progression of disease-associated structural damage as measured by X-ray.

Treatment of active polyarticular-course juvenile chronic arthritis in children aged 4 to 17 years who have had an inadequate response to, or who have proved intolerant of, methotrexate. Enbrel has not been studied in children aged less than 4 years.

Treatment of active and progressive psoriatic arthritis in adults when the response to previous disease-modifying antirheumatic drug therapy has been inadequate.

Treatment of adults with severe active ankylosing spondylitis who have had an inadequate response to conventional therapy.

Treatment of adults with moderate to severe plaque psoriasis who failed to respond to, or who have a contraindication to, or are intolerant to other systemic therapy including cyclosporine, methotrexate or PUVA (see Section 5.1).

4.2 Posology and method of administration
Enbrel treatment should be initiated and supervised by specialist physicians experienced in the diagnosis and treatment of rheumatoid arthritis, psoriatic arthritis, ankylosing spondylitis or psoriasis.

Each vial of Enbrel 25 mg must be reconstituted with 1 ml of water for injections before use and administered by subcutaneous injection.

Adults (18-64 years)

Rheumatoid arthritis

25 mg Enbrel administered twice weekly is the recommended dose, alternatively, 50 mg administered once weekly (as two 25 mg injections given at approximately the same time) has been shown to be safe and effective (see section 5.1).

Psoriatic arthritis and ankylosing spondylitis

25 mg Enbrel administered twice weekly is the recommended dose. Doses other than 25 mg administered twice weekly have not been studied.

Plaque psoriasis

The recommended dose of Enbrel is 25 mg administered twice weekly. Alternatively, 50 mg given twice weekly may be used for up to 12 weeks followed, if necessary, by a dose of 25 mg twice weekly. Treatment with Enbrel should continue until remission is achieved, for up to 24 weeks. Treatment should be discontinued in patients who show no response after 12 weeks.

If re-treatment with Enbrel is indicated, the above guidance on treatment duration should be followed. The dose should be 25 mg twice weekly.

Elderly patients (⩾ 65 years)
No dose adjustment is required. Posology and administration are the same as for adults 18-64 years of age.

Children and adolescents (⩾ 4 to <18 years)
0.4 mg/kg (up to a maximum of 25 mg per dose) after reconstitution of 25 mg Enbrel in 1 ml of water for injections, given twice weekly as a subcutaneous injection with an interval of 3-4 days between doses.

Renal and hepatic impairment
No dose adjustment is required.

4.3 Contraindications
Hypersensitivity to the active substance or to any of the excipients.

Sepsis or risk of sepsis.

Treatment with Enbrel should not be initiated in patients with active infections including chronic or localised infections.

4.4 Special warnings and special precautions for use

Infections

Sepsis and serious infections (fatal, life threatening, or requiring hospitalisation or intravenous antibiotics), have been reported with the use of Enbrel (see section 4.8). Many of these serious events have occurred in patients with underlying diseases that in addition to their rheumatoid arthritis could predispose them to infections. Patients who develop a new infection while undergoing treatment with Enbrel should be monitored closely. **Administration of Enbrel should be discontinued if a patient develops a serious infection.** Physicians should exercise caution when considering the use of Enbrel in patients with a history of recurring or chronic infections or with underlying conditions which may predispose patients to infections such as advanced or poorly controlled diabetes.

Concurrent Enbrel and anakinra treatment
Concurrent administration of Enbrel and anakinra has been associated with an increased risk of serious infections and neutropenia compared to Enbrel alone. This combination has not demonstrated increased clinical benefit. Thus the combined use of Enbrel and anakinra is not recommended (see sections 4.5 and 4.8).

Allergic reactions
Allergic reactions associated with Enbrel administration have been reported commonly. Allergic reactions have included angioedema and urticaria; serious reactions have occurred. If any serious allergic or anaphylactic reaction occurs, Enbrel therapy should be discontinued immediately and appropriate therapy initiated.

Immunosuppression

The possibility exists for anti-TNF therapies, including Enbrel, to affect host defences against infections and malignancies since TNF mediates inflammation and modulates cellular immune responses. Reports of various malignancies (including breast and lung carcinoma and lymphoma) have been received in the postmarketing period (see section 4.8). In a study of 49 patients with rheumatoid arthritis treated with Enbrel, there was no evidence of depression of delayed-type hypersensitivity, depression of immunoglobulin levels, or change in enumeration of effector cell populations. Whether treatment with Enbrel might influence the development and course of malignancies and active and/or chronic infections is unknown. The safety and efficacy of Enbrel in patients with immunosuppression or chronic infections have not been evaluated.

Two juvenile chronic arthritis patients developed varicella infection and signs and symptoms of aseptic meningitis which resolved without sequelae. Patients with a significant exposure to varicella virus should temporarily discontinue Enbrel therapy and be considered for prophylactic treatment with Varicella Zoster Immune Globulin.

Vaccinations

Live vaccines should not be given concurrently with Enbrel. No data are available on the secondary transmission of infection by live vaccines in patients receiving Enbrel. It is recommended that juvenile chronic arthritis patients, if possible, be brought up to date with all immunisations in agreement with current immunisation guidelines prior to initiating Enbrel therapy. In a double blind, placebo controlled, randomised clinical study in patients with psoriatic arthritis 184 patients also received a multivalent pneumococcal polysaccharide vaccine at week 4. In this study most psoriatic arthritis patients receiving Enbrel were able to mount effective B-cell immune response to pneumococcal polysaccharide vaccine, but titers in aggregate were moderately lower and few patients had two-fold rises in titers compared to patients not receiving Enbrel. The clinical significance of this is unknown.

Autoantibody formation

Treatment with Enbrel may result in the formation of autoimmune antibodies (see section 4.8).

Haematologic reactions

Rare cases of pancytopenia and very rare cases of aplastic anaemia, some with fatal outcome, have been reported in patients treated with Enbrel. Caution should be exercised in patients being treated with Enbrel who have a previous history of blood dyscrasias. All patients should be advised that if they develop signs and symptoms suggestive of blood dyscrasias or infections (e.g. persistent fever, sore throat, bruising, bleeding, paleness) whilst on Enbrel, they should seek immediate medical advice. Such patients should be investigated urgently, including full blood count; if blood dyscrasias are confirmed, Enbrel should be discontinued.

CNS disorders

There have been rare reports of CNS demyelinating disorders in patients treated with Enbrel (see section 4.8). Although no clinical trials have been performed evaluating Enbrel therapy in patients with multiple sclerosis, clinical trials of other TNF antagonists in patients with multiple sclerosis have shown increases in disease activity. A careful risk/benefit evaluation, including a neurological assessment, is recommended when prescribing Enbrel to patients with pre-existing or recent onset of CNS demyelinating disease, or to those who are considered to have an increased risk of developing demyelinating disease.

Combination therapy

In a controlled clinical trial of one year duration in rheumatoid arthritis patients, the combination of Enbrel and methotrexate did not result in unexpected safety findings, and the safety profile of Enbrel when given in combination with methotrexate was similar to the profiles reported in studies of Enbrel and methotrexate alone. Long-term studies to assess the safety of the combination are ongoing. The long-term safety of Enbrel in combination with other disease-modifying antirheumatic drugs has not been established.

The use of Enbrel in combination with other systemic therapies or phototherapy for the treatment of psoriasis has not been studied.

Renal and hepatic impairment

Based on pharmacokinetic data (see section 5.2), no dosage adjustment is needed in patients with renal or hepatic impairment; clinical experience in such patients is limited.

Congestive Heart Failure

Physicians should use caution when using Enbrel in patients who have congestive heart failure (CHF). There have been postmarketing reports of worsening of CHF, with and without identifiable precipitating factors, in patients taking Enbrel. Two large clinical trials evaluating the use of Enbrel in the treatment of CHF were terminated early due to lack of efficacy. Although not conclusive, data from one of these trials suggest a possible tendency toward worsening CHF in those patients assigned to Enbrel treatment.

Wegener's Granulomatosis

A placebo-controlled trial, in which 89 patients were treated with Enbrel in addition to standard therapy (including cyclophosphamide or methotrexate, and glucocorticoids) for a median duration of 25 months, has not shown Enbrel to be an effective treatment for Wegener's granulomatosis. The incidence of non-cutaneous malignancies of various types was significantly higher in patients treated with Enbrel than in the control group. Enbrel is not recommended for the treatment of Wegener's granulomatosis.

4.5 Interaction with other medicinal products and other forms of Interaction

In clinical trials, no interactions have been observed when Enbrel was administered with glucocorticoids, salicylates (except sulfasalazine), nonsteroidal anti-inflammatory drugs (NSAIDs), analgesics, or methotrexate. See section 4.4 for vaccination advice.

In a clinical study of patients who were receiving established doses of sulfasalazine, to which Enbrel was added, patients in the combination group experienced a statistically significant decrease in mean white blood cell counts in comparison to groups treated with Enbrel or sulfasalazine alone. The clinical significance of this interaction is unknown.

Concurrent Enbrel and anakinra treatment

Patients treated with Enbrel and anakinra were observed to have a higher rate of serious infection when compared with patients treated with either Enbrel or anakinra alone (historical data).

In addition, in a double-blind placebo-controlled trial in patients receiving background methotrexate, patients treated with Enbrel and anakinra were observed to have a higher rate of serious infections (7%) and neutropenia than patients treated with Enbrel (see sections 4.4 and 4.8). The combination Enbrel and anakinra has not demonstrated increased clinical benefit and is therefore not recommended.

4.6 Pregnancy and lactation

There are no studies of Enbrel in pregnant women. Developmental toxicity studies performed in rats and rabbits have revealed no evidence of harm to the foetus or neonatal rat due to etanercept. Preclinical data about peri- and postnatal toxicity of etanercept and of effects of etanercept on fertility and general reproductive performance are not available. Thus, the use of Enbrel in pregnant women is not recommended, and women of child-bearing potential should be advised not to get pregnant during Enbrel therapy.

Use during lactation

It is not known whether etanercept is excreted in human milk. Because immunoglobulins, in common with many medicinal products, can be excreted in human milk, a decision should be made whether to discontinue nursing or to discontinue Enbrel while nursing.

4.7 Effects on ability to drive and use machines

No studies on the effects on the ability to drive and use machines have been performed.

4.8 Undesirable effects

Enbrel has been studied in 2,680 patients with rheumatoid arthritis in double-blind and open-label trials. This experience includes 2 placebo-controlled studies (349 Enbrel patients and 152 placebo patients) and 2 active-controlled trials, one active-controlled trial comparing Enbrel to methotrexate (415 Enbrel patients and 217 methotrexate patients) and another active-controlled trial comparing Enbrel (223 patients), methotrexate (228 patients) and Enbrel in combination with methotrexate (231 patients). The proportion of patients who discontinued treatment due to adverse events was the same in both the Enbrel and placebo treatment groups; in the first active-controlled trial, the dropout rate was significantly higher for methotrexate (10%) than for Enbrel (5%). In the second active-controlled trial, the rate of discontinuation for adverse events was similar among all three treatment groups, Enbrel (11%), methotrexate (14%) and Enbrel in combination with methotrexate (10%). Additionally, Enbrel has been studied in 131 psoriatic arthritis patients who participated in 2 double-blind placebo-controlled studies and an open-label extension study. Two hundred and three (203) ankylosing spondylitis patients were treated with Enbrel in 3 double-blind placebo-controlled studies. Enbrel has also been studied in 1,084 patients with plaque psoriasis for up to 6 months in 3 double-blind placebo-controlled studies.

In double-blind clinical trials comparing Enbrel to placebo, injection site reactions were the most frequent adverse events among Enbrel-treated patients. Among patients with rheumatoid arthritis treated in placebo-controlled trials, serious adverse events occurred at a frequency of 4% in 349 patients treated with Enbrel compared with 5% of 152 placebo-treated patients. In the first active-controlled trial, serious adverse events occurred at a frequency of 6% in 415 patients treated with Enbrel compared with 8% of 217 methotrexate-treated patients. In the second active-controlled trial the rate of serious adverse events were similar among the three treatment groups (Enbrel 11%, methotrexate 12% and Enbrel in combination with methotrexate 8%). Among patients with plaque psoriasis treated in placebo-controlled trials, the frequency of serious adverse events was about 1% of 933 patients treated with Enbrel compared with 1% of 414 placebo-treated patients.

The following list of adverse reactions is based on experience from clinical trials in adults and on postmarketing experience.

Within the organ system classes, adverse reactions are listed under headings of frequency (number of patients expected to experience the reaction), using the following categories: very common (> 1/10); common (> 1/100, < 1/10); uncommon (> 1/1000, < 1/100); rare (> 1/10,000, < 1/1000); very rare (< 1/10,000).

Infections and infestations:

Very common: Infections (including upper respiratory tract infections, bronchitis, cystitis, skin infections)*

Uncommon: Serious infections (including pneumonia, cellulitis, septic arthritis, sepsis)*

Rare: Tuberculosis

Blood and lymphatic system disorders:

Uncommon: Thrombocytopenia

Rare: Anaemia, leukopenia, neutropenia, pancytopenia*

Very rare: Aplastic anaemia*

Immune system disorders:

Common: Allergic reactions (see Skin and subcutaneous tissue disorders), autoantibody formation*

Rare: Serious allergic/anaphylactic reactions (including angioedema, bronchospasm)

Nervous system disorders:

Rare: Seizures

CNS demyelinating events suggestive of multiple sclerosis or localised demyelinating conditions such as optic neuritis and transverse myelitis (see section 4.4)

Skin and subcutaneous tissue disorders:

Common: Pruritus

Uncommon: Angioedema, urticaria, rash

Rare: Cutaneous vasculitis (including leukocytoclastic vasculitis)

Musculoskeletal, connective tissue and bone disorders:

Rare: Subacute cutaneous lupus erythematosus, discoid lupus erythematosus, lupus-like syndrome

General disorders and administration site conditions:

Very common: Injection site reactions (including bleeding, bruising, erythema, itching, pain, swelling)*

Common: Fever

Cardiac Disorders:

There have been reports of worsening of congestive heart failure (see section 4.4).

*see Additional information, below.

Additional information

Serious adverse events reported in clinical trials

Among rheumatoid arthritis, psoriatic arthritis, ankylosing spondylitis and plaque psoriasis patients in placebo-controlled, active-controlled, and open-label trials of Enbrel, serious adverse events reported included malignancies (see below), asthma, infections, heart failure, myocardial infarction, myocardial ischaemia, chest pain, syncope, cerebral ischaemia, hypertension, hypotension, cholecystitis, pancreatitis, gastrointestinal haemorrhage, bursitis, confusion, depression, dyspnoea, abnormal healing, renal insufficiency, kidney calculus, deep vein thrombosis, pulmonary embolism, membranous glomerulonephropathy, polymyositis, thrombophlebitis, liver damage, leucopenia, paresis, paresthesia, vertigo, allergic alveolitis, angioedema, scleritis, bone fracture, lymphadenopathy, ulcerative colitis and intestinal obstruction.

Malignancies

One hundred and twenty-nine new malignancies of various types were observed in 4,114 rheumatoid arthritis patients treated in clinical trials with Enbrel for up to approximately 6 years, including 231 patients treated with Enbrel in combination with methotrexate in the 2-year active-controlled study. The observed rates and incidences in these clinical trials were similar to those expected for the population studied. A total of 2 malignancies were reported in clinical studies of approximately 2 years duration involving 240 Enbrel-treated psoriatic arthritis patients. In clinical studies conducted for more than 2 years with 351 ankylosing spondylitis patients, 6 malignancies were reported in Enbrel-treated patients. Twenty-three malignancies were reported in plaque psoriasis patients treated with Enbrel in double-blind and open-label studies of up to 15 months involving 1,261 Enbrel-treated patients.

There were a total of 15 lymphomas reported in 5,966 patients treated with Enbrel in rheumatoid arthritis, psoriatic arthritis, ankylosing spondylitis and psoriasis clinical trials.

Reports of various malignancies (including breast and lung carcinoma and lymphoma) have also been received in the postmarketing period (see section 4.4).

Injection Site Reactions

Compared to placebo, patients with rheumatic diseases treated with Enbrel had a significantly higher incidence of injection site reactions (36% vs. 9%). Injection site reactions usually occurred in the first month. Mean duration was approximately 3 to 5 days. No treatment was given for the majority of injection site reactions in the Enbrel treatment groups, and the majority of patients who were given treatment received topical preparations such as corticosteroids, or oral antihistamines. Additionally, some patients developed recall injection site reactions characterised by a skin reaction at the most recent site of injection along with the simultaneous appearance of injection site reactions at previous injection sites. These reactions were generally transient and did not recur with treatment.

In controlled trials in patients with plaque psoriasis, approximately 14% of patients treated with Enbrel developed injection site reactions compared with 6% of placebo-treated patients during the first 12 weeks of treatment.

Infections

In clinical trials in rheumatic disorders, upper respiratory infections ("colds") and sinusitis were the most frequently reported infections in patients receiving Enbrel or placebo. In placebo-controlled trials, the incidence of upper respiratory tract infections was 17% in the placebo treatment group and 22% in the group treated with Enbrel. In rheumatoid arthritis patients participating in placebo-controlled trials, there were 0.68 events per patient year in the placebo group and 0.82 events per patient year in the group treated with Enbrel when the longer observation of patients on Enbrel was accounted for. In placebo-controlled trials evaluating Enbrel, no increase in the incidence of serious infections (fatal, life threatening, or requiring hospitalisation or intravenous antibiotics) was observed. Among the 2,680 rheumatoid arthritis patients treated with Enbrel for up to 48 months, including 231 patients treated with Enbrel in combination with methotrexate in the 1-year active-controlled study, 170 serious infections were observed. These serious infections included abscess (at various sites), bacteraemia, bronchitis, bursitis, cellulitis, cholecystitis, diarrhoea, diverticulitis, endocarditis (suspected), gastroenteritis, hepatitis B, herpes zoster, leg ulcer, mouth infection, osteomyelitis, otitis, peritonitis, pneumonia, pyelonephritis, sepsis, septic arthritis, sinusitis, skin infection, skin ulcer, urinary tract infection, vasculitis, and wound infection. In the 1-year active-controlled study where patients were treated with either Enbrel alone, methotrexate alone or Enbrel in combination with methotrexate, the rates of serious infections were similar among the treatment groups. However, it cannot be excluded that the combination of Enbrel with methotrexate could be associated with an increase in the rate of infections.

In placebo-controlled psoriatic arthritis trials and plaque psoriasis trials, there were no differences in rates of infection among patients treated with Enbrel and those treated with placebo. In the psoriatic arthritis trials, no serious infections occurred in patients treated with Enbrel. In the double-blind and open-label plaque psoriasis trials of up to 15 months, serious infections experienced by Enbrel-treated patients included cellulitis, gastroenteritis, pneumonia, cholecystitis, osteomyelitis and abscess.

Serious and fatal infections have been reported during use of Enbrel; reported pathogens include bacteria, mycobacteria (including tuberculosis), viruses and fungi. Some have occurred within a few weeks after initiating treatment with Enbrel in patients who have underlying conditions (e.g. diabetes, congestive heart failure, history of active or chronic infections) in addition to their rheumatoid arthritis (see section 4.4). Data from a sepsis clinical trial not specifically in patients with rheumatoid arthritis suggest that Enbrel treatment may increase mortality in patients with established sepsis.

Autoantibodies

Patients had serum samples tested for autoantibodies at multiple timepoints. Of the rheumatoid arthritis patients evaluated for antinuclear antibodies (ANA), the percentage of patients who developed new positive ANA ($\geqslant$1:40) was higher in patients treated with Enbrel (11%) than in placebo-treated patients (5%). The percentage of patients who developed new positive anti-double-stranded DNA antibodies was also higher by radioimmunoassay (15% of patients treated with Enbrel compared to 4% of placebo-treated patients) and by *Crithidia luciliae* assay (3% of patients treated with Enbrel compared to none of placebo-treated patients). The proportion of patients treated with Enbrel who developed anticardiolipin antibodies was similarly increased compared to placebo-treated patients. The impact of long-term treatment with Enbrel on the development of autoimmune diseases is unknown.

There have been rare reports of patients, including rheumatoid factor positive patients, who have developed other autoantibodies in conjunction with a lupus-like syndrome or rashes that are compatible with subacute cutaneous lupus or discoid lupus by clinical presentation and biopsy.

Pancytopenia and aplastic anaemia

There have been postmarketing reports of pancytopenia and aplastic anaemia, some of which had fatal outcomes (see section 4.4).

Laboratory Evaluations

Based on the results of clinical studies, normally no special laboratory evaluations are necessary in addition to careful medical management and supervision of patients.

Concurrent Enbrel and anakinra treatment

In studies when patients received concurrent treatment with Enbrel plus anakinra, a higher rate of serious infections compared to Enbrel alone was observed and 2% of patients (3/139) developed neutropenia (absolute neutrophil count < 1000 / mm^3). While neutropenic, one patient developed cellulitis that resolved after hospitalisation (see sections 4.4 and 4.5).

Undesirable effects in paediatric patients with juvenile chronic arthritis

In general, the adverse events in paediatric patients were similar in frequency and type to those seen in adult patients. Differences from adults and other special considerations are discussed in the following paragraphs.

Severe adverse events reported in a trial in 69 juvenile chronic arthritis patients aged 4 to 17 years included varicella with signs and symptoms of aseptic meningitis which resolved without sequelae (see also 4.4), gastroenteritis, depression/personality disorder, cutaneous ulcer, oesophagitis/gastritis, group A streptococcal septic shock, type I diabetes mellitus, and soft tissue and post-operative wound infection.

Forty-three of 69 (62%) children with juvenile chronic arthritis experienced an infection while receiving Enbrel during 3 months of the study (part 1 open-label), and the frequency and severity of infections was similar in 58 patients completing 12 months of open-label extension therapy. The types of infections reported in juvenile chronic arthritis patients were generally mild and consistent with those commonly seen in outpatient paediatric populations. The types and proportion of adverse events in juvenile chronic arthritis patients were similar to those seen in trials of Enbrel in adult patients with rheumatoid arthritis, and the majority were mild. Several adverse events were reported more commonly in 69 juvenile chronic arthritis patients receiving 3 months of Enbrel compared to the 349 adult rheumatoid arthritis patients. These included headache (19% of patients, 1.7 events per patient year), nausea (9%, 1.0 event per patient year), abdominal pain (19%, 0.74 events per patient year), and vomiting (13%, 0.74 events per patient year).

4.9 Overdose

No dose-limiting toxicities were observed during clinical trials of rheumatoid arthritis patients. The highest dose level evaluated has been an intravenous loading dose of 32 mg/m^2 followed by subcutaneous doses of 16 mg/m^2 administered twice weekly. One rheumatoid arthritis patient mistakenly self-administered 62 mg Enbrel subcutaneously twice weekly for 3 weeks without experiencing undesirable effects. There is no known antidote to Enbrel.

5. PHARMACOLOGICAL PROPERTIES

5.1 Pharmacodynamic properties

Pharmacotherapeutic group: Selective immunosuppressant agents.

ATC code: L04AA11

Tumour necrosis factor (TNF) is a dominant cytokine in the inflammatory process of rheumatoid arthritis. Elevated levels of TNF are also found in the synovium and psoriatic plaques of patients with psoriatic arthritis and in serum and synovial tissue of patients with ankylosing spondylitis. In plaque psoriasis, infiltration by inflammatory cells including T-cells leads to increased TNF levels in psoriatic lesions compared with levels in uninvolved skin. Etanercept is a competitive inhibitor of TNF-binding to its cell surface receptors and thereby inhibits the biological activity of TNF. TNF and lymphotoxin are pro-inflammatory cytokines that bind to two distinct cell surface receptors: the 55-kilodalton (p55) and 75-kilodalton (p75) tumour necrosis factor receptors (TNFRs). Both TNFRs exist naturally in membrane-bound and soluble forms. Soluble TNFRs are thought to regulate TNF biological activity.

TNF and lymphotoxin exist predominantly as homotrimers, with their biological activity dependent on cross-linking of cell surface TNFRs. Dimeric soluble receptors such as etanercept possess a higher affinity for TNF than monomeric receptors and are considerably more potent competitive inhibitors of TNF binding to its cellular receptors. In addition, use of an immunoglobulin Fc region as a fusion element in the construction of a dimeric receptor imparts a longer serum half-life.

Mechanism of action

Much of the joint pathology in rheumatoid arthritis and ankylosing spondylitis and skin pathology in plaque psoriasis is mediated by pro-inflammatory molecules that are linked in a network controlled by TNF. The mechanism of action of etanercept is thought to be its competitive inhibition of TNF binding to cell surface TNFR, preventing TNF-mediated cellular responses by rendering TNF biologically inactive. Etanercept may also modulate biologic responses controlled by additional downstream molecules (e.g., cytokines, adhesion molecules, or proteinases) that are induced or regulated by TNF.

Clinical trials

This section presents data from four randomised controlled trials in rheumatoid arthritis, 1 study in polyarticular-course juvenile chronic arthritis, 1 study in psoriatic arthritis, 1 study in ankylosing spondylitis and 3 studies in plaque psoriasis.

Rheumatoid Arthritis

The efficacy of Enbrel was assessed in a randomised, double-blind, placebo-controlled study. The study evaluated 234 adult patients with active rheumatoid arthritis who had failed therapy with at least one but no more than four disease-modifying antirheumatic drugs (DMARDs). Doses of 10 mg or 25 mg Enbrel or placebo were administered subcutaneously twice a week for 6 consecutive months. The results of this controlled trial were expressed in percentage improvement in rheumatoid arthritis using American College of Rheumatology (ACR) response criteria.

ACR 20 and 50 responses were higher in patients treated with Enbrel at 3 and 6 months than in patients treated with placebo (ACR 20: Enbrel 62% and 59%, placebo 23% and 11% at 3 and 6 months respectively; ACR 50: Enbrel 41% and 40%, placebo 8% and 5% at months 3 and 6 respectively; $p < 0.01$ Enbrel vs Placebo at all time points for both ACR 20 and ACR 50 responses).

Approximately 15% of subjects who received Enbrel achieved an ACR 70 response at month 3 and month 6 compared to fewer than 5% of subjects in the placebo arm. Among patients receiving Enbrel, the clinical responses generally appeared within 1 to 2 weeks after initiation of therapy and nearly always occurred by 3 months. A dose response was seen; results with 10 mg were intermediate between placebo and 25 mg. Enbrel was significantly better than placebo in all components of the ACR criteria as well as other measures of rheumatoid arthritis disease activity not included in the ACR response criteria, such as morning stiffness. A Health Assessment Questionnaire (HAQ), which included disability, vitality, mental health, general health status, and arthritis-associated health status subdomains, was administered every 3 months during the trial. All subdomains of the HAQ were improved in patients treated with Enbrel compared to controls at 3 and 6 months.

After discontinuation of Enbrel, symptoms of arthritis generally returned within a month. Reintroduction of treatment with Enbrel after discontinuations of up to 24 months resulted in the same magnitudes of responses as patients who received Enbrel without interruption of therapy based on results of open-label studies. Continued durable responses have been seen for up to 48 months in open-label extension treatment trials when patients received Enbrel without interruption; longer-term experience is not available

The efficacy of Enbrel was compared to methotrexate in a third randomised, active-controlled study with blinded radiographic evaluations as a primary endpoint in 632 adult patients with active rheumatoid arthritis (<3 years duration) who had never received treatment with methotrexate. Doses of 10 mg or 25 mg Enbrel were administered SC twice a week for up to 24 months. Methotrexate doses were escalated from 7.5 mg/week to a maximum of 20 mg/week over the first 8 weeks of the trial and continued for up to 24 months. Clinical improvement including onset of action within 2 weeks with Enbrel 25 mg was similar to that seen in the previous trials, and was maintained for up to 24 months. At baseline, patients had a moderate degree of disability, with mean HAQ scores of 1.4 to 1.5. Treatment with Enbrel 25 mg resulted in substantial improvement at 12 months, with about 44% of patients achieving a normal HAQ score (less than 0.5). This benefit was maintained in Year 2 of this study.

In this study, structural joint damage was assessed radiographically and expressed as change in Total Sharp Score (TSS) and its components, the erosion score and joint space narrowing score (JSN). Radiographs of hands/wrists and feet were read at baseline and 6, 12, and 24 months. The 10 mg Enbrel dose had consistently less effect on structural damage than the 25 mg dose. Enbrel 25 mg was significantly superior to methotrexate for erosion scores at both 12 and 24 months. The differences in TSS and JSN were not statistically significant between methotrexate and Enbrel 25 mg. The results are shown in the figure below.

RADIOGRAPHIC PROGRESSION: COMPARISON OF ENBREL vs METHOTREXATE IN PATIENTS WITH RA OF <3 YEARS DURATION

(see Figure 1 on next page)

In another active-controlled, double-blind, randomised study, clinical efficacy, safety, and radiographic progression in RA patients treated with Enbrel alone (25 mg twice weekly), methotrexate alone (7.5 to 20 mg weekly, median dose 20 mg), and of the combination of Enbrel and methotrexate initiated concurrently were compared in 682 adult patients with active rheumatoid arthritis of 6 months to 20 years duration (median 5 years) who had a less than satisfactory response to at least 1 disease-modifying antirheumatic drug (DMARD) other than methotrexate.

Patients in the Enbrel in combination with methotrexate therapy group had significantly higher ACR 20, ACR 50, ACR 70 responses and improvement for DAS and HAQ scores at both 24 and 52 weeks than patients in either of the single therapy groups (results shown in table below).

(see Table 1 on next page)

Radiographic progression at week 52 was significantly less in the Enbrel group than in the methotrexate group, while the combination was significantly better than either monotherapy at slowing radiographic progression (see figure below).

Figure 1 RADIOGRAPHIC PROGRESSION: COMPARISON OF ENBREL vs METHOTREXATE IN PATIENTS WITH RA OF <3 YEARS DURATION

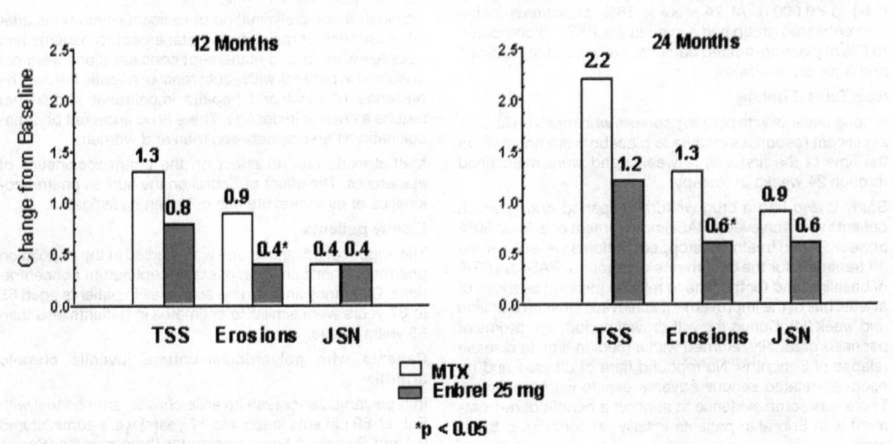

Table 1 CLINICAL EFFICACY RESULTS: COMPARISON OF ENBREL vs METHOTREXATE vs ENBREL IN COMBINATION WITH METHOTREXATE IN PATIENTS WITH RA OF 6 MONTHS to 20 YEARS DURATION

Endpoint	Methotrexate (n = 228)	Enbrel (n = 223)	Enbrel + Methotrexate (n = 231)
ACR Responses at week 52			
ACR 20	75.0%	75.8%	84.8% †,ϕ
ACR 50	42.5%	48.4%	69.3% †,ϕ
ACR 70	18.9%	24.2%	42.9% †,ϕ
DAS			
Baseline score[a]	5.5	5.7	5.5
Week 52 score[a]	3.0	3.0	2.3†,ϕ
Remission[b]	14%	18%	37%†,ϕ
HAQ			
Baseline			
Week 52	1.1	1.0	0.8†,ϕ

a: Values for Disease Activity Score (DAS) are means.
b: Remission is defined as DAS <1.6
Pairwise comparison p-values: † = $p < 0.05$ for comparisons of Enbrel + methotrexate vs methotrexate and ϕ = $p < 0.05$ for comparisons of Enbrel + methotrexate vs Enbrel

RADIOGRAPHIC PROGRESSION: COMPARISON OF ENBREL vs METHOTREXATE vs ENBREL IN COMBINATION WITH METHOTREXATE IN PATIENTS WITH RA OF 6 MONTHS TO 20 YEARS DURATION (52-WEEK RESULTS)

(see Figure 2 below)

Pairwise comparison p-values: * = $p < 0.05$ for comparisons of Enbrel vs methotrexate, † = $p < 0.05$ for comparisons of Enbrel + methotrexate vs methotrexate and ϕ = $p < 0.05$ for comparisons of Enbrel + methotrexate vs Enbrel

The percentage of patients without progression (TSS change ⩽ 0.5) was higher in the Enbrel in combination with methotrexate and Enbrel groups compared with methotrexate at week 24 (74%, 68%, and 56%, respectively; p<0.05) and week 52 (80%, 68%, and 57%, respectively; p<0.05).

The safety and efficacy of 50 mg Enbrel (two 25 mg SC injections) administered once weekly were evaluated in a double-blind, placebo-controlled study of 420 patients with active RA. In this study, 53 patients received placebo, 214 patients received 50 mg Enbrel once weekly and 153 patients received 25 mg Enbrel twice weekly. The safety and efficacy profiles of the two Enbrel treatment regimens were comparable at week 8 in their effect on signs and symptoms of RA; data at week 16 did not show comparability (non-inferiority) between the two regimens.

Polyarticular-Course Juvenile Chronic Arthritis

The safety and efficacy of Enbrel were assessed in a two-part study in 69 children with polyarticular-course juvenile chronic arthritis who had a variety of juvenile chronic arthritis onset types. Patients aged 4 to 17 years with moderately to severely active polyarticular-course juvenile chronic arthritis refractory to or intolerant of methotrexate were enrolled; patients remained on a stable dose of a single nonsteroidal anti-inflammatory drug and/or prednisone (< 0.2 mg/kg/day or 10 mg maximum). In part 1, all patients received 0.4 mg/kg (maximum 25 mg per dose) Enbrel subcutaneously twice weekly. In part 2, patients with a clinical response at day 90 were randomised to remain on Enbrel or receive placebo for four months and assessed for disease flare. Responses were measured using the JRA Definition of Improvement (DOI), defined as ⩾ 30% improvement in at least three of six and ⩾ 30% worsening in no more than one of six JRA core set criteria, including active joint count, limitation of motion, physician and patient/parent global assessments, functional assessment, and erythrocyte sedimentation rate (ESR). Disease flare was defined as a ⩾ 30% worsening in three of six JRA core set criteria and ⩾ 30% improvement in not more than one of the six JRA core set criteria and a minimum of two active joints.

In part 1 of the study, 51 of 69 (74%) patients demonstrated a clinical response and entered part 2. In part 2, 6 of 25 (24%) patients remaining on Enbrel experienced a disease flare compared to 20 of 26 (77%) patients receiving placebo (p=0.007). From the start of part 2, the median time to flare was ⩾ 116 days for patients who received Enbrel and 28 days for patients who received placebo. Of patients who demonstrated a clinical response at 90 days and entered part 2 of the study, some of the patients remaining on Enbrel continued to improve from month 3 through month 7, while those who received placebo did not improve.

Studies have not been done in patients with polyarticular-course juvenile chronic arthritis to assess the effects of continued Enbrel therapy in patients who do not respond within 3 months of initiating Enbrel therapy or to assess the combination of Enbrel with methotrexate.

Adults with Psoriatic Arthritis

The efficacy of Enbrel was assessed in a randomised, double-blind, placebo-controlled study in 205 patients with psoriatic arthritis. Patients were between 18 and 70 years of age and had active psoriatic arthritis (⩾ 3 swollen joints and ⩾ 3 tender joints) in at least one of the following forms: (1) distal interphalangeal (DIP) involvement; (2) polyarticular arthritis (absence of rheumatoid nodules and presence of psoriasis); (3) arthritis mutilans; (4) asymmetric psoriatic arthritis; or (5) spondylitis-like ankylosis. Patients also had plaque psoriasis with a qualifying target lesion ⩾ 2 cm in diameter. Patients had previously been treated with NSAIDs (86%), DMARDs (80%), and corticosteroids (24%). Patients currently on MTX therapy (stable for ⩾ 2 months) could continue at a stable dose of ⩽ 25 mg/week MTX. Doses of 25 mg Enbrel (based on dose-finding studies in patients with rheumatoid arthritis) or placebo were administered SC twice a week for 6 months.

The results were expressed as percentages of patients achieving the ACR 20, 50, and 70 response and percentages with improvement in Psoriatic Arthritis Response Criteria (PsARC). Results are summarised in the Table below.

RESPONSES OF PATIENTS WITH PSORIATIC ARTHRITIS IN PLACEBO-CONTROLLED TRIAL

	Percent of Patients	
	Placebo	Enbrel[a]
Psoriatic Arthritis Response	n = 104	n = 101
ACR 20		
Month 3	15	59[b]
Month 6	13	50[b]
ACR 50		
Month 3	4	38[b]
Month 6	4	37[b]
ACR 70		
Month 3	0	11[b]
Month 6	1	9[c]
PsARC		
Month 3	31	72[b]
Month 6	23	70[b]

a: 25 mg Enbrel SC twice weekly
b: $p < 0.001$, Enbrel vs. placebo
c: $p < 0.01$, Enbrel vs. placebo

Among patients with psoriatic arthritis who received Enbrel, the clinical responses were apparent at the time of the first visit (4 weeks) and were maintained through 6 months of therapy. Enbrel was significantly better than placebo in all measures of disease activity ($p < 0.001$), and responses were similar with and without concomitant methotrexate therapy. Quality of life in psoriatic arthritis patients was assessed at every timepoint using the disability index of the HAQ. The disability index score was significantly improved at all timepoints in psoriatic arthritis patients treated with Enbrel, relative to placebo ($p < 0.001$). There is insufficient evidence of the efficacy of Enbrel in patients with ankylosing spondylitis-like psoriatic arthropathy due to the small number of patients studied.

Adults with Ankylosing Spondylitis

The efficacy of Enbrel was assessed in 3 randomised, double-blind, placebo-controlled studies in 401 patients with ankylosing spondylitis from which 203 were treated with Enbrel. The largest of these trials (n= 277) enrolled patients who were between 18 and 70 years of age and had active ankylosing spondylitis defined as visual analog scale (VAS) scores of ⩾ 30 for average of duration and intensity of morning stiffness plus VAS scores of ⩾ 30 for

Figure 2 RADIOGRAPHIC PROGRESSION: COMPARISON OF ENBREL vs METHOTREXATE vs ENBREL IN COMBINATION WITH METHOTREXATE IN PATIENTS WITH RA OF 6 MONTHS TO 20 YEARS DURATION (52-WEEK RESULTS)

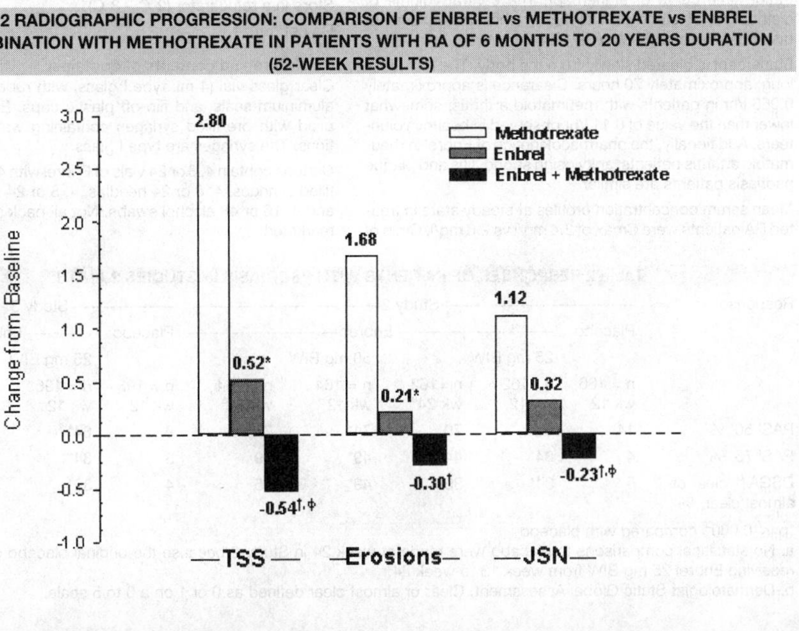

at least 2 of the following 3 parameters: patient global assessment; average of VAS values for nocturnal back pain and total back pain; average of 10 questions on the Bath Ankylosing Spondylitis Functional Index (BASFI). Patients receiving DMARDs, NSAIDS, or corticosteroids could continue them on stable doses. Patients with complete ankylosis of the spine were not included in the study. Doses of 25 mg of Enbrel (based on dose-finding studies in patients with rheumatoid arthritis) or placebo were administered subcutaneously twice a week for 6 months in 138 patients.

The primary measure of efficacy (ASAS 20) was a ⩾20% improvement in at least 3 of the 4 Assessment in Ankylosing Spondylitis (ASAS) domains (patient global assessments, back pain, BASFI, and inflammation) and absence of deterioration in the remaining domain. ASAS 50 and 70 responses used the same criteria with a 50% improvement or a 70% improvement, respectively.

Compared to placebo, treatment with Enbrel resulted in significant improvements in the ASAS 20, ASAS 50 and ASAS 70 as early as 2 weeks after the initiation of therapy.

RESPONSES OF PATIENTS WITH ANKYLOSING SPONDYLITIS IN A PLACEBO-CONTROLLED TRIAL

	Percent of Patients	
Ankylosing Spondylitis Response	Placebo N = 139	Enbrel N = 138
ASAS 20		
2 weeks	22	46[a]
3 months	27	60[a]
6 months	23	58[a]
ASAS 50		
2 weeks	7	24[a]
3 months	13	45[a]
6 months	10	42[a]
ASAS 70:		
2 weeks	2	12[b]
3 months	7	29[b]
6 months	5	28[b]

a: $p<0.001$, Enbrel vs. Placebo

b: $p = 0.002$, Enbrel vs. placebo

Among patients with ankylosing spondylitis who received Enbrel, the clinical responses were apparent at the time of the first visit (2 weeks) and were maintained through 6 months of therapy. Responses were similar in patients who were or were not receiving concomitant therapies at baseline.

Similar results were obtained in the 2 smaller ankylosing spondylitis trials.

Adults with Plaque Psoriasis

Enbrel is recommended for use in patients as defined in section 4.1. Patients who "failed to respond to" in the target population is defined by insufficient response (PASI<50 or PGA less than good), or worsening of the disease while on treatment, and who were adequately dosed for a sufficiently long duration to assess response with at least each of the three major systemic therapies as available.

The efficacy of Enbrel versus other systemic therapies in patients with moderate to severe psoriasis (responsive to other systemic therapies) has not been evaluated in studies directly comparing Enbrel with other systemic therapies. Instead, the safety and efficacy of Enbrel were assessed in three randomised, double-blind, placebo-controlled studies. The primary efficacy endpoint in all three studies was the proportion of patients in each treatment group who achieved the PASI 75 (i.e., at least a 75% improvement in the Psoriasis Area and Severity Index score from baseline) at 12 weeks.

Study 1 was a Phase 2 study in patients with active but clinically stable plaque psoriasis involving ⩾ 10% of the body surface area that were ⩾ 18 years old. One hundred and twelve (112) patients were randomised to receive a dose of 25 mg of Enbrel (n=57) or placebo (n=55) twice a week for 24 weeks.

Study 2 evaluated 652 patients with chronic plaque psoriasis using the same inclusion criteria as study 1 with the addition of a minimum psoriasis area and severity index (PASI) of 10 at screening. Enbrel was administered at doses of 25 mg once a week, 25 mg twice a week or 50 mg twice a week for 6 consecutive months. During the first 12 weeks of the double-blind treatment period, patients received placebo or one of the above three Enbrel doses. After 12 weeks of treatment, patients in the placebo group began treatment with blinded Enbrel (25 mg twice a week); patients in the active treatment groups continued to week 24 on the dose to which they were originally randomised.

Study 3 evaluated 583 patients and had the same inclusion criteria as study 2. Patients in this study received a dose of 25 mg or 50 mg Enbrel, or placebo twice a week for 12 weeks and then all patients received open-label 25 mg Enbrel twice weekly for an additional 24 weeks.

In study 1, the Enbrel-treated group had a significantly higher proportion of patients with a PASI 75 response at week 12 (30%) compared to the placebo-treated group (2%) ($p<0.0001$). At 24 weeks, 56% of patients in the Enbrel-treated group had achieved the PASI 75 compared to 5% of placebo-treated patients. Key results of studies 2 and 3 are shown below.

(see Table 2 below)

Among patients with plaque psoriasis who received Enbrel, significant responses relative to placebo were apparent at the time of the first visit (2 weeks) and were maintained through 24 weeks of therapy.

Study 2 also had a drug withdrawal period during which patients who achieved a PASI improvement of at least 50% at week 24 had treatment stopped. Patients were observed off treatment for the occurrence of rebound (PASI ⩾150% of baseline) and for the time to relapse (defined as a loss of at least half of the improvement achieved between baseline and week 24). During the withdrawal period, symptoms of psoriasis gradually returned with a median time to disease relapse of 3 months. No rebound flare of disease and no psoriasis-related serious adverse events were observed. There was some evidence to support a benefit of re-treatment with Enbrel in patients initially responding to treatment.

In study 3, the majority of patients (77%) who were initially randomised to 50 mg twice weekly and had their Enbrel dose decreased at week 12 to 25 mg twice weekly maintained their PASI 75 response through week 36. For patients who received 25 mg twice weekly throughout the study, the PASI 75 response continued to improve between weeks 12 and 36.

Antibodies to Enbrel

Antibodies to Enbrel, all non-neutralising, were detected in 4 out of 96 rheumatoid arthritis patients who received Enbrel at a dose of 25 mg twice a week for up to 3 months in a placebo-controlled trial. In the active-controlled trial, 11 (2.8%) of 400 etanercept-treated patients had at least one positive result but none of those patients had a positive neutralising antibody test. Results from JCA patients were similar to those seen in adult RA patients treated with Enbrel. Of 98 patients with psoriatic arthritis who have been tested, no patient has developed antibodies to Enbrel at 24 weeks. Among 175 ankylosing spondylitis patients treated with Enbrel, 3 patients were reported with antibodies to Enbrel, none were neutralising. In double-blind studies up to 6 months duration in plaque psoriasis, about 1% of the 1,084 patients developed antibodies to Enbrel, none were neutralising.

Although the experience does not exclude the possibility that a clinically relevant effect might occur, no apparent correlation of antibody development to clinical response or adverse events was seen.

5.2 Pharmacokinetic properties

Etanercept serum values were determined by an ELISA method, which may detect ELISA-reactive degradation products as well as the parent compound.

Etanercept is slowly absorbed from the site of subcutaneous injection, reaching maximum concentration approximately 48 hours after a single dose. The absolute bioavailability is 76%. With twice weekly doses, it is anticipated that steady-state concentrations are approximately twice as high as those observed after single doses. After a single subcutaneous dose of 25 mg Enbrel, the average maximum serum concentration observed in healthy volunteers was 1.65 ± 0.66 μg/ml, and the area under the curve was 235 ± 96.6 μg•hr/ml. Dose proportionality has not been formally evaluated, but there is no apparent saturation of clearance across the dosing range.

A biexponential curve is required to describe the concentration time curve of etanercept. The central volume of distribution of etanercept is 7.6 l, while the volume of distribution at steady-state is 10.4 l.

Etanercept is cleared slowly from the body. The half-life is long, approximately 70 hours. Clearance is approximately 0.066 l/hr in patients with rheumatoid arthritis, somewhat lower than the value of 0.11 l/hr observed in healthy volunteers. Additionally, the pharmacokinetics of Enbrel in rheumatoid arthritis patients, ankylosing spondylitis and plaque psoriasis patients are similar.

Mean serum concentration profiles at steady state in treated RA patients were Cmax of 2.4 mg/l vs 2.6 mg/l, Cmin of 1.2 mg/l vs 1.4 mg/l and partial AUC of 297 mgh/l vs 316 mgh/l for 50 mg Enbrel once weekly (n=21) vs 25 mg Enbrel twice weekly (n=16), respectively.

Although there is elimination of radioactivity in urine after administration of radiolabelled etanercept to patients and volunteers, increased etanercept concentrations were not observed in patients with acute renal or hepatic failure. The presence of renal and hepatic impairment should not require a change in dosage. There is no apparent pharmacokinetic difference between men and women.

Methotrexate has no effect on the pharmacokinetics of etanercept. The effect of Enbrel on the human pharmacokinetics of methotrexate has not been investigated.

Elderly patients

The impact of advanced age was studied in the population pharmacokinetic analysis of etanercept serum concentrations. Clearance and volume estimates in patients aged 65 to 87 years were similar to estimates in patients less than 65 years of age.

Patients with polyarticular-course juvenile chronic arthritis

In a polyarticular-course juvenile chronic arthritis trial with Enbrel, 69 patients (aged 4 to 17 years) were administered 0.4 mg Enbrel/kg twice weekly for three months. Serum concentration profiles were similar to those seen in adult rheumatoid arthritis patients. The youngest children (4 years of age) had reduced clearance (increased clearance when normalised by weight) compared with older children (12 years of age) and adults. Simulation of dosing suggests that while older children (10-17 years of age) will have serum levels close to those seen in adults, younger children will have appreciably lower levels.

5.3 Preclinical safety data

In the toxicological studies with Enbrel, no dose-limiting or target organ toxicity was evident. Enbrel was considered to be non-genotoxic from a battery of *in vitro* and *in vivo* studies. Carcinogenicity studies, and standard assessments of fertility and postnatal toxicity, were not performed with Enbrel due to the development of neutralising antibodies in rodents.

Enbrel did not induce lethality or notable signs of toxicity in mice or rats following a single subcutaneous dose of 2000 mg/kg or a single intravenous dose of 1000 mg/kg. Enbrel did not elicit dose-limiting or target organ toxicity in cynomolgus monkeys following twice weekly subcutaneous administration for 4 or 26 consecutive weeks at a dose (15 mg/kg) that resulted in AUC-based serum drug concentrations that were over 27-fold higher than that obtained in humans at the recommended dose of 25 mg.

6. PHARMACEUTICAL PARTICULARS

6.1 List of excipients

Powder: mannitol, sucrose, and trometamol.

Solvent: Water for injections

6.2 Incompatibilities

In the absence of incompatibility studies, this medicinal product must not be mixed with other medicinal products.

6.3 Shelf life

3 years.

After reconstitution, immediate use is recommended. Chemical and physical in-use stability has been demonstrated for 48 hours at 2° – 8°C. From a microbiological point of view, the product should be used immediately. If not used immediately, in-use storage times are the responsibility of the user and would normally not be longer than 6 hours at 2° – 8°C, unless reconstitution has taken place in controlled and validated aseptic conditions.

6.4 Special precautions for storage

Store in a refrigerator (2°C – 8°C).

Do not freeze

6.5 Nature and contents of container

Clear glass vial (4 ml, type I glass) with rubber stoppers, aluminium seals, and flip-off plastic caps. Enbrel is supplied with pre-filled syringes containing water for injections. The syringes are type I glass.

Cartons contain 4, 8 or 24 vials of Enbrel with 4, 8 or 24 pre-filled syringes, 4, 8 or 24 needles, 4, 8 or 24 vial adaptors and 8, 16 or 48 alcohol swabs. Not all pack sizes may be marketed.

Table 2 RESPONSES OF PATIENTS WITH PSORIASIS IN STUDIES 2 AND 3

Response	Study 2					Study 3		
	Placebo	Enbrel				Placebo	Enbrel	
		25 mg BIW		50 mg BIW			25 mg BIW	50 mg BIW
	n = 166 wk 12	n =162 wk 12	n =162 wk 24[a]	n = 164 wk 12	n = 164 wk 24[a]	n = 193 wk 12	n = 196 wk 12	n = 196 wk 12
PASI 50, %	14	58*	70	74*	77	9	64*	77*
PASI 75, %	4	34*	44	49*	59	3	34*	49*
DSGA [b], clear or almost clear, %	5	34*	39	49*	55	4	39*	57*

*$p \leqslant 0.0001$ compared with placebo

a. No statistical comparisons to placebo were made at week 24 in Study 2 because the original placebo group began receiving Enbrel 25 mg BIW from week 13 to week 24.

b. Dermatologist Static Global Assessment. Clear or almost clear defined as 0 or 1 on a 0 to 5 scale.

6.6 Instructions for use and handling
Enbrel 25 mg is reconstituted with 1 ml water for injections. Enbrel contains no antibacterial preservative, and therefore, solutions prepared with water for injections should be administered as soon as possible and within 6 hours following reconstitution. The solution should be clear and colourless with no lumps, flakes or particles. Some white foam may remain in the vial – this is normal. Do not use Enbrel if all the powder in the vial is not dissolved within 10 minutes. Start again with another vial.

Any unused product or waste material should be disposed of in accordance with local requirements.

7. MARKETING AUTHORISATION HOLDER
Wyeth Europa Ltd.

Huntercombe Lane South

Taplow, Maidenhead

Berkshire, SL6 0PH

United Kingdom

8. MARKETING AUTHORISATION NUMBER(S)
EU/1/99/126/003

9. DATE OF FIRST AUTHORISATION/RENEWAL OF THE AUTHORISATION
Date of first authorisation: 3 February 2000

Date of last renewal: 3 February 2005

10. DATE OF REVISION OF THE TEXT
1 August 2005

Enbrel 50mg

(Wyeth Pharmaceuticals)

1. NAME OF THE MEDICINAL PRODUCT
Enbrel▼ 50 mg powder and solvent for solution for injection.

2. QUALITATIVE AND QUANTITATIVE COMPOSITION
Each vial contains 50 mg of etanercept.

Etanercept is a human tumour necrosis factor receptor p75 Fc fusion protein produced by recombinant DNA technology in a Chinese hamster ovary (CHO) mammalian expression system. Etanercept is a dimer of a chimeric protein genetically engineered by fusing the extracellular ligand binding domain of human tumour necrosis factor receptor-2 (TNFR2/p75) to the Fc domain of human IgG1. This Fc component contains the hinge, CH_2 and CH_3 regions but not the CH_1 region of IgG1. Etanercept contains 934 amino acids and has an apparent molecular weight of approximately 150 kilodaltons. The potency is determined by measuring the ability of etanercept to neutralise the TNFα-mediated growth inhibition of A375 cells. The specific activity of etanercept is 1.7×10^6 units/mg.

For excipients, see section 6.1.

3. PHARMACEUTICAL FORM
Powder and solvent for solution for injection.

The white powder is supplied in a clear glass vial with rubber stopper, aluminium seal and green plastic cap. The solvent is a clear, colourless liquid supplied in a pre-filled glass syringe (see section 6.5).

4. CLINICAL PARTICULARS
4.1 Therapeutic indications
Enbrel can be used alone or in combination with methotrexate for the treatment of active rheumatoid arthritis in adults when the response to disease-modifying antirheumatic drugs, including methotrexate (unless contraindicated), has been inadequate.

Enbrel is also indicated in the treatment of severe, active and progressive rheumatoid arthritis in adults not previously treated with methotrexate.

In patients with rheumatoid arthritis, Enbrel used alone or in combination with methotrexate has been shown to slow the progression of disease-associated structural damage as measured by X-ray.

Treatment of adults with moderate to severe plaque psoriasis who failed to respond to, or who have a contraindication to, or are intolerant to other systemic therapy including cyclosporine, methotrexate or PUVA (see Section 5.1).

4.2 Posology and method of administration
Enbrel treatment should be initiated and supervised by specialist physicians experienced in the diagnosis and treatment of rheumatoid arthritis or psoriasis.

Each vial of Enbrel 50 mg must be reconstituted with 1 ml of water for injections before use and administered by subcutaneous injection.

Adults (18-64 years)
Rheumatoid arthritis

50 mg Enbrel administered once weekly

Plaque psoriasis

The recommended dose of Enbrel is 25 mg administered twice weekly. Alternatively, 50 mg given twice weekly may be used for up to 12 weeks followed, if necessary, by a dose of 25 mg twice weekly. Treatment with Enbrel should continue until remission is achieved, for up to 24 weeks. Treatment should be discontinued in patients who show no response after 12 weeks.

If re-treatment with Enbrel is indicated, the above guidance on treatment duration should be followed. The dose should be 25 mg twice weekly.

A 25 mg strength of Enbrel is available, and should be used for administration of 25 mg doses.

Elderly patients (⩾ 65 years)
No dose adjustment is required. Posology and administration are the same as for adults 18-64 years of age.

Renal and hepatic impairment
No dose adjustment is required.

4.3 Contraindications
Hypersensitivity to the active substance or to any of the excipients.

Sepsis or risk of sepsis.

Treatment with Enbrel should not be initiated in patients with active infections including chronic or localised infections.

4.4 Special warnings and special precautions for use
Infections
Sepsis and serious infections (fatal, life threatening, or requiring hospitalisation or intravenous antibiotics), have been reported with the use of Enbrel (see section 4.8). Many of these serious events have occurred in patients with underlying diseases that in addition to their rheumatoid arthritis could predispose them to infections. Patients who develop a new infection while undergoing treatment with Enbrel should be monitored closely. **Administration of Enbrel should be discontinued if a patient develops a serious infection.** Physicians should exercise caution when considering the use of Enbrel in patients with a history of recurring or chronic infections or with underlying conditions which may predispose patients to infections such as advanced or poorly controlled diabetes.

Concurrent Enbrel and anakinra treatment
Concurrent administration of Enbrel and anakinra has been associated with an increased risk of serious infections and neutropenia compared to Enbrel alone. This combination has not demonstrated increased clinical benefit. Thus the combined use of Enbrel and anakinra is not recommended (see sections 4.5 and 4.8).

Allergic reactions
Allergic reactions associated with Enbrel administration have been reported commonly. Allergic reactions have included angioedema and urticaria; serious reactions have occurred. If any serious allergic or anaphylactic reaction occurs, Enbrel therapy should be discontinued immediately and appropriate therapy initiated.

Immunosuppression
The possibility exists for anti-TNF therapies, including Enbrel, to affect host defences against infections and malignancies since TNF mediates inflammation and modulates cellular immune responses. Reports of various malignancies (including breast and lung carcinoma and lymphoma) have been received in the postmarketing period (see section 4.8). In a study of 49 patients with rheumatoid arthritis treated with Enbrel, there was no evidence of depression of delayed-type hypersensitivity, depression of immunoglobulin levels, or change in enumeration of effector cell populations. Whether treatment with Enbrel might influence the development and course of malignancies and active and/or chronic infections is unknown. The safety and efficacy of Enbrel in patients with immunosuppression or chronic infections have not been evaluated.

Two juvenile chronic arthritis patients developed varicella infection and signs and symptoms of aseptic meningitis which resolved without sequelae. Patients with a significant exposure to varicella virus should temporarily discontinue Enbrel therapy and be considered for prophylactic treatment with Varicella Zoster Immune Globulin.

Vaccinations
Live vaccines should not be given concurrently with Enbrel. No data are available on the secondary transmission of infection by live vaccines in patients receiving Enbrel. In a double blind, placebo controlled, randomised clinical study in patients with psoriatic arthritis 184 patients also received a multivalent pneumococcal polysaccharide vaccine at week 4. In this study most psoriatic arthritis patients receiving Enbrel were able to mount effective B-cell immune response to pneumococcal polysaccharide vaccine, but titers in aggregate were moderately lower and few patients had two-fold rises in titers compared to patients not receiving Enbrel. The clinical significance of this is unknown.

Autoantibody formation
Treatment with Enbrel may result in the formation of autoimmune antibodies (see section 4.8).

Haematologic reactions
Rare cases of pancytopenia and very rare cases of aplastic anaemia, some with fatal outcome, have been reported in patients treated with Enbrel. Caution should be exercised in patients being treated with Enbrel who have a previous history of blood dyscrasias. All patients should be advised that if they develop signs and symptoms suggestive of blood dyscrasias or infections (e.g. persistent fever, sore throat, bruising, bleeding, paleness) whilst on Enbrel, they should seek immediate medical advice. Such patients should be investigated urgently, including full blood count; if blood dyscrasias are confirmed, Enbrel should be discontinued.

CNS disorders
There have been rare reports of CNS demyelinating disorders in patients treated with Enbrel (see section 4.8). Although no clinical trials have been performed evaluating Enbrel therapy in patients with multiple sclerosis, clinical trials of other TNF antagonists in patients with multiple sclerosis have shown increases in disease activity. A careful risk/benefit evaluation, including a neurological assessment, is recommended when prescribing Enbrel to patients with pre-existing or recent onset of CNS demyelinating disease, or to those who are considered to have an increased risk of developing demyelinating disease.

Combination therapy
In a controlled clinical trial of one year duration in rheumatoid arthritis patients, the combination of Enbrel and methotrexate did not result in unexpected safety findings, and the safety profile of Enbrel when given in combination with methotrexate was similar to the profiles reported in studies of Enbrel and methotrexate alone. Long-term studies to assess the safety of the combination are ongoing. The long-term safety of Enbrel in combination with other disease-modifying antirheumatic drugs has not been established.

The use of Enbrel in combination with other systemic therapies or phototherapy for the treatment of psoriasis has not been studied.

Renal and hepatic impairment
Based on pharmacokinetic data (see section 5.2), no dosage adjustment is needed in patients with renal or hepatic impairment; clinical experience in such patients is limited.

Congestive Heart Failure
Physicians should use caution when using Enbrel in patients who have congestive heart failure (CHF). There have been postmarketing reports of worsening of CHF, with and without identifiable precipitating factors, in patients taking Enbrel. Two large clinical trials evaluating the use of Enbrel in the treatment of CHF were terminated early due to lack of efficacy. Although not conclusive, data from one of these trials suggest a possible tendency toward worsening CHF in those patients assigned to Enbrel treatment.

Wegener's Granulomatosis
A placebo-controlled trial, in which 89 patients were treated with Enbrel in addition to standard therapy (including cyclophosphamide or methotrexate, and glucocorticoids) for a median duration of 25 months, has not shown Enbrel to be an effective treatment for Wegener's granulomatosis. The incidence of non-cutaneous malignancies of various types was significantly higher in patients treated with Enbrel than in the control group. Enbrel is not recommended for the treatment of Wegener's granulomatosis.

4.5 Interaction with other medicinal products and other forms of Interaction
In clinical trials, no interactions have been observed when Enbrel was administered with glucocorticoids, salicylates (except sulfasalazine), nonsteroidal anti-inflammatory drugs (NSAIDs), analgesics, or methotrexate. See section 4.4 for vaccination advice.

In a clinical study of patients who were receiving established doses of sulfasalazine, to which Enbrel was added, patients in the combination group experienced a statistically significant decrease in mean white blood cell counts in comparison to groups treated with Enbrel or sulfasalazine alone. The clinical significance of this interaction is unknown.

Concurrent Enbrel and anakinra treatment
Patients treated with Enbrel and anakinra were observed to have a higher rate of serious infection when compared with patients treated with either Enbrel or anakinra alone (historical data).

In addition, in a double-blind placebo-controlled trial in patients receiving background methotrexate, patients treated with Enbrel and anakinra were observed to have a higher rate of serious infections (7%) and neutropenia than patients treated with Enbrel (see sections 4.4 and 4.8). The combination Enbrel and anakinra has not demonstrated increased clinical benefit and is therefore not recommended.

4.6 Pregnancy and lactation
There are no studies of Enbrel in pregnant women. Developmental toxicity studies performed in rats and rabbits have revealed no evidence of harm to the foetus or neonatal rat due to etanercept. Preclinical data about peri- and postnatal toxicity of etanercept and of effects of etanercept on fertility and general reproductive performance are not available. Thus, the use of Enbrel in pregnant women is not recommended, and women of child-bearing potential should be advised not to get pregnant during Enbrel therapy.

Use during lactation
It is not known whether etanercept is excreted in human milk. Because immunoglobulins, in common with many medicinal products, can be excreted in human milk, a

decision should be made whether to discontinue nursing or to discontinue Enbrel while nursing.

4.7 Effects on ability to drive and use machines

No studies on the effects on the ability to drive and use machines have been performed.

4.8 Undesirable effects

Enbrel has been studied in 2,680 patients with rheumatoid arthritis in double-blind and open-label trials. This experience includes 2 placebo-controlled studies (349 Enbrel patients and 152 placebo patients) and 2 active-controlled trials, one active-controlled trial comparing Enbrel to methotrexate (415 Enbrel patients and 217 methotrexate patients) and another active-controlled trial comparing Enbrel (223 patients), methotrexate (228 patients) and Enbrel in combination with methotrexate (231 patients). The proportion of patients who discontinued treatment due to adverse events was the same in both the Enbrel and placebo treatment groups; in the first active-controlled trial, the dropout rate was significantly higher for methotrexate (10%) than for Enbrel (5%). In the second active-controlled trial, the rate of discontinuation for adverse events was similar among all three treatment groups, Enbrel (11%), methotrexate (14%) and Enbrel in combination with methotrexate (10%). Additionally, Enbrel has also been studied in 1,084 patients with plaque psoriasis for up to 6 months in 3 double-blind placebo-controlled studies.

In double-blind clinical trials comparing Enbrel to placebo, injection site reactions were the most frequent adverse events among Enbrel-treated patients. Among patients with rheumatoid arthritis treated in placebo-controlled trials, serious adverse events occurred at a frequency of 4% in 349 patients treated with Enbrel compared with 5% of 152 placebo-treated patients. In the first active-controlled trial, serious adverse events occurred at a frequency of 6% in 415 patients treated with Enbrel compared with 8% of 217 methotrexate-treated patients. In the second active-controlled trial the rate of serious adverse events were similar among the three treatment groups (Enbrel 11%, methotrexate 12% and Enbrel in combination with methotrexate 8%). Among patients with plaque psoriasis treated in placebo-controlled trials, the frequency of serious adverse events was about 1% of 933 patients treated with Enbrel compared with 1% of 414 placebo-treated patients.

The following list of adverse reactions is based on experience from clinical trials in adults and on postmarketing experience.

Within the organ system classes, adverse reactions are listed under headings of frequency (number of patients expected to experience the reaction), using the following categories: very common (> 1/10); common (> 1/100, < 1/10); uncommon (> 1/1000, < 1/100); rare (> 1/10,000, < 1/1000); very rare (< 1/10,000).

Infections and infestations:

Very common: Infections (including upper respiratory tract infections, bronchitis, cystitis, skin infections)*

Uncommon: Serious infections (including pneumonia, cellulitis, septic arthritis, sepsis)*

Rare: Tuberculosis

Blood and lymphatic system disorders:

Uncommon: Thrombocytopenia

Rare: Anaemia, leukopenia, neutropenia, pancytopenia*

Very rare: Aplastic anaemia*

Immune system disorders:

Common: Allergic reactions (see Skin and subcutaneous tissue disorders), autoantibody formation*

Rare: Serious allergic/anaphylactic reactions (including angioedema, bronchospasm)

Nervous system disorders:

Rare: Seizures

CNS demyelinating events suggestive of multiple sclerosis or localised demyelinating conditions such as optic neuritis and transverse myelitis (see section 4.4)

Skin and subcutaneous tissue disorders:

Common: Pruritus

Uncommon: Angioedema, urticaria, rash

Rare: Cutaneous vasculitis (including leukocytoclastic vasculitis)

Musculoskeletal, connective tissue and bone disorders:

Rare: Subacute cutaneous lupus erythematosus, discoid lupus erythematosus, lupus-like syndrome

General disorders and administration site conditions:

Very common: Injection site reactions (including bleeding, bruising, erythema, itching, pain, swelling)*

Common: Fever

Cardiac Disorders:

There have been reports of worsening of congestive heart failure (see section 4.4).

*see Additional information, below.

Additional information

Serious adverse events reported in clinical trials

Among patients in placebo-controlled, active-controlled, and open-label trials of Enbrel, serious adverse events reported included malignancies (see below), asthma, infections, heart failure, myocardial infarction, myocardial ischaemia, chest pain, syncope, cerebral ischaemia, hypertension, hypotension, cholecystitis, pancreatitis, gastrointestinal haemorrhage, bursitis, confusion, depression, dyspnoea, abnormal healing, renal insufficiency, kidney calculus, deep vein thrombosis, pulmonary embolism, membranous glomerulonephropathy, polymyositis, thrombophlebitis, liver damage, leucopenia, paresis, paresthesia, vertigo, allergic alveolitis, angioedema, scleritis, bone fracture, lymphadenopathy, ulcerative colitis and intestinal obstruction.

Malignancies

One hundred and twenty-nine new malignancies of various types were observed in 4,114 rheumatoid arthritis patients treated in clinical trials with Enbrel for up to approximately 6 years, including 231 patients treated with Enbrel in combination with methotrexate in the 2-year active-controlled study. The observed rates and incidences in these clinical trials were similar to those expected for the population studied. A total of 2 malignancies were reported in clinical studies of approximately 2 years duration involving 240 Enbrel-treated psoriatic arthritis patients. In clinical studies conducted for more than 2 years with 351 ankylosing spondylitis patients, 6 malignancies were reported in Enbrel-treated patients. Twenty-three malignancies were reported in plaque psoriasis patients treated with Enbrel in double-blind and open-label studies of up to 15 months involving 1,261 Enbrel treated patients.

There were a total of 15 lymphomas reported in 5,966 patients treated with Enbrel in rheumatoid arthritis, psoriatic arthritis, ankylosing spondylitis and psoriasis clinical trials.

Reports of various malignancies (including breast and lung carcinoma and lymphoma) have also been received in the postmarketing period (see section 4.4).

Injection Site Reactions

Compared to placebo, patients with rheumatic diseases treated with Enbrel had a significantly higher incidence of injection site reactions (36% vs. 9%). Injection site reactions usually occurred in the first month. Mean duration was approximately 3 to 5 days. No treatment was given for the majority of injection site reactions in the Enbrel treatment groups, and the majority of patients who were given treatment received topical preparations such as corticosteroids, or oral antihistamines. Additionally, some patients developed recall injection site reactions characterised by a skin reaction at the most recent site of injection along with the simultaneous appearance of injection site reactions at previous injection sites. These reactions were generally transient and did not recur with treatment.

In controlled trials in patients with plaque psoriasis, approximately 14% of patients treated with Enbrel developed injection site reactions compared with 6% of placebo-treated patients during the first 12 weeks of treatment.

Infections

In clinical trials in rheumatic disorders, upper respiratory infections ("colds") and sinusitis were the most frequently reported infections in patients receiving Enbrel or placebo. In placebo-controlled trials, the incidence of upper respiratory tract infections was 17% in the placebo treatment group and 22% in the group treated with Enbrel. In rheumatoid arthritis patients participating in placebo-controlled trials, there were 0.68 events per patient year in the placebo group and 0.82 events per patient year in the group treated with Enbrel when the longer observation of patients on Enbrel was accounted for. In placebo-controlled trials evaluating Enbrel, no increase in the incidence of serious infections (fatal, life threatening, or requiring hospitalisation or intravenous antibiotics) was observed. Among the 2,680 rheumatoid arthritis patients treated with Enbrel for up to 48 months, including 231 patients treated with Enbrel in combination with methotrexate in the 1-year active-controlled study, 170 serious infections were observed. These serious infections included abscess (at various sites), bacteraemia, bronchitis, bursitis, cellulitis, cholecystitis, diarrhoea, diverticulitis, endocarditis (suspected), gastroenteritis, hepatitis B, herpes zoster, leg ulcer, mouth infection, osteomyelitis, otitis, peritonitis, pneumonia, pyelonephritis, sepsis, septic arthritis, sinusitis, skin infection, skin ulcer, urinary tract infection, vasculitis, and wound infection. In the 1-year active-controlled study where patients were treated with either Enbrel alone, methotrexate alone or Enbrel in combination with methotrexate, the rates of serious infections were similar among the treatment groups. However, it cannot be excluded that the combination of Enbrel with methotrexate could be associated with an increase in the rate of infections.

In placebo-controlled plaque psoriasis trials, there were no differences in rates of infection among patients treated with Enbrel and those treated with placebo. In the double-blind and open-label plaque psoriasis trials of up to 15 months, serious infections experienced by Enbrel-treated patients included cellulitis, gastroenteritis, pneumonia, cholecystitis, osteomyelitis and abscess.

Serious and fatal infections have been reported during use of Enbrel; reported pathogens include bacteria, mycobacteria (including tuberculosis), viruses and fungi. Some have occurred within a few weeks after initiating treatment with Enbrel in patients who have underlying conditions (e.g. diabetes, congestive heart failure, history of active or chronic infections) in addition to their rheumatoid arthritis (see section 4.4). Data from a sepsis clinical trial not specifically in patients with rheumatoid arthritis suggest that Enbrel treatment may increase mortality in patients with established sepsis.

Autoantibodies

Patients had serum samples tested for autoantibodies at multiple timepoints. Of the rheumatoid arthritis patients evaluated for antinuclear antibodies (ANA), the percentage of patients who developed new positive ANA (⩾1:40) was higher in patients treated with Enbrel (11%) than in placebo-treated patients (5%). The percentage of patients who developed new positive anti-double-stranded DNA antibodies was also higher by radioimmunoassay (15% of patients treated with Enbrel compared to 4% of placebo-treated patients) and by *Crithidia luciliae* assay (3% of patients treated with Enbrel compared to none of placebo-treated patients). The proportion of patients treated with Enbrel who developed anticardiolipin antibodies was similarly increased compared to placebo-treated patients. The impact of long-term treatment with Enbrel on the development of autoimmune diseases is unknown.

There have been rare reports of patients, including rheumatoid factor positive patients, who have developed other autoantibodies in conjunction with a lupus-like syndrome or rashes that are compatible with subacute cutaneous lupus or discoid lupus by clinical presentation and biopsy.

Pancytopenia and aplastic anaemia

There have been postmarketing reports of pancytopenia and aplastic anaemia, some of which had fatal outcomes (see section 4.4).

Laboratory Evaluations

Based on the results of clinical studies, normally no special laboratory evaluations are necessary in addition to careful medical management and supervision of patients.

Concurrent Enbrel and anakinra treatment

In studies when patients received concurrent treatment with Enbrel plus anakinra, a higher rate of serious infections compared to Enbrel alone was observed and 2% of patients (3/139) developed neutropenia (absolute neutrophil count < 1000 / mm^3). While neutropenic, one patient developed cellulitis that resolved after hospitalisation (see sections 4.4 and 4.5).

4.9 Overdose

No dose-limiting toxicities were observed during clinical trials of rheumatoid arthritis patients. The highest dose level evaluated has been an intravenous loading dose of 32 mg/m^2 followed by subcutaneous doses of 16 mg/m^2 administered twice weekly. One rheumatoid arthritis patient mistakenly self-administered 62 mg Enbrel subcutaneously twice weekly for 3 weeks without experiencing undesirable effects. There is no known antidote to Enbrel.

5. PHARMACOLOGICAL PROPERTIES

5.1 Pharmacodynamic properties

Pharmacotherapeutic group: Selective immunosuppressant agents.

ATC code: L04AA11

Tumour necrosis factor (TNF) is a dominant cytokine in the inflammatory process of rheumatoid arthritis. In plaque psoriasis, infiltration by inflammatory cells including T-cells leads to increased TNF levels in psoriatic lesions compared with levels in uninvolved skin. Etanercept is a competitive inhibitor of TNF-binding to its cell surface receptors and thereby inhibits the biological activity of TNF. TNF and lymphotoxin are pro-inflammatory cytokines that bind to two distinct cell surface receptors: the 55-kilodalton (p55) and 75-kilodalton (p75) tumour necrosis factor receptors (TNFRs). Both TNFRs exist naturally in membrane-bound and soluble forms. Soluble TNFRs are thought to regulate TNF biological activity.

TNF and lymphotoxin exist predominantly as homotrimers, with their biological activity dependent on cross-linking of cell surface TNFRs. Dimeric soluble receptors such as etanercept possess a higher affinity for TNF than monomeric receptors and are considerably more potent competitive inhibitors of TNF binding to its cellular receptors. In addition, use of an immunoglobulin Fc region as a fusion element in the construction of a dimeric receptor imparts a longer serum half-life.

Mechanism of action

Much of the joint pathology in rheumatoid arthritis and skin pathology in plaque psoriasis is mediated by pro-inflammatory molecules that are linked in a network controlled by TNF. The mechanism of action of etanercept is thought to be its competitive inhibition of TNF binding to cell surface TNFR, preventing TNF-mediated cellular responses by rendering TNF biologically inactive. Etanercept may also modulate biologic responses controlled by additional downstream molecules (e.g., cytokines, adhesion molecules, or proteinases) that are induced or regulated by TNF.

Clinical trials

This section presents data from four randomised controlled trials in rheumatoid arthritis and 3 studies in plaque psoriasis.

Rheumatoid Arthritis

The efficacy of Enbrel was assessed in a randomised, double-blind, placebo-controlled study. The study evaluated 234 adult patients with active rheumatoid arthritis who had failed therapy with at least one but no more than four disease-modifying antirheumatic drugs (DMARDs). Doses of 10 mg or 25 mg Enbrel or placebo were administered subcutaneously twice a week for 6 consecutive months. The results of this controlled trial were expressed in percentage improvement in rheumatoid arthritis using American College of Rheumatology (ACR) response criteria.

ACR 20 and 50 responses were higher in patients treated with Enbrel at 3 and 6 months than in patients treated with placebo (ACR 20: Enbrel 62% and 59%, placebo 23% and 11% at 3 and 6 months respectively; ACR 50: Enbrel 41% and 40%, placebo 8% and 5% at months 3 and 6 respectively; $p < 0.01$ Enbrel vs Placebo at all time points for both ACR 20 and ACR 50 responses).

Approximately 15% of subjects who received Enbrel achieved an ACR 70 response at month 3 and month 6 compared to fewer than 5% of subjects in the placebo arm. Among patients receiving Enbrel, the clinical responses generally appeared within 1 to 2 weeks after initiation of therapy and nearly always occurred by 3 months. A dose response was seen; results with 10 mg were intermediate between placebo and 25 mg. Enbrel was significantly better than placebo in all components of the ACR criteria as well as other measures of rheumatoid arthritis disease activity not included in the ACR response criteria, such as morning stiffness. A Health Assessment Questionnaire (HAQ), which included disability, vitality, mental health, general health status, and arthritis-associated health status subdomains, was administered every 3 months during the trial. All subdomains of the HAQ were improved in patients treated with Enbrel compared to controls at 3 and 6 months.

After discontinuation of Enbrel, symptoms of arthritis generally returned within a month. Reintroduction of treatment with Enbrel after discontinuations of up to 24 months resulted in the same magnitudes of responses as patients who received Enbrel without interruption of therapy based on results of open-label studies. Continued durable responses have been seen for up to 48 months in open-label extension treatment trials when patients received Enbrel without interruption; longer-term experience is not available.

The efficacy of Enbrel was compared to methotrexate in a third randomised, active-controlled study with blinded radiographic evaluations as a primary endpoint in 632 adult patients with active rheumatoid arthritis (<3 years duration) who had never received treatment with methotrexate. Doses of 10 mg or 25 mg Enbrel were administered SC twice a week for up to 24 months. Methotrexate doses were escalated from 7.5 mg/week to a maximum of 20 mg/week over the first 8 weeks of the trial and continued for up to 24 months. Clinical improvement including onset of action within 2 weeks with Enbrel 25 mg was similar to that seen in the previous trials, and was maintained for up to 24 months. At baseline, patients had a moderate degree of disability, with mean HAQ scores of 1.4 to 1.5. Treatment with Enbrel 25 mg resulted in substantial improvement at 12 months, with about 44% of patients achieving a normal HAQ score (less than 0.5). This benefit was maintained in Year 2 of this study.

In this study, structural joint damage was assessed radiographically and expressed as change in Total Sharp Score (TSS) and its components, the erosion score and joint space narrowing score (JSN). Radiographs of hands/wrists and feet were read at baseline and 6, 12, and 24 months. The 10 mg Enbrel dose had consistently less effect on structural damage than the 25 mg dose. Enbrel 25 mg was significantly superior to methotrexate for erosion scores at both 12 and 24 months. The differences in TSS and JSN were not statistically significant between methotrexate and Enbrel 25 mg. The results are shown in the figure below.

RADIOGRAPHIC PROGRESSION: COMPARISON OF ENBREL vs METHOTREXATE IN PATIENTS WITH RA OF <3 YEARS DURATION

(see Figure 1)

Figure 1 RADIOGRAPHIC PROGRESSION: COMPARISON OF ENBREL vs METHOTREXATE IN PATIENTS WITH RA OF <3 YEARS DURATION

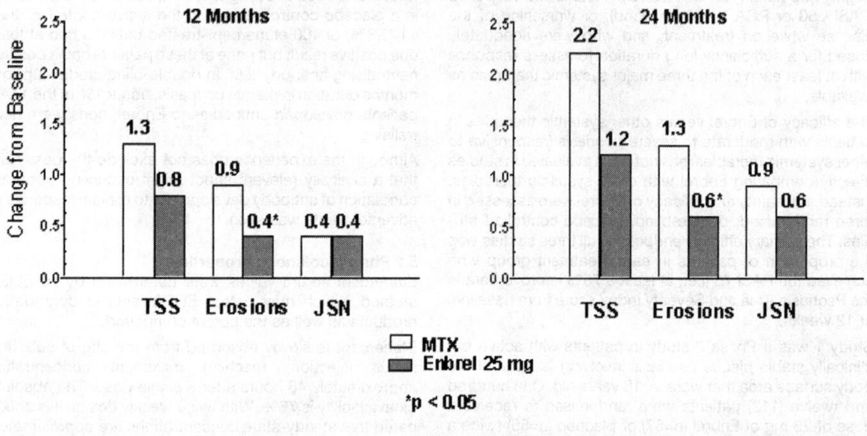

In another active-controlled, double-blind, randomised study, clinical efficacy, safety, and radiographic progression in RA patients treated with Enbrel alone (25 mg twice weekly), methotrexate alone (7.5 to 20 mg weekly, median dose 20 mg), and of the combination of Enbrel and methotrexate initiated concurrently were compared in 682 adult patients with active rheumatoid arthritis of 6 months to 20 years duration (median 5 years) who had a less than satisfactory response to at least 1 disease-modifying antirheumatic drug (DMARD) other than methotrexate.

Patients in the Enbrel in combination with methotrexate therapy group had significantly higher ACR 20, ACR 50, ACR 70 responses and improvement for DAS and HAQ scores at both 24 and 52 weeks than patients in either of the single therapy groups (results shown in table below).

(see Table 1)

Table 1 CLINCIAL EFFICACY RESULTS: COMPARISON OF ENBREL vs METHOTREXATE vs ENBREL IN COMBINATION WITH METHOTREXATE IN PATIENTS WITH RA OF 6 MONTHS to 20 YEARS DURATION

Endpoint	Methotrexate (n = 228)	Enbrel (n = 223)	Enbrel + Methotrexate (n = 231)
ACR Responses at week 52			
ACR 20	75.0%	75.8%	84.8% †,ϕ
ACR 50	42.5%	48.4%	69.3% †,ϕ
ACR 70	18.9%	24.2%	42.9% †,ϕ
DAS			
Baseline score[a]	5.5	5.7	5.5
Week 52 score[a]	3.0	3.0	2.3†,ϕ
Remission[b]	14%	18%	37%†,ϕ
HAQ			
Baseline	1.7	1.7	1.8
Week 52	1.1	1.0	0.8†,ϕ

a: Values for Disease Activity Score (DAS) are means.
b: Remission is defined as DAS <1.6

Pairwise comparison p-values: † = $p < 0.05$ for comparisons of Enbrel + methotrexate vs methotrexate and ϕ = $p < 0.05$ for comparisons of Enbrel + methotrexate vs Enbrel

Radiographic progression at week 52 was significantly less in the Enbrel group than in the methotrexate group, while the combination was significantly better than either monotherapy at slowing radiographic progression (see figure below).

Figure 2 RADIOGRAPHIC PROGRESSION: COMPARISON OF ENBREL vs METHOTREXATE vs ENBREL IN COMBINATION WITH METHOTREXATE IN PATIENTS WITH RA OF 6 MONTHS TO 20 YEARS DURATION (52-WEEK RESULTS)

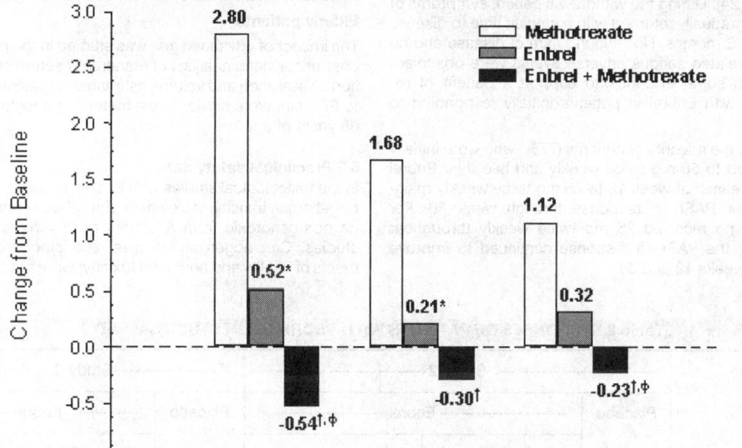

(see Figure 2 above)

Pairwise comparison p-values: * = $p < 0.05$ for comparisons of Enbrel vs methotrexate, † = $p < 0.05$ for comparisons of Enbrel + methotrexate vs methotrexate and ϕ = $p < 0.05$ for comparisons of Enbrel + methotrexate vs Enbrel

The percentage of patients without progression (TSS change ⩽ 0.5) was higher in the Enbrel in combination with methotrexate and Enbrel groups compared with methotrexate at week 24 (74%, 68%, and 56%, respectively; $p < 0.05$) and week 52 (80%, 68%, and 57%, respectively; $p < 0.05$).

The safety and efficacy of 50 mg Enbrel (two 25 mg SC injections) administered once weekly were evaluated in a double-blind, placebo-controlled study of 420 patients with active RA. In this study, 53 patients received placebo, 214 patients received 50 mg Enbrel once weekly and 153 patients received 25 mg Enbrel twice weekly. The safety and efficacy profiles of the two Enbrel treatment regimens were comparable at week 8 in their effect on signs and symptoms of RA; data at week 16 did not show comparability (non-inferiority) between the two regimens. A single 50 mg/ml injection of Enbrel was found to be bioequivalent to two simultaneous injections of 25 mg/ml.

Adults with Plaque Psoriasis

Enbrel is recommended for use in patients as defined in section 4.1. Patients who "failed to respond to" in the target population is defined by insufficient response (PASI < 50 or PGA less than good), or worsening of the disease while on treatment, and who were adequately dosed for a sufficiently long duration to assess response with at least each of the three major systemic therapies as available.

The efficacy of Enbrel versus other systemic therapies in patients with moderate to severe psoriasis (responsive to other systemic therapies) has not been evaluated in studies directly comparing Enbrel with other systemic therapies. Instead, the safety and efficacy of Enbrel were assessed in three randomised, double-blind, placebo-controlled studies. The primary efficacy endpoint in all three studies was the proportion of patients in each treatment group who achieved the PASI 75 (i.e., at least a 75% improvement in the Psoriasis Area and Severity Index score from baseline) at 12 weeks.

Study 1 was a Phase 2 study in patients with active but clinically stable plaque psoriasis involving ⩾ 10% of the body surface area that were ⩾ 18 years old. One hundred and twelve (112) patients were randomised to receive a dose of 25 mg of Enbrel (n=57) or placebo (n=55) twice a week for 24 weeks.

Study 2 evaluated 652 patients with chronic plaque psoriasis using the same inclusion criteria as study 1 with the addition of a minimum psoriasis area and severity index (PASI) of 10 at screening. Enbrel was administered at doses of 25 mg once a week, 25 mg twice a week or 50 mg twice a week for 6 consecutive months. During the first 12 weeks of the double-blind treatment period, patients received placebo or one of the above three Enbrel doses. After 12 weeks of treatment, patients in the placebo group began treatment with blinded Enbrel (25 mg twice a week); patients in the active treatment groups continued to week 24 on the dose to which they were originally randomised.

Study 3 evaluated 583 patients and had the same inclusion criteria as study 2. Patients in this study received a dose of 25 mg or 50 mg Enbrel, or placebo twice a week for 12 weeks and then all patients received open-label 25 mg Enbrel twice weekly for an additional 24 weeks.

In study 1, the Enbrel-treated group had a significantly higher proportion of patients with a PASI 75 response at week 12 (30%) compared to the placebo-treated group (2%) (p < 0.0001). At 24 weeks, 56% of patients in the Enbrel-treated group had achieved the PASI 75 compared to 5% of placebo-treated patients. Key results of studies 2 and 3 are shown below.

(see Table 2 below)

Among patients with plaque psoriasis who received Enbrel, significant responses relative to placebo were apparent at the time of the first visit (2 weeks) and were maintained through 24 weeks of therapy.

Study 2 also had a drug withdrawal period during which patients who achieved a PASI improvement of at least 50% at week 24 had treatment stopped. Patients were observed off treatment for the occurrence of rebound (PASI ⩾150% of baseline) and for the time to relapse (defined as a loss of at least half of the improvement achieved between baseline and week 24). During the withdrawal period, symptoms of psoriasis gradually returned with a median time to disease relapse of 3 months. No rebound flare of disease and no psoriasis-related serious adverse events were observed. There was some evidence to support a benefit of re-treatment with Enbrel in patients initially responding to treatment.

In study 3, the majority of patients (77%) who were initially randomised to 50 mg twice weekly and had their Enbrel dose decreased at week 12 to 25 mg twice weekly maintained their PASI 75 response through week 36. For patients who received 25 mg twice weekly throughout the study, the PASI 75 response continued to improve between weeks 12 and 36.

Antibodies to Enbrel

Antibodies to Enbrel, all non-neutralising, were detected in 4 out of 96 rheumatoid arthritis patients who received Enbrel at a dose of 25 mg twice a week for up to 3 months in a placebo-controlled trial. In the active-controlled trial, 11 (2.8%) of 400 etanercept-treated patients had at least one positive result but none of these patients had a positive neutralising antibody test. In double-blind studies up to 6 months duration in plaque psoriasis, about 1% of the 1,084 patients developed antibodies to Enbrel, none were neutralising.

Although the experience does not exclude the possibility that a clinically relevant effect might occur, no apparent correlation of antibody development to clinical response or adverse events was seen.

5.2 Pharmacokinetic properties

Etanercept serum values were determined by an ELISA method, which may detect ELISA-reactive degradation products as well as the parent compound.

Etanercept is slowly absorbed from the site of subcutaneous injection, reaching maximum concentration approximately 48 hours after a single dose. The absolute bioavailability is 76%. With twice weekly doses, it is anticipated that steady-state concentrations are approximately twice as high as those observed after single doses. After a single subcutaneous dose of 25 mg Enbrel, the average maximum serum concentration observed in healthy volunteers was 1.65 ± 0.66 μg/ml, and the area under the curve was 235 ± 96.6 μg•hr/ml. Dose proportionality has not been formally evaluated, but there is no apparent saturation of clearance across the dosing range.

A biexponential curve is required to describe the concentration time curve of etanercept. The central volume of distribution of etanercept is 7.6 l, while the volume of distribution at steady-state is 10.4 l.

Etanercept is cleared slowly from the body. The half-life is long, approximately 70 hours. Clearance is approximately 0.066 l/hr in patients with rheumatoid arthritis, somewhat lower than the value of 0.11 l/hr observed in healthy volunteers. Additionally, the pharmacokinetics of Enbrel in rheumatoid arthritis patients and plaque psoriasis patients are similar.

Mean serum concentration profiles at steady state i.e. Cmax (2.4 mg/l vs 2.6 mg/l), Cmin (1.2 mg/l vs 1.4 mg/l), and partial AUC (297 mgh/l vs 316 mgh/l), were shown to be comparable in RA patients treated with 50 mg etanercept once weekly (n=21) and 25 mg etanercept twice weekly (n=16), respectively. In an open-label, single-dose, two-treatment, crossover study in 28 healthy volunteers, etanercept administered as a single 50 mg/ml injection was found to be bioequivalent to two simultaneous injections of 25 mg/ml.

Although there is elimination of radioactivity in urine after administration of radiolabelled etanercept to patients and volunteers, increased etanercept concentrations were not observed in patients with acute renal or hepatic failure. The presence of renal and hepatic impairment should not require a change in dosage. There is no apparent pharmacokinetic difference between men and women.

Methotrexate has no effect on the pharmacokinetics of etanercept. The effect of Enbrel on the human pharmacokinetics of methotrexate has not been investigated.

Elderly patients

The impact of advanced age was studied in the population pharmacokinetic analysis of etanercept serum concentrations. Clearance and volume estimates in patients aged 65 to 87 years were similar to estimates in patients less than 65 years of age.

5.3 Preclinical safety data

In the toxicological studies with Enbrel, no dose-limiting or target organ toxicity was evident. Enbrel was considered to be non-genotoxic from a battery of *in vitro* and *in vivo* studies. Carcinogenicity studies, and standard assessments of fertility and postnatal toxicity, were not performed with Enbrel due to the development of neutralising antibodies in rodents.

Enbrel did not induce lethality or notable signs of toxicity in mice or rats following a single subcutaneous dose of 2000 mg/kg or a single intravenous dose of 1000 mg/kg. Enbrel did not elicit dose-limiting or target organ toxicity in cynomolgus monkeys following twice weekly subcutaneous administration for 4 or 26 consecutive weeks at a dose (15 mg/kg) that resulted in AUC-based serum drug concentrations that were over 27-fold higher than that obtained in humans at the recommended dose of 25 mg.

6. PHARMACEUTICAL PARTICULARS

6.1 List of excipients

Powder: Mannitol, sucrose, and trometamol.

Solvent: Water for injections

6.2 Incompatibilities

In the absence of incompatibility studies, this medicinal product must not be mixed with other medicinal products.

6.3 Shelf life

3 years.

After reconstitution, immediate use is recommended. Chemical and physical in-use stability has been demonstrated for 48 hours at 2° – 8°C. From a microbiological point of view, the product should be used immediately. If not used immediately, in-use storage times are the responsibility of the user and would normally not be longer than 6 hours at 2° – 8°C, unless reconstitution has taken place in controlled and validated aseptic conditions.

6.4 Special precautions for storage

Store in a refrigerator (2°C – 8°C).

Do not freeze

6.5 Nature and contents of container

Clear glass vial (4 ml, type I glass) with rubber stoppers, aluminium seals, and flip-off plastic caps. Enbrel is supplied with pre-filled syringes containing water for injections. The syringes are type I glass.

Cartons contain 2, 4 or 12 vials of Enbrel with 2, 4 or 12 pre-filled syringes, 2, 4 or 12 needles, 2, 4 or 12 vial adaptors and 4, 8 or 24 alcohol swabs. Not all pack sizes may be marketed.

6.6 Instructions for use and handling

Enbrel 50 mg is reconstituted with 1 ml water for injections. Enbrel contains no antibacterial preservative, and therefore, solutions prepared with water for injections should be administered as soon as possible and within 6 hours following reconstitution. The solution should be clear and colourless with no lumps, flakes or particles. Some white foam may remain in the vial – this is normal. Do not use Enbrel if all the powder in the vial is not dissolved within 10 minutes. Start again with another vial.

Any unused product or waste material should be disposed of in accordance with local requirements.

7. MARKETING AUTHORISATION HOLDER

Wyeth Europa Ltd.

Huntercombe Lane South

Taplow, Maidenhead

Berkshire, SL6 0PH

United Kingdom

8. MARKETING AUTHORISATION NUMBER(S)

EU/1/99/126/010

9. DATE OF FIRST AUTHORISATION/RENEWAL OF THE AUTHORISATION

Date of first authorisation: 28 April 2005

10. DATE OF REVISION OF THE TEXT

1st August 2005

[Wyeth logo]

Further information may be obtained from:

For the UK:

Wyeth Pharmaceuticals, Huntercombe Lane South, Taplow, Maidenhead, Berkshire, SL6 0PH, UK

Telephone: 01628 415330

For Ireland:

Wyeth Pharmaceuticals, M50 Business Park

Ballymount Road Upper, Walkinstown, Dublin 12

Ireland

Telephone: 01 449 3500

* Trade mark

Table 2 RESPONSES OF PATIENTS WITH PSORIASIS IN STUDIES 2 AND 3

Response	Study 2					Study 3		
	Placebo	Enbrel				Placebo	Enbrel	
		25 mg BIW		50 mg BIW			25 mg BIW	50 mg BIW
	n = 166 wk 12	n = 162 wk 12	n = 162 wk 24[a]	n = 164 wk 12	n = 164 wk 24[a]	n = 193 wk 12	n = 196 wk 12	n = 196 wk 12
PASI 50, %	14	58*	70	74*	77	9	64*	77*
PASI 75, %	4	34*	44	49*	59	3	34*	49*
DSGA[b], clear or almost clear, %	5	34*	39	49*	55	4	39*	57*

*p ⩽ 0.0001 compared with placebo

a. No statistical comparisons to placebo were made at week 24 in Study 2 because the original placebo group began receiving Enbrel 25 mg BIW from week 13 to week 24.

b. Dermatologist Static Global Assessment. Clear or almost clear defined as 0 or 1 on a 0 to 5 scale.

Engerix B syringe and Pre-filled syringe

(GlaxoSmithKline UK)

1. NAME OF THE MEDICINAL PRODUCT

Engerix B® 20 micrograms/1 ml

Suspension for injection in a vial or pre-filled syringe

Hepatitis B recombinant vaccine, adsorbed

2. QUALITATIVE AND QUANTITATIVE COMPOSITION

1 dose (0.5 ml) contains:

Hepatitis B surface antigen(rDNA)*, 10 micrograms

*adsorbed on aluminium oxide, hydrated Total: 0.25 milligrams Al^{3+} and produced on recombinant yeast cells (*Saccharomyces cerevisiae*)

1 dose (1 ml) contains:

Hepatitis B surface antigen(rDNA)*, 20 micrograms

* adsorbed on aluminium oxide, hydrated Total: 0.50 milligrams Al^{3+} and produced on recombinant yeast cells (*Saccharomyces cerevisiae*)

For excipients, see 6.1

3. PHARMACEUTICAL FORM

Suspension for injection in a vial or pre-filled syringe.

4. CLINICAL PARTICULARS

4.1 Therapeutic indications

Engerix B is indicated for active immunisation against hepatitis B virus infection (HBV) caused by all known subtypes in non immune subjects. The categories within the population to be immunised are determined on the basis of official recommendations.

It can be expected that hepatitis D will also be prevented by immunisation with Engerix B as hepatitis D (caused by the delta agent) does not occur in the absence of hepatitis B infection.

4.2 Posology and method of administration

Posology

Dosage

20μg dose vaccine: A 20 μg dose (in 1.0 ml suspension) is intended for use in adults and children older than 15 years of age.

10 μg dose vaccine: A 10 μg dose (in 0.5 ml suspension) is intended for use in children up to and including 15 years of age, including neonates.

Under normal conditions of use Engerix B 20 μg/1 ml is intended for adults and children older than 15 years of age and 10 μg/0.5 ml dose (0.5 ml suspension) is intended for use in children up to and including 15 years of age, including neonates. However, in children aged 10 to 15 years, the adult dose of 20 μg can be employed if low compliance is anticipated, since a higher percentage of vaccinees with protective antibody levels (10 IU/l) is obtained after two injections at this dosage.

Primary Immunisation schedule

A series of three intramuscular injections is required to achieve optimal protection.

Two primary immunisation schedules can be recommended:

An accelerated schedule, with immunisation at 0, 1 and 2 months, will confer protection more quickly and is expected to provide better patient compliance. A fourth dose should be administered at 12 months. In infants this schedule will allow for simultaneous administration of hepatitis B with other childhood vaccines.

Schedules which have more time between the second and third doses, such as immunisation at 0, 1 and 6 months, may take longer to confer protection, but will produce higher anti-HBs antibody titres.

These immunisation schedules may be adjusted to accommodate local immunisation practices with regard to the recommended age of administration of other childhood vaccines.

In exceptional circumstances in adults, where a more rapid induction of protection is required, e.g. persons travelling to areas of high endemicity and who commence a course of vaccination against hepatitis B within one month prior to departure, a schedule of three intramuscular injections given at 0, 7 and 21 days may be used. When this schedule is applied, a fourth dose is recommended 12 months after the first dose (see section 5.1 "Pharmacodynamic properties" for seroconversion rates).

Booster dose

The need for a booster dose in healthy individuals who have received a full primary vaccination course has not been established; however some official vaccination programmes currently include a recommendation for a booster dose and these should be respected.

For some categories of subjects or patients particularly exposed to the HBV (e.g. haemodialysis or immunocompromised patients) a precautionary attitude should be considered to ensure a protective antibody level > 10IU/l.

Interchangeability of hepatitis B vaccines

See 4.5. Interaction with other medicaments and other forms of interaction.

- Special dosage recommendations (see Dosage)

- Dosage recommendation for neonates born of mothers who are HBV carriers:

The immunisation with Engerix B (10 μg) of these neonates should start at birth, and two immunisation schedules have been followed. Either the 0, 1, 2 and 12 months or the 0, 1 and 6 months schedule can be used; however, the former schedule provides a more rapid immune response. When available, hepatitis B immune globulins (HBIg) should be given simultaneously with Engerix B at a separate injection site as this may increase the protective efficacy.

- Dosage recommendation for known or presumed exposure to HBV:

In circumstances where exposure to HBV has recently occurred (eg needlestick with contaminated needle) the first dose of Engerix B can be administered simultaneously with HBIg which however must be given at a separate injection site. The accelerated immunisation schedule should be advised.

- Dosage recommendation for chronic haemodialysis patients:

The primary immunisation schedule for chronic haemodialysis patients is four doses of 40 μg at elected date, 1 month, 2 months and 6 months from the date of the first dose. The immunisation schedule should be adapted in order to ensure that the anti-HBs antibody titre remains above the accepted protective level of 10 IU/l.

Method of Administration

Engerix B should be injected intramuscularly in the deltoid region in adults and children or in the anterolateral thigh in neonates, infants and young children.

Exceptionally the vaccine may be administered subcutaneously in patients with thrombocytopenia or bleeding disorders.

4.3 Contraindications

Engerix B should not be administered to subjects with known hypersensitivity to any component of the vaccine, or to subjects having shown signs of hypersensitivity after previous Engerix B administration.

As with other vaccines, the administration of Engerix B should be postponed in subjects suffering from acute severe febrile illness. The presence of a minor infection, however, is not a contra-indication for immunisation.

4.4 Special warnings and special precautions for use

Because of the long incubation period of hepatitis B it is possible for unrecognised infection to be present at the time of immunisation. The vaccine may not prevent hepatitis B infection in such cases.

The vaccine will not prevent infection caused by other agents such as hepatitis A, hepatitis C and hepatitis E and other pathogens known to infect the liver.

A number of factors have been observed to reduce the immune response to hepatitis B vaccines. These factors include older age, male gender, obesity, smoking, route of administration and some chronic underlying diseases. Consideration should be given to serological testing of those subjects who may be at risk of not achieving seroprotection following a complete course of Engerix B. Additional doses may need to be considered for persons who do not respond or have a sub-optimal response to a course of vaccinations.

Engerix B should not be administered in the buttock or intradermally since this may result in a lower immune response.

Engerix B should under no circumstances be administered intravenously.

Patients with chronic liver disease or with HIV infection or hepatitis C carriers should not be precluded from vaccination against hepatitis B. The vaccine could be advised since HBV infection can be severe in these patients: the HB vaccination should thus be considered on a case by case basis by the physician. In HIV infected patients, as also in haemodialysis patients and persons with an impaired immune system, adequate anti-HBs antibody titers may not be obtained after the primary immunisation course and such patients may therefore require administration of additional doses of vaccine. (see "Dosage recommendation for chronic haemodialysis patients.")

Thiomersal (an organomercuric compound) has been used in the manufacturing process of this medicinal product and residues of it are present in the final product. Therefore, sensitisation reactions may occur.

As with all injectable vaccines, appropriate medical treatment should always be readily available in case of rare anaphylactic reactions following the administration of the vaccine.

As with any vaccine, a protective immune response may not be elicited in all vaccinees.

4.5 Interaction with other medicinal products and other forms of Interaction

The simultaneous administration of Engerix B and a standard dose of HBIg does not result in lower anti-HBs antibody titres provided that they are administered at separate injection sites.

Engerix B can be given concomitantly with Haemophilus influenzae b, BCG, hepatitis A, polio, measles, mumps, rubella, diphtheria, tetanus and pertussis vaccines.

Different injectable vaccines should always be administered at different injection sites.

Engerix B may be used to complete a primary immunisation course started either with plasma-derived or with other genetically-engineered hepatitis B vaccines, or, if it is desired to administer a booster dose, it may be administered to subjects who have previously received a primary immunisation course with plasma-derived or with other genetically-engineered hepatitis B vaccines.

4.6 Pregnancy and lactation

Pregnancy

The effect of the HBsAg on foetal development has not been assessed.

However, as with all inactivated viral vaccines one does not expect harm for the foetus. Engerix B should be used during pregnancy only when clearly needed, and the possible advantages outweigh the possible risks for the foetus.

Lactation

The effect on breastfed infants of the administration of Engerix B to their mothers has not been evaluated in clinical studies, as information concerning the excretion into the breastmilk is not available.

No contra-indication has been established.

4.7 Effects on ability to drive and use machines

Some of the effects mentioned under section 4.8 "Undesirable Effects" may affect the ability to drive or operate machinery.

4.8 Undesirable effects

Engerix B is generally well tolerated.

The following undesirable events have been reported following the widespread use of the vaccine. As with other hepatitis B vaccines, in many instances the causal relationship to the vaccine has not been established.

Blood and lymphatic system disorders

Very rare: thrombocytopenia

Immune system disorders

Very rare: anaphylaxis, serum sickness, lymphadenopathy

Nervous system disorders

Rare: dizziness, headache, paraesthesia

Very rare: syncope, paralysis, neuropathy, neuritis (including Guillain-Barré syndrome, optic neuritis and multiple sclerosis), encephalitis, encephalophy, meningitis, convulsions

Vascular disorders

Very rare: hypotension, vasculitis

Respiratory, thoracic and mediastinal disorders

Very rare: bronchospasm

Gastrointestinal disorders

Rare: nausea, vomiting, diarrhoea, abdominal pain

Hepatobiliary disorders

Rare: hepatic function abnormal

Skin and subcutaneous tissue disorders

Rare: rash, pruritus, urticaria

Very rare: angioneurotic oedema, erythema multiforme

Musculoskeletal and connective tissue disorders

Rare: athralgia, myalgia

Very rare: arthritis

General disorders and administration site conditions

Common: injection site pain, injection site erythema, injection site induration

Rare: fatigue, fever, malaise, influenza-like symptoms

The booster dose is as well tolerated as the primary vaccination.

4.9 Overdose

Not applicable.

5. PHARMACOLOGICAL PROPERTIES

5.1 Pharmacodynamic properties

Engerix B, hepatitis B vaccine is a sterile suspension containing the purified major surface antigen of the virus manufactured by recombinant DNA technology, adsorbed onto aluminium oxide hydrated.

The antigen is produced by culture of genetically-engineered yeast cells (*Saccharomyces cerevisiae*) which carry the gene which codes for the major surface antigen of the hepatitis B virus (HBV). This hepatitis B surface antigen (HBsAg) expressed in yeast cells is purified by several physico-chemical steps.

The HBsAg assembles spontaneously, in the absence of chemical treatment, into spherical particles of 20 nm in average diameter containing non-glycosylated HBsAg polypeptides and a lipid matrix consisting mainly of phospholipids. Extensive tests have demonstrated that these particles display the characteristic properties of natural HBsAg.

The HBV component is formulated in phosphate buffered saline.

The vaccine is highly purified, and meets the WHO requirements for recombinant hepatitis B vaccines. No substances of human origin are used in its manufacture.

Engerix B induces specific humoral antibodies against HBsAg (anti-HBs antibodies). An anti-HBs antibody titre above 10 IU/l correlates with protection to HBV infection.

- Protective efficacy

- In risk groups:

In field studies, a protective efficacy between 95% and 100% was demonstrated in neonates, children and adults at risk.

A 95% protective efficacy was demonstrated in neonates of HBeAg positive mothers, immunised according to the 0, 1, 2 and 12 or 0, 1 and 6 schedules without the concomitant administration of HBIg at birth. However, simultaneous administration of HBIg and vaccine at birth increased the protective efficacy to 98%.

- In healthy subjects:

When the 0, 1 and 6 month schedule is followed, ≥96 % of vaccinees have seroprotective levels of antibody 7 months after the first dose.

When the 0, 1, 2 and 12 month schedule is followed, 15% and 89% of vaccinees have seroprotective levels of antibody one month after first dose and one month after the third dose respectively. One month after the fourth dose 95.8 % of vaccinees achieved seroprotective levels of antibody.

For use in exceptional circumstances, the 0, 7 and 21 day primary schedule plus a fourth dose at month 12 results in 65.2 % and 76% of vaccinees having seroprotective levels of antibody within 1 and 5 weeks respectively following the third dose. One month after the fourth dose 98.6 % of vaccinees achieved seroprotective levels of antibody.

Reduction in the incidence of hepatocellular carcinoma in children:

A clear link has been demonstrated between hepatitis B infection and the occurrence of hepatocellular carcinoma (HCC). The prevention of hepatitis B by vaccination results in a reduction of the incidence of HCC, as has been observed in Taiwan in children aged 6-14 years.

5.2 Pharmacokinetic properties
Not applicable.

5.3 Preclinical safety data
The preclinical safety data satisfy the requirements of the WHO.

6. PHARMACEUTICAL PARTICULARS

6.1 List of excipients
Sodium chloride,

Disodium phosphate dihydrate,

Sodium dihydrogen phosphate,

Water for injections.

For adsorbent, see 2

6.2 Incompatibilities
Engerix B should not be mixed with other medicinal products.

6.3 Shelf life
3 years.

6.4 Special precautions for storage
Store at 2 -°C to 8 -°C (in a refrigerator). Do not freeze; discard if vaccine has been frozen.

6.5 Nature and contents of container
0.5 ml or 1.0 ml of suspension in a vial (type I glass) with a stopper (rubber butyl). Pack of 1, 3, 10.

0.5 ml or 1.0 ml of suspension in a pre-filled syringe (type I glass). Pack of 1 & 10.

Disposable syringe(s) may be supplied.

Not all pack sizes may be marketed.

6.6 Instructions for use and handling
Upon storage, the content may present a fine white deposit with a clear colourless supernatant. Once shaken the vaccine is slightly opaque.

The vaccine should be inspected visually for any foreign particulate matter and/or coloration prior to administration. Discard if the content appears otherwise.

The vaccine must be administered immediately after either withdrawing the contents of the vial or opening the pre-filled syringe pack.

Administrative Data

7. MARKETING AUTHORISATION HOLDER
SmithKline Beecham plc

Trading as: GlaxoSmithKline UK,

Stockley Park West,

Uxbridge, Middlesex, UB11 1BT

8. MARKETING AUTHORISATION NUMBER(S)
Vial: PL 10592/0165

Pre-filled syringe: PL 10592/0166

9. DATE OF FIRST AUTHORISATION/RENEWAL OF THE AUTHORISATION
5 February 2001

10. DATE OF REVISION OF THE TEXT
14 November 2003

11. Legal Category
POM

Entocort CR 3mg Capsules

(AstraZeneca UK Limited)

1. NAME OF THE MEDICINAL PRODUCT
Entocort® CR 3mg Capsules.

2. QUALITATIVE AND QUANTITATIVE COMPOSITION
Each capsule contains budesonide 3mg

3. PHARMACEUTICAL FORM
Entocort CR 3mg Capsules: Hard gelatin capsules for oral administration with an opaque, light grey body and opaque, pink cap marked **CIR 3mg** in black radial print. Each capsule contains budesonide 3mg as gastro-resistant, prolonged release granules.

4. CLINICAL PARTICULARS

4.1 Therapeutic indications
Entocort CR Capsules are indicated for the induction of remission in patients with mild to moderate Crohn's disease affecting the ileum and/or the ascending colon.

4.2 Posology and method of administration
Adults:

Active Crohn's disease: The recommended daily dose for induction of remission is 9mg once daily in the morning, taken before breakfast, for up to eight weeks.

When treatment is to be discontinued, the dose should normally be reduced for the last 2 to 4 weeks of therapy.

Children:

There is presently no experience with Entocort CR Capsules in children. Entocort is not recommended for use in children.

Elderly:

No special dose adjustment is recommended. However, experience with Entocort CR Capsules in the elderly is limited.

4.3 Contraindications
Bacterial, fungal or viral infections. Known hypersensitivity to any of the ingredients.

4.4 Special warnings and special precautions for use
Treatment with Entocort CR Capsules results in lower systemic steroid levels than conventional oral steroid therapy. Transfer from other steroid therapy may result in symptoms related to the change in systemic steroid levels. The following warnings apply, in common with other oral steroids.

Use with caution in patients with tuberculosis, hypertension, diabetes mellitus, osteoporosis, peptic ulcer, glaucoma or cataracts or with a family history of diabetes or glaucoma or with any other condition where the use of glucocorticosteroids may have unwanted effects.

Chicken pox and measles may follow a more serious course in patients on oral glucocorticosteroids. Particular care should be taken to avoid exposure in patients who have not previously had these diseases.

Corticosteroids may cause suppression of the HPA axis and reduce the stress response. Where patients are subject to surgery or other stresses, supplementary systemic glucocorticoid treatment is recommended.

In patients with compromised liver function, blood levels of glucocorticosteroid may increase, as with other drugs which are metabolised via the liver.

When treatment is to be discontinued, the dose should normally be reduced for the last 2 to 4 weeks of therapy.

4.5 Interaction with other medicinal products and other forms of Interaction
Although not studied, concomitant administration of colestyramine may reduce Entocort uptake, in common with other drugs.

4.6 Pregnancy and lactation
Pregnancy
The ability of corticosteroids to cross the placenta varies between individual drugs, however, in mice, budesonide and/or its metabolites have been shown to cross the placenta.

Administration of corticosteroids to pregnant animals can cause abnormalities of foetal development including cleft palate, intra-uterine growth retardation and effects on brain growth and development. There is no evidence that corticosteroids result in an increased incidence of congenital abnormalities, such as cleft palate/lip in man. However, when administered for prolonged periods or repeatedly during pregnancy, corticosteroids may increase the risk of intra-uterine growth retardation.

Hypoadrenalism may, in theory, occur in the neonate following prenatal exposure to corticosteroids but usually resolves spontaneously following birth and is rarely clinically important. As with all drugs, corticosteroids should only be prescribed when the benefits to the mother and child outweigh the risks. When corticosteroids are essential however, patients with normal pregnancies may be treated as though they were in the non-gravid state.

Lactation
Corticosteroids are secreted in small amounts in breast milk, however, budesonide given at the clinically recommended dose is unlikely to cause systematic effects in the infant. Infants of mothers taking higher than recommended doses of budesonide may have a degree of adrenal suppression but the benefits of breast feeding are likely to outweigh any theoretical risk.

4.7 Effects on ability to drive and use machines
No effects are known.

4.8 Undesirable effects
Undesirable effects characteristic of systemic corticosteroid therapy, such as Cushingoid features, may occur.

In clinical trials other adverse events: dyspepsia, muscle cramps, tremor, palpitations, nervousness, blurred vision, skin reactions (rash, pruritus) and menstrual disorders have been reported. Most of these adverse events were classed as mild to moderate and were not considered serious. In clinical studies, at recommended doses, the incidence of adverse events was comparable to placebo.

Clinical studies showed the frequency of steroid associated side-effects for Entocort CR Capsules to be approximately half that of conventional prednisolone treatment, at equipotent doses. In studies of patients with active disease, receiving Entocort 9mg daily, the incidence of adverse events was comparable to placebo.

4.9 Overdose
Acute overdosage with Entocort CR Capsules even at very high doses, is not expected to lead to an acute clinical crisis. Use supportive therapy as required.

Chronic overdosage may lead to systemic corticosteroid effects, such as Cushingoid features. If such changes occur, the dose of Entocort CR Capsules should be gradually reduced until treatment is discontinued, in accordance with normal procedures for the discontinuation of prolonged oral steroid therapy.

5. PHARMACOLOGICAL PROPERTIES

5.1 Pharmacodynamic properties
The exact mechanism of budesonide in the treatment of Crohn's disease is not fully understood.

Data from clinical pharmacology studies and controlled clinical trials strongly indicate that the mode of action of Entocort CR Capsules is based, at least partly, on a local action in the gut. Budesonide is a glucocorticosteroid with a high local anti-inflammatory effect. At doses clinically equivalent to prednisolone, budesonide gives significantly less HPA axis suppression and has a lower impact on inflammatory markers.

At recommended doses, Entocort CR Capsules caused significantly less effect than prednisolone 20 - 40mg daily on: morning plasma cortisols; 24 hour plasma cortisol (AUC 0 - 24h) and 24 hour urine cortisol levels.

ACTH tests have shown Entocort CR Capsules to have significantly less effect than prednisolone on adrenal functions.

5.2 Pharmacokinetic properties
Budesonide has a high volume of distribution (about 3L/kg) and a high systemic clearance (about 1.2L/min). Plasma protein binding averages 85-90%. After oral dosing of plain micronized compound, absorption is rapid and seems to be complete. Budesonide then undergoes extensive biotransformation in the liver (approximately 90%) to metabolites of low glucocorticosteroid activity. The glucocorticosteroid activity of the major metabolites, 6β-hydroxybudesonide and 16α-hydroxy-prednisolone, is less than 1% of that of budesonide.

In healthy volunteers mean maximal plasma concentrations of 5 - 10 nmol/L were seen at 3 - 5 hours following a single oral dose of Entocort CR Capsules 9mg, taken before breakfast.

Systemic availability in healthy subjects is approximately 10% for Entocort CR Capsules similar to the systemic availability of plain micronised budesonide, indicating complete absorption.

In patients with active Crohn's disease systemic availability is approximately 20% at the start of treatment, and reduces to around 15% after 8 weeks treatment.

A large proportion of the drug is absorbed from the ileum and ascending colon. Elimination is rate limited by absorption. The average terminal half-life is 4 hours.

5.3 Preclinical safety data
Results from acute, subacute and chronic toxicity studies show that the systemic effects of budesonide are less severe or similar to those observed after administration of other glucocorticosteroids, e.g. decreased body-weight gain and atrophy of lymphoid tissues and adrenal cortex.

Budesonide, evaluated in six different test systems, did not show any mutagenic or clastogenic effects.

An increased incidence of brain gliomas in male rats in a carcinogenicity study could not be verified in a repeat study, in which the incidence of gliomas did not differ between any of the groups on active treatment (budesonide, prednisolone, triamcinolone acetonide) and the control groups.

Liver changes (primary hepatocellular neoplasms) found in male rats in the original carcinogenicity study were noted again in the repeat study with budesonide as well as the reference glucocorticosteroids. These effects are most probably related to a receptor effect and thus represent a class effect.

Available clinical experience shows that there are no indications that budesonide or other glucocorticosteroids induce brain gliomas or primary hepatocellular neoplasms in man.

The toxicity of Entocort CR Capsules, with focus on the gastro-intestinal tract, has been studied in cynomolgus monkeys in doses up to 5mg/kg after repeated oral administration for up to 6 months. No effects were observed in the gastrointestinal tract, neither at gross pathology nor in the histopathological examination.

6. PHARMACEUTICAL PARTICULARS

6.1 List of excipients
Ethylcellulose, Tributyl acetylcitrate, Methacrylic acid copolymer, Triethylcitrate, Antifoam M, Polysorbate 80, Talc, Sucrose, Maize starch, Gelatine, Titanium dioxide (E171), Iron-oxide (E172)

6.2 Incompatibilities
No known incompatibilities.

6.3 Shelf life
Entocort CR Capsules have a shelf-life of 3 years when stored not above 30°C in the original container.

6.4 Special precautions for storage
Store in the original container. Replace cap firmly after use. Store out of reach and sight of children.

6.5 Nature and contents of container
White polyethylene bottles of 100 capsules, having either a tamper evident or child resistant polypropylene screw cap, with an integral desiccant.

6.6 Instructions for use and handling
The capsules should be swallowed whole with water. The capsules must not be chewed.

7. MARKETING AUTHORISATION HOLDER
AstraZeneca UK Limited,

600 Capability Green,

Luton,

LU1 3LU,

UK.

8. MARKETING AUTHORISATION NUMBER(S)
PL 17901/0122

9. DATE OF FIRST AUTHORISATION/RENEWAL OF THE AUTHORISATION
4th June 2002

10. DATE OF REVISION OF THE TEXT
20th September 2004

Entocort Enema

(AstraZeneca UK Limited)

1. NAME OF THE MEDICINAL PRODUCT
Entocort® Enema.

2. QUALITATIVE AND QUANTITATIVE COMPOSITION
0.02 mg/ml budesonide (2 mg budesonide /100 ml).

3. PHARMACEUTICAL FORM
Enema.

4. CLINICAL PARTICULARS

4.1 Therapeutic indications
Ulcerative colitis involving rectal and recto-sigmoid disease.

4.2 Posology and method of administration
Adults: One Entocort Enema nightly for 4 weeks.

Children: Not recommended.

Elderly: Dosage as for adults.

No dosage reduction is necessary in patients with reduced liver function.

The route of administration is rectal.

4.3 Contraindications
Local bacterial and viral infection. Hypersensitivity to any of the ingredients.

4.4 Special warnings and special precautions for use
Special care is needed in treatment of patients transferred from systemic steroids to Entocort Enema, as disturbances in the hypothalamic-pituitary-adrenal axis could be expected in these patients.

4.5 Interaction with other medicinal products and other forms of Interaction
Information on possible interactions with rectal administration of budesonide is not available presently.

4.6 Pregnancy and lactation
Pregnancy

"The ability of corticosteroids to cross the placenta varies between individual drugs, however, in mice, budesonide and/or its metabolites have been shown to cross the placenta."

Administration of corticosteroids to pregnant animals can cause abnormalities of foetal development including cleft palate, intra-uterine growth retardation and affects on brain growth and development. There is no evidence that corticosteroids result in an increased incidence of congenital abnormalities, such as cleft palate/lip in man. However, when administered for prolonged periods or repeatedly during pregnancy, corticosteroids may increase the risk of intra-uterine growth retardation. Hypoadrenalism may, in theory, occur in the neonate following prenatal exposure to corticosteroids but usually resolves spontaneously following birth and is rarely clinically important. As with all drugs, corticosteroids should only be prescribed when the benefits to the mother and child outweigh the risks. When corticosteroids are essential however, patients with normal pregnancies may be treated as though they were in the non-gravid state.

Lactation

Corticosteroids are secreted in small amounts in breast milk, however, budesonide given at the clinically recommended dose is unlikely to cause systematic effects in the infant. Infants of mothers taking higher than recommended doses of budesonide may have a degree of adrenal suppression but the benefits of breast feeding are likely to outweigh any theoretical risk."

4.7 Effects on ability to drive and use machines
Entocort Enema does not affect the ability to drive and operate machinery.

4.8 Undesirable effects
The most common adverse reactions are gastrointestinal disturbances e.g. flatulence, nausea, diarrhoea. Skin reactions (e.g. rash, pruritus) may occur. Less common adverse reactions include agitation and insomnia.

4.9 Overdose
Acute overdosage with Entocort Enema, even in excessive doses, is not expected to be a clinical problem. The dosage form and route of administration make any prolonged overdosage unlikely.

5. PHARMACOLOGICAL PROPERTIES

5.1 Pharmacodynamic properties
Budesonide is a glucocorticosteroid with a high local anti-inflammatory effect. Budesonide undergoes an extensive degree (~90%) of biotransformation in the liver to metabolites of low glucocorticosteroid activity. The glucocorticosteroid activity of the major metabolites, 6-hydroxybudesonide and16-hydroxyprednisolone, is less than 1% of that of budesonide.

5.2 Pharmacokinetic properties
At recommended doses, budesonide causes no or small suppression of plasma cortisol.

The mean maximal plasma concentration after rectal administration of 2 mg budesonide is 3 nmol/L (range 1-9 nmol/L), reached within 1.5 hours.

5.3 Preclinical safety data
There are no other pre-clinical safety data of relevance to the prescriber apart from those already mentioned in the Summary of Product Characteristics.

6. PHARMACEUTICAL PARTICULARS

6.1 List of excipients
Tablet

Lactose anhydrous, riboflavine sodium phosphate, lactose, polyvidone, colloidal anhydrous silica and magnesium stearate.

Vehicle

Sodium chloride, methyl parahydroxybenzoate, propyl parahydroxybenzoate and water purified.

6.2 Incompatibilities
None stated.

6.3 Shelf life
24 months.

6.4 Special precautions for storage
Store below 30°C.

6.5 Nature and contents of container
Entocort Enema 0.02 mg/ml consists of 2 components: A dispersible tablet and a vehicle.

The primary package for the tablets is an aluminium blister package consisting of polyamide 25 m/ Al 43 m/ polyvinylchloride 60 m/ A1 20 m.

The primary package for the vehicle is a polyethylene bottle equipped with a combined seal gasket and non-return valve, a rectal nozzle and a protective cap for the nozzle.

The bottle, the nozzle and the protective cap are made of LD-polyethylene. The combined seal gasket and non-return valve is made of thermoplastic rubber.

Pack Size: 7 tablets

6.6 Instructions for use and handling
None stated.

7. MARKETING AUTHORISATION HOLDER
AstraZeneca UK Ltd.,

600 Capability Green,

Luton, LU1 3LU, UK.

8. MARKETING AUTHORISATION NUMBER(S)
PL 17901/0123

9. DATE OF FIRST AUTHORISATION/RENEWAL OF THE AUTHORISATION
4th June 2002

10. DATE OF REVISION OF THE TEXT
21st May 2003

Epanutin Capsules 25, 50, 100 and 300mg

(Pfizer Limited)

1. NAME OF THE MEDICINAL PRODUCT
EPANUTIN CAPSULES 25mg

EPANUTIN CAPSULES 50mg

EPANUTIN CAPSULES 100mg

EPANUTIN CAPSULES 300mg

2. QUALITATIVE AND QUANTITATIVE COMPOSITION
Epanutin Capsules 25mg containing Phenytoin Sodium PhEur 25mg

Epanutin Capsules 50mg containing Phenytoin Sodium PhEur 50mg

Epanutin Capsules 100mg containing Phenytoin Sodium PhEur 100mg

Epanutin Capsules 300mg containing Phenytoin Sodium PhEur 300mg

3. PHARMACEUTICAL FORM
Capsules, hard

Epanutin Capsules 25mg: A white powder in a No 4 hard gelatin capsule with a white opaque body and blue-violet cap, radially printed 'EPANUTIN 25'.

Epanutin Capsules 50mg: A white powder in a No 4 hard gelatin capsule with a white opaque body and a flesh-coloured transparent cap, radially printed 'EPANUTIN 50'.

Epanutin Capsules 100mg: A white powder in a No 3 hard gelatin capsule with a white opaque body and orange cap, radially printed 'EPANUTIN 100'.

Epanutin Capsules 300mg: A white powder in a No 1 hard gelatin capsule with a white opaque body and green cap, radially printed 'EPANUTIN 300'.

4. CLINICAL PARTICULARS

4.1 Therapeutic indications
Control of tonic-clonic seizures (grand mal epilepsy), partial seizures (focal including temporal lobe) or a combination of these, and the prevention and treatment of seizures occurring during or following neurosurgery and/or severe head injury. Epanutin has also been employed in the treatment of trigeminal neuralgia but it should only be used as second line therapy if carbamazepine is ineffective or patients are intolerant to carbamazepine.

4.2 Posology and method of administration
For oral administration only.

Dosage:

Dosage should be individualised as there may be wide interpatient variability in phenytoin serum levels with equivalent dosage. Epanutin should be introduced in small dosages with gradual increments until control is achieved or until toxic effects appear. In some cases serum level determinations may be necessary for optimal dosage adjustments - the clinically effective level is usually 10-20mg/l (40-80 micromoles/l) although some cases of tonic-clonic seizures may be controlled with lower serum levels of phenytoin. With recommended dosage a period of seven to ten days may be required to achieve steady state serum levels with Epanutin and changes in dosage should not be carried out at intervals shorter than seven to ten days. Maintenance of treatment should be the lowest dose of anticonvulsant consistent with control of seizures.

Epanutin Capsules, Suspension and Infatabs:

Epanutin Capsules contain phenytoin sodium whereas Epanutin Suspension and Epanutin Infatabs contain phenytoin. Although 100mg of phenytoin sodium is equivalent to 92mg of phenytoin on a molecular weight basis, these molecular equivalents are not necessarily biologically equivalent. Physicians should therefore exercise care in those situations where it is necessary to change the dosage form and serum level monitoring is advised.

Adults:

Initially 3 to 4mg/kg/day with subsequent dosage adjustment if necessary. For most adults a satisfactory maintenance dose will be 200 to 500mg daily in single or divided doses. Exceptionally, a daily dose outside this range may be indicated. Dosage should normally be adjusted according to serum levels where assay facilities exist.

Elderly:

Elderly (over 65 years): As with adults the dosage of Epanutin should be titrated to the patient's individual requirements using the same guidelines. As elderly patients tend to receive multiple drug therapies, the possibility of drug interactions should be borne in mind.

Infants and Children:

Initially, 5mg/kg/day in two divided doses, with subsequent dosage individualised to a maximum of 300mg daily. A recommended daily maintenance dosage is usually 4-8mg/kg.

Neonates:

The absorption of phenytoin following oral administration in neonates is unpredictable. Furthermore, the metabolism of phenytoin may be depressed. It is therefore especially important to monitor serum levels in the neonate.

4.3 Contraindications
Hypersensitivity to hydantoins.

4.4 Special warnings and special precautions for use

Abrupt withdrawal of phenytoin in epileptic patients may precipitate status epilepticus. When, in the judgement of the clinician, the need for dosage reduction, discontinuation, or substitution of alternative anti-epileptic medication arises, this should be done gradually. However, in the event of an allergic or hypersensitivity reaction, rapid substitution of alternative therapy may be necessary. In this case, alternative therapy should be an anti-epileptic drug not belonging to the hydantoin chemical class.

Phenytoin is highly protein bound and extensively metabolised by the liver. Reduced dosage to prevent accumulation and toxicity may therefore be required in patients with impaired liver function. Where protein binding is reduced, as in uraemia, total serum phenytoin levels will be reduced accordingly. However, the pharmacologically active free drug concentration is unlikely to be altered. Therefore, under these circumstances therapeutic control may be achieved with total phenytoin levels below the normal range of 10-20mg/l (40-80 micromoles/l). Patients with impaired liver function, elderly patients or those who are gravely ill may show early signs of toxicity.

Phenytoin should be discontinued if a skin rash appears. If the rash is exfoliative, purpuric, or bullous or if lupus erythematosus or Stevens-Johnson syndrome or toxic epidermal necrolysis is suspected, use of the drug should not be resumed (see Adverse Reactions). If the rash is of a milder type (measles-like or scarlatiniform), therapy may be resumed after the rash has completely disappeared. If the rash recurs upon reinstitution of therapy, further phenytoin medication is contra-indicated.

Phenytoin is not effective for absence (petit mal) seizures. If tonic-clonic (grand mal) and absence seizures are present together, combined drug therapy is needed.

Phenytoin may affect glucose metabolism and inhibit insulin release. Hyperglycaemia has been reported in association with toxic levels. Phenytoin is not indicated for seizures due to hypoglycaemia or other metabolic causes.

Serum levels of phenytoin sustained above the optimal range may produce confusional states referred to as "delirium", "psychosis", or "encephalopathy", or rarely irreversible cerebellar dysfunction. Accordingly, at the first sign of acute toxicity, serum drug level determinations are recommended. Dose reduction of phenytoin therapy is indicated if serum levels are excessive; if symptoms persist, termination of therapy with phenytoin is recommended.

Herbal preparations containing St John's wort (*Hypericum perforatum*) should not be used while taking phenytoin due to the risk of decreased plasma concentrations and reduced clinical effects of phenytoin (see Section 4.5).

Phenytoin therapy may interfere with Vitamin D metabolism. In the absence of an adequate dietary intake of Vitamin D or exposure to sunlight, osteomalacia, hypocalcaemia or rickets may develop.

In view of isolated reports associating phenytoin with exacerbation of porphyria, caution should be exercised in using the medication in patients suffering from this disease.

Patients with rare hereditary problems of galactose intolerance, the Lapp lactase deficiency or glucose-galactose metabolism should not take this medicine

4.5 Interaction with other medicinal products and other forms of Interaction

1. Drugs which may increase phenytoin serum levels include:

Amiodarone, antifungal agents (such as, but not limited to, amphotericin B, fluconazole, ketoconazole, miconazole and itraconazole), chloramphenicol, chlordiazepoxide, diazepam, dicoumarol, diltiazem, disulfiram, fluoxetine, H_2-antagonists, halothane, isoniazid, methylphenidate, nifedipine, omeprazole, oestrogens, phenothiazines, phenylbutazone, salicylates, succinimides, sulphonamides, tolbutamide, trazodone and viloxazine.

2. Drugs which may decrease phenytoin serum levels include:

Folic acid, reserpine, rifampicin, sucralfate, theophylline and vigabatrin.

Serum levels of phenytoin can be reduced by concomitant use of the herbal preparations containing St John's wort (*Hypericum perforatum*). This is due to induction of drug metabolising enzymes by St John's wort. Herbal preparations containing St John's wort should therefore not be combined with phenytoin. The inducing effect may persist for at least 2 weeks after cessation of treatment with St John's wort. If a patient is already taking St John's wort check the anticonvulsant levels and stop St John's wort. Anticonvulsant levels may increase on stopping St John's wort. The dose of anticonvulsant may need adjusting.

3. Drugs which may either increase or decrease phenytoin serum levels include:

Carbamazepine, phenobarbital, valproic acid, sodium valproate, antineoplastic agents, certain antacids and ciprofloxacin. Similarly, the effect of phenytoin on carbamazepine, phenobarbital, valproic acid and sodium valproate serum levels is unpredictable.

Acute alcohol intake may increase phenytoin serum levels while chronic alcoholism may decrease serum levels.

4. Although not a true pharmacokinetic interaction, tricyclic antidepressants and phenothiazines may precipitate seizures in susceptible patients and phenytoin dosage may need to be adjusted.

5. Drugs whose effect is impaired by phenytoin include:

Antifungal agents, antineoplastic agents, calcium channel blockers, clozapine, corticosteroids, ciclosporin, dicoumarol, digitoxin, doxycycline, furosemide, lamotrigine, methadone, neuromuscular blockers, oestrogens, oral contraceptives, paroxetine, quinidine, rifampicin, theophylline and vitamin D.

6. Drugs whose effect is altered by phenytoin include:

Warfarin. The effect of phenytoin on warfarin is variable and prothrombin times should be determined when these agents are combined.

Serum level determinations are especially helpful when possible drug interactions are suspected.

Drug/Laboratory Test Interactions:

Phenytoin may cause a slight decrease in serum levels of total and free thyroxine, possibly as a result of enhanced peripheral metabolism. These changes do not lead to clinical hypothyroidism and do not affect the levels of circulating TSH. The latter can therefore be used for diagnosing hypothyroidism in the patient on phenytoin. Phenytoin does not interfere with uptake and suppression tests used in the diagnosis of hypothyroidism. It may, however, produce lower than normal values for dexamethasone or metapyrone tests. Phenytoin may cause raised serum levels of glucose, alkaline phosphatase, and gamma glutamyl transpeptidase and lowered serum levels of calcium and folic acid. It is recommended that serum folate concentrations be measured at least once every 6 months, and folic acid supplements given if necessary. Phenytoin may affect blood sugar metabolism tests.

4.6 Pregnancy and lactation

There are intrinsic methodologic problems in obtaining adequate data on drug teratogenicity in humans. Genetic factors or the epileptic condition itself may be more important than drug therapy in leading to birth defects. The great majority of mothers on anticonvulsant medication deliver normal infants. It is important to note that anticonvulsant drugs should not be discontinued in patients in whom the drug is administered to prevent major seizures because of the strong possibility of precipitating status epilepticus with attendant hypoxia and threat to life. In individual cases where the severity and frequency of the seizure disorder are such that the removal of medication does not pose a serious threat to the patient, discontinuation of the drug may be considered prior to and during pregnancy although it cannot be said with any confidence that even minor seizures do not pose some hazard to the developing embryo or foetus.

Anticonvulsants including phenytoin may produce congenital abnormalities in the offspring of a small number of epileptic patients. The exact role of drug therapy in these abnormalities is unclear and genetic factors, in some studies, have also been shown to be important. Epanutin should only be used during pregnancy, especially early pregnancy, if in the judgement of the physician the potential benefits clearly outweigh the risk.

In addition to the reports of increased incidence of congenital malformations, such as cleft lip/palate and heart malformations in children of women receiving phenytoin and other antiepileptic drugs, there have more recently been reports of a foetal hydantoin syndrome. This consists of prenatal growth deficiency, micro-encephaly and mental deficiency in children born to mothers who have received phenytoin, barbiturates, alcohol, or trimethadione. However, these features are all interrelated and are frequently associated with intrauterine growth retardation from other causes.

There have been isolated reports of malignancies, including neuroblastoma, in children whose mothers received phenytoin during pregnancy.

An increase in seizure frequency during pregnancy occurs in a proportion of patients, and this may be due to altered phenytoin absorption or metabolism. Periodic measurement of serum phenytoin levels is particularly valuable in the management of a pregnant epileptic patient as a guide to an appropriate adjustment of dosage. However, postpartum restoration of the original dosage will probably be indicated.

Neonatal coagulation defects have been reported within the first 24 hours in babies born to epileptic mothers receiving phenytoin. Vitamin K_1 has been shown to prevent or correct this defect and may be given to the mother before delivery and to the neonate after birth.

Infant breast-feeding is not recommended for women taking phenytoin because phenytoin appears to be secreted in low concentrations in human milk.

4.7 Effects on ability to drive and use machines

None known.

4.8 Undesirable effects

Central Nervous System:

The most common manifestations encountered with phenytoin therapy are referable to this system and are usually dose-related. These include nystagmus, ataxia, slurred speech, decreased co-ordination, mental confusion, paraesthesia, drowsiness and vertigo. Dizziness, insomnia, transient nervousness, motor twitchings, and headaches have also been observed. There have also been rare reports of phenytoin induced dyskinesias, including chorea, dystonia, tremor and asterixis, similar to those induced by phenothiazine and other neuroleptic drugs. There are occasional reports of irreversible cerebellar dysfunction associated with severe phenytoin overdosage. A predominantly sensory peripheral polyneuropathy has been observed in patients receiving long-term phenytoin therapy.

Gastrointestinal:

Nausea, vomiting and constipation, toxic hepatitis, and liver damage.

Dermatological:

Dermatological manifestations sometimes accompanied by fever have included scarlatiniform or morbilliform rashes. A morbilliform rash is the most common; dermatitis is seen more rarely. Other more serious and rare forms have included bullous, exfoliative or purpuric dermatitis, lupus erythematosus, Stevens-Johnson syndrome and toxic epidermal necrolysis (see Section 4.4).

Connective Tissue:

Coarsening of the facial features, enlargement of the lips, gingival hyperplasia, hirsutism, hypertrichosis, Peyronie's Disease and Dupuytren's contracture may occur rarely.

Haemopoietic:

Haemopoietic complications, some fatal, have occasionally been reported in association with administration of phenytoin. These have included thrombocytopenia, leucopenia, granulocytopenia, agranulocytosis, pancytopenia with or without bone marrow suppression, and aplastic anaemia. While macrocytosis and megaloblastic anaemia have occurred, these conditions usually respond to folic acid therapy.

There have been a number of reports suggesting a relationship between phenytoin and the development of lymphadenopathy (local and generalised) including benign lymph node hyperplasia, pseudolymphoma, lymphoma, and Hodgkin's Disease. Although a cause and effect relationship has not been established, the occurrence of lymphadenopathy indicates the need to differentiate such a condition from other types of lymph node pathology. Lymph node involvement may occur with or without symptoms and signs resembling serum sickness, eg fever, rash and liver involvement. In all cases of lymphadenopathy, follow-up observation for an extended period is indicated and every effort should be made to achieve seizure control using alternative antiepileptic drugs.

Frequent blood counts should be carried out during treatment with phenytoin.

Immune System:

Hypersensitivity syndrome has been reported and may in rare cases be fatal (the syndrome may include, but is not limited to, symptoms such as arthralgias, eosinophilia, fever, liver dysfunction, lymphadenopathy or rash), systemic lupus erythematosus, polyarteritis nodosa, and immunoglobulin abnormalities may occur. Several individual case reports have suggested that there may be an increased, although still rare, incidence of hypersensitivity reactions, including skin rash and hepatotoxicity, in black patients.

Other:

Polyarthropathy, interstitial nephritis, pneumonitis.

4.9 Overdose

The lethal dose in children is not known. The mean lethal dose for adults is estimated to be 2 to 5g. The initial symptoms are nystagmus, ataxia and dysarthria. The patient then becomes comatose, the pupils are unresponsive and hypotension occurs followed by respiratory depression and apnoea. Death is due to respiratory and circulatory depression.

There are marked variations among individuals with respect to phenytoin serum levels where toxicity may occur. Nystagmus on lateral gaze usually appears at 20mg/l, and ataxia at 30mg/l, dysarthria and lethargy appear when the serum concentration is greater than 40mg/l, but a concentration as high as 50mg/l has been reported without evidence of toxicity.

As much as 25 times therapeutic dose has been taken to result in serum concentration over 100mg/l (400 micromoles/l) with complete recovery.

Treatment:

Treatment is non-specific since there is no known antidote. If ingested within the previous 4 hours the stomach should be emptied. If the gag reflex is absent, the airway should be supported. Oxygen, and assisted ventilation may be necessary for central nervous system, respiratory and cardiovascular depression. Haemodialysis can be considered since phenytoin is not completely bound to plasma proteins. Total exchange transfusion has been utilised in the treatment of severe intoxication in children.

In acute overdosage the possibility of the presence of other CNS depressants, including alcohol, should be borne in mind.

5. PHARMACOLOGICAL PROPERTIES

5.1 Pharmacodynamic properties

Phenytoin is effective in various animal models of generalised convulsive disorders, reasonably effective in models of partial seizures but relatively ineffective in models of myoclonic seizures.

It appears to stabilise rather than raise the seizure threshold and prevents spread of seizure activity rather than abolish the primary focus of seizure discharge.

The mechanism by which phenytoin exerts its anticonvulsant action has not been fully elucidated however, possible contributory effects include:

1. Non-synaptic effects to reduce sodium conductance, enhance active sodium extrusion, block repetitive firing and reduce post-tetanic potentiation

2. Post-synaptic action to enhance gaba-mediated inhibition and reduce excitatory synaptic transmission

3. Pre-synaptic actions to reduce calcium entry and block release of neurotransmitter.

5.2 Pharmacokinetic properties

Phenytoin is absorbed from the small intestine after oral administration. Various formulation factors may affect the bioavailability of phenytoin, however, non-linear techniques have estimated absorption to be essentially complete. After absorption it is distributed into body fluid including CSF. Its volume of distribution has been estimated to be between 0.52 and 1.19 litres/kg, and it is highly protein bound (usually 90% in adults).

The plasma half-life of phenytoin in man averages 22 hours with a range of 7 to 42 hours. Steady state therapeutic drug levels are achieved at least 7 to 10 days after initiation of therapy.

Phenytoin is hydroxylated in the liver by an enzyme system which is saturable. Small incremental doses may produce very substantial increases in serum levels when these are in the upper range of therapeutic concentrations.

The parameters controlling elimination are also subject to wide interpatient variation. The serum level achieved by a given dose is therefore also subject to wide variation.

5.3 Preclinical safety data

Pre-clinical safety data do not add anything of further significance to the prescriber.

6. PHARMACEUTICAL PARTICULARS

6.1 List of excipients

Each 25mg capsule contains lactose and magnesium stearate. The gelatin capsule shell also contains E127 (erythrosine), E131 (patent blue V), E171 (titanium dioxide) and sodiumlaurilsulfate. The printing ink contains shellac, E172 (black iron oxide), 2-ethoxyethanol, soya lecithin (E322) and dimethylpolysiloxane.

Each 50mg capsule contains lactose and magnesium stearate. The gelatin capsule shell also contains E127 (erythrosine), E104 (quinoline yellow), E171 (titanium dioxide) and sodium laurilsulfate. The printing ink contains shellac, black iron oxide (E172), 2-ethoxyethanol, soya lecithin (E322) and dimethylpolysiloxane.

Each 100mg capsule contains lactose and magnesium stearate. The gelatin capsule shell also contains E127 (erythrosine), E104 (quinoline yellow), E171 (titanium dioxide) and sodium laurilsulfate. The printing ink contains shellac, black iron oxide (E172), 2-ethoxyethanol, soya lecithin (E322) and dimethylpolysiloxane.

Each 300mg capsule contains lactose and magnesium stearate and silica. The gelatin capsule shell also contains E131 (patent blue V), E104 (quinoline yellow), E171 (titanium dioxide) and sodium laurilsulfate. The printing ink contains shellac, E172 (black iron oxide), 2-ethoxyethanol, soya lecithin (E322) and dimethylpolysiloxane.

6.2 Incompatibilities

None known

6.3 Shelf life

(a) 25mg Capsules: White HDPE container with white LDPE cap: 18 months

50mg, 100mg and 300mg Capsules White HDPE container with white LDPE cap: 36 months

(b) PVC/PVdC blister pack: 24 months

6.4 Special precautions for storage

Store at a temperature not exceeding 25°C

6.5 Nature and contents of container

Epanutin Capsules, 25mg and 50mg:

White HDPE container with white LDPE cap, containing 28 capsules

Epanutin Capsules 100mg:

White HDPE container with white LDPE cap, containing 84 capsules

Epanutin Capsules 300mg:

PVC/PVdC blister pack containing 28 capsules

6.6 Instructions for use and handling

No special requirements.

7. MARKETING AUTHORISATION HOLDER

Pfizer Limited

Ramsgate Road

Sandwich

Kent

CT13 9NJ

United Kingdom

8. MARKETING AUTHORISATION NUMBER(S)

PL 00057/0522 (25mg)

PL 00057/0523 (50mg)

PL 00057/0524 (100mg)

PL 00057/0525 (300mg)

9. DATE OF FIRST AUTHORISATION/RENEWAL OF THE AUTHORISATION

1st March 2004 (25mg)

1st March 2004 (50mg)

1st March 2004 (100mg)

1st February 2004 (300mg)

10. DATE OF REVISION OF THE TEXT

May 2005

Ref: EP_8_0

Epanutin Infatabs

(Pfizer Limited)

1. NAME OF THE MEDICINAL PRODUCT

EPANUTIN INFATABS

2. QUALITATIVE AND QUANTITATIVE COMPOSITION

Epanutin Infatabs containing Phenytoin BP 50mg

3. PHARMACEUTICAL FORM

Epanutin Infatabs: A yellow triangular tablet with a breaking line on one side.

4. CLINICAL PARTICULARS

4.1 Therapeutic indications

Control of tonic-clonic seizures (grand mal epilepsy), partial seizures (focal including temporal lobe) or a combination of these, and the prevention and treatment of seizures occurring during or following neurosurgery and/or severe head injury. Epanutin has also been employed in the treatment of trigeminal neuralgia but it should only be used as second line therapy if carbamazepine is ineffective or patients are intolerant to carbamazepine.

4.2 Posology and method of administration

For oral administration only.

Dosage:

Dosage should be individualised as there may be wide interpatient variability in phenytoin serum levels with equivalent dosage. Epanutin should be introduced in small dosages with gradual increments until control is achieved or until toxic effects appear. In some cases serum level determinations may be necessary for optimal dosage adjustments - the clinically effective level is usually 10-20mg/l (40-80 micromoles/l) although some cases of tonic-clonic seizures may be controlled with lower serum levels of phenytoin. With recommended dosage a period of seven to ten days may be required to achieve steady state serum levels with Epanutin and changes in dosage should not be carried out at intervals shorter than seven to ten days. Maintenance of treatment should be the lowest dose of anticonvulsant consistent with control of seizures.

Epanutin Capsules, Suspension and Infatabs:

Epanutin Capsules contain phenytoin sodium whereas Epanutin Suspension and Epanutin Infatabs contain phenytoin. Although 100mg of phenytoin sodium is equivalent to 92mg of phenytoin on a molecular weight basis, these molecular equivalents are not necessarily biologically equivalent. Physicians should therefore exercise care in those situations where it is necessary to change the dosage form and serum level monitoring is advised.

Adults:

Initially 3 to 4mg/kg/day with subsequent dosage adjustment if necessary. For most adults a satisfactory maintenance dose will be 200 to 500mg daily in single or divided doses. Exceptionally, a daily dose outside this range may be indicated. Dosage should normally be adjusted according to serum levels where assay facilities exist.

Elderly:

Elderly (over 65 years): As with adults the dosage of Epanutin should be titrated to the patient's individual requirements using the same guidelines. As elderly patients tend to receive multiple drug therapies, the possibility of drug interactions should be borne in mind.

Infants and Children:

Initially, 5mg/kg/day in two divided doses, with subsequent dosage individualised to a maximum of 300mg daily. A recommended daily maintenance dosage is usually 4-8mg/kg.

Epanutin Infatabs may be chewed.

Neonates:

The absorption of phenytoin following oral administration in neonates is unpredictable. Furthermore, the metabolism of phenytoin may be depressed. It is therefore especially important to monitor serum levels in the neonate.

4.3 Contraindications

Hypersensitivity to hydantoins.

4.4 Special warnings and special precautions for use

Abrupt withdrawal of phenytoin in epileptic patients may precipitate status epilepticus. When, in the judgement of the clinician, the need for dosage reduction, discontinuation, or substitution of alternative anti-epileptic medication arises, this should be done gradually. However, in the event of an allergic or hypersensitivity reaction, rapid substitution of alternative therapy may be necessary. In this case, alternative therapy should be an anti-epileptic drug not belonging to the hydantoin chemical class.

Phenytoin is highly protein bound and extensively metabolised by the liver. Reduced dosage to prevent accumulation and toxicity may therefore be required in patients with impaired liver function. Where protein binding is reduced, as in uraemia, total serum phenytoin levels will be reduced accordingly. However, the pharmacologically active free drug concentration is unlikely to be altered. Therefore, under these circumstances therapeutic control may be achieved with total phenytoin levels below the normal range of 10-20 mg/l (40-80 micromoles/l). Patients with impaired liver function, elderly patients or those who are gravely ill may show early signs of toxicity.

Phenytoin should be discontinued if a skin rash appears. If the rash is exfoliative, purpuric, or bullous or if lupus erythematosus or Stevens-Johnson syndrome or toxic epidermal necrolysis is suspected, use of the drug should not be resumed (see Adverse Reactions). If the rash is of a milder type (measles-like or scarlatiniform), therapy may be resumed after the rash has completely disappeared. If the rash recurs upon reinstitution of therapy, further phenytoin medication is contra-indicated.

Phenytoin is not effective for absence (petit mal) seizures. If tonic-clonic (grand mal) and absence seizures are present together, combined drug therapy is needed.

Phenytoin may affect glucose metabolism and inhibit insulin release. Hyperglycaemia has been reported in association with toxic levels. Phenytoin is not indicated for seizures due to hypoglycaemia or other metabolic causes.

Serum levels of phenytoin sustained above the optimal range may produce confusional states referred to as "delirium", "psychosis", or "encephalopathy", or rarely irreversible cerebellar dysfunction. Accordingly, at the first sign of acute toxicity, serum drug level determinations are recommended. Dose reduction of phenytoin therapy is indicated if serum levels are excessive; if symptoms persist, termination of therapy with phenytoin is recommended.

Herbal preparations containing St John's wort (*Hypericum perforatum*) should not be used while taking phenytoin due to the risk of decreased plasma concentrations and reduced clinical effects of phenytoin (see Section 4.5).

Phenytoin therapy may interfere with Vitamin D metabolism. In the absence of an adequate dietary intake of Vitamin D or exposure to sunlight, osteomalacia, hypocalcaemia or rickets may develop.

In view of isolated reports associating phenytoin with exacerbation of porphyria, caution should be exercised in using the medication in patients suffering from this disease.

4.5 Interaction with other medicinal products and other forms of Interaction

1. Drugs which may increase phenytoin serum levels include:

Amiodarone, antifungal agents (such as, but not limited to, amphotericin B, fluconazole, ketoconazole, miconazole and itraconazole), chloramphenicol, chlordiazepoxide, diazepam, dicoumarol, diltiazem, disulfiram, fluoxetine, H_2-antagonists, halothane, isoniazid, methylphenidate, nifedipine, omeprazole, oestrogens, phenothiazines, phenylbutazone, salicylates, succinimides, sulphonamides, tolbutamide, trazodone and viloxazine.

2. Drugs which may decrease phenytoin serum levels include:

Folic acid, reserpine, rifampicin, sucralfate, theophylline and vigabatrin.

Serum levels of phenytoin can be reduced by concomitant use of the herbal preparations containing St John's wort (*Hypericum perforatum*). This is due to induction of drug metabolising enzymes by St John's wort. Herbal preparations containing St John's wort should therefore not be combined with phenytoin. The inducing effect may persist for at least 2 weeks after cessation of treatment with St John's wort. If a patient is already taking St John's wort check the anticonvulsant levels and stop St John's wort. Anticonvulsant levels may increase on stopping St John's wort. The dose of anticonvulsant may need adjusting.

3. Drugs which may either increase or decrease phenytoin serum levels include:

Carbamazepine, phenobarbitone, valproic acid, sodium valproate, antineoplastic agents, certain antacids and ciprofloxacin. Similarly, the effect of phenytoin on carbamazepine, phenobarbitone, valproic acid and sodium valproate serum levels is unpredictable.

Acute alcohol intake may increase phenytoin serum levels while chronic alcoholism may decrease serum levels.

4. Although not a true pharmacokinetic interaction, tricylic antidepressants and phenothiazines may precipitate seizures in susceptible patients and phenytoin dosage may need to be adjusted.

5. Drugs whose effect is impaired by phenytoin include:

Antifungal agents, antineoplastic agents, calcium channel blockers, clozapine, corticosteroids, cyclosporin, dicoumarol, digitoxin, doxycycline, frusemide, lamotrigine, methadone, neuromuscular blockers, oestrogens, oral contraceptives, paroxetine, quinidine, rifampicin, theophylline and vitamin D.

6. Drugs whose effect is altered by phenytoin include:

Warfarin. The effect of phenytoin on warfarin is variable and prothrombin times should be determined when these agents are combined.

Serum level determinations are especially helpful when possible drug interactions are suspected.

Drug/Laboratory Test Interactions:

Phenytoin may cause a slight decrease in serum levels of total and free thyroxine, possibly as a result of enhanced peripheral metabolism. These changes do not lead to clinical hypothyroidism and do not affect the levels of circulating TSH. The latter can therefore be used for diagnosing hypothyroidism in the patient on phenytoin. Phenytoin does not interfere with uptake and suppression tests used in the diagnosis of hypothyroidism. It may, however, produce lower than normal values for dexamethasone or metapyrone tests. Phenytoin may cause raised serum levels of glucose, alkaline phosphatase, and gamma glutamyl transpeptidase and lowered serum levels of calcium and folic acid. It is recommended that serum folate concentrations be measured at least once every 6 months, and folic acid supplements given if necessary. Phenytoin may affect blood sugar metabolism tests.

4.6 Pregnancy and lactation

There are intrinsic methodologic problems in obtaining adequate data on drug teratogenicity in humans. Genetic factors or the epileptic condition itself may be more important than drug therapy in leading to birth defects. The great majority of mothers on anticonvulsant medication deliver normal infants. It is important to note that anticonvulsant drugs should not be discontinued in patients in whom the drug is administered to prevent major seizures because of the strong possibility of precipitating status epilepticus with attendant hypoxia and threat to life. In individual cases where the severity and frequency of the seizure disorder are such that the removal of medication does not pose a serious threat to the patient, discontinuation of the drug may be considered prior to and during pregnancy although it cannot be said with any confidence that even minor seizures do not pose some hazard to the developing embryo or foetus.

Anticonvulsants including phenytoin may produce congenital abnormalities in the offspring of a small number of epileptic patients. The exact role of drug therapy in these abnormalities is unclear and genetic factors, in some studies, have also been shown to be important. Epanutin should only be used during pregnancy, especially early pregnancy, if in the judgement of the physician the potential benefits clearly outweigh the risk.

In addition to the reports of increased incidence of congenital malformations, such as cleft lip/palate and heart malformations in children of women receiving phenytoin and other antiepileptic drugs, there have more recently been reports of a foetal hydantoin syndrome. This consists of prenatal growth deficiency, micro-encephaly and mental deficiency in children born to mothers who have received phenytoin, barbiturates, alcohol, or trimethadione. However, these features are all interrelated and are frequently associated with intrauterine growth retardation from other causes.

There have been isolated reports of malignancies, including neuroblastoma, in children whose mothers received phenytoin during pregnancy.

An increase in seizure frequency during pregnancy occurs in a proportion of patients, and this may be due to altered phenytoin absorption or metabolism. Periodic measurement of serum phenytoin levels is particularly valuable in the management of a pregnant epileptic patient as a guide to an appropriate adjustment of dosage. However, postpartum restoration of the original dosage will probably be indicated.

Neonatal coagulation defects have been reported within the first 24 hours in babies born to epileptic mothers receiving phenytoin. Vitamin K_1 has been shown to prevent or correct this defect and may be given to the mother before delivery and to the neonate after birth.

Infant breast-feeding is not recommended for women taking phenytoin because phenytoin appears to be secreted in low concentrations in human milk.

4.7 Effects on ability to drive and use machines

None known

4.8 Undesirable effects

Central Nervous System:

The most common manifestations encountered with phenytoin therapy are referable to this system and are usually dose-related. These include nystagmus, ataxia, slurred speech, decreased coordination, mental confusion, paraesthesia, drowsiness and vertigo. Dizziness, insomnia, transient nervousness, motor twitchings, and headaches have also been observed. There have also been rare reports of phenytoin induced dyskinesias, including chorea, dystonia, tremor and asterixis, similar to those induced by phenothiazine and other neuroleptic drugs. There are occasional reports of irreversible cerebellar dysfunction associated with severe phenytoin overdosage. A predominantly sensory peripheral polyneuropathy has been observed in patients receiving long-term phenytoin therapy.

Gastrointestinal:

Nausea, vomiting and constipation, toxic hepatitis, and liver damage.

Dermatological:

Dermatological manifestations sometimes accompanied by fever have included scarlatiniform or morbilliform rashes. A morbilliform rash is the most common; dermatitis is seen more rarely. Other more serious and rare forms have included bullous, exfoliative or purpuric dermatitis, lupus erythematosus, Stevens-Johnson syndrome and toxic epidermal necrolysis (see Section 4.4).

Connective Tissue:

Coarsening of the facial features, enlargement of the lips, gingival hyperplasia, hirsutism, hypertrichosis, Peyronie's Disease and Dupuytren's contracture may occur rarely.

Haemopoietic:

Haemopoietic complications, some fatal, have occasionally been reported in association with administration of phenytoin. These have included thrombocytopenia, leucopenia, granulocytopenia, agranulocytosis, pancytopenia with or without bone marrow suppression, and aplastic anaemia. While macrocytosis and megaloblastic anaemia have occurred, these conditions usually respond to folic acid therapy.

There have been a number of reports suggesting a relationship between phenytoin and the development of lymphadenopathy (local and generalised) including benign lymph node hyperplasia, pseudolymphoma, lymphoma, and Hodgkin's Disease. Although a cause and effect relationship has not been established, the occurrence of lymphadenopathy indicates the need to differentiate such a condition from other types of lymph node pathology. Lymph node involvement may occur with or without symptoms and signs resembling serum sickness, eg fever, rash and liver involvement. In all cases of lymphadenopathy, follow-up observation for an extended period is indicated and every effort should be made to achieve seizure control using alternative antiepileptic drugs.

Frequent blood counts should be carried out during treatment with phenytoin.

Immune System:

Hypersensitivity syndrome has been reported and may in rare cases be fatal (the syndrome may include, but is not limited to, symptoms such as arthralgias, eosinophilia, fever, liver dysfunction, lymphadenopathy or rash), systemic lupus erythematosus, polyarteritis nodosa, and immunoglobulin abnormalities may occur. Several individual case reports have suggested that there may be an increased, although still rare, incidence of hypersensitivity reactions, including skin rash and hepatotoxicity, in black patients.

Other:

Polyarthropathy, interstitial nephritis, pneumonitis.

4.9 Overdose

The lethal dose in children is not known. The mean lethal dose for adults is estimated to be 2 to 5g. The initial symptoms are nystagmus, ataxia and dysarthria. The patient then becomes comatose, the pupils are unresponsive and hypotension occurs followed by respiratory depression and apnoea. Death is due to respiratory and circulatory depression.

There are marked variations among individuals with respect to phenytoin serum levels where toxicity may occur. Nystagmus on lateral gaze usually appears at 20mg/l, and ataxia at 30mg/l, dysarthria and lethargy appear when the serum concentration is greater than 40mg/l, but a concentration as high as 50mg/l has been reported without evidence of toxicity.

As much as 25 times therapeutic dose has been taken to result in serum concentration over 100mg/l (400 micromoles/l) with complete recovery.

Treatment:

Treatment is non-specific since there is no known antidote. If ingested within the previous 4 hours the stomach should be emptied. If the gag reflex is absent, the airway should be supported. Oxygen, and assisted ventilation may be necessary for central nervous system, respiratory and cardiovascular depression. Haemodialysis can be considered since phenytoin is not completely bound to plasma proteins. Total exchange transfusion has been utilised in the treat-ment of severe intoxication in children.

In acute overdosage the possibility of the presence of other CNS depressants, including alcohol, should be borne in mind.

5. PHARMACOLOGICAL PROPERTIES

5.1 Pharmacodynamic properties

Phenytoin is effective in various animal models of generalised convulsive disorders, reasonably effective in models of partial seizures but relatively ineffective in models of myoclonic seizures.

It appears to stabilise rather than raise the seizure threshold and prevents spread of seizure activity rather than abolish the primary focus of seizure discharge.

The mechanism by which phenytoin exerts its anticonvulsant action has not been fully elucidated however, possible contributory effects include:

1. Non-synaptic effects to reduce sodium conductance, enhance active sodium extrusion, block repetitive firing and reduce post-tetanic potentiation

2. Post-synaptic action to enhance gaba-mediated inhibition and reduce excitatory synaptic transmission

3. Pre-synaptic actions to reduce calcium entry and block release of neurotransmitter.

5.2 Pharmacokinetic properties

Phenytoin is absorbed from the small intestine after oral administration. Various formulation factors may affect the bioavailability of phenytoin, however, non-linear techniques have estimated absorption to be essentially complete. After absorption it is distributed into body fluid including CSF. Its volume of distribution has been estimated to be between 0.52 and 1.19 litres/kg, and it is highly protein bound (usually 90% in adults).

The plasma half-life of phenytoin in man averages 22 hours with a range of 7 to 42 hours. Steady state therapeutic drug levels are achieved at least 7 to 10 days after initiation of therapy.

Phenytoin is hydroxylated in the liver by an enzyme system which is saturable. Small incremental doses may produce very substantial increases in serum levels when these are in the upper range of therapeutic concentrations.

The parameters controlling elimination are also subject to wide interpatient variation. The serum level achieved by a given dose is therefore also subject to wide variation.

5.3 Preclinical safety data

Pre-clinical safety data do not add anything of further significance to the prescriber.

6. PHARMACEUTICAL PARTICULARS

6.1 List of excipients

Sugar (icing sugar), maize starch, saccharin sodium, spearmint flavour, sugar solution (66.6% w/w), magnesium stearate, purified talc and E104 (quinoline yellow).

6.2 Incompatibilities

None known.

6.3 Shelf life

36 months

6.4 Special precautions for storage

Store at a temperature not exceeding 30°C

6.5 Nature and contents of container

White HDPE container with white LDPE cap, containing 112 tablets

6.6 Instructions for use and handling

No special requirements.

7. MARKETING AUTHORISATION HOLDER

Pfizer Limited

Sandwich

Kent, CT13 9NJ

United Kingdom

8. MARKETING AUTHORISATION NUMBER(S)

PL 00057/0526

9. DATE OF FIRST AUTHORISATION/RENEWAL OF THE AUTHORISATION

01/09/2003

10. DATE OF REVISION OF THE TEXT

September 2003

Ref: EPE3_0 UK

Epanutin Ready Mixed Parenteral

(Pfizer Limited)

1. NAME OF THE MEDICINAL PRODUCT

Epanutin Ready-Mixed Parenteral

2. QUALITATIVE AND QUANTITATIVE COMPOSITION

Each 5ml ampoule contains Phenytoin Sodium Ph Eur 250mg

3. PHARMACEUTICAL FORM

Solution for Injection.

Clear, colourless, sterile solution for injection.

4. CLINICAL PARTICULARS

4.1 Therapeutic indications

Parenteral Epanutin is indicated for the control of status epilepticus of the tonic-clonic (grand mal) type and prevention and treatment of seizures occurring during or following neurosurgery and/or severe head injury.

It is of use in the treatment of cardiac arrhythmias where first line therapy is not effective. It is of particular value when these are digitalis induced.

4.2 Posology and method of administration

For parenteral administration.

Parenteral drug products should be inspected visually for particulate matter and discolouration prior to administration, whenever solution and container permit. Parenteral Epanutin is suitable for use as long as it remains free of haziness and precipitate. Upon refrigeration or freezing a precipitate might form; this will dissolve again after the solution is allowed to stand at room temperature. The product is still suitable for use. Only a clear solution should be used. A faint yellow colouration may develop, however, this has no effect on the potency of this solution.

There is a relatively small margin between full therapeutic effect and minimally toxic doses of this drug. Optimum control without clinical signs of toxicity occurs most often with serum levels between 10 and 20mg/l (40-80 micromoles/l).

Parenteral Epanutin should be injected slowly directly into a large vein through a large-gauge needle or intravenous catheter.

Each injection or infusion of intravenous Epanutin should be preceded and followed by an injection of sterile saline through the same needle or catheter to avoid local venous irritation due to alkalinity of the solution. (See section 4.4.)

For infusion administration the parenteral phenytoin should be diluted in 50-100ml of normal saline, with the final concentration of phenytoin in the solution not exceeding 10mg/ml. Administration should commence immediately after the mixture has been prepared and must be completed within one hour (the infusion mixture should not be refrigerated). An in-line filter (0.22-0.50 microns) should be used.

The diluted form is suitable for use as long as it remains free of haziness and precipitate.

Continuous monitoring of the electrocardiogram and blood pressure is essential. Cardiac resuscitative equipment should be available. The patient should be observed for signs of respiratory depression. If administration of intravenous Epanutin does not terminate seizures, the use of other measures, including general anaesthesia, should be considered.

Epanutin Ready Mixed Parenteral contains phenytoin sodium whereas Epanutin Suspension and Epanutin Infatabs contain phenytoin. Although 100mg of phenytoin sodium is equivalent to 92mg of phenytoin on a molecular weight basis, these molecular equivalents are not necessarily biologically equivalent. Physicians should therefore exercise care in those situations where it is necessary to change the dosage form and serum level monitoring is advised.

Status Epilepticus:

In a patient having continuous seizure activity, as compared to the more common rapidly recurring seizures, i.e. serial epilepsy, injection of intravenous diazepam or a short acting barbiturate is recommended because of their rapid onset of action, prior to administration of Epanutin.

Following the use of diazepam in patients having continuous seizures and in the initial management of serial epilepsy a loading dose of Epanutin 10-15mg/kg should be injected slowly intravenously, at a rate not exceeding 50mg per minute in adults (this will require approximately 20 minutes in a 70kg patient). The loading dose should be followed by maintenance doses of 100mg orally or intravenously every 6 to 8 hours.

Recent work in neonates has shown that absorption of phenytoin is unreliable after oral administration, but a loading dose of 15-20mg/kg of Epanutin intravenously will usually produce serum concentrations of phenytoin within the generally accepted therapeutic range (10-20mg/l). The drug should be injected slowly intravenously at a rate of 1-3mg/kg/min.

Determination of phenytoin serum levels is advised when using Epanutin in the management of status epilepticus and in the subsequent establishing of maintenance dosage. The clinically effective level is usually 10-20mg/l although some cases of tonic-clonic seizures may be controlled with lower serum levels of phenytoin.

Intramuscular administration should not be used in the treatment of status epilepticus because the attainment of peak plasma levels may require up to 24 hours.

Use in Cardiac Arrhythmias:

3.5-5mg per kg of bodyweight intravenously initially, repeated once if necessary. The solution should be injected slowly, intravenously and at a uniform rate which should not exceed 1ml (50mg) per minute.

Other clinical conditions:

It is not possible to set forth a universally applicable dosage schedule. The intravenous route of administration is preferred. Dosage and dosing interval will, of necessity, be determined by the needs of the individual patient. Factors such as previous antiepileptic therapy, seizure control, age and general medical condition must be considered. Notwithstanding the slow absorption of Epanutin, when given intramuscularly, its use in certain conditions may be appropriate.

When short-term intramuscular administration is necessary for a patient previously stabilised orally, compensating dosage adjustments are essential to maintain therapeutic serum levels. An intramuscular dose 50% greater than the oral dose is necessary to maintain these levels. When returned to oral administration, the dose should be reduced by 50% of the original oral dose, for the same period of time the patient received Epanutin intramuscularly, to prevent excessive serum levels due to continued release from intramuscular tissue sites.

Neurosurgery:

In a patient who has not previously received the drug, Parenteral Epanutin 100-200mg (2-4ml) may be given intramuscularly at approximately 4-hour intervals prophylactically during neurosurgery and continued during the postoperative period for 48-72 hrs. The dosage should then be reduced to a maintenance dose of 300mg and adjusted according to serum level estimations.

If the patient requires more than a week of intramuscular Epanutin, alternative routes should be explored such as gastric intubation. For time periods less than one week, the patient switched from intramuscular administration should receive one half the original oral dose for the same period of time the patient received Epanutin intramuscularly. Measurement of serum levels is of value as a guide to an appropriate adjustment of dosage.

Elderly (over 65 years):

As for adults. However, complications may occur more readily in elderly patients.

Neonates:

Recent work in neonates has shown that absorption of phenytoin is unreliable after oral administration, but a loading dose of 15-20mg/kg of Epanutin intravenously will usually produce serum concentrations of phenytoin within the generally accepted therapeutic range (10-20mg/l). The drug should be injected slowly intravenously at a rate of 1-3mg/kg/min.

Infants and children:

As for adults. However, it has been shown that children tend to metabolise phenytoin more rapidly than adults. This should be borne in mind when determining dosage regimens; the use of serum level monitoring being particularly beneficial in such cases.

4.3 Contraindications

Phenytoin is contra-indicated in patients who are hypersensitive to phenytoin or other hydantoins. Intra-arterial administration must be avoided in view of the high pH of the preparation.

Because of its effect on ventricular automaticity, phenytoin is contra-indicated in sinus bradycardia, sino-atrial block, and second and third degree A-V block, and patients with Adams-Stokes syndrome.

4.4 Special warnings and special precautions for use

In adults, intravenous administration should not exceed 50mg per minute. In neonates, the drug should be administered at a rate of 1-3mg/kg/min.

The most notable signs of toxicity associated with the intravenous use of this drug are cardiovascular collapse and/or central nervous system depression. Severe cardiotoxic reactions and fatalities due to depression of atrial and ventricular conduction and ventricular fibrillation, respiratory arrest and tonic seizures have been reported particularly in elderly or gravely ill patients, if the preparation is given too rapidly or in excess.

Hypotension usually occurs when the drug is administered rapidly by the intravenous route.

Soft tissue irritation and inflammation has occurred at the site of injection with and without extravasation of intravenous phenytoin. Soft tissue irritation may vary from slight tenderness to extensive necrosis, sloughing and in rare instances has led to amputation. Subcutaneous or perivascular injection should be avoided because of the highly alkaline nature of the solution.

The intramuscular route is not recommended for the treatment of status epilepticus because of slow absorption. Serum levels of phenytoin in the therapeutic range cannot be rapidly achieved by this method.

General:

Intravenous Epanutin should be used with caution in patients with hypotension and severe myocardial insufficiency.

Phenytoin should be discontinued if a skin rash appears. If the rash is exfoliative, purpuric, or bullous or if lupus erythematosus, Stevens-Johnson syndrome, or toxic epidermal necrolysis is suspected, use of this drug should not be resumed and alternative therapy should be considered. If the rash is of a milder type (measles-like or scarlatiniform), therapy may be resumed after the rash has completely disappeared. If the rash recurs upon reinstitution of therapy, further phenytoin medication is contra-indicated.

Phenytoin is not effective for absence (petit mal) seizures. If tonic-clonic (grand mal) and absence (petit mal) seizures are present together, combined drug therapy is needed.

Serum levels of phenytoin sustained above the optimal range may produce confusional states referred to as "delirium", "psychosis", or "encephalopathy", or rarely irreversible cerebellar dysfunction. Accordingly, at the first sign of acute toxicity, serum drug level determinations are recommended. Dose reduction of phenytoin therapy is indicated if serum levels are excessive; if symptoms persist, termination of therapy with phenytoin is recommended.

Herbal preparations containing St John's wort (*Hypericum perforatum*) should not be used while taking phenytoin due to the risk of decreased plasma concentrations and reduced clinical effects of phenytoin (see Section 4.5).

Phenytoin is highly protein bound and extensively metabolised by the liver. Reduced maintenance dosage to prevent accumulation and toxicity may therefore be required in patients with impaired liver function. Where protein binding is reduced, as in uraemia, total serum phenytoin levels will be reduced accordingly. However, the pharmacologically active free drug concentration is unlikely to be altered. Therefore, under these circumstances therapeutic control may be achieved with total phenytoin levels below the normal range of 10-20mg/l. Dosage should not exceed the minimum necessary to control convulsions.

The liver is the chief site of biotransformation of phenytoin. Patients with impaired liver function, elderly patients, or those who are gravely ill may show early signs of toxicity.

Phenytoin may affect glucose metabolism and inhibit insulin release. Hyperglycaemia has been reported. Phenytoin is not indicated for seizures due to hypoglycaemia or other metabolic causes. Caution is advised when treating diabetic patients.

In view of isolated reports associating phenytoin with exacerbation of porphyria, caution should be exercised in using this medication in patients suffering from this disease.

Laboratory Tests:

Phenytoin serum level determinations may be necessary to achieve optimal dosage adjustments.

4.5 Interaction with other medicinal products and other forms of Interaction

Drugs which may increase phenytoin serum levels include: amiodarone, antifungal agents (such as, but not limited to, amphotericin B, fluconazole, ketoconazole, miconazole and itraconazole), chloramphenicol, chlordiazepoxide, diazepam, dicoumarol, diltiazem, disulfiram, oestrogens, fluoxetine, H_2-antagonists, halothane, isoniazid, methylphenidate, nifedipine, omeprazole, phenothiazines, phenylbutazone, salicylates, succinimides, sulphonamides, tolbutamide, trazodone, and viloxazine.

Drugs which may decrease phenytoin serum levels include: folic acid, reserpine, rifampicin, sucralfate, theophylline and vigabatrin.

Serum levels of phenytoin can be reduced by concomitant use of the herbal preparations containing St John's wort (*Hypericum perforatum*). This is due to induction of drug metabolising enzymes by St John's wort. Herbal preparations containing St John's wort should therefore not be combined with phenytoin. The inducing effect may persist for at least 2 weeks after cessation of treatment with St John's wort. If a patient is already taking St John's wort check the anticonvulsant levels and stop St John's wort. Anticonvulsant levels may increase on stopping St John's wort. The dose of anticonvulsant may need adjusting.

Drugs which may either increase or decrease phenytoin serum levels include: carbamazepine, phenobarbitone, valproic acid, sodium valproate, antineoplastic agents, certain antacids and ciprofloxacin. Similarly the effect of phenytoin on carbamazepine, phenobarbitone, valproic acid and sodium valproate serum levels is unpredictable.

Acute alcoholic intake may increase phenytoin serum levels while chronic alcoholic use may decrease serum levels.

Although not a true pharmacokinetic interaction, tricyclic antidepressants and phenothiazines may precipitate seizures in susceptible patients and phenytoin dosage may need to be adjusted.

Drugs whose effect is impaired by phenytoin include: antifungal agents, antineoplastic agents, calcium channel blockers, clozapine, corticosteroids, cyclosporin, dicoumarol, digitoxin, doxycycline, frusemide, lamotrigine, methadone, neuromuscular blockers, oestrogens, oral contraceptives, paroxetine, quinidine, rifampicin, theophylline and vitamin D.

Drugs whose effect is enhanced by phenytoin include: warfarin. The effect of phenytoin on warfarin is variable and prothrombin times should be determined when these agents are combined.

Serum level determinations are especially helpful when possible drug interactions are suspected.

Drug/Laboratory Test Interactions:

Phenytoin may cause a slight decrease in serum levels of total and free thyroxine, possibly as a result of enhanced peripheral metabolism. These changes do not lead to clinical hypothyroidism and do not affect the levels of circulating TSH. The latter can therefore be used for diagnosing hypothyroidism in the patient on phenytoin. Phenytoin does not interfere with uptake and suppression tests used in the diagnosis of hypothyroidism. It may, however, produce lower than normal values for dexamethasone or metapyrone tests. Phenytoin may cause raised serum levels of glucose, alkaline phosphatase, gamma glutamyl transpeptidase and lowered serum levels of calcium and folic acid. It is recommended that serum folate concentrations be measured at least every 6 months, and folic acid supplements given if necessary. Phenytoin may affect blood sugar metabolism tests.

4.6 Pregnancy and lactation

In considering the use of Epanutin intravenously in the management of status epilepticus in pregnancy, the following information should be weighed in assessing the risks and the benefits. The potential adverse effects upon the foetus of status epilepticus, specifically hypoxia, make it imperative to control the condition in the shortest possible time.

There are intrinsic methodologic problems in obtaining adequate data on drug teratogenicity in humans. Genetic factors or the epileptic condition itself may be more important than drug therapy in leading to birth defects. The great majority of mothers on anticonvulsant medication deliver normal infants. It is important to note that anticonvulsant drugs should not be discontinued in patients in whom the drug is administered to prevent major seizures because of the strong possibility of precipitating status epilepticus and attendant hypoxia and threat to life. In individual cases where the severity and frequency of the seizure disorder are such that the removal of medication does not pose a serious threat to the patient, discontinuation of the drug may be considered prior to and during pregnancy although it cannot be said with any confidence that even minor seizures do not pose some hazard to the developing embryo or foetus.

There is some evidence that phenytoin may produce congenital abnormalities in the offspring of a small number of epileptic patients, therefore it should not be used as the first drug during pregnancy, especially early pregnancy, unless in the judgement of the physician the potential benefits outweigh the risk.

In addition to the reports of increased incidence of congenital malformations, such as cleft lip/palate and heart malformations in children of women receiving phenytoin and other antiepileptic drugs, there have been recent reports of a foetal hydantoin syndrome. This consists of prenatal growth deficiency, microencephaly and mental deficiency in children born to mothers who have received phenytoin, barbiturates, alcohol, or trimethadione. However, these features are all interrelated and are frequently associated with intrauterine growth retardation from other causes.

There have been isolated reports of malignancies, including neuroblastoma, in children whose mothers received phenytoin during pregnancy.

An increase in seizure frequency during pregnancy occurs in a proportion of patients, because of altered phenytoin absorption or metabolism. Periodic measurement of serum phenytoin levels is particularly valuable in the management of a pregnant epileptic patient as a guide to an appropriate adjustment of dosage. However, post partum restoration of the original dosage will probably be indicated. Neonatal coagulation defects have been reported within the first 24 hours in babies born to epileptic mothers receiving phenytoin. Vitamin K has been shown to prevent or correct this defect and may be given to the mother before delivery and to the neonate after birth.

Infant breast-feeding is not recommended for women taking this drug because phenytoin appears to be secreted in low concentrations in human milk.

4.7 Effects on ability to drive and use machines

None known.

4.8 Undesirable effects

Signs of toxicity are associated with cardiovascular and central nervous system depression.

Central Nervous System:

The most common manifestations encountered with phenytoin therapy are referable to this system and are usually dose-related. These include nystagmus, ataxia, slurred speech, decreased coordination, mental confusion, paraesthesia, drowsiness and vertigo. Dizziness, insomnia, transient nervousness, motor twitching, and headache have also been observed. There have also been rare reports of phenytoin-induced dyskinesia, including chorea, dystonia, tremor, and asterixis, similar to those induced by phenothiazine and other neuroleptic drugs. A predominantly sensory peripheral polyneuropathy has been observed in patients receiving long-term phenytoin therapy. Tonic seizures have also been reported.

Cardiovascular:

Severe cardiotoxic reactions and fatalities have been reported with atrial and ventricular conduction depression and ventricular fibrillation. Severe complications are most commonly encountered in elderly or gravely ill patients.

Respiratory:

Alterations in respiratory function including respiratory arrest may occur.

Injection Site:

Local irritation, inflammation and tenderness. Necrosis and sloughing have been reported after subcutaneous or perivascular injection. Subcutaneous or perivascular injection should be avoided. Soft tissue irritation and inflammation have occurred at the site of injection with and without extravasation of intravenous phenytoin.

Dermatological System:

Dermatological manifestations sometimes accompanied by fever have included scarlatiniform or morbilliform rashes. A morbilliform rash (measles-like) is the most common. Other types of dermatitis are seen more rarely. Other more serious forms which may be fatal have included bullous, exfoliative or purpuric dermatitis, lupus erythematosus, Stevens-Johnson syndrome, and toxic epidermal necrolysis.

Haemopoietic System:

Haemopoietic complications, some fatal, have occasionally been reported in association with administration of phenytoin. These have included thrombocytopenia, leucopenia, granulocytopenia, agranulocytosis, and pancytopenia with or without bone marrow suppression and aplastic anaemia. While macrocytosis and megaloblastic anaemia have occurred, these conditions usually respond to folic acid therapy. There have been a number of reports suggesting a relationship between phenytoin and the development of lymphadenopathy (local or generalised) including benign lymph node hyperplasia, pseudolymphoma, lymphoma, and Hodgkin's Disease. Although a cause and effect relationship has not been established, the occurrence of lymphadenopathy indicates the need to differentiate such a condition from other types of lymph node pathology. Lymph node involvement may occur with or without symptoms and signs resembling serum sickness, e.g. fever, rash and liver involvement.

In all cases of lymphadenopathy, follow-up observation for an extended period is indicated and every effort should be made to achieve seizure control using alternative antiepileptic drugs.

Gastrointestinal System:

Nausea, vomiting, constipation, toxic hepatitis, and liver damage.

Connective Tissue System:

Coarsening of the facial features, enlargement of the lips, gingival hyperplasia, hirsutism, hypertrichosis, Peyronie's disease and Dupuytren's contracture may occur rarely.

Immune System:

Hypersensitivity syndrome has been reported and may in rare cases be fatal (the syndrome may include, but is not limited to, symptoms such as arthralgias, eosinophilia, fever, liver dysfunction, lymphadenopathy or rash), systemic lupus erythematosus, periarteritis nodosa, and immunoglobulin abnormalities may occur. Several individual case reports have suggested that there may be an increased, although still rare, incidence of hypersensitivity reactions, including skin rash and hepatotoxicity, in black patients.

Other:

Polyarthropathy, interstitial nephritis, pneumonitis.

4.9 Overdose

The lethal dose in children is not known. The mean lethal dose in adults is estimated to be 2 to 5 grams. The initial symptoms are nystagmus, ataxia, and dysarthria. Other signs are tremor, hyperflexia, lethargy, nausea, vomiting. The patient may become comatose and hypotensive. Death is due to respiratory and circulatory depression.

Attempts to relate serum levels of the drug to toxic effects have shown wide interpatient variation. Nystagmus on lateral gaze usually appears at 20mg/l, and ataxia at 30mg/l, dysarthria and lethargy appear when the serum concentration is >40mg/l, but a concentration as high as 50mg/l has been reported without evidence of toxicity.

As much as 25 times the therapeutic dose, which resulted in a serum concentration of 100mg/l, was taken with complete recovery.

Treatment:

Treatment is non-specific since there is no known antidote.

The adequacy of the respiratory and circulatory systems should be carefully observed and appropriate supportive measures employed. Haemodialysis can be considered since phenytoin is not completely bound to plasma proteins. Total exchange transfusion has been used in the treatment of severe intoxication in children.

In acute overdosage the possibility of the presence of other CNS depressants, including alcohol, should be borne in mind.

5. PHARMACOLOGICAL PROPERTIES

5.1 Pharmacodynamic properties

Phenytoin is effective in various animal models of generalised convulsive disorders and reasonably effective in models of partial seizures but relatively ineffective in models of myoclonic seizures.

It appears to stabilize rather than raise the seizure threshold and prevents spread of seizure activity rather than abolish the primary focus of seizure discharge.

The mechanism by which phenytoin exerts its anticonvulsant action has not been fully elucidated, however, possible contributory effects include:

1. Non-synaptic effects to reduce sodium conductance, enhance active sodium extrusion, block repetitive firing and reduce post-tetanic potentiation.

2. Post-synaptic action to enhance GABA-mediated inhibition and reduce excitory synaptic transmission.

3. Pre-synaptic actions to reduce calcium entry and block release of neurotransmitter.

5.2 Pharmacokinetic properties

After injection phenytoin is distributed into body fluids including CSF. Its volume of distribution has been estimated to be between 0.52 and 1.19 litres/kg, and it is highly protein bound (usually 90% in adults).

In serum, phenytoin binds rapidly and reversibly to proteins. About 90% of phenytoin in plasma is bound to albumin. The plasma half-life of phenytoin in man averages 22 hours with a range of 7 to 42 hours.

Phenytoin is hydroxylated in the liver by an enzyme system which is saturable. Small incremental doses may produce very substantial increases in serum levels when these are in the upper range of therapeutic concentrations.

The parameters controlling elimination are also subject to wide interpatient variation. The serum level achieved by a given dose is therefore also subject to wide variation.

5.3 Preclinical safety data

Pre-clinical safety data do not add anything of further significance to the prescriber.

6. PHARMACEUTICAL PARTICULARS

6.1 List of excipients

Each 5ml contains: propylene glycol, ethanol 96%, water for injection, sodium hydroxide

6.2 Incompatibilities

Epanutin Ready Mixed Parenteral should not be mixed with other drugs because of precipitation of phenytoin acid.

6.3 Shelf life

3 years.

6.4 Special precautions for storage

Do not store above 25°C. Keep the container in the outer carton. The product should not be used if a precipitate or haziness develops in the solution in the ampoule.

6.5 Nature and contents of container

5ml, colourless neutral glass, Type 1, Ph Eur, with a white colour break band. Each pack contains 10 ampoules.

6.6 Instructions for use and handling

Epanutin Ready Mixed Parenteral should be used immediately after opening. Discard any unused product once opened. See sections 4.2 and 6.2 for further information.

7. MARKETING AUTHORISATION HOLDER

Pfizer Limited,

Ramsgate Road,

Sandwich,

Kent,

CT13 9NJ,

United Kingdom

8. MARKETING AUTHORISATION NUMBER(S)

PL 00057/0527

9. DATE OF FIRST AUTHORISATION/RENEWAL OF THE AUTHORISATION

1st March 2004

10. DATE OF REVISION OF THE TEXT

December 2003

Ref: EPG_1_0

Epanutin Suspension

(Pfizer Limited)

1. NAME OF THE MEDICINAL PRODUCT

EPANUTIN SUSPENSION

2. QUALITATIVE AND QUANTITATIVE COMPOSITION

Epanutin Suspension containing Phenytoin Ph Eur 30mg/5ml

3. PHARMACEUTICAL FORM

Epanutin Suspension: Cherry red suspension.

4. CLINICAL PARTICULARS

4.1 Therapeutic indications

Control of tonic-clonic seizures (grand mal epilepsy), partial seizures (focal including temporal lobe) or a combination of these, and the prevention and treatment of seizures occurring during or following neurosurgery and/or severe head injury. Epanutin has also been employed in the treatment of trigeminal neuralgia but it should only be used as second line therapy if carbamazepine is ineffective or patients are intolerant to carbamazepine.

4.2 Posology and method of administration

For oral administration only.

Dosage:

Dosage should be individualised as there may be wide interpatient variability in phenytoin serum levels with equivalent dosage. Epanutin should be introduced in small dosages with gradual increments until control is achieved or until toxic effects appear. In some cases serum level determinations may be necessary for optimal dosage adjustments - the clinically effective level is usually 10-20mg/l (40-80 micromoles/l) although some cases of tonic-clonic seizures may be controlled with lower serum levels of phenytoin. With recommended dosage a period of seven to ten days may be required to achieve steady state serum levels with Epanutin and changes in dosage should not be carried out at intervals shorter than seven to ten days. Maintenance of treatment should be the lowest dose of anticonvulsant consistent with control of seizures.

Epanutin Capsules, Suspension and Infatabs:

Epanutin Capsules contain phenytoin sodium whereas Epanutin Suspension and Epanutin Infatabs contain phenytoin. Although 100mg of phenytoin sodium is equivalent to 92mg of phenytoin on a molecular weight basis, these molecular equivalents are not necessarily biologically equivalent. Physicians should therefore exercise care in those situations where it is necessary to change the dosage form and serum level monitoring is advised.

Adults:

Initially 3 to 4mg/kg/day with subsequent dosage adjustment if necessary. For most adults a satisfactory maintenance dose will be 200 to 500mg daily in single or divided doses. Exceptionally, a daily dose outside this range may be indicated. Dosage should normally be adjusted according to serum levels where assay facilities exist.

Elderly:

Elderly (over 65 years): As with adults the dosage of Epanutin should be titrated to the patient's individual requirements using the same guidelines. As elderly patients tend to receive multiple drug therapies, the possibility of drug interactions should be borne in mind.

Infants and Children:

Initially, 5mg/kg/day in two divided doses, with subsequent dosage individualised to a maximum of 300mg daily. A recommended daily maintenance dosage is usually 4-8mg/kg.

Neonates:

The absorption of phenytoin following oral administration in neonates is unpredictable. Furthermore, the metabolism of phenytoin may be depressed. It is therefore especially important to monitor serum levels in the neonate.

4.3 Contraindications

Hypersensitivity to hydantoins.

4.4 Special warnings and special precautions for use

Abrupt withdrawal of phenytoin in epileptic patients may precipitate status epilepticus. When, in the judgement of the clinician, the need for dosage reduction, discontinuation, or substitution of alternative anti-epileptic medication arises, this should be done gradually. However, in the event of an allergic or hypersensitivity reaction, rapid substitution of alternative therapy may be necessary. In this case, alternative therapy should be an anti-epileptic drug not belonging to the hydantoin chemical class.

Phenytoin is highly protein bound and extensively metabolised by the liver. Reduced dosage to prevent accumulation and toxicity may therefore be required in patients with impaired liver function. Where protein binding is reduced, as in uraemia, total serum phenytoin levels will be reduced accordingly. However, the pharmacologically active free drug concentration is unlikely to be altered. Therefore, under these circumstances therapeutic control may be achieved with total phenytoin levels below the normal range of 10-20 mg/l (40-80 micromoles/l). Patients with impaired liver function, elderly patients or those who are gravely ill may show early signs of toxicity.

Phenytoin should be discontinued if a skin rash appears. If the rash is exfoliative, purpuric, or bullous or if lupus erythematosus or Stevens-Johnson syndrome or toxic epidermal necrolysis is suspected, use of the drug should not be resumed (see Adverse Reactions). If the rash is of a milder type (measles-like or scarlatiniform), therapy may be resumed after the rash has completely disappeared. If the rash recurs upon reinstitution of therapy, further phenytoin medication is contra-indicated.

Phenytoin is not effective for absence (petit mal) seizures. If tonic-clonic (grand mal) and absence seizures are present together, combined drug therapy is needed.

Phenytoin may affect glucose metabolism and inhibit insulin release. Hyperglycaemia has been reported in association with toxic levels. Phenytoin is not indicated for seizures due to hypoglycaemia or other metabolic causes.

Serum levels of phenytoin sustained above the optimal range may produce confusional states referred to as "delirium", "psychosis", or "encephalopathy", or rarely irreversible cerebellar dysfunction. Accordingly, at the first sign of acute toxicity, serum drug level determinations are recommended. Dose reduction of phenytoin therapy is indicated if serum levels are excessive; if symptoms persist, termination of therapy with phenytoin is recommended.

Herbal preparations containing St John's wort (*Hypericum perforatum*) should not be used while taking phenytoin due to the risk of decreased plasma concentrations and reduced clinical effects of phenytoin (see Section 4.5).

Phenytoin therapy may interfere with Vitamin D metabolism. In the absence of an adequate dietary intake of Vitamin D or exposure to sunlight, osteomalacia, hypocalcaemia or rickets may develop.

In view of isolated reports associating phenytoin with exacerbation of porphyria, caution should be exercised in using the medication in patients suffering from this disease.

4.5 Interaction with other medicinal products and other forms of Interaction

1. Drugs which may increase phenytoin serum levels include:

Amiodarone, antifungal agents (such as, but not limited to, amphotericin B, fluconazole, ketoconazole, miconazole and itraconazole), chloramphenicol, chlordiazepoxide, diazepam, dicoumarol, diltiazem, disulfiram, fluoxetine, H_2-antagonists, halothane, isoniazid, methylphenidate, nifedipine, omeprazole, oestrogens, phenothiazines, phenylbutazone, salicylates, succinimides, sulphonamides, tolbutamide, trazodone and viloxazine.

2. Drugs which may decrease phenytoin serum levels include:

Folic acid, reserpine, rifampicin, sucralfate, theophylline and vigabatrin.

Serum levels of phenytoin can be reduced by concomitant use of the herbal preparations containing St John's wort (*Hypericum perforatum*). This is due to induction of drug metabolising enzymes by St John's wort. Herbal preparations containing St John's wort should therefore not be combined with phenytoin. The inducing effect may persist for at least 2 weeks after cessation of treatment with St John's wort. If a patient is already taking St John's wort check the anticonvulsant levels and stop St John's wort. Anticonvulsant levels may increase on stopping St John's wort. The dose of anticonvulsant may need adjusting.

3. Drugs which may either increase or decrease phenytoin serum levels include:

Carbamazepine, phenobarbitone, valproic acid, sodium valproate, antineoplastic agents, certain antacids and ciprofloxacin. Similarly, the effect of phenytoin on carbamazepine, phenobarbitone, valproic acid and sodium valproate serum levels is unpredictable.

Acute alcohol intake may increase phenytoin serum levels while chronic alcoholism may decrease serum levels.

4. Although not a true pharmacokinetic interaction, tricylic antidepressants and phenothiazines may precipitate seizures in susceptible patients and phenytoin dosage may need to be adjusted.

5. Drugs whose effect is impaired by phenytoin include:

Antifungal agents, antineoplastic agents, calcium channel blockers, clozapine, corticosteroids, cyclosporin, dicoumarol, digitoxin, doxycycline, frusemide, lamotrigine, methadone, neuromuscular blockers, oestrogens, oral contraceptives, paroxetine, quinidine, rifampicin, theophylline and vitamin D.

6. Drugs whose effect is altered by phenytoin include:

Warfarin. The effect of phenytoin on warfarin is variable and prothrombin times should be determined when these agents are combined.

Serum level determinations are especially helpful when possible drug interactions are suspected.

Drug-Enteral Feeding/Nutritional Preparations Interaction:

Literature reports suggest that patients who have received enteral feeding preparations and/or related nutritional supplements have lower than expected phenytoin plasma levels. It is therefore suggested that phenytoin should not be administered concomitantly with an enteral feeding preparation.

More frequent serum phenytoin level monitoring may be necessary in these patients.

There is some evidence that this effect is reduced if continuous feeding is stopped 2 hours before, and for 2 hours after, phenytoin suspension administration. However, it may still be necessary to monitor the serum phenytoin level and increase the dose of phenytoin.

Drug/Laboratory Test Interactions:

Phenytoin may cause a slight decrease in serum levels of total and free thyroxine, possibly as a result of enhanced peripheral metabolism. These changes do not lead to clinical hypothyroidism and do not affect the levels of circulating TSH. The latter can therefore be used for diagnosing hypothyroidism in the patient on phenytoin. Phenytoin does not interfere with uptake and suppression tests used in the diagnosis of hypothyroidism. It may, however, produce lower than normal values for dexamethasone or metapyrone tests. Phenytoin may cause raised serum levels of glucose, alkaline phosphatase, and gamma glutamyl transpeptidase and lowered serum levels of calcium and folic acid. It is recommended that serum folate concentrations be measured at least once every 6 months, and folic acid supplements given if necessary. Phenytoin may affect blood sugar metabolism tests.

4.6 Pregnancy and lactation

There are intrinsic methodologic problems in obtaining adequate data on drug teratogenicity in humans. Genetic factors or the epileptic condition itself may be more important than drug therapy in leading to birth defects. The great majority of mothers on anticonvulsant medication deliver normal infants. It is important to note that anticonvulsant drugs should not be discontinued in patients in whom the drug is administered to prevent major seizures because of the strong possibility of precipitating status epilepticus with attendant hypoxia and threat to life. In individual cases where the severity and frequency of the seizure disorder are such that the removal of medication does not pose a serious threat to the patient, discontinuation of the drug may be considered prior to and during pregnancy although it cannot be said with any confidence that even minor seizures do not pose some hazard to the developing embryo or foetus.

Anticonvulsants including phenytoin may produce congenital abnormalities in the offspring of a small number of epileptic patients. The exact role of drug therapy in these abnormalities is unclear and genetic factors, in some studies, have also been shown to be important. Epanutin should only be used during pregnancy, especially early pregnancy, if in the judgement of the physician the potential benefits clearly outweigh the risk.

In addition to the reports of increased incidence of congenital malformations, such as cleft lip/palate and heart malformations in children of women receiving phenytoin and other antiepileptic drugs, there have more recently been reports of a foetal hydantoin syndrome. This consists of prenatal growth deficiency, micro-encephaly and mental deficiency in children born to mothers who have received phenytoin, barbiturates, alcohol, or trimethadione. However, these features are all interrelated and are frequently associated with intrauterine growth retardation from other causes.

There have been isolated reports of malignancies, including neuroblastoma, in children whose mothers received phenytoin during pregnancy.

An increase in seizure frequency during pregnancy occurs in a proportion of patients, and this may be due to altered phenytoin absorption or metabolism. Periodic measurement of serum phenytoin levels is particularly valuable in the management of a pregnant epileptic patient as a guide to an appropriate adjustment of dosage. However, postpartum restoration of the original dosage will probably be indicated.

Neonatal coagulation defects have been reported within the first 24 hours in babies born to epileptic mothers receiving phenytoin. Vitamin K_1 has been shown to prevent or correct this defect and may be given to the mother before delivery and to the neonate after birth.

Infant breast-feeding is not recommended for women taking phenytoin because phenytoin appears to be secreted in low concentrations in human milk.

4.7 Effects on ability to drive and use machines

None known

4.8 Undesirable effects

Central Nervous System:

The most common manifestations encountered with phenytoin therapy are referable to this system and are usually dose-related. These include nystagmus, ataxia, slurred speech, decreased coordination, mental confusion, paraesthesia, drowsiness and vertigo. Dizziness, insomnia, transient nervousness, motor twitchings, and headaches have also been observed. There have also been rare reports of phenytoin induced dyskinesias, including chorea, dystonia, tremor and asterixis, similar to those induced by phenothiazine and other neuroleptic drugs. There are occasional reports of irreversible cerebellar dysfunction associated with severe phenytoin overdosage. A predominantly sensory peripheral polyneuropathy has been observed in patients receiving long-term phenytoin therapy.

Gastrointestinal:

Nausea, vomiting and constipation, toxic hepatitis, and liver damage.

Dermatological:

Dermatological manifestations sometimes accompanied by fever have included scarlatiniform or morbilliform rashes. A morbilliform rash is the most common; dermatitis is seen more rarely. Other more serious and rare forms have included bullous, exfoliative or purpuric dermatitis, lupus erythematosus, Stevens-Johnson syndrome and toxic epidermal necrolysis (see Section 4.4).

Connective Tissue:

Coarsening of the facial features, enlargement of the lips, gingival hyperplasia, hirsutism, hypertrichosis, Peyronie's Disease and Dupuytren's contracture may occur rarely.

Haemopoietic:

Haemopoietic complications, some fatal, have occasionally been reported in association with administration of phenytoin. These have included thrombocytopenia, leucopenia, granulocytopenia, agranulocytosis, pancytopenia with or without bone marrow suppression, and aplastic anaemia. While macrocytosis and megaloblastic anaemia have occurred, these conditions usually respond to folic acid therapy.

There have been a number of reports suggesting a relationship between phenytoin and the development of lymphadenopathy (local and generalised) including benign lymph node hyperplasia, pseudolymphoma, lymphoma, and

Hodgkin's Disease. Although a cause and effect relationship has not been established, the occurrence of lymphadenopathy indicates the need to differentiate such a condition from other types of lymph node pathology. Lymph node involvement may occur with or without symptoms and signs resembling serum sickness, eg fever, rash and liver involvement. In all cases of lymphadenopathy, follow-up observation for an extended period is indicated and every effort should be made to achieve seizure control using alternative antiepileptic drugs.

Frequent blood counts should be carried out during treatment with phenytoin.

Immune System:

Hypersensitivity syndrome has been reported and may in rare cases be fatal (the syndrome may include, but is not limited to, symptoms such as arthralgias, eosinophilia, fever, liver dysfunction, lymphadenopathy or rash), systemic lupus erythematosus, polyarteritis nodosa, and immunoglobulin abnormalities may occur. Several individual case reports have suggested that there may be an increased, although still rare, incidence of hypersensitivity reactions, including skin rash and hepatotoxicity, in black patients.

Other:

Polyarthropathy, interstitial nephritis, pneumonitis.

4.9 Overdose

The lethal dose in children is not known. The mean lethal dose for adults is estimated to be 2 to 5g. The initial symptoms are nystagmus, ataxia and dysarthria. The patient then becomes comatose, the pupils are unresponsive and hypotension occurs followed by respiratory depression and apnoea. Death is due to respiratory and circulatory depression.

There are marked variations among individuals with respect to phenytoin serum levels where toxicity may occur. Nystagmus on lateral gaze usually appears at 20mg/l, and ataxia at 30mg/l, dysarthria and lethargy appear when the serum concentration is greater than 40mg/l, but a concentration as high as 50mg/l has been reported without evidence of toxicity.

As much as 25 times therapeutic dose has been taken to result in serum concentration over 100mg/l (400 micromoles/l) with complete recovery.

Treatment:

Treatment is non-specific since there is no known antidote. If ingested within the previous 4 hours the stomach should be emptied. If the gag reflex is absent, the airway should be supported. Oxygen, and assisted ventilation may be necessary for central nervous system, respiratory and cardiovascular depression. Haemodialysis can be considered since phenytoin is not completely bound to plasma proteins. Total exchange transfusion has been utilised in the treatment of severe intoxication in children.

In acute overdosage the possibility of the presence of other CNS depressants, including alcohol, should be borne in mind.

5. PHARMACOLOGICAL PROPERTIES

5.1 Pharmacodynamic properties

Phenytoin is effective in various animal models of generalised convulsive disorders, reasonably effective in models of partial seizures but relatively ineffective in models of myoclonic seizures.

It appears to stabilise rather than raise the seizure threshold and prevents spread of seizure activity rather than abolish the primary focus of seizure discharge.

The mechanism by which phenytoin exerts its anticonvulsant action has not been fully elucidated however, possible contributory effects include:

1. Non-synaptic effects to reduce sodium conductance, enhance active sodium extrusion, block repetitive firing and reduce post-tetanic potentiation

2. Post-synaptic action to enhance gaba-mediated inhibition and reduce excitatory synaptic transmission

3. Pre-synaptic actions to reduce calcium entry and block release of neurotransmitter.

5.2 Pharmacokinetic properties

Phenytoin is absorbed from the small intestine after oral administration. Various formulation factors may affect the bioavailability of phenytoin, however, non-linear techniques have estimated absorption to be essentially complete. After absorption it is distributed into body fluid including CSF. Its volume of distribution has been estimated to be between 0.52 and 1.19 litres/kg, and it is highly protein bound (usually 90% in adults).

The plasma half-life of phenytoin in man averages 22 hours with a range of 7 to 42 hours. Steady state therapeutic drug levels are achieved at least 7 to 10 days after initiation of therapy.

Phenytoin is hydroxylated in the liver by an enzyme system which is saturable. Small incremental doses may produce very substantial increases in serum levels when these are in the upper range of therapeutic concentrations.

The parameters controlling elimination are also subject to wide interpatient variation. The serum level achieved by a given dose is therefore also subject to wide variation.

5.3 Preclinical safety data

Pre-clinical safety data do not add anything of further significance to the prescriber.

6. PHARMACEUTICAL PARTICULARS

6.1 List of excipients

Aluminium magnesium silicate, sodium benzoate, citric acid, sodium carboxymethylcellulose, glycerol, polysorbate 40, sucrose, ethanol, vanillin, banana flavour, orange oil, carmoisine (E122), sunset yellow (E110), water.

6.2 Incompatibilities

Refer to Enteral feeding/Nutritional Preparations Interaction in section 4.5.

6.3 Shelf life

36 months

6.4 Special precautions for storage

Store at a temperature not exceeding 25°C

6.5 Nature and contents of container

Amber glass bottle with 3 piece tamper evident child resistant closure fitted with a polyethylene faced liner containing 500ml. Finished pack will either have a label/leaflet or be enclosed in a carton with a separate PIL.

6.6 Instructions for use and handling

No special requirements.

7. MARKETING AUTHORISATION HOLDER

Pfizer Limited

Sandwich

Kent, CT13 9NJ

United Kingdom

8. MARKETING AUTHORISATION NUMBER(S)

PL 00057/0528

9. DATE OF FIRST AUTHORISATION/RENEWAL OF THE AUTHORISATION

1 April 2003

10. DATE OF REVISION OF THE TEXT

June 2003

Ref: EPF3_0 UK

Epaxal

(MASTA Ltd)

1. NAME OF THE MEDICINAL PRODUCT

Epaxal emulsion for injection in prefilled syringe

Hepatitis A vaccine (inactivated, virosome).

2. QUALITATIVE AND QUANTITATIVE COMPOSITION

1 vaccine dose (0.5 ml) contains at least 24 IU of inactivated hepatitis A virus (strain RG-SB), propagated in human diploid (MRC-5) cells.

The virus particles are adsorbed on virosomes as the adjuvant system, composed of highly purified influenza virus surface antigens (10 micrograms) of the A/Singapore/6/86 (H1N1) strain and the phospholipids lecithin (80 micrograms) and cephalin (20 micrograms).

For more information on the adjuvant, see 5.1.

For excipients, see 6.1.

3. PHARMACEUTICAL FORM

Emulsion for injection in prefilled syringe. Clear, colourless liquid.

4. CLINICAL PARTICULARS

4.1 Therapeutic indications

Active immunisation against hepatitis A of children from 1 year of age and adults.

4.2 Posology and method of administration

One dose of 0.5 ml is injected intramuscularly. To ensure optimal immune response, the vaccine should be injected into the deltoid muscle. In patients with coagulation disorders, the vaccine may be administered subcutaneously in the upper arm.

In order to provide long-term protection, a second (booster) dose of 0.5 ml should be administered. This is preferably given between 6-12 months after the first dose but may be given up to 4 years later based on experience in adult travellers.

Epaxal can be used interchangeably with other inactivated hepatitis A vaccines for the first and second (booster) dose.

Simultaneousactive and passive immunisation

If immediate protection against hepatitis A is necessary, Epaxal can be administered concomitantly with human gamma globulin at separate injection sites.

4.3 Contraindications

Hypersensitivity to any constituent of the vaccine.

Hypersensitivity to eggs, chicken protein or formaldehyde.

In cases of acute infectious disease with fever, vaccination with Epaxal should be postponed.

4.4 Special warnings and special precautions for use

As with all injectable vaccines, suitable treatment and medical supervision must always be promptly available in case there is a rare anaphylactic reaction following administration of the vaccine

Influenza haemagglutinin as contained in Epaxal does not provide an alternative for influenza vaccination.

Immunodeficiency disorders may impair the immune response. In splenectomised patients, the booster vaccination should be administered 1 to 6 months after primary immunisation, owing to the lower titres achieved in these subjects. This also applies to other categories of immunocompromised patients.

Experience of the vaccination of children under 1 year of age and in adults over 60 years of age is limited.

4.5 Interaction with other medicinal products and other forms of Interaction

A prospectively planned interaction study was performed with yellow fever vaccine in 55 subjects. In addition, concomitant vaccination against yellow fever, typhoid fever, poliomyelitis, diphtheria, tetanus, meningococci A + C, as well as concomitant malaria prophylaxis was studied as part of a travel prophylaxis program in 38 subjects.

A prospectively planned interaction study was performed with concomitant whole cell influenza vaccine in 163 subjects. Concomitant administration does not impair immune response to hepatitis A or influenza. In addition, the immune response to hepatitis A is independent of the level of influenza pre-immunisation titers.

The results indicated that Epaxal can be administered simultaneously with the above vaccines but in separate syringes, as well as with malaria prophylaxis.

4.6 Pregnancy and lactation

There are no adequate data from the use of Epaxal in pregnant women. The effect of Epaxal on foetal development has not been assessed. As with all inactivated vaccines, no harm to the foetus is expected. The vaccine should not be given to pregnant women unless the risk of hepatitis A is increased.

Whether the vaccine passes into the milk of a lactating mother is unknown. Breast-feeding women should use Epaxal with caution.

4.7 Effects on ability to drive and use machines

There is no evidence of any vaccine-related reduction in reaction times.

However, the occasional occurrence of dizziness or headache, as also observed occasionally with other vaccines, needs to be considered.

4.8 Undesirable effects

Possible undesirable effects are mild in nature and of short duration. The frequencies of adverse events provided below are derived from clinical studies. The most common adverse reactions are fatigue, local pain and headache, which have been shown in clinical studies to occur at frequencies of 6-32%, 5 – 25% and 6 – 25% respectively.

Very common (⩾1/10):

Nervous system disorders:

Headache

General disorders and administration site conditions:

Local pain, fatigue.

Common (⩾1/100 and <1/10):

Metabolism and nutrition disorders:

Anorexia

Gastrointestinal disorders:

Mild and transient diarrhoea, nausea

General disorders and administration site conditions:

Injection site reactions (induration, redness, swelling), malaise, fever

Uncommon (⩾1/1000 and <1/100):

Nervous system disorders:

Dizziness

Skin and subcutaneous tissue disorders:

Skin rash/pruritus

Gastrointestinal disorders:

Vomiting

Musculosceletal, connective tissue and bone disorders:

Arthralgia

The degree of dizziness is not more pronounced as compared to other vaccines in comparative trials.

A transient and mild rise in levels of liver enzymes was observed on single occasions at the time of vaccination.

As observed with other vaccines, occasional inflammatory diseases of the central and peripheral nervous system may occur, including ascending paralysis up to respiratory paralysis, e.g. Guillain-Barré Syndrome.

In very rare cases, anaphylactic shocks may occur.

4.9 Overdose

There are no reports of overdosage. Inadvertent administration of a second dose of 0.5 ml Epaxal has no adverse effects.

5. PHARMACOLOGICAL PROPERTIES

5.1 Pharmacodynamic properties

Pharmaceutical group: Vaccine against hepatitis A

ATC-code J07B C02.

Epaxal contains hepatitis A virus, strain RG-SB, propagated in MRC-5 human diploid cells and inactivated with formaldehyde. The isolated virus particles are bound to a new immunoadjuvant consisting of synthetic, spherical virosomes called IRIVs (IRIV = Immunopotentiating Reconstituted Influenza Virosome). IRIVs consist of a double membrane composed of the phospholipids lecithin (phosphatidylcholine) and cephalin (phosphatidylethanolamine) and of viral phospholipids. The double membrane contains the viral glycoproteins haemagglutinin and neuraminidase which have been isolated from inactivated influenza virus (A/Singapore/6/86 (H1N1)).

Presence of antibodies against the phospholipid of the IRIVs (i.e. antibodies against lecithin and cephalin) could not be detected by specific enzyme-linked immuno-sorbent assays (ELISAs) in sera of subject vaccinated and boosted with Epaxal.

After administration of Epaxal, the complexes of IRIV and hepatitis A virus actively bind to special receptors on macrophages and are then phagocytosed. Simultaneously, complexes of IRIV and hepatitis A virus bind to B lymphocytes, which are stimulated to proliferate. The membranes of the phagocytosed liposomes fuse with the membranes of the macrophage endosomes. Consequently, the hepatitis A virus antigen is presented on the surface of the macrophages. This potentiates the presentation of antigen and the stimulation of T lymphocytes which, in turn, stimulate the production of anti-hepatitis A antibodies by the B lymphocytes.

Immunogenicity and protective efficacy

Vaccination with one dose of 0.5 ml Epaxal results in protective antibody titres (min. 20 mIU/ml) in 80-97% of vaccinated subjects after 2 weeks, in 92-100% after 4 weeks, and in 78-100% after 12 months. More than 1,600 adults and children >10 years of age), more than 320 children (2-10 years of age), 61 children (1-2 years of age) and 30 children (6 months-1 year of age) have been followed in clinical trials. This includes a double-blind, placebo controlled field trial in 137 children (18 months-6 years of age) in a highly endemic area which showed a 96% protection rate against acute hepatitis A infection, based on IgM and IgG antibody titres, as well as clinical signs.

Duration of protection

The first vaccine dose with 0.5 ml Epaxal results in protective antibody titres (min. 20 mIU/ml) in 78-100% of vaccinated subjects for at least 12 months. A second (booster) vaccination with 0.5 ml Epaxal is estimated to prolong the protective efficacy to at least 20 years for at least 95% of the vaccinated subjects. This estimate is based on mathematical modelling and extrapolation of 3-6 years follow up data from subjects in the age range 16 to 45 years. A study among adult travellers demonstrated that a delay up to 48 months between the first and second vaccine dose had no effect on the magnitude of the booster response.

5.2 Pharmacokinetic properties
Pharmacokinetic studies are not required for vaccines.

5.3 Preclinical safety data
Preclinical safety data show no signs of toxicity after a single dose or after repeated doses. No tissue intolerance was observed after administration to rabbits.

6. PHARMACEUTICAL PARTICULARS

6.1 List of excipients
Sodium chloride

Water for injections

6.2 Incompatibilities
Epaxal must not be mixed with other vaccines or medicines in the same syringe.

6.3 Shelf life
2 years.

6.4 Special precautions for storage
Store at 2°C - 8°C. Do not freeze. Keep in original package in order to protect from light.

6.5 Nature and contents of container
Single-dose syringe

Container: 1 ml syringe of colourless glass type I with needle of stainless steel type 304

Closure: rubber plunger tip

Package sizes: 0.5 ml

10 × 0.5 ml

6.6 Instructions for use and handling
Before use, the syringe should be checked visually for integrity and any particulate matter in the syringe content. The vaccine should be clear and colourless. Any unused product or waste material should be disposed of in accordance with local requirements.

7. MARKETING AUTHORISATION HOLDER
Istituto Sieroterapico Berna s.r.l.

Via Bellinzona 39

IT-22100 Como

Italy

8. MARKETING AUTHORISATION NUMBER(S)
UK: PL 15747/0003; IR 941/1/1

9. DATE OF FIRST AUTHORISATION/RENEWAL OF THE AUTHORISATION
UK: 14 December 1999; IR: 21 January 2000; Renewal: 30 October 2002

10. DATE OF REVISION OF THE TEXT
5 January 2005

Epilim

(sanofi-aventis)

1. NAME OF THE MEDICINAL PRODUCT
Epilim 100mg Crushable Tablets

Epilim 200 Enteric Coated Tablets

Epilim 500 Enteric Coated Tablets

Epilim Liquid

Epilim Syrup

2. QUALITATIVE AND QUANTITATIVE COMPOSITION
Epilim 500 Enteric Coated: 500mg Sodium Valproate

Epilim 200 Enteric Coated: 200mg Sodium Valproate

Epilim 100mg Crushable: 100mg Sodium Valproate

Epilim Syrup and Liquid: 200mg Sodium Valproate per 5ml.

3. PHARMACEUTICAL FORM
Epilim 100mg Crushable: Tablets.

Epilim 500 Enteric Coated: Enteric coated tablets.

Epilim 200 Enteric Coated: Enteric coated tablets.

Epilim Syrup: Syrup.

Epilim Liquid: Liquid.

4. CLINICAL PARTICULARS

4.1 Therapeutic indications
Treatment of generalised, partial or other epilepsy.

4.2 Posology and method of administration
Epilim tablets, syrup & liquid are for oral administration.

Daily dosage requirements vary according to age and body weight.

Epilim tablets, syrup & liquid may be given twice daily. Uncoated tablets may be crushed if necessary

Epilim Liquid should not be diluted

In patients where adequate control has been achieved Epilim Chrono formulations are interchangeable with other conventional or prolonged release formulations on an equivalent daily dosage basis.

Monotherapy

Usual requirements are as follows:

Adults

Dosage should start at 600mg daily increasing by 200mg at three-day intervals until control is achieved. This is generally within the dosage range 1000mg to 2000mg per day, ie 20-30mg/kg body weight. Where adequate control is not achieved within this range the dose may be further increased to 2500mg per day.

Children over 20kg

Initial dosage should be 400mg/day (irrespective of weight) with spaced increases until control is achieved; this is usually within the range 20-30mg/kg body weight per day. Where adequate control is not achieved within this range the dose may be increased to 35mg/kg body weight per day.

Children under 20kg

20mg/kg of body weight per day; in severe cases this may be increased but only in patients in whom plasma valproic acid levels can be monitored. Above 40mg/kg/day, clinical chemistry and haematological parameters should be monitored.

Elderly

Although the pharmacokinetics of valproate are modified in the elderly, they have limited clinical significance and dosage should be determined by seizure control. The volume of distribution is increased in the elderly and because of decreased binding to serum albumin, the proportion of free drug is increased. This will affect the clinical interpretation of plasma valproic acid levels.

In patients with renal insufficiency

It may be necessary to decrease dosage. Dosage should be adjusted according to clinical monitoring since monitoring of plasma concentrations may be misleading (see section 5.2 Pharmacokinetic Properties).

In patients with hepatic insufficiency

Salicylates should not be used concomitantly with valproate since they employ the same metabolic pathway (see also sections 4.4 Special Warnings and Precautions for Use and 4.8 Undesirable Effects).

Liver dysfunction, including hepatic failure resulting in fatalities, has occurred in patients whose treatment included valproic acid (see sections 4.3 Contraindications and 4.4 Special Warnings and Precautions for Use).

Salicylates should not be used in children under 16 years (see aspirin/salicylate product information on Reye's syndrome). In addition in conjunction with Epilim, concomitant use in children under 3 years can increase the risk of liver toxicity (see section 4.4.1 Special warnings).

Combined Therapy

When starting Epilim in patients already on other anticonvulsants, these should be tapered slowly; initiation of Epilim therapy should then be gradual, with target dose being reached after about 2 weeks. In certain cases it may be necessary to raise the dose by 5 to 10mg/kg/day when used in combination with anticonvulsants which induce liver enzyme activity, eg phenytoin, phenobarbitone and carbamazepine. Once known enzyme inducers have been withdrawn it may be possible to maintain seizure control on a reduced dose of Epilim. When barbiturates are being administered concomitantly and particularly if sedation is observed (particularly in children) the dosage of barbiturate should be reduced.

NB: In children requiring doses higher than 40mg/kg/day clinical chemistry and haematological parameters should be monitored.

Optimum dosage is mainly determined by seizure control and routine measurement of plasma levels is unnecessary. However, a method for measurement of plasma levels is available and may be helpful where there is poor control or side effects are suspected (see section 5.2 Pharmacokinetic Properties).

4.3 Contraindications
- Active liver disease

- Personal or family history of severe hepatic dysfunction, especially drug related

- Hypersensitivity to sodium valproate

- Porphyria

4.4 Special warnings and special precautions for use
4.4.1 Special warnings

Liver dysfunction:

Conditions of occurrence:

Severe liver damage, including hepatic failure sometimes resulting in fatalities, has been very rarely reported. Experience in epilepsy has indicated that patients most at risk are infants, especially in cases of multiple anticonvulsant therapy, are infants and in particular young children under the age of 3 and those with severe seizure disorders, organic brain disease, and (or) congenital metabolic or degenerative disease associated with mental retardation.

After the age of 3, the incidence of occurrence is significantly reduced and progressively decreases with age.

The concomitant use of salicylates should be avoided in children under 3 due to the risk of liver toxicity. Additionally, salicylates should not be used in children under 16 years (see aspirin/salicylate product information on Reye's syndrome).

Monotherapy is recommended in children under the age of 3 years when prescribing Epilim, but the potential benefit of Epilim should be weighed against the risk of liver damage or pancreatitis in such patients prior to initiation of therapy

In most cases, such liver damage occurred during the first 6 months of therapy, the period of maximum risk being 2-12 weeks.

Suggestive signs:

Clinical symptoms are essential for early diagnosis. In particular the following conditions, which may precede jaundice, should be taken into consideration, especially in patients at risk (see above: 'Conditions of occurrence'):

- non specific symptoms, usually of sudden onset, such as asthenia, malaise, anorexia, lethargy, oedema and drowsiness, which are sometimes associated with repeated vomiting and abdominal pain.

- in patients with epilepsy, recurrence of seizures.

These are an indication for immediate withdrawal of the drug.

Patients (or their family for children) should be instructed to report immediately any such signs to a physician should they occur. Investigations including clinical examination and biological assessment of liver function should be undertaken immediately.

Detection:

Liver function should be measured before and then periodically monitored during the first 6 months of therapy, especially in those who seem most at risk, and those with a prior history of liver disease.

Amongst usual investigations, tests which reflect protein synthesis, particularly prothrombin rate, are most relevant.

Confirmation of an abnormally low prothrombin rate, particularly in association with other biological abnormalities (significant decrease in fibrinogen and coagulation factors; increased bilirubin level and raised transaminases) requires cessation of Epilim therapy.

As a matter of precaution and in case they are taken concomitantly salicylates should also be discontinued since they employ the same metabolic pathway.

As with most antiepileptic drugs, increased liver enzymes are common, particularly at the beginning of therapy; they are also transient.

More extensive biological investigations (including prothrombin rate) are recommended in these patients; a reduction in dosage may be considered when appropriate and tests should be repeated as necessary.

Pancreatitis: Pancreatitis, which may be severe and result in fatalities, has been very rarely reported. Patients experiencing nausea, vomiting or acute abdominal pain should have a prompt medical evaluation (including measurement of serum amylase). Young children are at particular risk;

this risk decreases with increasing age. Severe seizures and severe neurological impairment with combination anticonvulsant therapy may be risk factors. Hepatic failure with pancreatitis increases the risk of fatal outcome. In case of pancreatitis, valproate should be discontinued.

4.4.2 Precautions

Haematological: Blood tests (blood cell count, including platelet count, bleeding time and coagulation tests) are recommended prior to initiation of therapy or before surgery, and in case of spontaneous bruising or bleeding (see section 4.8 Undesirable Effects).

Renal insufficiency:

In patients with renal insufficiency, it may be necessary to decrease dosage. As monitoring of plasma concentrations may be misleading, dosage should be adjusted according to clinical monitoring (see sections 4.2 Posology and Method of Administration and 5.2. Pharmacokinetic Properties).

Systemic lupus erythematosus: Although immune disorders have only rarely been noted during the use of Epilim, the potential benefit of Epilim should be weighed against its potential risk in patients with systemic lupus erythematosus (see also section 4.8 Undesirable Effects).

Hyperammonaemia: When a urea cycle enzymatic deficiency is suspected, metabolic investigations should be performed prior to treatment because of the risk of hyperammonaemia with valproate.

Weight gain: Epilim very commonly causes weight gain, which may be marked and progressive. Patients should be warned of the risk of weight gain at the initiation of therapy and appropriate strategies should be adopted to minimise it (see section 4.8 Undesirable Effects).

Pregnancy: Women of childbearing potential should not be started on Epilim without specialist neurological advice. Epilim is the antiepileptic of choice in patients with certain types of epilepsy such as generalised epilepsy ± myoclonus/photosensitivity. For partial epilepsy, Epilim should be used only in patients resistant to other treatment. Women who are likely to get pregnant, should receive specialist advice because of the potential teratogenic risk to the foetus (see also section 4.6 Pregnancy and Lactation).

Diabetic patients: Valproate is eliminated mainly through the kidneys, partly in the form of ketone bodies; this may give false positives in the urine testing of possible diabetics.

4.5 Interaction with other medicinal products and other forms of Interaction

4.5.1 Effects of Valproate on other drugs

- Neuroleptics, MAO inhibitors, antidepressants and benzodiazepines

Valproate may potentiate the effect of other psychotropics such as neuroleptics, MAO inhibitors, antidepressants and benzodiazepines; therefore, clinical monitoring is advised and dosage should be adjusted when appropriate.

- ***Phenobarbital***

Valproate increases phenobarbital plasma concentrations (due to inhibition of hepatic catabolism) and sedation may occur, particularly in children. Therefore, clinical monitoring is recommended throughout the first 15 days of combined treatment with immediate reduction of phenobarbital doses if sedation occurs and determination of phenobarbital plasma levels when appropriate.

- ***Primidone***

Valproate increases primidone plasma levels with exacerbation of its adverse effects (such as sedation); these signs cease with long term treatment. Clinical monitoring is recommended especially at the beginning of combined therapy with dosage adjustment when appropriate.

- ***Phenytoin***

Valproate decreases phenytoin total plasma concentration. Moreover valproate increases phenytoin free form with possible overdosage symptoms (valproic acid displaces phenytoin from its plasma protein binding sites and reduces its hepatic catabolism). Therefore clinical monitoring is recommended; when phenytoin plasma levels are determined, the free form should be evaluated.

- ***Carbamazepine***

Clinical toxicity has been reported when valproate was administered with carbamazepine as valproate may potentiate toxic effects of carbamazepine. Clinical monitoring is recommended especially at the beginning of combined therapy with dosage adjustment when appropriate.

- ***Lamotrigine***

Valproate may reduce lamotrigine metabolism and increase its mean half-life, dosages should be adjusted (lamotrigine dosage decreased) when appropriate. Co-administration of lamotrigine and Epilim might increase the risk of rash.

- ***Zidovudine***

Valproate may raise zidovudine plasma concentration leading to increased zidovudine toxicity.

- ***Vitamin K-dependent anticoagulants***

The anticoagulant effect of warfarin and other coumarin anticoagulants may be increased following displacement from plasma protein binding sites by valproic acid. The prothrombin time should be closely monitored.

- ***Temozolomide***

Co-administration of temozolomide and valproate may cause a small decrease in the clearance of temozolomide that is not thought to be clinically relevant.

4.5.2 Effects of other drugs on Valproate

Antiepileptics with enzyme inducing effect (including ***phenytoin, phenobarbital, carbamazepine***) decrease valproic acid plasma concentrations. Dosages should be adjusted according to blood levels in case of combined therapy.

On the other hand, combination of ***felbamate*** and valproate may increase valproic acid plasma concentration. Valproate dosage should be monitored.

Mefloquine and ***chloroquine*** increase valproic acid metabolism and may lower the seizure threshold; therefore epileptic seizures may occur in cases of combined therapy. Accordingly, the dosage of Epilim may need adjustment.

In case of concomitant use of valproate and ***highly protein bound agents (e.g. aspirin)***, free valproic acid plasma levels may be increased.

Valproic acid plasma levels may be increased (as a result of reduced hepatic metabolism) in case of concomitant use with ***cimetidine*** or ***erythromycin***.

Carbapenem antibioticssuch as ***imipenem*** and ***meropenem***: Decrease in valproic acid blood level, sometimes associated with convulsions, has been observed when imipenem or meropenem were combined. If these antibiotics have to be administered, close monitoring of valproic acid blood levels is recommended.

Cholestyramine may decrease the absorption of valproate.

4.5.3 Other Interactions

Caution is advised when using Epilim in combination with newer anti-epileptics whose pharmacodynamics may not be well established.

Valproate usually has no enzyme-inducing effect; as a consequence, valproate does not reduce efficacy of oestroprogestative agents in women receiving hormonal contraception, including the oral contraceptive pill.

4.6 Pregnancy and lactation

4.6.1 Pregnancy

From experience in treating mothers with epilepsy, the risk associated with the use of valproate during pregnancy has been described as follows:

- Risk associated with epilepsy and antiepileptics

In offspring born to mothers with epilepsy receiving any anti-epileptic treatment, the overall rate of malformations has been demonstrated to be 2 to 3 times higher than the rate (approximately 3 %) reported in the general population. Although an increased number of children with malformations have been reported in cases of multiple drug therapy, the respective role of treatments and disease in causing the malformations has not been formally established. Malformations most frequently encountered are cleft lip and cardio-vascular malformations.

Epidemiological studies have suggested an association between in-utero exposure to sodium valproate and a risk of developmental delay. Many factors including maternal epilepsy may also contribute to this risk but it is difficult to quantify the relative contributions of these or of maternal anti-epileptic treatment. Notwithstanding those potential risks, no sudden discontinuation in the anti-epileptic therapy should be undertaken as this may lead to breakthrough seizures which could have serious consequences for both the mother and the foetus.

- Risk associated with valproate

In animals: teratogenic effects have been demonstrated in the mouse, rat and rabbit.

There is animal experimental evidence that high plasma peak levels and the size of an individual dose are associated with neural tube defects.

In humans: an increased incidence of congenital abnormalities (including cases of facial dysmorphia, hypospadias and multiple malformations, particularly of the limbs) has been demonstrated in offspring born to mothers with epilepsy treated with valproate.

Valproate use is associated with neural tube defects such as myelomeningocele and spina bifida. The frequency of this effect is estimated to be 1 to 2%.

- In view of the above data

When a woman is planning pregnancy, this provides an opportunity to review the need for anti-epileptic treatment. Women of childbearing age should be informed of the risks and benefits of continuing anti-epileptic treatment throughout pregnancy.

Folate supplementation, **prior** to pregnancy, has been demonstrated to reduce the incidence of neural tube defects in the offspring of women at high risk. Although no direct evidence exists of such effects in women receiving anti-epileptic drugs, women should be advised to start taking folic acid supplementation (5mg) as soon as contraception is discontinued.

The available evidence suggests that anticonvulsant monotherapy is preferred. Dosage should be reviewed before conception and the lowest effective dose used, in divided doses, as abnormal pregnancy outcome tends to be associated with higher total daily dosage and with the size of an individual dose. The incidence of neural tube defects rises with increasing dosage, particularly above 1000mg daily. The administration in several divided doses over the day and the use of a prolonged release formulation is preferable in order to avoid high peak plasma levels.

During pregnancy, valproate anti-epileptic treatment should not be discontinued if it has been effective.

Nevertheless, specialised prenatal monitoring should be instituted in order to detect the possible occurrence of a neural tube defect or any other malformation. Pregnancies should be carefully screened by ultrasound, and other techniques if appropriate (see Section 4.4 Special Warnings and Special Precautions for use).

- Risk in the neonate

Very rare cases of haemorrhagic syndrome have been reported in neonates whose mothers have taken valproate during pregnancy. This haemorrhagic syndrome is related to hypofibrinogenemia; afibrinogenemia has also been reported and may be fatal. These are possibly associated with a decrease of coagulation factors. However, this syndrome has to be distinguished from the decrease of the vitamin-K factors induced by phenobarbitone and other anti-epileptic enzyme inducing drugs.

Therefore, platelet count, fibrinogen plasma level, coagulation tests and coagulation factors should be investigated in neonates.

4.6.2

Lactation

Excretion of valproate in breast milk is low, with a concentration between 1 % to 10 % of total maternal serum levels; up to now children breast fed that have been monitored during the neonatal period have not experienced clinical effects. There appears to be no contra-indication to breast feeding by patients on valproate.

4.7 Effects on ability to drive and use machines

Use of Epilim may provide seizure control such that the patient may be eligible to hold a driving licence.

Patients should be warned of the risk of transient drowsiness, especially in cases of anticonvulsant polytherapy or association with benzodiazepines (see section 4.5 Interactions with Other Medicaments and Other Forms of Interaction).

4.8 Undesirable effects

Congenital and familial/genetic disorders: (see section 4.6 Pregnancy and Lactation)

Hepato-biliary disorders: rare cases of liver dysfunction (see section 4.4.1 Warnings)

Severe liver damage, including hepatic failure sometimes resulting in death, has been reported (see also sections 4.2, 4.3 and 4.4.1). Increased liver enzymes are common, particularly early in treatment, and may be transient (see section 4.4.1).

Gastrointestinal disorders (nausea, gastralgia, diarrhoea) frequently occur at the start of treatment. These problems can usually be overcome by taking Epilim with or after food or by using Enteric Coated Epilim.

Very rare cases of pancreatitis, sometimes lethal, have been reported (see section 4.4 Special Warnings and Special Precautions for Use).

Nervous system disorders:

Sedation has been reported occasionally, usually when in combination with other anticonvulsants. In monotherapy it occurred early in treatment on rare occasions and is usually transient. Rare cases of lethargy and confusion occasionally progressing to stupor, sometimes with associated hallucinations or convulsions have been reported. Encephalopathy and coma have very rarely been observed. These cases have often been associated with too high a starting dose or too rapid a dose escalation or concomitant use of other anticonvulsants, notably phenobarbitone. They have usually been reversible on withdrawal of treatment or reduction of dosage.

Very rare cases of reversible extrapyramidal symptoms including parkinsonism, or reversible dementia associated with reversible cerebral atrophy have been reported. Dose-related ataxia and fine postural tremor have occasionally been reported.

An increase in alertness may occur; this is generally beneficial but occasionally aggression, hyperactivity and behavioural deterioration have been reported.

Metabolic disorders:

Cases of isolated and moderate hyperammonaemia without change in liver function tests may occur frequently, are usually transient and should not cause treatment discontinuation. However, they may present clinically as vomiting, ataxia, and increasing clouding of consciousness. Should these symptoms occur Epilim should be discontinued.

Hyperammonaemia associated with neurological symptoms has also been reported (see section 4.4.2 Precautions). In such cases further investigations should be considered.

Blood and lymphatic system disorders:

Frequent occurrence of thrombocytopenia, rare cases of anaemia, leucopenia or pancytopenia. The blood picture returned to normal when the drug was discontinued.

Isolated reduction of fibrinogen or reversible increase in bleeding time have been reported, usually without associated clinical signs and particularly with high doses (sodium valproate has an inhibitory effect on the second phase of platelet aggregation). Spontaneous bruising or bleeding is an indication for withdrawal of medication pending investigations (see also section 4.6 Pregnancy and Lactation).

Skin and subcutaneous tissue disorders:

Cutaneous reactions such as exanthematous rash rarely occur with valproate. In very rare cases toxic epidermal necrolysis, Stevens-Johnson syndrome and erythema multiforme have been reported.

Transient hair loss, which may sometimes be dose-related, has often been reported. Regrowth normally begins within six months, although the hair may become more curly than previously. Hirsutism and acne have been very rarely reported.

Reproductive system and breast disorders:

Amenorrhoea and irregular periods have been reported. Very rarely gynaecomastia has occurred.

Vascular disorders: The occurrence of vasculitis has occasionally been reported.

Ear disorders:

Hearing loss, either reversible or irreversible has been reported rarely; however a cause and effect relationship has not been established.

Renal and urinary disorders:

There have been isolated reports of a reversible Fanconi's syndrome (a defect in proximal renal tubular function giving rise to glycosuria, amino aciduria, phosphaturia, and uricosuria) associated with valproate therapy, but the mode of action is as yet unclear.

Immune system disorders:

Allergic reactions (ranging from rash to hypersensitivity reactions) have been reported.

General disorders:

Very rare cases of non-severe peripheral oedema have been reported.

Increase in weight may also occur. Weight gain being a risk factor for polycystic ovary syndrome, it should be carefully monitored (see section 4.4 Special Warnings and Special Precautions for Use).

4.9 Overdose

Cases of accidental and deliberate valproate overdosage have been reported. At plasma concentrations of up to 5 to 6 times the maximum therapeutic levels, there are unlikely to be any symptoms other than nausea, vomiting and dizziness.

Clinical signs of massive overdose, i.e. plasma concentration 10 to 20 times maximum therapeutic levels, usually include CNS depression or coma with muscular hypotonia, hyporeflexia, miosis, impaired respiratory function.

Symptoms may however be variable and seizures have been reported in the presence of very high plasma levels (see also section 5.2 Pharmacokinetic Properties). Cases of intracranial hypertension related to cerebral oedema have been reported.

Hospital management of overdose should be symptomatic, including cardio-respiratory monitoring. Gastric lavage may be useful up to 10 to 12 hours following ingestion.

Haemodialysis and haemoperfusion have been used successfully.

Naloxone has been successfully used in a few isolated cases, sometimes in association with activated charcoal given orally. Deaths have occurred following massive overdose; nevertheless, a favourable outcome is usual.

5. PHARMACOLOGICAL PROPERTIES

5.1 Pharmacodynamic properties

Sodium valproate is an anticonvulsant.

The most likely mode of action for valproate is potentiation of the inhibitory action of gamma amino butyric acid (GABA) through an action on the further synthesis or further metabolism of GABA.

In certain *in-vitro* studies it was reported that sodium valproate could stimulate HIV replication but studies on peripheral blood mononuclear cells from HIV-infected subjects show that sodium valproate does not have a mitogen-like effect on inducing HIV replication. Indeed the effect of sodium valproate on HIV replication *ex-vivo* is highly variable, modest in quantity, appears to be unrelated to the dose and has not been documented in man.

5.2 Pharmacokinetic properties

The half-life of sodium valproate is usually reported to be within the range of 8-20 hours. It is usually shorter in children.

In patients with severe renal insufficiency it may be necessary to alter dosage in accordance with free plasma valproic acid levels.

The reported effective therapeutic range for plasma valproic acid levels is 40-100mg/litre (278-694 micromol/litre). This reported range may depend on time of sampling and presence of co-medication. The percentage of free (unbound) drug is usually between 6% and 15% of total plasma levels. An increased incidence of adverse effects may occur with plasma levels above the effective therapeutic range.

The pharmacological (or therapeutic) effects of Epilim may not be clearly correlated with the total or free (unbound) plasma valproic acid levels.

5.3 Preclinical safety data

There are no preclinical data of relevance to the prescriber which are additional to that already included in other sections of the SPC.

6. PHARMACEUTICAL PARTICULARS

6.1 List of excipients

Epilim Crushable Tablets; Maize Starch, Kaolin light (natural), Silica colloidal hydrated, Magnesium stearate and purified water*. (* not detected in final formulation).

Epilim Liquid: Hydroxyethyl cellulose, Sorbitol, Sodium methyl hydroxybenzoate, Sodium propyl hydroxybenzoate, Saccharin sodium, Ponceau 4R (E124), Flavour IFF cherry 740, Citric acid anhydrous and Purified water.

Epilim Enteric Coated Tablets; Povidone, talc, calcium silicate, magnesium stearate, hypromellose 6, citric acid anhydrous, macrogel 6000, polyvinyl acetate phthalate, diethyl phthalate, stearic acid, violet lake solids (containing titanium dioxide, amaranth lake, indigo carmine lake and hydroxypropyl cellulose), industrial methylated spirits, purified water.

6.2 Incompatibilities

None.

6.3 Shelf life

36 months.

6.4 Special precautions for storage

Epilim is hygroscopic. The tablets should not be removed from their foil until immediately before they are taken. Where possible, blister strips should not be cut. Store in a dry place below 30°C.

6.5 Nature and contents of container

Epilim Enteric Coated tablets are supplied in blister packs further packed into a cardboard carton. Pack size of 100 tablets.

Epilim 100mg Crushable Tablets are supplied in blister packs further packed into a cardboard carton. Pack size of 100 tablets.

Epilim Syrup and Liquid is supplied in amber glass bottles with polypropylene J-cap or aluminium tamper evident cap with extended polyethylene seal and amber polyethylene tetraphthalate bottles with polypropylene tamper evident closure. Bottle sizes of 300ml.

6.6 Instructions for use and handling

Not applicable.

7. MARKETING AUTHORISATION HOLDER

Sanofi-Synthelabo
PO Box 597
Guildford
Surrey

8. MARKETING AUTHORISATION NUMBER(S)

Epilim 500 Enteric Coated: PL 11723/0020.
Epilim 200 Enteric Coated: PL 11723/0018.
Epilim Crushable: PL 11723/0017.
Epilim Syrup: PL 11723/0025.
Epilim Liquid: PL 11723/0024.

9. DATE OF FIRST AUTHORISATION/RENEWAL OF THE AUTHORISATION

Epilim 500 Enteric Coated: 9 March 1998
Epilim 200 Enteric Coated: 17 July 2000
Epilim Crushable: 18 August 1993
Epilim Syrup: 17 August 2001
Epilim Liquid: 14 June 1999

10. DATE OF REVISION OF THE TEXT

Epilim 500 Enteric Coated: March 2004
Epilim 200 Enteric Coated: March 2004
Epilim Crushable: January 2004
Epilim Syrup: January 2004
Epilim Liquid: January 2004

Legal Category: POM

Epilim Chrono

(sanofi-aventis)

1. NAME OF THE MEDICINAL PRODUCT

Epilim Chrono 200 Controlled Release
Epilim Chrono 300 Controlled Release
Epilim Chrono 500 Controlled Release

2. QUALITATIVE AND QUANTITATIVE COMPOSITION

Active Constituents

Epilim Chrono 200 Controlled Release tablets contain 133.2mg Sodium Valproate and 58.0mg Valproic Acid equivalent to 200mg sodium valproate.

Epilim Chrono 300 Controlled Release tablets contain 199.8mg Sodium Valproate and 87.0mg Valproic Acid equivalent to 300mg sodium valproate.

Epilim Chrono 500 Controlled Release tablets contain 333mg Sodium Valproate and 145mg Valproic Acid equivalent to 500mg sodium valproate.

3. PHARMACEUTICAL FORM

Prolonged Release Tablet

4. CLINICAL PARTICULARS

4.1 Therapeutic indications

Treatment of generalised, partial or other epilepsy.

4.2 Posology and method of administration

Epilim Chrono Controlled Release tablets are for oral administration.

Epilim Chrono is a prolonged release formulation of Epilim which reduces peak concentration and ensures more even plasma concentrations throughout the day.

Epilim Chrono may be given once or twice daily. The tablets should be swallowed whole and not crushed or chewed.

Daily dosage requirements vary according to age and body weight.

In patients where adequate control has been achieved Epilim Chrono formulations are interchangeable with other conventional or prolonged release formulations on an equivalent daily dosage basis.

Monotherapy

Usual requirements are as follows:

Adults

Dosage should start at 600mg daily increasing by 200mg at three-day intervals until control is achieved. This is generally within the dosage range 1000mg to 2000mg per day, ie 20-30mg/kg body weight. Where adequate control is not achieved within this range the dose may be further increased to 2500mg per day.

Children over 20kg

Initial dosage should be 400mg/day (irrespective of weight) with spaced increases until control is achieved; this is usually within the range 20-30mg/kg body weight per day. Where adequate control is not achieved within this range the dose may be increased to 35mg/kg body weight per day.

Children under 20kg

An alternative formulation of Epilim should be used in this group of patients, due to the tablet size and need for dose titration. Epilim Liquid (sugar-free) or Epilim Syrup are alternatives.

Elderly

Although the pharmacokinetics of valproate are modified in the elderly, they have limited clinical significance and dosage should be determined by seizure control. The volume of distribution is increased in the elderly and because of decreased binding to serum albumin, the proportion of free drug is increased. This will affect the clinical interpretation of plasma valproic acid levels.

In patients with renal insufficiency

It may be necessary to decrease dosage. Dosage should be adjusted according to clinical monitoring since monitoring of plasma concentrations may be misleading (see section 5.2 Pharmacokinetic Properties).

In patients with hepatic insufficiency

Salicylates should not be used concomitantly with valproate since they employ the same metabolic pathway (see also sections 4.4 Special Warnings and Precautions for Use and 4.8 Undesirable Effects).

Liver dysfunction, including hepatic failure resulting in fatalities, has occurred in patients whose treatment included valproic acid (see sections 4.3 Containdications and 4.4 Special Warnings and Precautions for Use).

Salicylates should not be used in children under 16 years (see aspirin/salicylate product information on Reye's syndrome). In addition in conjunction with Epilim, concomitant use in children under 3 years can increase the risk of liver toxicity (see section 4.4.1 Special warnings).

Combined Therapy

When starting Epilim in patients already on other anticonvulsants, these should be tapered slowly; initiation of Epilim therapy should then be gradual, with target dose being reached after about 2 weeks. In certain cases it may be necessary to raise the dose by 5 to 10mg/kg/day when used in combination with anticonvulsants which induce liver enzyme activity, eg phenytoin, phenobarbitone and carbamazepine. Once known enzyme inducers have been withdrawn it may be possible to maintain seizure control on a reduced dose of Epilim. When barbiturates are being administered concomitantly and particularly if sedation is observed (particularly in children) the dosage of barbiturate should be reduced.

NB: In children requiring doses higher than 40mg/kg/day clinical chemistry and haematological parameters should be monitored.

Optimum dosage is mainly determined by seizure control and routine measurement of plasma levels is unnecessary. However, a method for measurement of plasma levels is available and may be helpful where there is poor control or side effects are suspected (see section 5.2 Pharmacokinetic Properties).

4.3 Contraindications

- Active liver disease
- Personal or family history of severe hepatic dysfunction, especially drug related
- Hypersensitivity to sodium valproate
- Porphyria

4.4 Special warnings and special precautions for use

4.4.1 Special warnings

Liver dysfunction:

Conditions of occurrence:

Severe liver damage, including hepatic failure sometimes resulting in fatalities, has been very rarely reported. Experience in epilepsy has indicated that patients most at risk are infants, especially in cases of multiple anticonvulsant therapy, are infants and in particular young children under the age of 3 and those with severe seizure disorders, organic brain disease, and (or) congenital metabolic or degenerative disease associated with mental retardation.

After the age of 3, the incidence of occurrence is significantly reduced and progressively decreases with age.

The concomitant use of salicylates should be avoided in children under 3 due to the risk of liver toxicity. Additionally, salicylates should not be used in children under 16 years (see aspirin/salicylate product information on Reye's syndrome).

Monotherapy is recommended in children under the age of 3 years when prescribing Epilim, but the potential benefit of Epilim should be weighed against the risk of liver damage or pancreatitis in such patients prior to initiation of therapy

In most cases, such liver damage occurred during the first 6 months of therapy, the period of maximum risk being 2-12 weeks.

Suggestive signs:

Clinical symptoms are essential for early diagnosis. In particular the following conditions, which may precede jaundice, should be taken into consideration, especially in patients at risk (see above: 'Conditions of occurrence'):

- non specific symptoms, usually of sudden onset, such as asthenia, malaise, anorexia, lethargy, oedema and drowsiness, which are sometimes associated with repeated vomiting and abdominal pain.

- in patients with epilepsy, recurrence of seizures.

These are an indication for immediate withdrawal of the drug.

Patients (or their family for children) should be instructed to report immediately any such signs to a physician should they occur. Investigations including clinical examination and biological assessment of liver function should be undertaken immediately.

Detection:

Liver function should be measured before and then periodically monitored during the first 6 months of therapy, especially in those who seem most at risk, and those with a prior history of liver disease.

Amongst usual investigations, tests which reflect protein synthesis, particularly prothrombin rate, are most relevant.

Confirmation of an abnormally low prothrombin rate, particularly in association with other biological abnormalities (significant decrease in fibrinogen and coagulation factors; increased bilirubin level and raised transaminases) requires cessation of Epilim therapy.

As a matter of precaution and in case they are taken concomitantly salicylates should also be discontinued since they employ the same metabolic pathway.

As with most antiepileptic drugs, increased liver enzymes are common, particularly at the beginning of therapy; they are also transient.

More extensive biological investigations (including prothrombin rate) are recommended in these patients; a reduction in dosage may be considered when appropriate and tests should be repeated as necessary.

Pancreatitis: Pancreatitis, which may be severe and result in fatalities, has been very rarely reported. Patients experiencing nausea, vomiting or acute abdominal pain should have a prompt medical evaluation (including measurement of serum amylase). Young children are at particular risk; this risk decreases with increasing age. Severe seizures and severe neurological impairment with combination anticonvulsant therapy may be risk factors. Hepatic failure with pancreatitis increases the risk of fatal outcome. In case of pancreatitis, valproate should be discontinued.

4.4.2 Precautions

Haematological: Blood tests (blood cell count, including platelet count, bleeding time and coagulation tests) are recommended prior to initiation of therapy or before surgery, and in case of spontaneous bruising or bleeding (see section 4.8 Undesirable Effects).

Renal insufficiency:

In patients with renal insufficiency, it may be necessary to decrease dosage. As monitoring of plasma concentrations may be misleading, dosage should be adjusted according to clinical monitoring (see sections 4.2 Posology and Method of Adminstration and 5.2. Pharmacokinetic Properties).

Systemic lupus erythematosus: Although immune disorders have only rarely been noted during the use of Epilim, the potential benefit of Epilim should be weighed against its potential risk in patients with systemic lupus erythematosus (see also section 4.8 Undesirable Effects).

Hyperammonaemia: When a urea cycle enzymatic deficiency is suspected, metabolic investigations should be performed prior to treatment because of the risk of hyperammonaemia with valproate.

Weight gain: Epilim very commonly causes weight gain, which may be marked and progressive. Patients should be warned of the risk of weight gain at the initiation of therapy and appropriate strategies should be adopted to minimise it (see section 4.8 Undesirable Effects).

Pregnancy: Women of childbearing potential should not be started on Epilim without specialist neurological advice. Epilim is the antiepileptic of choice in patients with certain types of epilepsy such as generalised epilepsy ± myoclonus/photosensitivity. For partial epilepsy, Epilim should be used only in patients resistant to other treatment. Women who are likely to get pregnant, should receive specialist advice because of the potential teratogenic risk to the foetus (see also section 4.6 Pregnancy and Lactation).

Diabetic patients: Valproate is eliminated mainly through the kidneys, partly in the form of ketone bodies; this may give false positives in the urine testing of possible diabetics.

4.5 Interaction with other medicinal products and other forms of Interaction

4.5.1 Effects of Valproate on other drugs

- Neuroleptics, MAO inhibitors, antidepressants and benzodiazepines

Valproate may potentiate the effect of other psychotropics such as neuroleptics, MAO inhibitors, antidepressants and benzodiazepines; therefore, clinical monitoring is advised and dosage should be adjusted when appropriate.

- Phenobarbital

Valproate increases phenobarbital plasma concentrations (due to inhibition of hepatic catabolism) and sedation may occur, particularly in children. Therefore, clinical monitoring is recommended throughout the first 15 days of combined treatment with immediate reduction of phenobarbital doses if sedation occurs and determination of phenobarbital plasma levels when appropriate.

- Primidone

Valproate increases primidone plasma levels with exacerbation of its adverse effects (such as sedation); these signs cease with long term treatment. Clinical monitoring is recommended especially at the beginning of combined therapy with dosage adjustment when appropriate.

- Phenytoin

Valproate decreases phenytoin total plasma concentration. Moreover valproate increases phenytoin free form with possible overdosage symptoms (valproic acid displaces phenytoin from its plasma protein binding sites and reduces its hepatic catabolism). Therefore clinical monitoring is recommended; when phenytoin plasma levels are determined, the free form should be evaluated.

- Carbamazepine

Clinical toxicity has been reported when valproate was administered with carbamazepine as valproate may potentiate toxic effects of carbamazepine. Clinical monitoring is recommended especially at the beginning of combined therapy with dosage adjustment when appropriate.

- Lamotrigine

Valproate may reduce lamotrigine metabolism and increase its mean half-life, dosages should be adjusted (lamotrigine dosage decreased) when appropriate. Co-administration of lamotrigine and Epilim might increase the risk of rash.

- Zidovudine

Valproate may raise zidovudine plasma concentration leading to increased zidovudine toxicity.

- Vitamin K-dependent anticoagulants

The anticoagulant effect of warfarin and other coumarin anticoagulants may be increased following displacement from plasma protein binding sites by valproic acid. The prothrombin time should be closely monitored.

- Temozolomide

Co-administration of temozolomide and valproate may cause a small decrease in the clearance of temozolomide that is not thought to be clinically relevant.

4.5.2 Effects of other drugs on Valproate

Antiepileptics with enzyme inducing effect (including ***phenytoin, phenobarbital, carbamazepine***) decrease valproic acid plasma concentrations. Dosages should be adjusted according to blood levels in case of combined therapy.

On the other hand, combination of ***felbamate*** and valproate may increase valproic acid plasma concentration. Valproate dosage should be monitored.

Mefloquine and ***chloroquine*** increase valproic acid metabolism and may lower the seizure threshold; therefore epileptic seizures may occur in cases of combined therapy. Accordingly, the dosage of Epilim may need adjustment.

In case of concomitant use of valproate and ***highly protein bound agents (e.g. aspirin)***, free valproic acid plasma levels may be increased.

Valproic acid plasma levels may be increased (as a result of reduced hepatic metabolism) in case of concomitant use with ***cimetidine*** or ***erythromycin***.

Carbapenem antibioticssuch as ***imipenem*** and ***meropenem***: Decrease in valproic acid blood level, sometimes associated with convulsions, has been observed when imipenem or meropenem were combined. If these antibiotics have to be administered, close monitoring of valproic acid blood levels is recommended.

Cholestyramine may decrease the absorption of valproate.

4.5.3 Other Interactions

Caution is advised when using Epilim in combination with newer anti-epileptics whose pharmacodynamics may not be well established.

Valproate usually has no enzyme-inducing effect; as a consequence, valproate does not reduce efficacy of oestroprogestative agents in women receiving hormonal contraception, including the oral contraceptive pill.

4.6 Pregnancy and lactation

4.6.1 Pregnancy

From experience in treating mothers with epilepsy, the risk associated with the use of valproate during pregnancy has been described as follows:

- Risk associated with epilepsy and antiepileptics

In offspring born to mothers with epilepsy receiving any anti-epileptic treatment, the overall rate of malformations has been demonstrated to be 2 to 3 times higher than the rate (approximately 3 %) reported in the general population. Although an increased number of children with malformations have been reported in cases of multiple drug therapy, the respective role of treatments and disease in causing the malformations has not been formally established. Malformations most frequently encountered are cleft lip and cardio-vascular malformations.

Epidemiological studies have suggested an association between in-utero exposure to sodium valproate and a risk of developmental delay. Many factors including maternal epilepsy may also contribute to this risk but it is difficult to quantify the relative contributions of these or of maternal anti-epileptic treatment. Notwithstanding those potential risks, no sudden discontinuation in the anti-epileptic therapy should be undertaken as this may lead to breakthrough seizures which could have serious consequences for both the mother and the foetus.

- Risk associated with valproate

In animals: teratogenic effects have been demonstrated in the mouse, rat and rabbit.

There is animal experimental evidence that high plasma peak levels and the size of an individual dose are associated with neural tube defects.

In humans: an increased incidence of congenital abnormalities (including cases of facial dysmorphia, hypospadias and multiple malformations, particularly of the limbs) has been demonstrated in offspring born to mothers with epilepsy treated with valproate.

Valproate use is associated with neural tube defects such as myelomeningocele and spina bifida. The frequency of this effect is estimated to be 1 to 2%.

- In view of the above data

When a woman is planning pregnancy, this provides an opportunity to review the need for anti-epileptic treatment. Women of childbearing age should be informed of the risks and benefits of continuing anti-epileptic treatment throughout pregnancy.

Folate supplementation, **prior** to pregnancy, has been demonstrated to reduce the incidence of neural tube defects in the offspring of women at high risk. Although no direct evidence exists of such effects in women receiving anti-epileptic drugs, women should be advised to start taking folic acid supplementation (5mg) as soon as contraception is discontinued.

The available evidence suggests that anticonvulsant monotherapy is preferred. Dosage should be reviewed before conception and the lowest effective dose used, in divided doses, as abnormal pregnancy outcome tends to be associated with higher total daily dosage and with the size of an individual dose. The incidence of neural tube defects rises with increasing dosage, particularly above 1000mg daily. The administration in several divided doses over the day and the use of a prolonged release formulation is preferable in order to avoid high peak plasma levels.

During pregnancy, valproate anti-epileptic treatment should not be discontinued if it has been effective.

Nevertheless, specialised prenatal monitoring should be instituted in order to detect the possible occurrence of a neural tube defect or any other malformation. Pregnancies should be carefully screened by ultrasound, and other techniques if appropriate (see Section 4.4 Special Warnings and Special Precautions for use).

- Risk in the neonate

Very rare cases of haemorrhagic syndrome have been reported in neonates whose mothers have taken valproate during pregnancy. This haemorrhagic syndrome is related to hypofibrinogenemia; afibrinogenemia has also been reported and may be fatal. These are possibly associated with a decrease of coagulation factors. However, this syndrome has to be distinguished from the decrease of the vitamin-K factors induced by phenobarbitone and other anti-epileptic enzyme inducing drugs.

Therefore, platelet count, fibrinogen plasma level, coagulation tests and coagulation factors should be investigated in neonates.

4.6.2

Lactation

Excretion of valproate in breast milk is low, with a concentration between 1 % to 10 % of total maternal serum levels; up to now children breast fed that have been monitored during the neonatal period have not experienced clinical effects. There appears to be no contra-indication to breast feeding by patients on valproate.

4.7 Effects on ability to drive and use machines

Use of Epilim may provide seizure control such that the patient may be eligible to hold a driving licence.

Patients should be warned of the risk of transient drowsiness, especially in cases of anticonvulsant polytherapy or association with benzodiazepines (see section 4.5 Interactions with Other Medicaments and Other Forms of Interaction).

4.8 Undesirable effects

Congenital and familial/genetic disorders: (see section 4.6 Pregnancy and Lactation)

Hepato-biliary disorders: rare cases of liver dysfunction (see section 4.4.1 Warnings)

Severe liver damage, including hepatic failure sometimes resulting in death, has been reported (see also sections 4.2, 4.3 and 4.4.1). Increased liver enzymes are common, particularly early in treatment, and may be transient (see section 4.4.1).

Gastrointestinal disorders (nausea, gastralgia, diarrhoea) frequently occur at the start of treatment. These problems can usually be overcome by taking Epilim with or after food or by using Enteric Coated Epilim.

Very rare cases of pancreatitis, sometimes lethal, have been reported (see section 4.4 Special Warnings and Special Precautions for Use).

Nervous system disorders:

Sedation has been reported occasionally, usually when in combination with other anticonvulsants. In monotherapy it occurred early in treatment on rare occasions and is usually transient. Rare cases of lethargy and confusion occasionally progressing to stupor, sometimes with associated hallucinations or convulsions have been reported. Encephalopathy and coma have very rarely been observed. These cases have often been associated with too high a starting dose or too rapid a dose escalation or concomitant use of other anticonvulsants, notably phenobarbitone. They have usually been reversible on withdrawal of treatment or reduction of dosage.

Very rare cases of reversible extrapyramidal symptoms including parkinsonism, or reversible dementia associated with reversible cerebral atrophy have been reported. Dose-related ataxia and fine postural tremor have occasionally been reported.

An increase in alertness may occur; this is generally beneficial but occasionally aggression, hyperactivity and behavioural deterioration have been reported.

Metabolic disorders:

Cases of isolated and moderate hyperammonaemia without change in liver function tests may occur frequently, are usually transient and should not cause treatment discontinuation. However, they may present clinically as vomiting, ataxia, and increasing clouding of consciousness. Should these symptoms occur Epilim should be discontinued.

Hyperammonaemia associated with neurological symptoms has also been reported (see section 4.4.2 Precautions). In such cases further investigations should be considered.

Blood and lymphatic system disorders:

Frequent occurrence of thrombocytopenia, rare cases of anaemia, leucopenia or pancytopenia. The blood picture returned to normal when the drug was discontinued.

Isolated reduction of fibrinogen or reversible increase in bleeding time have been reported, usually without associated clinical signs and particularly with high doses (sodium valproate has an inhibitory effect on the second phase of platelet aggregation). Spontaneous bruising or bleeding is an indication for withdrawal of medication pending investigations (see also section 4.6 Pregnancy and Lactation).

Skin and subcutaneous tissue disorders:

Cutaneous reactions such as exanthematous rash rarely occur with valproate. In very rare cases toxic epidermal necrolysis, Stevens-Johnson syndrome and erythema multiforme have been reported.

Transient hair loss, which may sometimes be dose-related, has often been reported. Regrowth normally begins within six months, although the hair may become more curly than previously. Hirsutism and acne have been very rarely reported.

Reproductive system and breast disorders:

Amenorrhoea and irregular periods have been reported. Very rarely gynaecomastia has occurred.

Vascular disorders: The occurrence of vasculitis has occasionally been reported.

Ear disorders:

Hearing loss, either reversible or irreversible has been reported rarely; however a cause and effect relationship has not been established.

Renal and urinary disorders:

There have been isolated reports of a reversible Fanconi's syndrome (a defect in proximal renal tubular function giving rise to glycosuria, amino aciduria, phosphaturia, and uricosuria) associated with valproate therapy, but the mode of action is as yet unclear.

Immune system disorders:

Allergic reactions (ranging from rash to hypersensitivity reactions) have been reported.

General disorders:

Very rare cases of non-severe peripheral oedema have been reported.

Increase in weight may also occur. Weight gain being a risk factor for polycystic ovary syndrome, it should be carefully monitored (see section 4.4 Special Warnings and Special Precautions for Use).

4.9 Overdose

Cases of accidental and deliberate valproate overdosage have been reported. At plasma concentrations of up to 5 to 6 times the maximum therapeutic levels, there are unlikely to be any symptoms other than nausea, vomiting and dizziness.

Clinical signs of massive overdose, i.e. plasma concentration 10 to 20 times maximum therapeutic levels, usually include CNS depression or coma with muscular hypotonia, hyporeflexia, miosis, impaired respiratory function.

Symptoms may however be variable and seizures have been reported in the presence of very high plasma levels (see also section 5.2 Pharmacokinetic Properties). Cases of intracranial hypertension related to cerebral oedema have been reported.

Hospital management of overdose should be symptomatic, including cardio-respiratory monitoring. Gastric lavage may be useful up to 10 to 12 hours following ingestion.

Haemodialysis and haemoperfusion have been used successfully.

Naloxone has been successfully used in a few isolated cases, sometimes in association with activated charcoal given orally. Deaths have occurred following massive overdose; nevertheless, a favourable outcome is usual.

5. PHARMACOLOGICAL PROPERTIES

5.1 Pharmacodynamic properties

Sodium valproate is an anticonvulsant.

The most likely mode of action for valproate is potentiation of the inhibitory action of gamma amino butyric acid (GABA) through an action on the further synthesis or further metabolism of GABA.

In certain *in-vitro* studies it was reported that sodium valproate could stimulate HIV replication but studies on peripheral blood mononuclear cells from HIV-infected subjects show that sodium valproate does not have a mitogen-like effect on inducing HIV replication. Indeed the effect of sodium valproate on HIV replication *ex-vivo* is highly variable, modest in quantity, appears to be unrelated to the dose and has not been documented in man.

5.2 Pharmacokinetic properties

The half-life of sodium valproate is usually reported to be within the range of 8-20 hours. It is usually shorter in children.

In patients with severe renal insufficiency it may be necessary to alter dosage in accordance with free plasma valproic acid levels.

The reported effective therapeutic range for plasma valproic acid levels is 40-100mg/litre (278-694 micromol/litre). This reported range may depend on time of sampling and presence of co-medication. The percentage of free (unbound) drug is usually between 6% and 15% of total plasma levels. An increased incidence of adverse effects may occur with plasma levels above the effective therapeutic range.

The pharmacological (or therapeutic) effects of Epilim Chrono may not be clearly correlated with the total or free (unbound) plasma valproic acid levels.

Epilim Chrono formulations are prolonged release formulations which demonstrate in pharmacokinetic studies less fluctuation in plasma concentration compared with other established conventional and modified release Epilim formulations.

In cases where measurement of plasma levels is considered necessary, the pharmacokinetics of Epilim Chrono make the measurement of plasma levels less dependent upon time of sampling.

The Epilim Chrono formulations are bioequivalent to Epilim Liquid and enteric coated (EC) formulations with respect to the mean areas under the plasma concentration time curves. Steady-state pharmacokinetic data indicate that the peak concentration (Cmax) and trough concentration (Cmin) of Epilim Chrono lie within the effective therapeutic range of plasma levels found in pharmacokinetic studies with Epilim EC.

5.3 Preclinical safety data

There are no preclinical data of relevance to the prescriber which are additional to that already included in other sections of the SPC.

6. PHARMACEUTICAL PARTICULARS

6.1 List of excipients

Film Coat

Violet coat (Opadry 04-S-6705), containing: Titanium dioxide (E171), Erythrosine BS aluminium lake (E127), Indigo Carmine aluminium lake FD and C Blue No 2 (E132), Iron Oxide Black (E172), Hypromellose (E464), Macrogol 400, Purified water*.

* Not detected in final formulation.

6.2 Incompatibilities

None.

6.3 Shelf life

36 months.

6.4 Special precautions for storage

Epilim is hygroscopic. The tablets should not be removed from their foil until immediately before they are taken. Where possible, blister strips should not be cut. Store in a dry place below 30°C.

6.5 Nature and contents of container

Epilim Chrono Controlled Release tablets are supplied in blister packs further packed into a cardboard carton. Pack size 100 tablets.

6.6 Instructions for use and handling

Not applicable.

7. MARKETING AUTHORISATION HOLDER

Sanofi-Synthelabo

PO Box 597

Guildford

Surrey

8. MARKETING AUTHORISATION NUMBER(S)

Epilim Chrono 200 Controlled Release - PL 11723/0078

Epilim Chrono 300 Controlled Release - PL 11723/0021

Epilim Chrono 500 Controlled Release - PL 11723/0079

9. DATE OF FIRST AUTHORISATION/RENEWAL OF THE AUTHORISATION

Epilim Chrono 200 Controlled Release - 25 November 1998

Epilim Chrono 500 Controlled Release - 28 January 2002

Epilim Chrono 500 Controlled Release - 25 November 1998

10. DATE OF REVISION OF THE TEXT

January 2004

Legal Category: POM

Epilim Intravenous

(sanofi-aventis)

1. NAME OF THE MEDICINAL PRODUCT

Epilim Intravenous

2. QUALITATIVE AND QUANTITATIVE COMPOSITION

Each vial contains 400mg of Sodium Valproate freeze-dried powder.

3. PHARMACEUTICAL FORM

Powder for Injection or Intravenous Infusions

4. CLINICAL PARTICULARS

4.1 Therapeutic indications

The treatment of epileptic patients who would normally be maintained on oral sodium valproate, and for whom oral therapy is temporarily not possible.

4.2 Posology and method of administration

Epilim Intravenous may be given by direct slow intravenous injection or by infusion using a separate intravenous line in normal saline, dextrose 5%, or dextrose saline.

Monotherapy

Daily dosage requirements vary according to age and body weight.

To reconstitute, inject the solvent provided (4ml) into the vial, allow to dissolve and extract the appropriate dose. Due to displacement of solvent by sodium valproate the concentration of reconstituted sodium valproate is 95mg/ml.

Each vial of Epilim Intravenous is for single dose injection only. It should be reconstituted immediately prior to use and infusion solutions containing it used within 24 hours. Any unused portion should be discarded. (See section 6.6).

Epilim Intravenous should not be administered via the same IV line as other IV additives. The intravenous solution is suitable for infusion by PVC, polyethylene or glass containers.

Patients already satisfactorily treated with Epilim may be continued at their current dosage using continuous or repeated infusion. Other patients may be given a slow intravenous injection over 3-5 minutes, usually 400-800mg depending on body weight (up to 10mg/kg) followed by continuous or repeated infusion up to a maximum of 2500mg/day.

Epilim Intravenous should be replaced by oral Epilim therapy as soon as practicable.

Use with children

Daily requirement for children is usually in the range 20-30mg/kg/day and method of administration is as above. Where adequate control is not achieved within this range the dose may be increased up to 40mg/kg/day but only in patients in whom plasma valproic acid levels can be monitored. Above 40mg/kg/day clinical chemistry and haematological parameters should be monitored.

Use in the elderly

Although the pharmacokinetics of valproate are modified in the elderly, they have limited clinical significance and dosage should be determined by seizure control. The volume of distribution is increased in the elderly and because of decreased binding to serum albumin, the proportion of free drug is increased. This will affect the clinical interpretation of plasma valproic acid levels.

In patients with renal insufficiency

It may be necessary to decrease dosage. Dosage should be adjusted according to clinical monitoring since monitoring of plasma concentrations may be misleading (see section 5.2 Pharmacokinetic Properties).

In patients with hepatic insufficiency

Salicylates should not be used concomitantly with valproate since they employ the same metabolic pathway (see also sections 4.4 Special Warnings and Precautions for Use and 4.8 Undesirable Effects).

Liver dysfunction, including hepatic failure resulting in fatalities, has occurred in patients whose treatment included valproic acid (see sections 4.3 Containdications and 4.4 Special Warnings and Precautions for Use).

Salicylates should not be used in children under 16 years (see aspirin/salicylate product information on Reye's syndrome). In addition in conjunction with Epilim, concomitant use in children under 3 years can increase the risk of liver toxicity (see section 4.4.1 Special warnings).

Combined Therapy

When starting Epilim in patients already on other anticonvulsants, these should be tapered slowly: initiation of Epilim therapy should then be gradual, with target dose being reached after about 2 weeks. In certain cases it may be necessary to raise the dose by 5 to 10mg/kg/day when used in combination with anticonvulsants which induce liver enzyme activity, eg phenytoin, phenobarbitone and carbamazepine. Once known enzyme inducers have been withdrawn it may be possible to maintain seizure control on a reduced dose of Epilim. When barbiturates are being administered concomitantly and particularly if sedation is observed (particularly in children) the dosage of barbiturate should be reduced.

NB: In children requiring doses higher than 40mg/kg/day clinical chemistry and haematological parameters should be monitored.

Optimum dosage is mainly determined by seizure control and routine measurement of plasma levels is unnecessary. However, a method for measurement of plasma levels is available and may be helpful where there is poor control or side effects are suspected (see section 5.2 Pharmacokinetic Properties).

4.3 Contraindications

- Active liver disease
- Personal or family history of severe hepatic dysfunction, especially drug related
- Hypersensitivity to sodium valproate
- Porphyria

4.4 Special warnings and special precautions for use

4.4.1 Special warnings

Liver dysfunction:

Conditions of occurrence:

Severe liver damage, including hepatic failure sometimes resulting in fatalities, has been very rarely reported. Experience in epilepsy has indicated that patients most at risk, especially in cases of multiple anticonvulsant therapy, are infants and in particular young children under the age of 3 and those with severe seizure disorders, organic brain disease, and (or) congenital metabolic or degenerative disease associated with mental retardation.

After the age of 3, the incidence of occurrence is significantly reduced and progressively decreases with age.

The concomitant use of salicylates should be avoided in children under 3 due to the risk of liver toxicity. Additionally, salicylates should not be used in children under 16 years (see aspirin/salicylate product information on Reye's syndrome).

Monotherapy is recommended in children under the age of 3 years when prescribing Epilim, but the potential benefit of Epilim should be weighed against the risk of liver damage or pancreatitis in such patients prior to initiation of therapy

In most cases, such liver damage occurred during the first 6 months of therapy, the period of maximum risk being 2-12 weeks.

Suggestive signs:

Clinical symptoms are essential for early diagnosis. In particular the following conditions, which may precede jaundice, should be taken into consideration, especially in patients at risk (see above: 'Conditions of occurrence'):

- non specific symptoms, usually of sudden onset, such as asthenia, malaise, anorexia, lethargy, oedema and drowsiness, which are sometimes associated with repeated vomiting and abdominal pain.

- in patients with epilepsy, recurrence of seizures.

These are an indication for immediate withdrawal of the drug.

Patients (or their family for children) should be instructed to report immediately any such signs to a physician should they occur. Investigations including clinical examination and biological assessment of liver function should be undertaken immediately.

Detection:

Liver function should be measured before and then periodically monitored during the first 6 months of therapy, especially in those who seem most at risk, and those with a prior history of liver disease.

Amongst usual investigations, tests which reflect protein synthesis, particularly prothrombin rate, are most relevant.

Confirmation of an abnormally low prothrombin rate, particularly in association with other biological abnormalities (significant decrease in fibrinogen and coagulation factors; increased bilirubin level and raised transaminases) requires cessation of Epilim therapy.

As a matter of precaution and in case they are taken concomitantly salicylates should also be discontinued since they employ the same metabolic pathway.

As with most antiepileptic drugs, increased liver enzymes are common, particularly at the beginning of therapy; they are also transient.

More extensive biological investigations (including prothrombin rate) are recommended in these patients; a reduction in dosage may be considered when appropriate and tests should be repeated as necessary.

Pancreatitis: Pancreatitis, which may be severe and result in fatalities, has been very rarely reported. Patients experiencing nausea, vomiting or acute abdominal pain should have a prompt medical evaluation (including measurement of serum amylase). Young children are at particular risk; this risk decreases with increasing age. Severe seizures and severe neurological impairment with combination anticonvulsant therapy may be risk factors. Hepatic failure with pancreatitis increases the risk of fatal outcome. In case of pancreatitis, valproate should be discontinued.

4.4.2 Precautions

Haematological: Blood tests (blood cell count, including platelet count, bleeding time and coagulation tests) are recommended prior to initiation of therapy or before surgery, and in case of spontaneous bruising or bleeding (see section 4.8 Undesirable Effects).

Renal insufficiency:

In patients with renal insufficiency, it may be necessary to decrease dosage. As monitoring of plasma concentrations may be misleading, dosage should be adjusted according to clinical monitoring (see sections 4.2 Posology and Method of Adminstration and 5.2. Pharmacokinetic Properties).

Systemic lupus erythematosus: Although immune disorders have only rarely been noted during the use of Epilim, the potential benefit of Epilim should be weighed against its potential risk in patients with systemic lupus erythematosus (see also section 4.8 Undesirable Effects).

Hyperammonaemia: When a urea cycle enzymatic deficiency is suspected, metabolic investigations should be performed prior to treatment because of the risk of hyperammonaemia with valproate.

Weight gain: Epilim very commonly causes weight gain, which may be marked and progressive. Patients should be warned of the risk of weight gain at the initiation of therapy and appropriate strategies should be adopted to minimise it (see section 4.8 Undesirable Effects).

Pregnancy: Women of childbearing potential should not be started on Epilim without specialist neurological advice. Epilim is the antiepileptic of choice in patients with certain types of epilepsy such as generalised epilepsy ± myoclonus/photosensitivity. For partial epilepsy, Epilim should be used only in patients resistant to other treatment. Women who are likely to get pregnant, should receive specialist advice because of the potential teratogenic risk to the foetus (see also section 4.6 Pregnancy and Lactation).

Diabetic patients: Valproate is eliminated mainly through the kidneys, partly in the form of ketone bodies; this may give false positives in the urine testing of possible diabetics.

4.5 Interaction with other medicinal products and other forms of Interaction

4.5.1 Effects of Valproate on other drugs

- Neuroleptics, MAO inhibitors, antidepressants and benzodiazepines

Valproate may potentiate the effect of other psychotropics such as neuroleptics, MAO inhibitors, antidepressants and benzodiazepines; therefore, clinical monitoring is advised and dosage should be adjusted when appropriate.

- Phenobarbital

Valproate increases phenobarbital plasma concentrations (due to inhibition of hepatic catabolism) and sedation may occur, particularly in children. Therefore, clinical monitoring is recommended throughout the first 15 days of combined treatment with immediate reduction of phenobarbital doses if sedation occurs and determination of phenobarbital plasma levels when appropriate.

- Primidone

Valproate increases primidone plasma levels with exacerbation of its adverse effects (such as sedation); these signs cease with long term treatment. Clinical monitoring is recommended especially at the beginning of combined therapy with dosage adjustment when appropriate.

- Phenytoin

Valproate decreases phenytoin total plasma concentration. Moreover valproate increases phenytoin free form with possible overdosage symptoms (valproic acid displaces phenytoin from its plasma protein binding sites and reduces its hepatic catabolism). Therefore clinical monitoring is recommended; when phenytoin plasma levels are determined, the free form should be evaluated.

- Carbamazepine

Clinical toxicity has been reported when valproate was administered with carbamazepine as valproate may potentiate toxic effects of carbamazepine. Clinical monitoring is recommended especially at the beginning of combined therapy with dosage adjustment when appropriate.

- Lamotrigine

Valproate may reduce lamotrigine metabolism and increase its mean half-life, dosages should be adjusted (lamotrigine dosage decreased) when appropriate. Co-administration of lamotrigine and Epilim might increase the risk of rash

- Zidovudine

Valproate may raise zidovudine plasma concentration leading to increased zidovudine toxicity.

- Vitamin K-dependent anticoagulants

The anticoagulant effect of warfarin and other coumarin anticoagulants may be increased following displacement from plasma protein binding sites by valproic acid. The prothrombin time should be closely monitored.

- Temozolomide

Co-administration of temozolomide and valproate may cause a small decrease in the clearance of temozolomide that is not thought to be clinically relevant.

4.5.2 Effects of other drugs on Valproate

Antiepileptics with enzyme inducing effect (including ***phenytoin, phenobarbital, carbamazepine***) decrease valproic acid plasma concentrations. Dosages should be adjusted according to blood levels in case of combined therapy.

On the other hand, combination of ***felbamate*** and valproate may increase valproic acid plasma concentration. Valproate dosage should be monitored.

Mefloquine and ***chloroquine*** increase valproic acid metabolism and may lower the seizure threshold; therefore epileptic seizures may occur in cases of combined therapy. Accordingly, the dosage of Epilim may need adjustment.

In case of concomitant use of valproate and ***highly protein bound agents (e.g. aspirin)***, free valproic acid plasma levels may be increased.

Valproic acid plasma levels may be increased (as a result of reduced hepatic metabolism) in case of concomitant use with ***cimetidine*** or ***erythromycin***.

Carbapenem antibioticssuch as ***imipenem*** and ***meropenem***: Decrease in valproic acid blood level, sometimes associated with convulsions, has been observed when imipenem or meropenem were combined. If these antibiotics have to be administered, close monitoring of valproic acid blood levels is recommended.

Cholestyramine may decrease the absorption of valproate.

4.5.3 Other Interactions

Caution is advised when using Epilim in combination with newer anti-epileptics whose pharmacodynamics may not be well established.

Valproate usually has no enzyme-inducing effect; as a consequence, valproate does not reduce efficacy of oestroprogestative agents in women receiving hormonal contraception, including the oral contraceptive pill.

4.6 Pregnancy and lactation

4.6.1 Pregnancy

From experience in treating mothers with epilepsy, the risk associated with the use of valproate during pregnancy has been described as follows:

- Risk associated with epilepsy and antiepileptics

In offspring born to mothers with epilepsy receiving any anti-epileptic treatment, the overall rate of malformations has been demonstrated to be 2 to 3 times higher than the rate (approximately 3 %) reported in the general population. Although an increased number of children with malformations have been reported in cases of multiple drug therapy, the respective role of treatments and disease in causing the malformations has not been formally established. Malformations most frequently encountered are cleft lip and cardio-vascular malformations.

Epidemiological studies have suggested an association between in-utero exposure to sodium valproate and a risk of developmental delay. Many factors including maternal epilepsy may also contribute to this risk but it is difficult to quantify the relative contributions of these or of maternal anti-epileptic treatment. Notwithstanding those potential risks, no sudden discontinuation in the anti-epileptic therapy should be undertaken as this may lead to breakthrough seizures which could have serious consequences for both the mother and the foetus.

- Risk associated with valproate

In animals: teratogenic effects have been demonstrated in the mouse, rat and rabbit.

There is animal experimental evidence that high plasma peak levels and the size of an individual dose are associated with neural tube defects.

In humans: an increased incidence of congenital abnormalities (including cases of facial dysmorphia, hypospadias and multiple malformations, particularly of the limbs) has been demonstrated in offspring born to mothers with epilepsy treated with valproate.

Valproate use is associated with neural tube defects such as myelomeningocele and spina bifida. The frequency of this effect is estimated to be 1 to 2%.

- In view of the above data

When a woman is planning pregnancy, this provides an opportunity to review the need for anti-epileptic treatment. Women of childbearing age should be informed of the risks and benefits of continuing anti-epileptic treatment throughout pregnancy.

Folate supplementation, **prior** to pregnancy, has been demonstrated to reduce the incidence of neural tube defects in the offspring of women at high risk. Although no direct evidence exists of such effects in women receiving anti-epileptic drugs, women should be advised to start taking folic acid supplementation (5mg) as soon as contraception is discontinued.

The available evidence suggests that anticonvulsant monotherapy is preferred. Dosage should be reviewed before conception and the lowest effective dose used, in divided doses, as abnormal pregnancy outcome tends to be associated with higher total daily dosage and with the size of an individual dose. The incidence of neural tube defects rises with increasing dosage, particularly above 1000mg daily. The administration in several divided doses over the day and the use of a prolonged release formulation is preferable in order to avoid high peak plasma levels.

During pregnancy, valproate anti-epileptic treatment should not be discontinued if it has been effective.

Nevertheless, specialised prenatal monitoring should be instituted in order to detect the possible occurrence of a neural tube defect or any other malformation. Pregnancies should be carefully screened by ultrasound, and other techniques if appropriate (see Section 4.4 Special Warnings and Special Precautions for use).

- Risk in the neonate

Very rare cases of haemorrhagic syndrome have been reported in neonates whose mothers have taken valproate during pregnancy. This haemorrhagic syndrome is related to hypofibrinogenemia; afibrinogenemia has also been reported and may be fatal. These are possibly associated with a decrease of coagulation factors. However, this syndrome has to be distinguished from the decrease of the vitamin-K factors induced by phenobarbitone and other anti-epileptic enzyme inducing drugs.

Therefore, platelet count, fibrinogen plasma level, coagulation tests and coagulation factors should be investigated in neonates.

4.6.2 Lactation

Excretion of valproate in breast milk is low, with a concentration between 1 % to 10 % of total maternal serum levels; up to now children breast fed that have been monitored during the neonatal period have not experienced clinical effects. There appears to be no contra-indication to breast feeding by patients on valproate.

4.7 Effects on ability to drive and use machines

Not applicable - use of intravenous formulation restricted to patients unable to take oral therapy. However, note use of Epilim may provide seizure control such that the patient may again be eligible to hold a driving licence.

Patients should be warned of the risk of transient drowsiness, especially in cases of anticonvulsant polytherapy or association with benzodiazepines (see section 4.5 Interactions with Other Medicaments and Other Forms of Interaction).

4.8 Undesirable effects

Congenital and familial/genetic disorders: (see section 4.6 Pregnancy and Lactation)

Hepato-biliary disorders: rare cases of liver dysfunction (see section 4.4.1 Warnings) Severe liver damage, including hepatic failure sometimes resulting in death, has been reported (see also sections 4.2, 4.3 and 4.4.1). Increased liver enzymes are common, particularly early in treatment, and may be transient (see section 4.4.1).

Gastrointestinal disorders (nausea, gastralgia, diarrhoea) frequently occur at the start of treatment. These problems can usually be overcome by taking Epilim with or after food or by using Enteric Coated Epilim.

Very rare cases of pancreatitis, sometimes lethal, have been reported (see section 4.4 Special Warnings and Special Precautions for Use).

Nervous system disorders:

Sedation has been reported occasionally, usually when in combination with other anticonvulsants. In monotherapy it occurred early in treatment on rare occasions and is usually transient. Rare cases of lethargy and confusion occasionally progressing to stupor, sometimes with associated hallucinations or convulsions have been reported. Encephalopathy and coma have very rarely been observed. These cases have often been associated with too high a starting dose or too rapid a dose escalation or concomitant use of other anticonvulsants, notably phenobarbitone. They have usually been reversible on withdrawal of treatment or reduction of dosage.

Very rare cases of reversible extrapyramidal symptoms including parkinsonism, or reversible dementia associated with reversible cerebral atrophy have been reported. Dose-related ataxia and fine postural tremor have occasionally been reported.

An increase in alertness may occur; this is generally beneficial but occasionally aggression, hyperactivity and behavioural deterioration have been reported.

Metabolic disorders:

Cases of isolated and moderate hyperammonaemia without change in liver function tests may occur frequently, are usually transient and should not cause treatment discontinuation. However, they may present clinically as vomiting, ataxia, and increasing clouding of consciousness. Should these symptoms occur Epilim should be discontinued.

Hyperammonaemia associated with neurological symptoms has also been reported (see section 4.4.2 Precautions). In such cases further investigations should be considered.

Blood and lymphatic system disorders:

Frequent occurrence of thrombocytopenia, rare cases of anaemia, leucopenia or pancytopenia. The blood picture returned to normal when the drug was discontinued.

Isolated reduction of fibrinogen or reversible increase in bleeding time have been reported, usually without associated clinical signs and particularly with high doses (sodium valproate has an inhibitory effect on the second phase of platelet aggregation). Spontaneous bruising or bleeding is an indication for withdrawal of medication pending investigations (see also section 4.6 Pregnancy and Lactation).

Skin and subcutaneous tissue disorders:

Cutaneous reactions such as exanthematous rash rarely occur with valproate. In very rare cases toxic epidermal necrolysis, Stevens-Johnson syndrome and erythema multiforme have been reported.

Transient hair loss, which may sometimes be dose-related, has often been reported. Regrowth normally begins within six months, although the hair may become more curly than previously. Hirsutism and acne have been very rarely reported.

Reproductive system and breast disorders:

Amenorrhoea and irregular periods have been reported. Very rarely gynaecomastia has occurred.

Vascular disorders: The occurrence of vasculitis has occasionally been reported.

Ear disorders:

Hearing loss, either reversible or irreversible has been reported rarely; however a cause and effect relationship has not been established.

Renal and urinary disorders:

There have been isolated reports of a reversible Fanconi's syndrome (a defect in proximal renal tubular function giving rise to glycosuria, amino aciduria, phosphaturia, and uricosuria) associated with valproate therapy, but the mode of action is as yet unclear.

Immune system disorders:

Allergic reactions (ranging from rash to hypersensitivity reactions) have been reported.

General disorders and administration site conditions:

Very rare cases of non-severe peripheral oedema have been reported.

Increase in weight may also occur. Weight gain being a risk factor for polycystic ovary syndrome, it should be carefully monitored (see section 4.4 Special Warnings and Special Precautions for Use).

When using Epilim intravenously, nausea or dizziness may occur a few minutes after injection; they disappear spontaneously within a few minutes.

4.9 Overdose

Cases of accidental and deliberate valproate overdosage have been reported. At plasma concentrations of up to 5 to 6 times the maximum therapeutic levels, there are unlikely to be any symptoms other than nausea, vomiting and dizziness.

Clinical signs of massive overdose, i.e. plasma concentration 10 to 20 times maximum therapeutic levels, usually include CNS depression or coma with muscular hypotonia, hyporeflexia, miosis, impaired respiratory function.

Symptoms may however be variable and seizures have been reported in the presence of very high plasma levels (see also section 5.2 Pharmacokinetic Properties).

Cases of intracranial hypertension related to cerebral oedema have been reported.

Hospital management of overdose should be symptomatic, including cardio-respiratory monitoring. Gastric lavage may be useful up to 10 to 12 hours following ingestion.

Haemodialysis and haemoperfusion have been used successfully.

Naloxone has been successfully used in a few isolated cases, sometimes in association with activated charcoal given orally. Deaths have occurred following massive overdose; nevertheless, a favourable outcome is usual.

5. PHARMACOLOGICAL PROPERTIES

5.1 Pharmacodynamic properties

Sodium valproate is an anticonvulsant.

In certain *in-vitro* studies it was reported that sodium valproate could stimulate HIV replication but studies on peripheral blood mononuclear cells from HIV-infected subjects show that sodium valproate does not have a mitogen-like effect on inducing HIV replication. Indeed the effect of sodium valproate on HIV replication *ex-vivo* is highly variable, modest in quantity, appears to be unrelated to the dose and has not been documented in man.

5.2 Pharmacokinetic properties

The half-life of sodium valproate is usually reported to be within the range 8-20 hours. It is usually shorter in children.

In patients with severe renal insufficiency it may be necessary to alter dosage in accordance with free plasma valproic acid levels.

The reported effective therapeutic range for plasma valproic acid levels is 40-100mg/litre (278-694 micromol/litre). This reported range may depend on time of sampling and presence of co-medication. The percentage of free (unbound) drug is usually between 6% and 15% of the total plasma levels. An increased incidence of adverse effects may occur with plasma levels above the effective therapeutic range.

The pharmacological (or therapeutic) effects of Epilim may not be clearly correlated with the total or free (unbound) plasma valproic acid levels.

5.3 Preclinical safety data

There are no pre-clinical data of relevance to the prescriber which are additional to that already included in other sections of the SPC.

6. PHARMACEUTICAL PARTICULARS

6.1 List of excipients

None.

6.2 Incompatibilities

Epilim Intravenous should not be administered via the same line as other IV additives.

6.3 Shelf life

36 months as unopened vial of freeze-dried powder. 24 hours after reconstitution and dilution for use as infusion solution (See Section 6.4 and 6.6).

6.4 Special precautions for storage

Epilim freeze-dried powder should be stored below 25°C. Reconstituted infusion solutions: at 2-8°C if stored before use, discarding any remaining solution after 24 hours.

6.5 Nature and contents of container

Colourless glass vial (Type I) with chlorobutyl rubber closure and crimped with an aluminium cap. The vial is supplied packed in a cardboard carton along with one ampoule containing 4ml of solvent (Water for Injection).

6.6 Instructions for use and handling

For intravenous use, the reconstituted solution should be used immediately and any unused portion discarded.

If the reconstituted solution is further diluted for use as an infusion solution, the dilute solution may be stored for up to 24 hours if kept at 2 to 8°C before use, discarding any remaining after 24 hours.

7. MARKETING AUTHORISATION HOLDER

Sanofi-Synthelabo
PO Box 597
Guildford
Surrey

8. MARKETING AUTHORISATION NUMBER(S)

PL 11723/0022

9. DATE OF FIRST AUTHORISATION/RENEWAL OF THE AUTHORISATION

18 August 1993

10. DATE OF REVISION OF THE TEXT

January 2004

Legal Category: POM

Epinephrine (Adrenaline) Injection 1,1000 Minijet

(International Medication Systems (UK) Ltd)

1. NAME OF THE MEDICINAL PRODUCT

Epinephrine (Adrenaline) Injection 1:1,000 Minijet.

2. QUALITATIVE AND QUANTITATIVE COMPOSITION

Epinephrine 1mg per ml.

3. PHARMACEUTICAL FORM

Sterile aqueous solution for intramuscular or subcutaneous administration.

4. CLINICAL PARTICULARS

4.1 Therapeutic indications

Emergency treatment of anaphylaxis or acute angioneurotic oedema with airways obstruction, or acute allergic reactions.

4.2 Posology and method of administration

For the relief of life-threatening angioneurotic oedema and anaphylactic shock, epinephrine should be administered by intramuscular injection.

For acute allergic reactions due to insect stings etc.: Intramuscular or subcutaneous injection.

The presentation with the 0.25″ integral needle is intended for self-administration by the subcutaneous route and the presentation with the 1.5″ integral needle is for paramedic use by subcutaneous or intramuscular injection.

Adults and children over 12 years: 0.5 ml (0.5 mg), administered slowly. The dose may be repeated every 5 to 15 minutes as needed.

This presentation may not be suitable for small or prepubertal patients over 12 years of age who require a smaller dose.

Elderly: as for adults, use with caution.

Children (up to age of 12): not recommended

4.3 Contraindications

Contraindications are relative as this product is intended for use in life-threatening emergencies.

Other than in the emergency situation, the following contraindications should be considered: hyperthyroidism, hypertension, ischaemic heart disease, diabetes mellitus, and closed angle glaucoma.

4.4 Special warnings and special precautions for use

These special warnings and precautions are relative as this product is intended for use in life-threatening situations.

Administer slowly with caution to elderly patients and to patients with ischaemic heart disease, hypertension, diabetes mellitus, hyperthyroidism or psychoneurosis. Anginal pain may be induced when coronary insufficiency is present. Use with caution in patients with closed angle glaucoma.

4.5 Interaction with other medicinal products and other forms of Interaction

The effects of epinephrine may be potentiated by tricyclic antidepressants. Halothane and other anaesthetics such as cyclopropane and trichloroethylene increase the risk of epinephrine -induced ventricular arrhythmias and acute pulmonary oedema if hypoxia is present. Severe hypertension and bradycardia may occur with non-selective beta-blocking drugs such as propranolol. Propranolol also inhibits the bronchodilator effect of epinephrine. The risk of cardiac arrhythmias is higher when epinephrine is given to patients receiving digoxin, quinidine, fluorohydrocarbons or cocaine. Epinephrine -induced hyperglycaemia may lead to loss of blood-sugar control in diabetic patients treated with hypoglycaemic agents.

The vasoconstrictor and pressor effects of epinephrine, mediated by its alpha-adrenergic action, may be enhanced by concomitant administration of drugs with similar effects, such as ergot alkaloids or oxytocin. Epinephrine specifically reverses the antihypertensive effects of adrenergic neurone blockers such as guanethidine with the risk of severe hypertension.

4.6 Pregnancy and lactation

Epinephrine crosses the placenta. There is some evidence of a slightly increased incidence of congenital abnormalities. Injection of epinephrine may cause foetal tachycardia, cardiac irregularities, extrasystoles and louder heart sounds. In labour, epinephrine may delay the second stage. Epinephrine should only be used in pregnancy if the potential benefits outweigh the risks to the foetus.

Epinephrine is excreted in breast milk, but as pharmacologically active plasma concentrations are not achieved by the oral route, the use of epinephrine in breast-feeding mothers is presumed to be safe.

4.7 Effects on ability to drive and use machines

Not applicable; this preparation is intended for use only in emergencies.

4.8 Undesirable effects

The potentially severe adverse effects of epinephrine arise from its effect upon blood pressure and cardiac rhythm. Ventricular fibrillation may occur and severe hypertension may lead to cerebral haemorrhage and pulmonary oedema. Symptomatic adverse effects are anxiety, dyspnoea, restlessness, palpitations, tachycardia, tremor, weakness, dizziness, headache, cold extremities, nausea, vomiting, sweating, local ischaemic necrosis. Biochemical effects include inhibition of insulin secretion and hyperglycaemia even with low doses, gluconeogenesis, glycolysis, lipolysis and ketogenesis.

4.9 Overdose

Symptoms: cardiac arrhythmias leading to ventricular fibrillation and death, severe hypertension leading to pulmonary oedema and cerebral haemorrhage.

Treatment: combined alpha- and beta-adrenergic blocking agents such as labetalol may counteract the effects of epinephrine, or a beta-blocking agent may be used to treat any supraventricular arrhythmias and phentolamine to control the alpha-mediated effects on the peripheral circulation. Rapidly acting vasodilators such as nitrates and sodium nitroprusside may also be helpful.

Immediate resuscitation support must be available.

5. PHARMACOLOGICAL PROPERTIES

5.1 Pharmacodynamic properties

Epinephrine is a direct-acting sympathomimetic agent exerting its effect on alpha- and beta-adrenoceptors. Major effects are increased systolic blood pressure, reduced diastolic pressure, tachycardia, hyperglycaemia and hypokalaemia. It is a powerful cardiac stimulant. It has vasopressor properties and is a bronchodilator.

5.2 Pharmacokinetic properties

Epinephrine is rapid in onset and of short duration and is rapidly distributed to the heart, spleen, several glandular tissues and adrenergic nerves. It crosses the placenta and is excreted in breast milk. It is approximately 50% bound to plasma proteins. The onset of action is rapid and after i.v. infusion the half-life is approximately 5-10 minutes.

Epinephrine is rapidly metabolised in the liver and tissues by oxidative deamination and O-methylation followed by reduction or by conjugation with glucuronic acid or sulphate. Up to 90% of the i.v. dose is excreted in the urine as metabolites.

5.3 Preclinical safety data

Not applicable since Epinephrine (Adrenaline) Injection has been used in clinical practice for many years and its effects in man are well known.

6. PHARMACEUTICAL PARTICULARS

6.1 List of excipients

Citric Acid Monohydrate
Sodium Citrate Dihydrate
Sodium Chloride
Sodium Bisulphite
Hydrochloric Acid 10% w/v
Water for Injection

6.2 Incompatibilities

Epinephrine should not be mixed with sodium bicarbonate; the solution is oxidised to adrenochrome and then forms polymers.

6.3 Shelf life

9 months.

6.4 Special precautions for storage

Store below 25°C. Protect from light.

6.5 Nature and contents of container

The solution is contained in a USP type I glass vial with an elastomeric closure which meets all the relevant USP specifications. Two presentations are available; one for patient self-administration with a 0.25″ integral needle and one for paramedic use with a 1.5″ integral needle. Both are 1ml presentations.

6.6 Instructions for use and handling

The container is specially designed for use with the IMS Minijet injector.

7. MARKETING AUTHORISATION HOLDER

International Medication Systems (UK) Limited
208 Bath Road
Slough
Berkshire
SL1 3WE
UK

8. MARKETING AUTHORISATION NUMBER(S)

PL 03265/0030

9. DATE OF FIRST AUTHORISATION/RENEWAL OF THE AUTHORISATION

Date first granted: 8 February 1978

Date renewed: 31 August 2000

10. DATE OF REVISION OF THE TEXT

August 2001

POM

Epinephrine (Adrenaline) Injection 1:10,000

(International Medication Systems (UK) Ltd)

1. NAME OF THE MEDICINAL PRODUCT

Adrenaline (Epinephrine) 1:10,000 Sterile Solution Minijet®.

2. QUALITATIVE AND QUANTITATIVE COMPOSITION

Adrenaline (Epinephrine) USP 0.1mg per ml.

3. PHARMACEUTICAL FORM

Sterile aqueous solution for parenteral administration.

4. CLINICAL PARTICULARS

4.1 Therapeutic indications

Adjunctive use in the management of cardiac arrest.

In cardiopulmonary resuscitation. Intracardiac puncture and intramyocardial injection of adrenaline may be effective when external cardiac compression and attempts to restore the circulation by electrical defibrillation or use of a pacemaker fail.

4.2 Posology and method of administration

Ventricular fibrillation (pulseless ventricular tachycardia)

Adults:

Intravenous injection: 10ml (1mg) by intravenous injection repeated every 2-3 minutes as necessary.

Endotracheal: 20-30ml (2-3mg) via an endotracheal tube, repeated as necessary.

Intracardiac injection: 1 to 10ml (0.1 to 1mg), direct into the atrium of the heart.

Intracardiac injection should only be considered if there is no other access available. It should be undertaken by personnel trained in the technique.

Children:

Intravenous injection: Initially 0.1ml/kg body weight (10mcg/kg); e.g. 2kg infant would receive 0.2ml of Adrenaline 1:10,000. Subsequent doses should be 1ml/kg (100mcg/kg).

Intraosseous: 0.1ml/kg body weight (10mcg/kg).

Endotracheal: A dose has not been established; 10 times the intravenous dose may be appropriate.

Asystole

Adults:

Intravenous: 10ml (1mg) by intravenous injection repeated every 2-3 minutes as necessary. If there is no response after three cycles, consider injections of adrenaline 5mg.

Endotracheal: 20-30 ml (2-3mg) via an endotracheal tube, repeated as necessary.

Children:

Intravenous: 0.1ml/kg initially (10mcg/kg). If no response give 1ml/kg (100mcg/kg). After 3 cycles consider alkalising or antiarrhythmic agents.

Intraosseus: 0.1 ml/kg initially (10mcg/kg). If no response give 1ml/kg (100mcg/kg). After 3 cycles consider alkalising or antiarrhythmic agents.

Electromechanical Dissociation (EMD)

Adults:

Intravenous: 10ml (1mg) by intravenous injection repeated every 2-3 minutes as necessary. If normal rhythm does not return after standard measures, consider adrenaline 5mg intravenous.

Children:

Intravenous: 0.1ml/kg initially (10mcg/kg) every 3 minutes, until underlying cause identified. Subsequent doses should be 1ml/kg (100mcg/kg).

4.3 Contraindications

Contraindications are relative as this product is intended for use in life-threatening emergencies.

Other than in the emergency situation, the following contraindications should be considered: hyperthyroidism, hypertension, ischaemic heart disease, diabetes mellitus and closed angle glaucoma.

4.4 Special warnings and special precautions for use

These special warnings and precautions are relative as this product is intended for use in life-threatening situations.

Administer slowly with caution to elderly patients and to patients with ischaemic heart disease, hypertension, diabetes mellitus, hyperthyroidism or psychoneurosis. Use with extreme caution in patients with long-standing bronchial asthma and emphysema who have developed degenerative heart disease. Anginal pain may be induced when coronary insufficiency is present.

4.5 Interaction with other medicinal products and other forms of Interaction

The effects of adrenaline may be potentiated by tricyclic antidepressants. Halothane can increase the risk of adrenaline-induced ventricular arrhythmias and acute pulmonary oedema if hypoxia is present. Severe hypertension and bradycardia may occur with non-selective beta-blocking drugs such as propranolol. Propranolol also inhibits the bronchodilator effect of adrenaline. The risk of cardiac arrhythmias is higher when adrenaline is given to patients receiving digoxin or quinidine. Adrenaline -induced hyperglycaemia may lead to loss of blood-sugar control in diabetic patients treated with hypoglycaemic agents.

4.6 Pregnancy and lactation

Adrenaline crosses the placenta. There is some evidence of a slightly increased incidence of congenital abnormalities. Injection of adrenaline may cause foetal tachycardia, cardiac irregularities, extrasystoles and louder heart sounds. In labour, adrenaline may delay the second stage. Adrenaline should only be used in pregnancy if the potential benefits outweigh the risks to the foetus.

Adrenaline is excreted in breast milk, but as pharmacologically active plasma concentrations are not achieved by the oral route, the use of adrenaline in breast feeding mothers is presumed to be safe.

4.7 Effects on ability to drive and use machines

Not applicable; this preparation is intended for use only in emergencies.

4.8 Undesirable effects

The potentially severe adverse effects of adrenaline arise from its effect upon blood pressure and cardiac rhythm. Ventricular fibrillation may occur and severe hypertension may lead to cerebral haemorrhage and pulmonary oedema. Symptomatic adverse effects are anxiety, dyspnoea, restlessness, palpitations, tachycardia, tremor, weakness, dizziness, headache and cold extremities. Biochemical effects include inhibition of insulin secretion, stimulation of growth hormone secretion, hyperglycaemia (even with low doses), gluconeogenesis, glycolysis, lipolysis and ketogenesis.

4.9 Overdose

Symptoms: cardiac arrhythmias leading to ventricular fibrillation and death; severe hypertension leading to pulmonary oedema and cerebral haemorrhage.

Treatment: combined alpha- and beta-adrenergic blocking agents such as labetalol may counteract the effects of adrenaline, or a beta-blocking agent may be used to treat any supraventricular arrhythmias and phentolamine to control the alpha-mediated effects on the peripheral circulation. Rapidly acting vasodilators such as nitrates and sodium nitroprusside may also be helpful.

Immediate resuscitation support must be available.

5. PHARMACOLOGICAL PROPERTIES

5.1 Pharmacodynamic properties

Adrenaline is a direct-acting sympathomimetic agent exerting its effect on alpha- and beta-adrenoceptors. The overall effect of adrenaline depends on the dose used, and may be complicated by the homeostatic reflex responses. In resuscitation procedures it is used to increase the efficacy of basic life support. It is a positive cardiac inotrope. Major effects are increased systolic blood pressure, reduced diastolic pressure(increased at higher doses), tachycardia, hyperglycaemia and hypokalaemia.

5.2 Pharmacokinetic properties

Adrenaline is rapid in onset and of short duration. After i.v. infusion the half-life is approximately 5-10 minutes. It is rapidly distributed to the heart, spleen, several glandular tissues and adrenergic nerves. It crosses the placenta and is excreted in breast milk. It is approximately 50% bound to plasma proteins.

Adrenaline is rapidly metabolised in the liver and tissues by oxidative deamination and O-methylation followed by reduction or by conjugation with glucuronic acid or sulphate. Up to 90% of the i.v. dose is excreted in the urine as metabolites.

5.3 Preclinical safety data

Not applicable since Adrenaline (Epinephrine) Injection has been used in clinical practice for many years and its effects in man are well known.

6. PHARMACEUTICAL PARTICULARS

6.1 List of excipients

Citric Acid Monohydrate
Sodium Citrate Dihydrate
Sodium Chloride
Sodium Bisulphite
Hydrochloric Acid 10%w/v
Water for Injection

6.2 Incompatibilities

Adrenaline should not be mixed with sodium bicarbonate; the solution is oxidised to adrenochrome and then forms polymers.

6.3 Shelf life

3ml - 18 months.

10ml - 24 months.

6.4 Special precautions for storage

Do not store above 25°C. Keep container in outer carton.

6.5 Nature and contents of container

The solution is contained in a USP type I glass vial with an elastomeric closure which meets all the relevant USP specifications. The product is available either as 3ml or 10ml.

6.6 Instructions for use and handling

The container is specially designed for use with the IMS Minijet injector.

7. MARKETING AUTHORISATION HOLDER

International Medication Systems (UK) Ltd
208 Bath Road
Slough
Berkshire
SL1 3WE
UK

8. MARKETING AUTHORISATION NUMBER(S)

PL 03265/0011R

9. DATE OF FIRST AUTHORISATION/RENEWAL OF THE AUTHORISATION

21 March 1991 / 30 August 2001

10. DATE OF REVISION OF THE TEXT

December 2004

POM

Epivir 150 mg film-coated tablets

(GlaxoSmithKline UK)

1. NAME OF THE MEDICINAL PRODUCT

Epivir 150 mg film-coated tablets

2. QUALITATIVE AND QUANTITATIVE COMPOSITION

Each film-coated tablet contains 150 mg lamivudine.

For excipients see section 6.1.

3. PHARMACEUTICAL FORM

Film-coated tablet

The film-coated tablets are white, diamond shaped and engraved with "GX CJ7" on one face.

4. CLINICAL PARTICULARS

4.1 Therapeutic indications

Epivir is indicated as part of antiretroviral combination therapy for the treatment of Human Immunodeficiency Virus (HIV) infected adults and children.

4.2 Posology and method of administration

The therapy should be initiated by a physician experienced in the management of HIV infection.

Adults and adolescents over 12 years of age: the recommended dose of Epivir is 300 mg daily. This may be administered as either 150 mg twice daily or 300 mg once daily (see section 4.4). The 300 mg tablet is only suitable for the once a day regimen.

Patients changing to the once daily regimen should take 150 mg twice a day and switch to 300 mg once a day the following morning. Where an evening once daily regimen is preferred, 150 mg of Epivir should be taken on the first morning only, followed by 300 mg in the evening. When changing back to a twice daily regimen patients should complete the days treatment and start 150 mg twice a day the following morning.

Children:

Three months to 12 years of age: the recommended dose is 4 mg/kg twice daily up to a maximum of 300 mg daily.

Less than three months of age: the limited data available are insufficient to propose specific dosage recommendations (see section 5.2).

Epivir is also available as an oral solution.

Epivir may be administered with or without food.

Renal impairment:- Lamivudine concentrations are increased in patients with moderate - severe renal impairment due to decreased clearance. The dose should therefore be adjusted, using oral solution presentation of Epivir for patients whose creatinine clearance falls below 30 ml/min (see tables).

Dosing Recommendations – Adults and adolescents over 12 years:

Creatinine Clearance (ml/min)	First Dose	Maintenance Dose
≥50	150 mg	150 mg Twice daily
30-<50	150 mg	150 mg Once daily
<30	As doses below 150 mg are needed the use of the oral solution is recommended	

There are no data available on the use of lamivudine in children with renal impairment. Based on the assumption that creatinine clearance and lamivudine clearance are correlated similarly in children as in adults it is recommended that the dosage in children with renal impairment be reduced according to their creatinine clearance by the same proportion as in adults.

Dosing Recommendations – Children from 3 months to 12 years:

Creatinine Clearance (ml/min)	First Dose	Maintenance Dose
≥50	4 mg/kg	4 mg/kg twice daily
30 to <50	4 mg/kg	4 mg/kg once daily
15 to <30	4 mg/kg	2.6 mg/kg once daily
5 to <15	4 mg/kg	1.3 mg/kg once daily
<5	1.3 mg/kg	0.7 mg/kg once daily

Hepatic Impairment: Data obtained in patients with moderate to severe hepatic impairment shows that lamivudine pharmacokinetics are not significantly affected by hepatic dysfunction. Based on these data, no dose adjustment is necessary in patients with moderate or severe hepatic impairment unless accompanied by renal impairment.

4.3 Contraindications

Hypersensitivity to lamivudine or to any of the excipients.

4.4 Special warnings and special precautions for use

Epivir is not recommended for use as monotherapy.

Renal impairment: In patients with moderate to severe renal impairment, the terminal plasma half-life of lamivudine is increased due to decreased clearance, therefore the dose should be adjusted (See section 4.2).

Once daily dosing (300 mg once a day): a clinical study has demonstrated the non inferiority between Epivir once a day and Epivir twice a day containing regimens. These, results were obtained in an antiretroviral naïve-population, primarily consisting of asymptomatic HIV infected patients (CDC stage A).

Triple nucleoside therapy: There have been reports of a high rate of virological failure and of emergence of resistance at an early stage when lamivudine was combined with tenofovir disoproxil fumarate and abacavir as well as with tenofovir disoproxil fumarate and didanosine as a once daily regimen.

Opportunistic infections: Patients receiving Epivir or any other antiretroviral therapy may continue to develop opportunistic infections and other complications of HIV infection, and therefore should remain under close clinical observation by physicians experienced in the treatment of patients with associated HIV diseases.

Transmission of HIV: Patients should be advised that current antiretroviral therapy, including Epivir, has not been proven to prevent the risk of transmission of HIV to others through sexual contact or blood contamination. Appropriate precautions should continue to be taken.

Pancreatitis: Cases of pancreatitis have occurred rarely. However it is not clear whether these cases were due to the antiretroviral treatment or to the underlying HIV disease. Treatment with Epivir should be stopped immediately if clinical signs, symptoms or laboratory abnormalities suggestive of pancreatitis occur.

Lactic acidosis: lactic acidosis, usually associated with hepatomegaly and hepatic steatosis, has been reported with the use of nucleoside analogues. Early symptoms (symptomatic hyperlactatemia) include benign digestive symptoms (nausea, vomiting and abdominal pain), non-specific malaise, loss of appetite, weight loss, respiratory symptoms (rapid and/or deep breathing) or neurological symptoms (including motor weakness).

Lactic acidosis has a high mortality and may be associated with pancreatitis, liver failure, or renal failure.

Lactic acidosis generally occurred after a few or several months of treatment.

Treatment with nucleoside analogues should be discontinued in the setting of symptomatic hyperlactatemia and metabolic/lactic acidosis, progressive hepatomegaly, or rapidly elevating aminotransferase levels.

Caution should be exercised when administering nucleoside analogues to any patient (particularly obese women) with hepatomegaly, hepatitis or other known risk factors for liver disease and hepatic steatosis (including certain medicinal products and alcohol). Patients co-infected with hepatitis C and treated with alpha interferon and ribavirin may constitute a special risk.

Patients at increased risk should be followed closely.

Mitochondrial dysfunction: Nucleoside and nucleotide analogues have been demonstrated *in vitro* and *in vivo* to cause a variable degree of mitochondrial damage. There have been reports of mitochondrial dysfunction in HIV-negative infants exposed *in utero* and/or post-natally to nucleoside analogues. The main adverse events reported are haematological disorders (anaemia, neutropenia), metabolic disorders (hyperlactatemia, hyperlipasemia). These events are often transitory. Some late-onset neurological disorders have been reported (hypertonia, convulsion, abnormal behaviour). Whether the neurological disorders are transient or permanent is currently unknown. Any child exposed *in utero* to nucleoside and nucleotide analogues, even HIV-negative children, should have clinical and laboratory follow-up and should be fully investigated for possible mitochondrial dysfunction in case of relevant signs or symptoms. These findings do not affect current national recommendations to use antiretroviral therapy in pregnant women to prevent vertical transmission of HIV.

Lipodystrophy: Combination antiretroviral therapy has been associated with the redistribution of body fat (lipodystrophy) in HIV patients. The long-term consequences of these events are currently unknown. Knowledge about the mechanism is incomplete. A connection between visceral lipomatosis and protease inhibitors (PIs) and lipoatrophy and nucleoside reverse transcriptase inhibitors (NRTIs) has been hypothesised. A higher risk of lipodystrophy has been associated with individual factors such as older age, and with drug related factors such as longer duration of antiretroviral treatment and associated metabolic disturbances. Clinical examination should include evaluation for physical signs of fat redistribution. Consideration should be given to the measurement of fasting serum lipids and blood glucose. Lipid disorders should be managed as clinically appropriate (see section 4.8).

Immune Reactivation Syndrome: In HIV-infected patients with severe immune deficiency at the time of institution of combination antiretroviral therapy (CART), an inflammatory reaction to asymptomatic or residual opportunistic pathogens may arise and cause serious clinical conditions, or aggravation of symptoms. Typically, such reactions have been observed within the first few weeks or months of initiation of CART. Relevant examples are cytomegalovirus retinitis, generalised and/or focal mycobacterium infections, and *Pneumocystis carinii* pneumonia. Any inflammatory symptoms should be evaluated and treatment instituted when necessary.

Liver disease: If lamivudine is being used concomitantly for the treatment of HIV and HBV, additional information relating to the use of lamivudine in the treatment of hepatitis B infection is available in the Zeffix SPC.

Patients with chronic hepatitis B or C and treated with combination antiretroviral therapy are at an increased risk of severe and potentially fatal hepatic adverse events. In case of concomitant antiviral therapy for hepatitis B or C, please refer also to the relevant product information for these medicinal products.

If Epivir is discontinued in patients co-infected with hepatitis B virus, periodic monitoring of liver function tests and markers of HBV replication is recommended, as withdrawal of lamivudine may result in an acute exacerbation of hepatitis (see Zeffix SPC).

Patients with pre-existing liver dysfunction, including chronic active hepatitis, have an increased frequency of liver function abnormalities during combination antiretroviral therapy, and should be monitored according to standard practice. If there is evidence of worsening liver disease in such patients, interruption or discontinuation of treatment must be considered.

4.5 Interaction with other medicinal products and other forms of Interaction

The likelihood of metabolic interactions is low due to limited metabolism and plasma protein binding and almost complete renal clearance.

A modest increase in C_{max} (28 %) was observed for zidovudine when administered with lamivudine, however overall exposure (AUC) is not significantly altered. Zidovudine has no effect on the pharmacokinetics of lamivudine (see section 5.2).

The possibility of interactions with other medicinal products administered concurrently should be considered, particularly when the main route of elimination is active renal secretion via the organic cationic transport system e.g. trimethoprim. Other medicinal products (e.g. ranitidine, cimetidine) are eliminated only in part by this mechanism and were shown not to interact with lamivudine. The nucleoside analogues (e.g. didanosine and zalcitabine) like zidovudine, are not eliminated by this mechanism and are unlikely to interact with lamivudine.

Administration of trimethoprim/sulfamethoxazole 160 mg/800 mg results in a 40 % increase in lamivudine exposure, because of the trimethoprim component; the sulfamethoxazole component did not interact. However, unless the patient has renal impairment, no dosage adjustment of lamivudine is necessary (see section 4.2). Lamivudine has no effect on the pharmacokinetics of trimethoprim or sulfamethoxazole. When concomitant administration is warranted, patients should be monitored clinically. Co-administration of lamivudine with high doses of co-trimoxazole for the treatment of *Pneumocystis carinii* pneumonia (PCP) and toxoplasmosis should be avoided.

Lamivudine metabolism does not involve CYP3A, making interactions with medicinal products metabolised by this system (e.g. PIs) unlikely.

Co-administration of lamivudine with intravenous ganciclovir or foscarnet is not recommended until further information is available.

Lamivudine may inhibit the intracellular phosphorylation of zalcitabine when the two medicinal products are used concurrently. Epivir is therefore not recommended to be used in combination with zalcitabine.

4.6 Pregnancy and lactation

Pregnancy: The safety of lamivudine in human pregnancy has not been established. Reproductive studies in animals have not shown evidence of teratogenicity, and showed no effect on male or female fertility. Lamivudine induces early embryonic death when administered to pregnant rabbits at exposure levels comparable to those achieved in man. In humans, consistent with passive transmission of lamivudine across the placenta, lamivudine concentrations in infant serum at birth were similar to those in maternal and cord serum at delivery.

Although animal reproductive studies are not always predictive of the human response, administration is not recommended during the first three months of pregnancy.

Lactation: Following oral administration lamivudine was excreted in breast milk at similar concentrations to those found in serum. Since lamivudine and the virus pass into breast milk, it is recommended that mothers taking Epivir do not breast-feed their infants. It is recommended that HIV infected women do not breast-feed their infants under any circumstances in order to avoid transmission of HIV.

4.7 Effects on ability to drive and use machines

No studies on the effects on the ability to drive and use machines have been performed.

4.8 Undesirable effects

The following adverse events have been reported during therapy for HIV disease with Epivir. With many it is unclear whether they are related to Epivir, other medications taken concurrently or are as a result of the underlying disease process.

The adverse events considered at least possibly related to the treatment are listed below by body system, organ class and absolute frequency. Frequencies are defined as very common (>1/10), common (>1/100, <1/10), uncommon (>1/1,000, <1/100), rare (>1/10,000, <1/1,000), very rare (<1/10,000).

Blood and lymphatic systems disorders

Uncommon: Neutropenia and anaemia (both occasionally severe), thrombocytopenia

Very rare: Pure red cell aplasia

Nervous system disorders

Common: Headache, insomnia

Very rare: Cases of peripheral neuropathy (or paraesthesia) have been reported.

Respiratory, thoracic and mediastinal disorders

Common: Cough, nasal symptoms

Gastrointestinal disorders

Common: Nausea, vomiting, abdominal pain or cramps, diarrhoea

Rare: Rises in serum amylase. Cases of pancreatitis have been reported.

Hepatobiliary disorders

Uncommon: Transient rises in liver enzymes (AST, ALT).

Rare: Hepatitis

Skin and subcutaneous tissue disorders

Common: Rash, alopecia

Musculoskeletal and connective tissue disorders

Common: Arthralgia, muscle disorders

Rare: Rhabdomyolysis

General disorders and administration site conditions

Common: Fatigue, malaise, fever.

Cases of lactic acidosis, sometimes fatal, usually associated with severe hepatomegaly and hepatic steatosis, have been reported with the use of nucleoside analogues (see section 4.4).

Combination antiretroviral therapy has been associated with redistribution of body fat (lipodystrophy) in HIV patients including the loss of peripheral and facial subcutaneous fat, increased intra-abdominal and visceral fat, breast hypertrophy and dorsocervical fat accumulation (buffalo hump).

Combination antiretroviral therapy has been associated with metabolic abnormalities such as hypertriglyceridaemia, hypercholesterolaemia, insulin resistance, hyperglycaemia and hyperlactataemia (see section 4.4).

In HIV-infected patients with severe immune deficiency at the time of initiation of combination antiretroviral therapy (CART), an inflammatory reaction to asymptomatic or residual opportunistic infections may arise (see section 4.4).

4.9 Overdose

Administration of lamivudine at very high dose levels in acute animal studies did not result in any organ toxicity. Limited data are available on the consequences of ingestion of acute overdoses in humans. No fatalities occurred, and the patients recovered. No specific signs or symptoms have been identified following such overdose.

If overdosage occurs the patient should be monitored, and standard supportive treatment applied as required. Since lamivudine is dialysable, continuous haemodialysis could be used in the treatment of overdosage, although this has not been studied.

5. PHARMACOLOGICAL PROPERTIES

5.1 Pharmacodynamic properties

Pharmacotherapeutic group: nucleoside analogue, ATC Code: J05A F05.

Lamivudine is a nucleoside analogue which has activity against human immunodeficiency virus (HIV) and hepatitis B virus (HBV). It is metabolised intracellularly to the active moiety, lamivudine 5'-triphosphate. Its main mode of action is as a chain terminator of viral reverse transcription. The triphosphate has selective inhibitory activity against HIV-1 and HIV-2 replication *in vitro*, it is also active against zidovudine-resistant clinical isolates of HIV. Lamivudine in combination with zidovudine exhibits synergistic anti-HIV activity against clinical isolates in cell culture.

HIV-1 resistance to lamivudine involves the development of a M184V amino acid change close to the active site of the viral reverse transcriptase (RT). This variant arises both *in vitro* and in HIV-1 infected patients treated with lamivudine-containing antiretroviral therapy. M184V mutants display greatly reduced susceptibility to lamivudine and show diminished viral replicative capacity *in vitro*. *In vitro* studies indicate that zidovudine-resistant virus isolates can become zidovudine sensitive when they simultaneously acquire resistance to lamivudine. The clinical relevance of such findings remains, however, not well defined.

Cross-resistance conferred by the M184V RT is limited within the nucleoside inhibitor class of antiretroviral agents. Zidovudine and stavudine maintain their antiretroviral activities against lamivudine-resistant HIV-1. Abacavir maintains its antiretroviral activities against lamivudine-resistant HIV-1 harbouring only the M184V mutation. The M184V RT mutant shows a <4-fold decrease in susceptibility to didanosine and zalcitabine; the clinical significance of these findings is unknown. *In vitro* susceptibility testing has not been standardised and results may vary according to methodological factors.

Lamivudine demonstrates low cytotoxicity to peripheral blood lymphocytes, to established lymphocyte and monocyte-macrophage cell lines, and to a variety of bone marrow progenitor cells *in vitro*.

Clinical experience:

In clinical trials, lamivudine in combination with zidovudine has been shown to reduce HIV-1 viral load and increase CD4 cell count. Clinical end-point data indicate that lamivudine in combination with zidovudine, results in a significant reduction in the risk of disease progression and mortality.

Evidence from clinical studies shows that lamivudine plus zidovudine delays the emergence of zidovudine resistant isolates in individuals with no prior antiretroviral therapy.

Lamivudine has been widely used as a component of antiretroviral combination therapy with other antiretroviral agents of the same class (NRTIs) or different classes (PIs, non-nucleoside reverse transcriptase inhibitors).

Multiple drug antiretroviral therapy containing lamivudine has been shown to be effective in antiretrovirally-naive patients as well as in patients presenting with viruses containing the M184V mutations.

The relationship between *in vitro* susceptibility of HIV to lamivudine and clinical response to lamivudine-containing therapy remains under investigation.

Lamivudine at a dose of 100 mg once daily has also been shown to be effective for the treatment of adult patients with chronic HBV infection (for details of clinical studies, see the prescribing information for Zeffix). However, for the treatment of HIV infection only a 300 mg daily dose of lamivudine (in combination with other antiretroviral agents) has been shown to be efficacious.

Lamivudine has not been specifically investigated in HIV patients co-infected with HBV.

5.2 Pharmacokinetic properties

Absorption: Lamivudine is well absorbed from the gastrointestinal tract, and the bioavailability of oral lamivudine in adults is normally between 80 and 85 %. Following oral administration, the mean time (t_{max}) to maximal serum concentrations (C_{max}) is about an hour. Based on data derived from a study in healthy volunteers, at a therapeutic dose of 150mg twice daily, mean (CV) steady-state C_{max} and C_{min} of lamivudine in plasma are 1.2 μg/ml (24%) and 0.09 μg/ml (27%), respectively. The mean (CV) AUC over a dosing interval of 12 hours is 4.7 μg.h/ml (18%). At a therapeutic dose of 300mg once daily, the mean (CV) steady-state C_{max}, C_{min} and 24h AUC are 2.0 μg/ml (26%), 0.04 μg/ml (34%) and 8.9 μg.h/ml (21%), respectively.

The 150 mg tablet is bioequivalent and dose proportional to the 300 mg tablet with respect to AUC_{∞}, C_{max}, and t_{max}.

Co-administration of lamivudine with food results in a delay of t_{max} and a lower C_{max} (decreased by 47 %). However, the extent (based on the AUC) of lamivudine absorbed is not influenced.

Co-administration of zidovudine results in a 13 % increase in zidovudine exposure and a 28 % increase in peak plasma levels. This is not considered to be of significance to patient safety and therefore no dosage adjustments are necessary.

Distribution: From intravenous studies, the mean volume of distribution is 1.3 l/kg. The observed half-life of elimination is 5 to 7 hours. The mean systemic clearance of lamivudine is approximately

0.32 l/h/kg, with predominantly renal clearance > 70 %) via the organic cationic transport system.

Lamivudine exhibits linear pharmacokinetics over the therapeutic dose range and displays limited binding to the major plasma protein albumin (< 16 % - 36 % to serum albumin in *in vitro* studies).

Limited data show that lamivudine penetrates the central nervous system and reaches the cerebro-spinal fluid (CSF). The mean ratio CSF/serum lamivudine concentration 2-4 hours after oral administration was approximately 0.12. The true extent of penetration or relationship with any clinical efficacy is unknown.

Metabolism: The active moiety, intracellular lamivudine triphosphate, has a prolonged terminal half-life in the cell (16 to 19 hours) compared to the plasma lamivudine half-life (5 to 7 hours). In 60 healthy adult volunteers, Epivir 300 mg once daily has been demonstrated to be pharmacokinetically equivalent at steady-state to Epivir 150 mg twice daily with respect to intracellular triphosphate AUC_{24} and C_{max}.

Lamivudine is predominately cleared unchanged by renal excretion. The likelihood of metabolic interactions of lamivudine with other medicinal products is low due to the small extent of hepatic metabolism (5-10 %) and low plasma protein binding.

Elimination: Studies in patients with renal impairment show lamivudine elimination is affected by renal dysfunction. A recommended dosage regimen for patients with creatinine clearance below 50 ml/min is shown in the dosage section (see section 4.2).

An interaction with trimethoprim, a constituent of co-trimoxazole, causes a 40 % increase in lamivudine exposure at therapeutic doses. This does not require dose adjustment unless the patient also has renal impairment (see sections 4.5 and 4.2). Administration of co-trimoxazole with lamivudine in patients with renal impairment should be carefully assessed.

Pharmacokinetics in children: In general, lamivudine pharmacokinetics in paediatric patients is similar to adults. However, absolute bioavailability (approximately 55-65 %) was reduced in paediatric patients below 12 years of age. In addition, systemic clearance values were greater in younger paediatric patients and decreased with age, approaching adult values around 12 years of age. Due to these differences, the recommended dose for children from three months to 12 years is 8 mg/kg/day, which will achieve similar adult and paediatric exposure (average AUC approximately 5,000 ng.h/ml).

There are limited pharmacokinetic data for patients less than three months of age. In neonates one week of age, lamivudine oral clearance was reduced when compared to paediatric patients and is likely to be due to immature renal function and variable absorption. Therefore to achieve similar adult and paediatric exposure, the recommended dose for neonates is 4 mg/kg/day. Glomerular filtration estimates suggests that to achieve similar adult and paediatric exposure, the recommended dose for children aged six weeks and older could be 8 mg/kg/day.

Pharmacokinetics in pregnancy: Following oral administration, lamivudine pharmacokinetics in late-pregnancy were similar to non-pregnant women.

5.3 Preclinical safety data

Administration of lamivudine in animal toxicity studies at high doses was not associated with any major organ toxicity. At the highest dosage levels, minor effects on indicators of liver and kidney function were seen together with occasional reductions in liver weight. The clinically relevant effects noted were a reduction in red blood cell count and neutropenia.

Lamivudine was not mutagenic in bacterial tests but, like many nucleoside analogues, showed activity in an *in vitro* cytogenetic assay and the mouse lymphoma assay. Lamivudine was not genotoxic *in vivo* at doses that gave plasma concentrations around 40-50 times higher than the anticipated clinical plasma levels. As the *in vitro* mutagenic activity of lamivudine could not be confirmed in *in vivo* tests, it is concluded that lamivudine should not represent a genotoxic hazard to patients undergoing treatment.

A transplacental genotoxicity study conducted in monkeys compared zidovudine alone with the combination of zidovudine and lamivudine at human-equivalent exposures. The study demonstrated that foetuses exposed *in utero* to the combination sustained a higher level of nucleoside analogue-DNA incorporation into multiple foetal organs, and showed evidence of more telomere shortening than in those exposed to zidovudine alone. The clinical significance of these findings is unknown.

The results of long-term carcinogenicity studies in rats and mice did not show any carcinogenic potential relevant for humans.

6. PHARMACEUTICAL PARTICULARS

6.1 List of excipients

Tablet Core:

Microcrystalline cellulose (E460),

Sodium starch glycollate

Magnesium stearate

Tablet film-coat:

Hypromellose (E464)

Titanium dioxide (E171),

Macrogol,

Polysorbate 80

6.2 Incompatibilities

Not applicable

6.3 Shelf life

HDPE bottles: 5 years

PVC/aluminium foil blister packs: 2 years

6.4 Special precautions for storage

Do not store above 30°C

6.5 Nature and contents of container

Epivir tablets are available in child resistant HDPE bottles or PVC/aluminium foil blister packs each containing 60 tablets.

6.6 Instructions for use and handling

No special requirements

Administrative Data

7. MARKETING AUTHORISATION HOLDER

Glaxo Group Ltd

Greenford Road

Greenford

Middlesex UB6 0NN

United Kingdom

8. MARKETING AUTHORISATION NUMBER(S)

EU/1/96/015/001 (Bottle)

EU/1/96/015/004 (Blister pack)

9. DATE OF FIRST AUTHORISATION/RENEWAL OF THE AUTHORISATION

Date of first authorisation: August 1996

Date of renewal: 8 November 2001

10. DATE OF REVISION OF THE TEXT

17 December 2004

Epivir 300mg Tablets

(GlaxoSmithKline UK)

1. NAME OF THE MEDICINAL PRODUCT

Epivir 300 mg film-coated tablets

2. QUALITATIVE AND QUANTITATIVE COMPOSITION

Each film-coated tablet contains 300 mg lamivudine.

For excipients see section 6.1.

3. PHARMACEUTICAL FORM

Film-coated tablet

The film-coated tablets are grey, diamond shaped and engraved with "GX EJ7" on one face.

4. CLINICAL PARTICULARS

4.1 Therapeutic indications

Epivir is indicated as part of antiretroviral combination therapy for the treatment of Human Immunodeficiency Virus (HIV) infected adults and children.

4.2 Posology and method of administration

The therapy should be initiated by a physician experienced in the management of HIV infection.

Adults and adolescents over 12 years of age: the recommended dose of Epivir is 300 mg daily. This may be administered as either 150 mg twice daily or 300 mg once daily (see section 4.4). The 300 mg tablet is only suitable for the once a day regimen.

Patients changing to the once daily regimen should take 150 mg twice a day and switch to 300 mg once a day the following morning. Where an evening once daily regimen is preferred, 150 mg of Epivir should be taken on the first morning only, followed by 300 mg in the evening. When changing back to a twice daily regimen patients should complete the days treatment and start 150 mg twice a day the following morning.

Children

Three months to 12 years of age: the recommended dose is 4 mg/kg twice daily up to a maximum of 300 mg daily.

Less than three months of age: the limited data available are insufficient to propose specific dosage recommendations (see section 5.2)

Epivir is also available as an oral solution.

Epivir may be administered with or without food.

Renal impairment- Lamivudine concentrations are increased in patients with moderate - severe renal impairment due to decreased clearance. The dose should therefore be adjusted, using oral solution presentation of Epivir for patients whose creatinine clearance falls below 30 ml/min (see tables).

Dosing Recommendations – Adults and adolescents over 12 years:

Creatinine Clearance (ml/min)	First Dose	Maintenance Dose
≥50	150 mg	150 mg Twice daily
30-<50	150 mg	150 mg Once daily
<30	As doses below 150 mg are needed the use of the oral solution is recommended	

There are no data available on the use of lamivudine in children with renal impairment. Based on the assumption that creatinine clearance and lamivudine clearance are correlated similarly in children as in adults it is recommended that the dosage in children with renal impairment be reduced according to their creatinine clearance by the same proportion as in adults.

Dosing Recommendations – Children from 3 months to 12 years:

Creatinine Clearance (ml/min)	First Dose	Maintenance Dose
≥50	4 mg/kg	4 mg/kg twice daily
30 to <50	4 mg/kg	4 mg/kg once daily
15 to <30	4 mg/kg	2.6 mg/kg once daily
5 to <15	4 mg/kg	1.3 mg/kg once daily
<5	1.3 mg/kg	0.7 mg/kg once daily

Hepatic Impairment: Data obtained in patients with moderate to severe hepatic impairment shows that lamivudine pharmacokinetics are not significantly affected by hepatic dysfunction. Based on these data, no dose adjustment is necessary in patients with moderate or severe hepatic impairment unless accompanied by renal impairment.

4.3 Contraindications

Hypersensitivity to lamivudine or to any of the excipients.

4.4 Special warnings and special precautions for use

Epivir is not recommended for use as monotherapy.

Renal impairment: In patients with moderate to severe renal impairment, the terminal plasma half-life of lamivudine is increased due to decreased clearance, therefore the dose should be adjusted (See section 4.2).

Once daily dosing (300 mg once a day): a clinical study has demonstrated the non inferiority between Epivir once a day and Epivir twice a day containing regimens. These results were obtained in an antiretroviral naïve-population, primarily consisting of asymptomatic HIV infected patients (CDC stage A).

Triple nucleoside therapy: There have been reports of a high rate of virological failure and of emergence of resistance at an early stage when lamivudine was combined with tenofovir disoproxil fumarate and abacavir as well as with tenofovir disoproxil fumarate and didanosine as a once daily regimen.

Opportunistic infections: Patients receiving Epivir or any other antiretroviral therapy may continue to develop opportunistic infections and other complications of HIV infection, and therefore should remain under close clinical observation by physicians experienced in the treatment of patients with associated HIV diseases.

Transmission of HIV: Patients should be advised that current antiretroviral therapy, including Epivir, has not been proven to prevent the risk of transmission of HIV to others through sexual contact or blood contamination. Appropriate precautions should continue to be taken.

Pancreatitis: Cases of pancreatitis have occurred rarely. However it is not clear whether these cases were due to the antiretroviral treatment or to the underlying HIV disease. Treatment with Epivir should be stopped immediately if clinical signs, symptoms or laboratory abnormalities suggestive of pancreatitis occur.

Lactic acidosis: lactic acidosis, usually associated with hepatomegaly and hepatic steatosis, has been reported with the use of nucleoside analogues. Early symptoms (symptomatic hyperlactatemia) include benign digestive symptoms (nausea, vomiting and abdominal pain), non-specific malaise, loss of appetite, weight loss, respiratory symptoms (rapid and/or deep breathing) or neurological symptoms (including motor weakness).

Lactic acidosis has a high mortality and may be associated with pancreatitis, liver failure, or renal failure.

Lactic acidosis generally occurred after a few or several months of treatment.

Treatment with nucleoside analogues should be discontinued in the setting of symptomatic hyperlactatemia and metabolic/lactic acidosis, progressive hepatomegaly, or rapidly elevating aminotransferase levels.

Caution should be exercised when administering nucleoside analogues to any patient (particularly obese women) with hepatomegaly, hepatitis or other known risk factors for liver disease and hepatic steatosis (including certain medicinal products and alcohol). Patients co-infected with hepatitis C and treated with alpha interferon and ribavirin may constitute a special risk.

Patients at increased risk should be followed closely.

Mitochondrial dysfunction: Nucleoside and nucleotide analogues have been demonstrated *in vitro* and *in vivo* to cause a variable degree of mitochondrial damage. There have been reports of mitochondrial dysfunction in HIV-negative infants exposed *in utero* and/or post-natally to nucleoside analogues. The main adverse events reported are haematological disorders (anaemia, neutropenia), metabolic disorders (hyperlactatemia, hyperlipasemia). These events are often transitory. Some late-onset neurological disorders have been reported (hypertonia, convulsion, abnormal behaviour). Whether the neurological disorders are transient or permanent is currently unknown. Any child exposed *in utero* to nucleoside and nucleotide analogues, even HIV-negative children, should have clinical and laboratory follow-up and should be fully investigated for possible mitochondrial dysfunction in case of relevant signs or symptoms. These findings do not affect current national recommendations to use antiretroviral therapy in pregnant women to prevent vertical transmission of HIV.

Lipodystrophy: Combination antiretroviral therapy has been associated with the redistribution of body fat (lipodystrophy) in HIV patients. The long-term consequences of these events are currently unknown. Knowledge about the mechanism is incomplete. A connection between visceral lipomatosis and protease inhibitors (PIs) and lipoatrophy and nucleoside reverse transcriptase inhibitors (NRTIs) has been hypothesised. A higher risk of lipodystrophy has been associated with individual factors such as older age, and with drug related factors such as longer duration of antiretroviral treatment and associated metabolic disturbances. Clinical examination should include evaluation for physical signs of fat redistribution. Consideration should be given to the measurement of fasting serum lipids and blood glucose. Lipid disorders should be managed as clinically appropriate (see section 4.8).

Immune Reactivation Syndrome: In HIV-infected patients with severe immune deficiency at the time of institution of combination antiretroviral therapy (CART), an inflammatory reaction to asymptomatic or residual opportunistic pathogens may arise and cause serious clinical conditions, or aggravation of symptoms. Typically, such reactions have been observed within the first few weeks or months of initiation of CART. Relevant examples are cytomegalovirus retinitis, generalised and/or focal mycobacterium infections, and *Pneumocystis carinii* pneumonia. Any inflammatory symptoms should be evaluated and treatment instituted when necessary.

Liver disease: If lamivudine is being used concomitantly for the treatment of HIV and HBV, additional information relating to the use of lamivudine in the treatment of hepatitis B infection is available in the Zeffix SPC.

Patients with chronic hepatitis B or C and treated with combination antiretroviral therapy are at an increased risk of severe and potentially fatal hepatic adverse events. In case of concomitant antiviral therapy for hepatitis B or C, please refer also to the relevant product information for these medicinal products.

If Epivir is discontinued in patients co-infected with hepatitis B virus, periodic monitoring of liver function tests and markers of HBV replication is recommended, as withdrawal of lamivudine may result in an acute exacerbation of hepatitis (see Zeffix SPC).

Patients with pre-existing liver dysfunction, including chronic active hepatitis, have an increased frequency of liver function abnormalities during combination antiretroviral therapy, and should be monitored according to standard practice. If there is evidence of worsening liver disease in such patients, interruption or discontinuation of treatment must be considered.

4.5 Interaction with other medicinal products and other forms of Interaction

The likelihood of metabolic interactions is low due to limited metabolism and plasma protein binding and almost complete renal clearance.

A modest increase in C_{max} (28 %) was observed for zidovudine when administered with lamivudine, however overall exposure (AUC) is not significantly altered. Zidovudine has no effect on the pharmacokinetics of lamivudine (see section 5.2).

The possibility of interactions with other medicinal products administered concurrently should be considered, particularly when the main route of elimination is active renal secretion via the organic cationic transport system e.g. trimethoprim. Other medicinal products (e.g. ranitidine, cimetidine) are eliminated only in part by this mechanism and were shown not to interact with lamivudine. The nucleoside analogues (e.g. didanosine and zalcitabine) like zidovudine, are not eliminated by this mechanism and are unlikely to interact with lamivudine.

Administration of trimethoprim/sulfamethoxazole 160 mg/800 mg results in a 40 % increase in lamivudine exposure, because of the trimethoprim component; the sulfamethoxazole component did not interact. However, unless the patient has renal impairment, no dosage adjustment of lamivudine is necessary (see section 4.2). Lamivudine has no effect on the pharmacokinetics of trimethoprim or sulfamethoxazole. When concomitant administration is warranted, patients should be monitored clinically. Co-administration of lamivudine with high doses of co-trimoxazole for the treatment of *Pneumocystis carinii* pneumonia (PCP) and toxoplasmosis should be avoided.

Lamivudine metabolism does not involve CYP3A, making interactions with medicinal products metabolised by this system (e.g. PIs) unlikely.

Co-administration of lamivudine with intravenous ganciclovir or foscarnet is not recommended until further information is available.

Lamivudine may inhibit the intracellular phosphorylation of zalcitabine when the two medicinal products are used concurrently. Epivir is therefore not recommended to be used in combination with zalcitabine.

4.6 Pregnancy and lactation

Pregnancy: The safety of lamivudine in human pregnancy has not been established. Reproductive studies in animals have not shown evidence of teratogenicity, and showed no effect on male or female fertility. Lamivudine induces early embryonic death when administered to pregnant rabbits at exposure levels comparable to those achieved in man. In humans, consistent with passive transmission of lamivudine across the placenta, lamivudine concentrations in infant serum at birth were similar to those in maternal and cord serum at delivery.

Although animal reproductive studies are not always predictive of the human response, administration is not recommended during the first three months of pregnancy.

Lactation: Following oral administration lamivudine was excreted in breast milk at similar concentrations to those found in serum. Since lamivudine and the virus pass into breast milk, it is recommended that mothers taking Epivir do not breast-feed their infants. It is recommended that HIV infected women do not breast-feed their infants under any circumstances in order to avoid transmission of HIV.

4.7 Effects on ability to drive and use machines

No studies on the effects on the ability to drive and use machines have been performed.

4.8 Undesirable effects

The following adverse events have been reported during therapy for HIV disease with Epivir. With many it is unclear whether they are related to Epivir, other medications taken concurrently or are as a result of the underlying disease process.

The adverse events considered at least possibly related to the treatment are listed below by body system, organ class and absolute frequency. Frequencies are defined as very common >1/10), common >1/100, <1/10), uncommon >1/1,000, <1/100), rare >1/10,000, <1/1,000), very rare (<1/10,000).

Blood and lymphatic systems disorders

Uncommon: Neutropenia and anaemia (both occasionally severe), thrombocytopenia

Very rare: Pure red cell aplasia

Nervous system disorders

Common: Headache, insomnia

Very rare: Cases of peripheral neuropathy (or paraesthesia) have been reported.

Respiratory, thoracic and mediastinal disorders

Common: Cough, nasal symptoms

Gastrointestinal disorders

Common: Nausea, vomiting, abdominal pain or cramps, diarrhoea

Rare: Rises in serum amylase. Cases of pancreatitis have been reported.

Hepatobiliary disorders

Uncommon: Transient rises in liver enzymes (AST, ALT).

Rare: Hepatitis

Skin and subcutaneous tissue disorders

Common: Rash, alopecia

Musculoskeletal and connective tissue disorders

Common: Arthralgia, muscle disorders

Rare: Rhabdomyolysis

General disorders and administration site conditions

Common: Fatigue, malaise, fever.

Cases of lactic acidosis, sometimes fatal, usually associated with severe hepatomegaly and hepatic steatosis, have been reported with the use of nucleoside analogues (see section 4.4).

Combination antiretroviral therapy has been associated with redistribution of body fat (lipodystrophy) in HIV patients including the loss of peripheral and facial subcutaneous fat, increased intra-abdominal and visceral fat, breast hypertrophy and dorsocervical fat accumulation (buffalo hump).

Combination antiretroviral therapy has been associated with metabolic abnormalities such as hypertriglyceridaemia, hypercholesterolaemia, insulin resistance, hyperglycaemia and hyperlactataemia (see section 4.4).

In HIV-infected patients with severe immune deficiency at the time of initiation of combination antiretroviral therapy (CART), an inflammatory reaction to asymptomatic or residual opportunistic infections may arise (see section 4.4).

4.9 Overdose

Administration of lamivudine at very high dose levels in acute animal studies did not result in any organ toxicity. Limited data are available on the consequences of ingestion of acute overdoses in humans. No fatalities occurred, and the patients recovered. No specific signs or symptoms have been identified following such overdose.

If overdosage occurs the patient should be monitored, and standard supportive treatment applied as required. Since lamivudine is dialysable, continuous haemodialysis could be used in the treatment of overdosage, although this has not been studied.

5. PHARMACOLOGICAL PROPERTIES

5.1 Pharmacodynamic properties

Pharmacotherapeutic group: nucleoside analogue, ATC Code: J05A F05.

Lamivudine is a nucleoside analogue which has activity against human immunodeficiency virus (HIV) and hepatitis B virus (HBV). It is metabolised intracellularly to the active moiety, lamivudine 5'-triphosphate. Its main mode of action is as a chain terminator of viral reverse transcription. The triphosphate has selective inhibitory activity against HIV-1 and HIV-2 replication *in vitro*; it is also active against zidovudine-resistant clinical isolates of HIV. Lamivudine in combination with zidovudine exhibits synergistic anti-HIV activity against clinical isolates in cell culture.

HIV-1 resistance to lamivudine involves the development of a M184V amino acid change close to the active site of the viral reverse transcriptase (RT). This variant arises both *in vitro* and in HIV-1 infected patients treated with lamivudine-containing antiretroviral therapy. M184V mutants display greatly reduced susceptibility to lamivudine and show diminished viral replicative capacity *in vitro*. *In vitro* studies indicate that zidovudine-resistant virus isolates can become zidovudine sensitive when they simultaneously acquire resistance to lamivudine. The clinical relevance of such findings remains, however, not well defined.

Cross-resistance conferred by the M184V RT is limited within the nucleoside inhibitor class of antiretroviral agents. Zidovudine and stavudine maintain their antiretroviral activities against lamivudine-resistant HIV-1. Abacavir maintains its antiretroviral activities against lamivudine-resistant HIV-1 harbouring only the M184V mutation. The M184V RT mutant shows a <4-fold decrease in susceptibility to didanosine and zalcitabine; the clinical significance of these findings is unknown. *In vitro* susceptibility testing has not been standardised and results may vary according to methodological factors.

Lamivudine demonstrates low cytotoxicity to peripheral blood lymphocytes, to established lymphocyte and monocyte-macrophage cell lines, and to a variety of bone marrow progenitor cells *in vitro*.

Clinical experience:

In clinical trials, lamivudine in combination with zidovudine has been shown to reduce HIV-1 viral load and increase CD4 cell count. Clinical end-point data indicate that lamivudine in combination with zidovudine, results in a significant reduction in the risk of disease progression and mortality.

Evidence from clinical studies shows that lamivudine plus zidovudine delays the emergence of zidovudine resistant isolates in individuals with no prior antiretroviral therapy.

Lamivudine has been widely used as a component of antiretroviral combination therapy with other antiretroviral agents of the same class (NRTIs) or different classes (PIs, non-nucleoside reverse transcriptase inhibitors).

Multiple drug antiretroviral therapy containing lamivudine has been shown to be effective in antiretrovirally-naive patients as well as in patients presenting with viruses containing the M184V mutations.

The relationship between *in vitro* susceptibility of HIV to lamivudine and clinical response to lamivudine-containing therapy remains under investigation.

Lamivudine at a dose of 100 mg once daily has also been shown to be effective for the treatment of adult patients with chronic HBV infection (for details of clinical studies, see the prescribing information for Zeffix). However, for the treatment of HIV infection, only a 300 mg daily dose of lamivudine (in combination with other antiretroviral agents) has been shown to be efficacious.

Lamivudine has not been specifically investigated in HIV patients co-infected with HBV.

5.2 Pharmacokinetic properties

Absorption: Lamivudine is well absorbed from the gastrointestinal tract, and the bioavailability of oral lamivudine in adults is normally between 80 and 85 %. Following oral administration, the mean time (t_{max}) to maximal serum concentrations (C_{max}) is about an hour. Based on data derived from a study in healthy volunteers, at a therapeutic dose of 150mg twice daily, mean (CV) steady-state C_{max} and C_{min} of lamivudine in plasma are 1.2 μg/ml (24%) and 0.09 μg/ml (27%), respectively. The mean (CV) AUC over a dosing interval of 12 hours is 4.7 μg.h/ml (18%). At a therapeutic dose of 300mg once daily, the mean (CV) steady-state C_{max}, C_{min} and 24h AUC are 2.0 μg/ml (26%), 0.04 μg/ml (34%) and 8.9 μg.h/ml (21%), respectively.

The 150 mg tablet is bioequivalent and dose proportional to the 300 mg tablet with respect to AUC_∞, C_{max}, and t_{max}.

Co-administration of lamivudine with food results in a delay of t_{max} and a lower C_{max} (decreased by 47 %). However, the extent (based on the AUC) of lamivudine absorbed is not influenced.

Co-administration of zidovudine results in a 13 % increase in zidovudine exposure and a 28 % increase in peak plasma levels. This is not considered to be of significance to patient safety and therefore no dosage adjustments are necessary.

Distribution: From intravenous studies, the mean volume of distribution is 1.3 l/kg. The observed half-life of elimination is 5 to 7 hours. The mean systemic clearance of lamivudine is approximately

0.32 l/h/kg, with predominantly renal clearance > 70 %) via the organic cationic transport system.

Lamivudine exhibits linear pharmacokinetics over the therapeutic dose range and displays limited binding to the major plasma protein albumin (< 16 % - 36 % to serum albumin in *in vitro* studies).

Limited data show that lamivudine penetrates the central nervous system and reaches the cerebro-spinal fluid (CSF). The mean ratio CSF/serum lamivudine concentration 2-4 hours after oral administration was approximately 0.12. The true extent of penetration or relationship with any clinical efficacy is unknown.

Metabolism: The active moiety, intracellular lamivudine triphosphate, has a prolonged terminal half-life in the cell (16 to 19 hours) compared to the plasma lamivudine half-life (5 to 7 hours). In 60 healthy adult volunteers, Epivir 300 mg once daily has been demonstrated to be pharmacokinetically equivalent at steady-state to Epivir 150 mg twice daily with respect to intracellular triphosphate AUC_{24} and C_{max}.

Lamivudine is predominately cleared unchanged by renal excretion. The likelihood of metabolic interactions of lamivudine with other medicinal products is low due to the small extent of hepatic metabolism (5-10 %) and low plasma protein binding.

Elimination: Studies in patients with renal impairment show lamivudine elimination is affected by renal dysfunction. A recommended dosage regimen for patients with creatinine clearance below 50 ml/min is shown in the dosage section (see section 4.2).

An interaction with trimethoprim, a constituent of co-trimoxazole, causes a 40 % increase in lamivudine exposure at therapeutic doses. This does not require dose adjustment unless the patient also has renal impairment (see sections 4.5 and 4.2). Administration of co-trimoxazole with lamivudine in patients with renal impairment should be carefully assessed.

Pharmacokinetics in children: In general, lamivudine pharmacokinetics in paediatric patients is similar to adults. However, absolute bioavailability (approximately 55-65 %) was reduced in paediatric patients below 12 years of age. In addition, systemic clearance values were greater in younger paediatric patients and decreased with age, approaching adult values around 12 years of age. Due to these differences, the recommended dose for children from three months to 12 years is 8 mg/kg/day, which will achieve similar adult and paediatric exposure (average AUC approximately 5,000 ng.h/ml).

There are limited pharmacokinetic data for patients less than three months of age. In neonates one week of age, lamivudine oral clearance was reduced when compared to paediatric patients and is likely to be due to immature renal function and variable absorption. Therefore to achieve similar adult and paediatric exposure, the recommended dose for neonates is 4 mg/kg/day. Glomerular filtration estimates suggests that to achieve similar adult and paediatric exposure, the recommended dose for children aged six weeks and older could be 8 mg/kg/day.

Pharmacokinetics in pregnancy: Following oral administration, lamivudine pharmacokinetics in late-pregnancy were similar to non-pregnant women.

5.3 Preclinical safety data

Administration of lamivudine in animal toxicity studies at high doses was not associated with any major organ toxicity. At the highest dosage levels, minor effects on indicators of liver and kidney function were seen together with occasional reductions in liver weight. The clinically relevant effects noted were a reduction in red blood cell count and neutropenia.

Lamivudine was not mutagenic in bacterial tests but, like many nucleoside analogues, showed activity in an *in vitro* cytogenetic assay and the mouse lymphoma assay. Lamivudine was not genotoxic *in vivo* at doses that gave plasma concentrations around 40-50 times higher than the anticipated clinical plasma levels. As the *in vitro* mutagenic activity of lamivudine could not be confirmed in *in vivo* tests, it is concluded that lamivudine should not represent a genotoxic hazard to patients undergoing treatment.

A transplacental genotoxicity study conducted in monkeys compared zidovudine alone with the combination of zidovudine and lamivudine at human-equivalent exposures. The study demonstrated that foetuses exposed *in utero* to the combination sustained a higher level of nucleoside analogue-DNA incorporation into multiple foetal organs, and showed evidence of more telomere shortening than in those exposed to zidovudine alone. The clinical significance of these findings is unknown.

The results of long-term carcinogenicity studies in rats and mice did not show any carcinogenic potential relevant for humans.

6. PHARMACEUTICAL PARTICULARS

6.1 List of excipients

Tablet Core:

Microcrystalline cellulose (E460),

Sodium starch glycollate

Magnesium stearate

Tablet film-coat:

Hypromellose (E464),

Titanium dioxide (E171),

Black iron oxide (E172),

Macrogol, Polysorbate 80

6.2 Incompatibilities

Not applicable

6.3 Shelf life

HDPE bottles: 3 years

PVC/aluminium foil blister packs: 2 years

6.4 Special precautions for storage

Do not store above 30°C

6.5 Nature and contents of container

Epivir tablets are available in child resistant HDPE bottles or PVC/aluminium foil blister packs each containing 30 tablets.

6.6 Instructions for use and handling

No special requirements

Administrative Data

7. MARKETING AUTHORISATION HOLDER

Glaxo Group Ltd

Greenford Road

Greenford

Middlesex UB6 0NN

United Kingdom

8. MARKETING AUTHORISATION NUMBER(S)

EU/1/96/015/003 (Bottle)

EU/1/96/015/005 (Blister pack)

9. DATE OF FIRST AUTHORISATION/RENEWAL OF THE AUTHORISATION

Date of first authorisation: 15 November 2001

10. DATE OF REVISION OF THE TEXT

17 December 2004

Epivir Oral Solution

(GlaxoSmithKline UK)

1. NAME OF THE MEDICINAL PRODUCT

Epivir 10 mg/ml oral solution

2. QUALITATIVE AND QUANTITATIVE COMPOSITION

Oral solution containing 10 mg/ml of lamivudine.

For excipients see section 6.1.

3. PHARMACEUTICAL FORM

Oral solution

It is a clear, colourless to pale yellow solution.

4. CLINICAL PARTICULARS

4.1 Therapeutic indications

Epivir is indicated as part of antiretroviral combination therapy for the treatment of Human Immunodeficiency Virus (HIV) infected adults and children.

4.2 Posology and method of administration

The therapy should be initiated by a physician experienced in the management of HIV infection.

Adults and adolescents over 12 years of age: the recommended dose of Epivir is 300 mg daily. This may be administered as either 150 mg (15 ml) twice daily or 300 mg (30 ml) once daily (see section 4.4).

Patients changing to the once daily regimen should take 150 mg (15 ml) twice a day and switch to 300 mg (30 ml) once a day the following morning. Where an evening once daily regimen is preferred, 150 mg (15 ml) of Epivir should be taken on the first morning only, followed by 300 mg (30 ml) in the evening. When changing back to a twice daily regimen, patients should complete the days treatment and start 150 mg (15 ml) twice a day the following morning.

Children

Three months to 12 years of age: the recommended dose is 4 mg/kg twice daily up to a maximum of 300 mg daily.

Less than three months of age the limited data available are insufficient to propose specific dosage recommendations (see section 5.2)

Epivir is also available as a tablet formulation.

Epivir may be administered with or without food.

Renal impairment:- Lamivudine concentrations are increased in patients with moderate - severe renal impairment due to decreased clearance. The dose should therefore be adjusted (see tables).

Dosing Recommendations – Adults and adolescents over 12 years:

Creatinine clearance (ml/min)	First Dose	Maintenance Dose
⩾50	150 mg (15 ml)	150 mg (15 ml) Twice daily
30 to <50	150 mg (15 ml)	150 mg (15 ml) Once daily
15 to <30	150 mg (15 ml)	100 mg (10 ml) Once daily
5 to <15	150 mg (15 ml)	50 mg (5 ml) Once daily
<5	50 mg (5 ml)	25 mg (2.5 ml) Once daily

There are no data available on the use of lamivudine in children with renal impairment. Based on the assumption that creatinine clearance and lamivudine clearance are correlated similarly in children as in adults it is recommended that the dosage in children with renal impairment be reduced according to their creatinine clearance by the same proportion as in adults.

Dosing Recommendations – Children from 3 months to 12 years:

Creatinine Clearance (ml/min)	First Dose	Maintenance Dose
⩾50	4 mg/kg	4 mg/kg twice daily
30 to <50	4 mg/kg	4 mg/kg once daily
15 to <30	4 mg/kg	2.6 mg/kg once daily
5 to <15	4 mg/kg	1.3 mg/kg once daily
<5	1.3 mg/kg	0.7 mg/kg once daily

Hepatic impairment: Data obtained in patients with moderate to severe hepatic impairment shows that lamivudine pharmacokinetics are not significantly affected by hepatic dysfunction. Based on these data, no dose adjustment is necessary in patients with moderate or severe hepatic impairment unless accompanied by renal impairment.

4.3 Contraindications

Hypersensitivity to lamivudine or to any of the excipients.

4.4 Special warnings and special precautions for use

Epivir is not recommended for use as monotherapy.

Diabetic patients should be advised that each dose (150 mg = 15 ml) contains 3 g of sucrose.

Renal impairment: In patients with moderate –to- severe renal impairment, the terminal plasma half-life of lamivudine is increased due to decreased clearance, therefore the dose should be adjusted (See section 4.2).

Once daily dosing (300 mg once a day): a clinical study has demonstrated the non inferiority between Epivir once a day and Epivir twice a day containing regimens. These results were obtained in an antiretroviral naïve-population, primarily consisting of asymptomatic HIV infected patients (CDC stage A).

Triple nucleoside therapy: There have been reports of a high rate of virological failure and of emergence of resistance at an early stage when lamivudine was combined with tenofovir disoproxil fumarate and abacavir as well as with tenofovir disoproxil fumarate and didanosine as a once daily regimen.

Opportunistic infections: Patients receiving Epivir or any other antiretroviral therapy may continue to develop opportunistic infections and other complications of HIV infection, and therefore should remain under close clinical observation by physicians experienced in the treatment of patients with associated HIV diseases.

Transmission of HIV: Patients should be advised that current antiretroviral therapy, including Epivir, has not been proven to prevent the risk of transmission of HIV to others through sexual contact or blood contamination. Appropriate precautions should continue to be taken.

Pancreatitis: Cases of pancreatitis have occurred rarely. However it is not clear whether these cases were due to the antiretroviral treatment or to the underlying HIV disease. Treatment with Epivir should be stopped immediately if clinical signs, symptoms or laboratory abnormalities suggestive of pancreatitis occur.

Lactic acidosis: lactic acidosis, usually associated with hepatomegaly and hepatic steatosis, has been reported with the use of nucleoside analogues. Early symptoms (symptomatic hyperlactatemia) include benign digestive symptoms (nausea, vomiting and abdominal pain), non-specific malaise, loss of appetite, weight loss, respiratory symptoms (rapid and/or deep breathing) or neurological symptoms (including motor weakness).

Lactic acidosis has a high mortality and may be associated with pancreatitis, liver failure, or renal failure.

Lactic acidosis generally occurred after a few or several months of treatment.

Treatment with nucleoside analogues should be discontinued in the setting of symptomatic hyperlactatemia and metabolic/lactic acidosis, progressive hepatomegaly, or rapidly elevating aminotransferase levels.

Caution should be exercised when administering nucleoside analogues to any patient (particularly obese women) with hepatomegaly, hepatitis or other known risk factors for liver disease and hepatic steatosis (including certain medicinal products and alcohol). Patients co-infected with hepatitis C and treated with alpha interferon and ribavirin may constitute a special risk.

Patients at increased risk should be followed closely.

Mitochondrial dysfunction: Nucleoside and nucleotide analogues have been demonstrated *in vitro* and *in vivo* to cause a variable degree of mitochondrial damage. There have been reports of mitochondrial dysfunction in HIV-negative infants exposed *in utero* and/or post-natally to nucleoside analogues. The main adverse events reported are haematological disorders (anaemia, neutropenia), metabolic disorders (hyperlactatemia, hyperlipasemia). These events are often transitory. Some late-onset neurological disorders have been reported (hypertonia, convulsion, abnormal behaviour). Whether the neurological disorders are transient or permanent is currently unknown. Any child exposed *in utero* to nucleoside and nucleotide analogues, even HIV-negative children, should have clinical and laboratory follow-up and should be fully investigated for possible mitochondrial dysfunction in case of relevant signs or symptoms. These findings do not affect current national recommendations to use antiretroviral therapy in pregnant women to prevent vertical transmission of HIV.

Lipodystrophy: Combination antiretroviral therapy has been associated with the redistribution of body fat (lipodystrophy) in HIV patients. The long-term consequences of these events are currently unknown. Knowledge about the mechanism is incomplete. A connection between visceral lipomatosis and protease inhibitors (PIs) and lipoatrophy and nucleoside analogue reverse transcriptase inhibitors (NRTIs) has been hypothesised. A higher risk of lipodystrophy has been associated with individual factors such as older age, and with drug related factors such as longer duration of antiretroviral treatment and associated metabolic disturbances. Clinical examination should include evaluation for physical signs of fat redistribution. Consideration should be given to the measurement of fasting serum lipids and blood glucose. Lipid disorders should be managed as clinically appropriate (see section 4.8).

Immune Reactivation Syndrome: In HIV-infected patients with severe immune deficiency at the time of institution of combination antiretroviral therapy (CART), an inflammatory reaction to asymptomatic or residual opportunistic pathogens may arise and cause serious clinical conditions, or aggravation of symptoms. Typically, such reactions have been observed within the first few weeks or months of initiation of CART. Relevant examples are cytomegalovirus retinitis, generalised and/or focal mycobacterium infections, and *Pneumocystis carinii* pneumonia. Any inflammatory symptoms should be evaluated and treatment instituted when necessary.

Liver disease: If lamivudine is being used concomitantly for the treatment of HIV and HBV, additional information relating to the use of lamivudine in the treatment of hepatitis B infection is available in the Zeffix SPC.

Patients with chronic hepatitis B or C and treated with combination antiretroviral therapy are at an increased risk of severe and potentially fatal hepatic adverse events. In case of concomitant antiviral therapy for hepatitis B or C, please refer also to the relevant product information for these medicinal products.

If Epivir is discontinued in patients co-infected with hepatitis B virus, periodic monitoring of liver function tests and markers of HBV replication is recommended, as withdrawal of lamivudine may result in an acute exacerbation of hepatitis (see Zeffix SPC).

Patients with pre-existing liver dysfunction, including chronic active hepatitis, have an increased frequency of liver function abnormalities during combination antiretroviral therapy, and should be monitored according to standard practice. If there is evidence of worsening liver disease in such patients, interruption or discontinuation of treatment must be considered.

4.5 Interaction with other medicinal products and other forms of Interaction

The likelihood of metabolic interactions is low due to limited metabolism and plasma protein binding and almost complete renal clearance.

A modest increase in C_{max} (28 %) was observed for zidovudine when administered with lamivudine, however overall exposure (AUC) is not significantly altered. Zidovudine has no effect on the pharmacokinetics of lamivudine (See section 5.2).

The possibility of interactions with other medicinal products administered concurrently should be considered, particularly when the main route of elimination is active renal secretion via the organic cationic transport system e.g. trimethoprim. Other medicinal products (e.g. ranitidine, cimetidine) are eliminated only in part by this mechanism and were shown not to interact with lamivudine. The nucleoside analogues (e.g. didanosine and zalcitabine) like zidovudine, are not eliminated by this mechanism and are unlikely to interact with lamivudine.

Administration of trimethoprim/sulfamethoxazole 160 mg/800 mg results in a 40 % increase in lamivudine exposure, because of the trimethoprim component; the sulfamethoxazole component did not interact. However, unless the patient has renal impairment, no dosage adjustment of lamivudine is necessary (see section 4.2). Lamivudine has no effect on the pharmacokinetics of trimethoprim or sulfamethoxazole. When concomitant administration is warranted, patients should be monitored clinically. Co-administration of lamivudine with high doses of co-trimoxazole for the treatment of *Pneumocystis carinii* pneumonia (PCP) and toxoplasmosis should be avoided.

Lamivudine metabolism does not involve CYP3A, making interactions with medicinal products metabolised by this system (e.g. PIs) unlikely.

Co-administration of lamivudine with intravenous ganciclovir or foscarnet is not recommended until further information is available.

Lamivudine may inhibit the intracellular phosphorylation of zalcitabine when the two medicinal products are used concurrently. Epivir is therefore not recommended to be used in combination with zalcitabine.

4.6 Pregnancy and lactation

Pregnancy: The safety of lamivudine in human pregnancy has not been established. Reproductive studies in animals have not shown evidence of teratogenicity, and showed no effect on male or female fertility. Lamivudine induces early embryonic death when administered to pregnant rabbits at exposure levels comparable to those achieved in man. In humans, consistent with passive transmission of lamivudine across the placenta, lamivudine concentrations in infant serum at birth were similar to those in maternal and cord serum at delivery.

Although animal reproductive studies are not always predictive of the human response, administration is not recommended during the first three months of pregnancy.

Lactation: Following oral administration lamivudine was excreted in breast milk at similar concentrations to those found in serum. Since lamivudine and the virus pass into breast milk, it is recommended that mothers taking Epivir do not breast-feed their infants. It is recommended that HIV infected women do not breast-feed their infants under any circumstances in order to avoid transmission of HIV.

4.7 Effects on ability to drive and use machines

No studies on the effects on the ability to drive and use machines have been performed.

4.8 Undesirable effects

The following adverse events have been reported during therapy for HIV disease with Epivir. With many it is unclear whether they are related to Epivir, other medications taken concurrently or are as a result of the underlying disease process.

The adverse events considered at least possibly related to the treatment are listed below by body system, organ class and absolute frequency. Frequencies are defined as very common >1/10), common >1/100, <1/10), uncommon >1/1,000, <1/100), rare >1/10,000, <1/1,000), very rare (<1/10,000).

Blood and lymphatic systems disorders

Uncommon: Neutropenia and anaemia (both occasionally severe), thrombocytopenia

Very rare: Pure red cell aplasia

Nervous system disorders

Common: Headache, insomnia

Very rare: Cases of peripheral neuropathy (or paraesthesia) have been reported.

Respiratory, thoracic and mediastinal disorders

Common: Cough, nasal symptoms

Gastrointestinal disorders

Common: Nausea, vomiting, abdominal pain or cramps, diarrhoea

Rare: Rises in serum amylase. Cases of pancreatitis have been reported.

Hepatobiliary disorders

Uncommon: Transient rises in liver enzymes (AST, ALT).

Rare: Hepatitis

Skin and subcutaneous tissue disorders

Common: Rash, alopecia

Musculoskeletal and connective tissue disorders

Common: Arthralgia, muscle disorders

Rare: Rhabdomyolysis

General disorders and administration site conditions

Common: Fatigue, malaise, fever.

Cases of lactic acidosis, sometimes fatal, usually associated with severe hepatomegaly and hepatic steatosis, have been reported with the use of nucleoside analogues (see section 4.4).

Combination antiretroviral therapy has been associated with redistribution of body fat (lipodystrophy) in HIV patients including the loss of peripheral and facial subcutaneous fat, increased intra-abdominal and visceral fat, breast hypertrophy and dorsocervical fat accumulation (buffalo hump).

Combination antiretroviral therapy has been associated with metabolic abnormalities such as hypertriglyceridaemia, hypercholesterolaemia, insulin resistance, hyperglycaemia and hyperlactataemia (see section 4.4).

In HIV-infected patients with severe immune deficiency at the time of initiation of combination antiretroviral therapy (CART), an inflammatory reaction to asymptomatic or residual opportunistic infections may arise (see section 4.4).

4.9 Overdose

Administration of lamivudine at very high dose levels in acute animal studies did not result in any organ toxicity. Limited data are available on the consequences of ingestion of acute overdoses in humans. No fatalities occurred, and the patients recovered. No specific signs or symptoms have been identified following such overdose.

If overdosage occurs the patient should be monitored, and standard supportive treatment applied as required. Since lamivudine is dialysable, continuous haemodialysis could be used in the treatment of overdosage, although this has not been studied.

5. PHARMACOLOGICAL PROPERTIES

5.1 Pharmacodynamic properties

Pharmacotherapeutic group: nucleoside analogue, ATC Code: J05A F05.

Lamivudine is a nucleoside analogue which has activity against human immunodeficiency virus (HIV) and hepatitis B virus (HBV). It is metabolised intracellularly to the active moiety, lamivudine 5'- triphosphate. Its main mode of action is as a chain terminator of viral reverse transcription. The triphosphate has selective inhibitory activity against HIV-1 and HIV-2 replication *in vitro*; it is also active against zidovudine-resistant clinical isolates of HIV. Lamivudine in combination with zidovudine exhibits synergistic anti-HIV activity against clinical isolates in cell culture.

HIV-1 resistance to lamivudine involves the development of a M184V amino acid change close to the active site of the viral reverse transcriptase (RT). This variant arises both *in vitro* and in HIV-1 infected patients treated with lamivudine-containing antiretroviral therapy. M184V mutants display greatly reduced susceptibility to lamivudine and show diminished viral replicative capacity *in vitro*. *In vitro* studies indicate that zidovudine-resistant virus isolates can become zidovudine sensitive when they simultaneously acquire resistance to lamivudine. The clinical relevance of such findings remains, however, not well defined.

Cross-resistance conferred by the M184V RT is limited within the nucleoside inhibitor class of antiretroviral agents. Zidovudine and stavudine maintain their antiretroviral activities against lamivudine-resistant HIV-1. Abacavir maintains its antiretroviral activities against lamivudine-resistant HIV-1 harbouring only the M184V mutation. The M184V RT mutant shows a <4-fold decrease in susceptibility to didanosine and zalcitabine; the clinical significance of these findings is unknown. *In vitro* susceptibility testing has not been standardised and results may vary according to methodological factors.

Lamivudine demonstrates low cytotoxicity to peripheral blood lymphocytes, to established lymphocyte and monocyte-macrophage cell lines, and to a variety of bone marrow progenitor cells *in vitro*.

Clinical experience

In clinical trials, lamivudine in combination with zidovudine has been shown to reduce HIV-1 viral load and increase CD4 cell count. Clinical end-point data indicate that lamivudine in combination with zidovudine, results in a significant reduction in the risk of disease progression and mortality.

Evidence from clinical studies shows that lamivudine plus zidovudine delays the emergence of zidovudine resistant isolates in individuals with no prior antiretroviral therapy.

Lamivudine has been widely used as a component of antiretroviral combination therapy with other antiretroviral agents of the same class (NRTIs) or different classes (PIs, non-nucleoside reverse transcriptase inhibitors).

Multiple drug antiretroviral therapy containing lamivudine has been shown to be effective in antiretrovirally-naive patients as well as in patients presenting with viruses containing the M184V mutations.

The relationship between *in vitro* susceptibility of HIV to lamivudine and clinical response to lamivudine-containing therapy remains under investigation.

Lamivudine at a dose of 100 mg once daily has also been shown to be effective for the treatment of adult patients with chronic HBV infection (for details of clinical studies, see the prescribing information for Zeffix). However, for the treatment of HIV infection, only a 300 mg daily dose of lamivudine (in combination with other antiretroviral agents) has been shown to be efficacious.

Lamivudine has not been specifically investigated in HIV patients co-infected with HBV.

5.2 Pharmacokinetic properties

Absorption: Lamivudine is well absorbed from the gastro-intestinal tract, and the bioavailability of oral lamivudine in adults is normally between 80 and 85 %. Following oral administration, the mean time (t_{max}) to maximal serum concentrations (C_{max}) is about an hour. Based on data derived from a study in healthy volunteers, at a therapeutic dose of 150mg twice daily, mean (CV) steady-state C_{max} and C_{min} of lamivudine in plasma are 1.2 μg/ml (24%) and 0.09 μg/ml (27%), respectively. The mean (CV) AUC over a dosing interval of 12 hours is 4.7 μg.h/ml (18%). At a therapeutic dose of 300mg once daily, the mean (CV) steady-state C_{max}, C_{min} and 24h AUC are 2.0 μg/ml (26%), 0.04 μg/ml (34%) and 8.9 μg.h/ml (21%), respectively.

Co-administration of lamivudine with food results in a delay of t_{max} and a lower C_{max} (decreased by 47 %). However, the extent (based on the AUC) of lamivudine absorbed is not influenced.

Co-administration of zidovudine results in a 13 % increase in zidovudine exposure and a 28 % increase in peak plasma levels. This is not considered to be of significance to patient safety and therefore no dosage adjustments are necessary.

Distribution: From intravenous studies, the mean volume of distribution is 1.3 l/kg. The observed half-life of elimination is 5 to 7 hours. The mean systemic clearance of lamivudine is approximately

0.32 l/h/kg, with predominantly renal clearance > 70 %) via the organic cationic transport system.

Lamivudine exhibits linear pharmacokinetics over the therapeutic dose range and displays limited binding to the major plasma protein albumin (< 16 % - 36 % to serum albumin in *in vitro* studies).

Limited data show that lamivudine penetrates the central nervous system and reaches the cerebro-spinal fluid (CSF). The mean ratio CSF/serum lamivudine concentration 2-4 hours after oral administration was approximately 0.12. The true extent of penetration or relationship with any clinical efficacy is unknown.

Metabolism: The active moiety, intracellular lamivudine triphosphate, has a prolonged terminal half-life in the cell (16 to 19 hours) compared to the plasma lamivudine half-life (5 to 7 hours). In 60 healthy adult volunteers, Epivir 300 mg once daily has been demonstrated to be pharmacokinetically equivalent at steady-state to Epivir 150 mg twice daily with respect to intracellular triphosphate AUC_{24} and C_{max}.

Lamivudine is predominately cleared unchanged by renal excretion. The likelihood of metabolic interactions of lamivudine with other medicinal products is low due to the small extent of hepatic metabolism (5-10 %) and low plasma protein binding.

Elimination: Studies in patients with renal impairment show lamivudine elimination is affected by renal dysfunction. A recommended dosage regimen for patients with creatinine clearance below 50 ml/min is shown in the dosage section (see section 4.2).

An interaction with trimethoprim, a constituent of co-trimoxazole, causes a 40 % increase in lamivudine exposure at therapeutic doses. This does not require dose adjustment unless the patient also has renal impairment (see sections 4.5 and 4.2). Administration of co-trimoxazole with lamivudine in patients with renal impairment should be carefully assessed.

Pharmacokinetics in children: In general, lamivudine pharmacokinetics in paediatric patients is similar to adults. However, absolute bioavailability (approximately 55-65 %) was reduced in paediatric patients below 12 years of age. In addition, systemic clearance values were greater in younger paediatric patients and decreased with age approaching adult values around 12 years of age. Due to these differences, the recommended dose for children from three months to 12 years is 8 mg/kg/day, which will achieve similar adult and paediatric exposure (average AUC approximately 5,000 ng.h/ml).

There are limited pharmacokinetic data for patients less than three months of age. In neonates one week of age, lamivudine oral clearance was reduced when compared to paediatric patients and is likely to be due to immature renal function and variable absorption. Therefore to achieve similar adult and paediatric exposure, the recommended dose for neonates is 4 mg/kg/day. Glomerular filtration estimates suggests that to achieve similar adult and paediatric exposure, the recommended dose for children aged six weeks and older could be 8 mg/kg/day.

Pharmacokinetics in pregnancy: Following oral administration, lamivudine pharmacokinetics in late-pregnancy were similar to non-pregnant women.

5.3 Preclinical safety data

Administration of lamivudine in animal toxicity studies at high doses was not associated with any major organ toxicity. At the highest dosage levels, minor effects on indicators of liver and kidney function were seen together with occasional reductions in liver weight. The clinically relevant effects noted were a reduction in red blood cell count and neutropenia.

Lamivudine was not mutagenic in bacterial tests but, like many nucleoside analogues, showed activity in an *in vitro* cytogenetic assay and the mouse lymphoma assay. Lamivudine was not genotoxic *in vivo* at doses that gave plasma concentrations around 40-50 times higher than the anticipated clinical plasma levels. As the *in vitro* mutagenic activity of lamivudine could not be confirmed in *in vivo* tests, it is concluded that lamivudine should not represent a genotoxic hazard to patients undergoing treatment.

A transplacental genotoxicity study conducted in monkeys compared zidovudine alone with the combination of zidovudine and lamivudine at human-equivalent exposures. The study demonstrated that foetuses exposed *in utero* to the combination sustained a higher level of nucleoside analogue-DNA incorporation into multiple foetal organs, and showed evidence of more telomere shortening than in those exposed to zidovudine alone. The clinical significance of these findings is unknown.

The results of long-term carcinogenicity studies in rats and mice did not show any carcinogenic potential relevant for humans.

6. PHARMACEUTICAL PARTICULARS

6.1 List of excipients

Sucrose 20 %(3 g/15 ml)

Methyl parahydroxybenzoate

Propyl parahydroxybenzoate

Citric acid Anhydrous

Propylene glycol

Sodium citrate

Artificial strawberry flavour

Artificial banana flavour

Purified water

6.2 Incompatibilities

Not applicable

6.3 Shelf life

2 years

Discard the oral solution one month after first opening.

6.4 Special precautions for storage

Do not store above 25°C.

6.5 Nature and contents of container

Cartons containing 240 ml oral solution in a white high density polyethylene (HDPE) bottle, with a child resistant closure. A 10 ml polypropylene oral dosing syringe and a polyethylene adapter are also included in the pack.

6.6 Instructions for use and handling

The oral dosing syringe is provided for accurate measurement of the prescribed dose of the oral solution. Instructions for use are included in the pack.

Administrative Data

7. MARKETING AUTHORISATION HOLDER

Glaxo Group Ltd

Greenford Road

Greenford

Middlesex UB6 0NN

United Kingdom

8. MARKETING AUTHORISATION NUMBER(S)

EU/1/96/015/002

9. DATE OF FIRST AUTHORISATION/RENEWAL OF THE AUTHORISATION

Date of first authorisation: 8 August 1996

Date of renewal: 8 November 2001

10. DATE OF REVISION OF THE TEXT

17 December 2004

Eposin

(medac GmbH)

1. NAME OF THE MEDICINAL PRODUCT

Eposin.

2. QUALITATIVE AND QUANTITATIVE COMPOSITION

1 vial with 5 ml concentrate for solution for infusion contains 100 mg etoposide, Ph.Eur.

1 vial with 25 ml concentrate for solution for infusion contains 500 mg etoposide, Ph.Eur.

1 ml concentrate for solution for infusion contains 20 mg etoposide.

3. PHARMACEUTICAL FORM

Concentrate for solution for infusion (to dilute).

4. CLINICAL PARTICULARS

4.1 Therapeutic indications

Etoposide is indicated for the management of:

- testicular tumours in combination with other chemotherapeutic agents
- small cell lung cancer, in combination with other chemotherapeutic agents
- monoblastic leukaemia (AML M5) and acute myelomonoblastic leukaemia (AML M4) when standard therapy has failed (in combination with other chemotherapeutic agents).

4.2 Posology and method of administration

Eposin, concentrate for solution for infusion 20 mg/ml must be diluted immediately prior to use with either 5 % dextrose in water, or 0.9 % sodium chloride solution to give a final concentration of 0.2 to 0.4 mg/ml. At higher concentrations precipitation of etoposide may occur. The usual dose of etoposide, in combination with other approved chemotherapeutic agents, ranges from 100-120mg/m²/day via continuous infusion over 30 minutes for 3-5 days, followed by a resting period of 10-20 days. Generally 3 to 4 chemotherapy cycles are administered. Dose and amount of cycles should be adjusted to the level of bone marrow suppression and the reaction of the tumour. In patients with renal function impairment the dose should be adjusted. Etoposide is intended for intravenous administration only. To prevent the occurrence of hypotension, the infusion should be given over at least 30 minutes.

4.3 Contraindications

Severe myelosuppression, unless when this is caused by the underlying disease. Liver impairment. Hypersensitivity to etoposide or one of the other constituents. Eposin must not be used in neonates because of the excipient benzyl alcohol.

4.4 Special warnings and special precautions for use

If Eposin is to be used as part of a chemotherapy regimen, the physician should weigh the necessity to use the drug against the potential risk and side effects (see "Undesirable effects"). Etoposide should only be administered under strict observation by a doctor specialised in oncology, preferable in institutions specialised in such therapies.

It should not be injected intraarterially, intrapleurally, or intraperitoneally. Etoposide vials are intended for intravenous administration only. Extravasation should be strictly avoided. If extravasation occurs, the administration should be terminated immediately and restarted in another vein. Cooling, flooding with normal saline and local infiltration with corticosteroids have been reported as therapeutic measures. Etoposide should be given by slow intravenous infusion over a period of 30-60 minutes; rapid intravenous administration may cause hypotension. One should be aware of the possible occurrence of an anaphylactic reaction manifested by flushing, tachycardia, bronchospasm, and hypotension (see "Undesirable effects" section).

The substance etoposide can have genotoxic effects. Therefore, men being treated with etoposide are advised not to father a child during and up to 6 months after treatment and to seek advice on cryo-conservation of sperm prior to treatment because of the possibility of irreversible infertility due to therapy with etoposide. Women should not become pregnant during treatment with etoposide.

The occurrence of a leucopenia with a leucocyte count below 2,000/mm³ is an indication to withhold further therapy until the blood counts have sufficiently recovered (usually after 10 days). The administration of etoposide should be terminated at the occurrence of thrombocytopenia. Bacterial infections should be treated before the start of the therapy with etoposide.

Great care should be taken on giving etoposide to patients who have, or have been exposed to infection with herpes zoster. The occurrence of bone marrow depression, caused by radiotherapy or chemotherapy, necessitates a resting period. It is advised not to restart treatment with etoposide until the platelet count has reached at least 100,000/mm³.

This product contains 24% m/v of ethanol. Each 5 ml vial contains up to 1,2 g of alcohol, each 25 ml vial contains up to 6 g of alcohol. This can be harmful for those suffering from liver disease, alcoholism, epilepsy, brain injury or disease as well as for children and pregnant women. Alcohol also may modify or increase the effect of other medicines.

Handling precautions: see "Instructions for Use/Handling" section.

4.5 Interaction with other medicinal products and other forms of Interaction

The action of oral anticoagulants can be increased.

Phenylbutazone, sodium salicylate and salicylic acid can affect protein binding of etoposide.

Etoposide may potentiate the cytotoxic and myelosuppressive action of other drugs.

4.6 Pregnancy and lactation

The substance etoposide can have genotoxic effects and can impair the development of embryos. Etoposide should not be given to patients who are pregnant. It is recommended that breastfeeding is discontinued prior to treatment with etoposide.

In cases of vital indication for treating a pregnant patient she should be informed about the risk of damage to the child connected with the treatment. Women of childbearing potential should avoid pregnancy during treatment with etoposide. No adequate studies are available on the possible adverse effects of etoposide during human pregnancy. Regarding the pharmacological action of etoposide adverse effects are possible. Etoposide has been shown to be teratogenic in animals, and has mutagenic properties. It is not known whether etoposide is excreted in human milk. Eposin concentrate for solution for infusion contains benzyl alcohol. Benzyl alcohol can cross the placental barrier. One should take into account the potential toxicity for the unborn child after administration of Eposin prior or during delivery or caesarean section.

4.7 Effects on ability to drive and use machines

Due to the frequent occurrence of nausea and vomiting, driving and operation of machinery should be discouraged.

4.8 Undesirable effects

Hematologic toxicity:

Myelosuppression is dose limiting, with granulocyte nadirs occurring 5 to 15 days after drug administration and platelet nadirs occurring 9 to 16 days after drug administration. Bone marrow recovery is usually complete by day 21, and no cumulative toxicity has been reported.

Secondary leukemia:

The risk of secondary leukaemia among patients with germ-cell tumours after treatment with etoposide is about 1%. This leukaemia is characterised with a relatively short latency period (mean 35 months), monocytic or myelomono-cytic FAB subtype, chromosomal abnormalities at 11q23 in about 50% and a good response to chemotherapy. A total cumulative dose (etoposide > 2 g/m²) is associated with increased risk. Etoposide is also associated with development of acute promyelocytic leukaemia (APL). High doses of etoposide > 4,000 mg/m²) appear to increase the risk of APL.

Gastrointestinal toxicity:

Nausea and vomiting are the major gastro-intestinal toxicities. The severity of such nausea and vomiting is generally mild to moderate with treatment discontinuation required in 1% of patients. Diarrhoea, anorexia and mucositis may occur. Constipation and swallowing disorder have been observed rarely.

Hypotension:

Transient hypotension following rapid intravenous administration has been reported in 1% to 2% of patients. It has not been associated with cardiac toxicity or electrocardiographic changes. To prevent this rare occurrence, it is recommended that etoposide is administered by slow intravenous infusion over a 30- to 60-minute period. If hypotension occurs, it usually responds to supportive therapy after cessation of the administration. When restarting the infusion, a slower administration rate should be used.

Allergic reactions:

Seldom hypersensitivity reactions caused by benzyl alcohol may occur. Anaphylactic-like reactions characterised by flushing, tachycardia, bronchospasm, and hypotension have been reported (incidence 0.7-2%), also apnoea followed by spontaneous recurrence of breathing after withdrawal of etoposide infusion, increase in blood pressure. The reactions can be managed by cessation of the infusion and administration of pressor agents, corticosteroids, antihistamines and/or volume expanders as appropriate.

Alopecia:

Reversible alopecia, sometimes progressing to total baldness was observed in up to 70% of patients.

Other toxicities:

The following adverse reactions have been infrequent-ly reported:

peripheral neuropathy, paresthesiae, increased liver function tests with high doses, radiation "recall" dermatitis, hand-foot syndrome, central nervous effects (fatigue, drowsiness) 0-3%, hyperuricemia, taste impairment, fever, rash, urticaria, skin discoloration, pruritus, abdominal pain. The following adverse events have been reported after administration of etoposide (a causal relationship has not been established): Stevens-Johnson syndrome, rhythm disorders, myocardial infarction, reversible loss of vision.

4.9 Overdose

Acute overdosage results in severe forms of normally occurring adverse reactions, in particular leucopenia and thrombopenia. Severe mucositis and elevated values of serum bilirubin, SGOT and alkaline phosphatase have been reported after administration of high doses of etoposide. The management of bone marrow depression is symptomatic, including antibiotics and transfusions. If hypersensitivity to etoposide occurs, antihistamines and intravenously administered corticosteroids are appropriate.

5. PHARMACOLOGICAL PROPERTIES

5.1 Pharmacodynamic properties

Pharmacotherapeutic classification: podophyllotoxine derivatives (ATC: L01CB01)

Etoposide is a semisynthetic derivative of podophyllotoxin used in the treatment of certain neoplastic diseases. Podophyllotoxins inhibit mitosis by blocking microtubular assembly. Etoposide inhibits cell cycle progression at a premitotic phase (late S and G2).

It does not interfere with the synthesis of nucleinic acids.

5.2 Pharmacokinetic properties

The concentration of etoposide in blood and organs is low with maximum values in the liver and the kidneys. Protein binding could be as high as 98%. On intravenous administration, the disposition of etoposide is best described as a biphasic process with an initial half-life of about 1.5 hours. After distribution, half-life is about 40 hours. The terminal half-life is 6-8 hours. Following a single intravenous dose etoposide is excreted in the urine for about 63% and in the faeces for about 31% after 80 hours.

5.3 Preclinical safety data

Reproductive toxicity/teratogenicity:

Etoposide has been shown to be embryotoxic and teratogenic in animal experiments with rats and mice.

Mutagenicity:

There are positive results from in vitro and in vivo test with regard to gene and chromosome mutations induced by etoposide. The results justify the suspicion of a mutagenic effect in humans.

Carcinogenicity:

No animal tests with regard to carcinogenicity were performed. Based on the DNA-damaging effect and the mutagenic properties, etoposide is potentially carcinogenic.

6. PHARMACEUTICAL PARTICULARS

6.1 List of excipients

Macrogol 300, polysorbate 80, benzyl alcohol, ethanol, citric acid, anhydrous.

6.2 Incompatibilities

Plastic devices made of acrylic or ABS polymers have been reported to crack when used with undiluted Eposin, concentrate for solution for infusion 20 mg/ml. This effect has not been reported with etoposide after dilution of the concentrate for solution for infusion according to instructions.

6.3 Shelf life

3 years.

6.4 Special precautions for storage

Unopened vials of Eposin, concentrate for solution for infusion 20 mg/ml are stable for 3 years when stored not above 25°C, protected from light (keep vials in the outer carton). Do not freeze.

After dilution to a concentration of 0.2 mg/ml or 0.4 mg/ml etoposide chemical and physical in use stability has been demonstrated for 24 hours at 15-25°C. From a microbiological point of view, the diluted product should be used immediately. If not used immediately, in-use storage times and conditions prior to use are the responsibility of the user and would normally not be longer than 12 hours at 15-25°C, unless dilution has taken place in controlled and validated aseptic conditions. Do not store the diluted product in a refrigerator (2-8°C) as this might cause precipitation.

Solutions showing any sign of precipitation should not be used.

6.5 Nature and contents of container

Each injection vial contains 100 mg (5 ml) of etoposide.

Each injection vial contains 500 mg (25 ml) of etoposide.

One package contains 1 (10) vial(s) of Eposin.

Not all pack sizes may be marketed.

6.6 Instructions for use and handling

Eposin should not be used without diluting! Dilute with 0,9% sodium chloride or 5% dextrose.

For waste-disposal and safety information guidelines on safe-handling of antineoplastic drugs should be followed.

Any contact with the fluid should be avoided. During preparation and reconstitution a strictly aseptic working technique should be used; protective measures should include the use of gloves, mask, safety goggles and protective clothing. Use of a vertical laminar airflow (LAF) hood is recommended. Gloves should be worn during administration. Waste-disposal procedures should take into account the cytotoxic nature of this substance. If etoposide contacts skin, mucosae or eyes, immediately wash thoroughly with water. Soap may be used for skin cleansing.

7. MARKETING AUTHORISATION HOLDER

Pharmachemie B.V.
P.O. Box 552
2003 RN Haarlem
The Netherlands.

8. MARKETING AUTHORISATION NUMBER(S)

PL 04946/0018

9. DATE OF FIRST AUTHORISATION/RENEWAL OF THE AUTHORISATION

17 December 1996

10. DATE OF REVISION OF THE TEXT

May 2001

Eprex solution for injection

(Janssen-Cilag Ltd)

1. NAME OF THE MEDICINAL PRODUCT

EPREX®

2. QUALITATIVE AND QUANTITATIVE COMPOSITION

Epoetinum alfa......... 2,000 IU or 16.8 micrograms per ml.

A pre-filled syringe of 0.5 ml contains 1,000 IU or 8.4 micrograms of epoetinum alfa.

Epoetinum alfa......... 4,000 IU or 33.6 micrograms per ml.

A pre-filled syringe of 0.5 ml contains 2,000 IU or 16.8 micrograms of epoetinum alfa.

Epoetinum alfa.......... 10,000 IU or 84 micrograms per ml.

A pre-filled syringe of 0.3 ml contains 3,000 IU or 25.2 micrograms of epoetinum alfa.

A pre-filled syringe of 0.4 ml contains 4,000 IU or 33.6 micrograms of epoetinum alfa.

A pre-filled syringe of 0.5 ml contains 5,000 IU or 42.0 micrograms of epoetinum alfa.

A pre-filled syringe of 0.6 ml contains 6,000 IU or 50.4 micrograms of epoetinum alfa.

A pre-filled syringe of 0.8 ml contains 8,000 IU or 67.2 micrograms of epoetinum alfa.

A pre-filled syringe of 1.0 ml contains 10,000 IU or 84.0 micrograms of epoetinum alfa.

Epoetinum alfa........ 40,000 IU or 336 micrograms per ml.

A vial of 1.0 ml contains 40,000 IU or 336 micrograms of epoetinum alfa.

For excipients, see 6.1

3. PHARMACEUTICAL FORM

Solution for injection.

Clear, colourless solution.

4. CLINICAL PARTICULARS

4.1 Therapeutic indications

• Treatment of anaemia associated with chronic renal failure in paediatric and adult patients on haemodialysis and adult patients on peritoneal dialysis.

• Treatment of severe anaemia of renal origin accompanied by clinical symptoms in adult patients with renal insufficiency not yet undergoing dialysis.

• Treatment of anaemia and reduction of transfusion requirements in adult patients receiving chemotherapy for solid tumours, malignant lymphoma or multiple myeloma, and at risk of transfusion as assessed by the patient's general status (e.g. cardiovascular status, pre-existing anaemia at the start of chemotherapy).

• Eprex can be used to increase the yield of autologous blood from patients in a predonation programme. Its use in this indication must be balanced against the reported risk of thrombo-embolic events. Treatment should only be given to patients with moderate anaemia (Hb 10-13 g/dl [6.2-8.1 mmol/l], no iron deficiency), if blood saving procedures are not available or insufficient when the scheduled major elective surgery requires a large volume of blood (4 or more units of blood for females or 5 or more units for males).

• Eprex can be used to reduce exposure to allogeneic blood transfusions in adult non-iron deficient patients prior to major elective orthopaedic surgery, having a high perceived risk for transfusion complications. Use should be restricted to patients with moderate anaemia (e.g. Hb 10-13 g/dl) who do not have an autologous predonation programme available and with expected moderate blood loss (900 to 1800 ml).

Good blood management practices should always be used in the perisurgical setting.

4.2 Posology and method of administration

Method of administration

As with any other injectable product, check that there are no particles in the solution or change in colour.

a. Intravenous injection: over at least one to five minutes, depending on the total dose. In haemodialysed patients, a bolus injection may be given during the dialysis session through a suitable venous port in the dialysis line. Alternatively, the injection can be given at the end of the dialysis session via the fistula needle tubing, followed by 10 ml of isotonic saline to rinse the tubing and ensure satisfactory injection of the product into the circulation.

   A slower injection is preferable in patients who react to the treatment with "flu-like" symptoms.

   Do not administer by intravenous infusion, or mixed with other drugs.

b. Subcutaneous injection: a maximum volume of 1 ml at one injection site should generally not be exceeded. In case of larger volumes, more than one site should be chosen for the injection.

   The injections are given in the limbs or the anterior abdominal wall.

Chronic renal failure patients:

In patients with chronic renal failure, the product must only be administered by the intravenous route (see sections 4.3 and 4.4 - Pure Red Cell Aplasia).

The haemoglobin concentration aimed for is between 10 and 12 g/dl (6.2-7.5 mmol/l), except in paediatric patients in whom the haemoglobin concentration should be between 9.5 and 11 g/dl (5.9-6.8 mmol/l).

In patients with chronic renal failure and clinically evident ischaemic heart disease or congestive heart failure, maintenance haemoglobin concentration should not exceed the upper limit of the target haemoglobin concentration.

Iron status should be evaluated prior to and during treatment and iron supplementation administered if necessary. In addition, other causes of anaemia, such as B_{12} or folate deficiency, should be excluded before instituting therapy with epoetinum alfa. Non response to epoetinum alfa therapy should prompt a search for causative factors. These include: iron, folate, or Vitamin B_{12} deficiency; aluminium intoxication; intercurrent infections; inflammatory or traumatic episodes; occult blood loss; haemolysis, and bone marrow fibrosis of any origin.

Adult haemodialysis patients:

In patients on haemodialysis, the product must only be administered by the intravenous route (see sections 4.3 and 4.4 - Pure Red Cell Aplasia).

The treatment is divided into two stages:

Correction phase:

50 IU/kg 3 times per week by the intravenous route.

When a dose adjustment is necessary, this should be done in steps of at least four weeks. At each step, the increase or reduction in dose should be of 25 IU/kg 3 times per week.

Maintenance phase:

Dosage adjustment in order to maintain haemoglobin values at the desired level: Hb between 10 and 12 g/dl (6.2-7.5 mmol/l).

The recommended total weekly dose is between 75 and 300 IU/kg.

The clinical data available suggest that those patients whose initial haemoglobin is very low (<6 g/dl or <3.75 mmol/l) may require higher maintenance doses than those whose initial anaemia is less severe >8 g/dl or >5 mmol/l).

Paediatric haemodialysis patients:

In paediatric patients on haemodialysis, the product must only be administered by the intravenous route (see sections 4.3 and 4.4 - Pure Red Cell Aplasia).

The treatment is divided into two stages:

Correction phase:

50 IU/kg 3 times per week by the intravenous route. When a dose adjustment is necessary, this should be done in steps of 25 IU/kg 3 times per week at intervals of at least 4 weeks until the desired goal is achieved.

Maintenance phase:

Dosage adjustment in order to maintain haemoglobin values at the desired level: Hb between 9.5 and 11 g/dl (5.9-6.8 mmol/l).

Generally, children under 30 kg require higher maintenance doses than children over 30 kg and adults. For example, the following maintenance doses were observed in clinical trials after 6 months of treatment.

	Dose (IU/kg given 3x week)	
Weight (kg)	Median	Usual maintenance dose
<10	100	75-150
10-30	75	60-150
>30	33	30-100

The clinical data available suggest that those patients whose initial haemoglobin is very low (<6.8 g/dl or <4.25 mmol/l) may require higher maintenance doses than those whose initial haemoglobin is higher >6.8 g/dl or >4.25 mmol/l).

Adult patients with renal insufficiency not yet undergoing dialysis:

EPREX must only be given by the intravenous route (see sections 4.3 and 4.4 - Pure Red Cell Aplasia).

The treatment is divided into two stages:

Correction phase:

Starting dose of 50 IU/kg 3 times per week, followed if necessary by a dosage increase with 25 IU/kg increments (3 times per week) until the desired goal is achieved (this should be done in steps of at least four weeks).

Maintenance phase:

Dosage adjustment in order to maintain haemoglobin values at the desired level: Hb between 10 and 12 g/dl (6.2-7.5 mmol/l) (maintenance dose between 17 and 33 IU/kg 3 times per week).

The maximum dosage should not exceed 200 IU/kg 3 times per week.

Adult peritoneal dialysis patients:

EPREX must only be given by the intravenous route (see sections 4.3 and 4.4 - Pure Red Cell Aplasia).

The treatment is divided into two stages:

Correction phase:

Starting dose of 50 IU/kg 2 times per week.

Maintenance phase:

Dosage adjustment in order to maintain haemoglobin values at the desired level: (Hb between 10 and 12 g/dl (6.2-7.5 mmol/l) (maintenance dose between 25 and 50 IU/kg 2 times per week into 2 equal injections).

Adult cancer patients receiving chemotherapy:

The subcutaneous route of administration should be used.

Epoetinum alfa therapy should be administered to patients with anaemia (e.g. Hb ≤10.5 g/dl [6.5 mmol/l]).

The target haemoglobin concentration is approximately 12 g/dl (7.5 mmol/l).

Epoetinum alfa therapy should continue until one month after the end of chemotherapy.

The initial dose is 150 IU/kg given subcutaneously 3 times per week. Alternatively, EPREX can be administered at an initial dose of 450 IU/kg subcutaneously once weekly. If the haemoglobin has increased by at least 1 g/dl (0.62 mmol/l) or the reticulocyte count has increased ≥40,000 cells/μl above baseline after 4 weeks of treatment, the dose should remain at 150 IU/kg 3 times per week or 450 IU/kg once weekly. If the haemoglobin increase is <1 g/dl (<0.62 mmol/l) and the reticulocyte count has increased <40,000 cells/μl above baseline, increase the dose to 300 IU/kg 3 times per week. If after an additional 4 weeks of therapy at 300 IU/kg 3 times per week, the haemoglobin has increased ≥1 g/dl (0.62 mmol/l) or the reticulocyte count has increased ≥40,000 cells/μl the dose should remain at 300 IU/kg 3 times per week. However, if the haemoglobin has increased <1 g/dl (<0.62 mmol/l) and the reticulocyte count has increased <40,000 cells/μl above baseline, response is unlikely and treatment should be discontinued. The recommended dosing regimen is described in the following diagram:

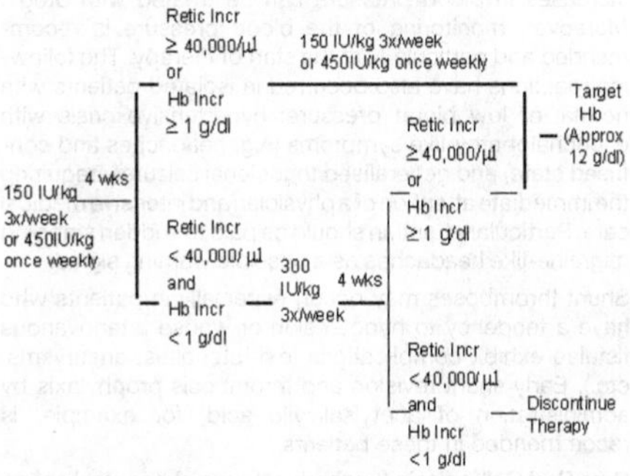

Dose adjustment:

A rate of rise in haemoglobin of greater than 2 g/dl (1.25 mmol/l) per month or haemoglobin levels of >13 g/dl >8.1 mmol/l) should be avoided. If the haemoglobin is rising by more than 2 g/dl (1.25 mmol/l) per month or haemoglobin is approaching 12 g/dl (7.4 mmol/l), reduce the epoetinum alfa dose by about 25-50% depending upon the rate of rise of haemoglobin. If the haemoglobin exceeds 13 g/dl (8.1 mmol/l), discontinue therapy until it falls to 12 g/dl (7.4 mmol/l) and then reinstitute epoetinum alfa therapy at a dose 25% below the previous dose.

Adult surgery patients in an autologous predonation programme:

The intravenous route of administration should be used. At the time of donating blood, epoetinum alfa should be administered after the completion of the blood donation procedure.

Mildly anaemic patients (haematocrit of 33-39%) requiring predeposit of ≥4 units of blood should be treated with epoetinum alfa at 600 IU/kg 2 times weekly for 3 weeks prior to surgery. Using this regimen, it was possible to withdraw ≥4 units of blood from 81% of epoetinum alfa-treated patients compared to 37% of placebo-treated patients. Epoetinum alfa therapy reduced the risk of exposure to homologous blood by 50% compared to patients not receiving epoetinum alfa.

All patients being treated with epoetinum alfa should receive adequate iron supplementation (e.g. 200 mg oral elemental iron daily) throughout the course of epoetinum alfa treatment. Iron supplementation should be started as soon as possible, even several weeks prior to initiating the autologous predeposit, in order to achieve high iron stores prior to starting epoetinum alfa therapy.

Adult patients scheduled for major elective orthopaedic surgery:

The subcutaneous route of administration should be used.

The recommended dose regimen is 600 IU/kg of epoetinum alfa, given weekly for three weeks (days -21, -14 and -7) prior to surgery and on the day of surgery. In cases where there is a medical need to shorten the lead time before surgery to less than three weeks, 300 IU/kg epoetinum alfa should be given daily for 10 consecutive days prior to surgery, on the day of surgery and for four days immediately thereafter. When performing haematologic assessments during the preoperative period, if the haemoglobin level reaches 15 g/dl, or higher, administration of epoetinum alfa should be stopped and further dosages should not be given.

Care should be taken to ensure that at the outset of the treatment patients are not iron-deficient. All patients being treated with epoetinum alfa should receive adequate iron supplementation (e.g. 200 mg oral elemental iron daily) throughout the course of epoetinum alfa treatment. If possible, iron supplementation should be started prior to epoetinum alfa therapy, to achieve adequate iron stores.

4.3 Contraindications

The subcutaneous route of administration is contra-indicated only in patients with chronic renal failure (see sections 4.4 - Pure Red Cell Aplasia and 4.8).

Patients who develop Pure Red Cell Aplasia (PRCA) following treatment with any erythropoietin should not receive EPREX or any other erythropoietin (see section 4.4 - Pure Red Cell Aplasia).

Uncontrolled hypertension.

All contra-indications associated with autologous blood predonation programmes should be respected in patients being supplemented with epoetinum alfa.

Hypersensitivity to the active substance or to any of the excipients.

The use of epoetinum alfa in patients scheduled for major elective orthopaedic surgery and not participating in an autologous blood predonation programme is contra-indicated in patients with severe coronary, peripheral arterial, carotid or cerebral vascular disease, including patients with recent myocardial infarction or cerebral vascular accident.

Patients who for any reason cannot receive adequate antithrombotic prophylaxis.

4.4 Special warnings and special precautions for use

Chronic renal failure and cancer patients on epoetinum alfa should have haemoglobin levels measured on a regular basis until a stable level is achieved, and periodically thereafter.

In chronic renal failure patients, therate of increase in haemoglobin should be approximately 1 g/dl (0.62 mmol/l) per month and should not exceed 2 g/dl (1.25 mmol/l) per month to minimise risks of an increase in hypertension.

As cases of PRCA have been reported in chronic renal failure patients with EPREX administered by the subcutaneous route, EPREX must only be administered by the intravenous route in these patients. In most of these patients, antibodies to erythropoietins have been observed. In patients developing sudden lack of efficacy, typical causes of non-response (e.g. iron, folate, or Vitamin B_{12} deficiency, aluminium intoxication, infection or inflammation, blood loss, and haemolysis) should be investigated. If no cause is identified, a bone marrow examination should be considered. If PRCA is diagnosed, therapy with EPREX must be immediately discontinued and testing for erythropoietin antibodies should be considered. Patients should not be switched to another product as anti-erythropoietin antibodies cross-react with other erythropoietins. Other causes of Pure Red Cell Aplasia should be excluded, and appropriate therapy instituted (see sections 4.2 and 4.3).

Monitoring of reticulocyte count on a regular basis is recommended to detect possible occurrence of lack of efficacy in chronic renal failure patients.

In all patients receiving epoetinum alfa, blood pressure should be closely monitored and controlled as necessary. Epoetinum alfa should be used with caution in the presence of untreated, inadequately treated or poorly controllable hypertension. It may be necessary to add or increase anti-hypertensive treatment. If blood pressure cannot be controlled, epoetinum alfa treatment should be discontinued.

Epoetinum alfa should also be used with caution in the presence of epilepsy and chronic liver failure.

Hyperkalaemia has been observed in isolated cases. In chronic renal failure patients, correction for anaemia may lead to increased appetite, and potassium and protein intake. Dialysis prescriptions may have to be adjusted periodically to maintain urea, creatinine and potassium in the desired range. Serum electrolytes should be monitored in chronic renal failure patients. If an elevated (or rising) serum potassium level is detected then consideration should be given to ceasing epoetinum alfa administration until hyperkalaemia has been corrected.

There may be a moderate dose-dependent rise in the platelet count within the normal range during treatment with epoetinum alfa. This regresses during the course of continued therapy. It is recommended that the platelet count is regularly monitored during the first 8 weeks of therapy.

An increase in heparin dose during haemodialysis is frequently required during the course of therapy with epoetinum alfa as a result of the increased packed cell volume. Occlusion of the dialysis system is possible if heparinisation is not optimum.

Based on information available to date, correction of anaemia with epoetinum alfa in adult patients with renal insufficiency not yet undergoing dialysis does not accelerate the rate of progression of renal insufficiency.

All other causes of anaemia (iron deficiency, haemolysis, blood loss, vitamin B_{12} or folate deficiencies) should be considered and treated prior to initiating therapy with epoetinum alfa. In most cases, the ferritin values in the serum fall simultaneously with the rise in packed cell volume. In order to ensure optimum response to epoetinum alfa, adequate iron stores should be assured:

- iron supplementation, e.g. 200-300 mg/day orally (100-200 mg/day for paediatric patients) is recommended for chronic renal failure patients whose serum ferritin levels are below 100 ng/ml.
- oral iron substitution of 200-300 mg/day is recommended for all cancer patients whose transferrin saturation is below 20%.

All of these additive factors of anaemia should also be carefully considered when deciding to increase the dose of epoetinum alfa in cancer patients.

In cancer patients receiving chemotherapy, the 2-3 week delay between erythropoietin administration and the appearance of erythropoietin-induced red cells should be taken into account when assessing if epoetinum alfa therapy is appropriate (patient at risk of being transfused).

In cancer patients receiving chemotherapy; should the rate of increase in haemoglobin exceed 2 g/dl (1.25 mmol/l) per month or the haemoglobin level exceed 13 g/dl (8.1 mmol/l) or haemoglobin is approaching 12 g/dl (7.4 mmol/l), the dose adjustment detailed in section 4.2 should be thoroughly performed to minimise potential risk factors of thrombotic events (see section 4.2 - Adult cancer patients receiving chemotherapy - Dose adjustment).

As an increased incidence of thrombotic vascular events (TVEs) has been observed in cancer patients receiving erythropoietic agents (see section 4.8 undesirable effects), this risk should be carefully weighed against the benefit to be derived from treatment (with epoetinum alfa) particularly in cancer patients with an increased risk of thrombotic vascular events, such as obesity and patients with a prior history of TVEs (e.g. deep venous thrombosis or pulmonary embolism).

All special warnings and special precautions associated with autologous predonation programs, especially routine volume replacement, should be respected.

In patients scheduled for major elective orthopaedic surgery the cause of anaemia should be established and treated, if possible, before the start of epoetinum alfa treatment. Thrombotic events can be a risk in this population and this possibility should be carefully weighed against the benefit to be derived from the treatment in this patient group.

Patients scheduled for major elective orthopaedic surgery should receive adequate antithrombotic prophylaxis, as thrombotic and vascular events may occur insurgical patients, especially in those with underlying cardiovascular disease. In addition, special precaution should be taken in patients with predisposition for development of DVTs. Moreover, in patients with a baseline haemoglobin of >13 g/dl, the possibility that epoetinum alfa treatment may be associated with an increased risk of postoperative thrombotic/vascular events cannot be excluded. Therefore, it should not be used in patients with baseline haemoglobin >13 g/dl.

In patients with chronic renal failure and clinically evident ischaemic heart disease or congestive heart failure, maintenance haemoglobin concentration should not exceed the upper limit of the target haemoglobin concentration as recommended under 4.2 Posology and Method of Administration.

Growth factor potential

Epoetinum alfa is a growth factor that primarily stimulates red blood cell production. However, the possibility that epoetinum alfa can act as a growth factor for any tumour type, particularly myeloid malignancies, cannot be excluded (see section 5.3).

Erythropoietin receptors are also found to be present on the surface of some malignant cell lines and tumour biopsy specimens. However, it is not known if these receptors are functional.

Clinical studies conducted with Epoetins have provided insufficient information to establish whether use of Epoetin products have an adverse effect on time to tumour progression or progression-free survival.

Until further information is available, the recommended target haemoglobin in cancer patients should not exceed 12 g/dl in men or women.

4.5 Interaction with other medicinal products and other forms of Interaction

No evidence exists that indicates that treatment with epoetinum alfa alters the metabolism of other drugs. However, since cyclosporin is bound by RBCs there is potential for a drug interaction. If epoetinum alfa is given concomitantly with cyclosporin, blood levels of cyclosporin should be monitored and the dose of cyclosporin adjusted as the haematocrit rises.

No evidence exists that indicates an interaction between epoetinum alfa and G-CSF or GM-CSF with regard to haematological differentiation or proliferation of tumour biopsy specimens *in vitro*.

4.6 Pregnancy and lactation

There are no adequate and well-controlled studies in pregnant women. Studies in animals have shown reproduction toxicity (see section 5.3). Consequently:

• In chronic renal failure patients, epoetinum alfa should be used in pregnancy only if the potential benefit outweighs the potential risk to the foetus.

• In pregnant or lactating surgical patients participating in an autologous blood predonation programme, the use of epoetinum alfa is not recommended.

4.7 Effects on ability to drive and use machines

None

4.8 Undesirable effects

General

Non-specific skin rashes have been described in association with epoetinum alfa.

"Flu-like" symptoms such as headaches, joint pains, feelings of weakness, dizziness and tiredness may occur, especially at the start of treatment.

Thrombocytosis has been observed but its occurrence is very rare. Refer to section 4.4 Special warnings and precautions for use.

Thrombotic/vascular events, such as myocardial ischaemia, myocardial infarction, cerebrovascular accidents (cerebral haemorrhage and cerebral infarction), transient ischaemic attacks, deep venous thrombosis, arterial thrombosis, pulmonary emboli, aneurysms, retinal thrombosis, and clotting of an artificial kidney have been reported in patients receiving erythropoietic agents, including patients receiving EPREX.

Hypersensitivity reactions have been rarely reported with epoetinum alfa including isolated cases of angioedema and anaphylactic reaction.

Adult and paediatric haemodialysis patients, adult peritoneal dialysis and adult patients with renal insufficiency not yet undergoing dialysis

The most frequent adverse reaction during treatment with epoetinum alfa is a dose-dependent increase in blood pressure or aggravation of existing hypertension. These increases in blood pressure can be treated with drugs. Moreover, monitoring of the blood pressure is recommended and particularly at the start of therapy. The following reactions have also occurred in isolated patients with normal or low blood pressure: hypertensive crisis with encephalopathy-like symptoms (e.g. headaches and confused state) and generalised tonoclonal seizures, requiring the immediate attention of a physician and intensive medical care. Particular attention should be paid to sudden stabbing migraine-like headaches as a possible warning signal.

Shunt thromboses may occur, especially in patients who have a tendency to hypotension or whose arteriovenous fistulae exhibit complications (e.g. stenoses, aneurysms, etc.). Early shunt revision and thrombosis prophylaxis by administration of acetylsalicylic acid, for example, is recommended in these patients.

Pure Red Cell Aplasia (erythroblastopenia) has rarely been reported in chronic renal failure patients after months to years of treatment with Eprex or other erythropoietins. In most of these patients, antibodies to erythropoietins have been observed (See sections 4.3 and 4.4 - Pure Red Cell Aplasia).

Anaemic adult cancer patients receiving chemotherapy

Hypertension may occur in epoetinum alfa treated patients. Consequently, haemoglobin and blood pressure should be closely monitored.

An increased incidence of thrombotic vascular events (see sections 4.4 Special warnings and precautions for use and 4.8 – General) has been observed in patients receiving erythropoietic agents.

In an investigational study in women with metastatic breast cancer, intended to determine whether erythropoeitin treatment beyond the correction of anaemia could improve treatment outcomes, overall mortality, mortality attributed to disease progression, and incidence of fatal thromboembolic events were all higher in patients receiving epoetinum alfa than in the placebo group.

Surgery patients in autologous predonation programs

Independent of epoetinum alfa treatment, thrombotic and vascular events may occur in surgical patients with underlying cardiovascular disease following repeated phlebotomy. Therefore, routine volume replacement should be performed in such patients.

Patients scheduled for major elective orthopaedic surgery

In patients scheduled for major elective orthopaedic surgery, with a baseline haemoglobin of 10 to 13 g/dl, the incidence of thrombotic/vascular events (most of which were DVTs), in the overall patient population of the clinical trials, appeared to be similar across the different epoetinum alfa dosing groups and placebo group, although the clinical experience is limited.

Moreover, in patients with a baseline haemoglobin of >13 g/dl, the possibility that epoetinum alfa treatment may be associated with an increased risk of postoperative thrombotic/vascular events cannot be excluded.

4.9 Overdose

The therapeutic margin of epoetinum alfa is very wide. Overdosage of epoetinum alfa may produce effects that are extensions of the pharmacological effects of the hormone. Phlebotomy may be performed if excessively high haemoglobin levels occur. Additional supportive care should be provided as necessary.

5. PHARMACOLOGICAL PROPERTIES

5.1 Pharmacodynamic properties

ATC Classification: B03XA01

Erythropoietin is a glycoprotein that stimulates, as a mitosis-stimulating factor and differentiating hormone, the formation of erythrocytes from precursors of the stem cell compartment.

The apparent molecular weight of erythropoietin is 32,000 to 40,000 dalton. The protein fraction of the molecule contributes about 58% and consists of 165 amino acids. The four carbohydrate chains are attached via three N-glycosidic bonds and one O-glycosidic bond to the protein. Epoetinum alfa obtained by gene technology is glycosylated and is identical in its amino acid and carbohydrate composition to endogenous human erythropoietin that has been isolated from the urine of anaemic patients.

Epoetinum alfa has the highest possible purity according to the present state of the art. In particular, no residues of the cell line used for the production are detectable at the concentrations of the active ingredient that are used in humans.

The biological efficacy of epoetinum alfa has been demonstrated in various animal models *in vivo* (normal and anaemic rats, polycythaemic mice). After administration of epoetinum alfa, the number of erythrocytes, the Hb values and reticulocyte counts increase as well as the ^{59}Fe-incorporation rate.

An increased ^{3}H-thymidine incorporation in the erythroid nucleated spleen cells has been found *in vitro* (mouse spleen cell culture) after incubation with epoetinum alfa.

It could be shown with the aid of cell cultures of human bone marrow cells that epoetinum alfa stimulates erythropoiesis specifically and does not affect leucopoiesis. Cytotoxic actions of epoetinum alfa on bone marrow cells could not be detected.

As with other haematopoietic growth factors, epoetinum alfa has shown *in vitro* stimulating properties on human endothelial cells. In more than ten years experience, no clinical consequences have been observed.

721 cancer patients receiving non-platinum chemotherapy were included in three placebo-controlled studies, 389 patients with haematological malignancies (221 multiple myeloma, 144 non-Hodgkin's lymphoma, and 24 other haematological malignancies) and 332 with solid tumours (172 breast, 64 gynaecological, 23 lung, 22 prostate, 21 gastro-intestinal, and 30 other tumour types). In two large, open-label studies, 2697 cancer patients receiving non-platinum chemotherapy were included, 1895 with solid tumours (683 breast, 260 lung, 174 gynaecological, 300 gastro-intestinal, and 478 other tumour types) and 802 with haematological malignancies.

In a prospective, randomised, double-blind, placebo-controlled trial conducted in 375 anaemic patients with various non-myeloid malignancies receiving non-platinum chemotherapy, there was a significant reduction of anaemia-related sequelae (e.g. fatigue, decreased energy, and activity reduction), as measured by the following instruments and scales: Functional Assessment of Cancer Therapy-Anemia (FACT-An) general scale, FACT-An fatigue scale, and Cancer Linear Analogue Scale (CLAS). Two other smaller, randomised, placebo-controlled trials failed to show a significant improvement in quality of life parameters on the EORTC-QLQ-C30 scale or CLAS, respectively.

5.2 Pharmacokinetic properties

I.V. route

Measurement of epoetinum alfa following multiple dose intravenous administration revealed a half-life of approximately 4 hours in normal volunteers and a somewhat more prolonged half-life in renal failure patients, approximately 5 hours. A half-life of approximately 6 hours has been reported in children.

S.C. route

Following subcutaneous injection, serum levels of epoetinum alfa are much lower than the levels achieved following i.v. injection, the levels increase slowly and reach a peak between 12 and 18 hours postdose. The peak is always well below the peak achieved using the i.v. route (approximately 1/20th of the value).

There is no accumulation: the levels remain the same, whether they are determined 24 hours after the first injection or 24 hours after the last injection.

The half-life is difficult to evaluate for the subcutaneous route and is estimated about 24 hours.

The bioavailability of subcutaneous injectable epoetinum alfa is much lower than that of the intravenous drug: approximately 20%.

5.3 Preclinical safety data

In some pre-clinical toxicological studies in dogs and rats, but not in monkeys, epoetinum alfa therapy was associated with subclinical bone marrow fibrosis (bone marrow fibrosis is a known complication of chronic renal failure in humans and may be related to secondary hyperparathyroidism or unknown factors. The incidence of bone marrow fibrosis was not increased in a study of haemodialysis patients who were treated with epoetinum alfa for 3 years compared to a matched control group of dialysis patients who had not been treated with epoetinum alfa).

In animal studies, epoetinum alfa has been shown to decrease foetal body weight, delay ossification and increase foetal mortality when given in weekly doses of approximately 20 times the recommended human weekly dose. These changes are interpreted as being secondary to decreased maternal body weight gain.

Epoetinum alfa did not show any changes in bacterial and mammalian cell culture mutagenicity tests and an *in vivo* micronucleus test in mice.

Long-term carcinogenicity studies have not been carried out. There are conflicting reports in the literature regarding whether erythropoietins may play a major role as tumour proliferators. These reports are based on *in vitro* findings from human tumour samples, but are of uncertain significance in the clinical situation.

6. PHARMACEUTICAL PARTICULARS

6.1 List of excipients

Sodium dihydrogen phosphate dihydrate

Disodium phosphate dihydrate

Sodium chloride

Polysorbate 80

Glycine

Water for injections

6.2 Incompatibilities

In the absence of compatibility studies, this medicinal product must not be mixed with other medicinal products.

6.3 Shelf life

Vials: 24 months

Syringes: 18 months

6.4 Special precautions for storage
Store at 2° to 8°C. This temperature range should be closely maintained until administration to the patient. Store in the original package in order to protect from light. Do not freeze or shake.

6.5 Nature and contents of container
Vials:
Pack of 1 vial with 40,000 IU/1.0 ml of epoetinum alfa,

a pack of 4 vials with 40,000 IU/1.0 ml of epoetinum alfa each,

and a pack of 6 vials with 40,000 IU/1.0 ml of epoetinum alfa each.

Pre-filled syringes

0.5 ml (1,000 IU) of solution in pre-filled syringe (type I glass) with plunger (teflon-faced rubber) and needle - pack of 6.

0.5 ml (2,000 IU) of solution in pre-filled syringe (type I glass) with plunger (teflon-faced rubber) and needle - pack of 6.

0.3 ml (3,000 IU) of solution in pre-filled syringe (type I glass) with plunger (teflon-faced rubber) and needle - pack of 6.

0.4 ml (4,000 IU) of solution in pre-filled syringe (type I glass) with plunger (teflon-faced rubber) and needle - pack of 6.

0.5 ml (5,000 IU) of solution in pre-filled syringe (type I glass) with plunger (teflon-faced rubber) and needle - pack of 6.

0.6 ml (6,000 IU) of solution in pre-filled syringe (type I glass) with plunger (teflon-faced rubber) and needle - pack of 6.

0.8 ml (8,000 IU) of solution in pre-filled syringe (type I glass) with plunger (teflon-faced rubber) and needle - pack of 6.

1.0 ml (10,000 IU) of solution in pre-filled syringe (type I glass) with plunger (teflon-faced rubber) and needle - pack of 6.

6.6 Instructions for use and handling
Do not administer by intravenous infusion or in conjunction with other drug solutions.

The product is for single use only.

The product should not be used, and discarded

- If the seal is broken,

- If the liquid if coloured or you can see particles floating in it,

- If you know, or think that it may have been accidentally frozen,

- If you know or suspect that the product has been left at room temperature for more than 60 minutes before injection, or

- If there has been a refrigerator failure.

Any waste material should be disposed of in accordance with local requirements.

7. MARKETING AUTHORISATION HOLDER
Janssen-Cilag Ltd
Saunderton
High Wycombe
Bucks
HP14 4HJ
UK

8. MARKETING AUTHORISATION NUMBER(S)
PL 0242/0297
PL 0242/0298
PL 0242/0299
PL 0242/0357

9. DATE OF FIRST AUTHORISATION/RENEWAL OF THE AUTHORISATION
Renewal of Authorisations: 04 August 2003

10. DATE OF REVISION OF THE TEXT
20 October 2004

Equasym 5mg,10mg and 20mg Tablets

(Celltech Pharmaceuticals Limited)

1. NAME OF THE MEDICINAL PRODUCT
Equasym® 5 mg, 10 mg, 20 mg tablets

2. QUALITATIVE AND QUANTITATIVE COMPOSITION
One tablet contains 5 mg, 10 mg, 20 mg of methylphenidate hydrochloride

For excipients, see section 6.1.

3. PHARMACEUTICAL FORM
Tablet.

Tablet with breakline, 'Medeva' and strength embossed on one side.

4. CLINICAL PARTICULARS

4.1 Therapeutic indications
Methylphenidate is indicated as part of a comprehensive treatment programme for attention-deficit hyperactivity disorder (ADHD) in children over 6 years of agewhen remedial measures alone prove insufficient. The decision to treat as well as follow-up must be under supervision of a specialist in childhood behavioural disorders. Diagnosis should be made according to DSM-IV criteria or the guidelines in ICD-10.

Additional information on the safe use of the product:
ADHD is also known as attention-deficit disorder (ADD).

A comprehensive treatment programme typically includes psychological, educational and social measures and is aimed at stabilising children with a behavioural syndrome characterised by symptoms which may include chronic history of short attention span, distractibility, emotional lability, impulsivity, moderate to severe hyperactivity, minor neurological signs and abnormal EEG. Learning may or may not be impaired.

Methylphenidate treatment is not indicated in all children with this syndrome and the decision to use the drug must be based on a very thorough assessment of the severity of the child's symptoms in relation to the child's age and the persistence of the symptoms.

4.2 Posology and method of administration
Adults: Not applicable.

Elderly: Not applicable

Children: (less than 6 years of age). Equasym is not indicated in children less than 6 years of age.

Children: (over 6 years). Begin with 5 mg once or twice daily (e.g. at breakfast and lunch), increasing the dose and frequency of administration if necessary by weekly increments of 5-10 mg in the daily dose. Doses above 60 mg daily are not recommended. The total daily dose should be administered in divided doses.

The last doses should, in general, not be given within 4 hours before bedtime in order to prevent disturbances in falling asleep. However, if the effect of the drug wears off too early in the evening, disturbed behaviour and/or inability to go to sleep may recur. A small evening dose may help to solve this problem. The pros and cons of a small evening dose versus disturbances in falling asleep should be considered.

Note: If improvement of symptoms is not observed after appropriate dosage adjustment over a one-month period, the drug should be discontinued. Methylphenidate should be discontinued periodically to assess the child's condition. Drug treatment is usually discontinued during or after puberty.

4.3 Contraindications
The presence of marked anxiety, agitation or tension is a contra-indication to the use of Equasym as it may aggravate these symptoms. Equasym is also contra-indicated in patients with diagnosis or a family history ofmotor tics, Tourette's syndrome or other movement disorders.

Methylphenidate is contra-indicated in patients with known drug dependence or history of drug dependence or alcoholism, severe depression, schizophrenic symptoms, anorexia nervosa, psychopathological personality structure, history of aggression, or suicidal tendency.

It is also contra-indicated in patients with severe hypertension, hyperthyroidism, angina pectoris, cardiac arrhythmia, glaucoma, thyrotoxicosis, or known hypersensitivity to the active substance or to any of the excipients.

Methylphenidate is contraindicated in concomitant use, or use within the last two weeks, of MAO inhibitors.

4.4 Special warnings and special precautions for use
Warnings: Equasym should not be used in children under 6 years of age, since safety and efficacy in this age group have not been established.

Clinical experience suggests that Equasym may exacerbate symptoms of behavioural disturbance and thought disorder in psychotic children.

Chronic abuse of Equasym can lead to marked tolerance and psychological dependence with varying degrees of abnormal behaviour. Frank psychotic episodes can occur, especially in response to parenteral abuse.

Whether treatment with methylphenidate during childhood does increase the likelihood of addiction for substances in later life is debated.

Precautions: Treatment with Equasym is not indicated in all cases of Attention-Deficit-Hyperactivity disorders, and should be considered only after detailed history taking and evaluation. The decision to prescribe Equasym should depend on an assessment of the severity and persistence of symptoms and their appropriateness to the child's age and not simply on the presence of one or more abnormal behavioural characteristics. Where these symptoms are associated with acute stress reactions, treatment with Equasym is usually not indicated.

Reduced weight gain and growth retardation have been reported with the long term use of stimulants in children. Careful monitoring of growth is recommended during extended treatment with methylphenidate. Usually patients catch up when treatment is discontinued. Whether drug holidays are beneficial in this respect is debated by experts.

Blood pressure should be monitored at appropriate intervals in all patients taking Equasym.

Caution is called for in emotionally unstable patients, such as those with a history of drug dependence or alcoholism, because such patients may increase the dosage on their own initiative.

Equasym should be used with caution in patients with epilepsy as clinical experience has shown that it can cause an increase in seizure frequency in a small number of patients. If seizure frequency rises, methylphenidate should be discontinued.

The long term safety and efficacy profiles of methylphenidate are not fully known. Patients requiring long term therapy should therefore be carefully monitored and complete and differential blood counts and a platelet count performed periodically.

Careful supervision is required during drug withdrawal, since this may unmask depression as well as chronic over-activity. Some patients may require long term follow up.

In theory, there is a possibility that the clearance of methylphenidate might be affected by urinary pH, either being increased with acidifying agents or decreased with alkalising agents. This should be considered when methylphenidate is given in combination with agents that alter urinary pH.

This medicinal product contains lactose. Therefore, patients with rare hereditary problems of galactose intolerance, the Lapp lactase deficiency or glucose-galactose malabsorption should not take this medicine.

Females of child-bearing potential should not use methylphenidate unless clearly necessary (see section 4.6, Pregnancy and Lactation,- (Section 5.3, Preclinical Safety Data).

4.5 Interaction with other medicinal products and other forms of Interaction
Human pharmacological studies have shown that methylphenidate may inhibit the metabolism of coumarin anticoagulants, some anticonvulsants (phenobarbitone, phenytoin, primidone), phenylbutazone and tricyclic antidepressants. The dosage of these drugs may have to be reduced. Equasym should be used cautiously in patients being treated with pressor agents. Equasym should not be used in patients being treated (currently or within the last 2 weeks) with MAO inhibitors.

Methylphenidate may also decrease the antihypertensive effect of guanethidine.

Alcohol may exacerbate the CNS adverse reactions of psychoactive drugs, including methylphenidate. It is therefore advisable for patients to abstain from alcohol during treatment.

4.6 Pregnancy and lactation
There are no adequate data from the use of methylphenidate in pregnant women.

Studies in animals have shown reproductive toxicity (teratogenic effects) of methylphenidate (see Section 5.3 Preclinical Safety Data). The potential risk for humans is unknown.

Methylphenidate should not be used during pregnancy unless clearly necessary.

It is not known whether methylphenidate or its metabolites pass into breast milk but for safety reasons breast-feeding mothers should not use Equasym.

4.7 Effects on ability to drive and use machines
Equasym may cause dizziness and drowsiness. It is therefore advisable to exercise caution when driving, operating machinery or engaging in other potentially hazardous activities.

4.8 Undesirable effects
Frequency estimate: very common $\geqslant$ 10%; common $\geqslant$ 1% to <10%; uncommon $\geqslant$ 0.1% to <1%; rare $\geqslant$ 0.01% to <0.1%; very rare <0.01%.

Nervousness and insomnia are very common adverse reactions occurring at the beginning of treatment but can usually be controlled by reducing the dosage and/or omitting the afternoon or evening dose.

Decreased appetite is also common but usually transient.

Central and peripheral nervous system:

Common: Headache, drowsiness, dizziness, dyskinesia, irritability.

Rare: Difficulties in visual accommodation, and blurred vision.

Very rare: Hyperactivity, convulsions, muscle cramps, choreo-athetoid movements, tics or exacerbation of pre-existing tics, and Tourette's syndrome have been reported. Isolated cases of toxic psychosis (some with visual and tactile hallucinations), transient depressed mood, cerebral arteritis and/or occlusion.

Very rare reports of poorly documented neuroleptic malignant syndrome (NMS) have been received. In most of these reports patients were also receiving other medications. It is uncertain what role methylphenidate played in these cases.

Gastro-intestinal tract:

Common: Abdominal pain, nausea and vomiting. These usually occur at the beginning of treatment and may be alleviated by concomitant food intake. Dry mouth.

Very rare: Abnormal liver function, ranging from transaminase elevation to hepatic coma.

Cardiovascular system:

Common: Tachycardia, palpitations, arrhythmias, changes in blood pressure and heart rate (usually an increase).

Rare: Angina pectoris.

Skin and appendages

Common: Rash, pruritus, urticaria, fever, arthralgia, scalp hair loss.

Very rare: Thrombocytopenic purpura, exfoliative dermatitis and erythema multiforme.

Blood:

Very rare: Leucopenia, thrombocytopenia, anaemia.

Miscellaneous:

Rare: Reduced weight gain and growth retardation during prolonged use with stimulants in children have been observed.

4.9 Overdose

Signs and symptoms: Acute overdose, mainly due to overstimulation of the central and sympathetic nervous systems, may result in vomiting, agitation, tremors, hyperreflexia, muscle twitching, convulsions (may be followed by coma), euphoria, confusion, hallucinations, delirium, sweating, flushing, headache, hyperpyrexia, tachycardia, palpitations, cardiac arrhythmias, hypertension, mydriasis and dryness of mucous membranes.

Treatment: There is no specific antidote to Equasym overdosage.

Management consists of appropriate supportive measures, preventing self-injury and protecting the patient from external stimuli that would aggravate over-stimulation already present. If the signs and symptoms are not too severe and the patient is conscious, gastric contents may be evacuated by induction of vomiting or gastric lavage. In the presence of severe intoxication, a carefully titrated dose of a short-acting barbiturate should be given before performing gastric lavage.

Intensive care must be provided to maintain adequate circulation and respiratory exchange; external cooling procedures may be required for hyperpyrexia.

Efficacy of peritoneal dialysis or extracorporeal haemodialysis for overdose of Equasym has not been established.

5. PHARMACOLOGICAL PROPERTIES

5.1 Pharmacodynamic properties

Pharmacotherapeutic group: Psychoanaleptics, Psychostimulants and Nootropics, Centrally acting Sympathomimetics, ATC code: N06B A04.

Mode of action: Methylphenidate is a CNS stimulant. The mode of action is not completely understood. Methylphenidate is an indirect sympatheticomimetic. The pharmacological properties are amphetamine-like.

MAO-enzyme inhibition may result in an increased catecholamine concentration.

5.2 Pharmacokinetic properties

Absorption: The active substance methylphenidate hydrochloride is rapidly and almost completely absorbed from the tablets. Owing to extensive first-pass metabolism its systemic availability amounts to only 30% (11-51%) of the dose. Ingestion together with food accelerates its absorption, but has no influence on the amount absorbed. Peak plasma concentrations of approximately 40 nmol/litre (11 ng/ml) are attained, on average, 1-2 hours after administration of 0.30 mg/kg. The peak plasma concentrations, however, show considerable intersubject variability. The area under the plasma concentration curve (AUC), as well as the peak plasma concentration, is proportional to the dose.

Distribution: In the blood, methylphenidate and its metabolites become distributed in the plasma (57%) and the erythrocytes (43%). Methylphenidate and its metabolites have a low plasma protein-building rate (10-33%). The apparent distribution volume has been calculated as 13.1 litres/kg.

Biotransformation: Biotransformation of methylphenidate is rapid and extensive. Peak plasma concentrations of 2-phenyl -2-piperidyl acetic acid (PPAA) are attained approximately 2 hours after administration of methylphenidate and are 30 - 50 times higher than those of the unchanged substance. The half-life of PPAA is roughly twice as long as that of methylphenidate, and the mean systemic clearance is

0.17 litres/h/kg. Only small amounts of hydroxylated metabolites (e.g. hydroxymethylphenidate and hydroxyritalinic acid) are detectable. Therapeutic activity seems to be principally due to the parent compound.

Elimination: Methylphenidate is eliminated from the plasma with a mean half-life of 2 hours, and the calculated mean systemic clearance is 10 litres/h/kg. Within 48-96 hours 78-97% of the dose administered is excreted in the urine and 1-3% in the faeces in the form of metabolites. Unchanged methylphenidate appears in the urine only in small quantities (<1%). The bulk of the dose is excreted in the urine as 2-phenyl-2-piperidyl acetic acid (PPAA, 60-86%).

Characteristics in patients: There are no apparent differences in the pharmacokinetic behaviour of methylphenidate in hyperactive children and healthy adult volunteers.

Elimination data from patients with normal renal function suggest that renal excretion of the unchanged methylphenidate would hardly be diminished at all in the presence of impaired renal function. However, renal excretion of PPAA may be reduced.

5.3 Preclinical safety data

There is evidence that methylphenidate may be a teratogen in two species. Spina bifida and limb malformations have been reported in rabbits whilst in the rat, equivocal evidence of induction of abnormalities of the vertebrae was found.

Methylphenidate did not affect reproductive performance or fertility at low multiples of the clinical dose.

In life-time rat and mouse carcinogenicity studies, increased numbers of malignant liver tumours were noted in male mice only. The significance of this finding to humans is unknown.

6. PHARMACEUTICAL PARTICULARS

6.1 List of excipients

Anhydrous Lactose

Magnesium Stearate

Microcrystalline Cellulose

Sodium Starch Glycollate

6.2 Incompatibilities

Not applicable.

6.3 Shelf life

3 years

6.4 Special precautions for storage

Do not store above 25°C. Store in the original package

6.5 Nature and contents of container

PVC/Aluminium blisters of 30 tablets.

PVC/Aluminium blisters of 20 and 50 tablets.

Not all pack sizes may be marketed.

6.6 Instructions for use and handling

No special requirements.

7. MARKETING AUTHORISATION HOLDER

Celltech Pharmaceuticals Ltd

208 Bath Road

Slough

Berkshire

SL1 3WE

UK

8. MARKETING AUTHORISATION NUMBER(S)

5 mg: 00039/0519, 10 mg: 00039/0514, 20 mg: 00039/0520

9. DATE OF FIRST AUTHORISATION/RENEWAL OF THE AUTHORISATION

22 February 2000 / 20 June 2005

10. DATE OF REVISION OF THE TEXT

Equasym XL 10 mg, 20 mg or 30 mg Capsules

(UCB Pharma Limited)

1. NAME OF THE MEDICINAL PRODUCT

Equasym XL® 10 mg, 20 mg or 30 mg Capsules

2. QUALITATIVE AND QUANTITATIVE COMPOSITION

Each capsule contains 10 mg, 20 mg or 30 mg Methylphenidate Hydrochloride

For excipients, see 6.1

3. PHARMACEUTICAL FORM

Modified release capsule, hard.

10 mg Capsule:

The capsule has a dark green opaque cap imprinted with "Celltech 574" in white and a white opaque body imprinted with "10mg" in black.

20 mg Capsule:

The capsule has a blue opaque cap imprinted with "Celltech 575" in white and a white opaque body imprinted with "20mg" in black.

30 mg Capsule:

The capsule has a reddish-brown opaque cap imprinted with "Celltech 576" in white and a white opaque body imprinted with "30mg" in black.

4. CLINICAL PARTICULARS

4.1 Therapeutic indications

Equasym XL is indicated as part of a comprehensive treatment programme for attention-deficit/hyperactivity disorder (ADHD) when remedial measures alone prove insufficient. Treatment must be under the supervision of a specialist in childhood behavioural disorders. Diagnosis should be made according to DSM-IV criteria or the guidelines in ICD-10.

Additional information on the safe use of the product:

ADHD is also known as attention-deficit disorder (ADD). Other terms used to describe this behavioural syndrome include: hyperkinetic disorder, minimal brain damage, minimal brain dysfunction in children, minor cerebral dysfunction and psycho-organic syndrome of children.

A comprehensive treatment programme typically includes psychological, educational and social measures and is aimed at stabilising children with a behavioural syndrome characterised by symptoms which may include chronic history of short attention span, distractibility, emotional lability, impulsivity, moderate to severe hyperactivity, minor neurological signs and abnormal EEG. Learning may or may not be impaired. Equasym XL treatment is not indicated in all children with this syndrome and the decision to use the drug must be based on a very thorough assessment of the severity of the child's symptoms.

4.2 Posology and method of administration

Adults: Not applicable.

Elderly: Not applicable

Children: (over 6 years).

Careful dose titration is necessary at the start of treatment with methylphenidate. This may be achieved using an immediate release formulation taken in divided doses. The recommended starting daily dose is 5mg once daily or twice daily (e.g. at breakfast and lunch), increasing if necessary by weekly increments of 5-10mg in the daily dose according to tolerability and degree of efficacy observed. Equasym XL 10mg once daily may be used in place of immediate release methylphenidate 5mg twice daily from the beginning of treatment where appropriate.

Patients Currently Using Methylphenidate: Patients established on an immediate release methylphenidate formulation may be switched to the milligram equivalent daily dose of Equasym XL. For example, 20mg of Equasym XL is regarded as equivalent to 10mg at breakfast and 10mg at lunchtime of immediate release methylphenidate.

Equasym XL consists of an immediate release component (30% of the dose) and a modified release component (70% of the dose). Hence Equasym XL 10mg yields an immediate-release dose of 3mg and an extended release dose of 7mg. The extended-release portion of each dose is designed to maintain a treatment response through the afternoon without the need for a midday dose. It is designed to deliver therapeutic plasma levels for a period which is consistent with the school day rather than the whole day.

If the effect of the drug wears off too early in the evening, disturbed behaviour and/or inability to go to sleep may recur. A small evening dose of an immediate-release methylphenidate tablet may help to solve this problem.

The maximum daily dose of methylphenidate is 60mg.

Equasym XL is not indicated in children less than 6 years of age.

Equasym XL should be given in the morning before breakfast. The capsules must be swallowed whole and not opened, crushed or chewed.

Note: If improvement of symptoms is not observed after appropriate dosage adjustment over a one-month period, the drug should be discontinued. Methylphenidate should be discontinued periodically to assess the child's condition. Drug treatment is usually discontinued during or after puberty.

4.3 Contraindications

The presence of marked anxiety, agitation or tension is a contra-indication to the use of Equasym XL as it may aggravate these symptoms. Equasym XL is also contra-indicated in patients with motor tics, tics in siblings, or a family history or diagnosis of Tourette's syndrome.

It is also contra-indicated in patients with hyperthyroidism, severe angina pectoris, cardiac arrhythmia, glaucoma, thyrotoxicosis, or known sensitivity to methylphenidate or to any of the excipients.

4.4 Special warnings and special precautions for use

Warnings: Equasym XL should not be used in children under 6 years of age since safety and efficacy in this age group have not been established.

Equasym XL should not be used to treat severe exogenous or endogenous depression.

Clinical experience suggests that Equasym XL may exacerbate symptoms of behavioural disturbance and thought disorder in psychotic children.

Available clinical evidence indicates that treatment with methylphenidate during childhood does not increase the likelihood of addiction in later life.

Chronic abuse of methylphenidate can lead to marked tolerance and psychological dependence with varying degrees of abnormal behaviour. Frank psychotic episodes can occur, especially in response to parenteral abuse.

Precautions: Treatment with methylphenidate is not indicated in all cases of ADHD, and should be considered only after detailed history taking and evaluation. The decision to prescribe methylphenidate should depend on an assessment of the severity of symptoms and their appropriateness to the child's age and not simply on the presence of one or more abnormal behavioural characteristics. Where these symptoms are associated with acute stress reactions, treatment with methylphenidate is usually not indicated.

Moderately reduced weight gain and slight growth retardation have been reported with the long term use of stimulants in children, although a causal relationship has not been confirmed. Careful monitoring of growth is recommended during extended treatment with methylphenidate.

Blood pressure should be monitored at appropriate intervals in all patients taking methylphenidate, especially those with hypertension.

Caution is called for in emotionally unstable patients, such as those with a history of drug dependence or alcoholism, because such patients may increase the dosage on their own initiative.

Equasym XL should be used with caution in patients with epilepsy as clinical experience has shown it can cause an increase in seizure frequency in a small number of patients. If seizure frequency rises, methylphenidate should be discontinued.

The long term safety and efficacy profiles of methylphenidate are not fully known. Patients requiring long term therapy should therefore be carefully monitored and complete and differential blood counts and a platelet count performed periodically.

Careful supervision is required during drug withdrawal, since this may unmask depression as well as chronic over-activity. Some patients may require long-term follow up.

Females of childbearing potential (females post menarche) should use effective contraception (see Section 4.6, Pregnancy and Lactation and Section 5.3, Preclinical Safety Data).

Patients with rare hereditary problems of fructose intolerance, glucose-galactose malabsorption or sucrase-isomaltase insufficiency should not take this medicine.

4.5 Interaction with other medicinal products and other forms of Interaction

Human pharmacological studies have shown that methylphenidate may inhibit the metabolism of coumarin anticoagulants, some anticonvulsants (phenobarbital, phenytoin, primidone), phenylbutazone and tricyclic antidepressants. The dosage of these drugs may have to be reduced. Equasym XL should be used cautiously in patients being treated with pressor agents and MAO inhibitors.

Methylphenidate may also decrease the antihypertensive effect of guanethidine.

Alcohol may exacerbate the CNS adverse reactions of psychoactive drugs, including methylphenidate. It is therefore advisable for patients to abstain from alcohol during treatment.

4.6 Pregnancy and lactation

There are no adequate data from the use of methylphenidate in pregnancy.

Studies in animals have shown reproductive toxicity of methylphenidate (see Section 5.3, Preclinical Safety Data). The potential risk for humans is unknown.

Methylphenidate should not be used during pregnancy unless clearly necessary.

It is not known whether methylphenidate or its metabolites pass into breast milk but for safety reasons breast feeding mothers should not use Equasym XL.

4.7 Effects on ability to drive and use machines

Equasym XL may cause dizziness and drowsiness. It is therefore advisable to exercise caution when driving, operating machinery or engaging in other potentially hazardous activities.

4.8 Undesirable effects

Frequency estimate: very common ⩾ 10%; common ⩾ 1% to <10%; uncommon ⩾0.1% to <1%; rare ⩾ 0.01% to <0.1%; very rare <0.01%.

Nervousness and insomnia are very common adverse reactions occurring at the beginning of treatment but can usually be controlled by reducing the dosage. Decreased appetite is also common but usually transient.

Central and peripheral nervous system:

Common: Headache, drowsiness, dizziness, dyskinesia.

Rare: Difficulties in visual accommodation, and blurred vision.

Very rare: Hyperactivity, convulsions, muscle cramps, choreo-athetoid movements, tics or exacerbation of pre-existing tics, and Tourette's syndrome have been reported. Isolated cases of toxic psychosis (some with visual and tactile hallucinations), transient depressed mood, cerebral arteritis and/or occlusion.

Very rare reports of poorly documented neuroleptic malignant syndrome (NMS) have been received. In most of these reports patients were also receiving other medications. It is uncertain what role methylphenidate played in these cases.

Gastro-intestinal tract:

Common: Abdominal pain, nausea and vomiting. These usually occur at the beginning of treatment and may be alleviated by concomitant food intake. Dry mouth.

Figure 1

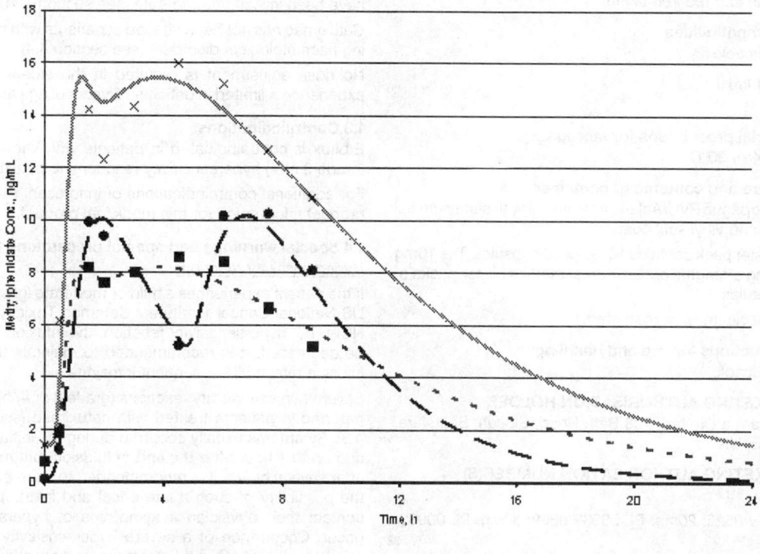

Very rare: Abnormal liver function, ranging from transaminase elevation to hepatic coma.

Cardiovascular system:

Common: Tachycardia, palpitations, arrhythmias, changes in blood pressure and heart rate (usually an increase).

Rare: Angina pectoris.

Skin and appendages:

Common: Rash, pruritus, urticaria, fever, arthralgia, scalp hair loss.

Very rare: Thrombocytopenic purpura, exfoliative dermatitis and erythema multiforme.

Blood:

Very rare: Leucopenia, thrombocytopenia, anaemia.

Miscellaneous:

Rare: Moderately reduced weight gain and slight growth retardation during prolonged use in children.

4.9 Overdose

Signs and symptoms: Acute overdose, mainly due to overstimulation of the central and sympathetic nervous systems, may result in vomiting, agitation, tremors, hyperreflexia, muscle twitching, convulsions (may be followed by coma), euphoria, confusion, hallucinations, delirium, sweating, flushing, headache, hyperpyrexia, tachycardia, palpitations, cardiac arrhythmias, hypertension, mydriasis and dryness of mucous membranes.

Treatment: There is no specific antidote to Equasym XL overdosage. Management consists of appropriate supportive measures, preventing self-injury and protecting the patient from external stimuli that would aggravate overstimulation already present. If the signs and symptoms are not too severe and the patient is conscious, gastric contents may be evacuated by induction of vomiting or gastric lavage. In the presence of severe intoxication, a carefully titrated dose of a short-acting barbiturate should be given before performing gastric lavage.

Intensive care must be provided to maintain adequate circulation and respiratory exchange; external cooling procedures may be required for hyperpyrexia.

Efficacy of peritoneal dialysis or extracorporeal haemodialysis for overdose of Equasym XL has not been established.

5. PHARMACOLOGICAL PROPERTIES

5.1 Pharmacodynamic properties

Mode of action: Equasym XL is a mild CNS stimulant with more prominent effects on mental than on motor activities. Its mode of action in man is not completely understood but its effects are thought to be due to cortical stimulation and possibly to stimulation of the reticular activating system.

The mechanism by which Equasym XL exerts its mental and behavioural effects in children is not clearly established, nor is there conclusive evidence showing how these effects relate to the condition of the central nervous system. It is thought to block the re-uptake of norepinephrine and dopamine into the presynaptic neurone and increase the release of these monoamines into the extraneuronal space. Equasym is a racemic mixture of the *d*- and *l-threo* enantiomers of methylphenidate. The *d*-enantiomer is more pharmacologically active than the *l*-enantiomer.

5.2 Pharmacokinetic properties

Absorption: Equasym XL has a plasma profile showing two phases of drug release, with a sharp, initial, upward slope similar to a methylphenidate immediate-release tablet, and a second rising portion approximately three hours later, followed by a gradual decline (See figure below for data in children with ADHD. Values beyond the 8.5 hour time point have been generated using pharmacokinetic modelling).

Mean observed and simulated methylphenidate plasma concentrations in children with ADHD after 7 days dosing with 40 mg Equasym XL (x) 20 mg Equasym XL (<) or 10 mg Ritalin twice daily (·).

(see Figure 1 above)

Peak plasma concentrations of approximately 40 nmol/litre (11 ng/ml) are attained, on average, 1-2 hours after administration of 0.30 mg/kg. The peak plasma concentrations, however, show considerable intersubject variability.

The range of concentrations at 1.5 hours was 3.2 – 13.3 ng/ml with a mean of 7.7 ng/ml. The second phase of release resulted in a second maximum observed concentration in most subjects at 4.5 hours after dosing, with the observed concentrations ranging from 4.9 – 15.5 ng/ml with a mean of 8.2 ng/ml.

The area under the plasma concentration curve (AUC), as well as the peak plasma concentration, is proportional to the dose.

Ingestion together with food with high fat content delays its absorption and increases the amount absorbed (AUC) by about 17%, on average.

Availability, systemic: Owing to extensive first-pass metabolism its systemic availability amounts to approximately 30% (11-51%) of the dose.

Distribution: In the blood, methylphenidate and its metabolites become distributed in the plasma (57%) and the erythrocytes (43%). Methylphenidate and its metabolites have a low plasma protein-building rate (10-33%). The apparent distribution has been calculated as 13.1 litres/kg.

Elimination: Methylphenidate is eliminated from the plasma with a mean half-life 2 hours, and the calculated mean systemic clearance is 10 litres/h/kg.

Within 48-96 hours 78-97% of the dose administered is excreted in the urine and 1-3% in the faeces in the form of metabolites.

The bulk of the dose is excreted in the urine as 2-phenyl-2-piperidyl acetic acid (PPAA, 60-86%).

5.3 Preclinical safety data

There is evidence that methylphenidate may be a teratogen in two species. Spina bifida and limb malformations have been reported in rabbits whilst in the rat, equivocal evidence of induction of abnormalities of the vertebrae was found.

Methylphenidate did not affect reproductive performance or fertility at low multiples of the clinical dose.

In life-time rat and mouse carcinogenicity studies, increased numbers of malignant liver tumours were noted in male mice only. The significance of this finding to humans is unknown.

The weight of evidence from the genotoxicity studies reveals no special hazard for humans.

6. PHARMACEUTICAL PARTICULARS

6.1 List of excipients

Sugar Spheres: Sucrose, maize starch

Povidone: Opadry Clear YS-1-7006 (hypromellose and macrogol), Ethylcellulose Aqueous Dispersion, Dibutyl Sebacate

Capsule shell: Gelatin, Titanium dioxide (E171) (10 mg, 20 mg, 30 mg capsules), FD&C blue No. 2 (E132) (10 mg, 20 mg, 30 mg capsules), Yellow iron oxide (E172) (10 mg capsules), Red iron oxide (E172) (30 mg capsules)

White printing ink: Shellac, propylene glycol, sodium hydroxide, povidone and titanium dioxide

Black printing ink: Pharmaceutical glaze, propylene glycol, ammonium hydroxide, simeticone, FD&C blue no. 2, yellow iron oxide and red iron oxide.

6.2 Incompatibilities
Not applicable.

6.3 Shelf life
18 months

6.4 Special precautions for storage
Store below 30°C.

6.5 Nature and contents of container
Clear or opaque PVC/Aclar blister packs with aluminum foil backing and vinyl seal coating.

Each blister pack contains 10, 30 or 60 capsules. The 10mg and 20mg strengths are also presented as blister packs of 100 capsules

Not all packs may be marketed.

6.6 Instructions for use and handling
Not applicable.

7. MARKETING AUTHORISATION HOLDER
UCB Pharma Limited, 208 Bath Road, Slough, Berkshire, SL1 3WE, UK

8. MARKETING AUTHORISATION NUMBER(S)
10 mg:

PL 00039/0528; *20mg:* PL 00039/0529; *30mg:* PL 00039/0530

9. DATE OF FIRST AUTHORISATION/RENEWAL OF THE AUTHORISATION
11 February 2005

10. DATE OF REVISION OF THE TEXT
17 May 2005.

11. LEGAL CATEGORY
POM

Erbitux 2 mg/ml solution for infusion

(Merck Pharmaceuticals)

1. NAME OF THE MEDICINAL PRODUCT
Erbitux▼ 2 mg/ml solution for infusion

2. QUALITATIVE AND QUANTITATIVE COMPOSITION
Each ml of solution for infusion contains 2 mg cetuximab. Each vial contains 50 ml.

Cetuximab is a chimeric monoclonal IgG1 antibody produced in a mammalian cell line (Sp2/0) by recombinant DNA technology.

For excipients, see section 6.1.

3. PHARMACEUTICAL FORM
Solution for infusion.

Erbitux is a colourless solution that may contain product-related whitish and amorphous visible particles.

4. CLINICAL PARTICULARS

4.1 Therapeutic indications
Erbitux in combination with irinotecan is indicated for the treatment of patients with epidermal growth factor receptor (EGFR)-expressing metastatic colorectal cancer after failure of irinotecan-including cytotoxic therapy.

4.2 Posology and method of administration
It is recommended that the detection of EGFR expression be performed by an experienced laboratory using a validated test method (see section 5.1).

Erbitux must be administered under the supervision of a physician experienced in the use of antineoplastic medicinal products. Close monitoring is required during the infusion and for at least 1 hour after the end of the infusion. Availability of resuscitation equipment must be ensured.

Prior to the first infusion, patients must receive premedication with an antihistamine. This premedication is recommended prior to all subsequent infusions.

Erbitux is administered once a week. The initial dose is 400 mg cetuximab per m^2 body surface area. The subsequent weekly doses are 250 mg/m^2 each.

For the dosage of concomitant irinotecan, refer to the product information for this medicinal product. Normally, the same dose of irinotecan is used as administered in the last cycles of the prior irinotecan-containing regimen. However, recommendations for dose modifications of irinotecan according to the product information for this medicinal product must be followed. Irinotecan must not be administered earlier than 1 hour after the end of the cetuximab infusion.

It is recommended that cetuximab treatment be continued until progression of the underlying disease.

Erbitux is administered intravenously via in-line filtration with an infusion pump, gravity drip or a syringe pump (for handling instructions, see section 6.6).

For the initial dose, the recommended infusion period is 120 minutes. For the subsequent weekly doses, the recommended infusion period is 60 minutes. The maximum infusion rate must not exceed 5 ml/min.

Special populations

Only patients with adequate renal and hepatic function have been investigated to date (see section 4.4).

Cetuximab has not been studied in patients with pre-existing haematological disorders (see section 4.4).

No dose adjustment is required in the elderly, but the experience is limited in patients 75 years of age and above.

4.3 Contraindications
Erbitux is contraindicated in patients with known severe (grade 3 or 4) hypersensitivity reactions to cetuximab.

For additional contraindications of irinotecan, refer to the product information for this medicinal product.

4.4 Special warnings and special precautions for use
Hypersensitivity reactions

If the patient experiences a mild or moderate (grade 1 or 2; US National Cancer Institute - Common Toxicity Criteria, NCI-CTC) hypersensitivity reaction, the infusion rate may be decreased. It is recommended to maintain this lower infusion rate in all subsequent infusions.

Severe hypersensitivity reactions (grade 3 or 4) have been reported in patients treated with cetuximab (see section 4.8). Symptoms usually occurred during the initial infusion and up to 1 hour after the end of infusion, but may occur after several hours. It is recommended to warn patients of the possibility of such a late onset and instruct them to contact their physician if symptoms of hypersensitivity occur. Occurrence of a severe hypersensitivity reaction requires immediate and permanent discontinuation of cetuximab therapy and may necessitate emergency treatment.

Special attention is recommended for patients with reduced performance status and pre-existing cardio-pulmonary disease.

Dyspnoea

Dyspnoea may occur in close temporal relationship to the cetuximab infusion as part of a hypersensitivity reaction, but has also been reported after several weeks of therapy, possibly related to the underlying disorder (see section 4.8). Patients with high age, impaired performance status and underlying pulmonary disorders may be at increased risk for dyspnoea, which may be severe and/or long-standing.

If patients develop dyspnoea during the course of cetuximab treatment, it is recommended to investigate them for signs of progressive pulmonary disorders as appropriate. Individual cases of interstitial lung disorders of unknown causal relationship to cetuximab have been reported.

Skin reactions

If a patient experiences a severe skin reaction (grade 3; NCI-CTC), cetuximab therapy must be interrupted. Treatment may only be resumed, if the reaction has resolved to grade 2 (see section 4.8).

If the severe skin reaction occurred for the first time, treatment may be resumed without any change in dose level.

With the second and third occurrences of severe skin reactions, cetuximab therapy must again be interrupted. Treatment may only be resumed at a lower dose level (200 mg/m^2 body surface area after the second occurrence and 150 mg/m^2 after the third occurrence), if the reaction has resolved to grade 2.

If severe skin reactions occur a fourth time or do not resolve to grade 2 during interruption of treatment, permanent discontinuation of cetuximab treatment is required.

Special populations

Only patients with adequate renal and hepatic function have been investigated to date (serum creatinine ⩽ 1.5fold, transaminases ⩽ 5fold and bilirubin ⩽ 1.5fold the upper limit of normal).

Cetuximab has not been studied in patients presenting with one or more of the following laboratory parameters:

- haemoglobin < 9 g/dl
- leukocyte count < 3000/mm^3
- absolute neutrophil count < 1500/mm^3
- platelet count < 100000/mm^3

The safety and effectiveness of cetuximab in paediatric patients have not been established.

There is limited experience in the use of cetuximab in combination with radiotherapy in colorectal cancer.

4.5 Interaction with other medicinal products and other forms of Interaction
There is no evidence that the safety profile of cetuximab is influenced by irinotecan or *vice versa*.

A formal interaction study showed that the pharmacokinetic characteristics of cetuximab remain unaltered after co-administration of a single dose of irinotecan (350 mg/m^2 body surface area). Similarly, the pharmacokinetics of irinotecan were unchanged when cetuximab was co-administered.

No other formal interaction studies with cetuximab have been performed in humans.

4.6 Pregnancy and lactation
The epidermal growth factor receptor (EGFR) is involved in foetal development and other IgG1 antibodies have been found to cross the placental barrier. Studies in animals or sufficient data from pregnant or lactating women are not available. It is strongly recommended that Erbitux be given only during pregnancy if the potential benefit justifies a potential risk to the foetus.

It is recommended that women do not breast-feed during treatment with Erbitux and for 1 month after the last dose, because it is not known whether cetuximab is excreted in breast milk.

4.7 Effects on ability to drive and use machines
No studies on the effects on ability to drive and use machines have been performed. If patients experience treatment-related symptoms affecting their ability to concentrate and react, it is recommended that they do not drive or use machines until the effect subsides.

4.8 Undesirable effects
Undesirable effects detailed in this section refer to cetuximab. There is no evidence that the safety profile of cetuximab is influenced by irinotecan or *vice versa*. In combination with irinotecan, additional reported undesirable effects were those expected with irinotecan (such as diarrhoea 72%, nausea 55%, vomiting 41%, mucositis, e.g. stomatitis 26%, fever 33%, leukopenia 25%, alopecia 22%). Therefore also refer to the product information for irinotecan.

Overall, no clinically relevant difference between genders was observed.

Immune system disorders

Common (>1/100, <1/10)

In approximately 5% of patients, hypersensitivity reactions may occur during treatment with cetuximab; approximately half of these reactions are severe.

Mild or moderate reactions (grade 1 or 2) include symptoms such as fever, chills, nausea, rash, or dyspnoea. Severe hypersensitivity reactions (grade 3 or 4) usually occur during or within 1 hour of the initial cetuximab infusion. Symptoms include the rapid onset of airway obstruction (bronchospasm, stridor, hoarseness, difficulty in speaking), urticaria, and/or hypotension.

For clinical management, see section 4.4.

Metabolism and nutrition disorders

Frequency not known (cannot be estimated from the available data)

Hypomagnesaemia has been reported.

Eye disorders

Common (>1/100, <1/10)

Conjunctivitis may be expected in approximately 5% of patients.

Respiratory, thoracic and mediastinal disorders

Very common (>1/10)

Dyspnoea has been reported in 25% of patients with end stage colorectal cancer. In elderly patients and in patients with reduced performance status or pre-existing pulmonary disorders, an increased incidence of dyspnoea, sometimes severe, was observed (see section 4.4).

Skin and subcutaneous tissue disorders

Very common (>1/10)

Skin reactions may develop in more than 80% of patients; approximately 15% of these are severe. They mainly present as acne-like rash and/or, less frequently, as nail disorders (e.g. paronychia). The majority of skin reactions develop within the first week of therapy. They generally resolve, without sequelae, over time following cessation of treatment if the recommended adjustments in dose regimen are followed (see section 4.4). According to NCI-CTC, grade 2 skin reactions are characterised by rash up to 50% of body surface area, while grade 3 reactions affect equal or more than 50% of body surface area.

4.9 Overdose
No case of overdose has been reported. However, there is no experience with single doses higher than 500 mg/m^2 body surface area to date.

5. PHARMACOLOGICAL PROPERTIES

5.1 Pharmacodynamic properties
Pharmacotherapeutic group: Antineoplastic agents, monoclonal antibodies, ATC code: L01XC06

Mechanism of action

Cetuximab is a chimeric monoclonal IgG1 antibody that is directed against the epidermal growth factor receptor (EGFR).

EGFR signalling pathways are involved in the control of cell survival, cell cycle progression, angiogenesis, cell migration and cellular invasion/metastasis.

Cetuximab binds to the EGFR with an affinity that is approximately 5- to 10fold higher than that of endogenous ligands. Cetuximab blocks binding of endogenous EGFR ligands resulting in inhibition of the function of the receptor. It further induces the internalisation of EGFR, which could lead to down-regulation of EGFR. Cetuximab also targets cytotoxic immune effector cells towards EGFR-expressing tumour cells (antibody dependent cell-mediated cytotoxicity, ADCC).

Pharmacodynamic effects

In both *in vitro* and *in vivo* assays, cetuximab inhibits the proliferation and induces apoptosis of human tumour cells that express EGFR. *In vitro* cetuximab inhibits the production of angiogenic factors by tumour cells and blocks endothelial cell migration. *In vivo* cetuximab inhibits expression of angiogenic factors by tumour cells and causes a reduction in tumour neo-vascularisation and metastasis.

Immunogenicity

The development of human anti-chimeric antibodies (HACA) is a class effect of monoclonal chimeric antibodies. Current data on the development of HACAs is limited. Overall, measurable HACA titres were noted in 3.7% of the patients studied, with incidences ranging from 0% to 8.5% in the target indication studies. No conclusive data on the neutralising effect of HACAs on cetuximab is available to date. The appearance of HACA did not correlate with the occurrence of hypersensitivity reactions or any other undesirable effect to cetuximab.

Clinical efficacy

A diagnostic assay (EGFR pharmDx) was used for immunohistochemical detection of EGFR expression in tumour material. A tumour was considered to be EGFR-positive, if one stained cell could be identified. Approximately 80% of the patients with metastatic colorectal cancer screened for clinical studies had an EGFR-expressing tumour and were therefore considered eligible for cetuximab treatment. The efficacy and safety of cetuximab have not been documented in EGFR-negative tumours.

Cetuximab in combination with irinotecan was investigated in 2 clinical studies. A total of 356 patients with EGFR-expressing metastatic colorectal cancer who had recently failed irinotecan-including cytotoxic therapy and who had a minimum Karnofsky performance status of 60, but the majority of whom had a Karnofsky performance status of ⩾ 80 received the combination treatment.

• EMR 62 202-007: This randomised study compared the combination of cetuximab and irinotecan (218 patients) with cetuximab monotherapy (111 patients). In the combination arm, irinotecan was administered as follows: 125 mg/m^2 body surface area weekly for 4 weeks followed by 2 weeks of rest, or 180 mg/m^2 every 2 weeks, or 350 mg/m^2 every 3 weeks, or modified doses according to the dosage recommendation given in the product information for irinotecan. More than half of the patients were treated with the 180 mg/m^2 irinotecan regimen given every 2 weeks.

Patients on cetuximab monotherapy who showed signs of disease progression were offered continuation of cetuximab treatment combined with the same regimen of irinotecan to which they had become refractory.

• IMCL CP02-9923: This single arm open-label study investigated the combination therapy in 138 patients. Almost 90% of patients received the irinotecan regimen of 125 mg/m^2 body surface area weekly for 4 weeks followed by 2 weeks of rest.

In both studies, cetuximab was administered at the doses described in section 4.2.

The efficacy data generated in these studies are summarised in the table below:

(see Table 1)

The efficacy of the combination of cetuximab with irinotecan was superior to that of cetuximab monotherapy, in terms of objective response rate (ORR), disease control rate (DCR) and progression-free survival (PFS). In the randomised trial, no effects on overall survival were demonstrated (Hazard ratio 0.91, p = 0.48).

5.2 Pharmacokinetic properties

Cetuximab pharmacokinetics were studied when cetuximab was administered as monotherapy or in combination with concomitant chemotherapy or radiotherapy in clinical studies. Intravenous infusions of cetuximab exhibited dose-dependent pharmacokinetics at weekly doses ranging from 5 to 500 mg/m^2 body surface area.

When cetuximab was administered at an initial dose of 400 mg/m^2 body surface area, the mean volume of distribution was approximately equivalent to the vascular space (2.9 l/m^2 with a range of 1.5 to 6.2 l/m^2). The mean C_{max} (± standard deviation) was 185±55 microgram per ml. The mean clearance was 0.022 l/h per m^2 body surface area. Cetuximab has a long elimination half-life with values ranging from 70 to 100 hours at the target dose.

Cetuximab serum concentrations reached stable levels after three weeks of cetuximab monotherapy. Mean peak cetuximab concentrations were 155.8 microgram per ml in week 3 and 151.6 microgram per ml in week 8, whereas the corresponding mean trough concentrations were 41.3 and 55.4 microgram per ml, respectively. In a study of cetuximab administered in combination with irinotecan, the mean cetuximab trough levels were 50.0 microgram per ml in week 12 and 49.4 microgram per ml in week 36.

Several pathways have been described that may contribute to the metabolism of antibodies. All of these pathways involve the biodegradation of the antibody to smaller molecules, i.e. small peptides or amino acids.

Pharmacokinetics in special populations

An integrated analysis across all clinical studies showed that the pharmacokinetic characteristics of cetuximab are not influenced by race, age, gender, renal or hepatic status.

Only patients with adequate renal and hepatic function have been investigated to date (serum creatinine ⩽ 1.5fold, transaminases ⩽ 5fold and bilirubin ⩽ 1.5fold the upper limit of normal).

5.3 Preclinical safety data

Skin toxicity was the major finding observed in a chronic repeat-dose toxicity study in Cynomolgus monkeys at clinically relevant levels. Cetuximab induced severe skin toxicity and lethal complications in monkeys, which exhibited blood levels of approximately 17-fold of those achieved under the standard human treatment regimen (see section 4.2).

Preclinical data on genotoxicity and local tolerability after accidental administration by routes other than the intended infusion revealed no special hazard for humans.

No formal animal studies have been performed to establish the carcinogenic potential of cetuximab or to determine its effects on male and female fertility or its teratogenic potential.

Toxicity studies with co-administration of cetuximab and irinotecan have not been performed.

No preclinical data on the effect of anti-EGFR antibodies on wound healing are available to date. However, in preclinical wound healing models EGFR selective tyrosine kinase inhibitors were shown to retard wound healing.

6. PHARMACEUTICAL PARTICULARS

6.1 List of excipients

Sodium dihydrogen phosphate

Disodium phosphate

Sodium chloride

Water for injections

6.2 Incompatibilities

In the absence of compatibility studies, this medicinal product must not be mixed with other medicinal products.

A separate infusion line must be used.

6.3 Shelf life

2 years.

Chemical and physical in-use stability has been demonstrated for 20 hours at 25°C.

Erbitux does not contain any antimicrobial preservative or bacteriostatic agent. From a microbiological point of view, the product shall be used immediately after opening. If not used immediately, in-use storage times and conditions prior to use are the responsibility of the user and would normally not be longer than 24 hours at 2 to 8°C, unless opening has taken place in controlled and validated aseptic conditions.

6.4 Special precautions for storage

Store in a refrigerator (2°C – 8°C). Do not freeze.

6.5 Nature and contents of container

50 ml of solution in a vial (Type I glass) with a stopper (teflon-coated bromobutyl rubber) and a seal (aluminium).

Pack size of 1.

6.6 Instructions for use and handling

Erbitux may be administered via a gravity drip, an infusion pump or a syringe pump. A separate infusion line must be used for the infusion, and the line must be flushed with sterile sodium chloride 9 mg/ml (0.9%) solution for injection at the end of infusion.

Erbitux is a colourless solution that may contain product-related whitish and amorphous visible particles. These particles do not affect the quality of the product. Nevertheless, the solution must be filtered with an in-line filter of 0.2 micrometer or 0.22 micrometer nominal pore size during administration.

Erbitux is compatible

• with polyethylene, ethyl vinyl acetate or polyvinyl chloride bags,

• with polyethylene, ethyl vinyl acetate, polyvinyl chloride, polybutadiene or polyurethane infusion sets,

• with polyethersulfone, polyamide or polysulfone in-line filters.

Care must be taken to ensure aseptic handling when preparing the infusion.

Erbitux must be prepared as follows:

• In-line filtration with an infusion pump or gravity drip: Take an appropriate sterile syringe (minimum 50 ml) and attach a suitable needle. Draw up the required volume of Erbitux from a vial. Transfer the Erbitux into a sterile evacuated container or bag. Repeat this procedure until the calculated volume has been reached. Insert a suitable in-line filter into the infusion line and prime it with Erbitux before starting the infusion. Use a gravity drip or an infusion pump for administration. Set and control the rate as explained in section 4.2.

• In-line filtration with a syringe pump: Take an appropriate sterile syringe (minimum 50 ml) and attach a suitable needle. Draw up the required volume of Erbitux from a vial. Remove the needle and put the syringe into the syringe pump. Take a suitable in-line filter and connect it to the application set. Connect the infusion line to the syringe, set and control the rate as explained in section 4.2 and start the infusion after priming the line with Erbitux. Repeat this procedure until the calculated volume has been infused.

Filters may occasionally clog up during the infusion. If there is evidence of filter clogging, the filter must be replaced.

7. MARKETING AUTHORISATION HOLDER

Merck KGaA, 64271 Darmstadt, Germany

8. MARKETING AUTHORISATION NUMBER(S)

EU/1/04/281/001

9. DATE OF FIRST AUTHORISATION/RENEWAL OF THE AUTHORISATION

29 June 2004

10. DATE OF REVISION OF THE TEXT

13 September 2005

Table 1

Study	N	ORR n (%)	ORR 95%CI	DCR n (%)	DCR 95%CI	PFS (months) Median	PFS 95%CI	OS (months) Median	OS 95%CI
Cetuximab +irinotecan									
EMR 62 202-007	218	50 (22.9)	17.5, 29.1	121 (55.5)	48.6, 62.2	4.1	2.8, 4.3	8.6	7.6, 9.6
IMCL CP02-923	138	21 (15.2)	9.7, 22.3	84 (60.9)	52.2, 69.1	2.9	2.6, 4.1	8.4	7.2, 10.3
Cetuximab									
EMR 62 202-007	111	12 (10.8)	5.7, 18.1	36 (32.4)	23.9, 42.0	1.5	1.4, 2.0	6.9	5.6, 9.1

CI = confidence interval, DCR = disease control rate (patients with complete response, partial response, or stable disease for at least 6 weeks), ORR = objective response rate (patients with complete response or partial response), OS = overall survival time, PFS = progression-free survival

Ergocalciferol Injection BP 300,000U and 600,000U

(UCB Pharma Limited)

1. NAME OF THE MEDICINAL PRODUCT

Ergocalciferol Injection BP 300,000U

Ergocalciferol Injection BP 600,000U

2. QUALITATIVE AND QUANTITATIVE COMPOSITION

Ergocalciferol BP 0.75% W/V

3. PHARMACEUTICAL FORM

Solution for Injection

4. CLINICAL PARTICULARS

4.1 Therapeutic indications

Intramuscular therapy with Ergocalciferol Injection is used in patients with gastrointestinal, liver or biliary disease associated with malabsorption of Vitamin D, resulting in hypophosphataemia, rickets, and osteomalacia.

4.2 Posology and method of administration

Route of Administration: IM injection

Adults, Children and Elderly:

Dosage should be individualised by the clinician for each patient. Serum and urinary calcium concentrations, phosphate and BUN should be monitored at regular intervals, initially weekly, in order to achieve optimum clinical response and to avoid hypercalcaemia.

Doses should not normally exceed 40,000 units/day (1.0mg/day) for adults and 10,000 units/day (0.25mg/day) for children.

Ergocalciferol Injection may be administered as a single dose or repeated daily, dependent upon clinical response and requirements. Calcium and phosphorous supplements should be administered where necessary.

4.3 Contraindications

Hypercalcaemia, evidence of vitamin D toxicity, hypervitaminosis D, abnormal sensitivity to the effect of vitamin D, decreased renal function.

4.4 Special warnings and special precautions for use

Adequate dietary calcium is necessary for clinical response to Ergocalciferol therapy.

Use with caution in patients with coronary disease, renal function impairment and arteriosclerosis, especially in the elderly.

Ergocalciferol is not recommended for use in hypoparathyroidism.

In the event of hypoparathyroidism when Ergocalciferol is used, calcium, parathyroid hormone or dihydrotachysterol may be required.

Dosage should be individualised. Frequent serum and urinary calcium, phosphate and urea nitrogen determinations should be carried out. Adequate fluid intake should be maintained.

Should hyperglycaemia develop, Ergocalciferol should be discontinued immediately.

Because of the effect on serum calcium, Ergocalciferol should only be administered to patients with renal stones when potential benefits outweigh possible hazards.

Paediatric doses should be individualised and monitored under close medical supervision.

4.5 Interaction with other medicinal products and other forms of Interaction

Ergocalciferol and:-

i) Magnesium-containing antacids: hypermagnesaemia may develop in patients on chronic renal dialysis.

ii) Digitalis glycosides: hypercalcaemia in patients on digitalis may precipitate cardiac arrhythmias.

iii) Verapamil atrial fibrillation has recurred when supplemental calcium and Ergocalciferol have induced hypercalcaemia.

iv) Phenytoin, barbiturates: half life of Ergocalciferol may be decreased.

v) Thiazide diuretics: hypoparathyroid patients on Ergocalciferol may develop hypercalcaemia due to increased Ergocalciferol (although Ergocalciferol is not recommended for use in hypoparathyroidism).

4.6 Pregnancy and lactation

Pregnancy: There are no adequate data on the use of Ergocalciferol in pregnant women. Ergocalciferol Injection should not be used in pregnancy unless the potential benefit outweighs the potential hazards to the foetus.

Animal studies have shown foetal abnormalities associated with hypervitaminosis D. Calcifediol and calcitriol are teratogenic in animals when given in doses several times the human dose. The offspring of a woman administered 17-144 times the recommended dose of calcitriol during pregnancy manifested mild hypercalcaemia in the first 2 days of life, which returned to normal at day 3.

Ergocalciferol should not be given in late pregnancy due to a risk of hypercalcaemia in the neonate.

Lactation: Ergocalciferol is excreted in breast milk in limited amounts. In a mother given large doses of Ergocalciferol, 25-hydroxycholecalciferol appeared in the milk and caused hypercalcaemia in the child. Monitoring of the infants serum calcium is required in such cases. Ergocalciferol should not be administered to breast-feeding mothers.

4.7 Effects on ability to drive and use machines

Ergocalciferol may cause drowsiness and, if affected, patients should not drive or operate machinery.

4.8 Undesirable effects

Early: weakness; headache; somnolence; nausea; dry mouth; constipation; muscle pain; bone pain; metallic taste.

Late: polyuria; polydipsia; anorexia; irritability; weight loss; nocturia; mild acidosis; reversible azotaemia; generalised vascular calcification; nephrocalcinosis; conjunctivitis (calcific); pancreatitis; photophobia; rhinorrhoea; pruritis; hyperthermia; decreased libido; elevated BUN; albuminuria; hypercholesterolaemia; elevated AST and ALT; ectopic calcification; hypertension; cardiac arrhythmias; overt psychosis (rare).

In clinical studies on hypoparathyroidism and pseudohypoparathyroidism, hypercalcaemia was noted on at least one occasion in about 1 in 3 patients and hypercalciuria in about 1 in 7. Elevated serum creatinine levels were observed in about 1 in 6 patients (approximately one half of whom had normal levels at baseline).

4.9 Overdose

Symptoms: administration to patients in excess of their daily requirement can cause hypercalcaemia, hypercalciuria and hyperphosphataemia. Concomitant high intake of calcium and phosphate may lead to similar abnormalities. Doses of 60,000 IU/day can cause hypercalcaemia.

Hypercalcaemia leads to anorexia, nausea, weakness, weight loss, vague aches and stiffness, constipation, diarrhoea, mental retardation, tinnitus, ataxia, hypotonia, depression, amnesia, disorientation, hallucinations, syncope, coma, anaemia and mild acidosis. Impairment of renal function may cause polyuria, nocturia, hypercalciuria, polydipsia, reversible azotaemia, hypertension, nephrocalcinosis, generalised vascular calcification, irreversible renal insufficiency or proteinuria, widespread calcification of soft tissues, including heart, blood vessels, renal tubules and lungs can occur. Bone demineralisation (osteoporosis) may occur in adults; decline in average linear growth rate and increased bone mineralisation may occur in infants and children (dwarfism). Effects can persist ⩾ 2 months after ergocalciferol treatment. Death can result from cardiovascular or renal failure.

Treatment of hypervitaminosis D with hypercalcaemia consists of immediate withdrawal of the vitamin, a low calcium diet, generous fluid intake and urine acidification along with symptomatic and supportive treatment.

Hypercalcaemic crisis with dehydration, stupor, coma and azotaemia requires more vigorous treatment. The first step in hydration; saline i.v. may quickly and significantly increase calcium excretion. A loop diuretic (e.g. Frusemide) may be given with administration of citrates, sulphates, phosphates, corticosteroids, EDTA and plicamycin. Persistent or markedly elevated serum calcium levels may be corrected by dialysis against a calcium-free dialysate. With appropriate therapy, and when no permanent damage has occurred, recovery is probable.

Treatment of accidental overdosage consists of general supportive measures. If ingestion is discovered within a short time, emesis or gastric lavage may be of benefit. Mineral oil may promote faecal elimination. Treat hypercalcaemia as outlined above.

5. PHARMACOLOGICAL PROPERTIES

5.1 Pharmacodynamic properties

Ergocalciferol (vitamin D) is a fat soluble vitamin. In conjunction with parathyroid hormone and calcitonin, it regulates calcium haemostasis. Ergocalciferol metabolites promote active absorption of calcium and phosphorous by the small intestine, increase rate of excretion and resorption of minerals in bone and promote resorption of minerals in bone and promote resorption of phosphate by renal tubules.

Ergocalciferol deficiency leads to rickets in children and osteomalacia in adults. Ergocalciferol reverses symptoms of nutritional rickets or osteomalacia unless permanent deformities have occurred.

5.2 Pharmacokinetic properties

Distribution - Stored chiefly in the liver, Ergocalciferol is also found in fat, muscle, skin and bones. In plasma, it is bound to alpha globulins and albumin.

Metabolism - There is a lag of 10 to 24 hours between administration of Ergocalciferol and initiation of its action in the body. Maximal hypercalcaemic effects occur about 4 weeks daily administration of a fixed dose and the duration of action can be ⩾ 2 months. Ergocalciferol is hydroxylated in the liver and further metabolism occurs in the kidney.

Excretion - The primary route of excretion of Ergocalciferol is in the bile. Additionally, some is excreted in the urine and faeces. There is also enterohepatic re-cycling.

5.3 Preclinical safety data

None stated.

6. PHARMACEUTICAL PARTICULARS

6.1 List of excipients

Ethyl oleate BP

6.2 Incompatibilities

None stated

6.3 Shelf life

36 months

6.4 Special precautions for storage

Store below 25°C

Protect from light

6.5 Nature and contents of container

Ergocalciferol Injection BP 300,000U - 1ml neutral glass (Type 1) ampoules

Ergocalciferol Injection BP 600,000U - 2ml neutral glass (Type 1) ampoules

6.6 Instructions for use and handling

Plastic syringes should not be used to administer Ergocalciferol Injection

7. MARKETING AUTHORISATION HOLDER

UCB Pharma Limited

208 Bath Road

Slough

Berkshire

SL1 3WE

UK

8. MARKETING AUTHORISATION NUMBER(S)

PL 00039/5655R - Ergocalciferol Injection BP 300,000U

PL 00039/5656R - Ergocalciferol Injection BP 600,000U

9. DATE OF FIRST AUTHORISATION/RENEWAL OF THE AUTHORISATION

25 July 1988 / 13 December 1994 / 04 August 2000

10. DATE OF REVISION OF THE TEXT

June 2005

POM

Ergocalciferol Tablets BP 0.25mg

(Celltech Manufacturing Services Limited)

1. NAME OF THE MEDICINAL PRODUCT

Ergocalciferol Tablets BP 0.25 mg

2. QUALITATIVE AND QUANTITATIVE COMPOSITION

Vitamin D_2 11.8 mg equivalent to 10,000 iu of Vitamin D. ≡ Ergocalciferol 0.25 mg.

For excipients, see 6.1.

3. PHARMACEUTICAL FORM

White biconvex sugar coated tablets with white cores.

4. CLINICAL PARTICULARS

4.1 Therapeutic indications

Simple Vitamin D deficiency

Vitamin D deficiency caused by intestinal malabsorption or chronic liver disease.

Hypocalcaemia of hypoparathyroidism.

4.2 Posology and method of administration

In the treatment of Vitamin D deficiency conditions 0.25 mg (10 000 units or one tablet) daily.

Vitamin D deficiency caused by intestinal malabsorption or chronic liver disease usually requires doses of up to 1 mg (40,000 iu or 4 tablets) daily in divided doses.

In the treatment of hypoparathyroidism 1.25 mg to 5 mg (50 000 to 200 000 units or 5 to 20 tablets) daily.

The hypocalcaemia of hypoparathyroidism often requires doses of up to 5 mg (200,000 iu or 20 tablets) daily in divided doses.

Patients with renal osteodystrophy may require as much as 5 mg (200 000 units or 20 tablets) daily.

For children and the elderly the adult dosage may require adjustment according to the severity of the condition.

This medicine is taken by mouth.

4.3 Contraindications

Renal insufficiency, Hypercalcaemia.

4.4 Special warnings and special precautions for use

All patients receiving pharmacological doses of vitamin D should have their plasma calcium concentration checked at intervals and whenever nausea and vomiting are present. Ergocalciferol appears to take slightly longer to act and slightly longer to cease acting than dihydrotachysterol, therefore it is even more important to avoid ergocalciferol overdosage than it is with the latter.

Absorption of calcium may be reduced by oral sodium sulphate or parenteral magnesium sulphate.

Vitamin D should be administered with caution to infants who may have an increased sensitivity to its effects and should be used with care in patients with calculi or heart disease, who may be at increased risk of organ damage if hypercalcaemia were to occur.

4.5 Interaction with other medicinal products and other forms of Interaction

Phosphate infusions should not be administered to lower hypercalcaemia of hypervitaminosis D because of the dangers of metastatic calcification.

Ergocalciferol is inactivated, probably through enzyme systems, by the continuous administration of anticonvulsants, for example by phenytoin.

There is an increased risk of hypercalcaemia if vitamin D is administered with thiazide diuretics and calcium.

4.6 Pregnancy and lactation

Ergocalciferol Tablets BP 0.25mg may be given to women in the third trimester of pregnancy if justified on medical grounds but the tablets should not be given to lactating mothers.

4.7 Effects on ability to drive and use machines

None documented.

4.8 Undesirable effects

Excessive doses may give rise to anorexia, nausea, vomiting, diarrhoea, loss of weight, headache, polyuria, thirst, vertigo, hypercalcaemia.

4.9 Overdose

If hypervitaminosis occurs:

Discontinue treatment with calciferol.

Reduce dietary calcium intake.

Correct dehydration and electrolyte disturbance.

Hypercalcaemia may be corrected by the administration of hydrocortisone or calcitonin.

5. PHARMACOLOGICAL PROPERTIES

5.1 Pharmacodynamic properties

Vitamin D_2 is a steroid derivative which controls the calcification of bones in both the young and old.

Although naturally produced under normal conditions, pharmacological doses are often required in disease states.

5.2 Pharmacokinetic properties

Vitamin D_2 is partly esterified during its absorption and is blood borne bound to α_2-globulins and albumin. About ½ of the ingested oral dose is excreted into the bile and lost with the faeces.

5.3 Preclinical safety data

Not applicable since ergocalciferol has been used in clinical practice for many years and its effects in man are well known.

6. PHARMACEUTICAL PARTICULARS

6.1 List of excipients

Avicel PH 101 (microcrystalline cellulose),

Magnesium Stearate,

Lactose DCL 11,

Acacia,

Sugar,

Talc,

Gelatin,

Titanium Dioxide,

Opaglos AG 7350.

6.2 Incompatibilities

None stated.

6.3 Shelf life

36 months.

6.4 Special precautions for storage

Store below 25°C in a well closed container protected from light.

6.5 Nature and contents of container

1.) Containers having snap-on Polythene lids, with integral tear-off security seals eg Jaycare "securitainer" or Wragby "snap-secure" container containing 100 tablets.

2.) Blister packs of 28 or 50 tablets in cartons which are white folding box board printed on white, the blister comprises 250 micron white rigid UPVC backed by 20 micron hard tempered aluminium foil, bearing a 6-8 gm^{-2} vinyl heat seal coating on the inner surface and printed / over lacquered on the reverse.

6.6 Instructions for use and handling

No special precautions are required.

7. MARKETING AUTHORISATION HOLDER

Celltech Manufacturing Services Limited

Vale of Bardsley

Ashton-under-Lyne

Lancashire

OL7 9RR

8. MARKETING AUTHORISATION NUMBER(S)

PL 18816/0002

9. DATE OF FIRST AUTHORISATION/RENEWAL OF THE AUTHORISATION

18 July 2001 / 17 May 2002

10. DATE OF REVISION OF THE TEXT

September 2001 / June 2002

Ergocalciferol Tablets BP 1.25mg

(Celltech Manufacturing Services Limited)

1. NAME OF THE MEDICINAL PRODUCT

Ergocalciferol Tablets BP 1.25mg

2. QUALITATIVE AND QUANTITATIVE COMPOSITION

Ergocalciferol 1.25 mg as Vitamin D_2 (gelatin coated) 62 mg

3. PHARMACEUTICAL FORM

White biconvex sugar coated tablets

4. CLINICAL PARTICULARS

4.1 Therapeutic indications

For the treatment of hypocalcaemia caused by of hypoparathyroidism or in patients with renal osteodystrophy.

4.2 Posology and method of administration

Adults, Children and Elderly

A dose of 1.25 to 5mg daily is recommended. The dose should be adjusted according to the severity of the condition.

This medicine is delivered by oral administration

4.3 Contraindications

Renal insufficiency, hypercalcaemia and metastatic calcification. Ergocalciferol Tablets BP 1.25mg are unsuitable for use in vitamin D deficiency diseases such as rickets.

4.4 Special warnings and special precautions for use

All patients receiving pharmacological doses of vitamin D should have their plasma calcium concentration checked regularly and monitored for symptoms of hypercalcaemia (anorexia, nausea, vomiting, lassitude, diarrhoea, weight loss, polyuria, sweating, headache, thirst, vertigo and raised concentrations of calcium and phosphate in plasma and urine) and therapy withdrawn or adjusted as appropriate. It is important to ensure correct dosage in infants.

4.5 Interaction with other medicinal products and other forms of Interaction

The effects of Vitamin D may be reduced in patients taking barbiturates or anti-convulsant, absorption of calcium may be reduced by oral sodium sulphate or parenteral magnesium sulphate.

4.6 Pregnancy and lactation

Ergocalciferol Tablets BP 1.25mg may be used in late pregnancy if justified on medical grounds. Use during very late pregnancy and breast feeding may lead to the development of hypercalcaemia in the infant, therefore use during this period is not recommended.

4.7 Effects on ability to drive and use machines

None documented.

4.8 Undesirable effects

Common side-effects include anorexia, nausea, vomiting, diarrhoea, loss of weight, headache, polyuria, thirst and vertigo.

4.9 Overdose

Symptoms of severe hypercalcaemia are constipation, abdominal pain, muscle weakness, mental disturbances, polydipsia, bone pain, nephrocalcinosis, renal calculi and in very severe cases cardiac arrhythmias and coma.

Cases of severe hypercalcaemia should be treated with IV infusion of sodium chloride to expand the extracellular fluid. This may be accompanied by administration of a suitable loop diuretic (such as frusemide) to increase calcium excretion. If unsuccessful, other drug therapy (such as calcitonin, bisphosphonates, plicamycin or corticosteroids) or, as a last resort, haemodialysis, may be considered. It is essential to monitor serum electrolyte therapy during overdose treatment.

5. PHARMACOLOGICAL PROPERTIES

5.1 Pharmacodynamic properties

Ergocalciferol, an oil soluble vitamin, increases the intestinal absorption of dietary calcium and increases the release of calcium from bone. These effects combine to raise the plasma calcium concentration.

Hyperparathyroidism causes a fall in plasma calcium concentration. Large doses of ergocalciferol control plasma calcium levels and is the preferred maintenance therapy of this disease.

5.2 Pharmacokinetic properties

Ergocalciferol is well absorbed after oral administration. The half-life is about 960 hours, with protein binding in the blood to alpha and beta-lipoproteins. It is secreted in milk and stored in the liver. Metabolism is by 25 hydroxylation in the liver, followed by hydroxylation at positions 12 or 24 by the kidney. The rate of kidney metabolism is controlled by parathyroid hormone. There is possible conjugation with sulphate or glucuronic acid and decreased absorption may result from impaired liver or biliary function.

5.3 Preclinical safety data

Not applicable.

6. PHARMACEUTICAL PARTICULARS

6.1 List of excipients

Tablet core: Avicel PH 101 BP (microcrystalline cellulose)

Magnesium Stearate BP

Lactose monohydrate EP

Tablet coats: Acacia EP

Sugar EP

Talc EP

Gelatin EP

Titanium Dioxide EP

Opaglos EP (containing: purified water EP, beeswax BP, carnuaba wax BP, polysorbate 20 BP, sorbic acid (E200)).

6.2 Incompatibilities

None stated.

6.3 Shelf life

36 months

6.4 Special precautions for storage

Store below 25° C in a well closed container.

6.5 Nature and contents of container

Containers of pigmented polypropylene having snap secure closure of pigmented low density polyethylene, containing 100 tablets.

6.6 Instructions for use and handling

No special precautions are required.

7. MARKETING AUTHORISATION HOLDER

Celltech Manufacturing Services Limited

Vale of Bardsley

Ashton-under-Lyne

Lancashire

OL7 9RR

8. MARKETING AUTHORISATION NUMBER(S)

PL 18816/0003

9. DATE OF FIRST AUTHORISATION/RENEWAL OF THE AUTHORISATION

18 July 2001

10. DATE OF REVISION OF THE TEXT

September 2001 / January 2003

Ergometrine Tabets BP 500mcg

(Celltech Manufacturing Services Limited)

1. NAME OF THE MEDICINAL PRODUCT

Ergometrine Maleate Tablets BP 500 micrograms.

2. QUALITATIVE AND QUANTITATIVE COMPOSITION

Ergometrine Maleate BP 0.5 mg.

3. PHARMACEUTICAL FORM

White, biconvex uncoated tablets, plain or engraved Evans 134, on one side.

4. CLINICAL PARTICULARS

4.1 Therapeutic indications

Ergometrine tablets are indicated in the treatment of mild secondary post partum haemorrhage.

4.2 Posology and method of administration

Women of child bearing age only.

Treatment of mild secondary post partum haemorrhage

500 mcg three times daily for 2-7 days.

Not appropriate for elderly or children.

4.3 Contraindications

Ergometrine is contra-indicated in the 1st and 2nd stages of labour, peripheral obliterative vascular disease, impaired pulmonary, hepatic and renal function. Ergometrine should not be used in patients with severe cardiac disease, arterial-venous shunts, ischaemic heart disease, a history of angina or a previous myocardial infarction. its use should be avoided in patients with eclampsia, hypertension of pregnancy or with sepsis.

Ergometrine should not be used for the induction of labour or in cases of threatened abortion.

4.4 Special warnings and special precautions for use

Prolonged use may give rise to gangrene.

Ergometrine should be used with caution in cases of multiple pregnancy or porphyria.

4.5 Interaction with other medicinal products and other forms of Interaction

The effects of Ergometrine on the parturient uterus are diminished by halothane. The vasoconstrictor effects of Ergometrine may be enhanced by sympathomimeticagents such as adrenaline.

Ergometrine should not be used concurrently with anti-viral agents (such as nelfinavir, ritonavir and possibly saquinavir), or macrolide antibiotics (such as erthromycin, azithromycin and clarithromycin) as potentially dangerous ergot toxicity may occur. Tetracycline antibiotics (including doxycline), in conjunction with ergot alkaloids, may also cause the same effect.

Prolonged vasospastic reactions have been reported between Ergotamine and $5ht_1$agonists and these effects may be additive. after taking Ergotamine, 24 hours should elapse before taking a $5ht_1$agonist. if a $5ht_1$agonist is taken first, at least 6 hours should elapse before taking.

4.6 Pregnancy and lactation

The use of Ergometrine is contraindicated during pregnancy and labour before delivery of the anterior shoulder. Ergometrine should not be used in lactating mothers as it may lower prolactin levels which may decrease lactation.

4.7 Effects on ability to drive and use machines

Patients should be advised not to drive or use machines while receiving Ergometrine.

4.8 Undesirable effects

The most common adverse effects are nausea and vomiting. hypertension, hypotension, chest pain, angina, palpitations, vasospasms, vasoconstrictions of extremities, headache, dizziness, confusion, tinnitus, abdominal pain, dyspnoea and bradycardia may also occur. Water intoxication, loss of consciousness, diarrhoea, stroke, myocardial infarction, pulmonary oedema and bronchospasm have been reported.

Ergometrine shows less tendency to produce gangrene than ergotamine but ergotism has been reported and symptoms of acute poisoning are similar.

4.9 Overdose

Acute overdosage causes convulsions and any of the effects listed under adverse effects. Gangrene results from chronic overdosage.

treatment

Empty stomach by gastric lavage or emesis. Delay absorption of ingested drug by giving activated charcoal followed by catharsis. Control hypercoagulability byadministering heparin. Nitroglycerin (sublingual or intravenous) is used for coronary vasospasm. Intravenous or intra-arterial nitroprusside is the drug of choice for severe vasospasm. Seizures should be treated with anti-convulsants and hypertension should be treated with nitrates, hydralazine or nitroprusside. Gangrene may require surgical amputation.

5. PHARMACOLOGICAL PROPERTIES

5.1 Pharmacodynamic properties

The main pharmacological action of ergometrine is uterine smooth muscle contraction. Ergometrine has a much more powerful action on the uterus than most of the other alkaloids of ergot, especially on the puerperal uterus. at low doses ergometrine causes intense uterine smooth muscle contraction followed by periods of relaxation. At high doses Ergometrine produces sustained contractions. This contrasts with the physiological rhythmic uterine contractions induced by oxytocin. Ergometrine's action is more prolonged than that of oxytocin but is less rapid in onset. Uterine stimulation is said to occur within about 10 minutes of administration by mouth.

Ergometrine produces vasoconstriction, mainly of capacitance vessels.

Ergometrine can lower prolactin levels.

When used after placental delivery, Ergometrine also decreases uterine bleeding.

5.2 Pharmacokinetic properties
Ergometrine is well absorbed after oral administration with peak plasma concentrations occurring 60 to 90 minutes after a dose. elimination is rapid, with a half life that is probably less than 2 hours.

Ergometrine is extensively metabolised in the liver. hydroxylation, glucuronic acid conjugation and possibly n-demethylation occur, with excretion in the faeces.

The distribution of Ergometrine has not been fully elucidated.

5.3 Preclinical safety data
Not applicable since Ergometrine tablets have been used in clinical practice for many years and its effects in man are well known.

6. PHARMACEUTICAL PARTICULARS

6.1 List of excipients
Maleic Acid BP

Mannitol BP

Magnesium Stearate BP

Acacia Powder BP

Purified Water BP

6.2 Incompatibilities
None.

6.3 Shelf life
36 months.

6.4 Special precautions for storage
Store below 25°C, protect from light and keep well closed.

6.5 Nature and contents of container
Amber glass bottles with wadded plastic screw cap closure containing either 21 or 100 tablets.

6.6 Instructions for use and handling
No special precautions are required.

Administrative Data

7. MARKETING AUTHORISATION HOLDER
Celltech Manufacturing Services Limited

Vale of Bardsley

Ashton under Lyne

Lancashire

OL7 9RR

United Kingdom

8. MARKETING AUTHORISATION NUMBER(S)
PL 18816/0006

9. DATE OF FIRST AUTHORISATION/RENEWAL OF THE AUTHORISATION
7 October 2001

10. DATE OF REVISION OF THE TEXT

Eryacne 4

(Galderma (U.K.) Ltd)

1. NAME OF THE MEDICINAL PRODUCT
Eryacne 4

2. QUALITATIVE AND QUANTITATIVE COMPOSITION
Eryacne 4 contains 4% w/w erythromycin Ph. Eur, expressed as erythromycin base with a potency of 1,000 IU/mg.

3. PHARMACEUTICAL FORM
Eryacne 4 is an alcohol-based gel for topical (cutaneous) use.

4. CLINICAL PARTICULARS

4.1 Therapeutic indications
Eryacne 4 is intended for the topical (cutaneous) treatment of *acne vulgaris*.

4.2 Posology and method of administration
Eryacne 4 is recommended for the first four weeks of treatment. If the condition has improved after four weeks, Eryacne 2 (containing 2% w/w erythromycin) may be substituted.

A thin film of Eryacne should be applied to the affected areas twice daily, morning and evening. These areas should be washed and dried before the product is used.

As a rule, treatment is continued for eight weeks, although this period may be extended to obtain a satisfactory response.

4.3 Contraindications
Eryacne 4 is contra-indicated in persons known to be sensitive to any of the ingredients.

4.4 Special warnings and special precautions for use
Eryacne 4 is for external use only and should be kept away from the eyes, nose, mouth and other mucous membranes. If accidental contact does occur, the area should be washed with lukewarm water.

If a reaction suggesting sensitivity or a severe reaction occurs, use of the product should be discontinued. Depending upon the degree of irritation, the patient should be advised to use the product less frequently, to discontinue its use temporarily or to discontinue its use altogether.

Cross-resistance could occur with other antibiotics of the macrolide group.

4.5 Interaction with other medicinal products and other forms of Interaction
Concurrent topical acne therapy should be used with caution because a cumulative irritant effect could occur.

Concurrent use of exfoliants or medicated soaps or cosmetics containing alcohol could also cause a cumulative irritant or drying effect in patients using Eryacne 4.

Erythromycin and clindamycin topical preparations should not be used concurrently.

4.6 Pregnancy and lactation
There is no evidence of risk from using erythromycin in human pregnancy. It has been in wide use for many years without apparent ill consequence. Animal reproduction studies have shown no risk.

If Eryacne 4 is used during lactation, it should not be applied on the chest to avoid accidental ingestion by the infant.

4.7 Effects on ability to drive and use machines
Performance related to driving and using machines should not be affected by the use of Eryacne 4.

4.8 Undesirable effects
Adverse reactions reported to date with topical erythromycin therapy include dryness, irritation, pruritis, erythema, desquamation, oiliness and a burning sensation.

Most of these reactions appear to be caused by alcohol or other excipients rather than by erythromycin and are reversible when the frequency of application is reduced or treatment is discontinued.

4.9 Overdose
Eryacne 4 is for cutaneous use only. If the product is applied excessively, no more rapid or better results will be obtained, and marked redness, peeling or discomfort could occur. If these effects should occur, the frequency of application could be reduced or treatment discontinued and appropriate symptomatic therapy instituted.

The acute oral toxicity in mice and rats is greater than $10ml.kg^{-1}$. Unless the amount accidentally ingested is small, an appropriate method of gastric emptying should be considered provided that this is carried out soon after ingestion. One unopened 30g tube of Eryacne 4 contains about 30ml of alcohol.

5. PHARMACOLOGICAL PROPERTIES

5.1 Pharmacodynamic properties
Erythromycin is a macrolide antibiotic active *in vivo* and *in vitro* against most aerobic and anaerobic gram-positive bacteria as well as some gram-negative bacilli.

Erythromycin is usually bacteriostatic in action, but may be bacteriocidal in high concentrations or against highly susceptible organisms.

Erythromycin appears to inhibit protein synthesis in susceptible organisms by reversible binding to 50S ribosomal subunits. Following application to the skin, the drug inhibits the growth of susceptible organisms (principally *Propionibacterium acnes*) on the surface of the skin and reduces the concentration of free fatty acids in the sebum. The reduction of free fatty acids in sebum may be an indirect result of the inhibition of lipase-producing organisms that convert triglycerides into free fatty acids. It may also be a direct result of interference with lipase production in these organisms.

Free fatty acids are comedogenic and are believed to be a positive cause of the inflammatory lesions of acne, e.g. papules, pustules, nodules and cysts. However, other mechanisms may be involved in the clinical improvement of *acne* as a direct result of the anti-inflammatory action of erythromycin applied topically to the skin.

5.2 Pharmacokinetic properties
Erythromycin does not appear to be absorbed systemically following application of Eryacne 4 to the skin, although it is not known whether it is absorbed from denuded or broken skin, wounds or mucous membranes.

5.3 Preclinical safety data
There is no evidence from toxicological studies that cutaneous application of the proposed clinical dose of erythromycin would be associated with the risk of significant adverse reactions in humans. Published data and information on the toxicity of erythromycin applied to the skin support this conclusion.

6. PHARMACEUTICAL PARTICULARS

6.1 List of excipients
Butylhydroxytoluene

Hydroxypropylcellulose

Alcohol

6.2 Incompatibilities
None known.

6.3 Shelf life
Twenty-four (24) months.

6.4 Special precautions for storage
Store below 25°C, and out of the sight and the reach of children.

6.5 Nature and contents of container
Eryacne 4 is presented in a collapsible aluminium tube. The tube has an internal coating of an epoxy-phenolic resin. It is closed with a polypropylene screw cap. This cap is used to pierce the tube before its first use. A tube of Eryacne 4 contains 30g of product.

6.6 Instructions for use and handling
On first use, the screw cap is removed and is used to pierce the neck of the tube. Unscrew the cap, remove the plastic collar and screw the cap back onto the tube.

7. MARKETING AUTHORISATION HOLDER
Galderma (UK) Limited,

Galderma House

Church lane

Kings Langley

Herts. WD4 8JP

England.

8. MARKETING AUTHORISATION NUMBER(S)
PL 10590/0022

9. DATE OF FIRST AUTHORISATION/RENEWAL OF THE AUTHORISATION
29 November 1996

10. DATE OF REVISION OF THE TEXT
May 2001

11. Legal Category
POM

Erymax Capsules

(Zeneus Pharma Ltd)

1. NAME OF THE MEDICINAL PRODUCT
Erymax 250mg Gastro-resistant Hard Capsules

2. QUALITATIVE AND QUANTITATIVE COMPOSITION
Each capsule contains 250mg of erythromycin.

For excipients, see 6.1.

3. PHARMACEUTICAL FORM
Gastro-resistant capsule, hard.

Hard gelatin capsule with opaque orange cap and clear orange body, imprinted with "Erymax 250mg", and containing white and orange enteric coated pellets of erythromycin base.

4. CLINICAL PARTICULARS

4.1 Therapeutic indications
Erythromycin is an antibiotic effective in the treatment of bacterial disease caused by susceptible organisms.

Examples of its use are in the treatment of upper and lower respiratory tract infections of mild to moderate severity; skin and soft tissue infections including pustular acne.

Erythromycin is usually active against the following organisms *in vitro* and in clinical infection: *Streptococcus pyogenes*; Alpha haemolytic streptococci; *Staphylococcus aureus*; *Streptococcus pneumoniae*; *Haemophilus influenzae*; *Mycoplasma pneumoniae*; *Treponema pallidum*; *Corynebacterium diphtheriae*; *Corynebacterium minutissimum*; *Entamoeba histolytica*; *Listeria monocytogenes*; *Neisseria gonorrhoeae*; *Bordetella pertussis*; *Legionella pneumophila*; *Chlamydia trachomatis*; *Propionibacterium acnes*.

4.2 Posology and method of administration
Oral use.

Adults and elderly

250 mg every six hours - before or with meals. 500 mg every twelve hours may be given if desired; b.i.d. dosage should not be used if dosage exceeds one gram.

Children

The usual dose is 30-50 mg/kg/day erythromycin, in divided doses given twice daily or every six hours. In severe infections, this dose may be doubled; elevated doses should be given every six hours. The drug should be given before or with meals.

Note: Erymax Capsules may be given to children of any age who can swallow the capsules whole.

The capsules should be swallowed whole either before or with food; they should not be chewed.

Streptococcal Infections:

For active infection - a full therapeutic dose is given for at least ten days.

For continuous prophylaxis against recurrences of streptococcal infections in patients with evidence of rheumatic fever or heart disease, the dose is 250 mg b.i.d.

For the prevention of bacterial endocarditis in patients with valvular disease scheduled for dental or surgical procedures of the upper respiratory tract, the adult dose is 1 gram (children 20 mg/kg) 2 hours before surgery. Following surgery, the dose is 500 mg for adults (children 10mg/kg) orally every six hours for 8 doses.

Primary Syphilis: 30-40 grams given in divided doses over a period of 10-15 days.

Intestinal Amoebiasis: 250 mg four times daily for 10 to 14 days for adults: 30 to 50 mg/kg/day in divided doses for 10 to 14 days for children.

Legionnaires' Disease: 1-4 g daily until clinical signs and symptoms indicate a clinical cure. Treatment may be prolonged.

Pertussis: 30-50 mg/kg/day given in divided doses for 5 - 14 days, depending upon eradication of a positive culture.

Acne: initially, 250 mg twice daily, which may be reduced to a maintenance dose of 250 mg once daily after one month according to response.

4.3 Contraindications

Use in patients hypersensitive to erythromycin or to any of the excipients, and in patients taking astemizole, terfenadine, cisapride, pimozide, ergotamine, dihydroergotamine or sertindole.

4.4 Special warnings and special precautions for use

In patients with impaired hepatic function, liver function should be monitored, since a few reports of hepatic dysfunction have been received in patients taking erythromycin as the estolate, base or stearate. Extended administration requires regular evaluation particularly of liver function. Therapy should be discontinued if significant hepatic dysfunction occurs.

Prolonged use of erythromycin has caused overgrowth of nonsusceptible bacteria or fungi; this is a rare occurrence.

It has been reported that erythromycin may aggravate the weakness of patients with myasthenia gravis.

Patients receiving erythromycin concurrently with drugs which can cause prolongation of the QT interval should be carefully monitored; the concomitant use of erythromycin with some of these drugs is contraindicated (see sections 4.3 and 4.5).

Owing to the presence of lactose, patients with rare hereditary problems of galactose intolerance, the Lapp lactase deficiency or glucose-galactose malabsorption should not take this medicine.

4.5 Interaction with other medicinal products and other forms of Interaction

Concomitant use of erythromycin with certain drugs metabolised by the cytochrome P450 system is likely to result in an increased frequency or seriousness of adverse effects associated with these drugs. The concomitant use of erythromycin with astemizole, cisapride, pimozide, sertindole and terfenadine is contraindicated due to the risk of QT prolongation and cardiac arrhythmias including ventricular tachycardia, ventricular fibrillation and Torsades de pointes. The concomitant use of erythromycin with ergotamine and dihydroergotamine is contraindicated due to the risk of ergot toxicity.

Other drugs metabolised by the cytochrome P450 system, such as acenocoumarol, atorvastatin, bromocriptine, buspirone, cabergoline, carbamazepine, ciclosporin, cilostazol, clozapine, digoxin, disopyramide, eletriptan, felodipine, hexobarbital, midazolam, mizolastine, phenytoin, quetiapine, quinidine, rifabutin, sildenafil, simvastatin, tacrolimus, tadalafil, theophylline, tolterodine, triazolam, valproate, warfarin and zopiclone, may be associated with elevated serum levels if administered concomitantly with erythromycin. Because of the risk of toxicity, appropriate monitoring should be undertaken, and dosage should be adjusted as necessary.

When oral erythromycin is given concurrently with theophylline, there is also a significant decrease in erythromycin serum concentrations, which could result in subtherapeutic concentrations of erythromycin.

Erythromycin should be used with caution if administered concomitantly with lincomycin, clindamycin or chloramphenicol, as competitive inhibition may occur.

The concomitant use of erythromycin with alfentanil can significantly inhibit the clearance of alfentanil and may increase the risk of prolonged or delayed respiratory depression.

Patients receiving concomitant lovastatin and erythromycin should be carefully monitored as cases of rhabdomyolysis have been reported in seriously ill patients. Rhabdomyolysis has also been reported with concomitant simvastatin and erythromycin, and caution is therefore recommended when erythromycin is used concurrently with other HMG-CoA reductase inhibitors.

An increased plasma concentration of erythromycin has been reported with concomitant cimetidine treatment, leading to increased risk of toxicity, including reversible deafness.

Erythromycin may interfere with the determination of urinary catecholamines and 17-hydroxycorticosteroids.

4.6 Pregnancy and lactation

Like all drugs erythromycin should be used in pregnancy only when clearly indicated. Erythromycin crosses the placental barrier.

Nursing mothers: erythromycin is excreted in human milk and should be used in lactating women only if clearly needed.

4.7 Effects on ability to drive and use machines

None known.

4.8 Undesirable effects

Serious allergic reaction, including anaphylaxis, has been reported.

There have been rare reports of skin rashes, including pruritus, urticaria and, very rarely, Stevens-Johnson syndrome.

Nausea and abdominal discomfort can occur at elevated doses; diarrhoea and vomiting are less common.

Hepatotoxicity: There have been reports of hepatic dysfunction, with or without jaundice, occurring in patients receiving erythromycin products and due to combined cholestatic and hepatocellular injury although less commonly than with erythromycin estolate.

Pancreatitis has been reported rarely.

Superinfections including pseudomembranous colitis have been occasionally reported to occur in association with erythromycin therapy.

Transient hearing disturbances and deafness have been reported with doses of erythromycin usually greater than 4g daily, and usually given intravenously.

There have been isolated reports of transient central nervous system side effects including confusion, hallucinations, seizures, and vertigo; however, a cause and effect relationship has not been established.

Cardiac arrhythmias have been reported rarely in patients receiving erythromycin.

4.9 Overdose

Nausea, vomiting and diarrhoea have been reported.

Treatment

Gastric lavage and general supportive therapy. Erythromycin is not removed by peritoneal dialysis or haemodialysis.

5. PHARMACOLOGICAL PROPERTIES

5.1 Pharmacodynamic properties

Erythromycin base and its salts are readily absorbed in the microbiologically active form. Erythromycin is largely bound to plasma proteins and after absorption erythromycin diffuses readily into most body fluids.

Erythromycin acts by inhibition of protein synthesis by binding 50s ribosomal subunits of susceptible organisms. It does not affect nucleic acid synthesis.

5.2 Pharmacokinetic properties

After administration of a single dose of Erymax 250 mg, peak serum levels are attained in approximately 3 hours.

In the presence of normal hepatic function, erythromycin is concentrated in the liver and is excreted in the bile. After oral administration, less than 5% of the administered dose can be recovered in the active form in the urine.

5.3 Preclinical safety data

Pre-clinical safety data does not add anything of further significance to the prescriber.

6. PHARMACEUTICAL PARTICULARS

6.1 List of excipients

Cellulose acetate phthalate, lactose, potassium phosphate monobasic, povidone, diethyl phthalate, purified water, sunset yellow, titanium dioxide, gelatin, erythrosine, quinoline yellow.

6.2 Incompatibilities

None known.

6.3 Shelf life

36 months.

6.4 Special precautions for storage

Do not store above 25°C. Store in the original package. Protect from moisture and light.

6.5 Nature and contents of container

Polypropylene Securitainers containing 100 capsules.

HDPE Tampertainers containing 28, 100 capsules.

Blister packs containing 4, 8, 28, 30, 100, 112 capsules.

6.6 Instructions for use and handling

No special requirements.

7. MARKETING AUTHORISATION HOLDER

Elan Pharma Ltd

Monksland

Athlone

Co. Westmeath

Ireland

Trading as

Elan Pharma

Abel Smith House

Gunnels Wood Road

Stevenage

Hertfordshire, SG1 2FG, UK

8. MARKETING AUTHORISATION NUMBER(S)

PL 10038/0030

9. DATE OF FIRST AUTHORISATION/RENEWAL OF THE AUTHORISATION

April 1998

10. DATE OF REVISION OF THE TEXT

March 2004

11. LEGAL CATEGORY

POM

Erythrocin 250

(Abbott Laboratories Limited)

1. NAME OF THE MEDICINAL PRODUCT

Erythrocin 250

2. QUALITATIVE AND QUANTITATIVE COMPOSITION

Erythromycin as erythromycin stearate 250 mg / tablet

3. PHARMACEUTICAL FORM

Film coated tablet

4. CLINICAL PARTICULARS

4.1 Therapeutic indications

For the prophylaxis and treatment of infections caused by erythromycin-sensitive organisms.

Erythromycin is highly effective in the treatment of a great variety of clinical infections such as:

1. Upper Respiratory Tract infections: tonsillitis, peritonsillar abscess, pharyngitis, laryngitis, sinusitis, secondary infections in influenza and common colds

2. Lower Respiratory Tract infections: tracheitis, acute and chronic bronchitis, pneumonia (lobar pneumonia, bronchopneumonia, primary atypical pneumonia), bronchiectasis, Legionnaire's disease

3. Ear infection: otitis media and otitis externa, mastoiditis

4. Oral infections: gingivitis, Vincent's angina

5. Eye infections: blepharitis

6. Skin and soft tissue infections: boils and carbuncles, paronychia, abscesses, pustular acne, impetigo, cellulitis, erysipelas

7. Gastrointestinal infections: cholecystitis, staphylococcal enterocolitis

8. Prophylaxis: pre- and post- operative trauma, burns, rheumatic fever, bacterial endocarditis in patients allergic to penicillin with congenital heart disease, or rheumatic or other acquired valvular heart disease when undergoing dental procedures or surgical procedures of the upper respiratory tract.

9. Other infections: osteomyelitis, urethritis, gonorrhoea, syphilis, lymphogranuloma venereum, diphtheria, prostatitis, scarlet fever

4.2 Posology and method of administration

Adults and children over 8 years: 1- 2g/day in divided doses. For severe infections up to 4g/day in divided doses.

Elderly: No special dosage recommendations

Children under 8 years: Erythroped suspension is recommended.

4.3 Contraindications

Known hypersensitivity to erythromycin. Erythromycin is contraindicated in patients taking astemizole, terfenadine, cisapride or pimozide.

Erythromycin is contraindicated with ergotamine and dihydroergotamine.

4.4 Special warnings and special precautions for use

Erythromycin is excreted principally by the liver, so caution should be exercised in administering the antibiotic to patients with impaired hepatic function or concomitantly receiving potentially hepatotoxic agents. Hepatic dysfunction including increased liver enzymes and/or cholestatic hepatitis, with or without jaundice, has been infrequently reported with erythromycin.

There have been reports suggesting erythromycin does not reach the foetus in adequate concentrations to prevent congenital syphilis. Infants born to women treated during pregnancy with oral erythromycin for early syphilis should be treated with an appropriate penicillin regimen.

There have been reports that erythromycin may aggravate the weakness of patients with myasthenia gravis.

Erythromycin interferes with the fluorometric determination of urinary catecholamines.

As with other broad spectrum antibiotics, pseudomembranous colitis has been reported rarely with erythromycin.

Rhabdomyolysis with or without renal impairment has been reported in seriously ill patients receiving erythromycin concomitantly with lovastatin.

4.5 Interaction with other medicinal products and other forms of Interaction

Concomitant use of erythromycin with terfenadine or astemizole is likely to result in an enhanced risk of cardiotoxicity with these drugs. The concomitant use of erythromycin with either astemizole or terfenadine is therefore contraindicated.

The metabolism of terfenadine and astemizole is significantly altered when either are taken concomitantly with erythromycin. Rare cases of serious cardiovascular events have been observed, including torsades de pointes, other ventricular arrhythmias and cardiac arrest. Death has been reported with the terfenadine / erythromycin combination.

Elevated cisapride levels have been reported in patients receiving erythromycin and cisapride concomitantly. This may result in QT prolongation and cardiac arrhythmias including ventricular trachycardia, ventricular fibrillation and Torsades de pointes. Similar effects have been observed with concomitant administration of pimozide and clarithromycin, another macrolide antibiotic.

Concurrent use of erythromycin and ergotamine or dihydroergotamine has been associated in some patients with acute ergot toxicity characterised by the rapid development of severe peripheral vasospasm and dysaesthesia.

Increases in serum concentrations of the following drugs metabolised by the cytochrome P450 system may occur when administered concurrently with erythromycin: alfentanil, astemizole, bromocriptine, carbamazepine, cyclosporin, digoxin, dihydroergotamine, disopyramide, ergotamine, hexobarbitone, midazolam, phenytoin, quinidine, tacrolimus, terfenadine, theophylline, triazolam, valproate, and warfarin. Appropriate monitoring should be undertaken and dosage should be adjusted as necessary.

Erythromycin has been reported to decrease the clearance of zopiclone and thus may increase the pharmacodynamic effects of this drug.

When oral erythromycin is given concurrently with theophylline, there is also a significant decrease in erythromycin serum concentrations. The decrease could result in subtherapeutic concentrations of erythromycin.

4.6 Pregnancy and lactation

There is no evidence of hazard from erythromycin in human pregnancy. It has been in widespread use for a number of years without apparent ill consequence. Animal studies have shown no hazard.

Erythromycin has been reported to cross the placental barrier in humans, but foetal plasma levels are generally low.

Erythromycin is excreted in breast milk, therefore, caution should be exercised when erythromycin is administered to a nursing mother.

4.7 Effects on ability to drive and use machines

None reported

4.8 Undesirable effects

Occasional side effects such as nausea, abdominal discomfort, vomiting and diarrhoea may be experienced. Reversible hearing loss associated with doses of erythromycin usually greater than 4g per day has been reported. Allergic reactions are rare and mild, although anaphylaxis has occurred. Skin reactions ranging from mild eruptions to erythema multiforme, Stevens-Johnson syndrome and toxic epidermal necrolysis have rarely been reported. There are no reports implicating erythromycin products with abnormal tooth development, and only rare reports of damage to the blood, kidneys or central nervous system.

Cardiac arrhythmias have been very rarely reported in patients receiving erythromycin therapy. There have been isolated reports of chest pain, dizziness and palpitations, however, a cause and effect relationship has not been established.

Symptoms of hepatitis, hepatic dysfunction and/or abnormal liver function test results may occur.

4.9 Overdose

Symptoms: hearing loss, severe nausea, vomiting and diarrhoea.

Treatment: gastric lavage, general supportive measures.

5. PHARMACOLOGICAL PROPERTIES

5.1 Pharmacodynamic properties

Erythromycin exerts its antimicrobial action by binding to the 50S ribosomal sub-unit of susceptible microorganisms and suppresses protein synthesis. Erythromycin is usually active against most strains of the following organisms both in vitro and in clinical infections:

Gram positive bacteria - Listeria monocytogenes, Corynebacterium diphtheriae (as an adjunct to antitoxin), Staphylococci *spp,* Streptococci *spp* (including Enterococci).

Gram negative bacteria - Haemophilus influenzae, Neisseria meningitidis, Neisseria gonorrhoeae, Legionella pneumophila, Moraxella (Branhamella) catarrhalis, Bordetella pertussis, Campylobacter spp.

Mycoplasma - Mycoplasma pneumoniae, Ureaplasma urealyticum.

Other organisms - Treponema pallidum, Chlamydia spp, Clostridia spp, L-forms, the agents causing trachoma and lymphogranuloma venereum.

Note: The majority of strains of Haemophilus influenzae are susceptible to the concentrations reached after ordinary doses.

5.2 Pharmacokinetic properties

None stated.

5.3 Preclinical safety data

There are no pre-clinical data of relevance to the prescriber which are additional to that already included in other sections of the SPC.

6. PHARMACEUTICAL PARTICULARS

6.1 List of excipients

Povidone, maize starch, magnesium hydroxide, polacrilin potassium, polyethylene glycol 8000, polyethylene glycol 400, hydroxypropyl methyl cellulose, sorbic acid.

6.2 Incompatibilities

None stated.

6.3 Shelf life

60 months.

6.4 Special precautions for storage

None stated.

6.5 Nature and contents of container

High density polyethlyene bottle with urea cap with 100 tablets, securitainer or snap-secure container with 50, 100 or 1000 tablets. Blister packs containing 28 tablets: PVC, heat sealed with 20 micron hard tamper aluminium foil.

6.6 Instructions for use and handling

Not applicable

7. MARKETING AUTHORISATION HOLDER

Abbott Laboratories Ltd., Queenborough, Kent. ME11 5EL.

8. MARKETING AUTHORISATION NUMBER(S)

PL 0037/5079R

9. DATE OF FIRST AUTHORISATION/RENEWAL OF THE AUTHORISATION

16/06/97

10. DATE OF REVISION OF THE TEXT

August 1997

Erythrocin 500

(Abbott Laboratories Limited)

1. NAME OF THE MEDICINAL PRODUCT

Erythrocin 500

2. QUALITATIVE AND QUANTITATIVE COMPOSITION

Erythromycin as erythromycin stearate 500 mg / tablet

3. PHARMACEUTICAL FORM

Film coated tablet

4. CLINICAL PARTICULARS

4.1 Therapeutic indications

For the prophylaxis and treatment of infections caused by erythromycin-sensitive organisms.

Erythromycin is highly effective in the treatment of a great variety of clinical infections such as:

1. Upper Respiratory Tract infections: tonsillitis, peritonsillar abscess, pharyngitis, laryngitis, sinusitis, secondary infections in influenza and common colds

2. Lower Respiratory Tract infections: tracheitis, acute and chronic bronchitis, pneumonia (lobar pneumonia, bronchopneumonia, primary atypical pneumonia), bronchiectasis, Legionnaire's disease

3. Ear infection: otitis media and otitis externa, mastoiditis

4. Oral infections: gingivitis, Vincent's angina

5. Eye infections: blepharitis

6. Skin and soft tissue infections: boils and carbuncles, paronychia, abscesses, pustular acne, impetigo, cellulitis, erysipelas

7. Gastrointestinal infections: cholecystitis, staphylococcal enterocolitis

8. Prophylaxis: pre- and post- operative trauma, burns, rheumatic fever, bacterial endocarditis in patients allergic to penicillin with congenital heart disease, or rheumatic or other acquired valvular heart disease when undergoing dental procedures or surgical procedures of the upper respiratory tract

9. Other infections: osteomyelitis, urethritis, gonorrhoea, syphilis, lymphogranuloma venereum, diphtheria, prostatitis, scarlet fever

4.2 Posology and method of administration

Adults and children over 8 years: 1-2g/day in divided doses. For severe infections up to 4g/day in divided doses.

Elderly: No special dosage recommendations

Children under 8 years: Erythroped suspension is recommended.

4.3 Contraindications

Known hypersensitivity to erythromycin. Erythromycin is contraindicated in patients taking astemizole, terfenadine, cisapride or pimozide.

Erythromycin is contraindicated with ergotamine and dihydroergotamine.

4.4 Special warnings and special precautions for use

Erythromycin is excreted principally by the liver, so caution should be exercised in administering the antibiotic to patients with impaired hepatic function or concomitantly receiving potentially hepatotoxic agents. Hepatic dysfunction including increased liver enzymes and/or cholestatic hepatitis, with or without jaundice, has been infrequently reported with erythromycin.

There have been reports suggesting erythromycin does not reach the foetus in adequate concentrations to prevent congenital syphilis. Infants born to women treated during pregnancy with oral erythromycin for early syphilis should be treated with an appropriate penicillin regimen.

There have been reports that erythromycin may aggravate the weakness of patients with myasthenia gravis.

Erythromycin interferes with the fluorometric determination of urinary catecholamines.

As with other broad spectrum antibiotics, pseudomembranous colitis has been reported rarely with erythromycin.

Rhabdomyolysis with or without renal impairment has been reported in seriously ill patients receiving erythromycin concomitantly with lovastatin.

4.5 Interaction with other medicinal products and other forms of Interaction

Concomitant use of erythromycin with terfenadine or astemizole is likely to result in an enhanced risk of cardiotoxicity with these drugs. The concomitant use of erythromycin with either astemizole or terfenadine is therefore contraindicated.

The metabolism of terfenadine and astemizole is significantly altered when either are taken concomitantly with erythromycin. Rare cases of serious cardiovascular events have been observed, including torsades de pointes, other ventricular arrhythmias and cardiac arrest. Death has been reported with the terfenadine / erythromycin combination.

Elevated cisapride levels have been reported in patients receiving erythromycin and cisapride concomitantly. This may result in QT prolongation and cardiac arrhythmias including ventricular trachycardia, ventricular fibrillation and Torsades de pointes. Similar effects have been observed with concomitant administration of pimozide and clarithromycin, another macrolide antibiotic.

Concurrent use of erythromycin and ergotamine or dihydroergotamine has been associated in some patients with acute ergot toxicity characterised by the rapid development of severe peripheral vasospasm and dysaesthesia.

Increases in serum concentrations of the following drugs metabolised by the cytochrome P450 system may occur when administered concurrently with erythromycin: alfentanil, astemizole, bromocriptine, carbamazepine, cyclosporin, digoxin, dihydroergotamine, disopyramide, ergotamine, hexobarbitone, midazolam, phenytoin, quinidine, tacrolimus, terfenadine, theophylline, triazolam, valproate, and warfarin. Appropriate monitoring should be undertaken and dosage should be adjusted as necessary.

Erythromycin has been reported to decrease the clearance of zopiclone and thus may increase the pharmacodynamic effects of this drug.

When oral erythromycin is given concurrently with theophylline, there is also a significant decrease in erythromycin serum concentrations. The decrease could result in subtherapeutic concentrations of erythromycin.

4.6 Pregnancy and lactation

There is no evidence of hazard from erythromycin in human pregnancy. It has been in widespread use for a number of years without apparent ill consequence. Animal studies have shown no hazard.

Erythromycin has been reported to cross the placental barrier in humans, but foetal plasma levels are generally low.

Erythromycin is excreted in breast milk, therefore, caution should be exercised when erythromycin is administered to a nursing mother.

4.7 Effects on ability to drive and use machines

None reported

4.8 Undesirable effects

Occasional side effects such as nausea, abdominal discomfort, vomiting and diarrhoea may be experienced. Reversible hearing loss associated with doses of erythromycin usually greater than 4g per day has been reported. Allergic reactions are rare and mild, although anaphylaxis has occurred. Skin reactions ranging from mild eruptions to erythema multiforme, Stevens-Johnson syndrome and toxic epidermal necrolysis have rarely been reported. There are no reports implicating erythromycin products with abnormal tooth development, and only rare reports of damage to the blood, kidneys or central nervous system.

Cardiac arrhythmias have been very rarely reported in patients receiving erythromycin therapy. There have been isolated reports of chest pain, dizziness and palpitations, however, a cause and effect relationship has not been established.

Symptoms of hepatitis, hepatic dysfunction and/or abnormal liver function test results may occur.

4.9 Overdose

Symptoms: hearing loss, severe nausea, vomiting and diarrhoea.

Treatment: gastric lavage, general supportive measures.

5. PHARMACOLOGICAL PROPERTIES

5.1 Pharmacodynamic properties

Erythromycin exerts its antimicrobial action by binding to the 50S ribosomal sub-unit of susceptible microorganisms and suppresses protein synthesis. Erythromycin is usually active against most strains of the following organisms both *in vitro* and in clinical infections:

Gram positive bacteria - *Listeria monocytogenes, Corynebacterium diphtheriae* (as an adjunct to antitoxin), Staphylococci *spp*, Streptococci *spp* (including Enterococci).

Gram negative bacteria - *Haemophilus influenzae, Neisseria meningitidis, Neisseria gonorrhoeae, Legionella pneumophila, Moraxella (Branhamella) catarrhalis, Bordetella pertussis*, Campylobacter spp.

Mycoplasma - *Mycoplasma pneumoniae, Ureaplasma urealyticum*.

Other organisms -*Treponema pallidum*, Chlamydia spp, Clostridia spp, L-forms, the agents causing trachoma and lymphogranuloma venereum.

Note: The majority of strains of *Haemophilus influenzae* are susceptible to the concentrations reached after ordinary doses.

5.2 Pharmacokinetic properties

None stated.

5.3 Preclinical safety data

There are no pre-clinical data of relevance to the prescriber which are additional to that already included in other sections of the SPC.

6. PHARMACEUTICAL PARTICULARS

6.1 List of excipients

Povidone, maize starch, magnesium hydroxide, polacrilin potassium, polyethylene glycol 8000, polyethylene glycol 400, hydroxypropyl methyl cellulose, sorbic acid.

6.2 Incompatibilities

None stated.

6.3 Shelf life

60 months.

6.4 Special precautions for storage

None stated.

6.5 Nature and contents of container

High density polyethylene bottle with urea cap with 100 tablets, securitainer or snap-secure container with 50, 100 or 1000 tablets. Blister packs containing 10, 14, 15, 28 or 56 tablets: PVC, heat sealed with 20 micron hard tamper aluminium foil.

6.6 Instructions for use and handling

Not applicable

7. MARKETING AUTHORISATION HOLDER

Abbott Laboratories Ltd., Queenborough, Kent. ME11 5EL.

8. MARKETING AUTHORISATION NUMBER(S)

PL 0037/5044R

9. DATE OF FIRST AUTHORISATION/RENEWAL OF THE AUTHORISATION

16/06/97

10. DATE OF REVISION OF THE TEXT

August 1997

Erythromid

(Abbott Laboratories Limited)

1. NAME OF THE MEDICINAL PRODUCT

Erythromid and Erythromycin Tablets BP

2. QUALITATIVE AND QUANTITATIVE COMPOSITION

Erythromycin BP 250 mg / tablet

3. PHARMACEUTICAL FORM

Enteric coated tablet

4. CLINICAL PARTICULARS

4.1 Therapeutic indications

For the prophylaxis and treatment of infections caused by erythromycin-sensitive organisms.

Erythromycin is highly effective in the treatment of a great variety of clinical infections such as:

1. Upper Respiratory Tract infections: tonsillitis, peritonsillar abscess, pharyngitis, laryngitis, sinusitis, secondary infections in influenza and common colds

2. Lower Respiratory Tract infections: tracheitis, acute and chronic bronchitis, pneumonia (lobar pneumonia, bronchopneumonia, primary atypical pneumonia), bronchiectasis, Legionnaire's disease

3. Ear infection: otitis media and otitis externa, mastoiditis

4. Oral infections: gingivitis, Vincent's angina

5. Eye infections: blepharitis

6. Skin and soft tissue infections: boils and carbuncles, paronychia, abscesses, pustular acne, impetigo, cellulitis, erysipelas

7. Gastrointestinal infections: cholecystitis, staphylococcal enterocolitis

8. Prophylaxis: pre- and post- operative trauma, burns, rheumatic fever

9. Other infections: osteomyelitis, urethritis, gonorrhoea, syphilis, lymphogranuloma venereum, diphtheria, prostatitis, scarlet fever

Note: Erythromycin has also proved to be of value in endocarditis and septicaemia, but in these conditions initial administration of erythromycin lactobionate by the intravenous route is advisable.

4.2 Posology and method of administration

Adults and older children: Usual oral dosage 1 tablet every four to six hours, increased to 4g per day in unusually severe infections.

4.3 Contraindications

Known hypersensitivity to erythromycin. Erythromycin is contraindicated in patients taking astemizole, terfenadine, cisapride or pimozide.

Erythromycin is contraindicated with ergotamine and dihydroergotamine.

4.4 Special warnings and special precautions for use

Erythromycin is excreted principally by the liver, so caution should be exercised in administering the antibiotic to patients with impaired hepatic function or concomitantly receiving potentially hepatotoxic agents. Hepatic dysfunction including increased liver enzymes and/or cholestatic hepatitis, with or without jaundice, has been infrequently reported with erythromycin.

There have been reports suggesting erythromycin does not reach the foetus in adequate concentrations to prevent congenital syphilis. Infants born to women treated during pregnancy with oral erythromycin for early syphilis should be treated with an appropriate penicillin regimen.

There have been reports that erythromycin may aggravate the weakness of patients with myasthenia gravis.

Erythromycin interferes with the fluorometric determination of urinary catecholamines.

As with other broad spectrum antibiotics, pseudomembranous colitis has been reported rarely with erythromycin.

Rhabdomyolysis with or without renal impairment has been reported in seriously ill patients receiving erythromycin concomitantly with lovastatin.

4.5 Interaction with other medicinal products and other forms of Interaction

Concomitant use of erythromycin with terfenadine or astemizole is likely to result in an enhanced risk of cardiotoxicity with these drugs. The concomitant use of erythromycin with either astemizole or terfenadine is therefore contraindicated.

The metabolism of terfenadine and astemizole is significantly altered when either are taken concomitantly with erythromycin. Rare cases of serious cardiovascular events have been observed, including torsades de pointes, other ventricular arrhythmias and cardiac arrest. Death has been reported with the terfenadine / erythromycin combination.

Elevated cisapride levels have been reported in patients receiving erythromycin and cisapride concomitantly. This may result in QT prolongation and cardiac arrhythmias including ventricular trachycardia, ventricular fibrillation and Torsades de pointes.

Similar effects have been observed with concomitant administration of pimozide and clarithromycin, another macrolide antibiotic.

Concurrent use of erythromycin and ergotamine or dihydroergotamine has been associated in some patients with acute ergot toxicity characterised by the rapid development of severe peripheral vasospasm and dysaesthesia.

Increases in serum concentrations of the following drugs metabolised by the cytochrome P450 system may occur when administered concurrently with erythromycin: alfentanil, astemizole, bromocriptine, carbamazepine, cyclosporin, digoxin, dihydroergotamine, disopyramide, ergotamine, hexobarbitone, midazolam, phenytoin, quinidine, tacrolimus, terfenadine, theophylline, triazolam, valproate, and warfarin. Appropriate monitoring should be undertaken and dosage should be adjusted as necessary.

Erythromycin has been reported to decrease the clearance of zopiclone and thus may increase the pharmacodynamic effects of this drug.

When oral erythromycin is given concurrently with theophylline, there is also a significant decrease in erythromycin serum concentrations. The decrease could result in subtherapeutic concentrations of erythromycin.

4.6 Pregnancy and lactation

There is no evidence of hazard from erythromycin in human pregnancy. It has been in widespread use for a number of years without apparent ill consequence. Animal studies have shown no hazard.

Erythromycin has been reported to cross the placental barrier in humans, but foetal plasma levels are generally low.

Erythromycin is excreted in breast milk, therefore, caution should be exercised when erythromycin is administered to a nursing mother.

4.7 Effects on ability to drive and use machines

None reported

4.8 Undesirable effects

Occasional side effects such as nausea, abdominal discomfort, vomiting and diarrhoea may be experienced. Reversible hearing loss associated with doses of erythromycin usually greater than 4g per day has been reported. Allergic reactions are rare and mild, although anaphylaxis has occurred. Skin reactions ranging from mild eruptions to erythema multiforme, Stevens-Johnson syndrome and toxic epidermal necrolysis have rarely been reported. There are no reports implicating erythromycin products with abnormal tooth development, and only rare reports of damage to the blood, kidneys or central nervous system.

Cardiac arrhythmias have been very rarely reported in patients receiving erythromycin therapy. There have been isolated reports of chest pain, dizziness and palpitations, however, a cause and effect relationship has not been established.

Symptoms of hepatitis, hepatic dysfunction and/or abnormal liver function test results may occur.

4.9 Overdose

Symptoms: hearing loss, severe nausea, vomiting and diarrhoea.

Treatment: gastric lavage, general supportive measures.

5. PHARMACOLOGICAL PROPERTIES

5.1 Pharmacodynamic properties

Erythromycin exerts its antimicrobial action by binding to the 50S ribosomal sub-unit of susceptible microorganisms and suppresses protein synthesis. Erythromycin is usually active against most strains of the following organisms both *in vitro* and in clinical infections:

Gram positive bacteria - *Listeria monocytogenes, Corynebacterium diphtheriae* (as an adjunct to antitoxin), Staphylococci *spp*, Streptococci *spp* (including Enterococci).

Gram negative bacteria - *Haemophilus influenzae, Neisseria meningitidis, Neisseria gonorrhoeae, Legionella pneumophila, Moraxella (Branhamella) catarrhalis, Bordetella pertussis*, Campylobacter spp.

Mycoplasma - *Mycoplasma pneumoniae, Ureaplasma urealyticum*.

Other organisms - *Treponema pallidum*, Chlamydia spp, Clostridia spp, L-forms, the agents causing trachoma and lymphogranuloma venereum.

Note: The majority of strains of *Haemophilus influenzae* are susceptible to the concentrations reached after ordinary doses.

5.2 Pharmacokinetic properties

Absorption and Fate

Erythromycin is adversely affected by gastric acid. For this reason erythromycin tablets are enteric coated.

It is absorbed from the small intestine. It is widely distributed throughout body tissues. Little metabolism occurs and only about 5% is eliminated in the urine. It is excreted principally by the liver.

5.3 Preclinical safety data

There are no pre-clinical data of relevance to the prescriber which are additional to that already included in other sections of the SPC.

6. PHARMACEUTICAL PARTICULARS

6.1 List of excipients

Sodium carboxymethylcellulose, microcrystalline cellulose, povidone, polacrilin potassium, talc, magnesium stearate, hypromellose, hydroxypropyl cellulose, proylene glycol, sorbitan oleate, methacrylic acid - ethyl acrylate copolymer, titanium dioxide, triethyl citrate, antifoam emulsion.

6.2 Incompatibilities

None Stated.

6.3 Shelf life

24 months.

6.4 Special precautions for storage

Protect from light, store below 25°C.

6.5 Nature and contents of container

Glass bottles, type III EP amber glass with a urea outer / aluminium liner cap, of 100 tablets.

Polypropylene bottles with either an LDPE or an HDPE closure, of 50, 100, 500 and 1000 tablets.

Blisters, clear or opaque PVC/PVDC 300μm / 60gsm film and 20μm hard tamper aluminium foil with 5 - 8gsm PVC/PVDC compatible heat seal lacquer on one side, of 28, 40 and 56 tablets.

6.6 Instructions for use and handling

Not applicable.

7. MARKETING AUTHORISATION HOLDER

Abbott Laboratories Ltd., Queenborough, Kent. ME11 5EL.

8. MARKETING AUTHORISATION NUMBER(S)

0037/5019R

9. DATE OF FIRST AUTHORISATION/RENEWAL OF THE AUTHORISATION

14/12/93

10. DATE OF REVISION OF THE TEXT

July 1997

Erythromycin Lactobionate I.V.

(Abbott Laboratories Limited)

1. NAME OF THE MEDICINAL PRODUCT

Erythrocin IV Lactobionate or Erythromycin Lactobionate

2. QUALITATIVE AND QUANTITATIVE COMPOSITION

Active: Erythromycin as Erythromycin lactobionate 1 g / vial

3. PHARMACEUTICAL FORM

Lyophilisate

4. CLINICAL PARTICULARS

4.1 Therapeutic indications

Erythromycin lactobionate is indicated in severe and immunocompromised cases of infections caused by sensitive organisms where high blood levels are required at the earliest opportunity or when the oral route is compromised.

1. Upper Respiratory Tract infections: tonsillitis, peritonsillar abscess, pharyngitis, laryngitis, sinusitis, secondary infections in influenza and common colds

2. Lower Respiratory Tract infections: tracheitis, acute and chronic bronchitis, pneumonia (lobar pneumonia, bronchopneumonia, primary atypical pneumonia), bronchiectasis, Legionnaire's disease

3. Ear infection: otitis media and otitis externa, mastoiditis

4. Oral infections: gingivitis, Vincent's angina

5. Eye infections: blepharitis

6. Skin and soft tissue infections: boils and carbuncles, paronychia, abscesses, pustular acne, impetigo, cellulitis, erysipelas

7. Gastrointestinal infections: cholecystitis, staphylococcal enterocolitis

8. Prophylaxis: peri-operative secondary infection prophylaxis, severe trauma and burns secondary infection prophylaxis, endocarditis prophylaxis (dental procedures)

9. Septicaemia

10. Endocarditis

11. Other infections: osteomyelitis, urethritis, gonorrhoea, syphilis, lymphogranuloma venereum, diphtheria, prostatitis, scarlet fever

4.2 Posology and method of administration

Adults: severe and immunocompromised infections, 50mg/kg/day, preferably by continuous infusion (equivalent to 4g per day for adults).

Mild to moderate infections (oral route compromised): 25mg/kg/day.

Newborn infant (birth to 1 month): 10-15mg/kg 3 times daily.

Children: 12.5mg/kg 4 times daily. Doses can be doubled in severe infections.

Elderly: No special dosage recommendations.

Recommended Administration

Continuous intravenous infusion with an erythromycin concentration of 1mg/ml (0.1% solution) is recommended. The infusion should be completed within 8 hours of preparation to ensure potency.

If required, solution strengths up to 5mg/ml (0.5% solution) may be used, but should not be exceeded. Higher concentrations may result in pain along the vein.

Bolus injection is not recommended.

However, if it is decided to administer the daily dose as 4 doses once every 6 hours, then the erythromycin concentration should not exceed 5mg/ml and the time of each infusion should be between 20 and 60 minutes.

4.3 Contraindications

Known hypersensitivity to erythromycin. Erythromycin is contraindicated in patients taking astemizole, terfenadine, cisapride or pimozide.

Erythromycin is contraindicated with ergotamine and dihydroergotamine.

4.4 Special warnings and special precautions for use

Erythromycin is excreted principally by the liver, so caution should be exercised in administering the antibiotic to patients with impaired hepatic function or concomitantly receiving potentially hepatotoxic agents. Hepatic dysfunction including increased liver enzymes and/or cholestatic hepatitis, with or without jaundice, has been infrequently reported with erythromycin.

There have been reports suggesting erythromycin does not reach the foetus in adequate concentrations to prevent congenital syphilis. Infants born to women treated during pregnancy with oral erythromycin for early syphilis should be treated with an appropriate penicillin regimen.

There have been reports that erythromycin may aggravate the weakness of patients with myasthenia gravis.

Erythromycin interferes with the fluorometric determination of urinary catecholamines.

As with other broad spectrum antibiotics, pseudomembranous colitis has been reported rarely with erythromycin.

Rhabdomyolysis with or without renal impairment has been reported in seriously ill patients receiving erythromycin concomitantly with lovastatin.

Prolonged QTc interval and ventricular arrhythmias have rarely been reported in patients receiving erythromycin IV.

4.5 Interaction with other medicinal products and other forms of Interaction

Concomitant use of erythromycin with terfenadine or astemizole is likely to result in an enhanced risk of cardiotoxicity with these drugs. The concomitant use of erythromycin with either astemizole or terfenadine is therefore contraindicated.

The metabolism of terfenadine and astemizole is significantly altered when either are taken concomitantly with erythromycin. Rare cases of serious cardiovascular events have been observed, including torsades de pointes, other ventricular arrhythmias and cardiac arrest. Death has been reported with the terfenadine / erythromycin combination.

Elevated cisapride levels have been reported in patients receiving erythromycin and cisapride concomitantly. This may result in QT prolongation and cardiac arrhythmias including ventricular trachycardia, ventricular fibrillation and Torsades de pointes. Similar effects have been observed with concomitant administration of pimozide and clarithromycin, another macrolide antibiotic.

Mizolastine has a weak potential to prolong QT interval and has not been associated with arrhythmias, however, the metabolism of mizolastine is inhibited by erythromycin, therefore concomitant use should be avoided.

Concurrent use of erythromycin and ergotamine or dihydroergotamine has been associated in some patients with acute ergot toxicity characterised by the rapid development of severe peripheral vasospasm and dysaesthesia.

Increases in serum concentrations of the following drugs metabolised by the cytochrome P450 system may occur when administered concurrently with erythromycin: alfentanil, astemizole, bromocriptine, carbamazepine, cyclosporin, digoxin, dihydroergotamine, disopyramide, ergotamine, hexobarbitone, midazolam, phenytoin, quinidine, tacrolimus, terfenadine, theophylline, triazolam, valproate, acenocoumarol, rifabutin, and warfarin. Appropriate monitoring should be undertaken and dosage should be adjusted as necessary.

Erythromycin has been reported to decrease the clearance of zopiclone and thus may increase the pharmacodynamic effects of this drug.

When oral erythromycin is given concurrently with theophylline, there is also a significant decrease in erythromycin serum concentrations. The decrease could result in subtherapeutic concentrations of erythromycin.

4.6 Pregnancy and lactation

There is no evidence of hazard from erythromycin in human pregnancy. It has been in widespread use for a number of years without apparent ill consequence. Animal studies have shown no hazard.

Erythromycin has been reported to cross the placental barrier in humans, but foetal plasma levels are generally low.

Erythromycin is excreted in breast milk, therefore, caution should be exercised when erythromycin is administered to a nursing mother.

4.7 Effects on ability to drive and use machines

None reported.

4.8 Undesirable effects

Occasional side effects such as nausea, abdominal discomfort, vomiting and diarrhoea may be experienced. Reversible hearing loss associated with doses of erythromycin usually greater than 4g per day has been reported. Allergic reactions are rare and mild, although anaphylaxis has occurred. Skin reactions ranging from mild eruptions to erythema multiforme, Stevens-Johnson syndrome and toxic epidermal necrolysis have rarely been reported. There are no reports implicating erythromycin products with abnormal tooth development, and only rare reports of damage to the blood, kidneys or central nervous system.

Cardiac arrhythmias have been very rarely reported in patients receiving erythromycin therapy. There have been isolated reports of chest pain, dizziness and palpitations, however, a cause and effect relationship has not been established.

Symptoms of hepatitis, hepatic dysfunction and/or abnormal liver function test results may occur.

4.9 Overdose

Symptoms: hearing loss, severe nausea, vomiting and diarrhoea.

Treatment: gastric lavage, general supportive measures.

5. PHARMACOLOGICAL PROPERTIES

5.1 Pharmacodynamic properties

Erythromycin exerts its antimicrobial action by binding to the 50S ribosomal sub-unit of susceptible microorganisms and suppresses protein synthesis. Erythromycin is usually active against most strains of the following organisms both in vitro and in clinical infections:

Gram positive bacteria - *Listeria monocytogenes, Corynebacterium diphtheriae* (as an adjunct to antitoxin), Staphylococci spp, Streptococci spp (including Enterococci).

Gram negative bacteria - *Haemophilus influenzae, Neisseria meningitidis, Neisseria gonorrhoeae, Legionella pneumophila, Moraxella (Branhamella) catarrhalis, Bordetella pertussis*, Campylobacter spp.

Mycoplasma - *Mycoplasma pneumoniae, Ureaplasma urealyticum*.

Other organisms - *Treponema pallidum*, Chlamydia spp, Clostridia spp, L-forms, the agents causing trachoma and lymphogranuloma venereum.

Note: The majority of strains of *Haemophilus influenzae* are susceptible to the concentrations reached after ordinary doses.

5.2 Pharmacokinetic properties

Following intravenous infusion, erythromycin is widely distributed throughout body tissues, including lung tissues.

5.3 Preclinical safety data

There are no pre-clinical data of relevance to the prescriber which are additional to that already included in other sections of the SPC.

6. PHARMACEUTICAL PARTICULARS

6.1 List of excipients

None.

6.2 Incompatibilities

None Stated.

6.3 Shelf life

36 months unopened, use within 1 day of opening.

6.4 Special precautions for storage

Once reconstituted, store in a refrigerator between 2° C and 8° C and use within 24 hours.

6.5 Nature and contents of container

Glass vial with rubber closure.

6.6 Instructions for use and handling

Continuous intravenous infusion with an erythromycin concentration of 1mg/ml (0.1% solution) is recommended. The infusion should be completed within 8 hours of preparation to ensure potency.

If required, solution strengths up to 5mg/ml (0.5% solution) may be used, but should not be exceeded. Higher concentrations may result in pain along the vein.

Bolus injection is not recommended.

7. MARKETING AUTHORISATION HOLDER

Abbott Laboratories Ltd

Queenborough

Kent

ME11 5EL

8. MARKETING AUTHORISATION NUMBER(S)

0037/0092

9. DATE OF FIRST AUTHORISATION/RENEWAL OF THE AUTHORISATION

26/6/79 / 30/01/95

10. DATE OF REVISION OF THE TEXT

January 2001

Erythroped A

(Abbott Laboratories Limited)

1. NAME OF THE MEDICINAL PRODUCT

Erythroped A Tablets

2. QUALITATIVE AND QUANTITATIVE COMPOSITION

Erythromycin as Erythromycin Ethylsuccinate Ph.Eur. 500mg/tablet

3. PHARMACEUTICAL FORM

Tablets

4. CLINICAL PARTICULARS

4.1 Therapeutic indications

For the prophylaxis and treatment of infections caused by erythromycin-sensitive organisms.

Erythromycin is highly effective in the treatment of a great variety of clinical infections such as:

1. Upper Respiratory Tract infections: tonsillitis, peritonsillar abscess, pharyngitis, laryngitis, sinusitis, secondary infections in influenza and common colds

2. Lower Respiratory Tract infections: tracheitis, acute and chronic bronchitis, pneumonia (lobar pneumonia, bronchopneumonia, primary atypical pneumonia), bronchiectasis, Legionnaire's disease

3. Ear infection: otitis media and otitis externa, mastoiditis

4. Oral infections: gingivitis, Vincent's angina

5. Eye infections: blepharitis

6. Skin and soft tissue infections: boils and carbuncles, paronychia, abscesses, pustular acne, impetigo, cellulitis, erysipelas

7. Gastrointestinal infections: cholecystitis, staphylococcal enterocolitis

8. Prophylaxis: pre- and post- operative trauma, burns, rheumatic fever

9. Other infections: osteomyelitis, urethritis, gonorrhoea, syphilis, lymphogranuloma venereum, diphtheria, prostatitis, scarlet fever

4.2 Posology and method of administration

For oral administration.

Adults and children over 8 years: For mild to moderate infections 2g daily in divided doses. Up to 4g daily in severe infections.

Elderly: No special dosage recommendations.

Note: For younger children, infants and babies, Erythroped, erythromycin ethylsuccinate suspensions, are normally recommended. The recommended dose for children age 2-8, for mild to moderate infections, is 1g daily in divided doses. The recommended dose for infants and babies, for mild to moderate infections, is 500 mg daily in divided doses. For severe infections doses may be doubled.

4.3 Contraindications

Known hypersensitivity to erythromycin. Erythromycin is contraindicated in patients taking astemizole, terfenadine, cisapride or pimozide.

Erythromycin is contraindicated with ergotamine and dihydroergotamine.

4.4 Special warnings and special precautions for use

Erythromycin is excreted principally by the liver, so caution should be exercised in administering the antibiotic to patients with impaired hepatic function or concomitantly receiving potentially hepatotoxic agents. Hepatic dysfunction including increased liver enzymes and/or cholestatic hepatitis, with or without jaundice, has been infrequently reported with erythromycin.

There have been reports suggesting erythromycin does not reach the foetus in adequate concentrations to prevent congenital syphilis. Infants born to women treated during pregnancy with oral erythromycin for early syphilis should be treated with an appropriate penicillin regimen.

There have been reports that erythromycin may aggravate the weakness of patients with myasthenia gravis.

Erythromycin interferes with the fluorometric determination of urinary catecholamines.

As with other broad spectrum antibiotics, pseudomembranous colitis has been reported rarely with erythromycin.

Rhabdomyolysis with or without renal impairment has been reported in seriously ill patients receiving erythromycin concomitantly with lovastatin.

4.5 Interaction with other medicinal products and other forms of Interaction

Concomitant use of erythromycin with terfenadine or astemizole is likely to result in an enhanced risk of cardiotoxicity with these drugs. The concomitant use of erythromycin with either astemizole or terfenadine is therefore contraindicated.

The metabolism of terfenadine and astemizole is significantly altered when either are taken concomitantly with erythromycin. Rare cases of serious cardiovascular events have been observed, including Torsades de pointes, other ventricular arrhythmias and cardiac arrest. Death has been reported with the terfenadine / erythromycin combination.

Mizolastine has a weak potential to prolong QT interval and has not been associated with arrhythmias, however the metabolism of mizolastine is inhibited by erythromycin, therefore concomitant use should be avoided.

Elevated cisapride levels have been reported in patients receiving erythromycin and cisapride concomitantly. This may result in QT prolongation and cardiac arrhythmias including ventricular tachycardia, ventricular fibrillation and Torsades de pointes. Similar effects have been observed with concomitant administration of pimozide and clarithromycin, another macrolide antibiotic.

Concurrent use of erythromycin and ergotamine or dihydroergotamine has been associated in some patients with acute ergot toxicity characterised by the rapid development of severe peripheral vasospasm and dysaesthesia.

Increases in serum concentrations of the following drugs metabolised by the cytochrome P450 system may occur when administered concurrently with erythromycin: acenocoumarol, alfentanil, astemizole, bromocriptine, carbamazepine, cyclosporin, digoxin, dihydroergotamine, disopyramide, ergotamine, hexobarbitone, midazolam, phenytoin, quinidine, rifabutin, tacrolimus, terfenadine, theophylline, triazolam, valproate, and warfarin. Appropriate monitoring should be undertaken and dosage should be adjusted as necessary.

Erythromycin has been reported to decrease the clearance of zopiclone and thus may increase the pharmacodynamic effects of this drug.

When oral erythromycin is given concurrently with theophylline, there is also a significant decrease in erythromycin serum concentrations. The decrease could result in subtherapeutic concentrations of erythromycin

4.6 Pregnancy and lactation

There is no evidence of hazard from erythromycin in human pregnancy. It has been in widespread use for a number of years without apparent ill consequence. Animal studies have shown no hazard.

Erythromycin has been reported to cross the placental barrier in humans, but foetal plasma levels are generally low.

Erythromycin is excreted in breast milk, therefore, caution should be exercised when erythromycin is administered to a nursing mother.

4.7 Effects on ability to drive and use machines

None stated

4.8 Undesirable effects

Occasional side effects such as nausea, abdominal discomfort, vomiting and diarrhoea may be experienced. Reversible hearing loss associated with doses of erythromycin usually greater than 4g per day has been reported. Allergic reactions are rare and mild, although anaphylaxis has occurred. Skin reactions ranging from mild eruptions to erythema multiforme, Stevens-Johnson syndrome and toxic epidermal necrolysis have rarely been reported. There are no reports implicating erythromycin products with abnormal tooth development, and only rare reports of damage to the blood, kidneys or central nervous system.

Cardiac arrhythmias have been very rarely reported in patients receiving erythromycin therapy. There have been isolated reports of chest pain, dizziness and palpitations, however, a cause and effect relationship has not been established.

Symptoms of hepatitis, hepatic dysfunction and/or abnormal liver function test results may occur.

4.9 Overdose

Symptoms: hearing loss, severe nausea, vomiting and diarrhoea.

Treatment: gastric lavage, general supportive measures

5. PHARMACOLOGICAL PROPERTIES

5.1 Pharmacodynamic properties

Erythromycin exerts its antimicrobial action by binding to the 50S ribosomal sub-unit of susceptible microorganisms and suppresses protein synthesis. Erythromycin is usually active against most strains of the following organisms both *in vitro* and in clinical infections:

Gram positive bacteria - *Listeria monocytogenes, Corynebacterium diphtheriae* (as an adjunct to antitoxin), Staphylococci spp, Streptococci spp (including Enterococci).

Gram negative bacteria - *Haemophilus influenzae, Neisseria meningitidis, Neisseria gonorrhoeae, Legionella pneumophila, Moraxella (Branhamella) catarrhalis, Bordetella pertussis*, Campylobacter spp.

Mycoplasma - *Mycoplasma pneumoniae, Ureaplasma urealyticum*.

Other organisms - Treponema pallidum, Clostridia spp, Chlamydia spp, L-forms, the agents causing trachoma and lymphogranuloma venereum.

Note: The majority of strains of *Haemophilus influenzae* are susceptible to the concentrations reached after ordinary doses.

5.2 Pharmacokinetic properties

Peak blood levels normally occur within 1 hour of dosing of erythromycin ethylsuccinate granules. The elimination half life is approximately 2 hours. Doses may be administered 2, 3 or 4 times a day.

Erythromycin ethylsuccinate is less susceptible than erythromycin to the adverse effect of gastric acid. It is absorbed from the small intestine. It is widely distributed throughout body tissues. Little metabolism occurs and only about 5% is excreted in the urine. It is excreted principally by the liver.

5.3 Preclinical safety data

There are no pre-clinical data of relevance to the prescriber which are additional to that already included in other sections of the SPC.

6. PHARMACEUTICAL PARTICULARS

6.1 List of excipients

Calcium hydrogen phosphate, sodium starch glycollate, starch maize, povidone, magnesium stearate, hydroxypropyl methylcellulose, polyethylene glycol, titanium dioxide, quinoline yellow(E104), sorbic acid.

6.2 Incompatibilities

None stated.

6.3 Shelf life

24 months

6.4 Special precautions for storage

None

6.5 Nature and contents of container

Polypropylene bottles of 50, 100 or 500 tablets.

Blister: PVC/aluminium of 4 or 28 tablets.

6.6 Instructions for use and handling

Not applicable

7. MARKETING AUTHORISATION HOLDER

Abbott Laboratories Ltd

Queenborough

Kent

ME11 5EL

8. MARKETING AUTHORISATION NUMBER(S)

0037/0137

9. DATE OF FIRST AUTHORISATION/RENEWAL OF THE AUTHORISATION

19/05/95

10. DATE OF REVISION OF THE TEXT

June 2000

Erythroped Forte SF

(Abbott Laboratories Limited)

1. NAME OF THE MEDICINAL PRODUCT

Erythroped Forte SF

Erythromycin Ethylsuccinate SF 500mg/5ml

Erythromycin SF 500mg/5ml

Erythromycin Suspension 500mg/5ml SF

Erythromycin Ethylsuccinate SF Suspension 500mg/5ml

2. QUALITATIVE AND QUANTITATIVE COMPOSITION

Active: Erythromycin as Erythromycin Ethylsuccinate 500 mg / 5 ml

3. PHARMACEUTICAL FORM

Granules for reconstitution

4. CLINICAL PARTICULARS

4.1 Therapeutic indications

For the prophylaxis and treatment of infections caused by erythromycin-sensitive organisms.

Erythromycin is highly effective in the treatment of a great variety of clinical infections such as:

1. Upper Respiratory Tract infections: tonsillitis, peritonsillar abscess, pharyngitis, laryngitis, sinusitis, secondary infections in influenza and common colds

2. Lower Respiratory Tract infections: tracheitis, acute and chronic bronchitis, pneumonia (lobar pneumonia, bronchopneumonia, primary atypical pneumonia), bronchiectasis, Legionnaire's disease

3. Ear infection: otitis media and otitis externa, mastoiditis

4. Oral infections: gingivitis, Vincent's angina

5. Eye infections: blepharitis

6. Skin and soft tissue infections: boils and carbuncles, paronychia, abscesses, pustular acne, impetigo, cellulitis, erysipelas

7. Gastrointestinal infections: cholecystitis, staphylococcal enterocolitis

8. Prophylaxis: pre- and post- operative trauma, burns, rheumatic fever

9. Other infections: osteomyelitis, urethritis, gonorrhoea, syphilis, lymphogranuloma venereum, diphtheria, prostatitis, scarlet fever

Note: Erythromycin has also proved to be of value in endocarditis and septicaemia, but in these conditions initial administration of erythromycin lactobionate by the intravenous route is advisable.

4.2 Posology and method of administration

Adults and children over 8 years: 2g/day in divided doses. For severe infections up to 4g/day in divided doses.

Children 2 - 8 years: 30 mg/kg/day in divided doses. For severe infections up to 50 mg/kg/day in divided doses. Normal dose: 250mg four times a day or 500mg twice daily.

Children up to 2 years: 30 mg/kg/day in divided doses. For severe infections up to 50 mg/kg/day in divided doses. Normal dose: 125mg four times a day or 250mg twice daily.

Presentations are available for adults and children over 8 years, children aged 2-8 years, and for children under 2 years.

4.3 Contraindications
Known hypersensitivity to erythromycin. Erythromycin is contraindicated in patients taking astemizole, terfenadine, cisapride or pimozide.

Erythromycin is contraindicated with ergotamine and dihydroergotamine.

4.4 Special warnings and special precautions for use
Erythromycin is excreted principally by the liver, so caution should be exercised in administering the antibiotic to patients with impaired hepatic function or concomitantly receiving potentially hepatotoxic agents. Hepatic dysfunction including increased liver enzymes and/or cholestatic hepatitis, with or without jaundice, has been infrequently reported with erythromycin.

There have been reports suggesting erythromycin does not reach the foetus in adequate concentrations to prevent congenital syphilis. Infants born to women treated during pregnancy with oral erythromycin for early syphilis should be treated with an appropriate penicillin regimen.

There have been reports that erythromycin may aggravate the weakness of patients with myasthenia gravis.

Erythromycin interferes with the fluorometric determination of urinary catecholamines.

As with other broad spectrum antibiotics, pseudomembranous colitis has been reported rarely with erythromycin.

Rhabdomyolysis with or without renal impairment has been reported in seriously ill patients receiving erythromycin concomitantly with lovastatin.

4.5 Interaction with other medicinal products and other forms of Interaction
Concomitant use of erythromycin with terfenadine or astemizole is likely to result in an enhanced risk of cardiotoxicity with these drugs. The concomitant use of erythromycin with either astemizole or terfenadine is therefore contraindicated.

The metabolism of terfenadine and astemizole is significantly altered when either are taken concomitantly with erythromycin. Rare cases of serious cardiovascular events have been observed, including torsades de pointes, other ventricular arrhythmias and cardiac arrest. Death has been reported with the terfenadine / erythromycin combination.

Elevated cisapride levels have been reported in patients receiving erythromycin and cisapride concomitantly. This may result in QT prolongation and cardiac arrhythmias including ventricular trachycardia, ventricular fibrillation and Torsades de pointes. Similar effects have been observed with concomitant administration of pimozide and clarithromycin, another macrolide antibiotic.

Concurrent use of erythromycin and ergotamine or dihydroergotamine has been associated in some patients with acute ergot toxicity characterised by the rapid development of severe peripheral vasospasm and dysaesthesia.

Increases in serum concentrations of the following drugs metabolised by the cytochrome P450 system may occur when administered concurrently with erythromycin: alfentanil, astemizole, bromocriptine, carbamazepine, cyclosporin, digoxin, dihydroergotamine, disopyramide, ergotamine, hexobarbitone, midazolam, phenytoin, quinidine, tacrolimus, terfenadine, theophylline, triazolam, valproate, and warfarin. Appropriate monitoring should be undertaken and dosage should be adjusted as necessary.

Erythromycin has been reported to decrease the clearance of zopiclone and thus may increase the pharmacodynamic effects of this drug.

When oral erythromycin is given concurrently with theophylline, there is also a significant decrease in erythromycin serum concentrations. The decrease could result in subtherapeutic concentrations of erythromycin.

4.6 Pregnancy and lactation
There is no evidence of hazard from erythromycin in human pregnancy. It has been in widespread use for a number of years without apparent ill consequence. Animal studies have shown no hazard.

Erythromycin has been reported to cross the placental barrier in humans, but foetal plasma levels are generally low.

Erythromycin is excreted in breast milk, therefore, caution should be exercised when erythromycin is administered to a nursing mother.

4.7 Effects on ability to drive and use machines
None reported

4.8 Undesirable effects
Occasional side effects such as nausea, abdominal discomfort, vomiting and diarrhoea may be experienced. Reversible hearing loss associated with doses of erythromycin usually greater than 4g per day has been reported. Allergic reactions are rare and mild, although anaphylaxis has occurred. Skin reactions ranging from mild eruptions to erythema multiforme, Stevens-Johnson syndrome and toxic epidermal necrolysis have rarely been reported. There are no reports implicating erythromycin products with abnormal tooth development, and only rare reports of damage to the blood, kidneys or central nervous system.

Cardiac arrhythmias have been very rarely reported in patients receiving erythromycin therapy. There have been isolated reports of chest pain, dizziness and palpitations, however, a cause and effect relationship has not been established.

Symptoms of hepatitis, hepatic dysfunction and/or abnormal liver function test results may occur.

4.9 Overdose
Symptoms: hearing loss, severe nausea, vomiting and diarrhoea.

Treatment: gastric lavage, general supportive measures.

5. PHARMACOLOGICAL PROPERTIES

5.1 Pharmacodynamic properties
Erythromycin exerts its antimicrobial action by binding to the 50S ribosomal sub-unit of susceptible microorganisms and suppresses protein synthesis. Erythromycin is usually active against most strains of the following organisms both *in vitro* and in clinical infections:

Gram positive bacteria - *Listeria monocytogenes, Corynebacterium diphtheriae* (as an adjunct to antitoxin), Staphylococci *spp*, Streptococci *spp* (including Enterococci).

Gram negative bacteria - *Haemophilus influenzae, Neisseria meningitidis, Neisseria gonorrhoeae, Legionella pneumophila, Moraxella (Branhamella) catarrhalis, Bordetella pertussis*, Campylobacter spp.

Mycoplasma - *Mycoplasma pneumoniae, Ureaplasma urealyticum*.

Other organisms - *Treponema pallidum*, Chlamydia spp, Clostridia spp, L-forms, the agents causing trachoma and lymphogranuloma venereum.

Note: The majority of strains of *Haemophilus influenzae* are susceptible to the concentrations reached after ordinary doses.

5.2 Pharmacokinetic properties
Peak blood levels normally occur within 1 hour of dosing of erythromycin ethylsuccinate granules. The elimination half life is approximately 2 hours. Doses may be administered 2, 3 or 4 times a day.

Erythromycin ethylsuccinate is less susceptible than erythromycin to the adverse effect of gastric acid. It is absorbed from the small intestine. It is widely distributed throughout body tissues. Little metabolism occurs and only about 5% is excreted in the urine. It is excreted principally by the liver.

5.3 Preclinical safety data
There are no pre-clinical data of relevance to the prescriber which are additional to that already included in other sections of the SPC.

6. PHARMACEUTICAL PARTICULARS

6.1 List of excipients
Sorbitol, xanthan gum, sodium citrate, surfactant poloxamer 188, acesulfame (K), sodium saccharin, purified water, sodium methylhydroxybenzoate, sodium propylhydroxybenzoate, colloidal silicon dioxide, imitation banana flavour entrapped No.2, entrapped artificial cream.

6.2 Incompatibilities
None stated.

6.3 Shelf life
24 months. Once reconstituted, Erythroped Forte SF should be used with 7 days.

6.4 Special precautions for storage
None

6.5 Nature and contents of container
High density polyethylene bottles, 100ml or 140ml, with polypropylene cap which may be a child resistant cap.

6.6 Instructions for use and handling
Not applicable

7. MARKETING AUTHORISATION HOLDER
Abbott Laboratories Ltd, Queenborough, Kent, ME11 5EL.

8. MARKETING AUTHORISATION NUMBER(S)
0037/0225

9. DATE OF FIRST AUTHORISATION/RENEWAL OF THE AUTHORISATION
25/03/97

10. DATE OF REVISION OF THE TEXT
August 1998

Erythroped PI SF

(Abbott Laboratories Limited)

1. NAME OF THE MEDICINAL PRODUCT
Erythroped PI SF

Erythromycin Ethylsuccinate SF 125mg/5ml

Erythromycin SF 125mg/5ml

Erythromycin Suspension 125mg/5ml SF

Erythromycin Ethylsuccinate SF Suspension 125mg/5ml

2. QUALITATIVE AND QUANTITATIVE COMPOSITION
Active: Erythromycin as Erythromycin Ethylsuccinate 125 mg / 5 ml

3. PHARMACEUTICAL FORM
Granules for reconstitution

4. CLINICAL PARTICULARS

4.1 Therapeutic indications
For the prophylaxis and treatment of infections caused by erythromycin-sensitive organisms.

Erythromycin is highly effective in the treatment of a great variety of clinical infections such as:

1. Upper Respiratory Tract infections: tonsillitis, peritonsillar abscess, pharyngitis, laryngitis, sinusitis, secondary infections in influenza and common colds

2. Lower Respiratory Tract infections: tracheitis, acute and chronic bronchitis, pneumonia (lobar pneumonia, bronchopneumonia, primary atypical pneumonia), bronchiectasis, Legionnaire's disease

3. Ear infection: otitis media and otitis externa, mastoiditis

4. Oral infections: gingivitis, Vincent's angina

5. Eye infections: blepharitis

6. Skin and soft tissue infections: boils and carbuncles, paronychia, abscesses, pustular acne, impetigo, cellulitis, erysipelas

7. Gastrointestinal infections: cholecystitis, staphylococcal enterocolitis

8. Prophylaxis: pre- and post- operative trauma, burns, rheumatic fever

9. Other infections: osteomyelitis, urethritis, gonorrhoea, syphilis, lymphogranuloma venereum, diphtheria, prostatitis, scarlet fever

Note: Erythromycin has also proved to be of value in endocarditis and septicaemia, but in these conditions initial administration of erythromycin lactobionate by the intravenous route is advisable.

4.2 Posology and method of administration
Adults and children over 8 years: 2g/day in divided doses. For severe infections up to 4g/day in divided doses.

Children 2 - 8 years: 30 mg/kg/day in divided doses. For severe infections up to 50 mg/kg/day in divided doses. Normal dose: 250mg four times a day or 500mg twice daily.

Children up to 2 years: 30 mg/kg/day in divided doses. For severe infections up to 50 mg/kg/day in divided doses. Normal dose: 125mg four times a day or 250mg twice daily.

Presentations are available for adults and children over 8 years, children aged 2-8 years, and for children under 2 years.

4.3 Contraindications
Known hypersensitivity to erythromycin. Erythromycin is contraindicated in patients taking astemizole, terfenadine, cisapride or pimozide.

Erythromycin is contraindicated with ergotamine and dihydroergotamine.

4.4 Special warnings and special precautions for use
Erythromycin is excreted principally by the liver, so caution should be exercised in administering the antibiotic to patients with impaired hepatic function or concomitantly receiving potentially hepatotoxic agents. Hepatic dysfunction including increased liver enzymes and/or cholestatic hepatitis, with or without jaundice, has been infrequently reported with erythromycin.

There have been reports suggesting erythromycin does not reach the foetus in adequate concentrations to prevent congenital syphilis. Infants born to women treated during pregnancy with oral erythromycin for early syphilis should be treated with an appropriate penicillin regimen.

There have been reports that erythromycin may aggravate the weakness of patients with myasthenia gravis.

Erythromycin interferes with the fluorometric determination of urinary catecholamines.

As with other broad spectrum antibiotics, pseudomembranous colitis has been reported rarely with erythromycin.

Rhabdomyolysis with or without renal impairment has been reported in seriously ill patients receiving erythromycin concomitantly with lovastatin.

4.5 Interaction with other medicinal products and other forms of Interaction
Concomitant use of erythromycin with terfenadine or astemizole is likely to result in an enhanced risk of cardiotoxicity with these drugs. The concomitant use of erythromycin with either astemizole or terfenadine is therefore contraindicated.

The metabolism of terfenadine and astemizole is significantly altered when either are taken concomitantly with erythromycin. Rare cases of serious cardiovascular events have been observed, including torsades de pointes, other ventricular arrhythmias and cardiac arrest. Death has been reported with the terfenadine / erythromycin combination.

Elevated cisapride levels have been reported in patients receiving erythromycin and cisapride concomitantly. This may result in QT prolongation and cardiac arrhythmias including ventricular trachycardia, ventricular fibrillation and Torsades de pointes. Similar effects have been observed with concomitant administration of pimozide and clarithromycin, another macrolide antibiotic.

Concurrent use of erythromycin and ergotamine or dihydroergotamine has been associated in some patients with acute ergot toxicity characterised by the rapid development of severe peripheral vasospasm and dysaesthesia.

Increases in serum concentrations of the following drugs metabolised by the cytochrome P450 system may occur when administered concurrently with erythromycin: alfentanil, astemizole, bromocriptine, carbamazepine, cyclosporin, digoxin, dihydroergotamine, disopyramide, ergotamine, hexobarbitone, midazolam, phenytoin, quinidine, tacrolimus, terfenadine, theophylline, triazolam, valproate, and warfarin. Appropriate monitoring should be undertaken and dosage should be adjusted as necessary.

Erythromycin has been reported to decrease the clearance of zopiclone and thus may increase the pharmacodynamic effects of this drug.

When oral erythromycin is given concurrently with theophylline, there is also a significant decrease in erythromycin serum concentrations. The decrease could result in sub-therapeutic concentrations of erythromycin.

4.6 Pregnancy and lactation

There is no evidence of hazard from erythromycin in human pregnancy. It has been in widespread use for a number of years without apparent ill consequence. Animal studies have shown no hazard.

Erythromycin has been reported to cross the placental barrier in humans, but foetal plasma levels are generally low.

Erythromycin is excreted in breast milk, therefore, caution should be exercised when erythromycin is administered to a nursing mother.

4.7 Effects on ability to drive and use machines

None reported

4.8 Undesirable effects

Occasional side effects such as nausea, abdominal discomfort, vomiting and diarrhoea may be experienced. Reversible hearing loss associated with doses of erythromycin usually greater than 4g per day has been reported. Allergic reactions are rare and mild, although anaphylaxis has occurred. Skin reactions ranging from mild eruptions to erythema multiforme, Stevens-Johnson syndrome and toxic epidermal necrolysis have rarely been reported. There are no reports implicating erythromycin products with abnormal tooth development, and only rare reports of damage to the blood, kidneys or central nervous system.

Cardiac arrhythmias have been very rarely reported in patients receiving erythromycin therapy. There have been isolated reports of chest pain, dizziness and palpitations, however, a cause and effect relationship has not been established.

Symptoms of hepatitis, hepatic dysfunction and/or abnormal liver function test results may occur.

4.9 Overdose

Symptoms: hearing loss, severe nausea, vomiting and diarrhoea.

Treatment: gastric lavage, general supportive measures.

5. PHARMACOLOGICAL PROPERTIES

5.1 Pharmacodynamic properties

Erythromycin exerts its antimicrobial action by binding to the 50S ribosomal sub-unit of susceptible microorganisms and suppresses protein synthesis. Erythromycin is usually active against most strains of the following organisms both *in vitro* and in clinical infections:

Gram positive bacteria - *Listeria monocytogenes, Corynebacterium diphtheriae* (as an adjunct to antitoxin), Staphylococci *spp*, Streptococci *spp* (including Enterococci).

Gram negative bacteria - *Haemophilus influenzae, Neisseria meningitidis, Neisseria gonorrhoeae, Legionella pneumophila, Moraxella (Branhamella) catarrhalis, Bordetella pertussis*, Campylobacter spp.

Mycoplasma - *Mycoplasma pneumoniae, Ureaplasma urealyticum*.

Other organisms - *Treponema pallidum*, Chlamydia spp, Clostridia spp, L-forms, the agents causing trachoma and lymphogranuloma venereum.

Note: The majority of strains of *Haemophilus influenzae* are susceptible to the concentrations reached after ordinary doses.

5.2 Pharmacokinetic properties

Peak blood levels normally occur within 1 hour of dosing of erythromycin ethylsuccinate granules. The elimination half life is approximately 2 hours. Doses may be administered 2, 3 or 4 times a day.

Erythromycin ethylsuccinate is less susceptible than erythromycin to the adverse effect of gastric acid. It is absorbed from the small intestine. It is widely distributed throughout body tissues. Little metabolism occurs and only about 5% is excreted in the urine. It is excreted principally by the liver.

5.3 Preclinical safety data

There are no pre-clinical data of relevance to the prescriber which are additional to that already included in other sections of the SPC.

6. PHARMACEUTICAL PARTICULARS

6.1 List of excipients

Sorbitol, xanthan gum, sodium citrate, surfactant poloxamer 188, acesulfame (K), sodium saccharin, purified water, sodium methylhydroxybenzoate, sodium propylhydroxybenzoate, colloidal silicon dioxide, imitation banana flavour entrapped No.2, entrapped artificial cream.

6.2 Incompatibilities

None stated.

6.3 Shelf life

Bottles: 24 months. Once reconstituted Erythroped PI SF should be used within 7 days.

Sachets: 24 months.

6.4 Special precautions for storage

None

6.5 Nature and contents of container

High density polyethylene bottles, 100ml or 140ml, with polypropylene cap which may be a child resistant cap.

Sachet: 44 GSM paper / 12 GSM LDPE / 9μm Al foil / 34 GSM LDPE.

6.6 Instructions for use and handling

Not applicable

7. MARKETING AUTHORISATION HOLDER

Abbott Laboratories Ltd, Queenborough, Kent, ME11 5EL

8. MARKETING AUTHORISATION NUMBER(S)

0037/0223

9. DATE OF FIRST AUTHORISATION/RENEWAL OF THE AUTHORISATION

25/03/97

10. DATE OF REVISION OF THE TEXT

August 1998

Erythroped SF

(Abbott Laboratories Limited)

1. NAME OF THE MEDICINAL PRODUCT

Erythroped SF

Erythromycin Ethylsuccinate SF 250mg/5ml

Erythromycin SF 250mg/5ml

Erythromycin Suspension 250mg/5ml SF

Erythromycin Ethylsuccinate SF Suspension 250mg/5ml

2. QUALITATIVE AND QUANTITATIVE COMPOSITION

Active: Erythromycin as Erythromycin Ethylsuccinate 250 mg / 5 ml

3. PHARMACEUTICAL FORM

Granules for reconstitution

4. CLINICAL PARTICULARS

4.1 Therapeutic indications

For the prophylaxis and treatment of infections caused by erythromycin-sensitive organisms.

Erythromycin is highly effective in the treatment of a great variety of clinical infections such as:

1. Upper Respiratory Tract infections: tonsillitis, peritonsillar abscess, pharyngitis, laryngitis, sinusitis, secondary infections in influenza and common colds

2. Lower Respiratory Tract infections: tracheitis, acute and chronic bronchitis, pneumonia (lobar pneumonia, bronchopneumonia, primary atypical pneumonia), bronchiectasis, Legionnaire's disease

3. Ear infection: otitis media and otitis externa, mastoiditis

4. Oral infections: gingivitis, Vincent's angina

5. Eye infections: blepharitis

6. Skin and soft tissue infections: boils and carbuncles, paronychia, abscesses, pustular acne, impetigo, cellulitis, erysipelas

7. Gastrointestinal infections: cholecystitis, staphylococcal enterocolitis

8. Prophylaxis: pre- and post- operative trauma, burns, rheumatic fever

9. Other infections: osteomyelitis, urethritis, gonorrhoea, syphilis, lymphogranuloma venereum, diphtheria, prostatitis, scarlet fever

Note: Erythromycin has also proved to be of value in endocarditis and septicaemia, but in these conditions initial administration of erythromycin lactobionate by the intravenous route is advisable.

4.2 Posology and method of administration

Adults and children over 8 years: 2g/day in divided doses. For severe infections up to 4g/day in divided doses.

Children 2 - 8 years: 30 mg/kg/day in divided doses. For severe infections up to 50 mg/kg/day in divided doses. Normal dose: 250mg four times a day or 500mg twice daily.

Children up to 2 years: 30 mg/kg/day in divided doses. For severe infections up to 50 mg/kg/day in divided doses. Normal dose: 125mg four times a day or 250mg twice daily.

Presentations are available for adults and children over 8 years, children aged 2-8 years, and for children under 2 years.

4.3 Contraindications

Known hypersensitivity to erythromycin. Erythromycin is contraindicated in patients taking astemizole, terfenadine, cisapride or pimozide.

Erythromycin is contraindicated with ergotamine and dihydroergotamine.

4.4 Special warnings and special precautions for use

Erythromycin is excreted principally by the liver, so caution should be exercised in administering the antibiotic to patients with impaired hepatic function or concomitantly receiving potentially hepatotoxic agents. Hepatic dysfunction including increased liver enzymes and/or cholestatic hepatitis, with or without jaundice, has been infrequently reported with erythromycin.

There have been reports suggesting erythromycin does not reach the foetus in adequate concentrations to prevent congenital syphilis. Infants born to women treated during pregnancy with oral erythromycin for early syphilis should be treated with an appropriate penicillin regimen.

There have been reports that erythromycin may aggravate the weakness of patients with myasthenia gravis.

Erythromycin interferes with the fluorometric determination of urinary catecholamines.

As with other broad spectrum antibiotics, pseudomembranous colitis has been reported rarely with erythromycin.

Rhabdomyolysis with or without renal impairment has been reported in seriously ill patients receiving erythromycin concomitantly with lovastatin.

4.5 Interaction with other medicinal products and other forms of Interaction

Concomitant use of erythromycin with terfenadine or astemizole is likely to result in an enhanced risk of cardiotoxicity with these drugs. The concomitant use of erythromycin with either astemizole or terfenadine is therefore contraindicated.

The metabolism of terfenadine and astemizole is significantly altered when either are taken concomitantly with erythromycin. Rare cases of serious cardiovascular events have been observed, including torsades de pointes, other ventricular arrhythmias and cardiac arrest. Death has been reported with the terfenadine / erythromycin combination.

Elevated cisapride levels have been reported in patients receiving erythromycin and cisapride concomitantly. This may result in QT prolongation and cardiac arrhythmias including ventricular trachycardia, ventricular fibrillation and Torsades de pointes. Similar effects have been observed with concomitant administration of pimozide and clarithromycin, another macrolide antibiotic.

Concurrent use of erythromycin and ergotamine or dihydroergotamine has been associated in some patients with acute ergot toxicity characterised by the rapid development of severe peripheral vasospasm and dysaesthesia.

Increases in serum concentrations of the following drugs metabolised by the cytochrome P450 system may occur when administered concurrently with erythromycin: alfentanil, astemizole, bromocriptine, carbamazepine, cyclosporin, digoxin, dihydroergotamine, disopyramide, ergotamine, hexobarbitone, midazolam, phenytoin, quinidine, tacrolimus, terfenadine, theophylline, triazolam, valproate, and warfarin. Appropriate monitoring should be undertaken and dosage should be adjusted as necessary.

Erythromycin has been reported to decrease the clearance of zopiclone and thus may increase the pharmacodynamic effects of this drug.

When oral erythromycin is given concurrently with theophylline, there is also a significant decrease in erythromycin serum concentrations. The decrease could result in sub-therapeutic concentrations of erythromycin.

4.6 Pregnancy and lactation

There is no evidence of hazard from erythromycin in human pregnancy. It has been in widespread use for a number of years without apparent ill consequence. Animal studies have shown no hazard.

Erythromycin has been reported to cross the placental barrier in humans, but foetal plasma levels are generally low.

Erythromycin is excreted in breast milk, therefore, caution should be exercised when erythromycin is administered to a nursing mother.

4.7 Effects on ability to drive and use machines

None reported

4.8 Undesirable effects

Occasional side effects such as nausea, abdominal discomfort, vomiting and diarrhoea may be experienced. Reversible hearing loss associated with doses of erythromycin usually greater than 4g per day has been reported. Allergic reactions are rare and mild, although anaphylaxis has occurred. Skin reactions ranging from mild eruptions to erythema multiforme, Stevens-Johnson syndrome and toxic epidermal necrolysis have rarely been reported. There are no reports implicating erythromycin products with abnormal tooth development, and only rare reports of damage to the blood, kidneys or central nervous system.

Cardiac arrhythmias have been very rarely reported in patients receiving erythromycin therapy. There have been isolated reports of chest pain, dizziness and palpitations, however, a cause and effect relationship has not been established.

Symptoms of hepatitis, hepatic dysfunction and/or abnormal liver function test results may occur.

4.9 Overdose

Symptoms: hearing loss, severe nausea, vomiting and diarrhoea.

Treatment: gastric lavage, general supportive measures.

5. PHARMACOLOGICAL PROPERTIES

5.1 Pharmacodynamic properties

Erythromycin exerts its antimicrobial action by binding to the 50S ribosomal sub-unit of susceptible microorganisms and suppresses protein synthesis. Erythromycin is usually active against most strains of the following organisms both *in vitro* and in clinical infections:

Gram positive bacteria - *Listeria monocytogenes, Corynebacterium diphtheriae* (as an adjunct to antitoxin), Staphylococci *spp*, Streptococci *spp* (including Enterococci).

Gram negative bacteria - *Haemophilus influenzae, Neisseria meningitidis, Neisseria gonorrhoeae, Legionella pneumophila, Moraxella (Branhamella) catarrhalis, Bordetella pertussis*, Campylobacter spp.

Mycoplasma - *Mycoplasma pneumoniae, Ureaplasma urealyticum.*

Other organisms - *Treponema pallidum*, Chlamydia spp, Clostridia spp, L-forms, the agents causing trachoma and lymphogranuloma venereum.

Note: The majority of strains of *Haemophilus influenzae* are susceptible to the concentrations reached after ordinary doses.

5.2 Pharmacokinetic properties

Peak blood levels normally occur within 1 hour of dosing of erythromycin ethylsuccinate granules. The elimination half life is approximately 2 hours. Doses may be administered 2, 3 or 4 times a day.

Erythromycin ethylsuccinate is less susceptible than erythromycin to the adverse effect of gastric acid. It is absorbed from the small intestine. It is widely distributed throughout body tissues. Little metabolism occurs and only about 5% is excreted in the urine. It is excreted principally by the liver.

5.3 Preclinical safety data

There are no pre-clinical data of relevance to the prescriber which are additional to that already included in other sections of the SPC.

6. PHARMACEUTICAL PARTICULARS

6.1 List of excipients

Sorbitol, xanthan gum, sodium citrate, surfactant poloxamer 188, acesulfame (K), sodium saccharin, purified water, sodium methylhydroxybenzoate, sodium propylhydroxybenzoate, colloidal silicon dioxide, imitation banana flavour entrapped No.2, entrapped artificial cream.

6.2 Incompatibilities

None stated.

6.3 Shelf life

Bottles: 24 months. Once reconstituted Erythroped SF should be used within 7 days.

Sachets: 24 months.

6.4 Special precautions for storage

None

6.5 Nature and contents of container

High density polyethylene bottles, 100ml or 140ml, with polypropylene cap which may be a child resistant cap.

Sachet: 44 GSM paper / 12 GSM LDPE / 9μm Al foil / 34 GSM LDPE

6.6 Instructions for use and handling

Not applicable

7. MARKETING AUTHORISATION HOLDER

Abbott Laboratories Ltd, Queenborough, Kent, ME11 5EL.

8. MARKETING AUTHORISATION NUMBER(S)

0037/0224

9. DATE OF FIRST AUTHORISATION/RENEWAL OF THE AUTHORISATION

25/03/97

10. DATE OF REVISION OF THE TEXT

August 1998

Estracombi TTS

(Novartis Pharmaceuticals UK Ltd)

1. NAME OF THE MEDICINAL PRODUCT

Estracombi TTS®

Estracombi TTS is a combination of Estraderm TTS 50 and Estragest TTS transdermal patches.

2. QUALITATIVE AND QUANTITATIVE COMPOSITION

Active substances: Estra-1,3,5(10)-triene-3, 17β-diol (estradiol) and 17-Hydroxy-19-nor-17α-pregn-4-en-20-yn-3-one-acetate (norethisterone acetate).

One package of Estracombi TTS comprises 4 Estraderm TTS 50 patches and 4 Estragest TTS (0.25/50) patches.

One Estraderm TTS 50 transdermal patch contains 4mg estradiol Ph.Eur. One Estragest TTS (0.25/50) transdermal patch contains 10mg estradiol Ph.Eur. and 30mg norethisterone acetate Ph.Eur.

3. PHARMACEUTICAL FORM

Estraderm TTS 50 is a thin, round, multilayer, transparent, transdermal patch, i.e. an adhesive patch for application to an area of intact skin.

Estragest TTS (0.25/50) is a thin, goggle-shaped, multilayer transparent transdermal patch, with two separate drug reservoir chambers, i.e. an adhesive patch for application to an area of intact skin.

4. CLINICAL PARTICULARS

4.1 Therapeutic indications

Hormone replacement therapy for patients with an intact uterus with disorders due to natural or surgically induced menopause, which may include, for example, vasomotor symptoms (hot flushes and nocturnal sweating), urogenital conditions such as atrophic vaginitis/vulvitis, and/or atrophic urethritis and trigonitis, sleep disturbances as well as accompanying mood changes.

Second line therapy for prevention of osteoporosis in postmenopausal women at high risk of future fractures who are intolerant of, or contraindicated for, other medicinal products approved for the prevention of osteoporosis.

4.2 Posology and method of administration

Estracombi TTS provides continuous estrogen and sequential progestogen therapy to women with an intact uterus.

One treatment cycle of Estracombi TTS consists of 4 patches of transdermal estradiol followed by 4 patches of transdermal estradiol and norethisterone acetate. Therapy is started with transdermal estradiol (Estraderm TTS 50) which should be applied twice weekly for 2 weeks, i.e. the patch should be changed once every 3 to 4 days. For the following 2 weeks, one transdermal estradiol plus norethisterone acetate patch (Estragest TTS) is applied twice weekly. The next treatment cycle should be started immediately after the removal of the last Estragest TTS patch.

Each fresh patch should be applied to a slightly different site. Recommended application sites are clean, dry and intact areas of skin on the trunk below the waistline. The site selected should be one at which little wrinkling of the skin occurs during movement of the body, e.g. buttock, hip, abdomen. Experience to date has shown that less irritation of the skin occurs on the buttocks than at other sites of application, and this site is preferred by patients. It is therefore recommended to apply Estracombi TTS to the buttock. Estracombi TTS should NOT be applied on or near the breasts.

Estracombi TTS incorporates a combined estrogen and progestogen patch to induce withdrawal bleeding, thereby minimising the risk of endometrial hyperplasia and carcinoma which can occur with unopposed estrogen therapy. Most patients will bleed towards the end of progestogen therapy. The first transdermal patch of the new cycle should be applied irrespective of the duration of bleeding. It is important that the patches be used in the correct sequence (i.e. 2 weeks Estraderm TTS 50 followed by 2 weeks Estragest TTS each cycle) to ensure regular cyclic bleeding.

For most postmenopausal women Estracombi TTS therapy may be started at any convenient time. However, if the patient is still menstruating commencement within 5 days of the onset of bleeding is recommended.

Some breakthrough bleeding or spotting may be seen until therapy has become established. Some effects, usually of estrogenic origin, e.g. breast discomfort, water retention or bloating, are often observed at the start of treatment, especially in patients receiving hormone replacement therapy for the first time. However, if symptoms persist for more than 6 weeks, treatment should be reconsidered.

The transdermal patch should not be exposed to sunlight.

The use of creams, oils or lotions should be avoided since these may reduce patch adhesion.

Children

Estracombi TTS is not indicated.

4.3 Contraindications

- Known or suspected cancer of the breast, genital tract, endometrium or other estrogen-dependent neoplasia
- Severe hepatic, renal or cardiac disease
- Undiagnosed vaginal bleeding
- Porphyria, confirmed active venous thromboembolism (deep venous thrombosis, pulmonary embolism) within the last 2 years
- A history of recurrent VTE or known thrombophilic disease in a patient who is not already on anticoagulant treatment (see Special Warnings and Special Precautions for Use)
- Dubin-Johnson syndrome
- Rotor syndrome
- Known hypersensitivity to the components of the patch
- Pregnancy and lactation.

4.4 Special warnings and special precautions for use

Assessment of each woman prior to taking hormone replacement therapy (and at regular intervals thereafter) should include a personal and family medical history. Physical examination should be guided by this and by the Contra-indications (section 4.3) and Warnings (section 4.4) for this product. During assessment of each individual woman, clinical examination of the breasts and pelvic examination should be performed where clinically indicated rather than as a routine procedure. Women should be encouraged to participate in the national breast cancer screening programme (mammography) and the national cervical cancer screening programme (cervical cytology) as appropriate for their age. Breast awareness should also be encouraged and women advised to report any changes in their breasts to their doctor or nurse.

Examinations to rule out endometrial abnormalities should be undertaken at regular intervals (e.g. every 6 to 12 months), including monitoring of the endometrium if thought necessary. In all cases of undiagnosed persistent or irregular vaginal bleeding, adequate diagnostic measures, including endometrial sampling when indicated should be undertaken to rule out abnormality and the treatment should be re-evaluated.

Contact sensitisation is known to occur with all topical applications. Although it is extremely rare, patients who develop contact sensitisation to any of the components of the patch should be warned that a severe hypersensitivity reaction may occur with continuing exposure to the causative agent.

A reanalysis of original data from 51 epidemiological studies (not necessarily including Estracombi TTS) reported a small or moderate increase in the probability of having breast cancer diagnosed in women currently or recently using HRT. The findings may be due to earlier diagnosis, an actual effect of HRT or a combination of both. The probability of diagnosing breast cancer increased with duration of treatment and returned to normal in the course of five years after stopping HRT. Breast cancers diagnosed in current or recent users of HRT are less likely to have spread outside the breast than those found in non-users.

Between the ages of 50 and 70, about 45 women in every 1000 not using HRT will have breast cancer diagnosed, the rate increasing with age. It is estimated that among those who use HRT for 5 to 15 years, depending on age of starting and duration of treatment, the number of additional cases of breast cancer diagnosed will be of the order of 2 to 12 cases per 1000 women.

Caution is advised in patients with a history of estrogen related jaundice and pruritus. If cholestatic jaundice develops during treatment, the treatment should be stopped and appropriate investigations carried out. Although observations to date suggest that estrogens, including transdermal estradiol do not impair carbohydrate metabolism diabetic patients should be monitored during initiation of therapy until further information is available. Pre-existing uterine leiomyomas or fibroids may become enlarged during estrogen therapy. Women with endometriosis should be carefully monitored.

If any of the following conditions are present, have occurred previously and/or have become aggravated during pregnancy or previous hormone treatment, the benefits of treatment should be weighed against the possible risks. In these cases the patient should be closely supervised. It should be taken into account that these conditions may, in rare cases, recur or be aggravated during treatment with Estracombi TTS:

- A history of thromboembolic disorders or the presence of risk factors (see below).

Epidemiological studies have suggested that hormone replacement therapy (HRT) is associated with a higher relative risk of developing venous thromboembolism (VTE), i.e. deep vein thrombosis or pulmonary embolism. The studies find a 2-3 fold higher risk for users compared with non-users, which for healthy women amounts to one or two additional cases of VTE in 10,000 patient-years of treatment with HRT. The occurrence of such an event is more likely in the first year of HRT than later.

Generally recognised risk factors for VTE include a personal history or family history, severe obesity (Body Mass Index > 30kg/m^2) and systemic lupus erythematosus (SLE). There is no consensus about the role of varicose veins in VTE.

Use of HRT in patients with a history of recurrent VTE or known thrombophilic states already on anticoagulant treatment require careful consideration of the benefit-risk of use of HRT (see also Contra-indications).

The presence of a personal or strong family history of recurrent thromboembolism or recurrent spontaneous abortion should be investigated in order to exclude a thrombophilic predisposition. Until a definitive diagnosis has been made or anticoagulant treatment initiated use of HRT in such patients should be viewed as contra-indicated.

The risk of VTE may be temporarily increased with prolonged immobilisation, major trauma or major surgery. As in all post-operative patients scrupulous attention should be given to prophylactic measures to prevent VTE following surgery. Where prolonged immobilisation is liable to follow elective surgery, particularly abdominal or orthopaedic surgery to the lower limbs, consideration should be given to temporarily stopping HRT four to six weeks earlier, if possible.

If VTE develops after initiating therapy, the drug should be discontinued.

Patients should be told to contact their doctors immediately when they are aware of a potential thromboembolic symptom (e.g. painful swelling of a leg, sudden pain in the chest, dyspnoea).

The following conditions may deteriorate on HRT:

- Hypertension
- Asthma
- Heart failure
- Disorders of renal or hepatic function
- Migraine or
- Epilepsy.

It is essential that affected patients be kept under surveillance and HRT be stopped if there is an increase in epileptic seizures. If worsening of any of the above mentioned conditions is diagnosed or suspected during HRT the benefits and risks of HRT should be reassessed on an individual case.

Women with familial hypertriglyceridaemia need special surveillance. Lipid lowering measures are recommended additionally before HRT is started.

Estracombi TTS is not a contraceptive.

4.5 Interaction with other medicinal products and other forms of Interaction

Preparations inducing microsomal liver enzymes e.g.

- Barbiturates
- Hydantoins
- Carbamazepine
- Meprobamate
- Phenylbutazone

Antibiotics (including rifampicin) and activated charcoal, may impair the activity of estrogens and progestogens (irregular bleeding and recurrence of symptoms may occur).

The extent of interference with transdermally administered estradiol and norethisterone acetate is not known; these problems should be minimised by the transdermal route of administration which avoids any first pass hepatic metabolism.

4.6 Pregnancy and lactation

Estracombi TTS is not indicated.

4.7 Effects on ability to drive and use machines

None stated.

4.8 Undesirable effects

Skin:

Frequently: Transient erythema and irritation at site of application with or without pruritus. This usually disappears 3-4 days after patch removal and is similar to the effect observed after occlusion of the skin with household medical adhesive plasters.

Very infrequently: Local swelling, papules/vesicles and scaling have been reported, which also resolved spontaneously and did not result in permanent skin damage.

Isolated cases: Allergic contact dermatitis, reversible post-inflammatory pigmentation; generalised pruritus and exanthema.

Urogenital tract:

Frequently: Breakthrough bleeding, spotting.

Occasionally: Heavy, sometimes prolonged bleeding, dysmenorrhoea, pre-menstrual syndrome-like symptoms; endometrial hyperplasia (incidence similar to that reported for other opposed HRT regimes). Amenorrhoea may occur during treatment.

Endocrine system:

Frequently: Breast discomfort.

Gastro-intestinal tract:

Occasionally: Nausea, abdominal cramps, bloating.

Very infrequently: Asymptomatic impaired liver function, cholestatic jaundice

Central nervous system:

Occasionally: Headache, migraine.

Rarely: Dizziness.

Cardiovascular system:

Venous thromboembolism, i.e. deep leg or pelvic venous thrombosis and pulmonary embolism, is more frequent among HRT users than among non-users. For further information see sections "4.3 Contra-indications" and "4.4 Warnings and Precautions for Use".

Very infrequently: Exacerbation of varicose veins, increase in blood pressure.

Miscellaneous:

Rarely: Oedema and/or weight changes,

Occasionally: Leg cramps (not related to thromboembolic disease and usually transient lasting 3-6 weeks; if symptoms persist treatment should be reviewed).

Very infrequently: Anaphylactoid reactions (history of previous allergy or allergic disorders in some cases)

4.9 Overdose

Due to the mode of administration overdosage is unlikely.

Signs and symptoms:

Signs of acute estrogen overdosage may be either one of, or a combination of, breast discomfort, fluid retention and bloating, or nausea.

Signs of progestogen overdosage may be nausea, vomiting, breast enlargement and vaginal bleeding.

Treatment:

Overdosage can if necessary be reversed by removal of the patch.

5. PHARMACOLOGICAL PROPERTIES

5.1 Pharmacodynamic properties

Estradiol

Estrogen substitution effectively prevents the symptomatic, metabolic and trophic changes due to loss of ovarian function associated with the menopause.

The patch formulation (transdermal therapeutic system, TTS) delivers hormone into the bloodstream via intact skin. Estraderm TTS and Estragest TTS are both designed to deliver estradiol at a low rate over several days.

Studies of bone mineral content have shown Estracombi TTS to be effective in the prevention of progressive bone loss following the menopause.

Adverse effects on lipid and non-lipid mediated markers of cardiovascular disease may contribute to the increased incidence of cardiovascular disease seen in women post-menopause.

An improved lipid profile may be one factor contributing to the beneficial effect of estrogen replacement therapy on the risk of coronary heart disease in postmenopausal women.

Studies have indicated beneficial effects of Estraderm TTS with progestogen on serum total cholesterol, low density lipoprotein (LDL), triglyceride and high density lipoprotein (HDL) levels. There have been few long-term studies of the effect of Estraderm TTS alone on these measurements and the results are thus less conclusive although generally favourable. Studies of Estraderm TTS incorporating progestogen treatment have demonstrated effects on arterial tone which may have a beneficial effect on cardiovascular risk, and have not shown deleterious effects on blood pressure, coagulation and insulin resistance.

Epidemiological studies indicate that a useful reduction in fracture frequency of approx. 50% is achieved with 5 to 6 years estrogen therapy.

Norethisterone Acetate

With Estragest TTS progestogen is added for the last 14 days in each cycle in order to prevent endometrial hyperstimulation. A regular cyclic bleed can be expected to start on day 24-26 of treatment.

5.2 Pharmacokinetic properties

Estradiol

Within four hours of application of the first Estraderm TTS 50 patch plasma estradiol levels reach the therapeutic range, and these are maintained throughout the dose interval (for up to four days).

After removal of the last patch plasma estrogen levels return to baseline values in less than 24 hours, and urinary estrogen conjugates within 2-3 days.

Mean plasma concentrations of estradiol are similar during both phases of the treatment (i.e. transdermal estradiol alone with Estraderm TTS 50, or transdermal estradiol plus norethisterone acetate with Estragest TTS).

Absorption rates of estradiol from both Estraderm TTS 50 and Estragest TTS may vary between individual patients.

Norethisterone Acetate

Norethisterone acetate is metabolised to the active progestogen, norethisterone, which reaches plasma levels of 0.5 - 1.0 ng/ml within 2 days after Estragest TTS application. These levels are maintained throughout the dose interval and are sufficient to prevent endometrial hyperstimulation. After removal of the transdermal patch, levels of norethisterone return to baseline within 2 days.

The absorption rate of norethisterone acetate may vary between individual patients.

5.3 Preclinical safety data

None relevant.

6. PHARMACEUTICAL PARTICULARS

6.1 List of excipients

The patches contain

- Ethanol
- Hydroxypropylcellulose
- Polyethylene terephthalate
- Ethylenevinylacetate copolymer
- Liquid paraffin
- Polyisobutylene
- Silicone-coating (on the inner side of the protective release liner which is removed before patch application).

6.2 Incompatibilities

None known.

6.3 Shelf life

2 years.

6.4 Special precautions for storage

Store below 25°C.

6.5 Nature and contents of container

Cartons containing four transdermal estradiol, marked CG EFE, and four transdermal estradiol and norethisterone acetate patches, marked CG FNF, each individually sealed in a protective pouch (sufficient for one month's treatment).

A three monthly pack containing twelve transdermal estradiol and twelve transdermal estradiol and norethisterone acetate patches each individually sealed in a protective pouch is also available.

6.6 Instructions for use and handling

None stated.

7. MARKETING AUTHORISATION HOLDER

Novartis Pharmaceuticals UK Limited
Trading as Ciba Laboratories
Frimley Business Park
Frimley
Camberley
Surrey
GU16 7SR
England.

8. MARKETING AUTHORISATION NUMBER(S)

PL 00101/0485

9. DATE OF FIRST AUTHORISATION/RENEWAL OF THE AUTHORISATION

12 September 1997

10. DATE OF REVISION OF THE TEXT

December 2003

Legal Category

POM

Estracyt Capsules

(Pharmacia Limited)

1. NAME OF THE MEDICINAL PRODUCT

Estracyt Capsules.

2. QUALITATIVE AND QUANTITATIVE COMPOSITION

Estramustine phosphate 140 mg as estramustine sodium phosphate.

3. PHARMACEUTICAL FORM

Gelatin capsules.

4. CLINICAL PARTICULARS

4.1 Therapeutic indications

Carcinoma of the prostate, especially in cases unresponsive to, or relapsing after, treatment by conventional oestrogens (stilboestrol, polyoestradiol phosphate etc.) or by orchidectomy.

4.2 Posology and method of administration

Adult and the elderly

Dosage range may be from 1 to 10 capsules a day by mouth. The capsules should be taken not less than 1 hour before or 2 hours after meals. The capsules should not be taken with milk or milk products. Standard starting dosage is 4-6 capsules a day in divided doses with later adjustment according to response and gastrointestinal tolerance.

Children

Estracyt should not be administered to children.

4.3 Contraindications

Use in patients with peptic ulceration, or those with severe liver dysfunction or myocardial insufficiency.

Use in children.

Use in patients hypersensitive to oestradiol or nitrogen mustard.

4.4 Special warnings and special precautions for use

Use with caution in patients with moderate to severe bone marrow depression, thrombophlebitis, thrombosis, thromboembolic disorders, cardiovascular disease, coronary artery disease and congestive heart failure.

Caution should also be exercised in patients with diabetes, hypertension, epilepsy, hepatic and renal impairment and diseases associated with hypercalcaemia. Blood counts, liver function tests and serum calcium in hypercalcaemia should be performed at regular intervals. Patients with prostate cancer and osteoblastic metastases are at risk of hypocalcaemia and should have calcium levels closely monitored.

4.5 Interaction with other medicinal products and other forms of Interaction

Milk, milk products or drugs containing calcium may impair the absorption of Estracyt and should not be taken simultaneously with Estracyt.

An interaction between Estracyt and ACE-inhibitors, possibly leading to an increased risk of angioneurotic oedema cannot be excluded.

4.6 Pregnancy and lactation

Not applicable.

4.7 Effects on ability to drive and use machines

No adverse effects on a patient's ability to drive or operate heavy machinery have been reported.

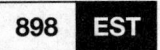

4.8 Undesirable effects
The most common adverse reactions include gynaecomastia and impotence, nausea/vomiting and fluid retention/oedema.

The most serious reactions are thromboembolism, ischaemic heart disease, congestive heart failure and, rarely, angioneurotic oedema.

Reported reactions arranged according to organ system are the following:

Cardiovascular

Fluid retention

Congestive heart failure.

Ischaemic heart disease, myocardial infarction.

Thromboembolism.

Hypertension

Gastrointestinal

Nausea and vomiting, particularly during the first two weeks of treatment.

Diarrhoea.

Hepato-biliary

Impairment of liver function.

Haematological

Anaemia, leukopaenia, thrombocytopaenia rarely occur.

Endocrine

Gynaecomastia and impotence.

Central Nervous System

Muscular weakness, depression, headache, confusion, lethargy rarely occur.

Hypersensitivity Reactions

Hypersensitivity reactions, including allergic skin rash have been reported. Angioneurotic oedema (Quincke oedema, larynx oedema) can rarely occur. In many reported cases, including a fatal one, patients were concomitantly receiving ACE-inhibitors. Therapy with Estracyt is to be immediately discontinued, should angioneurotic oedema occur.

4.9 Overdose
There is no specific antidote. Treatment is symptomatic and supportive and in the event of dangerously low red cell, white cell or platelet count, whole blood should be given as necessary. Liver function should be monitored.

5. PHARMACOLOGICAL PROPERTIES

5.1 Pharmacodynamic properties
Estracyt is a chemical compound of oestradiol and nitrogen mustard. It is effective in the treatment of advanced prostatic carcinoma.

Estracyt has a dual mode of action. The intact molecule acts as an anti-miotic agent; after hydrolysis of the carbamate ester, the metabolites act to bridge the released oestrogens and exert an anti-gonadotrophic effect. The low level of clinical side effects may be due to the fact that estramustine binds to a protein present in the tumour tissue, so resulting in accumulation of the drug at the target site. Estracyt also has weak oestrogenic and anti-gonadotrophic properties.

Estracyt causes little or no bone marrow depression at usual therapeutic dosage. Estracyt is effective in patients who have not previously received drug therapy, as well as in those who have shown no response to conventional hormone treatment.

5.2 Pharmacokinetic properties
Estramustine phosphate sodium is rapidly dephosphorylated in the intestine and prostate to estramustine and estromustine, which accumulate in the prostatic tissue. The plasma half-lives of these metabolites are 10 - 20 hours. Estramustine and estromustine are further metabolised before excretion.

5.3 Preclinical safety data
No particular information is presented given the experience gained with the use of estramustine phosphate sodium in humans over the past several years.

6. PHARMACEUTICAL PARTICULARS

6.1 List of excipients
Talcum, sodium lauryl sulphate, colloidal silicon dioxide, magnesium stearate, titanium dioxide (E171), hard gelatin capsule, black ink.

6.2 Incompatibilities
None that are relevant.

6.3 Shelf life
60 months in brown glass bottles.

6.4 Special precautions for storage
Store out of the sight and reach of children.

The product is stable at storage conditions of 25°C ± 2°C/60%RH (long term) and 40°C ± 2°C/75%RH (short term). Therefore the product does not require any special storage precautions within EU countries (Climactic zone 2).

6.5 Nature and contents of container
Brown glass bottle containing 100 capsules.

6.6 Instructions for use and handling
No special instructions.

7. MARKETING AUTHORISATION HOLDER
Pharmacia Limited

Davy Avenue

Milton Keynes

MK5 8PH

UK

8. MARKETING AUTHORISATION NUMBER(S)
PL 00032/0316

9. DATE OF FIRST AUTHORISATION/RENEWAL OF THE AUTHORISATION
25 May 2002

10. DATE OF REVISION OF THE TEXT
August 2003

Legal Category:
POM

Ref: ES 1_0

Estraderm MX 25, 50, 75, 100

(Novartis Pharmaceuticals UK Ltd)

1. NAME OF THE MEDICINAL PRODUCT
Estraderm MX 25®

Estraderm MX 50®

Estraderm MX 75®

Estraderm MX 100®

2. QUALITATIVE AND QUANTITATIVE COMPOSITION
The active ingredient is Estra-1, 3,5(10)-triene-3,17β-diol (estradiol).

Patches contain 0.75, 1.5, 2.25 and 3.0 mg estradiol Ph. Eur corresponding to surface areas of 11, 22, 33 and 44 cm^2 respectively.

3. PHARMACEUTICAL FORM
Estraderm MX is a square-shaped, self-adhesive, transparent, transdermal patch for application to the skin surface. Each patch comprises an impermeable polyester backing film, an adhesive matrix containing estradiol and an oversized protective liner which is removed prior to application of the patch to the skin. Estraderm MX releases estradiol into the circulation via intact skin at a low rate for up to 4 days.

Cross section:

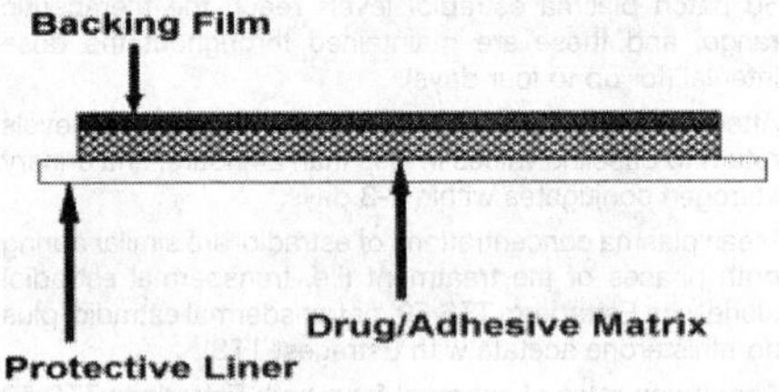

(see Table 1 below)

4. CLINICAL PARTICULARS

4.1 Therapeutic indications
Estrogen replacement therapy for patients with disorders due to natural or surgically induced menopause which may include, for example, vasomotor symptoms (hot flushes and nocturnal sweating), urogenital conditions such as atrophic vaginitis/ vulvitis, and/or atrophic urethritis and trigonitis, sleep disturbances as well as accompanying mood changes.

Second line therapy for prevention of osteoporosis in postmenopausal women at high risk of future fractures who are intolerant of, or contraindicated for, other medicinal products approved for the prevention of osteoporosis.

Estrogen therapy must not be used in patients with an intact uterus unless an appropriate dose of progestogen is administered for twelve days per month.

4.2 Posology and method of administration
Menopausal symptoms

Therapy should be initiated with one Estraderm MX 50 and the dose adjusted after the first treatment month depending on efficacy and signs of overdosage. Effects usually of estrogenic origin e.g. breast discomfort, water retention or bloating are often observed at the start of treatment especially in patients receiving hormone replacement therapy for the first time, however, if symptoms persist for more than six weeks the dose should be reduced. For maintenance therapy the lowest effective dose should be used; a maximum dose of 100 micrograms per day should not be exceeded. Unopposed estrogen therapy should not be used unless the patient has had a hysterectomy.

Postmenopausal osteoporosis
Estraderm MX 50 or Estraderm MX 75 is recommended as an effective bone-sparing dose. Estraderm MX 100 is not recommended as the risk/benefit of the higher dose in osteoporosis has not been assessed in clinical studies. However, it may be used if necessary to control concurrent menopausal symptoms. Estraderm MX 25 is not recommended as it has been shown to slow down but not completely halt the rate of bone loss.

Where a progestogen is considered necessary, the appropriate dose should be administered for 12 days per month. If the estrogen is adequately combined with a progestogen withdrawal bleeding occurs, in a way similar to normal menstrual bleeding. Breakthrough bleeding or spotting may be seen until therapy has become established. Signs of breakthrough bleeding early in the cycle should be investigated.

Estraderm MX is not indicated in children

Administration
Estraderm MX should be applied immediately after removal of the protective liner (see Figs.), to an area of clean, dry, and intact skin on the trunk below the waistline. The site chosen should be one at which little wrinkling of skin occurs during movement of the body, e.g. buttock. Estraderm MX should NOT be applied on or near the breasts.

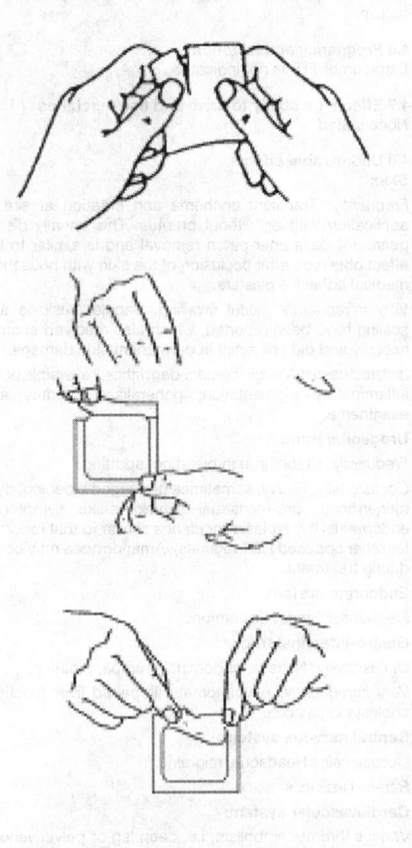

Estraderm MX should be applied twice weekly on a continuous basis, each used patch being removed after 3-4 days and a fresh transdermal patch applied to a slightly different site. The patch should not be exposed to sunlight.

Table 1

DOSAGE STRENGTHS	ESTRADERM MX 25	ESTRADERM MX 50	ESTRADERM MX 75	ESTRADERM MX 100
Nominal rate of estradiol release	25 μg/day	50 μg/day	75 μg/day	100 μg/day
Estradiol content	0.75mg	1.5mg	2.25mg	3.0mg
Drug-releasing area	11 cm^2	22 cm^2	33 cm^2	44 cm^2
Imprint (on backing film)	CG GRG	CG GSG	CG HKH	CG GTG

4.3 Contraindications

- Known or suspected cancer of the breast, genital tract, endometrium or other estrogen-dependent neoplasia
- Severe hepatic, renal or cardiac disease
- Undiagnosed vaginal bleeding
- Porphyria
- Confirmed active venous thromboembolism (deep venous thrombosis, pulmonary embolism) within the last 2 years
- A history of recurrent VTE or known thrombophilic disease in a patient who is not already on anticoagulant treatment (see Special Warnings and Special Precautions for Use)
- Dubin-Johnson syndrome
- Rotor syndrome
- Known hypersensitivity to the components of the patch
- Pregnancy and lactation.

4.4 Special warnings and special precautions for use

Assessment of each woman prior to taking hormone replacement therapy (and at regular intervals thereafter) should include a personal and family medical history. Physical examination should be guided by this and by the Contra-indications (section 4.3) and Warnings (section 4.4) for this product. During assessment of each individual woman, clinical examination of the breasts and pelvic examination should be performed where clinically indicated rather than as a routine procedure. Women should be encouraged to participate in the national breast cancer screening programme (mammography) and the national cervical cancer screening programme (cervical cytology) as appropriate for their age. Breast awareness should also be encouraged and women advised to report any changes in their breasts to their doctor or nurse.

Examinations to rule out endometrial abnormalities should be undertaken at regular intervals, including monitoring of the endometrium if thought necessary. In all cases of undiagnosed persistent or irregular vaginal bleeding, adequate diagnostic measures, including endometrial sampling when indicated should be undertaken to rule out abnormality and the treatment should be re-evaluated.

Prolonged monotherapy with estrogens increases the risk of endometrial hyperplasia and carcinoma in postmenopausal women unless supplemented by sequential administration of a progestogen to protect the endometrium.

Contact sensitisation is known to occur with all topical applications. Although it is extremely rare, patients who develop contact sensitisation to any of the components of the patch should be warned that a severe hypersensitivity reaction may occur with continuing exposure to the causative agent.

A reanalysis of original data from 51 epidemiological studies (not necessarily including Estraderm MX) reported a small or moderate increase in the probability of having breast cancer diagnosed in women currently or recently using HRT. The findings may be due to earlier diagnosis, an actual effect of HRT or a combination of both. The probability of diagnosing breast cancer increased with duration of treatment and returned to normal in the course of five years after stopping HRT. Breast cancers diagnosed in current or recent users of HRT are less likely to have spread outside the breast than those found in non-users.

Between the ages of 50 and 70, about 45 women in every 1000 not using HRT will have breast cancer diagnosed, the rate increasing with age. It is estimated that among those who use HRT for 5 to 15 years, depending on age of starting and duration of treatment, the number of additional cases of breast cancer diagnosed will be of the order of 2 to 12 cases per 1000 women.

The following conditions may deteriorate on HRT: Hypertension, asthma, heart failure, disorders of renal or hepatic function, migraine or epilepsy. It is essential that affected patients are kept under surveillance and HRT be stopped if there is an increase in epileptic seizures. If worsening of any of the above mentioned conditions is diagnosed or suspected during HRT, the benefits and risks of HRT should be reassessed based on the individual case.

Caution is advised in patients with a history of estrogen related jaundice and pruritus. If cholestatic jaundice develops during treatment the treatment should be stopped and appropriate investigations carried out. Although observations to date suggest that estrogens, including transdermal estradiol, do not impair carbohydrate metabolism diabetic patients should be monitored during initiation of therapy until further information is available. Preexisting uterine leiomyomas or fibroids may become enlarged during estrogen therapy. Women with endometriosis should be carefully monitored.

If any of the following conditions are present, have occurred previously and/or have become aggravated during pregnancy or previous hormone treatment, the benefits of treatment should be weighed against the possible risks. In these cases the patient should be closely supervised. It should be taken into account that these conditions may, in rare cases, recur or be aggravated during treatment with Estraderm MX:

- A history of thromboembolic disorders or the presence of risk factors (see below).

Epidemiological studies have suggested that hormone replacement therapy (HRT) is associated with a higher relative risk of developing venous thromboembolism (VTE), i.e. deep vein thrombosis or pulmonary embolism. The studies find a 2-3 fold higher risk for users compared with non-users, which for healthy women amounts to one or two additional cases of VTE in 10,000 patient-years of treatment with HRT. The occurrence of such an event is more likely in the first year of HRT than later.

Generally recognised risk factors for VTE include a personal history or family history, severe obesity (Body Mass Index > 30kg/m^2) and systemic lupus erythematosus (SLE). There is no consensus about the role of varicose veins in VTE.

Use of HRT in patients with a history of recurrent VTE or known thrombophilic states already on anticoagulant treatment require careful consideration of the benefit-risk of use of HRT (see also Contra-indications).

The presence of a personal or strong family history of recurrent thromboembolism or recurrent spontaneous abortion should be investigated in order to exclude a thrombophilic predisposition. Until a definitive diagnosis has been made or anticoagulant treatment initiated use of HRT in such patients should be viewed as contra-indicated.

The risk of VTE may be temporarily increased with prolonged immobilisation, major trauma or major surgery. As in all post-operative patients scrupulous attention should be given to prophylactic measures to prevent VTE following surgery. Where prolonged immobilisation is liable to follow elective surgery, particularly abdominal or orthopaedic surgery to the lower limbs, consideration should be given to temporarily stopping HRT four to six weeks earlier, if possible.

If VTE develops after initiating therapy, the drug should be discontinued.

Patients should be told to contact their doctors immediately when they are aware of a potential thromboembolic symptom (e.g. painful swelling of a leg, sudden pain in the chest, dyspnoea).

Women with familial hypertriglyceridaemia need special surveillance. Lipid lowering measures are recommended additionally, before HRT is started.

4.5 Interaction with other medicinal products and other forms of Interaction

Preparations inducing microsomal liver enzymes, e.g.

- Barbiturates
- Hydantoins
- Anticonvulsants
- Meprobamate
- Phenylbutazone

Antibiotics and activated charcoal, may impair the activity of estrogens (irregular bleeding and recurrence of symptoms may occur).

The extent of interference with transdermally administered estradiol is not known; these problems should be minimised by the transdermal route of administration which avoids any first pass hepatic metabolism.

4.6 Pregnancy and lactation

Estraderm MX should not be used during pregnancy and lactation.

4.7 Effects on ability to drive and use machines

None known.

4.8 Undesirable effects

Frequency estimates are as follows: *frequently > 10%; occasionally 1-10%; rarely 0.001-1%; isolated cases < 0.001%.*

The following systemic effects have been reported for Estraderm TTS, which is bioequivalent to Estraderm MX:

Urogenital tract

Frequently: Breakthrough bleeding (usually a sign of estrogen overdosage).

Endocrine system

Frequently: Breast discomfort

Gastrointestinal tract

Occasionally: Nausea, abdominal cramps, bloating.

Isolated cases: Asymptomatic impaired liver function, cholestatic jaundice

Central nervous system

Occasionally: Headache, migraine.

Rarely: Dizziness.

Cardiovascular system

Venous thromboembolism, i.e. deep leg or pelvic venous thrombosis and pulmonary embolism, is more frequent among HRT users than among non-users. For further information see sections "4.3 Contra-indications" and "4.4 Warnings and Precautions for Use".

Isolated cases: Exacerbation of varicose veins, increase in blood pressure.

Miscellaneous

Rarely: Oedema and/or weight changes, leg cramps (not related to thromboembolic disease and usually transient lasting 3-6 weeks; if symptoms persist the dose of estrogen should be reduced).

Skin

Very common: Transient erythema and irritation with or without pruritus.

Very rare: Allergic contact dermatitis, reversible post inflammatory pigmentation, generalised pruritus and exanthema

4.9 Overdose

This is not likely due to the mode of administration.

Signs and Symptoms

See "Dosage", section 4.2.

Treatment

Overdosage can if necessary be reversed by removal of the patch.

5. PHARMACOLOGICAL PROPERTIES

5.1 Pharmacodynamic properties

Like all steroid hormones, estrogens exert their metabolic effects intracellularly. In the cells of target organs estrogens interact with specific receptors to form a complex which stimulates both DNA and protein synthesis. Such receptors have been identified in various organs, e.g. the hypothalamus, pituitary, vagina, urethra, breast, and liver, and in osteoblasts.

Estradiol, which in women from the menarche to the menopause is produced mainly by the ovarian follicles, is the most active estrogen at the receptor level. After the menopause, when the ovaries have ceased to function, only small amounts of estradiol are still produced from aromatisation of androstenedione and to a lesser extent of testosterone by the aromatase enzyme, yielding estrone and estradiol, respectively.

Estrone is further transformed to estradiol by the enzyme 17β-hydroxysteroid dehydrogenase. Both enzymes are found in fat, liver, and muscle tissue.

In many women, the cessation of ovarian estradiol production results in vasomotor and thermoregulatory instability (hot flushes), sleep disturbances, and progressive atrophy of the urogenital system. These disorders can be largely eliminated by means of estrogen replacement therapy. Owing to the accelerated loss of bone substance induced by postmenopausal estrogen deficiency many women develop osteoporosis, particularly of the vertebral column, hip, and wrist. This can be prevented by estrogen replacement therapy, preferably initiated early in the menopause. Epidemiological studies indicate that a useful reduction in fracture frequency of approx. 50% is achieved with 5 to 6 years estrogen therapy.

Transdermal therapy with Estraderm MX delivers the physiological estrogen estradiol in unchanged form into the bloodstream via intact skin. Estraderm MX raises estradiol concentrations to levels similar to those found in the early to mid-follicular phase and maintains them over the application period of 3-4 days. The estradiol/estrone ratio is restored to premenopausal levels.

The following pharmacodynamic effects have been reported for Estraderm TTS, which is bioequivalent to Estraderm MX:

Estraderm TTS treatment for 28 days did not result in changes in circulating levels of fibrinopeptide A, high molecular weight fibrinogen, or antithrombin III. There were no changes in concentrations either of circulating renin substrate or of the sex-hormone-binding, thyroxine-binding, and cortisol-binding globulins.

After only a few weeks treatment Estraderm TTS has been shown to elicit a dose-dependent reduction in urinary excretion of calcium and hydroxyproline which is indicative of a slowing down of the rate of bone loss.

Adverse effects on lipid and non-lipid mediated markers of cardiovascular disease may contribute to the increased incidence of cardiovascular disease seen in women post-menopause. An improved lipid profile may be one factor contributing to the beneficial effect of estrogen replacement therapy on the risk of coronary heart disease in postmenopausal women. Studies have indicated beneficial effects of Estraderm TTS with progestogen on serum total cholesterol, low density lipoprotein (LDL), triglyceride and high density lipoprotein (HDL) levels. There have been few long-term studies of the effect of Estraderm TTS alone on these measurements and the results are thus less conclusive although generally favourable. Studies of Estraderm TTS incorporating progestogen treatment have demonstrated effects on arterial tone which may have a beneficial effect on cardiovascular risk, and have not shown deleterious effects on blood pressure, coagulation and insulin resistance.

Regardless of the route of administration, the estrogen doses required to relieve menopausal symptoms and conserve bone mass are also a potent stimulus for endometrial mitosis and proliferation. Unopposed estrogens increase the incidence of endometrial hyperplasia and the risk of endometrial carcinoma. Following 1 year of unopposed estrogen therapy endometrial hyperplasia has been found in up to 57% of biopsies. Endometrial hyperplasia is also possible as a result of unopposed transdermal estrogen therapy. A high rate of endometrial hyperplasia has been observed with the higher doses of Estraderm TTS.

5.2 Pharmacokinetic properties
Within 8 hours after application of Estraderm MX 25, 50, 75 and 100 steady-state plasma estradiol concentrations are reached and remain stable throughout the dose interval (up to 4 days). The average increase in estradiol concentration over baseline reached with Estraderm MX 50 is 37 pg/ml. The estradiol/estrone ratio increases from a postmenopausal value of 0.3 to a value of 1.3, similar to the physiological ratio observed before menopause in women with normally functioning ovaries. Following 12 weeks treatment with Estraderm MX 50 the average increase in estradiol concentration over baseline was 36 pg/ml, indicating an absence of estradiol accumulation.

Absorption rates may vary between individual patients. However, the plasma estradiol levels achieved with different sized transdermal patches have been shown to be proportional to the drug-releasing area of the dosage form.

After removal of the last transdermal patch plasma estradiol levels return to baseline values in less than 24 hours.

Estradiol

The plasma elimination half-life of estradiol is approx. 1 hour. The metabolic plasma clearance ranges from 650 to 900 l/(day × m^2). Estradiol is mainly metabolised in the liver. Its most important metabolites are estriol and estrone and their conjugates (glucuronides, sulphates); these are far less active than estradiol.

The bulk of the conjugates are excreted in urine. Estrogen metabolites are also subject to enterohepatic circulation.

5.3 Preclinical safety data
At low physiological doses of estradiol (similar to those delivered by Estraderm MX), the potential for neoplasia is negligible in experimental animals. Most of the documented effects of exogenously administered estradiol in animal studies have been consequences of the administration of higher doses and are consistent with an exaggerated pharmacological response (most notably the promotion of tumours in estrogen-responsive tissues). However, long term unopposed treatment with physiological doses of estradiol may potentially lead to hyperplastic changes in estrogen-dependent reproductive organs like the uterus.

Some dermal irritation associated with the patch has been observed in the rabbit.

6. PHARMACEUTICAL PARTICULARS
6.1 List of excipients
- Acrylate
- Methacrylate
- Isopropyl palmitate
- Polyethylene terephthalate
- Ethylenevinylacetate copolymer
- Silicone coating (on the inner side of the protective release liner which is removed before patch application).

6.2 Incompatibilities
None known

6.3 Shelf life
2 years.

6.4 Special precautions for storage
Store below 25°C.

Keep out of the reach of children both before and after use.

6.5 Nature and contents of container
Each system is individually heat sealed in a paper/aluminium/polyethylene foil pouch. Eight or twenty four Estraderm MX pouches are placed in an appropriately sized carton which comprises the finished product (one or three month's treatment respectively). A "hospital pack" of twenty Estraderm MX 50 (10 X 2 patch "starter packs") is also available.

6.6 Instructions for use and handling
See Section 4.2. Exposure of Estraderm MX patches to ultra-violet light results in degradation of estradiol. Patches should not be exposed to sunlight. They should be applied immediately after removal from the pouch to skin sites covered by clothing.

7. MARKETING AUTHORISATION HOLDER
Novartis Pharmaceuticals UK Ltd

Trading as Ciba Laboratories

Frimley Business Park

Frimley

Camberley

Surrey

GU16 7SR

England.

8. MARKETING AUTHORISATION NUMBER(S)
Estraderm MX 25: PL 00101/0486

Estraderm MX 50: PL 00101/0487

Estraderm MX 75: PL 00101/0549

Estraderm MX 100: PL 00101/0488

9. DATE OF FIRST AUTHORISATION/RENEWAL OF THE AUTHORISATION
Estraderm MX 25 and 50 12 September 1997 / 23 May 2001

Estraderm MX 75 9 November 1998

Estraderm MX 100 12 September 1997 / 24 May 2001

10. DATE OF REVISION OF THE TEXT
December 2003

Legal Category
POM

Estraderm TTS

(Novartis Pharmaceuticals UK Ltd)

1. NAME OF THE MEDICINAL PRODUCT
Estraderm® TTS

2. QUALITATIVE AND QUANTITATIVE COMPOSITION
The active ingredient is estra-1,3,5 (10)-triene-3, 17β-diol (estradiol).

One patch contains 2mg, 4mg or 8mg of estradiol Ph Eur. One month packs of Estraderm TTS 25, 50 or 100 contains 8 patches. Three month packs containing 24 patches are also available.

(see Table 1 below)

3. PHARMACEUTICAL FORM
Estraderm TTS® is a transdermal patch (transdermal therapeutic system). It is a thin multilayer transparent, transdermal therapeutic patch for application to an area of intact skin.

4. CLINICAL PARTICULARS
4.1 Therapeutic indications
Estrogen replacement therapy for patients with disorders due to natural or surgically induced menopause, which may include, for example, vasomotor symptoms (hot flushes and nocturnal sweating), urogenital conditions such as atrophic vaginitis/ vulvitis and/or atrophic urethritis and trigonitis, sleep disturbances, as well as accompanying mood changes.

Estrogen therapy must not be used in patients with an intact uterus unless an appropriate dose of progestogen is administered for twelve days per month.

Estraderm TTS 50 only

Second line therapy for prevention of osteoporosis in postmenopausal women at high risk of future fractures who are intolerant of, or contraindicated for, other medicinal products approved for the prevention of osteoporosis.

4.2 Posology and method of administration
Adults and Elderly

Menopausal Symptoms: Therapy should be initiated with one Estraderm TTS and the dose adjusted after the first treatment month depending on efficacy and signs of overdosage. Effects usually of estrogenic origin eg. breast discomfort, water retention or bloating are often observed at the start of treatment, especially in patients receiving hormone replacement therapy for the first time, however, if symptoms persist for more than six weeks the dose should be reduced. For maintenance therapy the lowest effective dose should be used; a maximum dose of 100 micrograms per day should not be exceeded. Unopposed estrogen therapy should not be used unless the patient has had a hysterectomy.

Postmenopausal osteoporosis: Estraderm TTS 50 is recommended as an effective bone-sparing dose. Estraderm TTS 100 is not recommended as the risk/benefit of the higher dose in osteoporosis has not been assessed in clinical studies. However, it may be used if necessary to control concurrent menopausal symptoms. Estraderm TTS 25 is not recommended as it has been shown to slow down but not completely halt the rate of bone loss.

Where a progestogen is considered necessary the appropriate dose should be administered for 12 days per month. If the estrogen is adequately combined with a progestogen withdrawal bleeding occurs, in a similar way to normal menstrual bleeding. Breakthrough bleeding or spotting may be seen until therapy has become established. Signs of breakthrough bleeding early in the cycle should be investigated.

Estraderm TTS should be applied twice weekly on a continuous basis, each used transdermal patch being removed after 3-4 days and a fresh transdermal patch applied to a slightly different site. Recommended application sites are clean, dry and intact areas of skin on the trunk below the waistline. The site selected should be one at which little wrinkling of the skin occurs during movement of the body, e.g. buttock, hip, abdomen. Experience to date has shown that less irritation of the skin occurs on the buttocks than on other sites of application. It is therefore advisable to apply Estraderm TTS to the buttock. Estraderm TTS should not be applied on or near the breasts.

The transdermal patch should not be exposed to sunlight.

Children

Estraderm TTS is not indicated in children.

4.3 Contraindications
- Known or suspected cancer of the breast, genital tract, endometrium or other estrogen-dependent neoplasia
- Severe hepatic, renal or cardiac disease
- Undiagnosed vaginal bleeding
- Porphyria
- Confirmed active venous thromboembolism (deep venous thrombosis, pulmonary embolism) within the last 2 years
- A history of recurrent VTE or known thrombophilic disease in a patient who is not already on anticoagulant treatment (see Special Warnings and Special Precautions for Use)
- Dubin-Johnson Syndrome
- Rotor Syndrome
- Known hypersensitivity to the components of the patch
- Pregnancy
- Lactation.

4.4 Special warnings and special precautions for use
Assessment of each woman prior to taking hormone replacement therapy (and at regular intervals thereafter) should include a personal and family medical history. Physical examination should be guided by this and by the Contra-indications (section 4.3) and Warnings (section 4.4) for this product. During assessment of each individual woman, clinical examination of the breasts and pelvic examination should be performed where clinically indicated rather than as a routine procedure. Women should be encouraged to participate in the national breast cancer screening programme (mammography) and the national cervical cancer screening programme (cervical cytology) as appropriate for their age. Breast awareness should also be encouraged and women advised to report any changes in their breasts to their doctor or nurse.

Examinations to rule out endometrial abnormalities should be undertaken at regular intervals, including monitoring of the endometrium if thought necessary. In all cases of undiagnosed persistent or irregular vaginal bleeding, adequate diagnostic measures, including endometrial sampling when indicated should be undertaken to rule out abnormality and the treatment should be re-evaluated.

Prolonged monotherapy with estrogens increases the risk of endometrial hyperplasia and carcinoma in postmenopausal women, unless supplemented by sequential administration of a progestogen to protect the endometrium.

Contact sensitisation is known to occur with all topical applications. Although it is extremely rare, patients who develop contact sensitisation to any of the components of the patch should be warned that a severe hypersensitivity reaction may occur with continuing exposure to the causative agent.

A reanalysis of original data from 51 epidemiological studies (not necessarily including Estraderm TTS) reported a small or moderate increase in the probability of having breast cancer diagnosed in women currently or recently using HRT. The findings may be due to earlier diagnosis, an actual effect of HRT or a combination of both. The probability of diagnosing breast cancer increased with duration of treatment and returned to normal in the course of five years after stopping HRT. Breast cancers diagnosed in current or recent users of HRT are less likely to have spread outside the breast than those found in non-users.

Between the ages of 50 and 70, about 45 women in every 1000 not using HRT will have breast cancer diagnosed, the rate increasing with age. It is estimated that among those who use HRT for 5 to 15 years, depending on age of starting and duration of treatment, the number of additional cases of breast cancer diagnosed will be of the order of 2 to 12 cases per 1000 women.

Caution is advised in patients with a history of estrogen related jaundice and pruritus. If cholestatic jaundice develops during treatment the treatment should be stopped and

Table 1

DOSAGE STRENGTHS	ESTRADERM TTS 25	ESTRADERM TTS 50	ESTRADERM TTS 100
Estradiol content	2.0mg	4.0mg	8.0mg
Drug-releasing area	5 cm^2	10 cm^2	20 cm^2
Imprint (on backing film)	CG DWD	CG EFE	CG FBF

appropriate investigations carried out. Although observations to date indicate that estrogens, including transdermal estradiol do not impair carbohydrate metabolism diabetic patients should be monitored during initiation of therapy until further information is available. Preexisting uterine leiomyomas or fibroids may become enlarged during estrogen therapy. Women with endometriosis should be carefully monitored.

If any of the following conditions are present, have occurred previously and/or have become aggravated during pregnancy or previous hormone treatment, the benefits of treatment should be weighed against the possible risks. In these cases the patient should be closely supervised. It should be taken into account that these conditions may, in rare cases, recur or be aggravated during treatment with Estraderm TTS:

- A history of thromboembolic disorders or the presence of risk factors (see below).

Epidemiological studies have suggested that hormone replacement therapy (HRT) is associated with a higher relative risk of developing venous thromboembolism (VTE), i.e. deep vein thrombosis or pulmonary embolism. The studies find a 2-3 fold higher risk for users compared with non-users, which for healthy women amounts to one or two additional cases of VTE in 10,000 patient-years of treatment with HRT. The occurrence of such an event is more likely in the first year of HRT than later.

Generally recognised risk factors for VTE include a personal history or family history, severe obesity (Body Mass Index > 30k/m^2) and systemic lupus erythematosus (SLE). There is no consensus about the role of varicose veins in VTE.

Use of HRT in patients with a history of recurrent VTE or known thrombophilic states already on anticoagulant treatment require careful consideration of the benefit-risk of use of HRT (see also Contra-indications).

The presence of a personal or strong family history of recurrent thromboembolism or recurrent spontaneous abortion should be investigated in order to exclude a thrombophilic predisposition. Until a definitive diagnosis has been made or anticoagulant treatment initiated use of HRT in such patients should be viewed as contra-indicated.

The risk of VTE may be temporarily increased with prolonged immobilisation, major trauma or major surgery. As in all post-operative patients scrupulous attention should be given to prophylactic measures to prevent VTE following surgery. Where prolonged immobilisation is liable to follow elective surgery, particularly abdominal or orthopaedic surgery to the lower limbs, consideration should be given to temporarily stopping HRT four to six weeks earlier, if possible.

If VTE develops after initiating therapy, the drug should be discontinued.

Patients should be told to contact their doctors immediately when they are aware of a potential thromboembolic symptom (e.g. painful swelling of a leg, sudden pain in the chest, dyspnoea).

The following conditions may deteriorate on HRT:

- Hypertension
- Asthma
- Heart failure
- Disorders of renal or hepatic function
- Migraine or
- Epilepsy.

It is essential that affected patients are kept under surveillance and HRT be stopped if there is an increase in epileptic seizures. If worsening of any of the above mentioned conditions is diagnosed or suspected during HRT, the benefits and risks of HRT should be reassessed based on the individual case.

Women with familial hypertriglyceridaemia need special surveillance. Lipid-lowering measures are recommended additionally before HRT is started.

4.5 Interaction with other medicinal products and other forms of Interaction

Preparations inducing microsomal liver enzymes e.g.

- Barbiturates
- Hydantoins
- Anti-convulsants (including carbamazepine)
- Meprobamate
- Phenylbutazone

Antibiotics (including rifampicin) and activated charcoal, may impair the activity of estrogens (irregular bleeding and recurrence of symptoms may occur).

The extent of interference with transdermally administered estradiol is not known; these problems should be minimised by the transdermal route of administration which avoids any first pass hepatic metabolism.

4.6 Pregnancy and lactation

Estraderm TTS should not be used during pregnancy and lactation.

4.7 Effects on ability to drive and use machines

None known

4.8 Undesirable effects

Skin

Frequently: Transient erythema and irritation at site of application with or without pruritus. This usually disappears 3-4 days after patch removal and is similar to the effect observed after occlusion of the skin with household medical adhesive plasters.

Very infrequently: Local swelling, papules/vesicles and scaling have been reported, which also resolved spontaneously and did not result in permanent skin damage.

Isolated cases: Allergic contact dermatitis, reversible post-inflammatory pigmentation; generalised pruritis and exanthema.

Urogenital Tract

Frequently: Breakthrough bleeding (usually a sign of estrogen overdosage see "Dosage and Administration")

Endocrine System

Frequently: Breast discomfort

Gastrointestinal Tract

Occasionally: Nausea, abdominal cramps, bloating.

Isolated cases: Asymptomatic impaired liver function, cholestatic jaundice.

Central Nervous System

Occasionally: Headache, migraine.

Rarely: Dizziness.

Cardiovascular System

Venous thromboembolism, i.e. deep leg or pelvic venous thrombosis and pulmonary embolism, is more frequent among HRT users than among non-users. For further information see sections "4.3 Contra-indications" and "4.4 Warnings and Precautions for Use".

Isolated cases: Exacerbation of varicose veins, increase in blood pressure.

Miscellaneous

Occasionally: Leg cramps (not related to thromboembolic disease and usually transient lasting 3-6 weeks, if symptoms persist, the dose of estrogen should be reduced).

Rarely: Oedema and/or weight changes.

Isolated cases: Anaphylactoid reactions (history of previous allergy or allergic disorders in some cases).

4.9 Overdose

This is not likely due to the method of administration.

Signs and Symptoms

(See Dosage and administration)

Treatment

Overdosage can if necessary be reversed by removal of the patch(es).

5. PHARMACOLOGICAL PROPERTIES

5.1 Pharmacodynamic properties

Estrogen substitution effectively prevents the characteristics symptomatic, metabolic and trophic changes due to loss of ovarian function associated with loss of ovarian function due to natural or surgical menopause.

The patch formulation (transdermal therapeutic system, TTS) delivers hormone directly into the bloodstream via intact skin. Estraderm TTS is designed to deliver estradiol at a low rate over several days.

Epidemiological studies indicate that a useful reduction in fracture frequency of approx. 50% is achieved with 5 to 6 years estrogen therapy.

Adverse effects on lipid and non-lipid mediated markers of cardiovascular disease may contribute to the increased incidence of cardiovascular disease seen in women post-menopause.

An improved lipid profile may be one factor contributing to the beneficial effect of estrogen replacement therapy on the risk of coronary heart disease in postmenopausal women. Studies have indicated beneficial effects of Estraderm TTS with progestogen on serum total cholesterol, low density lipoprotein (LDL), triglyceride and high density lipoprotein (HDL) levels. There have been few long-term studies of the effect of Estraderm TTS alone on these measurements and the results are thus less conclusive although generally favourable. Studies of Estraderm TTS incorporating progestogen treatment have demonstrated effects on arterial tone which may have a beneficial effect on cardiovascular risk, and have not shown deleterious effects on blood pressure, coagulation and insulin resistance.

5.2 Pharmacokinetic properties

Within four hours of application of the first transdermal patch, plasma estradiol levels reach the therapeutic range and these are maintained throughout the dose interval (for up to four days). After removal of the last transdermal patch plasma estrogen levels return to baseline values in less than 24 hours and urinary estrogen conjugates within 2-3 days. Absorption rates may vary between individual patients. However, the plasma estradiol levels achieved with different sized transdermal patches have been shown to be proportional to the drug-releasing area of the dosage form.

5.3 Preclinical safety data

None relevant.

6. PHARMACEUTICAL PARTICULARS

6.1 List of excipients

- Ethanol
- Hyroxypropylcellulose
- Polyethylene terephthalate
- Ethylenevinylacetate copolymer
- Liquid paraffin
- Polyisobutylene
- Silicone coating on the inner side of the protective liner (which is removed before application of the patch).

6.2 Incompatibilities

None known.

6.3 Shelf life

24 months.

6.4 Special precautions for storage

Store below 25°C

6.5 Nature and contents of container

Estraderm TTS is available in packs of 8 or 24 patches. Each patch is individually heat sealed in a Surlyn coated aluminium pouch and enclosed in a cardboard container.

6.6 Instructions for use and handling

None stated

7. MARKETING AUTHORISATION HOLDER

Novartis Pharmaceuticals UK Ltd

Trading as

Ciba Laboratories

Frimley Business Park

Frimley

Camberley

Surrey

GU16 7SR

8. MARKETING AUTHORISATION NUMBER(S)

Estraderm TTS 25	PL 00101/0489
Estraderm TTS 50	PL 00101/0490
Estraderm TTS 100	PL 00101/0491

9. DATE OF FIRST AUTHORISATION/RENEWAL OF THE AUTHORISATION

12 September 1997

10. DATE OF REVISION OF THE TEXT

December 2003

Legal Category

POM

ESTRADOT

(Novartis Pharmaceuticals UK Ltd)

1. NAME OF THE MEDICINAL PRODUCT

Estradot® 25 micrograms/24 hours, transdermal patch.

Estradot® 37.5 micrograms/24 hours, transdermal patch.

Estradot® 50 micrograms/24 hours, transdermal patch.

Estradot® 75 micrograms/24 hours, transdermal patch.

Estradot® 100 micrograms/24 hours, transdermal patch.

2. QUALITATIVE AND QUANTITATIVE COMPOSITION

2.5 cm^2 patch containing 0.39 mg estradiol (as hemihydrate) with a release rate of 25 microgram estradiol per 24 hours.

3.75 cm^2 patch containing 0.585 mg estradiol (as hemihydrate) with a release rate of 37.5 microgram estradiol per 24 hours.

5 cm^2 patch containing 0.78 mg estradiol (as hemihydrate) with a release rate of 50 microgram estradiol per 24 hours.

7.5 cm^2 patch containing 1.17 mg estradiol (as hemihydrate) with a release rate of 75 microgram estradiol per 24 hours.

10 cm^2 patch containing 1.56 mg estradiol (as hemihydrate) with a release rate 100 microgram estradiol per 24 hours.

For excipients, see 6.1.

3. PHARMACEUTICAL FORM

Transdermal patch.

Rectangular patch with rounded corners, comprising a pressure-sensitive adhesive layer containing estradiol, with a translucent polymeric backing on one side and a protective liner on the other.

4. CLINICAL PARTICULARS

4.1 Therapeutic indications

Hormone replacement therapy (HRT) for oestrogen deficiency symptoms in postmenopausal women.

Prevention of osteoporosis in postmenopausal women at high risk of future fractures who are intolerant of, or contra-indicated for, other medicinal products approved for the prevention of osteoporosis (for Estradot 50, 75 and 100 only).

The experience of treating women older than 65 years is limited.

4.2 Posology and method of administration

Dosage

The transdermal patch is applied twice weekly, i.e. every three to four days.

Oestrogen deficiency symptoms:

Estradot is available in five strengths: 25, 37.5, 50, 75 and 100. For initiation and continuation of treatment of post-menopausal symptoms, the lowest effective dose for the shortest duration (see also Section 4.4) should be used. Depending on the clinical response the dose can then be adjusted to the patient's individual needs. If, after three months, there is insufficient response in the form of alleviated symptoms, the dose can be increased. If symptoms of overdose arise (e.g. tender breasts) the dose must be decreased.

Prevention of postmenopausal osteoporosis:

Estradot is available in three strengths: 50, 75 and 100.

Treatment must be initiated with an Estradot 50 microgram/24 hours patch. Adjustments can be made by using Estradot 50, 75 and 100 microgram patches.

General instructions

Estradot is administered as continuous therapy (uninterrupted application twice weekly).

In women with an intact uterus, Estradot should be combined with a progestagen approved for addition to oestrogen treatment in a continuous sequential dosing scheme: the oestrogen is dosed continuously. The progestagen is added for at least 12 to 14 days of every 28-day cycle, in a sequential manner.

Unless there is a previous diagnosis of endometriosis, it is not recommended to add a progestagen in hysterectomised women.

In women who are not taking HRT or women transferring from a continuous combined HRT product, treatment may be started on any convenient day. In women transferring from a sequential HRT regimen, treatment should begin the day following completion of the prior regimen.

Method of administration

The adhesive side of Estradot should be placed on a clean, dry area of the abdomen.

Estradot should not be applied to the breasts.

Estradot should be replaced twice weekly. The site of application must be rotated, with an interval of at least 1 week allowed between applications to a particular site. The area selected should not be oily, damaged, or irritated. The waistline should be avoided, since tight clothing may dislodge the patch. The patch should be applied immediately after opening the sachet and removing the protective liner. The patch should be pressed firmly in place with the palm of the hand for about 10 seconds, making sure there is good contact, especially around the edges.

In the event that a patch should fall off, the same patch may be reapplied. If necessary, a new patch may be applied. In either case, the original treatment schedule should be continued. The patch may be worn during bathing.

If a woman has forgotten to apply a patch, she should apply a new patch as soon as possible. The subsequent patch should be applied according to the original treatment schedule. The interruption of treatment might increase the likelihood of irregular bleeding and spotting.

4.3 Contraindications

- Known, past or suspected breast cancer.
- Known or suspected oestrogen-dependent malignant tumours (e.g. endometrial cancer).
- Undiagnosed genital bleeding.
- Untreated endometrial hyperplasia.
- Previous idiopathic or current venous thromboembolism (deep venous thrombosis, pulmonary embolism).
- Active or recent arterial thromboembolic disease (e.g. angina, myocardial infarction).
- Acute liver disease, or a history of liver disease as long as liver function tests have failed to return to normal.
- Known hypersensitivity to estradiol or to any of the excipients.
- Porphyria.

4.4 Special warnings and special precautions for use

For the treatment of postmenopausal symptoms, HRT should only be initiated for symptoms that adversely affect quality of life. In all cases, a careful appraisal of the risks and benefits should be undertaken at least annually and HRT should only be continued as long as the benefit outweighs the risk.

Medical examination/follow-up

Before initiating or reinstituting HRT, a complete personal and family medical history should be taken. Physical (including pelvic and breast) examination should be guided by this and by the sections 4.3 "Contraindications" and 4.4 "Special warnings and precautions for use".

During treatment, periodic check-ups are recommended of a frequency and nature adapted to the individual woman. Women should be advised what changes in their breasts should be reported to their doctor or nurse (see "Breast cancer" below). Investigations, including mammography, should be carried out in accordance with currently accepted screening practices, modified to the clinical needs of the individual.

Conditions which need supervision

If any of the following conditions are present, have occurred previously, and/or have been aggravated during pregnancy or previous hormone treatment, the patient should be closely supervised. It should be taken into account that these conditions may recur or be aggravated during treatment with Estradot, in particular:

- Leiomyoma (uterine fibroids) or endometriosis
- A history of, or risk factors for, thromboembolic disorders (see below)
- Risk factors for oestrogen-dependent tumours, e.g. 1st-degree heredity for breast cancer
- Hypertension
- Liver disorders (e.g. liver adenoma)
- Diabetes mellitus with or without vascular involvement
- Cholelithiasis
- Migraine or (severe) headache
- Systemic lupus erythematosus (SLE)
- A history of endometrial hyperplasia (see below)
- Epilepsy
- Asthma
- Otosclerosis.

Reasons for immediate withdrawal of therapy:

Therapy should be discontinued in cases where a contra-indication is discovered and in the following situations:

- Jaundice or deterioration in liver function
- Significant increase in blood pressure
- New onset of migraine-type headache
- Pregnancy.

Endometrial hyperplasia

The risk of endometrial hyperplasia and carcinoma is increased when oestrogens are administered alone for prolonged periods (see section 4.8). The addition of a progestagen for at least 12 days per cycle in non-hysterectomised women greatly reduces this risk.

For Estradot 75 or 100 μg/day the endometrial safety of added progestagens has not been studied.

Break-through bleeding and spotting may occur during the first months of treatment. If break-through bleeding or spotting appears after some time on therapy or continues after treatment has been discontinued, the reason should be investigated, which may include endometrial biopsy to exclude endometrial malignancy.

Unopposed oestrogen stimulation may lead to pre-malignant or malignant transformation in the residual foci of endometriosis. Therefore, the addition of progestagens to oestrogen replacement therapy should be considered in women who have undergone hysterectomy because of endometriosis, if they are known to have residual endometriosis.

Breast cancer

A randomised placebo-controlled trial, the Women's Health Initiative study (WHI), and epidemiological studies, including the Million Women Study (MWS), have reported an increased risk of breast cancer in women taking oestrogens, oestrogen-progestagen combinations or tibolone for HRT for several years (see section 4.8).

For all HRT, an excess risk becomes apparent within a few years of use and increases with duration of intake, but returns to baseline within a few (at most five) years after stopping treatment.

In the MWS, the relative risk of breast cancer with conjugated equine oestrogens (CEE) or estradiol (E2) was greater when a progestagen was added, either sequentially or continuously, and regardless of type of progestagen. There was no evidence of a difference in risk between the different routes of administration.

In the WHI study, the continuous combined conjugated equine oestrogen and medroxyprogesterone acetate (CEE + MPA) product used was associated with breast cancers that were slightly larger in size and more frequently had local lymph node metastases compared to placebo.

HRT, especially oestrogen-progestagen combined treatment, increases the density of mammographic images which may adversely affect the radiological detection of breast cancer.

Venous thromboembolism

HRT is associated with a higher relative risk of developing venous thromboembolism (VTE), i.e. deep vein thrombosis or pulmonary embolism. One randomised controlled trial and epidemiological studies found a two- to threefold higher risk for users compared with non-users.

For non-users, it is estimated that the number of VTE cases that will occur over a 5 year period is about 3 per 1000 women aged 50-59 years and 8 per 1000 women aged between 60-69 years. It is estimated that in healthy women who use HRT for 5 years, the number of additional cases of VTE over a 5 year period will be between 2 and 6 (best estimate = 4) per 1000 women aged 50-59 years and between 5 and 15 (best estimate = 9) per 1000 women aged 60-69 years. The occurrence of such an event is more likely in the first year of HRT than later.

Generally recognised risk factors for VTE include a personal history or family history, severe obesity (BMI > 30 kg/m^2) and systemic lupus erythematosus (SLE). There is no consensus about the possible role of varicose veins in VTE.

Patients with a history of VTE or known thrombophilic states have an increased risk of VTE. HRT may add to this risk. Personal or strong family history of thromboembolism or recurrent spontaneous abortion should be investigated in order to exclude a thrombophilic predisposition. Until a thorough evaluation of thrombophilic factors has been made or anticoagulant treatment initiated, use of HRT in such patients should be viewed as contraindicated. Those women already on anticoagulant treatment require careful consideration of the benefit-risk of use of HRT.

The risk of VTE may be temporarily increased with prolonged immobilisation, major trauma or major surgery. As in all postoperative patients, scrupulous attention should be given to prophylactic measures to prevent VTE following surgery. Where prolonged immobilisation is liable to follow elective surgery, particularly abdominal or orthopaedic surgery to the lower limbs, consideration should be given to temporarily stopping HRT 4 to 6 weeks earlier, if possible. Treatment should not be restarted until the woman is completely mobilised.

If VTE develops after initiating therapy, the drug should be discontinued. Patients should be told to contact their doctors immediately when they are aware of a potential thromboembolic symptom (e.g., painful swelling of a leg, sudden pain in the chest, dyspnea).

Coronary artery disease (CAD)

There is no evidence from randomised controlled trials of cardiovascular benefit with continuous combined conjugated oestrogens and medroxyprogesterone acetate (MPA). Two large clinical trials (WHI and HERS i.e. Heart and Estrogen/progestin Replacement Study) showed a possible increased risk of cardiovascular morbidity in the first year of use and no overall benefit.

For other HRT products there are only limited data from randomised controlled trials examining effects in cardiovascular morbidity or mortality. Therefore, it is uncertain whether these findings also extend to other HRT products.

Stroke

One large randomised clinical trial (WHI-trial) found, as a secondary outcome, an increased risk of ischaemic stroke in healthy women during treatment with continuous combined conjugated oestrogens and MPA. For women who do not use HRT, it is estimated that the number of cases of stroke that will occur over a 5 year period is about 3 per 1000 women aged 50-59 years and 11 per 1000 women aged 60-69 years. It is estimated that for women who use conjugated oestrogens and MPA for 5 years, the number of additional cases will be between 0 and 3 (best estimate = 1) per 1000 users aged 50-59 years and between 1 and 9 (best estimate = 4) per 1000 users aged 60-69 years. It is unknown whether the increased risk also extends to other HRT products.

Ovarian cancer

Long-term (at least 5-10 years) use of oestrogen-only HRT products in hysterectomised women has been associated with an increased risk of ovarian cancer in some epidemiological studies. It is uncertain whether long-term use of combined HRTs confers a different risk than oestrogen-only products.

Other conditions

Oestrogens may cause fluid retention, and therefore patients with cardiac or renal dysfunction should be carefully observed. Patients with terminal renal insufficiency should be closely observed, since it is expected that the level of circulating active substance in Estradot is increased.

Women with pre-existing hypertriglyceridaemia should be followed closely during oestrogen replacement or hormone replacement therapy, since rare cases of large increases of plasma triglycerides leading to pancreatitis and other complications, have been reported with oestrogen therapy in this condition.

Oestrogens increase thyroid binding globulin (TBG), leading to increased circulating total thyroid hormone, as measured by protein-bound iodine (PBI), T4 levels (by column or by radio-immunoassay) or T3 levels (by radio-immunoassay). T3 resin uptake is decreased, reflecting the elevated TBG. Free T4 and free T3 concentrations are unaltered. Other binding proteins may be elevated in serum, i.e. corticoid binding globulin (CBG), sex-hormone-binding globulin (SHBG) leading to increased circulating corticosteroids and sex steroids, respectively. Free or biological active hormone concentrations are unchanged. Other plasma proteins may be increased (angiotensinogen/renin substrate, alpha-I-antitrypsin, ceruloplasmin).

There is no conclusive evidence for improvement of cognitive function. There is some evidence from the WHI trial of increased risk of probable dementia in women who start using continuous combined CEE and MPA after the age of 65. It is unknown whether the findings apply to younger postmenopausal women or other HRT products.

Contact sensitisation is known to occur with all topical applications. Although it is extremely rare, women who develop contact sensitisation to any of the components of the patch should be warned that a severe hypersensitivity reaction may occur with continuing exposure to the causative agent.

4.5 Interaction with other medicinal products and other forms of Interaction

The metabolism of oestrogens (and progestagens) may be increased by concomitant use of substances known to induce drug-metabolising enzymes, specifically cytochrome P450 enzymes, such as anticonvulsants (e.g. phenobarbital, phenytoin, carbamazepine), and anti-infectives (e.g. rifampicin, rifabutin, nevirapine, efavirenz).

Ritonavir and nelfinavir, although known as strong inhibitors, by contrast exhibit inducing properties when used concomitantly with steroid hormones. Herbal preparations containing St John's wort (*Hypericum Perforatum*) may induce the metabolism of oestrogens (and progestagens).

At transdermal administration, the first-pass effect in the liver is avoided and, thus, transdermally applied oestrogens might be less affected than oral hormones by enzyme inducers.

Clinically, an increased metabolism of oestrogens and progestagens may lead to decreased effect and changes in the uterine bleeding profile.

4.6 Pregnancy and lactation

Pregnancy

Estradot is not indicated during pregnancy. If pregnancy occurs during medication with Estradot, treatment should be withdrawn immediately.

The results of most epidemiological studies to date relevant to inadvertent foetal exposure to oestrogens indicate no teratogenic or foetotoxic effects.

Lactation

Estradot is not indicated during lactation.

4.7 Effects on ability to drive and use machines

Estradot has no or negligible influence on the ability to drive and use machines.

4.8 Undesirable effects

Mild erythema at the patch application site was the most reported undesirable effect (16.6%). The erythema was observed after removing the patch by peeling from the skin at the application site. Mild pruritus and rash were also reported around the application site.

The following adverse drug reactions have been reported with either Estradot or oestrogen therapy in general:

(see Table 1)

Breast cancer

According to evidence from a large number of epidemiological studies and one randomised placebo-controlled trial, the Women's Health Initiative (WHI), the overall risk of breast cancer increases with increasing duration of HRT use in current or recent HRT users.

For oestrogen-only HRT, estimates of relative risk (RR) from a reanalysis of original data from 51 epidemiological studies (in which >80% of HRT use was oestrogen-only HRT) and from the epidemiological Million Women Study (MWS) are similar at 1.35 (95% CI: 1.21 - 1.49) and 1.30 (95% CI: 1.21 – 1.40), respectively.

For oestrogen plus progestagen combined HRT, several epidemiological studies have reported an overall higher risk for breast cancer than with oestrogens alone.

The MWS reported that, compared to never users, the use of various types of oestrogen-progestagen combined HRT was associated with a higher risk of breast cancer (RR = 2.00, 95% CI: 1.88 – 2.12) than use of oestrogens alone (RR = 1.30, 95% CI: 1.21 – 1.40) or use of tibolone (RR=1.45; 95% CI: 1.25-1.68).

The WHI trial reported a risk estimate of 1.24 (95% CI: 1.01 – 1.54) after 5.6 years of use of oestrogen-progestagen combined HRT (CEE + MPA) in all users compared with placebo.

The absolute risks calculated from the MWS and the WHI trial are presented below:

The MWS has estimated, from the known average incidence of breast cancer in developed countries, that:

- For women not using HRT, about 32 in every 1000 are expected to have breast cancer diagnosed between the ages of 50 and 64 years.
- For 1000 current or recent users of HRT, the number of additional cases during the corresponding period will be:
- For users of oestrogen-only replacement therapy
  - between 0 and 3 (best estimate = 1.5) for 5 years' use
  - between 3 and 7 (best estimate = 5) for 10 years' use.
- For users of oestrogen plus progestagen combined HRT
  - between 5 and 7 (best estimate = 6) for 5 years' use
  - between 18 and 20 (best estimate = 19) for 10 years' use.

The WHI trial estimated that after 5.6 years of follow-up of women between the ages of 50 and 79 years, an additional 8 cases of invasive breast cancer would be due to oestrogen-progestagen combined HRT (CEE + MPA) per 10,000 women years.

According to calculations from the trial data, it is estimated that:

- For 1000 women in the placebo group, about 16 cases of invasive breast cancer would be diagnosed in 5 years.
- For 1000 women who used oestrogen + progestagen combined HRT (CEE + MPA), the number of additional cases would be between 0 and 9 (best estimate = 4) for 5 years' use.

The number of additional cases of breast cancer in women who use HRT is broadly similar for women who start HRT irrespective of age at start of use (between the ages of 45-65) (see section 4.4).

Endometrial cancer

In women with an intact uterus, the risk of endometrial hyperplasia and endometrial cancer increases with increasing duration of use of unopposed oestrogens. According to data from epidemiological studies, the best estimate of the risk of endometrial cancer is that for women not using HRT, about 5 in every 1000 are expected to have endometrial cancer diagnosed between the ages of 50 and 65. Depending on the duration of treatment and oestrogen dose, the reported increase in endometrial cancer risk among unopposed oestrogen users varies from 2- to 12-fold greater compared with non-users. Adding a progestagen to oestrogen-only therapy greatly reduces this increased risk.

Table 1

Organ Class	Very common > 1/10)	Common > 1/100 to < 1/10)	Uncommon > 1/1,000 to < 1/100)	Rare > 1/10,000 to 1/1,000)
Psychiatric disorders	-	Depression	-	-
Nervous system disorders	Headache	Nervousness, mood changes, insomnia	Migraine, dizziness	Paraesthesia
Vascular disorders	-	-	Increase in blood pressure	Venous thrombo-embolism
Gastro-intestinal disorders	-	Nausea, dyspepsia, diarrhoea, abdominal pain, bloating	Vomiting	Gallstones
Skin and subcutaneous tissue disorders	Application site reactions, erythema	Acne, rash, dry skin, pruritus	Skin discoloration	
Musculo-skeletal disorders	-	-	-	Myasthenia
Reproductive system and breast disorders	Breast tension and pain, dysmenorrhoea, menstrual disorders	Breast enlargement, menorrhagia, leukorrhoea, irregular vaginal bleeding, uterine spasms, vaginitis, endometrial hyperplasia		Uterine leiomyomata, paratubular cysts, endocervical polyps
General disorders	-	Pain, back pain, asthenia, peripheral oedema, weight changes	-	Libido changes, allergic reaction
Laboratory abnormalities	-	-	Transaminases increase	-

Other adverse reactions have been reported in association with oestrogen/progestagen treatment:

- Oestrogen-dependent neoplasms benign and malignant, e.g. endometrial cancer.
- Venous thromboembolism, i.e. deep leg or pelvic venous thrombosis and pulmonary embolism, is more frequent among hormone replacement therapy users than among non-users. For further information, see sections 4.3 "Contraindications" and 4.4 "Special warnings and precautions for use".
- Myocardial infarction and stroke.
- Gall bladder disease.
- Skin and subcutaneous tissue disorders: chloasma, erythema multiforme, erythema nodosum, vascular purpura.
- Probable dementia (see section 4.4).

4.9 Overdose

Acute overdose is unlikely due to the method of administration. The most common symptoms of overdose in clinical use are breast tenderness and/or vaginal bleeding. If such symptoms occur, a reduction in dosage should be considered. The effects of overdose can be rapidly reversed by removal of the patch.

5. PHARMACOLOGICAL PROPERTIES

5.1 Pharmacodynamic properties

Pharmacotherapeutic group: Oestrogens

ATC code: G03C A 03

The active substance in Estradot, synthetic 17β-estradiol, is chemically and biologically identical to endogenous human estradiol. It substitutes for the loss of oestrogen production in menopausal women and alleviates menopausal symptoms.

- *Relief of oestrogen-deficiency symptoms*

- Relief of menopausal symptoms was achieved during the first few weeks of treatment.

- *Prevention of osteoporosis (for Estradot 50, 75 and 100 only)*

- Oestrogens prevent bone loss following menopause or ovariectomy.

- Oestrogen deficiency at menopause is associated with an increasing bone turnover and decline in bone mass. The effect of oestrogens on the bone mineral density is dose-dependent.

Protection appears to be effective for as long as treatment is continued. After discontinuation of HRT, bone mass is lost at a rate similar to that in untreated women.

- Evidence from the WHI trial and meta-analysed trials show that current use of HRT, alone or in combination with a progestagen – given to predominantly healthy women – reduces the risk of hip, vertebral, and other osteoporotic fractures. HRT may also prevent fractures in women with low bone density and/or established osteoporosis, but the evidence for that is limited.

5.2 Pharmacokinetic properties

Transdermal administration of estradiol achieves therapeutic plasma concentrations using a lower total dose of estradiol than required with oral administration, whereas plasma levels of estrone and estrone conjugates are lower with the transdermal route.

Estradiol is more than 50% bound to plasma proteins such as sex hormone binding globulin and albumin. It is excreted in the urine as sulphate and glucuronide esters along with a small proportion of estradiol and several other metabolites. Only a small amount is excreted in faeces.

In studies in postmenopausal women with application of Estradot 37.5, 50, and 100 μg/24 hours patches, average peak estradiol serum levels (C_{max}) were approximately 35 pg/ml, 50-55 pg/ml and 95-105 pg/ml, respectively. Linear pharmacokinetics have been demonstrated for estradiol following transdermal administration.

Since estradiol has a short half-life (approximately one hour), serum concentrations of estradiol and estrone returned to baseline values within 24 hours following removal of the patch.

At steady state, after repeated applications of Estradot 50 μg/24 hours patches, C_{max} and C_{min} values were 57 and 28 pg/ml for estradiol and 42 and 31 pg/ml for estrone, respectively.

5.3 Preclinical safety data

The toxicity profile of estradiol is well known. There are no preclinical data of relevance to the prescriber which are additional to that already included in other sections of the SPC.

6. PHARMACEUTICAL PARTICULARS

6.1 List of excipients

Adhesive matrix:

- acrylic adhesive
- silicone adhesive
- oleyl alcohol
- dipropylene glycol
- povidone (E1201).

Backing layer:

- ethylene/vinyl acetate copolymer
- polyethylene
- vinylidene/vinyl chloride copolymer
- polyethylene
- ethylene/vinyl acetate copolymer co-extruded film.

Release liner:

- fluoropolymer-coated polyester film.

6.2 Incompatibilities

Not applicable.

6.3 Shelf life

2 years.

6.4 Special precautions for storage

Do not refrigerate or freeze.

6.5 Nature and contents of container

Each Estradot patch is individually sealed in an aluminium laminate sachet.

Sachets may be provided in cartons of 2, 8 and 24.

Not all pack sizes may be marketed.

6.6 Instructions for use and handling

No special requirements.

7. MARKETING AUTHORISATION HOLDER

Novartis Pharmaceuticals UK Limited

Frimley Business Park

Frimley

Camberley

Surrey

GU16 7SR

8. MARKETING AUTHORISATION NUMBER(S)

Estradot 25: PL 00101/0703

Estradot 37.5: PL 00101/0642

Estradot 50: PL 00101/0643

Estradot 75: PL 00101/0644

Estradot 100: PL 00101/0645

9. DATE OF FIRST AUTHORISATION/RENEWAL OF THE AUTHORISATION

Estradot 37.5 - 100: 3rd April 2002

Estradot 25: 16 September 2004

10. DATE OF REVISION OF THE TEXT

Estradot 37.5 - 100: 8 June 2004

Estradot 25: 16 September 2004

LEGAL CATEGORY

POM

Estring

(Pharmacia Limited)

1. NAME OF THE MEDICINAL PRODUCT

ESTRING vaginal ring

2. QUALITATIVE AND QUANTITATIVE COMPOSITION

Each vaginal ring contains:

Active ingredient

Estradiol Hemihydrate Ph.Eur. 2.0 mg

For excipients, see 6.1

3. PHARMACEUTICAL FORM

Estradiol vaginal ring is a slightly opaque ring, made of a silicone elastomer, with a whitish core, containing a drug reservoir of Estradiol Hemihydrate. The product has the following dimensions. Outer diameter - 55 mm; cross sectional diameter - 9 mm; core diameter - 2 mm.

4. CLINICAL PARTICULARS

4.1 Therapeutic indications

Hormone replacement therapy (HRT) for atrophic vaginitis, (due to estrogen deficiency) in postmenopausal women.

4.2 Posology and method of administration

Estring vaginal ring is an estrogen-only product for vaginal use.

Adults including the elderly

One ring to be inserted into the upper third of the vagina, to be worn continuously for 3 months, then replaced by a new ring as appropriate. For initiation and continuation of treatment of postmenopausal symptoms, the lowest effective dose for the shortest duration (See also Section 4.4) should be used. The maximum recommended duration of continuous therapy is two years.

Therapy may start at any time in women with established amenorrhoea or who are experiencing long intervals between spontaneous menses. Patients changing from a cyclical or continuous sequential preparation should complete the cycle, after a withdrawal bleed, and then change to Estring vaginal ring. Patients changing from a continuous combined preparation may start therapy at any time.

Estring vaginal ring is a local therapy and in women with an intact uterus, progestogen treatment is *not* necessary, (But see Section 4.4, Special Warnings and Precautions for Use, Endometrial Hyperplasia).

To put Estring into the vagina:

- A relaxed position must be found
- With one hand, the folds of skin around the vagina are opened.
- With the other hand, the ring is pressed into an oval.
- The ring is pushed into the vagina as far as it will go, upwards and backwards towards the small of the back.

To take out Estring

- A relaxed position must be found
- A finger is placed into the vagina and hooked around the ring.
- The ring is gently pulled out - downwards and forwards.

Comprehensive advice for removal and reinsertion of the ring are provided in the Patient Information Leaflet, which is included in every pack.

Children

Estring vaginal ring is not recommended for use in children.

4.3 Contraindications

Active or recent arterial thromboembolic disease (e.g. angina, myocardial infarction);

Known or suspected estrogen-dependent malignancy, (e.g. endometrial carcinoma)

Undiagnosed genital bleeding;

Untreated endometrial hyperplasia:

Acute liver disease, or a history of liver disease as long as liver function tests have failed to return to normal;

Porphyria;

Previous idiopathic or current venous thromboembolism (deep vein thrombosis, pulmonary embolism);

Known, past or suspected breast cancer.

Known hypersensitivity to the active substances or to any of the excipients.

4.4 Special warnings and special precautions for use

For the treatment of postmenopausal symptoms, HRT should only be initiated for symptoms that adversely affect quality of life. In all cases, a careful appraisal of the risks and benefits should be undertaken at least annually and HRT should only be continued as long as the benefit outweighs the risk

Assessment of each woman prior to taking hormone replacement therapy (and at regular intervals thereafter) should include a personal and family medical history. Physical examination should be guided by this and by the contraindications (see Section 4.3) and warnings (see Section 4.4) for this product. During assessment of each individual woman, clinical examination of the breasts and pelvic examination should be performed where clinically indicated rather than as a routine procedure. Women should be encouraged to participate in the national cervical cancer screening programme (cervical cytology) and the national breast cancer screening programme (mammography) as appropriate for their age. Breast awareness should also be encouraged and women advised to report any changes in their breasts to their doctor or nurse.

Patients on long-term corticosteroid treatment or those with conditions causing poor skin integrity, e.g Cushing's Disease, may be unsuitable for treatment as they may have vaginal atrophy unresponsive to estrogen therapy.

The pharmacokinetic profile shows that there is low systemic absorption of estradiol (see Section 5.2 Pharmacokinetic Properties), however, being a HRT product the following need to be considered, especially for long term or repeated use of this product.

Conditions which need supervision:

If any of the following conditions are present, have occurred previously, and/or have been aggravated during pregnancy or previous hormone treatment, the patient should be closely supervised. It should be taken into account that these conditions may recur or be aggravated during treatment with Estring vaginal ring, in particular:

Risk factors for estrogen dependent tumours, e.g. 1st degree heredity for breast cancer (see below)

Diabetes mellitus with or without vascular involvement

Migraine or (severe) headache

Epilepsy

A history of, or risk of factors for, thromboembolic disorders (see below)

Systemic lupus erythematosus

Liver disorders (e.g. liver adenoma)

Otosclerosis

Cholelithiasis

Leiomyoma (uterine fibroids)

Endometriosis

A history of endometrial hyperplasia (see below);

Hypertension;

Asthma.

Reasons for immediate withdrawal of therapy:

Therapy should be discontinued in case a contra-indication is discovered and in the following situations:

- Jaundice or deterioration in liver function
- ***Significant increase in blood pressure***
- New onset of migraine-type headache
- Pregnancy

Endometrial Hyperplasia

The risk of endometrial hyperplasia and carcinoma is increased when systemic estrogens are administered alone for prolonged periods of time, (See Section 4.8). The endometrial safety of long-term or repeated use of topical vaginal estrogens is uncertain. Therefore, if repeated, treatment should be reviewed at least annually, with special consideration given to any symptoms of endometrial hyperplasia or carcinoma.

If breakthrough bleeding or spotting appears at any time on therapy, the reason should be investigated, which may include endomentrial biopsy to exclude endometrial malignancy.

Unopposed estrogen stimulation may lead to premalignant or malignant transformation in the residual foci of endometriosis. Therefore, caution is advised when using this product in women who have undergone hysterectomy, because of endometriosis, especially if they are known to have residual endometriosis.

Breast Cancer

A randomised placebo-controlled trials, the Women's Health Initiative study (WHI), and epidemiological studies, including the Million Women Study (MWS), have reported an increased risk of breast cancer in women taking estrogens, estrogen-progestogen combinations or tibolone for HRT for several years (see Section 4.8). For all HRT, an excess risk becomes apparent within a few years of use and increases with duration of intake but returns to within a few (at most five) years after stopping treatment.

In the MWS, the relative risk of breast cancer with conjugated equine estrogens (CEE) or estradiol (E2) was greater when a progestogen was added, either sequentially or continuously, and regardless of type of progestogen. There was no evidence of a difference in risk between the different routes of administration.

In the WHI study, the continuous combined conjugated equine estrogen and medroxyprogesterone acetate (CEE + MPA) product used was associated with breast cancers that were slightly larger in size and more frequently had local lymph node metastases compared to placebo.

HRT, especially estrogen-progestogen combined treatment, increases the density of mammographic images which may adversely affect the radiological detection of breast cancer.

Venous Thromboembolism

HRT is associated with a higher relative risk of developing venous thromboembolism (VTE), i.e. deep vein thrombosis or pulmonary embolism. One randomised controlled trial and epidemiological studies found a two to threefold higher risk for users compared with non-users. For non-users, it is estimated that the number of cases of VTE that will occur over a 5 year period is about 3 per 1000 women aged 50-59 years and 8 per 1000 women aged between 60-69 years. It is estimated that in healthy women who use HRT for 5 years, the number of additional cases of VTE over a 5 year period will be between 2 and 6 (best estimate = 4) per 1000 women aged 50-59 years and between 5 and 15 (best estimate = 9) per 1000 women aged 60-69 years. The occurrence of such an event is more likely in the first year of HRT than later.

Generally recognised risk factors for VTE include a personal history or family history, severe obesity (BM $> 30\ kg/m^2$) and systemic lupus erythematosus (SLE). There is no consensus about the possible role of varicose veins in VTE.

Patients with a history of VTE or known thrombophilic states have an increased risk of VTE. HRT may add to this risk. Personal or strong family history of thromboembolism or recurrent spontaneous abortion should be investigated in order to exclude a thrombophilic predisposition. Until a thorough evaluation of thrombophilic factors has been made or anticoagulant treatment initiated, use of HRT in such patients should be viewed as contraindicated. Those women already on anticoagulant treatment require careful consideration of the benefit-risk of use of HRT.

The risk of VTE may be temporarily increased with prolonged immobilisation, major trauma or major surgery. As in all postoperative patients, scrupulous attention should be given to prophylactic measures to prevent VTE following surgery. Where prolonged immobilisation is liable to follow elective surgery, particularly abdominal or orthopaedic surgery to the lower limbs, consideration should be given to temporarily stopping HRT 4 to 6 weeks earlier, if possible. Treatment should not be restarted until the woman is completely mobilised.

If VTE develops after initiating therapy, the drug should be discontinued. Patients should be told to contact their doctor immediately when they are aware of a potential thromboembolic symptom (e.g. painful swelling of a leg, sudden pain in the chest, dyspnea).

Coronary Artery Disease

There is no evidence from randomised controlled trials of cardiovasular benefit with continuous combined conjugated estrogens and medroxyprogesterone acetate (MPA). Twp large clinical trials (WHI and HERS, i.e. Heart and Estrogen/progestin Replacement Study) showed a possible increased risk of cardiovascular morbidity in the first year of use and no overall benefit. For other HRT products there are only limited data from randomised controlled trials to date examining effects in cardiovascular morbidity or mortality. Therefore, it is uncertain whether these findings also extend to other HRT products.

Stroke

One large randomised clinical trial (WHI-trial) found, as a secondary outcome, an increased risk of ischaemic stroke in healthy women during treatment with continuous combined conjugated estrogens and medroxyprogesterone acetate. For women who do not use HRT, it is estimated that the number of cases of stroke that will occur over a 5 year period is about 3 per 1000 women aged 50-59 years and 11 per 1000 women aged 60-69 years. It is estimated that for women who use conjugated estrogens and medroxyprogesterone acetate for 5 years, the number of additional cases will be between 0 and 3 (best estimate = 1) per 1000 users aged 50-59 years and between 1 and 9 (best estimate = 4) per 1000 users aged 60-69 years. It is unknown whether the increased risk also extends to other HRT products.

Ovarian Cancer

Long-term (at least 5 to 10 years) use of estrogen-only HRT products in hysterectomised women has been associated with an increased risk of ovarian cancer in some epidemiological studies. It is uncertain whether long-term use of combined HRT confers a different risk than estrogen-only products.

Other Conditions

Some women may be unsuitable for treatment with Estring vaginal ring, in particular those with short narrow vaginas due to previous surgery or the effect of atrophy, or those with a degree of uterovaginal prolapse severe enough to prevent retention of the ring.

In addition, any woman with symptoms/signs of abnormal vaginal discharge, vaginal discomfort, or any vaginal bleeding should be examined fully, to exclude ulceration, infection, or unresponsive atrophic vaginitis. Minor signs of irritation are often transient.

Any woman experiencing persistent or severe discomfort due to the presence of the ring or excessive movement of the ring should be withdrawn from treatment. Patients with signs of ulceration or severe inflammation due to unresponsive atrophic vaginitis should also be withdrawn from treatment.

Patients with vaginal infection should be treated appropriately. In the case of systemic therapy, Estring vaginal ring treatment may continue without interruption. However, removal of Estring vaginal ring should be considered while using other vaginal preparations.

There have been incidences of both the ring falling out and movement of the ring, generally at defaecation. Therefore, if the woman is constipated she should remove the ring before defaecation. There may also be other instances when some women wish to remove the ring, e.g. prior to sexual intercourse.

Estrogens may cause fluid retention and therefore patients with cardiac or renal dysfunction should be carefully observed. Patients with terminal renal insufficiency should be closely observed, since it is expected that the level of circulating active ingredients in Estring vaginal ring are increased.

Women with pre-existing hypertriglyceridaemia should be followed closely during estrogen replacement or hormone replacement therapy, since rare cases of large increases of plasma triglycerides leading to pancreatitis have been reported with estrogen therapy in this condition.

Estrogens increase thyroid binding globulin (TBG), leading to increased circulating total thyroid hormone, as measured by protein-bound iodine (PBI), T4 levels (by column or by radio-immunoassay) or T3 levels (by radio-immunoassay). T3 resin uptake is decreased, reflecting the elevated TBG. Free T4 and free T3 concentrations are unaltered. Other binding proteins may be elevated in serum, i.e. corticoid binding globulin (CBG), sex-hormone-binding globulin (SHGB) leading to increased circulating corticosteroids and sex steroids, respectively. Free or biologically active hormone concentrations are unchanged. Other plasma proteins may be increased (angiotensinogen/renin substrate, alpha-1-antitrypsin, ceruloplasmin). The low systemic absorption of estradiol with vaginal administration (see Section 5.2 Pharmacokinetic Properties) may result in less pronounced effects on plasma binding proteins than with oral hormones.

There is no conclusive evidence for improvement of cognitive function. There is some evidence from the WHI trial of increased risk of probable dementia in women who start using continuous combined CEE and MPA after the age of 65. It is unknown whether the findings apply to younger post-menopausal women or other HRT products.

In rare cases benign, and in even rarer cases malignant liver tumours leading in isolated cases to life-threatening intra-abdominal haemorrhage have been observed after the use of hormonal substances such as those contained in Estring. If severe upper abdominal complaints, enlarged liver or signs of intra-abdominal haemorrhage occur, a liver tumour should be considered in the differential diagnosis.

Women who may be at risk of pregnancy should be advised to adhere to non-hormonal contraceptive methods.

The requirement for oral anti-diabetics or insulin can change as a result of the effect on glucose tolerance.

4.5 Interaction with other medicinal products and other forms of Interaction

As the estrogen is administered vaginally and due to the low levels released, it is unlikely that any clinically relevant drug interactions will occur with Estring vaginal ring.

However, the prescriber should be aware that the metabolism of estrogens may be increased by concomitant use of substances known to induce drug-metabolising enzymes, specifically cytochrome P450 enzymes, such as anticonvulsants (e.g. phenobarbital, phenytoin, carbamazepine) and anti-infectives (e.g. rifampicin, rifabutin, nevirapine, efavirenz).

Ritonavir and nelfinavir, although known as strong inhibitors, by contrast exhibit inducing properties when used concomitantly with steroid hormones. Herbal preparations containing St John's wort (Hypericum Perforatum) may induce the metabolism of estrogens.

Clinically, an increased metabolism of estrogens may lead to decreased effect and changes in the uterine bleeding profile.

Removal of Estring vaginal ring should be considered when using other vaginal preparations (See Section 4.4 Special Warnings and Precautions for Use).

4.6 Pregnancy and lactation

Pregnancy

Estring vaginal ring is not indicated during pregnancy. If pregnancy occurs during medication with Estring vaginal ring treatment should be withdrawn immediately. The results of most epidemiological studies to date relevant to inadvertent foetal exposure to estrogens indicate no teratogenic or foetotoxic effects

Lactation

Estring vaginal ring is not indicated during lactation.

4.7 Effects on ability to drive and use machines

Estring vaginal ring is unlikely to have any effect on alertness or coordination.

4.8 Undesirable effects

Adverse reactions with Estring vaginal ring are rare. Adverse reactions reported with a frequency of 1% or more in clinical trials, in order of decreasing frequency, were vaginal irritation, abdominal pain/lower abdominal pain/abdominal discomfort, vulvovaginal infection, urogenital pruritus, pressure symptoms in vagina/on bladder/on rectum, generalised pruritus, urinary tract infection and increased sweating (See Section 4.4 Special Warnings and Precautions for Use). However, some of these symptoms occur more frequently in untreated post-menopausal women, e.g. vaginal irritation, urinary tract infection, urogenital pruritus, vulvovaginal infection and increased sweating.

The following adverse reactions have been reported with estrogen therapy:

1. *Genito-urinary tract:* Endometrial neoplasia*, intermenstrual bleeding, increase in the size of uterine fibromyomata, endometrial proliferation or aggravation of endometriosis, changes in cervical eversion and excessive production of cervical mucus, thrush, vaginal ulceration;

2. *Breast:* Tenderness, pain, enlargement or secretion,; breast cancer* ‡ (uncommon)

3. *Gastro-intestinal tract*: Nausea, vomiting, abdominal cramp, bloating;

4. *Cardiovascular system*: Hypertension, thrombosis, thrombophlebitis, venous thromboembolism*, myocardial infarction* and stroke*;

5. *Liver/biliary system*: In rare cases benign, and in even rarer cases malignant liver tumours, gall bladder disease, cholelithiasis, cholestatic jaundice; aggravation of porphyria;

6. *Skin*: Chloasma which may persist when the drug is discontinued, erythema multiforme, erythema nodosum, candidal infections, vascular purpura, rash, loss of scalp hair, hirsutism;

7. *Eyes*: Steepening of corneal curvature, intolerance to contact lenses;

8. *CNS*: Headache, migraine, dizziness, mood changes (elation or depression), chorea;

9. *Miscellaneous:* Sodium and water retention, reduced glucose tolerance, change in body weight, changes in libido, muscle cramps.

* See sections 4.3, Contraindications and Section 4.4 Special Warnings and Special Precautions for Use.

Breast cancer

According to evidence from a large number of epidemiological studies and one randomised placebo-controlled trial, the Women's Health Initiative (WHI), the overall risk of breast cancer increases with increasing duration of HRT use in current or recent HRT users.

For *estrogen-only* HRT, estimates of relative risk (RR) from a reanalysis of original data from 51 epidemiological studies (in which >80% of HRT use was estrogen-only HRT) and from the epidemiological Million Women Study (MWS) are similar at 1.35 (95% CI 1.21 – 1.49) and 1.30 (95% CI 1.21 – 1.40), respectively.

For *estrogen plus progestogen* combined HRT, several epidemiological studies have reported an overall higher risk for breast cancer than with estrogens alone.

The MWS reported that, compared to never users, the use of various types of estrogen-progestogen combined HRT was associated with a higher risk of breast cancer (RR = 2.00, 95% CI: 1.88 – 2.12) than use of estrogens alone (RR = 1.30, 95% CI: 1.21 – 1.40) or use of tibolone (RR=1.45; 95%CI 1.25-1.68).

The WHI trial reported a risk estimate of 1.24 (95% CI 1.01 – 1.54) after 5.6 years of use of estrogen-progestogen combined HRT (CEE + MPA) in all users compared with placebo.

The absolute risks calculated from the MWS and the WHI trial are presented below:

The MWS has estimated, from the known average incidence of breast cancer in developed countries, that:

Ø *For women not using HRT, about 32 in every 1000 are expected to have breast cancer diagnosed between the ages of 50 and 64 years.*

Ø For 1000 current or recent users of HRT, the number of *additional* cases during the corresponding period will be

Ø For users of *estrogen-only* replacement therapy

• between 0 and 3 (best estimate = 1.5) for 5 years' use
• between 3 and 7 (best estimate = 5) for 10 years' use.

Ø For users of *estrogen plus progestogen* combined HRT,

• between 5 and 7 (best estimate = 6) for 5 years' use
• between 18 and 20 (best estimate = 19) for 10 years' use.

The WHI trial estimated that after 5.6 years of follow-up of women between the ages of 50 and 79 years, an *additional* 8 cases of invasive breast cancer would be due to *estrogen-progestogen combined* HRT (CEE + MPA) per 10,000 women years.

According to calculations from the trial data, it is estimated that:

Ø For 1000 women in the placebo group, about 16 cases of invasive breast cancer would be diagnosed in 5 years.

Ø For 1000 women who used estrogen + progestogen combined HRT (CEE + MPA), the number of *additional* cases would be between 0 and 9 (best estimate = 4) for 5 years' use.

The number of additional cases of breast cancer in women who use HRT is broadly similar for women who start HRT irrespective of age at start of use (between the ages of 45-65) (see section 4.4).

4.9 Overdose

This is not relevant due to the mode of administration.

5. PHARMACOLOGICAL PROPERTIES

5.1 Pharmacodynamic properties

Pharmacotherapeutic group: Natural and semisynthetic estrogens, plain.

ATC Code G03C A

Estring vaginal ringis a vaginal ring, which delivers approximately 7.5 μg/24 hours of 17 β-estradiol for 3 months. Estring vaginal ring is only suitable for the treatment of urogenital complaints due to estrogen deficiency. Its pharmacokinetic profile shows that it is not suitable for post-menopausal complaints which require a systemically active dose of estrogen (eg vasomotor symptoms), neither is it suitable for osteoporosis prevention.

The active ingredient, synthetic 17β-estradiol, is chemically and biologically identical to endogenous human estradiol. The estradiol from the vaginal ring substitutes for the loss of estrogen production in menopausal women, and alleviates menopausal symptoms. It acts locally to restore vaginal pH and to eliminate or reduce symptoms and signs of post-menopausal urogenital estrogen deficiency

Estring vaginal ring presumably increases local estradiol target concentrations, while maintaining very low and stable systemic plasma concentrations. The maximum duration of use during clinical trials was 2 years and, therefore, the maximum recommended duration of continuous therapy is 2 years.

5.2 Pharmacokinetic properties

After a brief initial peak, the release of estradiol from Estring vaginal ring is constant (7.5 μg/24 h), according to Fick's law, for at least 90 days. As a consequence of the initial release peak, plasma levels of estradiol reach about 200 pmol/l within 3 hours.

After this initial peak, plasma estradiol concentrations decline rapidly and constant levels are achieved after 2-3 days. These levels are maintained at, or near, the quantification limit (20-30 pmol/l) throughout the rest of the treatment period. The levels are considerably lower than the lowest levels commonly detected in pre-menopausal women, i.e during the early follicular phase.

Estradiol is mainly metabolized in the liver. Its main metabolites are estriol, estrone, and their conjugates. The plasma half life of estradiol is 1-2 hours. Metabolic plasma clearance varies between 450-625 ml/min/m^2. The metabolites are mainly excreted via the kidneys as glucuronides and sulphates. Estrogens also undergo enterohepatic circulation.

5.3 Preclinical safety data

Silicone elastomer in Estring vaginal ring

The biological safety of the silicone elastomer has been studied in various in-vitro and in-vivo test models.

The results show that the silicone elastomer was non-toxic in in-vitro studies, and non-pyrogenic, non-irritant, and non-sensitizing in short term in-vivo tests. Long-term implantation induced encapsulation equal to or less than the negative control (polyethylene) used in the prescribed USP test. No toxic reaction or further formation was observed with the silicone elastomer.

6. PHARMACEUTICAL PARTICULARS

6.1 List of excipients

Silicone elastomer Q7-4735 A, Silicone elastomer Q7-4735 B

Silicone Fluid, Barium sulphate

6.2 Incompatibilities

No incompatibilities are known.

6.3 Shelf life

Results from stability studies indicate that Estring vaginal ring is stable for at least 24 months when stored at room temperature (below 30°C).

6.4 Special precautions for storage

Keep out of the reach of children.

Do not store above 30°C.

6.5 Nature and contents of container

One ring is individually packed in a heat-sealed rectangular pouch consisting of, from outside to inside: Polyester/Aluminium foil/Low density Poly-ethylene. Each pouch is provided with a tear-off notch on one side and is packed into a cardboard carton. Each carton contains a Patient Information Leaflet.

6.6 Instructions for use and handling

Comprehensive details are provided in the Patient Information Leaflet.

Administrative Details

7. MARKETING AUTHORISATION HOLDER

Pharmacia Limited

Davy Avenue,

Milton Keynes,

MK5 8PH

UK

8. MARKETING AUTHORISATION NUMBER(S)

PL 00032/0340

9. DATE OF FIRST AUTHORISATION/RENEWAL OF THE AUTHORISATION

12 July 1994/18 October 2000

10. DATE OF REVISION OF THE TEXT

April 2004

Ref: 1_4

Ethanolamine Oleate Injection BP

(UCB Pharma Limited)

1. NAME OF THE MEDICINAL PRODUCT

Ethanolamine Oleate Injection (monoethanolamine oleate). Solution for injection.

2. QUALITATIVE AND QUANTITATIVE COMPOSITION

Oleic acid 4.23% w/v

Ethanolamine 0.910% w/v

For excipients see 6.1.

3. PHARMACEUTICAL FORM

Solution for injection.

5 ml neutral glass ampoule containing a clear solution.

4. CLINICAL PARTICULARS

4.1 Therapeutic indications

The injection is recommended for use as a sclerosing agent in the treatment of small, uncomplicated varicose veins in the lower extremities.

4.2 Posology and method of administration

Ethanolamine Oleate is administered by slow intravenous injection.

Adults Including The Elderly

The product is used only as a sclerosant and injected directly into the varicose vein. A dose of 2 to 5ml, divided between 3 or 4 sites, administered by slow injection into empty isolated segments of vein.

Children

The product is not recommended for use in children.

4.3 Contraindications

Inability to walk, acute phlebitis, oral contraceptive use, obese legs, known hypersensitivity to Ethanolamine Oleate or benzyl alcohol. Superficial thrombophlebitis and deep vein thrombosis in the region of the varicose veins. Marked arterial, cardiac or renal disease. Uncontrolled metabolic disorders such as diabetes mellitus. Patients with local or systemic infections.

4.4 Special warnings and special precautions for use

Care should be taken to ensure that the injection does not leak into perivenous tissue which could cause sloughing, ulceration and in severe cases, necrosis.

4.5 Interaction with other medicinal products and other forms of Interaction

None known.

4.6 Pregnancy and lactation

Safety during pregnancy has not been established. Use in pregnancy is not recommended.

4.7 Effects on ability to drive and use machines

None known.

4.8 Undesirable effects

Burning, cramping sensation, urticaria. Allergic reactions and anaphylaxis have been reported following use of sclerosing agents.

4.9 Overdose

Acute nephrotoxicity has been reported in two patients given 15-20ml of a solution containing 5% Ethanolamine with 2% Benzl Alcohol.

5. PHARMACOLOGICAL PROPERTIES

5.1 Pharmacodynamic properties

ATC Code: C05B B 01; sclerosing agent for local injection.

Ethanolamine Oleate is an irritant. An injection of Ethanolamine Oleate into a vein irritates the intimal endothelium resulting in the formation of a thrombus. The thrombus occludes the vein and fibrous tissue develops resulting in a permanent obliteration of the vein.

5.2 Pharmacokinetic properties

Ethanolamine Oleate is a locally acting agent. Absorption from the site of administration is not anticipated as its mode of action is to cause a permanent obstruction in the vein.

5.3 Preclinical safety data

None.

6. PHARMACEUTICAL PARTICULARS

6.1 List of excipients

Benzyl alcohol

Water for Injection

6.2 Incompatibilities

Not applicable.

6.3 Shelf life

36 months.

6.4 Special precautions for storage

Do not store above 25°C. Keep the ampoule in the outer carton.

6.5 Nature and contents of container

5 ml Neutral Glass (Type 1) Ampoules.

6.6 Instructions for use and handling

The product is used only as a sclerosant and injected directly into the varicose vein.

7. MARKETING AUTHORISATION HOLDER

UCB Pharma Limited

208 Bath Road

Slough

Berkshire

SL1 3WE

UK

8. MARKETING AUTHORISATION NUMBER(S)

PL 0039/5671R

9. DATE OF FIRST AUTHORISATION/RENEWAL OF THE AUTHORISATION

27 March 1987 / 26 May 1994 / 27 May 1999

10. DATE OF REVISION OF THE TEXT

June 2005

Ethinyloestradiol Tablets BP 10 mcg, 50 mcg, 1 mg

(UCB Pharma Limited)

1. NAME OF THE MEDICINAL PRODUCT

Ethinyloestradiol Tablets BP 10 mcg, 50mcg and 1mg

2. QUALITATIVE AND QUANTITATIVE COMPOSITION

Ethinylestradiol 10.5 mcg, 52.5mcg or 1.048mg

For excipients see 6.1.

3. PHARMACEUTICAL FORM

White uncoated tablets for oral administration

4. CLINICAL PARTICULARS

4.1 Therapeutic indications

Post menopausal symptoms due to oestrogen deficiency.

Second line therapy for prevention of osteoporosis in post-menopausal women at high risk of future fractures who are intolerant of, or contraindicated for, other medicinal products approved for the prevention of osteoporosis.

Palliative treatment of prostatic cancer.

Hormone replacement therapy for failure of ovarian development e.g. in patients with gonadal dysgenesis where initial oestrogen therapy is later followed by combined oestrogen/progestogen therapy.

Disorders of menstruation, given in conjunction with a progestogen.

4.2 Posology and method of administration

Ethinyloestradiol Tablets is an oestrogen-only preparation of hormone replacement therapy (HRT) for oral administration.

Post menopausal symptoms due to oestrogen deficiency including prevention of postmenopausal osteoporosis: the lowest dose that will control symptoms should be chosen. The usual dose range is 10 to 50 micrograms daily, usually on a cyclical basis (e.g., 3 weeks on and 1 week off).

For women without a uterus, who did not have endometriosis diagnosed, it is not recommended to add a progestogen.

In women with an intact uterus (or in endometriosis when endometrial foci may be present despite hysterectomy), where a progestogen is necessary, it should be added for at least 12-14 days every month/28 day cycle to reduce the risk to the endometrium.

The benefits of the lower risk of endometrial hyperplasia and endometrial cancer due to adding progestogen should be weighed against the increased risk of breast cancer (see sections 4.4 and 4.8).

Therapy with Ethinyloestradiol Tablets may start at any time in women with established amenorrhoea or who are experiencing long intervals between spontaneous menses. In women who are menstruating, it is advised that therapy starts on the first day of bleeding. As Ethinyloestradiol Tablets are usually taken on a cyclical basis direct switching from other oestrogen-only HRT preparations taken cyclically is possible.

HRT should only be continued as long as the benefit in alleviation of severe symptoms outweighs the risks of HRT.

Palliative treatment of prostatic cancer: 150 micrograms to 1.5 mg daily. Larger dose Ethinyloestradiol Tablets are available.

Hormone replacement therapy for failure of ovarian development e.g. in patients with gonadal dysgenesis: 10 to 50 micrograms daily, usually on a cyclical basis. Initial oestrogen therapy should be followed by combined oestrogen/progestogen therapy.

Disorders of menstruation: 20 to 50 micrograms daily from day 5 to day 25 of each cycle. A progestogen is given daily in addition, either throughout the cycle or from days 15 to 25 of the cycle.

If a dose is forgotten it should be taken as soon as it is remembered. If it is nearly time for the next dose then the patient should wait until then. Two doses should not be taken together. Forgetting a dose may increase the likelihood of break-through bleeding and spotting.

4.3 Contraindications

Active or recent arterial thromboembolic disease, e.g. angina, myocardial infarction

Current or previous idiopathic venous thromboembolism (deep venous thrombosis, pulmonary embolism)

Known, past or suspected breast cancer or other known or suspected oestrogen dependent tumours (e.g. endometrial cancer)

Untreated endometrial hyperplasia

Undiagnosed genital bleeding

Acute liver disease or a history of liver disease as long as liver function tests have failed to return to normal

Porphyria

Known hypersensitivity to the active substance or to any of the excipients

4.4 Special warnings and special precautions for use

Medical examination/follow-up

Before initiating or reinstituting HRT, a complete personal and family medical history should be taken. Physical (including pelvic and breast) examination should be guided by this and by the contraindications and warnings for use. During treatment, periodic check-ups are recommended of a frequency and nature adapted to the individual woman. Women should be advised what changes in their breasts should be reported to their doctor or nurse (see 'Breast cancer' below). Investigation, including mammography, should be carried out in accordance with currently accepted screening practices, modified to the clinical needs of the individual. A careful appraisal of the risks and benefits should be undertaken at least annually in women treated with hormone replacement therapy.

In women with an intact uterus, the benefits of the lower risk of endometrial hyperplasia and endometrial cancer due to adding a progestogen should be weighed against the increased risk of breast cancer (see below and Section 4.8).

Conditions which need supervision

If any of the following conditions are present, have occurred previously, and/or have been aggravated during pregnancy or previous hormone treatment, the patient should be closely supervised. It should be taken into account that these conditions may recur or be aggravated during treatment with ethinyloestradiol tablets, in particular:

Risk factors for oestrogen dependent tumours e.g. 1st degree heredity for breast cancer

Leimyoma (uterine fibroids) or endometriosis

A history of, or risk factors for, thromboembolic disorders (see below)

Hypertension

Liver disorders (e.g. liver adenoma)

Diabetes Mellitus with or without vascular involvement

Cholelithiasis

Otosclerosis

Asthma

Migraine or (severe) headache and epilepsy

Systemic Lupus erythematosis

Hyperplasia of the endometrium (see below)

Reasons for immediate withdrawal of therapy

Jaundice or deterioration in liver function

Significant increase in blood pressure

New onset of migraine-type headache

Pregnancy

Endometrial hyperplasia

The risk of endometrial hyperplasia and carcinoma is increased when oestrogens are administered alone for prolonged periods. The addition of a progestogen for at least 12 days of the cycle in non-hysterectomised women reduces, but may not eliminate, this risk (see section 4.8).

The reduction in risk to the endometrium should be weighed against the increase in the risk of breast cancer of added progestogen (see 'Breast cancer' below and in Section 4.8)

Break-through bleeding and spotting may occur during the first months of treatment. If break-through bleeding or spotting appears after some time on therapy, or continues after treatment has been discontinued, the reason should be investigated, which may include endometrial biopsy to exclude endometrial malignancy.

Unopposed oestrogen stimulation may lead to premalignant or malignant transformation in the residual foci of endometriosis. Therefore, the addition of progestogens to oestrogen replacement therapy should be considered in women who have undergone hysterectomy because of endometriosis, especially if they are known to have residual endometriosis (but see above).

Breast cancer

Randomised controlled trials and epidemiological studies have reported an increased risk of breast cancer in women taking oestrogens or oestrogen-progestogen combinations for HRT for several years (see section 4.8). An observational study of almost 829,000 women has shown that, compared to never-users, use of oestrogen-progestogen combined HRT is associated with a higher risk of breast cancer (RR = 2.00, 95%CI: 1.88 – 2.12) than use of oestrogens alone (RR = 1.30, 95%CI: 1.21 - 1.40). In this study the magnitude of the increase in breast cancer risk was similar for all oestrogen-only preparations, irrespective of the type, dose or route of administration of the oestrogen (oral, transdermal and implanted). Likewise the magnitude of the increased risk was similar for all oestrogen plus progestogen preparations, irrespective of the type of progestogen or the number of days of addition per cycle. For all HRT, an excess risk becomes apparent within 1-2 years of starting treatment and increases with duration of use of HRT but begins to decline when HRT is stopped and by 5 years reaches the same level as in women who have never taken HRT.

The increase in risk applies to all women studied, although the relative risk was significantly higher in those with a lean or normal body build (body mass index or BMI of < 25kg/m2) compared to those with a BMI of ≥25kg/m2.

At present the effect of HRT on the diagnosis of breast tumours remains unclear – all women should be encouraged to report any changes in their breasts to their doctor or nurse.

Ovarian Cancer

Long-term (at least 5 to 10 years) use of oestrogen-only HRT products in hysterectomised women has been associated with an increased risk of ovarian cancer in some epidemiological studies. It is uncertain whether long-term use of combined HRT confers a different risk than oestrogen-only products.

Venous thromboembolism

HRT is associated with a higher relative risk of developing venous thromboembolism (VTE), i.e. deep vein thrombosis or pulmonary embolism. One randomised controlled trial and epidemiological studies found a two- to three fold higher risk for users compared with non-users. For non-users, it is estimated that the number of cases of VTE that will occur over a 5 year period is about 3 per 1000 women aged 50 – 59 years and 8 per 1000 women aged between 60 – 69 years. It is estimated that in healthy women who use HRT for 5 years, the number of additional cases of VTE over a 5 year period will be between 2 and 6 (best estimate = 4) per 1000 women aged 50 – 59 years and between 5 and 15 (best estimate = 9) per 1000 women aged 60 – 69 years. The occurrence of such an event is more likely in the first year of HRT than later.

Generally recognised risk factors for VTE include a personal history or family history, severe obesity (BMI> 30 kg/m2) and systemic lupus erythematosus (SLE). There is no consensus about the possible role of varicose veins in VTE.

Patients with a history of VTE or known thrombophilic states have an increased risk of VTE. HRT may add further to this risk. Personal or strong family history of recurrent thromboembolism or recurrent spontaneous abortion, should be investigated in order to exclude a thrombophilic predisposition. Until a thorough evaluation of thrombophilic factors has been made or anticoagulant treatment initiated, use of HRT in such patients should be viewed as contraindicated. Those women already on anticoagulant treatment require careful consideration of the benefit-risk of use of HRT.

The risk of VTE may be temporarily increased with prolonged immobilisation, major trauma or major surgery. As in all postoperative patients, scrupulous attention should be given to prophylactic measures to prevent VTE following surgery. Where prolonged immobilisation is liable to follow elective surgery, particularly abdominal or orthopaedic surgery to the lower limbs, consideration should be given to temporarily stopping HRT 4 to 6 weeks earlier, if possible. Treatment should not be restarted until the woman is completely mobilised.

If VTE develops after initiating therapy, the drug should be discontinued. Patients should be told to contact their doctors immediately when they are aware of a potential thromboembolic symptom (e.g., painful swelling of a leg, sudden pain in the chest, dyspnoea).

Stroke

One large randomised clinical trial (WHI-trial) found, as a secondary outcome, an increased risk of stroke in healthy women during treatment with continuous combined conjugated oestrogens and medroxyprogesterone acetate (MPA). For women who do not use HRT, it is estimated that the number of cases of stroke that will occur over a 5 year period is about 3 per 1000 women aged 50 – 59 years and 11 per 1000 women aged 60 – 69 years. It is estimated that for women who use conjugated oestrogens and MPA for 5 years, the number of additional cases will be between 0 and 3 (best estimate = 1) per 1000 users aged 50 – 59 years and between 1 and 9 (best estimate = 4) per 1000 users aged 60 – 69 years. It is unknown whether the increased risk also extends to other HRT products.

Coronary Artery Disease (CAD)

There is no evidence from randomised controlled trials of cardiovascular benefit with continuous combined conjugated oestrogens and MPA. Large clinical trials showed a possible increased risk of cardiovascular morbidity in the first year of use and no benefit thereafter. For other HRT products there are as yet no randomised controlled trials to date examining benefit in cardiovascular morbidity or mortality. Therefore, it is uncertain whether these findings also extend to other HRT products.

Other conditions

Oestrogens may cause fluid retention, and therefore patients with cardiac or renal dysfunction should be carefully observed. Patients with terminal renal insufficiency should be closely observed, since it is expected that the level of circulating active ingredients in Ethinyloestradiol Tablets is increased.

Women with pre-existing hypertriglyceridemia should be followed closely during oestrogen replacement or hormone replacement therapy, since rare cases of large increases of plasma triglycerides leading to pancreatitis have been reported with oestrogen therapy in this condition.

Oestrogens increase thyroid binding globulin (TBG), leading to increased circulating total thyroid hormone, as measured by protein-bound iodine (PBI), T4 levels (by column or by radio-immunoassay) or T3 levels (by radio-immunoassay). T3 resin uptake is decreased, reflecting the elevated TBG. Free T4 and free T3 concentrations are unaltered. Other binding proteins may be elevated in serum, i.e. corticoid binding globulin (CBG), sex-hormone-binding globulin (SHBG) leading to increased circulating corticosteroids and sex steroids, respectively. Free or biological active hormone concentrations are unchanged. Other plasma proteins may be increased (angiotensinogen/renin substrate, alpha-I-antitrypsin, ceruloplasmin).

Patients with rare hereditary problems of galactose intolerance, the Lapp-lactose deficiency, or glucose-galactose malabsorption should not take this medicine.

4.5 Interaction with other medicinal products and other forms of Interaction

The metabolism of oestrogens may be increased by concomitant use of substances known to induce drug metabolising enzymes, specifically cytochrome P450 enzymes, such as anti-convulsants (e.g. phenobarbitol, phenytoin, carbamazepine) and anti-infectives (e.g. rifampicin, rifabutin, nevirapine, efavirenz).

Ritonavir and nelfinavir, although known as strong inhibitors, by contrast exhibit inducing properties when used concomitantly with steroid hormones. Herbal preparations containing St Johns Wort (Hypericum Perforatum) may induce the metabolism of oestrogens.

Clinically, an increased metabolism of oestrogens may lead to decreased effect and changes in the uterine bleeding profile.

Ethinyloestradiol doses greater than 50 micrograms per day may cause imipramine toxicity in patients on concomitant therapy.

Through its effects on the coagulation system, ethinyloestradiol may reduce the effects of anticoagulants such as warfarin, phenindione or nicoumalone.

The doses of insulin or hypoglycaemic drugs may need to be adjusted due to the mild diabetogenic effect of ethinyloestradiol.

Ethinyloestradiol may inhibit the metabolism of theophylline and reduce its clearance.

4.6 Pregnancy and lactation

Ethinyloestradiol Tablets are not indicated during pregnancy. If pregnancy occurs during medication with Ethinyloestradiol Tablets treatment should be withdrawn immediately. The results of most epidemiological studies to date relevant to inadvertent fetal exposure to oestrogens indicate no teratogenic or fetotoxic effects.

Ethinyloestradiol Tablets are not indicated during lactation.

4.7 Effects on ability to drive and use machines

None stated

4.8 Undesirable effects

Breast cancer

The risk of breast cancer increases with the number of years of HRT usage. According to data from a recent epidemiological study in about 829,000 postmenopausal women, the best estimate of the risk is that for women not using HRT, in total about 32 in every 1000 are expected to have breast cancer diagnosed between the ages of 50 and 65 years. Among those with current or recent use of oestrogen-only replacement therapy, it is estimated that the total number of additional cases during the corresponding period will be between 0 and 3 (best estimate = 1.5) per 1000 for 5 years' use and between 3 and 7 (best estimate = 5) per 1000 for 10 years' use (see table) Among those with current or recent use of oestrogen plus progestogen combined HRT, it is estimated that the total number of additional cases will be between 5 and 7 (best estimate = 6) per 1000 for 5 years' use and between 18 and 20 (best estimate = 19) per 1000 for 10 years' use (see section 4.4). The number of additional cases of breast cancer is broadly similar for women who start HRT irrespective of age at start of HRT use (between the ages of 45 and 65).

	No of additional cases of breast cancer diagnosed per 1000 users (95% confidence intervals)	
Type of HRT	5 years of use	10 years of use
Oestrogen-only	1.5 (0 – 3)	5 (3 – 7)
Combined	6 (5 – 7)	19 (18 – 20)

Endometrial cancer

In women with an intact uterus, the risk of endometrial hyperplasia and endometrial cancer increases with increasing duration of use of unopposed oestrogens and is substantially reduced by the addition of a progestogen (see section 4.4). According to the data from epidemiological studies, the best estimate of the risk of endometrial cancer is that for women not using HRT, about 5 in every 1000 are expected to have endometrial cancer diagnosed between the ages of 50 and 65. It is estimated that, among those who use oestrogen-only replacement therapy, there will be 4 additional cases per 1000 after 5 years' use and 10 additional cases per 1000 after 10 years' use. Adding a progestogen to oestrogen-only therapy substantially reduces, but may not eliminate, this increased risk.

Other adverse reactions have been reported in association with oestrogen treatment;

Genito-urinary tract: endometrial neoplasia, endometrial cancer, intermenstrual bleeding, increase in the size of uterine fibromyomata, endometrial proliferation or aggravation of endometriosis, excessive production of cervical mucus.

Breast: tenderness, pain, enlargement, secretion.

Gastro-intestinal tract: nausea, vomiting, cholelithiasis, cholestatic jaundice.

Cardiovascular system: hypertension, thrombosis, thrombophlebitis, thromboembolism, myocardial infarction, stroke.

Venous thromboembolism, i.e. deep leg or pelvic venous thrombosis and pulmonary embolism, is more frequent among hormone replacement therapy users than among non-users. For further information, see section 4.3 Contraindications and 4.4 Special warnings and precautions for use.

Skin: erythema nodosum, erythema multiforme, vascular purpura, rash, chloasma.

Eyes: corneal discomfort if contact lenses are used.

CNS: headache, migraine, mood changes (elation or depression).

Metabolic: sodium and water retention, reduced glucose tolerance and change in body weight, hypercalcaemia.

In men: feminisation, gynaecomastia, testicular atrophy and impotence.

4.9 Overdose

Acute overdose of ethinyloestradiol may cause nausea and vomiting and may result in withdrawal bleeding in females.

5. PHARMACOLOGICAL PROPERTIES

5.1 Pharmacodynamic properties

Oestrogen deficiency at menopause is associated with an increasing bone turnover and decline in bone mass. Therefore, if possible, treatment for prevention of osteoporosis should start as soon as possible after the onset of menopause in women with increased risk for future osteoporotic fractures. The effect of oestrogens on the bone mineral density is dose-dependent. Protection appears to be effective for as long as treatment is continued.

The active ingredient, ethinyloestradiol, is chemically and biologically identical to endogenous human oestradiol. It substitutes for the loss of oestrogen production in menopausal women, and alleviates menopausal symptoms. Oestrogens prevent bone loss following menopause or ovariectomy.

The main therapeutic use of exogenous oestrogens is replacement in deficiency states.

5.2 Pharmacokinetic properties

Ethinyloestradiol is rapidly and completely absorbed from the gut but it undergoes some first pass metabolism in the gut wall.

Ethinyloestradiol is rapidly distributed throughout most body tissues with the largest concentration found in adipose tissue. It distributes into breast milk in low concentrations. More than 80% of ethinyloestradiol in serum is conjugated as the sulphate and almost all the conjugated form is bound to albumin.

Ethinyloestradiol is metabolised in the liver. Hydroxylation appears to be the main metabolic pathway. 60% of a dose is excreted in the urine and 40% in the faeces. About 30% is excreted in the urine and bile as the glucuronide or sulphate conjugate.

The rate of metabolism of ethinyloestradiol is affected by several factors, including enzyme-inducing agents, antibiotics and cigarette smoking.

After oral administration, an initial peak occurs in plasma at 2 to 3 hours, with a secondary peak at about 12 hours after dosing; the second peak is interpreted as evidence for extensive enterohepatic circulation of ethinyloestradiol.

The elimination half-life of ethinyloestradiol ranges from 5 to 16 hours.

5.3 Preclinical safety data

None stated

6. PHARMACEUTICAL PARTICULARS

6.1 List of excipients

Lactose

Starch Maize

Magnesium Stearate

IMS 99%

Purified water

6.2 Incompatibilities

None stated

6.3 Shelf life

36 months

6.4 Special precautions for storage

Store below 25° C

6.5 Nature and contents of container

Pigmented polypropylene container fitted with a tamper evident closure containing 21, 28, 100, or 500 tablets. All pack sizes may not be marketed.

6.6 Instructions for use and handling

Not applicable

7. MARKETING AUTHORISATION HOLDER

UCB Pharma Ltd

208 Bath Road

Slough

Berkshire

SL1 3WE

8. MARKETING AUTHORISATION NUMBER(S)

10mcg: PL 00039/0548

50mcg: PL 00039/0549

1mg: PL 00039/0550

9. DATE OF FIRST AUTHORISATION/RENEWAL OF THE AUTHORISATION

4 July 2005

10. DATE OF REVISION OF THE TEXT

July 2005

Etopophos Injection

(Bristol-Myers Squibb Pharmaceuticals Ltd)

1. NAME OF THE MEDICINAL PRODUCT

ETOPOPHOS INJECTION

2. QUALITATIVE AND QUANTITATIVE COMPOSITION

Each vial contains 113.6 mg etoposide phosphate (equivalent to 100 mg etoposide).

3. PHARMACEUTICAL FORM

Lyophilised powder for injection.

4. CLINICAL PARTICULARS

4.1 Therapeutic indications

Etopophos is an anti-neoplastic drug for intravenous use, which can be used alone or in combination with other cytotoxic drugs.

Present data indicate that Etopophos is applicable in the therapy of: small cell lung cancer, resistant non-seminomatous testicular carcinoma.

4.2 Posology and method of administration

Etopophos should be administered by individuals experienced in the use of anti-neoplastic therapy.

The recommended course of Etopophos Injection is 60-120 mg/m^2, (etoposide equivalent) i.v daily for five consecutive days. As Etopophos produces myelosuppression, courses should not be repeated more frequently than at 21 day intervals. In any case, repeat courses of Etopophos should not be given until the blood picture has been checked for evidence of myelosuppression and found to be satisfactory.

When used as part of combination therapy, the dosage should be reduced toward the lower end of the dosage range to take into account the myelosuppressive effects of radiation therapy or chemotherapy which may have compromised bone marrow reserve.

Immediately prior to administration, the content of each vial must be reconstituted with either 5 ml or 10 ml Water for Injections B.P., 5% Glucose Intravenous Infusion B.P. or 0.9% Sodium Chloride Intravenous Infusion B.P. to a concentration equivalent to 20 mg/ml or 10 mg/ml etoposide (22.7 mg/ml or 11.4 mg/ml etoposide phosphate) respectively. Following reconstitution the solution may be administered without further dilution or it can be further diluted to concentrations as low as 0.1 mg/ml etoposide (0.14 mg/ml etoposide phosphate) with either 5% Glucose Intravenous Infusion B.P. or 0.9% Sodium Chloride Intravenous Infusion B.P.

Etopophos solutions may be infused over 5 minutes to 3.5 hours.

Care should be taken to avoid extravasation. Occasionally following extravasation of etoposide, soft tissue irritation and inflammation has occurred, ulceration was generally not seen.

<u>Elderly:</u>

No dosage adjustment is necessary.

<u>Paediatric use:</u>

Safety and effectiveness in children have not been established. Until further data are available, Etopophos should not be given to children under 12 years of age.

4.3 Contraindications

Etopophos is contra-indicated in patients with severe hepatic dysfunction or in those patients who have demonstrated hypersensitivity to etoposide, etoposide phosphate or any other component of the formulation.

4.4 Special warnings and special precautions for use

Since etoposide phosphate is rapidly and completely converted to etoposide, the WARNINGS and PRECAUTIONS that are considered when prescribing etoposide should be considered when prescribing Etopophos.

When Etopophos is administered intravenously care should be taken to avoid extravasation.

If radiotherapy and/or chemotherapy has been given prior to starting Etopophos treatment, an adequate interval should be allowed to enable the bone marrow to recover. If the leucocyte count falls below 2,000/mm^3, treatment should be suspended until the circulating blood elements have returned to acceptable levels (platelets above 100,000/mm^3, leucocytes above 4,000/mm^3), this is usually within 10 days.

Peripheral blood counts and liver function should be monitored. (See Undesirable Effects.)

Bacterial infections should be brought under control before treatment with Etopophos commences.

No data are available on the use of Etopophos in patients with renal and hepatic impairment.

The occurrence of acute leukaemia, which can occur with or without myelodysplasia has been reported rarely in patients treated with etoposide containing regimens.

4.5 Interaction with other medicinal products and other forms of Interaction

Caution should be exercised when administering Etopophos with drugs that are known to inhibit phosphatase activities (e.g., levamisole hydrochloride). High dose cyclosporin (resulting in concentrations >2000 ng/ml) administered with oral etoposide has led to an 80% increase in etoposide exposure (AUC) with a 38% decrease in total body clearance of etoposide, compared to etoposide alone.

In children, elevated SGPT levels are associated with reduced drug total body clearance. Prior use of cisplatin may also result in a decrease of etoposide total body clearance in children.

4.6 Pregnancy and lactation

Etopophos can cause foetal harm when administered to pregnant women. Etoposide is teratogenic in rats and mice at dose levels equivalent to those employed clinically and it is therefore assumed that Etopophos is also teratogenic in humans. There are no adequate and well-controlled studies in pregnant women.

Women of childbearing potential should be advised to avoid becoming pregnant. If Etopophos is used during pregnancy, or if the patient becomes pregnant while receiving this product, the patient should be appraised of the potential hazard to the foetus.

The influence of etoposide on human reproduction has not been determined (see 5.3 Preclinical Safety Data).

It is not known whether Etopophos is excreted in human milk. Because many drugs are excreted in human milk and because of the potential for serious adverse reactions in nursing infants from Etopophos, a decision should be made whether to discontinue nursing or to discontinue Etopophos, taking into account the importance of Etopophos to the mother.

4.7 Effects on ability to drive and use machines

None.

4.8 Undesirable effects

In clinical studies with Etopophos the most frequent clinically significant adverse experiences were leucopenia and neutropenia which occurred in almost all patients. The leucopenia was severe in approximately 20% of the patients, with neutropenia severe in about one third. Thrombocytopenia was reported in about a quarter of the patients and was severe in about 10% of the cases. Anaemia was observed in about three quarters of the patients and was severe in about 20%. Gastrointestinal adverse events were usually mild to moderate. Nausea and/or vomiting was seen in about a third of the patients. Anorexia and mucositis was reported by 10-20% of the patients and constipation, abdominal pain, diarrhoea and taste alteration was seen in between 5 to 10%. Asthenia or malaise affected about a third of the patients. Alopecia was also observed in a third of the patients. Chills and/or fever were reported in a quarter of the patients, dizziness and extravasation/phlebitis in about 5% of the patients. No cardiovascular symptoms including hypotension, have been observed during administration of 5 minute infusions of Etopophos.

Since etoposide phosphate is converted to etoposide, the adverse experiences reported below that are associated with etoposide may occur with Etopophos.

The following data on adverse reactions are based on both oral and intravenous administration of etoposide.

<u>Haematological:</u>

The dose limiting toxicity of etoposide is myelosuppression, predominantly leucopenia and thrombocytopenia. Anaemia occurs infrequently.

The leucocyte count nadir occurs approximately 21 days after treatment.

<u>Alopecia:</u>

Alopecia occurs in approximately two-thirds of patients and is reversible on cessation of therapy.

<u>Gastrointestinal:</u>

Nausea and vomiting are the major gastrointestinal toxicities and occur in over one-third of patients. Anti-emetics are useful in controlling these side effects. Abdominal pain, anorexia, diarrhoea, oesophagitis and stomatitis occur infrequently.

<u>Other Toxicities:</u>

Hypotension may occur following an excessively rapid infusion of etoposide and may be reversed by slowing the infusion rate. Symptomatic hypotension has not been seen with Etopophos.

Anaphylactoid reactions have been reported following administration of etoposide. Higher rates of anaphylactoid reactions have been reported in children who received infusions at concentrations higher than those recommended. The role that concentration of infusion (or rate of infusion) plays in the development of anaphylactoid reactions is uncertain. These reactions have usually responded to cessation of therapy and administration of pressor agents, corticosteroids, antihistamines or volume expanders as appropriate.

Apnoea with spontaneous resumption of breathing following discontinuation of etoposide injection has been reported. Sudden fatal reactions associated with bronchospasm have been reported. Hypertension and/or flushing have also been reported. Blood pressure usually returns to normal within a few hours after cessation of the infusion.

The use of etoposide has been reported infrequently to cause peripheral neuropathy.

Etoposide has been shown to reach high concentrations in the liver and kidney, thus presenting a potential for accumulation in cases of functional impairment.

Somnolence, fatigue, aftertaste, fever, rash, pigmentation, pruritus, urticaria, dysphagia, transient cortical blindness and a single case of radiation recall dermatitis have also been reported following the administration of etoposide.

4.9 Overdose

Total etoposide doses of 2.4 g/m^2 to 3.5 g/m^2 administered intravenously over three days have resulted in severe mucositis and myelotoxicity. Metabolic acidosis and cases of severe hepatic toxicity have been reported in patients receiving higher than recommended doses of etoposide.

No proven antidotes have been established for Etopophos overdosage. Treatment should therefore be symptomatic and supportive.

5. PHARMACOLOGICAL PROPERTIES

5.1 Pharmacodynamic properties

Etoposide phosphate is converted *in vivo* to the active moiety, etoposide, by dephosphorylation. The mechanism of action of etoposide phosphate is believed to be the same as that of etoposide.

Etoposide is a semi-synthetic derivative of podophyllotoxin. Experimental data indicate that etoposide arrests the cell cycle in the G^2 phase. Etoposide differs from the vinca alkaloids in that it does not cause an accumulation of cells in metaphase, but prevents cells from entering mitosis or destroys cells in the G^2 phase. The incorporation of thymidine into DNA is inhibited *in vitro* by etoposide.

5.2 Pharmacokinetic properties

Following intravenous administration of Etopophos, etoposide phosphate is rapidly and completely converted to etoposide in plasma. A direct comparison of the pharmacokinetic parameters (AUC and C_{MAX}) of etoposide following intravenous administration of molar equivalent doses of Etopophos and etoposide was made in two randomised cross-over studies in patients. Results from both studies demonstrated no statistically significant differences in the AUC and C_{MAX} for etoposide when administered as Etopophos or etoposide. In addition, there were no statistically significant differences in the pharmacodynamic parameters (haematologic toxicity) after administration of Etopophos or etoposide. Because of the pharmacokinetic and pharmacodynamic bioequeivalence of Etopophos to etoposide, the following information on etoposide should be considered.

In vitro, etoposide is highly protein bound (97%) to human plasma proteins. In a study of the effects of other therapeutic agents on *in vitro* binding of ^{14}C etoposide to human serum proteins, only sodium salicylate, and aspirin displaced protein-bound etoposide at concentrations generally achieved *in vivo.* Plasma decay kinetics follow a bi-exponential curve and correspond to a two compartmental model. The mean volume of distribution is approximately 32% of body weight. Etoposide demonstrates relatively poor penetration into the cerebrospinal fluid. Urinary excretion is approximately 45% of an administered dose, 29% being excreted unchanged in 72 hours.

Etoposide is cleared by both renal metabolism and biliary excretion. Patients with impaired renal function receiving etoposide have exhibited reduced total body clearance, increased AUC and lower steady state volume of distribution.

5.3 Preclinical safety data

The carcinogenic potential of Etopophos has not been studied. However, based upon its pharmacodynamic mechanism of action, Etopophos is a potential carcinogenic and genotoxic agent. Etoposide has been shown to be mutagenic in mammalian cells and Etopophos is expected to have similar mutagenic effects.

6. PHARMACEUTICAL PARTICULARS

6.1 List of excipients

Dextran 40, sodium citrate dihydrate.

6.2 Incompatibilities

Etopophos should not be physically mixed with any other drug.

6.3 Shelf life

18 months.

6.4 Special precautions for storage

Store between 2-8°C. Protect from light.

6.5 Nature and contents of container

20ml flint glass type I vial with a butyl rubber stopper and flip-off aluminium seal.

6.6 Instructions for use and handling

Immediately prior to administration, the content of each vial must be reconstituted with either 5 ml or 10 ml Water for Injection B.P., 5% Glucose Intravenous Infusion B.P. or 0.9% Sodium Chloride Intravenous Infusion BP to a concentration equivalent to 20 mg/ml or 10 mg/ml etoposide (22.7 mg/ml or 11.4 mg/ml etoposide phosphate), respectively. Following reconstitution the solution may be administered without further dilution or it can be further diluted to concentrations as low as 0.1 mg/mL etoposide (0.14 mg/ml etoposide phosphate) with either 5% Glucose Intravenous Infusion BP or 0.9% Sodium Chloride Intravenous Infusion BP.

When reconstituted and/or diluted as directed Etopophos solutions are chemically and physically stable for 48 hours at 37°C, 96 hours at 25°C and 7 days under refrigeration (2-8°C) under normal room fluorescent light in both glass and plastic containers. For microbiological reasons, the product should be stored for not more than 8 hours at room temperature or 24 hours in a refrigerator. Solutions of Etopophos should be prepared in an aseptic manner.

Etopophos should not be physically mixed with any other drug.

<u>Guidelines for the safe handling of anti-neoplastic agents</u>:

1. Trained personnel should reconstitute the drug.
2. This should be performed in a designated area.
3. Adequate protective gloves should be worn.
4. Precautions should be taken to avoid the drug accidentally coming into contact with the eyes. In the event of contact with the eyes, irrigate with large amounts of water and/or saline.
5. The cytotoxic preparation should not be handled by pregnant staff.
6. Adequate care and precautions should be taken in the disposal of items (syringes, needles etc) used to reconstitute cytotoxic drugs. Excess material and body waste may be disposed of by placing in double sealed polythene bags and incinerating at a temperature of 1,000°C. Liquid waste may be flushed with copious amounts of water.
7. The work surface should be covered with disposable plastic backed absorbent paper.
8. Use Luer-Lock fittings on all syringes and sets. Large bore needles are recommended to minimise pressure and the possible formation of aerosols. The latter may also be reduced by the use of a venting needle.

7. MARKETING AUTHORISATION HOLDER

Bristol-Myers Squibb Pharmaceuticals Limited
Uxbridge Business Park,
Sanderson Road,
Uxbridge,
Middlesex UB8 1DH

8. MARKETING AUTHORISATION NUMBER(S)

PL 11184/0052

9. DATE OF FIRST AUTHORISATION/RENEWAL OF THE AUTHORISATION

23rd May 1996

10. DATE OF REVISION OF THE TEXT

June 2005

Eucardic

(Roche Products Limited)

1. NAME OF THE MEDICINAL PRODUCT

Eucardic▼ 3.125
Eucardic▼ 6.25
Eucardic▼ 12.5
Eucardic▼ 25

2. QUALITATIVE AND QUANTITATIVE COMPOSITION

Each Eucardic 3.125 tablet contains 3.125mg carvedilol.

Each Eucardic 6.25 tablet contains 6.25mg carvedilol.

Each Eucardic 12.5 tablet contains 12.5mg carvedilol.

Each Eucardic 25 tablet contains 25mg carvedilol.

3. PHARMACEUTICAL FORM

Tablet for oral use.

4. CLINICAL PARTICULARS

4.1 Therapeutic indications

Symptomatic chronic heart failure (CHF)

Eucardic is indicated for the treatment of stable mild, moderate and severe chronic heart failure as adjunct to standard therapies e.g. diuretics, digoxin, and ACE inhibitors in patients with euvolemia.

Hypertension

Eucardic is indicated for the treatment of hypertension.

Angina

Eucardic is indicated for the prophylactic treatment of stable angina.

4.2 Posology and method of administration

The tablets should be taken with fluid. For CHF patients Eucardic should be given with food.

Symptomatic chronic heart failure

Initiation of therapy with Eucardic should only be under the supervision of a hospital physician, following a thorough assessment of the patient's condition.

Prior to any subsequent titration of the dose, the patient must be clinically evaluated on the day of up-titration by a health-care professional experienced in the management of heart failure to ensure that the clinical status has remained stable. The dose of carvedilol should not be increased in any patient with deteriorating heart failure since last visit or with signs of decompensated or unstable chronic heart failure.

The dosage must be titrated to individual requirements.

For those patients receiving diuretics and/or digoxin and/or ACE inhibitors, dosing of these other drugs should be stabilised prior to initiation of Eucardic treatment.

Adults

The recommended dose for the initiation of therapy is 3.125mg twice a day for two weeks. If this dose is tolerated, the dosage should be increased subsequently, at intervals of not less than two weeks, to 6.25mg twice daily, followed by 12.5mg twice daily and thereafter 25mg twice daily. Dosing should be increased to the highest level tolerated by the patient.

The recommended maximum daily dose is 25mg given twice daily for all patients with severe CHF and for patients with mild to moderate CHF weighing less than 85kg (187lbs). In patients with mild or moderate CHF weighing more than 85kg, the recommended maximum dose is 50mg twice daily.

During up-titration of the dose in patients with systolic blood pressure < 100mmHg, deterioration of renal and/or cardiac functions may occur. Therefore, before each dose increase these patients should be evaluated by the physician for renal function and symptoms of worsening heart failure or vasodilation. Transient worsening of heart failure, vasodilation or fluid retention may be treated by adjusting doses of diuretics or ACE inhibitors or by modifying or temporarily discontinuing Eucardic treatment. Under these circumstances, the dose of Eucardic should not be increased until symptoms of worsening heart failure or vasodilation have been stabilised.

If Eucardic is discontinued for more than two weeks, therapy should be recommenced at 3.125mg twice daily and up-titrated in line with the above dosing recommendation.

Elderly

As for adults.

Children

Safety and efficacy in children (under 18 years) has not been established.

Hypertension

Once daily dosing is recommended.

Adults

The recommended dose for initiation of therapy is 12.5mg once a day for the first two days. Thereafter the recommended dosage is 25mg once a day. Although this is an adequate dose in most patients, if necessary the dose may be titrated up to a recommended daily maximum dose of 50mg given once a day or in divided doses.

Dose titration should occur at intervals of at least two weeks.

Elderly

An initial dose of 12.5mg daily is recommended. This has provided satisfactory control in some cases. If the response is inadequate the dose may be titrated up to the recommended daily maximum dose of 50mg given once a day or in divided doses.

Children

Safety and efficacy in children (under 18 years) has not been established.

Angina

Adults

The recommended dose for initiation of therapy is 12.5mg twice a day for the first two days. Thereafter, the recommended dosage is 25mg twice a day.

Elderly

The recommended maximum daily dose is 50mg given in divided doses.

Children

Safety and efficacy in children (under 18 years) has not been established.

Patients with co-existing hepatic disease

Eucardic is contra-indicated in patients with hepatic dysfunction (see sections *4.3 Contra-indications* and *5.2 Pharmacokinetic properties*).

Patients with co-existing renal dysfunction

No dose adjustment is anticipated as long as systolic blood pressure is above 100mmHg (see also sections *4.4 Special warnings and precautions for use* and *5.2 Pharmacokinetic properties*).

4.3 Contraindications

Eucardic is contra-indicated in patients with marked fluid retention or overload requiring intravenous inotropic support.

Patients with obstructive airways disease, liver dysfunction, hypersensitivity to carvedilol or any other constituent of the tablets.

As with other beta-blocking agents: History of bronchospasm or asthma, 2nd and 3rd degree A-V heart block, (unless a permanent pacemaker is in place), severe bradycardia (< 50 bpm), cardiogenic shock, sick sinus syndrome (including sino-atrial block), severe hypotension (systolic blood pressure < 85mmHg), metabolic acidosis and phaeochromocytoma (unless adequately controlled by alpha blockade).

4.4 Special warnings and special precautions for use

In chronic heart failure patients, worsening cardiac failure or fluid retention may occur during up-titration of Eucardic. If such symptoms occur, the dose of diuretic should be adjusted and the Eucardic dose should not be advanced until clinical stability resumes. Occasionally it may be necessary to lower the Eucardic dose or temporarily discontinue it. Such episodes do not preclude subsequent successful titration of Eucardic.

In hypertensive patients who have chronic heart failure controlled with digoxin, diuretics and/or an ACE inhibitor, Eucardic should be used with caution since both digoxin and Eucardic may slow A-V conduction.

As with other drugs with beta-blocking activity, Eucardic may mask the early signs of acute hypoglycaemia in patients with diabetes mellitus. Alternatives to beta-blocking agents are generally preferred in insulin-dependent patients. In patients with diabetes, the use of Eucardic may be associated with worsening control of blood glucose. Therefore, regular monitoring of blood glucose is required in diabetics when Eucardic is initiated or up-titrated and hypoglycaemic therapy adjusted accordingly.

Reversible deterioration of renal function has been observed with Eucardic therapy in chronic heart failure patients with low blood pressure (systolic BP < 100mmHg), ischaemic heart disease and diffuse vascular disease, and/or underlying renal insufficiency. In CHF patients with these risk factors, renal function should be monitored during up-titration of Eucardic and the drug discontinued or dosage reduced if worsening of renal failure occurs.

Wearers of contact lenses should be advised of the possibility of reduced lacrimation.

Although angina has not been reported on stopping treatment, discontinuation should be gradual (1 - 2 weeks) particularly in patients with ischaemic heart disease, as Eucardic has beta-blocking activity.

Eucardic may be used in patients with peripheral vascular disease. Pure beta-blockers can precipitate or aggravate symptoms of arterial insufficiency. However as Eucardic also has alpha-blocking properties this effect is largely counterbalanced.

Eucardic, as with other agents with beta-blocking activity, may mask the symptoms of thyrotoxicosis.

If Eucardic induces bradycardia, with a decrease in pulse rate to less than 55 beats per minute, the dosage of Eucardic should be reduced.

Care should be taken in administering Eucardic to patients with a history of serious hypersensitivity reactions and in those undergoing desensitisation therapy as beta-blockers may increase both the sensitivity towards allergens and the seriousness of anaphylactic reactions.

In patients suffering from the peripheral circulatory disorder Raynaud's phenomenon, there may be exacerbation of symptoms.

Patients with a history of psoriasis associated with beta-blocker therapy should be given Eucardic only after consideration of the risk-benefit ratio.

In patients with phaeochromocytoma, an alpha-blocking agent should be initiated prior to the use of any beta-blocking agent. There is no experience of the use of carvedilol in this condition. Therefore, caution should be taken in the administration of Eucardic to patients suspected of having phaeochromocytoma.

Agents with non-selective beta-blocking activity may provoke chest pain in patients with Prinzmetal's variant angina. There is no clinical experience with Eucardic in these patients, although the alpha-blocking activity of Eucardic may prevent such symptoms. However, caution should be taken in the administration of Eucardic to patients suspected of having Prinzmetal's variant angina.

In patients with a tendency to bronchospastic reactions, respiratory distress can occur as a result of a possible increase in airway resistance. The following warnings will be included on the outer packaging and leaflet:

Packaging

Do not take this medicine if you have a history of wheezing due to asthma or other lung diseases.

Leaflet

Do not take this medicine if you have a history of wheezing due to asthma or other lung diseases. Consult your doctor or pharmacist first.

4.5 Interaction with other medicinal products and other forms of Interaction

As with other agents with beta-blocking activity, Eucardic may potentiate the effect of other concomitantly administered drugs that are anti-hypertensive in action (e.g. $alpha_1$-receptor antagonists) or have hypotension as part of their adverse effect profile.

Patients taking an agent with β-blocking properties and a drug that can deplete catecholamines (e.g. reserpine and monoamine oxidase inhibitors) should be observed closely for signs of hypotension and/or severe bradycardia.

Isolated cases of conduction disturbance (rarely with haemodynamic disruption) have been observed when Eucardic and diltiazem were given concomitantly. Therefore, as with other drugs with beta-blocking activity, careful monitoring of ECG and blood pressure should be undertaken when co-administering calcium channel blockers of the verapamil or diltiazem type, or class I antiarrhythmic drugs. These types of drugs should not be co-administered intravenously in patients receiving Eucardic.

The effects of insulin or oral hypoglycaemics may be intensified. Regular monitoring of blood glucose is therefore recommended.

Trough plasma digoxin levels may be increased by approximately 16% in hypertensive patients co-administered Eucardic and digoxin. Increased monitoring of digoxin levels is recommended when initiating, adjusting or discontinuing Eucardic. Concomitant administration of Eucardic and cardiac glycosides may prolong AV conduction time.

When treatment with Eucardic and clonidine together is to be terminated, Eucardic should be withdrawn first, several days before gradually decreasing the dosage of clonidine.

Care may be required in those receiving inducers of mixed function oxidases e.g. rifampicin, as serum levels of carvedilol may be reduced or inhibitors of mixed function oxidases e.g. cimetidine, as serum levels may be increased.

During general anaesthesia, attention should be paid to the potential synergistic negative inotropic effects of carvedilol and anaesthetic drugs.

Modest increases in mean trough cyclosporin concentrations were observed following initiation of carvedilol treatment in 21 renal transplant patients suffering from chronic vascular rejection. In about 30% of patients, the dose of cyclosporin had to be reduced in order to maintain cyclosporin concentrations within the therapeutic range, while in the remainder no adjustment was needed. On average, the dose of cyclosporin was reduced about 20% in these patients. Due to wide interindividual variability in the dose adjustment required, it is recommended that cyclosporin concentrations be monitored closely after initiation of carvedilol therapy and that the dose of cyclosporin be adjusted as appropriate.

4.6 Pregnancy and lactation

There is no adequate experience with Eucardic in pregnant women.

Eucardic should not be used in pregnancy or in breast feeding mothers unless the anticipated benefits outweigh the potential risks. There is no evidence from animal studies that Eucardic has any teratogenic effects. Embryotoxicity was observed only after large doses in rabbits. The relevance of these findings for humans is uncertain. Beta-blockers reduce placental perfusion which may result in intrauterine foetal death and immature and premature deliveries. In addition, animal studies have shown that carvedilol crosses the placental barrier and therefore the possible consequences of alpha and beta-blockade in the human foetus and neonate should also be borne in mind. With other alpha and beta-blocking agents, effects have included perinatal and neonatal distress (bradycardia, hypotension, respiratory depression, hypoglycaemia, hypothermia). There is an increased risk of cardiac and pulmonary complications in the neonate in the postnatal period.

Animal studies have shown that carvedilol or its metabolites are excreted in breast milk. It is not known whether carvedilol is excreted in human milk. Breast feeding is therefore not recommended during the administration of carvedilol.

4.7 Effects on ability to drive and use machines

As for other drugs which produce changes in blood pressure, patients taking Eucardic should be warned not to drive or operate machinery if they experience dizziness or related symptoms. This applies particularly when starting or changing treatment and in conjunction with alcohol.

4.8 Undesirable effects

Adverse events are listed separately for CHF because of differences in the background diseases.

__In chronic heart failure__

Haematological

Rare, thrombocytopenia.

Leucopenia has been reported in isolated cases.

Metabolic

Commonly: weight increase and hypercholesterolaemia. Hyperglycaemia, hypoglycaemia and worsening control of blood glucose are also common in patients with pre-existing diabetes mellitus (see section *4.5 Interaction with other medicinal products and other forms of interaction*).

Central nervous system

Very common: dizziness, headache are usually mild and occur particularly at the start of treatment. Asthenia (including fatigue).

Cardiovascular system

Common: bradycardia, postural hypotension, hypotension, oedema (including generalised, peripheral, dependent and genital oedema, oedema of the legs, hypervolaemia and fluid overload).

Uncommon: syncope (including presyncope), AV-block and cardiac failure during up-titration.

Gastro-intestinal system

Commonly: nausea, diarrhoea, and vomiting.

Skin and appendages

Dermatitis, and increased sweating.

Others

Commonly: vision abnormalities.

Rarely: acute renal failure and renal function abnormalities in patients with diffuse vascular disease and/or impaired renal function (see section *4.4 Special warnings and precautions for use*).

The frequency of adverse experiences is not dose dependent, with the exception of dizziness, abnormal vision and bradycardia.

__In hypertension and angina:__

The profile is similar to that observed in chronic heart failure although the incidence of events is generally lower in patients with hypertension or angina treated with Eucardic.

Blood chemistry and haematological

Isolated cases of changes in serum transaminases, thrombocytopenia and leucopenia have been reported.

Central nervous system

Commonly: dizziness, headaches and fatigue, which are usually mild and occur particularly at the beginning of treatment.

Uncommonly: depressed mood, sleep disturbance, paraesthesia, asthenia.

Metabolic

Due to the beta-blocking properties it is also possible for latent diabetes mellitus to become manifest, manifest diabetes to be aggravated, and blood glucose counter-regulation to be inhibited.

Cardiovascular system

Commonly: bradycardia, postural hypotension, especially at the beginning of treatment.

Uncommonly, syncope, hypotension, disturbances of peripheral circulation (cold extremities, PVD, exacerbation of intermittent claudication and Raynauds phenomenon). AV-block, angina pectoris (including chest pain), symptoms of heart failure and peripheral oedema.

Respiratory system

Commonly: asthma and dyspnoea in predisposed patients.

Rarely: stuffy nose. Wheezing and flu-like symptoms.

Gastro-intestinal system

Commonly: gastro-intestinal upset (with symptoms such as nausea, abdominal pain, diarrhoea).

Uncommonly: constipation and vomiting.

Skin and appendages

Uncommonly: skin reactions (eg allergic exanthema, dermatitis, urticaria, pruritus, lichen planus-like reactions, and increased sweating). Psoriatic skin lesions may occur or existing lesions exacerbated.

Others

Commonly: pain in the extremities, reduced lacrimation.

Uncommon: cases of sexual impotence and disturbed vision.

Rarely: dryness of the mouth and disturbances of micturition and eye irritation.

Isolated cases of allergic reactions have been reported.

4.9 Overdose

Symptoms and signs

Profound cardiovascular effects such as hypotension and bradycardia would be expected after massive overdose. Heart failure, cardiogenic shock and cardiac arrest may follow. There may also be respiratory problems, bronchospasm, vomiting, disturbed consciousness and generalised seizures.

Treatment

Gastric lavage or induced emesis may be useful in the first few hours after ingestion.

In addition to general procedures, vital signs must be monitored and corrected, if necessary under intensive care conditions.

Patients should be placed in the supine position. Atropine, 0.5mg to 2mg i.v. and/or glucagon 1 to 10mg i.v. (followed by a slow i.v. infusion of 2 to 5mg/hour if necessary) may be given when bradycardia is present. Pacemaker therapy may be necessary. For excessive hypotension, intravenous fluids may be administered. In addition, norepinephrine may be given, either 5 to 10 micrograms i.v., repeated according to blood pressure response, or 5 micrograms per minute by infusion titrated to blood pressure. Bronchospasm may be treated using salbutamol or other $beta_2$-agonists given as aerosol or, if necessary, by the intravenous route. In the event of seizures, slow i.v. injection of diazepam or clonazepam is recommended.

In cases of severe overdose with symptoms of shock, supportive treatment as described should be continued for a sufficiently long period of time, i.e. until the patient stabilises, since prolonged elimination half life and redistribution of carvedilol from deeper compartments can be expected.

5. PHARMACOLOGICAL PROPERTIES

5.1 Pharmacodynamic properties

Carvedilol is a vasodilating non-selective beta-blocking agent with antioxidant properties. Vasodilation is predominantly mediated through $alpha_1$ receptor antagonism.

Carvedilol reduces the peripheral vascular resistance through vasodilation and suppresses the renin-angiotensin-aldosterone system through beta-blockade. The activity of plasma renin is reduced and fluid retention is rare.

Carvedilol has no intrinsic sympathomimetic activity and like propranolol, it has membrane stabilising properties.

Carvedilol is a racemate of two stereoisomers. Beta-blockade is attributed to the S(-) enantiomer; in contrast, both enantiomers exhibit the same α_1-blocking activity.

Carvedilol is a potent antioxidant, a scavenger of reactive oxygen radicals and an anti-proliferative agent. The properties of carvedilol and its metabolites have been demonstrated in *in vitro* and *in vivo* animal studies and *in vitro* in a number of human cell types.

Clinical studies have shown that the balance of vasodilation and beta-blockade provided by carvedilol results in the following effects:

– In hypertensive patients, a reduction in blood pressure is not associated with a concomitant increase in total peripheral resistance, as observed with pure beta-blocking agents. Heart rate is slightly decreased. Renal blood flow and renal function are maintained. Peripheral blood flow is maintained, therefore, cold extremities, often observed with drugs possessing beta-blocking activity, are rarely seen.

– In patients with stable angina, Eucardic has demonstrated anti-ischaemic and anti-anginal properties. Acute haemodynamic studies demonstrated that Eucardic reduces ventricular pre- and after-load.

– In patients with left ventricular dysfunction or chronic heart failure, carvedilol has demonstrated favourable effects on haemodynamics and improvements in left ventricular ejection fraction and dimensions.

– In a large, multi-centre, double-blind, placebo-controlled mortality trial (COPERNICUS), 2289 patients with severe stable CHF of ischaemic or non-ischaemic origin, on standard therapy, were randomised to either carvedilol (1156 patients) or placebo (1133 patients). Patients had left ventricular systolic dysfunction with a mean ejection fraction of < 20%. All-cause mortality was reduced by 35% from 19.7% in the placebo group to 12.8% in the carvedilol group (Cox proportional hazards, p = 0.00013).

Combined secondary endpoints of mortality or hospitalisation for heart failure, mortality or cardiovascular hospitalisation and mortality or all-cause hospitalisation were all significantly lower in the carvedilol group than placebo (31%, 27% and 24% reductions, respectively, all p < 0.00004).

The incidence of serious adverse events during the study was lower in the carvedilol group (39.0% *vs* 45.4%). During initiation of treatment, the incidence of worsening heart failure was similar in both carvedilol and placebo groups. The incidence of serious worsening heart failure during the study was lower in the carvedilol group (14.6% *vs* 21.6%).

Serum lipid profile and electrolytes are not affected.

5.2 Pharmacokinetic properties

The absolute bioavailability of carvedilol is approximately 25% in humans. Bioavailability is stereo-selective, 30% for the R-form and 15% for the S-form. Serum levels peak at approximately 1 hour after an oral dose. There is a linear relationship between the dose and serum concentrations. Food does not affect bioavailability or the maximum serum concentration although the time to reach maximum serum concentration is delayed. Carvedilol is highly lipophilic, approximately 98% to 99% is bound to plasma proteins. The distribution volume is approximately 2 l/kg and increased in patients with liver cirrhosis. The first pass effect after oral administration is approximately 60 - 75%; enterohepatic circulation of the parent substance has been shown in animals.

Carvedilol exhibits a considerable first pass effect. The metabolite pattern reveals intensive metabolism with glucuronidation as one of the major steps. Demethylation and hydroxylation at the phenol ring produce 3 metabolites with beta-receptor blocking activity.

The average elimination half-life ranges from 6 to 10 hours. Plasma clearance is approximately 590ml/min. Elimination is mainly biliary. The primary route of excretion is via the faeces. A minor portion is eliminated via the kidneys in the form of various metabolites.

The pharmacokinetics of carvedilol are affected by age; plasma levels of carvedilol are approximately 50% higher in the elderly compared to young subjects. In a study in patients with cirrhotic liver disease, the bioavailability of carvedilol was four times greater and the peak plasma level five times higher than in healthy subjects. Since carvedilol is primarily excreted via the faeces, significant accumulation in patients with renal impairment is unlikely. In patients with impaired liver function, bioavailability is raised to as much as 80% due to a reduced first pass effect.

5.3 Preclinical safety data

Animal studies revealed no special findings relevant to clinical use (although see *Pregnancy and lactation*).

6. PHARMACEUTICAL PARTICULARS

6.1 List of excipients

Lactose, sucrose, povidone, crospovidone, colloidal silicon dioxide, magnesium stearate and red iron oxide E172 (3.125 and 12.5), yellow iron oxide E172 (6.25 and 12.5).

6.2 Incompatibilities

Not applicable.

6.3 Shelf life

3 years – 3.125 and 6.25 tablets.

4 years – 12.5 tablets.

5 years – 25 tablets.

6.4 Special precautions for storage

The tablets should be stored in a dry place below 25°C and protected from light.

6.5 Nature and contents of container

Blister packs, PVC/Aluminium of 28 or 56 tablets.

6.6 Instructions for use and handling

Not applicable.

7. MARKETING AUTHORISATION HOLDER

Roche Products Limited, 40 Broadwater Road, Welwyn Garden City, Hertfordshire, AL7 3AY.

8. MARKETING AUTHORISATION NUMBER(S)

PL 00031/0550 – Eucardic 3.125

PL 00031/0551 – Eucardic 6.25

PL 00031/0552 – Eucardic 12.5

PL 00031/0553 – Eucardic 25

9. DATE OF FIRST AUTHORISATION/RENEWAL OF THE AUTHORISATION

20 July 2003 (3.125/6.25)

7 Sep 2001 (12.5/25)

10. DATE OF REVISION OF THE TEXT

10 July 2002

Eucardic is a registered trade mark

Item Code

Eudemine Tablets

(UCB Pharma Limited)

1. NAME OF THE MEDICINAL PRODUCT

Eudemine Tablets

2. QUALITATIVE AND QUANTITATIVE COMPOSITION

Diazoxide 50mg

3. PHARMACEUTICAL FORM

White, sugar coated tablet.

4. CLINICAL PARTICULARS

4.1 Therapeutic indications

Eudemine Tablets are used orally in the treatment of intractable hypoglycaemia.

Diazoxide also causes salt and water retention.

Hypoglycaemia: Eudemine administered orally is indicated for the treatment of intractable hypoglycaemia with severe symptoms from a variety of causes including: idiopathic hypoglycaemia in infancy, leucine-sensitive or unclassified; functional islet cell tumours both malignant and benign if inoperable, extra-pancreatic neoplasms producing hypoglycaemia; glycogen storage disease; hypoglycaemia of unknown origin.

4.2 Posology and method of administration

Hypoglycaemia: In hypoglycaemia, the dosage schedule of Eudemine tablets is determined according to the clinical needs and the response of the individual patient. For both adults and children a starting oral dose of 5mg/kg body weight divided into 2 or 3 equal doses per 24 hours will establish the patient's response and thereafter the dose can be increased until the symptoms and blood glucose level respond satisfactorily. Regular determinations of the blood glucose in the initial days of treatment are essential. The usual maintenance dose is 3 - 8mg/kg/day given in two or three divided doses.

Reduced doses may be required in patients with impaired renal function.

In children with leucine-sensitive hypoglycaemia, a dosage range of 15-20mg/kg/day is suggested.

In adults with benign or malignant islet-cell tumours producing large quantities of insulin, high dosages of up to 1,000mg per day have been used.

4.3 Contraindications

In the treatment of hypoglycaemia, Eudemine is contraindicated in all cases which are amenable to surgery or other specific therapy.

Hypersensitivity to any component of the preparation or other thiazides.

4.4 Special warnings and special precautions for use

In the treatment of hypoglycaemia it is necessary that the blood pressure be monitored regularly.

Retention of sodium and water is likely to necessitate therapy with an oral diuretic such as frusemide or ethacrynic acid. The dosage of either of the diuretics mentioned may be up to 1g daily. It must be appreciated that if diuretics are employed then both the hypotensive and hyperglycaemic activities of diazoxide will be potentiated and it is likely that the dosage of diazoxide will require adjustment downwards. In patients with severe renal failure it is desirable to maintain, with diuretic therapy, urinary volumes in excess of 1 litre daily. Hypokalaemia should be avoided by adequate potassium replacement.

Diazoxide should be used with caution in patients with impaired cardiac reserve, in whom sodium and water retention may precipitate congestive heart failure (see section 4.8 "Undesirable Effects").

Diazoxide should be administered with caution to patients with hyperuricaemia or a history of gout, and it is advisable to monitor serum uric acid concentration.

Whenever Eudemine is given over a prolonged period regular haematological examinations are indicated to exclude changes in white blood cell and platelet counts.

Also in children there should be regular assessment of growth, bone and psychological maturation.

The very rapid, almost complete protein binding of diazoxide requires cautious dosage to be used in patients whose plasma proteins may be lower than normal.

4.5 Interaction with other medicinal products and other forms of Interaction

Drugs potentiated by diazoxide therapy include: oral diuretics, anti-hypertensive agents and anticoagulants.

Phenytoin levels should be monitored as increased dosage may be needed if administered concurrently with diazoxide.

The risk of hyperglycaemia may be increased by concurrent administration of corticosteroids or oestrogen-progestogen combinations.

4.6 Pregnancy and lactation

Eudemine Tablets are only to be used in pregnant women when the indicated condition is deemed to put the mother's life at risk.

Side Effects

Prolonged oral therapy of Eudemine during pregnancy has been reported to cause alopecia in the newborn.

Eudemine should not be given to nursing mothers as the safety of diazoxide during lactation has not been established.

4.7 Effects on ability to drive and use machines

None known.

4.8 Undesirable effects

With oral therapy, nausea is common in the first two or three weeks and may require relief with an anti-nauseant. Prolonged therapy has given rise to reports of hypertrichosis lanuginosa, anorexia and hyperuricaemia.

Extra-pyramidal side-effects have been reported with oral diazoxide. It was found that extra-pyramidal effects such as parkinsonian tremor, cogwheel rigidity and oculogyric crisis could be easily suppressed by intravenous injection of an antiparkinsonian drug such as procyclidine and that they could be prevented by maintenance therapy with such a drug given orally.

Other adverse effects of Eudemine which have been reported are hyperosmolar non-ketotic coma, cardiomegaly, leucopenia, thrombocytopenia, and hirsutism.

Sodium and water retention occur frequently in patients receiving multiple doses of diazoxide, and may precipitate cardiac failure in susceptible patients (e.g. those with impaired cardiac reserve). Symptoms of disturbed cardiac function (tachycardia, arrhythmias), inappropriate hypotension or hyperglycaemia (including ketoacidosis) have also been reported.

Diazoxide may cause gastrointestinal disturbances including nausea, vomiting, abdominal pain, anorexia, diarrhoea, ileus and constipation.

Changes in hepatic and renal function have been observed occasionally, including increased AST, alkaline phosphatase, azotemia, decreased creatinine clearance, reversible nephrotic syndrome, haematuria and albuminuria.

Disorders of blood components (decreased haemoglobin and/or haematocrit, eosinophilia, bleeding) have been reported. Hypogammaglobulinaemia may also occur.

Other reported side effects of diazoxide treatment include: headache, dyspnoea, musculoskeletal pain, hypersensitivity reactions (rash, fever, leucopenia), blurred vision, transient cataracts. Voice changes in children and abnormal facies in children on long term treatment have also been reported.

4.9 Overdose
Excessive dosage of Eudemine can result in hyperglycaemia. Severe hyperglycaemia may be corrected by giving insulin and less severe hyperglycaemia may respond to oral hypoglycaemics. Hypotension may be managed with intravenous fluids and in severe cases may require sympathomimetics.

5. PHARMACOLOGICAL PROPERTIES
5.1 Pharmacodynamic properties
None stated.

5.2 Pharmacokinetic properties
None stated.

5.3 Preclinical safety data
None stated.

6. PHARMACEUTICAL PARTICULARS
6.1 List of excipients
The tablet core consists of:
Lactose
Maize starch
Maize starch, pre-gelatinised
Magnesium stearate
Purified water
The tablet coating consists of:
Sugar (mineral water grade)
Gelatin coarse powder 200 bloom
Purified water
Opaglos AG-7350
Opaglos AG-7350 consists of:
Purified water
Carnauba wax (E903)
Beeswax, white (E901)
Polysorbate 20 (E432)
Sorbic acid (E200)

6.2 Incompatibilities
None stated.

6.3 Shelf life
36 months.

6.4 Special precautions for storage
None.

6.5 Nature and contents of container
Plastic containers with tamper evident closure containing 100 tablets.

6.6 Instructions for use and handling
None stated.

7. MARKETING AUTHORISATION HOLDER
UCB Pharma Limited
208 Bath Road
Slough
Berkshire
SL1 3WE
UK

8. MARKETING AUTHORISATION NUMBER(S)
PL 00039/0412

9. DATE OF FIRST AUTHORISATION/RENEWAL OF THE AUTHORISATION
17 December 1992 / 17 December 1997

10. DATE OF REVISION OF THE TEXT
June 2005
POM

Eumovate Cream

(GlaxoSmithKline UK)

1. NAME OF THE MEDICINAL PRODUCT
Eumovate Cream

2. QUALITATIVE AND QUANTITATIVE COMPOSITION
0.05% w/w clobetasone butyrate.

3. PHARMACEUTICAL FORM
Water miscible cream.

4. CLINICAL PARTICULARS
4.1 Therapeutic indications
Eumovate is suitable for the treatment of eczema and dermatitis of all types including atopic eczema, photodermatitis, otitis externa, primary irritant and allergic dermatitis (including napkin rash), intertrigo, prurigo nodularis, seborrhoeic dermatitis and insect bite reactions.

Eumovate may be used as maintenance therapy between courses of one of the more active topical steroids.

4.2 Posology and method of administration
Route of administration: Topical application

For all ages:

Eumovate should be applied to the affected area up to four times a day until improvement occurs, when the frequency of application may be reduced.

4.3 Contraindications
Skin lesions caused by infection with viruses (e.g. herpes simplex, chickenpox), fungi (e.g. candidiasis, tinea) or bacteria (e.g. impetigo).

4.4 Special warnings and special precautions for use
Hypersensitivity to the preparations.

Although generally regarded as safe, even for long-term administration in adults, there is a potential for overdosage, and in infants and children this may result in adrenal suppression. Extreme caution is required in dermatoses in such patients and treatment should not normally exceed seven days. In infants, the napkin may act as an occlusive dressing, and increase absorption.

Appropriate antimicrobial therapy should be used whenever treating inflammatory lesions which have become infected. Any spread of infection requires withdrawal of topical corticosteroid therapy, and systemic administration of antimicrobial agents.

As with all corticosteroids, prolonged application to the face is undesirable.

Topical corticosteroids may be hazardous in psoriasis for a number of reasons including rebound relapses, development of tolerance, risk of generalised pustular psoriasis and development of local or systemic toxicity due to impaired barrier function of the skin. If used in psoriasis, careful patient supervision is important.

If applied to the eyelids, care is needed to ensure that the preparation does not enter the eye as glaucoma might result.

4.5 Interaction with other medicinal products and other forms of Interaction
None stated.

4.6 Pregnancy and lactation
There is inadequate evidence of safety in human pregnancy. Topical administration of corticosteroids to pregnant animals can cause abnormalities of foetal development including cleft palate and intra-uterine growth retardation. There may therefore be a very small risk of such effects in the human foetus.

4.7 Effects on ability to drive and use machines
None stated.

4.8 Undesirable effects
In the unlikely event of signs of hypersensitivity appearing, application should stop immediately. When large areas of the body are being treated with Eumovate, it is possible that some patients will absorb sufficient steroid to cause transient adrenal suppression despite the low degree of systemic activity associated with clobetasone butyrate.

Local atrophic changes could possibly occur in situations where moisture increases absorption of clobetasone butyrate, but only after prolonged use.

There are reports of pigmentation changes and hypertrichosis with topical steroids.

Exacerbation of symptoms may occur.

4.9 Overdose
Acute overdosage is very unlikely to occur, however, in the case of chronic overdosage or misuse the features of hypercorticism may appear and in this situation topical steroids should be discontinued.

5. PHARMACOLOGICAL PROPERTIES
5.1 Pharmacodynamic properties
Clobetasone butyrate is a topically active corticosteroid.

Clobetasone butyrate has little effect on hypothalamo-pituitary-adrenal function. This was so even when Eumovate was applied to adults in large amounts under whole body occlusion.

Clobetasone butyrate is less potent than other available corticosteroid preparations and has been shown not to suppress the hypothalamo-pituitary-adrenal axis in patients treated for psoriasis or eczema.

Pharmacological studies in man and animals have shown that clobetasone butyrate has a relatively high level of topical activity accompanied by a low level of systemic activity.

5.2 Pharmacokinetic properties
A single application of 30g clobetasone butyrate 0.05% ointment to eight patients resulted in a measurable rise in plasma clobetasone butyrate levels during the first three hours but then the levels gradually decreased. The maximum plasma level reached in the first three hours was 0.6ng/ml. This rise in levels was followed by a more gradual decline with plasma levels of clobetasone butyrate falling below 0.1ng/ml (the lower limit of the assay) after 72 hours. The normal diurnal variation in plasma cortisol levels was not affected by the application of clobetasone butyrate ointment.

5.3 Preclinical safety data
No additional data included.

6. PHARMACEUTICAL PARTICULARS
6.1 List of excipients
Glycerol
Glycerol monostearate
Cetostearyl alcohol
Beeswax substitute 6621
Arlacel 165
Dimethicone 20
Chlorocresol
Sodium citrate
Citric acid monohydrate
Purified water

6.2 Incompatibilities
None stated.

6.3 Shelf life
36 months

6.4 Special precautions for storage
Store below 25°C.

6.5 Nature and contents of container
Internally lacquered aluminium tubes with latex band and wadless polypropylene cap.

30 and 100gm tubes are available (25gm pack is also registered).

6.6 Instructions for use and handling
None

Administrative Data
7. MARKETING AUTHORISATION HOLDER
Glaxo Wellcome UK Limited
trading as GlaxoSmithKline UK
Stockley Park West
Uxbridge
Middlesex UB11 1BT

8. MARKETING AUTHORISATION NUMBER(S)
PL 10949/0035

9. DATE OF FIRST AUTHORISATION/RENEWAL OF THE AUTHORISATION
1 April 1993

10. DATE OF REVISION OF THE TEXT
29 January 2003

Eumovate Ointment

(GlaxoSmithKline UK)

1. NAME OF THE MEDICINAL PRODUCT
Eumovate Ointment

2. QUALITATIVE AND QUANTITATIVE COMPOSITION
0.05% w/w clobetasone butyrate.

3. PHARMACEUTICAL FORM
Paraffin based ointment.

4. CLINICAL PARTICULARS
4.1 Therapeutic indications
Eumovate is suitable for the treatment of eczema and dermatitis of all types including atopic eczema, photodermatitis, otitis externa, primary irritant and allergic dermatitis (including napkin rash), intertrigo, prurigo nodularis, seborrhoeic dermatitis and insect bite reactions.

Eumovate may be used as maintenance therapy between courses of one of the more active topical steroids.

4.2 Posology and method of administration
Route of administration: Topical application

For all ages:

Eumovate should be applied to the affected area up to four times a day until improvement occurs, when the frequency of application may be reduced.

4.3 Contraindications
Skin lesions caused by infection with viruses (e.g. herpes simplex, chickenpox), fungi (e.g. candidiasis, tinea) or bacteria (e.g. impetigo).

Hypersensitivity to the preparation.

4.4 Special warnings and special precautions for use
Although generally regarded as safe, even for long-term administration in adults, there is a potential for overdosage, and in infants and children this may result in adrenal suppression. Extreme caution is required in dermatoses in such patients and treatment should not normally exceed seven days. In infants, the napkin may act as an occlusive dressing, and increase absorption.

Appropriate antimicrobial therapy should be used whenever treating inflammatory lesions which have become infected. Any spread of infection requires withdrawal of topical corticosteroid therapy, and systemic administration of antimicrobial agents.

As with all corticosteroids, prolonged application to the face is undesirable.

Topical corticosteroids may be hazardous in psoriasis for a number of reasons including rebound relapses, development of tolerance, risk of generalised pustular psoriasis and development of local or systemic toxicity due to impaired barrier function of the skin. If used in psoriasis, careful patient supervision is important.

If applied to the eyelids, care is needed to ensure that the preparation does not enter the eye as glaucoma might result.

4.5 Interaction with other medicinal products and other forms of Interaction
None stated.

4.6 Pregnancy and lactation
There is inadequate evidence of safety in human pregnancy. Topical administration of corticosteroids to pregnant animals can cause abnormalities of foetal development including cleft palate and intra-uterine growth retardation. There may therefore be a very small risk of such effects in the human foetus.

4.7 Effects on ability to drive and use machines
None stated.

4.8 Undesirable effects
In the unlikely event of signs of hypersensitivity appearing, application should stop immediately. When large areas of the body are being treated with Eumovate, it is possible that some patients will absorb sufficient steroid to cause transient adrenal suppression despite the low degree of systemic activity associated with clobetasone butyrate.

Local atrophic changes could possibly occur in situations where moisture increases absorption of clobetasone butyrate, but only after prolonged use.

There are reports of pigmentation changes and hypertrichosis with topical steroids.

Exacerbation of symptoms may occur.

4.9 Overdose
Acute overdosage is very unlikely to occur, however, in the case of chronic overdosage or misuse the features of hypercortisolism may appear and in this situation topical steroids should be discontinued.

5. PHARMACOLOGICAL PROPERTIES

5.1 Pharmacodynamic properties
Clobetasone butyrate is a topically active corticosteroid.

Clobetasone butyrate has little effect on hypothalamo-pituitary-adrenal function. This was so even when Eumovate was applied to adults in large amounts under whole body occlusion.

Clobetasone butyrate is less potent than other available corticosteroid preparations and has been shown not to suppress the hypothalamo-pituitary-adrenal axis in patients treated for psoriasis or eczema.

Pharmacological studies in man and animals have shown that clobetasone butyrate has a relatively high level of topical activity accompanied by a low level of systemic activity.

5.2 Pharmacokinetic properties
A single application of 30g clobetasone butyrate 0.05% ointment to eight patients resulted in a measurable rise in plasma clobetasone butyrate levels during the first three hours but then the levels gradually decreased. The maximum plasma level reached in the first three hours was 0.6ng/ml. This rise in levels was followed by a more gradual decline with plasma levels of clobetasone butyrate falling below 0.1ng/ml (the lower limit of the assay) after 72 hours. The normal diurnal variation in plasma cortisol levels was not affected by the application of clobetasone butyrate ointment.

5.3 Preclinical safety data
No additional data included.

6. PHARMACEUTICAL PARTICULARS

6.1 List of excipients
Liquid paraffin

White soft paraffin

6.2 Incompatibilities
None stated.

6.3 Shelf life
36 months

6.4 Special precautions for storage
Store below 25°C.

6.5 Nature and contents of container
Collapsible aluminium tube and wadless polypropylene cap.

30 and 100gm tubes are available (25gm pack is also registered).

6.6 Instructions for use and handling
None

Administrative Data

7. MARKETING AUTHORISATION HOLDER
Glaxo Wellcome UK Limited

Trading as GlaxoSmithKline UK

Stockley Park West

Uxbridge

Middlesex UB11 1BT

8. MARKETING AUTHORISATION NUMBER(S)
PL 10949/0037

9. DATE OF FIRST AUTHORISATION/RENEWAL OF THE AUTHORISATION
1 April 1993/11 March 1996

10. DATE OF REVISION OF THE TEXT
29 January 2003

Eurax Cream & Lotion

(Novartis Consumer Health)

1. NAME OF THE MEDICINAL PRODUCT
Eurax Cream and Lotion

2. QUALITATIVE AND QUANTITATIVE COMPOSITION
Crotamiton 10.00%

3. PHARMACEUTICAL FORM
Cream or Topical Emulsion

4. CLINICAL PARTICULARS

4.1 Therapeutic indications
1. For the relief of itching and skin irritation caused by, for example sunburn, dry eczema, itchy dermatitis, allergic rashes, hives, nettle rash, chickenpox, insect bites and stings, heat rashes and personal itching.

2. The treatment of scabies.

4.2 Posology and method of administration
For cutaneous use.

Recommended dose and dosage schedules

Pruritus

Adults (including the elderly) and children:

Apply to the affected area 2-3 times daily. Eurax will provide relief from irritation for 6-10 hours after each application. Eurax can be used in children. There are no special dosage recommendations in the elderly.

Scabies

Adults (including the elderly):

After the patient has taken a warm bath, the skin should be well dried and Eurax rubbed into the entire body surface (excluding the face and scalp) until no traces of the preparation remain visible on the surface. The application should be repeated once daily, preferably in the evening, for a total of 3-5 days. Depending on the response, special attention should be paid to sites that are particularly susceptibly to infestation by the mites (e.g. interdigital spaces, wrists, axillae and genitalia). Areas where there is pus formation should be covered with a dressing impregnated with Eurax. While the treatment is in progress the patient may take a bath shortly before the next application. After completion of the treatment, a cleansing bath should be taken followed by a change of bed linen and underclothing.

Children:

Application as described for adults but in children under 3 years of age Eurax should not be applied more than once a day.

4.3 Contraindications
Acute exudative dermatoses. Hypersensitivity to any of the ingredients. Eurax should not be used in or around the eyes since contact with the eyelids may give rise to conjunctival inflammation.

4.4 Special warnings and special precautions for use
Eurax can be used for children; consult your doctor before use on children under 3 years of age.

For external use only.

Do not use in or around the eyes, on broken skin, for weeping skin conditions or if you are sensitive to any of the ingredients.

Keep all medicines out of the reach of children.

Consult your doctor or pharmacist before using Eurax if you are pregnant or breast feeding, or suffering from genital itching.

If symptoms persist consult your doctor.

4.5 Interaction with other medicinal products and other forms of Interaction
None.

4.6 Pregnancy and lactation
There is no experience to judge the safety of Eurax in pregnancy, therefore Eurax is not recommended during pregnancy, especially in the first three months. It is not known whether the active substance passes into breast milk. Nursing mothers should avoid applying Eurax in the area of the nipples.

4.7 Effects on ability to drive and use machines
None.

4.8 Undesirable effects
Occasionally irritation of the skin or contact allergy may occur. In such cases the preparation should be discontinued.

4.9 Overdose
Eurax is for application to the skin only. Following accidental ingestion, nausea, vomiting and irritation of the buccal, oesophageal and gastric mucosa have been reported. If accidental ingestion of large quantities occurs, there is no specific antidote and general measures to eliminate the drug and reduce its absorption should be undertaken. Symptomatic treatment should be administered as appropriate. A risk of methaemoglobinaemia exists, which may be treated with methylene blue.

5. PHARMACOLOGICAL PROPERTIES

5.1 Pharmacodynamic properties
Eurax has a symptomatic action on pruritus and is an acaricide.

5.2 Pharmacokinetic properties
Eurax penetrates rapidly into human skin. Low but measurable concentrations of crotamiton are found in plasma, with a maximum level after 4-10 hours, declining rapidly thereafter.

5.3 Preclinical safety data
Eurax cream administered dermally once daily under occlusive dressing for 3 months to rabbits was tolerated at doses of up to 250mg/kg without signs of toxicity, apart from transient skin irritation. No sensitising or photo-sensitising potential has been observed in animal studies.

Crotamiton does not induce mutations in bacteria nor chromosomal damage in mammalian cells. Studies to detect a possible effect on fertility and reproductive behaviour also gave negative results.

6. PHARMACEUTICAL PARTICULARS

6.1 List of excipients

Eurax Cream	**Eurax Lotion**
Methyl hydroxybenzoate	Glyceryl monostearate
Phenylethyl alcohol	NSE
Glycerol	Cetomacrogol 1000
Triethanolamine	Eutanol G
Sodium lauryl sulphate	Lanette N
Ethylene glycol monostearate	Sorbic acid
Stearyl alcohol	Citric acid monohydrate
Strong ammonia solution 25%	Phenylethyl alcohol
Stearic acid	Propylene glycol
Hard paraffin	Perfume Givaudan no 45
White beeswax	Purified water
Perfume Givaudan no 45	
Purified water	

6.2 Incompatibilities
None.

6.3 Shelf life
5 years

6.4 Special precautions for storage
Protect from heat.

6.5 Nature and contents of container
Eurax Cream: Internally lacquered aluminium tube, with a screw cap, in a cardboard carton. Pack sizes: 30 and 100g

Eurax lotion: Amber glass bottle with wadless polypropylene cap in cardboard carton. Pack size 100 ml

6.6 Instructions for use and handling
Medicines should be kept out of the reach of children.

7. MARKETING AUTHORISATION HOLDER
Novartis Consumer Health UK Limited

T/A Novartis Consumer Health

Wimblehurst Road

Horsham

West Sussex

RH12 5AB

8. MARKETING AUTHORISATION NUMBER(S)
Eurax Cream: PL 00030/0092

Eurax Lotion: 00030/0095

9. DATE OF FIRST AUTHORISATION/RENEWAL OF THE AUTHORISATION
1 September 1997

10. DATE OF REVISION OF THE TEXT
Eurax Cream: 7 November 2001

Eurax Lotion: 18 October 2001

Legal category:
GSL

Eurax Hydrocortisone Cream

(Novartis Consumer Health)

1. NAME OF THE MEDICINAL PRODUCT
Eurax Hydrocortisone Cream

2. QUALITATIVE AND QUANTITATIVE COMPOSITION
Active ingredients:

Crotamiton 10.0% w/w

Hydrocortisone 0.25% w/w

3. PHARMACEUTICAL FORM
Cream

4. CLINICAL PARTICULARS

4.1 Therapeutic indications

Eczema and dermatitis of all types including atopic eczema, photodermatitis, otitis external, primary irritant and allergic dermatitis, intertrigo, prurigo nodularis, seborrhoeic dermatitis and insect bite reactions.

Route of Administration: Cutaneous use.

4.2 Posology and method of administration

Adults

A thin layer of Eurax Hydrocortisone Cream should be applied to the affected area 2-3 times a day. Occlusive dressings should not be used. Treatment should be limited to 10-14 days or up to 7 days if applied to the face.

Use in the Elderly

Clinical evidence would indicate that no special dosage regime is necessary.

Use in Children

Eurax Hydrocortisone should be used with caution in infants and for not more than 7 days. Eurax Hydrocortisone should not be applied more than once a day to large areas of the body surface in young children.

4.3 Contraindications

Hypersensitivity to any component of the formulation. Bacterial, viral or fungal infections of the skin. Acute exudative dermatoses. Application to ulcerated areas.

4.4 Special warnings and special precautions for use

Eurax Hydrocortisone should be used with caution in infants and for not more than 7 days; long-term continuous topical therapy should be avoided since this can lead to adrenal suppression even without occlusion.

Eurax Hydrocortisone should not be allowed to come into contact with the conjunctiva and mucous membranes.

4.5 Interaction with other medicinal products and other forms of Interaction

None known.

4.6 Pregnancy and lactation

There is inadequate evidence of safety in human pregnancy. Topical administration of corticosteroids to pregnant animals can cause abnormalities of foetal development, including cleft palate and intra-uterine growth retardation. There may therefore be a very small risk of such effects in the human foetus.

It is not known whether the active substances of Eurax Hydrocortisone and/or their metabolites pass into the breast milk after topical administration. Use in lactating mothers should only be at the doctor's discretion.

4.7 Effects on ability to drive and use machines

None known.

4.8 Undesirable effects

Occasionally at the site of application signs of irritation such as a burning sensation, itching, contact dermatitis/ contact allergy may occur. Treatment should be discontinued if patients experience severe irritation or sensitisation.

4.9 Overdose

Eurax Hydrocortisone is for application to the skin only. If accidental ingestion of large quantities occurs, there is no specific antidote and general measures to eliminate the drug and reduce its absorption should be undertaken. Symptomatic treatment should be administered as appropriate.

5. PHARMACOLOGICAL PROPERTIES

5.1 Pharmacodynamic properties

Eurax Hydrocortisone combines the antipruritic action of crotamiton with the anti-inflammatory and anti-allergic properties of hydrocortisone.

5.2 Pharmacokinetic properties

No pharmacokinetic data on Eurax Hydrocortisone Cream are available.

5.3 Preclinical safety data

Not applicable.

6. PHARMACEUTICAL PARTICULARS

6.1 List of excipients

Stearyl alcohol

White soft paraffin

Polyoxy 40 stearate

Propyl hydroxybenzoate

Propylene glycol

Methyl hydroxybenzoate

Perfume Givaudan no 45

Sulphuric acid

Purified water

6.2 Incompatibilities

None known.

6.3 Shelf life

30 months.

6.4 Special precautions for storage

Protect from heat.

6.5 Nature and contents of container

Collapsible aluminium tube

Pack Size: 30g.

6.6 Instructions for use and handling

Medicines should be kept out of the reach of children.

Administrative Data

7. MARKETING AUTHORISATION HOLDER

Novartis Consumer Health UK Ltd

Trading as

Novartis Consumer Health

Wimblehurst Road

Horsham

West Sussex

RH12 5AB

8. MARKETING AUTHORISATION NUMBER(S)

PL 00030/0094

9. DATE OF FIRST AUTHORISATION/RENEWAL OF THE AUTHORISATION

Original grant date: 17 January 1991

Date of renewal: 17 January 1996

10. DATE OF REVISION OF THE TEXT

October 2002

Legal Category:

POM

Evorel 100 Patch

(Janssen-Cilag Ltd)

1. NAME OF THE MEDICINAL PRODUCT

Evorel 100

2. QUALITATIVE AND QUANTITATIVE COMPOSITION

Each Evorel 100 patch contains estradiol 6.40 mg.

3. PHARMACEUTICAL FORM

Evorel is a square shaped, transparent, self-adhesive transdermal therapeutic system (patch) to skin. Evorel 100 has a surface area of 32 cm^2 and 0.2 mm thickness. It consists of a monolayered adhesive matrix throughout which 17β estradiol is uniformly distributed. The adhesive matrix is protected on the outside surface (from clothes etc.) by a polyethylene teraphthalate backing foil, while the adhesive surface of the patch is covered by a polyester sheet (the release liner) which is removed before placing the patch on the body surface. This release liner has an S-shaped incision which facilitates easy removal from the patch.

4. CLINICAL PARTICULARS

4.1 Therapeutic indications

Oestrogen replacement for the symptomatic relief of menopausal symptoms.

Second line therapy for prevention of osteoporosis in post-menopausal women at high risk of future fractures who are intolerant of, or contraindicated for, other medicinal products approved for the prevention of osteoporosis.

4.2 Posology and method of administration

Adults:

Menopausal symptoms

Therapy should be started with one Evorel 50 patch (delivering 50 micrograms of estradiol/24 hours) and the dose adjusted after the first month if necessary depending on efficacy and signs of over-oestrogenisation (eg breast tenderness). For maintenance therapy, the lowest effective dose should be used; a maximum dose of 100 micrograms of estradiol/24 hours should not be exceeded.

Post menopausal osteoporosis

Evorel 100 is recommended as an effective bone-sparing dose, with lower doses of estradiol slowing but not halting bone loss.

Evorel should be applied twice weekly on a continuous basis, each patch being renewed after 3 to 4 days and a fresh patch applied. Evorel should be applied to the skin as soon as it is removed from the wrapper. Recommended application sites are on clean, dry, healthy, intact skin and each application should be made to a slightly different area of skin on the trunk below waistline. Evorel should not be applied on or near the breasts. Evorel should remain in place during bathing and showering. Should it fall off during bathing or showering the patient should wait until cutaneous vasodilation ceases before applying a replacement patch to avoid potential excessive absorption. Should a patch fall off at other times it should be replaced immediately.

Patients can be advised to use baby oil to help remove any gum/glue which may remain on their skin after patch removal.

Unopposed oestrogen therapy is not recommended unless the patient has had hysterectomy. Where a progestogen is considered necessary, the appropriate dose should be administered for not less than 12 days each month.

Children: Evorel is not indicated in children.

4.3 Contraindications

Known or suspected malignant tumours of the breast, genital tract or other oestrogen dependent neoplasia. Undiagnosed vaginal bleeding, known or suspected pregnancy and lactation, severe hepatic, renal or cardiac disease, Rotor syndrome or Dubin-Johnson syndrome, active thrombophlebitis, active deep venous thrombosis, thrombo-embolic disorders, or a history of confirmed venous thrombo-embolism, endometriosis, hypersensitivity to any of the excipients.

4.4 Special warnings and special precautions for use

Assessment of each woman prior to using hormone replacement therapy (and at regular intervals thereafter) should include a personal and family medical history. Physical examination should be guided by this and by the Contraindications (Section 4.3) and Warnings (Section 4.4) for this product. During assessment of each individual woman clinical examination of the breasts and pelvic examination should be performed where clinically indicated rather than as a routine procedure. Women should be encouraged to participate in the national breast cancer screening programme (mammography) and the national cervical cancer screening programme (cervical cytology) as appropriate for their age. Breast awareness should also be encouraged and women advised to report any changes in their breasts to their doctor or nurse.

A re-analysis of original data from 51 epidemiological studies reported a small or moderate increase in the probability of having breast cancer *diagnosed* in women currently or recently using HRT. The findings may be due to biological effects of HRT, earlier diagnosis, or a combination of both. The relative risk increased with duration of treatment (by 2.3% per year of use) and returned to normal in the course of five years after cessation of HRT use. This is comparable to the increase in relative risk when natural menopause is delayed in the absence of HRT. Breast cancers diagnosed in current or recent users of HRT are more likely to be localised to the breast than those found in non-users. HRT use may not be associated with increased mortality from breast cancer.

Between the ages of 50 and 70, about 45 women in every 1,000 not using HRT will have breast cancer diagnosed. It is estimated that among those who use HRT for 5 years starting at age 50, 2 extra cases of breast cancer will be detected by age 70 in every 1,000 women. For those who use HRT for 10 years, there will be 6 extra cases of breast cancer, and for 15 years use, 12 extra cases of breast cancer in every 1,000 women during the 20 year period until age 70.

It is important that the increased risk of being diagnosed with breast cancer is discussed with the patient and weighed against the known benefits of HRT.

Administration of unopposed oestrogen therapy in patients with an intact uterus has been reported to increase the risk of endometrial hyperplasia. Repeated breakthrough bleeding should be investigated, including endometrial biopsy.

Close monitoring is recommended in patients with: epilepsy, diabetes or hypertension (as oestrogens may cause fluid retention), disturbances or impairment of liver function, mastopathy or a strong family history of breast cancer, fibrocystic disease, uterine fibromyomata, cholelithiasis, otosclerosis, multiple sclerosis, systemic lupus erythematosus, porphyria, melanoma, migraine, and asthma, as these conditions may be worsened by oestrogen therapy.

Consideration should be given to discontinuing treatment at least four weeks prior to surgery or during periods of prolonged immobilisation. Also, if hypertension develops after initiating therapy, consider discontinuing Evorel while the cause is investigated.

Epidemiological studies have suggested that hormone replacement therapy (HRT) is associated with an increased relative risk of developing venous thrombo-embolism (VTE), ie deep vein thrombosis or pulmonary embolism. The studies find a 2-3 fold increase for users compared with non-users which for healthy women amounts to a low risk for one extra case of VTE each year for every 5,000 patients taking HRT.

Generally recognised risk factors for VTE include a personal or family history and severe obesity (body mass index >30 kg/m2). In women with these factors the benefits of treatment with HRT need to be carefully weighed against risks.

The risk of VTE may be temporarily increased with prolonged immobilisation, major trauma or major surgery. In women on HRT scrupulous attention should be given to prophylactic measures to prevent VTE following surgery. Where prolonged immobilisation is liable to follow elective surgery, particularly abdominal or orthopaedic surgery to the lower limbs, consideration should be given to temporarily stopping HRT 4 weeks earlier, if this is possible.

If venous thrombo-embolism develops after initiating therapy the drug should be discontinued.

Evorel is not to be used for contraception.

4.5 Interaction with other medicinal products and other forms of Interaction

Drugs which cause microsomal liver enzyme activity may alter oestrogen action. Examples of such drugs include barbiturates, hydantoins, carbamazepine, meprobamate, phenylbutazole and rifampicin. In transdermal administration of estradiol, a first pass effect via the liver is avoided.

There have been no reports of interaction with Evorel although the clinical exposure has been very limited.

4.6 Pregnancy and lactation
Evorel in contra-indicated in pregnancy and lactation.

4.7 Effects on ability to drive and use machines
In normal use, Evorel would not be expected to have any effect on the ability to drive or use machinery.

4.8 Undesirable effects
Although side effects are rare, minor effects which do not usually preclude continuation of therapy include headaches, nausea, breast tenderness, and intermittent bleeding.

In clinical studies with Evorel (50 μg/24 hours) the following side effects were seen: breast tenderness (less than 2%), bleeding (less than 2%), and intermittent bleeding/spotting (less than 5%). None were serious, reflecting the known profile of oestrogen or oestrogen/progestogen therapy. Skin reactions were reported by less than 6% of patients over six treatment cycles. Rarely, dizziness, bloating, oedema, weight gain and leg cramps may occur.

4.9 Overdose
By virtue of the mode of administration of Evorel, overdosage is unlikely, but effects can if necessary be reversed by removal of the patch. The most commonly observed symptoms of overdose with oestrogen therapy are breast tenderness, nausea and breakthrough bleeding.

5. PHARMACOLOGICAL PROPERTIES

5.1 Pharmacodynamic properties
Estradiol is a naturally occurring oestrogenic hormone. It is formed in the ovarian follicles under the influence of the pituitary gland. In the female it stimulates the accessory reproductive organs and causes development of the secondary sexual changes in the endometrium during the first half of the menstrual cycle.

Estradiol is readily and completely absorbed from the gastro-intestinal tract and through the skin and mucous membranes. Metabolism is primarily in the liver. Excretion of the less active metabolites, primarily oestrone and oestriol is via the urine.

Evorel releases estradiol transdermally into the circulation in pre-menopausal physiological amounts.

In post-menopausal women, Evorel increased estradiol levels to early and mid-follicular phase levels. The transcutaneous route avoids the first pass hepatic effect seen with orally administered oestrogens.

In contrast with oral oestrogens, stimulation of hepatic protein synthesis is largely avoided with consequent lack of effect on circulating levels of renin substrate, thyroid binding globulin, sex hormone binding globulin and cortisol binding globulin. Similarly coagulation factors also appear to be unaffected (e.g. fibrinopeptide A etc.). Transdermal estradiol does not affect circulating levels of renin.

Studies with Evorel have shown a significant decrease in hot flushes, improvement in Kupperman Index and vaginal cytology.

Local tolerance with Evorel has been very good. The adhesive matrix used has a low irritation index.

5.2 Pharmacokinetic properties
General characteristics: Oestrogens are in general readily absorbed from the gastro-intestinal tract, through the skin and mucous membranes. Absorption from the gastro-intestinal tract is prompt and complete. Transdermal absorption of oestrogens is sufficient to cause a systemic effect. Inactivation of oestrogens in the body is mainly in the liver and consequently the limited oral effectiveness of oestrogens is related to first pass hepatic metabolism and not to poor absorption. A certain proportion of oestrogen is excreted into the bile and then reabsorbed from the intestine. During the enterohepatic circulation, estradiol is readily oxidised to the less pharmacologically active oestrone which may in turn then be hydrated to form oestriol (also pharmacologically less than estradiol). Estradiol circulates in the blood in association with sex hormone-binding globulin and albumin.

Characteristics in patients: With Evorel, therapeutic serum estradiol levels are achieved approximately four hours after application to the skin. From 10 hours onwards, the serum levels remain stable and at early to mid-follicular levels throughout the duration of the application (3 to 4 days).

Twenty four hours following removal of the transdermal therapeutic system estradiol levels return to baseline.

5.3 Preclinical safety data
Not applicable

6. PHARMACEUTICAL PARTICULARS

6.1 List of excipients
Adhesive acrylic polymer (Duro-Tak 387-2287)

Guar gum

Hostaphan MN19 (polyester film - removed before application)

6.2 Incompatibilities
None known.

6.3 Shelf life
36 months for the product as packed for sale.

6.4 Special precautions for storage
Do not store above 25°C.

6.5 Nature and contents of container
Each Evorel 100 patch is presented in a sealed protective pouch. The pouches are packed in a cardboard carton.

6.6 Instructions for use and handling
Not applicable.

7. MARKETING AUTHORISATION HOLDER
Janssen-Cilag Limited

Saunderton

High Wycombe

Buckinghamshire

HP14 4HJ

UK

8. MARKETING AUTHORISATION NUMBER(S)
00242/0295

9. DATE OF FIRST AUTHORISATION/RENEWAL OF THE AUTHORISATION
1 November 1995

10. DATE OF REVISION OF THE TEXT
December 2004

Evorel 25 Patch

(Janssen-Cilag Ltd)

1. NAME OF THE MEDICINAL PRODUCT
Evorel 25

2. QUALITATIVE AND QUANTITATIVE COMPOSITION
Each Evorel 25 patch contains estradiol 1.60 mg.

3. PHARMACEUTICAL FORM
Evorel is a square shaped, transparent, self-adhesive transdermal therapeutic system (patch) to skin. Evorel 25 has a surface area of 8 cm^2 and 0.2 mm thickness. It consists of a monolayered adhesive matrix throughout which 17β estradiol is uniformly distributed. The adhesive matrix is protected on the outside surface (from clothes etc.) by a polyethylene teraphthalate backing foil, while the adhesive surface of the patch is covered by a polyester sheet (the release liner) which is removed before placing the patch on the body surface. This release liner has an S-shaped incision which facilitates easy removal from the patch.

4. CLINICAL PARTICULARS

4.1 Therapeutic indications
Oestrogen replacement for the symptomatic relief of menopausal symptoms.

4.2 Posology and method of administration
Adults: Evorel should be applied twice weekly on a continuous basis, each patch being renewed after 3 to 4 days and a fresh patch applied. Therapy should be started with one Evorel 50 patch (delivering 50 micrograms of estradiol/24 hours) and the dose adjusted after the first month if necessary depending on efficacy and signs of over-oestrogenisation (e.g. breast tenderness). For maintenance therapy, the lowest effective dose should be used; a maximum dose of 100 micrograms of estradiol/24 hours should not be exceeded. Evorel should be applied to the skin as soon as it is removed from the wrapper.

Recommended application sites are on clean, dry, healthy, intact skin and each application should be made to a slightly different area of skin on the trunk below waistline. **Evorel should not be applied on or near the breasts.** Evorel should remain in place during bathing and showering. Should it fall off during bathing or showering the patient should wait until cutaneous vasodilation ceases before applying a replacement patch to avoid potential excessive absorption. Should a patch fall off at other times it should be replaced immediately.

Patients can be advised to use baby oil to help remove any gum/glue which may remain on their skin after patch removal.

Unopposed oestrogen therapy is not recommended unless the patient has had hysterectomy. Where a progestogen is considered necessary, the appropriate dose should be administered for not less than 12 days each month.

Children: Evorel is not indicated in children.

4.3 Contraindications
Known or suspected malignant tumours of the breast, genital tract or other oestrogen dependent neoplasia. Undiagnosed vaginal bleeding, known or suspected pregnancy and lactation, severe hepatic, renal or cardiac disease, Rotor syndrome or Dubin-Johnson syndrome, active thrombophlebitis, active deep venous thrombosis, thrombo-embolic disorders, or a history of confirmed venous thrombo-embolism, endometriosis, hypersensitivity to any of the excipients.

4.4 Special warnings and special precautions for use
Assessment of each woman prior to using hormone replacement therapy (and at regular intervals thereafter) should include a personal and family medical history. Physical examination should be guided by this and by the Contra-indications (Section 4.3) and Warnings (Section 4.4) for this product. During assessment of each individual woman clinical examination of the breasts and pelvic examination should be performed where clinically indicated rather than as a routine procedure. Women should be encouraged to participate in the national breast cancer screening programme (mammography) and the national cervical cancer screening programme (cervical cytology) as appropriate for their age. Breast awareness should also be encouraged and women advised to report any changes in their breasts to their doctor or nurse.

A re-analysis of original data from 51 epidemiological studies reported a small or moderate increase in the probability of having breast cancer *diagnosed* in women currently or recently using HRT. The findings may be due to biological effects of HRT, earlier diagnosis, or a combination of both. The relative risk increased with duration of treatment (by 2.3% per year of use) and returned to normal in the course of five years after cessation of HRT use. This is comparable to the increase in relative risk when natural menopause is delayed in the absence of HRT. Breast cancers diagnosed in current or recent users of HRT are more likely to be localised to the breast than those found in non-users. HRT use may not be associated with increased mortality from breast cancer.

Between the ages of 50 and 70, about 45 women in every 1,000 not using HRT will have breast cancer diagnosed. It is estimated that among those who use HRT for 5 years starting at age 50, 2 extra cases of breast cancer will be detected by age 70 in every 1,000 women. For those who use HRT for 10 years, there will be 6 extra cases of breast cancer, and for 15 years use, 12 extra cases of breast cancer in every 1,000 women during the 20 year period until age 70.

It is important that the increased risk of being diagnosed with breast cancer is discussed with the patient and weighed against the known benefits of HRT.

Administration of unopposed oestrogen therapy in patients with an intact uterus has been reported to increase the risk of endometrial hyperplasia. Repeated breakthrough bleeding should be investigated, including endometrial biopsy.

Close monitoring is recommended in patients with: epilepsy, diabetes or hypertension (as oestrogens may cause fluid retention), disturbances or impairment of liver function, mastopathy or a strong family history of breast cancer, fibrocystic disease, uterine fibromyomata, cholelithiasis, otosclerosis, multiple sclerosis, systemic lupus erythematosus, porphyria, melanoma, migraine, and asthma, as these conditions may be worsened by oestrogen therapy.

Consideration should be given to discontinuing treatment at least four weeks prior to surgery or during periods of prolonged immobilisation. Also, if hypertension develops after initiating therapy, consider discontinuing Evorel while the cause is investigated.

Epidemiological studies have suggested that hormone replacement therapy (HRT) is associated with an increased relative risk of developing venous thrombo-embolism (VTE), ie deep vein thrombosis or pulmonary embolism. The studies find a 2-3 fold increase for users compared with non-users which for healthy women amounts to a low risk for one extra case of VTE each year for every 5,000 patients taking HRT.

Generally recognised risk factors for VTE include a personal or family history and severe obesity (body mass index >30 kg/m^2). In women with these factors the benefits of treatment with HRT need to be carefully weighed against risks.

The risk of VTE may be temporarily increased with prolonged immobilisation, major trauma or major surgery. In women on HRT scrupulous attention should be given to prophylactic measures to prevent VTE following surgery. Where prolonged immobilisation is liable to follow elective surgery, particularly abdominal or orthopaedic surgery to the lower limbs, consideration should be given to temporarily stopping HRT 4 weeks earlier, if this is possible.

If venous thrombo-embolism develops after initiating therapy the drug should be discontinued.

Evorel is not to be used for contraception.

4.5 Interaction with other medicinal products and other forms of Interaction
Drugs which cause microsomal liver enzyme activity may alter oestrogen action. Examples of such drugs include barbiturates, hydantoins, carbamazepine, meprobamate, phenylbutazole and rifampicin. In transdermal administration of estradiol, a first pass effect via the liver is avoided.

There have been no reports of interaction with Evorel although the clinical exposure has been very limited.

4.6 Pregnancy and lactation
Evorel in contra-indicated in pregnancy and lactation.

4.7 Effects on ability to drive and use machines
In normal use, Evorel would not be expected to have any effect on the ability to drive or use machinery.

4.8 Undesirable effects
Although side effects are rare, minor effects which do not usually preclude continuation of therapy include headaches, nausea, breast tenderness, and intermittent bleeding.

In clinical studies with Evorel (50 μg/24 hours) the following side effects were seen: breast tenderness (less than 2%), bleeding (less than 2%), and intermittent bleeding/spotting (less than 5%). None were serious, reflecting the known profile of oestrogen or oestrogen/progestogen therapy. Skin reactions were reported by less than 6% of patients over six treatment cycles. Rarely, dizziness, bloating, oedema, weight gain and leg cramps may occur.

4.9 Overdose

By virtue of the mode of administration of Evorel, overdosage is unlikely, but effects can if necessary be reversed by removal of the patch. The most commonly observed symptoms of overdose with oestrogen therapy are breast tenderness, nausea and breakthrough bleeding.

5. PHARMACOLOGICAL PROPERTIES

5.1 Pharmacodynamic properties

Estradiol is a naturally occurring oestrogenic hormone. It is formed in the ovarian follicles under the influence of the pituitary gland. In the female it stimulates the accessory reproductive organs and causes development of the secondary sexual changes in the endometrium during the first half of the menstrual cycle.

Estradiol is readily and completely absorbed from the gastro-intestinal tract and through the skin and mucous membranes. Metabolism is primarily in the liver. Excretion of the less active metabolites, primarily oestrone and oestriol is via the urine.

Evorel releases estradiol transdermally into the circulation in pre-menopausal physiological amounts.

In post-menopausal women, Evorel increased estradiol levels to early and mid-follicular phase levels. The transcutaneous route avoids the first pass hepatic effect seen with orally administered oestrogens.

In contrast with oral oestrogens, stimulation of hepatic protein synthesis is largely avoided with consequent lack of effect on circulating levels of renin substrate, thyroid binding globulin, sex hormone binding globulin and cortisol binding globulin. Similarly coagulation factors also appear to be unaffected (e.g. fibrinopeptide A etc.). Transdermal estradiol does not affect circulating levels of renin.

Studies with Evorel have shown a significant decrease in hot flushes, improvement in Kupperman Index and vaginal cytology.

Local tolerance with Evorel has been very good. The adhesive matrix used has a low irritation index.

5.2 Pharmacokinetic properties

General characteristics: Oestrogens are in general readily absorbed from the gastro-intestinal tract, through the skin and mucous membranes. Absorption from the gastro-intestinal tract is prompt and complete. Transdermal absorption of oestrogens is sufficient to cause a systemic effect. Inactivation of oestrogens in the body is mainly in the liver and consequently the limited oral effectiveness of oestrogens is related to first pass hepatic metabolism and not to poor absorption. A certain proportion of oestrogen is excreted into the bile and then reabsorbed from the intestine. During the enterohepatic circulation, estradiol is readily oxidised to the less pharmacologically active oestrone which may in turn then be hydrated to form oestriol (also pharmacologically less than estradiol). Estradiol circulates in the blood in association with sex hormone-binding globulin and albumin.

Characteristics in patients: With Evorel, therapeutic serum estradiol levels are achieved approximately four hours after application to the skin. From 10 hours onwards, the serum levels remain stable and at early to mid-follicular levels throughout the duration of the application (3 to 4 days).

Twenty four hours following removal of the transdermal therapeutic system estradiol levels return to baseline.

5.3 Preclinical safety data

Not applicable

6. PHARMACEUTICAL PARTICULARS

6.1 List of excipients

Adhesive acrylic polymer (Duro-Tak 387-2287)

Guar gum

Hostaphan MN19 (polyester film - removed before application)

6.2 Incompatibilities

None known.

6.3 Shelf life

36 months for the product as packed for sale.

6.4 Special precautions for storage

Do not store above 25°C.

6.5 Nature and contents of container

Each Evorel 25 patch is presented in a sealed protective pouch. The pouches are packed in a cardboard carton.

6.6 Instructions for use and handling

Not applicable.

7. MARKETING AUTHORISATION HOLDER

Janssen-Cilag Limited
Saunderton
High Wycombe
Buckinghamshire
HP14 4HJ
UK

8. MARKETING AUTHORISATION NUMBER(S)

00242/0293

9. DATE OF FIRST AUTHORISATION/RENEWAL OF THE AUTHORISATION

1 November 1995

10. DATE OF REVISION OF THE TEXT

December 2004

Evorel 50 Patch

(Janssen-Cilag Ltd)

1. NAME OF THE MEDICINAL PRODUCT

Evorel 50

2. QUALITATIVE AND QUANTITATIVE COMPOSITION

Each Evorel 50 patch contains estradiol 3.20 mg.

3. PHARMACEUTICAL FORM

Evorel is a square shaped, transparent, self-adhesive transdermal therapeutic system (patch) of surface area 16 sq. cm and 0.2 mm thickness, for application to the skin surface. It consists of a monolayered adhesive matrix throughout which 17β estradiol is uniformly distributed. The adhesive matrix is protected on the outside surface (from clothes etc.) by a polyethylene teraphthalate backing foil, while the adhesive surface of the patch is covered by a polyester sheet (the release liner) which is removed before placing the patch on the body surface. This release liner has an S-shaped incision which facilitates easy removal from the patch.

4. CLINICAL PARTICULARS

4.1 Therapeutic indications

Oestrogen replacement for the symptomatic relief of menopausal symptoms.

Second line therapy for prevention of osteoporosis in postmenopausal women at high risk of future fractures who are intolerant of, or contraindicated for, other medicinal products approved for the prevention of osteoporosis.

4.2 Posology and method of administration

Adults:

Menopausal symptoms

Therapy should be started with one Evorel 50 patch (delivering 50 micrograms of estradiol/24 hours) and the dose adjusted after the first month if necessary depending on efficacy and signs of over-oestrogenisation (eg breast tenderness). For maintenance therapy, the lowest effective dose should be used; a maximum dose of 100 micrograms of estradiol/24 hours should not be exceeded.

Post menopausal osteoporosis

Evorel 50 is recommended as an effective bone-sparing dose, with lower doses of estradiol slowing but not halting bone loss.

Evorel should be applied twice weekly on a continuous basis, each patch being renewed after 3 to 4 days and a fresh patch applied. Evorel should be applied to the skin as soon as it is removed from the wrapper. Recommended application sites are on clean, dry, healthy, intact skin and each application should be made to a slightly different area of skin on the trunk below waistline. Evorel should not be applied on or near the breasts. Evorel should remain in place during bathing and showering. Should it fall off during bathing or showering the patient should wait until cutaneous vasodilation ceases before applying a replacement patch to avoid potential excessive absorption. Should a patch fall off at other times it should be replaced immediately.

Patients can be advised to use baby oil to help remove any gum/glue which may remain on their skin after patch removal.

Unopposed oestrogen therapy is not recommended unless the patient has had hysterectomy. Where a progestogen is considered necessary, the appropriate dose should be administered for not less than 12 days each month.

Children: Evorel is not indicated in children.

4.3 Contraindications

Known or suspected malignant tumours of the breast, genital tract or other oestrogen dependent neoplasia. Undiagnosed vaginal bleeding, known or suspected pregnancy and lactation, severe hepatic, renal or cardiac disease, Rotor syndrome or Dubin-Johnson syndrome, active thrombophlebitis, active deep venous thrombosis, thrombo-embolic disorders, or a history of confirmed venous thrombo-embolism, endometriosis, hypersensitivity to any of the excipients.

4.4 Special warnings and special precautions for use

Assessment of each woman prior to using hormone replacement therapy (and at regular intervals thereafter) should include a personal and family medical history. Physical examination should be guided by this and by the Contraindications (Section 4.3) and Warnings (Section 4.4) for this product. During assessment of each individual woman clinical examination of the breasts and pelvic examination should be performed where clinically indicated rather than as a routine procedure. Women should be encouraged to participate in the national breast cancer screening programme (mammography) and the national cervical cancer screening programme (cervical cytology) as appropriate for their age. Breast awareness should also be encouraged and women advised to report any changes in their breasts to their doctor or nurse.

A re-analysis of original data from 51 epidemiological studies reported a small or moderate increase in the probability of having breast cancer *diagnosed* in women currently or recently using HRT. The findings may be due to biological effects of HRT, earlier diagnosis, or a combination of both. The relative risk increased with duration of treatment (by 2.3% per year of use) and returned to normal in the course of five years after cessation of HRT use. This is comparable to the increase in relative risk when natural menopause is delayed in the absence of HRT. Breast cancers diagnosed in current or recent users of HRT are more likely to be localised to the breast than those found in non-users. HRT use may not be associated with increased mortality from breast cancer.

Between the ages of 50 and 70, about 45 women in every 1,000 not using HRT will have breast cancer diagnosed. It is estimated that among those who use HRT for 5 years starting at age 50, 2 extra cases of breast cancer will be detected by age 70 in every 1,000 women. For those who use HRT for 10 years, there will be 6 extra cases of breast cancer, and for 15 years use, 12 extra cases of breast cancer in every 1,000 women during the 20 year period until age 70.

It is important that the increased risk of being diagnosed with breast cancer is discussed with the patient and weighed against the known benefits of HRT.

Administration of unopposed oestrogen therapy in patients with an intact uterus has been reported to increase the risk of endometrial hyperplasia. Repeated breakthrough bleeding should be investigated, including endometrial biopsy.

Close monitoring is recommended in patients with: epilepsy, diabetes or hypertension (as oestrogens may cause fluid retention), disturbances or impairment of liver function, mastopathy or a strong family history of breast cancer, fibrocystic disease, uterine fibromyomata, cholelithiasis, otosclerosis, multiple sclerosis, systemic lupus erythematosus, porphyria, melanoma, migraine, and asthma, as these conditions may be worsened by oestrogen therapy.

Consideration should be given to discontinuing treatment at least four weeks prior to surgery or during periods of prolonged immobilisation. Also, if hypertension develops after initiating therapy, consider discontinuing Evorel while the cause is investigated.

Epidemiological studies have suggested that hormone replacement therapy (HRT) is associated with an increased relative risk of developing venous thrombo-embolism (VTE), ie deep vein thrombosis or pulmonary embolism. The studies find a 2-3 fold increase for users compared with non-users which for healthy women amounts to a low risk for one extra case of VTE each year for every 5,000 patients taking HRT.

Generally recognised risk factors for VTE include a personal or family history and severe obesity (body mass index >30 kg/m^2). In women with these factors the benefits of treatment with HRT need to be carefully weighed against risks.

The risk of VTE may be temporarily increased with prolonged immobilisation, major trauma or major surgery. In women on HRT scrupulous attention should be given to prophylactic measures to prevent VTE following surgery. Where prolonged immobilisation is liable to follow elective surgery, particularly abdominal or orthopaedic surgery to the lower limbs, consideration should be given to temporarily stopping HRT 4 weeks earlier, if this is possible.

If venous thrombo-embolism develops after initiating therapy the drug should be discontinued.

Evorel is not to be used for contraception.

4.5 Interaction with other medicinal products and other forms of interaction

Drugs which induce microsomal liver enzyme activity may alter oestrogen and progestogen metabolism. Examples of such drugs include barbiturates, hydantoins, carbamazepine, meprobamate, phenylbutazole and rifampicin. In transdermal administration of estradiol, a first pass effect via the liver is avoided.

There have been no reports of interaction with Evorel although the clinical exposure has been very limited.

4.6 Pregnancy and lactation

Evorel in contra-indicated in pregnancy and lactation.

4.7 Effects on ability to drive and use machines

In normal use, Evorel would not be expected to have any effect on the ability to drive or use machinery.

4.8 Undesirable effects

Although side effects are rare, minor effects which do not usually preclude continuation of therapy include headaches, nausea, breast tenderness, and intermittent bleeding.

In clinical studies with Evorel (50 μg/24 hours) the following side effects were seen: breast tenderness (less than 2%), bleeding (less than 21%), and intermittent bleeding/spotting (less than 5%). None were serious, reflecting the known profile of oestrogen or oestrogen/progestogen therapy. Skin reactions were reported by less than 6% of patients over six treatment cycles. Rarely, dizziness, bloating, oedema, weight gain and leg cramps may occur.

4.9 Overdose
By virtue of the mode of administration of Evorel, overdosage is unlikely, but effects can if necessary be reversed by removal of the patch. The most commonly observed symptoms of overdose with oestrogen therapy are breast tenderness, nausea and breakthrough bleeding.

5. PHARMACOLOGICAL PROPERTIES

5.1 Pharmacodynamic properties
Estradiol is a naturally occurring oestrogenic hormone. It is formed in the ovarian follicles under the influence of the pituitary gland. In the female it stimulates the accessory reproductive organs and causes development of the secondary sexual changes in the endometrium during the first half of the menstrual cycle.

Estradiol is readily and completely absorbed from the gastro-intestinal tract through the skin and mucous membranes. Metabolism is primarily in the liver. Excretion of the less active metabolites, primarily oestrone and oestriol is via the urine.

Evorel releases estradiol transdermally into the circulation in pre-menopausal physiological amounts.

In post-menopausal women, Evorel increased estradiol levels to early and mid-follicular phase levels. The transcutaneous route avoids the first pass hepatic effect seen with orally administered oestrogens.

In contrast with oral oestrogens, stimulation of hepatic protein synthesis is largely avoided with consequent lack of effect on circulating levels of renin substrate, thyroid binding globulin, sex hormone binding globulin and cortisol binding globulin. Similarly coagulation factors also appear to be unaffected (e.g. fibrinopeptide A etc.). Transdermal estradiol does not affect circulating levels of renin.

Studies with Evorel have shown a significant decrease in hot flushes, improvement in Kupperman Index and vaginal cytology.

Local tolerance with Evorel has been very good. The adhesive matrix used has a low irritation index.

5.2 Pharmacokinetic properties
General characteristics: Oestrogens are in general readily absorbed from the gastro-intestinal tract, through the skin and mucous membranes. Absorption from the gastro-intestinal tract is prompt and complete. Transdermal absorption of oestrogens is sufficient to cause a systemic effect. Inactivation of oestrogens is related to first pass hepatic metabolism and not to poor absorption. A certain proportion of oestrogen is excreted into the bile and then reabsorbed from the intestine. During the enterohepatic circulation, estradiol is readily oxidised to the less pharmacologically active oestrone which may in turn then be hydrated to form oestriol (also pharmacologically less than estradiol). Estradiol circulates in the blood in association with sex hormone-binding globulin and albumin.

Characteristics in patients: With Evorel, therapeutic serum estradiol levels are achieved approximately four hours after application to the skin. From 10 hours onwards, the serum levels remain stable and at early to mid-follicular levels throughout the duration of the application (3 to 4 days).

Twenty four hours following removal of the transdermal therapeutic system estradiol levels return to baseline.

5.3 Preclinical safety data
Not applicable

6. PHARMACEUTICAL PARTICULARS

6.1 List of excipients
Adhesive acrylic polymer (Duro-Tak 387-2287)

Guar gum

Hostaphan MN19 (polyester film - removed before application)

6.2 Incompatibilities
None known.

6.3 Shelf life
36 months for the product as packed for sale.

6.4 Special precautions for storage
Do not store above 25°C.

6.5 Nature and contents of container
Each Evorel 50 patch is presented in a sealed protective pouch. The pouches are packed in a cardboard carton. (Pack sizes 2, 8, 10, 24, 26, 30, 48, 60 patches).

Evorel 50 is also available in a combination pack as Evorel Pak. Evorel Pak contains 8 × Evorel 50 Patches (PL/0242/0223) and 12 × 1 mg Micronor HRT/norethisterone tablets (PL/0242/0241).

6.6 Instructions for use and handling
Not applicable

7. MARKETING AUTHORISATION HOLDER
Janssen-Cilag Limited

Saunderton

High Wycombe

Buckinghamshire

HP14 4HJ

UK

8. MARKETING AUTHORISATION NUMBER(S)
0242/0223

9. DATE OF FIRST AUTHORISATION/RENEWAL OF THE AUTHORISATION
1 November 1995

10. DATE OF REVISION OF THE TEXT
December 2004

11. Legal Category
POM.

Evorel 75 Patch

(Janssen-Cilag Ltd)

1. NAME OF THE MEDICINAL PRODUCT
Evorel 75

2. QUALITATIVE AND QUANTITATIVE COMPOSITION
Each Evorel 75 patch contains estradiol 4.80 mg.

3. PHARMACEUTICAL FORM
Evorel is a square shaped, transparent, self-adhesive transdermal therapeutic system (patch) to skin. Evorel 75 has a surface area of 16 cm^2 and 0.2 mm thickness. It consists of a monolayered adhesive matrix throughout which 17β estradiol is uniformly distributed. The adhesive matrix is protected on the outside surface (from clothes etc.) by a polyethylene teraphthalate backing foil, while the adhesive surface of the patch is covered by a polyester sheet (the release liner) which is removed before placing the patch on the body surface. This release liner has an S-shaped incision which facilitates easy removal from the patch.

4. CLINICAL PARTICULARS

4.1 Therapeutic indications
Oestrogen replacement for the symptomatic relief of menopausal symptoms.

Second line therapy for prevention of osteoporosis in post-menopausal women at high risk of future fractures who are intolerant of, or contraindicated for, other medicinal products approved for the prevention of osteoporosis.

4.2 Posology and method of administration
Adults:

Menopausal symptoms

Therapy should be started with one Evorel 50 patch (delivering 50 micrograms of estradiol/24 hours) and the dose adjusted after the first month if necessary depending on efficacy and signs of over-oestrogenisation (eg breast tenderness). For maintenance therapy, the lowest effective dose should be used; a maximum dose of 100 micrograms of estradiol/24 hours should not be exceeded.

Post menopausal osteoporosis

Evorel 75 is recommended as an effective bone-sparing dose, with lower doses of estradiol slowing but not halting bone loss.

Evorel should be applied twice weekly on a continuous basis, each patch being renewed after 3 to 4 days and a fresh patch applied. Evorel should be applied to the skin as soon as it is removed from the wrapper. Recommended application sites are on clean, dry, healthy, intact skin and each application should be made to a slightly different area of skin on the trunk below waistline. **Evorel should not be applied on or near the breasts.** Evorel should remain in place during bathing and showering. Should it fall off during bathing or showering the patient should wait until cutaneous vasodilation ceases before applying a replacement patch to avoid potential excessive absorption. Should a patch fall off at other times it should be replaced immediately.

Patients can be advised to use baby oil to help remove any gum/glue which may remain on their skin after patch removal.

Unopposed oestrogen therapy is not recommended unless the patient has had hysterectomy. Where a progestogen is considered necessary, the appropriate dose should be administered for not less than 12 days each month.

Children: Evorel is not indicated in children.

4.3 Contraindications
Known or suspected malignant tumours of the breast, genital tract or other oestrogen dependent neoplasia. Undiagnosed vaginal bleeding, known or suspected pregnancy and lactation, severe hepatic, renal or cardiac disease, Rotor syndrome or Dubin-Johnson syndrome, active thrombophlebitis, active deep venous thrombosis, thrombo-embolic disorders, or a history of confirmed venous thrombo-embolism, endometriosis, hypersensitivity to any of the excipients.

4.4 Special warnings and special precautions for use
Assessment of each woman prior to using hormone replacement therapy (and at regular intervals thereafter) should include a personal and family medical history. Physical examination should be guided by this and by the Contra-indications (Section 4.3) and Warnings (Section 4.4) for this product. During assessment of each individual woman clinical examination of the breasts and pelvic examination should be performed where clinically indicated rather than as a routine procedure. Women should be encouraged to participate in the national breast cancer screening programme (mammography) and the national cervical cancer screening programme (cervical cytology) as appropriate for their age. Breast awareness should also be encouraged and women advised to report any changes in their breasts to their doctor or nurse.

A re-analysis of original data from 51 epidemiological studies reported a small or moderate increase in the probability of having breast cancer *diagnosed* in women currently or recently using HRT. The findings may be due to biological effects of HRT, earlier diagnosis, or a combination of both. The relative risk increased with duration of treatment (by 2.3% per year of use) and returned to normal in the course of five years after cessation of HRT use. This is comparable to the increase in relative risk when natural menopause is delayed in the absence of HRT. Breast cancers diagnosed in current or recent users of HRT are more likely to be localised to the breast than those found in non-users. HRT use may not be associated with increased mortality from breast cancer.

Between the ages of 50 and 70, about 45 women in every 1,000 not using HRT will have breast cancer diagnosed. It is estimated that among those who use HRT for 5 years starting at age 50, 2 extra cases of breast cancer will be detected by age 70 in every 1,000 women. For those who use HRT for 10 years, there will be 6 extra cases of breast cancer, and for 15 years use, 12 extra cases of breast cancer in every 1,000 women during the 20 year period until age 70.

It is important that the increased risk of being diagnosed with breast cancer is discussed with the patient and weighed against the known benefits of HRT.

Administration of unopposed oestrogen therapy in patients with an intact uterus has been reported to increase the risk of endometrial hyperplasia. Repeated breakthrough bleeding should be investigated, including endometrial biopsy.

Close monitoring is recommended in patients with: epilepsy, diabetes or hypertension (as oestrogens may cause fluid retention), disturbances or impairment of liver function, mastopathy or a strong family history of breast cancer, fibrocystic disease, uterine fibromyomata, cholelithiasis, otosclerosis, multiple sclerosis, systemic lupus erythematosus, porphyria, melanoma, migraine, and asthma, as these conditions may be worsened by oestrogen therapy.

Consideration should be given to discontinuing treatment at least four weeks prior to surgery or during periods of prolonged immobilisation. Also, if hypertension develops after initiating therapy, consider discontinuing Evorel while the cause is investigated.

Epidemiological studies have suggested that hormone replacement therapy (HRT) is associated with an increased relative risk of developing venous thrombo-embolism (VTE), ie deep vein thrombosis or pulmonary embolism. The studies find a 2-3 fold increase for users compared with non-users which for healthy women amounts to a low risk for one extra case of VTE each year for every 5,000 patients taking HRT.

Generally recognised risk factors for VTE include a personal or family history and severe obesity (body mass index >30 kg/m^2). In women with these factors the benefits of treatment with HRT need to be carefully weighed against risks.

The risk of VTE may be temporarily increased with prolonged immobilisation, major trauma or major surgery. In women on HRT scrupulous attention should be given to prophylactic measures to prevent VTE following surgery. Where prolonged immobilisation is liable to follow elective surgery, particularly abdominal or orthopaedic surgery to the lower limbs, consideration should be given to temporarily stopping HRT 4 weeks earlier, if this is possible.

If venous thrombo-embolism develops after initiating therapy the drug should be discontinued.

Evorel is not to be used for contraception.

4.5 Interaction with other medicinal products and other forms of Interaction
Drugs which cause microsomal liver enzyme activity may alter oestrogen action. Examples of such drugs include barbiturates, hydantoins, carbamazepine, meprobamate, phenylbutazole and rifampicin. In transdermal administration of estradiol, a first pass effect via the liver is avoided.

There have been no reports of interaction with Evorel although the clinical exposure has been very limited.

4.6 Pregnancy and lactation
Evorel in contra-indicated in pregnancy and lactation.

4.7 Effects on ability to drive and use machines
In normal use, Evorel would not be expected to have any effect on the ability to drive or use machinery.

4.8 Undesirable effects
Although side effects are rare, minor effects which do not usually preclude continuation of therapy include headaches, nausea, breast tenderness, and intermittent bleeding.

In clinical studies with Evorel (50 μg/24 hours) the following side effects were seen: breast tenderness (less than 2%), bleeding (less than 2%), and intermittent bleeding/spotting (less than 5%). None were serious, reflecting the known profile of oestrogen or oestrogen/progestogen therapy. Skin reactions were reported by less than 6% of patients over six treatment cycles. Rarely, dizziness, bloating, oedema, weight gain and leg cramps may occur.

4.9 Overdose

By virtue of the mode of administration of Evorel, overdosage is unlikely, but effects can if necessary be reversed by removal of the patch. The most commonly observed symptoms of overdose with oestrogen therapy are breast tenderness, nausea and breakthrough bleeding.

5. PHARMACOLOGICAL PROPERTIES

5.1 Pharmacodynamic properties

Estradiol is a naturally occurring oestrogenic hormone. It is formed in the ovarian follicles under the influence of the pituitary gland. In the female it stimulates the accessory reproductive organs and causes development of the secondary sexual changes in the endometrium during the first half of the menstrual cycle.

Estradiol is readily and completely absorbed from the gastro-intestinal tract and through the skin and mucous membranes. Metabolism is primarily in the liver. Excretion of the less active metabolites, primarily oestrone and oestriol is via the urine.

Evorel releases estradiol transdermally into the circulation in pre-menopausal physiological amounts.

In post-menopausal women, Evorel increased estradiol levels to early and mid-follicular phase levels. The transcutaneous route avoids the first pass hepatic effect seen with orally administered oestrogens.

In contrast with oral oestrogens, stimulation of hepatic protein synthesis is largely avoided with consequent lack of effect on circulating levels of renin substrate, thyroid binding globulin, sex hormone binding globulin and cortisol binding globulin. Similarly coagulation factors also appear to be unaffected (e.g. fibrinopeptide A etc.). Transdermal estradiol does not affect circulating levels of renin.

Studies with Evorel have shown a significant decrease in hot flushes, improvement in Kupperman Index and vaginal cytology.

Local tolerance with Evorel has been very good. The adhesive matrix used has a low irritation index.

5.2 Pharmacokinetic properties

General characteristics: Oestrogens are in general readily absorbed from the gastro-intestinal tract, through the skin and mucous membranes. Absorption from the gastro-intestinal tract is prompt and complete. Transdermal absorption of oestrogens is sufficient to cause a systemic effect. Inactivation of oestrogens in the body is mainly in the liver and consequently the limited oral effectiveness of oestrogens is related to first pass hepatic metabolism and not to poor absorption. A certain proportion of oestrogen is excreted into the bile and then reabsorbed from the intestine. During the enterohepatic circulation, estradiol is readily oxidised to the less pharmacologically active oestrone which may in turn then be hydrated to form oestriol (also pharmacologically less than estradiol). Estradiol circulates in the blood in association with sex hormone-binding globulin and albumin.

Characteristics in patients: With Evorel, therapeutic serum estradiol levels are achieved approximately four hours after application to the skin. From 10 hours onwards, the serum levels remain stable and at early to mid-follicular levels throughout the duration of the application (3 to 4 days).

Twenty four hours following removal of the transdermal therapeutic system estradiol levels return to baseline.

5.3 Preclinical safety data

Not applicable

6. PHARMACEUTICAL PARTICULARS

6.1 List of excipients

Adhesive acrylic polymer (Duro-Tak 387-2287)

Guar gum

Hostaphan MN19 (polyester film - removed before application)

6.2 Incompatibilities

None known.

6.3 Shelf life

36 months for the product as packed for sale.

6.4 Special precautions for storage

Do not store above 25°C.

6.5 Nature and contents of container

Each Evorel 75 patch is presented in a sealed protective pouch. The pouches are packed in a cardboard carton.

6.6 Instructions for use and handling

Not applicable.

7. MARKETING AUTHORISATION HOLDER

Janssen-Cilag Limited

Saunderton

High Wycombe

Buckinghamshire

HP14 4HJ

UK

8. MARKETING AUTHORISATION NUMBER(S)

00242/0294

9. DATE OF FIRST AUTHORISATION/RENEWAL OF THE AUTHORISATION

1 November 1995

10. DATE OF REVISION OF THE TEXT

December 2004

Evorel Conti

(Janssen-Cilag Ltd)

1. NAME OF THE MEDICINAL PRODUCT

EVOREL® CONTI

estradiol

norethisterone acetate

2. QUALITATIVE AND QUANTITATIVE COMPOSITION

EVOREL® CONTI

3.2 mg of estradiol hemihydrate

11.2 mg of norethisterone acetate

3. PHARMACEUTICAL FORM

The EVOREL® CONTI Transdermal Delivery System (TDS), or transdermal patch, is a flat two-layer laminate which is 0.1 mm in thickness. The first layer is a flexible, translucent, and nearly colourless backing film. The second layer is a monolayer adhesive film (matrix) composed of acrylic adhesive and guar gum and contains the hormones. This system is protected by a polyester foil release liner, which is affixed to the adhesive matrix and is removed prior to application of the patch to the skin. The polyester foil used is coated with silicone on both sides. The release liner has an S-shaped opening to facilitate its removal prior to use. Each TDS is enclosed in a protective, hermetically-sealed sachet.

EVOREL® CONTI has a surface area of 16 sq cm and contains 3.2 mg of estradiol corresponding to a nominal release of 50 micrograms of estradiol per 24 hours and 11.2 mg of norethisterone acetate corresponding to a nominal release of 170 micrograms of norethisterone acetate per 24 hours. Each TDS is marked in the centre of the lower margin on the outside of the backing film: CEN1.

4. CLINICAL PARTICULARS

4.1 Therapeutic indications

Hormone replacement therapy for the relief of menopausal symptoms.

Second line therapy for prevention of osteoporosis in post-menopausal women at high risk of future fractures who are intolerant of, or contraindicated for, other medicinal products approved for the prevention of osteoporosis.

4.2 Posology and method of administration

Adults

Menopausal symptoms

EVOREL® CONTI TDS should be applied individually without interruption.

EVOREL CONTI TDS should be applied twice weekly, every three to four days, to the trunk below the waist.

Insufficient data are available to guide dose adjustments for patients with severe liver or kidney function impairment.

Post menopausal osteoporosis

Evorel Conti is recommended as an effective bone-sparing dose, with lower doses of estradiol slowing but not halting bone loss.

Children

EVOREL® CONTI is not indicated in children.

Elderly

Data are insufficient in regard to the use of EVOREL® CONTI in the elderly (>65 years old).

The sachet containing one TDS should be opened and one part of the protective foil removed at the S-shaped incision. The TDS should be applied to clean, dry, healthy, intact skin as soon as it is removed from the sachet.

The patient should avoid contact between fingers and the adhesive part of the TDS during application. Each application should be made to a different area of the skin, on the trunk below the waist. EVOREL® CONTI should not be applied on or near the breasts.

EVOREL® CONTI should remain in place during bathing and showering. Should a TDS fall off, it should be replaced immediately with a new patch. However the usual day of changing TDSs should be maintained.

4.3 Contraindications

- Hypersensitivity to any component of this product
- Known or suspected malignant tumours of the breast
- Genital tract or other oestrogen-dependent neoplasia
- Undiagnosed vaginal bleeding
- Pregnancy or lactation
- Severe hepatic or renal disease
- Active thrombophlebitis
- Active deep venous thrombosis, thrombo-embolic disorders, or a history of confirmed venous thrombo-embolism
- Endometriosis

4.4 Special warnings and special precautions for use

Assessment of each woman prior to using hormone replacement therapy (and at regular intervals thereafter) should include a personal and family medical history. Physical examination should be guided by this and by the Contra-indications (Section 4.3) and Warnings (Section 4.4) for this product. During assessment of each individual woman clinical examination of the breasts and pelvic examination should be performed where clinically indicated rather than as a routine procedure. Women should be encouraged to participate in the national breast cancer screening programme (mammography) and the national cervical cancer screening programme (cervical cytology) as appropriate for their age. Breast awareness should also be encouraged and women advised to report any changes in their breasts to their doctor or nurse. Repeated breakthrough bleeding, unexplained vaginal bleeding and changes noticed during breast examination require further evaluation.

A re-analysis of original data from 51 epidemiological studies reported a small or moderate increase in the probability of having breast cancer *diagnosed* in women currently or recently using HRT. The findings may be due to biological effects of HRT, earlier diagnosis, or a combination of both. The relative risk increased with duration of treatment (by 2.3% per year of use) and returned to normal in the course of five years after cessation of HRT use. This is comparable to the increase in relative risk when natural menopause is delayed in the absence of HRT. Breast cancers diagnosed in current or recent users of HRT are more likely to be localised to the breast than those found in non-users. HRT use may not be associated with increased mortality from breast cancer.

Between the ages of 50 and 70, about 45 women in every 1,000 not using HRT will have breast cancer diagnosed. It is estimated that among those who use HRT for 5 years starting at age 50, 2 extra cases of breast cancer will be detected by age 70 in every 1,000 women. For those who use HRT for 10 years, there will be 6 extra cases of breast cancer, and for 15 years use, 12 extra cases of breast cancer in every 1,000 women during the 20 year period until age 70.

It is important that the increased risk of being diagnosed with breast cancer is discussed with the patient and weighed against the known benefits of HRT.

Epidemiological studies have suggested that hormone replacement therapy (HRT) is associated with an increased relative risk of developing venous thromboembolism (VTE), ie deep vein thrombosis or pulmonary embolism. The studies find a 2-3 fold increase for users compared with non-users which for healthy women amounts to a low risk for one extra case of VTE each year for every 5,000 patients taking HRT.

Generally recognised risk factors for VTE include a personal or family history and severe obesity (body mass index >30 kg/m^2). In women with these factors the benefits of treatment with HRT need to be carefully weighed against risks.

The risk of VTE may be temporarily increased with prolonged immobilisation, major trauma or major surgery. In women on HRT scrupulous attention should be given to prophylactic measures to prevent VTE following surgery. Where prolonged immobilisation is liable to follow elective surgery, particularly abdominal or orthopaedic surgery to the lower limbs, consideration should be given to temporarily stopping HRT 4 weeks earlier, if this is possible.

If venous thrombo-embolism develops after initiating therapy the drug should be discontinued.

Appropriate monitoring is recommended in patients with cardiac impairment, epilepsy, diabetes, hypertension, disturbances or impairment of liver or kidney function, mastopathy, a family history of breast cancer, or a history of cholestatic jaundice.

Administration of unopposed oestrogen in patients with an intact uterus has been reported to increase the risk of endometrial hyperplasia and of endometrial carcinoma. Therefore, oestrogen in combination with progestogen as in EVOREL® CONTI is recommended in women with an intact uterus in order to reduce the risk of hyperplasia or endometrial carcinoma.

EVOREL® CONTI is not to be used as contraception.

The EVOREL® CONTI patches should be kept away from children and pets.

4.5 Interaction with other medicinal products and other forms of Interaction

Drugs which induce microsomal liver enzyme activity may alter oestrogen and progestogen metabolism. Examples of such drugs are barbiturates, hydantoins, carbamazepine, meprobamate, phenylbutazone and rifampicin. On a theoretical basis, the effects of liver enzyme induction on the metabolism of transdermally administered estradiol and norethisterone acetate should be minimised by the avoidance of the first pass liver metabolism.

4.6 Pregnancy and lactation

The use of EVOREL® CONTI is contra-indicated in pregnancy and lactation.

4.7 Effects on ability to drive and use machines

There are no known data on the effects of EVOREL® CONTI on the ability to drive or use machinery.

4.8 Undesirable effects

The most commonly reported adverse events reported in clinical trials with EVOREL® CONTI include vaginal bleeding, spotting, breast tenderness, headache and abdominal cramps/bloating. These adverse events reflect the known profile of oestrogen or oestrogen/progestogen therapy.

Skin reactions reported include transient erythema and irritation with or without pruritus at the site of TDS application. Very rarely, contact dermatitis, reversible post-inflammatory pigmentation, generalised pruritus and exanthema occurred in studies with EVOREL® 50.

Rare adverse events reported in association with oral progestogen or oestrogen replacement therapy include: thrombo-embolic events, cholestasis, benign or malignant breast disease, uterine carcinoma, aggravation of epilepsy, liver adenoma and galactorrhoea. If such events occur, EVOREL® CONTI should be discontinued immediately.

4.9 Overdose

Symptoms of overdose of oestrogen and progestogen therapy may include nausea, break-through bleeding, breast tenderness, abdominal cramps and/or bloating. These symptoms can be reversed by removing the TDS.

5. PHARMACOLOGICAL PROPERTIES

5.1 Pharmacodynamic properties

EVOREL® CONTI belongs to pharmacotherapeutic class G03 FA01, according to the ATC classification.

The active hormone of EVOREL® CONTI is 17β-estradiol, the biologically most potent oestrogen produced by the ovary. Its synthesis in the ovarian follicles is regulated by pituitary hormones. Like all steroid hormones, estradiol diffuses freely into target cells, where it binds to specific macromolecules (receptors). The estradiol-receptor complex then interacts with genomic DNA to alter transcriptional activity. This results in increases or decreases in protein synthesis and in changes of cellular functions.

Estradiol is secreted at different rates during the menstrual cycle. The endometrium is highly sensitive to estradiol, which regulates endometrial proliferation during the follicular phase of the cycle and together with progesterone, induces secretory changes during the luteal phase. Around the menopause, estradiol secretion becomes irregular and eventually ceases altogether. The absence of estradiol is associated with menopausal symptoms such as vasomotor instability, sleep disturbances, depressive mood, signs of vulvovaginal and urogenital atrophy and with increased bone loss. In addition, there is growing evidence for an increased incidence in cardiovascular disease in the absence of oestrogen.

Oestrogen replacement therapy has been found effective in most postmenopausal women to compensate for the endogenous oestrogen depletion. It has been demonstrated that transdermal estradiol administration of 50 micrograms per day is effective in the treatment of menopausal symptoms and of postmenopausal bone loss.

In postmenopausal women, EVOREL® CONTI increases estradiol to early follicular levels, with a consequent significant decrease in hot flushes, improvement in Kupperman Index and beneficial changes in vaginal cytology.

However, there is substantial evidence that oestrogen replacement therapy is associated with an increase in endometrial cancer. There is also compelling evidence that adjunctive progestogen treatment protects against oestrogen-induced endometrial cancer. Therefore, women with a uterus should receive combination oestrogen-progestogen hormone replacement therapy.

Norethisterone acetate, used in the EVOREL® CONTI TDS, is rapidly hydrolysed to norethisterone, a synthetic 19-nortestosterone derivative of the 13-methyl gonane group, with potent progestational activity. Transdermal norethisterone acetate administration prevents oestrogen-related endometrial proliferation. Combined 17β-estradiol-norethisterone acetate therapy is effective in treating the deficits associated with menopause.

5.2 Pharmacokinetic properties

Estradiol is readily absorbed from the gastro-intestinal tract and is extensively metabolised by the intestinal mucosa and the liver during the first hepatic passage. Transdermal delivery of estradiol is sufficient to cause a systemic effect.

Estradiol distributes widely in body tissues and is bound to albumin (~60-65%) and sex-hormone-binding globulin (~35-45%) in serum. Serum protein-binding fractions remain unaltered following transdermal delivery of estradiol. Estradiol is promptly eliminated from the systemic circulation. The elimination half-life is ~1 hour following intravenous administration. Estradiol is metabolised principally into the less pharmacologically active estrone and its conjugates. Estradiol, estrone and estrone sulphate are interconverted and are excreted in urine as glucuronides and sulphates. The skin metabolises estradiol only to a small extent.

In a single and multiple application study in postmenopausal women, serum estradiol concentrations increased rapidly from pretreatment levels (~ 5 pg/ml) after application of an EVOREL® CONTI TDS. At four hours after application, the mean serum estradiol concentration was ~19 pg/ml. A mean peak serum estradiol concentration of ~41 pg/ml above the pretreatment level was observed at about 23 hours following application. Serum estradiol concentrations remained elevated for the 3.5-day application period. Concentrations returned rapidly to pretreatment levels within 24 hours of removal of the TDS. A serum half-life of ~6.6 hours was determined following removal of the TDS, indicative of the skin depot effect. Multiple application of the TDS resulted in little or no accumulation of estradiol in the systemic circulation.

Prior to treatment, the mean serum estradiol to estrone concentration ratio (E_2/E_1) was less than 0.3 in the postmenopausal women studied. During use of EVOREL® CONTI TDS the E_2/E_1 ratios increased rapidly and were maintained at physiological levels that approximated 1. The E_2/E_1 ratios returned to pretreatment levels within 24 hours after removal of the TDS.

Norethisterone acetate is rapidly hydrolysed to the active progestogen, norethisterone. After oral administration, norethisterone is subject to pronounced first-pass metabolism which reduces the bioavailability. Transdermal delivery of norethisterone acetate produces a sustained and effective level of norethisterone in the systemic circulation.

Norethisterone distributes widely in body tissues and is bound to albumin (~61%) and sex-hormone-binding globulin (~36%) in serum. The elimination half-life is ~6 to 12 hours following oral administration which is not altered following long-term therapy. Norethisterone is primarily metabolised in the liver by reduction of the α,β-unsaturated ketone structure in ring A of the molecule. Among the four possible stereoisomeric tetrahydrosteroids, the 5β-, 3α-hydroxy-derivative appears to be the predominant metabolite. These compounds are primarily excreted in urine and faeces as sulphate and glucuronide conjugates.

In a single and multiple application study in postmenopausal women, serum norethisterone concentrations rose within 1 day after application of an EVOREL® CONTI TDS to a mean steady-state level of ~199 pg/ml. Mean steady-state serum norethisterone concentrations ranging between ~141 to 224 pg/ml were maintained for the entire 3.5-day application period following multiple application. Mean concentrations declined rapidly to the lower limit of assay quantitation at 24 hours after removal of the TDS. A serum half-life of ~15 hours was determined following removal of the TDS; indicative of the skin depot effect. As expected from transdermal delivery of most drugs, only a transient and limited increase in serum norethisterone concentrations was observed following multiple application of the TDS.

5.3 Preclinical safety data

Estradiol is a naturally occurring hormone and norethisterone acetate is a synthetic derivative of 19-nortestosterone. The pharmacology and toxicology of estradiol and norethisterone acetate are well documented.

Additional toxicity studies which include local tolerance studies in rabbits and dermal sensitisation studies in guinea pigs have been conducted to support registration of EVOREL® CONTI. These studies indicate that EVOREL® CONTI caused mild local skin irritation. It is recognised that test studies on rabbits over-predict skin irritation which occurs in humans. EVOREL® CONTI appeared to be a weak sensitiser to the guinea pig model. Clinical trial experience with a duration of TDS use over more than one year revealed no evidence of a clinically relevant sensitisation potential in humans.

6. PHARMACEUTICAL PARTICULARS

6.1 List of excipients

EVOREL® CONTI TDS

Adhesive: acrylate-vinylacetate copolymer (Duro-Tak 387-2287)

Guar gum

Backing film: polyethylene terephthalate foil (Hostaphan MN19)

Release liner: siliconised polyethylene terephthalate foil, is removed before application

6.2 Incompatibilities

No creams, lotions or powders should be applied to the skin area where the TDS is to be applied to prevent interference with the adhesive properties of EVOREL® CONTI TDS.

6.3 Shelf life

EVOREL® CONTI has a shelf-life of 24 months, when stored at or below 25°C. The product can be used until the expiration date mentioned on the container.

6.4 Special precautions for storage

Store at room temperature, at or below 25°C, within the original sachet and box.

Keep out of reach of children. This also applies to used and disposed patches.

6.5 Nature and contents of container

Each carton box has 2, 8 or 24 TDSs in individual foil-lined sachets. The sachet comprises a 4 layer laminate including:

– surlyn-ionomer film on the inside,

– then aluminium foil,

– then polyethylene film,

– with a layer of bleached reinforced paper on the outside.

6.6 Instructions for use and handling

The EVOREL® CONTI TDS should be placed on a clean, dry area of skin on the trunk of the body below the waist. Creams, lotions or powders may interfere with the adhesive properties of the EVOREL® CONTI TDS. The TDS should not be applied on or near to the breasts. The area of application should be changed, with an interval of at least one week allowed between applications to a particular site. The skin area selected should not be damaged or irritated. The waistline should not be used because excessive rubbing of the TDS may occur.

The TDS should be used immediately after opening the sachet. Remove one part of the protecting foil. Apply the exposed part of adhesive to the application site from the edge to the middle; avoid wrinkling of the TDS. The second part of the protective foil should now be removed and the freshly exposed adhesive applied. Wrinkling should again be avoided and the palm of the hand used to press the TDS onto the skin and to bring the TDS to skin temperature, at which the adhesive effect is optimised. Do not touch the adhesive part of the TDS.

To remove the EVOREL® TDS, peel away an edge of the patch and pull smoothly away from the skin.

Any gum that remains on the skin after removal of EVOREL® TDS may be removed by rubbing it off with the fingers, washing with soap and water or by using baby oil.

The TDSs should be disposed of in household waste (do not flush down the toilet).

7. MARKETING AUTHORISATION HOLDER

Janssen-Cilag Ltd

Saunderton

High Wycombe

Buckinghamshire

HP14 4HJ

UK

8. MARKETING AUTHORISATION NUMBER(S)

PL/0242/0319

9. DATE OF FIRST AUTHORISATION/RENEWAL OF THE AUTHORISATION

Date of First Authorisation 15 May 1997

10. DATE OF REVISION OF THE TEXT

December 2004

Legal category POM

EVOREL® Pak (transdermal oestradiol and norethisterone tablets)

(Janssen-Cilag Ltd)

Presentation:

EVOREL® Pak is a calendar pack comprising:

i. 8 "EVOREL 50" patches - each patch is a square shaped, transparent, self-adhesive transdermal delivery system of surface area 16 sq cm and 0.2 mm thickness, for application to the skin surface. Each consists of a monolayered adhesive matrix throughout which 17ß-oestradiol is uniformly distributed and each contains 3.2 mg of oestradiol corresponding to a release rate of 50 micrograms of oestradiol in 24 hours. Patches are marked 'CE 50'.

ii. 12 white tablets each containing 1 mg norethisterone. The tablets are round with C over 1 engraved on both faces.

Uses:

Hormone replacement therapy for the symptomatic relief of menopausal symptoms.

Prevention and management of post-menopausal osteoporosis in women considered at risk of developing fractures. Epidemiological studies have suggested that there are a number of risk factors associated with post-menopausal osteoporosis such as early menopause, a family history of osteoporosis, prolonged exposure to corticosteroid therapy, small and thin skeletal frame and excessive cigarette smoking.

Mode of action:

Oestrogen substitution effectively prevents the characteristic symptomatic, metabolic and atrophic changes associated with loss of ovarian function due to natural or surgical menopause.

EVOREL releases oestradiol transdermally into the circulation. In post-menopausal women EVOREL increases oestradiol levels to early and mid-follicular phase levels.

Norethisterone tablets, an oral progestogen, are used to oppose the oestrogenic effects on the endometrium by converting the oestrogen-primed proliferative endometrium into secretory endometrium which, on withdrawal of norethisterone at the end of each cycle, causes a withdrawal bleed in most patients thus eliminating the possibility of endometrial hyperplasia.

Pharmacokinetics:

With EVOREL, therapeutic serum oestradiol levels are achieved approximately four hours after application to the skin. From 10 hours onwards, the serum levels remain stable and at early to mid-follicular levels throughout the duration of the application (3 to 4 days).

Twenty four hours following removal of EVOREL oestradiol levels return to baseline.

Norethisterone is rapidly and completely absorbed from the gastro-intestinal tract; mean peak plasma levels are observed at 1 - 2 hours post-dose and the elimination half-life is 7-9 hours.

Dosage and Administration

Adults

Menopausal symptoms

Therapy should be started with one Evorel 50 patch (delivering 50 micrograms of estradiol/24 hours) and the dose adjusted after the first month if necessary depending on efficacy and signs of over-oestrogenisation (eg breast tenderness). For maintenance therapy the lowest effective dose should be used; a maximum dose of 100 micrograms of estradiol/24 hours should not be exceeded.

Post menopausal osteoporosis

Evorel 50 is recommended as an effective bone-sparing dose, with lower doses of estradiol slowing but not halting bone loss.

Evorel should be applied twice weekly on a continuous basis, each patch being renewed after 3 to 4 days and a fresh patch applied. Evorel should be applied to the skin as soon as it is removed from the wrapper. Recommended application sites are on clean, dry, healthy, intact skin and each application should be made to a slightly different area of skin on the trunk below waistline. Evorel should not be applied on or near the breasts. Evorel should remain in place during bathing and showering. Should it fall off during bathing or showering the patient should wait until cutaneous vasodilation ceases before applying a replacement patch to avoid potential excessive absorption. Should a patch fall off at other times it should be replaced immediately.

Patients can be advised to use baby oil to help remove any gum/glue which may remain on their skin after patch removal.

Children

EVOREL Pak is not indicated in children.

Use in pregnancy and lactation

EVOREL Pak is contra-indicated in pregnancy or lactation.

Contra-indications

Known or suspected malignant tumours of the breast, genital tract or other oestrogen dependent neoplasia. Undiagnosed vaginal bleeding, known or suspected pregnancy and lactation, severe hepatic, renal or cardiac disease, Rotor syndrome or Dubin-Johnson syndrome, active thrombophlebitis or thrombo-embolic disorders, endometriosis, hypersensitivity to any of the excipients. History during pregnancy of idiopathic jaundice, severe pruritus or pemphigoid gestationis.

Precautions and Warnings

A re-analysis of original data from 51 epidemiological studies reported a small or moderate increase in the probability of having breast cancer *diagnosed* in women currently or recently using HRT. The findings may be due to biological effects of HRT, earlier diagnosis, or a combination of both. The relative risk increased with duration of treatment (by 2.3% per year of use) and returned to normal in the course of five years after cessation of HRT use. This is comparable to the increase in relative risk when natural menopause is delayed in the absence of HRT. Breast cancers diagnosed in current or recent users of HRT are more likely to be localised to the breast than those found in non-users. HRT use may not be associated with increased mortality from breast cancer.

Between the ages of 50 and 70, about 45 women in every 1,000 not using HRT will have breast cancer diagnosed. It is estimated that among those who use HRT for 5 years starting at age 50, 2 extra cases of breast cancer will be detected by age 70 in every 1,000 women. For those who use HRT for 10 years, there will be 6 extra cases of breast cancer, and for 15 years use, 12 extra cases of breast cancer in every 1,000 women during the 20 year period until age 70.

It is important that the increased risk of being diagnosed with breast cancer is discussed with the patient and weighed against the known benefits of HRT.

Administration of unopposed oestrogen therapy in patients with an intact uterus has been reported to increase the risk of endometrial hyperplasia. Consequently, prior to commencing and periodically during oestrogen replacement therapy, it is recommended that the patient should be given a thorough physical and gynaecological examination and a complete medical and family history taken. Repeated breakthrough bleeding should be investigated, including endometrial biopsy.

Epidemiological studies have suggested that hormone replacement therapy (HRT) is associated with an increased relative risk of developing venous thrombo-embolism (VTE), ie deep vein thrombosis or pulmonary embolism. The studies find a 2-3 fold increase for users compared with non-users which for healthy women amounts to a low risk of one extra case of VTE each year for every 5,000 patients taking HRT.

Generally recognised risk factors for VTE include a personal or family history and severe obesity (body mass index >30 kg/m^2). In women with these factors the benefits of treatment with HRT need to be carefully weighed against risks.

The risk of VTE may be temporarily increased with prolonged immobilisation, major trauma or major surgery. In women on HRT scrupulous attention should be given to prophylactic measures to prevent VTE following surgery. Where prolonged immobilisation is liable to follow elective surgery, particularly abdominal or orthopaedic surgery to the lower limbs, consideration should be given to temporarily stopping HRT 4 weeks earlier, if this is possible.

If venous thrombo-embolism develops after initiating therapy the drug should be discontinued.

Consideration should be given to discontinuing treatment at least four weeks prior to surgery or during periods of prolonged immobilisation. Also, if hypertension develops after initiating therapy, consider discontinuing EVOREL Pak while the cause is investigated.

Close monitoring is recommended in patients with epilepsy, diabetes or hypertension (as oestrogens may cause fluid retention), disturbances or impairment of liver function, mastopathy or a strong family history of breast cancer, fibrocystic disease, uterine fibromyomata, cholelithiasis, otosclerosis, multiple sclerosis, systemic lupus erythematosus, porphyria, melanoma, migraine, asthma, as these conditions may be worsened by oestrogen therapy.

Drug Interactions:

Barbiturates, hydantoins, carbamazepine, meprobamate, phenylbutazone, antibiotics (including rifampicin) and activated charcoal, may impair the activity of oestrogen and progestogens (irregular bleeding and recurrence of symptoms may occur). In transdermal administration of oestradiol, a first pass effect via the liver is avoided.

EVOREL Pak is not to be used for contraception.

Side effects:

Minor effects of oestrogen and combined oestrogen/progestogen hormone replacement therapy which do not usually preclude continuation of therapy include headaches, nausea and breast-tenderness. The following side effects have been reported with oestrogen/progestogen therapy:-

Genito-urinary system:

Pre-menstrual-like syndrome, increase in size of uterine fibromyomata, vaginal candidiasis, change in cervical erosion and degree of cervical secretion, cystitis-like syndrome.

Breasts:

Tenderness, enlargement, secretion.

Gastro-intestinal:

Nausea, vomiting, abdominal cramps, bloating, cholestatic jaundice.

Skin:

Chloasma which may persist when drug is discontinued, erythema multiforme, erythema nodosum, haemorrhagic eruption, loss of scalp hair, hirsutism.

Eyes:

Steepening of corneal curvature, intolerance to contact lenses.

CNS:

Headaches, migraine, dizziness, mental depression, chorea.

Miscellaneous:

Increase or decrease in weight, reduced carbohydrate tolerance, aggravation of porphyria, oedema, changes in libido, leg cramps.

In clinical studies with "EVOREL 50" patches, the following side effects were seen: breast tenderness (less than 2%), bleeding (less than 2%) and intermittent bleeding/spotting (less than 5%). None were serious and they reflect the known profile of oestrogen or oestrogen/progestogen therapy. Skin reactions were reported by less than 6% of patients over six treatment cycles.

Overdosage:

There have been no reports of serious ill-effects from overdosage with EVOREL or norethisterone and treatment is usually unnecessary. Nausea and vomiting may occur in the event of a norethisterone overdosage. There is no special antidote and treatment should be symptomatic. The most commonly observed symptoms of overdose with oestrogen therapy are breast tenderness, nausea and breakthrough bleeding. Effects of EVOREL overdosage can be reversed by removal of the patch.

Pharmaceutical Precautions:

Protect from light.

Store below 25°C

Legal Category: POM

Package Quantities: EVOREL Pak contains

"EVOREL 50" patches, each presented in a sealed protective pouch

norethisterone 1 mg tablets

Patient Information Booklet

Product Licence Numbers:

PL/0242/0223 (EVOREL 50)

PL/0242/0241 (Norethisterone 1 mg tablets)

Product Licence Holder:

Janssen-Cilag Ltd

Saunderton

High Wycombe

Bucks

HP14 4HJ

UK

Date of Preparation:

August 1999

Evorel Sequi

(Janssen-Cilag Ltd)

1. NAME OF THE MEDICINAL PRODUCT

EVOREL® SEQUI

International non-proprietary names

estradiol

norethisterone acetate

2. QUALITATIVE AND QUANTITATIVE COMPOSITION

EVOREL® SEQUI is a transdermal therapy comprising

a) 4 EVOREL® 50 TDSs, each containing:

3.2 mg of estradiol hemihydrate

b) 4 EVOREL® CONTI TDSs, each containing:

3.2 mg of estradiol hemihydrate

11.2 mg of norethisterone acetate

3. PHARMACEUTICAL FORM

EVOREL® SEQUI is composed of EVOREL® 50 and EVOREL® CONTI. Both EVOREL® 50 and EVOREL® CONTI are a Transdermal Delivery System (TDS), or transdermal patch, composed of a flat two-layer laminate which is 0.1 mm in thickness. The first layer is a flexible, translucent, and nearly colourless backing film. The second layer is a monolayer adhesive film (matrix) composed of acrylic adhesive and guar gum and contains the hormones. This system is protected by a polyester foil release liner, which is affixed to the adhesive matrix and is removed prior to application of the patch to the skin. The polyester foil used is coated with silicone on both sides. The release liner has an S-shaped opening to facilitate its removal prior to use. Each TDS is enclosed in a protective, hermetically-sealed sachet.

EVOREL® CONTI has a surface area of 16 sq cm and contains 3.2 mg of estradiol corresponding to a nominal release of 50 micrograms of estradiol per 24 hours and 11.2 mg of norethisterone acetate corresponding to a nominal release of 170 micrograms of norethisterone acetate per 24 hours. Each EVOREL Conti patch is marked in the centre of the lower margin on the outside of the backing film: CEN1.

EVOREL® 50 has a surface area of 16 sq cm and contains 3.2 mg of estradiol corresponding to a nominal release of 50 micrograms of estradiol per 24 hours. The release liner of EVOREL® 50 is aluminised on one side. Each EVOREL® 50 patch is marked in the centre of the lower margin of the outside of the backing film: CE50.

4. CLINICAL PARTICULARS

4.1 Therapeutic indications

Hormone replacement therapy for the relief of menopausal symptoms.

Second line therapy for prevention of osteoporosis in post-menopausal women at high risk of future fractures who are intolerant of, or contraindicated for, other medicinal products approved for the prevention of osteoporosis.

4.2 Posology and method of administration

Adults

Menopausal symptoms

EVOREL® 50 and EVOREL® CONTI should be applied individually in the following sequence: four EVOREL® 50 TDSs followed by four EVOREL® CONTI TDSs. This cycle should be repeated without interruption. TDSs should be applied twice weekly, every three to four days, to the trunk below the waist.

Insufficient data are available to guide dose adjustments for patients with severe liver or kidney function impairment.

It is important that the TDS be used in the correct sequence to ensure regular cyclic bleeding. Most patients will experience vaginal bleeding after the start of the progestogen therapy.

Post menopausal osteoporosis

Evorel Sequi is recommended as an effective bone-sparing dose, with lower doses of estradiol slowing but not halting bone loss.

Children

EVOREL® SEQUI (EVOREL® 50 and EVOREL® CONTI) is not indicated in children.

Elderly

Data are insufficient in regard to the use of EVOREL® SEQUI in the elderly >65 years old).

Administration

The sachet containing one TDS should be opened and one part of the protective foil removed at the S-shaped incision. The TDS should be applied to clean, dry, healthy, intact skin as soon as it is removed from the sachet. The patient should avoid contact between fingers and the adhesive part of the TDS during application. Each application should be made to a different area of the skin, on the trunk below the waist. EVOREL® SEQUI should not be applied on or near the breasts.

Should a TDS fall off, it should be replaced immediately with a new equivalent EVOREL® 50 or EVOREL® CONTI TDS. However, the usual day of changing TDSs should be maintained.

4.3 Contraindications

- Hypersensitivity to any component of this product
- Known or suspected malignant tumours of the breast
- Genital tract or other oestrogen-dependent neoplasia
- Undiagnosed vaginal bleeding
- Pregnancy or lactation
- Severe hepatic or renal disease
- Active thrombophlebitis
- Active deep venous thrombosis, thrombo-embolic disorders, or a history of confirmed venous thrombo-embolism
- Endometriosis

4.4 Special warnings and special precautions for use

Assessment of each woman prior to using hormone replacement therapy (and at regular intervals thereafter) should include a personal and family medical history. Physical examination should be guided by this and by the Contraindications (Section 4.3) and Warnings (Section 4.4) for this product. During assessment of each individual woman clinical examination of the breasts and pelvic examination should be performed where clinically indicated rather than as a routine procedure. Women should be encouraged to participate in the national breast cancer screening programme (mammography) and the national cervical cancer screening programme (cervical cytology) as appropriate for their age. Breast awareness should also be encouraged and women advised to report any changes in their breasts to their doctor or nurse.

Repeated breakthrough bleeding, unexplained vaginal bleeding and changes noticed during breast examination require further evaluation.

A re-analysis of original data from 51 epidemiological studies reported a small or moderate increase in the probability of having breast cancer *diagnosed* in women currently or recently using HRT. The findings may be due to biological effects of HRT, earlier diagnosis, or a combination of both. The relative risk increased with duration of treatment (by 2.3% per year of use) and returned to normal in the course of five years after cessation of HRT use. This is comparable to the increase in relative risk when natural menopause is delayed in the absence of HRT. Breast cancers diagnosed in current or recent users of HRT are more likely to be localised to the breast than those found in non-users. HRT use may not be associated with increased mortality from breast cancer.

Between the ages of 50 and 70, about 45 women in every 1,000 not using HRT will have breast cancer diagnosed. It is estimated that among those who use HRT for 5 years starting at age 50, 2 extra cases of breast cancer will be detected by age 70 in every 1,000 women. For those who use HRT for 10 years, there will be 6 extra cases of breast cancer, and for 15 years use, 12 extra cases of breast cancer in every 1,000 women during the 20 year period until age 70.

It is important that the increased risk of being diagnosed with breast cancer is discussed with the patient and weighed against the known benefits of HRT.

Epidemiological studies have suggested that hormone replacement therapy (HRT) is associated with an increased relative risk of developing venous thrombo-embolism (VTE), ie deep vein thrombosis or pulmonary embolism. The studies find a 2-3 fold increase for users compared with non-users which for healthy women amounts to a low risk for one extra case of VTE each year for every 5,000 patients taking HRT.

Generally recognised risk factors for VTE include a personal or family history and severe obesity (body mass index >30 kg/m^2). In women with these factors the benefits of treatment with HRT need to be carefully weighed against risks.

The risk of VTE may be temporarily increased with prolonged immobilisation, major trauma or major surgery. In women on HRT scrupulous attention should be given to prophylactic measures to prevent VTE following surgery. Where prolonged immobilisation is liable to follow elective surgery, particularly abdominal or orthopaedic surgery to the lower limbs, consideration should be given to temporarily stopping HRT 4 weeks earlier, if this is possible.

If venous thrombo-embolism develops after initiating therapy the drug should be discontinued.

Appropriate monitoring is recommended in patients with cardiac impairment, epilepsy, diabetes mellitus, hypertension, disturbances or impairment of liver or kidney function, mastopathy, a family history of breast cancer, or a history of cholestatic jaundice.

Administration of unopposed oestrogen in patients with an intact uterus has been reported to increase the risk of endometrial hyperplasia and of endometrial carcinoma. Therefore oestrogen in combination with sequential administration of a progestogen as in EVOREL® SEQUI is recommended in women with an intact uterus in order to reduce the risk of hyperplasia or endometrial carcinoma.

EVOREL® SEQUI is not to be used as contraception.

The TDSs should be kept away from children and pets.

4.5 Interaction with other medicinal products and other forms of Interaction

Drugs which induce microsomal liver enzyme activity may alter oestrogen and progestogen metabolism. Examples of such drugs are barbiturates, hydantoins, carbamazepine, meprobamate, phenylbutazone and rifampicin. On a theoretical basis, the effects of liver enzyme induction on the metabolism of transdermally administered estradiol and norethisterone acetate should be minimised by the avoidance of the first pass liver metabolism.

4.6 Pregnancy and lactation

The use of EVOREL® SEQUI is contra-indicated in pregnancy and lactation.

4.7 Effects on ability to drive and use machines

There are no known data on the effects of EVOREL® SEQUI on the ability to drive or use machinery.

4.8 Undesirable effects

The most commonly reported adverse events reported in clinical trials with EVOREL® SEQUI include vaginal bleeding, spotting, breast tenderness, headache and abdominal cramps/bloating. These adverse events reflect the known profile of oestrogen or oestrogen/progestogen therapy.

Skin reactions reported include transient erythema and irritation with or without pruritus at the site of TDS application. Very rarely, contact dermatitis, reversible post-inflammatory pigmentation, generalised pruritus and exanthema occurred in studies with EVOREL® 50.

Rare adverse events reported in association with oral progestogen or oestrogen replacement therapy include: thrombo-embolic events, cholestasis, benign or malignant breast disease, uterine carcinoma, aggravation of epilepsy, liver adenoma and galactorrhoea. If such events occur, EVOREL® SEQUI should be discontinued immediately.

4.9 Overdose

Symptoms of overdose of oestrogen and progestogen therapy may include nausea, break-through bleeding, breast tenderness, abdominal cramps and/or bloating. These symptoms can be reversed by removing the TDS.

5. PHARMACOLOGICAL PROPERTIES

5.1 Pharmacodynamic properties

EVOREL® SEQUI belongs to pharmacotherapeutic class G03 FB05, according to the ATC classification.

The active hormone of EVOREL® SEQUI is 17β-estradiol, the biologically most potent oestrogen produced by the ovary. Its synthesis in the ovarian follicles is regulated by pituitary hormones. Like all steroid hormones, estradiol diffuses freely into target cells, where it binds to specific macromolecules (receptors). The estradiol-receptor complex then interacts with genomic DNA to alter transcriptional activity. This results in increases or decreases in protein synthesis and in changes of cellular functions.

Estradiol is secreted at different rates during the menstrual cycle. The endometrium is highly sensitive to estradiol, which regulates endometrial proliferation during the follicular phase of the cycle and together with progesterone, induces secretory changes during the luteal phase. Around the menopause, estradiol secretion becomes irregular and eventually ceases altogether. The absence of estradiol is associated with menopausal symptoms such as vasomotor instability, sleep disturbances, depressive mood, signs of vulvovaginal and urogenital atrophy and with increased bone loss. In addition, there is growing evidence for an increased incidence in cardiovascular disease in the absence of oestrogen.

Oestrogen replacement therapy has been found effective in most postmenopausal women to compensate for the endogenous oestrogen depletion. It has been demonstrated that transdermal estradiol administration of 50 micrograms/day is effective in the treatment of menopausal symptoms and of postmenopausal bone loss.

In postmenopausal women, EVOREL® SEQUI increases estradiol to early follicular levels, with a consequent significant decrease in hot flushes, improvement in Kupperman Index and beneficial changes in vaginal cytology.

However, there is substantial evidence that oestrogen replacement therapy is associated with an increase in endometrial cancer. There is also compelling evidence that adjunctive progestogen treatment protects against oestrogen-induced endometrial cancer. Therefore, women with a uterus should receive combination oestrogen-progestogen hormone replacement therapy.

Norethisterone acetate, used in the EVOREL® CONTI TDS of EVOREL® SEQUI, is rapidly hydrolysed to norethisterone, a synthetic 19-nortestosterone derivative of the 13-methyl gonane group, with potent progestational activity. Transdermal norethisterone acetate administration prevents oestrogen-related endometrial proliferation. Combined 17β-estradiol-norethisterone acetate therapy is effective in treating the deficits associated with menopause.

5.2 Pharmacokinetic properties

Estradiol is readily absorbed from the gastro-intestinal tract but is extensively metabolised by the intestinal mucosa and the liver during the first hepatic passage. Transdermal delivery of estradiol is sufficient to cause a systemic effect.

Estradiol distributes widely in body tissues and is bound to albumin (~60-65%) and sex-hormone-binding globulin (~35-45%) in serum. Serum protein-binding fractions remain unaltered following transdermal delivery of estradiol. Estradiol is promptly eliminated from the systemic circulation. The elimination half-life is ~1 hour following intravenous administration. Estradiol is metabolised principally into the less pharmacologically active estrone and its conjugates. Estradiol, estrone and estrone sulphate are interconverted to each other and are excreted in urine as glucuronides and sulphates. The skin metabolizes estradiol only to a small extent.

In a single and multiple application study in postmenopausal women, serum estradiol concentrations increased rapidly from pretreatment levels (~ 5 pg/ml) after application of an EVOREL® CONTI TDS. At four hours after application, the mean serum estradiol concentration was ~19 pg/ml. A mean peak serum estradiol concentration of ~41 pg/ml above the pretreatment level was observed at about 23 hours following application. Serum estradiol concentrations remained elevated for the 3.5-day application period. Concentrations returned rapidly to pretreatment levels within 24 hours of removal of the TDS. A serum half-life of ~6.6 hours was determined following removal of the TDS, indicative of the skin depot effect. Multiple application of the EVOREL® CONTI TDS resulted in little or no accumulation of estradiol in the systemic circulation. Higher circulating levels of estradiol were attained from EVOREL® 50. Both formulations were shown to be effective in achieving serum estradiol concentration typically seen in premenopausal women.

Prior to treatment, the mean serum estradiol to estrone concentration ratio (E_2/E_1) was less than 0.3 in the postmenopausal women studied. During use of EVOREL® CONTI TDS the E_2/E_1 ratios increased rapidly and were maintained at the physiological levels that approximated 1. The E_2/E_1 ratios returned to pretreatment levels within 24 hours after removal of the TDS. An average E_2/E_1 ratio that approximated 1 was also maintained over an entire 3.5-day application period following EVOREL® 50 application.

Norethisterone acetate is rapidly hydrolysed to the active progestogen, norethisterone. After oral administration, norethisterone is subject to pronounced first-pass metabolism which reduces the bioavailability. Transdermal delivery of norethisterone acetate produces a sustained and effective level of norethisterone in the systemic circulation.

Norethisterone distributes widely in body tissues and is bound to albumin (~61%) and sex-hormone-binding globulin (~36%) in serum. The elimination half-life is ~6 to 12 hours following oral administration which is not altered following long-term therapy. Norethisterone is primarily metabolised in the liver by reduction of the α,β-unsaturated ketone structure in ring A of the molecule. Among the four possible stereoisomeric tetrahydrosteroids, the 5β-, 3α-hydroxy-derivative appears to be the predominant metabolite. These compounds are primarily excreted in urine and faeces as sulphate and glucuronide conjugates.

In a single and multiple application study in postmenopausal women, serum norethisterone concentrations rose within 1 day after application of an EVOREL® CONTI TDS to a mean steady-state level of ~199 pg/ml. Mean steady-state serum norethisterone concentrations ranging between ~141 to 224 pg/ml were maintained for the entire 3.5-day application period following multiple application. Mean concentrations declined rapidly to the lower limit of assay quantitation at 24 hours after removal of the TDS. A serum half-life of ~15 hours was determined following removal of the TDS, indicative of the skin depot effect. As expected from transdermal delivery of most drugs, only a transient and limited increase in serum norethisterone concentrations was observed following multiple application of the TDS.

5.3 Preclinical safety data

Estradiol is a naturally occurring hormone and norethisterone acetate is a synthetic derivative of 19-nortestosterone. The pharmacology and toxicology of estradiol and norethisterone acetate are well documented.

Additional toxicity studies which include local tolerance studies in rabbits and dermal sensitisation studies in guinea pigs have been conducted to support registration of EVOREL® SEQUI. These studies indicate that the EVOREL® CONTI TDS caused mild local skin irritation. It is recognised that test studies on rabbits over-predict skin irritation which occurs in humans. EVOREL® CONTI appeared to be a weak sensitiser to the guinea pig model. Clinical trial experience with a duration of TDS use over more than one year revealed no evidence of a clinically relevant sensitisation potential in humans.

6. PHARMACEUTICAL PARTICULARS

6.1 List of excipients

EVOREL® 50

Adhesive: acrylate-vinylacetate copolymer (Duro-Tak 387-2287)

Guar gum

Backing film: polyethylene terephthalate foil (Hostaphan MN19)

Release liner: siliconised polyethylene terephthalate foil, is removed before application

EVOREL® CONTI

Adhesive: acrylate-vinylacetate copolymer (Duro-Tak 387-2287)

Guar gum

Backing film: polyethylene terephthalate foil (Hostaphan MN19)

Release liner: siliconised polyethylene terephthalate foil, is removed before application

6.2 Incompatibilities

No creams, lotions or powders should be applied to the skin area where the TDS is to be applied to prevent interference with the adhesive properties of EVOREL® 50 TDS and EVOREL® CONTI TDS.

6.3 Shelf life

EVOREL® SEQUI has a shelf-life of 24 months when stored at or below 25°C. The product can be used until the expiration date mentioned on the container.

6.4 Special precautions for storage

Store at room temperature, at or below 25°C within the original sachet and box.

Keep out of reach of children. This also applies to used and disposed TDSs.

6.5 Nature and contents of container

Each carton box has 8 TDSs in individual foil-lined sachets. The sachet comprises a 4 layer laminate including:-

- surlyn-ionomer film on the inside,
- then aluminium foil,
- then polyethylene film,
- with a layer of bleached reinforced paper on the outside.

One EVOREL® SEQUI box contains 4 EVOREL® 50 TDSs and 4 EVOREL® CONTI TDSs.

6.6 Instructions for use and handling

The EVOREL® SEQUI TDS should be placed on a clean, dry area of skin on the trunk of the body below the waist. Creams, lotions or powders may interfere with the adhesive properties of the EVOREL® SEQUI TDS. The TDS should not be applied on or near to the breasts. The area of application should be changed, with an interval of at least one week allowed between applications to a particular site. The skin area selected should not be damaged or irritated. The waistline should not be used because excessive rubbing of the TDS may occur.

The TDS should be used immediately after opening the sachet. Remove one part of the protecting foil. Apply the exposed part of adhesive to the application site from the edge to the middle; avoid wrinkling of the TDS. The second part of the protective foil should now be removed and the freshly exposed adhesive applied. Wrinkling should again be avoided and the palm of the hand used to press the TDS onto the skin and to bring the TDS to skin temperature at which the adhesive effect is optimised. Do not touch the adhesive part of the TDS.

When using EVOREL® SEQUI for the first two weeks, one of the EVOREL® 50 TDSs should be applied and changed twice weekly. During the following two weeks of EVOREL® SEQUI, one of the EVOREL® CONTI TDSs should be applied, also to be changed twice weekly. The patient then starts again with a new box of EVOREL® SEQUI.

To remove the EVOREL® TDS, peel away an edge of the patch and pull smoothly away from the skin.

Any gum that remains on the skin after removal of EVOREL® TDS may be removed by rubbing it off with the fingers, washing with soap and water or by using baby oil.

The EVOREL® TDS should be disposed of in household waste (do not flush down the toilet).

7. MARKETING AUTHORISATION HOLDER

Janssen-Cilag Limited

Saunderton

High Wycombe

Buckinghamshire

HP14 4HJ

UK

8. MARKETING AUTHORISATION NUMBER(S)

PL/0242/0320

9. DATE OF FIRST AUTHORISATION/RENEWAL OF THE AUTHORISATION

Date of First Authorisation: 15 May 1997

10. DATE OF REVISION OF THE TEXT

8 December 2003

Legal category POM

Evra transdermal patch

(Janssen-Cilag Ltd)

1. NAME OF THE MEDICINAL PRODUCT

EVRA▼ transdermal patch

2. QUALITATIVE AND QUANTITATIVE COMPOSITION

Each transdermal patch contains 6 mg norelgestromin (NGMN) and 600 micrograms ethinyl estradiol (EE).

Each transdermal patch releases 150 micrograms of NGMN and 20 micrograms of EE per 24 h.

For excipients, see Section 6.1.

3. PHARMACEUTICAL FORM

Transdermal patch.

EVRA is a thin, matrix-type transdermal patch consisting of three layers.

The outside of the backing layer is beige and heat-stamped "EVRA 150/20".

4. CLINICAL PARTICULARS

4.1 Therapeutic indications

Female contraception

EVRA is intended for women of fertile age. The safety and efficacy has been established in women aged 18 to 45 years.

4.2 Posology and method of administration

Posology

To achieve maximum contraceptive effectiveness, patients must be advised to use EVRA exactly as directed. For initiation instructions see 'How to start EVRA' below.

Only one patch is to be worn at a time.

Each used patch is removed and immediately replaced with a new one on the same day of the week (Change Day) on Day 8 and Day 15 of the cycle. Patch changes may occur at any time on the scheduled Change Day. The fourth week is patch-free starting on Day 22.

A new contraceptive cycle begins on the next day following patch-free week; the next EVRA patch should be applied even if there has been no bleeding or if bleeding has not yet stopped.

Under no circumstances should there be more than a 7-day patch-free interval between dosing cycles. If there are more than 7 patch-free days, the user may not be protected against pregnancy. A non-hormonal contraceptive must then be used concurrently for 7 days. As with combined oral contraceptives, the risk of ovulation increases with each day beyond the recommended contraceptive-free period. If intercourse has occurred during such an extended patch-free interval, the possibility of fertilisation should be considered.

Method of administration

EVRA should be applied to clean, dry, hairless, intact healthy skin on the buttock, abdomen, upper outer arm or upper torso, in a place where it will not be rubbed by tight clothing. EVRA should not be placed on the breasts or on skin that is red, irritated or cut. Each consecutive patch should be applied to a different place on the skin to help avoid potential irritation, although they may be kept within the same anatomic site.

The patch should be pressed down firmly until the edges stick well.

To prevent interference with the adhesive properties of the patch, no make-up, creams, lotions, powders or other topical products should be applied to the skin area where the patch is placed or where it will be applied shortly.

It is recommended that users visually check their patch daily to ensure continued proper adhesion. **Used patches should be discarded carefully in accordance with the instructions given in Section 6.6.**

How to start EVRA

When there has been no hormonal contraceptive use in the preceding cycle

Contraception with EVRA begins on the first day of menses. A single patch is applied and worn for one full week (7 days). The day the first patch is applied (Day 1/ Start Day) determines the subsequent Change Days. The patch Change Day will be on this day every week (cycle Days 8, 15, 22 and Day 1 of the next cycle) The fourth week is patch-free starting on Day 22.

If Cycle 1 therapy starts after first day of the menstrual cycle, a non-hormonal contraceptive should be used concurrently for the first 7 consecutive days of the first treatment cycle only.

When switching from an oral combined contraceptive

Treatment with EVRA should begin on the first day of withdrawal bleeding. If there is no withdrawal bleeding within 5 days of the last active (hormone containing) tablet, pregnancy must be ruled out prior to the start of treatment with EVRA. If therapy starts after the first day of withdrawal bleeding, a non-hormonal contraceptive must be used concurrently for 7 days.

If more than 7 days elapse after taking the last active oral contraceptive tablet, the woman may have ovulated and should, therefore, be advised to consult a physician before initiating treatment with EVRA. If intercourse has occurred during such an extended pill-free interval, the possibility of pregnancy should be considered.

When changing from a progestogen-only-method

The woman may switch any day from the minipill (from an implant on the day of its removal, from an injectable when the next injection would be due), but a back-up barrier method of birth control must be used during the first 7 days.

Following abortion or miscarriage

After an abortion or miscarriage that occurs before 20 weeks gestation, EVRA may be started immediately. An additional method of contraception is not needed if EVRA is started immediately. Be advised that ovulation may occur within 10 days of an abortion or miscarriage.

After an abortion or miscarriage that occurs at or after 20 weeks gestation, EVRA may be started either on Day 21 post-abortion or on the first day of the first spontaneous menstruation, whichever comes first. The incidence of ovulation on Day 21 post abortion (at 20 weeks gestation) is not known.

Following delivery

Users who choose not to breast-feed should start contraceptive therapy with EVRA no sooner than 4 weeks after child-birth. When starting later, the woman should be advised to additionally use a barrier method for the first 7 days. However, if intercourse has already occurred, pregnancy should be excluded before the actual start of EVRA or the woman has to wait for her first menstrual period.

For breast-feeding women, see section 4.6.

What to do if the patch comes off or partly detaches

If the EVRA patch partly or completely detaches and remains detached, insufficient medicinal product delivery occurs.

If EVRA remains even partly detached:

- for less than one day (up to 24 hours): it should be re-applied to the same place or replaced with a new EVRA patch immediately. No additional contraceptive is needed. The next EVRA patch should be applied on the usual "Change Day".

- for more than one day (24 hours or more) or if the user is not aware when the patch has lifted or become detached: the user may not be protected from pregnancy: The user should stop the current contraceptive cycle and start a new cycle immediately by applying a new EVRA patch. There is now a new "Day 1" and a new "Change Day". A non-hormonal contraceptive must be used concurrently for the first 7 days of the new cycle only.

A patch should not be reapplied if it is no longer sticky; a new patch should be applied immediately. Supplemental adhesives or bandages should not be used to hold the EVRA patch in place.

If subsequent EVRA patch change days are delayed

At the start of any patch cycle (Week One/Day 1):

The user may not be protected from pregnancy. The user should apply the first patch of the new cycle as soon as remembered. There is now a new patch "Change Day" and a new "Day 1". A non-hormonal contraceptive must be used concurrently for the first 7 days of the new cycle. If intercourse has occurred during such an extended patch-free interval, the possibility of fertilisation should be considered.

-In the middle of the cycle (Week Two/Day 8 or Week Three/ Day 15):

- for one or two days (up to 48 hours): The user should apply a new EVRA patch immediately. The next EVRA patch should be applied on the usual "Change Day". If during the 7 days preceding the first skipped day of patch application, the patch was worn correctly, no additional contraceptive use is required.

- for more than two days (48 hours or more): The user may not be protected from pregnancy. The user should stop the current contraceptive cycle and start a new four-week cycle immediately by putting on a new EVRA patch. There is now a new "Day 1" and a new "Change Day". A non-hormonal contraceptive must be used concurrently for the first 7 consecutive days of the new cycle.

- at the end of the cycle (Week Four/Day 22): If the EVRA patch is not removed at the beginning of Week 4 (Day 22), it should be removed as soon as possible. The next cycle should begin on the usual "Change Day", which is the day after Day 28. No additional contraceptive use is required.

Change Day adjustment

In order to postpone a menstrual period for one cycle, the woman must apply another patch at the beginning of Week 4 (Day 22) thus not observing the patch free interval. Breakthrough bleeding or spotting may occur. After 6 consecutive weeks of patch wear, there should be a patch free interval of 7 days. Following this, the regular application of EVRA is resumed.

If the user wishes to move the Change Day the current cycle should be completed, removing the third EVRA patch on the correct day. During the patch-free week a new Change Day may be selected by applying the first EVRA patch of the next cycle on the first occurrence of the desired day. In no case should there be more than 7 consecutive patch-free days. The shorter the patch-free interval, the higher the risk that the user does not have a withdrawal bleed and may experience breakthrough bleeding and spotting during the subsequent treatment cycle.

In case of minor skin irritation

If patch use results in uncomfortable irritation, a new patch may be applied to a new location until the next Change Day. Only one patch should be worn at a time.

Special populations

Body weight equal or greater than 90 kg: contraceptive efficacy may be decreased in women weighing equal or greater than 90 kg.

Renal impairment: EVRA has not been studied in women with renal impairment. No dose adjustment is necessary but as there is a suggestion in the literature that the unbound fraction of EE is higher, EVRA should be used with supervision in this population.

Hepatic impairment: EVRA has not been studied in women with hepatic impairment. EVRA is contraindicated in women with hepatic impairment (See section 4.3).

Post-menopausal women: EVRA is not intended for use as hormonal replacement therapy.

Children and adolescents: safety and efficacy of EVRA was only established in women between 18 and 45 years of age.

4.3 Contraindications

EVRA should not be used in the presence of one of the following disorders. If one of these disorders occurs for the first time during the use of EVRA, EVRA must be discontinued immediately.

- Hypersensitivity to the active substances or to any of the excipients
- Presence or history of venous thrombosis, with or without the involvement of pulmonary embolism
- Presence or history of arterial thrombosis (e.g. cerebrovascular accident, myocardial infarction, retinal thrombosis) or prodromi of a thrombosis (e.g. angina pectoris or transient ischaemic attack)
- Migraine with focal aura
- The presence of serious or multiple risk factor(s) for the occurrence of arterial thrombosis:

- Severe hypertension (persistent values of ⩾ 160+/100+ mmHg)

- Diabetes Mellitus with vascular involvement

- Hereditary dyslipoproteinemia

- Possible hereditary predisposition for venous or arterial thrombosis, such as activated protein C (APC-) resistance, antithrombin-III deficiency, protein C deficiency, protein S deficiency, hyperhomocysteinemia, and antiphospholipid antibodies (anticardiolipin antibodies, lupus anticoagulant)
- Known or suspected carcinoma of the breast
- Carcinoma of the endometrium or other known or suspected estrogen-dependent neoplasia
- Abnormal liver function related to acute or chronic hepatocellular disease
- Hepatic adenomas or carcinomas
- Undiagnosed abnormal genital bleeding

4.4 Special warnings and special precautions for use

There is no clinical evidence indicating that a transdermal patch is, in any aspect, safer than combined oral contraceptives.

If any of the conditions/risk factors mentioned below is present, the benefits of the use of EVRA should be weighed against the possible risks for each individual woman and discussed with the woman before she decides to start using EVRA. In the event of aggravation, exacerbation or first appearance of any of these conditions or risk factors, the woman should be emphatically told to contact her physician who will decide on whether its use should be discontinued.

Thromboembolic and other vascular disorders

Epidemiological studies have associated the use of combined oral contraceptives (COCs) with an increased risk for deep venous (deep venous thrombosis, pulmonary embolism) and arterial (myocardial infarction, transient ischaemic attack) thromboembolism. In these studies, the incidence of VTE in users of oral contraceptives with low estrogen content (< 50 μg ethinyl estradiol) ranges from about 20 to 40 cases per 100,000 women years, but this risk varies according to the progestagen (for COCs containing levonorgestrel, the incidence is about 20 cases per 100,000 women years). This compares with 5-10 cases per 100,000 women years for non-users.

The use of any combined oral contraceptive carries an increased risk of venous thromboembolism (VTE) compared to no use. The excess risk of VTE is highest during the first year a woman ever uses a combined oral contraceptive. This increased risk is less than the risk of VTE associated with pregnancy, which is estimated as 60 per 100,000 pregnant women years. VTE is fatal in 1%-2% of cases.

It is not yet known how EVRA influences the risk of VTE compared with combined oral contraceptives.

Extremely rarely, thrombosis has been reported to occur in other blood vessels e.g. hepatic, mesenteric, renal, cerebral or retinal veins and arteries, in COC users. There is no consensus as to whether the occurrence of these events is associated with the use of COCs.

Symptoms of venous or arterial thrombosis can include:

- Unilateral leg pain, and/or swelling
- Sudden severe pain in the chest with possible radiation to the left arm
- Sudden breathlessness, sudden onset of coughing without a clear cause
- Any unusual, severe, prolonged headache
- Sudden partial or complete loss of vision
- Diplopia
- Slurred speech or aphasia
- Vertigo; collapse with or without focal seizure
- Weakness or very marked numbness suddenly affecting one side or one part of the body
- Motor disturbances
- 'Acute' abdominal pain

-The risk of venous thromboembolism in combined contraceptives users increases with:

- Increasing age

- A positive family history (i.e. venous thromboembolism ever in a sibling or parent at relatively early age). If a hereditary predisposition is suspected, the woman should be referred to a specialist for advice before deciding about any hormonal contraceptive use

- Prolonged immobilisation, major surgery to the legs, or major trauma. In these situations it is advisable to discontinue use (in the case of elective surgery at least 4 weeks in advance) and not to resume until two weeks after complete remobilisation

- Obesity (body mass index over 30 kg/m^2)

- Possibly also with superficial thrombophlebitis and varicose veins. There is no consensus about the possible role of these conditions in the aetiology of venous thrombosis.

- The risk of arterial thromboembolic complications in combined contraceptives users increases with:

- Increasing age;

- Smoking (with heavier smoking and increasing age the risk further increases, especially in women over 35 years of age);

- Dyslipoproteinaemia;

- Obesity (body mass index over 30 kg/m^2);

- Hypertension;

- Valvular heart disease;

- Atrial fibrillation;

- A positive family history (arterial thrombosis ever in a sibling or parent at a relatively early age). If a hereditary predisposition is suspected, the woman should be referred to a specialist for advice before deciding about any hormonal contraceptive use.

Biochemical factors that may be indicative of hereditary or acquired predisposition for venous or arterial thrombosis include Activated Protein C (APC) resistance, hyper homocysteinaemia, antithrombin-III deficiency, protein C deficiency, protein S deficiency, antiphospholipid antibodies (anticardiolipin antibodies, lupus anticoagulant).

Other medical conditions, which have been associated with adverse circulatory events, included diabetes mellitus, systemic lupus erythematosus, haemolytic uraemic syndrome, chronic inflammatory bowel disease (e.g. Crohn's disease or ulcerative colitis).

The increased risk for thromboembolism in the puerperium must be considered (for information on 'pregnancy and lactation' see section 4.6.).

An increase in frequency or severity of headache (which may be prodromal of a cerebrovascular event) may be a reason for immediate discontinuation of combination contraceptives.

Women using combined contraceptives should be emphatically advised to contact their physician in case of possible symptoms of thrombosis. In case of suspected or confirmed thrombosis, hormonal contraceptive use should be discontinued. Adequate contraception should be initiated because of the teratogenicity of anti-coagulant therapy (coumarins).

Tumours

An increased risk of cervical cancer in long-term users of COCs has been reported in some epidemiological studies, but there continues to be controversy about the extent to which this finding is attributable to the compounding effects of sexual behaviour and other factors such as human papilloma virus (HPV).

A meta-analysis of 54 epidemiological studies reported that there is a slightly increased risk (RR = 1.24) of having breast cancer diagnosed in women who are currently using COCs. The excess risk gradually disappears during the course of the 10 years after cessation of COC use. Because breast cancer is rare in women under 40 years of age, the excess number of breast cancer diagnoses in current and recent COC users is small in relation to the overall risk of breast cancer. The breast cancers diagnosed in ever-users tend to be less advanced clinically than the cancers diagnosed in never-users. The observed pattern of increased risk may be due to an earlier diagnosis of breast cancer in COC users, the biological effects of COCs or a combination of both.

In rare cases, benign liver tumours, and even more rarely, malignant liver tumours have been reported in users of COCs. In isolated cases, these tumours have led to life-threatening intra-abdominal haemorrhages. Therefore a hepatic tumour should be considered in the differential diagnosis when severe upper abdominal pain, liver enlargement or signs of intra-abdominal haemorrhage occur in women using EVRA.

Other conditions

- Contraceptive efficacy may be reduced in women weighing equal or greater than 90 kg (See sections 4.2 and 5.1).
- Women with hypertriglyceridaemia, or a family history thereof, may be at an increased risk of pancreatitis when using combination hormonal contraceptives.
- Although small increases of blood pressure have been reported in many women using hormonal contraceptives, clinically relevant increases are rare. A definitive relationship between hormonal contraceptive use and clinical hypertension has not been established. If, during the use of a combination hormonal contraceptive in pre-existing hypertension, constantly elevated blood pressure values or a significant increase in blood pressure do not respond adequately to antihypertensive treatment, the combination hormonal contraceptive must be withdrawn. Combination hormonal contraceptive use may be resumed if normotensive values can be achieved with antihypertensive therapy.
- The following conditions have been reported to occur or deteriorate with both pregnancy and COC use, but the evidence of an association with COC use is inconclusive: Jaundice and/or pruritus related to cholestasis; gallstones; porphyria; systemic erythematosus; haemolytic uraemic syndrome; Sydenham's chorea; herpes gestationis; otosclerosis-related hearing loss.
- Acute or chronic disturbances of liver function may necessitate the discontinuation of combination hormonal contraceptives until markers of liver function return to normal. Recurrence of cholestatic-related pruritus, which occurred during a previous pregnancy or previous use of sex steroids necessitates the discontinuation of combination hormonal contraceptives.
- Although combined hormonal contraceptives may have an effect on peripheral insulin resistance and glucose tolerance there is no evidence for a need to alter the therapeutic regimen in diabetes during use of combined hormonal contraception. However, diabetic women should be carefully observed, particularly in the early stage of EVRA use.
- Worsening of endogenous depression, of epilepsy, of Crohn's disease and of ulcerative colitis has been reported during COC use.
- Chloasma may occasionally occur with the use of hormonal contraception, especially in users with a history of chloasma gravidarum. Users with a tendency to chloasma should avoid exposure to the sun or ultraviolet radiation while using EVRA. Chloasma is often not fully reversible.

Medical Examination/Consultation

Prior to the initiation or reinstitution of EVRA a complete medical history (including family history) should be taken and pregnancy should be ruled out. Blood pressure should be measured and a physical examination should be performed guided by the contraindications (See section 4.3) and warnings (See section 4.4). The woman should also be instructed to carefully read the package leaflet and to adhere to the advice given.

The frequency and nature of subsequent examinations should be based on established guidelines and be adapted to the individual woman on the basis of clinical impression.

Women should be advised that hormonal contraceptives do not protect against HIV infections (AIDS) and other sexually transmissible diseases.

Bleeding irregularities

With all combination hormonal contraceptives, irregular blood loss (spotting or breakthrough bleeding) can occur, especially during the initial months of usage. For this reason, a medical opinion on irregular blood loss will only be useful after an adjustment period of approximately three cycles. If breakthrough bleeding persists, or breakthrough bleeding occurs after previously regular cycles, while EVRA has been used according the recommended regimen, a cause other than EVRA should be considered. Non-hormonal causes should be considered and, if necessary, adequate diagnostic measures taken to rule out organic disease or pregnancy. This may include curettage. In some women withdrawal bleeding may not occur during this patch free period. If EVRA has been taken according the directions described in section 4.2, it is unlikely that the woman is pregnant. However, if EVRA has not been taken according to these directions prior to the first missed withdrawal bleed or if two withdrawal bleeds are missed, pregnancy must be ruled out before EVRA use is continued.

Some users may experience amenorrhoea or oligomenorrhoea after discontinuing hormonal contraception, especially when such a condition was pre-existent.

Herbal preparations containing St John's Wort (*Hypericum perforatum*) should not be used while taking EVRA (See 4.5 Interactions)

4.5 Interaction with other medicinal products and other forms of Interaction

Influence of other medications on EVRA

Medicinal product interactions, which result in an increased clearance of sex hormones can lead to breakthrough bleeding and hormonal contraceptive failure. This has been established with hydantoins, barbiturates, primidone, carbamazepine and rifampicin; oxcarbazepine, topiramate, felbamate, ritonavir, griseofulvin, modafinil and phenyl butazone are also suspected. The mechanism of these interactions appears to be based on the hepatic enzyme inducing properties of these medicinal products. Maximal enzyme induction is generally not seen for 2-3 weeks but may be sustained for at least 4 weeks after cessation of therapy.

The herbal preparation of St John's Wort (*Hypericum perforatum*) should not be taken concomitantly with this medicinal product as this could potentially lead to a loss of contraceptive effect. Breakthrough bleeding and unintended pregnancies have been reported. This is due to induction of metabolising enzymes by St John's Wort. The inducing effect may persist for at least 2 weeks after cessation of treatment with St John's Wort.

Contraceptive failures have also been reported with antibiotics, such as ampicillin and tetracyclines. The mechanism of this effect has not been elucidated. In a pharmacokinetic interaction study, oral administration of tetracycline hydrochloride, 500 mg four times daily for 3 days prior to and 7 days during wear of EVRA, did not significantly affect the pharmacokinetics of norelgestromin or EE.

Women on treatment with any of these medicinal products should temporarily use a barrier method in addition to EVRA or choose another method of contraception. With microsomal enzyme-inducing drugs, the barrier method should be used during the time of concomitant administration of these medicinal products and for 28 days after their discontinuation. Women on treatment with antibiotics (except tetracycline) should use the barrier method until 7 days after discontinuation. If concomitant medicinal product administration runs beyond the 3 weeks of patch treatment, a new treatment cycle should be started immediately without having the usual patch-free interval.

For women on long-term therapy with hepatic enzyme inducers, another method of contraception should be considered.

Influence of EVRA on other medications

Progestogens and estrogens inhibit a variety of P450 enzymes (e.g. CYP 3A4, CYP 2C19) in human liver microsomes. However, under the recommended dosing regimen, the *in vivo* concentrations of norelgestromin and its metabolites, even at the peak serum levels, are relatively low compared to the inhibitory constant (Ki), indicating a low potential for clinical interaction. Nevertheless, physicians are advised to refer to prescribing information for recommendations regarding management of concomitant therapy, especially for agents with a narrow therapeutic index metabolised by these enzymes (e.g. cyclosporin).

Laboratory tests

Certain endocrine and liver function tests and blood components may be affected by hormonal contraceptives:

- Increased prothrombin and factors VII, VIII, IX and X; decreased anti-thrombin III; decreased protein S; increased norepinephrine (noradrenaline)-induced platelet aggregability.

- Increased thyroid binding globulin (TBG) leading to increased circulating total thyroid hormone, as measured by protein-bound iodine (PBI), T4 by column or by radioimmunoassay. Free T3 resin uptake is decreased, reflecting the elevated TBG, free T4 concentration is unaltered.

Other binding proteins may be elevated in serum.

Sex hormone-binding globulins (SHBG) are increased and result in elevated levels of total circulating endogenous sex steroids. However, the free or biologically active levels of sex steroids either decrease or remain the same.

High-density lipoprotein (HDL-C), total cholesterol (Total-C), low-density lipoprotein (LDL-C) and triglycerides may all increase slightly with EVRA, while LDL-C/HDL-C ratio may remain unchanged.

Glucose tolerance may be decreased.

Serum folate levels may be depressed by hormonal contraceptive therapy. This has potential to be of clinical significance if a woman becomes pregnant shortly after discontinuing hormonal contraceptives. All women are now advised to take supplemental folic acid peri-conceptionally.

4.6 Pregnancy and lactation

EVRA is not indicated during pregnancy.

Epidemiological studies indicate no increased risk of birth defects in children born to women who used hormonal contraceptives prior to pregnancy. The majority of recent studies also do not indicate a teratogenic effect when hormonal contraceptives are used inadvertently during early pregnancy.

For EVRA there are no clinical data on exposed pregnancies, which allow conclusions about its safety during pregnancy.

Table 1

	Common Adverse Events ≥ 1/100 to < 1/10	Uncommon Adverse Events ≥ 1/1,000 to < 1/100	Rare Adverse Events > 1/10,000 to < 1/1,000
Application site disorders			Cellulitis
General disorders	Influenza-like symptoms Back pain Injury Fatigue Allergy	Allergic reaction Hot flushes Chest pain Leg pain Pain Asthenia Oedema Syncope	Abdomen enlarged Alcohol intolerance Crying abnormal
Cardiovascular disorders		Hypertension	Hypotension
Central & peripheral nervous systems disorders	Dizziness Migraine	Cramp legs Vertigo Paraesthesia Hypoaesthesia Convulsions Tremor	Hypertonia Coordination abnormal Dysphonia Hemiplegia Hypotonia Migraine aggravated Neuralgia Stupor
Endocrine disorders			Fat disorder Hyperprolactinaemia
Gastro-intestinal disorders	Abdominal Pain Vomiting Diarrhoea Gastroenteritis Flatulence Dyspepsia	Constipation Gastritis Haemorrhoids Tooth disorder Gingivitis	Enanthema Gastro-intestinal Disorder Mouth dry Saliva increased Colitis
Heart rate and rhythm disorders		Palpitation	
Liver and biliary system disorders			Cholecystitis SGPT increased Cholelithiasis SGOT increased Hepatic function abnormal
Metabolic and nutritional disorders	Weight increase	Hypertriglyceridaemia Hypercholesterolaemia	Xerophthalmia Weight decrease Obesity
Musculo-skeletal system disorders	Myalgia	Tendon disorder Arthralgia Muscle weakness	
Neoplasms	Breast fibroadenosis Cervical smear test positive	Ovarian cyst	Breast neoplasm benign female Cervix carcinoma in situ.
Platelet, bleeding and clotting disorders			Purpura Embolism pulmonary Thrombosis
Psychiatric disorders	Emotional lability Depression	Libido decreased Anxiety Appetite increased Insomnia Anorexia Dyspareunia Somnolence	Libido increased Depersonalisation Apathy Depression aggravated Paranoia
Red blood cell disorders		Anaemia	
Reproductive disorders	Dysmenorrhoea Vaginitis Intermenstrual bleeding Menorrhagia Breast enlargement Menstrual disorder	Vulva disorder Cervix lesion Lactation nonpuerperal Uterine spasm Ovarian disorder Vaginal haemorrhage Withdrawal bleeding Mastitis	Perineal pain female Genital ulceration Breast atrophy
Resistance mechanism disorders		Abscess	
Respiratory system disorders	Upper respiratory tract infection Sinusitis	Dyspnoea Asthma	
Skin and appendages disorders	Pruritus Acne Rash	Skin discoloration Skin disorder Eczema Sweating increased Urticaria Alopecia Photosensitivity reaction Skin dry Dermatitis contact Bullous eruption	Melanosis Pigmentation abnormal Skin depigmentation Chloasma Skin cold clammy
Urinary system disorders	Urinary tract infection		Pain on micturation
Vascular (extracardiac) disorders		Vein varicose	Flushing Deep venous thrombosis Pulmonary embolism* Thrombophlebitis Superficial vein disorder Vein pain
Vision disorders		Conjunctivitis Vision abnormal	Eye abnormality
White cell and reticuloendothelial system disorders		Lymphadenopathy	

* Currently there is no evidence to exclude that EVRA may be more thrombogenic than combined oral contraceptives.

Table 2

Study Group	CONT-002 EVRA	CONT-003 EVRA	CONT-003 COC*	CONT-004 EVRA	CONT-004 COC**	All EVRA Subjects
# of cycles	10,743	5831	4592	5095	4005	21,669
Overall Pearl Index (95% CI)	0.73 (0.15,1.31)	0.89 (0.02,1.76)	0.57 (0,1.35)	1.28 (0.16,2.39)	2.27 (0.59,3.96)	0.90 (0.44,1.35)
Method Failure Pearl Index (95% CI)	0.61 (0.0,1.14)	0.67 (0,1.42)	0.28 (0,0.84)	1.02 (0.02,2.02)	1.30 (0.03,2.57)	0.72 (0.31,1.13)

*: DSG 150 μg + 20 μg EE

**: 50 μg LNG + 30 μg for days 1 – 6, 75 μg LNG + 40 μg EE for days 7 – 11, 125 μg LNG + 30 μg EE for 12 – 21 days

Studies in animals have shown reproductive toxicity (See section 5.3). On the basis of available data, a potential risk of masculinisation as a consequence of an exaggerated hormonal action cannot be excluded.

If pregnancy occurs during use of EVRA, EVRA should be stopped immediately.

Lactation may be influenced by combination hormonal contraceptives as they may reduce the quantity and change the composition of breast milk. Therefore, the use of EVRA is not to be recommended until the nursing mother has completely weaned her child.

4.7 Effects on ability to drive and use machines

Evra has no or negligible influence on ability to drive and use machines.

4.8 Undesirable effects

The very common > 1/10) adverse events in the clinical trials with EVRA were breast symptoms, headache, application site reactions, and nausea.

The following adverse events have been reported in the clinical trials with EVRA among 3,330 women, and in some cases have been considered at least possibly related to treatment:

(see Table 1 on previous page)

4.9 Overdose

Serious ill effects have not been reported following accidental ingestion of large doses of oral contraceptives. Overdosage may cause nausea or vomiting. Vaginal bleeding may occur in some females. In cases of suspected overdose, all transdermal contraceptive systems should be removed and symptomatic treatment given.

5. PHARMACOLOGICAL PROPERTIES

5.1 Pharmacodynamic properties

Pharmacotherapeutic group: progestagens and estrogens; ATC-code: GO3AA.

EVRA acts through the mechanism of gonadotropin suppression by the estrogenic and progestational actions of ethinyl estradiol and norelgestromin. The primary mechanism of action is inhibition of the ovulation, but the alterations of the cervical mucus, and to the endometrium may also contribute to the efficacy of the product.

Pearl Indices (see table):

(see Table 2 above)

Exploratory analyses were performed to determine whether in the Phase III studies (n=3319) the population characteristics of age, race and weight were associated with pregnancy. The analyses indicated no association of age and race with pregnancy. With respect to weight, 5 of the 15 pregnancies reported with EVRA were among women with baseline body weight equal or greater than 90 kg, which constituted < 3 % of the study population. Below 90 kg there was no association between body weight and pregnancy. Although only 10-20 % of the variability in pharmacokinetic data can be explained by weight (see Pharmacokinetic Properties, Special Populations), the greater proportions of pregnancies among women at or above 90 kg was statistically significant and indicates the EVRA is less effective in these women.

With the use of higher dosed COCs (50 microgram ethinyl estradiol) the risk of endometrial and ovarian cancer is reduced. Whether this is also applies to the lower dosed combined hormonal contraceptives remains to be confirmed.

5.2 Pharmacokinetic properties

Absorption

Following application of EVRA, norelgestromin and ethinyl estradiol levels in serum reach a plateau by approximately 48 hours. Steady state concentrations of norelgestromin and EE during one week of patch wear are approximately 0.8 ng/ml and 50 pg/ml, respectively. In multiple-dose studies, serum concentrations and AUC for norelgestromin and EE were found to increase only slightly over time when compared to week 1 cycle 1.

The absorption of norelgestromin and ethinyl estradiol following application of EVRA was studied under conditions encountered in a health club (sauna, whirlpool, treadmill and other aerobic exercise) and in a cold water bath. The results indicated that for norelgestromin there were no significant treatment effects on C_{ss} or AUC when compared to normal wear. For EE, slight increases were observed due to treadmill and other aerobic exercise; however, the C_{ss} values following these treatments were within the reference range. There was no significant effect of cool water on these parameters.

Results from an EVRA study of extended wear of single contraceptive patch for 7 days and 10 days indicated that target C_{ss} of norelgestromin and ethinyl estradiol were maintained during a 3-day period of extended wear of EVRA (10 days). These findings suggest that clinical efficacy would be maintained even if a scheduled change is missed for as long as 2 full days.

Distribution

Norelgestromin and norgestrel (a serum metabolite of norelgestromin) are highly bound > 97 %) to serum proteins. Norelgestromin is bound to albumin and not to SHBG, while norgestrel is bound primarily to SHBG, which limits its biological activity. Ethinyl estradiol is extensively bound to serum albumin.

Biotransformation

Hepatic metabolism of norelgestromin occurs and metabolites include norgestrel, which is largely bound to SHBG, and various hydroxylated and conjugated metabolites. Ethinyl estradiol is also metabolised to various hydroxylated products and their glucuronide and sulfate conjugates.

Elimination

Following removal of a patch, the mean elimination half-lives of norelgestromin and ethinyl estradiol were approximately 28 hours and 17 hours, respectively. The metabolites of norelgestromin and ethinyl estradiol are eliminated by renal and fecal pathways.

Effects of age, body weight, and body surface area

The effects of age, body weight, and body surface area on the pharmacokinetics of norelgestromin and ethinyl estradiol were evaluated in 230 healthy women from nine pharmacokinetic studies of single 7-day applications of EVRA. For both norelgestromin and EE, increasing age, body weight and body surface area each were associated with slight decreases in C_{ss} and AUC values. However, only a small fraction (10 –20 %) of the overall variability in the pharmacokinetics of the norelgestromin and EE following application of EVRA may be associated with any or all of the above demographic parameters.

5.3 Preclinical safety data

Preclinical data reveal no special hazard for humans based on conventional studies of safety pharmacology, repeated dose toxicity, genotoxicity and carcinogenic potential. With respect to the reproductive toxicity norelgestromin showed foetal toxicity in rabbits, but the safety margin for this effect was sufficiently high. Data on reproductive toxicity of the combination of norelgestromin with ethinyl estradiol are not available. Data for combination of norgestimate (precursor of norelgestromin) with ethinyl estradiol indicate for female animals a decrease in fertility and implantation efficiency (rat), an increase in foetal resorption (rat, rabbit) and, with high dosages, a decrease in viability and fertility of female offspring (rat). The relevance of these data for human exposure is unknown as these effects have been seen as related to well-known pharmacodynamic or species-specific actions.

Studies conducted to examine the dermal effect of EVRA indicate this system has no potential to produce sensitisation and results in only mild irritation when applied to rabbits skin.

6. PHARMACEUTICAL PARTICULARS

6.1 List of excipients

Backing layer: low-density pigmented polyethylene outer layer and a polyester inner layer.

Middle layer: polyisobutylene/polybutene adhesive, crospovidone, non-woven polyester fabric, lauryl lactate.

Third layer: polyethylene terephthalate (PET) film, polydimethylsiloxane coating.

6.2 Incompatibilities

To prevent interference with the adhesive properties of EVRA, no creams, lotions or powders should be applied to the skin area where the EVRA transdermal patch is to be applied.

6.3 Shelf life

2 years

6.4 Special precautions for storage

Store in the original package.

Do not refrigerate or freeze

6.5 Nature and contents of container

Primary Packaging Material

A sachet is composed of four layers: a low-density polyethylene film (innermost layer), an aluminium foil, a low-density polyethylene film, and an outer layer of bleached paper.

Secondary Packaging Material

Sachets are packaged in a cardboard carton

Every carton has 9 EVRA transdermal patches in individual foil-lined sachets.

6.6 Instructions for use and handling

Apply immediately upon removal from the protective sachet. After use the patch still contains substantial quantities of active ingredients. Remaining hormonal active ingredients of the patch may have harmful effects if reaching the aquatic environment. Therefore, the used patch should be discarded carefully. The disposal label from the outside of the sachet should be peeled open. The used patch should be placed within the open disposal label so that the sticky surface covers the shaded area on the sachet. The disposal label should then be closed sealing the used patch within. Any used or unused patches should be discarded according to local requirements or returned to the pharmacy. Used patches should not be flushed down the toilet nor placed in liquid waste disposal systems.

7. MARKETING AUTHORISATION HOLDER

JANSSEN-CILAG INTERNATIONAL N.V.

Turnhoutseweg, 30

B-2340 Beerse

Belgium

8. MARKETING AUTHORISATION NUMBER(S)

EU/1/02/223/002

9. DATE OF FIRST AUTHORISATION/RENEWAL OF THE AUTHORISATION

22.08.2002

10. DATE OF REVISION OF THE TEXT

17.02.03

Exelon

(Novartis Pharmaceuticals UK Ltd)

1. NAME OF THE MEDICINAL PRODUCT

EXELON 1.5 mg hard capsules

EXELON 3 mg hard capsules

EXELON 4.5 mg hard capsules

EXELON 6 mg hard capsules

EXELON 2mg/ml Oral Solution

2. QUALITATIVE AND QUANTITATIVE COMPOSITION

Each capsule contains rivastigmine hydrogen tartrate corresponding to rivastigmine 1.5 mg, 3 mg, 4.5 mg or 6 mg.

Each ml contains rivastigmine hydrogen tartrate corresponding to rivastigmine base 2.0 mg.

For excipients, see 6.1.

3. PHARMACEUTICAL FORM

Capsule, hard.

EXELON 1.5 mg: Off-white to slightly yellow powder in a capsule with yellow cap and yellow body, with red imprint "EXELON 1.5 mg" on body.

EXELON 3 mg: Off-white to slightly yellow powder in a capsule with orange cap and orange body, with red imprint "EXELON 3 mg" on body.

EXELON 4.5 mg: Off-white to slightly yellow powder in a capsule with red cap and red body, with white imprint "EXELON 4.5 mg" on body.

EXELON 6 mg: Off-white to slightly yellow powder in a capsule with red cap and orange body, with red imprint "EXELON 6 mg" on body.

Oral Solution.

Clear, yellow solution.

4. CLINICAL PARTICULARS

4.1 Therapeutic indications

Symptomatic treatment of mild to moderately severe Alzheimer's dementia.

4.2 Posology and method of administration

Administration: Treatment should be initiated and supervised by a physician experienced in the diagnosis and treatment of Alzheimer's dementia. Diagnosis should be made according to current guidelines. Therapy with rivastigmine should only be started if a caregiver is available who will regularly monitor drug intake by the patient.

Rivastigmine should be administered twice a day, with morning and evening meals. The capsules should be swallowed whole. The prescribed amount of solution should be withdrawn from the container using the oral dosing syringe supplied. Rivastigmine oral solution may be swallowed directly from the syringe. Rivastigmine oral solution and rivastigmine capsules may be interchanged at equal doses.

Initial dose: 1.5 mg twice a day.

Dose titration: The starting dose is 1.5 mg twice a day. If this dose is well tolerated after a minimum of two weeks of treatment, the dose may be increased to 3 mg twice a day. Subsequent increases to 4.5 mg and then 6 mg twice a day should also be based on good tolerance of the current dose and may be considered after a minimum of two weeks of treatment at that dose level.

If adverse effects (e.g. nausea, vomiting, abdominal pain or loss of appetite) or weight decrease are observed during treatment, these may respond to omitting one or more doses. If adverse effects persist, the daily dose should be temporarily reduced to the previous well-tolerated dose.

Maintenance dose: The effective dose is 3 to 6 mg twice a day; to achieve maximum therapeutic benefit patients should be maintained on their highest well tolerated dose. The recommended maximum daily dose is 6 mg twice a day.

Maintenance treatment can be continued for as long as a therapeutic benefit for the patient exists. Therefore, the clinical benefit of rivastigmine should be reassessed on a regular basis, especially for patients treated at doses less than 3 mg twice a day. Discontinuation should be considered when evidence of a therapeutic effect is no longer present. Individual response to rivastigmine cannot be predicted.

Treatment effect has not been studied in placebo-controlled trials beyond 6 months.

Re-initiation of therapy: If treatment is interrupted for more than several days, it should be re-initiated at 1.5 mg twice daily. Dose titration should then be carried out as described above.

Renal and hepatic impairment:

Due to increased exposure in renal and mild to moderate hepatic impairment, dosing recommendations to titrate according to individual tolerability should be closely followed (see 5.2 Pharmacokinetics properties).

Children:

Rivastigmine is not recommended for use in children.

4.3 Contraindications

The use of this medicinal product is contraindicated in patients with known hypersensitivity to rivastigmine, other carbamate derivatives or to any excipients used in the formulation, severe liver impairment, as it has not been studied in this population

4.4 Special warnings and special precautions for use

The incidence and severity of adverse events generally increase with higher doses. If treatment is interrupted for more than several days, it should be re-initiated at 1.5 mg twice daily to reduce the possibility of adverse reactions (e.g. vomiting).

Dose titration: Adverse effects (e.g. hypertension, hallucinations) have been observed shortly after dose increase. They may respond to a dose reduction. In other cases, Exelon has been discontinued (see 4.8 Undesirable effects).

Gastrointestinal disorders such as nausea and vomiting may occur particularly when initiating treatment and/or increasing the dose. These adverse events occur more commonly in women. Patients with Alzheimer's disease may lose weight. Cholinesterase inhibitors, including rivastigmine, have been associated with weight loss in these patients. During therapy patient's weight should be monitored.

As with other cholinomimetics, care must be taken when using rivastigmine in patients with sick sinus syndrome or conduction defects (sino-atrial block, atrio-ventricular block) (see section 4.8).

As with other cholinergic substances, rivastigmine may cause increased gastric acid secretions. Care should be exercised in treating patients with active gastric or duodenal ulcers or patients predisposed to these conditions.

Cholinesterase inhibitors should be prescribed with care to patients with a history of asthma or obstructive pulmonary disease.

Cholinomimetics may induce or exacerbate urinary obstruction and seizures. Caution is recommended in treating patients predisposed to such diseases.

One of the excipients in Exelon oral solution is sodium benzoate. Benzoic acid is a mild irritant to the skin, eyes and mucous membrane.

The use of rivastigmine in patients with severe Alzheimer's dementia, other types of dementia or other types of memory impairment (e.g. age-related cognitive decline) has not been investigated.

Like other cholinomimetics, rivastigmine may exacerbate or induce extrapyramidal symptoms, including worsening in patients with Parkinson's disease.

4.5 Interaction with other medicinal products and other forms of Interaction

As a cholinesterase inhibitor, rivastigmine may exaggerate the effects of succinylcholine-type muscle relaxants during anaesthesia.

In view of its pharmacodynamic effects, rivastigmine should not be given concomitantly with other cholinomimetic drugs and might interfere with the activity of anticholinergic medications.

No pharmacokinetic interaction was observed between rivastigmine and digoxin, warfarin, diazepam or fluoxetine in studies in healthy volunteers. The increase in prothrombin time induced by warfarin is not affected by administration of rivastigmine. No untoward effects on cardiac conduction were observed following concomitant administration of digoxin and rivastigmine.

According to its metabolism, metabolic drug interactions appear unlikely, although rivastigmine may inhibit the butyrylcholinesterase mediated metabolism of other drugs.

4.6 Pregnancy and lactation

Pregnancy: No clinical data on exposed pregnancies are available. No effects on fertility or embryofoetal development were observed in rats and rabbits, except at doses related to maternal toxicity. In peri/postnatal studies in rats, an increased gestation time was observed. Rivastigmine should not be used during pregnancy unless clearly necessary.

Lactation: In animals, rivastigmine is excreted into milk. It is not known if rivastigmine is excreted into human milk. Therefore, women on rivastigmine should not breast-feed.

4.7 Effects on ability to drive and use machines

Alzheimer's disease may cause gradual impairment of driving performance or compromise the ability to use machinery. Furthermore, rivastigmine can induce dizziness and somnolence, mainly when initiating treatment or increasing the dose. Therefore, the ability of Alzheimer patients on rivastigmine to continue driving or operating complex machines should be routinely evaluated by the treating physician.

4.8 Undesirable effects

The most commonly reported adverse drug reactions are gastrointestinal, including nausea (38 %) and vomiting (23 %), especially during titration. Female patients in clinical studies were found to be more susceptible than male patients to gastrointestinal adverse drug reactions and weight loss.

The following adverse drug reactions, listed below in Table 1, have been accumulated both from clinical studies with Exelon and since the introduction of Exelon into the market.

Table 1*

Infections and infestation	
Very rare	Urinary infection
Psychiatric disorders	
Common	Agitation
Common	Confusion
Uncommon	Insomnia
Uncommon	Depression
Very rare	Hallucinations
Nervous system disorders	
Very common	Dizziness
Common	Headache
Common	Somnolence
Common	Tremor
Uncommon	Syncope
Rare	Seizures
Very rare	Extrapyramidal symptoms (including worsening of Parkinson's disease)
Cardiac disorders	
Rare	Angina pectoris
Very rare	Cardiac arrhythmia (e.g. bradycardia, atrio-ventricular block, atrial fibrillation and tachycardia)
Vascular disorders	
Very rare	Hypertension
Gastrointestinal disorders	
Very common	Nausea
Very common	Vomiting
Very common	Diarrhoea
Very common	Loss of appetite
Common	Abdominal pain and dyspepsia
Rare	Gastric and duodenal ulcers
Very rare	Gastrointestinal haemorrhage
Very rare	Pancreatitis
Hepato-biliary disorders	
Very rare	Elevated liver function tests
Skin and subcutaneous disorders	
Common	Sweating increased
Rare	Rashes
General disorders	
Common	Fatigue and asthenia
Common	Malaise
Uncommon	Accidental fall
Investigations	
Common	Weight loss

* Adverse reactions are ranked under headings of frequency, the most frequent first, using the following convention: Very common >1/10); common >1/100, <1/10); uncommon >1/1,000, <1/100); rare >1/10,000, <1/1,000); very rare (<1/10,000), including isolated reports.

4.9 Overdose

Symptoms: Most cases of accidental overdosage have not been associated with any clinical signs or symptoms and almost all of the patients concerned continued rivastigmine treatment. Where symptoms have occurred, they have included nausea, vomiting and diarrhoea, hypertension or hallucinations. Due to the known vagotonic effect of cholinesterase inhibitors on heart rate, bradycardia and/or syncope may also occur. Ingestion of 46 mg occurred in one case; following conservative management the patient fully recovered within 24 hours.

Treatment: As rivastigmine has a plasma half-life of about 1 hour and a duration of acetylcholinesterase inhibition of about 9 hours, it is recommended that in cases of asymptomatic overdose no further dose of rivastigmine should be administered for the next 24 hours. In overdose accompanied by severe nausea and vomiting, the use of antiemetics should be considered. Symptomatic treatment for other adverse events should be given as necessary.

In massive overdose, atropine can be used. An initial dose of 0.03 mg/kg intravenous atropine sulphate is recommended, with subsequent doses based on clinical response. Use of scopolamine as an antidote is not recommended.

5. PHARMACOLOGICAL PROPERTIES

5.1 Pharmacodynamic properties

Pharmacotherapeutic group: anticholinesterases; ATC-code: N06D A03

Rivastigmine is an acetyl- and butyrylcholinesterase inhibitor of the carbamate type, thought to facilitate cholinergic neurotransmission by slowing the degradation of acetylcholine released by functionally intact cholinergic neurones. Thus, rivastigmine may have an ameliorative effect on cholinergic-mediated cognitive deficits associated with Alzheimer's disease.

Rivastigmine interacts with its target enzymes by forming a covalently bound complex that temporarily inactivates the enzymes. In healthy young men, an oral 3 mg dose decreases acetylcholinesterase (AChE) activity in CSF by approximately 40% within the first 1.5 hours after administration. Activity of the enzyme returns to baseline levels about 9 hours after the maximum inhibitory effect has been achieved. In patients with Alzheimer's disease, inhibition of AChE in CSF by rivastigmine was dose-dependent up to 6 mg given twice daily, the highest dose tested. Inhibition of butyrylcholinesterase activity in CSF of 14 Alzheimer patients treated by rivastigmine was similar to that of AChE.

Clinical studies

The efficacy of rivastigmine has been established through the use of three independent, domain specific, assessment tools which were assessed at periodic intervals during 6 month treatment periods. These include the ADAS-Cog (a performance based measure of cognition), the CIBIC-Plus (a comprehensive global assessment of the patient by the physician incorporating caregiver input), and the PDS (a caregiver-rated assessment of the activities of daily living including personal hygiene, feeding, dressing, household chores such as shopping, retention of ability to orient oneself to surroundings as well as involvement in activities relating to finances, etc.).

The results for clinically relevant responders pooled from two flexible dose studies out of the three pivotal 26-week multicentre studies in patients with mild-to-moderately severe Alzheimer's Dementia, are provided in Table 2 below. Clinically relevant improvement in these studies was defined *a priori* as at least 4-point improvement on the ADAS-Cog, improvement on the CIBIC-Plus, or at least a 10% improvement on the PDS.

In addition, a post-hoc definition of response is provided in the same table. The secondary definition of response required a 4-point or greater improvement on the ADAS-Cog, no worsening on the CIBIC-Plus, and no worsening on the PDS. The mean actual daily dose for responders in the 6-12 mg group, corresponding to this definition, was 9.3 mg. It is important to note that the scales used in this indication vary and direct comparisons of results for different therapeutic agents are not valid.

Table 2

	Patients with Clinically Significant Response (%)			
	Intent to Treat		Last Observation Carried Forward	
Response Measure	Rivastigmine 6-12 mg N=473	Placebo N=472	Rivastigmine7 6-12 mg N=379	Placebo N=444
ADAS-Cog: improvement of at least 4 points	21***	12	25***	12
CIBIC-Plus: improvement	29***	18	32***	19
PDS: improvement of at least 10%	26***	17	30***	18
At least 4 points improvement on ADAS-Cog with no worsening on CIBIC-Plus and PDS	10*	6	12**	6

* $p<0.05$, ** $p<0.01$, *** $p<0.001$

Table 2

(see Table 2 above)

5.2 Pharmacokinetic properties

Absorption: Rivastigmine is rapidly and completely absorbed. Peak plasma concentrations are reached in approximately 1 hour. As a consequence of the drug's interaction with its target enzyme, the increase in bioavailability is about 1.5-fold greater than that expected from the increase in dose. Absolute bioavailability after a 3 mg dose is about 36%±13%. Administration of rivastigmine with food delays absorption (t_{max}) by 90 min and lowers C_{max} and increases AUC by approximately 30%. Administration of rivastigmine oral solution with food delays absorption (t_{max}) by 74 min and lowers C_{max} by 43% and increases AUC by approximately 9%.

Distribution: Rivastigmine is weakly bound to plasma proteins (approximately 40%). It readily crosses the blood brain barrier and has an apparent volume of distribution in the range of 1.8-2.7 l/kg.

Metabolism: Rivastigmine is rapidly and extensively metabolised (half-life in plasma approximately 1 hour), primarily via cholinesterase-mediated hydrolysis to the decarbamylated metabolite. *In vitro*, this metabolite shows minimal inhibition of acetylcholinesterase (<10%). Based on evidence from *in vitro* and animal studies the major cytochrome P450 isoenzymes are minimally involved in rivastigmine metabolism. Total plasma clearance of rivastigmine was approximately 130 l/h after a 0.2 mg intravenous dose and decreased to 70 l/h after a 2.7 mg intravenous dose.

Excretion: Unchanged rivastigmine is not found in the urine; renal excretion of the metabolites is the major route of elimination. Following administration of ^{14}C-rivastigmine, renal elimination was rapid and essentially complete (> 90 %) within 24 hours. Less than 1% of the administered dose is excreted in the faeces. There is no accumulation of rivastigmine or the decarbamylated metabolite in patients with Alzheimer's disease.

Elderly subjects: While bioavailability of rivastigmine is greater in elderly than in young healthy volunteers, studies in Alzheimer patients aged between 50 and 92 years showed no change in bioavailability with age.

Subjects with hepatic impairment: The C_{max} of rivastigmine was approximately 60% higher and the AUC of rivastigmine was more than twice as high in subjects with mild to moderate hepatic impairment than in to healthy subjects.

Subjects with renal impairment: C_{max} and AUC of rivastigmine were more than twice as high in subjects with moderate renal impairment compared with healthy subjects; however there were no changes in C_{max} and AUC of rivastigmine in subjects with severe renal impairment.

5.3 Preclinical safety data

Repeated-dose toxicity studies in rats, mice and dogs revealed only effects associated with an exaggerated pharmacological action. No target organ toxicity was observed. No safety margins to human exposure were achieved in the animal studies due to the sensitivity of the animal models used.

Rivastigmine was not mutagenic in a standard battery of *in vitro* and *in vivo* tests, except in a chromosomal aberration test in human peripheral lymphocytes at a dose 10^4 times the maximum clinical exposure. The *in vivo* micronucleus test was negative.

No evidence of carcinogenicity was found in studies in mice and rats at the maximum tolerated dose, although the exposure to rivastigmine and its metabolites was lower than the human exposure. When normalised to body surface area, the exposure to rivastigmine and its metabolites was approximately equivalent to the maximum recommended human dose of 12 mg/day; however, when compared to the maximum human dose, a multiple of approximately 6-fold was achieved in animals.

In animals, rivastigmine crosses the placenta and is excreted into milk. Oral studies in pregnant rats and rabbits gave no indication of teratogenic potential on the part of rivastigmine.

6. PHARMACEUTICAL PARTICULARS

6.1 List of excipients

EXELON Capsules:

Gelatin

Magnesium stearate

Hypromellose

Microcrystalline cellulose

Silica, colloidal anhydrous

Yellow iron oxide (E172)

Red iron oxide (E172)

Titanium dioxide (E171)

EXELON Oral Solution:

Sodium benzoate

Citric acid

Sodium citrate

Quinoline yellow WS dye E104

Purified water.

6.2 Incompatibilities

Not applicable

6.3 Shelf life

EXELON Capsules: 5 years

EXELON Oral Solution: 3 years

EXELON Oral Solution should be used within 1 month of opening the bottle.

6.4 Special precautions for storage

EXELON Capsules: Do not store above 30°C

EXELON Oral Solution: Do not store above 30°C. Do not refrigerate or freeze.

Store in an upright position.

6.5 Nature and contents of container

EXELON Capsules:

Blister with 14 capsules; clear PVC tray with blue lidding foil. Each box contains 2, 4 or 8 blisters.

EXELON Oral Solution:

120 ml Type III amber glass bottle with a child-resistant cap, dip tube and self aligning plug. The oral solution is packaged with an oral dosing syringe in a plastic tube container.

6.6 Instructions for use and handling

EXELON Capsules:

No special requirements.

EXELON Oral Solution:

The prescribed amount of solution should be withdrawn from the bottle using the oral dosing syringe supplied.

7. MARKETING AUTHORISATION HOLDER

Novartis Europharm Limited

Wimblehurst Road

Horsham

West Sussex, RH12 5AB

UNITED KINGDOM

8. MARKETING AUTHORISATION NUMBER(S)

EXELON 1.5 mg hard capsules:	EU/1/98/066/001-3
EXELON 3 mg hard capsules:	EU/1/98/066/004-6
EXELON 4.5 mg hard capsules:	EU/1/98/066/007-9
EXELON 6 mg hard capsules:	EU/1/98/066/010-12
EXELON 2mg/ml Oral Solution:	EU/1/98/066/013

9. DATE OF FIRST AUTHORISATION/RENEWAL OF THE AUTHORISATION

EXELON Capsules:	12.05.98 / 12.05.2003
EXELON Oral Solution:	02.06.99 / 12.05.2003

10. DATE OF REVISION OF THE TEXT

30.06.2003

LEGAL CATEGORY

POM

Exocin

(Allergan Ltd)

1. NAME OF THE MEDICINAL PRODUCT

EXOCIN.

2. QUALITATIVE AND QUANTITATIVE COMPOSITION

Ofloxacin 0.3% w/v.

3. PHARMACEUTICAL FORM

Eye drops.

4. CLINICAL PARTICULARS

4.1 Therapeutic indications

Exocin is indicated for the topical treatment of external ocular infections (such as conjunctivitis and keratoconjunctivitis) in adults and children caused by ofloxacin - sensitive organisms. Safety and efficacy in the treatment of ophthalmia neonatorum has not been established.

4.2 Posology and method of administration

Topical ocular instillation.

For all ages: one to two drops in the affected eye(s) every two to four hours for the first two days and then four times daily. The length of treatment should not exceed ten days.

4.3 Contraindications

Exocin is contra-indicated in patients sensitive to ofloxacin or any of its other components.

4.4 Special warnings and special precautions for use

Precautions

As with other anti-infectives, prolonged use may result in overgrowth of non-susceptible organisms. If worsening infection occurs, or if clinical improvement is not noted within a reasonable period, discontinue use and institute alternative therapy.

Use Exocin with caution in patients who have exhibited sensitivities to other quinolone antibacterial agents.

Exocin contains benzalkonium chloride and should not be used in patients continuing to wear hydrophilic (soft) contact lenses.

Use in elderly: No comparative data are available with topical dosing in elderly versus other age groups.

4.5 Interaction with other medicinal products and other forms of Interaction

None known

4.6 Pregnancy and lactation

Use in pregnancy: There have been no adequate and well-controlled studies performed in pregnant women. Since systemic quinolones have been shown to cause arthropathy in immature animals, it is recommended that Exocin be used in pregnant women only if the potential benefit justifies the potential risk to the foetus.

Use during lactation: Because ofloxacin and other quinolones taken systemically are excreted in breast milk, and there is potential for harm to nursing infants, a decision should be made whether to temporarily discontinue nursing or not to administer the drug, taking into account the importance of the drug to the mother.

4.7 Effects on ability to drive and use machines

None known.

4.8 Undesirable effects

Adverse reactions: Transient ocular irritation (burning, stinging, redness, itching or photophobia) has been reported. Extremely low incidence of dizziness, with numbness and nausea and of headache were reported from clinical trials. Since ofloxacin is systemically absorbed after topical administration, side-effects reported with systemic use could possibly occur.

4.9 Overdose

In the event of a topical overdosage, flush the eye with water.

5. PHARMACOLOGICAL PROPERTIES

5.1 Pharmacodynamic properties

Ofloxacin is a synthetic fluorinated 4-quinolone antibacterial agent with activity against a broad spectrum of Gram negative and to a lesser degree Gram positive organisms.

Ofloxacin has been shown to be active against most strains of the following organisms both in vitro and clinically in ophthalmic infections. Clinical trial evidence of the efficacy of Exocin against S. pneumoniae was based on a limited number of isolates.

Gram-negative bacteria: Acinetobacter calcoaceticus var. anitratum, and A. calcoaceticus var. iwoffi; Enterobacter Sp. including E. cloacae; Haemophilis Sp, including H. influenza and H. aegyptius; Klebsiella Sp., including K. Pneumoniae; Moraxella Sp., Morganella morganii; Proteus Sp., including P. Mirabilis; Pseudomonas Sp.; including P. Aeruginosa, P. cepacia, and P. fluoroscens; and Serratia Sp., including S. marcescens.

Gram-positive bacteria: Bacillus Sp.; Corynebacterium Sp.; Micrococcus Sp.; Staphylococcus Sp., including S. aureus and S. epidermidis; Streptococcus Sp., including S. Pneumoniae (see above), S. viridans and Beta-haemolytic.

The primary mechanisms of action is through inhibition of bacterial DNA gyrase, the enzyme responsible for maintaining the structure of DNA.

Ofloxacin is not subject to degradation by beta-lactamase enzymes nor is it modified by enzymes such as aminoglycoside adenylases or phosphorylases, or chloramphenicol acetyltransferase.

5.2 Pharmacokinetic properties

After ophthalmic instillation, ofloxacin is well maintained in the tear-film.

In a healthy volunteer study, mean tear film concentrations of ofloxacin measured four hours after topical dosing (9.2 μg/g) were higher than the 2μg/ml minimum concentration of ofloxacin necessary to inhibit 90% of most ocular bacterial strains (MIC_{90}) in-vitro.

Maximum serum ofloxacin concentrations after ten days of topical dosing were about 1000 times lower than those reported after standard oral doses of ofloxacin, and no systemic side-effects attributable to topical ofloxacin were observed.

5.3 Preclinical safety data

There are no toxicological safety issues with this product in man as the level of systemic absorption from topical ocular administration of ofloxacin is minimal.

Animal studies in the dog have found cases of arthropathy in weight bearing joints of juvenile animals after high oral doses of certain quinolones. However, these findings have not been seen in clinical studies and their relevance to man is unknown.

6. PHARMACEUTICAL PARTICULARS

6.1 List of excipients

Benzalkonium chloride (EP) 0.005% w/v

Sodium chloride (EP) 0.9% w/v

Purified water (EP)

6.2 Incompatibilities

None known.

6.3 Shelf life

24 months.

6.4 Special precautions for storage

Do not store above 25°C.

6.5 Nature and contents of container

5 ml or 10 ml low density polyethylene (LDPE) bottles with LDPE tip and medium or high impact polystyrene cap.

6.6 Instructions for use and handling

Discard bottle 28 days after opening.

7. MARKETING AUTHORISATION HOLDER

Allergan Ltd

Coronation Road

High Wycombe

Buckinghamshire

HP12 3SH

UK

8. MARKETING AUTHORISATION NUMBER(S)

PL 00426/0070

9. DATE OF FIRST AUTHORISATION/RENEWAL OF THE AUTHORISATION

26th October 1992/8th November 2004

10. DATE OF REVISION OF THE TEXT

8th November 2004

Exorex Lotion

(Forest Laboratories UK Limited)

1. NAME OF THE MEDICINAL PRODUCT

EXOREX LOTION

2. QUALITATIVE AND QUANTITATIVE COMPOSITION

The active ingredient is an alcoholic extract of prepared coal tar (BP 1973) 1% w/w (10 mg/g)

3. PHARMACEUTICAL FORM

Cutaneous emulsion

4. CLINICAL PARTICULARS

4.1 Therapeutic indications

Exorex is for the treatment of psoriasis of the skin and scalp.

4.2 Posology and method of administration

Adults and children over 12 years of age:

Ensure that the lesions are clean. Apply a thin layer of Exorex two or three times per day to the affected areas. Massage gently and leave to dry.

For young children under 12 years of age and the elderly:

The emulsion may be diluted by mixing with a few drops of freshly boiled and cooled water in the palm of the hand.

4.3 Contraindications

Do not use if sensitive to any of the ingredients.

Presence of folliculitis and acne vulgaris.

Exorex should not be used on patients who have disease characterised by photosensitivity such as lupus erythematosus or allergy to sunlight.

Exorex should not be applied to inflamed or broken skin (open exuding wounds or infection of the skin).

4.4 Special warnings and special precautions for use

Coal tar may cause skin irritation. If irritation occurs, the treatment should be reviewed and discontinued if necessary.

Coal tar enhances photosensitivity of the skin, and exposure to direct sunlight after application of Exorex should be avoided.

Use with care near the eyes and mucous membranes. If any emulsion should accidentally enter the eye, flush with normal saline solution or water.

Do not apply to genital and rectal areas.

Apply with caution to the face.

4.5 Interaction with other medicinal products and other forms of Interaction

None known.

4.6 Pregnancy and lactation

There is inadequate evidence of safety in pregnant and lactating women but coal tar preparations have been in use for many years without apparent ill-consequence and no harmful effects on the health of the child is anticipated with the proper use of this product. However it is recommended that the use of coal tar in pregnancy and lactation be restricted to intermittent use, in a low concentration on a relatively small percentage of body surface and that use during the first trimester be avoided.

4.7 Effects on ability to drive and use machines

None known.

4.8 Undesirable effects

Skin irritation, photosensitivity of the skin. In addition coal tar may cause acne-like eruptions of the skin.

An increased risk of skin cancer in psoriatic patients treated with a combination of coal tar and UVB radiation has been reported. However epidemiological studies of patients treated with coal tar alone are inconclusive. The risk of toxicity should be taken into account when considering the suitability of this product for the patient (see also Section 5.3).

4.9 Overdose

There is no evidence that overdose of topical Exorex would be harmful other than possibly inducing a hypersensitivity to coal tar. Ingestion of Exorex may require gastric lavage depending on the quantity taken and should be treated symptomatically.

5. PHARMACOLOGICAL PROPERTIES

5.1 Pharmacodynamic properties

Exorex contains coal tar, an antipruritic and keratoplastic. It is used in eczema, psoriasis and other skin conditions. Tar acids have also been shown to have disinfectant properties. Exorex may be used alone, or as part of a more extensive treatment regimen.

5.2 Pharmacokinetic properties

Not applicable.

5.3 Preclinical safety data

In animal studies coal tar has been shown to increase the incidence of epidermal carcinomas and self-limiting keratoacanthomas.

While the ingredients of coal tar have been shown to express genotoxic properties, epidemiological studies with patients have been shown to be inconclusive concerning the potential carcinogenic risks of coal tar products in human long term treatment. Nevertheless the possible risk of prolonged treatment should be taken into account when considering the usage of the product.

6. PHARMACEUTICAL PARTICULARS

6.1 List of excipients

Polysorbate 80

Industrial methylated spirits

DL-Alpha Tocopherol

Complex of esterified essential fatty acids

Xanthan gum

Sodium propyl paraben

Methyl paraben

PEG-40 hydrogenated castor oil

Water

6.2 Incompatibilities

None known

6.3 Shelf life

2 years

6.4 Special precautions for storage

Store at room temperature below 25°C.

6.5 Nature and contents of container

High density polyethylene bottle containing titanium dioxide.

Polypropylene green flip-top caps

Pack sizes: 100 and 250ml

A professional sales pack of 30ml is also available.

6.6 Instructions for use and handling

None

7. MARKETING AUTHORISATION HOLDER

Marketing Authorisation Holder	UK Distributor
Forest Tosara Limited Baldoyle Industrial Estate Dublin 13 Ireland	Forest Laboratories UK Limited Bourne Road Bexley Kent DA5 1NX

8. MARKETING AUTHORISATION NUMBER(S)

PL 06166/0001

9. DATE OF FIRST AUTHORISATION/RENEWAL OF THE AUTHORISATION

3 November 1999

10. DATE OF REVISION OF THE TEXT

October 1998

11. Legal Category

GSL

Exosurf Neonatal

(GlaxoSmithKline UK)

1. NAME OF THE MEDICINAL PRODUCT

Exosurf Neonatal

2. QUALITATIVE AND QUANTITATIVE COMPOSITION

Colfosceril Palmitate HSE 108.0mg or 67.5mg

3. PHARMACEUTICAL FORM

Lyophilised powder, for endotracheal administration after reconstitution.

4. CLINICAL PARTICULARS

4.1 Therapeutic indications

Exosurf neonatal is indicated for the treatment of newborn infants with or at risk of respiratory distress syndrome, who are undergoing mechanical ventilation and whose heart rate and arterial oxygenation are continuously monitored.

4.2 Posology and method of administration

Recommended doses and dosage schedules

A dose of 5ml/kg birthweight of reconstituted Exosurf Neonatal should be given via the endotracheal tube. If the baby is still intubated, a second equal dose should be given 12 hours later by the same route. Each dose corresponds to 67.5mg of colfosceril palmitate per kg birthweight.

Reconstitution

The contents of each vial of Exosurf Neonatal should be reconstituted with the diluent supplied. If this is not available, for the 108 mg vial use 8 ml of water for injections BP (i.e. sterile, preservative-free water) and for the 67.5 mg vial use 5 ml. This gives a white suspension containing 13.5 mg per ml colfosceril palmitate.

Exosurf Neonatal is physically and chemically stable for 24 hours after reconstitution if stored between 2 and 30 degrees centigrade. Exosurf Neonatal contains no antimicrobial preservative. Reconstitution should therefore be performed, either immediately before use, or, if storage is required, under sterile conditions. In either case, any unused suspension should be discarded.

Carry out the preparation as follows:-

1. Fill a syringe with the required volume of diluent.

2. Allow the vacuum in the vial of Exosurf Neonatal to draw the diluent into the vial through a needle.

3. Aspirate the resulting suspension back into the syringe and then release the syringe plunger to allow the suspension to return into the Exosurf Neonatal vial.

4. Repeat aspiration and return three or four times to ensure adequate mixing of the vial contents. If the suspension appears to separate, gently shake or swirl the vial to resuspend.

5. Withdraw the required volume of Exosurf Neonatal Suspension from the vial with the tip of the withdrawing needle well below the froth on the surface of the suspension.

Administration

Exosurf Neonatal should be administered only by those trained and experienced in the care and resuscitation of preterm infants.

Exosurf Neonatal can only be administered to endotracheally intubated infants undergoing mechanical ventilation. Infants should not be intubated solely for the administration of Exosurf Neonatal.

The infant's airway should be cleared by suction prior to the administration of Exosurf Neonatal.

Exosurf Neonatal is administered from a syringe into the endotracheal tube via the side-port on a special endotracheal adaptor, without interrupting mechanical ventilation. The part of the endotracheal tube outside the infant should be aligned vertically during administration.

The total dose should be administered at a rate slow enough to allow reconstituted Exosurf Neonatal suspension to pass into the lungs through the endotracheal tube without accumulation. The minimum recommended time for administration of the full dose is 4 minutes.

Dosing should be slowed or interrupted if the infant's skin colour deteriorates, the heart rate slows, arterial oxygen monitors indicate more than transitory depression of arterial oxygen concentration or Exosurf Neonatal accumulates in the endotracheal tube.

4.3 Contraindications

There are no known contra-indications to treatment with Exosurf Neonatal.

4.4 Special warnings and special precautions for use

Exosurf Neonatal is not for intravenous administration.

Exosurf Neonatal should only be administered with adequate facilities for ventilation and monitoring of babies with RDS.

Preterm birth is hazardous, surfactant administration can be expected to diminish the severity of respiratory distress syndrome and hence to diminish complications of the intensive care, especially of the ventilatory support required for the treatment of respiratory distress syndrome, but cannot be expected to eliminate entirely the mortality and morbidity associated with preterm delivery. Infants who but for the administration of surfactant might have died from RDS may be exposed to other complications of their immaturity.

As a consequence of the surfactant properties of Exosurf Neonatal, chest expansion may improve rapidly after dosing. To avoid the risk of pneumothorax and other forms of pulmonary air leak, rapid reduction in peak ventilatory pressure may therefore be necessary.

The improvement in lung mechanics resulting from Exosurf Neonatal administration may result in rapid improvement in arterial oxygen concentration. After any appropriate reduction in ventilator pressure, rapid reduction in inspired oxygen concentration may be needed to avoid hyperoxaemia.

Infants no longer requiring positive pressure ventilation may require treatment for apnoea of prematurity. In clinical trials, infants treated with Exosurf Neonatal had a higher incidence of apnoea, probably as a consequence of earlier ending of positive pressure ventilation. There were no adverse consequences in terms of increased mortality or long-term morbidity associated with this increased incidence.

Problems encountered during dosing in the clinical trials included reflux of Exosurf and changes in arterial oxygen partial pressure (rises and falls of greater than 20 mm Hg). These should be managed by careful attention to the dosing instructions (see Administration).

4.5 Interaction with other medicinal products and other forms of Interaction

No specific drug interactions have been identified.

4.6 Pregnancy and lactation

Not relevant with this product.

4.7 Effects on ability to drive and use machines

Not relevant with this product.

4.8 Undesirable effects

Pulmonary haemorrhage, the incidence of which increases the more immature the infant, is a rare but sometimes fatal complication of preterm delivery. In a placebo-controlled trial of single dose Exosurf Neonatal prophylaxis in babies with birth weight 500-700 G, the incidence of pulmonary haemorrhage was significantly increased in the Exosurf group (11% versus 2% in the placebo group). Although no other single trial of Exosurf Neonatal has demonstrated a significant increase in pulmonary haemorrhage, cross study analyses suggest that Exosurf Neonatal administration may be associated with an increase from 1 to 2% in the incidence of pulmonary haemorrhage. As might be expected, this association appears to be more marked the more immature the infant. In an open uncontrolled study of Exosurf Neonatal administration in 11,455 infants the reported incidence of pulmonary haemorrhage was 4%.

Pulmonary haemorrhage after surfactant administration is believed to be a consequence of increased pulmonary blood flow in the presence of a patent ductus arteriosus. Preventative measures, early diagnosis and the treatment of patent ductus arteriosus, especially during the first three days of life, may reduce the incidence of pulmonary haemorrhage.

In occasional infants (approximately 3 per thousand) Exosurf Neonatal administration has been associated with obstruction of the endotracheal tube by mucous secretions. If endotracheal tube obstruction is suspected this should be treated, according to normal practice, by suction of the tube, or by replacement of the tube if suction is unsuccessful.

Infants no longer requiring positive pressure ventilation may require treatment for apnoea of prematurity. In clinical trials, infants treated with Exosurf Neonatal had a higher incidence of apnoea, probably as a consequence of earlier ending of positive pressure ventilation. There were no adverse consequences in terms of increased mortality or long-term morbidity associated with this increased incidence.

4.9 Overdose

There have been no reports of overdosage with Exosurf Neonatal. In case of accidental overdosage, as much as possible of the suspension should be aspirated and the baby should then be managed with supportive treatment, with particular attention to fluid and electrolyte balance.

5. PHARMACOLOGICAL PROPERTIES

5.1 Pharmacodynamic properties

Exosurf Neonatal is designed to replace deficient surfactant in newborn infants with respiratory distress syndrome. The active component colfosceril palmitate (dipalmitoylphosphatidylcholine) is the major surface active component of natural lung surfactant and acts by forming a stable film that stabilises the terminal airways by lowering the surface tension of the pulmonary fluid lining them. The lowered surface tension prevents alveolar collapse at end-inspiration; the hysteresis effect equalises the distension of adjacent alveoli and hence prevents overdistension which might result in alveolar rupture and pulmonary air leak.

5.2 Pharmacokinetic properties

Dipalmitoylphosphatidylcholine is a naturally occurring saturated phospholipid. It can be absorbed from the alveolus into lung tissue then reutilised for further phospholipid synthesis and secretion into the alveolus as new surfactant. Metabolism by the normal metabolic pathways would be followed by incorporation of the products into the body pools.

5.3 Preclinical safety data

A. Mutagenicity

Exosurf Neonatal was non-mutagenic in the Ames Salmonella assay.

B. Carcinogenicity

No studies have been performed in animals to determine whether Exosurf Neonatal has carcinogenic potential.

C. Fertility

The effects of Exosurf Neonatal on fertility have not been studied.

6. PHARMACEUTICAL PARTICULARS

6.1 List of excipients

Cetyl alcohol 98% HSE

Hydrochloric acid EP - used to adjust pH

Sodium hydroxide BP - used to adjust pH

Sodium chloride EP

Tyloxapol USP

Water for injections EP

6.2 Incompatibilities

None known.

6.3 Shelf life

Exosurf Neonatal Sterile powder - 3 years

Reconstituted Exosurf Neonatal - 24 hours.

6.4 Special precautions for storage

For the sterile powder: Store below 30°C.

Once reconstituted, Exosurf Neonatal may be stored between 2 and 30°C and should be used within 24 hours. Do not freeze the reconstituted product. Any reconstituted product inadvertently frozen should be discarded. If stored in a refrigerator, the reconstituted product should be allowed to warm up to ambient temperature before use and should not be exposed to rapid heating.

6.5 Nature and contents of container

Neutral glass vials closed with a synthetic bromobutyl rubber stopper secured with an aluminium collar with a plastic flip top cover.

Each pack of Exosurf also contains a vial of water for injection (PL 0003/0284) and five different sizes of sterile endotracheal adaptors for use in administration of the product.

Pack sizes: 67.5mg or 108.0mg

6.6 Instructions for use and handling

No special instructions.

Administrative Data

7. MARKETING AUTHORISATION HOLDER

The Wellcome Foundation Ltd

Glaxo Wellcome House

Berkeley Avenue

Greenford

Middlesex

8. MARKETING AUTHORISATION NUMBER(S)

PL 00003/0283

9. DATE OF FIRST AUTHORISATION/RENEWAL OF THE AUTHORISATION

MAA: 14.12.90

Renewal: 14.12.95

10. DATE OF REVISION OF THE TEXT

21 November 2000

11. Legal Status

POM

Exterol Ear Drops

(Dermal Laboratories Limited)

1. NAME OF THE MEDICINAL PRODUCT

EXTEROL® EAR DROPS

2. QUALITATIVE AND QUANTITATIVE COMPOSITION

Urea Hydrogen Peroxide 5.0% w/w.

3. PHARMACEUTICAL FORM

Clear, straw-coloured, viscous ear drops.

4. CLINICAL PARTICULARS

4.1 Therapeutic indications

As an aid in the removal of hardened ear wax.

4.2 Posology and method of administration

For adults, children and the elderly: Instil up to 5 drops into the ear. Retain drops in ear for several minutes by keeping the head tilted and then wipe away any surplus. Repeat once or twice daily for at least 3 to 4 days, or as required.

4.3 Contraindications

Do not use if the eardrum is known or suspected to be damaged, in cases of dizziness, or if there is, or has been, any other ear disorder (such as pain, discharge, inflammation, infection or tinnitus). Do not use after ill-advised attempts to dislodge wax using fingernails, cotton buds or similar implements, as such mechanical efforts can cause the ear's delicate inner lining to become damaged, inflamed or infected, whereupon the use of ear drops can be painful. For similar reasons, it is inadvisable to use Exterol within 2 to 3 days of syringing. Do not use where there is a history of ear problems, unless under close medical supervision. Do not use if sensitive to any of the ingredients.

4.4 Special warnings and special precautions for use

Keep Exterol away from the eyes. For external use only.

4.5 Interaction with other medicinal products and other forms of Interaction

Exterol should not be used at the same time as anything else in the ear.

4.6 Pregnancy and lactation

No known side-effects.

4.7 Effects on ability to drive and use machines

None known.

4.8 Undesirable effects

Due to the release of oxygen, patients may experience a mild, temporary effervescence in the ear. Stop usage if irritation or pain occurs. Instillation of ear drops can aggravate the painful symptoms of excessive ear wax, including some loss of hearing, dizziness and tinnitus. Very rarely, unpleasant taste has been reported. If patients encounter any of these problems, or if their symptoms persist or worsen, they should discontinue treatment and consult a doctor.

4.9 Overdose

No adverse effects.

5. PHARMACOLOGICAL PROPERTIES

5.1 Pharmacodynamic properties

After insertion of the drops into the ear, the urea hydrogen peroxide complex liberates oxygen which acts to break up the hardened wax. The hydrogen peroxide component is also an antiseptic, especially in sites with relative anaerobiosis. The glycerol assists in softening the wax, so that it may more easily be removed from the ear, either with or without syringing. The urea acts as a mild keratolytic, helping to reduce the keratin-load in the wax debris, thereby assisting penetration of the other components.

5.2 Pharmacokinetic properties

Exterol is intended only for the treatment of impacted wax in the external auditory canal. The ingredients of the formulation are therefore readily available for intimate contact with the affected area, as the drops are instilled into the ear and retained therein for several minutes by tilting the head.

5.3 Preclinical safety data

No special information.

6. PHARMACEUTICAL PARTICULARS

6.1 List of excipients

8-Hydroxyquinoline; Glycerol.

6.2 Incompatibilities

None known.

6.3 Shelf life

24 months.

6.4 Special precautions for storage

Do not store above 25°C. Replace cap after use, and store bottle upright in carton.

6.5 Nature and contents of container

8 ml easy squeeze plastic dropper bottle with screw cap. This is supplied as an original pack (OP).

6.6 Instructions for use and handling

Not applicable.

7. MARKETING AUTHORISATION HOLDER

Dermal Laboratories

Tatmore Place, Gosmore

Hitchin, Herts SG4 7QR, UK.

8. MARKETING AUTHORISATION NUMBER(S)
0173/0037.

9. DATE OF FIRST AUTHORISATION/RENEWAL OF THE AUTHORISATION
28 January 2002.

10. DATE OF REVISION OF THE TEXT
September 2001.

Ezetrol 10mg Tablets

(MSD-SP LTD)

1. NAME OF THE MEDICINAL PRODUCT
EZETROL® ▼10 mg Tablets

2. QUALITATIVE AND QUANTITATIVE COMPOSITION
Each tablet contains 10 mg of ezetimibe.

For excipients see 6.1.

3. PHARMACEUTICAL FORM
Tablet.

White to off-white, capsule-shaped tablets debossed with '414' on one side.

4. CLINICAL PARTICULARS

4.1 Therapeutic indications
Primary hypercholesterolaemia

'Ezetrol', co-administered with an HMG-CoA reductase inhibitor (statin) is indicated as adjunctive therapy to diet for use in patients with primary (heterozygous familial and non-familial) hypercholesterolaemia who are not appropriately controlled with a statin alone.

'Ezetrol' monotherapy is indicated as adjunctive therapy to diet for use in patients with primary (heterozygous familial and non-familial) hypercholesterolaemia in whom a statin is considered inappropriate or is not tolerated.

Homozygous Familial Hypercholesterolaemia (HoFH)

'Ezetrol' co-administered with a statin, is indicated as adjunctive therapy to diet for use in patients with HoFH. Patients may also receive adjunctive treatments (e.g. LDL apheresis).

Homozygous sitosterolaemia (phytosterolaemia)

'Ezetrol' is indicated as adjunctive therapy to diet for use in patients with homozygous familial sitosterolaemia.

Studies to demonstrate the efficacy of 'Ezetrol' in the prevention of complications of atherosclerosis have not yet been completed.

4.2 Posology and method of administration
The patient should be on an appropriate lipid-lowering diet and should continue on this diet during treatment with 'Ezetrol'.

Route of administration is oral. The recommended dose is one 'Ezetrol' 10 mg tablet daily. 'Ezetrol' can be administered at any time of the day, with or without food.

When 'Ezetrol' is added to a statin, either the indicated usual initial dose of that particular statin or the already established higher statin dose should be continued. In this setting, the dosage instructions for that particular statin should be consulted.

Co-administration with bile acid sequestrants

Dosing of 'Ezetrol' should occur either ⩾2 hours before or ⩾4 hours after administration of a bile acid sequestrant.

Use in the elderly

No dosage adjustment is required for elderly patients (see section 5.2).

Use in paediatric patients

Children and adolescents ⩾10 years: No dosage adjustment is required (see section 5.2). However, clinical experience in paediatric and adolescent patients (ages 9 to 17) is limited.

Children <10 years: No sufficient clinical data are available, therefore treatment with 'Ezetrol' is not recommended.

Use in hepatic impairment

No dosage adjustment is required in patients with mild hepatic insufficiency (Child Pugh score 5 to 6). Treatment with 'Ezetrol' is not recommended in patients with moderate (Child Pugh score 7 to 9) or severe (Child Pugh score >9) liver dysfunction. (See sections 4.4 and 5.2.)

Use in renal impairment

No dosage adjustment is required for renally impaired patients (see section 5.2).

4.3 Contraindications
Hypersensitivity to the active substance or to any of the excipients.

When 'Ezetrol' is co-administered with a statin, please refer to the SPC for that particular statin.

Therapy with 'Ezetrol' co-administered with a statin is contra-indicated during pregnancy and lactation.

'Ezetrol' co-administered with a statin is contra-indicated in patients with active liver disease or unexplained persistent elevations in serum transaminases.

4.4 Special warnings and special precautions for use
When 'Ezetrol' is co-administered with a statin, please refer to the SPC for that particular statin.

Liver enzymes

In controlled co-administration trials in patients receiving 'Ezetrol' with a statin, consecutive transaminase elevations (⩾3 X the upper limit of normal [ULN]) have been observed. When 'Ezetrol' is co-administered with a statin, liver function tests should be performed at initiation of therapy and according to the recommendations of the statin. (See section 4.8.)

Skeletal muscle

In post-marketing experience with 'Ezetrol', cases of myopathy and rhabdomyolysis have been reported. Most patients who developed rhabdomyolysis were taking a statin concomitantly with 'Ezetrol'. However, rhabdomyolysis has been reported very rarely with 'Ezetrol' monotherapy and very rarely with the addition of 'Ezetrol' to other agents known to be associated with increased risk of rhabdomyolysis. If myopathy is suspected based on muscle symptoms or is confirmed by a creatinine phosphokinase (CPK) level >10 times the ULN, 'Ezetrol', any statin, and any of these other agents that the patient is taking concomitantly should be immediately discontinued. All patients starting therapy with 'Ezetrol' should be advised of the risk of myopathy and told to report promptly any unexplained muscle pain, tenderness or weakness (see section 4.8).

Hepatic insufficiency

Due to the unknown effects of the increased exposure to ezetimibe in patients with moderate or severe hepatic insufficiency, 'Ezetrol' is not recommended (see section 5.2).

Fibrates

The safety and efficacy of 'Ezetrol' administered with fibrates have not been established; therefore, co-administration of 'Ezetrol' and fibrates is not recommended (see section 4.5).

Ciclosporin

Caution should be exercised when initiating 'Ezetrol' in the setting of ciclosporin. Ciclosporin concentrations should be monitored in patients receiving 'Ezetrol' and ciclosporin (see section 4.5).

Warfarin

If 'Ezetrol' is added to warfarin, the International Normalised Ratio (INR) should be appropriately monitored (see section 4.5).

Excipient

Patients with rare hereditary problems of galactose intolerance, the Lapp lactase deficiency or glucose-galactose malabsorption should not take this medicine.

4.5 Interaction with other medicinal products and other forms of Interaction
In preclinical studies, it has been shown that ezetimibe does not induce cytochrome P450 drug metabolising enzymes. No clinically significant pharmacokinetic interactions have been observed between ezetimibe and drugs known to be metabolised by cytochromes P450 1A2, 2D6, 2C8, 2C9, and 3A4, or N-acetyltransferase.

In clinical interaction studies, ezetimibe had no effect on the pharmacokinetics of dapsone, dextromethorphan, digoxin, oral contraceptives (ethinyl estradiol and levonorgestrel), glipizide, tolbutamide, or midazolam, during co-administration. Cimetidine, co-administered with ezetimibe, had no effect on the bioavailability of ezetimibe.

Antacids: Concomitant antacid administration decreased the rate of absorption of ezetimibe but had no effect on the bioavailability of ezetimibe. This decreased rate of absorption is not considered clinically significant.

Colestyramine: Concomitant colestyramine administration decreased the mean area under the curve (AUC) of total ezetimibe (ezetimibe + ezetimibe glucuronide) approximately 55%. The incremental low-density lipoprotein cholesterol (LDL-C) reduction due to adding 'Ezetrol' to colestyramine may be lessened by this interaction (see section 4.2).

Fibrates: Concomitant fenofibrate or gemfibrozil administration increased total ezetimibe concentrations approximately 1.5- and 1.7-fold respectively, however these increases are not considered clinically significant.

Fibrates may increase cholesterol excretion into the bile, leading to cholelithiasis. In a preclinical study in dogs, ezetimibe increased cholesterol in the gallbladder bile (see section 5.3). Although the relevance of this preclinical finding to humans is unknown, co-administration of 'Ezetrol' with fibrates is not recommended until use in patients is studied (see section 4.4).

Statins: No clinically significant pharmacokinetic interactions were seen when ezetimibe was co-administered with atorvastatin, simvastatin, pravastatin, lovastatin, fluvastatin or rosuvastatin.

Ciclosporin: In a study of eight post-renal transplant patients with creatinine clearance of >50 ml/min on a stable dose of ciclosporin, a single 10-mg dose of 'Ezetrol' resulted in a 3.4-fold (range 2.3 to 7.9-fold) increase in the mean AUC for total ezetimibe compared to a healthy control population, receiving ezetimibe alone, from another study (n=17). In a different study, a renal transplant patient with severe renal insufficiency who was receiving ciclosporin and multiple other medications, demonstrated a 12-fold greater exposure to total ezetimibe compared to concurrent controls receiving ezetimibe alone. In a two-period crossover study in 12 healthy subjects, daily administration of 20 mg ezetimibe for 8 days with a single 100-mg dose of ciclosporin on Day 7 resulted in a mean 15 % increase in ciclosporin AUC (range 10 % decrease to 51 % increase) compared to a single 100-mg dose of ciclosporin alone. A controlled study on the effect of co-administered ezetimibe on ciclosporin exposure in renal transplant patients has not been conducted. Caution should be exercised when initiating Ezetrol in the setting of ciclosporin. Ciclosporin concentrations should be monitored in patients receiving Ezetrol and ciclosporin (see section 4.4).

Warfarin: Concomitant administration of ezetimibe (10 mg once daily) had no significant effect on bioavailability of warfarin and prothrombin time in a study of twelve healthy adult males. There have been post-marketing reports of increased International Normalised Ratio in patients who had 'Ezetrol' added to warfarin (see section 4.4).

4.6 Pregnancy and lactation
'Ezetrol' co-administered with a statin is contra-indicated during pregnancy and lactation (see section 4.3), please refer to the SPC for that particular statin.

Pregnancy:

'Ezetrol' should be given to pregnant women only if clearly necessary. No clinical data are available on the use of 'Ezetrol' during pregnancy. Animal studies on the use of ezetimibe in monotherapy have shown no evidence of direct or indirect harmful effects on pregnancy, embryofoetal development, birth or postnatal development (see section 5.3).

Lactation:

'Ezetrol' should not be used during lactation. Studies on rats have shown that ezetimibe is secreted into breast milk. It is not known if ezetimibe is secreted into human breast milk.

4.7 Effects on ability to drive and use machines
No studies of the effects on the ability to drive and use of machines have been performed. However, 'Ezetrol' is not expected to affect the ability to drive and use machines.

4.8 Undesirable effects
Clinical Studies

In clinical studies of 8 to 14 weeks duration, 'Ezetrol' 10 mg daily was administered alone or with a statin in 3,366 patients. Adverse reactions were usually mild and transient. The overall incidence of side effects reported with 'Ezetrol' was similar between 'Ezetrol' and placebo. Similarly, the discontinuation rate due to adverse experiences was comparable between 'Ezetrol' and placebo.

The following common (⩾1/100, <1/10) drug-related adverse experiences were reported in patients taking 'Ezetrol' alone (n=1,691) or co-administered with a statin (n=1,675):

'Ezetrol' administered alone:

Nervous system disorders: headache

Gastro-intestinal disorders: abdominal pain and diarrhoea.

'Ezetrol' co-administered with a statin:

Nervous system disorders: headache and fatigue

Gastro-intestinal disorders: abdominal pain, constipation, diarrhoea, flatulence and nausea

Musculoskeletal and connective tissue disorders: myalgia.

Laboratory values

In controlled clinical monotherapy trials, the incidence of clinically important elevations in serum transaminases (ALT and/or AST ⩾3 X ULN, consecutive) was similar between 'Ezetrol' (0.5%) and placebo (0.3%). In co-administration trials, the incidence was 1.3% for patients treated with 'Ezetrol' co-administered with a statin and 0.4% for patients treated with a statin alone. These elevations were generally asymptomatic, not associated with cholestasis, and returned to baseline after discontinuation of therapy or with continued treatment. (See section 4.4.)

In clinical trials, CPK > 10 X ULN was reported for 4 of 1,674 (0.2%) patients administered 'Ezetrol' alone vs 1 of 786 (0.1%) patients administered placebo, and for 1 of 917 (0.1%) patients co-administered 'Ezetrol' and a statin vs 4 of 929 (0.4%) patients administered a statin alone. There was no excess of myopathy or rhabdomyolysis associated with 'Ezetrol' compared with the relevant control arm (placebo or statin alone). (See section 4.4.)

Post-marketing Experience

The following additional rare (>1/10,000, <1/1,000) or very rare (<1/10,000) adverse reactions have been reported in post-marketing experience:

Blood and lymphatic system disorders: thrombocytopenia (very rare)

Immune system disorders: hypersensitivity, including rash (rare) and angioedema (very rare)

Gastro-intestinal disorders: nausea (rare); pancreatitis (very rare)

Hepatobiliary disorders: hepatitis (rare), cholelithiasis (very rare), cholecystitis (very rare)

Musculoskeletal and connective tissue disorders: myalgia (rare); myopathy/rhabdomyolysis (very rare; see section 4.4).

Laboratory values: increased transaminases (rare); increased CPK (rare).

4.9 Overdose

In clinical studies, administration of ezetimibe, 50 mg/day, to 15 healthy subjects for up to 14 days, or 40 mg/day to 18 patients with primary hypercholesterolaemia for up to 56 days, was generally well tolerated. In animals, no toxicity was observed after single oral doses of 5,000 mg/kg of ezetimibe in rats and mice and 3,000 mg/kg in dogs.

A few cases of overdosage with 'Ezetrol' have been reported: most have not been associated with adverse experiences. Reported adverse experiences have not been serious. In the event of an overdose, symptomatic and supportive measures should be employed.

5. PHARMACOLOGICAL PROPERTIES

5.1 Pharmacodynamic properties

Pharmacotherapeutic group: Other cholesterol and triglyceride reducers, ATC code: C10A X09

'Ezetrol' is in a new class of lipid-lowering compounds that selectively inhibit the intestinal absorption of cholesterol and related plant sterols. 'Ezetrol' is orally active, and has a mechanism of action that differs from other classes of cholesterol-reducing compounds (e.g. statins, bile acid sequestrants [resins], fibric acid derivatives, and plant stanols).

Ezetimibe localises at the brush border of the small intestine and inhibits the absorption of cholesterol, leading to a decrease in the delivery of intestinal cholesterol to the liver; statins reduce cholesterol synthesis in the liver and together these distinct mechanisms provide complementary cholesterol reduction. The molecular mechanism of action is not fully understood. In a 2-week clinical study in 18 hypercholesterolaemic patients, 'Ezetrol' inhibited intestinal cholesterol absorption by 54%, compared with placebo.

A series of preclinical studies was performed to determine the selectivity of ezetimibe for inhibiting cholesterol absorption. Ezetimibe inhibited the absorption of [^{14}C]-cholesterol with no effect on the absorption of triglycerides, fatty acids, bile acids, progesterone, ethinyl estradiol, or fat soluble vitamins A and D.

Epidemiologic studies have established that cardiovascular morbidity and mortality vary directly with the level of total-C and LDL-C and inversely with the level of HDL-C. Studies to demonstrate the efficacy of 'Ezetrol' in the prevention of complications of atherosclerosis have not yet been completed.

CLINICAL TRIALS

In controlled clinical studies, 'Ezetrol', either as monotherapy or co-administered with a statin significantly reduced total cholesterol (total-C), low-density lipoprotein cholesterol (LDL-C), apolipoprotein B (Apo B), and trigylcerides (TG) and increased high-density lipoprotein cholesterol (HDL-C) in patients with hypercholesterolaemia.

Primary hypercholesterolaemia

In a double-blind, placebo-controlled, 8-week study, 769 patients with hypercholesterolaemia already receiving statin monotherapy and not at National Cholesterol Education Program (NCEP) LDL-C goal (2.6 to 4.1 mmol/l [100 to 160 mg/dl], depending on baseline characteristics) were randomised to receive either 'Ezetrol' 10 mg or placebo in addition to their on-going statin therapy.

Among statin-treated patients not at LDL-C goal at baseline (~82%), significantly more patients randomised to 'Ezetrol' achieved their LDL-C goal at study endpoint compared to patients randomised to placebo, 72% and 19% respectively. The corresponding LDL-C reductions were significantly different (25% and 4% for 'Ezetrol' versus placebo, respectively). In addition, 'Ezetrol', added to on-going statin therapy, significantly decreased total-C, Apo B, TG and increased HDL-C, compared with placebo. 'Ezetrol' or placebo added to statin therapy reduced median C-reactive protein by 10% or 0% from baseline, respectively.

In two, double-blind, randomised placebo-controlled, 12-week studies in 1,719 patients with primary hypercholesterolaemia, 'Ezetrol' 10 mg significantly lowered total-C (13%), LDL-C (19%), Apo B (14%), and TG (8%) and increased HDL-C (3%) compared to placebo. In addition, 'Ezetrol' had no effect on the plasma concentrations of the fat-soluble vitamins A, D, and E, no effect on prothrombin time, and, like other lipid-lowering agents, did not impair adrenocortical steroid hormone production.

Homozygous Familial Hypercholesterolaemia (HoFH)

A double-blind, randomised, 12-week study enrolled 50 patients with a clinical and/or genotypic diagnosis of HoFH, who were receiving atorvastatin or simvastatin (40 mg) with or without concomitant LDL apheresis. 'Ezetrol' co-administered with atorvastatin (40 or 80 mg) or simvastatin (40 or 80 mg), significantly reduced LDL-C by 15% compared with increasing the dose of simvastatin or atorvastatin monotherapy from 40 to 80 mg.

Homozygous sitosterolaemia (phytosterolaemia)

In a double-blind, placebo-controlled, 8-week trial, 37 patients with homozygous sitosterolaemia were randomised to receive 'Ezetrol' 10 mg (n=30) or placebo (n=7). Some patients were receiving other treatments (e.g. statins, resins). 'Ezetrol' significantly lowered the two major plant sterols, sitosterol and campesterol, by 21% and 24% from baseline, respectively. The effects of decreasing sitosterol on morbidity and mortality in this population are not known.

5.2 Pharmacokinetic properties

Absorption: After oral administration, ezetimibe is rapidly absorbed and extensively conjugated to a pharmacologically-active phenolic glucuronide (ezetimibe-glucuronide). Mean maximum plasma concentrations (C_{max}) occur within 1 to 2 hours for ezetimibe-glucuronide and 4 to 12 hours for ezetimibe. The absolute bioavailability of ezetimibe cannot be determined as the compound is virtually insoluble in aqueous media suitable for injection.

Concomitant food administration (high fat or non-fat meals) had no effect on the oral bioavailability of ezetimibe when administered as 'Ezetrol' 10-mg tablets. 'Ezetrol' can be administered with or without food.

Distribution: Ezetimibe and ezetimibe-glucuronide are bound 99.7% and 88 to 92% to human plasma proteins, respectively.

Biotransformation: Ezetimibe is metabolised primarily in the small intestine and liver via glucuronide conjugation (a phase II reaction) with subsequent biliary excretion. Minimal oxidative metabolism (a phase I reaction) has been observed in all species evaluated. Ezetimibe and ezetimibe-glucuronide are the major drug-derived compounds detected in plasma, constituting approximately 10 to 20 % and 80 to 90 % of the total drug in plasma, respectively. Both ezetimibe and ezetimibe-glucuronide are slowly eliminated from plasma with evidence of significant enterohepatic recycling. The half-life for ezetimibe and ezetimibe-glucuronide is approximately 22 hours.

Elimination: Following oral administration of ^{14}C-ezetimibe (20 mg) to human subjects, total ezetimibe accounted for approximately 93% of the total radioactivity in plasma. Approximately 78% and 11% of the administered radioactivity were recovered in the faeces and urine, respectively, over a 10-day collection period. After 48 hours, there were no detectable levels of radioactivity in the plasma.

Special populations:

Paediatric patients

The absorption and metabolism of ezetimibe are similar between children and adolescents (10 to 18 years) and adults. Based on total ezetimibe, there are no pharmacokinetic differences between adolescents and adults. Pharmacokinetic data in the paediatric population $<$10 years of age are not available. Clinical experience in paediatric and adolescent patients (ages 9 to 17) has been limited to patients with HoFH or sitosterolaemia.

Geriatric patients

Plasma concentrations for total ezetimibe are about 2-fold higher in the elderly ($\geqslant$65 years) than in the young (18 to 45 years). LDL-C reduction and safety profile are comparable between elderly and young subjects treated with 'Ezetrol'. Therefore, no dosage adjustment is necessary in the elderly.

Hepatic insufficiency

After a single 10-mg dose of ezetimibe, the mean AUC for total ezetimibe was increased approximately 1.7-fold in patients with mild hepatic insufficiency (Child Pugh score 5 or 6), compared to healthy subjects. In a 14-day, multiple-dose study (10 mg daily) in patients with moderate hepatic insufficiency (Child Pugh score 7 to 9), the mean AUC for total ezetimibe was increased approximately 4-fold on Day 1 and Day 14 compared to healthy subjects. No dosage adjustment is necessary for patients with mild hepatic insufficiency. Due to the unknown effects of the increased exposure to ezetimibe in patients with moderate or severe (Child Pugh score $>$9) hepatic insufficiency, 'Ezetrol' is not recommended in these patients (see section 4.4).

Renal insufficiency

After a single 10-mg dose of ezetimibe in patients with severe renal disease (n=8; mean CrCl $\leqslant$30 ml/min/1.73m^2), the mean AUC for total ezetimibe was increased approximately 1.5-fold, compared to healthy subjects (n=9). This result is not considered clinically significant. No dosage adjustment is necessary for renally impaired patients.

An additional patient in this study (post-renal transplant and receiving multiple medications, including ciclosporin) had a 12-fold greater exposure to total ezetimibe.

Gender

Plasma concentrations for total ezetimibe are slightly higher (approximately 20%) in women than in men. LDL-C reduction and safety profile are comparable between men and women treated with 'Ezetrol'. Therefore, no dosage adjustment is necessary on the basis of gender.

5.3 Preclinical safety data

Animal studies on the chronic toxicity of ezetimibe identified no target organs for toxic effects. In dogs treated for four weeks with ezetimibe ($\geqslant$0.03 mg/kg/day) the cholesterol concentration in the cystic bile was increased by a factor of 2.5 to 3.5. However, in a one-year study on dogs given doses of up to 300 mg/kg/day no increased incidence of cholelithiasis or other hepatobiliary effects were observed. The significance of these data for humans is not known. A lithogenic risk associated with the therapeutic use of 'Ezetrol' cannot be ruled out.

In co-administration studies with ezetimibe and statins the toxic effects observed were essentially those typically associated with statins. Some of the toxic effects were more pronounced than observed during treatment with statins alone. This is attributed to pharmacokinetic and pharmacodynamic interactions in co-administration therapy. No such interactions occurred in the clinical studies. Myopathies occurred in rats only after exposure to doses that were several times higher than the human therapeutic dose (approximately 20 times the AUC level for statins and 500 to 2,000 times the AUC level for the active metabolites).

In a series of *in vivo* and *in vitro* assays ezetimibe, given alone or co-administered with statins, exhibited no genotoxic potential. Long-term carcinogenicity tests on ezetimibe were negative.

Ezetimibe had no effect on the fertility of male or female rats, nor was it found to be teratogenic in rats or rabbits, nor did it affect prenatal or postnatal development. Ezetimibe crossed the placental barrier in pregnant rats and rabbits given multiple doses of 1,000 mg/kg/day. The co-administration of ezetimibe and statins was not teratogenic in rats. In pregnant rabbits a small number of skeletal deformities (fused thoracic and caudal vertebrae, reduced number of caudal vertebrae) were observed. The co-administration of ezetimibe with lovastatin resulted in embryolethal effects.

6. PHARMACEUTICAL PARTICULARS

6.1 List of excipients

Croscarmellose sodium

Lactose monohydrate

Magnesium stearate

Microcrystalline cellulose

Povidone (K29-32)

Sodium laurylsulphate

6.2 Incompatibilities

Not applicable.

6.3 Shelf life

2 years.

6.4 Special precautions for storage

Do not store above 30°C.

Blisters: Store in the original package.

Bottles: Keep the bottle tightly closed.

6.5 Nature and contents of container

Unit Dose peelable blisters of clear polychlorotrifluoroethylene/PVC sealed to vinyl coated aluminium backed with paper and polyester in packs of 7, 10, 14, 20, 28, 30, 50, 98, 100, or 300 tablets.

Push through blisters of clear polychlorotrifluoroethylene/PVC sealed to vinyl coated aluminium in packs of 7, 10, 14, 20, 28, 30, 50, 98, 100, or 300 tablets.

Unit dose push through blisters of clear polychlorotrifluoroethylene/PVC coated aluminium in packs of 50, 100, or 300 tablets.

HDPE bottles with polypropylene cap, containing 100 tablets.

Not all pack sizes may be marketed.

6.6 Instructions for use and handling

No special requirements.

7. MARKETING AUTHORISATION HOLDER

MSD-SP Limited

Hertford Road, Hoddesdon, Hertfordshire EN11 9BU, UK

8. MARKETING AUTHORISATION NUMBER(S)

PL 19945/0001

9. DATE OF FIRST AUTHORISATION/RENEWAL OF THE AUTHORISATION

3 April 2003

10. DATE OF REVISION OF THE TEXT

June 2005

EZETROL SPC.EZE.04.UK-IRL.2102 II-/014

FAMVIR 125 mg, 250 mg, 500 mg, 750 mg Tablets

(Novartis Pharmaceuticals UK Ltd)

1. NAME OF THE MEDICINAL PRODUCT

Famvir® 125 mg Tablets

Famvir® 250 mg Tablets

Famvir® 500 mg Tablets

Famvir® 750 mg Tablets

2. QUALITATIVE AND QUANTITATIVE COMPOSITION

Each tablet contains 125 mg, 250 mg, 500 mg or 750 mg famciclovir.

For excipients, see 6.1

3. PHARMACEUTICAL FORM

Film-coated tablet.

125 mg tablets: White, round, biconvex tablets, debossed with 'FAMVIR' or 'FV' on one side and 125 on the reverse side.

250 mg tablets: White, round, biconvex tablets, debossed with 'FAMVIR' or 'FV' on one side and 250 on the reverse side.

500 mg tablets: White, oval, biconvex tablets debossed with 'FAMVIR 500' or 'ORAVIR 500' or 'FV 500' on one side and plain on the reverse side.

750 mg tablets: White, oval, biconvex tablets debossed with 'FAMVIR 750' or 'FV 750' on one side and plain on the reverse side.

4. CLINICAL PARTICULARS

4.1 Therapeutic indications

125 mg tablets: For the treatment of acute recurrent genital herpes infections.

250 mg tablets: For the treatment of *herpes zoster* (shingles) infections, first episode genital herpes infections and the suppression of recurrent genital herpes infections.

500 mg tablets: Treatment of *herpes zoster* infections and treatment and suppression of *herpes simplex* infections in immunocompromised patients.

750 mg tablets: For the treatment of *herpes zoster* (shingles) infections.

4.2 Posology and method of administration

Dosage: Adults:

Herpes zoster infections:

- One 750 mg tablet once daily for seven days, or
- One 250 mg tablet three times daily or three 250 mg tablets once daily for seven days

If the tablets are taken once a day they should be taken at approximately the same time each day.

In immunocompromised patients, one 500mg tablet three times daily for ten days.

Initiation of treatment is recommended as soon as possible after rash onset.

First-episode genital herpes infections: One 250 mg tablet three times daily for five days. Initiation of treatment is recommended as soon as possible after onset of lesions.

Recurrent genital herpes infections: Acute treatment: One 125 mg tablet twice daily for five days. Initiation of treatment is recommended during the prodromal period or as soon as possible after onset of lesions. In immunocompromised patients, one 500 mg tablet twice daily for seven days. Initiation of treatment is recommended as soon as possible after rash onset.

Suppression: One 250 mg tablet twice daily. A dose of 500 mg twice daily has been shown to be efficacious in HIV patients. Therapy should be interrupted periodically at intervals of six to twelve months in order to observe possible changes in the natural history of the disease.

Elderly: Dosage modification is not required unless renal function is impaired.

Renally impaired: As reduced clearance of penciclovir related to reduced renal function, special attention should be given to dosage in patients with impaired renal function (see section 4.9). The following modifications are recommended:

For the treatment of *herpes zoster* infections and first-episode genital herpes infections:

Creatinine clearance (ml/min/1.73m^2)	*Dosage*
30-59	250 mg twice daily
10-29	250 mg once daily

For the treatment of acute recurrent genital herpes infections:

Creatinine clearance (ml/min/1.73m^2)	*Dosage*
30-59	No dose adjustment necessary
10-29	125 mg once daily

For the suppression of recurrent genital herpes infections:

Creatinine clearance (ml/min/1.73m^2)	*Dosage*
≥30	250 mg twice daily
10-29	125 mg twice daily

In renally impaired patients who are also immunocompromised:

For the treatment of *herpes zoster* infections in immunocompromised patients:

Creatinine clearance (ml/min/1.73m^2)	*Dosage*
≥40	500 mg three times daily
30-39	250 mg three times daily
10-29	125 mg three times daily

For the treatment of *herpes simplex* infections in immunocompromised patients:

Creatinine clearance (ml/min/1.73m^2)	*Dosage*
≥40	500 mg twice daily
30-39	250 mg twice daily
10-29	125 mg twice daily

When only serum creatinine is available, a nomogram or the following formula (Cockcroft and Gault) should be used to estimate creatinine clearance.

Formula to estimate creatinine clearance (ml/min/1.73 m^2):

$$\frac{[140 - \text{age in years}] \times \text{weight (kg)}}{72 \times \text{serum creatinine } (\mu mol/l)} \times \textbf{either } 88.5 \text{ (for males) } \textbf{or } 75.2 \text{ (for females)}$$

Renally impaired patients on haemodialysis:

For a patient on haemodialysis, a dosage interval of 48 hours is recommended for periods between dialysis. Since four hours' haemodialysis results in approximately 75% reduction in plasma concentrations of penciclovir, a dose of famciclovir (250 mg for *herpes zoster* patients and 125 mg for *herpes simplex* patients) should be administered immediately following dialysis.

Hepatically Impaired:

Dosage modification is not required for patients with well compensated chronic liver disease. There is no information on patients with decompensated chronic liver disease; accordingly no precise dose recommendations can be made for this group of patients.

Children:

There are currently insufficient data on the safety and efficacy of Famvir in children and therefore its use in children is not recommended.

Administration:

Oral.

4.3 Contraindications

Famvir is contraindicated in patients with known hypersensitivity to famciclovir or other constituents of Famvir. It is also contraindicated in those patients who have shown hypersensitivity to penciclovir.

4.4 Special warnings and special precautions for use

Special attention should be paid to patients with impaired renal function as dosage adjustment is necessary (see sections 4.2 and 4.9). No special precautions are required for hepatically impaired or elderly patients with normal renal function.

125 mg, 250 mg and 500 mg tablets: Genital herpes is a sexually transmitted disease. The risk of transmission is increased during acute episodes. Patients should avoid sexual intercourse when symptoms are present even if treatment with an antiviral has been initiated.

250 mg and 500 mg tablets: During suppressive treatment with famciclovir, the frequency of viral shedding (both symptomatic and asymptomatic) may be reduced. However, the risk of viral transmission remains even during suppressive antiviral therapy and with protected intercourse, i.e. the use of condoms.

4.5 Interaction with other medicinal products and other forms of Interaction

No clinically significant interactions have been identified. Evidence from preclinical studies has shown no potential for induction of cytochrome P450. Probenecid and other drugs that affect renal physiology could affect plasma levels of penciclovir. In a Phase I study, no drug interactions were observed after co-administration of zidovudine and famciclovir.

4.6 Pregnancy and lactation

Although animal studies have not shown any embryotoxic or teratogenic effects with famciclovir or penciclovir, the safety of Famvir in human pregnancy has not been established. Famvir should therefore not be used during pregnancy or in nursing mothers unless the potential benefits of treatment outweigh any possible risk.

Studies in rats show that penciclovir is excreted in the breast milk of lactating females given oral famciclovir. There is no information on excretion in human milk.

4.7 Effects on ability to drive and use machines

Patients who experience dizziness, somnolence, confusion or other central nervous system disturbances while taking Famvir should refrain from driving or operating machinery.

4.8 Undesirable effects

Famciclovir has been well tolerated in human studies. Headache and nausea have been reported in clinical trials. These were generally mild or moderate in nature and occurred at a similar incidence in patients receiving placebo treatment.

The following table specifies the estimated frequency of adverse reactions based on all the spontaneous reports and literature cases that have been reported for Famvir since its introduction to the market.

Frequencies are defined as: common (> 1/100, ≤ 1/10), uncommon (> 1/1000, ≤ 1/100), rare (> 1/10000, ≤ 1/1000), very rare (< 1/10000).

Nervous system	
Rare	Headache, confusion (predominantly in the elderly)
Very rare	Dizziness, somnolence (predominantly in the elderly), hallucinations
Gastrointestinal disorders	
Rare	Nausea
Very rare	Vomiting
Hepatobiliary disorders	
Very rare	Jaundice
Skin and subcutaneous tissue disorders	
Very rare	Rash, pruritus, urticaria

500 mg tablets: Famciclovir has also been well tolerated in immunocompromised patients. Undesirable effects reported from clinical studies were similar to those reported in the immunocompetent population. Cases of abdominal pain, fever and rarely granulocytopenia and thrombocytopenia have been observed (granulocytopenia and thrombocytopenia have also been observed in immunocompromised patients not treated with famciclovir).

4.9 Overdose

Overdose experience with famciclovir is limited. A report of accidental acute overdosage (10.5 g) was asymptomatic. In a report of chronic use (10 g/day for two years), famciclovir was well tolerated. In the event of an overdose supportive and symptomatic therapy should be given as appropriate.

Acute renal failure has been reported rarely in patients with underlying renal disease where the Famvir dosage has not been appropriately reduced for the level of renal function.

Penciclovir is dialysable and plasma concentrations are reduced by approximately 75% following four hours' haemodialysis.

5. PHARMACOLOGICAL PROPERTIES

5.1 Pharmacodynamic properties

Pharmacotherapeutic group: Oral antiviral agent (ATC code J05A B09)

Famciclovir is the oral form of penciclovir. Famciclovir is rapidly converted *in vivo* into penciclovir, which has *in vivo* and *in vitro* activity against human herpes viruses including *varicella zoster* virus and *herpes simplex* types 1 and 2.

The antiviral effect of orally administered famciclovir has been demonstrated in several animal models; this effect is due to *in vivo* conversion to penciclovir. In virus-infected cells penciclovir is rapidly and efficiently converted into the triphosphate (mediated via virus-induced thymidine kinase). Penciclovir triphosphate persists in infected cells for more than 12 hours where it inhibits replication of viral DNA and has a half-life of 9, 10 and 20 hours in cells infected with *varicella zoster*, *herpes simplex* virus type 1 and *herpes simplex* virus type 2 respectively. In uninfected cells treated with penciclovir, concentrations of penciclovir-triphosphate are only barely detectable. Accordingly, uninfected cells are unlikely to be affected by therapeutic concentrations of penciclovir.

The most common form of resistance encountered with aciclovir among HSV strains is a deficiency in the production of the thymidine kinase (TK) enzyme. Such TK-deficient strains would be expected to be cross-resistant to both penciclovir and aciclovir. However, penciclovir has been shown to be active *in vitro* against a recently isolated aciclovir-resistant *herpes simplex* virus strain which has an altered DNA polymerase.

125 mg, 250 mg and 500 mg tablets: In a study in suppression of recurrent genital herpes in which immunocompetent patients were treated with famciclovir for 4 months, there was no evidence of resistance to famciclovir when isolates from 71 patients were analysed.

Results from penciclovir and famciclovir patient studies, including studies of up to four months' treatment with famciclovir, have shown a small overall frequency of penciclovir-resistant isolates: 0.3% in the 981 total isolates tested to date and 0.19% in the 529 virus isolates from immunocompromised patients. The resistant isolates were found at the start of treatment or in a placebo group, with no resistance occurring on or after treatment with famciclovir or penciclovir.

125 mg, 250 mg and 500 mg tablets: A placebo-controlled study in patients with immunodeficiency due to HIV has shown that famciclovir 500mg b.i.d. significantly decreased the proportion of days of both symptomatic and asymptomatic HSV shedding.

5.2 Pharmacokinetic properties

General characteristics

Following oral administration, famciclovir is rapidly and extensively absorbed and rapidly converted to the active compound, penciclovir. Bioavailability of penciclovir after oral administration of Famvir is 77%. Mean peak plasma concentrations of penciclovir, following 125 mg, 250 mg and 500 mg oral doses of famciclovir, were 0.8 micrograms/ml, 1.6 micrograms/ml and 3.3 micrograms/ml, respectively, and occurred at a median time of 45 minutes post-dose. Plasma concentration-time curves of penciclovir are similar following single and repeat (t.i.d. and b.i.d.) dosing. The terminal plasma half-life of penciclovir after both single and repeat dosing with famciclovir is approximately 2.0 hours. There is no accumulation of penciclovir on repeated dosing with famciclovir. Penciclovir and its 6-deoxy precursor are poorly (<20%) bound to plasma proteins.

Famciclovir is eliminated principally as penciclovir and its 6-deoxy precursor which are excreted in urine unchanged. Famciclovir has not been detected in urine. Tubular secretion contributes to the renal elimination of the compound.

Characteristics in patients

Uncomplicated *herpes zoster* infection does not significantly alter the pharmacokinetics of penciclovir measured after oral administration of Famvir.

5.3 Preclinical safety data

Famciclovir has no significant effects on spermatogenesis or sperm morphology and motility in man. At doses greatly in excess of those used therapeutically impaired fertility was observed in male rats - no such effects being observed in female rats.

At a dose level approximately 50 times the normal therapeutic dose there was an increased incidence of mammary adenocarcinoma in female rats. No such effect was seen in male rats or mice of either sex.

Additionally, famciclovir was not found to be genotoxic in a comprehensive battery of *in vivo* and *in vitro* tests designed to detect gene mutation, chromosomal damage and repairable damage to DNA. Penciclovir, in common with other drugs of this class, has been shown to cause chromosomal damage, but did not induce gene mutation in bacterial or mammalian cell systems, nor was there evidence of increased DNA repair *in vitro*.

These findings are not considered to have any clinical significance.

6. PHARMACEUTICAL PARTICULARS

6.1 List of excipients

Tablet core:

Hydroxypropyl Cellulose

Lactose Anhydrous*

Sodium Starch Glycollate

Magnesium Stearate

Tablet coat:

Hydroxypropyl Methyl Cellulose

Titanium Dioxide

Polyethylene Glycol

* Constituent of Famvir 125 mg and 250 mg tablets only

6.2 Incompatibilities

Not applicable.

6.3 Shelf life

3 years.

6.4 Special precautions for storage

Do not store above 30°C. Store in the original package.

6.5 Nature and contents of container

125 mg tablets:

Famvir is supplied in PVC/PVdC/Aluminium blister packs containing 10 tablets.

250 mg tablets:

Herpez zoster treatment – Famvir is supplied as a shingles patient pack in PVC/PVdC/Aluminium blister packs containing 21 × 250 mg tablets.

Genital herpes treatment – Famvir is supplied in PVC/PVdC/Aluminium blister packs containing 15 × 250 mg tablets for the treatment of first episode infection or 56 × 250 mg tablets for suppressive treatment.

500 mg tablets:

Herpes zoster treatment – For immunocompromised patients Famvir is supplied in PVC/PVdC/Aluminium blister packs containing 30 × 500 mg tablets.

Genital herpes treatment – For immunocompromised patients Famvir is supplied in PVC/PVdC/Aluminium blister packs containing 14 × 500 mg tablets for treatment of acute infections or 56 × 500 mg tablets for suppressive treatment.

750 mg tablets:

Famvir is supplied as a starter pack containing one tablet and as a shingles patient pack in PVC/PVdC/Aluminium blister packs containing seven tablets.

6.6 Instructions for use and handling

No special instructions

7. MARKETING AUTHORISATION HOLDER

Novartis Pharmaceuticals UK Ltd

Frimley Business Park

Frimley

Camberley

Surrey

GU16 7SR

United Kingdom

8. MARKETING AUTHORISATION NUMBER(S)

Famvir 125 mg Tablets: PL 00101/0625

Famvir 250 mg Tablets: PL 00101/0624

Famvir 500 mg Tablets: PL 00101/0623

Famvir 750 mg Tablets: PL 00101/0622

9. DATE OF FIRST AUTHORISATION/RENEWAL OF THE AUTHORISATION

Famvir 125 mg Tablets: 15 June 2001

Famvir 250 mg Tablets: 29 August 2001

Famvir 500 mg Tablets: 29 August 2001

Famvir 750 mg Tablets: 1 October 2001

10. DATE OF REVISION OF THE TEXT

6 December 2004

LEGAL CATEGORY

POM

Fansidar

(Roche Products Limited)

1. NAME OF THE MEDICINAL PRODUCT

Fansidar

2. QUALITATIVE AND QUANTITATIVE COMPOSITION

Fansidar tablets contain 500mg sulfadoxine and 25mg pyrimethamine.

3. PHARMACEUTICAL FORM

Tablets.

4. CLINICAL PARTICULARS

4.1 Therapeutic indications

Fansidar is indicated for the treatment of *Plasmodium falciparum* malaria and in restricted circumstances can be used for the prophylaxis of *Plasmodium falciparum* malaria.

Treatment of malaria

Fansidar is indicated for the treatment of malaria, particularly when caused by strains of *Plasmodium falciparum* resistant to other antimalarials.

Prophylaxis of malaria

Fansidar is not routinely recommended for malaria prophylaxis.

Malaria prophylaxis with Fansidar is indicated for travellers to areas where *Plasmodium falciparum* malaria is endemic and sensitive to Fansidar, and when alternative drugs are not available or contra-indicated. Whenever malaria prophylaxis is prescribed, the malaria situation and in particular, resistance trends at the traveller's destination and any stop-over point must be considered. At present, there is no antimalarial agent which provides absolute protection against malaria, but careful compliance to drug prophylaxis can usually prevent serious progression of the disease.

4.2 Posology and method of administration

The tablets should be swallowed with plenty of fluid after a meal.

Adults and children

Curative treatment of malaria

The appropriate amount of the drug is given in one single dose. This dose should not be repeated for at least seven days.

Adults (higher dose for persons over 60kg)		2 to 3 tablets
Children	10 - 14 years (> 30 - 45kg)	2 tablets
	5 - 10 years (> 20 - 30kg)	1 ½ tablets
	2 - 5 years (> 10 - 20kg)	1 tablet
	under 2 years (5 - 10kg)	½ tablet

In very severe cases, quinine may be added, preferably parenterally. An adequate supply of fluids and electrolytes should be maintained.

Prophylaxis of malaria

The malaria risk must be carefully weighed against the risk of serious adverse drug reactions. **If Fansidar is prescribed for prophylaxis, it is important that the physician inquires about sulfonamide intolerance and points out the risk and the need for immediate drug withdrawal if skin reactions do occur.**

The following dose of Fansidar should be taken every seven days:

Adults		1 tablet
Children	10 -14 years (> 30 - 45kg)	¾ tablet
	2 - 10 years (> 10 - 30kg)	½ tablet
	under 2 years (5 - 10kg)	¼ tablet

Regular dosage using the above schedule during the stay in the malarious area is important for continuous protection to be maintained. Routine measures to protect against mosquito bites should not be omitted.

Fansidar prophylaxis should be started about one week before entering the endemic area in order to assess tolerance; this will enable an alternative drug to be selected in the infrequent case where Fansidar is poorly tolerated.

IMPORTANT: Fansidar prophylaxis should be continued for four to six weeks after returning to a non-malarious area to ensure elimination of possible falciparum infections. However, as with other prophylactic drugs, infections of benign malaria (vivax and malariae infections) may give rise to clinical attacks up to several months after return, despite regular prophylaxis.

Prophylaxis with Fansidar should not be continued for more than two years since no experience of more prolonged administration is available to date.

All travellers should inform their doctor of their exposure to the risk of malaria, should they fall ill either during their stay, or upon their return home.

Elderly

Although no specific studies have been performed to establish the use of Fansidar in the elderly, it has been used extensively and the dosage requirements and side-effects appear to be similar to those of younger adults.

4.3 Contraindications

Patients with known sulphonamide or pyrimethamine hypersensitivity or hypersensitivity to any of the ingredients of Fansidar.

Prophylactic (prolonged) use of Fansidar is contra-indicated in patients with severe renal or hepatic failure, or blood dyscrasias.

Treatment must be immediately discontinued upon the appearance of any skin reactions or mucocutaneous signs or symptoms such as pruritus, erythema, rash, urogenital lesions or pharyngitis, and a medical practitioner consulted as these may be indicative of a life-threatening reaction to the drug. The possibility of an adverse drug reaction should be considered in patients developing a rash, jaundice, fever or severe generalised malaise during treatment with Fansidar.

Like all other preparations containing sulphonamides, Fansidar is contra-indicated in premature babies and during the first two months of life.

4.4 Special warnings and special precautions for use
Excessive exposure to the sun must be strictly avoided.

Patients should be advised that sore throat, fever, cough, dyspnoea or purpura may be first signs of serious side-effects. In particular, Fansidar must be immediately withdrawn at the first sign of a skin rash, a marked reduction in the blood cell count or in the presence of a bacterial or fungal superinfection.

On prolonged administration of high doses, folic acid deficiency can be prevented by administration of folinic acid.

Regular blood counts are recommended during long-term prophylactic use (over three months) of Fansidar.

4.5 Interaction with other medicinal products and other forms of Interaction
Concurrent administration of other preparations containing folate antagonists (e.g. trimethoprim, co-trimoxazole, methotrexate, anticonvulsants) can result in increased impairment of folic acid metabolism which leads to haematological side-effects. Such concomitant therapy should be avoided if possible.

There is evidence which may indicate an increase in incidence and severity of adverse reactions when chloroquine is used with Fansidar, as compared to the use of Fansidar alone.

4.6 Pregnancy and lactation
In experiments in rats, embryotoxic and teratogenic effects with Fansidar were abolished by administration of folinic acid.

In pregnant women, limited prophylactic and therapeutic use of Fansidar did not indicate a risk of foetal damage. Nevertheless, Fansidar should be used in pregnancy only if it is absolutely essential, and only after the expected benefit has been weighed against the potential risk to the foetus. Pregnant women should be made aware of the particular risks of contracting malaria during pregnancy, and should be advised not to undertake unnecessary journeys to endemic areas. A folate supplement should be given to pregnant women receiving Fansidar. Women of childbearing potential should be advised to practise contraception during prophylaxis with Fansidar and for three months after the last dose.

Although no cases have been documented to date, there is a possibility that use of Fansidar during pregnancy at term may produce kernicterus in the neonate.

Both pyrimethamine and sulfadoxine are secreted in maternal breast milk. Nursing mothers should not take Fansidar. In cases where the use of Fansidar is essential, women should abstain from breast feeding.

4.7 Effects on ability to drive and use machines
None known.

4.8 Undesirable effects
Fansidar is usually well tolerated at the recommended dosage.

As with other drugs containing sulphonamides and/or pyrimethamine, the following side-effects and hypersensitivity reactions may occur:

Skin reactions

Drug rash, pruritus, urticaria, photosensitisation and slight hair loss have been observed. These reactions are usually mild and regress spontaneously upon withdrawal of the drug. In very rare cases, particularly in hypersensitive patients, severe, possibly life-threatening skin reactions such as erythema multiforme, Stevens-Johnson syndrome and Lyell's syndrome have occurred.

Gastro-intestinal reactions

Feeling of fullness, nausea, rarely vomiting, diarrhoea, stomatitis. There have been isolated reports of a transient rise of liver enzymes as well as hepatitis occurring conjointly with administration of Fansidar.

Haematological changes

In rare cases, leucopenia, thrombocytopenia and megaloblastic anaemia have been observed, though these usually have been asymptomatic. In extremely rare cases, they take the form of agranulocytosis or purpura. As a rule, all these changes regress after withdrawal of the drug.

Other side-effects

Fatigue, headache, dizziness, fever and polyneuritis may occasionally occur. Pulmonary infiltrates resembling eosinophilic or allergic alveolitis have been reported in rare instances. If symptoms such as cough or shortness of breath should occur during Fansidar therapy, the drug should be discontinued. Isolated cases of serum sickness as well as allergic pericarditis have also been reported.

Adverse reactions occurring after the administration of the sulfadoxine component of Fansidar are not normally more prolonged than those occurring after shorter-acting sulphonamides despite the continued presence of the drug in the body.

4.9 Overdose
Possible symptoms of overdosage include headache, anorexia, nausea, vomiting, signs of excitation, and possibly convulsions and haematological changes (megaloblastic anaemia, leucopenia, thrombocytopenia).

In acute intoxication, induction of vomiting or gastric lavage as appropriate, as well as fluid replacement is recommended. Possible convulsions due to the pyrimethamine component of Fansidar should be watched for and may require anticonvulsant therapy with parenteral diazepam or a barbiturate. Monitoring of renal and hepatic function and repeated blood counts is recommended for up to four weeks after overdosage. If haematological changes are found, folinic acid should be administered intramuscularly.

5. PHARMACOLOGICAL PROPERTIES
5.1 Pharmacodynamic properties
Fansidar acts on the asexual intraerythrocytic forms of the human malaria parasites. By synergistic action of the two components, sulfadoxine and pyrimethamine, two enzymes involved in the biosynthesis of folinic acid in the parasites are inhibited.

Fansidar is also effective against strains of *P. falciparum* resistant to chloroquine. However, in parts of South-East Asia and South America the occurrence of *P. falciparum* malaria clinically resistant to Fansidar are frequent, resistant strains also occur in East and Central Africa. Fansidar should not be used where the prevalence of resistant strains is thought to be high.

5.2 Pharmacokinetic properties
Absorption: After administration of 1 tablet, peak plasma levels for pyrimethamine (approximately 0.2mg per litre) and for sulfadoxine (approximately 60mg per litre) are reached after about four hours.

Distribution: The volume of distribution for sulfadoxine and pyrimethamine is 0.14 litres per kg and 2.3 litres per kg respectively.

Patients taking 1 tablet a week (recommended adult dose for malaria prophylaxis) can be expected to have mean steady state plasma concentrations of 0.15mg per litre for pyrimethamine after about four weeks and 98mg per litre for sulfadoxine after about seven weeks. Plasma protein binding is about 90% for both pyrimethamine and sulfadoxine. Both pyrimethamine and sulfadoxine cross the placental barrier and pass into breast milk.

Metabolism: About 5% of sulfadoxine appear in the blood as acetylated metabolite, about 2 – 3% as the glucuronide. Pyrimethamine is transformed to several metabolites.

Elimination: A relatively long elimination half-life is characteristic of both components. The mean values are about 100 hours for pyrimethamine and about 200 hours for sulfadoxine. Both pyrimethamine and sulfadoxine are eliminated mainly via the kidneys.

Characteristics in patients: In malaria patients, single pharmacokinetic parameters may differ from those in healthy subjects, depending on the population concerned.

In patients with renal insufficiency delayed elimination of the components of Fansidar must be anticipated.

5.3 Preclinical safety data
There are no pre-clinical data of relevance to the prescriber which are additional to that already included in other sections of the SPC.

6. PHARMACEUTICAL PARTICULARS
6.1 List of excipients
Maize starch, lactose, gelatin, talc, magnesium stearate.

6.2 Incompatibilities
None known.

6.3 Shelf life
5 years.

6.4 Special precautions for storage
No special precautions are required.

6.5 Nature and contents of container
Fansidar tablets are available in amber glass/HDPE bottles and aluminium foil strips, in packs of 3, 10 and 150.

6.6 Instructions for use and handling
Not applicable.

7. MARKETING AUTHORISATION HOLDER
Roche Products Limited, 40 Broadwater Road, Welwyn Garden City, Hertfordshire, AL7 3AY.

8. MARKETING AUTHORISATION NUMBER(S)
PL 0031/5097R

9. DATE OF FIRST AUTHORISATION/RENEWAL OF THE AUTHORISATION
March 1992

10. DATE OF REVISION OF THE TEXT
November 2001

Fansidar is a registered trade mark

Item Code

Fareston

(Orion Pharma (UK) Limited)

1. NAME OF THE MEDICINAL PRODUCT
Fareston 60 mg tablets

2. QUALITATIVE AND QUANTITATIVE COMPOSITION
Each tablet contains 60 mg toremifene (as citrate)

For excipients see section 6.1

3. PHARMACEUTICAL FORM
Tablet.

White, round, flat, bevelled edge tablet with TO 60 on one side.

4. CLINICAL PARTICULARS
4.1 Therapeutic indications
First line hormone treatment of hormone-dependent metastatic breast cancer in postmenopausal patients. Fareston is not recommended for patients with oestrogen receptor negative tumours.

4.2 Posology and method of administration
The recommended dose is 60 mg, one tablet, daily.

Renal insufficiency: No dose adjustment is needed in patients with renal insufficiency.

Hepatic impairment: Toremifene should be used cautiously in patients with liver impairment (see also section 5.2. Pharmacokinetic properties, b) Characteristics in patients).

4.3 Contraindications
Pre-existing endometrial hyperplasia and severe hepatic failure are contra-indications in long-term use of toremifene.

Hypersensitivity to toremifene or any of the excipients.

4.4 Special warnings and special precautions for use
Gynaecological examination should be performed before treatment administration, closely looking at pre-existing endometrial abnormality. Afterwards gynaecological examination should be repeated at least once a year. Patients with additional risk of endometrial cancer, e.g. patients suffering from hypertension or diabetes, having high BMI (>30) or history of hormone replacement therapy should be closely monitored (see also section 4.8 Undesirable effects).

Patients with a history of severe thromboembolic disease should generally not be treated with toremifene (see also section 4.8 Undesirable effects).

Patients with non-compensated cardiac insufficiency or severe angina pectoris should be closely monitored.

Hypercalcemia may occur at the beginning of toremifene treatment in patients with bone metastasis and thus these patients should be closely monitored.

There are no systematic data available from patients with labile diabetes, from patients with severely altered performance status or from patients with cardiac failure.

4.5 Interaction with other medicinal products and other forms of Interaction
No specific interaction studies have been performed.

Drugs which decrease renal calcium excretion, e.g. thiazide diuretics, may increase the risk of hypercalcaemia.

Enzyme inducers, like phenobarbital, phenytoin and carbamazepine, may increase the rate of toremifene metabolism thus lowering the steady-state concentration in serum. In such cases doubling of the daily dose may be necessary.

There is a known interaction between anti-oestrogens and warfarin-type anticoagulants leading to a seriously increased bleeding time. Therefore, the concomitant use of toremifene with such drugs should be avoided.

Theoretically the metabolism of toremifene is inhibited by drugs known to inhibit the CYP 3A enzyme system which is reported to be responsible for its main metabolic pathways. Examples of such drugs are ketoconazole and similar antimycotics, erythromycin and troleandomycin. Concomitant use of those drugs with toremifene should be carefully considered.

4.6 Pregnancy and lactation
Toremifene is recommended for postmenopausal patients. Owing to the lack of specific data in humans toremifene should not be used during pregnancy and lactation.

In the animal reproduction studies toremifene has been shown to prevent implantation, to induce parturition failures, and to reduce perinatal survival. In addition, treatment during organogenesis induces changes in ossification, rib abnormalities, and oedematous foetuses.

In rats, decreased body weight gain of the offspring during lactation was observed.

4.7 Effects on ability to drive and use machines
None.

4.8 Undesirable effects
The most frequent adverse reactions are hot flushes, sweating, uterine bleeding, leukorrhea, fatigue, nausea, rash, itching, dizziness and depression. The reactions are usually mild and mostly due to the hormonal action of toremifene.

Adverse reactions according to system organ classes:

(see Table 1)

Thromboembolic events include deep venous thrombosis and pulmonary embolism (see also section 4.4 Special warnings and special precautions for use).

Toremifene treatment has been associated with changes in liver enzyme levels (increases of transaminases) and in very rare occasions with more severe liver function abnormalities (jaundice).

A few cases of hypercalcaemia have been reported in patients with bone metastases at the beginning of toremifene treatment.

Endometrial hypertrophy may develop during the treatment due to the partial oestrogenic effect of toremifene. There is a risk of increased endometrial changes including hyperplasia, polyps and cancer. This may be due to the underlying mechanism/estrogenic stimulation (see also section 4.4 Special warnings and special precautions for use).

4.9 Overdose
No overdose cases are known.

Vertigo, headache and dizziness were observed in healthy volunteer studies at daily dose of 680 mg. There is no specific antidote and the treatment is symptomatic.

5. PHARMACOLOGICAL PROPERTIES

5.1 Pharmacodynamic properties
Pharmacotherapeutic group: Anti-oestrogens, ATC code: L02BA02

Toremifene is a nonsteroidal triphenylethylene derivative. As other members of this class, e.g. tamoxifen and clomifene, toremifene binds to oestrogen receptors and may produce oestrogenic, anti-oestrogenic or both effects, depending upon the duration of treatment, animal species, gender, target organ and variable selected. In general, however, nonsteroidal triphenylethylene derivatives are predominantly anti-oestrogenic in rats and man and oestrogenic in mice.

In post-menopausal breast cancer patients toremifene treatment is associated with modest reductions in both total serum cholesterol and low density lipoprotein (LDL).

Toremifene binds specifically to oestrogen receptors, competitively with oestradiol, and inhibits oestrogen-induced stimulation of DNA synthesis and cell replication. In some experimental cancers and/or using high-dose, toremifene displays anti-tumour effects which are not oestrogen-dependent.

The anti-tumour effect of toremifene in breast cancer is mainly due to the anti-oestrogenic effect, although other mechanisms (changes in oncogene expression, growth factor secretion, induction of apoptosis and influence on cell cycle kinetics) may also be involved in the anti-tumour effect.

5.2 Pharmacokinetic properties
a) General characteristics

Toremifene is readily absorbed after oral administration. Peak concentrations in serum are obtained within 3 (range 2 - 5) hours. Food intake has no effect on the extent of absorption but may delay the peak concentrations by 1.5 - 2 hours. The changes due to food intake are not clinically significant.

The serum concentration curve can be described by a biexponential equation. The half-life of the first (distribution) phase is 4 (range 2 - 12) hours, and of the second (elimination) phase 5 (range 2 - 10) days. The basal disposition parameters (CL and V) could not be estimated due to the lack of intravenous study. Toremifene binds extensively (> 99.5 %) to serum proteins, mainly to albumin. Toremifene obeys linear serum kinetics at oral daily doses between 11 and 680 mg. The mean concentration of toremifene at steady-state is 0.9 (range 0.6 - 1.3) μg/ml at the recommended dose of 60 mg per day.

Toremifene is extensively metabolised. In human serum the main metabolite is N-demethyltoremifene with mean half-life of 11 (range 4 - 20) days. Its steady-state concentrations are about twice compared to those of the parent compound. It has similar anti-oestrogenic, albeit weaker anti-tumour activity than the parent compound.

It is bound to plasma proteins even more extensively than toremifene, the protein bound fraction being > 99.9 %. Three minor metabolites have been detected in human serum: (deaminohydroxy)toremifene, 4-hydroxytoremifene, and N,N-didemethyltoremifene. Although they have theoretically interesting hormonal effects, their concentrations during toremifene treatment are too low to have any major biological importance.

Toremifene is eliminated mainly as metabolites to the faeces. Enterohepatic circulation can be expected. About 10 % of the administered dose is eliminated via urine as metabolites. Owing to the slow elimination, steady-state concentrations in serum are reached in 4 to 6 weeks.

b) Characteristics in patients

Clinical anti-tumour efficacy and serum concentrations have no positive correlation at the recommended daily dose of 60 mg.

No information is available concerning polymorphic metabolism. Enzyme complex, known to be responsible for the metabolism of toremifene in humans, is cytochrome P450-dependent hepatic mixed function oxidase. The main metabolic pathway, N-demethylation, is mediated mainly by CYP 3A.

Pharmacokinetics of toremifene were investigated in an open study with four parallel groups of ten subjects: normal subjects, patients with impaired (mean AST 57 U/L - mean ALT 76 U/L - mean gamma GT 329 U/L) or activated liver function (mean AST 25 U/L - mean ALT 30 U/L - mean gamma GT 91 U/L - patients treated with antiepileptics) and patients with impaired renal function (creatinine: 176 μmol/L). In this study the kinetics of toremifene in patients with impaired renal function were not significantly altered as compared to normal subjects. The elimination of toremifene and its metabolites was significantly increased in patients with activated liver function and decreased in patients with impaired liver function.

5.3 Preclinical safety data
The acute toxicity of toremifene is low with LD-50 in rats and mice of more than 2000 mg/kg. In repeated toxicity studies the cause of death in rats is gastric dilatation. In the acute and chronic toxicity studies most of the findings are related to the hormonal effects of toremifene. The other findings are not toxicologically significant. Toremifene has not shown any genotoxicity and has not been found to be carcinogenic in rats. In mice, oestrogens induce ovarian and testicular tumours as well as hyperostosis and osteosarcomas. Toremifene has a species-specific oestrogen-like effect in mice and causes similar tumours. These findings are postulated to be of little relevance for the safety in man, where toremifene acts mainly as an anti-oestrogen.

6. PHARMACEUTICAL PARTICULARS

6.1 List of excipients
Maize starch

Lactose

Povidone

Purified water

Sodium starch glycolate

Magnesium stearate

Microcrystalline cellulose

Colloidal anhydrous silica

6.2 Incompatibilities
None.

6.3 Shelf life
5 years

6.4 Special precautions for storage
No special precautions for storage.

6.5 Nature and contents of container
Green PVC foil and aluminium foil blister in a cardboard box.

Package sizes: 30 and 100 tablets.

6.6 Instructions for use and handling
None.

7. MARKETING AUTHORISATION HOLDER
ORION CORPORATION
Orionintie 1
FIN-02200 ESPOO
FINLAND

8. MARKETING AUTHORISATION NUMBER(S)
EU/1/96/004/001
EU/1/96/004/002

9. DATE OF FIRST AUTHORISATION/RENEWAL OF THE AUTHORISATION
14 February 1996

10. DATE OF REVISION OF THE TEXT
18 May 2001

Table 1 Adverse reactions according to system organ classes

Organ Group	Very Common*	Common*	Uncommon*	Rare*	Very Rare*
Reproductive disorders, female		uterine bleeding, leukorrhea	endometrial hypertrophy	endometrial polyps	endometrial hyperplasia, endometrial cancer
General disorders	hot flushes, sweating	Fatigue, oedema	weight increase, headache,		
Gastrointestinal disorders		Nausea, vomiting	loss of appetite, constipation		
Skin and appendages disorders		rash, itching			alopecia
Central and peripheral nervous system disorders		dizziness	insomnia	vertigo	
Psychiatric disorders		depression			
Respiratory system disorders			dyspnoea		
Vision disorders					transient corneal opacity
Platelet, bleeding and clotting disorders			thromboembolic events		
Liver and biliary system disorders				increase of transaminases	jaundice

Adverse drug reactions are ordered under headings of frequency using the following convention: very common (> 1/10), common (> 1/100, < 1/10), uncommon (> 1/1,000, < 1/100), rare (> 1/10,000, < 1/1,000), very rare (< 1/10,000 including isolated reports)

Farlutal 100,250,500

(Pharmacia Limited)

1. NAME OF THE MEDICINAL PRODUCT
Farlutal 100, Farlutal 250, Farlutal 500

2. QUALITATIVE AND QUANTITATIVE COMPOSITION
Medroxyprogesterone acetate BP 100 mg, 250 mg and 500 mg respectively.

3. PHARMACEUTICAL FORM
Tablets

4. CLINICAL PARTICULARS

4.1 Therapeutic indications
Palliative treatment of hormone-sensitive malignancies. Farlutal has been successfully used to produce regressions in breast, endometrial, prostatic and renal cell carcinoma. High dose Farlutal treatment has proved especially useful in breast carcinoma and in achieving subjective improvements in terminally ill patients, notably pain relief and improved performance status.

4.2 Posology and method of administration
Route of administration: Oral

Adults and elderly

Suggested dosage schemes are as follows:-

Breast carcinoma

400 - 1500 mg daily is recommended, although doses of up to 2000 mg daily have been used. There is an alternative Farlutal formulation for injection. To be effective, daily oral administration must be at least 2-3 times the recommended i.m. dosage where the initial dose is 500-1000 mg/day i.m. for 4 weeks and maintenance dose 500 mg i.m. twice a week. The two treatment modalities, oral and i.m., may be mixed, especially in maintenance therapy to reduce the number of i.m. injections (and possible related adverse effects) and yet maintain high plasma levels with a minimum of oral therapy.

Other hormone dependent malignancies

The oral dose is 100-600 mg/day. For i.m. treatment of endometrial cancer the recommended initial dose is 400-1000 mg per week. If improvement is noted within a few weeks or months and the disease appears to be stabilised, it may be possible to maintain improvement with as little as 400 mg per month.

Children

None stated.

4.3 Contraindications

Medroxyprogesterone acetate is contraindicated in the following conditions:

- thrombophlebitis, thrombo-embolic disorders, and where there is a high risk of developing such manifestations [presence or history of atrial fibrillation, valvular disorders, endocarditis, heart failure, pulmonary embolism; thrombo-embolic ischaemic attack (TIA), cerebral infarction; atherosclerosis; immediate post surgery period]
- Previous idiopathic or current venous thromboembolism (deep vein thrombosis, pulmonary embolism)
- Active or recent arterial thrombo-embolic disease (e.g., angina, myocardial infarction)
- severe hepatic insufficiency
- hypercalcaemia in patients with osseous metastases
- suspected or early breast carcinoma
- missed abortion, metrorrhagia, known or suspected pregnancy
- undiagnosed vaginal bleeding
- known hypersensitivity to medroxyprogesterone acetate or any other component of Farlutal Tablets.

Progestogens are known to be porphyrogenic. Patients with a history of attacks or aged under 30 are at greatest risk of an acute attack while on progesterone treatment. A careful assessment of potential benefit should be made where this risk is present.

4.4 Special warnings and special precautions for use

Warnings

Farlutal should be used under the direction of those experienced in cancer chemotherapy.

Since medroxyprogesterone acetate appears to enhance blood clotting potential, treatment should be discontinued upon the appearance of thrombo-embolic episodes, migraine or associated ocular problems such as sudden or partial or total loss of vision, diplopia or vascular lesions of the retina.

Treatment with medroxyprogesterone acetate should be discontinued in the event of:

- jaundice or deterioration in liver function
- significant increase in blood pressure
- new onset of migraine-type headache

In the event of vaginal bleeding occurring, an accurate diagnosis should be made. If a histological examination is indicated, the laboratory should be informed that the patient has been receiving a progestogen.

The pathologist or laboratory should be advised that the patient is receiving medroxyprogesterone acetate as this can decrease the levels of the following endocrine biomarkers:

- Plasma/urinary steroids (e.g., cortisol, oestrogen, pregnanediol, progesterone, testosterone)
- Plasma/urinary gonadotrophins (e.g., LH and FSH)
- Sex-hormone-binding-globulin

Precautions

Animal studies have shown that medroxyprogesterone acetate possesses adrenocorticoid activity and this effect has also been observed in humans. Patients treated with high doses continuously over long periods should be carefully observed for signs normally associated with adrenocorticoid therapy, such as hypertension, sodium retention, oedema, etc. Care is needed in treating patients with diabetes and/or arterial hypertension.

When used in oncology indications, medroxyprogesterone acetate may cause partial adrenal insufficiency (decrease in pituitary-adrenal axis response) during metyrapone testing. Thus the ability of the adrenal cortex to respond to ACTH should be demonstrated before metyrapone is administrated. The pathologist/laboratory should be made aware that the patient is being treated with medroxyprogesterone acetate.

Patients with the following conditions should be carefully monitored while taking progestogens:

- Conditions which may be influenced by potential fluid retention
  - o Epilepsy
  - o Migraine
  - o Asthma
  - o Cardiac dysfunction
  - o Renal dysfunction
- Hyperlipidaemia
- History of mental depression
- Diabetes (a decrease in glucose tolerance has been observed in some patients)

Farlutal may raise plasma calcium levels; some cases of hypercalcaemia have been reported in the treatment of breast carcinoma.

Risk of venous thromboembolism (VTE)

The risk of VTE has not been assessed for progesterone alone. However, VTE is a known risk factor of oestrogen-only and combined hormone replacement therapy. When prescribing medroxyprogesterone acetate for oncology indications the following precautions and risk factors should be considered in the light of the patient's condition, the dose of medroxyprogesterone acetate and the duration of therapy:

- Generally recognised risk factors for VTE include a personal or family history of VTE or known thrombo-embolic states, severe obesity (BMI > 30 kg/m^2) and systemic lupus erythematosus
- The risk of VTE may be temporarily increased with prolonged immobilisation, major trauma or major surgery.

If VTE develops after initiating therapy, medroxyprogesterone acetate should be discontinued. Patients should be told to contact their doctor immediately if they become aware of a symptom suggestive of potential thromboembolism (e.g. painful swelling of a leg, sudden pain in the chest, dyspnoea).

4.5 Interaction with other medicinal products and other forms of Interaction

Interaction with other medicaments

The metabolism of progestogens may be increased by concomitant administration of compounds known to induce drug-metabolising enzymes, specifically cytochrome P450 enzymes. These compounds include anticonvulsants (e.g., phenobarbital, phenytoin, carbamezapine) and anti-infectives (e.g., rifampicin, rifabutin, nevirapine, efavirenz).

Ritonavir and nelfinavir, although known as strong inhibitors, by contrast exhibit inducing properties when used concomitantly with steroid hormones. Herbal preparations containing St John's Wort (Hypericum Perforatum) may induce the metabolism of progestogens. Progestogen levels may therefore be reduced.

Aminoglutethimide has been reported to decrease plasma levels of some progestogens.

When used in combination with cytotoxic drugs, it is possible that progestogens may reduce the haematological toxicity of chemotherapy.

Special care should be taken when progestogens are administered with other drugs which also cause fluid retention, such as NSAIDs and vasodilators.

Progestogens may inhibit the metabolism of cyclosporin, leading to increased plasma cyclosporin concentrations.

Interactions with other medicinal treatments (including oral anti-coagulants) have rarely been reported, but causality has not been determined. The possibility of interaction should be born in mind in patients receiving concurrent treatment with other drugs.

Other forms of interaction

Progestogens can influence certain laboratory tests (e.g., tests for hepatic function, thyroid function and coagulation).

4.6 Pregnancy and lactation

Pregnancy

Administration of progesterone during the first months of pregnancy may possibly be associated with the occurrence of congenital cardiac malformations in the neonate. In addition, instances of masculinisation of female foetuses have been reported following high dose therapy during pregnancy. For these reasons, Farlutal is contra-indicated during pregnancy.

It should be noted that long term administration of medroxyprogesterone acetate to beagle dogs has resulted in the development of mammary nodules which were occasionally found to be malignant. The relevance of these findings to humans has not been established.

Lactation

Medroxyprogesterone acetate and its metabolites are excreted in breast milk. Therefore, the use of Farlutal in breast-feeding is not recommended.

4.7 Effects on ability to drive and use machines

None known.

4.8 Undesirable effects

Genitourinary	Abnormal uterine bleeding (irregular, increase, decrease), amenorrhoea, alterations of cervical secretions, cervical erosions, prolonged anovulation
Breast	Galactorrhoea, mastodynia, tenderness
Central Nervous System	Confusion, depression, dizziness, euphoria, fatigue, headache, insomnia, loss of concentration, nervousness, somnolence, vision disorders
Gastrointestinal/ Hepatobiliary	Constipation, diarrhoea, dry mouth, disturbed liver function, jaundice, nausea, vomiting
Metabolic & Nutritional	Adrenergic-like effects (e.g., fine-hand tremors, sweating, cramps in calves at night), corticoid-like effects (e.g., facies lunaris, Cushingoid syndrome), decreased glucose tolerance, diabetic cataract, exacerbation of diabetes mellitus, glycosuria
Cardiovascular	Cerebral and myocardial infarction, congestive heart failure, increased blood pressure, palpitations, pulmonary embolism, retinal thrombosis, tachycardia, thrombo-embolic disorders, thrombophlebitis
Haematological	Elevation of white blood cells and platelet counts
Skin & Mucous Membranes	Acne, alopecia, hirsutism, pruritus, rash, urticaria
Allergy	Hypersensitivity reactions (e.g., anaphylaxis & anaphylactoid reactions, angioedema)
Miscellaneous	Changes in appetite, changes in libido, oedema/fluid retention, hypocalcaemia, malaise, pyrexia, weight change

4.9 Overdose

No treatment recommendations.

5. PHARMACOLOGICAL PROPERTIES

5.1 Pharmacodynamic properties

Medroxyprogesterone acetate is active when administered orally and displays a marked progestomimetic activity in animals and man. It has no oestrogenic activity but possesses antioestrogenic, anti-androgenic and antigonadotropic properties. Medroxyprogesterone acetate behaves both as a corticosteroid agonist and antagonist.

In man, medroxyprogesterone acetate lowers blood levels of FSH, LH, ACTH, testosterone and cortisol. Unlike progesterone it has a glucocorticoid action.

5.2 Pharmacokinetic properties

After oral administration of medroxyprogesterone acetate, absorption is rapid. The plasma half life is of the order of 2 days and with repeated dosing once daily a steady state concentration is reached in about 10 days. Plasma concentrations are usually proportional to the administered dose, but considerable individual variation occurs. In general, to obtain concentrations comparable to those achieved after 4 weeks i.m. administration, at least twice the daily i.m. dose should be given.

5.3 Preclinical safety data

No further preclinical safety data is available.

6. PHARMACEUTICAL PARTICULARS

6.1 List of excipients

Lactose

Crospovidone

Polyvinylpyrrolidone

Polysorbate 80

Microcrystalline cellulose

Magnesium stearate

Purified water

6.2 Incompatibilities

None stated.

6.3 Shelf life

60 months

6.4 Special precautions for storage

Store in a dry place.

6.5 Nature and contents of container

Farlutal 100: PVDC/Aluminium blister containing 100 tablets.

Farlutal 250: PVDC/Aluminium blister containing 50 tablets.

Farlutal 500: PVDC/Aluminium blister containing 56 tablets.

6.6 Instructions for use and handling

None.

7. MARKETING AUTHORISATION HOLDER
Pharmacia Limited

Davy Avenue

Milton Keynes

MK5 8PH

UK

8. MARKETING AUTHORISATION NUMBER(S)
Farlutal 100: PL 00032/0368

Farlutal 250: PL 00032/0369

Farlutal 500: PL 00032/0370

9. DATE OF FIRST AUTHORISATION/RENEWAL OF THE AUTHORISATION
14th January 2002

10. DATE OF REVISION OF THE TEXT
August 2004.

FL1_0

Farlutal 500 for Injection

(Pharmacia Limited)

1. NAME OF THE MEDICINAL PRODUCT
Farlutal 500 for injection

Farlutal 1000 for injection*

Not marketed in UK

2. QUALITATIVE AND QUANTITATIVE COMPOSITION
Medroxyprogesterone Acetate BP, 20.0 W/V

3. PHARMACEUTICAL FORM
White sterile suspension for injection which settles on standing but readily disperses on shaking.

4. CLINICAL PARTICULARS

4.1 Therapeutic indications
Palliative treatment of hormone-sensitive malignancies. Farlutal has been successfully used to produce regressions in breast, endometrial, prostatic and renal cell carcinoma. High dose Farlutal therapy has proved especially useful in breast carcinoma and in achieving subjective improvements in terminally ill patients, notably pain relief and improved performance status.

4.2 Posology and method of administration
Route of administration: Intramuscular injection

Suggested dosage schemes are as follows:

Breast Carcinoma:

Initial dose: 500 - 1000 mg/day i.m. for 4 weeks

Maintenance: 500 mg i.m. twice a week

Endometrial Carcinoma:

Initial dose: 500 mg i.m. twice weekly for 3 months

Maintenance: 500 mg i.m. weekly

Renal Adenocarcinoma:

Initial dose: 500 mg i.m. on alternate days for 30 days

Maintenance: 500 mg i.m. twice weekly until 60th day, then 250 mg i.m. weekly

Prostatic Adenocarcinoma:

Initial dose: 500 mg i.m. twice weekly

Maintenance: 500 mg i.m. weekly

Children and Elderly:

None stated.

4.3 Contraindications
Thrombophlebitis, thrombo-embolic disorders, severe hepatic insufficiency and hypercalcaemia as may occur in patients with osseous metastases; also, suspected or early breast carcinoma, missed abortion, metrorrhagia, pregnancy and known hypersensitivity to medroxyprogesterone acetate, or, for the injectable formulation, hydroxybenzoates (excipients).

4.4 Special warnings and special precautions for use
Farlutal should be used under the direction of those experienced in cancer chemotherapy.

Since medroxyprogesterone acetate appears to enhance blood clotting potential, treatment should be discontinued upon the appearance of thrombo-embolic episodes, migraine or associated ocular problems such as sudden partial or total loss of vision, diplopia or vascular lesions of the retina.

In the event of vaginal bleeding occurring, an accurate diagnosis should be made. If a histological examination is indicated, the laboratory should be informed that the patient has been receiving a progestogen.

Animal studies have shown that medroxyprogesterone acetate possesses adrenocorticoid activity and this effect has also been observed in humans. Patients treated with high doses continuously over long periods should be carefully observed for signs normally associated with adrenocorticoid therapy, such as hypertension, sodium retention, oedema, etc. and care is needed in treating patients with diabetes and/or arterial hypertension.

Farlutal may raise plasma calcium levels; some cases of hypercalcaemia have been reported in the treatment of breast carcinoma.

4.5 Interaction with other medicinal products and other forms of Interaction
None known.

4.6 Pregnancy and lactation
Administration of progesterone during the first months of pregnancy may possibly be associated with the occurrence of congenital cardiac malformations in the neonate. In addition, instances of masculinisation of female foetuses have been reported following high dose therapy during pregnancy. For these reasons, Farlutal is contra-indicated during pregnancy.

It should be noted that long term administration of medroxyprogesterone acetate to beagle dogs has resulted in the development of mammary nodules which were occasionally found to be malignant. The relevance of these findings to humans has, however, not been established.

4.7 Effects on ability to drive and use machines
Not applicable.

4.8 Undesirable effects
As is generally found after intramuscular administration of large volumes of suspension, the i.m. preparation may cause local lesions at the injection site, such as sterile abscesses or inflammatory infiltrates. Therefore, the suspension should be well shaken before use and injected deeply into healthy gluteal muscle.

In common with other progestogens, Farlutal may cause mastodynia, galactorrhoea, vaginal bleeding, changes in menstrual flow, amenorrhoea, cervical erosions and modifications of cervical secretions. Farlutal also exerts a corticoid-like effect which may lead to facies lunaris, cushingoid syndrome and weight changes; and an adrenergic-like action which may result in fine hand tremors, sweating and cramps in the calves at night. Cholestatic jaundice has occasionally been reported.

4.9 Overdose
No positive action is required.

5. PHARMACOLOGICAL PROPERTIES

5.1 Pharmacodynamic properties
MPA has an antigonadotrophic effect, it blocks the preovulatory intermenstrual oestrogen peak by direct action on the ovary. Its effects at low doses include contraceptive action, secretion by the endometrium, delay in the menstrual flow, a decrease in the viscosity of cervical mucus and a reduction in the vaginal karyopycnotic index.

At higher doses, oncological actions are evident. There is a direct cytotoxic action on tumour cells manifested by a decrease in DNA and RNA synthesis.

5.2 Pharmacokinetic properties
The absorption and metabolism of the MPA are affected by both the administration route used and the type of pharmaceutical preparation.

After i.m. administration of MPA in an aqueous solution, absorption is slow. The highest blood levels are found during the first 2 days, measurable amounts being found up to 100 days after treatment. Variations in plasma concentrations are interpreted as being due to irregular release from the injection site.

Only 3-6% of the administered dose is recovered in urine after 24 hours. After 6 days approximately 11% is found in the urine and 3% in the faeces, hence elimination is slow after i.m. administration. Traces of metabolites have been found in the urine up to 6 months after high doses of MPA. Only a slight increase in porter-silber steroids is found in the urine of patients treated by the i.m. route.

5.3 Preclinical safety data
No further preclinical safety data available.

6. PHARMACEUTICAL PARTICULARS

6.1 List of excipients
Polysorbate 80 BP

Sodium Chloride Ph. Eur.

Carbowax 400 BP

Methyl Hydroxybenzoate BP

Propyl Hydroxybenzoate BP

Water for Injections BP

6.2 Incompatibilities
None known.

6.3 Shelf life
48 months

6.4 Special precautions for storage
The vials should be stored between 15° - 30°C and should not be frozen.

6.5 Nature and contents of container
Colourless siliconised glass vial (Type I) with grey chlorobutyl rubber stopper and aluminium seal containing 2.5 or 5 ml of suspension.

6.6 Instructions for use and handling
None stated.

7. MARKETING AUTHORISATION HOLDER
Farmitalia Carlo Erba Limited

Davy Avenue

Milton Keynes

MK5 8PH

UK

8. MARKETING AUTHORISATION NUMBER(S)
PL 3433/0045

9. DATE OF FIRST AUTHORISATION/RENEWAL OF THE AUTHORISATION
Date of First Authorisation: 14 August 1981

Date of Renewal of Authorisation: 15 January 1993

10. DATE OF REVISION OF THE TEXT
4 September 1997

Legal Category
POM

Fasigyn

(Pfizer Limited)

1. NAME OF THE MEDICINAL PRODUCT
FASIGYN

2. QUALITATIVE AND QUANTITATIVE COMPOSITION
Tinidazole 500mg.

3. PHARMACEUTICAL FORM
Film-coated tablets.

White, round, biconvex film-coated tablet embossed on one side with "FAS 500".

4. CLINICAL PARTICULARS

4.1 Therapeutic indications
Treatment of the following infections:

1. Eradication of *Helicobacter pylori* associated with duodenal ulcers, in the presence of antibiotic and acid suppressant therapy. See Posology and Method of Administration section.

2. Anaerobic infections such as:

Intraperitoneal infections: peritonitis, abscess.

Gynaecological infections: endometritis, endomyometritis, tube-ovarian abscess.

Bacterial septicaemia.

Post-operative wound infections.

Skin and soft tissue infections.

Upper and lower respiratory tract infections: pneumonia, empyema, lung abscess.

3. Non-specific vaginitis.

4. Acute ulcerative gingivitis.

5. Urogenital trichomoniasis in both male and female patients.

6. Giardiasis.

7. Intestinal amoebiasis.

8. Amoebic involvement of the liver.

9. Prophylaxis: The prevention of post-operative infections caused by anaerobic bacteria, especially those associated with colonic, gastro-intestinal and gynaecological surgery.

4.2 Posology and method of administration
Route: Oral administration during or after a meal.

1. Eradication of

H.pylori associated with duodenal ulcers:

Adults: the usual dose of Fasigyn is 500mg twice daily coadministered with omeprazole 20mg twice daily and clarithromycin 250mg twice daily for 7 days.

Clinical studies using this 7 day regimen have shown similar *H.pylori* eradication rates when omeprazole 20mg once daily was used. For further information on the dosage for omeprazole see Astra data sheet.

2. Anaerobic infections:

Adults: an initial dose of 2g the first day followed by 1g daily given as a single dose or as 500mg twice daily. Treatment for 5 to 6 days will generally be adequate but clinical judgement must determine the duration of therapy, particularly when eradication of infection from certain sites may be difficult. Regular clinical and laboratory observation is advised if it is considered necessary to continue therapy for more than 7 days.

Children: < 12 years - data are not available.

3. Non-specific vaginitis:

Adults: non-specific vaginitis has been successfully treated with a single oral dose of 2g. Higher cure rates have been achieved with 2g single doses on 2 consecutive days (total dose 4g).

4. Acute Ulcerative Gingivitis:

Adults: a single oral dose of 2g.

5. Urogenital trichomoniasis:

(when infection with *Trichomonas vaginalis* is confirmed, simultaneous treatment of the consort is recommended).

Adults: a single dose of 2g.

Children: a single dose of 50 to 75mg/kg of body weight. It may be necessary to repeat this dose.

6. Giardiasis:

Adults: a single dose of 2g.

Children: a single dose of 50 to 75mg/kg of body weight. It may be necessary to repeat this dose.

7. Intestinal Amoebiasis:

Adults: a single daily dose of 2g for 2 to 3 days.

Children: a single daily dose of 50 to 60mg/kg of body weight on each of 3 successive days.

8. Amoebic involvement in the liver:

Adults: total dosage varies from 4.5 to 12g, depending on the virulence of the *Entamoeba histolytica*.

For amoebic involvement of the liver, the aspiration of pus may be required in addition to therapy with Fasigyn.

Initiate treatment with 1.5 to 2g as a single oral daily dose for three days. Occasionally when a three day course is ineffective, treatment may be continued for up to six days.

Children: a single dose of 50 to 60 mg/kg of body weight per day for five successive days.

9. Prevention of post-operative infection:

Adults: a single dose of 2g approximately 12 hours before surgery.

Children: < 12 years - data are not available.

Use in the elderly: there are no special recommendations for this age group.

4.3 Contraindications

As with other drugs of similar structure, Fasigyn is contraindicated in patients having, or with a history of, blood dyscrasia, although no persistent haematological abnormalities have been noted in clinical or animal studies.

Fasigyn should be avoided in patients with organic neurological disorders.

Fasigyn should not be administered to patients with known hypersensitivity to the drug.

See 4.6 Pregnancy and Lactation section.

4.4 Special warnings and special precautions for use

Fasigyn and related compounds when taken together with alcoholic beverages have caused abdominal cramps, flushing and vomiting.

Drugs of similar chemical structure have also produced various neurological disturbances such as dizziness, vertigo, inco-ordination and ataxia. If during therapy with Fasigyn abnormal neurological signs develop, therapy should be discontinued.

4.5 Interaction with other medicinal products and other forms of Interaction

As with related compounds, alcoholic beverages should be avoided during Fasigyn therapy because of the possibility of a disulfiram-like reaction (flushing, abdominal cramps, vomiting, tachycardia). Alcohol should be avoided until 72 hours after discontinuing Fasigyn.

4.6 Pregnancy and lactation

Use in pregnancy:

Fertility studies in rats receiving 100mg and 300mg tinidazole/kg had no effect on fertility, adult and pup weights, gestation, viability or lactation. There was a slight, not significant, increase in resorption rate at the 300mg/kg dose.

Tinidazole crosses the placental barrier. Since the effects of compounds of this class on foetal development are unknown, the use of tinidazole during the first trimester is contraindicated. There is no evidence that Fasigyn is harmful during the latter stages of pregnancy, but its use during the second and third trimesters requires that the potential benefits be weighed against possible hazards to mother or foetus.

Use in lactation:

Tinidazole is excreted in breast milk. Tinidazole may continue to appear in breast milk for more than 72 hours after administration. Women should not nurse until at least 3 days after having discontinued taking Fasigyn.

4.7 Effects on ability to drive and use machines

No special precautions should be necessary. However, drugs of similar chemical structure, including Fasigyn, have been associated with various neurological disturbances such as dizziness, vertigo, ataxia, peripheral neuropathy (paraesthesia, sensory disturbances, hypoaesthesia) and rarely convulsions. If any abnormal neurological signs develop during Fasigyn therapy, the drug should be discontinued.

4.8 Undesirable effects

Reported side effects have generally been infrequent, mild and self-limiting. Gastro-intestinal side effects include nausea, vomiting, anorexia, diarrhoea, metallic taste and abdominal pain.

Hypersensitivity reactions, occasionally severe, may occur in rare cases in the form of skin rash, pruritus, urticaria and angioneurotic oedema.

Neurological disturbances: See 'Effects on Ability to Drive and Use Machines' section.

As with related compounds, Fasigyn may produce transient leucopenia. Other rarely reported side-effects are headache, tiredness, furry tongue and dark urine.

4.9 Overdose

In acute animal studies with mice and rats, the LD_{50} for mice was >3600mg/kg and >2300mg/kg for oral and intraperitoneal administration respectively. For rats, the LD_{50} was >2000mg/kg for both oral and intraperitoneal administration.

Signs and symptoms of overdosage: There are no reported overdoses in humans with Fasigyn.

Treatment for overdosage: There is no specific antidote for treatment of overdosage with tinidazole. Treatment is symptomatic and supportive. Gastric lavage may be useful. Tinidazole is easily dialysable.

5. PHARMACOLOGICAL PROPERTIES

5.1 Pharmacodynamic properties

Fasigyn is active against both protozoa and obligate anaerobic bacteria. The activity against protozoa involves *Trichomonas vaginalis*, *Entamoeba histolytica* and *Giardia lamblia*.

The mode of action of Fasigyn against anaerobic bacteria and protozoa involves penetration of the drug into the cell of the micro-organism and subsequent damage of DNA strands or inhibition of their synthesis.

Fasigyn is active against *Helicobacter pylori*, *Gardnerella vaginalis* and most anaerobic bacteria including *Bacteroides fragilis*, *Bacteroides melaninogenicus*, Bacteroides spp., Clostridium spp., Eubacterium spp., Fusobacterium spp., Peptococcus spp., Peptostreptococcus spp. and Veillonella spp.

Helicobacter pylori (H.pylori) is associated with acid peptic disease including duodenal ulcer and gastric ulcer in which about 95% and 80% of patients respectively are infected with this agent. *H.pylori* is also implicated as a major contributing factor in the development of gastritis and ulcer recurrence in such patients. Evidence suggests a causative link between *H.pylori* and gastric carcinoma.

Clinical evidence has shown that the combination of Fasigyn with omeprazole and clarithromycin eradicates 91-96% of *H.pylori* isolates.

Various different *H.pylori* eradication regimens have shown that eradication of *H.pylori* heals duodenal ulcers and reduces the risk of ulcer recurrence.

5.2 Pharmacokinetic properties

Fasigyn is rapidly and completely absorbed following oral administration. In studies with healthy volunteers receiving 2g tinidazole orally, peak serum levels of 40-51 micrograms/ml were achieved within two hours and decreased to between 11-19 micrograms/ml at 24 hours. Healthy volunteers who received 800mg and 1.6g tinidazole IV over 10-15 minutes achieved peak plasma concentrations that ranged from 14 to 21mcg/ml for the 800mg dose and averaged 32mcg/ml for the 1.6g dose. At 24 hours post-infusion, plasma levels of tinidazole decreased to 4-5mcg/ml and 8.6mcg/ml respectively, justifying once daily dosing. Plasma levels decline slowly and tinidazole can be detected in plasma at concentrations of up to 1 microgram/ml at 72 hours after oral administration. The plasma elimination half-life for tinidazole is between 12-14.

Tinidazole is widely distributed in all body tissues and also crosses the blood brain barrier, obtaining clinically effective concentrations in all tissues. The apparent volume of distribution is about 50 litres. About 12% of plasma tinidazole is bound to plasma protein.

Tinidazole is excreted by the liver and kidneys. Studies in healthy patients have shown that over 5 days, 60-65% of an administered dose is excreted by the kidneys with 20-25% of the administered dose excreted as unchanged tinidazole. Approximately 12% of the administered dose is excreted in the faeces.

Studies in patients with renal failure (creatinine clearance <22ml/min) indicate that there is no statistically significant change in tinidazole pharmacokinetic parameters in these patients. Thus no adjustments in dosing are required in these patients.

5.3 Preclinical safety data

None.

6. PHARMACEUTICAL PARTICULARS

6.1 List of excipients

Fasigyn tablets contain the following ingredients:

Tablet Core: microcrystalline cellulose (Avicel PH 101), alginic acid, maize starch, magnesium stearate and sodium lauryl sulphate.

Film Coating: hydroxypropyl methyl cellulose, propylene glycol, titanium dioxide (E171).

6.2 Incompatibilities

No major incompatibilities have been noted.

6.3 Shelf life

3 years.

6.4 Special precautions for storage

Store below 25°C in a dry place in the absence of light.

6.5 Nature and contents of container

Fasigyn tablets will be supplied in aluminium foil backed blister packs of 20 (5 × 4) 500mg tablets consisting of:

a) 250 micron PVC blister coated with 40gsm of PVdC

b) 20 micron aluminium foil backing coated with 20gsm PVdC.

6.6 Instructions for use and handling

Fasigyn tablets should be swallowed whole.

Administrative Data

7. MARKETING AUTHORISATION HOLDER

Pfizer Limited
Ramsgate Road
Sandwich
Kent CT13 9NJ

8. MARKETING AUTHORISATION NUMBER(S)

PL 00057/0150

9. DATE OF FIRST AUTHORISATION/RENEWAL OF THE AUTHORISATION

22nd December 1994

10. DATE OF REVISION OF THE TEXT

November 1998

11. Legal Category

POM

Faslodex 250 mg/5 ml solution for injection

(AstraZeneca UK Limited)

1. NAME OF THE MEDICINAL PRODUCT

Faslodex 250 mg/5 ml solution for injection. ▼

2. QUALITATIVE AND QUANTITATIVE COMPOSITION

One pre-filled syringe contains 250 mg fulvestrant in 5 ml solution.

For excipients, see 6.1.

3. PHARMACEUTICAL FORM

Solution for injection.

Clear, colourless to yellow, viscous liquid.

4. CLINICAL PARTICULARS

4.1 Therapeutic indications

Faslodex is indicated for the treatment of postmenopausal women with oestrogen receptor positive, locally advanced or metastatic breast cancer for disease relapse on or after adjuvant antioestrogen therapy or disease progression on therapy with an antioestrogen.

4.2 Posology and method of administration

Adult females (including the elderly):

The recommended dose is 250 mg at intervals of 1 month.

Children and adolescents:

Faslodex is not recommended for use in children or adolescents, as safety and efficacy have not been established in this age group.

Patients with renal impairment:

No dose adjustments are recommended for patients with mild to moderate renal impairment (creatinine clearance ⩾ 30 ml/min). Safety and efficacy have not been evaluated in patients with severe renal impairment (creatinine clearance < 30 ml/min) (see 4.4).

Patients with hepatic impairment:

Use Faslodex with caution in treating patients with mild to moderate hepatic impairment. Safety and efficacy have not been evaluated in patients with hepatic impairment (see 4.3, 4.4 and 5.2).

Method of administration:

Administer intramuscularly slowly into the buttock. For full administration instructions see 6.6.

4.3 Contraindications

Faslodex is contraindicated in:

- patients with known hypersensitivity to the active substance or to any of the excipients
- pregnancy and in breast-feeding (see 4.6)
- severe hepatic impairment

4.4 Special warnings and special precautions for use

Use Faslodex with caution in patients with mild to moderate, hepatic impairment (see 4.2, 4.3 and 5.2).

Use Faslodex with caution in patients with severe renal impairment (creatinine clearance less than 30 ml/min) (see 5.2).

Due to the route of administration, use Faslodex with caution if treating patients with bleeding diatheses, thrombocytopenia or those taking anticoagulant treatment.

Thromboembolic events are commonly observed in women with advanced breast cancer and have been observed in clinical trials (see 4.8). This should be taken into consideration when prescribing Faslodex to patients at risk.

There are no long-term data on the effect of fulvestrant on bone. Due to the mode of action of fulvestrant, there is a potential risk of osteoporosis.

4.5 Interaction with other medicinal products and other forms of Interaction

A clinical interaction study with midazolam demonstrated that fulvestrant does not inhibit CYP 3A4.

Clinical interaction studies with rifampicin (inducer of CYP 3A4) and ketoconazole (inhibitor of CYP 3A4) showed no clinically relevant change in fulvestrant clearance. Dosage adjustment is therefore not necessary in patients who are co-prescribed fulvestrant and CYP 3A4 inhibitors or inducers.

4.6 Pregnancy and lactation

Faslodex is contraindicated in pregnancy (see 4.3). Fulvestrant has been shown to cross the placenta after single intramuscular doses in rat and rabbit. Studies in animals have shown reproductive toxicity including an increased incidence of foetal abnormalities and deaths (see 5.3). If pregnancy occurs while taking Faslodex the patient must be informed of the potential hazard to the foetus and potential risk for loss of pregnancy.

Fulvestrant is excreted in milk in lactating rats. It is not known whether fulvestrant is excreted in human milk. Considering the potential for serious adverse reactions due to fulvestrant in breast-fed infants, breast-feeding is contraindicated (see 4.3).

4.7 Effects on ability to drive and use machines

Faslodex has no or negligible influence on the ability to drive or use machines. However, during treatment with Faslodex, asthenia has been reported. Therefore caution must be observed by those patients who experience this symptom when driving or operating machinery.

4.8 Undesirable effects

Approximately 47% of patients experienced adverse reactions in the clinical trial programme. However, only 0.9% of patients stopped therapy because of an adverse reaction. The most commonly reported adverse reactions are hot flushes, nausea, and injection site reactions.

The adverse reactions are summarised as follows:

(see Table 1)

4.9 Overdose

There is no human experience of overdosage. Animal studies suggest that no effects other than those related directly or indirectly to anti-oestrogenic activity were evident with higher doses of fulvestrant. If overdose occurs, manage symptomatically.

5. PHARMACOLOGICAL PROPERTIES

5.1 Pharmacodynamic properties

Pharmacotherapeutic group: anti-oestrogen, ATC code: L02BA03

Fulvestrant is an oestrogen receptor antagonist and binds to oestrogen receptors in a competitive manner with an affinity comparable with that of oestradiol. Fulvestrant blocks the trophic actions of oestrogens without itself having any partial agonist (oestrogen-like) activity. The mode of action is associated with down-regulation of oestrogen receptor (ER) protein.

Clinical trials in postmenopausal women with primary breast cancer have shown that fulvestrant significantly down-regulates ER protein in ER positive tumours compared with placebo. There was also a significant decrease in progesterone receptor expression consistent with a lack of intrinsic oestrogen agonist effects.

Effects on advanced breast cancer

Two Phase III clinical trials were completed in a total of 851 postmenopausal women with advanced breast cancer who had disease recurrence on or after adjuvant endocrine therapy or progression following endocrine therapy for advanced disease. 77% of the study population had oestrogen receptor positive breast cancer. These trials compared the safety and efficacy of monthly administration of 250 mg fulvestrant with a third-generation aromatase inhibitor, anastrozole, at a daily dose of 1 mg.

Overall, fulvestrant at the 250 mg monthly dose was at least as effective as anastrozole in terms of time to progression, objective response, and time to death. There were no statistically significant differences in any of these end-points between the two treatment groups. Time to progression was the primary endpoint. Combined analysis of both trials showed that 83% of patients who received fulvestrant progressed, compared with 85% of patients who received anastrozole. The hazard ratio of fulvestrant to anastrozole for time to progression was 0.95 (95% CI 0.82 to 1.10). The objective response rate for fulvestrant was 19.2% compared with 16.5% for anastrozole. The median time to death was 27.4 months for patients treated with fulvestrant and 27.6 months for patients treated with anastrozole. The hazard ratio of fulvestrant to anastrozole for time to death was 1.01 (95% CI 0.86 to 1.19). Analysis of results by ER status showed that the use of fulvestrant should be restricted to patients with ER positive breast cancer.

Effects on the postmenopausal endometrium

Preclinical data suggest that fulvestrant will not have a stimulatory effect on the postmenopausal endometrium. A 2-week study in healthy postmenopausal volunteers showed that compared to placebo, pre-treatment with 250 mg fulvestrant resulted in significantly reduced stimulation of the postmenopausal endometrium, as judged by ultrasound measurement of endometrium thickness, in volunteers treated with 20 micrograms per day ethinyl oestradiol.

There are no data on the long-term effects of fulvestrant on the postmenopausal endometrium. No data are available regarding endometrial morphology.

In two studies with premenopausal patients with benign gynaecologic disease, no significant differences in endometrial thickness were observed (measured with ultrasound) between fulvestrant and placebo. However, the duration of treatment was short (1, and 12 weeks, respectively).

Effects on bone

There are no long-term data on the effect of fulvestrant on bone.

5.2 Pharmacokinetic properties

Absorption:

After administration of Faslodex long-acting intramuscular injection, fulvestrant is slowly absorbed and maximum plasma concentrations are reached after about 7 days. Absorption continues for over one month and monthly administration results in an approximate 2-fold accumulation. Steady-state levels are reached after about 6 doses during monthly injections with the major part of the accumulation achieved after 3-4 doses. The terminal half-life is governed by the absorption rate and was estimated to be 50 days. At steady state, fulvestrant plasma concentrations are maintained within a relatively narrow range with approximately 2- to 3-fold difference between maximum and trough concentrations.

After intramuscular administration, the exposure is approximately dose proportional in the dose range 50 to 250 mg.

Distribution:

Fulvestrant is subject to extensive and rapid distribution. The apparent volume of distribution at steady state is large (approximately 3 to 5 l/kg), which suggests that the compound distribution is largely extravascular. Fulvestrant is highly (99%) bound to plasma proteins. Very low density lipoprotein (VLDL), low density lipoprotein (LDL), and high density lipoprotein (HDL) fractions are the major binding components. Therefore no drug interaction studies were conducted on competitive protein binding. The role of sex hormone-binding globulin has not been determined.

Metabolism:

The metabolism of fulvestrant has not been fully evaluated, but involves combinations of a number of possible biotransformation pathways analogous to those of endogenous steroids (includes 17-ketone, sulphone, 3-sulphate, 3- and 17-glucuronide metabolites). Identified metabolites are either less active or exhibit similar activity to fulvestrant in anti-oestrogen models. Studies using human liver preparations and recombinant human enzymes indicate that CYP 3A4 is the only P450 isoenzyme involved in the oxidation of fulvestrant, however non-P450 routes appear to be more predominant *in vivo*. *In vitro* data suggest that fulvestrant does not inhibit CYP450 isoenzymes.

Elimination:

Fulvestrant is eliminated mainly by metabolism. The major route of excretion is via the faeces with less than 1% being excreted in the urine. Fulvestrant has a high clearance, 11±1.7 ml/min/kg, suggesting a high hepatic extraction ratio.

Special populations:

In a population pharmacokinetic analysis of data from Phase III studies, no difference in fulvestrant pharmacokinetic profile was detected with regard to age (range 33 to 89 years), weight (40-127 kg) or race.

Renal impairment

Mild to moderate impairment of renal function did not influence the pharmacokinetics of fulvestrant to any clinically relevant extent.

Hepatic impairment

The pharmacokinetics of fulvestrant have not been studied in patients with hepatic impairment.

5.3 Preclinical safety data

The acute toxicity of fulvestrant is low.

Faslodex and other formulations of fulvestrant were well tolerated in animal species used in multiple dose studies. Local reactions, including myositis and granulomatoma at the injection site were attributed to the vehicle but the severity of myositis in rabbits increased with fulvestrant, compared to the saline control. In toxicity studies with multiple intramuscular doses of fulvestrant in rats and dogs, the anti-oestrogenic activity of fulvestrant was responsible for most of the effects seen, particularly in the female reproductive system, but also in other organs sensitive to hormones in both sexes.

In dog studies following oral and intravenous administration, effects on the cardiovascular system (slight elevations of the S-T segment of the ECG [oral], and sinus arrest in one dog [intravenous]) were seen. These occurred at exposure levels higher than in patients (C_{max} >40 times) and are likely to be of limited significance for human safety at the clinical dose.

Fulvestrant showed no genotoxic potential.

Fulvestrant showed effects upon reproduction and embryo/foetal development consistent with its anti-oestrogenic activity, at doses similar to the clinical dose. In rats a reversible reduction in female fertility and embryonic survival, dystocia and an increased incidence of foetal abnormalities including tarsal flexure were observed. Rabbits given fulvestrant failed to maintain pregnancy. Increases in placental weight and post-implantation loss of foetuses were seen. There was an increased incidence of foetal variations in rabbits (backwards displacement of the pelvic girdle and 27 pre-sacral vertebrae).

A two-year oncogenicity study in rats (intramuscular administration of Faslodex) showed increased incidence of ovarian benign granulosa cell tumours in female rats at the high dose, 10 mg/rat/15 days and an increased incidence of testicular Leydig cell tumours in males. Induction of such tumours is consistent with pharmacology-related endocrine feedback alterations. These findings are not of clinical relevance for the use of fulvestrant in postmenopausal women with advanced breast cancer.

6. PHARMACEUTICAL PARTICULARS

6.1 List of excipients

Ethanol 96%

Benzyl alcohol

Benzyl benzoate

Castor oil

6.2 Incompatibilities

In the absence of incompatibility studies, this medicinal product must not be mixed with other medicinal products.

6.3 Shelf life

4 years.

6.4 Special precautions for storage

Store at 2°C-8°C (in a refrigerator).

Store in the original package in order to protect from light.

Table 1 The adverse reactions are summarised as follows

Body System/ Frequency	Very Common (>1/10)	Common (>1/100, <1/10)	Uncommon (>1/1000, <1/100
Cardiovascular	• Hot flushes		
Gastrointestinal		• Gastrointestinal disturbance including nausea, vomiting, diarrhoea and anorexia.	
Hepatobiliary disorders		• Elevated liver enzymes, the vast majority <2xULN	
Reproductive and breast			• Vaginal haemorrhage • Vaginal moniliasis • Leukorrhea
Skin		• Rash	• Hypersensitivity reactions, including angioedema and urticaria
Urogenital		• Urinary tract infections	
Vascular		• Venous thromboembolism	
Whole body		• Injection site reactions including transient pain and inflammation in 7% of patients (1% of injections) when given as a single 5 ml injection. • Headache • Asthenia • Back pain	

6.5 Nature and contents of container
One 5 ml clear neutral glass (Type 1) pre-filled syringe with polystyrene plunger rod. The syringe has a nominal content of 5 ml solution and is fitted with a tamper evident closure.

A safety needle (SafetyGlide) for connection to the barrel is also provided.

6.6 Instructions for use and handling
Remove glass syringe barrel from tray and check that it is not damaged.

Peel open the safety needle (SafetyGlide) outer packaging. (For safety needle instructions see below).

Break the seal of the white plastic cover on the syringe Luer connector to remove the cover with the attached rubber tip cap (see Figure 1). Twist to lock the needle to the Luer connector.

Remove needle sheath.

Parenteral solutions must be inspected visually for particulate matter and discolouration prior to administration.

Remove excess gas from the syringe (a small gas bubble may remain). Administer intramuscularly slowly into the buttock.

Immediately activate needle protection device upon withdrawal of the needle from patient by pushing lever arm completely forward until needle tip is fully covered (see Figure 2).

Visually confirm that the lever arm has fully advanced and the needle tip is covered. If unable to activate the safety needle, discard immediately into an approved sharps collector.

SafetyGlideInformation from Becton Dickinson

WARNING: - Do not autoclave safety needle before use. Hands must remain behind the needle at all times during use and disposal.

Directions for Use of safety needle

Peel apart packaging of the safety needle, break the seal of the white plastic cover on the syringe Luer connector and attach the safety needle to the Luer Lock of the syringe by twisting.

Transport filled syringe to point of administration.

Pull shield straight off needle to avoid damaging needle point.

Administer injection following package instruction.

For user convenience, the needle 'bevel up' position is orientated to the lever arm, as shown in Figure 3.

Immediately activate needle protection device upon withdrawal from patient by pushing lever arm completely forward until needle tip is fully covered (Figure 2).

Visually confirm that the lever arm has fully advanced and the needle tip is covered. If unable to activate, discard immediately into an approved sharps collector.

Activation of the protective mechanism may cause minimal splatter of fluid that may remain on the needle after injection.

For greatest safety, use a one-handed technique and activate away from self and others.

After single use, discard in an approved sharps collector in accordance with applicable regulations and institutional policy.

Figure 1

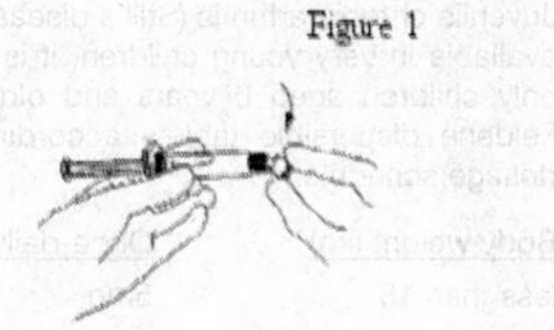

Figure 2

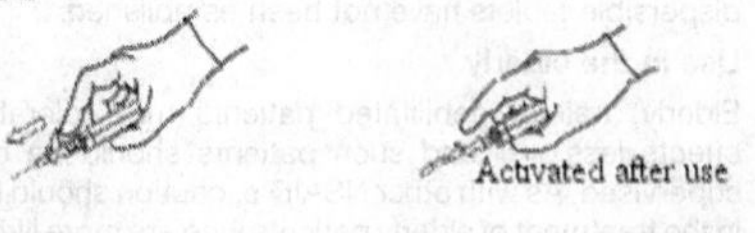

Figure 3

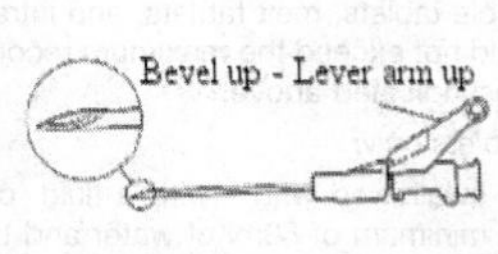

7. MARKETING AUTHORISATION HOLDER
AstraZeneca UK Limited

Alderley Park

Macclesfield

Cheshire

SK10 4TG

United Kingdom

8. MARKETING AUTHORISATION NUMBER(S)
EU/1/03/269/001

9. DATE OF FIRST AUTHORISATION/RENEWAL OF THE AUTHORISATION
10th March 2004

10. DATE OF REVISION OF THE TEXT
6th July 2005

Fasturtec

(sanofi-aventis)

1. NAME OF THE MEDICINAL PRODUCT
Fasturtec ▼1.5 mg/ml powder and solvent for concentrate for solution for infusion.

2. QUALITATIVE AND QUANTITATIVE COMPOSITION
After reconstitution, one ml of Fasturtec concentrate contains 1.5 mg rasburicase.

Fasturtec is a recombinant urate-oxidase enzyme produced by genetically modified *Saccharomyces cerevisiae* strain. Rasburicase is a tetrameric protein with identical subunits of a molecular mass of about 34 kDa.

1 mg corresponds to 18.2 EAU*.

*One enzyme activity unit (EAU) corresponds to the enzyme activity that converts 1 μmol of uric acid into allantoin per minute under the operating conditions described: +30°C±1°C TEA pH8.9 buffer.

For excipients, see 6.1

3. PHARMACEUTICAL FORM
Powder and solvent for concentrate for solution for infusion.

The reconstituted solution is clear and colourless.

4. CLINICAL PARTICULARS

4.1 Therapeutic indications
Treatment and prophylaxis of acute hyperuricaemia, in order to prevent acute renal failure, in patients with haematological malignancy with a high tumor burden and at risk of a rapid tumor lysis or shrinkage at initiation of chemotherapy.

4.2 Posology and method of administration
Fasturtec should be administered under the supervision of a physician trained in chemotherapy of haematological malignancies.

Fasturtec is to be used immediately prior to and during the initiation of chemotherapy only, as at the present, there is insufficient data to recommend multiple treatment courses.

The recommended dose for Fasturtec is 0.20 mg/kg/day. Fasturtec is administered as a once daily 30 minute intravenous infusion in 50 ml of a sodium chloride 9 mg/ml (0.9%) solution (see section 6.6 «Instructions for use and handling»).

The duration of treatment with Fasturtec may vary between 5 and 7 days.

No dose adjustment is necessary for special populations (renally or hepatically impaired patients).

Administration of rasburicase does not require any change in the timing or schedule of initiation of cytoreductive chemotherapy.

Rasburicase solution should be infused over 30 minutes. Rasburicase solution should be infused through a different line than that used for infusion of chemotherapeutic agents to prevent any possible drug incompatibility. If use of a separate line is not possible, the line should be flushed out with saline solution between infusion of chemotherapeutic agents and rasburicase. For instruction on use, see section 6.6 «Instruction for use and handling».

Because rasburicase may degrade uric acid in vitro, special precautions must be used during sample handling for plasma uric acid measurements, see section 6.6 «Instruction for use and handling».

4.3 Contraindications
Hypersensitivity to uricases or any of the excipients.

G6PD deficiency and other cellular metabolic disorders known to cause haemolytic anaemia. Hydrogen peroxide is a by-product of the conversion of uric acid to allantoin. In order to prevent possible haemolytic anaemia induced by hydrogen peroxide, rasburicase is contraindicated in patients with these disorders.

4.4 Special warnings and special precautions for use
Rasburicase like other proteins, has the potential to induce allergic responses in humans. Clinical experience with Fasturtec demonstrates that patients should be closely monitored for the onset of allergic-type undesirable effects, especially severe hypersensitivity reactions including anaphylaxis (see section 4.8 «Undesirable effects»). In such cases, treatment should immediately and permanently be discontinued and appropriate therapy initiated.

Caution should be used in patients with a history of atopic allergies.

At present, there is insufficient data available on patients being retreated to recommend multiple treatment courses.

Anti-rasburicase antibodies have been detected in treated patients and healthy volunteers administered rasburicase.

Methaemoglobinaemia has been reported in patients receiving Fasturtec. Fasturtec should immediately and permanently be discontinued in patients having developed methaemoglobinaemia, and appropriate measures initiated (see section 4.8 Undesirable Effects).

Haemolysis has been reported in patients receiving Fasturtec. In such case, treatment should immediately and permanently be discontinued and appropriate measures initiated (see section 4.8 Undesirable Effects).

Administration of Fasturtec reduces the uric acid levels to below normal levels and by this mechanism reduces the chance of development of renal failure due to precipitation of uric acid crystals in renal tubules as a consequence of hyperuricaemia. Tumor lysis can also result in hyperphosphataemia, hyperkalaemia and hypocalcaemia. Fasturtec is not directly effective in the treatment of these abnormalities. Therefore, patients must be monitored closely.

Fasturtec has not been investigated in the patients with hyperuricemia in the context of myeloproliferative disorders.

There is no data available to recommend the sequential use of Fasturtec and allopurinol.

To ensure accurate measurement of uric acid plasma level during treatment with Fasturtec, a strict sample handling procedure must be followed (see section 6.6 Instructions for use and handling).

4.5 Interaction with other medicinal products and other forms of Interaction
No metabolism studies have been carried out. Rasburicase being an enzyme itself, it would be an unlikely candidate for drug-drug interactions.

4.6 Pregnancy and lactation
For rasburicase no clinical data on exposed pregnancies are available. Animal studies with respect to effects on pregnancy, embryonic/fœtal development, parturition and postnatal development have not been performed (see section 5.3. «Preclinical safety data»). The potential risk for humans is unknown. Fasturtec should not be used during pregnancy or breast-feeding women.

It is unknown whether rasburicase is excreted in human milk.

4.7 Effects on ability to drive and use machines
No studies on the effect on the ability to drive and use machines have been performed.

4.8 Undesirable effects
Fasturtec is concomitantly administered as supportive care to cytoreductive chemotherapy of advanced malignancies, the causality of adverse events is therefore difficult to assess due to the significant burden of adverse events expected from the underlying disease and its treatment.

The most significant drug-related adverse events were allergic reactions, mainly rashes. Cases of bronchospasm (< 1%) and severe hypersensitivity reactions, including anaphylaxis (< 1%) have also been attributed to Fasturtec. Haematological disorders such as haemolysis and methaemoglobinaemia are uncommonly caused by Fasturtec. The enzymatic digestion of uric acid to allantoin by rasburicase produces hydrogen peroxide and haemolytic anaemia or methaemoglobinaemia have been observed in certain at risk populations such as those with G6PD deficiency. In clinical trials involving 347 subjects, 3 subjects (< 1%) developed haemolytic anaemia, one of these subjects was documented to have G6PD deficiency.

In addition, grade 3 or 4 adverse reactions possibly attributed to Fasturtec and reported in the clinical trials, are listed below, by system organ class and by frequency. Frequencies are defined as: common (> 1/100, ≤ 1/10), uncommon (> 1/1000, ≤ 1/100).

	Common	Uncommon
Gastro-intestinal disorders	Vomiting Nausea	Diarrhoea
Central nervous system disorders		Headache
Body as a whole	Fever	

4.9 Overdose
No cases of overdosage with Fasturtec have been reported. In view of the mechanism of action of Fasturtec, an overdose will lead to low or undetectable plasma uric acid concentrations and increased production of hydrogen peroxide. Thus patients suspected of receiving an overdose should be monitored for haemolysis, and general supportive measures should be initiated as no specific antidote for Fasturtec has been identified.

5. PHARMACOLOGICAL PROPERTIES

5.1 Pharmacodynamic properties
ATC code for rasburicase: V03AF07

In humans, uric acid is the final step in the catabolic pathway of purines. The acute increase in plasma levels of uric acid subsequent to the lysis of large numbers of malignant cells and during cytoreductive chemotherapy may lead to impairment of renal function and renal failure resulting from the precipitation of crystals of uric acid in renal tubules. Rasburicase is a highly potent uricolytic agent that catalyses enzymatic oxidation of uric acid into allantoin, a water soluble product, easily excreted by the kidneys in the urine.

The enzymatic oxidation of uric acid leads to stoichiometric formation of hydrogen peroxide. The increased of hydrogen peroxide over ambient levels can be eliminated by endogenous antioxidants and the only increased risk is for haemolysis in G6PD deficient and inherited anaemia patients.

In healthy volunteers, a marked dose-related decrease in plasma uric acid levels was observed across the dose range 0.05 mg/kg to 0.20 mg/kg of Fasturtec.

A randomised comparative phase III study, using the recommended dose, showed a significantly more rapid onset of action of Fasturtec in comparison with allopurinol. At 4 hours post first dose, there was a significant difference in the mean percentage change from baseline plasma uric acid concentration ($p<0.0001$) in the Fasturtec group (-86.0%) compared to that for the allopurinol group (-12.1%).

Time to first confirmation of normal levels of uric acid in hyperuricaemic patients is four hours for Fasturtec and 24 hours for allopurinol. In addition this rapid control of uric acid in this population is accompanied by improvements in renal function. In turn, this allows efficient excretion of the serum phosphate load preventing further deterioration of renal function from calcium/phosphorus precipitation.

5.2 Pharmacokinetic properties

After infusion of rasburicase at a dose of 0.20 mg/kg/day, steady state is achieved at day 2-3. No unexpected accumulation of rasburicase was observed. In patients, the volume of distribution ranged from 110 - 127 ml/kg, which is comparable to the physiological vascular volume. Clearance of rasburicase was ca. 3.5 ml/h/kg and the elimination half-life ca. 19 hours. The patients included in the pharmacokinetic studies were mainly children and adolescents. Based upon these limited data, it seems that clearance is increased (ca. 35%) in children and adolescents compared to adults, resulting in a lower systemic exposure.

Rasburicase is a protein, and therefore: 1) not expected to bind to proteins, 2) expected that metabolic degradation will follow the pathways of other proteins, i.e. peptide hydrolysis, 3) unlikely to be candidate for drug-drug interactions.

Renal elimination of rasburicase is considered to be a minor pathway for rasburicase clearance. As metabolism is expected to occur by peptide hydrolysis, an impaired liver function is not expected to affect the pharmacokinetics.

5.3 Preclinical safety data

Preclinical data reveal no special hazard for humans based on conventional studies of safety pharmacology, repeated dose toxicity and genotoxicity. The interpretation of the preclinical studies is hampered due to the presence of endogenous urate oxidase in standard animal models.

6. PHARMACEUTICAL PARTICULARS

6.1 List of excipients

Powder:

alanine

mannitol

disodium phosphate

sodium dihydrogen phosphate.

Solvent:

Poloxamer 188

water for injections.

6.2 Incompatibilities

This medicinal product must not be mixed with other medicinal products.

Rasburicase solution should be infused through a different line than that used for infusion of chemotherapeutic agents to prevent any possible drug incompatibility. If use of a separate line is not possible, the line should be flushed out with saline solution between chemotherapeutic agent infusions and rasburicase.

No filter should be used for infusion.

Do not use any glucose solution for dilution due to potential incompatibility.

6.3 Shelf life

3 years

- After reconstitution or dilution an immediate use is recommended. However, the in-use stability has been demonstrated for 24 hours between +2°C and 8°C.

6.4 Special precautions for storage

Powder in vial: store at 2°C - 8° C (in a refrigerator).

Store in the original package in order to protect from light.

Do not freeze.

6.5 Nature and contents of container

Fasturtec is supplied as a pack of:

3 vials of 1.5 mg rasburicase and 3 ampoules of 1 ml solvent. The powder is supplied in 3 ml clear glass (type I) vial with a rubber stopper and the solvent in a 2 ml clear glass (type I) ampoule.

1 vial of 7.5 mg rasburicase and 1 ampoule of 5 ml solvent. The powder is supplied in 10 ml clear glass (type I) vial with a rubber stopper and the solvent in a 5 ml clear glass (type I) ampoule.

6.6 Instructions for use and handling

Rasburicase must be reconstituted with the entire volume of the supplied solvent ampoule (1.5 mg rasburicase vial to be reconstituted with the 1 ml solvent ampoule; 7.5 mg rasburicase vial to be reconstituted with the 5 ml solvent ampoule). Reconstitution results in a solution with a concentration of 1.5 mg/ml rasburicase to be further diluted with sodium chloride 9 mg/ml (0.9%) intravenous solution.

Reconstitution of the solution:

Add the content of one ampoule of solvent to one vial containing rasburicase and mix by swirling very gently under controlled and validated aseptic conditions.

Do not shake.

Inspect visually prior to use. Only clear solutions without particles should be used.

For single-use only, any unused solution should be discarded.

The solvent contains no preservative. Therefore the reconstituted solution should be diluted under controlled and validated aseptic conditions.

Dilution before infusion:

The required volume of the reconstituted solution depends on the patient's body weight. The use of several vials may be necessary to obtain the quantity of rasburicase required for one administration. The required volume of the reconstituted solution, taken from one or more vials, is to be further diluted with sodium chloride 9 mg/ml (0.9%) solution to make a total volume of 50 ml. The concentration of rasburicase in the final solution for infusion depends on the patient's body weight.

The reconstituted solution contains no preservative. Therefore the diluted solution should be infused immediately.

Infusion:

The final solution should be infused over 30 minutes.

Sample handling:

If it is necessary to monitor a patient's uric acid level, a strict sample-handling procedure must be followed to minimise *ex vivo* degradation of the analyte. Blood must be collected into pre-chilled tubes containing heparin anticoagulant. Samples must be immersed in an ice/water bath. Plasma samples should immediately be prepared by centrifugation in a pre-cooled centrifuge (4°C). Finally, plasma must be maintained in an ice/water bath and analysed for uric acid within 4 hours.

7. MARKETING AUTHORISATION HOLDER

SANOFI-SYNTHELABO

174, avenue de France

F - 75013 Paris, France

8. MARKETING AUTHORISATION NUMBER(S)

EU/1/00/170/001-002

9. DATE OF FIRST AUTHORISATION/RENEWAL OF THE AUTHORISATION

February 2001

10. DATE OF REVISION OF THE TEXT

June 2003

Legal Category: POM

Feldene Capsules, Dispersible Tablets, Intramuscular Injection, and Melt Tablets

(Pfizer Limited)

1. NAME OF THE MEDICINAL PRODUCT

FELDENE™ CAPSULES

FELDENE™ DISPERSIBLE TABLETS

FELDENE™ I.M. INTRAMUSCULAR INJECTION

FELDENE™ MELT

2. QUALITATIVE AND QUANTITATIVE COMPOSITION

Active Ingredient: piroxicam

Capsules: piroxicam 10mg or 20mg (anhydrous)

Dispersible Tablets: piroxicam 10mg or 20mg (anhydrous)

I.M.: the intramuscular injection contains 1ml of piroxicam solution (20mg/ml) in ampoules of 1ml

Melt tablets: piroxicam 20mg

3. PHARMACEUTICAL FORM

Capsules (10mg and 20mg): capsules for oral administration.

Dispersible Tablets (10mg or 20mg): tablets for oral administration.

I.M.: solution for intramuscular injection.

Melt tablets: fast dissolving dosage form (tablet).

4. CLINICAL PARTICULARS

4.1 Therapeutic indications

Capsules, Dispersible tablets, Melt tablets: Feldene is a non-steroidal anti-inflammatory agent indicated for a variety of conditions requiring anti-inflammatory and/or analgesic activity, such as rheumatoid arthritis, osteoarthritis (arthrosis, degenerative joint disease) ankylosing spondylitis, acute musculo-skeletal disorders and acute gout. Pain following orthopaedic, dental and other minor surgery.

Dispersible tablets only:Children with definitely diagnosed juvenile chronic arthritis (Still's disease).

I.M. only: Feldene is a non-steroidal anti-inflammatory drug indicated for a variety of conditions requiring anti-inflammatory and/or analgesic activity. Feldene I.M. is indicated for initial treatment of acute conditions (acute gout, acute musculoskeletal disorders) and acute exacerbations of chronic conditions (rheumatoid arthritis, osteoarthritis, ankylosing spondylitis). Pain following orthopaedic, dental and other minor surgery.

4.2 Posology and method of administration

IM only: Feldene I.M. is for intramuscular administration only

Therapy should be initiated at the lowest recommended dose, especially in elderly patients.

Adults

Rheumatoid arthritis, osteoarthritis, ankylosing spondylitis: The recommended starting dose is 20mg given as a single dose. The majority of patients will be maintained on 20mg daily. A relatively small group of patients may require up to 30mg daily given in single or divided doses. Administration of doses exceeding 20mg daily (or more than several days duration) carries an increased risk of gastro-intestinal side-effects.

Acute gout: Therapy should be initiated by a single dose of 40mg followed by the next 4 to 6 days with 40mg daily, given in a single or divided daily dosage. Feldene is not indicated for the long-term management of gout.

Acute musculo-skeletal disorders: Therapy should be initiated with 40mg daily for the first 2 days, given in single or divided doses. For the remainder of the 7 to 14 day treatment period, the dose should be reduced to 20mg daily.

Post-operative pain

Dental and other minor surgery: The recommended starting and maintenance dose is 20mg once daily. Doses of 40mg daily, in single or divided doses, for the first two days of treatment may provide faster onset of action.

Orthopaedic surgery: Therapy should be initiated with 40mg daily for the first two days, given in single or divided doses. For the remainder of the treatment period, the dose should be reduced to 20mg daily.

Children

Capsules, IM and Melt tablets:

Dosage recommendations and indications for use in children other than in juvenile chronic arthritis using Feldene Dispersible Tablets have not been established.

Dispersible Tablets only:

Juvenile chronic arthritis (Still's disease): As little data are available in very young children, it is recommended that only children aged 6 years and older are treated with Feldene dispersible tablets according to the following dosage schedule:

Body weight (kg)	Once-daily dose
less than 15	5mg
16 - 25	10mg
26 - 45	15mg
46 and above	20mg

Dosage recommendations and indications for use in children other than in juvenile chronic arthritis using Feldene dispersible tablets have not been established.

Use in the elderly

Elderly, frail or debilitated patients may tolerate side-effects less well and such patients should be carefully supervised. As with other NSAID's, caution should be used in the treatment of elderly patients who are more likely to be suffering from impaired renal, hepatic or cardiac function.

Combined administration

The total daily dosage of Feldene administered as capsules, dispersible tablets, melt tablets, and intramuscular injection, should not exceed the maximum recommended daily dosage as indicated above.

Dispersible Tablets only:

These can be swallowed whole with a fluid, or may be dispersed in a minimum of 50ml of water and then swallowed.

I.M. only:

The dosage of Feldene I.M. intramuscular injection is identical to the dosage of oral Feldene. For continuation of treatment, oral (capsules or dispersible tablets) or suppository dose forms should be used. Feldene I.M. intramuscular injection should be administered by deep intramuscular injection into the upper, outer quadrant of the buttock. Feldene I.M. intramuscular injection should not be administered intravenously.

Melt tablets only:

The fast dissolving dosage form may be swallowed with water, or placed on the tongue to disperse and then swallowed with the saliva. The fast dissolving dosage form dissolves almost instantly in the mouth in the presence of water or saliva.

4.3 Contraindications

1. Active peptic ulceration or history of recurrent ulceration.

2. Feldene should not be used in those patients who have previously shown a hypersensitivity to the drug. The potential exists for cross-sensitivity to aspirin and other non-steroidal anti-inflammatory drugs.

3. Feldene should not be given to patients in whom aspirin and other non-steroidal anti-inflammatory drugs induce the symptoms of asthma, nasal polyps, angioedema or urticaria.

4.4 Special warnings and special precautions for use

Drug administration should be closely supervised in patients with a history of upper gastro-intestinal disease. Feldene should be withdrawn if peptic ulceration or gastro-intestinal bleeding occurs.

Feldene should be used with caution in patients with or a history of bronchial asthma (see also 'Contra-indications').

Feldene should be used with caution in patients with renal, hepatic and cardiac impairment. In rare cases, non-steroidal anti-inflammatory drugs may cause interstitial nephritis, glomerulitis, papillary necrosis and the nephrotic syndrome. Such agents inhibit the synthesis of the prostaglandin which plays a supportive role in the maintenance of renal perfusion in patients whose renal blood flow and blood volume are decreased. In these patients, administration of a non-steroidal anti-inflammatory drug may precipitate overt renal decompensation, which is typically followed by recovery to pretreatment state upon discontinuation of non-steroidal anti-inflammatory therapy. Patients at greatest risk of such a reaction are those with congestive heart failure, liver cirrhosis, nephrotic syndrome and overt renal disease, such patients should be carefully monitored whilst receiving NSAID therapy. Because of reports of adverse eye findings with non-steroidal anti-inflammatory drugs, it is recommended that patients who develop visual complaints during treatment with Feldene have ophthalmic evaluation.

Melt tablets only:

Patients with phenylketonuria:

Due to aspartame content of Feldene Melt, each tablet contains 0.07mg phenylalanine. Each 20mg tablet contains 0.14mg phenylalanine.

4.5 Interaction with other medicinal products and other forms of Interaction

Antacids: Concomitant administration of antacids had no effect on piroxicam plasma levels.

Anticoagulants: As with other non-steroidal anti-inflammatory drugs, bleeding has been reported rarely when Feldene has been administered to patients on coumarin-type anticoagulants. Patients should be monitored closely if Feldene oral anticoagulants are administered together.

Aspirin and other Non-Steroidal Anti-Inflammatory Drugs: Feldene, like other non-steroidal anti-inflammatory drugs decreases platelet aggregation and prolongs bleeding time. This effect should be kept in mind when bleeding times are determined.

As with other non-steroidal anti-inflammatory drugs, the use of Feldene with aspirin or the concomitant use of two non-steroidal anti-inflammatory drugs is not recommended because data are inadequate to demonstrate that the combination produces greater improvement than that with the drug alone and the potential for adverse reactions is increased.

Studies in man have shown that the concomitant administration of Feldene and aspirin resulted in a reduction of plasma levels of piroxicam to about 80% of the normal values.

Cimetidine: Results of two separate studies indicate a slight but significant increase in absorption of piroxicam following cimetidine administration but no significant changes in elimination rate constants or half-life. The small increase in absorption is unlikely to be clinically significant.

Digoxin, Digitoxin: Concurrent therapy with Feldene and digoxin, or Feldene and digitoxin, did not affect the plasma levels of either drug.

Diuretics: Non-steroidal anti-inflammatory drugs may cause sodium, potassium and fluid retention and may interfere with the natriuretic action of diuretic agents. These properties should be kept in mind when treating patients with compromised cardiac function or hypertension since they may be responsible for the worsening of those conditions.

Highly protein-bound drugs: Feldene is highly protein-bound and therefore might be expected to displace other protein-bound drugs. The physician should closely monitor patients for change when administering Feldene to patients on highly protein-bound drugs.

Lithium: Non-steroidal anti-inflammatory drugs, including Feldene, have been reported to increase steady state plasma lithium levels. It is recommended that these levels are monitored when initiating, adjusting and discontinuing Feldene.

Feldene, like other non-steroidal anti-inflammatory drugs, may interact with the following drugs / classes of therapeutic agents:

Antihypertensives -antagonism of the hypotensive effect

Methotrexate - reduced excretion of methotrexate, possibly leading to acute toxicity

Cyclosporin - possible increased risk of nephrotoxicity

Corticosteroids - increased risk of gastro-intestinal bleeding and ulceration

Quinolone antibiotics - possible increased risk of convulsions

Mifepristone - NSAIDs could interfere with mifepristone-mediated termination of pregnancy

4.6 Pregnancy and lactation

Use in pregnancy: Although no teratogenic effects were seen in animal testing, the safety of Feldene during pregnancy or during lactation has not yet been established. Feldene inhibits prostaglandin synthesis and release through a reversible inhibition of the cyclo-oxygenase enzyme. This effect, as with other non-steroidal anti-inflammatory drugs, has been associated with an increased incidence of dystocia and delayed parturition in pregnant animals when drug administration was continued in late pregnancy. Non-steroidal anti-inflammatory drugs are also known to induce closure of the ductus arteriosus in infants.

Nursing mothers: A study indicates that piroxicam appears in the breast milk at about 1% to 3% of the maternal plasma concentrations. No accumulation of piroxicam occurred in milk relative to that in plasma during treatment for up to 52 days. Feldene is not recommended for use in nursing mothers as clinical safety has not been established.

4.7 Effects on ability to drive and use machines

None known.

4.8 Undesirable effects

Gastro-intestinal: These are the most commonly encountered side-effects but in most instances do not interfere with the course of therapy. They include stomatitis, anorexia, epigastric distress, gastritis, nausea, vomiting, constipation, abdominal discomfort, flatulance, diarrhoea, abdominal pain and indigestion, rare cases of pancreatitis have been reported.

Objective evaluations of gastric mucosa appearances and intestinal blood loss show that 20mg/day of Feldene administered either in single or divided doses is significantly less irritating to the gastro-intestinal tract than aspirin. Peptic ulceration, perforation and gastro-intestinal bleeding (including haematemesis and melaena) in rare cases fatal, have been reported with Feldene.

Some epidemiological studies have suggested that piroxicam is associated with higher risk of gastro-intestinal adverse reactions compared with some NSAIDs, but this has not been confirmed in all studies. Administration of doses exceeding 20mg daily (of more than several days duration) carries an increased risk of gastro-intestinal side-effects, but they may also occur with lower doses. See section 4.2 Posology and method of administration.

Oedema: As with other non-steroidal anti-inflammatory drugs, oedema, mainly of the ankle, has been reported in a small percentage of patients and the possibility of precipitating congestive heart failure in elderly patients or those with compromised cardiac function should therefore be borne in mind.

CNS: Dizziness, headache, somnolence, insomnia, depression, nervousness, hallucinations, mood alterations, dream abnormalities, mental confusion, paraesthesiae and vertigo have been reported rarely.

Dermal hypersensitivity: Rash and pruritis. Onycholysis and analopoecia have rarely been reported. Photosensitivity reactions occur infrequently. As with other non-steroidal anti-inflammatory drugs, toxic epidermal necrolysis (Lyell's disease) and Stevens-Johnson syndrome may develop in rare cases. Vesiculo bullous reactions have been reported rarely.

Hypersensitivity reactions: Hypersensitivity reactions such as anaphylaxis, bronchospasm, urticaria/angioneurotic oedema, vasculitis and serum sickness have been reported rarely.

Renal function: Interstitial nephritis, nephrotic syndrome, renal failure and renal papillary necrosis have been reported rarely.

Haematological: Decreases in haemaglobin and haematocrit, unassociated with obvious gastro-intestinal bleeding have occurred. Anaemia, thrombocytopenia and non-thrombocytopenia purpura (Henoch-Schoenlein), leucopenia and eosinophilia have been reported. Cases of aplastic anaemia, haemolytic anaemia and epistaxis have rarely been reported.

Liver function: Changes in various liver function parameters have been observed. As with most other non-steroidal anti-inflammatory drugs, some patients may develop increased serum transaminase levels during treatment with Feldene. Severe hepatic reactions including jaundice and cases of fatal hepatitis have been reported with Feldene. Although such reactions are rare, if abnormal liver function tests persist or worsen, if clinical symptoms consistent with liver disease develop, or if systemic manifestations occur e.g.eosinophilia, rash etc., Feldene should be discontinued.

Other: The following have been reported rarely, palpitations and dyspnoea, anecdotal cases of positive ANA, anecdotal cases of hearing abnormalities, metabolic abnormalities such as hypoglycaemia, hyperglycaemia, weight increase or decrease. Swollen eyes, blurred vision and eye irritations have been reported. Routine ophthalmoscopy and slit-lamp examination have revealed no evidence of ocular changes. Malaise and tinnitus may occur.

I.M. only:

Intramuscular: Transient pain upon injection has occasionally been reported. Local adverse reactions (burning sensations) or tissue damage (sterile abscess formation, fatty tissue necrosis) may occasionally occur at the site of injection.

4.9 Overdose

In the event of overdosage with Feldene, supportive and symptomatic therapy is indicated. Studies indicate that administration of activated charcoal may result in reduced re-absorption of piroxicam, thus reducing the total amount of active drug available.

Although there are no studies to date, haemodialysis is probably not useful in enhancing elimination of piroxicam since the drug is highly protein bound.

5. PHARMACOLOGICAL PROPERTIES

5.1 Pharmacodynamic properties

Capsules, Dispersible Tablets and Melt tablets:

Piroxicam is a non-steroidal anti-inflammatory agent which also possesses analgesic and antipyretic properties. Oedema, erythema, tissue proliferation, fever and pain can all be inhibited in laboratory animals by the administration of piroxicam. It is effective regardless of the aetiology of the inflammation. While its mode of action is not fully understood, independent studies *in vitro* as well as *in vivo* have shown that piroxicam interacts at several steps in the immune and inflammation responses through:

Inhibition of prostanoid synthesis, including prostaglandins, through a reversible inhibition of the cyclo-oxygenase enzyme.

Inhibition of neutrophil aggregation.

Inhibition of polymorphonuclear cell and monocyte migration to the area of inflammation.

Inhibition of lyosomal enzyme release from stimulated leucocytes.

Reduction of both systemic and synovial fluid rheumatoid factor production in patients with seropositive rheumatoid arthritis.

It is established that piroxicam does not act by pituitary-adrenal axis stimulation. In-vitro studies have not revealed any negative effects on cartilage metabolism.

I.M. only:

Feldene is a non-steroidal anti-inflammatory agent useful in the treatment of inflammatory conditions. Although the mode of action for this agent is not precisely understood, Feldene inhibits prostaglandin synthesis and release through a reversible inhibition of the cyclo-oxygenase enzyme.

Transient pain upon injection has occasionally been reported. Local adverse reactions (burning sensations) or tissue damage (sterile abscess formation, fatty tissue necrosis) may occasionally occur at the site of injection.

5.2 Pharmacokinetic properties

Capsules, Dispersible Tablets and Melt tablets:

Piroxicam is well absorbed following oral administration. With food there is a slight delay in the rate but not the extent of absorption following administration. The plasma half-life is approximately 50 hours in man and stable plasma concentrations are maintained throughout the day on once-daily dosage. Continuous treatment with 20mg/day for periods of 1 year produces similar blood levels to those seen once steady state is first achieved.

Drug plasma concentrations are proportional for 10 and 20mg doses and generally peak within 3 to 5 hours after medication. A single 20mg dose generally produces peak piroxicam plasma levels of 1.5 to 2 microgram/ml while maximum plasma concentrations, after repeated daily ingestion of 20mg piroxicam, usually stabilise at 3 to 8 microgram/ml. Most patients approximate steady state plasma levels within 7 to 12 days.

Treatment with a loading dose regimen of 40mg daily for the first 2 days followed by 20mg daily thereafter allows a high percentage (approximately 76%) of steady state levels to be achieved immediately following the second dose. Steady state levels, area under the curves and elimination half-life are similar to that following a 20mg daily dose regimen.

A multiple dose comparative study of the bioavailability of the injectable forms with the oral capsule has shown that after intramuscular administration of piroxicam, plasma levels are significantly higher than those obtained after ingestion of capsules during the 45 minutes following administration the first day, during 30 minutes the second day and 15 minutes the seventh day. Bioequivalence exists between the two dosage forms.

A multiple dose comparative study of the pharmacokinetics and the bioavailability of Feldene FDDF with the oral capsule has shown that after once daily administration for 14 days, the mean plasma piroxicam concentration time profiles for capsules and Feldene FDDF were nearly superimposable. There were no significant differences between the mean steady state C_{max} values, C_{min} values, T½, or T_{max} values. This study concluded that Feldene FDDF (Fast Dissolving Dosage Form) is bioequivalent to the capsule after once daily dosing. Single dose studies have demonstrated bioequivalence as well when the tablet is taken with or without water.

Piroxicam is extensively metabolised and less than 5% of the daily dose is excreted unchanged in urine and faeces. One important metabolic pathway is hydroxylation of the pyridyl ring of the piroxicam side-chain, followed by conjugation with glucuronic acid and urinary elimination.

I.M. only:

Feldene I.M. and Feldene capsules are bioequivalent. However, Feldene I.M. provides significantly higher plasma levels of piroxicam during the first 45 minutes on the first day and 30 minutes on the second day.

The plasma half-life is approximately 50 hours in man and stable plasma concentrations are maintained throughout the day on once-daily dosage.

Feldene is extensively metabolised and less than 5% of the daily dose is excreted unchanged in urine and faeces. One important metabolic pathway is hydroxyiation of the pyridyl ring of the piroxicam side chain followed by conjugation with glucaronic acid and urinary elimination.

6. PHARMACEUTICAL PARTICULARS

6.1 List of excipients

Capsules 10mg and 20mg: lactose Ph.Eur., maize starch Ph.Eur., magnesium stearate NF, sodium lauryl sulphate Ph.Eur. 10mg capsule shell - cap (scarlet opaque) and body (powder blue opaque) gelatin, titanium dioxide (E171), indigocarmine (E132). The cap also contains erythrosine (E127). 20mg capsule shell - (cap and body scarlet opaque) gelatin, titanium dioxide (E171), indigocarmine (E132), erythrosine (E127).

Dispersible Tablets 10mg and 20mg: lactose Ph.Eur, microcrystalline cellulose NF, hydroxypropyl cellulose and sodium stearyl fumarate FCC.

I.M. Intramuscular Injection: sodium dihydrogen phosphate Ph.Eur., nicotinamide Ph.Eur, propylene glycol Ph.Eur, ethanol BP, benzyl alcohol Ph.Eur, sodium hydroxide BP, hydrochloric acid Ph.Eur, water for injection Ph.Eur.

Melt tablets: gelatin USNF., mannitol Ph.Eur., aspartame USNF., citric acid Ph.Eur., purified water Ph.Eur.

6.2 Incompatibilities

None stated.

6.3 Shelf life

Capsules	36 months
Dispersible Tablets	36 months
I.M. Intramuscular Injection	48 months
Melt tablets	60 months

6.4 Special precautions for storage

Capsules, Dispersible Tablets:

Store below 30°C.

I.M., Melt tablets:

Store below 25°C.

6.5 Nature and contents of container

Capsules 10mg: original pack of 56 capsules contained in a white HDPE bottle with a blue round ribbed cap.

Capsules 20mg: original pack of 28 capsules contained in a white HDPE bottle with a blue round ribbed cap. Physicians sample: 5 capsules contained in a light blue HDPE bottle with a blue round ribbed cap.

Dispersible Tablets 10mg: original pack of 56 tablets contained in a white HDPE screw capped bottle with cap.

Dispersible Tablets 20mg: original pack of 28 tablets contained in a white HDPE screw capped bottle with cap.

I.M.: Type I, 2ml amber glass ampoules containing 1ml.

Melt tablets 20mg: blister strip PVC/PVdC and paper foil laminate. Each pack contains 28 units.

6.6 Instructions for use and handling

No special requirements.

7. MARKETING AUTHORISATION HOLDER

Pfizer Limited

Ramsgate Road

Sandwich

Kent

CT13 9NJ

United Kingdom

8. MARKETING AUTHORISATION NUMBER(S)

Capsules 10mg	PL 00057/0145
Capsules 20mg	PL 00057/0146
Dispersible tablets 10mg	PL 00057/0240
Dispersible tablets 20mg	PL 00057/0242
I.M. intramuscular injection 20mg/ml	PL 00057/0320
Melt tablets 20mg	PL 00057/0352

9. DATE OF FIRST AUTHORISATION/RENEWAL OF THE AUTHORISATION

Capsules 10mg	07/02/96
Capsules 20mg	07/02/96
Dispersible Tablets 10mg	09/02/00
Dispersible Tablets 20mg	09/02/00
I.M. intramuscular injection 20mg/ml	11/02/00
Melt tablets 20mg	09/02/00

10. DATE OF REVISION OF THE TEXT

August 2002

LEGAL CATEGORY

POM

Ref (UK): Fe 3_0

Feldene Gel

(Pfizer Limited)

1. NAME OF THE MEDICINAL PRODUCT

FELDENE GEL

FELDENE SPORTS GEL

FELDENE GEL STARTER PACK.

2. QUALITATIVE AND QUANTITATIVE COMPOSITION

Active ingredient: Piroxicam

The Gel contains 5mg piroxicam in each gram in tubes of 7.5g - Feldene Gel starter Pack, 30g - Feldene Sports Gel, 60g and 112g - Feldene Gel.

3. PHARMACEUTICAL FORM

Gel for topical application.

4. CLINICAL PARTICULARS

4.1 Therapeutic indications

Feldene Gel is a non-steroidal anti-inflammatory agent indicated for a variety of conditions characterised by pain and inflammation, or stiffness. It is effective in the treatment of osteoarthritis of superficial joints such as the knee, acute musculoskeletal injuries, periarthritis, epicondylitis, tendinitis, and tenosynovitis.

4.2 Posology and method of administration

Dosage

Adults Feldene Gel, Feldene Sports Gel and Feldene Gel Starter Pack are for external use only. No occlusive dressings should be employed. Apply 1g of Gel, corresponding to 3cms, and rub into the affected site three to four times daily leaving no residual material on the skin. Therapy should be reviewed after 4 weeks.

Use in Children(See under 'Special warnings and special precautions for use').

Use in the Elderly(See under 'Special warnings and special precautions for use').

4.3 Contraindications

Feldene Gel, Feldene Sports Gel and Feldene Gel Starter Pack should not be used in those patients who have previously shown a hypersensitivity to the Gel or piroxicam in any of its forms. The potential exists for cross sensitivity to aspirin and other non-steroidal anti-inflammatory agents. Feldene Gel, Feldene Sports Gel and Feldene Gel Starter Pack should not be given to patients in whom aspirin and other non-steroidal anti-inflammatory agents induce the symptoms of asthma, nasal polyps, angioneurotic oedema or urticaria.

4.4 Special warnings and special precautions for use

If local irritation develops, the use of the Gel should be discontinued and appropriate therapy instituted as necessary.

Keep away from the eyes and mucosal surfaces. Do not apply to any sites affected by open skin lesions, dermatoses or infection.

Use in patients with impaired hepatic function

Use in patients with renal impairment

Use in the ElderlyNo special precautions are required.

Use in Children Dosage recommendations and indications for the use of Feldene Gel, Feldene Sports Gel and Feldene Gel Starter Pack in children under 12 years have not been established.

4.5 Interaction with other medicinal products and other forms of Interaction

None known.

4.6 Pregnancy and lactation

Use in pregnancy Although no teratogenic effects were seen when piroxicam was orally administered in animal testing, the use of Feldene Gel, Feldene Sports Gel and Feldene Gel Starter Pack during pregnancy or during lactation is not recommended.

Nursing mothers Feldene Gel, Feldene Sports Gel and Feldene Gel Starter Pack are not recommended for use in nursing mothers as clinical safety has not been established.

4.7 Effects on ability to drive and use machines

None known.

4.8 Undesirable effects

Feldene Gel is well tolerated. Mild to moderate local irritation, erythema, pruritus and dermatitis may occur at the application site. The systemic absorption of Feldene Gel, is very low. In common with other topical non-steroidal anti-inflammatory agents, systemic reactions occur infrequently and have included minor gastro-intestinal side-effects such as nausea and dyspepsia. Cases of abdominal pain and gastritis have been reported rarely. There have been isolated reports of bronchospasm and dyspnoea (see also Contra-indications).

Contact dermatitis, eczema and photosensitivity skin reaction have also been observed from post-marketing experience.

4.9 Overdose

Overdosage is unlikely to occur with this topical preparation.

5. PHARMACOLOGICAL PROPERTIES

5.1 Pharmacodynamic properties

Piroxicam is a non-steroidal anti-inflammatory agent useful in the treatment of inflammatory conditions. Although the mode of action for this agent is not precisely understood, piroxicam inhibits prostaglandin synthesis and release through a reversible inhibition of the cyclo-oxygenase enzyme. New data are presented on the anti-inflammatory and analgesic effects of Feldene Gel compared with its vehicle and indomethacin 1% Gel in rats and guinea pigs. Using established animal models of pain and inflammation, Feldene Gel was as effective as oral Feldene and indomethacin 1% Gel and significantly more effective than its vehicle.

5.2 Pharmacokinetic properties

On the basis of various pharmacokinetic and tissue distribution studies in animals, with piroxicam gel 0.5%, the highest concentrations of piroxicam were achieved in the tissues below the site of application with low concentrations being reached in the plasma. Piroxicam gel 0.5% was continuously and gradually released from the skin to underlying tissues, equilibrium between skin, and muscle or synovial fluid appeared to be reached rapidly, within a few hours of application.

From a pharmacokinetic study in man, 2g of the Gel was applied to the shoulders of normal volunteers twice daily (corresponding to 20mg piroxicam/day) for 14 days, plasma levels of piroxicam rose slowly, reaching steady state after about 11 days. The plasma levels at this time were between 300-400 ng/ml, or one-twentieth of those observed in subjects receiving 20mg orally.

The serum half-life of piroxicam is approximately 50 hours.

6. PHARMACEUTICAL PARTICULARS

6.1 List of excipients

Propylene Glycol EP, Carbopol 980 EP, Ethyl Alcohol EP, Benzyl Alcohol EP, di-isopropanolamine NF, Hydroxyethyl Cellulose EP, Purified Water EP.

6.2 Incompatibilities

None known.

6.3 Shelf life

3 years.

6.4 Special precautions for storage

Store below 30°C.

6.5 Nature and contents of container

Aluminium blind-ended tube incorporating epoxy-phenol internal lacquer with a white vinyl pressure sensitive polyethylene end seal, fitted with a polypropylene cap containing either 7.5g, 30g, 60g or 112g of Feldene Gel

6.6 Instructions for use and handling

No special requirements

7. MARKETING AUTHORISATION HOLDER

Pfizer Limited

Ramsgate Road

Sandwich

Kent

CT 13 9NJ

United Kingdom

8. MARKETING AUTHORISATION NUMBER(S)

Feldene Gel, Feldene Sports Gel and Feldene Gel Starter Pack PL 0057/0284

9. DATE OF FIRST AUTHORISATION/RENEWAL OF THE AUTHORISATION

13 January 2000

10. DATE OF REVISION OF THE TEXT

February 2003

11. LEGAL CATEGORY

POM

Ref (UK): FE 3_1

Felotens XL 10mg Prolonged Release Tablets

(Genus Pharmaceuticals)

1. NAME OF THE MEDICINAL PRODUCT
Felotens XL 10 mg Prolonged Release Tablets

2. QUALITATIVE AND QUANTITATIVE COMPOSITION
Felotens XL 10 mg Prolonged Release Tablets contain 10mg of felodipine.

3. PHARMACEUTICAL FORM
Reddish brown, round, biconvex, film coated prolonged-release tablets with imprint 10.

4. CLINICAL PARTICULARS
4.1 Therapeutic indications
In the management of hypertension and prophylaxis of chronic stable angina pectoris.

4.2 Posology and method of administration
For oral administration

Hypertension:

Adults (including elderly): The dose should be adjusted to the individual requirements of the patient. The recommended starting dose is 5 mg once daily. If necessary the dose may be further increased or another antihypertensive agent added. The usual maintenance dose is 5-10 mg once daily. Doses higher than 20 mg daily are not usually needed. For dose titration purposes a 2.5 mg tablet is available. In elderly patients an initial treatment with 2.5 mg daily should be considered.

Angina pectoris:

Adults: The dose should be adjusted individually. Treatment should be started with 5 mg once daily and if needed be increased to 10 mg once daily.

Administration: The tablets should regularly be taken in the morning without food or with a light meal. Felotens XL 10 mg Prolonged Release Tablets must not be chewed or crushed. They should be swallowed whole with half a glass of water.

Children: The safety and efficacy of Felotens XL 10 mg Prolonged Release Tablets in children has not been established.

Felotens XL 10 mg Prolonged Release Tablets can be used in combination with β-blockers, ACE inhibitors or diuretics. The effects on blood pressure are likely to be additive and combination therapy will usually enhance the antihypertensive effect. Care should be taken to avoid hypotension. In patients with severely impaired liver function the dose of felodipine should be low. The pharmacokinetics are not significantly affected in patients with impaired renal function.

4.3 Contraindications
Unstable angina pectoris.

Pregnancy.

Patient with a previous allergic reaction to Felotens XL 10 mg Prolonged Release Tablets or other dihydropyridines because of the theoretical risk of cross-reactivity.

Felotens XL 10 mg Prolonged Release Tablets should not be used in patients with clinically significant aortic stenosis, and during or within one month of a myocardial infarction.

As with other calcium channel blockers, Felotens XL 10 mg Prolonged Release Tablets should be discontinued in patients who develop cardiogenic shock.

4.4 Special warnings and special precautions for use
As with other vasodilators, Felotens XL 10 mg Prolonged Release Tablets may, in rare cases, precipitate significant hypotension with tachycardia which in susceptible individuals may result in myocardial ischaemia.

There is no evidence that Felotens XL 10 mg Prolonged Release Tablets are useful for secondary prevention of myocardial infarction.

The efficacy and safety of Felotens XL 10 mg Prolonged Release Tablets in the treatment of malignant hypertension has not been studied.

Felotens XL 10 mg Prolonged Release Tablets should be used with caution in patients with severe left ventricular dysfunction.

4.5 Interaction with other medicinal products and other forms of Interaction
Concomitant administration of substances which interfere with the cytochrome P450 system may affect plasma concentrations of felodipine. Enzyme inhibitors such as cimetidine, erythromycin and itraconazole impair the elimination of felodipine, and Felotens XL 10 mg Prolonged Release Tablets dosage may need to be reduced when drugs are given concomitantly. Conversely, powerful enzyme inducing agents such as some anticonvulsants (phenytoin, carbamazepine, phenobarbitone) can increase felodipine elimination and higher than normal Felotens XL 10 mg Prolonged Release Tablets doses may be required in patients taking the drugs.

No dosage adjustment is required when Felotens XL 10 mg Prolonged Release Tablets are given concomitantly with digoxin.

Felodipine does not appear to affect the unbound fraction of other extensively plasma protein bound drugs such as warfarin.

Grapefruit juice results in increased peak plasma levels and bioavailability possibly due to an interaction with flavonoids in the fruit juice. This interaction has been seen with other dihydropyridine calcium antagonists and represents a class effect. Therefore grapefruit juice should not be taken together with Felotens XL 10 mg Prolonged Release Tablets.

4.6 Pregnancy and lactation
Felodipine should not be given during pregnancy.

In a study on fertility and general reproductive performance in rats, a prolongation of parturition resulting in difficult labour, increased foetal deaths and early postnatal deaths were observed in the medium- and high-dose groups. Reproductive studies in rabbits have shown a dose-related reversible enlargement of the mammary glands of the parent animals and dose-related digital abnormalities in the foetuses when felodipine was administered during stages of early foetal development.

Felodipine has been detected in breast milk, but it is unknown whether it has harmful effects on the new-born.

4.7 Effects on ability to drive and use machines
None.

4.8 Undesirable effects
As with other calcium antagonists, flushing, headache, palpitations, dizziness and fatigue may occur. These reactions are usually transient and are most likely to occur at the start of treatment or after an increase in dosage.

As with other calcium antagonists ankle swelling, resulting from precapillary vasodilation, may occur. The degree of ankle swelling is dose related.

In patients with gingivitis/periodontitis, mild gingival enlargement has been reported with Felotens XL 10 mg Prolonged Release Tablets, as with other calcium antagonists. The enlargement can be avoided or reversed by careful dental hygiene.

As with other dihydropyridines, aggravation of angina has been reported in a small number of individuals especially after starting treatment. This is more likely to happen in patients with symptomatic ischaemic heart disease.

The following adverse events have been reported from clinical trials and from Post Marketing Surveillance. In the great majority of cases a causal relationship between these events and treatment with felodipine has not been established.

Skin: rarely - rash and/or pruritus, and isolated cases of photosensitivity.

Musculoskeletal: in isolated cases arthralgia and myalgia.

Central and peripheral nervous system: headache, dizziness. In isolated cases paraesthesia.

Gastrointestinal: in isolated cases nausea, gum hyperplasia.

Hepatic: in isolated cases increased liver enzymes.

Cardiovascular: rarely - tachycardia, palpitations and syncope.

Vascular (extracardiac): peripheral oedema, flush.

Other: rarely - fatigue, in isolated cases hypersensitivity reactions e.g. urticaria, angiooedema.

4.9 Overdose
Symptoms: Overdosage may cause excessive peripheral vasodilatation with marked hypotension, which may sometimes be accompanied by bradycardia.

Management: Severe hypotension should be treated symptomatically, with the patient placed supine and the legs elevated. Bradycardia, if present, should be treated with atropine 0.5-1 mg i.v. If this is not sufficient, plasma volume should be increased by infusion of e.g. glucose, saline or dextran. Sympathomimetic drugs with predominant effect on the α_1-adrenoceptor may be given e.g. metaraminol or phenylephrine.

5. PHARMACOLOGICAL PROPERTIES
5.1 Pharmacodynamic properties
Felodipine is a vascular selective calcium antagonist, which lowers arterial blood pressure by decreasing peripheral vascular residence. Due to the high degree of selectivity for smooth muscle in the arterioles, felodipine in therapeutic doses has no direct effect on cardiac contractility or conduction.

It can be used as monotherapy or in combination with other antihypertensive drugs, e.g. β-receptor blockers, diuretics or ACE-inhibitors, in order to achieve an increased antihypertensive effect. Felodipine reduces both systolic and diastolic blood pressure and can be used in isolated systolic hypertension. In a study of 12 patients, felodipine maintained its antihypertensive effect during concomitant therapy with indomethacin.

Because there is no effect on venous smooth muscle or adrenergic vasomotor control, felodipine is not associated with orthostatic hypotension.

Felodipine has anti-anginal and anti-ischaemic effects due to improved myocardial oxygen supply/ demand balance. Coronary vascular resistance is decreased and coronary blood flow as well as myocardial oxygen supply are increased by felodipine due to dilation of both epicardial arteries and arterioles. Felodipine effectively counteracts coronary vasospasm. The reduction in systemic blood pressure caused by felodipine leads to decreased left ventricular afterload.

Felodipine improves exercise tolerance and reduces anginal attacks in patients with stable effort induced angina pectoris. Both symptomatic and silent myocardial ischaemia are reduced by felodipine in patients with vasospastic angina. Felodipine can be used as monotherapy or in combination with β-receptor blockers in patients with stable angina pectoris.

Felodipine possesses a mild natriuretic/diuretic effect and generalised fluid retention does not occur.

Felodipine is well tolerated in patients with concomitant disease such as congestive heart failure well controlled on appropriate therapy, asthma and other obstructive pulmonary diseases, diabetes, gout, hyperlipidemia impaired renal function, renal transplant recipients and Raynaud's disease. Felodipine has no significant effect on bland glucose levels or lipid profiles.

Haemodynamic effects: The primary haemodynamic effect of felodipine is a reduction of total peripheral vascular resistance which leads to a decrease in blood pressure. These effects are dose- dependent. In patients with mild to moderate essential hypertension, a reduction in blood pressure usually occurs 2 hours after the first oral dose and lasts for at least 24 hours with a trough/peak ratio usually above 50%.

Plasma concentration of felodipine and decrease in total peripheral resistance and blood pressure are positively correlated.

Electrophysiological and other cardiac effects: Felodipine in therapeutic doses has no effect on cardiac contractility or atrioventricular conduction or refractoriness.

Renal effects: Felodipine has a natriuretic and diuretic effect. Studies have shown that the tubular reabsorption of filtered sodium is reduced. This counteracts the salt and water retention observed for other vasodilators. Felodipine does not affect the daily potassium excretion. The renal vascular resistance is decreased by felodipine. Normal glomerular filtration rate is unchanged. In patients with impaired renal function glomerular filtration rate may increase.

Felodipine is well tolerated in renal transplant recipients.

Site and mechanism of action: The predominant pharmacodynamic feature of felodipine is its pronounced vascular versus myocardial selectivity. Myogenically active smooth muscles in arterial resistance vessels are particularly sensitive to felodipine.

Felodipine inhibits electrical and contractile activity of vascular smooth muscle cells via an effect on the calcium channels in the cell membrane.

5.2 Pharmacokinetic properties
Absorption and distribution: Felodipine is completely absorbed from the gastrointestinal tract after administration of felodipine extended release tablets.

The systemic availability of felodipine is approximately 15% in man and is independent of dose in the therapeutic dose range.

With the extended-release tablets the absorption phase is prolonged. This results in even felodipine plasma concentrations within the therapeutic range for 24 hours.

The plasma protein binding of felodipine is approximately 99%. It is bound predominantly to the albumin fraction.

Elimination and metabolism: The average half-life of felodipine in the terminal phase is 25 hours. There is no significant accumulation during long-term treatment. Felodipine is extensively metabolised by the liver and all identified metabolites are inactive. Elderly patients and patients with reduced liver function have an average higher plasma concentration of felodipine than younger patients.

About 70% of a given dose is excreted as metabolites in the urine; the remaining fraction is excreted in the faeces. Less than 0.5% of a dose is recovered unchanged in the urine.

The kinetics of felodipine are not changed in patients with renal impairment.

5.3 Preclinical safety data
Felodipine is a calcium antagonist and lowers arterial blood pressure by decreasing vascular resistance. In general a reduction in blood pressure is evident 2 hours after the first oral dose and at steady state lasts for at least 24 hours after dose.

Felodipine exhibits a high degree of selectivity for smooth muscles in the arterioles and in therapeutic doses has no direct effect on cardiac contractility. Felodipine does not affect venous smooth muscle and adrenergic vasomotor control.

Electrophysiological studies have shown that felodipine has no direct effect on conduction in the specialised conducting system of the heart and no effect on the AV nodal refractories.

Felotens XL 10 mg Prolonged Release Tablets possess a mild natriuretic/diuretic effect and does not produce general fluid retention, nor affect daily potassium excretion. Felotens XL 10 mg Prolonged Release Tablets are well tolerated in patients with congestive heart failure.

6. PHARMACEUTICAL PARTICULARS

6.1 List of excipients

Lactose monohydrate, cellulose microcristalline, hypromellose, povidone, propyl gallate, silica colloidal anhydrous, magnesium stearate, ferric oxide yellow (E172), ferric oxide red (E172), titanium dioxide (E171), talc, propylene glycol.

6.2 Incompatibilities

None stated.

6.3 Shelf life

24 months.

6.4 Special precautions for storage

Do not store above 25 °C. Store in the original package.

6.5 Nature and contents of container

PVC/PE/PVDC Aluminium Blisters.

A single pack contains 10, 20, 28, 30, 50, 56 or 100 tablets.

6.6 Instructions for use and handling

None stated.

7. MARKETING AUTHORISATION HOLDER

STADA Arzneimittel AG

Stadastraße 2-18

D-61118 Bad Vilbel

Germany

8. MARKETING AUTHORISATION NUMBER(S)

11204/0055

9. DATE OF FIRST AUTHORISATION/RENEWAL OF THE AUTHORISATION

02 July 2002

10. DATE OF REVISION OF THE TEXT

11. LEGAL CATEGORY

POM

Felotens XL 5mg Prolonged Release Tablets

(Genus Pharmaceuticals)

1. NAME OF THE MEDICINAL PRODUCT

Felotens XL 5 mg Prolonged Release Tablets

2. QUALITATIVE AND QUANTITATIVE COMPOSITION

Felotens XL 5 mg Prolonged Release Tablets contain 5 mg of felodipine.

3. PHARMACEUTICAL FORM

Light pink, round, biconvex, film coated prolonged-release tablets with imprint 5.

4. CLINICAL PARTICULARS

4.1 Therapeutic indications

In the management of hypertension and prophylaxis of chronic stable angina pectoris.

4.2 Posology and method of administration

For oral administration

Hypertension:

Adults (including elderly): The dose should be adjusted to the individual requirements of the patient. The recommended starting dose is 5 mg once daily. If necessary the dose may be further increased or another antihypertensive agent added. The usual maintenance dose is 5-10 mg once daily. Doses higher than 20 mg daily are not usually needed. For dose titration purposes a 2.5 mg tablet is available. In elderly patients an initial treatment with 2.5 mg daily should be considered.

Angina pectoris:

Adults: The dose should be adjusted individually. Treatment should be started with 5 mg once daily and if needed be increased to 10 mg once daily.

Administration: The tablets should regularly be taken in the morning without food or with a light meal. Felotens XL 5 mg Prolonged Release Tablets must not be chewed or crushed. They should be swallowed whole with half a glass of water.

Children: The safety and efficacy of Felotens XL 5 mg Prolonged Release Tablets in children has not been established.

Felotens XL 5 mg Prolonged Release Tablets can be used in combination with β-blockers, ACE inhibitors or diuretics. The effects on blood pressure are likely to be additive and combination therapy will usually enhance the antihypertensive effect. Care should be taken to avoid hypotension. In patients with severely impaired liver function the dose of felodipine should be low. The pharmacokinetics are not significantly affected in patients with impaired renal function.

4.3 Contraindications

Unstable angina pectoris.

Pregnancy.

Patient with a previous allergic reaction to Felotens XL 5 mg Prolonged Release Tablets or other dihydropyridines because of the theoretical risk of cross-reactivity.

Felotens XL 5 mg Prolonged Release Tablets should not be used in patients with clinically significant aortic stenosis, and during or within one month of a myocardial infarction.

As with other calcium channel blockers, Felotens XL 5 mg Prolonged Release Tablets should be discontinued in patients who develop cardiogenic shock.

4.4 Special warnings and special precautions for use

As with other vasodilators, Felotens XL 5 mg Prolonged Release Tablets may, in rare cases, precipitate significant hypotension with tachycardia which in susceptible individuals may result in myocardial ischaemia.

There is no evidence that Felotens XL 5 mg Prolonged Release Tablets are useful for secondary prevention of myocardial infarction.

The efficacy and safety of Felotens XL 5 mg Prolonged Release Tablets in the treatment of malignant hypertension has not been studied.

Felotens XL 5 mg Prolonged Release Tablets should be used with caution in patients with severe left ventricular dysfunction.

4.5 Interaction with other medicinal products and other forms of Interaction

Concomitant administration of substances which interfere with the cytochrome P450 system may affect plasma concentrations of felodipine. Enzyme inhibitors such as cimetidine, erythromycin and itraconazole impair the elimination of felodipine, and Felotens XL 5 mg Prolonged Release Tablets dosage may need to be reduced when drugs are given concomitantly. Conversely, powerful enzyme inducing agents such as some anticonvulsants (phenytoin, carbamazepine, phenobarbitone) can increase felodipine elimination and higher than normal Felotens XL 5 mg Prolonged Release Tablets doses may be required in patients taking the drugs.

No dosage adjustment is required when Felotens XL 5 mg Prolonged Release Tablets are given concomitantly with digoxin.

Felodipine does not appear to affect the unbound fraction of other extensively plasma protein bound drugs such as warfarin.

Grapefruit juice results in increased peak plasma levels and bioavailability possibly due to an interaction with flavonoids in the fruit juice. This interaction has been seen with other dihydropyridine calcium antagonists and represents a class effect. Therefore grapefruit juice should not be taken together with Felotens XL 5 mg Prolonged Release Tablets.

4.6 Pregnancy and lactation

Felodipine should not be given during pregnancy.

In a study on fertility and general reproductive performance in rats, a prolongation of parturition resulting in difficult labour, increased foetal deaths and early postnatal deaths were observed in the medium- and high-dose groups. Reproductive studies in rabbits have shown a dose-related reversible enlargement of the mammary glands of the parent animals and dose-related digital abnormalities in the foetuses when felodipine was administered during stages of early foetal development.

Felodipine has been detected in breast milk, but it is unknown whether it has harmful effects on the new-born.

4.7 Effects on ability to drive and use machines

None.

4.8 Undesirable effects

As with other calcium antagonists, flushing, headache, palpitations, dizziness and fatigue may occur. These reactions are usually transient and are most likely to occur at the start of treatment or after an increase in dosage.

As with other calcium antagonists ankle swelling, resulting from precapillary vasodilation, may occur. The degree of ankle swelling is dose related.

In patients with gingivitis/periodontitis, mild gingival enlargement has been reported with Felotens XL 5 mg Prolonged Release Tablets, as with other calcium antagonists. The enlargement can be avoided or reversed by careful dental hygiene.

As with other dihydropyridines, aggravation of angina has been reported in a small number of individuals especially after starting treatment. This is more likely to happen in patients with symptomatic ischaemic heart disease.

The following adverse events have been reported from clinical trials and from Post Marketing Surveillance. In the great majority of cases a causal relationship between these events and treatment with felodipine has not been established.

Skin: rarely - rash and/or pruritus, and isolated cases of photosensitivity.

Musculoskeletal: in isolated cases arthralgia and myalgia.

Central and peripheral nervous system: headache, dizziness. In isolated cases paraesthesia.

Gastrointestinal: in isolated cases nausea, gum hyperplasia.

Hepatic: in isolated cases increased liver enzymes.

Cardiovascular: rarely - tachycardia, palpitations and syncope.

Vascular (extracardiac): peripheral oedema, flush.

Other: rarely - fatigue, in isolated cases hypersensitivity reactions e.g. urticaria, angiooedema.

4.9 Overdose

Symptoms: Overdosage may cause excessive peripheral vasodilatation with marked hypotension which may sometimes be accompanied by bradycardia.

Management: Severe hypotension should be treated symptomatically, with the patient placed supine and the legs elevated. Bradycardia, if present, should be treated with atropine 0.5-1 mg i.v. If this is not sufficient, plasma volume should be increased by infusion of e.g. glucose, saline or dextran. Sympathomimetic drugs with predominant effect on the α_1-adrenoceptor may be given e.g. metaraminol or phenylephrine.

5. PHARMACOLOGICAL PROPERTIES

5.1 Pharmacodynamic properties

Felodipine is a vascular selective calcium antagonist, which lowers arterial blood pressure by decreasing peripheral vascular residence. Due to the high degree of selectivity for smooth muscle in the arterioles, felodipine in therapeutic doses has no direct effect on cardiac contractility or conduction.

It can be used as monotherapy or in combination with other antihypertensive drugs, e.g. β-receptor blockers, diuretics or ACE-inhibitors, in order to achieve an increased antihypertensive effect. Felodipine reduces both systolic and diastolic blood pressure and can be used in isolated systolic hypertension. In a study of 12 patients, felodipine maintained its antihypertensive effect during concomitant therapy with indomethacin.

Because there is no effect on venous smooth muscle or adrenergic vasomotor control, felodipine is not associated with orthostatic hypotension.

Felodipine has anti-anginal and anti-ischaemic effects due to improved myocardial oxygen supply/ demand balance. Coronary vascular resistance is decreased and coronary blood flow as well as myocardial oxygen supply are increased by felodipine due to dilation of both epicardial arteries and arterioles. Felodipine effectively counteracts coronary vasospasm. The reduction in systemic blood pressure caused by felodipine leads to decreased left ventricular afterload.

Felodipine improves exercise tolerance and reduces anginal attacks in patients with stable effort induced angina pectoris. Both symptomatic and silent myocardial ischaemia are reduced by felodipine in patients with vasospastic angina. Felodipine can be used as monotherapy or in combination with β-receptor blockers in patients with stable angina pectoris.

Felodipine possesses a mild natriuretic/diuretic effect and generalised fluid retention does not occur.

Felodipine is well tolerated in patients with concomitant disease such as congestive heart failure well controlled on appropriate therapy, asthma and other obstructive pulmonary diseases, diabetes, gout, hyperlipidemia impaired renal function, renal transplant recipients and Raynaud's disease. Felodipine has no significant effect on bland glucose levels or lipid profiles.

Haemodynamic effects: The primary haemodynamic effect of felodipine is a reduction of total peripheral vascular resistance which leads to a decrease in blood pressure. These effects are dose- dependent. In patients with mild to moderate essential hypertension, a reduction in blood pressure usually occurs 2 hours after the first oral dose and lasts for at least 24 hours with a trough/peak ratio usually above 50%.

Plasma concentration of felodipine and decrease in total peripheral resistance and blood pressure are positively correlated.

Electrophysiological and other cardiac effects: Felodipine in therapeutic doses has no effect on cardiac contractility or atrioventricular conduction or refractoriness.

Renal effects: Felodipine has a natriuretic and diuretic effect. Studies have shown that the tubular reabsorption of filtered sodium is reduced. This counteracts the salt and water retention observed for other vasodilators. Felodipine does not affect the daily potassium excretion. The renal vascular resistance is decreased by felodipine. Normal glomerular filtration rate is unchanged. In patients with impaired renal function glomerular filtration rate may increase.

Felodipine is well tolerated in renal transplant recipients.

Site and mechanism of action: The predominant pharmacodynamic feature of felodipine is its pronounced vascular versus myocardial selectivity. Myogenically active smooth muscles in arterial resistance vessels are particularly sensitive to felodipine.

Felodipine inhibits electrical and contractile activity of vascular smooth muscle cells via an effect on the calcium channels in the cell membrane.

5.2 Pharmacokinetic properties

Absorption and distribution: Felodipine is completely absorbed from the gastrointestinal tract after administration of felodipine extended release tablets.

The systemic availability of felodipine is approximately 15% in man and is independent of dose in the therapeutic dose range.

With the extended-release tablets the absorption phase is prolonged. This results in even felodipine plasma concentrations within the therapeutic range for 24 hours.

The plasma protein binding of felodipine is approximately 99%. It is bound predominantly to the albumin fraction.

Elimination and metabolism: The average half-life of felodipine in the terminal phase is 25 hours. There is no significant accumulation during long-term treatment. Felodipine is extensively metabolised by the liver and all identified metabolites are inactive. Elderly patients and patients with reduced liver function have an average higher plasma concentration of felodipine than younger patients.

About 70% of a given dose is excreted as metabolites in the urine; the remaining fraction is excreted in the faeces. Less than 0.5% of a dose is recovered unchanged in the urine.

The kinetics of felodipine are not changed in patients with renal impairment.

5.3 Preclinical safety data

Felodipine is a calcium antagonist and lowers arterial blood pressure by decreasing vascular resistance. In general a reduction in blood pressure is evident 2 hours after the first oral dose and at steady state lasts for at least 24 hours after dose.

Felodipine exhibits a high degree of selectivity for smooth muscles in the arterioles and in therapeutic doses has no direct effect on cardiac contractility. Felodipine does not affect venous smooth muscle and adrenergic vasomotor control.

Electrophysiological studies have shown that felodipine has no direct effect on conduction in the specialised conducting system of the heart and no effect on the AV nodal refractories.

Felotens XL 5 mg Prolonged Release Tablets possess a mild natriuretic/diuretic effect and does not produce general fluid retention, nor affect daily potassium excretion. Felotens XL 5 mg Prolonged Release Tablets are well tolerated in patients with congestive heart failure.

6. PHARMACEUTICAL PARTICULARS

6.1 List of excipients

Lactose monohydrate, cellulose microcristalline, hypromellose, povidone, propyl gallate, silica colloidal anhydrous, magnesium stearate, ferric oxide yellow (E172), ferric oxide red (E172), titanium dioxide (E171), talc, propylene glycol.

6.2 Incompatibilities

None stated.

6.3 Shelf life

24 months.

6.4 Special precautions for storage

Do not store above 25 °C. Store in the original package.

6.5 Nature and contents of container

PVC/PE/PVDC Aluminium Blisters.

A single pack contains 10, 20, 28, 30, 50, 56 or 100 tablets.

6.6 Instructions for use and handling

None stated.

7. MARKETING AUTHORISATION HOLDER

STADA Arzneimittel AG

Stadastraβe 2-18

D-61118 Bad Vilbel

Germany

8. MARKETING AUTHORISATION NUMBER(S)

11204/0054

9. DATE OF FIRST AUTHORISATION/RENEWAL OF THE AUTHORISATION

02 July 2002

10. DATE OF REVISION OF THE TEXT

11. LEGAL CATEGORY

POM

Femapak 40 and Femapak 80

(Solvay Healthcare Limited)

1. NAME OF THE MEDICINAL PRODUCT

Femapak® 40

Femapak® 80

2. QUALITATIVE AND QUANTITATIVE COMPOSITION

Femapak 40 consists of a pack containing eight Fematrix 40 transdermal patches and a blister strip of 14 Duphaston tablets. Each Fematrix 40 patch contains 1.25 mg estradiol (each patch delivers approximately 40 micrograms of estradiol per 24 hours).

Femapak 80 consists of a pack containing eight Fematrix 80 transdermal patches and a blister strip of 14 Duphaston tablets. Each Fematrix 80 patch contains 2.5 mg estradiol (each patch delivers approximately 80 micrograms of estradiol per 24 hours).

Each Duphaston tablet contains 10mg Dydrogesterone BP.

3. PHARMACEUTICAL FORM

Fematrix is a self adhesive, flexible transdermal delivery system comprising a layer of clear adhesive sandwiched between a translucent patch and a metallised polyester backing.

Fematrix 40 is a rectangular shape with rounded corners and has an active surface area of 14.25 cm^2.

Fematrix 80 is a rectangular shape with rounded corners and has an active surface area of 28.5 cm^2.

Duphaston tablets are round and white, marked on one side with an 'S' and on the other scored and marked with '155' on each half of the tablet.

4. CLINICAL PARTICULARS

4.1 Therapeutic indications

Femapak 40: Hormone replacement therapy in female patients who have an intact uterus for the treatment of symptoms of oestrogen deficiency as a result of the natural menopause or oophorectomy. Dydrogesterone is provided to counteract the effects of estrogen during the second two weeks of each cycle.

Femapak 80: Hormone replacement therapy (HRT) for estrogen deficiency symptoms in peri and postmenopausal women.

Second line therapy for prevention of osteoporosis in postmenopausal women at high risk of future fractures who are intolerant of, or contraindicated for, other medicinal products approved for the prevention of osteoporosis.

The experience in treating women older than 65 years is limited.

4.2 Posology and method of administration

Climateric Symptoms

Therapy should be initiated with Femapak 40 in women who have menopausal symptoms, who have been oestrogen deficient for a prolonged time or who are likely to be intolerant of high levels of oestradiol. The dosage may be increased if required by using Femapak 80. For maintenance therapy the lowest effective dose should be used.

Prevention of Osteoporosis - Femapak 80 only

Treatment should be with Femapak 80, as the efficacy of Femapak 40 in this indication has yet to be established.

For optimum benefit treatment should continue for 5 to 10 years, protection appears to be effective for as long as treatment continues, however, data beyond 10 years is limited. For long term use see also Precautions and Warnings.

Dosage Schedule (for both indications)

One Fematrix transdermal patch should be applied twice weekly on a continuous basis. Each patch should be removed after 3 to 4 days and replaced with a new patch applied to a slightly different site. Patches should be applied to clean, dry and intact areas of skin below the waist on the lower back or buttocks. Fematrix should not be applied on or near the breasts.

Women who are having regular periods should commence therapy within five days of the start of bleeding. Women whose periods have stopped or have become very irregular may commence therapy at any time.

During the second two weeks of the cycle, that is from the 15th day after applying the first patch, one Duphaston tablet should be taken each day for the next 14 days. Most patients will commence bleeding towards the end of the Duphaston therapy.

Unopposed oestrogen therapy should not be used unless the patient has undergone a hysterectomy.

Children

Femapak is not indicated in children.

4.3 Contraindications

Femapak is contra-indicated in women with known or suspected pregnancy or cancer of the breast, cancer of the genital tract or other oestrogen-dependent neoplasia, undiagnosed vaginal bleeding, endometriosis, severe renal or cardiac disease; acute or chronic liver disease where liver function tests have failed to return to normal, active deep venous thrombosis, thromboembolic disorders, or a history of confirmed venous thromboembolism (see Special Precautions and Warnings), Dubin-Johnson syndrome or rotor syndrome or hypersensitivity to lactose or other ingredients of the tablet.

4.4 Special warnings and special precautions for use

Assessment of each woman prior to taking hormone replacement therapy (and at regular intervals thereafter) should include a personal and family medical history. Physical examination should be guided by this and by the contraindications (section 4.3) and warnings (section 4.4) for this product. During assessment of each individual woman clincial examination of the breasts and pelvic examination should be performed where clinically indicated rather than as a routine procedure. Women should be encouraged to participate in the national breast screening programme (mammography) amd the national cervical cancer screening programme (cervical cytology) as appropriate for their age. Breast awareness should also be encouraged and women advised to report any changes in their breasts to their doctor or nurse.

Unopposed oestradiol therapy should not be used in non-hysterectomised women because of the increased risk of endometrial hyperplasia or carcinoma.

A reanalysis of original data from 51 epidemiological studies reported a small or moderate increase in the probability of having breast cancer *diagnosed* in women currently or recently using HRT. The findings may be due to biological effects of HRT, earlier diagnosis, or a combination of both. The relative risk increased with duration of treatment (by 2.3% per year of use) and returned to normal in the course of five years of cessation of HRT use. This is comparable to the increase in relative risk when natural menopause is delayed in the absence of HRT. Breast cancers diagnosed in current or recent users of HRT are more likely to be localised to the breast than those found in non-users. HRT use may not be associated with increased mortality from breast cancer.

Between the ages of 50 and 70, about 45 women in every 1000 not using HRT will have breast cancer diagnosed. It is estimated that among those who use HRT for 5 years starting at age 50, 2 extra cases of breast cancer will be detected by age 70 in every 1000 women. For those who use HRT for 10 years there will be 6 extra cases of breast cancer, and for 15 years use, 12 extra cases of breast cancer in every 1000 women during the 20 year period until age 70.

It is important that the increased risk of being diagnosed with breast cancer is discussed with the patient and weighed against the known benefits of HRT.

Certain diseases may be made worse by hormone replacement therapy and patients with these conditions should be closely monitored. These include otosclerosis, multiple sclerosis, systemic lupus erythematosus, cholelithiasis, porphyria, melanoma, epilepsy, migraine, thyrotoxicosis, surgically confirmed gall bladder disease, asthma and diabetes (worsening of glucose tolerance). Pre-existing uterine fibroids may increase in size during oestrogen therapy and symptoms associated with endometriosis may be exacerbated.

Epidemiological studies have suggested that hormone replacement therapy (HRT) is associated with an increased relative risk of developing venous thromboembolism (VTE) i.e. deep vein thrombosis or pulmonary embolism. The studies find a 2-3 fold increase for users compared with non-users which for healthy women amounts to a low risk of one extra case of VTE each year for every 5000 patients taking HRT.

Generally recognised risk factors for VTE include a personal or family history and severe obesity (Body Mass Index $>30kg/m^2$). In women with these factors the benefits of treatment with HRT need to be carefully weighed against risks.

The risk of VTE may be temporarily increased with prolonged immobilisation, major trauma or major surgery. In women with HRT scrupulous attention should be given to prophylactic measures to prevent VTE following surgery. Where prolonged immobilisation is liable to follow elective surgery, particularly abdominal or orthopaedic surgery to the lower limbs, consideration should be given to temporarily stopping HRT 4 weeks earlier, if this is possible.

If venous thromboembolism develops after initiating therapy the drug should be discontinued.

If jaundice or significant hypertension develop, treatment should be discontinued whilst the cause is investigated.

As oestrogens may cause fluid retention, patients with cardiac or renal dysfunction should be closely observed. Regular monitoring of blood pressure should be carried out in hypertensive patients.

Women who may be at risk of pregnancy should be advised to adhere to non-hormonal contraceptive methods.

4.5 Interaction with other medicinal products and other forms of Interaction

Preparations inducing microsomal liver enzymes, e.g. barbiturates, hydantoins, anti-convulsants (including carbamazepine), meprobromate, phenylbutazone, antibiotics (including rifampicin), and activated charcoal may impair the activity of oestrogens. Transdermally applied oestrogens are less likely to be affected by such interactions than oral oestrogens since first pass hepatic metabolism is avoided.

Changes in oestrogen serum concentrations may affect the results of certain endocrine or liver function tests.

4.6 Pregnancy and lactation

Femapak is contraindicated.

4.7 Effects on ability to drive and use machines

None.

4.8 Undesirable effects

Fematrix is generally well tolerated. The most frequent side effects (reported in 10 to 20% of patients, on at least one occasion in clinical trials with Fematrix 80) which do not normally prevent continued treatment include: breast tenderness, headaches, and breakthrough bleeding. Some patients experience mild and transient local erythema at the site of patch application with or without itching; this usually disappears rapidly on removal of the patch. The overall incidence of general patch irritation in clinical studies is less than 5%. In a clinical study 3% of 102 patients showed well defined erythema (draize scale) 30 minutes after patch removal. No instances of permanent skin damage have been reported. If unacceptable topical side effects do occur discontinuation of treatment should be considered.

Other side effects associated with estrogen or estrogen/progestogen treatment have occasionally been reported (in 1 to 5% of patients in clinical trials with Fematrix 80) include: abdominal cramps, abdominal bloating, oedema, nausea, migraine and weight changes. Additional side effects of dydrogesterone include occasional reports of transient dizziness and skin reactions.

More rarely (less than 1% in clinical trials with Fematrix 80) dizziness, dysmenhorrhoea, leg cramps and visual disturbances have been reported.

Other side effects which have been rarely reported with oestrogen products include: changes in libido or changes in carbohydrate tolerance, vaginal candidiasis, change in vaginal secretions, cystitis like syndrome, cervical erosion, erythema multiforme, erythema nodosa, haemeorrhagic eruptions, chloasma or melasma which may be persistent when the drug is discontinued, steepening of corneal curvature, intolerance to contact lenses, mental depression and chorea minor. Cholestatis may be possible in predisposed patients.

4.9 Overdose

Fematrix

This is not likely due to the mode of administration. If it is necessary to stop delivery then the patch can be removed and plasma estradiol levels will fall rapidly.

Duphaston

Symptoms:

No reports of ill effects from overdosage have been recorded and remedial action is generally unnecessary.

Treatment:

If a large overdosage is discovered within 2-3 hours and treatment seems desirable, gastric lavage is recommended. There are no special antidotes and treatment should be symptomatic.

5. PHARMACOLOGICAL PROPERTIES

5.1 Pharmacodynamic properties

Estradiol

In the female, estradiol stimulates the accessory reproductive organs and causes development of the secondary sexual characteristics at puberty. It is also responsible for the hypertrophy of the uterus and for the changes in the endometrium during the first half of the menstrual cycle which, when acted on by progesterone, prepares it for the reception of a fertilized ovum. It furthermore promotes the growth of the ducts of the mammary glands. Large doses inhibit the gonadotropic secretion of the anterior pituitary, thus influencing the normal ovarian cycle.

It is of value in menstrual disorders, ovarian insufficiency, especially at the menopause, and for the treatment of infections of the vagina in children, where it promotes the growth of a cornified and more resistant epithelium; it is also used to terminate lactation, not very successfully, by inhibiting the release of prolactin.

Dydrogesterone

Dydrogesterone is an orally-active progestogen which produces a complete secretory endometrium in an oestrogen-primed uterus thereby providing protection for oestrogen-induced increased risk of endometrial hyperplasia and/or carcinogenesis. It is indicated in all cases of endogenous progesterone deficiency. Duphaston is non-androgenic, non-oestrogenic, non-corticoid and non-anabolic.

5.2 Pharmacokinetic properties

Fematrix

Absorption:

Estradiol is absorbed from the patch across the stratum corneum and is delivered systemically at a low but constant rate throughout the period of application (3 to 4 days). The estimated delivery of oestradiol is around 40 μg/day.

Distribution:

Oestrogens circulate in the blood bound to albumin, sex hormone binding globulin (SHBG), cortisol-binding globulin and alpha 1-glycoprotein. Following diffusion of free oestrogen into the cells of the target tissues in the hypothalamus, pituitary, vagina, urethra, uterus, breast and liver, binding to specific oestrogen receptors occurs. Very little information is currently available on the distribution of estradiol following transdermal administration.

Biotransformation:

Inactivation of oestrogens in the body is carried out mainly in the liver. Metabolism of 17β estradiol is by oxidation to oestrone, which in turn can be hydrated to form oestriol. There is free interconversion between oestrone and estradiol. Oestrone and oestriol may then undergo conversion to their corresponding sulphate and glucuronide derivatives for excretion in the urine. Oestrone sulphate has a long biologic half-life because of its enterohepatic recirculation and interconversion to oestrone and estradiol.

Elimination:

The plasma elimination half-life of estradiol is approximately 1 hour and is independent of the route of administration. The metabolic plasma clearance rate is between 650 and 900 L/day/m^2.

Steady state plasma estradiol concentrations have been demonstrated in the range of 34 pg/ml to 62 pg/ml and these are maintained throughout the dose interval (for up to four days). Absorption rate may vary between individual patients. After removal of the last patch plasma estradiol and oestrone concentrations return to baseline values in less than 24 hours. The median terminal half-life for estradiol following patch removal has been determined as 5.24h.

Dydrogesterone

After oral administration of labelled dydrogesterone on average 63% of the dose is excreted into the urine. Within 72 hours excretion is complete. Dydrogesterone is completely metabolised.

The main metabolite of dydrogesterone is 20 α-dihydrodydrogesterone (DHD) and is present in the urine predominantly as the glucuronic acid conjugate. A common feature of all metabolites characterized is the retention of the 4, 6 diene-3-one configuration of the parent compound and the absence of 17 α-hydroxylation. This explains the lack of oestrogenic and androgenic effects of dydrogesterone.

After oral administration of dydrogesterone, plasma concentrations of DHD are substantially higher as compared to the parent drug. The AUC and C_{max} ratios of DHD to dydrogesterone are in the order of 40 and 25, respectively.

Dydrogesterone is rapidly absorbed. The T_{max} values of dydrogesterone and DHD vary between 0.5 and 2.5 hours.

Mean terminal half lives of dydrogesterone and DHD vary between 5 to 7 and 14 to 17 hours, respectively.

Unlike progesterone, dydrogesterone is not excreted in the urine as pregnanediol. It is therefore possible to analyse production of endogenous progesterone even in the presence of dydrogesterone.

5.3 Preclinical safety data

Fematrix

No specific preclinical studies have been conducted on Fematrix. Supraphysiologically high doses (prolonged overdoses) of oestradiol have been associated with the induction of tumours in oestrogen dependent target organs in rodent species. Pronounced species differences in toxicology, pharmacology and pharmacodynamics exist.

Dydrogesterone

Dydrogesterone has been used in several animal models and has been proven to have low toxicity. It does not have mutagenic or carcinogenic properties. No effects were seen in reproduction experiments.

6. PHARMACEUTICAL PARTICULARS

6.1 List of excipients

Fematrix

Diethyltoluamide

Acrylic adhesive (Dow Corning MG-0560)

Acrylic thickener (Acrysol 33)

Backing: Polyester film

Release liner: Aluminised/Polyester

Duphaston

Lactose, maize starch, methylhydroxypropylcellulose, silica, magnesium stearate and titanium dioxide (E171)

6.2 Incompatibilities

None known.

6.3 Shelf life

The shelf life of the product as packaged for sale is 3 years.

6.4 Special precautions for storage

Femapak should be stored at room temperature below 25°C in a dry place. Duphaston tablets should also be protected from light.

6.5 Nature and contents of container

Fematrix: Sealed laminated sachet (paper/polyethylene/aluminium foil/polyethylene) containing one transdermal patch.

Duphaston: Blister strip containing 14 tablets. Each carton contains eight Fematrix patches and 14 Duphaston HRT tablets sufficient for one 28 day cycle.

6.6 Instructions for use and handling

Detailed instructions for use are given in the patient leaflet.

7. MARKETING AUTHORISATION HOLDER

Solvay Healthcare Ltd

Mansbridge Road

West End

Southampton

SO18 3JD

United Kingdom

8. MARKETING AUTHORISATION NUMBER(S)

Femapak 40: PL 00512/0175

Femapak 80: PL 00512/0174

9. DATE OF FIRST AUTHORISATION/RENEWAL OF THE AUTHORISATION

01 February 2002

10. DATE OF REVISION OF THE TEXT

October 2004

Femara

(Novartis Pharmaceuticals UK Ltd)

1. NAME OF THE MEDICINAL PRODUCT

Femara®

2. QUALITATIVE AND QUANTITATIVE COMPOSITION

Active substance: 4, 4'-[(1H-1, 2, 4-triazol-1-yl)-methylene]bis-benzonitrile (INN/USAN= letrozole).

Each film-coated tablet contains 2.5 mg letrozole.

3. PHARMACEUTICAL FORM

Film-coated tablets.

4. CLINICAL PARTICULARS

4.1 Therapeutic indications

Treatment of early invasive breast cancer in postmenopausal women who have received prior standard adjuvant tamoxifen therapy.

First-line treatment in postmenopausal women with advanced breast cancer.

Advanced breast cancer in postmenopausal women in whom tamoxifen or other anti-oestrogen therapy has failed.

Pre-operative therapy in postmenopausal women with localised hormone receptor positive breast cancer, to allow subsequent breast-conserving surgery in women not originally considered candidates for breast-conserving surgery. Subsequent treatment after surgery should be in accordance with standard of care.

4.2 Posology and method of administration

Adult and elderly patients

The recommended dose of Femara is 2.5 mg once daily. Following standard adjuvant tamoxifen therapy, treatment with Femara should continue for 3 years or until tumour relapse occurs, whichever comes first. Currently there is a lack of long-term data, therefore the optimal duration of therapy has not yet been established. In patients with metastatic disease, treatment with Femara should continue until tumour progression is evident. Regular monitoring to observe progression during the pre-operative treatment period is recommended (see Section 5.1 "Pharmacodynamic properties"). No dose adjustment is required for elderly patients.

Children

Not recommended for use in children.

Patients with hepatic and/or renal impairment

No dosage adjustment is required for patients with mild to moderate hepatic impairment (Child-Pugh grade A and B) or renal impairment (creatinine clearance 10 mL/min.), (see "Pharmacokinetic properties").

4.3 Contraindications

Hypersensitivity to the active substance or to any of the excipients. Premenopausal, pregnant or lactating women; patients with severe hepatic impairment (Child-Pugh grade C).

Pre-operative use of letrozole is contraindicated if the receptor status is negative or unknown.

4.4 Special warnings and special precautions for use

Femara is not recommended for use in children as efficacy and safety in this patient group have not been assessed in clinical studies. There are no efficacy data to support the use of Femara in men with breast cancer.

Femara has not been investigated in patients with creatinine clearance 10 mL/min. The potential risk/benefit to such patients should be carefully considered before administration of Femara.

Following standard adjuvant tamoxifen therapy, women with osteoporosis or at risk of osteoporosis should have their bone mineral density formally assessed by bone densitometry e.g. DEXA scanning at the commencement of treatment and at regular intervals thereafter. Treatment or prophylaxis for osteoporosis should be initiated as appropriate and carefully monitored.

4.5 Interaction with other medicinal products and other forms of Interaction

Clinical interaction studies with cimetidine and warfarin indicated that the coadministration of Femara with these drugs does not result in clinically significant drug interactions, even though cimetidine is a known inhibitor of one of the cytochrome P450 isoenzymes capable of metabolising letrozole *in vitro* (see also section 5.2, "Metabolism and elimination").

There was no evidence of other clinically relevant interaction in patients receiving other commonly prescribed drugs (e.g. benzodiazepines; barbiturates; NSAIDs such as diclofenac sodium, ibuprofen; paracetamol; furosemide; omeprazole).

There is no clinical experience to date on the use of Femara in combination with other anti-cancer agents.

Letrozole inhibits *in vitro* the cytochrome P450-isoenzymes 2A6 and moderately 2C19, however, CYP2A6 does not play a major role in drug metabolism. In *in vitro* experiments letrozole was not able to substantially inhibit the metabolism of diazepam (a substrate of CYP2C19) at concentrations approximately 100-fold higher than those observed in plasma at steady-state. Thus, clinically relevant interactions with CYP2C19 are unlikely to occur. Nevertheless, caution should be used in the concomitant administration of drugs whose disposition is mainly dependent on these isoenzymes and whose therapeutic index is narrow.

4.6 Pregnancy and lactation

There is no experience of the use of Femara in human pregnancy or lactation. Femara is contraindicated during pregnancy, lactation and in premenopausal women.

Embryotoxicity and foetotoxicity were seen in pregnant rats following oral administration of Femara, and there was an increase in the incidence of foetal malformation among the animals treated. However, it is not known whether this was an indirect consequence of the pharmacological activity of Femara (inhibition of oestrogen biosynthesis) or a direct drug effect.

4.7 Effects on ability to drive and use machines

Since fatigue and dizziness have been observed with the use of Femara and somnolence has been reported uncommonly, caution is advised when driving or using machines.

4.8 Undesirable effects

Femara was generally well tolerated across all studies as first-line and second-line treatment for advanced breast cancer as well as in the treatment of women who have received prior standard tamoxifen therapy. Approximately one third of the patients treated with Femara in the metastatic and neoadjuvant settings and approximately 40% of the patients treated following standard adjuvant tamoxifen (both Femara and placebo arms) can be expected to experience adverse reactions. Generally, the observed adverse reactions are mainly mild or moderate in nature.

In the metastatic and neoadjuvant settings, the most frequently reported adverse reactions in the clinical trials were hot flushes (10.8%), nausea (6.9%) and fatigue (5.0%). Many adverse reactions can be attributed to the normal pharmacological consequences of oestrogen deprivation (e.g. hot flushes, alopecia and vaginal bleeding).

After standard adjuvant tamoxifen, the following adverse events irrespective of causality were reported significantly more often with Femara than with placebo – hot flushes (49.7 % vs. 43.3 %), arthralgia/arthritis (27.7 % vs. 22.2 %) and myalgia (9.5 % vs. 6.7 %). The majority of these adverse events were observed during the first year of treatment. The incidence of self-reported osteoporosis was higher in patients who received Femara than in patients who received placebo (6.9 % vs. 5.5 %). The incidence of clinical fractures was only slightly higher in patients who received Femara than in placebo patients (5.9 % vs. 5.5 %). The fracture rate per 1000-women years in the letrozole group (24.6) is in the range of aged-matched postmenopausal healthy women.

The following adverse drug reactions, listed in Table 1, have been accumulated from clinical studies and from post marketing experience with Femara.

Table 1

Adverse reactions are ranked under headings of frequency, the most frequent first, using the following convention: *very common* ⩾ *10%; common* ⩾ *1% to* < *10%; uncommon* ⩾ *0.1% to* < *1%; rare* ⩾ *0.01% to* < *0.1%; very rare* < *0.01%*, including isolated report.

Infections and infestations	
Uncommon:	Urinary tract infection
Neoplasms, benign, malignant and unspecified (including cysts and polyps)	
Uncommon:	Tumour pain (6)
Blood and the lymphatic system disorders	
Uncommon:	Leukopenia
Metabolism and nutrition disorders	
Common:	Anorexia, appetite increase
Uncommon:	Hypercholesterolaemia, general oedema
Psychiatric disorders	
Uncommon:	Depression, anxiety (1)
Nervous system disorders	
Common:	Headache, dizziness
Uncommon:	Somnolence, insomnia, memory impairment, dysaesthesia (2), taste disturbance
Rare:	Cerebrovascular accident
Eye disorders	
Uncommon	Cataract, eye irritation, blurred vision
Cardiac disorders	
Uncommon:	Palpitations, tachycardia
Vascular disorders	
Uncommon:	Thrombophlebitis (3), hypertension
Rare:	Pulmonary embolism, arterial thrombosis, cerebrovascular infarction
Respiratory, thoracic and mediastinal disorders	
Uncommon:	Dyspnoea
Gastrointestinal disorders	
Common:	Nausea, vomiting, dyspepsia, constipation, diarrhoea
Uncommon:	Abdominal pain, stomatitis, dry mouth
Hepatobiliary disorders	
Uncommon:	Increased hepatic enzymes
Skin and subcutaneous tissue disorders	
Common:	Alopecia, increased sweating, rash (4)
Uncommon:	Pruritus, dry skin, urticaria
Musculoskeletal and connective tissue disorders	
Common:	Myalgia, bone pain, arthralgia, arthritis
Renal and urinary disorders	
Uncommon	Increased urinary frequency
Reproductive system and breast disorders	
Uncommon	Vaginal bleeding, vaginal discharge, vaginal dryness, breast pain
General disorders and administration site conditions	
Very common:	Hot flushes
Common:	Fatigue (5), peripheral oedema
Uncommon:	Pyrexia, mucosal dryness, thirst
Investigations	
Common:	Weight increase
Uncommon:	Weight loss,

*Including:
(1) including nervousness, irritability
(2) including paraesthesia, hypoaesthesia
(3) including superficial and deep thrombophlebitis
(4) including erythematous, maculopapular, psoriaform and vesicular rash
(5) including aesthenia and malaise
(6) in metastatic/neoadjuvant setting only

4.9 Overdose

There is no clinical experience of overdosage. In animal studies, Femara exhibits only a slight degree of acute toxicity. In clinical trials, the highest single and multiple dose tested in healthy volunteers was 30 mg and 5 mg, respectively, the latter also being the highest dose tested in postmenopausal breast cancer patients. Each of these doses was well tolerated. There is no clinical evidence for a particular dose of Femara resulting in life-threatening symptoms.

There is no specific antidote to Femara. In general, supportive care, symptomatic treatment and frequent monitoring of vital signs is appropriate.

5. PHARMACOLOGICAL PROPERTIES

5.1 Pharmacodynamic properties

Pharmacotherapeutic group

ATC Code: L02B G

Non-steroidal aromatase inhibitor (inhibitor of oestrogen biosynthesis); antineoplastic agent.

Pharmacodynamic effects

The elimination of oestrogen-mediated stimulatory effects is a prerequisite for tumour response in cases where the growth of tumour tissue depends on the presence of oestrogens. In postmenopausal women, oestrogens are mainly derived from the action of the aromatase enzyme, which converts adrenal androgens - primarily androstenedione and testosterone - to oestrone (E1) and oestradiol (E2). The suppression of oestrogen biosynthesis in peripheral tissues and the cancer tissue itself can therefore be achieved by specifically inhibiting the aromatase enzyme.

Letrozole is a non-steroidal aromatase inhibitor. It inhibits the aromatase enzyme by competitively binding to the haem of the cytochrome P450 subunit of the enzyme, resulting in a reduction of oestrogen biosynthesis in all tissues.

In healthy postmenopausal women, single doses of 0.1, 0.5, and 2.5 mg letrozole suppress serum oestrone and oestradiol by 75-78% and 78% from baseline respectively. Maximum suppression is achieved in 48-78 h.

In postmenopausal patients with advanced breast cancer, daily doses of 0.1 to 5 mg suppress plasma concentration of oestradiol, oestrone, and oestrone sulphate by 75 - 95% from baseline in all patients treated. With doses of 0.5 mg and higher, many values of oestrone and oestrone sulphate are below the limit of detection in the assays, indicating that higher oestrogen suppression is achieved with these doses. Oestrogen suppression was maintained throughout treatment in all these patients.

Letrozole is highly specific in inhibiting aromatase activity. Impairment of adrenal steroidogenesis has not been observed. No clinically relevant changes were found in the plasma concentrations of cortisol, aldosterone, 11-deoxycortisol, 17-hydroxy-progesterone, and ACTH or in plasma renin activity among postmenopausal patients treated with a daily dose of letrozole 0.1 to 5 mg. The ACTH stimulation test performed after 6 and 12 weeks of treatment with daily doses of 0.1, 0.25, 0.5, 1, 2.5, and 5 mg did not indicate any attenuation of aldosterone or cortisol production. Thus, glucocorticoid and mineralocorticoid supplementation is not necessary.

No changes were noted in plasma concentrations of androgens (androstenedione and testosterone) among healthy postmenopausal women after 0.1, 0.5, and 2.5 mg single doses of letrozole or in plasma concentrations of androstenedione among postmenopausal patients treated with daily doses of 0.1 to 5 mg, indicating that the blockade of oestrogen biosynthesis does not lead to accumulation of androgenic precursors. Plasma levels of LH and FSH are not affected by letrozole in patients, nor is thyroid function as evaluated by TSH, T4 and T3 uptake.

Treatment after standard adjuvant tamoxifen

In a multicentre, double-blind, randomised, placebo-controlled study, performed in over 5100 postmenopausal patients with receptor-positive or unknown primary breast cancer patients who had remained disease-free after completion of adjuvant treatment with tamoxifen (4.5 to 6 years) were randomly assigned either Femara or placebo.

Analysis conducted at a median follow-up of around 28 months (25% of the patients being followed-up for up to 38 months) showed that Femara reduced the risk of recurrence by 42% compared with placebo (hazard ratio 0.58; P=0.00003), an absolute reduction of 2.4%. This statistically significant benefit in DFS in favour of letrozole was observed regardless of nodal status or prior chemotherapy.

For the secondary endpoint overall survival (OS) a total 113 deaths were reported (51 Femara, 62 placebo). Overall, there was no significant difference between treatments in OS (hazard ratio 0.82; P=0.29). Table 1 summarises the results:

Table 2 Disease-free and overall survival (Modified ITT population)

(see Table 2 on next page)

The efficacy of Femara was not assessed in women who discontinued tamoxifen therapy more than 3 months earlier.

There was no difference in safety and efficacy between patients aged < 65 versus ⩾ 65 years.

Preliminary results (median duration of follow-up was 20 months) from the bone mineral density (BMD) sub-study (n=222) demonstrated that, at 2 years, compared to baseline, patients receiving letrozole had a mean decrease of 3 % in hip BMD compared to 0.4 % in the placebo group (P=0.048). There was no significant difference in terms of changes in lumbar spine BMD. Concomitant calcium and vitamin D supplementation was mandatory in the BMD substudy. Preliminary results (median duration of follow-up was 29 months) from the lipid sub-study (n=310) show no significant difference between the Femara and placebo groups. In the core study the incidence of cardiovascular ischemic events was comparable between treatment arms (6.8% vs. 6.5%).

First-line treatment

One large well-controlled double-blind trial was conducted comparing Femara 2.5 mg to tamoxifen 20 mg daily as first-line therapy in postmenopausal women with locally advanced or metastatic breast cancer. In this trial of 907 women, Femara was superior to tamoxifen in time to progression (primary endpoint) and in overall objective response, time to treatment failure and clinical benefit (CR+PR+NC≥24 weeks).

Femara treatment in the first line therapy of advanced breast cancer patients is associated with an early survival advantage over tamoxifen. A significantly greater number of patients were alive on Femara versus tamoxifen throughout the first 24 months of the study. As the study design allowed patients to cross-over upon progression to

Table 2 Disease-free and overall survival (Modified ITT population)

	Letrozole N=2582	Placebo N=2586	Hazard Ratio (95 % CI)	P-Value
Disease-free survival (primary)				
- events (protocol definition, total)	**92** (3.6%)	**155** (6.0%)	0.58 (0.45, 0.76) [1]	P=0.00003
Distant disease-free survival	**57**	**93**	0.61 (0.44, 0.84) [2]	P=0.003
Overall survival (secondary)				
- number of deaths (total)	**51**	**62**	0.82 (0.56, 1.19) [1]	P=0.292
Contralateral breast cancer (secondary)				
- including DCIS/LCIS	**19**	**30**	0.63 (0.36, 1.13) [3]	P=0.120
- invasive	**15**	**25**	0.60 (0.31, 1.14) [3]	P=0.117

CI = confidence interval, CLBC = contralateral breast cancer, DCIS = ductal carcinoma in situ, LCIS = lobular carcinoma in situ
1 Stratified by receptor status, nodal status and prior adjuvant chemotherapy
2 Non-stratified analysis
3 Odds ratio, non-stratified analysis

the other therapy the long-term survival could not be evaluated.

Pre-operative treatment:

A double blind trial was conducted in 337 postmenopausal breast cancer patients randomly allocated either Femara 2.5mg for 4 months or tamoxifen for 4 months. At baseline all patients had tumours stage T2-T4c, N0-2, M0, ER and/or PgR positive and none of the patients would have qualified for breast-conserving surgery. There were 55% objective responses in the Femara treated patients versus 36% for the tamoxifen treated patients ($p<0.001$) based on clinical assessment. This finding was consistently confirmed by ultrasound (p=0.042) and mammography ($p<0.001$) giving the most conservative assessment of response. This response was reflected in a statistically significantly higher number of patients in the Femara group who became suitable for and underwent breast-conserving therapy (45% of patients in the Femara group versus 35% of patients in the tamoxifen group, p=0.022). During the 4 month pre-operative treatment period, 12% of patients treated with Femara and 17% of patients treated with tamoxifen had disease progression on clinical assessment.

5.2 Pharmacokinetic properties

Absorption

Letrozole is rapidly and completely absorbed from the gastrointestinal tract (mean absolute bioavailability: 99.9%). Food slightly decreases the rate of absorption (median t_{max}: 1 hour fasted versus 2 hours fed; and mean C_{max}: 129 ± 20.3 nmol/L fasted versus 98.7 ± 18.6 nmol/L fed) but the extent of absorption (AUC) is not changed. The minor effect on the absorption rate is not considered to be of clinical relevance and therefore letrozole may be taken without regard to mealtimes.

Distribution

Plasma protein binding of letrozole is approximately 60%, mainly to albumin (55%). The concentration of letrozole in erythrocytes is about 80% of that in plasma. After administration of 2.5 mg ^{14}C-labelled letrozole, approximately 82% of the radioactivity in plasma was unchanged compound. Systemic exposure to metabolites is therefore low. Letrozole is rapidly and extensively distributed to tissues. Its apparent volume of distribution at steady state is about 1.87 0.47 L/kg.

Metabolism and elimination

Metabolic clearance to a pharmacologically inactive carbinol metabolite is the major elimination pathway of letrozole (CL_m= 2.1 L/h) but is relatively slow when compared to hepatic blood flow (about 90 L/h). The cytochrome P450 isoenzymes 3A4 and 2A6 were found to be capable of converting letrozole to this metabolite *in vitro*, but their individual contributions to letrozole clearance *in vivo* have not been established. In an interaction study co-administration with cimetidine, which is known to inhibit only the 3A4 isoenzyme, did not result in a decrease in letrozole clearance suggesting that *in vivo* the 2A6 isoenzyme plays an important part in total clearance. In this study a slight decrease in AUC and increase in C_{max} were observed.

Formation of minor unidentified metabolites and direct renal and faecal excretion play only a minor role in the overall elimination of letrozole. Within 2 weeks after administration of 2.5 mg ^{14}C-labelled letrozole to healthy postmenopausal volunteers, 88.2 ± 7.6% of the radioactivity was recovered in urine and 3.8 ± 0.9% in faeces. At least 75% of the radioactivity recovered in urine up to 216 hours (84.7 ± 7.8% of the dose) was attributed to the glucuronide of the carbinol metabolite, about 9% to two unidentified metabolites, and 6% to unchanged letrozole.

The apparent terminal elimination half-life in plasma is about 2 days. After daily administration of 2.5 mg steady-state levels are reached within 2 to 6 weeks. Plasma concentrations at steady state are approximately 7 times higher than concentrations measured after a single dose of 2.5 mg, while they are 1.5 to 2 times higher than the steady-state values predicted from the concentrations measured after a single dose, indicating a slight non-linearity in the pharmacokinetics of letrozole upon daily administration of 2.5 mg. Since steady-state levels are maintained over time, it can be concluded that no continuous accumulation of letrozole occurs.

Age had no effect on the pharmacokinetics of letrozole.

Special populations

In a study involving volunteers with varying degrees of renal function (24 hour creatinine clearance 9-116 mL/min) no effect on the pharmacokinetics of letrozole or the urinary excretion of the glucoronide of its carbinol metabolite was found after a single dose of 2.5 mg. The C_{max}, AUC and half-life of the metabolite have not been determined. In a similar study involving subjects with varying degrees of hepatic function, the mean AUC values of the volunteers with moderate hepatic impairment was 37 % higher than in normal subjects, but still within the range seen in subjects without impaired function.

5.3 Preclinical safety data

Femara showed a low degree of acute toxicity in rodents exposed up to 2000 mg/kg. In dogs Femara caused signs of moderate toxicity at 100 mg/kg.

In repeated-dose toxicity studies in rats and dogs up to 12 months, the main findings can be attributed to the pharmacological action of the compound. Effects on the liver (increased weight, hepatocellular hypertrophy, fatty changes) were observed, mainly at high dose levels. Increased incidences of hepatic vacuolation (both sexes, high dose) and necrosis (intermediate and high dose females) were also noted in rats treated for 104 weeks in a carcinogenicity study. They may have been associated with the endocrine effects and hepatic enzyme-inducing properties of Femara. However, a direct drug effect cannot be ruled out.

In a 104-week mouse carcinogenicity study, dermal and systemic inflammation occurred, particularly at the highest dose of 60 mg/kg, leading to increased mortality at this dose level. Again it is not known whether these findings were an indirect consequence of the pharmacological activity of Femara (i.e. linked to long-term oestrogen deprivation) or a direct drug effect.

Both *in vitro* and *in vivo* investigations on Femara's mutagenic potential revealed no indication of any genotoxicity.

In the carcinogenicity studies no treatment-related tumours were noted in male animals. In female animals, treatment-related changes in genital tract tumours (a reduced incidence of benign and malignant mammary tumours in rats, an increased incidence of benign ovarian stromal tumours in mice) were secondary to the pharmacological effect of the compound.

6. PHARMACEUTICAL PARTICULARS

6.1 List of excipients

Silica aerogel, cellulose, lactose, magnesium stearate, maize starch, sodium carboxymethyl starch, hydroxypropyl methylcellulose, polyethylene glycol, talc, titanium dioxide, iron oxide yellow.

6.2 Incompatibilities

None known.

6.3 Shelf life

Five years

6.4 Special precautions for storage

Do not store above 30°C. Store in the original package.

6.5 Nature and contents of container

PVC/PE/PVDC blister packs of 14 or 28 tablets.

6.6 Instructions for use and handling

No specific instructions for use/handling.

7. MARKETING AUTHORISATION HOLDER

Novartis Pharmaceuticals UK Limited
Trading as Ciba Laboratories
Frimley Business Park
Frimley
Camberley
Surrey
GU16 7SR.

8. MARKETING AUTHORISATION NUMBER(S)

PL 00101/0493

9. DATE OF FIRST AUTHORISATION/RENEWAL OF THE AUTHORISATION

18 November 1996

10. DATE OF REVISION OF THE TEXT

09 September 2004

LEGAL CATEGORY

POM

Fematrix 40 and Fematrix 80

(Solvay Healthcare Limited)

1. NAME OF THE MEDICINAL PRODUCT

Fematrix® 40
Fematrix® 80

2. QUALITATIVE AND QUANTITATIVE COMPOSITION

Fematrix 40 contains 1.25 mg of oestradiol (Estradiol INN) and each patch delivers approximately 40 micrograms of oestradiol per 24 hours.

Fematrix 80 contains 2.5 mg of oestradiol (Estradiol INN) and each patch delivers approximately 80 micrograms of oestradiol per 24 hours

3. PHARMACEUTICAL FORM

Fematrix is a self adhesive, flexible transdermal patch comprising a layer of clear adhesive sandwiched between a translucent patch and a metallised polyester backing.

Fematrix 40 is a rectangular shape with rounded corners and has an active surface area of 14.25 cm^2.

Fematrix 80 is a rectangular shape with rounded corners and has an active surface area of 28.5 cm^2.

4. CLINICAL PARTICULARS

4.1 Therapeutic indications

Fematrix 40: Oestrogen replacement therapy in female patients for the treatment of symptoms of oestrogen deficiency as a result of the natural menopause or oophorectomy.

Fematrix 80: Hormone replacement therapy (HRT) for estrogen deficiency symptoms in peri and postmenopausal women.

Second line therapy for prevention of osteoporosis in postmenopausal women at high risk of future fractures who are intolerant of, or contraindicated for, other medicinal products approved for the prevention of osteoporosis.

The experience in treating women older than 65 years is limited.

4.2 Posology and method of administration

Climacteric Symptoms: Fematrix 40, Fematrix 80

Therapy should be initiated with Fematrix 40 in women who have menopausal symptoms, who have been oestrogen deficient for a prolonged time or who are likely to be intolerant of high levels of oestradiol. The dosage may be increased if required by using Fematrix 80. For maintenance therapy the lowest effective dose should be used.

Prevention of Osteoporosis: Fematrix 80 only

Treatment should be with Fematrix 80, as the efficacy of Fematrix 40 in this indication has yet to be established.

For optimum benefit treatment should continue for 5 to 10 years, protection appears to be effective for as long as treatment continues, however data beyond 10 years is limited. For long term use see also Precautions and warnings.

Dosage Schedule (for both indications)

One Fematrix transdermal patch should be applied twice weekly on a continuous basis. Each patch should be removed after 3 to 4 days and replaced with a new patch applied to a slightly different site. Patches should be applied to clean, dry and intact areas of skin below the waist on the lower back or buttocks. Fematrix should not be applied on or near the breasts.

Women who are having regular periods should commence therapy within five days of the start of bleeding. Women whose periods have stopped or have become very irregular may commence therapy at any time.

In women with a uterus, a progestogen should be added for 12 to 14 days of each cycle. Most patients will commence bleeding towards the end of the progestogen therapy.

Unopposed oestrogen therapy should not be used unless the patient has undergone a hysterectomy.

Children

Fematrix is not indicated in children.

4.3 Contraindications

Fematrix is contraindicated in women with known or suspected pregnancy or cancer of the breast, cancer of the genital tract or other oestrogen-dependent neoplasia, undiagnosed vaginal bleeding, endometriosis, severe renal or cardiac disease, acute or chronic liver disease where liver function tests have failed to return to normal, active deep venous thrombosis, thromboembolic disorders, or a history of confirmed venous thromboembolism (see Special Precautions and Warnings), Dubin-Johnson syndrome or rotor syndrome.

4.4 Special warnings and special precautions for use

Assessment of each woman prior to taking hormone replacement therapy (and at regular intervals thereafter) should include a personal and family medical history. Physical examination should be guided by this and by the contraindications (section 4.3) and warnings (section 4.4) for this product. During assessment of each individual woman clincial examination of the breasts and pelvic examination should be performed where clinically indicated rather than as a routine procedure. Women should be encouraged to participate in the national breast screening programme (mammography) amd the national cervical cancer screening programme (cervical cytology) as appropriate for their age. Breast awareness should also be encouraged and women advised to report any changes in their breasts to their doctor or nurse.

Unopposed oestradiol therapy should not be used in non-hysterectomised women because of the increased risk of endometrial hyperplasia or carcinoma.

A reanalysis of original data from 51 epidemiological studies reported a small or moderate increase in the probability of having breast cancer *diagnosed* in women currently or recently using HRT. The findings may be due to biological effects of HRT, earlier diagnosis, or a combination of both. The relative risk increased with duration of treatment (by 2.3% per year of use) and returned to normal in the course of five years of cessation of HRT use. This is comparable to the increase in relative risk when natural menopause is delayed in the absence of HRT. Breast cancers diagnosed in current or recent users of HRT are more likely to be localised to the breast than those found in non-users. HRT use may not be associated with increased mortality from breast cancer.

Between the ages of 50 and 70, about 45 women in every 1000 not using HRT will have breast cancer diagnosed. It is estimated that among thosé who use HRT for 5 years starting at age 50, 2 extra cases of breast cancer will be detected by age 70 in every 1000 women. For those who use HRT for 10 years there will be 6 extra cases of breast cancer, and for 15 years use, 12 extra cases of breast cancer in every 1000 women during the 20 year period until age 70.

It is important that the increased risk of being diagnosed with breast cancer is discussed with the patient and weighed against the known benefits of HRT.

Certain diseases may be made worse by hormone replacement therapy and patients with these conditions should be closely monitored. These include otosclerosis, multiple sclerosis, systemic lupus erythematosus, cholelithiasis, porphyria, melanoma, epilepsy, migraine, thyrotoxicosis, surgically confirmed gall bladder disease, asthma and diabetes (worsening of glucose tolerance). Pre-existing uterine fibroids may increase in size during oestrogen therapy and symptoms associated with endometriosis may be exacerbated.

Epidemiological studies have suggested that hormone replacement therapy (HRT) is associated with an increased relative risk of developing venous thromboembolism (VTE)i.e. deep vein thrombosis or pulmonary embolism. The studies find a 2-3 fold increase for users compared with non-users which for healthy women amounts to a low risk of one extra case of VTE each year for every 5000 patients taking HRT.

Generally recognised risk factors for VTE include a personal or family history and severe obesity (Body Mass Index $>30kg/m^2$). In women with these factors the benefits of treatment with HRT need to be carefully weighed against risks.

The risk of VTE may be temporarily increased with prolonged immobilisation, major trauma or major surgery. In women with HRT scrupulous attention should be given to prophylactic measures to prevent VTE following surgery. Where prolonged immobilisation is liable to follow elective surgery, particularly abdominal or orthopaedic surgery to the lower limbs, consideration should be given to temporarily stopping HRT 4 weeks earlier, if this is possible.

If venous thromboembolism develops after initiating therapy the drug should be discontinued.

If jaundice or significant hypertension develop, treatment should be discontinued whilst the cause is investigated. As oestrogens may cause fluid retention, patients with cardiac or renal dysfunction should be closely observed. Regular monitoring of blood pressure should be carried out in hypertensive patients.

Women who may be at risk of pregnancy should be advised to adhere to non-hormonal contraceptive methods.

4.5 Interaction with other medicinal products and other forms of Interaction

Preparations inducing microsomal liver enzymes, eg barbituates, hydantoins, anti-convulsants (including carbamazepine), meprobromate, phenylbutazone, antibiotics (including rifampicin), and activated charcoal may impair the activity of oestrogens. Transdermally applied oestrogens are less likely to be affected by such interactions than oral oestrogens since first pass hepatic metabolism is avoided.

Changes in oestrogen serum concentrations may affect the results of certain endocrine or liver function tests.

4.6 Pregnancy and lactation

Fematrix is contraindicated.

4.7 Effects on ability to drive and use machines

None.

4.8 Undesirable effects

Fematrix is generally well tolerated. The most frequent side effects, (reported in 10 to 20% of patients, on at least one occasion, in clinical trials with Fematrix 80) which do not normally prevent continued treatment include: breast tenderness, headaches and breakthrough bleeding. Some patients experience mild and transient local erythema at the site of application with or without itching; this usually disappears rapidly on removal of the patch. The overall incidence of general patch irritation in clinical studies is less than 5%. In a clinical study 3% of 102 patients showed well defined erythema (Draize scale) 30 minutes after patch removal. No instances of permanent skin damage have been reported. If unacceptable topical side effects do occur discontinuation of treatment should be considered.

Other side effects associated with oestrogen or oestrogen/progestogen treatment have occasionally been reported (in 1% to 5% of patients in clinical trials with Fematrix 80) include: abdominal cramps, abdominal bloating, oedema, nausea, migraine and weight changes. More rarely (less than 1% in clinical trials with Fematrix 80) dizziness, dysmenorrhoea, leg cramps and visual disturbances have been reported.

Other side effects which have been rarely reported with oestrogen products include: changes in libido or changes in carbohydrate tolerance, vaginal candidiasis, change in vaginal secretions, cystitis like syndrome, cervical erosion, erythema multiforme, erythema nodosa, haemorrhagic eruptions, chloasma or melasma which may be persistent when the drug is discontinued, steepening of corneal curvature, intolerance to contact lenses, mental depression and chorea minor. Cholestasis may be possible in predisposed patients.

4.9 Overdose

This is not likely due to the mode of administration. If it is necessary to stop delivery then the patch can be removed and plasma oestradiol levels will fall rapidly.

5. PHARMACOLOGICAL PROPERTIES

5.1 Pharmacodynamic properties

Pharmacotherapeutic group

Natural oestrogen

Mechanism of action/pharmacodynamic effects

In the female, oestradiol stimulates the accessory reproductive organs and causes development of the secondary sexual characteristics at puberty. It is also responsible for the hypertrophy of the uterus and for the changes in the endometrium during the first half of the menstrual cycle which when acted on by progesterone prepares it for the reception of a fertilized ovum. It furthermore promotes the growth of the ducts of the mammary glands. Large doses inhibit the gonadotropic secretion of the anterior pituitary, thus influencing the normal ovarian cycle.

It is of value in menstrual disorders, ovarian insufficiency, especially at the menopause, and for the treatment of infections of the vagina in children, where it promotes the growth of a cornified and more resistant epithelium; it is also used to terminate lactation, not very successfully, by inhibiting the release of prolactin.

5.2 Pharmacokinetic properties

General characteristics of the active substance

Absorption Oestradiol is absorbed from the patch across the stratum corneum and is delivered systemically at a low but constant rate throughout the period of application (3 to 4 days). The estimated delivery of oestradiol is approximately 80 micrograms per day for Fematrix 80.

Distribution Oestrogens circulate in the blood bound to albumin, sex hormone binding globulin (SHBG), cortisol binding globulin and alpha1-glycoprotein. Following diffusion of free oestrogen into the cells of the target tissues in the hypothalamus, pituitary, vagina, urethra, uterus, breast and liver, binding to specific oestrogen receptors occurs. Very little information is currently available on the distribution of oestradiol following transdermal administration.

Biotransformation Inactivation of oestrogens in the body is carried out mainly in the liver. Metabolism of 17 β-oestradiol is by oxidation to oestrone, which in turn can be hydrated to form oestriol. There is free interconversion between oestrone and oestradiol. Oestrone and oestriol may then undergo conversion to their corresponding sulphate and glucuronide derivatives for excretion in the urine. Oestrone sulphate has a long biologic half-life because of its enterohepatic recirculation and interconversion to oestrone and oestradiol.

Elimination The plasma elimination half-life of oestradiol is approximately 1 hour and is independent of the route of administration. The metabolic plasma clearance rate is between 650 and 900 L/day/m2.

Steady state plasma oestradiol concentrations have been demonstrated in the range of 34 to 62 pg/ml for the Fematrix 80 patch (including baseline levels) and these are maintained throughout the dose interval (for up to four days). Absorption rate may vary between individual patients. After removal of the last patch plasma oestradiol and oestrone concentrations return to baseline values in less than 24 hours. The median terminal half-life for oestradiol following patch removal has been determined as 5.24h.

5.3 Preclinical safety data

No specific preclinical studies have been conducted on Fematrix. Supraphysiologically high doses (prolonged overdoses) of oestradiol have been associated with the induction of tumours in oestrogen-dependent target organs in rodent species. Pronounced species differences in toxicology, pharmacology and pharmacodynamics exist.

6. PHARMACEUTICAL PARTICULARS

6.1 List of excipients

Diethyltoluamide

Acrylic adhesive (Dow Corning MG-0560)

Acrylic thickener (Acrysol 33)

Backing: Polyester

Release liner: Aluminised/polyester

6.2 Incompatibilities

Not applicable.

6.3 Shelf life

The shelf-life of the product as packaged for sale is 3 years.

6.4 Special precautions for storage

Fematrix patches should be stored at below 25°C in a dry place.

6.5 Nature and contents of container

Sealed laminated sachet (paper/polyethylene/aluminium foil/polyethylene) containing one transdermal patch. Each carton contains eight patches, sufficient for one 28 day cycle and a patient leaflet. An additional pack containing two patches may also be available

6.6 Instructions for use and handling

Detailed instructions for use are provided in the patient leaflet.

7. MARKETING AUTHORISATION HOLDER

Solvay Healthcare Ltd

Mansbridge Road

West End

Southampton

SO18 3JD

United Kingdom

8. MARKETING AUTHORISATION NUMBER(S)

Fematrix 40: PL 00512/0173

Fematrix 80: PL 00512/0172

9. DATE OF FIRST AUTHORISATION/RENEWAL OF THE AUTHORISATION

12 November 2001

10. DATE OF REVISION OF THE TEXT

October 2004

Femodene

(Schering Health Care Limited)

1. NAME OF THE MEDICINAL PRODUCT

FEMODENE ®

2. QUALITATIVE AND QUANTITATIVE COMPOSITION

Each tablet contains 75 micrograms gestodene and 30 micrograms ethinylestradiol.

3. PHARMACEUTICAL FORM

Sugar-coated tablets

4. CLINICAL PARTICULARS

4.1 Therapeutic indications

Oral contraception and the recognised gynaecological indications for such oestrogen-progestogen combinations.

4.2 Posology and method of administration

First treatment cycle: 1 tablet daily for 21 days, starting on the first day of the menstrual cycle. Contraceptive protection begins immediately.

Subsequent cycles: Tablet taking from the next pack of Femodene is continued after a 7-day interval, beginning on the same day of the week as the first pack.

Changing from 21-day combined oral contraceptives: The first tablet of Femodene should be taken on the first day immediately after the end of the previous oral contraceptive course. Additional contraceptive precautions are not required.

Changing from a combined Every Day pill (28 day tablets): Femodene should be started after taking the last active tablet from the Every Day Pill pack. The first Femodene tablet is taken the next day. Additional contraceptive precautions are not then required.

Changing from a progestogen-only pill (POP): The first tablet of Femodene should be taken on the first day of bleeding, even if a POP has already been taken on that day. Additional contraceptive precautions are not then required. The remaining progestogen-only pills should be discarded.

Post-partum and post-abortum use: After pregnancy, oral contraception can be started 21 days after a vaginal delivery, provided that the patient is fully ambulant and there are no puerperal complications. Additional contraceptive precautions will be required for the first 7 days of tablet taking. Since the first post-partum ovulation may precede the first bleeding, another method of contraception should be used in the interval between childbirth and the first course of tablets. After a first-trimester abortion, oral contraception may be started immediately in which case no additional contraceptive precautions are required.

Special circumstances requiring additional contraception

Incorrect administration: A single delayed tablet should be taken as soon as possible, and if this can be done within 12 hours of the correct time, contraceptive protection is maintained. With longer delays, additional contraception is needed. Only the most recently delayed tablet should be taken, earlier missed tablets being omitted, and additional non-hormonal methods of contraception (except the rhythm or temperature methods) should be used for the next 7 days, while the next 7 tablets are being taken. Additionally, therefore, if tablet(s) have been missed during the last 7 days of a pack, there should be no break before the next pack is started. In this situation, a withdrawal bleed should not be expected until the end of the second pack. Some breakthrough bleeding may occur on tablet taking days but this is not clinically significant. If the patient does not have a withdrawal bleed during the tablet-free interval following the end of the second pack, the possibility of pregnancy must be ruled out before starting the next pack.

Gastro-intestinal upset: Vomiting or diarrhoea may reduce the efficacy of oral contraceptives by preventing full absorption. Tablet-taking from the current pack should be continued. Additional non-hormonal methods of contraception (except the rhythm or temperature methods) should be used during the gastro-intestinal upset and for 7 days following the upset. If these 7 days overrun the end of a pack, the next pack should be started without a break. In this situation, a withdrawal bleed should not be expected until the end of the second pack. If the patient does not have a withdrawal bleed during the tablet-free interval following the end of the second pack, the possibility of pregnancy must be ruled out before starting the next pack. Other methods of contraception should be considered if the gastro-intestinal disorder is likely to be prolonged.

4.3 Contraindications

1. Pregnancy
2. Severe disturbances of liver function, jaundice or persistent itching during a previous pregnancy, Dubin-Johnson syndrome, Rotor syndrome, previous or existing liver tumours.
3. History of confirmed venous thromboembolism (VTE). Family history of idiopathic VTE. Other known risk factors for VTE.
4. Existing or previous arterial thrombotic or embolic processes, conditions which predispose to them e.g. disorders of the clotting processes, valvular heart disease and atrial fibrillation.
5. Sickle-cell anaemia.
6. Mammary or endometrial carcinoma, or a history of these conditions.
7. Severe diabetes mellitus with vascular changes.
8. Disorders of lipid metabolism.
9. History of herpes gestationis.
10. Deterioration of otosclerosis during pregnancy.
11. Undiagnosed abnormal vaginal bleeding.
12. Hypersensitivity to any of the components of Femodene.

4.4 Special warnings and special precautions for use

Warnings: Some epidemiological studies have suggested an association between the use of combined oral contraceptives (COCs) and an increased risk of arterial and venous thrombotic and thromboembolic diseases such as myocardial infarction, stroke, deep venous thrombosis and pulmonary embolism. These events occur rarely. Full recovery from such disorders does not always occur, and it should be realised that in a few cases they are fatal.

The use of any combined oral contraceptive carries an increased risk of venous thromboembolism (VTE) compared with no use. The excess risk of VTE is highest during the first year a woman ever uses a combined oral contraceptive. This increased risk is less than the risk of VTE associated with pregnancy which is estimated as 60 cases per 100 000 pregnancies. Some epidemiological studies have reported a greater risk of VTE for women using combined oral contraceptives containing desogestrel or gestodene (the so-called third generation pills) than for women using pills containing levonorgestrel (the so-called second generation pills).

The spontaneous incidence of VTE in healthy non-pregnant women (not taking any oral contraceptive) is about 5 cases per 100,000 women per year. The incidence in users of second generation pills is about 15 per 100,000 women per year of use. The incidence in users of third generation pills is about 25 cases per 100,000 women per year of use; this excess incidence has not been satisfactorily explained by bias or confounding. The level of all of these risks of VTE increases with age and is likely to be further increased in women with other known risk factors for VTE such as obesity.

The risk of venous and/or arterial thrombosis associated with combined oral contraceptives increases with:

- age;
- smoking (with heavier smoking and increasing age the risk further increases, especially in women over 35 years of age);
- a positive family history (i.e. venous or arterial thromboembolism ever in a sibling or parent at a relatively early age). If a hereditary predisposition is suspected, the woman should be referred to a specialist for advice before deciding about any COC use;
- obesity (body mass index over 30 kg/m^2);
- dyslipoproteinaemia;
- hypertension;
- valvular heart disease;
- atrial fibrillation;
- prolonged immobilisation, major surgery, any surgery to the legs, or major trauma. In these situations it is advisable to discontinue COC use (in the case of elective surgery at least six weeks in advance) and not to resume until two weeks after complete remobilisation.
- There is no consensus about the possible role of varicose veins and superficial thrombophlebitis in venous thromboembolism.
- The increased risk of thromboembolism in the puerperium must be considered (for information on "Pregnancy and Lactation" see Section 4.6).
- Other medical conditions which have been associated with adverse circulatory events include diabetes mellitus, systemic lupus erythematosus, haemolytic uraemic syndrome, chronic inflammatory bowel disease (Crohn's disease or ulcerative colitis), sickle cell disease and subarachnoid haemorrhage.
- An increase in frequency or severity of migraine during COC use (which may be prodromal of a cerebrovascular event) may be a reason for immediate discontinuation of the COC.
- Biochemical factors that may be indicative of hereditary or acquired predisposition for venous or arterial thrombosis include Activated Protein C (APC) resistance, hyperhomocysteinaemia, antithrombin-III deficiency, protein C deficiency, protein S deficiency, antiphospholipid antibodies (anticardiolipin antibodies, lupus anticoagulant).

When considering risk/benefit, the physician should take into account that adequate treatment of a condition may reduce the associated risk of thrombosis and that the risk associated with pregnancy is higher than that associated with COC use.

Numerous epidemiological studies have been reported on the risks of ovarian, endometrial, cervical and breast cancer in women using combined oral contraceptives. The evidence is clear that combined oral contraceptives offer substantial protection against both ovarian and endometrial cancer.

An increased risk of cervical cancer in long-term users of combined oral contraceptives has been reported in some studies, but there continues to be controversy about the extent to which this is attributable to the confounding effects of sexual behaviour and other factors.

A meta-analysis from 54 epidemiological studies reported that there is a slightly increased relative risk (RR = 1.24) of having breast cancer diagnosed in women who are currently using combined oral contraceptives (COCs). The observed pattern of increased risk may be due to an earlier diagnosis of breast cancer in COC users, the biological effects of COCs or a combination of both. The additional breast cancers diagnosed in current users of COCs or in women who have used COCs in the last ten years are more likely to be localised to the breast than those in women who never used COCs.

Breast cancer is rare among women under 40 years of age whether or not they take COCs. Whilst this background risk increases with age, the excess number of breast cancer diagnoses in current and recent COC users is small in relation to the overall risk of breast cancer (see bar chart).

The most important risk factor for breast cancer in COC users is the age women discontinue the COC; the older the age at stopping, the more breast cancers are diagnosed. Duration of use is less important and the excess risk gradually disappears during the course of the 10 years after stopping COC use such that by 10 years there appears to be no excess.

The possible increase in risk of breast cancer should be discussed with the user and weighed against the benefits of COCs taking into account the evidence that they offer substantial protection against the risk of developing certain other cancers (e.g. ovarian and endometrial cancer).

(see Figure 1 above)

The possibility cannot be ruled out that certain chronic diseases may occasionally deteriorate during the use of combined oral contraceptives (see '*Precautions*').

The combination of ethinylestradiol and gestodene, like other contraceptive steroids, is associated with an increased incidence of neoplastic nodules in the rat liver, the relevance of which to man is unknown. Malignant liver tumours have been reported on rare occasions in long-term users of oral contraceptives.

In rare cases benign and, in even rarer cases, malignant liver tumours leading in isolated cases to life-threatening intra-abdominal haemorrhage have been observed after the use of hormonal substances such as those contained in Femodene. If severe upper abdominal complaints, liver enlargement or signs of intra-abdominal haemorrhage occur, the possibility of a liver tumour should be included in the differential diagnosis.

Figure 1

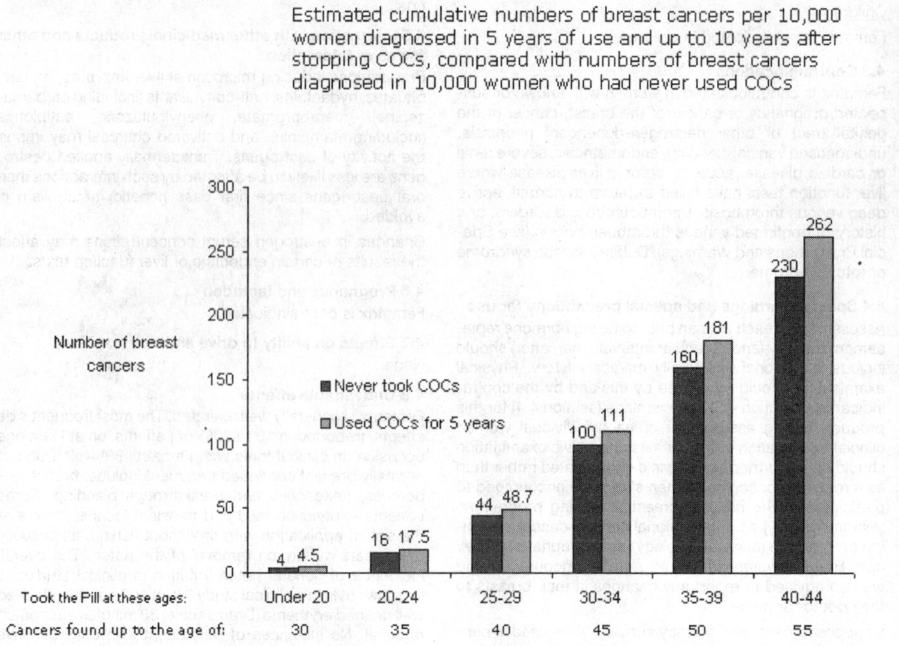

Reasons for stopping oral contraception immediately:

1. Occurrence for the first time, or exacerbation, of migrainous headaches or unusually frequent or unusually severe headaches.

2. Sudden disturbances of vision, of hearing or other perceptual disorders.

3. First signs of thrombophlebitis or thromboembolic symptoms (e.g. unusual pains in or swelling of the leg(s), stabbing pains on breathing or coughing for no apparent reason). Feeling of pain and tightness in the chest.

4. Six weeks before an elective major operation (e.g. abdominal, orthopaedic), any surgery to the legs, medical treatment for varicose veins or prolonged immobilisation, e.g. after accidents or surgery. Do not restart until 2 weeks after full ambulation. In case of emergency surgery, thrombotic prophylaxis is usually indicated e.g. subcutaneous heparin.

5. Onset of jaundice, hepatitis, itching of the whole body.

6. Increase in epileptic seizures.

7. Significant rise in blood pressure.

8. Onset of severe depression.

9. Severe upper abdominal pain or liver enlargement.

10. Clear exacerbation of conditions known to be capable of deteriorating during oral contraception or pregnancy.

11. Pregnancy is a reason for stopping immediately because it has been suggested by some investigations that oral contraceptives taken in early pregnancy may slightly increase the risk of foetal malformations. Other investigations have failed to support these findings. The possibility therefore cannot be excluded, but it is certain that if a risk exists at all, it is very small.

Precautions:

Assessment of women prior to starting oral contraceptives (and at regular intervals thereafter) should include a personal and family medical history of each woman. Physical examination should be guided by this and by the contraindications (section 4.3) and warnings (section 4.4) for this product. The frequency and nature of these assessments should be based upon relevant guidelines and should be adapted to the individual woman, but should include measurement of blood pressure and, if judged appropriate by the clinician, breast, abdominal and pelvic examination including cervical cytology.

The following conditions require strict medical supervision during medication with oral contraceptives. Deterioration or first appearance of any of these conditions may indicate that use of the oral contraceptive should be discontinued:

Diabetes mellitus, or a tendency towards diabetes mellitus (e.g. unexplained glycosuria), hypertension, varicose veins, a history of phlebitis, otosclerosis, multiple sclerosis, epilepsy, porphyria, tetany, disturbed liver function, Sydenham's chorea, renal dysfunction, family history of clotting disorders (see also contraindications), obesity, family history of breast cancer and patient history of benign breast disease, history of clinical depression, systemic lupus erythematosus, uterine fibroids, an intolerance of contact lenses, migraine, gall-stones, cardiovascular diseases, chloasma, asthma, or any disease that is prone to worsen during pregnancy.

Some women may experience amenorrhoea or oligomenorrhoea after discontinuation of oral contraceptives, especially when these conditions existed prior to use. Women should be informed of this possibility.

4.5 Interaction with other medicinal products and other forms of Interaction

Hepatic enzyme inducers such as barbiturates, primidone, phenobarbitone, phenytoin, phenylbutazone, rifampicin, carbamazepine and griseofulvin can impair the efficacy of Femodene. For women receiving long-term therapy with hepatic enzyme inducers, another method of contraception should be used. The use of antibiotics may also reduce the efficacy of Femodene, possibly by altering the intestinal flora.

Women receiving short courses of enzyme inducers or broad spectrum antibiotics should take additional, non-hormonal (except rhythm or temperature method) contraceptive precautions during the time of concurrent medication and for 7 days afterwards. If these 7 days overrun the end of a pack, the next pack should be started without a break. In this situation, a withdrawal bleed should not be expected until the end of the second pack. If the patient does not have a withdrawal bleed during the tablet-free interval following the end of the second pack, the possibility of pregnancy must be ruled out before resuming with the next pack. With rifampicin, additional contraceptive precautions should be continued for 4 weeks after treatment stops, even if only a short course was administered.

The requirement for oral antidiabetics or insulin can change as a result of the effect on glucose tolerance.

The herbal remedy St John's wort (Hypericum perforatum) should not be taken concomitantly with Femodene as this could potentially lead to a loss of contraceptive effect.

4.6 Pregnancy and lactation

If pregnancy occurs during medication with oral contraceptives, the preparation should be withdrawn immediately (see Section 4.4. 'Reasons for stopping oral contraception immediately').

The use of Femodene during lactation may lead to a reduction in the volume of milk produced and to a change in its composition. Minute amounts of the active substances are excreted with the milk. Mothers who are breast-feeding may be advised instead to use a progestogen-only pill.

4.7 Effects on ability to drive and use machines

None known.

4.8 Undesirable effects

In rare cases, headaches, gastric upsets, nausea, vomiting, breast tenderness, changes in body weight, changes in libido, depressive moods can occur.

In predisposed women, use of Femodene can sometimes cause chloasma which is exacerbated by exposure to sunlight. Such women should avoid prolonged exposure to sunlight.

Individual cases of poor tolerance of contact lenses have been reported with use of oral contraceptives. Contact lens wearers who develop changes in lens tolerance should be assessed by an ophthalmologist.

Menstrual changes:

1. Reduction of menstrual flow:

This is not abnormal and it is to be expected in some patients. Indeed, it may be beneficial where heavy periods were previously experienced.

2. Missed menstruation:

Occasionally, withdrawal bleeding may not occur at all. If the tablets have been taken correctly, pregnancy is very unlikely. If withdrawal bleeding fails to occur at the end of a second pack, the possibility of pregnancy must be ruled out before resuming with the next pack.

Intermenstrual bleeding: 'Spotting' or heavier 'breakthrough bleeding' sometimes occur during tablet taking, especially in the first few cycles, and normally cease spontaneously. Femodene should therefore, be continued even if irregular bleeding occurs. If irregular bleeding is persistent, appropriate diagnostic measures to exclude an organic cause are indicated and may include curettage. This also applies in the case of spotting which occurs at irregular intervals in several consecutive cycles or which occurs for the first time after long use of Femodene.

Effect on blood chemistry: The use of oral contraceptives may influence the results of certain laboratory tests including biochemical parameters of liver, thyroid, adrenal and renal function, plasma levels of carrier proteins and lipid/lipoprotein fractions, parameters of carbohydrate metabolism and parameters of coagulation and fibrinolysis. Laboratory staff should therefore be informed about oral contraceptive use when laboratory tests are requested.

Refer to Section 4.4. 'Special warnings and special precautions for use' for additional information.

4.9 Overdose

Overdosage may cause nausea, vomiting and, in females, withdrawal bleeding.

There are no specific antidotes and treatment should be symptomatic.

5. PHARMACOLOGICAL PROPERTIES

5.1 Pharmacodynamic properties

This oestrogen-progestogen combination acts by inhibiting ovulation by suppression of the mid-cycle surge of luteinising hormone, the inspissation of cervical mucus so as to constitute a barrier to sperm, and the rendering of the endometrium unreceptive to implantation.

5.2 Pharmacokinetic properties

Gestodene

Orally administered gestodene is rapidly and completely absorbed. Following single ingestion of Femodene, maximum drug serum levels of 4ng/ml are reached at about 1.0 hour. Thereafter, gestodene serum levels decrease in two phases. The terminal disposition phase is characterized by a half-life of 12 - 15 hours. For gestodene, an apparent volume of distribution of 0.7 l/kg and a metabolic clearance rate from serum of about 0.8 ml/min/kg were determined. Gestodene is not excreted in unchanged form but as metabolites, which are eliminated with a half-life of about 1 day. Gestodene metabolites are excreted at a urinary to biliary ratio of about 6:4. The biotransformation follows the known pathways of steroid metabolism. No pharmacologically active metabolites are known.

Gestodene is bound to serum albumin and to SHBG (sex hormone binding globulin). Only 1 - 2% of the total serum drug levels are present as free steroid, about 50 - 70% are specifically bound to SHBG. The relative distribution (free, albumin-bound, SHBG-bound) depends on the SHBG concentrations in the serum. Following induction of the binding protein, the SHBG-bound fraction increases while the unbound and the albumin-bound fractions decrease.

Following daily repeated administration of Femodene, gestodene concentrations in the serum increase by a factor of 2.8. Mean serum levels are fourfold higher at steady-state conditions which are reached during the second half of a treatment cycle. The pharmacokinetics of gestodene is influenced by SHBG serum levels. Under treatment with Femodene, a threefold increase in the serum SHBG levels has been observed for the first treatment cycle. Due to the specific binding of gestodene to SHBG, the increase in SHBG levels is accompanied by an almost parallel increase in gestodene serum levels. After three treatment cycles the extent of SHBG induction per cycle does not change any more. The absolute bioavailability of gestodene was determined to be 99% of the dose administered.

Ethinylestradiol

Orally administered ethinylestradiol is rapidly and completely absorbed. Following ingestion of Femodene, maximum drug serum levels of 82pg/ml are reached at 1.4 hours. Thereafter, ethinylestradiol serum levels decrease in two phases characterized by half-lives of 1 - 2 hours and about 20 hours. Because of analytical reasons, these parameters can only be calculated following the administration of higher doses. For ethinylestradiol, an apparent volume of distribution of about 5 l/kg and a metabolic clearance rate from serum of about 5ml/min/kg were determined. Ethinylestradiol is highly but non-specifically bound to serum albumin. About 2% of drug levels are present unbound. During absorption and first liver passage, ethinylestradiol is metabolized resulting in a reduced absolute and variable oral bioavailability. Unchanged drug is not excreted. Ethinylestradiol metabolites are excreted at a urinary to biliary ratio of 4:6 with a half-life of about 1 day.

According to the half-life of the terminal disposition phase from serum and the daily ingestion, steady-state serum levels are reached after 3 - 4 days and are higher by 30 - 40% as compared to a single dose.

During established lactation, 0.02% of the daily maternal dose could be transferred to the newborn via milk.

The systemic availability of ethinylestradiol might be influenced in both directions by other drugs. There is, however, no interaction with high doses of vitamin C. Ethinylestradiol induces the hepatic synthesis of SHBG and CBG (corticoid binding globulin) during continuous use. The extent of SHBG induction, however, depends on the chemical structure and the dose of the co-administered progestogen. During treatment with Femodene, SHBG concentrations in the serum increased from 69nmol/l to 198nmol/l in the first and to 210nmol/l in the third cycle. Serum concentrations of CBG were increased from 37μg/ml to 85μg/ml in the first cycle and remained constant thereafter.

5.3 Preclinical safety data

There are no preclinical safety data which could be of relevance to the prescriber and which are not already included in other relevant sections of the SPC.

6. PHARMACEUTICAL PARTICULARS

6.1 List of excipients

lactose

maize starch

povidone

magnesium stearate (E 572)

sodium calcium edetate

sucrose

macrogol 6000

calcium carbonate (E 170)

talc

montan glycol wax

6.2 Incompatibilities

None known.

6.3 Shelf life

5 years.

6.4 Special precautions for storage

Not applicable.

6.5 Nature and contents of container

Deep drawn strips made of polyvinyl chloride film with counter-sealing foil made of aluminium with heat sealable coating.

Presentation:

Carton containing memo-packs of either 1 × 21 tablets or 3 × 21 tablets.

6.6 Instructions for use and handling

Keep out of the reach of children.

7. MARKETING AUTHORISATION HOLDER

Schering Health Care Limited

The Brow

Burgess Hill

West Sussex RH15 9NE

8. MARKETING AUTHORISATION NUMBER(S)

0053/0179

9. DATE OF FIRST AUTHORISATION/RENEWAL OF THE AUTHORISATION

31 July 1991

10. DATE OF REVISION OF THE TEXT

24 November 2004

LEGAL CATEGORY

POM

Femodene ED

(Schering Health Care Limited)

1. NAME OF THE MEDICINAL PRODUCT
FEMODENE ® ED

2. QUALITATIVE AND QUANTITATIVE COMPOSITION
Each active tablet contains 75 micrograms gestodene and 30 micrograms ethinylestradiol. Each pack also contains seven placebo tablets which are larger.

3. PHARMACEUTICAL FORM
Sugar-coated tablets

4. CLINICAL PARTICULARS

4.1 Therapeutic indications
Oral contraception and the recognised gynaecological indications for such oestrogen-progestogen combinations.

4.2 Posology and method of administration
First treatment cycle: 1 tablet daily for 28 days, starting on the first day of the menstrual cycle. 21 (small) active tablets are taken followed by 7 (larger) placebo tablets. Contraceptive protection begins immediately.

Subsequent cycles: Tablet-taking is continuous, which means that the next pack of Femodene ED follows immediately without a break. A withdrawal bleed usually occurs when the placebo tablets are being taken.

Changing from 21-day combined oral contraceptives: The first tablet of Femodene ED should be taken on the first day immediately after the end of the previous oral contraceptive course. Additional contraceptive precautions are not required.

Changing from a combined Every Day pill (28 -day pill): Femodene ED should be started after taking the last active tablet from the previous Every Day pill pack. The first Femodene ED tablet is taken the next day. Additional contraceptive precautions are not then required.

Changing from a progestogen-only pill (POP):
The first tablet of Femodene ED should be taken on the first day of bleeding, even if a POP has already been taken on that day. Additional contraceptive precautions are not then required. The remaining progestogen-only pills should be discarded.

Post-partum and post-abortum use: After pregnancy, Femodene ED can be started 21 days after a vaginal delivery, provided that the patient is fully ambulant and there are no puerperal complications. Additional contraceptive precautions will be required for the first 7 days of tablet taking. Since the first post-partum ovulation may precede the first bleeding, another method of contraception should be used in the interval between childbirth and the first course of tablets. After a first-trimester abortion, oral contraception may be started immediately in which case no additional contraceptive precautions are required.

Special circumstances requiring additional contraception

Incorrect administration: Errors in taking the 7 placebo tablets (i.e. the larger white tablets in the last row) can be ignored. A single delayed active (small) tablet should be taken as soon as possible, and if this can be done within 12 hours of the correct time, contraceptive protection is maintained.

With longer delays in taking active tablets, additional contraception is needed. Only the most recently delayed tablet should be taken, earlier missed tablets being omitted, and additional non-hormonal methods of contraception (except the rhythm or temperature methods) should be used for *the next 7 days, while the next 7 active (small) tablets are being taken.* Therefore, if the 7 days additional contraception will extend beyond the last active (small) tablet, the user should finish taking all the active tablets, discard the placebo tablets and start a new pack of Femodene ED the next day with an appropriate active (small) tablet. Thus, active tablet follows active tablet with no 7 day break. In this situation, a withdrawal bleed should not be expected until the end of the second pack. Some breakthrough bleeding may occur on tablet taking days but this is not clinically significant. If the patient does not have a withdrawal bleed following the end of the second pack, the possibility of pregnancy must be ruled out before starting the next pack.

Gastro-intestinal upset: Vomiting or diarrhoea may reduce the efficacy of oral contraceptives by preventing full absorption. Tablet-taking from the current pack should be continued. Additional non-hormonal methods of contraception (except the rhythm or temperature methods) should be used during the gastro-intestinal upset and for 7 days following the upset. If these 7 days extend beyond the last active (small) tablet the user should finish taking all the active tablets, discard the placebo tablets and start a new pack of Femodene ED the next day with an appropriate active (small) tablet. In this situation, a withdrawal bleed should not be expected until the end of the second pack. If the patient does not have a withdrawal bleed at the end of the second pack, the possibility of pregnancy must be ruled out before starting the next pack. Other methods of contraception should be considered if the gastro-intestinal disorder is likely to be prolonged.

4.3 Contraindications
1. Pregnancy

2. Severe disturbances of liver function, jaundice or persistent itching during a previous pregnancy, Dubin-Johnson syndrome, Rotor syndrome, previous or existing liver tumours.

3. History of confirmed venous thromboembolism (VTE). Family history of idiopathic VTE. Other known risk factors for VTE.

4. Existing or previous arterial thrombotic or embolic processes, conditions which predispose to them e.g. disorders of the clotting processes, valvular heart disease and atrial fibrillation.

5. Sickle-cell anaemia.

6. Mammary or endometrial carcinoma, or a history of these conditions.

7. Severe diabetes mellitus with vascular changes.

8. Disorders of lipid metabolism.

9. History of herpes gestationis.

10. Deterioration of otosclerosis during pregnancy.

11. Undiagnosed abnormal vaginal bleeding.

12. Hypersensitivity to any of the components of Femodene ED.

4.4 Special warnings and special precautions for use
Warnings:

Some epidemiological studies have suggested an association between the use of combined oral contraceptives (COCs) and an increased risk of arterial and venous thrombotic and thromboembolic diseases such as myocardial infarction, stroke, deep venous thrombosis and pulmonary embolism. These events occur rarely. Full recovery from such disorders does not always occur, and it should be realised that in a few cases they are fatal.

The use of any combined oral contraceptive carries an increased risk of venous thromboembolism (VTE) compared with no use. The excess risk of VTE is highest during the first year a woman ever uses a combined oral contraceptive. This increased risk is less than the risk of VTE associated with pregnancy which is estimated as 60 cases per 100 000 pregnancies. Some epidemiological studies have reported a greater risk of VTE for women using combined oral contraceptives containing desogestrel or gestodene (the so-called third generation pills) than for women using pills containing levonorgestrel (the so-called second generation pills).

The spontaneous incidence of VTE in healthy non-pregnant women (not taking any oral contraceptive) is about 5 cases per 100,000 women per year. The incidence in users of second generation pills is about 15 per 100,000 women per year of use. The incidence in users of third generation pills is about 25 cases per 100,000 women per year of use; this excess incidence has not been satisfactorily explained by bias or confounding. The level of all of these risks of VTE increases with age and is likely to be further increased in women with other known risk factors for VTE such as obesity.

The risk of venous and/or arterial thrombosis associated with combined oral contraceptives increases with:

- age;
- smoking (with heavier smoking and increasing age the risk further increases, especially in women over 35 years of age);
- a positive family history (i.e. venous or arterial thromboembolism ever in a sibling or parent at a relatively early age). If a hereditary predisposition is suspected, the woman should be referred to a specialist for advice before deciding about any COC use;
- obesity (body mass index over 30 kg/m^2);
- dyslipoproteinaemia;
- hypertension;
- valvular heart disease;
- atrial fibrillation;
- prolonged immobilisation, major surgery, any surgery to the legs, or major trauma. In these situations it is advisable to discontinue COC use (in the case of elective surgery at least six weeks in advance) and not to resume until two weeks after complete remobilisation.
- There is no consensus about the possible role of varicose veins and superficial thrombophlebitis in venous thromboembolism.
- The increased risk of thromboembolism in the puerperium must be considered (for information on "Pregnancy and Lactation" see Section 4.6).
- Other medical conditions which have been associated with adverse circulatory events include diabetes mellitus, systemic lupus erythematosus, haemolytic uraemic syndrome, chronic inflammatory bowel disease (Crohn's disease or ulcerative colitis), sickle cell disease and subarachnoid haemorrhage.
- An increase in frequency or severity of migraine during COC use (which may be prodromal of a cerebrovascular event) may be a reason for immediate discontinuation of the COC.
- Biochemical factors that may be indicative of hereditary or acquired predisposition for venous or arterial thrombosis include Activated Protein C (APC) resistance, hyperhomocysteinaemia, antithrombin-III deficiency, protein C deficiency, protein S deficiency, antiphospholipid antibodies (anticardiolipin antibodies, lupus anticoagulant).

When considering risk/benefit, the physician should take into account that adequate treatment of a condition may reduce the associated risk of thrombosis and that the risk associated with pregnancy is higher than that associated with COC use.

Numerous epidemiological studies have been reported on the risks of ovarian, endometrial, cervical and breast cancer in women using combined oral contraceptives. The evidence is clear that combined oral contraceptives offer substantial protection against both ovarian and endometrial cancer.

An increased risk of cervical cancer in long-term users of combined oral contraceptives has been reported in some studies, but there continues to be controversy about the extent to which this is attributable to the confounding effects of sexual behaviour and other factors.

A meta-analysis from 54 epidemiological studies reported that there is a slightly increased relative risk (RR = 1.24) of having breast cancer diagnosed in women who are currently using combined oral contraceptives (COCs). The observed pattern of increased risk may be due to an earlier diagnosis of breast cancer in COC users, the biological effects of COCs or a combination of both. The additional breast cancers diagnosed in current users of COCs or in women who have used COCs in the last ten years are more likely to be localised to the breast than those in women who never used COCs.

Breast cancer is rare among women under 40 years of age whether or not they take COCs. Whilst this background risk increases with age, the excess number of breast cancer diagnoses in current and recent COC users is small in relation to the overall risk of breast cancer (see bar chart).

The most important risk factor for breast cancer in COC users is the age women discontinue the COC; the older the age at stopping, the more breast cancers are diagnosed. Duration of use is less important and the excess risk gradually disappears during the course of the 10 years after stopping COC use such that by 10 years there appears to be no excess.

The possible increase in risk of breast cancer should be discussed with the user and weighed against the benefits of COCs taking into account the evidence that they offer substantial protection against the risk of developing certain other cancers (e.g. ovarian and endometrial cancer).

(see Figure 1 on next page)

The possibility cannot be ruled out that certain chronic diseases may occasionally deteriorate during the use of combined oral contraceptives (see '*Precautions*').

The combination of ethinylestradiol and gestodene, like other contraceptive steroids, is associated with an increased incidence of neoplastic nodules in the rat liver, the relevance of which to man is unknown. Malignant liver tumours have been reported on rare occasions in long-term users of oral contraceptives.

In rare cases benign and, in even rarer cases, malignant liver tumours leading in isolated cases to life-threatening intra-abdominal haemorrhage have been observed after the use of hormonal substances such as those contained in Femodene ED. If severe upper abdominal complaints, liver enlargement or signs of intra-abdominal haemorrhage occur, the possibility of a liver tumour should be included in the differential diagnosis.

Reasons for stopping oral contraception immediately:

1. Occurrence for the first time, or exacerbation, of migrainous headaches or unusually frequent or unusually severe headaches.

2. Sudden disturbances of vision, of hearing or other perceptual disorders.

3. First signs of thrombophlebitis or thromboembolic symptoms (e.g. unusual pains in or swelling of the leg(s), stabbing pains on breathing or coughing for no apparent reason). Feeling of pain and tightness in the chest.

4. Six weeks before an elective major operation (e.g. abdominal, orthopaedic), any surgery to the legs, medical treatment for varicose veins or prolonged immobilisation, e.g. after accidents or surgery. Do not restart until 2 weeks after full ambulation. In case of emergency surgery, thrombotic prophylaxis is usually indicated e.g. subcutaneous heparin.

5. Onset of jaundice, hepatitis, itching of the whole body.

6. Increase in epileptic seizures.

7. Significant rise in blood pressure.

8. Onset of severe depression.

9. Severe upper abdominal pain or liver enlargement.

10. Clear exacerbation of conditions known to be capable of deteriorating during oral contraception or pregnancy.

11. Pregnancy is a reason for stopping immediately because it has been suggested by some investigations that oral contraceptives taken in early pregnancy may slightly increase the risk of foetal malformations. Other investigations have failed to support these findings. The possibility therefore cannot be excluded, but it is certain that if a risk exists at all, it is very small.

Figure 1

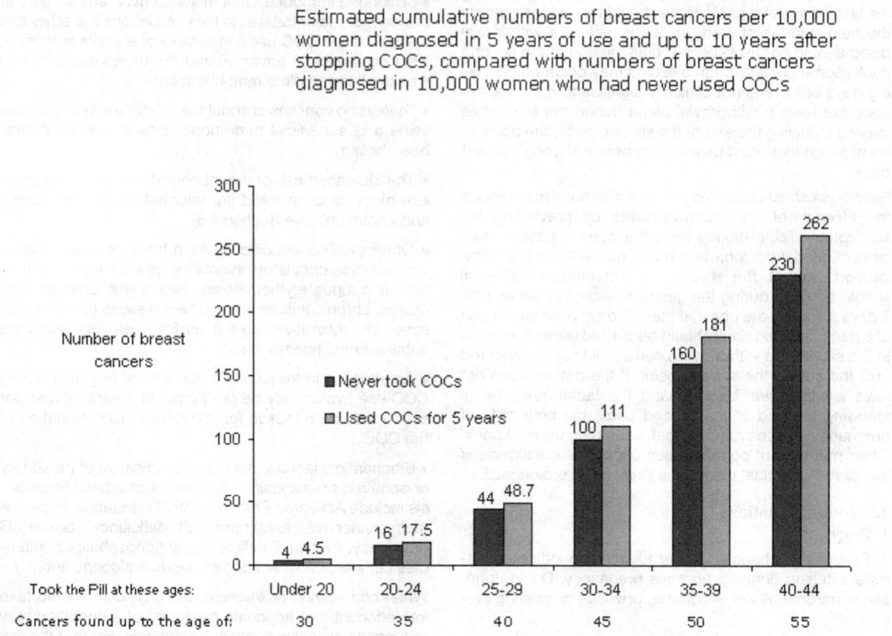

Precautions:

Assessment of women prior to starting oral contraceptives (and at regular intervals thereafter) should include a personal and family medical history of each woman. Physical examination should be guided by this and by the contraindications (section 4.3) and warnings (section 4.4) for this product. The frequency and nature of these assessments should be based upon relevant guidelines and should be adapted to the individual woman, but should include measurement of blood pressure and, if judged appropriate by the clinician, breast, abdominal and pelvic examination including cervical cytology.

The following conditions require strict medical supervision during medication with oral contraceptives. Deterioration or first appearance of any of these conditions may indicate that use of the oral contraceptive should be discontinued:

Diabetes mellitus, or a tendency towards diabetes mellitus (e.g. unexplained glycosuria), hypertension, varicose veins, a history of phlebitis, otosclerosis, multiple sclerosis, epilepsy, porphyria, tetany, disturbed liver function, Sydenham's chorea, renal dysfunction, family history of clotting disorders (see also contraindications), obesity, family history of breast cancer and patient history of benign breast disease, history of clinical depression, systemic lupus erythematosus, uterine fibroids and migraine, gallstones, cardiovascular diseases, chloasma, asthma, an intolerance to contact lenses, or any disease that is prone to worsen during pregnancy.

Some women may experience amenorrhoea or oligomenorrhoea after discontinuation of oral contraceptives, especially when these conditions existed prior to use. Women should be informed of this possibility.

4.5 Interaction with other medicinal products and other forms of Interaction

Hepatic enzyme inducers such as barbiturates, primidone, phenobarbitone, phenytoin, phenylbutazone, rifampicin, carbamazepine and griseofulvin can impair the efficacy of Femodene ED. For women receiving long-term therapy with hepatic enzyme inducers, another method of contraception should be used. The use of antibiotics may also reduce the efficacy of Femodene ED, possibly by altering the intestinal flora.

Women receiving short courses of enzyme inducers or broad spectrum antibiotics should take additional, non-hormonal (except rhythm or temperature method) contraceptive precautions during the time of concurrent medication and for 7 days afterwards. If these 7 days extend beyond the last active (small) tablet the user should finish taking all the active tablets, discard the placebo (large) tablets and start a new pack of Femodene ED the next day with an appropriate active (small) tablet. In this situation, a withdrawal bleed should not be expected until the end of the second pack. If the patient does not have a withdrawal bleed at the end of the second pack, the possibility of pregnancy must be ruled out before resuming with the next pack. With rifampicin, additional contraceptive precautions should be continued for 4 weeks after treatment stops, even if only a short course was administered.

The requirement for oral antidiabetics or insulin can change as a result of the effect on glucose tolerance.

The herbal remedy St John's wort (Hypericum perforatum) should not be taken concomitantly with Femodene ED as this could potentially lead to a loss of contraceptive effect.

4.6 Pregnancy and lactation

If pregnancy occurs during medication with oral contraceptives, the preparation should be withdrawn immediately (see Section 4.4. 'Reasons for stopping oral contraception immediately').

The use of Femodene ED during lactation may lead to a reduction in the volume of milk produced and to a change in its composition. Minute amounts of the active substances are excreted with the milk. Mothers who are breast-feeding may be advised instead to use a progestogen-only pill.

4.7 Effects on ability to drive and use machines

None known.

4.8 Undesirable effects

In rare cases, headaches, gastric upsets, nausea, vomiting, breast tenderness, changes in body weight, changes in libido, depressive moods can occur.

In predisposed women, use of Femodene ED can sometimes cause chloasma which is exacerbated by exposure to sunlight. Such women should avoid prolonged exposure to sunlight.

Individual cases of poor tolerance of contact lenses have been reported with use of oral contraceptives. Contact lens wearers who develop changes in lens tolerance should be assessed by an ophthalmologist.

Menstrual changes:

1. Reduction of menstrual flow:

This is not abnormal and it is to be expected in some patients. Indeed, it may be beneficial where heavy periods were previously experienced.

2. Missed menstruation:

Occasionally, withdrawal bleeding may not occur at all. If the tablets have been taken correctly, pregnancy is very unlikely. If withdrawal bleeding fails to occur at the end of a second pack, the possibility of pregnancy must be ruled out before resuming with the next pack.

Intermenstrual bleeding: 'Spotting' or heavier 'breakthrough bleeding' sometimes occur during tablet taking, especially in the first few cycles, and normally cease spontaneously. Femodene ED should therefore, be continued even if irregular bleeding occurs. If irregular bleeding is persistent, appropriate diagnostic measures to exclude an organic cause are indicated and may include curettage. This also applies in the case of spotting which occurs at irregular intervals in several consecutive cycles or which occurs for the first time after long use of Femodene ED.

Effect on blood chemistry: The use of oral contraceptives may influence the results of certain laboratory tests including biochemical parameters of liver, thyroid, adrenal and renal function, plasma levels of carrier proteins and lipid/lipoprotein fractions, parameters of carbohydrate metabolism and parameters of coagulation and fibrinolysis. Laboratory staff should therefore be informed about oral contraceptive use when laboratory tests are requested.

Refer to Section 4.4. 'Special warnings and special precautions for use' for additional information.

4.9 Overdose

Overdosage may cause nausea, vomiting and, in females, withdrawal bleeding.

There are no specific antidotes and treatment should be symptomatic.

5. PHARMACOLOGICAL PROPERTIES

5.1 Pharmacodynamic properties

This oestrogen-progestogen combination acts by inhibiting ovulation by suppression of the mid-cycle surge of luteinising hormone, the inspissation of cervical mucus so as to constitute a barrier to sperm, and the rendering of the endometrium unreceptive to implantation.

5.2 Pharmacokinetic properties

Gestodene

Orally administered gestodene is rapidly and completely absorbed. Following single ingestion of Femodene ED, maximum drug serum levels of 4ng/ml are reached at about 1.0 hour. Thereafter, gestodene serum levels decrease in two phases. The terminal disposition phase is characterised by a half-life of 12 - 15 hours. For gestodene, an apparent volume of distribution of 0.7 l/kg and a metabolic clearance rate from serum of about 0.8 ml/min/kg were determined. Gestodene is not excreted in unchanged form but as metabolites, which are eliminated with a half-life of about 1 day. Gestodene metabolites are excreted at an urinary to biliary ratio of about 6:4. The biotransformation follows the known pathways of steroid metabolism. No pharmacologically active metabolites are known.

Gestodene is bound to serum albumin and to SHBG (sex hormone binding globulin). Only 1 - 2% of the total serum drug levels are present as free steroid, about 50 - 70% are specifically bound to SHBG. The relative distribution (free, albumin-bound, SHBG-bound) depends on the SHBG concentrations in the serum. Following induction of the binding protein, the SHBG-bound fraction increases while the unbound and the albumin-bound fractions decrease.

Following daily repeated administration of Femodene ED, gestodene concentrations in the serum increase by a factor of 2.8. Mean serum levels are fourfold higher at steady-state conditions which are reached during the second half of a treatment cycle. The pharmacokinetics of gestodene is influenced by SHBG serum levels. Under treatment with Femodene ED, a threefold increase in the serum SHBG levels has been observed for the first treatment cycle. Due to the specific binding of gestodene to SHBG, the increase in SHBG levels is accompanied by an almost parallel increase in gestodene serum levels. After three treatment cycles the extent of SHBG induction per cycle does not change any more. The absolute bioavailability of gestodene was determined to be 99% of the dose administered.

Ethinylestradiol

Orally administered ethinylestradiol is rapidly and completely absorbed. Following ingestion of Femodene ED, maximum drug serum levels of 82pg/ml are reached at 1.4 hours. Thereafter, ethinylestradiol serum levels decrease in two phases characterised by half-lives of 1 - 2 hours and about 20 hours. Because of analytical reasons, these parameters can only be calculated following the administration of higher doses. For ethinylestradiol, an apparent volume of distribution of about 5 l/kg and a metabolic clearance rate from serum of about 5ml/min/kg were determined. Ethinylestradiol is highly but non-specifically bound to serum albumin. About 2% of drug levels are present unbound. During absorption and first liver passage, ethinylestradiol is metabolised resulting in a reduced absolute and variable oral bioavailability. Unchanged drug is not excreted. Ethinylestradiol metabolites are excreted at a urinary to biliary ratio of 4:6 with a half-life of about 1 day.

According to the half-life of the terminal disposition phase from serum and the daily ingestion, steady-state serum levels are reached after 3 - 4 days and are higher by 30 - 40% as compared to a single dose.

During established lactation, 0.02% of the daily maternal dose could be transferred to the newborn via milk.

The systemic availability of ethinylestradiol might be influenced in both directions by other drugs. There is, however, no interaction with high doses of vitamin C. Ethinylestradiol induces the hepatic synthesis of SHBG and CBG (corticoid binding globulin) during continuous use. The extent of SHBG induction, however, depends on the chemical structure and the dose of the co-administered progestogen. During treatment with Femodene ED, SHBG concentrations in the serum increased from 69nmol/l to 198nmol/l in the first and to 210nmol/l in the third cycle. Serum concentrations of CBG were increased from 37μg/ml to 85μg/ml in the first cycle and remained constant thereafter.

5.3 Preclinical safety data

There are no preclinical safety data which could be of relevance to the prescriber and which is not already included in other relevant sections of the SPC.

6. PHARMACEUTICAL PARTICULARS

6.1 List of excipients

Active tablets	Placebo tablets
lactose	lactose
maize starch	maize starch
povidone	povidone
sodium calcium edetate	magnesium stearate (E 572)
magnesium stearate (E 572)	sucrose
sucrose	polyethylene glycol 6000
macrogol 6000	calcium carbonate (E 170)
calcium carbonate (E 170)	talc
talc	montan glycol wax
montan glycol wax	

6.2 Incompatibilities
None known.

6.3 Shelf life
5 years.

6.4 Special precautions for storage
Not applicable.

6.5 Nature and contents of container
Deep drawn strips made of polyvinyl chloride film with counter-sealing foil made of aluminium with heat sealable coating.

Presentation

Each carton contains either 1 or 3 blister memo-packs. Each blister memo-pack contains 21 active tablets and 7 placebo tablets.

6.6 Instructions for use and handling
Keep out of the reach of children.

7. MARKETING AUTHORISATION HOLDER
Schering Health Care Limited
The Brow
Burgess Hill
West Sussex RH15 9NE

8. MARKETING AUTHORISATION NUMBER(S)
0053/0180

9. DATE OF FIRST AUTHORISATION/RENEWAL OF THE AUTHORISATION
31 July 1991

10. DATE OF REVISION OF THE TEXT
24 November 2004

LEGAL CATEGORY
POM

Femodette

(Schering Health Care Limited)

1. NAME OF THE MEDICINAL PRODUCT
Femodette®

2. QUALITATIVE AND QUANTITATIVE COMPOSITION
Each tablet contains 0.075mg gestodene and 0.02mg ethinylestradiol.

3. PHARMACEUTICAL FORM
Sugar - coated tablets.

4. CLINICAL PARTICULARS

4.1 Therapeutic indications
Oral contraception and the recognised gynaecological indications for such oestrogen-progestogen combinations.

4.2 Posology and method of administration
First treatment cycle: 1 tablet for 21 days, starting on the first day of the menstrual cycle. Contraceptive protection begins immediately.

Subsequent cycles: Tablet taking from the next pack of Femodette is continued after a 7-day interval, beginning on the same day of the week as the first pack.

Changing from 21 day combined oral contraceptives: The first tablet of Femodette should be taken on the first day immediately after the end of the previous oral contraceptive course. Additional contraceptive precautions are not required.

Changing from a combined Every Day pill (28 day tablets): Femodette should be started after taking the last active tablet from the Every Day Pill pack. The first Femodette tablet is taken the next day. Additional contraceptive precautions are not then required.

Changing from a progestogen-only pill (POP):
The first tablet of Femodette should be taken on the first day of bleeding, even if a POP has already been taken on that day. Additional contraceptive precautions are not then required. The remaining progestogen-only pills should be discarded.

Post-partum and post-abortum use: After pregnancy, oral contraception can be started 21 days after a vaginal delivery, provided that the patient is fully ambulant and there are no puerperal complications. Additional contraceptive precautions will be required for the first 7 days of pill taking. Since the first post-partum ovulation may precede the first bleeding, another method of contraception should be used in the interval between childbirth and the first course of tablets. After a first-trimester abortion, oral contraception may be started immediately in which case no additional contraceptive precautions are required.

Special circumstances requiring additional contraception

Incorrect administration: A single delayed tablet should be taken as soon as possible, and if this can be done within 12 hours of the correct time, contraceptive protection is maintained. With longer delays, additional contraception is needed. Only the most recently delayed tablet should be taken, earlier missed tablets being omitted, and additional non-hormonal methods of contraception (except the rhythm and temperature methods) should be used for the next 7 days, while the next 7 tablets are being taken. Additionally, therefore, if tablet(s) have been missed during the last 7 days of a pack, there should be no break before the next pack is started. In this situation, a withdrawal bleed should not be expected until the end of the second pack. Some breakthrough bleeding may occur on pill taking days but this is not clinically significant. If the patient does not have a withdrawal bleed during the tablet-free interval following the end of the second pack, the possibility of pregnancy must be ruled out before starting the next pack.

Gastro-intestinal upset: Vomiting or diarrhoea may reduce the efficacy of oral contraceptives by preventing full absorption. Tablet-taking from the current pack should be continued. Additional non-hormonal methods of contraception (except the rhythm or temperature methods) should be used during the gastro-intestinal upset and for 7 days following the upset. If these 7 days overrun the end of a pack, the next pack should be started without a break. In this situation, a withdrawal bleed should not be expected until the end of the second pack. If the patient does not have a withdrawal bleed during the tablet-free interval following the end of the second pack, the possibility of pregnancy must be ruled out before starting the next pack. Other methods of contraception should be considered if the gastro-intestinal disorder is likely to be prolonged.

4.3 Contraindications
1. Pregnancy.
2. Severe disturbances of liver function, jaundice or persistent itching during a previous pregnancy, Dubin-Johnson syndrome, Rotor syndrome, previous or existing liver tumours.
3. History of confirmed venous thromboembolism (VTE). Family history of idiopathic VTE. Other known risk factors for VTE.
4. Existing or previous arterial thrombotic or embolic processes, conditions which predispose to them e.g. disorders of the clotting processes, valvular heart disease and atrial fibrillation.
5. Sickle-cell anaemia.
6. Mammary or endometrial carcinoma, or a history of these conditions.
7. Severe diabetes mellitus with vascular changes.
8. Disorders of lipid metabolism.
9. History of herpes gestationis.
10. Deterioration of otosclerosis during pregnancy.
11. Undiagnosed abnormal vaginal bleeding.
12. Hypersensitivity to any of the components of Femodette.

4.4 Special warnings and special precautions for use
Warnings:

Some epidemiological studies have suggested an association between the use of combined oral contraceptives (COCs) and an increased risk of arterial and venous thrombotic and thromboembolic diseases such as myocardial infarction, stroke, deep venous thrombosis and pulmonary embolism. These events occur rarely. Full recovery from such disorders does not always occur, and it should be realised that in a few cases they are fatal.

The use of any combined oral contraceptive carries an increased risk of venous thromboembolism (VTE) compared with no use. The excess risk of VTE is highest during the first year a woman ever uses a combined oral contraceptive. This increased risk is less than the risk of VTE associated with pregnancy which is estimated as 60 cases per 100 000 pregnancies. Some epidemiological studies have reported a greater risk of VTE for women using combined oral contraceptives containing desogestrel or gestodene (the so-called third generation pills) than for women using pills containing levonorgestrel (the so-called second generation pills).

The spontaneous incidence of VTE in healthy non-pregnant women (not taking any oral contraceptive) is about 5 cases per 100,000 women per year. The incidence in users of second generation pills is about 15 per 100,000 women per year of use. The incidence in users of third generation pills is about 25 cases per 100,000 women per year of use; this excess incidence has not been satisfactorily explained by bias or confounding. The level of all of these risks of VTE increases with age and is likely to be further increased in women with other known risk factors for VTE such as obesity.

The risk of venous and/or arterial thrombosis associated with combined oral contraceptives increases with:

- age;
- smoking (with heavier smoking and increasing age the risk further increases, especially in women over 35 years of age);a positive family history (i.e. venous or arterial thromboembolism ever in a sibling or parent at a relatively early age). If a hereditary predisposition is suspected, the woman should be referred to a specialist for advice before deciding about any COC use;
- obesity (body mass index over 30 kg/m2);
- dyslipoproteinaemia;
- hypertension;
- valvular heart disease;
- atrial fibrillation;
- prolonged immobilisation, major surgery, any surgery to the legs, or major trauma. In these situations it is advisable to discontinue COC use (in the case of elective surgery at least six weeks in advance) and not to resume until two weeks after complete remobilisation.
- There is no consensus about the possible role of varicose veins and superficial thrombophlebitis in venous thromboembolism.
- The increased risk of thromboembolism in the puerperium must be considered (for information on "Pregnancy and Lactation" see Section 4.6).
- Other medical conditions which have been associated with adverse circulatory events include diabetes mellitus, systemic lupus erythematosus, haemolytic uraemic syndrome, chronic inflammatory bowel disease (Crohn's disease or ulcerative colitis) sickle cell disease and subarachnoid haemorrhage
- An increase in frequency or severity of migraine during COC use (which may be prodromal of a cerebrovascular event) may be a reason for immediate discontinuation of the COC.
- Biochemical factors that may be indicative of hereditary or acquired predisposition for venous or arterial thrombosis include Activated Protein C (APC) resistance, hyperhomocysteinaemia, antithrombin-III deficiency, protein C deficiency, protein S deficiency, antiphospholipid antibodies (anticardiolipin antibodies, lupus anticoagulant).

When considering risk/benefit, the physician should take into account that adequate treatment of a condition may reduce the associated risk of thrombosis and that the risk associated with pregnancy is higher than that associated with COC use.

Numerous epidemiological studies have been reported on the risks of ovarian, endometrial, cervical and breast cancer in women using combined oral contraceptives. The evidence is clear that combined oral contraceptives offer substantial protection against both ovarian and endometrial cancer.

An increased risk of cervical cancer in long-term users of combined oral contraceptives has been reported in some studies, but there continues to be controversy about the extent to which this is attributable to the confounding effects of sexual behaviour and other factors.

A meta-analysis from 54 epidemiological studies reported that there is a slightly increased relative risk (RR = 1.24) of having breast cancer diagnosed in women who are currently using combined oral contraceptives (COCs). The observed pattern of increased risk may be due to an earlier diagnosis of breast cancer in COC users, the biological effects of COCs or a combination of both. The additional breast cancers diagnosed in current users of COCs or in women who have used COCs in the last ten years are more likely to be localised to the breast than those in women who never used COCs.

Breast cancer is rare among women under 40 years of age whether or not they take COCs. Whilst this background risk increases with age, the excess number of breast cancer diagnoses in current and recent COC users is small in relation to the overall risk of breast cancer (see bar chart).

The most important risk factor for breast cancer in COC users is the age women discontinue the COC; the older the age at stopping, the more breast cancers are diagnosed. Duration of use is less important and the excess risk gradually disappears during the course of the 10 years after stopping COC use such that by 10 years there appears to be no excess.

The possible increase in risk of breast cancer should be discussed with the user and weighed against the benefits of COCs taking into account the evidence that they offer substantial protection against the risk of developing certain other cancers (e.g. ovarian and endometrial cancer).

Estimated cumulative numbers of breast cancers per 10 000 women diagnosed in 5 years of use and up to 10 years after stopping COCs, compared with numbers of breast cancers diagnosed in 10 000 women who had never used COCs.

(see Figure 1 on next page)

The possibility cannot be ruled out that certain chronic diseases may occasionally deteriorate during the use of combined oral contraceptives (see 'Precautions').

The combination of ethinylestradiol and gestodene, like other contraceptive steroids, is associated with an increased incidence of neoplastic nodules in the rat liver, the relevance of which to man is unknown. Malignant liver tumours have been reported on rare occasions in long-term users of oral contraceptives.

In rare cases benign and, in even rarer cases, malignant liver tumours leading in isolated cases to life-threatening intraabdominal haemorrhage have been observed after the use of hormonal substances such as those contained in Femodette. If severe upper abdominal complaints, liver enlargement or signs of intra-abdominal haemorrhage occur, the possibility of a liver tumour should be included in the differential diagnosis.

Figure 1 Estimated cumulative numbers of breast cancers per 10 000 women diagnosed in 5 years of use and up to 10 years after stopping COCs, compared with numbers of breast cancers diagnosed in 10 000 women who had never used COCs

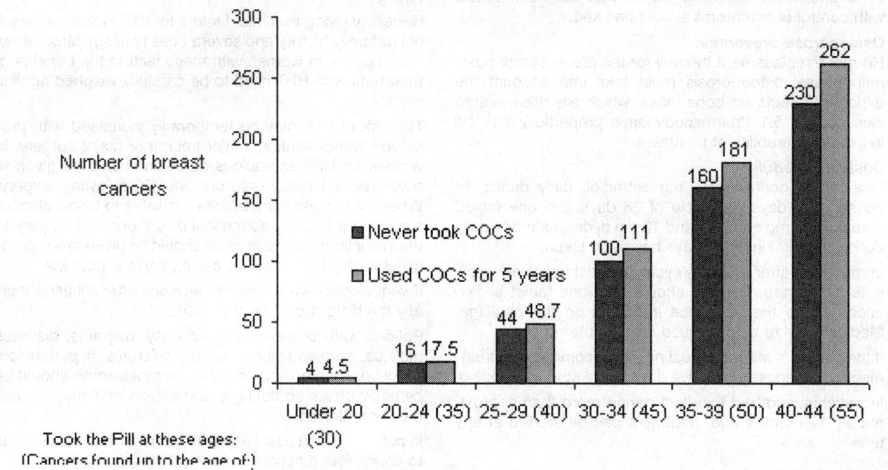

Reasons for stopping oral contraception immediately:

1. Occurrence for the first time, or exacerbation, of migrainous headaches or unusually frequent or unusually severe headaches.

2. Sudden disturbances of vision, of hearing or other perceptual disorders.

3. First signs of thrombophlebitis or thromboembolic symptoms (e.g. unusual pains in or swelling of the leg(s), stabbing pains on breathing or coughing for no apparent reason). Feeling of pain and tightness in the chest.

4. Six weeks before an elective major operation (e.g. abdominal, orthopaedic), any surgery to the legs, medical treatment for varicose veins or prolonged immobilisation, e.g. after accidents or surgery. Do not restart until 2 weeks after full ambulation. In case of emergency surgery, thrombotic prophylaxis is usually indicated e.g. subcutaneous heparin.

5. Onset of jaundice, hepatitis, itching of the whole body.

6. Increase in epileptic seizures.

7. Significant rise in blood pressure.

8. Onset of severe depression.

9. Severe upper abdominal pain or liver enlargement.

10. Clear exacerbation of conditions known to be capable of deteriorating during oral contraception or pregnancy.

11. Pregnancy is a reason for stopping immediately because it has been suggested by some investigations that oral contraceptives taken in early pregnancy may slightly increase the risk of foetal malformations. Other investigations have failed to support these findings. The possibility therefore cannot be excluded, but it is certain that if a risk exists at all, it is very small.

Precautions:

Assessment of women prior to starting oral contraceptives (and at regular intervals thereafter) should include a personal and family medical history of each woman. Physical examination should be guided by this and by the contraindications (section 4.3) and warnings (section 4.4) for this product. The frequency and nature of these assessments should be based upon relevant guidelines and should be adapted to the individual woman, but should include measurement of blood pressure and, if judged appropriate by the clinician, breast, abdominal and pelvic examination including cervical cytology.

<u>The following conditions require strict medical supervision during medication with oral contraceptives.</u> Deterioration or first appearance of any of these conditions may indicate that use of the oral contraceptive should be discontinued:

Diabetes mellitus, or a tendency towards diabetes mellitus (e.g. unexplained glycosuria), hypertension, varicose veins, a history of phlebitis, otosclerosis, multiple sclerosis, epilepsy, porphyria, tetany, disturbed liver function, Sydenham's chorea, renal dysfunction, family history of clotting disorders (see also contraindications), obesity, family history of breast cancer and patient history of benign breast disease, history of clinical depression, systemic lupus erythematosus, uterine fibroids and migraine, gallstones, cardiovascular diseases, chloasma, asthma, an intolerance of contact lenses, or any disease that is prone to worsen during pregnancy.

Some women may experience amenorrhoea or oligomenorrhoea after discontinuation of oral contraceptives, especially when these conditions existed prior to use. Women should be informed of this possibility.

4.5 Interaction with other medicinal products and other forms of Interaction

Hepatic enzyme inducers such a barbiturates, primidone, phenobarbitone, phenytoin, phenylbutazone, rifampicin, carbamazepine and griseofulvin can impair the efficacy of Femodette. For women receiving long-term therapy with hepatic enzyme inducers, another method of contraception should be used. The use of ampicillin and other antibiotics may also reduce the efficacy of Femodette, possibly by altering the intestinal flora.

Women receiving short courses of enzyme inducers or broad spectrum antibiotics should take additional, non-hormonal (except rhythm or temperature method) contraceptive precautions during the time of concurrent medication and for 7 days afterwards. If these 7 days overrun the end of a pack, the next pack should be started without a break. In this situation, a withdrawal bleed should not be expected until the end of the second pack. If the patient does not have a withdrawal bleed during the tablet-free interval following the end of the second pack, the possibility of pregnancy must be ruled out before resuming with the next pack. With rifampicin, additional contraceptive precautions should be continued for 4 weeks after treatment stops, even if only a short course was administered.

The requirement for oral antidiabetics or insulin can change as a result of the effect on glucose tolerance.

The herbal remedy St John's wort (Hypericum perforatum) should not be taken concomitantly with Femodette as this could potentially lead to a loss of contraceptive effect.

4.6 Pregnancy and lactation

If pregnancy occurs during medication with oral contraceptives, the preparation should be withdrawn immediately. (See Section 4.4. Reasons for stopping oral contraception immediately).

The use of Femodette during lactation may lead to a reduction in the volume of milk produced and to a change in its composition. Minute amounts of the active substances are excreted with the milk. Mothers who are breast-feeding may be advised instead to use a progestogen-only pill.

4.7 Effects on ability to drive and use machines

None known.

4.8 Undesirable effects

In rare cases, headaches, gastric upsets, nausea, vomiting, breast tenderness, changes in body weight, changes in libido, depressive moods can occur.

In predisposed women, use of Femodette can sometimes cause chloasma which is exacerbated by exposure to sunlight. Such women should avoid prolonged exposure to sunlight.

Individual cases of poor tolerance of contact lenses have been reported with use of oral contraceptives. Contact lens wearers who develop changes in lens tolerance should be assessed by an ophthalmologist.

Menstrual changes:

1. Reduction of menstrual flow:

This is not abnormal and it is to be expected in some patients. Indeed, it may be beneficial where heavy periods were previously experienced.

2. Missed menstruation:

Occasionally, withdrawal bleeding may not occur at all. If the tablets have been taken correctly, pregnancy is very unlikely. If withdrawal bleeding fails to occur at the end of a second pack, the possibility of pregnancy must be ruled out before resuming with the next pack.

Intermenstrual bleeding: 'Spotting' or heavier 'breakthrough bleeding' sometimes occur during tablet taking, especially in the first few cycles, and normally cease spontaneously. Femodette should therefore, be continued even if irregular bleeding occurs. If irregular bleeding is persistent, appropriate diagnostic measures to exclude an organic cause are indicated and may include curettage. This also applies in the case of spotting which occurs at irregular intervals in several consecutive cycles or which occurs for the first time after long use of Femodette.

Effect on blood chemistry: The use of oral contraceptives may influence the results of certain laboratory tests including biochemical parameters of liver, thyroid, adrenal and renal function, plasma levels of carrier proteins and lipid/lipoprotein fractions, parameters of carbohydrate metabolism and parameters of coagulation and fibrinolysis. Laboratory staff should therefore be informed about oral contraceptive use when laboratory tests are requested.

Refer to Section 4.4. "Special warnings and special precautions for use" for additional information.

4.9 Overdose

Overdosage may cause nausea, vomiting and withdrawal bleeding in females.

There are no specific antidotes and treatment should be symptomatic.

5. PHARMACOLOGICAL PROPERTIES

5.1 Pharmacodynamic properties

The contraceptive effect of Femodette is based on the interaction of various factors, the most important of which are seen as the inhibition of ovulation and the changes in the cervical secretion. Furthermore, the endometrium is rendered unreceptive to implantation.

5.2 Pharmacokinetic properties

Gestodene

Orally administered gestodene is rapidly and completely absorbed. Following ingestion of a single Femodette tablet, maximum drug serum levels of about 3.5 ng/ml are reached at about 1.0 hour. Thereafter, gestodene serum levels decrease in two phases. The terminal disposition phase is characterised by a half-life of about 12 hours. For gestodene, an apparent volume of distribution of 0.7 l/kg and a metabolic clearance rate from serum of about 0.8 ml/min/kg were determined.

Gestodene is not excreted in unchanged form, but as metabolites, which are eliminated with a half-life of about 1 day. Gestodene metabolites are excreted at a urinary to biliary ratio of about 6:4. The biotransformation follows the known pathways of steroid metabolism. No pharmacologically active metabolites are known.

Gestodene is bound to serum albumin and to sex hormone binding globulin (SHBG). Only about 1.3 % of the total serum drug levels are present as free steroid, but about 69 % are specifically bound to SHBG. The relative distribution (free, albumin-bound, SHBG-bound) depends on the SHBG concentrations in the serum. Following induction of the binding protein, the SHBG bound fraction increases to ca. 80 % while the unbound and the albumin-bound fraction decrease.

Following daily repeated administration of Femodette, an accumulation of gestodene concentration in the serum is observed. Mean serum levels are about fivefold higher at a steady-state, which is generally reached during the second half of a treatment cycle. The pharmacokinetics of gestodene are influenced by SHBG serum levels. Under treatment with Femodette a twofold increase in the serum SHBG levels has been observed for the first treatment cycle. Due to the specific binding of gestodene to SHBG, the increase in SHBG levels is accompanied by an almost parallel increase in gestodene serum levels. After three treatment cycles, the extent of SHBG induction per cycle does not seem to change further. The absolute bioavailability of gestodene was determined to be 99 % of the dose administered.

Ethinylestradiol

Orally administered ethinylestradiol is rapidly and completely absorbed. Following ingestion of a single Femodette tablet, maximum drug serum levels of about 65 pg/ml are reached at 1.7 hours.

Thereafter, ethinylestradiol serum levels decrease in two disposition phases, characterised by half-lives of about 2 hours and 21 hours, respectively. The terminal half-life of ethinylestradiol is subject to a large interindividual variation and a range of 5 to 30h has been reported in the literature. Due to analytical reasons, these parameters can only be calculated following the administration of higher doses. For ethinylestradiol, an apparent volume of distribution of about 5 l/kg and a metabolic clearance rate from plasma of about 5 ml/min/kg were determined. Ethinylestradiol is highly but non-specifically bound to albumin. About 2 % of drug levels are present unbound. During absorption and first-liver passage, ethinylestradiol is metabolized extensively, resulting in a mean oral bioavailability of about 45% with a large interindividual variation of about 20-65%. Unchanged drug is not excreted. Ethinylestradiol metabolites are excreted at a urinary to biliary ratio of 4:6 with a half-life of about 1 day.

According to the half-life of the terminal disposition phase from serum and the daily ingestion, steady-state serum levels of ethinylestradiol can be expected to be reached after 5 – 6 days. At the end of a treatment cycle, they were found to be higher by about 40-60% as compared to single dose administration.

During established lactation, 0.02 % of the daily maternal dose could be transferred to the newborn via milk.

The systemic availability of ethinylestradiol might be influenced in both directions by other drugs. There is, however, no interaction with high doses of Vitamin C. Ethinylestradiol induces the hepatic synthesis of SHBG and corticoid binding globulin (CBG) during continuous use. The extent of SHBG induction, however, depends on the chemical structure and the dose of the co-administered progestogen. During treatment with Femodette, SHBG concentrations in the serum increased from 107 nmol/l to 216 nmol/l in the first and to 223 nmol/l in the third cycle. Serum concentrations of CBG were increased from 42 μg/ml to 77 μg/ml in the first cycle and remained constant thereafter.

5.3 Preclinical safety data

There are no preclinical safety data which could be of relevance to the prescriber and which are not already included in other relevant sections of the SPC.

6. PHARMACEUTICAL PARTICULARS

6.1 List of excipients

lactose

maize starch

povidone 25 000

magnesium stearate (E572)

sucrose

povidone 700 000

polyethylene glycol 6000

calcium carbonate (E170)

talc

montan glycol wax

6.2 Incompatibilities

None known.

6.3 Shelf life

4 years.

6.4 Special precautions for storage

Do not store above 25°C.

6.5 Nature and contents of container

The blister packs consist of hard tempered aluminium foil of thickness 20μm and transparent PVC film of thickness 250μm.

Presentation

Cartons containing 1 or 3 blister memo-packs.

Each memo-pack contains 21 tablets.

6.6 Instructions for use and handling

Store all drugs properly and keep them out of reach of children.

7. MARKETING AUTHORISATION HOLDER

Schering Health Care Limited

The Brow

Burgess Hill

West Sussex RH15 9NE

8. MARKETING AUTHORISATION NUMBER(S)

0053/0250

9. DATE OF FIRST AUTHORISATION/RENEWAL OF THE AUTHORISATION

17th March 1995

10. DATE OF REVISION OF THE TEXT

12th October 2001

LEGAL CATEGORY

POM

Femoston 1/10mg

(Solvay Healthcare Limited)

1. NAME OF THE MEDICINAL PRODUCT

Femoston® 1/10 mg

2. QUALITATIVE AND QUANTITATIVE COMPOSITION

Each tablet contains 1 mg estradiol (as hemihydrate) or a combination of 1 mg estradiol (as hemihydrate) and 10 mg dydrogesterone.

3. PHARMACEUTICAL FORM

Coated tablets.

Estradiol only tablets: Round, biconvex, white film-coated tablets with inscriptions 'S' and '379'.

Estradiol/dydrogesterone combination tablets: Round, biconvex, grey film-coated tablets with inscriptions 'S' and '379'.

4. CLINICAL PARTICULARS

4.1 Therapeutic indications

Hormone replacement therapy (HRT) for estrogen deficiency symptoms in peri and postmenopausal women.

Second line therapy for prevention of osteoporosis in postmenopausal women at high risk of future fractures who are intolerant of, or contraindicated for, other medicinal products approved for the prevention of osteoporosis.

The experience in treating women older than 65 years is limited.

4.2 Posology and method of administration

Climacteric symptoms

Initial treatment should be with Femoston 1/10 mg. Femoston 2/10 mg should be substituted if control of climacteric symptoms is not achieved. The lowest dose compatible with control of symptoms should be used.

Osteoporosis prevention

Hormone replacement therapy for the prevention of postmenopausal osteoporosis must take into account the expected effects on bone mass, which are dose-related (see section 5.1 Pharmacodynamic properties) and the individual tolerability of treatment.

Dosage Schedule

One tablet, containing 1 mg estradiol, daily during 14 consecutive days per cycle of 28 days and one tablet, containing 1 mg estradiol and 10 mg dydrogesterone daily during the remaining 14 days has to be taken.

Immediately after a 28-day cycle, the next treatment cycle is to be started. Patients should take one tablet a day, according to the sequence indicated on the package. Medication is to be continued without interruption.

If the patient is still menstruating, it is recommended treatment commences within five days of the start of bleeding.

In patients who had their last period more than approximately 12 months ago, treatment can be started at any time.

4.3 Contraindications

Known or suspected carcinoma of the breast, endometrial carcinoma or other hormone dependent neoplasia.

Acute or chronic liver disease.

History of liver disease where the liver function tests have failed to return to normal.

Active deep venous thrombosis, thromboembolic disorders, or a history of confirmed venous thromboembolism.

Cerebral vascular accident.

Abnormal genital bleeding of unknown aetiology.

Known or suspected pregnancy.

4.4 Special warnings and special precautions for use

Assessment of each woman prior to taking hormone replacement therapy (and at regular intervals thereafter) should include a personal and family medical history. Physical examination should be guided by this and by the contra-indications (section 4.3) and warnings (section 4.4) for this product. During assessment of each individual woman clinical examination of the breasts and pelvic examination should be performed where clinically indicated rather than as a routine procedure. Women should be encouraged to participate in the national breast cancer screening programme (mammography) and the national cervical cancer screening programme (cervical cytology) as appropriate for their age. Breast awareness should also be encouraged and women advised to report any changes in their breasts to their doctor or nurse.

Patients who are, or have previously been treated with unopposed oestrogens should be examined with special care in order to investigate a possible hyperstimulation of the endometrium before commencing therapy.

There is an increased risk of endometrial hyperplasia or carcinoma associated with unopposed estrogen administered long-term. However, the appropriate addition of a progestogen as in Femoston lowers this additional risk.

In case of continuing abnormal and/or irregular bleeding, endometrial evaluation, including endometrial biopsy should be performed.

This oestrogen-progestogen combination treatment is not contraceptive. Patients in the peri-menopausal phase should be advised to take non-hormonal contraceptive precautions.

A reanalysis of original data from 51 epidemiological studies reported a small or moderate increase in the probability of having breast cancer *diagnosed* in women currently or recently using HRT. The findings may be due to biological effects of HRT, earlier diagnosis, or a combination of both. The relative risk increased with duration of treatment (by 2.3% per year of use) and returned to normal in the course of five years cessation of HRT use. This is comparable to the increase in relative risk when natural menopause is delayed in the absence of HRT. Breast cancers diagnosed in current or recent users of HRT are more likely to be localised to the breast than those found in non-users. HRT use may not be associated with increased mortality from breast cancer.

Between the ages of 50 and 70, about 45 women in every 1000 not using HRT will have breast cancer diagnosed. It is estimated that among those who use HRT for 5 years starting at 50, 2 extra cases of breast cancer will be detected by age 70 in every 1000 women. For those who use HRT for 10 years there will be 6 extra cases of breast cancer, and for 15 years use, 12 extra cases of breast cancer in every 1000 women during the 20 year period until age 70.

It is important that the increased risk of being diagnosed with breast cancer is discussed with the patient and weighed against the known benefits of HRT.

Epidemiological studies have suggested that hormone replacement therapy (HRT) is associated with an increased relative risk of developing venous thromboembolism (VTE) i.e. deep vein thrombosis or pulmonary embolism. The studies find a 2-3 fold increase for users compared with non-users which for healthy women amounts to a low risk of one extra case of VTE each year for every 5000 patients taking HRT.

Generally recognised risk factors for VTE include a personal or family history and severe obesity (Body Mass Index >30 kg/m^2). In women with these factors the benefits of treatment with HRT need to be carefully weighed against risks.

The risk of VTE may be temporarily increased with prolonged immobilisation, major trauma or major surgery. In women on HRT scrupulous attention should be given to prophylactic measures to prevent VTE following surgery. Where prolonged immobilisation is liable to follow elective surgery, particularly abdominal or orthopaedic surgery to the lower limbs, consideration should be given to temporarily stopping HRT 4 weeks earlier, if this is possible.

If venous thromboembolism develops after initiating therapy the drug should be discontinued.

Patients with or developing epilepsy, migraine, diabetes mellitus, cardiac failure, multiple sclerosis, hypertension, porphyria, haemoglobinopathies or otosclerosis should be carefully observed during treatment, as HRT may worsen these conditions.

In patients with a past history of liver disease it is advisable to check liver functions on a regular basis.

Special care should be taken in patients with uterine leiomyomata and patients with (a history of) endometriosis as oestrogens may influence these conditions.

The indications for immediate withdrawal of therapy are:

* deep venous thrombosis
* thromboembolic disorders
* the appearance of jaundice
* the emergence of migraine - type headache
* sudden visual disturbances
* significant increase in blood pressure
* pregnancy

4.5 Interaction with other medicinal products and other forms of Interaction

Oestrogens interact with liver enzyme inducing drugs with increased metabolism of oestrogens, which may reduce the oestrogen effect. Interactions are documented for the following liver enzyme inducing drugs: barbiturates, phenytoin, rifampicin, carbamazepine.

No drug interactions are known for dydrogesterone.

4.6 Pregnancy and lactation

Known, or suspected pregnancy is a contraindication.

Lactation: this product is not indicated during this period.

4.7 Effects on ability to drive and use machines

No effects known.

4.8 Undesirable effects

During the first few months of treatment breast tenderness may occur. Nausea, headache, abdominal pain, dysmenorrhoea, bloating, oedema and dizziness have been reported. Symptoms are normally transient. Skin reactions have also been reported.

4.9 Overdose

There have been no reports of ill-effects from overdosing. If overdosage is discovered within two or three hours and is so large that treatment seems desirable, gastric lavage can safely be used. There is no specific antidote and further treatment should be symptomatic.

5. PHARMACOLOGICAL PROPERTIES

5.1 Pharmacodynamic properties

Estradiol is chemically and biologically identical to the endogenous human estradiol and is, therefore, classified as a human oestrogen. Estradiol is the primary oestrogen and the most active of the ovarian hormones. The endogenous oestrogens are involved in certain functions of the uterus and accessory organs, including the proliferation of the endometrium and the cyclic changes in the cervix and vagina. Oestrogens are known to play an important role for bone and fat metabolism.

Estradiol plays an important part in maintaining bone mass, and has a preventative effect on the incidence of osteoporotic fractures.

The effects of estradiol on bone mineral density were examined in a two-year, randomised, double-blind, placebo-controlled clinical trial in 579 postmenopausal women (113 on placebo, 231 on 1 mg estradiol and 235 on 2 mg estradiol). The results show that dydrogesterone does not affect the increase in bone mass observed on estradiol and that the effect on the bone was dose-dependent. The percentage change from baseline in bone mineral density at lumbar spine, femoral neck and trochanter in women completing two years of treatment with 1 mg estradiol was 5.20 ± 3.76%, 2.65 ± 4.24% and 3.54 ± 5.02%, respectively. The corresponding results on 2 mg estradiol were 6.64 ± 3.83%, 2.56 ± 4.99% and 4.60 ± 5.01%. The difference in bone density compared to placebo was statistically highly significant at all sites ($p<0.001$). Changes on the lower dose of estradiol were smaller than on the higher dose in the lumbar spine and trochanter but were comparable in the femoral neck after two years treatment.

Furthermore, oestrogens also affect the autonomic nervous system and may have indirect positive psychotropic actions.

Dydrogesterone is an orally-active progestogen having an activity comparable to parenterally administered progesterone.

In the context of HRT, dydrogesterone produces a complete secretory endometrium in an oestrogen-primed uterus thereby providing protection for oestrogen induced increased risk of endometrial hyperplasia and/or carcinoma, without androgenic side-effects.

The beneficial effects of 17β-estradiol on lipoprotein, glucose and insulin metabolism are maintained in the presence of dydrogesterone.

5.2 Pharmacokinetic properties

Following oral administration, micronised estradiol, is readily absorbed, but extensively metabolised. The major unconjugated and conjugated metabolites are oestrone and oestrone sulphate. These metabolites can contribute to the oestrogen activity, either directly or after conversion to estradiol. Oestrone sulphate may undergo enterohepatic circulation. In urine, the major compounds are the glucuronides of oestrone and estradiol.

Oestrogens are secreted in the milk of nursing mothers.

After oral administration of labelled dydrogesterone, on average 63% of the dose is excreted into the urine. Within 72 hours excretion is complete.

In man, dydrogesterone is completely metabolised. The main metabolite of dydrogesterone is 20α-dihydrodydrogesterone (DHD) and is present in the urine predominantly as the glucoronic acid conjugate. A common feature of all metabolites characterised is the retention of the 4,6 diene-3-one configuration of the parent compound and the absence of 17α-hydroxylation. This explains the lack of oestrogenic and androgenic effects of dydrogesterone.

After oral administration of dydrogesterone, plasma concentrations of DHD are substantially higher as compared to the parent drug. The AUC and C_{max} ratios of DHD to dydrogesterone are in the order of 40 and 25, respectively. Dydrogesterone is rapidly absorbed. The T_{max} values of dydrogesterone and DHD vary between 0.5 and 2.5 hours.

Mean terminal half lives of dydrogesterone and DHD vary between 5 to 7 and 14 to 17 hours, respectively. Dydrogesterone is not excreted in urine as pregnanediol, like progesterone. Analysis of endogenous progesterone production based on pregnanediol excretion therefore remains possible. No pharmacokinetic interactions occur between estradiol and dydrogesterone.

5.3 Preclinical safety data

Supraphysiologically high doses (prolonged overdoses) of estradiol have been associated with the induction of tumours in oestrogen-dependent target organs for all rodent species tested. Pronounced species differences in toxicology, pharmacology and pharmacodynamics exist. The changes observed with dydrogesterone in animal toxicity studies are associated with the effects of progesterone-like compounds.

Doses administered to rats and mice sufficient to produce hormone mediated changes gave no evidence of carcinogenesis.

6. PHARMACEUTICAL PARTICULARS

6.1 List of excipients

Estradiol only tablets: Lactose, hypromellose, maize starch, colloidal anhydrous silica, magnesium stearate, Opadry Y-1-7000 white.

Opadry Y-1-7000 white: hypromellose, polyethylene glycol 400, titanium dioxide (E171).

Estradiol/dydrogesterone tablets: Lactose, hypromellose, maize starch, colloidal anhydrous silica, magnesium stearate, Opadry OY-8243 grey.

Opadry OY-8243 grey: hypromellose, polyethylene glycol 400, titanium dioxide (E171), iron oxide black (E172).

6.2 Incompatibilities

Not applicable.

6.3 Shelf life

Three years.

6.4 Special precautions for storage

Do not store above 30°C.

6.5 Nature and contents of container

The tablets are packed in blister strips of 28. The blister strips are made of PVC film with a covering aluminium foil. Each carton contains 84 tablets.

6.6 Instructions for use and handling

Not applicable.

Administrative Data

7. MARKETING AUTHORISATION HOLDER

Solvay Healthcare Limited
Mansbridge Road
West End
Southampton
SO18 3JD

8. MARKETING AUTHORISATION NUMBER(S)

PL 00512/0121

9. DATE OF FIRST AUTHORISATION/RENEWAL OF THE AUTHORISATION

27 September 1995

10. DATE OF REVISION OF THE TEXT

December 2003

Legal category

POM

Femoston 2/10mg

(Solvay Healthcare Limited)

1. NAME OF THE MEDICINAL PRODUCT

Femoston® 2/10 mg

2. QUALITATIVE AND QUANTITATIVE COMPOSITION

Femoston 2/10 mg contains 2 mg estradiol (as hemihydrate) for the first 14 days of a cycle (brick-red tablets). For the next 14 days of a 28-day cycle, the yellow tablets contain 2 mg estradiol and 10 mg dydrogesterone.

3. PHARMACEUTICAL FORM

Film-coated tablets for oral use.

4. CLINICAL PARTICULARS

4.1 Therapeutic indications

Hormone replacement therapy (HRT) for estrogen deficiency symptoms in peri and postmenopausal women.

Second line therapy for prevention of osteoporosis in postmenopausal women at high risk of future fractures who are intolerant of, or contraindicated for, other medicinal products approved for the prevention of osteoporosis.

The experience in treating women older than 65 years is limited.

4.2 Posology and method of administration

For oral administration.

Osteoporosis prevention

Treatment should be with Femoston 2/10.

Climacteric symptoms

Patients should be treated with Femoston 2/10 if they do not respond to a 1 mg estradiol dosage.

Dosage schedule

Adults (including the elderly):

One tablet, containing 2 mg estradiol, daily during 14 consecutive days per cycle of 28 days, and one tablet, containing 2 mg estradiol and 10 mg dydrogesterone, daily during the remaining 14 days of the cycle.

Femoston 2/20 may be prescribed if either early withdrawal bleeding occurs or if endometrial biopsy reveals inadequate progestational response.

Immediately after a 28-day cycle, the next treatment cycle is to be started. Patients should take one tablet a day orally, according to the sequence indicated on the package. Medication is to be continued without interruption.

If the patient is still menstruating, it is recommended that treatment commences within 5 days of the start of bleeding.

In patients who had their last period more than approximately 12 months ago, treatment can be started at any time.

Children: Not applicable.

4.3 Contraindications

Known or suspected carcinoma of the breast, endometrial carcinoma or other hormone dependent neoplasia.

Acute or chronic liver disease.

History of liver disease where the liver function tests have failed to return to normal.

Active deep venous thrombosis, thromboembolic disorders, or a history of confirmed venous thromboembolism.

Cerebral vascular accident.

Abnormal genital bleeding of unknown aetiology.

Known or suspected pregnancy.

4.4 Special warnings and special precautions for use

Assessment of each woman prior to taking hormone replacement therapy (and at regular intervals thereafter) should include a personal and family medical history. Physical examination should be guided by this and by the contra-indications (section 4.3) and warnings (section 4.4) for this product. During assessment of each individual woman clinical examination of the breasts and pelvic examination should be performed where clinically indicated rather than as a routine procedure. Women should be encouraged to participate in the national breast cancer screening programme (mammography) and the national cervical cancer screening programme (cervical cytology) as appropriate for their age). Breast awareness should also be encouraged and women advised to report any changes in their breasts to their doctor or nurse.

Patients who are, or have previously been treated with unopposed oestrogens should be examined with special care in order to investigate possible hyperstimulation of the endometrium before commencing therapy. There is an increased risk of endometrial hyperplasia or carcinoma associated with unopposed oestrogen long term. However, the appropriate addition of a progestogen as in Femoston lowers this risk

In case of continuing abnormal and/or irregular bleeding, endometrial evaluation, including endometrial biopsy, should be performed.

This oestrogen-progestogen combination treatment is not contraceptive. Patients in the peri-menopausal phase should be advised to take non-hormonal contraceptive precautions.

A reanalysis of original data from 51 epidemiological studies reported a small or moderate increase in the probability of having breast cancer *diagnosed* in women currently or recently using HRT. The findings may be due to biological effects of HRT, earlier diagnosis, or a combination of both. The relative risk increased with duration of treatment (by 2.3% per year of use) and returned to normal in the course of five years cessation of HRT use. This is comparable to the increase in relative risk when natural menopause is delayed in the absence of HRT. Breast cancers diagnosed in current or recent users of HRT are more likely to be localised to the breast than those found in non-users. HRT use may not be associated with increased mortality from breast cancer.

Between the ages of 50 and 70, about 45 women in every 1000 not using HRT will have breast cancer diagnosed. It is estimated that among those who use HRT for 5 years starting at 50, 2 extra cases of breast cancer will be detected by age 70 in every 1000 women. For those who use HRT for 10 years there will be 6 extra cases of breast cancer, and for 15 years use, 12 extra cases of breast cancer in every 1000 women during the 20 year period until age 70.

It is important that the increased risk of being diagnosed with breast cancer is discussed with the patient and weighed against the known benefits of HRT.

Epidemiological studies have suggested that hormone replacement therapy (HRT) is associated with an increased relative risk of developing venous thromboembolism (VTE) i.e. deep vein thrombosis or pulmonary embolism. The studies find a 2-3 fold increase for users compared with non-users which for healthy women amounts to a low risk of one extra case of VTE each year for every 5000 patients taking HRT.

Generally recognised risk factors for VTE include a personal or family history and severe obesity (Body Mass Index >30 kg/m^2). In women with these factors, the benefits of treatment with HRT need to be carefully weighed against risks.

The risk of VTE may be temporarily increased with prolonged immobilisation, major trauma or major surgery. In women on HRT, scrupulous attention should be given to prophylactic measures to prevent VTE following surgery. Where prolonged immobilisation is liable to follow elective surgery, particularly abdominal or orthopaedic surgery to the lower limbs, consideration should be given to temporarily stopping HRT 4 weeks earlier, if this is possible.

If venous thromboembolism develops after initiating therapy, the drug should be discontinued.

Patients with, or developing epilepsy, migraine, diabetes mellitus, cardiac failure, multiple sclerosis, hypertension, porphyria, haemoglobinopathies or otosclerosis should be carefully observed during treatment, as HRT may worsen these conditions.

In patients with a past history of liver disease, it is advisable to check liver functions on a regular basis.

Special care should be taken in patients with uterine leiomyomata and patients with a history of endometriosis as oestrogens may influence these conditions.

The indications for immediate withdrawal of therapy are:

* deep venous thrombosis
* thromboembolic disorders
* the appearance of jaundice
* the emergence of migraine - type headache
* sudden visual disturbances
* significant increase in blood pressure
* pregnancy

4.5 Interaction with other medicinal products and other forms of Interaction

Oestrogens interact with liver enzyme-inducing drugs with increased metabolism of oestrogens, which may reduce their effect. Interactions are documented for the following liver enzyme-inducing drugs: barbiturates, phenytoin, rifampicin, carbamazepine.

No drug interactions are known for dydrogesterone.

4.6 Pregnancy and lactation

Known, or suspected pregnancy is a contraindication.

Lactation: this product is not indicated during this period.

4.7 Effects on ability to drive and use machines

No effects known.

4.8 Undesirable effects

During the first few months of treatment breast tenderness may occur. Nausea, headache, abdominal pain, dysmenorrhoea, bloating, oedema and dizziness have been reported. Symptoms are normally transient. Furthermore, skin reactions have been reported.

4.9 Overdose
There have been no reports of ill-effects from overdosing. If overdosage is discovered within two to three hours and is so large that treatment seems desirable, gastric lavage can safely be used. There is no specific antidote and further treatment should be symptomatic.

5. PHARMACOLOGICAL PROPERTIES
5.1 Pharmacodynamic properties
Estradiol is chemically and biologically identical to the endogenous human estradiol and is therefore classified as a human oestrogen. Estradiol is the primary oestrogen and the most active of the ovarian hormones. The endogenous oestrogens are involved in certain functions of the uterus and accessory organs, including the proliferation of the endometrium and the cyclic changes in the cervix and vagina.

Oestrogens are known to play an important role for bone and fat metabolism. Furthermore, oestrogens also affect the autonomic nervous system and may have indirect positive psychotropic actions.

Dydrogesterone is an orally-active progestogen having an activity comparable to parenterally administered progesterone.

In the context of HRT, dydrogesterone produces a complete secretory endometrium in an oestrogen-primed uterus thereby providing protection for oestrogen induced increased risk of endometrial hyperplasia and/or carcinoma, without androgenic side-effects.

The beneficial effects of 17β-estradiol on lipoprotein, glucose and insulin metabolism are maintained in the presence of dydrogesterone.

5.2 Pharmacokinetic properties
Following oral administration, micronised estradiol is readily absorbed, but extensively metabolised. The major unconjugated and conjugated metabolites are estrone and estrone sulphate. These metabolites can contribute to the oestrogen activity, either directly or after conversion to estradiol. Estrone sulphate may undergo enterohepatic circulation. In urine, the major compounds are the glucuronides of estrone and estradiol.

Estrogens are secreted in the milk of nursing mothers.

After oral administration of labelled dydrogesterone, on average 63% of the dose is excreted into the urine. Within 72 hours, excretion is complete.

In man, dydrogesterone is completely metabolised. The main metabolite of dydrogesterone is 20α-dihydrodydrogesterone (DHD) and is present in the urine predominantly as the glucoronic acid conjugate. A common feature of all metabolites characterised is the retention of the 4,6 diene-3-one configuration of the parent compound and the absence of 17α-hydroxylation. This explains the lack of oestrogenic and androgenic effects of dydrogesterone.

After oral administration of dydrogesterone, plasma concentrations of DHD are substantially higher as compared to the parent drug. The AUC and C_{max} ratios of DHD to dydrogesterone are in the order of 40 and 25, respectively. Dydrogesterone is rapidly absorbed. The T_{max} values of dydrogesterone and DHD vary between 0.5 and 2.5 hours. Mean terminal half lives of dydrogesterone and DHD vary between 5 to 7 and 14 to 17 hours, respectively.

Dydrogesterone is not excreted in urine as pregnanediol, like progesterone. Analysis of endogenous progesterone production based on pregnanediol excretion therefore remains possible. No pharmacokinetic interactions occur between estradiol and dydrogesterone.

5.3 Preclinical safety data
Supraphysiologically high doses (prolonged overdoses) of estradiol have been associated with the induction of tumours in oestrogen-dependent target organs for all rodent species tested. Pronounced species differences in toxicology, pharmacology and pharmacodynamics exist. The changes observed with dydrogesterone in animal toxicity studies are associated with the effects of progesterone-like compounds.

Doses administered to rats and mice sufficient to produce hormone-mediated changes gave no evidence of carcinogenesis.

6. PHARMACEUTICAL PARTICULARS
6.1 List of excipients
Tablet cores: Lactose

Methylhydroxypropylcellulose

Maize starch

Colloidal anhydrous silica

Magnesium stearate

Film coats: Methylhydroxypropylcellulose

Polyethylene glycol 400

Titanium dioxide E171

Iron oxide red E172

Iron oxides black and yellow E172 (brick red tablets only)

6.2 Incompatibilities
Not applicable.

6.3 Shelf life
3 years.

6.4 Special precautions for storage
Do not store above 30°C.

6.5 Nature and contents of container
The tablets are packed in blister strips of 28. The blister packs are made of PVC/PVdC or PVC film with a covering aluminium foil. Each carton contains 28 or 84 tablets.

6.6 Instructions for use and handling
Not applicable.

Administrative Data
7. MARKETING AUTHORISATION HOLDER
Solvay Healthcare Limited

Mansbridge Road

West End

Southampton

SO18 3JD

8. MARKETING AUTHORISATION NUMBER(S)
PL 00512/0113

9. DATE OF FIRST AUTHORISATION/RENEWAL OF THE AUTHORISATION
17 January 1995

10. DATE OF REVISION OF THE TEXT
December 2003

Legal category
POM

Femoston-conti
(Solvay Healthcare Limited)

1. NAME OF THE MEDICINAL PRODUCT
Femoston-conti ® 1 mg/5 mg film-coated tablets

2. QUALITATIVE AND QUANTITATIVE COMPOSITION
Each film-coated tablet contains 1 mg estradiol as estradiol hemihydrate and 5 mg dydrogesterone.

For excipients, see 6.1.

3. PHARMACEUTICAL FORM
Film-coated tablet.

Salmon-coloured, round, biconvex, film-coated tablets imprinted '$' on one side and '379' on the other.

4. CLINICAL PARTICULARS
4.1 Therapeutic indications
Hormone replacement therapy (HRT) for estrogen deficiency symptoms in postmenopausal women. Femoston-conti should be used only in postmenopausal women more than 12 months after menopause.

Prevention of osteoporosis in postmenopausal women at high risk of future fractures who are intolerant of, or contra-indicated for, other medicinal products approved for the prevention of osteoporosis.

(See also section 4.4)

The experience in treating women older than 65 years is limited.

4.2 Posology and method of administration
Femoston-conti is a continuous combined HRT.

The dosage is one tablet per day. Femoston-conti should be taken continuously without a break between packs.

Femoston-conti can be taken with or without food.

<u>Starting Femoston-conti:</u>

Women experiencing a natural menopause should commence treatment with Femoston-conti 12 months after their last natural menstrual bleed. For surgically induced menopause, treatment may start immediately.

In women who are not taking hormone replacement therapy or women, who switch from a continuous combined hormone replacement therapy, treatment may be started on any convenient day. In women transferring from a cyclic or continuous sequential HRT regimen, treatment should begin the day following completion of the prior regimen.

If a dose has been forgotten, it should be taken as soon as possible. When more than 12 hours have elapsed, it is recommended to continue with the next dose without taking the forgotten tablet. The likelihood of breakthrough bleeding or spotting may be increased.

For initiation and continuation of treatment of postmenopausal symptoms, the lowest effective dose for the shortest duration (see also section 4.4) should be used.

4.3 Contraindications
Known, past or suspected breast cancer;

Known or suspected estrogen-dependent malignant tumours (e.g. endometrial cancer);

Undiagnosed genital bleeding;

Untreated endometrial hyperplasia;

Previous idiopathic or current venous thromboembolism (deep vein thrombosis, pulmonary embolism);

Active or recent arterial thromboembolic disease (e.g. angina, myocardial infarction);

Acute liver disease or a history of liver disease as long as liver function tests have failed to return to normal;

Known hypersensitivity to the active substances or to any of the excipients;

Porphyria.

4.4 Special warnings and special precautions for use
For the treatment of postmenopausal symptoms, HRT should only be initiated for symptoms that adversely affect quality of life. In all cases, a careful appraisal of the risks and benefits should be undertaken at least annually and HRT should only be continued as long as the benefit outweighs the risk.

<u>Medical examination/follow up</u>

Before initiating or reinstituting HRT, a complete personal and family medical history should be taken. Physical (including pelvic and breast) examination should be guided by this and by the contraindications and warnings for use. During treatment, periodic check-ups are recommended of a frequency and nature adapted to the individual woman. Women should be advised what changes in their breasts should be reported to their doctor or nurse. Investigations, including mammography, should be carried out in accordance with currently accepted screening practices, modified to the clinical needs of the individual.

<u>Conditions which need supervision</u>

If any of the following conditions are present, have occurred previously, and/or have been aggravated during pregnancy or previous hormone treatment, the patient should be closely supervised. It should be taken into account that these conditions may recur or be aggravated during treatment with Femoston-conti in particular:

- Leiomyoma (uterine fibroids) or endometriosis
- A history of, or risk factors for, thromboembolic disorders (see below)
- Risk factors for estrogen dependent tumours, e.g. 1st degree heredity for breast cancer
- Hypertension
- Liver disorders (e.g. liver adenoma)
- Diabetes mellitus with or without vascular involvement
- Cholelithiasis
- Migraine or (severe) headache
- Systemic lupus erythematosus
- A history of endometrial hyperplasia (see below)
- Epilepsy
- Asthma
- Otosclerosis

<u>Reasons for immediate withdrawal of therapy:</u>

<u>Therapy should be discontinued in cases where a contra-indication is discovered and in the following situations</u>:

- Jaundice or deterioration in liver function
- Significant increase in blood pressure
- New onset of migraine-type headache
- Pregnancy

<u>Endometrial hyperplasia</u>

The risk of endometrial hyperplasia and carcinoma is increased when estrogens are administered alone for prolonged periods (see section 4.8). The addition of a progestagen for at least 12 days per cycle in non-hysterectomised women greatly reduces this risk.

Break-through bleeding and spotting may occur during the first months of treatment. If break-through bleeding or spotting appears after some time on therapy, or continues after treatment has been discontinued, the reason should be investigated, which may include endometrial biopsy to exclude endometrial malignancy.

<u>Breast cancer</u>

A randomised placebo-controlled trial, the Womens Health Initiative study (WHI) and epidemiological studies, including the Million Women Study (MWS), have reported an increased risk of breast cancer in women taking estrogens, estrogen-progestagen combinations or tibolone for HRT for several years (see Section 4.8).

For all HRT, an excess risk becomes apparent within a few years of use and increases with duration of intake but returns to baseline within a few (at most five) years after stopping treatment.

In the MWS, the relative risk of breast cancer with conjugated equine estrogens (CEE) or estradiol (E2) was greater when a progestagen was added, either sequentially or continuously, and regardless of type of progestagen. There was no evidence of a difference in risk between the different routes of administration.

In the WHI study, the continuous combined conjugated equine estrogen and medroxyprogesterone acetate (CEE + MPA) product used was associated with breast cancers that were slightly larger in size and more frequently had local lymph node metastases compared to placebo.

HRT, especially estrogen-progestagen combined treatment, increases the density of mammographic images which may adversely affect the radiological detection of breast cancer.

Venous thromboembolism

HRT is associated with a higher relative risk of developing venous thromboembolism (VTE), i.e. deep vein thrombosis or pulmonary embolism. One randomised controlled trial and epidemiological studies found a two-to threefold higher risk for users compared with non-users. For non-users, it is estimated that the number of cases of VTE that will occur over a 5 year period is about 3 per 1000 women aged 50-59 years and 8 per 1000 women aged between 60-69 years. It is estimated that in healthy women who use HRT for 5 years, the number of additional cases of VTE over a 5 year period will be between 2 and 6 (best estimate = 4) per 1000 women aged 50-59 years and between 5 and 15 (best estimate = 9) per 1000 women aged 60-69 years. The occurrence of such an event is more likely in the first year of HRT than later.

• Generally recognised risk factors for VTE include a personal or family history; severe obesity (BMI > 30 kg/m^2) and systemic lupus erythematosus (SLE). There is no consensus about the possible role of varicose veins in VTE.

• Patients with a history of VTE or known thrombophilic states have an increased risk of VTE. HRT may add to this risk. Personal or strong family history of thromboembolism or recurrent spontaneous abortion should be investigated in order to exclude a thrombophilic predisposition. Until a thorough evaluation of thrombophilic factors has been made or anticoagulant treatment initiated, use of HRT in such patients should be viewed as contraindicated. Those women already on anticoagulant treatment require careful consideration of the benefit-risk of use of HRT.

• The risk of VTE may be temporarily increased with prolonged immobilisation, major trauma or major surgery. As in all postoperative patients, scrupulous attention should be given to prophylactic measures to prevent VTE following surgery. Where prolonged immobilisation is liable to follow elective surgery, particularly abdominal or orthopaedic surgery to the lower limbs, consideration should be given to temporarily stopping HRT 4 to 6 weeks earlier, if possible. Treatment should not be restarted until the women is completely mobilised.

• If VTE develops after initiating therapy, the drug should be discontinued. Patients should be told to contact their doctors immediately when they are aware of a potential thromboembolic symptom (e.g. painful swelling of a leg, sudden pain in the chest, dyspnea).

Coronary artery disease (CAD)

There is no evidence from randomised controlled trials of cardiovascular benefit with continuous combined conjugated estrogens and medroxyprogesterone acetate (MPA). Two large clinical trials (WHI and HERS i.e. Heart and Estrogen/progestin Replacement Study) showed a possible increased risk of cardiovascular morbidity in the first year of use and no overall benefit. For other HRT products there are only limited data from randomised controlled trials examining effects in cardiovascular morbidity or mortality. Therefore, it is uncertain whether these findings also extend to other HRT products.

Stroke

One large randomised clinical trial (WHI-trial) found, as a secondary outcome, an increased risk of ischaemic stroke in healthy women during treatment with continuous combined conjugated estrogens and MPA. For women who do not use HRT, it is estimated that the number of cases of stroke that will occur over a 5 year period is about 3 per 1000 women aged 50-59 and 11 per 1000 women aged 60-69 years. It is estimated that for women who use conjugated estrogens and MPA for 5 years, the number of additional cases will be between 0 and 3 (best estimate = 1) per 1000 users aged 50-59 years and between 1 and 9 (best estimate = 4) per 1000 users aged 60-69 years. It is unknown whether the increased risk also extends to other HRT products.

Ovarian cancer

Long-term (at least 5 to 10 years) use of estrogen-only HRT products in hysterectomised women has been associated with an increased risk of ovarian cancer in some epidemiological studies. It is uncertain whether long term use of combined HRT confers a different risk than estrogen-only products

Other conditions

– Estrogens may cause fluid retention and therefore patients with cardiac or renal dysfunction should be carefully observed. Patients with terminal renal insufficiency should be closely observed, since it is expected that the level of circulating active ingredients in Femoston-conti is increased.

– Women with pre-existing hypertriglyceridemia should be followed closely during estrogen replacement or hormone replacement therapy, since rare cases of large increases of plasma triglycerides leading to pancreatitis have been reported with estrogen therapy in this condition.

– Estrogens increase thyroid binding globulin (TBG), leading to increased circulating total thyroid hormone, as measured by protein-bound iodine (PBI), T4 levels (by column or by radio-immunoassay) or T3 levels (by radio-immunoassay). T3 resin uptake is decreased, reflecting the elevated TBG. Free T4 and free T3 concentrations are unaltered. Other binding proteins may be elevated in serum, i.e. corticoid binding globulin (CBG), sex -hormone—binding globulin (SHBG) leading to increased circulating corticosteroids and sex steroids, respectively. Free or biological active hormone concentrations are unchanged. Other plasma proteins may be increased (angiotensinogen/renin substrate, alpha-1-antitrypsin, ceruloplasmin).

– There is no conclusive evidence for improvement of cognitive function. There is some evidence from the WHI trial of increased risk of probable dementia in women who start using continuous combined CEE and MPA after the age of 65. It is unknown whether the findings apply to younger post-menopausal women or other HRT products.

This medicinal product contains lactose monohydrate and therefore should not be used by patients with rare hereditary problems of galactose intolerance, the Lapp lactase deficiency or glucose-galactose malabsorption.

4.5 Interaction with other medicinal products and other forms of Interaction

- The metabolism of estrogens and progestagens may be increased by concomitant use of substances known to induce drug-metabolising enzymes, specifically cytochrome P450 enzymes, such as anticonvulsants (eg. phenobarbital, phenytoin, carbamezapine) and anti-infectives (e.g. rifampicin, rifabutin, nevirapine, efavirenz).

- Ritonavir and nelfinavir, although known as strong inhibitors, by contrast exhibit inducing properties when used concomitantly with steroid hormones.

- Herbal preparations containing St John's wort (Hypericum perforatum) may induce the metabolism of estrogens and progestagens.

- Clinically an increased metabolism of estrogens and progestagens may lead to decreased effect and changes in the uterine bleeding profile.

4.6 Pregnancy and lactation

Pregnancy:

Femoston-conti is not indicated during pregnancy. If pregnancy occurs during medication with Femoston-conti, treatment should be withdrawn immediately.

Clinically, data based on an assumed large number of exposed pregnancies indicate no adverse effects of dydrogesterone on the foetus.

The results of most epidemiological studies to date relevant to inadvertent foetal exposure to combinations of estrogens and progestagens indicate no teratogenic or foetotoxic effect.

Lactation:

Femoston-conti is not indicated during lactation.

4.7 Effects on ability to drive and use machines

Femoston-conti does not affect the ability to drive or use machines.

4.8 Undesirable effects

Undesirable effects reported in clinical trials and in post-marketing experience are the following:

(see Table 1 on next page)

Breast cancer

According to evidence from a large number of epidemiological studies and one randomised placebo-controlled trial, the Women's Health Initiative (WHI), the overall risk of breast cancer increases with increasing duration of HRT use in current or recent HRT users.

For *estrogen-only* HRT, estimates of relative risk (RR) from a reanalysis of original data from 51 epidemiological studies (in which > 80% of HRT use was estrogen-only HRT) and from the epidemiological Million Women Study (MWS) are similar at 1.35 (95%CI 1.21 – 1.49) and 1.30 (95%CI 1.21 – 1.40), respectively.

For *estrogen plus progestagen* combined HRT, several epidemiological studies have reported an overall higher risk for breast cancer than with estrogens alone.

The MWS reported that, compared to never users, the use of various types of estrogen-progestagen combined HRT was associated with a higher risk of breast cancer (RR = 2.00, 95%CI: 1.88 – 2.12) than use of estrogens alone (RR = 1.30, 95%CI: 1.21 – 1.40) or use of tibolone (RR=1.45; 95%CI 1.25-1.68).

The WHI trial reported a risk estimate of 1.24 (95%CI 1.01 – 1.54) after 5.6 years of use of estrogen-progestagen combined HRT (CEE + MPA) in all users compared with placebo.

The absolute risks calculated from the MWS and the WHI trials are presented below:

The MWS has estimated, from the known average incidence of breast cancer in developed countries, that:

– For women not using HRT, about 32 in every 1000 are expected to have breast cancer diagnosed between the ages of 50 and 64 years.

- For 1000 current or recent users of HRT, the number of *additional* cases during the corresponding period will be

- For users of *estrogen-only* replacement therapy

• between 0 and 3 (best estimate = 1.5) for 5 years' use

• between 3 and 7 (best estimate = 5) for 10 years' use.

- For users of *estrogen plus progestagen* combined HRT,

• between 5 and 7 (best estimate = 6) for 5 years' use

• between 18 and 20 (best estimate = 19) for 10 years' use.

The WHI trial estimated that after 5.6 years of follow-up of women between the ages of 50 and 79 years, an *additional* 8 cases of invasive breast cancer would be due to *estrogen-progestagen combined* HRT (CEE + MPA) per 10,000 women years.

According to calculations from the trial data, it is estimated that:

- For 1000 women in the placebo group,

• about 16 cases of invasive breast cancer would be diagnosed in 5 years.

- For 1000 women who used estrogen + progestagen combined HRT (CEE + MPA), the number of *additional* cases would be

• between 0 and 9 (best estimate = 4) for 5 years' use.

The number of additional cases of breast cancer in women who use HRT is broadly similar for women who start HRT irrespective of age at start of use (between the ages of 45-65) (see section 4.4).'

Endometrial cancer

In women with an intact uterus, the risk of endometrial hyperplasia and endometrial cancer increases with increasing duration of use of unopposed estrogens. According to data from epidemiological studies, the best estimate of the risk is that for women not using HRT, about 5 in every 1000 are expected to have endometrial cancer diagnosed between the ages of 50 and 65. Depending on the duration of treatment and estrogen dose, the reported increase in endometrial cancer risk among unopposed estrogen users varies from 2-to 12-fold greater compared with non-users. Adding a progestagen to estrogen-only therapy greatly reduces this increased risk.

Other adverse reactions have been reported in association with estrogen/progestagen treatment:

- Estrogen-dependent neoplasms benign and malignant, e.g. endometrial cancer.

- Venous thromboembolism, i.e. deep leg or pelvic venous thrombosis and pulmonary embolism, is more frequent among hormone replacement therapy users than among non-users. For further information, see section 4.3 Contra-indications and 4.4 Special warnings and precautions for use.

- Probable dementia (see section 4.4)

4.9 Overdose

Both estradiol and dydrogesterone are substances with low toxicity. Theoretically, symptoms such as nausea, vomiting, sleepiness and dizziness could occur in cases of overdosing. It is unlikely that any specific or symptomatic treatment will be necessary.

Aforementioned information is applicable for overdosing by children also.

5. PHARMACOLOGICAL PROPERTIES

5.1 Pharmacodynamic properties

The ATC code is G03 F A14. (Estrogens: urogenital system and sex hormones).

Hormone replacement therapy (combined estradiol and dydrogesterone).

Estradiol

The active ingredient, synthetic 17β-estradiol, is chemically and biologically identical to endogenous human estradiol. It substitutes for the loss of estrogen production in menopausal women, and alleviates menopausal symptoms. Estrogens prevent bone loss following menopause or ovariectomy.

Dydrogesterone

As estrogens promote the growth of the endometrium, unopposed estrogens increase the risk of endometrial hyperplasia and cancer. The addition of a progestagen greatly reduces the estrogen-induced risk of endometrial hyperplasia in non-hysterectomised women.

- Clinical trial Information

- Relief of estrogen-deficiency symptoms and bleeding patterns

Relief of menopausal symptoms was achieved during the first few weeks of treatment.

Amenorrhoea (no bleeding or spotting) was seen in 76% of women during months 10 -12 of treatment.

Bleeding and/or spotting appeared in 29 % of the women during the first three months of treatment and in 24% during months 10 -12 of treatment.

- Prevention of osteoporosis

- Estrogen deficiency at menopause is associated with an increasing bone turnover and decline in bone mass. The effect of estrogens on the bone mineral density is dose-dependent. Protection appears to be effective for as long as treatment is continued. After discontinuation of HRT, bone mass is lost at a rate similar to that in untreated women.

- Evidence from the WHI trial and meta-analysed trials shows that current use of HRT, alone or in combination with a progestagen – given to predominantly healthy women – reduces the risk of hip, vertebral, and other osteoporotic fractures. HRT may also prevent fractures in women with low bone density and/or established osteoporosis, but the evidence for that is limited.

Table 1

MedDRA system organ class	Common >1/100, <1/10	Uncommon >1/1,000, <1/100	Rare >1/10,000, <1/1,000	Very rare <1/10,000 incl. isolated reports
Infections and infestations		Cystitis-like syndrome, Vaginal candidiasis		
Neoplasms benign, Malignant and unspecified		Increase in size of leiomyoma		
Blood and the lymphatic system disorders				Haemolytic anaemia
Psychiatric disorders		Depression, Change in libido, Nervousness		
Nervous system disorders	Headache, Migraine	Dizziness		Chorea
Eye disorders			Intolerance to contact lenses, Steepening of corneal curvature	
Cardiac disorders				Myocardial infarction
Vascular disorders		Hypertension, Peripheral vascular disease, Varicose vein, Venous thromboembolism		Stroke
Gastrointestinal disorders	Nausea, Abdominal pain, Flatulence	Dyspepsia		Vomiting
Hepatobiliary disorders		Gall bladder disease	Alterations in liver function, sometimes with asthenia or malaise, jaundice and abdominal pain	
Skin and subcutaneous tissue disorders		Allergic skin reactions, Rash, Urticaria, Pruritus		Chloasma or melasma, which may persist when drug is discontinued, Erythema multiforme, Erythema nodosum, Vascular purpura, Angioedema
Musculoskeletal and connective tissue disorders	Leg cramps	Back pain		
Reproductive system and breast disorders	Breast pain/ tenderness, Breakthrough bleeding and spotting, Pelvic pain	Change in cervical erosion, Change in cervical secretion, Dysmenorrhoea, Menorrhagia, Metrorrhagia	Breast enlargement, Premenstrual-like symptoms	
Congenital and familial/genetic disorders				Aggravation of porphyria
General disorders and administration site reactions	Asthenia	Peripheral oedema		
Investigations	Increase/decrease in weight			

After two years of treatment with Femoston-conti, the increase in lumbar spine bone mineral density (BMD) was 5.20% ± 3.76 % (mean ± SD). The percentage of women who maintained or gained BMD in lumbar zone during treatment was 95%.

Femoston-conti also had an effect on hip BMD. The increase after two years was 2.7% ± 4.2 % (mean ± SD) at femoral neck, 3.5% +/- 5.0% (mean ± SD) at trochanter and 2.7%±6.7% (mean ± SD) at Wards triangle. The percentage of women who maintained or gained BMD in the 3 hip areas during treatment was 67-78%.

5.2 Pharmacokinetic properties

Estradiol

Orally administered estradiol, comprising particles whose size has been reduced to less than 5 μm, is quickly and efficiently absorbed from the gastrointestinal tract. The primary unconjugated and conjugated metabolites are estrone and estrone sulphate. These metabolites can contribute to the estrogen effect, both directly and after conversion to estradiol. Estrogens are excreted in the bile and reabsorbed from the intestine. During this enterohepatic cycle the estrogens are broken down. Estrogens are excreted in the urine as biologically inactive glucuronide and sulphate compounds (90 to 95%), or in the faeces (5 to 10%), mostly unconjugated. Estrogens are secreted in the milk of nursing mothers.

The $C_{average}$ is 28 pg/ml, the C_{min} is 20 pg/ml and the C_{max} is 54 pg/ml. The E1/E2 (Estrone/Estradiol) ratio is 7.0.

Dydrogesterone

After oral administration of labelled dydrogesterone, on average 63% of the dose is excreted into the urine. Within 72 hours, excretion is complete.

In man, dydrogesterone is completely metabolised. The main metabolite of dydrogesterone is 20α-dihydrodydrogesterone (DHD) and is present in the urine predominantly as the glucoronic acid conjugate. A common feature of all metabolites characterised is the retention of the 4,6 diene-3-one configuration of the parent compound and the absence of 17α-hydroxylation. This explains the absence of estrogenic and androgenic activity.

After oral administration of dydrogesterone, plasma concentrations of DHD are higher as compared to the parent drug. The AUC and C_{max} ratios of DHD to dydrogesterone are in the order of 40 and 25, respectively. Dydrogesterone is rapidly absorbed. The T_{max} values of dydrogesterone and DHD vary between 0.5 and 2.5 hours.

Mean terminal half lives of dydrogesterone and DHD vary between 5 to 7 and 14 to 17 hours, respectively.

The dihydrodydrogesterone $C_{average}$ is 13 ng/ml, the C_{min} is 4.1 ng/ml and the C_{max} is 63 ng/ml. The dydrogesterone $C_{average}$ is 0.38 ng/ml the C_{min} is <0.1 ng/ml and the C_{max} is 2.5 ng/ml.

Dydrogesterone is not excreted in urine as pregnanediol, like progesterone. Analysis of endogenous progesterone production based on pregnanediol excretion therefore remains possible.

5.3 Preclinical safety data

Supraphysiologically high doses (prolonged application) of estradiol have been associated with the induction of tumours in estrogen-dependent target organs for all rodent species tested. Furthermore, inherent to its hormonal activity, estradiol displays untoward embryotoxic effects and feminisation of male fetuses was occasionally observed. The changes observed with dydrogesterone in animal toxicity studies are associated with the effects of progesterone-like compounds.

Doses administered to rats and mice sufficient to produce hormone mediated changes gave no evidence of carcinogenesis

6. PHARMACEUTICAL PARTICULARS

6.1 List of excipients

Tablet core: Lactose monohydrate

Hypromellose

Maize starch

Colloidal anhydrous silica

Magnesium stearate

Film coat: Hypromellose

Macrogol 400

Titanium dioxide (E171)

Iron oxides, yellow and red (E172)

6.2 Incompatibilities

Not applicable.

6.3 Shelf life

3 years.

6.4 Special precautions for storage

Do not store above 30°C. Keep blister in the outer carton.

6.5 Nature and contents of container

Calendar packs of 14, 28, 84 (3 × 28) or 280 (10 × 28) tablets in PVC-Aluminium blister strips.

Not all pack sizes may be marketed.

6.6 Instructions for use and handling

Not applicable.

7. MARKETING AUTHORISATION HOLDER

Solvay Healthcare Limited

Mansbridge Road

Southampton

SO18 3JD

United Kingdom

8. MARKETING AUTHORISATION NUMBER(S)

PL 00512/0157

9. DATE OF FIRST AUTHORISATION/RENEWAL OF THE AUTHORISATION

Date of First authorisation: 23 November 1999

Date of last renewal: December 2004

10. DATE OF REVISION OF THE TEXT

November 2004

Femseven 50, 75, 100

(Merck Pharmaceuticals)

1. NAME OF THE MEDICINAL PRODUCT

FemSeven 50, 50 microgram/24 hours, transdermal patch.

FemSeven 75, 75 microgram/24 hours, transdermal patch.

FemSeven 100, 100 microgram/24 hours, transdermal patch.

2. QUALITATIVE AND QUANTITATIVE COMPOSITION

One FemSeven 50 transdermal patch contains 1.5 mg estradiol hemihydrate delivering 50 microgram of estradiol in 24 hours. The area of the releasing surface is 15 cm^2.

One FemSeven 75 transdermal patch contains 2.25 mg estradiol hemihydrate delivering 75 microgram of estradiol in 24 hours. The area of the releasing surface is 22.5 cm^2.

One FemSeven 100 transdermal patch contains 3.00 mg estradiol hemihydrate delivering 100 microgram of estradiol in 24 hours. The area of the releasing surface is 30 cm^2.

3. PHARMACEUTICAL FORM

Transdermal patch.

4. CLINICAL PARTICULARS

4.1 Therapeutic indications

• Hormone replacement therapy for oestrogen deficiency symptoms in post-menopausal women.

• Prevention of osteoporosis in postmenopausal women at high risk of future fractures who are intolerant of, or contra-indicated for, other medicinal products approved for the prevention of osteoporosis.

(See also section 4.4)

The experience of treating women older than 65 years is limited.

4.2 Posology and method of administration

FemSeven is an oestrogen-only patch that should be applied to the skin once weekly on a continuous basis, i.e. each patch is replaced with a new one after 7 days.

In women with an intact uterus the addition of a progestogen for at least 12 to 14 days per cycle is essential to help prevent any endometrial hyperplasia induced by the oestrogen. For more detailed information, please refer to section 4.4 (Special warnings and precautions for use - "Endometrial hyperplasia").

Unless there is a previous diagnosis of endometriosis, the addition of a progestogen in hysterectomised women is not recommended.

For initiation and continuation of treatment of postmenopausal symptoms, the lowest effective dose for the shortest duration (see also section 4.4) should be used. Therefore, therapy should normally be started with one FemSeven 50 patch (delivering 50 micrograms of estradiol in 24 hours). If the prescribed dose does not eliminate the menopausal symptoms the dose should be adjusted stepwise after the first few months by using a transdermal patch delivering 75 or 100 micrograms estradiol per day. A maximum of 100 micrograms estradiol per day should not be exceeded. If there are persistent signs of overdose, such as breast tenderness, the dose should be reduced accordingly.

Hysterectomised women not taking HRT or transferring from another HRT product may start treatment with FemSeven on any convenient day. The same holds true for non-hysterectomised women not taking HRT or transferring from a continuous combined HRT product. In non-hysterectomised women switching from sequential HRT regimens, treatment with FemSeven should start after the previous treatment regimen has ended.

Consecutive new patches should be applied to different sites. It is recommended that sites are chosen below the waist where little wrinkling of the skin occurs e.g., buttocks, hip or abdomen. FemSeven must not be applied on or near the breasts. The patch should be applied to clean, dry, healthy and intact skin. The patch should be applied to the skin as soon as it is removed from its wrapping. The patch is applied by removing both parts of the protective liner and then holding it in contact with the skin for at least 30 seconds (warmth is essential to ensure maximal adhesive strength).

Should part or all of a patch detach prematurely (before 7 days) it should be removed and a new patch applied. To aid compliance it is recommended the patient then continues to change the patch on the usual day. This advice also applies if a patient forgets to change the patch on schedule. Forgetting a patch may increase the likelihood of break-through bleeding or spotting.

4.3 Contraindications

FemSeven is contra-indicated in:

- Known, past or suspected breast cancer;
- Known or suspected oestrogen-dependent malignant tumours (e.g. endometrial cancer);
- Undiagnosed genital bleeding;
- Untreated endometrial hyperplasia;
- Previous idiopathic or current venous thromboembolism (deep venous thrombosis, pulmonary embolism);
- Active or recent arterial thromboembolic disease (e.g. angina, myocardial infarction);
- Acute liver disease, or a history of liver disease as long as liver function tests have failed to return to normal;
- Known hypersensitivity to the active substances or to any of the excipients;
- Porphyria.

4.4 Special warnings and special precautions for use

For the treatment of postmenopausal symptoms, HRT should only be initiated for symptoms that adversely affect quality of life. In all cases, a careful appraisal of the risks and benefits should be undertaken at least annually and HRT should only be continued as long as the benefit outweighs the risk.

Medical examination/follow up

Before initiating or reinstituting HRT, a complete personal and family medical history should be taken. Physical (including pelvic and breast) examination should be guided by this and by the contraindications and warnings for use. During treatment, periodic check-ups are recommended of a frequency and nature adapted to the individual woman.

Women should be advised what changes in their breasts should be reported to their doctor or nurse (see "Breast cancer" below). Investigations, including mammography, should be carried out in accordance with currently accepted screening practices, modified to the clinical needs of the individual.

Conditions which need supervision

If any of the following conditions are present, have occurred previously and/or have been aggravated during pregnancy or previous hormone treatment, the patient should be closely supervised. It should be taken into account that these conditions may recur or be aggravated during treatment with FemSeven:

- Leiomyoma (uterine fibroids) or endometriosis
- A history of, or risk factors for, thromboembolic disorders (see below)
- Risk factors for oestrogen dependent tumours, e.g. 1st degree heredity for breast cancer
- Hypertension
- Liver disorders (e.g. liver adenoma)
- Diabetes mellitus with or without vascular involvement
- Cholelithiasis
- Migraine or severe headache
- Systemic lupus erythematosus
- A history of endometrial hyperplasia (see below)
- Epilepsy
- Asthma
- Otosclerosis.

Reasons for immediate withdrawal of therapy

-Therapy should be discontinued if a contra-indication is discovered and in the following situations:

- Jaundice or deterioration in liver function
- Significant increase in blood pressure
- New onset of migraine-type headache
- Pregnancy

Endometrial hyperplasia

• The risk of endometrial hyperplasia and carcinoma is increased when oestrogens are administered alone for prolonged periods (see section 4.8). The addition of a progestogen for at least 12 days per cycle in non-hysterectomised women greatly reduces this risk.

• For FemSeven 75 and 100, the endometrial safety of added progestogens has not been established.

• Break-through bleeding and spotting may occur during the first months of treatment. If break-through bleeding or spotting appears after some time on therapy, or continues after treatment has been discontinued, the reason should be investigated, which may include endometrial biopsy to exclude endometrial malignancy.

• Unopposed oestrogen stimulation may lead to premalignant or malignant transformation in the residual foci of endometriosis. Therefore, the addition of progestogens to oestrogen replacement therapy should be considered in women who have undergone hysterectomy because of endometriosis, if they are known to have residual endometriosis.

Breast cancer

A randomised placebo-controlled trial, the Women's Health Initative study (WHI), and epidemiological studies, including the Million Women Study (MWS), have reported an increased risk of breast cancer in women taking oestrogens, oestrogen-progestogen combinations or tibolone for HRT for several years (see section 4.8). For all HRT, an excess risk becomes apparent within a few years of use and increases with duration of intake but returns to baseline within a few (at most five) years after stopping treatment.

In the MWS, the relative risk of breast cancer with conjugated equine oestrogens (CEE) or estradiol (E2) was greater when a progestogen was added, either sequentially or continuously, and regardless of type of progestogen. There was no evidence of a difference in risk between the different routes of administration.

In the WHI study, the continuous combined conjugated equine oestrogen and medroxyprogesterone acetate (CEE + MPA) product used was associated with breast cancers that were slightly larger in size and more frequently had local lymph node metastases compared to placebo.

HRT, especially oestrogen-progestogen combined treatment, increases the density of mammographic images which may adversely affect the radiological detection of breast cancer.

Venous thromboembolism

• HRT is associated with a higher relative risk of developing venous thromboembolism (VTE), i.e. deep vein thrombosis or pulmonary embolism. One randomised controlled trial and epidemiological studies found a two to three fold higher risk for users compared with non-users. For non-users it is estimated that the number of cases of VTE that will occur over a 5 year period is about 3 per 1000 women aged 50-59 years and 8 per 1000 women aged between 60-69 years.

It is estimated that in healthy women who use HRT for 5 years the number of additional cases of VTE over a 5 year period will be between 2 and 6 (best estimate = 4) per 1000 women aged 50-59 years and between 5 and 15 (best estimate = 9) per 1000 women aged 60-69 years. The occurrence of such an event is more likely in the first year of HRT than later.

• Generally recognized risk factors for VTE include a personal history or family history, severe obesity (Body Mass Index > 30 kg/m^2) and systemic lupus erythematosus (SLE). There is no consensus about the possible role of varicose veins in VTE.

• Patients with a history of VTE or known thrombophilic states have an increased risk of VTE. HRT may add to this risk. Personal or strong family history of thromboembolism or recurrent spontaneous abortion should be investigated in order to exclude a thrombophilic predisposition. Until a thorough evaluation of thrombophilic factors has been made or anticoagulant treatment initiated, use of HRT in such patients should be viewed as contraindicated. Those women already on anticoagulant treatment require careful consideration of the benefit-risk of use of HRT.

• The risk of VTE may be temporarily increased with prolonged immobilisation, major trauma or major surgery. As in all post-operative patients, scrupulous attention should be given to prophylactic measures to prevent VTE following surgery. Where prolonged immobilisation is liable to follow elective surgery, particularly abdominal or orthopaedic surgery to the lower limbs, consideration should be given to temporarily stopping HRT four to six weeks earlier, if possible. Treatment should not be restarted until the woman is completely mobilised.

• If VTE develops after initiating therapy, the drug should be discontinued.

Patients should be told to contact their doctors immediately when they are aware of a potential thromboembolic symptom (e.g. painful swelling of a leg, sudden pain in the chest, dyspnoea).

Coronary artery disease (CAD)

There is no evidence from randomised controlled trials of cardiovascular benefit with continuous combined conjugated oestrogens and medroxyprogesterone acetate (MPA). Two large clinical trials (WHI and HERS i.e. Heart and Estrogen/progestin Replacement Study) showed a possible increased risk of cardiovascular morbidity in the first year of use and no overall benefit. For other HRT products there are only limited data from randomised controlled trials examining effects in cardiovascular morbidity or mortality. Therefore, it is uncertain whether these findings also extend to other HRT products.

Stroke

One large randomised clinical trial (WHI-trial) found, as a secondary outcome, an increased risk of ischaemic stroke in healthy women during treatment with continuous combined conjugated oestrogens and MPA. For women who do not use HRT, it is estimated that the number of cases of stroke that will occur over a 5 year period is about 3 per 1000 women aged 50-59 years and 11 per 1000 women aged 60-69 years.

It is estimated that for women who use conjugated oestrogens and MPA for 5 years, the number of additional cases will be between 0 and 3 (best estimate = 1) per 1000 users aged 50-59 years and between 1 and 9 (best estimate = 4) per 1000 users aged 60-69 years. It is unknown whether the increased risk also extends to other HRT products.

Ovarian cancer

Long-term (at least 5-10 years) use of oestrogen-only HRT products in hysterectomised women has been associated with an increased risk of ovarian cancer in some epidemiological studies. It is uncertain whether long-term use of combined HRT confers a different risk than oestrogen-only products.

Other conditions

• Oestrogens may cause fluid retention, and therefore patients with cardiac or renal dysfunction should be carefully observed. Patients with terminal renal insufficiency should be closely observed, since it is expected that the level of circulating active ingredients in FemSeven is increased.

• Women with pre-existing hypertriglyceridemia should be followed closely during oestrogen replacement or hormone replacement therapy, since rare cases of large increases of plasma triglycerides leading to pancreatitis have been reported with oestrogen therapy in this condition.

• Oestrogens increase thyroid binding globulin (TBG), leading to increased circulating total thyroid hormone, as measured by protein-bound iodine (PBI), T4 levels (by column or by radio-immunoassay) or T3 levels (by radio-immunoassay). T3 resin uptake is decreased, reflecting the

Table 1

Organ system class	Common ADRs > 1/100; < 1/10	Uncommon ADRs >1/1000; < 1/100	Rare ADRs >1/10000; < 1/1000
Skin and sub cutaneous tissue		Hair changes, sweating increased	
Muscular and skeletal		Arthralgia, leg cramps	
Central & peri. nervous system	Headache	Dizziness, paresthesia, migraine	
Psychiatric disorders		Anxiety, appetite increase, depression, insomnia, nervousness	
Gastrointestinal system dis.		Nausea, dyspepsia, abdominal pain, vomiting	
Cardiovasc.		Blood pressure changes	
Myo-, endo-, pericards		Chest pain	
Vascular (extracardial)		Vein disorders	
Reproductive disease female	Breast discomfort (e.g. Mastalgia/ mastopathies, breast tenderness, breast enlargement)	Vaginal discharge, breakthrough bleeding	Worsening of uterine fibroids
Body as a whole/general dis.		Edema, fatigue, weight changes	

elevated TBG. Free T4 and free T3 concentrations are unaltered. Other binding proteins may be elevated in serum, i.e. corticoid binding globulin (CBG), sex-hormone-binding globulin (SHBG) leading to increased circulating corticosteroids and sex steroids, respectively. Free or biological active hormone concentrations are unchanged. Other plasma proteins may be increased (angiotensinogen/renin substrate, alpha-I-antitrypsin, ceruloplasmin).

• There is no conclusive evidence for improvement of cognitive function. There is some evidence from the WHI trial of increased risk of probable dementia in women who start using continuous combined CEE and MPA after the age of 65. It is unknown whether the findings apply to younger post-menopausal women or other HRT products.

4.5 Interaction with other medicinal products and other forms of Interaction

The metabolism of oestrogens may be increased by concomitant use of substances known to induce drug-metabolising enzymes, specifically cytochrome P450 enzymes, such as anticonvulsants (e.g. phenobarbital, phenytoin, carbamazepine) and anti-infectives (e.g. rifampicin, rifabutin, nevirapine, efavirenz).

Ritonavir and nelfinavir, although known as strong inhibitors, by contrast exhibit inducing properties when used concomitantly with steroid hormones. Herbal preparations containing St John's wort (Hypericum Perforatum) may induce the metabolism of oestrogens.

With transdermal administration, the first-pass effect in the liver is avoided and, thus, transdermally applied oestrogens might be less affected than oral hormones by enzyme inducers.

Clinically, an increased metabolism of oestrogens may lead to decreased effect and changes in the uterine bleeding profile.

4.6 Pregnancy and lactation

• Pregnancy:

FemSeven is not indicated during pregnancy. If pregnancy occurs during medication with FemSeven, treatment should be withdrawn immediately.

The results of most epidemiological studies to date relevant to inadvertent fœtal exposure to oestrogens indicate no teratogenic or foetotoxic effects.

• Lactation:

FemSeven is not indicated during lactation.

4.7 Effects on ability to drive and use machines

There is no evidence from the clinical data available on oestrogen therapy to suggest that FemSeven should have any effect on a patient's ability to drive or operate machinery.

4.8 Undesirable effects

The most frequently reported undesirable effects (> 10 %) in clinical trials during treatment with FemSeven were application site reactions, e.g. pruritus, erythema, eczema, urticaria, oedema and changes in skin pigmentation. They were mostly mild skin reactions and usually disappeared 2 – 3 days after patch removal. These effects are usually observed with transdermal oestrogen replacement therapy.

All adverse events considered to be drug-related, which were observed during the Phase III (> 500 patients) and Phase IV (> 10,000 patients) clinical trials or from the spontaneous reporting system and literature, are summarised in the following table:

(see Table 1 above)

Breast cancer

According to evidence from a large number of epidemiological studies and one randomised placebo-controlled trial, the Women's Health Initiative (WHI), the overall risk of breast cancer increases with increasing duration of HRT use in current or recent HRT users.

For *oestrogen-only* HRT, estimates of relative risk (RR) from a reanalysis of original data from 51 epidemiological studies (in which >80% of HRT use was oestrogen-only HRT) and from the epidemiological Million Women Study (MWS) are similar at 1.35 (95%CI: 1.21 – 1.49) and 1.30 (95%CI: 1.21 – 1.40), respectively.

For *oestrogen plus progestogen* combined HRT, several epidemiological studies have reported an overall higher risk for breast cancer than with oestrogens alone.

The MWS reported that, compared to never users, the use of various types of oestrogen-progestogen combined HRT was associated with a higher risk of breast cancer (RR = 2.00, 95%CI: 1.88 – 2.12) than use of oestrogens alone (RR = 1.30, 95%CI: 1.21 – 1.40) or use of tibolone (RR = 1.45, 95%CI: 1.25-1.68).

The WHI trial reported a risk estimate of 1.24 (95%CI: 1.01 – 1.54) after 5.6 years of use of oestrogen-progestogen combined HRT (CEE + MPA) in all users compared with placebo.

The absolute risks calculated from the MWS and the WHI trial are presented below:

The MWS has estimated, from the known average incidence of breast cancer in developed countries, that:

♦ For women not using HRT, about 32 in every 1000 are expected to have breast cancer diagnosed between the ages of 50 and 64 years.

♦ For 1000 current or recent users of HRT, the number of *additional* cases during the corresponding period will be

• For users of *oestrogen-only* replacement therapy

- between 0 and 3 (best estimate = 1.5) for 5 years' use
- between 3 and 7 (best estimate = 5) for 10 years' use.

• For users of *oestrogen plus progestogen* combined HRT,

- between 5 and 7 (best estimate = 6) for 5 years' use
- between 18 and 20 (best estimate = 19) for 10 years' use.

The WHI trial estimated that after 5.6 years of follow-up of women between the ages of 50 and 79 years, an *additional* 8 cases of invasive breast cancer would be due to *oestrogen-progestogen combined* HRT (CEE + MPA) per 10,000 women years.

According to calculations from the trial data, it is estimated that:

♦ For 1000 women in the placebo group,

• about 16 cases of invasive breast cancer would be diagnosed in 5 years.

♦ For 1000 women who used oestrogen + progestogen combined HRT (CEE + MPA), the number of *additional* cases would be

• between 0 and 9 (best estimate = 4) for 5 years' use.

The number of additional cases of breast cancer in women who use HRT is broadly similar for women who start HRT irrespective of age at start of use (between the ages of 45-65) (see section 4.4).

Endometrial cancer

In women with an intact uterus, the risk of endometrial hyperplasia and endometrial cancer increases with increasing duration of use of unopposed oestrogens. According to data from epidemiological studies, the best estimate of the risk is that for women not using HRT, about 5 in every 1000 are expected to have endometrial cancer diagnosed between the ages of 50 and 65. Depending on the duration of treatment and oestrogen dose, the reported increase in endometrial cancer risk among unopposed oestrogen users varies from 2-to 12-fold greater compared with non-users. Adding a progestogen to oestrogen-only therapy greatly reduces this increased risk.

Other adverse reactions have been reported in association with oestrogen/progestogen treatment (class-effect):

- Oestrogen-dependent neoplasms benign and malignant, e.g. endometrial cancer.
- Venous thromboembolism, i.e. deep leg or pelvic venous thrombosis and pulmonary embolism, is more frequent among hormone replacement therapy users than among non-users. For further information, see section 4.3 Contra-indications and 4.4 Special warnings and precautions for use.
- Myocardial infarction and stroke
- Gall bladder disease
- Skin and subcutaneous disorders: chloasma, erythema multiforme, erythema nodosum, vascular purpura
- Deterioration of liver function
- Probable dementia (see section 4.4).

4.9 Overdose

The mode of administration makes significant overdose unlikely; removal of the patches is all that is required should it occur.

5. PHARMACOLOGICAL PROPERTIES

5.1 Pharmacodynamic properties

ATC code: G03 A03

Oestrogens

The active ingredient, synthetic 17β-estradiol, is chemically and biologically identical to endogenous human estradiol. It substitutes for the loss of oestrogen production in menopausal women, and alleviates menopausal symptoms. Oestrogens prevent bone loss following menopause or ovariectomy.

Clinical Trial Information:

• Relief of menopausal symptoms was achieved during the first few weeks of the treatment.

In non-hysterectomised women the bleeding profile depends on the type and dose of the progestogen and duration used in combination with FemSeven.

• Prevention of osteoporosis

- Oestrogen deficiency at menopause is associated with an increasing bone turnover and decline in bone mass. The effect of oestrogens on the bone mineral density is dose-dependent. Protection appears to be effective for as long as treatment is continued. After discontinuation of HRT, bone mass is lost at a rate similar to that in untreated women.

- Evidence from the WHI trial and meta-analysed trials shows that current use of HRT, alone or in combination with a progestogen – given to predominantly healthy women – reduces the risk of hip, vertebral, and other osteoporotic fractures. HRT may also prevent fractures in women with low bone density and/or established osteoporosis, but the evidence for that is limited.

5.2 Pharmacokinetic properties

After application of the transdermal system containing estradiol, therapeutic concentrations of estradiol are achieved within 3 hours and maintained throughout the entire application period of the transdermal patch (7 days). Estradiol peak plasma concentrations (C_{max}) range from 59 to 155 pg/ml (baseline corrected geometric mean 92 pg/ml) and $AUC_{0\text{-}168h}$ values were between 2478 and 10694 h*pg/ml (baseline corrected geometric mean 5188 h*pg/ml). The mean average plasma concentration (C_{av}) is 42 pg/ml (range: 20 to 145 pg/ml) and mean C_{pre} (trough concentration before next patch application) is 29 pg/ml. After removal of the transdermal patch, estradiol concentrations return to pre-treatment values (below 10 pg/ml) within 12 hours.

By transdermal administration of FemSeven, there is no hepatic first-pass effect and the estradiol reaches the bloodstream directly in unchanged form and in physiological amounts. With the use of FemSeven the estradiol concentrations are raised to values similar to those of the early to middle follicular phase.

The liver is the major site for estradiol metabolism. The primary metabolites are estrone and estriol and their conjugates (glucuronide and sulfate). Estradiol is excreted into the urine mostly as glucuronide and sulfate. The urinary excretion approaches pretreatment levels within 24 hours after patch removal.

5.3 Preclinical safety data
No adverse effects can be predicted from animal toxicology studies other than those documented from human use of estradiol.

6. PHARMACEUTICAL PARTICULARS

6.1 List of excipients
Backing layer: Transparent polyethylene terephthalate (PET) foil.

Adhesive matrix: Styrene-isoprene block copolymer, glycerine esters of completely hydrogenated resins.

6.2 Incompatibilities
None known.

6.3 Shelf life
2 years.

6.4 Special precautions for storage
Do not store above 30°C.

6.5 Nature and contents of container
The container (primary packaging) consists of a sealed laminated sachet. This comprises layers of food grade paper/polyethylene/aluminium/ethylene copolymer.

Package sizes:

FemSeven 50: Cartons of 4 and 12 patches.

FemSeven 75 & FemSeven 100: Cartons of 1, 4, 8, 9 and 12 patches.

6.6 Instructions for use and handling
After removal from the laminated sachet, peel off the two part protective liner. Try to avoid touching the adhesive. Stick the adhesive side down to the upper left or right buttock on a clean and dry area of skin. Hold the applied patch to the skin with the palm of the hand for at least 30 seconds, in order to ensure optimal adhesion to the skin.

Recommended application sites are clean, dry and intact areas of skin on the trunk below the waistline. FemSeven should not be applied on or near the breasts. After removal the used patch should be folded and disposed of with the normal household solid waste.

7. MARKETING AUTHORISATION HOLDER
Merck Ltd. (t/a Merck Pharmaceuticals (a division of Merck Ltd))

Harrier House

High Street

West Drayton

Middlesex

UB7 7QG

UK

8. MARKETING AUTHORISATION NUMBER(S)
FemSeven 50, 50 microgram/24 hours, transdermal patch. - PL 11648/0021

FemSeven 75, 75 microgram/24 hours, transdermal patch. - PL 11648/0023

FemSeven 100, 100 microgram/24 hours, transdermal patch. - PL 11648/0024

9. DATE OF FIRST AUTHORISATION/RENEWAL OF THE AUTHORISATION
14 December 2000

10. DATE OF REVISION OF THE TEXT
8 March 2004

FemSeven Conti

(Merck Pharmaceuticals)

1. NAME OF THE MEDICINAL PRODUCT
Femseven Conti,

50 micrograms / 7 micrograms / 24 hours,

transdermal patch

2. QUALITATIVE AND QUANTITATIVE COMPOSITION
Each patch contains 1.5 mg of estradiol hemihydrate and 0.525 mg levonorgestrel in a patch size of 15 cm^2, releasing 50 micrograms of estradiol and 7 micrograms of levonorgestrel per 24 hours.

For excipients, see 6.1.

3. PHARMACEUTICAL FORM
Transdermal patch

Octagonal, transparent, flexible, rounded-edge transdermal matrix patch located on an oversized removable protective liner.

4. CLINICAL PARTICULARS

4.1 Therapeutic indications
Hormone replacement therapy (HRT) for oestrogen deficiency symptoms in postmenopausal women more than one year after menopause.

Experience of treating women older than 65 years is limited.

4.2 Posology and method of administration
For transdermal use.

Femseven Conti has to be applied once a week, i.e. each patch is replaced every 7 days. Femseven Conti is a continuous combined hormone replacement therapy (HRT) treatment without a treatment-off phase: as one patch is removed, the next is applied immediately. Forgetting to change a patch on schedule may increase the likelihood of break-through bleeding or spotting.

In women with amenorrhoea and not taking HRT or women transferring from another continuous combined HRT product, treatment with Femseven Conti may be started on any convenient day.

In women transferring from sequential HRT regimens, treatment should start right after their withdrawal bleeding has ended.

For initiation and continuation of treatment of postmenopausal symptoms, the lowest effective dose for the shortest duration (see also section 4.4) should be used.

Method of administration

Femseven Conti should be applied to clean, dry, healthy skin (which is neither irritated nor grazed), free from any cream, lotion or other oily product.

Femseven Conti should be applied to an area of skin without major skin folds, i.e. the buttocks or hips, and not subject to chafing by clothing (avoid the waist and also avoid wearing tight clothing that could loosen the transdermal patch).

Femseven Conti must not be applied either on or near the breasts. It is advisable to avoid applying the patch to the same site twice running. At least one week should be allowed to elapse between applications to the same site.

After opening the sachet, one-half of the protective foil is peeled off, being careful not to touch the adhesive part of the transdermal patch with the fingers. Then the patch must be applied directly to the skin. After that the other half of the protective foil is peeled off, and the patch must be firmly pressed **with the palm of the hand for at least 30 seconds, concentrating on the edges. Pressure and the warmth of the hand are essential to ensure maximal adhesive strength of the patch.**

It is possible to take a shower or have a bath without removing the transdermal patch. In the event that the transdermal patch should become detached prematurely, i.e. before the seventh day (due to vigorous physical activity, excessive sweating, abnormal chafing of clothing), a new patch should be applied (to aid compliance it is recommended that the patient then continues to change the patch on the original scheduled day).

Once applied, the transdermal patch has to be covered by clothes to avoid direct exposure to sunlight.

Removal of the transdermal patch should be carried out slowly to avoid irritating the skin. In the event of some of the adhesive remaining on the skin, this can usually be removed by gently rubbing with a cream or an oily lotion.

After use, Femseven Conti is to be folded in two (with the adhesive surface to the inside) and disposed of with normal household solid waste.

4.3 Contraindications
- Known, past or suspected breast cancer;
- Known or suspected oestrogen-dependent malignant tumours (e.g. endometrial cancer);
- Undiagnosed genital bleeding;
- Untreated endometrial hyperplasia;
- Previous idiopathic or current venous thromboembolism (deep venous thrombosis, pulmonary embolism);
- Active or recent arterial thromboembolic disease, (e.g. angina, myocardial infarction);
- Acute liver disease, or a history of liver disease as long as liver function tests have failed to return to normal;
- Known hypersensitivity to the active substances or to any of the excipients;
- Porphyria.

4.4 Special warnings and special precautions for use
For the treatment of postmenopausal symptoms, HRT should only be initiated for symptoms that adversely affect quality of life. In all cases, a careful appraisal of the risks and benefits should be undertaken at least annually and HRT should only be continued as long as the benefit outweighs the risk.

Medical examination/follow-up

Before initiating or reinstituting HRT, a complete personal and family medical history should be taken. Physical (including pelvic and breast) examination should be guided by this and by the contraindications and warnings for use. During treatment, periodic check-ups are recommended of a frequency and nature adapted to the individual woman. Women should be advised what changes in their breasts should be reported to their doctor or nurse (see "Breast cancer" below). Investigations, including mammography, should be carried out in accordance with currently accepted screening practices, modified to the clinical needs of the individual.

Conditions which need supervision

If any of the following conditions are present, have occurred previously, and/or have been aggravated during pregnancy or previous hormone treatment, the patient should be closely supervised. It should be taken into account that these conditions may recur or be aggravated during treatment with Femseven Conti, in particular:

- Leiomyoma (uterine fibroids) or endometriosis
- A history of, or risk factors for, thromboembolic disorders (see below)
- Risk factors for oestrogen-dependent tumours, e.g. 1st degree heredity for breast cancer
- Hypertension
- Liver disorders (e.g. liver adenoma)
- Diabetes mellitus with or without vascular involvement
- Cholelithiasis
- Migraine or (severe) headache
- Systemic lupus erythematosus
- A history of endometrial hyperplasia (see below)
- Epilepsy
- Asthma
- Otosclerosis

Reasons for immediate withdrawal of therapy:

Therapy should be discontinued in case a contra-indication is discovered and in the following situations:
- Jaundice or deterioration in liver function
- Significant increase in blood pressure
- New onset of migraine-type headache
- Pregnancy

Endometrial hyperplasia

• The risk of endometrial hyperplasia and carcinoma is increased when oestrogens are administered alone for prolonged periods (see section 4.8). The addition of a progestagen for at least 12 days per cycle in non-hysterectomised women greatly reduces this risk.

• Break-through bleeding and spotting may occur during the first months of treatment. If break-through bleeding or spotting appears after some time on therapy, or continues after treatment has been discontinued, the reason should be investigated, which may include an endometrial biopsy to exclude endometrial malignancy.

Breast cancer

A randomised placebo-controlled trial, the Women's Health Initiative study (WHI), and epidemiological studies, including the Million Women Study (MWS), have reported an increased risk of breast cancer in women taking oestrogens, oestrogen-progestagen combinations or tibolone for HRT for several years (see Section 4.8). For all HRT, an excess risk becomes apparent within a few years of use and increases with duration of intake but returns to baseline within a few (at most five) years after stopping treatment.

In the MWS, the relative risk of breast cancer with conjugated equine oestrogens (CEE) or estradiol (E2) was greater when a progestagen was added, either sequentially or continuously, and regardless of type of progestagen. There was no evidence of a difference in risk between the different routes of administration.

In the WHI study, the continuous combined conjugated equine oestrogen and medroxyprogesterone acetate (CEE + MPA) product used was associated with breast cancers that were slightly larger in size and more frequently had local lymph node metastases compared to placebo.

HRT, especially oestrogen-progestagen combined treatment, increases the density of mammographic images which may adversely affect the radiological detection of breast cancer.

Venous thromboembolism

• HRT is associated with a higher relative risk of developing venous thromboembolism (VTE), i.e. deep vein thrombosis or pulmonary embolism. One randomised controlled trial and epidemiological studies found a two- to threefold higher risk for users compared with non-users. For non-users it is estimated that the number of cases of VTE that will occur over a 5 year period is about 3 per 1000 women aged 50-59 years and 8 per 1000 women aged between 60-69 years. It is estimated that in healthy women who use HRT for 5 years, the number of additional cases of VTE over a 5 year period will be between 2 and 6 (best estimate = 4) per 1000 women aged 50-59 years and between 5 and 15 (best estimate = 9) per 1000 women aged 60-69 years. The occurrence of such an event is more likely in the first year of HRT than later.

• Generally recognised risk factors for VTE include a personal history or family history, severe obesity (BMI > 30 kg/m^2) and systemic lupus erythematosus (SLE). There is no consensus about the possible role of varicose veins in VTE.

• Patients with a history of VTE or known thrombophilic states have an increased risk of VTE. HRT may add to this risk. A personal or strong family history of thromboembolism or recurrent spontaneous abortion should be investigated in order to exclude a thrombophilic predisposition. Until a thorough evaluation of thrombophilic factors has been made or anticoagulant treatment initiated, use of HRT in such patients should be viewed as contraindicated. Those women already on anticoagulant treatment require careful consideration of the benefit-risk of use of HRT.

• The risk of VTE may be temporarily increased with prolonged immobilisation, major trauma or major surgery. As in all post-operative patients, scrupulous attention should be given to prophylactic measures to prevent

VTE following surgery. Where prolonged immobilisation is liable to follow elective surgery, particularly abdominal or orthopaedic surgery to the lower limbs, consideration should be given to temporarily stopping HRT 4 to 6 weeks earlier, if possible. Treatment should not be restarted until the woman is completely mobilised.

• If VTE develops after initiating therapy, the drug should be discontinued. Patients should be told to contact their doctors immediately when they are aware of a potential thromboembolic symptom (e.g. painful swelling of a leg, sudden pain in the chest, dyspnea).

Coronary artery disease (CAD)

• There is no evidence from randomised controlled trials of cardiovascular benefit with continuous combined conjugated oestrogens and medroxyprogesterone acetate (MPA). Two large clinical trials (WHI and HERS i.e. Heart and Estrogen/progestin Replacement Study) showed a possible increased risk of cardiovascular morbidity in the first year of use and no overall benefit. For other HRT products there are only limited data from randomised controlled trials examining effects in cardiovascular morbidity or mortality. Therefore, it is uncertain whether these findings also extend to other HRT products.

Stroke

• One large randomised clinical trial (WHI-trial) found, as a secondary outcome, an increased risk of ischaemic stroke in healthy women during treatment with continuous combined conjugated oestrogens and MPA. For women who do not use HRT, it is estimated that the number of cases of stroke that will occur over a 5 year period is about 3 per 1000 women aged 50-59 years and 11 per 1000 women aged 60-69 years. It is estimated that for women who use conjugated oestrogens and MPA for 5 years, the number of additional cases will be between 0 and 3 (best estimate = 1) per 1000 users aged 50-59 years and between 1 and 9 (best estimate = 4) per 1000 users aged 60-69 years. It is unknown whether the increased risk also extends to other HRT products.

Ovarian cancer

• Long-term (at least 5-10 years) use of oestrogen-only HRT products in hysterectomised women has been associated with an increased risk of ovarian cancer in some epidemiological studies. It is uncertain whether long-term use of combined HRT confers a different risk than oestrogen-only products.

Other conditions

• Oestrogens may cause fluid retention, and therefore patients with cardiac or renal dysfunction should be carefully observed. Patients with terminal renal insufficiency should be closely observed, since it is expected that the level of circulating active ingredients in Femseven Conti is increased.

• Women with pre-existing hypertriglyceridemia should be followed closely during oestrogen replacement or hormone replacement therapy, since rare cases of large increases of plasma triglycerides leading to pancreatitis have been reported with oestrogen therapy in this condition.

• Oestrogens increase thyroid binding globulin (TBG), leading to increased circulating total thyroid hormone, as measured by protein-bound iodine (PBI), T4 levels (by column or by radio-immunoassay) or T3 levels (by radio-immunoassay). T3 resin uptake is decreased, reflecting the elevated TBG. Free T4 and free T3 concentrations are unaltered. Other binding proteins may be elevated in serum, i.e. corticoid binding globulin (CBG), sex hormone-binding globulin (SHBG) leading to increased circulating corticosteroids and sex steroids, respectively. Free or biological active hormone concentrations are unchanged. Other plasma proteins may be increased (angiotensinogen/renin substrate, alpha-I-antitrypsin, ceruloplasmin).

• There is no conclusive evidence for improvement of cognitive function. There is some evidence from the WHI trial of increased risk of probable dementia in women who start using continuous combined CEE and MPA after the age of 65. It is unknown whether the findings apply to younger post-menopausal women or other HRT products.

4.5 Interaction with other medicinal products and other forms of Interaction

The metabolism of oestrogens and progestagens may be increased by concomitant use of substances known to induce drug-metabolising enzymes, specifically cytochrome P450 enzymes, such as anticonvulsants (e.g. phenobarbital, phenytoin, carbamazepine) and anti-infectives (e.g. rifampicin, rifabutin, nevirapine, efavirenz).

Ritonavir and nelfinavir, although known as strong inhibitors, by contrast exhibit inducing properties when used concomitantly with steroid hormones.

Herbal preparations containing St John's wort (Hypericum Perforatum) may induce the metabolism of oestrogens and progestagens.

With transdermal administration, the first-pass effect in the liver is avoided and, thus, transdermally applied oestrogens and progestagens might be less affected than oral hormones by enzyme inducers.

Clinically, an increased metabolism of oestrogens and progestagens may lead to decreased effect and changes in the uterine bleeding profile.

4.6 Pregnancy and lactation

Pregnancy

Femseven Conti is not indicated during pregnancy. If pregnancy occurs during treatment with Femseven Conti, treatment should be withdrawn immediately.

Clinically, data on a large number of exposed pregnancies indicate no adverse effects of levonorgestrel on the foetus.

The results of most epidemiological studies to date that are relevant to inadvertent foetal exposure to combinations of oestrogens and progestagens indicate no teratogenic or foetotoxic effect.

Lactation

Femseven Conti is not indicated during lactation.

4.7 Effects on ability to drive and use machines

No effects on ability to drive and use machines have been observed.

4.8 Undesirable effects

The most frequently reported undesirable effects (> 10 %) in clinical trials during treatment with Femseven Conti were application site reactions, breast tenderness and bleeding or spotting. The application site reactions were mostly mild skin reactions and usually disappeared 2 – 3 days after patch removal. In the majority of cases breast tenderness was reported as mild or moderate and tend to decrease during treatment time.

Other potential systemic undesirable effects are those commonly observed with oestrogen and progestin treatments.

(see Table 1)

Breast cancer

According to evidence from a large number of epidemiological studies and one randomised placebo-controlled trial, the Women's Health Initiative (WHI), the overall risk of breast cancer increases with increasing duration of HRT use in current or recent HRT users.

For *oestrogen-only* HRT, estimates of relative risk (RR) from a reanalysis of original data from 51 epidemiological studies (in which >80% of HRT use was oestrogen-only HRT) and from the epidemiological Million Women Study (MWS) are similar at 1.35 (95%CI: 1.21 – 1.49) and 1.30 (95%CI: 1.21 - 1.40), respectively.

For *oestrogen plus progestagen* combined HRT, several epidemiological studies have reported an overall higher risk for breast cancer than with oestrogens alone.

The MWS reported that, compared to never users, the use of various types of oestrogen-progestagen combined HRT was associated with a higher risk of breast cancer (RR = 2.00, 95%CI: 1.88 – 2.12) than use of oestrogens alone (RR = 1.30, 95%CI: 1.21 – 1.40) or use of tibolone (RR = 1.45, 95%CI: 1.25 - 1.68).

The WHI trial reported a risk estimate of 1.24 (95%CI: 1.01 – 1.54) after 5.6 years of use of oestrogen-progestagen combined HRT (CEE + MPA) in all users compared with placebo.

The absolute risks calculated from the MWS and the WHI trial are presented below:

The MWS has estimated, from the known average incidence of breast cancer in developed countries, that:

◆ For women not using HRT, about 32 in every 1000 are expected to have breast cancer diagnosed between the ages of 50 and 64 years.

◆ For 1000 current or recent users of HRT, the number of *additional* cases during the corresponding period will be

• For users of *oestrogen-only* replacement therapy

- between 0 and 3 (best estimate = 1.5) for 5 years' use

- between 3 and 7 (best estimate = 5) for 10 years' use.

• For users of *oestrogen plus progestogen* combined HRT,

- between 5 and 7 (best estimate = 6) for 5 years' use

- between 18 and 20 (best estimate = 19) for 10 years' use.

The WHI trial estimated that after 5.6 years of follow-up of women between the ages of 50 and 79 years, an *additional* 8 cases of invasive breast cancer would be due to *oestrogen-progestogen combined* HRT (CEE + MPA) per 10,000 women years.

According to calculations from the trial data, it is estimated that:

◆ For 1000 women in the placebo group,

• about 16 cases of invasive breast cancer would be diagnosed in 5 years.

◆ For 1000 women who used oestrogen + progestogen combined HRT (CEE + MPA), the number of *additional* cases would be

• between 0 and 9 (best estimate = 4) for 5 years' use.

The number of additional cases of breast cancer in women who use HRT is broadly similar for women who start HRT irrespective of age at start of use (between the ages of 45-65) (see section 4.4).

Endometrial cancer

In women with an intact uterus, the risk of endometrial hyperplasia and endometrial cancer increases with increasing duration of use of unopposed oestrogens. According to data from epidemiological studies, the best estimate of the risk is that for women not using HRT, about 5 in every 1000 are expected to have endometrial cancer diagnosed between the ages of 50 and 65. Depending on the duration of treatment and oestrogen dose, the reported increase in endometrial cancer risk among unopposed oestrogen users varies from 2-to 12-fold greater compared with non-users. Adding a progestagen to oestrogen-only therapy greatly reduces this increased risk.

Other adverse reactions have been reported in association with oestrogen/progestagen treatment:

- Oestrogen-dependent neoplasms benign and malignant, e.g. endometrial cancer.

- Venous thromboembolism, i.e. deep leg or pelvic venous thrombosis and pulmonary embolism, is more frequent among hormone replacement therapy users than among non-users. For further information, see section 4.3 Contra-indications and 4.4 Special warnings and precautions for use.

- Myocardial infarction and stroke.

- Gall bladder disease.

- Skin and subcutaneous disorders: chloasma, erythema multiforme, erythema nodosum, vascular purpura.

- Probable dementia (see section 4.4).

4.9 Overdose

The method of administration makes significant overdose unlikely. Signs of an overdose are generally breast tenderness, swelling of the abdomen/pelvis, anxiety, irritability, nausea and vomiting. Removal of the transdermal patches is all that is required should it occur.

5. PHARMACOLOGICAL PROPERTIES

5.1 Pharmacodynamic properties

Pharmacotherapeutic group:

Progestagens and oestrogens, combinations, levonorgestrel and oestrogen

ATC code: G03F A11

Femseven Conti contains a continuous combined combination of oestrogen and progestagen for continuous use, combining estradiol hemihydrate and levonorgestrel.

Estradiol: The active substance, synthetic 17β-estradiol, is chemically and biologically identical to endogenous human estradiol. It substitutes for the loss of oestrogen production in menopausal women, and alleviates menopausal symptoms.

Levonorgestrel: As oestrogens promote the growth of the endometrium, unopposed oestrogens increase the risk of endometrial hyperplasia and cancer. The addition of levonorgestrel greatly reduces the oestrogen-induced risk of endometrial hyperplasia in non-hysterectomised women.

Table 1

Organ system	Common ADRs > 1/100, < 1/10	Uncommon ADRs > 1/1000, < 1/100	Rare ADRs > 1/10,000, < 1/1000
General disorders		Fluid retention/ oedema/ weight increase/loss, fatigue, leg cramps	
Nervous system disorders	Headache	Dizziness, migraine	
Gastrointestinal disorders	Dyspepsia	Bloating, abdominal cramps, nausea	Choletithiasis, cholestatic jaundice
Cardiovascular disorders		Hypertension	
Reproductive system and breast disorders	Mastodynia	Endometrial hyperplasia, benign breast tissue changes,	Increase in size of uterine fibrosis
Psychiatric disorders		Depression	

Clinical trial information

Relief of oestrogen-deficiency symptoms and bleeding patterns:

- Under treatment with Femseven Conti, relief of menopausal symptoms was achieved during the first weeks of treatment.
- Femseven Conti is a continuous-combined HRT given with the intent of avoiding the regular withdrawal bleeding associated with cyclic or sequential HRT.

Amenorrhoea (no bleeding or spotting) was seen in 59-68 % of the women during months 10-12 of treatment. Spottings were seen in 19-16 % of women within the same period. Break through bleeding and/or spotting appeared in 28-39 % of the women during the first three months of treatment and in 37 % during months 10-12 of treatment.

Women with longer-established menopause and with an atrophic endometrium will reach amenorrhoea earlier.

5.2 Pharmacokinetic properties

By transdermal administration there is no hepatic first-pass effect as observed with oral administration; estradiol reaches the bloodstream in unchanged form and in physiological amounts. Therapeutic estradiol concentrations are comparable to those observed in the follicular phase.

After continuous application of Femseven Conti, maximum plasma concentration of estradiol (C_{max}) reaches 82 pg/ml and average plasma concentration (C_{av}) is about 34 pg/ml. Trough plasma concentration (C_{trough}) at the end of a 7-day wearing period is 27 pg/ml. After removal of the transdermal patch, estradiol concentrations return to their baseline values within 12 to 24 hours.

The maximum plasma concentration of levonorgestrel is reached after three to four days and C_{max} is approximately 113 pg/ml at steady state. The average plasma concentration of levonorgestrel during a 7-day period is approximately 88 pg/ml and trough plasma concentration (C_{trough}) reaches 72 pg/ml.

After percutaneous absorption, levonorgestrel is bound to plasma proteins, i.e. albumin (50%), and sex hormone-binding globulin (SHBG) (47.5%). Affinity to SHBG is higher than for other commonly used progestagens.

5.3 Preclinical safety data

In experimental animals estradiol displayed an embryo-lethal effect already at relatively low doses; malformations of the urogenital tract and feminisation of male foetuses were observed. Levonorgestral displayed an embryolethal effect in animal experiments and, in high doses, a virilising effect on female fetuses.

Because of marked differences between animal species and between animals and humans, preclinical results are of limited predictive value for the treatment of humans with oestrogens.

6. PHARMACEUTICAL PARTICULARS

6.1 List of excipients

Backing layer: Polyethylene terephthalate (PET) foil.

Adhesive matrix: Styrene-isoprene-styrene block copolymer, glycerine esters of completely hydrogenated resins.

Protective liner: Siliconized polyethylene terephthalate (PET) foil.

6.2 Incompatibilities

Not applicable.

6.3 Shelf life

2 years.

6.4 Special precautions for storage

Do not store above 30°C.

6.5 Nature and contents of container

Sachet (Paper/PE/aluminium/ethylene copolymer). Ccarton of 4 or 12 sachets.

6.6 Instructions for use and handling

See 4.2 Posology and method of administration.

No special requirements.

7. MARKETING AUTHORISATION HOLDER

Merck Ltd

t/a Merck Pharmaceuticals (A division of Merck Ltd)

Harrier House

High Street

West Drayton

Middlesex

UB7 7QG

8. MARKETING AUTHORISATION NUMBER(S)

PL 11648/0050

9. DATE OF FIRST AUTHORISATION/RENEWAL OF THE AUTHORISATION

5 November 2002

10. DATE OF REVISION OF THE TEXT

22 August 2004

FemSeven Sequi

(Merck Pharmaceuticals)

1. NAME OF THE MEDICINAL PRODUCT

FemSeven Sequi,

50 micrograms/10 micrograms/24 hours,

transdermal patch

2. QUALITATIVE AND QUANTITATIVE COMPOSITION

Phase 1:

Each patch contains 1.5 mg of estradiol hemihydrate in a patch size of 15 cm^2, releasing 50 micrograms of estradiol per 24 hours.

Phase 2:

Each patch contains 1.5 mg of estradiol hemihydrate and 1.5 mg of levonorgestrel in a patch size of 15 cm^2, releasing 50 micrograms of estradiol and 10 micrograms of levonorgestrel per 24 hours.

For excipients, see 6.1.

3. PHARMACEUTICAL FORM

Transdermal patch

Octagonal, transparent, flexible, rounded-edge transdermal matrix patch located on an oversized removable protective liner.

4. CLINICAL PARTICULARS

4.1 Therapeutic indications

Hormone replacement therapy (HRT) for oestrogen deficiency symptoms in post-menopausal women.

Experience of treating women older than 65 years is limited.

4.2 Posology and method of administration

For transdermal use.

Apply FemSeven Sequi once a week, i.e. replace each patch every 7 days. FemSeven Sequi is a continuous sequential hormone replacement therapy (HRT) without a treatment-off phase: as one patch is removed, the next is applied immediately.

Each treatment cycle with FemSeven Sequi consists of the successive application of two transdermal patches containing estradiol (phase 1) and then two transdermal patches containing estradiol and levonorgestrel (phase 2).

Accordingly, the following treatment cycle should be observed:

- one phase 1 patch once a week for the first two weeks
- then one phase 2 patch once a week for the following two weeks.

In women who are not taking HRT or women who switch from a continuous combined HRT product, treatment may be started on any convenient day.

In women transferring from a sequential HRT regimen, treatment should begin the day following completion of the prior regimen.

For initiation and continuation of treatment of postmenopausal symptoms, the lowest effective dose for the shortest duration (see also section 4.4) should be used.

Method of administration

FemSeven Sequi should be applied to clean, dry, healthy skin (which is neither irritated nor grazed), free from any cream, lotion or other oily product.

FemSeven Sequi should be applied to an area of skin without major skin folds, e.g. the buttocks or hips, and not subject to chafing by clothing (avoid the waist and also avoid wearing tight clothing that could loosen the transdermal patch).

FemSeven Sequi must not be applied either on or near the breasts. It is advisable to avoid applying the patch to the same site twice. At least one week should be allowed to elapse between applications to the same site.

After opening the sachet, peel off one-half of the protective foil, being careful not to touch the adhesive part of the transdermal patch with the fingers. Apply directly to the skin. Now peel off the other half of the protective foil and press the patch on firmly with the palm of the hand for at least 30 seconds, concentrating on the edges. The pressure and the warmth of the hand are essential to ensure maximal adhesive strength of the patch.

It is possible to take a shower or have a bath without removing the transdermal patch.

Should a patch detach prematurely, before 7 days (due to vigorous physical activity, excessive sweating, abnormal chafing of clothing), it should be removed and a new patch of the same phase applied. To aid compliance it is recommended the patient then continues to change the patch on the usual day and according to the initial treatment cycle. This advice also applies if a patient forgets to change the patch on schedule. Forgetting a patch may increase the likelihood of break-through bleeding or spotting.

Once applied, the transdermal patch should not be exposed to sunlight.

Removal of the transdermal patch should be carried out slowly to avoid irritating the skin. In the event of some of the adhesive remaining on the skin, this can usually be removed by gently rubbing with a cream or an oily lotion.

After use, fold FemSeven Sequi in two (with the adhesive surface to the inside) and dispose of it with normal household solid waste.

4.3 Contraindications

- Known, past or suspected breast cancer;
- Known or suspected oestrogen-dependent malignant tumours (e.g. endometrial cancer);
- Undiagnosed genital bleeding;
- Untreated endometrial hyperplasia;
- Previous idiopathic or current venous thromboembolism (deep venous thrombosis, pulmonary embolism);
- Active or recent arterial thromboembolic disease (e.g. angina, myocardial infarction);
- Acute liver disease or a history of liver disease as long as liver function tests have failed to return to normal;
- Known hypersensitivity to the active substances or to any of the excipients;
- Porphyria.

4.4 Special warnings and special precautions for use

For the treatment of postmenopausal symptoms, HRT should only be initiated for symptoms that adversely affect quality of life. In all cases, a careful appraisal of the risks and benefits should be undertaken at least annually and HRT should only be continued as long as the benefit outweighs the risk.

Medical examination/follow-up

Before initiating or reinstituting HRT, a complete personal and family medical history should be taken. Physical (including pelvic and breast) examination should be guided by this and by the contraindications and warnings for use. During treatment, periodic check-ups are recommended of a frequency and nature adapted to the individual woman.

Women should be advised what changes in their breasts should be reported to their doctor or nurse (see "Breast cancer" below). Investigations, including mammography, should be carried out in accordance with currently accepted screening practices, modified according to the clinical needs of the individual.

Conditions which need supervision

If any of the following conditions are present, have occurred previously and/or have been aggravated during pregnancy or previous hormone treatment, the patient should be closely supervised. It should be taken into account that these conditions may recur or be aggravated during treatment with FemSeven Sequi, in particular:

- Leiomyoma (uterine fibroids) or endometriosis
- A history of, or risk factors for, thromboembolic disorders (see below)
- Risk factors for oestrogen dependent tumours, e.g. 1st degree heredity for breast cancer
- Hypertension
- Liver disorders (e.g. liver adenoma)
- Diabetes mellitus with or without vascular involvement
- Cholelithiasis
- Migraine or (severe) headache
- Systemic lupus erythematosus
- A history of endometrial hyperplasia (see below)
- Epilepsy
- Asthma
- Otosclerosis.

Reasons for immediate withdrawal of therapy:

-Therapy should be discontinued if a contra-indication is discovered and in the following situations:

- Jaundice or deterioration in liver function
- Significant increase in blood pressure
- New onset of migraine-type headache
- Pregnancy.

Endometrial hyperplasia

- The risk of endometrial hyperplasia and carcinoma is increased when oestrogens are administered alone for prolonged periods (see section 4.8). The addition of a progestagen for at least 12 days per cycle in non-hysterectomised women greatly reduces this risk.
- Break-through bleeding and spotting may occur during the first months of treatment. If break-through bleeding or spotting appears after some time on therapy, or continues after treatment has been discontinued, the reason should be investigated, which may include endometrial biopsy to exclude endometrial malignancy.

Breast cancer

A randomised placebo-controlled trial, the Women's Health Initiative study (WHI), and epidemiological studies, including the Million Women Study (MWS), have reported an increased risk of breast cancer in women taking oestrogens, oestrogen-progestagen combinations or tibolone for HRT for several years (see section 4.8). For all HRT, an excess risk becomes apparent within a few years of use and increases with duration of intake but returns to baseline within a few (at most five) years after stopping treatment.

In the MWS, the relative risk of breast cancer with conjugated equine oestrogens (CEE) or estradiol (E2) was greater when a progestagen was added, eithersequentially or continuously, and regardless of type of progestagen. There was no evidence of a difference in risk between the different routes of administration.

In the WHI study, the continuous combined conjugated equine oestrogen and medroxyprogesterone acetate (CEE + MPA) product used was associated with breast cancers that were slightly larger in size and more frequently had local lymph node metastases compared to placebo.

HRT, especially oestrogen-progestagen combined treatment, increases the density of mammographic images which may adversely affect the radiological detection of breast cancer.

Venous thromboembolism

- HRT is associated with a higher relative risk of developing venous thromboembolism (VTE), i.e. deep vein thrombosis or pulmonary embolism. One randomised controlled trial and epidemiological studies found a two- to threefold higher risk for users compared with non-users. For non-users it is estimated that the number of cases of VTE that will occur over a 5 year period is about 3 per 1000 women aged 50-59 years and 8 per 1000 women aged between 60-69 years. It is estimated that in healthy women who use HRT for 5 years the number of additional cases of VTE over a 5 year period will be between 2 and 6 (best estimate = 4) per 1000 women aged 50-59 years and between 5 and 15 (best estimate = 9) per 1000 women aged 60-69 years. The occurrence of such an event is more likely in the first year of HRT than later.
- Generally recognized risk factors for VTE include a personal history or family history, severe obesity (BMI > 30 kg/m^2) and systemic lupus erythematosus (SLE). There is no consensus about the possible role of varicose veins in VTE.
- Patients with a history of VTE or known thrombophilic states have an increased risk of VTE. HRT may add to this risk. Personal or strong family history of thromboembolism or recurrent spontaneous abortion should be investigated in order to exclude a thrombophilic predisposition. Until a thorough evaluation of thrombophilic factors has been made or anticoagulant treatment initiated, use of HRT in such patients should be viewed as contra-indicated. Those women already on anticoagulant treatment require careful consideration of the benefit-risk of use of HRT.
- The risk of VTE may be temporarily increased with prolonged immobilisation, major trauma or major surgery. As in all postoperative patients, scrupulous attention should be given to prophylactic measures to prevent VTE following surgery. Where prolonged immobilisation is liable to follow elective surgery, particularly abdominal or orthopaedic surgery to the lower limbs, consideration should be given to temporarily stopping HRT four to six weeks earlier, if possible. Treatment should not be restarted until the woman is completely mobilised.
- If VTE develops after initiating therapy, the drug should be discontinued.

Patients should be told to contact their doctors immediately when they are aware of a potential thromboembolic symptom (e.g. painful swelling of a leg, sudden pain in the chest, dyspnea).

Coronary artery disease (CAD)

There is no evidence from randomised controlled trials of cardiovascular benefit with continuous combined conjugated oestrogens and medroxyprogesterone acetate (MPA). Two large clinical trials (WHI and HERS i.e. Heart and Estrogen/progestin Replacement Study) showed a possible increased risk of cardiovascular morbidity in the first year of use and no overall benefit. For other HRT products there are only limited data from randomised controlled trials examining effects in cardiovascular morbidity or mortality. Therefore, it is uncertain whether these findings also extend to other HRT products.

Stroke

One large randomised clinical trial (WHI-trial) found, as a secondary outcome, an increased risk of ischaemic stroke in healthy women during treatment with continuous combined conjugated oestrogens and MPA. For women who do not use HRT, it is estimated that the number of cases of stroke that will occur over a 5 year period is about 3 per 1000 women aged 50-59 years and 11 per 1000 women aged 60-69 years. It is estimated that for women who use conjugated oestrogens and MPA for 5 years, the number of additional cases will be between 0 and 3 (best estimate = 1) per 1000 users aged 50-59 years and between 1 and 9 (best estimate = 4) per 1000 users aged 60-69 years. It is unknown whether the increased risk also extends to other HRT products.

Ovarian cancer

Long-term (at least 5-10 years) use of oestrogen-only HRT products in hysterectomised women has been associated with an increased risk of ovarian cancer in some epidemiological studies. It is uncertain whether long-term use of combined HRT confers a different risk than oestrogen-only products.

Other conditions

Oestrogens may cause fluid retention, and therefore patients with cardiac or renal dysfunction should be carefully observed. Patients with terminal renal insufficiency should be closely observed, since it is expected that the level of circulating active ingredients in FemSeven Sequi transdermal patch is increased.

Women with pre-existing hypertriglyceridemia should be followed closely during oestrogen replacement or hormone replacement therapy, since rare cases of large increases of plasma triglycerides leading to pancreatitis have been reported with oestrogen therapy in this condition.

Oestrogens increase thyroid binding globulin (TBG), leading to increased circulating total thyroid hormone, as measured by protein-bound iodine (PBI), T4 levels (by column or by radio-immunoassay) or T3 levels (by radio-immunoassay). T3 resin uptake is decreased, reflecting the elevated TBG. Free T4 and free T3 concentrations are unaltered. Other binding proteins may be elevated in serum, i.e. corticoid binding globulin (CBG), sex-hormone-binding globulin (SHBG) leading to increased circulating corticosteroids and sex steroids, respectively. Free or biological active hormone concentrations are unchanged. Other plasma proteins may be increased (angiotensinogen/renin substrate, alpha-I-antitrypsin, ceruloplasmin).

There is no conclusive evidence for improvement of cognitive function. There is some evidence from the WHI trial of increased risk of probable dementia in women who start using continuous combined CEE and MPA after the age of 65. It is unknown whether the findings apply to younger post-menopausal women or other HRT products.

4.5 Interaction with other medicinal products and other forms of Interaction

The metabolism of oestrogens and progestagens may be increased by concomitant use of substances known to induce drug-metabolising enzymes, specifically cytochrome P450 enzymes, such as anticonvulsants (e.g. phenobarbital, phenytoin, carbamazepine) and anti-infectives (e.g. rifampicin, rifabutin, nevirapine, efavirenz).

Ritonavir and nelfinavir, although known as strong inhibitors, by contrast exhibit inducing properties when used concomitantly with steroid hormones.

Herbal preparations containing St John's wort (*Hypericum Perforatum*) may induce the metabolism of oestrogens and progestagens.

At transdermal administration, the first-pass effect in the liver is avoided and, thus, transdermally applied oestrogens and progestagens might be less affected than oral hormones by enzyme inducers.

Clinically, an increased metabolism of oestrogens and progestagens may lead to decreased effect and changes in the uterine bleeding profile.

4.6 Pregnancy and lactation

Pregnancy:

FemSeven Sequi is not indicated during pregnancy. If pregnancy occurs during medication with FemSeven Sequi, treatment should be withdrawn immediately.

Clinically, data on a large number of exposed pregnancies indicate no adverse effects of levonorgestrel on the fœtus.

The results of most epidemiological studies to date relevant to inadvertent fœtal exposure to combinations of oestrogens and progestagens indicate no teratogenic or foetotoxic effects.

Lactation:

FemSeven Sequi is not indicated during lactation.

4.7 Effects on ability to drive and use machines

No effects on ability to drive and use machines have been observed.

4.8 Undesirable effects

The most frequently reported undesirable effects (> 10 %) in clinical trials during treatment with FemSeven Sequi were application site reactions. They usually disappeared 2 – 3 days after patch removal.

Other potential systemic undesirable effects are those commonly observed with oestrogen and progestin treatments.

(see Table 1)

Breast cancer

According to evidence from a large number of epidemiological studies and one randomised placebo-controlled trial, the Women's Health Initiative (WHI), the overall risk of breast cancer increases with increasing duration of HRT use in current or recent HRT users.

For *oestrogen-only* HRT, estimates of relative risk (RR) from a reanalysis of original data from 51 epidemiological studies (in which >80% of HRT use was oestrogen-only HRT) and from the epidemiological Million Women Study (MWS) are similar at 1.35 (95%CI: 1.21 – 1.49) and 1.30 (95%CI: 1.21 – 1.40), respectively.

For *oestrogen plus progestagen* combined HRT, several epidemiological studies have reported an overall higher risk for breast cancer than with oestrogens alone.

The MWS reported that, compared to never users, the use of various types of oestrogen-progestagen combined HRT was associated with a higher risk of breast cancer (RR = 2.00, 95%CI: 1.88 - 2.12) than use with oestrogens alone (RR = 1.30, 95%CI: 1.21 – 1.40) or use of tibolone (RR=1.45, 95%CI: 1.25 – 1.68).

The WHI trial reported a risk estimate of 1.24 (95%CI: 1.01 – 1.54) after 5.6 years of use of oestrogen-progestagen combined HRT (CEE + MPA) in all users compared with placebo.

The absolute risks calculated from the MWS and the WHI trial are presented below:

The MWS has estimated, from the known average incidence of breast cancer in developed countries that:

- For women not using HRT, about 32 in every 1000 are expected to have breast cancer diagnosed between the ages of 50 and 64 years.
- For 1000 current or recent users of HRT, the number of *additional* cases during the corresponding period will be
- For users of *oestrogen-only* replacement therapy
- between 0 and 3 (best estimate = 1.5) for 5 years' use
- between 3 and 7 (best estimate = 5) for 10 years' use.
- For users of *oestrogen plus progestogen* combined HRT,
- between 5 and 7 (best estimate = 6) for 5 years' use
- between 18 and 20 (best estimate = 19) for 10 years' use.

The WHI trial estimated that after 5.6 years of follow-up of women between the ages of 50 and 79 years, an *additional* 8 cases of invasive breast cancer would be due to *oestrogen-progestogen combined* HRT (CEE + MPA) per 10,000 women years.

According to calculations from the trial data, it is estimated that:

- For 1000 women in the placebo group,
- about 16 cases of invasive breast cancer would be diagnosed in 5 years.
- For 1000 women who used oestrogen + progestogen combined HRT (CEE + MPA), the number of *additional* cases would be
- between 0 and 9 (best estimate = 4) for 5 years' use.

The number of additional cases of breast cancer in women who use HRT is broadly similar for women who start HRT irrespective of age at start of use (between the ages of 45-65) (see section 4.4).

Endometrial cancer

In women with an intact uterus, the risk of endometrial hyperplasia and endometrial cancer increases with increasing duration of use of unopposed oestrogens. According to data from epidemiological studies, the best estimate of the risk is that for women not using HRT, about 5 in every 1000 are expected to have endometrial cancer diagnosed between the ages of 50 and 65. Depending on the duration of treatment and oestrogen dose, the reported increase in endometrial cancer risk among unopposed oestrogen users varies from 2-to 12-fold greater compared with non-users. Adding a progestagen to oestrogen-only therapy greatly reduces this increased risk.

Other adverse reactions have been reported in association with oestrogen/progestagen treatment:

- Oestrogen-dependent neoplasms benign and malignant: e.g. endometrial cancer.
- Venous thromboembolism, i.e. deep leg or pelvic venous thrombosis and pulmonary embolism, is more frequent among hormone replacement therapy users than among non-users. For further information see sections 4.3 Contra-indications and 4.4 Special warnings and precautions for use.
- Myocardial infarction and stroke.
- Gall bladder disease.
- Skin and subcutaneous disorders: chloasma, erythema multiforme, erythema nodosum, vascular purpura.
- Probable dementia (see section 4.4).

Table 1

Organ system	Common ADRs > 1/100, < 1/10	Uncommon ADRs > 1/1000, < 1/100	Rare ADRs > 1/10,000, < 1/1000
Body as a whole	Headache, Mastodynia	Fluid retention/oedema/weight increase/loss, fatigue, dizziness, leg cramps, migraine	
Gastro-intestinal	Nausea, Vomiting	Bloating, abdominal cramps	Cholelithiasis, cholestatic jaundice
Cardio-vascular		Hypertension	
Reproductive	Breakthrough bleeding, spotting	Dysmenorrhoea, endometrial hyperplasia, benign breast tumours,	Increase in size of uterine fibrosis
Psychiatric	Increase/ decrease in libido		Depression

4.9 Overdose

The mode of administration makes significant overdose unlikely. Signs of an overdose are generally breast tenderness, swelling of the abdomen/pelvis, anxiety, irritability, nausea and vomiting. Removal of the transdermal patches is all that is required should it occur.

5. PHARMACOLOGICAL PROPERTIES

5.1 Pharmacodynamic properties

Pharmacotherapeutic group:

Progestogens and oestrogens for sequential administration

ATC code: G03FB 09

Transdermal route.

Estradiol: the active ingredient, synthetic 17β-estradiol is chemically and biologically identical to endogenous human estradiol. It substitutes for the loss of oestrogen production in postmenopausal women, and alleviates menopausal symptoms.

Levonorgestrel: as oestrogens promote the growth of the endometrium, unopposed oestrogens increase the risk of endometrial hyperplasia and cancer. The addition of levonorgestrel, a synthetic progestin, greatly reduces the oestrogen-induced risk of endometrial hyperplasia in non-hysterectomised women.

Under treatment with FemSeven Sequi, relief of menopausal symptoms was achieved during the first weeks of treatment.

At the end of one year treatment, 82.7% of women with bleeding reported regular withdrawal bleeding. The day of onset was rather constant 1 – 2 days before the end of the cycle with a mean duration of 4 - 5 days. The percentage of women with breakthrough bleeding and/or spotting was 17.3%. During the 13 cycles of therapy, 19.4% of women treated presented with amenorrhoea.

5.2 Pharmacokinetic properties

With transdermal administration there is no hepatic first-pass effect as observed with oral administration; estradiol reaches the bloodstream in unchanged form and in physiological amounts. Therapeutic estradiol concentrations are comparable to those observed in the follicular phase.

After application of the transdermal system containing estradiol alone (phase 1), therapeutic concentrations of estradiol are achieved within 4 hours; these concentrations are maintained throughout the entire application period of the transdermal patch (7 days). When estradiol is administered simultaneously with levonorgestrel (phase 2), the pharmacokinetics of estradiol are unaltered by levonorgestrel. Peak plasma concentrations of estradiol (C_{max}) range from 58 to 71 pg/ml, average plasma concentration (C_{av}) is between 29 to 33 pg/ml and trough plasma concentration (C_{pre}) is about 21 pg/ml during both treatment phases. After removal of the transdermal patch, estradiol concentrations return to their baseline values within 12 to 24 hours.

After application of the transdermal system containing estradiol and levonorgestrel at a dose of 10 μg/day (phase 2), the maximum plasma concentration of levonorgestrel (C_{max}) range from 156 to 189 pg/ml and is reached within 63 to 91 hours (t_{max}). The average plasma concentration of levonorgestrel (C_{av}) during a 7-day period is between 121 and 156 pg/ml and the trough plasma concentration (C_{pre}) levels are 118 pg/ml. The half-life of levonorgestrel after transdermal application is approximately 28 hours (minimum: 16 hours, maximum: 42 hours).

After percutaneous absorption, levonorgestrel is bound to plasma proteins, i.e. albumin (50%), and SHBG (47.5%). Affinity to SHBG is higher than for other commonly used progestogens.

5.3 Preclinical safety data

Preclinical data reveal no special hazard for humans, beyond information included in other sections of the SmPC.

6. PHARMACEUTICAL PARTICULARS

6.1 List of excipients

Backing layer Transparent polyethylene terephthalate (PET) foil

Adhesive matrix: Styrene-isoprene-styrene block copolymer, glycerine esters of completely hydrogenated resins

Protective liner: Siliconized transparent polyethylene terephthalate (PET) foil.

6.2 Incompatibilities

Not applicable.

6.3 Shelf life

2 years

6.4 Special precautions for storage

Do not store above 30°C

6.5 Nature and contents of container

Each phase 1 or phase 2 transdermal patch is contained in an individual sachet (Paper/PE/aluminium/ethylene copolymer). Each carton contains 4 or 12 sachets consisting of 2 × phase 1 patches and 2 × phase 2 patches or 6 × phase 1 patches and 6 × phase 2 patches.

6.6 Instructions for use and handling

See 4.2 Posology and method of administration

7. MARKETING AUTHORISATION HOLDER

Merck Ltd. (t/a Merck Pharmaceuticals (A division of Merck Ltd.))

Harrier House

High Street

West Drayton

Middlesex

UB7 7QG

UK

8. MARKETING AUTHORISATION NUMBER(S)

PL 11648/0044

9. DATE OF FIRST AUTHORISATION/RENEWAL OF THE AUTHORISATION

15 May 2001

10. DATE OF REVISION OF THE TEXT

28 May 2004

FemTab 1 mg

(Merck Pharmaceuticals)

1. NAME OF THE MEDICINAL PRODUCT

FemTab 1mg

2. QUALITATIVE AND QUANTITATIVE COMPOSITION

Each memo pack contains 28 tablets each containing estradiol valerate 1.0 mg.

3. PHARMACEUTICAL FORM

Sugar coated tablet for oral administration.

4. CLINICAL PARTICULARS

4.1 Therapeutic indications

Hormone replacement therapy for the treatment of the climacteric syndrome in menopausal women. In women with a uterus, a progestogen should be added to FemTab for 12 days each month.

4.2 Posology and method of administration

Adults: One tablet of FemTab 1mg to be taken daily. For maintenance the lowest effective dose should be used.

Treatment is continuous, which means that the next pack follows immediately without a break.

Children: not recommended.

4.3 Contraindications

1. Pregnancy and lactation

2. Severe disturbances of liver function (including porphyria), previous or existing liver tumours, jaundice or general pruritus during a previous pregnancy, Dubin-Johnson syndrome, Rotor syndrome

3. Severe cardiac or severe renal disease.

4. Active deep venous thrombosis, thromboembolic disorders, or a history of confirmed venous thromboembolism. (See also Special Warnings and Special Precautions for Use).

5. Suspected or existing hormone-dependent disorders or tumours.

6. Tumours of the uterus or breast

7. Congenital disturbances of lipid metabolism

8. Severe diabetes with vascular changes

9. Hypersensitivity to any of the ingredients.

4.4 Special warnings and special precautions for use

Before starting treatment pregnancy must be excluded.

Assessment of each woman prior to taking hormone replacement therapy (and at regular intervals thereafter) should include a personal and family medical history. Physical examination should be guided by this and by the contra-indications (section 4.3) and warnings (section 4.4) for FemTab. During assessment of each individual woman clinical examination of the breasts and pelvic examination should be performed where clinically indicated rather than as a routine procedure. Women should be encouraged to participate in the national breast cancer screening programme (mammography) and the national cervical cancer screening programme (cervical cytology) as appropriate for their age. Breast awareness should also be encouraged and women advised to report any changes in their breasts to their doctor or nurse.

A reanalysis of original data from 51 epidemiological studies reported a small or moderate increase in the probability of having breast cancer *diagnosed* in women currently or recently using HRT. The findings may be due to biological effects of HRT, earlier diagnosis, or a combination of both. The relative risk increased with duration of treatment (by 2.3% per year of use) and returned to normal in the course of five years after cessation of HRT use. This increase in relative risk associated with duration of HRT use is comparable to the increase in relative risk when natural menopause is delayed in the absence of HRT (2.8% increase for each year older at menopause). Breast cancers diagnosed in current or recent users of HRT are more likely to be localised to the breast than those found in non-users. HRT use may not be associated with increased mortality from breast cancer.

Between the ages of 50 and 70, about 45 women in every 1000 not using HRT will have breast cancer diagnosed. It is estimated that among those who use HRT for 5 years starting at age 50, 2 extra cases of breast cancer will be detected by age 70 in every 1000 women. For those who use HRT for 10 years there will be 6 extra cases of breast cancer, and for 15 years use, 12 extra cases of breast cancer in every 1000 women during the 20 year period until age 70.

It is important that the increased risk of being diagnosed with breast cancer is discussed with the patient and weighed against the known benefits of HRT.

There is a need for caution when prescribing oestrogens in women who have a history of, or known, breast nodules or fibrocystic disease.

Treatment should be stopped at once if migrainous or frequent and unusually severe headaches occur for the first time, or if there are any other symptoms that are possible prodromata of vascular occlusion e.g. sudden visual disturbances.

Treatment should be stopped at once if jaundice, cholestasis, hepatitis, or pregnancy occurs or if there is a significant rise in blood-pressure or an increase in epileptic seizures.

Epidemiological studies have suggested that hormone replacement therapy (HRT) is associated with an increased relative risk of developing venous thromboembolism (VTE) i.e. deep vein thrombosis or pulmonary embolism. The studies find a 2-3 fold increase for users compared with non-users which for healthy women amounts to a low risk of one extra case of VTE each year for every 5000 patients taking HRT.

Generally recognised risk factors for VTE include a personal or family history and severe obesity (Body Mass Index >30 kg/m^2). In women with these factors the benefits of treatment with HRT need to be carefully weighed against risks. There is no consensus about the possible role of varicose veins in VTE.

The risk of VTE may be temporarily increased with prolonged immobilisation, major trauma or major surgery. In women on HRT scrupulous attention should be given to prophylactic measures to prevent VTE following surgery. Where prolonged immobilisation is liable to follow elective surgery, particularly abdominal or orthopaedic surgery to the lower limbs, consideration should be given to temporarily stopping HRT 4 weeks earlier, if this is possible.

If venous thromboembolism develops after initiating therapy the drug should be discontinued.

There is an increased risk of gall bladder disease in women receiving post menopausal oestrogens.

In women with an intact uterus, there is an increased risk of endometrial hyperplasia and carcinoma associated with unopposed oestrogen administered long term (for more than one year). However, the appropriate addition of a progestogen to the oestrogen regimen statistically lowers the risk.

Should endometriosis be reactivated under therapy with FemTab, therapy should be discontinued.

Diseases that are known to be subject to deterioration during pregnancy (e.g. multiple sclerosis, epilepsy, diabetes, benign breast disease, hypertension, cardiac or renal dysfunction, asthma, migraine, tetany, systemic lupus erythematosus and melanoma) and women with a strong family history of breast cancer should be carefully observed during treatment.

Because of the occurrence of herpes gestationis and the worsening of otosclerosis in pregnancy, it is thought that treatment with female hormones may have similar effects. Patients with these conditions should be carefully monitored. Similarly, patients with sickle-cell anaemia should be monitored because of the increased risk of thrombosis that accompanies this disease.

Patients with pre-existing fibroids should be closely monitored as fibroids may increase in size under the influence of oestrogens. If this is observed, treatment should be discontinued.

Oestrogens may cause fluid retention and therefore patients with renal or cardiac dysfunction should be carefully observed.

Most studies demonstrate that oestrogen replacement therapy has little effect on blood pressure. Some show that it may decrease blood pressure. In addition, studies on combined therapy show that the addition of a progestogen also has little effect on blood pressure. Rarely, idiosyncratic hypertension may occur. When oestrogens are administered to hypersensitive women, supervision is necessary and blood pressure should be monitored at regular intervals.

In patients with mild chronic liver disease, liver function should be checked every 8-12 weeks. Results of liver function tests may be affected by HRT.

In rare cases benign and in even rarer cases malignant liver tumours leading in isolated cases to life-threatening intra-abdominal haemorrhage have been observed after the use of hormonal substances such as the one contained in FemTab. A hepatic tumour should be considered in the differential diagnosis if upper abdominal pain, enlarged liver or signs of intra-abdominal haemorrhage occur.

Diabetes should be carefully observed when initiating HRT as worsening of the glucose tolerance may occur.

In women with a uterus, contraception should be practised with non-hormonal methods.

4.5 Interaction with other medicinal products and other forms of Interaction

Drugs which induce hepatic microsomal enzyme systems e.g. barbiturates, carbamazepine, phenytoin, rifampicin accelerate the metabolism of oestrogen products such as FemTab and may reduce their efficacy.

The requirement for oral antidiabetics or insulin can change as a result of the effect on glucose tolerance.

There are some laboratory tests that can be influenced by oestrogens, such as tests for glucose tolerance, liver function or thyroid function.

4.6 Pregnancy and lactation

Contra-indicated

4.7 Effects on ability to drive and use machines

None known.

4.8 Undesirable effects

During the first few months of treatment, breast tenderness or enlargement can occur. These are usually temporary and normally disappear after continued treatment. Other symptoms known to occur are dyspepsia, flatulence, nausea, vomiting, leg pains, anxiety, depressive symptoms, increased appetite, abdominal pain and bloating, altered weight, oedema, palpitations, altered libido, headache, dizziness, epistaxis, hypertension, rashes, thrombophlebitis, mucous vaginal discharge, general pruritus. Some women are predisposed to cholestasis during steroid therapy.

4.9 Overdose

Nausea and vomiting may occur with an overdose. There are no specific antidotes, and treatment should be symptomatic. Withdrawal bleeding may occur in females with a uterus.

5. PHARMACOLOGICAL PROPERTIES

5.1 Pharmacodynamic properties

FemTab contains estradiol valerate, (the valeric-acid ester of the endogenous female oestrogen, estradiol).

Estradiol valerate provides hormone replacement during the climacteric.

Most studies show that oral administration of estradiol valerate to post-menopausal women increases serum high density lipoprotein cholesterol (HDL-C) and decreases low density lipoprotein cholesterol (LDL-C). Although epidemiological data are limited such alterations are recognised as potentially protective against the development of arterial disease.

5.2 Pharmacokinetic properties

After oral administration estradiol valerate is quickly and completely absorbed.

Already after 0.5 - 3 hours peak plasma levels of estradiol, the active drug substance, are measured. As a rule, after 6 - 8 hours a second maximum appears, possibly indicating an entero-hepatic circulation of estradiol.

Esterases in plasma and the liver quickly decompose estradiol valerate into estradiol and valerianic acid. Further decomposition of valerianic acid through β-oxidation leads to C_2.units and results in CO_2 and water as end products. Estradiol itself undergoes several hydroxylating steps. Its metabolites as well as the unchanged substance are finally conjugated. Intermediate products of metabolism are oestrone and oestriol, which exhibit a weak oestrogenic activity of their own, although this activity is not so pronounced as with estradiol. The plasma concentration of conjugated oestrone is about 25 to 30 fold higher than the concentration of unconjugated oestrone. In a study using radioactive labelled estradiol valerate about 20% of radioactive substances in the plasma could be characterised as unconjugated steroids, 17% as glucuronized steroids and 33% as steroid sulphates. About 30% of all substances could not be extracted from the aqueous phase and, therefore, represent probably metabolites of high polarity.

Estradiol and its metabolites are mainly excreted by the kidneys (relation of urine:faeces = 9:1). Within 5 days about 78 - 96% of the administered dose are excreted with an excretion half-life of about 27 hours.

In plasma, estradiol is mainly found in its protein-bound form. About 37% are bound to SHBG and 61% to albumin. Cumulation of estradiol after daily repetitive intake of FemTab does not need to be expected.

The absolute bioavailability of estradiol amounts to 3 - 5% of the oral dose of estradiol valerate.

5.3 Preclinical safety data

There are no preclinical safety data which could be of relevance to the prescriber and which are not already included in other relevant sections of the SPC.

6. PHARMACEUTICAL PARTICULARS

6.1 List of excipients

Lactose monohydrate

Maize Starch

Povidone 25,000

Talc

Magnesium Stearate [E572]

Sucrose

Povidone 700,000

Macrogol 6,000

Calcium Carbonate [E170]

Titanium Dioxide [E171]

Glycerol 85% [E422]

Montan Glycol Wax

Ferric oxide pigment

Purified water

6.2 Incompatibilities

None known.

6.3 Shelf life

5 years.

6.4 Special precautions for storage

None.

6.5 Nature and contents of container

Container consists of aluminium foil and PVC blister strips packed in a cardboard carton.

Presentation: Carton containing memo-packs of either 1 × 28 tablets or 3 × 28 tablets.

6.6 Instructions for use and handling

None.

7. MARKETING AUTHORISATION HOLDER

Schering Health Care Limited

The Brow

Burgess Hill

West Sussex

RH15 9NE

8. MARKETING AUTHORISATION NUMBER(S)

PL 0053/0057.

9. DATE OF FIRST AUTHORISATION/RENEWAL OF THE AUTHORISATION

14 April 1972/24th May 1993.

10. DATE OF REVISION OF THE TEXT

20 March 2001

FemTab 2 mg

(Merck Pharmaceuticals)

1. NAME OF THE MEDICINAL PRODUCT

FemTab 2mg.

2. QUALITATIVE AND QUANTITATIVE COMPOSITION

Each memo pack contains 28 tablets each containing estradiol valerate 2.0 mg.

3. PHARMACEUTICAL FORM

Sugar coated tablet for oral administration.

4. CLINICAL PARTICULARS

4.1 Therapeutic indications

In menopausal women:

1. Hormone replacement therapy for the treatment of the climacteric syndrome.

2. Second line therapy for prevention of osteoporosis in postmenopausal women at high risk of future fractures who are intolerant of, or contraindicated for, other medicinal products approved for the prevention of osteoporosis.

In women with a uterus, a progestogen should be added to FemTab for 12 days each month.

4.2 Posology and method of administration

Adults:

Climacteric syndrome: One tablet to be taken daily. For maintenance the lowest effective dose should be used.

Prophylaxis of osteoporosis: One tablet to be taken daily.

For maximum prophylactic benefit, treatment should commence as soon as possible after onset of the menopause.

Bone mineral density measurements may help to confirm the presence of low bone mass.

Treatment is continuous, which means that the next pack follows immediately without a break.

Children: not recommended

4.3 Contraindications

1. Pregnancy and lactation.

2. Severe disturbances of liver function (including porphyria), previous or existing liver tumours, jaundice or general pruritus during a previous pregnancy, Dubin-Johnson syndrome, Rotor syndrome.

3. Severe cardiac or severe renal disease.

4. Active deep venous thrombosis, thromboembolic disorders, or a history of confirmed venous thromboembolism. (See also Special Warnings and Special Precautions for use).

5. Suspected or existing hormone-dependent disorders or tumours.

6. Tumours of the uterus or breast

7. Congenital disturbances of lipid metabolism.

8. Severe diabetes with vascular changes.

9. Hypersensitivity to any of the ingredients

4.4 Special warnings and special precautions for use

Before starting treatment pregnancy must be excluded.

Assessment of each woman prior to taking hormone replacement therapy (and at regular intervals thereafter) should include a personal and family medical history. Physical examination should be guided by this and by the contra-indications (section 4.3) and warnings (section 4.4) for FemTab. During assessment of each individual woman clinical examination of the breasts and pelvic examination should be performed where clinically indicated rather than as a routine procedure. Women should be encouraged to participate in the national breast cancer screening programme (mammography) and the national cervical cancer screening programme (cervical cytology) as appropriate for their age. Breast awareness should also be encouraged and women advised to report any changes in their breasts to their doctor or nurse.

A reanalysis of original data from 51 epidemiological studies reported a small or moderate increase in the probability of having breast cancer *diagnosed* in women currently or recently using HRT. The findings may be due to biological effects of HRT, earlier diagnosis, or a combination of both. The relative risk increased with duration of treatment (by 2.3% per year of use) and returned to normal in the course of five years after cessation of HRT use. This increase in relative risk associated with duration of HRT use is comparable to the increase in relative risk when natural menopause is delayed in the absence of HRT (2.8% increase for each year older at menopause). Breast cancers diagnosed in current or recent users of HRT are more likely to be localised to the breast than those found in non-users. HRT use may not be associated with increased mortality from breast cancer.

Between the ages of 50 and 70, about 45 women in every 1000 not using HRT will have breast cancer diagnosed. It is estimated that among those who use HRT for 5 years starting at age 50, 2 extra cases of breast cancer will be detected by age 70 in every 1000 women. For those who use HRT for 10 years there will be 6 extra cases of breast cancer, and for 15 years use, 12 extra cases of breast cancer in every 1000 women during the 20 year period until age 70.

It is important that the increased risk of being diagnosed with breast cancer is discussed with the patient and weighed against the known benefits of HRT.

There is a need for caution when prescribing oestrogens in women who have a history of, or known, breast nodules or fibrocystic disease.

Treatment should be stopped at once if migrainous or frequent and unusually severe headaches occur for the first time, or if there are any other symptoms that are possible prodromata of vascular occlusion e.g. sudden visual disturbances.

Treatment should be stopped at once if jaundice, cholestasis, hepatitis, or pregnancy occurs or if there is a significant rise in blood-pressure or an increase in epileptic seizures.

Epidemiological studies have suggested that hormone replacement therapy (HRT) is associated with an increased relative risk of developing venous thromboembolism (VTE) i.e. deep vein thrombosis or pulmonary embolism. The studies find a 2-3 fold increase for users compared with non-users which for healthy women amounts to a low risk of one extra case of VTE each year for every 5000 patients taking HRT.

Generally recognised risk factors for VTE include a personal or family history and severe obesity (Body Mass Index >30 kg/m^2). In women with these factors the benefits of treatment with HRT need to be carefully weighed against risks. There is no consensus about the possible role of varicose veins in VTE.

The risk of VTE may be temporarily increased with prolonged immobilisation, major trauma or major surgery. In women on HRT scrupulous attention should be given to prophylactic measures to prevent VTE following surgery. Where prolonged immobilisation is liable to follow elective surgery, particularly abdominal or orthopaedic surgery to the lower limbs, consideration should be given to temporarily stopping HRT 4 weeks earlier, if this is possible.

If venous thromboembolism develops after initiating therapy the drug should be discontinued.

There is an increased risk of gall bladder disease in women receiving post menopausal oestrogens.

In women with an intact uterus, there is an increased risk of endometrial hyperplasia and carcinoma associated with unopposed oestrogen administered long term (for more than one year). However, the appropriate addition of a progestogen to the oestrogen regimen statistically lowers the risk.

Should endometriosis be reactivated under therapy with FemTab, therapy should be discontinued.

Diseases that are known to be subject to deterioration during pregnancy (e.g. multiple sclerosis, epilepsy, diabetes, benign breast disease, hypertension, cardiac or renal dysfunction, asthma, migraine, tetany, systemic lupus erythematosus and melanoma) and women with a strong family history of breast cancer should be carefully observed during treatment.

Because of the occurrence of herpes gestationis and the worsening of otosclerosis in pregnancy, it is thought that treatment with female hormones may have similar effects. Patients with these conditions should be carefully monitored. Similarly, patients with sickle-cell anaemia should be monitored because of the increased risk of thrombosis that accompanies this disease.

Patients with pre-existing fibroids should be closely monitored as fibroids may increase in size under the influence of oestrogens. If this is observed, treatment should be discontinued.

Oestrogens may cause fluid retention and therefore patients with renal or cardiac dysfunction should be carefully observed.

Most studies demonstrate that oestrogen therapy has little effect on blood pressure. Some show that it may decrease blood pressure. In addition, studies on combined therapy show that the addition of a progestogen also has little effect on blood pressure. Rarely, idiosyncratic hypertension may occur. When oestrogens are administered to hypertensive women, supervision is necessary and blood pressure should be monitored at regular intervals.

In patients with mild chronic liver disease, liver function should be checked every 8-12 weeks. Results of liver function tests may be affected by HRT.

In rare cases benign and in even rarer cases malignant liver tumours leading in isolated cases to life-threatening intra-abdominal haemorrhage have been observed after the use of hormonal substances such as the one contained in FemTab. A hepatic tumour should be considered in the differential diagnosis if upper abdominal pain, enlarged liver or signs of intra-abdominal haemorrhage occur.

Diabetes should be carefully observed when initiating HRT as worsening of the glucose tolerance may occur.

In women with a uterus, contraception should be practised with non-hormonal methods.

4.5 Interaction with other medicinal products and other forms of Interaction

Drugs which induce hepatic microsomal enzyme systems e.g. barbiturates, carbamazepine, phenytoin, rifampicin accelerate the metabolism of oestrogen products such as FemTab and may reduce their efficacy.

The requirement for oral antidiabetics or insulin can change as a result of the effect on glucose tolerance.

There are some laboratory tests that can be influenced by oestrogens, such as tests for glucose tolerance, liver function or thyroid function.

4.6 Pregnancy and lactation

Contra-indicated

4.7 Effects on ability to drive and use machines

None known

4.8 Undesirable effects

During the first few months of treatment, breast tenderness or enlargement can occur. These are usually temporary and normally disappear after continued treatment. Other symptoms known to occur are dyspepsia, flatulence, nausea, vomiting, leg pains, anxiety, depressive symptoms, increased appetite, abdominal pain and bloating, altered weight, oedema, palpitations, altered libido, headache, dizziness, epistaxis, hypertension, rashes, thrombophlebitis, mucous vaginal discharge, general pruritus. Some women are predisposed to cholestasis during steroid therapy.

4.9 Overdose

Nausea and vomiting may occur with an overdose. There are no specific antidotes, and treatment should be symptomatic. Withdrawal bleeding may occur in females with a uterus.

5. PHARMACOLOGICAL PROPERTIES

5.1 Pharmacodynamic properties

FemTab contains estradiol valerate, (the valeric-acid ester of the endogenous female oestrogen, estradiol).

Estradiol valerate provides hormone replacement during the climacteric.

Most studies show that oral administration of estradiol valerate to post-menopausal women increases serum high density lipoprotein cholesterol (HDL-C) and decreases low density lipoprotein cholesterol (LDL-C). Although epidemiological data are limited such alterations are recognised as potentially protective against the development of arterial disease.

5.2 Pharmacokinetic properties

After oral administration estradiol valerate is quickly and completely absorbed.

Already after 0.5 - 3 hours peak plasma levels of estradiol, the active drug substance, are measured. As a rule, after 6 - 8 hours a second maximum appears, possibly indicating an entero-hepatic circulation of estradiol.

Esterases in plasma and the liver quickly decompose estradiol valerate into estradiol and valerianic acid. Further decomposition of valerianic acid through β-oxidation leads to C_2-units and results in CO_2 and water as end products. Estradiol itself undergoes several hydroxylating steps. Its metabolites as well as the unchanged substance are finally conjugated. Intermediate products of metabolism are oestrone and oestriol, which exhibit a weak oestrogenic activity of their own, although this activity is not so pronounced as with estradiol. The plasma concentration of conjugated oestrone is about 25 to 30 fold higher than the concentration of unconjugated oestrone. In a study using radioactive labelled estradiol valerate about 20% of radioactive substances in the plasma could be characterised as unconjugated steroids, 17% as glucuronized steroids and 33% as steroid sulphates. About 30% of all substances could not be extracted from the aqueous phase and, therefore, represent probably metabolites of high polarity.

Estradiol and its metabolites are mainly excreted by the kidneys (relation of urine:faeces = 9:1). Within 5 days about 78 - 96% of the administered dose are excreted with an excretion half-life of about 27 hours.

In plasma, estradiol is mainly found in its protein-bound form. About 37% are bound to SHBG and 61% to albumin. Cumulation of estradiol after daily repetitive intake of FemTab does not need to be expected.

The absolute bioavailability of estradiol amounts to 3 - 5% of the oral dose of estradiol valerate.

5.3 Preclinical safety data

There are no preclinical safety data which could be of relevance to the prescriber and which are not already included in other relevant sections of the SPC.

6. PHARMACEUTICAL PARTICULARS

6.1 List of excipients

Lactose monohydrate

Maize Starch

Povidone 25000

Talc

Magnesium Stearate [E572]

Sucrose

Povidone 700,000

Macrogol 6000

Calcium Carbonate [E170]

Titanium Dioxide [E171]

Glycerol 85% [E422]

Montan Glycol Wax

Indigo Carmine [E132]

Purified Water

6.2 Incompatibilities

None known.

6.3 Shelf life

5 years.

6.4 Special precautions for storage

None.

6.5 Nature and contents of container

Container consists of aluminium foil and PVC blister strips packed in a cardboard carton

Presentation: Carton containing memo-packs of either 1 × 28 tablets or 3 × 28 tablets.

6.6 Instructions for use and handling

None.

7. MARKETING AUTHORISATION HOLDER

Schering Health Care Limited

The Brow

Burgess Hill

West Sussex

RH15 9NE

8. MARKETING AUTHORISATION NUMBER(S)

PL 0053/0058

9. DATE OF FIRST AUTHORISATION/RENEWAL OF THE AUTHORISATION

14 April 1972/24th May 1993.

10. DATE OF REVISION OF THE TEXT

9 December 2003

FemTab Sequi

(Merck Pharmaceuticals)

1. NAME OF THE MEDICINAL PRODUCT

FemTab Sequi

2. QUALITATIVE AND QUANTITATIVE COMPOSITION

- Each white sugar-coated tablet contains:

Estradiol valerate 2.0mg

- Each pink sugar-coated tablet contains:

Estradiol valerate 2.0mg

Levonorgestrel 75 micrograms

3. PHARMACEUTICAL FORM

Sugar coated tablets for oral use.

4. CLINICAL PARTICULARS

4.1 Therapeutic indications

Hormone replacement therapy for the treatment of the climacteric syndrome.

Second line therapy for prevention of osteoporosis in post-menopausal women at high risk of future fractures who are intolerant of, or contraindicated for, other medicinal products approved for the prevention of osteoporosis.

For maximum prophylactic benefit treatment should commence as soon as possible after the menopause.

Bone mineral density measurements may help to confirm the presence of low bone mass.

FemTab Sequi is designed to provide hormone replacement therapy during and after the climacteric. The addition of a progestogen in the second half of each course helps to provide good control of the irregular cycles that are characteristic of the premenopausal phase and opposes the production of endometrial hyperplasia. Whilst ovarian hormone production is little affected, FemTab Sequi abolishes or improves the characteristic symptoms of the climacteric such as hot flushes, sweating attacks and sleep disorders.

Studies of bone mineral content have shown FemTab Sequi to be effective in the prevention of progressive bone loss following the menopause.

FemTab Sequi does not consistently inhibit ovulation and is therefore unsuitable for contraception.

4.2 Posology and method of administration

Adults, including the elderly:

If the patient is still menstruating, treatment should begin on the 5th day of menstruation. Patients whose periods are very infrequent or who are postmenopausal may start at any time, provided pregnancy has been excluded (see Section 4.4. Special warnings and special precautions for use).

One white tablet is taken daily for the first 16 days, followed by one pink tablet daily for 12 days. Thus, each pack contains 28 days treatment. Treatment is continuous, which means that the next pack follows immediately without a break. Bleeding usually occurs within the last few days of one pack and the first week of the next.

4.3 Contraindications

- Pregnancy (See Section 4.4. Special warnings and special precautions for use)
- severe disturbances of liver function
- previous or existing liver tumours
- jaundice or general pruritus during a previous pregnancy
- Dubin-Johnson syndrome
- Rotor syndrome
- active deep venous thrombosis, thromboembolic disorders, or a history of confirmed venous thromboembolism. (See also Special warnings and special precautions for use).
- sickle-cell anaemia
- suspected or existing hormone-dependent disorders or tumours of the uterus and breast
- undiagnosed irregular vaginal bleeding
- congenital disturbances of lipid metabolism
- a history of herpes gestationis
- otosclerosis with deterioration in previous pregnancies
- endometriosis
- severe diabetes with vascular changes
- mastopathy.

4.4 Special warnings and special precautions for use

Assessment of each woman prior to taking hormone replacement therapy (and at regular intervals thereafter) should include a personal and family medical history. Physical examination should be guided by this and by the contra-indications (section 4.3) and warnings (section 4.4) for FemTab Sequi. During assessment of each individual woman clinical examination of the breasts and pelvic examination should be performed where clinically indicated rather than as a routine procedure. Women should be encouraged to participate in the national breast cancer screening programme (mammography) and the national cervical cancer screening programme (cervical cytology) as appropriate for their age. Breast awareness should also be encouraged and women advised to report any changes in their breasts to their doctor or nurse.

Before starting treatment, pregnancy must be excluded. If the expected bleeding fails to occur at about 28-day intervals, treatment should be stopped until pregnancy has been ruled out.

Persistent breakthrough bleeding during treatment is an indication for endometrial assessment which may include biopsy.

Epidemiological studies have suggested that hormone replacement therapy (HRT) is associated with an increased relative risk of developing venous thromboembolism (VTE) i.e. deep vein thrombosis or pulmonary embolism. The studies find a 2-3 fold increase for users compared with non-users which for healthy women amounts to a low risk of one extra case of VTE each year for every 5000 patients taking HRT.

Generally recognised risk factors for VTE include a personal or family history and severe obesity (Body Mass Index >30 kg/m^2). In women with these factors the benefits of treatment with HRT need to be carefully weighed against risks. There is no consensus about the possible role of varicose veins in VTE.

The risk of VTE may be temporarily increased with prolonged immobilisation, major trauma or major surgery. In women on HRT scrupulous attention should be given to prophylactic measures to prevent VTE following surgery. Where prolonged immobilisation is liable to follow elective surgery, particularly abdominal or orthopaedic surgery to the lower limbs, consideration should be given to temporarily stopping HRT 4 weeks earlier, if this is possible.

If venous thromboembolism develops after initiating HRT the drug should be discontinued.

Prolonged exposure to unopposed oestrogens increases the risk of development of endometrial carcinoma. The general consensus of opinion is that the addition of 12 days progestogen towards the end of the cycle, as in FemTab Sequi, diminishes the possibility of such a risk, and some investigators consider that it might be protective.

A reanalysis of original data from 51 epidemiological studies reported a small or moderate increase in the probability of having breast cancer *diagnosed* in women currently or recently using HRT. The findings may be due to biological effects of HRT, earlier diagnosis, or a combination of both. The relative risk increased with duration of treatment (by 2.3% per year of use) and returned to normal in the course of five years after cessation of HRT use. This increase in relative risk associated with duration of HRT use is comparable to the increase in relative risk when natural menopause is delayed in the absence of HRT (2.8% increase for each year older at menopause). Breast cancers diagnosed in current or recent users of HRT are more likely to be localised to the breast than those found in non-users. HRT use may not be associated with increased mortality from breast cancer.

Between the ages of 50 and 70, about 45 women in every 1000 not using HRT will have breast cancer diagnosed. It is estimated that among those who use HRT for 5 years starting at age 50, 2 extra cases of breast cancer will be detected by age 70 in every 1000 women. For those who use HRT for 10 years there will be 6 extra cases of breast cancer, and for 15 years use, 12 extra cases of breast cancer in every 1000 women during the 20 year period until age 70.

It is important that the increased risk of being diagnosed with breast cancer is discussed with the patient and weighed against the known benefits of HRT.

Treatment should be stopped at once if migrainous or frequent and unusually severe headaches occur for the first time, or if there are other symptoms that are possible prodromata of vascular occlusion.

Treatment should be stopped at once if jaundice or pregnancy occurs, if there is a significant rise in blood pressure, or an increase in epileptic seizures.

Some women are predisposed to cholestasis during steroid therapy. Diseases that are known to be subject to deterioration during pregnancy (e.g. multiple sclerosis, epilepsy, diabetes, benign breast disease, hypertension, cardiac or renal dysfunction, asthma, porphyria, tetany and otosclerosis) and women with a strong family history of breast cancer should be carefully observed during treatment.

Pre-existing fibroids may increase in size under the influence of oestrogens. If this is observed treatment should be discontinued.

In patients with mild chronic liver disease, liver function should be checked every 8 - 12 weeks.

In rare cases benign and, in even rarer cases, malignant liver tumours leading in isolated cases to life-threatening intra-abdominal haemorrhage have been observed after the use of hormonal substances such as those contained in FemTab Sequi. If severe upper abdominal complaints, enlarged liver, or signs of intra-abdominal haemorrhage occur, a liver tumour should be included in the differential diagnostic considerations.

4.5 Interaction with other medicinal products and other forms of Interaction

Hormonal contraception should be stopped when treatment with FemTab Sequi is started and the patient should be advised to take non-hormonal contraceptive precautions.

Drugs which induce hepatic microsomal enzyme systems e.g. barbiturates, phenytoin, rifampicin, accelerate the metabolism of oestrogen/progestogen combinations such as FemTab Sequi and may reduce their efficacy.

The requirement for oral antidiabetics or insulin can change.

4.6 Pregnancy and lactation

Contra-indicated.

4.7 Effects on ability to drive and use machines

None known.

4.8 Undesirable effects

During the first few months of treatment, breakthrough bleeding, spotting and breast tenderness or enlargement can occur. These are usually temporary and normally disappear after continued treatment. Other symptoms known to occur are: anxiety; increased appetite; bloating; palpitations; depressive symptoms; headache; migraine; dizziness; dyspepsia; leg pains; oedema; altered libido; nausea; rashes; vomiting; altered weight; chloasma.

4.9 Overdose

There have been no reports of ill-effects from overdosage, which it is, therefore, generally unnecessary to treat. There are no specific antidotes, and treatment should be symptomatic.

5. PHARMACOLOGICAL PROPERTIES

5.1 Pharmacodynamic properties

FemTab Sequi contains estradiol valerate (the valeric acid ester of the endogenous female oestrogen, estradiol) and the synthetic progestogen, levonorgestrel. Estradiol valerate provides hormone replacement during and after the climacteric. The addition of levonorgestrel in the second half of each course of tablets helps to provide good cycle control and opposes the development of endometrial hyperplasia.

Most studies show that oral administration of estradiol valerate to post-menopausal women increases serum high density lipoprotein cholesterol (HDL-C) and decreases low density lipoprotein cholesterol (LDL-C). Although epidemiological data are limited such alterations are recognised as potentially protective against the development of arterial disease. A possible attenuation of these effects may occur with the addition of a progestogen. However, at the doses used in FemTab Sequi, the 12 days of combined therapy with estradiol valerate and levonorgestrel have not been observed to be associated with any unwanted lipid effects.

5.2 Pharmacokinetic properties

1. Levonorgestrel (LNG)

Orally administered LNG is rapidly and completely absorbed. Following ingestion of one tablet of FemTab Sequi maximum drug serum levels of 1.9ng/ml were found at 1.3 hours. Thereafter, LNG serum levels decrease in two disposition phases. The first phase is described by a half-life of 0.5-1.5 hours and the terminal phase by a half-life of 20-27 hours. For LNG, a metabolic clearance rate from serum of about 1.5 ml/min/kg was determined. LNG is not excreted in unchanged form but as metabolites. LNG metabolites are excreted at about equal proportions with urine and faeces. The biotransformation follows the known pathways of steroid metabolism. No pharmacologically active metabolites are known.

LNG is bound to serum albumin and to SHBG. Only about 1.5% of the total serum drug levels are present as free steroid, but 65% are specifically bound to SHBG. The relative distribution (free, albumin-bound, SHBG-bound) depends on the SHBG concentrations in the serum. Following induction of the binding protein, the SHBG bound fraction increases while the unbound and the albumin-bound fraction decrease.

Following daily repeated administration, LNG concentrations in the serum increase by a factor of about 2. Steady-state conditions are reached within a few days. The pharmacokinetics of LNG is influenced by SHBG serum levels. Under treatment with FemTab Sequi SHBG levels will rise by about 40% during the oestrogen phase and remain constant or slightly decrease thereafter. The absolute bioavailability of LNG was determined to be almost 100% of the dose administered. The relative bioavailability was tested against an aqueous microcrystalline suspension and was found to be complete (108%).

About 0.1% of the maternal dose can be transferred via milk to the nursed infant.

2. Estradiol valerate (E_2 val)

E_2 val is completely absorbed from the FemTab Sequi tablet. During absorption and the first passage through the liver the steroid ester is cleaved into estradiol (E_2) and valeric acid. At the same time E_2 undergoes extensive further metabolism yielding E_2 conjugates, estrone (E_1) and E_1 conjugates. The pharmacologically most active metabolites of E_2 val are E_2 and E_1. Maximum serum levels of 25 pg E_2/ml and 180 pg E_1/ml are reached 5-7 hours after the administration of one FemTab Sequi tablet.

Mean E1 serum levels are 10-12 fold higher than mean E_2 serum concentrations. Serum levels of E_1 conjugates are about 25 fold higher than the E_1 serum levels.

E_2 is rapidly metabolised and the metabolic clearance rate has been determined to 30ml/min/kg. After oral intake of E_2 the half-life of the terminal disposition phase was about 13 hours for E_2. The respective half-life for E_1 serum level decline was about 20 hours. The daily use of FemTab Sequi will lead to an about 50% increase in E_2 serum levels and to twofold E_1 levels at steady state.

Estradiol is bound to about 97% to serum proteins, about 35% are specifically bound to SHBG. E_2- val is not excreted in unchanged form. The metabolites of estradiol are excreted via urine and bile with a half-life of about 1 day at a ratio of 9:1.

The absolute bioavailability of E_2 from E_2 val is about 3% of oral dose and thus in the same range like oral E_2 (5% of dose).

The relative bioavailability of E_2 val (reference: aqueous microcrystalline suspension) from FemTab Sequi tablets was complete (111-112%).

Estradiol and its metabolites are excreted into milk only to a minor extent.

5.3 Preclinical safety data

There are no preclinical data which could be of relevance to the prescriber and which are not already included in other relevant sections of the SPC.

6. PHARMACEUTICAL PARTICULARS

6.1 List of excipients

FemTab Sequi contains the following excipients: lactose, maize starch, povidone 25 000, povidone 700 000, talcum, magnesium stearate (E572), sucrose, macrogol 6000 (polyethylene glycol 6000), calcium carbonate (E170), glycerol (E422), montan glycol wax, yellow and red ferric oxide pigments (E172), titanium dioxide (E171).

6.2 Incompatibilities

Not applicable.

6.3 Shelf life

5 years.

6.4 Special precautions for storage

None.

6.5 Nature and contents of container

Packs containing aluminium foil and PVC blister strips.

Presentation:

Carton containing memo-packs of either 1 × 28 tablets or 3 × 28 tablets.

6.6 Instructions for use and handling

Not applicable.

7. MARKETING AUTHORISATION HOLDER

Schering Health Care Limited
The Brow
Burgess Hill
West Sussex RH15 9NE

8. MARKETING AUTHORISATION NUMBER(S)

PL 0053/0219

9. DATE OF FIRST AUTHORISATION/RENEWAL OF THE AUTHORISATION

7th October 1991/26th March 1997

10. DATE OF REVISION OF THE TEXT

9 December 2003

Femulen Tablets

(Pharmacia Limited)

1. NAME OF THE MEDICINAL PRODUCT

Femulen.

2. QUALITATIVE AND QUANTITATIVE COMPOSITION

Each tablet contains 500 micrograms etynodiol diacetate.

3. PHARMACEUTICAL FORM

White tablet inscribed "SEARLE" on both sides.

4. CLINICAL PARTICULARS

4.1 Therapeutic indications

Oral contraception.

4.2 Posology and method of administration

Starting on the first day of menstruation, one pill every day without a break in medication for as long as contraception is required. Additional contraceptive precautions (such as a condom) should be used for the first 7 days of the first pack. Pills should be taken at the same time each day.

Missed Pills

If a pill is missed within 3 hours of the correct dosage time then the missed pill should be taken as soon as possible; this will ensure that contraceptive protection is maintained. If a pill is taken 3 or more hours late it is recommended that the woman takes the last missed pill as soon as possible and then continues to take the rest of the pills in the normal manner. However, to provide continued contraceptive protection it is recommended that an alternative method of contraception, such as a condom, is used for the next 7 days.

Changing from another oral contraceptive

In order to ensure that contraception is maintained it is advised that the first pill is taken on the day immediately after the patient has finished the previous pack.

Use after childbirth, miscarriage or abortion

The first pill should be taken on the 21st day after childbirth. This will ensure the patient is protected immediately. If there is any delay in taking the first pill, **contraception may not be established until 7 days after the first pill has been taken. In** these circumstances women should be advised that extra contraceptive methods will be necessary.

After a miscarriage or abortion patients can take the first pill on the next day; in this way they will be protected immediately.

Vomiting or diarrhoea

Gastrointestinal upsets, such as vomiting and diarrhoea, may interfere with the absorption of the pill leading to a reduction in contraceptive efficacy. Women should continue to take Femulen, but they should also be advised to use another contraceptive method during the period of gastrointestinal upset and for the next 7 days.

4.3 Contraindications

The contraindications for progestogen-only oral contraceptives are:

(i) Known, suspected, or a past history of breast, genital or hormone dependent cancer;

(ii) Acute or severe chronic liver diseases including past or present liver tumours, Dubin-Johnson or Rotor syndrome;

(iii) Active liver disease;

(iv) History during pregnancy of idiopathic jaundice or severe pruritus;

(v) Disorders of lipid metabolism;

(vi) Undiagnosed abnormal vaginal bleeding;

(vii) Known or suspected pregnancy;

(viii) Hypersensitivity to any component.

Combined oestrogen/progestogen preparations have been associated with an increase in the risk of thromboembolic and thrombotic disease. Risk has been reported to be related to both oestrogenic and progestogenic activity. In the absence of long term epidemiological studies with progestogen-only oral contraceptives, it is required that the existence, or history of thrombophlebitis, thromboembolic disorders, cerebral vascular disease, myocardial infarction, angina, coronary artery disease, or a haemoglobinopathy be described as a contraindication to Femulen as it is to oestrogen containing oral contraceptives.

4.4 Special warnings and special precautions for use

Assessment of women prior to starting oral contraceptives (and at regular intervals thereafter) should include a personal and family medical history of each woman. Physical examination should be guided by this and by the contraindications (section 4.3) and warnings (section 4.4) for this product. The frequency and nature of these assessments should be based upon relevant guidelines and should be adapted to the individual woman, but should include measurement of blood pressure and, if judged appropriate by the clinician, breast, abdominal and pelvic examination including cervical cytology.

Femulen should be discontinued if there is a gradual or sudden, partial or complete loss of vision or any evidence of ocular changes, onset or aggravation of migraine or development of headache of a new kind which is recurrent, persistent or severe, suspicion of thrombosis or infarction, significant rise in blood pressure or if jaundice occurs.

Malignant hepatic tumours have been reported on rare occasions in long-term users of contraceptives. Benign hepatic tumours have also been associated with oral contraceptive usage. A hepatic tumour should be considered in the differential diagnosis when upper abdominal pain, enlarged liver or signs of intra-abdominal haemorrhage occur.

Progestogen-only oral contraceptives may offer less protection against ectopic pregnancy, than against intrauterine pregnancy.

Femulen should be discontinued at least 4 weeks before elective surgery or during periods of prolonged immobilisation. It would be reasonable to resume Femulen two weeks after surgery provided the woman is ambulant. However, every woman, should be considered individually with regard to the nature of the operation, the extent of immobilisation, the presence of additional risk factors and the chance of unwanted conception.

Caution should be exercised where there is the possibility of an interaction between a pre-existing disorder and a known or suspected side effect. The use of Femulen in women suffering from epilepsy, or with a history of migraine or cardiac or renal dysfunction may result in exacerbation of these disorders because of fluid retention. Caution should also be observed in women who wear contact lenses, women with impaired carbohydrate tolerance, depression, gallstones, a past history of liver disease, varicose veins, hypertension, asthma or any disease that is prone to worsen during pregnancy (eg. multiple sclerosis, porphyria, tetany and otosclerosis). Progestogen-only oral contraceptives may offer less protection against ectopic pregnancy, than against intrauterine pregnancy.

A meta-analysis from 54 epidemiological studies reported that there is a slightly increased relative risk of having breast cancer diagnosed in women who are currently using oral contraceptives (OC). The observed pattern of increased risk may be due to an earlier diagnosis of breast cancer in OC users, the biological effects of OCs or a combination of both. The additional breast cancers diagnosed in current users of OCs or in women who have used OCs in the last ten years are more likely to be localised to the breast than those in women who never used OCs.

Breast cancer is rare among women under 40 years of age whether or not they take OCs. Whilst the background risk increases with age, the excess number of breast cancer diagnoses in current and recent progesterone-only pill (POP) users is small in relation to the overall risk of breast cancer, possibly of similar magnitude to that associated with combined OCs. However, for POPs, the evidence is based on much smaller populations of users and so is less conclusive than that for combined OCs.

The most important risk factor for breast cancer in POP users is the age women discontinue the POP; the older the age at stopping, the more breast cancers are diagnosed. Duration of use is less important and the excess risk gradually disappears during the course of the 10 years after stopping POP use, such that by 10 years there appears to be no excess.

The evidence suggests that compared with never-users, among 10,000 women who use POPs for up to 5 years but stop by age 20, there would be much less than 1 extra case of breast cancer diagnosed up to 10 years afterwards. For those stopping by age 30 after 5 years use of the POP, there would be an estimated 2-3 extra cases (additional to the 44 cases of breast cancer per 10,000 women in this age group never exposed to oral contraceptives). For those stopping by age 40 after 5 years use, there would be an estimated 10 extra cases diagnosed up to 10 years afterwards (additional to the 160 cases of breast cancer per 10,000 never-exposed women in this age group).

It is important to inform patients that users of all contraceptive pills appear to have a small increase in the risk of being diagnosed with breast cancer, compared with non-users of oral contraceptives, but this has to be weighed against the known benefits.

4.5 Interaction with other medicinal products and other forms of Interaction

Drug Interactions

The herbal remedy St John's wort (*Hypericum perforatum*) should not be taken concomitantly with this medicine as this could potentially lead to a loss of contraceptive effect.

Some drugs may modify the metabolism of Femulen reducing its effectiveness; these include certain sedatives, antibiotics, anti-epileptic and anti-arthritic drugs. During the time such agents are used concurrently, it is advised that mechanical contraceptives also be used.

4.6 Pregnancy and lactation

Pregnancy

Femulen is contraindicated in women with suspected pregnancy. Several reports suggest an association between foetal exposure to female sex hormones, including oral contraceptives, and congenital anomalies.

Lactation

There is no evidence that progestogen - only oral contraceptives diminish the yield of breast milk. In a study of nursing mothers taking Femulen, the median percentage of norethisterone, the principal metabolite of etynodiol diacetate given to the mother which was ingested by the infant was 0.02%. No adverse effect of the drug on the infants was noted.

4.7 Effects on ability to drive and use machines

None known.

4.8 Undesirable effects

Clinical investigations with Femulen indicate that side effects are infrequent and tend to decrease with time. Known or suspected side effects of progestogen-only oral contraceptives include gastrointestinal disorders such as nausea and vomiting, skin disorders including chloasma, breast changes, ocular changes, headache, migraine and depression, appetite and weight changes, changes in libido, increase in size of uterine myofibromata, and changes in carbohydrate, lipid or vitamin metabolism. Rarely dizziness, hirsutism and colitis have been reported in users of progestogen-only oral contraceptive.

The use of oral contraceptives has also been associated with a possible increased incidence of gallbladder disease.

Tests of endocrine, hepatic and thyroid function, as well as coagulation tests may be affected by Femulen.

Menstrual pattern: Women taking Femulen for the first time should be informed that they may initially experience menstrual irregularity. This may include amenorrhoea, prolonged bleeding and/or spotting but such irregularity tends to decrease with time. If a woman misses two consecutive periods, pregnancy should be ruled out before continuing the contraceptive regimen.

4.9 Overdose

Serious ill effects have not been reported following acute ingestion of large doses of oral contraceptives by young children. Nausea and vomiting may occur and vaginal withdrawal bleeding may present in pre-pubertal girls. There is no specific antidote and treatment should be symptomatic. Gastric lavage may be employed if the overdose is large and the patient is seen sufficiently early (within four hours).

5. PHARMACOLOGICAL PROPERTIES

5.1 Pharmacodynamic properties

Femulen does not necessarily inhibit ovulation but it is believed to discourage implantation of the fertilised ovum by altering the endometrium. Cervical mucus viscosity is also changed which may render the passage of sperm less likely.

5.2 Pharmacokinetic properties

Etynodiol diacetate is readily absorbed from the gastro-intestinal tract and rapidly metabolised, largely to norethisterone. Following administration of a radiolabelled dose of etynodiol diacetate about 60% of the radioactivity is stated to be excreted in urine and about 30% in faeces; half life in plasma was about 25 hours.

5.3 Preclinical safety data

The toxicity of norethisterone is very low. Reports of teratogenic effects in animals are uncommon. No carcinogenic effects have been found even in long-term studies. In subacute and chronic studies only minimal differences between treated and control animals are observed.

6. PHARMACEUTICAL PARTICULARS

6.1 List of excipients

Calcium phosphate dibasic anhydrous, maize starch, polyvinyl pyrrolidine, sodium phosphate dibasic anhydrous, calcium acetate anhydrous, thixcin R (hydrogenated castor oil).

6.2 Incompatibilities

None known.

6.3 Shelf life

The shelf life of Femulen is 5 years.

6.4 Special precautions for storage

Store in a dry place below 30°C.

6.5 Nature and contents of container

Femulen tablets are stored in PVC/foil blister packs of 28 and 84 tablets.

6.6 Instructions for use and handling

None.

7. MARKETING AUTHORISATION HOLDER

Pharmacia Limited
Davy Avenue
Milton Keynes
Buckinghamshire
MK5 8PH
United Kingdom

8. MARKETING AUTHORISATION NUMBER(S)

PL 00032/0406

9. DATE OF FIRST AUTHORISATION/RENEWAL OF THE AUTHORISATION

1st September 2002

10. DATE OF REVISION OF THE TEXT

1st December 2004

Fendrix

(GlaxoSmithKline UK)

1. NAME OF THE MEDICINAL PRODUCT

Fendrix suspension for injection. ▼

Hepatitis B (rDNA) vaccine (adjuvanted, adsorbed).

2. QUALITATIVE AND QUANTITATIVE COMPOSITION

1 dose (0.5 ml) of Fendrix contains:

Hepatitis B surface antigen [1, 2, 3] 20 micrograms

[1]adjuvanted by AS04C containing:

- 3-*O*-desacyl-4'- monophosphoryl lipid A (MPL)[2] 50 micrograms

[2]adsorbed on aluminium phosphate (0.5 milligrams Al^{3+} in total)

[3]produced in yeast cells (*Saccharomyces cerevisiae*) by recombinant DNA technology.

For excipients, see section 6.1

3. PHARMACEUTICAL FORM

Suspension for injection.

Turbid white suspension. Upon storage, a fine white deposit with a clear colourless supernatant can be observed.

4. CLINICAL PARTICULARS

4.1 Therapeutic indications

Fendrix is indicated for active immunisation against hepatitis B virus infection (HBV) caused by all known subtypes for patients with renal insufficiency (including pre-haemodialysis and haemodialysis patients), from the age of 15 years onwards.

4.2 Posology and method of administration

Posology

Primary Immunisation schedule:

A four dose schedule, with immunisations at the elected date, 1 month, 2 months and 6 months from the date of the first dose is recommended.

Once initiated, the primary course of vaccination at 0, 1, 2 and 6 months should be completed with Fendrix, and not with other commercially available HBV vaccine.

Booster dose:

As pre-haemodialysis and haemodialysis patients are particularly exposed to HBV and have a higher risk to become chronically infected, a precautionary attitude should be considered i.e. giving a booster dose in order to ensure a protective antibody level as defined by national recommendations and guidelines.

Fendrix can be used as a booster dose after a primary vaccination course with either Fendrix or any other commercial recombinant hepatitis B vaccine.

Special dosage recommendation for known or presumed exposure to HBV:

Data on concomitant administration of Fendrix with specific hepatitis B immunoglobulin (HBIg) have not been generated. However, in circumstances where exposure to HBV has recently occurred (e.g. stick with contaminated needle) and where simultaneous administration of Fendrix and a standard dose of HBIg is necessary, these should be given at separate injection sites.

Method of administration

Fendrix should be injected intramuscularly in the deltoid region.

4.3 Contraindications

Hypersensitivity to the active substance or to any of the excipients.

Hypersensitivity after previous administration of other hepatitis B vaccines.

Subjects suffering from acute severe febrile illness. The presence of a minor infection such as a cold, is not a contraindication for immunisation.

4.4 Special warnings and special precautions for use

Because of the long incubation period of hepatitis B, it is possible that patients could have been infected before the time of immunisation. The vaccine may not prevent hepatitis B infection in such cases.

The vaccine will not prevent infection caused by other agents such as hepatitis A, hepatitis C and hepatitis E or other pathogens known to infect the liver.

As with any vaccine, a protective immune response may not be elicited in all vaccinees.

A number of factors have been observed to reduce the immune response to hepatitis B vaccines. These factors include older age, male gender, obesity, smoking, route of administration, and some chronic underlying diseases. Consideration should be given to serological testing of those subjects who may be at risk of not achieving seroprotection following a complete course of Fendrix. Additional doses may need to be considered for persons who do not respond or have a sub-optimal response to a course of vaccinations.

Since intramuscular administration into the gluteal muscle could lead to a suboptimal response to the vaccine, this route should be avoided.

Fendrix should under no circumstances be administered intradermally or intravenously.

Patients with chronic liver disease or with HIV infection or hepatitis C carriers should not be precluded from vaccination against hepatitis B. The vaccine could be advised since HBV infection can be severe in these patients: the Hepatitis B vaccination should thus be considered on a casebycase basis by the physician.

Thiomersal (an organomercuric compound) has been used in the manufacturing process of this medicinal product and residues of it are present in the final product. Therefore, sensitisation reactions may occur.

Appropriate medical treatment should always be readily available in case of rare anaphylactic reactions following the administration of the vaccine.

4.5 Interaction with other medicinal products and other forms of Interaction

No data on the concomitant administration of Fendrix and other vaccines or with specific hepatitis B immunoglobulin have been generated. If concomitant administration of specific hepatitis B immunoglobulin and Fendrix is required, these should be given at different injection sites. As no data are available for the concomitant administration of this particular vaccine with other vaccines, an interval of 2 to 3 weeks should be respected.

4.6 Pregnancy and lactation

No clinical data on use during pregnancies are available with Fendrix.

Animal studies do not indicate direct or indirect harmful effects with respect to pregnancy, embryonal/foetal development, parturition or postnatal development.

Vaccination during pregnancy should only be performed if the risk-benefit ratio at individual level outweighs possible risks for the foetus.

Adequate human data on use during lactation are not available. In a reproductive toxicity study in animals which included post-natal follow-up until weaning (see 5.3), no effect on the development of the pups was observed. Vaccination should only be performed if the risk-benefit ratio at individual level outweighs possible risks for the infant.

4.7 Effects on ability to drive and use machines

Fendrix has a minor or moderate influence on the ability to drive and use machine.

Some of the undesirable effects mentioned under section 4.8 may affect the ability to drive or operate machinery.

4.8 Undesirable effects

• Clinical trials involving the administration of 2476 doses of Fendrix to 82 pre-haemodialysis and haemodialysis patients and to 713 healthy subjects ≥ 15 years of age allowed to document the reactogenicity of the vaccine.

Pre-haemodialysis and haemodialysis patients

The reactogenicity profile of Fendrix in a total of 82 pre-haemodialysis and haemodialysis patients was generally comparable to that seen in healthy subjects.

Adverse reactions reported in a clinical trial following primary vaccination with Fendrix and considered as being related or possibly related to vaccination have been categorised by frequency.

Frequencies are reported as:

Very common: >1/10

Common: >1/100, <1/10

Uncommon: >1/1000, <1/100

Rare: >1/10 000, <1/1000

Very rare: <1/10 000, including isolated reports

Nervous system disorders:

Very common: headache

Gastrointestinal disorders:

Common: gastrointestinal disorder

General disorders and administration site conditions

Very common: pain, fatigue

Common: fever, redness, injection site swelling

Unsolicited symptoms considered to be at least possibly related to vaccination were uncommonly reported and consisted of rigors, other injection site reaction and maculo-papular rash.

Healthy subjects

The reactogenicity profile of Fendrix in healthy subjects was generally comparable to that seen in pre-haemodialysis and haemodialysis patients.

In a large double-blind randomised comparative study, healthy subjects were enrolled to receive a three dose primary course of Fendrix (N= 713) or a commercially available hepatitis B vaccine (N= 238) at 0, 1, 2 months. Fendrix was generally well tolerated. The most common adverse events reported were local reactions at the injection site.

Vaccination with Fendrix induced more transient local symptoms as compared to the comparator vaccine, with pain at the injection site being the most frequently reported solicited local symptom. However, solicited general symptoms were observed with similar frequencies in both groups.

Adverse reactions reported in a clinical trial following primary vaccination with Fendrix and considered as being at least possibly related to vaccination have been categorised by frequency.

Infections and infestations:

Rare: viral infection

Metabolism and nutrition disorders:

Rare: thirst

Psychiatric disorders:

Rare: nervousness

Nervous system disorders:

Common: headache

Rare: vertigo

Gastrointestinal disorders:

Common: gastrointestinal disorder

Muskuloskeletal and connective tissue disorders:

Rare: back pain, tendinitis

General disorders and administration site conditions

Very common: fatigue, pain, redness, injection site swelling

Common: fever

Uncommon: other injection site reaction

Rare: allergy, asthenia, hot flushes, rigors

No increase in the incidence or severity of these undesirable events was seen with subsequent doses of the primary vaccination schedule.

No increase in the reactogenicity was observed after the booster vaccination with respect to the primary vaccination.

Allergic reactions, including anaphylactoid reactions, may occur very rarely.

• Experience with hepatitis B vaccine:

Following widespread use of hepatitis B vaccines, in very rare cases, syncope, paralysis, neuropathy, neuritis (including Guillain-Barré syndrome, optic neuritis and multiple sclerosis), encephalitis, encephalopathy, meningitis and convulsions have been reported. The causal relationship to the vaccine has not been established.

4.9 Overdose

No case of overdose has been reported.

5. PHARMACOLOGICAL PROPERTIES

5.1 Pharmacodynamic properties

Pharmaco-therapeutic group: Hepatitis vaccines, ATC code JO7AP.

Fendrix induces specific humoral antibodies against HBsAg (anti-HBs antibodies). An anti-HBs antibody titre ≥ 10 mIU/ml correlates with protection to HBV infection.

It can be expected that hepatitis D will also be prevented by immunisation with Fendrix as hepatitis D (caused by the delta agent) does not occur in the absence of hepatitis B infection.

Immunological data

In pre-haemodialysis and haemodialysis patients:

In a comparative clinical study in 165 pre-haemodialysis and haemodialysis patients (15 years and above), protective levels of specific humoral antibodies (anti-HBs titres ≥ 10 mIU/ml) were observed in 74.4% of Fendrix recipients (N = 82) one month after the third dose (i.e at month 3), as compared to 52.4% of patients in the control group who received a double dose of a commercially available hepatitis B vaccine (N = 83) for this population.

At month 3, Geometric Mean Titres (GMT) were 223.0 mIU/ml and 50.1 mIU/ml in the Fendrix and control groups respectively, with 41.0% and 15.9% of subjects with anti-HBs antibody titres ≥100 mIU/ml respectively.

After completion of a four dose primary course (i.e at month 7), 90.9% of Fendrix recipients were seroprotected (≥ 10 mIU/ml) against hepatitis B, in comparison with 84.4% in a control group who received the commercially available hepatitis B vaccine.

At month 7, GMTs were 3559.2 mIU/ml and 933.0 mIU/ml in the Fendrix and control groups who received the commercially available hepatitis B vaccine respectively, with 83.1% and 67.5% of subjects with anti-HBs antibody titres ≥100 mIU/ml respectively.

Antibody persistence

In pre-haemodialysis and haemodialysis patients:

Anti-HBs antibodies have been shown to persist for at least 36 months following a 0, 1, 2, 6 month primary course of Fendrix in pre-haemodialysis and haemodialysis patients. At month 36, 80.4% of these patients retained protective antibody levels (anti-HBs titres ≥ 10mIU/ml), as compared to 51.3% of patients who received a commercially available hepatitis B vaccine.

At month 36, GMTs were 154.1 mIU/ml and 111.9 mIU/ml in the Fendrix and control groups respectively, with 58.7% and 38.5% of subjects with anti-HBs antibody titres ≥100 mIU/ml respectively.

5.2 Pharmacokinetic properties

Pharmacokinetic properties of Fendrix or MPL alone has not been studied in humans.

5.3 Preclinical safety data

Preclinical data reveal no special hazard for humans based on conventional animal studies consisting of acute and repeated dose toxicity, cardiovascular and respiratory safety pharmacology and reproductive toxicity including pregnancy and peri and postnatal development of the pups till weaning.

6. PHARMACEUTICAL PARTICULARS

6.1 List of excipients

Sodium chloride

Water for injections

For adjuvants, see section 2.

6.2 Incompatibilities

In the absence of compatibility studies, this medicinal product must not be mixed with other medicinal products.

6.3 Shelf life

3 years.

6.4 Special precautions for storage

Store in a refrigerator (2°C – 8°C).

Do not freeze.

Store in the original package in order to protect from light.

6.5 Nature and contents of container

0.5 ml of suspension in pre-filled syringe (type I glass) with a plunger stopper (rubber butyl) with or without separate needle in a pack size of 1, or without needles in a pack size of 10.

Not all pack sizes may be marketed.

6.6 Instructions for use and handling

Upon storage, a fine white deposit with a clear colourless supernatant can be observed.

Before administration, the vaccine should be well shaken to obtain a slightly opaque, white suspension.

The vaccine should be visually inspected both before and after re-suspension for any foreign particulate matter and/or change in physical appearance. The vaccine must not be used if any change in the appearance of the vaccine has taken place.

Any unused vaccine or waste material should be disposed of in accordance with local requirements.

Administrative Data

7. MARKETING AUTHORISATION HOLDER

GlaxoSmithKline Biologicals s.a.

Rue de l'Institut 89

B-1330 Rixensart, Belgium

8. MARKETING AUTHORISATION NUMBER(S)

EU/1/04/0299/001-2-3

9. DATE OF FIRST AUTHORISATION/RENEWAL OF THE AUTHORISATION

2 February 2005

10. DATE OF REVISION OF THE TEXT

Ferrograd C Tablets

(Abbott Laboratories Limited)

1. NAME OF THE MEDICINAL PRODUCT

Ferrograd C Tablets

2. QUALITATIVE AND QUANTITATIVE COMPOSITION

Dried Ferrous sulphate BP 325 mg (elemental iron 105 mg).

Sodium ascorbate 562.4 mg (ascorbic acid 500 mg).

3. PHARMACEUTICAL FORM

Prolonged release, film coated tablets.

Ovoid, biconvex, two layered, red tablet.

4. CLINICAL PARTICULARS

4.1 Therapeutic indications

Prevention and treatment of iron deficiency anaemia and for the simultaneous treatment of vitamin C deficiency.

4.2 Posology and method of administration

Adults including the elderly

1 tablet daily. Take before food. Patients should be advised to swallow tablets whole.

Children

Not recommended for children under 12 years. Above this age, as for adults.

4.3 Contraindications

Intestinal diverticular disease or any intestinal obstruction.

Iron preparations are contra-indicated in patients with haemochromatosis and haemosiderosis.

Iron is contra-indicated in patients receiving repeated blood transfusions.

Oral iron preparations are contra-indicated when used concomitantly with parenteral iron therapy.

4.4 Special warnings and special precautions for use

Ferrograd C tablets should be kept out of children's reach. Acute iron poisoning occurs rarely in adults, however it could happen if children swallow this medication.

The label will state 'Important warning: Contains iron. Keep out of the reach and sight of children, as overdose may be fatal'. This will appear on the front of the pack within a rectangle in which there is no other information.

The prolonged release tablet and its inert plastic matrix may cause a safety hazard in some elderly or other patients suffering from delayed intestinal transit.

Iron preparations colour the faeces black, which may interfere with tests used for detection of occult blood in the stools. The guaiac test occasionally yields false positive tests for blood.

4.5 Interaction with other medicinal products and other forms of Interaction

Iron interacts with tetracyclines, magnesium trisilicate, trientine and zinc salts and absorption of all of these agents may be impaired.

Iron inhibits the absorption of tetracyclines from the gastrointestinal tract and tetracycline inhibits the absorption of iron. If both drugs must be given, tetracycline should be administered three hours after or two hours before oral iron supplements.

Concurrent administration of oral iron preparations with antacids, calcium supplements (calcium carbonate or phosphate), tea, coffee, eggs, food or medications containing bicarbonates, carbonate, oxalates or phosphates, milk or milk products, wholegrain breads and cereals and dietary fibre, may decrease iron absorption. Therefore, oral iron preparations should not be taken within one hour before or two hours after ingestion of such items.

Concurrent administration of oral iron preparations may interfere with the oral absorption of some quinolone anti-infective agents (e.g. ciprofloxacin, norfloxacin, ofloxacin), resulting in decreased serum and urine concentrations of the quinolones. Therefore, oral iron preparations should not be ingested with or within two hours of a dose of an oral quinolone.

Iron can decrease gastrointestinal absorption of penicillamines. Therefore, administration should be at least two hours apart if both drugs must be co-administered.

Chloramphenicol may delay response to iron therapy.

The administration of therapeutic doses of ascorbic acid may interfere with the Clinistix test for glucosuria giving a false negative result.

Ascorbic acid may enhance the absorption of iron from the gastrointestinal tract.

4.6 Pregnancy and lactation

Ferrograd tablets are inappropriate for use during pregnancy since they do not contain folic acid.

4.7 Effects on ability to drive and use machines

None

4.8 Undesirable effects

Side-effects reported are similar to those associated with conventional oral iron preparations, i.e. nausea, vomiting, abdominal pain or discomfort, blackening of stools, diarrhoea and/or constipation, but the incidence of side-effects is less owing to the prolonged release nature of the formulation.

Isolated cases of allergic reaction have been reported ranging from rash to anaphylaxis.

Ascorbic acid is usually well tolerated. However, large doses are reported to cause diarrhoea and other gastro-intestinal disturbances and are associated with the formation of renal calcium oxalate calculi.

4.9 Overdose

Symptoms: Initial symptoms of iron overdosage include nausea, vomiting, diarrhoea, abdominal pain, haematemesis, rectal bleeding, lethargy and circulatory collapse. Hyperglycaemia and metabolic acidosis may also occur. The prolonged release characteristic may delay excessive absorption of iron, and thus allow more time for counter measures to be implemented. However, initial symptoms of overdosage may be absent due to the prolonged release formulation. Therefore, if overdosage is suspected, treatment should be implemented immediately. In severe cases, after a latent phase, relapse may occur after 24-48 hours, manifested by hypotension, coma and hepatocellular necrosis and renal failure.

Vitamin C overdosage may cause acidosis and haemolytic anaemia in predisposed individuals (glucose-6-phosphate dehydrogenase deficiency). Renal failure may occur in massive vitamin C overdose.

Treatment: The following steps are recommended to minimise or prevent further absorption of the medication:

Children:

1. Administer an emetic such as syrup of ipecacuanha.

2. Emesis should be followed by gastric lavage with desferrioxamine solution (2g/l). This should then be followed by the instillation of desferrioxamine 5 g in 50-100 ml water, to be retained in the stomach. Inducing diarrhoea in children may be dangerous and should not be undertaken in young children. Keep the patient under constant surveillance to detect possible aspiration of vomitus - maintain suction apparatus and standby emergency oxygen in case of need.

3. Unleached tablets are radio-opaque. Therefore, an abdominal x-ray should be taken to determine the number of tablets retained in the stomach following emesis and gastric lavage.

4. Severe poisoning: in the presence of shock and/or coma with high serum iron levels (serum iron >90 μmol/l) immediate supportive measures plus i.v. infusion of desferrioxamine should be instituted. Desferrioxamine 15 mg/kg body weight should be administered every hour by slow i.v. infusion to a maximum 80 mg/kg/24 hours. Warning: hypotension may occur if the infusion rate is too rapid.

5. Less severe poisoning: i.m. desferrioxamine 1 g 4-6 hourly is recommended.

6. Serum iron levels should be monitored throughout.

Adults:

1. Administer an emetic.

2. Gastric lavage may be necessary to remove drug already released into the stomach. This should be undertaken using desferrioxamine solution (2g/l). Desferrioxamine 5 g in 50-100 ml water should be introduced into the stomach following gastric emptying. Keep the patient under constant surveillance to detect possible aspiration of vomitus; maintain suction apparatus and standby emergency oxygen in case of need.

3. Unleached tablets are radio-opaque. Therefore, an abdominal x-ray of the patient should be taken to determine the number of tablets retained in the stomach following emesis and gastric lavage. The risk/benefit ratio of x-raying pregnant women must be carefully weighed but should be avoided if possible.

4. A drink of mannitol or sorbitol should be given to induce small bowel emptying.

5. Severe poisoning: in the presence of shock and/or coma with high serum iron levels >142 μmol/l) immediate supportive measures plus i.v. infusion of desferrioxamine should be instituted. The recommended dose of desferrioxamine is 5 mg/kg/h by slow i.v. infusion up to a maximum of 80 mg/kg/24 hours. Warning: hypotension may occur if the infusion rate is too rapid.

6. Less severe poisoning: i.m. desferrioxamine 50 mg/kg up to a maximum dose of 4 g should be given.

7. Serum iron levels should be monitored throughout.

5. PHARMACOLOGICAL PROPERTIES

5.1 Pharmacodynamic properties

Ferrograd C combines the advantages of ferrous sulphate in the Gradumet® matrix with a large dose of vitamin C to further enhance absorption. It is indicated in iron-deficiency anaemia, especially when poor absorption is a problem, and to promote haemopoiesis in patients where an underlying vitamin C deficiency limits optimal haemoglobin formation. In patients whose haemoglobin has returned to normal, Ferrograd C may be of particular value in replenishing the depleted stores of iron.

5.2 Pharmacokinetic properties

The Gradumet device allows controlled release of ferrous sulphate over a number of hours and reduces gastro-intestinal intolerance. The device consists of an inert plastic matrix, honeycombed by thousands of narrow passages which contain ferrous sulphate together with a water soluble channelling agent. As the tablet passes down the gastro-intestinal tract the iron is leached out. The spent matrix is finally excreted in the stools.

Oral iron is absorbed better when administered between meals. However, conventional iron preparations often cause gastric irritation when taken on an empty stomach.

5.3 Preclinical safety data

There are no preclinical data of relevance to the prescriber which are additional to that already included in other sections of the SPC.

6. PHARMACEUTICAL PARTICULARS

6.1 List of excipients

Tablet core:

Methylacrylate methylmethacrylate copolymer,

Magnesium stearate,

Povidone,

Macrogol 8000

Maize starch,

Purified talc,

Film coating:

Subcoat:

Povidone

Ethylcellulose,

Macrogol 400

Colour coating:

Hydroxypropylmethylcellulose,

Macrogol 8000

Macrogol 400

Titanium dioxide

Dye Red Ponceau 4R Lake (E124).

Glossing:

Purified talc

Macrogol 8000

6.2 Incompatibilities

None.

6.3 Shelf life

5 years.

6.4 Special precautions for storage

Store in a cool dry place at or below 25°C.

6.5 Nature and contents of container

Carton containing 30 (3x10) tablets in a blister (OP).

6.6 Instructions for use and handling

None

7. MARKETING AUTHORISATION HOLDER

Abbott Laboratories Limited, Queenborough, Kent ME11 5EL

8. MARKETING AUTHORISATION NUMBER(S)

0037/5001R

9. DATE OF FIRST AUTHORISATION/RENEWAL OF THE AUTHORISATION

16/12/88; 18/02/99

10. DATE OF REVISION OF THE TEXT

April 2002

Ferrograd Folic Tablets

(Abbott Laboratories Limited)

1. NAME OF THE MEDICINAL PRODUCT

Ferrograd Folic Tablets

2. QUALITATIVE AND QUANTITATIVE COMPOSITION

Dried Ferrous sulphate BP 325 mg (elemental iron 105 mg)

Folic acid BP 350 micrograms

3. PHARMACEUTICAL FORM

Prolonged release, film coated tablets.

Circular, biconvex, two layered, red and yellow tablet with the Abbott impressed on the red surface.

4. CLINICAL PARTICULARS

4.1 Therapeutic indications

Prevention and treatment of iron deficiency anaemia of pregnancy.

Prophylaxis of megaloblastic anaemia of pregnancy.

4.2 Posology and method of administration

Adults including the elderly

1 tablet daily throughout pregnancy and the first month of the puerperium. Take before food. Patients should be advised to swallow tablets whole.

Children

Not recommended for children under 12 years.

4.3 Contraindications

Megaloblastic anaemia due to primary vitamin B_{12} deficiency.

Ferrograd Folic is contraindicated in patients with pernicious anaemia.

Intestinal diverticular disease or any intestinal obstruction.

Iron preparations are contra-indicated in patients with haemochromatosis and haemosiderosis.

Iron is contra-indicated in patients receiving repeated blood transfusions.

Oral iron preparations are contra-indicated when used concomitantly with parenteral iron therapy.

Ferrograd Folic is contraindicated in the rare instance of hypersensitivity to folic acid.

4.4 Special warnings and special precautions for use

Ferrograd Folic tablets should be kept out of children's reach. Acute iron poisoning occurs rarely in adults, however it could happen if children swallow this medication.

The label will state 'Important warning: Contains iron. Keep out of the reach and sight of children, as overdose may be fatal'. This will appear on the front of the pack within a rectangle in which there is no other information.

The controlled release tablet and its inert plastic matrix may cause a safety hazard in some elderly or other patients suffering from delayed intestinal transit.

Pernicious anaemia is rare in women of childbearing age and is less likely in pregnancy as vitamin B_{12} deficiency reduces fertility. However, folic acid, at the recommended dosage, may obscure the neurological manifestations of pernicious anaemia.

Iron preparations colour the faeces black, which may interfere with tests used for detection of occult blood in the stools. The guaiac test occasionally yields false positive tests for blood.

4.5 Interaction with other medicinal products and other forms of Interaction

Iron interacts with tetracyclines, magnesium trisilicate, trientine and zinc salts and absorption of all of these agents may be impaired.

Iron inhibits the absorption of tetracyclines from the gastrointestinal tract and tetracycline inhibits the absorption of iron. If both drugs must be given, tetracycline should be administered three hours after or two hours before oral iron supplements.

Concurrent administration of oral iron preparations with antacids, calcium supplements (calcium carbonate or phosphate), tea, coffee, eggs, food or medications containing bicarbonates, carbonate, oxalates or phosphates, milk or milk products, wholegrain breads and cereals and dietary fibre, may decrease iron absorption. Therefore, oral iron preparations should not be taken within one hour before or two hours after ingestion of such items.

Concurrent administration of oral iron preparations may interfere with the oral absorption of some quinolone anti-infective agents (e.g. ciprofloxacin, norfloxacin, ofloxacin), resulting in decreased serum and urine concentrations of the quinolones. Therefore, oral iron preparations should not be ingested with or within two hours of a dose of an oral quinolone.

Iron can decrease gastrointestinal absorption of penicillamines. Therefore, administration should be at least two hours apart if both drugs must be co-administered.

Chloramphenicol may delay response to iron therapy.

4.6 Pregnancy and lactation

Ferrograd Folic is indicated for prevention and treatment of iron deficiency anaemia of pregnancy, and prophylaxis of megaloblastic anaemia of pregnancy.

Folic acid is excreted in breast milk.

4.7 Effects on ability to drive and use machines

None

4.8 Undesirable effects

Side-effects reported are similar to those associated with conventional oral iron preparations, i.e. nausea, vomiting, abdominal pain or discomfort, blackening of stools, diarrhoea and/or constipation, but the incidence of side-effects is less owing to the prolonged release nature of the formulation.

Isolated cases of allergic reaction have been reported ranging from rash to anaphylaxis. Allergy is more common in those people who are allergic to asprin.

Allergic sensitisation has been reported following both oral and parenteral administration of folic acid.

4.9 Overdose

Symptoms: Initial symptoms of iron overdosage include nausea, vomiting, diarrhoea, abdominal pain, haematemesis, rectal bleeding, lethargy and circulatory collapse. Hyperglycaemia and metabolic acidosis may also occur. The prolonged release characteristic may delay excessive absorption of iron, and thus allow more time for counter measures to be implemented. However, initial symptoms of overdosage may be absent due to the prolonged release formulation. Therefore, if overdosage is suspected, treatment should be implemented immediately. In severe cases, after a latent phase, relapse may occur after 24-48 hours, manifested by hypotension, coma and hepatocellular necrosis and renal failure.

Treatment: The following steps are recommended to minimise or prevent further absorption of the medication:

Children:

1. Administer an emetic such as syrup of ipecacuanha.

2. Emesis should be followed by gastric lavage with desferrioxamine solution (2g/l). This should then be followed by the instillation of desferrioxamine 5 g in 50-100 ml water, to be retained in the stomach. Inducing diarrhoea in children may be dangerous and should not be undertaken in young children. Keep the patient under constant surveillance to detect possible aspiration of vomitus - maintain suction apparatus and standby emergency oxygen in case of need.

3. Unleached tablets are radio-opaque. Therefore, an abdominal x-ray should be taken to determine the number of tablets retained in the stomach following emesis and gastric lavage.

4. Severe poisoning: in the presence of shock and/or coma with high serum iron levels (serum iron >90 μmol/l) immediate supportive measures plus i.v. infusion of desferrioxamine should be instituted. Desferrioxamine 15 mg/kg body weight should be administered every hour by slow i.v. infusion to a maximum 80 mg/kg/24 hours. Warning: hypotension may occur if the infusion rate is too rapid.

5. Less severe poisoning: i.m. desferrioxamine 1 g 4-6 hourly is recommended.

6. Serum iron levels should be monitored throughout.

Adults:

1. Administer an emetic.

2. Gastric lavage may be necessary to remove drug already released into the stomach. This should be undertaken using desferrioxamine solution (2g/l). Desferrioxamine 5 g in 50-100 ml water should be introduced into the stomach following gastric emptying. Keep the patient under constant surveillance to detect possible aspiration of vomitus; maintain suction apparatus and standby emergency oxygen in case of need.

3. Unleached tablets are radio-opaque. Therefore, an abdominal x-ray of the patient should be taken to determine the number of tablets retained in the stomach following emesis and gastric lavage. The risk/benefit ratio of x-raying pregnant women must be carefully weighed but should be avoided if possible.

4. A drink of mannitol or sorbitol should be given to induce small bowel emptying.

5. Severe poisoning: in the presence of shock and/or coma with high serum iron levels >142 μmol/l) immediate supportive measures plus i.v. infusion of desferrioxamine should be instituted. The recommended dose of desferrioxamine is 5 mg/kg/h by slow i.v. infusion up to a maximum of 80 mg/kg/24 hours. Warning: hypotension may occur if the infusion rate is too rapid.

6. Less severe poisoning: i.m. desferrioxamine 50 mg/kg up to a maximum dose of 4 g should be given.

7. Serum iron levels should be monitored throughout.

5. PHARMACOLOGICAL PROPERTIES

5.1 Pharmacodynamic properties

Folic acid requirements in pregnancy can be met with supplements of between 300 and 400 micrograms daily. Without such supplements, folate deficiency may develop, leading to megaloblastic anaemia with attendant obstetric risks. Doses over 400 micrograms may mask undiagnosed vitamin B_{12} deficiency. In the extremely unlikely event of this condition occurring in a pregnant woman, the safe prophylactic dose is considered to be 350 micrograms.

Iron provided by Ferrograd Folic aids haemoglobin regeneration. Once haemoglobin returns to normal, continuing iron therapy for 3 months will help replenish the iron stores in the body.

5.2 Pharmacokinetic properties

The Gradumet® device allows controlled release of ferrous sulphate over a number of hours and reduces gastro-intestinal intolerance. The device consists of an inert plastic matrix, honeycombed by thousands of narrow passages which contain ferrous sulphate together with a water soluble channelling agent. As the tablet passes down the gastro-intestinal tract the iron is leached out. The spent matrix is finally excreted in the stools.

Iron is found in the body principally as haemoglobin. Storage in the form of ferritin occurs in the liver, spleen, and bone marrow. Concentrations of plasma iron and the total iron-binding capacity of the plasma vary greatly in different physiological conditions and disease states.

Folic acid and iron are absorbed in the proximal small intestine, particularly the duodenum. Folic acid is absorbed maximally and rapidly at this site, and iron is absorbed in a descending gradient from the duodenum distally.

After absorption, folic acid is rapidly converted into its metabolically active forms. Approximately two-thirds is bound to plasma protein. Half of the folic acid stored in the body is found in the liver. Folic acid is also concentrated in spinal fluid.

5.3 Preclinical safety data

There are no preclinical data of relevance to the prescriber which are additional to that already included in other sections of the SPC.

6. PHARMACEUTICAL PARTICULARS

6.1 List of excipients

Tablet core:

Methylacrylate methylmethacrylate copolymer,

Magnesium stearate,

Povidone,

Polyethylene glycol 8000,

Colloidal silicon dioxide,

Lactose,

Sucrose,

Acacia powder,

Maize starch,

Tablet coat:

Cellulose acetate phthalate,

Propylene glycol,

Sorbitan monooleate,

Castor oil,

Titanium dioxide

Dye Red Ponceau 4R Lake (E124).

6.2 Incompatibilities

None.

6.3 Shelf life

3 years

6.4 Special precautions for storage

Store in a cool dry place at or below 25°C.

6.5 Nature and contents of container

Carton containing 30 (3x10) tablets in a blister (OP), and a sample blister of 4 tablets.

6.6 Instructions for use and handling

None

7. MARKETING AUTHORISATION HOLDER

Abbott Laboratories Limited, Queenborough, Kent ME11 5EL

8. MARKETING AUTHORISATION NUMBER(S)

0037/5002R

9. DATE OF FIRST AUTHORISATION/RENEWAL OF THE AUTHORISATION

21/12/88; 12/02/99

10. DATE OF REVISION OF THE TEXT

April 2002

Ferrograd Tablets

(Abbott Laboratories Limited)

1. NAME OF THE MEDICINAL PRODUCT

Ferrograd Tablets

2. QUALITATIVE AND QUANTITATIVE COMPOSITION

Dried Ferrous sulphate 325 mg (elemental iron 105 mg).

3. PHARMACEUTICAL FORM

Prolonged release, film coated tablets.

Circular, biconvex, red tablet with the Abbott impressed on one surface.

4. CLINICAL PARTICULARS

4.1 Therapeutic indications

Prevention and treatment of iron deficiency anaemia.

4.2 Posology and method of administration

Adults including the elderly

1 tablet daily. Take before food. Patients should be advised to swallow tablets whole.

Children

Not recommended for children under 12 years. Above this age, as for adults.

4.3 Contraindications

Intestinal diverticular disease or any intestinal obstruction.

Iron preparations are contra-indicated in patients with haemochromatosis and haemosiderosis.

Iron is contra-indicated in patients receiving repeated blood transfusions.

Oral iron preparations are contra-indicated when used concomitantly with parenteral iron therapy.

4.4 Special warnings and special precautions for use

Ferrograd tablets should be kept out of children's reach. Acute iron poisoning occurs rarely in adults, however it could happen if children swallow this medication.

The label will state 'Important warning: Contains iron. Keep out of the reach and sight of children, as overdose may be fatal'. This will appear on the front of the pack within a rectangle in which there is no other information.

The prolonged release tablet and its inert plastic matrix may cause a safety hazard in some elderly or other patients suffering from delayed intestinal transit.

Iron preparations colour the faeces black, which may interfere with tests used for detection of occult blood in the stools. The guaiac test occasionally yields false positive tests for blood.

4.5 Interaction with other medicinal products and other forms of Interaction
Iron interacts with tetracyclines, magnesium trisilicate, trientine and zinc salts and absorption of all of these agents may be impaired.

Iron inhibits the absorption of tetracyclines from the gastrointestinal tract and tetracycline inhibits the absorption of iron. If both drugs must be given, tetracycline should be administered three hours after or two hours before oral iron supplements.

Concurrent administration of oral iron preparations with antacids, calcium supplements (calcium carbonate or phosphate), tea, coffee, eggs, food or medications containing bicarbonates, carbonate, oxalates or phosphates, milk or milk products, wholegrain breads and cereals and dietary fibre, may decrease iron absorption. Therefore, oral iron preparations should not be taken within one hour before or two hours after ingestion of such items.

Concurrent administration of oral iron preparations may interfere with the oral absorption of some quinolone anti-infective agents (e.g. ciprofloxacin, norfloxacin, ofloxacin), resulting in decreased serum and urine concentrations of the quinolones. Therefore, oral iron preparations should not be ingested with or within two hours of a dose of an oral quinolone.

Iron can decrease gastrointestinal absorption of penicillamines. Therefore, administration should be at least two hours apart if both drugs must be co-administered.

Chloramphenicol may delay response to iron therapy.

4.6 Pregnancy and lactation
Ferrograd tablets are inappropriate for use during pregnancy since they do not contain folic acid.

4.7 Effects on ability to drive and use machines
None

4.8 Undesirable effects
Side-effects reported are similar to those associated with conventional oral iron preparations, i.e. nausea, vomiting, abdominal pain or discomfort, blackening of stools, diarrhoea and/or constipation, but the incidence of side-effects is less owing to the prolonged release nature of the formulation.

Isolated cases of allergic reaction have been reported ranging from rash to anaphylaxis.

4.9 Overdose
Symptoms: Initial symptoms of iron overdosage include nausea, vomiting, diarrhoea, abdominal pain, haematemesis, rectal bleeding, lethargy and circulatory collapse. Hyperglycaemia and metabolic acidosis may also occur. The prolonged release characteristic may delay excessive absorption of iron, and thus allow more time for counter measures to be implemented. However, initial symptoms of overdosage may be absent due to the prolonged release formulation. Therefore, if overdosage is suspected, treatment should be implemented immediately. In severe cases, after a latent phase, relapse may occur after 24-48 hours, manifested by hypotension, coma and hepatocellular necrosis and renal failure.

Treatment: The following steps are recommended to minimise or prevent further absorption of the medication:

Children:

1. Administer an emetic such as syrup of ipecacuanha.

2. Emesis should be followed by gastric lavage with desferrioxamine solution (2g/l). This should then be followed by the instillation of desferrioxamine 5 g in 50-100 ml water, to be retained in the stomach. Inducing diarrhoea in children may be dangerous and should not be undertaken in young children. Keep the patient under constant surveillance to detect possible aspiration of vomitus - maintain suction apparatus and standby emergency oxygen in case of need.

3. Unleached tablets are radio-opaque. Therefore, an abdominal x-ray should be taken to determine the number of tablets retained in the stomach following emesis and gastric lavage.

4. Severe poisoning: in the presence of shock and/or coma with high serum iron levels (serum iron >90 μmol/l) immediate supportive measures plus i.v. infusion of desferrioxamine should be instituted. Desferrioxamine 15 mg/kg body weight should be administered every hour by slow i.v. infusion to a maximum 80 mg/kg/24 hours. Warning: hypotension may occur if the infusion rate is too rapid.

5. Less severe poisoning: i.m. desferrioxamine 1 g 4-6 hourly is recommended.

6. Serum iron levels should be monitored throughout.

Adults:

1. Administer an emetic.

2. Gastric lavage may be necessary to remove drug already released into the stomach. This should be undertaken using desferrioxamine solution (2g/l). Desferrioxamine 5 g in 50-100 ml water should be introduced into the stomach following gastric emptying. Keep the patient under constant surveillance to detect possible aspiration of vomitus; maintain suction apparatus and standby emergency oxygen in case of need.

3. Unleached tablets are radio-opaque. Therefore, an abdominal x-ray of the patient should be taken to determine the number of tablets retained in the stomach following emesis and gastric lavage. The risk/benefit ratio of x-raying pregnant women must be carefully weighed but should be avoided if possible.

4. A drink of mannitol or sorbitol should be given to induce small bowel emptying.

5. Severe poisoning: in the presence of shock and/or coma with high serum iron levels >142 μmol/l) immediate supportive measures plus i.v. infusion of desferrioxamine should be instituted. The recommended dose of desferrioxamine is 5 mg/kg/h by slow i.v. infusion up to a maximum of 80 mg/kg/24 hours. Warning: hypotension may occur if the infusion rate is too rapid.

6. Less severe poisoning: i.m. desferrioxamine 50 mg/kg up to a maximum dose of 4 g should be given.

7. Serum iron levels should be monitored throughout.

5. PHARMACOLOGICAL PROPERTIES

5.1 Pharmacodynamic properties
Iron provided by Ferrograd aids haemoglobin regeneration. Once haemoglobin returns to normal, continuing iron therapy for 3 months will help replenish the iron stores in the body.

5.2 Pharmacokinetic properties
Oral iron is absorbed better when administered between meals. However, conventional iron preparations often cause gastric irritation when taken on an empty stomach. Studies with Gradumet iron have indicated that relatively little of the iron is released in the stomach, the major portion being released in the upper intestinal tract. Thus, the possibility of gastric irritation is minimised when iron is administered in the Gradumet form in comparison with conventional iron preparations.

5.3 Preclinical safety data
There are no preclinical data of relevance to the prescriber which are additional to that already included in other sections of the SPC.

6. PHARMACEUTICAL PARTICULARS

6.1 List of excipients
Tablet core:

Methylacrylate methylmethacrylate copolymer,

Lactose,

Povidone,

Magnesium stearate,

Film coating:

Hydroxypropylmethylcellulose,

Ethylcellulose,

Sodium saccharin,

Triethyl citrate,

Sorbitan monooleate,

Castor oil,

Titanium dioxide,

Dye Red FD & C No.3 (E127)

Dye Yellow FD & C No.6 (E110)

6.2 Incompatibilities
None.

6.3 Shelf life
5 years.

6.4 Special precautions for storage
Store in a cool dry place at or below 25°C.

6.5 Nature and contents of container
Ferrograd is supplied in 5 carton packs, each containing 30 (3x10) tablets in a blister (OP), a sample blister of 4 tablets, and securitainers of 1000 tablets.

6.6 Instructions for use and handling
None.

7. MARKETING AUTHORISATION HOLDER
Abbott Laboratories Limited, Queenborough, Kent ME11 5EL

8. MARKETING AUTHORISATION NUMBER(S)
0037/5000R

9. DATE OF FIRST AUTHORISATION/RENEWAL OF THE AUTHORISATION
16/12/88; 13/03/2000

10. DATE OF REVISION OF THE TEXT
April 2002

Fibrogammin P

(ZLB Behring UK Limited)

1. NAME OF THE MEDICINAL PRODUCT
Fibrogammin® P

2. QUALITATIVE AND QUANTITATIVE COMPOSITION

2.1 Qualitative Composition
Human plasma coagulation factor XIII

2.2 Quantitative Composition

Fibrogammin P	250 U	1250 U
Dried substance	68 - 135 mg	340 - 673 mg
Human plasma fraction with a factor XIII activity of	250 U*	1250 U*
Total protein	24 - 64 mg	120 – 320 mg

* 1 Unit (U) is equivalent to the factor-XIII-activity of 1 ml fresh citrated plasma

(pooled plasma) of healthy donors.

3. PHARMACEUTICAL FORM
Powder and solvent for solution for injection or infusion.

Fibrogammin P is a purified concentrate of blood coagulation factor XIII. It is derived from human plasma, presented as a white powder and contains no preservatives.

4. CLINICAL PARTICULARS

4.1 Therapeutic indications
Congenital deficiency of Factor XIII and resultant haemorrhagic syndromes, haemorrhages and disturbances in wound healing.

4.2 Posology and method of administration
Posology
1 ml is equivalent to 62.5 U, and 100 U are equivalent to 1.6 ml, respectively.

Important:
The amount to be administered and the frequency of administration should always be orientated towards clinical efficacy in the individual case.

The following table can be used to guide dosing in bleeding episodes and surgery:

	Dosage Units [U] per kg body weight [b.w.]	Type of Haemorrhage
Congenital F XIII deficiency	10	*Prophylaxis of haemorrhages:* approx. once every month. The interval is to be shortened if spontaneous haemorrhages develop.
	Up to 35	*Before surgical operations:* immediately before surgery in adults plus approx. 10U/kg body weight on each of the following 5 days or until the wound has healed completely.
	10-20	*Therapy:* daily, for severe haemorrhages and extensive haematomas until bleeding has stopped.

Due to the different pathogenesis of factor-XIII-deficiencies the data available on half-lives differ considerably.

Thus, monitoring the increase in factor- XIII-activity with a factor-XIII-assay is recommended. In the case of major surgery and severe haemorrhages the aim is to obtain normal values.

Method of administration
Reconstitute the preparation as described under 6.6. The preparation should be warmed to room or body temperature before administration. Slowly inject or infuse intravenously at a rate which the patient finds comfortable. The injection or infusion rate should not exceed approx. 4 ml per minute.

Observe the patient for any immediate reaction. If any reaction takes place during the administration of Fibrogammin P, the rate of infusion should be decreased or the infusion stopped, as required by the clinical condition of the patient (see also Section 4.4.).

4.3 Contraindications
Known hypersensitivity to constituents of the product.

In cases of recent thrombosis caution should be exercised on account of the fibrin-stabilizing effect of factor XIII.

4.4 Special warnings and special precautions for use

In the case of patients with known allergies to the product, antihistaminics and corticosteroids may be administered prophylactically.

In case of existing thrombosis a stabilization of the thrombus might occur, consecutively resulting in increased risk of vessel occlusions.

After repeated Fibrogammin P treatment, patients should be carefully monitored for the development of inhibitors to F XIII by appropriate clinical observation and laboratory tests.

If allergic-anaphylactic reactions occur (see also section 4.8), the administration of Fibrogammin P has to be discontinued immediately (e.g. by interruption of the injection) and an appropriate treatment has to be initiated. The current medical standards for shock treatment are to be observed.

Note for diabetic patients

Fibrogammin P contains glucose (96 mg per 1000 U). When administering a dose of 10 U/kg body weight to a patient with 75 kg body weight, 72 mg of glucose will be supplied. In cases of the maximum daily dose of 35 U/kg body weight (assuming the same body weight), 252 mg glucose would be supplied.

Note for patients on a low sodium diet

Fibrogammin P contains sodium chloride and may therefore be harmful to patients on a low sodium diet.

Virus safety

When medicinal products prepared from human blood or plasma are administered, infectious diseasesdue to the transmission of infective agents cannot be totally excluded. This also applies to pathogens of hitherto unknown nature.

Some viruses, such as parvovirus B 19 or hepatitis A virus, are particularly difficult to remove or inactivate at this time. Parvovirus B 19 may most seriously affect seronegative pregnant women, or immune-compromised individuals.

To reduce the risk of transmission of infective agents, stringent controls are applied to the selection of donors and donations. In addition, virus elimination / inactivation procedures are included in the production process of Fibrogammin P.

Fibrogammin P is prepared exclusively from plasma donations, which have been tested negative for antibodies to HIV-1, HIV-2, HCV and HBs antigen. The levels of ALT (GPT) in the plasma are also determined and must not exceed twice the normal value specified in the test.

In addition, the plasma pool is tested for antibodies to HIV-1, HIV-2, HCV and HBs antigen as well as for virus genetic material of HCV. The plasma pool is used for further processing only if the results of all these tests are negative.

The production process of Fibrogammin P contains various steps which contribute towards the elimination / inactivation of viruses. These include chromatographic procedures and the heat-treatment of the preparation in aqueous solution at 60 °C for 10 hours.

Appropriate hepatitis vaccination (hepatitis A and hepatitis B) for patients in regular receipt of medicinal products derived from human blood or plasma (including Fibrogammin P), is recommended.

4.5 Interaction with other medicinal products and other forms of Interaction

No interactions of Fibrogammin P with other medicinal products are known so far.

4.6 Pregnancy and lactation

The safety of Fibrogammin P for use in human pregnancy or breastfeeding has not been established in controlled clinical trials.

Experimental animal studies are insufficient to assess the safety with respect to reproduction, development of the embryo or foetus, the course of gestation and peri- and postnatal development.

The clinical use of Fibrogammin P in pregnancy did not show any negative effects on the course of gestation and the peri- or postnatal development. The efficacy of Fibrogammin P in pregnant women with congenital factor XIII deficiency has been described.

Therefore, Fibrogammin P should only be used if clearly needed during pregnancy and lactation.

4.7 Effects on ability to drive and use machines

There are no indications that Fibrogammin P may impair the ability to drive or to operate machines.

4.8 Undesirable effects

In rare cases allergic reactions and/or rise in temperature are observed. The treatment required depends on the nature and severity of the side-effects.

In very rare cases the development of inhibitors to Factor XIII may occur.

4.9 Overdose

No symptoms of overdose with Fibrogammin P are known so far.

5. PHARMACOLOGICAL PROPERTIES

5.1 Pharmacodynamic properties

5.1.1 Pharmaco-therapeutic group

Haemostyptics/Antihaemorrhagics

ATC-code: B02B D07

5.1.2 Pharmacodynamics

Biochemically factor XIII acts as transglutaminase. Physiologically, this corresponds to cross-linking of fibrin-monomers representing the final steps of blood coagulation. Fibrin cross-linking and stabilization promote penetration of fibroblasts. Thus, factor XIII is essentially involved in the principal steps of wound healing and tissue repair.

5.2 Pharmacokinetic properties

The product is administered intravenously, and is thus immediately bioavailable resulting in a plasma concentration corresponding to the applied dose.

In congenital factor-XIII-deficiency the biological half-life of Fibrogammin P was determined to be 9.2 days (median). Fibrogammin P is metabolised in the same way as is the endogenous coagulation factor XIII.

5.3 Preclinical safety data

Concentrate of human factor XIII as a normal constituent of the human plasma acts like the physiological factor XIII. Single dose toxicity testing revealed no adverse findings in different species even at dose levels several times higher than the recommended human dose.

Repeated dose toxicity testing is impracticable due to the development of antibodies in animal models.

To date, Fibrogammin P has not been reported to be associated with embryo-foetal toxicity, oncogenic or mutagenic potential.

6. PHARMACEUTICAL PARTICULARS

6.1 List of excipients

Fibrogammin P	**250 U**	**1250 U**
Human albumin	24 – 40 mg	120–200 mg
Glucose*	16 – 24 mg	80 – 120 mg
Sodium chloride*	28 – 44 mg	140–220 mg
HCl or NaOH (in small amounts for pH adjustment)		
*see also section 4.4		
Supplied diluent		
Water for injections	4 ml	20 ml

6.2 Incompatibilities

Fibrogammin P should not be mixed with other medicinal products and should be administered by a separate infusion line.

6.3 Shelf life

When stored in the unopened container Fibrogammin P has a shelf-life of 2 years.

Do not use after the expiry date given on the pack and container.

From a microbiological point of view, and as Fibrogammin P contains no preservative, the reconstituted product should be used immediately. If it is not administered immediately, storage shall not exceed 8 hours at +2 to +8 °C.

6.4 Special precautions for storage

Fibrogammin P should be stored at +2 to +8 °C. Do not freeze.

Keep container in the outer carton.

Keep out of the reach of children!

6.5 Nature and contents of container

Vials:

250 U: 6 ml injection vial of colourless tube glass, Type I (Ph.Eur.)

1250 U: 30 ml injection vial of colourless blow moulded glass, Type II (Ph.Eur.)

Vials are sealed with a rubber stopper, a plastic disc and an aluminium cap

Presentations:

Pack with 250 U

1 vial with dried substance

1 ampoule with 4 ml water for injections

Pack with 1250 U

1 vial with dried substance

1 vial with 20 ml water for injections

1 transfer device

6.6 Instructions for use and handling

6.6.1 General instructions

Reconstitution and withdrawal must be carried out under aseptic conditions.

Do not use solutions which are cloudy or contain residues (deposits/particles).

After administration, any unused solution and the administration equipment must be discarded appropriately.

6.6.2 Reconstitution of the pack with Fibrogammin P 250 U:

Warm both the diluent and Fibrogammin P vial in unopened vials to room or body temperature (not above 37 °C).

Take the diluent ampoule upright in your hand and shake down the diluent from the ampoule tip.

Break off the ampoule tip with thumb and forefinger. Withdraw the diluent into a syringe.

Remove the cap from the substance vial. Treat the surface of the rubber stopper with antiseptic solution and allow to dry.

Insert the cannula of the syringe filled with the diluent into the rubber stopper of the substance vial.

Do not squirt the diluent directly onto the powder. The diluent should rinse down at the inner face of the vial.

After complete transfer of the diluent to the substance vial gently swirl the vial until the powder is reconstituted and the solution is ready for administration. Avoid vigorous shaking causing formation of foam. A colourless, clear to slightly opalescent solution of neutral pH is obtained.

The reconstituted product should be administered immediately (see section 6.3).

Reconstitution of the pack with Fibrogammin P 1250 U:

Warm both the diluent and Fibrogammin P vial in unopened vials to room or body temperature (not above 37 °C).

Remove the caps from both vials to expose the central portions of the infusion stoppers.

Treat the surface of the infusion stoppers with antiseptic solution and allow them to dry.

Remove the protective sheath from one end of the transfer device.

Using aseptic technique, insert the transfer device into the infusion stopper of the diluent vial. Assure that the red valve at the transfer device is open. Remove the protective sheath from the other end of the transfer device. Assure that the red valve at the transfer device remains open. Invert the diluent vial and insert the transfer device – without touching it – into the infusion stopper of the substance vial. Do not squirt the diluent directly onto the powder. The diluent should rinse down at the inner face of the vial.

Close the red valve at the transfer device.

Remove diluent vial and the transfer device from the substance vial.

Gently swirl the vial until the powder is reconstituted and the solution is ready for administration. Avoid vigorous shaking causing formation of foam. A colourless, clear to slightly opalescent solution of neutral pH is obtained.

The reconstituted product should be administered immediately (see section 6.3).

7. MARKETING AUTHORISATION HOLDER

ZLB Behring GmbH

Emil-von-Behring-Str. 76

P.O. Box 1230

D-35002 Marburg

Germany

8. MARKETING AUTHORISATION NUMBER(S)

PL 15036/0006

9. DATE OF FIRST AUTHORISATION/RENEWAL OF THE AUTHORISATION

22 June 1998 / 15 January 2004

10. DATE OF REVISION OF THE TEXT

14 July 2004

Fibro-Vein 3.0%, 1.0%, 0.5%, 0.2%

(STD Pharmaceutical Products Ltd)

1. NAME OF THE MEDICINAL PRODUCT

Fibro-vein 3.0%, 1.0%, 0.5%, 0.2%

2. QUALITATIVE AND QUANTITATIVE COMPOSITION

Active ingredient

Fibro-vein 3% Sodium Tetradecyl Sulphate BP 3.0% w/v

Fibro-vein 1% Sodium Tetradecyl Sulphate BP 1.0% w/v

Fibro-vein 0.5% Sodium Tetradecyl Sulphate BP 0.5% w/v

Fibrovein 0.2% Sodium Tetradecyl Sulphate BP 0.2% w/v

For excipients, see 6.1

3. PHARMACEUTICAL FORM

Intravenous injection

4. CLINICAL PARTICULARS

4.1 Therapeutic indications

Fibro-vein 3%

For the treatment of varicose veins of the leg by injection sclerotherapy.

Fibro-vein 1%

For the treatment of small varicose veins and the larger venules of the leg by injection sclerotherapy.

Fibro-vein 0.5%

For the treatment of minor venules and spider veins (venous flares) of the leg by injection sclerotherapy.

Fibro-vein 0.2%

For the treatment of minor venules and spider veins (venous flares) by injection sclerotherapy.

4.2 Posology and method of administration

Route of administration

For intravenous administration into the lumen of an isolated segment of emptied vein followed by immediate continuous compression.

Recommended doses and dosage schedules.

Adults

Fibro-vein 3%

0.5 to 1.0ml of 3.0% Fibro-vein injected intravenously at each of 4 sites (maximum 4ml).

Fibro-vein 1%

0.25 to 1.0ml of 1.0% Fibro-vein injected intravenously at each of 10 sites (maximum 10ml).

Fibro-vein 0.5%

0.25 to 1.0ml of 0.5% Fibro-vein injected intravenously at each of 10 sites (maximum 10ml).

Fibro-vein 0.2%

0.1 to 1.0ml of Fibro-vein 0.2% injected intravenously at each of 10 sites (maximum 10ml).

The smallest of needles (30 gauge) should be used to perform the injection which should be made slowly so that the blood content of these veins is expelled. In the treatment of spider veins an air block technique may be used.

Children

Not recommended in children

The elderly

As for adults

4.3 Contraindications

1. Allergy to sodium tetradecyl sulphate or to any component of the preparation.
2. Patients unable to walk due to any cause.
3. Patients currently taking oral contraceptives.
4. Significant obesity.
5. Acute superficial thrombophlebitis.
6. Local or systemic infection.
7. Varicosities caused by pelvic or abdominal tumours.
8. Uncontrolled systemic disease eg diabetes mellitus.
9. Surgical valvular incompetence requiring surgical treatment.

4.4 Special warnings and special precautions for use

1. Fibro-vein should only be administered by practitioners familiar with an acceptable injection technique. Thorough pre-injection assessment for valvular competence and deep vein patency must be carried out.

Extreme care in needle placement and slow injection of the minimal effective volume at each injection site are essential for safe and efficient use.

2. A history of allergy should be taken from all patients prior to treatment. Where special caution is indicated a test dose of 0.25 to 0.5ml Fibro-vein should be given up to 24 hours before any further therapy.

3. Treatment of anaphylaxis may require, depending on the severity of attack, some or all of the following: injection of adrenaline, injection of hydrocortisone, injection of antihistamine, endotracheal intubation with use of a laryngoscope and suction.

The treatment of varicose veins by Fibro-vein should not be undertaken in clinics where these items are not readily available.

4. Extreme caution in use is required in patients with arterial disease such as severe peripheral atherosclerosis or thromboangiitis obliterans (Buerger's disease).

5. Special care is required when injecting above and posterior to the medial malleolus where the posterior tibial artery may be at risk.

6. Pigmentation may be more likely to result if blood is extravasated at the injection site (particularly when treating smaller surface veins) and compression is not used.

4.5 Interaction with other medicinal products and other forms of Interaction

Do not use with heparin in the same syringe

4.6 Pregnancy and lactation

Safety for use in pregnancy has not been established. Use only when clearly needed for symptomatic relief and when the potential benefits outweigh the potential hazards to the foetus.

It is not known whether sodium tetradecyl sulphate is excreted in human milk. Caution should be exercised when used in nursing mothers.

4.7 Effects on ability to drive and use machines

None known

4.8 Undesirable effects

1. Local: Pain or burning. Skin pigmentation. Tissue necrosis and ulceration may occur with extravasation. Paraesthesia and anaesthesia may occur if an injection effects a cutaneous nerve.

2. Vascular: Superficial thrombophlebitis. Deep vein thrombosis and pulmonary embolism are very rare. Inadvertent intra-arterial injection is very rare but may lead to gangrene. Most cases have involved the posterior tibial artery above the medial malleolus.

3. Systemic reactions: Allergic reactions are rare, presenting as local or generalised rash, urticaria, nausea or vomiting, asthma, vascular collapse. Anaphylactic shock, which may potentially be fatal, is extremely rare.

4.9 Overdose

Not applicable.

5. PHARMACOLOGICAL PROPERTIES

5.1 Pharmacodynamic properties

Sodium tetradecyl sulphate damages the endothelium cells within the lumen of the injected vein. The object of compression sclerotherapy is then to compress the vein so that the resulting thrombus is kept to the minimum and the subsequent formation of scar tissue within the vein produces a fibrous cord and permanent obliteration. Non-compressed veins permit the formation of a large thrombus and produce less fibrosis within the vein.

5.2 Pharmacokinetic properties

Not applicable.

5.3 Preclinical safety data

Not applicable

6. PHARMACEUTICAL PARTICULARS

6.1 List of excipients

Benzyl Alcohol BP 2.0% w/v

Di-Sodium Hydrogen Phosphate BP 0.75% w/v

Potassium Di-Hydrogen Phosphate BP 0.1% w/v

Water For Injection BP to 100%

Potassium Di-Hydrogen Phosphate* BP qs

Sodium Carbonate (anhydrous)* BP qs

Sodium Hydroxide (5% soln)* BP qs

* Either sodium carbonate or sodium hydroxide is used for adjustment of pH

6.2 Incompatibilities

Do not use with heparin in the same syringe

6.3 Shelf life

36 months

6.4 Special precautions for storage

Store below 25°C away from direct sunlight

6.5 Nature and contents of container

2ml ampoules type 1 neutral hydrolytic glass conforming with EP requirements for injectable preparations. Five 2ml ampoules per pack.

5ml glass vials type 1 neutral hydrolytic glass conforming with EP requirements for injectable preparations. Sealed with a chlorobutyl rubber bung and silver aluminium "tear off" seal conforming with the European Pharmacopoeia requirements. Ten 5ml vials per pack.

Fibro-vein 3.0% available as 5 × 2ml ampoules and 10 × 5ml vials

Fibro-vein 1.0% available as 5 × 2ml ampoules

Fibro-vein 0.5% available as 5 × 2ml ampoules

Fibro-vein 0.2% available as 5 × 2ml ampoules and 10 × 5ml vials

6.6 Instructions for use and handling

The in use period of each 5ml multidose vial is a single session of therapy and for use in the treatment of a single patient. Unused vial contents should be discarded immediately afterwards.

7. MARKETING AUTHORISATION HOLDER

STD Pharmaceutical Products Ltd

Fields Yard

Plough Lane

Hereford

HR4 0EL

United Kingdom

8. MARKETING AUTHORISATION NUMBER(S)

Fibro-vein 3.0% PL 0398/5000R

Fibro-vein 1.0% PL 0398/0003

Fibro-vein 0.5% PL 0398/0002

Fibro-vein 0.2% PL 0398/0004

9. DATE OF FIRST AUTHORISATION/RENEWAL OF THE AUTHORISATION

Fibro-vein 3.0% 03/11/2000

Fibro-vein 1.0% 15/06/2001

Fibro-vein 0.5% 15/06/2001

Fibro-vein 0.2% 27/02/2001

10. DATE OF REVISION OF THE TEXT

09/01/2003

Filair 100 Inhaler

(3M Health Care Limited)

1. NAME OF THE MEDICINAL PRODUCT

Filair 100 Inhaler and Beclometasone Dipropionate 100 micrograms Inhaler

(Throughout the text Filair 100 Inhaler may be replaced by Beclometasone Dipropionate 100 micrograms Inhaler)

2. QUALITATIVE AND QUANTITATIVE COMPOSITION

Each actuation delivers beclometasone dipropionate 100 micrograms (as propellant solvate) into the mouthpiece of the adapter.

3. PHARMACEUTICAL FORM

Pressurised aerosol for inhalation therapy.

4. CLINICAL PARTICULARS

4.1 Therapeutic indications

Filair 100 Inhaler is indicated for the prophylactic treatment of chronic reversible obstructive airways disease.

4.2 Posology and method of administration

The dose should be titrated to the lowest dose at which effective control of asthma is maintained.

ADULTS: for maintenance: 1 inhalation (100 micrograms), three or four times daily or 2 inhalations (200 micrograms), twice daily. In more severe cases a dose of 600-800 micrograms (6-8 inhalations) daily is recommended, with subsequent reductions. The maximum recommended daily dose of this preparation is 1 mg. In patients receiving doses of 1500 micrograms or more daily, adrenal suppression may occur.

CHILDREN: 1 inhalation (100 micrograms), two to four times daily.

ELDERLY: No special dosage recommendations are made for elderly patients.

4.3 Contraindications

Hypersensitivity to beclometasone is a contra-indication. Caution should be observed in patients with pulmonary tuberculosis.

4.4 Special warnings and special precautions for use

Patients should be instructed on the proper use of the inhaler. They should be made aware of the prophylactic nature of Filair 100 Inhaler therapy and that it should be used regularly at the intervals recommended and not when immediate relief is required.

In patients who have been transferred to inhalation therapy, systemic steroid therapy may need to be re-instated rapidly during periods of stress or where airways obstruction or mucus prevents absorption from the inhalation.

Systemic effects of inhaled corticosteroids may occur, particularly at high doses prescribed for prolonged periods. These effects are much less likely to occur than with oral corticosteroids. Possible systemic effects include adrenal suppression, growth retardation in children and adolescents, decrease in bone mineral density, cataract and glaucoma. It is important therefore that the dose of inhaled steroid is titrated to the lowest dose at which effective control of asthma is maintained.

It is recommended that the height of children receiving prolonged treatment with inhaled corticosteroids is regularly monitored. If growth is slowed, therapy should be reviewed with the aim of reducing the dose of inhaled corticosteroid, if possible, to the lowest dose at which effective control of asthma is maintained. In addition, consideration should be given to referring the patient to a paediatric respiratory specialist.

Prolonged treatment with high doses of inhaled corticosteroids, particularly higher than the recommended doses, may result in clinically significant adrenal suppression. Additional systemic corticosteroid cover should be considered during periods of stress or elective surgery.

Patients who have received systemic steroids for long periods of time or at high doses, or both, need special care and subsequent management when transferred to beclometasone therapy. Recovery from impaired adrenocortical function, caused by prolonged systemic steroid therapy, is slow. The patient should be in a reasonably stable state before being given Filair 100 Inhaler in addition to his usual maintenance dose of systemic steroid. Withdrawal of the systemic steroid should be gradual, starting after about seven days by reducing the daily oral dose by 1 mg prednisolone, or equivalent, at intervals not less than one week. Adrenocortical function should be monitored regularly.

Most patients can be successfully transferred to Filair 100 Inhaler with maintenance of good respiratory function, but special care is necessary for the first months after the transfer until the hypothalamic-pituitary-adrenal (HPA) system has sufficiently recovered to enable the patient to cope with emergencies such as trauma, surgery or infections.

Patients who have been transferred to inhalation therapy should carry a warning card indicating that systemic steroid therapy may need to be re-instated without delay during periods of stress. It may be advisable to provide such patients with a supply of oral steroid to use in emergency, for example when the asthma worsens as a result of a chest infection. The dose of Filair 100 Inhaler should be increased at this time and then gradually reduced to the maintenance level after the systemic steroid has been discontinued.

Discontinuation of systemic steroids may cause exacerbation of allergic diseases such as atopic eczema and rhinitis. These should be treated as required with antihistamine and topical therapy.

4.5 Interaction with other medicinal products and other forms of Interaction

None known

4.6 Pregnancy and lactation
There is inadequate evidence of safety in human pregnancy. In animals, systemic administration of relatively high doses can cause abnormalities of foetal development including growth retardation and cleft palate. There may therefore be a very small risk of such effects in the human foetus. However, inhalation of beclometasone dipropionate into the lungs avoids the high level of exposure that occurs with administration by systemic routes.

The use of beclometasone in pregnancy requires that the possible benefits of the drug be weighed against the possible hazards. The drug has been in widespread use for many years without apparent ill consequence.

It is probable that beclometasone is excreted in milk. However, given the relatively low doses used by the inhalation route, the levels are likely to be low. In mothers breast feeding their baby the therapeutic benefits of the drug should be weighed against the potential hazards to mother and baby.

4.7 Effects on ability to drive and use machines
None

4.8 Undesirable effects
Candidiasis of the throat and mouth may develop in some patients, but this can be treated without discontinuation of beclometasone therapy. Hoarseness may also occur.

As with other inhaled therapy, paradoxical bronchospasm with wheezing may occur immediately after dosing. Immediate treatment with an inhaled short-acting bronchodilator is required. Filair 100 Inhaler should be discontinued immediately and alternative prophylactic therapy introduced.

Systemic effects of inhaled corticosteroids may occur particularly at high doses prescribed for prolonged periods. These may include adrenal suppression, growth retardation in children and adolescents, decrease in bone mineral density, cataract and glaucoma.

Hypersensitivity reactions including rashes, urticaria, pruritus and erthyema and oedema of the eyes, face, lips and throat (angioedema) have been reported.

4.9 Overdose
Acute overdosage is unlikely to cause problems. The only harmful effect that follows inhalation of large amounts of the drug over a short time period is suppression of HPA function. Specific emergency action need not be taken. Treatment with Filair 100 Inhaler should be continued at the recommended dose to control the asthma; HPA function recovers in a day or two.

If grossly excessive doses of beclometasone dipropionate were taken over a prolonged period a degree of atrophy of the adrenal cortex could occur in addition to HPA suppression. In this event the patient should be treated as steroid-dependent and transferred to a suitable maintenance dose of a systemic steroid such as prednisolone. Once the condition is stabilised the patient should be returned to Filair 100 Inhaler by the method recommended above.

5. PHARMACOLOGICAL PROPERTIES

5.1 Pharmacodynamic properties
Inhaled beclometasone dipropionate is now well established in the management of asthma. It is a synthetic glucocorticoid and exerts a topical, anti-inflammatory effect on the lungs, without significant systemic activity.

5.2 Pharmacokinetic properties
The beclometasone dipropionate absorbed directly from the lungs is converted to less active metabolites during its passage through the liver. Peak plasma concentrations are reached 3-5 hours following ingestion. Excretion is via the urine.

5.3 Preclinical safety data
Not applicable.

6. PHARMACEUTICAL PARTICULARS

6.1 List of excipients
Sorbitan trioleate Ph Eur

Trichlorofluoromethane (Propellant 11) BP (1988)

Dichlorodifluoromethane (Propellant 12) BP (1988)

Dichlorotetrafluoroethane (Propellant 114) BP (1988)

6.2 Incompatibilities
None known.

6.3 Shelf life
3 years

6.4 Special precautions for storage
Do not store above 30°C. Avoid storage in direct sunlight or heat. Protect from frost.

6.5 Nature and contents of container
10ml Aluminium vial closed with a 50μl metering valve containing 200 doses.

6.6 Instructions for use and handling
Pressurised vial. Do not puncture. Do not burn, even when empty.

Administrative Data

7. MARKETING AUTHORISATION HOLDER
3M Health Care Limited

3M House

Morley Street

Loughborough

Leicestershire

LE11 1EP

8. MARKETING AUTHORISATION NUMBER(S)
0068/0144

9. DATE OF FIRST AUTHORISATION/RENEWAL OF THE AUTHORISATION
January 1992

10. DATE OF REVISION OF THE TEXT
October 2004.

Filair 50 Inhaler

(3M Health Care Limited)

1. NAME OF THE MEDICINAL PRODUCT
Filair 50 Inhaler or Beclometasone Dipropionate 50 micrograms Inhaler

(Throughout the text Filair 50 Inhaler may be replaced by Beclometasone Dipropionate 50 micrograms Inhaler)

2. QUALITATIVE AND QUANTITATIVE COMPOSITION
Each actuation delivers beclometasone dipropionate 50 micrograms (as propellant solvate) into the mouthpiece of the adapter.

3. PHARMACEUTICAL FORM
Pressurised aerosol for inhalation therapy.

4. CLINICAL PARTICULARS

4.1 Therapeutic indications
Filair 50 Inhaler is indicated for the prophylactic treatment of chronic reversible obstructive airways disease.

4.2 Posology and method of administration
The dose should be titrated to the lowest dose at which effective control of asthma is maintained.

ADULTS: for maintenance: 4 inhalations (200 micrograms), twice daily or 2 inhalations (100 micrograms), three or four times daily. In more severe cases a dose of 600-800 micrograms (12-16 inhalations) daily is recommended, with subsequent reductions. The maximum recommended daily dose of this preparation is 1 mg. In patients receiving doses of 1500 micrograms or more daily, adrenal suppression may occur.

CHILDREN: 1 or 2 inhalations (50-100 micrograms), two to four times daily.

ELDERLY: No special dosage recommendations are made for elderly patients.

4.3 Contraindications
Hypersensitivity to beclometasone is a contra-indication. Caution should be observed in patients with pulmonary tuberculosis.

4.4 Special warnings and special precautions for use
Patients should be instructed on the proper use of the inhaler. They should be made aware of the prophylactic nature of Filair therapy and that it should be used regularly at the intervals recommended and not when immediate relief is required.

In patients who have been transferred to inhalation therapy, systemic steroid therapy may need to be re-instated rapidly during periods of stress or where airways obstruction or mucus prevents absorption from the inhalation.

Systemic effects of inhaled corticosteroids may occur, particularly at high doses prescribed for prolonged periods. These effects are much less likely to occur than with oral corticosteroids. Possible systemic effects include adrenal suppression, growth retardation in children and adolescents, decrease in bone mineral density, cataract and glaucoma. It is important therefore that the dose of inhaled steroid is titrated to the lowest dose at which effective control of asthma is maintained.

It is recommended that the height of children receiving prolonged treatment with inhaled corticosteroids is regularly monitored. If growth is slowed, therapy should be reviewed with the aim of reducing the dose of inhaled corticosteroid, if possible, to the lowest dose at which effective control of asthma is maintained. In addition, consideration should be given to referring the patient to a paediatric respiratory specialist.

Prolonged treatment with high doses of inhaled corticosteroids, particularly higher than the recommended doses, may result in clinically significant adrenal suppression. Additional systemic corticosteroid cover should be considered during periods of stress or elective surgery.

Patients who have received systemic steroids for long periods of time or at high doses, or both, need special care and subsequent management when transferred to beclometasone therapy. Recovery from impaired adrenocortical function, caused by prolonged systemic steroid therapy, is slow. The patient should be in a reasonably stable state before being given Filair Inhaler in addition to his usual maintenance dose of systemic steroid. Withdrawal of the systemic steroid should be gradual, starting after about seven days by reducing the daily oral dose by 1 mg prednisolone, or equivalent, at intervals not less than one week. Adrenocortical function should be monitored regularly.

Most patients can be successfully transferred to Filair Inhaler with maintenance of good respiratory function, but special care is necessary for the first months after the transfer until the hypothalamic-pituitary-adrenal (HPA) system has sufficiently recovered to enable the patient to cope with emergencies such as trauma, surgery or infections.

Patients who have been transferred to inhalation therapy should carry a warning card indicating that systemic steroid therapy may need to be re-instated without delay during periods of stress. It may be advisable to provide such patients with a supply of oral steroid to use in emergency, for example when the asthma worsens as a result of a chest infection. The dose of Filair Inhaler should be increased at this time and then gradually reduced to the maintenance level after the systemic steroid has been discontinued.

Discontinuation of systemic steroids may cause exacerbation of allergic diseases such as atopic eczema and rhinitis. These should be treated as required with antihistamine and topical therapy.

4.5 Interaction with other medicinal products and other forms of Interaction
None known

4.6 Pregnancy and lactation
There is inadequate evidence of safety in human pregnancy. In animals, systemic administration of relatively high doses can cause abnormalities of foetal development including growth retardation and cleft palate. There may therefore be a very small risk of such effects in the human foetus. However, inhalation of beclometasone dipropionate into the lungs avoids the high level of exposure that occurs with administration by systemic routes.

The use of beclometasone in pregnancy requires that the possible benefits of the drug be weighed against the possible hazards. The drug has been in widespread use for many years without apparent ill consequence.

It is probable that beclometasone is excreted in milk. However, given the relatively low doses used by the inhalation route, the levels are likely to be low. In mothers breast feeding their baby the therapeutic benefits of the drug should be weighed against the potential hazards to mother and baby.

4.7 Effects on ability to drive and use machines
None

4.8 Undesirable effects
Candidiasis of the throat and mouth may develop in some patients, but this can be treated without discontinuation of beclometasone therapy. Hoarseness may also occur.

As with other inhaled therapy, paradoxical bronchospasm with wheezing may occur immediately after dosing. Immediate treatment with an inhaled short-acting bronchodilator is required. Filair Inhaler should be discontinued immediately and alternative prophylactic therapy introduced.

Systemic effects of inhaled corticosteroids may occur particularly at high doses prescribed for prolonged periods. These may include adrenal suppression, growth retardation in children and adolescents, decrease in bone mineral density, cataract and glaucoma.

Hypersensitivity.reactions including rashes, uticaria, pruritus and erthyema and oedema of the eyes, face, lips and throat (angioedema) have been reported.

4.9 Overdose
Acute overdosage is unlikely to cause problems. The only harmful effect that follows inhalation of large amounts of the drug over a short time period is suppression of HPA function. Specific emergency action need not be taken. Treatment with Filair Inhaler should be continued at the recommended dose to control the asthma; HPA function recovers in a day or two.

If grossly excessive doses of beclometasone dipropionate were taken over a prolonged period a degree of atrophy of the adrenal cortex could occur in addition to HPA suppression. In this event the patient should be treated as steroid-dependent and transferred to a suitable maintenance dose of a systemic steroid such as prednisolone. Once the condition is stabilised the patient should be returned to Filair Inhaler by the method recommended above.

5. PHARMACOLOGICAL PROPERTIES

5.1 Pharmacodynamic properties
Inhaled beclometasone dipropionate is now well established in the management of asthma. It is a synthetic glucocorticoid and exerts a topical, anti-inflammatory effect on the lungs, without significant systemic activity.

5.2 Pharmacokinetic properties
The beclometasone dipropionate absorbed directly from the lungs is converted to less active metabolites during its passage through the liver. Peak plasma concentrations are

reached 3-5 hours following ingestion. Excretion is via the urine.

5.3 Preclinical safety data
Not applicable.

6. PHARMACEUTICAL PARTICULARS

6.1 List of excipients
Sorbitan trioleate Ph Eur
Trichlorofluoromethane (Propellant 11) BP (1988)
Dichlorodifluoromethane (Propellant 12) BP (1988)
Dichlorotetrafluoroethane (Propellant 114) BP (1988)

6.2 Incompatibilities
None known

6.3 Shelf life
3 years

6.4 Special precautions for storage
Do not store above 30°C. Avoid storage in direct sunlight or heat. Protect from frost.

6.5 Nature and contents of container
10ml Aluminium vial closed with a 50μl metering valve containing 200 doses.

6.6 Instructions for use and handling
Pressurised vial. Do not puncture. Do not burn, even when empty.

Administrative Data

7. MARKETING AUTHORISATION HOLDER
3M Health Care Limited
3M House
Morley Street
Loughborough
Leicestershire
LE11 1EP

8. MARKETING AUTHORISATION NUMBER(S)
0068/0121

9. DATE OF FIRST AUTHORISATION/RENEWAL OF THE AUTHORISATION
October 1991

10. DATE OF REVISION OF THE TEXT
October 2004

Filair Forte Inhaler

(3M Health Care Limited)

1. NAME OF THE MEDICINAL PRODUCT
Filair Forte Inhaler and Beclometasone Dipropionate 250 micrograms Inhaler

(Throughout the text Filair Forte Inhaler may be replaced by Beclometasone Dipropionate 250 micrograms Inhaler)

2. QUALITATIVE AND QUANTITATIVE COMPOSITION
Each actuation delivers beclometasone dipropionate 250 micrograms (as propellant solvate) into the mouthpiece of the adapter.

3. PHARMACEUTICAL FORM
Pressurised aerosol for inhalation therapy.

4. CLINICAL PARTICULARS

4.1 Therapeutic indications
Filair Forte Inhaler is indicated for the prophylactic treatment of chronic reversible obstructive airways disease in those patients who require high doses of beclometasone to control their symptoms.

4.2 Posology and method of administration
The dose should be titrated to the lowest dose at which effective control of asthma is maintained.

ADULTS: for maintenance: 2 inhalations (500 micrograms), twice daily or 1 inhalation (250 micrograms), four times daily; may be increased to 2 inhalations four times daily if necessary.

In patients receiving doses of 1500 micrograms or more daily, adrenal suppression may occur. The degree of suppression may not always be clinically significant but it is advisable to provide such patients with a supply of oral steroid to use in stressful situations. The risk of adrenal suppression occurring should be balanced against the therapeutic advantages.

CHILDREN: Filair Forte Inhaler is not recommended for use in children.

ELDERLY: No special dosage recommendations are made for elderly patients.

4.3 Contraindications
Hypersensitivity to beclometasone is a contra-indication. Caution should be observed in patients with pulmonary tuberculosis.

4.4 Special warnings and special precautions for use
Patients should be instructed on the proper use of the inhaler. They should be made aware of the prophylactic nature of Filair therapy and that it should be used regularly at the intervals recommended and not when immediate relief is required.

In patients who have been transferred to inhalation therapy, systemic steroid therapy may need to be re-instated rapidly during periods of stress or where airways obstruction or mucus prevents absorption from the inhalation.

Systemic effects of inhaled corticosteroids may occur, particularly at high doses prescribed for prolonged periods. These effects are much less likely to occur than with oral corticosteroids. Possible systemic effects include adrenal suppression, growth retardation in adolescents, decrease in bone mineral density, cataract and glaucoma. It is important therefore that the dose of inhaled steroid is titrated to the lowest dose at which effective control of asthma is maintained.

It is recommended that the height of adolescents receiving prolonged treatment with inhaled corticosteroids is regularly monitored. If growth is slowed, therapy should be reviewed with the aim of reducing the dose of inhaled corticosteroid, if possible, to the lowest dose at which effective control of asthma is maintained.

Prolonged treatment with high doses of inhaled corticosteroids, particularly higher than the recommended doses, may result in clinically significant adrenal suppression. Additional systemic corticosteroid cover should be considered during periods of stress or elective surgery.

Patients who have received systemic steroids for long periods of time or at high doses, or both, need special care and subsequent management when transferred to beclometasone therapy. Recovery from impaired adrenocortical function, caused by prolonged systemic steroid therapy, is slow. The patient should be in a reasonably stable state before being given Filair Forte Inhaler in addition to his usual maintenance dose of systemic steroid. Withdrawal of the systemic steroid should be gradual, starting after about seven days by reducing the daily oral dose by 1 mg prednisolone, or equivalent, at intervals not less than one week. Adrenocortical function should be monitored regularly.

Most patients can be successfully transferred to Filair Forte Inhaler with maintenance of good respiratory function, but special care is necessary for the first months after the transfer until the hypothalamic-pituitary-adrenal (HPA) system has sufficiently recovered to enable the patient to cope with emergencies such as trauma, surgery or infections.

Patients who have been transferred to inhalation therapy should carry a warning card indicating that systemic steroid therapy may need to be re-instated without delay during periods of stress. It may be advisable to provide such patients with a supply of oral steroid to use in emergency, for example when the asthma worsens as a result of a chest infection. The dose of Filair Forte Inhaler should be increased at this time and then gradually reduced to the maintenance level after the systemic steroid has been discontinued.

Discontinuation of systemic steroids may cause exacerbation of allergic diseases such as atopic eczema and rhinitis. These should be treated as required with antihistamine and topical therapy.

4.5 Interaction with other medicinal products and other forms of Interaction
None known

4.6 Pregnancy and lactation
There is inadequate evidence of safety in human pregnancy. In animals, systemic administration of relatively high doses can cause abnormalities of foetal development including growth retardation and cleft palate. There may therefore be a very small risk of such effects in the human foetus. However, inhalation of beclometasone dipropionate into the lungs avoids the high level of exposure that occurs with administration by systemic routes.

The use of beclometasone in pregnancy requires that the possible benefits of the drug be weighed against the possible hazards. The drug has been in widespread use for many years without apparent ill consequence.

It is probable that beclometasone is excreted in milk. However, given the relatively low doses used by the inhalation route, the levels are likely to be low. In mothers breast feeding their baby the therapeutic benefits of the drug should be weighed against the potential hazards to mother and baby.

4.7 Effects on ability to drive and use machines
None

4.8 Undesirable effects
Candidiasis of the throat and mouth may develop in some patients, but this can be treated without discontinuation of beclometasone therapy. Hoarseness may also occur.

As with other inhaled therapy, paradoxical bronchospasm with wheezing may occur immediately after dosing. Immediate treatment with an inhaled short-acting bronchodilator is required. Filair Forte Inhaler should be discontinued immediately and alternative prophylactic therapy introduced.

Systemic effects of inhaled corticosteroids may occur particularly at high doses prescribed for prolonged periods. These may include adrenal suppression, growth retardation in adolescents, decrease in bone mineral density, cataract and glaucoma.

Hypersensitivity reactions including rashes, urticaria, pruritus and erthyema and oedema of the eyes, face, lips and throat (angioedema) have been reported.

4.9 Overdose
If grossly excessive doses of beclometasone dipropionate were taken over a prolonged period a degree of atrophy of the adrenal cortex could occur in addition to HPA suppression. In this event the patient should be treated as steroid-dependent and transferred to a suitable maintenance dose of a systemic steroid such as prednisolone. Once the condition is stabilised the patient should be returned to Filair Forte Inhaler by the method recommended above. To guard against the unexpected occurrence of adrenal suppression regular tests of adrenal function are advised.

5. PHARMACOLOGICAL PROPERTIES

5.1 Pharmacodynamic properties
Inhaled beclometasone dipropionate is now well established in the management of asthma. It is a synthetic glucocorticoid and exerts a topical, anti-inflammatory effect on the lungs, without significant systemic activity.

5.2 Pharmacokinetic properties
The beclometasone dipropionate absorbed directly from the lungs is converted to less active metabolites during its passage through the liver. Peak plasma concentrations are reached 3-5 hours following ingestion. Excretion is via the urine.

5.3 Preclinical safety data
Not applicable

6. PHARMACEUTICAL PARTICULARS

6.1 List of excipients
Sorbitan trioleate Ph Eur
Trichlorofluoromethane (Propellant 11) BP (1988)
Dichlorodifluoromethane (Propellant 12) BP (1988)
Dichlorotetrafluoroethane (Propellant 114) BP (1988)

6.2 Incompatibilities
None known.

6.3 Shelf life
3 years

6.4 Special precautions for storage
Do not store above 30°C. Avoid storage in direct sunlight or heat. Protect from frost.

6.5 Nature and contents of container
10ml Aluminium vial closed with a 50μl metering valve containing 200 doses.

6.6 Instructions for use and handling
Pressurised vial. Do not puncture. Do not burn, even when empty.

Administrative Data

7. MARKETING AUTHORISATION HOLDER
3M Health Care Limited
3M House
Morley Street
Loughborough
Leicestershire
LE11 1EP

8. MARKETING AUTHORISATION NUMBER(S)
0068/0139

9. DATE OF FIRST AUTHORISATION/RENEWAL OF THE AUTHORISATION
October 1991

10. DATE OF REVISION OF THE TEXT
October 2004.

Flagyl Injection (100ml)

(sanofi-aventis)

1. NAME OF THE MEDICINAL PRODUCT
Flagyl Injection 0.5% w/v (100 ml).
Flagyl Injection - Minibag Plus 0.5% w/v (100 ml).

2. QUALITATIVE AND QUANTITATIVE COMPOSITION
The active component of this injection is metronidazole BP 0.5% w/v.

3. PHARMACEUTICAL FORM
A clean, bright, pale yellow sterile isotonic solution for intravenous infusion.

4. CLINICAL PARTICULARS

4.1 Therapeutic indications
Flagyl is indicated in the prophylaxis and treatment of infections in which anaerobic bacteria have been identified or are suspected to be the cause.

Flagyl is active against a wide range of pathogenic micro-organisms notably species of *Bacteroides, Fusobacteria, Clostridia, Eubacteria*, anaerobic cocci and *Gardnerella vaginalis.*

It is indicated in:

1. The prevention of postoperative infections due to anaerobic bacteria, particularly species of *Bacteroides* and anaerobic Streptococci.

2. The treatment of septicaemia, bacteraemia, peritonitis, brain abscess, necrotising pneumonia, osteomyelitis, puerperal sepsis, pelvic abscess, pelvic cellulitis, and post-operative wound infections from which pathogenic anaerobes have been isolated.

4.2 Posology and method of administration

Flagyl injection should be infused intravenously at an approximate rate of 5 ml/min. Oral medication should be substituted as soon as feasible.

ANAEROBIC INFECTIONS:Treatment for seven days should be satisfactory for most patients but, depending upon clinical and bacteriological assessments, the physician might decide to prolong treatment e.g. for the eradication of infection from sites which cannot be drained or are liable to endogenous recontamination by anaerobic pathogens from the gut, oropharynx or genital tract.

PROPHYLAXIS AGAINST ANAEROBIC INFECTION:Chiefly in the context of abdominal (especially colorectal) and gynaecological surgery.

Adults

500mg shortly before operation, repeated 8 hourly. Oral doses of 200 mg or 400 mg 8 hourly to be started as soon as feasible

Children

7.5 mg/kg (1.5 ml/kg) 8 hourly.

TREATMENT OF ESTABLISHED ANAEROBIC INFECTIONS: Intravenous route is to be used initially if patient's symptoms preclude oral therapy.

Adults

500 mg 8 hourly.

Children

7.5 mg/kg 8 hourly.

Elderly

Caution is advised in the elderly. Particularly at high doses although there is limited information available on modification of dosage.

4.3 Contraindications

Known hypersensitivity to metronidazole.

4.4 Special warnings and special precautions for use

Metronidazole has no direct activity against aerobic or facultative anaerobic bacteria.

Regular clinical and laboratory monitoring are advised if administration of Flagyl for more than 10 days is considered to be necessary.

There is a possibility that after *Trichomonas vaginalis* has been eliminated a gonococcal infection might persist.

The elimination half-life of metronidazole remains unchanged in the presence of renal failure. Therefore the dosage of metronidazole needs no reduction. Such patients however retain the metabolites of metronidazole. The clinical significance of this is not known at present.

In patients undergoing haemodialysis metronidazole and metabolites are efficiently removed during an eight hour period of dialysis. Metronidazole should therefore be re-administered immediately after haemodialysis.

No routine adjustment in the dosage of Flagyl need be made in patients with renal failure undergoing intermittent peritoneal dialysis (IDP) or continuous ambulatory peritoneal dialysis (CAPD).

Metronidazole is mainly metabolised by hepatic oxidation. Substantial impairment of metronidazole clearance may occur in the presence of advanced hepatic insufficiency. Significant cumulation may occur in patients with hepatic encephalopathy and the resulting high plasma concentrations of metronidazole may contribute to the symptoms of the encephalopathy. Flagyl should therefore, be administered with caution to patients with hepatic encephalopathy. The daily dosage should be reduced to one third and may be administered once daily.

Aspartate amino transferase assays may give spuriously low values in patients being treated with metronidzole depending on the method used.

Flagyl should be used with caution in patients with active disease of the CNS.

Cefuroxime is physically and chemically compatible with Flagyl. The following drugs have been shown to be physically compatible in terms of pH and appearance with Flagyl injection over the normal period of administration, although there is no evidence of chemical stability: amikacin sulphate, ampicillin sodium, carbenicillin sodium, cephazolin sodium, cefotaxime sodium, cephalothin sodium, chloramphenicol sodium succinate, clindamycin phosphate, gentamicin sulphate, hydrocortisone sodium succinate, latamoxef disodium, netilmicin sulphate and tobramycin sulphate. In patients maintained on intravenous fluids, Flagyl injection may be diluted with appropriate volumes of normal saline, dextrose-saline, dextrose 5% w/v or potassium chloride infusions (20 and 40 mmol/litre). Apart from the above, Flagyl should on no account be mixed with any other substance.

4.5 Interaction with other medicinal products and other forms of Interaction

Patients should be advised not to take alcohol during metronidazole therapy and for at least 48 hours afterwards because of the possibility of a disulfiram-like (antabuse effect) reaction.

Some potentiation of anticoagulant therapy has been reported when metronidazole has been used with the warfarin type oral anticoagulants. Dosage of the latter may require reducing. Prothrombin times should be monitored. There is no interaction with heparin.

Lithium retention accompanied by evidence of possible renal damage has been reported in patients treated simultaneously with lithium and metronidazole. Lithium treatment should be tapered or withdrawn before administering metronidazole. Plasma concentrations of lithium, creatinine and electrolytes should be monitored in patients under treatment with lithium while they receive metronidazole.

Patients receiving phenobarbitone metabolise metronidazole at a much greater rate than normally, reducing the half-life to approximately 3 hours.

Metronidazole reduces the clearance of 5 fluorouracil and can therefore result in increased toxicity of 5 fluorouracil.

Patients receiving cyclosporin are at risk of elevated cyclosporin serum levels. Serum cyclosporin and serum creatinine should be closely monitored when coadministration is necessary..

4.6 Pregnancy and lactation

There is inadequate evidence of the safety of metronidazole in pregnancy. Flagyl should not therefore be given during pregnancy or during lactation unless the physician considers it essential; in these circumstances the short, high-dosage regimens are not recommended.

4.7 Effects on ability to drive and use machines

Patients should be warned about the potential for drowsiness, dizziness, confusion, hallucinations, convulsions or transient visual disorders, and advised not to drive or operate machinery if these symptoms occur.

4.8 Undesirable effects

During intensive and/or prolonged metronidazole therapy, a few instances of peripheral neuropathy or transient epileptiform seizures have been reported. In most cases neuropathy disappeared after treatment was stopped or when dosage was reduced. A moderate leucopenia has been reported in some patients but the white cell count has always returned to normal before or after treatment has been completed.

Clinicians who contemplate continuous therapy for the relief of chronic conditions, for periods longer than those recommended, are advised to consider the possible therapeutic benefit against the risk of peripheral neuropathy.

Serious adverse reactions occur rarely with standard recommended regimens. Taste disorders, oral mucositis, furred tongue, nausea, vomiting, gastro-intestinal disturbances, anorexia, urticaria and angioedema occur occasionally. Anaphylaxis may occur rarely. Erythema multiforme may occur, which may be reversed on drug withdrawal.

Abnormal liver function tests, cholestatic hepatitis, jaundice and pancreatitis, reversible on drug withdrawal, have been reported very rarely.

Agranulocytosis, neutropenia, thrombocytopenia and pancytopenia, often reversible on drug withdrawal, have very rarely been reported, although fatalities have occurred.

Drowsiness, dizziness, headaches, ataxia, skin rashes, pustular eruptions, pruritus, inco-ordination of movement, darkening of urine (due to metronidazole metabolite) myalgia arthralgia and transient visual disorders such as diplopia and myopia have been reported but very rarely.

Psychotic disorders, including confusion and hallucinations, have been reported very rarely.

4.9 Overdose

There is no specific treatment for gross overdosage of Flagyl.

5. PHARMACOLOGICAL PROPERTIES

5.1 Pharmacodynamic properties

Metronidazole has antiprotozoal and antibacterial actions and is effective against *Trichomonas vaginalis* and other protozoa including *Entamoeba histolytica* and *Giardia lamblia* and against anaerobic bacteria.

5.2 Pharmacokinetic properties

Metronidazole is widely distributed in body tissues after injection. At least half the dose is excreted in the urine as metronidazole and its metabolites, including an acid oxidation product, a hydroxy derivative and glucuronide. Metronidazole diffuses across the placenta, and is found in breast milk of nursing mothers in concentrations equivalent to those in serum.

10% of the dose is bound in plasma.

Clearance: 1.3 ± 0.3 ml/min/kg.

Volume of distribution: 1.1 ± 0.4 litres/kg.

Half-life: 8.5 ± 2.9 hours.

Effective concentration: 3-6 micrograms/ml.

5.3 Preclinical safety data

There are no preclinical data of relevance to the prescriber which are additional to that already included in other sections of the SPC.

6. PHARMACEUTICAL PARTICULARS

6.1 List of excipients

Flagyl injection also contains the following excipients: sodium phosphate (pyrogen free) PhEur, citric acid anhydrous (pyrogen free) PhEur, sodium chloride (pyrogen free) PhEur and water for injections (non-sterilised) BP.

6.2 Incompatibilities

Flagyl injection should not be mixed with cefamandole nafate, cefoxitin sodium, dextrose 10% w/v, compound sodium lactate injection, penicillin G potassium.

6.3 Shelf life

Glass bottles containing 100 ml - 36 months.

Viaflex minibags containing 100 ml - 24 months

6.4 Special precautions for storage

100 ml bottle: store below 30°C, protect from light.

100 ml Viaflex minibags: store below 25°C, protect from light.

6.5 Nature and contents of container

Flagyl injection 0.5% w/v (100 ml) is available in type I glass or type II glass DIN bottles closed with a chlorobutyl or bromobutyl rubber plug.

Flagyl injection 0.5% w/v (100 ml) is available in Viaflex minibags.

Flagyl injection - Minibag Plus 0.5% w/v (100 ml) is available in Viaflex minibags incorporating a combination device.

6.6 Instructions for use and handling

The Viaflex containers are for single use only. Discard any unused portion. Do not reconnect partially used containers.

7. MARKETING AUTHORISATION HOLDER

May and Baker Limited

trading as

May & Baker or Rorer Pharmaceuticals or Rhône-Poulenc Rorer or Pharmuka or Theraplix or APS or Berk Pharmaceuticals

RPR House

50 Kings Hill Avenue

Kings Hill

West Malling

Kent ME19 4AH

8. MARKETING AUTHORISATION NUMBER(S)

PL 00012/0107

9. DATE OF FIRST AUTHORISATION/RENEWAL OF THE AUTHORISATION

24 September 1996

10. DATE OF REVISION OF THE TEXT

May 2001

11 LEGAL CLASSIFICATION

POM

Flagyl S Suspension

(sanofi-aventis)

1. NAME OF THE MEDICINAL PRODUCT

Flagyl S Suspension

2. QUALITATIVE AND QUANTITATIVE COMPOSITION

In terms of the active ingredient

The active component of this suspension is 320 mg/5ml metronidazole benzoate equivalent to 200 mg/5 ml metronidazole.

3. PHARMACEUTICAL FORM

Flagyl S suspension is a white to cream suspension with a slight yellow tinge and an odour of orange and lemon.

4. CLINICAL PARTICULARS

4.1 Therapeutic indications

Flagyl S is administered orally for:

1. The prevention of post-operative infections due to anaerobic bacteria, particularly species of *Bacteroides*, and anaerobic streptococci.

2. Treatment of urogenital trichomonas in the female (trichomonal vaginitis) and in the male.

3. Treatment of all forms of amoebiasis (intestinal and extra-intestinal disease and that of symptomless cyst passers).

4. Treatment of giardiasis.

5. Treatment of acute ulcerative gingivitis (Vincent's).

6. Treatment of anaerobically-infected leg ulcers and pressure sores.

7. Treatment of acute dental infections (e.g. acute pericoronitis and acute apical infections).

8. Treatment of septicaemia, bacteraemia, brain abscess, necrotising pneumonia, osteomyelitis, puerperal sepsis,

pelvic abscess, pelvic cellulitis, peritonitis, and post-operative wound infections from which pathogenic anaerobes have been isolated.

9. Non specific vaginitis.

4.2 Posology and method of administration

For oral administration.

Suspension can be diluted with syrup BP.

Dosage is given in terms of metronidazole or metronidazole equivalent.

Treatment of anaerobic infections:

Treatment for seven days should be satisfactory for most patients but, depending on the clinical and bacteriological assessments, the physician might decide to prolong treatment. The tablets or suspension may be given alone or concurrently with other appropriate antibacterial agents.

Adults and children over 10 years - 400 mg orally three times daily.

Children and infants - 7.5 mg/kg bodyweight three times daily.

Protozoal and other infections:

(see Table 1)

(see Table 2)

4.3 Contraindications

Known hypersensitivity to metronidazole.

4.4 Special warnings and special precautions for use

Regular clinical and laboratory monitoring are advised if administration of Flagyl for more than 10 days is considered to be necessary.

There is a possibility that after *Trichomonas vaginalis* has been eliminated a gonococcal infection might persist.

The elimination half-life of metronidazole remains unchanged in the presence of renal failure. The dosage of metronidazole therefore needs no reduction. Such patients however retain the metabolites of metronidazole. The clinical significance of this is not known at present.

In patients undergoing haemodialysis metronidazole and metabolites are efficiently removed during an eight hour period of dialysis. Metronidazole should therefore be re-administered immediately after haemodialysis.

No routine adjustment in the dosage of Flagyl need be made in patients with renal failure undergoing intermittent peritoneal dialysis (IDP) or continuous ambulatory peritoneal dialysis (CAPD).

Metronidazole is mainly metabolised by hepatic oxidation. Substantial impairment of metronidazole clearance may occur in the presence of advanced hepatic insufficiency. Significant cumulation may occur in patients with hepatic encephalopathy and the resulting high plasma concentrations of metronidazole may contribute to the symptoms of the encephalopathy. Flagyl should therefore, be administered with caution to patients with hepatic encephalopathy. The daily dosage should be reduced to one third and may be administered once daily.

4.5 Interaction with other medicinal products and other forms of Interaction

Patients should be advised not to take alcohol during metronidazole therapy and for at least 48 hours afterwards because of the possibility of a disulfiram-like (antabuse effect) reaction.

Some potentiation of anticoagulant therapy has been reported when metronidazole has been used with the warfarin type oral anticoagulants. Dosage of the latter may require reducing. Prothrombin times should be monitored. There is no interaction with heparin.

Lithium retention accompanied by evidence of possible renal damage has been reported in patients treated simultaneously with lithium and metronidazole. Lithium treatment should be tapered or withdrawn before administering metronidazole. Plasma concentrations of lithium, creatinine and electrolytes should be monitored in patients under treatment with lithium while they receive metronidazole.

Patients receiving phenobarbitone metabolise metronidazole at a much greater rate than normally, reducing the half-life to approximately 3 hours.

Metronidazole reduces the clearance of 5 fluorouracil and can therefore result in increased toxicity of 5 fluorouracil.

Patients receiving cyclosporin are at risk of elevated cyclosporin serum levels. Serum cyclosporin and serum creatinine should be closely monitored when coadministration is necessary.

4.6 Pregnancy and lactation

There is inadequate evidence of the safety of metronidazole in pregnancy. Flagyl should not be given during pregnancy or during lactation unless the physician considers it essential; in these circumstances the short, high-dosage regimens are not recommended.

4.7 Effects on ability to drive and use machines

Patients should be warned about the potential for drowsiness, dizziness, confusion, hallucinations, convulsions or transient visual disorders, and advised not to drive or operate machinery if these symptoms occur.

4.8 Undesirable effects

During intensive and/or prolonged metronidazole therapy, a few instances of peripheral neuropathy or transient epileptiform seizures have been reported. In most cases neuropathy disappeared after treatment was stopped or when dosage was reduced. A moderate leucopenia has been reported in some patients but the white cell count has always returned to normal before or after treatment has been completed.

Clinicians who contemplate continuous therapy for the relief of chronic conditions, for periods longer than those recommended, are advised to consider the possible therapeutic benefit against the risk of peripheral neuropathy.

Serious adverse reactions occur rarely with standard recommended regimens. Taste disorders, oral mucositis, furred tongue, nausea, vomiting, gastro-intestinal disturbances, anorexia, urticaria and angioedema occur occasionally. Anaphylaxis may occur rarely. Erythema multiforme may occur, which may be reversed on drug withdrawal.

Abnormal liver function tests, cholestatic hepatitis, jaundice and pancreatitis, reversible on drug withdrawal have been reported but very rarely.

Agranulocytosis, neutropenia, thrombocytopenia and pancytopenia, often reversible on drug withdrawal have been very rarely reported, although fatalities have occurred.

Drowsiness, dizziness, headaches, ataxia, skin rashes, pustular eruptions, pruritus, inco-ordination of movement, darkening of urine (due to metronidazole metabolite), myalgia, arthralgia and transient visual disorders such as diplopia and myopia have been reported but very rarely.

Psychotic disorders, including confusion and hallucinations, have been reported very rarely.

4.9 Overdose

There is no specific treatment for gross overdosage of Flagyl

5. PHARMACOLOGICAL PROPERTIES

5.1 Pharmacodynamic properties

Metronidazole is active against a wide range of pathogenic micro-organisms notably species of *Bacteroides*, *Fusobacteria*, *Clostridia*, *Eubacteria*, anaerobic cocci and *Gardnerella vaginalis*. It is also active against *Trichomonas*, *Entamoeba histolytica*, *Giardia lamblia* and *Balantidium coli*.

5.2 Pharmacokinetic properties

Metronidazole is rapidly absorbed after oral administration of Flagyl with peak plasma concentrations occur after 20 min to 3 hours.

The elimination half-life of metronidazole is 7 - 8 hours. Metronidazole is excreted in milk but the intake of a suckling infant of a mother receiving normal dose would be considerably less than the therapeutic dosage for infants.

5.3 Preclinical safety data

There are no preclinical data of relevance to the prescriber which are additional to that already included in other sections of the SPC.

6. PHARMACEUTICAL PARTICULARS

6.1 List of excipients

Liquid sugar granular liquors (sucrose)

sodium dihydrogen phosphate LC BP or sodium acid phosphate crystalline BP

Veegum HV

methyl hydroxybenzoate BP (E218)

propyl hydroxybenzoate BP (E216)

ethanol 96% v/v BP

lemon No. 1 NA

oil orange terpenless BP

demineralised water BP

6.2 Incompatibilities

None known.

Table 1 Protozoal and other infections

Dosage is given in terms of metronidazole or metronidazole equivalent

	Duration of dosage in days	Adults and children over 10 years	Children 7 to 10 years	Children 3 to 7 years	Children 1 to 3 years
Urogenital trichomoniasis	7	200 mg three times daily	100 mg three times daily	100 mg twice daily	50 mg three times daily
Where re-infection is likely, in adults the consort should receive a similar course of treatment concurrently	or 2	800 mg in the morning and 1,200 mg in the evening			
		2.0 g as a single dose			
Non-specific vaginitis	7	400 mg twice daily			
	or				
	1	2.0g as a single dose			

Table 2 Protozoal and other infections

Dosage is given in terms of metronidazole or metronidazole equivalent

	Duration of dosage in days	Adults and children over 10 years	Children 7 to 10 years	Children 3 to 7 years	Children 1 to 3 years
Amoebiasis (a) Invasive intestinal disease in susceptible subjects	5	800 mg three times daily	400 mg three times daily	200 mg four times daily	200 mg three times daily
(b) Intestinal disease in less susceptible subjects and chronic amoebic hepatitis	5-10	400mg three times daily	200mg three times daily	100mg four times daily	100mg three times daily
(c) Amoebic liver abscess also other forms of extra-intestinal amoebiasis	5	400mg three times daily	200mg three times daily	100mg four times daily	100mg three times daily
(d) Symptomless cyst passers	5-10	400-800 mg three times daily	200-400 mg three times daily	100-200 mg four times daily	100-200 mg three times daily
Giardiasis	3	2.0 g once daily	1.0 g once daily	600-800 mg once daily	500 mg once daily
Acute ulcerative gingivitis	3	200 mg three times daily	100 mg three times daily	100 mg twice daily	50 mg three times daily
Acute dental infections	3-7	200 mg three times daily			
Leg ulcers and pressure sores	7	400 mg three times daily			

Immature children and infants weighing less than 10 kg should receive proportionally smaller dosages.

6.3 Shelf life
36 months.

After dilution with syrup BP the shelf life is 14 days.

6.4 Special precautions for storage
Store below 25°C. Protect from light.

6.5 Nature and contents of container
Flagyl S suspension is available in amber glass bottles containing 50, 100 or 125 ml with either a rolled on pilfer proof aluminium cap and a PVDC emulsion coated wad or a HDPE/polypropylene child resistant cap with a tamper evident band.

6.6 Instructions for use and handling
None stated.

7. MARKETING AUTHORISATION HOLDER
Hawgreen Limited
4 Priory Hall
Stillorgan Road
Stillorgan
Dublin
Eire

8. MARKETING AUTHORISATION NUMBER(S)
PL 17077/0001

9. DATE OF FIRST AUTHORISATION/RENEWAL OF THE AUTHORISATION
September 1998

10. DATE OF REVISION OF THE TEXT
July 2005

11. Legal Classification
POM

Flagyl Suppositories

(sanofi-aventis)

1. NAME OF THE MEDICINAL PRODUCT
Flagyl Suppositories 500 mg.
Flagyl Suppositories 1g

2. QUALITATIVE AND QUANTITATIVE COMPOSITION
In terms of the active ingredient;

Flagyl Suppositories 500 mg: The active component of the suppository is metronidazole BP 500 mg.

Flagyl Suppositories 1g: The active component of the suppository is metronidazole BP 1.0 g.

3. PHARMACEUTICAL FORM
A cream coloured, smooth, torpedo-shaped suppository.

4. CLINICAL PARTICULARS
4.1 Therapeutic indications
1. Treatment of infections in which anaerobic bacteria have been identified or are suspected as pathogens, particularly *Bacteroides fragilis* and other species of *Bacteroides* and including other species for which metronidazole is bactericidal, such as *Fusobacteria*, *Eubacteria*, *Clostridia* and anaerobic cocci.

Flagyl has been used successfully in: septicaemia, bacteraemia, brain abscess, necrotising pneumonia, osteomyelitis, puerperal sepsis, pelvic abscess, pelvic cellulitis, peritonitis and post-operative wound infection from which one or more of these anaerobes have been isolated.

2. Prevention of post-operative infections due to an anaerobic bacteria, particularly species of *Bacteroides* and anaerobic Streptococci.

4.2 Posology and method of administration
Route of administration: Rectal

1. Treatment of Anaerobic Infections:

Adults and children over 10 years: 1 gram suppository inserted into the rectum eight hourly for three days. Oral medication with 400 mg three times daily should be substituted as soon as this becomes feasible. If rectal medication must be continued for more than three days, the suppositories should be inserted at 12 hourly intervals.

Children (5 -10 years): As for adults but with 500 mg suppositories and oral medication with 7.5 mg/kg bodyweight three times daily.

Infants and children under 5 years: As for children of 5-10 years but with appropriate reduction in dosage of suppositories (one half of a 500 mg suppository for 1 to 5 years and one quarter of a 500 mg suppository for under 1 year).

2. Prevention of Anaerobic Infections:

In appendectomy and post-operative medication for elective colonic surgery.

Adults and children over 10 years: 1 gram suppository inserted into the rectum two hours before surgery and repeated at eight hourly intervals until oral medication (200 to 400 mg three times daily) can be given to complete a seven day course.

If rectal medication is necessary after the third post-operative day, the frequency of administration should be reduced to 12 hourly.

Children (5-10 years): 500 mg suppositories administered as for adults until oral medication (3.7 to 7.5 mg/kg bodyweight three times daily) becomes possible.

4.3 Contraindications
Known hypersensitivity to metronidazole.

4.4 Special warnings and special precautions for use
Metronidazole has no direct activity against aerobic or facultative anaerobic bacteria.

Regular clinical and laboratory monitoring are advised if administration of Flagyl for more than 10 days is considered to be necessary.

There is a possibility that after *Trichomonas vaginalis* has been eliminated a gonococcal infection might persist.

The elimination half-life of metronidazole remains unchanged in the presence of renal failure. The dosage of metronidazole therefore needs no reduction. Such patients however retain the metabolites of metronidazole. The clinical significance of this is not known at present.

In patients undergoing haemodialysis metronidazole and metabolites are efficiently removed during an eight hour period of dialysis. Metronidazole should therefore be re-administered immediately after haemodialysis.

No routine adjustment in the dosage of Flagyl need be made in patients with renal failure undergoing intermittent peritoneal dialysis (IDP) or continuous ambulatory peritoneal dialysis (CAPD).

Metronidazole is mainly metabolised by hepatic oxidation. Substantial impairment of metronidazole clearance may occur in the presence of advanced hepatic insufficiency. Significant cumulation may occur in patients with hepatic encephalopathy and the resulting high plasma concentrations of metronidazole may contribute to the symptoms of the encephalopathy. Flagyl should therefore, be administered with caution to patients with hepatic encephalopathy. The daily dosage should be reduced to one third and may be administered once daily.

4.5 Interaction with other medicinal products and other forms of Interaction
Patients should be advised not to take alcohol during metronidazole therapy and for at least 48 hours afterwards because of the possibility of a disulfiram-like (antabuse effect) reaction.

Some potentiation of anticoagulant therapy has been reported when metronidazole has been used with the warfarin type oral anticoagulants. Dosage of the latter may require reducing. Prothrombin times should be monitored. There is no interaction with heparin.

Lithium retention accompanied by evidence of possible renal damage has been reported in patients treated simultaneously with lithium and metronidazole. Lithium treatment should be tapered or withdrawn before administering metronidazole. Plasma concentrations of lithium, creatinine and electrolytes should be monitored in patients under treatment with lithium while they receive metronidazole.

Patients receiving phenobarbitone metabolise metronidazole at a much greater rate than normally, reducing the half-life to approximately 3 hours.

Metronidazole reduces the clearance of 5 fluorouracil and can therefore result in increased toxicity of 5 fluorouracil.

Patients receiving cyclosporin are at risk of elevated cyclosporin serum levels. Serum cyclosporin and serum creatinine should be closely monitored when coadministration is necessary.

4.6 Pregnancy and lactation
There is inadequate evidence of the safety of metronidazole in pregnancy. Flagyl should not be given during pregnancy or during lactation unless the physician considers it essential; in these circumstances the short, high-dosage regimens are not recommended.

4.7 Effects on ability to drive and use machines
Patients should be warned about the potential for drowsiness, dizziness, confusion, hallucinations, convulsions or transient visual disorders, and advised not to drive or operate machinery if these symptoms occur.

4.8 Undesirable effects
During intensive and/or prolonged metronidazole therapy, a few instances of peripheral neuropathy or transient epileptiform seizures have been reported. In most cases neuropathy disappeared after treatment was stopped or when dosage was reduced.

A moderate leucopenia has been reported in some patients but the white cell count has always returned to normal before or after treatment has been completed.

Clinicians who contemplate continuous therapy for the relief of chronic conditions, for periods longer than those recommended, are advised to consider the possible therapeutic benefit against the risk of peripheral neuropathy.

Serious adverse reactions occur rarely with standard recommended regimens. Taste disorders, oral mucositis, furred tongue, nausea, vomiting, gastro-intestinal disturbances, anorexia, urticaria and angioedema occur occasionally. Anaphylaxis may occur rarely. Erythema multiforme may occur, which may be reversed on drug withdrawal.

Abnormal liver function tests, cholestatic hepatitis, jaundice and pancreatitis, reversible on drug withdrawal have been reported but very rarely.

Agranulocytosis, neutropenia, thrombocytopenia and pancytopenia, often reversible on drug withdrawal, have been very rarely reported, although fatalities have occurred.

Drowsiness, dizziness, headaches, ataxia, skin rashes, pustular eruptions, pruritus, inco-ordination of movement, darkening of urine (due to metronidazole metabolite), myalgia, arthralgia and transient visual disorders such as diplopia and myopia have been reported but very rarely.

Psychotic disorders, including confusion and hallucinations, have been reported very rarely.

4.9 Overdose
There is no specific treatment for gross overdosage of Flagyl

5. PHARMACOLOGICAL PROPERTIES
5.1 Pharmacodynamic properties
Metronidazole has antiprotozoal and antibacterial actions and is effective against *Trichomonas vaginalis* and other protozoa including *Entamoeba histolytica* and *Giardia lamblia* and against anaerobic bacteria.

5.2 Pharmacokinetic properties
Metronidazole is readily absorbed from the rectal mucosa and widely distributed in body tissues. Maximum concentrations occur in the serum after about 1 hour and traces are detected after 24 hours.

At least half the dose is excreted in the urine as metronidazole and its metabolites, including an acid oxidation product, a hydroxy derivative and glucoronide. Metronidazole diffuses across the placenta, and is found in breast milk of nursing mothers in concentrations equivalent to those in serum.

5.3 Preclinical safety data
There are no preclinical data of relevance to the prescriber which are additional to that already included in other sections of the SPC.

6. PHARMACEUTICAL PARTICULARS
6.1 List of excipients
Flagyl suppository also contain the following excipients: suppository base E75 and suppository base W35.

6.2 Incompatibilities
None stated.

6.3 Shelf life
36 months.

6.4 Special precautions for storage
Store below 20°C, protect from light.

6.5 Nature and contents of container
Flagyl suppositories are available PVC/polyethylene bandoliers containing 10 suppositories.

6.6 Instructions for use and handling
None stated.

7. MARKETING AUTHORISATION HOLDER
Hawgreen Limited
4, Priory Hall
Stillorgan Road
Stillorgan
Dublin
Eire

8. MARKETING AUTHORISATION NUMBER(S)
Flagyl Suppositories 500 mg: PL 17077/0004

Flagyl Suppositories 1g: PL 17077/0005

9. DATE OF FIRST AUTHORISATION/RENEWAL OF THE AUTHORISATION
September 1998

10. DATE OF REVISION OF THE TEXT
January 2002

11. Legal Classification
POM

Flagyl Tablets 200 mg & 400mg

(sanofi-aventis)

1. NAME OF THE MEDICINAL PRODUCT
Flagyl Tablets 200 mg
Flagyl Tablets 400 mg

2. QUALITATIVE AND QUANTITATIVE COMPOSITION
Flagyl Tablets 200 mg: The active component of these tablets is metronidazole BP 200 mg.

Flagyl Tablets 400 mg: The active component of these tablets is metronidazole BP 400 mg.

3. PHARMACEUTICAL FORM
Flagyl tablets 200 mg:

White to off-white, biconvex, capsule shaped, film coated tablets impressed 'FLAGYL 200' on one face, plain reverse.

Flagyl tablets 400 mg:

White to off-white, biconvex, capsule shaped, film coated tablets impressed 'FLAGYL 400' on one face, plain revers

4. CLINICAL PARTICULARS

4.1 Therapeutic indications

Flagyl is indicated in the prophylaxis and treatment of infections in which anaerobic bacteria have been identified or are suspected to be the cause.

Flagyl is active against a wide range of pathogenic micro-organisms notably species of *Bacteroides*, *Fusobacteria*, *Clostridia*, *Eubacteria*, anaerobic cocci and *Gardnerella vaginalis*.

It is also active against *Trichomonas*, *Entamoeba histolytica*, *Giardia lamblia* and *Balantidium coli*.

It is indicated in:

1. The prevention of post-operative infections due to anaerobic bacteria, particularly species of *Bacteroides* and anaerobic streptococci.
2. The treatment of septicaemia, bacteraemia, peritonitis, brain abscess, necrotising pneumonia, osteomyelitis, puerperal sepsis, pelvic abscess, pelvic cellulitis, and post-operative wound infections from which pathogenic anaerobes have been isolated.
3. Urogenital trichomoniasis in the female (trichomonal vaginitis) and in the male.
4. Bacterial vaginosis (also known as non-specific vaginitis, anaerobic vaginosis or Gardnerella vaginitis).
5. All forms of amoebiasis (intestinal and extra-intestinal disease and that of symptomless cyst passers).
6. Giardiasis.
7. Acute ulcerative gingivitis.
8. Anaerobically-infected leg ulcers and pressure sores.
9. Acute dental infections (e.g. acute pericoronitis and acute apical infections).

4.2 Posology and method of administration

Oral route of administration.

Flagyl tablets should be swallowed with water (not chewed). It is recommended that the tablets be taken during or after a meal.

Anaerobic infections: The duration of a course of Flagyl treatment is about 7 days but it will depend upon the seriousness of the patient's condition as assessed clinically and bacteriologically.

Prophylaxis against anaerobic infection: Chiefly in the context of abdominal (especially colorectal) and gynaecological surgery.

ADULTS

400 mg 8 hourly during 24 hours immediately preceding operation followed by postoperative intravenous or rectal administration until the patient is able to take tablets.

CHILDREN

7.5 mg/kg 8 hourly.

Treatment of established anaerobic infection:

ADULTS

800 mg followed by 400 mg 8 hourly.

CHILDREN

7.5 mg/kg 8 hourly

Protozoal and other infections:

(see Table 1 below)

(see Table 2 above)

Table 2 Protozoal and other infections

Dosage is given in terms of metronidazole or metronidazole equivalent

	Duration of dosage in days	Adults and children over 10 years	Children 7 to 10 years	3 to 7 years	1 to 3 years
Acute ulcerative gingivitis	3	200 mg three times daily	100 mg three times daily	100 mg twice daily	50 mg three times daily
Acute dental infections	3-7	200 mg three times daily			
Leg ulcers and pressure sores	7	400 mg three times daily			

Children and infants weighing less than 10 kg should receive proportionally smaller dosages.

Elderly: Flagyl is well tolerated by the elderly but a pharmacokinetic study suggests cautious use of high dosage regimens in this age group.

4.3 Contraindications

Known hypersensitivity to metronidazole.

4.4 Special warnings and special precautions for use

Regular clinical and laboratory monitoring are advised if administration of Flagyl for more than 10 days is considered to be necessary.

There is a possibility that after *Trichomonas vaginalis* has been eliminated a gonococcal infection might persist.

The elimination half-life of metronidazole remains unchanged in the presence of renal failure. The dosage of metronidazole therefore needs no reduction. Such patients however retain the metabolites of metronidazole. The clinical significance of this is not known at present.

In patients undergoing haemodialysis metronidazole and metabolites are efficiently removed during an eight hour period of dialysis. Metronidazole should therefore be re-administered immediately after haemodialysis.

No routine adjustment in the dosage of Flagyl need be made in patients with renal failure undergoing intermittent peritoneal dialysis (IDP) or continuous ambulatory peritoneal dialysis (CAPD).

Metronidazole is mainly metabolised by hepatic oxidation. Substantial impairment of metronidazole clearance may occur in the presence of advanced hepatic insufficiency. Significant cumulation may occur in patients with hepatic encephalopathy and the resulting high plasma concentrations of metronidazole may contribute to the symptoms of the encephalopathy. Flagyl should therefore, be administered with caution to patients with hepatic encephalopathy. The daily dosage should be reduced to one third and may be administered once daily.

Table 1 Protozoal and other infections

Dosage is given in terms of metronidazole or metronidazole equivalent

	Duration of dosage in days	Adults and children over 10 years	Children 7 to 10 years	3 to 7 years	1 to 3 years
Urogenital trichomoniasis	7	200 mg three times daily	100 mg three times daily	100 mg twice daily	50 mg three times daily
		or			
Where re-infection is likely, in adults the consort should receive a similar course of treatment concurrently		400 mg twice daily			
	or				
	2	800 mg in the morning and 1,200 mg in the evening			
		2.0 g as a single dose			
Bacterial vaginosis	7	400 mg twice daily			
	or				
	1	2.0g as a single dose			
Amoebiasis (a) Invasive intestinal disease in susceptible subjects	5	800 mg three times daily	400 mg three times daily	200 mg four times daily	200 mg three times daily
(b) Intestinal disease in less susceptible subjects and chronic amoebic hepatitis	5-10	400 mg three times daily	200 mg three times daily	100 mg four times daily	100 mg three times daily
(c) Amoebic liver abscess also other forms of extra-intestinal amoebiasis	5	400 mg three times daily	200 mg three times daily	100 mg four times daily	100 mg three times daily
(d) Symptomless cyst passers	5-10	400-800 mg three times daily	200-400 mg three times daily	100-200 mg four times daily	100-200 mg three times daily
Giardiasis	3	2.0 g once daily	1.0 g once daily	600-800 mg once daily	500 mg once daily

4.5 Interaction with other medicinal products and other forms of Interaction

Patients should be advised not to take alcohol during metronidazole therapy and for at least 48 hours afterwards because of the possibility of a disulfiram-like (antabuse effect) reaction.

Some potentiation of anticoagulant therapy has been reported when metronidazole has been used with the warfarin type oral anticoagulants. Dosage of the latter may require reducing. Prothrombin times should be monitored. There is no interaction with heparin.

Lithium retention accompanied by evidence of possible renal damage has been reported in patients treated simultaneously with lithium and metronidazole. Lithium treatment should be tapered or withdrawn before administering metronidazole. Plasma concentrations of lithium, creatinine and electrolytes should be monitored in patients under treatment with lithium while they receive metronidazole.

Patients receiving phenobarbitone metabolise metronidazole at a much greater rate than normally, reducing the half-life to approximately 3 hours.

Metronidazole reduces the clearance of 5 fluorouracil and can therefore result in increased toxicity of 5 fluorouracil.

Patients receiving cyclosporin are at risk of elevated cyclosporin serum levels. Serum cyclosporin and serum creatinine should be closely monitored when coadministration is necessary.

4.6 Pregnancy and lactation

There is inadequate evidence of the safety of metronidazole in pregnancy but it has been in wide use for many years without apparent ill consequence. Nevertheless Flagyl, like other medicines, should not be given during pregnancy or during lactation unless the physician considers it essential; in these circumstances the short, high-dosage regimens are not recommended.

4.7 Effects on ability to drive and use machines

Patients should be warned about the potential for drowsiness, dizziness, confusion, hallucinations, convulsions or transient visual disorders, and advised not to drive or operate machinery if these symptoms occur.

4.8 Undesirable effects

During intensive and/or prolonged metronidazole therapy, a few instances of peripheral neuropathy or transient epileptiform seizures have been reported. In most cases neuropathy disappeared after treatment was stopped or when dosage was reduced. A moderate leucopenia has been reported in some patients but the white cell count has always returned to normal before or after treatment has been completed.

Clinicians who contemplate continuous therapy for the relief of chronic conditions, for periods longer than those recommended, are advised to consider the possible therapeutic benefit against the risk of peripheral neuropathy.

Serious adverse reactions occur rarely with standard recommended regimens. Taste disorders, oral mucositis, furred tongue, nausea, vomiting, gastro-intestinal disturbances, anorexia, urticaria and angioedema occur occasionally. Anaphylaxis may occur rarely. Erythema multiforme may occur, which may be reversed on drug withdrawal.

Abnormal liver function tests, cholestatic hepatitis, jaundice and pancreatitis, reversible on drug withdrawal have been reported but very rarely.

Agranulocytosis, neutropenia, thrombocytopenia and pancytopenia, often reversible on drug withdrawal, have been very rarely reported, although fatalities have occurred.

Drowsiness, dizziness, headaches, ataxia, skin rashes, pustular eruptions, pruritus, inco-ordination of movement, darkening of urine (due to metronidazole metabolite) myalgia, arthralgia and transient visual disorders such as diplopia and myopia have been reported but very rarely.

Psychotic disorders, including confusion and hallucinations, have been reported very rarely.

4.9 Overdose
There is no specific treatment for gross overdosage of Flagyl

5. PHARMACOLOGICAL PROPERTIES

5.1 Pharmacodynamic properties
Metronidazole has antiprotozoal and antibacterial actions and is effective against *Trichomonas vaginalis* and other protozoa including *Entamoeba histolytica* and *Giardia lamblia* and against anaerobic bacteria.

5.2 Pharmacokinetic properties
Metronidazole is rapidly and almost completely absorbed on administration of Flagyl tablets; peak plasma concentrations occur after 20 min to 3 hours.

The half-life of metronidazole is 8.5 ± 2.9 hours. Metronidazole can be used in chronic renal failure; it is rapidly removed from the plasma by dialysis. Metronidazole is excreted in milk but the intake of a suckling infant of a mother receiving normal dosage would be considerably less than the therapeutic dosage for infants.

5.3 Preclinical safety data
There are no preclinical data of relevance to the prescriber which are additional to that already included in other sections of the SPC.

6. PHARMACEUTICAL PARTICULARS

6.1 List of excipients
Flagyl 200mg & 400mg tablets also contain the following excipients:

calcium hydrogen phosphate BP (E341), starch maize BP, Povidone K30 BP (E1201), magnesium stearate BP (E572), Pharmacoat 615 (E464), macrogol 400 Ph. Eur., French chalk powdered (E533(b)) and demineralised water.

6.2 Incompatibilities
None known.

6.3 Shelf life
60 months.

6.4 Special precautions for storage
Store protected from light.

6.5 Nature and contents of container
Flagyl tablets 200 mg are available in aluminium/plastic blisters of 21 tablets and HDPE bottles of 100 and 250 tablets.

Flagyl tablets 400 mg are available in aluminium/plastic blisters of 14 tablets and HDPE bottles of 100 tablets.

6.6 Instructions for use and handling
None stated.

7. MARKETING AUTHORISATION HOLDER
Hawgreen Limited

4 Priory Hall

Stillorgan Road

Stillorgan

Dublin

Eire

8. MARKETING AUTHORISATION NUMBER(S)
Flagyl 200mg tablets: PL 17077/0002

Flagyl 400mg tablets: PL 17077/0003

9. DATE OF FIRST AUTHORISATION/RENEWAL OF THE AUTHORISATION
September 1998

10. DATE OF REVISION OF THE TEXT
July 2005

11. Legal Classification
POM

Flamatak MR

(Alpharma Limited)

1. NAME OF THE MEDICINAL PRODUCT
FLAMATAK MR TABLETS 75mg

2. QUALITATIVE AND QUANTITATIVE COMPOSITION
Diclofenac Sodium PhEur 75mg

3. PHARMACEUTICAL FORM
Prolonged release tablet.

4. CLINICAL PARTICULARS

4.1 Therapeutic indications
Adults:

Relief of all grades of pain and inflammation in a wide range of conditions, including:

(i) arthritic conditions: rheumatoid arthritis, osteoarthritis, ankylosing spondylitis, acute gout.

(ii) acute musculo-skeletal disorders such as periarthritis (for example frozen shoulder), tendinitis, tenosynovitis, bursitis.

(iii) other painful conditions resulting from trauma, including fracture, low back pain, sprains, strains, dislocations, orthopaedic, dental and other minor surgery.

4.2 Posology and method of administration

4.2.1 Dosage
Adults: One tablet once or twice daily, taken whole with liquid, preferably at meal times.

Elderly: Although the pharmacokinetics of diclofenac sodium are not impaired to any clinically relevant extent in elderly patients, non-steroidal anti-inflammatory drugs should be used with particular caution in such patients who generally are more prone to adverse reactions. In particular it is recommended that the lowest effective dosage be used in frail elderly patients or those with a low body weight (see also precautions).

Children: Diclofenac sodium is not recommended for use in children as dosage recommendations and indications for use in this group of patients have not been established.

4.2.2 Administration

For oral use only.

4.3 Contraindications
Active or suspected peptic ulcer or gastro-intestinal bleeding.

Previous sensitivity to diclofenac sodium.

Patients in whom attacks of asthma, urticaria or acute rhinitis are precipitated by aspirin or other non-steroidal anti-inflammatory agents.

4.4 Special warnings and special precautions for use
Gastro-intestinal:

Close medical surveillance is imperative in patients with symptoms indicative of gastro-intestinal disorders, with a history suggestive of gastro-intestinal ulceration, with ulcerative colitis or with Crohn's disease, bleeding diathesis or haematological abnormalities.

Gastro-intestinal bleeding ulceration/perforation, haematemesis and melaena have in general more serious consequences in the elderly. They can occur at any time during treatment with or without warning symptoms or a previous history. In the rare instances where gastro-intestinal bleeding or ulceration occurs in patients receiving diclofenac sodium the drug should be withdrawn.

Hypersensitivity reactions:

As with other nonsteroidal anti-inflammatory drugs, allergic reactions, including anaphylactic/anaphylactoid reactions, can also occur without earlier exposure to the drug.

Renal:

Patients with renal, cardiac or hepatic impairment and the elderly should be kept under surveillance, since the use of NSAIDS may result in deterioration of renal function. The lowest effective dose should be used and renal function monitored.

The importance of prostaglandins in maintaining renal blood flow should be taken into account in patients with impaired cardiac or renal function, those being treated with diuretics or recovering from major surgery. Effects on renal function are usually reversible on withdrawal of diclofenac sodium.

Hepatic:

Close medical surveillance is imperative in patients suffering from severe impairment of hepatic function. If abnormal liver function tests persist or worsen, clinical signs or symptoms consistent with liver disease develop or if other manifestations occur (eosinophilia, rash), Diclofenac sodium should be discontinued. Hepatitis may occur without prodromal symptoms. Use of diclofenac sodium in patients with hepatic porphyria may trigger an attack.

Hematological:

Diclofenac sodium may reversibly inhibit platelet aggregation (see anticoagulants in 'drug interactions'). Patients with defects of haemostasis, bleeding diathesis or hematological abnormalities should be closely monitored.

Long-term treatment:

All patients who are receiving non-steroidal anti-inflammatory agents should be monitored as a precautionary measure e.g. renal function, hepatic function (elevation of liver enzymes may occur) and blood counts. This is particularly important in the elderly.

4.5 Interaction with other medicinal products and other forms of Interaction
Lithium and digoxin:

Diclofenac sodium may increase plasma concentrations of lithium and digoxin.

Anticoagulants:

Although clinical investigations do not appear to indicate that diclofenac sodium has an influence on the effect of anticoagulants, there are isolated reports of an increased risk of haemorrhage with the combined use of diclofenac sodium and anticoagulant therapy. Therefore, to be certain that no change in anticoagulant dosage is required, close monitoring of such patients is required. As with other non-steroidal anti-inflammatory agents, Diclofenac sodium in high doses can reversibly inhibit platelet aggregation.

Antidiabetic agents:

Clinical studies have shown that diclofenac sodium can be given together with oral antidiabetic agents without influencing their clinical effect. However there have been isolated reports of hypoglycaemic and hyperglycaemic effects which have required adjustment to the dosage of hypoglycaemic agents.

Cyclosporin:

Cases of nephrotoxicity have been reported in patients receiving concomitant cyclosporin and NSAIDS, including diclofenac sodium. This might be mediated through combined renal antiprostaglandin effects of both the NSAIDS and cyclosporin.

Methotrexate:

Cases of serious toxicity have been reported when methotrexate and NSAIDS are given within 24 hours of each other. This interaction is mediated through accumulation of methotrexate resulting from impairment of renal excretion in the presence of the NSAID.

Quinolone antimicrobials:

Convulsions may occur due to an interaction between quinolones and NSAIDS. This may occur in patients with or without a previous history of epilepsy or convulsions. Therefore, caution should be exercised when considering the use of a quinolone in patients who are already receiving an NSAID.

Other NSAIDS and steroids:

Co-administration of diclofenac sodium with other systemic NSAIDS and steroids may increase the frequency of unwanted effects. Concomitant therapy with aspirin lowers the plasma levels of each, although no clinical significance is known.

Diuretics:

Various NSAIDS are liable to inhibit the activity of diuretics. Concomitant treatment with potassium-sparing diuretics may be associated with increased serum potassium levels, hence serum potassium should be monitored.

4.6 Pregnancy and lactation
Although animal studies have not demonstrated teratogenic effects, diclofenac sodium should not be prescribed during pregnancy, unless there are compelling reasons for doing so. The lowest effective dosage should be used.

Use of prostaglandin synthetase inhibitors may result in premature closure of the ductus arteriosus or uterine inertia; such drugs are therefore not recommended during the last trimester of pregnancy.

Following doses of 50mg enteric coated tablets every 8 hours, traces of active substance have been detected in breast milk, but in quantities so small that no undesirable effects on the infant are to be expected.

4.7 Effects on ability to drive and use machines
Patients who experience dizziness or other central nervous system disturbances while taking NSAIDS should refrain from driving or operating machinery.

4.8 Undesirable effects
If serious side-effects occur, diclofenac sodium should be withdrawn.

Gastro-intestinal tract:

Occasional: Epigastric pain, other gastro-intestinal disorders (e.g. nausea, vomiting, diarrhoea, abdominal cramps, dyspepsia, flatulence, anorexia).

Rare: Gastro-intestinal bleeding, peptic ulcer (with or without bleeding or perforation), bloody diarrhoea.

In isolated cases: Lower gut disorders (e.g. non-specific haemorrhagic colitis and exacerbations of ulcerative colitis or crohn's proctocolitis), pancreatitis, aphthous stomatitis, glossitis, oesophageal lesions, constipation.

Central nervous system:

Occasional: Headache, dizziness, or vertigo.

Rare: Drowsiness, tiredness.

In isolated cases: Disturbances of sensation, paraesthesia, memory disturbance, disorientation, disturbance of vision (blurred vision, diplopia), impaired hearing, tinnitus, insomnia, irritability, convulsions, depression, anxiety, nightmares, tremor, psychotic reactions. Taste alteration disorders.

Skin:

Occasional: Rashes or skin eruptions.

Rare: Urticaria.

In isolated cases: Bullous eruptions, eczema, erythema multiforme, Stevens-Johnson syndrome, Lyell's syndrome, (acute toxic epidermolysis), erythroderma (exfoliative dermatitis), loss of hair, photosensitivity reactions, purpura including allergic purpura.

Kidney:

In isolated cases: Acute renal insufficiency, urinary abnormalities (e.g. haematuria, proteinuria), interstitial nephritis, nephrotic syndrome, papillary necrosis.

Liver:

Occasional: Elevation of serum aminotransferase enzymes (ALT, AST).

Rare: Liver function disorders including hepatitis (in isolated cases fulminant) with or without jaundice.

Blood:

In isolated cases: Thrombocytopenia, leucopenia, agranulocytosis, haemolytic anaemia, aplastic anaemia.

Other organ systems:

Rare: Oedema, hypersensitivity reactions (e.g. bronchospasm, anaphylactic/anaphylactoid systemic reactions including hypotension).

Isolated cases: Impotence (association with diclofenac sodium intake is doubtful), palpitation, chest pain, hypertension.

4.9 Overdose

Management of acute poisoning with NSAIDS essentially consists of supportive and symptomatic measures. There is no typical clinical picture resulting from diclofenac sodium overdosage. The therapeutic measures to be taken are: absorption should be prevented as soon as possible after overdosage by means of gastric lavage and treatment with activated charcoal; supportive and symptomatic treatment should be given for complications such as hypotension, renal failure, convulsions, gastro-intestinal irritation, and respiratory depression; specific therapies such as forced diuresis, dialysis or haemoperfusion are probably of no help in eliminating NSAIDS due to their high rate of protein binding and extensive metabolism.

5. PHARMACOLOGICAL PROPERTIES

5.1 Pharmacodynamic properties

Diclofenac sodium is a non-steroidal agent with marked analgesic/anti-inflammatory properties. It is an inhibitor of prostaglandin synthetase, (cyclo-oxygenase). Diclofenac sodium in vitro does not suppress proteoglycan biosynthesis in cartilage at concentrations equivalent to the concentrations reached in human beings.

5.2 Pharmacokinetic properties

Diclofenac sodium is rapidly absorbed from the gut and is subject to first-pass metabolism.

The active substances is 99.7% protein bound and plasma half-life for the terminal elimination phase is 1-2 hours.

Diclofenac sodium enters the synovial fluid, where maximum concentrations are measured 2-4 hours after the peak plasma values have been obtained. The apparent half-life for elimination from the synovial fluid is 3-6 hours. Two hours after reaching the peak plasma values, concentrations of the active substance are already higher in the synovial fluid than they are in the plasma, and they remain higher for up to 12 hours.

Approximately 60% of the administered dose is excreted via the kidneys in the form of metabolites and less than 1% in unchanged form. The remainder of the dose is excreted via the bile in metabolised form. In patients with impaired renal function, no accumulation of diclofenac sodium has been reported.

A single dose of two Flamatak MR Tablets 75mg (150mg diclofenac) resulted in a peak plasma concentration of 639ng/ml after 2.6 hours. Following repeated administration of a single Flamatak MR Tablet 75mg twice a day for 6 days, maximum plasma levels of 353ng/ml were recorded. Peak levels were reached 3.6 hours after the morning dose and 6.3 hours after the evening dose. The minimum diclofenac plasma concentration recorded at steady state was 142.5ng/ml.

5.3 Preclinical safety data

There are no pre-clinical data of relevance to the prescriber which are additional to that already included in other sections of the SPC.

6. PHARMACEUTICAL PARTICULARS

6.1 List of excipients

Also contains: lactose monohydrate, magnesium stearate (E572), methylhydroxypropylcellulose (E464), microcrystalline cellulose (E460), povidone, talc (E553) and Iron Oxide Red (E172).

6.2 Incompatibilities

None known.

6.3 Shelf life

2 years.

6.4 Special precautions for storage

Do not store above 25°C.

6.5 Nature and contents of container

Al/Al blisters

7s, 10s, 14s, 20s, 21s, 28s, 30s, 40s, 56s, 60s, 80s, 84s,100s, 250s, 500s, 1000s

Al/PVDC blisters

7s, 10s, 14s, 20s, 21s, 28s, 30s, 40s, 56s, 60s, 80s, 84s,100s, 250s, 500s, 1000s

PP-container and PE lids

7s, 10s, 14s, 20s, 21s, 28s, 30s, 40s, 56s, 60s, 80s, 84s,100s, 250s, 500s, 1000s

HDPE-container and PE lids

7s, 10s, 14s, 20s, 21s, 28s, 30s, 40s, 56s, 60s, 80s, 84s,100s, 250s, 500s, 1000s

6.6 Instructions for use and handling

Not relevant.

7. MARKETING AUTHORISATION HOLDER

Alpharma Limited

(Trading styles: Alpharma, Cox Pharmaceuticals)

Whiddon Valley

BARNSTAPLE

N Devon EX32 8NS

8. MARKETING AUTHORISATION NUMBER(S)

PL 0142/0435

9. DATE OF FIRST AUTHORISATION/RENEWAL OF THE AUTHORISATION

September 1999

10. DATE OF REVISION OF THE TEXT

April 2001

Fleet Phospho-Soda

(E. C. De Witt & Company Limited)

1. NAME OF THE MEDICINAL PRODUCT

Fleet® Phospho-soda® oral solution

2. QUALITATIVE AND QUANTITATIVE COMPOSITION

	per 45ml dose	per 1ml
Disodium phosphate dodecahydrate	10.8g	0.24g
Sodium dihydrogen phosphate dihydrate	24.4g	0.542g

Each 45ml bottle contains 5.0g sodium.

For excipients, see section 6.1.

3. PHARMACEUTICAL FORM

Oral solution.

4. CLINICAL PARTICULARS

4.1 Therapeutic indications

As a bowel cleanser in preparing the patient for colon surgery or for preparing the colon for x-ray or for endoscopic examination.

Bowel cleansing agents are not to be considered as treatments for constipation.

4.2 Posology and method of administration

Adults Only: Not to be given to children under the age of 15 years.

Elderly patients: As for Adults.

The taking of Fleet Phospho-soda should be started the day before the hospital appointment.

If the hospital appointment is before 12 noon the dosage instructions for morning appointments should be followed and for appointments after 12 noon the dosage instructions for an afternoon appointment should be followed.

Morning Appointment

Day before appointment

7am – In place of breakfast drink at least one full glass of "clear liquid" or water, more if desired.

"Clear liquids" include water, clear soup, strained fruit juices without pulp, black tea or black coffee, clear carbonated and non-carbonated soft drinks.

1st dose – straight after breakfast. Dilute the contents of one bottle (45ml) in half a glass (120ml) cold water. Drink this solution followed by one full glass (240ml) cold water, more if desired.

1pm lunch – In place of lunch drink at least three full glasses (720ml) of "clear liquid" or water, more if desired.

7pm supper – In place of supper drink at least one full glass of "clear liquid" or water, more if desired.

2nd dose – Straight after supper. Dilute the contents of the second bottle (45ml) in half a glass (120ml) cold water.

Drink this solution followed by one full glass (240ml) cold water, more if desired. Additional water or "clear liquids" may be taken up until midnight if necessary.

Afternoon appointment

Day before appointment

1pm lunch – A light snack may be taken. After lunch no more solid food must be taken until after the hospital appointment.

7pm supper – In place of supper drink at least one full glass of "clear liquid" or water, more if desired.

1st dose – Straight after supper. Dilute the contents of one bottle (45ml) in half a glass (120ml) cold water.

Drink this solution followed by one full glass (240ml) cold water, more if desired.

During the evening drink at least three full glasses of water or "clear liquid" before going to bed.

Day of appointment

7am breakfast – In place of breakfast drink at least one full glass of "clear liquid" or water, more if desired.

2nd dose - Straight after breakfast. Dilute the contents of the second bottle (45ml) in half a glass (120ml) cold water.

Drink this solution followed by one full glass (240ml) cold water. More water or "clear liquid" may be taken up until 8am.

This product normally produces a bowel movement in 1/2 to 6 hours.

4.3 Contraindications

Do not use in patients with known or suspected gastro-intestinal obstruction, perforation or ileus. Do not use in patients with congestive heart failure, megacolon (congenital or acquired) or renal failure.

Do not use in patients with active inflammatory bowel disease.

Do not use when nausea, vomiting or abdominal pain are present.

Do not use when there is a hypersensitivity to the active ingredients or any of excipients.

Do not use in children under the age of 15 years.

4.4 Special warnings and special precautions for use

Use with caution in the frail and elderly, in patients with impaired renal function, heart disease, colostomy, on a low salt diet or with pre-existing electrolyte disturbances as hyperphosphataemia, hypocalcaemia, hypokalaemia, hypernatraemic dehydration and acidosis may occur, see section 4.8 below.

Patients should be warned to expect frequent, liquid stools.

Very rarely, single or multiple aphthoid-like punctiform lesions located in the rectosigmoid region have been observed by endoscopy. These were either lymphoid follicles or discrete inflammatory infiltrates or epithelial congestions/changes revealed by the colonic preparation. These abnormalities are not clinically significant and disappear spontaneously without any treatment.

Slight QT interval prolongation may rarely occur as a result of electrolyte imbalances such as hypocalcaemia or hypokalaemia. These changes are clinically insignificant.

4.5 Interaction with other medicinal products and other forms of Interaction

Use with caution in patients taking calcium channel blockers, diuretics, lithium treatment or other medications that might affect electrolyte levels as hyperphosphataemia, hypocalcaemia, hypokalaemia, hypernatraemic dehydration and acidosis may occur.

During the intake of Fleet Phospho-soda the absorption of drugs from the gastrointestinal tract may be delayed or even completely prevented. The efficacy of regularly taken oral drugs (e.g. oral contraceptives, antiepileptic drugs, antidiabetics, antibiotics) may be reduced or completely absent.

4.6 Pregnancy and lactation

There is no reliable data on teratogenesis in animals.

Due to there being no relevant data available to evaluate a potential malformative or foetotoxic effect when administered during pregnancy, this product should not be used during pregnancy.

4.7 Effects on ability to drive and use machines

Not applicable.

4.8 Undesirable effects

The most common adverse events reported post marketing have been nausea, vomiting, abdominal pain, bloating and diarrhoea, asthenia, chills, headache, dizziness, allergic reactions with/without rash, fatigue and gastrointestinal cramping.

Dehydration and/or electrolyte disturbances, including hyperphosphataemia, hypocalcaemia, hypokalaemia, hypernatraemia and acidosis, may occur in some 'at risk' patients.

Very rarely, single or multiple aphthoid-like punctiform lesions located in the rectosigmoid region have been observed by endoscopy. These abnormalities are not clinically significant and disappear spontaneously without any treatment (see Section 4.4 Special warning and precautions for use).

4.9 Overdose

There have been fatal cases of hyperphosphataemia with concomitant hypocalcaemia, hypernatraemia and acidosis when Fleet Phospho-soda has been used in excessive doses, given to children or to obstructed patients.

There are also documented cases of complete recovery from overdoses in both children accidentally given Fleet Phospho-soda, and also in patients with obstruction, one of whom received a six-fold overdose.

Recovery from the toxic effect of excess ingestion can normally be achieved by rehydration, though the intravenous administration of 10% calcium gluconate may be necessary.

5. PHARMACOLOGICAL PROPERTIES

5.1 Pharmacodynamic properties

A06AD – osmotically acting laxative.

Fleet Phospho-soda is a saline laxative which acts by osmotic processes to increase fluid retention in the lumen of the small intestine. Fluid accumulation in the ileum produces distension and, in turn, promotes peristalsis and bowel evacuation.

5.2 Pharmacokinetic properties

Not applicable.

5.3 Preclinical safety data

No particular remarks.

6. PHARMACEUTICAL PARTICULARS

6.1 List of excipients
Glycerol

Saccharin Sodium

Sodium Benzoate (E211)

Ginger Lemon Flavour*

Purified Water

*Ginger Lemon Flavour:

Oleoresin Ginger

Alcohol

Oil Lemon

Partially Deterpinated Oil Lemon

Citric Acid

Water

6.2 Incompatibilities
None known.

6.3 Shelf life
3 years

6.4 Special precautions for storage
Do not store above 25°C.

6.5 Nature and contents of container
Fleet Phospho-soda is supplied in cartons containing 2 × 45ml or 100 × 45ml (hospital pack) polyethylene bottles with polypropylene, aluminium foil-lined screw caps.

Not all pack sizes may be marketed.

6.6 Instructions for use and handling
No special instructions.

7. MARKETING AUTHORISATION HOLDER
E. C. De Witt & Company Limited

Tudor Road

Manor Park

Runcorn

WA7 1SZ

England

8. MARKETING AUTHORISATION NUMBER(S)
PL 0083/0044

9. DATE OF FIRST AUTHORISATION/RENEWAL OF THE AUTHORISATION
6th July 1995

10. DATE OF REVISION OF THE TEXT
April 2003

Fleet Ready-to-Use Enema

(E. C. De Witt & Company Limited)

1. NAME OF THE MEDICINAL PRODUCT
Fleet Ready-to-Use Enema

2. QUALITATIVE AND QUANTITATIVE COMPOSITION

Name of ingredients	Per 118ml delivered dose
Sodium Acid Phosphate	18.1% w/v
Sodium Phosphate	8.0% w/v

The delivered dose contains 4.4g sodium

3. PHARMACEUTICAL FORM
Solution

4. CLINICAL PARTICULARS

4.1 Therapeutic indications
For use in the relief of occasional constipation, pre and post-operative bowel cleansing, obstetrics and prior to proctoscopy, sigmoidoscopy and x-ray examination.

4.2 Posology and method of administration
Adults and children over 12 years of age: 1 Bottle (118ml delivered dose) no more than once daily or as directed by a physician.

Children 3 years to under 12 years: As directed by a physician.

Do not administer to children under 3 years of age.

For rectal use only.

4.3 Contraindications
Do not use in patients with congenital megacolon, Hirschsprung's Disease, imperforate anus or congestive heart failure.

4.4 Special warnings and special precautions for use
Use with caution in patients with impaired renal function, heart disease, colostomy or pre-existing electrolyte disturbances as hypocalcaemia, hyperphosphataemia, hypernatraemia and acidosis may occur.

Keep all medicines out of the reach of children.

Do not use Fleet Ready-to-use enema when nausea, vomiting or abdominal pain is present unless directed by a physician.

Prolonged repeated use of Fleet Ready-to-use enema is not recommended and may lead to dependence. Unless directed by a physician, Fleet Ready-to-use enema should not be used for more than two weeks.

Fleet Ready-to-use enema should be administered following the instructions on the carton. Discontinue use if resistance is encountered, forcing the enema may result in injury.

4.5 Interaction with other medicinal products and other forms of Interaction
Use with caution in patients taking calcium channel blockers, diuretics or other medications that might affect electrolyte levels as hypocalcaemia, hyperphosphataemia, hypernatraemia and acidosis may result.

4.6 Pregnancy and lactation
Use only under medical supervision.

4.7 Effects on ability to drive and use machines
Not applicable

4.8 Undesirable effects
Rectal bleeding or failure to have a bowel movement after use of a laxative may indicate a serious condition.

Discontinue use and consult a physician.

4.9 Overdose
In the case of accidental ingestion or overdose, seek professional assistance.

5. PHARMACOLOGICAL PROPERTIES

5.1 Pharmacodynamic properties
Phosphates act as saline laxatives when administered by the rectal route.

Peristalsis is stimulated and an approximately normal bowel movement occurs with only the rectum, sigmoid and part or all of the descending colon being evacuated.

When used in patients with abnormal bowel anatomy, renal insufficiency or heart failure electrolyte disturbances have been noted. Hypocalcaemia, hyperphosphataemia, hypernatraemia and acidosis have been reported.

5.2 Pharmacokinetic properties
Not applicable

5.3 Preclinical safety data
Not applicable

6. PHARMACEUTICAL PARTICULARS

6.1 List of excipients
Disodium Edetate

Benzalkonium Chloride

Purified Water

Nozzle lubricant: White Soft Paraffin

6.2 Incompatibilities
None known

6.3 Shelf life
3 Years

6.4 Special precautions for storage
Store below 25°C

Do not refrigerate

6.5 Nature and contents of container
Fleet Ready-to-use enema is supplied in a 133ml disposable LDPE squeeze bottle with a soft, pre-lubricated Comfortip with protective sheath and gives a delivered single dose of 118ml. Cap and sheath made from LDPE.

6.6 Instructions for use and handling
Lie on left side with both knees bent, arms at rest.

Remove orange protective shield.

With steady pressure, gently insert enema Comfortip into anus with nozzle pointing towards navel.

Squeeze bottle until nearly all liquid is expelled.

Discontinue use if resistance is encountered. Forcing the enema can result in injury.

Return enema to carton for disposal.

7. MARKETING AUTHORISATION HOLDER
E. C. De Witt & Company Limited

Tudor Road

Manor Park

Runcorn

Cheshire

England WA7 1SZ

8. MARKETING AUTHORISATION NUMBER(S)
PL 0083/0043

9. DATE OF FIRST AUTHORISATION/RENEWAL OF THE AUTHORISATION
07/10/93; 09/02/99

10. DATE OF REVISION OF THE TEXT
October 1998

Fletchers' Arachis Oil Retention Enema

(Forest Laboratories UK Limited)

1. NAME OF THE MEDICINAL PRODUCT
FLETCHERS' ARACHIS OIL RETENTION ENEMA

2. QUALITATIVE AND QUANTITATIVE COMPOSITION
The 130ml enema contains:

Arachis Oil BP 100%

3. PHARMACEUTICAL FORM
Single dose disposable retention enema for rectal administration

4. CLINICAL PARTICULARS

4.1 Therapeutic indications
To soften impacted faeces.

4.2 Posology and method of administration
Adults and elderly:

1 enema as required

Children:

In proportion, according to body weight.

Method of administration – rectal administration.

4.3 Contraindications
Hypersensitivity to Arachis oil or peanuts.

Inflammatory bowel disease, except under the instruction of a medical practitioner.

4.4 Special warnings and special precautions for use
Fletchers' Arachis Oil Retention Enema contains Arachis oil (peanut oil) and should not be used by patients known to be allergic to peanut. As there is a possible relationship between allergy to peanut and allergy to soya, patients with soya allergy should also avoid Fletchers' Arachis Oil Retention Enema.

Not for use in children unless under medical supervision. Use with caution in patients with intestinal obstruction. Care should be taken not to use undue force in administration of the enema especially in the elderly or debilitated patients or those with neurological disorders. The enema should be warmed before use by placing in warm water.

4.5 Interaction with other medicinal products and other forms of Interaction
None known

4.6 Pregnancy and lactation
The use of enemas is not recommended during pregnancy except under medical advice.

4.7 Effects on ability to drive and use machines
Not applicable

4.8 Undesirable effects
Like other rectally applied substances, Arachis oil may produce local irritation.

4.9 Overdose
No cases of overdosages have been reported.

5. PHARMACOLOGICAL PROPERTIES

5.1 Pharmacodynamic properties
Arachis oil is utilised in this product to soften impacted faeces.

5.2 Pharmacokinetic properties
Arachis oil is not known to be absorbed and acts purely locally.

5.3 Preclinical safety data
There are no preclinical data of relevance to the prescriber which are additional to that already included in other sections of the SPC.

6. PHARMACEUTICAL PARTICULARS

6.1 List of excipients
None

6.2 Incompatibilities
None known

6.3 Shelf life
2 years

6.4 Special precautions for storage
Store at room temperature (25°C).

6.5 Nature and contents of container
Blue PVC bag with clear plastic nozzle and cap.

OR

Blue LDPE bottle with clear PVC nozzle and blue overcap.

Pack size 130ml.

6.6 Instructions for use and handling
None stated.

7. MARKETING AUTHORISATION HOLDER
Forest Laboratories UK Limited

Bourne Road

Bexley

Kent DA5 1NX

8. MARKETING AUTHORISATION NUMBER(S)
PL 0108/5016R

9. DATE OF FIRST AUTHORISATION/RENEWAL OF THE AUTHORISATION
25th July 1988 / 24 November 1998

10. DATE OF REVISION OF THE TEXT
June 2003

11. Legal Category
P

Fletchers' Phosphate Enema

(Forest Laboratories UK Limited)

1. NAME OF THE MEDICINAL PRODUCT
Fletchers' Phosphate Enema
Alternative name: Phosphates Enema BP Formula B

2. QUALITATIVE AND QUANTITATIVE COMPOSITION
Each 128ml enema contains:

Sodium Dihydrogen Phosphate Dihydrate	10% w/v
Disodium Phosphate Dodecahydrate	8% w/v

3. PHARMACEUTICAL FORM
Rectal solution

4. CLINICAL PARTICULARS

4.1 Therapeutic indications
Routine treatment of constipation. Pre- and post-operative cleansing of the bowel, in obstetrics and prior to proctoscopy, sigmoidoscopy or X-ray examination.

4.2 Posology and method of administration
Adults including the elderly:
1 enema as required.
Children over 3 years of age:
Reduce adult dosage in proportion to body weight.
Children under 3 years of age:
Not recommended.

For rectal administration only. The enema may be administered at room temperature or warmed in water before use.

4.3 Contraindications
Hypersensitivity to any of the constituents. Use in patients with inflammatory or ulcerative conditions of the large bowel, in those with increased colonic absorptive capacity e.g. Hirschsprung's disease and in those with acute gastrointestinal conditions.

4.4 Special warnings and special precautions for use
Prolonged use may lead to irritation of the anal canal. Use with caution in patients requiring a reduced sodium intake and electrolyte balance should be maintained during extended use. Use with caution in patients with intestinal obstruction. Care should be taken not to use undue force in administration of the enema especially in the elderly or debilitated patients or those with neurological disorders.

4.5 Interaction with other medicinal products and other forms of Interaction
None known

4.6 Pregnancy and lactation
No special warnings

4.7 Effects on ability to drive and use machines
Not applicable

4.8 Undesirable effects
Local irritation.

There have been occasional reports of apparent vasovagal attacks occurring in elderly patients following administration of phosphate enemata.

4.9 Overdose
There have been no cases of overdosage. In the event of overdosage, electrolyte levels should be monitored and balance restored where appropriate.

5. PHARMACOLOGICAL PROPERTIES

5.1 Pharmacodynamic properties
Fletchers' Phosphate Enema is a solution of sodium dihydrogen phosphate dihydrate and disodium phosphate dodecahydrate. The formulation is equivalent to Phosphates Enema BP Formula B. Following rectal administration the active ingredients exert their laxative effect via their osmotic properties. The resulting fluid retention in the bowel encourages evacuation.

5.2 Pharmacokinetic properties
Saline laxatives are poorly and slowly absorbed following rectal administration. Under normal usage only minimal absorption is likely to occur.

5.3 Preclinical safety data
There are no preclinical data of relevance to the prescriber which are additional to that already included in other sections of the SPC.

6. PHARMACEUTICAL PARTICULARS

6.1 List of excipients

Benzalkonium chloride
Disodium Edetate
Purified Water

6.2 Incompatibilities
Not applicable

6.3 Shelf life
3 years

6.4 Special precautions for storage
Do not store above 25°C.

6.5 Nature and contents of container
Translucent LDPE bottle with rubber non-return valve, plastic nozzle and nozzle plug containing 128 ml solution packed singly in a cardboard carton, or alternatively long-tube version with separate applicator with extension tube for attachment before use.

6.6 Instructions for use and handling
None stated.

7. MARKETING AUTHORISATION HOLDER
Forest Laboratories UK Limited
Bourne Road
Bexley
Kent DA5 1NX

8. MARKETING AUTHORISATION NUMBER(S)
PL 0108/5015R

9. DATE OF FIRST AUTHORISATION/RENEWAL OF THE AUTHORISATION
12 August 1985 / 27 July 2005

10. DATE OF REVISION OF THE TEXT
June 2005

11. Legal Category
P

Flixonase Aqueous Nasal Spray

(Allen & Hanburys)

1. NAME OF THE MEDICINAL PRODUCT
Flixonase Aqueous Nasal Spray

2. QUALITATIVE AND QUANTITATIVE COMPOSITION
Aqueous suspension of 0.05% w/w micronised fluticasone propionate. Each metered dose contains 50 micrograms of fluticasone propionate.

3. PHARMACEUTICAL FORM
Aqueous suspension for intranasal inhalation via metered dose atomising pump.

4. CLINICAL PARTICULARS

4.1 Therapeutic indications
The prophylaxis and treatment of seasonal allergic rhinitis (including hay fever) and perennial rhinitis. Fluticasone propionate has potent anti-inflammatory activity but when used topically on the nasal mucosa has no detectable systemic activity.

4.2 Posology and method of administration
Flixonase Aqueous Nasal Spray is for administration by the intranasal route only.

Adults and children over 12 years of age:

For the prophylaxis and treatment of seasonal allergic rhinitis and perennial rhinitis. Two sprays into each nostril once a day, preferably in the morning. In some cases two sprays into each nostril twice daily may be required. Once symptoms are under control a maintenance dose of one spray per nostril once a day may be used. If symptoms recur the dosage may be increased accordingly. The minimum dose should be used at which effective control of symptoms is maintained. The maximum daily dose should not exceed four sprays into each nostril.

Elderly patients:

The normal adult dosage is applicable.

Children under 12 years of age:

For the prophylaxis and treatment of seasonal allergic rhinitis and perennal rhinitis in children aged 4-11 years a dose of one spray into each nostril once daily preferably in the morning is recommended. In some cases one spray into each nostril twice daily may be required. The maximum daily dose should not exceed two sprays into each nostril. The minimum dose should be used at which effective control of symptoms is maintained.

For full therapeutic benefit regular usage is essential. The absence of an immediate effect should be explained to the patient, as maximum relief may not be obtained until after 3 to 4 days of treatment.

4.3 Contraindications
Hypersensitivity to any of its ingredients.

4.4 Special warnings and special precautions for use
Local infections: infections of the nasal airways should be appropriately treated but do not constitute a specific contra-indication to treatment with Flixonase Aqueous Nasal Spray.

The full benefit of Flixonase Aqueous Nasal Spray may not be achieved until treatment has been administered for several days.

Care must be taken while transferring patients from systemic steroid treatment to Flixonase Aqueous Nasal Spray if there is any reason to suppose that their adrenal function is impaired.

Although Flixonase Aqueous Nasal Spray will control seasonal allergic rhinitis in most cases, an abnormally heavy challenge of summer allergens may in certain instances necessitate appropriate additional therapy.

Systemic effects of nasal corticosteroids may occur particularly at high doses prescribed for prolonged periods. These effects vary between patients and different corticosteroids (please refer to pharmacokinetic and pharmacodynamic information).

Growth retardation has been reported in children receiving some nasal corticosteroids at licensed doses. It is recommended that the height of children receiving prolonged treatment with nasal corticosteroids is regularly monitored. If growth is slowed, therapy should be reviewed with the aim of reducing the dose of nasal corticosteroid, if possible, to the lowest dose at which effective control of symptoms is maintained. In addition, consideration should be given to referring the patient to a paediatric specialist.

Treatment with higher than recommended doses of nasal corticosteroids may result in clinically significant adrenal suppression. If there is evidence for higher than recommended doses being used then additional systemic corticosteroid cover should be considered during periods of stress or elective surgery.

Ritonavir can greatly increase the concentration of fluticasone propionate in plasma. Therefore, concomitant use should be avoided, unless the potential benefit to the patient outweighs the risk of systemic corticosteroid side effects. There is also an increased risk of systemic side effects when combining fluticasone propionate with other potent CYP3A inhibitors (see 4.5 Interaction with Other Medicinal Products and Other Forms of Interaction).

4.5 Interaction with other medicinal products and other forms of Interaction
Under normal circumstances, low plasma concentrations of fluticasone propionate are achieved after inhaled dosing, due to extensive first pass metabolism and high systemic clearance mediated by cytochrome P450 3A4 in the gut and liver. Hence, clinically significant drug interactions mediated by fluticasone propionate are unlikely.

In an interaction study in healthy subjects with intranasal fluticasone propionate, ritonavir (a highly potent cytochrome P450 3A4 inhibitor) 100 mg b.i.d. increased the fluticasone propionate plasma concentrations several hundred fold, resulting in markedly reduced serum cortisol concentrations. Cases of Cushing's syndrome and adrenal suppression have been reported. The combination should be avoided unless the benefit outweighs the increased risk of systemic glucocorticoid side-effects.

In a small study using inhaled fluticasone propionate in healthy volunteers, the slightly less potent CYP3A inhibitor ketoconazole increased the exposure of fluticasone propionate after a single inhalation by 150%. This resulted in a greater reduction of plasma cortisol as compared with fluticasone propionate alone. Co-treatment with other potent CYP3A inhibitors, such as itraconazole, is also expected to increase the systemic fluticasone propionate exposure and the risk of systemic side-effects. Caution is recommended and long-term treatment with such drugs should if possible be avoided.

4.6 Pregnancy and lactation
There is inadequate evidence of safety in human pregnancy. Administration of corticosteroids to pregnant animals can cause abnormalities of foetal development, including cleft palate and intra-uterine growth retardation. There may therefore be a very small risk of such effects in the human foetus. It should be noted, however, that the foetal changes in animals occur after relatively high systemic exposure; direct intranasal application ensures minimal systemic exposure.

As with other drugs the use of Flixonase Aqueous Nasal Spray during human pregnancy requires that the possible benefits of the drug be weighed against the possible hazards.

The secretion of fluticasone propionate in human breast milk has not been investigated. Subcutaneous administration of fluticasone propionate to lactating laboratory rats produced measurable plasma levels and evidence of fluticasone propionate in the milk. However, following intranasal administration to primates, no drug was detected in the plasma, and it is therefore unlikely that the drug would be detectable in milk. When Flixonase Aqueous Nasal Spray is used in breast feeding mothers the therapeutic benefits must be weighed against the potential hazards to mother and baby.

4.7 Effects on ability to drive and use machines
None reported.

4.8 Undesirable effects
Adverse events are listed below by system organ class and frequency. Frequencies are defined as: very common ($\geqslant$1/10), common ($\geqslant$1/100 and <1/10), uncommon ($\geqslant$1/1000 and <1/100), rare ($\geqslant$1/10,000 and <1/1000) and very rare (<1/10,000) including isolated reports. Very common, common and uncommon events were generally determined from clinical trial data. Rare and very rare events were generally determined from spontaneous data. In assigning adverse event frequencies, the background rates in placebo groups were not taken into account.

System Organ Class	Adverse Event	Frequency
Immune system disorders	Hypersensitivity reactions with the following manifestations:	
	Cutaneous hypersensitivity reactions	Very rare
	Angioedema (mainly facial and oropharyngeal oedema)	Very rare
	Respiratory symptoms (bronchospasm)	Very rare
	Anaphylactic reactions	Very rare
Nervous system disorders	Headache, unpleasant taste, unpleasant smell.	Common
Eye disorders	Glaucoma, raised intraocular pressure, cataract	Very rare
	These events have been identified from spontaneous reports following prolonged treatment.	
Respiratory, Thoracic & Mediastinal disorders	Epistaxis	Very common
	Nasal dryness, nasal irritation, throat dryness, throat irritation.	Common
	Nasal septal perforation.	Very rare

As with other nasal sprays, unpleasant taste and smell and headache have been reported.

As with other nasal sprays, dryness and irritation of the nose and throat, and epistaxis have been reported. Nasal septal perforation has also been reported following the use of intranasal corticosteroids.

Systemic effects of some nasal corticosteroids may occur, particularly when prescribed at high doses for prolonged periods.

4.9 Overdose

There are no data available on the effects of acute or chronic overdosage with Flixonase Aqueous Nasal Spray. Intranasal administration of 2 mg fluticasone propionate twice daily for seven days to healthy human volunteers has no effect on hypothalamo-pituitary-adrenal (HPA) axis function.

Inhalation or oral administration of high doses of corticosteroids over a long period may lead to suppression of HPA axis function.

5. PHARMACOLOGICAL PROPERTIES

5.1 Pharmacodynamic properties

Fluticasone propionate causes little or no hypothalamic-pituitary-adrenal axis suppression following intranasal administration.

Following intranasal dosing of fluticasone propionate, (200mcg/day) no significant change in 24h serum cortisol AUC was found compared to placebo (ratio1.01, 90%CI 0.9-1.14).

5.2 Pharmacokinetic properties

Absorption: Following intranasal dosing of fluticasone propionate, (200mcg/day) steady-state maximum plasma concentrations were not quantifiable in most subjects (<0.01ng/mL). The highest Cmax observed was 0.017ng/mL. Direct absorption in the nose is negligible due to the low aqueous solubility with the majority of the dose being eventually swallowed. When administered orally the systemic exposure is <1% due to poor absorption and pre-systemic metabolism. The total systemic absorption arising from both nasal and oral absorption of the swallowed dose is therefore negligible.

Distribution: Fluticasone propionate has a large volume of distribution at steady-state (approximately 318L). Plasma protein binding is moderately high (91%).

Metabolism: Fluticasone propionate is cleared rapidly from the systemic circulation, principally by hepatic metabolism to an inactive carboxylic acid metabolite, by the cytochrome P450 enzyme CYP3A4. Swallowed fluticasone propionate is also subject to extensive first pass metabolism. Care should be taken when co-administering potent CYP3A4 inhibitors such as ketoconazole and ritonavir as there is potential for increased systemic exposure to fluticasone propionate.

Elimination: The elimination rate of intravenous administered fluticasone propionate is linear over the 250-1000mcg dose range and are characterized by a high plasma clearance (CL=1.1L/min). Peak plasma concentrations are reduced by approximately 98% within 3-4 hours and only low plasma concentrations were associated with the 7.8h terminal half-life. The renal clearance of fluticasone propionate is negligible (<0.2%) and less than 5% as the carboxylic acid metabolite. The major route of elimination is the excretion of fluticasone propionate and its metabolites in the bile.

5.3 Preclinical safety data

There are no preclinical data of relevance to the prescriber which are additional to that already included in other sections of the SPC.

6. PHARMACEUTICAL PARTICULARS

6.1 List of excipients

Dextrose (Anhydrous) PhEur

Microcrystalline Celluose NF

Carboxymethylcellulose Sodium NF

Phenylethyl Alcohol USP

Benzalkonium Chloride PhEur

Polysorbate 80 PhEur

Purified Water PhEur

6.2 Incompatibilities

None reported.

6.3 Shelf life

24 months

6.4 Special precautions for storage

Flixonase Aqueous Nasal Spray should not be stored above 30°C

6.5 Nature and contents of container

Flixonase Aqueous Nasal Spray is supplied in an amber glass bottle fitted with a metering, atomising pump. Pack size of 120 and 150 metered sprays.

Not all pack sizes may be marketed.

6.6 Instructions for use and handling

Shake gently before use.

Administrative Data

7. MARKETING AUTHORISATION HOLDER

Glaxo Wellcome UK Limited trading as:

Allen & Hanburys

Stockley Park West

Uxbridge

Middlesex UB11 1BT

8. MARKETING AUTHORISATION NUMBER(S)

PL 10949/0036

9. DATE OF FIRST AUTHORISATION/RENEWAL OF THE AUTHORISATION

13 September 2005

10. DATE OF REVISION OF THE TEXT

13 September 2005

11. Legal Category

POM

Flixonase Nasule Drops

(Allen & Hanburys)

1. NAME OF THE MEDICINAL PRODUCT

Flixonase Nasule Drops 400micrograms (1 milligram/millilitre), nasal drops suspension.

2. QUALITATIVE AND QUANTITATIVE COMPOSITION

Each single dose of Flixonase Nasal Drops contains:

Fluticasone propionate 400 micrograms (1milligram/millilitre).

For excipients see section 6.1

3. PHARMACEUTICAL FORM

Nasal drops

Single dose aqueous suspension.

4. CLINICAL PARTICULARS

4.1 Therapeutic indications

Flixonase Nasule Drops are indicated for the regular treatment of nasal polyps and associated symptoms of nasal obstruction.

4.2 Posology and method of administration

Adults:

The contents of one container (400 micrograms) to be instilled once or twice daily. The dose should be divided between the affected nostrils.

After shaking and opening the container, the patient should adopt one of the positions outlined in the patient information leaflet. The dose should be divided between the nostrils by either counting approximately 6 drops into each nostril or by holding the dimpled sides of the container and squeezing once into each nostril (one squeeze delivers approximately half the dose).

Full instructions for use are given in the patient information leaflet.

Elderly: The normal adult dosage is applicable.

Children: There are insufficient data at present to recommend the use of fluticasone propionate for the treatment of nasal polyps in children less than 16 years.

The dose should be titrated to the lowest dose at which effective control of disease is maintained.

For full therapeutic benefit regular usage is essential. The absence of an immediate effect should be explained to the patient as maximum relief may not be obtained until after several weeks of treatment. However, if no improvement in symptoms is seen after four to six weeks, alternative therapies should be considered.

4.3 Contraindications

Flixonase Nasule Drops are contra-indicated in patients with a history of hypersensitivity to the active substance or to any of the excipients.

4.4 Special warnings and special precautions for use

Local infection: Infections of the nasal airways should be appropriately treated but do not constitute a specific contra-indication to treatment with Flixonase Nasule Drops.

Unilateral polyposis rarely occurs, and could be indicative of other conditions. Diagnosis should be confirmed by a specialist.

Nasal polyps require regular medical assessment to monitor severity of the condition.

Contact with the eyes and broken skin should be avoided.

Care must be taken when withdrawing patients from systemic steroid treatment, and commencing therapy with Flixonase Nasule Drops, particularly if there is any reason to suppose that their adrenal function is impaired.

Systemic effects of nasal corticosteroids may occur, particularly at high doses prescribed for prolonged periods.

It is possible that long term treatment with higher than recommended doses of nasal corticosteroids could result in clinically significant adrenal suppression. If there is evidence of higher than recommended doses being used then additional systemic corticosteroid cover should be considered during periods of stress or elective surgery.

Ritonavir can greatly increase the concentration of fluticasone propionate in plasma. Therefore, concomitant use should be avoided, unless the potential benefit to the patient outweighs the risk of systemic corticosteroid side-effects. There is also an increased risk of systemic side effects when combining fluticasone propionate with other potent CYP3A inhibitors (see 4.5 Interaction with Other Medicinal Products and Other Forms of Interaction).

4.5 Interaction with other medicinal products and other forms of Interaction

Under normal circumstances, low plasma concentrations of fluticasone propionate are achieved after intranasal dosing, due to extensive first pass metabolism and high systemic clearance mediated by cytochrome P450 3A4 in the gut and liver. Hence, clinically significant drug interactions mediated by fluticasone propionate are unlikely.

In an interaction study in healthy subjects with intranasal fluticasone propionate, ritonavir (a highly potent cytochrome P450 3A4 inhibitor) 100 mg b.i.d. increased the fluticasone propionate plasma concentrations several hundred fold, resulting in markedly reduced serum cortisol concentrations. Cases of Cushing's syndrome and adrenal suppression have been reported. The combination should be avoided unless the benefit outweighs the increased risk of systemic glucocorticoid side-effects.

Other inhibitors of cytochrome P450 3A4 produce negligible (erythromycin) and minor (ketoconazole) increases in systemic exposure to fluticasone propionate without notable reductions in serum cortisol concentrations. Care is advised when co-administering cytochrome P450 3A4 inhibitors, especially in long-term use and in case of potent inhibitors as there is potential for increased systemic exposure to fluticasone propionate.

4.6 Pregnancy and lactation

The use of Flixonase Nasule Drops during pregnancy and lactation requires that the benefits be weighed against possible risks associated with the product or with any alternative therapy.

Pregnancy: There is inadequate evidence of safety in human pregnancy. In animal reproduction studies adverse effects typical of potent corticosteroids are only seen at high systemic exposure levels; direct intranasal application ensures minimal systemic exposure.

Lactation: The excretion of fluticasone propionate into human breast milk has not been investigated. Following subcutaneous administration in lactating laboratory rats, there was evidence of fluticasone propionate in the breast milk, however plasma levels in patients following intranasal application of fluticasone propionate at recommended doses are low.

4.7 Effects on ability to drive and use machines
Not applicable.

4.8 Undesirable effects
Adverse events are listed below by system organ class and frequency. Frequencies are defined as: very common (⩾1/10), common (⩾1/100 and <1/10), uncommon (⩾1/1000 and <1/100), rare (⩾1/10,000 and <1/1000) and very rare (<1/10,000) including isolated reports. Very common, common and uncommon events were generally determined from clinical trial data. Rare and very rare events were generally determined from spontaneous data. In assigning adverse event frequencies, the background rates in placebo groups were not taken into account, since these rates were generally comparable to or higher than those in the active treatment group.

Immune system disorders

Very rare: Hypersensitivity reactions, anaphylaxis/anaphylactic reactions, bronchospasm.

Respiratory, thoracic and mediastinal disorders

Very common: Epistaxis

Common: Nasal dryness, nasal irritation, throat dryness, throat irritation.

Very rare: Nasal septal perforation.

As with other intranasal products, dryness and irritation of the nose and throat, and epistaxis may occur. There have also been cases of nasal septal perforation following the use of intranasal corticosteroids.

Eye Disorders

Very rare: Glaucoma, raised intraocular pressure, cataract. These have been identified from spontaneous reports following prolonged treatment.

4.9 Overdose
There are no data available from patients on the effects of acute or chronic overdosage with Flixonase Nasule Drops.

In healthy volunteers, intranasal administration of 2mg fluticasone propionate twice daily for seven days had no effect on hypothalamic-pituitary-adrenal axis (HPA) function. Administration of doses higher than those recommended over a long period of time may lead to temporary suppression of the adrenal function. In these patients, treatment with fluticasone propionate should be continued at a dose sufficient to control symptoms; the adrenal function will recover in a few days and can be verified by measuring plasma cortisol.

5. PHARMACOLOGICAL PROPERTIES

5.1 Pharmacodynamic properties
Pharmacotherapeutic Group: Nasal preparations, Corticosteroids

ATC Code: R01AD08

Fluticasone propionate has potent anti-inflammatory activity when used topically on the nasal mucosa.

Fluticasone propionate causes little or no HPA axis suppression following intranasal administration.

5.2 Pharmacokinetic properties
After recommended doses of intranasal fluticasone propionate plasma levels are low. Systemic bioavailability for the nasal drop formula is extremely low (mean value 0.06%).

Following intravenous administration the pharmacokinetics of fluticasone propionate are proportional to the dose, and can be described by three exponentials.

Absolute oral bio-availability is negligible (<1%) due to a combination of incomplete absorption from the gastro-intestinal tract and extensive first pass metabolism.

Fluticasone propionate is extensively distributed within the body (Vss is approximately 300 litre). Plasma protein binding is 91%.

After intravenous administration, fluticasone propionate has a very high clearance (estimated Cl 1.1 litre/min) indicating extensive hepatic extraction. It is extensively metabolised by CYP3A4 enzyme to an inactive carboxylic derivative.

Peak plasma concentrations are reduced by approximately 98% within 3-4 hours, and only low plasma concentrations are associated with the terminal half life, which is approximately 8 hours.

Following oral administration of fluticasone propionate, 87-100% of the dose is excreted in the faeces as parent compound or as metabolites.

5.3 Preclinical safety data
At doses in excess of those recommended for therapeutic use, only class effects typical of potent corticosteroids have been shown in repeat dose toxicity tests, reproductive toxicology and teratology studies. Fluticasone propionate has no mutagenic effect in vitro or in vivo, no tumorigenic potential in rodents and is non-irritant and non-sensitising in animals.

6. PHARMACEUTICAL PARTICULARS

6.1 List of excipients
Polysorbate 20, sorbitan laurate, sodium dihydrogen phosphate dihydrate, disodium phosphate anhydrous, sodium chloride, water for injections.

6.2 Incompatibilities
None reported.

6.3 Shelf life
3 years.

After removal of foil: 28 days.

6.4 Special precautions for storage
Do not freeze.

Keep containers in outer carton.

Store upright.

Do not store above 30 degrees Centigrade.

6.5 Nature and contents of container
Strips of polyethylene single dose (400micrograms) containers, within foil wrapping are available in the following pack sizes.

28 containers (4 strips of 7 nasules)
84 containers (12 strips of 7 nasules)

Not all pack sizes may be marketed

6.6 Instructions for use and handling
Full instructions for use are given in the patient information leaflet.

Administrative Data

7. MARKETING AUTHORISATION HOLDER
Glaxo Wellcome UK Limited trading as Allen & Hanburys

Stockley Park West

Uxbridge

Middlesex

UB11 1BT

8. MARKETING AUTHORISATION NUMBER(S)
PL 10949/0323

9. DATE OF FIRST AUTHORISATION/RENEWAL OF THE AUTHORISATION
27 January 1999 / 23 October 2003

10. DATE OF REVISION OF THE TEXT
26 November 2004

11. Legal Status
POM

Flixotide 50, 125, 250 micrograms Evohaler

(Allen & Hanburys)

1. NAME OF THE MEDICINAL PRODUCT
Flixotide™ 50 micrograms Evohaler™

Flixotide™ 125 micrograms Evohaler™

Flixotide™ 250 micrograms Evohaler™

2. QUALITATIVE AND QUANTITATIVE COMPOSITION
Flixotide 50 micrograms Evohaler, Flixotide 125 micrograms Evohaler and Flixotide 250 micrograms Evohaler are pressurised inhalation, suspensions, delivering either 50, 125 or 250 micrograms of fluticasone propionate per actuation, respectively.

3. PHARMACEUTICAL FORM
Pressurised inhalation, suspension

Flixotide Evohaler does not contain any chlorofluorocarbons (CFCs).

4. CLINICAL PARTICULARS

4.1 Therapeutic indications
Fluticasone propionate given by inhalation offers prophylactic treatment for asthma.

Adults:

Mild asthma: Patients requiring intermittent symptomatic bronchodilator asthma medication on a regular daily basis.

Moderate asthma:Patients with unstable or worsening asthma despite prophylactic therapy or bronchodilator alone.

Severe asthma:Patients with severe chronic asthma and those who are dependent on systemic corticosteroids for adequate control of symptoms. On introduction of inhaled fluticasone propionate many of these patients may be able to reduce significantly, or to eliminate, their requirement for oral corticosteroids.

Children:

Any child who requires prophylactic medication, including patients not controlled on currently available prophylactic medication.

4.2 Posology and method of administration
Flixotide Evohaler is for oral inhalation use only. A spacer device may be used in patients who find it difficult to synchronise aerosol actuation with inspiration of breath.

Patients should be made aware of the prophylactic nature of therapy with Flixotide Evohaler and that it should be taken regularly even when they are asymptomatic. The onset of therapeutic effect is within 4 to 7 days.

Adults and children over 16 years: 100 to 1,000 micrograms twice daily, usually as two twice daily inhalations.

Prescribers should be aware that fluticasone propionate is as effective as other inhaled steroids approximately at half the microgram daily dose. For example, a 100mcg of fluticasone propionate is approximately equivalent to 200mcg dose of beclometasone dipropionate (CFC containing) or budesonide.

Due to the risk of systemic effects, doses above 500 micrograms twice daily should be prescribed only for adult patients with severe asthma where additional clinical benefit is expected, demonstrated by either an improvement in pulmonary function and/or symptom control, or by a reduction in oral corticosteroid therapy (see 4.4 Special Warnings and Precautions for Use and 4.8 Undesirable Effects).

Patients should be given a starting dose of inhaled fluticasone propionate which is appropriate to the severity of their disease.

Typical Adult Starting Doses:

For patients with mild asthma, a typical starting dose is 100 micrograms twice daily. In moderate and more severe asthma, starting doses may need to be 250 to 500 micrograms twice daily. Where additional clinical benefit is expected, doses of up to 1000 micrograms twice daily may be used. Initiation of such doses should be prescribed only by a specialist in the management of asthma (such as a consultant physician or general practitioner with appropriate experience).

The dose should be titrated down to the lowest dose at which effective control of asthma is maintained

Typical starting doses for children over 4years of age:

50 to 100 micrograms twice daily.

Many children's asthma will be well controlled using the 50 to 100 microgram twice daily dosing regime. For those patients whose asthma is not sufficiently controlled, additional benefit may be obtained by increasing the dose up to 200 micrograms twice daily. **The maximum licensed dose in children is 200 micrograms twice daily.**

The starting dose should be appropriate to the severity of the disease. The dose should be titrated down to the lowest dose at which effective control of asthma is maintained.

Should Flixotide 50 microgram Evohaler presentation not offer the exact paediatric dose prescribed by the physician, please see data sheets of alternative Flixotide presentation (Accuhaler, Diskhaler, Inhaler).

Administration of doses above 1000 micrograms (500 micrograms twice daily) should be via a spacer device to help reduce side-effects in the mouth and throat. (See section 4.4)

Special patient groups:

There is no need to adjust the dose in elderly patients or those with hepatic or renal impairment.

4.3 Contraindications
Hypersensitivity to any ingredient of the preparation.

4.4 Special warnings and special precautions for use
Patients' inhaler technique should be checked regularly to make sure that inhaler actuation is synchronised with inspiration to ensure optimum delivery to the lungs.

Flixotide Evohaler is not designed to relieve acute symptoms for which an inhaled short-acting bronchodilator is required. Patients should be advised to have such rescue medication available.

Severe asthma requires regular medical assessment, including lung-function testing, as patients are at risk of severe attacks and even death. Increasing use of short-acting inhaled β_2-agonists to relieve symptoms indicates deterioration of asthma control. If patients find that short-acting relief bronchodilator treatment becomes less effective, or they need more inhalations than usual, medical attention must be sought. In this situation patients should be reassessed and consideration given to the need for increased anti-inflammatory therapy (e.g. higher doses of inhaled corticosteroids or a course of oral corticosteroids). Severe exacerbations of asthma must be treated in the normal way.

As with other inhalation therapy, paradoxical bronchospasm may occur with an immediate increase in wheezing after dosing. Flixotide Evohaler should be discontinued immediately, the patient assessed and alternative therapy instituted if necessary.

Systemic effects of inhaled corticosteroids may occur, particularly at high doses prescribed for prolonged periods. These effects are much less likely to occur than with oral corticosteroids. Possible systemic effects include Cushing's syndrome, Cushingoid features, adrenal suppression, growth retardation in children and adolescents, decrease in bone mineral density, cataract and glaucoma. **It is important therefore that the dose of inhaled corticosteroid is reviewed regularly and reduced to the lowest dose at which effective control of asthma is maintained.**

Prolonged treatment with high doses of inhaled corticosteroids may result in adrenal suppression and acute adrenal crisis. Children aged < 16 years taking higher than licensed doses of fluticasone (typically ⩾1000mcg/day) may be at particular risk. Situations, which could potentially trigger acute adrenal crisis, include trauma, surgery, infection or any rapid reduction in dosage. Presenting symptoms are typically vague and may include anorexia, abdominal pain, weight loss, tiredness, headache, nausea, vomiting, decreased level of consciousness, hypoglycaemia, and seizures. Additional systemic corticosteroid cover should be considered during periods of stress or elective surgery.

It is recommended that the height of children receiving prolonged treatment with inhaled corticosteroids is regularly monitored. If growth is slowed, therapy should be reviewed with the aim of reducing the dose of inhaled corticosteroid, if possible, to the lowest dose at which effective control of asthma is maintained. In addition, consideration should be given to referring the patient to a paediatric respiratory specialist.

Administration of high doses, above 1000 mcg daily is recommended through a spacer to reduce side effects in the mouth and throat. However, as systemic absorption is largely through the lungs, the use of a spacer plus metered dose inhaler may increase drug delivery to the lungs. It should be noted that this could potentially lead to an increase in the risk of systemic adverse effects. A lower dose may be required.(See section 4.2)

The benefits of inhaled fluticasone propionate should minimise the need for oral steroids. However, patients transferred from oral steroids, remain at risk of impaired adrenal reserve for a considerable time after transferring to inhaled fluticasone propionate. The possibility of adverse effects may persist for some time. These patients may require specialised advice to determine the extent of adrenal impairment before elective procedures. The possibility of residual impaired adrenal response should always be considered in emergency (medical or surgical) and elective situations likely to produce stress, and appropriate corticosteroid treatment considered.

Lack of response or severe exacerbations of asthma should be treated by increasing the dose of inhaled fluticasone propionate and, if necessary, by giving a systemic steroid and/or an antibiotic if there is an infection.

Replacement of systemic steroid treatment with inhaled therapy sometimes unmasks allergies such as allergic rhinitis or eczema previously controlled by the systemic drug. These allergies should be symptomatically treated with antihistamine and/or topical preparations, including topical steroids.

As with all inhaled corticosteroids, special care is necessary in patients with active or quiescent pulmonary tuberculosis.

Treatment with Flixotide Evohaler should not be stopped abruptly.

For the transfer of patients being treated with oral corticosteroids: The transfer of oral steroid-dependent patients to Flixotide Evohaler and their subsequent management needs special care as recovery from impaired adrenocortical function, caused by prolonged systemic steroid therapy, may take a considerable time.

Patients who have been treated with systemic steroids for long periods of time or at a high dose may have adrenocortical suppression. With these patients adrenocortical function should be monitored regularly and their dose of systemic steroid reduced cautiously.

After approximately a week, gradual withdrawal of the systemic steroid is commenced. Decrements in dosages should be appropriate to the level of maintenance systemic steroid, and introduced at not less than weekly intervals. For maintenance doses of prednisolone (or equivalent) of 10mg daily or less, the decrements in dose should not be greater than 1mg per day, at not less than weekly intervals. For maintenance doses of prednisolone in excess of 10mg daily, it may be appropriate to employ cautiously, larger decrements in dose at weekly intervals.

Some patients feel unwell in a non-specific way during the withdrawal phase despite maintenance or even improvement of the respiratory function. They should be encouraged to persevere with inhaled fluticasone propionate and to continue withdrawal of systemic steroid, unless there are objective signs of adrenal insufficiency.

Patients weaned off oral steroids whose adrenocortical function is still impaired should carry a steroid warning card indicating that they need supplementary systemic steroid during periods of stress, e.g. worsening asthma attacks, chest infections, major intercurrent illness, surgery, trauma, etc.

Ritonavir can greatly increase the concentration of fluticasone propionate in plasma. Therefore, concomitant use should be avoided, unless the potential benefit to the patient outweighs the risk of systemic corticosteroid side-effects. There is also an increased risk of systemic side effects when combining fluticasone propionate with other potent CYP3A inhibitors (see 4.5 Interaction with Other Medicinal Products and Other Forms of Interaction).

4.5 Interaction with other medicinal products and other forms of Interaction

Under normal circumstances, low plasma concentrations of fluticasone propionate are achieved after inhaled dosing, due to extensive first pass metabolism and high systemic clearance mediated by cytochrome P450 3A4 in the gut and liver. Hence, clinically significant drug interactions mediated by fluticasone propionate are unlikely.

In an interaction study in healthy subjects with intranasal fluticasone propionate, ritonavir (a highly potent cytochrome P450 3A4 inhibitor) 100 mg b.i.d. increased the fluticasone propionate plasma concentrations several hundred fold, resulting in markedly reduced serum cortisol concentrations. Information about this interaction is lacking for inhaled fluticasone propionate, but a marked increase in fluticasone propionate plasma levels is expected. Cases of Cushing's syndrome and adrenal suppression have been reported. The combination should be avoided unless the benefit outweighs the increased risk of systemic glucocorticoid side-effects.

In a small study in healthy volunteers, the slightly less potent CYP3A inhibitor ketoconazole increased the exposure of fluticasone propionate after a single inhalation by 150%. This resulted in a greater reduction of plasma cortisol as compared with fluticasone propionate alone. Co-treatment with other potent CYP3A inhibitors, such as itraconazole, is also expected to increase the systemic fluticasone propionate exposure and the risk of systemic side-effects. Caution is recommended and long-term treatment with such drugs should, if possible, be avoided.

4.6 Pregnancy and lactation

There is inadequate evidence of safety of fluticasone propionate in human pregnancy. Data on a limited number (200) of exposed pregnancies indicate no adverse effects of Flixotide Evohaler on pregnancy or the health of the foetus/new born child. To date no other relevant epidemiological data are available. Administration of corticosteroids to pregnant animals can cause abnormalities of fetal development, including cleft palate and intra-uterine growth retardation. There may therefore be a very small risk of such effects in the human fetus. It should be noted, however, that the fetal changes in animals occur after relatively high systemic exposure. Because Flixotide Evohaler delivers fluticasone propionate directly to the lungs by the inhaled route it avoids the high level of exposure that occurs when corticosteroids are given by systemic routes. Administration of fluticasone propionate during pregnancy should only be considered if the expected benefit to the mother is greater than any possible risk to the fetus.

The secretion of fluticasone propionate in human breast milk has not been investigated. Subcutaneous administration of fluticasone propionate to lactating laboratory rats produced measurable plasma levels and evidence of fluticasone propionate in the milk. However, plasma levels in humans after inhalation at recommended doses are likely to be low. When fluticasone propionate is used in breast-feeding mothers the therapeutic benefits must be weighed against the potential hazards to mother and baby.

4.7 Effects on ability to drive and use machines

Fluticasone propionate is unlikely to produce an effect.

4.8 Undesirable effects

Adverse events are listed below by system organ class and frequency. Frequencies are defined as: very common (⩾1/10), common (⩾1/100 and <1/10), uncommon (⩾1/1000 and <1/100), rare (⩾1/10,000 and <1/1000) and very rare (<1/10,000) including isolated reports. Very common, common and uncommon events were generally determined from clinical trial data. Rare and very rare events were generally determined from spontaneous data.

System Organ Class	Adverse Event	Frequency
Infections & Infestations	Candidiasis of the mouth and throat	Very Common
Immune System Disorders	Hypersensitivity reactions with the following manifestations:	
	Cutaneous hypersensitivity reactions	Uncommon
	Angioedema (mainly facial and oropharyngeal oedema)	Very Rare
	Respiratory symptoms (dyspnoea and/ or bronchospasm)	Very Rare
	Anaphylactic reactions	Very Rare
Endocrine Disorders	Cushing's syndrome, Cushingoid features, adrenal suppression, growth retardation in children and adolescents, decreased bone mineral density, cataract, glaucoma	Very Rare
Gastrointestinal Disorders	Dyspepsia	Very Rare
Musculoskeletal & Connective Tissue Disorders	Arthralgia	Very Rare
Psychiatric Disorders	Anxiety, sleep disorders, behavioural changes, including hyperactivity and irritability (predominantly in children)	Very Rare
Respiratory, Thoracic & Mediastinal Disorders	Hoarseness/ dysphonia	Common
	Paradoxical bronchospasm	Very Rare

Hoarseness and candidiasis of the mouth and throat (thrush) occurs in some patients. Such patients may find it helpful to rinse out their mouth with water after using the inhaler. Symptomatic candidiasis can be treated with topical anti-fungal therapy whilst still continuing with Flixotide Evohaler.

Possible systemic effects include Cushing's syndrome, Cushingoid features, adrenal suppression, growth retardation, decreased bone mineral density, cataract, glaucoma (see 4.4 Special Warning and Special Precautions for Use).

As with other inhalation therapy, paradoxical bronchospasm may occur (see 4.4 'Special Warnings and Precautions for Use'). This should be treated immediately with a fast-acting inhaled bronchodilator. Flixotide Evohaler should be discontinued immediately, the patient assessed, and if necessary alternative therapy instituted.

4.9 Overdose

Acute: Inhalation of the drug in doses in excess of those recommended may lead to temporary suppression of adrenal function. This does not necessitate emergency action being taken. In these patients treatment with fluticasone propionate by inhalation should be continued at a dose sufficient to control asthma adrenal function recovers in a few days and can be verified by measuring plasma cortisol.

Chronic: refer to section 4.4: risk of adrenal suppression.

Monitoring of adrenal reserve may be indicated. Treatment with inhaled fluticasone propionate should be continued at a dose sufficient to control asthma.

5. PHARMACOLOGICAL PROPERTIES

5.1 Pharmacodynamic properties

Fluticasone propionate given by inhalation at recommended doses has a potent glucocorticoid anti-inflammatory action within the lungs, resulting in a reduction of both symptoms and exacerbations of asthma, with a lower incidence and severity of adverse effects than those observed when corticosteroids are administered systemically.

5.2 Pharmacokinetic properties

In healthy subjects the mean systemic bioavailability of Flixotide Evohaler is 28.6%. In patients with asthma (FEV_1 < 75% predicted) the mean systemic absolute bioavailability was reduced by 62%. Systemic absorption occurs mainly through the lungs and has been shown to be linearly related to dose over the dose range 500 to 2000 micrograms. Absorption is initially rapid then prolonged and the remainder of the dose may be swallowed.

Absolute oral bioavailability is negligible (<1%) due to a combination of incomplete absorption from the GI tract and extensive first-pass metabolism.

87-100% of an oral dose is excreted in the faeces, up to 75% as parent compound. There is also a non-active major metabolite.

After an intravenous dose, fluticasone propionate is extensively distributed in the body. The very high clearance rate indicates extensive hepatic clearance.

5.3 Preclinical safety data

Toxicology has shown only those class effects typical of potent corticosteroids, and these only at doses greatly in excess of that proposed for therapeutic use. No novel effects were identified in repeat dose toxicity tests, reproductive studies or teratology studies. Fluticasone propionate is devoid of mutagenic activity *in vitro* and *in vivo* and showed no tumorigenic potential in rodents. It is both non-irritant and non-sensitising in animal models.

The non-CFC propellant, HFA 134a, has been shown to have no toxic effect at very high vapour concentrations, far in excess of those likely to be experienced by patients, in a wide range of animal species exposed daily for periods of two years.

The use of HFA 134a as a propellant has not altered the toxicity profile of fluticasone propionate compared to that using the conventional CFC propellant.

6. PHARMACEUTICAL PARTICULARS

6.1 List of excipients

HFA 134a.

6.2 Incompatibilities

None reported.

6.3 Shelf life

24 months

6.4 Special precautions for storage

Do not store above 30°C (86°F). Do not refrigerate or freeze. Protect from frost and direct sunlight.

As with most medicines in pressurised canisters, the therapeutic effect of this medication may decrease when the canister is cold.

The canister should not be punctured, broken or burnt even when apparently empty.

6.5 Nature and contents of container

An inhaler comprising an aluminium alloy can sealed with a metering valve, actuator and dust cap. Each canister contains 120 metered actuations of either 50, 125 or 250 micrograms of fluticasone propionate. (60 metered actuation hospital packs are available in the 125 or 250 microgram products).

6.6 Instructions for use and handling

The aerosol spray is inhaled through the mouth into the lungs. After shaking the inhaler the patient should exhale, the mouthpiece should be placed in the mouth and the lips closed around it. The actuator is depressed to release a spray, which must coincide with inspiration of breath.

For detailed instructions for use refer to the Patient Information Leaflet in every pack.

Administrative Data

7. MARKETING AUTHORISATION HOLDER

Glaxo Wellcome UK Ltd, trading as

Allen & Hanburys, Stockley Park West, Uxbridge, Middlesex, UB11 1BT

8. MARKETING AUTHORISATION NUMBER(S)

Flixotide 50 micrograms Evohaler	PL 10949/0324
Flixotide 125 micrograms Evohaler	PL 10949/0265
Flixotide 250 micrograms Evohaler	PL 10949/0266

9. DATE OF FIRST AUTHORISATION/RENEWAL OF THE AUTHORISATION

Flixotide Evohaler 50 micrograms	27 June 2000
Flixotide Evohaler 125/250 micrograms	14 March 2000

10. DATE OF REVISION OF THE TEXT

24 March 2005

11. Legal Category

POM.

Flixotide Accuhaler

(Allen & Hanburys)

1. NAME OF THE MEDICINAL PRODUCT

Flixotide$_{TM}$ Accuhaler$_{TM}$

2. QUALITATIVE AND QUANTITATIVE COMPOSITION

Flixotide Accuhaler is a moulded plastic device containing a foil strip with 28 or 60 regularly placed blisters each containing a mixture of microfine fluticasone propionate (50 micrograms, 100 micrograms, 250 micrograms or 500 micrograms) and larger particle size lactose.

3. PHARMACEUTICAL FORM

Multi-dose dry powder inhalation device.

4. CLINICAL PARTICULARS

4.1 Therapeutic indications

Fluticasone propionate given by inhalation offers preventative treatment for asthma. At recommended doses it has a potent glucocorticoid anti-inflammatory action within the lungs, with a lower incidence and severity of adverse effects than those observed when corticosteroids are administered systemically.

Adults: Prophylactic management in:

Mild asthma: Patients requiring intermittent symptomatic bronchodilator asthma medication on a regular daily basis.

Moderate asthma:Patients with unstable or worsening asthma despite prophylactic therapy or bronchodilator alone.

Severe asthma:Patients with severe chronic asthma and those who are dependent on systemic corticosteroids for adequate control of symptoms. On introduction of inhaled fluticasone propionate many of these patients may be able to reduce significantly, or to eliminate, their requirement for oral corticosteroids.

Children: Any child who requires prophylactic medication, including patients not controlled on currently available prophylactic medication.

4.2 Posology and method of administration

Flixotide Accuhaler is for oral inhalation use only. Flixotide Accuhaler is suitable for many patients, including those who cannot use a metered-dose inhaler successfully.

Patients should be made aware of the prophylactic nature of therapy with Flixotide Accuhaler and that it should be taken regularly even when they are asymptomatic. The onset of therapeutic effect is within 4 to 7 days.

Adults and children over 16 years: 100 to 1,000 micrograms twice daily.

Prescribers should be aware that fluticasone propionate is as effective as other inhaled steroids approximately at half the microgram daily dose. For example, a 100mcg of fluticasone propionate is approximately equivalent to 200mcg dose of beclometasone dipropionate (CFC containing) or budesonide.

Due to the risk of systemic effects, doses above 500 micrograms twice daily should be prescribed only for adult patients with severe asthma where additional clinical benefit is expected, demonstrated by either an improvement in pulmonary function and/or symptom control, or by a reduction in oral corticosteroid therapy (see 4.4 Special Warnings and Precautions for Use and 4.8 Undesirable Effects).

Patients should be given a starting dose of inhaled fluticasone propionate which is appropriate to the severity of their disease.

Typical Adult Starting Doses:

For patients with mild asthma, a typical starting dose is 100 micrograms twice daily. In moderate and more severe asthma, starting doses may need to be 250 to 500 micrograms twice daily. Where additional clinical benefit is expected, doses of up to 1000 micrograms twice daily may be used. Initiation of such doses should be prescribed only by a specialist in the management of asthma (such as a consultant physician or general practitioner with appropriate experience).

The dose should be titrated down to the lowest dose at which effective control of asthma is maintained.

Typical starting doses for children over 4 years of age:

50 to 100 micrograms twice daily.

Many children's asthma will be well controlled using the 50 to100 microgram twice daily dosing regime. For those patients whose asthma is not sufficiently controlled, additional benefit may be obtained by increasing the dose up to 200 micrograms twice daily. **The maximum licensed dose in children is 200 micrograms twice daily.**

The starting dose should be appropriate to the severity of the disease.

The dose should be titrated down to the lowest dose at which effective control of asthma is maintained.

Special patient groups:

There is no need to adjust the dose in elderly patients or in those with hepatic or renal impairment.

4.3 Contraindications

Hypersensitivity to any ingredient of the preparation. (See Pharmaceutical Particulars – List of Excipients).

4.4 Special warnings and special precautions for use

Flixotide Accuhaler is not designed to relieve acute symptoms for which an inhaled short acting bronchodilator is required. Patients should be advised to have such rescue medication available.

Severe asthma requires regular medical assessment, including lung-function testing, as patients are at risk of severe attacks and even death. Increasing use of short-acting inhaled β_2-agonists to relieve symptoms indicates deterioration of asthma control. If patients find that short-acting relief bronchodilator treatment becomes less effective, or they need more inhalations than usual, medical attention must be sought. In this situation patients should be reassessed and consideration given to the need for increased anti-inflammatory therapy (e.g. higher doses of inhaled corticosteroids or a course of oral corticosteroids). Severe exacerbations of asthma must be treated in the normal way.

As with other inhalation therapy, paradoxical bronchospasm may occur with an immediate increase in wheezing after dosing. Flixotide Accuhaler should be discontinued immediately, the patient assessed and alternative therapy instituted if necessary

Systemic effects of inhaled corticosteroids may occur, particularly at high doses prescribed for prolonged periods. These effects are much less likely to occur than with oral corticosteroids. Possible systemic effects include Cushing's syndrome, Cushingoid features, adrenal suppression, growth retardation in children and adolescents, decrease in bone mineral density, cataract and glaucoma. **It is important therefore that the dose of inhaled corticosteroid is reviewed regularly and reduced to the lowest dose at which effective control of asthma is maintained.**

Prolonged treatment with high doses of inhaled corticosteroids may result in adrenal suppression and acute adrenal crisis. Children aged < 16 years taking higher than licensed doses of fluticasone (typically ≥1000mcg/day) may be at particular risk. Situations, which could potentially trigger acute adrenal crisis, include trauma, surgery, infection or any rapid reduction in dosage. Presentingsymptoms are typically vague and may include anorexia, abdominal pain, weight loss, tiredness, headache, nausea, vomiting, decreased level of consciousness, hypoglycaemia, and seizures. Additional systemic corticosteroid cover should be considered during periods of stress or elective surgery.

It is recommended that the height of children receiving prolonged treatment with inhaled corticosteroids is regularly monitored. If growth is slowed, therapy should be reviewed with the aim of reducing the dose of inhaled corticosteroid, if possible, to the lowest dose at which effective control of asthma is maintained. In addition, consideration should be given to referring the patient to a paediatric respiratory specialist.

When changing from a dry powder inhaler to a metered dose inhaler, administration of high doses, above 1000 mcg daily, is recommended through a spacer to reduce side effects in the mouth and throat. However, this may increase drug delivery to the lungs. As systemic absorption is largely through the lungs, there may be an increase in the risk of systemic adverse effects. A lower dose may be required.

The benefits of inhaled fluticasone propionate should minimise the need for oral steroids. However, patients transferred from oral steroids, remain at risk of impaired adrenal reserve for a considerable time after transferring to inhaled fluticasone propionate. The possibility of adverse effects may persist for some time. These patients may require specialised advice to determine the extent of adrenal impairment before elective procedures. The possibility of residual impaired adrenal response should always be considered in emergency (medical or surgical) and elective situations likely to produce stress, and appropriate corticosteroid treatment considered.

Lack of response or severe exacerbations of asthma should be treated by increasing the dose of inhaled fluticasone propionate and, if necessary, by giving a systemic steroid and/or an antibiotic if there is an infection.

Replacement of systemic steroid treatment with inhaled therapy sometimes unmasks allergies such as allergic rhinitis or eczema previously controlled by the systemic drug. These allergies should be symptomatically treated with antihistamine and/or topical preparations, including topical steroids.

As with all inhaled corticosteroids, special care is necessary in patients with active or quiescent pulmonary tuberculosis.

Treatment with Flixotide Accuhaler should not be stopped abruptly.

For the transfer of patients being treated with oral corticosteroids: The transfer of oral steroid-dependent patients to Flixotide Accuhaler and their subsequent management needs special care as recovery from impaired adrenocortical function, caused by prolonged systemic steroid therapy, may take a considerable time.

Patients who have been treated with systemic steroids for long periods of time or at a high dose may have adrenocortical suppression. With these patients adrenocortical function should be monitored regularly and their dose of systemic steroid reduced cautiously.

After approximately a week, gradual withdrawal of the systemic steroid is commenced. Decrements in dosages should be appropriate to the level of maintenance systemic steroid, and introduced at not less than weekly intervals. For maintenance doses of prednisolone (or equivalent) of 10mg daily or less, the decrements in dose should not be greater than 1mg per day, at not less than weekly intervals. For maintenance doses of prednisolone in excess of 10mg daily, it may be appropriate to employ cautiously, larger decrements in dose at weekly intervals.

Some patients feel unwell in a non-specific way during the withdrawal phase despite maintenance or even improvement of the respiratory function. They should be encouraged to persevere with inhaled fluticasone propionate and to continue withdrawal of systemic steroid, unless there are objective signs of adrenal insufficiency.

Patients weaned off oral steroids whose adrenocortical function is still impaired should carry a steroid warning card indicating that they need supplementary systemic steroid during periods of stress, e.g. worsening asthma attacks, chest infections, major intercurrent illness, surgery, trauma, etc.

Ritonavir can greatly increase the concentration of fluticasone propionate in plasma. Therefore, concomitant use should be avoided, unless the potential benefit to the patient outweighs the risk of systemic corticosteroid side-effects. There is also an increased risk of systemic side effects when combining fluticasone propionate with other potent CYP3A inhibitors (see 4.5 Interaction with Other Medicinal Products and Other Forms of Interaction).

4.5 Interaction with other medicinal products and other forms of Interaction
Under normal circumstances, low plasma concentrations of fluticasone propionate are achieved after inhaled dosing, due to extensive first pass metabolism and high systemic clearance mediated by cytochrome P450 3A4 in the gut and liver. Hence, clinically significant drug interactions mediated by fluticasone propionate are unlikely.

In an interaction study in healthy subjects with intranasal fluticasone propionate, ritonavir (a highly potent cytochrome P450 3A4 inhibitor) 100 mg b.i.d. increased the fluticasone propionate plasma concentrations several hundred fold, resulting in markedly reduced serum cortisol concentrations. Information about this interaction is lacking for inhaled fluticasone propionate, but a marked increase in fluticasone propionate plasma levels is expected. Cases of Cushing's syndrome and adrenal suppression have been reported. The combination should be avoided unless the benefit outweighs the increased risk of systemic glucocorticoid side-effects.

In a small study in healthy volunteers, the slightly less potent CYP3A inhibitor ketoconazole increased the exposure of fluticasone propionate after a single inhalation by 150%. This resulted in a greater reduction of plasma cortisol as compared with fluticasone propionate alone. Co-treatment with other potent CYP3A inhibitors, such as itraconazole, is also expected to increase the systemic fluticasone propionate exposure and the risk of systemic side-effects. Caution is recommended and long-term treatment with such drugs should, if possible, be avoided.

4.6 Pregnancy and lactation
There is inadequate evidence of safety of fluticasone propionate in human pregnancy. Administration of corticosteroids to pregnant animals can cause abnormalities of fetal development, including cleft palate and intra-uterine growth retardation. There may therefore be a very small risk of such effects in the human fetus. It should be noted, however, that the fetal changes in animals occur after relatively high systemic exposure. Because Flixotide Accuhaler delivers fluticasone propionate directly to the lungs by the inhaled route it avoids the high level of exposure that occurs when corticosteroids are given by systemic routes. Administration of fluticasone propionate during pregnancy should only be considered if the expected benefit to the mother is greater than any possible risk to the fetus.

The secretion of fluticasone propionate in human breast milk has not been investigated. Subcutaneous administration of fluticasone propionate to lactating laboratory rats produced measurable plasma levels and evidence of fluticasone propionate in the milk. However, plasma levels in humans after inhalation at recommended doses are likely to be low.

When fluticasone propionate is used in breast feeding mothers the therapeutic benefits must be weighed against the potential hazards to mother and baby.

4.7 Effects on ability to drive and use machines
Fluticasone propionate is unlikely to produce an effect.

4.8 Undesirable effects
Adverse events are listed below by system organ class and frequency. Frequencies are defined as: very common (≥1/10), common (≥1/100 and <1/10), uncommon (≥1/1000 and <1/100), rare (≥1/10,000 and <1/1000) and very rare (<1/10,000) including isolated reports. Very common, common and uncommon events were generally determined from clinical trial data. Rare and very rare events were generally determined from spontaneous data.

System Organ Class	Adverse Event	Frequency
Infections & Infestations	Candidiasis of the mouth and throat	Very Common
Immune System Disorders	Hypersensitivity reactions with the following manifestations:	
	Cutaneous hypersensitivity reactions	Uncommon
	Angioedema (mainly facial and oropharyngeal oedema)	Very Rare
	Respiratory symptoms (dyspnoea and/or bronchospasm)	Very Rare
	Anaphylactic reactions	Very Rare
Endocrine Disorders	Cushing's syndrome, Cushingoid features, adrenal suppression, growth retardation in children and adolescents, decreased bone mineral density, cataract, glaucoma	Very Rare
Gastrointestinal Disorders	Dyspepsia	Very Rare
Musculoskeletal & Connective Tissue Disorders	Arthralgia	Very Rare
Psychiatric Disorders	Anxiety, sleep disorders, behavioural changes, including hyperactivity and irritability (predominantly in children)	Very Rare
Respiratory, Thoracic & Mediastinal Disorders	Hoarseness/dysphonia	Common
	Paradoxical bronchospasm	Very Rare

Hoarseness and candidiasis of the mouth and throat (thrush) occurs in some patients. Such patients may find it helpful to rinse out their mouth with water after using the Accuhaler. Symptomatic candidiasis can be treated with topical anti-fungal therapy whilst still continuing with the Flixotide Accuhaler.

Possible systemic effects include Cushing's syndrome, Cushingoid features, adrenal suppression, growth retardation, decreased bone mineral density, cataract, glaucoma (see 4.4 Special Warnings and Special Precautions for Use).

As with other inhalation therapy, paradoxical bronchospasm may occur (see 4.4 'Special Warnings and Precautions for Use'). This should be treated immediately with a fast-acting inhaled bronchodilator. Flixotide Accuhaler should be discontinued immediately, the patient assessed, and if necessary alternative therapy instituted.

4.9 Overdose
Acute: Inhalation of the drug in doses in excess of those recommended may lead to temporary suppression of adrenal function. This does not necessitate emergency action being taken. In these patients treatment with fluticasone propionate by inhalation should be continued at a dose sufficient to control asthma; adrenal function recovers in a few days and can be verified by measuring plasma cortisol.

Chronic: refer to section 4.4: risk of adrenal suppression.

Monitoring of adrenal reserve may be indicated. Treatment with inhaled fluticasone propionate should be continued at a dose sufficient to control asthma.

5. PHARMACOLOGICAL PROPERTIES

5.1 Pharmacodynamic properties
Fluticasone propionate given by inhalation at recommended doses has a potent glucocorticoid anti-inflammatory action within the lungs, resulting in reduced symptoms and exacerbations of asthma, with a lower incidence and severity of adverse effects than those observed when corticosteroids are administered systemically.

5.2 Pharmacokinetic properties
Systemic absolute bioavailability of fluticasone propionate is estimated at 12-26% of an inhaled dose, dependent on presentation. Systemic absorption occurs mainly through the lungs and is initially rapid then prolonged. The remainder of the dose may be swallowed.

Absolute oral bioavailability is negligible (<1%) due to a combination of incomplete absorption from the GI tract and extensive first-pass metabolism.

87-100% of an oral dose is excreted in the faeces, up to 75% as parent compound. There is also a non-active major metabolite.

After an intravenous dose, fluticasone propionate is extensively distributed in the body. The very high clearance rate indicates extensive hepatic clearance.

5.3 Preclinical safety data
Toxicology has shown only those class effects typical of potent corticosteroids, and these only at doses greatly in excess of that proposed for therapeutic use. No novel effects were identified in repeat dose toxicity tests, reproductive studies or teratology studies. Fluticasone propionate is devoid of mutagenic activity *in vitro* and *in vivo* and showed no tumorigenic potential in rodents. It is both non-irritant and non-sensitising in animal models.

6. PHARMACEUTICAL PARTICULARS

6.1 List of excipients
Lactose (which contains milk protein)

6.2 Incompatibilities
None reported.

6.3 Shelf life
Flixotide 50 Accuhaler 18 months when notstored above 30°C.

Flixotide 100 Accuhaler 24 months when not stored above 30°C.

Flixotide 250/500 Accuhaler 36 months when not stored above 30°C.

6.4 Special precautions for storage
Do not store above 30°C (86°F). Store in the original package.

6.5 Nature and contents of container
The powder mix of fluticasone propionate and lactose is filled into a blister strip consisting of a formed base foil with a peelable foil laminate lid. The foil strip is contained within the Accuhaler device.

6.6 Instructions for use and handling
The powdered medicine is inhaled through the mouth into the lungs.

The Accuhaler device contains the medicine in individual blisters which are opened as the device is manipulated.

For detailed instructions for use refer to the Patient Information Leaflet in every pack.

Administrative Data

7. MARKETING AUTHORISATION HOLDER
Glaxo Wellcome UK Ltd,
trading as Allen & Hanburys,
Stockley Park West,
Uxbridge,
Middlesex, UB11 1BT

8. MARKETING AUTHORISATION NUMBER(S)

Flixotide Accuhaler 50 micrograms	10949/0226
Flixotide Accuhaler 100 micrograms	10949/0227
Flixotide Accuhaler 250 micrograms	10949/0228
Flixotide Accuhaler 500 micrograms	10949/0229

9. DATE OF FIRST AUTHORISATION/RENEWAL OF THE AUTHORISATION
April 1995.

10. DATE OF REVISION OF THE TEXT
24 March 2005

11. Legal Status
POM.

Flixotide Diskhaler
(Allen & Hanburys)

1. NAME OF THE MEDICINAL PRODUCT
Flixotide$_{TM}$ Diskhaler$_{TM}$ 50 Micrograms
Flixotide$_{TM}$ Diskhaler$_{TM}$ 100 Micrograms
Flixotide$_{TM}$ Diskhaler$_{TM}$ 250 Micrograms
Flixotide$_{TM}$ Diskhaler$_{TM}$ 500 Micrograms

2. QUALITATIVE AND QUANTITATIVE COMPOSITION
Fluticasone Propionate (micronised) 50, 100, 250 or 500 micrograms

3. PHARMACEUTICAL FORM
Inhalation Powder.

4. CLINICAL PARTICULARS

4.1 Therapeutic indications
Fluticasone propionate given by inhalation offers preventative treatment for asthma. At recommended doses it has a potent glucocorticoid anti-inflammatory action within the lungs, with a lower incidence and severity of adverse effects than those observed when corticosteroids are administered systemically.

Prophylactic management in:-
Adults
Moderate asthma:

Patients with unstable or worsening asthma despite prophylactic therapy or bronchodilator alone.

Severe asthma:

Patients with severe chronic asthma and those who are dependent on systemic corticosteroids for adequate control of symptoms. On introduction of inhaled fluticasone propionate many of these patients may be able to reduce significantly, or to eliminate, their requirement for oral corticosteroids.

Children

Any child who requires prophylactic medication, including patients not controlled on currently available prophylactic medication.

Route of administration: by inhalation.

4.2 Posology and method of administration

The onset of therapeutic effect is within 4 to 7 days.

Adults and children over 16 years: 100 to 1,000 micrograms twice daily.

Patients should be given a starting dose of inhaled fluticasone propionate, which is appropriate to the severity of their disease.

Prescribers should be aware that fluticasone propionate is as effective as other inhaled steroids approximately at half the microgram daily dose. For example, a 100mcg of fluticasone propionate is approximately equivalent to 200mcg dose of beclometasone dipropionate (CFC containing) or budesonide

Due to the risk of systemic effects, doses above 500 micrograms twice daily should be prescribed only for adult patients with severe asthma where additional clinical benefit is expected, demonstrated by either an improvement in pulmonary function and/or symptom control, or by a reduction in oral corticosteroid therapy (see 4.4 Special Warnings and Precautions for Use and 4.8 Undesirable Effects).

***Typical Adult Starting Doses*:**

For patients with mild asthma, a typical starting dose is 100 micrograms twice daily. In moderate and more severe asthma, starting doses may need to be 250 to 500 micrograms twice daily. Where additional clinical benefit is expected, doses of up to 1000 micrograms twice daily may be used. Initiation of such doses should be prescribed only by a specialist in the management of asthma (such as a consultant physician or general practitioner with appropriate experience).

The dose should be titrated down to the lowest dose at which effective control of asthma is maintained.

Typical starting doses for children over 4years of age:

50 to 100 micrograms twice daily.

Many children's asthma will be well controlled using the 50 to 100 microgram twice daily dosing regime. For those patients whose asthma is not sufficiently controlled, additional benefit may be obtained by increasing the dose up to 200 micrograms twice daily. **The maximum licensed dose in children is 200 micrograms twice daily.**

The starting dose should be appropriate to the severity of the disease. The dose should be titrated down to the lowest dose at which effective control of asthma is maintained.

Special patient groups:

There is no need to adjust the dose in elderly patients or those with hepatic or renal impairment.

4.3 Contraindications

Flixotide preparations are contra-indicated in patients with a history of hypersensitivity to any of their components. (see Pharmaceutical Particulars – List of Excipients).

4.4 Special warnings and special precautions for use

Flixotide Diskhalers are not designed to relieve acute symptoms for which an inhaled short acting bronchodilator is required. Patients should be advised to have such rescue medication available.

Severe asthma requires regular medical assessment, including lung-function testing, as patients are at risk of severe attacks and even death. Increasing use of short-acting inhaled β_2-agonists to relieve symptoms indicates deterioration of asthma control. If patients find that short-acting relief bronchodilator treatment becomes less effective, or they need more inhalations than usual, medical attention must be sought.

In this situation patients should be reassessed and consideration given to the need for increased anti-inflammatory therapy (e.g. higher doses of inhaled corticosteroids or a course of oral corticosteroids). Severe exacerbations of asthma must be treated in the normal way.

As with other inhalation therapy, paradoxical bronchospasm may occur with an immediate increase in wheezing after dosing. Flixotide Diskhaler should be discontinued immediately, the patient assessed and alternative therapy instituted if necessary.

Systemic effects of inhaled corticosteroids may occur, particularly at high doses prescribed for prolonged periods. These effects are much less likely to occur than with oral corticosteroids. Possible systemic effects include Cushing's syndrome, Cushingoid features, adrenal suppression, growth retardation in children and adolescents, decrease in bone mineral density, cataract and glaucoma. **It is important therefore that the dose of inhaled corticosteroid is reviewed regularly and reduced to the lowest dose at which effective control of asthma is maintained.**

Prolonged treatment with high doses of inhaled corticosteroids may result in adrenal suppression and acute adrenal crisis. Children aged < 16 years taking higher than licensed doses of fluticasone(typically ≥1000mcg/day) may be at particular risk. Situations, which could potentially trigger acute adrenal crisis, include trauma, surgery, infection or any rapid reduction in dosage. Presenting symptoms are typically vague and may include anorexia, abdominal pain, weight loss, tiredness, headache, nausea, vomiting, decreased level of consciousness, hypoglycaemia, and seizures. Additional systemic corticosteroid cover should be considered during periods of stress or elective surgery.

It is recommended that the height of children receiving prolonged treatment with inhaled corticosteroids is regularly monitored. If growth is slowed, therapy should be reviewed with the aim of reducing the dose of inhaled corticosteroid, if possible, to the lowest dose at which effective control of asthma is maintained. In addition, consideration should be given to referring the patient to a paediatric respiratory specialist.

When changing from a dry powder inhaler to a metered dose inhaler, administration of high doses, above 1000 mcg daily, is recommended through a spacer to reduce side effects in the mouth and throat. However, this may increase drug delivery to the lungs. As systemic absorption is largely through the lungs, there may be an increase in the risk of systemic adverse effects. A lower dose may be required.

The benefits of inhaled fluticasone propionate should minimise the need for oral steroids. However, patients transferred from oral steroids, remain at risk of impaired adrenal reserve for a considerable time after transferring to inhaled fluticasone propionate. The possibility of adverse effects may persist for some time.

These patients may require specialised advice to determine the extent of adrenal impairment before elective procedures. The possibility of residual impaired adrenal response should always be considered in emergency (medical or surgical) and elective situations likely to produce stress, and appropriate corticosteroid treatment considered.

Lack of response or severe exacerbations of asthma should be treated by increasing the dose of inhaled fluticasone propionate and, if necessary, by giving a systemic steroid and/or an antibiotic if there is an infection.

For the transfer of patients being treated with oral corticosteroids:

The transfer of oral steroid-dependent patients to Flixotide and their subsequent management needs special care as recovery from impaired adrenocortical function, caused by prolonged systemic steroid therapy, may take a considerable time.

Patients who have been treated with systemic steroids for long periods of time or at a high dose may have adrenocortical suppression. With these patients adrenocortical function should be monitored regularly and their dose of systemic steroid reduced cautiously.

After approximately a week, gradual withdrawal of the systemic steroid is started by reducing the daily dose by one milligram prednisolone, or its equivalent. For maintenance doses of prednisolone in excess of 10mg daily, it may be appropriate to cautiously use larger reductions in dose at weekly intervals.

Some patients feel unwell in a non-specific way during the withdrawal phase despite maintenance or even improvement of the respiratory function. They should be encouraged to persevere with inhaled fluticasone propionate and to continue withdrawal of systemic steroid, unless there are objective signs of adrenal insufficiency.

Patients transferred from oral steroids whose adrenocortical function is still impaired should carry a steroid warning card indicating that they need supplementary systemic steroid during periods of stress, e.g. worsening asthma attacks, chest infections, major intercurrent illness, surgery, trauma, etc.

Replacement of systemic steroid treatment with inhaled therapy sometimes unmasks allergies such as allergic rhinitis or eczema previously controlled by the systemic drug. These allergies should be symptomatically treated with antihistamine and/or topical preparations, including topical steroids.

Treatment with Flixotide Diskhalers should not be stopped abruptly.

Special care is necessary in patients with active or quiescent pulmonary tuberculosis.

Ritonavir can greatly increase the concentration of fluticasone propionate in plasma. Therefore, concomitant use should be avoided, unless the potential benefit to the patient outweighs the risk of systemic corticosteroid side-effects. There is also an increased risk of systemic side effects when combining fluticasone propionate with other potent CYP3A inhibitors (see 4.5 Interaction with Other Medicinal Products and Other Forms of Interaction).

4.5 Interaction with other medicinal products and other forms of Interaction

Under normal circumstances, low plasma concentrations of fluticasone propionate are achieved after inhaled dosing, due to extensive first pass metabolism and high systemic clearance mediated by cytochrome P450 3A4 in the gut and liver. Hence, clinically significant drug interactions mediated by fluticasone propionate are unlikely.

In an interaction study in healthy subjects with intranasal fluticasone propionate, ritonavir (a highly potent cytochrome P450 3A4 inhibitor) 100 mg b.i.d. increased the fluticasone propionate plasma concentrations several hundred fold, resulting in markedly reduced serum cortisol concentrations. Information about this interaction is lacking for inhaled fluticasone propionate, but a marked increase in fluticasone propionate plasma levels is expected. Cases of Cushing's syndrome and adrenal suppression have been reported. The combination should be avoided unless the benefit outweighs the increased risk of systemic glucocorticoid side-effects.

In a small study in healthy volunteers, the slightly less potent CYP3A inhibitor ketoconazole increased the exposure of fluticasone propionate after a single inhalation by 150%. This resulted in a greater reduction of plasma cortisol as compared with fluticasone propionate alone. Co-treatment with other potent CYP3A inhibitors, such as itraconazole, is also expected to increase the systemic fluticasone propionate exposure and the risk of systemic side-effects. Caution is recommended and long-term treatment with such drugs should if possible be avoided.

4.6 Pregnancy and lactation

There is inadequate evidence of safety of fluticasone propionate in human pregnancy. Administration of corticosteroids to pregnant animals can cause abnormalities of fetal development, including cleft palate and intra-uterine growth retardation. There may therefore be a very small risk of such effects in the human fetus. It should be noted, however, that the fetal changes in animals occur after relatively high systemic exposure. Because fluticasone propionate is delivered directly to the lungs by the inhaled route it avoids the high level of exposure that occurs when corticosteroids are given by systemic routes.

Administration of fluticasone propionate during pregnancy should only be considered if the expected benefit to the mother is greater than any possible risk to the fetus.

The secretion of fluticasone propionate in human breast milk has not been investigated. Subcutaneous administration of fluticasone propionate to lactating laboratory rats produced measurable plasma levels and evidence of fluticasone propionate in the milk. However, plasma levels in humans after inhalation at recommended doses are likely to be low.

When fluticasone propionate is used in breast feeding mothers the therapeutic benefits must be weighed against the potential hazards to mother and baby.

4.7 Effects on ability to drive and use machines

Fluticasone propionate is unlikely to produce an effect.

4.8 Undesirable effects

Adverse events are listed below by system organ class and frequency. Frequencies are defined as: very common (≥1/10), common (≥1/100 and <1/10), uncommon (≥1/1000 and <1/100), rare (≥1/10,000 and <1/1000) and very rare (<1/10,000) including isolated reports. Very common, common and uncommon events were generally determined from spontaneous data.

System Organ Class	Adverse Event	Frequency
Infections & Infestations	Candidiasis of the mouth and throat	Vey Common
Immune System Disorders	Hypersensitivity reactions with the following manifestations:	
	Cutaneous hypersensitivity reactions	Uncommon
	Angioedema (mainly facial and oropharyngeal oedema)	Very Rare
	Respiratory symptoms (dyspnoea and/or bronchospasm)	Very Rare
	Anaphylactic reactions	Very Rare
Endocrine Disorders	Cushing's syndrome, Cushingoid features, adrenal suppression, growth retardation in children and adolescents, decreased bone mineral density, cataract, glaucoma	Very Rare
Gastrointestinal Disorders	Dyspepsia	Very Rare

Musculoskeletal & Connective Tissue Disorders	Arthralgia	Very Rare
Psychiatric Disorders	Anxiety, sleep disorders, behavioural changes, including hyperactivity and irritability (predominantly in children)	Very Rare
Respiratory, Thoracic & Mediastinal Disorders	Hoarseness/ dysphonia	Common
	Paradoxical bronchospasm	Very Rare

Hoarseness and candidiasis of the mouth and throat (thrush) occurs in some patients. Such patients may find it helpful to rinse out their mouth with water after using the Diskhaler. Symptomatic candidiasis can be treated with topical anti-fungal therapy whilst still continuing with the Flixotide Diskhaler.

Possible systemic effects include Cushing's syndrome, Cushingoid features, adrenal suppression, growth retardation, decreased bone mineral density, cataract, glaucoma. (see 4.4 Special Warnings and Special Precautions for Use).

As with other inhalation therapy, paradoxical bronchospasm may occur (see 4.4 'Special Warnings and Precautions for Use'). This should be treated immediately with a fast-acting inhaled bronchodilator. FlixotideDiskhaler should be discontinued immediately, the patient assessed, and if necessary alternative therapy instituted.

4.9 Overdose

Acute: Inhalation of the drug in doses in excess of those recommended may lead to temporary suppression of adrenal function. This does not necessitate emergency action being taken.

In these patients treatment with fluticasone propionate by inhalation should be continued at a dose sufficient to control asthma; adrenal function recovers in a few days and can be verified by measuring plasma cortisol.

Chronic: refer to section 4.4: risk of adrenal suppression.

Monitoring of adrenal reserve may be indicated. Treatment with inhaled fluticasone propionate should be continued at a dose sufficient to control asthma.

5. PHARMACOLOGICAL PROPERTIES

5.1 Pharmacodynamic properties

Fluticasone propionate given by inhalation at recommended doses has a potent glucocorticoid anti-inflammatory action within the lungs, with a lower incidence and severity of adverse effects than those observed when corticosteroids are administered systemically.

5.2 Pharmacokinetic properties

Systemic absolute bioavailability of fluticasone propionate is estimated at 12-26% of an inhaled dose, dependent on presentation. Systemic absorption occurs mainly through the lungs and is initially rapid then prolonged. The remainder of the dose may be swallowed.

Absolute oral bioavailability is negligible (<1%) due to a combination of incomplete absorption from the GI tract and extensive first-pass metabolism.

87-100% of an oral dose is excreted in the faeces, up to 75% as parent compound. There is also a non-active major metabolite.

After an intravenous dose, fluticasone propionate is extensively distributed in the body. The very high clearance rate indicates extensive hepatic clearance.

5.3 Preclinical safety data

No clinically relevant findings were observed in preclinical studies.

6. PHARMACEUTICAL PARTICULARS

6.1 List of excipients

Lactose (which contains milk protein)

6.2 Incompatibilities

None known

6.3 Shelf life

24 months

6.4 Special precautions for storage

Whilst the disks provide good protection to the blister contents from the effects of the atmosphere, they should not be exposed to extremes of temperature and should not be stored above 30°C. A disk may be kept in the diskhaler at all times but a blister should only be pierced immediately prior to use. Failure to observe this instruction will affect the operation of the diskhaler.

6.5 Nature and contents of container

A circular double-foil (PVC/Aluminium) disk with four blisters, containing a mixture of fluticasone propionate and lactose. The foil disk is inserted into the Diskhaler device.

Flixotide Diskhaler has the following packs are registered:

- 5, 7, 10, 14 or 15 disks with or without a diskhaler.
- Refill packs of 5, 7, 10, 14 or 15 disks.
- A starter pack consisting of diskhaler pre-loaded with one disk (with or without a peak flow meter and diary card).
- A starter pack plus a spare disk (with or without a peak flow meter and diary card).

Not all pack sizes may be marketed

6.6 Instructions for use and handling

See Patient Information Leaflet for detailed instructions.

Administrative Data

7. MARKETING AUTHORISATION HOLDER

Glaxo Wellcome UK Ltd
trading as Allen & Hanburys
Stockley Park West
Uxbridge,
Middlesex
UB11 1BT

8. MARKETING AUTHORISATION NUMBER(S)

Flixotide Diskhaler 50 microgram	PL 10949/0005
Flixotide Diskhaler 100 microgram	PL 10949/0006
Flixotide Diskhaler 250 microgram	PL 10949/0007
Flixotide Diskhaler 500 microgram	PL 10949/0008

9. DATE OF FIRST AUTHORISATION/RENEWAL OF THE AUTHORISATION

25 February 1993

10. DATE OF REVISION OF THE TEXT

24 March 2005

11. Legal Status

POM.

Flixotide Nebules 0.5mg/2ml

(Allen & Hanburys)

1. NAME OF THE MEDICINAL PRODUCT

Flixotide Nebules 0.5mg/2ml.

2. QUALITATIVE AND QUANTITATIVE COMPOSITION

Plastic ampoules containing 2ml of a buffered, isotonic saline suspension containing 0.5mg fluticasone propionate

3. PHARMACEUTICAL FORM

Inhalation suspension for nebulisation.

4. CLINICAL PARTICULARS

4.1 Therapeutic indications

In adults and adolescents over 16 years Flixotide Nebules can be used:

For prophylactic management of severe chronic asthma in patients requiring high dose inhaled or oral corticosteroid therapy. On introduction of inhaled fluticasone propionate many patients currently treated with oral corticosteroids may be able to reduce significantly, or eliminate, their oral dose.

Children and adolescents from 4 to 16 years of age:

Treatment of acute exacerbations of asthma. Subsequent maintenance dosing may be more conveniently accomplished using a pressurised metered dose inhaler or powder formulation.

Fluticasone propionate given by inhalation has a potent glucocorticoid anti-inflammatory action within the lungs. It reduces symptoms and exacerbations of asthma in patients previously treated with bronchodilators alone or with other prophylactic therapy. Relatively brief symptomatic episodes can generally be relieved by the use of fast-acting bronchodilators, but longer-lasting exacerbations require, in addition, the use of corticosteroid therapy as soon as possible to control the inflammation.

4.2 Posology and method of administration

Adults and adolescents over 16 years: 500-2,000 micrograms twice daily.

Prescribers should be aware that fluticasone propionate is as effective as other inhaled steroids approximately at half the microgram daily dose. For example, a 100mcg of fluticasone propionate is approximately equivalent to 200mcg dose of beclometasone dipropionate (CFC containing) or budesonide

Prescribers should be aware of the risks of systemic effects when using high doses of corticosteroids (see 4.4 special warnings and precautions for use and 4.8 undesirable effects).

Patients should be given a starting dose of inhaled fluticasone propionate, which is appropriate to the severity of their disease.

The dose should be titrated down to the lowest dose at which effective control of asthma is maintained.

Children and adolescents from 4 to 16 years of age: 1000 mcg twice daily

Special patient groups: There is no need to adjust the dose in elderly patients or those with hepatic or renal impairment.

Flixotide Nebules are for inhalation use only. They should be administered as an aerosol produced by a jet nebuliser, as directed by a physician. As drug delivery from nebulisers is variable, the manufacturer's instructions for using the nebuliser must be followed.

Use of Flixotide Nebules with ultrasonic nebulisers is not generally recommended.

Flixotide Nebules should not be injected or administered orally.

Patients should be made aware of the prophylactic nature of therapy with inhaled fluticasone propionate and that it should be taken regularly.

It is advisable to administer Flixotide Nebules via a mouthpiece to avoid the possibility of atrophic changes to facial skin which may occur with prolonged use with a face-mask. When a face-mask is used, the exposed skin should be protected using a barrier cream, or the face should be thoroughly washed after treatment.

4.3 Contraindications

Hypersensitivity to any ingredient of the preparation.

4.4 Special warnings and special precautions for use

Flixotide Nebules are not designed to relieve acute symptoms for which an inhaled short-acting bronchodilator is required. Patients should be advised to have such rescue medication available. Flixotide Nebules are intended for regular daily prophylactic treatment.

Flixotide Nebules are not a substitute for injectable or oral corticosteroids in an emergency (i.e. life threatening asthma).

Severe asthma requires regular medical assessment, including lung function testing, as patients are at risk of severe attacks and even death. Increasing use of short-acting inhaled β_2-agonists to relieve symptoms indicates deterioration of asthma control. If patients find that short-acting relief bronchodilator treatment becomes less effective, or they need more inhalations than usual, medical attention must be sought. In this situation patients should be reassessed and consideration given to the need for increased anti-inflammatory therapy (e.g. higher doses of inhaled corticosteroids or a course of oral corticosteroids). Severe exacerbations of asthma must be treated in the normal way.

As with other inhalation therapy, paradoxical bronchospasm may occur with an immediate increase in wheezing after dosing. Flixotide Nebules should be discontinued immediately, the patient assessed and alternative therapy instituted if necessary.

Systemic effects of inhaled corticosteroids may occur, particularly at high doses prescribed for prolonged periods. These effects are much less likely to occur than with oral steroids. Possible systemic effects include Cushing's syndrome, Cushingoid features, adrenal suppression, growth retardation in children and adolescents, decrease in bone mineral density, cataract and glaucoma. **It is important therefore that the dose of inhaled corticosteroid is reviewed regularly and reduced to the lowest dose at which effective control of asthma is maintained.**

Prolonged treatment with high doses of inhaled corticosteroids may result in adrenal suppression and acute adrenal crisis. Children aged < 16 years taking higher than licensed doses of fluticasone (typically ≥1000mcg/day) may be at particular risk. Situations, which could potentially trigger acute adrenal crisis, include trauma, surgery, infection or any rapid reduction in dosage. Presenting symptoms are typically vague and may include anorexia, abdominal pain, weight loss, tiredness, headache, nausea, vomiting, decreased level of consciousness, hypoglycaemia, and seizures. Additional systemic corticosteroid cover should be considered during periods of stress or elective surgery.

It is recommended that the height of children receiving prolonged treatment with inhaled corticosteroids is regularly monitored. If growth is slowed, therapy should be reviewed with the aim of reducing the dose of inhaled corticosteroid, if possible to the lowest dose at which effective control of asthma is maintained. In addition, consideration should be given to referring the patient to a paediatric respiratory specialist.

The benefits of inhaled fluticasone propionate should minimise the need for oral steroids. However, patients transferred from oral steroids, remain at risk of impaired adrenal reserve for a considerable time after transferring to inhaled fluticasone propionate. The possibility of adverse effects may persist for some time. These patients may require specialised advice to determine the extent of adrenal impairment before elective procedures. The possibility of residual impaired adrenal response should always be considered in emergency (medical or surgical) and elective situations likely to produce stress, and appropriate corticosteroid treatment considered.

Patients should receive a dose appropriate to the severity of their disease; the dose should be titrated to the lowest dose at which effective control of asthma is maintained. If control cannot be maintained, the use of a systemic steroid and/or an antibiotic may be necessary.

Replacement of systemic steroid treatment with inhaled therapy sometimes unmasks allergies such as allergic rhinitis or eczema previously controlled by the systemic drug. These allergies should be symptomatically treated with antihistamine and/or topical preparations, including topical steroids.

As with all inhaled corticosteroids, special care is necessary in patients with active or quiescent pulmonary tuberculosis.

Treatment with Flixotide Nebules should not be stopped abruptly.

For the transfer of patients being treated with oral corticosteroids: The transfer of oral steroid-dependent patients to Flixotide Nebules and their subsequent management needs special care as recovery from impaired adrenocortical function, caused by prolonged systemic steroid therapy, may take a considerable time.

Patients who have been treated with systemic steroids for long periods of time or at a high dose may have adrenocortical suppression. With these patients adrenocortical function should be monitored regularly and their dose of systemic steroid reduced cautiously.

After approximately a week, gradual withdrawal of the systemic steroid is commenced. Dosage reductions should be appropriate to the level of maintenance systemic steroid, and introduced at not less than weekly intervals. In general, for maintenance doses of prednisolone (or equivalent) of 10mg daily or less, the dosage reductions should not be greater than 1mg per day, at not less than weekly intervals. For maintenance doses of prednisolone in excess of 10mg daily, it may be appropriate to employ cautiously, larger reductions in dose at weekly intervals.

Some patients feel unwell in a non-specific way during the withdrawal phase despite maintenance or even improvement of the respiratory function. They should be encouraged to persevere with inhaled fluticasone propionate and to continue withdrawal of systemic steroid, unless there are objective signs of adrenal insufficiency.

Patients weaned off oral steroids whose adrenocortical function is still impaired should carry a steroid warning card indicating that they need supplementary systemic steroid during periods of stress, e.g. worsening asthma attacks, chest infections, major intercurrent illness, surgery, trauma, etc.

Ritonavir can greatly increase the concentration of fluticasone propionate in plasma. Therefore, concomitant use should be avoided, unless the potential benefit to the patient outweighs the risk of systemic corticosteroid side-effects. There is also an increased risk of systemic side effects when combining fluticasone propionate with other potent CYP3A inhibitors (see 4.5 Interaction with Other Medicinal Products and Other Forms of Interaction).

4.5 Interaction with other medicinal products and other forms of Interaction

Under normal circumstances, low plasma concentrations of fluticasone propionate are achieved after inhaled dosing, due to extensive first pass metabolism and high systemic clearance mediated by cytochrome P450 3A4 in the gut and liver. Hence, clinically significant drug interactions mediated by fluticasone propionate are unlikely.

In an interaction study in healthy subjects with intranasal fluticasone propionate, ritonavir (a highly potent cytochrome P450 3A4 inhibitor) 100 mg b.i.d. increased the fluticasone propionate plasma concentrations several hundred fold, resulting in markedly reduced serum cortisol concentrations. Information about this interaction is lacking for inhaled fluticasone propionate, but a marked increase in fluticasone propionate plasma levels is expected. Cases of Cushing's syndrome and adrenal suppression have been reported. The combination should be avoided unless the benefit outweighs the increased risk of systemic glucocorticoid side-effects.

In a small study in healthy volunteers, the slightly less potent CYP3A inhibitor ketoconazole increased the exposure of fluticasone propionate after a single inhalation by 150%. This resulted in a greater reduction of plasma cortisol as compared with fluticasone propionate alone. Co-treatment with other potent CYP3A inhibitors, such as itraconazole, is also expected to increase the systemic fluticasone propionate exposure and the risk of systemic side-effects. Caution is recommended and long-term treatment with such drugs should if possible be avoided.

4.6 Pregnancy and lactation

There is inadequate evidence of safety of fluticasone propionate in human pregnancy. Administration of corticosteroids to pregnant animals can cause abnormalities of fetal development, including cleft palate and intra-uterine growth retardation. There may therefore be a very small risk of such effects in the human fetus. It should be noted, however, that the fetal changes in animals occur after relatively high systemic exposure. Because Flixotide Nebules deliver fluticasone propionate directly to the lungs by the inhaled route the high level of exposure that occurs when corticosteroids are given by systemic routes is avoided. Administration of fluticasone propionate during pregnancy should only be considered if the expected benefit to the mother is greater than any possible risk to the fetus.

The secretion of fluticasone propionate in human breast milk has not been investigated. Subcutaneous administration of fluticasone propionate to lactating laboratory rats produced measurable plasma levels and evidence of fluticasone propionate in the milk. However, plasma levels in humans after inhalation at recommended doses are likely to be low. When fluticasone propionate is used in breast-feeding mothers the therapeutic benefits must be weighed against the potential hazards to mother and baby.

4.7 Effects on ability to drive and use machines

Fluticasone propionate is unlikely to produce an effect.

4.8 Undesirable effects

Adverse events are listed below by system organ class and frequency. Frequencies are defined as: very common ($\geq$1/10), common ($\geq$1/100 and <1/10), uncommon ($\geq$1/1000 and <1/100), rare ($\geq$1/10,000 and <1/1000) and very rare (<1/10,000) including isolated reports. Very common, common and uncommon events were generally determined from clinical trial data. Rare and very rare events were generally determined from spontaneous data.

System Organ Class	Adverse Event	Frequency
Infections & Infestations	Candidiasis of the mouth and throat	Very Common
Immune System Disorders	Hypersensitivity reactions with the following manifestations:	
	Cutaneous hypersensitivity reactions	Uncommon
	Angioedema (mainly facial and oropharyngeal oedema),	Very Rare
	Respiratory symptoms (dyspnoea and/ or bronchospasm)	Very Rare
	Anaphylactic reactions	Very Rare
Endocrine Disorders	Cushing's syndrome, Cushingoid features, adrenal suppression, growth retardation in children and adolescents, decreased bone mineral density, cataract, glaucoma	Very Rare
Gastrointestinal Disorders	Dyspepsia	Very Rare
Musculoskeletal & Connective Tissue Disorders	Arthralgia	Very Rare
Psychiatric Disorders	Anxiety, sleep disorders, behavioural changes, including hyperactivity and irritability (predominantly in children)	Very Rare
Respiratory, Thoracic & Mediastinal Disorders	Hoarseness/ dysphonia Paradoxical bronchospasm	Common Very Rare

Hoarseness and candidiasis of the mouth and throat (thrush) occurs in some patients. Such patients may find it helpful to rinse out their mouth with water after inhalation from the nebuliser. Symptomatic candidiasis can be treated with topical anti-fungal therapy whilst still continuing with Flixotide Nebules.

Possible systemic effects include Cushing's syndrome, Cushingoid features, adrenal suppression, growth retardation, decreased bone mineral density, cataract, glaucoma (see 4.4 Special Warnings and Special Precautions for Use).

As with other inhalation therapy, paradoxical bronchospasm may occur (see 4.4 'Special Warnings and Precautions for Use'). This should be treated immediately with a fast acting inhaled bronchodilators. Flixotide Nebules should be discontinued immediately, the patient assessed, and if necessary alternative therapy instituted.

4.9 Overdose

Acute: Inhalation of the drug in doses in excess of those recommended may lead to temporary suppression of adrenal function. This does not necessitate emergency action being taken. In these patients treatment with fluticasone propionate by inhalation should be continued at a dose sufficient to control asthma adrenal function recovers in a few days and can be verified by measuring plasma cortisol.

Chronic: refer to section 4.4: risk of adrenal suppression.

Monitoring of adrenal reserve may be indicated. Treatment with inhaled fluticasone propionate should be continued at a dose sufficient to control asthma.

5. PHARMACOLOGICAL PROPERTIES

5.1 Pharmacodynamic properties

Fluticasone propionate given by inhalation at recommended doses has a potent glucocorticoid anti-inflammatory action within the lungs, which results in reduced symptoms and exacerbations of asthma.

5.2 Pharmacokinetic properties

Following inhaled dosing, systemic availability of the nebulised fluticasone propionate in healthy volunteers is estimated at 8% as compared with up to 26% received from the metered dose inhaler presentation. Systemic absorption occurs mainly through the lungs and is initially rapid then prolonged. The remainder of the dose may be swallowed.

Absolute oral bioavailability is negligible (<1%) due to a combination of incomplete absorption from the GI tract and extensive first-pass metabolism.

87-100% of an oral dose is excreted in the faeces, up to 75% as parent compound. There is also a non-active major metabolite.

After an intravenous dose, fluticasone propionate is extensively distributed in the body. The very high clearance rate indicates extensive hepatic clearance.

5.3 Preclinical safety data

Generally, toxicology has shown only those class effects typical of potent corticosteroids, and these only at doses greatly in excess of that proposed for therapeutic use. However, corticosteroid overdosage effects were produced in juvenile rats at systemic fluticasone propionate doses similar to the maximum paediatric dose. No novel effects were identified in repeat dose toxicity tests, reproductive studies or teratology studies. Fluticasone propionate is devoid of mutagenic activity *in vitro* and *in vivo* and showed no tumorigenic potential in rodents. It is both non-irritant and non-sensitising in animal models.

6. PHARMACEUTICAL PARTICULARS

6.1 List of excipients

Polysorbate 20

Sorbitan laurate

Monosodium phosphate dihydrate

Dibasic sodium phosphate anhydrous

Sodium Chloride

Water for Injection

6.2 Incompatibilities

None reported.

6.3 Shelf life

36 months unopened.

6.4 Special precautions for storage

Flixotide Nebules should not be stored above 30°C. Keep container in the outer carton. Protect from freezing. Store upright.

The blister pack should be opened immediately before use. Opened Nebules should be refrigerated and used within 12 hours of opening.

6.5 Nature and contents of container

2.5ml low density polyethylene ampoules wrapped in a double foil blister, in boxes of 10 or 20.

The foil blister pack consists of a base and lidding foil. The base foil of the blister consists of aluminium (60 microns) coated on the outside with polyamide and on the inside with polyvinylchloride. The lidding consists of paper bonded to polyethyleneterephthalate bonded to aluminium (20 microns), with a coating of vinyl/acrylate lacquer on the inner surface.

6.6 Instructions for use and handling

It is important to ensure that the contents of the Nebule are well mixed before use. While holding the Nebule horizontally by the labelled tab, 'flick' the other end a few times and shake. Repeat this process several times until the entire contents of the Nebule are completely mixed. To open the Nebule, twist off the tab.

Dilution: Flixotide Nebules may be diluted with Sodium Chloride Injection BP if required, to aid administration of small volumes or if a prolonged delivery time is desirable.

Any unused suspension remaining in the nebuliser should be discarded.

For detailed instructions please refer to the Patient Information Leaflet in every pack.

The nebuliser must be used according to the manufacturer's instructions. It is advisable to administer Flixotide Nebules via a mouthpiece (see *Posology and method of administration*).

As many nebulisers operate on a continuous flow basis, it is likely that some nebulised drug will be released into the local environment. Flixotide Nebules should therefore be administered in a well-ventilated room, particularly in hospitals where several patients may be using nebulisers at the same time.

Administrative Data

7. MARKETING AUTHORISATION HOLDER

Glaxo Wellcome UK Ltd,
trading as Allen & Hanburys,
Stockley Park West,
Uxbridge,
Middlesex, UB11 1BT.

8. MARKETING AUTHORISATION NUMBER(S)

PL 10949/0297

9. DATE OF FIRST AUTHORISATION/RENEWAL OF THE AUTHORISATION

21 August 1998

10. DATE OF REVISION OF THE TEXT

24 March 2005

11. Legal Category

POM.

Flixotide Nebules 2mg/2ml

(Allen & Hanburys)

1. NAME OF THE MEDICINAL PRODUCT

Flixotide Nebules 2mg/2ml.

2. QUALITATIVE AND QUANTITATIVE COMPOSITION

Plastic ampoules containing 2ml of a buffered, isotonic saline suspension containing 2mg fluticasone propionate

3. PHARMACEUTICAL FORM

Inhalation suspension for nebulisation.

4. CLINICAL PARTICULARS

4.1 Therapeutic indications

In adults and adolescents over 16 years Flixotide Nebules can be used:

For prophylactic management of severe chronic asthma in patients requiring high dose inhaled or oral corticosteroid therapy. On introduction of inhaled fluticasone propionate many patients currently treated with oral corticosteroids may be able to reduce significantly, or eliminate, their oral dose.

Flixotide Nebules 2mg/2ml are not licensed for use in children under 16 years and therefore should not be used in this patient population. Current clinical data do not allow appropriate dosage recommendations to be made in this patient population.

Fluticasone propionate given by inhalation has a potent glucocorticoid anti-inflammatory action within the lungs. It reduces symptoms and exacerbations of asthma in patients previously treated with bronchodilators alone or with other prophylactic therapy. Relatively brief symptomatic episodes can generally be relieved by the use of fast-acting bronchodilators, but longer-lasting exacerbations require, in addition, the use of corticosteroid therapy as soon as possible to control the inflammation.

4.2 Posology and method of administration

Adults and adolescents over 16 years: 500-2,000 micrograms twice daily.

Prescribers should be aware that fluticasone propionate is as effective as other inhaled steroids approximately at half the microgram daily dose. For example, a 100mcg of fluticasone propionate is approximately equivalent to 200mcg dose of beclometasone dipropionate (CFC containing) or budesonide.

Prescribers should be aware of the risks of systemic effects when using high doses of corticosteroids (see 4.4 special warnings and precautions for use and 4.8 undesirable effects).

Patients should be given a starting dose of inhaled fluticasone propionate, which is appropriate to the severity of their disease.

The dose should be titrated down to the lowest dose at which effective control of asthma is maintained.

Children 16 years and under: Flixotide Nebules 2mg/2ml are not licensed for use in children under 16 years and therefore should not be used in this patient population. Current clinical data do not allow appropriate dosage recommendations to be made in this patient population.

Special patient groups: There is no need to adjust the dose in elderly patients or those with hepatic or renal impairment.

Flixotide Nebules are for inhalation use only. They should be administered as an aerosol produced by a jet nebuliser, as directed by a physician. As drug delivery from nebulisers is variable, the manufacturer's instructions for using the nebuliser must be followed.

Use of Flixotide Nebules with ultrasonic nebulisers is not generally recommended.

Flixotide Nebules should not be injected or administered orally.

Patients should be made aware of the prophylactic nature of therapy with inhaled fluticasone propionate and that it should be taken regularly.

It is advisable to administer Flixotide Nebules via a mouthpiece to avoid the possibility of atrophic changes to facial skin, which may occur with prolonged use with a face-mask. When a face-mask is used, the exposed skin should be protected using a barrier cream, or the face should be thoroughly washed after treatment.

4.3 Contraindications

Hypersensitivity to any ingredient of the preparation.

4.4 Special warnings and special precautions for use

Flixotide Nebules are not designed to relieve acute symptoms for which an inhaled short-acting bronchodilator is required. Patients should be advised to have such rescue medication available. Flixotide Nebules are intended for regular daily prophylactic treatment.

Flixotide Nebules are not a substitute for injectable or oral corticosteroids in an emergency (i.e. life threatening asthma).

Severe asthma requires regular medical assessment, including lung function testing, as patients are at risk of severe attacks and even death. Increasing use of short-acting inhaled β_2-agonists to relieve symptoms indicates deterioration of asthma control. If patients find that short-acting relief bronchodilator treatment becomes less effective, or they need more inhalations than usual, medical attention must be sought. In this situation patients should be reassessed and consideration given to the need for increased anti-inflammatory therapy (e.g. higher doses of inhaled corticosteroids or a course of oral corticosteroids). Severe exacerbations of asthma must be treated in the normal way.

As with other inhalation therapy, paradoxical bronchospasm may occur with an immediate increase in wheezing after dosing. Flixotide Nebules should be discontinued immediately, the patient assessed and alternative therapy instituted if necessary.

Systemic effects of inhaled corticosteroids may occur, particularly at high doses prescribed for prolonged periods. These effects are much less likely to occur than with oral steroids. Possible systemic effects include Cushing's syndrome, Cushingoid features, adrenal suppression, growth retardation in children and adolescents, decrease in bone mineral density, cataract and glaucoma. **It is important therefore that the dose of inhaled corticosteroid is reviewed regularly and reduced to the lowest dose at which effective control of asthma is maintained.**

Prolonged treatment with high doses of inhaled corticosteroids may result in adrenal suppression and acute adrenal crisis. Children aged $<$ 16 years taking higher than licensed doses of fluticasone (typically $\geqslant$1000mcg/day) may be at particular risk. Situations, which could potentially trigger acute adrenal crisis, include trauma, surgery, infection or any rapid reduction in dosage. Presenting symptoms are typically vague and may include anorexia, abdominal pain, weight loss, tiredness, headache, nausea, vomiting, decreased level of consciousness, hypoglycaemia, and seizures. Additional systemic corticosteroid cover should be considered during periods of stress or elective surgery.

It is recommended that the height of children receiving prolonged treatment with inhaled corticosteroids is regularly monitored. If growth is slowed, therapy should be reviewed with the aim of reducing the dose of inhaled corticosteroid, if possible to the lowest dose at which effective control of asthma is maintained. In addition, consideration should be given to referring the patient to a paediatric respiratory specialist.

The benefits of inhaled fluticasone propionate should minimise the need for oral steroids. However, patients transferred from oral steroids, remain at risk of impaired adrenal reserve for a considerable time after transferring to inhaled fluticasone propionate. The possibility of adverse effects may persist for some time. These patients may require specialised advice to determine the extent of adrenal impairment before elective procedures. The possibility of residual impaired adrenal response should always be considered in emergency (medical or surgical) and elective situations likely to produce stress, and appropriate corticosteroid treatment considered.

Patients should receive a dose appropriate to the severity of their disease; the dose should be titrated to the lowest dose at which effective control of asthma is maintained. If control cannot be maintained, the use of a systemic steroid and/or an antibiotic may be necessary.

Replacement of systemic steroid treatment with inhaled therapy sometimes unmasks allergies such as allergic rhinitis or eczema previously controlled by the systemic drug. These allergies should be symptomatically treated with antihistamine and/or topical preparations, including topical steroids.

As with all inhaled corticosteroids, special care is necessary in patients with active or quiescent pulmonary tuberculosis.

Treatment with Flixotide Nebules should not be stopped abruptly.

For the transfer of patients being treated with oral corticosteroids: The transfer of oral steroid-dependent patients to Flixotide Nebules and their subsequent management needs special care as recovery from impaired adrenocortical function, caused by prolonged systemic steroid therapy, may take a considerable time.

Patients who have been treated with systemic steroids for long periods of time or at a high dose may have adrenocortical suppression. With these patients adrenocortical function should be monitored regularly and their dose of systemic steroid reduced cautiously.

After approximately a week, gradual withdrawal of the systemic steroid is commenced. Dosage reductions should be appropriate to the level of maintenance systemic steroid, and introduced at not less than weekly intervals. In general, for maintenance doses of prednisolone (or equivalent) of 10mg daily or less, the dosage reductions should not be greater than 1mg per day, at not less than weekly intervals. For maintenance doses of prednisolone in excess of 10mg daily, it may be appropriate to employ cautiously, larger reductions in dose at weekly intervals.

Some patients feel unwell in a non-specific way during the withdrawal phase despite maintenance or even improvement of the respiratory function. They should be encouraged to persevere with inhaled fluticasone propionate and to continue withdrawal of systemic steroid, unless there are objective signs of adrenal insufficiency.

Patients weaned off oral steroids whose adrenocortical function is still impaired should carry a steroid warning card indicating that they need supplementary systemic steroid during periods of stress, e.g. worsening asthma attacks, chest infections, major intercurrent illness, surgery, trauma, etc.

Ritonavir can greatly increase the concentration of fluticasone propionate in plasma. Therefore, concomitant use should be avoided, unless the potential benefit to the patient outweighs the risk of systemic corticosteroid side-effects. There is also an increased risk of systemic side effects when combining fluticasone propionate with other potent CYP3A inhibitors (see 4.5 Interaction with Other Medicinal Products and Other Forms of Interaction).

4.5 Interaction with other medicinal products and other forms of Interaction

Under normal circumstances, low plasma concentrations of fluticasone propionate are achieved after inhaled dosing, due to extensive first pass metabolism and high systemic clearance mediated by cytochrome P450 3A4 in the gut and liver. Hence, clinically significant drug interactions mediated by fluticasone propionate are unlikely.

In an interaction study in healthy subjects with intranasal fluticasone propionate, ritonavir (a highly potent cytochrome P450 3A4 inhibitor) 100 mg b.i.d. increased the fluticasone propionate plasma concentrations several hundred fold, resulting in markedly reduced serum cortisol concentrations. Information about this interaction is lacking for inhaled fluticasone propionate, but a marked increase in fluticasone propionate plasma levels is expected. Cases of Cushing's syndrome and adrenal suppression have been reported. The combination should be avoided unless the benefit outweighs the increased risk of systemic glucocorticoid side-effects.

In a small study in healthy volunteers, the slightly less potent CYP3A inhibitor ketoconazole increased the exposure of fluticasone propionate after a single inhalation by 150%. This resulted in a greater reduction of plasma cortisol as compared with fluticasone propionate alone. Co-treatment with other potent CYP3A inhibitors, such as itraconazole, is also expected to increase the systemic fluticasone propionate exposure and the risk of systemic side-effects. Caution is recommended and long-term treatment with such drugs should if possible be avoided.

4.6 Pregnancy and lactation

There is inadequate evidence of safety of fluticasone propionate in human pregnancy. Administration of corticosteroids to pregnant animals can cause abnormalities of fetal development, including cleft palate and intra-uterine growth retardation. There may therefore be a very small risk of such effects in the human fetus. It should be noted, however, that the fetal changes in animals occur after relatively high systemic exposure. Because Flixotide Nebules deliver fluticasone propionate directly to the lungs by the inhaled route the high level of exposure that occurs when corticosteroids are given by systemic routes is avoided. Administration of fluticasone propionate during pregnancy should only be considered if the expected benefit to the mother is greater than any possible risk to the fetus.

The secretion of fluticasone propionate in human breast milk has not been investigated. Subcutaneous administration of fluticasone propionate to lactating laboratory rats produced measurable plasma levels and evidence of fluticasone propionate in the milk. However, plasma levels in humans after inhalation at recommended doses are likely to be low. When fluticasone propionate is used in breast-feeding mothers the therapeutic benefits must be weighed against the potential hazards to mother and baby.

4.7 Effects on ability to drive and use machines
Fluticasone propionate is unlikely to produce an effect.

4.8 Undesirable effects
Adverse events are listed below by system organ class and frequency. Frequencies are defined as: very common (≥1/10), common (≥1/100 and <1/10), uncommon (≥1/1000 and <1/100), rare (≥1/10,000 and <1/1000) and very rare (<1/10,000) including isolated reports. Very common, common and uncommon events were generally determined from clinical trial data. Rare and very rare events were generally determined from spontaneous data.

System Organ Class	Adverse Event	Frequency
Infections & Infestations	Candidiasis of the mouth and throat	Very Common
Immune System Disorders	Hypersensitivity reactions with the following manifestations:	
	Cutaneous hypersensitivity reactions	Uncommon
	Angioedema (mainly facial and oropharyngeal oedema),	Very Rare
	Respiratory symptoms (dyspnoea and/or bronchospasm)	Very Rare
	Anaphylactic reactions	Very Rare
Endocrine Disorders	Cushing's syndrome, Cushingoid features, adrenal suppression, growth retardation in children and adolescents, decreased bone mineral density, cataract, glaucoma	Very Rare
Gastrointestinal Disorders	Dyspepsia	Very Rare
Musculoskeletal & Connective Tissue Disorders	Arthralgia	Very Rare
Psychiatric Disorders	Anxiety, sleep disorders, behavioural changes, including hyperactivity and irritability (predominantly in children)	Very Rare
Respiratory, Thoracic & Mediastinal Disorders	Hoarseness/dysphonia Paradoxical bronchospasm	Common Very Rare

Hoarseness and candidiasis of the mouth and throat (thrush) occurs in some patients. Such patients may find it helpful to rinse out their mouth with water after inhalation from the nebuliser. Symptomatic candidiasis can be treated with topical anti-fungal therapy whilst still continuing with Flixotide Nebules.

Possible systemic effects include Cushing's syndrome, Cushingoid features, adrenal suppression, growth retardation, decreased bone mineral density, cataract, glaucoma (see 4.4 Special Warnings and Special Precautions for Use).

As with other inhalation therapy, paradoxical bronchospasm may occur (see 4.4 'Special Warnings and Precautions for Use'). This should be treated immediately with a fast acting inhaled bronchodilators. Flixotide Nebules should be discontinued immediately, the patient assessed, and if necessary alternative therapy instituted.

4.9 Overdose
Acute: Inhalation of the drug in doses in excess of those recommended may lead to temporary suppression of adrenal function. This does not necessitate emergency action being taken. In these patients treatment with fluticasone propionate by inhalation should be continued at a dose sufficient to control asthma adrenal function recovers in a few days and can be verified by measuring plasma cortisol.

Chronic: refer to section 4.4: risk of adrenal suppression.

Monitoring of adrenal reserve may be indicated. Treatment with inhaled fluticasone propionate should be continued at a dose sufficient to control asthma.

5. PHARMACOLOGICAL PROPERTIES

5.1 Pharmacodynamic properties
Fluticasone propionate given by inhalation at recommended doses has a potent glucocorticoid anti-inflammatory action within the lungs, which results in reduced symptoms and exacerbations of asthma.

5.2 Pharmacokinetic properties
Following inhaled dosing, systemic availability of the nebulised fluticasone propionate in healthy volunteers is estimated at 8% as compared with up to 26% received from the metered dose inhaler presentation. Systemic absorption occurs mainly through the lungs and is initially rapid then prolonged. The remainder of the dose may be swallowed.

Absolute oral bioavailability is negligible (<1%) due to a combination of incomplete absorption from the GI tract and extensive first-pass metabolism.

87-100% of an oral dose is excreted in the faeces, up to 75% as parent compound. There is also a non-active major metabolite.

After an intravenous dose, fluticasone propionate is extensively distributed in the body. The very high clearance rate indicates extensive hepatic clearance.

5.3 Preclinical safety data
Toxicology has shown only those class effects typical of potent corticosteroids, and these only at doses greatly in excess of that proposed for therapeutic use. No novel effects were identified in repeat dose toxicity tests, reproductive studies or teratology studies. Fluticasone propionate is devoid of mutagenic activity *in vitro* and *in vivo* and showed no tumorigenic potential in rodents. It is both non-irritant and non-sensitising in animal models.

6. PHARMACEUTICAL PARTICULARS

6.1 List of excipients
Polysorbate 20 Ph. Eur

Sorbitan laurate Ph. Eur

Monosodium phosphate dihydrate Ph. Eur

Dibasic sodium phosphate anhydrous USP

Sodium Chloride Ph. Eur

Water for Injection Ph. Eur

6.2 Incompatibilities
None reported.

6.3 Shelf life
36 months unopened.

6.4 Special precautions for storage
Flixotide Nebules should not be stored above 30°C. Keep container in the outer carton. Protect from freezing. Store upright.

The blister pack should be opened immediately before use. Opened Nebules should be refrigerated and used within 12 hours of opening.

6.5 Nature and contents of container
2.5ml low density polyethylene ampoules wrapped in a double foil blister, in boxes of 10 or 20.

The foil blister pack consists of a base and lidding foil. The base foil of the blister consists of aluminium (60 microns) coated on the outside with polyamide and on the inside with polyvinylchloride. The lidding consists of paper bonded to polyethyleneterephthalate bonded to aluminium (20 microns), with a coating of vinyl/acrylate lacquer on the inner surface.

6.6 Instructions for use and handling
It is important to ensure that the contents of the Nebule are well mixed before use. While holding the Nebule horizontally by the labelled tab, 'flick' the other end a few times and shake. Repeat this process several times until the entire contents of the Nebule are completely mixed. To open the Nebule, twist off the tab.

Dilution: Flixotide Nebules may be diluted with Sodium Chloride Injection BP if required, to aid administration of small volumes or if a prolonged delivery time is desirable. Any unused suspension remaining in the nebuliser should be discarded.

For detailed instructions please refer to the Patient Information Leaflet in every pack.

The nebuliser must be used according to the manufacturer's instructions. It is advisable to administer Flixotide Nebules via a mouthpiece (see *Posology and method of administration*).

As many nebulisers operate on a continuous flow basis, it is likely that some nebulised drug will be released into the local environment. Flixotide Nebules should therefore be administered in a well-ventilated room, particularly in hospitals where several patients may be using nebulisers at the same time.

Administrative Data

7. MARKETING AUTHORISATION HOLDER
Glaxo Wellcome UK Ltd,
trading as Allen & Hanburys,
Stockley Park West,
Uxbridge,
Middlesex, UB11 1BT.

8. MARKETING AUTHORISATION NUMBER(S)
PL 10949/0298

9. DATE OF FIRST AUTHORISATION/RENEWAL OF THE AUTHORISATION
21 August 1998

10. DATE OF REVISION OF THE TEXT
24 March 2005

11. Legal Status
POM.

Flolan 0.5mg Injection

(GlaxoSmithKline UK)

1. NAME OF THE MEDICINAL PRODUCT
Flolan 0.5mg Injection

2. QUALITATIVE AND QUANTITATIVE COMPOSITION
Epoprostenol Sodium 0.5mg

3. PHARMACEUTICAL FORM
Freeze-Dried Powder

4. CLINICAL PARTICULARS

4.1 Therapeutic indications
Flolan is indicated for use in renal dialysis when use of heparin carries a high risk of causing or exacerbating bleeding or when heparin is otherwise contra-indicated.

Route of administration

By continuous infusion, either intravascularly or into the blood supplying the dialyser.

4.2 Posology and method of administration
Flolan is suitable for continuous infusion only, either intravascularly or into the blood supplying the dialyser.

The following schedule of infusion has been found effective in adults:

Prior to dialysis: 4 nanogram/kg/min intravenously.

During dialysis: 4 nanogram/kg/min into the arterial inlet of the dialyser.

The infusion should be stopped at the end of dialysis.

The recommended doses should be exceeded only with careful monitoring of patient blood pressure.

Use in children: There is no specific information on the use of Flolan in children.

Use in the elderly: There is no specific information available on the use of Flolan in elderly patients.

Reconstitution: Only the GlaxoSmithKline Glycine Buffer Diluent provided for the purpose should be used. The enclosed filter unit must be used once only and then discarded after use.

To reconstitute Flolan, a strict aseptic technique must be used. Particular care should be taken in calculating dilutions, and in diluting Flolan the following procedure is recommended:

1. Withdraw approximately 10 ml of the sterile GlaxoSmithKline Glycine Buffer Diluent into a sterile syringe.

2. Inject the contents of the syringe into the vial containing Flolan and shake gently until the powder has dissolved.

3. Draw up all the Flolan solution into the syringe.

4. Re-inject the entire contents into the residue of the original 50 ml of sterile GlaxoSmithKline Glycine Buffer Diluent.

5. Mix well. This solution is now referred to as the *concentrated solution* and contains Flolan 10,000 nanograms per millilitre. When 0.5mg Flolan powder for intravenous infusion is reconstituted with 50 ml sterile GlaxoSmithKline Glycine Buffer Diluent solution, the final injection has a pH of approximately 10.5 and a sodium ion content of approximately 56mg. The *concentrated solution* is normally further diluted before use. It may be diluted with physiological saline (0.9%), provided a ratio of 6 volumes of saline to 1 volume of *concentrated solution* is not exceeded; e.g. 50 ml of *concentrated solution* further diluted with a maximum of 300 ml saline. Other common intravenous fluids are unsatisfactory for the dilution of the *concentrated solution* as the required pH is not attained. Flolan solutions are less stable at low pH. For administration using a pump capable of delivering small volume constant infusions, suitable aliquots of concentrated solution may be diluted with sterile physiological saline.

6. Before further dilution, draw up the *concentrated solution* into a larger syringe.

7. The filter provided should then be attached to the syringe and the *concentrated solution* is dispensed by filtration using firm but not excessive pressure. The typical time taken for filtration of 50 ml of of solution is 70 seconds.

When reconstituted and diluted as directed, Flolan infusion solutions have a pH of approximately 10 and will retain 90% of their initial potency for approximately 12 hours at 25°C.

Infusion rate guidance In general, the infusion rate may be calculated by the following formula:

$$\text{Infusion rate (ml/min)} = \frac{\text{Dosage (ng/kg/min)} \times \text{body weight (kg)}}{\text{Concentration of infusion (ng/ml)}}$$

Examples:

Flolan may be administered in diluted form (1) or as the *concentrated solution* (2)

1. *Diluted*: A commonly used dilution is:

10ml *concentrated solution* + 40 ml physiological saline (0.9%).

Resultant concentration = 2,000 nanogram/ml epoprostenol.

Body weight (kilograms)

(see Table 1)

2. Using *concentrated solution* ie 10,000 ng/ml epoprostenol.

Bodyweight (kilograms)

(see Table 2)

4.3 Contraindications

Flolan is contra-indicated in patients with known hypersensitivity to the drug.

4.4 Special warnings and special precautions for use

Because of the high pH of the final infusion solutions, care should be taken to avoid extravasation during their administration and consequent risk of tissue damage.

Flolan is a potent vasodilator. The cardiovascular effects during infusion disappear within 30 minutes of the end of administration.

Flolan is not a conventional anticoagulant. Flolan has been successfully used instead of heparin in renal dialysis, but in a small proportion of dialyses clotting has developed in the dialysis circuit, requiring termination of dialysis.

Haemorrhagic complications have not been encountered with Flolan but the possibility should be considered when the drug is administered to patients with spontaneous or drug-induced haemorrhagic diatheses. When Flolan is used alone, measurements such as activated whole blood clotting time may not be reliable.

Blood pressure and heart rate should be monitored during administration of Flolan. Flolan may either decrease or increase heart rate. The change is thought to depend on the concentration of epoprostenol administered. Hypotension may occur during infusions of Flolan.

The effects of Flolan on heart-rate may be masked by concomitant use of drugs which affect cardiovascular reflexes.

If excessive hypotension occurs during administration of Flolan, the dose should be reduced or the infusion discontinued. Hypotension may be profound in overdose and may result in loss of consciousness. (See section 4.9, Overdose.)

The hypotensive effect of Flolan may be enhanced by the use of acetate buffer in the dialysis bath during renal dialysis.

During renal dialysis with Flolan there is a need for careful haematological monitoring and it should be ensured that cardiac output is adequately maintained so that delivery of oxygen to peripheral tissues is not diminished.

Elevated serum glucose levels have been reported during infusion of Flolan in man but these are not inevitable.

The pack for this product will contain the following statements:

Keep out reach of children

Store below 25°C

Do not freeze

Protect from light

Keep dry

Reconstitute only with the GlaxoSmithKline Glycine Buffer Diluent provided

Prepare immediately prior to use

Discard any unused solution after 12 hours

4.5 Interaction with other medicinal products and other forms of Interaction

When Flolan is administered to patients receiving concomitant anticoagulants standard anticoagulant monitoring is advisable as there may be potentiation of effect.

The vasodilator effect of Flolan may augment or be augmented by concomitant use of other vasodilators.

Flolan may reduce the thrombolytic efficacy of tissue plasminogen activator (t-PA) by increasing hepatic clearance of t-PA.

4.6 Pregnancy and lactation

For epoprostenol sodium no clinical data on exposed pregnancies are available. Animal studies do not indicate direct or indirect harmful effects with respect to pregnancy, embryonal/foetal development, parturition or postnatal development. Caution should be exercised when prescribing to pregnant women.

Lactation:

There is no information on the use of Flolan during lactation.

4.7 Effects on ability to drive and use machines

Not applicable.

4.8 Undesirable effects

Facial flushing is commonly seen, even in the anaesthetised patient.

Headache and gastro-intestinal symptoms including nausea, vomiting and abdominal colic have occurred in some conscious individuals.

Jaw pain, dry mouth, lassitude, reddening over the infusion site, chest pain and tightness and decreased platelet count have been reported with varying frequency.

Tachycardia has frequently been reported as a response to Flolan at doses of 5 ng/kg/min and below.

Bradycardia, accompanied by pallor, nausea, sweating and sometimes abdominal discomfort and orthostatic hypotension, have occurred in healthy volunteers at doses of epoprostenol sodium greater than 5 nanogram/kg/min. Bradycardia associated with a considerable fall in systolic and diastolic blood pressure has followed intravenous administration of a dose of epoprostenol sodium equivalent to 30 nanogram/kg/min in healthy conscious volunteers.

4.9 Overdose

The main feature of overdosage is likely to be hypotension.

In general, events seen after overdose of epoprostenol represent exaggerated pharmacological effects of the drug. If overdose occurs reduce the dose or discontinue the infusion and initiate appropriate supportive measures as necessary; for example, plasma volume expansion and/or adjustment to pump flow.

5. PHARMACOLOGICAL PROPERTIES

5.1 Pharmacodynamic properties

Flolan is epoprostenol sodium, the monosodium salt of epoprostenol, a naturally occurring prostaglandin produced by the intima of blood vessels. Epoprostenol is the most potent inhibitor of platelet aggregation known. It is also a potent vasodilator.

Infusions of 4ng/kg/min for 30 minutes have been shown to have no significant effect on heart rate or blood pressure, although facial flushing may occur at these levels.

Many of the actions of epoprostenol are exerted via the stimulation of adenylate cyclase, which leads to increased intracellular levels of cyclic adenosine 3'5' monophosphate (cAMP). A sequential stimulation of adenylate cyclase, followed by activation of phosphodiesterase, has been described in human platelets. Elevated cAMP levels regulate intracellular calcium concentrations by stimulating calcium removal, and this platelet aggregation is ultimately inhibited by the reduction of cytoplasmic calcium, upon which platelet shape change, aggregation and the release reaction depend.

The effect of epoprostenol on platelet aggregation is dose-related when between 2 and 16 ng/kg/min is administered intravenously, and significant inhibition of aggregation induced by adenosine diphosphate is observed at doses 4ng/kg/min and above.

Effects on platelets have been found to disappear within 2 hours of discontinuing the infusion, and haemodynamic changes due to epoprostenol to return to baseline within 10 minutes of termination of 60-minute infusions at 1-16 ng/kg/min.

Higher doses of epoprostenol sodium (20 nanograms/kg/min) disperse circulating platelet aggregates and increase by up to two fold the cutaneous bleeding time.

Epoprostenol potentiates the anticoagulant activty of heparin by approximately 50%, possibly reducing the release of heparin neutralising factor.

5.2 Pharmacokinetic properties

Intravenously administered epoprostenol sodium is rapidly distributed from blood to tissue. At normal physiological pH and temperature, it breaks down spontaneously to 6-oxo-prostaglandin $F_{1\alpha}$, although there is some enzymatic degradation to other products. The half-life for this process in man is expected to be no more than 6 minutes, and may be as short as 2-3 minutes, as estimated from in vitro rates of degradation of epoprostenol in human whole blood.

Pharmacokinetic studies in animals have shown the whole body distribution to be 1015ml/kg, and the whole body clearance to be 4.27ml/kg/sec. Following intravenous injection of radiolabelled epoprostenol, the highest concentrations are found in the liver, kidneys and small intestine. Steady-state plasma concentrations are reached within 15 minutes and are proportional to infusion rates. Extensive clearance by the liver has been demonstrated, with approximately 80% being removed in a single pass. Urinary excretion of the metabolites of epoprostenol accounts for between 40% and 90% of the administered dose, with biliary excretion accounting for the remainder. Urinary excretion is greater than 95% complete within 25 hours of dosing. Tissue levels decline rapidly with no evidence of accumulation.

Following the administration of radiolabelled epoprostenol to humans, the urinary and faecal recoveries of radioactivity were 82% and 4% respectively. At least 16 compounds were found, 10 of which were structurally identified. Unlike many other prostaglandins, epoprostenol is not metabolised during passage through the pulmonary circulation.

Due to the chemical instability, high potency and short half-life of epoprostenol, no precise and accurate assay has been identified as appropriate for quantifying epoprostenol in biological fluids.

5.3 Preclinical safety data

Fertility:

A study in which male and female rats were dosed subcutaneously for 74 or 63 days respectively, with 0, 10, 30 or 100mg/kg/day, showed no effects on fertility.

6. PHARMACEUTICAL PARTICULARS

6.1 List of excipients

FREEZE-DRIED POWDER

Glycine BP 3.76 mg

Sodium chloride EP 2-932 mg

Mannitol BP 50.0 mg

Sodium hydroxide BP (quantity not fixed - used to adjust pH)

*Water for injections EP

*Water for injections is used during manufacture but is not present in the finished product, but removed during the freeze-drying process.

6.2 Incompatibilities

None known.

6.3 Shelf life

2 years - freeze dried powder

0.5 day - reconstituted solution for injection

6.4 Special precautions for storage

Freeze dried powder:

Keep dry

Protect from light

Store below 25°C

Table 1 Body weight (kilograms)

		30	40	50	60	70	80	90	100
Dosage (ng/kg/min)	1	0.90	1.20	1.50	1.80	2.10	2.40	2.70	3.00
	2	1.80	2.40	3.00	3.60	4.20	4.80	5.40	6.00
	3	2.70	3.60	4.50	5.40	6.30	7.20	8.10	9.00
	4	3.60	4.80	6.00	7.20	8.40	9.60	10.80	12.00
	5	4.50	6.00	7.50	9.00	10.50	12.00	13.50	15.00

Flow rates in mls/hr

Table 2 Bodyweight (kilograms)

		30	40	50	60	70	80	90	100
Dosage (ng/kg/min)	1	0.18	0.24	0.30	0.36	0.42	0.48	0.54	0.60
	2	0.36	0.48	0.60	0.72	0.84	0.96	1.08	1.20
	3	0.54	0.72	0.90	1.08	1.26	1.44	1.62	1.80
	4	0.72	0.96	1.20	1.44	1.68	1.92	2.16	2.40
	5	0.90	1.20	1.50	1.80	2.10	2.40	2.70	3.00

Flow rates in mls/hr

6.5 Nature and contents of container

0.5 mg freeze dried powder is contained in glass vials with synthetic butyl rubber plugs and aluminium collars.

6.6 Instructions for use and handling

No special instructions.

Administrative Data

7. MARKETING AUTHORISATION HOLDER

Glaxo Wellcome UK Ltd

Trading as GlaxoSmithKline UK

Stockley Park West

Uxbridge

Middlesex

UB11 1BT

United Kingdom

8. MARKETING AUTHORISATION NUMBER(S)

PL 10949/0310

9. DATE OF FIRST AUTHORISATION/RENEWAL OF THE AUTHORISATION

MAA 18.03.81

Renewal: 13.08.87, 23.04.91, 03.08.02

10. DATE OF REVISION OF THE TEXT

30 December 2004

11. Legal Status

POM

Flolan Injection 1.5mg

(GlaxoSmithKline UK)

1. NAME OF THE MEDICINAL PRODUCT

Flolan 1.5mg Injection ▼

2. QUALITATIVE AND QUANTITATIVE COMPOSITION

Epoprostenol sodium equivalent to 1.5 mg epoprostenol.

3. PHARMACEUTICAL FORM

Sterile freeze-dried powder for solution for infusion.

4. CLINICAL PARTICULARS

4.1 Therapeutic indications

Flolan is indicated for use in renal dialysis when use of heparin carries a high risk of causing or exacerbating bleeding or when heparin is otherwise contraindicated.

Flolan is also indicated for the intravenous treatment of primary pulmonary hypertension (PPH) in New York Heart Association (NYHA) functional Class III and Class IV patients who do not respond adequately to conventional therapy. There are limited data on long term use.

4.2 Posology and method of administration

Flolan is not to be used for bolus administration.

Flolan (epoprostenol sodium) must be reconstituted only with specific sterile diluent for Flolan. (*See section 6.6 Instructions for use/handling).*

Renal Dialysis:

Flolan is suitable for continuous infusion only, either intravascularly or into the blood supplying the dialyser.

The following general schedule of infusion has been found effective in adults:

Prior to dialysis: 4 nanogram/kg/min intravenously.

During dialysis: 4 nanogram/kg/min into the arterial inlet of the dialyser.

The infusion should be stopped at the end of dialysis.

The recommended dose for renal dialysis should be exceeded only with careful monitoring of patient blood pressure.

Children and the elderly:

There is no specific information available on the use of Flolan for renal dialysis in children or in elderly patients.

Primary Pulmonary Hypertension:

The following schedules have been found effective:

Adults

Short-term (acute) dose ranging:

A short-term dose-ranging procedure administered via either a peripheral or central venous line is required to determine the long-term infusion rate. The infusion rate is initiated at 2 nanogram/kg/min and increased by increments of 2 nanogram/kg/min every 15 minutes or longer until maximum haemodynamic benefit or dose-limiting pharmacological effects are elicited.

During acute dose ranging in clinical trials, the mean maximum tolerated dose was 8.6±0.3 nanogram/kg/min.

Long-term continuous infusion:

Long-term continuous infusion of Flolan should be administered through a central venous catheter. Temporary peripheral intravenous infusions may be used until central access is established. Long-term infusions should be initiated at 4 nanogram/kg/min less than the maximum tolerated infusion rate determined during short-term dose-ranging. If the maximum tolerated infusion rate is less than 5 nanogram/kg/min; the long-term infusion should be started at one-half the maximum tolerated infusion rate.

Dosage adjustments:

Changes in the long-term infusion rate should be based on persistence, recurrence or worsening of the patient's symptoms of PPH or the occurrence of adverse events due to excessive doses of Flolan.

In general, the need for increases in dose from the initial long-term dose should be expected over time. Increases in dose should be considered if symptoms of PPH persist, or recur after improving. The infusion rate should be increased by 1 to 2 nanogram/kg/min increments at intervals sufficient to allow assessment of clinical response; these intervals should be of at least 15 minutes. Following establishment of a new infusion rate, the patient should be observed, and erect and supine blood pressure and heart rate monitored for several hours to ensure that the new dose is tolerated.

During long-term infusion, the occurrence of dose-related pharmacological events similar to those observed during the dose-ranging period may necessitate a decrease in infusion rate, but the adverse event may occasionally resolve without dosage adjustment. Dosage decreases should be made gradually in 2 nanogram/kg/min decrements every 15 minutes or longer until the dose-limiting effects resolve. Abrupt withdrawal of Flolan or sudden large reductions in infusion rates should be avoided. Except in life-threatening situations (eg. unconsciousness, collapse, etc) infusion rates of Flolan should be adjusted only under the direction of a physician.

Oral anticoagulation was continued in the PPH clinical trial population in addition to continuous intravenous Flolan administration and was well tolerated. Concurrent oral anticoagulation is recommended.

Children

There is limited information on the use of Flolan for PPH in children.

Elderly

There is limited information on the use of Flolan in patients over 65. In general, dose selection for an elderly patient should be made carefully, reflecting the greater frequency of decreased hepatic, renal or cardiac function and of concomitant disease or other drug therapy.

4.3 Contraindications

Flolan is contraindicated in patients with known hypersensitivity to the drug.

Flolan is contraindicated in patients with congestive heart failure arising from severe left ventricular dysfunction.

Flolan should not be used chronically in patients who develop pulmonary oedema during dose-ranging.

4.4 Special warnings and special precautions for use

Because of the high pH of the final infusion solutions, care should be taken to avoid extravasation during their administration and consequent risk of tissue damage

Flolan is a potent pulmonary and systemic vasodilator. The cardiovascular effects during infusion disappear within 30 minutes of the end of administration.

Blood pressure and heart rate should be monitored during administration of Flolan. Flolan may either decrease or increase heart rate. The change is thought to depend on the concentration of epoprostenol administered.

The effects of Flolan on heart-rate may be masked by concomitant use of drugs which affect cardiovascular reflexes.

If excessive hypotension occurs during administration of Flolan, the dose should be reduced or the infusion discontinued. Hypotension may be profound in overdose and may result in loss of consciousness. (See section 4.9, Overdose.)

Elevated serum glucose levels have been reported during infusion of Flolan in man but these are not inevitable.

Renal Dialysis:

The hypotensive effect of Flolan may be enhanced by the use of acetate buffer in the dialysis bath during renal dialysis.

Flolan is not a conventional anticoagulant. Flolan has been successfully used instead of heparin in renal dialysis, but in a small proportion of dialyses clotting has developed in the dialysis circuit, requiring termination of dialysis.

During renal dialysis with Flolan there is a need for careful haematological monitoring and it should be ensured that cardiac output is adequately maintained so that delivery of oxygen to peripheral tissues is not diminished.

Haemorrhagic complications have not been encountered with Flolan but the possibility should be considered when the drug is administered to patients with spontaneous or drug-induced haemorrhagic diatheses. When Flolan is used alone, measurements such as activated whole blood clotting time may not be reliable.

Primary Pulmonary Hypertension:

The hazards of Flolan treatment are considered to outweigh the risks of the disease in patients with functional capacity of New York Heart Association (NYHA) Class I and Class II. Flolan therapy should therefore not be initiated in these patients.

Flolan should be used only by clinicians experienced in the diagnosis and treatment of this disorder.

Short-term dose-ranging with Flolan must be performed in a hospital setting with adequate personnel and equipment for haemodynamic monitoring and emergency care.

Some patients with primary pulmonary hypertension have developed pulmonary oedema during dose-ranging, which may be associated with pulmonary veno-occlusive disease.

Flolan is infused continuously through a permanent indwelling central venous catheter via a small, portable infusion pump. Thus, therapy with Flolan requires commitment by the patient to sterile drug reconstitution, drug administration, care of the permanent central venous catheter, and access to intense and ongoing patient education.

Sterile technique must be adhered to in preparing the drug and in the care of the catheter. Even brief interruptions in the delivery of Flolan may result in rapid symptomatic deterioration. The decision to receive Flolan for PPH should be based upon the understanding that there is a high likelihood that therapy with Flolan will be needed for prolonged periods, possibly years, and the patient's ability to accept and care for a permanent intravenous catheter and infusion pump should be carefully considered.

GlaxoSmithKline Glycine Buffer Diluent contains no preservative, consequently a vial should be used once only and then discarded.

4.5 Interaction with other medicinal products and other forms of Interaction

When Flolan is administered to patients receiving concomitant anticoagulants standard anticoagulant monitoring is advisable as there may be potentiation of effect.

The vasodilator effects of Flolan may augment or be augmented by concomitant use of vasodilators.

Flolan may reduce the thrombolytic efficacy of tissue plasminogen activator (t-PA) by increasing hepatic clearance of t-PA.

When NSAIDS or other drugs affecting platelets aggregation are used concomitantly, there is the potential for Flolan to increase the risk of bleeding.

4.6 Pregnancy and lactation

No teratogenic effects have been seen in rats or rabbits. However, as animal studies are not always predictive of human response, administration of this drug should only be considered if the expected benefit to the mother is greater than any risk to the foetus.

For epoprostenol sodium no clinical data on exposed pregnancies are available. Animal studies do not indicate direct or indirect harmful effects with respect to pregnancy, embryonal/foetal development, parturition or postnatal development. Caution should be exercised when prescribing to pregnant women.

It is not known whether epoprostenol is excreted in breast milk. Nursing mothers should be advised to discontinue breast feeding during treatment with Flolan.

4.7 Effects on ability to drive and use machines

There are no data regarding the effect of Flolan used in renal dialysis on the ability to drive or operate machinery.

PPH and its therapeutic management may affect the ability to drive and operate machinery.

4.8 Undesirable effects

Facial flushing is commonly seen, even in the anaesthetised patient.

Headache and gastrointestinal symptoms including nausea, vomiting and abdominal colic have occurred in some conscious individuals.

Jaw pain, dry mouth, lassitude, reddening over the infusion site, chest pain and tightness and decreased platelet count have been reported with varying frequency.

Tachycardia has frequently been reported as a response to Flolan at doses of 5nanograms/kg/min and below.

Bradycardia, accompanied by pallor, nausea, sweating and occasionally abdominal discomfort and orthostatic hypotension, has occurred in healthy volunteers at doses of epoprostenol sodium greater than 5 nanogram/kg/min. Bradycardia associated with a considerable fall in systolic and diastolic blood pressure has followed intravenous administration of a dose of epoprostenol sodium equivalent to 30 nanogram/kg/min in healthy conscious volunteers.

Additional adverse events reported during the clinical trials of Flolan in PPH include anxiety, nervousness and agitation. The interpretation of adverse events during long term administration of Flolan is complicated by the clinical features of PPH.

In patients receiving Flolan for PPH local infection, pain at the injection site, occlusion of the long intravenous catheter and sepsis/septicaemia have been reported.

4.9 Overdose

The main feature of overdosage is likely to be hypotension.

In general, events seen after overdose of epoprostenol represent exaggerated pharmacological effects of the drug. If overdose occurs reduce the dose or discontinue the infusion and initiate appropriate supportive measures as necessary; for example plasma volume expansion and/or adjustment to pump flow.

5. PHARMACOLOGICAL PROPERTIES

5.1 Pharmacodynamic properties

Flolan is epoprostenol sodium, the monosodium salt of epoprostenol, a naturally occurring prostaglandin produced by the intima of blood vessels. Epoprostenol is a potent inhibitor of platelet aggregation. It is also a potent vasodilator.

Infusions of 4 nanogram/kg/min for 30 minutes have been shown to have no significant effect on heart rate or blood pressure, although facial flushing may occur at these levels.

Renal Dialysis:

Many of the actions of epoprostenol are exerted via the stimulation of adenylate cyclase, which leads to increased intracellular levels of cyclic adenosine 3'5' monophosphate (cAMP). A sequential stimulation of adenylate cyclase, followed by activation of phosphodiesterase, has been described in human platelets. Elevated cAMP levels regulate intracellular calcium concentrations by stimulating calcium removal, and this platelet aggregation is ultimately inhibited by the reduction of cytoplasmic calcium, upon which platelet shape change, aggregation and the release reaction depend.

The effect of epoprostenol on platelet aggregation is dose-related when between 2 and 16 ng/kg/min is administered intravenously, and significant inhibition of aggregation induced by adenosine diphosphate is observed at doses 4ng/kg/min and above.

Effects on platelets have been found to disappear within 2 hours of discontinuing the infusion, and haemodynamic changes due to epoprostenol to return to baseline within 10 minutes of termination of 60-minute infusions at 1-16 ng/kg/min.

Higher doses of epoprostenol sodium (20 nanograms/kg/min) disperse circulating platelet aggregates and increase by up to two fold the cutaneous bleeding time.

Epoprostenol potentiates the anticoagulant activty of heparin by approximately 50%, possibly reducing the release of heparin neutralising factor.

Primary Pulmonary Hypertension:

Intravenous Flolan infusions of up to 15 minutes have been found to produce dose-related increases in cardiac index (CI) and stroke volume (SV), and dose-related decreases in pulmonary vascular resistance (PVR), total pulmonary resistance (TPR), and mean systemic arterial pressure (SAPm). The effects of Flolan on mean pulmonary artery pressure (PAPm) in patients with PPH were variable and minor.

Chronic haemodynamic effects are generally similar to acute effects. During chronic infusion cardiac index (CI), stroke volume (SV) and arterial oxygen saturation are increased and mean systemic arterial pressure (SAPm), right atrial pressure, total pulmonary resistance (TPR) and systemic vascular resistance are decreased.

5.2 Pharmacokinetic properties

Intravenously administered epoprostenol sodium is rapidly distributed from blood to tissue. At normal physiological pH and temperature, it breaks down spontaneously to 6-oxo-prostaglandin $F_1\alpha$, although there is some enzymatic degradation to other products. The half-life for this process in man is expected to be no more than 6 minutes, and may be as short as 2-3 minutes, as estimated from in vitro rates of degradation of epoprostenol in human whole blood.

Pharmacokinetic studies in animals have shown the whole body distribution to be 1015ml/kg, and the whole body clearance to be 4.27ml/kg/sec. Following intravenous injection of radiolabelled epoprostenol, the highest concentrations are found in the liver, kidneys and small intestine. Steady-state plasma concentrations are reached within 15 minutes and are proportional to infusion rates. Extensive clearance by the liver has been demonstrated, with approximately 80% being removed in a single pass. Urinary excretion of the metabolites of epoprostenol accounts for between 40% and 90% of the administered dose, with biliary excretion accounting for the remainder. Urinary excretion is greater than 95% complete within 25 hours of dosing. Tissue levels decline rapidly with no evidence of accumulation.

Following the administration of radiolabelled epoprostenol to humans, the urinary and faecal recoveries of radioactivity were 82% and 4% respectively. At least 16 compounds were found, 10 of which were structurally identified. Unlike many other prostaglandins, epoprostenol is not metabolised during passage through the pulmonary circulation.

Due to the chemical instability, high potency and short half-life of epoprostenol, no precise and accurate assay has been identified as appropriate for quantifying epoprostenol in biological fluids.

5.3 Preclinical safety data

Fertility: A study in which male and female rats were dosed subcutaneously for 74 or 63 days respectively, with 0, 10, 30 or 100mg/kg/day, showed no effects on fertility.

There was no evidence of mutagenicity in the Ames test, micronucleus assay or DNA elution.

Carcinogenicity: Oncology studies have not been performed.

6. PHARMACEUTICAL PARTICULARS

6.1 List of excipients

Freeze-dried powder:

Glycine

Sodium Chloride

Mannitol

Sodium hydroxide

6.2 Incompatibilities

Flolan must be reconstituted using only the sterile buffer provided. Any further dilution must be performed using only the recommended solutions *(see 6.6, instructions for use/handling)*

6.3 Shelf life

FLOLAN freeze dried powder: 3 years.

Renal Dialysis: When reconstituted with GlaxoSmithKline Glycine Buffer Diluent and diluted with physiological saline as instructed (see 6.6, Instructions for Use/Handling, Renal Dialysis), freshly prepared Flolan solutions should be used within 12 hours at 25°C.

Primary Pulmonary Hypertension: When reconstituted and diluted with GlaxoSmithKline Glycine Buffer Diluent as instructed (see 6.6, Instructions for Use/Handling, Primary Pulmonary Hypertension), freshly prepared Flolan solutions should be infused immediately. If not used immediately, in-use storage times are the responsibilty of the user and should not be longer than 24 hours at 2-8°C.

Where the solution is held in an ambulatory infusion pump system, a cold pouch must be used to maintain the temperature of the solution at 2-8°C for the full administration period. Flolan solution may then be used over a 24 hour period provided that the cold pouch is changed as necessary throughout the day.

Where an ambulatory cold pouch system cannot be used the maximum administration time at 25°C is 12 hours for freshly prepared solutions and 8 hours for solutions that have been stored prior to use.

6.4 Special precautions for storage

Do not store above 25°C. Protect from light. Keep dry. Do not freeze. Keep container in the outer carton. Under these conditions, freeze-dried Flolan in an unopened vial should not be affected by moisture present in the atmosphere.

Any cold pouch used must be capable of maintaining the temperature of reconstituted Flolan between 2°C and 8°C for the full administration period.

The stability of solutions of Flolan is pH dependent. Only the diluent supplied should be used for reconstitution of freeze-dried Flolan and only the recommended infusion solutions, in the stated ratio, should be used for further dilution, otherwise the required pH may not be maintained.

Reconstitution and dilution should be carried out immediately prior to use *(see Posology and method of administration, and instructions for use/handling).*

GlaxoSmithKline Glycine Buffer Diluent contains no preservative, consequently a vial should be used once only and then discarded.

6.5 Nature and contents of container

Freeze dried powder in glass vials with synthetic butyl rubber plugs and aluminium collars.

Pack presentations:

Single 1.5 mg vial mg of freeze dried powder (Non-marketed)

Single 1.5 mg vial of freeze dried powder plus single vial of diluent

Single 1.5 mg vial of freeze dried powder plus two vials of diluent (Non-marketed)

6.6 Instructions for use and handling

Reconstitution and dilution:-

Particular care should be taken in the preparation of the infusion and in calculating the rate of infusion. The procedure given below should be closely followed.

Reconstitution and dilution of Flolan must be carried out using sterile techniques, immediately prior to clinical use.

Renal dialysis

Reconstitution:-

1. Use only the GlaxoSmithKline Glycine Buffer Diluent provided for reconstitution.

2. Withdraw approximately 10 ml of the GlaxoSmithKline Glycine Buffer Diluent into a sterile syringe, inject the contents of the syringe into the vial containing 1.5 mg freeze-dried Flolan and shake gently until the powder has dissolved.

3. Draw up the resulting Flolan solution into the syringe, re-inject it into the remaining volume of the GlaxoSmithKline Glycine Buffer Diluent solution and mix thoroughly.

This solution is now referred to as the concentrated solution and contains 30,000 nanograms per ml epoprostenol. Only this concentrated solution is suitable for further dilution prior to use.

When 0.5 mg Flolan powder is reconstituted with 50 ml of GlaxoSmithKline Glycine Buffer Diluent, the final injection has a pH of approximately 10.5 and a sodium ion content of approximately 56 mg.

Dilution:-

For administration using a pump capable of delivering small volume constant infusions, suitable aliquots of concentrated solution may be diluted with sterile physiological saline.

It may be diluted with physiological saline (0.9%), provided a ratio of 6 volumes of saline to 1 volume of concentrated solution is not exceeded; e.g. 50 ml of concentrated solution further diluted with a maximum of 300 ml saline.

Other common intravenous fluids are unsatisfactory for the dilution of the concentrated solution as the required pH is not attained. Flolan solutions are less stable at low pH.

Prior to using the concentrated solution, or the diluted form, a filtration step is needed. To filter, draw the reconstituted product into a large syringe and then attach the sterile filter provided to the syringe.

Dispense the concentrated solution directly into the chosen infusion solution using firm but not excessive pressure; the typical time taken for filtration of 50 ml of concentrated solution is 70 seconds. Mix well.

The filter unit must be used once only and then discarded.

When reconstituted and diluted as directed above, Flolan infusion solutions have a pH of approximately 10 and will retain 90% of their initial potency for approximately 12 hours at 25°C.

CALCULATION OF INFUSION RATE:-

The infusion rate may be calculated from the following formula:-

$$\text{Infusion rate (ml/min)} = \frac{\text{dosage (ng /kg/min) X bodyweight (kg)}}{\text{concentration of solution (ng/ml)}}$$

Infusion rate (ml/hr) = Infusion rate (ml/min) × 60

Infusion rate formulae - examples

When used in renal dialysis Flolan may be administered as the concentrated solution (a) or in diluted form (b).

a. Using concentrated solution, i.e. 30 000 nanogram/ml epoprostenol:

(see Table 1 on next page)

b. *Diluted*: A commonly used dilution is: -

10 ml concentrated solution plus50 ml physiological saline (0.9%). To give a final total volume of 60 ml.

Resultant concentration = 5000 nanogram/ml epoprostenol:

(see Table 2 on next page)

Primary Pulmonary Hypertension

The following packs are available for use in the treatment of primary pulmonary hypertension:

One vial containing sterile freeze-dried epoprostenol sodium equivalent to 1.5 mg epoprostenol supplied with one 50 ml vial of sterile GlaxoSmithKline Glycine Buffer Diluent solution.

One vial containing sterile freeze-dried epoprostenol sodium equivalent to 1.5 mg epoprostenol supplied with two 50 ml vials of sterile GlaxoSmithKline Glycine Buffer Diluent (Non-Marketed).

One vial containing sterile freeze-dried epoprostenol sodium equivalent to 1.5 mg epoprostenol supplied alone (Non-Marketed).

Initially a pack containing diluent buffer must be used. During chronic Flolan therapy the final concentration of solution may be increased by the addition of a 1.5 mg vial of freeze dried epoprostenol.

Only vials of the same amount as that included in the initial starter pack may be used to increase the final concentration of solution.

Reconstitution:

This should be carried out according to the instructions given for renal dialysis. Where a pack containing 1.5 mg epoprostenol is reconstituted with 50 ml sterile diluent the resultant concentration is 30,000 nanograms per ml.

Dilution:

Flolan may be used either as concentrated solution or in a diluted form for the treatment of PPH. Only GlaxoSmithKline Glycine Buffer Diluent provided may be used for the further dilution of reconstituted Flolan. Physiological saline must not be used when Flolan is to be used for the treatment of primary pulmonary hypertension.

Concentrations commonly used in the treatment of primary pulmonary hypertension are as follows:

30,000ng/ml - 1.5mg epoprostenol reconstituted to a total volume of 50 ml in GlaxoSmithKline Glycine Buffer Diluent

15,000ng/ml – 1.5mg epoprostenol reconstituted and diluted to a total volume of 100ml in GlaxoSmithKline Glycine Buffer Diluent.

The maximum recommended concentration for administration in primary pulmonary hypertension is 60,000ng/ml.

Flolan must not be administered with other parenteral solutions or medications when used for primary pulmonary hypertension.

To dilute the concentrated solution, draw it up into a larger syringe and then attach the sterile filter provided to the syringe.

Table 1

Concentration of solution = 30 000ng/ml epoprostenol								
Dosage (ng/kg/min)	Bodyweight (kilograms)							
	30	40	50	60	70	80	90	100
1	n/a*	n/a*	n/a*	n/a*	n/a*	n/a*	0.18	0.20
2	n/a*	n/a*	0.20	0.24	0.28	0.32	0.36	0.40
3	0.18	0.24	0.30	0.36	0.42	0.48	0.54	0.60
4	0.24	0.32	0.40	0.48	0.56	0.64	0.72	0.80
5	0.30	0.40	0.50	0.60	0.70	0.80	0.90	1.00
	Flow rates in **ml/hr**							

* Very low flow rates required. Diluted solutions in physiological saline should be considered.

Table 2

Concentration of solution = 5000ng/ml epoprostenol								
Dosage (ng/kg/ min)	Bodyweight (kilograms)							
	30	40	50	60	70	80	90	100
1	0.4	0.5	0.6	0.7	0.9	1.0	1.1	1.2
2	0.7	1.0	1.2	1.4	1.7	1.9	2.2	2.4
3	1.1	1.5	1.8	2.2	2.5	2.9	3.2	3.6
4	1.4	1.9	2.4	2.9	3.4	3.8	4.3	4.8
5	1.8	2.4	3.0	3.6	4.2	4.8	5.4	6.0
	Flow rates in **ml/hr**							

Dispense the concentrated solution directly into the pump cassette using firm but not excessive pressure; the typical time taken for filtration of 50 ml of concentrated solution is 70 seconds.

Remove the filter from the syringe and draw up the additional volume of GlaxoSmithKline Glycine Buffer Diluent required to achieve the desired dilution.

Refit the filter to the syringe and dispense the additional buffer through this into the concentrated Flolan solution in the cassette.

Mix well.

The filter unit must be used for the dilution of one pack only and then discarded.

The ambulatory pump used to administer Flolan should (1) be small and lightweight, (2) be able to adjust infusion rates in ng/kg/min increments, (3) have occlusion, end of infusion, and low battery alarms, (4) be accurate to ± 6% of the programmed rate (5) be positive pressure driven (continuous or pulsatile) with intervals between pulses not exceeding 3 minutes at infusion rates used to deliver Flolan, and (6) include a cold pouch system The reservoir should be made of polyvinyl chloride, polypropylene, or glass.

CALCULATION OF INFUSION RATE: -

The infusion rate may be calculated from the formula given above for renal dialysis. An example of a concentration commonly used in primary pulmonary hypertension is shown below.

Infusion rates for a concentration of 15,000 nanogram/ml ***(see Table 3 below)***

Administrative Data

7. MARKETING AUTHORISATION HOLDER

GlaxoWellcome UK Ltd

Trading as GlaxoSmithKline UK

Stockley Park West

Uxbridge

Middlesex

UB11 1BT

8. MARKETING AUTHORISATION NUMBER(S)

PL10949/0312

9. DATE OF FIRST AUTHORISATION/RENEWAL OF THE AUTHORISATION

7th March 2001

10. DATE OF REVISION OF THE TEXT

30 December 2004

Table 3 Infusion rates for a concentration of 15,000 nanogram/ml

Concentration of solution = 15 000ng/ml epoprostenol								
Dosage (ng/kg/ min)	Bodyweight (kilograms)							
	30	40	50	60	70	80	90	100
4				1.0	1.1	1.3	1.4	1.6
6		1.0	1.2	1.4	1.7	1.9	2.2	2.4
8	1.0	1.3	1.6	1.9	2.2	2.6	2.9	3.2
10	1.2	1.6	2.0	2.4	2.8	3.2	3.6	4.0
12	1.4	1.9	2.4	2.9	3.4	3.8	4.3	4.8
14	1.7	2.2	2.8	3.4	3.9	4.5	5.0	5.6
16	1.9	2.6	3.2	3.8	4.5	5.1	5.8	6.4
	Flow rates in **ml/hr**							

11. Legal Status

POM

Flomaxtra XL, 400 micrograms, film-coated prolonged release tablet

(Astellas Pharma Limited)

1. NAME OF THE MEDICINAL PRODUCT

Flomaxtra® XL, 400 micrograms, film-coated prolonged release tablet

2. QUALITATIVE AND QUANTITATIVE COMPOSITION

Each tablet contains as active ingredient tamsulosin hydrochloride 400 micrograms, equivalent to 367 micrograms tamsulosin.

For excipients, see section 6.1.

3. PHARMACEUTICAL FORM

Film coated, prolonged release tablet.

Approximately 9 mm, round, bi-convex, yellow, film-coated tablets debossed with the code '04'.

4. CLINICAL PARTICULARS

4.1 Therapeutic indications

Treatment of functional symptoms of benign prostatic hyperplasia (BPH).

4.2 Posology and method of administration

Posology

One tablet daily, to be taken with or without food.

Method of administration

For oral use.

The tablet should be swallowed whole and should not be crunched or chewed as this will interfere with the prolonged release of the active ingredient.

4.3 Contraindications

A history of orthostatic hypotension; severe hepatic insufficiency.

Hypersensitivity to tamsulosin hydrochloride or any other component of the product.

4.4 Special warnings and special precautions for use

As with other $alpha_1$ blockers, a reduction in blood pressure can occur in individual cases during treatment with Flomaxtra XL, as a result of which, rarely, syncope can occur. At the first signs of orthostatic hypotension (dizziness, weakness), the patient should sit or lie down until the symptoms have disappeared.

Before therapy with Flomaxtra XL is initiated, the patient should be examined in order to exclude the presence of other conditions which can cause the same symptoms as benign prostatic hyperplasia. Digital rectal examination and, when necessary, determination of prostate specific antigen (PSA) should be performed before treatment and at regular intervals afterwards.

The treatment of severely renally impaired patients (creatinine clearance of less than 10 ml/min) should be approached with caution as these patients have not been studied.

4.5 Interaction with other medicinal products and other forms of Interaction

No interactions have been seen when tamsulosin was given concomitantly with atenolol, enalapril, nifedipine or theophylline. Concomitant cimetidine brings about a rise in plasma levels of tamsulosin, and furosemide a fall, but as levels remain within the normal range, posology need not be changed.

In vitro, neither diazepam nor propranolol, trichlormethiazide, chlormadinon, amitryptyline, diclofenac, glibenclamide, simvastatin and warfarin change the free fraction of tamsulosin in human plasma. Neither does tamsulosin change the free fractions of diazepam, propranolol, trichlormethiazide, and chlormadinon.

No interactions at the level of hepatic metabolism have been seen during *in vitro* studies with liver microsomal fractions (representative of the cytochrome P_{450}-linked drug metabolising enzyme system), involving amitriptyline, salbutamol, glibenclamide and finasteride. Diclofenac and warfarin, however, may increase the elimination rate of tamsulosin.

There is a theoretical risk of enhanced hypotensive effect when given concurrently with drugs which may reduce blood pressure, including anaesthetic agents and other α_1-adrenoceptor antagonists.

4.6 Pregnancy and lactation

Not applicable, as Flomaxtra XL is intended for male patients only.

4.7 Effects on ability to drive and use machines

No data is available on whether Flomaxtra XL adversely affects the ability to drive or operate machines. However, in this respect patients should be aware of the fact that drowsiness, blurred vision, dizziness and syncope can occur.

4.8 Undesirable effects

Flomaxtra XL was evaluated in two double - blind placebo controlled trials. Adverse events were mostly mild and their incidence was generally low. The most commonly reported ADR was abnormal ejaculation occurring in approximately 2% of patients.

Suspected adverse reactions reported with Flomaxtra XL or an alternative formulation of tamsulosin, were:-

Nervous systems disorders

Common: dizziness, headache

Uncommon: syncope

Cardiac disorders

Uncommon: palpitations

Vascular disorders

Uncommon: postural hypotension

Respiratory disorders

Uncommon: rhinitis

Gastrointestinal disorders

Uncommon: nausea, vomiting, constipation, diarrhoea

Skin and subcutaneous tissue disorders

Uncommon: rash, pruritus, urticaria

Very rare: angioedema

Reproductive system disorders

Common: abnormal ejaculation

Very rare: priapism

General disorders

Common: asthenia

As with other alpha-blockers, drowsiness, blurred vision, dry mouth or oedema can occur.

4.9 Overdose

Acute overdose with 5 mg tamsulosin hydrochloride has been reported. Acute hypotension (systolic blood pressure 70 mm Hg), vomiting and diarrhoea were observed, which were treated with fluid replacement and the patient was able to be discharged the same day. In case of acute hypotension occurring after overdose, cardiovascular support should be given. Blood pressure can be restored and heart rate brought back to normal by lying the patient down. If this does not help, then volume expanders, and when necessary, vasopressors could be employed. Renal function should be monitored and general supportive measures applied. Dialysis is unlikely to be of help, as tamsulosin is very highly bound to plasma proteins.

Measures, such as emesis, can be taken to impede absorption. When large quantities are involved, gastric lavage can be applied and activated charcoal and an osmotic laxative, such as sodium sulphate, can be administered.

5. PHARMACOLOGICAL PROPERTIES

5.1 Pharmacodynamic properties

Pharmacotherapeutic group:

Alpha$_1$-adrenoceptor antagonist.

ATC code: G04C A02. Preparations for the exclusive treatment of prostatic disease.

Mechanism of action:

Tamsulosin binds selectively and competitively to postsynaptic alpha$_1$-receptors, in particular to the subtype alpha$_{1A}$, which bring about relaxation of the smooth muscle of the prostate, whereby tension is reduced.

Pharmacodynamic effects:

Flomaxtra XL increases maximum urinary flow rate by reducing smooth muscle tension in the prostate and urethra, thereby relieving obstruction.

It also improves the complex of irritative and obstructive symptoms in which bladder instability and tension of the smooth muscles of the lower urinary tract play an important role. Alpha$_1$-blockers can reduce blood pressure by lowering peripheral resistance. No reduction in blood pressure of any clinical significance was observed during studies with Flomaxtra XL.

5.2 Pharmacokinetic properties

Absorption:

Flomaxtra XL is formulated as an Oral Controlled Absorption System (OCAS) and is a prolonged release tablet of the non-ionic gel matrix type.

Tamsulosin administered as Flomaxtra XL is absorbed from the intestine and is approximately 55 - 59% bioavailable. A consistent slow release of tamsulosin is maintained over the whole pH range encountered in the gastro-intestinal tract with little fluctuation over 24 hours. The rate and extent of absorption of tamsulosin administered as Flomaxtra XL is not affected by food.

Tamsulosin shows linear kinetics.

After a single dose of Flomaxtra in the fasted state, plasma levels of tamsulosin peak at a median time of 6 hours. In steady state, which is reached by day 4 of multiple dosing, plasma levels of tamsulosin peak at 4 to 6 hours in the fasted and fed state. Peak plasma levels increase from approximately 6 ng/ml after the first dose to 11 ng/ml in steady state.

As a result of the prolonged release characteristics of Flomaxtra XL, the trough concentration of tamsulosin in plasma amounts to 40% of the peak plasma concentration under fasted and fed conditions.

There is a considerable inter-patient variation in plasma levels, both after single and multiple dosing.

Distribution:

In man, tamsulosin is about 99% bound to plasma proteins and volume of distribution is small (about 0.2l/kg).

Metabolism:

Tamsulosin has a low first pass effect, being metabolised slowly. Most tamsulosin is present in plasma in the form of unchanged drug. It is metabolised in the liver.

In rats, hardly any induction of microsomal liver enzymes was seen to be caused by tamsulosin.

No dose adjustment is warranted in hepatic insufficiency.

None of the metabolites are more active than the original compound.

Excretion:

Tamsulosin and its metabolites are mainly excreted in the urine. The amount excreted as unchanged drug is estimated to be about 4 - 6% of the dose, administered as Flomaxtra XL.

After a single dose of Flomaxtra XL, and in steady state, elimination half-lives of about 19 and 15 hours, respectively, have been measured.

No dose adjustment is necessary in patients with renal impairment.

5.3 Preclinical safety data

Single and repeat dose toxicity studies were performed in mice, rats and dogs. In addition, reproduction toxicity studies were performed in rats, carcinogenicity in mice and rats, and *in vivo* and *in vitro* genotoxicity were examined. The general toxicity profile, as seen with high doses of tamsulosin, is consistent with the known pharmacological actions of the alpha-adrenergic blocking agents. At very high dose levels, the ECG was altered in dogs. This response is considered to be not clinically relevant. Tamsulosin showed no relevant genotoxic properties.

Increased incidences of proliferative changes of mammary glands of female rats and mice have been reported. These findings, which are probably mediated by hyperprolactinaemia and only occurred at high dose levels, are regarded as irrelevant.

6. PHARMACEUTICAL PARTICULARS

6.1 List of excipients

Core

Macrogol (containing butylhydroxytoluene)

Magnesium stearate

Film-coat

Hypromellose

Macrogol

Yellow iron oxide (E172)

6.2 Incompatibilities

None known.

6.3 Shelf life

2 years

6.4 Special precautions for storage

There are no special storage instructions

6.5 Nature and contents of container

Aluminium foil blister packs containing 30 tablets.

6.6 Instructions for use and handling

No special instructions.

7. MARKETING AUTHORISATION HOLDER

Yamanouchi Pharma Ltd

Yamanouchi House

Pyrford Road

West Byfleet

Surrey

KT14 6RA

8. MARKETING AUTHORISATION NUMBER(S)

PL 00166/ 0199

9. DATE OF FIRST AUTHORISATION/RENEWAL OF THE AUTHORISATION

11th July 2005

10. DATE OF REVISION OF THE TEXT

11. LEGAL CATEGORY

POM

Florinef 0.1 mg Tablets

(E. R. Squibb & Sons Limited)

1. NAME OF THE MEDICINAL PRODUCT

FLORINEF 0.1MG TABLETS

2. QUALITATIVE AND QUANTITATIVE COMPOSITION

Each tablet contains fludrocortisone acetate Ph.Eur 0.1mg

For excipients, see 6.1.

3. PHARMACEUTICAL FORM

Oral tablet.

Light pink coloured, round, flat faced, uncoated, bevel-edged tablet with "Squibb" and "429" on one side and scored on the other.

4. CLINICAL PARTICULARS

4.1 Therapeutic indications

For partial replacement therapy for primary and secondary adrenocortical insufficiency in Addison's disease and for the treatment of salt-losing adrenogenital syndrome.

4.2 Posology and method of administration

Adults:

A daily dosage range of 0.05-0.3mg Florinef tablets orally. Supplementary parenteral administration of sodium-retaining hormones is not necessary. When an enhanced glucocorticoid effect is desirable, cortisone or hydrocortisone by mouth should be given concomitantly with Florinef tablets.

Elderly:

No specific dosage recommendations. (See Precautions).

Children:

May be used adjusted to the age and weight of the child according to the severity of the condition. Caution should be used in the event of exposure to chickenpox, measles or other communicable diseases. (See 4.3 Contraindications).

4.3 Contraindications

Hypersensitivity to any of the ingredients.

Systemic infections unless specific anti-infective therapy is employed.

Because of its marked effect on sodium retention, the use of Florinef in the treatment of conditions other than those indicated, is not advised.

Since Florinef is a potent mineralocorticoid both the dosage and salt intake should be carefully monitored to avoid the development of hypertension, oedema or weight gain. Periodic checking of serum electrolyte levels is advisable during prolonged therapy.

Precautions:

Florinef is a potent mineralocorticoid and is used predominantly for replacement therapy. Although glucocorticoid side effects may occur, these can be reduced by reducing the dosage.

Undesirable effects may be minimised using the lowest effective dose for the minimum period. Frequent patient review is required to titrate the dose appropriately against disease activity (See dosage section).

Adrenal cortical atrophy develops during prolonged therapy and may persist for years after stopping treatment. Withdrawal of corticosteroids after prolonged therapy must, therefore, always be gradual to avoid acute adrenal insufficiency and should be tapered off over weeks or months according to the dose and duration of treatment. Patients on long-term systemic therapy with Florinef may require supportive corticosteroid therapy in times of stress (such as trauma, surgery or severe illness) both during the treatment period and up to a year afterwards. If corticosteroids have been stopped following prolonged therapy they may need to be reintroduced temporarily.

Patients should carry steroid treatment cards which give clear guidance on the precautions to be taken to minimise risk and which provides details of prescriber, drug, dosage and the duration of treatment.

Anti-inflammatory/immunosuppressive effects:

Suppression of the inflammatory response and immune function increases the susceptibility to infections and their severity. The clinical presentation may often be atypical and serious infections such as septicaemia and tuberculosis may be masked and may reach an advanced stage before being recognised.

Chickenpox, shingles and measles are of particular concern since these illnesses may be fatal in immunosuppressed patients. Patients should be advised to avoid exposure to these diseases, and to seek medical advice without delay if exposure occurs.

Chickenpox: Unless they have had chickenpox, patients receiving oral corticosteroids for purposes other than replacement should be regarded as being *at risk of severe chickenpox.* Manifestations of fulminant illness include pneumonia, hepatitis and disseminated intravascular coagulation; rash is not necessarily a prominent feature. Passive immunisation with varicella zoster immunoglobulin (VZIG) is needed by exposed non-immune patients who are receiving systemic corticosteroids or who have used them within the previous 3 months; this should preferably be given within 3 days of exposure, and not later than 10 days after exposure to chickenpox. Confirmed chickenpox warrants specialist care and urgent treatment. Corticosteroids should not be stopped and the dose may need to be increased.

Measles: Prophylaxis with normal immunoglobulin may be needed.

During corticosteroid therapy antibody response will be reduced and therefore affect the patient's response to vaccines. Live vaccines should not be administered.

4.4 Special warnings and special precautions for use

Particular care is required when considering use of systemic corticosteroids in patients with the following conditions and frequent patient monitoring is necessary.

Recent intestinal anastomoses, diverticulitis, thrombophlebitis, existing or previous history of severe affective disorders (especially previous steroid psychosis), exanthematous disease, chronic nephritis, or renal insufficiency, metastatic carcinoma, osteoporosis (post-menopausal females are particularly at risk); in patients with an active peptic ulcer (or a history of peptic ulcer). Myasthenia gravis. Latent or healed tuberculosis; in the presence of local or systemic viral infection, systemic fungal infections or in active infections not controlled by antibiotics. In acute psychoses; in acute glomerulonephritis. Hypertension; congestive heart failure; glaucoma (or a family history of glaucoma), previous steroid myopathy or epilepsy. Liver failure.

Corticosteroid effects may be enhanced in patients with hypothyroidism or cirrhosis.

Diabetes may be aggravated, necessitating a higher insulin dosage. Latent diabetes mellitus may be precipitated.

Menstrual irregularities may occur, and this possibility should be mentioned to female patients.

Rare instances of anaphylactoid reactions have occurred in patients receiving corticosteroids, especially when a patient has a history of drug allergies.

Aspirin should be used cautiously in conjunction with corticosteroids in patients with hypoprothrombinaemia.

Children:

Growth and development of children on prolonged corticosteroid therapy should be carefully observed. Corticosteroids cause dose-related growth retardation in infancy, childhood and adolescence which may be irreversible.

Elderly:

The common adverse effects of systemic corticosteroids may be associated with more serious consequences in old age, especially osteoporosis, hypertension, hypokalaemia, diabetes, susceptibility to infection and thinning of the skin. Close clinical supervision is required to avoid life-threatening reactions.

4.5 Interaction with other medicinal products and other forms of Interaction

Barbiturates, phenytoin, rifampicin, rifabutin, carbamazepine, primidone and aminoglutethimide may enhance the metabolic clearance of corticosteroids, resulting in decreased therapeutic effects.

Corticosteroids antagonise the effects of hypoglycaemic agents (including insulin), anti-hypertensives and diuretics. The hypokalaemic effects of acetazolamide, loop diuretics, thiazide diuretics and carbenoxolone are enhanced.

The efficacy of coumarin anticoagulants may be enhanced by concurrent corticosteroid therapy and close monitoring of the INR or prothrombin time is required to avoid spontaneous bleeding.

The renal clearance of salicylates is increased by corticosteroids and steroid withdrawal may result in salicylate intoxication.

4.6 Pregnancy and lactation

It may be decided to continue a pregnancy in a woman requiring replacement mineralocorticoid therapy, despite the risk to the foetus. When corticosteroids are essential however, patients with normal pregnancies may be treated as though they were in the non-gravid state.

There is evidence of harmful effects in pregnancy in animals. There may be a small risk of cleft palate and intrauterine growth retardation. Hypoadrenalism may occur in the neonate. Patients with pre-eclampsia or fluid retention require close monitoring.

Corticosteroids are found in breast milk.

Infants born of mothers who have received substantial doses of corticosteroids during pregnancy or during breast feeding should be carefully observed for signs of hypoadrenalism. Maternal treatment should be carefully documented in the infant's medical records to assist in follow up.

4.7 Effects on ability to drive and use machines

None known.

4.8 Undesirable effects

Where adverse reactions occur they are usually reversible on cessation of therapy. The incidence of predictable side-effects, including hypothalamic-pituitary-adrenal suppression correlate with the relative potency of the drug, dosage, timing of administration and duration of treatment (See Warnings and Precautions).

Patients should be watched closely for the following adverse reactions which may be associated with any corticosteroid therapy:

Anti-inflammatory and immunosuppressive effects: Increased susceptibility and severity of infections with suppression of clinical symptoms and signs, opportunistic infections, recurrence of dormant tuberculosis (See Warnings and Precautions).

Fluid and electrolyte disturbances: sodium retention, fluid retention, congestive heart failure in susceptible patients, potassium loss, cardiac arrhythmias or ECG changes due to potassium deficiency, hypokalaemic alkalosis, increased calcium excretion and hypertension.

Musculoskeletal: muscle weakness, fatigue, steroid myopathy, loss of muscle mass, osteoporosis, avascular osteonecrosis, vertebral compression fractures, delayed healing of fractures, aseptic necrosis of femoral and humeral heads, pathological fractures of long bones and spontaneous fractures, tendon rupture.

Gastrointestinal: dyspepsia, peptic ulcer with possible subsequent perforation and haemorrhage, pancreatitis, abdominal distension and ulcerative oesophagitis, candidiasis.

Dermatologic: impaired wound healing, thin fragile skin, petechiae and ecchymoses, facial erythema, increased sweating, purpura, striae, hirsutism, acneiform eruptions, lupus erythematosus-like lesions and suppressed reactions to skin tests.

Neurological: euphoria, psychological dependence, depression, insomnia, convulsions, increased intracranial pressure with papilloedema (pseudo-tumour cerebri) usually after treatment, vertigo, headache, neuritis or paraesthesias and aggravation of pre-existing psychiatric conditions and epilepsy.

Endocrine/metabolic: menstrual irregularities and amenorrhoea; development of the Cushingoid state; suppression of growth in childhood and adolescence; secondary adrenocortical and pituitary unresponsiveness, particularly in times of stress (eg. trauma, surgery or illness); decreased carbohydrate tolerance; manifestations of latent diabetes mellitus and increased requirements for insulin or oral hypoglycaemic agents in diabetes, weight gain. Negative protein and calcium balance. Increased appetite.

Ophthalmic: posterior subcapsular cataracts, increased intraocular pressure, glaucoma, exophthalmos, papilloedema, corneal or scleral thinning, exacerbation of ophthalmic viral or fungal diseases.

Others: necrotising angiitis, thrombophlebitis, thromboembolism, leucocytosis, insomnia, syncopal episodes and anaphylactoid reactions, particularly where there is a history of drug allergies.

Withdrawal Symptoms and Signs:

On withdrawal, fever, myalgia, arthralgia, rhinitis, conjunctivitis, painful itchy skin nodules and weight loss may occur. Too rapid a reduction in dose following prolonged treatment can lead to acute adrenal insufficiency, hypotension and death (See Warnings and Precautions).

4.9 Overdose

A single large dose should be treated with plenty of water by mouth. Careful monitoring of serum electrolytes is essential, with particular consideration being given to the need for administration of potassium chloride and restriction of dietary sodium intake.

5. PHARMACOLOGICAL PROPERTIES

5.1 Pharmacodynamic properties

Qualitatively, the physiological action of fludrocortisone acetate is similar to hydrocortisone. In very small doses, fludrocortisone maintains life in adrenalectomised animals, enhances the deposition of liver glycogen and produces thymic involution, eosinopenia, retention of sodium and increased urinary excretion of potassium.

5.2 Pharmacokinetic properties

Fludrocortisone is rapidly and completely absorbed after oral administration. Man, dog, rat, monkey and guinea-pig were studied after i.v. and intraduodenal administration. Depending on species, 50% or more of the steroid remained unchanged 30 minutes after administration. Fludrocortisone is hydrolysed to produce the non-esterified alcohol; after administration of the acetate, only the non-esterified alcohol is detectable in blood. The blood level reaches a peak between 4 and 8 hours. The highest blood level after i.v. administration to human volunteers was 1.7 hours.

Elimination half life after i.v. administration was 30 minutes in dogs and in human volunteers. Following administration of the acetate to dogs, the blood concentration shows a triphasic decline and each phase may represent the elimination of a metabolite.

Fludrocortisone is widely distributed throughout the body. It is 70 to 80% bound to serum proteins, mainly to the globulin fractions. The concentrations ratio of the drug in CSF to that in plasma was 1:6 in human volunteers.

In rats, most of a dose is excreted in the bile, and in dogs and guinea-pigs most of the dose is excreted in the urine. In human volunteers, excretion through urine was about 80%, and it was concluded that about 20% were excreted by a different route. It is likely that, as for the metabolism of other steroids, excretion into the bile is balanced by reabsorption in the intestine and some part is excreted with the faeces.

5.3 Preclinical safety data

Nothing further of relevance to the prescriber.

6. PHARMACEUTICAL PARTICULARS

6.1 List of excipients

Maize starch, dicalcium phosphate, lactose, talc, erythrosine (E127), industrial methylated spirits, sodium benzoate, purified water, magnesium stearate.

6.2 Incompatibilities

None known.

6.3 Shelf life

12 months.

6.4 Special precautions for storage

Do not store above 25°C.

6.5 Nature and contents of container

Amber glass bottles with aluminium ropp cap with saran PVDC lined expanded polyethylene wad containing 56 tablets.

6.6 Instructions for use and handling

None.

7. MARKETING AUTHORISATION HOLDER

E.R. Squibb & Sons Limited

Uxbridge Business Park

Sanderson Road

Uxbridge,

Middlesex UB8 1DH

8. MARKETING AUTHORISATION NUMBER(S)

PL 0034/5027R

9. DATE OF FIRST AUTHORISATION/RENEWAL OF THE AUTHORISATION

16 November 1988 / 27 January 2004

10. DATE OF REVISION OF THE TEXT

24 June 2005

Floxapen Capsules, Syrups, Vials for Injection

(GlaxoSmithKline UK)

1. NAME OF THE MEDICINAL PRODUCT

Floxapen® Capsules

Floxapen® Syrups

Floxapen® Vials for Injection

2. QUALITATIVE AND QUANTITATIVE COMPOSITION

Floxapen Capsules (Flucloxacillin Capsules BP) containing 250 mg or 500 mg flucloxacillin as Flucloxacillin Sodium BP.

Floxapen Syrups (Flucloxacillin Oral Suspension BP) when reconstituted each 5 ml contains 125 mg or 250 mg flucloxacillin as Flucloxacillin Magnesium BP.

Floxapen Vials for Injection (Flucloxacillin Injection BP). Each vial contains 250 mg, 500 mg or 1 g flucloxacillin as Flucloxacillin Sodium BP.

3. PHARMACEUTICAL FORM

Floxapen Capsules: Black and caramel capsules overprinted with Floxapen.

Floxapen Syrups: Bottles containing powder for the preparation of suspension.

Floxapen Injection: Vials containing sterile powder for reconstitution.

4. CLINICAL PARTICULARS

Flucloxacillin is an isoxazolyl penicillin of the β-lactam group of antibiotics which exerts a bactericidal effect upon many Gram-positive organisms including β-lactamase-producing staphylococci and streptococci.

4.1 Therapeutic indications

Floxapen is indicated for the treatment of infections due to sensitive Gram-positive organisms, including β-lactamase-producing staphyloccoci and streptococci. Typical indications include:

Skin and soft tissue infections:

Boils Cellulitis Infected burns

Abscesses Infected skin conditions, Protection for skin grafts

Carbuncles e.g. ulcer, eczema, and acne Impetigo

Furunculosis Infected wounds

Respiratory tract infections:

Pneumonia Lung abscess Empyema

Sinusitis Pharyngitis Otitis media and externa

Tonsillitis Quinsy

Other infections caused by Floxapen-sensitive organisms:

Osteomyelitis Urinary tract infection

Enteritis Meningitis

Endocarditis Septicaemia

Floxapen is also indicated for use as a prophylactic agent during major surgical procedures when appropriate; for example cardiothoracic and orthopaedic surgery.

Parenteral usage is indicated where oral dosage is inappropriate.

4.2 Posology and method of administration

Depends on the age, weight and renal function of the patient, as well as the severity of the infection.

Usual adult dosage (including elderly patients)

Oral - 250 mg four times a day.

Intramuscular - 250 mg four times a day.

Intravenous - 250 mg to 1 g four times a day.

The above systemic dosages may be doubled where necessary.

Osteomyelitis, endocarditis - Up to 8 g daily, in divided doses six to eight hourly.

Surgical prophylaxis - 1 to 2 g IV at induction of anaesthesia followed by 500 mg six hourly IV, IM or orally for up to 72 hours.

Floxapen may be administered by other routes in conjunction with systemic therapy. (Proportionately lower doses should be given in children.)

Intrapleural - 250 mg once daily.

By nebuliser - 125 to 250 mg four times a day.

Intra-articular - 250 to 500 mg once daily.

Usual children's dosage

2-10 years: half adult dose

Under 2 years: quarter adult dose.

Abnormal renal function: In common with other penicillins, Floxapen usage in patients with renal impairment does not usually require dosage reduction. However, in the presence of severe renal failure (creatinine clearance < 10 ml/min) a reduction in dose or an extension of dose interval should be considered. Floxapen is not significantly removed by dialysis and hence no supplementary dosages need to be administered either during, or at the end of the dialysis period.

Administration

Oral: Oral doses should be administered half to one hour before meals.

Intramuscular: Add 1.5 ml Water for Injections BP to 250 mg vial contents or 2 ml Water for Injections BP to 500 mg vial contents.

Intravenous: Dissolve 250-500 mg in 5-10 ml Water for Injections BP or 1 g in 15-20 ml Water for Injections BP. Administer by slow intravenous injection (three to four minutes). Floxapen may also be added to infusion fluids or injected, suitably diluted, into the drip tube over a period of three to four minutes.

Interpleural: Dissolve 250 mg in 5-10 ml Water for Injections BP.

Intra-articular: Dissolve 250-500 mg in up to 5 ml Water for Injections BP or 0.5% lignocaine hydrochloride solution.

Nebuliser solution: Dissolve 125-250 mg of the vial contents in 3 ml sterile water.

4.3 Contraindications

Flucloxacillin should not be given to patients with a history of hypersensitivity to β-lactam antibiotics (e.g. penicillins, cephalosporins) or excipients.

Flucloxacillin is contra-indicated in patients with a previous history of flucloxacillin-associated jaundice/hepatic dysfunction.

Ocular administration.

4.4 Special warnings and special precautions for use

Before initiating therapy with flucloxacillin, careful enquiry should be made concerning previous hypersensitivity reactions to β-lactams.

Serious and occasionally fatal hypersensitivity reactions (anaphylaxis) have been reported in patients receiving β-lactam antibiotics. Although anaphylaxis is more frequent following parenteral therapy, it has occurred in patients on oral therapy. These reactions are more likely to occur in individuals with a history of β-lactam hypersensitivity.

Flucloxacillin should be used with caution in patients with evidence of hepatic dysfunction (see section 4.8).

Special caution is essential in the newborn because of the risk of hyperbilirubinaemia. Studies have shown that, at high dose following parenteral administration, flucloxacillin can displace bilirubin from plasma protein binding sites, and may therefore predispose to kernicterus in a jaundiced baby. In addition, special caution is essential in the newborn because of the potential for high serum levels of flucloxacillin due to a reduced rate of renal excretion.

During prolonged treatments (e.g. osteomyelitis, endocarditis), regular monitoring of hepatic and renal functions is recommended.

Prolonged use may occasionally result in overgrowth of non-susceptible organisms.

Sodium Content: Floxapen capsules and injection contain approximately 51 mg sodium per g. This should be included in the daily allowance of patients on sodium restricted diets.

4.5 Interaction with other medicinal products and other forms of Interaction

Probenecid decreases the renal tubular secretion of flucloxacillin. Concurrent administration of probenecid delays the renal excretion of flucloxacillin.

4.6 Pregnancy and lactation

Pregnancy: Animal studies with flucloxacillin have shown no teratogenic effects. The product has been in clinical use since 1970 and the limited number of reported cases of use in human pregnancy have shown no evidence of untoward effects. The decision to administer any drug during pregnancy should be taken with the utmost care. Therefore flucloxacillin should only be used in pregnancy when the potential benefits outweigh the potential risks associated with treatment.

Lactation: Trace quantities of flucloxacillin can be detected in breast milk. The possibility of hypersensitivity reactions must be considered in breast-feeding infants. Therefore flucloxacillin should only be administered to a breast-feeding mother when the potential benefits outweigh the potential risks associated with the treatment.

4.7 Effects on ability to drive and use machines

Adverse effects on the ability to drive or operate machinery have not been observed.

4.8 Undesirable effects

The following convention has been utilised for the classification of undesirable effects:- Very common >1/10), common >1/100, <1/10), uncommon >1/1000, <1/100), rare >1/10,000, <1/1000), very rare (<1/10,000).

Unless otherwise stated, the frequency of the adverse events has been derived from more than 30 years of post-marketing reports.

Blood and lymphatic system disorders

Very rare: Neutropenia (including agranulocytosis) and thrombocytopenia. These are reversible when treatment is discontinued.

Immune system disorders

Very rare:Anaphylactic shock (exceptional with oral administration) (see Section 4.4 Special Warnings and Precautions for Use), angioneurotic oedema.

If any hypersensitivity reaction occurs, the treatment should be discontinued. (See also Skin and subcutaneous tissue disorders).

Nervous system disorders

Very rare: In patients suffering from renal failure, neurological disorders with convulsions are possible with the I.V. injection of high doses.

Gastrointestinal disorders

Clinical Trial Data

***Common:** Minor gastrointestinal disturbances.

Post Marketing Data

Very rare: Pseudomembranous colitis.

If pseudomembranous colitis develops, flucloxacillin treatment should be discontinued and appropriate therapy, e.g. oral vancomycin should be initiated.

Hepato-biliary disorders

Very rare: Hepatitis and cholestatic jaundice. (See Section 4.4 Special Warnings and Special Precautions for Use). Changes in liver function test results (reversible when treatment is discontinued).

Hepatitis and cholestatic jaundice may be delayed for up to two months post-treatment. In some cases the course has been protracted and lasted for several months. Very rarely, deaths have been reported, almost always in patients with serious underlying disease.

Skin and subcutaneous tissue disorders

Clinical Trial Data

***Uncommon:** Rash, urticaria and purpura.

Post Marketing Data

Very rare: Erythema multiforme, Stevens-Johnson syndrome and toxic epidermal necrolysis.

(See also Immune system disorders).

Musculoskeletal and connective tissue disorders

Very rare:Arthralgia and myalgia sometimes develop more than 48 hours after the start of the treatment.

Renal and urinary disorders

Very rare: Interstitial nephritis.

This is reversible when treatment is discontinued.

General disorders and administration site conditions

Very rare: Fever sometimes develops more than 48 hours after the start of the treatment.

*The incidence of these AEs was derived from clinical studies involving a total of approximately 929 adult and paediatric patients taking flucloxacillin.

4.9 Overdose

Gastrointestinal effects such as nausea, vomiting and diarrhoea may be evident and should be treated symptomatically.

Flucloxacillin is not removed from the circulation by haemodialysis.

5. PHARMACOLOGICAL PROPERTIES

5.1 Pharmacodynamic properties

Properties: Flucloxacillin is a narrow-spectrum antibiotic of the group of isoxazolyl penicillins; it is not inactivated by staphylococcal β-lactamases.

Activity: Flucloxacillin, by its action on the synthesis of the bacterial wall, exerts a bactericidal effect on streptococci, except those of group D (*Streptococcus faecalis*), staphylococci, including the β-lactamase-producing strains, Clostridia and Neisseria. It is not active against methicillin-resistant staphylococci.

5.2 Pharmacokinetic properties

Absorption: Flucloxacillin is stable in acid media and can therefore be administered either by the oral or parenteral route. The peak serum levels of flucloxacillin reached after one hour are as follows.

- After 250 mg by the oral route (in fasting subjects): Approximately 8.8 mg/l.

- After 500 mg by the oral route (in fasting subjects): Approximately 14.5 mg/l.

- After 500 mg by the IM route: Approximately 16.5 mg/l.

The total quantity absorbed by the oral route represents approximately 79% of the quantity administered.

Distribution: Flucloxacillin diffuses well into most tissue. Specifically, active concentrations of flucloxacillin have been recovered in bones: 11.6 mg/l (compact bone) and 15.6 mg/l (spongy bone), with a mean serum level of 8.9 mg/l.

Crossing the meningeal barrier: Flucloxacillin diffuses in only small proportion into the cerebrospinal fluid of subjects whose meninges are not inflamed.

Crossing into mothers' milk: Flucloxacillin is excreted in small quantities in mothers' milk.

Metabolism: In normal subjects approximately 10% of the flucloxacillin administered is metabolised to penicilloic acid. The elimination half-life of flucloxacillin is in the order of 53 minutes.

Excretion: Excretion occurs mainly through the kidney. Between 65.5% (oral route) and 76.1% (parenteral route) of the dose administered is recovered in unaltered active form in the urine within 8 hours. A small portion of the dose administered is excreted in the bile. The excretion of flucloxacillin is slowed in cases of renal failure.

Protein binding: The serum protein-binding rate is 95%.

5.3 Preclinical safety data

No further information of relevance to add.

6. PHARMACEUTICAL PARTICULARS

6.1 List of excipients

Floxapen Capsules: Magnesium stearate, black iron oxide (E172), titanium dioxide (E171), red iron oxide (E172), yellow iron oxide (E172)

Floxapen Syrups: Saccharin sodium, xanthan gum, citric acid, sodium citrate, sodium benzoate, blood orange, tutti fruitti and menthol dry flavours, erythrosine CI 45430, quinoline yellow (E104), sucrose.

Floxapen Injection: None

6.2 Incompatibilities

It is advisable not to combine flucloxacillin with other drugs in solution for parenteral administration.

Floxapen should not be mixed with blood products or other proteinaceous fluids (e.g. protein hydrolysates) or with intravenous lipid emulsions.

If Floxapen is prescribed concurrently with an aminoglycoside, the two antibiotics should not be mixed in the syringe, intravenous fluid container or giving set; precipitation may occur.

6.3 Shelf life

Floxapen Capsules: Three years (except in fibreboard drums - 12 months).

Floxapen Syrups: Three years (following reconstitution: 14 days).

Floxapen Vials: Three years. After opening 24 hours.

6.4 Special precautions for storage

Floxapen Capsules in Original Packs should be stored in a dry place. Floxapen Capsules in reclosable containers should be stored in a cool, dry place. Fibreboard drums should be kept tightly closed in a cool, dry place.

Floxapen Syrups should be stored in a dry place. Once dispensed, Floxapen Syrups (bottles) remain stable for 14 days stored in a refrigerator (5°C).

Floxapen Vials for Injection should be stored in a cool, dry place. Once reconstituted Floxapen solutions should be stored in a refrigerator (2-8°C) and used within 24 hours.

6.5 Nature and contents of container

Floxapen Capsules 250 mg: Aluminium canister - 20, 50, 100 and 500; Glass bottle with screwcap - 20, 50, 100 and 500; Polypropylene tube with polyethylene closure - 20, 50, 100 and 500; Aluminium foil - 12; Aluminium/PVC/PVdC blister - 28; Fibreboard drum with metal or HDPE lid - 50,000.

Floxapen Capsules 500 mg: Aluminium canister - 50 and 100; Glass bottle with screwcap - 50 and 100; Polypropylene tube with polyethylene closure - 50 and 100; Aluminium foil - 12; Aluminium/PVC/PVdC blister - 28.

Floxapen Syrup 125 mg/5 ml and Floxapen Syrup 250 mg/5 ml: Clear glass bottles, reconstituted volume of 60 ml or 100 ml.

Floxapen Injection 250 mg or 500 mg: Clear glass vials with butyl rubber plug and aluminium seal, boxes of 10.

Floxapen Vials 1 g: Clear glass vials with butyl rubber plug or polypropylene flip-top lid and aluminium seal, boxes of 10.

6.6 Instructions for use and handling

If a dilution of the reconstituted syrup is required, Syrup BP should be used.

Reconstituted solutions for IM or direct IV injection should normally be administered within 30 minutes of preparation. However, aqueous solutions of Floxapen Injection retain their activity for up to 24 hours when stored in a refrigerator (2°-8°C).

Floxapen may be added to most intravenous fluids (e.g. Water for Injections, sodium chloride 0.9%, glucose 5%, sodium chloride 0.18% with glucose 4%). Once reconstituted, Floxapen solutions should be stored in a refrigerator (2°-8°C) and used within 24 hours of preparation. Full particulars are given in the Package Enclosure Leaflet.

Reconstitution of Floxapen injections and preparation of Floxapen infusion solutions must be carried out under appropriate aseptic conditions if the extended storage periods are required.

N.B. FLOXAPEN VIALS ARE NOT SUITABLE FOR MULTI-DOSE USE.

Any residual Floxapen should be discarded.

Administrative Data

7. MARKETING AUTHORISATION HOLDER

Beecham Group plc

Great West Road

Brentford

Middlesex TW8 9GS

trading as:

GlaxoSmithKline UK, Stockley Park West, Uxbridge, Middlesex UB11 1BT

8. MARKETING AUTHORISATION NUMBER(S)

Floxapen Capsules 250 mg: PL 0038/5055R

Floxapen Capsules 500 mg: PL 0038/5056R

Floxapen Syrup 125 mg/5 ml: PL 0038/0309

Floxapen Syrup 250 mg/5 ml: PL 0038/0310

Floxapen Vials for Injection 250 mg: PL 0038/5051R

Floxapen Vials for Injection 500 mg: PL 0038/5052R

Floxapen Vials for Injection 1 g: PL 0038/5053R

9. DATE OF FIRST AUTHORISATION/RENEWAL OF THE AUTHORISATION

Floxapen Capsules 250 mg: 12.12.97

Floxapen Capsules 500 mg: 12.12.97

Floxapen Syrup 125 mg/5 ml: 20.12.94

Floxapen Syrup 250 mg/5 ml: 20.12.94

Floxapen Vials for Injection 250 mg: 13.01.94

Floxapen Vials for Injection 500 mg: 13.01.94

Floxapen Vials for Injection 1 g: 13.01.94

10. DATE OF REVISION OF THE TEXT

20th April 2005

11. Legal Status

POM

Fluanxol Tablets

(Lundbeck Limited)

1. NAME OF THE MEDICINAL PRODUCT

Fluanxol® Tablets 0.5 mg and 1 mg

2. QUALITATIVE AND QUANTITATIVE COMPOSITION

0.5 mg tablets (containing 0.584 mg flupentixol dihydrochloride equivalent to 0.5 mg flupentixol base).

1 mg tablets (containing 1.168 mg flupentixol dihydrochloride equivalent to 1 mg flupentixol base).

3. PHARMACEUTICAL FORM

Round, biconvex, red, sugar-coated tablets.

4. CLINICAL PARTICULARS

4.1 Therapeutic indications

Symptomatic treatment of depression (with or without anxiety).

4.2 Posology and method of administration

Route of administration: Oral.

Adults: The standard initial dosage is 1 mg as a single morning dose. After one week the dose may be increased to 2 mg if there is inadequate clinical response. Daily dosage of more than 2 mg should be in divided doses up to a maximum of 3 mg daily.

Elderly: The standard initial dosage is 0.5 mg as a single morning dose. After one week, if response is inadequate, dosage may be increased to 1 mg once a day. Caution should be exercised in further increasing the dosage but occasional patients may require up to a maximum of 2 mg a day which should be given in divided doses.

Children: Not recommended for children.

Patients often respond within 2-3 days. If no effect has been observed within one week at maximum dosage the drug should be withdrawn.

4.3 Contraindications

Severe depression requiring ECT or hospitalisation, states of excitement or overactivity, including mania.

4.4 Special warnings and special precautions for use

Caution should be exercised in patients having: liver disease; cardiac disease or arrhythmias; severe respiratory disease; renal failure; epilepsy (and conditions predisposing to epilepsy e.g. alcohol withdrawal or brain damage); Parkinson's disease; narrow angle glaucoma; prostatic hypertrophy; hypothyroidism; hyperthyroidism; myasthenia gravis; phaeochromocytoma and patients who have shown hypersensitivity to thioxanthenes or other antipsychotics.

The elderly require close supervision because they are specially prone to experience such adverse effects as sedation, hypotension, confusion and temperature changes.

Recurrence of depressive symptoms on abrupt withdrawal is rare. Acute withdrawal symptoms, including nausea, vomiting, sweating and insomnia have been described after abrupt cessation of thioxanthenes and similar drugs. The emergence of involuntary movement disorders (such as akathisia, dystonia and dyskinesia) has been reported. Therefore, gradual withdrawal is advisable.

Dependence has not been reported to date.

4.5 Interaction with other medicinal products and other forms of Interaction

In common with other similar drugs, flupentixol enhances the response to alcohol, the effects of barbiturates and other CNS depressants. Flupentixol may potentiate the effects of general anaesthetics and anticoagulants and prolong the action of neuromuscular blocking agents.

The anticholinergic effects of atropine or other drugs with anticholinergic properties may be increased. Concomitant use of drugs such as metoclopramide, piperazine or antiparkinson drugs may increase the risk of extrapyramidal effects such as tardive dyskinesia. Combined use of antipsychotics and lithium or sibutramine has been associated with an increased risk of neurotoxicity.

Antipsychotics may enhance the cardiac depressant effects of quinidine; the absorption of corticosteroids and digoxin. The hypotensive effect of vasodilator antihypertensive agents such as hydralazine and α-blockers (e.g. doxazosin), or methyl-dopa may be enhanced. Concomitant use of flupentixol and drugs known to cause QT prolongation or cardiac arrhythmias, such as tricyclic antidepressants, other antipsychotics or terfenadine should be avoided.

Antipsychotics may antagonise the effects of adrenaline and other sympathomimetic agents, and reverse the antihypertensive effects of guanethidine, possibly clonidine and similar adrenergic-blocking agents. Antipsychotics may also impair the effect of levodopa, adrenergic drugs and anticonvulsants.

The metabolism of tricyclic antidepressants may be inhibited and the control of diabetes may be impaired.

4.6 Pregnancy and lactation

As the safety of Fluanxol in human pregnancy has not been established, use during pregnancy, especially the first and last trimesters, should be avoided unless the expected benefit to the patient outweighs the potential risk to the foetus.

Flupentixol is excreted into the breast milk. If the use of Fluanxol is considered essential, nursing mothers should be advised to stop breast feeding.

The newborn of mothers treated with antipsychotics in late pregnancy, or labour, may show signs of intoxication such as lethargy, tremor and hyperexcitability, and have a low apgar score.

4.7 Effects on ability to drive and use machines

Alertness may be impaired, especially at the start of treatment, or following the consumption of alcohol; patients should be warned of this risk and advised not to drive or operate machinery until their susceptibility is known. Patients should not drive if they have blurred vision.

4.8 Undesirable effects

Drowsiness and sedation are unusual. Sedation, if it occurs, is more often seen with high dosage and at the start of treatment, particularly in the elderly. Other adverse effects include blurring of vision, tachycardia and urinary incontinence and frequency. Dose-related postural hypotension may occur, particularly in the elderly.

Extrapyramidal reactions in the form of acute dystonias (including oculogyric crisis), parkinsonian rigidity, tremor, akinesia and akathisia have been reported and may occur even at lower dosage in susceptible patients. Such effects would usually be encountered early in treatment, but delayed reactions may also occur. If they do occur, treatment with Fluanxol should be withdrawn. Antiparkinson agents should not be prescribed routinely because of the possible risk of precipitating toxic-confusional states, impairing therapeutic efficacy or causing anticholinergic side-effects. They should only be given if required and their requirement reassessed at regular intervals. Precipitation of hypomania has been occasionally reported.

Tardive dyskinesia can occur with antipsychotic treatment. It is more common at high doses for prolonged periods but has been reported at lower dosage for short periods. The risk seems to be greater in the elderly, especially females. It has been reported that fine vermicular movements of the tongue are an early sign. It has been observed occasionally in patients receiving Fluanxol. The concurrent use of anticholinergic antiparkinson drugs may exacerbate this effect. The potential irreversibility and seriousness, as well as the unpredictability of the syndrome, requires especially careful assessment of the risk versus benefit, and the lowest possible dosage and duration of treatment consistent with therapeutic efficacy. Short-lived dyskinesia may occur after abrupt withdrawal of the drug (see section 4.4).

The neuroleptic malignant syndrome has rarely been reported in patients receiving antipsychotics, including flupentixol. This potentially fatal syndrome is characterised by hyperthermia, a fluctuating level of consciousness, muscular rigidity and autonomic dysfunction with pallor, tachycardia, labile blood pressure, sweating and urinary incontinence. Antipsychotic therapy should be discontinued immediately and vigorous symptomatic treatment implemented.

Epileptic fits have occasionally been reported. Confusional states can occur.

The hormonal effects of antipsychotic drugs include hyperprolactinaemia, which may be associated with galactorrhoea, gynaecomastia, oligomenorrhoea or amenorrhoea. Sexual function, including erection and ejaculation may be impaired; but increased libido has also been reported.

Flupentixol may impair body temperature control, and cases of hyperthermia have occurred rarely. The possible development of hypothermia, particularly in the elderly and hypothyroid, should be borne in mind.

Blood dyscrasias, including thrombocytopenia, have occasionally been reported. Blood counts should be carried out if a patient develops signs of persistent infection. Jaundice and other liver abnormalities have been reported rarely.

Weight gain and less commonly weight loss have been reported; oedema has occasionally been reported and has been considered to be allergic in origin. Rashes have occurred rarely. Although less likely than with phenothiazines, flupentixol can rarely cause increased susceptibility to sunburn.

Other reactions that have been reported rarely at low doses include nausea, dizziness or headache, migraine, excitement, agitation, or unpleasant subjective feelings of being mentally dulled or slowed down. Other occasional side effects are restlessness and insomnia.

4.9 Overdose

ECG changes with prolongation of the QT interval and T-wave changes may occur with moderate to high doses; they are reversible on reducing the dose.

Overdosage may cause somnolence, or even coma, extrapyramidal symptoms, convulsions, hypotension, shock, hyper- or hypothermia. Treatment is symptomatic and supportive, with measures aimed at supporting the respiratory and cardiovascular systems. The following specific measures may be employed if required.

- anticholinergic antiparkinson drugs if extrapyramidal symptoms occur.
- sedation (with benzodiazepines) in the unlikely event of agitation or excitement or convulsions.
- noradrenaline in saline intravenous drip if the patient is in shock. Adrenaline must not be given.
- gastric lavage should be considered.

5. PHARMACOLOGICAL PROPERTIES

5.1 Pharmacodynamic properties

The precise pharmacological mode of action of flupentixol has not been determined. It has been postulated that at low dosages flupentixol binds to presynaptic dopamine receptors causing increased neurotransmitter release. There is evidence that postsynaptic aminergic receptors become down regulated in response to increased levels of neurotransmitter and this is responsible for the observed improvement in depressive symptoms.

5.2 Pharmacokinetic properties

Mean oral bioavailability is about 55%. Maximum drug serum concentrations occur about 4 hours after dosing and the biological half-life is about 35 hours. Flupentixol is widely distributed in the body. Metabolism is by sulphoxidation, N-dealkylation and glucuronic acid conjugation. Excretion is via the urine and faeces.

5.3 Preclinical safety data

Nil of relevance

6. PHARMACEUTICAL PARTICULARS

6.1 List of excipients

Potato starch, lactose, gelatin, talc, magnesium stearate, sucrose and ultralake ponceau 4R (E124)

6.2 Incompatibilities

None known.

6.3 Shelf life

Fluanxol tablets are stable for 3 years.

6.4 Special precautions for storage

Do not store above 30°C.

6.5 Nature and contents of container

PVC/PVdC blister strips of 60 tablets per box.

6.6 Instructions for use and handling

Nil.

7. MARKETING AUTHORISATION HOLDER

Lundbeck Limited

Lundbeck House

Caldecotte Lake Business Park

Caldecotte

Milton Keynes

MK7 8LF

8. MARKETING AUTHORISATION NUMBER(S)

Fluanxol Tablets 0.5 mg	PL 0458/0011R
Fluanxol Tablets 1 mg	PL 0458/0037

9. DATE OF FIRST AUTHORISATION/RENEWAL OF THE AUTHORISATION

First Authorisation	November 1982
Renewal of Authorisation	17 March 2002

10. DATE OF REVISION OF THE TEXT

17 September 2004

® Registered trademark

Fluarix

(GlaxoSmithKline UK)

1. NAME OF THE MEDICINAL PRODUCT

Fluarix®, suspension for injection in a pre-filled syringe.

Influenza vaccine (split virion, inactivated)

2. QUALITATIVE AND QUANTITATIVE COMPOSITION

Split Influenza virus, inactivated, containing antigens* equivalent to:

A/California/7/2004 (H_3N_2)-like strain: A/New York/55/2004 (NYMC X-157)	15 micrograms**
A/New Caledonia/20/99 (H_1N_1)-like strain: A/New Caledonia/20/99 (IVR-116)	15 micrograms**
B/Shanghai/361/2002-like strain: B/Jiangsu/10/2003	15 micrograms**
	per 0.5 ml dose

* propagated in eggs

** haemagglutinin

This vaccine complies with the WHO recommendation (northern hemisphere) and EU decision for the year season (2005/2006).

For excipients see section 6.1.

3. PHARMACEUTICAL FORM

Suspension for injection in a pre-filled syringe.

Fluarix is colourless to slightly opalescent.

4. CLINICAL PARTICULARS

4.1 Therapeutic indications

Prophylaxis of influenza, especially in those who run an increased risk of associated complications.

4.2 Posology and method of administration

Posology

Adults and children from 36 months: 0.5 ml.

Children from 6 months to 35 months: Clinical data are limited. Dosages of 0.25 ml or 0.5 ml have been used.

For children who have not previously been vaccinated, a second dose should be given after an interval of at least 4 weeks.

Method of administration

Immunisation should be carried out by intramuscular or deep subcutaneous injection.

4.3 Contraindications

Hypersensitivity to the active substances, to any of the excipients, to egg, to chicken protein, formaldehyde, gentamicin sulphate and sodium deoxycholate.

Immunisation shall be postponed in patients with febrile illness or acute infection.

4.4 Special warnings and special precautions for use

As with all injectable vaccines, appropriate medical treatment and supervision should always be readily available in case of a rare anaphylactic event following the administration of the vaccine.

Fluarix should under no circumstances be administered intravascularly.

Antibody response in patients with endogenous or iatrogenic immunosuppression may be insufficient.

Thiomersal (an organomercuric compound) has been used in the manufacturing process of this medicinal product and residues of it are present in the final product. Therefore, sensitisation reactions may occur.

4.5 Interaction with other medicinal products and other forms of Interaction

Fluarix may be given at the same time as other vaccines. Immunisation should be carried out on separate limbs. It should be noted that the adverse reactions may be intensified.

The immunological response may be diminished if the patient is undergoing immunosuppressant treatment.

Following influenza vaccination, false positive results in serology tests using the ELISA method to detect antibodies against HIV1, Hepatitis C and especially HTLV1 have been observed. The Western Blot technique disproves the results. The transient false positive reactions could be due to the IgM response by the vaccine.

4.6 Pregnancy and lactation

Limited data from vaccinations in pregnant women do not indicate that adverse fetal and maternal outcomes were attributable to the vaccine. The use of this vaccine may be considered from the second trimester of pregnancy. For pregnant women with medical conditions that increase their risk of complications from influenza, administration of the vaccine is recommended, irrespective of their stage of pregnancy.

Fluarix may be used during lactation.

4.7 Effects on ability to drive and use machines

The vaccine is unlikely to produce an effect on the ability to drive and use machines.

4.8 Undesirable effects

Adverse reactions from clinical trials

The safety of trivalent inactivated influenza vaccines is assessed in open label, uncontrolled clinical trials performed as annual update requirement, including at least 50 adults aged 18 – 60 years of age and at least 50 elderly aged 60 years or older. Safety evaluation is performed during the first 3 days following vaccination.

Undesirable effects reported are listed according to the following frequency:

Adverse events from clinical trials:

Common >1/100, <1/10):

Local reactions: redness, swelling, pain, ecchymosis, induration

Systemic reactions: fever, malaise, shivering, fatigue, headache, sweating, myalgia, arthralgia.

These reactions usually disappear within 1-2 days without treatment.

From Post-marketing surveillance additionally, the following adverse events have been reported:

Uncommon >1/1,000, <1/100):

Generalised skin reactions including pruritis, urticaria or non specific rash.

Rare >1/10,000, <1/1,000):

Neuralgia, paraesthesia, convulsions, transient thrombocytopenia.

Allergic reactions, in rare cases leading to shock, have been reported.

Very rare (<1/10,000)

Vasculitis with transient renal involvement.

Neurological disorders, such as encephalomyelitis, neuritis and Guillain Barré syndrome.

4.9 Overdose

Overdosage is unlikely to have any untoward effect.

5. PHARMACOLOGICAL PROPERTIES

5.1 Pharmacodynamic properties

Seroprotection is generally obtained within 2 to 3 weeks. The duration of postvaccinal immunity to homologous strains or to strains closely related to the vaccine strains varies but is usually 6-12 months.

5.2 Pharmacokinetic properties

Not applicable.

5.3 Preclinical safety data

Not applicable.

6. PHARMACEUTICAL PARTICULARS

6.1 List of excipients

Sodium chloride, disodium phosphate dodecahydrate, potassium dihydrogen phosphate, potassium chloride, magnesium chloride hexahydrate, RRR-α-tocopheryl hydrogen succinate, polysorbate 80, octoxinol 10 and water for injections.

6.2 Incompatibilities

In the absence of compatibility studies, this medicinal product must not be mixed with other medicinal products.

6.3 Shelf life

1 year

6.4 Special precautions for storage

Store at 2°C – 8°C (in a refrigerator).

Do not freeze.

Store in the original package in order to protect from light.

6.5 Nature and contents of container

0.5 ml suspension for injection in prefilled syringe (Type I glass) with a plunger stopper (butyl) with or without needles – pack of 1, 10 or 20.

Not all pack sizes may be marketed.

6.6 Instructions for use and handling

The vaccine should be allowed to reach room temperature before use. Shake before use.

When a dose of 0.25 ml is indicated, the prefilled syringe should be held in upright position and half of the volume should be eliminated. The remaining volume should be injected.

Administrative Data

7. MARKETING AUTHORISATION HOLDER

SmithKline Beecham plc

980 Great West Road

Brentford

Middlesex TW8 9GS

Trading as:

GlaxoSmithKline UK,

Stockley Park West,

Uxbridge,

Middlesex, UB11 1BT

8. MARKETING AUTHORISATION NUMBER(S)

PL 10592/0118

9. DATE OF FIRST AUTHORISATION/RENEWAL OF THE AUTHORISATION

27 February 1998

10. DATE OF REVISION OF THE TEXT

15 August 2005

11. Legal Category

POM

Flucloxacillin for Injection 1g

(Wockhardt UK Ltd)

1. NAME OF THE MEDICINAL PRODUCT

Flucloxacillin for Injection 1g

2. QUALITATIVE AND QUANTITATIVE COMPOSITION

Sodium flucloxacillin monohydrate equivalent to flucloxacillin 1g

For excipients, see 6.1

3. PHARMACEUTICAL FORM

Powder for solution for injection/infusion

Flucloxacillin sodium is supplied as a white or almost white crystalline powder

4. CLINICAL PARTICULARS

4.1 Therapeutic indications

Flucloxacillin is indicated for the treatment of infections due to penicillinase producing staphylococci and other gram positive organisms susceptible to this anti-infective (see Section 5.1).

Indications include: osteomyelitis and endocarditis.

Flucloxacillin is also indicated for use as a prophylactic agent during major surgical procedures when appropriate; for example cardiothoracic and orthopaedic surgery.

Consideration should be given to official guidance on the appropriate use of antibacterial agents.

4.2 Posology and method of administration

The dosage depends on the severity and nature of the infection.

The usual routes of administration are by intramuscular injection, slow intravenous injection and intravenous infusion. Flucloxacillin may also be administered by intra-articular or intrapleural injection or inhaled by nebuliser. The solutions must be prepared as follows:

Intramuscular: Add 1.5ml of water for injections to 250mg vial contents or 2ml of water for injections to 500mg vial contents.

Intravenous: Dissolve 250 to 500mg in 5 to 10ml of water for injections or 1g in 15 to 20ml of water for injections. Administer by slow intravenous injection (over three to four minutes). Flucloxacillin may also be added to infusion fluids or injected (suitably diluted) into the drip tube over three to four minutes. Flucloxacillin may be added to most intravenous fluids (eg water for injections, sodium chloride 0.9%, glucose 5%, sodium chloride 0.18% with glucose 4%).

Intrapleural: Dissolve 250mg in 5 to 10ml of water for injections.

Intra-articular: Dissolve 250 to 500mg in up to 5ml of water for injections or 0.5% lignocaine hydrochloride solution for injection.

Nebuliser Solution: Dissolve 125mg to 250mg of the vial contents in 3ml of water for injections.

The usual adult dosage (including the elderly) is as follows:

By intramuscular injection: 250mg every six hours

By slow intravenous injection or by infusion: 250mg to 1g every six hours

These doses may be doubled in severe infections. Doses of up to 8g daily have been suggested for endocarditis or osteomyelitis.

During surgical prophylaxis, doses of 1 to 2g should be given intravenously at induction of anaesthesia followed by 500mg six hourly intravenously or intramuscularly.

By intrapleural injection: 250mg once daily

By intra-articular injection: 250mg to 500mg once daily

By nebuliser: 125mg to 250mg every six hours

Children

Any route of administration may be used. For children under two years old, a quarter of the adult dose should be administered. For children two to ten years old, half of the adult dose should be administered.

Impaired renal function:

Dosage reduction is not usually required. In severe renal failure, however, (creatinine clearance less than 10ml/min) a reduction in dose or extension of dose interval should be considered.

No supplementary dosages need be administered during or at the end of the dialysis period, as flucloxacillin is not significantly removed by dialysis.

4.3 Contraindications
Flucloxacillin should not be given to patients with a history of hypersensitivity to β-lactam antibiotics (e.g. penicillins, cephalosporins).

Flucloxacillin is contraindicated in patients with a previous history of flucloxacillin-associated jaundice/hepatic dysfunction.

Ocular or subconjunctival administration is contraindicated.

4.4 Special warnings and special precautions for use
Flucloxacillin should be given with caution to patients with a history of allergy, especially to drugs. Before initiating therapy with flucloxacillin, careful enquiry should be made concerning previous hypersensitivity reactions to β-lactams. Cross sensitivity between penicillins and cephalosporins is well documented. Serious and occasionally fatal hypersensitivity reactions (anaphylaxis) have been reported in patients receiving β-lactam antibiotics. These reactions are more likely to occur in individuals with a history of β-lactam hypersensitivity. Desensitisation may be necessary if treatment is essential.

Care is necessary if very high doses of flucloxacillin are given, especially if renal function is poor, because of the risk of nephrotoxicity. The intrathecal route should be avoided. Care is also necessary if large doses of sodium salts are given to patients with impaired renal function or heart failure. Flucloxacillin should be used with caution in patients with evidence of hepatic dysfunction (see section 4.8). Renal, hepatic and haematological status should be monitored during prolonged and high-dose therapy (e.g. osteomyelitis, endocarditis). Prolonged use may occasionally result in overgrowth of non-susceptible organisms.

Care is required when treating some patients with syphilis because of the Jarisch- Herxheimer reaction.

Contact with flucloxacillin should be avoided since skin sensitisation may occur.

Caution is advised in patients with porphyria.

Special caution is essential in the newborn because of the risk of hyperbilirubinemia. Studies have shown that, at high dose following parenteral administration, flucloxacillin can displace bilirubin from plasma protein binding sites, and may therefore predispose to kernicterus in a jaundiced baby. In addition, special caution is essential in the newborn because of the potential for high serum levels of flucloxacillin due to a reduced rate of renal excretion.

Sodium content: Flucloxacillin for Injection 1g contains approximately 2.26mmol sodium per vial. This should be included in the daily allowance of patients on sodium restricted diets.

4.5 Interaction with other medicinal products and other forms of Interaction
Flucloxacillin may decrease the efficacy of oestrogen-containing oral contraceptives. Plasma concentrations of flucloxacillin are enhanced if probenecid is given concurrently. There is reduced excretion of methotrexate (increased risk of toxicity).

4.6 Pregnancy and lactation
There has been no evidence of a teratogenic effect in animals or untoward effect in humans. However, use in pregnancy should be reserved for essential cases.

Trace quantities of penicillin can be detected in breast milk.

4.7 Effects on ability to drive and use machines
None.

4.8 Undesirable effects
The most common adverse effects are sensitivity reactions including urticaria, maculo- papular rashes, fever, joint pains and angioedema. Anaphylaxis occasionally occurs and has sometimes been fatal. Late sensitivity reactions may include serum sickness-like reactions, haemolytic anaemia and acute interstitial nephritis, which is reversible whentreatment is discontinued.

Other adverse effects are generally associated with large intravenous doses of flucloxacillin or impaired renal function. These include transient leucopenia and thrombocytopenia, haemolytic anaemia and neutropenia (which might have some immunological basis); prolongation of bleeding time and defective platelet function; convulsions and other signs of central nervous system toxicity (encephalopathy has been reported following intrathecal administration and can be fatal); electrolyte disturbances due to administration of large amounts of sodium (see Section 4.4).

Hepatic effects: Changes in liver function test results may occur, but are reversible when treatment is discontinued. Hepatitis and cholestatic jaundice have been reported. These reactions are related neither to the dose nor to the route of administration; administration for more than two weeks and increasing age are risk factors. The onset of these effects may be delayed for up to two months post-treatment; in several cases the course of the reactions has been protracted and lasted for some months. In very rare cases, a fatal outcome has been reported, almost always in patients with serious underlying disease.

Some patients with syphilis may experience a Jarisch - Herxheimer reaction shortly after treatment is started. Symptoms include fever, chills, headache and reaction at the site of lesions. The reaction can be dangerous in cardiovascular syphilis or where there is a serious risk of increased local damage such as with optic atrophy.

Gastrointestinal effects (diarrhoea and nausea) reported with flucloxacillin commonly occur after oral administration, not parenteral administration. Pseudomembranous colitis has been reported with most antibiotics.

Phlebitis has followed intravenous infusion.

4.9 Overdose
Problems with overdosage are unlikely to occur. If they do occur, treatment is symptomatic.

5. PHARMACOLOGICAL PROPERTIES

5.1 Pharmacodynamic properties
Flucloxacillin is bactericidal with a similar mode of action to benzylpenicillin. It is resistant to staphylococcal penicillinase and therefore active against penicillinase-producing and non-penicillinase-producing staphylococci. It has minimum inhibitory concentrations in the range of 0.25 to 0.5μg per ml. Its activity against streptococci such as *Streptococcus pneumoniae* and *Str. pyogenes* is less than that of benzylpenicillin but sufficient to be useful when these organisms are present with penicillin-resistant staphylococci. It is virtually ineffective against *Enterococcus faecalis*.

5.2 Pharmacokinetic properties
After the intramuscular administration of a single 250 or 500mg dose of flucloxacillin to volunteers, mean peak concentrations of the drug in serum were approximately 10.5 and 16mg.l^{-1} respectively. Mean urinary excretion of flucloxacillin following its intramuscular use is 61% of the administered dose.

Flucloxacillin may also be administered by intravenous bolus injection or by slow intravenous infusion. High serum levels of the drug are achieved by these modes of administration: 30 minutes and 2 hours after a single 500mg intravenous bolus injection of flucloxacillin the mean serum concentration of the drug was 38 and 7.5mg.l^{-1}, respectively; 30 minutes and 3 hours after a single 1g intravenous bolus injection of flucloxacillin, the mean serum concentrations were 60 and 4mg.l^{-1} respectively. The administration of 2g flucloxacillin by intravenous infusion over 20 minutes resulted in mean serum concentrations of 244 and 27.7mg.l^{-1} 15 minutes and 120 minutes respectively after the end of the infusion.

The percentage of a dose of intravenous flucloxacillin recovered in urine in an 8 hour collection period varies from 60 to 76%.

About 95% of flucloxacillin in the circulation is bound to plasma proteins. Flucloxacillin has been reported to have a plasma half-life of approximately one hour. The half-life is prolonged in neonates.

The serum half-life of flucloxacillin in patients with severe kidney disease has been reported as 135 to 173 minutes. No significant difference in the half-life was found between patients on or off haemodialysis. Flucloxacillin is not removed by haemodialysis.

Flucloxacillin is metabolised to a limited extent and the unchanged drug and metabolites are excreted in the urine by glomerular filtration and renal tubular secretion. Up to 90% of an intramuscular dose is excreted in the urine within six hours. Only small amounts are excreted in the bile.

Flucloxacillin is unlikely to be excreted in breast milk to any significant extent. Similarly, placental transfer is unlikely to occur to any appreciable extent.

5.3 Preclinical safety data
There are no pre-clinical data of relevance to the prescriber which are additional to those included in other sections.

6. PHARMACEUTICAL PARTICULARS

6.1 List of excipients
None

6.2 Incompatibilities
Flucloxacillin may be administered in combination with other antibiotics including ampicillin to produce a wider spectrum of antibacterial activity. If used concurrently with an aminoglycoside the two antibiotics should not be mixed in the syringe, container or giving set as precipitation may occur.

Flucloxacillin should not be mixed with blood products or other proteinaceous fluids (eg protein hydrolysates) or with intravenous lipid emulsions.

6.3 Shelf life
3 years.

The unreconstituted dry powder is stable for 3 years. For the reconstituted solution, chemical and physical in-use stability has been demonstrated for 24 hours at 2-8°C. From a microbiological point of view, once opened, the product should be used immediately. If not used immediately, in-use storage times and conditions prior to use are the responsibility of the user and would normally not be longer than 24 hours at 2-8°C, unless reconstitution has taken place in controlled and validated aseptic conditions.

6.4 Special precautions for storage
Do not store above 25°C

6.5 Nature and contents of container
Flucloxacillin for Injection is supplied in Type II clear glass vials containing 1g of flucloxacillin equivalent. The vials are closed with a Type I chlorobutyl rubber stopper, sealed with an aluminium ring. The vials are packed in cartons of 10 vials.

6.6 Instructions for use and handling
None

Administrative Data

7. MARKETING AUTHORISATION HOLDER
CP Pharmaceuticals Ltd
Ash Road North
Wrexham
LL13 9UF
UK.

8. MARKETING AUTHORISATION NUMBER(S)
UK - PL 4543/0403
Ireland - PA 409/22/3

9. DATE OF FIRST AUTHORISATION/RENEWAL OF THE AUTHORISATION
30 October 1998 – UK
16 June 2003 – Ireland

10. DATE OF REVISION OF THE TEXT
26th August 2003

Flucloxacillin for Injection 250mg

(Wockhardt UK Ltd)

1. NAME OF THE MEDICINAL PRODUCT
Flucloxacillin for Injection 250mg

2. QUALITATIVE AND QUANTITATIVE COMPOSITION
Sodium flucloxacillin monohydrate equivalent to flucloxacillin 250mg

For excipients, see 6.1

3. PHARMACEUTICAL FORM
Powder for solution for injection/infusion

Flucloxacillin sodium is supplied as a white or almost white crystalline powder

4. CLINICAL PARTICULARS

4.1 Therapeutic indications
Flucloxacillin is indicated for the treatment of infections due to penicillinase producing staphylococci and other gram positive organisms susceptible to this anti-infective (see Section 5.1).

Indications include: osteomyelitis and endocarditis.

Flucloxacillin is also indicated for use as a prophylactic agent during major surgical procedures when appropriate; for example cardiothoracic and orthopaedic surgery.

Consideration should be given to official guidance on the appropriate use of antibacterial agents.

4.2 Posology and method of administration
The dosage depends on the severity and nature of the infection.

The usual routes of administration are by intramuscular injection, slow intravenous injection and intravenous infusion. Flucloxacillin may also be administered by intra-articular or intrapleural injection or inhaled by nebuliser. The solutions must be prepared as follows:

Intramuscular: Add 1.5ml of water for injections to 250mg vial contents or 2ml of water for injections to 500mg vial contents.

Intravenous: Dissolve 250 to 500mg in 5 to 10ml of water for injections or 1g in 15 to 20ml of water for injections. Administer by slow intravenous injection (over three to four minutes). Flucloxacillin may also be added to infusion fluids or injected (suitably diluted) into the drip tube over three to four minutes. Flucloxacillin may be added to most intravenous fluids (eg water for injections, sodium chloride 0.9%, glucose 5%, sodium chloride 0.18% with glucose 4%).

Intrapleural: Dissolve 250mg in 5 to 10ml of water for injections.

Intra-articular: Dissolve 250 to 500mg in up to 5ml of water for injections or 0.5% lignocaine hydrochloride solution for injection.

Nebuliser Solution: Dissolve 125mg to 250mg of the vial contents in 3ml of water for injections.

The usual adult dosage (including the elderly) is as follows:

By intramuscular injection: 250mg every six hours

By slow intravenous injection or by infusion: 250mg to 1g every six hours

These doses may be doubled in severe infections. Doses of up to 8g daily have been suggested for endocarditis or osteomyelitis.

During surgical prophylaxis, doses of 1 to 2g should be given intravenously at induction of anaesthesia followed by 500mg six hourly intravenously or intramuscularly.

By intrapleural injection: 250mg once daily

By intra-articular injection: 250mg to 500mg once daily

By nebuliser: 125mg to 250mg every six hours

Children

Any route of administration may be used. For children under two years old, a quarter of the adult dose should be administered. For children two to ten years old, half of the adult dose should be administered.

Impaired renal function:

Dosage reduction is not usually required. In severe renal failure, however, (creatinine clearance less than 10ml/min) a reduction in dose or extension of dose interval should be considered.

No supplementary dosages need be administered during or at the end of the dialysis period, as flucloxacillin is not significantly removed by dialysis.

4.3 Contraindications
Flucloxacillin should not be given to patients with a history of hypersensitivity to β-lactam antibiotics (e.g. penicillins, cephalosporins).

Flucloxacillin is contraindicated in patients with a previous history of flucloxacillin-associated jaundice/hepatic dysfunction.

Ocular or subconjunctival administration is contraindicated.

4.4 Special warnings and special precautions for use
Flucloxacillin should be given with caution to patients with a history of allergy, especially to drugs. Before initiating therapy with flucloxacillin, careful enquiry should be made concerning previous hypersensitivity reactions to β-lactams. Cross sensitivity between penicillins and cephalosporins is well documented. Serious and occasionally fatal hypersensitivity reactions (anaphylaxis) have been reported in patients receiving β-lactam antibiotics. These reactions are more likely to occur in individuals with a history of β-lactam hypersensitivity. Desensitisation may be necessary if treatment is essential.

Care is necessary if very high doses of flucloxacillin are given, especially if renal function is poor, because of the risk of nephrotoxicity. The intrathecal route should be avoided. Care is also necessary if large doses of sodium salts are given to patients with impaired renal function or heart failure. Flucloxacillin should be used with caution in patients with evidence of hepatic dysfunction (see section 4.8). Renal, hepatic and haematological status should be monitored during prolonged and high-dose therapy (e.g. osteomyelitis, endocarditis). Prolonged use may occasionally result in overgrowth of non-susceptible organisms.

Care is required when treating some patients with syphilis because of the Jarisch- Herxheimer reaction.

Contact with flucloxacillin should be avoided since skin sensitisation may occur.

Caution is advised in patients with porphyria.

Special caution is essential in the newborn because of the risk of hyperbilirubinemia. Studies have shown that, at high dose following parenteral administration, flucloxacillin can displace bilirubin from plasma protein binding sites, and may therefore predispose to kernicterus in a jaundiced baby. In addition, special caution is essential in the newborn because of the potential for high serum levels of flucloxacillin due to a reduced rate of renal excretion.

Sodium content: Flucloxacillin for Injection 250mg contains approximately 0.57mmol sodium per vial. This should be included in the daily allowance of patients on sodium restricted diets.

4.5 Interaction with other medicinal products and other forms of Interaction
Flucloxacillin may decrease the efficacy of oestrogen-containing oral contraceptives. Plasma concentrations of flucloxacillin are enhanced if probenecid is given concurrently. There is reduced excretion of methotrexate (increased risk of toxicity).

4.6 Pregnancy and lactation
There has been no evidence of a teratogenic effect in animals or untoward effect in humans. However, use in pregnancy should be reserved for essential cases.

Trace quantities of penicillin can be detected in breast milk.

4.7 Effects on ability to drive and use machines
None.

4.8 Undesirable effects
The most common adverse effects are sensitivity reactions including urticaria, maculo- papular rashes, fever, joint pains and angioedema. Anaphylaxis occasionally occurs and has sometimes been fatal. Late sensitivity reactions may include serum sickness-like reactions, haemolytic anaemia and acute interstitial nephritis, which is reversible when treatment is discontinued.

Other adverse effects are generally associated with large intravenous doses of flucloxacillin or impaired renal function. These include transient leucopenia and thrombocytopenia, haemolytic anaemia and neutropenia (which might have some immunological basis); prolongation of bleeding time and defective platelet function; convulsions and other signs of central nervous system toxicity (encephalopathy has been reported following intrathecal administration and can be fatal); electrolyte disturbances due to administration of large amounts of sodium (see Section 4.4).

Hepatic effects: Changes in liver function test results may occur, but are reversible when treatment is discontinued. Hepatitis and cholestatic jaundice have been reported. These reactions are related neither to the dose nor to the route of administration; administration for more than two weeks and increasing age are risk factors. The onset of these effects may be delayed for up to two months post-treatment; in several cases the course of the reactions has been protracted and lasted for some months. In very rare cases, a fatal outcome has been reported, almost always in patients with serious underlying disease.

Some patients with syphilis may experience a Jarisch - Herxheimer reaction shortly after treatment is started. Symptoms include fever, chills, headache and reaction at the site of lesions. The reaction can be dangerous in cardiovascular syphilis or where there is a serious risk of increased local damage such as with optic atrophy.

Gastrointestinal effects (diarrhoea and nausea) reported with flucloxacillin commonly occur after oral administration, not parenteral administration. Pseudomembranous colitis has been reported with most antibiotics.

Phlebitis has followed intravenous infusion.

4.9 Overdose
Problems with overdosage are unlikely to occur. If they do occur, treatment is symptomatic.

5. PHARMACOLOGICAL PROPERTIES

5.1 Pharmacodynamic properties
Flucloxacillin is bactericidal with a similar mode of action to benzylpenicillin. It is resistant to staphylococcal penicillinase and therefore active against penicillinase-producing and non-penicillinase-producing staphylococci. It has minimum inhibitory concentrations in the range of 0.25 to 0.5μg per ml. Its activity against streptococci such as *Streptococcus pneumoniae* and *Str. pyogenes* is less than that of benzylpenicillin but sufficient to be useful when these organisms are present with penicillin-resistant staphylococci. It is virtually ineffective against *Enterococcus faecalis*.

5.2 Pharmacokinetic properties
After the intramuscular administration of a single 250 or 500mg dose of flucloxacillin to volunteers, mean peak concentrations of the drug in serum were approximately 10.5 and 16mg.l^{-1} respectively. Mean urinary excretion of flucloxacillin following its intramuscular use is 61% of the administered dose.

Flucloxacillin may also be administered by intravenous bolus injection or by slow intravenous infusion. High serum levels of the drug are achieved by these modes of administration: 30 minutes and 2 hours after a single 500mg intravenous bolus injection of flucloxacillin the mean serum concentration of the drug was 38 and 7.5mg.l^{-1}, respectively; 30 minutes and 3 hours after a single 1g intravenous bolus injection of flucloxacillin, the mean serum concentrations were 60 and 4mg.l^{-1} respectively. The administration of 2g flucloxacillin by intravenous infusion over 20 minutes resulted in mean serum concentrations of 244 and 27.7mg.l^{-1} 15 minutes and 120 minutes respectively after the end of the infusion.

The percentage of a dose of intravenous flucloxacillin recovered in urine in an 8 hour collection period varies from 60 to 76%.

About 95% of flucloxacillin in the circulation is bound to plasma proteins. Flucloxacillin has been reported to have a plasma half-life of approximately one hour. The half-life is prolonged in neonates.

The serum half-life of flucloxacillin in patients with severe kidney disease has been reported as 135 to 173 minutes. No significant difference in the half-life was found between patients on or off haemodialysis. Flucloxacillin is not removed by haemodialysis.

Flucloxacillin is metabolised to a limited extent and the unchanged drug and metabolites are excreted in the urine by glomerular filtration and renal tubular secretion. Up to 90% of an intramuscular dose is excreted in the urine within six hours. Only small amounts are excreted in the bile.

Flucloxacillin is unlikely to be excreted in breast milk to any significant extent. Similarly, placental transfer is unlikely to occur to any appreciable extent.

5.3 Preclinical safety data
There are no pre-clinical data of relevance to the prescriber which are additional to those included in other sections.

6. PHARMACEUTICAL PARTICULARS

6.1 List of excipients
None

6.2 Incompatibilities
Flucloxacillin may be administered in combination with other antibiotics including ampicillin to produce a wider spectrum of antibacterial activity. If used concurrently with an aminoglycoside the two antibiotics should not be mixed in the syringe, container or giving set as precipitation may occur.

Flucloxacillin should not be mixed with blood products or other proteinaceous fluids (eg protein hydrolysates) or with intravenous lipid emulsions.

6.3 Shelf life
3 years.

The unreconstituted dry powder is stable for 3 years. For the reconstituted solution, chemical and physical in-use stability has been demonstrated for 24 hours at 2-8°C. From a microbiological point of view, once opened, the product should be used immediately. If not used immediately, in-use storage times and conditions prior to use are the responsibility of the user and would normally not be longer than 24 hours at 2-8°C, unless reconstitution has taken place in controlled and validated aseptic conditions.

6.4 Special precautions for storage
Do not store above 25°C

6.5 Nature and contents of container
Flucloxacillin for Injection is supplied in Type II clear glass vials containing 250mg of flucloxacillin equivalent. The vials are closed with a Type I chlorobutyl rubber stopper, sealed with an aluminium ring. The vials are packed in cartons of 10 vials.

6.6 Instructions for use and handling
None

Administrative Data

7. MARKETING AUTHORISATION HOLDER
CP Pharmaceuticals Ltd
Ash Road North
Wrexham
LL13 9UF
UK.

8. MARKETING AUTHORISATION NUMBER(S)
UK - PL 4543/0401
Ireland - PA 409/22/1

9. DATE OF FIRST AUTHORISATION/RENEWAL OF THE AUTHORISATION
30 October 1998 – UK
16 June 2003 – Ireland

10. DATE OF REVISION OF THE TEXT
26th August 2003

Flucloxacillin for Injection 500mg

(Wockhardt UK Ltd)

1. NAME OF THE MEDICINAL PRODUCT
Flucloxacillin for Injection 500mg

2. QUALITATIVE AND QUANTITATIVE COMPOSITION
Sodium flucloxacillin monohydrate equivalent to flucloxacillin 500mg

For excipients, see 6.1

3. PHARMACEUTICAL FORM
Powder for solution for injection/infusion

Flucloxacillin sodium is supplied as a white or almost white crystalline powder

4. CLINICAL PARTICULARS

4.1 Therapeutic indications
Flucloxacillin is indicated for the treatment of infections due to penicillinase producing staphylococci and other gram positive organisms susceptible to this anti-infective (see Section 5.1).

Indications include: osteomyelitis and endocarditis.

Flucloxacillin is also indicated for use as a prophylactic agent during major surgical procedures when appropriate; for example cardiothoracic and orthopaedic surgery.

Consideration should be given to official guidance on the appropriate use of antibacterial agents.

4.2 Posology and method of administration
The dosage depends on the severity and nature of the infection.

The usual routes of administration are by intramuscular injection, slow intravenous injection and intravenous infusion. Flucloxacillin may also be administered by intra-articular or intrapleural injection or inhaled by nebuliser. The solutions must be prepared as follows:

Intramuscular: Add 1.5ml of water for injections to 250mg vial contents or 2ml of water for injections to 500mg vial contents.

Intravenous: Dissolve 250 to 500mg in 5 to 10ml of water for injections or 1g in 15 to 20ml of water for injections. Administer by slow intravenous injection (over three to four minutes). Flucloxacillin may also be added to infusion fluids or injected (suitably diluted) into the drip tube over three to four minutes. Flucloxacillin may be added to most intravenous fluids (eg water for injections, sodium chloride 0.9%, glucose 5%, sodium chloride 0.18% with glucose 4%).

Intrapleural: Dissolve 250mg in 5 to 10ml of water for injections.

Intra-articular: Dissolve 250 to 500mg in up to 5ml of water for injections or 0.5% lignocaine hydrochloride solution for injection.

Nebuliser Solution: Dissolve 125mg to 250mg of the vial contents in 3ml of water for injections.

The usual adult dosage (including the elderly) is as follows:

By intramuscular injection: 250mg every six hours

By slow intravenous injection or by infusion: 250mg to 1g every six hours

These doses may be doubled in severe infections. Doses of up to 8g daily have been suggested for endocarditis or osteomyelitis.

During surgical prophylaxis, doses of 1 to 2g should be given intravenously at induction of anaesthesia followed by 500mg six hourly intravenously or intramuscularly.

By intrapleural injection: 250mg once daily

By intra-articular injection: 250mg to 500mg once daily

By nebuliser: 125mg to 250mg every six hours

Children

Any route of administration may be used. For children under two years old, a quarter of the adult dose should be administered. For children two to ten years old, half of the adult dose should be administered.

Impaired renal function:

Dosage reduction is not usually required. In severe renal failure, however, (creatinine clearance less than 10ml/min) a reduction in dose or extension of dose interval should be considered.

No supplementary dosages need be administered during or at the end of the dialysis period, as flucloxacillin is not significantly removed by dialysis.

4.3 Contraindications

Flucloxacillin should not be given to patients with a history of hypersensitivity to β-lactam antibiotics (e.g. penicillins, cephalosporins).

Flucloxacillin is contraindicated in patients with a previous history of flucloxacillin-associated jaundice/hepatic dysfunction.

Ocular or subconjunctival administration is contraindicated.

4.4 Special warnings and special precautions for use

Flucloxacillin should be given with caution to patients with a history of allergy, especially to drugs. Before initiating therapy with flucloxacillin, careful enquiry should be made concerning previous hypersensitivity reactions to β-lactams. Cross sensitivity between penicillins and cephalosporins is well documented. Serious and occasionally fatal hypersensitivity reactions (anaphylaxis) have been reported in patients receiving β-lactam antibiotics. These reactions are more likely to occur in individuals with a history of β-lactam hypersensitivity. Desensitisation may be necessary if treatment is essential.

Care is necessary if very high doses of flucloxacillin are given, especially if renal function is poor, because of the risk of nephrotoxicity. The intrathecal route should be avoided. Care is also necessary if large doses of sodium salts are given to patients with impaired renal function or heart failure. Flucloxacillin should be used with caution in patients with evidence of hepatic dysfunction (see section 4.8). Renal, hepatic and haematological status should be monitored during prolonged and high-dose therapy (e.g. osteomyelitis, endocarditis). Prolonged use may occasionally result in overgrowth of non-susceptible organisms.

Care is required when treating some patients with syphilis because of the Jarisch- Herxheimer reaction.

Contact with flucloxacillin should be avoided since skin sensitisation may occur.

Caution is advised in patients with porphyria.

Special caution is essential in the newborn because of the risk of hyperbilirubinemia. Studies have shown that, at high dose following parenteral administration, flucloxacillin can displace bilirubin from plasma protein binding sites, and may therefore predispose to kernicterus in a jaundiced baby. In addition, special caution is essential in the newborn because of the potential for high serum levels of flucloxacillin due to a reduced rate of renal excretion.

Sodium content: Flucloxacillin for Injection 500mg contains approximately 1.13mmol sodium per vial. This should be included in the daily allowance of patients on sodium restricted diets.

4.5 Interaction with other medicinal products and other forms of Interaction

Flucloxacillin may decrease the efficacy of oestrogen-containing oral contraceptives. Plasma concentrations of flucloxacillin are enhanced if probenecid is given concurrently. There is reduced excretion of methotrexate (increased risk of toxicity).

4.6 Pregnancy and lactation

There has been no evidence of a teratogenic effect in animals or untoward effect in humans. However, use in pregnancy should be reserved for essential cases.

Trace quantities of penicillin can be detected in breast milk.

4.7 Effects on ability to drive and use machines

None.

4.8 Undesirable effects

The most common adverse effects are sensitivity reactions including urticaria, maculo- papular rashes, fever, joint pains and angioedema. Anaphylaxis occasionally occurs and has sometimes been fatal. Late sensitivity reactions may include serum sickness-like reactions, haemolytic anaemia and acute interstitial nephritis, which is reversible when treatment is discontinued.

Other adverse effects are generally associated with large intravenous doses of flucloxacillin or impaired renal function. These include transient leucopenia and thrombocytopenia, haemolytic anaemia and neutropenia (which might have some immunological basis); prolongation of bleeding time and defective platelet function; convulsions and other signs of central nervous system toxicity (encephalopathy has been reported following intrathecal administration and can be fatal); electrolyte disturbances due to administration of large amounts of sodium (see Section 4.4).

Hepatic effects: Changes in liver function test results may occur, but are reversible when treatment is discontinued. Hepatitis and cholestatic jaundice have been reported. These reactions are related neither to the dose nor to the route of administration; administration for more than two weeks and increasing age are risk factors. The onset of these effects may be delayed for up to two months post-treatment; in several cases the course of the reactions has been protracted and lasted for some months. In very rare cases, a fatal outcome has been reported, almost always in patients with serious underlying disease.

Some patients with syphilis may experience a Jarisch - Herxheimer reaction shortly after treatment is started. Symptoms include fever, chills, headache and reaction at the site of lesions. The reaction can be dangerous in cardiovascular syphilis or where there is a serious risk of increased local damage such as with optic atrophy.

Gastrointestinal effects (diarrhoea and nausea) reported with flucloxacillin commonly occur after oral administration, not parenteral administration. Pseudomembranous colitis has been reported with most antibiotics.

Phlebitis has followed intravenous infusion.

4.9 Overdose

Problems with overdosage are unlikely to occur. If they do occur, treatment is symptomatic.

5. PHARMACOLOGICAL PROPERTIES

5.1 Pharmacodynamic properties

Flucloxacillin is bactericidal with a similar mode of action to benzylpenicillin. It is resistant to staphylococcal penicillinase and therefore active against penicillinase-producing and non-penicillinase-producing staphylococci. It has minimum inhibitory concentrations in the range of 0.25 to 0.5μg per ml. Its activity against streptococci such as *Streptococcus pneumoniae* and *Str. pyogenes* is less than that of benzylpenicillin but sufficient to be useful when these organisms are present with penicillin-resistant staphylococci. It is virtually ineffective against *Enterococcus faecalis.*

5.2 Pharmacokinetic properties

After the intramuscular administration of a single 250 or 500mg dose of flucloxacillin to volunteers, mean peak concentrations of the drug in serum were approximately 10.5 and 16mg.l^{-1} respectively. Mean urinary excretion of flucloxacillin following its intramuscular use is 61% of the administered dose.

Flucloxacillin may also be administered by intravenous bolus injection or by slow intravenous infusion. High serum levels of the drug are achieved by these modes of administration: 30 minutes and 2 hours after a single 500mg intravenous bolus injection of flucloxacillin the mean serum concentration of the drug was 38 and 7.5mg.l^{-1}, respectively; 30 minutes and 3 hours after a single 1g intravenous bolus injection of flucloxacillin, the mean serum concentrations were 60 and 4mg.l^{-1} respectively. The administration of 2g flucloxacillin by intravenous infusion over 20 minutes resulted in mean serum concentrations of 244 and 27.7mg.l^{-1} 15 minutes and 120 minutes respectively after the end of the infusion.

The percentage of a dose of intravenous flucloxacillin recovered in urine in an 8 hour collection period varies from 60 to 76%.

About 95% of flucloxacillin in the circulation is bound to plasma proteins. Flucloxacillin has been reported to have a plasma half-life of approximately one hour. The half-life is prolonged in neonates.

The serum half-life of flucloxacillin in patients with severe kidney disease has been reported as 135 to 173 minutes. No significant difference in the half-life was found between patients on or off haemodialysis. Flucloxacillin is not removed by haemodialysis.

Flucloxacillin is metabolised to a limited extent and the unchanged drug and metabolites are excreted in the urine by glomerular filtration and renal tubular secretion. Up to 90% of an intramuscular dose is excreted in the urine within six hours. Only small amounts are excreted in the bile.

Flucloxacillin is unlikely to be excreted in breast milk to any significant extent. Similarly, placental transfer is unlikely to occur to any appreciable extent.

5.3 Preclinical safety data

There are no pre-clinical data of relevance to the prescriber which are additional to those included in other sections.

6. PHARMACEUTICAL PARTICULARS

6.1 List of excipients

None

6.2 Incompatibilities

Flucloxacillin may be administered in combination with other antibiotics including ampicillin to produce a wider spectrum of antibacterial activity. If used concurrently with an aminoglycoside the two antibiotics should not be mixed in the syringe, container or giving set as precipitation may occur.

Flucloxacillin should not be mixed with blood products or other proteinaceous fluids (eg protein hydrolysates) or with intravenous lipid emulsions.

6.3 Shelf life

3 years.

The unreconstituted dry powder is stable for 3 years. For the reconstituted solution, chemical and physical in-use stability has been demonstrated for 24 hours at 2-8°C. From a microbiological point of view, once opened, the product should be used immediately. If not used immediately, in-use storage times and conditions prior to use are the responsibility of the user and would normally not be longer than 24 hours at 2-8°C, unless reconstitution has taken place in controlled and validated aseptic conditions.

6.4 Special precautions for storage

Do not store above 25°C

6.5 Nature and contents of container

Flucloxacillin for Injection is supplied in Type II clear glass vials containing 500mg of flucloxacillin equivalent. The vials are closed with a Type I chlorobutyl rubber stopper, sealed with an aluminium ring. The vials are packed in cartons of 10 vials.

6.6 Instructions for use and handling

None

Administrative Data

7. MARKETING AUTHORISATION HOLDER

CP Pharmaceuticals Ltd

Ash Road North

Wrexham

LL13 9UF

UK.

8. MARKETING AUTHORISATION NUMBER(S)

UK - PL 4543/0402

Ireland - PA 409/22/2

9. DATE OF FIRST AUTHORISATION/RENEWAL OF THE AUTHORISATION

30 October 1998 – UK

16 June 2003 – Ireland

10. DATE OF REVISION OF THE TEXT

26th August 2003

Fludara

(Schering Health Care Limited)

1. NAME OF THE MEDICINAL PRODUCT

Fludara® 50mg powder for solution for injection or infusion

2. QUALITATIVE AND QUANTITATIVE COMPOSITION

Each vial contains 50mg fludarabine phosphate

1ml of reconstituted solution contains 25mg fludarabine phosphate.

For excipients, see section 6.1.

3. PHARMACEUTICAL FORM

Powder for solution for injection or infusion.

White lyophilisate.

4. CLINICAL PARTICULARS

4.1 Therapeutic indications

Treatment of B-cell chronic lymphocytic leukaemia (CLL) in patients with sufficient bone marrow reserves.

First line treatment with Fludara should only be initiated in patients with advanced disease, Rai stages III/IV (Binet stage C), or Rai stages I/II (Binet stage A/B) where the patient has disease related symptoms or evidence of progressive disease.

4.2 Posology and method of administration

Fludara should be administered under the supervision of a qualified physician experienced in the use of antineoplastic therapy.

It is strongly recommended that Fludara should be only administered intravenously. No cases have been reported in which paravenously administered Fludara led to severe local adverse reactions. However, the unintentional paravenous administration must be avoided.

• Adults

The recommended dose is 25 mg fludarabine phosphate/ m^2 body surface given daily for 5 consecutive days every

28 days by the intravenous route. Each vial is to be made up in 2 ml water for injection. Each ml of the resulting reconstituted solution will contain 25 mg fludarabine phosphate. The required dose (calculated on the basis of the patient's body surface) of the reconstituted solution is drawn up into a syringe. For intravenous bolus injection this dose is further diluted in10 ml of 0.9 % sodium chloride. Alternatively, for infusion, the required dose may be diluted in 100 ml 0.9 % sodium chloride and infused over approximately 30 minutes (see also section 6.6).

The optimal duration of treatment has not been clearly established. The duration of treatment depends on the treatment success and the tolerability of the drug.

It is recommended that Fludara be administered up to the achievement of response (usually 6 cycles) and then the drug should be discontinued.

• Hepatic impairment

No data are available concerning the use of Fludara in patients with hepatic impairment. In this group of patients, Fludara should be used with caution and administered if the perceived benefit outweighs any potential risk.

• Renal impairment

The total body clearance of the principle plasma metabolite 2-F-ara-A shows a correlation with creatinine clearance, indicating the importance of the renal excretion pathway for the elimination of the compound. Patients with reduced kidney function demonstrated an increased total body exposure (AUC of 2F-ara-A). Limited clinical data are available in patients with impairment of renal function (creatinine clearance below 70 ml/min). Therefore, if renal impairment is clinically suspected, or in patients over the age of 70 years, creatinine clearance should be measured. If creatinine clearance is between 30 and 70 ml/min, the dose should be reduced by up to 50% and close haematological monitoring should be used to assess toxicity. Fludara treatment is contraindicated, if creatinine clearance is < 30 ml/min.

• Children

The safety and effectiveness of Fludara in children has not been established.

4.3 Contraindications

Fludara is contraindicated

- in those patients who are hypersensitive to the active substance or any of the excipients
- in renally impaired patients with creatinine clearance < 30 ml/min
- in patients with decompensated haemolytic anaemia
- during pregnancy and lactation.

4.4 Special warnings and special precautions for use

When used at high doses in dose-ranging studies in patients with acute leukaemia, Fludara was associated with severe neurological effects, including blindness, coma and death. This severe central nervous system toxicity occurred in 36 % of patients treated with doses approximately four times greater (96 mg/m^2/day for 5 - 7 days) than the dose recommended for treatment of CLL. In patients treated at doses in the range of the dose recommended for CLL, severe central nervous system toxicity occurred rarely (coma, seizures and agitation) or uncommonly (confusion). Patients should be closely observed for signs of neurological side effects.

The effect of chronic administration of Fludara on the central nervous system is unknown. However, patients tolerated the recommended dose, in some studies for relatively long term treatment times, whereby up to 26 courses of therapy were administered.

In patients with impaired state of health, Fludara should be given with caution and after careful risk/benefit consideration. This applies especially for patients with severe impairment of bone marrow function (thrombocytopenia, anaemia, and/or granulocytopenia), immunodeficiency or with a history of opportunistic infection.

Severe bone marrow suppression, notably anaemia, thrombocytopenia and neutropenia, has been reported in patients treated with Fludara. In a Phase I study in solid tumour patients, the median time to nadir counts was 13 days (range, 3 - 25 days) for granulocytes and 16 days (range, 2 - 32) for platelets. Most patients had haematological impairment at baseline either as a result of disease or as a result of prior myelosuppressive therapy. Cumulative myelosuppression may be seen. While chemotherapy-induced myelosuppression is often reversible, administration of fludarabine phosphate requires careful haematological monitoring.

Fludara is a potent antineoplastic agent with potentially significant toxic side effects. Patients undergoing therapy should be closely observed for signs of haematological and non-haematological toxicity. Periodic assessment of peripheral blood counts is recommended to detect the development of anaemia, neutropenia and thrombocytopenia.

As with other cytotoxics, caution should be exercised with fludarabine phosphate, when further haematopoietic stem sampling is considered.

Transfusion-associated graft-versus-host disease (reaction by the transfused immunocompetent lymphocytes to the host) has been observed after transfusion of non-irradiated blood in Fludara-treated patients. Fatal outcome as a consequence of this disease has been reported with a high frequency. Therefore, patients who require blood transfusion and who are undergoing, or who have received, treatment with Fludara should receive irradiated blood only.

Reversible worsening or flare up of pre-existing skin cancer lesions has been reported in some patients to occur during or after Fludara therapy.

Tumour lysis syndrome associated with Fludara treatment has been reported in CLL patients with large tumour burdens. Since Fludara can induce a response as early as the first week of treatment, precautions should be taken in those patients at risk of developing this complication.

Irrespective of any previous history of autoimmune processes or Coombs test status, life-threatening and sometimes fatal autoimmune phenomena (e.g. autoimmune haemolytic anaemia, autoimmune thrombocytopenia, thrombocytopenic purpura, pemphigus, Evans' syndrome) have been reported to occur during or after treatment with Fludara. The majority of patients experiencing haemolytic anaemia developed a recurrence in the haemolytic process after rechallenge with Fludara. Patients treated with Fludara should be closely monitored for haemolysis.

Patients undergoing treatment with Fludara should be closely monitored for signs of autoimmune haemolytic anaemia (decline in haemoglobin linked with haemolysis and positive Coombs test). Discontinuation of therapy with Fludara is recommended in case of haemolysis. Blood transfusion (irradiated, see above) and adrenocorticoid preparations are the most common treatment measures for autoimmune haemolytic anaemia.

Since there are limited data for the use of Fludara in elderly persons > 75 years), caution should be exercised with the administration of Fludara in these patients.

No data are available concerning the use of Fludara in children. Therefore, treatment with Fludara in children is not recommended.

Females of child-bearing potential or males must take contraceptive measures during and at least for 6 months after cessation of therapy.

During and after treatment with Fludara vaccination with live vaccines should be avoided.

A crossover from initial treatment with Fludara to chlorambucil for non responders to Fludara should be avoided because most patients who have been resistant to Fludara have shown resistance to chlorambucil.

4.5 Interaction with other medicinal products and other forms of Interaction

In a clinical investigation using Fludara in combination with pentostatin (deoxycoformycin) for the treatment of refractory chronic lymphocytic leukaemia (CLL), there was an unacceptably high incidence of fatal pulmonary toxicity. Therefore, the use of Fludara in combination with pentostatin is not recommended.

The therapeutic efficacy of Fludara may be reduced by dipyridamole and other inhibitors of adenosine uptake.

A pharmacokinetic drug interaction was observed in CLL and AML patients during combination therapy with fludarabine phosphate and Ara-C. Clinical studies and in vitro experiments with cancer cell lines demonstrated elevated intracellular Ara-CTP levels in leukaemic cells in terms of intracellular peak concentrations as well as of intracellular exposure (AUC) in combination of Fludara and subsequent Ara-C treatment. Plasma concentrations of Ara-C and the elimination rate of Ara-CTP were not affected.

4.6 Pregnancy and lactation

• Pregnancy

Fludara should not be used during pregnancy.

Women of child-bearing potential should be advised to avoid becoming pregnant and to inform the treating physician immediately should this occur.

Very limited human experience supports the findings of embryotoxicity studies in animals demonstrating an embryotoxic and/or teratogenic potential at the therapeutic dose. Preclinical data in rats demonstrated a transfer of fludarabine phosphate and/or metabolites through the foeto-placental barrier.

• Lactation

Breast-feeding should be discontinued for the duration of Fludara therapy.

It is not known whether this drug is excreted in human milk.

However, there is evidence from preclinical data that fludarabine phosphate and/or metabolites transfer from maternal blood to milk.

4.7 Effects on ability to drive and use machines

The effect of treatment with Fludara on the patient's ability to drive or operate machinery has not been evaluated.

4.8 Undesirable effects

The most common adverse events include myelosuppression (neutropenia, thrombocytopenia and anaemia), infection including pneumonia, fever, nausea, vomiting and diarrhoea. Other commonly reported events include fatigue, weakness, stomatitis, malaise, anorexia, oedema, chills, peripheral neuropathy, visual disturbances and skin rashes. Serious opportunistic infections have occurred in patients treated with Fludara. Fatalities as a consequence of serious adverse events have been reported.

The most frequently reported adverse events and those reactions which are more clearly related to the drug are arranged below according to body system regardless of their seriousness. Their frequencies (common ≥ 1%, uncommon ≥ 0.1% and < 1%) are based on clinical trial data regardless of the causal relationship with Fludara. The rare events (< 0.1%) were mainly identified from the post-marketing experience.

• Body as a whole

Infection, fever, fatigue, weakness, malaise, and chills have been commonly reported.

• Haemic and lymphatic system

Haematological events (neutropenia, thrombocytopenia, and anaemia) have been reported in the majority of patients treated with Fludara. Myelosuppression may be severe and cumulative. Fludarás prolonged effect on the decrease in the number of T-lymphocytes may lead to increased risk of opportunistic infections, including those due to latent viral reactivation, e.g. Herpes zoster, Epstein-Barr Virus (EBV) or progressive multifocal leucoencephalopathy (see 4.4. "Special warnings and special precautions for use"). Evolution of EBV-infection/reactivation into EBV-associated lymphoproliferative disorders has been observed in immunocompromised patients.

In rare cases, the occurrence of myelodysplastic syndrome (MDS) has been described in patients treated with Fludara. The majority of these patients also received prior, concomitant or subsequent treatment with alkylating agents or irradiation. Monotherapy with Fludara has not been associated with an increased risk for the development of MDS.

Clinically significant autoimmune phenomena have been reported to occur uncommonly in patients receiving Fludara (see section 4.4).

• Metabolic and nutritional disorders

Tumour lysis syndrome has been reported uncommonly in patients treated with Fludara. This complication may include hyperuricaemia, hyperphosphataemia, hypocalcaemia, metabolic acidosis, hyperkalaemia, haematuria, urate crystalluria, and renal failure. The onset of this syndrome may be heralded by flank pain and haematuria.

Oedema has been commonly reported.

Changes in hepatic and pancreatic enzyme levels are uncommon.

• Nervous system

Peripheral neuropathy has been commonly observed. Confusion is uncommon. Coma, agitation and seizures occur rarely.

• Special senses

Visual disturbances are commonly reported events in patients treated with Fludara. In rare cases, optic neuritis, optic neuropathy and blindness have occurred.

• Respiratory system

Pneumonia commonly occurs in association with Fludara treatment. Pulmonary hypersensitivity reactions to Fludara (pulmonary infiltrates/pneumonitis/fibrosis) associated with dyspnoea and cough have been uncommonly observed.

• Digestive system

Gastrointestinal disturbances such as nausea and vomiting, diarrhoea, stomatitis, and anorexia are common events. Gastrointestinal bleeding, mainly related to thrombocytopenia has been uncommonly reported in patients treated with Fludara.

• Cardiovascular system

In rare cases, heart failure and arrhythmia have been reported in patients treated with Fludara.

• Urogenital system

Rare cases of haemorrhagic cystitis have been reported in patients treated with Fludara.

• Skin and appendages

Skin rashes have been commonly reported in patients treated with Fludara.

In rare cases a Stevens-Johnson syndrome or a toxic epidermal necrolysis (Lyell's syndrome) may develop.

4.9 Overdose

High doses of Fludara have been associated with an irreversible central nervous system toxicity characterised by delayed blindness, coma, and death. High doses are also associated with severe thrombocytopenia and neutropenia due to bone marrow suppression. There is no known specific antidote for Fludara overdosage. Treatment consists of drug discontinuation and supportive therapy.

5. PHARMACOLOGICAL PROPERTIES

5.1 Pharmacodynamic properties

• Pharmacotherapeutic group: Antineoplastic agents

ATC-code L01B B05

Fludara contains fludarabine phosphate, a water-soluble fluorinated nucleotide analogue of the antiviral agent vidarabine, 9-β-D-arabinofuranosyladenine (ara-A) that is relatively resistant to deamination by adenosine deaminase.

Fludarabine phosphate is rapidly dephosphorylated to 2F-ara-A which is taken up by cells and then phosphorylated intracellularly by deoxycytidine kinase to the active triphosphate, 2F-ara-ATP. This metabolite has been shown to inhibit ribonucleotide reductase, DNA polymerase a/dand ε, DNA primase and DNA ligase thereby inhibiting DNA synthesis. Furthermore, partial inhibition of RNA polymerase II and consequent reduction in protein synthesis occur.

While some aspects of the mechanism of action of 2F-ara-ATP are as yet unclear, it is assumed that effects on DNA, RNA and protein synthesis all contribute to inhibition of cell growth with inhibition of DNA synthesis being the dominant factor. In addition, in vitro studies have shown that exposure of CLL lymphocytes to 2F-ara-A triggers extensive DNA fragmentation and cell death characteristic of apoptosis.

A phase III trial in patients with previously untreated B-chronic lymphocytic leukaemia comparing treatment with Fludara vs. chlorambucil (40mg / m^2 q4 weeks) in 195 and 199 patients respectively showed the following outcome: statistically significant higher overall response rates and complete response rates after 1st line treatment with Fludara compared to chlorambucil (61.1% vs. 37.6% and 14.9% vs. 3.4%, respectively); statistically significant longer duration of response (19 vs. 12.2 months) and time to progression (17 vs. 13.2 months) for the patients in the Fludara group. The median survival of the two patient groups was 56.1 months for Fludara and 55.1 months for chlorambucil, a non-significant difference was also shown with performance status. The proportion of patients reported to have toxicities were comparable between Fludara patients (89.7%) and chlorambucil patients (89.9%). While the difference in the overall incidence of haematological toxicities was not significant between the two treatment groups, significantly greater proportions of Fludara patients experienced white blood cell (p=0.0054) and lymphocyte (p=0.0240) toxicities than chlorambucil patients. The proportions of patients who experienced nausea, vomiting, and diarrhoea were significantly lower for Fludara patients ($p<0.0001$, $p<0.0001$, and $p=0.0489$, respectively) than chlorambucil patients. Toxicities of the liver were also reported for significantly (p=0.0487) less proportions of patients in the Fludara group than in the chlorambucil group.

Patients who initially respond to Fludara have a chance of responding again to Fludara monotherapy.

A randomised trial of Fludara vs. cyclophosphamide, adriamycin and prednisone (CAP) in 208 patients with CLL Binet stage B or C revealed the following results in the subgroup of 103 previously treated patients: the overall response rate and the complete response rate were higher with Fludara compared to CAP (45% vs. 26% and 13% vs. 6%, respectively); response duration and overall survival were similar with Fludara and CAP. Within the stipulated treatment period of 6 months the number of deaths was 9 (Fludara) vs. 4 (CAP).

Post-hoc analyses using only data of up to 6 months after start of treatment revealed a difference between survival curves of Fludara and CAP in favour of CAP in the subgroup of pretreated Binet stage C patients.

5.2 Pharmacokinetic properties

• Plasma and urinary pharmacokinetics of fludarabine (2F-ara-A)

The pharmacokinetics of fludarabine (2F-ara-A) have been studied after intravenous administration by rapid bolus injection and short-term infusion as well as following continuous infusion of fludarabine phosphate (Fludara, 2F-ara-AMP).

2F-ara-AMP is a water-soluble prodrug, which is rapidly and quantitatively dephosphorylated in the human organism to the nucleoside fludarabine (2F-ara-A). After single dose infusion of 25 mg 2F-ara-AMP per m^2 to cancer patients for 30 minutes 2F-ara-A reached mean maximum concentrations in the plasma of 3.5 - 3.7 μM at the end of the infusion. Corresponding 2F-ara-A levels after the fifth dose showed a moderate accumulation with mean maximum levels of 4.4 - 4.8 μM at the end of infusion. During a 5-day treatment schedule 2F-ara-A plasma trough levels increased by a factor of about 2. An accumulation of 2F-ara-A over several treatment cycles can be excluded. Postmaximum levels decayed in three disposition phases with an initial half-life of approx. 5 minutes, an intermediate half-life of 1 - 2 hours and a terminal half-life of approx. 20 hours.

An interstudy comparison of 2F-ara-A pharmacokinetics resulted in a mean total plasma clearance (CL) of 79 ± 40 ml/min/m^2 (2.2 ± 1.2 ml/min/kg) and a mean volume of distribution (Vss) of 83 ± 55 l/m^2 (2.4 ± 1.6 l/kg). Data showed a high interindividual variability. Plasma levels of 2F-ara-A and areas under the plasma level time curves increased linearly with the dose, whereas half-lives, plasma clearance and volumes of distribution remained constant independent of the dose indicating a dose linear behaviour.

Occurrence of neutropenia and haematocrit changes indicated that the cytotoxicity of fludarabine phosphate depresses the haematopoiesis in a dose dependent manner.

2F-ara-A elimination is largely by renal excretion. 40 to 60 % of the administered i.v. dose was excreted in the urine. Mass balance studies in laboratory animals with ^{3}H-2F-ara-AMP showed a complete recovery of radio-labelled substances in the urine. Another metabolite, 2F-ara-hypoxanthine, which represents the major metabolite in the dog, was observed in humans only to a minor extent. Individuals with impaired renal function exhibit a reduced total body clearance, indicating the need for a dose reduction. In vitro investigations with human plasma proteins revealed no pronounced tendency of 2F-ara-A protein binding.

• Cellular pharmacokinetics of fludarabine triphosphate

2F-ara-A is actively transported into leukaemic cells, whereupon it is rephosphorylated to the monophosphate and subsequently to the di- and triphosphate. The triphosphate 2F-ara-ATP is the major intracellular metabolite and the only metabolite known to have cytotoxic activity. Maximum 2F-ara-ATP levels in leukaemic lymphocytes of CLL patients were observed at a median of 4 hours and exhibited a considerable variation with a median peak concentration of approx. 20 μM. 2F-ara-ATP levels in leukaemic cells were always considerably higher than maximum 2F-ara-A levels in the plasma indicating an accumulation at the target sites. In-vitro incubation of leukaemic lymphocytes showed a linear relationship between extracellular 2F-ara-A exposure (product of 2F-ara-A concentration and duration of incubation) and intracellular 2F-ara-ATP enrichment. 2F-ara-ATP elimination from target cells showed median half-life values of 15 and 23 hours.

No clear correlation was found between 2F-ara-A pharmacokinetics and treatment efficacy in cancer patients.

5.3 Preclinical safety data

In acute toxicity studies, single doses of fludarabine phosphate produced severe intoxication symptoms or death at dosages about two orders of magnitude above the therapeutic dose. As expected for a cytotoxic compound, the bone marrow, lymphoid organs, gastrointestinal mucosa, kidneys and male gonads were affected. In patients, severe side effects were observed closer to the recommended therapeutic dose (factor 3 to 4) and included severe neurotoxicity partly with lethal outcome (see section 4.9).

Systemic toxicity studies following repeated administration of fludarabine phosphate showed also the expected effects on rapidly proliferating tissues above a threshold dose. The severity of morphological manifestations increased with dose levels and duration of dosing and the observed changes were generally considered to be reversible. In principle, the available experience from the therapeutic use of Fludara points to a comparable toxicological profile in humans, although additional undesirable effects such as neurotoxicity were observed in patients (see section 4.8).

The results from animal embryotoxicity studies indicated a teratogenic potential of fludarabine phosphate. In view of the small safety margin between the teratogenic doses in animals and the human therapeutic dose as well as in analogy to other antimetabolites which are assumed to interfere with the process of differentiation, the therapeutic use of Fludara is associated with a relevant risk of teratogenic effects in humans (see section 4.6).

Fludarabine phosphate has been shown to induce chromosomal aberrations in an in vitro cytogenetic assay, to cause DNA-damage in a sister chromatid exchange test and to increase the rate of micronuclei in the mouse micronucleus test in vivo, but was negative in gene mutation assays and in the dominant lethal test in male mice. Thus, the mutagenic potential was demonstrated in somatic cells but could not be shown in germ cells.

The known activity of fludarabine phosphate at the DNA-level and the mutagenicity test results form the basis for the suspicion of a tumorigenic potential. No animal studies which directly address the question of tumorigenicity have been conducted, because the suspicion of an increased risk of second tumours due to Fludara therapy can exclusively be verified by epidemiological data.

According to the results from animal experiments following intravenous administration of fludarabine phosphate, no remarkable local irritation has to be expected at the injection site. Even in case of misplaced injections, no relevant local irritation was observed after paravenous, intraarterial, and intramuscular administration of an aqueous solution containing 7.5 mg fludarabine phosphate/ml.

6. PHARMACEUTICAL PARTICULARS

6.1 List of excipients

Mannitol

Sodium hydroxide (to adjust the pH to 7.7).

6.2 Incompatibilities

Must not be mixed with other drugs.

6.3 Shelf life

As packaged for sale: 3 years.

Chemical and physical in-use stability after reconstitution has been demonstrated for 7 days at 4 °C.

From a microbiological point of view, the product should be used immediately. If not used immediately, in-use storage times and conditions prior to use are the responsibility of the user and should not be longer than 24 hours at 2 to 8 °C or 8 hours at room temperature.

6.4 Special precautions for storage

This medicinal product does not require any special storage conditions.

For storage after reconstitution or dilution, see Section 6.3

6.5 Nature and contents of container

10 ml colourless type I glass vials containing 50 mg fludarabine phosphate.

Each package contains 5 vials.

6.6 Instructions for use and handling

• Reconstitution

Fludara should be prepared for parenteral use by aseptically adding sterile water for injection. When reconstituted with 2 ml of sterile water for injection, the powder should fully dissolve in 15 seconds or less. Each ml of the resulting solution will contain 25 mg of fludarabine phosphate, 25 mg of mannitol, and sodium hydroxide to adjust the pH to 7.7. The pH range for the final product is 7.2 - 8.2.

• Dilution

The required dose (calculated on the basis of the patient's body surface) is drawn up into a syringe.

For intravenous bolus injection this dose is further diluted in 10 ml of 0.9 % sodium chloride. Alternatively, for infusion, the required dose may be diluted in 100 ml of 0.9 % sodium chloride and infused over approximately 30 minutes.

In clinical studies, the product has been diluted in 100 ml or 125 ml of 5 % dextrose injection or 0.9 % sodium chloride.

• Inspection prior to use

The reconstituted solution is clear and colourless. It should be visually inspected before use.

Only clear and colourless solutions without particles should be used. Fludara should not be used in case of a defective container.

• Handling and disposal

Fludara should not be handled by pregnant staff.

Procedures for proper handling should be followed according to local requirements for cytotoxic drugs. Caution should be exercised in the handling and preparation of the Fludara solution. The use of latex gloves and safety glasses is recommended to avoid exposure in case of breakage of the vial or other accidental spillage. If the solution comes into contact with the skin or mucous membranes, the area should be washed thoroughly with soap and water. In the event of contact with the eyes, rinse them thoroughly with copious amounts of water. Exposure by inhalation should be avoided.

The medicinal product is for single use only. Any unused product or waste material should be disposed of in accordance with local requirements.

7. MARKETING AUTHORISATION HOLDER

Schering Health Care Limited

The Brow

Burgess Hill

West Sussex RH15 9NE

8. MARKETING AUTHORISATION NUMBER(S)

PL/0053/0239

9. DATE OF FIRST AUTHORISATION/RENEWAL OF THE AUTHORISATION

11 August 1999

10. DATE OF REVISION OF THE TEXT

August 2005

LEGAL CATEGORY

POM

Fludara oral 10 mg film-coated tablet

(Schering Health Care Limited)

1. NAME OF THE MEDICINAL PRODUCT

Fludara® ▼ oral 10 mg film-coated tablet

2. QUALITATIVE AND QUANTITATIVE COMPOSITION

Each film-coated tablet contains fludarabine phosphate 10mg.

For excipients, see 6.1

3. PHARMACEUTICAL FORM

Film-coated tablet.

Salmon-pink, capsule-shaped tablet marked with 'LN' in a regular hexagon on one side

4. CLINICAL PARTICULARS

4.1 Therapeutic indications

Treatment of B-cell chronic lymphocytic leukaemia (CLL) in patients with sufficient bone marrow reserves.

First line treatment with Fludara oral should only be initiated in patients with advanced disease, Rai stages III/IV (Binet stage C) or Rai stages I/II (Binet stage A/B) where the patient has disease related symptoms or evidence of progressive disease.

4.2 Posology and method of administration

Fludara oral should be prescribed by a qualified physician experienced in the use of antineoplastic therapy.

• Adults

The recommended dose is 40 mg fludarabine phosphate/ m^2 body surface given daily for 5 consecutive days every 28 days by the oral route. This dose corresponds to 1.6

times the recommended intravenous dose of fludarabine phosphate (25 mg/m² body surface per day).

The following table provides guidance for determining the number of tablets of Fludara oral to be administered:

Body Surface Area (BSA) [m²]	Calculated total daily dose based on BSA (rounded up or down to whole number) [mg/day]	Number of tablets per day (total daily dose)
0.75 - 0.88	30 – 35	3 (30 mg)
0.89 - 1.13	36 – 45	4 (40 mg)
1.14 - 1.38	46 – 55	5 (50 mg)
1.39 - 1.63	56 – 65	6 (60 mg)
1.64 - 1.88	66 – 75	7 (70 mg)
1.89 - 2.13	76 – 85	8 (80 mg)
2.14 - 2.38	86 – 95	9 (90 mg)
2.39 - 2.50	96 – 100	10 (100 mg)

Fludara oral can be taken either on an empty stomach or together with food. The tablets have to be swallowed whole with water, they should not be chewed or broken.

The duration of treatment depends on the success of treatment and the tolerability of the drug. Fludara oral should be administered until best response is achieved (complete or partial remission, usually 6 cycles) and then the drug should be discontinued.

Patients undergoing treatment with Fludara should be closely monitored for response and toxicity. Individual dosing should be carefully adjusted according to the observed haematological toxicity.

Dose adjustments for the first treatment cycle (start of therapy with Fludara) are not recommended (except in patients with impairment of renal function – see 4.2).

If at the start of a subsequent cycle cell numbers are too low to administer the recommended dosage and there is evidence of treatment associated myelosuppression, the planned treatment cycle should be postponed until granulocyte count is above 1.0×10^9/l and platelet count is above 100×10^9/l. Treatment should only be postponed up to a maximum of two weeks. If granulocyte and platelet counts have not recovered after two weeks of postponement, the dose should be reduced according to the suggested dose adjustments in the table below.

Granulocytes and / or Platelets [10^9/l]		Fludarabine phosphate dose
0.5 - 1.0	50 - 100	**30**mg/m²/day
<0.5	<50	**20**mg/m²/day

Dose should not be reduced if thrombocytopenia is disease related.

If a patient does not respond to treatment after two cycles and shows no or little haematological toxicity a careful dose adjustment towards higher fludarabine phosphate doses in subsequent treatment cycles could be considered

• Patients with reduced kidney or liver function

Doses should be adjusted for patients with reduced kidney function. If creatinine clearance is between 30 and 70 ml/min, the dose should be reduced by up to 50 % and close haematological monitoring should be used to assess toxicity. For further information see section 4.4. Fludara oral treatment is contraindicated if creatinine clearance is < 30 ml/min (see 4.3).

No data are available concerning the use of Fludara in patients with hepatic impairment. In this group of patients, Fludara should be used with caution and administered if the perceived benefit outweighs any potential risk (see 4.4).

• Children

The safety and effectiveness of Fludara oral in children has not been established.

• Elderly patients

Since there are limited data for the use of Fludara in elderly persons (> 75 years), caution should be exercised with the administration of Fludara in these patients.

In patients over the age of 70 years, creatinine clearance should be measured. If creatinine clearance is between 30 and 70 ml/min, the dose should be reduced by up to 50% and close haematological monitoring should be used to assess toxicity (see 4.4).

4.3 Contraindications

Hypersensitivity to fludarabine phosphate or to any of the excipients

Renal impairment with creatinine clearance < 30 ml/min

Decompensated haemolytic anaemia

Pregnancy and lactation

4.4 Special warnings and special precautions for use

When used at high doses in dose-ranging studies in patients with acute leukaemia, intravenous Fludara was associated with severe neurological effects, including blindness, coma and death. This severe central nervous system toxicity occurred in 36 % of patients treated intravenously with doses approximately four times greater (96 mg/m²/day for 5 - 7 days) than the dose recommended for treatment of CLL. In patients treated at doses in the range of the dose recommended for CLL, severe central nervous system toxicity occurred rarely (coma, seizures and agitation) or uncommonly (confusion). Patients should be closely observed for signs of neurological side effects.

The effect of chronic administration of Fludara on the central nervous system is unknown. However, patients tolerated the recommended intravenous dose, in some studies for relatively long treatment times, whereby up to 26 courses of therapy were administered.

In patients with impaired state of health, Fludara oral should be given with caution and after careful risk/benefit consideration. This applies especially for patients with severe impairment of bone marrow function (thrombocytopenia, anaemia, and/or granulocytopenia), immunodeficiency or with a history of opportunistic infection.

Severe bone marrow suppression, notably anaemia, thrombocytopenia and neutropenia, has been reported in patients treated with Fludara. In a Phase I intravenous study in solid tumour patients, the median time to nadir counts was 13 days (range, 3 - 25 days) for granulocytes and 16 days (range, 2 - 32) for platelets. Most patients had haematological impairment at baseline either as a result of disease or as a result of prior myelosuppressive therapy.

No data are available concerning the use of Fludara in patients with hepatic impairment. In this group of patients, Fludara should be used with caution and administered if the perceived benefit outweighs any potential risk.

Cumulative myelosuppression may be seen. While chemotherapy-induced myelosuppression is often reversible, administration of fludarabine phosphate requires careful haematological monitoring.

Fludara is a potent antineoplastic agent with potentially significant toxic side effects. Patients undergoing therapy should be closely observed for signs of haematological and non-haematological toxicity. Periodic assessment of peripheral blood counts is recommended to detect the development of anaemia, neutropenia and thrombocytopenia.

As with other cytotoxics, caution should be exercised with fludarabine phosphate, when further haematopoietic stem sampling is considered.

Transfusion-associated graft-versus-host disease (reaction by the transfused immunocompetent lymphocytes to the host) has been observed after transfusion of non-irradiated blood in patients treated with intravenous Fludara. Fatal outcome as a consequence of this disease has been reported with a high frequency. Therefore, patients who require blood transfusion and who are undergoing, or who have received, treatment with Fludara should receive irradiated blood only.

Reversible worsening or flare up of pre-existing skin cancer lesions has been reported in some patients to occur during or after intravenous Fludara therapy.

Tumour lysis syndrome associated with intravenous Fludara treatment has been reported in patients with large tumour burdens. Since Fludara can induce a response as early as the first week of treatment, precautions should be taken in those patients at risk of developing this complication, and hospitalisation may be recommended for these patients during the first course of treatment.

Irrespective of any previous history of autoimmune processes or Coombs test status, life-threatening and sometimes fatal autoimmune phenomena (e.g. autoimmune haemolytic anaemia, autoimmune thrombocytopenia, thrombocytopenic purpura, pemphigus, Evans' syndrome) have been reported to occur during or after treatment with intravenous Fludara. The majority of patients experiencing haemolytic anaemia developed a recurrence in the haemolytic process after rechallenge with Fludara.

Patients undergoing treatment with Fludara should be closely monitored for signs of autoimmune haemolytic anaemia (decline in haemoglobin linked with haemolysis and positive Coombs test). Discontinuation of therapy with Fludara is recommended in case of haemolysis. Blood transfusion (irradiated, see above) and adrenocorticoid preparations are the most common treatment measures for autoimmune haemolytic anaemia.

The total body clearance of the principle plasma metabolite 2-F-ara-A shows a correlation with creatinine clearance, indicating the importance of the renal excretion pathway for the elimination of the compound. Patients with reduced kidney function demonstrated an increased total body exposure (AUC of 2F-ara-A). Limited clinical data are available in patients with impairment of renal function (creatinine clearance below 70 ml/min). Therefore, if renal impairment is clinically suspected, or in patients over the age of 70 years, creatinine clearance should be measured. If creatinine clearance is between 30 and 70 ml/min, the dose should be reduced by up to 50% and close haematological monitoring should be used to assess toxicity (see 4.2).

Since there are limited data for the use of Fludara in elderly persons (> 75 years), caution should be exercised with the administration of Fludara in these patients.

No data are available concerning the use of Fludara in children. Therefore, treatment with Fludara in children is not recommended.

Females of child-bearing potential or males must take contraceptive measures during and at least for 6 months after cessation of therapy.

During and after treatment with Fludara, vaccination with live vaccines should be avoided.

The reported incidence of nausea/vomiting was higher with the oral than the i.v. formulation. If this presents a persistent clinical problem it is recommended to switch to the i.v. formulation.

A crossover from initial treatment with Fludara to chlorambucil for non responders to Fludara should be avoided because most patients who have been resistant to Fludara have shown resistance to chlorambucil.

4.5 Interaction with other medicinal products and other forms of Interaction

In a clinical investigation using intravenous Fludara in combination with pentostatin (deoxycoformycin) for the treatment of refractory chronic lymphocytic leukaemia (CLL), there was an unacceptably high incidence of fatal pulmonary toxicity. Therefore, the use of Fludara in combination with pentostatin is not recommended.

The therapeutic efficacy of Fludara may be reduced by dipyridamole and other inhibitors of adenosine uptake.

A pharmacokinetic drug interaction was observed in CLL and AML patients during combination therapy with fludarabine phosphate and Ara-C. Clinical studies and in vitro experiments with cancer cell lines demonstrated elevated intracellular Ara-CTP levels in leukaemic cells in terms of intracellular peak concentrations as well as of intracellular exposure (AUC) in combination of Fludara and subsequent Ara-C treatment. Plasma concentrations of Ara-C and the elimination rate of Ara-CTP were not affected.

In a clinical investigation, pharmacokinetic parameters after peroral administration were not significantly affected by concomitant food intake (see 5.2).

4.6 Pregnancy and lactation

• Pregnancy

Fludara should not be used during pregnancy.

Women of child-bearing potential should be advised to avoid becoming pregnant and to inform the treating physician immediately should this occur.

Very limited human experience supports the findings of embryotoxicity studies in animals demonstrating an embryotoxic and/or teratogenic potential at the therapeutic dose. Preclinical data in rats demonstrated a transfer of fludarabine phosphate and/or metabolites through the feto-placental barrier.

• Lactation

Breast-feeding should be discontinued for the duration of Fludara therapy.

It is not known whether this drug is excreted in human milk. However, there is evidence from preclinical data that fludarabine phosphate and/or metabolites transfer from maternal blood to milk.

4.7 Effects on ability to drive and use machines

No studies on the effects on the ability to drive and use machines have been performed.

However, Fludara treatment may be associated with fatigue or visual disturbances. Patients experiencing such adverse events should avoid driving and using machines.

4.8 Undesirable effects

Based on the experience with the intravenous use of Fludara, the most common adverse events include myelosuppression (neutropenia, thrombocytopenia and anaemia), infection including pneumonia, fever, nausea, vomiting and diarrhoea. Other commonly reported events include fatigue, weakness, stomatitis, malaise, anorexia, oedema, chills, peripheral neuropathy, visual disturbances, and skin rashes. Serious opportunistic infections have occurred in patients treated with Fludara. Fatalities as a consequence of serious adverse events have been reported.

The most frequently reported adverse events and those reactions which are more clearly related to the drug are arranged below according to body system regardless of their seriousness. Their frequencies (common ⩾ 1%, uncommon ⩾ 0.1% and < 1%) are based on clinical trial data regardless of the causal relationship with intravenous Fludara. The rare events (< 0.1%) were mainly identified from the post-marketing experience.

• Body as a whole

Infection, fever, fatigue, weakness, malaise, and chills have been commonly reported.

• Haemic and lymphatic system

Haematological events (neutropenia, thrombocytopenia, and anaemia) have been reported in the majority of patients treated with Fludara. Myelosuppression may be severe and cumulative. Fludara's prolonged effect on the decrease in the number of T-lymphocytes may lead to increased risk of opportunistic infections, including those due to latent viral reactivation, e.g. Herpes zoster, Epstein-Barr Virus (EBV) or progressive multifocal leucoencephalopathy (see 4.4. "Special warnings and special precautions for use"). Evolution of EBV-infection/reactivation into EBV-associated lymphoproliferative disorders has been observed in immunocompromised patients.

In rare cases, the occurrence of myelodysplastic syndrome (MDS) has been described in patients treated with Fludara. The majority of these patients also received prior, concomitant or subsequent treatment with alkylating agents or irradiation. Monotherapy with Fludara has not been associated with an increased risk for the development of MDS.

Clinically significant autoimmune phenomena have been reported to occur uncommonly in patients receiving Fludara (see section 4.4).

• Metabolic and nutritional disorders

Tumour lysis syndrome has been reported uncommonly in patients treated with Fludara. This complication may include hyperuricaemia, hyperphosphataemia, hypocalcaemia, metabolic acidosis, hyperkalaemia, haematuria, urate crystalluria, and renal failure. The onset of this syndrome may be heralded by flank pain and haematuria.

Oedema has been commonly reported.

Changes in hepatic and pancreatic enzyme levels are uncommon.

• Nervous system

Peripheral neuropathy has been commonly observed.

Confusion is uncommon. Coma, agitation and seizures occur rarely.

• Special senses

Visual disturbances are commonly reported events in patients treated with Fludara. In rare cases, optic neuritis, optic neuropathy and blindness have occurred.

• Cardiovascular system

In rare cases, heart failure and arrhythmia have been reported in patients treated with Fludara.

• Respiratory system

Pneumonia commonly occurs in association with Fludara treatment. Pulmonary hypersensitivity reactions to Fludara (pulmonary infiltrates/pneumonitis/fibrosis) associated with dyspnoea and cough have been uncommonly observed.

• Digestive system

Gastrointestinal disturbances such as nausea and vomiting, diarrhoea, stomatitis and anorexia, are common events. Gastrointestinal bleeding, mainly related to thrombocytopenia has been uncommonly reported in patients treated with Fludara.

• Skin and appendages

Skin rashes have been commonly reported in patients treated with Fludara.

In rare cases a Stevens-Johnson syndrome or a toxic epidermal necrolysis (Lyell's syndrome) may develop.

• Urogenital system

Rare cases of haemorrhagic cystitis have been reported in patients treated with Fludara.

4.9 Overdose

High doses of Fludara given intravenously have been associated with an irreversible central nervous system toxicity characterised by delayed blindness, coma, and death. High doses are also associated with severe thrombocytopenia and neutropenia due to bone marrow suppression. There is no known specific antidote for Fludara overdosage. Treatment consists of drug discontinuation and supportive therapy.

5. PHARMACOLOGICAL PROPERTIES

5.1 Pharmacodynamic properties

Pharmacotherapeutic group: Antineoplastic and immunomodulating agents

ATC Code: L01B B05

Fludara contains fludarabine phosphate, a water-soluble fluorinated nucleotide that is relatively resistant to deamination by adenosine deaminase.

Fludarabine phosphate is rapidly dephosphorylated to 2F-ara-A which is taken up by cells and then phosphorylated intracellularly by deoxycytidine kinase to the active triphosphate, 2F-ara-ATP. This metabolite is a potent inhibitor of DNA synthesis and also reduces RNA and protein synthesis.

Inhibition of DNA synthesis leads to a reduction in cell division and induction of apoptosis. This is believed to be the dominant mechanism of action of the compound.

A randomised trial of intravenous Fludara vs. cyclophosphamide, adriamycin and prednisone (CAP) in 208 patients with CLL Binet stage B or C revealed the following results in the subgroup of 103 previously treated patients: the overall response rate and the complete response rate were higher with Fludara compared to CAP (45% vs. 26% and 13% vs. 6%, respectively); response duration and overall survival were similar with Fludara and CAP. Within the stipulated treatment period of 6 months the number of deaths was 9 (Fludara) vs. 4 (CAP).

Post-hoc analyses using only data of up to 6 months after start of treatment revealed a difference between survival curves of Fludara and CAP in favour of CAP in the subgroup of pretreated Binet stage C patients.

5.2 Pharmacokinetic properties

• Plasma and urinary pharmacokinetics of fludarabine (2F-ara-A)

The pharmacokinetics of fludarabine (2F-ara-A) have been studied after intravenous administration by rapid bolus injection and short-term infusion as well as following continuous infusion and after peroral dosing of fludarabine phosphate (Fludara, 2F-ara-AMP).

2F-ara-AMP is a water-soluble prodrug, which is rapidly and quantitatively dephosphorylated in the human organism to the nucleoside fludarabine (2F-ara-A). After single dose infusion of 25 mg 2F-ara-AMP per m^2 to cancer patients for 30 minutes 2F-ara-A reached mean maximum concentrations in the plasma of 3.5 - 3.7 μM at the end of the infusion. Corresponding 2F-ara-A levels after the fifth dose showed a moderate accumulation with mean maximum levels of 4.4 -4.8 μM at the end of infusion. During a 5-day treatment schedule 2F-ara-A plasma trough levels increased by a factor of about 2. An accumulation of 2F-ara-A over several treatment cycles can be excluded. Postmaximum levels decayed in three disposition phases with an initial half-life of approx. 5 minutes, an intermediate half-life of 1 - 2 hours and a terminal half-life of approx. 20 hours.

An interstudy comparison of 2F-ara-A pharmacokinetics resulted in a mean total plasma clearance (CL) of 79 ± 40 ml/min/m^2 (2.2 ± 1.2 ml/min/kg) and a mean volume of distribution (Vss) of 83 ± 55 l/m^2 (2.4 ± 1.6 l/kg). Data showed a high interindividual variability. After intravenous and peroral administration of fludarabine phosphate, plasma levels of 2F-ara-A and areas under the plasma level time curves increased linearly with the dose, whereas half-lives, plasma clearance and volumes of distribution remained constant independent of the dose indicating a dose linear behaviour.

After peroral fludarabine phosphate doses, maximum 2F-ara-A plasma levels reached approximately 20 - 30 % of corresponding intravenous levels at the end of infusion and occurred 1 – 2 hours postdose. The systemic 2F-ara-A availability was 50 - 65 % following single and repeated doses and was similar after ingestion of a solution or immediate release tablet formulation. After oral dose of 2F-ara-AMP with concomitant food intake a slight increase (<10 %) of systemic availability (AUC), a slight decrease of maximum plasma levels (C_{max}) of 2F-ara-A and a delayed time of occurrence of C_{max} was observed; terminal half-lives were unaffected.

Occurrence of neutropenia and haematocrit changes indicated that the cytotoxicity of fludarabine phosphate depresses the haematopoiesis in a dose dependent manner.

2F-ara-A elimination is largely by renal excretion. 40 to 60 % of the administered intravenous dose was excreted in the urine. Mass balance studies in laboratory animals with ^{3}H-2F-ara-AMP showed a complete recovery of radio-labelled substances in the urine. Another metabolite, 2F-ara-hypoxanthine, which represents the major metabolite in the dog, was observed in humans only to a minor extent. Individuals with impaired renal function exhibit a reduced total body clearance, indicating the need for a dose reduction. *In vitro* investigations with human plasma proteins revealed no pronounced tendency of 2F-ara-A protein binding.

• Cellular pharmacokinetics of fludarabine triphosphate

2F-ara-A is actively transported into leukaemic cells, whereupon it is rephosphorylated to the monophosphate and subsequently to the di- and triphosphate. The triphosphate 2F-ara-ATP is the major intracellular metabolite and the only metabolite known to have cytotoxic activity. Maximum 2F-ara-ATP levels in leukaemic lymphocytes of CLL patients were observed at a median of 4 hours and exhibited a considerable variation with a median peak concentration of approx. 20 μM. 2F-ara-ATP levels in leukaemic cells were always considerably higher than maximum 2F-ara-A levels in the plasma indicating an accumulation at the target sites. In-vitro incubation of leukaemic lymphocytes showed a linear relationship between extracellular 2F-ara-A exposure (product of 2F-ara-A concentration and duration of incubation) and intracellular 2F-ara-ATP enrichment. 2F-ara-ATP elimination from target cells showed median half-life values of 15 and 23 hours.

No clear correlation was found between 2F-ara-A pharmacokinetics and treatment efficacy in cancer patients.

5.3 Preclinical safety data

In acute toxicity studies, single doses of fludarabine phosphate produced severe intoxication symptoms or death at dosages about two orders of magnitude above the therapeutic dose. As expected for a cytotoxic compound, the bone marrow, lymphoid organs, gastrointestinal mucosa, kidneys and male gonads were affected. In patients, severe side effects were observed closer to the recommended therapeutic dose (factor 3 to 4) and included severe neurotoxicity partly with lethal outcome (cf. section 4.9).

Systemic toxicity studies following repeated administration of fludarabine phosphate showed also the expected effects on rapidly proliferating tissues above a threshold dose. The severity of morphological manifestations increased with dose levels and duration of dosing and the observed changes were generally considered to be reversible. In principle, the available experience from the therapeutic use of Fludara points to a comparable toxicological profile in humans, although additional undesirable effects such as neurotoxicity were observed in patients (cf. section 4.8).

The results from animal embryotoxicity studies indicated a teratogenic potential of fludarabine phosphate. In view of the small safety margin between the teratogenic doses in animals and the human therapeutic dose as well as in analogy to other antimetabolites which are assumed to interfere with the process of differentiation, the therapeutic use of Fludara is associated with a relevant risk of teratogenic effects in humans (cf. section 4.6).

Fludarabine phosphate has been shown to induce chromosomal aberrations in an *in vitro* cytogenetic assay, to cause DNA-damage in a sister chromatid exchange test and to increase the rate of micronuclei in the mouse micronucleus test *in vivo*, but was negative in gene mutation assays and in the dominant lethal test in male mice. Thus, the mutagenic potential was demonstrated in somatic cells but could not be shown in germ cells.

The known activity of fludarabine phosphate at the DNA-level and the mutagenicity test results form the basis for the suspicion of a tumorigenic potential. No animal studies which directly address the question of tumorigenicity have been conducted, because the suspicion of an increased risk of second tumours due to Fludara therapy can exclusively be verified by epidemiological data.

According to the results from animal experiments following intravenous administration of fludarabine phosphate, no remarkable local irritation is to be expected at the injection site. Even in case of misplaced injections, no relevant local irritation was observed after paravenous, intraarterial, and intramuscular administration of an aqueous solution containing 7.5 mg fludarabine phosphate/ml. The similarity in nature of the observed lesions in the gastrointestinal tract after intravenous or intragastric dosing in animal experiments supports the assumption that the fludarabine phosphate induced enteritis is a systemic effect.

6. PHARMACEUTICAL PARTICULARS

6.1 List of excipients

Tablet core: Cellulose, microcrystalline

Lactose, monohydrate

Silica, colloidal anhydrous

Croscarmellose sodium

Magnesium stearate

Film-coat: Hypromellose

Talc

Titanium dioxide (E171)

Ferric oxide pigment, yellow (E172)

Ferric oxide pigment, red (E172)

6.2 Incompatibilities

Not Applicable

6.3 Shelf life

2 years.

6.4 Special precautions for storage

Store in the original package

6.5 Nature and contents of container

Blisters of 5 tablets each, comprising polyamide/aluminium/polypropylene thermoformable foil with a lidding foil of aluminium. The blisters are packed in a polyethylene tablet container with a child-resistant polypropylene screw cap.

Pack sizes: 15 or 20 film-coated tablets per tablet container

6.6 Instructions for use and handling

Fludara should not be handled by pregnant staff.

Procedures for proper handling and disposal should be observed. Consideration should be given to handling and disposal according to guidelines used for cytotoxic drugs. Waste material may be disposed of by incineration.

7. MARKETING AUTHORISATION HOLDER

Schering Health Care Limited

The Brow

Burgess Hill

West Sussex RH15 9NE

United Kingdom

8. MARKETING AUTHORISATION NUMBER(S)

PL 00053/0290

9. DATE OF FIRST AUTHORISATION/RENEWAL OF THE AUTHORISATION

24 October 2000

10. DATE OF REVISION OF THE TEXT

October 2004

LEGAL CATEGORY

POM

Fluorets

(Chauvin Pharmaceuticals Ltd)

1. NAME OF THE MEDICINAL PRODUCT
Fluorets

2. QUALITATIVE AND QUANTITATIVE COMPOSITION
Paper strips each impregnated with approximately 1mg Fluorescein Sodium BP.

3. PHARMACEUTICAL FORM
Sterile, individually wrapped paper strips.

4. CLINICAL PARTICULARS
4.1 Therapeutic indications
Fluorescein is a corneal stain and can be used in diagnostic examinations of the eye including Goldmann tonometry and in the fitting of contact lenses.

4.2 Posology and method of administration
One Fluoret moistened with tear fluid, sterile water or sterile ophthalmic solution applied topically to the eye should be sufficient to provide adequate corneal staining.

4.3 Contraindications
Not for use in patients with a known hypersensitivity to fluorescein.

Not to be used with soft contact lenses.

4.4 Special warnings and special precautions for use
Care should be taken to handle the strip by the non-impregnated end. The applicator should be used once and discarded.

4.5 Interaction with other medicinal products and other forms of Interaction
None known.

4.6 Pregnancy and lactation
Safety for use in pregnancy and lactation has not been established, therefore, use only when considered essential by a physician.

4.7 Effects on ability to drive and use machines
May cause transient blurring of vision when applied. Warn patients not to drive or operate hazardous machinery unless vision is clear.

4.8 Undesirable effects
None.

4.9 Overdose
Not applicable.

5. PHARMACOLOGICAL PROPERTIES
5.1 Pharmacodynamic properties
Fluorescein sodium acts as a diagnostic stain.

5.2 Pharmacokinetic properties
Fluorescein will resist penetration of a normal cornea and most excess solution will, therefore, be carried with the tear film away from the conjunctival sac. The majority will be lost through the naso-lacrimal ducts and absorbed via the gastro-intestinal tract from where it is converted rapidly to its glucuronide and excreted via the urine.

If fluorescein crosses the cornea it will enter the Bowman's membrane, stroma and possibly the anterior chamber. Aqueous flow and diffusion into the blood in the anterior chamber finally removes fluorescein from the eye and it is excreted unchanged in the urine.

5.3 Preclinical safety data
There are no preclinical data of relevance to the prescriber which are additional to that already included in other sections of this SPC.

6. PHARMACEUTICAL PARTICULARS
6.1 List of excipients
None.

6.2 Incompatibilities
None.

6.3 Shelf life
5 years.

6.4 Special precautions for storage
Store below 25°C

6.5 Nature and contents of container
Individually wrapped sterile paper strips, supplied in cartons containing 100 Fluorets.

6.6 Instructions for use and handling
Each Fluoret should be handled by the non-impregnated end. Fluorets should be used once and discarded.

7. MARKETING AUTHORISATION HOLDER
Chauvin Pharmaceuticals Ltd
106 London Road
Kingston-upon-Thames
Surrey
KT2 6TN.

8. MARKETING AUTHORISATION NUMBER(S)
PL 0033/5095R

9. DATE OF FIRST AUTHORISATION/RENEWAL OF THE AUTHORISATION
Date of First Authorisation: 1 October 1987
Date of Renewal of Authorisation: 25 January 1998

10. DATE OF REVISION OF THE TEXT
January 1998
December 2002

Fluorouracil Injection, 25 mg / ml, solution for injection

(medac GmbH)

1. NAME OF THE MEDICINAL PRODUCT
Fluorouracil Injection, 25 mg / ml, solution for injection

2. QUALITATIVE AND QUANTITATIVE COMPOSITION
One vial of Fluorouracil Injection contains:
2500 mg Fluorouracil in 100 ml solution (25 mg/ml)
For excipients, see 6.1

3. PHARMACEUTICAL FORM
Solution for injection
Fluorouracil Injection, 25 mg / ml, solution for injection is a clear, colourless or almost colourless solution.

4. CLINICAL PARTICULARS
4.1 Therapeutic indications
Fluorouracil Injection 25 mg/ml, solution for injection, may be used alone or in combination, for its palliative action in the management of common malignancies particularly cancer of the colon and breast, either as single agent or in combination with other cytotoxic agents.

4.2 Posology and method of administration
Routes of administration:
Fluorouracil Injection can be given by intravenous injection or intravenous or intra-arterial infusion.

Adults:
Selection of an appropriate dose and treatment regime depends upon the condition of the patient, the type of carcinoma being treated and whether Fluorouracil is to be administered alone or in combination with other therapy. Initial treatment should be given in hospital and the total daily dose should not exceed 0.8 - 1 gram. It is customary to calculate the dose in accordance with the patient's actual bodyweight unless there is obesity, oedema or some other form of abnormal fluid retention such as ascites. In this case, ideal weight is used as the basis for calculation.

Reduction of the dose is advisable in patients with any of the following:
1. Cachexia.
2. Major surgery within preceding 30 days.
3. Reduced bone marrow function.
4. Impaired hepatic or renal function.

ADULT DOSE
The following regimen have been recommended for use as a single agent-
Initial Treatment:
this may be in the form of an infusion or an injection, the former usually being preferred because of lesser toxicity.

Intravenous Infusion:
15 mg/kg bodyweight but not more than 1 g per infusion, diluted in 300 - 500 ml of 5% glucose or 0.9% NaCl injection and given over 4 hours. Alternatively the daily dose may be infused over 30-60 minutes or may be given as a continuous infusion over 24 hours. The infusion may be repeated daily until there is evidence of toxicity or a total dose of 12-15 g has been reached.

Intravenous Injection:
12 mg/kg bodyweight may be given daily for 3 days and then, if there is no evidence of toxicity, 6 mg/kg on alternate days for 3 further doses. An alternative regime is 15 mg/kg as a single intravenous injection once a week throughout the course.

Intra-arterial Infusion:
5 - 7.5 mg/kg bodyweight daily may be given by 24 hour continuous intra-arterial infusion.

Maintenance Therapy:
An initial intensive course may be followed by maintenance therapy providing there are no significant toxic effects.

In all instances, toxic side effects must disappear before maintenance therapy is started.

The initial course of Fluorouracil can be repeated after an interval of 4 to 6 weeks from the last dose or, alternatively, treatment can be continued with intravenous injections of 5-15 mg/kg bodyweight at weekly intervals.

This sequence constitutes a course of therapy. Some patients have received up to 30 g at a maximum rate of 1 g daily. A more recent alternative method is to give 15 mg/kg IV once a week throughout the course of treatment. This obviates the need for an initial period of daily administration.

In combination with Irradiation:
Irradiation combined with 5-FU has been found to be useful in the treatment of certain types of metastatic lesions in the lungs and for the relief of pain caused by recurrent, inoperable growth. The standard dose of 5-FU should be used.

CHILDREN:
No recommendations are made regarding the use of Fluorouracil in children.

ELDERLY:
Fluorouracil should be used in the elderly with similar considerations as with normal adult doses.

4.3 Contraindications
Fluorouracil is contraindicated in seriously debilitated patients or those with bone marrow depression after radiotherapy or treatment with other antineoplastic agents.

Fluorouracil is strictly contraindicated in pregnant or breast feeding women.

Fluorouracil should not be used in the management of non-malignant disease.

4.4 Special warnings and special precautions for use
It is recommended that Fluorouracil should only be given by, or under the strict supervision of, a qualified physician who is conversant with the use of potent antimetabolites.

All patients should be admitted to hospital for initial treatment.

Adequate treatment with Fluorouracil is usually followed by leucopenia, the lowest white blood cell (W.B.C.) count commonly being observed between the 7th and 14th day of the first course, but occasionally being delayed for as long as 20 days.

The count usually returns to normal by the 30th day. Daily monitoring of platelet and W.B.C. count is recommended and treatment should be stopped if platelets fall below 100,000 per mm^3 or the W.B.C. count falls below 3,500 per mm^3. If the total count is less than 2000 per mm^3, and especially if there is granulocytopenia, it is recommended that the patient be placed in protective isolation in the hospital and treated with appropriate measures to prevent systemic infection.

Treatment should also be stopped at the first sign of oral ulceration or if there is evidence of gastrointestinal side effects such as stomatitis, diarrhoea, bleeding from the G.I. tract or haemorrhage at any site. The ratio between effective and toxic dose is small and therapeutic response is unlikely without some degree of toxicity. Care must be taken therefore, in the selection of patients and adjustment of dosage.

Fluorouracil should be used with caution in patients with reduced renal or liver function or jaundice. Isolated cases of angina, ECG abnormalities and rarely, myocardial infarction have been reported following administration of Fluorouracil. Caution should therefore be exercised in treating patients who experience chest pain during courses of treatment, or patients with a history of heart disease.

4.5 Interaction with other medicinal products and other forms of Interaction
Drug Interactions
Various agents have been reported to biochemically modulate the antitumour efficacy or toxicity of Fluorouracil, common drugs include Methotrexate, Metronidazole, Leucovorin as well as Allopurinol and Cimetidine which can affect the availability of the active drug.

4.6 Pregnancy and lactation
Fluorouracil is strictly contraindicated in pregnant and breast feeding women.

4.7 Effects on ability to drive and use machines
Not applicable

4.8 Undesirable effects
Diarrhoea, nausea and vomiting are observed quite commonly during therapy and may be treated symptomatically. An anti-emetic may be given for nausea and vomiting.

Alopecia may be seen in a substantial number of cases, particularly in females, but is reversible. Other side effects include dermatitis, pigmentation, changes in the nails, ataxia and fever.

There have been reports of chest pain, tachycardia, breathlessness and E.C.G. changes after administration of Fluorouracil. Special attention is therefore advisable in treating patients with a history of heart disease or those who develop chest pain during treatment.

Leucopenia is common and the precautions described above should be followed.

Systemic Fluorouracil treatment has been associated with various types of ocular toxicity.

Additionally several other reports have been noted including:

Incidences of excessive lacrimation, dacryostenosis, visual changes and photophobia.

A transient reversible cerebellar syndrome can occur after the use of 5-Fluorouracil. Rarely, a reversible confusional state may occur. Both neurological conditions usually respond to withdrawal of 5-fluorouracil.

Palmar-Plantar Erythrodysesthesia Syndrome has been reported as an unusual complication of high dose bolus or protracted continuous therapy with Fluorouracil.

Thrombophlebitis/Vein tracking.

4.9 Overdose

The symptoms and signs of overdosage are qualitatively similar to the adverse reactions and should be managed as indicated under *'Other Undesirable effects'* and *'Precautions and Special Warnings'*.

5. PHARMACOLOGICAL PROPERTIES

5.1 Pharmacodynamic properties

Fluorouracil is an analogue of uracil, a component of ribonucleic acid. The drug is believed to function as an antimetabolite. After intracellular conversion to the active deoxynucleotide, it interferes with the synthesis of DNA by blocking the conversion of deoxyuridylic acid to thymidylic acid by the cellular enzyme thymidylate synthetase. Fluorouracil may also interfere with RNA synthesis.

Pharmacotherapeutic group: Antimetabolite

ATC code: L01BC02

5.2 Pharmacokinetic properties

After intravenous administration, Fluorouracil is distributed through the body water and disappears from the blood within 3 hours. It is preferentially taken up by actively dividing tissues and tumours after conversion to its nucleotide. Fluorouracil readily enters the C.S.F. and brain tissue.

Following IV administration, the plasma elimination half-life averages about 16 minutes and is dose dependant. Following a single IV dose of Fluorouracil approximately 15 % of the dose is excreted unchanged in the urine within 6 hours; over 90% of this is excreted in the first hour. The remainder is mostly metabolised in the liver by the usual body mechanisms for uracil.

5.3 Preclinical safety data

not applicable

6. PHARMACEUTICAL PARTICULARS

6.1 List of excipients

Sodium hydroxide, water for injections

6.2 Incompatibilities

5-Fluorouracil is incompatible with Carboplatin, Cisplatin, Cytarabine, Diazepam, Doxorubicin, other Anthracyclines and possibly Methotrexate.

Formulated solutions are alkaline and it is recommended that admixture with acidic drug preparations should be avoided.

6.3 Shelf life

18 months

Fluorouracil Injection 25 mg/ml, solution for injection, is intended for single use only.

The Chemical and physical in-use stability of the solution diluted with Glucose 5% or Sodium Chloride 0.9% Injection has been demonstrated for 24 hours at a temperature not exceeding 25°C.

From a microbiological point of view, the product should be used immediately. If not used immediately, in use storage times and conditions prior to use are the responsibility of the user and would normally not be longer than 24 hours at 2 - 8°C, unless dilution has taken place in controlled and validated aseptic conditions.

6.4 Special precautions for storage

Do not store Fluorouracil Injection 25 mg/ml, solution for injection above 25°C.

Do not refrigerate or freeze.

Keep container in outer carton.

If a precipitate has formed as a result of exposure to low temperatures, redissolve by heating to 40°C accompanied by vigorous shaking. Allow to cool to body temperature prior to use.

6.5 Nature and contents of container

Type I conventional clear glass vials, rubber closures. The rubber stopper is protected by a flanged aluminium cap with a flip-off top.

2500 mg/ 100 ml: Pack Size: Singles, 10

6.6 Instructions for use and handling

Fluorouracil Injection 25 mg/ml, solution for injection, should only be opened by trained staff and as with all cytotoxic agents, precautions should be taken to avoid exposing staff during pregnancy. Preparation of solution for administration should be carried out in a designated handling area and working over a washable tray or disposable plastic-backed absorbent paper.

Suitable eye protection, disposable gloves, face mask and disposable apron should be worn. Syringes and infusion sets should be assembled carefully to avoid leakage (use of Luer lock fittings is recommended).

On completion, any exposed surface should be thoroughly cleaned and hands and face washed.

Fluorouracil is an irritant, contact with skin and mucous membranes should be avoided.

In the event of spillage, operators should put on gloves, face masks, eye-protection and disposable apron and mop up the spilled material with an absorbent material tapped in the area for that purpose. The area should then be cleaned and all contaminated material transferred to a cytotoxic spillage bag or bin or sealed for incineration.

Disposal:

All materials that have been utilised for dilution and administration should be disposed of according to standard procedures (incineration).

Diluents:

Fluorouracil injection, 25 mg/ml, solution for injection may be diluted with 5% glucose or 0.9% sodium chloride intravenous infusions immediately before parenteral use. The remainder of solutions should be discarded after use; do not make up into multi-dose preparations.

First aid:

Eye contact: Irrigate immediately with water and seek medical advice.

Skin contact: Wash thoroughly with soap and water and remove contaminated clothing.

Inhalation, Ingestion: Seek medical advice.

7. MARKETING AUTHORISATION HOLDER

medac

Gesellschaft fur klinische Spezialpraparate mbH

Fehlandtstrasse 3

D-20354 Hamburg

8. MARKETING AUTHORISATION NUMBER(S)

PL 11587 / 0021

9. DATE OF FIRST AUTHORISATION/RENEWAL OF THE AUTHORISATION

21 February 2003

10. DATE OF REVISION OF THE TEXT

21 January 2003

Fluorouracil Injection, 50 mg / ml, solution for injection

(medac GmbH)

1. NAME OF THE MEDICINAL PRODUCT

Fluorouracil Injection, 50 mg / ml, solution for injection

2. QUALITATIVE AND QUANTITATIVE COMPOSITION

One vial of Fluorouracil Injection contains:

500 mg Fluorouracil in 10 ml solution (50 mg/ml)

1000 mg Fluorouracil in 20 ml solution (50 mg/ml)

2500 mg Fluorouracil in 50 ml solution (50 mg/ml)

5000 mg Fluorouracil in 100 ml solution (50 mg/ml)

3. PHARMACEUTICAL FORM

Solution for injection

Fluorouracil Injection, 50 mg / ml, solution for injection is a clear, colourless or almost colourless solution.

4. CLINICAL PARTICULARS

4.1 Therapeutic indications

Fluorouracil Injection 50 mg/ml, solution for injection, may be used alone or in combination, for its palliative action in the management of common malignancies particularly cancer of the colon and breast, either as single agent or in combination with other cytotoxic agents.

4.2 Posology and method of administration

Routes of administration:

Fluorouracil Injection can be given by intravenous injection or intravenous or intra-arterial infusion.

Adults:

Selection of an appropriate dose and treatment regime depends upon the condition of the patient, the type of carcinoma being treated and whether Fluorouracil is to be administered alone or in combination with other therapy. Initial treatment should be given in hospital and the total daily dose should not exceed 1 gram. It is customary to calculate the dose in accordance with the patient's actual bodyweight unless there is obesity, oedema or some other form of abnormal fluid retention such as ascites. In this case, ideal weight is used as the basis for calculation.

Reduction of the dose is advisable in patients with any of the following:

1. Cachexia.
2. Major surgery within preceding 30 days.
3. Reduced bone marrow function.
4. Impaired hepatic or renal function.

ADULT DOSE

The following regimen has been recommended for use as a single agent-

Initial Treatment:

this may be in the form of an infusion or an injection, the former usually being preferred because of lesser toxicity.

Intravenous Infusion:

15 mg/kg bodyweight but not more than 1 g per infusion, diluted in 500 ml of 5% glucose or 0.9% NaCl injection and given by intravenous infusion at a rate of 40 drops per minute over 4 hours. Alternatively the daily dose may be infused over 30-60 minutes or may be given as a continuous infusion over 24 hours. The infusion may be repeated daily until there is evidence of toxicity or a total dose of 12-15 g has been reached.

Intravenous Injection:

12 mg/kg bodyweight may be given daily for 3 days and then, if there is no evidence of toxicity, 6 mg/kg on alternate days for 3 further doses. An alternative regime is 15 mg/kg as a single intravenous injection once a week throughout the course.

Intra-arterial Infusion:

5-7.5 mg/kg bodyweight daily may be given by 24 hour continuous intra-arterial infusion.

Maintenance Therapy:

An initial intensive course may be followed by maintenance therapy providing there are no significant toxic effects. In all instances, toxic side effects must disappear before maintenance therapy is started.

The initial course of Fluorouracil can be repeated after an interval of 4 to 6 weeks from the last dose or, alternatively, treatment can be continued with intravenous injections of 5-15 mg/kg bodyweight at weekly intervals.

This sequence constitutes a course of therapy. Some patients have received up to 30 g at a maximum rate of 1 g daily. A more recent alternative method is to give 15 mg/kg IV once a week throughout the course of treatment. This obviates the need for an initial period of daily administration.

In combination with Irradiation: Irradiation combined with 5-FU has been found to be useful in the treatment of certain types of metastatic lesions in the lungs and for the relief of pain caused by recurrent, inoperable growth. The standard dose of 5-FU should be used.

CHILDREN:

No recommendations are made regarding the use of Fluorouracil in children.

ELDERLY:

Fluorouracil should be used in the elderly with similar considerations as with normal adult doses.

4.3 Contraindications

Fluorouracil is contraindicated in seriously debilitated patients or those with bone marrow depression after radiotherapy or treatment with other antineoplastic agents.

Fluorouracil is strictly contraindicated in pregnant or breast feeding women.

Fluorouracil should not be used in the management of non-malignant disease.

4.4 Special warnings and special precautions for use

It is recommended that Fluorouracil should only be given by, or under the strict supervision of, a qualified physician who is conversant with the use of potent antimetabolites.

All patients should be admitted to hospital for initial treatment.

Adequate treatment with Fluorouracil is usually followed by leucopenia, the lowest white blood cell (W.B.C.) count commonly being observed between the 7th and 14th day of the first course, but occasionally being delayed for as long as 20 days.

The count usually returns to normal by the 30th day. Daily monitoring of platelet and W.B.C. count is recommended and treatment should be stopped if platelets fall below 100,000 per mm^3 or the W.B.C. count falls below 3,500 per mm^3. If the total count is less than 2000 per mm^3, and especially if there is granulocytopenia, it is recommended that the patient be placed in protective isolation in the hospital and treated with appropriate measures to prevent systemic infection.

Treatment should also be stopped at the first sign of oral ulceration or if there is evidence of gastrointestinal side effects such as stomatitis, diarrhoea, bleeding from the G.I. tract or haemorrhage at any site. The ratio between effective and toxic dose is small and therapeutic response is unlikely without some degree of toxicity. Care must be taken therefore, in the selection of patients and adjustment of dosage.

Fluorouracil should be used with caution in patients with reduced renal or liver function or jaundice. Isolated cases of angina, ECG abnormalities and rarely, myocardial infarction have been reported following administration of Fluorouracil. Caution should therefore be exercised in treating patients who experience chest pain during courses of treatment, or patients with a history of heart disease.

4.5 Interaction with other medicinal products and other forms of Interaction

Drug Interactions

Various agents have been reported to biochemically modulate the antitumour efficacy or toxicity of Fluorouracil, common drugs include Methotrexate, Metronidazole, Leucovorin as well as Allopurinol and Cimetidine which can affect the availability of the active drug.

4.6 Pregnancy and lactation
Fluorouracil is strictly contraindicated in pregnant and breast feeding women.

4.7 Effects on ability to drive and use machines
Not applicable

4.8 Undesirable effects
Diarrhoea, nausea and vomiting are observed quite commonly during therapy and may be treated symptomatically. An antiemetic may be given for nausea and vomiting.

Alopecia may be seen in a substantial number of cases, particularly in females, but is reversible. Other side effects include dermatitis, pigmentation, changes in the nails, ataxia and fever.

There have been reports of chest pain, tachycardia, breathlessness and E.C.G. changes after administration of Fluorouracil. Special attention is therefore advisable in treating patients with a history of heart disease or those who develop chest pain during treatment.

Leucopenia is common and the precautions described above should be followed.

Systemic Fluorouracil treatment has been associated with various types of ocular toxicity.

A transient reversible cerebellar syndrome can occur after the use of 5-Fluorouracil. Rarely, a reversible confusional state may occur. Both neurological conditions usually respond to withdrawal of 5-fluorouracil.

Additionally several other reports have been noted including:

Incidences of excessive lacrimation, dacryostenosis, visual changes and photophobia.

Palmar-Plantar Erythrodysesthesia Syndrome has been reported as an unusual complication of high dose bolus or protracted continuous therapy with Fluorouracil.

Thrombophlebitis/Vein tracking.

4.9 Overdose
The symptoms and signs of overdosage are qualitatively similar to the adverse reactions and should be managed as indicated under *'Other Undesirable effects'* and *'Precautions and Special Warnings'*.

5. PHARMACOLOGICAL PROPERTIES

5.1 Pharmacodynamic properties
Fluorouracil is an analogue of uracil, a component of ribonucleic acid. The drug is believed to function as an antimetabolite. After intracellular conversion to the active deoxynucleotide, it interferes with the synthesis of DNA by blocking the conversion of deoxyuridylic acid to thymidylic acid by the cellular enzyme thymidylate synthetase. Fluorouracil may also interfere with RNA synthesis.

Pharmacotherapeutic group: Antimetabolite

ATC code: L01B C02

5.2 Pharmacokinetic properties
After intravenous administration, Fluorouracil is distributed through the body water and disappears from the blood within 3 hours. It is preferentially taken up by actively dividing tissues and tumours after conversion to its nucleotide. Fluorouracil ready enters the C.S.F. and brain tissue.

Following IV administration, the plasma elimination half-life averages about 16 minutes and is dose dependant. Following a single IV dose of Fluorouracil approximately 15 % of the dose is excreted unchanged in the urine within 6 hours; over 90% of this is excreted in the first hour. The remainder is mostly metabolised in the liver by the usual body mechanisms for uracil.

5.3 Preclinical safety data
not applicable

6. PHARMACEUTICAL PARTICULARS

6.1 List of excipients
Sodium hydroxide, water for injections

6.2 Incompatibilities
5-Fluorouracil is incompatible with Carboplatin, Cisplatin, Cytarabine, Diazepam, Doxorubicin, other Anthracyclines and possibly Methotrexate.

Formulated solutions are alkaline and it is recommended that admixture with acidic drug preparations should be avoided.

6.3 Shelf life
2 years

Fluorouracil Injection 50 mg/ml, solution for injection, is intended for single use only.

The Chemical and physical in-use stability of the solution diluted with Glucose or Sodium Chloride Injection has been demonstrated for 24 hours at a temperature not exceeding 25°C.

From a microbiological point of view, the product should be used immediately. If not used immediately, in use storage times and conditions prior to use are the responsibility of the user and would normally not be longer than 24 hours at 2 - 8°C, unless dilution has taken place in controlled and validated aseptic conditions.

6.4 Special precautions for storage
Do not store Fluorouracil Injection 50 mg/ml, solution for injection above 25°C.

Do not refrigerate or freeze.

Keep container in outer carton.

If a precipitate has formed as a result of exposure to low temperatures, redissolve by heating to 40°C accompanied by vigorous shaking. Allow to cool to body temperature prior to use.

6.5 Nature and contents of container
Type I conventional clear glass vials, rubber closures. The rubber stopper is protected by a flanged aluminium cap with a flip-off top.

500 mg/ 10 ml: Pack Size: Singles, 10

1000 mg/ 20 ml: Pack Size: Singles, 10

2500 mg/ 50 ml: Pack Size: Singles, 10

5000 mg/100 ml: Pack Size: Singles, 10

6.6 Instructions for use and handling
Fluorouracil Injection 50 mg/ml, solution for injection, should only be opened by trained staff and as with all cytotoxic agents, precautions should be taken to avoid exposing staff during pregnancy. Preparation of solution for administration should be carried out in a designated handling area and working over a washable tray or disposable plastic-backed absorbent paper.

Suitable eye protection, disposable gloves, face mask and disposable apron should be worn. Syringes and infusion sets should be assembled carefully to avoid leakage (use of Luer lock fittings is recommended).

On completion, any exposed surface should be thoroughly cleaned and hands and face washed.

Fluorouracil is an irritant, contact with skin and mucous membranes should be avoided.

In the event of spillage, operators should put on gloves, face masks, eye-protection and disposable apron and mob up the spilled material with an absorbent material tapped in the area for that purpose. The area should then be cleaned and all contaminated material transferred to a cytotoxic spillage bag or bin or sealed for incineration.

Disposal:

All materials that have been utilised for dilution and administration should be disposed of according to standard procedures (incineration).

Diluents:

Fluorouracil may be diluted with 5% glucose or 0.9% sodium chloride intravenous infusions immediately before parenteral use. The remainder of solutions should be discarded after use; do not make up into multi-dose preparations.

First aid:

Eye contact: Irrigate immediately with water and seek medical advice.

Skin contact: Wash thoroughly with soap and water and remove contaminated clothing.

Inhalation, Ingestion: Seek medical advice.

7. MARKETING AUTHORISATION HOLDER
medac

Gesellschaft fur klinische Spezialpraparate mbH

Fehlandtstrasse 3

D-20354 Hamburg

Germany

8. MARKETING AUTHORISATION NUMBER(S)
PL 11587/0015

9. DATE OF FIRST AUTHORISATION/RENEWAL OF THE AUTHORISATION
6 July 2000

10. DATE OF REVISION OF THE TEXT
15 October 2001

FML

(Allergan Ltd)

1. NAME OF THE MEDICINAL PRODUCT
FML Liquifilm Ophthalmic Suspension

2. QUALITATIVE AND QUANTITATIVE COMPOSITION
Fluorometholone 0.10% w/v

3. PHARMACEUTICAL FORM
Sterile Ophthalmic Suspension

4. CLINICAL PARTICULARS

4.1 Therapeutic indications
For steroid-responsive inflammation of the palpebral and bulbar conjunctiva, cornea and anterior segment of the globe.

4.2 Posology and method of administration
Route of administration: topical ophthalmic administration.

Adults: One to two drops instilled into the conjunctival sac two to four times daily. During the initial 24 to 48 hours the dosage may be safely increased to 2 drops every hour. Care should be taken not to discontinue therapy prematurely.

Children: Not recommended for children aged two and under.

4.3 Contraindications
Acute superficial herpes simplex (dendritic) keratitis, vaccinia, varicella and most other viral diseases of the conjunctiva and cornea. Ocular tuberculosis. Fungal diseases of the eye. Hypersensitivity to any of the constituents of the medication.

4.4 Special warnings and special precautions for use
Steroid medication in the treatment of herpes simplex keratitis (involving the stroma) requires great caution: frequent slit-lamp microscopy is mandatory. Prolonged use may result in glaucoma, damage to the optic nerve, defects in visual acuity and fields of vision, posterior subcapsular cataract formation, or may aid in the establishment of secondary ocular infections from fungi or viruses liberated from ocular tissue.

In those diseases causing thinning of the cornea or sclera, perforation has been known to occur with use of topical steroids.

Safety and effectiveness have not been demonstrated in children of the age group two years or below.

This preparation contains benzalkonium chloride and should not be used by patients continuing to wear soft (hydrophilic) contact lenses.

As fungal infections of the cornea are particularly prone to develop coincidentally with long term local steroid applications, fungus invasion must be suspected in any persistent corneal ulceration where a steroid has been or is in use.

Intraocular pressure should be checked frequently.

4.5 Interaction with other medicinal products and other forms of Interaction
None known.

4.6 Pregnancy and lactation
There is inadequate evidence of safety in human pregnancy. Administration of corticosteroids to pregnant animals can cause abnormalities of foetal development including cleft palate and intra-uterine growth retardation. There may therefore be a very small risk of such effects in the human foetus.

4.7 Effects on ability to drive and use machines
None known.

4.8 Undesirable effects
Glaucoma with optic nerve damage, visual acuity or field defects, posterior subcapsular cataract formation, secondary ocular infection from pathogens liberated from ocular tissues, perforation of the globe.

Local side-effects of steroid therapy, i.e. skin atrophy, striae and telangiectasia, are especially likely to affect facial skin.

4.9 Overdose
Not likely to occur.

5. PHARMACOLOGICAL PROPERTIES

5.1 Pharmacodynamic properties
FML is a synthetic adrenocorticosteroid (glucocorticoid), a derivative of desoxyprednisolone. It forms part of a well-known group of steroids used to treat ocular inflammation. Glucocorticosteroids complex with cytoplasmic receptors and subsequently stimulate synthesis of proteins with anti-inflammatory effects. They inhibit early phenomena of the inflammatory response (oedema, fibrin deposition, capillary dilation, phagocytic migration) as well as capillary proliferation, collagen deposition and scar formation.

Whilst topical corticosteroid therapy frequently increases intraocular pressure in normal eyes and in ocular hypertensive subjects, fluorometholone has a substantially lower propensity to elevate IOP than, for example, dexamethasone.

5.2 Pharmacokinetic properties
Topical application of a 0.1% tritium-labelled-fluorometholone suspension gave rise to peak radioactivity levels in the aqueous humour 30 minutes post-instillation. A high concentration of rapidly-produced metabolite was found both in aqueous humour and corneal extracts, indicating that fluorometholone undergoes metabolic change as it penetrates into the cornea and aqueous humour.

5.3 Preclinical safety data
No information.

6. PHARMACEUTICAL PARTICULARS

6.1 List of excipients
Polyvinyl alcohol

Benzalkonium chloride

Edetate Disodium

Sodium chloride

Sodium phosphate, dibasic, heptahydrate

Sodium phosphate, monobasic, monohydrate

Polysorbate 80

Sodium hydroxide to adjust pH

Purified water

6.2 Incompatibilities
None known.

6.3 Shelf life
36 months unopened.

28 days after first opening.

6.4 Special precautions for storage
Do not store above 25°C. Do not freeze.

6.5 Nature and contents of container
5 ml and 10 ml bottles and dropper tips composed of low density polyethylene. Caps are impact polystyrene.

6.6 Instructions for use and handling
No information.

Administrative Data

7. MARKETING AUTHORISATION HOLDER
Allergan Limited
Coronation Road
High Wycombe
Buckinghamshire HP12 3SH

8. MARKETING AUTHORISATION NUMBER(S)
PL 00426/0028

9. DATE OF FIRST AUTHORISATION/RENEWAL OF THE AUTHORISATION
15th July 2003

10. DATE OF REVISION OF THE TEXT
15th July 2003

Foradil

(Novartis Pharmaceuticals UK Ltd)

1. NAME OF THE MEDICINAL PRODUCT
Foradil ®

2. QUALITATIVE AND QUANTITATIVE COMPOSITION
Active substance: (±)-2'-Hydroxy-5'-[(RS)-1-hydroxy-2-[[(RS)-p-methoxy-a-methylphenethyl]-amino] ethyl] formanilide fumarate dihydrate (= formoterol fumarate).

One capsule contains 12 micrograms formoterol fumarate.

3. PHARMACEUTICAL FORM
Inhalation powder in capsules.

4. CLINICAL PARTICULARS

4.1 Therapeutic indications
Foradil is indicated in asthma (including nocturnal asthma and exercise-induced symptoms) for those treated with inhaled corticosteroids who also require a long-acting beta agonist in accordance with current treatment guidelines.

Foradil is indicated for the relief of reversible airways obstruction in patients with chronic obstructive pulmonary disease (COPD) requiring long-term bronchodilatory therapy.

4.2 Posology and method of administration

<u>**For use in adults (including the elderly)**</u>

Asthma
Regular maintenance therapy: 1 inhalation capsule (12 micrograms) to be inhaled twice daily. For more severe cases 2 inhalation capsules to be inhaled twice daily. This dosing regimen provides symptomatic relief throughout day and night.

Chronic Obstructive Pulmonary Disease
1 inhalation capsule to be inhaled twice daily.

<u>**For use in children aged 5 and above**</u>

Asthma
Regular maintenance therapy: 1 inhalation capsule (12 micrograms) to be inhaled twice daily. For more severe cases the dose may be increased to 2 inhalation capsules to be inhaled twice daily after assessment by a physician.

Foradil should be taken twice daily. The maximum daily dose is 24 micrograms b.i.d. (4 capsules).

Although Foradil has a rapid onset of action, current asthma management guidelines recommend that long-acting inhaled bronchodilators should be used for maintenance bronchodilator therapy. They further recommend that in the event of an acute attack, a β-agonist with a short duration of action should be used.

In accordance with the current management Guidelines, long-acting β2-agonists may be added to the treatment regimen in patients experiencing problems with high dose inhaled steroids. Alternatively, where regular symptomatic treatment of asthma is required in addition to inhaled steroids, then long-acting β2-agonists can be used. Patients should be advised not to stop or change their steroid therapy when Foradil is introduced.

If the symptoms persist or worsen, or if the recommended dose of Foradil fails to control symptoms (maintain effective relief), this is usually an indication of a worsening of the underlying condition.

Chronic Obstructive Pulmonary Disease
Not appropriate

<u>**Children under 5 years**</u>
Foradil is not recommended in children under the age of 5 years

<u>**Renal and hepatic impairment**</u>
There is no theoretical reason to suggest that Foradil dosage requires adjustment in patients with renal or hepatic impairment, however no clinical data have been generated to support its use in these groups.

4.3 Contraindications
Hypersensitivity to formoterol fumarate or lactose.

4.4 Special warnings and special precautions for use

Anti-inflammatory therapy:
Asthmatic patients who require regular therapy with a β2-agonist should also receive regular and adequate doses of an inhaled anti-inflammatory agent (e.g. corticosteroids, and/or sodium cromoglicate) or oral corticosteroids. Whenever Foradil is prescribed, patients should be evaluated for the adequacy of the anti-inflammatory therapy they receive. Patients must be advised to continue taking anti-inflammatory therapy unchanged after the introduction of Foradil, even when the symptoms improve. Should symptoms persist, or should the number of doses of Foradil required to control symptoms increase, this usually indicates a worsening of the underlying condition and warrants a reassessment of asthma therapy by a physician.

Concomitant conditions
Special care and supervision, with particular emphasis on dosage limits, is required in patients receiving Foradil when the following conditions may exist:

Ischaemic heart disease, cardiac arrhythmias, especially third degree atrioventricular block, severe cardiac decompensation, idiopathic subvalvular aortic stenosis, hypertrophic obstructive cardiomyopathy, thyrotoxicosis, known or suspected prolongation of the QT interval (QTc > 0.44 sec.; see section 4.5).

Caution should be used when co-administering theophylline and formoterol in patients with pre-existing cardiac conditions

Due to the hyperglycaemic effect of β2-stimulants, additional blood glucose controls are recommended in diabetic patients.

Hypokalaemia
Potentially serious hypokalaemia may result from β2-agonist therapy. Particular caution is advised in severe asthma as this effect may be potentiated by hypoxia and concomitant treatment (see section 4.5). It is recommended that serum potassium levels be monitored in such situations.

Paradoxical bronchospasm
As with other inhalation therapy, the potential for paradoxical bronchospasm should be kept in mind. If it occurs, the preparation should be discontinued immediately and alternative therapy substituted.

4.5 Interaction with other medicinal products and other forms of Interaction
There are no clinical data to support the advice given below, but from consideration of first principles one might expect the following interactions:

Drugs such as quinidine, disopyramide, procainamide, phenothiazines, antihistamines, and tricyclic antidepressants may be associated with QT-interval prolongation and an increased risk of ventricular arrhythmia (see section 4.3).

Concomitant administration of other sympathomimetic agents may potentiate the undesirable effects of Foradil.

Administration of Foradil to patients being treated with monoamine oxidase inhibitors or tricyclic antidepressants should be performed with caution, since the action of β2-adrenergic stimulants on the cardiovascular system may be potentiated.

Concomitant treatment with xanthine derivatives, steroids, or diuretics may potentiate a possible hypokalaemic effect of β2-agonists. Hypokalaemia may increase susceptibility to cardiac arrhythmias in patients treated with digitalis (see section 4.4).

β-adrenergic blockers may weaken or antagonise the effect of Foradil. Therefore Foradil should not be given together with β-adrenergic blockers (including eye drops) unless there are compelling reasons for their use.

4.6 Pregnancy and lactation
There were no teratogenic effects revealed in animal tests. However, until further experience is gained, Foradil is not recommended for use during pregnancy (particularly at the end of pregnancy or during labour) unless there is no more established alternative. As with any medicine, use during pregnancy should only be considered if the expected benefit to the mother is greater than any risk to the foetus. The substance has been detected in the milk of lactating rats, but it is not known whether formoterol passes into human breast milk, therefore mothers using Foradil should refrain from breast feeding their infants.

4.7 Effects on ability to drive and use machines
Foradil is unlikely to have any effect on the ability to drive and operate machinery.

4.8 Undesirable effects
Frequency estimate: Frequent =>10%, occasional =>1%-10%, rare =>0.001% - 1%, isolated cases = < 0.001%

Musculoskeletal system:
Occasional: tremor
Rare: muscle cramps, myalgia

Cardiovascular system:
Occasional: palpitations
Rare: tachycardia

Central nervous system:
Occasional: headache
Rare: agitation, dizziness, anxiety, nervousness, insomnia

Respiratory tract:
Rare: aggravated bronchospasm

Local irritation:
Rare: oropharyngeal irritation

Others:
Isolated cases: hypersensitivity reactions such as severe hypotension urticaria, angioedema, pruritus, exanthema, periphera oedema, taste disturbance, nausea.

4.9 Overdose

Symptoms
There is no clinical experience to date on the management of overdose, however, an overdosage of Foradil would be likely to lead to effects that are typical of β2-adrenergic agonists: nausea, vomiting, headache, tremor, somnolence, palpitations, tachycardia, ventricular arrhythmias, metabolic acidosis, hypokalaemia, hyperglycaemia.

Treatment
Supportive and symptomatic treatment is indicated. Serious cases should be hospitalised.

Use of cardioselective beta-blockers may be considered, but only subject to extreme caution since the use of β-adrenergic blocker medication may provoke bronchospasm.

Serum potassium should be monitored.

5. PHARMACOLOGICAL PROPERTIES

5.1 Pharmacodynamic properties
Formoterol is a potent selective β2-adrenergic stimulant. It exerts a bronchodilator effect in patients with reversible airways obstruction. The effect sets in rapidly (within 1-3 minutes) and is still significant 12 hours after inhalation.

In man, Foradil has been shown to be effective in preventing bronchospasm induced by exercise and methacholine.

Formoterol has been studied in the treatment of conditions associated with COPD, and has been shown to improve symptoms and pulmonary function and quality of life. Formoterol acts on the reversible component of the disease.

5.2 Pharmacokinetic properties

Absorption
As reported for other inhaled drugs, it is likely that about 90% of formoterol administered from an inhaler will be swallowed and then absorbed from the gastrointestinal tract. This means that the pharmacokinetic characteristics of the oral formulation largely apply also to the inhalation powder. Following inhalation of therapeutic doses, formoterol cannot be detected in the plasma using current analytical methods.

Absorption is both rapid and extensive: At a higher than therapeutic dose (120 micrograms), the peak plasma concentration is observed at 5 minutes post inhalation whilst at least 65% of a radiolabeled 80 micrograms oral dose is absorbed, and oral doses of up to 300 micrograms are readily absorbed with the peak concentrations of unchanged formoterol at 0.5-1 hour. In COPD patients treated for 12 weeks with formoterol fumarate 12 or 24 micrograms b.i.d. the plasma concentrations of formoterol ranged between 11.5 and 25.7 pmol/L and 23.3 and 50.3 pmol/L respectively at 10 minutes, 2 hours and 6 hours post inhalation.

The pharmacokinetics of formoterol appear linear in the range of oral doses investigated, i.e. 20-300 micrograms. Repeated oral administration of 40-160 micrograms daily does not lead to significant accumulation of the drug. The maximum excretion rate after administration of 12-96 micrograms is reached within 1-2 hours of inhalation.

After 12 weeks administration of 12 micrograms or 24 micrograms formoterol powder b.i.d., the urinary excretion of unchanged formoterol increased by 63-73% in adult patients and by 18-84% in children, suggesting a modest and self-limiting accumulation of formoterol in plasma after repeated dosing.

Studies investigating the cumulative urinary excretion of formoterol and/or its (R,R) and (S,S)-enantiomers, after inhalation of dry powder (12-96 micrograms) or aerosol formulations (12-96 micrograms), showed that absorption increased linearly with the dose.

Distribution
The plasma protein binding of formoterol is 61-64% (34% primarily to albumin).

There is no saturation of binding sites in the concentration range reached with therapeutic doses.

Biotransformation
Formoterol is eliminated primarily by metabolism, direct glucuronidation being the major pathway of biotransformation, with O-demethylation followed by further glucuronidation being another pathway. Multiple CYP450 isozymes catalyze the transformation (2D6, 2C19, 2C9, and 2A6) and so consequently the potential for metabolic drug-drug interaction is low. The kinetics of formoterol are similar after single and repeated administration, indicating no auto-induction or inhibition of metabolism.

Elimination

Elimination of formoterol from the circulation seems to be polyphasic; the apparent half-life depends on the time interval considered. On the basis of plasma or blood concentrations up to 6, 8 or 12 hours after oral administration, an elimination half-life of about 2-3 hours was determined. From urinary excretion rates between 3 and 16 hours after inhalation, a half-life of about 5 hours was calculated.

After inhalation, plasma formoterol kinetics and urinary excretion rate data in healthy volunteers indicate a biphasic elimination, with the terminal elimination half-lives of the (R,R)- and (S,S)-enantiomers being 13.9 and 12.3 hours, respectively. Approximately 6.4-8% of the dose was recovered in the urine as unchanged formoterol, with the (R,R) and (S,S)-enantiomers contributing 40% and 60% respectively.

After a single oral dose of ^{3}H-formoterol, 59-62% of the dose was recovered in the urine and 32-34% in the faeces. Renal clearance of formoterol is 150 mL/min.

In adult asthmatics, approximately 10% and 15-18% of the dose was recovered in the urine as unchanged and conjugated formoterol, respectively, after multiple doses of 12 and 24 micrograms. In children, approximately 6% and 6.5-9% of the dose was recovered in the urine as unchanged and conjugated formoterol, respectively, after multiple doses of 12 and 24 micrograms. As in healthy volunteers, the (R,R) and (S,S)-enantiomers contributed approximately 40% and 60% of unchanged drug excreted in the urine of adults, respectively, and there was no relative accumulation of one enantiomer over the other after repeated dosing.

5.3 Preclinical safety data

Mutagenicity

Mutagenicity tests covering a broad range of experimental endpoints have been conducted. No genotoxic effects were found in any of the *in vitro* or *in vivo* tests performed.

Carcinogenicity

Two-year studies in rats and mice did not show any carcinogenic potential.

Male mice treated at very high dose levels showed a slightly higher incidence of benign adrenal subcapsular cell tumours, which are considered to reflect alterations in the physiological ageing process.

Two studies in rats, covering different dose ranges, showed an increase in mesovarial leiomyomas. These benign neoplasms are typically associated with long-term treatment of rats at high doses of β2-adrenergic drugs. Increased incidences of ovarian cysts and benign granulosa/theca cell tumours were also seen; β-agonists are known to have effects on the ovary in rats in which are very likely specific to rodents. A few other tumour types noted in the first study using the higher doses were within the incidences of the historical control population, and were not seen in the lower-dose experiment.

None of the tumour incidences were increased to a statistically significant extent at the lowest dose of the second study, a dose leading to a systemic exposure 10 times higher than that expected from the maximum recommended dose of formoterol.

On the basis of these findings and the absence of a mutagenic potential, it is concluded that use of formoterol at therapeutic doses does not present a carcinogenic risk.

Reproduction toxicity

Animal tests showed no teratogenic effects; after oral administration, formoterol was excreted in the milk of lactating rats.

6. PHARMACEUTICAL PARTICULARS

6.1 List of excipients

Lactose EP/USP NF/JP (150 mesh).

6.2 Incompatibilities

None known.

6.3 Shelf life

2 years in Alu/Alu blisters

6.4 Special precautions for storage

In Alu/Alu blisters: protect from moisture (store below 25°C).

6.5 Nature and contents of container

Blister calendar packs of 60 capsules, with an inhaler device in each pack.

6.6 Instructions for use and handling

To ensure proper administration of the drug, the patient should be shown how to use the inhaler by a physician or other health professional.

It is important for the patient to understand that the gelatin capsule may very occasionally break up and small pieces of gelatin might reach the mouth or throat after inhalation. The patient may be reassured that gelatin is harmless and will soften in the mouth and can be swallowed. The tendency for the capsule to break up is minimised by not piercing the capsule more than once.

The capsules should be removed from the blister strip **only** immediately before use.

7. MARKETING AUTHORISATION HOLDER

Novartis Pharmaceuticals UK Ltd
Trading as Geigy Pharmaceuticals
Frimley Business Park,
Frimley, Camberley
Surrey, GU16 7SR
UK

8. MARKETING AUTHORISATION NUMBER(S)

PL 00101/0494

9. DATE OF FIRST AUTHORISATION/RENEWAL OF THE AUTHORISATION

20 March 2003

10. DATE OF REVISION OF THE TEXT

17 December 2004

LEGAL CATEGORY:

POM

Forceval Capsules

(Alliance Pharmaceuticals)

1. NAME OF THE MEDICINAL PRODUCT

Forceval Capsules

2. QUALITATIVE AND QUANTITATIVE COMPOSITION

Each capsule contains:

Vitamin A (as β-Carotene) HSE 2,500.0 iu
Vitamin D2 (Ergocalciferol) HSE 400.0 iu
Vitamin B1 (Thiamine) USP 1.2 mg
Vitamin B2 (Riboflavin) BP 1.6 mg
Vitamin B6 (Pyridoxine) BP 2.0 mg
Vitamin B12 (Cyanocobalamin) PhEur 3.0 mcg
Vitamin C (Ascorbic Acid) BP 60.0 mg
Vitamin E (dl-α-Tocopheryl Acetate) USP 10.0 mg
d-Biotin (Vitamin H) FCC 100.0 mcg
Nicotinamide (Vitamin B3) BP 18.0 mg
Pantothenic Acid (Vitamin B5) USP 4.0 mg
Folic Acid (Vitamin B Complex) BP 400.0 mcg
Calcium FCC 100.0 mg
Iron BP 12.0 mg
Copper HSE 2.0 mg
Phosphorus HSE 77.0 mg
Magnesium BP 30.0 mg
Potassium HSE 4.0 mg
Zinc HSE 15.0 mg
Iodine BP 140.0 mcg
Manganese HSE 3.0 mg
Selenium BP 50.0 mcg
Chromium HSE 200.0 mcg
Molybdenum HSE 250.0 mcg

3. PHARMACEUTICAL FORM

Brown and maroon, oblong, soft gelatin capsule printed with **FORCEVAL** in white on one side and with **6377** in white on the other side.

4. CLINICAL PARTICULARS

4.1 Therapeutic indications

1. As a therapeutic nutritional adjunct where the intake of vitamins and minerals is suboptimal, e.g. in the presence of organic disease such as malignancy and immune deficiency syndromes, such as AIDS.

2. As a therapeutic nutritional adjunct in conditions where the absorption of vitamins and minerals is suboptimal, e.g. malabsorption, inflammatory bowel disease and fistulae, short bowel syndrome and Crohn's disease, and where concurrent medication decreases vitamin and mineral absorption.

3. As a therapeutic nutritional adjunct in convalescence from illness, e.g. where anorexia or cachexia exists and following chemo- or radio-therapy.

4. As a therapeutic nutritional adjunct in convalescence from surgery, e.g. where nutritional intake continues to be inadequate.

5. As a therapeutic nutritional adjunct for patients on special or restricted diets, e.g. in renal diets and where several food groups are restricted in therapeutic weight reducing diets.

6. As a therapeutic nutritional adjunct where food intolerance exists, e.g. exclusion diets.

7. As an adjunct in synthetic diets, e.g. in phenylketonuria, galactosaemia and ketogenic diets.

4.2 Posology and method of administration

Adults and the Elderly

One capsule daily, preferably taken one hour after meals. Do not exceed the stated dose. The capsule should be swallowed whole with water.

Children under 12 years of age

Forceval Capsules are not recommended for this age group.

4.3 Contraindications

Hypercalcaemia, haemochromatosis and other iron storage disorders.

4.4 Special warnings and special precautions for use

Whilst taking Forceval Capsules both protein and energy are also required to provide complete nutrition in the daily diet. No other vitamins, minerals or supplements with or without vitamin A should be taken with this preparation except under medical supervision.

Do not take Forceval Capsules on an empty stomach. Do not exceed the stated dose. Keep out of the reach of children. If symptoms persist, consult your doctor.

Important warning: Contains iron. Keep out of the reach and sight of children, as overdose may be fatal.

This medicine contains E123 (amaranth) and E124 (ponceau 4R red) which may cause allergic reactions.

Evidence from Randomised Control Trials suggests that high doses (20-30 mg/day) b-carotene intake may increase the risk of lung cancer in current smokers and those previously exposed to asbestos. This high-risk population should consider the potential risks and benefits of Forceval Capsules, which contain 4.5mg per recommended daily dose, before use.

4.5 Interaction with other medicinal products and other forms of Interaction

Folic acid can reduce the plasma concentration of phenytoin. Oral iron and zinc sulphate reduce the absorption of tetracyclines.

4.6 Pregnancy and lactation

Forceval Capsules may be administered during pregnancy and lactation at the recommendation of the physician.

4.7 Effects on ability to drive and use machines

None anticipated.

4.8 Undesirable effects

No undesirable effects due to Forceval therapy have been reported and none can be expected if the dosage schedule is adhered to.

4.9 Overdose

No cases of overdosage due to Forceval therapy have been reported. Any symptoms which may be observed due to the ingestion of large quantities of Forceval capsules will be due to the fat soluble vitamin content. If iron overdosage is suspected, symptoms may include nausea, vomiting, diarrhoea, abdominal pain, haematemesis, rectal bleeding, lethargy and circulatory collapse. Hyperglycaemia and metabolic acidosis may also occur. Treatment should be implemented immediately. In severe cases, after a latent phase, relapse may occur after 24 - 48 hours, manifest by hypotension coma and hepatocellular necrosis and renal failure.

Treatment

The following steps are recommended to minimise or prevent further absorption of the medication:

1. Administer an emetic.

2. Gastric lavage may be necessary to remove drug already released into the stomach. This should be undertaken using desferrioxamine solution (2 g/l). Desferrioxamine 5 g in 50 - 100 ml water should be introduced into the stomach following gastric emptying. Keep the patient under constant surveillance to detect possible aspiration of vomitus; maintain suction apparatus and standby emergency oxygen in case of need.

3. A drink of mannitol or sorbitol should be given to induce small bowel emptying.

4. Severe poisoning: in the presence of shock and/or coma with high serum iron levels >142 μmol/l) immediate supportive measures plus i.v. infusion of desferrioxamine should be instituted. The recommended dose of desferrioxamine is 5 mg/kg/h by slow i.v. infusion up to a maximum of 80 mg/kg/24 hours. Warning: hypotension may occur if the infusion rate is too rapid.

5. Less severe poisoning: i.m. desferrioxamine 50 mg/kg up to a maximum dose of 4 g should be given.

6. Serum iron levels should be monitored throughout.

7. Any fluid or electrolyte imbalance should be corrected.

5. PHARMACOLOGICAL PROPERTIES

5.1 Pharmacodynamic properties

The following account summarises the pharmacological effects of the vitamins and minerals in Forceval Capsules and describes the conditions caused by deficiency of these.

Vitamin A

Vitamin A plays an important role in the visual process. It is isomerised to the 11-cis isomer and subsequently bound to the opsin to form the photoreceptor for vision under subdued light. One of the earliest symptoms of deficiency is night blindness which may develop into the more serious condition xerophthalmia. Vitamin A also participates in the formation and maintenance of the integrity of epithelial tissues and mucous membranes. Deficiency may cause skin changes resulting in a dry rough skin with lowered resistance to minor skin infections. Deficiency of Vitamin A, usually accompanied by protein-energy malnutrition, is linked with a frequency of infection and with defective immunological defence mechanisms.

Vitamin D

Vitamin D is required for the absorption of calcium and phosphate from the gastro-intestinal tract and for their transport. Its involvement in the control of calcium metabolism and hence the normal calcification of bones is well documented. Deficiency of Vitamin D in children may result in the development of rickets.

Vitamin B_1 (Thiamine)

Thiamine (as the coenzyme, thiamine pyrophosphate) is associated with carbohydrate metabolism. Thiamine pyrophosphate also acts as a co-enzyme in the direct oxidative pathway of glucose metabolism. In thiamine deficiency, pyruvic and lactic acids accumulate in the tissues. The pyruvate ion is involved in the biosynthesis of acetylcholine via its conversion to acetyl co-enzyme A through a thiamine-dependent process. In thiamine deficiency, therefore, there are effects on the central nervous system due either to the effect on acetylcholine synthesis or to the lactate and pyruvate accumulation. Deficiency of thiamine results in fatigue, anorexia, gastro-intestinal disturbances, tachycardia, irritability and neurological symptoms. Gross deficiency of thiamine (and other Vitamin B group factors) leads to the condition beri-beri.

Vitamin B_2 (Riboflavine)

Riboflavine is phosphorylated to flavine mononucleotide and flavine adenine dinucleotide which act as co-enzymes in the respiratory chain and in oxidative phosphorylation. Riboflavine deficiency presents with ocular symptoms, as well as lesions on the lips and at angles of the mouth.

Vitamin B_6 (Pyridoxine)

Pyridoxine, once absorbed, is rapidly converted to the co-enzymes pyridoxal phosphate and pyridoxamine phosphate which play an essential role in protein metabolism. Convulsions and hypochromic anaemia have occurred in infants deficient in pyridoxine.

Vitamin B_{12} (Cyanocobalamin)

Vitamin B_{12} is present in the body mainly as methylcobalamin and as adenosylcobalamin and hydroxocobalamin. These act as co-enzymes in the trans methylation of homocysteine to methionine; in the isomerisation of methylmalonyl co-enzyme to succinyl co-enzyme and with folate in several metabolic pathways respectively. Deficiency of Vitamin B_{12} interferes with haemopoiesis and produces megaloblastic anaemia.

Vitamin C (Ascorbic Acid)

Vitamin C cannot be synthesised by man therefore a dietary source is necessary. It acts as a cofactor in numerous biological processes including the hydroxylation of proline to hydroxyproline. In deficiency, the formation of collagen is, therefore, impaired. Ascorbic acid is important in the hydroxylation of dopamine to noradrenaline and in hydroxylations occurring in steroid synthesis in the adrenals. It is a reducing agent in tyrosine metabolism and by acting as an electron donor in the conversion of folic acid to tetrahydrofolic acid is indirectly involved in the synthesis of purine and thymine. Vitamin C is also necessary for the incorporation of iron into ferritin. Vitamin C increases the phagocytic function of leucocytes; it possesses anti-inflammatory activity and it promotes wound healing. Deficiency can produce scurvy. Features include swollen inflamed gums, petechial haemorrhages and subcutaneous bruising. The deficiency of collagen leads to development of thin watery ground substances in which blood vessels are insecurely fixed and readily ruptured. The supportive components of bone and cartilage are also deficient causing bones to fracture easily and teeth to become loose. Anaemia commonly occurs probably due to Vitamin C's role in iron metabolism.

Vitamin E

Vitamin E deficiency has been linked to disorders such as cystic fibrosis where fat absorption is impaired. It is essential for the normal function of the muscular system and the blood.

Nicotinamide

The biochemical functions of nicotinamide as NAD and NADP (nicotinamide adenine dinucleotide phosphate) include the degradation and synthesis of fatty acids, carbohydrates and amino acids as well as hydrogen transfer. Deficiency produces pellagra and mental neurological changes.

Calcium (Dicalcium Phosphate)

Calcium is an essential body electrolyte. It is involved in the maintenance of normal muscle and nerve function and essential for normal cardiac function and the clotting of blood. Calcium is mainly found in the bones and teeth. Deficiency of calcium leads to rickets, osteomalacia in children and osteoporosis in the elderly.

Phosphorus (Dicalcium Phosphate)

Phosphate plays important roles in the osteoblastic and osteoclastic reactions. It interacts with calcium to modify the balance between these two processes. Organic phosphate esters play a key role in the metabolism of carbohydrates, fats and proteins and in the formation of 'high energy phosphate' compounds. Phosphate also acts as a buffer and plays a role in the renal excretion of sodium and hydrogen ions.

Pantothenic Acid

Pantothenic acid is incorporated into co-enzyme A and is involved in metabolic pathways involving acetylation which includes detoxification of drug molecules and biosynthesis of cholesterol, steroid hormones, mucopolysaccharides and acetylcholine. CoA has an essential function in lipid metabolism.

Folic Acid

Folic acid is reduced in the body to tetrahydrofolate which is a co-enzyme for various metabolic processes, including the synthesis of purine and pyrimidine nucleotides and hence in the synthesis of DNA. It is also involved in some amino acid conversion and in the formation and utilisation of formate. Deficiency of folic acid leads to megaloblastic anaemia.

Vitamin H (d-Biotin)

Biotin is a co-enzyme for carboxylation during the metabolism of proteins and carbohydrates.

Selenium

Selenium is an essential trace element, deficiency of which has been reported in man. It is thought to be involved in the functioning of membranes and the synthesis of amino acids. Deficiency of selenium in the diet of experimental animals produces fatty liver followed by necrosis.

Iron

Iron, as a constituent of haemoglobin, plays an essential role in oxygen transport. It is also present in the muscle protein myoglobin and in the liver. Deficiency of iron leads to anaemia.

Copper (Copper Sulphate)

Traces of copper are essential to the body as constituents of enzyme systems involved in oxidation reactions.

Magnesium (Magnesium Oxide)

Magnesium is essential to the body as a constituent of skeletal structures and in maintaining cell integrity and fluid balance. It is utilised in many of the functions in which calcium is concerned but often exerts the opposite effect. Some enzymes require the magnesium ion as a co-factor.

Potassium (Potassium Sulphate)

Potassium is the principle cation of intracellular fluid and is intimately involved in the cell function and metabolism. It is essential for carbohydrate metabolism and glycogen storage and protein synthesis and is involved in transmembrane potential where it is necessary to maintain the resting potential in excitable cells. Potassium ions maintain intracellular pH and osmotic pressure. Prolonged or severe diarrhoea may lead to potassium deficiency.

Zinc (Zinc Sulphate)

Zinc is a constituent of many enzymes and is, therefore, essential to the body. It is present with insulin in the pancreas. It plays a role in DNA synthesis and cell division. Reported effects of deficiency include delayed puberty and hypogonadal dwarfism.

Manganese (Manganese Sulphate)

Manganese is a constituent of enzyme systems including those involved in lipid synthesis, the tricarboxylic acid cycle and purine and pyrimidine metabolism. It is bound to arginase of the liver and activates many enzymes.

Iodine (Potassium Iodide)

Iodine is an essential constituent of the thyroid hormones.

Chromium (Chromium Amino Acid Chelate 10%)

Chromium is an essential trace element involved in carbohydrate metabolism.

Molybdenum (Sodium Molybdate)

Molybdenum is an essential trace element although there have been no reports of deficiency states in man. Molybdenum salts have been used to treat copper poisoning in sheep.

5.2 Pharmacokinetic properties

The following account describes the absorption and fate of each of the active constituents of Forceval Capsules.

Vitamin A

Except when liver function is impaired, Vitamin A is readily absorbed. β-carotene (as in Forceval Capsules) is Provitamin A and is the biological precursor to Vitamin A. It is converted to Vitamin A (Retinol) in the liver; retinol is emulsified by bile salts and phospholipids and absorbed in a micellar form. Part is conjugated with glucuronic acid in the kidney and part is metabolised in the liver and kidney, leaving 30 to 50% of the dose for storage in the liver. It is bound to a globulin in the blood. Metabolites of Vitamin A are excreted in the faeces and the urine.

Vitamin D

The metabolism of ergocalciferol is similar to that of cholecalciferol. Cholecalciferol is absorbed from the gastro-intestinal tract into the circulation. In the liver, it is hydroxylated to 25-hydroxycholecalciferol, is subject to enterohepatic circulation and is further hydroxylated to 1,25-dihydroxycholecalciferol in the renal tubule cells. Vitamin D metabolites are bound to specific plasma proteins.

Vitamin B_1 (Thiamine)

Thiamine is absorbed from the gastro-intestinal tract and is widely distributed to most body tissues. Amounts in excess of the body's requirements are not stored but excreted in the urine as unchanged thiamine or its metabolites.

Vitamin B_2 (Riboflavine)

Riboflavine is absorbed from the gastro-intestinal tract and in the circulation is bound to plasma proteins. It is widely distributed. Little is stored and excess amounts are excreted in the urine. In the body riboflavine is converted to flavine mononucleotide (FMN) and then to flavine adenine dinucleotide (FAD).

Vitamin B_6 (Pyridoxine)

Pyridoxine is absorbed from the gastro-intestinal tract and converted to the active pyridoxal phosphate which is bound to plasma proteins. It is excreted in the urine as 4-pyridoxic acid.

Vitamin B_{12} (Cyanocobalamin)

Cyanocobalamin is absorbed from the gastro-intestinal tract and is extensively bound to specific plasma proteins. A study with labelled Vitamin B_{12} showed it was quickly taken up by the intestinal mucosa and held there for 2 - 3 hours. Peak concentrations in the blood and tissues did not occur until 8 - 12 hours after dosage with maximum concentrations in the liver within 24 hours. Cobalamins are stored in the liver, excreted in the bile and undergo enterohepatic recycling. Part of a dose is excreted in the urine, most of it in the first eight hours.

Vitamin C (Ascorbic Acid)

Ascorbic acid is readily absorbed from the gastro-intestinal tract and is widely distributed in the body tissues. Ascorbic acid in excess of the body's needs is rapidly eliminated in the urine and this elimination is usually accompanied by a mild diuresis.

Vitamin E

Vitamin E is absorbed from the gastro-intestinal tract. Most appears in the lymph and is then widely distributed to all tissues. Most of a dose is slowly excreted in the bile and the remainder is eliminated in the urine as glucuronides of tocopheronic acid or other metabolites.

Nicotinamide (Nicotinic Acid Amide)

Nicotinic acid is absorbed from the gastro-intestinal tract, is widely distributed in the body tissues and has a short half-life.

Calcium (Dicalcium Phosphate)

A third of ingested calcium is absorbed from the small intestine. Absorption of calcium decreases with age.

Phosphorus (Dicalcium Phosphate)

The body contains from 600 - 800 g of phosphorus, over 80% of which is present in the bone as phosphate salts, mainly hydroxyapatite crystals. The phosphate in these crystals is available for exchange with phosphate ions in the extra-cellular fluids.

Calcium Pantothenate

Pantothenic acid is readily absorbed from the gastro-intestinal tract and is widely distributed in the body tissues. About 70% of pantothenic acid is excreted unchanged in the urine and about 30% in the faeces.

Folic Acid

Folic acid is absorbed mainly from the proximal part of the small intestine. Folate polyglutamates are considered to be deconjugated to monoglutamates during absorption. Folic acid rapidly appears in the blood where it is extensively bound to plasma proteins. Some folic acid is distributed in body tissues, some is excreted as folate in the urine and some is stored in the liver as folate.

Vitamin H (d-Biotin)

Following absorption, biotin is stored in the liver, kidney and pancreas.

Selenium

Although it has been established that selenium is essential to human life, very little information is available on its function and metabolism.

Ferrous Fumarate (Iron)

Iron is absorbed chiefly in the duodenum and jejunum. Absorption is aided by the acid secretion of the stomach and if the iron is in the ferrous state as in ferrous fumarate. In conditions of iron deficiency, absorption is increased and, conversely, it is decreased in iron overload. Iron is stored as ferritin.

Copper Sulphate (Copper)

Copper is absorbed from the gastro-intestinal tract and its major route of excretion is in the bile.

Magnesium Oxide (Magnesium)

Magnesium salts are poorly absorbed from the gastro-intestinal tract; however, sufficient magnesium will normally be absorbed to replace deficiency states. Magnesium is excreted in both the urine and the faeces but excretion is reduced in deficiency states.

Potassium Sulphate (Potassium)

Potassium salts are absorbed from the gastro-intestinal tract. Potassium is excreted in the urine, the faeces and in perspiration. Urinary excretion of potassium continues even when intake is low.

Zinc Sulphate (Zinc)

Zinc is poorly absorbed from the gastro-intestinal tract. It is widely distributed throughout the body. It is excreted in the faeces with traces appearing in the urine.

Manganese Sulphate (Manganese)

Manganese salts are poorly absorbed.

Potassium Iodide (Iodine)

Iodides are absorbed and stored in the thyroid gland as thyroglobulin. Iodides are excreted in the urine with smaller amounts appearing in the faeces, saliva and sweat.

Chromium Amino Acid Chelate 10% (Chromium)

Although it has been established that chromium is essential to human life, little information is available on its function and metabolism.

Sodium Molybdate (Molybdenum)

Although it has been established that molybdenum is essential to human life, little information is available on its function and metabolism.

5.3 Preclinical safety data

There are no pre-clinical data of relevance to the prescriber which are additional to that already included in other sections of the SPC.

6. PHARMACEUTICAL PARTICULARS

6.1 List of excipients

Soya Bean Oil BP

Soya Lecithin HSE

Hard Vegetable Fat (Loders 7) HSE

Yellow Beeswax BP

Purified Water PhEur

Gelatin BP

Glycerine BP

Ponceau 4R (E124) HSE

Amaranth (E123) HSE

Titanium Dioxide (E171) BP

Red Iron Oxide Paste (E172) HSE

Vegetable Black Paste (E153) HSE

6.2 Incompatibilities

No major incompatibilities are known.

6.3 Shelf life

24 months, as packaged for sale..

6.4 Special precautions for storage

Store in a cool dry place at a temperature not exceeding 25°C.

Protect from light.

6.5 Nature and contents of container

The product is presented in press-thru blister packs, each blister strip containing 15 Forceval capsules. The blister strip is composed of PVC/PVdC with a printed aluminium foil lidding. The foil is printed (red on gold) with the name and PL number of the product, the number of vitamins and minerals per capsule and the daily dose.

The product is available in packs of 30, 45 or 90 capsules.

6.6 Instructions for use and handling

Not applicable.

7. MARKETING AUTHORISATION HOLDER

Alliance Pharmaceuticals Ltd
Avonbridge House
2 Bath Road
Chippenham
Wiltshire
SN15 2BB
United Kingdom

8. MARKETING AUTHORISATION NUMBER(S)

PL 16853/0079

9. DATE OF FIRST AUTHORISATION/RENEWAL OF THE AUTHORISATION

18th April 2005

10. DATE OF REVISION OF THE TEXT

April 2005

Forceval Junior Capsules

(Alliance Pharmaceuticals)

1. NAME OF THE MEDICINAL PRODUCT

Forceval Junior Capsules

2. QUALITATIVE AND QUANTITATIVE COMPOSITION

Each capsule contains:

Vitamin A (as β-Carotene) HSE 1,250.0 iu

Vitamin D2 (Ergocalciferol) HSE 200.0 iu

Vitamin B1 (Thiamine) USP 1.5 mg

Vitamin B2 (Riboflavin) BP 1.0 mg

Vitamin B6 (Pyridoxine) BP 1.0 mg

Vitamin B12 (Cyanocobalamin) PhEur 2.0 mcg

Vitamin C (Ascorbic Acid) BP 25.0 mg

Vitamin E (dl-α-Tocopheryl Acetate) USP 5.0 mg

d-Biotin (Vitamin H) FCC 50.0 mcg

Nicotinamide (Vitamin B3) BP 7.5 mg

Pantothenic Acid (Vitamin B5) USP 2.0 mg

Vitamin K1 (Phytomenadione) BP 25.0 mcg

Folic Acid (Vitamin B Complex) BP 100.0 mcg

Iron BP 5.0 mg

Copper HSE 1.0 mg

Magnesium BP 1.0 mg

Zinc HSE 5.0 mg

Iodine BP 75.0 mcg

Manganese HSE 1.25 mg

Selenium BP 25.0 mcg

Chromium HSE 50.0 mcg

Molybdenum HSE 50.0 mcg

3. PHARMACEUTICAL FORM

Small, opaque, brown, oval, soft gelatin capsule printed in white with **571**.

4. CLINICAL PARTICULARS

4.1 Therapeutic indications

1. As a therapeutic nutritional adjunct where the intake of vitamins and minerals is suboptimal, e.g. in the presence of organic disease such as malignancy and immune deficiency syndromes, such as AIDS.

2. As a therapeutic nutritional adjunct in conditions where the absorption of vitamins and minerals is suboptimal, e.g. malabsorption, inflammatory bowel disease and fistulae, short bowel syndrome and Crohn's disease, and where concurrent medication decreases vitamin and mineral absorption.

3. As a therapeutic nutritional adjunct in convalescence from illness, e.g. where anorexia or cachexia exists and following chemo- or radio-therapy.

4. As a therapeutic nutritional adjunct in convalescence from surgery, e.g. where nutritional intake continues to be inadequate.

5. As a therapeutic nutritional adjunct for patients on special or restricted diets, e.g. in renal diets and where several food groups are restricted in therapeutic weight reducing diets.

6. As a therapeutic nutritional adjunct where food intolerance exists, e.g. exclusion diets.

7. As an adjunct in synthetic diets, e.g. in phenylketonuria, galactosaemia and ketogenic diets.

4.2 Posology and method of administration

Children over 5 years of age

2 capsules per day or as recommended by the doctor.

Do not exceed the stated dose.

Adults and the Elderly

Not recommended - use Forceval Capsules.

4.3 Contraindications

Haemochromatosis and other iron storage disorders.

4.4 Special warnings and special precautions for use

Forceval Junior Capsules should be used as a vitamin and mineral source in conjunction with an energy-providing diet suitable for individual patient requirements. No other vitamins, minerals or supplements with or without vitamin A should be taken with this preparation except under medical supervision.

Do not exceed the stated dose. Keep out of the reach of children.

The label will state:

Important warning: Contains iron. Keep out of the reach and sight of children, as overdose may be fatal.

This warning will appear on the front of pack, enclosed in a rectangle, in which there is no other information of any kind.

This medicine contains sorbitol. Patients with rare hereditary problems of fructose intolerance should not take this medicine.

Evidence from Randomised Control Trials suggests that high doses (20-30 mg/day) b-carotene intake may increase the risk of lung cancer in current smokers and those previously exposed to asbestos. This high-risk population should consider the potential risks and benefits of Forceval Junior Capsules, which contain 4.5mg per recommended daily dose, before use.

4.5 Interaction with other medicinal products and other forms of Interaction

Vitamin K may interact with anticoagulants such as phenindione, warfarin and nicoumalone inhibiting their effect. Folic acid can reduce the plasma concentration of phenytoin. Oral iron and zinc sulphate reduce the absorption of tetracyclines.

4.6 Pregnancy and lactation

Forceval Junior Capsules can be given to pregnant and lactating women, provided the product is administered with the approval of their clinician.

4.7 Effects on ability to drive and use machines

None anticipated.

4.8 Undesirable effects

No undesirable effects due to Forceval Junior therapy have been reported and none can be expected if the dosage schedule is adhered to.

4.9 Overdose

No cases of overdosage due to Forceval Junior therapy have been reported. Any symptoms which may be observed due to ingestion of large quantities of Forceval Junior capsules will be due to the fat soluble vitamin content. If iron overdosage is suspected, symptoms may include nausea, vomiting, diarrhoea, abdominal pain, haematemesis, rectal bleeding, lethargy and circulatory collapse. Hyperglycaemia and metabolic acidosis may also occur. Treatment should be implemented immediately. In severe cases, after a latent phase, relapse may occur after 24 - 48 hours, manifest by hypotension coma and hepatocellular necrosis and renal failure.

Treatment

The following steps are recommended to minimise or prevent further absorption of the medication:

1. Administer an emetic.

2. Gastric lavage may be necessary to remove drug already released into the stomach. This should be undertaken using desferrioxamine solution (2 g/l). Desferrioxamine 5 g in 50-100 ml water should be introduced into the stomach following gastric emptying. Keep the patient under constant surveillance to detect possible aspiration of vomitus; maintain suction apparatus and standby emergency oxygen in case of need.

3. A drink of mannitol or sorbitol should be given to induce small bowel emptying.

4. Severe poisoning: in the presence of shock and/or coma with high serum iron levels >142 μmol/l) immediate supportive measures plus i.v. infusion of desferrioxamine should be instituted. The recommended dose of desferrioxamine is 5 mg/kg/h by slow i.v. infusion up to a maximum of 80 mg/kg/24 hours. Warning: hypotension may occur if the infusion rate is too rapid.

5. Less severe poisoning: i.m. desferrioxamine 50 mg/kg up to a maximum dose of 4 g should be given.

6. Serum iron levels should be monitored throughout.

7. Any fluid or electrolyte imbalance should be corrected.

5. PHARMACOLOGICAL PROPERTIES

5.1 Pharmacodynamic properties

The following account summarises the pharmacological effects of the vitamins and minerals in Forceval Junior Capsules and describes the conditions caused by deficiency of these.

Vitamin A

Vitamin A plays an important role in the visual process. It is isomerised to the 11-cis isomer and subsequently bound to the opsin to form the photoreceptor for vision under subdued light. One of the earliest symptoms of deficiency is night blindness which may develop into the more serious condition xerophthalmia. Vitamin A also participates in the formation and maintenance of the integrity of epithelial tissues and mucous membranes. Deficiency may cause skin changes resulting in a dry rough skin with lowered resistance to minor skin infections. Deficiency of Vitamin A, usually accompanied by protein-energy malnutrition, is linked with a frequency of infection and with defective immunological defence mechanisms.

Vitamin D

Vitamin D is required for the absorption of calcium and phosphate from the gastro-intestinal tract and for their transport. Its involvement in the control of calcium metabolism and hence the normal calcification of bones is well documented. Deficiency of Vitamin D in children may result in the development of rickets.

Vitamin B_1 (Thiamine)

Thiamine (as the coenzyme, thiamine pyrophosphate) is associated with carbohydrate metabolism. Thiamine pyrophosphate also acts as a co-enzyme in the direct oxidative pathway of glucose metabolism. In thiamine deficiency, pyruvic and lactic acids accumulate in the tissues. The pyruvate ion is involved in the biosynthesis of acetylcholine via its conversion to acetyl co-enzyme A through a thiamine-dependent process. In thiamine deficiency, therefore, there are effects on the central nervous system due either to the effect on acetylcholine synthesis or to the lactate and pyruvate accumulation. Deficiency of thiamine results in fatigue, anorexia, gastro-intestinal disturbances, tachycardia, irritability and neurological symptoms. Gross deficiency of thiamine (and other Vitamin B group factors) leads to the condition beri-beri.

Vitamin B_2 (Riboflavine)

Riboflavine is phosphorylated to flavine mononucleotide and flavine adenine dinucleotide which act as co-enzymes in the respiratory chain and in oxidative phosphorylation. Riboflavine deficiency presents with ocular symptoms, as well as lesions on the lips and at angles of the mouth.

Vitamin B_6 (Pyridoxine)

Pyridoxine, once absorbed, is rapidly converted to the co-enzymes pyridoxal phosphate and pyridoxamine phosphate which play an essential role in protein metabolism. Convulsions and hypochromic anaemia have occurred in infants deficient in pyridoxine.

Vitamin B_{12} (Cyanocobalamin)

Vitamin B_{12} is present in the body mainly as methylcobalamin and as adenosylcobalamin and hydroxocobalamin. These act as co-enzymes in the trans methylation of homocysteine to methionine; in the isomerisation of methylmalonyl co-enzyme to succinyl co-enzyme and with folate in several metabolic pathways respectively. Deficiency of Vitamin B_{12} interferes with haemopoiesis and produces megaloblastic anaemia.

Vitamin C (Ascorbic Acid)

Vitamin C cannot be synthesised by man therefore a dietary source is necessary. It acts as a cofactor in numerous biological processes including the hydroxylation of proline to hydroxyproline. In deficiency, the formation of collagen is, therefore, impaired. Ascorbic acid is important in the hydroxylation of dopamine to noradrenaline and in hydroxylations occurring in steroid synthesis in the adrenals. It is a reducing agent in tyrosine metabolism and by acting as an electron donor in the conversion of folic acid to tetrahydrofolic acid is indirectly involved in the synthesis of purine and thymine. Vitamin C is also necessary for the incorporation of iron into ferritin. Vitamin C increases the phagocytic function of leucocytes; it possesses anti-inflammatory activity and it promotes wound healing. Deficiency can produce scurvy. Features include swollen inflamed gums, petechial haemorrhages and subcutaneous bruising. The deficiency of collagen leads to development of thin watery ground substances in which blood vessels are insecurely fixed and readily ruptured. The supportive components of bone and cartilage are also deficient causing bones to fracture easily and teeth to become loose. Anaemia commonly occurs probably due to Vitamin C's role in iron metabolism.

Vitamin E

Vitamin E deficiency has been linked to disorders such as cystic fibrosis where fat absorbtion is impaired. It is essential for the normal function of the muscular system and the blood.

Nicotinamide

The biochemical functions of nicotinamide as NAD and NADP (nicotinamide adenine dinucleotide phosphate) include the degradation and synthesis of fatty acids, carbohydrates and amino acids as well as hydrogen transfer. Deficiency produces pellagra and mental neurological changes.

Pantothenic Acid

Pantothenic acid is incorporated into co-enzyme A and is involved in metabolic pathways involving acetylation which includes detoxification of drug molecules and biosynthesis of cholesterol, steroid hormones, mucopolysaccharides and acetylcholine. CoA has an essential function in lipid metabolism.

Vitamin K1 (Phytomenadione)

Phytomenadione is a provitamin; following activation it exerts Vitamin K effects. Vitamin K is essential for the formation of prothrombin (Factor II) and other clotting factors (Factors VII, IX and X) in the liver. Deficiency of Vitamin K produces hypoprothrombinaemia, in which the clotting time of the blood is prolonged and spontaneous haemorrhage may occur.

Folic Acid

Folic acid is reduced in the body to tetrahydrofolate which is a co-enzyme for various metabolic processes, including the synthesis of purine and pyrimidine nucleotides and hence in the synthesis of DNA. It is also involved in some amino acid conversion and in the formation and utilisation of formate. Deficiency of folic acid leads to megaloblastic anaemia.

Vitamin H (d-Biotin)

Biotin is a co-enzyme for carboxylation during the metabolism of proteins and carbohydrates.

Selenium

Selenium is an essential trace element, deficiency of which has been reported in man. It is thought to be involved in the functioning of membranes and the synthesis of amino acids. Deficiency of selenium in the diet of experimental animals produces fatty liver followed by necrosis.

Iron

Iron, as a constituent of haemoglobin, plays an essential role in oxygen transport. It is also present in the muscle protein myoglobin and in the liver. Deficiency of iron leads to anaemia.

Copper (Copper Sulphate)

Traces of copper are essential to the body as constituents of enzyme systems involved in oxidation reactions.

Magnesium (Magnesium Sulphate)

Magnesium is essential to the body as a constituent of skeletal structures and in maintaining cell integrity and fluid balance. It is utilised in many of the functions in which calcium is concerned but often exerts the opposite effect. Some enzymes require the magnesium ion as a co-factor.

Zinc (Zinc Sulphate)

Zinc is a constituent of many enzymes and is, therefore, essential to the body. It is present with insulin in the pancreas. It plays a role in DNA synthesis and cell division. Reported effects of deficiency include delayed puberty and hypogonadal dwarfism.

Manganese (Manganese Sulphate)

Manganese is a constituent of enzyme systems including those involved in lipid synthesis, the tricarboxylic acid cycle and purine and pyrimidine metabolism. It is bound to arginase of the liver and activates many enzymes.

Iodine (Potassium Iodide)

Iodine is an essential constituent of the thyroid hormones.

Chromium (Chromium Amino Acid Chelate 10%)

Chromium is an essential trace element involved in carbohydrate metabolism.

Molybdenum (Sodium Molybdate)

Molybdenum is an essential trace element although there have been no reports of deficiency states in man. Molybdenum salts have been used to treat copper poisoning in sheep.

5.2 Pharmacokinetic properties

The following account describes the absorption and fate of each of the active constituents of Forceval Junior Capsules.

Vitamin A

Except when liver function is impaired, Vitamin A is readily absorbed. β-carotene (as in Forceval Junior Capsules) is Provitamin A and is the biological precursor to Vitamin A. It is converted to Vitamin A (Retinol) in the liver; retinol is emulsified by bile salts and phospholipids and absorbed in a micellar form. Part is conjugated with glucuronic acid in the kidney and part is metabolised in the liver and kidney, leaving 30 to 50% of the dose for storage in the liver. It is bound to a globulin in the blood. Metabolites of Vitamin A are excreted in the faeces and the urine.

Vitamin D

The metabolism of ergocalciferol is similar to that of cholecalciferol. Cholecalciferol is absorbed from the gastro-intestinal tract into the circulation. In the liver, it is hydroxylated to 25-hydroxycholecalciferol, is subject to entero-hepatic circulation and is further hydroxylated to 1,25-dihydroxycholecalciferol in the renal tubule cells. Vitamin D metabolites are bound to specific plasma proteins.

Vitamin B_1 (Thiamine)

Thiamine is absorbed from the gastro-intestinal tract and is widely distributed to most body tissues. Amounts in excess of the body's requirements are not stored but excreted in the urine as unchanged thiamine or its metabolites.

Vitamin B_2 (Riboflavine)

Riboflavine is absorbed from the gastro-intestinal tract and in the circulation is bound to plasma proteins. It is widely distributed. Little is stored and excess amounts are excreted in the urine. In the body riboflavine is converted to flavine mononucleotide (FMN) and then to flavine adenine dinucleotide (FAD).

Vitamin B_6 (Pyridoxine)

Pyridoxine is absorbed from the gastro-intestinal tract and converted to the active pyridoxal phosphate which is bound to plasma proteins. It is excreted in the urine as 4-pyridoxic acid.

Vitamin B_{12} (Cyanocobalamin)

Cyanocobalamin is absorbed from the gastro-intestinal tract and is extensively bound to specific plasma proteins. Vitamin B_{12} is taken up by the intestinal mucosa and held there for 2 - 3 hours. Peak concentrations in the blood and tissues occur 8 - 12 hours after dosage with maximum concentrations in the liver within 24 hours. Cobalamins are stored in the liver, excreted in the bile and undergo enterohepatic recycling. Part of a dose is excreted in the urine, most of it in the first eight hours.

Vitamin C (Ascorbic Acid)

Ascorbic acid is readily absorbed from the gastro-intestinal tract and is widely distributed in the body tissues. Ascorbic acid in excess of the body's needs is rapidly eliminated in the urine.

Vitamin E

Vitamin E is absorbed from the gastro-intestinal tract. Most appears in the lymph and is then widely distributed to all tissues. Most of a dose is slowly excreted in the bile and the remainder is eliminated in the urine as glucuronides of tocopheronic acid or other metabolites.

Nicotinamide (Nicotinic Acid Amide)

Nicotinamide is absorbed from the gastro-intestinal tract, is widely distributed in the body tissues and has a short half-life.

Calcium Pantothenate

Pantothenic acid is readily absorbed from the gastro-intestinal tract and is widely distributed in the body tissues. About 70% of pantothenic acid is excreted unchanged in the urine and about 30% in the faeces.

Vitamin K1 (Phytomenadione)

Phytomenadione is absorbed from the gastro-intestinal tract. It is rapidly metabolised and excreted and is not significantly stored in the body.

Folic Acid

Folic acid is absorbed mainly from the proximal part of the small intestine. Folate polyglutamates are considered to be deconjugated to monoglutamates during absorption. Folic acid rapidly appears in the blood where it is extensively bound to plasma proteins. Some folic acid is distributed in body tissues, some is excreted as folate in the urine and some is stored in the liver as folate.

Vitamin H (d-Biotin)

Following absorption, biotin is stored in the liver, kidney and pancreas.

Selenium

Although it has been established that selenium is essential to human life, very little information is available on its function and metabolism.

Ferrous Fumarate (Iron)

Iron is absorbed chiefly in the duodenum and jejunum. Absorption is aided by the acid secretion of the stomach and if the iron is in the ferrous state as in ferrous fumarate. In iron deficiency, absorption is increased and, conversely, it is decreased in iron overload. Iron is stored as ferritin.

Copper Sulphate (Copper)

Copper is absorbed from the gastro-intestinal tract and its major route of excretion is in the bile.

Magnesium Sulphate (Magnesium)

Magnesium salts are poorly absorbed from the gastro-intestinal tract; however, sufficient magnesium will normally be absorbed to replace deficiency states. It is excreted in both the urine and the faeces but excretion in the urine is reduced in deficiency states.

Zinc Sulphate (Zinc)

Zinc is poorly absorbed from the gastro-intestinal tract. It is widely distributed throughout the body. It is excreted in the faeces with traces appearing in the urine.

Manganese Sulphate (Manganese)

Manganese salts are poorly absorbed.

Potassium Iodide (Iodine)

Iodides are absorbed and stored in the thyroid gland as thyroglobulin. Iodides are excreted in the urine with smaller amounts appearing in the faeces, saliva and sweat.

Chromium Amino Acid Chelate 10% (Chromium)

Although it has been established that chromium is essential to human life, little information is available on its function and metabolism.

Sodium Molybdate (Molybdenum)

Although it has been established that molybdenum is essential to human life, little information is available on its function and metabolism.

5.3 Preclinical safety data

There are no pre-clinical data of relevance to the prescriber which are additional to that already included in other sections of the SPC.

6. PHARMACEUTICAL PARTICULARS

6.1 List of excipients

Soya Bean Oil BP

Soya Lecithin HSE

Fat Mix HSE

Purified Water PhEur

Gelatin BP

Glycerine BP

Black Iron Oxide Pigment (E172) HSE

Red Iron Oxide Pigment (E172) HSE

Sorbitol Solution 70% BP

6.2 Incompatibilities

No major incompatibilities are known.

6.3 Shelf life

24 months, as packaged for sale.

6.4 Special precautions for storage

Store in a cool dry place at a temperature not exceeding 25°C.

Protect from light.

6.5 Nature and contents of container

The product is presented in press-thru blister packs, each blister strip containing 10 Forceval Junior capsules. The blister strip is composed of PVC/PVdC with a printed aluminium foil lidding. The foil is printed (red on gold) with the name and PL number of the product, the number of vitamins and minerals per capsule and the daily dose.

The product is available in packs of 30, 60 or 120 capsules.

6.6 Instructions for use and handling

Not applicable.

7. MARKETING AUTHORISATION HOLDER

Alliance Pharmaceuticals Ltd

Avonbridge House

2 Bath Road

Chippenham

Wiltshire

SN15 2BB

United Kingdom

8. MARKETING AUTHORISATION NUMBER(S)

PL 16853/0080

9. DATE OF FIRST AUTHORISATION/RENEWAL OF THE AUTHORISATION

18th April 2005

10. DATE OF REVISION OF THE TEXT

April 2005

Forceval Protein Powder - Chocolate

(Alliance Pharmaceuticals)

1. NAME OF THE MEDICINAL PRODUCT

Forceval Protein Powder (Chocolate Flavour)

2. QUALITATIVE AND QUANTITATIVE COMPOSITION

Each 72 g of product provide:

Vitamin A	HSE	2500.0 iu (750 mcg)
Vitamin B1 (Thiamin)	HSE	1.5 mg
Vitamin B2 (Riboflavin)	BP	1.5 mg
Vitamin B3 (Nicotinamide)	HSE	18.0 mg
Vitamin B5 (Pantothenic Acid)	PhEur	6.0 mg
Vitamin B6 (Pyridoxine)	BP	2.0 mg
Vitamin B12 (Cyanocobalamin)	HSE	2.0 mcg
Vitamin B Complex (Folic Acid)	HSE	400.0 mcg
Vitamin C (Ascorbic Acid)	HSE	120.0 mg
Vitamin D3 (Cholecalciferol)	HSE	400.0 iu (10 mcg)
Vitamin E	HSE	10.0 mg
Vitamin H (Biotin)	HSE	100.0 mcg
Calcium	HSE	550.0 mg*
Magnesium	BP	360.0 mg
Iron	FCC	15.0 mg
Zinc	HSE	15.0 mg
Manganese	USP	4.0 mg
Copper	USP	2.5 mg
Iodine	BP	150.0 mcg
Selenium	HSE	55.0 mcg
Chromium	BP	200.0 mcg
Molybdenum	HSE	250.0 mcg
Calcium Caseinate (Instant) providing:	HSE	
Calcium		550.0 mg*
Phosphorus†		293.0 mg (9.45 mmol)
Protein‡		32.0 g
Potassium§		10.0 mg Max (0.26 mmol)
Fat		2.16 g Max
Carbohydrate		21.6 g
Energy (calories)		259.0 kcal (1084 kJ)
Sodium		166.0 mg Max (7.2 mmol)
Potassium (total)§		226.0 mg Max (5.8 mmol)
Phosphorus (total) †		369.0 mg (11.9 mmol)

‡ Amino Acid Profile of Forceval Protein Powder:

Arginine #	1.2 g
Histidine #	1.0 g
Leucine #	3.2 g
Isoleucine #	1.8 g
Valine #	2.3 g
Lysine #	2.7 g
Methionine #	1.0 g
Phenylalanine #	1.7 g
Threonine #	1.5 g
Tryptophan #	0.4 g
Cystine	0.1 g
Tyrosine	1.8 g
Alanine	1.0 g
Aspartic Acid	2.3 g
Glutamic Acid	7.1 g
Glycine	0.6 g
Serine	2.0 g
Proline	3.4 g

= essential amino acids.

3. PHARMACEUTICAL FORM

Brown, speckled, fine powder with an odour of chocolate.

4. CLINICAL PARTICULARS

4.1 Therapeutic indications

Forceval Protein Powder may be used as the Protein, Vitamin, Mineral and Trace Elements source in the following situations:-

- As a therapeutic nutritional adjunct in malabsorptive states such as short bowel syndrome, intestinal fistulas, abdominal sepsis and inflammatory bowel disease.

- As a therapeutic nutritional adjunct in conditions leading to hypoproteinaemia such as trauma and burns.

- As a peri-operative therapeutic nutritional support for undernourished patients and patients with sepsis.

RECOMMENDED USES

1. FORCEVAL PROTEIN POWDER is recommended for children over two years of age, adults and the elderly with an inadequate protein, vitamin, mineral and trace element intake resulting from their inability to maintain a well balanced diet.

2. FORCEVAL PROTEIN POWDER is suitable for patients suffering from Protein, Vitamin, Mineral and Trace Element deficiency as a result of failure to absorb their diet, eg. in malabsorption conditions such as Crohn's disease, Inflammatory Bowel disease and in the presence of Bowel Fistulae or following surgery of the bowel.

3. FORCEVAL PROTEIN POWDER is recommended before and after surgery where a balanced nutritional intake is required to ensure rapid healing, prevention of malnutrition and to reduce the likelihood of infection.

4. FORCEVAL PROTEIN POWDER is recommended where additional protein is required following trauma, eg. burns, infection and multiple injuries.

5. FORCEVAL PROTEIN POWDER is recommended where a high protein intake is required, yet other dietary factors need also to be modified, eg. where a low fat diet is needed; where a reduced carbohydrate diet is needed, as in the case of diabetics; and where electrolytes such as sodium, potassium and phosphorus may need to be reduced eg. in certain heart or kidney conditions.

6. FORCEVAL PROTEIN POWDER is recommended for patients who develop a condition called hypoproteinaemia; this is a condition where the level of protein in the blood is substantially reduced. This can occur in many medical and surgical conditions such as malabsorption, anorexia, carcinoma, following injury or surgery etc. In the case of injury or surgery, damaged tissue needs replacing with new tissue; this requires considerable additional protein. Many of these conditions are accompanied by loss of appetite and possibly altered taste sensations and subclinical Vitamin, Mineral and Trace Element deficiency.

7. FORCEVAL PROTEIN POWDER can be used in conjunction with a calorie controlled, high protein diet under medical supervision - 72g will provide 25 essential Vitamins, Minerals and Trace Elements in line with the UK Dietary Reference Values and US Recommended Dietary Allowances.

4.2 Posology and method of administration

The route of administration is oral or naso-gastric.

ADULTS AND ELDERLY PATIENTS

Sachets: 1-2 × 36g Sachet or 2-4 × 18g (36g-72g) Sachets daily or as prescribed by the doctor.

360 g tins: 2-4 level scoops (36g-72g approx) daily or as prescribed by the doctor.

CHILDREN (ABOVE 2 YEARS OF AGE)

Sachets: 1-2 × 18g Sachets (18g-36g) daily or as prescribed by the doctor.

1 × 36g Sachet daily or as prescribed by the doctor.

360 g tins: 1-2 level scoops (18g-36g) daily or as prescribed by the doctor.

1 level scoop of powder = 18g approx.

Each tin contains a 45ml plastic scoop.

72g of Forceval Protein Powder will provide Vitamins and Minerals in line with the UK Dietary Reference Values and US Recommended Dietary Allowances

Recommended Dilution

18g of Forceval Protein Powder in 125 ml liquid (¼ pint)

36g of Forceval Protein Powder in 250 ml liquid (½ pint)

Extra liquid can be added if a thinner consistency is required

Do not exceed the stated dose.

4.3 Contraindications

Forceval Protein Powder is contra-indicated in patients with renal or hepatic failure and in children below 2 years of age.

4.4 Special warnings and special precautions for use

Forceval Protein Powder is formulated as a nutritional supplement. It is not a total feed or total food replacement and must not be used as such.

It should be used as the protein, vitamin and mineral source in total feed systems, combined with an additional energy source, carbohydrate (such as Caloreen, a glucose polymer) and/or fat (LCT or MCT emulsions), to give energy: N, osmolality and calorific values suitable for individual patient requirements.

Ideally the energy: N ratio should be between 100 and 200 kcal/g N and the osmolality of the total feed as near as possible to 300 m osmol/kg.

Patients on lactose-free diets should not use milk or diluents containing milk or milk products to mix with Forceval Protein Powder.

Prepared drinks should not be heated as the nutritional values of the essential proteins and vitamins will be impaired.

When Forceval Protein is mixed with milk, osmolality problems should be anticipated at the extremes of age.

No other vitamins, minerals or supplements with vitamin A should be taken with this preparation except under close medical supervision.

Do not exceed the stated dose.

The label will state:

Important warning: Contains iron. Keep out of the reach and sight of children, as overdose may be fatal.

This will appear on the front of the pack and on the sachet in a rectangle in which there is no other information.

This product contains 10g sucrose per sachet. This should be taken into account in patients with diabetes mellitus.

4.5 Interaction with other medicinal products and other forms of Interaction

Folic acid can reduce the plasma concentration of phenytoin. Oral iron and zinc sulphate reduce the absorption of tetracyclines.

4.6 Pregnancy and lactation

Forceval Protein Powder may be administered during pregnancy and lactation at the recommendation of the physician.

4.7 Effects on ability to drive and use machines

Not applicable.

4.8 Undesirable effects

If the product is re-constituted as described, together with an additional energy source, to give the required energy:-nitrogen ratio and osmolality, it is unlikely that undesirable effects will occur. However, prescribers should be aware of the potential risks of diarrhoea, dehydration, electrolyte imbalance, hyperglycaemia and osmolal disorders.

Care should be taken when administering some medications concurrently with Forceval Protein Powder, or shortly thereafter.

The possibility of infection risk should be noted if the nutritional supplement is prepared in unsatisfactory conditions.

4.9 Overdose

No cases of overdosage due to Forceval Protein Powder have been reported. Overdosage is extremely unlikely if the dosage recommendations are followed. Any symptoms which may be observed due to ingestion of large quantities of Forceval Protein Powder will be due to hyperproteinaemia.

5. PHARMACOLOGICAL PROPERTIES

5.1 Pharmacodynamic properties

Vitamin A

Vitamin A plays an important role in the visual process. It is isomerised to the 11-cis isomer and subsequently bound to the opsin to form the photoreceptor for vision under subdued light. One of the earliest symptoms of deficiency is night blindness which may develop into the more serious condition xerophthalmia. Vitamin A also participates in the formation and maintenance of the integrity of epithelial tissues and mucous membranes. Deficiency may cause skin changes resulting in a dry rough skin with lowered resistance to minor skin infections. Deficiency of Vitamin A, usually accompanied by protein-energy malnutrition, is linked with a frequency of infection and with defective immunological defence mechanisms.

Vitamin D

Vitamin D is required for the absorption of calcium and phosphate from the gastro-intestinal tract and for their transport. Its involvement in the control of calcium metabolism and hence the normal calcification of bones is well documented. Deficiency of Vitamin D in children may result in the development of rickets.

Vitamin B_1 (Thiamine)

Thiamine (as the coenzyme, thiamine pyrophosphate) is associated with carbohydrate metabolism. Thiamine pyrophosphate also acts as a co-enzyme in the direct oxidative pathway of glucose metabolism. In thiamine deficiency, pyruvic and lactic acids accumulate in the tissues. The pyruvate ion is involved in the biosynthesis of acetylcholine via its conversion to acetyl co-enzyme A through a thiamine-dependent process. In thiamine deficiency, therefore, there are effects on the central nervous system due either to the effect on acetylcholine synthesis or to the lactate and pyruvate accumulation. Deficiency of thiamine results in fatigue, anorexia, gastro-intestinal disturbances, tachycardia, irritability and neurological symptoms. Gross deficiency of thiamine (and other Vitamin B group factors) leads to the condition beri-beri.

Vitamin B_2 (Riboflavine)

Riboflavine is phosphorylated to flavine mononucleotide and flavine adenine dinucleotide, which act as co-enzymes in the respiratory chain and in oxidative phosphorylation. Riboflavine deficiency presents with ocular symptoms, as well as lesions on the lips and at the angles of the mouth.

Vitamin B_6 (Pyridoxine)

Pyridoxine, once absorbed, is rapidly converted to the co-enzymes, pyridoxal phosphate and pyridoxamine phosphate which play an essential role in protein metabolism. Convulsions and hypochromic anaemia have occurred in infants deficient in pyridoxine.

Vitamin B_{12} (Cyanocobalamin)

Vitamin B_{12} is present in the body mainly as methylcobalamin and as adenosylcobalamin and hydroxocobalamin. These act as co-enzymes in the trans methylation of homocysteine to methionine; in the isomerization of methylmalonyl co-enzyme to succinyl co-enzyme and with folate in several metabolic pathways respectively. Deficiency of Vitamin B_{12} interferes with haemopoiesis and produces megaloblastic anaemia.

Vitamin C (Ascorbic Acid)

Vitamin C cannot be synthesised by man, therefore, a dietary source is necessary. It acts as a cofactor in numerous biological processes including the hydroxylation of proline to hydroxyproline. In deficiency, the formation of collagen is, therefore, impaired. Ascorbic acid is important in the hydroxylation of dopamine to noradrenaline and in hydroxylations occurring in steroid synthesis in the adrenals. It is a reducing agent in tyrosine metabolism and by acting as an electron donor in the conversion of folic acid to tetrahydrofolic acid is indirectly involved in the synthesis of purine and thymine. Vitamin C is also necessary for the incorporation of iron into ferritin. Vitamin C increases the phagocytic function of leucocytes; it possesses anti-inflammatory activity and it promotes wound healing. Deficiency can produce scurvy. Features include swollen inflamed gums, petechial haemorrhages and subcutaneous bruising. The deficiency of collagen leads to development of thin watery ground substances in which blood vessels are insecurely fixed and readily ruptured. The supportive components of bone and cartilage are also deficient causing bones to fracture easily and teeth to become loose. Anaemia commonly occurs probably due to Vitamin C's role in the iron metabolism.

Vitamin E

Vitamin E deficiency has been linked to disorders such as cystic fibrosis where fat absorption is impaired. It is essential for the normal function of the muscular system and the blood.

Nicotinamide

The biochemical functions of nicotinamide as NAD and NADP (nicotinamide adenine dinucleotide phosphate) include the degradation and synthesis of fatty acids, carbohydrates and amino acids as well as hydrogen transfer. Deficiency produces pellagra and mental and neurological changes.

Calcium

Calcium is an essential body electrolyte. It is involved in the maintenance of normal muscle and nerve function and essential for normal cardiac function and the clotting of blood. Calcium is mainly found in the bones and teeth. Deficiency of calcium leads to rickets, osteomalacia in children and osteoporosis in the elderly.

Phosphorus

Phosphate plays important roles in the osteoblastic and osteoclastic reactions. It interacts with calcium to modify the balance between these two processes. Organic phosphate esters play a key role in the metabolism of carbohydrates, fats and proteins and in the formation of 'high energy phosphate' compounds. Phosphate also acts as a buffer and plays a role in the renal excretion of sodium and hydrogen ions.

Pantothenic Acid

Pantothenic acid is incorporated into co-enzyme A and is involved in metabolic pathways involving acetylation which includes detoxification of drug molecules and biosynthesis of cholesterol, steroid hormones, mucopolysaccharides and acetylcholine. CoA has an essential function in lipid metabolism.

Folic Acid

Folic acid is reduced in the body to tetrahydrofolate which is a co-enzyme for various metabolic processes, including the synthesis of purine and pyrimidine nucleotides and hence in the synthesis of DNA. It is also involved in some amino acid conversion and in the formation and utilisation of formate. Deficiency of folic acid leads to megaloblastic anaemia.

Vitamin H (d-Biotin)

Biotin is a co-enzyme for carboxylation during the metabolism of proteins and carbohydrates.

Selenium

Selenium is an essential trace element, deficiency of which has been reported in man. It is thought to be involved in the functioning of membranes and the synthesis of amino acids. Deficiency of selenium in the diet of experimental animals produces fatty liver followed by necrosis.

Iron

Iron, as a constituent of haemoglobin, plays an essential role in oxygen transport. It is also present in the muscle protein myoglobin and in the liver. Deficiency of iron leads to anaemia.

Copper

Traces of copper are essential to the body as constituents of enzyme systems involved in oxidation reactions.

Magnesium

Magnesium is essential to the body as a constituent of skeletal structures and in maintaining cell integrity and fluid balance. It is utilised in many of the functions in which calcium is concerned but often exerts the opposite effect. Some enzymes require the magnesium ion as a co-factor.

Potassium

Potassium is the principle cation of intracellular fluid and is intimately involved in the cell function and metabolism. It is essential for carbohydrate metabolism and glycogen storage and protein synthesis and is involved in transmembrane potential where it is necessary to maintain the resting potential in excitable cells. Potassium ions maintain intracellular pH and osmotic pressure. Prolonged or severe diarrhoea may lead to potassium deficiency.

Zinc

Zinc is a constituent of many enzymes and is, therefore, essential to the body. It is present with insulin in the pancreas. It plays a role in DNA synthesis and cell division. Reported effects of deficiency include delayed puberty and hypogonadal dwarfism.

Manganese

Manganese is a constituent of enzyme systems including those involved in lipid synthesis, the tricarboxylic acid cycle and purine and pyrimidine metabolism. It is bound to arginase of the liver and activates many enzymes.

Iodine

Iodine is an essential constituent of the thyroid hormones.

Chromium

Chromium is an essential trace element involved in carbohydrate metabolism.

Molybdenum

Molybdenum is an essential trace element although there have been no reports of deficiency states in man. Molybdenum salts have been used to treat copper poisoning in sheep.

Calcium Caseinate

Calcium caseinate is the sole protein source in Forceval Protein Powder. It is a high biological value protein containing all ten essential and eight other nutritionally important amino acids.

Essential amino acids cannot be synthesised by the body and are necessary for the synthesis of most proteins and some non-protein substances e.g. phenylalanine is required to produce the hormones adrenaline and thyroxine. Insulin has more than 50% of its constituent amino acids as essential amino acids. Because these hormones are removed from the body once their effect is exerted, there is a constant need for their renewal, hence a constant need for a source of essential amino acids in the diet. If amino acids are not available in the diet they have to be supplied by the breakdown of other body proteins. During starvation and malnutrition and following surgical operations or in patients with severe burns, a negative nitrogen balance occurs in which the nitrogen (from proteins and amino acids) lost from the body exceeds the intake.

5.2 Pharmacokinetic properties

Vitamin A

Except when liver function is impaired, Vitamin A is readily absorbed. Vitamin A esters (such as Vitamin A Acetate in Forceval Protein Powder) are largely hydrolysed to retinol which is emulsified by bile salts and phospholipids and absorbed in a micellar form. Part is conjugated with glucuronic acid in the kidney and part is metabolised in the liver and kidney, leaving 30 to 50% of the dose for storage in the liver. It is bound to a globulin in the blood. Metabolites of Vitamin A are excreted in the faeces and the urine.

Vitamin D

Cholecalciferol is absorbed from the gastro-intestinal tract into the circulation. In the liver, it is hydroxylated to 25-hydroxycholecalciferol, is subject to entero-hepatic circulation and is further hydroxylated to 1,25-dihydroxycholecalciferol in the renal tubule cells. Vitamin D metabolites are bound to specific plasma proteins.

Vitamin B_1 (Thiamide)

Thiamine is absorbed from the gastro-intestinal tract and is widely distributed to most body tissues. Amounts in excess of the body's requirements are not stored but excreted in the urine as unchanged thiamine or its metabolites.

Vitamin B_2 (Riboflavine)

Riboflavine is absorbed from the gastro-intestinal tract and in the circulation is bound to plasma proteins. It is widely distributed. Little is stored and excess amounts are excreted in the urine. In the body riboflavine is converted to flavine mononucleotide (FMN) and then to flavine adenine dinucleotide (FAD).

Vitamin B_6 (Pyridoxine)

Pyridoxine is absorbed from the gastro-intestinal tract and converted to the active pyridoxal phosphate which is bound to plasma proteins. It is excreted in the urine as 4-pyridoxic acid.

Vitamin B_{12} (Cyanocobalamin)

Cyanocobalamin is absorbed from the gastro-intestinal tract and is extensively bound to specific plasma proteins. A study with labelled Vitamin B_{12} showed it was quickly taken up by the intestinal mucosa and held there for 2-3 hours. Peak concentrations in the blood and tissues did not occur until 8-12 hours after dosage with maximum concentrations in the liver within 24 hours. Cobalamins are stored in the liver, excreted in the bile and undergo enterohepatic recycling. Part of a dose is excreted in the urine, most of it in the first eight hours.

Vitamin C (Ascorbic Acid)

Ascorbic acid is readily absorbed from the gastro-intestinal tract and is widely distributed in the body tissues. Ascorbic acid in excess of the body's needs is rapidly eliminated in the urine and this elimination is usually accompanied by a mild diuresis.

Vitamin E

Vitamin E is absorbed from the gastro-intestinal tract. Most appears in the lymph and is then widely distributed to all tissues. Most of a dose is slowly excreted in the bile and the remainder is eliminated in the urine as glucuronides of tocopheronic acid or other metabolites.

Nicotinamide (Nicotinic Acid Amide)

Nicotinic acid is absorbed from the gastro-intestinal tract, is widely distributed in the body tissues and has a short half-life.

Calcium

A third of ingested calcium is absorbed from the small intestine. Absorption of calcium decreases with age.

Phosphorus

The body contains from 600-800 g of phosphorus, over 80% of which is present in bone as phosphate salts, mainly hydroxyapatite crystals. The phosphate in these crystals is available for exchange with phosphate ions in the extracellular fluids.

Calcium Pantothenate

Pantothenic acid is readily absorbed from the gastrointestinal tract and is widely distributed in the body tissues. About 70% of pantothenic acid is excreted unchanged in the urine and about 30% in the faeces.

Folic Acid

Folic acid is absorbed mainly from the proximal part of the small intestine. Folate polyglutamates are considered to be deconjugated to monoglutamates during absorption. Folic acid rapidly appears in the blood where it is extensively bound to plasma proteins. Some Folic acid is distributed in body tissues, some is excreted as folate in the urine and some is stored in the liver as folate.

Vitamin H (d-Biotin)

Following absorption, biotin is stored in the liver, kidney and pancreas.

Selenium

Although it has been established that selenium is essential to human life, very little information is available on its function and metabolism.

Iron

Iron is absorbed chiefly in the duodenum and jejunum. Absorption is aided by the acid secretion of the stomach. In conditions of iron deficiency, absorption is increased and, conversely, it is decreased in iron overload. Iron is stored as ferritin.

Copper

Copper is absorbed from the gastro-intestinal tract and its major route of excretion is in the bile.

Magnesium

Magnesium salts are poorly absorbed from the gastrointestinal tract; however, sufficient magnesium will normally be absorbed to replace deficiency states. Magnesium is excreted in both the urine and the faeces but excretion is reduced in deficiency states.

Potassium

Potassium salts are absorbed from the gastro-intestinal tract. Potassium is excreted in the urine, the faeces and in perspiration. Urinary excretion of potassium continues even when intake is low.

Zinc

Zinc is poorly absorbed from the gastro-intestinal tract. It is widely distributed throughout the body. It is excreted in the faeces with traces appearing in the urine.

Manganese

Manganese salts are poorly absorbed.

Iodine

Iodides are absorbed and stored in the thyroid gland as thyroglobulin. Iodides are excreted in the urine with smaller amounts appearing in the faeces, saliva and sweat.

Chromium

Although it has been established that chromium is essential to human life, little information is available on its function and metabolism.

Molybdenum

Although it has been established that molybdenum is essential to human life, little information is available on its function and metabolism.

Calcium Caseinate

Calcium caseinate is metabolised by the body to its constituent amino acids, as are other proteins.

5.3 Preclinical safety data

There are no pre-clinical data of relevance to the prescriber which are additional to that already included in other sections of the SPC.

6. PHARMACEUTICAL PARTICULARS

6.1 List of excipients

Butylated Hydroxyanisole BP

Sodium Benzoate BP

Cocoa Powder SF11HT HSE

Vanilla Flavour HSE

Sucrose BP

6.2 Incompatibilities

No major incompatibilities are known.

6.3 Shelf life

36 months, as packaged for sale.

6.4 Special precautions for storage

Store in a cool, dry place at a temperature not exceeding 25°C (77°F) protected from light.

6.5 Nature and contents of container

a) Composite cans (aluminium lined cardboard cylinder sealed with a solid metal base and aluminium pull tab diaphragm) with resealable plastic plug lid. 45 ml opaque scoop included in can with leaflet under plastic plug lid.

b) Sachets - paper/polythene/aluminium foil laminated. Leaflet in carton with sachets.

The product may be available in three pack sizes:

i) 360 g cans

ii) 18 g sachets in a carton

iii) 36 g sachets in a carton

6.6 Instructions for use and handling

Please refer to the patient information leaflet for detailed use of the product, including mixing instructions and use of the scoop.

7. MARKETING AUTHORISATION HOLDER

Alliance Pharmaceuticals Limited

Avonbridge House

2 Bath Road

Chippenham

Wiltshire

SN15 2BB

United Kingdom

8. MARKETING AUTHORISATION NUMBER(S)

PL 16853/0084

9. DATE OF FIRST AUTHORISATION/RENEWAL OF THE AUTHORISATION

18th April 2005

10. DATE OF REVISION OF THE TEXT

April 2005

Forceval Protein Powder - Natural

(Alliance Pharmaceuticals)

1. NAME OF THE MEDICINAL PRODUCT

Forceval Protein Powder (Natural Flavour)

2. QUALITATIVE AND QUANTITATIVE COMPOSITION

Each 60 g of product provide:

Vitamin A	HSE	2500.0 iu (750 mcg)
Vitamin B1 (Thiamin)	HSE	1.5 mg
Vitamin B2 (Riboflavin)	BP	1.5 mg
Vitamin B3 (Nicotinamide)	HSE	18.0 mg
Vitamin B5 (Pantothenic Acid)	PhEur	6.0 mg
Vitamin B6 (Pyridoxine)	BP	2.0 mg
Vitamin B12 (Cyanocobalamin)	HSE	2.0 mcg
Vitamin B Complex (Folic Acid)	HSE	400.0 mcg
Vitamin C (Ascorbic Acid)	HSE	120.0 mg
Vitamin D3 (Cholecalciferol)	HSE	400.0 iu (10 mcg)
Vitamin E	HSE	10.0 mg
Vitamin H (Biotin)	HSE	100.0 mcg
Calcium	HSE	550.0 mg*
Magnesium	BP	300.0 mg
Iron	FCC	12.0 mg
Zinc	HSE	15.0 mg
Manganese	USP	4.0 mg
Copper	USP	2.0 mg
Iodine	BP	150.0 mcg
Selenium	HSE	55.0 mcg
Chromium	BP	200.0 mcg
Molybdenum	HSE	250.0 mcg
Calcium Caseinate (Instant) providing:	HSE	
Calcium		550.0 mg*
Phosphorus†		293.0 mg (9.45 mmol)
Protein‡		33.0 g
Potassium§		10.0 mg Max (0.26 mmol)
Fat		0.6 g Max
Carbohydrate		18.0 g
Energy (calories)		200.0 kcal (837 kJ)
Sodium		72.0 mg Max (3.1 mmol)
Potassium (total)§		10.0 mg Max (0.26 mmol)
Phosphorus (total) †		300.0 mg (9.7 mmol)

‡ Amino Acid Profile of Forceval

Protein Powder:

Arginine #	1.2 g
Histidine #	1.0 g
Leucine #	3.2 g
Isoleucine #	1.8 g
Valine #	2.3 g
Lysine #	2.7 g
Methionine #	1.0 g
Phenylalanine #	1.7 g
Threonine #	1.5 g
Tryptophan #	0.4 g
Cystine	0.1 g
Tyrosine	1.8 g
Alanine	1.0 g
Aspartic Acid	2.3 g
Glutamic Acid	7.1 g
Glycine	0.6 g
Serine	2.0 g
Proline	3.4 g

= essential amino acids.

3. PHARMACEUTICAL FORM

White to off-white, speckled, fine powder with a slight odour of vanilla.

4. CLINICAL PARTICULARS

4.1 Therapeutic indications

Forceval Protein Powder may be used as the Protein, Vitamin, Mineral and Trace Elements source in the following situations:-

- As a therapeutic nutritional adjunct in malabsorptive states such as short bowel syndrome, intestinal fistulas, abdominal sepsis and inflammatory bowel disease.

- As a therapeutic nutritional adjunct in conditions leading to hypoproteinaemia such as trauma and burns.

- As a peri-operative therapeutic nutritional support for undernourished patients and patients with sepsis.

RECOMMENDED USES

1. FORCEVAL PROTEIN POWDER is recommended for children over two years of age, adults and the elderly with an inadequate protein, vitamin, mineral and trace element intake resulting from their inability to maintain a well balanced diet.

2. FORCEVAL PROTEIN POWDER is suitable for patients suffering from Protein, Vitamin, Mineral and Trace Element deficiency as a result of failure to absorb their diet, eg. in malabsorption conditions such as Crohn's disease, Inflammatory Bowel disease and in the presence of Bowel Fistulae or following surgery of the bowel.

3. FORCEVAL PROTEIN POWDER is recommended before and after surgery where a balanced nutritional intake is required to ensure rapid healing, prevention of malnutrition and to reduce the likelihood of infection.

4. FORCEVAL PROTEIN POWDER is recommended where additional protein is required following trauma, eg. burns, infection and multiple injuries.

5. FORCEVAL PROTEIN POWDER is recommended where a high protein intake is required, yet other dietary factors need also to be modified, eg. where a low fat diet is needed; where a reduced carbohydrate diet is needed, as in the case of diabetics; and where electrolytes such as sodium, potassium and phosphorus may need to be reduced eg. in certain heart or kidney conditions.

6. FORCEVAL PROTEIN POWDER is recommended for patients who develop a condition called hypoproteinaemia; this is a condition where the level of protein in the blood is substantially reduced. This can occur in many medical and surgical conditions such as malabsorption, anorexia, carcinoma, following injury or surgery etc. In the case of injury or surgery, damaged tissue needs replacing with new tissue; this requires considerable additional protein. Many of these conditions are accompanied by loss of appetite and possibly altered taste sensations and subclinical Vitamin, Mineral and Trace Element deficiency.

7. FORCEVAL PROTEIN POWDER can be used in conjunction with a calorie controlled, high protein diet under medical supervision - 60g will provide 25 essential Vitamins, Minerals and Trace Elements in line with the UK Dietary Reference Values and US Recommended Dietary Allowances.

4.2 Posology and method of administration

The route of administration is oral or naso-gastric.

ADULTS AND ELDERLY PATIENTS

Sachets: 1-2 × 30g Sachet or 2-4 × 15g (30g-60g) Sachets daily or as prescribed by the doctor.

300 g tins: 2-4 level scoops (30g-60g approx) daily or as prescribed by the doctor.

CHILDREN (ABOVE 2 YEARS OF AGE)

Sachets: 1-2 × 15g Sachets (15g-30g) daily or as prescribed by the doctor.

1 × 30g Sachet daily or as prescribed by the doctor.

300 g tins: 1-2 level scoops (15g-30g) daily or as prescribed by the doctor.

1 level scoop of powder = 15g approx.

Each tin contains a 38ml plastic scoop.

60g of Forceval Protein Powder will provide Vitamins and Minerals in line with the UK Dietary Reference Values and US Recommended Dietary Allowances.

Recommended Dilution

15g of Forceval Protein Powder in 125 ml liquid (¼ pint)

30g of Forceval Protein Powder in 250 ml liquid (½ pint)

Extra liquid can be added if a thinner consistency is required.

Do not exceed the stated dose.

4.3 Contraindications

Forceval Protein Powder is contra-indicated in patients with renal or hepatic failure and in children below 2 years of age.

4.4 Special warnings and special precautions for use

Forceval Protein Powder is formulated as a nutritional supplement. It is not a total feed or total food replacement and must not be used as such.

It should be used as the protein, vitamin and mineral source in total feed systems, combined with an additional energy source, carbohydrate (such as Caloreen, a glucose polymer) and/or fat (LCT or MCT emulsions), to give energy: N, osmolality and calorific values suitable for individual patient requirements.

Ideally the energy: N ratio should be between 100 and 200 kcal/g N and the osmolality of the total feed as near as possible to 300 m osmol/kg.

Patients on lactose-free diets should not use milk or diluents containing milk or milk products to mix with Forceval Protein Powder.

Prepared drinks should not be heated as the nutritional values of the essential proteins and vitamins will be impaired.

When Forceval Protein is mixed with milk, osmolality problems should be anticipated at the extremes of age.

No other vitamins, minerals or supplements with vitamin A should be taken with this preparation except under close medical supervision.

Do not exceed the stated dose.

The label will state:

Important warning: Contains iron. Keep out of the reach and sight of children, as overdose may be fatal.

This will appear on the front of the pack and on the sachet in a rectangle in which there is no other information.

This medicine contains 8g sucrose per sachet. This should be taken into account in patients with diabetes mellitus.

4.5 Interaction with other medicinal products and other forms of Interaction

Folic acid can reduce the plasma concentration of phenytoin. Oral iron and zinc sulphate reduce the absorption of tetracyclines.

4.6 Pregnancy and lactation

Forceval Protein Powder may be administered during pregnancy and lactation at the recommendation of the physician.

4.7 Effects on ability to drive and use machines

Not applicable.

4.8 Undesirable effects

If the product is re-constituted as described, together with an additional energy source, to give the required energy:-nitrogen ratio and osmolality, it is unlikely that undesirable effects will occur. However, prescribers should be aware of the potential risks of diarrhoea, dehydration, electrolyte imbalance, hyperglycaemia and osmolal disorders.

Care should be taken when administering some medications concurrently with Forceval Protein Powder, or shortly thereafter.

The possibility of infection risk should be noted if the nutritional supplement is prepared in unsatisfactory conditions.

4.9 Overdose

No cases of overdosage due to Forceval Protein Powder have been reported. Overdosage is extremely unlikely if the dosage recommendations are followed. Any symptoms which may be observed due to ingestion of large quantities of Forceval Protein Powder will be due to hyperproteinaemia.

5. PHARMACOLOGICAL PROPERTIES

5.1 Pharmacodynamic properties

Vitamin A

Vitamin A plays an important role in the visual process. It is isomerised to the 11-cis isomer and subsequently bound to the opsin to form the photoreceptor for vision under subdued light. One of the earliest symptoms of deficiency is night blindness which may develop into the more serious condition xerophthalmia. Vitamin A also participates in the formation and maintenance of the integrity of epithelial tissues and mucous membranes. Deficiency may cause skin changes resulting in a dry rough skin with lowered resistance to minor skin infections. Deficiency of Vitamin A, usually accompanied by protein-energy malnutrition, is linked with a frequency of infection and with defective immunological defence mechanisms.

Vitamin D

Vitamin D is required for the absorption of calcium and phosphate from the gastro-intestinal tract and for their transport. Its involvement in the control of calcium metabolism and hence the normal calcification of bones is well documented. Deficiency of Vitamin D in children may result in the development of rickets.

Vitamin B_1 (Thiamine)

Thiamine (as the coenzyme, thiamine pyrophosphate) is associated with carbohydrate metabolism. Thiamine pyrophosphate also acts as a co-enzyme in the direct oxidative pathway of glucose metabolism. In thiamine deficiency, pyruvic and lactic acids accumulate in the tissues. The pyruvate ion is involved in the biosynthesis of acetylcholine via its conversion to acetyl co-enzyme A through a thiamine-dependent process. In thiamine deficiency, therefore, there are effects on the central nervous system due either to the effect on acetylcholine synthesis or to the lactate and pyruvate accumulation. Deficiency of thiamine results in fatigue, anorexia, gastro-intestinal disturbances, tachycardia, irritability and neurological symptoms. Gross deficiency of thiamine (and other Vitamin B group factors) leads to the condition beri-beri.

Vitamin B_2 (Riboflavine)

Riboflavine is phosphorylated to flavine mononucleotide and flavine adenine dinucleotide, which act as co-enzymes in the respiratory chain and in oxidative phosphorylation. Riboflavine deficiency presents with ocular symptoms, as well as lesions on the lips and at the angles of the mouth.

Vitamin B_6 (Pyridoxine)

Pyridoxine, once absorbed, is rapidly converted to the co-enzymes, pyridoxal phosphate and pyridoxamine phosphate which play an essential role in protein metabolism. Convulsions and hypochromic anaemia have occurred in infants deficient in pyridoxine.

Vitamin B_{12} (Cyanocobalamin)

Vitamin B_{12} is present in the body mainly as methylcobalamin and as adenosylcobalamin and hydroxocobalamin. These act as co-enzymes in the trans methylation of homocysteine to methionine; in the isomerization of methylmalonyl co-enzyme to succinyl co-enzyme and with folate in several metabolic pathways respectively. Deficiency of Vitamin B_{12} interferes with haemopoiesis and produces megaloblastic anaemia.

Vitamin C (Ascorbic Acid)

Vitamin C cannot be synthesised by man, therefore, a dietary source is necessary. It acts as a cofactor in numerous biological processes including the hydroxylation of proline to hydroxyproline. In deficiency, the formation of collagen is, therefore, impaired. Ascorbic acid is important in the hydroxylation of dopamine to noradrenaline and in hydroxylations occurring in steroid synthesis in the adrenals. It is a reducing agent in tyrosine metabolism and by acting as an electron donor in the conversion of folic acid to tetrahydrofolic acid is indirectly involved in the synthesis of purine and thymine. Vitamin C is also necessary for the incorporation of iron into ferritin. Vitamin C increases the phagocytic function of leucocytes; it possesses anti-inflammatory activity and it promotes wound healing. Deficiency can produce scurvy. Features include swollen inflamed gums, petechial haemorrhages and subcutaneous bruising. The deficiency of collagen leads to development of thin watery ground substances in which blood vessels are insecurely fixed and readily ruptured. The supportive components of bone and cartilage are also deficient causing bones to fracture easily and teeth to become loose. Anaemia commonly occurs probably due to Vitamin C's role in the iron metabolism.

Vitamin E

Vitamin E deficiency has been linked to disorders such as cystic fibrosis where fat absorption is impaired. It is essential for the normal function of the muscular system and the blood.

Nicotinamide

The biochemical functions of nicotinamide as NAD and NADP (nicotinamide adenine dinucleotide phosphate) include the degradation and synthesis of fatty acids, carbohydrates and amino acids as well as hydrogen transfer. Deficiency produces pellagra and mental and neurological changes.

Calcium

Calcium is an essential body electrolyte. It is involved in the maintenance of normal muscle and nerve function and essential for normal cardiac function and the clotting of blood. Calcium is mainly found in the bones and teeth. Deficiency of calcium leads to rickets, osteomalacia in children and osteoporosis in the elderly.

Phosphorus

Phosphate plays important roles in the osteoblastic and osteoclastic reactions. It interacts with calcium to modify the balance between these two processes. Organic phosphate esters play a key role in the metabolism of carbohydrates, fats and proteins and in the formation of 'high energy phosphate' compounds. Phosphate also acts as a buffer and plays a role in the renal excretion of sodium and hydrogen ions.

Pantothenic Acid

Pantothenic acid is incorporated into co-enzyme A and is involved in metabolic pathways involving acetylation which includes detoxification of drug molecules and biosynthesis of cholesterol, steroid hormones, mucopolysaccharides and acetylcholine. CoA has an essential function in lipid metabolism.

Folic Acid

Folic acid is reduced in the body to tetrahydrofolate which is a co-enzyme for various metabolic processes, including the synthesis of purine and pyrimidine nucleotides and hence in the synthesis of DNA. It is also involved in some amino acid conversion and in the formation and utilisation of formate. Deficiency of folic acid leads to megaloblastic anaemia.

Vitamin H (d-Biotin)

Biotin is a co-enzyme for carboxylation during the metabolism of proteins and carbohydrates.

Selenium

Selenium is an essential trace element, deficiency of which has been reported in man. It is thought to be involved in the functioning of membranes and the synthesis of amino acids. Deficiency of selenium in the diet of experimental animals produces fatty liver followed by necrosis.

Iron

Iron, as a constituent of haemoglobin, plays an essential role in oxygen transport. It is also present in the muscle protein myoglobin and in the liver. Deficiency of iron leads to anaemia.

Copper

Traces of copper are essential to the body as constituents of enzyme systems involved in oxidation reactions.

Magnesium

Magnesium is essential to the body as a constituent of skeletal structures and in maintaining cell integrity and fluid balance. It is utilised in many of the functions in which calcium is concerned but often exerts the opposite effect. Some enzymes require the magnesium ion as a co-factor.

Potassium

Potassium is the principle cation of intracellular fluid and is intimately involved in the cell function and metabolism. It is essential for carbohydrate metabolism and glycogen storage and protein synthesis and is involved in transmembrane potential where it is necessary to maintain the resting potential in excitable cells. Potassium ions maintain intracellular pH and osmotic pressure. Prolonged or severe diarrhoea may lead to potassium deficiency.

Zinc

Zinc is a constituent of many enzymes and is, therefore, essential to the body. It is present with insulin in the pancreas. It plays a role in DNA synthesis and cell division. Reported effects of deficiency include delayed puberty and hypogonadal dwarfism.

Manganese

Manganese is a constituent of enzyme systems including those involved in lipid synthesis, the tricarboxylic acid cycle and purine and pyrimidine metabolism. It is bound to arginase of the liver and activates many enzymes.

Iodine

Iodine is an essential constituent of the thyroid hormones.

Chromium

Chromium is an essential trace element involved in carbohydrate metabolism.

Molybdenum

Molybdenum is an essential trace element although there have been no reports of deficiency states in man. Molybdenum salts have been used to treat copper poisoning in sheep.

Calcium Caseinate

Calcium caseinate is the sole protein source in Forceval Protein Powder. It is a high biological value protein containing all ten essential and eight other nutritionally important amino acids.

Essential amino acids cannot be synthesised by the body and are necessary for the synthesis of most proteins and some non-protein substances e.g. phenylalanine is required to produce the hormones adrenaline and thyroxine. Insulin has more than 50% of its constituent amino acids as essential amino acids. Because these hormones are removed from the body once their effect is exerted, there is a constant need for their renewal, hence a constant need for a source of essential amino acids in the diet. If amino acids are not available in the diet they have to be supplied by the breakdown of other body proteins. During starvation and malnutrition and following surgical operations or in patients with severe burns, a negative nitrogen balance occurs in which the nitrogen (from proteins and amino acids) lost from the body exceeds the intake.

5.2 Pharmacokinetic properties

Vitamin A

Except when liver function is impaired, Vitamin A is readily absorbed. Vitamin A esters (such as Vitamin A Acetate in Forceval Protein Powder) are largely hydrolysed to retinol which is emulsified by bile salts and phospholipids and absorbed in a micellar form. Part is conjugated with glucuronic acid in the kidney and part is metabolised in the liver and kidney, leaving 30 to 50% of the dose for storage in the liver. It is bound to a globulin in the blood. Metabolites of Vitamin A are excreted in the faeces and the urine.

Vitamin D

Cholecalciferol is absorbed from the gastro-intestinal tract into the circulation. In the liver, it is hydroxylated to 25-hydroxycholecalciferol, is subject to entero-hepatic circulation and is further hydroxylated to 1,25-dihydroxycholecalciferol in the renal tubule cells. Vitamin D metabolites are bound to specific plasma proteins.

Vitamin B_1 (Thiamine)

Thiamine is absorbed from the gastro-intestinal tract and is widely distributed to most body tissues. Amounts in excess of the body's requirements are not stored but excreted in the urine as unchanged thiamine or its metabolites.

Vitamin B_2 (Riboflavine)

Riboflavine is absorbed from the gastro-intestinal tract and in the circulation is bound to plasma proteins. It is widely distributed. Little is stored and excess amounts are excreted in the urine. In the body riboflavine is converted to flavine mononucleotide (FMN) and then to flavine adenine dinucleotide (FAD).

Vitamin B_6 (Pyridoxine)

Pyridoxine is absorbed from the gastro-intestinal tract and converted to the active pyridoxal phosphate which is bound to plasma proteins. It is excreted in the urine as 4-pyridoxic acid.

Vitamin B_{12} (Cyanocobalamin)

Cyanocobalamin is absorbed from the gastro-intestinal tract and is extensively bound to specific plasma proteins. A study with labelled Vitamin B_{12} showed it was quickly taken up by the intestinal mucosa and held there for 2-3 hours. Peak concentrations in the blood and tissues did not occur until 8-12 hours after dosage with maximum concentrations in the liver within 24 hours. Cobalamins are stored in the liver, excreted in the bile and undergo enterohepatic recycling. Part of a dose is excreted in the urine, most of it in the first eight hours.

Vitamin C (Ascorbic Acid)

Ascorbic acid is readily absorbed from the gastro-intestinal tract and is widely distributed in the body tissues. Ascorbic acid in excess of the body's needs is rapidly eliminated in the urine and this elimination is usually accompanied by a mild diuresis.

Vitamin E

Vitamin E is absorbed from the gastro-intestinal tract. Most appears in the lymph and is then widely distributed to all tissues. Most of a dose is slowly excreted in the bile and the remainder is eliminated in the urine as glucuronides of tocopheronic acid or other metabolites.

Nicotinamide (Nicotinic Acid Amide)

Nicotinic acid is absorbed from the gastro-intestinal tract, is widely distributed in the body tissues and has a short half-life.

Calcium

A third of ingested calcium is absorbed from the small intestine. Absorption of calcium decreases with age.

Phosphorus

The body contains from 600-800 g of phosphorus, over 80% of which is present in bone as phosphate salts, mainly hydroxyapatite crystals. The phosphate in these crystals is available for exchange with phosphate ions in the extracellular fluids.

Calcium Pantothenate

Pantothenic acid is readily absorbed from the gastro-intestinal tract and is widely distributed in the body tissues. About 70% of pantothenic acid is excreted unchanged in the urine and about 30% in the faeces.

Folic Acid

Folic acid is absorbed mainly from the proximal part of the small intestine. Folate polyglutamates are considered to be deconjugated to monoglutamates during absorption. Folic acid rapidly appears in the blood where it is extensively bound to plasma proteins. Some Folic acid is distributed in body tissues, some is excreted as folate in the urine and some is stored in the liver as folate.

Vitamin H (d-Biotin)

Following absorption, biotin is stored in the liver, kidney and pancreas.

Selenium

Although it has been established that selenium is essential to human life, very little information is available on its function and metabolism.

Iron

Iron is absorbed chiefly in the duodenum and jejunum. Absorption is aided by the acid secretion of the stomach. In conditions of iron deficiency, absorption is increased and, conversely, it is decreased in iron overload. Iron is stored as ferritin.

Copper

Copper is absorbed from the gastro-intestinal tract and its major route of excretion is in the bile.

Magnesium

Magnesium salts are poorly absorbed from the gastro-intestinal tract; however, sufficient magnesium will normally be absorbed to replace deficiency states. Magnesium is excreted in both the urine and the faeces but excretion is reduced in deficiency states.

Potassium

Potassium salts are absorbed from the gastro-intestinal tract. Potassium is excreted in the urine, the faeces and in perspiration. Urinary excretion of potassium continues even when intake is low.

Zinc

Zinc is poorly absorbed from the gastro-intestinal tract. It is widely distributed throughout the body. It is excreted in the faeces with traces appearing in the urine.

Manganese

Manganese salts are poorly absorbed.

Iodine

Iodides are absorbed and stored in the thyroid gland as thyroglobulin. Iodides are excreted in the urine with smaller amounts appearing in the faeces, saliva and sweat.

Chromium

Although it has been established that chromium is essential to human life, little information is available on its function and metabolism.

Molybdenum

Although it has been established that molybdenum is essential to human life, little information is available on its function and metabolism.

Calcium Caseinate

Calcium caseinate is metabolised by the body to its constituent amino acids, as are other proteins.

5.3 Preclinical safety data

There are no pre-clinical data of relevance to the prescriber which are additional to that already included in other sections of the SPC.

6. PHARMACEUTICAL PARTICULARS

6.1 List of excipients

Butylated Hydroxyanisole BP

Sodium Benzoate BP

Vanilla Flavour HSE

Sucrose BP

Dextrose Monohydrate BP

6.2 Incompatibilities

No major incompatibilities are known.

6.3 Shelf life

36 months, as packaged for sale.

6.4 Special precautions for storage

Store in a cool, dry place at a temperature not exceeding 25°C (77°F) protected from light.

6.5 Nature and contents of container

a) Composite cans (aluminium lined cardboard cylinder sealed with a solid metal base and aluminium pull tab diaphragm) with resealable plastic plug lid. 38 ml opaque scoop included in can with leaflet under plastic plug lid.

b) Sachets - paper/polythene/aluminium foil laminated. Leaflet in carton with sachets.

The product may be available in three pack sizes:

i) 300 g cans

ii) 15 g sachets in a carton

iii) 30 g sachets in a carton

6.6 Instructions for use and handling

Please refer to the patient information leaflet for detailed use of the product, including mixing instructions and use of the scoop.

7. MARKETING AUTHORISATION HOLDER

Alliance Pharmaceuticals Ltd

Avonbridge House

2 Bath Road

Chippenham

Wiltshire

SN15 2BB

United Kingdom

8. MARKETING AUTHORISATION NUMBER(S)

PL 16853/0081

9. DATE OF FIRST AUTHORISATION/RENEWAL OF THE AUTHORISATION

18th April 2005

10. DATE OF REVISION OF THE TEXT

April 2005

Forceval Protein Powder - Strawberry

(Alliance Pharmaceuticals)

1. NAME OF THE MEDICINAL PRODUCT

Forceval Protein Powder (Strawberry Flavour)

2. QUALITATIVE AND QUANTITATIVE COMPOSITION

Each 60 g of product provide:

Vitamin A	HSE	2500.0 iu (750 mcg)
Vitamin B1 (Thiamin)	HSE	1.5 mg
Vitamin B2 (Riboflavin)	BP	1.5 mg
Vitamin B3 (Nicotinamide)	HSE	18.0 mg
Vitamin B5 (Pantothenic Acid)	PhEur	6.0 mg
Vitamin B6 (Pyridoxine)	BP	2.0 mg
Vitamin B12 (Cyanocobalamin)	HSE	2.0 mcg
Vitamin B Complex (Folic Acid)	HSE	400.0 mcg
Vitamin C (Ascorbic Acid)	HSE	120.0 mg
Vitamin D3 (Cholecalciferol)	HSE	400.0 iu (10 mcg)
Vitamin E	HSE	10.0 mg
Vitamin H (Biotin)	HSE	100.0 mcg
Calcium	HSE	550.0 mg*
Magnesium	BP	300.0 mg
Iron	FCC	12.0 mg
Zinc	HSE	15.0 mg
Manganese	USP	4.0 mg
Copper	USP	2.0 mg
Iodine	BP	150.0 mcg
Selenium	HSE	55.0 mcg
Chromium	BP	200.0 mcg
Molybdenum	HSE	250.0 mcg
Calcium Caseinate (Instant)	HSE	
providing:		
Calcium		550.0 mg*
Phosphorus†		293.0 mg (9.45 mmol)
Protein‡		33.0 g
Potassium§		10.0 mg Max (0.26 mmol)
Fat		0.6 g Max
Carbohydrate		18.0 g
Energy (calories)		200.0 kcal (837 kJ)
Sodium		72.0 mg Max (3.1 mmol)
Potassium (total)§		10.0 mg Max (0.26 mmol)
Phosphorus (total) †		300.0 mg (9.7 mmol)

‡ Amino Acid Profile of Forceval Protein Powder:

Arginine #	1.2 g
Histidine #	1.0 g
Leucine #	3.2 g
Isoleucine #	1.8 g
Valine #	2.3 g
Lysine #	2.7 g
Methionine #	1.0 g
Phenylalanine #	1.7 g
Threonine #	1.5 g
Tryptophan #	0.4 g
Cystine	0.1 g
Tyrosine	1.8 g
Alanine	1.0 g
Aspartic Acid	2.3 g
Glutamic Acid	7.1 g
Glycine	0.6 g
Serine	2.0 g
Proline	3.4 g

= essential amino acids.

3. PHARMACEUTICAL FORM

Pink, speckled, fine powder with an odour of strawberry.

4. CLINICAL PARTICULARS

4.1 Therapeutic indications

Forceval Protein Powder may be used as the Protein, Vitamin, Mineral and Trace Elements source in the following situations:-

- As a therapeutic nutritional adjunct in malabsorptive states such as short bowel syndrome, intestinal fistulas, abdominal sepsis and inflammatory bowel disease.

- As a therapeutic nutritional adjunct in conditions leading to hypoproteinaemia such as trauma and burns.

- As a peri-operative therapeutic nutritional support for undernourished patients and patients with sepsis.

RECOMMENDED USES

1. FORCEVAL PROTEIN POWDER is recommended for children over two years of age, adults and the elderly with an inadequate protein, vitamin, mineral and trace element intake resulting from their inability to maintain a well balanced diet.

2. FORCEVAL PROTEIN POWDER is suitable for patients suffering from Protein, Vitamin, Mineral and Trace Element deficiency as a result of failure to absorb their diet, eg. in malabsorption conditions such as Crohn's disease, Inflammatory Bowel disease and in the presence of Bowel Fistulae or following surgery of the bowel.

3. FORCEVAL PROTEIN POWDER is recommended before and after surgery where a balanced nutritional intake is required to ensure rapid healing, prevention of malnutrition and to reduce the likelihood of infection.

4. FORCEVAL PROTEIN POWDER is recommended where additional protein is required following trauma, eg. burns, infection and multiple injuries.

5. FORCEVAL PROTEIN POWDER is recommended where a high protein intake is required, yet other dietary factors need also to be modified, eg. where a low fat diet is needed; where a reduced carbohydrate diet is needed, as in the case of diabetics; and where electrolytes such as sodium, potassium and phosphorus may need to be reduced eg. in certain heart or kidney conditions.

6. FORCEVAL PROTEIN POWDER is recommended for patients who develop a condition called hypoproteinaemia; this is a condition where the level of protein in the blood is substantially reduced. This can occur in many medical and surgical conditions such as malabsorption, anorexia, carcinoma, following injury or surgery etc. In the case of injury or surgery, damaged tissue needs replacing with new tissue; this requires considerable additional protein. Many of these conditions are accompanied by loss of appetite and possibly altered taste sensations and subclinical Vitamin, Mineral and Trace Element deficiency.

7. FORCEVAL PROTEIN POWDER can be used in conjunction with a calorie controlled, high protein diet under medical supervision - 60g will provide 25 essential Vitamins, Minerals and Trace Elements in line with the UK Dietary Reference Values and US Recommended Dietary Allowances.

4.2 Posology and method of administration

The route of administration is oral or naso-gastric.

ADULTS AND ELDERLY PATIENTS

Sachets: 1-2 × 30g Sachet or 2-4 × 15g (30g-60g) Sachets daily or as prescribed by the doctor.

300 g tins: 2-4 level scoops (30g-60g approx) daily or as prescribed by the doctor.

CHILDREN (ABOVE 2 YEARS OF AGE)

Sachets: 1-2 × 15g Sachets (15g-30g) daily or as prescribed by the doctor.

1 × 30g Sachet daily or as prescribed by the doctor.

300 g tins: 1-2 level scoops (15g-30g) daily or as prescribed by the doctor.

1 level scoop of powder = 15g approx.

Each tin contains a 38ml plastic scoop.

60g of Forceval Protein Powder will provide Vitamins and Minerals in line with the UK Dietary Reference Values and US Recommended Dietary Allowances

Recommended Dilution

15g of Forceval Protein Powder in 125 ml liquid (¼ pint)

30g of Forceval Protein Powder in 250 ml liquid (½ pint)

Extra liquid can be added if a thinner consistency is required

Do not exceed the stated dose.

4.3 Contraindications

Forceval Protein Powder is contra-indicated in patients with renal or hepatic failure and in children below 2 years of age.

4.4 Special warnings and special precautions for use

Forceval Protein Powder is formulated as a nutritional supplement. It is not a total feed or total food replacement and must not be used as such.

It should be used as the protein, vitamin and mineral source in total feed systems, combined with an additional energy source, carbohydrate (such as Caloreen, a glucose polymer) and/or fat (LCT or MCT emulsions), to give energy: N, osmolality and calorific values suitable for individual patient requirements.

Ideally the energy: N ratio should be between 100 and 200 kcal/g N and the osmolality of the total feed as near as possible to 300 m osmol/kg.

Patients on lactose-free diets should not use milk or dilu-ents containing milk or milk products to mix with Forceval Protein Powder.

Prepared drinks should not be heated as the nutritional values of the essential proteins and vitamins will be impaired.

When Forceval Protein is mixed with milk, osmolality pro-blems should be anticipated at the extremes of age.

No other vitamins, minerals or supplements with vitamin A should be taken with this preparation except under close medical supervision.

Do not exceed the stated dose.

The label will state:

Important warning: Contains iron. Keep out of the reach and sight of children, as overdose may be fatal.

This will appear on the front of the pack and on the sachet in a rectangle in which there is no other information.

This product contains 8g sucrose per sachet. This should be taken into account in patients with diabetes mellitus.

4.5 Interaction with other medicinal products and other forms of Interaction

Folic acid can reduce the plasma concentration of pheny-toin. Oral iron and zinc sulphate reduce the absorption of tetracyclines.

4.6 Pregnancy and lactation

Forceval Protein Powder may be administered during pregnancy and lactation at the recommendation of the physician.

4.7 Effects on ability to drive and use machines

Not applicable.

4.8 Undesirable effects

If the product is re-constituted as described, together with an additional energy source, to give the required energy:-nitrogen ratio and osmolality, it is unlikely that undesirable effects will occur. However, prescribers should be aware of the potential risks of diarrhoea, dehydration, electrolyte imbalance, hyperglycaemia and osmolal disorders.

Care should be taken when administering some medica-tions concurrently with Forceval Protein Powder, or shortly thereafter.

The possibility of infection risk should be noted if the nutritional supplement is prepared in unsatisfactory con-ditions.

4.9 Overdose

No cases of overdosage due to Forceval Protein Powder have been reported. Overdosage is extremely unlikely if the dosage recommendations are followed. Any symptoms which may be observed due to ingestion of large quantities of Forceval Protein Powder will be due to hyperproteinae-mia.

5. PHARMACOLOGICAL PROPERTIES

5.1 Pharmacodynamic properties

Vitamin A

Vitamin A plays an important role in the visual process. It is isomerised to the 11-cis isomer and subsequently bound to the opsin to form the photoreceptor for vision under subdued light. One of the earliest symptoms of deficiency is night blindness which may develop into the more serious condition xerophthalmia. Vitamin A also participates in the formation and maintenance of the integrity of epithelial tissues and mucous membranes. Deficiency may cause skin changes resulting in a dry rough skin with lowered resistance to minor skin infections. Deficiency of Vitamin A, usually accompanied by protein-energy malnutrition, is linked with a frequency of infection and with defective immunological defence mechanisms.

Vitamin D

Vitamin D is required for the absorption of calcium and phosphate from the gastro-intestinal tract and for their transport. Its involvement in the control of calcium meta-bolism and hence the normal calcification of bones is well documented. Deficiency of Vitamin D in children may result in the development of rickets.

Vitamin B_1 (Thiamine)

Thiamine (as the coenzyme, thiamine pyrophosphate) is associated with carbohydrate metabolism. Thiamine pyr-ophosphate also acts as a co-enzyme in the direct oxida-tive pathway of glucose metabolism. In thiamine deficiency, pyruvic and lactic acids accumulate in the tissues. The pyruvate ion is involved in the biosynthesis of acetylcholine via its conversion to acetyl co-enzyme A through a thiamine-dependent process. In thiamine defi-ciency, therefore, there are effects on the central nervous system due either to the effect on acetylcholine synthesis or to the lactate and pyruvate accumulation. Deficiency of thiamine results in fatigue, anorexia, gastro-intestinal dis-turbances, tachycardia, irritability and neurological symp-toms. Gross deficiency of thiamine (and other Vitamin B group factors) leads to the condition beri-beri.

Vitamin B_2 (Riboflavine)

Riboflavine is phosphorylated to flavine mononucleotide and flavine adenine dinucleotide, which act as co-enzymes in the respiratory chain and in oxidative phosphorylation. Riboflavine deficiency presents with ocular symptoms, as well as lesions on the lips and at the angles of the mouth.

Vitamin B_6 (Pyridoxine)

Pyridoxine, once absorbed, is rapidly converted to the co-enzymes, pyridoxal phosphate and pyridoxamine phos-phate which play an essential role in protein metabolism. Convulsions and hypochromic anaemia have occurred in infants deficient in pyridoxine.

Vitamin B_{12} (Cyanocobalamin)

Vitamin B_{12} is present in the body mainly as methylcoba-lamin and as adenosylcobalamin and hydroxocobalamin. These act as co-enzymes in the trans methylation of homo-cysteine to methionine; in the isomerization of methylma-lonyl co-enzyme to succinyl co-enzyme and with folate in several metabolic pathways respectively. Deficiency of Vitamin B_{12} interferes with haemopoiesis and produces megaloblastic anaemia.

Vitamin C (Ascorbic Acid)

Vitamin C cannot be synthesised by man, therefore, a dietary source is necessary. It acts as a cofactor in numer-ous biological processes including the hydroxylation of proline to hydroxyproline. In deficiency, the formation of collagen is, therefore, impaired. Ascorbic acid is important in the hydroxylation of dopamine to noradrenaline and in hydroxylations occurring in steroid synthesis in the adre-nals. It is a reducing agent in tyrosine metabolism and by acting as an electron donor in the conversion of folic acid to tetrahydrofolic acid is indirectly involved in the synthesis of purine and thymine. Vitamin C is also necessary for the incorporation of iron into ferritin. Vitamin C increases the phagocytic function of leucocytes; it possesses anti-inflammatory activity and it promotes wound healing. Defi-ciency can produce scurvy. Features include swollen inflamed gums, petechial haemorrhages and subcuta-neous bruising. The deficiency of collagen leads to devel-opment of thin watery ground substances in which blood vessels are insecurely fixed and readily ruptured. The supportive components of bone and cartilage are also deficient causing bones to fracture easily and teeth to become loose. Anaemia commonly occurs probably due to Vitamin C's role in the iron metabolism.

Vitamin E

Vitamin E deficiency has been linked to disorders such as cystic fibrosis where fat absorption is impaired. It is essen-tial for the normal function of the muscular system and the blood.

Nicotinamide

The biochemical functions of nicotinamide as NAD and NADP (nicotinamide adenine dinucleotide phosphate) include the degradation and synthesis of fatty acids, car-bohydrates and amino acids as well as hydrogen transfer. Deficiency produces pellagra and mental and neurological changes.

Calcium

Calcium is an essential body electrolyte. It is involved in the maintenance of normal muscle and nerve function and essential for normal cardiac function and the clotting of blood. Calcium is mainly found in the bones and teeth. Deficiency of calcium leads to rickets, osteomalacia in children and osteoporosis in the elderly.

Phosphorus

Phosphate plays important roles in the osteoblastic and osteoclastic reactions. It interacts with calcium to modify the balance between these two processes. Organic phos-phate esters play a key role in the metabolism of carbohy-drates, fats and proteins and in the formation of 'high energy phosphate' compounds. Phosphate also acts as a buffer and plays a role in the renal excretion of sodium and hydrogen ions.

Pantothenic Acid

Pantothenic acid is incorporated into co-enzyme A and is involved in metabolic pathways involving acetylation which includes detoxification of drug molecules and biosynthesis of cholesterol, steroid hormones, mucopolysaccharides and acetylcholine. CoA has an essential function in lipid metabolism.

Folic Acid

Folic acid is reduced in the body to tetrahydrofolate which is a co-enzyme for various metabolic processes, including the synthesis of purine and pyrimidine nucleotides and hence in the synthesis of DNA. It is also involved in some amino acid conversion and in the formation and utilisation of formate. Deficiency of folic acid leads to megaloblastic anaemia.

Vitamin H (d-Biotin)

Biotin is a co-enzyme for carboxylation during the meta-bolism of proteins and carbohydrates.

Selenium

Selenium is an essential trace element, deficiency of which has been reported in man. It is thought to be involved in the functioning of membranes and the synthesis of amino acids. Deficiency of selenium in the diet of experimental animals produces fatty liver followed by necrosis.

Iron

Iron, as a constituent of haemoglobin, plays an essential role in oxygen transport. It is also present in the muscle protein myoglobin and in the liver. Deficiency of iron leads to anaemia.

Copper

Traces of copper are essential to the body as constituents of enzyme systems involved in oxidation reactions.

Magnesium

Magnesium is essential to the body as a constituent of skeletal structures and in maintaining cell integrity and fluid balance. It is utilised in many of the functions in which calcium is concerned but often exerts the opposite effect. Some enzymes require the magnesium ion as a co-factor.

Potassium

Potassium is the principle cation of intracellular fluid and is intimately involved in the cell function and metabolism. It is essential for carbohydrate metabolism and glycogen sto-rage and protein synthesis and is involved in transmem-brane potential where it is necessary to maintain the resting potential in excitable cells. Potassium ions maintain intra-cellular pH and osmotic pressure. Prolonged or severe diarrhoea may lead to potassium deficiency.

Zinc

Zinc is a constituent of many enzymes and is, therefore, essential to the body. It is present with insulin in the pancreas. It plays a role in DNA synthesis and cell division. Reported effects of deficiency include delayed puberty and hypogonadal dwarfism.

Manganese

Manganese is a constituent of enzyme systems including those involved in lipid synthesis, the tricarboxylic acid cycle and purine and pyrimidine metabolism. It is bound to arginase of the liver and activates many enzymes.

Iodine

Iodine is an essential constituent of the thyroid hormones.

Chromium

Chromium is an essential trace element involved in carbo-hydrate metabolism.

Molybdenum

Molybdenum is an essential trace element although there have been no reports of deficiency states in man. Molyb-denum salts have been used to treat copper poisoning in sheep.

Calcium Caseinate

Calcium caseinate is the sole protein source in Forceval Protein Powder. It is a high biological value protein contain-ing all ten essential and eight other nutritionally important amino acids.

Essential amino acids cannot be synthesised by the body and are necessary for the synthesis of most proteins and some non-protein substances e.g. phenylalanine is required to produce the hormones adrenaline and thyrox-ine. Insulin has more than 50% of its constituent amino acids as essential amino acids. Because these hormones are removed from the body once their effect is exerted, there is a constant need for their renewal, hence a constant need for a source of essential amino acids in the diet. If amino acids are not available in the diet they have to be supplied by the breakdown of other body proteins. During starvation and malnutrition and following surgical opera-tions or in patients with severe burns, a negative nitrogen balance occurs in which the nitrogen (from proteins and amino acids) lost from the body exceeds the intake.

5.2 Pharmacokinetic properties

Vitamin A

Except when liver function is impaired, Vitamin A is readily absorbed. Vitamin A esters (such as Vitamin A Acetate in Forceval Protein Powder) are largely hydrolysed to retinol which is emulsified by bile salts and phospholipids and absorbed in a micellar form. Part is conjugated with glu-curonic acid in the kidney and part is metabolised in the liver and kidney, leaving 30 to 50% of the dose for storage in the liver. It is bound to a globulin in the blood. Metabo-lites of Vitamin A are excreted in the faeces and the urine.

Vitamin D

Cholecalciferol is absorbed from the gastro-intestinal tract into the circulation. In the liver, it is hydroxylated to 25-hydroxycholecalciferol, is subject to entero-hepatic circu-lation and is further hydroxylated to 1,25-dihydroxychole-calciferol in the renal tubule cells. Vitamin D metabolites are bound to specific plasma proteins.

Vitamin B_1 (Thiamine)

Thiamine is absorbed from the gastro-intestinal tract and is widely distributed to most body tissues. Amounts in excess of the body's requirements are not stored but excreted in the urine as unchanged thiamine or its metabolites.

Vitamin B_2 (Riboflavine)

Riboflavine is absorbed from the gastro-intestinal tract and in the circulation is bound to plasma proteins. It is widely distributed. Little is stored and excess amounts are excreted in the urine. In the body riboflavine is converted to flavine mononucleotide (FMN) and then to flavine ade-nine dinucleotide (FAD).

Vitamin B_6 (Pyridoxine)

Pyridoxine is absorbed from the gastro-intestinal tract and converted to the active pyridoxal phosphate which is bound to plasma proteins. It is excreted in the urine as 4-pyridoxic acid.

Vitamin B_{12} (Cyanocobalamin)

Cyanocobalamin is absorbed from the gastro-intestinal tract and is extensively bound to specific plasma proteins. A study with labelled Vitamin B_{12} showed it was quickly taken up by the intestinal mucosa and held there for 2-3 hours. Peak concentrations in the blood and tissues did not occur until 8-12 hours after dosage with maximum concentrations in the liver within 24 hours. Cobalamins are stored in the liver, excreted in the bile and undergo enterohepatic recycling. Part of a dose is excreted in the urine, most of it in the first eight hours.

Vitamin C (Ascorbic Acid)

Ascorbic acid is readily absorbed from the gastro-intestinal tract and is widely distributed in the body tissues. Ascorbic acid in excess of the body's needs is rapidly eliminated in the urine and this elimination is usually accompanied by a mild diuresis.

Vitamin E

Vitamin E is absorbed from the gastro-intestinal tract. Most appears in the lymph and is then widely distributed to all tissues. Most of a dose is slowly excreted in the bile and the remainder is eliminated in the urine as glucuronides of tocopheronic acid or other metabolites.

Nicotinamide (Nicotinic Acid Amide)

Nicotinic acid is absorbed from the gastro-intestinal tract, is widely distributed in the body tissues and has a short half-life.

Calcium

A third of ingested calcium is absorbed from the small intestine. Absorption of calcium decreases with age.

Phosphorus

The body contains from 600-800 g of phosphorus, over 80% of which is present in bone as phosphate salts, mainly hydroxyapatite crystals. The phosphate in these crystals is available for exchange with phosphate ions in the extracellular fluids.

Calcium Pantothenate

Pantothenic acid is readily absorbed from the gastro-intestinal tract and is widely distributed in the body tissues. About 70% of pantothenic acid is excreted unchanged in the urine and about 30% in the faeces.

Folic Acid

Folic acid is absorbed mainly from the proximal part of the small intestine. Folate polyglutamates are considered to be deconjugated to monoglutamates during absorption. Folic acid rapidly appears in the blood where it is extensively bound to plasma proteins. Some Folic acid is distributed in body tissues, some is excreted as folate in the urine and some is stored in the liver as folate.

Vitamin H (d-Biotin)

Following absorption, biotin is stored in the liver, kidney and pancreas.

Selenium

Although it has been established that selenium is essential to human life, very little information is available on its function and metabolism.

Iron

Iron is absorbed chiefly in the duodenum and jejunum. Absorption is aided by the acid secretion of the stomach. In conditions of iron deficiency, absorption is increased and, conversely, it is decreased in iron overload. Iron is stored as ferritin.

Copper

Copper is absorbed from the gastro-intestinal tract and its major route of excretion is in the bile.

Magnesium

Magnesium salts are poorly absorbed from the gastro-intestinal tract; however, sufficient magnesium will normally be absorbed to replace deficiency states. Magnesium is excreted in both the urine and the faeces but excretion is reduced in deficiency states.

Potassium

Potassium salts are absorbed from the gastro-intestinal tract. Potassium is excreted in the urine, the faeces and in perspiration. Urinary excretion of potassium continues even when intake is low.

Zinc

Zinc is poorly absorbed from the gastro-intestinal tract. It is widely distributed throughout the body. It is excreted in the faeces with traces appearing in the urine.

Manganese

Manganese salts are poorly absorbed.

Iodine

Iodides are absorbed and stored in the thyroid gland as thyroglobulin. Iodides are excreted in the urine with smaller amounts appearing in the faeces, saliva and sweat.

Chromium

Although it has been established that chromium is essential to human life, little information is available on its function and metabolism.

Molybdenum

Although it has been established that molybdenum is essential to human life, little information is available on its function and metabolism.

Calcium Caseinate

Calcium caseinate is metabolised by the body to its constituent amino acids, as are other proteins.

5.3 Preclinical safety data

There are no pre-clinical data of relevance to the prescriber which are additional to that already included in other sections of the SPC.

6. PHARMACEUTICAL PARTICULARS

6.1 List of excipients

Butylated Hydroxyanisole BP

Sodium Benzoate BP

Strawberry Flavour HSE

Pink Colour (E127) HSE

Sucrose BP

6.2 Incompatibilities

No major incompatibilities are known.

6.3 Shelf life

36 months, as packaged for sale.

6.4 Special precautions for storage

Store in a cool, dry place at a temperature not exceeding 25°C (77°F) protected from light.

6.5 Nature and contents of container

a) Composite cans (aluminium lined cardboard cylinder sealed with a solid metal base and aluminium pull tab diaphragm) with resealable plastic plug lid. 38 ml opaque scoop included in can with leaflet under plastic plug lid.

b) Sachets - paper/polythene/aluminium foil laminated. Leaflet in carton with sachets.

The product may be available in three pack sizes:

i) 300 g cans

ii) 15 g sachets in a carton

iii) 30 g sachets in a carton

6.6 Instructions for use and handling

Please refer to the patient information leaflet for detailed use of the product, including mixing instructions and use of the scoop.

7. MARKETING AUTHORISATION HOLDER

Alliance Pharmaceuticals Ltd

Avonbridge House

2 Bath Road

Chippenham

Wiltshire

SN15 2BB

United Kingdom

8. MARKETING AUTHORISATION NUMBER(S)

PL 16853/0083

9. DATE OF FIRST AUTHORISATION/RENEWAL OF THE AUTHORISATION

18th April 2005

10. DATE OF REVISION OF THE TEXT

April 2005

Forceval Protein Powder - Vanilla

(Alliance Pharmaceuticals)

1. NAME OF THE MEDICINAL PRODUCT

Forceval Protein Powder (Vanilla Flavour)

2. QUALITATIVE AND QUANTITATIVE COMPOSITION

Each 60 g of product provide:

Vitamin A	HSE	2500.0 iu (750 mcg)
Vitamin B1 (Thiamin)	HSE	1.5 mg
Vitamin B2 (Riboflavin)	BP	1.5 mg
Vitamin B3 (Nicotinamide)	HSE	18.0 mg
Vitamin B5 (Pantothenic Acid)	PhEur	6.0 mg
Vitamin B6 (Pyridoxine)	BP	2.0 mg
Vitamin B12 (Cyanocobalamin)	HSE	2.0 mcg
Vitamin B Complex (Folic Acid)	HSE	400.0 mcg
Vitamin C (Ascorbic Acid)	HSE	120.0 mg
Vitamin D3 (Cholecalciferol)	HSE	400.0 iu (10 mcg)
Vitamin E	HSE	10.0 mg
Vitamin H (Biotin)	HSE	100.0 mcg
Calcium	HSE	550.0 mg*
Magnesium	BP	300.0 mg
Iron	FCC	12.0 mg
Zinc	HSE	15.0 mg
Manganese	USP	4.0 mg
Copper	USP	2.0 mg
Iodine	BP	150.0 mcg
Selenium	HSE	55.0 mcg
Chromium	BP	200.0 mcg
Molybdenum	HSE	250.0 mcg
Calcium Caseinate (Instant)	HSE	
providing:		
Calcium		550.0 mg*
Phosphorus†		293.0 mg (9.45 mmol)
Protein‡		33.0 g
Potassium§		10.0 mg Max (0.26 mmol)
Fat		0.6 g Max
Carbohydrate		18.0 g
Energy (calories)		200.0 kcal (837 kJ)
Sodium		72.0 mg Max (3.1 mmol)
Potassium (total)§		10.0 mg Max (0.26 mmol)
Phosphorus (total) †		300.0 mg (9.7 mmol)

‡ Amino Acid Profile of Forceval Protein Powder:

Arginine #	1.2 g
Histidine #	1.0 g
Leucine #	3.2 g
Isoleucine #	1.8 g
Valine #	2.3 g
Lysine #	2.7 g
Methionine #	1.0 g
Phenylalanine #	1.7 g
Threonine #	1.5 g
Tryptophan #	0.4 g
Cystine	0.1 g
Tyrosine	1.8 g
Alanine	1.0 g
Aspartic Acid	2.3 g
Glutamic Acid	7.1 g
Glycine	0.6 g
Serine	2.0 g
Proline	3.4 g

= essential amino acids.

3. PHARMACEUTICAL FORM

White to off-white, speckled, fine powder with an odour of vanilla.

4. CLINICAL PARTICULARS

4.1 Therapeutic indications

Forceval Protein Powder may be used as the Protein, Vitamin, Mineral and Trace Elements source in the following situations:-

- As a therapeutic nutritional adjunct in malabsorptive states such as short bowel syndrome, intestinal fistulas, abdominal sepsis and inflammatory bowel disease.

- As a therapeutic nutritional adjunct in conditions leading to hypoproteinaemia such as trauma and burns.

- As a peri-operative therapeutic nutritional support for undernourished patients and patients with sepsis.

RECOMMENDED USES

1. FORCEVAL PROTEIN POWDER is recommended for children over two years of age, adults and the elderly with an inadequate protein, vitamin, mineral and trace element intake resulting from their inability to maintain a well balanced diet.

2. FORCEVAL PROTEIN POWDER is suitable for patients suffering from Protein, Vitamin, Mineral and Trace Element deficiency as a result of failure to absorb their diet, eg. in malabsorption conditions such as Crohn's disease, Inflammatory Bowel disease and in the presence of Bowel Fistulae or following surgery of the bowel.

3. FORCEVAL PROTEIN POWDER is recommended before and after surgery where a balanced nutritional intake is required to ensure rapid healing, prevention of malnutrition and to reduce the likelihood of infection.

4. FORCEVAL PROTEIN POWDER is recommended where additional protein is required following trauma, eg. burns, infection and multiple injuries.

5. FORCEVAL PROTEIN POWDER is recommended where a high protein intake is required, yet other dietary factors need also to be modified, eg. where a low fat diet is needed; where a reduced carbohydrate diet is needed, as in the case of diabetics; and where electrolytes such as sodium, potassium and phosphorus may need to be reduced eg. in certain heart or kidney conditions.

6. FORCEVAL PROTEIN POWDER is recommended for patients who develop a condition called hypoproteinaemia; this is a condition where the level of protein in the blood is substantially reduced. This can occur in many medical and surgical conditions such as malabsorption, anorexia, carcinoma, following injury or surgery etc. In the case of injury or surgery, damaged tissue needs replacing with new tissue; this requires considerable additional

protein. Many of these conditions are accompanied by loss of appetite and possibly altered taste sensations and subclinical Vitamin, Mineral and Trace Element deficiency.

7. FORCEVAL PROTEIN POWDER can be used in conjunction with a calorie controlled, high protein diet under medical supervision - 60g will provide 25 essential Vitamins, Minerals and Trace Elements in line with the UK Dietary Reference Values and US Recommended Dietary Allowances.

4.2 Posology and method of administration

The route of administration is oral or naso-gastric.

ADULTS AND ELDERLY PATIENTS

Sachets: 1-2 × 30g Sachet or 2-4 × 15g (30g-60g) Sachets daily or as prescribed by the doctor.

300 g tins: 2-4 level scoops (30g-60g approx) daily or as prescribed by the doctor.

CHILDREN (ABOVE 2 YEARS OF AGE)

Sachets: 1-2 × 15g Sachets (15g-30g) daily or as prescribed by the doctor.

1 × 30g Sachet daily or as prescribed by the doctor.

300 g tins: 1-2 level scoops (15g-30g) daily or as prescribed by the doctor.

1 level scoop of powder = 15g approx.

Each tin contains a 38ml plastic scoop.

60g of Forceval Protein Powder will provide Vitamins and Minerals in line with the UK Dietary Reference Values and US Recommended Dietary Allowances

Recommended Dilution

15g of Forceval Protein Powder in 125 ml liquid (¼ pint)

30g of Forceval Protein Powder in 250 ml liquid (½ pint)

Extra liquid can be added if a thinner consistency is required

Do not exceed the stated dose.

4.3 Contraindications

Forceval Protein Powder is contra-indicated in patients with renal or hepatic failure and in children below 2 years of age.

4.4 Special warnings and special precautions for use

Forceval Protein Powder is formulated as a nutritional supplement. It is not a total feed or total food replacement and must not be used as such.

It should be used as the protein, vitamin and mineral source in total feed systems, combined with an additional energy source, carbohydrate (such as Caloreen, a glucose polymer) and/or fat (LCT or MCT emulsions), to give energy: N, osmolality and calorific values suitable for individual patient requirements.

Ideally the energy: N ratio should be between 100 and 200 kcal/g N and the osmolality of the total feed as near as possible to 300 m osmol/kg.

Patients on lactose-free diets should not use milk or diluents containing milk or milk products to mix with Forceval Protein Powder.

Prepared drinks should not be heated as the nutritional values of the essential proteins and vitamins will be impaired.

When Forceval Protein is mixed with milk, osmolality problems should be anticipated at the extremes of age.

No other vitamins, minerals or supplements with vitamin A should be taken with this preparation except under close medical supervision.

Do not exceed the stated dose.

The label will state:

Important warning: Contains iron. Keep out of the reach and sight of children, as overdose may be fatal.

This will appear on the front of the pack and on the sachet in a rectangle in which there is no other information.

This product contains 8g sucrose per dose. This should be taken into account in patients with diabetes mellitus.

4.5 Interaction with other medicinal products and other forms of Interaction

Folic acid can reduce the plasma concentration of phenytoin. Oral iron and zinc sulphate reduce the absorption of tetracyclines.

4.6 Pregnancy and lactation

Forceval Protein Powder may be administered during pregnancy and lactation at the recommendation of the physician.

4.7 Effects on ability to drive and use machines

Not applicable.

4.8 Undesirable effects

If the product is re-constituted as described, together with an additional energy source, to give the required energy:-nitrogen ratio and osmolality, it is unlikely that undesirable effects will occur. However, prescribers should be aware of the potential risks of diarrhoea, dehydration, electrolyte imbalance, hyperglycaemia and osmolal disorders.

Care should be taken when administering some medications concurrently with Forceval Protein Powder, or shortly thereafter.

The possibility of infection risk should be noted if the nutritional supplement is prepared in unsatisfactory conditions.

4.9 Overdose

No cases of overdosage due to Forceval Protein Powder have been reported. Overdosage is extremely unlikely if the dosage recommendations are followed. Any symptoms which may be observed due to ingestion of large quantities of Forceval Protein Powder will be due to hyperproteinaemia.

5. PHARMACOLOGICAL PROPERTIES

5.1 Pharmacodynamic properties

Vitamin A

Vitamin A plays an important role in the visual process. It is isomerised to the 11-cis isomer and subsequently bound to the opsin to form the photoreceptor for vision under subdued light. One of the earliest symptoms of deficiency is night blindness which may develop into the more serious condition xerophthalmia. Vitamin A also participates in the formation and maintenance of the integrity of epithelial tissues and mucous membranes. Deficiency may cause skin changes resulting in a dry rough skin with lowered resistance to minor skin infections. Deficiency of Vitamin A, usually accompanied by protein-energy malnutrition, is linked with a frequency of infection and with defective immunological defence mechanisms.

Vitamin D

Vitamin D is required for the absorption of calcium and phosphate from the gastro-intestinal tract and for their transport. Its involvement in the control of calcium metabolism and hence the normal calcification of bones is well documented. Deficiency of Vitamin D in children may result in the development of rickets.

Vitamin B_1 (Thiamine)

Thiamine (as the coenzyme, thiamine pyrophosphate) is associated with carbohydrate metabolism. Thiamine pyrophosphate also acts as a co-enzyme in the direct oxidative pathway of glucose metabolism. In thiamine deficiency, pyruvic and lactic acids accumulate in the tissues. The pyruvate ion is involved in the biosynthesis of acetylcholine via its conversion to acetyl co-enzyme A through a thiamine-dependent process. In thiamine deficiency, therefore, there are effects on the central nervous system due either to the effect on acetylcholine synthesis or to the lactate and pyruvate accumulation. Deficiency of thiamine results in fatigue, anorexia, gastro-intestinal disturbances, tachycardia, irritability and neurological symptoms. Gross deficiency of thiamine (and other Vitamin B group factors) leads to the condition beri-beri.

Vitamin B_2 (Riboflavine)

Riboflavine is phosphorylated to flavine mononucleotide and flavine adenine dinucleotide, which act as co-enzymes in the respiratory chain and in oxidative phosphorylation. Riboflavine deficiency presents with ocular symptoms, as well as lesions on the lips and at the angles of the mouth.

Vitamin B_6 (Pyridoxine)

Pyridoxine, once absorbed, is rapidly converted to the co-enzymes, pyridoxal phosphate and pyridoxamine phosphate which play an essential role in protein metabolism. Convulsions and hypochromic anaemia have occurred in infants deficient in pyridoxine.

Vitamin B_{12} (Cyanocobalamin)

Vitamin B_{12} is present in the body mainly as methylcobalamin and as adenosylcobalamin and hydroxocobalamin. These act as co-enzymes in the trans methylation of homocysteine to methionine; in the isomerization of methylmalonyl co-enzyme to succinyl co-enzyme and with folate in several metabolic pathways respectively. Deficiency of Vitamin B_{12} interferes with haemopoiesis and produces megaloblastic anaemia.

Vitamin C (Ascorbic Acid)

Vitamin C cannot be synthesised by man, therefore, a dietary source is necessary. It acts as a cofactor in numerous biological processes including the hydroxylation of proline to hydroxyproline. In deficiency, the formation of collagen is, therefore, impaired. Ascorbic acid is important in the hydroxylation of dopamine to noradrenaline and in hydroxylations occurring in steroid synthesis in the adrenals. It is a reducing agent in tyrosine metabolism and by acting as an electron donor in the conversion of folic acid to tetrahydrofolic acid is indirectly involved in the synthesis of purine and thymine. Vitamin C is also necessary for the incorporation of iron into ferritin. Vitamin C increases the phagocytic function of leucocytes; it possesses anti-inflammatory activity and it promotes wound healing. Deficiency can produce scurvy. Features include swollen inflamed gums, petechial haemorrhages and subcutaneous bruising. The deficiency of collagen leads to development of thin watery ground substances in which blood vessels are insecurely fixed and readily ruptured. The supportive components of bone and cartilage are also deficient causing bones to fracture easily and teeth to become loose. Anaemia commonly occurs probably due to Vitamin C's role in the iron metabolism.

Vitamin E

Vitamin E deficiency has been linked to disorders such as cystic fibrosis where fat absorption is impaired. It is essential for the normal function of the muscular system and the blood.

Nicotinamide

The biochemical functions of nicotinamide as NAD and NADP (nicotinamide adenine dinucleotide phosphate) include the degradation and synthesis of fatty acids, carbohydrates and amino acids as well as hydrogen transfer. Deficiency produces pellagra and mental and neurological changes.

Calcium

Calcium is an essential body electrolyte. It is involved in the maintenance of normal muscle and nerve function and essential for normal cardiac function and the clotting of blood. Calcium is mainly found in the bones and teeth. Deficiency of calcium leads to rickets, osteomalacia in children and osteoporosis in the elderly.

Phosphorus

Phosphate plays important roles in the osteoblastic and osteoclastic reactions. It interacts with calcium to modify the balance between these two processes. Organic phosphate esters play a key role in the metabolism of carbohydrates, fats and proteins and in the formation of 'high energy phosphate' compounds. Phosphate also acts as a buffer and plays a role in the renal excretion of sodium and hydrogen ions.

Pantothenic Acid

Pantothenic acid is incorporated into co-enzyme A and is involved in metabolic pathways involving acetylation which includes detoxification of drug molecules and biosynthesis of cholesterol, steroid hormones, mucopolysaccharides and acetylcholine. CoA has an essential function in lipid metabolism.

Folic Acid

Folic acid is reduced in the body to tetrahydrofolate which is a co-enzyme for various metabolic processes, including the synthesis of purine and pyrimidine nucleotides and hence in the synthesis of DNA. It is also involved in some amino acid conversion and in the formation and utilisation of formate. Deficiency of folic acid leads to megaloblastic anaemia.

Vitamin H (d-Biotin)

Biotin is a co-enzyme for carboxylation during the metabolism of proteins and carbohydrates.

Selenium

Selenium is an essential trace element, deficiency of which has been reported in man. It is thought to be involved in the functioning of membranes and the synthesis of amino acids. Deficiency of selenium in the diet of experimental animals produces fatty liver followed by necrosis.

Iron

Iron, as a constituent of haemoglobin, plays an essential role in oxygen transport. It is also present in the muscle protein myoglobin and in the liver. Deficiency of iron leads to anaemia.

Copper

Traces of copper are essential to the body as constituents of enzyme systems involved in oxidation reactions.

Magnesium

Magnesium is essential to the body as a constituent of skeletal structures and in maintaining cell integrity and fluid balance. It is utilised in many of the functions in which calcium is concerned but often exerts the opposite effect. Some enzymes require the magnesium ion as a co-factor.

Potassium

Potassium is the principle cation of intracellular fluid and is intimately involved in the cell function and metabolism. It is essential for carbohydrate metabolism and glycogen storage and protein synthesis and is involved in transmembrane potential where it is necessary to maintain the resting potential in excitable cells. Potassium ions maintain intracellular pH and osmotic pressure. Prolonged or severe diarrhoea may lead to potassium deficiency.

Zinc

Zinc is a constituent of many enzymes and is, therefore, essential to the body. It is present with insulin in the pancreas. It plays a role in DNA synthesis and cell division. Reported effects of deficiency include delayed puberty and hypogonadal dwarfism.

Manganese

Manganese is a constituent of enzyme systems including those involved in lipid synthesis, the tricarboxylic acid cycle and purine and pyrimidine metabolism. It is bound to arginase of the liver and activates many enzymes.

Iodine

Iodine is an essential constituent of the thyroid hormones.

Chromium

Chromium is an essential trace element involved in carbohydrate metabolism.

Molybdenum

Molybdenum is an essential trace element although there have been no reports of deficiency states in man. Molybdenum salts have been used to treat copper poisoning in sheep.

Calcium Caseinate

Calcium caseinate is the sole protein source in Forceval Protein Powder. It is a high biological value protein containing all ten essential and eight other nutritionally important amino acids.

Essential amino acids cannot be synthesised by the body and are necessary for the synthesis of most proteins and some non-protein substances e.g. phenylalanine is required to produce the hormones adrenaline and thyroxine. Insulin has more than 50% of its constituent amino acids as essential amino acids. Because these hormones are removed from the body once their effect is exerted, there is a constant need for their renewal, hence a constant need for a source of essential amino acids in the diet. If amino acids are not available in the diet they have to be supplied by the breakdown of other body proteins. During starvation and malnutrition and following surgical operations or in patients with severe burns, a negative nitrogen balance occurs in which the nitrogen (from proteins and amino acids) lost from the body exceeds the intake.

5.2 Pharmacokinetic properties

Vitamin A

Except when liver function is impaired, Vitamin A is readily absorbed. Vitamin A esters (such as Vitamin A Acetate in Forceval Protein Powder) are largely hydrolysed to retinol which is emulsified by bile salts and phospholipids and absorbed in a micellar form. Part is conjugated with glucuronic acid in the kidney and part is metabolised in the liver and kidney, leaving 30 to 50% of the dose for storage in the liver. It is bound to a globulin in the blood. Metabolites of Vitamin A are excreted in the faeces and the urine.

Vitamin D

Cholecalciferol is absorbed from the gastro-intestinal tract into the circulation. In the liver, it is hydroxylated to 25-hydroxycholecalciferol, is subject to entero-hepatic circulation and is further hydroxylated to 1,25-dihydroxycholecalciferol in the renal tubule cells. Vitamin D metabolites are bound to specific plasma proteins.

Vitamin B_1 (Thiamine)

Thiamine is absorbed from the gastro-intestinal tract and is widely distributed to most body tissues. Amounts in excess of the body's requirements are not stored but excreted in the urine as unchanged thiamine or its metabolites.

Vitamin B_2 (Riboflavine)

Riboflavine is absorbed from the gastro-intestinal tract and in the circulation is bound to plasma proteins. It is widely distributed. Little is stored and excess amounts are excreted in the urine. In the body riboflavine is converted to flavine mononucleotide (FMN) and then to flavine adenine dinucleotide (FAD).

Vitamin B_6 (Pyridoxine)

Pyridoxine is absorbed from the gastro-intestinal tract and converted to the active pyridoxal phosphate which is bound to plasma proteins. It is excreted in the urine as 4-pyridoxic acid.

Vitamin B_{12} (Cyanocobalamin)

Cyanocobalamin is absorbed from the gastro-intestinal tract and is extensively bound to specific plasma proteins. A study with labelled Vitamin B_{12} showed it was quickly taken up by the intestinal mucosa and held there for 2-3 hours. Peak concentrations in the blood and tissues did not occur until 8-12 hours after dosage with maximum concentrations in the liver within 24 hours. Cobalamins are stored in the liver, excreted in the bile and undergo enterohepatic recycling. Part of a dose is excreted in the urine, most of it in the first eight hours.

Vitamin C (Ascorbic Acid)

Ascorbic acid is readily absorbed from the gastro-intestinal tract and is widely distributed in the body tissues. Ascorbic acid in excess of the body's needs is rapidly eliminated in the urine and this elimination is usually accompanied by a mild diuresis.

Vitamin E

Vitamin E is absorbed from the gastro-intestinal tract. Most appears in the lymph and is then widely distributed to all tissues. Most of a dose is slowly excreted in the bile and the remainder is eliminated in the urine as glucuronides of tocopheronic acid or other metabolites.

Nicotinamide (Nicotinic Acid Amide)

Nicotinic acid is absorbed from the gastro-intestinal tract, is widely distributed in the body tissues and has a short half-life.

Calcium

A third of ingested calcium is absorbed from the small intestine. Absorption of calcium decreases with age.

Phosphorus

The body contains from 600-800 g of phosphorus, over 80% of which is present in bone as phosphate salts, mainly hydroxyapatite crystals. The phosphate in these crystals is available for exchange with phosphate ions in the extracellular fluids.

Calcium Pantothenate

Pantothenic acid is readily absorbed from the gastro-intestinal tract and is widely distributed in the body tissues. About 70% of pantothenic acid is excreted unchanged in the urine and about 30% in the faeces.

Folic Acid

Folic acid is absorbed mainly from the proximal part of the small intestine. Folate polyglutamates are considered to be deconjugated to monoglutamates during absorption. Folic acid rapidly appears in the blood where it is extensively bound to plasma proteins. Some Folic acid is distributed in body tissues, some is excreted as folate in the urine and some is stored in the liver as folate.

Vitamin H (d-Biotin)

Following absorption, biotin is stored in the liver, kidney and pancreas.

Selenium

Although it has been established that selenium is essential to human life, very little information is available on its function and metabolism.

Iron

Iron is absorbed chiefly in the duodenum and jejunum. Absorption is aided by the acid secretion of the stomach. In conditions of iron deficiency, absorption is increased and, conversely, it is decreased in iron overload. Iron is stored as ferritin.

Copper

Copper is absorbed from the gastro-intestinal tract and its major route of excretion is in the bile.

Magnesium

Magnesium salts are poorly absorbed from the gastro-intestinal tract; however, sufficient magnesium will normally be absorbed to replace deficiency states. Magnesium is excreted in both the urine and the faeces but excretion is reduced in deficiency states.

Potassium

Potassium salts are absorbed from the gastro-intestinal tract. Potassium is excreted in the urine, the faeces and in perspiration. Urinary excretion of potassium continues even when intake is low.

Zinc

Zinc is poorly absorbed from the gastro-intestinal tract. It is widely distributed throughout the body. It is excreted in the faeces with traces appearing in the urine.

Manganese

Manganese salts are poorly absorbed.

Iodine

Iodides are absorbed and stored in the thyroid gland as thyroglobulin. Iodides are excreted in the urine with smaller amounts appearing in the faeces, saliva and sweat.

Chromium

Although it has been established that chromium is essential to human life, little information is available on its function and metabolism.

Molybdenum

Although it has been established that molybdenum is essential to human life, little information is available on its function and metabolism.

Calcium Caseinate

Calcium caseinate is metabolised by the body to its constituent amino acids, as are other proteins.

5.3 Preclinical safety data

There are no pre-clinical data of relevance to the prescriber which are additional to that already included in other sections of the SPC.

6. PHARMACEUTICAL PARTICULARS

6.1 List of excipients

Butylated Hydroxyanisole BP

Sodium Benzoate BP

Vanilla Flavour HSE

Sucrose BP

6.2 Incompatibilities

No major incompatibilities are known.

6.3 Shelf life

36 months, as packaged for sale.

6.4 Special precautions for storage

Store in a cool, dry place at a temperature not exceeding 25°C (77°F) protected from light.

6.5 Nature and contents of container

a) Composite cans (aluminium lined cardboard cylinder sealed with a solid metal base and aluminium pull tab diaphragm) with resealable plastic plug lid. 38 ml opaque scoop included in can with leaflet under plastic plug lid.

b) Sachets - paper/polythene/aluminium foil laminated. Leaflet in carton with sachets.

The product may be available in three pack sizes:

i) 300 g cans

ii) 15 g sachets in a carton

iii) 30 g sachets in a carton

6.6 Instructions for use and handling

Please refer to the patient information leaflet for detailed use of the product, including mixing instructions and use of the scoop.

7. MARKETING AUTHORISATION HOLDER

Alliance Pharmaceuticals Ltd

Avonbridge House

2 Bath Road

Chippenham

Wiltshire

SN15 2BB

United Kingdom

8. MARKETING AUTHORISATION NUMBER(S)

PL 16853/0082

9. DATE OF FIRST AUTHORISATION/RENEWAL OF THE AUTHORISATION

18th April 2005

10. DATE OF REVISION OF THE TEXT

April 2005

Forsteo 20 micrograms/80 microlitres, solution for injection, in pre-filled pen

(Eli Lilly and Company Limited)

1. NAME OF THE MEDICINAL PRODUCT

Forsteo*▼, 20 micrograms/80 microlitres, solution for injection, in pre-filled pen.

2. QUALITATIVE AND QUANTITATIVE COMPOSITION

One pre-filled pen of 3ml contains 750 micrograms of teriparatide (corresponding to 250 micrograms per ml). Each dose contains 20 micrograms of teriparatide. The pre-filled pen is intended for 28 days of dosing.

Teriparatide, rhPTH(1-34), (Forsteo), produced in *E. coli*, using recombinant DNA technology, is identical to the 34 N-terminal amino acid sequence of endogenous human parathyroid hormone.

For excipients, see section 6.1.

3. PHARMACEUTICAL FORM

Solution for injection in a pre-filled pen. Colourless, clear solution.

4. CLINICAL PARTICULARS

4.1 Therapeutic indications

Treatment of established osteoporosis in postmenopausal women. A significant reduction in the incidence of vertebral, but not hip, fractures has been demonstrated.

4.2 Posology and method of administration

The recommended dose of Forsteo is 20 micrograms administered once daily by subcutaneous injection in the thigh or abdomen.

Patients must be trained to use the proper injection techniques (see section 6.6). A User Manual is also available to instruct patients on the correct use of the pen.

The maximum total duration of treatment with Forsteo should be 18 months (see section 4.4, 'Special warnings and special precautions for use').

Patients should receive supplemental calcium and vitamin D supplements if dietary intake is inadequate.

Following cessation of Forsteo therapy, patients may be continued on other osteoporosis therapies.

Use in renal impairment: Forsteo should not be used in patients with severe renal impairment (see section 4.3, 'Contra-indications'). In patients with moderate renal impairment, Forsteo should be used with caution.

Use in hepatic impairment: No data are available in patients with impaired hepatic function (see section 5.3, 'Preclinical safety data').

Specific Populations

Children: Forsteo has not been studied in paediatric populations. Forsteo should not be used in paediatric patients or young adults with open epiphyses.

Elderly patients: Dosage adjustment based on age is not required (see section 5.2, 'Pharmacokinetic properties').

4.3 Contraindications

- Hypersensitivity to teriparatide or any of its excipients.
- Pre-existing hypercalcaemia.
- Severe renal impairment.
- Metabolic bone diseases other than primary osteoporosis (including hyperparathyroidism and Paget's disease of the bone).
- Unexplained elevations of alkaline phosphatase.
- Prior radiation therapy to the skeleton.

4.4 Special warnings and special precautions for use

In normocalcaemic patients, slight and transient elevations of serum calcium concentrations have been observed following teriparatide injection. Serum calcium concentrations reach a maximum between 4 and 6 hours and return to baseline by 16 to 24 hours after each dose of teriparatide. Routine calcium monitoring during therapy is not required.

Therefore if any blood samples are taken from a patient, this should be done at least 16 hours after the most recent Forsteo injection.

Table 1 Very Common Adverse Events (≥10%)

System Organ Class	Adverse Event	Forsteo n = 691 (%)	Placebo n = 691 (%)
Musculoskeletal and connective tissue and bone disorders	Pain in limb	10.0	9.0

Table 2 Common Adverse Events (≥1%, <10%)

System Organ Class	Adverse Event	Forsteo n = 691 (%)	Placebo n = 691 (%)
Blood and lymphatic system disorders	Anaemia	1.7	1.3
Metabolism and nutrition disorders	Hypercholesterolaemia	2.6	2.3
Psychiatric disorders	Depression	4.1	2.5
Nervous system disorders	Headache Dizziness Sciatica	7.7 8.0 1.3	7.4 5.2 0.7
Ear and labyrinth disorders	Vertigo	3.6	2.5
Cardiac disorders	Palpitations	1.4	1.2
Vascular disorders	Hypotension	1.0	1.0
Respiratory, thoracic, and mediastinal disorders	Dyspnoea	3.3	2.3
Gastro-intestinal disorders	Nausea Vomiting Hiatus hernia Gastro-oesophageal reflux disease	8.5 3.3 1.0 1.0	6.2 2.6 0.9 0.4
Skin and subcutaneous tissue disorders	Sweating increased	1.9	1.3
Musculoskeletal and connective tissue and bone disorders	Muscle cramps	3.6	2.9
General disorders and administration site conditions	Fatigue Chest pain Asthenia	4.8 3.8 1.6	4.3 3.5 1.2

Forsteo may cause small increases in urinary calcium excretion, but the incidence of hypercalciuria did not differ from that in the placebo-treated patients in clinical trials.

Forsteo has not been studied in patients with active urolithiasis. Forsteo should be used with caution in patients with active or recent urolithiasis because of the potential to exacerbate this condition.

In short-term clinical studies with Forsteo, isolated episodes of transient orthostatic hypotension were observed. Typically, an event began within 4 hours of dosing and spontaneously resolved within a few minutes to a few hours. When transient orthostatic hypotension occurred, it happened within the first several doses, was relieved by placing subjects in a reclining position, and did not preclude continued treatment.

Caution should be exercised in patients with moderate renal impairment.

Studies in rats indicate an increased incidence of osteosarcoma with long-term administration of teriparatide (see section 5.3). Until further clinical data become available, the recommended treatment time of 18 months should not be exceeded.

4.5 Interaction with other medicinal products and other forms of Interaction

Forsteo has been evaluated in pharmacodynamic interaction studies with hydrochlorothiazide. No clinically significant interactions were noted.

Co-administration of raloxifene or hormone replacement therapy with Forsteo did not alter the effects of Forsteo on serum or urine calcium or on clinical adverse events.

In a study of 15 healthy subjects administered digoxin daily to steady state, a single Forsteo dose did not alter the cardiac effect of digoxin. However, sporadic case reports have suggested that hypercalcaemia may predispose patients to digitalis toxicity. Because Forsteo transiently increases serum calcium, Forsteo should be used with caution in patients taking digitalis.

4.6 Pregnancy and lactation

Studies in rabbits have shown reproductive toxicity (see section 5.3). The potential risk for humans is unknown. Given the indication, Forsteo should not be used during pregnancy or by breast-feeding women.

4.7 Effects on ability to drive and use machines

No studies on the effects on the ability to drive and use machines have been performed. However, transient, orthostatic hypotension or dizziness was observed in some patients. These patients should refrain from driving or the use of machines until symptoms have subsided.

4.8 Undesirable effects

Of patients in the teriparatide trials, 82.8% of the Forsteo patients and 84.5% of the placebo patients reported at least 1 adverse event.

The most commonly reported adverse events in patients treated with Forsteo are nausea, pain in limb, headache, and dizziness. Tables 1, 2, and 3 give an overview of all treatment emergent adverse events that were observed in the trial populations, irrespective of causal relationship. The following events were observed in clinical trials in 1,382 patients.

Table 1

Very Common Adverse Events (≥10%)

(see Table 1 above)

Table 2

Common Adverse Events (≥1%, <10%)

(see Table 2 above)

Table 3

Uncommon Adverse Events (≥ 0.1%, <1%)

(see Table 3 below)

Forsteo increases serum uric acid concentrations. In clinical trials, 2.8% of Forsteo patients had serum uric acid concentrations above the upper limit of normal compared with 0.7% of placebo patients. However, the hyperuricaemia did not result in an increase in gout, arthralgia, or urolithiasis.

In a large clinical trial, antibodies that cross-reacted with teriparatide were detected in 2.8% of women receiving Forsteo. Generally, antibodies were first detected following 12 months of treatment and diminished after withdrawal of therapy. There was no evidence of hypersensitivity reactions, allergic reactions, effects on serum calcium, or effects on bone mineral density (BMD) response.

4.9 Overdose

Signs and symptoms: No cases of overdose were reported during clinical trials. Forsteo has been administered in single doses of up to 100 micrograms and in repeated doses of up to 60 micrograms/day for 6 weeks.

The effects of overdose that might be expected include delayed hypercalcaemia and risk of orthostatic hypotension. Nausea, vomiting, dizziness, and headache can also occur.

Overdose management: There is no specific antidote for Forsteo. Treatment of suspected overdose should include transitory discontinuation of Forsteo, monitoring of serum calcium, and implementation of appropriate supportive measures, such as hydration.

5. PHARMACOLOGICAL PROPERTIES

5.1 Pharmacodynamic properties

Pharmaco-therapeutic group: Calcium homeostasis, ATC code: H05 AA02.

Mechanism of action: Endogenous 84-amino-acid parathyroid hormone (PTH) is the primary regulator of calcium and phosphate metabolism in bone and kidney. Forsteo (rhPTH[1-34]) is the active fragment (1-34) of endogenous human parathyroid hormone. Physiological actions of PTH include stimulation of bone formation by direct effects on bone forming cells (osteoblasts) indirectly increasing the intestinal absorption of calcium and increasing the tubular re-absorption of calcium and excretion of phosphate by the kidney.

Pharmacodynamic effects: Forsteo is a bone formation agent to treat osteoporosis. The skeletal effects of Forsteo depend upon the pattern of systemic exposure. Once-daily administration of Forsteo increases apposition of new bone on trabecular and cortical bone surfaces by preferential stimulation of osteoblastic activity over osteoclastic activity.

Clinical Efficacy

Postmenopausal women with established osteoporosis (T-score below -2.5 in the presence of one or more fragility fracture): The pivotal study included 1,637 postmenopausal women (mean age 69.5 years). Ninety percent of the patients had one or more vertebral fractures at baseline. All patients were offered 1,000mg calcium per day and at least 400IU vitamin D per day. Results from up to 24 months (median: 19 months) treatment with Forsteo demonstrate statistically significant fracture reduction (Table 4). To prevent one or more new vertebral fractures, 11 women had to be treated for a median of 19 months.

Table 4

Vertebral Fracture Incidence in Postmenopausal Women

(see Table 4 on next page)

After 19 months (median) treatment, BMD had increased in the lumbar spine and total hip, respectively, by 9% and 4% compared with placebo ($P<0.001$).

Post-treatment management: Following treatment with Forsteo, 1,262 postmenopausal women from the pivotal trial enrolled in a post-treatment follow-up study. The primary objective of the study was to collect safety data on Forsteo. During this observational period, other osteoporosis treatments were allowed and additional assessment of vertebral fractures was performed.

During a median of 18 months following discontinuation of Forsteo, there was a 41% reduction ($P = 0.004$) compared

Table 3 Uncommon Adverse Events (≥ 0.1%, <1%)

System Organ Class	Adverse Event	Forsteo n = 691 (%)	Placebo n = 691 (%)
Cardiac disorders	Tachycardia	0.9	0.9
Respiratory, thoracic, and mediastinal disorders	Emphysema	0.3	0
Gastro-intestinal disorders	Haemorrhoids	0.9	0.4
Renal and urinary disorders	Urinary incontinence Polyuria Micturition urgency	0.6 0.3 0.3	0.3 0.1 0
General disorders and administration site conditions	Injection site erythema Injection site reaction	0.7 0.3	0 0.1
Investigations	Weight increased Cardiac murmur	0.7 0.4	0.3 0.1

Table 4 Vertebral Fracture Incidence in Postmenopausal Women

	Placebo n = 448 (%)	Forsteo n = 444 (%)	Relative Risk (95% CI) vs Placebo
New fracture (⩾1)	14.3	5.0 [a]	0.35 (0.22, 0.55)
Multiple fractures (⩾2)	4.9	1.1 [a]	0.23 (0.09, 0.60)

[a]*P*⩽0.001 compared with placebo; CI = Confidence Interval.

with placebo in the number of patients with a minimum of one new vertebral fracture.

Male osteoporosis: 437 patients were enrolled in a clinical trial for men with hypogonadal or idiopathic osteoporosis. All patients were offered 1,000mg calcium per day and at least 400IU vitamin D per day. Lumbar spine BMD significantly increased by 3 months. After 12 months, BMD had increased in the lumbar spine and total hip by 5% and 1%, respectively, compared with placebo. However, no significant effect on fracture rates was demonstrated.

5.2 Pharmacokinetic properties

Forsteo is eliminated through hepatic and extra-hepatic clearance (approximately 62 l/hr in women and 94 l/hr in men). The volume of distribution is approximately 1.7 l/kg. The half-life of Forsteo is approximately 1 hour when administered subcutaneously, which reflects the time required for absorption from the injection site. No metabolism or excretion studies have been performed with Forsteo but the peripheral metabolism of parathyroid hormone is believed to occur predominantly in liver and kidney.

Patient Characteristics

Geriatrics: No differences in Forsteo pharmacokinetics were detected with regard to age (range 31 to 85 years). Dosage adjustment based on age is not required.

5.3 Preclinical safety data

Teriparatide was not genotoxic in a standard battery of tests. It produced no teratogenic effects in rats, mice or rabbits.

Rats treated with near-life-time daily injections had dose-dependent exaggerated bone formation and increased incidence of osteosarcoma most probably due to an epigenetic mechanism. Teriparatide did not increase the incidence of any other type of neoplasia in rats. Due to the differences in bone physiology in rats and humans, the clinical relevance of these findings is probably minor. No bone tumours were observed in ovariectomised monkeys treated for 18 months. In addition, no osteosarcomas have been observed in clinical trials or during the post-treatment follow-up study.

Animal studies have shown that severely reduced hepatic blood flow decreases exposure of PTH to the principal cleavage system (Kupffer cells) and consequently clearance of PTH(1-84).

6. PHARMACEUTICAL PARTICULARS

6.1 List of excipients

Glacial acetic acid

Sodium acetate (anhydrous)

Mannitol, metacresol (preservative)

Hydrochloric acid

Sodium hydroxide

Water for injections

Hydrochloric acid and/or sodium hydroxide solution may be added to adjust pH.

6.2 Incompatibilities

In the absence of compatibility studies, this medicinal product must not be mixed with other medicinal products.

6.3 Shelf life

Two years.

Chemical, physical, and microbiological in-use stability has been demonstrated for 28 days at 2°C-8°C. Once opened, the product may be stored for a maximum of 28 days at 2°C-8°C. Other in-use storage times and conditions are the responsibility of the user.

6.4 Special precautions for storage

Store at 2°C-8°C at all times. The pen should be returned to the refrigerator immediately after use. Do not freeze.

Do not store the injection device with the needle attached.

6.5 Nature and contents of container

3ml solution in cartridge (siliconised Type I glass) with a plunger (halobutyl rubber), disc seal (polyisoprene/bromobutyl rubber laminate), and crimp cap (aluminium), assembled into a disposable pen.

Forsteo is available in pack sizes of 1 or 3 pens. Each pen contains 28 doses of 20 micrograms (per 80 microlitres). Not all pack sizes may be marketed.

6.6 Instructions for use and handling

Forsteo is a pre-filled pen and is intended for single patient use only. A new, sterile needle must be used for every injection. Each Forsteo pack is provided with a User Manual that fully describes the use of the pen. No needles are supplied with the product. The device can be used with insulin pen injection needles (Becton Dickinson). After each injection, the Forsteo pen should be returned to the refrigerator.

Forsteo should not be used if the solution is cloudy, coloured or contains particles.

Please also refer to the User Manual for instructions on how to use the pen.

7. MARKETING AUTHORISATION HOLDER

Eli Lilly Nederland BV, Grootslag 1-5, NL-3991 RA Houten, The Netherlands.

8. MARKETING AUTHORISATION NUMBER(S)

EU/1/03/247/001: 1 pre-filled pen

EU/1/03/247/002: 3 pre-filled pens

9. DATE OF FIRST AUTHORISATION/RENEWAL OF THE AUTHORISATION

June 2003

10. DATE OF REVISION OF THE TEXT

-

LEGAL CATEGORY

POM

*FORSTEO (teriparatide) is a trademark of Eli Lilly and Company.

FS1M

Fortum for Injection

(GlaxoSmithKline UK)

1. NAME OF THE MEDICINAL PRODUCT

Fortum for Injection

Ceftazidime (as pentahydrate) (INN) Injection

2. QUALITATIVE AND QUANTITATIVE COMPOSITION

Fortum for Injection: Vials contain either 250mg, 500mg, 1g, 2g or 3g ceftazidime (as pentahydrate) with sodium carbonate (118mg per gram of ceftazidime).

Fortum Monovial in a vial containing 2g ceftazidime pentahydrate.

3. PHARMACEUTICAL FORM

Sterile Powder for constitution for Injection

4. CLINICAL PARTICULARS

4.1 Therapeutic indications

Single infections

Mixed infections caused by two or more susceptible organisms

Severe infections in general

Respiratory tract infections

Ear, nose and throat infections

Urinary tract infections

Skin and soft tissue infections

Gastrointestinal, biliary and abdominal infections

Bone and joint infections

Dialysis: infections associated with haemo - and peritoneal dialysis and with continuous peritoneal dialysis (CAPD)

In meningitis it is recommended that the results of a sensitivity test are known before treatment with ceftazidime as a single agent. It may be used for infections caused by organisms resistant to other antibiotics including aminoglycosides and many cephalosporins. When appropriate, however, it may be used in combination with an aminoglycoside or other beta-lactam antibiotic for example, in the presence of severe neutropenia, or with an antibiotic active against anaerobes when the presence of bacteroides fragilis is suspected. In addition, ceftazidime is indicated in the perioperative prophylaxis of transurethral prostatectomy.

Bacteriology: Ceftazidime is bactericidal in action, exerting its effect on target cell wall proteins and causing inhibition of cell wall synthesis. A wide range of pathogenic strains and isolates associated with hospital-acquired infections are susceptible to ceftazidime *in vitro*, including strains resistant to gentamicin and other aminoglycosides. It is highly stable to most clinically important beta-lactamases produced by both gram-positive and gram-negative organisms and consequently is active against many ampicillin- and cephalothin-resistant strains. Ceftazidime has high intrinsic activity *in vitro* and acts within a narrow mic range for most genera with minimal changes in mic at varied inoculum levels. Ceftazidime has been shown to have *in vitro* activity against the following organisms:

Gram-negative: pseudomonas aeruginosa, pseudomonas spp (other), klebsiella pneumoniae, klebsiella spp (other), proteus mirabilis, proteus vulgaris, morganella morganii (formerly proteus morganii), proteus rettgeri, providencia spp, escherichia coli, enterobacter spp, citrobacter spp, serratia spp, salmonella spp, shigella spp, yersinia enterocolitica, pasteurella multocida, acinetobacter spp, neisseria gonorrhoeae, neisseria meningitidis, haemophilus influenzae (including ampicillin-resistant strains), haemophilus parainfluenzae (including ampicillin-resistant strains).

Gram-positive: staphylococcus aureus (methicillin-sensitive strains), staphylococcus epidermidis (methicillin-sensitive strains), micrococcus spp, streptococcus pyogenes, streptococcus group b, streptococcus pneumoniae, streptococcus mitis, streptococcus spp (excluding enterococcus (streptococcus) faecalis).

Anaerobic strains: peptococcus spp, peptostreptococcus spp, streptococcus spp, propionibacterium spp, clostridium perfringens, fusobacterium spp, bacteroides spp (many strains of bact fragilis are resistant).

Ceftazidime is not active *in vitro* against methicillin-resistant staphylococci, enterococcus (streptococcus) faecalis and many other enterococci, listeria monocytogenes, campylobacter spp or clostridium difficile.

In vitro the activities of ceftazidime and aminoglycoside antibiotics in combination have been shown to be at least additive; there is evidence of synergy in some strains tested. This property may be important in the treatment of febrile neutropenic patients.

4.2 Posology and method of administration

Ceftazidime is to be used by the parenteral route, the dosage depending upon the severity, sensitivity and type of infection and the age, weight and renal function of the patient.

Adults: The adult dosage range for ceftazidime is 1 to 6g per day 8 or 12 hourly (im or iv). In the majority of infections, 1g 8-hourly or 2g 12-hourly should be given. In urinary tract infections and in many less serious infections, 500mg or 1g 12-hourly is usually adequate. In very severe infections, especially immunocompromised patients, including those with neutropenia, 2g 8 or 12-hourly or 3g 12-hourly should be administered.

When used as a prophylactic agent in prostatic surgery 1g (from the 1g vial) should be given at the induction of anaesthesia. A second dose should be considered at the time of catheter removal.

Elderly: In view of the reduced clearance of ceftazidime in acutely ill elderly patients, the daily dosage should not normally exceed 3g, especially in those over 80 years of age.

Cystic fibrosis: In fibrocystic adults with normal renal function who have pseudomonal lung infections, high doses of 100 to 150mg/kg/day as three divided doses should be used. In adults with normal renal function 9g/day has been used.

Infants and children: The usual dosage range for children aged over two months is 30 to 100mg/kg/day, given as two or three divided doses.

Doses up to 150mg/kg/day (maximum 6g daily) in three divided doses may be given to infected immunocompromised or fibrocystic children or children with meningitis.

Neonates and children up to 2 months of age: Whilst clinical experience is limited, a dose of 25 to 60mg/kg/day given as two divided doses has proved to be effective. In the neonate the serum half-life of ceftazidime can be three to four times that in adults.

Dosage in impaired renal function: Ceftazidime is excreted by the kidneys almost exclusively by glomerular filtration. Therefore, in patients with impaired renal function it is recommended that the dosage of ceftazidime should be reduced to compensate for its slower excretion, except in mild impairment, i.e. glomerular filtration rate (GFR) greater than 50ml/min. In patients with suspected renal insufficiency, an initial loading dose of 1g of ceftazidime may be given. An estimate of GFR should be made to determine the appropriate maintenance dose.

Renal impairment: For patients in renal failure on continuous arteriovenous haemodialysis or high-flux haemofiltration in intensive therapy units, it is recommended that the dosage should be 1g daily in divided doses. For low-flux haemofiltration it is recommended that the dosage should be that suggested under impaired renal function.

Recommended maintenance doses are shown below:

RECOMMENDED MAINTENANCE DOSES OF CEFTAZIDIME IN RENAL insufficiency

(see Table 1 on next page)

In patients with severe infections, especially in neutropenics, who would normally receive 6g of ceftazidime daily were it not for renal insufficiency, the unit dose given in the table above may be increased by 50% or the dosing frequency increased appropriately. In such patients it is recommended that ceftazidime serum levels should be monitored and trough levels should not exceed 40mg/litre.

When only serum creatinine is available, the following formula (Cockcroft's equation) may be used to estimate

Table 1 RECOMMENDED MAINTENANCE DOSES OF CEFTAZIDIME IN RENAL insufficiency

Creatinine clearance ml/min	Approx. serum creatinine* µmol/l(mg/dl)	Recommended unit dose of ceftazidime (g)	Frequency of dosing (hourly)
50-31	150-200 (1.7-2.3)	1	12
30-16	200-350 (2.3-4.0)	1	24
15-6	350-500 (4.0-5.6)	0.5	24
<5	>500 >5.6)	0.5	48

* These values are guidelines and may not accurately predict renal function in all patients especially in the elderly in whom the serum creatinine concentration may overestimate renal function.

creatinine clearance. The serum creatinine should represent a steady state of renal function:

Males:

Creatinine clearance = Weight (kg) × (140 - age in years)

(ml/min) 72 × serum creatinine (mg/dl)

Females:

0.85 × above value.

To convert serum creatinine in mol/litre into mg/dl divide by 88.4.

In children the creatinine clearance should be adjusted for body surface area or lean body mass and the dosing frequency reduced in cases of renal insufficiency as for adults.

The serum half-life of ceftazidime during haemodialysis ranges from 3 to 5 hours. The appropriate maintenance dose of ceftazidime should be repeated following each haemodialysis period.

Dosage in peritoneal dialysis: Ceftazidime may also be used in peritoneal dialysis and continuous ambulatory peritoneal dialysis (CAPD). As well as using ceftazidime intravenously, it can be incorporated into the dialysis fluid (usually 125 to 250mg for 2L of dialysis fluid).

Administration: Ceftazidime may be given intravenously or by deep intramuscular injection into a large muscle mass such as the upper outer quadrant of the gluteus maximus or lateral part of the thigh.

4.3 Contraindications

Ceftazidime is contraindicated in patients with known hypersensitivity to cephalosporin antibiotics.

4.4 Special warnings and special precautions for use

Hypersensitivity reactions:

As with other beta-lactam antibiotics, before therapy with ceftazidime is instituted, careful inquiry should be made for a history of hypersensitivity reactions to ceftazidime, cephalosporins, penicillins or other drugs. Special care is indicated in patients who have experienced an allergic reaction to penicillins or beta-lactams. Ceftazidime should be given only with special caution to patients with type I or immediate hypersensitivity reactions to penicillin. If an allergic reaction to ceftazidime occurs, discontinue the drug. Serious hypersensitivity reactions may require epinephrine (adrenaline), hydrocortisone, antihistamine or other emergency measures.

Renal function:

Cephalosporin antibiotics at high dosage should be given with caution to patients receiving concurrent treatment with nephrotoxic drugs, e.g. aminoglycoside antibiotics, or potent diuretics such as frusemide, as these combinations are suspected of affecting renal function adversely. Clinical experience with ceftazidime has shown that this is not likely to be a problem at the recommended dose levels. There is no evidence that ceftazidime adversely affects renal function at normal therapeutic doses: however, as for all antibiotics eliminated via the kidneys, it is necessary to reduce the dosage according to the degree of reduction in renal function to avoid the clinical consequences of elevated antibiotic levels, e.g. neurological sequelae, which have occasionally been reported when the dose has not been reduced appropriately (see 4.2 Dosage in Impaired Renal Function and 4.8 Undesirable Effects).

Overgrowth of non-susceptible organisms:

As with other broad spectrum antibiotics, prolonged use of ceftazidime may result in the overgrowth of non-susceptible organisms (e.g. Candida, Enterococci and Serratia spp.) which may require interruption of treatment or adoption of appropriate measures. Repeated evaluation of the patient's condition is essential.

4.5 Interaction with other medicinal products and other forms of Interaction

Ceftazidime does not interfere with enzyme-based tests for glycosuria. Slight interference with copper reduction methods (Benedict's, Fehling's, Clinitest) may be observed. Ceftazidime does not interfere in the alkaline picrate assay for creatinine. The development of a positive Coombs' test associated with the use of ceftazidime in about 5% of patients may interfere with the cross-matching of blood.

Chloramphenicol is antagonistic *in vitro* with ceftazidime and other cephalosporins. The clinical relevance of this finding is unknown, but if concurrent administration of ceftazidime with chloramphenicol is proposed, the possibility of antagonism should be considered.

4.6 Pregnancy and lactation

There is no experimental evidence of embryopathic or teratogenic effects attributable to ceftazidime but, as with all drugs, it should be administered with caution during the early months of pregnancy and in early infancy. Use in pregnancy requires that the anticipated benefit be weighed against the possible risks.

Ceftazidime is excreted in human milk in low concentrations and consequently caution should be exercised when ceftazidime is administered to a nursing mother.

4.7 Effects on ability to drive and use machines

None reported.

4.8 Undesirable effects

Clinical trial experience has shown that ceftazidime is generally well tolerated.

Hypersensitivity: maculopapular or urticarial rash, fever, pruritus, and very rarely angioedema and anaphylaxis (including bronchospasm and/or hypotension).

Adverse reactions are infrequent and include:

Nervous system disorders: Headache, dizziness, paraesthesiae and bad taste. There have been reports of neurological sequelae including tremor, myoclonia, convulsions, and encephalopathy in patients with renal impairment in whom the dose of ceftazidime has not been appropriately reduced.

Gastrointestinal disorders: diarrhoea, nausea, vomiting, abdominal pain, and very rarely oral thrush or colitis. As with other cephalosporins, colitis may be associated with *Clostridium difficile* and may present as pseudomembranous colitis.

Hepato - biliary disorders: very rarely jaundice.

Skin and subcutaneous tissue disorders: As with other cephalosporins, there have been rare reports of erythema multiforme, Stevens-Johnson syndrome and toxic epidermal necrolysis.

Reproductive system disorders: Candidiasis, vaginitis.

General disorders and administration site conditions: phlebitis or thrombophlebitis with i.v. administration, pain and/or inflammation after i.m. injection.

Investigations: Laboratory test changes noted transiently during ceftazidime therapy include: eosinophilia, positive Coombs' test, very rarely haemolytic anaemia, thrombocytosis and elevations in one or more of the hepatic enzymes, ALT (SGPT), AST (SGOT), LDH, GGT and alkaline phosphatase.

As with some other cephalosporins, transient elevation of blood urea, blood urea nitrogen and/or serum creatinine have been observed occasionally. Very rarely, leucopenia, neutropenia, agranulocytosis, thrombocytopenia and lymphocytosis have been seen.

4.9 Overdose

Overdosage can lead to neurological sequelae including encephalopathy, convulsions and coma.

Serum levels of ceftazidime can be reduced by dialysis.

5. PHARMACOLOGICAL PROPERTIES

5.1 Pharmacodynamic properties

Ceftazidime is a bactericidal cephalosporin antibiotic which is resistant to most beta-lactamases and is active against a wide range of gram-positive and gram-negative bacteria.

5.2 Pharmacokinetic properties

Ceftazidime administered by the parenteral route reaches high and prolonged serum levels in man. After intramuscular administration of 500mg and 1g serum mean peak levels of 18 and 37mg/litre respectively are rapidly achieved. Five minutes after an intravenous bolus injection of 500mg, 1g or 2g, serum mean levels are respectively 46, 87 and 170mg/litre.

Therapeutically effective concentrations are still found in the serum 8 to 12 hours after both intravenous and intramuscular administration. The serum half-life is about 1.8 hours in normal volunteers and about 2.2 hours in patients with apparently normal renal function. The serum protein binding of ceftazidime is low at about 10%.

Ceftazidime is not metabolised in the body and is excreted unchanged in the active form into the urine by glomerular filtration. Approximately 80 to 90% of the dose is recovered in the urine within 24 hours. Less than 1% is excreted via the bile, significantly limiting the amount entering the bowel.

Concentrations of ceftazidime in excess of the minimum inhibitory levels for common pathogens can be achieved in tissues such as bone, heart, bile, sputum, aqueous humour, synovial and pleural and peritoneal fluids. Transplacental transfer of the antibiotic readily occurs. Ceftazidime penetrates the intact blood brain barrier poorly and low levels are achieved in the csf in the absence of inflammation. Therapeutic levels of 4 to 20mg/litre or more are achieved in the csf when the meninges are inflamed.

5.3 Preclinical safety data

No additional data of relevance.

6. PHARMACEUTICAL PARTICULARS

6.1 List of excipients

Sodium carbonate (anhydrous sterile)

6.2 Incompatibilities

Ceftazidime is less stable in Sodium Bicarbonate Injection than other intravenous fluids. It is not recommended as a diluent.

Ceftazidime and aminoglycosides should not be mixed in the same giving set or syringe.

Precipitation has been reported when vancomycin has been added to ceftazidime in solution. It is recommended that giving sets and intravenous lines are flushed been administration of these two agents.

6.3 Shelf life

Three years when stored below 25°C and protected from light.

Two years for Fortum Monovials when stored below 30°C and protected from light.

6.4 Special precautions for storage

Fortum for Injection should be below 25°C and Fortum Monovial should be stored below 30°C. Protect from light.

6.5 Nature and contents of container

Individually cartoned vials containing 250mg, 500mg or 1g ceftazidime (as pentahydrate) for intramuscular or intravenous use in packs of 5.

Individually cartoned vials containing 2g ceftazidime (as pentahydrate) for intravenous use in packs of 5.

Individually cartoned vials containing 2g ceftazidime (as pentahydrate) for intravenous infusion in packs of 5.

Individually cartoned Monovials containing 2g ceftazidime (as pentahydrate) for intravenous infusion.

Individually cartoned vials containing 3g ceftazidime (as pentahydrate) for intravenous and intravenous infusion use.

6.6 Instructions for use and handling

Instructions for constitution: See table for addition volumes and solution concentrations, which may be useful when fractional doses are required.

PREPARATION OF SOLUTION

(see Table 2 below)

All sizes of vials as supplied are under reduced pressure. As the product dissolves, carbon dioxide is released and a positive pressure develops. For ease of use, it is recommended that the following techniques of reconstitution are adopted.

Table 2 PREPARATION OF SOLUTION

Vial size		Amount of Diluent to be added (ml)	Approximate Concentration (mg/ml)
250mg	Intramuscular	1.0	210
250mg	Intravenous	2.5	90
500mg	Intramuscular	1.5	260
500mg	Intravenous	5.0	90
1g	Intramuscular	3.0	260
1g	Intravenous	10.0	90
2g	Intravenous bolus	10.0	170
2g	Intravenous Infusion	50.0*	40‡
3g	Intravenous bolus	15.0	170
3g	Intravenous Infusion	75.0*	40‡

*Note: Addition should be in two stages.

‡Note: Use Sodium Chloride Injection 0.9%, Dextrose Injection 5% or other approved diluent (see pharmaceutical precautions) as Water for Injections produces hypotonic solutions at this concentration.

250mg i.m./i.v., 500mg i.m./i.v., 1g i.m./i.v., and 2g and 3g i.v. bolus vials:

1. Insert the syringe needle through the vial closure and inject the recommended volume of diluent. The vacuum may assist entry of the diluent. Remove the syringe needle.

2. Shake to dissolve: carbon dioxide is released and a clear solution will be obtained in about 1 to 2 minutes.

3. Invert the vial. With the syringe plunger fully depressed, insert the needle through the vial closure and withdraw the total volume of solution into the syringe (the pressure in the vial may aid withdrawal). Ensure that the needle remains within the solution and does not enter the head space. The withdrawn solution may contain small bubbles of carbon dioxide; they may be disregarded.

2g and 3g i.v. infusion vials:

This vial may be constituted for short intravenous infusion (e.g. up to 30 minutes) as follows:

1. Insert the syringe needle through the vial closure and inject 10ml of diluent for 2g vial and 15ml for 3g vial. The vacuum may assist entry of the diluent. Remove the syringe needle.

2. Shake to dissolve: carbon dioxide is released and a clear solution obtained in about 1 to 2 minutes.

3. Insert a gas relief needle through the vial closure to relieve the internal pressure and, with the gas relief in position, add a further 40ml of diluent for 2g vial and 60ml for 3g vial. Remove the gas relief needle and syringe needle; shake the vial and set up for infusion use in the normal way.

NOTE: To preserve product sterility, it is important that a gas relief needle is not inserted through the vial closure before the product has dissolved.

Fortum Monovial:

The contents of the Monovial are added to small volume infusion bags containing 0.9% Sodium Chloride Injection or 5% Dextrose Injection, or another compatible fluid.

The 2g presentation must be constituted in not less than 100mL infusion bag.

1) Peel off the removable top part of the label and remove the cap.

2) Insert the needle of the Monovial into the additive port of the infusion bag.

3) To activate, push the plastic needle holder of the Monovial down onto the vial shoulder until a "click" is heard.

4) Holding it upright, fill the vial to approximately two-thirds capacity by squeezing the bag several times.

5) Shake the vial to reconstitute the Fortum.

6) On constitution, the Fortum will effervesce slightly.

7) With the vial uppermost, transfer the reconstituted Fortum into the infusion bag by squeezing and releasing the bag.

8) Repeat the steps 4 to 7 to rinse the inside of the vial. Dispose of the empty Monovial safely. Check that the powder is completely dissolved and that the bag has no leaks.

Fortum Monovial is for i.v. infusion only.

These solutions may be given directly into the vein or introduced into the tubing of a giving set if the patient is receiving parenteral fluids. Ceftazidime is compatible with the most commonly used intravenous fluids.

Vials of Fortum for Injection and Fortum Monovials as supplied are under reduced pressure; a positive pressure is produced on constitution due to the release of carbon dioxide.

Vials of Fortum for Injection should be stored at a temperature below 25°C.

Vials of Fortum for Injection do not contain any preservatives and should be used as single-dose preparations.

In keeping with good pharmaceutical practice, it is preferable to use freshly constituted solutions of Fortum for Injection. If this is not practicable, satisfactory potency is retained for 24 hours in the refrigerator (2 - 8°C) when prepared in Water for Injection BP or any of the injections listed below.

At ceftazidime concentrations between 1mg/ml and 40mg/ml in:

0.9% Sodium Chloride Injection BP

M/6 Sodium Lactate Injection BP

Compound Sodium Lactate Injection BP (Hartmann's Solution)

5% Dextrose Injection BP

0.225% Sodium Chloride and 5% Dextrose Injection BP

0.45% Sodium Chloride and 5% Dextrose Injection BP

0.9% Sodium Chloride and 5% Dextrose Injection BP

0.18% Sodium Chloride and 4% Dextrose Injection BP

10% Dextrose Injection BP

Dextran 40 Injection BP 10% in 0.9% Sodium Chloride Injection BP

Dextran 40 Injection BP 10% in 5% Dextrose Injection BP

Dextran 70 Injection BP 6% in 0.9% Sodium Chloride Injection BP

Dextran 70 Injection BP 6% in 5% Dextrose Injection BP

(Ceftazidime is less stable in Sodium Bicarbonate Injection than in other intravenous fluids. It is not recommended as a diluent)

At concentrations of between 0.05mg/ml and 0.25mg/ml in Intraperitoneal Dialysis Fluid (Lactate) BPC 1973.

When reconstituted for intramuscular use with: 0.5% or 1% Lignocaine Hydrochloride Injection BP

When admixed at 4mg/ml with (both components retain satisfactory potency):

Hydrocortisone (hydrocortisone sodium phosphate) 1mg/ml in 0.9% Sodium Chloride Injection BP or 5% Dextrose Injection BP

Cefuroxime (cefuroxime sodium) 3mg/ml in 0.9% Sodium Chloride Injection BP

Cloxacillin (cloxacillin sodium) 4mg/ml in 0.9% Sodium Chloride Injection BP

Heparin 10u/ml or 50u/ml in 0.9% Sodium Chloride Injection BP

Potassium Chloride 10mEq/L or 40 Eq/L in 0.9% Sodium Chloride Injection BP

The contents of a 500mg vial of Fortum for Injection, constituted with 1.5ml water for injections, may be added to metronidazole injection (500mg in 100ml) and both retain their activity.

Solutions range from light yellow to amber depending on concentration, diluent and storage conditions used. Within the stated recommendations, product potency is not adversely affected by such colour variations.

Administrative Data

7. MARKETING AUTHORISATION HOLDER

Glaxo Operations UK Ltd

Greenford

Middlesex

UB6 OHE

Trading as

GlaxoSmithKline UK

Stockley Park West

Uxbridge

Middlesex UB11 1BT

8. MARKETING AUTHORISATION NUMBER(S)

250mg vials	0004/0304
500mg vials	0004/0292
1 gram vials	0004/0293
2 and 3 gram vials	0004/0294

9. DATE OF FIRST AUTHORISATION/RENEWAL OF THE AUTHORISATION

250mg vials	12.02.99
500mg vials	18.05.01
1 gram vials	18.05.01
2 and 3 gram vials	18.05.01

10. DATE OF REVISION OF THE TEXT

24 February 2003

11. Legal Status

POM

Fosamax

(Merck Sharp & Dohme Limited)

1. NAME OF THE MEDICINAL PRODUCT

FOSAMAX® 5 mg Tablets

FOSAMAX® 10 mg Tablets

2. QUALITATIVE AND QUANTITATIVE COMPOSITION

5 mg tablets: 6.53 mg of alendronate sodium, which is the molar equivalent to 5 mg of alendronic acid.

10 mg tablets: 13.05 mg of alendronate sodium, which is the molar equivalent to 10 mg of alendronic acid.

3. PHARMACEUTICAL FORM

Tablets

5 mg tablets: round white tablets, with an outline of a bone image on one side, and 'MSD 925' on the other.

10 mg tablets: oval white tablets marked with '936' on one side, and plain on the other.

4. CLINICAL PARTICULARS

4.1 Therapeutic indications

'Fosamax' is indicated for the treatment of osteoporosis in post-menopausal women to prevent fractures.

'Fosamax' is indicated for the treatment of osteoporosis in men to prevent fractures.

'Fosamax' is indicated for the treatment of glucocorticoid-induced osteoporosis and prevention of bone loss in men and women considered at risk of developing the disease.

'Fosamax' is indicated for the prevention of osteoporosis in those post-menopausal women considered at risk of developing the disease.

Risk factors often associated with the development of osteoporosis include thin body build, family history of osteoporosis, early menopause, moderately low bone mass and long-term glucocorticoid therapy, especially with high doses (⩾15 mg/day).

4.2 Posology and method of administration

Treatment of osteoporosis in post-menopausal women: The recommended dosage is 10 mg once a day.

Treatment of osteoporosis in men: The recommended dosage is 10 mg once a day.

Treatment and prevention of glucocorticoid-induced osteoporosis: For post-menopausal women not receiving hormone replacement therapy (HRT) with an oestrogen, the recommended dosage is 10 mg once a day.

For other patients (i.e. men, pre-menopausal women and post-menopausal women receiving HRT with an oestrogen), the recommended dosage is 5 mg once a day.

Prevention of osteoporosis in post-menopausal women: The recommended dosage is 5 mg once a day.

To permit adequate absorption of 'Fosamax':

'Fosamax' must be taken at least 30 minutes before the first food, beverage, or medication of the day with plain water only. Other beverages (including mineral water), food and some medications are likely to reduce the absorption of 'Fosamax' (see 4.5 'Interaction with other medicinal products and other forms of interaction').

To facilitate delivery to the stomach and thus reduce the potential for local and oesophageal irritation/adverse experiences (see 4.4 'Special warnings and precautions for use'):

• 'Fosamax' should only be swallowed upon arising for the day with a full glass of water (not less than 200 mls or 7 fl.oz.).

• Patients should not chew the tablet or allow the tablet to dissolve in their mouths because of a potential for oropharyngeal ulceration.

• Patients should not lie down until after their first food of the day which should be at least 30 minutes after taking the tablet.

• Patients should not lie down for at least 30 minutes after taking 'Fosamax'.

• 'Fosamax' should not be taken at bedtime or before arising for the day.

Patients should receive supplemental calcium and vitamin D if dietary intake is inadequate (see 4.4 'Special warnings and precautions for use').

Use in the elderly: In clinical studies there was no age-related difference in the efficacy or safety profiles of 'Fosamax'. Therefore no dosage adjustment is necessary for the elderly.

Use in renal impairment: No dosage adjustment is necessary for patients with GFR greater than 35 ml/min. 'Fosamax' is not recommended for patients with renal impairment where GFR is less than 35 ml/min, due to lack of experience.

Use in children: 'Fosamax' has not been studied in children and should not be given to them.

4.3 Contraindications

• Abnormalities of the oesophagus and other factors which delay oesophageal emptying such as stricture or achalasia.

• Inability to stand or sit upright for at least 30 minutes.

• Hypersensitivity to any component of this product.

• Hypocalcaemia (see 4.4 'Special warnings and precautions for use').

4.4 Special warnings and special precautions for use

'Fosamax' can cause local irritation of the upper gastro-intestinal mucosa. Because there is a potential for worsening of the underlying disease, caution should be used when 'Fosamax' is given to patients with active upper gastro-intestinal problems, such as dysphagia, oesophageal disease, gastritis, duodenitis, or ulcers (see 4.3 'Contraindications').

Oesophageal reactions (sometimes severe and requiring hospitalisation), such as oesophagitis, oesophageal ulcers and oesophageal erosions, rarely followed by oesophageal stricture or perforation, have been reported in patients receiving 'Fosamax'. Physicians should therefore be alert to any signs or symptoms signalling a possible oesophageal reaction and patients should be instructed to discontinue 'Fosamax' and seek medical attention if they develop symptoms of oesophageal irritation such as dysphagia, pain on swallowing or retrosternal pain, new or worsening heartburn.

The risk of severe oesophageal adverse experiences appears to be greater in patients who fail to take 'Fosamax' properly and/or who continue to take 'Fosamax' after developing symptoms suggestive of oesophageal irritation. It is very important that the full dosing instructions are provided to, and understood by the patient (see 4.2 'Posology and method of administration'). Patients should be informed that failure to follow these instructions may increase their risk of oesophageal problems.

While no increased risk was observed in extensive clinical trials, there have been rare (post-marketing) reports of gastric and duodenal ulcers, some severe and with complications. However a causal relationship has not been established.

'Fosamax' is not recommended for patients with renal impairment where GFR is less than 35 ml/min, (see 4.2 'Posology and method of administration').

Causes of osteoporosis other than oestrogen deficiency, ageing and glucocorticoid use should be considered.

Hypocalcaemia must be corrected before initiating therapy with alendronate (see 4.3 'Contraindications'). Other disorders affecting mineral metabolism (such as vitamin D deficiency and hypoparathyroidism) should also be effectively treated. In patients with these conditions, serum calcium and symptoms of hypocalcaemia should be monitored during therapy with 'Fosamax'.

Due to the positive effects of alendronate in increasing bone mineral, decreases in serum calcium and phosphate may occur. These are usually small and asymptomatic. However, there have been rare reports of symptomatic hypocalcaemia, which have occasionally been severe and often occurred in patients with predisposing conditions (e.g. hypoparathyroidism, vitamin D deficiency and calcium malabsorption).

Ensuring adequate calcium and vitamin D intake is particularly important in patients receiving glucocorticoids.

4.5 Interaction with other medicinal products and other forms of Interaction

If taken at the same time, it is likely that calcium supplements, antacids, and some oral medications will interfere with absorption of 'Fosamax'. Therefore, patients must wait at least 30 minutes after taking 'Fosamax' before taking any other oral medication.

No other drug interactions of clinical significance are anticipated. Concomitant use of HRT (oestrogen ± progestin) and 'Fosamax' was assessed in two clinical studies of one or two years duration in post-menopausal osteoporotic women (5.1 'Pharmacodynamic properties, *concomitant use with oestrogen/hormone replacement therapy (HRT)*').

Combined use of 'Fosamax' and HRT resulted in greater increases in bone mass, together with greater decreases in bone turnover, than seen with either treatment alone. In these studies, the safety and tolerability profile of the combination was consistent with those of the individual treatments.

Although specific interaction studies were not performed, in clinical studies 'Fosamax' was used concomitantly with a wide range of commonly prescribed drugs without evidence of clinical adverse interactions.

4.6 Pregnancy and lactation

Use during pregnancy

'Fosamax' has not been studied in pregnant women and should not be given to them.

In developmental toxicity studies in animals, there were no adverse effects at doses up to 25 mg/kg/day in rats and 35 mg/kg/day in rabbits.

Use during lactation

'Fosamax' has not been studied in breast-feeding women and should not be given to them.

4.7 Effects on ability to drive and use machines

There are no data to suggest that 'Fosamax' affects the ability to drive or use machines.

4.8 Undesirable effects

'Fosamax' has been studied in nine major clinical studies (n=5,886). In the longest running trials in post-menopausal women up to five years experience has been collected. Two years safety data are available in both men with osteoporosis and men and women on glucocorticoids.

The following adverse experiences have been reported during clinical studies and/or post-marketing use:

Common (≥ 1.0% and < 10%)

Gastro-intestinal:	abdominal pain, dyspepsia, constipation, diarrhoea, flatulence, oesophageal ulcer*, melaena, dysphagia*, abdominal distension, acid regurgitation.
Musculoskeletal:	musculoskeletal (bone, muscle or joint) pain.
Neurological:	headache.

Uncommon (≥ 0.1% and < 1%)

Gastro-intestinal:	nausea, vomiting, gastritis, oesophagitis*, oesophageal erosions*.
Skin	rash, pruritus, erythema.

Rare (≥ 0.01% and < 0.1%)

Body as a whole:	hypersensitivity reactions including urticaria and angioedema. Transient symptoms as in an acute-phase response (myalgia, malaise and rarely, fever), typically in association with initiation of treatment. Symptomatic hypocalcaemia, occasionally severe, often in association with predisposing conditions (see 4.4 'Special warnings and precautions for use')
Gastro-intestinal:	oesophageal stricture*, oropharyngeal ulceration*, upper gastrointestinal PUBs (perforation, ulcers, bleeding), although a causal relationship cannot be ruled out.
Skin	rash with photosensitivity.
Special senses:	uveitis, scleritis.

Very rare, including isolated cases:

Skin	severe skin reactions including Stevens-Johnson syndrome and toxic epidermal necrolysis.

* See 4.4 'Special warnings and precautions for use' and 4.2 'Posology and method of administration'.

Laboratory test findings

In clinical studies, asymptomatic, mild and transient decreases in serum calcium and phosphate were observed in approximately 18 and 10%, respectively, of patients taking 'Fosamax' versus approximately 12 and 3% of those taking placebo. However, the incidences of decreases in serum calcium to <8.0 mg/dl (2.0 mmol/l) and serum phosphate to ⩽2.0 mg/dl (0.65 mmol/l) were similar in both treatment groups.

4.9 Overdose

No specific information is available on the treatment of overdosage with 'Fosamax'. Hypocalcaemia, hypophosphataemia and upper gastro-intestinal adverse events, such as upset stomach, heartburn, oesophagitis, gastritis, or ulcer, may result from oral overdosage. Milk or antacids should be given to bind alendronate. Owing to the risk of oesophageal irritation, vomiting should not be induced and the patient should remain fully upright.

5. PHARMACOLOGICAL PROPERTIES

5.1 Pharmacodynamic properties

'Fosamax' is a bisphosphonate that inhibits osteoclastic bone resorption with no direct effect on bone formation. The bone formed during treatment with 'Fosamax' is of normal quality.

Treatment of post-menopausal osteoporosis

The effects of 'Fosamax' on bone mass and fracture incidence in post-menopausal women were examined in two initial efficacy studies of identical design (n=994) as well as in the Fracture Intervention Trial (FIT: n=6,459).

In the initial efficacy studies, the mean bone mineral density (BMD) increases with 'Fosamax' 10 mg/day relative to placebo at three years were 8.8%, 5.9% and 7.8% at the spine, femoral neck and trochanter, respectively. Total body BMD also increased significantly. There was a 48% reduction in the proportion of patients treated with 'Fosamax' experiencing one or more vertebral fractures relative to those treated with placebo. In the two-year extension of these studies BMD at the spine and trochanter continued to increase and BMD at the femoral neck and total body were maintained.

FIT consisted of two placebo-controlled studies: a three-year study of 2,027 patients who had at least one baseline vertebral (compression) fracture and a four-year study of 4,432 patients with low bone mass but without a baseline vertebral fracture, 37% of whom had osteoporosis as defined by a baseline femoral neck BMD at least 2.5 standard deviations below the mean for young, adult women. In all FIT patients with osteoporosis from both studies, 'Fosamax' reduced the incidence of: ⩾1 vertebral fracture by 48%, multiple vertebral fractures by 87%, ⩾1 painful vertebral fracture by 45%, any painful fracture by 31% and hip fracture by 54%.

Overall these results demonstrate the consistent effect of 'Fosamax' to reduce the incidence of fractures, including those of the spine and hip, which are the sites of osteoporotic fracture associated with the greatest morbidity.

Prevention of post-menopausal osteoporosis

The effects of 'Fosamax' to prevent bone loss were examined in two studies of post-menopausal women aged ⩽60 years. In the larger study of 1,609 women (⩾6 months post-menopausal) those receiving 'Fosamax' 5 mg daily for two years had BMD increases of 3.5%, 1.3%, 3.0% and 0.7% at the spine, femoral neck, trochanter and total body, respectively. In the smaller study (n=447), similar results were observed in women (6 to 36 months post-menopausal) treated with 'Fosamax' 5 mg daily for three years. In contrast, in both studies, women receiving placebo lost bone mass at a rate of approximately 1% per year. The longer term effects of 'Fosamax' in an osteoporosis prevention population are not known but clinical trial extensions of up to 10 years of continuous treatment are currently in progress.

Concomitant use with oestrogen/hormone replacement therapy (HRT)

The effects on BMD of treatment with 'Fosamax' 10 mg once-daily and conjugated oestrogen (0.625 mg/day) either alone or in combination were assessed in a two-year study of hysterectomised, post-menopausal, osteoporotic women. At two years, the increases in lumbar spine BMD from baseline were significantly greater with the combination (8.3%) than with either oestrogen or 'Fosamax' alone (both 6.0%).

The effects on BMD when 'Fosamax' was added to stable doses (for at least one year) of HRT (oestrogen ± progestin) were assessed in a one-year study in post-menopausal, osteoporotic women. The addition of 'Fosamax' 10 mg once-daily to HRT produced, at one year, significantly greater increases in lumbar spine BMD (3.7%) vs. HRT alone (1.1%).

In these studies, significant increases or favourable trends in BMD for combined therapy compared with HRT alone were seen at the total hip, femoral neck and trochanter. No significant effect was seen for total body BMD.

Treatment of osteoporosis in men

The efficacy of 'Fosamax' 10 mg once daily in men (ages 31 to 87; mean, 63) with osteoporosis was demonstrated in a two-year study. At two years, the mean increases relative to placebo in BMD in men receiving 'Fosamax' 10 mg/day were: lumbar spine, 5.3%; femoral neck, 2.6%; trochanter, 3.1%; and total body, 1.6%. 'Fosamax' was effective regardless of age, race, gonadal function, baseline rate of bone turnover, or baseline BMD. Consistent with much larger studies in post-menopausal women, in these 127 men, 'Fosamax' 10 mg/day reduced the incidence of new vertebral fracture (assessed by quantitative radiography) relative to placebo (0.8% vs. 7.1%) and, correspondingly, also reduced height loss (-0.6 vs. -2.4 mm).

Glucocorticoid-induced osteoporosis

The efficacy of 'Fosamax' 5 and 10 mg once-daily in men and women receiving at least 7.5 mg/day of prednisone (or equivalent) was demonstrated in two studies. At two years of treatment, spine BMD increased by 3.7% and 5.0% (relative to placebo) with 'Fosamax' 5 and 10 mg/day respectively. Significant increases in BMD were also observed at the femoral neck, trochanter, and total body. In post-menopausal women not receiving oestrogen, greater increases in lumbar spine and trochanter BMD were seen in those receiving 10 mg 'Fosamax' than those receiving 5 mg. 'Fosamax' was effective regardless of dose or duration of glucocorticoid use. Data pooled from three dosage groups (5 or 10 mg for two years or 2.5 mg for one year followed by 10 mg for one year) showed a significant reduction in the incidence of patients with a new vertebral fracture at two years ('Fosamax' 0.7% vs. placebo 6.8%).

5.2 Pharmacokinetic properties

Absorption

Relative to an intravenous (IV) reference dose, the oral bioavailability of alendronate in women was 0.7% for doses ranging from 5 to 40 mg when administered after an overnight fast and two hours before a standardised breakfast. Oral bioavailability in men (0.6%) was similar to that in women. Bioavailability was decreased similarly to an estimated 0.46% and 0.39% when alendronate was administered one hour or half an hour before a standardised breakfast. In osteoporosis studies, 'Fosamax' was effective when administered at least 30 minutes before the first food or beverage of the day.

Bioavailability was negligible whether alendronate was administered with, or up to two hours after, a standardised breakfast. Concomitant administration of alendronate with coffee or orange juice reduced bioavailability by approximately 60%.

In healthy subjects, oral prednisone (20 mg three times daily for five days) did not produce a clinically meaningful change in oral bioavailability of alendronate (a mean increase ranging from 20% to 44%).

Distribution

Studies in rats show that alendronate transiently distributes to soft tissues following 1 mg/kg IV administration but is then rapidly redistributed to bone or excreted in the urine. The mean steady-state volume of distribution, exclusive of bone, is at least 28 litres in humans. Concentrations of drug in plasma following therapeutic oral doses are too low for analytical detection (<5 ng/ml). Protein binding in human plasma is approximately 78%.

Biotransformation

There is no evidence that alendronate is metabolised in animals or humans.

Elimination

Following a single IV dose of [^{14}C]alendronate, approximately 50% of the radioactivity was excreted in the urine within 72 hours and little or no radioactivity was recovered in the faeces. Following a single 10 mg IV dose, the renal clearance of alendronate was 71 ml/min, and systemic clearance did not exceed 200 ml/min. Plasma concentrations fell by more than 95% within six hours following IV administration. The terminal half-life in humans is estimated to exceed ten years, reflecting release of alendronate from the skeleton. Alendronate is not excreted through the acidic or basic transport systems of the kidney in rats, and thus it is not anticipated to interfere with the excretion of other drugs by those systems in humans.

Characteristics in patients

Preclinical studies show that the drug that is not deposited in bone is rapidly excreted in the urine. No evidence of saturation of bone uptake was found after chronic dosing with cumulative IV doses up to 35 mg/kg in animals. Although no clinical information is available, it is likely that, as in animals, elimination of alendronate via the kidney will be reduced in patients with impaired renal function. Therefore, somewhat greater accumulation of alendronate in bone might be expected in patients with impaired renal function (see 4.2 'Posology and method of administration').

5.3 Preclinical safety data

In test animal species the main target organs for toxicity were kidneys and gastro-intestinal tract. Renal toxicity was seen only at doses >2 mg/kg/day orally (ten times the recommended dose) and was evident only on histological examination as small widely scattered foci of nephritis, with no evidence of effect on renal function. The gastro-intestinal toxicity, seen in rodents only, occurred at doses >2.5 mg/kg/day and appears to be due to a direct effect on the mucosa. There is no additional relevant information.

Significant lethality after single oral doses was seen in female rats and mice at 552 mg/kg (3,256 mg/m^2) and 966 mg/kg (2,898 mg/m^2) (equivalent to human oral doses* of 27,600 and 48,300 mg), respectively. In males, these values were slightly higher, 626 and 1,280 mg/kg, respectively. There was no lethality in dogs at oral doses up to 200 mg/kg (4,000 mg/m^2) (equivalent to a human oral dose* of 10,000 mg).

* Based on a patient weight of 50 kg.

6. PHARMACEUTICAL PARTICULARS

6.1 List of excipients

5 mg tablets: microcrystalline cellulose, anhydrous lactose, croscarmellose sodium and magnesium stearate.

10 mg tablets: microcrystalline cellulose, anhydrous lactose, croscarmellose sodium, magnesium stearate and carnauba wax.

6.2 Incompatibilities

None known.

6.3 Shelf life

24 months.

6.4 Special precautions for storage

Do not store above 30°C.

6.5 Nature and contents of container

Blisters of opaque white PVC lidded with aluminium foil.

Pack size: 28 tablets.

6.6 Instructions for use and handling

None.

7. MARKETING AUTHORISATION HOLDER

Merck Sharp & Dohme Limited

Hertford Road, Hoddesdon, Hertfordshire EN11 9BU, UK

8. MARKETING AUTHORISATION NUMBER(S)

5 mg tablets: PL 0025/0360

10 mg tablets: PL 0025/0326

9. DATE OF FIRST AUTHORISATION/RENEWAL OF THE AUTHORISATION

5 mg tablets: 6 May 1999

10 mg tablets: 28 July 1995

10. DATE OF REVISION OF THE TEXT

April 2004

LEGAL CATEGORY

POM

MSD (logo)

Merck Sharp & Dohme Limited

Hertford Road, Hoddesdon, Hertfordshire EN11 9BU, UK

SPC.FSM5&10.03.UK.0917

Fosamax Once Weekly 70mg Tablets

(Merck Sharp & Dohme Limited)

1. NAME OF THE MEDICINAL PRODUCT

'Fosamax'® Once Weekly 70 mg Tablets

2. QUALITATIVE AND QUANTITATIVE COMPOSITION

Each tablet contains the equivalent of 70 mg of alendronic acid as 91.37 mg alendronate sodium trihydrate.

For excipients, see 6.1.

3. PHARMACEUTICAL FORM

Tablet.

Oval white tablets, marked with an outline of a bone image on one side, and '31' on the other.

4. CLINICAL PARTICULARS

4.1 Therapeutic indications

Treatment of postmenopausal osteoporosis. 'Fosamax' reduces the risk of vertebral and hip fractures.

4.2 Posology and method of administration

The recommended dosage is one 70 mg tablet once weekly.

To permit adequate absorption of alendronate:

'Fosamax' must be taken at least 30 minutes before the first food, beverage, or medicinal product of the day with plain water only. Other beverages (including mineral water), food and some medicinal products are likely to reduce the absorption of alendronate (see 4.5 'Interaction with other medicinal products and other forms of interaction').

To facilitate delivery to the stomach and thus reduce the potential for local and oesophageal irritation/adverse experiences (see 4.4 'Special warnings and precautions for use'):

- 'Fosamax' should only be swallowed upon arising for the day with a full glass of water (not less than 200 ml or 7 fl.oz.).
- Patients should not chew the tablet or allow the tablet to dissolve in their mouths because of a potential for oropharyngeal ulceration.
- Patients should not lie down until after their first food of the day which should be at least 30 minutes after taking the tablet.
- Patients should not lie down for at least 30 minutes after taking 'Fosamax'.
- 'Fosamax' should not be taken at bedtime or before arising for the day.

Patients should receive supplemental calcium and vitamin D if dietary intake is inadequate (see 4.4 'Special warnings and precautions for use').

Use in the elderly: In clinical studies there was no age-related difference in the efficacy or safety profiles of alendronate. Therefore no dosage adjustment is necessary for the elderly.

Use in renal impairment: No dosage adjustment is necessary for patients with GFR greater than 35 ml/min. Alendronate is not recommended for patients with renal impairment where GFR is less than 35 ml/min, due to lack of experience.

Use in children: Alendronate has not been studied in children and should not be given to them.

'Fosamax' Once Weekly 70 mg has not been investigated in the treatment of glucocorticoid-induced osteoporosis.

4.3 Contraindications

- Abnormalities of the oesophagus and other factors which delay oesophageal emptying such as stricture or achalasia.
- Inability to stand or sit upright for at least 30 minutes.
- Hypersensitivity to alendronate or to any of the excipients.
- Hypocalcaemia.
- See also 4.4 'Special warnings and precautions for use'.

4.4 Special warnings and special precautions for use

Alendronate can cause local irritation of the upper gastro-intestinal mucosa. Because there is a potential for worsening of the underlying disease, caution should be used when alendronate is given to patients with active upper gastro-intestinal problems, such as dysphagia, oesophageal disease, gastritis, duodenitis, ulcers, or with a recent history (within the previous year) of major gastro-intestinal disease such as peptic ulcer, or active gastro-intestinal bleeding, or surgery of the upper gastro-intestinal tract other than pyloroplasty (see 4.3 'Contra-indications').

Oesophageal reactions (sometimes severe and requiring hospitalisation), such as oesophagitis, oesophageal ulcers and oesophageal erosions, rarely followed by oesophageal stricture, have been reported in patients receiving alendronate. Physicians should therefore be alert to any signs or symptoms signalling a possible oesophageal reaction and patients should be instructed to discontinue alendronate and seek medical attention if they develop symptoms of oesophageal irritation such as dysphagia, pain on swallowing or retrosternal pain, new or worsening heartburn.

The risk of severe oesophageal adverse experiences appears to be greater in patients who fail to take alendronate properly and/or who continue to take alendronate after developing symptoms suggestive of oesophageal irritation. It is very important that the full dosing instructions are provided to, and understood by the patient (see 4.2 'Posology and method of administration'). Patients should be informed that failure to follow these instructions may increase their risk of oesophageal problems.

While no increased risk was observed in extensive clinical trials, there have been rare (post-marketing) reports of gastric and duodenal ulcers, some severe and with complications. A causal relationship cannot be ruled out.

Patients should be instructed that if they miss a dose of 'Fosamax' Once Weekly, they should take one tablet on the morning after they remember. They should not take two tablets on the same day but should return to taking one tablet once a week, as originally scheduled on their chosen day.

Alendronate is not recommended for patients with renal impairment where GFR is less than 35 ml/min, (see 4.2 'Posology and method of administration').

Causes of osteoporosis other than oestrogen deficiency and ageing should be considered.

Hypocalcaemia must be corrected before initiating therapy with alendronate (see 4.3 'Contra-indications'). Other disorders affecting mineral metabolism (such as vitamin D deficiency and hypoparathyroidism) should also be effectively treated. In patients with these conditions, serum calcium and symptoms of hypocalcaemia should be monitored during therapy with 'Fosamax'.

Due to positive effects of alendronate in increasing bone mineral, decreases in serum calcium and phosphate may occur. These are usually small and asymptomatic. However, there have been reports of symptomatic hypocalcaemia, which occasionally have been severe and often occurred in patients with predisposing conditions (e.g. hypoparathyroidism, vitamin D deficiency and calcium malabsorption). Ensuring adequate calcium and vitamin D intake is therefore particularly important in patients receiving glucocorticoids.

4.5 Interaction with other medicinal products and other forms of Interaction

If taken at the same time, it is likely that food and beverages (including mineral water), calcium supplements, antacids, and some oral medicinal products will interfere with absorption of alendronate. Therefore, patients must wait at least 30 minutes after taking alendronate before taking any other oral medicinal product (see 4.2 'Posology and method of administration' and 5.2 'Pharmacokinetic properties').

No other interactions with medicinal products of clinical significance are anticipated. A number of patients in the clinical trials received oestrogen (intravaginal, transdermal, or oral) while taking alendronate. No adverse experiences attributable to their concomitant use were identified.

Although specific interaction studies were not performed, in clinical studies alendronate was used concomitantly with a wide range of commonly prescribed medicinal products without evidence of clinical adverse interactions.

4.6 Pregnancy and lactation

Use during pregnancy

There are no adequate data from the use of alendronate in pregnant women. Animal studies do not indicate direct harmful effects with respect to pregnancy, embryonal/foetal development, or postnatal development. Alendronate given during pregnancy in rats caused dystocia related to hypocalcemia (see 5.3 'Preclinical safety data'). Given the indication, alendronate should not be used during pregnancy.

Use during lactation

It is not known whether alendronate is excreted into human breast milk. Given the indication, alendronate should not be used by breast-feeding women.

4.7 Effects on ability to drive and use machines

No effects on ability to drive and use machines have been observed.

4.8 Undesirable effects

In a one-year study in post-menopausal women with osteoporosis the overall safety profiles of 'Fosamax' Once Weekly 70 mg (n=519) and alendronate 10 mg/day (n=370) were similar.

In two three-year studies of virtually identical design, in post-menopausal women (alendronate 10 mg: n=196, placebo: n=397) the overall safety profiles of alendronate 10 mg/day and placebo were similar.

Adverse experiences reported by the investigators as possibly, probably or definitely drug-related are presented below if they occurred in ⩾1% in either treatment group in the one-year study, or in ⩾1% of patients treated with alendronate 10 mg/day and at a greater incidence than in patients given placebo in the three-year studies:

(see Table 1 on next page)

The following adverse experiences have also been reported during clinical studies and/or post-marketing use:

Common (⩾1/100, <1/10)

Gastro-intestinal: abdominal pain, dyspepsia, constipation, diarrhoea, flatulence, oesophageal ulcer*, dysphagia*, abdominal distension, acid regurgitation.

Musculoskeletal: musculoskeletal (bone, muscle or joint) pain.

Neurological: headache.

Uncommon (⩾1/1,000, <1/100)

Body as a whole: rash, pruritus, erythema

Gastro-intestinal: nausea, vomiting, gastritis, oesophagitis*, oesophageal erosions*, melaena.

Rare (⩾1/10,000, <1/1,000)

Body as a whole: hypersensitivity reactions including urticaria and angioedema. Transient symptoms as in an acute-phase response (myalgia, malaise and rarely, fever), typically in association with initiation of treatment. Rash with photosensitivity. Symptomatic hypocalcaemia, often in association with predisposing conditions (see 4.4 'Special warnings and precautions for use').

Gastro-intestinal: oesophageal stricture*, oropharyngeal ulceration*, upper gastrointestinal PUBs (perforation, ulcers, bleeding), although a causal relationship cannot be ruled out.

Special senses: uveitis, scleritis, episcleritis.

Isolated cases of severe skin reactions, including Stevens-Johnson syndrome and toxic epidermal necrolysis have been reported.

* See 4.4 'Special warnings and precautions for use' and 4.2 'Posology and method of administration'.

Table 1

	One-Year Study		Three-Year Studies	
	'Fosamax' Once Weekly 70 mg (n = 519)	Alendronate 10 mg/day (n = 370)	Alendronate 10 mg/day (n = 196)	Placebo(n = 397)
	%	%	%	%
Gastro-intestinal				
abdominal pain	3.7	3.0	6.6	4.8
dyspepsia	2.7	2.2	3.6	3.5
acid regurgitation	1.9	2.4	2.0	4.3
Nausea	1.9	2.4	3.6	4.0
abdominal distention	1.0	1.4	1.0	0.8
constipation	0.8	1.6	3.1	1.8
diarrhoea	0.6	0.5	3.1	1.8
dysphagia	0.4	0.5	1.0	0.0
flatulence	0.4	1.6	2.6	0.5
Gastritis	0.2	1.1	0.5	1.3
gastric ulcer	0.0	1.1	0.0	0.0
oesophageal ulcer	0.0	0.0	1.5	0.0
Musculoskeletal				
musculoskeletal (bone, muscle or joint) pain	2.9	3.2	4.1	2.5
muscle cramp	0.2	1.1	0.0	1.0
Neurological				
headache	0.4	0.3	2.6	1.5

Laboratory test findings

In clinical studies, asymptomatic, mild and transient decreases in serum calcium and phosphate were observed in approximately 18 and 10%, respectively, of patients taking alendronate 10 mg/day versus approximately 12 and 3% of those taking placebo. However, the incidences of decreases in serum calcium to <8.0 mg/dl (2.0 mmol/l) and serum phosphate to ≤2.0 mg/dl (0.65 mmol/l) were similar in both treatment groups.

4.9 Overdose

Hypocalcaemia, hypophosphataemia and upper gastro-intestinal adverse events, such as upset stomach, heartburn, oesophagitis, gastritis, or ulcer, may result from oral overdosage.

No specific information is available on the treatment of overdosage with alendronate. Milk or antacids should be given to bind alendronate. Owing to the risk of oesophageal irritation, vomiting should not be induced and the patient should remain fully upright.

5. PHARMACOLOGICAL PROPERTIES

5.1 Pharmacodynamic properties

Pharmacotherapeutic group: Bisphosphonate, for the treatment of bone diseases.

ATC Code: M05B A04

The active ingredient of 'Fosamax', alendronate sodium trihydrate, is a bisphosphonate that inhibits osteoclastic bone resorption with no direct effect on bone formation. Preclinical studies have shown preferential localisation of alendronate to sites of active resorption. Activity of osteoclasts is inhibited, but recruitment or attachment of osteoclasts is not affected. The bone formed during treatment with alendronate is of normal quality.

Treatment of post-menopausal osteoporosis

Osteoporosis is defined as BMD of the spine or hip 2.5 SD below the mean value of a normal young population or as a previous fragility fracture, irrespective of BMD.

The therapeutic equivalence of 'Fosamax' Once Weekly 70 mg (n=519) and alendronate 10 mg daily (n=370) was demonstrated in a one-year multicentre study of post-menopausal women with osteoporosis. The mean increases from baseline in lumbar spine BMD at one year were 5.1% (95% CI: 4.8, 5.4%) in the 70 mg once-weekly group and 5.4% (95% CI: 5.0, 5.8%) in the 10 mg daily group. The mean BMD increases were 2.3% and 2.9% at the femoral neck and 2.9% and 3.1% at the total hip in the 70 mg once weekly and 10 mg daily groups, respectively. The two treatment groups were also similar with regard to BMD increases at other skeletal sites.

The effects of alendronate on bone mass and fracture incidence in post-menopausal women were examined in two initial efficacy studies of identical design (n=994) as well as in the Fracture Intervention Trial (FIT: n=6,459).

In the initial efficacy studies, the mean bone mineral density (BMD) increases with alendronate 10 mg/day relative to placebo at three years were 8.8%, 5.9% and 7.8% at the spine, femoral neck and trochanter, respectively. Total body BMD also increased significantly. There was a 48% reduction (alendronate 3.2% vs placebo 6.2%) in the proportion of patients treated with alendronate experiencing one or more vertebral fractures relative to those treated with placebo. In the two-year extension of these studies BMD at the spine and trochanter continued to increase and BMD at the femoral neck and total body were maintained.

FIT consisted of two placebo-controlled studies using alendronate daily (5 mg daily for two years and 10 mg daily for either one or two additional years):

- FIT 1: A three-year study of 2,027 patients who had at least one baseline vertebral (compression) fracture. In this study alendronate daily reduced the incidence of ≥1 new vertebral fracture by 47% (alendronate 7.9% vs. placebo 15.0%). In addition, a statistically significant reduction was found in the incidence of hip fractures (1.1% vs. 2.2%, a reduction of 51%).
- FIT 2: A four-year study of 4,432 patients with low bone mass but without a baseline vertebral fracture. In this study, a significant difference was observed in the analysis of the subgroup of osteoporotic women (37% of the global population who correspond with the above definition of osteoporosis) in the incidence of hip fractures (alendronate 1.0% vs. placebo 2.2%, a reduction of 56%) and in the incidence of ≥1 vertebral fracture (2.9% vs. 5.8%, a reduction of 50%).

5.2 Pharmacokinetic properties

Absorption

Relative to an intravenous reference dose, the oral mean bioavailability of alendronate in women was 0.64% for doses ranging from 5 to 70 mg when administered after an overnight fast and two hours before a standardised breakfast. Bioavailability was decreased similarly to an estimated 0.46% and 0.39% when alendronate was administered one hour or half an hour before a standardised breakfast. In osteoporosis studies, alendronate was effective when administered at least 30 minutes before the first food or beverage of the day.

Bioavailability was negligible whether alendronate was administered with, or up to two hours after, a standardised breakfast. Concomitant administration of alendronate with coffee or orange juice reduced bioavailability by approximately 60%.

In healthy subjects, oral prednisone (20 mg three times daily for five days) did not produce a clinically meaningful change in oral bioavailability of alendronate (a mean increase ranging from 20% to 44%).

Distribution

Studies in rats show that alendronate transiently distributes to soft tissues following 1 mg/kg intravenous administration but is then rapidly redistributed to bone or excreted in the urine. The mean steady-state volume of distribution, exclusive of bone, is at least 28 litres in humans. Concentrations of drug in plasma following therapeutic oral doses are too low for analytical detection (<5 ng/ml). Protein binding in human plasma is approximately 78%.

Biotransformation

There is no evidence that alendronate is metabolised in animals or humans.

Elimination

Following a single intravenous dose of [^{14}C]alendronate, approximately 50% of the radioactivity was excreted in the urine within 72 hours and little or no radioactivity was recovered in the faeces. Following a single 10 mg intravenous dose, the renal clearance of alendronate was 71 ml/min, and systemic clearance did not exceed 200 ml/min. Plasma concentrations fell by more than 95% within six hours following intravenous administration. The terminal half-life in humans is estimated to exceed ten years, reflecting release of alendronate from the skeleton. Alendronate is not excreted through the acidic or basic transport systems of the kidney in rats, and thus it is not anticipated to interfere with the excretion of other medicinal products by those systems in humans.

Characteristics in patients

Preclinical studies show that the drug that is not deposited in bone is rapidly excreted in the urine. No evidence of saturation of bone uptake was found after chronic dosing with cumulative intravenous doses up to 35 mg/kg in animals. Although no clinical information is available, it is likely that, as in animals, elimination of alendronate via the kidney will be reduced in patients with impaired renal function. Therefore, somewhat greater accumulation of alendronate in bone might be expected in patients with impaired renal function (see 4.2 'Posology and method of administration').

5.3 Preclinical safety data

Preclinical data reveal no special hazard for humans based on conventional studies of safety pharmacology, repeated dose toxicity, genotoxicity and carcinogenic potential. Studies in rats have shown that treatment with alendronate during pregnancy was associated with dystocia in dams during parturition which was related to hypocalcaemia. In studies, rats given high doses showed an increased incidence of incomplete foetal ossification. The relevance to humans is unknown.

6. PHARMACEUTICAL PARTICULARS

6.1 List of excipients

Microcrystalline cellulose

Lactose anhydrous

Croscarmellose sodium

Magnesium stearate

6.2 Incompatibilities

Not applicable.

6.3 Shelf life

3 years.

6.4 Special precautions for storage

No special precautions for storage.

6.5 Nature and contents of container

Aluminum/aluminum blisters in packs containing 4 tablets.

6.6 Instructions for use and handling

No special requirements.

7. MARKETING AUTHORISATION HOLDER

Merck Sharp and Dohme Limited

Hertford Road, Hoddesdon, Hertfordshire EN11 9BU, UK

8. MARKETING AUTHORISATION NUMBER(S)

PL 0025/0399

9. DATE OF FIRST AUTHORISATION/RENEWAL OF THE AUTHORISATION

10 November 2000

10. DATE OF REVISION OF THE TEXT

January 2005

LEGAL CATEGORY

POM

® denotes registered trademark of Merck and Co., Inc., Whitehouse Station, NJ, USA.

FSM70.04.UK-IRL.2098   II-015

FOSAVANCE Tablets

(Merck Sharp & Dohme Limited)

1. NAME OF THE MEDICINAL PRODUCT

FOSAVANCE tablets

2. QUALITATIVE AND QUANTITATIVE COMPOSITION

Each tablet contains 70 mg alendronic acid as alendronate sodium trihydrate and 70 micrograms (2800 IU) colecalciferol (vitamin D_3).

For excipients, see section 6.1.

3. PHARMACEUTICAL FORM

Tablet.

Capsule-shaped, white to off-white tablets, marked with an outline of a bone image on one side, and '710' on the other.

4. CLINICAL PARTICULARS

4.1 Therapeutic indications

Treatment of postmenopausal osteoporosis in patients at risk of vitamin D insufficiency.

FOSAVANCE reduces the risk of vertebral and hip fractures.

4.2 Posology and method of administration

The recommended dosage is one (70 mg/70 microgram) tablet once weekly.

Due to the nature of the disease process in osteoporosis, FOSAVANCE is intended for long-term use.

To permit adequate absorption of alendronate:

FOSAVANCE must be taken with water only (**not** mineral water) at least 30 minutes before the first food, beverage, or medicinal product (including antacids, calcium supplements and vitamins) of the day. Other beverages (including mineral water), food and some medicinal products are likely to reduce the absorption of alendronate (see section 4.5).

The following instructions should be followed exactly in order to minimize the risk of oesophageal irritation and related adverse reactions (see section 4.4):

• FOSAVANCE should only be swallowed upon arising for the day with a full glass of water (not less than 200ml or 7fl.oz.).

• Patients should not chew the tablet or allow the tablet to dissolve in their mouths because of a potential for oropharyngeal ulceration.

• Patients should not lie down until after their first food of the day which should be at least 30 minutes after taking the tablet.

• Patients should not lie down for at least 30 minutes after taking FOSAVANCE.

• FOSAVANCE should not be taken at bedtime or before arising for the day.

Patients should receive supplemental calcium if intake is inadequate (see section 4.4). Additional supplementation with vitamin D should be considered on an individual basis taking into account any vitamin D intake from vitamins and dietary supplements. Equivalence of 2800 IU of vitamin D_3 weekly in FOSAVANCE to daily dosing of vitamin D 400 IU has not been studied.

Use in the elderly:

In clinical studies there was no age-related difference in the efficacy or safety profiles of alendronate. Therefore no dosage adjustment is necessary for the elderly.

Use in renal impairment:

No dosage adjustment is necessary for patients with glomerular filtration rate (GFR) greater than 35 ml/min. FOSAVANCE is not recommended for patients with renal impairment where GFR is less than 35 ml/min, due to lack of experience.

Use in children and adolescents:

FOSAVANCE has not been studied in children and adolescents and therefore should not be given to them.

4.3 Contraindications

• Hypersensitivity to the active substances or to any of the excipients.

• Abnormalities of the oesophagus and other factors which delay oesophageal emptying such as stricture or achalasia.

• Inability to stand or sit upright for at least 30 minutes.

• Hypocalcaemia.

4.4 Special warnings and special precautions for use

Alendronate

Alendronate can cause local irritation of the upper gastro-intestinal mucosa. Because there is a potential for worsening of the underlying disease, caution should be used when alendronate is given to patients with active upper gastro-intestinal problems, such as dysphagia, oesophageal disease, gastritis, duodenitis, ulcers, or with a recent history (within the previous year) of major gastrointestinal disease such as peptic ulcer, or active gastrointestinal bleeding, or surgery of the upper gastrointestinal tract other than pyloroplasty (see section 4.3).

Oesophageal reactions (sometimes severe and requiring hospitalisation), such as oesophagitis, oesophageal ulcers and oesophageal erosions, rarely followed by oesophageal stricture, have been reported in patients receiving alendronate. Physicians should therefore be alert to any signs or symptoms signalling a possible oesophageal reaction and patients should be instructed to discontinue alendronate and seek medical attention if they develop symptoms of oesophageal irritation such as dysphagia, pain on swallowing or retrosternal pain, new or worsening heartburn (see section 4.8).

The risk of severe oesophageal adverse reactions appears to be greater in patients who fail to take alendronate properly and/or who continue to take alendronate after developing symptoms suggestive of oesophageal irritation. It is very important that the full dosing instructions are provided to, and understood by the patient (see section 4.2). Patients should be informed that failure to follow these instructions may increase their risk of oesophageal problems.

While no increased risk was observed in extensive clinical trials with alendronate, there have been rare (post-marketing) reports of gastric and duodenal ulcers, some severe and with complications. A causal relationship cannot be ruled out (see section 4.8).

Bone, joint, and/or muscle pain has been reported in patients taking bisphosphonates. In post-marketing experience, these symptoms have rarely been severe and/or incapacitating (see section 4.8). The time to onset of symptoms varied from one day to several months after starting treatment. Most patients had relief of symptoms after stopping treatment. A subset had recurrence of symptoms when rechallenged with the same medicinal product or another bisphosphonate.

Patients should be instructed that if they miss a dose of FOSAVANCE they should take one tablet on the morning after they remember. They should not take two tablets on the same day but should return to taking one tablet once a week, as originally scheduled on their chosen day.

FOSAVANCE is not recommended for patients with renal impairment where GFR is less than 35 ml/min (see section 4.2).

Causes of osteoporosis other than oestrogen deficiency and ageing should be considered.

Hypocalcaemia must be corrected before initiating therapy with FOSAVANCE (see section 4.3). Other disorders affecting mineral metabolism (such as vitamin D deficiency and hypoparathyroidism) should also be effectively treated before starting FOSAVANCE. The content of vitamin D in FOSAVANCE is not suitable for correction of vitamin D deficiency. In patients with these conditions, serum calcium and symptoms of hypocalcaemia should be monitored during therapy with FOSAVANCE.

Due to the positive effects of alendronate in increasing bone mineral, decreases in serum calcium and phosphate may occur. These are usually small and asymptomatic. However, there have been rare reports of symptomatic hypocalcaemia, which have occasionally been severe and often occurred in patients with predisposing conditions (e.g. hypoparathyroidism, vitamin D deficiency and calcium malabsorption) (see section 4.8).

Colecalciferol

Vitamin D_3 may increase the magnitude of hypercalcaemia and/or hypercalciuria when administered to patients with disease associated with unregulated overproduction of calcitriol (e.g. leukaemia, lymphoma, sarcoidosis). Urine and serum calcium should be monitored in these patients.

Patients with malabsorption may not adequately absorb vitamin D_3.

Excipients

This medicinal product contains lactose and sucrose. Patients with rare hereditary problems of fructose intolerance, galactose intolerance, the Lapp lactase deficiency, glucose-galactose malabsorption or sucrase-isomaltase insufficiency should not take this medicinal product.

4.5 Interaction with other medicinal products and other forms of Interaction

Alendronate

If taken at the same time, it is likely that food and beverages (including mineral water), calcium supplements, antacids, and some oral medicinal products will interfere with absorption of alendronate. Therefore, patients must wait at least 30 minutes after taking alendronate before taking any other oral medicinal product (see sections 4.2 and 5.2).

No other interactions with medicinal products of clinical significance are anticipated. A number of patients in the clinical trials received oestrogen (intravaginal, transdermal, or oral) while taking alendronate. No adverse reactions attributable to their concomitant use were identified.

Although specific interaction studies were not performed, in clinical studies alendronate was used concomitantly with a wide range of commonly prescribed medicinal products without evidence of interactions of clinical relevance.

Colecalciferol

Olestra, mineral oils, orlistat, and bile acid sequestrants (e.g. cholestyramine, colestipol) may impair the absorption of vitamin D. Anticonvulsants, cimetidine and thiazides may increase the catabolism of vitamin D. Additional vitamin D supplements may be considered on an individual basis.

4.6 Pregnancy and lactation

FOSAVANCE is only intended for use in postmenopausal women and therefore it should not be used during pregnancy or in breast-feeding women.

There are no adequate data from the use of FOSAVANCE in pregnant women. Animal studies with alendronate do not indicate direct harmful effects with respect to pregnancy, embryonal/foetal development, or postnatal development. Alendronate given during pregnancy in rats caused dystocia related to hypocalcaemia (see section 5.3). Studies in animals have shown hypercalcaemia and reproductive toxicity with high doses of vitamin D (see section 5.3).

It is not known whether alendronate is excreted into human breast milk. Colecalciferol and some of its active metabolites pass into breast milk.

4.7 Effects on ability to drive and use machines

No studies on the effects on the ability to drive and use machines have been performed.

However, there is no information to indicate that FOSAVANCE affects a patient's ability to drive or operate machines.

4.8 Undesirable effects

The following adverse reactions have been reported during clinical studies and/or post-marketing use with alendronate.

No new adverse reactions have been identified for FOSAVANCE.

[Common (⩾ 1/100, < 1/10), Uncommon (⩾ 1/1000, < 1/100), Rare (⩾ 1/10,000, < 1/1000), Very rare (< 1/10,000 including isolated cases)]

Immune system disorders:

Rare: hypersensitivity reactions including urticaria and angioedema

Metabolism and nutrition disorders:

Rare: symptomatic hypocalcaemia, often in association with predisposing conditions. (see section 4.4)

Nervous system disorders:

Common: headache

Eye disorders:

Rare: uveitis, scleritis, episcleritis

Gastrointestinal disorders:

Common: abdominal pain, dyspepsia, constipation, diarrhoea, flatulence, oesophageal ulcer*, dysphagia*, abdominal distension, acid regurgitation

Uncommon: nausea, vomiting, gastritis, oesophagitis*, oesophageal erosions*, melena

Rare: oesophageal stricture*, oropharyngeal ulceration*, upper gastrointestinal PUBs (perforation, ulcers, bleeding) see section 4.4); localised osteonecrosis of the jaw, generally associated with tooth extraction and/or local infection, often with delayed healing.

*See sections 4.2 and 4.4

Skin and subcutaneous tissue disorders:

Uncommon: rash, pruritus, erythema

Rare: rash with photosensitivity

Very rare and isolated cases: isolated cases of severe skin reactions including Stevens-Johnson syndrome and toxic epidermal necrolysis

Musculoskeletal, connective tissue and bone disorders:

Common: musculoskeletal (bone, muscle or joint) pain

Rare: severe musculoskeletal (bone, muscle or joint) pain (see section 4.4)

General disorders and administration site conditions:

Rare: transient symptoms as in an acute-phase response (myalgia, malaise and rarely, fever), typically in association with initiation of treatment.

Laboratory test findings

In clinical studies, asymptomatic, mild and transient decreases in serum calcium and phosphate were observed in approximately 18% and 10%, respectively, of patients taking alendronate 10 mg/day versus approximately 12% and 3% of those taking placebo. However, the incidences of decreases in serum calcium to < 8.0 mg/dl (2.0 mmol/l) and serum phosphate to ⩽ 2.0 mg/dl (0.65 mmol/l) were similar in both treatment groups.

4.9 Overdose

Alendronate

Hypocalcaemia, hypophosphataemia and upper gastrointestinal adverse reactions, such as upset stomach, heartburn, oesophagitis, gastritis, or ulcer, may result from oral overdosage.

No specific information is available on the treatment of overdosage with alendronate. In case of overdosage with FOSAVANCE, milk or antacids should be given to bind alendronate. Owing to the risk of oesophageal irritation, vomiting should not be induced and the patient should remain fully upright.

Colecalciferol

Vitamin D toxicity has not been documented during chronic therapy in generally healthy adults at a dose less than 10,000 IU/day. In a clinical study of healthy adults a 4000

IU daily dose of vitamin D_3 for up to five months was not associated with hypercalciuria or hypercalcaemia.

5. PHARMACOLOGICAL PROPERTIES

5.1 Pharmacodynamic properties

Pharmacotherapeutic group: Drugs for treatment of bone diseases [pending]

ATC code: M05XX ***[pending]***

FOSAVANCE is a combination tablet containing the two active substances alendronate sodium trihydrate and colecalciferol (vitamin D_3).

Alendronate

Alendronate sodium is a bisphosphonate that inhibits osteoclastic bone resorption with no direct effect on bone formation. Preclinical studies have shown preferential localisation of alendronate to sites of active resorption. Activity of osteoclasts is inhibited, but recruitment or attachment of osteoclasts is not affected. The bone formed during treatment with alendronate is of normal quality.

Colecalciferol (vitamin D_3)

Vitamin D_3 is produced in the skin by conversion of 7-dehydrocholesterol to vitamin D_3 by ultraviolet light. In the absence of adequate sunlight exposure, vitamin D_3 is an essential dietary nutrient. Vitamin D_3 is converted to 25-hydroxyvitamin D_3 in the liver, and stored until needed. Conversion to the active calcium-mobilizing hormone 1,25-dihydroxyvitamin D_3 (calcitriol) in the kidney is tightly regulated. The principal action of 1,25-dihydroxyvitamin D_3 is to increase intestinal absorption of both calcium and phosphate as well as regulate serum calcium, renal calcium and phosphate excretion, bone formation and bone resorption.

Vitamin D_3 is required for normal bone formation. Vitamin D insufficiency develops when both sunlight exposure and dietary intake are inadequate. Insufficiency is associated with negative calcium balance, bone loss, and increased risk of skeletal fracture. In severe cases, deficiency results in secondary hyperparathyroidism, hypophosphataemia, proximal muscle weakness and osteomalacia, further increasing the risk of falls and fractures in osteoporotic individuals.

Osteoporosis is defined as bone mineral density (BMD) of the spine or hip 2.5 standard deviations (SD) below the mean value of a normal young population or as a previous fragility fracture, irrespective of BMD.

FOSAVANCE study

The effect of FOSAVANCE on vitamin D status was demonstrated in a 15-week, multinational study that enrolled 682 osteoporotic post-menopausal women (serum 25-hydroxyvitamin D at baseline: mean, 56 nmol/l [22.3 ng/ml]; range, 22.5-225 nmol/l [9-90 ng/ml]). Patients received FOSAVANCE (alendronate 70 mg/vitamin D_3 2800 IU) (n=350) or FOSAMAX (alendronate) 70 mg (n=332) once a week; additional vitamin D supplements were prohibited. After 15 weeks of treatment, the mean serum 25-hydroxyvitamin D levels were significantly higher (26%) in the FOSAVANCE group (56 nmol/l [23 ng/ml]) than in the alendronate-only group (46 nmol/l [18.2 ng/ml]). The percentage of patients with vitamin D insufficiency (serum 25-hydroxyvitamin D < 37.5 nmol/l [< 15 ng/ml]) was significantly reduced by 62.5% with FOSAVANCE vs. alendronate-only (12% vs. 32%, respectively), through week 15. The percentage of patients with vitamin D deficiency (serum 25-hydroxyvitamin D <22.5 nmol/l [<9 ng/ml]) was significantly reduced by 92% with FOSAVANCE vs. alendronate-only (1% vs 13%, respectively). In this study, mean 25-hydroxyvitamin D levels in patients with vitamin D insufficiency at baseline (25- hydroxyvitamin D, 22.5 to 37.5 nmol/l [9 to < 15 ng/ml]) increased from 30 nmol/l (12.1 ng/ml) to 40 nmol/l (15.9 ng/ml) at week 15 in the FOSAVANCE group (n=75) and decreased from 30 nmol/l (12.0 ng/ml) at baseline to 26 nmol/l (10.4 ng/ml) at week 15 in the alendronate-only group (n=70). There were no differences in mean serum calcium, phosphate, or 24-hour urine calcium between treatment groups.

Alendronate studies

The therapeutic equivalence of alendronate once weekly 70 mg (n=519) and alendronate 10 mg daily (n=370) was demonstrated in a one-year multicentre study of post-menopausal women with osteoporosis. The mean increases from baseline in lumbar spine BMD at one year were 5.1% (95% CI: 4.8, 5.4%) in the 70 mg once-weekly group and 5.4 % (95 % CI: 5.0, 5.8 %) in the 10 mg daily group. The mean BMD increases were 2.3% and 2.9% at the femoral neck and 2.9% and 3.1% at the total hip in the 70 mg once weekly and 10 mg daily groups, respectively. The two treatment groups were also similar with regard to BMD increases at other skeletal sites.

The effects of alendronate on bone mass and fracture incidence in post-menopausal women were examined in two initial efficacy studies of identical design (n=994) as well as in the Fracture Intervention Trial (FIT: n=6,459).

In the initial efficacy studies, the mean BMD increases with alendronate 10 mg/day relative to placebo at three years were 8.8%, 5.9% and 7.8% at the spine, femoral neck and trochanter, respectively. Total body BMD also increased significantly. There was a 48% reduction (alendronate 3.2% vs placebo 6.2%) in the proportion of patients treated with alendronate experiencing one or more vertebral fractures relative to those treated with placebo. In the two-year extension of these studies BMD at the spine and trochanter continued to increase and BMD at the femoral neck and total body were maintained.

FIT consisted of two placebo-controlled studies using alendronate daily (5 mg daily for two years and 10 mg daily for either one or two additional years):

• FIT 1: A three-year study of 2,027 patients who had at least one baseline vertebral (compression) fracture. In this study alendronate daily reduced the incidence of $\geqslant$ 1 new vertebral fracture by 47 % (alendronate 7.9% vs. placebo 15.0%). In addition, a statistically significant reduction was found in the incidence of hip fractures (1.1% vs. 2.2%, a reduction of 51 %).

• FIT 2: A four-year study of 4,432 patients with low bone mass but without a baseline vertebral fracture. In this study, a significant difference was observed in the analysis of the subgroup of osteoporotic women (37% of the global population who correspond with the above definition of osteoporosis) in the incidence of hip fractures (alendronate 1.0% vs. placebo 2.2%, a reduction of 56%) and in the incidence of $\geqslant$ 1 vertebral fracture (2.9% vs. 5.8%, a reduction of 50%).

5.2 Pharmacokinetic properties

Alendronate

Absorption

Relative to an intravenous reference dose, the oral mean bioavailability of alendronate in women was 0.64% for doses ranging from 5 to 70 mg when administered after an overnight fast and two hours before a standardised breakfast. Bioavailability was decreased similarly to an estimated 0.46% and 0.39% when alendronate was administered one hour or half an hour before a standardised breakfast. In osteoporosis studies, alendronate was effective when administered at least 30 minutes before the first food or beverage of the day.

The alendronate component in the FOSAVANCE combination tablet is bioequivalent to the alendronate 70 mg tablet.

Bioavailability was negligible whether alendronate was administered with, or up to two hours after, a standardised breakfast. Concomitant administration of alendronate with coffee or orange juice reduced bioavailability by approximately 60%.

In healthy subjects, oral prednisone (20 mg three times daily for five days) did not produce a clinically meaningful change in oral bioavailability of alendronate (a mean increase ranging from 20% to 44%).

Distribution

Studies in rats show that alendronate transiently distributes to soft tissues following 1 mg/kg intravenous administration but is then rapidly redistributed to bone or excreted in the urine. The mean steady-state volume of distribution, exclusive of bone, is at least 28 litres in humans. Concentrations of alendronate in plasma following therapeutic oral doses are too low for analytical detection (< 5 ng/ml). Protein binding in human plasma is approximately 78%.

Biotransformation

There is no evidence that alendronate is metabolised in animals or humans.

Elimination

Following a single intravenous dose of [^{14}C]alendronate, approximately 50% of the radioactivity was excreted in the urine within 72 hours and little or no radioactivity was recovered in the faeces. Following a single 10 mg intravenous dose, the renal clearance of alendronate was 71 ml/min, and systemic clearance did not exceed 200 ml/min. Plasma concentrations fell by more than 95 % within six hours following intravenous administration. The terminal half-life in humans is estimated to exceed ten years, reflecting release of alendronate from the skeleton. Alendronate is not excreted through the acidic or basic transport systems of the kidney in rats, and thus it is not anticipated to interfere with the excretion of other medicinal products by those systems in humans.

Colecalciferol

Absorption

In healthy adult subjects (males and females), following administration of FOSAVANCE after an overnight fast and two hours before a meal, the mean area under the serum-concentration-time curve ($AUC_{0\text{-}120\ hrs}$) for vitamin D_3 (unadjusted for endogenous vitamin D_3 levels) was 296.4 ng•hr/ml. The mean maximal serum concentration (C_{max}) of vitamin D_3 was 5.9 ng/ml, and the median time to maximal serum concentration (T_{max}) was 12 hours. The bioavailability of the 2800 IU vitamin D_3 in FOSAVANCE is similar to 2800 IU vitamin D_3 administered alone.

Distribution

Following absorption, vitamin D_3 enters the blood as part of chylomicrons. Vitamin D_3 is rapidly distributed mostly to the liver where it undergoes metabolism to 25-hydroxyvitamin D_3, the major storage form. Lesser amounts are distributed to adipose and muscle tissue and stored as vitamin D_3 at these sites for later release into the circulation. Circulating vitamin D_3 is bound to vitamin D-binding protein.

Biotransformation

Vitamin D_3 is rapidly metabolized by hydroxylation in the liver to 25-hydroxyvitamin D_3, and subsequently metabolized in the kidney to 1,25-dihydroxyvitamin D_3, which represents the biologically active form. Further hydroxylation occurs prior to elimination. A small percentage of vitamin D_3 undergoes glucuronidation prior to elimination.

Elimination

When radioactive vitamin D_3 was administered to healthy subjects, the mean urinary excretion of radioactivity after 48 hours was 2.4%, and the mean faecal excretion of radioactivity after 4 days was 4.9%. In both cases, the excreted radioactivity was almost exclusively as metabolites of the parent. The mean half-life of vitamin D_3 in the serum following an oral dose of FOSAVANCE is approximately 24 hours.

Characteristics in patients

Preclinical studies show that alendronate that is not deposited in bone is rapidly excreted in the urine. No evidence of saturation of bone uptake was found after chronic dosing with cumulative intravenous doses up to 35 mg/kg in animals. Although no clinical information is available, it is likely that, as in animals, elimination of alendronate via the kidney will be reduced in patients with impaired renal function. Therefore, somewhat greater accumulation of alendronate in bone might be expected in patients with impaired renal function (see section 4.2).

5.3 Preclinical safety data

No preclinical studies with the combination of alendronate and colecalciferol have been conducted.

Alendronate

Preclinical data reveal no special hazard for humans based on conventional studies of safety pharmacology, repeated dose toxicity, genotoxicity and carcinogenic potential. Studies in rats have shown that treatment with alendronate during pregnancy was associated with dystocia in dams during parturition which was related to hypocalcaemia. In studies, rats given high doses showed an increased incidence of incomplete foetal ossification. The relevance to humans is unknown.

Colecalciferol

At doses far higher than the human therapeutic range, reproductive toxicity has been observed in animal studies.

6. PHARMACEUTICAL PARTICULARS

6.1 List of excipients

Microcrystalline cellulose (E460)

Lactose anhydrous

Medium chain triglycerides

Gelatin

Croscarmellose sodium

Sucrose

Colloidal silicon dioxide

Magnesium stearate (E572)

Butylated hydroxytoluene (E321)

Modified starch (maize)

Sodium aluminium silicate (E554)

6.2 Incompatibilities

Not applicable.

6.3 Shelf life

18 months.

6.4 Special precautions for storage

Store in the original blister in order to protect from moisture and light.

6.5 Nature and contents of container

Wallet with sealed aluminium/aluminium blisters, in cartons containing 2, 4, 6 (3 wallets × 2 tablets), 12 (3 wallets × 4 tablets) or 40 (10 wallets × 4 tablets) tablets.

Not all pack sizes may be marketed.

6.6 Instructions for use and handling

No special requirements.

7. MARKETING AUTHORISATION HOLDER

Merck Sharp & Dohme Ltd.

Hertford Road, Hoddesdon

Hertfordshire EN11 9BU

United Kingdom

8. MARKETING AUTHORISATION NUMBER(S)

EU/1/05/310/001 – 2 tablets

EU/1/05/310/002 – 4 tablets

EU/1/05/310/003 – 6 tablets

EU/1/05/310/004 – 12 tablets

EU/1/05/310/005 – 40 tablets

9. DATE OF FIRST AUTHORISATION/RENEWAL OF THE AUTHORISATION

24 August 2005

10. DATE OF REVISION OF THE TEXT
24 August 2005

SPC.FOS.05.UK-IRL.2234 F.T. 26 Aug 2005

Foscavir

(AstraZeneca UK Limited)

1. NAME OF THE MEDICINAL PRODUCT
Brand name: Foscavir

Non-proprietary name: Foscarnet trisodium hexahydrate

2. QUALITATIVE AND QUANTITATIVE COMPOSITION
Foscarnet trisodium hexahydrate 24mg/ml.

3. PHARMACEUTICAL FORM
Intravenous infusion.

4. CLINICAL PARTICULARS

4.1 Therapeutic indications
Foscavir is indicated for induction and maintenance therapy of cytomegalovirus (CMV) retinitis in patients with AIDS. Induction therapy of mucocutaneous Herpes Simplex Virus (HSV) infections, unresponsive to acyclovir in immunocompromised patients.

Following induction therapy over 2-3 weeks Foscavir produced stabilisation of retinal lesions in approximately 80% of cases treated. However, since CMV causes latent infections and since Foscavir exerts a virustatic activity, relapses are likely in the majority of patients with persistent immunodeficiency once treatment is discontinued. Following completion of induction therapy, maintenance therapy should be instituted with a once daily regimen at an initial dose of 60 mg/kg increasing to 90-120 mg/kg if tolerated. A number of patients have received 90 mg/kg over a two hour period as a maintenance therapy starting dose. Maintenance therapy has produced a delay in time to retinitis progression. In patients experiencing progression of retinitis while receiving maintenance therapy or off therapy, reinstitution of induction therapy has shown equal efficacy equivalent to that of the initial course.

Foscavir is also indicated for the treatment of mucocutaneous HSV infections, clinically unresponsive to acyclovir in immunocompromised patients. The safety and efficacy of Foscavir for the treatment of other HSV infection (e.g. retinitis, encephalitis); congenital or neonatal disease; or HSV in immunocompetent individuals has not been established.

The diagnosis of acyclovir unresponsiveness can be made either clinically by treatment with intravenous acyclovir (5-10mg/kg t.i.d) for 10 days without response or by *in vitro* testing.

For treatment of acyclovir unresponsive mucocutaneous infections Foscavir was administered at 40mg/kg every 8 hours over 2-3 weeks or until healing. In a prospective randomised study in patients with AIDS, Foscavir treated patients healed within 11-25 days, had a complete relief of pain within 9 days and stopped shedding HSV virus within 7 days.

Foscavir is not recommended for treatment of CMV infections other than retinitis or HSV or for use in non-AIDS or non-immunocompromised patients.

4.2 Posology and method of administration
Method of administration: Foscarnet should be administered by the intravenous route only, either by a central venous line or in a peripheral vein.

When peripheral veins are used, the solution of foscarnet 24mg/ml must be diluted. Individually dispensed doses of foscarnet should be aseptically transferred and diluted with equal parts of 0.9% sodium chloride (9mg/ml) or 5% dextrose (50mg/ml) by the hospital pharmacy. The diluted solutions should be used as soon as possible after preparation but can be stored for up to 24 hours if kept refrigerated.

The solution of foscarnet 24mg/ml may be given without dilution via a central vein.

Adults: Induction therapy for CMV retinitis: Foscavir is administered over 2-3 weeks depending on the clinical response, as intermittent infusions every 8 hours at a dose of 60mg/kg in patients with normal renal function. Dosage must be individualised for patient's renal function (see dosing chart below). The infusion time should not be shorter than 1 hour.

Maintenance therapy: For maintenance therapy, following induction therapy of CMV retinitis, Foscavir is administered seven days a week as long as therapy is considered appropriate. In patients with normal renal function it is recommended to initiate therapy at 60 mg/kg. Increase to a dose of 90-120 mg/kg may then be considered in patients tolerating the initial dose level and/or those with progressive retinitis. A number of patients have received 90 mg/kg over a 2 hour period as a starting dose for maintenance therapy. Dosage must be reduced in patients with renal insufficiency (see dosage chart at end of dosage section).

Patients who experience progression of retinitis while receiving maintenance therapy may be re-treated with the induction regimen.

Induction therapy of mucocutaneous HSV infections unresponsive to acyclovir: Foscavir is administered for 2-3 weeks or until healing of lesions, as intermittent infusions at a dose of 40mg/kg over one hour every 8 hours in patients with normal renal function. Dosage must be individualised for patients renal function (see dosing chart below). The infusion time should not be shorter than 1 hour.

Efficacy of Foscavir maintenance therapy following induction therapy of acyclovir unresponsive HSV infections has not been established.

Caution: Do not administer Foscavir by rapid intravenous injection.

Foscavir Dosing Chart

Induction Therapy

Creatinine Clearance (ml/kg/min)	CMV Every 8 Hours (mg/kg)	HSV Every 8 Hours (mg/kg)
> 1.6	60	40
1.6 – 1.4	55	37
1.4 – 1.2	49	33
1.2 – 1.0	42	28
1.0 – 0.8	35	24
0.8 – 0.6	28	19
0.6 – 0.4	21	14
< 0.4	Treatment not recommended	

CMV Maintenance Therapy

Creatinine Clearance (ml/kg/min)	One Infusion Dose (mg/kg/day in not less than one hour)
> 1.6	60*
1.6 – 1.4	55
1.4 – 1.2	49
1.2 – 1.0	42
1.0 – 0.8	35
0.8 – 0.6	28
0.6 – 0.4	21
< 0.4	Treatment not recommended

*A number of patients have received 90 mg/kg as a starting dose for maintenance therapy.

Foscavir is not recommended in patients undergoing haemodialysis since dosage guidelines have not been established.

Hydration: Renal toxicity of Foscavir can be reduced by adequate hydration of the patient. It is recommended to establish diuresis by hydration with 0.5-1.0 L of normal saline at each infusion.

Elderly: As for adults.

Children: There is very limited experience in treating children.

Renal or hepatic insufficiency: The dose must be reduced in patients with renal insufficiency, according to the creatinine clearance level as described in the table above. Dose adjustment is not required in patients with hepatic insufficiency.

4.3 Contraindications
Hypersensitivity to Foscavir, pregnancy and lactation.

4.4 Special warnings and special precautions for use
Foscavir should be used with caution in patients with reduced renal function. Since renal functional impairment may occur at any time during Foscavir administration, serum creatinine should be monitored every second day during induction therapy and once weekly during maintenance therapy and appropriate dose adjustments should be performed according to renal function. Adequate hydration should be maintained in all patients. (See Dosage and Administration).

Due to Foscavir's propensity to chelate bivalent metal ions, such as calcium, Foscavir administration may be associated with an acute decrease of ionised serum calcium, which may not be reflected in total serum calcium levels. The electrolytes, especially calcium and magnesium, should be assessed prior to and during Foscavir therapy and deficiencies corrected.

Foscavir has local irritating properties and when excreted in high concentrations in the urine it may induce genital irritation or even ulcerations. Close attention to personal hygiene is recommended after micturition to lessen the potential of local irritation.

When diuretics are indicated thiazides are recommended.

Following treatment with foscarnet, clinical unresponsiveness can appear which may be due to appearance of virus strains with decreased sensitivity towards foscarnet. Termination of treatment with foscarnet should then be considered.

Mutagenicity studies showed that foscarnet has a genotoxic potential. The possible explanation for the observed effect in the mutagenicity studies is an inhibition of the DNA polymerase in the cell line used. Foscarnet therapeutically acts by inhibition of the herpes virus specific DNA polymerase. The human cellular polymerase α is about 100 times less sensitive to foscarnet. The carcinogenicity studies performed did not disclose any oncogenic potential.

4.5 Interaction with other medicinal products and other forms of Interaction
Since Foscavir can impair renal function, additive toxicity may occur when used in combination with other nephrotoxic drugs such as aminoglycoside antibiotics, amphotericin B and cyclosporin A. Moreover, since Foscavir can reduce serum levels of ionised calcium, extreme caution is advised when used concurrently with other drugs known to influence serum calcium levels, like *i.v.* pentamidine. Renal impairment and symptomatic hypocalcaemia (Trousseau's and Chvostek's signs) have been observed during concurrent treatment with Foscavir and *i.v.* pentamidine. Abnormal renal function has been reported in connection with the use of foscarnet in combination with protease inhibitors associated with impaired renal function e.g. ritonavir and saquinavir.

The elimination of Foscavir may be impaired by drugs which inhibit renal tubular secretion.

There is no evidence of an increased myelotoxicity when foscarnet is used in combination with zidovudine (AZT). Neither is there any pharmacokinetic interaction between the two drugs.

4.6 Pregnancy and lactation
Foscavir is contra-indicated in pregnancy. Breast feeding should be discontinued before starting Foscavir treatment.

4.7 Effects on ability to drive and use machines
Adverse effects such as dizziness and convulsions may occur during Foscavir therapy. The physician is advised to discuss this issue with the patient, and based upon the condition of the disease and the tolerance of medication, give his recommendation in the individual case.

4.8 Undesirable effects
In different patient populations Foscavir has been administered to more than 11,500 patients, the majority severely immunocompromised and suffering from serious viral infections.

The patient's physical status, the severity of the underlying disease, other infections and concurrent therapy also contribute to the observed adverse event profile of Foscavir.

Consistent findings associated with Foscavir administration are renal function impairment, impact on serum electrolytes and haemoglobin concentration, convulsions and local genital irritation/ulceration.

The adverse events discussed and tabulated below refer to results for 188 AIDS patients in prospective clinical trials and include those events related, unrelated and of unknown relationship to Foscavir. The adverse event profile from the market is similar to that reported in clinical studies.

Renal function impairment: Twenty-seven percent of the above 188 study patients experienced renal functional impairment recorded as a rise in serum creatinine (19%), decreases in creatinine clearance (6%), abnormal renal function (9%), acute renal failure (2%), uraemia (1%) and polyuria in 2%. Metabolic acidosis was seen in 1%. The overall pattern of these symptoms is consistent with previous experiences although the incidence may vary. Most patients with increased serum creatinine have shown normalisation or return to pre-treatment levels within 1-10 weeks of treatment discontinuation.

Electrolytes: Among the above 188 patients, hypocalcaemia was recorded in 14%. Also, hypomagnesaemia was recorded in 15%. Frequently recorded were also hypokalaemia in 16% and hypophosphataemia and hyperphosphataemia in 8 and 6% respectively. Foscarnet chelates with metal ions (Ca^{2+}. Mg^{2+}, Fe^{2+}, Zn^{2+}) and acute hypocalcaemia, sometimes symptomatic, has been a common observation in some 30% of AIDS patients receiving foscarnet. Experimental and clinical data have shown that foscarnet acutely decreases ionised calcium in a dose-related manner. The drop in serum calcium is reversible. It is reasonable to assume that the infusion rate significantly affects the decrease rate of ionised calcium.

Convulsions: Among the AIDS patients referred to above, convulsions including grand mal were recorded in 10%. Based on the occurrence of convulsions among immunocompromised patients receiving foscarnet, an association between foscarnet induced hypocalcaemia or a direct action of foscarnet per se and convulsions has been discussed. Although many of the patients experiencing convulsions had pre-existing CNS abnormalities such as cryptococcal meningitis, space occupying lesions or other CNS tumours, an association with foscarnet can not be excluded.

Haemoglobin concentration: Decreases of the haemoglobin concentration have been observed in 25-33% of patients. Generally, there has been no consistent pattern of simultaneous decreases in white blood cell and platelet counts. Some 30% of the above study patients were also on concurrent AZT treatment. Many AIDS patients were anaemic already before foscarnet administration.

Local irritation in terms of thrombophlebitis in peripheral veins following infusion of undiluted foscarnet solution and genital irritation/ulcerations have been observed. Since foscarnet is excreted in high concentrations in the urine local irritation/ulceration may ensue especially during induction therapy when high doses of foscarnet are being administered.

Other Adverse Events: Other adverse events that were recorded in the 188 study patients include a variety of symptoms varying in frequency from 1% to approximately 60%, the latter being the incidence for fever. Subgrouped by body system the following adverse events, related, unrelated or of unknown relationship to foscarnet therapy were recorded.

Body as a whole: Asthenia, fatigue, malaise and chills were observed in 12, 20, 7 and 13% respectively and sepsis in 7%.

Gastro-intestinal system disorders: Nausea and vomiting were observed in 45 and 25% respectively and diarrhoea in 32%. Abdominal pain and occasionally dyspepsia and constipation were observed in 10, 3 and 6% respectively. Isolated cases of pancreatitis have been reported from marketed use.

Metabolic and nutritional disorders: Hyponatraemia and oedema in legs were seen in 4 and 1% respectively and increase in LDH and alkaline phosphatases in 2 and 3% respectively. Increased levels of amylase have been reported from marketed use.

Central/Peripheral nervous system disorders: Paraesthesia was observed in 18%, headache in 25% and dizziness in 12%. Involuntary muscle contractions and tremor were seen in 9 and 5% respectively. Hypoaesthesia, ataxia and neuropathy were observed in 7, 4 and 6% respectively.

Psychiatric disorders: Anorexia, anxiety and nervousness were observed in 15 and 5% respectively and depression in 10%, confusion in 7%, psychosis in 1%, agitation in 3% and aggressive reaction in 2%.

White blood cells: Adverse events related to white blood cells included leukopenia 9%, granulocytopenia 17%. In these patients over 90% had some degree of leukopenia already before foscarnet administration, in 8% severe or even life-threatening. Moreover in some patients, it is noteworthy that mean WBC counts increased during treatment with foscarnet. Although a few patients worsened in this respect, there is no clear evidence to indicate that foscarnet is myelosuppressive.

Platelet, bleeding, clotting disorders: Thrombocytopenia was observed in 4%.

Skin and appendages: Rash was observed in 16%.

Liver and biliary system disorders: Abnormal liver function was observed in 4% and increase in serum ALAT and ASAT in 3 and 2% respectively and gamma GT in 2%.

Cardiovascular disorders: Abnormal ECG, hypertension and hypotension were observed in 1, 4 and 2% respectively.

Heart rate and rhythm disorders: Ventricular arrhythmia has been reported in 2 patients from marketed use.

Urinary system disorders: A few cases of diabetes insipidus, usually of the nephrogenic type, have been reported from marketed use.

Musculo-skeletal disorders: Muscle weakness has been reported from marketed use.

4.9 Overdose

Overdose has been reported in 33 patients, the highest dose being about 10 times the prescribed dose. Twenty-eight of the patients experienced adverse events and five patients suffered no ill effects in connection with foscarnet overdosing. Four patients died, one from respiratory/cardiac arrest 3 days after stopping foscarnet, one from progressive AIDS and renal failure approximately 2 months after the last foscarnet dose, one from end stage AIDS and bacteraemia 2 weeks after overdosing and one from multi-organ failure 11 days after stop of foscarnet. The pattern of adverse events reported in connection with overdose was in correspondence with the symptoms previously observed during foscarnet therapy.

Haemodialysis increases foscarnet elimination and may be of benefit in severe overdosage.

5. PHARMACOLOGICAL PROPERTIES

5.1 Pharmacodynamic properties

Foscarnet is an antiviral agent with a broad spectrum inhibiting all known human viruses of the herpes group, herpes simplex virus type 1 and 2, human herpes virus 6, varicella zoster virus, Epstein-Barr virus and cytomegalovirus (CMV) and some retroviruses, including human immunodeficiency virus (HIV) at concentrations not affecting normal cell growth. Foscarnet also inhibits the viral DNA polymerase from hepatitis B virus.

Foscarnet exerts its antiviral activity by a direct inhibition of viral specific DNA polymerase a reverse transcriptase at concentrations that do not affect cellular DNA polymerases. Foscarnet does not require activation (phosphorylation) by thymidine kinase or other kinases and therefore is active in vitro against HSV mutants deficient in thymidine kinase. CMV strains resistant to ganciclovir may be sensitive to foscarnet. Sensitivity test results expressed as concentration of the drug required to inhibit growth of virus by 50% in cell culture (IC_{50}) vary greatly depending on the assay method used and cell type employed. A number of sensitive viruses and their IC_{50} are listed below.

FOSCARNET Inhibition of virus multiplication cell culture	
Virus	$IC_{50}(\mu m)$
CMV	50 - 800 *
HSV-1, HSV-2	10 - 130
VZV	48 - 90
EBV	<500**
HHV-6	49
Ganciclovir resistant CMV	190
HSV - TK Minus Mutant	67
HSV - DNA Polymerase Mutant	5 - 443
HIV-1	11 - 32
Zidovudine resistant HIV-1	10 - 32

* Mean = 269μm

** 97% of viral antigen synthesis inhibited at 500μm.

If no clinical response to foscarnet is observed, viral isolates should be tested for sensitivity to foscarnet since naturally resistant mutants may exist or emerge under selective pressure both in vitro and in vivo.

The mean foscarnet 50% inhibition value for more than one hundred clinical CMV isolates was approximately 270μmol/L, while a reversible inhibition of normal cell growth was observed at about 1000μmol/L.

5.2 Pharmacokinetic properties

Foscarnet is eliminated by the kidneys mainly through glomerular filtration. The plasma clearance after intravenous administration to man varies between 130-160ml/min and the renal clearance is about 130ml/min. The half-life is in the order of 2-4 hours in patients with normal renal function.

The mean volume of distribution of foscarnet at steady state varies between 0.4-0.6 l/kg. There is no metabolic conversion of foscarnet and the binding to human plasma proteins is low (<20%). Foscarnet is distributed to the cerebrospinal fluid and concentrations ranging from 10 to 70% of the concurrent plasma concentrations have been observed in HIV infected patients.

5.3 Preclinical safety data

The most pronounced effects noted during general toxicity studies performed with foscarnet are perturbation of some serum electrolytes, and kidney and bone changes.

An observed reduction of serum electrolytes such as calcium and magnesium can be explained by the property of foscarnet to form chelate with divalent metal ions. The reduction of ionised calcium and magnesium is, most probably the explanation to seizures/convulsions seen during and shortly after the infusion of high doses of foscarnet. This reduction may also have a bearing on heart function (e.g. ECG) although the toxicological studies performed did not disclose any such effects. The rate of infusion of foscarnet is critical to disturbances in the homeostasis of some serum divalent cations.

The mechanism behind the kidney changes e.g. tubular atrophy, mainly confined to juxtamedullary nephrons, is less clear. The changes were noted in all species investigated. It is known that other complex binders of divalent cations (EDTA and biphosphonates) can cause changes of the kidney similar to those of foscarnet. It has been shown that hydration, to induce diuresis, significantly reduces kidney changes during foscarnet treatment.

The bone changes were characterised as increased osteoclast activity and bone resorption. This effect has only been seen in the dog. The reason to these changes may be that foscarnet, due to the structural similarity to phosphate is incorporated into the hydroxyapatite. Autoradiographic studies showed that foscarnet has a pronounced affinity to bone tissue. Recovery studies revealed that the bone changes were reversible.

Mutagenicity studies showed that foscarnet has a genotoxic potential. The possible explanation for the observed effect in the mutagenicity studies is an inhibition of the DNA polymerase in the cell line used. Foscarnet therapeutically acts by inhibition of the herpes virus specific DNA polymerase. The human cellular polymerase is about 100 times less sensitive to foscarnet. The carcinogenicity studies performed did not disclose any oncogenic potential. The information gained from teratogenicity and fertility studies did not reveal any adverse events upon the reproductive process. However, the results are of limited value since the dose levels used in these studies are below or at most similar (75-150mg/kg sc) to those used in man for treatment of CMV retinitis.

6. PHARMACEUTICAL PARTICULARS

6.1 List of excipients

Water for injection, hydrochloric acid.

6.2 Incompatibilities

Foscarnet is not compatible with dextrose 30% solution, amphotericin B, acyclovir sodium, ganciclovir, pentamidine isethionate, trimethoprimsulfamtoxazole and vancomycin hydrochloride. Neither is foscarnet compatible with solutions containing calcium. It is recommended that other drugs should not be infused concomitantly in the same line until further experience is gained.

6.3 Shelf life

3 years.

6.4 Special precautions for storage

Do not store above 30 °C. Do not refrigerate. If refrigerated or exposed to temperatures below freezing point precipitation may occur. By keeping the bottle at room temperature with repeated shaking, the precipitate can be brought into solution again.

6.5 Nature and contents of container

Infusion glass bottles of 250ml and 500ml.

6.6 Instructions for use and handling

Foscarnet contains no preservatives and once the sterility seal of a bottle has been broken the solution should be used within 24 hours.

Individually dispensed doses of foscarnet can be aseptically transferred to plastic infusion bags by the hospital pharmacy. The physico-chemical stability of foscarnet and dilutions thereof in equal parts with 0.9% sodium chloride (9mg/ml) or 5% dextrose (50mg/ml) in PVC bags is 7 days. However, diluted solutions should be refrigerated and storage restricted to 24 hours.

Each bottle of Foscavir should only be used to treat one patient with a single infusion. Unused solution should be discarded.

Accidental skin and eye contact with the foscarnet sodium solution may cause local irritation and burning sensation. If accidental contact occurs the exposed area should be rinsed with water.

7. MARKETING AUTHORISATION HOLDER

AstraZeneca UK Ltd.,

600 Capability Green,

Luton, LU1 3LU, UK.

8. MARKETING AUTHORISATION NUMBER(S)

PL 17901/0124

9. DATE OF FIRST AUTHORISATION/RENEWAL OF THE AUTHORISATION

16th October 2002

10. DATE OF REVISION OF THE TEXT

16th October 2002

Fragmin - Haemodialysis/Haemofiltration

(Pharmacia Limited)

1. NAME OF THE MEDICINAL PRODUCT

1. Fragmin 10,000 IU/1 ml

2. Fragmin 10,000 IU/4ml

2. QUALITATIVE AND QUANTITATIVE COMPOSITION

Active ingredient

Dalteparin sodium (INN)

Quality according to Ph Eur and in-house specification.

Potency is described in International anti-Factor Xa units (IU) of the 1st International Standard for Low Molecular Weight Heparin.

Content of active ingredient

1. Ampoules containing dalteparin sodium, 10,000 IU (anti-Factor Xa) in 1 ml.

2. Fragmin 10,000 IU/4ml: Ampoules containing dalteparin sodium corresponding to 2,500 IU (anti-Factor Xa)/ml.

3. PHARMACEUTICAL FORM

Solution for injection for intravenous or subcutaneous administration.

4. CLINICAL PARTICULARS

4.1 Therapeutic indications

Prevention of clotting in the extracorporeal circulation during haemodialysis or haemofiltration, in patients with chronic renal insufficiency or acute renal failure.

4.2 Posology and method of administration

Recommended dosage for adults

(i) Prevention of clotting during haemodialysis and haemofiltration

In chronic renal insufficiency for patients with no known additional bleeding risk, the dosage is:

(a) Long-term haemodialysis or haemofiltration - duration of haemodialysis/haemofiltration more than 4 hours;

An I.V. bolus injection of Fragmin 30-40 IU (anti-Factor Xa)/kg bodyweight, followed by an infusion of 10-15 IU (anti-Factor Xa)/kg bodyweight/hour.

(b) Short-term haemodialysis or haemofiltration - duration of haemodialysis/haemofiltration less than 4 hours:

Either as above, or, a single IV bolus injection of Fragmin 5000 IU (anti-Factor Xa).

Both for long and short-term haemodialysis and haemofiltration, the plasma anti-Factor Xa levels should be within the range 0.5-1.0 IU (anti-Factor Xa)/ml.

In acute renal failure, or chronic renal failure in patients with a high risk of bleeding, the dosage is:

An I.V. bolus injection of Fragmin 5-10 IU (anti-Factor Xa)/kg bodyweight, followed by an infusion of 4-5 IU (anti-Factor Xa)/kg bodyweight/hour.

The plasma anti-Factor Xa levels should be within the range 0.2-0.4 IU (anti-Factor Xa)/ml.

When considered necessary, it is recommended that the antithrombotic effect of Fragmin be monitored by analysing anti-Factor Xa activity using a suitable chromogenic substrate assay. This is because Fragmin has only a moderate prolonging effect on clotting time assays such as APTT or thrombin time.

Children

Not recommended for children.

Elderly

Fragmin has been used safely in elderly patients without the need for dosage adjustment.

4.3 Contraindications

Known hypersensitivity to Fragmin or other low molecular weight heparins and/or heparins e.g. history of confirmed or suspected immunologically mediated heparin induced thrombocytopenia, acute gastroduodenal ulcer; cerebral haemorrhage; known haemorrhagic diathesis; subacute endocarditis; injuries to and operations on the central nervous system, eyes and ears.

In patients receiving Fragmin for treatment rather than prophylaxis, local and/or regional anaesthesia in elective surgical procedures is contra-indicated.

4.4 Special warnings and special precautions for use

Do not administer by the intramuscular route.

Caution should be exercised in patients in whom there is an increased risk of bleeding complications, e.g. following surgery or trauma, haemorrhagic stroke, severe liver or renal failure, thrombocytopenia or defective platelet function, uncontrolled hypertension, hypertensive or diabetic retinopathy, patients receiving concurrent anticoagulant/antiplatelet agents (see interactions section).

It is recommended that platelets be counted before starting treatment with Fragmin and monitored regularly. Special caution is necessary in rapidly developing thrombocytopenia and severe thrombocytopenia ($<100,000/\mu l$) associated with positive or unknown results of in-vitro tests for anti-platelet antibody in the presence of Fragmin or other low molecular weight (mass) heparins and/or heparin

Fragmin induces only a moderate prolongation of the APTT and thrombin time. Accordingly, dosage increments based upon prolongation of the APTT may cause overdosage and bleeding. Therefore, prolongation of the APTT should only be used as a test of overdosage.

Anti-Factor Xa levels should be regularly monitored in new patients on chronic haemodialysis during the first weeks, later less frequent monitoring is generally required. Patients undergoing acute haemodialysis have a narrower therapeutic dose range and should be monitored frequently in accordance with the individual course of the disease.

Patients with severely disturbed hepatic function may need a reduction in dosage and should be monitored accordingly.

As individual low molecular weight (mass) heparins have differing characteristics, switching to an alternative low molecular weight heparin should be avoided. The directions for use relating to each specific product must be observed as different dosages may be required.

Heparin can suppress adrenal secretion of aldosterone leading to hyperkalaemia, particularly in patients such as those with diabetes mellitus, chronic renal failure, pre-existing metabolic acidosis, a raised plasma potassium or taking potassium sparing drugs. The risk of hyperkalaemia appears to increase with duration of therapy but is usually reversible. Plasma potassium should be measured in patients at risk before starting heparin therapy and monitored regularly thereafter particularly if treatment is prolonged beyond about 7 days.

In patients undergoing spinal or epidural anaesthesia, the prophylactic use of heparin may be very rarely associated with spinal haematomas resulting in prolonged or permanent paralysis. The risk is increased by use of an epidural or spinal catheter for anaesthesia, by the concomitant use of drugs (NSAIDs), platelet inhibitors or anti-coagulants and by traumatic or repeated puncture.

In decision-making on the interval between the last administration of Fragmin at prophylactic doses and the placement or removal of a peridural or spinal catheter for anaesthesia, the product characteristics and the patient profile should be taken into account. Readministration should be delayed until at least four hours after the surgical procedure is completed.

Should a physician, as a clinical judgement, decide to administer anticoagulation in the context of peridual or spinal anaesthesia, extreme vigilance and frequent monitoring must be exercised to detect any signs and symptoms of neurologic impairment such as back pain, sensory or motor deficits (numbness and weakness in lower limbs) and bowel or bladder dysfunction. Nurses should be trained to detect such signs and symptoms. Patients should be instructed to inform immediately a nurse or a clinician if they experience any of these.

If signs or symptoms of epidural or spinal haematoma are suspected, urgent diagnosis and treatment may include spinal cord decompression.

There have been no adequate studies to assess the safe and effective use of Fragmin in preventing valve thrombosis in patients with prosthetic heart valves. Prophylactic doses of Fragmin are not sufficient to prevent valve thrombosis in patients with prosthetic heart valves. The use of Fragmin cannot be recommended for this purpose

4.5 Interaction with other medicinal products and other forms of Interaction

The possibility of the following interactions with Fragmin should be considered:

(i) An enhancement of the anticoagulant effect by anticoagulant/antiplatelet agents e.g. aspirin/ dipyridamole, vitamin K antagonists, NSAIDs e.g. indomethacin, cytostatics, dextran, sulphinpyrazone, probenecid, and ethacrynic acid.

(ii) A reduction of the anticoagulant effect may occur with concomitant administration of antihistamines, cardiac glycosides, tetracycline and ascorbic acid.

4.6 Pregnancy and lactation

This medicinal product has been assessed in pregnant women and no harmful effects are known with respect to the course of pregnancy and the health of the unborn and neonate.

No information is available as to whether Fragmin passes into breast milk.

Therapeutic failures have been reported in pregnant women with prosthetic heart valves on full anti-coagulant doses of low molecular weight heparin. In the absence of clear dosing, efficacy and safety information in this circumstance, Fragmin is not recommended for use in pregnant women with prosthetic heart valves.

4.7 Effects on ability to drive and use machines

Fragmin does not affect the ability to drive or operate machinery.

4.8 Undesirable effects

Bleeding may be provoked, especially at high dosages corresponding with anti-Factor Xa levels greater than 1.5 IU/ml. However, at recommended dosages bleedings rarely occur.

Transient, slight to moderate, elevation of liver transaminases (ASAT, ALAT) has been observed, but no clinical significance has been demonstrated.

Commonly reported side-effects include subcutaneous haematomas at the injection site;

Mild thrombocytopenia (type I) which is usually reversible during treatment.

Allergic reactions (urticaria, pruritus, hair loss and skin necrosis) occur rarely.

A few cases of anaphylactoid reactions and of severe immunologically mediated thrombocytopenia (type II) with arterial and/or venous thrombosis or thromboembolism have been observed.

Osteoporosis has been associated with long-term heparin treatment and therefore cannot be excluded with Fragmin.

Heparin products can cause hypoaldosteronism which may result in an increase in plasma potassium. Rarely, clinically significant hyperkalaemia may occur, particularly in patients with chronic renal failure and diabetes mellitus (see Special Warnings and Precautions for Use)

Valve thrombosis in patients with prosthetic heart valves have been reported rarely, usually associated with inadequate dosing, (see Special Warnings and Precautions for Use).

Very rare cases of epidural and spinal haematoma have been reported in association with prophylactic use of heparin in the context of spinal or epidural anaesthesia and of spinal puncture. These haematomas have caused various degrees of neurological impairment, including prolonged or permanent paralysis (cross reference to section 4.4 Special Warnings and Precautions for Use").

4.9 Overdose

The anticoagulant effect (i.e. prolongation of the APTT) induced by Fragmin is inhibited by protamine. Since protamine itself has an inhibiting effect on primary haemostasis it should be used only in an emergency.

The prolongation of the clotting time induced by Fragmin may be fully neutralised by protamine, but the anti-Factor Xa activity is only neutralised to about 25-50%. 1 mg of protamine inhibits the effect of 100 IU (anti-Factor Xa) of Fragmin.

5. PHARMACOLOGICAL PROPERTIES

5.1 Pharmacodynamic properties

Dalteparin sodium is a low molecular weight heparin fraction (average molecular weight 4000-6000 Daltons) produced from porcine-derived sodium heparin.

Dalteparin sodium is an antithrombotic agent, which acts mainly through its ability to potentiate the inhibition of Factor Xa and thrombin by antithrombin. It has a relatively higher ability to potentiate Factor Xa inhibition than to prolong plasma clotting time (APTT).

Compared with standard, unfractionated heparin, dalteparin sodium has a reduced adverse effect on platelet function and platelet adhesion, and thus has only a minimal effect on primary haemostasis. Some of the antithrombotic properties of dalteparin sodium are thought to be mediated through the effects on vessel walls or the fibrinolytic system.

5.2 Pharmacokinetic properties

The half life following iv and sc. administration is 2 hours and 3.5-4 hours respectively, twice that of unfractionated heparin.

The bioavailability following sc. injection is approximately 87 per cent and the pharmacokinetics are not dose dependent. The half life is prolonged in uraemic patients as dalteparin sodium is eliminated primarily through the kidneys.

5.3 Preclinical safety data

The acute toxicity of dalteparin sodium is considerably lower than that of heparin. The only significant finding, which occurred consistently throughout the toxicity studies after subcutaneous administration of the higher dose levels was local haemorrhage at the injection site, dose-related in incidence and severity. There was no cumulative effect on injection site haemorrhages.

The haemorrhagic reaction was reflected in dose related changes in the anticoagulant effects as measured by APTT and anti-Factor Xa activities.

It was concluded that dalteparin sodium did not have a greater osteopenic effect than heparin since at equivalent doses the osteopenic effect was comparable.

The results revealed no organ toxicity irrespective of the route of administration, doses or the duration of treatment. No mutagenic effect was found. No embryotoxic or teratogenic effects and no effect on fertility reproductive capacity or peri- and postnatal development was shown.

6. PHARMACEUTICAL PARTICULARS

6.1 List of excipients

10,000 IU/ml and 10,000 IU/4ml

Sodium chloride (Ph Eur)

Water for injections (Ph Eur)

6.2 Incompatibilities

The compatibility of Fragmin with products other than those mentioned under 6.6 has not been investigated.

6.3 Shelf life

10,000 IU/ml and 10,000 IU/4ml

36 months.

6.4 Special precautions for storage

10,000 IU/ml and 10,000 IU/4ml

Store at room temperature (below 30°C).

6.5 Nature and contents of container

1. Clear glass ampoules (Ph Eur Type 1) containing dalteparin sodium, 10,000 IU (anti-factor Xa) in 1 ml.

2. Clear glass ampoules (Ph Eur Type 1) containing dalteparin sodium, 10,000 IU (anti-factor Xa) in 4 ml.

6.6 Instructions for use and handling

10,000 IU/ml and 10,000 IU/4ml

Fragmin solution for injection is compatible with isotonic sodium chloride (9 mg/ml) or isotonic glucose (50 mg/ml) infusion solutions in glass bottles and plastic containers for up to 24 hours. Compatibility between Fragmin and other products has not been studied.

7. MARKETING AUTHORISATION HOLDER

Pharmacia Limited

Davy Avenue

Milton Keynes

MK5 8PH

UK

8. MARKETING AUTHORISATION NUMBER(S)

PL 0032/0376: 10,000 IU/ml

PL 0032/0377: 10,000 IU/4ml

9. DATE OF FIRST AUTHORISATION/RENEWAL OF THE AUTHORISATION

5 April 2002: 10,000 IU/ml

27 March 2002: 10,000 IU/4ml

10. DATE OF REVISION OF THE TEXT

January 2004

Legal Category: POM: 10,000 IU/ml

10,000 IU/4ml

Ref: FR 1_0

Fragmin - Surgical and Medical Thromboprophylaxis

(Pharmacia Limited)

1. NAME OF THE MEDICINAL PRODUCT
Fragmin® 2500IU/5000 IU

2. QUALITATIVE AND QUANTITATIVE COMPOSITION
Active ingredient

Dalteparin sodium (INN)

Quality according to Ph.Eur. and in-house specification.

Potency is described in International anti-Factor Xa units (IU) of the 1st International Standard for Low Molecular Weight Heparin.

Content of active ingredient

Fragmin 2500 IU: single dose syringe containing dalteparin sodium 2,500 IU (anti-Factor Xa) in 0.2 ml solution.

Fragmin 5000 IU: single dose syringe containing dalteparin sodium 5000 IU (anti-Factor Xa) in 0.2 ml solution.

Fragmin syringes do not contain preservatives.

3. PHARMACEUTICAL FORM
Solution for injection for subcutaneous administration.

4. CLINICAL PARTICULARS
4.1 Therapeutic indications
Peri- and post-operative surgical thromboprophylaxis.

For the 5000 IU Presentation Only:

The prophylaxis of proximal deep venous thrombosis in patients bedridden due to a medical condition, including, but not limited to; congestive cardiac failure (NYHA class III or IV), acute respiratory failure or acute infection, who also have a predisposing risk factor for venous thromboembolism such as age over 75 years, obesity, cancer or previous history of VTE.

4.2 Posology and method of administration
Adults

a) Surgical thromboprophylaxis in patients at moderate risk of thrombosis

2,500IU is administered subcutaneously 1-2 hours before the surgical procedure and thereafter 2,500 IU subcutaneously each morning until the patient is mobilised, in general 5-7 days or longer.

b) Surgical thromboprophylaxis in patients at high risk of thrombosis

2,500 IU is administered subcutaneously 1-2 hours before the surgical procedure and 2,500 IU subcutaneously 8-12 hours later. On the following days, 5,000 IU subcutaneously each morning.

As an alternative, 5,000 IU is administered subcutaneously the evening before the surgical procedure and 5,000 IU subcutaneously the following evenings.

Treatment is continued until the patient is mobilised, in general 5-7 days or longer.

c) Prolonged thromboprophylaxis in hip replacement surgery

5,000IU is given subcutaneously the evening before the operation and 5,000IU subcutaneously the following evenings. Treatment is continued for five post-operative weeks.

If pre-operative administration of Fragmin is not considered appropriate because the patient is at high risk of haemorrhage during the procedure, post-operative Fragmin may be administered (see Section 5.1).

d) Prophylaxis of venous thromboembolism in medical patients: The recommended dose of dalteparin sodium is 5,000 IU once daily. Treatment with dalteparin sodium is prescribed for up to 14 days or longer.

Children

Not recommended for children.

Elderly

Fragmin has been used safely in elderly patients without the need for dosage adjustment.

Method of Administration

By subcutaneous injection, preferably into the abdominal subcutaneous tissue anterolaterally or posterolaterally, or into the lateral part of the thigh. Patients should be supine and the total length of the needle should be introduced vertically, not at an angle, into the thick part of a skin fold, produced by squeezing the skin between the thumb and forefinger; the skin fold should be held throughout the injection.

4.3 Contraindications
Known hypersensitivity to Fragmin or other low molecular weight heparins and/or heparins e.g. history of confirmed or suspected immunologically mediated heparin induced thrombocytopenia; acute gastroduodenal ulcer; cerebral haemorrhage; known haemorrhagic diathesis; subacute endocarditis; injuries to and operations on the central nervous system, eyes and ears.

In patients receiving Fragmin for treatment rather than prophylaxis, local and/or regional anaesthesia in elective surgical procedures is contra-indicated.

For the 5000 IU Presentation Only:

Dalteparin should not be used in patients who have suffered a recent (within 3 months) stroke unless due to systemic emboli.

4.4 Special warnings and special precautions for use
Caution should be exercised in patients in whom there is an increased risk of bleeding complications, e.g. following trauma, haemorrhagic stroke, severe liver or renal failure, thrombocytopenia or defective platelet function, uncontrolled hypertension, hypertensive or diabetic retinopathy, patients receiving concurrent anticoagulant/antiplatelet agents (see Interactions Section).

It is recommended that platelets be counted before starting treatment with Fragmin and monitored regularly. Special caution is necessary in rapidly developing thrombocytopenia and severe thrombocytopenia ($<100{,}000/\mu l$) associated with positive or unknown results of in-vitro tests for anti-platelet antibody in the presence of Fragmin or other low molecular weight (mass) heparins and/or heparin.

Fragmin when administered in a dose of 2,500-5,000 IU (anti-Factor Xa)/day does not generally accumulate, and therefore monitoring of the effect is not usually required. However, if considered necessary, chromogenic substrate assays can be used to measure anti-Factor Xa activity (Fragmin has only a moderate prolonging effect on clotting time assays such as APTT or thrombin time).

As individual low molecular weight (mass) heparins have differing characteristics, switching to an alternative low molecular weight heparin should be avoided. The directions for use relating to each specific product must be observed as different dosages may be required.

Do not administer by the intramuscular route.

Heparin can suppress adrenal secretion of aldosterone leading to hyperkalaemia, particularly in patients such as those with diabetes mellitus, chronic renal failure, preexisting metabolic acidosis, a raised plasma potassium or taking potassium sparing drugs. The risk of hyperkalaemia appears to increase with duration of therapy but is usually reversible. Plasma potassium should be measured in patients at risk before starting heparin therapy and monitored regularly thereafter particularly if treatment is prolonged beyond about 7 days.

In patients undergoing spinal or epidural anaesthesia, the prophylactic use of heparin maybe very rarely associated with spinal haematomas resulting in prolonged or permanent paralysis. The risk is increased by use of an epidural or spinal catheter for anaesthesia, by the concomitant use of drugs (NSAIDs), platelet inhibitors or anti-coagulants and by traumatic or repeated puncture.

In decision-making on the interval between the last administration of Fragmin at prophylactic doses and the placement or removal of a peridural or spinal catheter for anaesthesia, the product characteristics and the patient profile should be taken into account. Readministration should be delayed until at least four hours after the surgical procedure is completed.

Should a physician, as a clinical judgement, decide to administer anticoagulation in the context of peridural or spinal anaesthesia, extreme vigilance and frequent monitoring must be exercised to detect any signs and symptoms of neurologic impairment such as back pain, sensory or motor deficits (numbness and weakness in lower limbs) and bowel or bladder dysfunction. Nurses should be trained to detect such signs and symptoms. Patients should be instructed to inform immediately a nurse or a clinician if they experience any of these.

If signs or symptoms of epidural or spinal haematoma are suspected, urgent diagnosis and treatment may include spinal cord decompression.

There have been no adequate studies to assess the safe and effective use of Fragmin in preventing valve thrombosis in patients with prosthetic heart valves. Prophylactic doses of Fragmin are not sufficient to prevent valve thrombosis in patients with prosthetic heart valves. The use of Fragmin cannot be recommended for this purpose

4.5 Interaction with other medicinal products and other forms of Interaction
The possibility of the following interactions with Fragmin should be considered:

i) An enhancement of the anticoagulant effect by anticoagulant/antiplatelet agents e.g. aspirin/dipyridamole, Vitamin K antagonists, NSAIDs e.g. indomethacin, cytostatics, dextran, sulphinpyrazone, probenecid, and ethacrynic acid.

ii) A reduction of the anticoagulant effect may occur with concomitant administration of antihistamines, cardiac glycosides, tetracycline and ascorbic acid.

4.6 Pregnancy and lactation
This medicinal product has been assessed in pregnant women and no harmful effects are known with respect to the course of pregnancy and the health of the unborn and neonate.

No information is available as to whether Fragmin passes into breast milk.

Therapeutic failures have been reported in pregnant women with prosthetic heart valves on full anti-coagulant doses of low molecular weight heparin. In the absence of clear dosing, efficacy and safety information in this circumstance, Fragmin is not recommended for use in pregnant women with prosthetic heart valves.

4.7 Effects on ability to drive and use machines
Fragmin does not affect the ability to drive or operate machinery.

4.8 Undesirable effects
Bleeding may be provoked, especially at high dosages corresponding with anti-Factor Xa levels greater than 1.5 IU/ml. However, at recommended dosages bleeding rarely occurs.

Transient, slight to moderate, elevation of liver transaminases (ASAT, ALAT) has been observed, but no clinical significance has been demonstrated.

Commonly reported side-effects include subcutaneous haematomas at the injection site, mild thrombocytopenia (type I) which is usually reversible during treatment

Allergic reactions (urticaria, pruritus, hair loss and skin necrosis) occur rarely.

A few cases of anaphylactoid reactions and of severe immunologically mediated thrombocytopenia (type II) with arterial and/or venous thrombosis or thromboembolism have been observed.

Osteoporosis has been associated with long-term heparin treatment and therefore cannot be excluded with Fragmin.

Heparin products can cause hypoaldosteronism which may result in an increase in plasma potassium. Rarely, clinically significant hyperkalaemia may occur, particularly in patients with chronic renal failure and diabetes mellitus (see Special warnings and precautions for use)

Valve thrombosis in patients with prosthetic heart valves have been reported rarely, usually associated with inadequate dosing, (See Special warnings and precautions for Use).

Very rare cases of epidural and spinal haematoma have been reported in association with prophylactic use of heparin in the context of spinal or epidural anaesthesia and of spinal puncture. These haematomas have caused various degrees of neurological impairment, including prolonged or permanent paralysis (cross reference to section 4.4 "Special warnings and precautions for use").

4.9 Overdose
The anticoagulant effect (i.e. prolongation of the APTT) induced by Fragmin is inhibited by protamine. Since protamine itself has an inhibiting effect on primary haemostasis it should be used only in an emergency. The prolongation of the clotting time induced by Fragmin may be fully neutralised by protamine, but the anti-Factor Xa activity is only neutralised to about 25-50%. 1 mg of protamine inhibits the effect of 100 IU (anti-Factor Xa) of Fragmin.

5. PHARMACOLOGICAL PROPERTIES
5.1 Pharmacodynamic properties
Dalteparin sodium is a low molecular weight heparin fraction (average molecular weight 4000-6000 daltons) produced from porcine-derived sodium heparin.

Dalteparin sodium is an antithrombotic agent, which acts mainly through its ability to potentiate the inhibition of Factor Xa and thrombin by antithrombin.

It has a relatively higher ability to potentiate Factor Xa inhibition than to prolong plasma clotting time (APTT)

Compared with standard, unfractionated heparin, dalteparin sodium has a reduced adverse effect on platelet function and platelet adhesion, and thus has only a minimal effect on primary haemostasis. Still some of the antithrombotic properties of dalteparin sodium are thought to be mediated through the effects on vessel walls or the fibrinolytic system.

In a randomised, actively controlled, double –bliond trial in 1500 patients undergoing hip replacement surgery (North American Fragmin Trial), both pre-operative and post operative Fragmin were found to be superior to warfarin (see table below). There was a numerical superiority for pre-operative Fragmin over post-operative Fragmin. Thus in patients wehre the risk of bleeding is perceived to be too great for pre-operative Fragmin administration other means of reducing thromboembolic risk such as post-oeprative Fragmin administration may be considered.

Incidence of verified thromboembolic events in ITT efficacy population within 6 ± 2 post operative days

(see Table 1 on next page)

In a randomised; placebo-controlled double-blind trial (PREVENT) in 3700 patients with acute medical conditions requiring a projected stay in hospital of >4 days and with recent (<3 days) immobilisation (defined as patients mainly confined to bed during waking hours), the incidence of clinically relevant thromboembolic events was reduced by 45% in patients randomised to receive Fragmin compared with those who received placebo. The incidence of the events comprising the primary endpoint was 2.77% compared with 4.96% in placebo treated patients (difference: - 2.19; 95% CI: - 3.57 to - 0.81; p=0.0015. Therefore, a clinically meaningful reduction in the incidence of venous thromboembolism was seen in this study.

Table 1

Phase 1	Pre-op Dalteparin		Post-op Dalteparin		Warfarin	
	n/N	%	n/N	%	n/N	%
DVT and or PE	37/338*	10.9	44/336*	13.1	81/338	24.0
Proximal DVT	3/354	0.8	3/358	0.8	11/363	3.0

*p 0.001 vs warfarin (Cocharan-Mantel-Haenszel test, two-sided)

Abbreviations: n/N = number of patients affected/number of efficacy-evaluable patients; post-op = treatment at earliest 4 hours after surgery;
Pre-op, = treatment within 2 hours before surgery

5.2 Pharmacokinetic properties

The half-life following i.v. and s.c. administration is 2 hours and 3.5-4 hours respectively, twice that of unfractionated heparin.

The bioavailability following s.c. injection is approximately 87 per cent and the pharmacokinetics are not dose dependent. The half life is prolonged in uraemic patients as dalteparin sodium is eliminated primarily through the kidneys.

5.3 Preclinical safety data

The acute toxicity of dalteparin sodium is considerably lower than that of heparin. The only significant finding, which occurred consistently throughout the toxicity studies after subcutaneous administration of the higher dose levels was local haemorrhage at the injection sites, dose-related in incidence and severity. There was no cumulative effect on injection site haemorrhages.

The haemorrhagic reaction was reflected in dose related changes in the anticoagulant effects as measured by APTT and anti-Factor Xa activities.

It was concluded that dalteparin sodium did not have a greater osteopenic effect than heparin since at equivalent doses the osteopenic effect was comparable.

The results revealed no organ toxicity irrespective of the route of administration, doses or duration of treatment. No mutagenic effect was found. No embryotoxic or teratogenic effects and no effect on fertility, reproductive capacity or peri- and post natal development was shown.

6. PHARMACEUTICAL PARTICULARS

6.1 List of excipients

Sodium Chloride (Ph.Eur)

(2,500 IU presentation only)

Water for Injections (Ph. Eur.)

(2,500IU and 5,000IU presentations)

6.2 Incompatibilities

Not applicable.

6.3 Shelf life

36 months

6.4 Special precautions for storage

Do not store above 25°C

6.5 Nature and contents of container

Single dose syringe (glass Ph. Eur. Type I) with chlorobutyl rubber stopper containing dalteparin sodium 2500 IU (anti-Factor Xa) in 0.2 ml

Single dose syringe (glass Ph. Eur. Type I) with chlorobutyl rubber stopper containing dalteparin sodium 5000 IU (anti-Factor Xa) in 0.2 ml.

6.6 Instructions for use and handling

Not applicable

7. MARKETING AUTHORISATION HOLDER

Pharmacia Limited

Davy Avenue

Milton Keynes

MK5 8PH

United Kingdom

8. MARKETING AUTHORISATION NUMBER(S)

Fragmin 2500 IU:PL 00032/0382

Fragmin 5000 IU:PL 00032/0383

9. DATE OF FIRST AUTHORISATION/RENEWAL OF THE AUTHORISATION

18 March 2002

10. DATE OF REVISION OF THE TEXT

January 2004

11. LEGAL CATEGORY

POM

Ref: FR 3_0

Fragmin - Treatment of VTE

(Pharmacia Limited)

1. NAME OF THE MEDICINAL PRODUCT

Single Dose Syringes

1. Fragmin 7,500 IU/0.3ml Solution for Injection
2. Fragmin 10,000 IU/0.4ml Solution for Injection
3. Fragmin 12,500 IU/0.5ml Solution for Injection
4. Fragmin 15,000 IU/0.6ml Solution for Injection
5. Fragmin 18,000 IU/0.72ml Solution for Injection

Ampoules/Vials

6. Fragmin 10,000 IU/1 ml Ampoule
7. Fragmin 100,000 IU/4ml Multidose-Vial

2. QUALITATIVE AND QUANTITATIVE COMPOSITION

Active ingredient

Dalteparin sodium (INN)

Quality according to Ph Eur and in-house specification

1. Fragmin 7,500 IU: Single dose syringe containing dalteparin sodium 7,500IU (anti-Factor Xa*) in 0.3ml solution for injection equivalent to 25,000 IU/ml.

2. Fragmin 10,000 IU: Single dose syringe containing dalteparin sodium 10,000IU (anti-Factor Xa*) in 0.4ml solution for injection equivalent to 25,000 IU/ml.

3. Fragmin 12,500 IU: Single dose syringe containing dalteparin sodium 12,500IU (anti-Factor Xa*) in 0.5ml solution for injection equivalent to 25,000 IU/ml.

4. Fragmin 15,000 IU: Single dose syringe containing dalteparin sodium 15,000IU (anti-Factor Xa*) in 0.3ml solution for injection equivalent to 25,000 IU/ml.

5. Fragmin 18,000 IU: Single dose syringe containing dalteparin sodium 18,000IU (anti-Factor Xa*) in 0.72ml solution for injection equivalent to 25,000 IU/ml.

6. Ampoules containing dalteparin sodium 10,000 IU (anti-Factor Xa*) in 1ml

7. Fragmin 100,000 IU/4ml: Multidose vial containing dalteparin sodium corresponding to 25,000 IU (anti-Factor Xa*)/ml.

For excipients see section 6.1.

1 – 6: Fragmin does not contain preservatives

7: Contains a preservative (Benzyl alcohol (Ph. Eur))

*Potency is described in International anti-Factor Xa units (IU) of the 1st International Standard for Low Molecular Weight Heparin.

3. PHARMACEUTICAL FORM

Solution for injection for subcutaneous administration.

4. CLINICAL PARTICULARS

4.1 Therapeutic indications

Treatment of venous thromboembolism (VTE) presenting clinically as deep vein thrombosis (DVT), pulmonary embolism (PE) or both.

4.2 Posology and method of administration

Recommended dosage for adults: Single Dose Syringes

1 – 5: A single daily dose of Fragmin is administered subcutaneously, once daily according to the following weight ranges. Monitoring of the anticoagulant effect is not usually necessary:

Weight (kg)	Dose
<46	7,500 IU (1)
46-56	10,000 IU (2)
57-68	12,500 IU (3)
69-82	15,000 IU (4)
83 and over	18,000 IU (5)

The single daily dose should not exceed 18,000 IU.

For patients with an increased risk of bleeding, it is recommended that Fragmin be administered according to the twice daily regimen detailed for Fragmin 10,000 IU/ml ampoules or Fragmin Multidose Vial.

Recommended dosage for adults: Ampoule and Multidose Vial:

Fragmin can be administered subcutaneously either as a single daily injection or as twice daily injections:

(a) Once daily administration

200 IU/kg body weight is administered sc. once daily. Monitoring of the anticoagulant effect is not necessary. The single daily dose should not exceed 18,000 IU.

(b) Twice daily administration

A dose of 100 IU/kg body weight administered sc. twice daily can be used for patients with increased risk of bleeding. Monitoring of the treatment is generally not necessary but can be performed with a functional anti-Factor Xa assay. Maximum plasma levels are obtained 3-4 hours after sc. injection, when samples should be taken. Recommended plasma levels are between 0.5-1.0 IU (anti-Factor Xa)/ml.

Simultaneous anticoagulation with oral vitamin K antagonists can be started immediately. Treatment with Fragmin is continued until the prothrombin complex levels (factor II, VII, IX and X) have decreased to a therapeutic level. At least five days of combined treatment is normally required.

Children

Not recommended for children.

Elderly

Fragmin has been used safely in elderly patients without the need for dosage adjustment.

Method of Administration

By subcutaneous injection, preferably into the abdominal subcutaneous tissue anterolaterally or posterolaterally, or into the lateral part of the thigh. Patients should be supine and the total length of the needle should be introduced vertically, not at an angle, into the thick part of a skin fold, produced by squeezing the skin between thumb and forefinger; the skin fold should be held throughout the injection.

4.3 Contraindications

Known hypersensitivity to Fragmin or other low molecular weight heparins and/or heparins e.g. history of confirmed or suspected immunologically mediated heparin induced thrombocytopenia, acute gastroduodenal ulcer; cerebral haemorrhage; known haemorrhagic diathesis; subacute endocarditis; injuries to and operations on the central nervous system, eyes and ears.

In patients receiving Fragmin for treatment rather than prophylaxis, local and/or regional anaesthesia in elective surgical procedures is contra-indicated.

4.4 Special warnings and special precautions for use

Do not administer by the intramuscular route.

Caution should be exercised in patients in whom there is an increased risk of bleeding complications, e.g. following surgery or trauma, haemorrhagic stroke, severe liver or renal failure, thrombocytopenia or defective platelet function, uncontrolled hypertension, hypertensive or diabetic retinopathy, patients receiving concurrent anticoagulant/antiplatelet agents (see interactions section).

It is recommended that platelets be counted before starting treatment with Fragmin and monitored regularly. Special caution is necessary in rapidly developing thrombocytopenia and severe thrombocytopenia (<100,000/μl) associated with positive or unknown results of in-vitro tests for anti-platelet antibody in the presence of Fragmin or other low molecular weight (mass) heparins and/or heparin

Fragmin induces only a moderate prolongation of the APTT and thrombin time. Accordingly, dosage increments based upon prolongation of the APTT may cause overdosage and bleeding. Therefore, prolongation of the APTT should only be used as a test of overdosage.

Patients with severely disturbed hepatic function may need a reduction in dosage and should be monitored accordingly.

As individual low molecular weight (mass) heparins have differing characteristics, switching to an alternative low molecular weight heparin should be avoided. The directions for use relating to each specific product must be observed as different dosages may be required.

Heparin can suppress adrenal secretion of aldosterone leading to hyperkalaemia, particularly in patients such as those with diabetes mellitus, chronic renal failure, pre-existing metabolic acidosis, a raised plasma potassium or taking potassium sparing drugs. The risk of hyperkalaemia appears to increase with duration of therapy but is usually reversible. Plasma potassium should be measured in patients at risk before starting heparin therapy and monitored regularly thereafter particularly if treatment is prolonged beyond about 7 days.

In patients undergoing spinal or epidural anaesthesia, the prophylactic use of heparin may be very rarely associated with spinal haematomas resulting in prolonged or permanent paralysis. The risk is increased by use of an epidural or spinal catheter for anaesthesia, by the concomitant use of drugs (NSAIDs), platelet inhibitors or anti-coagulants and by traumatic or repeated puncture.

In decision-making on the interval between the last administration of Fragmin at prophylactic doses and the placement or removal of a peridural or spinal catheter for anaesthesia, the product characteristics and the patient profile should be taken into account. Readministration should be delayed until at least four hours after the surgical procedure is completed.

Should a physician, as a clinical judgement, decide to administer anticoagulation in the context of peridual spinal anaesthesia, extreme vigilance and frequent monitoring must be exercised to detect any signs and symptoms of neurologic impairment such as back pain, sensory or motor deficits (numbness and weakness in lower limbs) and bowel or bladder dysfunction. Nurses should be trained to detect such signs and symptoms. Patients should be instructed to inform immediately a nurse or a clinician if they experience any of these.

If signs or symptoms of epidural or spinal haematoma are suspected, urgent diagnosis and treatment may include spinal cord decompression.

There have been no adequate studies to assess the safe and effective use of Fragmin in preventing valve thrombosis in patients with prosthetic heart valves. Prophylactic doses of Fragmin are not sufficient to prevent valve thrombosis in patients with prosthetic heart valves. The use of Fragmin cannot be recommended for this purpose

4.5 Interaction with other medicinal products and other forms of Interaction

The possibility of the following interactions with Fragmin should be considered:

(i) An enhancement of the anticoagulant effect by anticoagulant/antiplatelet agents e.g. aspirin/ dipyridamole, vitamin K antagonists, NSAIDs e.g. indomethacin, cytostatics, dextran, sulphinpyrazone, probenecid, and ethacrynic acid.

(ii) A reduction of the anticoagulant effect may occur with concomitant administration of antihistamines, cardiac glycosides, tetracycline and ascorbic acid.

4.6 Pregnancy and lactation

1 – 6

This medicinal product has been assessed in pregnant women and no harmful effects are known with respect to the course of pregnancy and the health of the unborn and neonate.

7 Only

Fragmin multidose vial contains benzyl alcohol as a preservative and is not recommended for use during pregnancy. Benzyl alcohol may cross the placenta. One should bear in mind the potential toxicity for premature infants.

(1-7)

No information is available as to whether Fragmin passes into breast milk.

Therapeutic failures have been reported in pregnant women with prosthetic heart valves on full anti-coagulant doses of low molecular weight heparin. In the absence of clear dosing, efficacy and safety information in this circumstance, Fragmin is not recommended for use in pregnant women with prosthetic heart valves.

4.7 Effects on ability to drive and use machines

Fragmin does not affect the ability to drive or operate machinery.

4.8 Undesirable effects

Bleeding may be provoked, especially at high dosages corresponding with anti-Factor Xa levels greater than 1.5 IU/ml. However, at recommended dosages bleedings rarely occur.

Transient, slight to moderate, elevation of liver transaminases (ASAT, ALAT) has been observed, but no clinical significance has been demonstrated.

Commonly reported side-effects include subcutaneous haematomas at the injection site;

Mild thrombocytopenia (type I) which is usually reversible during treatment.

Allergic reactions (urticaria, pruritus, hair loss and skin necrosis) occur rarely.

A few cases of anaphylactoid reactions and of severe immunologically mediated thrombocytopenia (type II) with arterial and/or venous thrombosis or thromboembolism have been observed.

Osteoporosis has been associated with long-term heparin treatment and therefore cannot be excluded with Fragmin.

Heparin products can cause hypoaldosteronism which may result in an increase in plasma potassium. Rarely, clinically significant hyperkalaemia may occur, particularly in patients with chronic renal failure and diabetes mellitus (see Special warnings and precautions for use)

Valve thrombosis in patients with prosthetic heart valves have been reported rarely, usually associated with inadequate dosing, (see Special warnings and precautions for use).

Very rare cases of epidural and spinal haematoma have been reported in association with prophylactic use of heparin in the context of spinal or epidural anaesthesia and of spinal puncture. These haematomas have caused various degrees of neurological impairment, including prolonged or permanent paralysis (cross reference to section 4.4 "Special warnings and precautions for use").

4.9 Overdose

The anticoagulant effect (i.e. prolongation of the APTT) induced by Fragmin is inhibited by protamine. Since protamine itself has an inhibiting effect on primary haemostasis it should be used only in an emergency.

The prolongation of the clotting time induced by Fragmin may be fully neutralised by protamine, but the anti-Factor Xa activity is only neutralised to about 25-50%. 1 mg of protamine inhibits the effect of 100 IU (anti-Factor Xa) of Fragmin.

Protamine should be given by intravenous injection over approximately 10 minutes.

5. PHARMACOLOGICAL PROPERTIES

5.1 Pharmacodynamic properties

ATC Code BO1A B

Dalteparin sodium is a low molecular weight heparin fraction (average molecular weight 4000-6000 Daltons) produced from porcine-derived sodium heparin.

Dalteparin sodium is an antithrombotic agent, which acts mainly through its ability to potentiate the inhibition of Factor Xa and thrombin by antithrombin. It has a relatively higher ability to potentiate Factor Xa inhibition than to prolong plasma clotting time (APTT).

Compared with standard, unfractionated heparin, dalteparin sodium has a reduced adverse effect on platelet function and platelet adhesion, and thus has only a minimal effect on primary haemostasis. Some of the antithrombotic properties of dalteparin sodium are thought to be mediated through the effects on vessel walls or the fibrinolytic system.

5.2 Pharmacokinetic properties

The half life following iv and sc. administration is 2 hours and 3.5-4 hours respectively, twice that of unfractionated heparin.

The bioavailability following sc. injection is approximately 87 per cent and the pharmacokinetics are not dose dependent. The half life is prolonged in uraemic patients as dalteparin sodium is eliminated primarily through the kidneys.

5.3 Preclinical safety data

The acute toxicity of dalteparin sodium is considerably lower than that of heparin. The only significant finding, which occurred consistently throughout the toxicity studies after subcutaneous administration of the higher dose levels was local haemorrhage at the injection site, dose-related in incidence and severity. There was no cumulative effect on injection site haemorrhages.

The haemorrhagic reaction was reflected in dose related changes in the anticoagulant effects as measured by APTT and anti-Factor Xa activities.

It was concluded that dalteparin sodium did not have a greater osteopenic effect than heparin since at equivalent doses the osteopenic effect was comparable.

The results revealed no organ toxicity irrespective of the route of administration, doses or the duration of treatment. No mutagenic effect was found. No embryotoxic or teratogenic effects and no effect on fertility reproductive capacity or peri- and postnatal development was shown.

6. PHARMACEUTICAL PARTICULARS

6.1 List of excipients

1	Fragmin 7,500 IU/0.3ml (1) Water for injections (Ph. Eur) Sodium hydroxide or hydrochloric acid for pH adjustment
2 – 5	Fragmin 10,000 IU/0.4ml (2) Fragmin 12,500 IU/0.5ml (3) Fragmin 15,000 IU/0.6ml (4) Framgin 18,000 IU/0.72ml (5) Water for Injections (Ph. Eur) Sodium Chloride (Ph. Eur) Sodium hydroxide or hydrochloric acid for pH adjustment
6	Fragmin 10,000 IU/ml Ampoule (6) Sodium chloride (Ph. Eur) Water for Injections (Ph. Eur)
7	Fragmin 100,000 IU/4ml Multidose Vial (7) Benzyl Alcohol (Ph. Eur) Water for Injections (Ph. Eur)

6.2 Incompatibilities

Not applicable.

6.3 Shelf life

1	Fragmin 7,500 IU/0.3ml	36 months
2	Fragmin 10,000 IU/0.4ml	24 months
3	Fragmin 12,500 IU/0.5ml	24 months
4	Fragmin 15,000 IU/0.6ml	24 months
5	Fragmin 18,000 IU/0.72ml	24 months
6	Fragmin 10,000 IU/ml Ampoule	36 months
7	Fragmin 100,000 IU/4ml Multidose Vial	24 months Once opened the solution should be used within 14 days

6.4 Special precautions for storage

1 – 5: Do no store above 25°C

6 – 7: Store at room temperature (below 30°C)

6.5 Nature and contents of container

1	Fragmin 7,500 IU/0.3ml Solution for Injection is supplied in 0.5ml glass Ph.Eur type I single dose syringes with chlorobutyl (Type I) rubber and polypropylene rod. Each pack contains 10 syringes.
2	Fragmin 10,000 IU/0.4 ml Solution for Injection is supplied in 1 ml glass Ph. Eur. Type I single dose syringes with chlorobutyl (Type I) rubber stopper and polypropylene rod. Each pack contains 5 syringes.
3	Fragmin 12,500 IU/0.5 ml solution for injection is supplied in 1 ml glass Ph. Eur. Type I single dose syringes with chlorobutyl (Type I) rubber stopper and polypropylene rod. Each pack contains 5 syringes.
4	Fragmin 15 000 IU/0.6 ml solution for injection is supplied in 1 ml glass Ph. Eur. Type I single dose syringes with chlorobutyl (Type I) rubber stopper and polypropylene rod. Each pack contains 5 syringes.
5	1 ml single dose syringe (glass Ph. Eur. Type I) with chlorobutyl rubber stopper containing dalteparin sodium 18,000 IU (anti-Factor Xa) in 0.72 ml. Each pack contains 5 syringes.
6	Clear glass ampoules (Ph Eur Type 1) containing dalteparin sodium, 10,000 IU (anti-factor Xa) in 1 ml
7	Multidose vial (Ph Eur Type 1) with bromobutyl rubber stopper, secured with aluminium overseal with flip off cap, containing dalteparin sodium 100,000 IU (anti-Factor Xa) in 4 ml.

6.6 Instructions for use and handling

1 – 6: Not applicable

7: As with other multidose preparations, care should be taken to avoid any risk of cross-contamination during use.

7. MARKETING AUTHORISATION HOLDER

Pharmacia Limited

Davy Avenue

Milton Keynes

MK5 8PH

UK

8. MARKETING AUTHORISATION NUMBER(S)

1	PL 0022/0206
2	PL 0032/0375
3	PL 0032/0379
4	PL 0032/0380
5	PL 0032/0381
6	PL 0032/0376
7	PL 0032/0378

9. DATE OF FIRST AUTHORISATION/RENEWAL OF THE AUTHORISATION

1: 24 April 2001

2 – 5: 18 March 2002

6: 5 April 2002

7: 27 march 2002

10. DATE OF REVISION OF THE TEXT

January 2004

Legal Category: POM (1-7)

Ref: FR 1_0

Fragmin - Unstable Angina

(Pharmacia Limited)

1. NAME OF THE MEDICINAL PRODUCT
Fragmin Graduated Syringe 10,000 IU/1 ml solution for Injection

Fragmin 7,500 IU/0.3 ml solution for injection

Fragmin 10,000 IU/1 ml Ampoule

2. QUALITATIVE AND QUANTITATIVE COMPOSITION
Pre-filled, single dose syringes containing dalteparin sodium 10,000 IU (anti-Factor Xa*) in 1.0ml solution for injection

Fragmin 7,500 IU: single dose syringe containing dalteparin sodium 7,500 IU (anti-Factor Xa*) in 0.3 ml solution for injection equivalent to 25,000 IU/ml

Fragmin Syringes do not contain preservatives

Ampoules containing dalteparin sodium, 10,000 IU (anti-Factor Xa*) in 1 ml.

*Potency is described in International anti-Factor Xa units (IU) of the 1st International Standard for Low Molecular Weight Heparin.

3. PHARMACEUTICAL FORM
Solution for injection for intravenous or subcutaneous administration.

4. CLINICAL PARTICULARS

4.1 Therapeutic indications
Unstable angina and non-Q wave myocardial infarction (unstable coronary artery disease-UCAD), administered concurrently with aspirin.

Extended Use

Fragmin may be used beyond 8 days in patients awaiting angiography/revascularisation procedures (see Section 5.1)

4.2 Posology and method of administration
Recommended dosage for adults
120 IU/kg body weight are administered subcutaneously 12 hourly for up to 8 days if considered of benefit by the physician. Maximum dose is 10,000 IU/12 hours.

Patients needing treatment beyond 8 days, while awaiting angiography/revascularisation, should receive a fixed dose of either 5,000 IU (women < 80 kg and men <70 kg) or 7,500 IU (women ≥80 kg and men ≥70 kg) 12 hourly. Treatment is recommended to be given until the day of the revascularisation procedure (PTCA or CA BG) but not for more than 45 days.

Children
Not recommended for children.

Elderly
Fragmin has been used safely in elderly patients without the need for dosage adjustment.

Method of Administration

Following the determination of the required dose, excess solution should be ejected from the syringe.

Administration is by subcutaneous injection, prefereably into the addomin subcutaneous tissue anterolaterally or poterolaterally, or into the lateral part of the thigh. Patients should be supine and the total length of the needle should be introduced vertically, not at an angle, into the thick part of a skin fold, produced by squeezing the skin between thumb and forefinger; the skin fold should be held throughout the injection.

Syringes should be discarded after use

4.3 Contraindications
Known hypersensitivity to Fragmin or other low molecular weight heparins and/or heparins e.g. history of confirmed or suspected immunologically mediated heparin induced thrombocytopenia, acute gastroduodenal ulcer; cerebral haemorrhage; known haemorrhagic diathesis; subacute endocarditis; injuries to and operations on the central nervous system, eyes and ears.

In patients receiving Fragmin for treatment rather than prophylaxis, local and/or regional anaesthesia in elective surgical procedures is contra-indicated.

4.4 Special warnings and special precautions for use
Do not administer by the intramuscular route.

Caution should be exercised in patients in whom there is an increased risk of bleeding complications, e.g. following surgery or trauma, haemorrhagic stroke, severe liver or renal failure, thrombocytopenia or defective platelet function, uncontrolled hypertension, hypertensive or diabetic retinopathy, patients receiving concurrent anticoagulant/antiplatelet agents (see interactions section).

It is recommended that platelets be counted before starting treatment with Fragmin and monitored regularly. Special caution is necessary in rapidly developing thrombocytopenia and severe thrombocytopenia (<100,000/μl) associated with positive or unknown results of in-vitro tests for anti-platelet antibody in the presence of Fragmin or other low molecular weight (mass) heparins and/or heparin

Fragmin induces only a moderate prolongation of the APTT and thrombin time. Accordingly, dosage increments based upon prolongation of the APTT may cause overdosage and bleeding. Therefore, prolongation of the APTT should only be used as a test of overdosage.

Patients with severely disturbed hepatic function may need a reduction in dosage and should be monitored accordingly.

If a transmural myocardial infarction occurs in patients with unstable coronary artery disease, thrombolytic treatment might be appropriate. This does not necessitate discontinuation of treatment with Fragmin, but might increase the risk of bleeding.

As individual low molecular weight (mass) heparins have differing characteristics, switching to an alternative low molecular weight heparin should be avoided. The directions for use relating to each specific product must be observed as different dosages may be required.

Heparin can suppress adrenal secretion of aldosterone leading to hyperkalaemia, particularly in patients such as those with diabetes mellitus, chronic renal failure, pre-existing metabolic acidosis, a raised plasma potassium or taking potassium sparing drugs. The risk of hyperkalaemia appears to increase with duration of therapy but is usually reversible. Plasma potassium should be measured in patients at risk before starting heparin therapy and monitored regularly thereafter particularly if treatment is prolonged beyond about 7 days.

In patients undergoing spinal or epidural anaesthesia, the prophylactic use of heparin may be very rarely associated with spinal haematomas resulting in prolonged or permanent paralysis. The risk is increased by use of an epidural or spinal catheter for anaesthesia, by the concomitant use of drugs (NSAIDs), platelet inhibitors or anti-coagulants and by traumatic or repeated puncture.

In decision-making on the interval between the last administration of Fragmin at prophylactic doses and the placement or removal of a peridural or spinal catheter for anaesthesia, the product characteristics and the patient profile should be taken into account. Readministration should be delayed until at least four hours after the surgical procedure is completed.

Should a physician, as a clinical judgement, decide to administer anticoagulation in the context of peridual or spinal anaesthesia, extreme vigilance and frequent monitoring must be exercised to detect any signs and symptoms of neurologic impairment such as back pain, sensory or motor deficits (numbness and weakness in lower limbs) and bowel or bladder dysfunction. Nurses should be trained to detect such signs and symptoms. Patients should be instructed to inform immediately a nurse or a clinician if they experience any of these.

If signs or symptoms of epidural or spinal haematoma are suspected, urgent diagnosis and treatment may include spinal cord decompression.

There have been no adequate studies to assess the safe and effective use of Fragmin in preventing valve thrombosis in patients with prosthetic heart valves. Prophylactic doses of Fragmin are not sufficient to prevent valve thrombosis in patients with prosthetic heart valves. The use of Fragmin cannot be recommended for this purpose

4.5 Interaction with other medicinal products and other forms of Interaction
The possibility of the following interactions with Fragmin should be considered:

(i) An enhancement of the anticoagulant effect by anticoagulant/antiplatelet agents e.g. aspirin/ dipyridamole, vitamin K antagonists, NSAIDs e.g. indomethacin, cytostatics, dextran, sulphinpyrazone, probenecid, and ethacrynic acid.

However, unless specifically contraindicated, patients with unstable coronary artery disease should receive oral low dose aspirin.

(ii) A reduction of the anticoagulant effect may occur with concomitant administration of antihistamines, cardiac glycosides, tetracycline and ascorbic acid.

4.6 Pregnancy and lactation
This medicinal product has been assessed in pregnant women and no harmful effects are known with respect to the course of pregnancy and the health of the unborn and neonate.

No information is available as to whether Fragmin passes into breast milk.

Therapeutic failures have been reported in pregnant women with prosthetic heart valves on full anti-coagulant doses of low molecular weight heparin. In the absence of clear dosing, efficacy and safety information in this circumstance, Fragmin is not recommended for use in pregnant women with prosthetic heart valves.

4.7 Effects on ability to drive and use machines
Fragmin does not affect the ability to drive or operate machinery.

4.8 Undesirable effects
Bleeding may be provoked, especially at high dosages corresponding with anti-Factor Xa levels greater than 1.5 IU/ml. However, at recommended dosages bleedings rarely occur.

Transient, slight to moderate, elevation of liver transaminases (ASAT, ALAT) has been observed, but no clinical significance has been demonstrated.

Commonly reported side-effects include, subcutaneous haematomas at the injection site;

Mild thrombocytopenia (type I) which is usually reversible during treatment.

Allergic reactions (urticaria, pruritus, hair loss and skin necrosis) occur rarely.

A few cases of anaphylactoid reactions and of severe immunologically mediated thrombocytopenia (type II) with arterial and/or venous thrombosis or thromboembolism have been observed.

Osteoporosis has been associated with long-term heparin treatment and therefore cannot be excluded with Fragmin.

Heparin products can cause hypoaldosteronism which may result in an increase in plasma potassium. Rarely, clinically significant hyperkalaemia may occur, particularly in patients with chronic renal failure and diabetes mellitus (see Special Warnings and Precautions for Use)

Valve thrombosis in patients with prosthetic heart valves have been reported rarely, usually associated with inadequate dosing, (See Special Warnings and Special Precautions for Use).

Very rare cases of epidural and spinal haematoma have been reported in association with prophylactic use of heparin in the context of spinal or epidural anaesthesia and of spinal puncture. These haematomas have caused various degrees of neurological impairment, including prolonged or permanent paralysis (cross reference to section 4.4 "Special warnings and precautions for use").

4.9 Overdose
The anticoagulant effect (i.e. prolongation of the APTT) induced by Fragmin is inhibited by protamine. Since protamine itself has an inhibiting effect on primary haemostasis it should be used only in an emergency.

The prolongation of the clotting time induced by Fragmin may be fully neutralised by protamine, but the anti-Factor Xa activity is only neutralised to about 25-50%. 1 mg of protamine inhibits the effect of 100 IU (anti-Factor Xa) of Fragmin. Protamine should be given by intravenous injection over approximately 10 minutes.

5. PHARMACOLOGICAL PROPERTIES

5.1 Pharmacodynamic properties
ATC Code BO1A B

Dalteparin sodium is a low molecular weight heparin fraction (average molecular weight 4000-6000 Daltons) produced from porcine-derived sodium heparin.

Dalteparin sodium is an antithrombotic agent, which acts mainly through its ability to potentiate the inhibition of Factor Xa and thrombin by antithrombin. It has a relatively higher ability to potentiate Factor Xa inhibition than to prolong plasma clotting time (APTT).

Compared with standard, unfractionated heparin, dalteparin sodium has a reduced adverse effect on platelet function and platelet adhesion, and thus has only a minimal effect on primary haemostasis. Some of the antithrombotic properties of dalteparin sodium are thought to be mediated through the effects on vessel walls or the fibrinolytic system.

In a prospectively randomised study in 3489 patients (FRISC II) with acute coronary syndromes, early invasive strategy was clearly superior to non –invasive strategy.

In a post-hoc analysis, the extended use of Fragmin, up to Day 45 reduced the incidence of death and/or MI compared with placebo in the non-invasive group (revascularisation only if necessary).

The use of Fragmin beyond 8 days did not significantly reduce the incidence of death and/or MI, compared to placebo, in patients who were contraindicated to early angiography and revascularisation.

5.2 Pharmacokinetic properties
The half life following iv and sc. administration is 2 hours and 3.5-4 hours respectively, twice that of unfractionated heparin.

The bioavailability following sc. injection is approximately 87 per cent and the pharmacokinetics are not dose dependent. The half life is prolonged in uraemic patients as dalteparin sodium is eliminated primarily through the kidneys.

5.3 Preclinical safety data
The acute toxicity of dalteparin sodium is considerably lower than that of heparin. The only significant finding, which occurred consistently throughout the toxicity studies after subcutaneous administration of the higher dose levels was local haemorrhage at the injection site, dose-related in incidence and severity. There was no cumulative effect on injection site haemorrhages.

The haemorrhagic reaction was reflected in dose related changes in the anticoagulant effects as measured by APTT and anti-Factor Xa activities.

It was concluded that dalteparin sodium did not have a greater osteopenic effect than heparin since at equivalent doses the osteopenic effect was comparable.

The results revealed no organ toxicity irrespective of the route of administration, doses or the duration of treatment. No mutagenic effect was found. No embryotoxic or teratogenic effects and no effect on fertility reproductive capacity or peri- and postnatal development was shown.

6. PHARMACEUTICAL PARTICULARS

6.1 List of excipients

Graduated Syringe 10,000 IU/ml

Sodium chloride (Ph Eur)

Water for injections (Ph Eur)

Sodium Hydroxide or hydrochloric acid for pH adjustment

7,500 IU/0.3 ml solution for injection

Water for injections (Ph Eur)

Sodium Hydroxide or hydrochloric acid for pH adjustment

Fragmin 10,000 IU/ml Ampoule

Sodium chloride (Ph Eur)

Water for injections (Ph Eur)

6.2 Incompatibilities

Not applicable.

6.3 Shelf life

36 months.

6.4 Special precautions for storage

Store at room temperature (below 30°C).

6.5 Nature and contents of container

Clear glass ampoules (Ph Eur Type 1) containing dalteparin sodium, 10,000 IU (anti-factor Xa) in 1 ml

6.6 Instructions for use and handling

Not applicable

7. MARKETING AUTHORISATION HOLDER

Pharmacia Limited

Davy Avenue

Milton Keynes

MK5 8PH

UK

8. MARKETING AUTHORISATION NUMBER(S)

Graduated Syringe 10,000 IU/ml

PL 0032/0384

7,500 IU/0.3 ml solution for injection

PL 0032/0483

Fragmin 10,000 IU/ml Ampoule

PL 0032/0376

9. DATE OF FIRST AUTHORISATION/RENEWAL OF THE AUTHORISATION

Graduated Syringe 10,000 IU/ml

29 April 2002

7,500 IU/0.3 ml solution for injection

26 June 2002

Fragmin 10,000 IU/ml Ampoule

5 April 2002

10. DATE OF REVISION OF THE TEXT

January 2004

Legal Category: POM

Ref: FR 1_0

Franol Plus

(sanofi-aventis)

1. NAME OF THE MEDICINAL PRODUCT

Franol Plus Tablets

2. QUALITATIVE AND QUANTITATIVE COMPOSITION

Theophylline EP 120.0mg

Ephedrine sulphate USP 15.0mg

3. PHARMACEUTICAL FORM

Tablet

4. CLINICAL PARTICULARS

4.1 Therapeutic indications

Franol Plus Tablets are recommended for the management of bronchospasm in reversible airway-obstruction associated with stable asthma or chronic bronchitis.

4.2 Posology and method of administration

Route of administration: Oral.

Adults

Dosage varies with individual requirements and should be adjusted accordingly. The usual dosage is 3 tablets daily (morning, midday and evening). For the patient who suffers nocturnal attacks, an extra tablet taken at bedtime is recommended.

Elderly

As for adults but see 4.4 Special Warnings and Precautions for Use.

Children

Not recommended for children under 12 years of age.

If more than four tablets a day are required, it is advisable to monitor plasma theophylline levels during dose titration to ensure that levels are kept below 20μg/ml.

4.3 Contraindications

Franol Plus should not be given to patients who are sensitive to either of its ingredients or to patients with unstable angina, cardiac arrhythmias, severe hypertension, severe coronary artery disease, porphyria or to those receiving other xanthines. Franol Plus should not be used during pregnancy.

4.4 Special warnings and special precautions for use

Hepatic dysfunction: Theophylline is eliminated primarily by metabolism in the liver. Thus in patients with severe liver disease, theophylline clearance may be decreased. If Franol Plus is used in such patients, dosage may need to be reduced.

Renal dysfunction: Ephedrine is excreted largely unchanged in the urine, therefore Franol Plus should be used with caution in patients with severe renal impairment.

Cardiac dysfunction: Theophylline clearance may be decreased in patients with congestive cardiac failure, acute pulmonary oedema or cor pulmonale, and theophylline may cause arrhythmias or worsen existing arrhythmias, thus caution should be exercised if Franol Plus is used in such patients.

Elderly (over 65 years): Theophylline clearance decreases slightly with age. Elderly patients will tend therefore to have higher serum theophylline levels than younger adults at a given dose. They should be monitored closely for signs of toxicity during dose adjustment.

Others: Theophylline clearance may be increased in heavy smokers, decreased in patients with respiratory infection, or those on a high carbohydrate - low protein diet therefore the dose of Franol Plus may need to be adjusted appropriately in these groups.

Avoid or use with special caution in patients with cardiovascular disease, hypertension, agitation, phaeochromocytoma, hyperthyroidism, closed-angle glaucoma, prostatic hypertrophy, peptic ulceration, underlying seizure disorders, patients receiving anti-depressant drugs, or patients on MAO inhibitors within the previous 14 days. Special caution is also needed in the elderly, those with hepatic, renal, or cardiac dysfunction and during lactation.

Ephedrine has a potential for tachyphylaxis, and abuse with dependence has been reported. Potentially serious hypokalaemia can result from the use of $beta_2$ agonists and xanthines in combination particularly when hypoxia is present. The effect may be enhanced by concomitant diuretics or corticosteroids. Care should be observed and serum potassium levels monitored in patients receiving Franol Plus who develop severe asthma, particularly if concomitant diuretic, corticosteroid or $beta_2$ agonist therapy is being employed.

4.5 Interaction with other medicinal products and other forms of Interaction

Theophylline clearance may be decreased by concurrent administration of cimetidine, macrolide antibiotics, oral contraceptives, interferons, diltiazem, verapamil and viloxazine. Ciprofloxacin also increases plasma theophylline concentrations and if concomitant use is essential, the dose of theophylline should be reduced and plasma concentrations closely monitored to avoid toxicity. Theophylline clearance may be increased by concurrent administration of barbiturates, carbamazepine, phenytoin, rifampicin, sulphinpyrazone, aminoglutethimide, phenobarbitone and primidone.

The effects of ephedrine are diminished by guanethidine, reserpine, and probably methyldopa, and may be diminished or enhance by tricyclic anti-depressants. Ephedrine may also diminish the effects of guanethidine and may increase the possibility of arrhythmias in digitalised patients. Lithium excretion is accelerated by theophylline.

The concomitant use of theophylline and fluvoxamine should usually be avoided. Where this is not possible, patients should have their theophylline dose halved and plasma theophylline should be monitored closely.

Plasma concentrations of theophylline can be reduced by concomitant use of the herbal remedy St John's Wort (Hypericum perforatum).

4.6 Pregnancy and lactation

Pregnancy: Although caffeine has been implicated as a teratogen, adequate animal teratogenic studies have not been conducted with theophylline nor with ephedrine. The safety of ephedrine and of theophylline, which crosses the placental barrier have not been established in human pregnancy. Franol Plus should not therefore be prescribed for patients who are pregnant.

Lactation: Theophylline distributes readily into breast milk therefore Franol Plus should be used with caution in nursing women.

4.7 Effects on ability to drive and use machines

No known effects.

4.8 Undesirable effects

Large doses of Franol Plus may give rise to the following side effects: arrhythmias, tachycardia, palpitation, flushing, giddiness, headache, tremor, anxiety, restlessness, insomnia, muscular weakness, nausea, vomiting, dyspepsia, thirst, sweating, difficulty in micturition.

Some patients may exhibit one or more such symptoms with therapeutic doses.

4.9 Overdose

The symptoms and signs of overdose with Franol Plus are likely to include, excessive irritability, sweating, nausea and vomiting, tachycardia, arrhythmias, hypertension, profuse diuresis with fever, flushing and hyperglycaemia, opisthotonos, hallucinations, convulsions and respiratory difficulty.

In general, the management of overdose with Franol Plus involves supportive and symptomatic therapy with particular attention being paid to the detection and correction of hypokalaemia and should include serial assay of plasma potassium and theophylline levels, cardiac monitoring with electro-cardiogram and maintenance of fluid and electrolyte balance.

Gastric aspiration and lavage may be employed. Convulsions and other CNS stimulation can usually be controlled by intravenous diazepam, or if that fails anti-convulsants may be used. Marked excitement or hallucinations may be managed with chlorpromazine. Severe hypertensions may necessitate the use of an alpha-adrenoceptor blocking agent and a beta-adrenoceptor blocking agent may be required to control arrhythmias. $Beta_1$ -receptor agonist agents such as dopamine should be avoided. Charcoal haemoperfusion may be indicated to remove theophylline, but forced diuresis or peritoneal dialysis are inadequate for this purpose.

5. PHARMACOLOGICAL PROPERTIES

5.1 Pharmacodynamic properties

The action of ephedrine as a dilator of the bronchioles is mediated via a direct agonist effect on beta-adrenoceptors and by release of sympathomimetic amines. Theophylline has been shown to relieve bronchospasm and achieve subjective relief during an acute attack of bronchial asthma of allergic origin. The mechanism of action of theophylline has not yet been fully elucidated but may be by blockade of adenosine receptors or by phosphodiesterase inhibition.

5.2 Pharmacokinetic properties

Theophylline is variably absorbed from the gastrointestinal tract. It is excreted in the urine as metabolites, mainly 1, 3-dimethyluric acid, and about 10% is unchanged.

Ephedrine is readily absorbed from the gastrointestinal tract, its effect becoming apparent within one hour. It does not appear to be subject to enzyme inactivation by either monoamine oxidase or catechol-o-methyl transferase, and about 60-75% is excreted in the urine unchanged. The half-life in the circulation is about 4 hours.

5.3 Preclinical safety data

There are no preclinical data of relevance to the prescriber which are additional to that already included in other sections of the SPC.

6. PHARMACEUTICAL PARTICULARS

6.1 List of excipients

Maize starch, Talc, Magnesium stearate, Stearic acid.

6.2 Incompatibilities

Not applicable.

6.3 Shelf life

60 months.

6.4 Special precautions for storage

None.

6.5 Nature and contents of container

Amber glass bottles fitted with tin-plate caps or polypropylene lids.

Pack size: 90

6.6 Instructions for use and handling

None.

7. MARKETING AUTHORISATION HOLDER

Sanofi-Synthelabo

PO Box 597

Guildford

Surrey

8. MARKETING AUTHORISATION NUMBER(S)

11723/0034

9. DATE OF FIRST AUTHORISATION/RENEWAL OF THE AUTHORISATION

1 August 1993/ 5 March 2001

10. DATE OF REVISION OF THE TEXT

November 2001

Legal Category P

Franol Tablets

(sanofi-aventis)

1. NAME OF THE MEDICINAL PRODUCT

Franol Tablets

2. QUALITATIVE AND QUANTITATIVE COMPOSITION

Theophylline (anhydrous) EP 120.0mg

Ephedrine hydrochloride EP 11.0mg

3. PHARMACEUTICAL FORM

Tablet

4. CLINICAL PARTICULARS

4.1 Therapeutic indications
Franol Tablets are recommended for the management of bronchospasm in reversible airway-obstruction associated with stable asthma or chronic bronchitis.

4.2 Posology and method of administration
Route of administration: Oral.

Adults

Dosage varies with individual requirements and should be adjusted accordingly. The usual dosage is 3 tablets daily (morning, midday and evening). For the patient who suffers nocturnal attacks, an extra tablet taken at bedtime is recommended.

Elderly

As for adults but see 4.4 Special Warnings and Precautions for Use.

Children

Not recommended for children under 12 years of age.

If more than four tablets a day are required, it is advisable to monitor plasma theophylline levels during dose titration to ensure that levels are kept below 20μg/ml.

4.3 Contraindications
Franol should not be given to patients who are sensitive to either of its ingredients or to patients with unstable angina, cardiac arrhythmias, severe hypertension, severe coronary artery disease, porphyria or to those receiving other xanthines. Franol should not be used during pregnancy.

4.4 Special warnings and special precautions for use
Hepatic dysfunction: Theophylline is eliminated primarily by metabolism in the liver. Thus in patients with severe liver disease, theophylline clearance may be decreased. If Franol is used in such patients, dosage may need to be reduced.

Renal dysfunction: Ephedrine is excreted largely unchanged in the urine, therefore Franol should be used with caution in patients with severe renal impairment.

Cardiac dysfunction: Theophylline clearance may be decreased in patients with congestive cardiac failure, acute pulmonary oedema or cor pulmonale, and theophylline may cause arrhythmias or worsen existing arrhythmias, thus caution should be exercised if Franol is used in such patients.

Elderly (over 65 years): Theophylline clearance decreases slightly with age. Elderly patients will tend therefore to have higher serum theophylline levels than younger adults at a given dose. They should be monitored closely for signs of toxicity during dose adjustment.

Others: Theophylline clearance may be increased in heavy smokers, decreased in patients with respiratory infection, or those on a high carbohydrate - low protein diet therefore the dose of Franol may need to be adjusted appropriately in these groups.

Avoid or use with special caution in patients with cardiovascular disease, hypertension, agitation, phaeochromocytoma, hyperthyroidism, closed-angle glaucoma, prostatic hypertrophy, peptic ulceration, underlying seizure disorders, patients receiving anti-depressant drugs, or patients on MAO inhibitors within the previous 14 days. Special caution is also needed in the elderly, those with hepatic, renal, or cardiac dysfunction and during lactation.

Ephedrine has a potential for tachyphylaxis, and abuse with dependence has been reported. Potentially serious hypokalaemia can result from the use of $beta_2$ agonists and xanthines in combination particularly when hypoxia is present. The effect may be enhanced by concomitant diuretics or corticosteroids. Care should be observed and serum potassium levels monitored in patients receiving Franol who develop severe asthma, particularly if concomitant diuretic, corticosteroid or $beta_2$ agonist therapy is being employed.

4.5 Interaction with other medicinal products and other forms of Interaction
Theophylline clearance may be decreased by concurrent administration of cimetidine, macrolide antibiotics, oral contraceptives, interferons, diltiazem, verapamil and viloxazine. Ciprofloxacin also increases plasma theophylline concentrations and if concomitant use is essential, the dose of theophylline should be reduced and plasma concentrations closely monitored to avoid toxicity. Theophylline clearance may be increased by concurrent administration of barbiturates, carbamazepine, phenytoin, rifampicin, sulphinpyrazone, aminoglutethimide, phenobarbitone and primidone.

Plasma concentrations of theophylline can be reduced by concomitant use of the herbal remedy St John's Wort (Hypericum perforatum).

The effects of ephedrine are diminished by guanethidine, reserpine, and probably methyldopa, and may be diminished or enhance by tricyclic anti-depressants. Ephedrine may also diminish the effects of guanethidine and may increase the possibility of arrhythmias in digitalised patients.

The concomitant use of theophylline and fluvoxamine should usually be avoided. Where this is not possible, patients should have their theophylline dose halved and plasma theophylline should be monitored closely.

4.6 Pregnancy and lactation
Pregnancy: Although caffeine has been implicated as a teratogen, adequate animal teratogenic studies have not been conducted with theophylline nor with ephedrine. The safety of ephedrine and of theophylline, which crosses the placental barrier have not been established in human pregnancy. Franol should not therefore be prescribed for patients who are pregnant.

Lactation: Theophylline distributes readily into breast milk therefore Franol should be used with caution in nursing women.

4.7 Effects on ability to drive and use machines
No known effects.

4.8 Undesirable effects
Large doses of Franol may give rise to the following side effects: arrhythmias, tachycardia, palpitation, flushing, giddiness, headache, tremor, anxiety, restlessness, insomnia, muscular weakness, nausea, vomiting, dyspepsia, thirst, sweating, difficulty in micturition.

Some patients may exhibit one or more such symptoms with therapeutic doses.

4.9 Overdose
The symptoms and signs of overdose with Franol are likely to include, excessive irritability, sweating, nausea and vomiting, tachycardia, arrhythmias, hypertension, profuse diuresis with fever, flushing and hyperglycaemia, opisthotonos, hallucinations, convulsions and respiratory difficulty.

In general, the management of overdose with Franol involves supportive and symptomatic therapy with particular attention being paid to the detection and correction of hypokalaemia and should include serial assay of plasma potassium and theophylline levels, cardiac monitoring with electro-cardiogram and maintenance of fluid and electrolyte balance.

Gastric aspiration and lavage may be employed. Convulsions and other CNS stimulation can usually be controlled by intravenous diazepam, or if that fails anti-convulsants may be used. Marked excitement or hallucinations may be managed with chlorpromazine. Severe hypertensions may necessitate the use of an alpha-adrenoceptor blocking agent and a beta-adrenoceptor blocking agent may be required to control arrhythmias. $Beta_1$ -receptor agonist agents such as dopamine should be avoided. Charcoal haemoperfusion may be indicated to remove theophylline, but forced diuresis or peritoneal dialysis are inadequate for this purpose.

5. PHARMACOLOGICAL PROPERTIES

5.1 Pharmacodynamic properties
The action of ephedrine as a dilator of the bronchioles is mediated via a direct agonist effect on beta-adrenoceptors and by release of sympathomimetic amines. Theophylline has been shown to relieve bronchospasm and achieve subjective relief during an acute attack of bronchial asthma of allergic origin. The mechanism of action of theophylline has not yet been fully elucidated but may be by blockade of adenosine receptors or by phosphodiesterase inhibition.

5.2 Pharmacokinetic properties
Theophylline is variably absorbed from the gastrointestinal tract. It is excreted in the urine as metabolites, mainly 1, 3-dimethyluric acid, and about 10% is unchanged.

Ephedrine is readily absorbed from the gastrointestinal tract, its effect becoming apparent within one hour. It does not appear to be subject to enzyme inactivation by either monoamine oxidase or catechol-o-methyl transferase, and about 60-75% is excreted in the urine unchanged. The half-life in the circulation is about 4 hours.

5.3 Preclinical safety data
There are no preclinical data of relevance to the prescriber which are additional to that already included in other sections of the SPC.

6. PHARMACEUTICAL PARTICULARS

6.1 List of excipients
Calcium phosphate, Starch (maize), Magnesium stearate, Talc.

6.2 Incompatibilities
Not applicable.

6.3 Shelf life
60 months.

6.4 Special precautions for storage
Store below 25°C.

6.5 Nature and contents of container
Amber glass bottles fitted with tin-plate caps.

Pack size: 100.

6.6 Instructions for use and handling
None.

7. MARKETING AUTHORISATION HOLDER
Sanofi-Synthelabo

PO Box 597

Guildford

Surrey

8. MARKETING AUTHORISATION NUMBER(S)
11723/0035

9. DATE OF FIRST AUTHORISATION/RENEWAL OF THE AUTHORISATION
August 1993

10. DATE OF REVISION OF THE TEXT
November 2001

Legal Category P

Frisium Tablets 10 mg

(sanofi-aventis)

1. NAME OF THE MEDICINAL PRODUCT
Frisium™.

2. QUALITATIVE AND QUANTITATIVE COMPOSITION
Clobazam 10 mg.

3. PHARMACEUTICAL FORM
Tablet.

4. CLINICAL PARTICULARS

4.1 Therapeutic indications
Frisium is a 1,5-benzodiazepine indicated for the short-term relief (2-4 weeks) only of anxiety that is severe, disabling or subjecting the individual to unacceptable distress, occurring alone or in association with insomnia or short term psychosomatic, organic or psychotic illness. The use of Frisium to treat short-term "mild" anxiety is inappropriate and unsuitable.

Before treatment of anxiety states associated with emotional instability, it must first be determined whether the patient suffers from a depressive disorder requiring adjunctive or different treatment. Indeed, in patients with anxiety associated with depression, Frisium must be used only in conjunction with adequate concomitant treatment. Use of benzodiazepine (such as Frisium) alone, can precipitate suicide in such patients.

In patients with schizophrenic or other psychotic illnesses, use of benzodiazepines is recommended only for adjunctive, i.e. not for primary treatment.

Frisium may be used as adjunctive therapy in epilepsy.

4.2 Posology and method of administration
Treatment of anxiety

The usual anxiolytic dose for adults and adolescents over 15 years of age is 20-30 mg daily in divided doses or as a single dose given at night. Doses up to 60mg daily have been used in the treatment of adult in-patients with severe anxiety.

The lowest dose that can control symptoms should be used. After improvement of the symptoms, the dose may be reduced.

It should not be used for longer than 4 weeks. Long term chronic use as an anxiolytic is not recommended. In certain cases, extension beyond the maximum treatment period may be necessary; treatment must not be extended without re-evaluation of the patient's status using special expertise. It is strongly recommended that prolonged periods of uninterrupted treatment be avoided, since they may lead to dependence. Treatment should always be withdrawn gradually. Patients who have taken Frisium for a long time may require a longer period during which doses are reduced.

Treatment of epilepsy in association with one or more other anticonvulsants

In epilepsy a starting dose of 20-30 mg/day is recommended, increasing as necessary up to a maximum of 60 mg daily. The patient must be re-assessed after a period not exceeding 4 weeks and regularly thereafter in order to evaluate the need for continued treatment. A break in therapy may be beneficial if drug exhaustion develops, recommencing therapy at a low dose. At the end of treatment (including in poor-responding patients), since the risk of withdrawal phenomena/rebound phenomena is greater after abrupt discontinuation of treatment, it is recommended to gradually decrease the dosage.

Elderly: Doses of 10-20 mg daily in anxiety may be used in the elderly, who are more sensitive to the effects of psychoactive agents. Treatment requires low initial doses and gradual dose increments under careful observation.

Children: When prescribed for children over three years of age, dosage should not exceed half the recommended adult dose. Treatment requires low initial doses and gradual dose increments under careful observation. There is insufficient experience of the use of Frisium in children under three years of age to enable any dosage recommendation to be made.

Tablets should to be swallowed without chewing with sufficient amount of liquid (1/2 glass).

4.3 Contraindications
Frisium must not be used:

- In patients with hypersensitivity to benzodiazepines or any of the excipients of Frisium.

- In patients with any history of drug or alcohol dependence (increased risk of development of dependence).

- In patients with myasthenia gravis (risk of aggravation of muscle weakness).

- In patients with severe respiratory insufficiency (risk of deterioration).

- In patients with sleep apnoea syndrome (risk of deterioration).

- In patients with severe hepatic insufficiencies (risk of precipitating encephalopathy).

- During the first trimester of pregnancy (for use during second and third trimester, see section 4.6 Pregnancy and Lactation).

- In breast-feeding women.

Benzodiazepines must not be given to children without careful assessment of the need for their use. Frisium must not be used in children between the ages of 6 months and 3 years, other than in exceptional cases for anticonvulsant treatment where there is a compelling indication.

4.4 Special warnings and special precautions for use

Amnesia may occur with benzodiazepines. In case of loss or bereavement psychological adjustment may be inhibited by benzodiazepines.

Special caution is necessary if clobazam is used in patients with myasthenia gravis, spinal or cerebellar ataxia or sleep apnoea. A dose reduction may be necessary.

Disinhibiting effects may be manifested in various ways. Suicide may be precipitated in patients who are depressed and aggressive behaviour towards self and others may be precipitated. Extreme caution should therefore be used in prescribing benzodiazepines in patients with personality disorders.

Use of benzodiazepines - including clobazam - may lead to the development of physical and psychic dependence upon these products. The risk of dependence increases with dose and duration of treatment; it is also greater in patients with a history of alcohol or drug abuse. Therefore the duration of treatment should be as short as possible (see Posology).

Once physical dependence has developed, abrupt termination of treatment will be accompanied by withdrawal symptoms (or rebound phenomena). Rebound phenomena are characterised by a recurrence in enhanced form of the symptoms which originally led to clobazam treatment. This may be accompanied by other reactions including mood changes, anxiety or sleep disturbances and restlessness.

A withdrawal syndrome may also occur when abruptly changing over from a benzodiazepine with a long duration of action (for example, Frisium) to one with a short duration of action.

Respiratory function should be monitored in patients with chronic or acute severe respiratory insufficiency and a dose reduction of clobazam may be necessary.

In patients with impairment of renal or hepatic function, responsiveness to clobazam and susceptibility to adverse effects are increased, and a dose reduction may be necessary. In long-term treatment renal and hepatic function must be checked regularly.

In the treatment of epilepsy with benzodiazepines - including clobazam - consideration must be given to the possibility of a decrease in anticonvulsant efficacy (development of tolerance) in the course of treatment.

4.5 Interaction with other medicinal products and other forms of Interaction

Especially when clobazam is administered at higher doses, an enhancement of the central depressive effect may occur in cases of concomitant use with antipsychotics (neuroleptics), hypnotics, anxiolytics/sedatives, antidepressant agents, narcotic analgesics, anticonvulsant drugs, anaesthetics and sedative antihistamines. Special caution is also necessary when clobazam is administered in cases of intoxication with such substances or with lithium.

Concomitant consumption of alcohol can increase the bioavailability of clobazam by 50% and therefore increase the effects of clobazam(e.g.; sedation). This affects the ability to drive or use machines.

Addition of clobazam to established anticonvulsant medication (eg, phenytoin, valproic acid) may cause a change in plasma levels of these drugs. If used as an adjuvant in epilepsy the dosage of Frisium should be determined by monitoring the EEG and the plasma levels of the other drugs checked.

Phenytoin and carbamazepine may cause an increase in the metabolic conversion of clobazam to the active metabolite N-desmethyl clobazam.

The effects of muscle relaxants, analgesics and nitrous oxide may be enhanced. If clobazam is used concomitantly with narcotic analgesics, possible euphoria may be enhanced; this may lead to increased psychological dependence.

Concurrent treatment with drugs that inhibit the cytochrome P-450 enzyme (mono-oxygenase) system (eg cimetidine) may enhance and prolong the effect of clobazam.

4.6 Pregnancy and lactation

If the product is prescribed to a woman of childbearing potential, she should be warned to contact her physician regarding discontinuation of the product if she intends to become pregnant or suspects that she is pregnant.

If, for compelling medical reasons, the product is administered during the late phase of pregnancy, or during labour at high doses, effects on the neonate such as hypothermia, hypotonia, moderate respiratory depression and difficulties in drinking (signs and symptoms of so-called "floppy infant syndrome"), can be expected due to the pharmacological action of the compound.

Moreover, infants born to mothers who took benzodiazepines during the latter stage of pregnancy may have developed physical dependence and may be at some risk for developing withdrawal symptoms in the postnatal period.

Since benzodiazepines are found in the breast milk, benzodiazepines should not be given to breast feeding mothers.

4.7 Effects on ability to drive and use machines

Sedation, amnesia, impaired concentration and impaired muscular function may adversely affect the ability to drive or to use machines. If insufficient sleep duration occurs, the likelihood of impaired alertness may be increased (see also Interactions).

4.8 Undesirable effects

Clobazam may cause sedation, leading to fatigue and sleepiness, especially at the beginning of treatment and when higher doses are used. Side-effects such as drowsiness, dizziness or dryness of the mouth, constipation, loss of appetite, nausea, or a fine tremor of the fingers have been reported. These are more likely to occur at the beginning of treatment and often disappear with continued treatment or a reduction in dose.

Paradoxical reactions, such as restlessness, irritability, difficulty in sleeping, anxiety, delusion, nightmare, hallucinations or suicidal tendencies may occur, especially in elderly and in children. In the event of such reactions, treatment with clobazam must be discontinued.

Anterograde amnesia may occur, especially at higher dose levels. Amnesia effects may be associated with inappropriate behaviour.

Clobazam may cause respiratory depression, especially if administered in high doses. Therefore, particularly in patients with pre-existing compromised respiratory function (i.e., in patients with bronchial asthma) or brain damage, respiratory insufficiency may occur or deteriorate.

Isolated cases of skin reactions, such as rashes or urticaria, have been observed.

Slowing of reaction time, ataxia, confusion and headaches may occasionally occur.

Disorders of articulation, unsteadiness of gait and other motor functions, visual disorders (e.g., double vision), weight gain, or loss of libido may occur, particularly with high doses or in long-term treatment. These reactions are reversible.

Pre-existing depression may be unmasked during benzodiazepine use.

After prolonged use of benzodiazepines, impairment of consciousness, sometimes combined with respiratory disorders, has been reported in very rare cases, particularly in elderly patients: it sometimes persists for some length of time. These disorders have not been seen so far under clobazam treatment.

Tolerance and physical and/or psychic dependence may develop, especially during prolonged use. Discontinuation of the therapy may result in withdrawal or rebound phenomena (see Warnings and Precautions). Abuse of benzodiazepines has been reported.

When used as an adjuvant in the treatment of epilepsy, this preparation may in rare cases cause restlessness and muscle weakness.

As with other benzodiazepines, the therapeutic benefit must be balanced against the risk of habituation and dependence during prolonged use.

4.9 Overdose

Overdose of benzodiazepines is usually manifested by degrees of central nervous system depression ranging from drowsiness to coma. In mild cases, symptoms include drowsiness, mental confusion and lethargy, in more serious cases, symptoms may include ataxia, hypotonia, hypotension, respiratory depression, rarely coma and very rarely death. As with other benzodiazepines, overdose should not present a threat to life unless combined with other CNS depressants (including alcohol).

In the management of overdose, it is recommended that the possible involvement of multiple agents be taken into consideration.

Following overdose with oral benzodiazepines, vomiting should be induced (within one hour) if the patient is conscious, or gastric lavage undertaken with the airway protected if the patient is unconscious. If there is no advantage in emptying the stomach, activated charcoal should be given to reduce absorption. Special attention should be paid to respiratory and cardiovascular functions in intensive care.

Secondary elimination of clobazam (by forced diuresis or haemodialysis) is ineffective.

Consideration should be given to the use of flumazenil as a benzodiazepine antagonist.

5. PHARMACOLOGICAL PROPERTIES

5.1 Pharmacodynamic properties

Clobazam is a 1,5-benzodiazepine. In single doses up to 20mg or in divided doses up to 30mg, clobazam does not affect psychomotor function, skilled performance, memory or higher mental functions.

5.2 Pharmacokinetic properties

Absorption of clobazam is virtually complete after oral administration. Approximately 85% is protein bound in man. It is metabolised by demethylation and hydroxylation. It is excreted unchanged and as metabolites in the urine (87%) and feces.

5.3 Preclinical safety data

None applicable.

6. PHARMACEUTICAL PARTICULARS

6.1 List of excipients

Lactose monohydrate, maize starch, colloidal silicon dioxide, talc, magnesium stearate.

6.2 Incompatibilities

None.

6.3 Shelf life

Five years.

6.4 Special precautions for storage

Store below 25°C.

6.5 Nature and contents of container

Blister pack (Alufoil/PVC) containing 30 tablets.

6.6 Instructions for use and handling

None.

7. MARKETING AUTHORISATION HOLDER

Aventis Pharma Limited
50 Kings Hill Avenue
Kings Hill
West Malling
Kent ME19 4AH
UK

8. MARKETING AUTHORISATION NUMBER(S)

PL 04425/0214

9. DATE OF FIRST AUTHORISATION/RENEWAL OF THE AUTHORISATION

15 January 2002

10. DATE OF REVISION OF THE TEXT

January 2002

11. Legal Category

POM

Froben SR

(Abbott Laboratories Limited)

1. NAME OF THE MEDICINAL PRODUCT

Froben SR 200 mg

2. QUALITATIVE AND QUANTITATIVE COMPOSITION

Each Froben SR capsule contains 200 mg Flurbiprofen in a sustained-release form.

3. PHARMACEUTICAL FORM

A hard gelatin capsule with a yellow opaque cap and a transparent yellow body.

4. CLINICAL PARTICULARS

4.1 Therapeutic indications

Froben SR is indicated for the treatment of rheumatoid disease, osteoarthritis, ankylosing spondylitis, musculoskeletal disorders and trauma such as periarthritis, frozen shoulder, bursitis, tendinitis, tenosynovitis, low back pain, sprains and strains.

4.2 Posology and method of administration

For oral administration.

Adults: The recommended daily dose is one 200 mg capsule, taken preferably in the evening after food.

Children: Paediatric dosage has not been established.

Elderly: Although flurbiprofen is well tolerated in the elderly, some patients, especially those with impaired renal function, may eliminate NSAIDs more slowly than normal. In these cases, Froben SR should be used with caution and dosage should be assessed individually, using the standard formulation if necessary.

4.3 Contraindications

Froben SR is contra-indicated in patients with peptic ulceration, gastrointestinal haemorrhage or ulcerative colitis. Froben SR should not be given to patients with a history of asthma or to patients who have experienced bronchospasm, anaphylactic reactions, angioedema or other hypersensitivity-type reactions from the use of aspirin or other NSAIDs.

4.4 Special warnings and special precautions for use

Caution is necessary if Froben SR is given to patients with a history of cardiac decompensation, hypertension or non-allergic asthma. As it has been shown that flurbiprofen may prolong bleeding time, Froben SR should be used with caution in patients with a potential for abnormal bleeding.

NSAIDs have been reported to cause nephrotoxicity in various forms: interstitial nephritis, nephrotic syndrome and renal failure. In patients with renal, cardiac or hepatic impairment, caution is required since the use of NSAIDs may result in deterioration of renal function. The dose should be kept as low as possible and renal function should be monitored in these patients.

4.5 Interaction with other medicinal products and other forms of Interaction
Special clinical studies have shown that the diuretic response to frusemide can occasionally be reduced by flurbiprofen. Similarly, interference with the action of anticoagulants has occasionally been reported.

Other studies have failed to show any interaction between flurbiprofen and digoxin, tolbutamide or antacids. There is no evidence so far that flurbiprofen interferes with standard laboratory tests.

4.6 Pregnancy and lactation
Preclinical studies have not revealed any teratogenic effects, although Froben SR should not be prescribed during pregnancy unless the benefits outweigh the possible risks. If Froben SR is used during early pregnancy, the lowest effective dose should be employed. During the third trimester of pregnancy, regular use of NSAIDs has been associated with delayed and prolonged parturition and premature closure of the foetal ductus arteriosus *in utero* and possibly persistent pulmonary hypertension of the newborn.

The amount of flurbiprofen secreted into the breast milk during lactation is considered too small to be harmful. For this reason, breast-feeding would not be contra-indicated.

4.7 Effects on ability to drive and use machines
No adverse effects known.

4.8 Undesirable effects
Dyspepsia, nausea, vomiting, gastrointestinal haemorrhage, diarrhoea, ulcers of the mouth, fluid retention, oedema, and exacerbation of peptic ulceration and perforation have been reported.

Urticaria, angioedema and rashes of varying description may occur. Very rarely, cholestatic jaundice and thrombocytopenia have been reported; these are usually reversible on withdrawal of the drug. Very rarely, aplastic anaemia and agranulocytosis have been associated with the use of flurbiprofen but causality has not been established.

4.9 Overdose
Symptoms of overdosage may include nausea, vomiting and gastrointestinal irritation. Treatment should consist of gastric lavage and if necessary, correction of serum electrolytes. There is no specific antidote to flurbiprofen.

5. PHARMACOLOGICAL PROPERTIES

5.1 Pharmacodynamic properties
Flurbiprofen has analgesic, anti-inflammatory and antipyretic properties. These are thought to result from the drug's ability to inhibit prostaglandin synthesis.

5.2 Pharmacokinetic properties
Following oral administration, flurbiprofen in sustained-release formulation is readily absorbed from the gastro-intestinal tract, with peak plasma concentrations occurring 4 to 6 hours after ingestion. It is approximately 99% protein-bound and has an elimination half-life of about three to four hours.

The rate of urinary excretion of flurbiprofen and its two major metabolites ([2-(2-fluoro-4'hydroxy-4-biphenylyl) propionic acid] and [2-(2-fluoro-3'hydroxy-4'methoxy-4-biphenylyl) propionic acid]) in both free and conjugated states is the same for Froben SR as for the other oral forms of flurbiprofen. Metabolic patterns are the same for Froben SR as for the other oral forms of flurbiprofen.

5.3 Preclinical safety data
Not applicable.

6. PHARMACEUTICAL PARTICULARS

6.1 List of excipients
Microcrystalline cellulose, gelatin, acrylic/methacrylic acid ester copolymer, magnesium stearate, colloidal silicon dioxide, quinoline yellow, polyethylene glycol 6000, titanium dioxide, shellac, black iron oxide, red iron oxide, glycerin, soya lecithin, polydimethylsiloxane.

6.2 Incompatibilities
None.

6.3 Shelf life
36 months.

6.4 Special precautions for storage
None.

6.5 Nature and contents of container
White HDPE bottles containing 4, 30 or 210 capsules.

6.6 Instructions for use and handling
None.

7. MARKETING AUTHORISATION HOLDER
Abbott Laboratories Limited
Queenborough
Kent
ME11 5EL
United Kingdom

8. MARKETING AUTHORISATION NUMBER(S)
PL 00037/0353

9. DATE OF FIRST AUTHORISATION/RENEWAL OF THE AUTHORISATION
31 December 2001

10. DATE OF REVISION OF THE TEXT

Froben Suppositories 100mg

(Abbott Laboratories Limited)

1. NAME OF THE MEDICINAL PRODUCT
Froben Suppositories 100 mg

2. QUALITATIVE AND QUANTITATIVE COMPOSITION
Each suppository contains 100 mg flurbiprofen (Pfive) milled HSE.

3. PHARMACEUTICAL FORM
Froben Suppositories are wax-based and white in colour.

4. CLINICAL PARTICULARS

4.1 Therapeutic indications
Froben Suppositories are indicated for the treatment of rheumatoid disease, osteoarthritis, ankylosing spondylitis, musculoskeletal disorders and trauma such as periarthritis, frozen shoulder, bursitis, tendinitis, tenosynovitis, low back pain, sprains and strains.

Also indicated for its analgesic effect in the relief of mild to moderate pain in conditions such as dental pain, post-operative pain, dysmenorrhoea and migraine.

4.2 Posology and method of administration
Froben Suppositories are for rectal administration.

Adults and children over 12 years:

One suppository may be administered twice daily or may replace the equivalent dose of oral therapy to give a total daily dosage of 150 to 200 mg. In patients with severe disease or disease of recent origin, or during acute exacerbations, the total daily dosage may be increased to 300 mg in divided doses.

Dysmenorrhoea.

A suppository can be administered at the start of symptoms, followed by 50 or 100 mg (in the form of tablets) given at four- to six-hourly intervals. The maximum total daily dosage should not exceed 300 mg.

Children:

Froben Suppositories are not indicated for use in children.

Elderly:

The elderly are at increased risk of the serious consequences of adverse reactions. If an NSAID is considered necessary, the lowest dose should be used and the patient should be monitored for GI bleeding for four weeks following initiation of NSAID therapy.

4.3 Contraindications
Froben Suppositories should not be administered to patients with a history of, or active, peptic ulceration. Froben Suppositories are also contra-indicated in patients who have previously shown hypersensitivity reactions (*e.g.* asthma, rhinitis or urticaria) in response to flurbiprofen, aspirin or other NSAIDs.

Froben Suppositories are contra-indicated in patients with inflammatory diseases of the rectum and perianal area.

4.4 Special warnings and special precautions for use
Caution is required if Froben Suppositories are administered to patients suffering from, or with a previous history of, bronchial asthma since flurbiprofen has been reported to cause bronchospasm in such patients. Froben Suppositories should only be given with care to patients with a history of gastrointestinal disease.

Caution is required in patients with renal, hepatic or cardiac impairment since the use of NSAIDs may result in deterioration of renal function. The dose should be kept as low as possible and renal function should be monitored in these patients.

Froben Suppositories should be given with care to patients with a history of heart failure or hypertension since oedema has been reported in association with flurbiprofen administration.

As it has been shown that flurbiprofen may prolong bleeding time, Froben Suppositories should be used with caution in patients with a potential for abnormal bleeding.

4.5 Interaction with other medicinal products and other forms of Interaction
Care should be taken in patients treated with any of the following drugs as interactions have been reported in some patients.

Anti-hypertensives: Reduced antihypertensive effect.

Diuretics: Reduced diuretic effect. Diuretics can increase the risk of nephrotoxicity of NSAIDs.

Cardiac glycosides: NSAIDs may exacerbate cardiac failure, reduce GFR and increase plasma cardiac glycoside levels.

Lithium: Decreased elimination of lithium.

Methotrexate: Decreased elimination of methotrexate.

Cyclosporin: Increased risk of nephrotoxicity with NSAIDs.

Mifepristone: NSAIDs should not be used for 8-12 days after mifepristone administration as NSAIDs can reduce the effects of mifepristone.

Other analgesics: Avoid concomitant use of two or more NSAIDs.

Corticosteroids: Increased risk of gastrointestinal bleeding.

Anticoagulants: Enhanced anticoagulant effect.

Quinolone antibiotics: Animal data indicate that NSAIDs can increase the risk of convulsions associated with quinolone antibiotics. Patients taking NSAIDs and quinolones may have an increased risk of developing convulsions.

Studies have failed to show any interaction between flurbiprofen and tolbutamide or antacids. There is no evidence so far that flurbiprofen interferes with standard laboratory tests.

4.6 Pregnancy and lactation
Whilst no teratogenic effects have been demonstrated in animal toxicology studies, the use of flurbiprofen during pregnancy should, if possible, be avoided. Congenital abnormalities have been reported in association with flurbiprofen administration in man; however, these are low in frequency and do not appear to follow any discernible pattern. In view of the known effects of NSAIDs on the foetal cardiovascular system (closure of ductus arteriosus), use in late pregnancy should be avoided.

In the limited studies so far available, flurbiprofen appears in the breast milk in very low concentrations and is unlikely to adversely affect the breast-fed infant.

4.7 Effects on ability to drive and use machines
No adverse effects known.

4.8 Undesirable effects
Gastrointestinal: The most commonly-observed adverse events are gastrointestinal in nature. Nausea, vomiting, diarrhoea, dyspepsia, abdominal pain, melaena, haematemesis, ulcerative stomatitis and gastrointestinal haemorrhage have been reported following flurbiprofen administration. Less frequently, gastritis, duodenal ulcer, gastric ulcer and gastrointestinal perforation have been observed.

Hypersensitivity: Hypersensitivity reactions have been reported following treatment with NSAIDs. These may consist of (a) non-specific allergic reactions and anaphylaxis, (b) respiratory tract reactivity comprising asthma, aggravated asthma, bronchospasm or dyspnoea, or (c) assorted skin disorders, including rashes of various types, pruritus, urticaria, purpura, angioedema and, less commonly, bullous dermatoses (including epidermal necrolysis and erythema multiforme).

Cardiovascular: Oedema has been reported in association with NSAID treatment.

Other adverse events reported less commonly and for which causality has not necessarily been established include:

Renal: Nephrotoxicity in various forms, including interstitial nephritis, nephrotic syndrome and renal failure.

Hepatic: Abnormal liver function, hepatitis and jaundice.

Neurological &

special senses: Visual disturbances, optic neuritis, headaches, paraesthesia, depression, confusion, hallucinations, tinnitus, vertigo, dizziness, malaise, fatigue and drowsiness.

Haematological: Thrombocytopenia, neutropenia, agranulocytosis, aplastic anaemia and haemolytic anaemia.

Dermatological: Photosensitivity (see 'hypersensitivity' for other skin reactions).

4.9 Overdose
Symptoms of overdosage may include nausea, vomiting and gastrointestinal irritation. Treatment should consist of gastric lavage and if necessary, correction of serum electrolytes. There is no specific antidote to flurbiprofen.

5. PHARMACOLOGICAL PROPERTIES

5.1 Pharmacodynamic properties
Flurbiprofen has analgesic, anti-inflammatory and antipyretic properties. These are thought to result from the drug's ability to inhibit prostaglandin synthesis.

5.2 Pharmacokinetic properties
Bioavailability of flurbiprofen from the suppositories is comparable with that from the tablets. Absorption from the suppository formulation may be more rapid but the peak serum concentration is lower than with the tablet formulation.

The rate of urinary excretion of flurbiprofen and its two major metabolites ([2-(2-fluoro-4'-hydroxy-4-biphenylyl) propionic acid] and [2-(2-fluoro-3'-hydroxy-4'-methoxy-4-biphenylyl) propionic acid]) in both the free and conjugated states is similar for both the oral and rectal routes of administration. Metabolic patterns are also quantitatively similar for both routes of administration.

5.3 Preclinical safety data
Not applicable.

6. PHARMACEUTICAL PARTICULARS

6.1 List of excipients
Hard fat.

6.2 Incompatibilities
None.

6.3 Shelf life
36 months.

6.4 Special precautions for storage
Store in a cool place.

6.5 Nature and contents of container
A white moulded strip containing 12 suppositories.

6.6 Instructions for use and handling
None.

7. MARKETING AUTHORISATION HOLDER
Abbott Laboratories Limited, Queenborough, Kent, ME11 5EL, United Kingdom

8. MARKETING AUTHORISATION NUMBER(S)
PL 00037/0345

9. DATE OF FIRST AUTHORISATION/RENEWAL OF THE AUTHORISATION
4 September 2002

10. DATE OF REVISION OF THE TEXT

Froben Tablets 50 & 100 mg

(Abbott Laboratories Limited)

1. NAME OF THE MEDICINAL PRODUCT
Froben Tablets 50 mg

Froben Tablets 100 mg

2. QUALITATIVE AND QUANTITATIVE COMPOSITION
Froben Tablets 50 mg contain 50 mg Flurbiprofen BP.

Froben Tablets 100 mg contain 100 mg Flurbiprofen BP.

3. PHARMACEUTICAL FORM
The tablets are sugar-coated and yellow in colour. They may be either unprinted or printed in black with an identifying motif.

4. CLINICAL PARTICULARS

4.1 Therapeutic indications
For the treatment of rheumatoid disease, osteoarthritis, ankylosing spondylitis, musculoskeletal disorders and trauma such as periarthritis, frozen shoulder, bursitis, tendinitis, tenosynovitis, low back pain, sprains and strains.

Froben is also indicated for its analgesic effect in the relief of mild to moderate pain in conditions such as dental pain, post-operative pain, dysmenorrhoea and migraine.

4.2 Posology and method of administration
For oral administration.

Adults:

150 to 200 mg daily in two, three or four divided doses. In patients with severe symptoms or disease of recent origin, or during acute exacerbations, the total daily dosage may be increased to 300 mg in divided doses.

Dysmenorrhoea:

A dosage of 100 mg may be administered at the start of symptoms followed by 50 or 100 mg given at four- to six-hour intervals. The maximum total daily dosage not to exceed 300 mg.

Children:

Not recommended for use in children under 12 years.

Elderly:

The elderly are at increased risk of the serious consequences of adverse reactions. If an NSAID is considered necessary, the lowest dose should be used and the patient should be monitored for GI bleeding for four weeks following initiation of NSAID therapy.

4.3 Contraindications
Froben should not be administered to patients with a history of, or active, peptic ulceration. Froben is also contra-indicated in patients who have previously shown hypersensitivity reactions (*e.g.* asthma, rhinitis or urticaria) in response to flurbiprofen, aspirin or other NSAIDs.

4.4 Special warnings and special precautions for use
Caution is required if Froben is administered to patients suffering from, or with a previous history of, bronchial asthma since flurbiprofen has been reported to cause bronchospasm in such patients. Froben should only be given with care to patients with a history of gastrointestinal disease.

Caution is required in patients with renal, hepatic or cardiac impairment since the use of NSAIDs may result in deterioration of renal function. The dose should be kept as low as possible and renal function should be monitored in these patients.

Froben should be given with care to patients with a history of heart failure or hypertension since oedema has been reported in association with flurbiprofen administration.

As it has been shown that flurbiprofen may prolong bleeding time, Froben should be used with caution in patients with a potential for abnormal bleeding.

4.5 Interaction with other medicinal products and other forms of Interaction
Care should be taken in patients treated with any of the following drugs as interactions have been reported in some patients.

Antihypertensives: Reduced antihypertensive effect.

Diuretics: Reduced diuretic effect. Diuretics can increase the risk of nephrotoxicity of NSAIDs.

Cardiac glycosides: NSAIDs may exacerbate cardiac failure, reduce GFR and increase plasma cardiac glycoside levels.

Lithium: Decreased elimination of lithium.

Methotrexate: Decreased elimination of methotrexate.

Cyclosporin: Increased risk of nephrotoxicity with NSAIDs.

Mifepristone: NSAIDs should not be used for 8-12 days after mifepristone administration as NSAIDs can reduce the effects of mifepristone.

Other analgesics: Avoid concomitant use of two or more NSAIDs.

Corticosteroids: Increased risk of gastrointestinal bleeding.

Anticoagulants: Enhanced anticoagulant effect.

Quinolone antibiotics: Animal data indicate that NSAIDs can increase the risk of convulsions associated with quinolone antibiotics. Patients taking NSAIDs and quinolones may have an increased risk of developing convulsions.

Studies have failed to show any interaction between flurbiprofen and tolbutamide or antacids. There is no evidence so far that flurbiprofen interferes with standard laboratory tests.

4.6 Pregnancy and lactation
Whilst no teratogenic effects have been demonstrated in animal toxicology studies, the use of flurbiprofen during pregnancy should, if possible, be avoided. Congenital abnormalities have been reported in association with flurbiprofen administration in man; however, these are low in frequency and do not appear to follow any discernible pattern. In view of the known effects of NSAIDs on the foetal cardiovascular system (closure of ductus arteriosus), use in late pregnancy should be avoided.

In the limited studies so far available, flurbiprofen appears in the breast milk in very low concentrations and is unlikely to adversely affect the breast-fed infant.

4.7 Effects on ability to drive and use machines
No adverse effects known.

4.8 Undesirable effects
Gastrointestinal: The most commonly-observed adverse events are gastrointestinal in nature. Nausea, vomiting, diarrhoea, dyspepsia, abdominal pain, melaena, haematemesis, ulcerative stomatitis and gastrointestinal haemorrhage have been reported following flurbiprofen administration. Less frequently, gastritis, duodenal ulcer, gastric ulcer and gastrointestinal perforation have been observed.

Hypersensitivity: Hypersensitivity reactions have been reported following treatment with NSAIDs. These may consist of (a) non-specific allergic reactions and anaphylaxis, (b) respiratory tract reactivity comprising asthma, aggravated asthma, bronchospasm or dyspnoea, or (c) assorted skin disorders, including rashes of various types, pruritus, urticaria, purpura, angioedema and, less commonly, bullous dermatoses (including epidermal necrolysis and erythema multiforme).

Cardiovascular: Oedema has been reported in association with NSAID treatment.

Other adverse events reported less commonly and for which causality has not necessarily been established include:

Renal: Nephrotoxicity in various forms, including interstitial nephritis, nephrotic syndrome and renal failure.

Hepatic: Abnormal liver function, hepatitis and jaundice.

Neurological & special senses: Visual disturbances, optic neuritis, headaches, paraesthesia, depression, confusion, hallucinations, tinnitus, vertigo, dizziness, malaise, fatigue and drowsiness.

Haematological: Thrombocytopenia, neutropenia, agranulocytosis, aplastic anaemia and haemolytic anaemia.

Dermatological: Photosensitivity (see 'hypersensitivity' for other skin reactions).

4.9 Overdose
Symptoms of overdosage may include nausea, vomiting and gastrointestinal irritation. Treatment should consist of gastric lavage and if necessary, correction of serum electrolytes. There is no specific antidote to flurbiprofen.

5. PHARMACOLOGICAL PROPERTIES

5.1 Pharmacodynamic properties
Flurbiprofen has analgesic, anti-inflammatory and antipyretic properties. These are thought to result from the drug's ability to inhibit prostaglandin synthesis.

5.2 Pharmacokinetic properties
Flurbiprofen is readily absorbed from the gastrointestinal tract, with peak plasma concentrations occurring about 90 minutes after ingestion. It is about 99% protein-bound and has an elimination half-life of about three to four hours.

The rate of urinary excretion of flurbiprofen and its two major metabolites ([2-(2-fluoro-4'-hydroxy-4-biphenylyl) propionic acid] and [2-(2-fluoro-3'-hydroxy-4'-methoxy-4-biphenylyl) propionic acid]) in both free and conjugated states is similar for both the oral and rectal routes of administration. Metabolic patterns are quantitatively similar for both routes of administration.

5.3 Preclinical safety data
Not applicable.

6. PHARMACEUTICAL PARTICULARS

6.1 List of excipients
Maize starch powder EP, lactose NF anhydrous, povidone BPC, industrial alcohol FRP, magnesium stearate EP, stearic acid PDR BPC, *sandarac BPC 49 tablet varnish WMR, isopropyl alcohol, sucrose, purified water

Coat

Liquid glucose BPC 63, French chalk for tablets HSE, titanium dioxide BP, colloidal silicon dioxide NF, opalux yellow ASF 2230 HSE, carnauba wax PDR BP, **opacode S-1-8152HV black HSE

* Alternatively sandarac tablet varnish BPC 49

** Alternatively fine black ink markem

6.2 Incompatibilities
None known.

6.3 Shelf life
Blister pack: 36 months (unopened)

Bulk pack: 12 months (unopened)

6.4 Special precautions for storage
None for the blister pack.

Store in a cool, dry place for the bulk pack.

6.5 Nature and contents of container
A blister pack consisting of a PVC blister heat sealed to hard temper aluminium foil packed in a cardboard carton. Each blister contains 10 tablets.

Pack sizes: 10, 20, 30, 100 and 500 tablets. Also a sample pack of 5 tablets in a blister.

A bulk pack of a low density polyethylene bag in a rectangular white plastic tub having a snap-on lid.

Pack sizes: Approx. 25,000 or 50,000 tablets.

6.6 Instructions for use and handling
None stated.

7. MARKETING AUTHORISATION HOLDER
Abbott Laboratories Limited

Queenborough

Kent

ME11 5EL

United Kingdom

8. MARKETING AUTHORISATION NUMBER(S)
Froben Tablets 50 mg: PL 00037/0349

Froben Tablets 100 mg: PL 00037/0347

9. DATE OF FIRST AUTHORISATION/RENEWAL OF THE AUTHORISATION
31 December 2001

10. DATE OF REVISION OF THE TEXT

Frumil Forte

(sanofi-aventis)

1. NAME OF THE MEDICINAL PRODUCT
FRUMIL FORTE ™

2. QUALITATIVE AND QUANTITATIVE COMPOSITION
in terms of the active ingredient

The active ingredient is Furosemide 80.0mg and amiloride hydrochloride equivalent to 10mg anhydrous amiloride hydrochloride.

3. PHARMACEUTICAL FORM
Tablets for oral administration.

4. CLINICAL PARTICULARS

4.1 Therapeutic indications
Frumil Forte is a potassium sparing diuretic which is indicated where a prompt diuresis is required. It is of particular value in conditions where potassium conservation is important: congestive cardiac failure, nephrosis, corticosteriod therapy, oestrogen therapy and for ascites associated with cirrhosis.

4.2 Posology and method of administration
Adults: One tablet to be taken in the morning.

Children: Not recommended for children under 18 years of age as safety and efficacy have not been established.

Elderly: The dosage should be adjusted according to the diuretic response; serum electrolytes and urea should be carefully monitored.

4.3 Contraindications

Hyperkalaemia (serum potassium >5.3mmol/litre), Addison's disease, acute renal failure, anuria, severe progressive renal disease, electrolyte imbalance, precomatose states associated with cirrhosis, concomitant potassium supplements or potassium sparing diuretics, known sensitivity to furosemide or amiloride.

Frumil Forte is contra-indicated in children under 18 years of age as safety has not been established.

4.4 Special warnings and special precautions for use

Frumil Forte should be discontinued before a glucose tolerance test.

Patients who are being treated with this preparation require regular supervision, with monitoring of fluid electrolyte states to avoid excessive loss of fluid

Frumil Forte should be used with particular caution in elderly patients or those with potential obstruction of the urinary tract or disorders rendering electrolyte balance precarious.

4.5 Interaction with other medicinal products and other forms of Interaction

Frumil Forte may enhance the nephrotoxicity of cephalosporin antibacterials such as cephalothin, NSAID's or cisplatin, and enhance the ototoxicity of aminoglycoside antibacterials and other ototoxic drugs.

Concurrent use of other diuretics, reboxetine, sympathomimetic agents, corticosteroids, ampotericin and carbenoxolone may lead to an increased risk of hypokalaemia.

The diuretic effect of Frumil Forte may be reduced by concurrent use of phenytoin or NSAID's, notably indometacin and ketorolac. Severe diuresis may occur if metolazone is administered concomitantly.

Hyperkalaemia may occur in patients receiving potassium salts, ACE Inhibitors, indometacin and possibly other NSAID's, ciclosporin or trilostane.

Potentially serious hypokalaemia may result from beta$_2$-adreno-receptor stimulant therapy. Particular caution is required with concomitant therapy with diuretics.

If other antihypertensives or drugs which can lead to a reduction in blood pressure are taken concurrently with Frumil Forte, a more pronounced fall in blood pressure must be anticipated. Profound first-dose hypotension may occur when ACE inhibitors are introduced to patients with heart failure who are already taking a high dose of a loop diuretic (e.g. furosemide 80mg daily or more). Temporary withdrawal of the loop diuretic reduces the risk, but may cause severe rebound pulmonary oedema. The ACE inhibitor should, therefore, be started at a very low dosage (e.g. captopril 6.25mg), with the patient recumbent and under close medical supervision and with facilities to treat profound hypotension. In these circumstances the patient should be admitted to hospital for initiation of therapy.

Frumil Forte may antagonise the effects of antidiabetic drugs and pressor amines and potentiate the effects of lithium and curare-type muscle relaxants.

Concomitant administration of carbamazepine or aminoglutethimide may increase the risk of hyponatraemia.

The dosage of concurrently administered cardiac glycosides may also require adjustment.

4.6 Pregnancy and lactation

The safety of Frumil Forte during pregnancy and lactation has not been established.

4.7 Effects on ability to drive and use machines

None stated.

4.8 Undesirable effects

Serum uric acid levels may rise during treatment with Frumil Forte and acute attacks of gout may be precipitated.

Malaise, dry mouth, gastric upset, nausea, vomiting, diarrhoea and constipation may occur.

If skin rashes or pruritus occur treatment should be withdrawn.

Rare complications may include minor psychiatric disturbances, disturbances in liver function tests and ototoxicity. Bone marrow depression occasionally complicates treatment, necessitating withdrawal of the product. The haematopoietic state should be regularly monitored during treatment.

Hyponatraemia, hypochloraemia and raised blood urea nitrogen may occur during vigorous diuresis, especially in seriously ill patients. Careful monitoring of serum electrolytes and urea should therefore be undertaken in these patients. Hyperkalaemia has been observed in patients receiving amiloride hydrochloride.

As ACE inhibitors may elevate serum potassium levels, especially in the presence of renal impairment, combination with Frumil Forte is best avoided in elderly patients or in any others in whom renal function may be compromised. If use of the combination is deemed essential clinical condition and serum electrolytes must be continuously monitored.

Furosemide may cause latent diabetes to become manifest. It may be necessary to increase the dose of hypoglycaemic agents in diabetic patients.

Patients with prostatic hypertrophy or impairment of micturition have an increased risk of developing acute urinary retention during diuretic therapy.

4.9 Overdose

Treatment of overdosage should be aimed at reversing dehydration and correcting electrolyte imbalance, particularly hyperkalaemia. Emesis should be induced or gastric lavage performed. Treatment should be symptomatic and supportive. If hyperkalaemia is seen, appropriate measures to reduce serum potassium must be instituted.

5. PHARMACOLOGICAL PROPERTIES

5.1 Pharmacodynamic properties

FUROSEMIDE:

Furosemide is a loop diuretic which acts primarily to inhibit electrolyte reabsorption in the thick ascending Loop of Henle. Excretion of sodium, potassium and chloride ions is increased and water excretion enhanced.

AMILORIDE:

Amiloride is a mild diuretic which moderately increases the excretion of sodium and chloride and reduces potassium excretion, and appears to act mainly on the distal renal tubules. It does not appear to act by inhibition of aldosterone and does not inhibit carbonic anhydrase. Amiloride adds to the natiuretic but diminishes the kaliuretic effect of other diuretics.

A combination of Furosemide and Amiloride is a diuretic which reduces the potassium loss of furosemide alone while avoiding the possible gastro-intestinal disturbances of potassium supplements.

5.2 Pharmacokinetic properties

FUROSEMIDE:

Approximately 65% of the dose is absorbed after oral administration. The plasma half-life is biphasic with a terminal elimination phase of about 1 ½ hours. Furosemide is up to 99% bound to plasma proteins and is mainly excreted in the urine, largely unchanged, but also excreted in the bile, non-renal elimination being considerably increased in renal failure. Furosemide crosses the placental barrier and is excreted in the milk.

AMILORIDE:

Approximately 50% of the dose is absorbed after oral administration and peak serum concentrations are achieved by about 3 - 4 hours. The serum half-life is estimated to be about 6 hours. Amiloride is not bound to plasma proteins. Amiloride is not metabolised and is excreted unchanged in the urine.

5.3 Preclinical safety data

No further information available

6. PHARMACEUTICAL PARTICULARS

6.1 List of excipients

Frumil Forte tablets contain the following excipients:

Lactose

Starch Maize

Microcrystalline Cellulose

Sodium Starch Glycollate

Sunset Yellow Dye (E110)

French Chalk Powdered

Colloidal Anhydrous Silica

Magnesium Stearate

6.2 Incompatibilities

None stated

6.3 Shelf life

The shelf-life of Frumil Forte is 36 months

6.4 Special precautions for storage

Store below 25°C in a dry place. Protect from light.

6.5 Nature and contents of container

Blister packs of 28 and 56

6.6 Instructions for use and handling

None

7. MARKETING AUTHORISATION HOLDER

Helios Healthcare Limited

11A Ferraidy Street

Peyki - Attikas,

Greece

8. MARKETING AUTHORISATION NUMBER(S)

PL 17076/0003

9. DATE OF FIRST AUTHORISATION/RENEWAL OF THE AUTHORISATION

September 1998

10. DATE OF REVISION OF THE TEXT

November 2004

Legal category: POM

Frumil, Frumil LS

(sanofi-aventis)

1. NAME OF THE MEDICINAL PRODUCT

Frumil

Frumil LS

2. QUALITATIVE AND QUANTITATIVE COMPOSITION

In terms of the active ingredient

Frumil: The active ingredient is Furosemide 40.0mg and amiloride hydrochloride equivalent to 5.0mg anhydrous amiloride hydrochloride.

Frumil LS: The active ingredient is Furosemide 20.0mg and amiloride hydrochloride equivalent to 2.5mg anhydrous amiloride hydrochloride.

3. PHARMACEUTICAL FORM

Tablets for oral administration.

4. CLINICAL PARTICULARS

4.1 Therapeutic indications

Frumil/Frumil LS is a potassium sparing diuretic which is indicated where a prompt diuresis is required. It is of particular value in conditions where potassium conservation is important: congestive cardiac failure, nephrosis, corticosteroid therapy, oestrogen therapy and for ascites associated with cirrhosis.

4.2 Posology and method of administration

Adults: One or two tablets to be taken in the morning.

Children: Not recommended for children under 18 years of age as safety and efficacy have not been established.

Elderly: The dosage should be adjusted according to the diuretic response; serum electrolytes and urea should be carefully monitored.

4.3 Contraindications

Hyperkalaemia (serum potassium >5.3mmol/litre), Addison's disease, acute renal failure, anuria, severe progressive renal disease, electrolyte imbalance, precomatose states associated with cirrhosis, concomitant potassium supplements or potassium sparing diuretics, known sensitivity to furosemide or amiloride.

Frumil/Frumil LS is contra-indicated in children under 18 years of age as safety in this age group has not been established.

4.4 Special warnings and special precautions for use

Frumil/Frumil LS should be discontinued before a glucose tolerance test.

Patients who are being treated with this preparation require regular supervision, with monitoring of fluid electrolyte states to avoid excessive loss of fluid.

Frumil/Frumil LS should be used with particular caution in elderly patients or those with potential obstruction of the urinary tract or disorders rendering electrolyte balance precarious.

4.5 Interaction with other medicinal products and other forms of Interaction

Frumil/Frumil LS may enhance the nephrotoxicity of cephalosporin antibacterials such as cephalothin, NSAID's or cisplatin, and enhance the ototoxicity of aminoglycoside antibacterials and other ototoxic drugs.

Concurrent use of other diuretics, reboxetine, sympathomimetic agents, corticosteroids, ampotericin and carbenoxolone may lead to an increased risk of hypokalaemia.

The diuretic effect of Frumil/Frumil LS may be reduced by concurrent use of phenytoin or NSAID's, notably indometacin and ketorolac. Severe diuresis may occur if metolazone is administered concomitantly.

Hyperkalaemia may occur in patients receiving potassium salts, ACE Inhibitors, indometacin and possibly other NSAID's, ciclosporin or trilostane.

Potentially serious hypokalaemia may result from beta$_2$-adreno-receptor stimulant therapy. Particular caution is required with concomitant therapy with diuretics.

If other antihypertensives or drugs which can lead to a reduction in blood pressure are taken concurrently with Frumil/Frumil LS, a more pronounced fall in blood pressure must be anticipated. Profound first-dose hypotension may occur when ACE inhibitors are introduced to patients with heart failure who are already taking a high dose of a loop diuretic (e.g. furosemide 80mg daily or more). Temporary withdrawal of the loop diuretic reduces the risk, but may cause severe rebound pulmonary oedema. The ACE inhibitor should, therefore, be started at a very low dosage (e.g. captopril 6.25mg), with the patient recumbent and under close medical supervision and with facilities to treat profound hypotension. In these circumstances the patient should be admitted to hospital for initiation of therapy.

Frumil/Frumil LS may antagonise the effects of antidiabetic drugs and pressor amines and potentiate the effects of lithium and curare-type muscle relaxants.

Concomitant administration of carbamazepine or aminoglutethimide may increase the risk of hyponatraemia.

The dosage of concurrently administered cardiac glycosides may also require adjustment.

4.6 Pregnancy and lactation

The safety of Frumil/Frumil LS during pregnancy and lactation has not been established.

4.7 Effects on ability to drive and use machines

None stated.

4.8 Undesirable effects

Serum uric acid levels may rise during treatment with Frumil/Frumil LS and acute attacks of gout may be precipitated.

Malaise, dry mouth, gastric upset, nausea, vomiting, diarrhoea and constipation may occur.

If skin rashes or pruritus occur treatment should be withdrawn. Rare complications may include minor psychiatric disturbances, disturbances in liver function tests and ototoxicity. Bone marrow depression occasionally complicates treatment, necessitating withdrawal of the product. The haematopoietic state should be regularly monitored during treatment.

Hyponatraemia, hypochloraemia and raised blood urea nitrogen may occur during vigorous diuresis, especially in seriously ill patients. Careful monitoring of serum electrolytes and urea should therefore be undertaken in these patients. Hyperkalaemia has been observed in patients receiving amiloride hydrochloride.

As ACE inhibitors may elevate serum potassium levels, especially in the presence of renal impairment, combination with Frumil/Frumil LS is best avoided in elderly patients or in any others in whom renal function may be compromised. If use of the combination is deemed essential clinical condition and serum electrolytes must be continuously monitored.

Furosemidemay cause latent diabetes to become manifest. It may be necessary to increase the dose of hypoglycaemic agents in diabetic patients.

Patients with prostatic hypertrophy or impairment of micturition have an increased risk of developing acute urinary retention during diuretic therapy.

4.9 Overdose
Treatment of overdosage should be aimed at reversing dehydration and correcting electrolyte imbalance, particularly hyperkalaemia. Emesis should be induced or gastric lavage performed. Treatment should be symptomatic and supportive. If hyperkalaemia is seen, appropriate measures to reduce serum potassium must be instituted.

5. PHARMACOLOGICAL PROPERTIES

5.1 Pharmacodynamic properties

FUROSEMIDE:

Furosemide is a loop diuretic which acts primarily to inhibit electrolyte reabsorption in the thick ascending Loop of Henle. Excretion of sodium, potassium and chloride ions is increased and water excretion enhanced.

AMILORIDE:

Amiloride is a mild diuretic which moderately increases the excretion of sodium and chloride and reduces potassium excretion, and appears to act mainly on the distal renal tubules. It does not appear to act by inhibition of aldosterone and does not inhibit carbonic anhydrase. Amiloride adds to the natiuretic but diminishes the kaliuretic effect of other diuretics.

A combination of Furosemide and Amiloride is a diuretic which reduces the potassium loss of furosemidealone while avoiding the possible gastro-intestinal disturbances of potassium supplements.

5.2 Pharmacokinetic properties

FUROSEMIDE:

Approximately 65% of the dose is absorbed after oral administration. The plasma half-life is biphasic with a terminal elimination phase of about 1 ½ hours. Furosemideis up to 99% bound to plasma proteins and is mainly excreted in the urine, largely unchanged, but also excreted in the bile, non-renal elimination being considerably increased in renal failure. Furosemide crosses the placental barrier and is excreted in the milk.

AMILORIDE:

Approximately 50% of the dose is absorbed after oral administration and peak serum concentrations are achieved by about 3 - 4 hours. The serum half-life is estimated to be about 6 hours. Amiloride is not bound to plasma proteins. Amiloride is not metabolised and is excreted unchanged in the urine.

Pharmacokinetic studies have been completed on Frumil.

FUROSEMIDE	AMILORIDE
Cp MAX = 1/14 μg/ml SD = 0.67	Cp MAX = 13.42 ng/ml SD = 5.74
Tmax = 3.0 hours	Tmax = 4.0 hours
AUC = 3.17μg/ml hr SD = ± 1.25	AUC = 154 ng/ml hr SD = ± 65.2

5.3 Preclinical safety data
No further information available

6. PHARMACEUTICAL PARTICULARS

6.1 List of excipients
Frumil/Frumil LS tablets contain the following excipients:

Lactose

Starch Maize

Microcrystalline Cellulose

Sodium Starch Glycollate

Sunset Yellow Dye (E110)

French Chalk Powdered

Colloidal Anhydrous Silica

Magnesium Stearate

6.2 Incompatibilities
None stated.

6.3 Shelf life
The shelf-life of Frumil/Frumil LS is 3 years.

6.4 Special precautions for storage
Store below 25°C in a dry place. Protect from light.

6.5 Nature and contents of container
Blister packs of 28 and 56 tablets.

6.6 Instructions for use and handling
None

Administrative Data

7. MARKETING AUTHORISATION HOLDER
Helios Healthcare Limited

11A Ferraidy Street

Peyki-Attikis

Greece

8. MARKETING AUTHORISATION NUMBER(S)
Frumil: PL17076/0001

Frumil LS: PL17076/0002

9. DATE OF FIRST AUTHORISATION/RENEWAL OF THE AUTHORISATION
01 September 1998

10. DATE OF REVISION OF THE TEXT
November 2004

Legal Category:POM

Frusene Tablets

(Orion Pharma (UK) Limited)

1. NAME OF THE MEDICINAL PRODUCT
Frusene

2. QUALITATIVE AND QUANTITATIVE COMPOSITION
Furosemide 40.0mg

Triamterene 50.0mg

For excipients, refer to 6.1.

3. PHARMACEUTICAL FORM
Tablet.

Pale yellowish, convex, scored, uncoated tablet, diameter 9 mm.

4. CLINICAL PARTICULARS

4.1 Therapeutic indications
For the treatment of oedematous conditions, where a prompt diuresis is required and where potassium conservation is important: congestive heart failure, pulmonary oedema, cardiac oedema, hepatic oedema, and ascites.

A fixed ratio combination should only be used if titration with component drugs separately indicates that this product is appropriate.

4.2 Posology and method of administration
The dosage depends on individual requirements.

Tablets should be taken with a sufficient quantity of liquid, preferably one hour before food because concomitant intake of food can reduce the absorption of furosemide by 30%.

Adults:

The usual adult dose is ½ to 2 tablets, taken in the morning. Maximum daily dose is 6 tablets.

Children:

Not recommended for use in children.

Hepatic insufficiency:

Treatment must be initiated using a small dose with careful monitoring of the serum electrolyte concentrations (refer to section 4.4 Special warnings and precautions for use). The natriuretic potency of Furosemide may be weakened in patients with hepatic insufficiency but the kaliuretic potency usually remains. Elimination of triamterene is slowed down and its efficacy is increased in severe hepatic insufficiency.

4.3 Contraindications
Moderate or severe renal impairment (Creatinine Clearance < 25 ml/min). Hepatic coma and severe hepatic insufficiency. Anuria. Hyperkalaemia. Sodium depletion and accompanying hypovolemia.

Hypersensitivity to Furosemide, triamterene or to the excipients of the preparation. Hypersensitivity to sulphonamides (because of cross-sensitivity between sulphonamides and furosemide.

4.4 Special warnings and special precautions for use
Electrolyte balance of the patients receiving furosemide and triamterene must be monitored. More frequent and careful monitoring is required for the following patient groups: diabetics, patients with cardiac, renal or hepatic impairment and elderly patients. Of note, the risk of electrolyte disturbances can be increased even in mild renal failure. Hepatic failure and alcoholic cirrhosis particularly predispose to hypokalaemia and hypomagnesaemia. Refer to section 4.8 for details of electrolyte and metabolic abnormalities.

In elderly patients there is no requirement for dosage adjustments unless a clinically significant impairment of renal or hepatic function also exists. Creatinine and serum electrolytes should be monitored.

Diuretics must be administered carefully to avoid hypotension and circulatory collapse in patients with pulmonary oedema caused by acute myocardial infarction.

Daily weight loss should not exceed 1 kg daily to avoid relative intravascular dehydration; particular care is required in hepatic failure and ascites. Caution should also be exercised in the presence of liver disease as hepatic coma may be precipitated in susceptible cases.

Development of megaloblastic anaemia is possible in patients having folic acid deficiency (e.g. in hepatic cirrhosis). Triamterene may worsen this condition as it is a weak folic acid antagonist. In patients considered at risk, red cell folate levels should be measured and replacement given as appropriate.

Furosemide and, to a lesser extent, triamterene may predispose the patient to the development of hyperuricaemia and precipitate gout attacks (refer to section 4.8).

Acute diuresis may cause urinary retention in patients with urinary outflow obstruction (such as prostatic hyperplasia). Urinary output must be monitored in these patients.

Co-administration with nonsteriodal anti-inflammatory analgesics (NSAIDs) should be avoided wherever possible. Where this is not possible particularly careful monitoring is required to ensure that the diuretic effect is not attenuated (Refer to section 4.5)

Triamterene may cause blue discolouration of the urine.

4.5 Interaction with other medicinal products and other forms of Interaction
Triamterene reduces the risk of hypokalaemia induced by the use of furosemide. This is the rationale for using the two medications in a combination product.

Effect of drugs and other substances on Frusene

Drugs likely to increase the hypotensive effect:

ACE inhibitors, angiotensin receptor antagonists, beta-blockers, calcium-channel blockers, diuretics, nitrates, other antihypertensive drugs and other drugs such as dipyridamole, moxisylate, tizanidine, alprostadil.

Drugs likely to exacerbate hyponatraemia:

Diuretics, carbamazepine, aminoglutethamide, trimethoprim.

Drugs and other substances likely to exacerbate hypokalaemia

Thiazide and loop diuretics, corticosteroids, glycyrrhizin (contained in liquorice), amphotericin B.

Drugs and other substances likely to exacerbate hyperkalaemia:

Potassium salts or supplements, potassium-sparing diuretics (such as amiloride and spironolactone), ACE inhibitors, angiotensin receptor antagonists, ciclosporin, tacrolimus, trilostane and drosperinone.

Drugs and other substances likely to decrease the hypotensive and natriuretic effect:

Nonsteroidal anti-inflammatory analgesics (NSAIDs), probenecid, phenytoin, tobacco smoking. Cholestyramine and cholestipol prevent the absorption of Frusene, so they should be taken at different times, preferably 4 to 6 hours after Frusene administration.

Drugs likely to exacerbate nephrotoxicity:

Aminoglycoside and cephalosporin antibiotics, amphotericin B. Concomitant use of NSAIDs and Frusene increases the risk of acute renal failure (refer to section 4.4).

Drugs likely to exacerbate ototoxicity:

Aminoglycoside antibiotics, cisplatin.

Concomitant intake of food may reduce the absorption of furosemide by approximately 30%.

Effect of Frusene on other drugs

Frusene induced electrolyte disturbances (such as hypokalaemia) may predispose the patient to arrhythmogenic effect of other drugs (such as digoxin and drugs that prolong the QT interval). Effect of competitive muscle relaxants may also be reduced in hypokalaemia.

Frusene may reduce the elimination of lithium, phenobarbital, and amantadine causing toxic drug concentrations. Drug concentrations and/or signs of toxicity should be monitored in concomitant use and if Frusene is discontinued.

Frusene may reduce the efficacy of antihyperglycaemic medications. Adjustment of the dose of antihyperglycaemic medications may be needed in concomitant use.

Warfarin and clofibrate compete with Furosemide in the binding to serum albumin. This may have clinical significance in patients with low serum albumin levels (e.g. in nephrotic syndrome). Furosemide does not change the pharmacokinetics of warfarin to a significant extent, but the strong diuresis with associated dehydration may weaken the antithrombotic effect of warfarin.

4.6 Pregnancy and lactation
Furosemide crosses the placenta and has been shown to reduce placental circulation. It may predispose the foetus to hypercalciuria, nephrocalcinosis, and secondary hyperparathyroidism. Closure of the patent arterial duct can also be hindered after birth. Use of Furosemide in premature infants has led to development of sensorineural hearing

loss. Triamterene crosses the placenta, but has not been associated with causing birth defects.

Furosemide and triamterene are excreted in the breast milk in small quantities and Furosemide may impair lactation.

Frusene Tablets should be used during pregnancy or lactation only if clearly needed.

4.7 Effects on ability to drive and use machines
Occasionally Frusene may cause hypotension, especially at the start of therapy. This may manifest itself as dizziness or faintness. If affected, avoid driving or the use of machinery.

4.8 Undesirable effects
Of the adverse events caused by Furosemide and triamterene, most are linked to the pharmacological effects of the compounds, and they are more common in patients with multiple illnesses or compromised physical condition.

Furosemide:

(see Table 1)

Triamterene:

(see Table 2)

4.9 Overdose
Symptoms of overdose include increased diuresis, natriuresis, hypovolaemia, and decrease of blood pressure (refer to section 4.8 Undesirable effects). After an overdose, activated charcoal should be administered as soon as possible to decrease absorption of the drug. Fluid and electrolyte balance must be monitored. Sodium chloride-infusion can be used to sustain blood pressure. Otherwise, the treatment is symptomatic.

5. PHARMACOLOGICAL PROPERTIES

5.1 Pharmacodynamic properties
Furosemide:

Furosemide is a potent diuretic with a rapid action. Its effects are evident within 1 hour after a dose by mouth and lasts for about 4 to 6 hours. It has been reported to exert inhibiting effects on electrolyte reabsorption in the proximal and distal renal tubules and in the ascending Loop of Henle.

Excretion of sodium, potassium and chloride ions is increased and water excretion enhanced.

Unlike thiazide diuretics where, owing to their flat dose-response curve, very little is gained by increasing the dose, furosemide has a steep dose-response curve, which gives it a wide therapeutic range.

Triamterene:

Triamterene is a mild diuretic which appears to mainly act on the distal renal tubules. It produces a diuresis in about 2 to 4 hours, reaching a maximum effect in about 6 hours. Triamterene adds to the natriuretic but diminishes the kaliuretic affects of other diuretics and is used as an adjunct to furosemide to conserve potassium, in the treatment of refractory oedema associated with hepatic cirrhosis, congestive heart failure and the nephrotic syndrome.

5.2 Pharmacokinetic properties
Furosemide:

Furosemide is incompletely but fairly rapidly absorbed from the gastrointestinal tract. It has a biphasic half-life in the plasma with a terminal elimination phase that has been estimated to range up to about 1 ½ hours. It is up to 99% bound to plasma proteins and is mainly excreted in the urine, largely unchanged, but also in the form of the glucuronide and free amine metabolites. Variable amounts are also excreted in the bile, non renal elimination being considerably increased in renal failure. Furosemide crosses the placental barrier and is excreted in the breast milk.

Triamterene:

Triamterene is incompletely but fairly rapidly absorbed from the gastrointestinal tract. It has been estimated to have a plasma half-life of about 2 hours. It is extensively metabolised and is excreted in the urine in the form of metabolites with some unchanged triamterene. Variable amounts are also excreted in the bile. Animal studies have indicated that triamterene crosses the placental barrier and is excreted in the breast milk.

5.3 Preclinical safety data
None stated.

6. PHARMACEUTICAL PARTICULARS

6.1 List of excipients
Lactose monohydrate

Corn starch

Starch, pregelatinised

Polysorbate 80

Gelatin

Sodium starch glycolate

Magnesium stearate.

6.2 Incompatibilities
Not applicable.

6.3 Shelf life
5 years.

6.4 Special precautions for storage
Store below 30°C. Store in the original container.

Table 1

Blood and lymphatic system disorders	Rare or very rare (<1/1000, including case reports)	Bone marrow depression, aplastic anaemia, agranulocytosis, thrombocytopenia, haemolytic anaemia
Metabolism and nutrition disorders	Very common or common (> 1/100)	Dehydration*, hyponatraemia*, hypochloremic metabolic alkalosis*, hypokalaemia*, hypocalcaemia*, hypomagnesemia* (incidences of the last three are reduced by triamterene)
	Uncommon (> 1/1,000, < 1/100)	Impaired glucose tolerance (by hypokalaemia)*, hyperuricaemia, gout, reduction of serum HDL-cholesterol, elevation of serum LDL-cholesterol, elevation of serum triglycerides
Nervous system disorders	Uncommon (> 1/1,000, < 1/100)	Tiredness*, dizziness*, headache*, paresthesias*, restlessness*
Eye disorders	Uncommon (> 1/1,000, < 1/100)	Visual disturbance*
Ear and labyrinth disorders	Rare or very rare (< 1/1000, including case reports)	Tinnitus, reversible or irreversible loss of hearing (after large doses or prolonged use of Furosemide)
Cardiac disorders	Uncommon (> 1/1,000, < 1/100)	Cardiac arrhythmias*
Vascular disorders	Very common or common (> 1/100)	Decreased blood pressure*
	Uncommon (> 1/1,000, < 1/100)	Hypotension*, hypovolaemia
	Rare or very rare (< 1/1000, including case reports)	Vasculitis
Gastro-intestinal disorders	Uncommon (> 1/1,000, < 1/100)	Dry mouth*, thirst*, nausea*, bowel motility disturbances*
	Rare or very rare (< 1/1000, including case reports)	Pancreatitis
Hepato-biliary disorders	Rare or very rare (< 1/1,000, including case reports)	Cholestasis
Skin and subcutaneous tissue disorders	Rare or very rare (< 1/1,000, including case reports)	Urticaria, purpura, *erythema multiforme*, exfoliative dermatitis, photosensitivity reactions
Musculoskeletal, connective tissue and bone disorders	Uncommon (> 1/1,000, < 1/100)	Muscle cramps*
Renal and urinary disorders	Uncommon (> 1/1,000, < 1/100)	Reduced diuresis*, urinary incontinence, urinary obstruction (in patients with hyperplasia of the prostate)
	Rare or very rare (< 1/1000, including case reports)	Nephrocalcinosis (in pre-term infants treated with Furosemide), interstitial nephritis, acute renal failure
General disorders and administration site conditions	Uncommon (> 1/ 1,000, < 1/100)	Fatigue*
	Rare or very rare (1/1000, including case reports)	Fever

Table 2

Blood and lymphatic system disorders	Rare or very rare (< 1/1000, including case reports)	Megaloblastic anaemia, pancytopenia
Metabolism and nutrition disorders	Very common or common (> 1/100)	Hyperkalaemia (incidence is reduced by Furosemide)
	Uncommon (> 1/1,000, < 1/100)	Hyperuricaemia
Nervous system disorders	Uncommon (> 1/1,000, < 1/100)	Headache
Vascular disorders	Uncommon (> 1/1,000, < 1/100)	Hypovolaemia
Gastrointestinal disorders	Very common or common (> 1/100)	Nausea, vomiting, diarrhoea
	Uncommon (> 1/1,000, < 1/100)	Dry mouth
Skin and subcutaneous tissue disorders	Uncommon (> 1/1,000, < 1/100)	Rashes
	Rare or very rare (< 1/1000, including case reports)	Photosensitivity reactions, pseudoporphyria
Renal and urinary disorders	Uncommon (> 1/1,000, < 1/100)	Elevation of s-creatinine, transient renal insufficiency
	Rare or very rare (< 1/1000, including case reports)	Interstitial nephritis, urinary stones
General disorders and administration site conditions	Rare or very rare (< 1/1000, including case reports)	Serum sickness

6.5 Nature and contents of container
PVC-Al-foil blister strip, 14 or 56 tablets.

PE-bottle with LDPE snap cap, 28, 100, or 1000 tablets.

PE-bottle with HDPE screw cap, 100 tablets.

6.6 Instructions for use and handling
No special instructions.

7. MARKETING AUTHORISATION HOLDER
Orion Corporation
P.O. Box 65
02101 Espoo
Finland

8. MARKETING AUTHORISATION NUMBER(S)
PL 06043/0020

9. DATE OF FIRST AUTHORISATION/RENEWAL OF THE AUTHORISATION
20 December 1996

10. DATE OF REVISION OF THE TEXT
24th May 2004

Frusol 20mg/5ml

(Rosemont Pharmaceuticals Limited)

1. NAME OF THE MEDICINAL PRODUCT
Frusol 20mg/5ml
Furosemide Oral Solution 20mg/5ml

2. QUALITATIVE AND QUANTITATIVE COMPOSITION
Furosemide Ph.Eur 20mg/5ml

3. PHARMACEUTICAL FORM
Oral Solution

4. CLINICAL PARTICULARS

4.1 Therapeutic indications
Furosemide is indicated in all conditions requiring prompt diuresis, including cardiac, pulmonary, hepatic and renal oedema, peripheral oedema due to mechanical obstruction or venous insufficiency and hypertension.

It is also indicated for the maintenance therapy of mild oedema of any origin.

4.2 Posology and method of administration
This liquid should only be taken orally.

The medication should be administered in the morning to avoid nocturnal diuresis.

Adults: The usual initial daily dose is 40mg. This may be adjusted until an effective dose is achieved.

Children: 1 to 3mg/Kg body weight daily up to a maximum total dose of 40mg/day.

Elderly: In the elderly, Furosemide is generally eliminated more slowly. Dosage should be titrated until the required response is achieved.

4.3 Contraindications
Furosemide is contra-indicated in pre-comatose states associated with liver cirrhosis, anuria and electrolyte deficiency.

Contra-indicated in hypersensitivity to Furosemide, sulphonamides or any of the excipients listed.

4.4 Special warnings and special precautions for use
Patients with prostatic hypertrophy or impairment of micturition have an increased risk of developing acute retention. Caution is required in patients liable to electrolyte deficiency. Where indicated, steps should be taken to correct hypotension or hypovolaemia before commencing therapy.

Latent diabetes may become manifest or the insulin requirements of diabetic patients may increase.

Excipient Warnings
This product contains:

Ethanol 10%v/v (alcohol) – each dose contains up to 0.4g of alcohol.

It is harmful to those suffering from alcoholism. It should be taken into account in pregnant and lactating women, children and other high-risk groups (those suffering from liver disease, epilepsy, brain injury or disease). It may modify or increase the effect of other medicines.

Liquid maltitol – patients with a rare hereditary problem of fructose intolerance should not take this medicine.

Quinoline Yellow (E104) – can cause allergic-type reactions including asthma. The allergy is more common in people who are allergic to aspirin.

4.5 Interaction with other medicinal products and other forms of Interaction
The toxic effects of nephrotoxic antibiotics may be increased by concomitant administration of potent diuretics e.g. Furosemide

Serum lithium levels may be increased when Furosemide is given with lithium and therefore lithium levels should be monitored and adjusted when necessary.

A marked fall in blood pressure may occur when Furosemide is given with ACE inhibitors. The Furosemide dose should be reduced or stopped, and salt and water depletion corrected before commencing the ACE inhibitor therapy.

If cardiac glycosides or anti-hypertensives are concurrently administered with Furosemide their dosages may require adjustment.

Certain non-steroidal anti-inflammatory agents (e.g. indometacin, acetylsalicylic acid) may attenuate the action of Furosemide and may cause renal failure in cases of pre-existing hypovolaemia.

Furosemide may sometimes attenuate the effects of other drugs (e.g. antidiabetics and pressor amines) or it may potentiate effects of other drugs (e.g. salicylates, theophylline, lithium and curariform muscle relaxants.)

Interactions have been reported with ototoxic antibiotics leading to enhanced ototoxicity.

In cases of concomitant glucocorticoid therapy or abuse of laxatives, the risk of an increased potassium loss should be noted.

4.6 Pregnancy and lactation
Furosemide should be used with caution during pregnancy and whilst breast-feeding.

It is advisable that Furosemide should only be used in pregnancy if strictly indicated and for short term treatment.

Furosemide may inhibit lactation and may pass into breast milk and therefore it should be used with caution in nursing mothers.

4.7 Effects on ability to drive and use machines
Mental alertness may be reduced and the ability to drive or operate machinery may be impaired.

4.8 Undesirable effects
The side effects are generally minor and Furosemide is well tolerated.

General

Nausea, malaise, gastric upset

Haematological

Electrolytes and water balance may be disturbed as a result of diuresis after prolonged therapy. This may cause symptoms such as headache, hypotension or muscle cramps.

A transient rise in creatinine levels and urea levels has also been reported with Furosemide.

Serum cholesterol and triglyceride levels may rise during Furosemide treatment. During long term therapy they will usually return to normal within six months.

Bone marrow depression has been reported as a rare complication and necessitates withdrawal of treatment.

Pre-existing metabolic alkalosis (e.g. in decompensated cirrhosis of the liver) may be aggravated by Furosemide therapy

Organ Specific

Serum calcium levels may be reduced; in very rare cases tetany has been observed. Nephrocalcinosis has been reported in premature infants.

As with other sulphonamide-based diuretics, furosemide may bring about hyperuricaemia and, in rare cases, clinical gout may be precipitated.

Isolated cases of acute pancreatitis and jaundice have been reported after long term diuretic therapy.

Disorders of hearing after Furosemide are rare and in most cases reversible.

Allergic

The reports of allergic reactions such as skin rashes, photosensitivity, vasculitis or interstitial nephritis are low, but if they do occur the Furosemide treatment should be stopped.

4.9 Overdose
Overdosing may lead to dehydration and electrolyte depletion through excessive diuresis. Severe potassium loss may lead to serious cardiac arrhythmias.

Treatment of overdose consists of fluid replacement and electrolyte imbalance correction.

5. PHARMACOLOGICAL PROPERTIES

5.1 Pharmacodynamic properties
Pharmacotherapeutic group:

High-Ceiling Diuretic Sulfonamide - CO3C A 01

Furosemide is a potent loop diuretic which inhibits sodium and chloride reabsorption at the Loop of Henlé. The drug eliminates both positive and negative free water production. Furosemide acts at the luminal face of the epithelial cells by inhibiting co-transport mechanisms for the entry of sodium and chloride. Furosemide gains access to its site of action by being transported through the secretory pathway for organic acids in the proximal tubule. It reduces the renal excretion of uric acid. Furosemide causes an increased loss of potassium in the urine and also increases the excretion of ammonia by the kidney.

5.2 Pharmacokinetic properties
When oral doses of Furosemide are given to normal subjects the mean bioavailability of the drug is approximately 52% but the range is wide. In plasma, Furosemide is extensively bound to proteins mainly to albumin. The unbound fraction in plasma averages 2 - 4% at therapeutic concentrations. The volume of distribution ranges between 170 - 270ml/Kg. The half life of the β phase ranges from 45 - 60 min. The total plasma clearance is about 200ml/min. Renal excretion of unchanged drug and elimination by metabolism plus faecal excretion contribute almost equally to the total plasma clearance. Furosemide is in part cleared by the kidneys in the form of the glucuronide conjugate.

5.3 Preclinical safety data
Furosemide is a widely used diuretic which has been available for over thirty years and its safety profile in man is well established.

6. PHARMACEUTICAL PARTICULARS

6.1 List of excipients
Ethanol, sodium hydroxide (E524), quinoline yellow (E104), cherry flavour (containing propylene glycol), liquid maltitol (E965), disodium hydrogen phosphate (E339), citric acid monohydrate (E330) and purified water.

6.2 Incompatibilities
None known

6.3 Shelf life
24 months

3 months once open

6.4 Special precautions for storage
Store at or below 25°C.

6.5 Nature and contents of container
Bottles: Amber (Type III) glass

Closures: a) Aluminium, EPE wadded, Roll-On Pilfer Proof Closures (ROPP)

b) HDPE, EPE wadded, tamper evident

c) HDPE, EPE wadded, tamper evident, child resistant

Capacity:150ml, 200ml or 300ml.

6.6 Instructions for use and handling
Keep out of the reach of children.

Administrative Data

7. MARKETING AUTHORISATION HOLDER
Rosemont Pharmaceuticals Ltd, Yorkdale Industrial Park, Braithwaite Street, Leeds, LS11 9XE, UK

8. MARKETING AUTHORISATION NUMBER(S)
00427/0109

9. DATE OF FIRST AUTHORISATION/RENEWAL OF THE AUTHORISATION
6 April 1998

10. DATE OF REVISION OF THE TEXT
November 2003

Frusol 40mg/5ml

(Rosemont Pharmaceuticals Limited)

1. NAME OF THE MEDICINAL PRODUCT
Frusol 40mg/5ml

Furosemide Oral Solution 40mg/5ml

2. QUALITATIVE AND QUANTITATIVE COMPOSITION
Furosemide Ph.Eur 40mg/5ml

3. PHARMACEUTICAL FORM
Oral Solution

4. CLINICAL PARTICULARS

4.1 Therapeutic indications
Furosemide is indicated in all conditions requiring prompt diuresis, including cardiac, pulmonary, hepatic and renal oedema, peripheral oedema due to mechanical obstruction or venous insufficiency and hypertension.

It is also indicated for the maintenance therapy of mild oedema of any origin.

4.2 Posology and method of administration
This liquid should only be taken orally.

The medication should be administered in the morning to avoid nocturnal diuresis.

Adults: The usual initial daily dose is 40mg. This may be adjusted until an effective dose is achieved.

Children: 1 to 3mg/Kg body weight daily up to a maximum total dose of 40mg/day.

Elderly: In the elderly, Furosemide is generally eliminated more slowly. Dosage should be titrated until the required response is achieved.

4.3 Contraindications
Furosemide is contra-indicated in pre-comatose states associated with liver cirrhosis, anuria and electrolyte deficiency.

Contra-indicated in hypersensitivity to Furosemide, sulphonamides or any of the excipients listed

4.4 Special warnings and special precautions for use
Patients with prostatic hypertrophy or impairment of micturition have an increased risk of developing acute retention. Caution is required in patients liable to electrolyte deficiency. Where indicated, steps should be taken to correct hypotension or hypovolaemia before commencing therapy.

Latent diabetes may become manifest or the insulin requirements of diabetic patients may increase.

Excipient Warnings

This product contains:

Ethanol 10%v/v (alcohol) – each dose contains up to 0.4g of alcohol.

It is harmful to those suffering from alcoholism. It should be taken into account in pregnant and lactating women, children and other high-risk groups (those suffering from liver disease, epilepsy, brain injury or disease). It may modify or increase the effect of other medicines.

Liquid maltitol – patients with a rare hereditary problem of fructose intolerance should not take this medicine.

4.5 Interaction with other medicinal products and other forms of Interaction

The toxic effects of nephrotoxic antibiotics may be increased by concomitant administration of potent diuretics e.g. Furosemide

Serum lithium levels may be increased when Furosemide is given with lithium and therefore lithium levels should be monitored and adjusted when necessary.

A marked fall in blood pressure may occur when Furosemide is given with ACE inhibitors. The Furosemide dose should be reduced or stopped, and salt and water depletion corrected before commencing the ACE inhibitor therapy.

If cardiac glycosides or anti-hypertensives are concurrently administered with furosemide their dosages may require adjustment.

Certain non-steroidal anti-inflammatory agents (e.g. indometacin, acetylsalicylic acid) may attenuate the action of Furosemide and may cause renal failure in cases of pre-existing hypovolaemia.

Furosemide may sometimes attenuate the effects of other drugs (e.g. antidiabetics and pressor amines) or it may potentiate effects of other drugs (e.g. salicylates, theophylline, lithium and curariform muscle relaxants.)

Interactions have been reported with ototoxic antibiotics leading to enhanced ototoxicity.

In cases of concomitant glucocorticoid therapy or abuse of laxatives, the risk of an increased potassium loss should be noted.

4.6 Pregnancy and lactation

Furosemide should be used with caution during pregnancy and whilst breast-feeding.

It is advisable that Furosemide should only be used in pregnancy if strictly indicated and for short term treatment.

Furosemide may inhibit lactation and may pass into breast milk and therefore it should be used with caution in nursing mothers.

4.7 Effects on ability to drive and use machines

Mental alertness may be reduced and the ability to drive or operate machinery may be impaired.

4.8 Undesirable effects

The side effects are generally minor and Furosemide is well tolerated.

General

Nausea, malaise, gastric upset

Haematological

Electrolytes and water balance may be disturbed as a result of diuresis after prolonged therapy. This may cause symptoms such as headache, hypotension or muscle cramps.

A transient rise in creatinine levels and urea levels has also been reported with furosemide.

Serum cholesterol and triglyceride levels may rise during Furosemide treatment. During long term therapy they will usually return to normal within six months.

Bone marrow depression has been reported as a rare complication and necessitates withdrawal of treatment.

Pre-existing metabolic alkalosis (e.g. in decompensated cirrhosis of the liver) may be aggravated by Furosemide therapy.

Organ Specific

Serum calcium levels may be reduced; in very rare cases tetany has been observed. Nephrocalcinosis has been reported in premature infants.

As with other sulphonamide-based diuretics, Furosemide may bring about hyperuricaemia and, in rare cases, clinical gout may be precipitated.

Isolated cases of acute pancreatitis and jaundice have been reported after long term diuretic therapy.

Disorders of hearing after furosemide are rare and in most cases reversible.

Allergic

The reports of allergic reactions such as skin rashes, photosensitivity, vasculitis or interstitial nephritis are low, but if they do occur the Furosemide treatment should be stopped.

4.9 Overdose

Overdosing may lead to dehydration and electrolyte depletion through excessive diuresis. Severe potassium loss may lead to serious cardiac arrhythmias.

Treatment of overdose consists of fluid replacement and electrolyte imbalance correction.

5. PHARMACOLOGICAL PROPERTIES

5.1 Pharmacodynamic properties

Pharmacotherapeutic group:

High-Ceiling Diuretic Sulfonamide - CO3C A 01

Furosemide is a potent loop diuretic which inhibits sodium and chloride reabsorption at the Loop of Henlé. The drug eliminates both positive and negative free water production. Furosemide acts at the luminal face of the epithelial cells by inhibiting co-transport mechanisms for the entry of sodium and chloride. Furosemide gains access to its site of action by being transported through the secretory pathway for organic acids in the proximal tubule. It reduces the renal excretion of uric acid. Furosemide causes an increased loss of potassium in the urine and also increases the excretion of ammonia by the kidney.

5.2 Pharmacokinetic properties

When oral doses of Furosemide are given to normal subjects the mean bioavailability of the drug is approximately 52% but the range is wide. In plasma, Furosemide is extensively bound to proteins mainly to albumin. The unbound fraction in plasma averages 2 - 4% at therapeutic concentrations. The volume of distribution ranges between 170 - 270ml/Kg. The half life of the β phase ranges from 45 - 60 min. The total plasma clearance is about 200ml/min. Renal excretion of unchanged drug and elimination by metabolism plus faecal excretion contribute almost equally to the total plasma clearance. Furosemide is in part cleared by the kidneys in the form of the glucuronide conjugate.

5.3 Preclinical safety data

Furosemide is a widely used diuretic which has been available for over thirty years and its safety profile in man is well established.

6. PHARMACEUTICAL PARTICULARS

6.1 List of excipients

Ethanol, sodium hydroxide (E524), cherry flavour (containing propylene glycol), liquid maltitol (E965), disodium hydrogen phosphate (E339), citric acid monohydrate (E330) and purified water.

6.2 Incompatibilities

None known

6.3 Shelf life

24 months

3 months after opening

6.4 Special precautions for storage

Store at or below 25°C.

6.5 Nature and contents of container

Bottles: Amber (Type III) glass

Closures: a) Aluminium, EPE wadded, Roll-On Pilfer Proof Closures (ROPP)

b) HDPE, EPE wadded, tamper evident

c) HDPE, EPE wadded, tamper evident, child resistant

Capacity:150ml, 200ml or 300ml.

6.6 Instructions for use and handling

Keep out of the reach of children.

Administrative Data

7. MARKETING AUTHORISATION HOLDER

Rosemont Pharmaceuticals Ltd, Yorkdale Industrial Park, Braithwaite Street, Leeds, LS11 9XE, UK

8. MARKETING AUTHORISATION NUMBER(S)

00427/0110

9. DATE OF FIRST AUTHORISATION/RENEWAL OF THE AUTHORISATION

6 April 1998

10. DATE OF REVISION OF THE TEXT

November 2003

Frusol 50mg/5ml

(Rosemont Pharmaceuticals Limited)

1. NAME OF THE MEDICINAL PRODUCT

Frusol 50mg/5ml

Furosemide Oral Solution 50mg/5ml

2. QUALITATIVE AND QUANTITATIVE COMPOSITION

Furosemide Ph.Eur 50mg/5ml

3. PHARMACEUTICAL FORM

Oral Solution

4. CLINICAL PARTICULARS

4.1 Therapeutic indications

Furosemide is indicated in all conditions requiring prompt diuresis, including cardiac, pulmonary, hepatic and renal oedema, peripheral oedema due to mechanical obstruction or venous insufficiency and hypertension.

It is also indicated for the maintenance therapy of mild oedema of any origin.

4.2 Posology and method of administration

This liquid should only be taken orally.

The medication should be administered in the morning to avoid nocturnal diuresis.

Adults: The usual initial daily dose is 40mg. This may be adjusted until an effective dose is achieved.

Children: 1 to 3mg/Kg body weight daily up to a maximum total dose of 40mg/day.

Elderly: In the elderly, Furosemide is generally eliminated more slowly. Dosage should be titrated until the required response is achieved.

4.3 Contraindications

Furosemide is contra-indicated in pre-comatose states associated with liver cirrhosis, anuria and electrolyte deficiency.

Contra-indicated in hypersensitivity to Furosemide, sulphonamides or any of the excipients listed

4.4 Special warnings and special precautions for use

Patients with prostatic hypertrophy or impairment of micturition have an increased risk of developing acute retention. Caution is required in patients liable to electrolyte deficiency. Where indicated, steps should be taken to correct hypotension or hypovolaemia before commencing therapy.

Latent diabetes may become manifest or the insulin requirements of diabetic patients may increase.

Excipient Warnings

This product contains:

Ethanol 10%v/v (alcohol) – each dose contains up to 0.4g of alcohol.

It is harmful to those suffering from alcoholism. It should be taken into account in pregnant and lactating women, children and other high-risk groups (those suffering from liver disease, epilepsy, brain injury or disease). It may modify or increase the effect of other medicines.

Liquid maltitol – patients with a rare hereditary problem of fructose intolerance should not take this medicine.

4.5 Interaction with other medicinal products and other forms of Interaction

The toxic effects of nephrotoxic antibiotics may be increased by concomitant administration of potent diuretics e.g. Furosemide

Serum lithium levels may be increased when Furosemide is given with lithium and therefore lithium levels should be monitored and adjusted when necessary.

A marked fall in blood pressure may occur when Furosemide is given with ACE inhibitors. The Furosemide dose should be reduced or stopped, and salt and water depletion corrected before commencing the ACE inhibitor therapy.

If cardiac glycosides or anti-hypertensives are concurrently administered with furosemide their dosages may require adjustment.

Certain non-steroidal anti-inflammatory agents (e.g. indometacin, acetylsalicylic acid) may attenuate the action of Furosemide and may cause renal failure in cases of pre-existing hypovolaemia.

Furosemide may sometimes attenuate the effects of other drugs (e.g. antidiabetics and pressor amines) or it may potentiate effects of other drugs (e.g. salicylates, theophylline, lithium and curariform muscle relaxants.)

Interactions have been reported with ototoxic antibiotics leading to enhanced ototoxicity.

In cases of concomitant glucocorticoid therapy or abuse of laxatives, the risk of an increased potassium loss should be noted.

4.6 Pregnancy and lactation

Furosemide should be used with caution during pregnancy and whilst breast-feeding.

It is advisable that Furosemide should only be used in pregnancy if strictly indicated and for short term treatment.

Furosemide may inhibit lactation and may pass into breast milk and therefore it should be used with caution in nursing mothers.

4.7 Effects on ability to drive and use machines

Mental alertness may be reduced and the ability to drive or operate machinery may be impaired.

4.8 Undesirable effects

The side effects are generally minor and furosemide is well tolerated.

General

Nausea, malaise, gastric upset

Haematological

Electrolytes and water balance may be disturbed as a result of diuresis after prolonged therapy. This may cause symptoms such as headache, hypotension or muscle cramps.

A transient rise in creatinine levels and urea levels has also been reported with furosemide.

Serum cholesterol and triglyceride levels may rise during Furosemide treatment. During long term therapy they will usually return to normal within six months.

Bone marrow depression has been reported as a rare complication and necessitates withdrawal of treatment.

Pre-existing metabolic alkalosis (e.g. in decompensated cirrhosis of the liver) may be aggravated by Furosemide therapy.

Organ Specific

Serum calcium levels may be reduced; in very rare cases tetany has been observed. Nephrocalcinosis has been reported in premature infants.

As with other sulphonamide-based diuretics, Furosemide may bring about hyperuricaemia and, in rare cases, clinical gout may be precipitated.

Isolated cases of acute pancreatitis and jaundice have been reported after long term diuretic therapy.

Disorders of hearing after Furosemide are rare and in most cases reversible.

Allergic

The reports of allergic reactions such as skin rashes, photosensitivity, vasculitis or interstitial nephritis are low, but if they do occur the Furosemide treatment should be stopped.

4.9 Overdose

Overdosing may lead to dehydration and electrolyte depletion through excessive diuresis. Severe potassium loss may lead to serious cardiac arrhythmias.

Treatment of overdose consists of fluid replacement and electrolyte imbalance correction.

5. PHARMACOLOGICAL PROPERTIES

5.1 Pharmacodynamic properties

Pharmacotherapeutic group:

High-Ceiling Diuretic Sulfonamide - CO3C A 01

Furosemide is a potent loop diuretic which inhibits sodium and chloride reabsorption at the Loop of Henlé. The drug eliminates both positive and negative free water production. Furosemide acts at the luminal face of the epithelial cells by inhibiting co-transport mechanisms for the entry of sodium and chloride. Furosemide gains access to its site of action by being transported through the secretory pathway for organic acids in the proximal tubule. It reduces the renal excretion of uric acid. Furosemide causes an increased loss of potassium in the urine and also increases the excretion of ammonia by the kidney.

5.2 Pharmacokinetic properties

When oral doses of Furosemide are given to normal subjects the mean bioavailability of the drug is approximately 52% but the range is wide. In plasma, Furosemide is extensively bound to proteins mainly to albumin. The unbound fraction in plasma averages 2 - 4% at therapeutic concentrations. The volume of distribution ranges between 170 - 270ml/Kg. The half life of the β phase ranges from 45 - 60 min. The total plasma clearance is about 200ml/min. Renal excretion of unchanged drug and elimination by metabolism plus faecal excretion contribute almost equally to the total plasma clearance. Furosemide is in part cleared by the kidneys in the form of the glucuronide conjugate.

5.3 Preclinical safety data

Furosemide is a widely used diuretic which has been available for over thirty years and its safety profile in man is well established.

6. PHARMACEUTICAL PARTICULARS

6.1 List of excipients

Ethanol, sodium hydroxide (E524), cherry flavour (containing propylene glycol), liquid maltitol (E965), disodium hydrogen phosphate (E339), citric acid monohydrate (E330) and purified water.

6.2 Incompatibilities

None known

6.3 Shelf life

24 months

3 months after opening

6.4 Special precautions for storage

Store at or below 25°C.

6.5 Nature and contents of container

Bottles: Amber (Type III) glass

Closures: a) Aluminium, EPE wadded, Roll-On Pilfer Proof Closures (ROPP)

b) HDPE, EPE wadded, tamper evident

c) HDPE, EPE wadded, tamper evident, child resistant

Capacity:150ml, 200ml or 300ml.

6.6 Instructions for use and handling

Keep out of the reach of children.

Administrative Data

7. MARKETING AUTHORISATION HOLDER

Rosemont Pharmaceuticals Ltd, Yorkdale Industrial Park, Braithwaite Street, Leeds, LS11 9XE, UK

8. MARKETING AUTHORISATION NUMBER(S)

00427/0111

9. DATE OF FIRST AUTHORISATION/RENEWAL OF THE AUTHORISATION

6 April 1998

10. DATE OF REVISION OF THE TEXT

November 2003

FuciBET Cream

(Leo Laboratories Limited)

1. NAME OF THE MEDICINAL PRODUCT

Fucibet® cream

2. QUALITATIVE AND QUANTITATIVE COMPOSITION

Fucibet® cream contains Fusidic acid Ph.Eur. 2% and Betamethasone 0.1% (as the valerate ester Ph.Eur)

3. PHARMACEUTICAL FORM

Cream for topical administration

4. CLINICAL PARTICULARS

4.1 Therapeutic indications

Fucibet® cream is indicated for the treatment of eczematous dermatoses including atopic eczema, infantile eczema, discoid eczema, stasis eczema, contact eczema and seborrhoeic eczema when secondary bacterial infection is confirmed or suspected.

4.2 Posology and method of administration

A small quantity should be applied to the affected area twice daily until a satisfactory response is obtained. A single treatment course should not normally exceed 2 weeks. In the more resistant lesions the effect of Fucibet® cream can be enhanced by occlusion with polythene film. Overnight occlusion is usually adequate.

4.3 Contraindications

Acne rosacea and perioral dermatitis. Skin lesions of viral, fungal or bacterial origin. Hypersensitivity to the preparation.

4.4 Special warnings and special precautions for use

Long-term continuous topical therapy should be avoided, particularly in infants and children. Adrenal suppression can occur even without occlusion. Atrophic changes may occur on the face and to a lesser degree in other parts of the body, after prolonged treatment with potent topical steroids. Caution should be exercised if Fucibet® cream is used near the eye. Glaucoma might result if the preparation enters the eye. Systemic chemotherapy is required if bacterial infection persists.

Bacterial resistance has been reported to occur with the use of fusidic acid applied topically. As with all topical antibiotics, extended or recurrent application may increase the risk of contact sensitisation and the development of antibiotic resistance.

Steroid-antibiotic combinations should not be continued for more than 7 days in the absence of any clinical improvement since in this situation occult extension of the infection may occur due to the masking of the steroid. Similarly, steroids may also mask hypersensitivity reactions.

4.5 Interaction with other medicinal products and other forms of Interaction

None known

4.6 Pregnancy and lactation

Topical administration of any corticosteroid to pregnant animals can cause abnormalities of foetal development. The relevance of this finding to human beings has not been established; however, topical steroids should not be used extensively in pregnancy, i.e. in large amounts or for prolonged periods.

4.7 Effects on ability to drive and use machines

Not applicable

4.8 Undesirable effects

Prolonged and intensive treatment with potent corticosteroids may cause local atrophic changes in the skin, including striae, thinning and dilation of superficial blood vessels, particularly when applied to the flexures or when occlusion is employed. As with other topical corticosteroids sufficient systemic absorption to produce hypercorticism can occur with prolonged or extensive use. Infants and children are at particular risk, more so if occlusive dressings are used. A napkin may act as an occlusive dressing in infants. Hypersensitivity reactions to fusidic acid are rare and Fucibet® cream does not contain lanolin. However, if signs of hypersensitivity occur, treatment should be withdrawn.

4.9 Overdose

Not applicable

5. PHARMACOLOGICAL PROPERTIES

5.1 Pharmacodynamic properties

Fucibet® cream combines the well-known anti-inflammatory and antipruritic effects of betamethasone with the potent topical antibacterial action of fusidic acid. Betamethasone valerate is a topical steroid rapidly effective in those inflammatory dermatoses which normally respond to this form of therapy. More refractory conditions can often be treated successfully. When applied topically, fusidic acid is effective against *Staphyloccus aureus,* Streptococci, Corynebacteria, Neisseria and certain Clostridia and Bacteroides. Concentrations of 0.03 to 0.12 microgram per ml inhibit nearly all strains of *S. aureus*. The antibacterial activity of fusidic acid is not diminished in the presence of betamethasone.

5.2 Pharmacokinetic properties

There are no data which define the pharmacokinetics of Fucibet® cream, following topical administration in man.

However, *in vitro* studies show that fusidic acid can penetrate intact human skin. The degree of penetration depends on factors such as the duration of exposure to fusidic acid and the condition of the skin. Fusidic acid is excreted mainly in the bile with little excreted in the urine.

Betamethasone is absorbed following topical administration. The degree of absorption is dependent on various factors including skin condition and site of application. Betamethasone is metabolised largely in the liver but also to a limited extent in the kidneys, and the inactive metabolites are excreted with the urine.

5.3 Preclinical safety data

There are no pre-clinical data of relevance to the prescriber which are additional to that already included in other sections of the SPC.

6. PHARMACEUTICAL PARTICULARS

6.1 List of excipients

Macrogol cetostearyl ether, cetostearyl alcohol, chlorocresol, liquid paraffin, sodium dihydrogen phosphate, white soft paraffin, purified water, sodium hydroxide.

6.2 Incompatibilities

Not applicable

6.3 Shelf life

3 years

6.4 Special precautions for storage

Nil

6.5 Nature and contents of container

Aluminium tube of 30 gram and 60 gram.

6.6 Instructions for use and handling

None

7. MARKETING AUTHORISATION HOLDER

LEO Laboratories Limited

Princes Risborough

Bucks

HP27 9RR

8. MARKETING AUTHORISATION NUMBER(S)

PL 0043/0091

9. DATE OF FIRST AUTHORISATION/RENEWAL OF THE AUTHORISATION

27.10.83

10. DATE OF REVISION OF THE TEXT

March 2005

11. Legal Category

POM

Fucidin Cream

(Leo Laboratories Limited)

1. NAME OF THE MEDICINAL PRODUCT

Fucidin® Cream

2. QUALITATIVE AND QUANTITATIVE COMPOSITION

Fucidin Cream contains fusidic acid Ph.Eur. 2%.

3. PHARMACEUTICAL FORM

Cream for topical administration

4. CLINICAL PARTICULARS

4.1 Therapeutic indications

Indicated either alone or in combination with systemic therapy, in the treatment of primary and secondary skin infections caused by sensitive strains of *Staphylococcus aureus,* Streptococcus spp and *Corynebacterium minutissimum*. Primary skin infections that may be expected to respond to treatment with fusidic acid applied topically include: impetigo contagiosa, superficial folliculitis, sycosis barbae, paronychia and erythrasma; also such secondary skin infections as infected eczematoid dermatitis, infected contact dermatitis and infected cuts / abrasions.

4.2 Posology and method of administration

Adults and Children:

Uncovered lesions - apply gently three or four times daily.

Covered lesions - less frequent applications may be adequate.

4.3 Contraindications

Infection caused by non-susceptible organisms, in particular, Pseudomonas aeruginosa.

Fucidin Cream is contraindicated in patients with hypersensitivity to fusidic acid and its salts.

4.4 Special warnings and special precautions for use

Bacterial resistance has been reported to occur with the use of fusidic acid applied topically. As with all topical antibiotics, extended or recurrent application may increase the risk of contact sensitisation and the development of antibiotic resistance.

Fusidic acid does not appear to cause conjunctival irritation in experimental animals. Caution should still be exercised, however, when Fucidin Cream is used near the eyes.

4.5 Interaction with other medicinal products and other forms of Interaction
Not applicable.

4.6 Pregnancy and lactation
There is inadequate evidence of safety in human pregnancy. Animal studies and many years of clinical experience have suggested that fusidic acid is devoid of teratogenic effect. There is evidence to suggest that when given systemically, fusidic acid can penetrate the placental barrier. The use of topical Fucidin in pregnancy requires that the potential benefits be weighed against the possible hazards to the foetus.

Safety in nursing mothers has not been established. When fusidic acid (as the sodium salt) has been given systemically, levels have been detected in breast milk, but with topical use the possible amount of drug present is unlikely to affect the infant.

4.7 Effects on ability to drive and use machines
Not applicable

4.8 Undesirable effects
Hypersensitivity reactions to the active ingredient in the form of skin rashes; mild stinging and irritation on application have been reported rarely.

4.9 Overdose
Not applicable

5. PHARMACOLOGICAL PROPERTIES

5.1 Pharmacodynamic properties
Fusidic acid is a potent antibacterial agent. Fusidic acid and its salts show fat and water solubility and strong surface activity and exhibit unusual ability to penetrate intact skin. Concentrations of 0.03 - 0.12 mcg fusidic acid per ml inhibit nearly all strains of *Staphylococcus aureus.* Topical application of fusidic acid is also effective against streptococci, corynebacteria, neisseria and certain clostridia.

5.2 Pharmacokinetic properties
In Vitro studies show that fusidic acid can penetrate intact human skin. The degree of penetration depends on factors such as the duration of exposure to fusidic acid and the condition of the skin. Fusidic acid is excreted mainly in the bile with little excreted in the urine.

5.3 Preclinical safety data
There are no pre-clinical data of relevance to the prescribe which are additional to that already included in other sections of the SPC.

6. PHARMACEUTICAL PARTICULARS

6.1 List of excipients
Butylated hydroxyanisole, cetanol, glycerol, liquid paraffin, potassium sorbate, Tween 60, white soft paraffin, purified water.

6.2 Incompatibilities
Not applicable

6.3 Shelf life
3 years

6.4 Special precautions for storage
Nil

6.5 Nature and contents of container
Aluminium tubes of 15 gram and 30 gram.

6.6 Instructions for use and handling
None

7. MARKETING AUTHORISATION HOLDER
Leo Laboratories Limited

Princes Risborough

Bucks

HP27 9RR

8. MARKETING AUTHORISATION NUMBER(S)
PL 0043/0065

9. DATE OF FIRST AUTHORISATION/RENEWAL OF THE AUTHORISATION
14 August 1979.

10. DATE OF REVISION OF THE TEXT
June 1999

11. Legal Category
POM

Fucidin H Cream

(Leo Laboratories Limited)

1. NAME OF THE MEDICINAL PRODUCT
Fucidin® H Cream

2. QUALITATIVE AND QUANTITATIVE COMPOSITION
Fucidin H Cream contains Fusidic acid Ph.Eur.2% and Hydrocortisone acetate Ph.Eur.1%.

3. PHARMACEUTICAL FORM
Cream for topical administration

4. CLINICAL PARTICULARS

4.1 Therapeutic indications
Fucidin H Cream is indicated in eczema and dermatitis with secondary bacterial infections, including atopic eczema, primary irritant dermatitis and allergic and seborrhoeic dermatitis where the organisms responsible are known to be or believed to be sensitive to fusidic acid.

4.2 Posology and method of administration
Adults and Children:

Uncovered lesions - apply gently three or four times daily.

Covered lesions - less frequent applications may be adequate.

4.3 Contraindications
As with other topical corticosteroid preparations, Fucidin H Cream is contraindicated in primary bacterial, viral and fungal skin infections.

Fucidin H Cream is contraindicated in patients with hypersensitivity to fusidic acid and its salts.

4.4 Special warnings and special precautions for use
Bacterial resistance has been reported to occur with the use of fusidic acid applied topically. As with all topical antibiotics, extended or recurrent application may increase the risk of contact sensitisation and the development of antibiotic resistance.

Fusidic acid does not appear to cause conjunctival irritation in experimental animals. Caution should still be exercised, however, when Fucidin H Cream is used near the eyes.

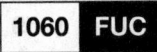

In infants, long-term continuous topical therapy with corticosteroids should be avoided. Adrenal suppression can occur even without occlusion.

4.5 Interaction with other medicinal products and other forms of Interaction
Steroid-antibiotic combinations should not be continued for more than 7 days in the absence of any clinical improvement since in this situation occult extension of the infection may occur due to the masking of the steroid. Similarly, steroids may also mask hypersensitivity reactions.

4.6 Pregnancy and lactation
There is inadequate evidence of safety in human pregnancy. Topical administration of corticosteroids to pregnant animals can cause abnormalities of foetal development including cleft palate and intra-uterine growth retardation. There may, therefore, be a very small risk of such effects in the human foetus.

Animal studies and many years of clinical experience have suggested that fusidic acid is devoid of teratogenic effect. There is evidence to suggest that when given systemically, fusidic acid can penetrate the placental barrier. The use of topical Fucidin in pregnancy requires that the potential benefits be weighed against the possible hazards to the foetus.

Safety in nursing mothers has not been established.

When fusidic acid (as the sodium salt) has been given systemically, levels have been detected in breast milk, but with topical use the possible amount of drug present is unlikely to affect the infant.

4.7 Effects on ability to drive and use machines
Not applicable

4.8 Undesirable effects
Hypersensitivity reactions to the active ingredient in the form of skin rashes; mild stinging and irritation on application have been reported rarely.

4.9 Overdose
Not applicable

5. PHARMACOLOGICAL PROPERTIES

5.1 Pharmacodynamic properties
Fucidin H Cream combines the potent topical antibacterial action of fusidic acid with the anti-inflammatory and antipruritic effects of hydrocortisone. Concentrations of 0.03 - 0.12 mcg fusidic acid per ml inhibit nearly all strains of *Staphylococcus aureus.* Topical application of fusidic acid is also effective against streptococci, corynebacteria, neisseria and certain clostridia.

5.2 Pharmacokinetic properties
There are no data which define the pharmacokinetics of Fucidin H Cream, following topical administration in man.

However, in Vitro studies show that fusidic acid can penetrate intact human skin. The degree of penetration depends on factors such as the duration of exposure to fusidic acid and the condition of the skin. Fusidic acid is excreted mainly in the bile with little excreted in the urine.

Hydrocortisone is absorbed following topical administration. The degree of absorption is dependent on various factors including skin condition and site of application. Absorbed hydrocortisone is extensively metabolised and rapidly eliminated in the urine.

5.3 Preclinical safety data
There are no pre-clinical data of relevance to the prescribe which are additional to that already included in other sections of the SPC.

6. PHARMACEUTICAL PARTICULARS

6.1 List of excipients
Butylated hydroxyanisole, cetanol, glycerol, liquid paraffin, potassium sorbate, Tween 60, white soft paraffin, deionised water.

6.2 Incompatibilities
Not applicable

6.3 Shelf life
3 years

6.4 Special precautions for storage
Nil

6.5 Nature and contents of container
Aluminium tube of 30 gram and 60 gram.

6.6 Instructions for use and handling
None

7. MARKETING AUTHORISATION HOLDER
Leo Laboratories Limited

Princes Risborough

Bucks

HP27 9RR

8. MARKETING AUTHORISATION NUMBER(S)
PL 0043/0093

9. DATE OF FIRST AUTHORISATION/RENEWAL OF THE AUTHORISATION
1 November 1983/26 May 1994.

10. DATE OF REVISION OF THE TEXT
May 2000

LEGAL CATEGORY
POM

Fucidin H Ointment

(Leo Laboratories Limited)

1. NAME OF THE MEDICINAL PRODUCT
Fucidin® H Ointment

2. QUALITATIVE AND QUANTITATIVE COMPOSITION
Fucidin® H Ointment contains Sodium Fusidate Ph. Eur. 2% and Hydrocortisone Acetate Ph.Eur. 1%.

3. PHARMACEUTICAL FORM
Ointment for topical administration.

4. CLINICAL PARTICULARS

4.1 Therapeutic indications
Fucidin® H Ointment is indicated in eczema and dermatitis with secondary bacterial infections, including atopic eczema, primary irritant dermatitis and allergic and seborrhoeic dermatitis where the organisms responsible are known to be or believed to be sensitive to fusidic acid.

4.2 Posology and method of administration
Adults and Children: Uncovered lesions - apply gently three or four times daily.

Covered lesions - less frequent applications may be adequate.

4.3 Contraindications
Hypersensitivity to fusidic acid and its salts. As with other topical corticosteroid preparations, Fucidin® H Ointment is contra-indicated in primary bacterial, viral and fungal skin infections, skin manifestations in relation to tuberculosis or syphilis, perioral dermatitis and rosacea.

4.4 Special warnings and special precautions for use
Fucidin® H Ointment should not be used in or near the eye as sodium fusidate causes conjunctival irritation.

Bacterial resistance has been reported to occur with the use of fusidic acid applied topically. As with all topical antibiotics, extended or recurrent application may increase the risk of contact sensitisation and the development of antibiotic resistance.

Steroid-antibiotic combinations should not be continued for more than 7 days in the absence of any clinical improvement since in this situation occult extension of the infection may occur due to the masking of the steroid. Similarly, steroids may also mask hypersensitivity reactions.

As Fucidin® H Ointment contains a corticosteroid it is not recommended in the following conditions: atrophic skin, cutaneous ulcer, acne vulgaris, fragile skin veins and perianal and genital pruritus. Contact with open wounds and mucous membranes should be avoided. As with all corticosteroids, prolonged use on the face should be avoided.

In infants and children, long-term continuous topical therapy with corticosteroids should be avoided. Adrenal suppression can occur even without occlusion.

4.5 Interaction with other medicinal products and other forms of Interaction
None known.

4.6 Pregnancy and lactation
There is inadequate evidence of safety in human pregnancy. Topical administration of corticosteroids to pregnant animals can cause abnormalities of foetal development including cleft palate and intra-uterine

growth retardation. There may, therefore, be a very small risk of such effects in the human foetus. Animal studies and many years of clinical experience have suggested that fusidic acid is devoid of teratogenic effect. There is evidence to suggest that when given systemically, fusidic acid can penetrate the placental barrier. The use of topical Fucidin® in pregnancy requires that the potential benefits be weighed against the possible hazards to the foetus.

Safety in nursing mothers has not been established.

When fusidic acid (as the sodium salt) has been given systemically, levels have been detected in breast milk, but with topical use the possible amount of drug present is unlikely to affect the infant.

4.7 Effects on ability to drive and use machines

Not known.

4.8 Undesirable effects

Very common > 1/10

Common > 1/100 and < 1/10

Uncommon > 1/1,000 and < 1/100

Rare > 1/10,000 and < 1/1,000

Very rare < 1/10,000

The most frequently reported undesirable effects on Fucidin® H are various symptoms of application site irritation. Allergic reactions have been reported.

Based on clinical data for Fucidin® H approximately 5% of patients can be expected to experience an undesirable effect. Pruritus, skin irritation, skin rash, worsening of eczema, transient stinging and burning sensation were uncommon.

Although it has not been observed in the clinical studies for Fucidin® H, topical use of steroids may result in skin atrophy, telangiectasia or skin striae, especially during prolonged application.

As with all other corticosteroids folliculitis, hypertrichosis, perioral dermatitis, allergic contact dermatitis, depigmentation and systemic activity, although rare, may occur.

Based on post-marketing data the total 'reporting rate' of undesirable effect is very rare being approximately 1:1,000,000 treatment courses.

The undesirable effects are listed by MedDRA SOC and the individual undesirable effects are listed starting with the most frequently reported.

• **Skin and subcutaneous tissue disorders**

Pruritus

Skin irritation

Skin burning sensation

Skin stinging sensation

Rash

Eczema aggravated

• **Immune system disorders**

Allergic reaction

4.9 Overdose

Acute overdosage is very unlikely to occur. However, chronic overdosage or misuse may result in increased risk of topical or systemic side effects.

5. PHARMACOLOGICAL PROPERTIES

5.1 Pharmacodynamic properties

Fucidin® H Ointment combines the potent topical antibacterial action of fusidic acid with the anti-inflammatory and antipruritic effects of hydrocortisone. Concentrations of 0.03 - 0.12 microgram fusidic acid per ml inhibit nearly all strains of *staphylococcus aureus*. Topical application of fusidic acid is also effective against streptococci, corynebacteria, neisseria and certain clostridia.

5.2 Pharmacokinetic properties

There are no data which define the pharmacokinetics of Fucidin® H Ointment following topical administration in man.

However, *in vitro* studies show that fusidic acid can penetrate intact human skin. The degree of penetration depends on factors such as the duration of exposure to fusidic acid and the condition of the skin. Fusidic acid is excreted mainly in the bile with little excreted in the urine.

Hydrocortisone is absorbed following topical administration. The degree of absorption is dependent on various factors including skin condition and site of application. Absorbed hydrocortisone is extensively metabolised and rapidly eliminated in the urine.

5.3 Preclinical safety data

There are no pre-clinical data of relevance to the prescriber which are additional to that already included in other sections of the SPC.

6. PHARMACEUTICAL PARTICULARS

6.1 List of excipients

Cetyl alcohol, lanolin, white soft paraffin, liquid paraffin.

6.2 Incompatibilities

Not applicable.

6.3 Shelf life

3 years.

6.4 Special precautions for storage

None.

6.5 Nature and contents of container

Aluminium tubes of 30 gram and 60 gram.

6.6 Instructions for use and handling

None.

7. MARKETING AUTHORISATION HOLDER

LEO Laboratories Limited

Longwick Road

Princes Risborough

Bucks

HP27 9RR

8. MARKETING AUTHORISATION NUMBER(S)

PL 0043/5012R

9. DATE OF FIRST AUTHORISATION/RENEWAL OF THE AUTHORISATION

24 October 1986 / 24 October 1991

10. DATE OF REVISION OF THE TEXT

September 2004.

11. Legal Category

POM

Fucidin Ointment

(Leo Laboratories Limited)

1. NAME OF THE MEDICINAL PRODUCT

Fucidin® Ointment.

2. QUALITATIVE AND QUANTITATIVE COMPOSITION

Fucidin Ointment contains Sodium Fusidate Ph. Eur. 2%.

3. PHARMACEUTICAL FORM

Ointment for topical administration.

4. CLINICAL PARTICULARS

4.1 Therapeutic indications

Indicated either alone or in combination with systemic therapy, in the treatment of primary and secondary skin infections caused by sensitive strains of *Staphylococcus aureus, streptococcus spp* and *Corynebacterium minutissimum*. Primary skin infections that may be expected to respond to treatment with fusidic acid applied topically include: impetigo contagiosa, superficial folliculitis, sycosis barbae, paronychia and erythrasma; also such secondary skin infections as infected eczematoid dermatitis, infected contact dermatitis and infected cuts /abrasions.

4.2 Posology and method of administration

Adults and Children: Uncovered lesions - apply gently, three or four times daily. Covered lesions - less frequent applications may be adequate.

4.3 Contraindications

Infection caused by non-susceptible organisms, in particular, Pseudomonas aeruginosa.

Fucidin ointment is contra-indicated in patients with hypersensitivity to fusidic acid and its salts.

4.4 Special warnings and special precautions for use

The sodium salt of fusidic acid has been shown to cause conjunctival irritation. The ointment should not be used in or near the eye. Bacterial resistance has been reported to occur with the use of fusidic acid applied topically. As with all topical antibiotics, extended or recurrent application may increase the risk of contact sensitisation and the development of antibiotic resistance.

4.5 Interaction with other medicinal products and other forms of Interaction

Not applicable.

4.6 Pregnancy and lactation

There is inadequate evidence of safety in human pregnancy. Animal studies and many years of clinical experience have suggested that fusidic acid is devoid of teratogenic effects.

There is evidence to suggest that when given systemically, fusidic acid can penetrate the placental barrier. The use of topical fucidin in pregnancy requires that the potential benefits be weighed against the possible hazards to the foetus.

Safety in nursing mothers has not been established. When fusidic acid (as the sodium salt) has been given systemically, levels have been detected in breast milk but with topical use the possible amount of drug present is unlikely to affect the infant.

4.7 Effects on ability to drive and use machines

Not applicable.

4.8 Undesirable effects

Hypersensitivity reactions to the active ingredient in the form of skin rashes, mild stinging and irritation on application have been reported rarely.

4.9 Overdose

Not applicable.

5. PHARMACOLOGICAL PROPERTIES

5.1 Pharmacodynamic properties

Fusidic acid is a potent topical antibacterial agent. Fusidic acid and its salts show fat and water solubility and strong surface activity and exhibit unusual ability to penetrate intact skin. Concentrations of 0.03-0.12 microgram/ml inhibit nearly all strains of *Staphylococcus aureus*. Topical application of fusidic acid is also effective against streptococci, corynebacteria, neisseria and certain clostridia.

5.2 Pharmacokinetic properties

In vitro studies show that fusidic acid can penetrate intact human skin. The degree of penetration depends on factors such as the duration of exposure to fusidic acid and the condition of the skin. Fusidic acid is excreted mainly in the bile with little excreted in the urine.

5.3 Preclinical safety data

There are no pre-clinical data of relevance to the prescriber which are additional to that already included in other sections of the SPC.

6. PHARMACEUTICAL PARTICULARS

6.1 List of excipients

Cetyl alcohol, lanolin, white soft paraffin, liquid paraffin.

6.2 Incompatibilities

Not applicable.

6.3 Shelf life

3 years.

6.4 Special precautions for storage

None.

6.5 Nature and contents of container

Aluminium tubes of 15 gram and 30 gram.

6.6 Instructions for use and handling

None.

7. MARKETING AUTHORISATION HOLDER

LEO Laboratories Limited

Longwick Road

Princes Risborough

Bucks

HP27 9RR

8. MARKETING AUTHORISATION NUMBER(S)

PL 0043/5005R

9. DATE OF FIRST AUTHORISATION/RENEWAL OF THE AUTHORISATION

24.10.1986.

10. DATE OF REVISION OF THE TEXT

May 1998

LEGAL CATEGORY

POM

Fucidin Suspension

(Leo Laboratories Limited)

1. NAME OF THE MEDICINAL PRODUCT

FUCIDIN® SUSPENSION

2. QUALITATIVE AND QUANTITATIVE COMPOSITION

Each 5ml of Suspension contains 250mg Fusidic Acid Ph.Eur. (therapeutically equivalent to 175mg Sodium Fusidate Ph.Eur.).

3. PHARMACEUTICAL FORM

Suspension for oral administration.

4. CLINICAL PARTICULARS

4.1 Therapeutic indications

Fucidin® is indicated in the treatment of all staphylococcal infections due to susceptible organisms such as: osteomyelitis, pneumonia, septicaemia, wound infections, endocarditis, superinfected cystic fibrosis, cutaneous infections.

Fucidin® should be administered intravenously whenever oral therapy is inappropriate, which includes cases where absorption from the gastro-intestinal tract is unpredictable.

4.2 Posology and method of administration

Each 5ml of Fucidin® Suspension is therapeutically equivalent to 175mg of sodium fusidate owing to its lower oral bioavailability. Therefore the following dosages are recommended:

Adults: 15ml three times daily

Children:

• 0-1 year: 1ml/kg bodyweight daily, divided into 3 equal doses

• 1-5 years: 5ml three times daily

• 5-12 years: 10ml three times daily

Elderly: No dosage alterations are necessary in the elderly.

Since Fucidin® is excreted in the bile, no dosage modifications are needed in renal impairment.

The dosage in patients undergoing haemodialysis needs no adjustment as Fucidin® is not significantly dialysed.

The Suspension should be shaken before use and dilution is not recommended.

4.3 Contraindications

Contra-indicated in patients with known hypersensitivity to fusidic acid and its salts.

4.4 Special warnings and special precautions for use

Caution should be exercised with other antibiotics which have similar biliary excretion pathways, e.g. lincomycin and rifampicin. Periodic liver function tests should be carried out when high oral doses are used, when the drug is given for prolonged periods and in patients with liver dysfunction.

Fucidin® displaces bilirubin from its albumin binding site in vitro. The clinical significance of this finding is uncertain and kernicterus has not been observed in neonates receiving Fucidin®. However, this observation should be borne in mind when the drug is given to pre-term, jaundiced, acidotic or seriously ill neonates.

The use of Fucidin® in combination with drugs that are CYP-3A4 biotransformed should be avoided. See Section 4.5

Patients given Fucidin® systemically in combination with HMG-CoA reductase inhibitors should be closely clinically monitored. See Section 4.5

4.5 Interaction with other medicinal products and other forms of Interaction

Specific pathways of Fucidin® metabolism in the liver are not known, however, an interaction between Fucidin® and drugs being CYP-3A4 biotransformed can be suspected. The mechanism of this interaction is presumed to be a mutual inhibition of metabolism. There is insufficient data to characterise the effect of fusidic acid on CYPs *in-vitro*. The use of Fucidin® systemically should be avoided in patients treated with CYP-3A4 biotransformed drugs.

Fucidin® administered systemically and concomitantly with oral anticoagulants such as coumarin derivatives or anticoagulants with similar actions may increase the plasma concentration of these agents enhancing the anticoagulant effect. Anticoagulation should be closely monitored and a decrease of the oral anticoagulant dose may be necessary in order to maintain the desired level of anticoagulation. Similarly, discontinuation of Fucidin® may require the maintenance dose of anticoagulant to be re-assessed. The mechanism of this suspected interaction remains unknown.

Co-administration of Fucidin® systemically and HMG-CoA reductase inhibitors such as statins may cause increased plasma concentrations of both agents and rare cases of rhabdomyolysis have been reported for this combination. Patients on this combination should be closely clinically monitored.

Co-administration of Fucidin® systemically and ciclosporin has been reported to cause increased plasma concentration of ciclosporin.

4.6 Pregnancy and lactation

There is inadequate evidence of safety in human pregnancy. Animal studies and many years of clinical experience suggest that fusidic acid is devoid of teratogenic effects. There is evidence to suggest that when given systemically, fusidic acid can cross the placental barrier. If the administration of Fucidin® to pregnant patients is considered essential, its use requires that the potential benefits be weighed against the possible hazards to the foetus.

Safety in nursing mothers has not been established. When fusidic acid (as the sodium salt) has been given systemically, levels have been detected in the breast milk. Caution is therefore required when Fucidin® is used in mothers who wish to breast feed.

4.7 Effects on ability to drive and use machines

None known.

4.8 Undesirable effects

In some patients, given Fucidin®, particularly in the young and elderly, a reversible jaundice has been reported. Jaundice has been seen most frequently in patients receiving intravenous Fucidin® in high dosage, or where the drug has been infused too rapidly or at too high a concentration in the infusion fluid. In some instances instituting oral therapy may be beneficial. If the jaundice persists Fucidin® should be withdrawn, following which the serum bilirubin will invariably return to normal. Reported reactions are gastro-intestinal upsets and, rarely, skin rashes and other allergic reactions including anaphylaxis. Isolated cases of haematological abnormalities which can affect the 3 blood cell lines but mainly white blood cells e.g. bone marrow depression, neutropenia, granulocytopenia, agranulocytosis and pancytopenia have been reported. Reported less often is a depressive effect on the platelets and red blood cells with reports of thrombocytopenia and various anaemias. These abnormalities have been observed especially with treatment of more than 15 days. Acute renal failure has been described in patients with jaundice, particularly in the presence of other factors predisposing to renal failure.

4.9 Overdose

There has been no experience of overdosage with Fucidin®. Treatment should be restricted to symptomatic and supportive measures. Dialysis is of no benefit since the drug is not significantly dialysed.

5. PHARMACOLOGICAL PROPERTIES

5.1 Pharmacodynamic properties

Fusidic acid and its salts are potent anti-staphylococcal agents with unusual ability to penetrate tissue. Bactericidal levels have been assayed in bone and necrotic tissue. Concentrations of 0.03-0.12 mcg/ml inhibit nearly all strains of *staphylococcus aureus*. Fusidic acid is active against *staphylococcus epidermidis* and methicillin resistant staphylococci.

5.2 Pharmacokinetic properties

Blood levels are cumulative, reaching concentrations of 50-100 mcg/ml after oral administration of 1.5g daily for three to four days.

Fucidin® is excreted mainly in the bile, little or none being excreted in the urine.

In severe or deep-seated infections and when prolonged therapy may be required, systemic Fucidin® should generally be given concurrently with other anti-staphylococcal antibiotic therapy.

5.3 Preclinical safety data

There are no pre-clinical data of relevance to the prescriber which are additional to that already included in other sections of the SPC.

6. PHARMACEUTICAL PARTICULARS

6.1 List of excipients

Acesulfame potassium, banana flavour, citric acid, disodium phosphate dihydrate, hydroxyethylcellulose, glucose liquid, methylcellulose, orange dry flavour, sodium benzoate, sorbitol, purified water.

6.2 Incompatibilities

Not applicable.

6.3 Shelf life

3 years.

6.4 Special precautions for storage

Protect from direct sunlight and heat.

6.5 Nature and contents of container

Bottles of 50ml.

6.6 Instructions for use and handling

None.

7. MARKETING AUTHORISATION HOLDER

LEO Laboratories Limited
Longwick Road
Princes Risborough
Bucks
HP27 9RR

8. MARKETING AUTHORISATION NUMBER(S)

PL 0043/5014R

9. DATE OF FIRST AUTHORISATION/RENEWAL OF THE AUTHORISATION

United Kingdom 11.11.1986.

10. DATE OF REVISION OF THE TEXT

January 2004

Fucidin Tablets

(Leo Laboratories Limited)

1. NAME OF THE MEDICINAL PRODUCT

Fucidin® Tablets

2. QUALITATIVE AND QUANTITATIVE COMPOSITION

Each tablet contains Sodium Fusidate Ph.Eur.250mg

3. PHARMACEUTICAL FORM

Tablet.

4. CLINICAL PARTICULARS

4.1 Therapeutic indications

Fucidin® is indicated in the treatment of all staphylococcal infections due to susceptible organisms such as: cutaneous infections, osteomyelitis, pneumonia, septicaemia, wound infections, endocarditis, superinfected cystic fibrosis.

Fucidin® should be administered intravenously whenever oral therapy is inappropriate, which includes cases where absorption from the gastro-intestinal tract is unpredictable.

4.2 Posology and method of administration

For staphylococcal cutaneous infections:

Adults: Standard Dose: 250mg (one tablet) sodium fusidate (equivalent to 240mg fusidic acid) twice daily for 5-10 days.

For staphylococcal infections such as osteomyelitis, pneumonia, septicaemia, wound infections, endocarditis, superinfected cystic fibrosis.

Adults: Standard dose: 500mg (two tablets) sodium fusidate (equivalent to 480mg fusidic acid) three times daily.

In severe cases of fulminating infections, the dosage may be doubled or appropriate combined therapy may be used.

Elderly: No dosage alterations are necessary in the elderly.

Since Fucidin® is excreted in the bile, no dosage modifications are needed in renal impairment.

The dosage in patients undergoing haemodialysis needs no adjustment as Fucidin® is not significantly dialysed.

4.3 Contraindications

Contra-indicated in patients with known hypersensitivity to fusidic acid and its salts.

4.4 Special warnings and special precautions for use

Caution should be exercised with other antibiotics which have similar biliary excretion pathways e.g. lincomycin and rifampicin. Periodic liver function tests should be carried out when high oral doses are used, when the drug is given for prolonged periods and in patients with liver dysfunction.

Fucidin® displaces bilirubin from its albumin binding site *in vitro*. The clinical significance of this finding is uncertain and kernicterus has not been observed in neonates receiving Fucidin®. However, this observation should be borne in mind when the drug is given to pre-term, jaundiced, acidotic or seriously ill neonates.

The use of Fucidin® in combination with drugs that are CYP-3A4 biotransformed should be avoided. See Section 4.5

Patients given Fucidin® systemically in combination with HMG-CoA reductase inhibitors should be closely clinically monitored. See Section 4.5

4.5 Interaction with other medicinal products and other forms of Interaction

Specific pathways of Fucidin® metabolism in the liver are not known, however, an interaction between Fucidin® and drugs being CYP-3A4 biotransformed can be suspected. The mechanism of this interaction is presumed to be a mutual inhibition of metabolism. There is insufficient data to characterise the effect of fusidic acid on CYPs *in-vitro*. The use of Fucidin® systemically should be avoided in patients treated with CYP-3A4 biotransformed drugs.

Fucidin® administered systemically and concomitantly with oral anticoagulants such as coumarin derivatives or anticoagulants with similar actions may increase the plasma concentration of these agents enhancing the anticoagulant effect. Anticoagulation should be closely monitored and a decrease of the oral anticoagulant dose may be necessary in order to maintain the desired level of anticoagulation. Similarly, discontinuation of Fucidin® may require the maintenance dose of anticoagulant to be re-assessed. The mechanism of this suspected interaction remains unknown.

Co-administration of Fucidin® systemically and HMG-CoA reductase inhibitors such as statins may cause increased plasma concentrations of both agents and rare cases of rhabdomyolysis have been reported for this combination. Patients on this combination should be closely clinically monitored.

Co-administration of Fucidin® systemically and ciclosporin has been reported to cause increased plasma concentration of ciclosporin.

4.6 Pregnancy and lactation

There is inadequate evidence of safety in human pregnancy. Animal studies and many years of clinical experience suggest that fusidic acid is devoid of teratogenic effects. There is evidence to suggest that when given systemically, fusidic acid can cross the placental barrier. If the administration of Fucidin® to pregnant patients is considered essential, its use requires that the potential benefits be weighed against the possible hazards to the foetus.

Safety in nursing mothers has not been established. When fusidic acid (as the sodium salt) has been given systemically, levels have been detected in the breast milk. Caution is therefore required when Fucidin® is used in mothers who wish to breast feed.

4.7 Effects on ability to drive and use machines

None known.

4.8 Undesirable effects

In some patients, given Fucidin®, particularly in the young and elderly, a reversible jaundice has been reported. Jaundice has been seen most frequently in patients receiving intravenous Fucidin® in high dosage, or where the drug has been infused too rapidly or at too high a concentration in the infusion fluid. In some instances instituting oral therapy may be beneficial. If the jaundice persists Fucidin® should be withdrawn, following which the serum bilirubin will invariably return to normal. Reported reactions are gastro-intestinal upsets and, rarely, skin rashes and other allergic reactions including anaphylaxis. Isolated cases of haematological abnormalities which can affect the 3 blood cell lines but mainly white blood cells e.g. bone marrow depression, neutropenia, granulocytopenia, agranulocytosis and pancytopenia have been reported. Reported less often is a depressive effect on the platelets and red blood cells with reports of thrombocytopenia and various anaemias. These abnormalities have been observed especially with treatment of more than 15 days. Acute renal failure has been described in patients with jaundice, particularly in the presence of other factors predisposing to renal failure.

4.9 Overdose

There has been no experience of overdosage with Fucidin®. Treatment should be restricted to symptomatic and supportive measures. Dialysis is of no benefit, since the drug is not significantly dialysed.

5. PHARMACOLOGICAL PROPERTIES

5.1 Pharmacodynamic properties

Fusidic acid and its salts are potent anti-staphylococcal agents with unusual ability to penetrate tissue. Bactericidal levels have been assayed in bone and necrotic tissue. Concentrations of 0.03 - 0.12 micrograms/ml inhibit nearly all strains of *Staphylococcus aureus*. Fusidic acid is active against *Staphylococcus epidermidis* and methicillin resistant staphylococci.

5.2 Pharmacokinetic properties

Blood levels are cumulative, reaching concentrations of 20-35 micrograms/ml after oral administration of 250mg twice daily for seven days and 50-100 micrograms/ml after oral administration of 500mg three times daily for three to four days.

Fucidin® is excreted mainly in the bile, little or none being excreted in the urine.

In severe or deep-seated infections and when prolonged therapy may be required, Fucidin® should generally be given concurrently with other anti-staphylococcal antibiotic therapy.

5.3 Preclinical safety data

There are no pre-clinical data of relevance to the prescriber which are additional to that already included in other sections of the SPC.

6. PHARMACEUTICAL PARTICULARS

6.1 List of excipients

Cellulose microcrystalline, crospovidone, gelatin, hydroxypropylmethylcellulose, lactose, magnesium stearate, polyvinylpyrolidone, silicon dioxide, talc, titanium dioxide.

6.2 Incompatibilities

None.

6.3 Shelf life

3 years.

6.4 Special precautions for storage

Do not store above 25°C.

6.5 Nature and contents of container

Blister packs of 10 and 10 × 10 tablets.

6.6 Instructions for use and handling

None.

7. MARKETING AUTHORISATION HOLDER

LEO Laboratories Limited, Longwick Road, Princes Risborough, Bucks. HP27 9RR.

8. MARKETING AUTHORISATION NUMBER(S)

0043/5000R

9. DATE OF FIRST AUTHORISATION/RENEWAL OF THE AUTHORISATION

4.6.87 (after review).

10. DATE OF REVISION OF THE TEXT

January 2004.

LEGAL CATEGORY

POM

Fucithalmic

(Leo Laboratories Limited)

1. NAME OF THE MEDICINAL PRODUCT

Fucithalmic®

2. QUALITATIVE AND QUANTITATIVE COMPOSITION

Each gram contains fusidic acid, hemihydrate Ph.Eur. 10mg.

3. PHARMACEUTICAL FORM

Sterile viscous eye drops.

4. CLINICAL PARTICULARS

4.1 Therapeutic indications

Fucithalmic is indicated for the topical treatment of bacterial conjunctivitis where the organism is known to be sensitive to the antibiotic.

4.2 Posology and method of administration

For all ages: One Fucithalmic drop to be instilled into the eye twice daily. Treatment should be continued for at least 48 hours after the eye returns to normal.

4.3 Contraindications

Hypersensitivity to any of its components.

4.4 Special warnings and special precautions for use

Should not be used when contact lenses are being worn.

4.5 Interaction with other medicinal products and other forms of Interaction

Not applicable.

4.6 Pregnancy and lactation

Not applicable.

4.7 Effects on ability to drive and use machines

Not applicable.

4.8 Undesirable effects

Transient stinging after application has been encountered. Hypersensitivity may occur.

4.9 Overdose

Not applicable.

5. PHARMACOLOGICAL PROPERTIES

5.1 Pharmacodynamic properties

Fucithalmic is active against a wide range of gram-positive organisms, particularly *Staphylococcus aureus*. Other species against which Fucithalmic has been shown to have *in vitro* activity include *Streptococcus*, *Neisseria*, *Haemophilus*, *Moraxella* and *Corynebacteria*.

5.2 Pharmacokinetic properties

The sustained release formulation of Fucithalmic ensures a prolonged contact with the conjunctival sac. Twice daily application provides sufficient fusidic acid concentrations in all relevant tissues of the eye. Fusidic acid penetrates well into the aqueous humour.

5.3 Preclinical safety data

There are no pre-clinical data of relevance to the prescriber which are additional to that already included in other sections of the SPC.

6. PHARMACEUTICAL PARTICULARS

6.1 List of excipients

Benzalkonium chloride, disodium edetate, mannitol, carbomer, sodium hydroxide, water for injections.

6.2 Incompatibilities

None known.

6.3 Shelf life

3 years.

6.4 Special precautions for storage

Store below 25°C. Keep the tube tightly closed. The tube should be discarded one month after opening.

6.5 Nature and contents of container

Available in 5g tubes.

6.6 Instructions for use and handling

None.

7. MARKETING AUTHORISATION HOLDER

Leo Laboratories Limited, Longwick Road, Princes Risborough, Bucks. HP27 9RR.

8. MARKETING AUTHORISATION NUMBER(S)

0043/0137

9. DATE OF FIRST AUTHORISATION/RENEWAL OF THE AUTHORISATION

10.8.1987

10. DATE OF REVISION OF THE TEXT

June 1997.

LEGAL CATEGORY

POM

Full Marks Liquid

(SSL International plc)

1. NAME OF THE MEDICINAL PRODUCT

Full Marks Phenothrin Liquid.

2. QUALITATIVE AND QUANTITATIVE COMPOSITION

Phenothrin 0.5% w/w.

3. PHARMACEUTICAL FORM

Cutaneous emulsion.

4. CLINICAL PARTICULARS

4.1 Therapeutic indications

For the treatment of head louse infestations.

4.2 Posology and method of administration

Adults, the elderly and children aged 6 months and over: For topical external use only. The source of infestation should be sought and treated. Rub the emulsion into the scalp until all the hair and scalp are thoroughly moistened. Leave the hair to dry naturally in a warm but well ventilated room. After 12 hours, or the next day, if preferred, shampoo the hair in the normal way. Rinse the hair and comb whilst wet to remove dead lice and eggs (nits) using a nit comb.

4.3 Contraindications

Known sensitivity to pyrethroid insecticides. Not to be used on infants less than 6 months of age except on medical advice.

4.4 Special warnings and special precautions for use

Avoid contact with the eyes. For external use only. Keep out of the reach of children. If inadvertently swallowed, a doctor or casualty department should be contacted at once. When used by a school nurse or other health officer in the mass treatment of large numbers of children, it is advisable that protective plastic or rubber gloves be worn. Continued prolonged treatment with this product should be avoided. It should not be used more than once a week for more than three consecutive weeks. The treatment may affect permed, pre-rinsed or coloured hair.

4.5 Interaction with other medicinal products and other forms of Interaction

None stated.

4.6 Pregnancy and lactation

No known effects in pregnancy and lactation. However, as with all medicines, use with caution.

4.7 Effects on ability to drive and use machines

None stated.

4.8 Undesirable effects

Very rarely, skin irritation has been reported.

4.9 Overdose

It is most unlikely that a toxic dose will be ingested. Treatment consists of gastric lavage, assisted respiration and, if necessary in the event of massive ingestion, administration of atropine together with pralidoxime.

5. PHARMACOLOGICAL PROPERTIES

5.1 Pharmacodynamic properties

Phenothrin is a synthetic pyrethroid insecticide, highly effective against human lice but with an exceptionally low mammalian toxicity.

5.2 Pharmacokinetic properties

Full Marks Phenothrin Liquid is applied topically to the affected area. A pharmacokinetic study has shown absorption of its active constituent is negligible.

5.3 Preclinical safety data

None stated.

6. PHARMACEUTICAL PARTICULARS

6.1 List of excipients

Potassium Citrate Ph Eur; Citric Acid Monohydrate Ph Eur; Emulsifying Wax (Lanette Wax SX) BP; Methylhydroxybenzoate Ph Eur; Propylhydroxybenzoate Ph Eur; Perfume HT 52; Diethylene Glycol; Dimethyl Phthalate Ph Eur; Purified Water Ph Eur.

6.2 Incompatibilities

None stated.

6.3 Shelf life

36 months.

6.4 Special precautions for storage

Store below 25°C and do not refrigerate.

6.5 Nature and contents of container

Amber glass sirop bottle fitted with a polypropylene tamper evident lined cap containing 50 or 200ml of product.

6.6 Instructions for use and handling

Shake the bottle before use.

7. MARKETING AUTHORISATION HOLDER

Seton Products Limited, Tubiton House, Oldham, OL1 3HS.

8. MARKETING AUTHORISATION NUMBER(S)

PL 11314/0093.

9. DATE OF FIRST AUTHORISATION/RENEWAL OF THE AUTHORISATION

20th January 1998.

10. DATE OF REVISION OF THE TEXT

January 1998.

Full Marks Lotion

(SSL International plc)

1. NAME OF THE MEDICINAL PRODUCT

Full Marks Lotion.

2. QUALITATIVE AND QUANTITATIVE COMPOSITION

Phenothrin 0.2% w/v.

3. PHARMACEUTICAL FORM

Lotion.

4. CLINICAL PARTICULARS

4.1 Therapeutic indications

For the treatment of head and pubic louse infestations.

4.2 Posology and method of administration

For topical external use only. The source of infestation should be sought and treated. Adults and children aged 6 months and over: *For head lice:* Sprinkle the lotion on the hair and rub gently onto the head until the entire scalp is moistened. Pay special attention to the back of the neck and the area behind the ears. Take care to avoid the eyes. Allow to dry naturally. Use no heat. The hair may be washed with a standard shampoo 2 hours after application. Whilst still wet, comb the hair with an ordinary comb. A fine toothed louse comb can then be used to remove the dead lice and eggs. *For crab (pubic) lice:* Application and dosage etc are as for the head. Apply the lotion to the pubic hair and the hair between the legs and around the anus. Allow to dry naturally, using no heat. Not to be used on infants under the age of 6 months except under medical supervision.

4.3 Contraindications

A history of sensitivity to pyrethroid insecticides.

4.4 Special warnings and special precautions for use

Full Marks Lotion contains isopropyl alcohol which may cause wheezing in asthmatic patients or cause inflammation of the skin in patients with severe eczema. If such effects are apparent, patients should use a water-based formulation. Contains flammable alcohol. Apply and dry with care. Avoid naked flames or lighted objects. Do not use artificial heat (e.g. electric hairdryers). Dry in a well ventilated room. Do not cover the head before the lotion has dried completely. The hair should be dry before retiring to bed. When Full Marks Lotion is used by a school nurse or other health officer in the mass treatment of large numbers of children, it is advisable that protective plastic or rubber gloves be worn.

4.5 Interaction with other medicinal products and other forms of Interaction
None stated.

4.6 Pregnancy and lactation
There are no known effects in pregnancy and lactation. However, as with all drugs, Full Marks Lotion should be used with caution in pregnant and lactating women.

4.7 Effects on ability to drive and use machines
None stated.

4.8 Undesirable effects
Some patients may experience stinging or inflammation of the skin due to the alcohol content.

4.9 Overdose
In the event of deliberate or accidental ingestion, as for ethyl alcohol, empty the stomach by gastric lavage and treat symptomatically.

5. PHARMACOLOGICAL PROPERTIES

5.1 Pharmacodynamic properties
Phenothrin is a synthetic pyrethroid insecticide, highly effective against human lice but with an exceptionally low mammalian toxicity.

5.2 Pharmacokinetic properties
Full Marks Lotion is applied topically to the affected area. A pharmacokinetic study has shown absorption of its active constituent is negligible.

5.3 Preclinical safety data
None stated.

6. PHARMACEUTICAL PARTICULARS

6.1 List of excipients
Herbal Green Bouquet P15312; Isopropanol; Purified Water.

6.2 Incompatibilities
None stated.

6.3 Shelf life
Three years.

6.4 Special precautions for storage
Store bottle in carton at or below 30°C protected from light.

6.5 Nature and contents of container
Cartoned, clear or amber glass bottles with polyethylene caps and polypropylene sprinkler inserts containing 50 or 200 ml of product.

6.6 Instructions for use and handling
None stated.

7. MARKETING AUTHORISATION HOLDER
Seton Products Limited, Tubiton House, Oldham, OL1 3HS.

8. MARKETING AUTHORISATION NUMBER(S)
PL 11314/0047.

9. DATE OF FIRST AUTHORISATION/RENEWAL OF THE AUTHORISATION
27th November 1995.

10. DATE OF REVISION OF THE TEXT
May 1998.

Full Marks Mousse

(SSL International plc)

1. NAME OF THE MEDICINAL PRODUCT
Full Marks Mousse.

2. QUALITATIVE AND QUANTITATIVE COMPOSITION
Phenothrin 0.5% w/w.

3. PHARMACEUTICAL FORM
Topical mousse.

4. CLINICAL PARTICULARS

4.1 Therapeutic indications
For the treatment of head louse infestations.

4.2 Posology and method of administration
Apply the product in a well ventilated room away from naked flames and lighted objects. Adults, the elderly and children aged 6 months and over: For topical external use only. The source of infestation should be sought and treated. Family members and close contacts should be inspected and, if found to be infected, treated simultaneously. Shake the can well and invert to expel the mousse. Apply sufficient mousse to dry hair at several points on the scalp; massage into the scalp ensuring no part of the scalp is left uncovered. Pay special attention to the temples and crown of the head. Take care to avoid the eyes. Leave on the head for 30 minutes; do not attempt to dry the hair by artificial means (for example, electric hair dryers). Wash hair with normal shampoo. While the hair is still wet, comb with an ordinary comb. A fine-toothed louse comb can then be used to remove the dead or dying lice and eggs. Infants: Not to be used on infants under 6 months of age except under medical supervision.

4.3 Contraindications
Known sensitivity to phenothrin.

4.4 Special warnings and special precautions for use
Children under six months of age should only be treated under medical supervision. Avoid contact with the eyes. When Full Marks Mousse is used by a school nurse or other health officer in the mass treatment of large numbers of children, it is advisable that protective plastic or rubber gloves be worn. Prolonged and repeated application should be avoided. Contains flammable alcohol. Avoid naked flames or lighted objects. Do not use artificial heat (for example, electric hair dryers). Full Marks Mousse contains alcohol which may cause wheezing in asthmatic patients or cause inflammation of the skin in patients with severe eczema. If such effects are apparent, patients should use a non alcohol based formulation. The treatment may affect permed, pre-rinsed, bleached or coloured hair. For external use only.

4.5 Interaction with other medicinal products and other forms of Interaction
None stated.

4.6 Pregnancy and lactation
Long term studies have not been performed in humans, therefore as with all medicines, Full Marks Mousse should be used with caution in pregnant and lactating women.

4.7 Effects on ability to drive and use machines
None stated.

4.8 Undesirable effects
Very rarely, skin irritation may occur. The treatment may affect pre-rinsed, permed, coloured or bleached hair. The alcohol content of the mousse may cause stinging or inflammation in patients with eczema.

4.9 Overdose
This product contains 30% alcohol. In the event of deliberate or accidental consumption, particularly by a child, empty stomach contents by gastric lavage and treat symptomatically as hypoglycaemia may occur.

5. PHARMACOLOGICAL PROPERTIES

5.1 Pharmacodynamic properties
Phenothrin is a synthetic pyrethroid insecticide, highly effective against human lice but with an exceptionally low mammalian toxicity.

5.2 Pharmacokinetic properties
Full Marks Mousse is applied topically to the affected area.

5.3 Preclinical safety data
Dermal irritation and eye irritation tests carried out in rabbits showed Full Marks Mousse to be a minimal irritant and did not produce positive criteria in any rabbit.

6. PHARMACEUTICAL PARTICULARS

6.1 List of excipients
Potassium Citrate Ph Eur; Citric Acid Anhydrous Ph Eur; Emulsifying Wax (non-ionic)HSE; Purified Water Ph Eur; Ethanol (denatured)HSE; Butane 30 HSE.

6.2 Incompatibilities
None stated.

6.3 Shelf life
36 months.

6.4 Special precautions for storage
Store at or below 25°C. Do not puncture the can or expose to direct sunlight. Avoid naked flames or lighted objects. Do not use artificial heat (for example, electric hair dryers). When empty, dispose of safely as normal household waste.

6.5 Nature and contents of container
Aluminium monobloc aerosol cans with a mousse valve assembly, and a vertical foam spout and cap containing either 50g of product to treat one person or 150g of product to treat four persons.

6.6 Instructions for use and handling
Not applicable.

7. MARKETING AUTHORISATION HOLDER
Seton Products Limited, Tubiton House, Oldham, OL1 3HS.

8. MARKETING AUTHORISATION NUMBER(S)
PL 11314/0102.

9. DATE OF FIRST AUTHORISATION/RENEWAL OF THE AUTHORISATION
1st April 1998.

10. DATE OF REVISION OF THE TEXT
April 1998.

Fungilin Lozenge, Oral Suspension, Oral Tablets

(E. R. Squibb & Sons Limited)

1. NAME OF THE MEDICINAL PRODUCT
Fungilin Lozenge, Oral Suspension And Oral Tablets

2. QUALITATIVE AND QUANTITATIVE COMPOSITION

Fungilin Lozenge:	Round, pale yellow, engraved "929" and "Squibb" containing 10,000 units (10mg) amphotericin.
Fungilin Oral Suspension:	Orange-flavoured, viscous suspension containing 100,000 units (100mg) amphotericin per ml.
Fungilin Oral Tablets:	Yellow to tan, scored one side and engraved "Squibb" and "430" on reverse, containing 100,000 (100mg) amphotericin.

3. PHARMACEUTICAL FORM
Lozenge
Oral Suspension
Oral Tablets.

4. CLINICAL PARTICULARS

4.1 Therapeutic indications
<u>Lozenge/Suspension:</u>
For the treatment of candidal lesions (thrush) of the oral and perioral areas. The suspension may be used in the treatment of denture stomatitis.

<u>Suspension/Tablets:</u>
For the treatment of intestinal candidosis and the suppression of the intestinal reservoir of *C. albicans* which may precipitate cutaneous or vaginal candidosis.

4.2 Posology and method of administration
<u>Adults:</u>
<u>*Lozenge:*</u> Dissolve one lozenge slowly in the mouth four times a day. Depending on the severity of infection, the dose may be increased to 8 lozenges daily.

To clear the condition fully may require 10-15 days' treatment.

<u>*Suspension:*</u> For denture stomatitis and oral infections caused by *C. albicans*, 1ml should be placed in the mouth four times daily; it should be kept in contact with lesions for as long as possible.

For the treatment of suppression of intestinal candidosis, 2ml four times daily.

<u>*Tablets:*</u> 1 or 2 tablets four times daily.

Administration of Fungilin for oral and intestinal candidosis should be continued for 48 hours after clinical cure to prevent relapse.

<u>Infants and Children:</u>
<u>*Lozenge/Tablets:*</u> Not recommended

<u>*Suspension:*</u> For intestinal and oral candidosis, 1ml should be dropped into the mouth four times daily. The suspension should be held in contact with oral lesions for as long as possible before swallowing.

For prophylaxis in the newborn, the suggested dose is 1ml daily.

<u>Elderly:</u>
No specific dosage recommendations or precautions.

4.3 Contraindications
Fungilin is contraindicated in patients with known hypersensitivity to amphotericin or to any of the other ingredients.

4.4 Special warnings and special precautions for use
No specific warnings or precautions apply.

4.5 Interaction with other medicinal products and other forms of Interaction
None known

4.6 Pregnancy and lactation
No special precautions apply; absorption of amphotericin from the gastrointestinal tract is negligible.

4.7 Effects on ability to drive and use machines
Not applicable.

4.8 Undesirable effects
Since amphotericin B is not appreciably absorbed when taken orally, even at high dose, adverse effects following oral administration of up to 3g daily have been uncommon. Rash, glossitis and gastrointestinal distress, including nausea, vomiting and diarrhoea have been reported occasionally. Transient yellowing of the teeth may occur with use of the suspension and lozenge formulations, which can easily be removed by brushing. Urticaria, angioedema, Stevens-Johnson syndrome and toxic epidermal necrolysis have been reported rarely; an association between these events and administration of Fungilin is unclear.

4.9 Overdose
Since absorption of amphotericin from the gastro-intestinal tract is negligible, overdosage causes no systemic toxicity.

5. PHARMACOLOGICAL PROPERTIES

5.1 Pharmacodynamic properties

Actions:

Amphotericin is an antifungal antibiotic active against a wide range of yeasts and yeast-like fungi including Candida albicans. Extensive clinical experience has not shown problems of toxicity or sensitisation.

5.2 Pharmacokinetic properties

Absorption from the gastro-intestinal tract is negligible even with very large doses.

5.3 Preclinical safety data

No further relevant information.

6. PHARMACEUTICAL PARTICULARS

6.1 List of excipients

Lozenge:	Acacia powder, d-mannitol, flavours, magnesium stearate, polyvinyl alcohol, talc.
Suspension:	Citric acid, ethanol, flavours, glycerol, methyl and propyl parahydroxybenzoates, potassium chloride, sodium benzoate, sodium carboxymethylcellulose, sodium phosphate, sodium metabisulphite, water.
Tablets:	Ethyl cellulose, lactose, maize starch, magnesium stearate, talc.

6.2 Incompatibilities

None known.

6.3 Shelf life

Lozenge:	18 months
Suspension:	48 months
Tablets:	24 months

6.4 Special precautions for storage

Lozenge/ Tablets:	Do not store above 25°C.
Suspension:	Do not store above 25°C. Keep container in the outer carton. Discard any unused suspension 4 days after opening. Dilution: Fungilin Suspension should not be diluted prior to use; it is formulated to coat and adhere to the oral lesions being treated.

6.5 Nature and contents of container

Lozenge:	Aluminium tube, foil or blister pack of 60 lozenges.
Suspension:	12ml bottles with graduated dropper.
Tablets:	Bottles of 56 tablets.

6.6 Instructions for use and handling

No special handling instructions.

7. MARKETING AUTHORISATION HOLDER

E. R. Squibb & Sons Limited
Uxbridge Business Park
Sanderson Road
Uxbridge
Middlesex UB8 1DH

8. MARKETING AUTHORISATION NUMBER(S)

Lozenge:	PL 0034/5034R
Suspension:	PL 0034/5038R
Tablets:	PL 0034/5039R

9. DATE OF FIRST AUTHORISATION/RENEWAL OF THE AUTHORISATION

Lozenge:	30 January 1991 / 25 January 2005
Suspension:	20 March 1991 / 25 January 2005
Tablets:	20 March 1991 / 25 January 2005

10. DATE OF REVISION OF THE TEXT

24 June 2005

Fungizone Intravenous

(E. R. Squibb & Sons Limited)

1. NAME OF THE MEDICINAL PRODUCT

FUNGIZONE INTRAVENOUS

2. QUALITATIVE AND QUANTITATIVE COMPOSITION

Each vial contains as a yellow, fluffy powder: amphotericin 50,000 units (50mg).

3. PHARMACEUTICAL FORM

Powder for Injection

4. CLINICAL PARTICULARS

4.1 Therapeutic indications

Fungizone Intravenous should be administered primarily to patients with progressive, potentially fatal infections. This potent drug should not be used to treat the common forms of fungal disease which show only positive skin or serological tests.

Fungizone Intravenous is specifically intended to treat cryptococcosis (torulosis); North American blastomycosis; the disseminated forms of candidosis, coccidioidomycosis and histoplasmosis; mucormycosis (phycomycosis) caused by species of the genera *Mucor*, *Rhizopus*, *Absidia*, *Entomophthora*, and *Basidiobolus* sporotrichosis (*Sporotrichum schenckii*), aspergillosis (*Aspergillus fumigatus*).

Amphotericin may be helpful in the treatment of American mucocutaneous leishmaniasis but is not the drug of choice in primary therapy.

4.2 Posology and method of administration

Adults and children:

Fungizone should be administerd by intravenous infusion over a period of 2-4 hours. Reduction of the infusion rate may reduce the incidence of side-effects. In rare instances infusion times of up to 6 hours may be necessary. Initial daily dose should be 0.25mg/kg of body weight gradually increasing to a level of 1.0mg/kg of body weight depending on individual response and tolerance. Within the range of 0.25-1.0mg/kg the daily dose should be maintained at the highest level which is not accompanied by unacceptable toxicity.

In seriously ill patients the daily dose may be gradually increased up to a total of 1.5mg/kg. Since amphotericin is excreted slowly, therapy may be given on alternate days in patients on the higher dosage schedule. Several months of therapy are usually necessary; a shorter period of therapy may produce an inadequate response and lead to relapse.

When commencing all new courses of treatment, it is advisable to administer a test dose immediately preceding the first dose. A volume of the infusion containing 1mg (i.e. 10ml) should be infused over 20-30 minutes and the patient carefully observed for at least a further 30 minutes. It should be noted that patient responses to the test dose may not be predictive of subsequent severe side effects.

Whenever medication is interrupted for a period longer than seven days, therapy should be resumed by starting with the lowest dosage level, i.e. 0.25mg/kg of body weight and increased gradually.

CAUTION:

Under no circumstances should a total daily dose of 1.5mg/kg be exceeded. The recommended concentration for intravenous infusion is 10mg/100ml.

Elderly:

No specific dosage recommendations or precautions.

Preparation of solutions:

Reconstitute as follows: An initial concentrate of 5mg amphotericin per ml is first prepared by rapidly expressing 10ml sterile water for injection, without a bacteriostatic agent, directly into the lyophilized cake, using a sterile needle (minimum diameter: 20 gauge) and syringe. Shake the vial immediately until the colloidal solution is clear. The infusion solution, providing 10mg/100ml is obtained by further dilution (1:50) with 5% Glucose Injection of pH above 4.2. The pH of each container of Glucose Injection should be ascertained before use. Commercial Glucose Injection usually has a pH above 4.2; however, if it is below 4.2 then 1 or 2 ml of buffer should be added to the Glucose Injection before it is used to dilute a concentrated solution of amphotericin. The recommended buffer has the following composition:

Dibasic sodium phosphate (anhydrous)	1.59g
Monobasic sodium phosphate (anhydrous)	0.96g
Water for Injections BP	q.s. to 100ml

The buffer should be sterilised before it is added to the Glucose Injection, either by filtration through a bacterial filter, or by autoclaving for 30 mins at 15lb pressure (121°C).

CAUTION:

Aseptic technique must be strictly observed in all handling, since no preservative or bacteriostatic agent is present. Do not reconstitute with saline solutions. The use of any diluent other than the ones recommended or the presence of a bacteriostatic agent in the diluent may cause precipitation of the amphotericin. Do not use the initial concentrate or the infusion solution if there is any evidence of precipitation of foreign matter.

An in-line membrane filter may be used for intravenous infusion of amphotericin; however the mean pore diameter of the filter should not be less than 1.0 micron in order to assure passage of the amphotericin dispersion.

Other preparations for injection should not be added to the infusion solution or administered via the cannula being used to administer Fungizone Intravenous.

The use of Fungizone Intravenous by other routes has been documented in the published literature:

Bladder irrigation/instillation (eg candiduria): Continuous irrigation with 50mg Fungizone in 1 litre sterile water each day until urinary cultures are negative. Intermittent use of volumes of 100-400ml (concentrations of 37.5-200mcg/ml) has also been reported. The urine should be alkalinized (with potassium citrate) and antifungal ointment applied to the perineal area.

Lung inhalation (eg pulmonary aspergillosis): 8-40mg amphotericin (nebulized in sterile water or 5% Glucose) has been given daily in divided doses. Concurrent eradication of oral and intestinal yeast reservoirs is recommended.

Intrathecal (eg coccidiodal meningitis): Current published dosage recommendations are for maintenance 0.25-1.0mg amphotericin 2-4 times weekly following intitiation with a low dose (0.025mg) and cautious increases. Amphotericin is irritating when injected into the CSF.

Other: Other uses of solutions prepared using Fungizone Intravenous include local instillations for the treatment of fungal infections of the ear, eye, peritoneum, lung cavities and joint spaces.

4.3 Contraindications

Those patients who are hypersensitive to amphotericin, unless, in the opinion of the physician, the condition requiring treatment is life-threatening and amenable only to such therapy.

4.4 Special warnings and special precautions for use

Prolonged therapy with amphotericin is usually necessary. Unpleasant reactions are quite common when the drug is given parenterally at therapeutic dosage levels. Some of these reactions are potentially dangerous. Hence amphotericin should be used parenterally only in hospitalised patients, or those under close clinical observation. If serum creatinine exceeds 260 micromol/l the drug should be discontinued or the dosage markedly reduced until renal function is improved. Weekly blood counts and serum potassium determinations are also advisable. Low serum magnesium levels have also been noted during treatment with amphotericin. Therapy should be discontinued if liver function test results (elevated bromsulphalein, alkaline phosphatase and bilirubin) are abnormal.

Leucoencephalopathy has been reported very occasionally following the use of amphotericin injection in patients who received total body irradiation. Most of these patients received high cumulative doses of amphotericin.

Rapid intravenous infusion, over less than one hour, particularly in patients with renal insufficiency, has been associated with hyperkalaemia and arrhythmias and should therefore be avoided.

Corticosteroids should not be administered concomitantly unless they are necessary to control drug reactions. Other nephrotoxic antibiotics and antineoplastic agents should not be given concomitantly except with great caution.

4.5 Interaction with other medicinal products and other forms of Interaction

Concomitant administration of nephrotoxic drugs or antineoplastics should be avoided if at all possible.

The hypokalaemia following amphotericin therapy may potentiate the toxicity of digitalis glycosides or enhance the curariform actions of skeletal muscle relaxants.

Corticosteroids may increase the potassium loss due to amphotericin. Flucytosine toxicity may be enhanced during concomitant administration, possibly due to an increase in its cellular uptake and/or impairment of its renal excretion.

Acute pulmonary reactions have occasionally been observed in patients given amphotericin during or shortly after leukocyte transfusions. It is advisable to separate these infusions as far as possible and to monitor pulmonary function.

4.6 Pregnancy and lactation

Safety for use in pregnancy has not been established; therefore it should be used during pregnancy only if the possible benefits to be derived outweigh the potential risks involved.

4.7 Effects on ability to drive and use machines

Not applicable.

4.8 Undesirable effects

While some patients may tolerate full intravenous doses of amphotericin without difficulty, most will exhibit some intolerance. In patients experiencing adverse reactions these may be made less severe by giving aspirin, antihistamines or anti-emetics. Febrile reactions may be decreased by the intravenous administration of small doses of adrenal corticosteroids, e.g. 25mg hydrocortisone. This may be administered just prior to or during amphotericin infusion. The dosage and duration of such corticosteroid therapy should be kept to a minimum. Administration of the drug on alternate days may decrease anorexia and phlebitis. Adding a small amount of heparin to the infusion may lessen the incidence of thrombophlebitis and coagulation problems. Extravasation may cause chemical irritation. The adverse reactions that are most commonly observed are: fever (sometimes with shaking chills), headache, anorexia, weight loss, nausea and vomiting, malaise, muscle and joint pains, dyspepsia, cramping epigastric pain, diarrhoea, local venous pain at the injection site with phlebitis and thrombophlebitis, normochromic normocytic anaemia and hypokalaemia. Abnormal renal function including hypokalaemia, azotaemia, hyposthenuria, renal tubular acidosis or nephrocalcinosis, is also commonly observed and usually improves upon interruption of therapy; however, some permanent impairment often occurs, especially in those patients receiving large amounts (over 5g) of amphotericin.

The following adverse reactions occur less frequently or rarely; anuria (oliguria); cardiovascular toxicity including arrhythmias, ventricular fibrillation, cardiac arrest, hypotension, hypertension; coagulation defects; thrombocytopenia; leucopenia; agranulocytosis; eosinophilia; leucocytosis; melaena or haemorrhagic gastroenteritis; maculopapular rash and pruritus; hearing loss, tinnitus; transient vertigo; blurred vision, or diplopia; encephalopathy (see precautions); peripheral neuropathy, convulsions and other neurologic symptoms; anaphylactoid reactions, acute liver failure and flushing.

4.9 Overdose
Amphotericin overdoses can result in cardio-respiratory arrest. If an overdose is suspected, discontinue therapy and monitor the patient's clinical status (e.g., cardio-respiratory, renal, and liver function, haematologic status serum electrolytes) and administer supportive therapy as required. Amphotericin is not haemodialysable. Prior to reinstituting therapy, the patient's condition should be stabilised (including correction of electrolyte deficiencies, etc.)

5. PHARMACOLOGICAL PROPERTIES

5.1 Pharmacodynamic properties
Amphotericin is a polyene antifungal antibiotic active against a wide range of yeasts and yeast-like fungi including Candida albicans. Crystalline amphotericin is insoluble in water; therefore, the antibiotic is solubilised by the addition of sodium desoxycholate to form a mixture which provides a colloidal dispersion for parenteral administration. Amphotericin is fungistatic rather than fungicidal in concentrations obtainable in body fluids. It probably acts by binding to sterols in the fungal cell membrane with a resultant change in membrane permeability which allows leakage of intracellular components. Mammalian cell membranes also contain sterols and it has been suggested that the damage to human and fungal cells may share common mechanisms. No strains of Candida resistant to amphotericin have been reported in clinical use, and although in vitro testing does produce a small number of resistant isolates this occurs only following repeated subcultures.

5.2 Pharmacokinetic properties
An initial intravenous infusion of 1 to 5mg of amphotericin per day, gradually increased to 0.65mg/kg daily, produces peak plasma concentrations of approximately 2 to 4mg/l which can persist between doses since the plasma half-life of amphotericin is about 24 hours. It has been reported that amphotericin is highly bound (more than 90%) to plasma proteins and is poorly dialysable.

Amphotericin is excreted very slowly by the kidneys with 2 to 5% of a given dose being excreted in biologically active form. After treatment is discontinued the drug can be detected in the urine for at least seven weeks. The cumulative urinary output over a seven day period amounts to approximately 40% of the amount of drug infused.

Details of tissue distribution and possible metabolic pathways are not known.

5.3 Preclinical safety data
No further relevant data.

6. PHARMACEUTICAL PARTICULARS

6.1 List of excipients
Other ingredients: desoxycholic acid, phosphoric acid, sodium hydroxide, sodium phosphate, water.

6.2 Incompatibilities
None known.

6.3 Shelf life
24 months

6.4 Special precautions for storage
Vials of powder for reconstitution should be stored in a refrigerator. The concentrate (5mg per ml after reconstitution with 10ml sterile Water for Injections) should be stored protected from light. The absence of any microbial preservative and the risk of contamination during reconstitution mean that the product should be stored for no more than 8 hours at room temperature (25°C) or 24 hours in a refrigerator (2-8°C). Should the need arise and a validated aseptic reconstitution technique is applied, the product is chemically stable when stored for 24 hours at room temperature or one week in a refrigerator. It is not intended as a multidose vial. Any unused material should be discarded. Solutions prepared for intravenous infusion (i.e. 10mg or less amphotericin per 100ml) should be used promptly after preparation.

6.5 Nature and contents of container
Amber glass vials closed with a grey butyl rubber stopper. Vials of 50mg

6.6 Instructions for use and handling
See Section 4.2. Aseptic technique must be strictly observed during the preparation of the concentrate, the buffer and the infusion.

7. MARKETING AUTHORISATION HOLDER
E. R. Squibb & Sons Limited

Uxbridge Business Park

Sanderson Road

Uxbridge

Middlesex UB8 1DH

8. MARKETING AUTHORISATION NUMBER(S)
PL 0034/5041R

9. DATE OF FIRST AUTHORISATION/RENEWAL OF THE AUTHORISATION
21 March 1991

10. DATE OF REVISION OF THE TEXT
24 June 2005

Furosemide Injection BP Minijet

(International Medication Systems (UK) Ltd)

1. NAME OF THE MEDICINAL PRODUCT
Furosemide (Frusemide) Injection BP Minijet. 10mg/ml. Solution for Injection.

2. QUALITATIVE AND QUANTITATIVE COMPOSITION
Furosemide (Frusemide) 10mg per ml. 80mg per vial.

For excipients see section 6.1.

3. PHARMACEUTICAL FORM
Solution for Injection.

Sterile aqueous solution for intravenous or intramuscular administration.

4. CLINICAL PARTICULARS

4.1 Therapeutic indications
Conditions requiring prompt diuresis, where oral therapy is precluded.

Indications include oedema of cardiac, pulmonary, hepatic or renal origin, forced diuresis and severe hypercalcaemia.

4.2 Posology and method of administration
Parenteral administration should be replaced with oral therapy as soon as possible.

The intravenous injection should be given slowly (maximum 4mg/minute). Usually a prompt diuresis ensues.

Adults:

Acute pulmonary oedema: 40mg should be given immediately by slow intravenous injection, followed by further doses depending upon the patient's response. If there is no satisfactory response within 1 hour, 80mg may be given slowly intravenously.

Oedema: The usual initial dose of furosemide is 20 to 40mg given as a single dose, injected intravenously or intramuscularly.

If the diuretic response with a single dose of 20 to 40mg is not satisfactory, the dose may be increased in 20mg increments at 2 hourly intervals until the desired diuretic effect is obtained.

Very high doses may be required in patients with renal failure (see below).

Hypercalcaemia: Doses ranging from 20-240mg daily have been used. The aim is to increase diuresis to about 6 litres daily.

Forced diuresis: intravenous isotonic fluid at the rate of 500ml/hour is administered together with repeated doses of 20-80mg furosemide to produce a diuresis of 11-12 litres daily.

Acute or chronic renal failure: To avoid ototoxicity furosemide should be administered by intravenous infusion at a rate not exceeding 4mg/minute. The recommended initial dose in patients with acute or chronic renal failure is 25ml (250mg), diluted in approximately 225ml Sodium Chloride Injection BP or Ringer's Solution for Injection, administered over one hour. This gives an approximate drip rate of 80 drops/minute ensuring that the infusion is at the rate of 4mg/minute.

If a satisfactory increase in urine output, such as 40-50ml/hour, is not attained within the next hour, a second infusion of 50ml (500mg) in an appropriate infusion fluid should be given over 2 hours, the total volume of the infusion being governed by the patient's state of hydration. If a satisfactory output is still not achieved within one hour of the end of the second infusion, a third infusion of 100ml (1000mg) can be given over 4 hours. If the third infusion is not effective, then dialysis will probably be required.

In oliguric or anuric patients with significant fluid overload it may not be practicable to administer high dose furosemide by the above method. Under these circumstances the use of a constant rate infusion pump with micrometer screw-gauge adjustment may be considered for direct administration of the injection into the vein.

If the furosemide infusion produces a satisfactory response of 40-50ml/hour, the effective dose (up to 1000mg) can be repeated every 24 hours. Alternatively maintenance therapy can be continued with oral furosemide. Approximate dosage adjustments may then be made according to the observed clinical response.

Elderly: As for adults; the dose should be kept as low as possible.

Children: The usual initial dose is 0.5-1.5mg/kg up to 20mg/day. If the diuretic response after the initial dose is not satisfactory, the dose may be increased by 1mg/kg at 2 hourly intervals until the desired effect has been obtained. Doses greater than 6mg/kg are not recommended. For maintenance therapy, the dosage should be adjusted to the minimum effective level.

4.3 Contraindications
Furosemide is contra-indicated in women of child-bearing potential because animal reproductive studies have shown that it may cause foetal abnormalities. Exceptions to the above are life-threatening situations where the use of a diuretic such as furosemide is especially indicated as opposed to the use of alternative drugs. The physician of course should balance this efficacy potential against teratogenic and embryotoxic potential demonstrated to occur in animal studies.

Furosemide is contraindicated in patients with known hypersensitivity to the drug or to sulphonamides, renal failure associated with anuria or hepatic coma and in the presence of severe sodium and fluid depletion.

4.4 Special warnings and special precautions for use
Fluid balance should be carefully monitored. Furosemide may cause profound diuresis, resulting in fluid and electrolyte depletion. Serum electrolytes (especially sodium, potassium, chloride and bicarbonate) should be determined, and abnormalities corrected or the drug withdrawn. If increasing azotemia and oliguria occur during the treatment of progressive renal disease, the drug should be discontinued.

Initiation of furosemide therapy in patients with hepatic cirrhosis and ascites is best carried out in hospital. Sudden alteration of fluid and electrolyte balance in patients with cirrhosis may precipitate hepatic coma, therefore strict observation is necessary during the period of diuresis.

Patients should be regularly observed for the possible occurrence of blood dyscrasias, liver damage or other idiosyncratic reactions.

Periodic checks on urine and blood glucose should be made in diabetics and those suspected of latent diabetes when receiving furosemide. Increases in blood glucose and alterations in glucose tolerance test, with abnormalities of the fasting and 2-hour post-prandial sugar have been observed and rare cases of precipitation of diabetes mellitus have been reported.

Furosemide may lower serum calcium levels and rare cases of tetany have been reported. Accordingly, calcium should be determined periodically.

Patients with prostatic hypertrophy or impaired micturition have an increased risk of developing acute retention.

Care is advised when prescribing Furosemide to patients with either gout or porphyria.

4.5 Interaction with other medicinal products and other forms of Interaction
Furosemide -induced hypokalaemia may induce potentially fatal cardiac arrhythmias during treatment with cardiac glycosides. Furosemide may increase the ototoxicity of aminoglycoside antibiotics. Furosemide may enhance the nephrotoxicity of cephalosporins. Due to diuretic-induced sodium depletion, renal clearance of lithium is reduced, which may result in increased lithium concentrations leading to lithium toxicity. Fluid retention caused by steroids may potentially antagonise the diuretic effect but potentiate the potassium loss. In oedematous hypertensive patients being treated with antihypertensive agents, care should be taken to reduce the dose of these drugs since furosemide potentiates the hypotensive effect.

Severe hypotension and/or renal failure may occur if treatment with angiotensin-coverting enzyme-inhibitors is initiated while patients are receiving high doses of loop diuretics. The dose of furosemide should be reduced and severe salt and water depletion corrected before starting the ACE-inhibitor.

Sulphonamide diuretics have been reported to decrease arterial responsiveness to pressor amines and to enhance the effect of tubocurarine. Great caution should be exercised in administering curare or its derivatives to patients undergoing therapy with furosemide and it is advisable to discontinue furosemide two days before elective surgery.

Non-steroidal anti-inflammatory drugs may partially antagonise the action of furosemide. Because of competition for renal excretion, patients receiving high doses of salicylates together with furosemide may experience salicylate toxicity.

The following drugs have been reported to result in a disturbance in the electrolyte balance if given concurrently with furosemide: hormone antagonists, sympathetomimetics, carbamazepine, ulcer healing drugs e.g. carbenoxolone and metalozone.

Estrogens, antiepileptics, probenicid and lipid lowering resins may result in reduction in the diuretic effects of furosemide if administered concurrently.

Flushing, tachycardia, elevated blood pressure and severe diaphoresis have been seen in patients receiving intravenous furosemide having taken oral chloral hydrate in the preceding 24 hours.

Concurrent administration of furosemide and clofibrate may result in marked diuresis and muscle symptoms in patients with marked nephrotic syndrome.

The muscle relaxants baclofen and tizanidine may increase the hypotensive effect of furosemide.

4.6 Pregnancy and lactation
Animal teratology studies indicate that furosemide may cause foetal abnormalities. Therefore, furosemide should only be used in women of child-bearing age when

appropriate contraceptive measures are taken or if the potential benefits justify the potential risks to the foetus.

Furosemide is excreted in breast milk and breast-feeding should be discontinued if treatment is essential.

4.7 Effects on ability to drive and use machines
Furosemide may reduce mental alertness. Patients should be warned not to drive or operate machinery if affected.

4.8 Undesirable effects
Excessive diuresis may result in dehydration and reduction in blood volume, with circulatory collapse and with the possibility of vascular thrombosis and embolism, particularly in elderly patients. Serious depletion of potassium and magnesium may lead to cardiac arrhythmias.

Electrolyte depletion may manifest itself by weakness, fatigue, light-headedness or dizziness, muscle cramps, thirst, increased perspiration, urinary bladder spasm and symptoms of urinary frequency.

Transient pain after intramuscular injection has been reported at the injection site. Thrombophlebitis has occurred with intravenous administration.

Various forms of dermatitis, including urticaria and rare cases of exfoliative dermatitis, erythema multiforme, pruritus, paraesthesia, blurring of vision, postural hypotension, nausea, vomiting or diarrhoea, photosensitivity, or hypersensitivity reactions, including vasculitis/arteritis may occur. Anaemia, leucopenia, aplastic anaemia and thrombocytopenia (with purpura) may occur. Very rarely, agranulocytosis has occurred which has responded to treatment. If a rash or thrombocytopenia occur, furosemide should be stopped immediately.

Cases of tinnitus and reversible hearing impairment have been reported. There have also been some reports of cases in which hearing impairment was irreversible. Usually ototoxicity is associated with rapid injection in patients with severe renal impairment at doses several times more than the usual recommended dose and in whom other drugs of known ototoxicity were given.

Acute diuresis in male patients with prostatic obstruction may cause acute retention of urine.

In addition, the following rare adverse events have been reported although the relationship to the drug has not been confirmed: sweet taste, oral and gastric burning, paradoxical swelling, headache, jaundice and acute pancreatitis.

In children, complaints of mild to moderate abdominal pain and cramping have been reported after intravenous furosemide. Nephrocalcaemia has been reported in premature infants.

Asymptomatic hyperuricaemia can occur and rarely gout may be precipitated. These are associated with dehydration which should be avoided particularly in patients with renal insufficiency.

4.9 Overdose
Symptoms: Overdose with furosemide may lead to excessive loss of water and electrolytes. Severe potassium loss may cause serious cardiac arrhythmias.

Treatment: Restoration of fluid and electrolytes balance by administration of sodium chloride and water, intravenously if necessary.

5. PHARMACOLOGICAL PROPERTIES
5.1 Pharmacodynamic properties
Furosemide is a short-acting sulphonamide diuretic, chemically similar to the thiazides. With parenteral administration, the diuretic effect is immediate and lasts approximately two hours. Furosemide primarily inhibits the reabsorption of sodium in the proximal and distal tubules as well as in the Loop of Henle, thus increasing the urinary excretion of sodium, chloride and water. Urinary excretion of potassium, calcium and magnesium are also increased, together with bicarbonate; urinary pH rises.

5.2 Pharmacokinetic properties
Furosemide is 91% to 99% bound to serum albumin but protein binding is reduced in patients with uraemia and nephrosis. The plasma half life ranges from 45 to 60 minutes. Furosemide crosses the placenta and enters breast milk. It is eliminated by renal excretion of unchanged drug, metabolism to a glucuronide conjugate and faecal excretion.

5.3 Preclinical safety data
Toxicity studies in animals have not demonstrated toxic effects relevant to clinical use. There is no evidence of mutagenic or carcinogenic potential.

6. PHARMACEUTICAL PARTICULARS
6.1 List of excipients
Sodium Hydroxide

Sodium Chloride

Water for Injections

6.2 Incompatibilities
Furosemide is soluble in alkaline solutions. The injection is a mildly buffered alkaline solution which should not be mixed with highly acidic solutions.

6.3 Shelf life
36 months.

6.4 Special precautions for storage
Do not store above 25°C.

6.5 Nature and contents of container
The solution is contained in a USP type I glass vial with an elastomeric closure which meets all the relevant USP specifications. The product is available as 8ml.

6.6 Instructions for use and handling
The container is specially designed for use with the IMS Minijet injector.

7. MARKETING AUTHORISATION HOLDER
International Medication Systems (UK) Limited

208 Bath Road

Slough

Berkshire

SL1 3WE

UK

8. MARKETING AUTHORISATION NUMBER(S)
PL 03265/0025

9. DATE OF FIRST AUTHORISATION/RENEWAL OF THE AUTHORISATION
28 June 2003

10. DATE OF REVISION OF THE TEXT
January 2004

POM

Fuzeon

(Roche Products Limited)

1. NAME OF THE MEDICINAL PRODUCT
Fuzeon®▼ 90 mg/ ml powder and solvent for solution for injection

2. QUALITATIVE AND QUANTITATIVE COMPOSITION
Each vial contains 108 mg enfuvirtide. 1 ml of reconstituted solution contains 90 mg enfuvirtide.

For excipients, see section 6.1.

3. PHARMACEUTICAL FORM
Powder and solvent for solution for injection.

Fuzeon is a white to off-white lyophilised powder.

4. CLINICAL PARTICULARS
4.1 Therapeutic indications
Fuzeon is indicated in combination with other antiretroviral medicinal products for the treatment of HIV-1 infected patients who have received treatment with and failed on regimens containing at least one medicinal product from each of the following antiretroviral classes, protease inhibitors, non-nucleoside reverse transcriptase inhibitors and nucleoside reverse transcriptase inhibitors, or who have intolerance to previous antiretroviral regimens. (See section 5.1)

In deciding on a new regimen for patients who have failed an antiretroviral regimen, careful consideration should be given to the treatment history of the individual patient and the patterns of mutations associated with different medicinal products. Where available, resistance testing may be appropriate. (See sections 4.4 and 5.1)

4.2 Posology and method of administration
Fuzeon should be prescribed by physicians who are experienced in the treatment of HIV infection.

Fuzeon is only to be administered by subcutaneous injection.

Adults and adolescents ⩾ 16 years: The recommended dose of Fuzeon is 90 mg twice daily injected subcutaneously into the upper arm, anterior thigh or abdomen.

Elderly: There is no experience in patients > 65 years old.

Children ⩾ 6 years and adolescents: The experience is based on a very limited number of children. (See section 5.2). In ongoing clinical trials the dosage regimen in Table 1 below is being used.

Table 1: Paediatric Dosing

Weight (kg)	Dose per bid Injection (mg/ dose)	Injection Volume (90 mg enfuvirtide per ml)
11.0 to 15.5	27	0.3 ml
15.6 to 20.0	36	0.4 ml
20.1 to 24.5	45	0.5 ml
24.6 to 29.0	54	0.6 ml
29.1 to 33.5	63	0.7 ml
33.6 to 38.0	72	0.8 ml
38.1 to 42.5	81	0.9 ml
⩾42.6	90	1.0 ml

No data are available to establish dose recommendations of Fuzeon in children below the age of 6 years.

Renal impairment: No dose adjustment is required for patients with creatinine clearance above 35 ml/min. No data are available to establish a dose recommendation for patients with creatinine clearance below 35 ml/min or those receiving dialysis. (See sections 4.4 and 5.2)

Hepatic Impairment: No data are available to establish a dose recommendation for patients with hepatic impairment. (See sections 4.4 and 5.2)

4.3 Contraindications
Systemic hypersensitivity reactions to the active substance or to any of the excipients.

4.4 Special warnings and special precautions for use
Fuzeon must be taken as part of a combination regimen. Please also refer to the respective summary of product characteristics of the other antiretroviral medicinal products used in the combination. As with other antiretrovirals, enfuvirtide should optimally be combined with other antiretrovirals to which the patient's virus is sensitive. (See section 5.1)

Patients must be advised that antiretroviral therapies including enfuvirtide have not been proved to prevent the risk of transmission of HIV to others through sexual contact or blood contamination. They must continue to use appropriate precautions. Patients should also be informed that Fuzeon is not a cure for HIV-1 infection.

An increased rate of some bacterial infections, most notably a higher rate of pneumonia, has been seen in patients treated with Fuzeon. Patients should be monitored closely for signs and symptoms of pneumonia. (See section 4.8)

Hypersensitivity reactions have occasionally been associated with therapy with enfuvirtide and in rare cases hypersensitivity reactions have recurred on rechallenge. Events included rash, fever, nausea and vomiting, chills, rigors, low blood pressure and elevated serum liver transaminases in various combinations, and possibly primary immune complex reaction, respiratory distress and glomerulonephritis. Patients developing signs/symptoms of a systemic hypersensitivity reaction should discontinue enfuvirtide treatment and should seek medical evaluation immediately. Therapy with enfuvirtide should not be restarted following systemic signs and symptoms consistent with a hypersensitivity reaction considered related to enfuvirtide. Risk factors that may predict the occurrence or severity of hypersensitivity to enfuvirtide have not been identified.

Liver Disease: The safety and efficacy of enfuvirtide has not been specifically studied in patients with significant underlying liver disorders. Patients with chronic hepatitis B and C and treated with antiretroviral therapy are at an increased risk for severe and potentially fatal hepatic adverse events. Few patients included in the phase III trials were co-infected with hepatitis B/C. In these the addition of Fuzeon did not increase the incidence of hepatic events. In case of concomitant antiviral therapy for hepatitis B or C, please refer also to the relevant product information for these medicinal products.

Administration of Fuzeon to non-HIV-1 infected individuals may induce anti-enfuvirtide antibodies that cross-react with HIV gp41. This may result in a false positive HIV test with the anti-HIV ELISA test.

There is no experience in patients with reduced hepatic function or in patients with severe renal impairment and only limited data in patients with moderate renal impairment. Fuzeon should be used with caution in these populations. (See sections 4.2 and 5.2)

Immune Reactivation Syndrome: In HIV-infected patients with severe immune deficiency at the time of institution of combination antiretroviral therapy (CART), an inflammatory reaction to asymptomatic or residual opportunistic pathogens may arise and cause serious clinical conditions, or aggravation of symptoms. Typically, such reactions have been observed within the first few weeks or months of initiation of CART. Relevant examples are cytomegalovirus retinitis, generalised and/or focal mycobacterial infections, and Pneumocystis carinii pneumonia. Any inflammatory symptoms should be evaluated and treatment instituted when necessary.

4.5 Interaction with other medicinal products and other forms of Interaction
No clinically significant pharmacokinetic interactions are expected between enfuvirtide and concomitantly given medicinal products metabolised by CYP450 enzymes.

Influence of Enfuvirtide on Metabolism of Concomitant Medicinal Products: In an in-vivo human metabolism study enfuvirtide, at the recommended dose of 90 mg twice daily, did not inhibit the metabolism of substrates by CYP3A4 (dapsone), CYP2D6 (debrisoquine), CYP1A2 (caffeine), CYP2C19 (mephenytoin), and CYP2E1 (chlorzoxazone).

Influence of Concomitant Medicinal Products on Enfuvirtide Metabolism: In separate pharmacokinetic interaction studies, co-administration of ritonavir (potent CYP3A4 inhibitor) or saquinavir in combination with a booster dose of ritonavir or rifampicin (potent CYP34A inducer) did not result in clinically significant changes of the pharmacokinetics of enfuvirtide.

Table 2 Summary of Individual Signs/Symptoms Characterising Local Injection Site Reactions in studies TORO 1 and TORO 2 combined (% of patients)

	n=663		
Withdrawal Rate due to ISRs	4%		
Event Category	**FUZEON +Optimised background**[a]	**% of Event comprising Grade 3 reactions**	**% of Event comprising Grade 4 reactions**
Pain / discomfort	96.1%	11.0%[b]	0%[b]
Erythema	90.8%	23.8%[c]	10.5%[c]
Induration	90.2%	43.5%[d]	19.4%[d]
Nodules and cysts	80.4%	29.1%[e]	0.2%[e]
Pruritus	65.2%	3.9%[f]	NA
Ecchymosis	51.9%	8.7%[g]	4.7%[g]

[a]Any severity grade.

[b]Grade 3= severe pain requiring analgesics (or narcotic analgesics for ⩽ 72 hours) and/or limiting usual activities; Grade 4= severe pain requiring hospitalisation or prolongation of hospitalisation, resulting in death, or persistent or significant disability/incapacity, or life-threatening, or medically significant.

[c]Grade 3= ⩾ 50 mm but < 85 mm average diameter; Grade 4= ⩾ 85 mm average diameter.

[d]Grade 3= ⩾ 25 mm but < 50 mm average diameter; Grade 4= ⩾ 50 mm average diameter.

[e]Grade 3= ⩾ 3 cm; Grade 4= If draining.

[f]Grade 3= refractory to topical treatment or requiring oral or parenteral treatment; Grade 4= not defined.

[g]Grade 3= > 3 cm but ⩽ 5 cm; Grade 4= > 5 cm.

4.6 Pregnancy and lactation

There are no adequate and well-controlled studies in pregnant women. Animal studies do not indicate harmful effects with respect to foetal development. Enfuvirtide should be used during pregnancy only if the potential benefit justifies the potential risk to the foetus.

It is not known whether enfuvirtide is secreted in human milk. Mothers should be instructed not to breast-feed if they are receiving enfuvirtide because of the potential for HIV transmission and any possible undesirable effects in breast-fed infants.

4.7 Effects on ability to drive and use machines

No studies on the effects on ability to drive and use machines have been performed. There is no evidence that enfuvirtide may alter the patient's ability to drive and use machines, however, the adverse event profile of enfuvirtide should be taken into account. (See section 4.8)

4.8 Undesirable effects

Safety data mainly refer to 48-week data from studies TORO 1 and TORO 2 combined (see section 5.1). Safety results are expressed as the number of patients with an adverse event per 100 patient-years of exposure (except for injection site reactions).

Injection site reactions

Injection site reactions (ISRs) were the most frequently reported adverse reaction and occurred in 98% of the patients (Table 2). The vast majority of ISRs occurred within the first week of Fuzeon administration and were associated with mild to moderate pain or discomfort at the injection site without limitation of usual activities. The severity of the pain and discomfort did not increase with treatment duration. The signs and symptoms generally lasted equal to or less than 7 days. Infections at the injection site (including abscess and cellulitis) occurred in 1.5% of patients.

Table 2: Summary of Individual Signs/Symptoms Characterising Local Injection Site Reactions in studies TORO 1 and TORO 2 combined (% of patients)

(see Table 2 above)

Other adverse reactions

The addition of Fuzeon to background antiretroviral therapy generally did not increase the frequency or severity of most adverse events. The most frequently reported events occurring in the TORO 1 and TORO 2 studies were diarrhoea (38 versus 73 patients with event per 100 patient years for Fuzeon + OB versus OB) and nausea (27 versus 50 patients with event per 100 patient years for Fuzeon + OB versus OB).

The following list presents events seen at a higher rate among patients receiving Fuzeon+OB regimen than among patients on the OB alone regimen with an exposure adjusted increase of at least 2 patients with event per 100 patient-years. These events are then designated frequency estimation ("very common" or "common"). A statistically significant increase was seen for pneumonia and lymphadenopathy. Most adverse events were of mild or moderate intensity.

Infections and Infestations

Common (>1/100, <1/10): - sinusitis, skin papilloma, influenza, pneumonia, ear infection.

Blood and Lymphatic System Disorders

Common (>1/100, <1/10): - lymphadenopathy.

Metabolism and Nutrition Disorders

Common (>1/100, <1/10): - appetite decreased, anorexia, hypertriglyceridaemia, diabetes mellitus.

Psychiatric Disorders

Common (>1/100, <1/10): - anxiety, nightmare, irritability.

Nervous System Disorders

Very Common (>1/10): - peripheral neuropathy.

Common (>1/100, <1/10): -hypoaesthesia, disturbance in attention, tremor.

Eye Disorders

Common (>1/100, <1/10): - conjunctivitis.

Ear and Labyrinth disorders

Common (>1/100, <1/10): - vertigo.

Respiratory, Thoracic and Mediastinal Disorders

Common (>1/100, <1/10): - nasal congestion.

Gastrointestinal Disorders

Common (>1/100, <1/10): - pancreatitis, gastro-oesophageal reflux disease.

Skin and Subcutaneous Tissue Disorders

Common (>1/100, <1/10): - dry skin, eczema seborrhoeic, erythema, acne.

Musculoskeletal, Connective Tissue and Bone Disorders

Common (>1/100, <1/10): - myalgia.

Renal and Urinary Disorders

Common (>1/100, <1/10): - calculus renal.

General Disorders and Administration Site Conditions

Common (>1/100, <1/10): - influenza like illness, weakness.

Investigations

Very Common (>1/10): - weight decreased.

Common (>1/100, <1/10): - blood triglycerides increased, haematuria present.

In addition there have been a small number of hypersensitivity reactions attributed to enfuvirtide and in some cases recurrence has occurred upon re-challenge. (See section 4.4).

In HIV-infected patients with severe immune deficiency at the time of initiation of combination antiretroviral therapy (CART), an inflammatory reaction to asymptomatic or residual opportunistic infections may arise (see section 4.4).

Laboratory abnormalities

The majority of patients had no change in the toxicity grade of any laboratory parameter during the study except for those listed in Table 3. Through week 48, eosinophilia [greater than the Upper Limit of Normal of $> 0.7 \times 10^9$/l] occurred at a higher rate amongst patients in the Fuzeon containing group (12.4 patients with event per 100 patient-years) compared with OB alone regimen (5.6 patients with event per 100 patient-years). When using a higher threshold for eosinophilia ($>1.4 \times 10^9$/l), the patient exposure adjusted rate of eosinophilia is equal in both groups (1.8 patients with event per 100 patient-years).

Table 3: Exposure adjusted Grade 3 & 4 laboratory abnormalities among patients on Fuzeon+OB and OB alone regimens, reported at more than 2 patients with event per 100 patient years

Laboratory Parameters Grading	**Fuzeon+OB regimen Per 100 patient years**	**OB alone regimen Per 100 patient years**
N (Total Exposure patient years)	**663 (557.0)**	**334 (162.1)**
ALAT		
Gr. 3 (>5-10 × ULN)	4.8	4.3
Gr. 4 (>10 × ULN)	1.4	1.2
Haemoglobin		
Gr. 3 (6.5-7.9 g/dL)	2.0	1.9
Gr. 4 (<6.5 g/dL)	0.7	1.2
Creatinine phosphokinase		
Gr. 3 (>5-10 × ULN)	8.3	8.0
Gr. 4 (>10 × ULN)	3.1	8.6

4.9 Overdose

No case of overdose has been reported. The highest dose administered to 12 patients in a clinical trial was 180 mg as a single dose subcutaneously. These patients did not experience any adverse events that were not seen with the recommended dose. In an Early Access Program study, one patient administered 180 mg of Fuzeon as a single dose on one occasion. He did not experience an adverse event as a result.

There is no specific antidote for overdose with enfuvirtide. Treatment of overdose should consist of general supportive measures.

5. PHARMACOLOGICAL PROPERTIES

5.1 Pharmacodynamic properties

Pharmacotherapeutic group: Antivirals for systemic use, other antivirals.

ATC code: J05A X07.

Mechanism of Action: Enfuvirtide is a member of the therapeutic class called fusion inhibitors. It is an inhibitor of the structural rearrangement of HIV-1 gp41 and functions by specifically binding to this virus protein extracellularly thereby blocking fusion between the viral cell membrane and the target cell membrane, preventing the viral RNA from entering into the target cell.

Antiviral activity *in vitro*: The susceptibility to enfuvirtide of 612 HIV recombinants containing the env genes from HIV RNA samples taken at baseline from patients in Phase III studies gave a geometric mean EC_{50} of 0.259 µg/ml (geometric mean + 2SD = 1.96 µg/ml) in a recombinant phenotype HIV entry assay. Enfuvirtide also inhibited HIV-1 envelope mediated cell-cell fusion. Combination studies of enfuvirtide with representative members of the various antiretroviral classes exhibited additive to synergistic antiviral activities and an absence of antagonism. The relationship between the *in vitro* susceptibility of HIV-1 to enfuvirtide and inhibition of HIV-1 replication in humans has not been established.

Antiretroviral drug resistance: Incomplete viral suppression may lead to the development of drug resistance to one or more components of the regimen.

In Vitro resistance to enfuvirtide: HIV-1 isolates with reduced susceptibility to enfuvirtide have been selected *in vitro* which harbour substitutions in amino acids (aa) 36-38 of the gp41 ectodomain. These substitutions were correlated with varying levels of reduced enfuvirtide susceptibility in HIV site-directed mutants.

In Vivo resistance to enfuvirtide: In phase III clinical studies HIV recombinants containing the env genes from HIV RNA samples taken up to week 24 from 187 patients showed > 4 fold reduced susceptibility to enfuvirtide compared with the corresponding pre-treatment samples. Of these, 185 (98.9%) env genes carried specific substitutions in region of aa 36 - 45 of gp41. The substitutions observed in decreasing frequency were at aa positions 38, 43, 36, 40, 42 and 45. Specific single substitutions at these residues in gp41 each resulted in a range of decreases from baseline in recombinant viral susceptibility to enfuvirtide. The geometric mean changes ranged from 15.2 fold for V38M to 41.6 fold for V38A. There were insufficient examples of multiple substitutions to determine any consistent patterns of substitutions or their effect on viral susceptibility to enfuvirtide. The relationship of these substitutions to *in vivo* effectiveness of enfuvirtide has not been established. Decrease in viral sensitivity was correlated to the degree of pre-treatment resistance to background therapy. (See Table 5)

Table 4 Outcomes of Randomised Treatment at Week 48 (Pooled Studies TORO 1 and TORO 2, ITT)

Outcomes	FUZEON +OB 90 mg bid (N=661)	OB (N=334)	Treatment Difference	95% Confidence Interval	p-value
HIV-1 RNA Log Change from baseline (log_{10} copies/ml)*	-1.48	-0.63	LSM -0.85	-1.073, -0.628	<.0001
CD4+ cell count Change from baseline ($cells/mm^3$)#	+91	+45	LSM 46.4	25.1, 67.8	<.0001
HIV RNA ⩾1 log below Baseline**	247 (37.4%)	57 (17.1%)	Odds Ratio 3.02	2.16, 4.20	<.0001
HIV RNA <400 copies/ml**	201 (30.4%)	40 (12.0%)	Odds Ratio 3.45	2.36, 5.06	<.0001
HIV RNA <50 copies/ml**	121 (18.3%)	26 (7.8%)	Odds Ratio 2.77	1.76, 4.37	<.0001
Discontinued due to adverse reactions/intercurrent illness/ labs†	9%	11%			
Discontinued due to injection site reactions†	4%	N/A			
Discontinued due to other reasons† φ §	13%	25%			

* Based on results from pooled data of TORO 1 and TORO 2 on ITT population, week 48 viral load for subjects who were lost to follow-up, discontinued therapy, or had virological failure replaced by their last observation (LOCF).

\# Last value carried forward.

** M-H test: Discontinuations or virological failure considered as failures.

† Percentages based on safety population Fuzeon+background (N=663) and background (N=334). Denominator for non-switch patients: N=112.

φ As per the judgment of the investigator.

§ Includes discontinuations from loss to follow-up, treatment refusal, and other reasons.

Cross-resistance: Due to its novel viral target enfuvirtide is equally active *in vitro* against both wild-type laboratory and clinical isolates and those with resistance to 1, 2 or 3 other classes of antiretrovirals (nucleoside reverse transcriptase inhibitors, non-nucleoside reverse transcriptase inhibitors and protease inhibitors). Conversely, mutations in aa 36-45 of gp41 which give resistance to enfuvirtide would not be expected to give cross resistance to other classes of antiretrovirals.

Clinical Pharmacodynamic data

Studies in Antiretroviral Experienced Patients: The clinical activity of Fuzeon (in combination with other antiretroviral agents) on plasma HIV RNA levels and CD4 counts have been investigated in two randomised, multicentre, controlled studies (TORO 1 and TORO 2) of Fuzeon of 48 weeks duration. 995 patients comprised the intent-to-treat population. Patient demographics include a median baseline HIV-1 RNA of 5.2 log_{10} copies/ml and 5.1 log_{10} copies/ml and median baseline CD4 cell count of 88 $cells/mm^3$ and 97 $cells/mm^3$ for Fuzeon + OB and OB, respectively. Patients had prior exposure to a median of 12 antiretrovirals for a median of 7 years. All patients received an optimised background (OB) regimen consisting of 3 to 5 antiretroviral agents selected on the basis of the patient's prior treatment history, as well as baseline genotypic and phenotypic viral resistance measurements.

The proportion of patients achieving viral load of <400 copies/ml at week 48 was 30.4% among patients on the Fuzeon+OB regimen compared to 12% among patients receiving OB regimen only. The mean CD4 cell count increase was greater in patients on the Fuzeon + OB regimen than in patients on OB regimen only. (see Table 4)

Table 4 Outcomes of Randomised Treatment at Week 48 (Pooled Studies TORO 1 and TORO 2, ITT)

(see Table 4 above)

Fuzeon+OB therapy was associated with a higher proportion of patients reaching < 400 copies/ml (or < 50 copies/ml) across all subgroups based on baseline CD4, baseline HIV-1 RNA, number of prior antiretrovirals (ARVs) or number of active ARVs in the OB regimen. However, subjects with baseline CD4 >100 $cells/mm^3$, baseline HIV-1 RNA < 5.0 log_{10} copies/ml, ⩽ 10 prior ARVs, and/or other active ARVs in their OB regimen were more likely to achieve a HIV-1 RNA of < 400 copies/ml (or < 50 copies/ml) on either treatment. (see Table 5)

Table 5 Proportion of Patients achieving < 400 copies/ml and < 50 copies/ml at Week 48 by subgroup (pooled TORO 1 and TORO 2, ITT)

Subgroups	HIV-1 RNA < 400 copies/ml		HIV-1 RNA < 50 copies/ml	
	FUZEON + OB 90 mg bid (N=661)	OB (N=334)	FUZEON + OB 90 mg bid (N=661)	OB (N=334)
BL HIV-1 RNA < 5.0 log_{10}[1] copies/ml	118/269 (43.9%)	26/144 (18.1%)	77/269 (28.6%)	18/144 (12.5%)
BL HIV-1 RNA ⩾ 5.0 log_{10}[1] copies/ml	83/392 (21.2%)	14/190 (7.4%)	44/392 (11.2%)	8/190 (4.2%)
Total prior ARVs ⩽ 10^1	100/215 (46.5%)	29/120 (24.2%)	64/215 (29.8%)	19/120 (15.8%)
Total prior ARVs > 10^1	101/446 (22.6%)	11/214 (5.1%)	57/446 (12.8%)	7/214 (3.3%)
0 Active ARVs in background[1,2]	9/112 (8.0%)	0/53 (0%)	4/112 (3.5%)	0/53 (0%)
1 Active ARV in background[1,2]	56/194 (28.9%)	7/95 (7.4%)	34/194 (17.5%)	3/95 (3.2%)
⩾ 2 Active ARVs in background[1,2]	130/344 (37.8%)	32/183 (17.5%)	77/334 (22.4%)	22/183 (12.0%)

[1]Discontinuations or virological failures considered as failures.

[2]Based on GSS score.

Table 5 Proportion of Patients achieving < 400 copies/ml and < 50 copies/ml at Week 48 by subgroup (pooled TORO 1 and TORO 2, ITT)

(see Table 5 below)

5.2 Pharmacokinetic properties

The pharmacokinetic properties of enfuvirtide have been evaluated in HIV-1-infected adult and paediatric patients.

Absorption: The absolute bioavailability after subcutaneous administration of enfuvirtide 90 mg in the abdomen was 84.3 ± 15.5%. Mean (± SD) C_{max} was 4.59 ± 1.5 μg/ml, AUC was 55.8 ± 12.1 μg*hr/ml. The subcutaneous absorption of enfuvirtide is proportional to the administered dose over the 45 to 180 mg dose range. Subcutaneous absorption at the 90 mg dose is comparable when injected into abdomen, thigh or arm. In four separate studies (N = 9 to 12) the mean steady state trough plasma concentration ranged from 2.6 to 3.4 μg/ml.

Distribution: The steady state volume of distribution with intravenous administration of a 90 mg dose of enfuvirtide was 5.5 ± 1.1 l. Enfuvirtide is 92% bound to plasma proteins in HIV infected plasma over a plasma concentration range of 2 to 10 μg/ml. It is bound predominantly to albumin and to a lower extent to α-1 acid glycoprotein. In *in vitro* studies, enfuvirtide was not displaced from its binding sites by other medicinal products, nor did enfuvirtide displace other medicinal products from their binding sites.

Metabolism: As a peptide, enfuvirtide is expected to undergo catabolism to its constituent amino acids, with subsequent recycling of the amino acids in the body pool. *In vitro* human microsomal studies and in *in vivo* studies indicate that enfuvirtide is not an inhibitor of CYP450 enzymes. In *in vitro* human microsomal and hepatocyte studies, hydrolysis of the amide group of the C-terminus amino acid, phenylalanine results in a deamidated metabolite and the formation of this metabolite is not NADPH dependent. This metabolite is detected in human plasma following administration of enfuvirtide, with an AUC ranging from 2.4 to 15% of the enfuvirtide AUC.

Elimination: Clearance of enfuvirtide after intravenous administration 90 mg was 1.4 ± 0.28 l/h and the elimination half-life was 3.2 ± 0.42 h. Following a 90 mg subcutaneous dose of enfuvirtide the half-life of enfuvirtide is 3.8 ± 0.6 h. Mass balance studies to determine elimination pathway(s) of enfuvirtide have not been performed in humans.

Hepatic Insufficiency: The pharmacokinetics of enfuvirtide have not been studied in patients with hepatic impairment.

Renal Insufficiency: A specific pharmacokinetic study has not been conducted in patients with renal impairment or those receiving dialysis. However analysis of plasma concentration data from patients in clinical trials indicated that the clearance of enfuvirtide is not affected to any clinically relevant extent in patients with creatinine clearance above 35 ml/min.

Elderly: The pharmacokinetics of enfuvirtide have not been formally studied in elderly patients over 65 years of age.

Gender and Weight: Analysis of plasma concentration data from patients in clinical trials indicated that the clearance of enfuvirtide is 20% lower in females than males irrespective of weight and is increased with increased body weight irrespective of gender (20% higher in a 100 kg and 20% lower in a 40 kg body weight patient relative to a 70 kg reference patient). However, these changes are not clinically significant and no dose adjustment is required.

Race: Analysis of plasma concentration data from patients in clinical trials indicated that the clearance of enfuvirtide was not different in Blacks compared to Whites. Other PK studies suggest no difference between Asians and Whites after adjusting exposure for body weight.

Paediatric Patients: The pharmacokinetics of enfuvirtide have been studied in 37 paediatric patients. A dose of 2 mg/kg bid (maximum 90 mg bid) provided enfuvirtide plasma concentrations similar to those obtained in adult patients receiving 90 mg bid dosage. In 25 paediatric patients ranging in age from 5 to 16 years and receiving the 2 mg/kg bid dose into the upper arm, anterior thigh or abdomen, the mean steady-state AUC was 54.3 ± 23.5 μg*h/ml, C_{max} was 6.14 ± 2.48 μg/ml, and C_{trough} was 2.93 ± 1.55 μg/ml.

5.3 Preclinical safety data

Preclinical data reveal no special hazard for humans based on conventional studies of safety pharmacology, repeated dose toxicity, genotoxicity and late embryonal development. Long-term animal carcinogenicity studies have not been performed.

Studies in guinea pigs indicated a potential for enfuvirtide to produce delayed contact hypersensitivity. *In vitro* studies have shown that enfuvirtide may act as an agonist on the formyl peptide receptor, a receptor on leukocytes believed to be important for the early defense against infection. The clinical relevance of these findings is unknown.

6. PHARMACEUTICAL PARTICULARS

6.1 List of excipients

Powder

Sodium carbonate

Mannitol

Sodium hydroxide

Hydrochloric Acid

Solvent

Water for Injections

6.2 Incompatibilities
This medicinal product must not be mixed with other medicinal products except those mentioned in section 6.6.

6.3 Shelf life
Powder

3 years.

Solvent

3 years.

Shelf life after reconstitution

Chemical and physical in-use stability has been demonstrated for 48 hours at 5°C when protected from light.

From a microbiological point of view, the product should be used immediately. If not used immediately, in-use storage times and conditions prior to use are the responsibility of the user and would normally not be longer than 24 hours at 2°C to 8°C, unless reconstitution has taken place in controlled and validated aseptic conditions.

6.4 Special precautions for storage
Powder

This medicinal product does not require any special storage conditions.

After reconstitution: Store in a refrigerator (2°C - 8°C). Keep the vial in the outer carton in order to protect from light.

Solvent

This medicinal product does not require any special storage conditions.

6.5 Nature and contents of container
Powder

Vial: 3 ml vial, colourless glass type 1.

Closure: lyophilisate stopper, rubber (latex free).

Seal: aluminum seal with flip-off cap.

Solvent

Volume: 2 ml.

Vial: 2 ml vial, colourless glass type 1.

Closure: rubber stopper (latex free).

Seal: aluminum seal with flip-off cap.

Pack sizes

Pack 1

60 vials powder for solution for injection.

60 vials solvent.

60 3 ml syringes.

60 1 ml syringes.

180 alcohol swabs.

Pack 2

60 vials powder for solution for injection.

60 vials solvent.

6.6 Instructions for use and handling
Patients should be instructed on the use and administration of Fuzeon by a healthcare professional before using for the first time.

Fuzeon must only be reconstituted with 1.1 ml of Water for Injections. Patients must be instructed to add the water for injections and then gently tap the vial with their fingertip until the powder begins to dissolve. **They must never shake the vial or turn it upside down to mix—this will cause excessive foaming.** After the powder begins to dissolve they can set the vial aside to allow it to completely dissolve. The powder may take up to 45 minutes to dissolve into solution. The patient can gently roll the vial between their hands after adding the water for injections until it is fully dissolved and this may reduce the time it takes for the powder to dissolve. Before the solution is withdrawn for administration, the patient should inspect the vial visually to ensure that the contents are fully in solution, and that the solution is clear and without bubbles or particulate matter. If there is evidence of particulate matter, the vial must not be used and should be discarded or returned to the pharmacy.

The solvent vials contain 2 ml Water for Injections, of which 1.1 ml must be withdrawn for the reconstitution of the powder. Patients should be instructed to discard the remaining volume in the solvent vials.

Fuzeon contains no preservative. Once reconstituted, the solution should be injected immediately. If the reconstituted solution cannot be injected immediately, it must be kept refrigerated until use and used within 24 hours. Refrigerated reconstituted solution should be brought to room temperature before injection.

1 ml of the reconstituted solution should be injected subcutaneously in the upper arm, abdomen or anterior thigh. The injection should be given at a site different from the preceding injection site and where there is no current injection site reaction. A vial is suitable for single use only; unused portions must be discarded.

7. MARKETING AUTHORISATION HOLDER
Roche Registration Limited

40 Broadwater Road

Welwyn Garden City

Hertfordshire

AL7 3AY

United Kingdom

8. MARKETING AUTHORISATION NUMBER(S)
EU/1/03/252/001-002

9. DATE OF FIRST AUTHORISATION/RENEWAL OF THE AUTHORISATION
27.05.2003

10. DATE OF REVISION OF THE TEXT
April 2005

Gabitril 5mg, Gabitril 10mg, Gabitril 15mg

(Cephalon UK Limited)

1. NAME OF THE MEDICINAL PRODUCT

Gabitril 5 mg

Gabitril 10 mg

Gabitril 15 mg

2. QUALITATIVE AND QUANTITATIVE COMPOSITION

Each Gabitril 5 mg tablet contains:

Tiagabine anhydrous, INN 5 mg (as hydrochloride monohydrate)

Each Gabitril 10 mg tablet contains:

Tiagabine anhydrous, INN 10 mg (as hydrochloride monohydrate)

Each Gabitril 15 mg tablet contains

Tiagabine anhydrous, INN 15 mg (as hydrochloride monohydrate)

3. PHARMACEUTICAL FORM

White film-coated scored tablet for oral administration. Gabitril 5, 10 and 15 mg tablets are marked 251, 252 and 253 respectively.

4. CLINICAL PARTICULARS

4.1 Therapeutic indications

Gabitril is an antiepileptic drug indicated as add-on therapy for partial seizures with or without secondary generalisation where control is not achieved by optimal doses of at least one other antiepileptic drug.

4.2 Posology and method of administration

Adults and children over 12 years: Gabitril should be taken orally with meals. The initial dose for those taking enzyme-inducing antiepileptic drugs is 5 mg twice daily for one week followed by weekly increments of 5-10 mg/day.

The following titration schedule is suggested:

(see Table 1)

Table 1

Week	Breakfast	Evening meal	Total daily dose
1	5 mg	5 mg	10 mg
2	5 mg	10 mg	15 mg
3	10 mg	10 mg	20 mg
4	15 mg	15 mg	30 mg

The usual maintenance dose is 30-45 mg/day. Doses above 30 mg should be given in three divided doses.

The above regimen is appropriate for patients who are also taking other antiepileptic agents that induce hepatic enzymes (such as phenytoin, carbamazepine, phenobarbital and primidone); most patients in clinical trials of tiagabine were in this category.

In patients not taking enzyme-inducing drugs, the maintenance dosage initially should be lower at 15-30 mg/day. This is based on population kinetics analysis, which suggested that the clearance of tiagabine in non-induced patients is 60% of that in patients taking enzyme-inducing drugs.

Children under 12 years: There is no experience with Gabitril in children under 12 years of age and as such Gabitril should not be used in this age group.

Use in the elderly: There is limited information available on the use of Gabitril in elderly patients, but pharmacokinetics of tiagabine are unchanged, hence there should be no need for dose modification.

Use in patients with impaired liver function: In patients with mild to moderate hepatic dysfunction (Child Pugh Score 5 - 9) the initial daily maintenance dosage should be 5-10 mg given once or twice daily. Gabitril should not be used in patients with severely impaired hepatic function.

4.3 Contraindications

Gabitril should not be given to patients with a history of hypersensitivity to tiagabine or one of the excipients.

4.4 Special warnings and special precautions for use

Gabitril is eliminated by hepatic metabolism and therefore caution should be exercised when administering the product to patients with impaired hepatic function. Reduced doses and/or dose intervals should be used and patients should be monitored closely for adverse events such as dizziness and tiredness.

Gabitril should not be used in patients with severely impaired hepatic function.

Although Gabitril may slightly prolong the CNS depressant effect of triazolam, this interaction is unlikely to be relevant to clinical practice.

Antiepileptic agents that induce hepatic enzymes (such as phenytoin, carbamazepine, phenobarbital and primidone) enhance the metabolism of tiagabine. Consequently, patients not taking enzyme-inducing drugs may require doses below the usual dose range.

Although there is no evidence of withdrawal seizures following Gabitril, it is recommended to taper off treatment over a period of 2-3 weeks.

Spontaneous bruising has been reported. Therefore, if bruising is observed, full blood count including platelet count is to be performed.

Rare cases of visual field defects have been reported with tiagabine. If visual symptoms develop, the patient should be referred to an ophthalmologist for further evaluation including perimetry.

4.5 Interaction with other medicinal products and other forms of Interaction

Antiepileptic agents that induce hepatic enzymes (such as phenytoin, carbamazepine, phenobarbital and primidone) enhance the metabolism of tiagabine. The plasma concentration of tiagabine may be reduced by a factor of 1.5-3 by concomitant use of these drugs.

Gabitril does not have any clinically significant effect on the plasma concentrations of phenytoin, carbamazepine, phenobarbital, warfarin, digoxin, theophylline and hormones from oral contraceptive pills. Gabitril reduces the plasma concentration of valproate by about 10%, and cimetidine increases the bioavailability of tiagabine by about 5%. Neither of these findings are considered clinically important and do not warrant a dose modification.

4.6 Pregnancy and lactation

Animal experiments have not shown a teratogenic effect of tiagabine. Studies in animals have, however, revealed peri- and post-natal toxicity of tiagabine at very high doses.

Clinical experience of the use of Gabitril in pregnant women is limited.

No information on Gabitril during breast-feeding is available.

Consequently, as a precautionary measure, it is preferable not to use Gabitril during pregnancy or breast-feeding unless, in the opinion of the physician, the potential benefits of treatment outweigh the potential risks.

4.7 Effects on ability to drive and use machines

Gabitril may cause dizziness or other CNS related symptoms especially during initial treatment. Therefore caution should be shown by patients driving vehicles or operating machinery.

4.8 Undesirable effects

Adverse events are mainly CNS related.

In placebo controlled parallel group add-on epilepsy trials of Gabitril in combination with other antiepileptic drugs, the adverse events that occurred statistically more frequently with Gabitril than with placebo are tabulated below.

	Gabitril (n=493) %	Placebo (n=276) %
Dizziness	29	16
Tiredness	22	15
Nervousness (non-specific)	11	4
Tremor	10	4
Diarrhoea	8	3
Concentration difficulties	6	3
Depressed mood	4	1
Emotional lability	4	1
Slowness in speech	2	0

In clinical trials, about 15% of patients receiving Gabitril reported serious adverse events; the causal relationship of these events with Gabitril treatment has not been established and some may be associated with the underlying condition or concomitant treatment. Accidental injury (2.8%) was the only adverse event which occurred with a frequency of more than 1%; others included confusion (1.0%), depression (0.8%), somnolence (0.8%) and psychosis (0.7%). However, none of these adverse events led to the withdrawal of more than 0.2% of patients.

In patients with a history of serious behavioural problems there is a risk of recurrence of these symptoms during treatment with Gabitril, as occurs with certain other antiepileptic drugs.

Although not statistically significant, routine laboratory screening during placebo controlled trials showed a low white blood cell count ($<2.5 \times 10^9$ per litre) more frequently during Gabitril treatment (4.1%) than placebo (1.5%).

Rarely, cases of non-convulsive status epilepticus, hallucination and delusion have been reported.

Infrequent cases of bruising can occur.

Rare cases of visual field defects have been reported (see section 4.4 Special Warnings and Special Precautions for use).

4.9 Overdose

Reports on overdosage with Gabitril are few. Symptoms of overdosage are somnolence, dizziness, ataxia or incoordination and, in more severe instances, mute and withdrawn appearance of the patient, or risk of convulsion. In one patient an overdose of about 300 mg of Gabitril in combination with phenytoin resulted in coma. In all episodes of overdosage with Gabitril the patients have recovered within 24 hours without any sequelae.

Standard medical observation and supportive care should be given.

5. PHARMACOLOGICAL PROPERTIES

5.1 Pharmacodynamic properties

Gabitril is an antiepileptic drug.

Tiagabine is a potent and selective inhibitor of both neuronal and glial GABA uptake, which results in an increase in GABAergic mediated inhibition in the brain.

Tiagabine lacks significant affinity for other neurotransmitter receptor binding sites and/or uptake sites.

5.2 Pharmacokinetic properties

Tiagabine is rapidly and virtually completely absorbed from Gabitril tablets, with an absolute bioavailability of 89%. Administration with food results in a decreased rate and not extent of absorption.

The volume of distribution is approximately 1 L/kg.

Plasma protein binding of tiagabine is about 96%.

Renal clearance is negligible. Hepatic metabolism is the principal route for elimination of tiagabine. Less than 2% of the dose is excreted unchanged in urine and faeces. No active metabolites have been identified. Other antiepileptic drugs such as phenytoin, carbamazepine, phenobarbital and primidone induce hepatic drug metabolism and the hepatic clearance of tiagabine is increased when given concomitantly with these drugs.

There is no evidence that tiagabine causes clinically significant induction or inhibition of hepatic drug metabolising enzymes at clinical doses.

The plasma elimination half-life of tiagabine is 7-9 hours, except in induced patients where it is 2-3 hours.

Absorption and elimination of tiagabine are linear within the therapeutic dose range.

5.3 Preclinical safety data

Animal safety data carried out in the rat, mouse and dog gave no clear evidence of specific organ toxicity nor any findings of concern for the therapeutic use of tiagabine. The dog appears to be particularly sensitive to the pharmacological actions of tiagabine as clinical signs such as sedation, insensibility, ataxia and visual impairment reflecting CNS effects were seen at daily doses of 0.5 mg/kg and above in a dose related manner. The results of a wide range of mutagenicity tests showed that tiagabine is unlikely to be genotoxic to humans. Clastogenic activity was seen only at cytotoxic concentrations (>>200-fold human plasma levels) in the *in-vitro* human lymphocyte test in the absence of a metabolising system. In long-term carcinogenicity studies conducted in the rat and mouse, only the rat study revealed slightly increased incidences of hepatocellular adenomas in females and benign Leydig cell tumours in the high-dose (200 mg/kg/day) group only. These changes are considered to be rat-specific and of little clinical importance to humans. In rats treated with 100 mg/kg/day or more, pulmonary macrophages and inflammation were seen at a higher incidence than normal. The significance of this latter finding is unknown.

6. PHARMACEUTICAL PARTICULARS

6.1 List of excipients

α-Tocopherol

Macrogol 6000

Lactose, anhydrous

Talc

Hypromellose

Titanium dioxide, E171

6.2 Incompatibilities

None.

6.3 Shelf life

3 years.

6.4 Special precautions for storage

Do not refrigerate. Keep out of reach of children.

6.5 Nature and contents of container

Child resistant, white polyethylene container with white polypropylene screw closure. Available as packs of 100 tablets in 5, 10 or 15 mg strengths.

6.6 Instructions for use and handling

No special instructions.

7. MARKETING AUTHORISATION HOLDER

Cephalon UK Limited

11/13 Frederick Sanger Road

Surrey Research Park

Guildford

Surrey

GU2 7YD

UK

8. MARKETING AUTHORISATION NUMBER(S)

Gabitril 5 mg PL 16260/0009

Gabitril 10 mg PL 16260/0010

Gabitril 15 mg PL 16260/0011

9. DATE OF FIRST AUTHORISATION/RENEWAL OF THE AUTHORISATION

30 September 2002

10. DATE OF REVISION OF THE TEXT

November 2003

11. Legal Category

POM

Gamanil

(Merck Pharmaceuticals)

1. NAME OF THE MEDICINAL PRODUCT

Gamanil 70mg

2. QUALITATIVE AND QUANTITATIVE COMPOSITION

Lofepramine hydrochloride 76.10mg

equivalent to lofepramine 70mg

3. PHARMACEUTICAL FORM

Oral tablet

4. CLINICAL PARTICULARS

4.1 Therapeutic indications

In the treatment of symptoms of depressive illness

4.2 Posology and method of administration

Route of administration:

Oral

Recommended dosage:

The usual dose is 70mg twice daily (140mg) or three times daily (210mg) depending upon patient response.

Children: Not recommended

Elderly: May respond to lower doses in some cases

4.3 Contraindications

Lofepramine should not be used in patients hypersensitive to dibenzazepines, in mania, severe liver impairment and/or severe renal impairment, heart block, cardiac arrhythmias or during the recovery phase following a myocardial infarction.

Lofepramine should not be administered with or within 2 weeks of cessation of therapy with monoamine oxidase inhibitors (see Section 4.5).

Use of lofepramine with amiodarone should be avoided (see Section 4.5).

Use of lofepramine with terfenadine should be avoided (see Section 4.5).

4.4 Special warnings and special precautions for use

It should be remembered that severely depressed patients are at risk of suicide. An improvement in depression may not occur immediately upon initiation of treatment, therefore the patient should be closely monitored until symptoms improve.

Lofepramine may lower the convulsion threshold, therefore it should be used with extreme caution in patients with a history of epilepsy or recent convulsions or other predisposing factors, or during withdrawal from alcohol or other drugs with anticonvulsant properties.

Concurrent electroconvulsive therapy should only be undertaken with careful supervision.

Caution is needed in patients with hyperthyroidism, or during concomitant treatment with thyroid preparations, since aggravation of unwanted cardiac effects may occur.

Lofepramine should be used with caution in patients with cardiovascular disease, impaired liver function, impaired renal function, blood dyscrasias or porphyria.

Caution is called for where there is a history of prostatic hypertrophy, narrow angle glaucoma or increased intraocular pressure, because of lofepramine's anticholinergic properties.

In chronic constipation, tricyclic antidepressants may cause paralytic ileus, particularly in elderly and bedridden patients.

Care should be exercised in patients with tumours of the adrenal medulla (eg phaeochromocytoma, neuroblastoma) in whom tricyclic antidepressants may provoke antihypertensive crises.

Blood pressure should be checked before initiating treatment because individuals with hypertension, or an unstable circulation, may react to lofepramine with a fall in blood pressure.

Anaesthetics may increase the risks of arrhythmias and hypotension (see Interactions), therefore before local or general anaesthesia, the anaesthetist should be informed that the patient has been taking lofepramine.

Lofepramine should be used with caution where there is a history of mania. Psychotic symptoms may be aggravated. There have also been reports of hypomanic or manic episodes during a depressive phase in patients with cyclic affective disorders receiving tricyclic antidepressants.

Abrupt withdrawal of lofepramine should be avoided if possible.

4.5 Interaction with other medicinal products and other forms of Interaction

MAO Inhibitors: Lofepramine should not be administered with or within 2 weeks of cessation of therapy with monoamine oxidase inhibitors (See Section 4.3). It should be introduced cautiously using a low initial dose and the effects monitored.

SSRI Inhibitors: co-medication may lead to additive effects on the serotonergic system. Fluvoxamine and fluoxetine may also increase plasma concentrations of lofepramine resulting in a lowered convulsion threshold and seizures.

Anti-arrhythmic drugs: There is an increased risk of ventricular arrhythmias if lofepramine is given with drugs which prolong the Q-T interval e.g. disopyramide, procainamide, propafenone, quinidine and amiodarone. Concomitant use with amiodarone should be avoided (See Section 4.3)

Sympathomimetic drugs: Lofepramine should not be given with sympathomimetic agents (e.g. adrenalin, ephedrine, isoprenaline, noradrenaline, phenylephedrine, phenylpropanolamine) since their cardiovascular effects may be potentiated.

CNS depressants: Lofepramine's effects may be potentiated when administered with CNS depressant substances e.g. barbiturates, general anaesthetics and alcohol. If surgery is necessary, the anaesthetist should be informed that a patient is being so treated because of the increased risk of arrhythmias and hypotension.

Neuroleptics: There is an increased risk of arrhythmias; there may be an increased plasma level of the tricyclic antidepressant, a lowered convulsion threshold and seizures.

Adrenergic neurone blockers: Lofepramine may decrease or abolish the antihypertensive effects of some adrenergic neurone blocking drugs eg guanethidine, betanidine, reserpine, clonidine and a-methyl-dopa. Antihypertensives of a different type eg diuretics, vasodilators or β-blockers should be given therefore where patients require co-medication for hypertension.

Anticoagulants: Lofepramine may inhibit hepatic metabolism leading to an enhancement of anticoagulant effect. Careful monitoring of plasma prothrombin is advised.

Anti-cholinergic agents: Lofepramine may potentiate the effects of these drugs (e.g. phenothiazine, antiparkinson agents, antihistamines, atropine, beperiden) on the central nervous system, eye, bowel and bladder.

Analgesics: There is an increased risk of ventricular arrhythmias.

Anti-epileptics: Antagonism can lead to a lowering of the convulsive threshold. Plasma levels of some tricyclic antidepressants, and therefore the therapeutic effect, may be reduced.

Calcium channel blockers: diltiazem and verapamil increase the plasma concentration of lofepramine.

Diuretics: There is an increased risk of postural hypotension.

Terfenadine: There is an increased risk of ventricular arrhythmias therefore concomitant use should be avoided.

Rifampicin: The metabolism of lofepramine is accelerated by rifampicin leading to a reduced plasma concentration

Digitalis glycosides: With digitalis glycosides there is a higher risk of arrhythmias.

Sotalol: The risk of ventricular arrhythmias associated with sotalol is increased.

Cimetidine: Cimetidine can increase the plasma concentration of lofepramine.

Clonidine:The effect of antihypertensive agents of the clonidine type can be weakened.

Altretamine: There is a risk of severe postural hypotension when co-administered with tricyclic antidepressants

Disulfiram and alprazolam: Co-medication with either disulfiram or alprazolam may require a reduction in the dose of lofepramine

Nitrates: The effectiveness of sublingual nitrates may be reduced where the tricyclic antidepressant's anticholinergic effect has lead to dryness of the mouth

Ritonavir: There may be an increased plasma concentration of lofepramine.

Thyroid hormone therapy: During concomitant treatment, there may be aggravation of unwanted cardiac effects.

Oral contraceptives: Oestrogens and progestogens may antagonise the therapeutic effect of tricyclic antidepressants whilst the latter's side effects may be exacerbated due to an increased plasma concentration.

4.6 Pregnancy and lactation

The safety of lofepramine for use during pregnancy has not been established and there is evidence of harmful effects in pregnancy in animals when high doses are given. Lofepramine has been shown to be excreted in breast milk. The administration of lofepramine in pregnancy and during breast feeding therefore is not advised unless there are compelling medical reasons.

4.7 Effects on ability to drive and use machines

As with other antidepressants, ability to drive a car and operate machinery may be affected, especially in conjunction with alcohol. Therefore caution should be exercised initially until the individual reaction to treatment is known.

4.8 Undesirable effects

The following side effects have been reported with lofepramine:

Cardiovascular: hypotension, tachycardia, cardiac conduction disorders, increase in cardiac insufficiency, arrhythmias.

CNS & Neuromuscular: dizziness, sleep disturbances, agitation, confusion, headache, malaise, paraesthesia; rarely, drowsiness, hypomania and convulsions; very rarely, uncoordinated movement.

Anticholinergic: dryness of mouth, constipation, disturbances of accommodation, urinary hesitancy, urinary retention, sweating and tremor, induction of glaucoma; rarely, impairment of the sense of taste; very rarely, tinnitus.

Urinogenital: testicular disorders eg pain.

Allergic: skin rash, allergic skin reactions, "photosensitivity reactions", facial oedema; rarely, cutaneous bleeding, inflammation of mucosal membranes.

Gastrointestinal: nausea, vomiting.

Endocrine: rarely, hyponatraemia (inappropriate secretion of antidiuretic hormone), interference with sexual function, changes of blood sugar level, gynaecomastia, galactorrhoea.

Haematological/biochemical: rarely, bone marrow depression including isolated reports of: agranulocytosis, eosinophilia, granulocytopenia, leucopenia, pancytopenia, thrombocytopenia.

Increases in liver enzymes, sometimes progressing to clinical hepatitis and jaundice, have been reported in some patients, usually occurring within the first 3 months of starting therapy.

The following adverse effects have been encountered in patients under treatment with tricyclic antidepressants and should therefore be considered as theoretical hazards of lofepramine even in the absence of substantiation: psychotic manifestations, including mania and paranoid delusions may be exacerbated during treatment with tricyclic antidepressants; withdrawal symptoms may occur on abrupt cessation of therapy and include insomnia, irritability and excessive perspiration; adverse effects such as withdrawal symptoms, respiratory depression and agitation have been reported in neonates whose mothers have taken tricyclic antidepressants during the last trimester of pregnancy.

4.9 Overdose

The treatment of overdosage is symptomatic and supportive. It should include immediate gastric lavage and routine close monitoring of cardiac function.

5. PHARMACOLOGICAL PROPERTIES

5.1 Pharmacodynamic properties

Lofepramine is a tricyclic antidepressant. It exerts its therapeutic effect by blocking the uptake of noradrenaline by the nerve cell thus increasing the amine in the synaptic cleft and hence the effect on the receptors. There is evidence to suggest that serotonin may also be involved. Other pharmacological effects are due to anti-cholinergic activity, but less sedation is observed than with other tricyclics.

5.2 Pharmacokinetic properties

Lofepramine is a tertiary amine, similar in structure to imipramine but with improved lipophilicity and lower base strength. It is readily absorbed when given orally. From the plasma it is distributed throughout the body notably to the brain, lungs, liver and kidney. It is metabolised in the liver by cleavage of the p-chlorophenacyl group from the lofepramine molecule leaving desmethylimipramine (DMI).

The latter is pharmacologically active. The p-chlorobenzoyl portion is mainly metabolised to p-chlorobenzoic acid which is then conjugated with glycine. The conjugate is excreted mostly in the urine. DMI has been found excreted in the faeces. In a study of protein binding capability it has been found that lofepramine is up to 99% protein bound.

5.3 Preclinical safety data

N/A

6. PHARMACEUTICAL PARTICULARS

6.1 List of excipients

Excipients

Lactose

Corn starch

L(+) ascorbic acid

Talcum

Glycerol

Glycerol monostearate

Ethylene dinitriletetra acetic acid disodium salt (dihydrate) [titriplex III]

Dimethicone

Silicone dioxide

Hydroxypropyl methyl cellulose

Coating

1,2-Propanediol

Hydroxypropyl methyl cellulose

Ponceau 4R aluminium lake E124

Talc

Titanium dioxide

Indigotine lake E132

6.2 Incompatibilities

None

6.3 Shelf life

3 years

6.4 Special precautions for storage

Protect from light and moisture

6.5 Nature and contents of container

Containers

1. PVDC/Al foil blister calendar packs containing 28, 56, 1008 or 2016 tablets
2. Polypropylene containers containing 56, 250, 500 or 1000 tablets
3. Amber glass bottles containing 56 tablets

6.6 Instructions for use and handling

None

7. MARKETING AUTHORISATION HOLDER

E Merck Limited

Harrier House

High Street

West Drayton

Middlesex

UB7 7QG

Trading as:

E Merck Pharmaceuticals (a division of Merck Limited)

or

Merck Pharmaceuticals (a division of Merck Limited)

8. MARKETING AUTHORISATION NUMBER(S)

0493/0060

9. DATE OF FIRST AUTHORISATION/RENEWAL OF THE AUTHORISATION

30 July 1982/ 01 December 1998

10. DATE OF REVISION OF THE TEXT

12 October 2001

Gaviscon Advance

(Britannia Pharmaceuticals Limited)

1. NAME OF THE MEDICINAL PRODUCT

Gaviscon Advance.

2. QUALITATIVE AND QUANTITATIVE COMPOSITION

Active Substances	mg/10 ml	Specification
Sodium alginate	1000.0	Ph Eur
Potassium bicarbonate	200.0	Ph Eur

For excipients, see Section 6.1.

3. PHARMACEUTICAL FORM

Oral suspension.

Off-white, viscous suspension.

4. CLINICAL PARTICULARS

4.1 Therapeutic indications

Treatment of symptoms of gastro-oesophageal reflux such as acid regurgitation, heartburn, indigestion occurring due to the reflux of stomach contents, for instance, after gastric surgery, as a result of hiatus hernia, during pregnancy or accompanying reflux oesophagitis.

4.2 Posology and method of administration

Adults and children 12 years and over: 5-10 ml after meals and at bedtime.

Children under 12 years: Should be given only on medical advice.

Elderly: No dose modification is required for this age group.

4.3 Contraindications

Hypersensitivity to any of the ingredients, including the esters of hydroxybenzoates (parabens).

4.4 Special warnings and special precautions for use

Each 10 ml dose has a sodium content of 106 mg (4.6 mmol) and a potassium content of 78 mg (2.0 mmol). This should be taken into account when a highly restricted salt diet is recommended, e.g. in some cases of congestive cardiac failure and renal impairment or when taking drugs which can increase plasma potassium levels.

Each 10 ml contains 200 mg (2.0 mmol) of calcium carbonate. Care needs to be taken in treating patients with hypercalcaemia, nephrocalcinosis and recurrent calcium containing renal calculi.

There is a possibility of reduced efficacy in patients with very low levels of gastric acid.

Treatment of children younger than 12 years of age is not generally recommended, except on medical advice.

If symptoms do not improve after seven days, the clinical situation should be reviewed.

4.5 Interaction with other medicinal products and other forms of Interaction

None known.

4.6 Pregnancy and lactation

An open, uncontrolled study in 146 pregnant women did not demonstrate any significant adverse effects of this product on the course of pregnancy or on the health of the foetus/new-born child. Based on this and previous experience this product may be used during pregnancy and lactation.

4.7 Effects on ability to drive and use machines

None.

4.8 Undesirable effects

Very rarely (<1/10,000) patients sensitive to the ingredients may develop allergic manifestations such as urticaria or bronchospasm, anaphylactic or anaphylactoid reactions.

4.9 Overdose

In the event of overdosage, symptomatic treatment should be given. The patient may notice abdominal distension.

5. PHARMACOLOGICAL PROPERTIES

5.1 Pharmacodynamic properties

Pharmacotherapeutic classification: A02E A01 Anti-regurgitant.

On ingestion the suspension reacts with gastric acid to form a raft of alginic acid gel having a near-neutral pH and which floats on the stomach contents effectively impeding gastro-oesophageal reflux. In severe cases the raft itself may be refluxed into the oesophagus in preference to the stomach contents and exert a demulcent effect.

5.2 Pharmacokinetic properties

The mode of action of this product is physical and does not depend on absorption into the systemic circulation.

5.3 Preclinical safety data

No preclinical findings of relevance to the prescriber have been reported.

6. PHARMACEUTICAL PARTICULARS

6.1 List of excipients

Calcium carbonate, carbomer, methyl hydroxybenzoate, propyl hydroxybenzoate, saccharin sodium, fennel flavour, sodium hydroxide and purified water.

6.2 Incompatibilities

Not applicable.

6.3 Shelf life

Shelf life: 2 years.

Shelf life after opening: 3 months.

6.4 Special precautions for storage

Do not refrigerate.

6.5 Nature and contents of container

Amber glass bottles with moulded polypropylene cap having a tamper evident strip and lined with an expanded polyethylene wad with either a measuring device (natural polypropylene) containing 5, 10, 15 and 20 ml graduations, or a measuring spoon (crystal polystyrene) containing 2.5 ml and 5 ml measure and containing 80, 100, 125, 140, 150, 180, 200, 250, 300, 400, 500, 560 or 600 ml suspension.

Not all pack sizes may be marketed. The carton and measuring device or spoon may not be made available in all markets/pack sizes.

6.6 Instructions for use and handling

To be taken orally. Shake well before use. Check that the cap seal is unbroken before first taking the product.

7. MARKETING AUTHORISATION HOLDER

Reckitt Benckiser Healthcare (UK) Limited, Dansom Lane, Hull, HU8 7DS, United Kingdom.

8. MARKETING AUTHORISATION NUMBER(S)

PL 00063/0097.

9. DATE OF FIRST AUTHORISATION/RENEWAL OF THE AUTHORISATION

31st October, 1996.

10. DATE OF REVISION OF THE TEXT

November 2004.

Gaviscon Advance - Peppermint

(Britannia Pharmaceuticals Limited)

1. NAME OF THE MEDICINAL PRODUCT

Gaviscon Advance - Peppermint Flavour.

Oral suspension.

2. QUALITATIVE AND QUANTITATIVE COMPOSITION

Each 10 ml dose contains sodium alginate 1000 mg and potassium hydrogen carbonate 200 mg. 1 ml contains sodium alginate 100 mg and potassium carbonate 20.0 mg.

For excipients, see 6.1.

3. PHARMACEUTICAL FORM

Oral suspension.

Off-white viscous suspension.

4. CLINICAL PARTICULARS

4.1 Therapeutic indications

Treatment of symptoms of gastro-oesophageal reflux such as acid regurgitation, heartburn, indigestion occurring due to the reflux of stomach contents, for instance, after gastric surgery, as a result of hiatus hernia, during pregnancy or accompanying reflux oesophagitis.

4.2 Posology and method of administration

Adults and children 12 years and over: 5-10 ml after meals and at bedtime (one to two 5 ml measuring spoons).

Children under 12 years: Should be given only on medical advice.

Elderly: No dose modification is required for this age group.

4.3 Contraindications

Hypersensitivity to the active substances or to any of the excipients, including the esters of hydroxybenzoates (parabens).

4.4 Special warnings and special precautions for use

Each 10 ml dose has a sodium content of 106 mg (4.6 mmol) and a potassium content of 78 mg (2.0 mmol). This should be taken into account when a highly restricted salt diet is recommended, e.g. in some cases of congestive cardiac failure and renal impairment or when taking drugs which can increase plasma potassium levels.

Each 10 ml contains 200 mg (2.0 mmol) of calcium carbonate. Care needs to be taken in treating patients with hypercalcaemia, nephrocalcinosis and recurrent calcium containing renal calculi.

There is a possibility of reduced efficacy in patients with very low levels of gastric acid.

Treatment of children younger than 12 years of age is not generally recommended, except on medical advice.

If symptoms do not improve after seven days, the clinical situation should be reviewed.

This medicinal product contains Methyl hydroxybenzoate and Propyl hydroxybenzoate, which may cause allergic reactions (possibly delayed).

4.5 Interaction with other medicinal products and other forms of Interaction

None known.

4.6 Pregnancy and lactation
An open, uncontrolled study in 146 pregnant women did not demonstrate any significant undesirable effects of Gaviscon Advance on the course of the pregnancy or on the health of the foetus/new-born child. Based on this and previous experience, Gaviscon Advance - Peppermint Flavour may be used during pregnancy and lactation.

4.7 Effects on ability to drive and use machines
Not relevant.

4.8 Undesirable effects
Very rarely (< 1/10,000) patients sensitive to the excipients may develop allergic manifestations such as urticaria or bronchospasm, anaphylactic or anaphylactoid reactions.

4.9 Overdose
In the event of overdose, symptomatic treatment should be given. The patient may notice abdominal distension.

5. PHARMACOLOGICAL PROPERTIES

5.1 Pharmacodynamic properties
Pharmacotherapeutic group: Other drugs for peptic ulcer and gastro-oesophageal reflux disease (GORD).

ATC code: A02BX.

On ingestion the suspension reacts with gastric acid to form a raft of alginic acid gel having a near-neutral pH and which floats on the stomach contents effectively impeding gastro-oesophageal reflux. In severe cases the raft itself may be refluxed into the oesophagus in preference to the stomach contents and exert a demulcent effect.

5.2 Pharmacokinetic properties
The mechanism of action of the medicinal product is physical and does not depend on absorption into the systemic circulation.

5.3 Preclinical safety data
No preclinical findings of relevance to the prescriber have been reported.

6. PHARMACEUTICAL PARTICULARS

6.1 List of excipients
Calcium carbonate

Carbomer

Methyl parahydroxybenzoate E218

Propyl parahydroxybenzoate E216

Saccharin sodium

Peppermint flavour

Sodium hydroxide for pH adjustment

Purified water

6.2 Incompatibilities
Not applicable.

6.3 Shelf life
Shelf life: 2 years.

Shelf-life after opening: 3 months.

6.4 Special precautions for storage
Do not refrigerate.

6.5 Nature and contents of container
Amber glass bottles with moulded polypropylene cap having a tamper evident strip and lined with an expanded polyethylene wad. The bottles are enclosed in a cardboard outer containing a clear injection moulded crystal polystyrene measuring spoon with one bowl containing 2.5 ml and 5 ml measure. The pack sizes are 80, 100, 125, 140, 150, 180, 200, 250, 300, 400, 500, 560 or 600 ml suspension. Not all pack sizes may be marketed. The carton and spoon may not be made available in all markets/pack sizes.

6.6 Instructions for use and handling
No special requirements.

7. MARKETING AUTHORISATION HOLDER
Reckitt Benckiser Healthcare (UK) Limited, Dansom Lane, Hull, HU8 7DS, United Kingdom.

8. MARKETING AUTHORISATION NUMBER(S)
PL 00063/0103.

9. DATE OF FIRST AUTHORISATION/RENEWAL OF THE AUTHORISATION
15th March, 2001.

10. DATE OF REVISION OF THE TEXT
November 2004.

Gaviscon Advance Liquid Sachets

(Reckitt Benckiser Healthcare (UK) Ltd)

1. NAME OF THE MEDICINAL PRODUCT
Gaviscon Advance Liquid Sachets.

Oral suspension.

2. QUALITATIVE AND QUANTITATIVE COMPOSITION
Each 5 ml dose contains sodium alginate 500 mg and potassium hydrogen carbonate 100 mg. 1 ml contains sodium alginate 100 mg and potassium hydrogen carbonate 20 mg.

For excipients, see 6.1.

3. PHARMACEUTICAL FORM
Oral suspension.

Off-white viscous suspension.

4. CLINICAL PARTICULARS

4.1 Therapeutic indications
Treatment of symptoms of gastro-oesophageal reflux such as acid regurgitation, heartburn, indigestion occurring due to the reflux of stomach contents, for instance, after gastric surgery, as a result of hiatus hernia, during pregnancy or accompanying reflux oesophagitis.

4.2 Posology and method of administration
Adults and children 12 years and over: One to two 5 ml measuring spoons after meals and at bedtime.

Children under 12 years: Should be given only on medical advice.

Elderly: No dose modification is required for this age group.

Any unused solution should be discarded.

4.3 Contraindications
Hypersensitivity to the active substances or to any of the excipients, including the esters of hydroxybenzoates (parabens).

4.4 Special warnings and special precautions for use
Each 5 ml dose has a sodium content of 53 mg (2.3 mmol) and a potassium content of 39 mg (1.0 mmol). This should be taken into account when a highly restricted salt diet is recommended, e.g. in some cases of congestive cardiac failure and renal impairment or when taking drugs which can increase plasma potassium levels.

Each 5 ml contains 100 mg (1.0 mmol) of calcium carbonate. Care needs to be taken in treating patients with hypercalcaemia, nephrocalcinosis and recurrent calcium containing renal calculi.

There is a possibility of reduced efficacy in patients with very low levels of gastric acid.

Treatment of children younger than 12 years of age is not generally recommended, except on medical advice.

If symptoms do not improve after seven days, the clinical situation should be reviewed.

This medicinal product contains Methyl hydroxybenzoate and Propyl hydroxybenzoate, which may cause allergic reactions (possibly delayed).

4.5 Interaction with other medicinal products and other forms of Interaction
None known.

4.6 Pregnancy and lactation
An open, uncontrolled study in 146 pregnant women did not demonstrate any significant undesirable effects of Gaviscon Advance on the course of the pregnancy or on the health of the foetus/new-born child. Based on this and previous experience, Gaviscon Advance Liquid Sachets may be used during pregnancy and lactation.

4.7 Effects on ability to drive and use machines
Not relevant.

4.8 Undesirable effects
Very rarely (< 1/10,000) patients sensitive to the excipients may develop allergic manifestations such as urticaria or bronchospasm, anaphylactic or anaphylactoid reactions.

4.9 Overdose
In the event of overdose, symptomatic treatment should be given. The patient may notice abdominal distension.

5. PHARMACOLOGICAL PROPERTIES

5.1 Pharmacodynamic properties
Pharmacotherapeutic group: Other drugs for peptic ulcer and gastro-oesophageal reflux disease (GORD).

ATC code: A02BX.

On ingestion the suspension reacts with gastric acid to form a raft of alginic acid gel having a near-neutral pH and which floats on the stomach contents effectively impeding gastro-oesophageal reflux. In severe cases the raft itself may be refluxed into the oesophagus in preference to the stomach contents and exert a demulcent effect.

5.2 Pharmacokinetic properties
The mechanism of action of the medicinal product is physical and does not depend on absorption into the systemic circulation.

5.3 Preclinical safety data
No preclinical findings of relevance to the prescriber have been reported.

6. PHARMACEUTICAL PARTICULARS

6.1 List of excipients
Calcium carbonate

Carbomer

Methyl parahydroxybenzoate E218

Propyl parahydroxybenzoate E216

Saccharin sodium

Peppermint flavour

Sodium hydroxide for pH adjustment

Purified water

6.2 Incompatibilities
Not applicable.

6.3 Shelf life
2 years.

6.4 Special precautions for storage
Do not refrigerate.

6.5 Nature and contents of container
A cardboard outer carton containing unit dose stick pack style sachets and a clear injection moulded crystal polystyrene measuring spoon with one bowl containing 2.5 ml and 5 ml measure. The pack sizes are 10, 20, 24 or 48. Not all pack sizes may be marketed. The spoon may not be made available in all markets/pack sizes. The sachets are composed of polyester, aluminium and polyethylene. A single sachet or dual sachets, enclosed in an outer cardboard carton, are also available. Each sachet contains either 5 or 10 ml of medicinal product.

6.6 Instructions for use and handling
No special requirements.

7. MARKETING AUTHORISATION HOLDER
Reckitt Benckiser Healthcare (UK) Limited, Dansom Lane, Hull, HU8 7DS, United Kingdom.

8. MARKETING AUTHORISATION NUMBER(S)
PL 00063/0112.

9. DATE OF FIRST AUTHORISATION/RENEWAL OF THE AUTHORISATION
27th June, 2002.

10. DATE OF REVISION OF THE TEXT
November 2004.

Gaviscon Advance Tablets

(Britannia Pharmaceuticals Limited)

1. NAME OF THE MEDICINAL PRODUCT
Gaviscon Advance Tablets.

2. QUALITATIVE AND QUANTITATIVE COMPOSITION
Each tablet contains sodium alginate 500 mg and potassium bicarbonate 100 mg.

For excipients, see Section 6.1.

3. PHARMACEUTICAL FORM
Chewable tablet.

An off-white to cream, circular, flat with bevelled edges tablet with the odour and flavour of peppermint.

4. CLINICAL PARTICULARS

4.1 Therapeutic indications
Treatment of symptoms of gastro-oesophageal reflux such as acid regurgitation, heartburn, indigestion occurring due to the reflux of stomach contents, for instance, after gastric surgery, as a result of hiatus hernia, during pregnancy or accompanying reflux oesophagitis.

4.2 Posology and method of administration
For oral administration, after being thoroughly chewed.

Adults and children 12 years and over: One to two tablets after meals and at bedtime.

Children under 12 years: Should be given only on medical advice.

Elderly: No dose modifications necessary for this age group.

4.3 Contraindications
Hypersensitivity to any of the ingredients.

4.4 Special warnings and special precautions for use
The sodium content of a two-tablet dose is 103 mg (4.5 mmol) and a potassium content of 78 mg (2.0 mmol). This should be taken into account when a highly restricted salt diet is recommended, e.g. in some cases of congestive cardiac failure and renal impairment or when taking drugs which can increase plasma potassium levels.

Each two-tablet dose contains 200 mg (2.0 mmol) of calcium carbonate. Care needs to be taken in treating patients with hypercalcaemia, nephrocalcinosis and recurrent calcium containing renal calculi.

Due to its aspartame content this product should not be given to patients with phenylketonuria.

There is a possibility of reduced efficacy in patients with very low levels of gastric acid.

If symptoms do not improve after seven days, the clinical situation should be reviewed.

Treatment of children younger than 12 years of age is not generally recommended, except on medical advice.

4.5 Interaction with other medicinal products and other forms of Interaction
None known.

4.6 Pregnancy and lactation
An open controlled study in 146 pregnant women did not demonstrate any significant adverse effects of Gaviscon Advance on the course of pregnancy or on the health of the foetus/new-born child.

Based on this and previous experience, Gaviscon Advance Tablets may be used during pregnancy and lactation.

4.7 Effects on ability to drive and use machines
None.

4.8 Undesirable effects
Very rarely (<1/10,000) patients sensitive to the ingredients may develop allergic manifestations such as urticaria or bronchospasm, anaphylactic or anaphylactoid reactions.

4.9 Overdose
In the event of overdosage symptomatic treatment should be given. The patient may notice abdominal distension.

5. PHARMACOLOGICAL PROPERTIES
Pharmacotherapeutic classification: A02BX 13. Other drugs for peptic ulcer and gastro-oesophageal reflux disease.

5.1 Pharmacodynamic properties
On ingestion Gaviscon Advance Tablets react rapidly with gastric acid to form a raft of alginic acid gel having a near neutral pH and which floats on the stomach contents effectively impeding gastro-oesophageal reflux. In severe cases the raft itself may be refluxed into the oesophagus, in preference to the stomach contents, and exert a demulcent effect.

5.2 Pharmacokinetic properties
The mode of action of Gaviscon Advance Tablets is physical and does not depend on absorption into the systemic circulation.

5.3 Preclinical safety data
No pre-clinical findings of any relevance to the prescriber have been reported.

6. PHARMACEUTICAL PARTICULARS

6.1 List of excipients
Mannitol

Calcium carbonate

Polyethylene glycol 20,000

Magnesium stearate

Aspartame

Mint flavour no. 3

Acesulfame potassium

6.2 Incompatibilities
Not applicable.

6.3 Shelf life
Two years.

6.4 Special precautions for storage
Do not store above 30°C. Store in the original package.

6.5 Nature and contents of container
White, rigid, injection-moulded, polypropylene cylindrical tube with snap-bead neck finish packed into cartons.

Tube containing 20 tablets. One, two, three or four tubes in a carton.

Unprinted, glass-clear, thermoformable laminate of uPVC/PE/PVdC with aluminium foil lidding blisters packed into cartons.

Blister tray containing six individually sealed tablets. Two or four blister trays in a carton.

Not all pack sizes may be marketed.

6.6 Instructions for use and handling
No special instructions.

7. MARKETING AUTHORISATION HOLDER
Reckitt Benckiser Healthcare (UK) Limited, Dansom Lane, Hull, HU8 7DS, United Kingdom.

8. MARKETING AUTHORISATION NUMBER(S)
PL 00063/0144.

9. DATE OF FIRST AUTHORISATION/RENEWAL OF THE AUTHORISATION
15th January 2005.

10. DATE OF REVISION OF THE TEXT
15th January 2005

Gaviscon Cool Liquid

(Reckitt Benckiser Healthcare (UK) Ltd)

1. NAME OF THE MEDICINAL PRODUCT
Gaviscon Cool Liquid.

2. QUALITATIVE AND QUANTITATIVE COMPOSITION
Gaviscon Cool Liquid contains 250 mg sodium alginate Ph Eur, 133.5 mg sodium bicarbonate Ph Eur and 80 mg calcium carbonate Ph Eur per 5 ml.

3. PHARMACEUTICAL FORM
Oral suspension.

4. CLINICAL PARTICULARS

4.1 Therapeutic indications
Gastric reflux, heartburn, flatulence associated with gastric reflux, heartburn of pregnancy, all cases of epigastric and retrosternal distress where the underlying cause is gastric reflux.

4.2 Posology and method of administration
For oral administration.

Adults and children over 12: 10-20 ml after meals and at bedtime.

Elderly: No dose modification is required in this age group.

Children 6-12 years: 5-10 ml after meals and at bedtime.

Children under 6 years: Not recommended.

If symptoms persist consult your doctor.

4.3 Contraindications
None known.

4.4 Special warnings and special precautions for use
The sodium content of a 10 ml dose is 141 mg (6.2 mmol). This should be taken into account when a highly restricted salt diet is recommended as in some renal and cardiovascular conditions.

4.5 Interaction with other medicinal products and other forms of Interaction
None known.

4.6 Pregnancy and lactation
This medicine can be used as directed during pregnancy and lactation.

4.7 Effects on ability to drive and use machines
None.

4.8 Undesirable effects
Very rarely patients sensitive to the ingredients may develop allergic manifestations such as urticaria or bronchospasm.

4.9 Overdose
In the event of overdosage, symptomatic treatment should be given. The patient may notice abdominal distension.

5. PHARMACOLOGICAL PROPERTIES

5.1 Pharmacodynamic properties
On ingestion Gaviscon Cool Liquid reacts with gastric acid to form a raft of alginic acid gel having a near neutral pH and which floats on the stomach contents effectively (up to 4 hours) impeding gastro-oesophageal reflux. In severe cases the raft itself may be refluxed into the oesophagus in preference to the stomach contents and exert a demulcent effect.

5.2 Pharmacokinetic properties
The mode of action of Gaviscon Cool Liquid is physical and does not depend on absorption into the systemic circulation.

5.3 Preclinical safety data
No preclinical findings of relevance to the prescriber have been reported.

6. PHARMACEUTICAL PARTICULARS

6.1 List of excipients
Carbomer

E218 (Methyl parahydroxybenzoate)

E216 (Propyl parahydroxybenzoate)

Saccharin sodium

Mint flavour no. 4

Mint flavour no. 5

Sodium hydroxide

Purified water

6.2 Incompatibilities
None known.

6.3 Shelf life
Two years.

6.4 Special precautions for storage
Do not store above 30°C. Do not refrigerate or freeze.

6.5 Nature and contents of container
Amber glass bottles with a polypropylene cap with a polyethylene tamper-evident band lined with expanded polyethylene wad and containing 100, 150, 200, 300, 500 or 600 ml.

6.6 Instructions for use and handling
To be taken orally. If desired the standard dose of Gaviscon Cool Liquid may be taken diluted with not more than an equal quantity of water well stirred.

7. MARKETING AUTHORISATION HOLDER
Hamol Limited, 103-105 Bath Road, Slough, Berkshire, SL1 3UH, United Kingdom.

8. MARKETING AUTHORISATION NUMBER(S)
PL 01839/0003.

9. DATE OF FIRST AUTHORISATION/RENEWAL OF THE AUTHORISATION
6th December, 2001.

10. DATE OF REVISION OF THE TEXT
February 2004.

Gaviscon Cool Tablets

(Reckitt Benckiser Healthcare (UK) Ltd)

1. NAME OF THE MEDICINAL PRODUCT
Gaviscon Cool Tablets.

2. QUALITATIVE AND QUANTITATIVE COMPOSITION
Each tablet contains sodium alginate 250 mg, sodium bicarbonate 133.5 mg and calcium carbonate 80 mg.

For excipients, see Section 6.1.

3. PHARMACEUTICAL FORM
Chewable tablet.

A pale blue, circular, flat with bevelled edges tablet with the odour and flavour of peppermint.

4. CLINICAL PARTICULARS

4.1 Therapeutic indications
Treatment of symptoms of gastro-oesophageal reflux such as acid regurgitation, heartburn and indigestion, for example, following meals or during pregnancy.

4.2 Posology and method of administration
For oral administration, after being thoroughly chewed.

Adults and children 12 years and over: Two to four tablets after meals and at bedtime.

Children under 12 years: Should be given only on medical advice.

Elderly: No dose modifications necessary for this age group.

4.3 Contraindications
None.

4.4 Special warnings and special precautions for use
The sodium content of a four-tablet dose is 246 mg (10.6 mmol). This should be taken into account when a highly restricted salt diet is recommended, e.g. in some cases of congestive cardiac failure and renal impairment.

Each four-tablet dose contains 320 mg (3.2 mmol) of calcium carbonate. Care needs to be taken in treating patients with hypercalcaemia, nephrocalcinosis and recurrent calcium containing renal calculi.

Due to its aspartame content this product should not be given to patients with phenylketonuria.

There is a possibility of reduced efficacy in patients with very low levels of gastric acid.

If symptoms do not improve after seven days, the clinical situation should be reviewed.

Treatment of children younger than 12 years of age is not generally recommended, except on medical advice.

4.5 Interaction with other medicinal products and other forms of Interaction
None known.

4.6 Pregnancy and lactation
Open controlled studies in 281 pregnant women did not demonstrate any significant adverse effects of Gaviscon on the course of pregnancy or on the health of the foetus/new-born child. Based on this and previous experience Gaviscon Cool Tablets may be used during pregnancy and lactation.

4.7 Effects on ability to drive and use machines
None.

4.8 Undesirable effects
Very rarely patients sensitive to the ingredients may develop allergic manifestations such as urticaria or bronchospasm.

4.9 Overdose
In the event of overdosage symptomatic treatment should be given. The patient may notice abdominal distension.

5. PHARMACOLOGICAL PROPERTIES
Pharmacotherapeutic classification: A02BX 13. Other drugs for peptic ulcer and gastro-oesophageal reflux disease.

5.1 Pharmacodynamic properties
On ingestion Gaviscon Cool Tablets react rapidly with gastric acid to form a raft of alginic acid gel having a near neutral pH and which floats on the stomach contents effectively impeding gastro-oesophageal reflux. In severe cases the raft itself may be refluxed into the oesophagus, in preference to the stomach contents, and exert a demulcent effect.

5.2 Pharmacokinetic properties
The mode of action of Gaviscon Cool Tablets is physical and does not depend on absorption into the systemic circulation.

5.3 Preclinical safety data
No pre-clinical findings of any relevance to the prescriber have been reported.

6. PHARMACEUTICAL PARTICULARS

6.1 List of excipients
Peppermint flavour (Trusil coolmint flavour 108406)

Polyethylene glycol 20,000

Mannitol

Aspartame

Magnesium stearate

Xylitol DC

Indigo carmine

6.2 Incompatibilities
Not applicable.

6.3 Shelf life
Two years.

6.4 Special precautions for storage
Do not store above 30°C. Store in the original package.

6.5 Nature and contents of container
Unprinted, glass-clear, thermoformable laminate of uPVC/PE/PVdC with aluminium foil lidding blisters packed into cartons.

Blister tray containing two, four, six or eight sealed tablets. Larger packs (e.g. 16, 24, 32, 48, 60, 64, 72 and 80) will be made up of multiples of the above units.

Polypropylene container containing 8, 12 or 16 tablets. Larger packs will be made up of multiples of the above units.

Not all pack sizes may be marketed.

6.6 Instructions for use and handling
No special instructions.

7. MARKETING AUTHORISATION HOLDER
Reckitt Benckiser Healthcare (UK) Limited, Dansom Lane, Hull, HU8 7DS, United Kingdom.

8. MARKETING AUTHORISATION NUMBER(S)
PL 00063/0140.

9. DATE OF FIRST AUTHORISATION/RENEWAL OF THE AUTHORISATION
7th October, 2003.

10. DATE OF REVISION OF THE TEXT
November 2004.

Gaviscon Peppermint Liquid Relief

(Reckitt Benckiser Healthcare (UK) Ltd)

1. NAME OF THE MEDICINAL PRODUCT
Gaviscon Peppermint Liquid Relief.

2. QUALITATIVE AND QUANTITATIVE COMPOSITION
Gaviscon Peppermint Liquid Relief contains 250 mg sodium alginate, 133.5 mg sodium hydrogen carbonate and 80 mg calcium carbonate per 5 ml.

For excipients, see Section 6.1.

3. PHARMACEUTICAL FORM
Oral suspension.

An opaque, off-white to cream suspension with the odour and flavour of peppermint.

4. CLINICAL PARTICULARS

4.1 Therapeutic indications
Gastric reflux, heartburn, flatulence associated with gastric reflux, heartburn of pregnancy, all cases of epigastric and retrosternal distress where the underlying cause is gastric reflux.

4.2 Posology and method of administration
For oral administration.

Adults and children over 12 years: 10-20 ml after meals and at bedtime.

Elderly: No dosage modification is required in this age group.

Children 6 to 12 years: 5-10 ml after meals and at bedtime.

Children under 6 years: Not recommended.

4.3 Contraindications
None known.

4.4 Special warnings and special precautions for use
The sodium content of a 10 ml dose is 141 mg (6.2 mmol). Care to be exercised when a highly restricted salt diet is required as in some renal and cardiovascular conditions.

4.5 Interaction with other medicinal products and other forms of Interaction
None known.

4.6 Pregnancy and lactation
Open uncontrolled studies in 281 pregnant women did not demonstrate any significant adverse effects of Gaviscon on the course of pregnancy or on the health of the foetus/new-born child. Based on this and previous experience Liquid Gaviscon may be used during pregnancy and lactation.

4.7 Effects on ability to drive and use machines
None.

4.8 Undesirable effects
Very rarely (<1/10,000) patients sensitive to the ingredients may develop allergic manifestations such as urticaria or bronchospasm, anaphylactic or anaphylactoid reactions.

4.9 Overdose
In the event of overdosage symptomatic treatment should be given. The patient may notice abdominal distension.

5. PHARMACOLOGICAL PROPERTIES

5.1 Pharmacodynamic properties
On ingestion the product reacts rapidly with gastric acid to form a raft of alginic acid gel having a near neutral pH and which floats on the stomach contents effectively (up to 4 hours) impeding gastro-oesophageal reflux. In severe cases the raft itself may be refluxed into the oesophagus in preference to the stomach contents and exert a demulcent effect.

5.2 Pharmacokinetic properties
The mode of action of the product is physical and does not depend on absorption into the systemic circulation.

5.3 Preclinical safety data
No preclinical findings relevant to the prescriber have been reported.

6. PHARMACEUTICAL PARTICULARS

6.1 List of excipients
Carbomer

Methyl parahydroxybenzoate

Propyl parahydroxybenzoate

Saccharin sodium

Peppermint oil

Sodium hydroxide

Water

6.2 Incompatibilities
Not applicable.

6.3 Shelf life
Three years.

6.4 Special precautions for storage
Do not store above 30°C. Do not refrigerate or freeze.

6.5 Nature and contents of container
Amber glass Winchester bottle with a polypropylene cap with a polyethylene tamper-evident band lined with expanded polyethylene wad containing 100, 150, 200, 300 and 600 ml.

6.6 Instructions for use and handling
No special instructions.

7. MARKETING AUTHORISATION HOLDER
Reckitt Benckiser Healthcare (UK) Limited, Dansom Lane, Hull, HU8 7DS.

8. MARKETING AUTHORISATION NUMBER(S)
PL 00063/0127.

9. DATE OF FIRST AUTHORISATION/RENEWAL OF THE AUTHORISATION
3rd February, 2003.

10. DATE OF REVISION OF THE TEXT
January 2005.

Gaviscon Peppermint Tablets

(Reckitt Benckiser Healthcare (UK) Ltd)

1. NAME OF THE MEDICINAL PRODUCT
Gaviscon Peppermint Tablets.

2. QUALITATIVE AND QUANTITATIVE COMPOSITION
Each tablet contains sodium alginate 250 mg, sodium hydrogen carbonate 133.5 mg and calcium carbonate 80 mg.

For excipients, see Section 6.1.

3. PHARMACEUTICAL FORM
Chewable tablet.

An off-white to cream, slightly mottled tablet.

4. CLINICAL PARTICULARS

4.1 Therapeutic indications
Treatment of symptoms of gastro-oesophageal reflux such as acid regurgitation, heartburn and indigestion (related to reflux), for example, following meals or during pregnancy, or in patients with symptoms related to oesophagitis.

4.2 Posology and method of administration
For oral use, after being thoroughly chewed.

Adults and children 12 years and over: Two to four tablets after meals and at bedtime.

Elderly: No dose modifications necessary for this age group.

4.3 Contraindications
This medicinal product is contraindicated in patients with known or suspected hypersensitivity to the active substances or to any of the excipients.

4.4 Special warnings and special precautions for use
The sodium content of a four-tablet dose is 246 mg (10.6 mmol). This should be taken into account when a highly restricted salt diet is recommended, e.g. in some cases of congestive cardiac failure and renal impairment.

Each four-tablet dose contains 320 mg (3.2 mmol) of calcium carbonate. Care needs to be taken in treating patients with hypercalcaemia, nephrocalcinosis and recurrent calcium containing renal calculi.

Due to its aspartame content this medicinal product should not be given to patients with phenylketonuria.

There is a possibility of reduced efficacy in patients with very low levels of gastric acid.

If symptoms do not improve after seven days, the clinical situation should be reviewed.

Treatment of children younger than 12 years of age is not generally recommended, except on medical advice.

4.5 Interaction with other medicinal products and other forms of Interaction
Due to the presence of calcium carbonate which acts as an antacid, a time-interval of 2 hours should be considered between Gaviscon intake and the administration of other medicinal products, especially H2-antihistaminics, tetracyclines, digoxine, fluoroquinolone, iron salt, ketoconazole, neuroleptics, thyroxine, penicilamine, beta-blockers (atenolol, metoprolol, propanolol), glucocorticoid, chloroquine and diphosphonates.

4.6 Pregnancy and lactation
Open controlled studies in 281 pregnant women did not demonstrate any significant adverse effects of Gaviscon on the course of pregnancy or on the health of the foetus/new-born child. Based on this and previous experience the medicinal product may be used during pregnancy and lactation. Nevertheless, taking into account the presence of calcium carbonate (see Section 5.3) it is recommended to limit the treatment duration as much as possible.

4.7 Effects on ability to drive and use machines
Not relevant.

4.8 Undesirable effects
Very rarely patients sensitive to the ingredients may develop allergic manifestations such as urticaria or bronchospasm.

4.9 Overdose
In the event of overdose symptomatic treatment should be given. The patient may notice abdominal distension.

5. PHARMACOLOGICAL PROPERTIES

5.1 Pharmacodynamic properties
Pharmacotherapeutic group: Other drugs for peptic ulcer and gastro-oesophageal reflux disease (GORD) ATC code: A02BX.

On ingestion the medicinal product reacts rapidly with gastric acid to form a raft of alginic acid gel having a near neutral pH and which floats on the stomach contents effectively impeding gastro-oesophageal reflux. In severe cases the raft itself may be refluxed into the oesophagus, in preference to the stomach contents, and exert a demulcent effect.

5.2 Pharmacokinetic properties
The mechanism of action of the medicinal product is physical and does not depend on absorption into the systemic circulation.

5.3 Preclinical safety data
There is limited evidence in some reports in animals of delay in calcification of foetal skeleton/bone abnormalities relating to calcium carbonate.

6. PHARMACEUTICAL PARTICULARS

6.1 List of excipients
Peppermint flavour

Macrogol 20,000

Mannitol (E421)

Aspartame (E951)

Magnesium stearate

6.2 Incompatibilities
Not applicable.

6.3 Shelf life
2 years.

6.4 Special precautions for storage
This medicinal product does not require any special storage conditions.

6.5 Nature and contents of container
Unprinted, glass-clear, thermoformable laminate of uPVC/PE/PVdC with aluminium foil lidding blisters packed into cartons.

Blister containing four, six or eight sealed tablets. Pack sizes: 4, 6,8, 16, 24, 32 48 and 64 chewable tablets.

Not all pack sizes may be marketed.

6.6 Instructions for use and handling
No special requirements.

7. MARKETING AUTHORISATION HOLDER
Reckitt Benckiser Healthcare (UK) Limited, Dansom Lane, Hull, HU8 7DS, United Kingdom.

8. MARKETING AUTHORISATION NUMBER(S)
PL 00063/0134.

9. DATE OF FIRST AUTHORISATION/RENEWAL OF THE AUTHORISATION
7th October, 2003.

10. DATE OF REVISION OF THE TEXT
December 2004.

Gel Tears

(Chauvin Pharmaceuticals Ltd)

1. NAME OF THE MEDICINAL PRODUCT
GelTears.

2. QUALITATIVE AND QUANTITATIVE COMPOSITION
Clear, colourless gel containing 0.2% w/w carbomer 980 Ph.Eur.

3. PHARMACEUTICAL FORM
Eye gel.

4. CLINICAL PARTICULARS
4.1 Therapeutic indications
Substitution of tear fluid in the management of dry eye conditions, including keratoconjunctivitis sicca and unstable tear film.

4.2 Posology and method of administration
Adults (including the elderly) and children:

One drop to be instilled into the conjunctival fold of each affected eye 3 - 4 times daily or as required, depending on the degree of discomfort.

4.3 Contraindications
Use in patients with a known hypersensitivity to any component of the preparation.

4.4 Special warnings and special precautions for use
Blurred vision can occur if too much gel is instilled at one time, or if the gel is used too frequently. This effect can last for up to an hour. Recovery can be aided by blinking vigorously for a few seconds. If this fails, the lower eyelid should be manipulated until the gel returns to the lower fornix and normal vision is restored.

Contact lenses should be removed during treatment with GelTears.

4.5 Interaction with other medicinal products and other forms of Interaction
No significant interactions have been reported.

4.6 Pregnancy and lactation
Safety for use in pregnancy and lactation has not been established, therefore, Geltears should not be used in these circumstances.

4.7 Effects on ability to drive and use machines
As with other ophthalmic preparations, transient blurring of vision may occur on instillation. If affected, the patient should be advised not to drive or operate hazardous machinery until normal vision is restored.

4.8 Undesirable effects
Corneal irritation due to benzalkonium chloride could possibly occur with prolonged use.

4.9 Overdose
Not applicable.

5. PHARMACOLOGICAL PROPERTIES
5.1 Pharmacodynamic properties
GelTears contains Carbomer 980, a hydrophilic, high molecular weight polymer of carboxyvinylic acid. The gel forms a transparent lubricating and moistening film on the surface of the eye. The preparation has a pH similar to that found in the normal tear film and is slightly hypotonic with respect to tears. GelTears relieves the symptoms of irritation linked with dry eye syndromes and protects the cornea against drying out.

The use of vital stains has provided objective evidence that the corneal and conjunctival epithelial lesions associated with dry eye syndromes show improvement on treatment with GelTears. The gel remains on the surface of the eye for longer than low viscosity artificial tears and hence, less frequent application is required.

5.2 Pharmacokinetic properties
No human pharmacokinetic studies are available, however, absorption or accumulation in ocular tissues is likely to be negligible due to the high molecular weight of the active ingredient.

5.3 Preclinical safety data
No adverse safety issues were detected during the development of this formulation. The ingredients are well established in clinical ophthalmology.

6. PHARMACEUTICAL PARTICULARS
6.1 List of excipients
Benzalkonium chloride 0.01% w/w (as a preservative)

Purified water

Sorbitol

Sodium hydroxide

6.2 Incompatibilities
None known.

6.3 Shelf life
The shelf life expiry date shall not exceed 3 years from the date of its manufacture when stored below 25°C. Any remaining gel should be discarded 28 days after first opening the tube.

6.4 Special precautions for storage
The product should be transported in the original packaging. It should be stored below 25°C.

6.5 Nature and contents of container
Sterile ophthalmic gel presented in 5g and 10g plasticised, lacquered aluminium tubes, closed with a tamper evident polyethylene cap. Each tube is individually cartonned with a patient information leaflet.

6.6 Instructions for use and handling
Not applicable.

7. MARKETING AUTHORISATION HOLDER
Chauvin Pharmaceuticals Ltd

106 London Road

Kingston-Upon-Thames

Surrey

KT2 6TN

8. MARKETING AUTHORISATION NUMBER(S)
PL 0033/0149

9. DATE OF FIRST AUTHORISATION/RENEWAL OF THE AUTHORISATION
05 August 1996.

10. DATE OF REVISION OF THE TEXT
September 2002

November 2002

Gemeprost

(sanofi-aventis)

1. NAME OF THE MEDICINAL PRODUCT
Gemeprost Pessary 1.0mg

2. QUALITATIVE AND QUANTITATIVE COMPOSITION
Each pessary contains gemeprost 1.0mg

3. PHARMACEUTICAL FORM
White to yellowish-white spindle shaped vaginal pessary.

4. CLINICAL PARTICULARS
4.1 Therapeutic indications
• Softening and dilation of the cervix uteri to trans-cervical intra-uterine operative procedures in pregnant patients in the first trimester of gestation.

• Therapeutic termination of pregnancy conducted in licensed premises during the second trimester of pregnancy.

• Induction of abortion of second trimester pregnancy complicated by intrauterine foetal death.

Gemeprost is not indicated in the induction of labour or for cervical dilatation at term as foetal effects have not yet been sufficiently studied.

4.2 Posology and method of administration
Adults

• *Softening & dilatation of cervix uteri:* one pessary to be inserted into the posterior vaginal fornix 3 hours before surgery.

• *Therapeutic termination of pregnancy:* one pessary to be inserted into the posterior vaginal fornix at 3 hourly intervals to a maximum of 5 administrations. A second course of treatment may be instituted starting 24 hours after the initial commencement of treatment. If abortion is not well established after 10 pessaries, a further course of Gemeprost treatment is not recommended and alternative means should be employed to effect uterine emptying.

• *Intra-uterine foetal death:* one pessary to be inserted into the posterior vaginal fornix at 3 hourly intervals up to a maximum of 5 administrations.

Elderly Not applicable

Children Not applicable

4.3 Contraindications
Known hypersensitivity to prostaglandins, renal function disturbances. Gemeprost is also contraindicated in women experiencing uterine fragility related to uterine scarring, and in placenta previa.

Gemeprost pessaries should not be used for the induction of labour or cervical softening at term as foetal effects have not been ascertained.

4.4 Special warnings and special precautions for use
Gemeprost should be used with caution in patients with obstructive airways disease, those with cardiovascular insufficiency, elevated intraocular pressure, cervicitis or vaginitis. Serious, potentially fatal, cardiovascular accidents (myocardial infarction and/or spasm of the coronary arteries and severe hypotension) have been reported with prostaglandins including gemeprost. Cardiac and vascular parameters should be monitored by taking regular measurements of the patient's pulse and blood pressure.

Coagulopathy may occur following intra-uterine foetal death and should be monitored and managed actively according to current clinical standard practice. Adequate follow up of a patient having a pregnancy terminated is essential to ensure that the process has been completed, as the embryopathic hazards of gemeprost have not been determined.

Patients with the following diseases have not been studied: ulcerative colitis; diabetes mellitus; sickle-cell anaemia; epilepsy; disorders of blood coagulation; cardiovascular or pulmonary disease.

When used for cervical dilatation, if it is necessary to postpone surgery much beyond the recommended 3 hour interval patients should be kept under observation, as there is a possibility that spontaneous abortion may occur.

4.5 Interaction with other medicinal products and other forms of Interaction
Oxytocin and other labour inducers or accelerators can potentiate the action of Gemeprost

4.6 Pregnancy and lactation
Not applicable

4.7 Effects on ability to drive and use machines
Not applicable.

4.8 Undesirable effects
Vaginal bleeding and mild uterine pain, similar to menstrual pain, may occur in the interval between the administration of the pessary and surgery, especially if this interval is prolonged beyond the recommended 3 hours. Nausea, vomiting, loose stools or diarrhoea may occur but are rarely severe enough to require treatment. However, standard anti-emetic or anti-diarrhoeal agents may be administered if required. Other reported side effects include: headache, muscle weakness; dizziness; flushing; chills; backache; dyspnoea; chest pain; palpitations and mild pyrexia. Uterine rupture has been reported on rare occasions, most commonly in multiparous women and in those women with a history of uterine surgery. Anaphylactic reactions have not occurred with gemeprost but such reactions have very rarely been noted with other prostaglandins. In very rare cases, severe hypotension and coronary spasms with subsequent myocardial infarctions have been reported.

4.9 Overdose
The toxic dose of gemeprost in women has not been established. Cumulative dosage of 10mg in 24 hours was accompanied by a significant increase in incidence and severity of side-effects. In animals the acute toxic effects are similar to those of prostaglandin E1 and include relaxation of smooth muscle, leading to hypotension and depression of the CNS. Clinically valuable signs of impending toxicity are likely to be sedation; tremor; convulsion; dyspnoea; abdominal pain and diarrhoea, which may be bloody; palpitations or bradycardia. Treatment should be symptomatic. A vaginal douche may be of value depending on elapsed time since insertion of pessary.

5. PHARMACOLOGICAL PROPERTIES
5.1 Pharmacodynamic properties
Gemeprost (16, 16-dimethyl-trans-delta^2 PGE1 methyl ester) is a prostaglandin E1 analogue. Both in pregnant and non-pregnant animals, it causes contraction of the uterus and causes softening and decreases resistance of cervical tissue. Gemeprost depresses placental and uterine blood flow but those actions are secondary to the main uterine stimulation. In women, Gemeprost is an effective cervical dilator in the first trimester in pregnancy, Gemeprost is also effective at terminating pregnancy in the second trimester of gestation.

5.2 Pharmacokinetic properties
In pregnant women, although plasma levels of both the active drug and the main metabolite (de-esterified gemeprost) are very low, Gemeprost induces cervical softening within three hours of insertion. Between 12 and 28% of the vaginal dose is eventually absorbed into the circulation, and 50% of this is excreted in the urine. The unabsorbed dose is largely recovered from the genital area, either washed out in the urine or from pads used to absorb post-operative blood loss.

5.3 Preclinical safety data
No drug related toxicity has been observed in rodents given 6 times the therapeutic dose (3.2mmol Kg^{-1} daily) for up to 26 weeks.

In cynomolgus monkeys subcutaneous administration of doses up to 40 times the human therapeutic dose for 1 month caused effects such as muscular tremor, excessive salivation, poorly formed faeces and mild local reactions at the injection sites.

No teratogenic effects observed in either rats or rabbits receiving intra vaginal doses 10 to 40 times the human therapeutic dose.

No Mutagenic effects have been observed.

6. PHARMACEUTICAL PARTICULARS
6.1 List of excipients
Witepsol S 52

Dehydrated Ethanol

6.2 Incompatibilities
None known

6.3 Shelf life
The shelf-life of Gemeprost pessaries is 3 years. Once the foil sachet has been opened, any pessary not used within 12 hours should be destroyed.

6.4 Special precautions for storage
Store below minus 10°C in original pack. Temperature cycling should be avoided

6.5 Nature and contents of container
Container of 5 dose foil pessaries.

6.6 Instructions for use and handling
Before administration, the pessary should be allowed to warm to room temperature for 30 minutes away from direct heat and sunlight in the unopened foil sachet.

7. MARKETING AUTHORISATION HOLDER
Beacon Pharmaceuticals Ltd
85 High Street
Tunbridge Wells
Kent
TN1 1YG
United Kingdom

8. MARKETING AUTHORISATION NUMBER(S)
PL 18157/0001

9. DATE OF FIRST AUTHORISATION/RENEWAL OF THE AUTHORISATION
11th September 2000

10. DATE OF REVISION OF THE TEXT
August 2001

Gemzar

(Eli Lilly and Company Limited)

1. NAME OF THE MEDICINAL PRODUCT
Gemzar* 200mg Powder for Solution for Infusion.
Gemzar 1g Powder for Solution for Infusion.

2. QUALITATIVE AND QUANTITATIVE COMPOSITION
Gemcitabine hydrochloride equivalent to 200mg gemcitabine.
Gemcitabine hydrochloride equivalent to 1g gemcitabine.
Gemcitabine (INN) is a pyrimidine analogue.

3. PHARMACEUTICAL FORM
Vials containing powder for solution for infusion.

4. CLINICAL PARTICULARS

4.1 Therapeutic indications
Non-Small Cell Lung Cancer:
Gemcitabine in combination with cisplatin is indicated as a first line treatment of patients with locally advanced (inoperable Stage IIIA or IIIB) or metastatic (Stage IV) non-small cell lung cancer.

Gemcitabine is indicated for the palliative treatment of adult patients with locally advanced or metastatic non-small cell lung cancer.

Pancreatic Cancer:
Gemcitabine is indicated for the treatment of adult patients with locally advanced or metastatic adenocarcinoma of the pancreas. Gemcitabine is indicated for patients with 5-FU refractory pancreatic cancer.

Bladder Cancer:
Gemcitabine is indicated for treatment of advanced bladder cancer (muscle invasive Stage IV tumours with or without metastases) in combination with cisplatin therapy.

Breast Cancer:
Gemcitabine, in combination with paclitaxel, is indicated for the treatment of patients with metastatic breast cancer who have relapsed following adjuvant/neoadjuvant chemotherapy. Prior chemotherapy should have included an anthracycline, unless clinically contra-indicated.

4.2 Posology and method of administration
Non-Small Cell Lung Cancer:
Combination use: Adults: Gemcitabine in combination with cisplatin has been investigated using two dosing regimens. One regimen used a three week schedule and the other used a four week schedule.

The three week schedule used gemcitabine 1,250mg/m^2, given by 30 minute intravenous infusion, on days 1 and 8 of each 21 day cycle. Dosage reduction with each cycle or within a cycle may be applied based upon the amount of toxicity experienced by the patient.

The four week schedule used gemcitabine 1,000mg/m^2, given by 30 minute intravenous infusion, on days 1, 8, and 15 of each 28 day cycle. Dosage reduction with each cycle or within a cycle may be applied based upon the amount of toxicity experienced by the patient.

Cisplatin has been used at doses between 75-100mg/m^2 once every 3 or 4 weeks.

Single-agent use: Adults: The recommended dose of gemcitabine is 1,000mg/m^2, given by 30 minute intravenous infusion. This should be repeated once weekly for three weeks, followed by a one week rest period. This four week cycle is then repeated. Dosage reduction is applied based upon the amount of toxicity experienced by the patient.

Pancreatic Cancer:
Adults: The recommended dose of gemcitabine is 1,000mg/m^2, given by 30 minute intravenous infusion. This should be repeated once weekly for up to 7 weeks, followed by a week of rest. Subsequent cycles should consist of injections once weekly for 3 consecutive weeks out of every 4 weeks. Dosage reduction is applied based upon the amount of toxicity experienced by the patient.

Bladder Cancer:
Combination use: Adults: The recommended dose for gemcitabine is 1,000mg/m^2, given by 30 minute infusion. The dose should be given on days 1, 8, and 15 of each 28 day cycle in combination with cisplatin. Cisplatin is given at a recommended dose of 70mg/m^2 on day 1 following gemcitabine or day 2 of each 28 day cycle. This four week cycle is then repeated. Dosage reduction with each cycle or within a cycle may be applied based upon the amount of toxicity experienced by the patient. A clinical trial showed more myelosuppression when cisplatin was used in doses of 100mg/m^2.

Breast Cancer:
Combination use: Adults: Gemcitabine in combination with paclitaxel is recommended using paclitaxel (175mg/m^2) administered on day 1 over 3 hours as an intravenous infusion, followed by gemcitabine (1,250mg/m^2) as a 30-60 minute intravenous infusion on days 1 and 8 of each 21 day cycle. Dose reduction with each cycle or within a cycle may be applied based upon the amount of toxicity experienced by the patient. Patients should have an absolute granulocyte count of at least 1,500 (x 10^6/l) prior to initiation of gemcitabine + paclitaxel combination.

Patients receiving gemcitabine should be monitored prior to each dose for platelet, leucocyte, and granulocyte counts, and, if necessary, the dose of gemcitabine may be either reduced or withheld in the presence of haematological toxicity, according to the following scale:

(see Table 1)

For cisplatin dosage adjustment in combination therapy, see the manufacturers' prescribing information.

Periodic checks of liver and kidney functions, including transaminases and serum creatinine, should also be performed in patients receiving gemcitabine.

Gemcitabine is well tolerated during the infusion, with only a few cases of injection site reaction reported. There have been no reports of injection site necrosis. Gemcitabine can be easily administered on an outpatient basis.

Elderly patients: Gemcitabine has been well tolerated in patients over the age of 65. There is no evidence to suggest that dose adjustments are necessary in the elderly, although gemcitabine clearance and half-life are affected by age.

Children: Gemcitabine has not been studied in children.

Hepatic and renal impairment: Gemcitabine should be used with caution in patients with hepatic insufficiency or with impaired renal function. No studies have been done in patients with significant hepatic or renal impairment.

4.3 Contraindications
Gemcitabine is contra-indicated in those patients with a known hypersensitivity to the drug.

4.4 Special warnings and special precautions for use
Warnings:
Prolongation of the infusion time and increased dosing frequency have been shown to increase toxicity.

Gemcitabine can suppress bone marrow function as manifested by leucopenia, thrombocytopenia, and anaemia. However, myelosuppression is short lived and usually does not result in dose reductions and rarely in discontinuation (see sections 4.2 and 4.8).

Gemcitabine should be discontinued at the first signs of any evidence of microangiopathic haemolytic anaemia, such as rapidly falling haemoglobin with concomitant thrombocytopenia, elevation of serum bilirubin, serum creatinine, blood urea nitrogen, or LDH, which may indicate development of haemolytic uraemic syndrome (see section 4.8). Renal failure may not be reversible, even with discontinuation of therapy, and dialysis may be required.

Radiotherapy:
Concurrent (given together or ≤7 days apart):
Based on the result of preclinical studies and clinical trials, gemcitabine has radiosensitising activity. In a single trial, where gemcitabine at a dose of 1,000mg/m^2 was administered concurrently for up to 6 consecutive weeks with therapeutic thoracic radiation to patients with non-small cell lung cancer, significant toxicity in the form of severe and potentially life-threatening mucositis, especially oesophagitis, and pneumonitis was observed, particularly in patients receiving large volumes of radiotherapy (median treatment volumes 4,795 cm^3). Studies done subsequently have suggested that it is feasible to administer gemcitabine at lower doses with concurrent radiotherapy with predictable toxicity, such as a Phase II study in non-small cell lung cancer. Thoracic radiation doses of 66Gy were administered with gemcitabine (600mg/m^2, four times) and cisplatin (80mg/m^2, twice) during 6 weeks. The optimum regimen for safe administration of gemcitabine with therapeutic doses of radiation has not yet been determined.

Sequential (given >7 days apart):
Available information does not indicate any enhanced toxicity with administration of gemcitabine in patients who receive prior radiation, other than radiation recall. Data suggest that gemcitabine can be started after the acute effects of radiation have resolved or at least one week after radiation. Available information does not indicate any enhanced toxicity from radiation therapy following gemcitabine exposure.

Precautions:
General: Patients receiving therapy with gemcitabine must be monitored closely. Laboratory facilities should be available to monitor patient status. Treatment for a patient compromised by drug toxicity may be required.

Laboratory tests: Therapy should be started cautiously in patients with compromised bone marrow function. As with other oncolytics, the possibility of cumulative bone marrow suppression when using combination or sequential chemotherapy should be considered.

Patients receiving gemcitabine should be monitored prior to each dose for platelet, leucocyte, and granulocyte counts. Suspension or modification of therapy should be considered when drug-induced marrow depression is detected. Guidelines regarding dose modifications are provided in section 4.2 above. Peripheral blood counts may continue to fall after the drug is stopped.

4.5 Interaction with other medicinal products and other forms of Interaction
No interactions have been reported.

4.6 Pregnancy and lactation
The safety of this medicinal product for use in human pregnancy has not been established. Evaluation of experimental animal studies has shown reproductive toxicity, eg, birth defects or other effects on the development of the embryo or foetus, the course of gestation, or perinatal and postnatal development. The use of gemcitabine should be avoided in pregnant or nursing women because of the potential hazard to the foetus or infant.

4.7 Effects on ability to drive and use machines
Gemcitabine has been reported to cause mild to moderate somnolence. Patients should be cautioned against driving or operating machinery until it is established that they do not become somnolent.

4.8 Undesirable effects
The most commonly reported adverse drug reactions associated with Gemzar treatment include: nausea with or without vomiting, raised liver transaminases (AST/ALT) and alkaline phosphatase, reported in approximately 60% of patients; proteinuria and haematuria reported in approximately 50% patients; dyspnoea reported in 10-40% of patients (highest incidence in lung cancer patients); allergic skin rashes occur in approximately 25% of patients and are associated with itching in 10% of patients. The frequency and severity of the adverse reactions are affected by the dose, infusion rate, and intervals between doses (see section 4.4). Dose-limiting adverse reactions are reductions in thrombocyte, leucocyte, and granulocyte counts (see section 4.2).

The following table of undesirable effects and frequencies is based on clinical trial and post-marketing spontaneous reports.

Blood and Lymphatic System Disorders
Very common (>1/10):
- Leucopenia
- Thrombocytopenia
- Neutropenia - frequency of Grade 3 is 19.3%, and of Grade 4 6%. Bone-marrow suppression is usually mild to moderate and mostly affects the granulocyte count (see section 4.2).
- Anaemia

Very rare (<1/10,000):
- Thrombocythaemia

Table 1

Absolute granulocyte count (x 10^6/l)		Platelet count (x 10^6/l)	% of full dose
>1,000	and	>100,000	100
500-1,000	or	50,000-100,000	75
<500	or	<50,000	hold

Immune System Disorders
Very rare (<1/10,000):
• Anaphylactoid reaction

Nervous System Disorders
Common (>1/100, <1/10):
• Somnolence

Cardiac Disorders
Very rare (<1/10,000):
• Myocardial infarct
• Congestive heart failure
• Arrhythmia - predominantly supraventricular in nature

Vascular Disorders
Rare (<1/1000):
• Hypotension

Respiratory, Thoracic, and Mediastinal Disorders
Very common (>1/10):
• Dyspnoea - usually mild and passes rapidly without treatment
Uncommon (<1/100->1/1000):
• Bronchospasm - usually mild and transient but may require parenteral treatment
Rare (<1/1000):
• Adult respiratory distress syndrome (ARDS)
• Interstitial pneumonitis together with pulmonary infiltrates - symptoms may be relieved with steroid treatment
• Pulmonary oedema
In the event of ARDS, interstitial pneumonitis, or pulmonary oedema, Gemzar treatment must be stopped. Initiating supportive treatment early may improve the situation.

Gastro-intestinal Disorders
Very common (>1/10):
• Nausea
• Vomiting
Common (>1/100, <1/10):
• Stomatitis and ulceration of mouth
• Diarrhoea
• Constipation

Skin and Subcutaneous Tissue Disorders
Very common (>1/10):
• Allergic skin rash often associated with pruritus
• Alopecia - usually mild with minimal hair loss
Rare (<1/1000):
• Vesicle formation and ulceration
• Scaling

Renal and Urinary Disorders
Very common (>1/10):
• Haematuria
• Proteinuria
Rarely of clinical importance and do not usually change serum creatinine or urea levels.
Rare (<1/1000):
• Renal failure, aetiology unknown
• Haemolytic uraemic syndrome
Gemcitabine should be administered with caution to patients with impaired renal function (see section 4.4). Gemzar treatment should be withdrawn if there is any sign of microangiopathic haemolytic anaemia, such as rapidly falling haemoglobin levels with simultaneous thrombocytopenia, elevation of serum bilirubin, serum creatinine, urea or LDH. Renal failure may be irreversible despito withdrawal of the Gemzar treatment and may require dialysis.

General Disorders and Administration Site Conditions
Very common (>1/10):
• Oedema/peripheral oedema - reported in approximately 30% of patients. A few cases of facial oedema have been reported. The reaction is not associated with signs of cardiac, hepatic, or renal insufficiency and is usually reversible after stopping treatment.
• Influenza like symptoms - the most commonly reported symptoms include fever, headache, back pain, shivering, muscle pain, asthenia, and anorexia. Cough, rhinitis, malaise, perspiration, and sleeping difficulties have also been reported.
Common (>1/100, <1/10):
• Fever
• Asthenia

Investigations
Very common (>1/10):
• Elevation of liver transaminases and alkaline phosphatase - usually mild, transient, and non-progressive
Common (>1/100, <1/10):
• Increased bilirubin
• Gemcitabine should be given with caution to patients with impaired hepatic function

Injury and Poisoning
• Radiation toxicity (see section 4.4).

Haemolytic-uraemic syndrome (HUS) and/or thrombotic thrombocytopenic purpura and/or renal failure have been reported following one or more doses of Gemzar. Renal failure leading to death or requiring dialysis, despite discontinuation of therapy, has been rarely reported. The majority of the cases of renal failure leading to death were due to HUS.

Pulmonary effects, sometimes severe (such as pulmonary oedema, interstitial pneumonitis, or adult respiratory distress syndrome [ARDS]), have been reported rarely in association with gemcitabine therapy. The aetiology of these effects is unknown. If such effects develop, consideration should be made to discontinuing gemcitabine. Early use of supportive care measures may help ameliorate the condition.

A few cases of facial oedema have occurred.

Combination Use in Breast Cancer:

The frequency of Grade 3 and 4 haematological toxicities, particularly neutropenia, increases when gemcitabine is used in combination with paclitaxel. However, the increase in these adverse reactions is not associated with an increased incidence of infections or haemorrhagic events.

Fatigue and febrile neutropenia occur more frequently when gemcitabine is used in combination with paclitaxel. Fatigue, which is not associated with anaemia, usually resolves after the first cycle.

Grade 3 and 4 Adverse Events

Paclitaxel Versus Gemcitabine Plus Paclitaxel

(see Table 2 below)

4.9 Overdose

There is no antidote for overdosage of gemcitabine. Single doses as high as 5.7g/m^2 have been administered by IV infusion over 30 minutes every two weeks with clinically acceptable toxicity. In the event of suspected overdose, the patient should be monitored with appropriate blood counts and should receive supportive therapy, as necessary.

5. PHARMACOLOGICAL PROPERTIES

5.1 Pharmacodynamic properties

Cytotoxic Activity in Cell Culture Models:

Gemcitabine exhibits significant cytotoxicity activity against a variety of cultured murine and human tumour cells. It exhibits cell phase specificity, primarily killing cells undergoing DNA synthesis (S-phase) and under certain conditions blocking the progression of cells through the G1/S-phase boundary. *In vitro* the cytotoxic action of gemcitabine is both concentration and time dependent.

Antitumour Activity in Preclinical Models:

In animal tumour models, the antitumour activity of gemcitabine is schedule dependent. When administered daily, gemcitabine causes death in animals with minimal antitumour activity. However, when an every third or fourth day dosing schedule is used, gemcitabine can be given at non-lethal doses that have excellent antitumour activity against a broad range of mouse tumours.

Cellular Metabolism and Mechanisms of Action:

Gemcitabine (dFdC) is metabolised intracellularly by nucleoside kinases to the active diphosphate (dFdCDP) and triphosphate (dFdCTP) nucleosides. The cytotoxic action of gemcitabine appears to be due to inhibition of DNA synthesis by two actions of dFdCDP and dFdCTP. First, dFdCDP inhibits ribonucleotide reductase, which is uniquely responsible for catalysing the reactions that generate the deoxynucleoside triphosphates for DNA synthesis. Inhibition of this enzyme by dFdCDP causes a reduction in the concentrations of deoxynucleosides in general, and especially in that of dCTP. Second, dFdCTP competes with dCTP for incorporation into DNA (self-potentiation). Likewise, a small amount of gemcitabine may also be incorporated into RNA. Thus, the reduction in the intracellular concentration of dCTP potentiates the incorporation of dFdCTP into DNA. DNA polymerase epsilon is essentially unable to remove gemcitabine and repair the growing DNA strands. After gemcitabine is incorporated into DNA, one additional nucleotide is added to the growing DNA strands. After this addition there is essentially a complete inhibition in further DNA synthesis (masked chain termination). After incorporation into DNA, gemcitabine then appears to induce the programmed cellular death process known as apoptosis.

Gemcitabine and Paclitaxel Combination:

The combination of gemcitabine and paclitaxel was shown to be synergistic in a Calu-6 human lung xenograft model, which compared single-agent gemcitabine or paclitaxel versus the combination. In this model, minimal activity was seen with the paclitaxel monotherapy, while synergy was demonstrated with the combination of gemcitabine and paclitaxel. There is pharmacodynamic evidence, when paclitaxel is administered prior to gemcitabine in patients with NSCLC, that paclitaxel increases accumulation of the active metabolite, gemcitabine triphosphate (dFdCTP). The increased concentration of dFdCTP allows the metabolite to be effectively incorporated into RNA, resulting in an increased apoptotic index. This study also identified an increase in ribonucleotide levels with the combination of gemcitabine and paclitaxel, in which the author suggests that paclitaxel may enhance the antitumour activity of gemcitabine.

5.2 Pharmacokinetic properties

Gemcitabine Pharmacokinetics:

The pharmacokinetics of gemcitabine have been examined in 353 patients in seven studies. The 121 women and 232 men ranged in age from 29 to 79 years. Of these patients, approximately 45% had non-small cell lung cancer and 35% were diagnosed with pancreatic cancer. The following pharmacokinetic parameters were obtained for doses ranging from 500 to 2,592mg/m^2 that were infused from 0.4 to 1.2 hours.

Peak plasma concentrations (obtained within 5 minutes of the end of the infusion): 3.2 to 45.5μg/ml.

Volume of distribution of the central compartment: 12.4 l/m^2 for women and 17.5 l/m^2 for men (inter-individual variability was 91.9%).

Volume of distribution of the peripheral compartment: 47.4 l/m^2. The volume of the peripheral compartment was not sensitive to gender.

Plasma protein binding: Negligible.

Systemic clearance: Ranged from 29.2 l/hr/m^2 to 92.2 l/hr/m^2 depending on gender and age (inter-individual variability was 52.2%). Clearance for women is approximately 25% lower than the values for men. Although rapid, clearance for both men and women appears to decrease with age. For the recommended gemcitabine dose of 1,000mg/m^2 given as a 30 minute infusion, lower clearance values for women and men should not necessitate a decrease in the gemcitabine dose.

Urinary excretion: Less than 10% is excreted as unchanged drug.

Renal clearance: 2 to 7 l/hr/m^2.

Half-life: Ranged from 42 to 94 minutes depending on age and gender. For the recommended dosing schedule, gemcitabine elimination should be virtually complete within 5 to

Table 2 Grade 3 and 4 Adverse Events - Paclitaxel Versus Gemcitabine Plus Paclitaxel

	Number (%) of Patients			
	Paclitaxel Arm (n = 259)		Gemcitabine Plus Paclitaxel Arm (n = 262)	
	Grade 3	Grade 4	Grade 3	Grade 4
Blood and Lymphatic				
Haemoglobin	5 (1.9)	1 (0.4)	15 (5.7)	3 (1.1)
Platelets	0	0	14 (5.3)	1 (0.4)
Neutrophils/granulocytes	11 (4.2)	17 (6.6)*	82 (31.3)	45 (17.2)*
Febrile neutropenia	3 (1.2)	0	12 (4.6)	1 (0.4)
General Disorders and Administration Site Conditions				
Fatigue	3 (1.2)	1 (0.4)	15 (5.7)	2 (0.8)
Gastro-intestinal Disorders				
Diarrhoea	5 (1.9)	0	8 (3.1)	0

*Grade 4 neutropenia lasting for more than 7 days occurred in 12.6% of patients in the combination arm and 5.0% of patients in the paclitaxel arm.

11 hours of the start of the infusion. Gemcitabine does not accumulate when administered once weekly.

Metabolism:

Gemcitabine is rapidly metabolised by cytidine deaminase in the liver, kidney, blood, and other tissues.

Intracellular metabolism of gemcitabine produces the gemcitabine mono, di, and triphosphates (dFdCMP, dFdCDP, and dFdCTP), of which dFdCDP and dFdCTP are considered active. These intracellular metabolites have not been detected in plasma or urine.

The primary metabolite, 2'-deoxy-2',2'-difluorouridine (dFdU), is not active and is found in plasma and urine.

dFdCTP Kinetics:

This metabolite can be found in peripheral blood mononuclear cells and the information below refers to these cells.

Half-life of terminal elimination: 0.7-12 hours.

Intracellular concentrations increase in proportion to gemcitabine doses of 35-350mg/m^2/30 min, which give steady-state concentrations of 0.4-5μg/ml. At gemcitabine plasma concentrations above 5μg/ml, dFdCTP levels do not increase, suggesting that the formation is saturable in these cells. Parent plasma concentrations following a dose of 1,000mg/m^2/30 min are greater than 5μg/ml for approximately 30 minutes after the end of the infusion, and greater than 0.4μg/ml for an additional hour.

dFdU Kinetics:

Peak plasma concentrations (3-15 minutes after end of 30 minute infusion, 1,000mg/m^2): 28-52μg/ml.

Trough concentration following once weekly dosing: 0.07-1.12μg/ml, with no apparent accumulation.

Triphasic plasma concentration versus time curve, mean half-life of terminal phase: 65 hours (range 33-84 hours).

Formation of dFdU from parent compound: 91%-98%.

Mean volume of distribution of central compartment: 18 l/m^2 (range 11-22 l/m^2).

Mean steady-state volume of distribution (Vss): 150 l/m^2 (range 96-228 l/m^2).

Tissue distribution: Extensive.

Mean apparent clearance: 2.5 l/hr/m^2 (range 1-4 l/hr/m^2).

Urinary excretion: All.

Overall Elimination:

Amount recovered in one week: 92%-98%, of which 99% is dFdU, 1% of the dose is excreted in faeces.

Gemcitabine and Paclitaxel Combination Therapy:

Combination therapy did not alter the pharmacokinetics of either gemcitabine or paclitaxel.

5.3 Preclinical safety data

In repeat dose studies of up to 6 months in duration in mice and dogs, the principal finding was haematopoietic suppression. These effects were related to the cytotoxic properties of the drug and were reversible when treatment was withdrawn. The degree of the effect was schedule and dose-dependent.

Carcinogenesis, Mutagenesis, Fertility:

Cytogenetic damage has been produced by gemcitabine in an *in vivo* assay. Gemcitabine induced forward mutation *in vitro* in a mouse lymphoma (L5178Y) assay. Gemcitabine caused a reversible, dose and schedule dependent hypospermatogenesis in male mice. Although animal studies have shown an effect of gemcitabine on male fertility, no effect has been seen on female fertility. Long-term animal studies have not been conducted to evaluate the carcinogenic potential of gemcitabine.

6. PHARMACEUTICAL PARTICULARS

6.1 List of excipients

Mannitol

Sodium acetate

Hydrochloric acid

Sodium hydroxide

6.2 Incompatibilities

Compatibility with other drugs has not been studied.

6.3 Shelf life

3 years for the lyophilised powder.

6.4 Special precautions for storage

Store at room temperature (15 to 25°C).

Solutions of reconstituted gemcitabine, in sterile Sodium Chloride Injection BP, should be kept at controlled room temperature (15 to 25°C). Reconstituted solutions should be used immediately or may be stored for 6 hours if prepared in an appropriately controlled aseptic environment. Solutions should not be refrigerated, as crystallisation may occur.

6.5 Nature and contents of container

The product is contained in either 10ml or 50ml sterile Type I flint glass vials, which meet the requirements of the PhEur, and are closed with halobutyl rubber stoppers and sealed with aluminium seals with polypropylene caps.

1 vial per pack.

6.6 Instructions for use and handling

Reconstitution:

Gemzar has only been shown to be compatible with Sodium Chloride Injection BP. Accordingly, only this diluent should be used for reconstitution. Compatibility with other drugs has not been studied; therefore, it is not recommended to mix Gemzar with other drugs when reconstituted. Due to solubility considerations, the maximum concentration for gemcitabine upon reconstitution is 40mg/ml. Reconstitution at concentrations greater than 40mg/ml may result in incomplete dissolution, and should be avoided.

To reconstitute, add 5ml of Sodium Chloride Injection BP to the 200mg vial or 25ml of Sodium Chloride Injection BP to the 1g vial. Shake to dissolve. These dilutions each yield a gemcitabine concentration of 38mg/ml, which includes accounting for the displacement volume of the lyophilised powder (0.26ml for the 200mg vial or 1.3ml for the 1g vial). The total volume upon reconstitution will be 5.26ml or 26.3ml, respectively. Complete withdrawal of the vial contents will provide 200mg or 1g of gemcitabine, respectively. The appropriate amount of drug may be administered as prepared or further diluted with Sodium Chloride Injection BP. Reconstituted solutions should be used immediately or may be stored for 6 hours if prepared in an appropriately controlled aseptic environment.

Parenteral drugs should be inspected visually for particulate matter and discolouration, prior to administration, whenever solution and container permit.

Guidelines for the Safe Handling of Antineoplastic Agents:

Cytotoxic preparations should not be handled by pregnant staff. Trained personnel should reconstitute the drug. This should be performed in a designated area. The work surface should be covered with disposable plastic-backed absorbent paper.

Adequate protective gloves, masks, and clothing should be worn. Precautions should be taken to avoid the drug accidentally coming into contact with the eyes. If accidental contamination occurs, the eye should be washed with water thoroughly and immediately.

Use Luer-lock fittings on all syringes and sets. Large bore needles are recommended to minimise pressure and the possible formation of aerosols. The latter may also be reduced by the use of a venting needle.

Adequate care and precaution should be taken in the disposal of items used to reconstitute Gemzar. Any unused dry product or contaminated materials should be placed in a high-risk waste bag. Sharp objects (needles, syringes, vials, etc) should be placed in a suitable rigid container. Personnel concerned with the collection and disposal of this waste should be aware of the hazard involved. Waste material should be destroyed by incineration. Any excess drug solution should be flushed directly into a drain with copious amounts of water.

7. MARKETING AUTHORISATION HOLDER

Eli Lilly and Company Limited

Kingsclere Road

Basingstoke

Hampshire

RG21 6XA

8. MARKETING AUTHORISATION NUMBER(S)

200mg vial: PL 0006/0301

1g vial: PL 0006/0302

9. DATE OF FIRST AUTHORISATION/RENEWAL OF THE AUTHORISATION

Date of first authorisation: 26 October 1995

Date of last renewal of authorisation: 26 October 2000

10. DATE OF REVISION OF THE TEXT

12 November 2004

LEGAL CATEGORY

POM

PACKAGE QUANTITIES

Vials 200mg: Single vials

Vials 1g: Single vials

*GEMZAR (gemcitabine hydrochloride) is a trademark of Eli Lilly and Company.

GE19M

Genotropin 5.3mg, 12mg

(Pharmacia Limited)

1. NAME OF THE MEDICINAL PRODUCT

Genotropin 5.3 mg

Genotropin 12 mg

2. QUALITATIVE AND QUANTITATIVE COMPOSITION

Somatropin (INN) recombinant DNA-derived human growth hormone produced in E.coli.

Presentations
Powder and solvent for solution for injection with preservative One cartridge contains 5.3 mg somatropin. After reconstitution one cartridge contains 5.3mg somatropin in 1ml.
Powder and solvent for solution for injection with preservative One cartridge contains 12 mg somatropin. After reconstitution one cartridge contains 12 mg somatropin in 1ml.

For excipients, see 6.1

3. PHARMACEUTICAL FORM

Powder and solvent for solution for injection. In the two-chamber cartridge there is a white powder in the front compartment and a clear solution in the rear compartment.

4. CLINICAL PARTICULARS

4.1 Therapeutic indications

Children

Growth disturbance due to insufficient secretion of growth hormone and growth disturbance associated with Turner syndrome or chronic renal insufficiency.

Growth disturbance (current height SDS < -2.5 and parental adjusted height SDS < -1) in short children born small for gestational age (SGA), with a birth weight and/or length below –2SD, who failed to show catch-up growth (HV SDS < 0 during the last year) by 4 years of age or later.

Prader-Willi syndrome (PWS), for improvement of growth and body composition. The diagnosis of PWS should be confirmed by appropriate genetic testing.

Adults

Replacement therapy in adults with pronounced growth hormone deficiency. Patients with severe growth hormone deficiency in adulthood are defined as patients with known hypothalamic pituitary pathology and at least one known deficiency of a pituitary hormone not being prolactin. These patients should undergo a single dynamic test in order to diagnose or exclude a growth hormone deficiency. In patients with childhood onset isolated GH deficiency (no evidence of hypothalamic-pituitary disease or cranial irradiation), two dynamic tests should be recommended, except for those having low IGF-I concentrations (< 2 SDS) who may be considered for one test. The cut off point of the dynamic test should be strict.

4.2 Posology and method of administration

The dosage and administration schedule should be individualised.

The injection should be given subcutaneously and the site varied to prevent lipoatrophy.

Growth disturbance due to insufficient secretion of growth hormone in children: Generally a dose of 0.025 - 0.035 mg/kg body weight per day or 0.7 - 1.0 mg/m^2 body surface area per day is recommended. Even higher doses have been used.

Prader-Willi syndrome, for improvement of growth and body composition in children: Generally a dose of 0.035 mg/kg body weight per day or 1.0 mg/m^2 body surface area per day is recommended. Daily doses of 2.7 mg should not be exceeded. Treatment should not be used in children with a growth velocity less than 1 cm per year and near closure of epiphyses.

Growth disturbance due to Turner syndrome: A dose of 0.045 - 0.050 mg/kg body weight per day or 1.4 mg/m^2 body surface area per day is recommended.

Growth disturbance in chronic renal insufficiency: A dose of 1.4 mg/m^2 body surface area per day (approximately 0.045 - 0.050 mg/kg body weight per day) is recommended. Higher doses can be needed if growth velocity is too low. A dose correction can be needed after six months of treatment.

Growth disturbance in short children born small for gestational age (SGA): A dose of 0.035 mg/kg body weight per day (1 mg/m^2 body surface area per day) is usually recommended until final height is reached (see section 5.1). Treatment should be discontinued after the first year of treatment if the height velocity SDS is below +1. Treatment should be discontinued if the height velocity is < 2 cm/year and, if confirmation is required, bone age is > 14 years (girls) or > 16 years (boys), corresponding to closure of the epiphyseal growth plates.

Dosage Recommendations for Paediatric Patients

Indication	mg/kg body weight	mg/m^2 body surface area
	dose per day	dose per day
Growth hormone deficiency in children	0.025 - 0.035	0.7 - 1.0
Prader-Willi Syndrome in children	0.035	1.0
Turner syndrome	0.045 - 0.050	1.4

Chronic renal insufficiency	0.045 - 0.050	1.4
Children born small for gestational age (SGA)	0.035	1.0

Growth hormone deficient adult patients: Therapy should start with a low dose, 0.15 - 0.3 mg per day. The dose should be gradually increased according to individual patient requirements as determined by the IGF-I concentration. Treatment goal should be insulin-like growth factor (IGF-I) concentrations within 2 SDS from the age corrected mean. Patients with normal IGF-I concentrations at the start of the treatment should be administered growth hormone up to an IGF-I level into upper range of normal, not exceeding the 2 SDS. Clinical response and side effects may also be used as guidance for dose titration. The daily maintenance dose seldom exceeds 1.0 mg per day. Women may require higher doses than men, with men showing an increasing IGF-I sensitivity over time. This means that there is a risk that women, especially those on oral oestrogen replacement are under-treated while men are over-treated. The accuracy of the growth hormone dose should therefore be controlled every 6 months. As normal physiological growth hormone production decreases with age, dose requirements may be reduced. The minimum effective dose should be used.

4.3 Contraindications

Genotropin should not be used when there is any evidence of tumour activity and anti-tumour therapy must be completed prior to starting therapy.

Genotropin should not be used for growth promotion in children with closed epiphyses.

Genotropin should not be used in patients with Prader-Willi syndrome who are severely obese or have severe respiratory impairment (see 4.4 "Special Warnings and Precautions for Use").

Patients with acute critical illness suffering complications following open heart surgery, abdominal surgery, multiple accidental trauma, acute respiratory failure or similar conditions should not be treated with Genotropin. (Regarding patients undergoing substitution therapy, see 4.4 "Special Warnings and Precautions for Use".)

4.4 Special warnings and special precautions for use

Diagnosis and therapy with Genotropin should be initiated and monitored by physicians who are appropriately qualified and experienced in the diagnosis and management of patients with the therapeutic indication of use.

Myositis is a very rare adverse event that may be related to the preservative m-cresol. In the case of myalgia or disproportionate pain at the injection site, myositis should be considered and, if confirmed, a Genotropin presentation without m-cresol should be used.

Somatropin may induce a state of insulin resistance and in some patients hyperglycaemia. Therefore patients should be observed for evidence of glucose intolerance. In rare cases the diagnostic criteria for diabetes mellitus type II may be fulfilled as a result of the somatropin therapy, but risk factors such as obesity (including obese PWS patients), family history, steroid treatment, or pre-existing impaired glucose tolerance have been present in most cases where this has occurred. In patients with an already manifest diabetes mellitus, the anti-diabetic therapy might require adjustment when somatropin is instituted.

During treatment with somatropin, an enhanced T4 to T3 conversion has been found which may result in a reduction in serum T4 and an increase in serum T3 concentrations. In general, the peripheral thyroid hormone levels have remained within the reference ranges for healthy subjects. The effects of somatropin on thyroid hormone levels may be of clinical relevance in patients with central subclinical hypothyroidism in whom hypothyroidism theoretically may develop. Conversely, in patients receiving replacement therapy with thyroxin, mild hyperthyroidism may occur. It is therefore particularly advisable to test thyroid function after starting treatment with somatropin and after dose adjustments.

In growth hormone deficiency secondary to treatment of malignant disease, it is recommended to pay attention to signs of relapse of the malignancy.

In patients with endocrine disorders, including growth hormone deficiency, slipped epiphyses of the hip may occur more frequently than in the general population. Children limping during treatment with somatropin should be examined clinically.

In case of severe or recurrent headache, visual problems, nausea and/or vomiting, a funduscopy for papilloedema is recommended. If papilloedema is confirmed, a diagnosis of benign intracranial hypertension should be considered and, if appropriate, the growth hormone treatment should be discontinued. At present there is insufficient evidence to give specific advice on the continuation of growth hormone treatment in patients with resolved intracranial hypertension. However, clinical experience has shown that reinstitution of the therapy is often possible without recurrence of the intracranial hypertension. If growth hormone treatment is restarted, careful monitoring for symptoms of intracranial hypertension is necessary.

Experience in patients above 60 years is limited.

In patients with PWS, treatment should always be in combination with a calorie-restricted diet.

There have been reports of fatalities associated with the use of growth hormone in paediatric patients with Prader-Willi syndrome who had one or more of the following risk factors: severe obesity (those patients exceeding a weight/height of 200%), history of respiratory impairment or sleep apnoea, or unidentified respiratory infection. Male patients with one or more of these factors may be at increased risk.

Before initiation of treatment with somatropin in patients with Prader-Willi syndrome, signs for upper airway obstruction, sleep apnoea, or respiratory infections should be assessed.

If during the evaluation of upper airway obstruction, pathological findings are observed, the child should be referred to an ENT specialist for treatment and resolution of the respiratory disorder prior to initiating growth hormone treatment.

Sleep apnoea should be assessed before onset of growth hormone treatment by recognised methods such as polysomnography or overnight oxymetry, and monitored if sleep apnoea is suspected.

If during treatment with somatropin patients show signs of upper airway obstruction (including onset of or increased snoring), treatment should be interrupted, and a new ENT assessment performed.

All patients with Prader-Willi syndrome should be monitored if sleep apnoea is suspected.

Patients should be monitored for signs of respiratory infections, which should be diagnosed as early as possible and treated aggressively. Genotropin is contraindicated in patients who have severe respiratory impairment (see 4.3, "Contraindications").

All patients with Prader-Willi syndrome should also have effective weight control before and during growth hormone treatment (see 4.3, "Contraindications").

Scoliosis is common in patients with PWS. Scoliosis may progress in any child during rapid growth. Signs of scoliosis should be monitored during treatment. However, growth hormone treatment has not been shown to increase the incidence or severity of scoliosis.

Experience with prolonged treatment in adults and in patients with PWS is limited.

In short children born SGA other medical reasons or treatments that could explain growth disturbance should be ruled out before starting treatment.

In SGA children it is recommended to measure fasting insulin and blood glucose before start of treatment and annually thereafter. In patients with increased risk of diabetes mellitus (e.g. familial history of diabetes, obesity, severe insulin resistance, acanthosis nigricans) oral glucose tolerance testing (OGTT) should be performed. If overt diabetes occurs, growth hormone should not be administered.

In SGA children it is recommended to measure the IGF-I level before start of treatment and twice a year thereafter. If on repeated measurements IGF-I levels exceed +2 SD compared to references for age and pubertal status, the IGF-I / IGFBP-3 ratio could be taken into account to consider dose adjustment.

Experience in initiating treatment in SGA patients near onset of puberty is limited. It is therefore not recommended to initiate treatment near onset of puberty. Experience in patients with Silver-Russell syndrome is limited.

Some of the height gain obtained with treating short children born SGA with growth hormone may be lost if treatment is stopped before final height is reached.

In chronic renal insufficiency, renal function should be below 50 percent of normal before institution of therapy. To verify growth disturbance, growth should be followed for a year preceding institution of therapy. During this period, conservative treatment for renal insufficiency (which includes control of acidosis, hyperparathyroidism and nutritional status) should have been established and should be maintained during treatment. The treatment should be discontinued at renal transplantation. To date, no data on final height in patients with chronic renal insufficiency treated with Genotropin are available.

The effects of Genotropin on recovery were studied in two placebo controlled trials involving 522 critically ill adult patients suffering complications following open heart surgery, abdominal surgery, multiple accidental trauma or acute respiratory failure. Mortality was higher in patients treated with 5.3 or 8 mg Genotropin daily compared to patients receiving placebo, 42% vs. 19%. Based on this information, these types of patients should not be treated with Genotropin. As there is no information available on the safety of growth hormone substitution therapy in acutely critically ill patients, the benefits of continued treatment in this situation should be weighed against the potential risks involved. In all patients developing other or similar acute critical illness, the possible benefit of treatment with Genotropin must be weighed against the potential risk involved.

4.5 Interaction with other medicinal products and other forms of Interaction

Data from an interaction study performed in growth hormone deficient adults suggests that somatropin administration may increase the clearance of compounds known to be metabolised by cytochrome P450 isoenzymes. The clearance of compounds metabolised by cytochrome P450 3A4 (e.g. sex steroids, corticosteroids, anticonvulsants and cyclosporin) may be especially increased resulting in lower plasma levels of these compounds. The clinical significance of this is unknown.

Also see Section 4.4 for statements regarding diabetes mellitus and thyroid disorder and Section 4.2 for statement on oral oestrogen replacement therapy.

4.6 Pregnancy and lactation

No clinical experience of use in pregnant women is available. Animal experimental data are incomplete. Treatment with Genotropin should be interrupted if pregnancy occurs.

During normal pregnancy, levels of pituitary growth hormone fall markedly after 20 gestation weeks, being replaced almost entirely by placental growth hormone by 30 weeks. In view of this, it is unlikely that continued replacement therapy with somatropin would be necessary in growth hormone deficient women in the third trimester of pregnancy.

It is not known if somatropin is excreted into breast milk, but absorption of intact protein from the gastrointestinal tract of the infant is extremely unlikely.

4.7 Effects on ability to drive and use machines

No effects on the ability to drive and use machines have been observed.

4.8 Undesirable effects

Patients with growth hormone deficiency are characterised by extracellular volume deficit. When treatment with somatropin is started, this deficit is rapidly corrected. In adult patients, adverse effects related to fluid retention such as peripheral oedema, stiffness in the extremities, arthralgia, myalgia and paraesthesia are common. In general, these adverse effects are mild to moderate, arise within the first months of treatment and subside spontaneously or with dose reduction.

The incidence of these adverse effects is related to the administered dose, the age of patients and possibly inversely related to the age of patients at the onset of growth hormone deficiency. In children, such adverse effects are uncommon.

Transient local skin reactions at the injection site in children are common.

Rare cases of diabetes mellitus type II have been reported.

Rare cases of benign intracranial hypertension have been reported.

Carpal tunnel syndrome is an uncommon event among adults.

Somatropin has given rise to the formation of antibodies in approximately 1% of patients. The binding capacity of these antibodies has been low and no clinical changes have been associated with their formation.

(see Table 1 on next page)

Somatropin has been reported to reduce serum cortisol levels, possibly by affecting carrier proteins or by increased hepatic clearance. The clinical relevance of these findings may be limited. Nevertheless, corticosteroid replacement therapy should be optimised before initiation of Genotropin therapy.

Very rare cases of leukaemia have been reported in growth hormone deficient children treated with somatropin, but the incidence appears to be similar to that in children without growth hormone deficiency.

4.9 Overdose

No case of overdose or intoxication has been reported.

Acute overdosage could lead initially to hypoglycaemia and subsequently to hyperglycaemia. Long term overdosage could result in signs and symptoms consistent with the known effects of human growth hormone excess.

5. PHARMACOLOGICAL PROPERTIES

5.1 Pharmacodynamic properties

ATC code: H 01 A C 01

Somatropin is a potent metabolic hormone of importance for the metabolism of lipids, carbohydrates and proteins. In children with inadequate endogenous growth hormone, somatropin stimulates linear growth and increases growth rate. In adults, as well as in children, somatropin maintains a normal body composition by increasing nitrogen retention and stimulation of skeletal muscle growth, and by mobilisation of body fat. Visceral adipose tissue is particularly responsive to somatropin. In addition to enhanced lipolysis, somatropin decreases the uptake of triglycerides into body fat stores. Serum concentrations of IGF-I (Insulin-like Growth Factor-I) and IGFBP3 (Insulin-like Growth Factor Binding Protein 3) are increased by somatropin. In addition, the following actions have been demonstrated:

- Lipid metabolism: Somatropin induces hepatic LDL cholesterol receptors, and affects the profile of serum lipids and lipoproteins. In general, administration of somatropin to growth hormone deficient patients results in reductions in serum LDL and apolipoprotein B. A reduction in serum total cholesterol may also be observed.

Table 3

	Common >1/100, <1/10	Uncommon >1/1000, <1/100	Rare >1/10,000, < 1/1000	Very rare <1/10,000
Neoplasms, benign and malignant				Leukaemia
Immune system disorders	Formation of antibodies			
Endocrine disorders			Diabetes mellitus type II	
Nervous system disorders	In adults paraesthesia	In adults carpal tunnel syndrome. In children paraesthesia	Benign intracranial hypertension	
Skin and subcutaneous tissue disorders	In children transient local skin reactions			
Musculoskeletal, connective tissue and bone disorders	In adults stiffness in the extremities, arthralgia, myalgia	In children stiffness in the extremities, arthralgia, myalgia		
General disorders and administration site disorders	In adults peripheral oedema	In children peripheral oedema		

- Carbohydrate metabolism: Somatropin increases insulin but fasting blood glucose is commonly unchanged. Children with hypopituitarism may experience fasting hypoglycaemia. This condition is reversed by somatropin.

- Water and mineral metabolism: Growth hormone deficiency is associated with decreased plasma and extracellular volumes. Both are rapidly increased after treatment with somatropin. Somatropin induces the retention of sodium, potassium and phosphorus.

- Bone metabolism: Somatropin stimulates the turnover of skeletal bone. Long-term administration of somatropin to growth hormone deficient patients with osteopenia results in an increase in bone mineral content and density at weight bearing sites.

- Physical capacity: Muscle strength and physical exercise capacity are improved after long-term treatment with somatropin. Somatropin also increases cardiac output, but the mechanism has yet to be clarified. A decrease in peripheral vascular resistance may contribute to this effect.

In clinical trials in short children born SGA doses of 0.033 and 0.067 mg/kg body weight per day have been used for treatment until final height. In 56 patients who were continuously treated and have reached (near) final height, the mean change from height at start of treatment was +1.90 SDS (0.033 mg/kg body weight per day) and +2.19 SDS (0.067 mg/kg body weight per day). Literature data from untreated SGA children without early spontaneous catch-up suggest a late growth of 0.5 SDS. Long-term safety data are still limited.

5.2 Pharmacokinetic properties

Absorption: The bioavailability of subcutaneously administered somatropin is approximately 80% in both healthy subjects and growth hormone deficient patients. A subcutaneous dose of 0.035 mg/kg of somatropin results in plasma C_{max} and t_{max} values in the range of 13-35 ng/ml and 3-6 hours, respectively.

Elimination: The mean terminal half-life of somatropin after intravenous administration in growth hormone deficient adults is about 0.4 hours. However, after subcutaneous administration, half-lives of 2-3 hours are achieved. The observed difference is likely due to slow absorption from the injection site following subcutaneous administration.

Sub-populations: The absolute bioavailability of somatropin seems to be similar in males and females following s.c. administration.

Information about the pharmacokinetics of somatropin in geriatric and paediatric populations, in different races and in patients with renal, hepatic or cardiac insufficiency is either lacking or incomplete.

5.3 Preclinical safety data

In studies regarding general toxicity, local tolerance and reproduction toxicity no clinically relevant effects have been observed.

In vitro and in vivo genotoxicity studies on gene mutations and induction of chromosome aberrations have been negative.

An increased chromosome fragility has been observed in one in-vitro study on lymphocytes taken from patients after long term treatment with somatropin and following the addition of the radiomimetic drug bleomycin. The clinical significance of this finding is unclear.

In another study, no increase in chromosomal abnormalities was found in the lymphocytes of patients who had received long term somatropin therapy.

6. PHARMACEUTICAL PARTICULARS

6.1 List of excipients

Powder: Front compartment	Solvent: Rear compartment
Glycine, Sodium dihydrogen phosphate anhydrous, Disodium phosphate anhydrous, Mannitol	Water for injections, m-Cresol, Mannitol

6.2 Incompatibilities

This medical product must not be mixed with other medical products and should only be reconstituted in the supplied solvent.

6.3 Shelf life

24 months.

After reconstitution, chemical and physical in-use stability has been demonstrated for:

5.3 mg: 4 weeks

12 mg: 3 weeks

6.4 Special precautions for storage

Before reconstitution: Store at 2°C – 8°C, with up to 1 month at or below 25°C allowed. Keep container in the outer carton.

After reconstitution: Store at 2°C – 8°C, protected from light. Do not freeze.

6.5 Nature and contents of container

Two-chamber glass cartridge, in a reconstitution device, KabiVial, or for use in an injection device, Genotropin Pen, or reconstitution device, Genotropin Mixer, Ph.Eur. Type I with bromobutyl rubber plungers and an aluminium cap with a bromobutyl rubber disc.

Pack size:

Presentation	Package Size
1. Genotropin 5.3 mg	1 × 5.3 mg 5 × 5.3 mg
2. Genotropin 12 mg	1 × 12 mg 5 × 12 mg

6.6 Instructions for use and handling

Two-chamber cartridge: The solution is prepared by screwing the reconstitution device or injection device together so that the solvent will be mixed with the powder in the two chamber cartridge. Gently dissolve the drug with a slow, swirling motion. Do not shake vigorously; this might cause denaturation of the active ingredient. The reconstituted solution is almost colourless or slightly opalescent. The reconstituted solution for injection is to be inspected prior to use and only clear solutions without particles should be used.

When using an injection device, the injection needle should be screwed on before reconstitution.

In adults Genotropin cartridges 5.0 mg, 5.3 mg and 12 mg for use in an injection device or in a reconstitution device as well as Genotropin 5.0 mg, 5.3 mg and 12 mg KabiVial can also be administered by using JETEX, a jet injection device without use of a needle. Moreover, in adults as well as children, Genotropin cartridges 5.0mg, 5.3mg and 12mg can also be administered by using ZIPTIP, a jet injection device without the use of a needle. The instructions for use of these devices are enclosed in the ZIPTIP and JETEX packages. The devices can be obtained from Pharmacia.

7. MARKETING AUTHORISATION HOLDER

Pharmacia Laboratories Limited

Davy Avenue
Milton Keynes
MK5 8PH
UK

8. MARKETING AUTHORISATION NUMBER(S)

Genotropin 5.3 mg PL 0022/0085

Genotropin 12 mg PL 0022/0098

9. DATE OF FIRST AUTHORISATION/RENEWAL OF THE AUTHORISATION

1 February 1995/ 1 February 2000

10. DATE OF REVISION OF THE TEXT

February 2004

Legal Category

CD (Sch 4, Part I), POM

Ref: GN2_0 UK

Genotropin Miniquick

(Pharmacia Limited)

1. NAME OF THE MEDICINAL PRODUCT

1. Genotropin Miniquick 0.2 mg
2. Genotropin Miniquick 0.4 mg
3. Genotropin Miniquick 0.6 mg
4. Genotropin Miniquick 0.8 mg
5. Genotropin Miniquick 1 mg
6. Genotropin Miniquick 1.2 mg
7. Genotropin Miniquick 1.4 mg
8. Genotropin Miniquick 1.6 mg
9. Genotropin Miniquick 1.8 mg
10. Genotropin Miniquick 2 mg

2. QUALITATIVE AND QUANTITATIVE COMPOSITION

Somatropin (INN) recombinant DNA-derived human growth hormone produced in E.coli. Powder and solvent for solution for injection.

Presentation

1. Genotropin MiniQuick 0.2 mg. One cartridge contains 0.2 mg somatropin. After reconstitution one cartridge contains 0.2 mg somatropin in 0.25 ml.

2. Genotropin MiniQuick 0.4 mg. One cartridge contains 0.4 mg somatropin. After reconstitution one cartridge contains 0.4 mg somatropin in 0.25 ml.

3. Genotropin MiniQuick 0.6 mg. One cartridge contains 0.6 mg somatropin. After reconstitution one cartridge contains 0.6 mg somatropin in 0.25 ml.

4. Genotropin MiniQuick 0.8 mg. One cartridge contains 0.8 mg somatropin. After reconstitution one cartridge contains 0.8 mg somatropin in 0.25 ml.

5. Genotropin MiniQuick 1 mg. One cartridge contains 1 mg somatropin. After reconstitution one cartridge contains 1.0 mg somatropin in 0.25 ml.

6. Genotropin MiniQuick 1.2 mg. One cartridge contains 1.2 mg somatropin. After reconstitution one cartridge contains 1.2 mg somatropin in 0.25 ml.

7. Genotropin MiniQuick 1.4 mg. One cartridge contains 1.4 mg somatropin. After reconstitution one cartridge contains 1.4 mg somatropin in 0.25 ml.

8. Genotropin MiniQuick 1.6 mg. One cartridge contains 1.6 mg somatropin. After reconstitution one cartridge contains 1.6 mg somatropin in 0.25 ml.

9. Genotropin MiniQuick 1.8 mg. One cartridge contains 1.8 mg somatropin. After reconstitution one cartridge contains 1.8 mg somatropin in 0.25 ml.

10. Genotropin MiniQuick 2 mg. One cartridge contains 2 mg somatropin. After reconstitution one cartridge contains 2 mg somatropin in 0.25 ml.

For excipients, see 6.1

3. PHARMACEUTICAL FORM

Powder and solvent for solution for injection. A two chamber cartridge with a white powder in the front compartment and a clear solution in the rear compartment.

4. CLINICAL PARTICULARS

4.1 Therapeutic indications

Children

Growth disturbance due to insufficient secretion of growth hormone and growth disturbance associated with Turner syndrome or chronic renal insufficiency.

Growth disturbance (current height SDS < -2.5 and parental adjusted height SDS <-1) in short children born small for gestational age (SGA), with a birth weight and/or length below –2SD, who failed to show catch-up growth (HV SDS < 0 during the last year) by 4 years of age or later.

Prader-Willi syndrome (PWS), for improvement of growth and body composition. The diagnosis of PWS should be confirmed by appropriate genetic testing.

Adults

Replacement therapy in adults with pronounced growth hormone deficiency. Patients with severe growth hormone deficiency in adulthood are defined as patients with known hypothalamic pituitary pathology and at least one known deficiency of a pituitary hormone not being prolactin. These patients should undergo a single dynamic test in order to diagnose or exclude a growth hormone deficiency. In patients with childhood onset isolated GH deficiency (no evidence of hypothalamic-pituitary disease or cranial irradiation), two dynamic tests should be recommended, except for those having low IGF-I concentrations (< 2 SDS) who may be considered for one test. The cut off point of the dynamic test should be strict.

4.2 Posology and method of administration

The dosage and administration schedule should be individualised.

The injection should be given subcutaneously and the site varied to prevent lipoatrophy.

Growth disturbance due to insufficient secretion of growth hormone in children: Generally a dose of 0.025 - 0.035 mg/kg body weight per day or 0.7 - 1.0 mg/m^2 body surface area per day is recommended. Even higher doses have been used.

Prader-Willi syndrome, for improvement of growth and body composition in children: Generally a dose of 0.035 mg/kg body weight per day or 1.0 mg/m^2 body surface area per day is recommended. Daily doses of 2.7 mg should not be exceeded. Treatment should not be used in children with a growth velocity less than 1 cm per year and near closure of epiphyses.

Growth disturbance due to Turner syndrome: A dose of 0.045 - 0.050 mg/kg body weight per day or 1.4 mg/m^2 body surface area per day is recommended.

Growth disturbance in chronic renal insufficiency: A dose of 1.4 mg/m^2 body surface area per day (approximately 0.045 - 0.050 mg/kg body weight per day) is recommended. Higher doses can be needed if growth velocity is too low. A dose correction can be needed after six months of treatment.

Growth disturbance in short children born small for gestational age (SGA): A dose of 0.035 mg/kg body weight per day (1 mg/m^2 body surface area per day) is usually recommended until final height is reached (see section 5.1). Treatment should be discontinued after the first year of treatment if the height velocity SDS is below +1. Treatment should be discontinued if the height velocity is < 2 cm/year and, if confirmation is required, bone age is > 14 years (girls) or > 16 years (boys), corresponding to closure of the epiphyseal growth plates.

Dosage Recommendations In Paediatric Patients

Indication	mg/kg body weight	mg/m^2 body surface area
	dose per day	dose per day
Growth hormone deficiency in children	0.025 - 0.035	0.7 - 1.0
Prader-Willi Syndrome in children	0.035	1.0
Turner syndrome	0.045 - 0.050	1.4
Chronic renal insufficiency	0.045 - 0.050	1.4
Children born small for gestational age (SGA)	0.035	1.0

Growth hormone deficient adult patients: Therapy should start with a low dose, 0.15 - 0.3 mg per day. The dose should be gradually increased according to individual patient requirements as determined by the IGF-I concentration. Treatment goal should be insulin-like growth factor (IGF-I) concentrations within 2 SDS from the age corrected mean. Patients with normal IGF-I concentrations at the start of the treatment should be administered growth hormone up to an IGF-I level into upper range of normal, not exceeding the 2 SDS. Clinical response and side effects may also be used as guidance for dose titration. The daily maintenance dose seldom exceeds 1.0 mg per day. Women may require higher doses than men, with men showing an increasing IGF-I sensitivity over time. This means that there is a risk that women, especially those on oral oestrogen replacement are under-treated while men are over-treated. The accuracy of the growth hormone dose should therefore be controlled every 6 months. As normal physiological growth hormone production decreases with age, dose requirements may be reduced. The minimum effective dose should be used.

4.3 Contraindications

Genotropin MiniQuick should not be used when there is any evidence of tumour activity and anti-tumour therapy must be completed prior to starting therapy.

Genotropin MiniQuick should not be used for growth promotion in children with closed epiphyses.

Genotropin should not be used in patients with Prader-Willi syndrome who are severely obese or have severe respiratory impairment (see 4.4 "Special Warnings and Precautions for Use").

Patients with acute critical illness suffering complications following open heart surgery, abdominal surgery, multiple accidental trauma, acute respiratory failure or similar conditions should not be treated with Genotropin MiniQuick. (Regarding patients undergoing substitution therapy, see 4.4 "Special Warnings and Precautions for Use".)

4.4 Special warnings and special precautions for use

Diagnosis and therapy with Genotropin MiniQuick should be initiated and monitored by physicians who are appropriately qualified and experienced in the diagnosis and management of patients with the therapeutic indication of use.

Somatropin may induce a state of insulin resistance and in some patients hyperglycaemia. Therefore patients should be observed for evidence of glucose intolerance. In rare cases the diagnostic criteria for diabetes mellitus type II may be fulfilled as a result of the somatropin therapy, but risk factors such as obesity (including obese PWS patients), family history, steroid treatment, or pre-existing impaired glucose tolerance have been present in most cases where this has occurred. In patients with an already manifest diabetes mellitus, the anti-diabetic therapy might require adjustment when somatropin is instituted.

During treatment with somatropin, an enhanced T4 to T3 conversion has been found which may result in a reduction in serum T4 and an increase in serum T3 concentrations. In general, the peripheral thyroid hormone levels have remained within the reference ranges for healthy subjects. The effects of somatropin on thyroid hormone levels may be of clinical relevance in patients with central subclinical hypothyroidism in whom hypothyroidism theoretically may develop. Conversely, in patients receiving replacement therapy with thyroxin, mild hyperthyroidism may occur. It is therefore particularly advisable to test thyroid function after starting treatment with somatropin and after dose adjustments.

In growth hormone deficiency secondary to treatment of malignant disease, it is recommended to pay attention to signs of relapse of the malignancy.

In patients with endocrine disorders, including growth hormone deficiency, slipped epiphyses of the hip may occur more frequently than in the general population. Children limping during treatment with somatropin should be examined clinically.

In case of severe or recurrent headache, visual problems, nausea and/or vomiting, a funduscopy for papilloedema is recommended. If papilloedema is confirmed, a diagnosis of benign intracranial hypertension should be considered and, if appropriate, the growth hormone treatment should be discontinued. At present there is insufficient evidence to give specific advice on the continuation of growth hormone treatment in patients with resolved intracranial hypertension. However, clinical experience has shown that reinstitution of the therapy is often possible without recurrence of the intracranial hypertension. If growth hormone treatment is restarted, careful monitoring for symptoms of intracranial hypertension is necessary.

Experience in patients above 60 years is limited.

In patients with PWS, treatment should always be in combination with a calorie-restricted diet.

There have been reports of fatalities associated with the use of growth hormone in paediatric patients with Prader-Willi syndrome who had one or more of the following risk factors: severe obesity (those patients exceeding a weight/height of 200%), history of respiratory impairment or sleep apnoea, or unidentified respiratory infection. Male patients with one or more of these factors may be at increased risk.

Before initiation of treatment with somatropin in patients with Prader-Willi syndrome, signs for upper airway obstruction, sleep apnoea, or respiratory infections should be assessed.

If during the evaluation of upper airway obstruction, pathological findings are observed, the child should be referred to an ENT specialist for treatment and resolution of the respiratory disorder prior to initiating growth hormone treatment.

Sleep apnoea should be assessed before onset of growth hormone treatment by recognised methods such as polysomnography or overnight oxymetry, and monitored if sleep apnoea is suspected.

If during treatment with somatropin patients show signs of upper airway obstruction (including onset of or increased snoring), treatment should be interrupted, and a new ENT assessment performed.

All patients with Prader-Willi syndrome should be monitored if sleep apnoea is suspected.

Patients should be monitored for signs of respiratory infections, which should be diagnosed as early as possible and treated aggressively. Genotropin is contraindicated in patients who have severe respiratory impairment (see 4.3, "Contraindications").

All patients with Prader-Willi syndrome should also have effective weight control before and during growth hormone treatment (see 4.3, "Contraindications").

Scoliosis is common in patients with PWS. Scoliosis may progress in any child during rapid growth. Signs of scoliosis should be monitored during treatment. However, growth hormone treatment has not been shown to increase the incidence or severity of scoliosis.

Experience with prolonged treatment in adults and in patients with PWS is limited.

In short children born SGA other medical reasons or treatments that could explain growth disturbance should be ruled out before starting treatment.

In SGA children it is recommended to measure fasting insulin and blood glucose before start of treatment and annually thereafter. In patients with increased risk of diabetes mellitus (e.g. familial history of diabetes, obesity, severe insulin resistance, acanthosis nigricans) oral glucose tolerance testing (OGTT) should be performed. If overt diabetes occurs, growth hormone should not be administered.

In SGA children it is recommended to measure the IGF-I level before start of treatment and twice a year thereafter. If on repeated measurements IGF-I levels exceed +2 SD compared to references for age and pubertal status, the IGF-I / IGFBP-3 ratio could be taken into account to consider dose adjustment.

Experience in initiating treatment in SGA patients near onset of puberty is limited. It is therefore not recommended to initiate treatment near onset of puberty. Experience in patients with Silver-Russell syndrome is limited.

Some of the height gain obtained with treating short children born SGA with growth hormone may be lost if treatment is stopped before final height is reached.

In chronic renal insufficiency, renal function should be below 50 percent of normal before institution of therapy. To verify growth disturbance, growth should be followed for a year preceding institution of therapy. During this period, conservative treatment for renal insufficiency (which includes control of acidosis, hyperparathyroidism and nutritional status) should have been established and should be maintained during treatment. The treatment should be discontinued at renal transplantation. To date, no data on final height in patients with chronic renal insufficiency treated with Genotropin are available.

The effects of Genotropin on recovery were studied in two placebo controlled trials involving 522 critically ill adult patients suffering complications following open heart surgery, abdominal surgery, multiple accidental trauma or acute respiratory failure. Mortality was higher in patients treated with 5.3 or 8 mg Genotropin daily compared to patients receiving placebo, 42% vs. 19%. Based on this information, these types of patients should not be treated with Genotropin. As there is no information available on the safety of growth hormone substitution therapy in acutely critically ill patients, the benefits of continued treatment in this situation should be weighed against the potential risks involved. In all patients developing other or similar acute critical illness, the possible benefit of treatment with Genotropin must be weighed against the potential risk involved.

4.5 Interaction with other medicinal products and other forms of Interaction

Data from an interaction study performed in growth hormone deficient adults suggests that somatropin administration may increase the clearance of compounds known to be metabolised by cytochrome P450 isoenzymes. The clearance of compounds metabolised by cytochrome P450 3A4 (e.g. sex steroids, corticosteroids, anticonvulsants and cyclosporin) may be especially increased resulting in lower plasma levels of these compounds. The clinical significance of this is unknown.

Also see Section 4.4 for statements regarding diabetes mellitus and thyroid disorder and Section 4.2 for statement on oral oestrogen replacement therapy.

4.6 Pregnancy and lactation

No clinical experience of use in pregnant women is available. Animal experimental data are incomplete. Treatment with Genotropin should be interrupted if pregnancy occurs.

During normal pregnancy, levels of pituitary growth hormone fall markedly after 20 gestation weeks, being replaced almost entirely by placental growth hormone by 30 weeks. In view of this, it is unlikely that continued replacement therapy with somatropin would be necessary in growth hormone deficient women in the third trimester of pregnancy.

It is not known if somatropin is excreted into breast milk, but absorption of intact protein from the gastrointestinal tract of the infant is extremely unlikely.

4.7 Effects on ability to drive and use machines

No effects on the ability to drive and use machines have been observed.

4.8 Undesirable effects

Patients with growth hormone deficiency are characterised by extracellular volume deficit. When treatment with somatropin is started, this deficit is rapidly corrected. In adult patients, adverse effects related to fluid retention such as peripheral oedema, stiffness in the extremities, arthralgia, myalgia and paraesthesia are common. In general, these adverse effects are mild to moderate, arise within the first months of treatment and subside spontaneously or with dose reduction.

The incidence of these adverse effects is related to the administered dose, the age of patients and possibly inversely related to the age of patients at the onset of growth hormone deficiency. In children, such adverse effects are uncommon.

Transient local skin reactions at the injection site in children are common.

Rare cases of diabetes mellitus type II have been reported.

Rare cases of benign intracranial hypertension have been reported.

Carpal tunnel syndrome is an uncommon event among adults.

Somatropin has given rise to the formation of antibodies in approximately 1% of patients. The binding capacity of these antibodies has been low and no clinical changes have been associated with their formation.

(see Table 1)

Somatropin has been reported to reduce serum cortisol levels, possibly by affecting carrier proteins or by increased hepatic clearance. The clinical relevance of these findings may be limited. Nevertheless, corticosteroid replacement therapy should be optimised before initiation of Genotropin therapy.

Very rare cases of leukaemia have been reported in growth hormone deficient children treated with somatropin, but the incidence appears to be similar to that in children without growth hormone deficiency.

4.9 Overdose

No case of overdose or intoxication has been reported.

Acute overdosage could lead initially to hypoglycaemia and subsequently to hyperglycaemia. Long term overdosage could result in signs and symptoms consistent with the known effects of human growth hormone excess.

5. PHARMACOLOGICAL PROPERTIES

5.1 Pharmacodynamic properties

ATC code: H 01 A C 01

Somatropin is a potent metabolic hormone of importance for the metabolism of lipids, carbohydrates and proteins. In children with inadequate endogenous growth hormone, somatropin stimulates linear growth and increases growth rate. In adults, as well as in children, somatropin maintains a normal body composition by increasing nitrogen retention and stimulation of skeletal muscle growth, and by mobilisation of body fat. Visceral adipose tissue is particularly responsive to somatropin. In addition to enhanced lipolysis, somatropin decreases the uptake of triglycerides into body fat stores. Serum concentrations of IGF-I (Insulin-like Growth Factor-I) and IGFBP3 (Insulin-like Growth Factor Binding Protein 3) are increased by somatropin. In addition, the following actions have been demonstrated:

– Lipid metabolism: Somatropin induces hepatic LDL cholesterol receptors, and affects the profile of serum lipids and lipoproteins. In general, administration of somatropin to growth hormone deficient patients results in reductions in serum LDL and apolipoprotein B. A reduction in serum total cholesterol may also be observed.

– Carbohydrate metabolism: Somatropin increases insulin but fasting blood glucose is commonly unchanged. Children with hypopituitarism may experience fasting hypoglycaemia. This condition is reversed by somatropin.

– Water and mineral metabolism: Growth hormone deficiency is associated with decreased plasma and extracellular volumes. Both are rapidly increased after treatment with somatropin. Somatropin induces the retention of sodium, potassium and phosphorus.

– Bone metabolism: Somatropin stimulates the turnover of skeletal bone. Long-term administration of somatropin to growth hormone deficient patients with osteopenia results in an increase in bone mineral content and density at weight bearing sites.

– Physical capacity: Muscle strength and physical exercise capacity are improved after long-term treatment with somatropin. Somatropin also increases cardiac output, but the mechanism has yet to be clarified. A decrease in peripheral vascular resistance may contribute to this effect.

In clinical trials in short children born SGA doses of 0.033 and 0.067 mg/kg body weight per day have been used for treatment until final height. In 56 patients who were continuously treated and have reached (near) final height, the mean change from height at start of treatment was +1.90 SDS (0.033 mg/kg body weight per day) and +2.19 SDS (0.067 mg/kg body weight per day). Literature data from untreated SGA children without early spontaneous catch-up suggest a late growth of 0.5 SDS. Long-term safety data are still limited.

5.2 Pharmacokinetic properties

Absorption: The bioavailability of subcutaneously administered somatropin is approximately 80% in both healthy subjects and growth hormone deficient patients. A subcutaneous dose of 0.035 mg/kg of somatropin results in plasma C_{max} and t_{max} values in the range of 13-35 ng/ml and 3-6 hours, respectively.

Elimination: The mean terminal half-life of somatropin after intravenous administration in growth hormone deficient adults is about 0.4 hours. However, after subcutaneous administration, half-lives of 2-3 hours are achieved. The observed difference is likely due to slow absorption from the injection site following subcutaneous administration.

Sub-populations: The absolute bioavailability of somatropin seems to be similar in males and females following s.c. administration.

Information about the pharmacokinetics of somatropin in geriatric and paediatric populations, in different races and in patients with renal, hepatic or cardiac insufficiency is either lacking or incomplete.

5.3 Preclinical safety data

In studies regarding general toxicity, local tolerance and reproduction toxicity no clinically relevant effects have been observed.

In vitro and in vivo genotoxicity studies on gene mutations and induction of chromosome aberrations have been negative.

An increased chromosome fragility has been observed in one in-vitro study on lymphocytes taken from patients after long term treatment with somatropin and following the addition of the radiomimetic drug bleomycin. The clinical significance of this finding is unclear.

In another study, no increase in chromosomal abnormalities was found in the lymphocytes of patients who had received long term somatropin therapy.

Table 3

	Common >1/100, <1/10	Uncommon >1/1000, <1/100	Rare >1/10,000, < 1/1000	Very rare <1/10,000
Neoplasms, benign and malignant				**Leukaemia**
Immune system disorders	**Formation of antibodies**			
Endocrine disorders			**Diabetes mellitus type II**	
Nervous system disorders	**In adults paraesthesia**	**In adults carpal tunnel syndrome. In children paraesthesia**	**Benign intracranial hypertension**	
Skin and subcutaneous tissue disorders	**In children transient local skin reactions**			
Musculoskeletal, connective tissue and bone disorders	**In adults stiffness in the extremities, arthralgia, myalgia**	**In children stiffness in the extremities, arthralgia, myalgia**		
General disorders and administration site disorders	**In adults peripheral oedema**	**In children peripheral oedema**		

6. PHARMACEUTICAL PARTICULARS

6.1 List of excipients

Powder: front compartment	Solvent: rear compartment
Glycine Sodium dihydrogen phosphate anhydrous Disodium phosphate anhydrous Mannitol	Water for Injections mannitol

6.2 Incompatibilities

This medical product must not be mixed with other medical products should only be reconstituted in the supplied solvent.

6.3 Shelf life

24 months. Chemical and physical in-use stability has been demonstrated for 24 hours for the reconstituted solution.

6.4 Special precautions for storage

Before reconstitution: Store at 2°C - 8°C. Keep the container in the outer carton. For the only purpose of ambulatory use, the product may be stored at or below 25°C by the end user for a single period of not more than 6 months. During and/or at the end of this 6 months period, the product should not be put back in the refrigerator. The reconstituted solution should be stored at a temperature of 2°C - 8°C protected from light. Do not freeze.

6.5 Nature and contents of container

Two chamber glass cartridge, in a single dose syringe, Ph. Eur. Type 1, with separating bromobutyl rubber stoppers in a plastic sleeve with a bromobutyl plunger rod and a finger grip.

Presentation (See 2. Qualitative and quantitative composition)	Package size
1	7 × 0.2 mg
2	7 × 0.4 mg
3	7 × 0.6 mg
4	7 × 0.8 mg
5	7 × 1 mg
6	7 × 1.2 mg
7	7 × 1.4 mg
8	7 × 1.6 mg
9	7 × 1.8 mg
10	7 × 2 mg

6.6 Instructions for use and handling

The solution is prepared by screwing the plunger rod inwards so that the solvent will be mixed with the powder in the two chamber cartridge. Do not shake vigorously; this might cause denaturation of the active ingredient. The injection needle should be screwed on before reconstitution. The reconstituted solution is colourless or slightly opalescent. The reconstituted solution for injection is to be inspected prior to use and only clear solutions without particles should be used.

In adults as well as children, Genotropin MiniQuick can also be administered by using ZIPTIP, a jet injection device without the use of a needle. The instructions for use of this device is enclosed in the ZIPTIP package. The device can be obtained from Pharmacia.

7. MARKETING AUTHORISATION HOLDER

Pharmacia Laboratories Limited

Davy Avenue

Milton Keynes

MK5 8PH

UK

8. MARKETING AUTHORISATION NUMBER(S)

Presentation	PL number
1. Genotropin MiniQuick 0.2 mg	PL 0022/0186
2. Genotropin MiniQuick 0.4 mg	PL 0022/0187
3. Genotropin MiniQuick 0.6 mg	PL 0022/0188
4. Genotropin MiniQuick 0.8 mg	PL 0022/0189
5. Genotropin MiniQuick 1 mg	PL 0022/0190
6. Genotropin MiniQuick 1.2 mg	PL 0022/0191
7. Genotropin MiniQuick 1.4 mg	PL 0022/0192
8. Genotropin MiniQuick 1.6 mg	PL 0022/0193
9. Genotropin MiniQuick 1.8 mg	PL 0022/0194
10. Genotropin MiniQuick 2 mg	PL 0022/0195

9. DATE OF FIRST AUTHORISATION/RENEWAL OF THE AUTHORISATION

14 September 1998/1 February 2000

10. DATE OF REVISION OF THE TEXT

February 2004

Legal Category

CD (Sch 4, Part I), POM

Ref: GN 2_0 UK

Gentamicin Intrathecal 5mg/ml Solution for Injection

(sanofi-aventis)

1. NAME OF THE MEDICINAL PRODUCT
Gentamicin Intrathecal 5mg/ml Solution for Injection.

2. QUALITATIVE AND QUANTITATIVE COMPOSITION
Each ampoule (1ml) contains Gentamicin Sulphate Ph Eur equivalent to 5mg Gentamicin base.

3. PHARMACEUTICAL FORM
Injection.

4. CLINICAL PARTICULARS
4.1 Therapeutic indications
Gentamicin is an aminoglycoside antibiotic with broad-spectrum bactericidal activity. It is usually active against most strains of the following organisms: Escherichia coli, Klebsiella spp., Proteus spp. (indole positive and indole negative), Pseudomonas aeruginosa, Staphylococci, Enterobacter spp., Citrobacter spp. and Providencia spp.

Gentamicin Intrathecal Injection is indicated as a supplement to systemic therapy in bacterial meningitis, ventriculitis and other bacterial infections of the central nervous system.

4.2 Posology and method of administration
Bacterial meningitis and ventriculitis:

The starting dose of Gentamicin Intrathecal Injection for both children and adults is 1mg daily, intrathecally or intraventricularly, together with 1mg/kg every eight hours intramuscularly.

The MIC of the infecting organism in the C.S.F. should be assessed and, if necessary, the intrathecal/intraventricular dose increased to 5mg daily, whilst keeping the intramuscular dose at 1mg/kg eight-hourly.

Treatment should be continued for at least 7 days but longer if necessary.

Periodic serum and C.S.F. gentamicin assays should be carried out to ensure that adequate antibiotic levels are maintained and that serum and C.S.F. levels do not exceed 10mg/l.

Route of Administration

Intrathecal or intraventricular.

4.3 Contraindications
Gentamicin is contra-indicated in patients with a known allergy to it and other aminoglycosides. Evidence exists that gentamicin may cause neuromuscular blockade and is therefore contra-indicated in myasthenia gravis and related conditions.

4.4 Special warnings and special precautions for use
Ototoxicity has been recorded following the use of gentamicin. Groups at special risk include patients with impaired renal function and possibly the elderly. Consequently, renal, auditory and vestibular functions should be monitored in these patients and serum levels determined so as to avoid peak concentrations above 10mg/l and troughs above 2mg/l. As there is some evidence that risk of both ototoxicity and nephrotoxicity is related to the level of total exposure, duration of therapy should be the shortest possible compatible with clinical recovery. In some patients with impaired renal function there has been a transient rise in blood-urea-nitrogen which has usually reverted to normal during or following cessation of therapy. It is important to adjust the frequency of dosage according to the degree of renal function.

4.5 Interaction with other medicinal products and other forms of Interaction
Concurrent administration of gentamicin and other potentially ototoxic or nephrotoxic drugs should be avoided. Potent diuretics such as etacrynic acid and furosemide are believed to enhance the risk of ototoxicity whilst amphotericin B, cisplatin and ciclosporin are potential enhancers of nephrotoxicity.

Any potential nephrotoxicity of cephalosporins, and in particular cephaloridine, may also be increased in the presence of gentamicin. Consequently, if this combination is used monitoring of kidney function is advised.

Neuromuscular blockade and respiratory paralysis have been reported from administration of aminoglycosides to patients who have received curare-type muscle relaxants during anaesthesia.

4.6 Pregnancy and lactation
There are no proven cases of intrauterine damage caused by gentamicin. However, in common with most drugs known to cross the placenta, usage in pregnancy should only be considered in life threatening situations where expected benefits outweigh possible risks. In the absence of gastro-intestinal inflammation, the amount of gentamicin ingested from the milk is unlikely to result in significant blood levels in breast-fed infants.

4.7 Effects on ability to drive and use machines
Not known.

4.8 Undesirable effects
See "Special Warnings and Precautions for use".

4.9 Overdose
Haemodialysis and peritoneal dialysis will aid the removal from blood but the former is probably more efficient. Calcium salts given intravenously have been used to counter the neuromuscular blockade caused by gentamicin.

5. PHARMACOLOGICAL PROPERTIES
5.1 Pharmacodynamic properties
Gentamicin is a mixture of antibiotic substances produced by the growth of micromonospora purpurea. It is bactericidal with greater antibacterial activity than streptomycin, neomycin or kanamycin.

Gentamicin exerts a number of effects on cells of susceptible bacteria. It affects the integrity of the plasma membrane and the metabolism of RNA, but its most important effects is inhibition of protein synthesis at the level of the 30s ribosomal subunit.

5.2 Pharmacokinetic properties
Gentamicin is not readily absorbed from the gastro-intestinal tract. Gentamicin is 70-85% bound to plasma albumin following administration and is excreted 90% unchanged in urine. The half-life for its elimination in normal patients is 2 to 3 hours.

Effective plasma concentration is 4-8 μg/ml.

The volume of distribution (vd) is 0.3 l/kg.

The elimination rate constant is:

0.02 hr^{-1} for anuric patients *

0.30 hr^{-1} normal

* Therefore in those with anuria care must be exercised following the usual initial dose, any subsequent administration being reduced in-line with plasma concentrations of gentamicin.

5.3 Preclinical safety data
Not applicable.

6. PHARMACEUTICAL PARTICULARS
6.1 List of excipients
Sodium Chloride BP

Water for Injections BP

6.2 Incompatibilities
In general, gentamicin injection should not be mixed. In particular the following are incompatible in mixed solution with gentamicin injection: penicillins, cephalosporins, erythromycin, heparins, sodium bicarbonate. * Dilution in the body will obviate the danger of physical and chemical incompatibility and enable gentamicin to be given concurrently with the drugs listed above either as a bolus injection into the drip tubing, with adequate flushing, or at separate sites. In the case of carbenicillin, administration should only be at a separate site.

* Carbon dioxide may be liberated on addition of the two solutions. Normally this will dissolve in the solution but under some circumstances small bubbles may form.

6.3 Shelf life
36 months

6.4 Special precautions for storage
Store in a cold place.

6.5 Nature and contents of container
Gentamicin Intrathecal Injection is supplied in 1ml neutral glass ampoules in packs of 5.

6.6 Instructions for use and handling
Not applicable.

7. MARKETING AUTHORISATION HOLDER
Aventis Pharma

Broadwater Park

Denham

Uxbridge

Middlesex

UB9 5HP

8. MARKETING AUTHORISATION NUMBER(S)
PL 0109/0057R

9. DATE OF FIRST AUTHORISATION/RENEWAL OF THE AUTHORISATION
October 1999

10. DATE OF REVISION OF THE TEXT
July 2005

Legal category: POM

Gentamicin Paediatric 20mg/2ml Solution for Injection

(sanofi-aventis)

1. NAME OF THE MEDICINAL PRODUCT
Gentamicin Paediatric 20mg/2ml Solution for Injection.

2. QUALITATIVE AND QUANTITATIVE COMPOSITION
Each vial (2ml) contains Gentamicin Sulphate Ph Eur equivalent to 20mg Gentamicin base.

3. PHARMACEUTICAL FORM
Injectable.

4. CLINICAL PARTICULARS
4.1 Therapeutic indications
Gentamicin is an aminoglycoside antibiotic with broad-spectrum bactericidal activity. It is usually active against most strains of the following organisms: escherichia coli, klebsiella spp., Proteus spp. (indole positive and indole negative), pseudomonas aeruginosa, staphylococci, enterobacer spp., Citrobacter spp. and providencia spp.

Indications: gentamicin injection and gentamicin paediatric injection are indicated in bacteraemia, septicaemia, urinary tract infections, chest infections, severe neonatal infections and other serious systemic infections due to susceptible organisms.

4.2 Posology and method of administration
Adults:

Serious infections: if renal function is not impaired, 5mg/kg daily in divided doses at six or eight hourly intervals. The total daily dose may be subsequently increased or decreased as clinically indicated.

Systemic infections: if renal function is not impaired, 3-5 mg/kg/day in divided doses according to severity of infection, adjusting according to clinical response and body weight.

Urinary tract infections: as 'systemic infections'. Or, if renal function is not impaired, 160mg once daily may be used.

Children:

Premature infants or full - term neonates up to 2 weeks of age: 3mg/kg/12 hourly. 2 week to 12 years: 2mg/kg/8 hourly.

Elderly:

There is some evidence that elderly patients may be more susceptible to aminoglycoside toxicity whether secondary to previous eighth nerve impairment or borderline renal dysfunction.

Accordingly, therapy should be closely monitored by frequent determination of gentamicin serum levels, assessment of renal function and signs of toxicity.

Renal impairment

Gentamicin is excreted by simple glomerular filtration and therefore reduced dosage is necessary where renal function is impaired.

Nomograms are available for the calculation of the dose, which depends on the patient's age, weight, and renal function

The following table may be useful when treating adults.

(see Table 1 on next page)

The recommended dose and precautions for intramuscular and intravenous administration are identical. Gentamicin when given intravenously should be injected directly into a vein or into the drip set tubing over no less than three minutes. If administered by infusion, this should be over no longer than 20 minutes and in no greater volume of fluid than 100ml.

4.3 Contraindications
Hypersensitivity; maysthenia gravis.

4.4 Special warnings and special precautions for use
Ototoxicity has been recorded following the use of gentamicin. Groups at special risk include patients with impaired renal function and possibly the elderly. Consequently, renal, auditory and vastibular functions should be monitored in these patients and serum levels determined so as to avoid peak concentrations above 10mg/1 and troughs above 2mg/l. As there is some evidence that risk of both ototixicity and nephrotoxicity is related to the level of total exposure, duration of therapy should be the shortest possible compatible with clinical recovery. In some patients with impaired with impaired renal function there has been a transient rise in blood-urea-nitrogen which has usually reverted to normal during or following cessation of therapy. It is important to adjust the frequency of dosage according to the degree of renal function.

4.5 Interaction with other medicinal products and other forms of Interaction
Concurrent administration of gentamicin and other potentially ototoxic or nephrotoxic drugs should be avoided. Potent diuretics such as etacrynic acid and furosemide are believed to enhance the risk of otoxicity whilst amphotericin b, cis-platinumand ciclosporin are potential enhancers of nephortoxicity.

Any potential nephrotoxicity of cephalosporins, and in particular cephaloridine, may also be increased in the presence of gentamicin. Consequently, if this combination is used monitoring of kidney function is advised.

Neuromuscular blockade and respiratory paralysis have been reported from administration of aminoglycosides to patients who have received curare-type muscle relaxants during anaesthesia.

4.6 Pregnancy and lactation
There are no proven cases of intrauterine damage caused by gentamicin. However, in common with most drugs known to cross the placenta, usage in pregnancy should only be considered in life-threatening situations where the expected benefits outweigh possible risks. In the absence of gastro-intestinal inflammation, the amount of gentamcin ingested from the milk is unlikely to result in significant blood levels in breast -fed infants

Table 1

Blood Urea (mg/100ml)	(mmol/l)	Creatine clearance (GFR) (ml/min)	Dose and frequency of administration
<40	6-7	>70	80mg* 8 hourly
40-100	6-17	30-70	80mg* 12 hourly
100-200	17-34	10-30	80mg* daily
>200	>34	5-10	80mg* every 48 hours
Twice weekly intermittent haemodialysis		<5	80mg* after dialysis

*60mg if body weight <60kg. Frequency of dosage in hours may also be approximated as serum creatine (mg%) × eight or in SI units, as serum creatine (μmol/l) divided by 11. If these dosage guides are used peak serum levels must be measured. Peak levels of genamicin occur approximately one hour after intramuscular injectable and intravenous injectable. Trough levels are measured just prior to the next injectable. Assay of peak serum levels gives confirmation of adequacy of dosage and also serves to detect levels above 10mg/l, at which the possibility of ototoxicity should be considered. One hour concentrations of gentamicin should not exceed 10mg/l (but should reach 4mg/l), while the pre-dose trough concentration should be less than 2mg/l

4.7 Effects on ability to drive and use machines
Not known.

4.8 Undesirable effects
See section 4.4 "Special warnings & precautions for use"

4.9 Overdose
Haemodialysis and peritoneal dialysis will aid removal from the blood but the former is probably more efficient. Calcium salts given intravenously have been used to counter the neuromuscular blockade caused by gentamicin.

5. PHARMACOLOGICAL PROPERTIES

5.1 Pharmacodynamic properties
Gentamicin is a mixture of antibiotic substances produced by the growth of micromonospora purpurea. It is bactericidal with greater antibacterial activity than streptomycin, neomycin or kanamycin.

Gentamicin exerts a number of effects on cells of susceptible bacteria. It affects the integrity of the plasma membrane and the metabolism of RNA, but its most important effects is inhibition of protein synthesis at the level of the 30s ribosomal subunit.

5.2 Pharmacokinetic properties
Gentamicin is not readily absorbed from the gastro-intestinal tract. Gentamicin is 70-85% bound to plasma albumin following administration and is excreted 90% unchanged in urine. The half-life for its elimination in normal patients is 2 to 3 hours.

- Effective plasma concentration is 4-8μg/ml.
- The volume of distribution (VD) is 0.31kg.
- The elimination rate constant is:

1. $0.02hr^{-1}$ for anuric patients*
2. $0.30hr^{-1}$ normal

* Therefore in those with anuria care must be exercised following the initial dose, any subsequent administration being reduced in-line with plasma concentrations of gentamicin.

5.3 Preclinical safety data
Not applicable

6. PHARMACEUTICAL PARTICULARS

6.1 List of excipients
Methyl parahydroxybenzoate Ph.Eur.
Propyl parahydroxybenzoate Ph.Eur.
Disodium Edetate BP
Water for Injections BP

6.2 Incompatibilities
In general, gentamicin injection should not be mixed. In particular the following are incompatible in mixed solution with gentamicin injection: penicillins, cephalosporins, erythromycin, heparins, sodium bicarbonate. * Dilution in the body will obviate the danger of physical and chemical incompatibility and enable gentamicin to be given concurrently with the drugs listed above either as a bolus injection into the drip tubing, with adequate flushing, or at separate sites. In the case of carbenicillin, administration should only be at a separate site.

* Carbon Dioxide may be liberated on addition of the two solutions. Normally this will dissolve in the solution but under some circumstances small bubbles may form.

6.3 Shelf life
36 months.

6.4 Special precautions for storage
Store below 25°C. Do not refrigerate.

6.5 Nature and contents of container
Gentamicin Paediatric Injectable is supplied in vials.

6.6 Instructions for use and handling
Not applicable.

7. MARKETING AUTHORISATION HOLDER
Aventis Pharma
Broadwater Park
Denham
Uxbridge
Middlesex UB9 5HP

8. MARKETING AUTHORISATION NUMBER(S)
PL 00109/5066R

9. DATE OF FIRST AUTHORISATION/RENEWAL OF THE AUTHORISATION
24th January 1991 / 11th June 1999

10. DATE OF REVISION OF THE TEXT
July 2005

Legal category: POM

Genticin Eye/Ear Drops

(Roche Products Limited)

1. NAME OF THE MEDICINAL PRODUCT
Genticin eye/ear drops.

2. QUALITATIVE AND QUANTITATIVE COMPOSITION
Gentamicin Sulphate Ph. Eur. ≡ 0.3% w/v gentamicin base.

3. PHARMACEUTICAL FORM
Sterile, isotonic solution in dropper bottles.

4. CLINICAL PARTICULARS

4.1 Therapeutic indications
Genticin eye/ear drops are indicated:

1. For the treatment of superficial eye and ear infections caused by organisms sensitive to gentamicin.
2. For prophylaxis against infection in trauma of the eye or ear.

4.2 Posology and method of administration
Adults, including the elderly and children

Eyes: 1 or 2 drops should be instilled in the affected eye up to six times a day, or more frequently if required. (Severe infections may require 1 or 2 drops every fifteen to twenty minutes initially, reducing the frequency of instillation gradually as the infection is controlled).

Ears: The area should be cleaned and 2 - 3 drops instilled in the affected ear three to four times a day and at night, or more frequently if required.

4.3 Contraindications
Hypersensitivity to gentamicin or to any of the ingredients. Known or suspected perforation of the ear drum is a contra-indication to use in otitis externa only.

4.4 Special warnings and special precautions for use
Long-term continuous topical therapy should be avoided. Prolonged use may lead to skin sensitisation and the emergence of resistant organisms. Cross sensitivity with other aminoglycoside antibiotics may occur.

In severe infections, topical use of gentamicin should be supplemented with appropriate systemic antibiotic treatment.

Gentamicin may cause irreversible partial or total deafness when given systemically or when applied topically to open wounds or damaged skin. This effect is dose-related and is enhanced by renal and/or hepatic impairment and is more likely in the elderly.

Topical application of aminoglycoside antibiotics into the middle ear carries a theoretical risk of causing hearing loss due to ototoxicity. The benefits of gentamicin therapy should be considered against the risk of infection itself causing hearing loss.

Contact lenses should be removed during the period of treatment of ocular infections.

4.5 Interaction with other medicinal products and other forms of Interaction
Concurrent use with other potentially nephrotoxic or ototoxic drugs should be avoided unless considered essential by the physician.

4.6 Pregnancy and lactation
Safety for use in pregnancy and lactation has not been established. Gentamicin should only be used in pregnancy or lactation when considered essential by the physician, after careful assessment of the potential risks and benefits.

4.7 Effects on ability to drive and use machines
Patients should be advised that the use of Genticin in the eye may cause transient blurring of vision. If affected, patients should not drive or operate machinery until vision has cleared.

4.8 Undesirable effects
Irritation, burning, stinging, itching and dermatitis may occur. In the event of irritation, sensitisation or super-infection, treatment should be discontinued and appropriate therapy instituted.

Gentamicin may cause nephrotoxicity when given systemically. However, it is likely that systemic absorption following topical administration does not constitute a comparable risk.

4.9 Overdose
The oral ingestion of the contents of one bottle is unlikely to cause any significant adverse effect.

5. PHARMACOLOGICAL PROPERTIES

5.1 Pharmacodynamic properties
Gentamicin is a bactericidal antibiotic which acts by inhibiting protein synthesis.

5.2 Pharmacokinetic properties
Topical application of gentamicin can result in some systemic absorption. Treatment of large areas can result in plasma concentrations of up to 1μg/ml.

> 90% Gentamicin is excreted in the urine by glomerular filtration.

< 10% is bound to plasma protein.

$T_{½}$ = 2 - 3 hours in individuals with normal kidney function, but can be increased in cases of renal insufficiency.

5.3 Preclinical safety data
Not relevant.

6. PHARMACEUTICAL PARTICULARS

6.1 List of excipients
Benzalkonium chloride BP, Borax Ph. Eur., Sodium chloride Ph. Eur., Water, purified Ph. Eur.

6.2 Incompatibilities
None known.

6.3 Shelf life
3 years. Discard contents 4 weeks after opening.

6.4 Special precautions for storage
Store below 25°C. Do not freeze.

6.5 Nature and contents of container
Genticin eye/ear drops are available in 10ml dropper bottles.

6.6 Instructions for use and handling
Not applicable.

7. MARKETING AUTHORISATION HOLDER
Roche Products Limited, 40 Broadwater Road, Welwyn Garden City, Hertfordshire, AL7 3AY.

8. MARKETING AUTHORISATION NUMBER(S)
PL 0031/0380

9. DATE OF FIRST AUTHORISATION/RENEWAL OF THE AUTHORISATION
20 December 1994

10. DATE OF REVISION OF THE TEXT
October 2001

Genticin is a registered trade mark

P999650/1101

Genticin Injectable

(Roche Products Limited)

1. NAME OF THE MEDICINAL PRODUCT
Genticin® Injectable.

2. QUALITATIVE AND QUANTITATIVE COMPOSITION
Gentamicin sulphate Ph. Eur. ≡ 4.0% w/v (80mg) gentamicin base.

3. PHARMACEUTICAL FORM
Solution for injection.

Each ampoule contains a sterile, clear, colourless to pale yellow liquid. The solution is preservative free.

4. CLINICAL PARTICULARS

4.1 Therapeutic indications
Genticin Injectable ampoules are indicated for the treatment of systemic infections due to susceptible bacteria

such as, bacteraemia, septicaemia, urinary-tract infections and severe chest infections.

4.2 Posology and method of administration

Genticin is normally administered intramuscularly but may be given intravenously as a slow intravenous injection over at least 3 minutes or short infusion if required. Genticin should not be given as a slow infusion or mixed with other drugs before use (see *Incompatibilities*).

With either intramuscular or intravenous administration the following dosage applies for patients with normal renal function:

Adults

3 - 4mg/kg body weight daily in divided doses. Typical doses are 80mg 8-hourly for patients over 60kg and 60mg 8-hourly for patients less than 60kg.

In cases of impaired renal function a reduction in dosage frequency is recommended. The following table is a guide to recommended dosage schedules:

Blood urea (mg/100ml)	Creatinine clearance (GFR) (ml/min)	Dose and frequency of administration
< 40	> 70	80mg† 8-hourly
40 – 100	30 - 70	80mg† 12-hourly
100 – 200	10 - 30	80mg† daily
> 200	5 - 10	80mg† every 48 hours
Twice-weekly intermittent haemodialysis	< 5	80mg† after dialysis
† 60mg if body weight < 60kg		

In life-threatening infections the frequency of dosage may need to be increased to 6-hourly and the quantity of each dose may also be increased at the discretion of the clinician up to a total dosage of 5mg/kg in 24 hours. In such cases it is advisable to monitor gentamicin serum levels.

If renal function is not impaired, 160mg once daily may be used in some cases.

Elderly

Adjust dosage according to weight and renal function. Periodic serum monitoring is desirable.

Children

In children and in neonates, it can be expected that serum levels will be lower than those found in adults at equivalent dosage per kg body weight.

The recommended paediatric dosage is therefore as follows:

Up to 12 years:

6mg/kg in 24 hours in three equally divided doses (i.e. 2mg/kg 8-hourly).

In infants up to 2 weeks this dosage should be given in two equally divided doses (i.e. 3mg/kg 12-hourly).

Serum peak and trough levels should be monitored regularly. Peak levels should be measured about 1 hour after intramuscular or intravenous injection and should reach 4 micrograms/ml, but not exceed 10 micrograms/ml. Trough levels should be measured just prior to a dose and should be below 2 micrograms/ml.

Prolonged use should be avoided and whenever possible the treatment should not exceed 7 days.

Caution is advised in significant obesity as gentamicin is poorly distributed into fatty tissue. The dosage calculation should be based on an estimate of lean body weight. Serum levels should be monitored closely and the dose possibly adjusted (see *4.4*).

4.3 Contraindications

Hypersensitivity to gentamicin, any other ingredient or to other aminoglycosides.

Myasthenia gravis.

4.4 Special warnings and special precautions for use

Where renal function is impaired through disease or old age the frequency, but not the amount, of each dose should be reduced according to the degree of impairment. Gentamicin is excreted by simple glomerular filtration, and dosage frequency may be predicted by assessing creatinine clearance rates or blood urea and reducing the frequency accordingly.

It is also advisable to check serum levels to confirm that peak (1 hour) levels do not exceed 10 micrograms/ml and that trough levels (before next injection) do not exceed 2 micrograms/ml.

Caution is required in Parkinsonism and other conditions characterised by muscular weakness.

Regular assessment of auditory, vestibular and renal function is particularly necessary in patients with additional risk factors. Impaired hepatic function or auditory function, bacteraemia and fever have been reported to increase the risk of ototoxicity. Volume depletion or hypotension and liver disease have been reported as additional risk factors for nephrotoxicity.

Caution is advised in significant obesity (see *4.2*).

4.5 Interaction with other medicinal products and other forms of Interaction

Gentamicin should not be used concurrently with other potentially nephrotoxic or ototoxic drug substances unless considered essential by the physician. The potential nephrotoxicity of other aminoglycosides, vancomycin and some cephalosporins, ciclosporin, cisplatin, fludarabine and amphotericin may be increased in the presence of gentamicin and monitoring of renal function is therefore recommended.

Furosemide (frusemide) and piretanide may potentiate the ototoxicity of gentamicin, and etacrynic acid, which is ototoxic in its own right, should be avoided with gentamicin.

Aminoglycosides, including gentamicin, may induce neuromuscular blockade and respiratory paralysis and should therefore only be used with great caution in patients receiving curare-type muscle relaxants.

Aminoglycosides antagonise the effects of cholinergic agents such as neostigmine and pyridostigmine.

Indometacin has been reported to increase the plasma concentrations of aminoglycosides when given concomitantly.

Bacteriostatic antibiotics may give an antagonistic interaction, but in some cases (e.g. with clindamycin and lincomycin) the disadvantage of antagonism may be outweighed by the addition of activity against anaerobic organisms. Synergistic action has been demonstrated with penicillin. However, if penicillins (such as ticarcillin) are used with gentamicin the drugs should not be physically mixed and patients with poor renal function should be monitored for effectiveness of the gentamicin. Cross-sensitivity with aminoglycosides may occur.

4.6 Pregnancy and lactation

Safety for use in pregnancy and lactation has not been established. Gentamicin crosses the placenta and there is a risk of ototoxicity (auditory or vestibular nerve damage) in the foetus. Gentamicin should only be used where the seriousness of the mother's condition justifies the risk and use is considered essential by the physician. In such cases, serum gentamicin concentration monitoring is essential. Some animal studies have shown a teratogenic effect.

Gentamicin is excreted in breast milk, but is unlikely to be a hazard to the infant except in the presence of maternal renal insufficiency when breast-feeding should be avoided, as the levels in breast milk then rise appreciably.

4.7 Effects on ability to drive and use machines

None.

4.8 Undesirable effects

As with all aminoglycosides, at critical levels gentamicin exhibits toxicity.

Blood and lymphatic system disorders

Blood dyscrasias have been reported infrequently.

Electrolyte disturbances (e.g. hypomagnesaemia) have occurred rarely.

Immune system disorders

Hypersensitivity reactions and allergic rashes have occurred. Very rarely, anaphylactic reactions to gentamicin have occurred.

Nervous system disorders

Vestibular damage or hearing loss may occur, particularly after exposure to ototoxic drugs or in the presence of renal dysfunction. With gentamicin the vestibular mechanism may be affected when peak serum levels of 10 micrograms/ml or trough levels of 2 micrograms/ml are exceeded. This is usually reversible if observed promptly and the dose adjusted. In patients with normal renal function these levels are unlikely at standard dosage.

Gentamicin can cause neuromuscular blockade which may unmask or aggravate myasthenia gravis and cause postoperative respiratory distress.

Central neurotoxicity, including encephalopathy, convulsions, confusion, hallucinations and mental depression has been reported with gentamicin therapy, but this is extremely rare.

Gastrointestinal disorders

Infrequent effects reported include nausea, vomiting and stomatitis.

Gentamicin has rarely been associated with pseudomembranous colitis and usually in these cases other antibiotics are also involved.

Hepatobiliary disorders

Signs of liver dysfunction such as transient elevation of serum aminotransferase values and increased serum bilirubin concentration have been reported infrequently.

Renal and urinary disorders

Nephrotoxicity may occur, resulting in a gradual reduction in creatinine clearance after several days of treatment. This is usually reversible if the drug is withdrawn. Nephrotoxicity is more common if trough serum concentrations exceed 2 micrograms/ml and where there is pre-existing renal disease or concomitant treatment with other nephrotoxic agents.

4.9 Overdose

Symptoms include dizziness, vertigo and hearing loss if overdose accidentally given parenterally.

If the reaction is severe consider haemodialysis as treatment.

Gentamicin may be removed from the body by haemodialysis or peritoneal dialysis. Calcium salts given intravenously have been used to counter the neuromuscular blockade caused by gentamicin.

5. PHARMACOLOGICAL PROPERTIES

5.1 Pharmacodynamic properties

Gentamicin is a bactericidal aminoglycoside antibiotic which acts by inhibiting protein synthesis.

5.2 Pharmacokinetic properties

Gentamicin is rapidly absorbed following intramuscular injection, giving peak plasma concentrations after 30 minutes - 1 hour. Effective concentrations are still present 4 hours after injection. An injection of 1mg/kg body weight results in a peak plasma concentration of approximately 4 micrograms/ml.

> 90% gentamicin is excreted in the urine by glomerular filtration.

< 10% is bound to plasma protein.

$T_{½}$ = 2 - 3 hours in individuals with normal kidney function, but can be increased in individuals with renal insufficiency.

5.3 Preclinical safety data

There are no preclinical data of relevance to the prescriber which are additional to that already included in other sections of the SPC.

6. PHARMACEUTICAL PARTICULARS

6.1 List of excipients

Water for Injections, Sulphuric acid.

6.2 Incompatibilities

In general, mixing Genticin Injectable with other drugs prior to administration is not advised. In particular the following are incompatible in mixed solution: penicillins, cephalosporins, erythromycin, lipiphysan, heparins and sodium bicarbonate. In the latter case carbon dioxide may be liberated on addition of the two solutions. Normally this will dissolve in the solution, but under some circumstances small bubbles may form.

Dilution in the body will obviate the danger of physical and chemical incompatibility and enable Genticin Injectable to be given concurrently with the drugs listed above either as a bolus injection into the drip tubing with adequate flushing, or at separate sites. However, in the case of carbenicillin and gentamicin they should only be given at separate sites.

6.3 Shelf life

4 years.

6.4 Special precautions for storage

Do not store above 25°C. Do not freeze.

6.5 Nature and contents of container

Genticin Injectable is available in colourless, Type I glass ampoules containing 2ml, in boxes of 10 ampoules.

6.6 Instructions for use and handling

Discard any portion of the contents remaining after use.

Administrative Data

7. MARKETING AUTHORISATION HOLDER

Roche Products Limited, 40 Broadwater Road, Welwyn Garden City, Hertfordshire, AL7 3AY.

8. MARKETING AUTHORISATION NUMBER(S)

PL 0031/0381

PA 50/122/2

9. DATE OF FIRST AUTHORISATION/RENEWAL OF THE AUTHORISATION

28 May 2002 (UK)

20 April 2000 (Ireland)

10. DATE OF REVISION OF THE TEXT

August 2004

Genticin is a registered trade mark Item Code

Gentisone HC Ear Drops

(Roche Products Limited)

1. NAME OF THE MEDICINAL PRODUCT

Gentisone® HC Ear Drops.

2. QUALITATIVE AND QUANTITATIVE COMPOSITION

Gentisone HC ear drops is a sterile aqueous suspension in 10ml dropper bottles containing gentamicin sulphate, equivalent to 0.3% w/v gentamicin base and 1.0% w/v hydrocortisone acetate.

3. PHARMACEUTICAL FORM

Sterile aqueous suspension.

4. CLINICAL PARTICULARS

4.1 Therapeutic indications

Gentisone HC ear drops are indicated:

1. For the treatment of eczema and infection of the outer ear (otitis externa).

2. For prophylaxis against otitis externa following trauma.

3. For post-operative local use in surgery to infected mastoid cavities.

4.2 Posology and method of administration

For all ages

The area should be cleaned and 2 - 4 drops instilled in the affected ear three to four times a day and at night. Alternatively, wicks medicated with Gentisone HC drops may be placed in the external ear or mastoid cavity.

4.3 Contraindications

Hypersensitivity to gentamicin or to any of the ingredients. Known or suspected perforation of the ear drum is a contra-indication to use in otitis externa only.

4.4 Special warnings and special precautions for use

Long-term continuous topical therapy should be avoided. Prolonged use may lead to skin sensitisation and the emergence of resistant organisms. Cross sensitivity with other aminoglycoside antibiotics may occur.

In severe infections, topical use of Gentisone HC should be supplemented with appropriate systemic antibiotic treatment.

Gentamicin may cause irreversible partial or total deafness when given systemically or when applied topically to open wounds or damaged skin. This effect is dose-related and is enhanced by renal and/or hepatic impairment and is more likely in the elderly.

Topical application of aminoglycoside antibiotics into the middle ear carries a theoretical risk of causing hearing loss due to ototoxicity. The benefits of gentamicin therapy should be considered against the risk of infection itself causing hearing loss.

In infants there is a theoretical risk that sufficient steroid may be absorbed to cause adrenal suppression.

4.5 Interaction with other medicinal products and other forms of Interaction

None relevant to topical use.

4.6 Pregnancy and lactation

Safety for use in pregnancy and lactation has not been established. Topical administration of any corticosteroid to pregnant animals can cause abnormalities of foetal development. Gentisone HC drops should only be used in pregnancy or lactation when considered essential by the physician, after careful assessment of the potential risks and benefits.

4.7 Effects on ability to drive and use machines

Not applicable.

4.8 Undesirable effects

In the event of irritation, sensitisation or super-infection, treatment with Gentisone HC should be discontinued and appropriate therapy instituted.

4.9 Overdose

Not applicable.

5. PHARMACOLOGICAL PROPERTIES

5.1 Pharmacodynamic properties

Gentamicin is a bactericidal antibiotic which acts by inhibiting protein synthesis.

Corticosteroids, such as hydrocortisone acetate, are used in pharmacological doses for their anti—inflammatory and immuno-suppressant glucocorticoid properties which suppress the clinical manifestation of disease in a wide range of disorders.

5.2 Pharmacokinetic properties

Topical application of gentamicin can result in some systemic absorption. Treatment of large areas can result in plasma concentrations of up to 1μg/ml.

> 90% gentamicin is excreted in the urine by glomerular filtration.

< 10% is bound to plasma protein.

$T_{½}$ = 2 - 3 hours in individuals with normal kidney function, but can be increased in cases of renal insufficiency.

Hydrocortisone acetate is not absorbed through the skin as rapidly as hydrocortisone and therefore has a prolonged action. Some is absorbed systemically, where greater than 90% is protein bound.

> 70% hydrocortisone acetate is metabolised by the liver. The metabolites are excreted in the urine.

Plasma $T_{½}$ = 1½ hours.

5.3 Preclinical safety data

See *Pregnancy and lactation*.

6. PHARMACEUTICAL PARTICULARS

6.1 List of excipients

Benzalkonium chloride (preservative), povidone, polyethylene glycol 4000, sodium chloride, borax, disodium edetate and purified water.

6.2 Incompatibilities

None known.

6.3 Shelf life

3 years. Discard contents 4 weeks after opening.

6.4 Special precautions for storage

Store below 25°C. Do not freeze or mix with other liquids.

6.5 Nature and contents of container

10ml dropper bottles.

6.6 Instructions for use and handling

Not applicable.

7. MARKETING AUTHORISATION HOLDER

Roche Products Limited, 40 Broadwater Road, Welwyn Garden City, Hertfordshire, AL7 3AY.

8. MARKETING AUTHORISATION NUMBER(S)

PL 0031/0382

9. DATE OF FIRST AUTHORISATION/RENEWAL OF THE AUTHORISATION

20 December 1994

10. DATE OF REVISION OF THE TEXT

May 2000

Gentisone is a registered trade mark P037450/401

Germolene Antiseptic Cream

(Bayer plc)

1. NAME OF THE MEDICINAL PRODUCT

Germolene Antiseptic Cream

2. QUALITATIVE AND QUANTITATIVE COMPOSITION

Phenol Ph. Eur. 1.2% w/w

Chlorhexidine Digluconate Solution Ph. Eur.

to give Chlorhexidine Digluconate 0.25% w/w

3. PHARMACEUTICAL FORM

Cream for topical administration.

4. CLINICAL PARTICULARS

4.1 Therapeutic indications

The product will be recommended as an antiseptic (to help prevent secondary infection), local anaesthetic and emollient for minor cuts and grazes, minor burns and scalds and blisters, stings and insect bites, spots and other minor skin conditions, chapped or rough skin.

4.2 Posology and method of administration

All age groups:

Thoroughly clean the affected area of skin, apply the cream and rub gently. In the case of cuts or particularly tender areas, rubbing may be avoided by applying on a piece of white lint or gauze.

4.3 Contraindications

Known hypersensitivity to any of the constituents.

4.4 Special warnings and special precautions for use

Consult your doctor if symptoms persist.

Keep out of the reach of children

For external use only

Replace cap firmly after use

4.5 Interaction with other medicinal products and other forms of Interaction

Chlorhexidine is incompatible with anionic agents.

4.6 Pregnancy and lactation

The product is not contraindicated during pregnancy and lactation. However, as with all medicines during pregnancy, caution should be exercised.

4.7 Effects on ability to drive and use machines

None known.

4.8 Undesirable effects

Rarely irritancy, rashes and other skin conditions may occur.

4.9 Overdose

Repeated Topical Application

Frequently repeated topical application on the same site could theoretically lead to skin irritation. However, since the product is only intended for minor skin trauma, extensive exposure is unlikely.

Accidental or Deliberate Ingestion

The product would only be expected to be harmful if orally ingested in very large quantities. This is unlikely due to the unpleasant taste of the product. In such a case the primary concern would be the phenol intake which can cause nausea, vomiting, diarrhoea and headache.

Treatment

Gastric lavage with water and charcoal. Administration of demulcents such as egg white or milk and supportive measures.

5. PHARMACOLOGICAL PROPERTIES

5.1 Pharmacodynamic properties

Phenol – antiseptic and local anaesthetic.

Chlorhexidine digluconate – antiseptic.

5.2 Pharmacokinetic properties

The product has a local action with minimal risk of systemic effects.

5.3 Preclinical safety data

Preclinical safety data on these active ingredients in the literature have not revealed any pertinent and conclusive findings which are of relevance to the recommended dosage and use of the product.

6. PHARMACEUTICAL PARTICULARS

6.1 List of excipients

Cetostearyl alcohol

Light liquid paraffin

Polyoxyethylene - (21) - stearyl ether

Polyoxyethylene - (2) - stearyl ether

Dimeticone

Methyl salicylate

Sunset yellow (E110)

Ponceau 4R (E124)

Deionised water.

6.2 Incompatibilities

Chlorhexidine is incompatible with anionic agents.

6.3 Shelf life

Three years

6.4 Special precautions for storage

Do not store above 25°C.

6.5 Nature and contents of container

Flexible aluminium tubes internally lacquered, fitted with an integral nozzle and a polypropylene cap. 5 g, 30 g, 33 g, 55 g or 120 g tubes are contained in boxboard carton.

6.6 Instructions for use and handling

Not applicable.

7. MARKETING AUTHORISATION HOLDER

Bayer plc

Trading as: Bayer plc; Consumer Care Division

Bayer House

Strawberry Hill

Newbury

Berkshire

RG14 1JA

United Kingdom

8. MARKETING AUTHORISATION NUMBER(S)

PL 00010/0263

9. DATE OF FIRST AUTHORISATION/RENEWAL OF THE AUTHORISATION

1st July 2000

10. DATE OF REVISION OF THE TEXT

November 2004

Germolene Antiseptic First Aid Wash

(Bayer plc)

1. NAME OF THE MEDICINAL PRODUCT

Germolene Antiseptic First Aid Wash

also available as Germolene Bites and Stings Spray

2. QUALITATIVE AND QUANTITATIVE COMPOSITION

Phenol 1.20% w/v, chlorhexidine digluconate solution 1.33% w/v equivalent to chlorhexidine digluconate 0.25% w/v.

For excipients, see 6.1

3. PHARMACEUTICAL FORM

Cutaneous spray, solution

4. CLINICAL PARTICULARS

4.1 Therapeutic indications

As an antiseptic and cleansing agent (to help prevent secondary infection) and local anaesthetic for symptomatic relief of minor cuts and grazes, minor burns and scalds and blisters, stings and insect bites, spots and other minor skin disorders.

4.2 Posology and method of administration

Route of administration: External application to the skin.

All age groups: Use undiluted. Spray onto the affected area to wash away debris and dirt. If necessary use cotton wool or a clean tissue to remove dirt and excess liquid. Repeat procedure if necessary.

4.3 Contraindications

Known hypersensitivity to any of the constituents.

4.4 Special warnings and special precautions for use

If symptoms persist or if skin irritation occurs, stop using and consult your doctor.

Keep out of the reach and sight of children.

For external use only.

Keep away from eyes, ears and mouth.

If you accidentally spray this product in your eye, wash thoroughly with water.

Consult a doctor promptly if contact is made with eyes or if product is swallowed.

Do not use as a mouth wash or gargle.

4.5 Interaction with other medicinal products and other forms of Interaction

None stated.

4.6 Pregnancy and lactation
The product is not contra-indicated during pregnancy and lactation. However, as with all medicines during pregnancy, caution should be exercised.

4.7 Effects on ability to drive and use machines
None stated.

4.8 Undesirable effects
Rarely local irritation, rashes and other skin reactions may occur.

4.9 Overdose
Repeated topical application
Frequently repeated topical application on the same site could theoretically lead to skin irritation. However, since the product is only intended for minor skin trauma, extensive exposure is unlikely.
Accidental or deliberate oral ingestion
The product would only be expected to be harmful if orally ingested in very large quantities. This is unlikely due to the unpleasant taste of the product. In such a case, the primary concern would be the phenol intake which can cause nausea, vomiting, diarrhoea, headache and, in large amounts, excitement of respiratory stimulation leading to drowsiness and coma. The lethal dose of phenol has been estimated to be 15 grams.
Treatment
Gastric lavage with water and charcoal. Administration of demulcents such as egg white or milk and supportive measures.

5. PHARMACOLOGICAL PROPERTIES
5.1 Pharmacodynamic properties
Phenol - antiseptic and local anaesthetic.
Chlorhexidine digluconate - antiseptic.

5.2 Pharmacokinetic properties
Not applicable.

5.3 Preclinical safety data
There are no preclinical data of relevance to the prescriber, which are additional to those already included in other sections of the SPC.

6. PHARMACEUTICAL PARTICULARS
6.1 List of excipients
Cocamidopropylamine oxide solution (30%)
Denatured ethanol B
Perfume Medic 9884
Bitrex solution (0.25%)
Ponceau 4R (E124)
Purified water

6.2 Incompatibilities
None stated.

6.3 Shelf life
36 months

6.4 Special precautions for storage
None.

6.5 Nature and contents of container
A clear, straight-sided, oval, PVC bottle with a pump spray, containing 50, 100, 150 or 200 ml. Each bottle may be contained in a boxboard carton.

6.6 Instructions for use and handling
None

7. MARKETING AUTHORISATION HOLDER
Bayer plc
Bayer House
Strawberry Hill
Newbury
Berkshire
RG14 1JA
Trading as Bayer plc, Consumer Care Division

8. MARKETING AUTHORISATION NUMBER(S)
PL 0010/0261

9. DATE OF FIRST AUTHORISATION/RENEWAL OF THE AUTHORISATION
Date of first authorisation: 1 July 2000
Date of renewal of authorisation: 16 October 2000

10. DATE OF REVISION OF THE TEXT
November 2004

Germolene Antiseptic Gel

(Bayer plc)

1. NAME OF THE MEDICINAL PRODUCT
Germolene Antiseptic Gel

2. QUALITATIVE AND QUANTITATIVE COMPOSITION
Active ingredient%w/w
Cetylpyridinium chloride 0.025%

3. PHARMACEUTICAL FORM
Gel

4. CLINICAL PARTICULARS
4.1 Therapeutic indications
For cuts, grazes, insect bites, minor wounds, spots, minor burns and scalds.

4.2 Posology and method of administration
Adults and children: Apply to the affected area two or three times a day.
For topical application.

4.3 Contraindications
Hypersensitivity to any of the ingredients.

4.4 Special warnings and special precautions for use
Prolonged and repeated application is inadvisable as hypersensitivity may occur.
Do not use if the skin is weeping or badly inflamed.
Avoid contact with the eyes.
For external use only.
Keep all medicines out of the reach of children.

4.5 Interaction with other medicinal products and other forms of Interaction
There are no clinically significant interactions.

4.6 Pregnancy and lactation
The safety of Children's Antiseptic Gel during pregnancy and lactation has not been established but is not considered to constitute a hazard during these periods.

4.7 Effects on ability to drive and use machines
No adverse effects known.

4.8 Undesirable effects
Skin irritation may occasionally occur and hypersensitivity reactions may develop in certain individuals.

4.9 Overdose
It is unlikely that systemic toxicity will result from the ingestion of Children's Antiseptic Gel, although it may give rise to nausea, vomiting and diarrhoea. Treatment should be symptomatic.

5. PHARMACOLOGICAL PROPERTIES
5.1 Pharmacodynamic properties
Cetylpyridinium chloride is a quaternary ammonium disinfectant having bactericidal activity against both Gram-positive and Gram-negative organisms.

5.2 Pharmacokinetic properties
None stated.

5.3 Preclinical safety data
Not applicable.

6. PHARMACEUTICAL PARTICULARS
6.1 List of excipients
Hydroxypropyl methyl cellulose
Glycerin
Sodium citrate
Anhydrous citric acid
Purified water

6.2 Incompatibilities
None stated.

6.3 Shelf life
24 months.

6.4 Special precautions for storage
None

6.5 Nature and contents of container
Laminated tube with polythene lined tamper evident seal, fitted with a PP cap or a laminate tube with polythene ionomer (Surlyn) lined tamper evident seal fitted with a PP cap or a polythene tube consisting of LLDPE and LDPE fitted with a PP cap.

6.6 Instructions for use and handling
Not applicable.

7. MARKETING AUTHORISATION HOLDER
The Boots Company PLC
1 Thane Road West
Nottingham NG2 3AA
Trading as: BCM

8. MARKETING AUTHORISATION NUMBER(S)
PL 00014/0556

9. DATE OF FIRST AUTHORISATION/RENEWAL OF THE AUTHORISATION
29 October 1996

10. DATE OF REVISION OF THE TEXT
July 2004

Germolene Antiseptic Ointment

(Bayer plc)

1. NAME OF THE MEDICINAL PRODUCT
Germolene Antiseptic Ointment

2. QUALITATIVE AND QUANTITATIVE COMPOSITION
Wool fat Ph. Eur. 35%, Yellow Soft Paraffin B. P. 34.8%, White Soft Paraffin B. P. 1.13%, Light Liquid Paraffin Ph. Eur. 7.9%, Starch Ph. Eur. 10%, Zinc Oxide Ph. Eur. 6.55%, Methyl Salicylate Ph. Eur. 3%, Phenol Ph. Eur. 1.19% and Octaphonium Chloride 0.3%.

3. PHARMACEUTICAL FORM
Ointment for topical administration.

4. CLINICAL PARTICULARS
4.1 Therapeutic indications
For minor cuts and grazes, minor burns and scalds and blisters, sore or rough skin, wash-day hands, sunburn and the symptomatic relief of muscular pain and stiffness.

4.2 Posology and method of administration
Minor cuts and grazes etc.: Clean the wound and apply directly or on a dressing.
Minor burns, scalds and blisters: Apply liberally and cover with a light bandage.
Sore, rough skin, wash-day hands, sunburn etc.: Apply directly and rub in gently.
Stiff, aching muscles: Apply liberally and massage in thoroughly.

4.3 Contraindications
Hypersensitivity to any of the ingredients.

4.4 Special warnings and special precautions for use
For external use only.
Keep out of the reach of children.
If symptoms persist, consult your doctor.

4.5 Interaction with other medicinal products and other forms of Interaction
None known.

4.6 Pregnancy and lactation
Use in pregnancy and lactation is not contraindicated. However, as with all medicines during pregnancy, caution should be exercised.

4.7 Effects on ability to drive and use machines
None.

4.8 Undesirable effects
Local allergic reactions may occur. Very rarely, contact dermatitis may occur.

4.9 Overdose
It is very unlikely that overdose would occur with this pharmaceutical form. Theoretically, frequently repeated topical application on the same site could lead to skin irritation. However, since the product is only intended for minor skin trauma, extensive exposure is unlikely.

5. PHARMACOLOGICAL PROPERTIES
5.1 Pharmacodynamic properties
Zinc oxide is a mild astringent. Methyl salicylate is a topical analgesic and anti-inflammatory. Phenol is an antiseptic and local anaesthetic. Octafonium chloride is an antiseptic. Wool fat, yellow soft paraffin, white soft paraffin, light liquid paraffin and starch all have emollient properties.

5.2 Pharmacokinetic properties
Not applicable.

5.3 Preclinical safety data
There are no preclinical data of any relevance additional to that already included in other sections of the SmPC.

6. PHARMACEUTICAL PARTICULARS
6.1 List of excipients
Also contains menthol and colours: ponceau 4R (E124) & tartrazine (E102).

6.2 Incompatibilities
None.

6.3 Shelf life
Three years.

6.4 Special precautions for storage
None.

6.5 Nature and contents of container
Flexible aluminium tube, unlacquered internally, fitted with an integral nozzle and a polypropylene cap, containing 27g of ointment.

6.6 Instructions for use and handling
Replace closure firmly after use.

7. MARKETING AUTHORISATION HOLDER
Bayer plc
Trading as: Bayer plc; Consumer Care Division
Bayer House
Strawberry Hill
Newbury
Berkshire
RG14 1JA
United Kingdom

8. MARKETING AUTHORISATION NUMBER(S)
PL 00010/0262

9. DATE OF FIRST AUTHORISATION/RENEWAL OF THE AUTHORISATION
1st July 2000

10. DATE OF REVISION OF THE TEXT
December 2004

Germoloids Cream

(Bayer plc)

1. NAME OF THE MEDICINAL PRODUCT
Germoloids Cream

2. QUALITATIVE AND QUANTITATIVE COMPOSITION
Zinc oxide Ph. Eur. 6.6% w/w

Lidocaine hydrochloride Ph. Eur. 0.7% w/w

3. PHARMACEUTICAL FORM
Cream for topical and rectal administration.

4. CLINICAL PARTICULARS

4.1 Therapeutic indications
The symptomatic relief of pain, swelling, irritation and itching associated with haemorrhoids and pruritus ani.

4.2 Posology and method of administration
Adults and children aged 12 years and over:

Apply at least twice a day with a minimum of three to four hours between applications. Further applications can be made at any time of day and are particularly recommended after bowel movement.

Do not use more than four times in any 24 hour period.

External piles and pruritus ani:

Apply to the affected area.

Internal piles:

Gently insert applicator into the anal opening and expel a small amount of the cream by squeezing the tube gently.

Children under 12 years:

Only as directed by a doctor

The elderly:

Use as per adult directions.

4.3 Contraindications
Hypersensitivity to any of the constituents.

4.4 Special warnings and special precautions for use
Persons who continually suffer from haemorrhoids or who have severe haemorrhoids or who experience excessive bleeding, are advised to consult a doctor.

4.5 Interaction with other medicinal products and other forms of Interaction
None known for topical preparations.

4.6 Pregnancy and lactation
There is a lack of definitive evidence of safety of the product in human pregnancy and lactation. However, lidocaine hydrochloride and zinc oxide have been in wide use for many years without apparent ill consequence. It is not necessary to contraindicate this product in pregnancy and lactation provided caution is exercised and the directions for use are followed. However, as with all medicines, the advice of a doctor should be sought.

4.7 Effects on ability to drive and use machines
None.

4.8 Undesirable effects
Very rarely increased irritation may occur at the site of application.

4.9 Overdose
It is very unlikely that overdosage would occur from this pharmaceutical form. Symptoms of lidocaine overdosage would be unlikely to occur even after anal insertion of 25g of cream.

Normally there should be no systemic adverse effects, but at worst CNS and cardiovascular effects are possible. Treatment would be symptomatic after withdrawal of product.

In the case of accidental oral ingestion, the advice of a doctor should be sought.

5. PHARMACOLOGICAL PROPERTIES

5.1 Pharmacodynamic properties
Zinc oxide has astringent, antiseptic, soothing and protective properties.

Lidocaine hydrochloride has a local anaesthetic action.

The cream base has emollient properties.

5.2 Pharmacokinetic properties
The product has a local action with minimal risk of systemic effects. Lidocaine has a fast onset and intermediate duration of action. It is partially absorbed but plasma levels will be low in view of the concentration of lidocaine in the product. It undergoes de-ethylation in the liver where clearance approaches the rate of hepatic flow.

5.3 Preclinical safety data
Preclinical safety data on these active ingredients in the literature, have not revealed any pertinent and conclusive findings which are of relevance to the recommended dosage and use of the product.

6. PHARMACEUTICAL PARTICULARS

6.1 List of excipients
Polawax

White soft paraffin

Methyl salicylate

Methyl hydroxybenzoate (E218)

Butyl hydroxybenzoate

Deionised water.

6.2 Incompatibilities
None known.

6.3 Shelf life
Three years

6.4 Special precautions for storage
Do not store above 25°C.

6.5 Nature and contents of container
a) Flexible aluminium tubes internally lacquered, fitted with a polypropylene screw cap. 25, 27.5 or 55g tubes are contained in boxboard cartons, together with a polyethylene screw-on applicator nozzle.

b) Aluminium laminate tube consisting of 150μm Polyethylene /5μm polyacrylate outer layer, 30μm alumininum and an inner layer of 30μm polyacrylate / 60μm polyethylene, fitted with a HD polyethylene shoulder, an aluminium/surlyn tamper evident seal, polypropylene cap and a loose polyethylene screw-on applicator nozzle.

6.6 Instructions for use and handling
Not applicable.

Administrative Data

7. MARKETING AUTHORISATION HOLDER
Bayer plc

Trading style: Bayer plc; Consumer Care Division

Bayer House

Strawberry Hill

Newbury

Berkshire

RG14 1JA

United Kingdom

8. MARKETING AUTHORISATION NUMBER(S)
PL 00010/0265

9. DATE OF FIRST AUTHORISATION/RENEWAL OF THE AUTHORISATION
1st July 2000

10. DATE OF REVISION OF THE TEXT
16th June 2005

Germoloids HC Spray

(Bayer plc)

1. NAME OF THE MEDICINAL PRODUCT
Germoloids® HC Spray

2. QUALITATIVE AND QUANTITATIVE COMPOSITION
Hydrocortisone 0.2% w/w

Lidocaine Hydrochloride 1.0% w/w

For excipients, see 6.1.

3. PHARMACEUTICAL FORM
Cutaneous spray solution

Colourless to pale yellow

4. CLINICAL PARTICULARS

4.1 Therapeutic indications
For the symptomatic relief of anal and perianal itch, irritation and pain, associated with external haemorrhoids.

4.2 Posology and method of administration
The product is for cutaneous use.

Prime pump before initial use by depressing its top once or twice.

Adults

The product is applied by parting the buttocks if necessary, spraying once over the affected area, up to three times daily depending on the severity of the condition. The spray will operate in any orientation.

Wash hands and replace cap after use.

Elderly

The same dose applies to the elderly.

Children

The spray should not be used in children under 16 years.

4.3 Contraindications
Not to be used if sensitive to lidocaine or any of the other ingredients. Not to be used on broken or infected skin. Not to be used internally (inside the anus), or anywhere other than the anal area.

4.4 Special warnings and special precautions for use
Germoloids HC Spray is intended for use for limited periods and should not be used continuously for longer than 7 days. Patients should be instructed to seek medical advice if they experience persistent pain or bleeding from the anus, especially where associated with a change in bowel habit, abdominal pain, if the stomach is distended or if they are losing weight. Prompt medical treatment may be very important under such circumstances. Germoloids HC Spray should be kept away from the eyes, nose and mouth.

4.5 Interaction with other medicinal products and other forms of Interaction
No known interactions. Medical supervision is required if used in conjunction with other medicines containing steroids, owing to possible additive effects.

4.6 Pregnancy and lactation
This product should not be used during pregnancy or breast-feeding. There is inadequate evidence of safety in human pregnancy. Topical administration of corticosteroids to pregnant animals can cause abnormalities of foetal development including cleft palate and intra-uterine growth retardation. There may therefore be a very small risk of such effects in the human foetus.

4.7 Effects on ability to drive and use machines
None known.

4.8 Undesirable effects
A temporary tingling sensation may be experienced locally after initial application. Hypersensitivity to lidocaine has rarely been reported.

4.9 Overdose
Under exceptional circumstances, if Germoloids HC Spray is used excessively, particularly in young children, it is theoretically possible that adrenal suppression and skin thinning may occur. The symptoms are normally reversible on cessation of treatment.

5. PHARMACOLOGICAL PROPERTIES

5.1 Pharmacodynamic properties
ATC Code: C05A A Antihaemorrhoidals for topical use – products containing corticosteroids

The preparation combines the well-known local anti-inflammatory and anti-pruritic properties of hydrocortisone and the analgesic effect of lidocaine in an aqueous spray formulation. On application, finger contact with the affected area can be avoided which makes for improved hygiene, and lessens the risk of infection.

5.2 Pharmacokinetic properties
The active ingredients of the formulation are readily available for intimate contact with the skin and mucous membranes, as the preparation is sprayed in small droplets which dry after application to leave the active ingredients in close contact with the affected area.

Because the preparation is a clear solution, it is entirely homogeneous, and the availability of the active ingredient is optimal.

5.3 Preclinical safety data
There are no pre-clinical data of relevance to the prescriber, which are additional to that already included in other sections of the SPC.

6. PHARMACEUTICAL PARTICULARS

6.1 List of excipients
Cetomacrogol 1000

Citric Acid Monohydrate

Sodium Citrate

Propyl Gallate

Phenoxyethanol

Purified Water

6.2 Incompatibilities
Not applicable

6.3 Shelf life
30 months.

6.4 Special precautions for storage
Do not store above 25°C.

6.5 Nature and contents of container
High density polyethylene/aluminium/EAA copolymer collapsible laminate tube with metering spray pump.

Pack size: 25ml, 30ml.

The spray operates when held in any direction. The container is ozone-friendly. It is *not* an aerosol and does *not* contain any potentially irritant propellants.

6.6 Instructions for use and handling
Not applicable.

7. MARKETING AUTHORISATION HOLDER
Bayer plc

Bayer House

Strawberry Hill

Newbury, Berkshire

RG14 1JA

United Kingdom

Trading as Bayer plc, Consumer Care Division.

8. MARKETING AUTHORISATION NUMBER(S)
PL 0010/0274

9. DATE OF FIRST AUTHORISATION/RENEWAL OF THE AUTHORISATION
October 2004

10. DATE OF REVISION OF THE TEXT
July 2005

Legal Status: GSL

Germoloids Ointment

(Bayer plc)

1. NAME OF THE MEDICINAL PRODUCT
Germoloids Ointment.

2. QUALITATIVE AND QUANTITATIVE COMPOSITION
Zinc oxide Ph. Eur. 6.6% w/w

Lidocaine hydrochloride Ph. Eur. 0.7% w/w

3. PHARMACEUTICAL FORM
Ointment for topical and rectal administration.

4. CLINICAL PARTICULARS

4.1 Therapeutic indications
The symptomatic relief of pain, swelling, irritation and itching associated with haemorrhoids, and pruritus ani.

4.2 Posology and method of administration
Adults and children aged 12 years and over:

Apply at least twice a day with a minimum of three to four hours between applications. Further applications can be made at any time of day and are particularly recommended after a bowel movement.

Do not use more than four times in any 24-hour period.

External piles and pruritus ani:

Apply to the affected area.

Internal piles:

Gently insert applicator into the anal opening and expel a small amount of the ointment by squeezing the tube gently.

Children under 12 years:

Only as directed by a doctor.

The elderly:

Use as per adult directions.

4.3 Contraindications
Hypersensitivity to any of the constituents.

4.4 Special warnings and special precautions for use
Persons who continually suffer from haemorrhoids or who have severe haemorrhoids or who experience excessive bleeding, are advised to consult a doctor.

4.5 Interaction with other medicinal products and other forms of Interaction
None known for topical preparations.

4.6 Pregnancy and lactation
There is a lack of definitive evidence of safety of the product in human pregnancy and lactation. However, lidocaine hydrochloride and zinc oxide have been in wide use for many years without apparent ill consequence. It is not necessary to contraindicate this product in pregnancy and lactation provided caution is exercised and the directions for use are followed. However, as with all medicines, the advice of a doctor should be sought.

4.7 Effects on ability to drive and use machines
None.

4.8 Undesirable effects
Very rarely increased irritation and burning sensations may occur at the site of application. Rarely rashes may occur.

4.9 Overdose
It is very unlikely that overdosage would occur from this pharmaceutical form. Symptoms of lidocaine overdosage would be unlikely to occur even after anal insertion of 25g of ointment.

Normally there should be no systemic adverse effects, but at worst CNS and cardiovascular effects are possible. Treatment would be symptomatic after withdrawal of the product.

In the case of accidental oral ingestion, the advice of a doctor should be sought.

5. PHARMACOLOGICAL PROPERTIES

5.1 Pharmacodynamic properties
Zinc oxide has astringent, antiseptic, soothing and protectant properties.

Lidocaine hydrochloride has a local anaesthetic action.

The ointment base has lubricant and emollient properties.

5.2 Pharmacokinetic properties
The product has a local action with minimal risk of systemic effects. Lidocaine has a fast onset and intermediate duration of action. It is partially absorbed but plasma levels will be low, in view of the concentration of lidocaine in the product. It undergoes de-ethylation in the liver, where clearance approaches the rate of hepatic flow.

5.3 Preclinical safety data
Preclinical safety data on these active ingredients in the literature have not revealed any pertinent and conclusive findings which are of relevance to the recommended dosage and use of the product.

6. PHARMACEUTICAL PARTICULARS

6.1 List of excipients
Yellow soft paraffin

Anhydrous lanolin

Methyl salicylate

Propylene glycol

Menthol crystals

6.2 Incompatibilities
None known.

6.3 Shelf life
5 years for packaging option a

36 months for packaging option b

6.4 Special precautions for storage
None.

6.5 Nature and contents of container
a) Flexible aluminium tubes, internally lacquered, fitted with a polypropylene cap. 25 or 55ml tubes are contained in a boxboard carton, together with a polyethylene applicator.

b) Aluminium laminate tube consisting of 150μm Polyethylene /5μm polyacrylate outer layer, 30μm alumininum and an inner layer of 30μm polyacrylate / 60μm polyethylene, fitted with a HD polyethylene shoulder, an aluminium/surlyn tamper evident seal, polypropylene cap and a loose polyethylene screw-on applicator nozzle.

6.6 Instructions for use and handling
Not applicable.

Administrative Data

7. MARKETING AUTHORISATION HOLDER
Bayer plc

Trading as: Bayer plc; Consumer Care Division

Bayer House

Strawberry Hill

Newbury

Berkshire

RG14 1JA

United Kingdom

8. MARKETING AUTHORISATION NUMBER(S)
PL 00010/0266

9. DATE OF FIRST AUTHORISATION/RENEWAL OF THE AUTHORISATION
1st July 2000

10. DATE OF REVISION OF THE TEXT
16th June 2005

Germoloids Suppositories

(Bayer plc)

1. NAME OF THE MEDICINAL PRODUCT
Germoloids Suppositories

2. QUALITATIVE AND QUANTITATIVE COMPOSITION
Zinc oxide Ph. Eur. 283.5 mg

Lidocaine hydrochloride Ph. Eur. 13.2 mg

3. PHARMACEUTICAL FORM
Suppository for rectal administration.

4. CLINICAL PARTICULARS

4.1 Therapeutic indications
The symptomatic relief of pain, swelling, irritation and itching associated with haemorrhoids, and pruritus ani.

4.2 Posology and method of administration
Adults and children 12 years and over:

One suppository to be inserted into the rectum on retiring at night and in the morning, preferably after bowel movement.

If necessary Germoloids Suppositories may be used at any time during the day with a minimum 3 - 4 hours between suppositories.

Do not use more than 4 suppositories in any 24-hour period.

Children under 12 years:

Only as directed by a doctor.

The elderly:

The normal adult dose may be used.

4.3 Contraindications
Hypersensitivity to any of the constituents.

4.4 Special warnings and special precautions for use
Persons who continually suffer from haemorrhoids or who have severe haemorrhoids or who experience excessive bleeding, are advised to consult a doctor.

4.5 Interaction with other medicinal products and other forms of Interaction
None known for suppositories.

4.6 Pregnancy and lactation
There is a lack of definitive evidence of safety of the product in human pregnancy and lactation. However, lidocaine hydrochloride and zinc oxide have been in wide use for many years without apparent ill consequence. It is not necessary to contraindicate this product in pregnancy and lactation provided caution is exercised and the directions for use are followed. However, as with all medicines, the advice of a doctor should be sought.

4.7 Effects on ability to drive and use machines
None stated.

4.8 Undesirable effects
Very rarely increased irritation may occur at the site of application.

4.9 Overdose
It is very unlikely that overdosage would occur from this pharmaceutical form. Symptoms of lidocaine overdosage would be unlikely to occur even after rectal administration of large quantities (up to 30-fold greater doses).

Normally there should be no systemic adverse effects, but at worst CNS and cardiovascular effects are possible. Treatment would be symptomatic after withdrawal of the product.

In the case of accidental oral ingestion, the advice of a doctor should be sought.

5. PHARMACOLOGICAL PROPERTIES

5.1 Pharmacodynamic properties
Zinc oxide has astringent, antiseptic, soothing and protectant properties.

Lidocaine hydrochloride has a local anaesthetic action.

The suppository base has lubricant and emollient properties.

5.2 Pharmacokinetic properties
The product has a local action with minimal risk of systemic effects. Lidocaine has a fast onset and intermediate duration of action. It is partially absorbed but plasma levels will be low, in view of the concentration of lidocaine in the product. It undergoes de-ethylation in the liver, where clearance approaches the rate of hepatic flow.

5.3 Preclinical safety data
Preclinical safety data on these active ingredients in the literature have not revealed any pertinent and conclusive findings which are of relevance to the recommended dosage and use of the product.

6. PHARMACEUTICAL PARTICULARS

6.1 List of excipients
Hard fat

Methyl salicylate

Glyceryl tristearate

6.2 Incompatibilities
None known.

6.3 Shelf life
36 months

6.4 Special precautions for storage
Do not store above 25°C.

6.5 Nature and contents of container
Pre-formed, PVC/polyethylene laminate moulds. Strips of suppositories are packed in boxboard cartons. Six suppositories per strip, two or four strips per carton, to give pack sizes of 12 or 24 suppositories.

6.6 Instructions for use and handling
Not applicable.

7. MARKETING AUTHORISATION HOLDER
Bayer plc

Trading as: Bayer plc; Consumer Care Division

Bayer House

Strawberry Hill

Newbury

Berkshire

RG14 1JA

United Kingdom

8. MARKETING AUTHORISATION NUMBER(S)
PL 00010/0264

9. DATE OF FIRST AUTHORISATION/RENEWAL OF THE AUTHORISATION
1st July 2000

10. DATE OF REVISION OF THE TEXT
February 2003

Germoloids Suppositories & Ointment Duo Pack

(Bayer plc)

1. NAME OF THE MEDICINAL PRODUCT
Germoloids Suppositories & Ointment Duo Pack

2. QUALITATIVE AND QUANTITATIVE COMPOSITION
Suppositories:

Zinc Oxide 283.5 mg

Lidocaine Hydrochloride 13.2 mg

Ointment:

Zinc Oxide 6.6% w/w

Lidocaine Hydrochloride 0.7% w/w

For excipients, see section 6.1.

3. PHARMACEUTICAL FORM
Suppository for rectal administration.

Ointment for topical administration.

4. CLINICAL PARTICULARS
4.1 Therapeutic indications
The symptomatic relief of pain, swelling, irritation and itching associated with haemorrhoids and pruritus ani.

4.2 Posology and method of administration
Adults and children aged 12 years and over:

Suppositories:

One suppository to be inserted into the rectum on retiring at night and in the morning, preferably after a bowel movement. If necessary the suppository may be used at any time during the day with a minimum of three to four hours between suppositories. Do not use more than four suppositories in any 24-hour period.

Ointment:

Apply to the affected area at least twice a day with a minimum of three to four hours between applications. Further applications can be made at any time of day and are particularly recommended after a bowel movement. Do not use more than four times in any 24-hour period.

Children under 12:

Only as directed by a doctor.

The elderly:

The normal adult dose may be used.

4.3 Contraindications
Hypersensitivity to any of the ingredients.

4.4 Special warnings and special precautions for use
Persons who continually suffer from haemorrhoids, have severe haemorrhoids or experience excessive bleeding, are advised to consult a doctor.

4.5 Interaction with other medicinal products and other forms of Interaction
None known.

4.6 Pregnancy and lactation
There is a lack of definitive evidence of safety of the product in human pregnancy and lactation. However, lidocaine hydrochloride and zinc oxide have been in wide use for many years without apparent ill consequence. It is not necessary to contraindicate this product in pregnancy and lactation provided caution is exercised and the directions for use are followed. However, as with all medicines, the advice of a doctor should be sought.

4.7 Effects on ability to drive and use machines
None.

4.8 Undesirable effects
Very rarely increased irritation may occur at the site of application when using the suppositories or the ointment.

Very rarely burning sensations may occur at the site of application when using the ointment. Rarely rashes may occur.

4.9 Overdose
It is very unlikely that overdosage would occur from these pharmaceutical forms. Symptoms of lidocaine overdosage would be unlikely to occur even after rectal insertion of large quantities.

Normally there should be no systemic adverse effects, but at worst CNS and cardiovascular effects are possible. Treatment would be symptomatic after withdrawal of the product.

In the case of accidental oral ingestion, the advice of a doctor should be sought.

5. PHARMACOLOGICAL PROPERTIES
5.1 Pharmacodynamic properties
Zinc oxide has astringent, antiseptic, soothing and protectant properties.

Lidocaine hydrochloride has a local anaesthetic action.

The suppository and ointment bases have lubricant and emollient properties.

5.2 Pharmacokinetic properties
The product has a local action with minimal risk of systemic effects. Lidocaine has a fast onset and intermediate duration of action. It is partially absorbed but plasma levels will be low, in view of the concentration of lidocaine in the product. It undergoes de-ethylation in the liver, where clearance approaches the rate of hepatic flow.

5.3 Preclinical safety data
Preclinical safety data on the active ingredients in the literature have not revealed any pertinent and conclusive findings which are of relevance to the recommended dosage and use of the product.

6. PHARMACEUTICAL PARTICULARS
6.1 List of excipients
Suppository:

Hard fat

Methyl salicylate

Glyceryl tristearate

Ointment:

Yellow soft paraffin

Wool fat

Methyl salicylate

Propylene glycol

Menthol crystals

6.2 Incompatibilities
None known.

6.3 Shelf life
36 months.

6.4 Special precautions for storage
Do not store above 25°C.

6.5 Nature and contents of container
Suppository:

Preformed PVC/polyethylene laminate moulds. Strips of suppositories are packed in a boxboard carton. Six suppositories per strip, two strips per carton.

Ointment:

a) Flexible aluminium tubes, internally lacquered, fitted with a polypropylene cap contained in a boxboard carton.

b) Aluminium laminate tube consisting of 150μm Polyethylene /5μm polyacrylate outer layer, 30μm alumininum and an inner layer of 30μm polyacrylate / 60μm polyethylene, fitted with a HD polyethylene shoulder, an aluminium/surlyn tamper evident seal, HD polypropylene cap.

Pack size: Each carton contains 12 suppositories and 15ml ointment.

6.6 Instructions for use and handling
Not applicable.

Administrative Data
7. MARKETING AUTHORISATION HOLDER
Bayer plc,

Bayer House

Strawberry Hill

Newbury

Berkshire

RG14 1JA

Trading as Bayer plc, Consumer Care Division.

8. MARKETING AUTHORISATION NUMBER(S)
PL 0010/0277

9. DATE OF FIRST AUTHORISATION/RENEWAL OF THE AUTHORISATION
26 July 2001

10. DATE OF REVISION OF THE TEXT
16th June 2005

GHRH Ferring

(Ferring Pharmaceuticals Ltd)

1. NAME OF THE MEDICINAL PRODUCT
GHRH Ferring

2. QUALITATIVE AND QUANTITATIVE COMPOSITION
Active Ingredient

Somatorelin as acetate, 50 micrograms per ampoule.

3. PHARMACEUTICAL FORM
Lyophilised powder for injection.

Sterile solution for reconstitution of an injectable preparation.

4. CLINICAL PARTICULARS
4.1 Therapeutic indications
The product is applied to determine the somatotropic function of the anterior pituitary gland in cases of suspected growth hormone deficiency. The test distinguishes between hypophysic and hypothalamic disorders but is not suitable as a screening test for growth hormone deficiencies.

The diluent is supplied for the reconstitution of an injectable preparation.

4.2 Posology and method of administration
The recommended dosage for adult patients of standard weight is the content of one ampoule of GHRH Ferring (50 micrograms somatorelin) dissolved in 1ml of the supplied solvent. The solution is administered intravenously as a bolus injection.

In cases of highly overweight adult patients and in children, a dosage of 1 microgram per kg body weight is indicated.

GHRH Test: After withdrawal of approximately 2ml of venous blood from the fasted patient, the increase of basal growth hormone levels in plasma or serum after a single intravenous injection of the product is measured. For this procedure, the content of one ampoule is dissolved in 1ml of solvent (0.9% NaCl), or a volume corresponding to 1 microgram per kg body weight if appropriate, is administered intravenously to the fasted patient as a bolus injection (within 30 seconds).

To evaluate the growth hormone increment in plasma or serum, a second blood sample is taken 30 minutes after the injection. Peak growth hormone values may occasionally occur sooner or later. Therefore, additional blood samples may be taken 15, 45, 60 and 90 minutes after GHRH injection for better assessment of growth hormone release.

4.3 Contraindications
Hypersensitivity to growth hormone releasing hormone.

4.4 Special warnings and special precautions for use
Because of possible inhibitory influence of human growth hormone on the somatotropic function of the pituitary gland, the GHRH Ferring test should not be carried out earlier than one week after discontinuation of treatment with human growth hormone.

The test results may be affected in conditions such as:

– untreated hyperthyroidism

– obesity, hyperglycaemia, elevated plasma fatty acids

– high levels of somatostatin

Although no hypersensitivity reactions have yet been reported, the possibility of this kind of adverse event cannot be completely ruled out because of the peptide nature of this product and the intravenous route of administration. It is recommended that emergency facilities should be available to treat such a reaction if it occurs.

4.5 Interaction with other medicinal products and other forms of Interaction
The concomitant administration of substances which influence the release of growth hormone, such as growth hormone itself, somatostatin or its analogues, atropine, levodopa, dopamine, clonidine, arginine, ornithine, glycine, glucagon, insulin, oral glucose, anti thyroid drugs and propranolol should be avoided. High levels of glucocorticoids as well as somatostatin may inhibit the growth hormone response.

4.6 Pregnancy and lactation
GHRH Ferring is not indicated during pregnancy and lactation.

4.7 Effects on ability to drive and use machines
None.

4.8 Undesirable effects
Occasionally, a mild sensation of warmth may appear in the head, neck and upper part of the body, and there may be disturbances of smell and taste. These side effects are short lasting and will fade rapidly. In combination with "hot flush", a slight increase or decrease in blood pressure may occur occasionally in conjunction with the corresponding alterations in heart rate. The described side effects are insignificant when the suggested dose is applied and they do not need any special treatment.

4.9 Overdose
In cases of higher dosage, the known side effects may occur. The undesirable effects fade rapidly and do not need any special treatment.

5. PHARMACOLOGICAL PROPERTIES
5.1 Pharmacodynamic properties
Somatorelin is normally synthesised in the hypothalamus and stimulates the secretion of growth hormone from the pituitary gland.

GHRH Ferring is the synthetic form of somatorelin and is identical in structure and function to the somatorelin released by the hypothalamus.

Somatorelin physiologically increases plasma growth hormone levels.

5.2 Pharmacokinetic properties
After intravenous application of different doses of somatorelin in man, the concentrations of somatorelin in plasma increase within 5 minutes to the maximum value, followed by a rapid decrease. The basal values are reached again after 30-40 minutes.

5.3 Preclinical safety data
Not applicable.

6. PHARMACEUTICAL PARTICULARS
6.1 List of excipients
GHRH Ferring

None.

Diluent for GHRH Ferring

Each diluent ampoule contains:

Sodium chloride Ph. Eur. 9mg

Water for injection Ph. Eur. to 1.0ml

6.2 Incompatibilities
GHRH Ferring should not be administered together with other preparations for parenteral use (e.g. mixed injections or infusion solutions).

6.3 Shelf life
Shelf life of the unopened powder and diluent ampoule is 33 months.

6.4 Special precautions for storage
Do not store above 25°C.

6.5 Nature and contents of container
GHRH Ferring is supplied in clear glass ampoules of high hydrolytic resistance (hydrolytic Class 1 according to Ph. Eur.).

The diluent is supplied in clear glass ampoules of high hydrolytic resistance (hydrolytic Class 1 according to Ph. Eur.).

6.6 Instructions for use and handling
Reconstitute GHRH Ferring with the solvent supplied, immediately prior to use.

7. MARKETING AUTHORISATION HOLDER
Ferring Pharmaceuticals Limited

The Courtyard

Waterside Drive

Langley

Berkshire SL3 6EZ.

8. MARKETING AUTHORISATION NUMBER(S)
GHRH Ferring PL 03194/0050

Diluent for GHRH Ferring PL 03194/0051

9. DATE OF FIRST AUTHORISATION/RENEWAL OF THE AUTHORISATION
28th June 2002

10. DATE OF REVISION OF THE TEXT
May 2005

11. LEGAL CATEGORY
POM

Gliadel 7.7mg Implant

(Link Pharmaceuticals Ltd)

1. NAME OF THE MEDICINAL PRODUCT
GLIADEL® 7.7mg Implant

2. QUALITATIVE AND QUANTITATIVE COMPOSITION
Each implant of GLIADEL Implant contains 7.7mg of carmustine.

3. PHARMACEUTICAL FORM
Implant

4. CLINICAL PARTICULARS

4.1 Therapeutic indications
GLIADEL Implant is indicated in newly-diagnosed high-grade malignant glioma patients as an adjunct to surgery and radiation.

GLIADEL Implant is indicated for use as an adjunct to surgery in patients with recurrent histologically proved glioblastoma multiforme for whom surgical resection is indicated.

4.2 Posology and method of administration
For intralesional use in adults only.

Each GLIADEL Implant contains 7.7mg of carmustine, resulting in a dose of 61.6mg when eight implants are placed in the tumour resection cavity.

It is recommended that a maximum of eight implants be placed if the size and shape of the resection cavity allows it. Implants broken in half may be used, but implants broken in more than two pieces should be discarded in the dedicated biohazard waste containers (see Section 6.6, Instructions for Use, Handling and Disposal).

It is recommended that the placement of the implants should be directly from the product's inner sterile packaging into the resection cavity. Oxidised regenerated cellulose may be placed over the implants to secure them to the cavity surface (see Section 6.6, Instructions for Use, Handling and Disposal).

4.3 Contraindications
GLIADEL Implant is contraindicated in patients with a history of hypersensitivity to the active substance, carmustine, or to any of the excipients of GLIADEL Implant.

4.4 Special warnings and special precautions for use
Patients undergoing craniotomy for glioblastoma and implantation of GLIADEL Implant should be monitored closely in view of known complications of craniotomy which includes convulsions, intracranial infections, abnormal wound healing, and brain oedema (see Section 4.8, Undesirable Effects). Cases of intracerebral mass effect unresponsive to corticosteroids have been described in patients treated with GLIADEL Implant, including one case leading to brain herniation. Careful monitoring of GLIADEL Implant-treated patients for cerebral oedema/intracranial hypertension with consequent steroid use is warranted (see Section 4.8, Undesirable Effects). CSF leak was more common in GLIADEL Implant-treated patients. Attention to a water-tight dural closure and local wound care is indicated (see Section 4.8, Undesirable Effects).

Development of brain oedema with mass effect (due to tumour recurrence, intracranial infection or necrosis) may necessitate re-operation and, in some cases, removal of GLIADEL Implant or its remnants.

Communication between the surgical resection cavity and the ventricular system should be avoided to prevent the implants from migrating into the ventricular system and possibly causing obstructive hydrocephalus. If a communication larger than the diameter of the implant exists it should be closed prior to GLIADEL implantation.

Computed topography and magnetic resonance imaging may demonstrate enhancement in the brain tissue surrounding the resection cavity after placement of GLIADEL Implants. This enhancement may represent oedema and inflammation caused by GLIADEL Implants or tumour progression.

4.5 Interaction with other medicinal products and other forms of Interaction
Interactions of GLIADEL Implant with other drugs or chemotherapy have not been formally evaluated.

4.6 Pregnancy and lactation
Pregnancy:

There are no studies of GLIADEL Implant in pregnant women and no studies assessing the reproductive toxicity of GLIADEL Implant. Carmustine, the active component of GLIADEL Implant, when administered systemically can have genotoxic effects and can adversely affect foetal development. GLIADEL Implant, therefore, should not normally be administered to pregnant women. If the use of GLIADEL Implant during pregnancy is still considered, the patient should be informed of the potential risk to the foetus. Women of childbearing potential should be advised to avoid pregnancy while receiving GLIADEL Implant. In case of patients getting pregnant during treatment with GLIADEL Implant the opportunity for genetic advice should be seized.

Lactation:

It is not known if GLIADEL Implant components are excreted in human milk. Since some drugs are excreted in human milk, and because of the potential risk of serious adverse reactions of carmustine in nursing infants, breast-feeding is contraindicated.

4.7 Effects on ability to drive and use machines
No effects on ability to drive and use machines have been observed. However, driving is not advisable following treatment.

4.8 Undesirable effects
The spectrum of undesirable effects observed in patients with newly-diagnosed high-grade malignant glioma and recurrent malignant gliomas was generally consistent with that encountered in patients undergoing craniotomy for malignant gliomas.

Primary Surgery
The following data are the most frequently occurring adverse events observed in 5% or more of the 120 newly-diagnosed malignant glioma patients receiving GLIADEL Implant during the trial.

Common Adverse Events Observed in > 5% of Patients Receiving Gliadel Implant at Initial Surgery

(see Table 1)

Intracranial hypertension was present in more GLIADEL Implant-treated patients than in placebo patients (9.2% vs. 1.7%). It was typically observed late, at the time of tumour recurrence, and was unlikely to be associated with GLIADEL Implant use (see Section 4.4, Special Warnings and Precautions for Use).

CSF leak was more common in GLIADEL Implant-treated patients than in placebo patients. However intracranial infections and other healing abnormalities were not increased (see Section 4.4, Special Warnings and Precautions for Use).

Surgery for Recurrent Disease
The following post-operative adverse events were observed in 4% or more of the 110 patients receiving GLIADEL Implant at recurrent surgery in a controlled clinical trial. Except for nervous system effects, where there is a possibility that the placebo implants could have been responsible, only events more common in the GLIADEL Implant group are listed. These adverse events were either not present pre-operatively or worsened post-operatively during the follow-up period. The follow-up period was up to 71 months.

Common Adverse Events in ≥4% of Patients Receiving GLIADEL Implant at Recurrent Surgery

(see Table 2 on next page)

The following adverse events, not listed in the table above, were reported in less than 4% but at least 1% of patients treated with GLIADEL Implant in all studies. The events listed were either not present pre-operatively or worsened post-operatively. Whether GLIADEL Implant caused these events cannot be determined.

Common Adverse Events in 1% to 4% of Patients Receiving GLIADEL Implant

(see Table 3 on next page)

The following four categories of adverse events are possibly related to treatment with GLIADEL Implant.

Seizures:

In the initial surgery trial, the incidence of seizures within the first 5 days after implantation was 2.5% in the GLIADEL Implant group.

In the surgery for recurrent disease trial, the incidence of post-operative seizures was 19% in patients receiving GLIADEL Implant. 12/22 (54%) of patients treated with GLIADEL Implant experienced the first new or worsened seizure within the first five post-operative days. The median time to onset of the first new or worsened post-operative seizure was 3.5 days in patients treated with GLIADEL Implant.

Brain Oedema:

Development of brain oedema with mass effect (due to tumour recurrence, intracranial infection or necrosis) may necessitate re-operation and, in some cases, removal of GLIADEL Implant or its remnants (see Section 4.4, Special Warnings and Precautions for Use).

Table 1 Common Adverse Events Observed in > 5% of Patients Receiving Gliadel Implant at Initial Surgery

Class organ		Adverse events
Body as a whole	≥10%	Aggravation reaction, headache, asthenia, infection, fever, pain
	1-<10%	Abdominal pain, back pain, face oedema, chest pain, abscess, accidental injury
Cardiovascular system	≥10%	Deep thrombophlebitis
	1-<10%	Pulmonary embolism, haemorrhage
Digestive system	≥10%	Nausea, vomiting, constipation
	1-<10%	Diarrhoea
Endocrine system	1-<10%	Diabetes mellitus
Metabolic and nutritional disorders	≥10%	Healing abnormal
	1-<10%	Peripheral oedema
Nervous system	≥10%	Hemiplegia, convulsion, confusion, brain oedema, aphasia, depression, somnolence, speech disorder
	1-<10%	Amnesia, intracranial hypertension, personality disorder, anxiety, facial paralysis, neuropathy, ataxia, hypoesthesia, paresthesia, thinking abnormal, abnormal gait, dizziness, grand mal convulsion, hallucinations, insomnia, tremor
Respiratory system	1-<10%	Pneumonia
Skin and appendages	≥10%	Rash, alopecia
Special senses	1-<10%	Conjunctival oedema, abnormal vision, visual field defect
Urogenital system	1-<10%	Urinary tract infection, urinary incontinence

≥10%: very common and 1-<10%: common

Table 2 Common Adverse Events in ⩾4% of Patients Receiving GLIADEL Implant at Recurrent Surgery

Class organ		Adverse events
Body as a whole	⩾10%	Fever
	1-<10%	Infection, pain
Cardiovascular system	1-<10%	Deep thrombophlebitis, pulmonary embolism
Digestive system	1-<10%	Nausea, nausea and vomiting, oral moniliasis
Haemic and lymphatic system	1-<10%	Anaemia
Metabolic and nutritional disorders	⩾10%	Healing abnormal
	1-<10%	Hyponatraemia
Nervous system	⩾10%	Convulsion, hemiplegia, headache, somnolence, confusion
	1-<10%	Aphasia, stupor, brain oedema, intracranial hypertension, meningitis or abscess
Respiratory system	1-<10%	Pneumonia
Skin and appendages	1-<10%	Rash
Urogenital system	⩾10%	Urinary tract infection

Table 3 Common Adverse Events in 1% to 4% of Patients Receiving GLIADEL Implant

Class organ		Adverse events
Body as a whole	1-<10%	Peripheral oedema, neck pain, accidental injury, back pain, allergic reaction, asthenia, chest pain, sepsis
Cardiovascular system	1-<10%	Hypertension, hypotension
Digestive system	1-<10%	Diarrhoea, constipation, dysphagia, gastrointestinal haemorrhage, faecal incontinence
Haemic and lymphatic system	1-<10%	Thrombocytopenia, leukocytosis
Metabolic and nutritional disorders	1-<10%	Hyponatraemia, hyperglycaemia, hypokalaemia
Musculoskeletal system	1-<10%	Infection
Nervous system	1-<10%	Hydrocephalus, depression, abnormal thinking, ataxia, dizziness, insomnia, hemiplegia, coma, amnesia, diplopia, paranoid reaction
	0,1-<1%	Cerebral haemorrhage, cerebral infarct
Respiratory system	1-<10%	Infection, aspiration pneumonia
Skin and appendages	1-<10%	Rash
Special senses	1-<10%	Visual defect, eye pain
Urogenital system	1-<10%	Urinary incontinence

Healing Abnormalities:

The following healing abnormalities have been reported in clinical trials of GLIADEL Implant: wound dehiscence, delayed wound healing, subdural, subgaleal or wound effusions and cerebrospinal fluid leak.

In the initial surgery trial, cerebrospinal fluid leaks occurred in 5% of GLIADEL Implant recipients. During surgery a water-tight dural closure should be obtained to minimise the risk of cerebrospinal fluid leak (see Section 4.4, Special Warnings and Precautions for Use).

Intracranial Infection:

In the initial surgery trial the incidence of brain abscess or meningitis was 5% in patients treated with GLIADEL Implant.

In the recurrent setting, the incidence of brain abscess or meningitis was 4% in patients treated with GLIADEL Implant.

In a published clinical study cyst formation after GLIADEL Implant treatment has been reported. This reaction occurred in 10% of the patients observed in the study, however the formation of cysts is possible after resection of a malignant glioma.

4.9 Overdose

Not applicable

5. PHARMACOLOGICAL PROPERTIES

5.1 Pharmacodynamic properties

Pharmaco-therapeutic group: Antineoplastic agents, ATC Code: LO1ADO1

Pre-clinical data

GLIADEL Implant delivers carmustine directly into the surgical cavity created after tumoural resection. On exposure to the aqueous environment of the cavity the anhydride bonds in the copolymer are hydrolysed, releasing carmustine, carboxyphenoxypropane and sebacic acid. The carmustine released from GLIADEL Implant diffuses into the surrounding brain tissue and produces an antineoplastic effect by alkylating DNA and RNA.

Carmustine is spontaneously both degraded and metabolised. The alkylating moiety thus produced, and presumed to be chloroethyl carbonium ion, leads to the formation of irreversible DNA cross-links.

The tumourcidal activity of GLIADEL Implant is dependent on release of carmustine into the tumour cavity in concentrations sufficient for effective cytotoxicity.

More than 70% of the copolymer degrades by three weeks. The metabolic disposition and excretion of the monomers differ. Carboxyphenoxypropane is predominantly eliminated by the kidney and sebacic acid, an endogenous fatty acid, is metabolised by the liver and expired as CO_2 in animals.

Clinical data

Primary Surgery

In a randomised, double-blind, placebo-controlled clinical trial in 240 adults with newly-diagnosed high grade malignant glioma undergoing initial craniotomy for tumour resection median survival increased from 11.6 months with placebo to 13.9 months with GLIADEL Implant (p-value 0.079, unstratified log-rank test) in the original study phase. The most common tumour type was Glioblastoma Multiforme (GBM) (n=207), followed by anaplastic oligoastrocytoma (n=11), anaplastic oligodendroglioma (n=11) and anaplastic astrocytoma (n=2). The hazard ratio for GLIADEL Implant was 0.77 (95% CI: 0.57 to 1.03). In the long-term follow-up phase, patients still alive at the completion of the original phase were followed for up to at least three years or until death. Median survival increased from 11.6 months with placebo to 13.9 months with GLIADEL Implant (p-value <0.05, log-rank test). The hazard ratio for GLIADEL Implant treatment was 0.73 (95% CI: 0.56 to 0.95).

Surgery for Recurrent Disease

In a randomised, double-blind, placebo-controlled clinical trial in 145 adults with recurrent glioblastoma (GBM), GLIADEL Implant prolonged survival in these patients. Ninety-five percent of the patients treated with GLIADEL Implant received 7 to 8 implants.

The six-month survival rate was 36% (26/73) with placebo compared to 56% (40/72) with GLIADEL Implant treatment. Median survival of GBM patients is 20 weeks with placebo versus 28 weeks with GLIADEL Implant treatment.

5.2 Pharmacokinetic properties

The absorption, distribution, metabolism, and excretion of the copolymer in humans is unknown. Carmustine concentrations delivered by GLIADEL Implant in human brain tissue have not been determined. Plasma levels of carmustine after GLIADEL Implant implantation cannot be assayed. In rabbits that had implants containing 3.85% carmustine placed, carmustine is not detected in the blood or cerebrospinal fluid.

Following an intravenous infusion of carmustine at doses ranging from 30 to 170mg/m^2, the average terminal half-life, clearance, and steady-state volume of distribution are 22 minutes, 56mL/min/kg and 3.25L/kg, respectively. Approximately 60% of the intravenous 200mg/m^2 dose of ^{14}C-carmustine is excreted in the urine over 96 hours and 6% is expired as CO_2.

GLIADEL Implants are biodegradable in human brain when placed into the cavity after tumour resection. The rate of biodegradation is variable from patient to patient. During the biodegradation process an implant remnant may be observed on brain imaging scans or at re-operation even though extensive degradation of all components has occurred.

5.3 Preclinical safety data

No carcinogenicity, embryo-foetal toxicity, pre- and post-natal toxicity and impairment of fertility studies have been conducted with GLIADEL Implant.

Carmustine, the active component of GLIADEL Implant, when administered systemically, has embryotoxic, genotoxic and carcinogenic effects and can cause testicular degeneration in several animal models.

6. PHARMACEUTICAL PARTICULARS

6.1 List of excipients

Polifeprosan 20

6.2 Incompatibilities

None known.

6.3 Shelf life

3 years

6.4 Special precautions for storage

Store in a freezer at or below -20°C.

Unopened outer sachets may be kept at a temperature of not more than 22°C for a maximum of six hours.

The product may be refrozen only once if the sachets have been unopened and kept for a maximum of 6 hours at a temperature of not more than 22°C. After refreezing, the product should be used within 30 days.

6.5 Nature and contents of container

GLIADEL Implant is available in a box containing eight implants. Each implant is individually packaged in two aluminium foil laminate sachets.

6.6 Instructions for use and handling

Implants should be handled by personnel wearing surgical gloves because exposure to carmustine can cause severe burning and hyperpigmentation of the skin. Use of double gloves is recommended and the outer gloves should be discarded into a dedicated biohazard waste container after use. A surgical instrument dedicated to the handling of the implants should be used for implant placement. If repeat neurosurgical intervention is indicated, any implant or implant remnant should be handled as a potentially cytotoxic agent.

GLIADEL Implants should be handled with care. The sachets containing GLIADEL Implant should be delivered to the operating room and remain unopened until ready to place the implants in the resection cavity. Only the outside surface of the outer sachet is not sterile. In any case, if an implant is dropped, it should be discarded accordingly.

Instructions for opening sachets containing the implant:

- To open the outer sachet, locate the folded corner and slowly pull in an outward motion. Do not pull in a downward motion rolling knuckles over the sachet. This may exert pressure on the implant and cause it to break.
- Remove the inner sachet by grabbing with the aid of forceps and pulling upward.
- To open the inner sachet, gently hold it and cut in an arc-like fashion around the implant.
- To remove the implant, gently grasp the implant with the aid of forceps and place it directly into the resection cavity.

In any case, if an implant is dropped, it should be discarded accordingly.

Once the tumour is resected, tumour pathology is confirmed and haemostasis is obtained, up to eight implants may be placed to cover as much of the resection cavity as possible. Slight overlapping of the implants is acceptable. Implants broken in half may be used, but implants broken in more than two pieces should be discarded in the dedicated biohazard waste containers.

Oxidised regenerated cellulose may be placed over the implants to secure them to the cavity surface. After placement of the implants, the resection cavity should be irrigated and the dura closed in a water-tight fashion.

Any unused product or waste material should be disposed of in accordance with local requirements for biohazardous waste.

7. MARKETING AUTHORISATION HOLDER
Guilford Pharmaceuticals Limited, 193 Sparrows Herne, Bushey Heath, Hertfordshire, WD2 1AJ, United Kingdom

Distributed in the UK and Republic of Ireland by:

Link Pharmaceuticals Limited, Bishops Weald House, Albion Way, Horsham, West Sussex, RH12 1AH, United Kingdom

8. MARKETING AUTHORISATION NUMBER(S)
PL 18753/0001

PA 1018/1/1

9. DATE OF FIRST AUTHORISATION/RENEWAL OF THE AUTHORISATION
29 May 1999

10. DATE OF REVISION OF THE TEXT
June 2005

11. Legal Category
POM

® Gliadel is a registered trade mark

SPC0105

Glibenese

(Pfizer Limited)

1. NAME OF THE MEDICINAL PRODUCT
GLIBENESE® TABLETS 5mg.

2. QUALITATIVE AND QUANTITATIVE COMPOSITION
Each tablet contains 5mg glipizide as the active ingredient.

3. PHARMACEUTICAL FORM
Tablets.

4. CLINICAL PARTICULARS

4.1 Therapeutic indications
As an adjunct to diet, in Type 2 diabetes, when proper dietary management alone has failed.

4.2 Posology and method of administration
Route of administration: Oral.

There is no fixed dosage regimen for the management of diabetes mellitus with Glibenese or any other hypoglycaemic agent. In addition to the usual monitoring of urinary glucose, the patient's blood glucose must also be monitored periodically to determine the minimum effective dose for the patient, to detect primary failure: i.e. inadequate lowering of blood glucose at the maximum recommended dose of medication, and to detect secondary failure, i.e. loss of adequate blood-glucose-lowering response after an initial period of effectiveness. Glycosylated haemoglobin levels may also be of value in monitoring the patient's response to therapy.

Short term administration of Glibenese may be sufficient during periods of transient loss of control in patients usually controlled well on diet.

In general, Glibenese should be given approximately 30 minutes before a meal to achieve the greatest reduction in post-prandial hyperglycaemia.

Initial dose: The recommended starting dose is 5mg, given before breakfast or the midday meal. Elderly patients and other patients at risk for hypoglycaemia may be started on 2.5mg (see Use in Elderly and in High Risk Patients).

Titration: Dosage adjustments should ordinarily be in increments of 2.5 or 5mg, as determined by blood glucose response. At least several days should elapse between titration steps. The maximum recommended single dose is 15mg. Doses above 15mg should ordinarily be divided.

Maintenance: Some patients may be effectively controlled on a once-a-day regimen. Total daily dosage above 15mg should ordinarily be divided. Patients can usually be stabilized on a dosage ranging from 2.5 to 20mg daily. The maximum recommended daily dosage is 20mg.

Use in elderly and in high risk patients: Elderly diabetics are more sensitive to the hypoglycaemic effects of sulphonylurea drugs and should therefore be prescribed a low starting dose of 2.5mg daily. The elderly are also particularly susceptible to the effects of hypoglycaemia. Hypoglycaemia may be difficult to recognise in the elderly.

To decrease the risk of hypoglycaemia in patients at risk including elderly, debilitated or malnourished patients, patients with irregular calorie intake and patients with an impaired renal or hepatic function, the initial maintenance dosing should be conservative to avoid hypoglycaemic reactions (see 'Initial Dose' and Section 4.4 'Special warnings and special precautions for use').

Use in children: Safety and effectiveness in children have not been established.

Patients receiving insulin: As with other sulphonylurea-class hypoglycaemics, many stable non-insulin-dependent diabetic patients receiving insulin may be safely placed on Glibenese. When transferring patients from insulin to Glibenese, the following general guidelines should be considered:

For patients whose daily insulin requirement is 20 units or less, insulin may be discontinued and Glibenese therapy begun at usual dosages. Several days should elapse between Glibenese titration steps.

For patients whose daily insulin requirement is greater than 20 units, the insulin dose should be reduced by 50% and Glibenese therapy initiated at usual dosages. Subsequent reductions in insulin dosage should depend on individual patient response. Several days should elapse between Glibenese titration steps.

During the insulin withdrawal period, the patient should self-monitor glucose levels. Patients should be instructed to contact the prescriber immediately if these tests are abnormal. In some cases, especially when the patient has been receiving greater than 40 units of insulin daily, it may be advisable to consider hospitalisation during the transition period.

Patients receiving other oral hypoglycaemic agents: As with other sulphonylurea class hypoglycaemics, no transition period is necessary when transferring patients to Glibenese. Patients should be observed carefully (1-2 weeks) for hypoglycaemia when being transferred from longer half-life sulphonylureas (e.g. chlorpropamide) to Glibenese due to potential overlapping of drug effect.

Combination Use: When adding other blood-glucose-lowering agents to glipizide for combination therapy, the agent should be initiated at the lowest recommended dose and patients should be observed carefully for hypoglycaemia. Refer to the product information supplied with the oral agent for additional information.

When adding glipizide to other blood-glucose-lowering agents, glipizide can be initiated at 5mg. Those patients who may be more sensitive to hypoglycaemic drugs may be started at a lower dose. Titration should be based on clinical judgement.

4.3 Contraindications
Glipizide is contra-indicated in patients with:

1. Hypersensitivity to glipizide or any excipients in the tablets.

2. Type 1 diabetes, diabetic ketoacidosis, diabetic coma.

3. Severe renal, hepatic or thyroid impairment; co-existent renal and hepatic disease.

4. Pregnancy and lactation.

5. Patients treated with miconazole (see 4.5 Interactions)

4.4 Special warnings and special precautions for use
General

Hypoglycaemia: All sulphonylurea drugs including glipizide are capable of producing severe hypoglycaemia which may result in coma, and may require hospitalization. Patients experiencing severe hypoglycaemia should be managed with appropriate glucose therapy and be monitored for a minimum of 24 to 48 hours. Proper patient selection, dosage and instructions are important to avoid hypoglycaemic episodes. Regular, timely carbohydrate intake is important to avoid hypoglycaemic events occurring when a meal is delayed or insufficient food is eaten or carbohydrate intake is unbalanced. Renal or hepatic insufficiency may affect the disposition of glipizide and the latter may also diminish gluconeogenic capacity, both of which increase the risk of serious hypoglycaemic reactions. Elderly, debilitated or malnourished patients and those with adrenal or pituitary insufficiency are particularly susceptible to the hypoglycaemic action of glucose-lowering drugs. Hypoglycaemia may be difficult to recognise in the elderly and in people who are taking beta-adrenergic blocking drugs. Hypoglycaemia is more likely to occur when calorific intake is deficient, after severe or prolonged exercise, when alcohol is ingested or when more than one glucose-lowering drug is used.

Loss of control of blood glucose: When a patient stabilised on any diabetic regimen is exposed to stress such as fever, trauma, infection or surgery, a loss of control may occur. At such times, it may be necessary to discontinue glipizide and administer insulin.

The effectiveness of any oral hypoglycaemic drug, including glipizide, in lowering blood glucose to a desired level decreases in many patients over a period of time. This may be due to progression of the severity of the diabetes or to diminished responsiveness to the drug. This phenomenon is known as secondary failure, to distinguish it from primary failure in which the drug is ineffective in an individual patient when first given. Adequate adjustment of dose and adherence to diet should be assessed before classifying a patient as a secondary failure.

Renal and hepatic disease: The pharmacokinetics and/or pharmacodynamics of glipizide may be affected in patients with impaired renal or hepatic function. If hypoglycaemia should occur in such patients, it may be prolonged and appropriate management should be instituted.

Information for patients: Patients should be informed of the potential risks and advantages of glipizide and of alternative modes of therapy. They should also be informed about the importance of adherence to dietary instructions, of a regular exercise programme and of regular testing of blood glucose.

The risk of hypoglycaemia, its symptoms and treatment and conditions that predispose to its development should be explained to patients and responsible family members. Primary and secondary failure should also be explained.

Laboratory tests: Blood glucose should be monitored periodically. Measurement of glycosylated haemoglobin should be performed and goals assessed by the current standard of care.

4.5 Interaction with other medicinal products and other forms of Interaction
The following products are likely to increase the hypoglycaemic effect:

Miconazole: Increase in hypoglycaemic effect, possibly leading to symptoms of hypoglycaemia or even coma.

Fluconazole: There have been reports of hypoglycaemia following the co-administration of glipizide and fluconazole, possibly the result of an increased half-life of glipizide.

Nonsteroidal anti-inflammatory agents (NSAIDS) (e.g. phenylbutazone): increase in hypoglycaemic effect of sulphonylureas (displacement of sulphonylurea binding to plasma proteins and /or decrease in sulphonylurea elimination).

Salicylates (acetylsalicylic acid): Increase in hypoglycaemic effect by high doses of acetylsalicylic acid (hypoglycaemic action of the acetylsalicylic acid).

Alcohol: Increase in hypoglycaemic reaction which can lead to hypoglyaemic coma.

Beta-blockers: All beta-blockers mask some of the symptoms of hypoglycaemia, e.g., palpitations and tachycardia. Most noncardioselective beta-blockers increase the incidence and severity of hypoglycaemia.

Angiotensin converting enzyme inhibitors: The use of angiotensin converting enzyme inhibitors may lead to an increased hypoglycaemic effect in diabetic patients treated with sulphonylureas, including glipizide. Therefore, a reduction in glipizide dosage may be required.

H_2 Receptor Antagonists: The use of H_2 receptor antagonists may potentiate the hypoglycaemic effects of sulphonylureas, including glipizide.

The hypoglycaemic action of sulphonylureas in general may also be potentiated by monoamine oxidase inhibitors and drugs that are highly protein bound, such as sulphonamides, chloramphenicol, probenecid and coumarins.

When such drugs are administered to (or withdrawn from) a patient receiving glipizide, the patient should be observed closely for hypoglycaemia (or loss of control).

In vitro binding studies with human serum proteins indicate that glipizide binds to different sites on albumin than does tolbutamide and does not interact with salicylate or dicoumarol. However, caution must be exercised in extrapolating these findings to the clinical situation in the use of glipizide with these drugs.

The following products could lead to hyperglycaemia:

Danazol: diabetogenic effect of danazol.

If it cannot be avoided, warn the patient and step up self-monitoring of blood glucose and urine Possibly adjust the dosage of antidiabetic agent during treatment with danazol and after its discontinuation

Phenothiazines (e.g. chlorpromazine) at high doses > 100mg per day of chlorpromazine): elevation in blood glucose (reduction in insulin release).

Corticosteroids elevation in blood glucose.

Sympathomimetics (e.g., ritodrine, salbutamol, terbutaline): elevation in blood glucose due to beta-2-adrenoceptor stimulation.

Other drugs that may produce hyperglycaemia and lead to a loss of control include the thiazides and other diuretics, thyroid products, oestrogens, progestogens, oral contraceptives, phenytoin, nicotinic acid, calcium channel blocking drugs and isoniazid.

When such drugs are withdrawn from (or administered to) a patient receiving glipizide, the patient should be observed closely for hypoglycaemia (or loss of control).

4.6 Pregnancy and lactation

Use in pregnancy: Glipizide is contra-indicated during pregnancy. Diabetes in pregnancy should be treated with insulin and not sulphonylureas. Recent evidence suggests that hyperglycaemia in pregnancy is associated with a higher incidence of congenital abnormalities.

Lactation: Although it is not known whether glipizide is excreted in human milk, some sulphonylurea drugs are known to be excreted in human milk. Therefore glipizide is contra-indicated during lactation.

4.7 Effects on ability to drive and use machines
The effect of glipizide on the ability to drive or operate machinery has not been studied, however, there is no

evidence to suggest that glipizide may affect these abilities. Patients should be aware of the symptoms of hypoglycaemia and be careful about driving and the use of machinery.

4.8 Undesirable effects

The majority of side-effects have been dose related, transient, and have responded to dose reduction or withdrawal of the medication. However, clinical experience thus far has shown that, as with other sulphonylureas some side-effects associated with hypersensitivity may be severe and deaths have been reported in some instances.

Side effects listed in this section marked with * are usually transient and do not require discontinuance of therapy; however, they may also be symptoms of hypoglycaemia.

Blood and Lymphatic System Disorders: leucopenia, thrombocytopenia, haemolytic anaemia and pancytopenia have been reported. Aplastic anaemia and agranulocytosis have been reported with other sulphonylureas.

Metabolism and Nutritional Disorders: Hypoglycaemia (see 'Special warnings and precautions for use' section 4.4 and 'Overdose' section 4.9). Hyponatraemia has been reported. Disulfiram-like reactions have been reported with other sulphonylureas.

Psychiatric Disorders: Confusion*

Nervous System Disorders: Dizziness*, drowsiness, headache* and tremor*

Eye Disorders: Visual disturbances such as blurred vision*, diplopia* and abnormal vision* including visual impairment* and decreased vision* have each been reported in patients treated with glipizide.

Gastrointestinal Disorders: Nausea, diarrhoea, constipation and gastralgia. They appear to be dose related and usually disappear on division or reduction of dosage. Abdominal pain and vomiting.

Hepatobiliary disorders: Cholestatic jaundice, impaired hepatic function and hepatitis have been reported. Discontinue treatment if jaundice occurs. Hepatic porphyria and porphyria cutanea tarda have been reported.

Skin and Subcutaneous Tissue Disorders: Allergic skin reactions including erythema, morbilliform or maculopapular reactions, urticaria, pruritus and eczema have been reported. They frequently disappear with continued therapy. However, if they persist, the drug should be discontinued. As with other sulphonylureas, photosensitivity reactions have been reported.

General Disorders and Administration Site Conditions: Malaise*.

Laboratory Investigations: Occasional mild to moderate elevations of AST (SGOT), LDH, alkaline phosphatase, BUN and creatinine were noted. The relationship of these abnormalities to glipizide is uncertain and they have rarely been associated with clinical symptoms.

4.9 Overdose

There is no well documented experience with glipizide overdosage.

Overdosage of sulphonylureas including glipizide can produce hypoglycaemia. Mild hypoglycaemic symptoms without loss of consciousness or neurological findings should be treated aggressively with oral glucose and adjustments in drug dosage and/or meal patterns. Close monitoring should continue until the physician is assured that the patient is out of danger. Severe hypoglycaemic reactions with coma, seizure or other neurological impairment occur infrequently but constitute medical emergencies requiring immediate hospitalisation. If hypoglycaemic coma is diagnosed or suspected, the patient should be given a rapid intravenous injection of concentrated (50%) glucose solution. This should be followed by continuous infusion of a more dilute (10%) glucose solution at a rate that will maintain the blood glucose at a level above 5.6mmol/1 (100mg/dl).

Patients should be closely monitored for a minimum of 48 hours and depending on the status of the patient at this time the physician should decide whether further monitoring is required. Clearance of glipizide from plasma would be prolonged in persons with liver disease. Because of the extensive protein binding of glipizide, dialysis is unlikely to be of benefit.

5. PHARMACOLOGICAL PROPERTIES

5.1 Pharmacodynamic properties

Glipizide is an oral blood glucose lowering drug of the sulphonylurea class.

The primary mode of action of glipizide is the stimulation of insulin secretion from the beta-cells of pancreatic islet tissue. Stimulation of insulin secretion by glipizide in response to a meal is of major importance. Fasting insulin levels are not elevated even on long-term glipizide administration but the post-prandial insulin response continues to be enhanced after at least 6 months of treatment. The insulinotropic response to a meal occurs within 30 minutes after an oral dose of glipizide in diabetic patients but elevated insulin levels do not persist beyond the time of the meal challenge. There is also increasing evidence that extrapancreatic effects involving potentiation of insulin action form a significant component of the activity of glipizide.

Blood sugar control persists for up to 24 hours after a single dose of glipizide, even though plasma levels have declined to a small fraction of peak levels by that time. See 'Pharmacokinetic properties' (section 5.2).

Some patients fail to respond initially, or gradually lose their responsiveness to sulphonylurea drugs, including glipizide. Alternatively, glipizide may be effective in some patients who have not responded or have ceased to respond to other sulphonylureas.

5.2 Pharmacokinetic properties

Gastrointestinal absorption of glipizide in man is uniform, rapid and essentially complete. Peak plasma concentrations occur 1-3 hours after a single oral dose. The half-life of elimination ranges from 2-4 hours in normal subjects, whether given intravenously or orally. The metabolic and excretory patterns are similar with the two routes of administration, indicating that first-pass metabolism is not significant. glipizide does not accumulate in plasma on repeated oral administration. Total absorption and disposition of an oral dose was unaffected by food in normal volunteers but absorption was delayed by about 40 minutes. Thus, glipizide was more effective when administered about 30 minutes before, rather than with a test meal in diabetic patients. Protein binding was studied in serum from volunteers who received either oral or intravenous glipizide and found to be 98%-99% one hour after either route of administration. The apparent volume of distribution of glipizide after intravenous administration was 11 litres, indicative of localisation within the extracellular fluid compartment.

The metabolism of glipizide is extensive and occurs mainly in the liver. The primary metabolites are inactive hydroxylation products and polar conjugates and are excreted mainly in the urine. Less than 10% unchanged glipizide is found in the urine.

5.3 Preclinical safety data

Acute toxicity studies showed no specific susceptibility. The acute oral toxicity of glipizide was extremely low in all species tested (LD_{50} greater than 4 g/kg). Chronic toxicity tests in rats and dogs at doses up to 8.0 mg/kg did not show any evidence of toxic effects.

A 20-month study in rats and an 18-month study in mice at doses up to 75 times the maximum human dose revealed no evidence of drug related carcinogenicity. Bacterial and *in vivo* mutagenicity tests were uniformly negative. Studies in rats of both sexes at doses up to 75 times the human dose showed no effects on fertility.

6. PHARMACEUTICAL PARTICULARS

6.1 List of excipients

The tablets contain the following ingredients: lactose, maize starch, microcrystalline cellulose and stearic acid.

6.2 Incompatibilities

None known.

6.3 Shelf life

2 years.

6.4 Special precautions for storage

Store below 25°C.

6.5 Nature and contents of container

Original packs of 56 tablets per carton. Blister pack formed from 250 μm white opaque PVC, coated 40g/m² PVdC and backed with 20μm hard tempered aluminium foil, coated with 5-6g/m² sealing lacquer.

6.6 Instructions for use and handling

None.

7. MARKETING AUTHORISATION HOLDER

Pfizer Limited
Ramsgate Road
Sandwich
CT13 9NJ
United Kingdom.

8. MARKETING AUTHORISATION NUMBER(S)

PL 00057/0113R.

9. DATE OF FIRST AUTHORISATION/RENEWAL OF THE AUTHORISATION

2 September 1997.

10. DATE OF REVISION OF THE TEXT

October 2004

11. Legal Category

POM

Ref: GL_5_2

GLIVEC Tablets

(Novartis Pharmaceuticals UK Ltd)

1. NAME OF THE MEDICINAL PRODUCT

▼Glivec® 100 mg film-coated tablets
▼Glivec® 400 mg film-coated tablets

2. QUALITATIVE AND QUANTITATIVE COMPOSITION

Glivec 100 mg film-coated tablets: Each film-coated tablet contains 100 mg imatinib (as mesilate).

Glivec 400 mg film-coated tablets: Each film-coated tablet contains 400 mg imatinib (as mesilate).

For excipients, see 6.1.

3. PHARMACEUTICAL FORM

Glivec 100 mg film-coated tablets: Very dark yellow to brownish-orange film-coated tablet, round with "NVR" on one side and "SA" and score on the other side.

Glivec 400 mg film-coated tablets: Very dark yellow to brownish-orange, ovaloid, biconvex film-coated tablet with bevelled edges, debossed with "NVR" on one side and "SL" on the other side.

4. CLINICAL PARTICULARS

4.1 Therapeutic indications

Glivec is indicated for the treatment of patients with newly diagnosed Philadelphia chromosome (bcr-abl) positive (Ph+) chronic myeloid leukaemia (CML) for whom bone marrow transplantation is not considered as the first line of treatment.

Glivec is also indicated for the treatment of patients with Ph+ CML in chronic phase after failure of interferon-alpha therapy, or in accelerated phase or blast crisis.

The effect of Glivec on the outcome of bone marrow transplantation has not been determined.

Glivec is also indicated for the treatment of adult patients with Kit (CD 117) positive unresectable and/or metastatic malignant gastrointestinal stromal tumours (GIST).

In adult patients, the effectiveness of Glivec is based on overall haematological and cytogenetic response rates and progression-free survival in CML and objective response rates in GIST. The experience with Glivec in children with CML is very limited (see section 5.1). There are no controlled trials demonstrating a clinical benefit or increased survival for either of the two diseases.

4.2 Posology and method of administration

Therapy should be initiated by a physician experienced in the treatment of patients with CML or GIST.

For doses of 400 mg and above (see dosage recommendation below) a 400 mg tablet (not divisible) is available.

For doses other than 400 mg and 800 mg (see dosage recommendation below) a 100 mg divisible tablet is available.

The prescribed dose should be administered orally with a meal and a large glass of water to minimise the risk of gastrointestinal irritations. Doses of 400 mg or 600 mg should be administered once daily, whereas a daily dose of 800 mg should be administered as 400 mg twice a day, in the morning and in the evening.

For patients unable to swallow the film-coated tablets, the tablets may be dispersed in a glass of mineral water or apple juice. The required number of tablets should be placed in the appropriate volume of beverage (approximately 50 ml for a 100 mg tablet, and 200 ml for a 400 mg tablet) and stirred with a spoon. The suspension should be administered immediately after complete disintegration of the tablet(s).

Posology for CML

The recommended dosage of Glivec is 400 mg/day for patients in chronic phase CML. Chronic phase CML is defined when all of the following criteria are met: blasts < 15% in blood and bone marrow, peripheral blood basophils < 20%, platelets > 100 × 10^9/l.

The recommended dosage of Glivec is 600 mg/day for patients in accelerated phase. Accelerated phase is defined by the presence of any of the following: blasts ⩾ 15% but < 30% in blood or bone marrow, blasts plus promyelocytes ⩾ 30% in blood or bone marrow (providing < 30% blasts), peripheral blood basophils ⩾ 20%, platelets < 100 × 10^9/l unrelated to therapy.

The recommended dose of Glivec is 600 mg/day for patients in blast crisis. Blast crisis is defined as blasts ⩾ 30% in blood or bone marrow or extramedullary disease other than hepatosplenomegaly.

Treatment duration: In clinical trials, treatment with Glivec was continued until disease progression. The effect of stopping treatment after the achievement of a complete cytogenetic response has not been investigated.

Dose increases from 400 mg to 600 mg or 800 mg in patients with chronic phase disease, or from 600 mg to a maximum of 800 mg (given as 400 mg twice daily) in patients with accelerated phase or blast crisis may be considered in the absence of severe adverse drug reaction and severe non-leukaemia-related neutropenia or thrombocytopenia in the following circumstances: disease progression (at any time); failure to achieve a satisfactory haematological response after at least 3 months of treatment; failure to achieve a cytogenetic response after 12 months of treatment; or loss of a previously achieved haematological and/or cytogenetic response. Patients should be monitored closely following dose escalation given the potential for an increased incidence of adverse reactions at higher dosages.

Dosing for children should be on the basis of body surface area (mg/m^2). Doses of 260 mg/m^2 and 340 mg/m^2 daily are recommended for children with chronic phase CML and advanced phases CML, respectively. However, the total daily dose in children should not exceed adult equivalent doses of 400 and 600 mg, respectively. Treatment can be given as a once daily dose or alternatively the daily dose may be split into two administrations – one in the morning and one in the evening. The dose recommendation is currently based on a small number of paediatric patients (see sections 5.1 and 5.2). There is no experience with the treatment of children below 3 years of age.

Posology for GIST

The recommended dose of Glivec is 400 mg/day for patients with unresectable and/or metastatic malignant GIST.

Limited data exist on the effect of dose increases from 400 mg to 600 mg or 800 mg in patients progressing at the lower dose (see section 5.1).

There are currently no data available to support specific dosing recommendations for GIST patients based on prior gastrointestinal resection. The majority (98%) of patients in the clinical trial (see section 5.2) had had prior resection. For all patients on the study, there was at least a two-week interval between resection and the first dose of Glivec administered; however, no additional recommendations can be made based on this study.

Treatment duration: In clinical trials in GIST patients, treatment with Glivec was continued until disease progression. At the time of analysis, the treatment duration was a median of 7 months (7 days to 13 months). The effect of stopping treatment after achieving a response has not been investigated.

Dose adjustment for adverse reactions in CML and GIST patients

Non-haematological adverse reactions

If a severe non-haematological adverse reaction develops with Glivec use, treatment must be withheld until the event has resolved. Thereafter, treatment can be resumed as appropriate depending on the initial severity of the event.

If elevations in bilirubin $> 3 \times$ institutional upper limit of normal (IULN) or in liver transaminases $> 5 \times$ IULN occur, Glivec should be withheld until bilirubin levels have returned to $< 1.5 \times$ IULN and transaminase levels to $< 2.5 \times$ IULN. Treatment with Glivec may then be continued at a reduced daily dose. In adults the dose should be reduced from 400 to 300 mg or from 600 to 400 mg and in children from 260 to 200 mg/m^2/day or from 340 to 260 mg/m^2/day.

Haematological adverse reactions

Dose reduction or treatment interruption for severe neutropenia and thrombocytopenia are recommended as indicated in the table below.

Dose adjustments for neutropenia and thrombocytopenia

(see Table 1 below)

Paediatric use: There is no experience with the use of Glivec in children below 3 years of age. The experience with Glivec in paediatric population with CML is limited to 14 patients with CML in chronic phase and 4 patients with CML in blast crisis. There is no experience in children or adolescents with GIST.

Hepatic insufficiency: Imatinib is mainly metabolised through the liver. Patients with mild, moderate or severe liver dysfunction should be given the minimum recommended dose of 400 mg daily. The dose can be reduced if the patient develops unacceptable toxicity (see sections 4.4, 4.8 and 5.2).

Liver dysfunction classification

Liver dysfunction	Liver function tests
Mild	Total bilirubin: = 1.5 ULN AST: >ULN (can be normal or <ULN if total bilirubin is >ULN)
Moderate	Total bilirubin: >1.5–3.0 ULN AST: any
Severe	Total bilirubin: >3–10 ULN AST: any

ULN = upper limit of normal for the institution

AST = aspartate aminotransferase

Renal insufficiency: No clinical studies were conducted with Glivec in patients with decreased renal function (studies excluded patients with serum creatinine concentration more than 2 times the upper limit of the normal range). Imatinib and its metabolites are not significantly excreted via the kidney. Since the renal clearance of imatinib is negligible, a decrease in total body clearance is not expected in patients with renal insufficiency. However, in severe renal insufficiency caution is recommended.

Elderly patients: Imatinib pharmacokinetics have not been specifically studied in the elderly. No significant age related pharmacokinetic differences have been observed in adult patients in clinical trials which included over 20% of patients age 65 and older. No specific dose recommendation is necessary in the elderly.

4.3 Contraindications

Hypersensitivity to the active substance or to any of the excipients.

4.4 Special warnings and special precautions for use

When Glivec is co-administered with other medicinal products, there is a potential for drug interactions (see section 4.5).

Concomitant use of imatinib and medicinal products that induce CYP3A4 (e.g. dexamethasone, phenytoin, carbamazepine, rifampicin, phenobarbital or Hypericum perforatum, also known as St. John's Wort) may significantly reduce exposure to Glivec, potentially increasing the risk of therapeutic failure. Therefore, concomitant use of strong CYP3A4 inducers and imatinib should be avoided (see section 4.5).

Metabolism of Glivec is mainly hepatic, and only 13% of excretion is through the kidneys. In patients with hepatic dysfunction (mild, moderate or severe), peripheral blood counts and liver enzymes should be carefully monitored (see sections 4.2, 4.8 and 5.2). It should be noted that GIST patients may have hepatic metastases which could lead to hepatic impairment.

Occurrences of severe fluid retention (pleural effusion, oedema, pulmonary oedema, ascites) have been reported in approximately 1 to 2% of patients taking Glivec. Therefore, it is highly recommended that patients be weighed regularly. An unexpected rapid weight gain should be carefully investigated and if necessary appropriate supportive care and therapeutic measures should be undertaken. In clinical trials, there was an increased incidence of these events in elderly patients and those with a prior history of cardiac disease. Therefore, caution should be exercised in patients with cardiac dysfunction.

In the GIST clinical trial, both gastrointestinal and intratumoural haemorrhages were reported (see section 4.8). Based on the available data, no predisposing factors (e.g. tumour size, tumour location, coagulation disorders) have been identified that place patients with GIST at a higher risk of either type of haemorrhage. Since increased vascularity and propensity for bleeding is a part of the nature and clinical course of GIST, standard practices and procedures for the monitoring and management of haemorrhage in all patients should be applied.

Laboratory tests

Complete blood counts must be performed regularly during therapy with Glivec. Treatment of CML patients with Glivec has been associated with neutropenia or thrombocytopenia. However, the occurrence of these cytopenias is likely to be related to the stage of the disease being treated and they were more frequent in patients with accelerated phase CML or blast crisis as compared to patients with chronic phase CML. Treatment with Glivec may be interrupted or the dose may be reduced, as recommended in section 4.2.

Liver function (transaminases, bilirubin, alkaline phosphatase) should be monitored regularly in patients receiving Glivec.

Glivec and its metabolites are not excreted via the kidney to a significant extent (13%). Creatinine clearance is known to decrease with age, and age did not significantly affect Glivec kinetics.

4.5 Interaction with other medicinal products and other forms of Interaction

Active substances that may **increase** imatinib plasma concentrations:

Substances that inhibit the cytochrome P450 isoenzyme CYP3A4 activity (e.g. ketoconazole, itraconazole, erythromycin, clarithromycin) could decrease metabolism and increase imatinib concentrations. There was a significant increase in exposure to imatinib (the mean C_{max} and AUC of imatinib rose by 26% and 40%, respectively) in healthy subjects when it was co-administered with a single dose of ketoconazole (a CYP3A4 inhibitor). Caution should be taken when administering Glivec with inhibitors of the CYP3A4 family.

Active substances that may **decrease** imatinib plasma concentrations:

Substances that are inducers of CYP3A4 activity could increase metabolism and decrease imatinib plasma concentrations. Co-medications which induce CYP3A4 (e.g. dexamethasone, phenytoin, carbamazepine, rifampicin, phenobarbital or Hypericum perforatum, also known as St. John's Wort) may significantly reduce exposure to Glivec, potentially increasing the risk of therapeutic failure. Pretreatment with multiple doses of rifampicin 600 mg followed by a single 400 mg dose of Glivec resulted in decrease in C_{max} and $AUC_{(0-\infty)}$ by at least 54% and 74%, of the respective values without rifampicin treatment. Concomitant use of rifampicin or other strong CYP3A4 inducers and imatinib should be avoided.

Active substances that may have their plasma concentration altered by Glivec

Imatinib increases the mean C_{max} and AUC of simvastatin (CYP3A4 substrate) 2- and 3.5-fold, respectively, indicating an inhibition of the CYP3A4 by imatinib. Therefore, caution is recommended when administering Glivec with CYP3A4 substrates with a narrow therapeutic window (e.g. cyclosporin or pimozide). Glivec may increase plasma concentration of other CYP3A4 metabolised drugs (e.g. triazolo-benzodiazepines, dihydropyridine calcium channel blockers, certain HMG-CoA reductase inhibitors, i.e. statins, etc.).

Because warfarin is metabolised by CYP2C9, patients who require anticoagulation should receive low-molecular-weight or standard heparin.

In vitro Glivec inhibits the cytochrome P450 isoenzyme CYP2D6 activity at concentrations similar to those that affect CYP3A4 activity. Systemic exposure to substrates of CYP2D6 is therefore potentially increased when co-administered with Glivec. No specific studies have been performed however and caution is recommended.

In vitro, Glivec inhibits paracetamol O-glucuronidation (Ki value of 58.5 micromol/l at therapeutic levels).

Caution should therefore be exercised when using Glivec and paracetamol concomitantly, especially with high doses of paracetamol.

4.6 Pregnancy and lactation

Pregnancy

There are no adequate data on the use of imatinib in pregnant women. Studies in animals have however shown reproductive toxicity (see section 5.3) and the potential risk for the foetus is unknown. Glivec should not be used during pregnancy unless clearly necessary. If it is used during pregnancy, the patient must be informed of the potential risk to the foetus. Women of childbearing potential must be advised to use effective contraception during treatment.

Lactation

It is not known whether imatinib is excreted in human milk. In animals, imatinib and/or its metabolites were extensively excreted in milk. Women who are taking Glivec should therefore not breast-feed.

4.7 Effects on ability to drive and use machines

While no specific reports have been received, patients should be advised that they may experience undesirable effects such as dizziness or blurred vision during treatment

Table 1 Dose adjustments for neutropenia and thrombocytopenia

Chronic phase CML and GIST (starting dose 400 mg[1])	ANC $< 1.0 \times 10^9$/l and/or platelets $< 50 \times 10^9$/l	1. Stop Glivec until ANC $\geqslant 1.5 \times 10^9$/l and platelets $\geqslant 75 \times 10^9$/l. 2. Resume treatment with Glivec at previous dose (i.e. before severe adverse reaction). 3. In the event of recurrence of ANC $< 1.0 \times 10^9$/l and/or platelets $< 50 \times 10^9$/l, repeat step 1 and resume Glivec at reduced dose of 300 mg[2].
Accelerated phase CML and blast crisis (starting dose 600 mg[3])	[4] ANC $< 0.5 \times 10^9$/l and/or platelets $< 10 \times 10^9$/l	1. Check whether cytopenia is related to leukaemia (marrow aspirate or biopsy). 2. If cytopenia is unrelated to leukaemia, reduce dose of Glivec to 400 mg[1]. 3. If cytopenia persists for 2 weeks, reduce further to 300 mg[2]. 4. If cytopenia persists for 4 weeks and is still unrelated to leukaemia, stop Glivec until ANC $\geqslant 1 \times 10^9$/l and platelets $\geqslant 20 \times 10^9$/l, then resume treatment at 300 mg[2].
ANC = absolute neutrophil count		

[1] or 260 mg/m^2 in children
[2] or 200 mg/m^2 in children
[3] or 340 mg/m^2 in children
[4] occurring after at least 1 month of treatment

with imatinib. Therefore, caution should be recommended when driving a car or operating machinery.

4.8 Undesirable effects

Patients with advanced stages of CML or malignant GIST may have numerous confounding medical conditions that make causality of adverse reactions difficult to assess due to the variety of symptoms related to the underlying disease, its progression, and the co-administration of numerous medicinal products.

In clinical trials in CML drug discontinuation for drug-related adverse reactions was observed in 2% of newly diagnosed patients, 4 % of patients in late chronic phase after failure of interferon therapy, 4% of patients in accelerated phase after failure of interferon therapy and 5% of blast crisis patients after failure of interferon therapy. In GIST the study drug was discontinued for drug-related adverse reactions in 4% of patients.

The adverse reactions were similar in CML and GIST patients, with two exceptions. There was more myelosuppression seen in CML patients than in GIST, which is probably due to the underlying disease. In the GIST clinical trial, 7 (5%) patients experienced CTC grade 3/4 GI bleeds (3 patients), intra-tumoural bleeds (3 patients) or both (1 patient). GI tumour sites may have been the source of the GI bleeds (see section 4.4). GI and tumoural bleeding may be serious and sometimes fatal. The most commonly reported (⩾ 10%) drug-related adverse reactions in both settings were mild nausea, vomiting, diarrhoea, abdominal pain, fatigue, myalgia, muscle cramps and rash. Superficial oedemas were a common finding in all studies and were described primarily as periorbital or lower limb oedemas. However, these oedemas were rarely severe and may be managed with diuretics, other supportive measures, or by reducing the dose of Glivec.

Miscellaneous adverse reactions such as pleural effusion, ascites, pulmonary oedema and rapid weight gain with or without superficial oedema may be collectively described as "fluid retention". These reactions can usually be managed by withholding Glivec temporarily and with diuretics and other appropriate supportive care measures. However, some of these reactions may be serious or life-threatening and several patients with blast crisis died with a complex clinical history of pleural effusion, congestive heart failure and renal failure. There were no special safety findings in paediatric clinical trials.

Adverse reactions

Adverse reactions reported as more than an isolated case are listed below, by system organ class and by frequency. Frequencies are defined as: very common (> 1/10), common (> 1/100, ⩽ 1/10), uncommon (> 1/1,000, ⩽ 1/100), rare (⩽ 1/1,000)

(see Table 2)

Laboratory test abnormalities

Haematology

In CML, cytopenias, particularly neutropenia and thrombocytopenia, have been a consistent finding in all studies, with the suggestion of a higher frequency at high doses ⩾ 750 mg (phase I study). However, the occurrence of cytopenias was also clearly dependent on the stage of the disease, the frequency of grade 3 or 4 neutropenias (ANC < 1.0 x10^9/l) and thrombocytopenias (platelet count < 50 x10^9/l) being between 4 and 6 times higher in blast crisis and accelerated phase (59-64% and 44-63% for neutropenia and thrombocytopenia, respectively) as compared to newly diagnosed patients in chronic phase CML (15% neutropenia and 8.5% thrombocytopenia). In newly diagnosed chronic phase CML grade 4 neutropenia (ANC < 0.5 x10^9/l) and thrombocytopenia (platelet count < 10 x10^9/l) were observed in 3% and < 1% of patients, respectively. The median duration of the neutropenic and thrombocytopenic episodes usually ranged from 2 to 3 weeks, and from 3 to 4 weeks, respectively. These events can usually be managed with either a reduction of the dose or an interruption of treatment with Glivec, but can in rare cases lead to permanent discontinuation of treatment.

In patients with GIST, grade 3 and 4 anaemia was reported in 5.4% and 0.7% of patients, respectively, and may have been related to gastrointestinal or intra-tumoural bleeding in at least some of these patients. Grade 3 and 4 neutropenia was seen in 7.5% and 2.7% of patients, respectively, and grade 3 thrombocytopenia in 0.7% of patients. No patient developed grade 4 thrombocytopenia. The decreases in white blood cell (WBC) and neutrophil counts occurred mainly during the first six weeks of therapy, with values remaining relatively stable thereafter.

Biochemistry

Severe elevation of transaminases or bilirubin was uncommon (< 3% of patients) in CML patients and was usually managed with dose reduction or interruption (the median duration of these episodes was approximately one week). Treatment was discontinued permanently because of liver laboratory abnormalities in less than 0.5% of CML patients. In GIST patients (study B2222), 6.8% of grade 3 or 4 ALT (alanine aminotransferase)elevations and 4.8% of grade 3 or 4 AST (aspartate aminotransferase) elevations were observed. Bilirubin elevation was below 3%.

There have been cases of cytolytic and cholestatic hepatitis and hepatic failure; in some of them outcome was fatal, including one patient on high dose paracetamol.

Table 2

	Very Common	**Common**	**Uncommon**	**Rare**
Infections and infestations			Sepsis, pneumonia, herpes simplex, herpes zoster, upper respiratory tract infection, gastroenteritis	
Blood and lymphatic system disorders	Neutropenia, thrombocytopenia, anaemia	Febrile neutropenia	Pancytopenia, bone marrow depression	
Metabolism and nutrition disorders		Anorexia	Dehydration, hyperuricaemia, hypokalaemia, appetite increased, appetite decreased, gout, hypophosphataemia	Hyperkalaemia, hyponatraemia
Psychiatric disorders			Depression, anxiety, libido decreased	Confusion
Nervous system disorders	Headache	Dizziness, taste disturbance, paraesthesia, insomnia	Cerebral haemorrhage, syncope, peripheral neuropathy, hypoaesthesia, somnolence, migraine, memory impairment	Cerebral oedema, increased intracranial pressure, convulsions
Eye disorders		Conjunctivitis, lacrimation increased, vision blurred	Eye irritation, conjunctival haemorrhage, dry eye, orbital oedema	Macular oedema, papilloedema, retinal haemorrhage, vitreous haemorrhage, glaucoma
Ear and labyrinth disorders			Vertigo, tinnitus	
Cardiac disorders			Cardiac failure, pulmonary oedema, tachycardia	Pericardial effusion, pericarditis, cardiac tamponade
Vascular disorders			Haematoma, hypertension, hypotension, flushing, peripheral coldness	Thrombosis, embolism
Respiratory, thoracic and mediastinal disorders		Epistaxis, dyspnoea	Pleural effusion, cough, pharyngolaryngeal pain	Pulmonary fibrosis, interstitial pneumonitis
Gastrointestinal disorders	Nausea, vomiting, diarrhoea, dyspepsia, abdominal pain	Abdominal distension, flatulence, constipation, gastro-oesophageal reflux, mouth ulceration	Gastrointestinal haemorrhage, melaena, ascites, gastric ulcer, gastritis, eructation, dry mouth	Colitis, ileus, intestinal obstruction, pancreatitis
Hepato-biliary disorders		Increased hepatic enzymes	Jaundice, hepatitis, hyperbilirubinaemia	Hepatic failure
Skin and subcutaneous tissue disorders	Periorbital oedema, dermatitis/eczema/ rash	Face oedema, eyelid oedema, pruritus, erythema, dry skin, alopecia, night sweats	Petechiae, contusion, sweating increased, urticaria, onychoclasis, photosensitivity reaction, purpura, hypotrichosis, cheilitis, skin hyperpigmentation, skin hypopigmentation, psoriasis, exfoliative dermatitis and bullous eruptions	Angioedema, vesicular rash, Stevens-Johnson syndrome, acute febrile neutrophilic dermatosis (Sweet's syndrome)
Musculoskeletal, connective tissue and bone disorders	Muscle spasm and cramps, musculoskeletal pain, including arthralgia	Joint swelling	Sciatica, joint and muscle stiffness	
Renal and urinary disorders			Renal failure, renal pain, urinary frequency increased, haematuria	
Reproductive system and breast disorders			Gynaecomastia, breast enlargement, scrotal oedema, menorrhagia, nipple pain, sexual dysfunction	
General disorders and administration site conditions	Fluid retention and oedema, fatigue	Pyrexia, weakness, rigors	Malaise, haemorrhage	Anasarca, tumour haemorrhage, tumour necrosis
Investigations		Weight increased	Blood alkaline phosphatase increased, blood creatinine increased, weight decreased, blood creatine phosphokinase increased, blood lactate dehydrogenase increased	

4.9 Overdose

Experience with doses greater than 800 mg is limited. Isolated cases of Glivec overdose have been reported.

A patient with myeloid blast crisis inadvertently took Glivec 1200 mg for 6 days and experienced Grade 1 elevations of serum creatinine, Grade 2 ascites and elevated liver transaminase levels, and Grade 3 elevations of bilirubin. Treatment was temporarily interrupted and there was complete reversal of all abnormalities within one week. Treatment was resumed at a dose of 400 mg without recurrence of problems. Another patient developed severe muscle cramps after taking Glivec 1,600 mg daily for six days. Following interruption of treatment, complete resolution of muscle cramps occurred, treatment was subsequently resumed.

In the event of overdose, the patient should be observed and appropriate supportive treatment given.

5. PHARMACOLOGICAL PROPERTIES

5.1 Pharmacodynamic properties

Pharmacotherapeutic group: protein-tyrosine kinase inhibitor, ATC code: L01XX28

Imatinib is a protein-tyrosine kinase inhibitor which potently inhibits the Bcr-Abl tyrosine kinase at the *in vitro*, cellular and *in vivo* levels. The compound selectively inhibits proliferation and induces apoptosis in Bcr-Abl positive cell lines as well as fresh leukaemic cells from Philadelphia chromosome positive CML and acute lymphoblastic leukaemia (ALL) patients.

In vivo the compound shows anti-tumour activity as a single agent in animal models using Bcr-Abl positive tumour cells.

Imatinib is also an inhibitor of the receptor tyrosine kinases for platelet-derived growth factor (PDGF), PDGF-R, and stem cell factor (SCF), c-Kit, and inhibits PDGF- and SCF-mediated cellular events. *In vitro*, imatinib inhibits proliferation and induces apoptosis in gastrointestinal stromal tumour (GIST) cells, which express an activating *kit* mutation.

Clinical studies in chronic myeloid leukaemia

The effectiveness of Glivec is based on overall haematological and cytogenetic response rates. There are no controlled trials demonstrating a clinical benefit, such as improvement in disease-related symptoms or increased survival.

Three large, international, open-label, non-controlled phase II studies were conducted in patients with Philadelphia chromosome positive (Ph+) CML in advanced, blast or accelerated phase disease, other Ph+ leukaemias or with CML in the chronic phase but failing prior interferon-alpha (IFN) therapy. One large, open-label, multicentre, international randomised phase III study has been conducted in patients with newly diagnosed Ph+ CML. In addition, children have been treated in two phase I studies.

In all clinical studies 38–40% of patients were ⩾ 60 years of age and 10–12% of patients were ⩾ 70 years of age.

Chronic phase, newly diagnosed: This phase III study compared treatment with either single-agent Glivec or a combination of interferon-alfa (IFN) plus cytarabine (Ara-C). Patients showing lack of response (lack of complete haematological response (CHR) at 6 months, increasing WBC, no major cytogenetic response (MCyR) at 24 months), loss of response (loss of CHR or MCyR) or severe intolerance to treatment were allowed to cross over to the alternative treatment arm. In the Glivec arm, patients were treated with 400 mg daily. In the IFN arm, patients were treated with a target dose of IFN of 5 MIU/m^2/day subcutaneously in combination with subcutaneous Ara-C 20 mg/m^2/day for 10 days/month.

A total of 1106 patients were randomised, 553 to each arm. Baseline characteristics were well balanced between the two arms. Median age was 51 years (range 18–70 years), with 21.9% of patients ⩾ 60 years of age. There were 59% males and 41% females; 89.9% caucasian and 4.7% black patients. The median follow-up for all patients was 31 and 30 months in the Glivec and IFN arms, respectively. The primary efficacy endpoint of the study is progression-free survival. Progression was defined as any of the following events: progression to accelerated phase or blast crisis, death, loss of CHR or MCyR, or in patients not achieving a CHR an increasing WBC despite appropriate therapeutic management. Major cytogenetic response, haematological response, molecular response (evaluation of minimal residual disease), time to accelerated phase or blast crisis and survival are main secondary endpoints. Response data are shown in Table 3. Complete haematological response, major cytogenetic response and complete cytogenetic response as well as major molecular response were significantly higher in the Glivec arm compared to the IFN + Ara-C arm.

With the follow-up currently available, the estimated rate of patients free of progression to accelerated phase or blast crisis at 30 months was significantly higher in the Glivec arm compared to the IFN arm (94.8% versus 89.6%, $p<0.0016$). The estimated rate of progression-free survival at 30 months was 87.8% in the Glivec arm and 68.3% in the control arm. There were 33 and 46 deaths reported in the Glivec and IFN arms, with an estimated 30-month survival rate of 94.6% and 91.6%, respectively (difference not significant). The probability of remaining progression-free at 30 months was 100% for patients who were in complete cytogenetic response with major molecular response (⩾ 3-logarithms reduction) at 12 months, compared to 93% for patients in complete cytogenetic response but without a major molecular response, and 82% for patients who were not in complete cytogenetic response at this time point ($p<0.001$).

In this study, dose escalations were allowed from 400 mg daily to 600 mg daily, then from 600 mg daily to 800 mg daily. After 42 months of follow-up, 11 patients experienced a confirmed loss (within 4 weeks) of their cytogenetic response. Of these 11 patients, 4 patients escalated up to 800 mg daily, 2 of whom regained a cytogenetic response (1 partial and 1 complete, the latter also achieving a molecular response), while of the 7 patients who did not escalate the dose, only one regained a complete cytogenetic response. The percentage of some adverse reactions was higher in the 40 patients in whom the dose was increased to 800 mg daily compared to the population of patients before dose increase (n=551). The more frequent adverse reactions included gastrointestinal haemorrhages, conjunctivitis and elevation of transaminases or bilirubin. Other adverse reactions were reported with lower or equal frequency.

Table 3. Response in newly diagnosed CML Study (30-month data)

	Glivec	IFN+Ara-C
(Best response rates)	n=553	n=553
Haematological response		
CHR rate n (%)	527 (95.3%)	308 (55.7%)
[95% CI]	[93.2%, 96.9%]	[51.4%, 59.9%]
Cytogenetic response		
Major response n (%)	482 (87.2%)*	127 (23.0%)*
[95% CI]	[84.1%, 89.8%]	[19.5%, 26.7%]
Complete CyR n (%)	436 (78.8%)*	59 (10.7%)*
Partial CyR n (%)	46 (8.3%)	68 (12.3%)
Molecular response		
Major response at 12 months (%)	40%*	2%*
Major response at 24 months (%)	54%	NA**

* $p<0.001$, Fischer's exact test

** insufficient data, only two patients available with samples

Haematological response criteria (all responses to be confirmed after ⩾ 4 weeks):

WBC < 10 x10^9/l, platelet < 450 x10^9/l, myelocyte+metamyelocyte < 5% in blood, no blasts and promyelocytes in blood, basophils < 20%, no extramedullary involvement

Cytogenetic response criteria:

complete (0% Ph+ metaphases), partial (1–35%), minor (36–65%) or minimal (66–95%). A major response (0–35%) combines both complete and partial responses.

Major molecular response criteria: in the peripheral blood, after 12 months of therapy, reduction of ⩾ 3 logarithms in the amount of BCR-ABL transcripts (measured by real-time quantitative reverse transcriptase PCR assay) over a standardised baseline.

Chronic phase, Interferon failure: 532 patients were treated at a starting dose of 400 mg. The patients were distributed in three main categories: haematological failure (29%), cytogenetic failure (35%), or intolerance to interferon (36%). Patients had received a median of 14 months of prior IFN therapy at doses ⩾ 25 x10^6 IU/week and were all in late chronic phase, with a median time from diagnosis of 32 months. The primary efficacy variable of the study was the rate of major cytogenetic response (complete plus partial response, 0 to 35% Ph+ metaphases in the bone marrow).

In this study 65% of the patients achieved a major cytogenetic response that was complete in 53% (confirmed 43%) of patients (Table 4). A complete haematological response was achieved in 95% of patients.

Accelerated phase: 235 patients with accelerated phase disease were enrolled. The first 77 patients were started at 400 mg, the protocol was subsequently amended to allow higher dosing and the remaining 158 patients were started at 600 mg.

The primary efficacy variable was the rate of haematological response, reported as either complete haematological response, no evidence of leukaemia (i.e. clearance of blasts from the marrow and the blood, but without a full peripheral blood recovery as for complete responses), or return to chronic phase CML. A confirmed haematological response was achieved in 71.5% of patients (Table 4). Importantly, 27.7% of patients also achieved a major cytogenetic response, which was complete in 20.4% (confirmed 16%) of patients. For the patients treated at 600 mg, the current estimates for median progression-free-survival and overall survival were 22.9 and 42.5 months, respectively.

Myeloid blast crisis: 260 patients with myeloid blast crisis were enrolled. 95 (37%) had received prior chemotherapy for treatment of either accelerated phase or blast crisis ("pretreated patients") whereas 165 (63%) had not ("untreated patients"). The first 37 patients were started at 400 mg, the protocol was subsequently amended to allow higher dosing and the remaining 223 patients were started at 600 mg.

The primary efficacy variable was the rate of haematological response, reported as either complete haematological response, no evidence of leukaemia, or return to chronic phase CML using the same criteria as for the study in accelerated phase. In this study, 31% of patients achieved a haematological response (36% in previously untreated patients and 22% in previously treated patients). The rate of response was also higher in the patients treated at 600 mg (33%) as compared to the patients treated at 400 mg (16%, p=0.0220). The current estimate of the median survival of the previously untreated and treated patients was 7.7 and 4.7 months, respectively.

Lymphoid blast crisis: a limited number of patients were enrolled in phase I studies (n=10). The rate of haematological response was 70% with a duration of 2-3 months.

Table 4 Response in CML studies

(see Table 4 on next page)

Paediatric patients: A total of 26 paediatric patients of age < 18 years with either chronic phase CML (n=11) or CML in blast crisis or Ph+ acute leukaemias (n=15) were enrolled in a dose-escalation phase I trial. This was a population of heavily pretreated patients, as 46% had received prior BMT and 73% a prior multi-agent chemotherapy. The median age was 12 years (range 3 to 17). Among the chronic phase CML patients, 27% were between 3–12 years of age and 60% of the acute phase patients were between 3–12 years of age. Patients were treated at doses of Glivec of 260 mg/m^2/day (n=5), 340 mg/m^2/day (n=9), 440 mg/m^2/day (n=7) and 570 mg/m^2/day (n=5). Out of 9 patients with chronic phase CML and cytogenetic data available, 4 (44%) and 3 (33%) achieved a complete and partial cytogenetic response, respectively, for a rate of MCyR of 77%. Eight additional children (3 CML, 4 acute leukaemias, 1 lymphoid blast crisis) were treated in another phase I study. Three received a dose of 173 to 200 mg/m^2/day, four a dose of approximately 260 mg/m^2/day, and one a dose of 360 mg/m^2/day. Two out of the three chronic phase CML patients achieved a complete cytogenetic response. Among the total of 34 patients, there were no special safety findings in comparison with adult trials.

Clinical studies in GIST

One phase II, open-label, randomised, uncontrolled multinational study was conducted in patients with unresectable or metastatic malignant gastrointestinal stromal tumours (GIST). In this study 147 patients were enrolled and randomised to receive either 400 mg or 600 mg orally q.d. for up to 36 months. These patients ranged in age from 18 to 83 years old and had a pathologic diagnosis of Kit-positive malignant GIST that was unresectable and/or metastatic. Immunohistochemistry was routinely performed with Kit antibody (A-4502, rabbit polyclonal antiserum, 1:100; DAKO Corporation, Carpinteria, CA) according to analysis by an avidin-biotin-peroxidase complex method after antigen retrieval.

The primary evidence of efficacy was based on objective response rates. Tumours were required to be measurable in at least one site of disease, and response characterisation based on Southwestern Oncology Group (SWOG) criteria. Results are provided in Table 5.

Table 5 Best tumour response in trial STIB2222 (GIST)

Best response	All doses (n=147) 400 mg (n=73) 600 mg (n=74) n (%)
Complete response	1(0.7)
Partial response	98 (66.7)
Stable disease	23 (15.6)
Progressive disease	18 (12.2)
Not evaluable	5 (3.4)
Unknown	2 (1.4)

There were no differences in response rates between the two dose groups. A significant number of patients who had stable disease at the time of the interim analysis achieved a partial response with longer treatment (median follow-up

Table 4 Response in CML studies

	Study 0110 37-month data Chronic phase, IFN failure (n=532)	Study 0109 40.5-month data Accelerated phase (n=235)	Study 0102 38-month data Myeloid blast crisis (n=260)
	% of patients ($CI_{95\%}$)		
Haematological response[1]	95% (92.3-96.3)	71% (65.3-77.2)	31% (25.2-36.8)
Complete haematological response (CHR)	95%	42%	8%
No evidence of leukaemia (NEL)	Not applicable	12%	5%
Return to chronic phase (RTC)	Not applicable	17%	18%
Major cytogenetic response[2]	65% (61.2-69.5)	28% (22.0-33.9)	15% (11.2-20.4)
Complete	53%	20%	7%
(Confirmed[3]) [95% CI]	(43%) [38.6-47.2]	(16%) [11.3-21.0]	(2%) [0.6-4.4]
Partial	12%	7%	8%

[1] **Haematological response criteria (all responses to be confirmed after ⩾ 4 weeks):**
CHR: Study 0110 [WBC < 10 x10^9/l, platelets < 450 x10^9/l, myelocyte+metamyelocyte < 5% in blood, no blasts and promyelocytes in blood, basophils < 20%, no extramedullary involvement] and in studies 0102 and 0109 [ANC ⩾ 1.5 x10^9/l, platelets ⩾ 100 x10^9/l, no blood blasts, BM blasts < 5% and no extramedullary disease]
NEL Same criteria as for CHR but ANC ⩾ 1 x10^9/l and platelets ⩾ 20 x10^9/l (0102 and 0109 only)
RTC < 15% blasts BM and PB, < 30% blasts+promyelocytes in BM and PB, < 20% basophils in PB, no extramedullary disease other than spleen and liver (only for 0102 and 0109).
BM = bone marrow, PB = peripheral blood
[2] **Cytogenetic response criteria:**
A major response combines both complete and partial responses: complete (0% Ph+ metaphases), partial (1–35%)
[3] Complete cytogenetic response confirmed by a second bone marrow cytogenetic evaluation performed at least one month after the initial bone marrow study.

31 months). Median time to response was 13 weeks (95% C.I. 12–23). Median time to treatment failure in responders was 122 weeks (95% C.I 106–147), while in the overall study population it was 84 weeks (95% C.I 71–109). The median overall survival has not been reached. The Kaplan-Meier estimate for survival after 36-month follow-up is 68%.

In two clinical studies (study B2222 and an intergroup study S0033) the daily dose of Glivec was escalated to 800 mg in patients progressing at the lower daily doses of 400 mg or 600 mg. The daily dose was escalated to 800 mg in a total of 103 patients; 6 patients achieved a partial response and 21 stabilisation of their disease after dose escalation for an overall clinical benefit of 26%. From the safety data available, escalating the dose to 800 mg daily in patients progressing at lower doses of 400 mg or 600 mg daily does not seem to affect the safety profile of Glivec.

5.2 Pharmacokinetic properties

Pharmacokinetics of Glivec

The pharmacokinetics of Glivec have been evaluated over a dosage range of 25 to 1000 mg. Plasma pharmacokinetic profiles were analysed on day 1 and on either day 7 or day 28, by which time plasma concentrations had reached steady state.

Absorption

Mean absolute bioavailability for imatinib is 98%. There was high between-patient variability in plasma imatinib AUC levels after an oral dose. When given with a high-fat meal, the rate of absorption of imatinib was minimally reduced (11% decrease in C_{max} and prolongation of t_{max} by 1.5 h), with a small reduction in AUC (7.4%) compared to fasting conditions. The effect of prior gastrointestinal surgery on drug absorption has not been investigated.

Distribution

At clinically relevant concentrations of imatinib, binding to plasma proteins was approximately 95% on the basis of *in vitro* experiments, mostly to albumin and alpha-acid-glycoprotein, with little binding to lipoprotein.

Metabolism

The main circulating metabolite in humans is the N-demethylated piperazine derivative, which shows similar *in vitro* potency to the parent. The plasma AUC for this metabolite was found to be only 16% of the AUC for imatinib. The plasma protein binding of the N-demethylated metabolite is similar to that of the parent compound.

Imatinib and the N-demethyl metabolite together accounted for about 65% of the circulating radioactivity ($AUC_{(0-48h)}$). The remaining circulating radioactivity consisted of a number of minor metabolites.

The *in vitro* results showed that CYP3A4 was the major human P450 enzyme catalysing the biotransformation of imatinib. Of a panel of potential comedications (acetaminophen, aciclovir, allopurinol, amphotericin, cytarabine, erythromycin, fluconazole, hydroxyurea, norfloxacin, penicillin V) only erythromycin (IC_{50} 50 μM) and fluconazole (IC_{50} 118 μM) showed inhibition of imatinib metabolism which could have clinical relevance.

Imatinib was shown *in vitro* to be a competitive inhibitor of marker substrates for CYP2C9, CYP2D6 and CYP3A4/5. K_i values in human liver microsomes were 27, 7.5 and 7.9 μmol/l, respectively. Maximal plasma concentrations of imatinib in patients are 2 - 4 μmol/l, consequently an inhibition of CYP2D6 and/or CYP3A4/5-mediated metabolism of co-administered drugs is possible. Imatinib did not interfere with the biotransformation of 5-fluorouracil, but it inhibited paclitaxel metabolism as a result of competitive inhibition of CYP2C8 (K_i = 34.7 μM). This K_i value is far higher than the expected plasma levels of imatinib in patients, consequently no interaction is expected upon co-administration of either 5-fluorouracil or paclitaxel and imatinib.

Elimination

Based on the recovery of compound(s) after an oral ^{14}C-labelled dose of imatinib, approximately 81% of the dose was recovered within 7 days in faeces (68% of dose) and urine (13% of dose). Unchanged imatinib accounted for 25% of the dose (5% urine, 20% faeces), the remainder being metabolites.

Plasma pharmacokinetics

Following oral administration in healthy volunteers, the $t_{1/2}$ was approximately 18 h, suggesting that once-daily dosing is appropriate. The increase in mean AUC with increasing dose was linear and dose proportional in the range of 25–1000 mg imatinib after oral administration. There was no change in the kinetics of imatinib on repeated dosing, and accumulation was 1.5–2.5-fold at steady state when dosed once daily.

Pharmacokinetics in GIST patients

In patients with GIST steady-state exposure was 1.5-fold higher than that observed for CML patients for the same dosage (400 mg daily). Based on preliminary population pharmacokinetic analysis in GIST patients, there were three variables (albumin, WBC and bilirubin) found to have a statistically significant relationship with imatinib pharmacokinetics. Decreased values of albumin caused a reduced clearance (CL/f); and higher levels of WBC led to a reduction of CL/f. However, these associations are not sufficiently pronounced to warrant dose adjustment. In this patient population, the presence of hepatic metastases could potentially lead to hepatic insufficiency and reduced metabolism.

Population pharmacokinetics

Based on population pharmacokinetic analysis in CML patients, there was a small effect of age on the volume of distribution (12% increase in patients > 65 years old). This change is not thought to be clinically significant. The effect of bodyweight on the clearance of imatinib is such that for a patient weighing 50 kg the mean clearance is expected to be 8.5 l/h, while for a patient weighing 100 kg the clearance will rise to 11.8 l/h. These changes are not considered sufficient to warrant dose adjustment based on kg bodyweight. There is no effect of gender on the kinetics of imatinib.

Pharmacokinetics in children

As in adult patients, imatinib was rapidly absorbed after oral administration in paediatric patients in a phase I study. Dosing in children at 260 and 340 mg/m^2/day achieved the same exposure, respectively, as doses of 400 mg and 600 mg in adult patients. The comparison of $AUC_{(0-24)}$ on day 8 and day 1 at the 340 mg/m^2/day dose level revealed a 1.7-fold drug accumulation after repeated once-daily dosing.

Organ function impairment

Imatinib and its metabolites are not excreted via the kidney to a significant extent. Although the results of pharmacokinetic analysis showed that there is considerable intersubject variation, the mean exposure to imatinib did not increase in patients with varying degrees of liver dysfunction as compared to patients with normal liver function (see sections 4.2, 4.4 and 4.8).

5.3 Preclinical safety data

The preclinical safety profile of imatinib was assessed in rats, dogs, monkeys and rabbits.

Multiple dose toxicity studies revealed mild to moderate haematological changes in rats, dogs and monkeys, accompanied by bone marrow changes in rats and dogs.

The liver was a target organ in rats and dogs. Mild to moderate increases in transaminases and slight decreases in cholesterol, triglycerides, total protein and albumin levels were observed in both species. No histopathological changes were seen in rat liver. Severe liver toxicity was observed in dogs treated for 2 weeks, with elevated liver enzymes, hepatocellular necrosis, bile duct necrosis, and bile duct hyperplasia.

Renal toxicity was observed in monkeys treated for 2 weeks, with focal mineralisation and dilation of the renal tubules and tubular nephrosis. Increased blood urea nitrogen (BUN) and creatinine were observed in several of these animals. In rats, hyperplasia of the transitional epithelium in the renal papilla and in the urinary bladder was observed at doses ⩾ 6 mg/kg in the 13-week study, without changes in serum or urinary parameters. An increased rate of opportunistic infections was observed with chronic imatinib treatment.

In a 39-week monkey study, no NOAEL (no observed adverse effect level) was established at the lowest dose of 15 mg/kg, approximately one-third the maximum human dose of 800 mg based on body surface. Treatment resulted in worsening of normally suppressed malarial infections in these animals.

Imatinib was not considered genotoxic when tested in an *in vitro* bacterial cell assay (Ames test), an *in vitro* mammalian cell assay (mouse lymphoma) and an *in vivo* rat micronucleus test. Positive genotoxic effects were obtained for imatinib in an *in vitro* mammalian cell assay (Chinese hamster ovary) for clastogenicity (chromosome aberration) in the presence of metabolic activation. Two intermediates of the manufacturing process, which are also present in the final product, are positive for mutagenesis in the Ames assay. One of these intermediates was also positive in the mouse lymphoma assay.

In a study of fertility, in male rats dosed for 70 days prior to mating, testicular and epididymal weights and percent motile sperm were decreased at 60 mg/kg, approximately equal to the maximum clinical dose of 800 mg/day, based on body surface area. This was not seen at doses ⩽ 20 mg/kg. A slight to moderate reduction in spermatogenesis was also observed in the dog at oral doses ⩾ 30 mg/kg. When female rats were dosed 14 days prior to mating and through to gestational day 6, there was no effect on mating or on number of pregnant females. At a dose of 60 mg/kg, female rats had significant post-implantation foetal loss and a reduced number of live foetuses. This was not seen at doses ⩽ 20 mg/kg.

In an oral pre- and postnatal development study in rats, red vaginal discharge was noted in the 45 mg/kg/day group on either day 14 or day 15 of gestation. At the same dose, the number of stillborn pups as well as those dying between postpartum days 0 and 4 was increased. In the F_1 offspring, at the same dose level, mean body weights were reduced from birth until terminal sacrifice and the number of litters achieving criterion for preputial separation was slightly decreased. F_1 fertility was not affected, while an increased number of resorptions and a decreased number of viable foetuses was noted at 45 mg/kg/day. The no observed effect level (NOEL) for both the maternal animals and the F_1 generation was 15 mg/kg/day (one quarter of the maximum human dose of 800 mg).

Imatinib was teratogenic in rats when administered during organogenesis at doses ⩾ 100 mg/kg, approximately equal to the maximum clinical dose of 800 mg/day, based on body surface area. Teratogenic effects included exencephaly or encephalocele, absent/reduced frontal and absent parietal bones. These effects were not seen at doses ⩽ 30 mg/kg.

The urogenital tract findings from a 2-year carcinogenicity study in rats receiving doses of 15, 30 and 60 mg/kg/day of imatinib showed renal adenomas/carcinomas, urinary bladder papillomas and papillomas/carcinomas of the preputial and clitoral gland. Evaluation of other organs in rats is ongoing.

The papilloma/carcinoma of the preputial/clitoral gland were noted at 30 and 60 mg/kg/day, representing approximately 0.5 to 4 or 0.3 to 2.4 times the human daily exposure (based on AUC) at 400 mg/day or 800 mg/day, respectively, and 0.4 to 3.0 times the daily exposure in children (based on AUC) at 340 mg/m^2. The renal adenoma/carcinoma and the urinary bladder papilloma were noted at

60 mg/kg/day. The no observed effect levels (NOEL) for the various target organs with neoplastic lesions were 15 mg/kg/day for preputial and clitoral gland, and 30 mg/kg/day for kidney and urinary bladder.

The mechanism and relevance of these findings in the rat carcinogenicity study for humans are not yet clarified.

6. PHARMACEUTICAL PARTICULARS

6.1 List of excipients

Tablet core:

Cellulose microcrystalline

Crospovidone

Hypromellose

Magnesium stearate

Silica, colloidal anhydrous

Tablet coat:

Iron oxide, red (E172)

Iron oxide, yellow (E172)

6.2 Incompatibilities

Not applicable

6.3 Shelf life

2 years

6.4 Special precautions for storage

Do not store above 30°C.

Store in the original package in order to protect from moisture.

6.5 Nature and contents of container

PVC/alu blisters

Glivec 100 mg film-coated tablets: Packs containing 20, 60, 120 or 180 film-coated tablets

Glivec 400 mg film-coated tablets: Packs containing 10, 30 or 90 film-coated tablets

Not all pack sizes may be marketed.

6.6 Instructions for use and handling

No special requirements

7. MARKETING AUTHORISATION HOLDER

Novartis Europharm Limited

Wimblehurst Road

Horsham

West Sussex, RH12 5AB

UNITED KINGDOM

8. MARKETING AUTHORISATION NUMBER(S)

Glivec 100 mg film-coated tablets:

EU/1/01/198/007

EU/1/01/198/008

EU/1/01/198/011

EU/1/01/198/012

Glivec 400 mg film-coated tablets:

EU/1/01/198/009

EU/1/01/198/010

EU/1/01/198/013

9. DATE OF FIRST AUTHORISATION/RENEWAL OF THE AUTHORISATION

11.11.2003

10. DATE OF REVISION OF THE TEXT

08.07.2005

LEGAL CATEGORY

POM

GlucaGen Hypokit 1 mg

(Novo Nordisk Limited)

1. NAME OF THE MEDICINAL PRODUCT

GlucaGen HypoKit 1mg

Powder and solvent for solution for injection in pre-filled syringe.

2. QUALITATIVE AND QUANTITATIVE COMPOSITION

GlucaGen HypoKit 1mg consists of a vial containing 1mg (1iu) glucagon (rys) and a pre-filled syringe containing 1.1ml Water for Injections.

Active substance: Glucagon (biosynthetic (rys), structurally identical to human glucagon).

Glucagon 1 mg (1 IU) (as hydrochloride).

One vial contains 1 mg glucagon corresponding to 1 mg glucagon/ml after reconstitution.

For excipients, see 6.1.

3. PHARMACEUTICAL FORM

Powder and solvent for solution for injection in pre-filled syringe

4. CLINICAL PARTICULARS

4.1 Therapeutic indications

Treatment of severe hypoglycaemic reactions which may occur in the management of diabetic patients receiving insulin.

4.1.1 Diagnostic Indications

***Inhibition of motility*:**

(i) As a motility inhibitor in examinations of the gastrointestinal tract, e.g. double contrast radiography and endoscopy.

(ii) As a motility inhibitor in computerised tomography (CT), nuclear magnetic resonance scanning (NMR) and digital subtraction angiography (DSA).

4.2 Posology and method of administration

Dissolve the freeze-dried product in the accompanying solvent, as described under item 6.6. The reconstituted solution may be administered by intravenous, intramuscular or subcutaneous injection.

4.2.1 Severe Hypoglycaemia

(a) Administration by Medical Personnel

Administer 1.0mg (adults and children above 25kg or 6 - 8 years) or 0.5mg (children below 25kg or 6 - 8 years) by subcutaneous, intramuscular or intravenous injection. The patient will normally respond within 10 minutes. When the patient has responded to the treatment, give oral carbohydrate to restore the liver glycogen and prevent relapse of hypoglycaemia. If the patient does not respond within 10 minutes, intravenous glucose should be given.

(b) Administration to the Patient by a Relative

Inject GlucaGen as indicated below.

Administer 1.0mg (adults and children above 25kg or 6 - 8 years) or 0.5mg (children below 25kg or 6 - 8 years) by subcutaneous or intramuscular injection. The patient will normally respond within 10 minutes. When the patient has responded to the treatment, give oral carbohydrate to restore the liver glycogen and prevent relapse of hypoglycaemia.

Medical assistance is required for all patients with severe hypoglycaemia.

4.2.2. Diagnostic Indications

Inhibition of Motility:

Onset of action after an intravenous injection of 0.2 - 0.5mg occurs within one minute and the duration of effect is between 5 and 20 minutes depending on the organ under examination. The onset of action after an intramuscular injection of 1 - 2mg occurs after 5-15 minutes and lasts approximately 10-40 minutes depending on the organ.

(i) Dose ranges from 0.2 - 2mg depending on the diagnostic technique used and the route of administration. The usual diagnostic dose for relaxation of the stomach, duodenal bulb, duodenum and small bowel is 0.2 - 0.5mg given intravenously or 1mg given intramuscularly; the usual dose to relax the colon is 0.5 - 0.75mg intravenously or 1 - 2mg intramuscularly.

(ii) In CT-scanning, NMR and DSA intravenous doses of up to 1mg are used.

4.3 Contraindications

Hypersensitivity to glucagon or any of the excipients. GlucaGen is contraindicated in phaeocromocytoma.

4.4 Special warnings and special precautions for use

To prevent the occurrence of secondary hypoglycaemia, oral carbohydrates should be given to restore the liver glycogen when the patient has responded to the treatment or if used for diagnostic procedure, when the procedure has ended. In case of severe hypoglycaemia, intravenous glucose may be required.

Glucagon reacts antagonistically towards insulin and caution should be observed if GlucaGen is used in patients with insulinoma or glucagonoma. Caution should also be observed when GlucaGen is used as an adjunct in endoscopic or radiographic procedures in diabetic patients or in elderly patients with known cardiac disease. If fibril formation (viscous appearance) or solid particles are present in the solution, it must not be used.

4.5 Interaction with other medicinal products and other forms of Interaction

Insulin: Reacts antagonistically towards glucagon.

Indomethacin: Glucagon may lose its ability to raise blood glucose or, paradoxically, may even produce hypoglycaemia.

Warfarin: Glucagon may increase the anticoagulant effect of warfarin.

Interactions between GlucaGen and other drugs are not known when GlucaGen is used in the approved indications.

4.6 Pregnancy and lactation

Glucagon does not cross the human placenta barrier. The use of glucagon has been reported in pregnant women with diabetes and no harmful effects are known with respect to the course of pregnancy and the health of the unborn and the neonate.

Glucagon is cleared from the bloodstream very fast (mainly by the liver) (T/2 = 3-6 min.), thus the amount excreted in the milk of nursing mothers following treatment of severe hypoglycaemic reactions will be extremely small. As glucagon is degraded in the digestive tract and cannot be absorbed in its intact form, it will not exert any metabolic effect in the child.

4.7 Effects on ability to drive and use machines

GlucaGen is not known to produce any effect on the ability to drive and to operate machines.

4.8 Undesirable effects

a)

Based on post marketing experience adverse drug reactions are very rare (<1/10,000) – the estimated number of treatment episodes is 14 million over an 11 year period).

b)

Skin and appendages disorders

Body as a whole – general disorders

Hypersensitivity reactions including generalised hypersensitivity reactions has been reported in isolated cases (<1/10,000).

Gastro-intestinal system disorders

Abdominal pain, nausea and vomiting may occur in very rare cases (<1/10,000) especially with dosages higher than 1 mg or with rapid injection (less than 1 minute).

Cardiovascular disorders, general

Hypotension has been reported up to 2 hours after administration in patients receiving GlucaGen as premedication for upper GI endoscopy procedures.

c)

Metabolic effects:

Secondary hypoglycaemia, sometimes severe may occur when the patients have responded to the treatment. it can be more pronounced in patients having fasted before a diagnostic procedure (see section 4.4. Precautions for use).

Cardiovascular effects: Glucagon exerts positive inotropic and chronotropic effects (tachycardia).

4.9 Overdose

Adverse effects of overdose have not been reported. See 4.8.

In case of suspected overdosing (i.e. above therapeutic dosages) the serum potassium may decrease and should be monitored and corrected, if needed.

5. PHARMACOLOGICAL PROPERTIES

5.1 Pharmacodynamic properties

Pharmacotherapeutic Group: H 04 AA 01.

Glucagon is a hyperglycaemic agent that mobilises hepatic glycogen which is released into the blood as glucose. Glucagon will not be effective in patients whose liver glycogen is depleted. For that reason, glucagon has little or no effect when the patient is fasting or is suffering from adrenal insufficiency, chronic hypoglycaemia or alcohol-induced hypoglycaemia.

Glucagon, unlike adrenaline, has no effect upon muscle phosphorylase and therefore cannot assist in the transference of carbohydrate from the much larger stores of glycogen that are present in the skeletal muscle.

Glucagon stimulates the release of catecholamines. In the presence of phaeo-chromocytoma, glucagon can cause the tumour to release large amounts of catecholamines which will cause an acute hypertensive reaction.

Glucagon inhibits the tone and motility of the smooth muscle in the gastrointestinal tract.

5.2 Pharmacokinetic properties

Metabolic clearance rate of glucagon in humans is approximately 10ml/kg/min. It is degraded enzymatically in the blood plasma and in the organs to which it is distributed. The liver and kidney are major sites of glucagon clearance, each organ contributing about 30% to the overall metabolic clearance rate.

Glucagon has a short half-life in the blood of about 3-6 minutes.

Onset of effect occurs within 1 min. after an intravenous injection. Duration of action is in the range of 5-20 min. depending upon dose and the organ under examination. The onset of effect occurs within 5-15 minutes after an intramuscular injection, with a duration of 10-40 min. depending upon dose and organ.

When used in treatment of severe hypoglycaemia, an effect on blood glucose is usually seen within 10 minutes.

5.3 Preclinical safety data

No relevant preclinical data exist that provide information useful to the prescriber.

6. PHARMACEUTICAL PARTICULARS

6.1 List of excipients

Lactose Monohydrate

Hydrochloric Acid (pH adjuster)

Sodium Hydroxide (pH adjuster)

Water for Injections

After reconstitution with the solvent provided (Sterilised Water for Injections), the solution contains glucagon 1mg/ml and lactose monohydrate 107mg/ml.

6.2 Incompatibilities

There are no known incompatibilities with GlucaGen.

6.3 Shelf life

3 years

The reconstituted GlucaGen should be used immediately after preparation.

6.4 Special precautions for storage

The sealed container should be protected from light and stored between 2°C and 8°C. Freezing should be avoided. Packs can be stored at room temperature (up to 25°C) for 18 months provided that the expiry date is not exceeded.

If in rare cases it shows any signs of fibril formation (viscous appearance) or insoluble matter it should be discarded.

6.5 Nature and contents of container

Container for GlucaGen:

Vial made of glass type 1, Ph.Eur., closed with a bromobutyl stopper and covered with an aluminium cap. The vials are provided with a tamper-evident plastic cap which must be removed before use.

Container for diluent:

Syringe made of glass type I, Ph.Eur. and closed with a bromobutyl plunger.

6.6 Instructions for use and handling

Reconstitution

Inject the Sterilised Water for Injections (1.1ml) into the vial containing the freeze-dried glucagon. Shake the vial gently until the glucagon is completely dissolved and the solution is clear. Withdraw the solution back into the syringe.

The reconstituted solution forms an injection of 1mg (1 IU) per ml to be administered subcutaneously, intramuscularly or intravenously.

Any unused product or waste material should be disposed of in accordance with local requirements.

7. MARKETING AUTHORISATION HOLDER

Novo Nordisk A/S

Novo Allē

DK-2880 Bagsvaerd

Denmark

8. MARKETING AUTHORISATION NUMBER(S)

PL 4668/0027 GlucaGen 1mg

PL 4668/0028 Diluent for GlucaGen. 1mg

9. DATE OF FIRST AUTHORISATION/RENEWAL OF THE AUTHORISATION

30 September 1991 / 15 October 2001

10. DATE OF REVISION OF THE TEXT

June 2002

Legal Category

POM.

Glucobay 50, Glucobay 100

(Bayer plc)

1. NAME OF THE MEDICINAL PRODUCT

Glucobay 50

Glucobay 100

2. QUALITATIVE AND QUANTITATIVE COMPOSITION

Acarbose 50mg tablets.

Acarbose 100mg tablets

3. PHARMACEUTICAL FORM

Tablet for oral administration.

4. CLINICAL PARTICULARS

4.1 Therapeutic indications

Indications

Glucobay is recommended for the treatment of non-insulin dependent (NIDDM) diabetes mellitus in patients inadequately controlled on diet alone, or on diet and oral hypoglycaemic agents.

Mode of action

Glucobay is a competitive inhibitor of intestinal alpha-glucosidases with maximum specific inhibitory activity against sucrase. Under the influence of Glucobay, the digestion of starch and sucrose into absorbable monosaccharides in the small intestine is dose-dependently delayed. In diabetic subjects, this results in a lowering of postprandial hyperglycaemia and a smoothing effect on fluctuations in the daily blood glucose profile.

In contrast to sulphonylureas Glucobay has no stimulatory action on the pancreas.

Treatment with Glucobay also results in a reduction of fasting blood glucose and to modest changes in levels of glycated haemoglobin (HbA_1, HbA_{1c}). The changes may be a reduction or reduced deterioration in HbA_1 or HbA_{1c} levels, depending upon the patient's clinical status and disease progression. These parameters are affected in a dose-dependent manner by Glucobay.

Following oral administration, only 1-2% of the active inhibitor is absorbed.

4.2 Posology and method of administration

Glucobay tablets are taken orally and should be chewed with the first mouthful of food, or swallowed whole with a little liquid directly before the meal. Owing to the great individual variation of glucosidase activity in the intestinal mucosa, there is no fixed dosage regimen, and patients should be treated according to clinical response and tolerance of intestinal side-effects.

Adults

The recommended initial dose is 50mg three times a day. However, some patients may benefit from more gradual initial dose titration to minimise gastrointestinal side-effects. This may be achieved by initiating treatment at 50mg once or twice a day, with subsequent titration to a three times a day regimen.

If after six to eight weeks' treatment patients show an inadequate clinical response, the dosage may be increased to 100mg three times a day. A further increase in dosage to a maximum of 200mg three times a day may occasionally be necessary.

Glucobay is intended for continuous long-term treatment.

Elderly patients

No modification of the normal adult dosage regimen is necessary.

4.3 Contraindications

Hypersensitivity to acarbose or any of the excipients, use in children less than 12 years of age, pregnancy and in nursing mothers. Glucobay is also contra-indicated in patients with inflammatory bowel disease, colonic ulceration, partial intestinal obstruction or in patients predisposed to intestinal obstruction. In addition, Glucobay should not be used in patients who have chronic intestinal diseases associated with marked disorders of digestion or absorption and in patients who suffer from states which may deteriorate as a result of increased gas formation in the intestine, e.g. larger hernias.

Glucobay is contra-indicated in patients with hepatic impairment.

As Glucobay has not been studied in patients with severe renal impairment, it should not be used in patients with a creatinine clearance < 25 ml/min/1.73m^2.

4.4 Special warnings and special precautions for use

Hypoglycaemia: When administered alone, Glucobay does not cause hypoglycaemia. It may, however, act to potentiate the hypoglycaemic effects of insulin and sulphonylurea drugs, and the dosages of these agents may need to be modified accordingly. In individual cases hypoglycaemic shock may occur (i.e. clinical sequelae of glucose levels < 1 mmol/L such as altered conscious levels, confusion or convulsions).

Episodes of hypoglycaemia occurring during therapy must, where appropriate, be treated by the administration of glucose, not sucrose. This is because acarbose will delay the digestion and absorption of disaccharides, but not monosaccharides.

Transaminases: Patients treated with acarbose may, on rare occasions, experience an idiosyncratic response with either symptomatic or asymptomatic hepatic dysfunction. In the majority of cases this dysfunction is reversible on discontinuation of acarbose therapy. It is recommended that liver enzyme monitoring is considered during the first six to twelve months of treatment. If elevated transaminases are observed, withdrawal of therapy may be warranted, particularly if the elevations persist. In such circumstances, patients should be monitored at weekly intervals until normal values are established.

4.5 Interaction with other medicinal products and other forms of Interaction

Intestinal adsorbents (e.g. charcoal) and digestive enzyme preparations containing carbohydrate splitting enzymes (e.g. amylase, pancreatin) may reduce the effect of Glucobay and should not therefore be taken concomitantly.

The concomitant administration of neomycin may lead to enhanced reductions of postprandial blood glucose and to an increase in the frequency and severity of gastro-intestinal side-effects. If the symptoms are severe, a temporary dose reduction of Glucobay may be warranted.

The concomitant administration of cholestyramine may enhance the effects of Glucobay, particularly with respect to reducing postprandial insulin levels. In the rare circumstance that both acarbose and cholestyramine therapy are withdrawn simultaneously, care is needed as a rebound phenomenon has been observed with respect to insulin levels in non-diabetic subjects.

In individual cases acarbose may affect digoxin bioavailability, which may require dose adjustment of digoxin. Monitoring of serum digoxin levels should be considered.

In a pilot study to investigate a possible interaction between Glucobay and nifedipine, no significant or reproducible changes were observed in the plasma nifedipine profiles.

4.6 Pregnancy and lactation

The use of Glucobay is contra-indicated in pregnancy and in nursing mothers.

The safety of this medicinal product for use in human pregnancy has not been established. An evaluation of experimental animal studies does not indicate direct or indirect harmful effects with respect to reproduction, development of the embryo or foetus, the course of gestation, and peri- and postnatal development.

4.7 Effects on ability to drive and use machines

None known.

4.8 Undesirable effects

Owing to its mode of action, Glucobay results in a greater proportion of dietary carbohydrate being digested in the large bowel. This carbohydrate may also be utilised by the intestinal flora, resulting in the increased formation of intestinal gas. The majority of patients are therefore likely to experience one or more symptoms related to this, particularly flatulence, borborygmi, and a feeling of fullness. Abdominal distension, abdominal pain, softer stools and diarrhoea may occur, particularly after sugar or sucrose-containing foods have been ingested. Uncommonly nausea may occur. Very rarely subileus/ileus may occur.

The symptoms are both dose and dietary substrate related, and may subside with continued treatment. Symptoms can be reduced by adherence to the prescribed diabetic diet and the avoidance of sucrose or foodstuffs containing sugar. If symptoms are poorly tolerated, a reduction in dosage is recommended.

Should diarrhoea persist, patients should be closely monitored and the dosage reduced, or therapy withdrawn, if necessary.

The administration of antacid preparations containing magnesium and aluminium salts, e.g. hydrotalcite, has been shown not to ameliorate the acute gastro-intestinal symptoms of Glucobay in higher dosage and should therefore not be recommended to patients for this purpose.

Rarely, a transient elevation of serum hepatic transaminases may be observed. Very rarely, jaundice and hepatitis have been reported. Individual cases of fulminant hepatitis with fatal outcome have been reported in Japan. The relationship to acarbose is unclear.

Skin reactions may occur rarely. Very rarely oedema has been reported.

4.9 Overdose

No information on overdosage is available. No specific antidotes to Glucobay are known.

Intake of carbohydrate-containing meals or beverages should be avoided for 4-6 hours.

Diarrhoea should be treated by standard conservative measures.

5. PHARMACOLOGICAL PROPERTIES

5.1 Pharmacodynamic properties

In all species tested, acarbose exerts its activity in the intestinal tract. The action of acarbose is based on the competitive inhibition of intestinal enzymes (α-glucosidases) involved in the degradation of disaccharides, oligosaccharides, and polysaccharides. This leads to a dose-dependent delay in the digestion of these carbohydrates. Glucose derived from these carbohydrates is released and taken up into the blood more slowly. In this way, acarbose reduces the postprandial rise in blood glucose, thus reducing blood glucose fluctuations.

5.2 Pharmacokinetic properties

Following administration, only 1-2% of the active inhibitor is absorbed.

The pharmacokinetics of Glucobay were investigated after oral administration of the ^{14}C-labelled substance (200mg) to healthy volunteers. On average, 35% of the total radioactivity (sum of the inhibitory substance and any degradation products) was excreted by the kidneys within 96 h. The proportion of inhibitory substance excreted in the urine was 1.7% of the administered dose. 50% of the activity was eliminated within 96 hours in the faeces. The course of the total radioactivity concentration in plasma was comprised of two peaks. The first peak, with an average acarbose-equivalent concentration of $52.2 \pm 15.7\mu g/l$ after 1.1 ± 0.3 h, is in agreement with corresponding data for the concentration course of the inhibitor substance ($49.5 \pm 26.9\mu g/l$ after 2.1 ± 1.6 h). The second peak is on average $586.3 \pm 282.7\mu g/l$ and is reached after 20.7 ± 5.2 h. The second, higher peak is due to the absorption of bacterial degradation products from distal parts of the intestine. In contrast to the total radioactivity, the maximum plasma concentrations of the inhibitory substance are lower by a factor of 10-20. The plasma elimination half-lives of the inhibitory substance are 3.7 ± 2.7 h for the distribution phase and 9.6 ± 4.4 h for the elimination phase.

A relative volume of distribution of 0.32 l/kg body-weight has been calculated in healthy volunteers from the concentration course in the plasma.

5.3 Preclinical safety data

Acute toxicity

LD_{50} studies were performed in mice, rats and dogs. Oral LD_{50} values were estimated to be $>$ 10g/kg body-weight. Intravenous LD_{50} values ranged from 3.8g/kg (dog) to 7.7g/kg (mouse).

Sub-chronic toxicity

Three month studies have been conducted in rats and dogs in which acarbose was administered orally by gavage.

In rats, daily doses of up to 450mg/kg body-weight were tolerated without drug-related toxicity.

In the dog study, daily doses of 50-450mg/kg were associated with decreases in body-weight. This occurred because dosing of the animals took place shortly before the feed was administered, resulting in the presence of acarbose in the gastro-intestinal tract at the time of feeding. The pharmacodynamic action of acarbose led to a reduced availability of carbohydrate from the feed, and hence to weight loss in the animals. A greater time interval between dosing and feeding in the rat study resulted in most of the drug being eliminated prior to feed intake, and hence no effect on body-weight development was observed.

Owing to a shift in the intestinal α-amylase synthesis feedback mechanism a reduction in serum α-amylase activity was also observed in the dog study. Increases in blood urea concentrations in acarbose-treated dogs also occurred, probably as a result of increased catabolic metabolism associated with the weight loss.

Chronic toxicity

In rats treated for one year with up to 4500ppm acarbose in their feed, no drug-related toxicity was observed. In dogs, also treated for one year with daily doses of up to 400mg/kg by gavage, a pronounced reduction in body-weight development was observed, as seen in the sub-chronic study. Again this effect was due to an excessive pharmacodynamic activity of acarbose and was reversed by increasing the quantity of feed.

Carcinogenicity studies

In a study in which Sprague-Dawley rats received up to 4500ppm acarbose in their feed for 24-26 months, malnutrition was observed in animals receiving the drug substance. A dose-dependent increase in tumours of the renal parenchyma (adenoma, hypernephroid carcinoma) was also observed against a background of a decrease in the overall tumour rate. When this study was repeated, an increase in benign tumours of testicular Leydig cells was also observed. Owing to the malnutrition and excessive decrease in bodyweight gain these studies were considered inadequate to assess the carcinogenic potential of acarbose.

In further studies with Sprague-Dawley rats in which the malnutrition and glucose deprivation were avoided by either dietary glucose supplementation or administration of acarbose by gavage, no drug-related increases in the incidences of renal or Leydig cell tumours were observed.

In an additional study using Wistar rats and doses of up to 4500ppm acarbose in the feed, neither drug-induced malnutrition nor changes in the tumour profile occurred. Tumour incidences were also unaffected in hamsters receiving up to 4000ppm acarbose in the feed for 80 weeks (with and without dietary glucose supplementation).

Reproductive toxicity

There was no evidence of a teratogenic effect of acarbose in studies with oral doses of up to 480mg/kg/day in rats and rabbits.

In rats no impairment of fertility was observed in males or females at doses of up to 540mg/kg/day. The oral administration of up to 540mg/kg/day to rats during foetal development and lactation had no effect on parturition or on the young.

Mutagenicity

The results of a number of mutagenicity studies show no evidence of a genotoxic potential of acarbose.

6. PHARMACEUTICAL PARTICULARS

6.1 List of excipients

Glucobay tablets contain the following excipients:

Microcrystalline cellulose

Highly dispersed silicon dioxide

Magnesium stearate

Maize starch

6.2 Incompatibilities

None stated.

6.3 Shelf life

36 months.

6.4 Special precautions for storage

The tablets should be stored in the manufacturer's original container in a dry place at temperatures below 25°C.

6.5 Nature and contents of container

Blister strips comprising 300μm polypropylene foil (colourless) with a 20μm soft aluminium backing foil, in cardboard outers.

Pack sizes:

10, 30, 90, 100, 500

21, 42, 84, 420

6.6 Instructions for use and handling

None stated.

7. MARKETING AUTHORISATION HOLDER

Bayer plc

Bayer House

Strawberry Hill

Newbury

Berkshire

RG14 1JA

Trading as Baypharm or Baymet.

8. MARKETING AUTHORISATION NUMBER(S)

PL 0010/0171

PL 0010/0172

9. DATE OF FIRST AUTHORISATION/RENEWAL OF THE AUTHORISATION

28 May 1993/17 February 1999

10. DATE OF REVISION OF THE TEXT

March 2004

Glucophage

(Merck Pharmaceuticals)

1. NAME OF THE MEDICINAL PRODUCT

Glucophage 500 mg film-coated tablet

Glucophage 850 mg film-coated tablet

2. QUALITATIVE AND QUANTITATIVE COMPOSITION

Each Glucophage 500mg film-coated tablet contains metformin hydrochloride 500mg corresponding to metformin base 390 mg.

Each Glucophage 850mg film-coated tablet contains metformin hydrochloride 850 mg corresponding to metformin base 662.9 mg.

For excipients, see 6.1.

3. PHARMACEUTICAL FORM

Film-coated tablet.

White, circular, convex film-coated tablet.

4. CLINICAL PARTICULARS

4.1 Therapeutic indications

Treatment of type 2 diabetes mellitus, particularly in overweight patients, when dietary management and exercise alone does not result in adequate glycaemic control.

• In adults, Glucophage film-coated tablets may be used as monotherapy or in combination with other oral anti-diabetic agents or with insulin.

• In children from 10 years of age and adolescents, Glucophage film-coated tablets may be used as monotherapy or in combination with insulin.

A reduction of diabetic complications has been shown in overweight type 2 diabetic adult patients treated with metformin as first-line therapy after diet failure (see 5.1. Pharmacodynamic properties).

4.2 Posology and method of administration

Adults:

Monotherapy and combination with other oral antidiabetic agents:

• The usual starting dose is one tablet 2 or 3 times daily given during or after meals.

• After 10 to 15 days the dose should be adjusted on the basis of blood glucose measurements. A slow increase of dose may improve gastrointestinal tolerability. The maximum recommended dose of metformin is 3 g daily.

• If transfer from another oral antidiabetic agent is intended: discontinue the other agent and initiate metformin at the dose indicated above.

Combination with insulin:

Metformin and insulin may be used in combination therapy to achieve better blood glucose control. Metformin is given at the usual starting dose of one tablet 2-3 times daily, while insulin dosage is adjusted on the basis of blood glucose measurements.

Elderly: due to the potential for decreased renal function in elderly subjects, the metformin dosage should be adjusted based on renal function. Regular assessment of renal function is necessary (see section 4.4).

Children and adolescents:

Monotherapy and combination with insulin

• Glucophage film-coated tablets can be used in children from 10 years of age and adolescents.

• The usual starting dose is one tablet of 500 mg or 850 mg once daily, given during meals or after meals.

• After 10 to 15 days the dose should be adjusted on the basis of blood glucose measurements. A slow increase of dose may improve gastrointestinal tolerability. The maximum recommended dose of metformin is 2 g daily, taken as 2 or 3 divided doses.

4.3 Contraindications

• Hypersensitivity to metformin hydrochloride or to any of the excipients.

• Diabetic ketoacidosis, diabetic pre-coma.

• Renal failure or renal dysfunction (creatinine clearance < 60 mL/min).

• Acute conditions with the potential to alter renal function such as:

- dehydration
- severe infection
- shock
- Intravascular administration of iodinated contrast agents (see 4.4 Warnings and special precautions for use).

• Acute or chronic disease which may cause tissue hypoxia such as:

- cardiac or respiratory failure
- recent myocardial infarction
- shock

• Hepatic insufficiency, acute alcohol intoxication, alcoholism

• Lactation

4.4 Special warnings and special precautions for use

Lactic acidosis.

Lactic acidosis is a rare, but serious (high mortality in the absence of prompt treatment), metabolic complication that can occur due to metformin accumulation. Reported cases of lactic acidosis in patients on metformin have occurred primarily in diabetic patients with significant renal failure. The incidence of lactic acidosis can and should be reduced by assessing also other associated risk factors such as poorly controlled diabetes, ketosis, prolonged fasting, excessive alcohol intake, hepatic insufficiency and any condition associated with hypoxia.

Diagnosis:

Lactic acidosis is characterised by acidotic dyspnea, abdominal pain and hypothermia followed by coma. Diagnostic laboratory findings are decreased blood pH, plasma lactate levels above 5 mmol/L, and an increased anion gap and lactate/pyruvate ratio. If metabolic acidosis is suspected, metformin should be discontinued and the patient should be hospitalised immediately (see section 4.9).

Renal function:

As metformin is excreted by the kidney, serum creatinine levels should be determined before initiating treatment and regularly thereafter:

* at least annually in patients with normal renal function,

* at least two to four times a year in patients with serum creatinine levels at the upper limit of normal and in elderly subjects.

Decreased renal function in elderly subjects is frequent and asymptomatic. Special caution should be exercised in situations where renal function may become impaired, for example when initiating antihypertensive therapy or diuretic therapy and when starting therapy with an NSAID.

Administration of iodinated contrast agent

As the intravascular administration of iodinated contrast materials in radiologic studies can lead to renal failure, metformin should be discontinued prior to, or at the time of the test and not reinstituted until 48 hours afterwards, and only after renal function has been re-evaluated and found to be normal.

Surgery

Metformin hydrochloride should be discontinued 48 hours before elective surgery with general anaesthesia and should not be usually resumed earlier than 48 hours afterwards.

Children and adolescents:

The diagnosis of type 2 diabetes mellitus should be confirmed before treatment with metformin is initiated.

No effect of metformin on growth and puberty has been detected during controlled clinical studies of one-year duration but no long-term data on these specific points are available. Therefore, a careful follow-up of the effect of metformin on these parameters in metformin-treated children, especially pre-pubescent children, is recommended.

Children aged between 10 and 12 years:

Only 15 subjects aged between 10 and 12 years were included in the controlled clinical studies conducted in children and adolescents. Although metformin efficacy and safety in children below 12 did not differ from efficacy and safety in older children, particular caution is recommended when prescribing to children aged between 10 and 12 years.

- Other precautions:

- All patients should continue their diet with a regular distribution of carbohydrate intake during the day. Overweight patients should continue their energy-restricted diet.

- The usual laboratory tests for diabetes monitoring should be performed regularly.

- Metformin alone never causes hypoglycaemia, although caution is advised when it is used in combination with insulin or sulphonylureas.

4.5 Interaction with other medicinal products and other forms of Interaction

Concomitant use not recommended

Alcohol

Increased risk of lactic acidosis in acute alcohol intoxication, particularly in case of:

- fasting or malnutrition
- hepatic insufficiency

Avoid consumption of alcohol and alcohol-containing medications.

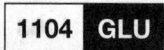

Iodinated contrast agents (see section 4.4)
Intravascular administration of iodinated contrast agents may lead to renal failure, resulting in metformin accumulation and a risk of lactic acidosis.

Metformin should be discontinued prior to, or at the time of the test and not reinstituted until 48 hours afterwards, and only after renal function has been re-evaluated and found to be normal.

Combinations requiring precautions for use
Glucocorticoids (systemic and local routes), beta-2-agonists, and diuretics have intrinsic hyperglycaemic activity. Inform the patient and perform more frequent blood glucose monitoring, especially at the beginning of treatment. If necessary, adjust the dosage of the antidiabetic drug during therapy with the other drug and upon its discontinuation.

ACE-inhibitors may decrease the blood glucose levels. If necessary, adjust the dosage of the antidiabetic drug during therapy with the other drug and upon its discontinuation.

4.6 Pregnancy and lactation
To date, no relevant epidemiological data are available. Animal studies do not indicate harmful effects with respect to pregnancy, embryonal or foetal development, parturition or postnatal development (see also section 5.3).

When the patient plans to become pregnant and during pregnancy, diabetes should not be treated with metformin but insulin should be used to maintain blood glucose levels as close to normal as possible in order to lower the risk of foetal malformations associated with abnormal blood glucose levels.

Metformin is excreted into milk in lactating rats. Similar data are not available in humans and a decision should be made whether to discontinue nursing or to discontinue metformin, taking into account the importance of the compound to the mother.

4.7 Effects on ability to drive and use machines
Glucophage monotherapy does not cause hypoglycaemia and therefore has no effect on the ability to drive or to use machines.

However, patients should be alerted to the risk of hypoglycaemia when metformin is used in combination with other antidiabetic agents (sulphonylureas, insulin, repaglinide).

4.8 Undesirable effects
The following undesirable effects may occur under treatment with metformin. Frequencies are defined as follows: very common: >1/10; common >1/100, <1/10; uncommon >1/1,000, <1/100; rare >1/10,000, <1/1,000; very rare <1/10,000 and isolated reports.

Metabolism and nutrition disorders:

Very rare: Decrease of vitamin B12 absorption with decrease of serum levels during long-term use of metformin. Consideration of such aetiology is recommended if a patient presents with megaloplastic anaemia.

Very rare: Lactic acidosis (see 4.4. Special warnings and precautions for use).

Nervous system disorders:

Common: Taste disturbance

Gastrointestinal disorders:

Very common: Gastrointestinal disorders such as nausea, vomiting, diarrhoea, abdominal pain and loss of appetite. These undesirable effects occur most frequently during initiation of therapy and resolve spontaneously in most cases. To prevent them, it is recommended that metformin be taken in 2 or 3 daily doses during or after meals. A slow increase of the dose may also improve gastrointestinal tolerability.

Hepatobiliary disorders:

Isolated reports: Liver function tests abnormalities or hepatitis resolving upon metformin discontinuation.

Skin and subcutaneous tissue disorders:

Very rare: Skin reactions such as erythema, pruritus, urticaria

In published and post marketing data and in controlled clinical studies in a limited paediatric population aged 10-16 years treated during 1 year, adverse event reporting was similar in nature and severity to that reported in adults.

4.9 Overdose
Hypoglycaemia has not been seen with metformin doses of up to 85g, although lactic acidosis has occurred in such circumstances. High overdose or concomitant risks of metformin may lead to lactic acidosis. Lactic acidosis is a medical emergency and must be treated in hospital. The most effective method to remove lactate and metformin is haemodialysis.

5. PHARMACOLOGICAL PROPERTIES
5.1 Pharmacodynamic properties
ORAL ANTI-DIABETICS

(A10BA02: Gastrointestinal tract and metabolism)

Metformin is a biguanide with antihyperglycaemic effects, lowering both basal and postprandial plasma glucose. It does not stimulate insulin secretion and therefore does not produce hypoglycaemia.

Metformin may act via 3 mechanisms:

(1) reduction of hepatic glucose production by inhibiting gluconeogenesis and glycogenolysis (2) in muscle, by increasing insulin sensitivity, improving peripheral glucose uptake and utilisation (3) and delay of intestinal glucose absorption.

Metformin stimulates intracellular glycogen synthesis by acting on glycogen synthase.

Metformin increases the transport capacity of all types of membrane glucose transporters (GLUT).

In humans, independently of its action on glycaemia, metformin has favourable effects on lipid metabolism. This has been shown at therapeutic doses in controlled, medium-term or long-term clinical studies: metformin reduces total cholesterol, LDL cholesterol and triglyceride levels.

Clinical efficacy:

The prospective randomised (UKPDS) study has established the long-term benefit of intensive blood glucose control in type 2 diabetes.

Analysis of the results for overweight patients treated with metformin after failure of diet alone showed:

- a significant reduction of the absolute risk of any diabetes-related complication in the metformin group (29.8 events/1000 patient-years) versus diet alone (43.3 events/1000 patient-years), p=0.0023, and versus the combined sulphonylurea and insulin monotherapy groups (40.1 events/1000 patient-years), p=0.0034.

- a significant reduction of the absolute risk of diabetes-related mortality: metformin 7.5 events/1000 patient-years, diet alone 12.7 events/1000 patient-years, p=0.017;

- a significant reduction of the absolute risk of overall mortality: metformin 13.5 events/1000 patient-years versus diet alone 20.6 events/1000 patient-years (p=0.011), and versus the combined sulphonylurea and insulin monotherapy groups 18.9 events/1000 patient-years (p=0.021);

- a significant reduction in the absolute risk of myocardial infarction: metformin 11 events/1000 patient-years, diet alone 18 events/1000 patient-years (p=0.01)

For metformin used as second-line therapy, in combination with a sulphonylurea, benefit regarding clinical outcome has not been shown.

In type 1 diabetes, the combination of metformin and insulin has been used in selected patients, but the clinical benefit of this combination has not been formally established.

Controlled clinical studies in a limited paediatric population aged 10-16 years treated during 1 year demonstrated a similar response in glycaemic control to that seen in adults.

5.2 Pharmacokinetic properties
Absorption:
After an oral dose of metformin, Tmax is reached in 2.5 hours. Absolute bioavailability of a 500mg or 850mg metformin tablet is approximately 50-60% in healthy subjects. After an oral dose, the non-absorbed fraction recovered in faeces was 20-30%.

After oral administration, metformin absorption is saturable and incomplete. It is assumed that the pharmacokinetics of metformin absorption are non-linear.

At the usual metformin doses and dosing schedules, steady state plasma concentrations are reached within 24 to 48 hours and are generally less than 1 μg/ml. In controlled clinical trials, maximum metformin plasma levels (Cmax) did not exceed 4 μg/ml, even at maximum doses.

Food decreases the extent and slightly delays the absorption of metformin. Following administration of a dose of 850 mg, a 40% lower plasma peak concentration, a 25% decrease in AUC (area under the curve) and a 35 minute prolongation of time to peak plasma concentration were observed. The clinical relevance of these decreases is unknown.

Distribution:

Plasma protein binding is negligible. Metformin partitions into erythrocytes. The blood peak is lower than the plasma peak and appears at approximately the same time. The red blood cells most likely represent a secondary compartment of distribution. The mean Vd ranged between 63-276 L.

Metabolism:

Metformin is excreted unchanged in the urine. No metabolites have been identified in humans.

Elimination:

Renal clearance of metformin is > 400 ml/min, indicating that metformin is eliminated by glomerular filtration and tubular secretion. Following an oral dose, the apparent terminal elimination half-life is approximately 6.5 hours.

When renal function is impaired, renal clearance is decreased in proportion to that of creatinine and thus the elimination half-life is prolonged, leading to increased levels of metformin in plasma.

Paediatrics:

Single dose study: After single doses of metformin 500 mg, paediatric patients have shown similar pharmacokinetic profile to that observed in healthy adults.

Multiple dose study: Data are restricted to one study. After repeated doses of 500 mg BID for 7 days in paediatric patients the peak plasma concentration (Cmax) and systemic exposure (AUC0-t) were reduced by approximately 33% and 40%, respectively compared to diabetic adults who received repeated doses of 500 mg BID for 14 days. As the dose is individually titratedbased on glycaemic control, this is of limited clinical relevance.

5.3 Preclinical safety data
Preclinical data reveal no special hazard for humans based on conventional studies on safety pharmacology, repeated dose toxicity, genotoxicity, carcinogenic potential, toxicity reproduction.

6. PHARMACEUTICAL PARTICULARS
6.1 List of excipients
Tablet core:

Povidone K 30

magnesium stearate

Film-coat:

Hypromellose

6.2 Incompatibilities
Not applicable

6.3 Shelf life
5 years

6.4 Special precautions for storage
No special precautions for storage.

6.5 Nature and contents of container
500 mg tablets

84 tablets in blister packs (PVC-aluminium)

850 mg tablets:

56 tablets in blister packs (PVC-aluminium)

6.6 Instructions for use and handling
No special requirements.

7. MARKETING AUTHORISATION HOLDER
Lipha Pharmaceuticals Limited
Harrier House
High Street
West Drayton
Middlesex
UB7 7QG

8. MARKETING AUTHORISATION NUMBER(S)
PL 03759/0012-0013

9. DATE OF FIRST AUTHORISATION/RENEWAL OF THE AUTHORISATION
01/10/2002

10. DATE OF REVISION OF THE TEXT
18/10/2004

Glucophage SR 500 mg Prolonged release tablets

(Merck Pharmaceuticals)

1. NAME OF THE MEDICINAL PRODUCT
Glucophage SR 500mg prolonged release tablet

2. QUALITATIVE AND QUANTITATIVE COMPOSITION
One prolonged release tablet contains 500mg metformin hydrochloride corresponding to 390mg metformin base.

For excipients, see section 6.1.

3. PHARMACEUTICAL FORM
Prolonged release tablet

White to off-white, capsule-shaped, biconvex tablet, debossed on one side with '500'.

4. CLINICAL PARTICULARS
4.1 Therapeutic indications
Treatment of type 2 diabetes mellitus in adults, particularly in overweight patients, when dietary management and exercise alone does not result in adequate glycaemic control. Glucophage SR may be used as monotherapy or in combination with other oral antidiabetic agents, or with insulin.

4.2 Posology and method of administration
Monotherapy and combination with other oral antidiabetic agents:

- The usual starting dose is one tablet once daily.
- After 10 to 15 days the dose should be adjusted on the basis of blood glucose measurements. A slow increase of dose may improve gastro-intestinal tolerability. The maximum recommended dose is 4 tablets daily.
- Dosage increases should be made in increments of 500mg every 10-15 days, up to a maximum of 2000mg once daily with the evening meal. If glycaemic control is not achieved on Glucophage SR 2000mg once daily, Glucophage SR 1000mg twice daily should be considered, with both doses being given with food. If glycaemic control is still not achieved, patients may be switched to standard metformin tablets to a maximum dose of 3000 mg daily.
- In patients already treated with metformin tablets, the starting dose of Glucophage SR should be equivalent to

the daily dose of metformin immediate release tablets. In patients treated with metformin at a dose above 2000 mg daily, switching to Glucophage SR is not recommended.

• If transfer from another oral antidiabetic agent is intended: discontinue the other agent and initiate Glucophage SR at the dose indicated above.

Combination with insulin:

Metformin and insulin may be used in combination therapy to achieve better blood glucose control. The usual starting dose of Glucophage SR is one tablet once daily, while insulin dosage is adjusted on the basis of blood glucose measurements.

Elderly: due to the potential for decreased renal function in elderly subjects, the metformin dosage should be adjusted based on renal function. Regular assessment of renal function is necessary (see section 4.4).

Children: In the absence of available data, Glucophage SR should not be used in children.

4.3 Contraindications

• Hypersensitivity to metformin hydrochloride or to any of the excipients.

• Diabetic ketoacidosis, diabetic pre-coma.

• Renal failure or renal dysfunction (e.g., serum creatinine levels > 135 μmol/L in males and > 110 μmol/L in females).

• Acute conditions with the potential to alter renal function such as:

- Dehydration,
- severe infection,
- shock,
- intravascular administration of iodinated contrast agents (see 4.4 Special warnings and precautions for use).

• Acute or chronic disease which may cause tissue hypoxia such as:

- cardiac or respiratory failure,
- recent myocardial infarction,
- shock

• Hepatic insufficiency, acute alcohol intoxication, alcoholism

• Lactation (see section 4.6).

4.4 Special warnings and special precautions for use

Lactic acidosis:

Lactic acidosis is a rare, but serious (high mortality in the absence of prompt treatment), metabolic complication that can occur due to metformin accumulation. Reported cases of lactic acidosis in patients on metformin have occurred primarily in diabetic patients with significant renal failure. The incidence of lactic acidosis can and should be reduced by assessing also other associated risk factors such as poorly controlled diabetes, ketosis, prolonged fasting, excessive alcohol intake, hepatic insufficiency and any condition associated with hypoxia.

Diagnosis:

Lactic acidosis is characterised by acidotic dyspnea, abdominal pain and hypothermia followed by coma. Diagnostic laboratory findings are decreased blood pH, plasma lactate levels above 5 mmol/L, and an increased anion gap and lactate/pyruvate ratio. If metabolic acidosis is suspected, metformin should be discontinued and the patient should be hospitalised immediately (see section 4.9).

Renal function:

As metformin is excreted by the kidney, serum creatinine levels should be determined before initiating treatment and regularly thereafter:

• at least annually in patients with normal renal function,

• at least two to four times a year in patients with serum creatinine levels at the upper limit of normal and in elderly subjects.

Decreased renal function in elderly subjects is frequent and asymptomatic. Special caution should be exercised in situations where renal function may become impaired, for example when initiating antihypertensive therapy or diuretic therapy and when starting therapy with an NSAID.

Administration of iodinated contrast agent:

As the intravascular administration of iodinated contrast materials in radiologic studies can lead to renal failure, metformin should be discontinued prior to, or at the time of the test and not reinstituted until 48 hours afterwards, and only after renal function has been re-evaluated and found to be normal.

Surgery:

Metformin hydrochloride should be discontinued 48 hours before elective surgery with general anaesthesia and should not be usually resumed earlier than 48 hours afterwards.

Other precautions:

• All patients should continue their diet with a regular distribution of carbohydrate intake during the day. Overweight patients should continue their energy-restricted diet.

• The usual laboratory tests for diabetes monitoring should be performed regularly.

• Metformin alone never causes hypoglycaemia, although caution is advised when it is used in combination with insulin or sulphonylureas.

• The tablet shells may be present in the faeces. Patients should be advised that this is normal.

4.5 Interaction with other medicinal products and other forms of Interaction

Inadvisable combinations

Alcohol

Increased risk of lactic acidosis in acute alcohol intoxication, particularly in case of:

• fasting or malnutrition,

• hepatic insufficiency.

Avoid consumption of alcohol and alcohol-containing medications.

Iodinated contrast agents

Intravascular administration of iodinated contrast agents may lead to renal failure, resulting in metformin accumulation and a risk of lactic acidosis.

Metformin should be discontinued prior to, or at the time of the test and not reinstituted until 48 hours afterwards, and only after renal function has been re-evaluated and found to be normal

(see 4.4 special warnings and precautions for use).

Associations requiring precautions for use

Glucocorticoids (systemic and local routes), beta-2-agonists, and diuretics have intrinsic hyperglycaemic activity. Inform the patient and perform more frequent blood glucose monitoring, especially at the beginning of treatment. If necessary, adjust the dosage of the antidiabetic drug during therapy with the other drug and upon its discontinuation.

ACE-inhibitors may decrease the blood glucose levels. If necessary, adjust the dosage of the antidiabetic drug during therapy with the other drug and upon its discontinuation.

4.6 Pregnancy and lactation

Pregnancy

To date, no relevant epidemiological data are available. Animal studies do not indicate harmful effects with respect to pregnancy, embryonal or fœtal development, parturition or postnatal development (see also section 5.3)

When the patient plans to become pregnant and during pregnancy, diabetes should not be treated with metformin but insulin should be used to maintain blood glucose levels as close to normal as possible in order to lower the risk of foetal malformations associated with abnormal blood glucose levels.

Lactation

Metformin is excreted into milk in lactating rats. Similar data is not available in humans and a decision should be made whether to discontinue nursing or to discontinue metformin, taking into account the importance of the compound to the mother.

4.7 Effects on ability to drive and use machines

Glucophage SR monotherapy does not cause hypoglycaemia and therefore has no effect on the ability to drive or to use machines.

However, patients should be alerted to the risk of hypoglycaemia when metformin is used in combination with other antidiabetic agents (sulphonylureas, insulin, repaglinide).

4.8 Undesirable effects

In post marketing data and in controlled clinical studies, adverse event reporting in patients treated with Glucophage SR was similar in nature and severity to that reported in patients treated with Glucophage immediate release.

The following undesirable effects may occur with Glucophage SR.

Frequencies are defined as follows: very common: >1/10; common $\geq$1/100, <1/10; uncommon $\geq$1/1,000, <1/100; rare $\geq$1/10,000, <1/1,000; very rare <1/10,000 and isolated reports.

Metabolism and nutrition disorders

very rare: Decrease of vitamin B12 absorption with decrease of serum levels during long-term use of metformin. This change is generally without clinical significance.

Lactic acidosis (see 4.4. Special warnings and precautions for use).

Nervous system disorders

Common: Metallic taste

Gastrointestinal disorders

very common: Gastrointestinal disorders such as nausea, vomiting, diarrhoea, abdominal pain and loss of appetite. These undesirable effects occur most frequently during initiation of therapy and resolve spontaneously in most cases. A slow increase of the dose may also improve gastrointestinal tolerability.

Skin and subcutaneous tissue disorders

very rare: Mild erythema in some hypersensitive individuals

4.9 Overdose

Hypoglycaemia has not been seen with metformin doses of up to 85 g, although lactic acidosis has occurred in such circumstances. High overdose or concomitant risks of metformin may lead to lactic acidosis. Lactic acidosis is a medical emergency and must be treated in hospital. The most effective method to remove lactate and metformin is haemodialysis.

5. PHARMACOLOGICAL PROPERTIES

5.1 Pharmacodynamic properties

ORAL ANTI-DIABETICS

(A10BA02: Gastrointestinal tract and metabolism)

Metformin is a biguanide with antihyperglycaemic effects, lowering both basal and postprandial plasma glucose. It does not stimulate insulin secretion and therefore does not produce hypoglycaemia.

Metformin may act via 3 mechanisms:

(1) reduction of hepatic glucose production by inhibiting gluconeogenesis and glycogenolysis

(2) in muscle, by increasing insulin sensitivity, improving peripheral glucose uptake and utilisation

(3) and delay of intestinal glucose absorption.

Metformin stimulates intracellular glycogen synthesis by acting on glycogen synthase.

Metformin increases the transport capacity of all types of membrane glucose transporters (GLUT).

In humans, independently of its action on glycaemia, immediate release metformin has favourable effects on lipid metabolism. This has been shown at therapeutic doses in controlled, medium-term or long-term clinical studies: immediate release metformin reduces total cholesterol, LDL cholesterol and triglyceride levels. A similar action has not been demonstrated with the prolonged release formulation, possibly due to the evening administration, and an increase in triglycerides may occur.

Clinical efficacy:

The prospective randomised (UKPDS) study has established the long-term benefit of intensive blood glucose control in overweight type 2 diabetic patients treated with immediate release metformin as first-line therapy after diet failure. Analysis of the results for overweight patients treated with metformin after failure of diet alone showed:

• a significant reduction of the absolute risk of any diabetes-related complication in the metformin group (29.8 events/ 1000 patient-years) versus diet alone (43.3 events/ 1000 patient-years), p=0.0023, and versus the combined sulphonylurea and insulin monotherapy groups (40.1 events/ 1000 patient-years), p=0.0034.

• a significant reduction of the absolute risk of diabetes-related mortality: metformin 7.5 events/1000 patient-years, diet alone 12.7 events/ 1000 patient-years, p=0.017;

• a significant reduction of the absolute risk of overall mortality: metformin 13.5 events/ 1000 patient-years versus diet alone 20.6 events/ 1000 patient-years (p=0.011), and versus the combined sulphonylurea and insulin monotherapy groups 18.9 events/ 1000 patient-years (p=0.021);

• a significant reduction in the absolute risk of myocardial infarction: metformin 11 events/ 1000 patient-years, diet alone 18 events/ 1000 patient-years (p=0.01)

For metformin used as second-line therapy, in combination with a sulphonylurea, benefit regarding clinical outcome has not been shown.

In type 1 diabetes, the combination of metformin and insulin has been used in selected patients, but the clinical benefit of this combination has not been formally established.

5.2 Pharmacokinetic properties

Absorption

After an oral dose of the prolonged release tablet, metformin absorption is significantly delayed compared to the immediate release tablet with a Tmax at 7 hours (Tmax for the immediate release tablet is 2.5 hours).

At steady state, similar to the immediate release formulation, Cmax and AUC are not proportionally increased to the administered dose. The AUC after a single oral administration of 2000mg of metformin prolonged release tablets is similar to that observed after administration of 1000mg of metformin immediate release tablets b.i.d.

Intrasubject variability of Cmax and AUC of metformin prolonged release is comparable to that observed with metformin immediate release tablets.

When the prolonged release tablet is administered in fasting conditions the AUC is decreased by 30% (both Cmax and Tmax are unaffected).

Metformin absorption from the prolonged release formulation is not altered by meal composition.

No accumulation is observed after repeated administration of up to 2000mg of metformin as prolonged release tablets.

Distribution

Plasma protein binding is negligible. Metformin partitions into erythrocytes. The blood peak is lower than the plasma peak and appears at approximately the same time. The red blood cells most likely represent a secondary compartment of distribution. The mean Vd ranged between 63-276 L.

Metabolism

Metformin is excreted unchanged in the urine. No metabolites have been identified in humans.

Elimination

Renal clearance of metformin is > 400 ml/min, indicating that metformin is eliminated by glomerular filtration and tubular secretion. Following an oral dose, the apparent terminal elimination half-life is approximately 6.5 hours.

When renal function is impaired, renal clearance is decreased in proportion to that of creatinine and thus the elimination half-life is prolonged, leading to increased levels of metformin in plasma.

5.3 Preclinical safety data

Preclinical data reveal no special hazard for humans based on conventional studies on safety pharmacology, repeated dose toxicity, genotoxicity, carcinogenic potential, toxicity reproduction.

6. PHARMACEUTICAL PARTICULARS

6.1 List of excipients

Magnesium stearate, sodium carboxymethylcellulose, hypromellose, microcrystalline cellulose.

6.2 Incompatibilities

None

6.3 Shelf life

36 months

6.4 Special precautions for storage

No special precautions for storage

6.5 Nature and contents of container

28 or 56 tablets in blister strips composed of PVC/PVDC 90g or PVC-Aclar aluminium.

6.6 Instructions for use and handling

Not applicable

7. MARKETING AUTHORISATION HOLDER

Merck Ltd

t/a Merck Pharmaceuticals (A division of Merck Ltd.)

Harrier House

High Street

West Drayton

Middlesex

UB7 7QG

United Kingdom

8. MARKETING AUTHORISATION NUMBER(S)

PL 11648/0054

9. DATE OF FIRST AUTHORISATION/RENEWAL OF THE AUTHORISATION

26th November 2004

10. DATE OF REVISION OF THE TEXT

Legal Category

POM

Glucose Injection BP Minijet

(International Medication Systems (UK) Ltd)

1. NAME OF THE MEDICINAL PRODUCT

Glucose Injection BP Minijet 50%w/v

2. QUALITATIVE AND QUANTITATIVE COMPOSITION

Glucose anhydrous Ph. Eur. 500 mg in 1ml.

3. PHARMACEUTICAL FORM

Sterile solution for injection. The clear, colourless solution is contained in a USP Type I glass vial with an elastomeric closure. The container is specially designed for use with the IMS Minijet injector supplied.

4. CLINICAL PARTICULARS

4.1 Therapeutic indications

a) As a source of energy in parenteral nutrition.

b) In severe hypoglycaemia due to insulin excess or other causes.

c) For reduction of cerebrospinal pressure and/or cerebral oedema due to *delirium tremens* or acute alcohol intoxication.

Glucose injection 50% w/v is strongly hypertonic and is used partly because of its dehydrating effects.

4.2 Posology and method of administration

Hypertonic solutions of glucose should be administered via a central vein. The dose is variable and depends upon the indication, clinical condition and size of the individual.

The rate of utilisation of glucose varies considerably from patient to patient. In general, the maximal rate has been estimated at 500-800mg/kg body weight/hour. If the patient's capacity to utilise glucose is exceeded, glycosuria and diuresis will occur.

Adults, elderly, children over 6 years:

Hypoglycaemia:

20-50ml of a 50% w/v solution, repeated as necessary according to the patient's response, by slow intravenous injection, e.g. 3ml/minute. After 25g of glucose has been given, it is advisable to interrupt the injection and evaluate the effect. The exact dose required to relieve hypoglycaemia will vary. After the patient responds, supplemental oral feeding is indicated to avoid relapse, especially after insulin shock therapy.

Acute alcoholism:

50ml of glucose 50% w/v solution should be administered intravenously. Unmodified insulin (20 units) and thiamine hydrochloride (100mg) should be added to the infusion.

4.3 Contraindications

The intravenous use of strongly hypertonic solutions of glucose is contraindicated in patients with anuria, intracranial or intraspinal haemorrhage, or delirium tremens *if the patient is already dehydrated*.

Known sensitivity to corn or corn products, hyperglycaemic coma, or ischaemic stroke.

4.4 Special warnings and special precautions for use

Hypertonic solutions of glucose should be administered via a large central vein to minimise the damage at the site of injection.

Use with caution in patients with diabetes mellitus, severe undernutrition, carbohydrate intolerance, thiamine deficiency, hypophosphataemia, haemodilution, sepsis and trauma. Rapid infusion of hypertonic glucose solution may lead to hyperglycaemia. Patients should be observed for signs of mental confusion or loss of consciousness.

Prolonged use in parenteral nutrition may affect insulin production; blood and urine glucose should be monitored. Fluid and acid-base balance and electrolyte status should also be determined during therapy with dextrose.

4.5 Interaction with other medicinal products and other forms of Interaction

None known.

4.6 Pregnancy and lactation

Intravenous glucose may result in considerable foetal insulin production, with an associated risk of rebound hypoglycaemia in the new-born. Infusion should not exceed 5-10g/hour during labour or Caesarean section.

4.7 Effects on ability to drive and use machines

This preparation is intended for use only in emergencies.

4.8 Undesirable effects

Anaphylactoid reactions have been reported in patients with asthma and diabetes mellitus.

Local pain, inflammation, irritation, thrombophlebitis and fever may occur.

Hypokalaemia, hypomagnesaemia or hypophosphataemia may result from the use of hypertonic solutions via the intravenous route.

Prolonged or rapid administration of hyperosmotic >5%) solutions may lead to dehydration.

The administration of glucose without adequate levels of thiamine (which form the coenzyme systems in its metabolism), may precipitate overt deficiency states, e.g. Wernicke's encephalopathy.

Excess glucose infusion produces increased CO_2, which may be important in respiratory failure, and stimulates catecholamine secretion.

4.9 Overdose

The patient becomes hyperglycaemic and glycosuria may occur. This can lead to dehydration, hyperosmolar coma and death.

Treatment: The infusion should be discontinued and the patient evaluated. Insulin may be administered and appropriate supportive measures taken.

5. PHARMACOLOGICAL PROPERTIES

5.1 Pharmacodynamic properties

Glucose, the natural sugar occurring in the blood, is the principle source of energy for the body. It is readily converted to fat and is also stored in the liver and muscles as glycogen. When a rapid rise in blood sugar is demanded by the body, glycogen is quickly liberated as d-glucose. When the supply of glucose is insufficient, the body mobilises fat stores which are converted to acetate with production of energy by the same oxidative pathways employed in the combustion of glucose.

It may decrease body protein and nitrogen losses. Glucose is also the probable source of glucuronic acid with which many foreign substances and their metabolites combine to form excretion products. It probably provides the basic substances required for the formation of hyalluronates and chondroitin sulphates, the supporting structures of the organism. It can be converted to a pentose essential for the formation of nucleic acids by the cells.

5.2 Pharmacokinetic properties

Glucose is metabolised to carbon dioxide and water with the release of energy.

5.3 Preclinical safety data

Not applicable since glucose has been used in clinical practice for many years and its effects in man are well known.

6. PHARMACEUTICAL PARTICULARS

6.1 List of excipients

Water for Injection Ph. Eur./USP

6.2 Incompatibilities

Glucose solutions which do not contain electrolytes should not be administered concomitantly with blood through the same infusion set as haemolysis and clumping may occur.

6.3 Shelf life

3 years.

6.4 Special precautions for storage

Store below 25°C.

6.5 Nature and contents of container

The solution is contained in a USP type I glass vial with an elastomeric closure which meets all the relevant USP specifications. The product is available as 10ml and 50ml.

6.6 Instructions for use and handling

The container is specially designed for use with the IMS Minijet injector. Do not use the injection if crystals have separated.

Administrative Data

7. MARKETING AUTHORISATION HOLDER

International Medication Systems (UK) Ltd

208 Bath Road

Slough

Berkshire

SL1 3WE

UK

8. MARKETING AUTHORISATION NUMBER(S)

PL 03265/0008R

9. DATE OF FIRST AUTHORISATION/RENEWAL OF THE AUTHORISATION

Date first granted: 28 February 1991

Date renewed: 28 February 1996

10. DATE OF REVISION OF THE TEXT

April 2001

POM

Glurenorm

(sanofi-aventis)

1. NAME OF THE MEDICINAL PRODUCT

Glurenorm 30mg Tablets.

2. QUALITATIVE AND QUANTITATIVE COMPOSITION

Gliquidone HSE 30mg.

For excipients, see 6.1.

3. PHARMACEUTICAL FORM

Tablet.

Tablets are white with a 'G' on one side.

4. CLINICAL PARTICULARS

4.1 Therapeutic indications

Glurenorm tablets are indicated for the treatment of non-insulin dependent diabetics who do not respond adequately to dietary control.

4.2 Posology and method of administration

Glurenorm tablets are for oral administration.

Glurenorm should be taken up to half an hour before a meal. The dose and frequency of administration should be adjusted, together with the diet, to obtain the best possible control of the diabetes throughout the day.

Adults (including the elderly)

Most patients respond to a total daily dose of 45-60mg given in two or three divided doses, of which the largest dose is usually taken in the morning with breakfast. The recommended maximum single dose is 60mg (2 tablets) and the maximum daily dose 180mg (6 tablets). During stabilisation, dosage adjustment should be based on frequent blood (random and postprandial) and urinary glucose determination.

Stabilisation of previously untreated cases:

Normally treatment should begin with 15mg (half a tablet) before breakfast and this should be gradually increased by 15mg increments prior to mealtimes.

Change-over in patients previously treated with other oral antidiabetic agents: Patients can be changed over from other sulphonylureas to Glurenorm without interruption. It is usual to start with 30mg Glurenorm before breakfast, increasing as necessary by increments of 15mg at mealtimes. In terms of comparative potency of single doses, 30mg Glurenorm corresponds approximately to 1000mg tolbutamide, 5mg glibenclamide, 250mg chlorpropamide or 500mg acetohexamide.

However, in estimating equivalent total daily doses, the half-lives and duration of action of the respective sulphonylureas must be taken into consideration. Thus it will usually be necessary to administer Glurenorm more frequently than a long-acting sulphonylurea.

Change-over in non-insulin dependent diabetics previously treated with insulin:

In patients treated with up to 30 IU of insulin daily, change-over to Glurenorm may be attempted with an initial dose of 30mg accompanied by a simultaneous gradual reduction of the amount of insulin, provided the pancreas still contains some functioning beta cells. Patients who change from insulin to Glurenorm should be strictly supervised and response assessed by frequent and regular blood glucose determinations.

It may be possible to reduce the insulin requirements of patients who require more than 30 IU daily by the concurrent administration of Glurenorm. Blood glucose should be monitored frequently during the change-over period.

Combined treatment:

The administration of metformin with Glurenorm to patients who cannot be adequately controlled by Glurenorm alone may achieve satisfactory stabilisation of blood glucose levels.

Children:

Dosage recommendation is not appropriate.

4.3 Contraindications

Do not use for diabetes complicated by acidosis or ketosis nor in patients subject to the stress of surgery or acute infections. Glurenorm should not be used in pregnancy or during breast feeding, nor in patients with severe hepatic or renal failure, or porphyria.

4.4 Special warnings and special precautions for use

Patients who miss a meal (particularly the elderly or debilitated) should be warned not to take their dose of Glurenorm, in order to reduce the risk of a hypoglycaemic reaction.

Special care should be observed in the concomitant use of Glurenorm with many other medications because interactions with sulphonylureas are common.

The effect of Glurenorm may be increased by physical exertion.

4.5 Interaction with other medicinal products and other forms of Interaction

The effects of Glurenorm may be increased by physical exertion, alcohol, salicylates, sulphonamides, phenylbutazone, ethionamide, coumarin, anti-coagulants, chloramphenicol, tetracyclines, cyclophosphamide, MAO inhibitors, tuberculostatics and beta-adrenergic blocking agents, azapropazone, co-trimoxazole, miconazole, fluconazole and sulphinpyrazone.

It may be necessary to increase the dose of Glurenorm when any of the following are administered concurrently: oral contraceptives, chlorpromazine, sympathomimetic agents, corticosteroids, thyroid hormones and nicotinic acid preparations, rifampicin, diazoxide and loop or thiazide diuretics.

The effects of barbiturates, vasopressin and oral anti-coagulants are potentiated by the administration of Glurenorm.

4.6 Pregnancy and lactation

Glurenorm should not be used in pregnancy or during breast feeding.

4.7 Effects on ability to drive and use machines

Not known.

4.8 Undesirable effects

Glurenorm is generally well tolerated, but minor skin allergies, gastric upsets and other non-specific symptoms have been noted. Reversible leucopenia has been reported on one occasion and reversible thrombocytopenia twice, but a causal connection with Glurenorm was not established.

Hypoglycaemic reactions are infrequent, but may be accompanied by malaise, impaired concentration and altered consciousness. They may be treated with oral carbohydrate, or with intravenous dextrose if the oral route is impractical. Glucagon (1mg subcutaneously) could also be given.

4.9 Overdose

In the conscious patient, hypoglycaemia may be managed by the oral administration of glucose. In the comatose patient, parenteral administration of glucose by intravenous infusion should be instituted. The patients should be kept under observation for further signs of hypoglycaemia. Consideration may be given to the recovery of ingested tablets by gastric lavage.

5. PHARMACOLOGICAL PROPERTIES

5.1 Pharmacodynamic properties

Pharmacotherapeutic group: Sulfonamides, Urea Derivatives Other Oral Hypoglycaemic Agents: ATC code: A10B B08

Glurenorm is a sulphonylurea compound which causes an increase in plasma insulin levels in normal subjects, and in non-insulin dependant diabetic patients there is a corresponding decrease in plasma glucose levels. The onset of activity is normally within one hour of oral dosing, and the optimum effect normally lasts 2-3 hours.

5.2 Pharmacokinetic properties

Glurenorm is rapidly absorbed, and quickly attains therapeutic blood levels. Plasma half-life is approximately 1.4 hours. It is almost completely metabolised in the liver by hydroxylation and demethylation. Only 5% of the pharmacologically inactive metabolites are excreted by the kidneys, the remainder are eliminated in the faeces via the bile. There is thus little risk of hypoglycaemia due to drug accumulation in patients with impaired renal function.

5.3 Preclinical safety data

There are no pre-clinical safety data of relevance to the prescriber which are additional to that already included in other sections of the SPC.

6. PHARMACEUTICAL PARTICULARS

6.1 List of excipients

Lactose, maize starch, soluble starch, magnesium stearate.

6.2 Incompatibilities

Not applicable.

6.3 Shelf life

60 months.

6.4 Special precautions for storage

None.

6.5 Nature and contents of container

Amber glass bottles with wadless polypropylene screw caps. Pack size of 100 tablets.

6.6 Instructions for use and handling

No Special requirements.

7. MARKETING AUTHORISATION HOLDER

Sanofi-Synthelabo Limited (*trading as Sanofi Winthrop*)

One Onslow Street

Guildford

Surrey GU1 4YS

or trading as:

Sanofi-Synthelabo

PO Box 597

Guildford

Surrey

8. MARKETING AUTHORISATION NUMBER(S)

PL 11723/0037

9. DATE OF FIRST AUTHORISATION/RENEWAL OF THE AUTHORISATION

5 February 2003

10. DATE OF REVISION OF THE TEXT

February 2004

Legal Category: POM

Glutarol

(Dermal Laboratories Limited)

1. NAME OF THE MEDICINAL PRODUCT

GLUTAROL®

2. QUALITATIVE AND QUANTITATIVE COMPOSITION

Glutaraldehyde 10.0% w/v.

3. PHARMACEUTICAL FORM

Colourless, evaporative wart paint.

4. CLINICAL PARTICULARS

4.1 Therapeutic indications

For the topical treatment of warts, especially plantar warts.

4.2 Posology and method of administration

For adults, children and the elderly:

1. Gently rub the surface of the wart with a piece of pumice stone or manicure emery board, or pare down any hard skin.

2. Using the applicator provided, carefully apply a few drops of the paint to the wart, taking care to localise the application to the affected area. Allow each drop to dry before the next is applied.

3. Repeat twice daily.

4. On subsequent days, repeat steps 1 to 3.

It is not necessary to cover the treated wart(s) with an adhesive plaster.

4.3 Contraindications

Not to be used in cases of sensitivity to any of the ingredients. Not to be used on the face, anal or perineal region. Not to be used on moles or on any other skin lesion for which it is not indicated.

4.4 Special warnings and special precautions for use

Keep away from the eyes and mucous membranes. Avoid spreading onto surrounding uninvolved skin. Avoid spillage. Avoid inhaling vapour. Replace cap tightly after use. For external use only.

4.5 Interaction with other medicinal products and other forms of Interaction

None known.

4.6 Pregnancy and lactation

No special precautions.

4.7 Effects on ability to drive and use machines

None known.

4.8 Undesirable effects

Undesirable effects occur very occasionally and mostly involve mild local skin rashes and irritation. Very rarely, a severe reaction may occur particularly on the hands or when the product is used excessively and allowed to spread onto surrounding normal skin. If mild irritation should occur, apply a reduced amount (taking special care to avoid spreading beyond the wart or verruca) and apply less often. If the irritation is severe, patients should stop treatment immediately and seek medical advice.

4.9 Overdose

Accidental oral ingestion should be treated immediately by gastric lavage with 2 to 5% aqueous sodium bicarbonate solution. Fluid and electrolyte balance should be monitored and appropriate supportive measures should be provided. Symptoms include headache, nausea, vomiting, diarrhoea and respiratory depression.

5. PHARMACOLOGICAL PROPERTIES

5.1 Pharmacodynamic properties

Glutaraldehyde is virucidal and thus inactivates the wart virus. On the skin, it also acts as an anhidrotic, drying the warts and surrounding skin, thus reducing the spread of lesions and simplifying the removal of persistent warts by curettage.

As glutaraldehyde stains the outer layer of the skin brown, treatment can be seen to be carried out. This stain soon disappears after cessation of treatment.

5.2 Pharmacokinetic properties

Addition of ethanol to the formulation stabilises the glutaraldehyde against irreversible polymerisation during storage but at the same time diminishes its activity. However, when the aqueous ethanolic solution is applied to the skin, the alcohol rapidly evaporates leaving a concentrated aqueous solution of glutaraldehyde which is highly reactive and attacks the wart before it has time to polymerise. Thus, the ethanolic formulation is stable in storage, as confirmed by stability tests, but is immediately activated when applied to the skin and the alcohol is allowed to evaporate.

5.3 Preclinical safety data

No relevant information additional to that contained elsewhere in the SPC.

6. PHARMACEUTICAL PARTICULARS

6.1 List of excipients

IMS; Purified Water.

6.2 Incompatibilities

None known.

6.3 Shelf life

24 months.

6.4 Special precautions for storage

Flammable. Keep away from flames. Keep upright. Do not store above 25°C.

6.5 Nature and contents of container

10 ml amber glass bottle incorporating a specially designed spatula for ease of application. This is supplied as an original pack (OP).

6.6 Instructions for use and handling

Not applicable.

7. MARKETING AUTHORISATION HOLDER

Dermal Laboratories

Tatmore Place, Gosmore

Hitchin, Herts SG4 7QR, UK.

8. MARKETING AUTHORISATION NUMBER(S)

0173/0022.

9. DATE OF FIRST AUTHORISATION/RENEWAL OF THE AUTHORISATION

15 September 2000.

10. DATE OF REVISION OF THE TEXT

November 2002.

Glypressin Injection

(Ferring Pharmaceuticals Ltd)

1. NAME OF THE MEDICINAL PRODUCT

Glypressin® Injection

2. QUALITATIVE AND QUANTITATIVE COMPOSITION

Each vial contains 1mg Terlipressin Acetate

For excipients, see 6.1

3. PHARMACEUTICAL FORM

Powder and solvent for solution for injection

Vial contains white, freeze-dried powder.

Ampoule contains solvent.

4. CLINICAL PARTICULARS

4.1 Therapeutic indications

Glypressin® is indicated in the treatment of bleeding oesophageal varices.

4.2 Posology and method of administration

In acute variceal bleeding, 2mg Glypressin® should be administered by intravenous bolus, followed by 1 - 2mg every 4 - 6 hours until bleeding is controlled, up to a maximum of 72 hours.

Administration is by intravenous injection.

4.3 Contraindications
Pregnancy

4.4 Special warnings and special precautions for use
Since Glypressin® has antidiuretic and pressor activity it should be used with great caution in patients with hypertension, atherosclerosis, cardiac dysrhythmias or coronary insufficiency. Constant monitoring of blood pressure, serum sodium and potassium and fluid balance is essential.

4.5 Interaction with other medicinal products and other forms of Interaction
None known

4.6 Pregnancy and lactation
Glypressin® may stimulate contraction of smooth muscle and is therefore contraindicated in pregnancy. There is no data concerning its use in lactation.

4.7 Effects on ability to drive and use machines
Not applicable

4.8 Undesirable effects
Glypressin® is only recommended for the short-term treatment of bleeding oesophageal varices, so few side effects have been reported. Those noted have included abdominal cramps, headache, transient blanching and increased arterial blood pressure.

4.9 Overdose
Increase in blood pressure in patients with known hypertension has been controlled with clonidine, 150mcg iv.

5. PHARMACOLOGICAL PROPERTIES

5.1 Pharmacodynamic properties
Glypressin® may be regarded as a circulating depot of lysine vasopressin. Following intravenous injection, three glycyl moieties are enzymatically cleaved from the N-terminus to release lysine vasopressin.

The slowly released vasopressin reduces blood flow in the splanchnic circulation in a prolonged manner, thereby helping to control bleeding from ruptured oesophageal varices.

5.2 Pharmacokinetic properties
Glypressin® is administered by bolus iv injection. It shows a biphasic plasma level curve which indicates that a two compartment model can be applied.

The half-life of distribution is about 8 -10 minutes.

The half-life of elimination is about 50 -70 minutes.

Lysine vasopressin reaches maximum plasma levels about 1 - 2 hours following iv administration and has a duration of activity of 4 - 6 hours.

5.3 Preclinical safety data
There are no pre-clinical data of relevance to the prescriber which are additional to that already included in other sections of the SPC.

6. PHARMACEUTICAL PARTICULARS

6.1 List of excipients
Vial:

Mannitol

Hydrochloric Acid 1M

Solvent Ampoule:

Sodium Chloride

Hydrochloric Acid 1M

Water for Injection

6.2 Incompatibilities
None known

6.3 Shelf life
36 months

6.4 Special precautions for storage
Do not store above 25°C. Keep container in the outer carton.

6.5 Nature and contents of container
Powder: Type I glass vial

Solvent: Type I glass ampoule

Pack size: Cartons containing 5 packs, each with one vial of powder and one ampoule of 5ml solvent.

6.6 Instructions for use and handling
Prior to injection, the powder should be reconstituted with the solvent provided. Use immediately after reconstitution.

7. MARKETING AUTHORISATION HOLDER
Ferring Pharmaceuticals Limited, The Courtyard, Waterside Drive, Langley, Berkshire SL3 6EZ (UK)

8. MARKETING AUTHORISATION NUMBER(S)
PL 3194/0018

9. DATE OF FIRST AUTHORISATION/RENEWAL OF THE AUTHORISATION
18th July 2001

10. DATE OF REVISION OF THE TEXT
June 2002

11. Legal Category
POM

Glytrin

(sanofi-aventis)

1. NAME OF THE MEDICINAL PRODUCT
Glytrin Spray

2. QUALITATIVE AND QUANTITATIVE COMPOSITION
Active Ingredient

Glyceryl Trinitrate: 400 micrograms/metered dose

(One metered dose with 8.8mg solution contains 400 micrograms glyceryl trinitrate)

3. PHARMACEUTICAL FORM
Sublingual spray.

4. CLINICAL PARTICULARS

4.1 Therapeutic indications
Treatment of acute angina pectoris.

Prevention of inducible angina (e.g. physical effort, emotional stress, exposure to cold).

4.2 Posology and method of administration
Route of administration

Oromucosal Dosage

Adults including the Elderly

At the onset of an attack: one or two metered doses (400 to 800 micrograms glyceryl trinitrate) to be sprayed under the tongue for the relief of anginal pain while the breath is held. No more than three doses are recommended at any one time.

For the prevention of inducible angina (e,g., physical effort, emotional stress, exposure to cold): one or two 400 microgram metered doses sprayed under the tongue within 2-3 minutes of the event starting.

Children

Glytrin Spray is not recommended for children.

Administration

During application the patient should rest, ideally in the sitting position. The canister should be held vertically with the valve head uppermost and the spray orifice as close to the mouth as possible. The dose should be sprayed under the tongue and the mouth should be closed immediately after each dose. The spray should not be inhaled. Patients should be instructed to familiarise themselves with the position of the spray orifice, which can be identified by the finger rest on top of the valve, in order to facilitate orientation for administration at night.

4.3 Contraindications
Hypersensitivity to nitrates. Severe hypotension (systolic blood pressure lower than 90mm Hg). Hypotensive shock, severe anaemia, constrictive pericarditis, extreme bradycardia, Glucose-6-phosphate- Dehydrogenase-deficiency, cerebral haemorrhage and brain trauma, aortic and/or mitral stenosis and angina caused by hypertrophic obstructive cardiomyopathy. Circulatory collapse, cardiogenic shock and toxic pulmonary oedema.

Sildenafil has been shown to potentiate the hypotensive effects of nitrates, and its co-administration with nitrates or nitric oxide donors is therefore contra-indicated.

4.4 Special warnings and special precautions for use
Tolerance to this drug and cross-tolerance to other nitrates may occur.

Glytrin Spray should be administered with particular caution in:

- pericardial tamponade
- low filling pressures (e.g. acute myocardial infarction, left ventricular failure)
- tendency to dysregulation of orthostatic blood pressure
- diseases accompanied by an increase intracranial pressure (so far further pressure increase has been observed solely in high doses of glyceryl trinitrate).

Alcohol should be avoided because of the hypotensive effect and medical controls of the intraocular pressure of glaucoma patients are advisable.

Particular caution should also be exercised when using Glytrin in patients with volume depletion from diuretic therapy, severe hepatic or renal impairment and hypothyroidism.

4.5 Interaction with other medicinal products and other forms of Interaction
Alcohol may potentiate the hypotensive effect. Vasodilators, antihypertensives, β-blockers, calcium antagonists, neuroleptics, tricyclic antidepressants and diuretics can increase nitrate induced hypotension.

The hypotensive effects of nitrates are potentiated by the concurrent administration of sildenafil.

The bioavialability of dihydroergotamine may be increased by concomitant use of Glytrin, which can result in vasoconstiction since dihyroergotamine can antagonise the effects of nitroglycerin. The concomitant administration of Glytrin and heparin can reduce the antithrombotic effect of heparin. Regular monitoring of coagulation parameters and adjustment of the heparin dose may be necessary.

In patients pre-treated with organic nitrates a higher dose of glyceryl trinitrate may be necessary to achieve the desired haemodynamic effect.

4.6 Pregnancy and lactation
The safety of glyceryl trinitrate in human pregnancy, especially during the first trimester has not been established. It is not known whether glyceryl trinitrate is excreted into human breast milk. Glytrin Spray should be used only after weighing the benefit for the mother against possible risks for the child. Nursing should be discontinued during treatment with this product.

4.7 Effects on ability to drive and use machines
The ability to react may be diminished because of the side effects or interactions due to the nitrates. This effect is potentiated by alcohol consumption. Therefore, driving and/or using machines should be avoided during treatment with Glytrin Spray.

4.8 Undesirable effects
Frequent headache, facial flushing, vertigo, dizziness, weakness and nausea have been reported.

Postural hypotension, tachycardia and paradoxical bradycardia have been reported occasionally.

Rarely collapse states with bradycardia and syncope, a severe fall in blood pressure accompanied by an enhancement of the anginal symptoms may occur.

Use of Glytrin may give rise to transient hypoxaemia and, in patients with coronary heart disease, ischaemia as a result of a relative redistribution of the bloodstream which is to hypoventilated alveolar areas.

Allergic skin reactions may occasionally occur and there have been isolated reports of burning sensation in the buccal cavity and stinging sensation in the throat.

Exfoliative dermatitis may occur rarely.

Tolerance development and the occurrence of crossed tolerance of other nitro compounds have been found in chronic, continuous treatment using high doses. To avoid a decrease in efficacy or a loss of efficacy high continuous doses should be avoided.

4.9 Overdose
Signs and Symptoms

Flushing, severe headache, vertigo, tachycardia, a feeling of suffocation, hypotension, fainting and rarely cyanosis and methaemoglobinaemia may occur. In a few patients, there may be a reaction comparable to shock with nausea, vomiting, weakness, sweating and syncope.

Treatment

Recovery often occurs without special treatment. Hypotension may be corrected by elevation of the legs to promote venous return. Methaemoglobinaemia should be treated by intravenous methylene blue and/or toluidine blue. Symptomatic treatment should be given for respiratory and circulatory defects in more serious cases.

5. PHARMACOLOGICAL PROPERTIES

5.1 Pharmacodynamic properties
ATC-Code: CO1DA02

Glyceryl trinitrate acts on vascular smooth muscles to produce arterial and venous vasodilation. The vasodilation results in a reduction of venous return and an improvement in myocardial perfusion with the result of a reduction in the work performed by the heart and hence reduced oxygen demand.

5.2 Pharmacokinetic properties
Glyceryl trinitrate is rapidly absorbed through the buccal and sublingual mucosa, and in man peak concentrations in plasma are observed within four minutes of sublingual administration.

The absolute bioavailability after sublingual administration is approximately 39%. After sublingual administration the plasma levels have shown a wide range of intra and inter-individual variability.

The compound is extensively metabolised by liver enzymes and has a plasma half-life of 1-3 minutes. The principle mechanism of metabolism involves denitration.

5.3 Preclinical safety data
Reproductive toxicity

Animal studies conducted with various routes of administration have not shown teratogenicity, other embryotoxic effects or impairment of fertility with dosages inducing parental toxicity.

Data from in-vitro mutagenicity testing as well as from studies in animals indicate that glyceryl trinitrate will not exert mutagenic or carcinogenic effects under conditions of clinical use.

6. PHARMACEUTICAL PARTICULARS

6.1 List of excipients
Peppermint oil Ph. Eur

Propellant HFC 134A (1,1,1.2 Tetrafluoroethane)

Ethanol BP

6.2 Incompatibilities
None.

6.3 Shelf life
Two years

6.4 Special precautions for storage
Do not store above 25°C. Protect from frost and direct heat or sunlight.

6.5 Nature and contents of container
Internally lacquered monobloc aluminium pressurised container sealed with a metered spray valve.

The product is presented in packs with one metered dose spray.

One metered dose spray (= one aluminium container) contains 1760.0mg of solution (according to 11400.0mg of solution and propellant) providing 200 single metered doses.

6.6 Instructions for use and handling
Glytrin Spray is a pressurised container, which must not be pierced or burnt even after use. It should not be sprayed at a naked flame or any incandescent material. Patients, especially those who smoke should be warned not to use Glytrin Spray near a naked flame.

7. MARKETING AUTHORISATION HOLDER
Ayrton Saunders Ltd

Peninsular Business Park

Reeds Lane

Moretons

Wirral

CH46 1DW

United Kingdom

8. MARKETING AUTHORISATION NUMBER(S)
PL 16431/0017

9. DATE OF FIRST AUTHORISATION/RENEWAL OF THE AUTHORISATION
25 February 2003

10. DATE OF REVISION OF THE TEXT
Legal Category: P

GONAL-f 1050 IU/1.75 ml (77mcg/1.75 ml)

(Serono Ltd)

1. NAME OF THE MEDICINAL PRODUCT
GONAL-f 1050 IU/1.75ml (77 micrograms/1.75ml), powder and solvent for solution for injection.

2. QUALITATIVE AND QUANTITATIVE COMPOSITION
One multidose vial contains 87 micrograms follitropin alfa, recombinant human follicle stimulating hormone (FSH) in order to deliver 77 micrograms, equivalent to 1050 IU. Follitropin alfa is produced in genetically engineered Chinese Hamster Ovary (CHO) cells.

For excipients, see 6.1.

3. PHARMACEUTICAL FORM
Powder and solvent for solution for injection in a pre-filled syringe.

Appearance of the powder: white lyophilised pellet.

Appearance of the solvent: clear colourless solution.

4. CLINICAL PARTICULARS
4.1 Therapeutic indications
Anovulation (including polycystic ovarian disease, PCOD) in women who have been unresponsive to treatment with clomiphene citrate.

Stimulation of multifollicular development in patients undergoing superovulation for assisted reproductive technologies (ART) such as *in vitro* fertilisation (IVF), gamete intra-fallopian transfer (GIFT) and zygote intra-fallopian transfer (ZIFT).

GONAL-f in association with a luteinising hormone (LH) preparation is recommended for the stimulation of follicular development in women with severe LH and FSH deficiency. In clinical trials these patients were defined by an endogenous serum LH level < 1.2 IU/l.

GONAL-f is indicated for the stimulation of spermatogenesis in men who have congenital or acquired hypogonadotrophic hypogonadism with concomitant human Chorionic Gonadotrophin (hCG) therapy.

4.2 Posology and method of administration
Treatment with GONAL-f should be initiated under the supervision of a physician experienced in the treatment of fertility problems.

GONAL-f is intended for subcutaneous administration. The powder should be reconstituted prior to the first use with the solvent provided. GONAL-f 1050 IU/1.75ml (77 micrograms/1.75ml) preparation must not be reconstituted with any other GONAL-f container.

The dosage recommendations given for GONAL-f are those in use for urinary FSH. Clinical assessment of GONAL-f indicates that its daily doses, regimens of administration, and treatment monitoring procedures should not be different from those currently used for urinary FSH-containing preparations. However, when these doses were used in a clinical study comparing GONAL-f and urinary FSH, GONAL-f was more effective than urinary FSH in terms of a lower total dose and a shorter treatment period needed to achieve pre-ovulatory conditions. Bioequivalence has been demonstrated between equivalent doses of the monodose presentation and the multidose presentation of GONAL-f. It is advised to adhere to the recommended starting doses indicated below.

<u>Women with anovulation (including PCOD)</u>:

The object of GONAL-f therapy is to develop a single mature Graafian follicle from which the ovum will be liberated after the administration of hCG.

GONAL-f may be given as a course of daily injections. In menstruating patients treatment should commence within the first 7 days of the menstrual cycle.

Treatment should be tailored to the individual patient's response as assessed by measuring follicle size by ultrasound and/or oestrogen secretion. A commonly used regimen commences at 75-150 IU FSH daily and is increased preferably by 37.5 IU, or 75 IU at 7 or preferably 14 day intervals if necessary, to obtain an adequate, but not excessive, response. The maximal daily dose is usually not higher than 225 IU FSH. If a patient fails to respond adequately after 4 weeks of treatment, that cycle should be abandoned and the patient should recommence treatment at a higher starting dose than in the abandoned cycle.

When an optimal response is obtained, a single injection of 5 000 IU, up to 10 000 IU hCG should be administered 24-48 hours after the last GONAL-f injection. The patient is recommended to have coitus on the day of, and the day following, hCG administration. Alternatively intrauterine insemination (IUI) may be performed.

If an excessive response is obtained, treatment should be stopped and hCG withheld (see warnings). Treatment should recommence in the next cycle at a dosage lower than that of the previous cycle.

<u>Women undergoing ovarian stimulation for multiple follicular development prior to *in vitro* fertilisation or other assisted reproductive technologies</u>:

A commonly used regimen for superovulation involves the administration of 150-225 IU of GONAL-f daily, commencing on days 2 or 3 of the cycle. Treatment is continued until adequate follicular development has been achieved (as assessed by monitoring of serum oestrogen concentrations and/or ultrasound examination), with the dose adjusted according to the patient's response, to usually not higher than 450 IU daily. In general adequate follicular development is achieved on average by the tenth day of treatment (range 5 to 20 days).

A single injection of up to 10 000 IU hCG is administered 24-48 hours after the last GONAL-f injection to induce final follicular maturation.

Down-regulation with a gonadotrophin-releasing hormone (GnRH) agonist is now commonly used in order to suppress the endogenous LH surge and to control tonic levels of LH. In a commonly used protocol, GONAL-f is started approximately 2 weeks after the start of agonist treatment, both being continued until adequate follicular development is achieved. For example, following two weeks of treatment with an agonist, 150-225 IU GONAL-f are administered for the first 7 days. The dose is then adjusted according to the ovarian response.

Overall experience with IVF indicates that in general the treatment success rate remains stable during the first four attempts and gradually declines thereafter.

<u>Women with anovulation resulting from severe LH and FSH deficiency</u>

In LH and FSH deficient women (hypogonadotrophic hypogonadism), the objective of GONAL-f therapy in association with lutropin alfa is to develop a single mature Graafian follicle from which the oocyte will be liberated after the administration of human chorionic gonadotrophin (hCG). GONAL-f should be given as a course of daily injections simultaneously with lutropin alfa. Since these patients are amenorrhoeic and have low endogenous oestrogen secretion, treatment can commence at any time.

Treatment should be tailored to the individual patient's response as assessed by measuring follicle size by ultrasound and oestrogen response. A recommended regimen commences at 75 IU of lutropin alfa daily with 75-150 IU FSH.

If an FSH dose increase is deemed appropriate, dose adaptation should preferably be after 7-14 day intervals and preferably by 37.5 IU-75 IU increments. It may be acceptable to extend the duration of stimulation in any one cycle to up to 5 weeks.

When an optimal response is obtained, a single injection of 5,000 IU to 10,000 IU hCG should be administered 24-48 hours after the last GONAL-f and lutropin alfa injections. The patient is recommended to have coitus on the day of, and on the day following, hCG administration. Alternatively, intrauterine insemination (IUI) may be performed.

Luteal phase support may be considered since lack of substances with luteotrophic activity (LH/hCG) after ovulation may lead to premature failure of the corpus luteum.

If an excessive response is obtained, treatment should be stopped and hCG withheld. Treatment should recommence in the next cycle at a dose of FSH lower than that of the previous cycle.

<u>Men with hypogonadotrophic hypogonadism.</u>

GONAL-f should be given at a dosage of 150 IU three times a week, concomitantly with hCG, for a minimum of 4 months. If after this period, the patient has not responded, the combination treatment may be continued; current clinical experience indicates that treatment for at least 18 months may be necessary to achieve spermatogenesis.

4.3 Contraindications
GONAL-f must not be used in:

hypersensitivity to follitropin alfa, FSH or to any of the excipients

case of tumours of the hypothalamus and pituitary gland and in women:

ovarian enlargement or cyst not due to polycystic ovarian disease

gynaecological haemorrhages of unknown aetiology

ovarian, uterine or mammary carcinoma

GONAL-f should not be used when an effective response cannot be obtained, such as:

In women:

primary ovarian failure

malformations of sexual organs incompatible with pregnancy

fibroid tumours of the uterus incompatible with pregnancy

In men:

primary testicular insufficiency

4.4 Special warnings and special precautions for use
GONAL-f is a potent gonadotrophic substance capable of causing mild to severe adverse reactions, and should only be used by physicians who are thoroughly familiar with infertility problems and their management.

Gonadotrophin therapy requires a certain time commitment by physicians and supportive health professionals, as well as the availability of appropriate monitoring facilities. In women, safe and effective use of GONAL-f calls for monitoring of ovarian response with ultrasound, alone or preferably in combination with measurement of serum oestradiol levels, on a regular basis. There may be a degree of interpatient variability in response to FSH administration, with a poor response to FSH in some patients. The lowest effective dose in relation to the treatment objective should be used in both men and women.

Self-administration of GONAL-f should only be performed by patients who are well motivated, adequately trained and with access to expert advice. During training of the patient for self-administration, special attention should be given to specific instructions for the use of the multidose and/or the monodose presentation(s).

Due to a local reactivity to benzyl alcohol, the same site of injection should not be used on consecutive days.

The first injection of GONAL-f should be performed under direct medical supervision.

<u>**Treatment in women**</u>

Before starting treatment, the couple's infertility should be assessed as appropriate and putative contraindications for pregnancy evaluated. In particular, patients should be evaluated for hypothyroidism, adrenocortical deficiency, hyperprolactinemia and pituitary or hypothalamic tumours, and appropriate specific treatment given.

Patients undergoing stimulation of follicular growth, whether in the frame of a treatment for anovulatory infertility or ART procedures, may experience ovarian enlargement or develop hyperstimulation. Adherence to recommended GONAL-f dosage and regimen of administration, and careful monitoring of therapy will minimise the incidence of such events. Acute interpretation of the indices of follicle development and maturation require a physician whom is experienced in the interpretation of the relevant tests.

In clinical trials, an increase of the ovarian sensitivity to GONAL-f was shown when administered with lutropin alfa. If an FSH dose increase is deemed appropriate, dose adaptation should preferably be at 7-14 day intervals and preferably with 37.5-75 IU increments.

No direct comparison of GONAL-f/LH versus human menopausal gonadotrophin (hMG) has been performed. Comparison with historical data suggests that the ovulation rate obtained with GONAL-f/LH is similar to what can be obtained with hMG.

Ovarian Hyperstimulation Syndrome (OHSS)

OHSS is a medical event distinct from uncomplicated ovarian enlargement. OHSS is a syndrome that can manifest itself with increasing degrees of severity. It comprises marked ovarian enlargement, high serum sex steroids, and an increase in vascular permeability which can result in an accumulation of fluid in the peritoneal, pleural and, rarely, in the pericardial cavities.

The following symptomatology may be observed in severe cases of OHSS: abdominal pain, abdominal distension, severe ovarian enlargement, weight gain, dyspnoea, oliguria and gastrointestinal symptoms including nausea, vomiting and diarrhoea. Clinical evaluation may reveal hypovolaemia, haemoconcentration, electrolyte imbalances, ascites, haemoperitoneum, pleural effusions, hydrothorax, acute pulmonary distress, and thromboembolic events.

Excessive ovarian response to gonadotrophin treatment seldom gives rise to OHSS unless hCG is administered to trigger ovulation. Therefore in cases of ovarian hyperstimulation it is prudent to withhold hCG and advise the patient to refrain from coitus or to use barrier methods for at least 4 days. OHSS may progress rapidly (within 24 hours to several days) to become a serious medical event, therefore patients should be followed for at least two weeks after hCG administration.

To minimise the risk of OHSS or of multiple pregnancy, ultrasound scans as well as oestradiol measurements are recommended. In anovulation the risk of OHSS and multiple pregnancy is increased by a serum oestradiol > 900 pg/ml (3300 pmol/l) and more than 3 follicles of 14 mm or more in diameter. In ART there is an increased risk of OHSS with a serum oestradiol > 3000 pg/ml (11000 pmol/l) and 20 or more follicles of 12 mm or more in diameter. When the oestradiol level is > 5500 pg/ml (20200 pmol/l) and where there are 40 or more follicles in total, it may be necessary to withhold hCG administration.

Adherence to recommended GONAL-f dosage, regimen of administration and careful monitoring of therapy will minimise the incidence of ovarian hyperstimulation and multiple pregnancy (see Sections 4.2 'Posology and method of administration' and 4.8 'Undesirable effects').

In ART, aspiration of all follicles prior to ovulation may reduce the occurrence of hyperstimulation.

OHSS may be more severe and more protracted if pregnancy occurs. Most often, OHSS occurs after hormonal treatment has been discontinued and reaches its maximum at about seven to ten days following treatment. Usually, OHSS resolves spontaneously with the onset of menses.

If severe OHSS occurs, gonadotrophin treatment should be stopped if still ongoing, the patient hospitalised and specific therapy for OHSS started.

This syndrome occurs with higher incidence in patients with polycystic ovarian disease.

Multiple pregnancy

Multiple pregnancy, specially high order, carries an increase risk in adverse maternal and perinatal outcomes.

In patients undergoing ovulation induction with GONAL-f, the incidence of multiple pregnancies is increased as compared with natural conception. The majority of multiple conceptions are twins. To minimise the risk of multiple pregnancy, careful monitoring of ovarian response is recommended.

In patients undergoing ART procedures the risk of multiple pregnancy is related mainly to the number of embryos replaced, their quality and the patient age.

The patients should be advised of the potential risk of multiple births before starting treatment.

Pregnancy wastage

The incidence of pregnancy wastage by miscarriage or abortion is higher in patients undergoing stimulation of follicular growth for ovulation induction or ART than in the normal population.

Ectopic pregnancy

Women with a history of tubal disease are at risk of ectopic pregnancy, whether the pregnancy is obtained by spontaneous conception of with fertility treatments. The prevalence of ectopic pregnancy after IVF was reported to be 2 to 5%, as compared to 1 to 1.5% in the general population.

Reproductive system neoplasms

There have been reports of ovarian and other reproductive system neoplasms, both benign and malignant, in women who have undergone multiple drug regimens for intertility treatment. It is not yet established whether or not treatment with gonadotrophins increases the baseline risk of these tumors in infertile women.

Congenital malformation

The prevalence of congenital malformations after ART may be slightly higher than after spontaneous conceptions. This is thought to be due to differences in parental characteristics (e.g. maternal age, sperm characteristics) and multiple pregnancies.

Thromboembolic events

In women with generally recognised risk factors for thrombo-embolic events, such as personal or family history, treatment with gonadotrophins may further increase the risk. In these women, the benefits of gonadotrophin administration need to be weighed against the risks. It should be noted however, that pregnancy itself also carries an increased risk of thrombo-embolic events.

Treatment in men

Elevated endogenous FSH levels are indicative of primary testicular failure. Such patients are unresponsive to GONAL-f/hCG therapy.

Semen analysis is recommended 4 to 6 months after the beginning of treatment in assessing the response.

4.5 Interaction with other medicinal products and other forms of Interaction

Concomitant use of GONAL-f with other agents used to stimulate ovulation (e.g. hCG, clomiphene citrate) may potentiate the follicular response, whereas concurrent use of a GnRH agonist to induce pituitary desensitisation may increase the dosage of GONAL-f needed to elicit an adequate ovarian response. No other clinically significant drug interaction has been reported during GONAL-f therapy.

GONAL-f should not be administered as mixture with other medicinal products in the same injection.

4.6 Pregnancy and lactation

Use during pregnancy

There is no indication for use of GONAL-f during pregnancy. No teratogenic risk has been reported, following controlled ovarian hyperstimulation, in clinical use with gonadotrophins. In case of exposure during pregnancy, clinical data are not sufficient to exclude a teratogenic effect of recombinant hFSH. However, to date, no particular malformative effect has been reported. No teratogenic effect has been observed in animal studies.

Use during lactation

GONAL-f is not indicated during lactation. During lactation, the secretion of prolactin can entail a poor prognosis to ovarian stimulation.

4.7 Effects on ability to drive and use machines

No studies on the effects on ability to drive and use machines have been performed.

4.8 Undesirable effects

Treatment in women

Very Common (> 1/10)

Ovarian cysts;

Mild to severe injection site reaction (pain, redness, bruising, swelling and/or irritation at the site of injection);

Headache.

Common (1/100 – 1/10)

Mild to moderate OHSS (see section 4.4);

Abdominal pain and gastrointestinal symptoms such as nausea, vomiting, diarrhoea, abdominal cramps and bloating.

Uncommon (1/1000 – 1/100)

Severe OHSS (see section 4.4).

Rare (1/10 000 – 1/1000)

Ovarian torsion, a complication of OHSS

Very rare (< 1/10 000)

Thromboembolism, usually associated with severe OHSS;

Mild systemic allergic reactions (erythema, rash or facial swelling).

Treatment in men

Common (1/100 – 1/10)

Gynaecomastia, acne and weight gain.

4.9 Overdose

The effects of an overdose of GONAL-f are unknown, nevertheless one could expect ovarian hyperstimulation syndrome to occur, which is further described in Special Warnings and Special Precautions for Use.

5. PHARMACOLOGICAL PROPERTIES

5.1 Pharmacodynamic properties

Pharmacotherapeutic group: gonadotrophins, ATC code: G03GA05.

GONAL-f is a preparation of follicle stimulating hormone produced by genetically engineered Chinese Hamster Ovary (CHO) cells.

In women, the most important effect resulting from parenteral administration of FSH is the development of mature Graafian follicles.

In clinical trials, patients with severe FSH and LH deficiency were defined by an endogenous serum LH level <1.2 IU/l as measured in a central laboratory. However, it should be taken into account that there are variations between LH measurements performed in different laboratories.

In men deficient in FSH, GONAL-f administered concomitantly with hCG for at least 4 months induces spermatogenesis.

5.2 Pharmacokinetic properties

Following intravenous administration, GONAL-f is distributed to the extracellular fluid space with an initial half-life of around 2 hours and eliminated from the body with a terminal half-life of about one day. The steady state volume of distribution and total clearance are 10 L and 0.6 L/h, respectively. One-eighth of the GONAL-f dose is excreted in the urine.

Following subcutaneous administration, the absolute bioavailability is about 70%. Following repeated administration, GONAL-f accumulates 3-fold achieving a steady-state within 3-4 days. In women whose endogenous gonadotrophin secretion is suppressed, GONAL-f has nevertheless been shown to effectively stimulate follicular development and steroidogenesis, despite unmeasurable LH levels.

5.3 Preclinical safety data

In an extensive range of toxicological, mutagenicity and animal studies (dogs, rats, monkeys), acute and chronic (up to 13 weeks and 52 weeks), no significant findings were observed.

In rabbits, the formulation reconstituted with 0.9% benzyl alcohol and 0.9% benzyl alcohol alone, both resulted in a slight haemorrhage and subacute inflammation after single subcutaneous injection or mild inflammatory and degenerative changes after single intramuscular injection respectively.

Impaired fertility has been reported in rats exposed to pharmacological doses of follitropin alfa (⩾ 40 IU/kg/day) for extended periods, through reduced fecundity.

Given in high doses (⩾ 5 IU/kg/day) follitropin alfa caused a decrease in the number of viable foetuses without being a teratogen, and dystocia similar to that observed with urinary hMG. However, since GONAL-f is not indicated in pregnancy, these data are of limited clinical relevance.

6. PHARMACEUTICAL PARTICULARS

6.1 List of excipients

Powder:

Sucrose

Sodium dihydrogen phosphate monohydrate

Disodium phosphate dihydrate

Phosphoric acid, concentrated

Sodium hydroxide

Solvent:

Water for Injections

Benzyl alcohol

6.2 Incompatibilities

In the absence of incompatibility studies, this medicinal product must not be mixed with other medicinal products.

6.3 Shelf life

2 years.

The reconstituted solution is stable for 28 days

Do not store above 25°C. Do not freeze.

6.4 Special precautions for storage

Prior to reconstitution, do not store above 25°C. Store in the original package.

After reconstitution, do not store above 25°C. Do not freeze. Store in the original container.

6.5 Nature and contents of container

GONAL-f is presented as a powder and solvent for injection. The powder is presented in 3ml vials (Type I glass), with rubber stopper (bromobutyl rubber) and aluminium flip-off cap. The solvent for reconstitution is presented in 2ml pre-filled syringes (Type I glass) with a rubber stopper. The Administration syringes made of polypropylene with a stainless steel pre-fixed needle are also provided.

The product is supplied as a pack of 1 vial of powder with 1 pre-filled syringe of solvent for reconstitution and 15 disposable syringes for administration graduated in FSH units.

6.6 Instructions for use and handling

GONAL-f 1050 IU/1.75ml (77 micrograms/1.75ml) must be reconstituted with the 2 ml solvent provided before use.

GONAL-f 1050 IU/1.75ml (77 micrograms/1.75ml) preparation must not be reconstituted with any other GONAL-f containers.

The solvent pre-filled syringe provided should be used for reconstitution only and then disposed of in accordance with local requirements. A set of administration syringes graduated in FSH units is supplied in the GONAL-f Multidose box. Alternatively, a 1 ml syringe, graduated in ml, with pre-fixed needle for subcutaneous administration could be used. Each ml of reconstituted solution contains 600 IU r-hFSH.

The following table states the volume to be administered to deliver the prescribed dose:

Dose (IU)	Volume to be injected (ml)
75	0.13
150	0.25
225	0.38
300	0.50
375	0.63
450	0.75

Individual reconstituted vials should be for single patient use only. The patient should reconstitute the product and inject it immediately. The next injection should be done at the same time the next day.

The reconstituted solution should not be administered if it contains particles or is not clear.

7. MARKETING AUTHORISATION HOLDER

SERONO EUROPE LIMITED

56 Marsh Wall

London E14 9TP

United Kingdom

8. MARKETING AUTHORISATION NUMBER(S)

EU/1/95/001/021

9. DATE OF FIRST AUTHORISATION/RENEWAL OF THE AUTHORISATION

29 January 2001

10. DATE OF REVISION OF THE TEXT

2nd October 2002

LEGAL STATUS

POM

NAME AND ADDRESS OF DISTRIBUTOR IN UK
Serono Limited
Bedfont Cross
Stanwell Road
Feltham
Middlesex
TW14 8NX

NAME AND ADDRESS OF DISTRIBUTOR IN IRELAND
Allphar Services Limited
Pharmaceutical Agents and Distributors
Belgard Road
Tallaght
Dublin 24

GONAL-f 300IU (22 mcg) pen

(Serono Ltd)

1. NAME OF THE MEDICINAL PRODUCT
GONAL-f 300 IU/0.5ml (22 micrograms/0.5ml), solution for injection in a pre-filled pen.

2. QUALITATIVE AND QUANTITATIVE COMPOSITION
Follitropin alfa*, 600IU/ml (equivalent to 44 micrograms/ml).

Each cartridge delivers 300IU (equivalent to 22 micrograms/ml) in 0.5ml.

*Follitropin alfa is recombinant human follicle stimulating hormone (FSH) produced by recombinant DNA technology in Chinese Hamster Ovary (CHO) cell line.

For excipients, see 6.1.

3. PHARMACEUTICAL FORM
Solution for injection in a pre-filled pen.

Clear colourless solution.

4. CLINICAL PARTICULARS

4.1 Therapeutic indications
• Anovulation (including polycystic ovarian disease, PCOD) in women who have been unresponsive to treatment with clomiphene citrate.

• Stimulation of multifollicular development in patients undergoing superovulation for assisted reproductive technologies (ART) such as *in vitro* fertilisation (IVF), gamete intra-fallopian transfer (GIFT) and zygote intra-fallopian transfer (ZIFT).

• GONAL-f in association with a luteinising hormone (LH) preparation is recommended for the stimulation of follicular development in women with severe LH and FSH deficiency. In clinical trials these patients were defined by an endogenous serum LH level <1.2 IU/l.

• GONAL-f is indicated for the stimulation of spermatogenesis in men who have congenital or acquired hypogonadotrophic hypogonadism with concomitant human Chorionic Gonadotrophin (hCG) therapy.

4.2 Posology and method of administration
Treatment with GONAL-f should be initiated under the supervision of a physician experienced in the treatment of fertility problems.

GONAL-f is intended for subcutaneous administration.

The dosage recommendations given for GONAL-f are those in use for urinary FSH. Clinical assessment of GONAL-f indicates that its daily doses, regimens of administration, and treatment monitoring procedures should not be different from those currently used for urinary FSH-containing preparations. However, when these doses were used in a clinical study comparing GONAL-f and urinary FSH, GONAL-f was more effective than urinary FSH in terms of a lower total dose and a shorter treatment period needed to achieve pre-ovulatory conditions. Bioequivalence has been demonstrated between equivalent doses of the monodose presentation and the multidose presentation of GONAL-f. It is advised to adhere to the recommended starting doses indicated below.

<u>Women with anovulation (including PCOD):</u>

The object of GONAL-f therapy is to develop a single mature Graafian follicle from which the ovum will be liberated after the administration of hCG.

GONAL-f may be given as a course of daily injections. In menstruating patients treatment should commence within the first 7 days of the menstrual cycle.

Treatment should be tailored to the individual patient's response as assessed by measuring follicle size by ultrasound and/or oestrogen secretion. A commonly used regimen commences at 75-150 IU FSH daily and is increased preferably by 37.5 IU, or 75 IU at 7 or preferably 14 day intervals if necessary, to obtain an adequate, but not excessive, response. The maximal daily dose is usually not higher than 225 IU FSH. If a patient fails to respond adequately after 4 weeks of treatment, that cycle should be abandoned and the patient should recommence treatment at a higher starting dose than in the abandoned cycle.

When an optimal response is obtained, a single injection of 250 micrograms r-hCG or 5 000 IU, up to 10 000 IU hCG should be administered 24-48 hours after the last GONAL-f injection. The patient is recommended to have coitus on the day of, and the day following, hCG administration. Alternatively intrauterine insemination (IUI) may be performed.

If an excessive response is obtained, treatment should be stopped and hCG withheld (see section 4.4). Treatment should recommence in the next cycle at a dosage lower than that of the previous cycle.

<u>Women undergoing ovarian stimulation for multiple follicular development prior to *in vitro* fertilisation or other assisted reproductive technologies:</u>

A commonly used regimen for superovulation involves the administration of 150-225 IU of GONAL-f daily, commencing on days 2 or 3 of the cycle. Treatment is continued until adequate follicular development has been achieved (as assessed by monitoring of serum oestrogen concentrations and/or ultrasound examination), with the dose adjusted according to the patient's response, to usually not higher than 450 IU daily. In general adequate follicular development is achieved on average by the tenth day of treatment (range 5 to 20 days).

A single injection of 250 micrograms r-hCG or 5 000 IU up to 10 000 IU hCG is administered 24-48 hours after the last GONAL-f injection to induce final follicular maturation.

Down-regulation with a gonadotrophin-releasing hormone (GnRH) agonist or antagonist is now commonly used in order to suppress the endogenous LH surge and to control tonic levels of LH. In a commonly used protocol, GONAL-f is started approximately 2 weeks after the start of agonist treatment, both being continued until adequate follicular development is achieved. For example, following two weeks of treatment with an agonist, 150-225 IU GONAL-f are administered for the first 7 days. The dose is then adjusted according to the ovarian response.

Overall experience with IVF indicates that in general the treatment success rate remains stable during the first four attempts and gradually declines thereafter.

<u>Women with anovulation resulting from severe LH and FSH deficiency</u>

In LH and FSH deficient women (hypogonadotrophic hypogonadism), the objective of GONAL-f therapy in association with lutropin alfa is to develop a single mature Graafian follicle from which the oocyte will be liberated after the administration of human chorionic gonadotrophin (hCG). GONAL-f should be given as a course of daily injections simultaneously with lutropin alfa. Since these patients are amenorrhoeic and have low endogenous oestrogen secretion, treatment can commence at any time.

Treatment should be tailored to the individual patient's response as assessed by measuring follicle size by ultrasound and oestrogen response. A recommended regimen commences at 75 IU of lutropin alfa daily with 75-150 IU FSH.

If an FSH dose increase is deemed appropriate, dose adaptation should preferably be after 7-14 day intervals and preferably by 37.5 IU-75 IU increments. It may be acceptable to extend the duration of stimulation in any one cycle to up to 5 weeks.

When an optimal response is obtained, a single injection of 250 micrograms r-hCG or 5,000 IU up to 10,000 IU hCG should be administered 24-48 hours after the last GONAL-f and lutropin alfa injections. The patient is recommended to have coitus on the day of, and on the day following, hCG administration. Alternatively, intrauterine insemination (IUI) may be performed.

Luteal phase support may be considered since lack of substances with luteotrophic activity (LH/hCG) after ovulation may lead to premature failure of the corpus luteum.

If an excessive response is obtained, treatment should be stopped and hCG withheld. Treatment should recommence in the next cycle at a dose of FSH lower than that of the previous cycle.

<u>Men with hypogonadotrophic hypogonadism.</u>

GONAL-f should be given at a dosage of 150 IU three times a week, concomitantly with hCG, for a minimum of 4 months. If after this period, the patient has not responded, the combination treatment may be continued; current clinical experience indicates that treatment for at least 18 months may be necessary to achieve spermatogenesis.

4.3 Contraindications
Hypersensitivity to follitropin alfa, FSH or to any of the excipients

Tumours of the hypothalamus and pituitary gland

In women:

ovarian enlargement or cyst not due to polycystic ovarian disease

gynaecological haemorrhages of unknown aetiology

ovarian, uterine or mammary carcinoma

Must not be used when an effective response cannot be obtained, such as:

In women:

primary ovarian failure

malformations of sexual organs incompatible with pregnancy

fibroid tumours of the uterus incompatible with pregnancy

In men:

• primary testicular insufficiency

4.4 Special warnings and special precautions for use
GONAL-f is a potent gonadotrophic substance capable of causing mild to severe adverse reactions, and should only be used by physicians who are thoroughly familiar with infertility problems and their management.

Gonadotrophin therapy requires a certain time commitment by physicians and supportive health professionals, as well as the availability of appropriate monitoring facilities. In women, safe and effective use of GONAL-f calls for monitoring of ovarian response with ultrasound, alone or preferably in combination with measurement of serum oestradiol levels, on a regular basis. There may be a degree of interpatient variability in response to FSH administration, with a poor response to FSH in some patients. The lowest effective dose in relation to the treatment objective should be used in both men and women.

Self-administration of GONAL-f should only be performed by patients who are well motivated, adequately trained and have access to expert advice. During training of the patient for self-administration, special attention should be given to specific instructions for the use of the pre-filled pen.

The first injection of GONAL-f should be performed under direct medical supervision.

Treatment in women
Before starting treatment, the couple's infertility should be assessed as appropriate and putative contraindications for pregnancy evaluated. In particular, patients should be evaluated for hypothyroidism, adrenocortical deficiency, hyperprolactinemia and pituitary or hypothalamic tumours, and appropriate specific treatment given.

Patients undergoing stimulation of follicular growth, whether as treatment for anovulatory infertility or ART procedures, may experience ovarian enlargement or develop hyperstimulation. Adherence to the recommended GONAL-f dosage and regimen of administration, and careful monitoring of therapy will minimise the incidence of such events. Acute interpretation of the indices of follicle development and maturation, the physician should be experienced in the interpretation of the relevant tests.

In clinical trials, an increase of the ovarian sensitivity to GONAL-f was shown when administered with lutropin alfa. If an FSH dose increase is deemed appropriate, dose adaptation should preferably be at 7-14 day intervals and preferably with 37.5-75 IU increments.

No direct comparison of GONAL-f/LH versus human menopausal gonadotrophin (hMG) has been performed. Comparison with historical data suggests that the ovulation rate obtained with GONAL-f/LH is similar to that obtained with hMG.

Ovarian Hyperstimulation Syndrome (OHSS)
OHSS is a medical event distinct from uncomplicated ovarian enlargement. OHSS is a syndrome that can manifest itself with increasing degrees of severity. It comprises marked ovarian enlargement, high serum sex steroids, and an increase in vascular permeability which can result in an accumulation of fluid in the peritoneal, pleural and, rarely, in the pericardial cavities.

The following symptomatology may be observed in severe cases of OHSS: abdominal pain, abdominal distension, severe ovarian enlargement, weight gain, dyspnoea, oliguria and gastrointestinal symptoms including nausea, vomiting and diarrhoea. Clinical evaluation may reveal hypovolaemia, haemoconcentration, electrolyte imbalances, ascites, haemoperitoneum, pleural effusions, hydrothorax, acute pulmonary distress, and thromboembolic events.

Excessive ovarian response to gonadotrophin treatment seldom gives rise to OHSS unless hCG is administered to trigger ovulation. Therefore in cases of ovarian hyperstimulation it is prudent to withhold hCG and advise the patient to refrain from coitus or to use barrier methods for at least 4 days. OHSS may progress rapidly (within 24 hours to several days) to become a serious medical event, therefore patients should be followed for at least two weeks after hCG administration.

To minimise the risk of OHSS or of multiple pregnancy, ultrasound scans as well as oestradiol measurements are recommended. In anovulation the risk of OHSS and multiple pregnancy is increased by a serum oestradiol > 900 pg/ml (3300 pmol/l) and more than 3 follicles of 14 mm or more in diameter. In ART there is an increased risk of OHSS with a serum oestradiol > 3000 pg/ml (11000 pmol/l) and 20 or more follicles of 12 mm or more in diameter. When the oestradiol level is > 5500 pg/ml (20200 pmol/l) and where there are 40 or more follicles in total, it may be necessary to withhold hCG administration.

Adherence to recommended GONAL-f dosage, regimen of administration and careful monitoring of therapy will minimise the incidence of ovarian hyperstimulation and multiple pregnancy (see Sections 4.2 and 4.8).

In ART, aspiration of all follicles prior to ovulation may reduce the occurrence of hyperstimulation.

OHSS may be more severe and more protracted if pregnancy occurs. Most often, OHSS occurs after hormonal treatment has been discontinued and reaches its maximum at about seven to ten days following treatment. Usually, OHSS resolves spontaneously with the onset of menses.

If severe OHSS occurs, gonadotrophin treatment should be stopped if still ongoing, the patient hospitalised and specific therapy for OHSS started.

This syndrome occurs with higher incidence in patients with polycystic ovarian disease.

Multiple pregnancy

Multiple pregnancy, specially high order, carries an increased risk in adverse maternal and perinatal outcomes.

In patients undergoing ovulation induction with GONAL-f, the incidence of multiple pregnancies is increased as compared with natural conception. The majority of multiple conceptions are twins. To minimise the risk of multiple pregnancy, careful monitoring of ovarian response is recommended.

In patients undergoing ART procedures the risk of multiple pregnancy is related mainly to the number of embryos replaced, their quality and the patient age.

The patients should be advised of the potential risk of multiple births before starting treatment.

Pregnancy wastage

The incidence of pregnancy wastage by miscarriage or abortion is higher in patients undergoing stimulation of follicular growth for ovulation induction or ART than in the normal population.

Ectopic pregnancy

Women with a history of tubal disease are at risk of ectopic pregnancy, whether the pregnancy is obtained by spontaneous conception or with fertility treatments. The prevalence of ectopic pregnancy after IVF was reported to be 2 to 5%, as compared to 1 to 1.5% in the general population.

Reproductive system neoplasms

There have been reports of ovarian and other reproductive system neoplasms, both benign and malignant, in women who have undergone multiple drug regimens for infertility treatment. It is not yet established whether or not treatment with gonadotropins increases the baseline risk of these tumors in infertile women.

Congenital malformation

The prevalence of congenital malformations after ART may be slightly higher than after spontaneous conceptions. This is thought to be due to differences in parental characteristics (e.g. maternal age, sperm characteristics) and multiple pregnancies.

Thromboembolic events

In women with generally recognised risk factors for thrombo-embolic events, such as personal or family history, treatment with gonadotrophins may further increase the risk. In these women, the benefits of gonadotrophin administration need to be weighed against the risks. It should be noted however, that pregnancy itself also carries an increased risk of thrombo-embolic events.

Treatment in men

Elevated endogenous FSH levels are indicative of primary testicular failure. Such patients are unresponsive to GONAL-f/hCG therapy.

Semen analysis is recommended 4 to 6 months after the beginning of treatment as part of the assessment of the response.

4.5 Interaction with other medicinal products and other forms of Interaction

Concomitant use of GONAL-f with other agents used to stimulate ovulation (e.g. hCG, clomiphene citrate) may potentiate the follicular response, whereas concurrent use of a GnRH agonist or antagonist to induce pituitary desensitisation may increase the dosage of GONAL-f needed to elicit an adequate ovarian response. No other clinically significant drug interaction has been reported during GONAL-f therapy.

4.6 Pregnancy and lactation

Use during pregnancy

There is no indication for use of GONAL-f during pregnancy. No teratogenic risk has been reported, following controlled ovarian hyperstimulation, in clinical use with gonadotrophins. In case of exposure during pregnancy, clinical data are not sufficient to exclude a teratogenic effect of recombinant hFSH. However, to date, no particular malformative effect has been reported. No teratogenic effect has been observed in animal studies.

Use during lactation

GONAL-f is not indicated during lactation. During lactation, the secretion of prolactin can entail a poor prognosis to ovarian stimulation.

4.7 Effects on ability to drive and use machines

No studies on the effects on ability to drive and use machines have been performed.

4.8 Undesirable effects

Treatment in women

Very Common > 1/10)

• Ovarian cysts;

• Mild to severe injection site reaction (pain, redness, bruising, swelling and/or irritation at the site of injection);

• Headache.

Common >1/100, <1/10)

• Mild to moderate OHSS (see section 4.4);

• Abdominal pain and gastrointestinal symptoms such as nausea, vomiting, diarrhoea, abdominal cramps and bloating.

Uncommon >1/1000, <1/100)

• Severe OHSS (see section 4.4).

Rare >1/10 000, <1/1000)

• Ovarian torsion, a complication of OHSS

Very rare (< 1/10 000)

• Thromboembolism, usually associated with severe OHSS;

• Mild systemic allergic reactions (erythema, rash or facial swelling).

Treatment in men

Common >1/100, <1/10)

• Gynaecomastia, acne and weight gain.

4.9 Overdose

The effects of an overdose of GONAL-f are unknown, nevertheless one could expect ovarian hyperstimulation syndrome to occur (see section 4.4).

5. PHARMACOLOGICAL PROPERTIES

5.1 Pharmacodynamic properties

Pharmacotherapeutic group: gonadotrophins, ATC code: G03GA05.

GONAL-f is a preparation of follicle stimulating hormone produced by genetically engineered Chinese Hamster Ovary (CHO) cells.

In women, the most important effect resulting from parenteral administration of FSH is the development of mature Graafian follicles.

In clinical trials, patients with severe FSH and LH deficiency were defined by an endogenous serum LH level <1.2 IU/l as measured in a central laboratory. However, it should be taken into account that there are variations between LH measurements performed in different laboratories.

In men deficient in FSH, GONAL-f administered concomitantly with hCG for at least 4 months induces spermatogenesis.

5.2 Pharmacokinetic properties

Following intravenous administration, follitropin alfa is distributed to the extracellular fluid space with an initial half-life of around 2 hours and eliminated from the body with a terminal half-life of about one day. The steady state volume of distribution and total clearance are 10 L and 0.6 L/h, respectively. One-eighth of the follitropin alfa dose is excreted in the urine.

Following subcutaneous administration, the absolute bioavailability is about 70%. Following repeated administration, follitropin alfa accumulates 3-fold achieving asteady-state within 3-4 days. In women whose endogenous gonadotrophin secretion is suppressed, follitropin alfa has nevertheless been shown to effectively stimulate follicular development and steroidogenesis, despite unmeasurable LH levels.

5.3 Preclinical safety data

In an extensive range of toxicological, mutagenicity and animal studies (dogs, rats, monkeys), acute and chronic (up to 13 weeks and 52 weeks), no significant findings were observed.

Impaired fertility has been reported in rats exposed to pharmacological doses of follitropin alfa (⩾ 40 IU/kg/day) for extended periods, through reduced fecundity.

Given in high doses (5 IU/kg/day) follitropin alfa caused a decrease in the number of viable foetuses without being a teratogen, and dystocia similar to that observed with urinary hMG. However, since GONAL-F is not indicated in pregnancy, these data are of limited clinical relevance.

6. PHARMACEUTICAL PARTICULARS

6.1 List of excipients

Poloxamer 188

Sucrose

Methionine

Sodium dihydrogen phosphate monohydrate

Disodium phosphate dihydrate

m-Cresol

Phosphoric acid, concentrated

Sodium hydroxide

Water for Injections

6.2 Incompatibilities

Not applicable.

6.3 Shelf life

2 year.

After first use: 28 days (within the 2 year shelf-life)

6.4 Special precautions for storage

Store at 2°C - 8°C (in a refrigerator). Do not freeze.

Within its shelf-life, the product may be stored at or below 25°C for up to 28 days and must be discarded if not used.

Store in the original package in order to protect from light.

6.5 Nature and contents of container

0.5ml of solution for injection in 3ml cartridge (Type I glass), with a plunger stopper (halobutyl rubber) and a crimp cap (halobutyl rubber).

Pack of one pre-filled pen and 5 needles to be used with the pen for administration.

6.6 Instructions for use and handling

The solution should not be administered if it contains particles or is not clear.

Any unused solution must be discarded not later than 28 days after first opening.

GONAL-f 300IU/0.5ml (22 micrograms/0.5ml) is not designed to allow the cartridge to be removed.

Discard used needles immediately after injection.

Any unused product or waste material should be disposed of in accordance with local requirements.

7. MARKETING AUTHORISATION HOLDER

SERONO EUROPE LIMITED

56 Marsh Wall

London E14 9TP

United Kingdom

8. MARKETING AUTHORISATION NUMBER(S)

EU/1/95/001/033

9. DATE OF FIRST AUTHORISATION/RENEWAL OF THE AUTHORISATION

23rd February 2004

10. DATE OF REVISION OF THE TEXT

29th June 2004

LEGAL STATUS

POM

NAME AND ADDRESS OF DISTRIBUTOR IN UK

Serono Limited

Bedfont Cross

Stanwell Road

Feltham

Middlesex

TW14 8NX

NAME AND ADDRESS OF DISTRIBUTOR IN IRELAND

Allphar Services Limited

Pharmaceutical Agents and Distributors

Belgard Road

Tallaght

Dublin 24

GONAL-f 450 IU (33 mcg) pen

(Serono Ltd)

1. NAME OF THE MEDICINAL PRODUCT

GONAL-f 450 IU/0.75ml (33 micrograms/0.75ml), solution for injection in a pre-filled pen.

2. QUALITATIVE AND QUANTITATIVE COMPOSITION

Follitropin alfa*, 600IU/ml (equivalent to 44 micrograms/ml).

Each cartridge delivers 450IU (equivalent to 33 micrograms/ml) in 0.75ml.

*Follitropin alfa is recombinant human follicle stimulating hormone (FSH) produced by recombinant DNA technology in Chinese Hamster Ovary (CHO) cell line.

For excipients, see 6.1.

3. PHARMACEUTICAL FORM

Solution for injection in a pre-filled pen.

Clear colourless solution.

4. CLINICAL PARTICULARS

4.1 Therapeutic indications

• Anovulation (including polycystic ovarian disease, PCOD) in women who have been unresponsive to treatment with clomiphene citrate.

• Stimulation of multifollicular development in patients undergoing superovulation for assisted reproductive technologies (ART) such as *in vitro* fertilisation (IVF), gamete intra-fallopian transfer (GIFT) and zygote intra-fallopian transfer (ZIFT).

• GONAL-f in association with a luteinising hormone (LH) preparation is recommended for the stimulation of follicular development in women with severe LH and FSH deficiency. In clinical trials these patients were defined by an endogenous serum LH level <1.2 IU/l.

• GONAL-f is indicated for the stimulation of spermatogenesis in men who have congenital or acquired hypogonadotrophic hypogonadism with concomitant human Chorionic Gonadotrophin (hCG) therapy.

4.2 Posology and method of administration

Treatment with GONAL-f should be initiated under the supervision of a physician experienced in the treatment of fertility problems.

GONAL-f is intended for subcutaneous administration.

The dosage recommendations given for GONAL-f are those in use for urinary FSH. Clinical assessment of GONAL-f indicates that its daily doses, regimens of administration, and treatment monitoring procedures should not be different from those currently used for urinary FSH-containing preparations. However, when these doses were used in a clinical study comparing GONAL-f and urinary FSH, GONAL-f was more effective than urinary FSH in terms of a lower total dose and a shorter treatment period needed to achieve pre-ovulatory conditions. Bioequivalence has been demonstrated between equivalent doses of the monodose presentation and the multidose presentation of GONAL-f. It is advised to adhere to the recommended starting doses indicated below.

Women with anovulation (including PCOD):

The object of GONAL-f therapy is to develop a single mature Graafian follicle from which the ovum will be liberated after the administration of hCG.

GONAL-f may be given as a course of daily injections. In menstruating patients treatment should commence within the first 7 days of the menstrual cycle.

Treatment should be tailored to the individual patient's response as assessed by measuring follicle size by ultrasound and/or oestrogen secretion. A commonly used regimen commences at 75-150 IU FSH daily and is increased preferably by 37.5 IU, or 75 IU at 7 or preferably 14 day intervals if necessary, to obtain an adequate, but not excessive, response. The maximal daily dose is usually not higher than 225 IU FSH. If a patient fails to respond adequately after 4 weeks of treatment, that cycle should be abandoned and the patient should recommence treatment at a higher starting dose than in the abandoned cycle.

When an optimal response is obtained, a single injection of 250 micrograms r-hCG or 5 000 IU, up to 10 000 IU hCG should be administered 24-48 hours after the last GONAL-f injection. The patient is recommended to have coitus on the day of, and the day following, hCG administration. Alternatively intrauterine insemination (IUI) may be performed.

If an excessive response is obtained, treatment should be stopped and hCG withheld (see section 4.4). Treatment should recommence in the next cycle at a dosage lower than that of the previous cycle.

Women undergoing ovarian stimulation for multiple follicular development prior to *in vitro* fertilisation or other assisted reproductive technologies:

A commonly used regimen for superovulation involves the administration of 150-225 IU of GONAL-f daily, commencing on days 2 or 3 of the cycle. Treatment is continued until adequate follicular development has been achieved (as assessed by monitoring of serum oestrogen concentrations and/or ultrasound examination), with the dose adjusted according to the patient's response, to usually not higher than 450 IU daily. In general adequate follicular development is achieved on average by the tenth day of treatment (range 5 to 20 days).

A single injection of 250 micrograms r-hCG or 5 000 IU up to 10 000 IU hCG is administered 24-48 hours after the last GONAL-f injection to induce final follicular maturation.

Down-regulation with a gonadotrophin-releasing hormone (GnRH) agonist or antagonist is now commonly used in order to suppress the endogenous LH surge and to control tonic levels of LH. In a commonly used protocol, GONAL-f is started approximately 2 weeks after the start of agonist treatment, both being continued until adequate follicular development is achieved. For example, following two weeks of treatment with an agonist, 150-225 IU GONAL-f are administered for the first 7 days. The dose is then adjusted according to the ovarian response.

Overall experience with IVF indicates that in general the treatment success rate remains stable during the first four attempts and gradually declines thereafter.

Women with anovulation resulting from severe LH and FSH deficiency

In LH and FSH deficient women (hypogonadotrophic hypogonadism), the objective of GONAL-f therapy in association with lutropin alfa is to develop a single mature Graafian follicle from which the oocyte will be liberated after the administration of human chorionic gonadotrophin (hCG). GONAL-f should be given as a course of daily injections simultaneously with lutropin alfa. Since these patients are amenorrhoeic and have low endogenous oestrogen secretion, treatment can commence at any time.

Treatment should be tailored to the individual patient's response as assessed by measuring follicle size by ultrasound and oestrogen response. A recommended regimen commences at 75 IU of lutropin alfa daily with 75-150 IU FSH.

If an FSH dose increase is deemed appropriate, dose adaptation should preferably be after 7-14 day intervals and preferably by 37.5 IU-75 IU increments. It may be acceptable to extend the duration of stimulation in any one cycle to up to 5 weeks.

When an optimal response is obtained, a single injection of 250 micrograms r-hCG or 5,000 IU up to 10,000 IU hCG should be administered 24-48 hours after the last GONAL-f and lutropin alfa injections. The patient is recommended to have coitus on the day of, and on the day following, hCG administration. Alternatively, intrauterine insemination (IUI) may be performed.

Luteal phase support may be considered since lack of substances with luteotrophic activity (LH/hCG) after ovulation may lead to premature failure of the corpus luteum.

If an excessive response is obtained, treatment should be stopped and hCG withheld. Treatment should recommence in the next cycle at a dose of FSH lower than that of the previous cycle.

Men with hypogonadotrophic hypogonadism.

GONAL-f should be given at a dosage of 150 IU three times a week, concomitantly with hCG, for a minimum of 4 months. If after this period, the patient has not responded, the combination treatment may be continued; current clinical experience indicates that treatment for at least 18 months may be necessary to achieve spermatogenesis.

4.3 Contraindications

Hypersensitivity to follitropin alfa, FSH or to any of the excipients

Tumours of the hypothalamus and pituitary gland

In women:

ovarian enlargement or cyst not due to polycystic ovarian disease

gynaecological haemorrhages of unknown aetiology

ovarian, uterine or mammary carcinoma

Must not be used when an effective response cannot be obtained, such as:

In women:

primary ovarian failure

malformations of sexual organs incompatible with pregnancy

fibroid tumours of the uterus incompatible with pregnancy

In men:

- primary testicular insufficiency

4.4 Special warnings and special precautions for use

GONAL-f is a potent gonadotrophic substance capable of causing mild to severe adverse reactions, and should only be used by physicians who are thoroughly familiar with infertility problems and their management.

Gonadotrophin therapy requires a certain time commitment by physicians and supportive health professionals, as well as the availability of appropriate monitoring facilities. In women, safe and effective use of GONAL-f calls for monitoring of ovarian response with ultrasound, alone or preferably in combination with measurement of serum oestradiol levels, on a regular basis. There may be a degree of interpatient variability in response to FSH administration, with a poor response to FSH in some patients. The lowest effective dose in relation to the treatment objective should be used in both men and women.

Self-administration of GONAL-f should only be performed by patients who are well motivated, adequately trained and have access to expert advice. During training of the patient for self-administration, special attention should be given to specific instructions for the use of the pre-filled pen.

The first injection of GONAL-f should be performed under direct medical supervision.

Treatment in women

Before starting treatment, the couple's infertility should be assessed as appropriate and putative contraindications for pregnancy evaluated. In particular, patients should be evaluated for hypothyroidism, adrenocortical deficiency, hyperprolactinemia and pituitary or hypothalamic tumours, and appropriate specific treatment given.

Patients undergoing stimulation of follicular growth, whether as treatment for anovulatory infertility or ART procedures, may experience ovarian enlargement or develop hyperstimulation. Adherence to the recommended GONAL-f dosage and regimen of administration, and careful monitoring of therapy will minimise the incidence of such events. Acute interpretation of the indices of follicle development and maturation, the physician should be experienced in the interpretation of the relevant tests.

In clinical trials, an increase of the ovarian sensitivity to GONAL-f was shown when administered with lutropin alfa. If an FSH dose increase is deemed appropriate, dose adaptation should preferably be at 7-14 day intervals and preferably with 37.5-75 IU increments.

No direct comparison of GONAL-f/LH versus human menopausal gonadotrophin (hMG) has been performed. Comparison with historical data suggests that the ovulation rate obtained with GONAL-f/LH is similar to that obtained with hMG.

Ovarian Hyperstimulation Syndrome (OHSS)

OHSS is a medical event distinct from uncomplicated ovarian enlargement. OHSS is a syndrome that can manifest itself with increasing degrees of severity. It comprises marked ovarian enlargement, high serum sex steroids, and an increase in vascular permeability which can result in an accumulation of fluid in the peritoneal, pleural and, rarely, in the pericardial cavities.

The following symptomatology may be observed in severe cases of OHSS: abdominal pain, abdominal distension, severe ovarian enlargement, weight gain, dyspnoea, oliguria and gastrointestinal symptoms including nausea, vomiting and diarrhoea. Clinical evaluation may reveal hypovolaemia, haemoconcentration, electrolyte imbalances, ascites, haemoperitoneum, pleural effusions, hydrothorax, acute pulmonary distress, and thromboembolic events.

Excessive ovarian response to gonadotrophin treatment seldom gives rise to OHSS unless hCG is administered to trigger ovulation. Therefore in cases of ovarian hyperstimulation it is prudent to withhold hCG and advise the patient to refrain from coitus or to use barrier methods for at least 4 days. OHSS may progress rapidly (within 24 hours to several days) to become a serious medical event, therefore patients should be followed for at least two weeks after hCG administration.

To minimise the risk of OHSS or of multiple pregnancy, ultrasound scans as well as oestradiol measurements are recommended. In anovulation the risk of OHSS and multiple pregnancy is increased by a serum oestradiol > 900 pg/ml (3300 pmol/l) and more than 3 follicles of 14 mm or more in diameter. In ART there is an increased risk of OHSS with a serum oestradiol > 3000 pg/ml (11000 pmol/l) and 20 or more follicles of 12 mm or more in diameter. When the oestradiol level is > 5500 pg/ml (20200 pmol/l) and where there are 40 or more follicles in total, it may be necessary to withhold hCG administration.

Adherence to recommended GONAL-f dosage, regimen of administration and careful monitoring of therapy will minimise the incidence of ovarian hyperstimulation and multiple pregnancy (see Sections 4.2 and 4.8).

In ART, aspiration of all follicles prior to ovulation may reduce the occurrence of hyperstimulation.

OHSS may be more severe and more protracted if pregnancy occurs. Most often, OHSS occurs after hormonal treatment has been discontinued and reaches its maximum at about seven to ten days following treatment. Usually, OHSS resolves spontaneously with the onset of menses.

If severe OHSS occurs, gonadotrophin treatment should be stopped if still ongoing, the patient hospitalised and specific therapy for OHSS started.

This syndrome occurs with higher incidence in patients with polycystic ovarian disease.

Multiple pregnancy

Multiple pregnancy, specially high order, carries an increased risk in adverse maternal and perinatal outcomes.

In patients undergoing ovulation induction with GONAL-f, the incidence of multiple pregnancies is increased as compared with natural conception. The majority of multiple conceptions are twins. To minimise the risk of multiple pregnancy, careful monitoring of ovarian response is recommended.

In patients undergoing ART procedures the risk of multiple pregnancy is related mainly to the number of embryos replaced, their quality and the patient age.

The patients should be advised of the potential risk of multiple births before starting treatment.

Pregnancy wastage

The incidence of pregnancy wastage by miscarriage or abortion is higher in patients undergoing stimulation of follicular growth for ovulation induction or ART than in the normal population.

Ectopic pregnancy

Women with a history of tubal disease are at risk of ectopic pregnancy, whether the pregnancy is obtained by spontaneous conception or with fertility treatments. The prevalence of ectopic pregnancy after IVF was reported to be 2 to 5%, as compared to 1 to 1.5% in the general population.

Reproductive system neoplasms

There have been reports of ovarian and other reproductive system neoplasms, both benign and malignant, in women who have undergone multiple drug regimens for infertility treatment. It is not yet established whether or not treatment with gonadotropins increases the baseline risk of these tumors in infertile women.

Congenital malformation

The prevalence of congenital malformations after ART may be slightly higher than after spontaneous conceptions. This is thought to be due to differences in parental characteristics (e.g. maternal age, sperm characteristics) and multiple pregnancies.

Thromboembolic events

In women with generally recognised risk factors for thrombo-embolic events, such as personal or family history, treatment with gonadotrophins may further increase the risk. In these women, the benefits of gonadotrophin administration need to be weighed against the risks. It should be noted however, that pregnancy itself also carries an increased risk of thrombo-embolic events.

Treatment in men

Elevated endogenous FSH levels are indicative of primary testicular failure. Such patients are unresponsive to GONAL-f/hCG therapy.

Semen analysis is recommended 4 to 6 months after the beginning of treatment in assessing the response.

4.5 Interaction with other medicinal products and other forms of Interaction
Concomitant use of GONAL-f with other agents used to stimulate ovulation (e.g. hCG, clomiphene citrate) may potentiate the follicular response, whereas concurrent use of a GnRH agonist or antagonist to induce pituitary desensitisation may increase the dosage of GONAL-f needed to elicit an adequate ovarian response. No other clinically significant drug interaction has been reported during GONAL-f therapy.

4.6 Pregnancy and lactation
Use during pregnancy
There is no indication for use of GONAL-f during pregnancy. No teratogenic risk has been reported, following controlled ovarian hyperstimulation, in clinical use with gonadotrophins. In case of exposure during pregnancy, clinical data are not sufficient to exclude a teratogenic effect of recombinant hFSH. However, to date, no particular malformative effect has been reported. No teratogenic effect has been observed in animal studies.

Use during lactation
GONAL-f is not indicated during lactation. During lactation, the secretion of prolactin can entail a poor prognosis to ovarian stimulation.

4.7 Effects on ability to drive and use machines
No studies on the effects on ability to drive and use machines have been performed.

4.8 Undesirable effects
Treatment in women

Very Common > 1/10)

- Ovarian cysts;
- Mild to severe injection site reaction (pain, redness, bruising, swelling and/or irritation at the site of injection);
- Headache.

Common >1/100, <1/10)

- Mild to moderate OHSS (see section 4.4);
- Abdominal pain and gastrointestinal symptoms such as nausea, vomiting, diarrhoea, abdominal cramps and bloating.

Uncommon >1/1000, <1/100)

- Severe OHSS (see section 4.4).

Rare >1/10 000, <1/1000)

- Ovarian torsion, a complication of OHSS

Very rare (< 1/10 000)

- Thromboembolism, usually associated with severe OHSS;
- Mild systemic allergic reactions (erythema, rash or facial swelling).

Treatment in men

Common >1/100, <1/10)

- Gynaecomastia, acne and weight gain.

4.9 Overdose
The effects of an overdose of GONAL-f are unknown, nevertheless one could expect ovarian hyperstimulation syndrome to occur (see section 4.4).

5. PHARMACOLOGICAL PROPERTIES
5.1 Pharmacodynamic properties
Pharmacotherapeutic group: gonadotrophins, ATC code: G03GA05.

GONAL-f is a preparation of follicle stimulating hormone produced by genetically engineered Chinese Hamster Ovary (CHO) cells.

In women, the most important effect resulting from parenteral administration of FSH is the development of mature Graafian follicles.

In clinical trials, patients with severe FSH and LH deficiency were defined by an endogenous serum LH level <1.2 IU/l as measured in a central laboratory. However, it should be taken into account that there are variations between LH measurements performed in different laboratories.

In men deficient in FSH, GONAL-f administered concomitantly with hCG for at least 4 months induces spermatogenesis.

5.2 Pharmacokinetic properties
Following intravenous administration, follitropin alfa is distributed to the extracellular fluid space with an initial half-life of around 2 hours and eliminated from the body with a terminal half-life of about one day. The steady state volume of distribution and total clearance are 10 L and 0.6 L/h, respectively. One-eighth of the follitropin alfa dose is excreted in the urine.

Following subcutaneous administration, the absolute bioavailability is about 70%. Following repeated administration, follitropin alfa accumulates 3-fold achieving asteady-state within 3-4 days. In women whose endogenous gonadotrophin secretion is suppressed, follitropin alfa has nevertheless been shown to effectively stimulate follicular development and steroidogenesis, despite unmeasurable LH levels.

5.3 Preclinical safety data
In an extensive range of toxicological, mutagenicity and animal studies (dogs, rats, monkeys), acute and chronic (up to 13 weeks and 52 weeks), no significant findings were observed.

Impaired fertility has been reported in rats exposed to pharmacological doses of follitropin alfa (≥ 40 IU/kg/day) for extended periods, through reduced fecundity.

Given in high doses (5 IU/kg/day) follitropin alfa caused a decrease in the number of viable foetuses without being a teratogen, and dystocia similar to that observed with urinary hMG. However, since GONAL-F is not indicated in pregnancy, these data are of limited clinical relevance.

6. PHARMACEUTICAL PARTICULARS
6.1 List of excipients
Poloxamer 188

Sucrose

Methionine

Sodium dihydrogen phosphate monohydrate

Disodium phosphate dihydrate

m-Cresol

Phosphoric acid, concentrated

Sodium hydroxide

Water for Injections

6.2 Incompatibilities
Not applicable.

6.3 Shelf life
2 year.

After first use: 28 days (within the 2 year shelf-life)

6.4 Special precautions for storage
Store at 2°C - 8°C (in a refrigerator). Do not freeze.

Within its shelf-life, the product may be stored at or below 25°C for up to 28 days and must be discarded if not used.

Store in the original package in order to protect from light.

6.5 Nature and contents of container
0.75ml of solution for injection in 3ml cartridge (Type I glass), with a plunger stopper (halobutyl rubber) and a crimp cap (halobutyl rubber).

Pack of one pre-filled pen and 7 needles to be used with the pen for administration.

6.6 Instructions for use and handling
The solution should not be administered if it contains particles or is not clear.

Any unused solution must be discarded not later than 28 days after first opening.

GONAL-f 450IU/0.75ml (33 micrograms/0.75ml) is not designed to allow the cartridge to be removed.

Discard used needles immediately after injection.

Any unused product or waste material should be disposed of in accordance with local requirements.

7. MARKETING AUTHORISATION HOLDER
SERONO EUROPE LIMITED

56 Marsh Wall

London E14 9TP

United Kingdom

8. MARKETING AUTHORISATION NUMBER(S)
EU/1/95/001/034

9. DATE OF FIRST AUTHORISATION/RENEWAL OF THE AUTHORISATION
23rd February 2004

10. DATE OF REVISION OF THE TEXT
29th June 2004

LEGAL STATUS
POM

NAME AND ADDRESS OF DISTRIBUTOR IN UK
Serono Limited

Bedfont Cross

Stanwell Road

Feltham

Middlesex

TW14 8NX

NAME AND ADDRESS OF DISTRIBUTOR IN IRELAND
Allphar Services Limited

Pharmaceutical Agents and Distributors

Belgard Road

Tallaght

Dublin 24

GONAL-f 450 IU/0.75 ml (33 mcg/0.75ml)

(Serono Ltd)

1. NAME OF THE MEDICINAL PRODUCT
GONAL-f 450 IU/0.75ml (33 micrograms/0.75ml), powder and solvent for solution for injection.

2. QUALITATIVE AND QUANTITATIVE COMPOSITION
One multidose vial contains 44 micrograms follitropin alfa, recombinant human follicle stimulating hormone (FSH) in order to deliver 33 micrograms, equivalent to 450 IU.

Follitropin alfa is produced in genetically engineered Chinese Hamster Ovary (CHO) cells.

For excipients, see 6.1.

3. PHARMACEUTICAL FORM
Powder and solvent for solution for injection in a pre-filled syringe.

Appearance of the powder: white lyophilised pellet.

Appearance of the solvent: clear colourless solution.

4. CLINICAL PARTICULARS
4.1 Therapeutic indications
Anovulation (including polycystic ovarian disease, PCOD) in women who have been unresponsive to treatment with clomiphene citrate.

Stimulation of multifollicular development in patients undergoing superovulation for assisted reproductive technologies (ART) such as *in vitro* fertilisation (IVF), gamete intra-fallopian transfer (GIFT) and zygote intra-fallopian transfer (ZIFT).

GONAL-f in association with a luteinising hormone (LH) preparation is recommended for the stimulation of follicular development in women with severe LH and FSH deficiency. In clinical trials these patients were defined by an endogenous serum LH level <1.2 IU/l.

GONAL-f is indicated for the stimulation of spermatogenesis in men who have congenital or acquired hypogonadotrophic hypogonadism with concomitant human Chorionic Gonadotrophin (hCG) therapy.

4.2 Posology and method of administration
Treatment with GONAL-f should be initiated under the supervision of a physician experienced in the treatment of fertility problems.

GONAL-f is intended for subcutaneous administration. The powder should be reconstituted prior to the first use with the solvent provided. GONAL-f 450 IU/0.75ml (33 micrograms/0.75ml) preparation must not be reconstituted with any other GONAL-f containers.

The dosage recommendations given for GONAL-f are those in use for urinary FSH. Clinical assessment of GONAL-f indicates that its daily doses, regimens of administration, and treatment monitoring procedures should not be different from those currently used for urinary FSH-containing preparations. However, when these doses were used in a clinical study comparing GONAL-f and urinary FSH, GONAL-f was more effective than urinary FSH in terms of a lower total dose and a shorter treatment period needed to achieve pre-ovulatory conditions. Bioequivalence has been demonstrated between equivalent doses of the monodose presentation and the multidose presentation of GONAL-f. It is advised to adhere to the recommended starting doses indicated below.

Women with anovulation (including PCOD):

The object of GONAL-f therapy is to develop a single mature Graafian follicle from which the ovum will be liberated after the administration of hCG.

GONAL-f may be given as a course of daily injections. In menstruating patients treatment should commence within the first 7 days of the menstrual cycle.

Treatment should be tailored to the individual patient's response as assessed by measuring follicle size by ultrasound and/or oestrogen secretion. A commonly used regimen commences at 75-150 IU FSH daily and is increased preferably by 37.5 IU, or 75 IU at 7 or preferably 14 day intervals if necessary, to obtain an adequate, but not excessive, response. The maximal daily dose is usually not higher than 225 IU FSH. If a patient fails to respond adequately after 4 weeks of treatment, that cycle should be abandoned and the patient should recommence treatment at a higher starting dose than in the abandoned cycle.

When an optimal response is obtained, a single injection of 5 000 IU, up to 10 000 IU hCG should be administered 24-48 hours after the last GONAL-f injection. The patient is recommended to have coitus on the day of, and the day following, hCG administration. Alternatively intrauterine insemination (IUI) may be performed.

If an excessive response is obtained, treatment should be stopped and hCG withheld (see warnings). Treatment should recommence in the next cycle at a dosage lower than that of the previous cycle.

Women undergoing ovarian stimulation for multiple follicular development prior to *in vitro* fertilisation or other assisted reproductive technologies:

A commonly used regimen for superovulation involves the administration of 150-225 IU of GONAL-f daily, commencing on days 2 or 3 of the cycle. Treatment is continued until adequate follicular development has been achieved (as assessed by monitoring of serum oestrogen concentrations and/or ultrasound examination), with the dose adjusted according to the patient's response, to usually not higher than 450 IU daily. In general adequate follicular development is achieved on average by the tenth day of treatment (range 5 to 20 days).

A single injection of up to 10 000 IU hCG is administered 24-48 hours after the last GONAL-f injection to induce final follicular maturation.

Down-regulation with a gonadotrophin-releasing hormone (GnRH) agonist is now commonly used in order to suppress the endogenous LH surge and to control tonic levels of LH.

In a commonly used protocol, GONAL-f is started approximately 2 weeks after the start of agonist treatment, both being continued until adequate follicular development is achieved. For example, following two weeks of treatment with an agonist, 150-225 IU GONAL-f are administered for the first 7 days. The dose is then adjusted according to the ovarian response.

Overall experience with IVF indicates that in general the treatment success rate remains stable during the first four attempts and gradually declines thereafter.

Women with anovulation resulting from severe LH and FSH deficiency

In LH and FSH deficient women (hypogonadotrophic hypogonadism), the objective of GONAL-f therapy in association with lutropin alfa is to develop a single mature Graafian follicle from which the oocyte will be liberated after the administration of human chorionic gonadotrophin (hCG). GONAL-f should be given as a course of daily injections simultaneously with lutropin alfa. Since these patients are amenorrhoeic and have low endogenous oestrogen secretion, treatment can commence at any time.

Treatment should be tailored to the individual patient's response as assessed by measuring follicle size by ultrasound and oestrogen response. A recommended regimen commences at 75 IU of lutropin alfa daily with 75-150 IU FSH.

If an FSH dose increase is deemed appropriate, dose adaptation should preferably be after 7-14 day intervals and preferably by 37.5 IU-75 IU increments. It may be acceptable to extend the duration of stimulation in any one cycle to up to 5 weeks.

When an optimal response is obtained, a single injection of 5,000 IU to 10,000 IU hCG should be administered 24-48 hours after the last GONAL-f and lutropin alfa injections. The patient is recommended to have coitus on the day of, and on the day following, hCG administration. Alternatively, intrauterine insemination (IUI) may be performed.

Luteal phase support may be considered since lack of substances with luteotrophic activity (LH/hCG) after ovulation may lead to premature failure of the corpus luteum.

If an excessive response is obtained, treatment should be stopped and hCG withheld. Treatment should recommence in the next cycle at a dose of FSH lower than that of the previous cycle.

Men with hypogonadotrophic hypogonadism.

GONAL-f should be given at a dosage of 150 IU three times a week, concomitantly with hCG, for a minimum of 4 months. If after this period, the patient has not responded, the combination treatment may be continued; current clinical experience indicates that treatment for at least 18 months may be necessary to achieve spermatogenesis.

4.3 Contraindications

GONAL-f must not be used in:

hypersensitivity to follitropin alfa, FSH or to any of the excipients

case of tumours of the hypothalamus and pituitary gland

and in women:

ovarian enlargement or cyst not due to polycystic ovarian disease

gynaecological haemorrhages of unknown aetiology

ovarian, uterine or mammary carcinoma

GONAL-f should not be used when an effective response cannot be obtained, such as:

In women:

primary ovarian failure

malformations of sexual organs incompatible with pregnancy

fibroid tumours of the uterus incompatible with pregnancy

In men:

primary testicular insufficiency

4.4 Special warnings and special precautions for use

GONAL-f is a potent gonadotrophic substance capable of causing mild to severe adverse reactions, and should only be used by physicians who are thoroughly familiar with infertility problems and their management.

Gonadotrophin therapy requires a certain time commitment by physicians and supportive health professionals, as well as the availability of appropriate monitoring facilities. In women, safe and effective use of GONAL-f calls for monitoring of ovarian response with ultrasound, alone or preferably in combination with measurement of serum oestradiol levels, on a regular basis. There may be a degree of interpatient variability in response to FSH administration, with a poor response to FSH in some patients. The lowest effective dose in relation to the treatment objective should be used in both men and women.

Self-administration of GONAL-f should only be performed by patients who are well motivated, adequately trained and with access to expert advice. During training of the patient for self-administration, special attention should be given to specific instructions for the use of the multidose and/or the monodose presentation(s).

Due to a local reactivity to benzyl alcohol, the same site of injection should not be used on consecutive days.

The first injection of GONAL-f should be performed under direct medical supervision.

Treatment in women

Before starting treatment, the couple's infertility should be assessed as appropriate and putative contraindications for pregnancy evaluated. In particular, patients should be evaluated for hypothyroidism, adrenocortical deficiency, hyperprolactinemia and pituitary or hypothalamic tumours, and appropriate specific treatment given.

Patients undergoing stimulation of follicular growth, whether in the frame of a treatment for anovulatory infertility or ART procedures, may experience ovarian enlargement or develop hyperstimulation. Adherence to recommended GONAL-f dosage and regimen of administration, and careful monitoring of therapy will minimise the incidence of such events. Acute interpretation of the indices of follicle development and maturation require a physician whom is experienced in the interpretation of the relevant tests.

In clinical trials, an increase of the ovarian sensitivity to GONAL-f was shown when administered with lutropin alfa. If an FSH dose increase is deemed appropriate, dose adaptation should preferably be at 7-14 day intervals and preferably with 37.5-75 IU increments.

No direct comparison of GONAL-f/LH versus human menopausal gonadotrophin (hMG) has been performed. Comparison with historical data suggests that the ovulation rate obtained with GONAL-f/LH is similar to what can be obtained with hMG.

Ovarian Hyperstimulation Syndrome (OHSS)

OHSS is a medical event distinct from uncomplicated ovarian enlargement. OHSS is a syndrome that can manifest itself with increasing degrees of severity. It comprises marked ovarian enlargement, high serum sex steroids, and an increase in vascular permeability which can result in an accumulation of fluid in the peritoneal, pleural and, rarely, in the pericardial cavities.

The following symptomatology may be observed in severe cases of OHSS: abdominal pain, abdominal distension, severe ovarian enlargement, weight gain, dyspnoea, oliguria and gastrointestinal symptoms including nausea, vomiting and diarrhoea. Clinical evaluation may reveal hypovolaemia, haemoconcentration, electrolyte imbalances, ascites, haemoperitoneum, pleural effusions, hydrothorax, acute pulmonary distress, and thromboembolic events.

Excessive ovarian response to gonadotrophin treatment seldom gives rise to OHSS unless hCG is administered to trigger ovulation. Therefore in cases of ovarian hyperstimulation it is prudent to withhold hCG and advise the patient to refrain from coitus or to use barrier methods for at least 4 days. OHSS may progress rapidly (within 24 hours to several days) to become a serious medical event, therefore patients should be followed for at least two weeks after hCG administration.

To minimise the risk of OHSS or of multiple pregnancy, ultrasound scans as well as oestradiol measurements are recommended. In anovulation the risk of OHSS and multiple pregnancy is increased by a serum oestradiol > 900 pg/ml (3300 pmol/l) and more than 3 follicles of 14 mm or more in diameter. In ART there is an increased risk of OHSS with a serum oestradiol > 3000 pg/ml (11000 pmol/l) and 20 or more follicles of 12 mm or more in diameter. When the oestradiol level is > 5500 pg/ml (20200 pmol/l) and where there are 40 or more follicles in total, it may be necessary to withhold hCG administration.

Adherence to recommended GONAL-f dosage, regimen of administration and careful monitoring of therapy will minimise the incidence of ovarian hyperstimulation and multiple pregnancy (see Sections 4.2 'Posology and method of administration' and 4.8 'Undesirable effects').

In ART, aspiration of all follicles prior to ovulation may reduce the occurrence of hyperstimulation.

OHSS may be more severe and more protracted if pregnancy occurs. Most often, OHSS occurs after hormonal treatment has been discontinued and reaches its maximum at about seven to ten days following treatment. Usually, OHSS resolves spontaneously with the onset of menses.

If severe OHSS occurs, gonadotrophin treatment should be stopped if still ongoing, the patient hospitalised and specific therapy for OHSS started.

This syndrome occurs with higher incidence in patients with polycystic ovarian disease.

Multiple pregnancy

Multiple pregnancy, specially high order, carries an increase risk in adverse maternal and perinatal outcomes.

In patients undergoing ovulation induction with GONAL-f, the incidence of multiple pregnancies is increased as compared with natural conception. The majority of multiple conceptions are twins. To minimise the risk of multiple pregnancy, careful monitoring of ovarian response is recommended.

In patients undergoing ART procedures the risk of multiple pregnancy is related mainly to the number of embryos replaced, their quality and the patient age.

The patients should be advised of the potential risk of multiple births before starting treatment.

Pregnancy wastage

The incidence of pregnancy wastage by miscarriage or abortion is higher in patients undergoing stimulation of follicular growth for ovulation induction or ART than in the normal population.

Ectopic pregnancy

Women with a history of tubal disease are at risk of ectopic pregnancy, whether the pregnancy is obtained by spontaneous conception or with fertility treatments. The prevalence of ectopic pregnancy after IVF was reported to be 2 to 5%, as compared to 1 to 1.5% in the general population.

Reproductive system neoplasms

There have been reports of ovarian and other reproductive system neoplasms, both benign and malignant, in women who have undergone multiple drug regimens for infertility treatment. It is not yet established whether or not treatment with gonadotropins increases the baseline risk of these tumors in infertile women.

Congenital malformation

The prevalence of congenital malformations after ART may be slightly higher than after spontaneous conceptions. This is thought to be due to differences in parental characteristics (e.g. maternal age, sperm characteristics) and multiple pregnancies.

Thromboembolic events

In women with generally recognised risk factors for thrombo-embolic events, such as personal or family history, treatment with gonadotrophins may further increase the risk. In these women, the benefits of gonadotrophin administration need to be weighed against the risks. It should be noted however, that pregnancy itself also carries an increased risk of thrombo-embolic events.

Treatment in men

Elevated endogenous FSH levels are indicative of primary testicular failure. Such patients are unresponsive to GONAL-f/hCG therapy.

Semen analysis is recommended 4 to 6 months after the beginning of treatment in assessing the response.

4.5 Interaction with other medicinal products and other forms of Interaction

Concomitant use of GONAL-f with other agents used to stimulate ovulation (e.g. hCG, clomiphene citrate) may potentiate the follicular response, whereas concurrent use of a GnRH agonist to induce pituitary desensitisation may increase the dosage of GONAL-f needed to elicit an adequate ovarian response. No other clinically significant drug interaction has been reported during GONAL-f therapy.

GONAL-f should not be administered as mixture with other medicinal products in the same injection.

4.6 Pregnancy and lactation

Use during pregnancy

There is no indication for use of GONAL-f during pregnancy. No teratogenic risk has been reported, following controlled ovarian hyperstimulation, in clinical use with gonadotrophins. In case of exposure during pregnancy, clinical data are not sufficient to exclude a teratogenic effect of recombinant hFSH. However, to date, no particular malformative effect has been reported. No teratogenic effect has been observed in animal studies.

Use during lactation

GONAL-f is not indicated during lactation. During lactation, the secretion of prolactin can entail a poor prognosis to ovarian stimulation.

4.7 Effects on ability to drive and use machines

No studies on the effects on ability to drive and use machines have been performed.

4.8 Undesirable effects

Treatment in women

Very Common (> 1/10)

Ovarian cysts;

Mild to severe injection site reaction (pain, redness, bruising, swelling and/or irritation at the site of injection);

Headache.

Common (1/100 – 1/10)

Mild to moderate OHSS (see section 4.4);

Abdominal pain and gastrointestinal symptoms such as nausea, vomiting, diarrhoea, abdominal cramps and bloating.

Uncommon (1/1000 – 1/100)

Severe OHSS (see section 4.4).

Rare (1/10 000 – 1/1000)

Ovarian torsion, a complication of OHSS

Very rare (< 1/10 000)

Thromboembolism, usually associated with severe OHSS;

Mild systemic allergic reactions (erythema, rash or facial swelling).

Treatment in men

Common (1/100 – 1/10)

Gynaecomastia, acne and weight gain.

4.9 Overdose

The effects of an overdose of GONAL-f are unknown, nevertheless one could expect ovarian hyperstimulation syndrome to occur, which is further described in Special Warnings and Special Precautions for Use.

5. PHARMACOLOGICAL PROPERTIES

5.1 Pharmacodynamic properties

Pharmacotherapeutic group: gonadotrophins, ATC code: G03GA05.

GONAL-f is a preparation of follicle stimulating hormone produced by genetically engineered Chinese Hamster Ovary (CHO) cells.

In women, the most important effect resulting from parenteral administration of FSH is the development of mature Graafian follicles.

In clinical trials, patients with severe FSH and LH deficiency were defined by an endogenous serum LH level <1.2 IU/l as measured in a central laboratory. However, it should be taken into account that there are variations between LH measurements performed in different laboratories.

In men deficient in FSH, GONAL-f administered concomitantly with hCG for at least 4 months induces spermatogenesis.

5.2 Pharmacokinetic properties

Following intravenous administration, GONAL-f is distributed to the extracellular fluid space with an initial half-life of around 2 hours and eliminated from the body with a terminal half-life of about one day. The steady state volume of distribution and total clearance are 10 L and 0.6 L/h, respectively. One-eighth of the GONAL-f dose is excreted in the urine.

Following subcutaneous administration, the absolute bioavailability is about 70%. Following repeated administration, GONAL-f accumulates 3-fold achieving a steady-state within 3-4 days. In women whose endogenous gonadotrophin secretion is suppressed, GONAL-F has nevertheless been shown to effectively stimulate follicular development and steroidogenesis, despite unmeasurable LH levels.

5.3 Preclinical safety data

In an extensive range of toxicological, mutagenicity and animal studies (dogs, rats, monkeys), acute and chronic (up to 13 weeks and 52 weeks), no significant findings were observed.

In rabbits, the formulation reconstituted with 0.9% benzyl alcohol and 0.9% benzyl alcohol alone, both resulted in a slight haemorrhage and subacute inflammation after single subcutaneous injection or mild inflammatory and degenerative changes after single intramuscular injection respectively.

Impaired fertility has been reported in rats exposed to pharmacological doses of follitropin alfa (⩾ 40 IU/kg/day) for extended periods, through reduced fecundity.

Given in high doses (⩾ 5 IU/kg/day) follitropin alfa caused a decrease in the number of viable foetuses without being a teratogen, and dystocia similar to that observed with urinary hMG. However, since GONAL-F is not indicated in pregnancy, these data are of limited clinical relevance.

6. PHARMACEUTICAL PARTICULARS

6.1 List of excipients

Powder:

Sucrose

Sodium dihydrogen phosphate monohydrate

Disodium phosphate dihydrate

Phosphoric acid, concentrated

Sodium hydroxide

Solvent:

Water for Injections

Benzyl alcohol

6.2 Incompatibilities

In the absence of incompatibility studies, this medicinal product must not be mixed with other medicinal products.

6.3 Shelf life

2 years.

The reconstituted solution is stable for 28 days

Do not store above 25°C. Do not freeze.

6.4 Special precautions for storage

Prior to reconstitution, do not store above 25°C. Store in the original package.

After reconstitution, do not store above 25°C. Do not freeze. Store in the original container.

6.5 Nature and contents of container

GONAL-f is presented as a powder and solvent for injection. The powder is presented in 3ml vials (Type I glass), with rubber stopper (bromobutyl rubber) and aluminium flip-off cap. The solvent for reconstitution is presented in 1ml pre-filled syringes (Type I glass) with a rubber stopper. The Administration syringes made of polypropylene with a stainless steel pre-fixed needle are also provided.

The product is supplied as a pack of 1 vial of powder with 1 pre-filled syringe of solvent for reconstitution and 6 disposable syringes for administration graduated in FSH units.

6.6 Instructions for use and handling

GONAL-f 450 IU/0.75ml (33 micrograms/0.75ml) must be reconstituted with the 1 ml solvent provided before use. GONAL-f 450 IU/0.75ml (33 micrograms/0.75ml) preparation must not be reconstituted with any other GONAL-f containers.

The solvent pre-filled syringe provided should be used for reconstitution only and then disposed of in accordance with local requirements. A set of administration syringes graduated in FSH units is supplied in the GONAL-f Multidose box. Alternatively, a 1 ml syringe, graduated in ml, with pre-fixed needle for subcutaneous administration could be used. Each ml of reconstituted solution contains 600 IU r-hFSH.

The following table states the volume to be administered to deliver the prescribed dose:

Dose (IU)	Volume to be injected (ml)
75	0.13
150	0.25
225	0.38
300	0.50
375	0.63
450	0.75

Individual reconstituted vials should be for single patient use only. The patient should reconstitute the product and inject it immediately. The next injection should be done at the same time the next day.

The reconstituted solution should not be administered if it contains particles or is not clear.

7. MARKETING AUTHORISATION HOLDER

SERONO EUROPE LIMITED

56 Marsh Wall

London E14 9TP

United Kingdom

8. MARKETING AUTHORISATION NUMBER(S)

EU/1/95/001/031

9. DATE OF FIRST AUTHORISATION/RENEWAL OF THE AUTHORISATION

7 June 2002

10. DATE OF REVISION OF THE TEXT

2nd October 2002

LEGAL STATUS

POM

NAME AND ADDRESS OF DISTRIBUTOR IN UK

Serono Limited

Bedfont Cross

Stanwell Road

Feltham

Middlesex

TW14 8NX

NAME AND ADDRESS OF DISTRIBUTOR IN IRELAND

Allphar Services Limited

Pharmaceutical Agents and Distributors

Belgard Road

Tallaght

Dublin 24

GONAL-f 75 IU (5.5 micrograms)

(Serono Ltd)

1. NAME OF THE MEDICINAL PRODUCT

GONAL-f 75 IU (5.5 micrograms), powder and solvent for solution for injection.

2. QUALITATIVE AND QUANTITATIVE COMPOSITION

One vial contains 6 micrograms follitropin alfa, recombinant human follicle stimulating hormone (FSH) in order to deliver 5.5 micrograms, equivalent to 75 IU. The reconstituted solution contains 75 IU/ml. Follitropin alfa is produced in genetically engineered Chinese Hamster Ovary (CHO) cells.

For excipients, see 6.1.

3. PHARMACEUTICAL FORM

Powder and solvent for solution for injection.

Appearance of the powder: white lyophilised pellet.

Appearance of the solvent: clear colourless solution.

4. CLINICAL PARTICULARS

4.1 Therapeutic indications

Anovulation (including polycystic ovarian disease, PCOD) in women who have been unresponsive to treatment with clomiphene citrate.

Stimulation of multifollicular development in patients undergoing superovulation for assisted reproductive technologies (ART) such as *in vitro* fertilisation (IVF), gamete intra-fallopian transfer (GIFT) and zygote intra-fallopian transfer (ZIFT).

GONAL-f in association with a luteinising hormone (LH) preparation is recommended for the stimulation of follicular development in women with severe LH and FSH deficiency. In clinical trials these patients were defined by an endogenous serum LH level <1.2 IU/l.

GONAL-f is indicated for the stimulation of spermatogenesis in men who have congenital or acquired hypogonadotrophic hypogonadism with concomitant human Chorionic Gonadotrophin (hCG) therapy.

4.2 Posology and method of administration

Treatment with GONAL-f should be initiated under the supervision of a physician experienced in the treatment of fertility problems.

GONAL-f is intended for subcutaneous administration. The powder should be reconstituted immediately prior to use with the solvent provided. In order to avoid the injection of large volumes, up to 3 vials of product may be dissolved in 1 ml of solvent.

The dosage recommendations given for GONAL-f are those in use for urinary FSH. Clinical assessment of GONAL-f indicates that its daily doses, regimens of administration, and treatment monitoring procedures should not be different from those currently used for urinary FSH-containing preparations. However, when these doses were used in a clinical study comparing GONAL-f and urinary FSH, GONAL-f was more effective than urinary FSH in terms of a lower total dose and a shorter treatment period needed to achieve pre-ovulatory conditions. It is advised to adhere to the recommended starting doses indicated below.

Women with anovulation (including PCOD):

The object of GONAL-f therapy is to develop a single mature Graafian follicle from which the ovum will be liberated after the administration of hCG.

GONAL-f may be given as a course of daily injections. In menstruating patients treatment should commence within the first 7 days of the menstrual cycle.

Treatment should be tailored to the individual patient's response as assessed by measuring follicle size by ultrasound and/or oestrogen secretion. A commonly used regimen commences at 75-150 IU FSH daily and is increased preferably by 37.5 IU, or 75 IU at 7 or preferably 14 day intervals if necessary, to obtain an adequate, but not excessive, response. The maximal daily dose is usually not higher than 225 IU FSH. If a patient fails to respond adequately after 4 weeks of treatment, that cycle should be abandoned and the patient should recommence treatment at a higher starting dose than in the abandoned cycle.

When an optimal response is obtained, a single injection of 5 000 IU, up to 10 000 IU hCG should be administered 24-48 hours after the last GONAL-f injection. The patient is recommended to have coitus on the day of, and the day following, hCG administration. Alternatively intrauterine insemination (IUI) may be performed.

If an excessive response is obtained, treatment should be stopped and hCG withheld (see warnings). Treatment should recommence in the next cycle at a dosage lower than that of the previous cycle.

Women undergoing ovarian stimulation for multiple follicular development prior to *in vitro* fertilisation or other assisted reproductive technologies:

A commonly used regimen for superovulation involves the administration of 150-225 IU of GONAL-f daily, commencing on days 2 or 3 of the cycle. Treatment is continued until adequate follicular development has been achieved (as assessed by monitoring of serum oestrogen concentrations and/or ultrasound examination), with the dose adjusted according to the patient's response, to usually not higher than 450 IU daily. In general adequate follicular development is achieved on average by the tenth day of treatment (range 5 to 20 days).

A single injection of up to 10 000 IU hCG is administered 24-48 hours after the last GONAL-f injection to induce final follicular maturation.

Down-regulation with a gonadotrophin-releasing hormone (GnRH) agonist is now commonly used in order to suppress the endogenous LH surge and to control tonic levels of LH. In a commonly used protocol, GONAL-f is started approximately 2 weeks after the start of agonist treatment, both being continued until adequate follicular development is achieved. For example, following two weeks of treatment with an agonist, 150-225 IU GONAL-f are administered for the first 7 days. The dose is then adjusted according to the ovarian response.

Overall experience with IVF indicates that in general the treatment success rate remains stable during the first four attempts and gradually declines thereafter.

Women with anovulation resulting from severe LH and FSH deficiency

In LH and FSH deficient women (hypogonadotrophic hypogonadism), the objective of GONAL-f therapy in association with lutropin alfa is to develop a single mature Graafian follicle from which the oocyte will be liberated after the administration of human chorionic gonadotrophin (hCG). GONAL-f should be given as a course of daily injections simultaneously with lutropin alfa. Since these patients are amenorrhoeic and have low endogenous oestrogen secretion, treatment can commence at any time.

Treatment should be tailored to the individual patient's response as assessed by measuring follicle size by ultrasound and oestrogen response. A recommended regimen commences at 75 IU of lutropin alfa daily with 75-150 IU FSH.

If an FSH dose increase is deemed appropriate, dose adaptation should preferably be after 7-14 day intervals and preferably by 37.5 IU-75 IU increments. It may be acceptable to extend the duration of stimulation in any one cycle to up to 5 weeks.

When an optimal response is obtained, a single injection of 5,000 IU to 10,000 IU hCG should be administered 24-48 hours after the last GONAL-f and lutropin alfa injections. The patient is recommended to have coitus on the day of, and on the day following, hCG administration.

Alternatively, intrauterine insemination (IUI) may be performed.

Luteal phase support may be considered since lack of substances with luteotrophic activity (LH/hCG) after ovulation may lead to premature failure of the corpus luteum.

If an excessive response is obtained, treatment should be stopped and hCG withheld. Treatment should recommence in the next cycle at a dose of FSH lower than that of the previous cycle.

Men with hypogonadotrophic hypogonadism.

GONAL-f should be given at a dosage of 150 IU three times a week, concomitantly with hCG, for a minimum of 4 months. If after this period, the patient has not responded, the combination treatment may be continued; current clinical experience indicates that treatment for at least 18 months may be necessary to achieve spermatogenesis.

4.3 Contraindications

GONAL-f must not be used in:

hypersensitivity to follitropin alfa, FSH or to any of the excipients

case of tumours of the hypothalamus and pituitary gland

and in women:

ovarian enlargement or cyst not due to polycystic ovarian disease

gynaecological haemorrhages of unknown aetiology

ovarian, uterine or mammary carcinoma

GONAL-f should not be used when an effective response cannot be obtained, such as:

In women:

primary ovarian failure

malformations of sexual organs incompatible with pregnancy

fibroid tumours of the uterus incompatible with pregnancy

In men:

primary testicular insufficiency

4.4 Special warnings and special precautions for use

GONAL-f is a potent gonadotropic substance capable of causing mild to severe adverse reactions, and should only be used by physicians who are thoroughly familiar with infertility problems and their management.

Gonadotropin therapy requires a certain time commitment by physicians and supportive health professionals, as well as the availability of appropriate monitoring facilities. In women, safe and effective use of GONAL-f calls for monitoring of ovarian response with ultrasound, alone or preferably in combination with measurement of serum oestradiol levels, on a regular basis. There may be a degree of interpatient variability in response to FSH administration, with a poor response to FSH in some patients. The lowest effective dose in relation to the treatment objective should be used in both men and women.

Self-administration of GONAL-f should only be performed by patients who are well motivated, adequately trained and with access to expert advice.

The first injection of GONAL-f should be performed under direct medical supervision.

Treatment in women

Before starting treatment, the couple's infertility should be assessed as appropriate and putative contraindications for pregnancy evaluated. In particular, patients should be evaluated for hypothyroidism, adrenocortical deficiency, hyperprolactinemia and pituitary or hypothalamic tumours, and appropriate specific treatment given.

Patients undergoing stimulation of follicular growth, whether in the frame of a treatment for anovulatory infertility or ART procedures, may experience ovarian enlargement or develop hyperstimulation. Adherence to recommended GONAL-f dosage and regimen of administration, and careful monitoring of therapy will minimise the incidence of such events. Acute interpretation of the indices of follicle development and maturation require a physician whom is experienced in the interpretation of the relevant tests.

In clinical trials, an increase of the ovarian sensitivity to GONAL-f was shown when administered with lutropin alfa. If an FSH dose increase is deemed appropriate, dose adaptation should preferably be at 7-14 day intervals and preferably with 37.5-75 IU increments.

No direct comparison of GONAL-f/LH versus human menopausal gonadotrophin (hMG) has been performed. Comparison with historical data suggests that the ovulation rate obtained with GONAL-f/LH is similar to what can be obtained with hMG.

Ovarian Hyperstimulation Syndrome (OHSS)

OHSS is a medical event distinct from uncomplicated ovarian enlargement. OHSS is a syndrome that can manifest itself with increasing degrees of severity. It comprises marked ovarian enlargement, high serum sex steroids, and an increase in vascular permeability which can result in an accumulation of fluid in the peritoneal, pleural and, rarely, in the pericardial cavities.

The following symptomatology may be observed in severe cases of OHSS: abdominal pain, abdominal distension, severe ovarian enlargement, weight gain, dyspnoea, oliguria and gastrointestinal symptoms including nausea, vomiting and diarrhoea. Clinical evaluation may reveal hypovolaemia, haemoconcentration, electrolyte imbalances, ascites, haemoperitoneum, pleural effusions, hydrothorax, acute pulmonary distress, and thromboembolic events.

Excessive ovarian response to gonadotropin treatment seldom gives rise to OHSS unless hCG is administered to trigger ovulation. Therefore in cases of ovarian hyperstimulation it is prudent to withhold hCG and advise the patient to refrain from coitus or to use barrier methods for at least 4 days. OHSS may progress rapidly (within 24 hours to several days) to become a serious medical event, therefore patients should be followed for at least two weeks after hCG administration.

To minimise the risk of OHSS or of multiple pregnancy, ultrasound scans as well as oestradiol measurements are recommended. In anovulation the risk of OHSS and multiple pregnancy is increased by a serum oestradiol > 900 pg/ml (3300 pmol/l) and more than 3 follicles of 14 mm or more in diameter. In ART there is an increased risk of OHSS with a serum oestradiol > 3000 pg/ml (11000 pmol/l) and 20 or more follicles of 12 mm or more in diameter. When the oestradiol level is > 5500 pg/ml (20200 pmol/l) and where there are 40 or more follicles in total, it may be necessary to withhold hCG administration.

Adherence to recommended GONAL-f dosage, regimen of administration and careful monitoring of therapy will minimise the incidence of ovarian hyperstimulation and multiple pregnancy (see Sections 4.2 'Posology and method of administration' and 4.8 'Undesirable effects').

In ART, aspiration of all follicles prior to ovulation may reduce the occurrence of hyperstimulation.

OHSS may be more severe and more protracted if pregnancy occurs. Most often, OHSS occurs after hormonal treatment has been discontinued and reaches its maximum at about seven to ten days following treatment. Usually, OHSS resolves spontaneously with the onset of menses.

If severe OHSS occurs, gonadotrophin treatment should be stopped if still ongoing, the patient hospitalised and specific therapy for OHSS started.

This syndrome occurs with higher incidence in patients with polycystic ovarian disease.

Multiple pregnancy

Multiple pregnancy, specially high order, carries an increase risk in adverse maternal and perinatal outcomes.

In patients undergoing ovulation induction with GONAL-f, the incidence of multiple pregnancies is increased as compared with natural conception. The majority of multiple conceptions are twins. To minimise the risk of multiple pregnancy, careful monitoring of ovarian response is recommended.

In patients undergoing ART procedures the risk of multiple pregnancy is related mainly to the number of embryos replaced, their quality and the patient age.

The patients should be advised of the potential risk of multiple births before starting treatment.

Pregnancy wastage

The incidence of pregnancy wastage by miscarriage or abortion is higher in patients undergoing stimulation of follicular growth for ovulation induction or ART than in the normal population.

Ectopic pregnancy

Women with a history of tubal disease are at risk of ectopic pregnancy, whether the pregnancy is obtained by spontaneous conception or with fertility treatments. The prevalence of ectopic pregnancy after IVF was reported to be 2 to 5%, as compared to 1 to 1.5% in the general population.

Reproductive system neoplasms

There have been reports of ovarian and other reproductive system neoplasms, both benign and malignant, in women who have undergone multiple drug regimens for intertility treatment. It is not yet established whether or not treatment with gonadotrophins increases the baseline risk of these tumors in infertile women.

Congenital malformation

The prevalence of congenital malformations after ART may be slightly higher than after spontaneous conceptions. This is thought to be due to differences in parental characteristics (e.g. maternal age, sperm characteristics) and multiple pregnancies.

Thromboembolic events

In women with generally recognised risk factors for thrombo-embolic events, such as personal or family history, treatment with gonadotrophins may further increase the risk. In these women, the benefits of gonadotrophin administration need to be weighed against the risks. It should be noted however, that pregnancy itself also carries an increased risk of thrombo-embolic events.

Treatment in men

Elevated endogenous FSH levels are indicative of primary testicular failure. Such patients are unresponsive to GONAL-f/hCG therapy.

Semen analysis is recommended 4 to 6 months after the beginning of treatment in assessing the response.

4.5 Interaction with other medicinal products and other forms of Interaction

Concomitant use of GONAL-f with other agents used to stimulate ovulation (e.g. hCG, clomiphene citrate) may potentiate the follicular response, whereas concurrent use of a GnRH agonist to induce pituitary desensitisation may increase the dosage of GONAL-f needed to elicit an adequate ovarian response. No other clinically significant drug interaction has been reported during GONAL-f therapy.

4.6 Pregnancy and lactation

Use during pregnancy

There is no indication for use of GONAL-f during pregnancy. No teratogenic risk has been reported, following controlled ovarian hyperstimulation, in clinical use with gonatrophins. In case of exposure during pregnancy, clinical data are not sufficient to exclude a teratogenic effect of recombinant hFSH. However, to date, no particular malformative effect has been reported. No teratogenic effect has been observed in animal studies.

Use during lactation

GONAL-f is not indicated during lactation. During lactation, the secretion of prolactin can entail a poor prognosis to ovarian stimulation.

4.7 Effects on ability to drive and use machines

No studies on the effects on ability to drive and use machines have been performed.

4.8 Undesirable effects

Treatment in women

Very Common (> 1/10)

Ovarian cysts;

Mild to severe injection site reaction (pain, redness, bruising, swelling and/or irritation at the site of injection);

Headache.

Common (1/100 – 1/10)

Mild to moderate OHSS (see section 4.4);

Abdominal pain and gastrointestinal symptoms such as nausea, vomiting, diarrhoea, abdominal cramps and bloating.

Uncommon (1/1000 – 1/100)

Severe OHSS (see section 4.4).

Rare (1/10 000 – 1/1000)

Ovarian torsion, a complication of OHSS

Very rare (< 1/10 000)

Thromboembolism, usually associated with severe OHSS;

Mild systemic allergic reactions (erythema, rash or facial swelling).

Treatment in men

Common (1/100 – 1/10)

Gynaecomastia, acne and weight gain.

4.9 Overdose

The effects of an overdose of GONAL-f are unknown, nevertheless one could expect ovarian hyperstimulation syndrome to occur, which is further described in Special Warnings and Special Precautions for Use.

5. PHARMACOLOGICAL PROPERTIES

5.1 Pharmacodynamic properties

Pharmacotherapeutic group: gonadotrophins, ATC code: G03GA05.

GONAL-f is a preparation of follicle stimulating hormone produced by genetically engineered Chinese Hamster Ovary (CHO) cells.

In women, the most important effect resulting from parenteral administration of FSH is the development of mature Graafian follicles.

In clinical trials, patients with severe FSH and LH deficiency were defined by an endogenous serum LH level < 1.2 IU/l as measured in a central laboratory. However, it should be taken into account that there are variations between LH measurements performed in different laboratories.

In men deficient in FSH, GONAL-f administered concomitantly with hCG for at least 4 months induces spermatogenesis.

5.2 Pharmacokinetic properties

Following intravenous administration, GONAL-f is distributed to the extra cellular fluid space with an initial half-life of around 2 hours and eliminated from the body with a terminal half-life of about one day. The steady state volume of distribution and total clearance are 10 L and 0.6 L/h, respectively. One-eighth of the GONAL-f dose is excreted in the urine.

Following subcutaneous administration, the absolute bioavailability is about 70%. Following repeated administration, GONAL-f accumulates 3-fold achieving within 3-4 days. In women whose endogenous gonadotrophin a steady-state secretion is suppressed, GONAL-f has nevertheless been shown to effectively stimulate follicular development and steroidogenesis, despite unmeasurable LH levels.

5.3 Preclinical safety data

In an extensive range of toxicological, mutagenicity and animal studies (dogs, rats, monkeys), acute and chronic (up to 13 weeks and 52 weeks), no significant findings were observed.

Impaired fertility has been reported in rats exposed to pharmacological doses of follitropin alfa (≥ 40 IU/kg/day) for extended periods, through reduced fecundity.

Given in high doses (≥ 5 IU/kg/day) follitropin alfa caused a decrease in the number of viable foetuses without being a teratogen, and dystocia similar to that observed with urinary hMG. However, since GONAL-f is not indicated in pregnancy, these data are of limited clinical relevance.

6. PHARMACEUTICAL PARTICULARS

6.1 List of excipients

Powder:

Sucrose

Sodium dihydrogen phosphate monohydrate

Disodium phosphate dihydrate

Methionine

Polysorbate 20

Phosphoric acid, concentrated

Sodium hydroxide

Solvent:

Water for Injections

6.2 Incompatibilities

This medicinal product must not be mixed with other medicinal products except those mentioned in 6.6.

6.3 Shelf life

2 years.

For immediate and single use following first opening and reconstitution.

6.4 Special precautions for storage

Do not store above 25°C.

Store in the original package.

6.5 Nature and contents of container

GONAL-f is presented as a powder and solvent for injection. The powder is presented in 3ml vials (Type I glass), with stopper (bromobutyl rubber) and aluminium flip-off cap. The solvent for reconstitution is presented in either 2ml vials (Type I glass) with stopper (Teflon-coated rubber) or in 1ml pre-filled syringes (Type I glass) with a rubber stopper.

The product is supplied in packs of 1, 3, 5, 10 vials with the corresponding number of solvent vials or packs of 1, 5 or 10 vials with the corresponding number of solvent pre-filled syringes. Not all pack sizes may be marketed.

6.6 Instructions for use and handling

For single use only.

GONAL-f must be reconstituted with the solvent before use.

GONAL-f may be co-reconstituted with lutropin alfa and co-administered as a single injection. In this case lutropin alfa should be reconstituted first and then used to reconstitute GONAL-f powder.

The reconstituted solution should not be administered if it contains particles or is not clear.

Any unused product or waste material should be disposed of in accordance with local requirements.

7. MARKETING AUTHORISATION HOLDER

SERONO EUROPE LIMITED

56 Marsh Wall

London E14 9TP

United Kingdom

8. MARKETING AUTHORISATION NUMBER(S)

EU/1/95/001/005

EU/1/95/001/006

EU/1/95/001/007

EU/1/95/001/008

EU/1/95/001/025

EU/1/95/001/026

EU/1/95/001/027

9. DATE OF FIRST AUTHORISATION/RENEWAL OF THE AUTHORISATION

December 29, 2000.

10. DATE OF REVISION OF THE TEXT

2nd October 2002.

LEGAL STATUS

POM

NAME AND ADDRESS OF DISTRIBUTOR IN UK

Serono Limited

Bedfont Cross

Stanwell Road

Feltham

Middlesex

TW14 8NX

NAME AND ADDRESS OF DISTRIBUTOR IN IRELAND

Allphar Services Limited

Pharmaceutical Agents and Distributors

Belgard Road

Tallaght

Dublin 24

GONAL-f 900 IU (66mcg) pen

(Serono Ltd)

1. NAME OF THE MEDICINAL PRODUCT

GONAL-f 900 IU/1.5ml (66 micrograms/1.5ml), solution for injection in a pre-filled pen.

2. QUALITATIVE AND QUANTITATIVE COMPOSITION

Follitropin alfa*, 600IU/ml (equivalent to 44 micrograms/ml).

Each cartridge delivers 900IU (equivalent to 66 micrograms/ml) in 1.5ml.

*Follitropin alfa is recombinant human follicle stimulating hormone (FSH) produced by recombinant DNA technology in Chinese Hamster Ovary (CHO) cell line.

For excipients, see 6.1.

3. PHARMACEUTICAL FORM

Solution for injection in a pre-filled pen.

Clear colourless solution.

4. CLINICAL PARTICULARS

4.1 Therapeutic indications

• Anovulation (including polycystic ovarian disease, PCOD) in women who have been unresponsive to treatment with clomiphene citrate.

• Stimulation of multifollicular development in patients undergoing superovulation for assisted reproductive technologies (ART) such as *in vitro* fertilisation (IVF), gamete intra-fallopian transfer (GIFT) and zygote intra-fallopian transfer (ZIFT).

• GONAL-f in association with a luteinising hormone (LH) preparation is recommended for the stimulation of follicular development in women with severe LH and FSH deficiency. In clinical trials these patients were defined by an endogenous serum LH level < 1.2 IU/l.

• GONAL-f is indicated for the stimulation of spermatogenesis in men who have congenital or acquired hypogonadotrophic hypogonadism with concomitant human Chorionic Gonadotrophin (hCG) therapy.

4.2 Posology and method of administration

Treatment with GONAL-f should be initiated under the supervision of a physician experienced in the treatment of fertility problems.

GONAL-f is intended for subcutaneous administration.

The dosage recommendations given for GONAL-f are those in use for urinary FSH. Clinical assessment of GONAL-f indicates that its daily doses, regimens of administration, and treatment monitoring procedures should not be different from those currently used for urinary FSH-containing preparations. However, when these doses were used in a clinical study comparing GONAL-f and urinary FSH, GONAL-f was more effective than urinary FSH in terms of a lower total dose and a shorter treatment period needed to achieve pre-ovulatory conditions. Bioequivalence has been demonstrated between equivalent doses of the monodose presentation and the multidose presentation of GONAL-f. It is advised to adhere to the recommended starting doses indicated below.

Women with anovulation (including PCOD):

The object of GONAL-f therapy is to develop a single mature Graafian follicle from which the ovum will be liberated after the administration of hCG.

GONAL-f may be given as a course of daily injections. In menstruating patients treatment should commence within the first 7 days of the menstrual cycle.

Treatment should be tailored to the individual patient's response as assessed by measuring follicle size by ultrasound and/or oestrogen secretion. A commonly used regimen commences at 75-150 IU FSH daily and is increased preferably by 37.5 IU, or 75 IU at 7 or preferably 14 day intervals if necessary, to obtain an adequate, but not excessive, response. The maximal daily dose is usually not higher than 225 IU FSH. If a patient fails to respond adequately after 4 weeks of treatment, that cycle should be abandoned and the patient should recommence treatment at a higher starting dose than in the abandoned cycle.

When an optimal response is obtained, a single injection of 250 micrograms r-hCG or 5 000 IU, up to 10 000 IU hCG should be administered 24-48 hours after the last GONAL-f injection. The patient is recommended to have coitus on the day of, and the day following, hCG administration. Alternatively intrauterine insemination (IUI) may be performed.

If an excessive response is obtained, treatment should be stopped and hCG withheld (see section 4.4). Treatment should recommence in the next cycle at a dosage lower than that of the previous cycle.

Women undergoing ovarian stimulation for multiple follicular development prior to *in vitro* fertilisation or other assisted reproductive technologies:

A commonly used regimen for superovulation involves the administration of 150-225 IU of GONAL-f daily, commencing on days 2 or 3 of the cycle. Treatment is continued until adequate follicular development has been achieved (as assessed by monitoring of serum oestrogen concentrations and/or ultrasound examination), with the dose adjusted according to the patient's response, to usually not higher than 450 IU daily. In general adequate follicular development is achieved on average by the tenth day of treatment (range 5 to 20 days).

A single injection of 250 micrograms r-hCG or 5 000 IU up to 10 000 IU hCG is administered 24-48 hours after the last GONAL-f injection to induce final follicular maturation.

Down-regulation with a gonadotrophin-releasing hormone (GnRH) agonist or antagonist is now commonly used in order to suppress the endogenous LH surge and to control tonic levels of LH. In a commonly used protocol, GONAL-f is started approximately 2 weeks after the start of agonist treatment, both being continued until adequate follicular development is achieved. For example, following two weeks of treatment with an agonist, 150-225 IU GONAL-f are administered for the first 7 days. The dose is then adjusted according to the ovarian response.

Overall experience with IVF indicates that in general the treatment success rate remains stable during the first four attempts and gradually declines thereafter.

Women with anovulation resulting from severe LH and FSH deficiency

In LH and FSH deficient women (hypogonadotrophic hypogonadism), the objective of GONAL-f therapy in association with lutropin alfa is to develop a single mature Graafian follicle from which the oocyte will be liberated after the administration of human chorionic gonadotrophin (hCG). GONAL-f should be given as a course of daily injections simultaneously with lutropin alfa. Since these patients are amenorrhoeic and have low endogenous oestrogen secretion, treatment can commence at any time.

Treatment should be tailored to the individual patient's response as assessed by measuring follicle size by ultrasound and oestrogen response. A recommended regimen commences at 75 IU of lutropin alfa daily with 75-150 IU FSH.

If an FSH dose increase is deemed appropriate, dose adaptation should preferably be after 7-14 day intervals and preferably by 37.5 IU-75 IU increments. It may be acceptable to extend the duration of stimulation in any one cycle to up to 5 weeks.

When an optimal response is obtained, a single injection of 250 micrograms r-hCG or 5,000 IU up to 10,000 IU hCG should be administered 24-48 hours after the last GONAL-f and lutropin alfa injections. The patient is recommended to have coitus on the day of, and on the day following, hCG administration. Alternatively, intrauterine insemination (IUI) may be performed.

Luteal phase support may be considered since lack of substances with luteotrophic activity (LH/hCG) after ovulation may lead to premature failure of the corpus luteum.

If an excessive response is obtained, treatment should be stopped and hCG withheld. Treatment should recommence in the next cycle at a dose of FSH lower than that of the previous cycle.

Men with hypogonadotrophic hypogonadism.

GONAL-f should be given at a dosage of 150 IU three times a week, concomitantly with hCG, for a minimum of 4 months. If after this period, the patient has not responded, the combination treatment may be continued; current clinical experience indicates that treatment for at least 18 months may be necessary to achieve spermatogenesis.

4.3 Contraindications

Hypersensitivity to follitropin alfa, FSH or to any of the excipients

Tumours of the hypothalamus and pituitary gland

In women:

ovarian enlargement or cyst not due to polycystic ovarian disease

gynaecological haemorrhages of unknown aetiology

ovarian, uterine or mammary carcinoma

Must not be used when an effective response cannot be obtained, such as:

In women:

primary ovarian failure

malformations of sexual organs incompatible with pregnancy

fibroid tumours of the uterus incompatible with pregnancy

In men:

• primary testicular insufficiency

4.4 Special warnings and special precautions for use

GONAL-f is a potent gonadotrophic substance capable of causing mild to severe adverse reactions, and should only be used by physicians who are thoroughly familiar with infertility problems and their management.

Gonadotrophin therapy requires a certain time commitment by physicians and supportive health professionals, as well as the availability of appropriate monitoring facilities. In women, safe and effective use of GONAL-f calls for monitoring of ovarian response with ultrasound, alone or preferably in combination with measurement of serum oestradiol levels, on a regular basis. There may be a degree of interpatient variability in response to FSH administration, with a poor response to FSH in some patients. The lowest effective dose in relation to the treatment objective should be used in both men and women.

Self-administration of GONAL-f should only be performed by patients who are well motivated, adequately trained and have access to expert advice. During training of the patient for self-administration, special attention should be given to specific instructions for the use of the pre-filled pen.

The first injection of GONAL-f should be performed under direct medical supervision.

Treatment in women

Before starting treatment, the couple's infertility should be assessed as appropriate and putative contraindications for pregnancy evaluated. In particular, patients should be evaluated for hypothyroidism, adrenocortical deficiency, hyperprolactinemia and pituitary or hypothalamic tumours, and appropriate specific treatment given.

Patients undergoing stimulation of follicular growth, whether as treatment for anovulatory infertility or ART procedures, may experience ovarian enlargement or develop hyperstimulation. Adherence to the recommended GONAL-f dosage and regimen of administration, and careful monitoring of therapy will minimise the incidence of such events. Acute interpretation of the indices of follicle development and maturation, the physician should be experienced in the interpretation of the relevant tests.

In clinical trials, an increase of the ovarian sensitivity to GONAL-f was shown when administered with lutropin alfa. If an FSH dose increase is deemed appropriate, dose adaptation should preferably be at 7-14 day intervals and preferably with 37.5-75 IU increments.

No direct comparison of GONAL-f/LH versus human menopausal gonadotrophin (hMG) has been performed. Comparison with historical data suggests that the ovulation rate obtained with GONAL-f/LH is similar to that can be obtained with hMG.

Ovarian Hyperstimulation Syndrome (OHSS)

OHSS is a medical event distinct from uncomplicated ovarian enlargement. OHSS is a syndrome that can manifest itself with increasing degrees of severity. It comprises marked ovarian enlargement, high serum sex steroids, and an increase in vascular permeability which can result in an accumulation of fluid in the peritoneal, pleural and, rarely, in the pericardial cavities.

The following symptomatology may be observed in severe cases of OHSS: abdominal pain, abdominal distension, severe ovarian enlargement, weight gain, dyspnoea, oliguria and gastrointestinal symptoms including nausea, vomiting and diarrhoea. Clinical evaluation may reveal hypovolaemia, haemoconcentration, electrolyte imbalances, ascites, haemoperitoneum, pleural effusions, hydrothorax, acute pulmonary distress, and thromboembolic events.

Excessive ovarian response to gonadotrophin treatment seldom gives rise to OHSS unless hCG is administered to trigger ovulation. Therefore in cases of ovarian hyperstimulation it is prudent to withhold hCG and advise the patient to refrain from coitus or to use barrier methods for at least 4 days. OHSS may progress rapidly (within 24 hours to several days) to become a serious medical event, therefore patients should be followed for at least two weeks after hCG administration.

To minimise the risk of OHSS or of multiple pregnancy, ultrasound scans as well as oestradiol measurements are recommended. In anovulation the risk of OHSS and multiple pregnancy is increased by a serum oestradiol > 900 pg/ml (3300 pmol/l) and more than 3 follicles of 14 mm or more in diameter. In ART there is an increased risk of OHSS with a serum oestradiol > 3000 pg/ml (11000 pmol/l) and 20 or more follicles of 12 mm or more in diameter. When the oestradiol level is > 5500 pg/ml (20200 pmol/l) and where there are 40 or more follicles in total, it may be necessary to withhold hCG administration.

Adherence to recommended GONAL-f dosage, regimen of administration and careful monitoring of therapy will minimise the incidence of ovarian hyperstimulation and multiple pregnancy (see Sections 4.2 and 4.8).

In ART, aspiration of all follicles prior to ovulation may reduce the occurrence of hyperstimulation.

OHSS may be more severe and more protracted if pregnancy occurs. Most often, OHSS occurs after hormonal treatment has been discontinued and reaches its maximum at about seven to ten days following treatment. Usually, OHSS resolves spontaneously with the onset of menses.

If severe OHSS occurs, gonadotrophin treatment should be stopped if still ongoing, the patient hospitalised and specific therapy for OHSS started.

This syndrome occurs with higher incidence in patients with polycystic ovarian disease.

Multiple pregnancy

Multiple pregnancy, specially high order, carries an increased risk in adverse maternal and perinatal outcomes.

In patients undergoing ovulation induction with GONAL-f, the incidence of multiple pregnancies is increased as compared with natural conception. The majority of multiple conceptions are twins. To minimise the risk of multiple pregnancy, careful monitoring of ovarian response is recommended.

In patients undergoing ART procedures the risk of multiple pregnancy is related mainly to the number of embryos replaced, their quality and the patient age.

The patients should be advised of the potential risk of multiple births before starting treatment.

Pregnancy wastage

The incidence of pregnancy wastage by miscarriage or abortion is higher in patients undergoing stimulation of follicular growth for ovulation induction or ART than in the normal population.

Ectopic pregnancy

Women with a history of tubal disease are at risk of ectopic pregnancy, whether the pregnancy is obtained by spontaneous conception or with fertility treatments. The prevalence of ectopic pregnancy after IVF was reported to be 2 to 5%, as compared to 1 to 1.5% in the general population.

Reproductive system neoplasms

There have been reports of ovarian and other reproductive system neoplasms, both benign and malignant, in women who have undergone multiple drug regimens for infertility treatment. It is not yet established whether or not treatment with gonadotropins increases the baseline risk of these tumors in infertile women.

Congenital malformation

The prevalence of congenital malformations after ART may be slightly higher than after spontaneous conceptions. This is thought to be due to differences in parental characteristics (e.g. maternal age, sperm characteristics) and multiple pregnancies.

Thromboembolic events

In women with generally recognised risk factors for thrombo-embolic events, such as personal or family history, treatment with gonadotrophins may further increase the risk. In these women, the benefits of gonadotrophin administration need to be weighed against the risks. It should be noted however, that pregnancy itself also carries an increased risk of thrombo-embolic events.

Treatment in men

Elevated endogenous FSH levels are indicative of primary testicular failure. Such patients are unresponsive to GONAL-f/hCG therapy.

Semen analysis is recommended 4 to 6 months after the beginning of treatment as part of the assessment of the response.

4.5 Interaction with other medicinal products and other forms of Interaction

Concomitant use of GONAL-f with other agents used to stimulate ovulation (e.g. hCG, clomiphene citrate) may potentiate the follicular response, whereas concurrent use of a GnRH agonist or antagonist to induce pituitary desensitisation may increase the dosage of GONAL-f needed to elicit an adequate ovarian response. No other clinically significant drug interaction has been reported during GONAL-f therapy.

4.6 Pregnancy and lactation

Use during pregnancy

There is no indication for use of GONAL-f during pregnancy. No teratogenic risk has been reported, following controlled ovarian hyperstimulation, in clinical use with gonadotrophins. In case of exposure during pregnancy, clinical data are not sufficient to exclude a teratogenic effect of recombinant hFSH. However, to date, no particular malformative effect has been reported. No teratogenic effect has been observed in animal studies.

Use during lactation

GONAL-f is not indicated during lactation. During lactation, the secretion of prolactin can entail a poor prognosis to ovarian stimulation.

4.7 Effects on ability to drive and use machines

No studies on the effects on ability to drive and use machines have been performed.

4.8 Undesirable effects

Treatment in women

Very Common > 1/10)

- Ovarian cysts;
- Mild to severe injection site reaction (pain, redness, bruising, swelling and/or irritation at the site of injection);
- Headache.

Common >1/100, <1/10)

- Mild to moderate OHSS (see section 4.4);
- Abdominal pain and gastrointestinal symptoms such as nausea, vomiting, diarrhoea, abdominal cramps and bloating.

Uncommon >1/1000, <1/100)

- Severe OHSS (see section 4.4).

Rare >1/10 000, <1/1000)

- Ovarian torsion, a complication of OHSS

Very rare (< 1/10 000)

- Thromboembolism, usually associated with severe OHSS;

Mild systemic allergic reactions (erythema, rash or facial swelling).

Treatment in men

Common >1/100, <1/10)

Gynaecomastia, acne and weight gain.

4.9 Overdose

The effects of an overdose of GONAL-f are unknown, nevertheless one could expect ovarian hyperstimulation syndrome to occur (see section 4.4).

5. PHARMACOLOGICAL PROPERTIES

5.1 Pharmacodynamic properties

Pharmacotherapeutic group: gonadotrophins, ATC code: G03GA05.

GONAL-f is a preparation of follicle stimulating hormone produced by genetically engineered Chinese Hamster Ovary (CHO) cells.

In women, the most important effect resulting from parenteral administration of FSH is the development of mature Graafian follicles.

In clinical trials, patients with severe FSH and LH deficiency were defined by an endogenous serum LH level < 1.2 IU/l as measured in a central laboratory. However, it should be taken into account that there are variations between LH measurements performed in different laboratories.

In men deficient in FSH, GONAL-f administered concomitantly with hCG for at least 4 months induces spermatogenesis.

5.2 Pharmacokinetic properties

Following intravenous administration, follitropin alfa is distributed to the extracellular fluid space with an initial half-life of around 2 hours and eliminated from the body with a terminal half-life of about one day. The steady state volume of distribution and total clearance are 10 L and 0.6 L/h, respectively. One-eighth of the follitropin alfa dose is excreted in the urine.

Following subcutaneous administration, the absolute bioavailability is about 70%. Following repeated administration, follitropin alfa accumulates 3-fold achieving asteady-state within 3-4 days. In women whose endogenous gonadotrophin secretion is suppressed, follitropin alfa has nevertheless been shown to effectively stimulate follicular development and steroidogenesis, despite unmeasurable LH levels.

5.3 Preclinical safety data

In an extensive range of toxicological, mutagenicity and animal studies (dogs, rats, monkeys), acute and chronic (up to 13 weeks and 52 weeks), no significant findings were observed.

Impaired fertility has been reported in rats exposed to pharmacological doses of follitropin alfa (⩾ 40 IU/kg/day) for extended periods, through reduced fecundity.

Given in high doses (5 IU/kg/day) follitropin alfa caused a decrease in the number of viable foetuses without being a teratogen, and dystocia similar to that observed with urinary hMG. However, since GONAL-F is not indicated in pregnancy, these data are of limited clinical relevance.

6. PHARMACEUTICAL PARTICULARS

6.1 List of excipients

Poloxamer 188

Sucrose

Methionine

Sodium dihydrogen phosphate monohydrate

Disodium phosphate dihydrate

m-Cresol

Phosphoric acid, concentrated

Sodium hydroxide

Water for Injections

6.2 Incompatibilities

Not applicable.

6.3 Shelf life

2 year.

After first use: 28 days (within the 2 year shelf-life)

6.4 Special precautions for storage

Store at 2°C - 8°C (in a refrigerator). Do not freeze.

Within its shelf-life, the product may be stored at or below 25°C for up to 28 days and must be discarded if not used.

Store in the original package in order to protect from light.

6.5 Nature and contents of container

1.5ml of solution for injection in 3ml cartridge (Type I glass), with a plunger stopper (halobutyl rubber) and a crimp cap (halobutyl rubber).

Pack of one pre-filled pen and 14 needles to be used with the pen for administration.

6.6 Instructions for use and handling

The solution should not be administered if it contains particles or is not clear.

Any unused solution must be discarded not later than 28 days after first opening.

GONAL-f 900IU/1.5ml (66 micrograms/1.5ml) is not designed to allow the cartridge to be removed.

Discard used needles immediately after injection.

Any unused product or waste material should be disposed of in accordance with local requirements.

7. MARKETING AUTHORISATION HOLDER

SERONO EUROPE LIMITED

56 Marsh Wall

London E14 9TP

United Kingdom

8. MARKETING AUTHORISATION NUMBER(S)

EU/1/95/001/035

9. DATE OF FIRST AUTHORISATION/RENEWAL OF THE AUTHORISATION

23rd February 2004

10. DATE OF REVISION OF THE TEXT

29th June 2004

LEGAL STATUS

POM

NAME AND ADDRESS OF DISTRIBUTOR IN UK

Serono Limited

Bedfont Cross

Stanwell Road

Feltham

Middlesex

TW14 8NX

NAME AND ADDRESS OF DISTRIBUTOR IN IRELAND

Allphar Services Limited

Pharmaceutical Agents and Distributors

Belgard Road

Tallaght

Dublin 24

Gonapeptyl Depot 3.75 mg

(Ferring Pharmaceuticals Ltd)

1. NAME OF THE MEDICINAL PRODUCT

GONAPEPTYL DEPOT

3.75 mg

Powder and solvent for suspension for injection.

2. QUALITATIVE AND QUANTITATIVE COMPOSITION

One pre-filled syringe contains 3.75 mg triptorelin (as acetate) to be suspended in one ml suspension agent.

For excipients, see 6.1.

3. PHARMACEUTICAL FORM

Powder and solvent for suspension for injection

prolonged release in pre-filled syringes.

4. CLINICAL PARTICULARS

4.1 Therapeutic indications

Men:

Treatment of advanced, hormone-dependent prostate carcinoma.

Women:

Preoperative reduction of myoma size to reduce the symptoms of bleeding and pain in women with symptomatic uterine myomas.

Symptomatic endometriosis confirmed by laparoscopy when suppression of the ovarian hormonogenesis is indicated to the extent that surgical therapy is not primarily indicated.

Children:

Treatment of confirmed central precocious puberty (girls under 9 years, boys under 10 years).

4.2 Posology and method of administration

The product should only be used under the supervision of an appropriate specialist having requisite facilities for regular monitoring of response.

It is important that the injection of the sustained release form be performed strictly in accordance with the instructions given in section 6.6.

Following reconstitution, the suspension has to be injected immediately.

Dosage and method of administration

The dosage of one syringe, equivalent to 3.75 mg triptorelin, is injected every 28 days either subcutaneously (e.g. into the skin of the abdomen, the buttock or thigh) or deep intramuscularly. The injection site should be changed each time.

Men:

Once every four weeks an injection with one syringe, equivalent to 3.75 mg triptorelin. In order to continually suppress testosterone levels, it is important to comply with a 4-weekly administration.

Women:

– *Uterine myomas and endometriosis:*

Once every four weeks an injection with one syringe, equivalent to 3.75 mg triptorelin. The treatment must be initiated in the first 5 days of the cycle.

Children:

At the beginning of treatment one injection with one syringe, equivalent to 3.75 mg triptorelin, on days 0, 14, and 28. Thereafter one injection every 4 weeks. Should the effect be insufficient, the injections may be given every 3 weeks. Dosing should be based on body weight. Children weighing less than 20 kg are injected with 1.875 mg (half dose), children between 20 and 30 kg receive 2.5 mg (2/3 dose), and children with more than 30 kg body weight are injected with 3.75 mg triptorelin (full dose).

Note for specific patient groups:

– There is no need to adjust the dose for the elderly.

– According to current data, dose reduction or prolongation of the dosage interval in patients with impaired renal function is not necessary.

Duration of administration

– *Prostate carcinoma:*

Treatment with *Gonapeptyl Depot* is usually a long-term therapy.

- *Uterine myomas and endometriosis:*

The duration of treatment depends on the initial degree of severity of endometriosis and on the evolution of its clinical manifestations (functional and anatomical) and on the evolution of the volume of the uterine myomas, determined by ultrasonography during treatment. Normally, the maximum attainable result is achieved after 3 to 4 injections.

In view of the possible effect on bone density, therapy should not exceed a duration of 6 months (see 4.4).

- *Central precocious puberty (CPP):*

Treatment should be stopped if a bone maturation of older than 12 years in girls and older than 13 years in boys has been achieved.

4.3 Contraindications

General:

Known hypersensitivity to triptorelin, poly-(d,l lactide coglycolide), dextran, or to any of the excipients.

In men:

– Hormone independent prostate carcinoma

– As sole treatment in prostate cancer patients with spinal cord compression or evidence of spinal metastases (see also section 4.4)

– After orchiectomy (in case of surgical castration *Gonapeptyl Depot* does not cause further decrease of serum testosterone)

In women:

– Pregnancy

– Clinically manifest osteoporosis

– Lactation period

In children:

– Progressive brain tumours

4.4 Special warnings and special precautions for use

Men:

The initial transient increase of serum testosterone has, in few patients, been associated with a temporary aggravation of symptoms of the disease (see 4.8). The patient should be advised to consult the physician, if any of these symptoms aggravates. For that reason, the use of *Gonapeptyl Depot* has to be carefully evaluated in patients with premonitory signs of medullary compression and the medical surveillance has to be closer in the first weeks of treatment, particularly in patients with urinary tract obstructions due to metastases and/or in patients with spinal metastases.

In order to prevent accentuation of the clinical symptoms, supplementary administration of an appropriate antiandrogen agent should be considered in the initial phase of the treatment.

In order to control the therapeutic effect, the prostate-specific antigen (PSA) and the testosterone plasma levels should be regularly monitored during treatment. Testosterone levels should not exceed 1 ng/ml.

Women:

Gonapeptyl Depot should only be prescribed after careful diagnosis (e.g. laparoscopy). Pregnancy should be precluded prior to treatment.

- *Uterine myomas and endometriosis:*

Menstruation does not occur during treatment. A supervening metrorrhagia in the course of treatment is abnormal (apart from the first month), and should lead to verification of plasma oestrogen level. Should this level be less than 50 pg/ml, possible associated organic lesions should be sought. After withdrawal of treatment, ovarian function resumes, e.g. menstrual bleeding will resume after 7-12 weeks after the final injection.

Non-hormonal contraception should be used during the initial month of treatment as ovulation may be triggered by the initial release of gonadotrophins. It should also be used from 4 weeks after the last injection until resumption of menstruation or until another contraceptive method has been established.

During treatment of uterine myomas the size of uterus and myoma should be determined regularly, e.g. by means of ultrasonography. Disproportionally fast reduction of uterus size in comparison with the reduction of myoma tissue has in isolated cases led to bleeding and sepsis.

Treatment with *Gonapeptyl Depot* over several months can lead to a decrease of bone density (see 4.8). For this reason, therapy should not exceed a duration of 6 months. After withdrawal of treatment, the bone loss is generally reversible within 6 - 9 months.

Particular caution is therefore advised in patients with additional risk factors in view of osteoporosis.

Children:

The chronological age at the beginning of therapy should be under 9 years in girls and under 10 years in boys.

After finalising the therapy, development of puberty characteristics will occur. Information with regards to future fertility is still limited. In most girls menses will start on average one year after ending the therapy, which in most cases is regular.

Pseudo-precocious puberty (gonadal or adrenal tumour or hyperplasia) and gonadotropin-independent precocious puberty (testicular toxicosis, familial Leydig cell hyperplasia) should be precluded.

Allergic and anaphylactic reactions have been reported in adults and children. These include both local site reactions and systemic symptoms. The pathogenesis could not be elucidated. A higher reporting rate was seen in children.

General:

When triptorelin is co-administered with drugs affecting pituitary secretion of gonadotrophins caution should be given and the patient's hormonal status should be supervised.

4.5 Interaction with other medicinal products and other forms of Interaction

Oestrogen containing medicinal products should not be used during treatment with Gonapeptyl Depot.

4.6 Pregnancy and lactation

Very limited data on the use of triptorelin during pregnancy do not indicate an increased risk of congenital malformations. However, long-term follow-up studies on development are far too limited. Animal data do not indicate direct or indirect harmful effects with respect to pregnancies or postnatal developments, but there are indications for foetotoxicity and delayed parturition. Based on the pharmacological effects disadvantageous influence on the pregnancy and the offspring cannot be excluded and *Gonapeptyl Depot* should not be used during pregnancy. Women of childbearing potential should use effective non-hormonal contraception. It is not known whether triptorelin is excreted in human milk. Because of the potential for adverse reactions from triptorelin in nursing infants, breast-feeding should be discontinued prior to and throughout administration.

4.7 Effects on ability to drive and use machines

Gonapeptyl Depot has no or negligible influence on the ability to drive and use machines.

4.8 Undesirable effects

Adverse experiences reported among patients treated with triptorelin during clinical trials and from post-marketing surveillance are shown below. As a consequence of decreased testosterone or oestrogen levels, most patients are expected to experience adverse reactions, with hot flushes being the most frequently reported (30% in men and 75-100% in women). Additionally, impotence and decreased libido should be expected in 30-40% of male patients, while bleeding/spotting, sweating, vaginal dryness and/or dyspareunia, decrease in libido and mood changes are expected in more than 10% of women.

Due to the fact that the testosterone levels normally increase during the first week of treatment, worsening of symptoms and complaints may occur (e.g. urinary obstruction, skeletal pain due to metastases, compression of the spinal cord, muscular fatigue and lymphatic oedema of the legs). In some cases urinary tract obstruction decreases the kidney function. Neurological compression with asthenia and paraesthesia in the legs has been observed.

Organ class	Common Adverse Reactions (> 1/100, < 1/10)	Uncommon Adverse Reactions (> 1/1000, < 1/100)
Men and women		
Endocrine	Depressive mood; irritation	
Metabolic and nutritional		Elevated enzyme levels (LDH, γGT, SGOT, SGPT)
Gastrointestinal	Nausea	
Musculo-skeletal system	Myalgia; arthralgia	
Body as a whole – general:	Tiredness; sleep disturbances; hypersensitivity reactions (itching; skin rash; fever)	Anaphylaxis
Application site disorders	Temporary pain at injection site	Foreign body reaction at injection site
Men		
Platelet, bleeding and clotting disorders		Thrombo-embolic disorder
Endocrine	Gynecomastia; headache; perspiration	Testicular atrophy; reduced growth of beard; hair loss on chest, arms and legs
Cardiovascular		Hypertension
Gastro-intestinal		Loss of appetite; gastralgia; dry mouth
Respiratory system disorders		Recurrence of asthma
General		Weight changes
Women		
Metabolic and nutritional		Slight rise in serum cholesterol
Central and peripheral nervous system		Visual disturbances; paraesthesia
General		Aching of back
Children		
Endocrine		Vaginal bleeding and discharge
Gastrointestinal		Vomiting; nausea
Body as a whole – general		Anaphylaxis

Slight trabecular bone loss may occur. This is generally reversible within 6-9 months after treatment discontinuation (see section 4.4).

Two cases of epiphysiolysis capitis femoris have been reported during use with triptorelin. Whether or not a causal relationship exists is unknown.

4.9 Overdose

There is insufficient experience of overdosing with triptorelin to draw conclusions on possible adverse effects. Considering the package form and the pharmaceutical form, overdosing is not expected.

5. PHARMACOLOGICAL PROPERTIES

5.1 Pharmacodynamic properties

Pharmacotherapeutic group: Gonadorelinanaloga

ATC code: L02AE04

Triptorelin is a synthetic decapeptide analogue of the natural gonadotrophin-releasing hormone (GnRH). GnRH is a decapeptide, which is synthesised in the hypothalamus and regulates the biosynthesis and release of the gonadotrophins LH (luteinising hormone) and FSH (follicle stimulating hormone) by the pituitary. Triptorelin stimulates the pituitary more strongly to secretion of LH and FSH than a comparable dose of gonadorelin, whereas the duration of action is longer. The increase of LH and FSH levels will initially lead to an increase of serum testosterone concentrations in men or serum oestrogen concentrations in women. Chronic administration of a GnRH agonist results in an inhibition of pituitary LH- and FSH-secretion. This inhibition leads to a reduction in steroidogenesis, by which the serum estradiol concentration in women and the serum testosterone concentration in men fall to within the postmenopausal or castrate range, respectively, i.e. a hypogonadotrophic hypogonadal state. In children with precocious puberty, the concentration of estradiol or testosterone will decrease to within the prepubertal range. Plasma DHEAS (dihydroepiandrostenedion sulphate) levels are not influenced. Therapeutically, this leads to a decrease in growth of testosterone-sensitive prostate tumours in men, and to reduction of endometriosis foci and oestrogen-dependent uterus myomas in women. Regarding uterine myoma, maximal benefit of treatment is observed in women with anaemia (haemoglobin inferior or equal to 8 g/dl). In children suffering from CPP triptorelin treatment leads to a suppression of the secretion of gonadotropins, estradiol, and testosterone to prepubertal levels. This results in arrest or even regression of pubertal signs and an increase in adult height prediction in CPP patients.

5.2 Pharmacokinetic properties

After intramuscular administration of *Gonapeptyl Depot*, the plasma concentrations of triptorelin are determined by the (slow) degradation of the poly-(d,l lactide coglycolide) polymer. The mechanism inherent to this administration form enables this slow release of triptorelin from the polymer.

After I.M. or S.C. application of a triptorelin depot-formulation (sustained-release microcapsules), a rapid increase in the concentration of triptorelin in plasma is recorded, with a maximum in the first hours. Then the triptorelin concentration declines notably within 24 hours. On day 4 the value reaches a second maximum, falling below the detection limit in a biexponential course after 44 days. After S.C. injections the triptorelin increase is more gradual and in a somewhat lower concentration than after I.M. injections. After S.C. injection, the decline in the triptorelin concentration takes longer, with values falling below the detection limit after 65 days.

During treatment over a period of 6 months and an administration every 28 days, there was no evidence of triptorelin accumulation in both modes of administration. Plasma triptorelin values decreased to approx. 100 pg/ml before the next application after I.M. or S.C. application (median values). It is to be assumed that the non-systemically available proportion of triptorelin is metabolized at the injection site, e.g. by macrophages.

In the pituitary, the systemically available triptorelin is inactivated by N-terminal cleavage via pyroglutamyl-peptidase and a neutral endopeptidase. In the liver and the kidneys, triptorelin is degraded to biologically inactive peptides and amino acids.

40 minutes after the end of an infusion of 100 μg triptorelin (over 1 hour) 3-14% of the administered dose has already been eliminated by the kidney.

For patients with an impaired renal function, adaptation and individualization of therapy with the triptorelin depot-formulation seems to be unnecessary, on account of the subordinate significance of the renal elimination route and the broad therapeutic range of triptorelin as an active component.

Bioavailability:

Men:

The systemic bioavailability of the active component triptorelin from the intramuscular depot is 38.3% in the first 13 days. Further release is linear at 0.92% of the dose per day on average. Bioavailability after S.C. application is 69% of I.M. availability.

Women:

After 27 test days, 35.7% of the applied dose can be detected on average, with 25.5% being released in the first 13 days and further release being linear at 0.73% of the dose per day on average.

General:

Calculation of the model-depending kinetic parameters ($t_{½}$, K_{el}, etc.) is inapplicable in presentations with a strongly protracted release of the active component.

5.3 Preclinical safety data

In rats, but not in mice treated over a long period of time with triptorelin, an increase in pituitary tumors has been detected. The influence of triptorelin on pituitary abnormalities in humans is unknown. The observation is considered not to be relevant to humans. Pituitary tumors in rodents in connection with other LHRH analogues have also been known to occur. Triptorelin has been shown to be embryo-/foetotoxic and to cause a delay in embryo-/foetal development as well as delay in parturition in rats. Preclinical data reveal no special hazard to humans based on repeat dose toxicity and genotoxicity studies. Single I.M. or S.C. injection of *Gonapeptyl Depot* or its suspension agent produced delayed foreign body reactions at the injection site. Within 8 weeks, these late reactions were nearly reversed after I.M. injection but only slightly reversed after S.C. injection. Local tolerance of *Gonapeptyl Depot* after I.V. injection was limited

6. PHARMACEUTICAL PARTICULARS

6.1 List of excipients

One pre-filledsyringe with powder contains:

Poly-(d,l lactide coglycolide)

Propyleneglycol octanoate decanoate

One pre-filledsyringe with one ml suspension agent contains:

Dextran 70

Polysorbate 80

Sodium chloride

Sodium hydrogen phosphate dihydrate

Sodium hydroxide

Water for injection

6.2 Incompatibilities

In the absence of compatibility studies this medicinal product should not be mixed with other medicinal products.

6.3 Shelf life

3 years

Reconstituted suspension: 3 minutes

6.4 Special precautions for storage

Store at 2°C - 8°C (in a refrigerator). Keep the container in the outer carton.

6.5 Nature and contents of container

Powder: Pre-filled syringe

Solvent: Pre-filled syringe

Pre-filled syringes (borosilicate glass type I, clear) with a connector (polypropylene), black chlorobutyl rubber stopper (plunger stopper, type I) and injection needle.

Pack sizes:

1 pre-filled syringe (powder) plus

1 pre-filled syringe (solvent)

3 pre-filled syringes (powder) plus

3 pre-filled syringes (solvent)

6.6 Instructions for use and handling

GonapeptylDepot is for single use only and any unused suspension should be discarded.

1. Preparation

Instructions for the physician how to prepare the suspension.

Since successful treatment depends upon correct preparation of the suspension, the following instructions must be strictly followed.

- Take the package of *Gonapeptyl Depot* from the refrigerator.

- Remove the cap from the disposable syringe containing the powder. Keep upright to prevent spilling.

- Open the package with the connector without removing the connector.

- Screw the syringe containing the sustained release microparticles on the connector in the package, then remove it.

Screw the syringe containing the suspension agent tightly on the free end of the connector and ensure that it fits tightly.

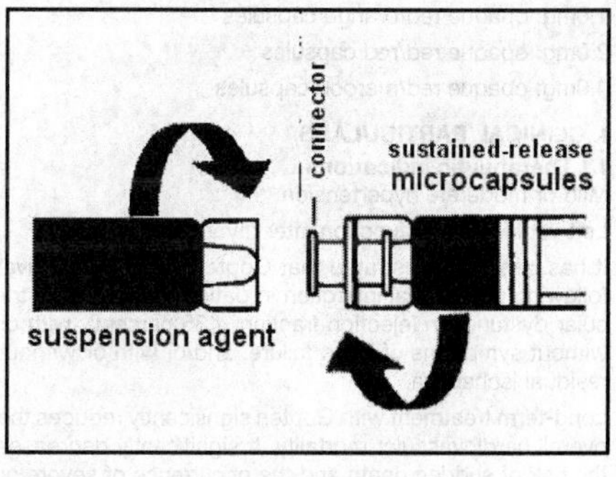

2. Reconstitution of a suspension

Empty the liquid into the syringe with the powder, then shoot it back and forth into the first syringe – the first two or three times without pushing the injection rod all the way in. Repeat this about 10 times or until you have a homogeneous milky-like suspension. While preparing the suspension, you might possibly create some foam. It is important that the foam be dissolved or removed from the syringe before giving the injection.

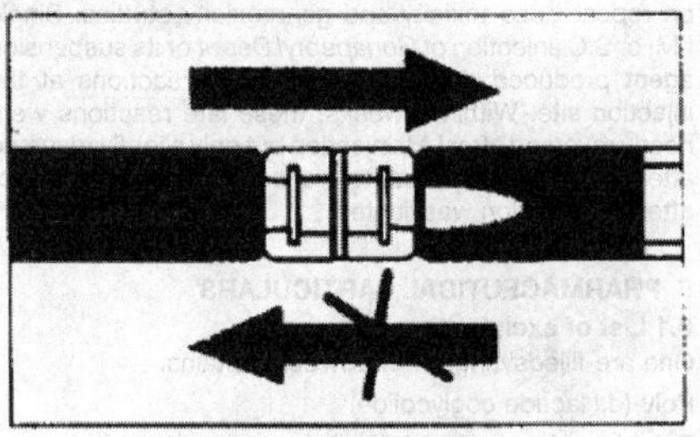

Mixing

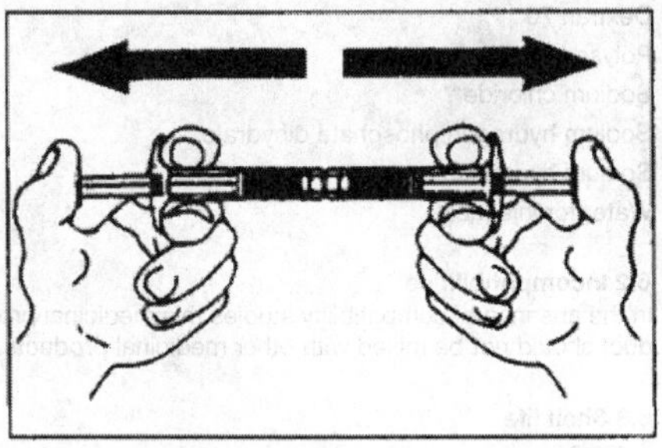

Mix approximately 10 times

3. Injection

- Remove the connector together with the empty syringe.

- Mount the injection needle on the syringe with the ready-to-use suspension.

- Inject subcutaneously or deep into the muscle immediately.

7. MARKETING AUTHORISATION HOLDER

Ferring Pharmaceuticals Ltd.

The Courtyard

Waterside Drive

Langley

Berkshire SL3 6EZ

United Kingdom

8. MARKETING AUTHORISATION NUMBER(S)

PL 03194/0085

9. DATE OF FIRST AUTHORISATION/RENEWAL OF THE AUTHORISATION

14th May 2003

10. DATE OF REVISION OF THE TEXT

Gopten

(Abbott Laboratories Limited)

1. NAME OF THE MEDICINAL PRODUCT

Gopten®

2. QUALITATIVE AND QUANTITATIVE COMPOSITION

Trandolapril, 0.5mg

Trandolapril, 1.0mg

Trandolapril, 2.0mg

Trandolapril, 4.0mg

For excipients see section 6.1

3. PHARMACEUTICAL FORM

Capsules, Hard

0.5mg: opaque red/yellow capsules

1.0mg: opaque red/orange capsules

2.0mg: opaque red/red capsules

4.0mg: opaque red/maroon capsules

4. CLINICAL PARTICULARS

4.1 Therapeutic indications

Mild or moderate hypertension.

Left ventricular dysfunction after myocardial infarction.

It has been demonstrated that Gopten improves survival following myocardial infarction in patients with left ventricular dysfunction (ejection fraction ⩽35 percent), with or without symptoms of heart failure, and/or with or without residual ischaemia.

Long-term treatment with Gopten significantly reduces the overall cardiovascular mortality. It significantly decreases the risk of sudden death and the occurrence of severe or resistant heart failure.

4.2 Posology and method of administration

Adults

Hypertension

For adults not taking diuretics, without congestive heart failure and without renal or hepatic insufficiency, the recommended initial dosage is 0.5mg as a single daily dose. A 0.5mg dose will only achieve a therapeutic response in a minority of patients. Dosage should be doubled incrementally at intervals of 2 to 4 weeks, based on patient response, up to a maximum of 4mg as a single daily dose.

The usual maintenance dose range is 1 to 2mg as a single daily dose. If the patient response is still unsatisfactory at a dose of 4mg Gopten, combination therapy should be considered.

Left ventricular dysfunction after myocardial infarction

Following a myocardial infarction, therapy may be initiated as early as the third day. Treatment should be initiated at a daily dose of 0.5mg. The dose should be progressively increased to a maximum of 4mg as a single daily dose. Depending upon the tolerability such as symptomatic hypotension, this forced titration can be temporarily suspended.

In the event of hypotension, all concomitant hypotensive therapies such as vasodilators, including nitrates and diuretics must be carefully checked and if possible, their dose reduced.

The dose of Gopten should be lowered only if the previous measures are not effective or not feasible.

Elderly

The dose in elderly patients is the same as in adults. There is no need to reduce the dose in elderly patients with normal renal and hepatic function. Caution is required in elderly patients with concomitant use of diuretics, congestive heart failure or renal or hepatic insufficiency. The dose should be titrated according to the need to control blood pressure.

Prior diuretic treatment

In patients who are at risk from a stimulated renin-angiotensin system (e.g. patients with water and sodium depletion), the diuretic should be discontinued 2-3 days before beginning therapy with 0.5mg trandolapril to reduce the likelihood of symptomatic hypotension. The diuretic may be resumed later if required.

Cardiac failure

In hypertensive patients who also have congestive heart failure, with or without associated renal insufficiency, symptomatic hypotension has been observed after treatment with ACE inhibitors. In these patients, therapy should be started at a dose of 0.5mg Gopten once daily under close medical supervision in hospital.

Dosage adjustment in renal impairment

For patients with mild or moderate renal impairment (creatinine clearance of 10-70ml/min), the usual adult and elderly doses are recommended.

For patients with severe renal impairment (creatinine clearance of <10ml/min), the usual adult and elderly starting doses are also recommended but the maximum daily dose should not exceed 2mg. In these patients, therapy should be under close medical supervision.

Dialysis: It is not known for certain if trandolapril or trandolaprilat are removed by dialysis. However, it would be expected that dialysis could remove the active moiety, trandolaprilat, from the circulation, resulting in a possible loss of control of blood pressure. Therefore careful monitoring of the patient's blood pressure during dialysis is required, and the dosage of trandolapril adjusted if needed.

Dosage adjustment in hepatic impairment

In patients with severely impaired liver function, a decrease in the metabolic clearance of the parent compound, trandolapril and the active metabolite, trandolaprilat results in a large increase in plasma trandolapril levels and to a lesser extent, an increase in trandolaprilat levels. Treatment with Gopten should therefore be initiated at a dose of 0.5mg once daily under close medical supervision.

Children

Gopten has not been studied in children and therefore use in this age group is not recommended.

4.3 Contraindications

Known hypersensitivity to trandolapril.

History of angioneurotic oedema associated with administration of an ACE inhibitor.

Hereditary/idiopathic angioneurotic oedema.

Pregnancy or lactation.

Use in children.

4.4 Special warnings and special precautions for use

Gopten should not be used in patients with aortic stenosis or outflow obstruction.

Assessment of renal function

Evaluation of the patient should include assessment of renal function prior to initiation of therapy and during treatment. Proteinuria may occur if renal impairment is present prior to therapy or relatively high doses are used.

Impaired renal function

Patients with severe renal insufficiency may require reduced doses of Gopten; their renal function should be closely monitored. In the majority, renal function will not alter. In patients with renal insufficiency, congestive heart failure or unilateral or bilateral renal artery stenosis, in the single kidney as well as after renal transplantation, there is a risk of impairment of renal function.

If recognised early, such impairment of renal function is reversible upon discontinuation of therapy.

Some hypertensive patients with no apparent pre-existing renal disease may develop minor and usually transient increases in blood urea nitrogen and serum creatinine when Gopten is given concomitantly with a diuretic. Dosage reduction of Gopten and/or discontinuation of the diuretic may be required. Additionally, in patients with renal insufficiency, the risk of hyperkalaemia should be considered and the patient's electrolyte status checked regularly.

Impaired liver function

As trandolapril is a prodrug metabolised to its active moiety in the liver, particular caution and close monitoring should be applied to patients with impaired liver function.

Symptomatic hypotension

In patients with uncomplicated hypertension, symptomatic hypotension has been observed rarely after the initial dose of Gopten, as well as after increasing the dose of Gopten. It is more likely to occur in patients who have been volume- and salt-depleted by prolonged diuretic therapy, dietary salt restriction, dialysis, diarrhoea or vomiting. Therefore, in these patients, diuretic therapy should be discontinued and volume and/or salt depletion should be corrected before initiating therapy with Gopten.

If symptomatic hypotension occurs, the patient should be placed in a supine position and, if necessary, receive an intravenous infusion of physiological saline. Intravenous atropine may be necessary if there is associated bradycardia. Treatment with Gopten may usually be continued following restoration of effective blood volume and blood pressure.

Surgery/anaesthesia

In patients undergoing surgery or during anaesthesia with agents producing hypotension, Gopten may block angiotensin II formation secondary to compensatory renin release. If hypotension occurs and is considered to be due to this mechanism, it can be corrected by appropriate treatment.

Agranulocytosis and bone marrow depression

In patients on ACE inhibitors, agranulocytosis and bone marrow depression have been seen rarely. They are more frequent in patients with renal impairment, especially if they have a collagen vascular disease. However, regular monitoring of white blood cell counts and protein levels in urine should be considered in patients with collagen vascular disease (e.g. lupus erythematosus and scleroderma), especially associated with impaired renal function and concomitant therapy, particularly with corticosteroids and antimetabolites.

Hyperkalaemia

Elevated serum potassium has been observed very rarely in hypertensive patients. Risk factors for the development of hyperkalaemia include renal insufficiency, potassium-sparing diuretics, the concomitant use of agents to treat hypokalaemia, diabetes mellitus and/or left ventricular dysfunction after myocardial infarction.

Angioneurotic oedema:

Rarely, ACE inhibitors (such as trandolapril) may cause angioneurotic oedema that includes swelling of the face, extremities, tongue, glottis, and/or larynx. Patients experiencing angioneurotic oedema must immediately discontinue Gopten therapy and be monitored until oedema resolution.

Angioneurotic oedema of the face will usually resolve spontaneously. Oedema involving not only the face but also the glottis may be life-threatening because of the risk of airway obstruction.

Angioneurotic oedema involving the tongue, glottis or larynx requires immediate subcutaneous administration of 0.3-0.5ml of adrenaline solution (1:1000) along with other therapeutic measures as appropriate.

Caution must be exercised in patients with a history of idiopathic angioneurotic oedema, and Gopten is contra-indicated if angioneurotic oedema was an adverse reaction to an ACE inhibitor (see Contra-indications, section 4.3).

Cough:

During treatment with an ACE inhibitor, a dry and non-productive cough may occur which disappears after discontinuation.

Hereditary disorders:

Patients with rare hereditary problems of galactose intolerance, the Lapp lactase deficiency or glucose-galactose malabsorption should not take this medicine.

4.5 Interaction with other medicinal products and other forms of Interaction

Drug interactions

Combination with diuretics or other antihypertensive agents may potentiate the antihypertensive response to Gopten. Adrenergic-blocking drugs should only be combined with trandolapril under careful supervision.

Potassium-sparing diuretics (spironolactone, amiloride, triamterene) or potassium supplements may increase the risk of hyperkalaemia, particularly in renal failure. Gopten may attenuate the potassium loss caused by thiazide-type diuretics. If concomitant use of these agents is indicated, they should be given with caution and serum potassium should be monitored regularly.

Antidiabetic agents

As with all ACE inhibitors, concomitant use of antidiabetic medicines (insulin or oral hypoglycaemic agents) may cause an increased blood glucose lowering effect with greater risk of hypoglycaemia. Therefore, blood glucose should be closely monitored in diabetics treated with a hypoglycaemic agent and Gopten, particularly when starting or increasing the dose of ACE inhibitor, or in patients with impaired renal function.

Combinations necessitating a warning

In some patients already receiving diuretic treatment, particularly if this treatment has been recently instituted, the fall in blood pressure on initiation of treatment with Gopten may be excessive. The risk of symptomatic hypotension may be reduced by stopping the diuretic a few days before starting treatment with Gopten. If it is necessary to continue the diuretic treatment, the patient should be monitored, at least after the initial administration of Gopten. As with all antihypertensives, combination with a neuroleptic or tricyclic antidepressant increases the risk of orthostatic hypotension. Gopten may reduce the elimination of lithium and serum levels of lithium should be monitored.

Anaphylactoid reactions to high-flux polyacrylonitrile membranes used in haemodialysis have been reported in patients treated with ACE inhibitors. As with other antihypertensives of this chemical class, this combination should be avoided when prescribing ACE inhibitors to renal dialysis patients.

The effects of certain anaesthetics may be enhanced by ACE inhibitors.

Allopurinol, cytostatic or immunosuppressive agents, systemic corticosteroids or procainamide may increase the risk of leucopenia, if used concomitantly with ACE inhibitors.

The antihypertensive effect of ACE inhibitors may be reduced by the administration of NSAIDs. An additive effect on serum potassium increase has been described when NSAIDs and ACE inhibitors have been used concomitantly, while renal function may be reduced.

Antacids cause reduced bioavailability of ACE inhibitors.

The antihypertensive effects of ACE inhibitors may be reduced by sympathomimetics; patients should be carefully monitored.

No clinical interaction has been observed in patients with left ventricular dysfunction after myocardial infarction when Gopten has been concomitantly administered with thrombolytics, aspirin, beta-blockers, calcium channel blockers, nitrates, anticoagulants, diuretics or digoxin.

4.6 Pregnancy and lactation

The use of Gopten is contra-indicated in pregnancy and lactation. Pregnancy should be excluded before start of treatment and avoided during treatment. Exposure of the mother to ACE inhibitors in mid or late pregnancy has been associated with oligohydramnios and neonatal hypotension with anuria or renal failure.

In the rat and particularly in the rabbit, trandolapril caused maternal toxicity together with foetotoxicity at high doses. Neither embryotoxicity nor teratogenicity was observed in the rat, rabbit or monkey.

4.7 Effects on ability to drive and use machines

Given the pharmacological properties of Gopten, no particular effect is expected. However, in some individuals, ACE inhibitors may affect the ability to drive or operate machinery, particularly at the start of treatment, when changing over from other medication or during concomitant use of alcohol. Therefore, after the first dose or subsequent increases in dose, it is not advisable to drive or operate machinery for several hours.

4.8 Undesirable effects

The following adverse events have been reported with ACE inhibitors as a class. Not all will have been reported in association with Gopten. The events are displayed by system organ class and frequency: common > 1/100 ⩽ 1/10; uncommon >1/1000 ⩽ 1/100.

Body System	Preferred Term	Frequency
Nervous system disorders	Headache Dizziness	Common (2.3%) Common (1.7%)
Cardiac disorders	Palpitations	Uncommon (0.7%)
Respiratory, thoracic and mediastinal disorders	Cough	Common (3.9%)
Gastrointestinal disorders	Nausea	Uncommon (0.5%)
Skin and subcutaneous tissue disorders	Pruritus Rash	Uncommon (0.5%) Uncommon (0.4%)
General disorders and administration site conditions	Asthenia Malaise	Common (2.1%) Uncommon (0.5%)

Respiratory

Dyspnoea, sinusitis, rhinitis, glossitis, bronchitis and bronchospasm have been reported, but rarely in association with treatment with ACE inhibitors.

Cardiovascular

Tachycardia, palpitations, arrhythmias, angina pectoris, myocardial infarction, transient ischaemic attacks and cerebral haemorrhage have been reported in association with hypotension during treatment with ACE inhibitors.

Gastrointestinal

Nausea, vomiting, abdominal pain, indigestion, diarrhoea, constipation and dry mouth have occurred occasionally during treatment with ACE inhibitors.

There have been reports of individual incidents of cholestatic jaundice, hepatitis, pancreatitis and ileus connected with the use of ACE inhibitors.

Hypersensitivity

Allergic hypersensitivity reactions such as pruritus and rash have been reported. Urticaria, erythema multiforme, Stevens-Johnson syndrome, toxic epidermal necrolysis, psoriasis-like efflorescences and alopecia, which may be accompanied by fever, myalgia, arthralgia, eosinophilia and/or increased ANA (anti-nuclear antibody) -titres have been occasionally reported with ACE inhibitor treatment.

Angioneurotic oedema

In very rare cases, angioneurotic oedema has occurred. If laryngeal stridor or angioedema of the face, tongue or glottis occurs, treatment with Gopten must be discontinued and appropriate therapy instituted immediately.

Renal

Deterioration of renal function and acute renal failure have been reported with the use of ACE inhibitors.

Drug/Laboratory parameters:

Reversible (on stopping treatment) increases in blood urea and plasma creatinine may result, particularly if renal insufficiency, severe heart failure or renovascular hypertension are present.

Decreased haemoglobin, haematocrit, platelets and white cell count, and individual cases of agranulocytosis or pancytopenia, have been reported with ACE inhibitor treatment; also evaluate liver enzymes and serum bilirubin. Haemolytic anaemia has been reported in some patients with a congenital deficiency concerning G-6 PDH (glucose-6-phosphate dehydrogenase) during treatment with ACE inhibitors.

4.9 Overdose

Symptoms expected with ACE inhibitors are severe hypotension, shock, stupor, bradycardia, electrolyte disturbance and renal failure. In the event of overdosage following recent ingestion, consideration should be given to emptying the stomach contents. Blood pressure should be monitored and if hypotension develops, volume expansion should be considered.

5. PHARMACOLOGICAL PROPERTIES

5.1 Pharmacodynamic properties

ATC Code: C 09A A10

Gopten capsules contain the prodrug, trandolapril, a non-peptide ACE inhibitor with a carboxyl group but without a sulphydryl group. Trandolapril is rapidly absorbed and then non-specifically hydrolysed to its potent, long-acting active metabolite, trandolaprilat.

Trandolaprilat binds tightly and in a saturable manner to ACE.

The administration of trandolapril causes decreases in the concentrations of angiotensin II, aldosterone and atrial natriuretic factor and increases in plasma renin activity and concentrations of angiotensin I. Gopten thus modulates the renin-angiotensin-aldosterone system which plays a major part in regulating blood volume and blood pressure and consequently has a beneficial antihypertensive effect.

The administration of usual therapeutic doses of Gopten to hypertensive patients produces a marked reduction in both supine and erect blood pressure. The antihypertensive effect is evident after 1 hour, with a peak effect between 8 and 12 hours, persisting for at least 24 hours.

The properties of trandolapril might explain the results obtained in the regression of cardiac hypertrophy with improvement of diastolic function, and improvement of arterial compliance in humans. In addition, a decrease in vascular hypertrophy has been shown in animals.

5.2 Pharmacokinetic properties

Trandolapril is very rapidly absorbed after oral administration. The amount absorbed is equivalent to 40 to 60% of the administered dose and is not affected by food consumption.

The peak plasma concentration of trandolapril is observed 30 minutes after administration. Trandolapril disappears rapidly from the plasma with a half-life of less than one hour.

Trandolapril is hydrolysed to trandolaprilat, a specific ACE inhibitor. The amount of trandolaprilat formed is not modified by food consumption. The peak plasma concentration of trandolaprilat is reached after 4 to 6 hours.

In the plasma, trandolaprilat is more than 80% protein-bound. It binds saturably, with a high affinity, to ACE. The major proportion of circulating trandolaprilat is also non-saturably bound to albumin.

After repeated administration of Gopten in a single daily dose, steady state is reached on average in four days, both in healthy volunteers and in young or elderly hypertensives. The effective half-life of trandolaprilat is between 16 and 24 hours. The terminal half-life of elimination is between 47 hours and 98 hours depending on dose. This terminal phase probably represent s binding/dissociation kinetics of the trandolaprilat/ACE complex.

Trandolaprilat eliminated in the urine in the unchanged form accounts for 10 to 15% of the dose of trandolapril administered. After oral administration of the labelled product in man, 33% of the radioactivity is found in the urine and 66% in the faeces.

The renal clearance of trandolaprilat is proportional to the creatinine clearance. The plasma concentrations of trandolaprilat are significantly higher in patients with a creatinine clearance less than or equal to 30ml/min. However, after repeated dosing in patients with chronic renal failure, steady state is also reached on average in four days, whatever the degree of renal failure.

5.3 Preclinical safety data

There are no relevant pre-clinical findings which are additional to those already included in other section of the SPC.

6. PHARMACEUTICAL PARTICULARS

6.1 List of excipients

Excipients

Maize starch

Lactose monohydrate

Povidone

Sodium stearyl fumarate

Capsule Shell

Gelatin

Titanium dioxide (E171)

Erythrosine (E127)

Black iron oxide (E172)

Yellow iron oxide (E172)

Sodium laurylsulphate

6.2 Incompatibilities

None

6.3 Shelf life

Gopten 0.5mg, 1.0mg and 2.0mg: 60 months

Gopten 4.0mg: 24 months

6.4 Special precautions for storage

Do not store above 25 °C.

6.5 Nature and contents of container

Gopten 0.5mg: PVC/PVDC/AL calendar pack containing 14 capsules or 56 capsules.

Gopten 1.0mg, 2.0mg and 4.0mg: PVC/PVDC/AL calendar pack containing 28 capsules or 56 capsules.

6.6 Instructions for use and handling

None

7. MARKETING AUTHORISATION HOLDER

Abbott Laboratories Limited

Queenborough

Kent

ME11 5EL

United Kingdom

8. MARKETING AUTHORISATION NUMBER(S)

PL 00037/0356

PL 00037/0357

PL 00037/0358

PL 00037/0406

9. DATE OF FIRST AUTHORISATION/RENEWAL OF THE AUTHORISATION

Gopten 0.5mg, 1.0mg and 2.0mg: 31 December 2001

Gopten 4.0mg: 12 January 2004

10. DATE OF REVISION OF THE TEXT

29 September 2004

Graneodin Ointment

(E. R. Squibb & Sons Limited)

1. NAME OF THE MEDICINAL PRODUCT

GRANEODIN OINTMENT

2. QUALITATIVE AND QUANTITATIVE COMPOSITION

Soft, slightly opaque, colourless ointment, containing neomycin (as sulphate) 1625 units (0.25%) and gramicidin 0.025% in Plastibase* (liquid paraffin and polyethylene resin).

3. PHARMACEUTICAL FORM

Ointment

4. CLINICAL PARTICULARS

4.1 Therapeutic indications

Superficial bacterial infections such as impetigo; impetiginised eczema; infected eczema; bacterial infections of the ear. (See Contra-indications).

4.2 Posology and method of administration

Adults and Children:

To be applied two to four times a day. Any crusts should be removed and the ointment rubbed well in.

Elderly:

No specific dosage recommendations or precautions.

If a satisfactory response has not been achieved after 7 days, treatment should be stopped and the organism identified.

4.3 Contraindications

Fungal or viral infections of the skin or for the treatment of deep-seated infections.

Persons with known sensitivity to neomycin.

Should not be applied to the external auditory canal in patients with perforated eardrums.

Should not be used for extensive areas because of possible risk of systemic absorption and neomycin-induced ototoxicity.

4.4 Special warnings and special precautions for use

The possibility of sensitivity to neomycin should be taken into consideration during treatment. Since the use of occlusive dressings may increase the risk of sensitivity reactions, such dressings should be avoided.

Children: No specific precautions apply.

4.5 Interaction with other medicinal products and other forms of Interaction

None stated.

4.6 Pregnancy and lactation

There are theoretical risks of neomycin-induced foetal ototoxicity; therefore the product should be used with caution only when the benefit outweighs the potential risk.

4.7 Effects on ability to drive and use machines

None stated.

4.8 Undesirable effects

Neomycin: Sensitivity reactions may occur especially with prolonged use. Ototoxicity and nephrotoxicity have been reported. The product should be used with caution and in small amounts in the treatment of skin infections following extensive burns, open lesion and other conditions where absorption of neomycin is possible particularly in children and elderly. The product should also be used with care in patients with established hearing loss and those with renal impairment.

Gramicidin: Sensitivity has occasionally been reported.

4.9 Overdose

In the event of accidental ingestion, the patient should be observed and treated symptomatically.

5. PHARMACOLOGICAL PROPERTIES

5.1 Pharmacodynamic properties

Actions:

Neomycin is active against a wide range of Gram-positive and Gram-negative bacteria, including many of the organisms responsible for bacterial skin infections.

Gramicidin is active against Gram-positive bacteria and supplements the action of neomycin against the many common skin pathogens found in this group.

5.2 Pharmacokinetic properties

Not applicable.

5.3 Preclinical safety data

No further relevant data.

6. PHARMACEUTICAL PARTICULARS

6.1 List of excipients

Liquid paraffin and polyethylene resin.

6.2 Incompatibilities

None known.

6.3 Shelf life

48 months

6.4 Special precautions for storage

Storage: Do not store above 25°C.

Dilution: Not recommended.

6.5 Nature and contents of container

Aluminium tubes of 25g.

6.6 Instructions for use and handling

Not applicable.

7. MARKETING AUTHORISATION HOLDER

E. R. Squibb & Sons Limited

Uxbridge Business Park

Sanderson Road,

Uxbridge,

Middlesex UB8 1DH

8. MARKETING AUTHORISATION NUMBER(S)

PL 0034/5042R

9. DATE OF FIRST AUTHORISATION/RENEWAL OF THE AUTHORISATION

24 April 1991 / 10 January 2002

10. DATE OF REVISION OF THE TEXT

24 th June 2005

Granocyte 13 million IU, and 34 million IU

(Chugai Pharma UK Limited)

1. NAME OF THE MEDICINAL PRODUCT

GRANOCYTE®13 million IU and GRANOCYTE®34 million IU, powder and solvent for solution for injection or infusion.

2. QUALITATIVE AND QUANTITATIVE COMPOSITION

Lenograstim* (rHuG-CSF)13.4 million IU (equivalent to 105 micrograms)

per mL after reconstitution

Lenograstim* (rHuG-CSF)33.6 million IU (equivalent to 263 micrograms)

per mL after reconstitution

*Produced by recombinant DNA technology in Chinese Hamster Ovary (CHO) cells.

For excipients, see 6.1.

3. PHARMACEUTICAL FORM

Powder and solvent for solution for injection or infusion.

- White lyophilised powder
- Solvent (water for injections)

4. CLINICAL PARTICULARS

4.1 Therapeutic indications

- Reduction in the duration of neutropenia in patients (with non-myeloid malignancy) undergoing myeloablative therapy followed by bone marrow transplantation (BMT) in patients considered to be at increased risk of prolonged severe neutropenia.
- Reduction of duration of severe neutropenia and its associated complications in patients undergoing established cytotoxic chemotherapy associated with a significant incidence of febrile neutropenia.
- Mobilisation of peripheral blood progenitor cells (PBPCs).

Note: The safety of the use of Granocyte with antineoplastic agents characterized by cumulative or predominant myelotoxicity *vis-à-vis* the platelet lineage (nitrosourea, mitomycin) has not been established. Administration of Granocyte might even enhance the toxicities of these agents, particularly *vis-à-vis* platelets.

4.2 Posology and method of administration

- The recommended dose of Granocyte is 150 μg (19.2 MIU) per m^2 per day, therapeutically equivalent to 5 μg (0.64 MIU) per kg per day for:

bone marrow transplantation,

established cytotoxic chemotherapy,

PBPC mobilisation after chemotherapy,

Granocyte 13.4 MIU/vial can be used in patients with body surface area up to 0.7 m^2, Granocyte 33.6 MIU/vial can be used in patients with body surface area up to 1.8 m^2.

- For PBPC mobilisation with Granocyte alone, the recommended dose is 10 μg (1.28 MIU) per kg per day.

4.2.1 Adults

- In Bone Marrow Transplantation

Granocyte should be administered daily at the recommended dose of 150 μg (19.2 MIU) per m^2 per day as a 30-minute intravenous infusion diluted in isotonic saline solution or as a subcutaneous injection, starting the day following transplantation (see 4.4 and 4.5). Dosing should continue until the expected nadir has passed and the neutrophil count returns to a stable level compatible with treatment discontinuation, with, if necessary, a maximum of 28 consecutive days of treatment.

It is anticipated that by day 14 following bone marrow transplantation, 50% of patients will achieve neutrophil recovery.

- In Established Cytotoxic Chemotherapy

Granocyte should be administered daily at the recommended dose of 150 μg (19.2 MIU) per m^2 per day as a subcutaneous injection starting on the day following completion of chemotherapy (see 4.4 and 4.5). Daily administration of Granocyte should continue until the expected nadir has passed and the neutrophil count returns to a stable level compatible with treatment discontinuation, with, if necessary, a maximum of 28 consecutive days of treatment.

A transient increase in neutrophil count may occur within the first 2 days of treatment, however Granocyte treatment should not be stopped, since the subsequent nadir usually occurs earlier and recovers more quickly if treatment continues.

- In Peripheral Blood Progenitor Cell (PBPC) Mobilisation

After chemotherapy, Granocyte should be administered daily, at the recommended dose of 150 μg (19.2 MIU) per m^2 per day as a subcutaneous injection starting on the day after completion of chemotherapy until the expected nadir has passed and neutrophil count returns to a normal range compatible with treatment discontinuation.

Leukapheresis should be performed when the post nadir leukocyte count is rising or after assessment of $CD34^+$ cells in blood with a validated method. For patients who have not had extensive chemotherapy, one leukapheresis is often sufficient to obtain the acceptable minimum yield ($\geqslant 2.0 \times 10^6$ $CD34^+$ cells per kg).

In PBPC mobilisation with Granocyte alone, Granocyte should be administered daily at the recommended dose of 10 μg (1.28 MIU) per kg per day as a subcutaneous injection for 4 to 6 days. Leukapheresis should be performed between day 5 and 7.

In patients who have not had extensive chemotherapy one leukapheresis is often sufficient to obtain the acceptable minimum yield ($\geqslant 2.0 \times 10^6$ $CD34^+$ cells per kg).

In healthy donors, a 10 μg/kg daily dose administered subcutaneously for 5-6 days allows a $CD34^+$ cells collection $\geqslant 3 \times 10^6$ /kg body weight with a single leukapheresis in 83% of subjects and with 2 leukapheresis in 97%.

Therapy should only be given in collaboration with an experienced oncology and/or haematology centre.

4.2.2 Elderly

Clinical trials with Granocyte have included a small number of patients up to the age of 70 years but special studies have not been performed in the elderly and therefore specific dosage recommendations cannot be made.

4.2.3 Children

The safety and efficacy of Granocyte have been established in patients older than 2 years in BMT.

4.3 Contraindications

Granocyte should not be administered to patients or subjects with known hypersensitivity to the product or its constituents.

Granocyte should not be used to increase the dose intensity of cytotoxic chemotherapy beyond established doses and dosage regimens since the drug could reduce myelotoxicity but not overall toxicity of cytotoxic drugs.

Granocyte should not be administered concurrently with cytotoxic chemotherapy.

Granocyte should not be administered to patients:

- with myeloid malignancy other than *de novo* acute myeloid leukaemia
- with *de novo* acute myeloid leukaemia aged below 55 years, and/or
- with *de novo* acute myeloid leukaemia with good cytogenetics, i.e. t(8;21), t(15;17) and inv (16)

4.4 Special warnings and special precautions for use

- Malignant Cell Growth

Granulocyte colony stimulating factor can promote growth of myeloid cells *in vitro* and similar effects may be seen on some non-myeloid cells *in vitro*.

The safety and efficacy of Granocyte administration in patients with myelodysplasia or secondary AML or chronic myelogenous leukemia have not been established. Therefore Granocyte should not be used in these indications. Particular care should be taken to distinguish the diagnosis of blast transformation of chronic myeloid leukaemia from acute myeloid leukaemia.

Clinical trials have not established whether Granocyte influences the progression of myelodysplastic syndrome to acute myeloid leukemia. Caution should be exercised in using Granocyte in any pre-malignant myeloid condition. As some tumours with non-specific characteristics can exceptionally express a G-CSF receptor, caution should be exerted in the event of unexpected tumour regrowth concomitantly observed with rHuG-CSF therapy.

- Leukocytosis

A leukocyte count greater than 50×10^9/L has not been observed in any of the 174 clinical trials patients treated with 5 μg/kg/day (0.64 million units/kg/day) following bone marrow transplantation. White blood cell counts of 70×10^9/L or greater have been observed in less than 5% of patients who received cytotoxic chemotherapy and were treated by Granocyte at 5 μg/kg/day (0.64 million units/kg/day). No adverse events directly attributable to this degree of leukocytosis have been reported. In view of the potential risks associated with severe leukocytosis, a white blood cell count should, however, be performed at regular intervals during Granocyte therapy. If leukocyte counts exceed 50×10^9/L after the expected nadir, Granocyte should be discontinued immediately.

During PBPC mobilisation, Granocyte should be discontinued if the leukocyte counts rise to $> 70 \times 10^9$/L.

- Pulmonary adverse effect

Rare ($>$0.01% and $<$0.1%) pulmonary adverse effects, in particular interstitial pneumonia, have been reported after G-CSFs administration. Patients with a recent history of pulmonary infiltrates or pneumonia may be at higher risk.

The onset of pulmonary symptoms or signs, such as cough, fever and dyspnoea, in association with radiological signs of pulmonary infiltrates and deterioration in pulmonary function may be preliminary signs of acute respiratory distress syndrome (ARDS). Granocyte should be immediately discontinued and appropriate treatment given.

• In Bone Marrow Transplantation

Special attention should be paid to platelet recovery since in double-blind placebo-controlled trials the mean platelet count was lower in patients treated with Granocyte as compared with placebo.

The effect of Granocyte on the incidence and severity of acute and chronic graft-versus-host disease has not been accurately determined.

• In Established Cytotoxic Chemotherapy

The use of Granocyte is not recommended from 24 hours before, until 24 hours after chemotherapy ends (see 4.5).

• Risks Associated with Increased Doses of Chemotherapy

The safety and efficacy of Granocyte have yet to be established in the context of intensified chemotherapy. Granocyte should not be used to decrease, beyond the established limits, intervals between chemotherapy courses and/or to increase the doses of chemotherapy. Non-myeloid toxicities were limiting factors in a phase II chemotherapy intensification trial with Granocyte.

• Special precautions in Peripheral Blood Progenitor Cell mobilisation

Choice of the Mobilisation Method

Clinical trials carried out among the same patient population have shown that PBPC mobilisation, as assessed within the same laboratory, was higher when Granocyte was used after chemotherapy than when used alone. Nevertheless the choice between the two mobilisation methods should be considered in relation to the overall objectives of treatment for an individual patient.

Prior exposure to radiotherapy and/or cytotoxic agents

Patients, who have undergone extensive prior myelosuppressive therapy and/or radiotherapy, may not show sufficient PBPC mobilisation to achieve the acceptable minimum yield ($\geqslant 2 \times 10^6$ $CD34^+$ /kg) and therefore adequate haematological reconstitution.

A PBPC transplantation program should be defined early in the treatment course of the patient and particular attention should be paid to the number of PBPC mobilised before the administration of high-dose chemotherapy. If yields are low, other forms of treatment should replace the PBPC transplantation program.

Assessment of progenitor cell yields

Particular attention should be paid to the method of quantification of progenitor cell yields as the results of flow cytometric analysis of $CD34^+$ cell number vary among laboratories.

The minimum yield of $CD34^+$ cells is not well defined. The recommendation of a minimum yield of $\geqslant 2.0 \times 10^6$ $CD34^+$ cells/kg is based on published experience in order to achieve adequate haematological reconstitution. Yields higher than $\geqslant 2.0 \times 10^6$ $CD34^+$ cells/kg are associated with more rapid recovery, including platelets, while lower yields result in slower recovery.

• In healthy donors

The PBPC mobilisation, which is a procedure without direct benefit for healthy people, should only be considered through a clear regular delimitation in accordance with local regulations as for bone marrow donation when applicable.

The efficacy and safety of Granocyte has not been assessed in donors aged over 60 years, therefore the procedure cannot be recommended. Based on some local regulations and lack of studies, minor donors should not be considered.

PBPC mobilisation procedure should be considered for donors who fit usual clinical and laboratory eligibility criteria for bone marrow donation especially normal haematological values.

Marked leukocytosis (WBC $\geqslant 50 \times 10^9$/L) was observed in 24% of subjects studied.

Apheresis-related thrombocytopenia (platelets $< 100 \times 10^9$/L) was observed in 42% of subjects studied and values $< 50 \times 10^9$/L were occasionally noted following leukapheresis without related clinical adverse events, all recovered.

Therefore leukapheresis should not be performed in donors who are anticoagulated or who have known defects in haemostasis. If more than one leukapheresis is required particular attention should be paid to donors with platelets $< 100 \times 10^9$/L prior to apheresis; in general apheresis should not be performed if platelets $< 75 \times 10^9$/L.

Insertion of a central venous catheter should be avoided if possible with consideration given to venous access in selection of donors.

Data on long-term follow-up of donors are available on a small number of subjects. Up to six years, no emerging long-term sequelae have been reported. Nevertheless, a risk of promotion of a malignant myeloid clone is possible. Therefore, it is recommended that systematic record and tracking of the stem-cell gifts be made by the apheresis centres.

• In recipients of allogenic peripheral blood stem-cells mobilised with Granocyte

Allogeneic stem-cell grafting may be associated with an increased risk for chronic GVHD (Graft Versus Host Disease), and long-term data of graft functioning are sparse.

• Other Special Precautions

In patients with severe impairment of hepatic or renal function, the safety and efficacy of Granocyte have not been established.

In patients with substantially reduced myeloid progenitor cells (e.g. due to prior intensive radiotherapy/chemotherapy), neutrophil response is sometimes diminished and the safety of Granocyte has not been established.

Common but generally asymptomatic cases of splenomegaly and very rare cases of splenic rupture in either healthy donors or patients following administration of Granulocyte-colony stimulating factors (G-CSFs). Therefore, spleen size should be carefully monitored (e.g. clinical examination, ultrasound). A diagnosis of splenic rupture should be considered when left upper abdominal pain or shoulder tip pain is reported.

4.5 Interaction with other medicinal products and other forms of Interaction

In view of the sensitivity of rapidly dividing myeloid cells to cytotoxic chemotherapy, the use of Granocyte is not recommended from 24 hours before until 24 hours after chemotherapy ends (see 4.4). Possible interactions with other haematopoietic growth factors and cytokines have yet to be investigated in clinical trials.

4.6 Pregnancy and lactation

• Pregnancy

There are no adequate data from the use of lenograstim in pregnant women.

Studies in animals have shown reproductive toxicity (see 5.3). The potential risk in humans is unknown.

Granocyte should not be used during pregnancy unless clearly necessary.

• Lactation

Granocyte is not recommended for use in nursing women, as it is not known whether Granocyte is excreted in human breast milk.

4.7 Effects on ability to drive and use machines

None.

4.8 Undesirable effects

• In Bone Marrow Transplantation

In double-blind placebo-controlled trials the mean platelet count was lower in patients treated with Granocyte as compared with placebo without an increase in incidence of adverse events related to blood loss, and the median number of days following BMT to last platelet infusion was similar in both groups.

In placebo-controlled trials, the most frequently reported adverse events (15% in at least one treatment group) occurred with equal frequency in patients treated with Granocyte or placebo. These adverse events were those usually encountered with conditioning regimens. The events consisted of infection/inflammatory disorder of the buccal cavity, fever, diarrhoea, rash, abdominal pain, vomiting, alopecia, sepsis and infection.

• In Chemotherapy-Induced Neutropenia

The safety of Granocyte use with antineoplastic agents with cumulative bone marrow toxicity or predominant toxicity to the platelet lineage (nitrosourea, mitomycin) has not been established. Granocyte use may even result in enhanced toxicity particularly vis-à-vis platelets.

In trials, the most frequently reported adverse events were the same in patients treated with either Granocyte or placebo. The most commonly reported adverse events were alopecia, nausea, vomiting, fever and headache, similar to those observed in cancer patients treated with chemotherapy.

A slightly higher incidence of bone pain (approximately 10% higher) and injection site reaction (approximately 5% higher) were reported in Granocyte -treated patients.

• In peripheral blood progenitor cell mobilisation

When Granocyte is administered to healthy subjects, the most commonly reported clinical adverse events were headache in 30%, bone pain in 23%, back pain in 17.5%, asthenia in 11%, abdominal pain in 6% and pain in 6% of subjects. The risk of occurrence of pain is increased in subjects with high peak WBC values, especially when WBC $\geqslant 50 \times 10^9$/L. Leukocytosis $\geqslant 50 \times 10^9$/L was reported in 24 % of donors and thrombocytopenia (platelets $< 100 \times 10^9$/L) apheresis-related in 42%.

Transient increase of ASAT and/or ALAT was observed in 12% of subjects and alkaline phosphatase in 16%.

• Other undesirable effects

Immune system disorders: In very rare cases, allergic reactions including isolated cases of anaphylactic shock have been reported during the course of Granocyte treatment.

Respiratory, thoracic and mediastinal disorders: Rare pulmonary adverse effects including interstitial pneumonia, pulmonary oedema, pulmonary infiltrates and pulmonary fibrosis have been reported. Some of the reported cases have resulted in respiratory failure or acute respiratory distress syndrome (ARDS), which may be fatal (see 4.4).

Skin and subcutaneous tissue disorders: Very rare cases of cutaneous vasculitis have been reported in patients treated with Granocyte.

Very rare cases of Sweet's syndrome, erythema nodosum and pyoderma gangrenosum have been reported. They were mainly described in patients with haematological malignancies, a condition known to be associated with neutrophilic dermatosis, but also in non-malignant related neutropenia.

Very rare cases of Lyell's syndrome have also been reported.

Investigations: Transient LDH increases have been reported very commonly. Increases of ASAT, ALAT and/or alkaline phosphatase have been commonly reported during lenograstim treatment. In most cases, liver function abnormalities improved after lenograstim discontinuation.

Spleen: Common but generally asymptomatic cases of splenomegaly and very rare cases of splenic rupture in either healthy donors or patients receiving G-CSFs (see 4.4).

4.9 Overdose

The effects of Granocyte overdosage have not been established (see section 5.3). Discontinuation of Granocyte therapy usually results in a 50% decrease in circulating, neutrophils within 1 to 2 days, with a return to normal levels in 1 to 7 days.

A white blood cell count of approximately 50×10^9/L was observed in one patient out of three receiving the highest Granocyte dose of 40 μg/kg/day (5.12 MIU/kg/day) on the 5th day of treatment.

In humans, doses up to 40 μg/kg/day were not associated with toxic side effects except musculoskeletal pain.

5. PHARMACOLOGICAL PROPERTIES

5.1 Pharmacodynamic properties

Granocyte (rHuG-CSF) listed in the therapeutic classification as L03 A A10, belongs to the cytokine group of biologically active proteins which regulate cell differentiation and cell growth.

rHuG-CSF is a factor that stimulates neutrophil precursor cells as demonstrated by the CFU-S and CFU-GM cell count which increases in peripheral blood.

Granocyte induces a marked increase in peripheral blood neutrophil counts within 24 hours of administration.

Elevations of neutrophil count are dose-dependent over the 1-10 μg/kg/day range. At the recommended dose, repeated doses induce an enhancement of the neutrophil response. Neutrophils produced in response to Granocyte show normal chemotactic and phagocytic functions.

As with other haematopoietic growth factors, G-CSF has shown in vitro stimulating properties on human endothelial cells.

Use of Granocyte in patients who underwent Bone Marrow Transplantation or who are treated with cytotoxic chemotherapy leads to significant reductions in duration of neutropenia and its associated complications.

Use of Granocyte, either alone or after chemotherapy mobilises haematopoietic progenitor cells into the peripheral blood. These autologous Peripheral Blood Progenitor Cells (PBPCs) can be harvested and infused after high dose cytotoxic chemotherapy, either in place of, or in addition to bone marrow transplantation.

Reinfused PBPCs, as obtained following mobilisation with Granocyte, have been shown to reconstitute haemopoiesis and reduce the time to engraftment, leading to a marked decrease of the days to platelets independence when compared to autologous bone marrow transplantation.

A pooled analysis of data from 3 double-blind placebo-controlled studies conducted in 861 patients (n = 411 $\geqslant$ 55 years) demonstrated a favourable benefit/risk ratio of lenograstim administration in patients over 55 years of age undergoing conventional chemotherapy for *de novo* acute myeloid leukaemia, in the exception of AML with good cytogenetics, i.e. t(8;21), t(15;17) and inv (16).

The benefit in the sub-group of patients over 55 years appeared in terms of lenograstim-induced acceleration of neutrophil recovery, increase in the percentage of patients without infectious episode, reduction in infection duration, reduction in the duration of hospitalisation, reduction in the duration of IV antibiotherapy. However, these beneficial results were not associated with decreased severe or life-threatening infections incidence, nor with decreased infection-related mortality.

Data from a double-blind placebo-controlled study conducted in 446 patients with *de novo* AML showed that, in the 99 patients subgroup with good cytogenetics, the event-free survival was significantly lower in the lenograstim arm than in the placebo arm, and there was a trend towards a lower overall survival in the lenograstim arm when compared to data from the not good cytogenetics subgroup.

5.2 Pharmacokinetic properties

The pharmacokinetics of Granocyte are dose and time dependent.

During repeated dosing (IV and SC routes), peak serum concentration (immediately after IV infusion or after SC injection) is proportional to the injected dose. Repeated dosing with Granocyte by the two administration routes showed no evidence of drug accumulation.

At the recommended dose, the absolute bioavailability of Granocyte is 30%. The apparent volume of distribution (Vd) is approximatively 1 L/kg body weight and the mean residence time close to 7 h following subcutaneous dosing.

The apparent serum elimination half-life of Granocyte (SC route) is approximatively 3-4 h, at steady state (repeated dosing) and is shorter (1-1.5 h) following repeated IV infusion.

Plasma clearance of rHuG-CSF increased 3-fold (from 50 up to 150 mL/min) during repeated SC dosing. Less than 1% of Granocyte is excreted in urine unchanged and Granocyte is considered to be metabolised to peptides. During multiple SC dosing, peak serum concentrations of Granocyte are close to 100 pg/mL/kg body weight at the recommended dosage. There is a positive correlation between the dose and the serum concentration of Granocyte and between the neutrophil response and the total amount of Granocyte recovered in serum.

5.3 Preclinical safety data
In animals, acute toxicity studies (up to 1000 μg/kg/day in mice) and sub-acute toxicity studies (up to 100 μg/kg/day in monkey) showed the effects of overdose were restricted to an exaggerated and reversible pharmacological effect.

There is no evidence from studies in rats and rabbits that Granocyte is teratogenic. An increased incidence of embryo-loss has been observed in rabbits, but no malformation has been seen.

6. PHARMACEUTICAL PARTICULARS
6.1 List of excipients
Powder

Arginine

Phenylalnine

Methionine

Mannitol

Polysorbate 20

Hydrochloric acid diluted

Solvent

Water for injections

6.2 Incompatibilities
Dilution of Granocyte-13 (13.4 MIU/vial) to a final concentration of less than 0.26 Million International Units/ml (2 μg/mL) is not recommended.

Dilution of Granocyte-34 (33.6 MIU/vial) to a final concentration of less than 0.32 Million International Units/ml (2.5 μg/mL) is not recommended.

6.3 Shelf life
2 years.

After reconstitution or dilution, an immediate use is recommended.

However, in-use stability has been demonstrated for 24 hours between +2°C and +8°C (in a refrigerator) for solution at a concentration not less than 0.26 million IU/mL (2 μg/mL) for Granocyte 13 (13.4 MIU/vial) or not less than 0.32 million IU/mL (2.5 μg/mL) for Granocyte 34 (33.6 MIU/vial).

6.4 Special precautions for storage
- Do not store above +30°C.
- Do not freeze.
- After reconstitution or dilution, store at +2°C - +8°C (in a refrigerator).
- Any unused solution must be discarded.

6.5 Nature and contents of container
105 micrograms (Granocyte 13) or 263 micrograms (Granocyte 34) of powder in vial (type I glass) with a rubber stopper (type I butyl rubber)

+ 1 mL of solvent in pre-filled syringe (type I glass)

+ 2 needles; pack of 1 or 5.

or

105 micrograms (Granocyte 13) or 263 micrograms (Granocyte 34) of powder in vial (type I glass) with a rubber stopper (type I butyl rubber)

+ 1 mL of solvent in ampoule (type I glass); pack of 1 or 5.

Not all pack sizes may be marketed.

6.6 Instructions for use and handling
Granocyte vials are for single-dose use only.

Preparation of subcutaneous injection solution

- Aseptically add the extractable contents of one ampoule or of one prefilled syringe of solvent (Water for Injection) using the 19G needle to the Granocyte vial.
- Agitate gently until complete dissolution (about 5 seconds). Do not shake vigorously.
- Withdraw the required volume from the vial using the 19G needle.
- Administer immediately, using the 26G needle by SC injection.

Preparation of infusion

- Aseptically add the extractable contents of one ampoule or of one prefilled syringe of solvent (Water for Injection) to the Granocyte vial.
- Agitate gently until complete dissolution (about 5 seconds). Do not shake vigorously.
- Withdraw the required volume from the vial, using the 19G needle.
- Dilute the resulting solution in 0.9% sodium chloride or in 5% dextrose solution.
- Administer by IV route.
- Dilution of Granocyte 13 (13.4 MIU/vial) to a final concentration of less than 0.26 million International Units/mL (2 μg/mL) is not recommended.

At all events 1 vial of reconstituted Granocyte13 should be diluted in not more than 50 mL.

Dilution of Granocyte 34 (33.6 MIU/vial) to a final concentration of less than 0.32 million International Units/mL (2.5 μg/mL) is not recommended.

At all events 1 vial of reconstituted Granocyte 34 should be diluted in not more than 100 mL.

Granocyte is compatible with the commonly used giving-sets for injection when diluted:

- in a 0.9% saline solution (polyvinyl chloride bags and glass bottles)
- or in a 5% dextrose solution (glass bottles)

7. MARKETING AUTHORISATION HOLDER
Chugai Pharma UK Ltd, Mulliner House, Flanders Road, Turnham Green, London W4 1NN.

8. MARKETING AUTHORISATION NUMBER(S)
PL 12185/0002

PL 12185/0005 (Water for Injections in prefilled syringe).

9. DATE OF FIRST AUTHORISATION/RENEWAL OF THE AUTHORISATION
November 1993.

10. DATE OF REVISION OF THE TEXT
29 October 2004.

Gregovite C Tablets

(Alliance Pharmaceuticals)

1. NAME OF THE MEDICINAL PRODUCT
Gregovite 'C' Tablets

2. QUALITATIVE AND QUANTITATIVE COMPOSITION
Sodium Ascorbate SA99 HSE 176.74 mg

(equivalent to ascorbic acid 155.54 mg)

Ascorbic acid C97 HSE 148.93 mg

(equivalent to ascorbic acid 144.46 mg)

3. PHARMACEUTICAL FORM
Yellow, biconvex, circular, plain, lemon flavoured chewable tablet.

4. CLINICAL PARTICULARS
4.1 Therapeutic indications
For use as a vitamin C supplement during cold and influenza infections.

4.2 Posology and method of administration
Adults: One Gregovite 'C' tablet to be swallowed whole, sucked or chewed every six hours.

Elderly: As adult dose.

Children: Over 12 years - One tablet to be swallowed whole, sucked or chewed every eight hours.

Under 12 years - Not recommended.

4.3 Contraindications
There are no known contraindications.

4.4 Special warnings and special precautions for use
Not applicable.

4.5 Interaction with other medicinal products and other forms of Interaction
There are no known clinically significant interactions with other medicaments.

4.6 Pregnancy and lactation
Gregovite 'C' may be administered to pregnant and lactating women under the supervision of a doctor.

4.7 Effects on ability to drive and use machines
Not applicable.

4.8 Undesirable effects
No undesirable effects have been reported.

4.9 Overdose
No cases of overdosage have been reported.

5. PHARMACOLOGICAL PROPERTIES
5.1 Pharmacodynamic properties
Ascorbic acid (vitamin C) cannot be synthesised by man, therefore a dietary source is necessary.

Ascorbic acid (vitamin C) acts as a cofactor in numerous biological processes including the hydroxylation of proline to hydroxyproline. In deficiency, the formation of collagen is therefore impaired.

Ascorbic acid (vitamin C) is important in the hydroxylation of dopamine to noradrenaline and in hydroxylations occurring in steroid synthesis in the adrenals.

Ascorbic acid (vitamin C) is a reducing agent in tyrosine metabolism and by acting as an electron donor in the conversion of folic acid to tetrahydrofolic acid is directly involved in the synthesis of purine to thymine.

Ascorbic acid (vitamin C) is also necessary for the incorporation of iron into ferritin.

Ascorbic acid (vitamin C) increases the phagocytic function of leucocytes; it possesses anti-inflammatory activity and promotes wound healing.

Deficiency can produce scurvy. Features include swollen inflamed gums, petechial haemorrhages and subcutaneous bruising.

The deficiency of collagen leads to development of thin watery ground substances in which blood vessels are insecurely fixed and readily ruptured. The supportive components of bone and cartilage are also deficient causing bones to fracture easily and teeth to become loose.

Anaemia commonly occurs probably due to the role of ascorbic acid (vitamin C) in iron metabolism.

5.2 Pharmacokinetic properties
Ascorbic acid (vitamin C) is a water soluble vitamin which is readily absorbed from the gastro-intestinal tract and is widely distributed in the body tissues.

Ascorbic acid (vitamin C) is reversibly oxidised to dehydroascorbic acid; some is metabolised to ascorbate-2-sulphate, which is inactive, and oxalic acid which are excreted in the urine. Ascorbic acid (vitamin C) in excess of the body's needs is also rapidly eliminated unchanged in the urine.

5.3 Preclinical safety data
There are no pre-clinical data of relevance to the prescriber which are additional to that already included in other sections of the SPC.

6. PHARMACEUTICAL PARTICULARS
6.1 List of excipients
Saccharin sodium BP

Stearic acid BPC (1973)

Magnesium stearate BP

Compressible sugar (Microtal) NF

Lemon flavour E2954 HSE

(includes Maltodextrin, Acacia, Lactose)

Quinoline yellow lake 19248 (E104) HSE

Maize starch Ph Eur

6.2 Incompatibilities
No major incompatibilities have been reported.

6.3 Shelf life
36 months, as packaged for sale.

6.4 Special precautions for storage
Gregovite 'C' Tablets should be stored in a cool, dry place, temperature not exceeding 25°C (77°F).

6.5 Nature and contents of container
The product is presented in press through blisters containing six Uniflu tablets with six Gregovite 'C' tablets. The blister pack is made from PVC/PVdC with a printed aluminium foil lidding. The foil is printed (red on gold) with the name and PL number of both products, together with the company name.

The product is available in two pack sizes:

i. 12 tablet box containing 1 blister strip

ii. 24 tablet box containing 2 blister strips

6.6 Instructions for use and handling
Not applicable.

7. MARKETING AUTHORISATION HOLDER
Alliance Pharmaceuticals Ltd

Avonbridge House

Chippenham

Wiltshire

SN15 2BB

United Kingdom

8. MARKETING AUTHORISATION NUMBER(S)
PL 16853/0087

9. DATE OF FIRST AUTHORISATION/RENEWAL OF THE AUTHORISATION
18th April 2005

10. DATE OF REVISION OF THE TEXT
April 2005

Gyno-Daktarin 1

(Janssen-Cilag Ltd)

1. NAME OF THE MEDICINAL PRODUCT
GYNO-DAKTARIN 1

2. QUALITATIVE AND QUANTITATIVE COMPOSITION
Miconazole nitrate 1200 mg.

3. PHARMACEUTICAL FORM
White, egg-shaped soft gelatin Scherer capsule.

4. CLINICAL PARTICULARS

4.1 Therapeutic indications

For the local treatment of vulvovaginal candidosis and superinfections due to Gram-positive bacteria.

4.2 Posology and method of administration

GYNO-DAKTARIN 1 is for intravaginal administration.

Adults and Elderly

One ovule to be inserted high in the vagina at night, as a single dose.

Children

Not recommended.

4.3 Contraindications

None known.

4.4 Special warnings and special precautions for use

None.

4.5 Interaction with other medicinal products and other forms of Interaction

Contact should be avoided between contraceptive diaphragms or sheaths and GYNO-DAKTARIN 1 since the rubber may be damaged by the emollient base.

4.6 Pregnancy and lactation

In animals, miconazole nitrate has shown no teratogenic effects but is foetotoxic at high oral doses. The significance of this to man is unknown as there is no evidence of increased risk when taken in human pregnancy. However, as with other imidazoles, GYNO-DAKTARIN 1 should be used in pregnant women only if the practitioner considers it to be necessary.

4.7 Effects on ability to drive and use machines

None.

4.8 Undesirable effects

Occasionally, irritation has been reported. Rarely, local sensitisation may occur requiring discontinuation of treatment.

4.9 Overdose

GYNO-DAKTARIN 1 is for intravaginal use only. If accidental ingestion of large quantities occurs, an appropriate method of gastric emptying may be used if considered desirable.

5. PHARMACOLOGICAL PROPERTIES

5.1 Pharmacodynamic properties

Miconazole is a synthetic imidazole antifungal agent with a broad spectrum of activity against pathogenic fungi (including yeasts and dermatophytes) and gram-positive bacteria (staphylococcus and streptococcus spp).

5.2 Pharmacokinetic properties

There is little absorption through mucous membranes when miconazole nitrate is applied topically.

5.3 Preclinical safety data

No relevant information additional to that contained elsewhere in the Summary of

Product Characteristics.

6. PHARMACEUTICAL PARTICULARS

6.1 List of excipients

Liquid paraffin, white petrolatum and lecithin. The capsule itself contains gelatin, glycerol, titanium dioxide, sodium ethylparahydroxybenzoate, sodium propyl parahydroxybenzoate and medium chain triglycerides.

6.2 Incompatibilities

None known.

6.3 Shelf life

60 months.

6.4 Special precautions for storage

Do not store above 25°C.

6.5 Nature and contents of container

One ovule packed in a blister pack.

6.6 Instructions for use and handling

None stated.

7. MARKETING AUTHORISATION HOLDER

Janssen-Cilag Ltd

Saunderton

High Wycombe

Buckinghamshire

HP14 4HJ

UK

8. MARKETING AUTHORISATION NUMBER(S)

PL 0242/0121

9. DATE OF FIRST AUTHORISATION/RENEWAL OF THE AUTHORISATION

Date of first authorisation: 30/01/86. Renewal of the authorisation: 07/01/02

10. DATE OF REVISION OF THE TEXT

20 June 2002

Gyno-Daktarin Cream

(Janssen-Cilag Ltd)

1. NAME OF THE MEDICINAL PRODUCT

Gyno-Daktarin® Cream

2. QUALITATIVE AND QUANTITATIVE COMPOSITION

Miconazole nitrate 2% w/w.

3. PHARMACEUTICAL FORM

White homogeneous vaginal cream.

4. CLINICAL PARTICULARS

4.1 Therapeutic indications

For the treatment of mycotic vulvovaginitis and superinfections due to Gram-positive bacteria.

4.2 Posology and method of administration

Route of administration:

Vaginal use.

Recommended dosage:

5 g once daily into vagina for 10 – 14 days or twice daily for 7 days. For vulvitis the cream should be applied topically twice daily. Continue treatment for a few days after symptomatic relief has been achieved.

4.3 Contraindications

None known.

4.4 Special warnings and special precautions for use

None.

4.5 Interaction with other medicinal products and other forms of Interaction

Contact between contraceptive diaphragms or condoms and this product must be avoided since the rubber may be damaged by this preparation.

4.6 Pregnancy and lactation

In animals, miconazole nitrate has shown no teratogenic effects, but is foetotoxic at high oral doses. Only small amounts of miconazole nitrate are absorbed following topical administration. However, as with other imidazoles, miconazole nitrate should be used with caution during pregnancy.

4.7 Effects on ability to drive and use machines

None known.

4.8 Undesirable effects

Occasionally irritation has been reported. Rarely local sensitisation or hypersensitivity may occur in which case administration of the product should be discontinued.

4.9 Overdose

Gyno-Daktarin cream is intended for vaginal use. If accidental ingestion of the product occurs, an appropriate method of gastric emptying may be used if considered advisable.

5. PHARMACOLOGICAL PROPERTIES

5.1 Pharmacodynamic properties

Miconazole is an imidazole antifungal agent and may act by interfering with the permeability of the fungal cell membrane. It possesses a wide antifungal spectrum and has some antibacterial activity.

5.2 Pharmacokinetic properties

There is little absorption through skin or mucous membranes when miconazole nitrate is applied topically.

When administered orally, miconazole is incompletely absorbed from the gastro-intestinal tract. Peak plasma concentrations occur at about 4 hours after administration. Miconazole nitrate disappears from the plasma in a triphasic manner with a biological half-life of about 24 hours. Over 90% is reported to be bound to plasma proteins.

5.3 Preclinical safety data

No relevant information additional to that contained elsewhere in the Summary of Product Characteristics.

6. PHARMACEUTICAL PARTICULARS

6.1 List of excipients

Macrogol 6-32 stearate and glycol stearate

Unsaturated polyglycolysed glycerides

Liquid paraffin

Benzoic acid (E210)

Butylated hydroxyanisole (E320)

Purified water

6.2 Incompatibilities

None known.

6.3 Shelf life

24 months.

6.4 Special precautions for storage

Do not store above 25°C.

6.5 Nature and contents of container

Aluminium tube inner lined with heat polymerised epoxyphenol resin with a white polypropylene cap containing 15 g, 40 g, or 78 g of cream.

6.6 Instructions for use and handling

Not applicable.

7. MARKETING AUTHORISATION HOLDER

Janssen-Cilag Ltd

Saunderton

High Wycombe

Buckinghamshire

HP14 4HJ

UK

8. MARKETING AUTHORISATION NUMBER(S)

PL 0242/0015

9. DATE OF FIRST AUTHORISATION/RENEWAL OF THE AUTHORISATION

Date of First Authorisation: 13 May 1974

Date of Renewal of Authorisation: 11 August 1995

10. DATE OF REVISION OF THE TEXT

June 2000

Legal Category: POM

Gyno-Daktarin Pessaries

(Janssen-Cilag Ltd)

1. NAME OF THE MEDICINAL PRODUCT

GYNO-DAKTARIN® Pessaries.

2. QUALITATIVE AND QUANTITATIVE COMPOSITION

Miconazole nitrate 100 mg.

3. PHARMACEUTICAL FORM

Vaginal pessary.

4. CLINICAL PARTICULARS

4.1 Therapeutic indications

For the local treatment of vulvovaginal candidosis and superinfections due to gram-positive bacteria.

4.2 Posology and method of administration

Adults and elderly

One pessary to be inserted in the vagina once daily for 14 days or 1 pessary twice daily for 7 days.

Children

Not recommended.

Method of administration

Vaginal administration.

4.3 Contraindications

None known.

4.4 Special warnings and special precautions for use

None.

4.5 Interaction with other medicinal products and other forms of Interaction

Contact should be avoided between contraceptive diaphragms or sheaths and Gyno-Daktarin pessaries since the rubber may be damaged by the emollient base.

4.6 Pregnancy and lactation

In animals, miconazole nitrate has shown no teratogenic effects but is foetotoxic at high oral doses. The significance of this to man is unknown as there is no evidence of increased risk when taken in human pregnancy. However, as with other imidazoles, Gyno-Daktarin should be used in pregnant women only if the practitioner considers it to be necessary.

4.7 Effects on ability to drive and use machines

None.

4.8 Undesirable effects

Occasionally, irritation has been reported. Rarely, local sensitisation may occur requiring discontinuation of treatment.

4.9 Overdose

Gyno-Daktarin pessaries are for intravaginal use only. In the unlikely event of oral ingestion, an appropriate method of gastric emptying may be used if considered desirable.

5. PHARMACOLOGICAL PROPERTIES

5.1 Pharmacodynamic properties

Miconazole is a synthetic imidazole antifungal agent with a broad spectrum of activity against pathogenic fungi (including yeasts and dermatophytes) and gram-positive bacteria (*Staphylococcus* and *Streptococcus spp*).

5.2 Pharmacokinetic properties

There is little absorption through mucous membranes when miconazole nitrate is applied topically.

5.3 Preclinical safety data

Not applicable.

6. PHARMACEUTICAL PARTICULARS

6.1 List of excipients

Hard fat.

6.2 Incompatibilities

Not applicable.

6.3 Shelf life

60 months.

6.4 Special precautions for storage

Store at or below 25°C.

6.5 Nature and contents of container
Cardboard cartons containing 14 pessaries packed in PVC-polyethylene strips.

Combination Pack: 1 × pessary pack as above and Gyno-Daktarin Cream pack(s) as for PL 0242/0015.

6.6 Instructions for use and handling
1. Each of the Gyno-Daktarin pessaries is individually wrapped to protect it and keep it clean. To remove a pessary, tear down the groove separating two pessaries and peel back the plastic wrapping, starting at the smooth end.

2. Lie on your back with your knees up and your legs apart. Holding the pessary between your thumb and first finger, insert the pessary as high into the vagina as possible with your finger.

3. Always wash your hands with soap and warm water after inserting the pessary.

7. MARKETING AUTHORISATION HOLDER
Janssen-Cilag Limited
Saunderton
High Wycombe
Buckinghamshire
HP14 4HJ

8. MARKETING AUTHORISATION NUMBER(S)
PL 0242/0037

9. DATE OF FIRST AUTHORISATION/RENEWAL OF THE AUTHORISATION
Date of First Authorisation: 9 July 1975
Date of Renewal of Authorisation: 28 September 1995

10. DATE OF REVISION OF THE TEXT
April 1997

Legal category POM

Gynol II Contraceptive Jelly

(Janssen-Cilag Ltd)

1. NAME OF THE MEDICINAL PRODUCT
GYNOL-II® Contraceptive Jelly

2. QUALITATIVE AND QUANTITATIVE COMPOSITION
The gel contains 2.0% w/w of nonoxinol-9.

3. PHARMACEUTICAL FORM
Vaginal gel.

4. CLINICAL PARTICULARS
4.1 Therapeutic indications
For use as a spermicidal contraceptive in conjunction with barrier methods of contraception.

4.2 Posology and method of administration
Method of Administration

For vaginal use.

For use by adult females only.

Posology
The gel should be spread over the surface of the diaphragm which will be in contact with the cervix, and on the rim. The diaphragm and spermicide must be allowed to remain undisturbed for at least six to eight hours after coitus. A fresh application of gel or other spermicides, e.g. Orthoforms® Contraceptive Pessaries must be made prior to any subsequent acts of coitus within this period of time, without removing the diaphragm. (A vaginal applicator should be used for inserting more jelly.)

Douching is not recommended, but if desired it should be deferred for at least six hours after intercourse.

4.3 Contraindications
Hypersensitivity to nonoxinol-9 or to any component of the preparation.

Patients with absent vaginal sensation e.g. paraplegics and quadriplegics.

4.4 Special warnings and special precautions for use
Spermicidal intravaginal preparations are intended for use in conjunction with barrier methods of contraception such as condoms, diaphragms and caps.

Where avoidance of pregnancy is important, the choice of contraceptive method should be made in consultation with a doctor or a family planning clinic.

This product does not protect against HIV (AIDS) or other sexually transmitted diseases (STDs). A latex condom should be used to protect against the spread of STDs. High frequency use of nonoxinol-9 has been reported to cause epithelial damage and increase the risk of HIV infection. Therefore women at risk of HIV/STD infection and who have multiple daily acts of intercourse should be advised to choose another method of contraception. Sexually active women should consider their individual HIV/STD infection risk when choosing a method of contraception.

If vaginal or penile irritation occurs, discontinue use. If symptoms worsen or continue for more than 48 hours, medical advice should be sought.

4.5 Interaction with other medicinal products and other forms of Interaction
None known.

4.6 Pregnancy and lactation
There is no evidence from animal and human studies that nonoxinol-9 is teratogenic. Human epidemiological studies have not shown any firm evidence of adverse effects on the foetus, however some studies have shown that nonoxinol-9 may be embryotoxic in animals. This product should not be used if pregnancy is suspected or confirmed. Animal studies have detected nonoxinol-9 in milk after intravaginal administration. Use by lactating women has not been studied.

4.7 Effects on ability to drive and use machines
None known.

4.8 Undesirable effects
May cause irritation of the vagina or penis.

4.9 Overdose
If taken orally, the surfactant properties of this preparation may cause gastric irritation. General supportive therapy should be carried out. Hepatic and renal function should be monitored if medically indicated.

5. PHARMACOLOGICAL PROPERTIES
5.1 Pharmacodynamic properties
The standard *in vitro* test (Sander-Cramer) evaluating the effect of nonoxinol-9 on animal sperm motility has shown the compound to be a potent spermicide.

The site of action of nonoxinol-9 has been determined as the sperm cell membrane. The lipoprotein membrane is disrupted, increasing permeability, with subsequent loss of cell components and decreased motility. A similar effect on vaginal epithelial and bacterial cells is also found.

5.2 Pharmacokinetic properties
The intravaginal absorption and excretion of radiolabelled (^{14}C) nonoxinol-9 has been studied in non-pregnant rats and rabbits and in pregnant rats. No appreciable difference was found in the extent or rate of absorption in pregnant and non-pregnant animals. Plasma levels peaked at about one hour and recovery from urine as unchanged nonoxinol-9 accounted for approximately 15-25% and faeces approximately 70% of the administered dose as unchanged nonoxinol-9. Less than 0.3% was found in the milk of lactating rats. No metabolites were detected in any of the samples analysed.

5.3 Preclinical safety data
No relevant information additional to that contained elsewhere in the Summary of Product Characteristics.

6. PHARMACEUTICAL PARTICULARS
6.1 List of excipients
Methyl parahydroxybenzoate (E 218)
Sorbitol solution (E 420)
Lactic acid
Povidone K30
Propylene glycol
Sodium carboxymethylcellulose
Sorbic acid (E 200)
Purified water

6.2 Incompatibilities
Not applicable.

6.3 Shelf life
2 years.

6.4 Special precautions for storage
Do not store above 25°C.

6.5 Nature and contents of container
Epoxy resin lined aluminium tubes with polyethylene caps. Available in 81 gram packs; an applicator is available separately if required.

6.6 Instructions for use and handling
Not applicable.

7. MARKETING AUTHORISATION HOLDER
Janssen-Cilag Limited
Saunderton
High Wycombe
Buckinghamshire
HP14 4HJ
UK

8. MARKETING AUTHORISATION NUMBER(S)
PL 0242/0225

9. DATE OF FIRST AUTHORISATION/RENEWAL OF THE AUTHORISATION
12 September 1995/17 July 1996

10. DATE OF REVISION OF THE TEXT
23 October 2002

Legal category GSL

Gyno-Pevaryl 1 Vaginal Pessary

(Janssen-Cilag Ltd)

1. NAME OF THE MEDICINAL PRODUCT
Gyno-Pevaryl 1 Vaginal Pessary.

2. QUALITATIVE AND QUANTITATIVE COMPOSITION
Each pessary contains econazole nitrate PhEur 150 mg.

3. PHARMACEUTICAL FORM
Pessary.

The pessary is light beige and bullet shaped, with a fat-like odour.

4. CLINICAL PARTICULARS
4.1 Therapeutic indications
Vaginitis due to *Candida Albicans* and other yeasts.

4.2 Posology and method of administration
For vaginal administration.

Adults:

Insert one pessary high into the vagina at night prior to retiring.

Children:

Gyno-Pevaryl 1 pessary is not indicated for use in children under the age of 16 years.

Elderly:

No specific dosage recommendations or precautions apply.

4.3 Contraindications
Hypersensitivity to any imidazole preparation (or other vaginal antifungal products).

4.4 Special warnings and special precautions for use
Hypersensitivity has rarely been recorded; if it should occur administration should be discontinued.

4.5 Interaction with other medicinal products and other forms of Interaction
Contact between contraceptive diaphragms or condoms and this product must be avoided since the rubber may be damaged by the preparation.

Although not studied, based on the chemical similarity of econazole with other imidazole compounds, a theoretical potential for competitive interaction with compounds metabolized by CYP3A4/2C9 exists. Due to the limited systemic availability after vaginal application (see 5.2. Pharmacokinetic Properties), clinically relevant interactions are unlikely to occur. In patients on oral anticoagulants, such as warfarin and acenocoumarol, caution should be exercised and monitoring of the anticoagulant effect should be considered.

4.6 Pregnancy and lactation
In animals, econazole nitrate has shown no teratogenic effects but is foetotoxic at high doses. The significance of this to man is unknown as there is no evidence of an increased risk when taken in human pregnancy. However, as with other imidazoles, econazole should be used in pregnancy only if the practitioner considers it to be necessary.

4.7 Effects on ability to drive and use machines
None known.

4.8 Undesirable effects
The most frequently reported adverse events in clinical trials were application site reactions, such as burning and stinging sensations, pruritus, and erythema.

Based on post-marketing experience, the following adverse reactions have also been reported:

Skin and subcutaneous tissue disorders; general disorders and administration site conditions

Very rare (< 1/10,000): Localized application site (mucocutaneous) reactions, such as erythema, rash, burning and pruritus.

Isolated reports of localized allergic reactions. Isolated reports of generalized allergic reactions, including angioedema and urticaria.

4.9 Overdose
This product is intended for vaginal use. If accidental ingestion of large quantities of the product occurs, an appropriate method of gastric emptying may be used if considered desirable.

5. PHARMACOLOGICAL PROPERTIES
5.1 Pharmacodynamic properties
Pharmacotherapeutic classification: (Antiinfectives and antiseptics, excl. combinations with corticosteroids, imidazole derivatives)

ATC code: G01A F05

Econazole is an imidazole derivative. The compound acts by damaging the membranes of bacterial and fungal cells; both the cellular and subcellular membranes are affected. Econazole apparently disturbs the permeability characteristics of the membrane which allow leakage of potassium and sodium ions and other intra cellular components. Macro-molecular synthesis may also be inhibited. Econazole is active against dermatophytes, yeast, moulds and Gram positive bacteria. Gram negative bacteria are generally resistant to econazole.

5.2 Pharmacokinetic properties
Econazole nitrate is poorly absorbed after vaginal application. Using radiolabelled techniques, it has been determined that between 2.5% and 7% of vaginally applied econazole nitrate is absorbed. However, no antimycotic activity could be detected in the serum after vaginal application of 5 g or 1% econazole nitrate cream or a suppository containing 50 mg econazole nitrate.

5.3 Preclinical safety data
No relevant information other than that contained elsewhere in the Summary of Product Characteristics.

6. PHARMACEUTICAL PARTICULARS

6.1 List of excipients
Polygel

Colloidal silicon dioxide

Witepsol H19

Wecobee FS

Stearyl heptanoate

6.2 Incompatibilities
None stated.

6.3 Shelf life
3 years.

6.4 Special precautions for storage
Do not store above 25°C.

6.5 Nature and contents of container
Multi-plast strip or PVC/PE moulds, containing one pessary.

1 applicator

Gyno-Pevaryl 1 Vaginal Pessary (PL 0242/0226) is also contained in:

Gyno-Pevaryl 1 C.P. PACK Vaginal Pessary and Cream (PL 0242/0226 & PL 0242/0229)

6.6 Instructions for use and handling
Not applicable.

7. MARKETING AUTHORISATION HOLDER
Janssen-Cilag Limited

Saunderton

High Wycombe

Buckinghamshire

HP14 4HJ

UK

8. MARKETING AUTHORISATION NUMBER(S)
PL 00242/0226

9. DATE OF FIRST AUTHORISATION/RENEWAL OF THE AUTHORISATION
1 October 1995/June 2003

10. DATE OF REVISION OF THE TEXT
October 2003

Legal category POM

Gyno-Pevaryl 150 mg Vaginal Pessaries

(Janssen-Cilag Ltd)

1. NAME OF THE MEDICINAL PRODUCT
GYNO-PEVARYL® 150 mg Vaginal Pessaries

2. QUALITATIVE AND QUANTITATIVE COMPOSITION
Vaginal pessaries each containing 150 mg econazole nitrate.

3. PHARMACEUTICAL FORM
Pessaries (creamy, white to yellowish, bullet-shaped).

4. CLINICAL PARTICULARS

4.1 Therapeutic indications
Vaginitis due to *Candida albicans* and other yeasts.

4.2 Posology and method of administration
For vaginal administration.

Adults:

One pessary should be inserted high into the vagina each evening for three consecutive days.

Children:

Gyno-Pevaryl 150 mg pessary is not indicated for use in children under the age of 16 years.

Elderly:

No specific dosage recommendations or precautions apply.

4.3 Contraindications
Hypersensitivity to any imidazole preparation or other vaginal antifungal products.

4.4 Special warnings and special precautions for use
Hypersensitivity has rarely been recorded; if it should occur administration should be discontinued.

4.5 Interaction with other medicinal products and other forms of Interaction
Contact between contraceptive diaphragms or condoms and this product must be avoided since the rubber may be damaged by this preparation.

Although not studied, based on the chemical similarity of econazole with other imidazole compounds, a theoretical potential for competitive interaction with compounds metabolized by CYP3A4/2C9 exists. Due to the limited systemic availability after vaginal application (see 5.2. Pharmacokinetic Properties), clinically relevant interactions are unlikely to occur. In patients on oral anticoagulants, such as warfarin and acenocoumarol, caution should be exercised and monitoring of the anticoagulant effect should be considered.

4.6 Pregnancy and lactation
In animals, econazole nitrate has shown no teratogenic effects but is foetotoxic at high doses. The significance of this to man is unknown as there is no evidence of an increased risk when taken in human pregnancy. However, as with other imidazoles, econazole should be used in pregnancy only if the practitioner considers it to be necessary.

4.7 Effects on ability to drive and use machines
None known.

4.8 Undesirable effects
The most frequently reported adverse events in clinical trials were application site reactions, such as burning and stinging sensations, pruritus, and erythema.

Based on post-marketing experience, the following adverse reactions have also been reported:

Skin and subcutaneous tissue disorders; general disorders and administration site conditions

Very rare (< 1/10,000): Localized application site (mucocutaneous) reactions, such as erythema, rash, burning and pruritus.

Isolated reports of localized allergic reactions. Isolated reports of generalized allergic reactions, including angioedema and urticaria.

4.9 Overdose
Gyno-Pevaryl 150 mg Vaginal Pessaries are intended for intra-vaginal use and by that route overdose is extremely unlikely. If accidental ingestion of large quantities of the product occurs an appropriate method of gastric emptying may be used if considered desirable.

5. PHARMACOLOGICAL PROPERTIES

5.1 Pharmacodynamic properties
Pharmacotherapeutic classification: (Antiinfectives and antiseptics, excl. combinations with corticosteroids, imidazole derivatives)

ATC code: G01A F05

Econazole nitrate has no anti-inflammatory action, no effects on the circulation, no central or autonomic nervous effects, no effects on respiration, no effect on α or β receptors, no anticholinergic or antiserotonic reactions.

A broad spectrum of antimycotic activity has been demonstrated against dermatophytes, yeasts and moulds. A clinically relevant action against Gram positive bacteria has also been found.

Econazole acts by damaging cell membranes. The permeability of the fungal cell is increased. Sub-cellular membranes in the cytoplasm are damaged. The site of action is most probably the unsaturated fatty acid acyl moiety of membrane phospholipids.

5.2 Pharmacokinetic properties
Econazole nitrate is poorly absorbed from the vagina and skin. If given orally, peak plasma levels occur six hours after dosing. About 90% of the absorbed dose is bound to plasma proteins. Metabolism is limited, but primarily occurs in the liver. Metabolites are excreted in the urine. Five major and two minor metabolites have been identified.

5.3 Preclinical safety data
No relevant information other than that contained elsewhere in the Summary of Product Characteristics.

6. PHARMACEUTICAL PARTICULARS

6.1 List of excipients
Wecobee M

Wecobee FS

6.2 Incompatibilities
None stated.

6.3 Shelf life
Five years.

6.4 Special precautions for storage
Do not store above 25°C.

Keep out of reach and sight of children.

6.5 Nature and contents of container
Available in PVC/PE strips containing three pessaries.

Gyno-Pevaryl 150 Vaginal Pessaries (PL 0242/0227) are also contained in:

Gyno-Pevaryl 150 Combined Vaginal Pessaries and Cream

(PL 0242/0227 & PL 0242/0229).

6.6 Instructions for use and handling
Not applicable.

7. MARKETING AUTHORISATION HOLDER
Janssen-Cilag Ltd

Saunderton

High Wycombe

Buckinghamshire

HP14 4HJ

UK

8. MARKETING AUTHORISATION NUMBER(S)
PL 00242/0227

9. DATE OF FIRST AUTHORISATION/RENEWAL OF THE AUTHORISATION
1st October 1995/June 2003

10. DATE OF REVISION OF THE TEXT
October 2003

Legal Category
POM

Gyno-Pevaryl Cream

(Janssen-Cilag Ltd)

1. NAME OF THE MEDICINAL PRODUCT
Gyno-Pevaryl® Cream.

2. QUALITATIVE AND QUANTITATIVE COMPOSITION
Each 100 g of cream contains 1 g econazole nitrate Ph.Eur. (1% w/w).

3. PHARMACEUTICAL FORM
Vaginal Cream.

4. CLINICAL PARTICULARS

4.1 Therapeutic indications
For the treatment of mycotic vulvovaginitis and mycotic balanitis.

4.2 Posology and method of administration
Route of Administration
For vaginal/penile administration.

Females: One applicator full (approximately 5 g) intravaginally once daily at night for not less than 14 days. The cream should also be applied to the vulva. The full 14 days treatment should be carried out even if the symptoms of vaginal itching or discharge have disappeared.

Males: Apply the cream to the penis, including under the foreskin, once daily for not less than 14 days.

The sexual partner should also be treated.

4.3 Contraindications
Hypersensitivity to any imidazole preparation (or other vaginal antifungal products).

4.4 Special warnings and special precautions for use
Hypersensitivity has rarely been recorded; if it should occur administration should be discontinued.

Gyno-Pevaryl Cream is not indicated for use in children under the age of 16 years.

4.5 Interaction with other medicinal products and other forms of Interaction
Contact between contraceptive diaphragms or condoms and this product must be avoided since the rubber may be damaged by this preparation.

Although not studied, based on the chemical similarity of econazole with other imidazole compounds, a theoretical potential for competitive interaction with compounds metabolized by CYP3A4/2C9 exists. Due to the limited systemic availability after vaginal application (see 5.2. Pharmacokinetic Properties), clinically relevant interactions are unlikely to occur. In patients on oral anticoagulants, such as warfarin and acenocoumarol, caution should be exercised and monitoring of the anticoagulant effect should be considered.

4.6 Pregnancy and lactation
In animals, econazole nitrate has shown no teratogenic effects but is foetotoxic at high doses. The significance of this to man is unknown as there is no evidence of an increased risk when taken in human pregnancy. However, as with other imidazoles, econazole should be used in pregnancy only if the practitioner considers it to be necessary.

4.7 Effects on ability to drive and use machines
None known.

4.8 Undesirable effects
The most frequently reported adverse events in clinical trials were application site reactions, such as burning and stinging sensations, pruritus, and erythema.

Based on post-marketing experience, the following adverse reactions have also been reported:

Skin and subcutaneous tissue disorders; general disorders and administration site conditions

Very rare (< 1/10,000): Localized application site (mucocutaneous) reactions, such as erythema, rash, burning and pruritus.

Isolated reports of localized allergic reactions. Isolated reports of generalized allergic reactions, including angioedema and urticaria.

4.9 Overdose
This product is intended for vaginal/penile use. If accidental ingestion of large quantities of the product occurs, an appropriate method of gastric emptying may be used if considered desirable.

5. PHARMACOLOGICAL PROPERTIES

5.1 Pharmacodynamic properties
Pharmacotherapeutic classification: (Antiinfectives and antiseptics, excl. combinations with corticosteroids, imidazole derivatives)

ATC code: G01A F05

Econazole nitrate has no anti-inflammatory action, no effect on circulation, no central or autonomic nervous effects, no effects on respiration, no effect on α or β receptors, no anticholinergic or antiserotonergic reactions.

A broad spectrum of antimycotic activity has been demonstrated against dermatophytes, yeasts and moulds. A clinically relevant action against Gram positive bacteria has also been found.

Econazole acts by damaging cell membranes. The permeability of the fungal cell is increased. Sub-cellular membranes in the cytoplasm are damaged. The site of action is most probably the unsaturated fatty acid acyl moiety of membrane phospholipids.

5.2 Pharmacokinetic properties
Econazole nitrate is poorly absorbed from the vagina and skin. If given orally, peak plasma levels occur six hours after dosing. About 90% of the absorbed dose is bound to plasma proteins. Metabolism is limited, but primarily occurs in the liver, the metabolites excreted in the urine.

Five major and two minor metabolites have been identified.

5.3 Preclinical safety data
No relevant information additional to that contained elsewhere in the Summary of Product Characteristics.

6. PHARMACEUTICAL PARTICULARS

6.1 List of excipients
Tefose 63

Labrafil M 1944 CS

Mineral oil

Butylated hydroxyanisole

Benzoic acid

Purified water

6.2 Incompatibilities
None stated.

6.3 Shelf life
36 months.

6.4 Special precautions for storage
Do not store above 25°C.

6.5 Nature and contents of container
Aluminium lacquered tubes.

Pack sizes 78 g, 30g, 15g.

Gyno-Pevaryl Cream (PL 0242/0229) is also contained in:

Gyno-Pevaryl 150 Combined Vaginal Pessaries and Cream

(PL 0242/0227 & PL 0242/0229)

Gyno-Pevaryl 1 C.P. PACK Vaginal Pessary and Cream
(PL 0242/0226 & PL 0242/0229)

6.6 Instructions for use and handling
None stated.

Administrative Data

7. MARKETING AUTHORISATION HOLDER
Janssen-Cilag Limited

Saunderton

High Wycombe

Buckinghamshire

HP14 4HJ

UK

8. MARKETING AUTHORISATION NUMBER(S)
PL 00242/0229

9. DATE OF FIRST AUTHORISATION/RENEWAL OF THE AUTHORISATION
22 September 1995/June 2003

10. DATE OF REVISION OF THE TEXT
October 2003.

LEGAL CATEGORY POM.

Haemate P 500 and 1000 IU

(ZLB Behring UK Limited)

1. NAME OF THE MEDICINAL PRODUCT
Haemate® P 500 and 1000 IU

2. QUALITATIVE AND QUANTITATIVE COMPOSITION
Haemate® P is prepared as a powder and solvent for solution for injection.

Haemate® P 500 IU: The product reconstituted with 20 ml of water for injection contains approximately 500 IU human coagulation factor VIII and 1100 IU of vWF:RCof per vial. Each vial contains 510-960 mg of dried substance. Each vial has a total protein content of 100-220 mg.

Haemate® P 1000 IU: The product reconstituted with 30 ml of water for injection contains approximately 1000 IU human coagulation factor VIII and 2200 IU of vWF:RCof per vial. Each vial contains 1020-1920mg of dried substance. Each vial has a total protein content of 200-440mg.

The potency (IU) for human coagulation factor VIII is determined using the European Pharmacopoeia chromogenic assay against the World Health Organisation (WHO) international standard.

For excipients, see 6.1

3. PHARMACEUTICAL FORM
Powder and solvent for solution for injection.

4. CLINICAL PARTICULARS

4.1 Therapeutic indications

- Prophylaxis and treatment of bleedings in:

- haemophilia A (congenital factor VIII deficiency) and other diseases with factor VIII deficiency

- Prophylaxis and treatment of bleedings in von Willebrand's disease

4.2 Posology and method of administration

4.2.1

Posology

Treatment should be initiated under the supervision of a physician experienced in the treatment of haemophilia.

- Haemophilia A:

The dosage and duration of the substitution therapy depends on the severity of factor VIII deficiency, on the location and extent of the bleeding and on the clinical condition.

The number of units of factor VIII administered is expressed in International Units (IU), which are related to the current WHO standard for factor VIII products. Factor VIII activity in plasma is expressed either as a percentage (relative to normal human plasma) or in International Units (relative to an International Standard for factor VIII in plasma).

One International Unit (IU) of factor VIII activity is equivalent to that quantity of factor VIII in one ml of normal human plasma.

The calculation of the required dosage of factor VIII is based on the empirical finding that 1 IU factor VIII:C per kg body weight raises the plasma factor VIII activity by about 1.5% to 2 % of normal activity (1.5 – 2 IU/dl). The required dosage is determined using the following formula:

Required units = body weight (kg) × desired F VIII:C rise (% or IU/dl) × 0.5 IU/Kg.

The amount to be administered and the frequency of administration should always be tailored to the clinical effectiveness the individual case.

In the case of the following haemorrhagic events, the factor VIII activity should not fall below the given plasma activity level (in % of norm) in the corresponding period. The following table can be used to guide dosing in bleeding episodes and surgery:

Degree of haemorrhage/ Type of Surgical Procedure	Factor VIII Level required (% or IU/dl)	Frequency of Doses (hours)/ Duration of Therapy (days)
Haemorrhage:		
Early haemarthrosis, muscle bleed or oral bleed	20-40	Repeat every 12 to 24 hours. At least 1 day, until the bleeding episode as indicated by pain is resolved or healing is achieved.
More extensive haemarthrosis, muscle bleed or haematoma	30-60	Repeat infusion every 12-24 hours for 3-4 days or more until pain and disability are resolved.
Life threatening bleeds such as head surgery, throat bleed, severe abdominal bleed	60-100	Repeat infusion every 8 to 24 hours until threat is resolved.
Surgery:		
Minor Including tooth extraction	30-60	Every 24 hours, at least 1 day, until healing is achieved.
Major	80-100 (pre- and post-operative)	Repeat infusion every 8-24 hours until adequate wound healing, then therapy for at least another 7 days to maintain a FVIII activity of 30% to 60% (IU/dl).

Under certain circumstances larger amounts than those calculated can be required, especially in the case of the initial dose.

During the course of treatment, appropriate determination of factor VIII levels is advised to guide the dose to be administered and the frequency of repeated infusions. In the case of major surgical interventions in particular, precise monitoring of the substitution therapy by means of coagulation analysis (plasma factor VIII activity) is indispensable. Individual patients may vary in their response to factor VIII, achieving different levels of in-vivo recovery and demonstrating different half-lives.

For long term prophylaxis against bleeds in patients with severe haemophilia A, doses of 20 to 60 IU of factor VIII:C per kg body weight should be given at intervals of 2 to 3 days. In some cases, especially in younger patients, shorter dosage intervals or higher doses may be necessary.

Patients should be monitored for the development of factor VIII inhibitors. If the expected factor VIII activity plasma levels are not attained, or if bleeding is not controlled with an appropriate dose, an assay should be performed to determine if a factor VIII inhibitor is present. If the inhibitor is present at levels less than 10 Bethesda Units (BU) per ml, administration of additional human coagulation factor VIII may neutralise the inhibitor. In patients with inhibitor titres above 10 BU or with high anamnestic response, the use of (activated) prothrombin complex concentrate (PCC) or recombinant activated factor VII (FVIIa) preparations has to be considered. These therapies should be directed by physicians with experience in the care of patients with haemophilia.

- von Willebrand's disease:

The dosage should be adjusted according to the extent and source of the bleeding. As a rule, 40 IU to 80 IU vWF:RCof per kilogram body weight (corresponds to 16-32 IU factor VIII per kilogram body weight) are administered every 8 to 12 hours.

Repeat doses are administered for as long as needed based on repeat monitoring of appropriate clinical and laboratory measures. Expected levels of vWF:RCof are based on an expected in-vivo recovery of 1.5 IU/dl rise per IU/kg vWF:RCof administered. The administration of 1 IU of Factor VIII per kg body weight can be expected to lead to a rise in circulating vWF:RCof of approximately 3.5 to 4 IU/dl.

The following table provides dosing guidelines for paediatric and adult patients.

(see Table 1 below)

4.2.2

Method of administration

Injection:

Reconstitute the preparation as described at 6.6. The product should be administered via the intravenous route. The injection or infusion rate should not exceed 4 ml per minute (approx 100 IU).

4.3 Contraindications

Hypersensitivity to the active substance or to any of the excipients.

4.4 Special warnings and special precautions for use

As with any intravenous protein product, allergic type hypersensitivity reactions are possible. The product contains traces of human proteins other than FVIII. Patients should be informed of the early signs of hypersensitivity reactions including hives, generalised urticaria, tightness of the chest, wheezing, hypotension and anaphylaxis. If these symptoms occur, they should be advised to discontinue use of the product immediately and contact their physician.

In case of shock, the current medical standards for shock treatment are to be observed.

When medicinal products prepared from human blood or plasma are administered, infectious diseases due to the transmission of infective agents cannot be totally

Table 1

Classification of vWD	Haemorrhage	Dosage (IU vWD:RCof / Kg body weight)
Type I		
Mild, (where use of desmopressin is known or suspected to be inadequate) Baseline vWF:RCof activity typically >30% of normal (i.e.>30 IU/dl)	**Major:** (e.g. severe or refractory epistaxis, GI bleeding, CNS trauma, or traumatic haemorrhage)	Loading dose 40 to 60 IU/kg, then 40 to 50 IU/kg every 8 to 12 hours for 3 days to keep the minimum level of vWF:RCof > 50% of normal (i.e.> 50 IU/dl); then 40 to 50 IU/kg daily for a total of up to 7 days of treatment
Moderate or Severe Baseline vWF:RCof activity typically < 30% (i.e. < 30 IU/dl)	**Minor:** (e.g. epistaxis, oral bleeding, menorrhagia)	40 to 50 IU/kg (1 or 2 doses)
	Major: (e.g. severe or refractory epistaxis, GI bleeding, CNS trauma, haemarthrosis or traumatic haemorrhage)	Loading dose of 50 to 75 IU/kg, then 40 to 60 IU/kg every 8 to 12 hours for 3 days to keep the minimum level of vWF:RCof>50% of normal (i.e.>50 IU/dl); then 40 to 60 IU/kg daily for a total of up to 7 days of treatment *Factor VIII:C levels should be monitored according to the guidelines for haemophilia A therapy in instances where both factor VIII and vWF must be monitored.*
Types 2 (all variants) and 3		
	Minor: (clinical indications above)	40 to 50 IU/kg (1 or 2 doses)
	Major: (clinical indications above)	Loading dose of 60 to 80 IU/kg, then 40 to 60 IU/kg every 8 to 12 hours for 3 days to keep the minimum level of vWF:RCof > 50% of normal (i.e. > 50 IU/dl); then 40 to 60 IU/kg daily for a total of up to 7 days of treatment *Factor VIII:C levels should be monitored according to the guidelines for haemophilia A therapy in instances where both factor VIII and vWF must be monitored*

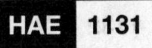

excluded. This also applies to pathogens of hitherto unknown nature.

Some viruses, such as parvovirus B19 or hepatitis A, are particularly difficult to remove or inactivate at this time. Parvovirus B19 may most seriously affect seronegative pregnant women, or immune-compromised individuals.

To reduce the risk of transmission of infective agents, stringent controls are applied to the selection of donors and donations. In addition, virus elimination/inactivation procedures are included in the production process of Haemate® P:

- Haemate® P is prepared exclusively from plasma donations which have been tested negative for antibodies to HIV-1, HIV-2, HCV and the HBs antigen. The levels of ALT (GPT) in the plasma are also determined and must not exceed twice the normal value specified in the test.

- In addition, the plasma pool is tested for antibodies to HIV-1, HIV-2, HCV and for HBs antigen as well as for virus genetic material of HBV, HCV and HIV-1 using Nucleic acid Amplification Technology (NAT), e.g., Polymerase Chain Reaction (PCR). The latter is a very sensitive test method by which – in contrast to the antibody testing – a direct test on virus genetic material is possible. The plasma pool is used for further processing only if the results of all these tests are negative.

- The production process of Haemate® P contains various steps which contribute towards the elimination/inactivation of viruses. These include chromatographic procedures, fractionation steps and the heat treatment of the preparation in aqueous solution at 60°C for 10 hours (pasteurisation).

These procedures have been validated with regard to the inactivation and/or removal of enveloped viruses (such as HIV, HBV, HCV and HAV). They may be of limited value against especially resistant, non-enveloped viruses, such as parvovirus B19.

Appropriate hepatitis vaccination (hepatitis A and hepatitis B) for patients in regular receipt of medicinal products derived from human blood or plasma, including Haemate® P, is recommended.

The formation of neutralising antibodies, inhibitors, to Factor VIII is a known complication in the management of individuals with haemophilia A. These inhibitors are invariably IgG immunoglobulins directed against the factor VIII procoagulant activity, which are quantified in Modified Bethesda Units (BU) per ml of plasma. The risk of developing inhibitors is correlated to the exposure to anti-haemophilic factor VIII, this risk being highest within the first 20 exposure days. Rarely, inhibitors may develop after the first 100 exposure days. Patients treated with human coagulation factor VIII should be carefully monitored for the development of inhibitory antibodies by appropriate clinical observations and laboratory test. See also 4.8 Undesirable Effects.

The product should be used with caution in children less than 6 years, who have limited exposure to factor VIII products.

4.5 Interaction with other medicinal products and other forms of Interaction
No interactions of human coagulation factor VIII products with other medicinal products are known.

4.6 Pregnancy and lactation
No animal reproduction and lactation studies have been conducted with Haemate® P. The safety of Haemate® P for use in human pregnancy has not been established. Therefore, Haemate® P should be administered to pregnant and lactating women only if clearly indicated and the benefit outweighs the risk.

4.7 Effects on ability to drive and use machines
No effects on ability to drive and use of machines have been observed.

4.8 Undesirable effects
Hypersensitivity or allergic reactions (which may include angioedema, burning and stinging at the infusion site, chills, flushing, generalised urticaria, headache, hives, hypotension, lethargy, nausea, restlessness, tachycardia, tightness of the chest, tingling, vomiting, wheezing) have been observed in rare cases. In some cases these reactions may progress to severe anaphylaxis (allergic shock). The treatment required depends on the nature and severity of the reaction.

Increase in body temperature is observed in rare cases.

Patients with haemophilia A may develop antibodies (inhibitors) to factor VIII. If such inhibitors occur, the condition will manifest as an insufficient clinical response. In such cases, it is recommended that a specialised haemophilia centre be contacted. (See also Section 4.2).

4.9 Overdose
No symptoms of overdose with human coagulation factor VIII have been reported.

5. PHARMACOLOGICAL PROPERTIES

5.1 Pharmacodynamic properties
Pharmacotherapeutic Group: Antihemorrhagics: blood coagulation factor VIII. ATC code: B02BD06.

The factor VIII/von Willebrand factor complex consists of two molecules (F VIII and vWF) with different physiological functions.

- Activated factor VIII acts as a cofactor for factor IX, accelerating the conversion of factor X to activated factor X. Activated factor X converts prothrombin into thrombin. Thrombin then converts fibrinogen into fibrin and a clot can be formed. Haemophilia A is a sex-linked hereditary disorder of blood coagulation due to decreased levels of factor VIII:C and results in profuse bleeding into joints, muscles or internal organs, either spontaneously or as a result of accidental or surgical trauma. By replacement therapy the plasma levels of factor VIII are increased, thereby enabling a temporary correction of the factor deficiency and correction of the bleeding tendencies.

- In addition to the role as a FVIII protecting protein, vWF mediates platelet adhesion to sites of vascular injury, plays a role in platelet aggregation and is indispensable for substitution therapy in patients with von Willebrand's disease. The activity of vWF is measured as von Willebrand factor: ristocetin cofactor (vWF:RCof). In severe cases of vWD the factor VIII activity is considerably reduced.

No fibrinogen can be detected by the Claus method.

5.2 Pharmacokinetic properties
After injection of the product approximately two thirds to three quarters of the factor VIII remains in the circulation. The factor VIII recovery should be between 80% - 120%.

Plasma factor VIII activity decreases by a two-phase exponential decay. In the initial phase, distribution between the intravascular and other compartments (body fluids) occurs with a half-life of elimination from the plasma of 3 to 6 hours. In the subsequent phase the half-life varies between 8 - 20 hours, with an average of 12 hours. This corresponds to the physiological half-life.

In a clinical study in patients with haemophilia A the in-vivo recovery of F VIII was determinated to be 101.5%. With reference to the administration of 1 IU Factor VIII:C/kg body weight, the mean F VIII increase was 2.3% of the norm. The biological half-life was determined to be 15.3 ± 5.5 hours. In individual cases the biological half-life may vary.

In clinical studies in patients with all types of von Willebrand's Disease, the mean RCof in-vivo recovery was 68.1 – 81% and the mean biological half-life proved to be a range between 8.1 and 10.3 hours. There were insufficient numbers of patients with each type of von Willebrand's Disease to distinguish possible differences in half-life and recovery.

Following the substitution with Haemate® P a quite normal multimeric structure is seen in the patient plasma lasting over several hours.

Intravenous administration means that the preparation is available immediately and with 100% bioavailability.

5.3 Preclinical safety data
Toxicological properties

Human plasma coagulation factor VIII (from the concentrate) is a normal constituent of the human plasma and acts like the endogenous factor VIII. Single dose toxicity testing revealed no adverse findings in different species even at dose levels several times higher than the recommended human dose.

Repeated dose toxicity testing is impracticable due to the development of antibodies to heterologous protein.

To date Haemate® P has not been reported to be associated with embryo – foetal toxicity, oncogenic or mutagenic potential.

6. PHARMACEUTICAL PARTICULARS

6.1 List of excipients
Human albumin 80-120 mg (500 IU), 160-240 mg (1000 IU)

Glycine

Sodium chloride

Sodium citrate

Water for injections, pyrogen free

6.2 Incompatibilities
This medicinal product must not be mixed with other medicinal products. Only the provided injection/infusion sets should be used because treatment failure can occur as a consequence of human factor VIII adsorption to the internal surfaces of some infusion equipment.

6.3 Shelf life
Haemate® P has a shelf-life of 36 months, when stored at + 2 to + 8 °C.

Reconstituted preparations should be used up within 8 hours.

6.4 Special precautions for storage
Haemate® P should be stored at +2 to +8 °C.

It may also be stored at room temperature for up to 6 months before the expiry date, but not at above 30 °C.

Do not freeze.

6.5 Nature and contents of container
Vials:

- Injection vial of colourless glass sealed with rubber infusion stopper, plastic disc and aluminium cap.

Haemate® P 500 IU: 1 vial (hermetically sealed under vacuum) with dried substance

1 vial with 20 ml water for injections, pyrogen-free

Haemate® P 1000 IU: 1 vial (hermetically sealed under vacuum) with dried substance

1 vial with 30 ml water for injections, pyrogen-free

6.6 Instructions for use and handling
Do not use after the expiry date given on the label. Usually the solution is clear or slightly opalescent. Do not use solutions that are cloudy or have deposits.

Preparation of the solution:

1. Bring the solvent to 20 to 37 °C.

2 Remove the caps from the vials of dried substance and solvent.

3. Disinfect the surface of both rubber stoppers.

4. Insert the needle at the corrugated side of the transfer set into the solvent vial. Remove the protective sheath from the other end of the transfer set. Invert the solvent vial and insert the needle into the preparation vial without touching the needle.

The solvent is then suctioned into the preparation vial by the vacuum. Finally, remove solvent vial and transfer set.

5. Slowly swirl the vial to dissolve the dried substance completely. Avoid vigorous shaking. A clear to slightly opalescent solution is obtained. Do not use solutions which are cloudy or have deposits.

The reconstitution time is approx. 2 minutes.

Any unused product or waste material should be disposed of in accordance with local requirements.

7. MARKETING AUTHORISATION HOLDER
ZLB Behring GmbH

P.O. Box 1230

35002 Marburg

Germany

8. MARKETING AUTHORISATION NUMBER(S)
Haemate® P 500 IU: PL 15036/0009

Haemate® P 1000 IU: PL 15036/0010

9. DATE OF FIRST AUTHORISATION/RENEWAL OF THE AUTHORISATION
12 April 2005

10. DATE OF REVISION OF THE TEXT
16 November 2004

Halciderm Topical

(E. R. Squibb & Sons Limited)

1. NAME OF THE MEDICINAL PRODUCT
HALCIDERM㊞ TOPICAL

2. QUALITATIVE AND QUANTITATIVE COMPOSITION
A white topical preparation containing halcinonide 0.1% in a water-miscible base.

3. PHARMACEUTICAL FORM
Topical Cream

4. CLINICAL PARTICULARS

4.1 Therapeutic indications
Halciderm is indicated in acute and chronic corticosteroid-responsive conditions which may include: psoriasis, atopic eczema, contact eczema, follicular eczema, infantile eczema, neurodermatitis, anogenital eczema, nummular eczema, seborrhoeic or flexural eczema, otitis externa without frank infection.

4.2 Posology and method of administration
Adults:

Halciderm should be applied to the affected area two, or occasionally three, times daily. In long-term therapy, or where lower strength preparations are required, do not dilute but use intermittently.

Elderly:

Natural thinning of the skin occurs in the elderly; hence corticosteroids should be used sparingly and for short periods of time.

Children:

In infants, long-term continuous topical steroid therapy should be avoided. Courses should be limited to 5 days and occlusion should not be used.

4.3 Contraindications
Contra-indicated in patients with a history of hypersensitivity to the product components.

Halciderm is not intended for ophthalmic use, nor should it be applied in the external auditory canal of patients with perforated eardrums.

Halciderm is contraindicated in tuberculous and most viral lesions of the skin, particularly herpes simplex, vacinnia, varicella. The product should not be used in fungal or bacterial skin infections without suitable concomitant anti-infective therapy. It should not be used for facial rosacea, acne vulgaris, perioral dermatitis or napkin eruptions.

4.4 Special warnings and special precautions for use
Adrenal suppression can occur with prolonged use of topical corticosteroids or treatment of extensive areas. These effects are more likely to occur in infants and children and if occlusive dressings are used. If used in childhood, or on the face, courses should be limited to 5 days and occlusion should not be used.

Topical corticosteroids may be hazardous in psoriasis for a number of reasons including rebound relapses following development of tolerance, risk of generalised pustular psoriasis and local and systemic toxicity due to impaired barrier function of the skin. Steroids may have a place in psoriasis of the scalp and chronic plaque psoriasis of the hands and feet. Careful patient supervision is important.

4.5 Interaction with other medicinal products and other forms of Interaction
None known.

4.6 Pregnancy and lactation
There is inadequate evidence of safety in human pregnancy. Topical administration of corticosteroids to pregnant animals can cause abnormalities of foetal development including cleft palate and intra-uterine growth retardation. There may, therefore, be a very small risk of such effects in the human foetus. Caution should be exercised when topical corticosteroids are administered to nursing women.

4.7 Effects on ability to drive and use machines
None known.

4.8 Undesirable effects
Halcinonide is well tolerated. Where adverse reactions occur they are usually reversible on cessation of therapy. However the following side effects have been reported usually with prolonged usage:

Dermatologic - impaired wound healing, thinning of the skin, petechiae and ecchymoses, facial erythema and telangiectasia, increased sweating, purpura, striae, hirsutism, acneiform eruptions, lupus erythematosus-like lesions and suppressed reaction to skin tests. These effects may be enhanced with occlusive dressings.

Oedema and electrolyte imbalance have not been observed even when high topical dosage has been used. The possibility of the systemic effects which are associated with all steroid therapy should be considered.

4.9 Overdose
Topically applied corticosteroids can be absorbed in sufficient amounts to produce systemic effects (see Undesirable Effects).

In the event of accidental ingestion, the patient should be observed and treated symptomatically.

5. PHARMACOLOGICAL PROPERTIES
5.1 Pharmacodynamic properties
Halcinonide is a potent corticosteroid with anti-inflammatory, antipruritic and anti-allergic actions. Halciderm is suitable for both wet and dry lesions.

5.2 Pharmacokinetic properties
The absorption of topically applied corticosteroids is determined by several factors such as the vehicle, the integrity of the skin and the use of occlusive dressings. Once absorbed, Halcinonide is handled in a similar way to other topically and systemically administered corticosteroids. They are primarily metabolised in the liver and the metabolites are excreted mainly via the kidneys.

5.3 Preclinical safety data
No further relevant data available.

6. PHARMACEUTICAL PARTICULARS
6.1 List of excipients
Benzyl alcohol, castor oil, silicone fluid, macrogol ether, propylene glycol, propylene glycol stearates, water, white soft paraffin.

6.2 Incompatibilities
None known.

6.3 Shelf life
48 months.

6.4 Special precautions for storage
Do not store above 25°C.

6.5 Nature and contents of container
Open end epoxy-lined aluminium tube of 30g.

6.6 Instructions for use and handling
Not applicable.

7. MARKETING AUTHORISATION HOLDER
E. R. Squibb & Sons Limited
Uxbridge Business Park,
Sanderson Road,
Uxbridge,
Middlesex UB8 1DH

8. MARKETING AUTHORISATION NUMBER(S)
PL 0034/0160

9. DATE OF FIRST AUTHORISATION/RENEWAL OF THE AUTHORISATION
10 June 1974 / 18 March 2002

10. DATE OF REVISION OF THE TEXT
24th June 2005

Haldol Decanoate
(Janssen-Cilag Ltd)

1. NAME OF THE MEDICINAL PRODUCT
HALDOL® decanoate 50 mg/ml
HALDOL® decanoate 100 mg/ml

2. QUALITATIVE AND QUANTITATIVE COMPOSITION
HALDOL® decanoate 50 mg/ml

Haloperidol decanoate 70.52 mg, equivalent to 50 mg haloperidol base, per millilitre.

HALDOL® decanoate 100 mg/ml

Haloperidol decanoate 141.04 mg, equivalent to 100 mg haloperidol base, per millilitre.

3. PHARMACEUTICAL FORM
Straw-coloured viscous solution for intramuscular injection.

4. CLINICAL PARTICULARS
4.1 Therapeutic indications
Haldol decanoate is indicated for long term maintenance treatment where a neuroleptic is required; for example in schizophrenia, other psychoses (especially paranoid), and other mental or behavioural problems where maintenance treatment is clearly indicated.

4.2 Posology and method of administration
By intramuscular administration.

Haldol decanoate is for use in adults only and has been formulated to provide one month's therapy for most patients following a single deep intramuscular injection in the gluteal region. Haldol decanoate should not be administered intravenously.

Since individual response to neuroleptic drugs is variable, dosage should be individually determined and is best initiated and titrated under close clinical supervision.

The size of the initial dose will depend on both the severity of the symptomatology and the amount of oral medication required to maintain the patient before starting depot treatment.

An initial dose of 50 mg every four weeks is recommended, increasing if necessary by 50 mg increments to 300 mg every four weeks. If, for clinical reasons, two-weekly administration is preferred, these doses should be halved.

In patients with severe symptomatology, or in those who require large oral doses as maintenance therapy, higher doses of Haldol decanoate will be required. However, clinical experience with Haldol decanoate at doses greater than 300 mg per month is limited.

Routine administration of volumes greater than 3 mls at any one injection site is not recommended as larger volumes of injection are uncomfortable for the patient.

Haldol decanoate should be administered by deep intramuscular injection using an appropriate needle, preferably 2-2.5 inches long, of at least 21 gauge. Local reactions and medication oozing from the injection site may be reduced by the use of a good injection technique, eg the 'Z-track' method. As with all oily injections, it is important to ensure, by aspiration before injection, that intravenous entry has not occurred.

For patients previously maintained on oral neuroleptics, an approximate guide to the starting dose of Haldol decanoate is as follows: 500 mg of chlorpromazine a day is equivalent to 100 mg of Haldol decanoate monthly.

The approximate equivalence for transferring patients previously maintained on fluphenazine decanoate or flupenthixol decanoate is as follows: 25 mg of fluphenazine decanoate 2-weekly or 40 mg of flupenthixol decanoate 2-weekly is equivalent to 100 mg of Haldol decanoate monthly. This dose should be adjusted to suit the individual patient's response.

Use in elderly:

It is recommended to start with low doses, for example 12.5 mg - 25 mg every four weeks, only increasing the dose according to the individual patient's response.

4.3 Contraindications
Comatose states, CNS depression, Parkinson's disease, known hypersensitivity to haloperidol, lesions of basal ganglia.

4.4 Special warnings and special precautions for use
Caution is advised in patients with liver disease, renal failure, phaeochromocytoma, epilepsy, and conditions predisposing to epilepsy (eg alcohol withdrawal and brain damage) or convulsions. Haloperidol should only be used with great caution in patients with disturbed thyroid function. Antipsychotic therapy in those patients must always be accompanied by adequate management of the underlying thyroid dysfunction.

Cases of sudden death have been reported in psychiatric patients receiving antipsychotic drugs, including haloperidol.

The risk-benefit of haloperidol treatment should be fully assessed before treatment is commenced and patients with risk factors for ventricular arrhythmias such as cardiac disease, subarachnoid haemorrhage, metabolic abnormalities such as hypokalaemia, hypocalcaemia or hypomagnesemia, starvation, alcohol abuse or those receiving concomitant therapy with other drugs known to prolong the QT interval, should be monitored carefully (ECGs and potassium levels), particularly during the initial phase of treatment, to obtain steady plasma levels.

In schizophrenia, the response to antipsychotic drug treatment may be delayed. If drugs are withdrawn, recurrence of symptoms may not become apparent for several weeks or months.

As with all antipsychotic agents, haloperidol should not be used alone where depression is predominant. It may be combined with antidepressants to treat those conditions in which depression and psychosis coexist. Haloperidol may impair the metabolism of tricyclic antidepressants (clinical significance unknown).

If concomitant anti-Parkinson medication is required, it may have to be continued after haloperidol is discontinued to take account of any differences in excretion rates. The physician should keep in mind the possible anticholinergic effects associated with anti-Parkinson agents.

4.5 Interaction with other medicinal products and other forms of Interaction
In common with all neuroleptics, haloperidol can increase the central nervous system depression produced by other CNS-depressant drugs, including alcohol, hypnotics, sedatives or strong analgesics. An enhanced CNS effect, when combined with methyldopa, has been reported.

Haloperidol may antagonise the action of adrenaline and other sympathomimetic agents and reverses the blood pressure lowering effects of adrenergic-blocking agents such as guanethidine.

Haloperidol may impair the metabolism of tricyclic antidepressants (clinical significance unknown) and the anti-Parkinson effects of levodopa. In pharmacokinetic studies, increased haloperidol levels have been reported when haloperidol was given concomitantly with the following drugs: quinidine, buspirone and fluoxetine. Haloperidol plasma levels should therefore be monitored and reduced if necessary. The dosage of anticonvulsants may need to be increased to take account of the lowered seizure threshold.

Co-administration of enzyme-inducing drugs such as carbamazepine, phenobarbitone and rifampicin with haloperidol may result in a significant reduction of haloperidol plasma levels. The haloperidol dose may therefore need to be increased or the dosage interval reduced, according to the patient's response. After stopping such drugs, it may be necessary to readjust the dosage of haloperidol.

Antagonism of the effect of phenindione has been reported.

In rare cases, an encephalopathy-like syndrome has been reported in combination with lithium and Haldol decanoate. It remains controversial whether these cases represent a distinct clinical entity or whether they are in fact cases of NMS and/or lithium toxicity. Signs of encephalopathy-like syndrome include confusion, disorientation, headache, disturbances of balance and drowsiness. One report showing symptomless EEG abnormalities on the combination has suggested that EEG monitoring might be advisable. When lithium and haloperidol therapy are used concomitantly, haloperidol should be given in the lowest effective dosage and lithium levels should be monitored and kept below 1 mmol/l. If symptoms of encephalopathy-like syndrome occur, therapy should be stopped immediately.

4.6 Pregnancy and lactation
The safety of haloperidol in pregnancy has not been established. There is some evidence of harmful effects in some, but not all, animal studies There have been a number of reports of birth defects following foetal exposure to haloperidol for which a causal role for haloperidol cannot be excluded. Haldol decanoate should be used during pregnancy only if the anticipated benefit outweighs the risk and the administered dose and duration of treatment should be as low and as short as possible.

Haloperidol is excreted in breast milk. There have been isolated cases of extrapyramidal symptoms in breast-fed children. If the use of Haldol decanoate is essential, the benefits of breast feeding should be balanced against its potential risks.

4.7 Effects on ability to drive and use machines
Some degree of sedation or impairment of alertness may occur, particularly with higher doses and at the start of treatment, and may be potentiated by alcohol or other CNS depressants. Patients should be advised not to undertake activities requiring alertness such as driving or operating machinery during treatment, until their susceptibility is known.

4.8 Undesirable effects
Central nervous system

In common with all neuroleptics, extrapyramidal symptoms may occur, eg tremor, rigidity, hypersalivation, bradykinesia, akathisia, acute dystonia, oculogyric crisis and laryngeal dystonia. Anti-Parkinson agents should not be prescribed routinely. Preliminary results suggest that withdrawal of anti-Parkinson medication may be attempted following transfer from oral medication to monthly depot injections of Haldol decanoate.

As with all antipsychotic agents, tardive dyskinesia may appear in some patients on long-term therapy or after drug discontinuation.

The syndrome is mainly characterised by rhythmical involuntary movements of the tongue, face, mouth or jaw. The manifestations may be permanent in some patients. The syndrome may be masked when treatment is reinstituted, when the dosage is increased or when a switch is made to a different antipsychotic drug. Treatment should be discontinued as soon as possible.

However, since its occurrence may be related to duration of treatment, as well as dose, haloperidol should be given in the minimum effective dose for the minimum possible time, unless it is established that long term administration for the treatment of schizophrenia is required.

It has been reported that fine vermicular movements of the tongue may be an early sign of tardive dyskinesia and that the full syndrome may not develop if the medication is stopped at that time.

The following effects have been reported rarely with haloperidol: confusional states or epileptic fits, depression, sedation, agitation, drowsiness, insomnia, headache, vertigo and apparent exacerbation of psychotic symptoms.

In common with other antipsychotic drugs, haloperidol has been associated with neuroleptic malignant syndrome (NMS), an idiosyncratic response characterised by hyperthermia, generalised muscle rigidity, autonomic instability, altered consciousness, coma and elevated CPK. Signs of autonomic dysfunction such as tachycardia, labile arterial pressure and sweating may precede the onset of hyperthermia, acting as early warning signs. Antipsychotic treatment should be withdrawn immediately and appropriate supportive therapy and careful monitoring instituted.

Haloperidol, even in low dosage in susceptible (especially non-psychotic) individuals, may cause unpleasant subjective feelings of being mentally dulled or slowed down, dizziness, headache or paradoxical effects of excitement, agitation or insomnia.

Gastro-intestinal system

Gastro-intestinal symptoms, nausea, loss of appetite, constipation and dyspepsia have been reported with haloperidol.

Endocrinological system

Hormonal effects of antipsychotic neuroleptic drugs include hyperprolactinaemia, which may cause galactorrhoea, gynaecomastia and oligo- or amenorrhoea. Hypoglycaemia and the Syndrome of Inappropriate Antidiuretic Hormone Secretion have been reported rarely. Impairment of sexual function including erection and ejaculation has also been occasionally reported.

Cardiovascular system

Tachycardia and dose related hypotension is uncommon, but can occur with haloperidol, particularly in the elderly, who are more susceptible to the sedative and hypotensive effects. Less commonly hypertension has also been reported. Cardiac effects such as QT-interval prolongation, Torsade de Pointes and/or ventricular arrhythmias have been reported rarely. They may occur more frequently with high doses, intravenous administration and in predisposed patients (see Precautions and Warnings).

Autonomic nervous system

Dry mouth as well as excessive salivation, blurred vision, urinary retention and hyperhidrosis have been reported with haloperidol.

Dermatological system

The following effects have been reported rarely with haloperidol: oedema, various skin rashes and reactions, including urticaria, exfoliative dermatitis and erythema multiforme. Photosensitive skin reactions have been reported very rarely.

Other adverse reactions

The following effects have been reported rarely with haloperidol: jaundice, cholestatic hepatitis or transient abnormalities of liver function in the absence of jaundice; priapism and weight changes may occur. Temperature disorders may also occur, characteristically hyperthermia associated with NMS, although hypothermia has also been reported.

The following have been reported very rarely with haloperidol: blood dyscrasias, including agranulocytosis, thrombocytopenia and transient leucopenia; hypersensitivity reactions including anaphylaxis. Occasional local reactions such as erythema, swelling or tender lumps have been reported.

4.9 Overdose

Symptoms

In general, the manifestations of haloperidol overdosage are an extension of its pharmacological actions, the most prominent of which would be severe extrapyramidal symptoms, hypotension and psychic indifference with a transition to sleep. The risk of ventricular arrhythmias possibly associated with QT-prolongation should be considered. The patient may appear comatose with respiratory depression and hypotension which could be severe enough to produce a shock-like state. Paradoxically, hypertension rather than hypotension may occur. Convulsions may also occur.

Treatment

There is no specific antidote to haloperidol. A patent airway should be established and maintained with mechanically assisted ventilation if necessary. In view of isolated reports of arrhythmia, ECG monitoring is strongly advised. Hypotension and circulatory collapse should be treated by plasma volume expansion and other appropriate measures. Adrenaline should not be used. The patient should be monitored, body temperature and adequate fluid intake should be maintained.

In cases of severe extrapyramidal symptoms, appropriate anti-Parkinson medication should be administered.

5. PHARMACOLOGICAL PROPERTIES

5.1 Pharmacodynamic properties

The antipsychotic activity of haloperidol is principally due to its central dopamine blocking activity.

It has some activity against noradrenaline and less against serotonin. There is only very minimal activity against histamine and acetylcholine receptors.

5.2 Pharmacokinetic properties

Haloperidol decanoate in solution is slowly released from the injection site and enters the systemic circulation, where it is hydrolysed by esterases to haloperidol. After an initial dose of 30-300 mg of haloperidol decanoate, plasma concentrations ranged from 0.8-3.2 ng/ml. After the second dose they were raised to 2.8 ng/ml which was steady state. A monthly dose of approximately 20 times the previous oral maintenance dose has been shown to be approximately clinically equivalent. Blood levels will vary considerably between patients.

5.3 Preclinical safety data

No relevant information additional to that contained elsewhere in the Summary of Product Characteristics.

6. PHARMACEUTICAL PARTICULARS

6.1 List of excipients

Benzyl alcohol Ph Eur

Sesame oil Ph Eur

6.2 Incompatibilities

None known.

6.3 Shelf life

5 years.

6.4 Special precautions for storage

Do not store above 25°C.

Do not refrigerate or freeze.

Keep ampoule in the outer carton to protect from light.

Lengthy storage in the cold may produce precipitation; if this does not clear after further storage at room temperature, the contents of the ampoule should be discarded.

6.5 Nature and contents of container

1 ml amber glass ampoule, in packs containing 5 ampoules.

6.6 Instructions for use and handling

Before use warm the ampoule in the hands to aid withdrawal of the contents.

1. Hold the body of the ampoule between the thumb and the index finger with the spot facing you.

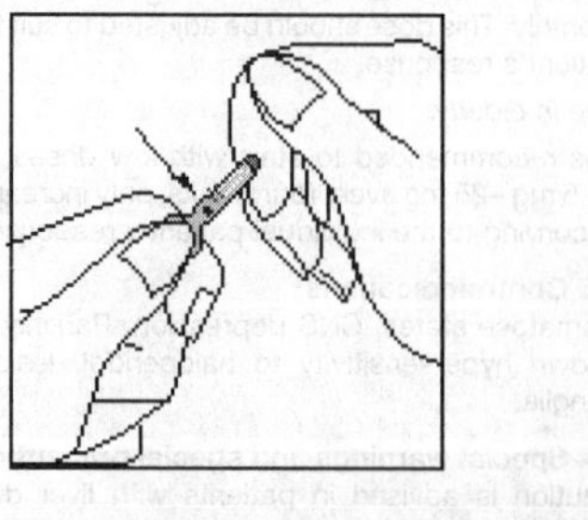

2. Position the index finger of the other hand so that it is supporting the neck of the ampoule. Position the thumb so that it covers the spot as shown below.

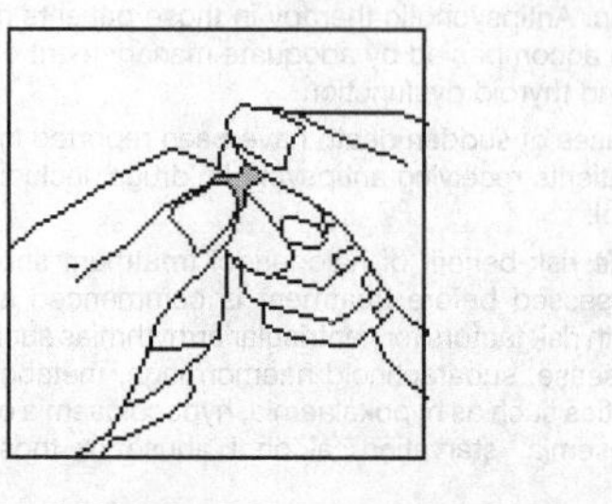

3. With the index fingers close together, apply firm downward pressure on the spot to snap the ampoule open.

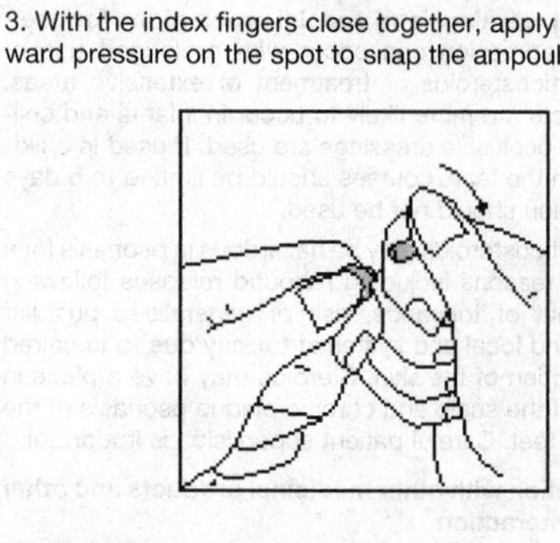

7. MARKETING AUTHORISATION HOLDER

Janssen-Cilag Limited

Saunderton

High Wycombe

Buckinghamshire

HP14 4HJ

UK

8. MARKETING AUTHORISATION NUMBER(S)

HALDOL DECANOATE 50 mg/ml: PL 0242/0094

HALDOL DECANOATE 100 mg/ml: PL 0242/0095

9. DATE OF FIRST AUTHORISATION/RENEWAL OF THE AUTHORISATION

Date of First Authorisation: 23 July 1982

Date of Renewal of Authorisation: 07 January 1998

10. DATE OF REVISION OF THE TEXT

26 Sept 2001

Legal category POM.

Haldol Injection

(Janssen-Cilag Ltd)

1. NAME OF THE MEDICINAL PRODUCT

HALDOL Injection

2. QUALITATIVE AND QUANTITATIVE COMPOSITION

Haloperidol 5 mg/ml

3. PHARMACEUTICAL FORM

Solution for injection

4. CLINICAL PARTICULARS

4.1 Therapeutic indications

Adults:

- Schizophrenia: treatment of symptoms and prevention of relapse.
- Other psychoses; especially paranoid.
- Mania and hypomania.
- Mental or behavioural problems such as aggression, hyperactivity and self-mutilation in the mentally retarded and in patients with organic brain damage.
- As an adjunct to short term management of moderate to severe psychomotor agitation, excitement, violent or dangerously impulsive behaviour.
- Nausea and vomiting.

4.2 Posology and method of administration

For intramuscular administration

Dosage for all indications should be individually determined and is best initiated and titrated under close clinical supervision. To determine the initial dose, consideration should be given to the patient's age, severity of symptoms and previous response to other neuroleptics.

Patients who are elderly or debilitated or those with previously reported adverse reactions to neuroleptic drugs may require less haloperidol. The normal starting dose should be halved, followed by a gradual titration to achieve optimal response.

Adults:

Schizophrenia, psychoses, mania and hypomania, mental or behavioural problems, psychomotor agitation, excitement, violent or dangerously impulsive behaviour, organic brain damage:

For control of acutely agitated patients with moderate symptoms: 2-10 mg IM. Depending on the response of the patient, subsequent doses may be given every 4-8 hours, up to a maximum of 18 mg/day.

Infrequently, severely disturbed patients may require an initial dose of up to 18 mg.

Oral treatment should succeed intramuscular administration as soon as practicable. Bioavailability from the oral route is about 60% of that from the IM route, and readjustment of dose may be required.

Haldol can also be administered by the IV route.

Nausea and vomiting

1-2 mg IM

Children:

Not recommended for parenteral use in children.

4.3 Contraindications

Comatose states, CNS depression, Parkinson's disease, known hypersensitivity to haloperidol, lesions of basal ganglia.

4.4 Special warnings and special precautions for use

Please also refer to section 4.5-Interactions with other Medicaments and other forms of Interaction. Caution is advised in patients with liver disease, renal failure, phaeochromocytoma, epilepsy, and conditions predisposing to epilepsy (eg alcohol withdrawal and brain damage) or convulsions. Haloperidol should only be used with great caution in patients with disturbed thyroid function. Antipsychotic therapy in those patients must always be accompanied by adequate management of the underlying thyroid dysfunction.

Cases of sudden death have been reported in psychiatric patients receiving antipsychotic drugs, including haloperidol.

The risk-benefit of haloperidol treatment should be fully assessed before treatment is commenced and patients with risk factors for ventricular arrhythmias such as cardiac disease; subarachnoid haemorrhage; metabolic abnormalities such as hypokalaemia, hypocalcaemia or hypomagnesemia; starvation; alcohol abuse or those receiving concomitant therapy with other drugs known to prolong the QT interval, should be monitored carefully (ECGs and potassium levels), particularly during the initial phase of treatment, to obtain steady plasma levels.

Acute withdrawal symptoms including nausea, vomiting and insomnia have very rarely been described after abrupt cessation of high doses of antipsychotic drugs. Relapse may also occur and gradual withdrawal is advisable.

In schizophrenia, the response to antipsychotic drug treatment may be delayed. If drugs are withdrawn, recurrence of symptoms may not become apparent for several weeks or months. As with all antipsychotic agents, haloperidol should not be used alone where depression is predominant. It may be combined with antidepressants to treat those conditions in which depression and psychosis coexist. Haloperidol may impair the metabolism of tricyclic antidepressants (clinical significance unknown). If concomitant anti-Parkinson medication is required, it may have to be continued after haloperidol is discontinued to take account of any differences in excretion rates. The physician should keep in mind the possible anticholinergic effects associated with anti-Parkinson agents.

4.5 Interaction with other medicinal products and other forms of Interaction

In common with all neuroleptics, haloperidol can increase the central nervous system depression produced by other CNS-depressant drugs, including alcohol, hypnotics, sedatives or strong analgesics.

An enhanced CNS effect, when combined with methyldopa, has been reported.

Haloperidol may antagonise the action of adrenaline and other sypathomimetic agents and reverses the blood pressure lowering effects of adrenergic-blocking agents such as guanethidine. The dosage of anticonvulsants may need to be increased to take account of the lowered seizure threshold. Co-administration of enzyme-inducing drugs such as carbamazepine, phenobarbitone and rifampicin with haloperidol may result in a significant reduction of haloperidol plasma levels. The haloperidol dose may therefore need to be increased, according to the patient's response. After stopping such drugs, it may be necessary to readjust the dosage of haloperidol. Haloperidol may impair the metabolism of tricyclic antidepressants (clinical significance unknown) and the anti-Parkinson effects of levodopa.

In pharmacokinetic studies, increased haloperidol levels have been reported when haloperidol was given concomitantly with the following drugs: quinidine, buspirone and fluoxetine. Haloperidol plasma levels should therefore be monitored and reduced if necessary.

Antagonism of the effect of phenindione has been reported.

In rare cases, an encephalopathy-like syndrome has been reported in combination with lithium and haloperidol. It remains controversial whether these cases represent a distinct clinical entity or whether they are in fact cases of NMS and/or lithium toxicity. Signs of encephalopathy-like syndrome include confusion, disorientation, headache, disturbances of balance and drowsiness. One report showing symptomless EEG abnormalities on the combination has suggested that EEG monitoring might be advisable. When lithium and haloperidol therapy are used concomitantly, haloperidol should be given in the lowest effective dose and lithium levels should be monitored and kept below 1mmol/L. If symptoms of encephalopathy-like syndrome occur, therapy should be stopped immediately.

4.6 Pregnancy and lactation

The safety of haloperidol in pregnancy has not been established. There is some evidence of harmful effects in some but not all animal studies. There have been a number of reports of birth defects following foetal exposure to haloperidol for which a causal role for haloperidol cannot be excluded. Haldol should be used during pregnancy only if the anticipated benefit outweighs the risk and the administered dose and duration of treatment should be as low and as short as possible.

Haloperidol is excreted in breast milk. There have been isolated cases of extrapyramidal symptoms in breast-fed children. If the use of Haldol is essential, the benefits of breast feeding should be balanced against its potential risks.

4.7 Effects on ability to drive and use machines

Some degree of sedation or impairment of alertness may occur, particularly with higher doses and at the start of treatment, and may be potentiated by alcohol or other CNS depressants. Patients should be advised not to undertake activities requiring alertness such as driving or operating machinery during treatment, until their susceptibility is known.

4.8 Undesirable effects

Central nervous system: In common with all neuroleptics, extrapyramidal symptoms may occur, eg tremor, rigidity, hypersalivation, bradykinesia, akathisia, acute dystonia, oculogyric crisis and laryngeal dystonia. Anti-Parkinson agents should not be prescribed routinely.

As with all antipsychotic agents, tardive dyskinesia may appear in some patients on long-term therapy or after drug discontinuation.

The syndrome is mainly characterised by rhythmical involuntary movements of the tongue, face, mouth or jaw. The manifestations may be permanent in some patients. The syndrome may be masked when treatment is re-instituted, when the dosage is increased or when a switch is made to a different antipsychotic drug. Treatment should be discontinued as soon as possible.

However, since its occurrence may be related to duration of treatment, as well as daily dose, Haldol should be given in the minimum effective dose for the minimum possible time, unless it is established that long term administration for the treatment of schizophrenia is required.

It has been reported that fine vermicular movements of the tongue may be an early warning sign of tardive dyskinesia and that the full syndrome may not develop if the medication is stopped at that time.

The following effects have been reported rarely: confusional states or epileptic fits, depression, sedation, agitation, drowsiness, insomnia, headache, vertigo and apparent exacerbation of psychotic symptoms.

In common with other antipsychotic drugs, haloperidol has been associated with neuroleptic malignant syndrome (NMS), an idiosyncratic response characterised by hyperthermia, generalised muscle rigidity, autonomic instability, altered consciousness, coma and elevated CPK. Signs of autonomic dysfunction such as tachycardia, labile arterial pressure and sweating may precede onset of hyperthermia, acting as early warning signs. Antipsychotic treatment should be withdrawn immediately and appropriate supportive therapy and careful monitoring instituted. Haloperidol, even in low dosage in susceptible (especially non-psychotic) individuals, may cause unpleasant subjective feelings of being mentally dulled or slowed down, dizziness, headache or paradoxical effects of excitement, agitation or insomnia.

Gastro-intestinal System: Gastro-intestinal symptoms, nausea, loss of appetite, constipation and dyspepsia have been reported.

Endocrinological System: Hormonal effects of antipsychotic neuroleptic drugs include hyperprolactinaemia, which may cause galactorrhoea, gynaecomastia and oligo- or amenorrhoea. Hypoglycaemia and the syndrome of inappropriate antidiuretic hormone secretion have been reported rarely. Impairment of sexual function including erection and ejaculation has also been occasionally reported.

Cardiovascular System: Tachycardia and dose related hypotension are uncommon, but can occur, particularly in the elderly, who are more susceptible to the sedative and hypotensive effects. Less commonly hypertension has also been reported.

Cardiac effects such as QT-interval prolongation, Torsade de Pointes and/or ventricular arrhythmias have been reported rarely. They may occur more frequently with high doses, intravenous administration and in predisposed patients (see Section 4.4-Special Warnings and Precautions for Use).

Autonomic nervous system: Dry mouth as well as excessive salivation, blurred vision, urinary retention and hyperhidrosis have been reported.

Dermatological system: The following effects have been reported rarely: oedema, various skin rashes and reactions including urticaria, exfoliative dermatitis and erythema multiforme. Photosensitive skin reactions have been reported very rarely.

Other adverse reactions: The following effects have been reported rarely: jaundice, cholestatic hepatitis or transient abnormalities of liver function in the absence of jaundice; priapism and weight changes. Temperature disorders may also occur, characteristically hyperthermia associated with NMS, although hypothermia has also been reported.

The following have been reported very rarely: blood dyscrasias, including agranulocytosis, thrombocytopenia and transient leucopenia; hypersensitivity reactions including anaphylaxis.

4.9 Overdose

Symptoms: In general, the manifestations of haloperidol overdosage are an extension of its pharmacological actions, the most prominent of which would be severe extrapyramidal symptoms, hypotension and psychic indifference with a transition to sleep. The risk of ventricular arrhythmias possibly associated with QT-prolongation should be considered. The patient may appear comatose with respiratory depression and hypotension which could be severe enough to produce a shock-like state. Paradoxically hypertension rather than hypotension may occur. Convulsions may also occur.

Treatment: There is no specific antidote to haloperidol. A patent airway should be established and maintained with mechanically assisted ventilation if necessary. In view of isolated reports of arrhythmia, ECG monitoring is strongly advised. Hypotension and circulatory collapse should be treated by plasma volume expansion and other appropriate measures. Adrenaline should not be used. The patient should be monitored carefully for 24 hours or longer, body temperature and adequate fluid intake should be maintained.

In cases of severe extrapyramidal symptoms, appropriate anti-Parkinson medication should be administered.

5. PHARMACOLOGICAL PROPERTIES

5.1 Pharmacodynamic properties

Haloperidol is a central dopamine antagonist. It also has some anticholinergic properties and is an opiate receptor antagonist, and acts at peripheral dopamine receptors.

5.2 Pharmacokinetic properties

A 10 mg IV dose of haloperidol given over 2 mins produced a peak serum concentration of u 34μg/ml at the end of infusion, declining to u 1μg/ml by 40 hours. Following IM administration of 2 mg, peak plasma concentrations were similar to after oral ie. 10μg/ml but are reached within 20 minutes.

Haloperidol is rapidly distributed throughout the body.

Haloperidol is excreted in human breast milk, milk concentrations being 59-69% of maternal plasma.

Haloperidol is extensively metabolised by oxidative dealkylation. Metabolites are ultimately conjugated with glycine.

5.3 Preclinical safety data

No relevant information additional to that contained elsewhere in the Summary of Product Characteristics.

6. PHARMACEUTICAL PARTICULARS

6.1 List of excipients

Lactic Acid

Water for Injections

6.2 Incompatibilities

None known.

6.3 Shelf life

5 years

6.4 Special precautions for storage

Protect from light

6.5 Nature and contents of container

Amber glass ampoules containing 1 or 2ml of solution for injection. Boxes of 5 ampoules.

6.6 Instructions for use and handling

None stated.

7. MARKETING AUTHORISATION HOLDER

Janssen-Cilag Limited

Saunderton

High Wycombe

Buckinghamshire

HP14 4HJ

UK

8. MARKETING AUTHORISATION NUMBER(S)

PL 00242/0036R

9. DATE OF FIRST AUTHORISATION/RENEWAL OF THE AUTHORISATION

23 November 1988/26 May 1999

10. DATE OF REVISION OF THE TEXT

March 1999

11. Legal category

POM

Haldol Tabs & Oral Solution

(Janssen-Cilag Ltd)

1. NAME OF THE MEDICINAL PRODUCT

HALDOL Tablets 5 mg

HALDOL Tablets 10 mg

HALDOL 2 mg/ml

2. QUALITATIVE AND QUANTITATIVE COMPOSITION

Haloperidol 5 mg

Haloperidol 10 mg

Haloperidol 2mg/ml

3. PHARMACEUTICAL FORM

Tablets.

Oral solution

4. CLINICAL PARTICULARS

4.1 Therapeutic indications

Adults:

• Schizophrenia: treatment of symptoms and prevention of relapse

• Other psychoses: especially paranoid

• Mania and hypomania

• Mental or behavioural problems such as aggression, hyperactivity and self mutilation in the mentally retarded and in patients with organic brain damage

• As an adjunct to short term management of moderate to severe psychomotor agitation, excitement, violent or dangerously impulsive behaviour

• Intractable hiccup

• Restlessness and agitation in the elderly

• Gilles de la Tourette syndrome and severe tics.

Children:

• Childhood behavioural disorders, especially when associated with hyperactivity and aggression

• Gilles de la Tourette syndrome

• Childhood schizophrenia.

4.2 Posology and method of administration

For oral administration.

Since the oral solution is not intended for administration in multiples of 5 ml, the quantities given are expressed per ml.

Dosage for all indications should be individually determined and is best initiated and titrated under close clinical supervision. To determine the initial dose, consideration should be given to the patient's age, severity of symptoms and previous response to other neuroleptic drugs.

Patients who are elderly or debilitated or those with previously reported adverse reactions to neuroleptic drugs may require less Haldol. The normal starting dose should be halved, followed by a gradual titration to achieve optimal response.

Adults

Schizophrenia, psychoses, mania and hypomania, mental or behavioural problems, psychomotor agitation, excitement, violent or dangerously impulsive behaviour, organic brain damage

Initial dose:

Moderate symptomatology 1.5-3.0 mg bd or tds

Severe symptomatology/resistant patients 3.0-5.0 mg bd or tds

The same starting doses may be employed in adolescents and resistant schizophrenics who may require up to 30 mg/day.

Maintenance dosage:

Once satisfactory control of symptoms has been achieved, dosage should be gradually reduced to the lowest effective maintenance dose, often as low as 5 or 10 mg/day. Too rapid a dosage reduction should be avoided.

Restlessness or agitation in the elderly

Initial dose 1.5-3.0 mg bd or tds titrated as required, to attain an effective maintenance dose (1.5 –30 mg daily).

Gilles de la Tourette syndrome, severe tics, intractable hiccup

Starting dose 1.5 mg tds adjusted according to response. A daily maintenance dose of 10 mg may be required in Gilles de la Tourette syndrome.

Children

Childhood behavioural disorders and schizophrenia

Total daily maintenance dose of 0.025-0.05 mg/kg/day. Half the dose should be given in the morning and the other half in the evening, up to a maximum of 10 mg daily.

Gilles de la Tourette syndrome

Oral maintenance doses of up to 10 mg/day in most patients.

4.3 Contraindications

Comatose states, CNS depression, Parkinson's disease, known hypersensitivity to haloperidol, lesions of basal ganglia.

4.4 Special warnings and special precautions for use

Please also refer to section 4.5. Interactions with other Medicinal Products and other forms of Interaction.

Caution is advised in patients with liver disease, renal failure, phaeochromocytoma, epilepsy and conditions predisposing to epilepsy (eg alcohol withdrawal and brain damage) or convulsions. Haloperidol should only be used with great caution in patients with disturbed thyroid function. Antipsychotic therapy in those patients must always be accompanied by adequate management of the underlying thyroid dysfunction.

Cases of sudden death have been reported in psychiatric patients receiving antipsychotic drugs, including haloperidol.

The risk-benefit of haloperidol treatment should be fully assessed before treatment is commenced and patients with risk factors for ventricular arrhythmias such as cardiac disease, subarachnoid haemorrhage, metabolic abnormalities such as hypokalaemia, hypocalcaemia or hypomagnesaemia, starvation, alcohol abuse or those receiving concomitant therapy with other drugs known to prolong the QT interval, should be monitored carefully (ECGs and potassium levels), particularly during the initial phase of treatment, to obtain steady plasma levels.

Acute withdrawal symptoms including nausea, vomiting and insomnia have very rarely been described after abrupt cessation of high doses of antipsychotic drugs. Relapse may also occur and gradual withdrawal is advisable.

In schizophrenia, the response to antipsychotic drug treatment may be delayed. If drugs are withdrawn, recurrence of symptoms may not become apparent for several weeks or months.

As with all antipsychotic agents, haloperidol should not be used alone where depression is predominant. It may be combined with antidepressants to treat those conditions in which depression and psychosis co-exist. Haloperidol may impair the metabolism of tricyclic antidepressants (clinical significance unknown).

If concomitant anti-Parkinson medication is required, it may have to be continued after haloperidol is discontinued to take account of any differences in excretion rates. The physician should keep in mind the possible anticholinergic effects associated with anti-Parkinson agents.

4.5 Interaction with other medicinal products and other forms of Interaction

In common with all neuroleptics, haloperidol can increase the central nervous system depression produced by other CNS-depressant drugs, including alcohol, hypnotics, sedatives or strong analgesics.

An enhanced CNS effect, when combined with methyldopa, has been reported.

Haloperidol may antagonise the action of adrenaline and other sympathomimetic agents and reverses the blood pressure lowering effects of adrenergic-blocking agents such as guanethidine.

The dosage of anticonvulsants may need to be increased to take account of the lowered seizure threshold.

Co-administration of enzyme-inducing drugs such as carbamazepine, phenobarbitone and rifampicin with haloperidol may result in a significant reduction of haloperidol plasma levels. The haloperidol dose may therefore need to be increased, according to the patient's response. After stopping such drugs, it may be necessary to re-adjust the dosage of haloperidol.

Haloperidol may impair the metabolism of tricyclic antidepressants (clinical significance unknown) and the anti-Parkinson effects of levodopa.

In pharmacokinetic studies, increased haloperidol levels have been reported when haloperidol was given concomitantly with the following drugs: quinidine, buspirone and fluoxetine. Haloperidol plasma levels should therefore be monitored and reduced if necessary.

Antagonism of the effect of phenindione has been reported.

In rare cases, an encephalopathy-like syndrome has been reported in combination with lithium and haloperidol. It remains controversial whether these cases represent a distinct clinical entity or whether they are in fact cases of NMS and/or lithium toxicity. Signs of encephalopathy-like syndrome include confusion, disorientation, headache, disturbances of balance and drowsiness. One report showing symptomless EEG abnormalities on the combination has suggested that EEG monitoring might be advisable. When lithium and haloperidol therapy are used concomitantly, haloperidol should be given in the lowest effective dose and lithium levels should be monitored and kept below 1 mmol/l. If symptoms of encephalopathy-like syndrome occur, therapy should be stopped immediately.

4.6 Pregnancy and lactation

The safety of haloperidol in pregnancy has not been established. There is some evidence of harmful effects in some but not all animal studies. There have been a number of reports of birth defects following foetal exposure to haloperidol for which a causal role for haloperidol cannot be excluded. Haldol should be used during pregnancy only if the anticipated benefit outweighs the risk and the administered dose and duration of treatment should be as low and as short as possible.

Haloperidol is excreted in breast milk. There have been isolated cases of extrapyramidal symptoms in breast-fed children. If the use of Haldol is essential, the benefits of breast feeding should be balanced against its potential risks.

4.7 Effects on ability to drive and use machines

Some degree of sedation or impairment of alertness may occur, particularly with higher doses and at the start of treatment, and may be potentiated by alcohol or other CNS depressants. Patients should be advised not to undertake activities requiring alertness such as driving or operating machinery during treatment, until their susceptibility is known.

4.8 Undesirable effects

Central nervous system

In common with all neuroleptics, extrapyramidal symptoms may occur, eg tremor, rigidity, hypersalivation, bradykinesia, akathisia, acute dystonia, oculogyric crisis and laryngeal dystonia. Anti-Parkinson agents should not be prescribed routinely.

As with all antipsychotic agents, tardive dyskinesia may appear in some patients on long term therapy or after drug discontinuation. The syndrome is mainly characterised by rhythmical involuntary movements of the tongue, face, mouth or jaw. The manifestations may be permanent in some patients. The syndrome may be masked when treatment is reinstituted, when the dosage is increased or when a switch is made to a different antipsychotic drug. Treatment should be discontinued as soon as possible.

However, since its occurrence may be related to duration of treatment, as well as daily dose, Haldol should be given in the minimum effective dose for the minimum possible time, unless it is established that long term administration for the treatment of schizophrenia is required.

It has been reported that fine vermicular movements of the tongue may be an early warning sign of tardive dyskinesia and that the full syndrome may not develop if the medication is stopped at that time.

The following effects have been reported rarely; confusional states or epileptic fits, depression, sedation, agitation, drowsiness, insomnia, headache, vertigo and apparent exacerbation of psychotic symptoms.

In common with other antipsychotic drugs, haloperidol has been associated with neuroleptic malignant syndrome (NMS), an idiosyncratic response characterised by hyperthermia, generalised muscle rigidity, autonomic instability, altered consciousness, coma and elevated CPK. Signs of autonomic dysfunction such as tachycardia, labile arterial pressure and sweating may precede onset of hyperthermia, acting as early warning signs. Antipsychotic treatment should be withdrawn immediately and appropriate supportive therapy and careful monitoring instituted.

Haloperidol, even in low dosage in susceptible (especially non-psychotic) individuals, may cause unpleasant subjective feelings of being mentally dulled or slowed down, dizziness, headache or paradoxical effects of excitement, agitation or insomnia.

Gastro-intestinal system

Gastro-intestinal symptoms, nausea, loss of appetite, constipation and dyspepsia have been reported.

Endocrinological system

Hormonal effects of antipsychotic neuroleptic drugs include hyperprolactinaemia, which may cause galactorrhoea, gynaecomastia and oligo- or amenorrhoea. Hypoglycaemia and the syndrome of inappropriate antidiuretic hormone secretion have been reported rarely. Impairment of sexual function including erection and ejaculation has also been occasionally reported.

Cardiovascular system

Tachycardia and dose related hypotension are uncommon, but can occur, particularly in the elderly, who are more susceptible to the sedative and hypotensive effects. Less commonly, hypertension has also been reported.

Cardiac effects such as QT-interval prolongation, Torsade de Pointes and/or ventricular arrhythmias have been reported rarely. They may occur more frequently with high doses, intravenous administration and in predisposed patients (see 4.4. Special Warnings and Special Precautions for Use).

Autonomic nervous system

Dry mouth as well as excessive salivation, blurred vision, urinary retention and hyperhidrosis have been reported.

Dermatological system

The following effects have been reported rarely: oedema, various skin rashes and reactions including urticaria, exfoliative dermatitis and erythema multiforme. Photosensitive skin reactions have been reported very rarely.

Other adverse reactions

The following effects have been reported rarely: jaundice, cholestatic hepatitis or transient abnormalities of liver function in the absence of jaundice; priapism and weight changes. Temperature disorders may also occur, characteristically hyperthermia associated with NMS, although hypothermia has also been reported.

The following have been reported very rarely: blood dyscrasia, including agranulocytosis, thrombocytopenia and transient leucopenia; hypersensitivity reactions including anaphylaxis.

4.9 Overdose

Symptoms

In general, the manifestations of haloperidol overdosage are an extension of its pharmacological actions, the most prominent of which would be severe extrapyramidal symptoms, hypotension and psychic indifference with a transition to sleep. The risk of ventricular arrhythmias possibly associated with QT-prolongation should be considered. The patient may appear comatose with respiratory depression and hypotension which could be severe enough to produce a shock-like state. Paradoxically hypertension rather than hypotension may occur. Convulsions may also occur.

Treatment

There is no specific antidote to haloperidol. A patent airway should be established and maintained with mechanically assisted ventilation if necessary. In view of isolated reports of arrhythmia ECG monitoring is strongly advised. Hypotension and circulatory collapse should be treated by plasma volume expansion and other appropriate measures. Adrenaline should not be used. The patient should be monitored carefully for 24 hours or longer, body temperature and adequate fluid intake should be maintained.

In cases of severe extrapyramidal symptoms, appropriate anti-Parkinson medication should be administered.

5. PHARMACOLOGICAL PROPERTIES

5.1 Pharmacodynamic properties

Haloperidol acts as a central dopamine receptor antagonist. It also has some anticholinergic activity and binds to opiate receptors. It also acts at peripheral dopamine receptors.

5.2 Pharmacokinetic properties

Pharmacotherapeutic group: Butyrophenone Derivatives: ATC code: NP5A DO1

Haloperidol is absorbed rapidly with a bioavailability of 44-74% (mean 60%) after tablets and a bioavailability of 38-86% (mean 58%) after oral solution. Variable bioavailability is likely to be due to interindividual differences in gastro-intestinal absorption and extent of first-pass hepatic metabolism.

Haloperidol is rapidly distributed to extravascular tissues especially liver and adipose tissue. Haloperidol crosses the blood-brain barrier and is excreted in human breast milk. It is approximately 92% bound to plasma proteins.

Metabolism is by oxidative dealkylation. The elimination half-life is approximately 20 hours, with considerable diurnal variation.

5.3 Preclinical safety data

No relevant information other than that contained elsewhere in the Summary of Product Characteristics.

6. PHARMACEUTICAL PARTICULARS

6.1 List of excipients

Haldol 5 mg

Lactose monohydrate

Maize starch

Talc

Cottonseed oil - hydrogenated

Indigotindisulphonate sodium (E132)

Purified water (not in final product)

Haldol 10 mg

Calcium hydrogen phosphate dihydrate

Maize starch

Calcium stearate

Quinoline yellow (E104)

Purified water (not in final product)

Haldol 2mg/ml

Lactic acid

Methyl parahydroxybenzoate

Purified water

6.2 Incompatibilities

None known.

6.3 Shelf life

60 months.

6.4 Special precautions for storage

5 mg, 10 mg tablets:	Do not store above 25°C.
2 mg/ml oral solution:	Do not store above 25°C
	Do not refrigerate or freeze

Keep out of reach and sight of children.

6.5 Nature and contents of container

5,10mg tablets: Blister packs of aluminium foil and polyvinylchloride genotherm glass clear. The strips are packed in cardboard cartons containing 100 tablets per pack.

2mg/ml oral solution: Bottle: Amber glass (Type III, Ph.Eur); 100 ml

Closure:

Aluminium screw cap, tamper resistant, coated on the inner side with polyvinylchloride.

OR

Child resistant, polypropylene screw cap with low density polyethylene insert.

Dosing Device:

2.5 ml glass pipette with 0.5 ml graduations fitted on a butyl rubber bulb with a polypropylene screw cap.

OR

2.5 ml glass pipette with 0.5 ml graduations fitted on a black siliconised rubber bulb. The pipette has a white polypropylene child-resistant screw cap and polypropylene sheath.

6.6 Instructions for use and handling

None.

7. MARKETING AUTHORISATION HOLDER

Janssen-Cilag Limited

Saunderton

High Wycombe

Buckinghamshire

HP14 4HJ

UK

8. MARKETING AUTHORISATION NUMBER(S)

Haldol 5 mg:	0242/0031R
Haldol 10 mg:	0242/0039R
Haldol 2 mg/ml:	0242/0035R

9. DATE OF FIRST AUTHORISATION/RENEWAL OF THE AUTHORISATION

Haldol 5 mg:	20 June 1986/12 January 1998
Haldol 10 mg:	17 June 1986/4 February 2002
Haldol 2 mg/ml:	7 June 1989/30 March 2000

10. DATE OF REVISION OF THE TEXT

Haldol 5 mg:	28 July 2003
Haldol 10 mg:	29 July 2003
Haldol 2 mg/ml:	15 June 2001

Legal status POM

Half Inderal LA 80mg

(AstraZeneca UK Limited)

1. NAME OF THE MEDICINAL PRODUCT

Half Inderal LA 80mg

2. QUALITATIVE AND QUANTITATIVE COMPOSITION

Propranolol hydrochloride Ph Eur 80 mg

3. PHARMACEUTICAL FORM

Pink/lavender prolonged release capsules, marked Half-Inderal LA in black.

4. CLINICAL PARTICULARS

4.1 Therapeutic indications

a) Management of angina

b) Prophylaxis of migraine

c) Management of essential tremor

d) Relief of situational anxiety and generalised anxiety, particularly those of somatic type

e) Adjunctive management of thyrotoxicosis

f) Prophylaxis of upper gastro-intestinal bleeding in patients with portal hypertension and oesophageal varices

g) Control of hypertension

4.2 Posology and method of administration

For oral administration.

Adults

Hypertension: The usual starting dose is one 160 mg Inderal LA capsule daily, taken either morning or evening. An adequate response is seen in most patients at this dosage. If necessary, it can be increased in 80 mg Half-Inderal LA increments until an adequate response is achieved. A further reduction in blood pressure can be obtained if a diuretic or other antihypertensive agent is given in addition to Inderal LA and Half-Inderal LA.

Angina, essential tremor, thyrotoxicosis and the prophylaxis of migraine: One Half-Inderal LA capsule daily, taken either morning or evening, may be sufficient to provide adequate control in many patients. If necessary the dose may be increased to one Inderal LA capsule per day and an additional Half-Inderal LA increment may be given.

Situational and generalised anxiety: One Half-Inderal LA capsule taken daily should be sufficient to provide short-term relief of acute situational anxiety. Generalised anxiety, requiring longer term therapy, usually responds adequately at the same dosage. In individual cases, the dosage may be increased to one Inderal LA capsule per day. Treatment should be continued according to response. Patients should be reviewed after 6 to 12 months' treatment.

Portal hypertension: Dosage should be titrated to achieve approximately 25% reduction in resting heart rate. Dosing should begin with one 80 mg Half-Inderal LA capsule daily, increasing to one 160 mg Inderal LA capsule daily depending on heart rate response. Further 80 mg Half-Inderal LA increments may be added up to a maximum dose of 320 mg once daily.

Patients who are already established on equivalent daily doses of Inderal tablets should be transferred to the equivalent doses of Half-Inderal LA or Inderal LA daily, taken either morning or evening.

Children

Inderal LA and Half-Inderal LA are not intended for use in children.

Elderly Patients

Evidence concerning the relation between blood level and age is conflicting. It is suggested that treatment should start with one Half-Inderal LA capsule once daily. The dose may be increased to one Inderal LA capsule daily or higher as appropriate.

4.3 Contraindications

Inderal LA and Half-Inderal LA must not be used if there is a history of bronchial asthma or bronchospasm. The product label states the following warning: "Do not take Inderal LA if you have a history of asthma or wheezing". A similar warning appears in the Patient Information Leaflet.

Bronchospasm can usually be reversed by beta$_2$- agonist bronchodilators such as salbutamol. Large doses of the beta$_2$- agonist bronchodilator may be required to overcome the beta-blockade produced by propranolol and the dose should be titrated according to the clinical response; both intravenous and inhalational administration should be considered. The use of intravenous aminophylline and/or the use of ipratropium (given by nebuliser) may also be considered. Glucagon (1 to 2 mg given intravenously) has also been reported to produce a bronchodilator effect in asthmatic patients. Oxygen or artificial ventilation may be required in severe cases.

Inderal LA and Half-Inderal LA, as with other beta-adrenoceptor blocking drugs, must not be used in patients with any of the following conditions: known hypersensitivity to the substance, bradycardia, cardiogenic shock, hypotension, metabolic acidosis, after prolonged fasting, severe peripheral arterial circulatory disturbances, second or third degree heart block, sick sinus syndrome, untreated phaeochromocytoma, uncontrolled heart failure or Prinzmetal's angina.

Inderal LA and Half-Inderal LA must not be used in patients prone to hypoglycaemia, i.e. patients after prolonged fasting or patients with restricted counter-regulatory reserves.

4.4 Special warnings and special precautions for use

Inderal LA and Half-Inderal LA as with other beta-adrenoceptor blocking drugs:

- although contra-indicated in uncontrolled heart failure (see Section 4.3) may be used in patients whose signs of heart failure have been controlled. Caution must be exercised in patients whose cardiac reserve is poor.
- should not be used in combination with calcium channel blockers with negative inotropic effects (e.g. verapamil, diltiazem), as it can lead to an exaggeration of these effects particularly in patients with impaired ventricular function and/or SA or AV conduction abnormalities. This may result in severe hypotension, bradycardia and cardiac failure. Neither the beta-blocker nor the calcium channel blocker should be administered intravenously within 48 hours of discontinuing the other.
- should not be used in patients with Prinzmetal's angina and beta-1 selective agents should be used with care (see section 4.3).
- although contra-indicated in severe peripheral arterial circulatory disturbances (see section 4.3) may also aggravate less severe peripheral arterial circulatory disturbances.
- due to its negative effect on conduction time, caution must be exercised if it is given to patients with first degree heart block.
- may block/modify the signs and symptoms of the hypoglycaemia (especially tachycardia). Inderal LA and Half-Inderal LA occasionally causes hypoglycaemia, even in non-diabetic patients, e.g., neonates, infants, children, elderly patients, patients on haemodialysis or patients suffering from chronic liver disease and patients suffering from overdose. Severe hypoglycaemia associated with Inderal LA and Half-Inderal LA has rarely presented with seizures and/or coma in isolated patients. Caution must be exercised in the concurrent use of Inderal LA and Half-Inderal LA and hypoglycaemic therapy in diabetic patients. Inderal LA and Half-Inderal LA may prolong the hypoglycaemic response to insulin (see section 4.3).
- may mask the signs of thyrotoxicosis.
- should not be used in untreated phaeochromocytoma. However, in patients with phaeochromocytoma, an alpha-blocker may be given concomitantly.
- should be used to treat the elderly with caution starting with a lower dose (see section 4.2).
- will reduce heart rate as a result of its pharmacological action. In the rare instances when a treated patient develops symptoms that may be attributable to a slow heart rate, the dose may be reduced.
- may cause a more severe reaction to a variety of allergens, when given to patients with a history of anaphylactic reaction to such allergens. Such patients may be unresponsive to the usual doses of adrenaline used to treat the allergic reactions.

Abrupt withdrawal of beta-blockers is to be avoided. The dosage should be withdrawn gradually over a period of 7 to 14 days. An equivalent dosage of another beta-blocker may be substituted during the withdrawal period to facilitate a reduction in dosage below Inderal LA 80mg.

Patients should be followed during withdrawal especially those with ischaemic heart disease.

When a patient is scheduled for surgery and a decision is made to discontinue beta-blocker therapy, this should be done at least 24 hours prior to the procedure. The risk/benefit of stopping beta blockade should be made for each patient.

Since the half-life may be increased in patients with significant hepatic or renal impairment, caution must be exercised when starting treatment and selecting the initial dose.

Inderal LA and Half-Inderal LA must be used with caution in patients with decompensated cirrhosis (see section 4.2).

In patients with portal hypertension, liver function may deteriorate and hepatic encephalopathy may develop. There have been reports suggesting that treatment with propranolol may increase the risk of developing hepatic encephalopathy (see section 4.2).

Interference with laboratory tests: Inderal LA and Half-Inderal LA have been reported to interfere with the estimation of serum bilirubin by the diazo method and with the determination of catecholamines by methods using fluorescence.

4.5 Interaction with other medicinal products and other forms of Interaction

Inderal LA and Half-Inderal LA modify the tachycardia of hypoglycaemia. Caution must be exercised in the concurrent use of Inderal LA or Half-Inderal LA and hypoglycaemic therapy in diabetic patients. Propranolol may prolong the hypoglycaemic response to insulin (see section 4.3 and 4.4).

Caution must be exercised when prescribing a beta-adrenoceptor blocking drug with Class 1 antiarrhythmic agents such as disopyramide.

Digitalis glycosides, in association with beta-adrenoceptor blocking drugs, may increase atrio-ventricular conduction time.

Combined use of beta-adrenoceptor blocking drugs and calcium channel blockers with negative inotropic effects eg, verapamil, diltiazem, can lead to an exaggeration of these effects, particularly in patients with impaired ventricular function and/or sino-atrial or atrio-ventricular conduction abnormalities. This may result in severe hypotension, bradycardia and cardiac failure. Neither the beta-adrenoceptor blocking drug nor the calcium channel blocker should be administered intravenously within 48 hours of discontinuing the other.

Concomitant therapy with dihydropyridine calcium channel blockers eg, nifedipine, may increase the risk of hypotension, and cardiac failure may occur in patients with latent cardiac insufficiency.

Concomitant use of sympathomimetic agents, eg, adrenaline, may counteract the effect of beta-adrenoceptor blocking drugs. Caution must be exercised in the parenteral administration of preparations containing adrenaline to patients taking beta-adrenoceptor blocking drugs as, in rare cases, vasoconstriction, hypertension and bradycardia may result.

Administration of propranolol during infusion of lignocaine may increase the plasma concentration of lignocaine by approximately 30%. Patients already receiving propranolol tend to have higher lignocaine levels than controls. The combination should be avoided.

Concomitant use of cimetidine will increase, whereas concomitant use of alcohol will decrease, the plasma levels of propranolol.

Beta-adrenoceptor blocking drugs may exacerbate the rebound hypertension which can follow the withdrawal of clonidine. If the two drugs are co-administered, the beta-adrenoceptor blocking drug should be withdrawn several days before discontinuing clonidine. If replacing clonidine by beta-adrenoceptor blocking drug therapy, the introduction of beta-adrenoceptor blocking drugs should be delayed for several days after clonidine administration has stopped.

Caution must be exercised if ergotamine, dihydroergotamine or related compounds are given in combination with propranolol since vasospastic reactions have been reported in a few patients.

Concomitant use of prostaglandin synthetase inhibiting drugs, e.g. ibuprofen or indomethacin, may decrease the hypotensive effects of propranolol.

Concomitant administration of propranolol and chlorpromazine may result in an increase in plasma levels of both drugs. This may lead to an enhanced antipsychotic effect for chlorpromazine and an increased antihypertensive effect for propranolol.

Caution must be exercised when using anaesthetic agents with Inderal LA and Half-Inderal LA. The anaesthetist should be informed and the choice of anaesthetic should be the agent with as little negative inotropic activity as possible. Use of beta-adrenoceptor blocking drugs with anaesthetic drugs may result in attenuation of the reflex tachycardia and increase the risk of hypotension. Anaesthetic agents causing myocardial depression are best avoided.

Pharmacokinetic studies have shown that the following agents may interact with propranolol due to effects on enzyme systems in the liver which metabolise propranolol and these agents: quinidine, propafenone, rifampicin, theophylline, warfarin, thioridazine and dihydropyridine calcium channel blockers such as nifedipine, nisoldipine, nicardipine, isradipine and lacidipine. Owing to the fact that blood concentrations of either agent may be affected, dosage adjustments may be needed according to clinical judgement, (see also the interaction above concerning concomitant therapy with dihydropyridine calcium channel blockers).

4.6 Pregnancy and lactation

Pregnancy: As with all drugs, Inderal LA and Half-Inderal LA should not be given during pregnancy unless their use is essential. There is no evidence of teratogenicity with Inderal.

However beta-adrenoceptor blocking drugs reduce placental perfusion, which may result in intra-uterine foetal death, immature and premature deliveries. In addition, adverse effects (especially hypoglycaemia and bradycardia in the neonate and bradycardia in the foetus) may occur. There is an increased risk of cardiac and pulmonary complications in the neonate in the post-natal period.

Lactation: Most beta-adrenoceptor blocking drugs particularly lipophilic compounds, will pass into breast milk although to a variable extent. Breast feeding is therefore not recommended following administration of these compounds.

4.7 Effects on ability to drive and use machines

The use of Inderal LA or Half-Inderal LA is unlikely to result in any impairment of the ability of patients to drive or operate machinery. However, it should be taken into account that occasionally dizziness or fatigue may occur.

4.8 Undesirable effects

Inderal LA and Half-Inderal LA are usually well tolerated. In clinical studies, the undesired events reported are usually attributable to the pharmacological actions of propranolol.

The following undesired events, listed by body system, have been reported.

Cardiovascular: bradycardia, heart failure deterioration, postural hypotension which may be associated with syncope, cold cyanotic extremities. In susceptible patients: precipitation of heart block, exacerbation of intermittent claudication, Raynaud's phenomenon.

CNS: confusion, dizziness, mood changes, nightmares, psychoses and hallucinations, sleep disturbances.

Endocrine: Hypoglycaemia in neonates, infants, children, elderly patients, patients on haemodialysis, patients on concomitant antidiabetic therapy, patients with prolonged fasting and patients with chronic liver disease has been reported (see section 4.3, 4.4 and 4.5).

Gastrointestinal: gastrointestinal disturbance.

Haematological: purpura, thrombocytopenia.

Integumentary: alopecia, dry eyes, psoriasiform skin reactions, exacerbation of psoriasis, skin rashes.

Neurological: paraesthesia.

Respiratory: bronchospasm may occur in patients with bronchial asthma or a history of asthmatic complaints, sometimes with fatal outcome (see Section 4.3).

Special senses: visual disturbances.

Others: fatigue and/or lassitude (often transient), an increase in ANA (antinuclear antibodies) has been observed, however the clinical relevance of this is not clear; isolated reports of myasthenia gravis like syndrome or exacerbation of myasthenia gravis have been reported in patients administered propranolol.

Discontinuance of the drug should be considered if, according to clinical judgement, the well being of the patient is adversely affected by any of the above reactions. Cessation of therapy with a beta-adrenoceptor blocking drug should be gradual. In the rare event of intolerance manifested as bradycardia and hypotension, the drug should be withdrawn and, if necessary, treatment for overdosage instituted.

4.9 Overdose

The symptoms of overdosage may include bradycardia, hypotension, acute cardiac insufficiency and bronchospasm.

General treatment should include: close supervision, treatment in an intensive care ward, the use of gastric lavage, activated charcoal and a laxative to prevent absorption of any drug still present in the gastrointestinal tract, the use of plasma or plasma substitutes to treat hypotension and shock.

Excessive bradycardia can be countered with atropine 1 to 2 mg intravenously and/or a cardiac pacemaker. If necessary, this may be followed by a bolus dose of glucagon 10 mg intravenously. If required, this may be repeated or followed by an intravenous infusion of glucagon 1 to 10 mg/hour depending on response. If no response to glucagon occurs or if glucagon is unavailable, a beta-adrenoceptor stimulant such as dobutamine 2.5 to 10 microgram/kg/minute by intravenous infusion may be given. Dobutamine, because of its positive inotropic effect, could also be used to treat hypotension and acute cardiac insufficiency. It is likely that these doses would be inadequate to reverse the cardiac effects of beta-blockade if a large overdose has been taken. The dose of dobutamine should therefore be increased if necessary to achieve the required response according to the clinical condition of the patient.

5. PHARMACOLOGICAL PROPERTIES

5.1 Pharmacodynamic properties

Propranolol is a competitive antagonist at both $beta_1$ and $beta_2$-adrenoceptors. It has no agonist activity at the beta-adrenoceptor, but has membrane stabilising activity at concentrations exceeding 1 to 3 mg/litre, though such concentrations are rarely achieved during oral therapy. Competitive beta-adrenoceptor blockade has been demonstrated in man by a parallel shift to the right in the dose-heart rate response curve to beta-agonists such as isoprenaline.

Propranolol, as with other beta-adrenoceptor blocking drugs, has negative inotropic effects, and is therefore contra-indicated in uncontrolled heart failure.

Propranolol is a racemic mixture and the active form is the S (-) isomer. With the exception of inhibition of the conversion of thyroxine to triiodothyronine it is unlikely that any additional ancillary properties possessed by R (+) propranolol, in comparison with the racemic mixture will give rise to different therapeutic effects.

Propranolol is effective and well tolerated in most ethnic populations, although the response may be less in black patients.

The sustained release preparation of propranolol maintains a higher degree of $beta_1$-blockade 24 hours after dosing compared with conventional propranolol.

5.2 Pharmacokinetic properties

Propranolol is completely absorbed after oral administration and peak plasma concentrations occur 1-2 hours after dosing in fasting patients. Following oral dosing with the sustained release preparation of propranolol, the blood profile is flatter than after conventional Inderal but the half-life is increased to between 10 and 20 hours. The liver removes up to 90% of an oral dose with an elimination half-life of 3 to 6 hours. Propranolol is widely and rapidly distributed throughout the body with highest levels occurring in the lungs, liver, kidney, brain and heart. Propranolol is highly protein bound (80 to 95%).

5.3 Preclinical safety data

Propranolol is a drug on which extensive clinical experience has been obtained. Relevant information for the prescriber is provided elsewhere in this Summary of Product Characteristics.

6. PHARMACEUTICAL PARTICULARS

6.1 List of excipients

Erythrosine (E127)

Ethyl cellulose

Gelatin

Iron oxide, red (E172)

Iron oxide, black (E172)

Methylhydroxypropylcellulose

Microcrystalline cellulose

Titanium dioxide (E171)

6.2 Incompatibilities

None known.

6.3 Shelf life

5 years.

6.4 Special precautions for storage

Store below 30°C, protected from light and moisture.

6.5 Nature and contents of container

Patient calendar pack of 28 capsules.

6.6 Instructions for use and handling

Use as directed by the prescriber.

Administrative Data

7. MARKETING AUTHORISATION HOLDER

AstraZeneca UK Limited

600 Capability Green

Luton

LU1 3LU

UK

8. MARKETING AUTHORISATION NUMBER(S)

PL 17901/0020

9. DATE OF FIRST AUTHORISATION/RENEWAL OF THE AUTHORISATION

11th June 2000

10. DATE OF REVISION OF THE TEXT

25th October 2001

Harmogen 1.5mg Tablets

(Pharmacia Limited)

1. NAME OF THE MEDICINAL PRODUCT

Harmogen 1.5 mg

2. QUALITATIVE AND QUANTITATIVE COMPOSITION

Each tablet contains Estropipate USP (piperazine estrone sulphate) equivalent to 0.93 mg estrone.

For excipients, see 6.1

3. PHARMACEUTICAL FORM

Tablets for oral administration

4. CLINICAL PARTICULARS

4.1 Therapeutic indications

Hormone Replacement Therapy (HRT) for estrogen deficiency symptoms in post- and peri-menopausal women.

Prevention of osteoporosis in postmenopausal women at high risk of future fractures who are intolerant of, or contraindicated for, other medicinal products approved for the prevention of osteoporosis, (See also Section 4.4).

4.2 Posology and method of administration

Harmogen is an estrogen-only product for oral use.

Adults and the Elderly:

Post-menopausal osteoporosis: 1.5 mg daily.

Estrogen-deficiency symptoms: 1.5 mg - 3.0 mg daily taken as a single or divided dose.

For initiation and continuation of treatment of peri- and postmenopausal symptoms, the lowest effective dose for the shortest duration (see also Section 4.4) should be used.

Dosage Schedule (for both indications):

Therapy may start at any time in women with established amenorrhoea or who are experiencing long intervals between spontaneous menses. In women who are menstruating, it is advised that therapy starts within five days of the start of bleeding. Patients changing from a cyclical or continuous sequential preparation should complete the cycle, and after a withdrawal bleed, may then change to Harmogen 1.5mg. Patients changing from a continuous combined preparation may start therapy at any time if amenorrhoea is established, or otherwise start within five days of the start of bleeding.

Harmogen should be given continuously and, in women with an intact uterus, a progestogen is recommended and should be added for at least 12-14 days each cycle. The benefits of the lower risk of endometrial hyperplasia and endometrial cancer, due to adding progestogen, should be weighed against the increased risk of Breast cancer, (See Sections 4.4 and 4.8). Unless there is a previous diagnosis of endometriosis, it is not recommended to add a progestogen in hysterectomised women.

If a tablet is missed it should be taken within a few hours of when normally taken, otherwise the forgotten tablet should be discarded, and the usual tablet should be taken at the next scheduled time. If one extra tablet is taken inadvertently, the usual tablet should be taken at the next scheduled time. There is an increased likelihood of break-through bleeding and spotting when a dose is missed.

4.3 Contraindications

Known, past or suspected breast cancer;

Known or suspected estrogen-dependent malignant tumours, (e.g. endometrial cancer);

Undiagnosed genital bleeding;

Untreated endometrial hyperplasia;

Previous idiopathic or current venous thromboembolism (deep vein thrombosis, pulmonary embolism);

Active or recent arterial thromboembolic disease (e.g. angina, myocardial infarction);

Acute liver disease, or a history of liver disease as long as liver function tests have failed to return to normal;

Known hypersensitivity to the active substances or to any of the excipients;

Porphyria.

4.4 Special warnings and special precautions for use

For the treatment of menopausal symptoms, HRT should only be initiated for symptoms that adversely affect quality of life. In all cases, a careful appraisal of the risks and benefits should be undertaken at least annually and HRT should only be continued as long as the benefit outweighs the risk

Medical Examination/Follow Up

Assessment of each woman prior to taking hormone replacement therapy (and at regular intervals thereafter) should include a personal and family medical history. Physical examination should be guided by this and by the contra-indications (see Section 4.3) and warnings (see Section 4.4) for this product. During assessment of each individual woman, clinical examination of the breasts and pelvic examination should be performed where clinically indicated rather than as a routine procedure. Women should be encouraged to participate in the national breast screening programme (mammography) and the national cervical screening programme (cervical cytology) as appropriate for their age. Breast awareness should also be encouraged and women advised to report any changes in their breasts to their doctor or nurse, (see "Breast Cancer" below).

Conditions which need supervision:

If any of the following conditions are present, have occurred previously, and/or have been aggravated during pregnancy or previous hormone treatment, the patient should be closely supervised. It should be taken into account that these conditions may recur or be aggravated during treatment with Harmogen, in particular:

Risk factors for estrogen dependent tumours, e.g. 1st degree heredity for breast cancer (see below);

Diabetes mellitus with or without vascular involvement;

Migraine or (severe) headache;

Epilepsy;

A history of, or risk of factors for, thromboembolic disorders (see below);

Systemic lupus erythematosus, SLE;

Liver disorders (e.g. liver adenoma);

Leiomyoma (uterine fibroids) or endometriosis;

Otosclerosis;

Cholelithiasis;

A history of endometrial hyperplasia (see below);

Hypertension;

Asthma.

Reasons for immediate withdrawal of therapy:

Therapy should be discontinued in case a contra-indication is discovered and in the following situations:

- Jaundice or deterioration in liver function
- Significant increase in blood pressure
- New onset of migraine-type headache
- Pregnancy

Endometrial Hyperplasia

The risk of endometrial hyperplasia and carcinoma is increased when estrogens are administered alone for prolonged periods, (see Section 4.8). The addition of progestogen for at least 12 days per cycle in non-hysterectomised women greatly reduces this risk (See Section 4.8).

The endometrial safety of added progestogen has not been studied for Harmogen 1.5mg.

The reduction in risk to the endometrium should be weighed against the increase in the risk of breast cancer of added progestogen (See 'Breast cancer' below, and in Section 4.8)

Breakthrough bleeding and spotting may occur during the first months of treatment. If breakthrough bleeding or spotting appears after some time on therapy or continues after treatment has been discontinued, the reason should be investigated which may include endometrial biopsy to exclude endometrial malignancy.

Unopposed estrogen stimulation may lead to premalignant transformation in the residual foci of endometriosis. Therefore, the addition of progestogens to estrogen replacement therapy should be considered in women who have undergone hysterectomy because of endometriosis, if they are known to have residual endometriosis (but see above).

Breast Cancer

A randomised placebo-controlled trial, the Women's Health Initiative study (WHI), and epidemiological studies, including the Million Women Study (MWS), have reported an increased risk of breast cancer in women taking estrogens, estrogen-progestogen combinations or tibolone for HRT for several years (see Section 4.8). For all HRT, an excess risk becomes apparent within a few years of use and increases with duration of intake but returns to baseline within a few (at most five) years after stopping treatment.

In the MWS, the relative risk of breast cancer with conjugated equine estrogens (CEE) or estradiol (E2) was greater when a progestogen was added, either sequentially or continuously, and regardless of type of progestogen. There was no evidence of a difference in risk between the different routes of administration.

In the WHI study, the continuous combined conjugated equine estrogen and medroxyprogesterone acetate (CEE + MPA) product used was associated with breast cancers that were slightly larger in size and more frequently had local lymph node metastases compared to placebo.

HRT, especially estrogen-progestogen combined treatment, increases the density of mammographic images which may adversely affect the radiological detection of breast cancer.

Venous Thromboembolism

HRT is associated with a higher relative risk of developing venous thromboembolism (VTE), i.e. deep vein thrombosis or pulmonary embolism. One randomised controlled trial and epidemiological studies found a two to threefold higher risk for users compared with non-users. For non-users, it is estimated that the number of cases of VTE that will occur over a 5 year period is about 3 per 1000 women aged 50-59 years and 8 per 1000 women aged between 60-69 years. It is estimated that in healthy women who use HRT for 5 years, the number of additional cases of VTE over a 5 year period will be between 2 and 6 (best estimate = 4) per 1000 women aged 50-59 years and between 5 and 15 (best estimate = 9) per 1000 women aged 60-69 years. The occurrence of such an event is more likely in the first year of HRT than later.

Generally recognised risk factors for VTE include a personal history or family history, severe obesity (BM > 30 kg/m^2) and systemic lupus erythematosus (SLE). There is no consensus about the possible role of varicose veins in VTE.

Patients with a history of VTE or known thrombophilic states have an increased risk of VTE. HRT may add to this risk. Personal or strong family history of thromboembolism or recurrent spontaneous abortion should be investigated in order to exclude a thrombophilic predisposition. Until a thorough evaluation of thrombophilic factors has been made or anticoagulant treatment initiated, use of HRT in such patients should be viewed as contraindicated. Those women already on anticoagulant treatment require careful consideration of the benefit-risk of use of HRT.

The risk of VTE may be temporarily increased with prolonged immobilisation, major trauma or major surgery. As in all postoperative patients, scrupulous attention should be given to prophylactic measures to prevent VTE following surgery. Where prolonged immobilisation is liable to follow elective surgery, particularly abdominal or orthopaedic surgery to the lower limbs, consideration should be given to temporarily stopping HRT 4 to 6 weeks earlier, if possible. Treatment should not be restarted until the woman is completely mobilised.

If VTE develops after initiating therapy, the drug should be discontinued. Patients should be told to contact their doctor immediately when they are aware of a potential thromboembolic symptom (e.g. painful swelling of a leg, sudden pain in the chest, dyspnoea).

Coronary Artery Disease

There is no evidence from randomised controlled trials of cardiovasular benefit with continuous combined conjugated estrogens and medroxyprogesterone acetate (MPA). Two large clinical trials (WHI and HERS, i.e. Heart and Estrogen/progestin Replacement Study) showed a possible increased risk of cardiovascular morbidity in the first year of use and no overall benefit. For other HRT products there are only limited data from randomised controlled trials examining effects in cardiovascular morbidity or mortality. Therefore, it is uncertain whether these findings also extend to other HRT products.

Stroke

One large randomised clinical trial (WHI-trial) found, as a secondary outcome, an increased risk of ischaemic stroke in healthy women during treatment with continuous combined conjugated estrogens and medroxyprogesterone acetate. For women who do not use HRT, it is estimated that the number of cases of stroke that will occur over a 5 year period is about 3 per 1000 women aged 50-59 years and 11 per 1000 women aged 60-69 years. It is estimated that for women who use conjugated estrogens and medroxyprogesterone acetate for 5 years, the number of additional cases will be between 0 and 3 (best estimate = 1) per 1000 users aged 50-59 years and between 1 and 9 (best estimate = 4) per 1000 users aged 60-69 years. It is unknown whether the increased risk also extends to other HRT products.

Ovarian Cancer

Long-term (at least 5 to 10 years) use of estrogen-only HRT products in hysterectomised women has been associated with an increased risk of ovarian cancer in some epidemiological studies. It is uncertain whether long-term use of combined HRT confers a different risk than estrogen-only products.

Other Conditions

Estrogens may cause fluid retention and therefore patients with cardiac or renal dysfunction should be carefully observed. Patients with terminal renal insufficiency should be closely observed, since it is expected that the level of circulating active ingredients in Harmogen 1.5 mg tablets is increased.

Women with pre-existing hypertriglyceridaemia should be followed closely during estrogen replacement or hormone replacement therapy, since rare cases of large increases of plasma triglycerides leading to pancreatitis have been reported with estrogen therapy in this condition.

Estrogens increase thyroid binding globulin (TBG), leading to increased circulating total thyroid hormone, as measured by protein-bound iodine (PBI), T4 levels (by column or by radio-immunoassay) or T3 levels (by radio-immunoassay). T3 resin uptake is decreased, reflecting the elevated TBG. Free T4 and free T3 concentrations are unaltered. Other binding proteins may be elevated in serum, i.e. corticoid binding globulin (CBG), sex-hormone-binding globulin (SHBG) leading to increased circulating corticosteroids and sex steroids, respectively. Free or biologically active hormone concentrations are unchanged. Other plasma proteins may be increased (angiotensinogen/renin substrate, alpha-1-antitrypsin, ceruloplasmin).

There is no conclusive evidence for improvement of cognitive function. There is some evidence from the WHI trial of increased risk of probable dementia in women who start using continuous combined CEE and MPA after the age of 65. It is unknown whether the findings apply to younger post-menopausal women or other HRT products.

In rare cases benign, and in even rarer cases malignant liver tumours leading in isolated cases to life-threatening intra-abdominal haemorrhage have been observed after the use of hormonal substances such as those contained in Harmogen 1.5mg. If severe upper abdominal complaints, enlarged liver or signs of intra-abdominal haemorrhage occur, a liver tumour should be considered in the differential diagnosis.

Women who may be at risk of pregnancy should be advised to adhere to non-hormonal contraceptive methods.

The requirement for oral anti-diabetics or insulin can change as a result of the effect on glucose tolerance.

4.5 Interaction with other medicinal products and other forms of Interaction

The metabolism of estrogen may be increased by concomitant use of substances known to induce drug-metabolising enzymes, specifically cytochrome P450 enzymes, such as anticonvulsants (e.g. phenobarbital, phenytoin, carbamazepine) and anti-infectives (e.g. rifampicin, rifabutin, nevirapine, efavirenz).

Ritonavir and nelfinavir, although known as strong inhibitors by contrast exhibit inducing properties when used concomitantly with steroid hormones. Herbal preparations containing St John's Wort (Hypericum Perforatum) may induce the metabolism of estrogens.

Clinically, an increased metabolism of estrogens and progestogens may lead to decreased effect and changes in the uterine bleeding profile.

Some laboratory tests can be influenced by estrogens such as tests for thyroid function (see Section 4.4).

4.6 Pregnancy and lactation

Pregnancy

Harmogen 1.5 mg is not indicated during pregnancy. If pregnancy occurs during medication with Harmogen 1.5 mg treatment should be withdrawn immediately.

The results of most epidemiological studies to date relevant to inadvertent foetal exposure to estrogens indicate no teratogenic or foetoxic effects.

Lactation

Harmogen 1.5mg is not indicated during lactation.

4.7 Effects on ability to drive and use machines

None known

4.8 Undesirable effects

The following adverse reactions have been reported with Harmogen 1.5 mg estrogen therapy:

1. *Genito-urinary tract:* Endometrial neoplasia*, intermenstrual bleeding, increase in the size of uterine fibromyomata, endometrial proliferation or aggravation of endometriosis, changes in cervical eversion and excessive production of cervical mucus, candidal infections, thrush;

2. *Breast:* Tenderness, pain, enlargement or secretion, breast cancer*

3. *Gastro-intestinal tract*: Nausea, vomiting, abdominal cramp, bloating;

4. *Cardiovascular system*: Hypertension, thrombosis, thrombophlebitis, venous thromboembolism*, myocardial infarction* and stroke*;

5. *Liver/biliary system*: In rare cases benign, and in even rarer cases malignant liver tumours, cholelithiasis, cholestatic jaundice, gall bladder disease;

6. *Skin*: Chloasma which may persist when the drug is discontinued, erythema multiforme, erythema nodosum,, vascular purpura, rash, loss of scalp hair, hirsutism;

7. *Eyes*: Steepening of corneal curvature, intolerance to contact lenses;

8. *CNS*: Headache, migraine, dizziness, mood changes (elation or depression), chorea, probable dementia (see Section 4.4);

9. Miscellaneous: Sodium and water retention, reduced glucose tolerance, change in body weight, muscle cramps, aggravation of porphyria, changes in libido.

* See sections 4.3, Contraindications and Section 4.4 Special Warnings and Special Precautions for Use.

Breast cancer

According to evidence from a large number of epidemiological studies and one randomised placebo-controlled trial, the Women's Health Initiative (WHI), the overall risk of breast cancer increases with increasing duration of HRT use in current or recent HRT users.

For *estrogen-only* HRT, estimates of relative risk (RR) from a reanalysis of original data from 51 epidemiological studies (in which >80% of HRT use was estrogen-only HRT) and from the epidemiological Million Women Study (MWS) are similar at 1.35 (95% CI 1.21 – 1.49) and 1.30 (95% CI 1.21 – 1.40), respectively.

For *estrogen plus progestogen* combined HRT, several epidemiological studies have reported an overall higher risk for breast cancer than with estrogens alone.

The MWS reported that, compared to never users, the use of various types of estrogen-progestogen combined HRT was associated with a higher risk of breast cancer (RR = 2.00, 95% CI: 1.88 – 2.12) than use of estrogens alone (RR = 1.30, 95% CI: 1.21 – 1.40) or use of tibolone (RR=1.45; 95%CI 1.25-1.68).

The WHI trial reported a risk estimate of 1.24 (95% CI 1.01 – 1.54) after 5.6 years of use of estrogen-progestogen combined HRT (CEE + MPA) in all users compared with placebo.

The absolute risks calculated from the MWS and the WHI trial are presented below:

The MWS has estimated, from the known average incidence of breast cancer in developed countries, that:

Ø *For women not using HRT, about 32 in every 1000 are expected to have breast cancer diagnosed between the ages of 50 and 64 years.*

Ø For 1000 current or recent users of HRT, the number of *additional* cases during the corresponding period will be

Ø For users of *estrogen-only* replacement therapy

- between 0 and 3 (best estimate = 1.5) for 5 years' use
- between 3 and 7 (best estimate = 5) for 10 years' use.

Ø For users of *estrogen plus progestogen* combined HRT,

- between 5 and 7 (best estimate = 6) for 5 years' use
- between 18 and 20 (best estimate = 19) for 10 years' use.

The WHI trial estimated that after 5.6 years of follow-up of women between the ages of 50 and 79 years, an *additional* 8 cases of invasive breast cancer would be due to *estrogen-progestogen combined* HRT (CEE + MPA) per 10,000 women years.

According to calculations from the trial data, it is estimated that:

Ø For 1000 women in the placebo group,

- about 16 cases of invasive breast cancer would be diagnosed in 5 years.

Ø For 1000 women who used estrogen + progestogen combined HRT (CEE + MPA), the number of *additional* cases would be

- between 0 and 9 (best estimate = 4) for 5 years' use.

The number of additional cases of breast cancer in women who use HRT is broadly similar for women who start HRT irrespective of age at start of use (between the ages of 45-65) (see Section 4.4).

Endometrial cancer

In women with an intact uterus, the risk of endometrial hyperplasia and endometrial cancer increases with increasing duration of use of unopposed estrogens. According to data from epidemiological studies, the best estimate of the risk is that for women not using HRT, about 5 in every 1000 are expected to have endometrial cancer diagnosed between the ages of 50 and 65. Depending on the duration of treatment and estrogen dose, the reported increase in endometrial cancer risk among unopposed estrogen users varies from 2-to 12-fold greater compared with non-users. Adding a progestogen to estrogen-only therapy greatly reduces this increased risk.

4.9 Overdose

Overdosage is unlikely to cause serious problems, although the following symptoms may be present, i.e. nausea and withdrawal bleeding in women. However gastric lavage or emesis may be used when considered appropriate.

5. PHARMACOLOGICAL PROPERTIES

5.1 Pharmacodynamic properties

Pharmacotherapeutic group: Natural and semisynthetic estrogens, plain.

ATC Code G03C A

Estropipate is a semi-synthetic estrogen conjugate, sulphate ester of estrone. This substitutes for the loss of estrogen production in menopausal women, and alleviates menopausal symptoms. Estrogens prevent bone loss following menopause or ovariectomy.

Estrogen deficiency at menopause is associated with an increasing bone turnover and decline in bone mass. The effect of estrogens on the bone mineral density is dose-dependent. Protection appears to be effective for as long as treatment is continued. After discontinuation of HRT, bone mass is lost at a rate similar to that in untreated women.

Evidence from the WHI trial and meta-analysed trials shows that current use of HRT, alone or in combination with a progestagen – given to predominantly healthy women – reduces the risk of hip, vertebral, and other osteoporotic fractures. HRT may also prevent fractures in women with low bone density and/or established osteoporosis, but the evidence for that is limited.

Women with an increased risk of osteoporosis include those suffering from an early menopause, receiving recent prolonged corticosteroid therapy, having a family history of osteoporosis, of small frame, who are thin, smokers and those with an excess alcohol intake.

5.2 Pharmacokinetic properties

Estropipate is metabolised in the liver, so any form of liver impairment will result in reduced metabolism.

Gastro-intestinal absorption of orally administered (tablets) estrogens is usually prompt and complete, inactivation of estrogens in the body occurs mainly in the liver. During cyclic passage through the liver, estrogens in the body are degraded to less active estrogenic compounds and conjugated with sulphuric and glucuronic acids. Estrone is 50-80% bound as it circulates in the blood, primarily as a conjugate with sulphate.

5.3 Preclinical safety data

No additional information is available.

6. PHARMACEUTICAL PARTICULARS

6.1 List of excipients

Lactose (monohydrate) NF

Lactose (anhydrous) NF

Dibasic potassium phosphate USP

Tromethamine USP

Hydroxypropyl cellulose NF

Sodium starch glycollate NF

Microcrystalline cellulose NF

Colloidal silicon dioxide NF

Magnesium stearate NF

Hydrogenated vegetable oil wax

Dye E110

Purified water USP

Alcohol 200 proof

6.2 Incompatibilities

None known

6.3 Shelf life

Two years

6.4 Special precautions for storage

None

6.5 Nature and contents of container

The containers comprise an HDPE container with tamper-evident cap or securitainer holding 100 estropipate tablets or a PVC/Aluminium foil blister pack, holding 28 tablets, which, together with a Patient Information Leaflet are packed in a carton.

6.6 Instructions for use and handling

No special instructions

Administrative Data

7. MARKETING AUTHORISATION HOLDER

Pharmacia Limited

Davy Avenue

Milton Keynes

MK5 8PH

UK

8. MARKETING AUTHORISATION NUMBER(S)

PL 0032/0252

9. DATE OF FIRST AUTHORISATION/RENEWAL OF THE AUTHORISATION

7th June 2001/7th June 2003

10. DATE OF REVISION OF THE TEXT

March 2004

Legal category: POM

Ref: HA 3_3

Havrix Junior Monodose Vaccine

(GlaxoSmithKline UK)

1. NAME OF THE MEDICINAL PRODUCT

Havrix® Junior Monodose® vaccine

2. QUALITATIVE AND QUANTITATIVE COMPOSITION

Hepatitis A virus antigen, 720 ELISA units/0.5 ml dose.

For excipients, see Section 6.1.

3. PHARMACEUTICAL FORM

Vaccine for injection

4. CLINICAL PARTICULARS

4.1 Therapeutic indications

Havrix Junior Monodose vaccine is indicated for active immunisation against HAV infection. The vaccine is particularly indicated for those at increased risk of infection or transmission. It is also indicated for use during outbreaks of hepatitis A infection.

4.2 Posology and method of administration

Havrix Junior Monodose vaccine should be injected intramuscularly in the deltoid region. The vaccine should never be administered intravenously.

Dosage

Children/adolescents (1-15 years)

Primary immunisation consists of a single dose of Havrix Junior Monodose vaccine (720 ELISA units/0.5 ml) given intramuscularly. This provides anti-HAV antibodies for at least one year.

Havrix Junior Monodose confers protection against hepatitis A within two to four weeks.

In order to obtain more persistent immunity, for at least 10 years, a booster dose is recommended between 6 and 12 months after primary immunisation.

Booster vaccination with Havrix Junior Monodose delayed up to 3 years after the primary dose induces similar antibody levels as a booster dose administered within the recommended time interval. That is, immunity is also expected to persist for at least 10 years after boosting. However to maintain continuous protection, boosting should take place between 6 and 12 months after primary immunisation.

Havrix Junior Monodose can be used as a booster in subjects previously immunised with any inactivated hepatitis A vaccine.

In the event of a subject being exposed to a high risk of contracting hepatitis A within two weeks of the primary immunisation dose, human normal immunoglobulin may be given simultaneously with Havrix Junior Monodose at different injection sites.

4.3 Contraindications

Hypersensitivity to any component of the vaccine.

Severe febrile illness.

4.4 Special warnings and special precautions for use

As with all vaccinations, appropriate medication (e.g. adrenaline) should be readily available for immediate use in case of anaphylaxis.

It is possible that subjects may be in the incubation period of a hepatitis A infection at the time of immunisation. It is not known whether Havrix Junior Monodose will prevent hepatitis A in such cases.

In haemodialysis patients and in subjects with an impaired immune system, adequate anti-HAV antibody titres may not be obtained after the primary immunisation and such patients may therefore require administration of additional doses of vaccine.

4.5 Interaction with other medicinal products and other forms of Interaction

Simultaneous administration of Havrix with normal immunoglobulin does not influence the seroconversion rate to Havrix, however, it may result in a lower antibody titre. A similar effect could be observed with Havrix Junior Monodose.

Preliminary data on the concomitant administration of Havrix, at a dose of 720 ELISA units/ml, with recombinant hepatitis B virus vaccine suggests that there is no interference in the immune response to either antigen. On this basis and since it is an inactivated vaccine interference with immune response is unlikely to occur when Havrix Junior Monodose is administered with other inactivated or live vaccines. When concomitant administration is considered necessary the vaccines must be given at different injection sites.

Havrix Junior Monodose must not be mixed with other vaccines in the same syringe.

4.6 Pregnancy and lactation

The effect of Havrix Junior Monodose on foetal development has not been assessed. However, as with all inactivated viral vaccines the risks to the foetus are considered to be negligible. Havrix Junior Monodose should be used during pregnancy only when clearly needed.

The effect on breast-fed infants of the administration of Havrix Junior Monodose to their mothers has not been evaluated in clinical studies. Havrix Junior Monodose should therefore be used with caution in breast-feeding women.

4.7 Effects on ability to drive and use machines

Not applicable.

4.8 Undesirable effects

These are usually mild and confined to the first few days after vaccination. The most common reactions are mild transient soreness, erythema and induration at the injection site. Less common general complaints, not necessarily related to the vaccination, include headache, fever, malaise, fatigue, nausea, vomiting, diarrhoea and loss of appetite and rash. Arthralgia, myalgia, convulsions and allergic reactions including anaphylactoid reactions have been reported very rarely. Elevations of serum liver enzymes (usually transient) have been reported occasionally. However, a causal relationship with the vaccine has not been established.

Neurological manifestations occurring in temporal association have been reported extremely rarely with the vaccine and include transverse myelitis, Guillain-Barré syndrome and neuralgic amyotrophy. No causal relationship has been established.

4.9 Overdose

Not applicable.

5. PHARMACOLOGICAL PROPERTIES

5.1 Pharmacodynamic properties

Not applicable.

5.2 Pharmacokinetic properties

Not applicable.

5.3 Preclinical safety data

Not applicable.

6. PHARMACEUTICAL PARTICULARS

6.1 List of excipients

Aluminium hydroxide gel (3% w/w)

2 Phenoxyethanol

Polysorbate 20

Amino acids for injection

Disodium phosphate

Monopotassium phosphate

Sodium chloride

Potassium Chloride

Water for injections

6.2 Incompatibilities

Not applicable.

6.3 Shelf life

Havrix Junior Monodose vaccine has a shelf-life of three years from the date of manufacture when stored at 2-8°C.

6.4 Special precautions for storage

Store at 2-8°C.

Protect from light.

Do not freeze.

6.5 Nature and contents of container

Neutral glass vials (type 1, PhEur) with grey butyl rubber stoppers and aluminium overcaps fitted with flip-off tops.

0.5 ml of suspension in prefilled syringe (type I glass) with a plunger stopper (rubber butyl) with or without needles - pack size of 1 or 10.

Not all pack sizes may be marketed.

6.6 Instructions for use and handling

The vaccine should be inspected visually for any foreign particulate matter and/or variation of physical aspect prior to administration. Before use, the vaccine should be well shaken to obtain a slightly opaque white suspension. Discard the vaccine if the content appears otherwise.

Administrative Data

7. MARKETING AUTHORISATION HOLDER

SmithKline Beecham plc

980 Great West Road, Brentford, Middlesex TW8 9GS

Trading as:

GlaxoSmithKline UK

Stockley Park West

Uxbridge

Middlesex UB11 1BT

8. MARKETING AUTHORISATION NUMBER(S)

PL 10592/0080.

9. DATE OF FIRST AUTHORISATION/RENEWAL OF THE AUTHORISATION

14 March 2003

10. DATE OF REVISION OF THE TEXT

25th June 2002

11. Legal Status

POM

Havrix Monodose Vaccine

(GlaxoSmithKline UK)

1. NAME OF THE MEDICINAL PRODUCT

Havrix® Monodose® Vaccine

2. QUALITATIVE AND QUANTITATIVE COMPOSITION

Each vial or syringe contains 1440 ELISA units/1 ml dose of hepatitis A virus antigen.

3. PHARMACEUTICAL FORM

Vaccine suspension for injection.

4. CLINICAL PARTICULARS

4.1 Therapeutic indications

Active immunisation against infections caused by hepatitis A virus. The vaccine is particularly indicated for those at increased risk of infection or transmission. For example immunisation should be considered for the following risk groups:

travellers visiting areas of medium or high endemicity, i.e. anywhere outside northern or western Europe, Australia, North America and New Zealand.

military and diplomatic personnel, haemophiliacs and patients, intravenous drug abusers, homosexual men, laboratory workers working directly with the hepatitis A virus, sanitation workers in contact with untreated sewage.

patients with chronic liver disease (including alcoholic cirrhosis, chronic hepatitis B, chronic hepatitis C, autoimmune hepatitis, primary biliary cirrhosis).

close contacts of hepatitis A cases.

Since virus shedding from infected persons may occur for a prolonged period, active immunisation of close contacts may be considered.

Under certain circumstances additional groups could be at increased risk of infection or transmission. Immunisation of such groups should be considered in the light of local circumstances. Such groups might include:

staff and inmates of residential institutions for the mentally handicapped and other institutions where standards of personal hygiene are poor.

staff working in day care centres and other settings with children who are not yet toilet trained.

food packagers or handlers.

In addition there may be other groups at risk or specific circumstances such as an outbreak of hepatitis A infection when immunisation should be given.

4.2 Posology and method of administration

Posology

Adults (16 years and over)

Primary immunisation consists of a single dose of Havrix Monodose vaccine (1440 ELISA units/ml) given intramuscularly. This provides anti-HAV antibodies for at least one year.

Havrix Monodose confers protection against hepatitis A within 2-4 weeks.

In order to obtain more persistent, immunity, for at least 10 years, a booster dose is recommended between 6 and 12 months after primary immunisation.

Booster vaccination with Havrix Monodose delayed up to 3 years after the primary dose induces similar antibody levels as a booster dose administered within the recommended time interval. That is, immunity is also expected to persist for at least 10 years after boosting. However to maintain continuous protection, boosting should take place between 6 and 12 months after primary immunisation.

Havrix Monodose can be used as a booster in subjects previously immunised with any inactivated hepatitis A vaccine.

In the event of a subject being exposed to a high risk of contracting hepatitis A within 2 weeks of the primary immunisation dose human normal immunoglobulin may be given simultaneously with Havrix Monodose at different injection sites.

Children/adolescents (1-15 years)

Havrix Monodose is not recommended (Havrix Junior Monodose should be used).

Method of administration

Havrix Monodose vaccine should be injected intramuscularly in the deltoid region.

The vaccine should never be administered intravenously.

4.3 Contraindications

Hypersensitivity to any component of the vaccine. Severe febrile illness.

4.4 Special warnings and special precautions for use

As for all vaccinations, appropriate medication (e.g. adrenaline) should be readily available for immediate use in case of anaphylaxis.

It is possible that subjects may be in the incubation period of a hepatitis A infection at the time of immunisation. It is not known whether Havrix Monodose will prevent hepatitis A in such cases.

In haemodialysis patients and in subjects with an impaired immune system, adequate anti-HAV antibody titres may not be obtained after the primary immunisation and such patients may therefore require administration of additional doses of vaccine.

4.5 Interaction with other medicinal products and other forms of Interaction

Simultaneous administration of Havrix at a dose of 720 ELISA units/ml with ISG does not influence the seroconversion rate to Havrix, however, it may result in a lower antibody titre. A similar effect could be observed with Havrix Monodose.

Preliminary data on the concomitant administration of Havrix at a dose of 720 ELISA units/ml, with recombinant hepatitis B virus vaccine suggest that there is no interference in the immune response to either antigen. On this basis and since it is an inactivated vaccine interference with immune response is unlikely to occur when Havrix Monodose is administered with other inactivated or live vaccines. When concomitant administration is considered necessary the vaccines must be given at different injection sites.

Havrix Monodose must not be mixed with other vaccines in the same syringe.

4.6 Pregnancy and lactation

The effect of Havrix Monodose on foetal development has not been assessed. However, as with all inactivated viral vaccines the risks to the foetus are considered negligible. Havrix Monodose should be used during pregnancy only when clearly needed.

The effect on breast fed infants of the administration of Havrix Monodose to their mothers has not been evaluated in clinical studies. Havrix Monodose should therefore be used with caution in breast feeding women.

4.7 Effects on ability to drive and use machines

Not applicable.

4.8 Undesirable effects

These are usually mild and confined to the first few days after vaccination. The most common reactions are mild transient soreness, erythema and induration at the injection site. Less common general complaints, not necessarily related to the vaccination, include headache, fever, malaise, fatigue, nausea, diarrhoea and loss of appetite and rash. Arthralgia, myalgia, convulsions and allergic reactions including anaphylactoid reactions have been reported very rarely. Elevations of serum liver enzymes (usually transient) have been reported occasionally. However, a causal relationship with the vaccine has not been established.

Neurological manifestations occurring in temporal association have been reported extremely rarely with the vaccine and included transverse myelitis, Guillain-Barre syndrome and neuralgic amyotrophy. No causal relationship has been established.

4.9 Overdose
Not applicable.

5. PHARMACOLOGICAL PROPERTIES

5.1 Pharmacodynamic properties
Active immunisation against hepatitis A virus.

5.2 Pharmacokinetic properties
Not applicable to vaccine products.

5.3 Preclinical safety data
Not applicable to vaccine products.

6. PHARMACEUTICAL PARTICULARS

6.1 List of excipients
Aluminium hydroxide, 2 phenoxyethanol, polysorbate 20, amino acids for injection, disodium phosphate, monopotassium phosphate, sodium chloride, potassium chloride, water for injections and also a trace of neomycin B sulphate (maximum 40 ng, 0.028 IU/ml).

6.2 Incompatibilities
Not applicable.

6.3 Shelf life
36 months.

6.4 Special precautions for storage
Store at 2°C-8°C. Protect from light. Do not freeze.

6.5 Nature and contents of container
Colourless glass vials (Type I, Ph Eur) with grey butyl rubber stoppers and aluminium overcaps fitted with avocado coloured flip-off tops containing 1 ml of suspension in packs of one and 10.

1 ml of suspension in prefilled syringe (type I glass) with a plunger stopper (rubber butyl) with or without needles - pack size of 1 or 10.

Not all pack sizes may be marketed.

6.6 Instructions for use and handling
The vaccine should be inspected visually for any foreign particulate matter and/or variation of physical aspect prior to administration. Before use, the vaccine should be well shaken to obtain a slightly opaque white suspension. Discard the vaccine if the content appears otherwise.

Administrative Data

7. MARKETING AUTHORISATION HOLDER
SmithKline Beecham plc

Great West Road, Brentford, Middlesex TW8 9GS

Trading as:

GlaxoSmithKline UK

Stockley Park West

Uxbridge

Middlesex

UB11 1BT

8. MARKETING AUTHORISATION NUMBER(S)
PL 10592/0037

9. DATE OF FIRST AUTHORISATION/RENEWAL OF THE AUTHORISATION
18.05.94

10. DATE OF REVISION OF THE TEXT
25th June 2002

11. Legal category
POM

Haymine Tablets

(Forest Laboratories UK Limited)

1. NAME OF THE MEDICINAL PRODUCT
HAYMINE TABLETS

2. QUALITATIVE AND QUANTITATIVE COMPOSITION
Each tablet contains:

Chlorphenamine maleate Ph.Eur. 10mg

Ephedrine hydrochloride Ph.Eur. 15mg

3. PHARMACEUTICAL FORM
Sustained release tablet

4. CLINICAL PARTICULARS

4.1 Therapeutic indications
Relief of symptoms caused by allergic conditions such as hay fever, allergic rhinitis, perennial rhinitis, urticaria etc., which are responsive to antihistamine.

4.2 Posology and method of administration
Adults, elderly and children over 12 years of age:

One or two tablets daily. One tablet should be taken in the morning on rising and a further tablet may be taken at night if required.

Children under 12 years of age:

Not recommended.

Method of administration - oral use

4.3 Contraindications
Coronary thrombosis, hypertension, thyrotoxicosis and those on treatment with monoamine oxidase inhibitors.

4.4 Special warnings and special precautions for use
Tablets should be swallowed whole and not sucked or chewed. Do not exceed the stated dose. Asthmatics should consult their doctor before using this product. May cause drowsiness, if affected do not drive or operate machinery. Avoid alcoholic drink.

4.5 Interaction with other medicinal products and other forms of Interaction
Alcoholic drinks and certain other central nervous system depressants can potentiate any sedative effect.

4.6 Pregnancy and lactation
Contra-indicated

4.7 Effects on ability to drive and use machines
Caution should be employed when driving or operating machinery.

4.8 Undesirable effects
Although the combination of ephedrine with the anti-histamine chlorphenamine is intended to reduce side-effects, slight drowsiness may occur. Side-effects of ephedrine are rare at the low dose employed in this preparation, however in particularly susceptible patients, effects such as giddiness, palpitations and muscular weakness may be experienced transiently.

4.9 Overdose
Treatment should include gastric lavage. In the event of convulsions sedate with intramuscular paraldehyde. Respiratory depression may necessitate mechanical ventilation. Symptomatic treatment of cardiovascular dysfunction should be given with careful patient monitoring. The physician should be aware that tablets in the intestine will continue to release the active ingredients for a period of hours.

5. PHARMACOLOGICAL PROPERTIES

5.1 Pharmacodynamic properties
Chlorphenamine is a potent H_1-blocking drug. It antagonises the pharmacological actions of histamine released by antigen-antibody reaction in allergic diseases, thus providing symptomatic relief. Chlorphenamine alone is less effective when pollen counts are high, allergen exposure is prolonged and nasal congestion has become prominent.

Ephedrine has mild CNS stimulant properties that counteract any drowsiness produced by chlorphenamine. In addition it produces a decongestant action on nasal mucosal surfaces relieving mucosal congestion in conditions such as hay fever and allergic rhinitis.

5.2 Pharmacokinetic properties
Chlorphenamine is readily absorbed after oral administration and may undergo enterohepatic re-circulation in man. It is eliminated with a t½ of 12-15 hours. Ephedrine is completely absorbed following oral administration and is eliminated with a t½ of 3-6 hours.

5.3 Preclinical safety data
There are no preclinical data of relevance to the prescriber which are additional to that already included in other sections of the SPC.

6. PHARMACEUTICAL PARTICULARS

6.1 List of excipients
Hydroxypropylmethylcellulose

Quinoline yellow

Hardened castor oil

Magnesium stearate

Nipastat

6.2 Incompatibilities
None known

6.3 Shelf life
4 years

6.4 Special precautions for storage
None

6.5 Nature and contents of container
Strip packed in soft tempered aluminium foil laminated to polyethylene or blister packed in PVC/polyvinyl dichloride on hard tempered aluminium foil in 10's or 30's in cardboard cartons.

6.6 Instructions for use and handling
None stated

7. MARKETING AUTHORISATION HOLDER
Forest Laboratories UK Limited

Bourne Road

Bexley

Kent DA5 1NX

8. MARKETING AUTHORISATION NUMBER(S)
PL 0108/0054

9. DATE OF FIRST AUTHORISATION/RENEWAL OF THE AUTHORISATION
9th March 1978 / 22 May 1998

10. DATE OF REVISION OF THE TEXT
August 1997

11. Legal Category
P

HBVAXPRO 10mcg

(Sanofi Pasteur MSD)

1. NAME OF THE MEDICINAL PRODUCT
HBVAXPRO 10 micrograms/ml, suspension for injection in vial

Hepatitis B (Recombinant) vaccine for adults and adolescents

2. QUALITATIVE AND QUANTITATIVE COMPOSITION
One dose of ml contains:

Hepatitis B virus surface antigen, recombinant (HBsAg) * 10.00 micrograms, adsorbed on amorphous aluminium hydroxyphosphate sulfate (0.50 milligram)

* produced from recombinant strain of the yeast Saccharomyces cerevisiae (strain 2150-2-3)

For excipients, see 6.1

3. PHARMACEUTICAL FORM
Suspension for injection in vial

4. CLINICAL PARTICULARS

4.1 Therapeutic indications
This vaccine is indicated for active immunisation against hepatitis B virus infection caused by all known subtypes in adults and adolescents (16 years of age and older) considered at risk of exposure to hepatitis B virus.

The specific at risk categories to be immunised are to be determined on the basis of the official recommendations.

It can be expected that hepatitis D will also be prevented by immunisation with HBVAXPRO as hepatitis D (caused by the delta agent) does not occur in the absence of hepatitis B infection.

4.2 Posology and method of administration
Posology

Adults and adolescents (16 years of age and older): 1 dose (10 μg) of 1 ml at each injection is intended for use.

Primary vaccination:

A course of vaccination should include at least three injections.

Two primary immunisation schedules can be recommended:

0, 1, 6 months: two injections with an interval of one month; a third injection 6 months after the first administration.

0, 1, 2,12 months: three injections with an interval of one month; a fourth dose should be administered at 12 months.

This accelerated schedule may induce protective antibody levels earlier in a slightly larger proportion of vaccinees.

These immunisation schedules may be adjusted to accommodate local immunisation practises.

Booster:

Immunocompetent vaccinees

The need for a booster dose in healthy individuals who have received a full primary vaccination course has not been established. However, some local vaccination schedules currently include a recommendation for a booster dose and these should be respected.

Immunocompromised vaccinees (e.g. dialysis patients, transplant patients)

In vaccinees with an impaired immune system, administration of additional doses of vaccine may be considered if the antibody level against hepatitis B virus surface antigen (anti-HBsAg) is less than 10 IU/l.

Revaccination of nonresponders

When persons who do not respond to the primary vaccine series are revaccinated, 15-25 % produce an adequate antibody response after one additional dose and 30-50 % after three additional doses. However, because data are insufficient concerning the safety of hepatitis B vaccine when additional doses in excess of the recommended series are administered, revaccination following completion of the primary series is not routinely recommended. Revaccination should only be considered for high-risk individuals, after weighing the benefits of vaccination against the potential risk of experiencing increased local or systemic adverse reactions.

Special dosage recommendations for known or presumed exposure to hepatitis B virus (e.g needlestick with contaminated needle):

Hepatitis B immunoglobulin should be given as soon as possible after exposure (within 24 hours).

The first dose of the vaccine should be given within 7 days of exposure and can be administered simultaneously with hepatitis B immunoglobulin, but at a separate injection site.

Subsequent doses of vaccine, if necessary, (i.e according to the serologic status of the patient)

should be given as in the recommended immunisation schedule. The accelerated schedule can be proposed.

Method of administration

This vaccine should be administered intramuscularly.

The deltoid muscle is the preferred site for injection in adults and adolescents.

The intravascular route must not be used.

Exceptionally, the vaccine may be administered subcutaneously in patients with thrombocytopenia or bleeding disorders.

4.3 Contraindications

Hypersensitivity to the active substance or to any of the excipients

Severe febrile illness

4.4 Special warnings and special precautions for use

Because of the long incubation period of hepatitis B, it is possible for unrecognised hepatitis B infection to be present at the time of vaccination. The vaccine may not prevent hepatitis B infection in such cases.

The vaccine will not prevent infection caused by other agents such as hepatitis A, hepatitis C and hepatitis E and other pathogens known to infect the liver.

As with all injectable vaccines, appropriate medical treatment should always be readily available in case of rare anaphylactic reactions following the administration of the vaccine.

This vaccine may contain traces of formaldehyde and potassium thiocyanate which are used during the manufacturing process. Therefore, sensitisation reactions may occur.

4.5 Interaction with other medicinal products and other forms of Interaction

This vaccine can be administered:

- with hepatitis B immunoglobulin, at a separate injection site.

- to complete a primary immunisation course or as a booster dose in subjects who have previously received another hepatitis B vaccine.

- concomitantly with other vaccines, using separate sites and syringes.

4.6 Pregnancy and lactation

For the hepatitis B virus surface antigen (HBsAg) no clinical data on exposed pregnancies are available. However, as with all inactivated viral vaccines, one does not expect harm for the foetus. Utilisation during pregnancy requires that the potential benefit justifies the potential risk to the foetus. Caution should be exercised when prescribing to pregnant women.

The effect on breastfed infants of the administration of this vaccine has not been assessed; no contraindication has been established.

4.7 Effects on ability to drive and use machines

No studies on the effects on the ability to drive and use machines have been performed. However, some of the rare effects mentioned under "Undesirable effects" may affect the ability to drive or operate machinery.

4.8 Undesirable effects

The following undesirable effects have been reported following the widespread use of the vaccine.

As with other hepatitis B vaccines, in many instances, the causal relationship to the vaccine has not been established.

Blood and lymphatic system disorders

Very rare (<1/10,000)

Thrombocytopenia, lymphadenopathy

Immune system disorders

Very rare (<1/10,000)

Serum sickness, anaphylaxis

Nervous system disorders

Very rare (<1/10,000)

Paresthesia, paralysis (Bell's palsy), peripheral neuropathies (polyradiculoneuritis, facial paralysis), neuritis (including Guillain Barre Syndrome, optical neuritis, myelitis including transverse myelitis), encephalitis, demyelinating disease of the central nervous system, exacerbation of multiple sclerosis, multiple sclerosis, seizure, headache, dizziness, syncope

Vascular disorders

Very rare (<1/10,000)

Hypotension, vasculitis

Respiratory, thoracic and mediastinal disorders

Very rare (<1/10,000)

Bronchospasm-like symptoms

Gastrointestinal disorders

Very rare (<1/10,000)

Vomiting, nausea, diarrhoea, abdominal pain

Skin and subcutaneous tissue disorders

Very rare (<1/10,000)

Rash, alopecia, pruritus, urticaria, erythema multiforme, angioedema

Musculoskeleta, connective tissue and bone disorders

Very rare (<1/10,000)

Arthralgia, arthritis, myalgia, pain in extremity

General disorders and administration site conditions

Common >1/100, <1/10)

Local reactions (injection site): transient soreness, erythema, induration

Very rare (<1/10,000)

Fatigue, fever, malaise, influenza-like symptoms

Investigations

Very rare (<1/10,000)

Elevation of liver enzymes

4.9 Overdose

No case of overdose has been reported.

5. PHARMACOLOGICAL PROPERTIES

5.1 Pharmacodynamic properties

Pharmacotherapeutic group: anti-infectious, ATC code: J07BC01

The vaccine induces specific humoral antibodies against hepatitis B virus surface antigen (anti-HBsAg). Development of an antibody titre against hepatitis B (anti-HBsAg) equal to or greater than 10 IU/l measured 1 to 2 months after the last injection correlates with protection to hepatitis B virus infection.

In clinical trials, 96 % of 1,497 healthy infants, children, adolescents and adults given a 3 dose course of a previous formulation of Merck's recombinant hepatitis B vaccine developed a protective level of antibodies against hepatitis B virus surface antigen (⩾ 10 IU/l).

Although the duration of the protective effect of a previous formulation of Merck's recombinant hepatitis B vaccine in healthy vaccinees is unknown, follow-up over 5-9 years of approximately 3,000 high-risk subjects given a similar plasma-derived vaccine has revealed no cases of clinically apparent hepatitis B infection.

In addition, persistence of vaccine-induced immunologic memory for hepatitis B virus surface antigen (HBsAg) has been demonstrated through an anamnestic antibody response to a booster dose of a previous formulation of Merck's recombinant hepatitis B vaccine in healthy adults given plasma-derived vaccine 5 to 7 years earlier.

Reduced risk of Hepatocellular Carcinoma

Hepatocellular carcinoma is a serious complication of hepatitis B virus infection. Studies have demonstrated the link between chronic hepatitis B infection and hepatocellular carcinoma and 80 % of hepatocellular carcinomas are caused by hepatitis B virus infection. Hepatitis B vaccine has been recognized as the first anti-cancer vaccine because it can prevent primary liver cancer.

5.2 Pharmacokinetic properties

Not applicable.

5.3 Preclinical safety data

Animal reproduction studies have not been conducted.

6. PHARMACEUTICAL PARTICULARS

6.1 List of excipients

Sodium chloride, borax and water for injections.

6.2 Incompatibilities

The vaccine should not be mixed in the same syringe with other vaccines or parenterally administered medicinal products.

6.3 Shelf life

3 years.

6.4 Special precautions for storage

Store at 2 °C – 8 °C (in a refrigerator).

Do not freeze.

6.5 Nature and contents of container

1 ml of suspension in vial (Type I glass). Pack of 1, 10

6.6 Instructions for use and handling

Before use, the vaccine should be well shaken to obtain a slightly opaque white suspension.

7. MARKETING AUTHORISATION HOLDER

SANOFI PASTEUR MSD SNC

8, rue Jonas Salk

F-69007 Lyon

France

8. MARKETING AUTHORISATION NUMBER(S)

EU/1/01/183/007

EU/1/01/183/008

9. DATE OF FIRST AUTHORISATION/RENEWAL OF THE AUTHORISATION

27/04/2001

10. DATE OF REVISION OF THE TEXT

May 2005

HBVAXPRO 40mcg

(Sanofi Pasteur MSD)

1. NAME OF THE MEDICINAL PRODUCT

HBVAXPRO 40 micrograms/ml, suspension for injection in vial

Hepatitis B (Recombinant) vaccine for predialysis and dialysis patients

2. QUALITATIVE AND QUANTITATIVE COMPOSITION

One dose of 1 ml contains:

Hepatitis B virus surface antigen, recombinant (HBsAg) * 40.00 micrograms, adsorbed on amorphous aluminium hydroxyphosphate sulfate (0.50 milligram)

* produced from recombinant strain of the yeast Saccharomyces cerevisiae (strain 2150-2-3)

For excipients, see 6.1

3. PHARMACEUTICAL FORM

Suspension for injection in vial

4. CLINICAL PARTICULARS

4.1 Therapeutic indications

This vaccine is indicated for the active immunisation against hepatitis B virus infection caused by all known subtypes in predialysis and dialysis adult patients.

It can be expected that hepatitis D will also be prevented by immunisation with HBVAXPRO as hepatitis D (caused by the delta agent) does not occur in the absence of hepatitis B infection.

4.2 Posology and method of administration

Posology

Predialysis and dialysis adult patients: 1 dose (40 µg) of 1 ml at each injection is intended for use.

Primary vaccination:

A course of vaccination should include three injections:

Schedule 0, 1, 6 months: two injections with an interval of one month; a third injection 6 months after the first administration.

Booster:

A booster dose may be considered in these vaccinees if the antibody level against hepatitis B virus surface antigen (anti-HBsAg) is less than 10 IU/l.

Special dosage recommendations for known or presumed exposure to hepatitis B virus (e.g needlestick with contaminated needle):

Hepatitis B immunoglobulin should be given as soon as possible after exposure (within 24 hours).

The first dose of the vaccine should be given within 7 days of exposure and can be administered simultaneously with hepatitis B immunoglobulin but at a separate injection site.

Subsequent doses of vaccine, if necessary, (i.e according to the serologic status of the patient) should be given as in the recommended immunisation schedule.

Method of administration

This vaccine should be administered intramuscularly.

The deltoid muscle is the preferred site for injection in adults.

The intravascular route must not be used.

Exceptionally, the vaccine may be administered subcutaneously in patients with thrombocytopenia or bleeding disorders.

4.3 Contraindications

- Hypersensitivity to the active substance or to any of the excipients

- Severe febrile illness

4.4 Special warnings and special precautions for use

Because of the long incubation period of hepatitis B, it is possible for unrecognised hepatitis B infection to be present at the time of vaccination. The vaccine may not prevent hepatitis B infection in such cases.

The vaccine will not prevent infection caused by other agents such as hepatitis A, hepatitis C and hepatitis E and other pathogens known to infect the liver.

As with all injectable vaccines, appropriate medical treatment should always be readily available in case of rare anaphylactic reactions following the administration of the vaccine.

This vaccine may contain traces of formaldehyde and potassium thiocyanate which are used during the manufacturing process. Therefore, sensitisation reactions may occur.

4.5 Interaction with other medicinal products and other forms of Interaction

This vaccine can be administered:

- with hepatitis B immunoglobulin, at a separate injection site.

- to complete a primary immunisation course or as a booster dose in subjects who have previously received another hepatitis B vaccine.

- concomitantly with other vaccines, using separate sites and syringes.

4.6 Pregnancy and lactation
For the hepatitis B virus surface antigen (HBsAg) no clinical data on exposed pregnancies are available. However, as with all inactivated viral vaccines, one does not expect harm for the foetus. Utilisation during pregnancy requires that the potential benefit justifies the potential risk to the foetus. Caution should be exercised when prescribing to pregnant women.

The effect on breast-fed infants of the administration of this vaccine has not been assessed; no contraindication has been established.

4.7 Effects on ability to drive and use machines
No studies on the effects on the ability to drive and use machines have been performed. However, some of the rare effects mentioned under "Undesirable effects" may affect the ability to drive or operate machinery.

4.8 Undesirable effects
The following undesirable effects have been reported following the widespread use of the vaccine.

As with other hepatitis B vaccines, in many instances, the causal relationship to the vaccine has not been established.

Blood and the lymphatic system disorders

Very rare (<1/10,000)

Thrombocytopenia, lymphadenopathy

Immune system disorders

Very rare (<1/10,000)

Serum sickness, anaphylaxis

Nervous system disorders

Very rare (<1/10,000)

Paresthesia, paralysis (Bell's palsy), peripheral neuropathies (polyradiculoneuritis, facial paralysis), neuritis (including Guillain Barre Syndrome, optical neuritis, myelitis including transverse myelitis), encephalitis, demyelinating disease of the central nervous system, exacerbation of multiple sclerosis, multiple sclerosis, seizure, headache, dizziness, syncope

Vascular disorders

Very rare (<1/10,000)

Hypotension, vasculitis

Respiratory, thoracic and mediastinal disorders

Very rare (<1/10,000)

Bronchospasm-like symptoms

Gastrointestinal disorders

Very rare (<1/10,000)

Vomiting, nausea, diarrhoea, abdominal pain

Skin and subcutaneous tissue disorders

Very rare (<1/10,000)

Rash, alopecia, pruritus, urticaria, erythema multiforme, angioedema

Musculoskeletal, connective tissue and bone disorders

Very rare (<1/10,000)

Arthralgia, arthritis, myalgia, pain in extremity

General disorders and administration site conditions

Common >1/100, <1/10)

Local reactions (injection site): transient soreness, erythema, induration

Very rare (<1/10,000)

Fatigue, fever, malaise, influenza-like symptoms

Investigations

Very rare (<1/10,000)

Elevation of liver enzymes

4.9 Overdose
No case of overdose has been reported.

5. PHARMACOLOGICAL PROPERTIES

5.1 Pharmacodynamic properties
Pharmacotherapeutic group: anti-infectious, ATC code: J07BC01

The vaccine induces specific humoral antibodies against hepatitis B virus surface antigen (anti-HBsAg). Development of an antibody titre against hepatitis B virus surface antigen (anti-HBsAg) equal to or greater than 10 IU/l measured 1 to 2 months after the last injection correlates with protection to hepatitis B virus infection.

In clinical trials, 96 % of 1,497 healthy infants, children, adolescents and adults given a 3 dose course of a previous formulation of Merck's recombinant hepatitis B vaccine developed a protective level of antibodies against hepatitis B virus surface antigen ($\geqslant$ 10 IU/l).

Although the duration of the protective effect of a previous formulation of Merck's recombinant hepatitis B vaccine in healthy vaccinees is unknown, follow-up over 5-9 years of approximately 3,000 high-risk subjects given a similar plasma-derived vaccine has revealed no cases of clinically apparent hepatitis B infection.

In addition, persistence of vaccine-induced immunologic memory for hepatitis B virus surface antigen (HBsAg) has been demonstrated through an anamnestic antibody response to a booster dose of a previous formulation of Merck's recombinant hepatitis B vaccine in healthy adults given plasma-derived vaccine 5 to 7 years earlier.

Reduced risk of Hepatocellular Carcinoma

Hepatocellular carcinoma is a serious complication of hepatitis B virus infection. Studies have demonstrated the link between chronic hepatitis B infection and hepatocellular carcinoma and 80 % of hepatocellular carcinomas are caused by hepatitis B virus infection. Hepatitis B vaccine has been recognized as the first anti-cancer vaccine because it can prevent primary liver cancer.

5.2 Pharmacokinetic properties
Not applicable.

5.3 Preclinical safety data
Animal reproduction studies have not been conducted.

6. PHARMACEUTICAL PARTICULARS

6.1 List of excipients
Sodium chloride, borax and water for injections.

6.2 Incompatibilities
The vaccine should not be mixed in the same syringe with other vaccines or parenterally administered medicinal products.

6.3 Shelf life
3 years.

6.4 Special precautions for storage
Store at 2 °C – 8 °C (in a refrigerator).

Do not freeze.

6.5 Nature and contents of container
1 ml of suspension in vial (Type I glass) - Pack of 1

6.6 Instructions for use and handling
Before use, the vaccine should be well shaken to obtain a slightly opaque white suspension.

7. MARKETING AUTHORISATION HOLDER
SANOFI PASTEUR MSD SNC

8, rue Jonas Salk

F-69007 Lyon

France

8. MARKETING AUTHORISATION NUMBER(S)
EU/1/01/183/015

9. DATE OF FIRST AUTHORISATION/RENEWAL OF THE AUTHORISATION
27/04/2001

10. DATE OF REVISION OF THE TEXT
May 2005

HBVAXPRO 5mcg

(Sanofi Pasteur MSD)

1. NAME OF THE MEDICINAL PRODUCT
HBVAXPRO 5 micrograms/0.5 ml, suspension for injection in vial

Hepatitis B (Recombinant) vaccine for children and adolescents

2. QUALITATIVE AND QUANTITATIVE COMPOSITION
One dose of 0.5 ml contains:

Hepatitis B virus surface antigen, recombinant (HBsAg) * 5.00 micrograms, adsorbed on amorphous aluminium hydroxyphosphate sulfate (0.25 milligram)

* produced from recombinant strain of the yeast Saccharomyces cerevisiae (strain 2150-2-3)

For excipients, see 6.1

3. PHARMACEUTICAL FORM
Suspension for injection in vial

4. CLINICAL PARTICULARS

4.1 Therapeutic indications
This vaccine is indicated for active immunisation against hepatitis B virus infection caused by all known subtypes in children and adolescents (from birth through 15 years of age) considered at risk of exposure to hepatitis B virus.

The specific at risk categories to be immunised are to be determined on the basis of the official recommendations.

It can be expected that hepatitis D will also be prevented by immunisation with HBVAXPRO as hepatitis D (caused by the delta agent) does not occur in the absence of hepatitis B infection.

4.2 Posology and method of administration
Posology

Children and adolescents (birth through 15 years of age): 1 dose (5 μg) of 0.5 ml at each injection is intended for use.

Primary vaccination:

A course of vaccination should include at least three injections.

Two primary immunisation schedules can be recommended:

0, 1, 6 months: two injections with an interval of one month; a third injection 6 months after the first administration.

0, 1, 2,12 months: three injections with an interval of one month; a fourth dose should be administered at 12 months.

This accelerated schedule may induce protective antibody levels earlier in a slightly larger proportion of vaccinees.

The timing of successive injections in a vaccination series may need to be adjusted to local programs, especially where hepatitis B vaccine is integrated with the administration of other paediatric vaccines.

Booster:

Immunocompetent vaccinees

The need for a booster dose in healthy individuals who have received a full primary vaccination course has not been established. However, some local vaccination schedules currently include a recommendation for a booster dose and these should be respected.

Immunocompromised vaccinees (e.g. dialysis patients, transplant patients)

In vaccinees with an impaired immune system, administration of additional doses of vaccine may be considered if the antibody level against hepatitis B virus surface antigen (anti-HBsAg) is less than 10 IU/l.

Revaccination of nonresponders

When persons who do not respond to the primary vaccine series are revaccinated, 15-25 % produce an adequate antibody response after one additional dose and 30-50 % after three additional doses. However, because data are insufficient concerning the safety of hepatitis B vaccine when additional doses in excess of the recommended series are administered, revaccination following completion of the primary series is not routinely recommended. Revaccination should only be considered for high-risk individuals, after weighing the benefits of vaccination against the potential risk of experiencing increased local or systemic adverse reactions.

Special dosage recommendations:

Dosage recommendation for neonates of mothers who are hepatitis B virus carriers

- At birth, one dose of hepatitis B immunoglobulin (within 24 hours).

The first dose of the vaccine should be given within 7 days of birth and can be administered simultaneously with hepatitis B immunoglobulin but at a separate injection site.

- Subsequent doses of vaccine should be given according to the locally recommended vaccination schedule.

Dosage recommendation for known or presumed exposure to hepatitis B virus (e.g needlestick with contaminated needle)

Hepatitis B immunoglobulin should be given as soon as possible after exposure (within 24 hours).

The first dose of the vaccine should be given within 7 days of exposure and can be administered simultaneously with hepatitis B immunoglobulin but at a separate injection site.

Subsequent doses of vaccine, if necessary, (i.e according to the serologic status of the patient) should be given as in the recommended immunisation schedule. The accelerated schedule can be proposed.

Method of administration

This vaccine should be administered intramuscularly.

The anterolateral thigh is the preferred site for injection in neonates and infants. The deltoid muscle is the preferred site for injection in children and adolescents.

The intravascular route must not be used.

Exceptionally, the vaccine may be administered subcutaneously in patients with thrombocytopoenia or bleeding disorders.

4.3 Contraindications
Hypersensitivity to the active substance or to any of the excipients

Severe febrile illness

4.4 Special warnings and special precautions for use
Because of the long incubation period of hepatitis B, it is possible for unrecognised hepatitis B infection to be present at the time of vaccination. The vaccine may not prevent hepatitis B infection in such cases.

The vaccine will not prevent infection caused by other agents such as hepatitis A, hepatitis C and hepatitis E and other pathogens known to infect the liver.

As with all injectable vaccines, appropriate medical treatment should always be readily available in case of rare anaphylactic reactions following the administration of the vaccine.

This vaccine may contain traces of formaldehyde and potassium thiocyanate, which are used during the manufacturing process. Therefore, sensitisation reactions may occur.

4.5 Interaction with other medicinal products and other forms of Interaction
This vaccine can be administered:

- with hepatitis B immunoglobulin, at a separate injection site.

- to complete a primary immunisation course or as a booster dose in subjects who have previously received another hepatitis B vaccine.

- concomitantly with other vaccines, using separate sites and syringes.

4.6 Pregnancy and lactation
Not applicable.

4.7 Effects on ability to drive and use machines
Not applicable.

4.8 Undesirable effects
The following undesirable effects have been reported following the widespread use of the vaccine.

As with other hepatitis B vaccines, in many instances, the causal relationship to the vaccine has not been established.

Blood and the lymphatic system disorders

Very rare (<1/10,000)

Thrombocytopenia, lymphadenopathy

Immune system disorders

Very rare (<1/10,000)

Serum sickness, anaphylaxis

Nervous system disorders

Very rare (<1/10,000)

Paresthesia, paralysis (Bell's palsy), peripheral neuropathies (polyradiculoneuritis, facial paralysis), neuritis (including Guillain Barre Syndrome, optical neuritis, myelitis including transverse myelitis), encephalitis, demyelinating disease of the central nervous system, exacerbation of multiple sclerosis, multiple sclerosis, seizure, headache, dizziness, syncope

Vascular disorders

Very rare (<1/10,000)

Hypotension, vasculitis

Respiratory, thoracic and mediastinal disorders

Very rare (<1/10,000)

Bronchospasm-like symptoms

Gastrointestinal disorders

Very rare (<1/10,000)

Vomiting, nausea, diarrhoea, abdominal pain

Skin and subcutaneous tissue disorders

Very rare (<1/10,000)

Rash, alopecia, pruritus, urticaria, erythema multiforme, angioedema

Musculoskeletal, connective tissue and bone disorders

Very rare (<1/10,000)

Arthralgia, arthritis, myalgia, pain in extremity

General disorders and administration site conditions

Common >1/100, <1/10)

Local reactions (injection site): transient soreness, erythema, induration

Very rare (<1/10,000)

Fatigue, fever, malaise, influenza-like symptoms

Investigations

Very rare (<1/10,000)

Elevation of liver enzymes

4.9 Overdose
No case of overdose has been reported.

5. PHARMACOLOGICAL PROPERTIES

5.1 Pharmacodynamic properties
Pharmacotherapeutic group: anti-infectious, ATC code: J07BC01

The vaccine induces specific humoral antibodies against hepatitis B virus surface antigen (anti-HBsAg). Development of an antibody titre against hepatitis B virus surface antigen (anti-HBsAg) equal to or greater than 10 IU/l measured 1 to 2 months after the last injection correlates with protection to hepatitis B virus infection.

In clinical trials, 96 % of 1,497 healthy infants, children, adolescents and adults given a 3 dose course of a previous formulation of Merck's recombinant hepatitis B vaccine developed a protective level of antibodies against hepatitis B virus surface antigen (≥ 10 IU/l).

The protective efficacy of a dose of hepatitis B immunoglobulin at birth followed by 3 doses of a previous formulation of Merck's recombinant hepatitis B vaccine has been demonstrated for neonates born to mothers positive for both hepatitis B virus surface antigen (HBsAg) and hepatitis B virus e antigen (HBeAg). Among 130 vaccinated infants, the estimated efficacy in prevention of chronic hepatitis B infection was 95 % as compared to the infection rate in untreated historical controls.

Although the duration of the protective effect of a previous formulation of Merck's recombinant hepatitis B vaccine in healthy vaccinees is unknown, follow-up over 5-9 years of approximately 3,000 high-risk subjects given a similar plasma-derived vaccine has revealed no cases of clinically apparent hepatitis B infection.

In addition, persistence of vaccine-induced immunologic memory for hepatitis B virus surface antigen (HBsAg) has been demonstrated through an anamnestic antibody response to a booster dose of a previous formulation of Merck's recombinant hepatitis B vaccine in healthy adults given plasma-derived vaccine 5 to 7 years earlier.

Reduced risk of Hepatocellular Carcinoma

Hepatocellular carcinoma is a serious complication of hepatitis B virus infection. Studies have demonstrated the link between chronic hepatitis B infection and hepatocellular carcinoma and 80 % of hepatocellular carcinomas are caused by hepatitis B virus infection. Hepatitis B vaccine has been recognized as the first anti-cancer vaccine because it can prevent primary liver cancer.

5.2 Pharmacokinetic properties
Not applicable.

5.3 Preclinical safety data
Animal reproduction studies have not been conducted.

6. PHARMACEUTICAL PARTICULARS

6.1 List of excipients
Sodium chloride, borax and water for injections.

6.2 Incompatibilities
The vaccine should not be mixed in the same syringe with other vaccines or parenterally administered medicinal products.

6.3 Shelf life
3 years.

6.4 Special precautions for storage
Store at 2 °C – 8 °C (in a refrigerator).

Do not freeze.

6.5 Nature and contents of container
0.5 ml of suspension in vial (Type I glass). Pack of 1, 10

0.5 ml of suspension in vial (Type I glass) and an empty sterile injection syringe with needle. Pack of 1.

Not all pack sizes may be marketed.

6.6 Instructions for use and handling
Before use, the vaccine should be well shaken to obtain a slightly opaque white suspension.

Once the vial has been penetrated, the withdrawn vaccine should be used promptly, and the vial must be discarded.

7. MARKETING AUTHORISATION HOLDER
SANOFI PASTEUR MSD SNC
8, rue Jonas Salk
F-69007 Lyon
France

8. MARKETING AUTHORISATION NUMBER(S)
EU/1/01/183/001
EU/1/01/183/018
EU/1/01/183/019

9. DATE OF FIRST AUTHORISATION/RENEWAL OF THE AUTHORISATION
27/04/2001

10. DATE OF REVISION OF THE TEXT
May 2005

Heliclear

(Wyeth Pharmaceuticals)

1. NAME OF THE MEDICINAL PRODUCT
HeliClear®

2. QUALITATIVE AND QUANTITATIVE COMPOSITION
Klaricid 500 tablets: Clarithromycin 500mg/tablet

Zoton* capsules: Lansoprazole 30mg/capsule

Amoxicillin capsules: Amoxicillin Trihydrate BP equivalent to Amoxicillin 500mg/capsule

3. PHARMACEUTICAL FORM
Each pack of HeliClear contains

Klaricid 500 - Film Coated Tablets

Zoton Capsules 30mg - Gastro-resistant Capsules

Amoxicillin - Capsules

4. CLINICAL PARTICULARS

4.1 Therapeutic indications
Eradication of *Helicobacter pylori (H. pylori)* from the upper gastrointestinal tract in patients with duodenal ulcer, leading to the healing and prevention of relapse of the ulcer.

4.2 Posology and method of administration
Dosage:

Adults: Zoton Capsules 30mg twice daily plus Klaricid 500mg twice daily and Amoxicillin Capsules 1000mg (2 × 500mg) twice daily for 7-14 days. A patient pack of HeliClear provides a complete 7 day eradication regimen.

Eradication of *H. pylori* with the HeliClear regimen has been shown to result in the healing of duodenal ulcers, without the need for continued anti-ulcer drug therapy. The risk of reinfection is low and relapse following successful eradication is, therefore, unlikely.

HeliClear should be taken before the morning and evening meals. All dosage forms should be swallowed whole. Do not crush or chew.

Elderly: Dose adjustment is not required in the elderly. The normal daily dosage should be given.

Children: There is no experience of the use of this combination in children.

Impaired Hepatic and Renal Function: Dosage adjustment information is provided under section 4.4 Special Warnings and Precautions for Use.

4.3 Contraindications
Patients with known hypersensitivity to lansoprazole, clarithromycin, other macrolides or any of the other ingredients in HeliClear. Patients with known or suspected hypersensitivity to penicillins, semi-synthetic penicillins or cephalosporins.

Clarithromycin and ergot derivatives should not be co-administered.

Concomitant administration of clarithromycin and any of the following drugs is contraindicated: cisapride, pimozide and terfenadine. Elevated cisapride, pimozide and terfenadine levels have been reported in patients receiving either of these drugs and clarithromycin concomitantly. This may result in QT prolongation and cardiac arrhythmias including ventricular tachycardia, ventricular fibrillation and Torsade de Pointes. Similar effects have been observed with concomitant administration of astemizole and other macrolides.

4.4 Special warnings and special precautions for use
Clarithromycin is principally excreted by the liver and kidney. Caution should be exercised in administering this antibiotic to patients with impaired hepatic or renal function. HeliClear should not be prescribed for patients with severe renal impairment (creatinine clearance (CL_{CR}) <30ml/min).

Lansoprazole is metabolised substantially by the liver. Clinical trials in patients with liver disease indicate that metabolism of lansoprazole is prolonged in patients with severe hepatic impairment. However, no dose adjustment is necessary.

In common with other anti-ulcer therapies, the possibility of malignancy should be excluded when gastric ulcer is suspected, as symptoms may be alleviated and diagnosis delayed. Similarly, the possibility of serious underlying disease such as malignancy should be excluded before treatment for dyspepsia commences, particularly in patients of middle age or older who have new or recently changed dyspeptic symptoms.

In patients with renal impairment, it may be necessary to reduce the total daily dosage of amoxicillin.

Prolonged use of an anti-infective may result in the development of superinfection due to organisms resistant to that anti-infective. Decreased gastric acidity due to any means, including proton pump inhibitors, increases gastric counts of bacteria normally present in the gastrointestinal tract. Treatment with acid-reducing drugs may lead to a slightly increased risk of gastrointestinal infections such as *Salmonella* and *Campylobacter*.

H. pylori organisms may develop resistance to clarithromycin in a small number of patients.

4.5 Interaction with other medicinal products and other forms of Interaction
As with other macrolide antibiotics the use of clarithromycin in patients concurrently taking drugs metabolised by the cytochrome P450 system, e.g. cilostazol, methylprednisolone, oral anticoagulants (e.g.warfarin), quinidine, sildenafil, ergot alkaloids, alprazolam, triazolam, midazolam, disopyramide, lovastatin, rifabutin, phenytoin, cyclosporin, vinblastine, valproate and tacrolimus, may be associated with elevations in serum levels of these other drugs. Rhabdomyolysis, co-incident with the co-administration of clarithromycin, and HMG-CoA reductase inhibitors, such as lovastatin and simvastatin has been reported.

The administration of clarithromycin to patients who are receiving theophylline has been associated with an increase in serum theophylline levels and potential theophylline toxicity.

The use of clarithromycin in patients receiving warfarin may result in potentiation of the effects of warfarin. Prothrombin time should be frequently monitored in these patients. The effects of digoxin may be potentiated with concomitant administration of clarithromycin. Monitoring of serum digoxin levels should be considered.

Clarithromycin may potentiate the effects of carbamazepine due to a reduction in the rate of excretion.

Simultaneous oral administration of clarithromycin tablets and zidovudine to HIV infected adult patients may result in decreased steady-state zidovudine levels. This can be largely avoided by staggering the doses of clarithromycin and zidovudine by 1-2 hours. No such reaction has been reported in children.

Ritonavir increases the area under the curve (AUC), C_{max} and C_{min} of clarithromycin when administered concurrently. Because of the large therapeutic window for clarithromycin, no dosage reduction should be necessary in patients with normal renal function. However, for patients with renal impairment, the following dosage adjustments should be considered: For patients with CL_{CR} 30 to 60 ml/min the dose of clarithromycin should be reduced by 50%. For patients with CL_{CR}<30ml/min the dose of clarithromycin should be decreased by 75%.

Doses of clarithromycin greater than 1g/day should not be coadministered with ritonavir.

At the dosages recommended, there is no clinically significant interaction between clarithromycin and lansoprazole. Increased plasma concentrations of clarithromycin may occur when it is co-administered with Maalox or ranitidine. No adjustment to the dosage is necessary.

There have been postmarketed reports of Torsade de Pointes occurring with the concurrent use of clarithromycin and quinidine or disopyramide. Levels of these medications should be monitored during clarithromycin therapy.

Lansoprazole is hepatically metabolised and studies indicate that it is a weak inducer of cytochrome P450. There is the possibility of interaction with drugs which are metabolised by the liver. Caution should be exercised when oral contraceptives and preparations such as phenytoin, carbamazepine, theophylline, or warfarin are taken concomitantly with the administration of lansoprazole.

No clinically significant effects of lansoprazole on non-steroidal anti-inflammatory drugs (NSAIDs) or diazepam have been found.

Antacids and sucralfate should not be taken within an hour of lansoprazole as they may reduce its bioavailability.

Amoxicillin may decrease the efficacy of combined oral contraceptives. Methotrexate excretion is reduced by penicillins.

4.6 Pregnancy and lactation

The safety of clarithromycin during pregnancy and breast feeding of infants has not been established. Some animal studies with clarithromycin have suggested an embryotoxic effect, but only at dose levels which are clearly toxic to mothers.

There is insufficient experience to recommend the use of lansoprazole in pregnancy. Animal studies do not reveal any teratogenic effect. Reproduction studies indicate slightly reduced litter survival and weights in rats and rabbits given very high doses of lansoprazole.

HeliClear therapy should be avoided during pregnancy.

Lansoprazole and clarithromycin have been found in human breast milk and/or in the milk of lactating animals.

HeliClear therapy should be avoided during breast feeding unless the clinical benefit is considered to outweigh the risk.

4.7 Effects on ability to drive and use machines

None known.

4.8 Undesirable effects

Clarithromycin is generally well tolerated. Side effects reported include nausea, dyspepsia, diarrhoea, vomiting, abdominal pain and paraesthesia. Stomatitis, glossitis, oral monilia and tongue discolouration have been reported. Other side-effects include headache, arthralgia, myalgia and allergic reactions ranging from urticaria and mild skin eruptions and angioedema to anaphylaxis have beenreported. There have been reports of Stevens-Johnson syndrome/toxic epidermal necrolysis with orally administered clarithromycin. Reports of alteration of the sense of smell, usually in conjunction with taste perversion, have also been received. There have been reports of tooth discolouration in patients treated with clarithromycin. Tooth discolouration is usually reversible with professional dental cleaning. There have been reports of transient central nervous system side-effects including dizziness, vertigo, anxiety, insomnia, bad dreams, tinnitus, confusion, disorientation, hallucinations, psychosis and depersonalisation. There have been reports of hearing loss with clarithromycin which is usually reversible on withdrawal of therapy. Pseudomembranous colitis has been reported rarely with clarithromycin, and may range in severity from mild to life threatening. There have been rare reports of hypoglycaemia, some of which have occurred in patients on concomitant oral hypoglycaemic agents or insulin. There have been rare reports of uveitis reported mainly in patients treated with concomitant rifabutin, most of these were reversible. Isolated cases of leucopenia and thrombocytopenia have been reported. As with other macrolides, hepatic dysfunction (which is usually reversible) including altered liver function tests, hepatitis and cholestasis with or without jaundice, has been reported. Dysfunction may be severe and very rarely fatal hepatic failure has been reported. Cases of increased serum creatinine, interstitial nephritis, renal failure, pancreatitis and convulsions have been reported rarely. As with other macrolides, QT prolongation, ventricular tachycardia and Torsade de Pointes have been reported rarely with clarithromycin.

Lansoprazole is well-tolerated, with adverse events generally being mild and transient. The most commonly reported adverse events are headache, dizziness, fatigue and malaise. Gastrointestinal effects include diarrhoea, constipation, abdominal pain, nausea, vomiting, flatulence and dry or sore mouth or throat. As with other PPIs, very rarely, cases of colitis have been reported. In severe and/or protracted cases of diarrhoea, discontinuation of therapy should be considered. In the majority of cases symptoms resolve on discontinuation of therapy. Alterations in liver function test values and, rarely, jaundice or hepatitis, have been reported. Dermatological reactions include skin rashes, urticaria and pruritus. These generally resolve on discontinuation of drug therapy. Serious dermatological reactions are rare but there have been occasional reports of Stevens-Johnson Syndrome, toxic epidermal necrolysis and erythematous or bullous rashes including erythema multiforme. Cases of hair thinning and photosensitivity have also been reported. Other hypersensitivity reactions include angioedema, wheezing, and very rarely, anaphylaxis. Cases of interstitial nephritis have been reported which have sometimes resulted in renal failure. Haematological effects (thrombocytopenia, eosinophilia, leucopenia and pancytopenia) have occurred rarely. Bruising, purpura and petechiae have also been reported. Other reactions include arthralgia, myalgia, depression, peripheral oedema and, rarely, paraesthesia, blurred vision, taste disturbances, vertigo, confusion and hallucinations. Gynaecomastia and impotence have been reported rarely.

The side-effects of amoxicillin are uncommon and mainly of a mild and transitory nature. These may include diarrhoea, indigestion, and occasionally an urticarial or erythematous type rash. An urticarial rash is usually indicative of true penicillin hypersensitivity and an erythematous-type rash may arise if amoxicillin is administered to patients with infectious mononucleosis. If a rash develops, discontinuation of amoxicillin therapy is advised. Hypersensitivity can also give rise to reactions such as anaphylaxis, angioneurotic oedema, erythema multiforme and interstitial nephritis. Pseudomembranous colitis has been reported rarely.

4.9 Overdose

Reports indicate that the ingestion of large amounts of clarithromycin can be expected to produce gastro-intestinal symptoms. One patient who had a history of bipolar disorder ingested 8 grams of clarithromycin and showed altered mental status, paranoid behaviour, hypokalemia and hypoxemia. Adverse reactions accompanying overdosage should be treated by gastric lavage and supportive measures. As with other macrolides, clarithromycin serum levels are not expected to be appreciably affected by haemodialysis or peritoneal dialysis.

There is no information on the effect of overdosage with lansoprazole. However, it has been given at doses up to 120mg/day without significant adverse effects. Symptomatic and supportive therapy should be given as appropriate.

Gross overdosage with amoxicillin will produce very high urinary concentrations. Problems are unlikely if adequate fluid intake and urinary output are maintained; however, crystalluria is a possibility. More specific measures may be necessary in patients with impaired renal function; the antibiotic is removed by haemodialysis.

5. PHARMACOLOGICAL PROPERTIES

5.1 Pharmacodynamic properties

Clarithromycin is a semi-synthetic derivative of erythromycin A and highly potent against a wide variety of aerobic and anaerobic gram-positive and gram-negative organisms. Amoxicillin is a broad spectrum, semi-synthetic penicillin and is bactericidal against a wide variety of Gram-positive and Gram-negative organisms. Lansoprazole is a proton pump inhibitor, it specifically inhibits the H^+/K^+ ATPase (proton pump) of the parietal cell in the stomach, the terminal step in acid production. By reducing gastric acidity, lansoprazole creates an environment in which clarithromycin and amoxicillin can be effective against *H. pylori*.

H. pylori is associated with acid peptic disease including duodenal and gastric ulceration in which about 95% and 80% of patients respectively are infected with the bacterium. Clinical studies using various different *H. pylori* eradication regimens have shown that eradication of *H. pylori* prevents ulcer recurrence. *H. pylori* is also implicated as a major contributory factor in the development of gastritis and ulcer recurrence in such patients. Recent evidence further suggests a causative link between *H. pylori* and gastric carcinoma.

5.2 Pharmacokinetic properties

Clarithromycin penetrates the gastric mucus. Clarithromycin is 80% bound to plasma proteins at therapeutic levels. At 500mg b.i.d., urinary excretion is approximately 36%. The microbiologically active metabolite 14-hydroxyclarithromycin is the major urinary metabolite and accounts for 10-15% of the dose. Most of the remainder of the dose is eliminated in the faeces, primarily via the bile. 5-10% of the parent drug is recovered from the faeces.

The plasma protein binding of lansoprazole is 97%. Following absorption, lansoprazole is extensively metabolised and is excreted by both the renal and biliary route. A study with ^{14}C-labelled lansoprazole indicated that up to 50% of the dose was excreted in the urine. Lansoprazole is metabolised substantially by the liver.

Amoxicillin trihydrate is resistant to inactivation by gastric acid secretions and is rapidly absorbed when given orally. Amoxicillin is approximately 20% bound to plasma proteins. It is excreted mainly unchanged in the urine by glomerular filtration and tubular excretion. There is limited metabolism of amoxicillin to penicilloic acid which is also excreted in the urine.

5.3 Preclinical safety data

In acute mouse and rat studies with clarithromycin, the median lethal dose was greater than the highest feasible dose for administration (5g/kg). In repeated dose studies, toxicity was related to dose, duration of treatment and species. Dogs were more sensitive than primates or rats. The major clinical signs at toxic doses included emesis, weakness, reduced food consumption and weight gain, salivation, dehydration and hyperactivity. In all species the liver was the primary target organ at toxic doses. Hepatotoxicity was detectable by early elevations of liver function tests. Discontinuation of clarithromycin generally resulted in a return to or toward normal results. Other tissues less commonly affected included the stomach, thymus and other lymphoid tissues and the kidneys. At near therapeutic doses, conjunctival injection and lacrimation occurred only in dogs. At a massive dose of 400mg/kg/day, some dogs and monkeys developed corneal opacities and/or oedema.

Fertility and reproduction studies with clarithromycin in rats have shown no adverse events. Teratogenicity studies with clarithromycin in rats (Wistar (p.o.) and Sprague-Dawley (p.o. and i.v.)), New Zealand White rabbits and cynomolgous monkeys failed to demonstrate any teratogenicity from clarithromycin. However, a further similar study in Sprague-Dawley rats indicated a low (6%) incidence of cardiovascular abnormalities which appeared to be due to spontaneous expression of genetic changes. Two mouse studies revealed a variable incidence (3-30%) of cleft palate and embryonic loss was seen in monkeys but only at dose levels which were clearly toxic to the mothers.

Gastric tumours have been observed in life-long studies with lansoprazole in rats. An increased incidence of spontaneous retinal atrophy has been observed in life-long studies with lansoprazole in rats. These lesions which are common to albino laboratory rats have not been observed in monkeys or dogs or life-long studies in mice. They are considered to be rat specific. No such treatment related changes have been observed in patients treated continuously for long periods.

Amoxicillin has been used for many years without proof of any relevant acute toxicity, chronic toxicity, mutagenic or carcinogenic potential or toxicity in reproduction.

6. PHARMACEUTICAL PARTICULARS

6.1 List of excipients

Klaricid 500 Tablets: Croscarmellose sodium, cellulose microcrystalline, silicon dioxide, povidone, stearic acid, magnesium stearate, talc, hypromellose, hydroxypropylcellulose, propylene glycol, sorbitan monooleate, titanium dioxide, sorbic acid, vanillin, quinoline yellow (E104).

Zoton Capsules: Gastro-resistant Granules: Magnesium Carbonate, Sugar Spheres, Sucrose, Maize Starch, Low Substituted Hydroxypropyl Cellulose, Hydroxypropylcellulose, Methacrylic Acid – Ethyl Acrylate Copolymer (1:1) Dispersion 30 per cent, Talc, Macrogol 8000, Titanium Dioxide, Polysorbate 80, Colloidal Anhydrous Silica, Purified Water.

Capsule Shells: Gelatin, opacode black 1007, titanium dioxide (E171), erythrosine (E127), indigo carmine (E132).

Amoxicillin Capsules: Sodium lauryl sulphate, magnesium stearate, gelatin, erythrosine (E127), red iron oxide (E172), titanium dioxide (E171).

6.2 Incompatibilities

None known.

6.3 Shelf life

The recommended shelf life is 36 months.

6.4 Special precautions for storage

Do not store above 25°C. Store in the original package. Keep containers in the outer carton.

6.5 Nature and contents of container

14 Klaricid 500 tablets, 14 Zoton Capsules 30mg and 28 Amoxicillin Capsules in a blister patient pack. The blisters are packaged in a carton with a pack insert.

Blister material: PVC/PVdC/Aluminium foil.

6.6 Instructions for use and handling

Not applicable

7. MARKETING AUTHORISATION HOLDER

John Wyeth and Brother Ltd
Trading as Wyeth Laboratories
Huntercombe Lane South
Taplow, Maidenhead
Berkshire
SL6 0PH

8. MARKETING AUTHORISATION NUMBER(S)

PL 0011/0240

9. DATE OF FIRST AUTHORISATION/RENEWAL OF THE AUTHORISATION

4 January 1999

10. DATE OF REVISION OF THE TEXT

8 November 2004

* Trademark of and under Licence Agreement from Takeda Chemical Industries Ltd., Japan.

HeliMet

(Wyeth Pharmaceuticals)

1. NAME OF THE MEDICINAL PRODUCT

HeliMet

2. QUALITATIVE AND QUANTITATIVE COMPOSITION

Zoton capsules: lansoprazole 30 mg/capsule

Klaricid 500 tablets: clarithromycin 500 mg/tablet

Metronidazole tablets: metronidazole 400 mg/tablet

For excipients, see Section 6.1 List of Excipients.

3. PHARMACEUTICAL FORM

Each pack of HeliMet contains:

Zoton Capsules 30 mg - Gastro-resistant capsules

Opaque, lilac/purple, size No. 1 elongated hard shell Zoton capsules; printed "Zoton" and "30mg" in black ink

Klaricid 500 - Film coated tablets

Pale yellow, ovaloid, tablets; plain or marked with the Abbott logo on one surface.

Metronidazole Tablets 400 mg – Tablets

White, biconvex tablets; 12.5mm in diameter, indented MZL 400 and marked with a breakline on one side and twin triangle logo on the reverse.

4. CLINICAL PARTICULARS

4.1 Therapeutic indications

Eradication of *Helicobacter pylori (H. pylori)* from the upper gastrointestinal tract in patients with duodenal ulcer, leading to the healing and prevention of relapse of the ulcer.

4.2 Posology and method of administration

Dosage:

Adults: Zoton Capsules 30 mg twice daily plus Klaricid 500 mg twice daily and Metronidazole Tablets 400 mg twice daily for 7 days. A patient pack of HeliMet provides a complete 7 day eradication regimen.

Eradication of *H. pylori* with the HeliMet regimen has been shown to result in the healing of duodenal ulcers, without the need for continued anti-ulcer drug therapy. The risk of reinfection is low and relapse following successful eradication is, therefore, unlikely.

HeliMet should be taken before the morning and evening meals. All dosage forms should be swallowed whole. Do not crush or chew.

Elderly: Dose adjustment is not required in the elderly. The normal daily dosage should be given.

Children: There is no experience of the use of this combination in children.

Impaired Hepatic and Renal Function: Dosage adjustment information is provided under section 4.4 Special Warnings and Precautions for Use.

4.3 Contraindications

Patients with known hypersensitivity to lansoprazole, clarithromycin or other macrolides, metronidazole or any of the other ingredients in HeliMet.

Clarithromycin and ergot derivatives should not be co-administered.

Concomitant administration of clarithromycin and any of the following drugs is contraindicated: cisapride, pimozide and terfenadine. Elevated cisapride, pimozide and terfenadine levels have been reported in patients receiving either of these drugs and clarithromycin concomitantly. This may result in QT prolongation and cardiac arrhythmias including ventricular tachycardia, ventricular fibrillation and Torsade de Pointes. Similar effects have been observed with concomitant administration of astemizole and other macrolides.

4.4 Special warnings and special precautions for use

Lansoprazole is metabolised substantially by the liver. Clinical trials in patients with liver disease indicate that metabolism of lansoprazole is prolonged in patients with severe hepatic impairment. However, no dose adjustment is necessary.

In common with other anti-ulcer therapies, the possibility of malignancy should be excluded when gastric ulcer is suspected, as symptoms may be alleviated and diagnosis delayed. Similarly, the possibility of serious underlying disease such as malignancy should be excluded before treatment for dyspepsia commences, particularly in patients of middle age or older who have new or recently changed dyspeptic symptoms.

Clarithromycin is principally excreted by the liver and kidney. Caution should be exercised in administering this antibiotic to patients with impaired hepatic or renal function. HeliMet should not be prescribed for patients with severe renal impairment (creatinine clearance (CL_{CR}) <30ml/min).

In patients with renal failure, there is no need to reduce the dosage of metronidazole as the elimination half-life remains unchanged. Such patients, however, retain the metabolites of metronidazole. The clinical significance of this is not known at present. In patients undergoing haemodialysis, metronidazole and metabolites are efficiently removed during an eight-hour period of dialysis. Metronidazole should therefore be readministered immediately after haemodialysis.

No routine adjustment in the dosage of metronidazole is needed in patients with renal failure undergoing intermittent peritoneal dialysis (IPD) or continuous ambulatory peritoneal dialysis (CAPD).

Metronidazole is mainly metabolised by hepatic oxidation. Substantial impairment of metronidazole clearance may occur in the presence of advanced hepatic insufficiency. Significant accumulation may occur in patients with hepatic encephalopathy and the resulting high plasma concentrations of metronidazole may contribute to symptoms of the encephalopathy. The daily dosage should be reduced to one-third and may be administered once daily.

Caution is advised in patients with active disease of the central nervous system other than brain abscess.

Prolonged use of an anti-infective may result in the development of superinfection due to organisms resistant to that anti-infective. Decreased gastric acidity due to any means, including proton pump inhibitors, increases gastric counts of bacteria normally present in the gastrointestinal tract. Treatment with acid-reducing drugs may lead to a slightly increased risk of gastrointestinal infections such as *Salmonella* and *Campylobacter*.

H. pylori organisms may develop resistance to clarithromycin in a small number of patients.

4.5 Interaction with other medicinal products and other forms of Interaction

Lansoprazole is hepatically metabolised and studies indicate that it is a weak inducer of cytochrome P450. There is the possibility of interaction with drugs which are metabolised by the liver. Caution should be exercised when oral contraceptives and preparations such as phenytoin, carbamazepine, theophylline, or warfarin are taken concomitantly with the administration of lansoprazole.

No clinically significant effects of lansoprazole on non-steroidal anti-inflammatory drugs (NSAIDs) or diazepam have been found.

Antacids and sucralfate should not be taken within an hour of lansoprazole as they may reduce its bioavailability.

As with other macrolide antibiotics the use of clarithromycin in patients concurrently taking drugs metabolised by the cytochrome P450 system, e.g. cilostazol, methylprednisolone, oral anticoagulants (e.g.warfarin), quinidine, sildenafil, ergot alkaloids, alprazolam, triazolam, midazolam, disopyramide, lovastatin, rifabutin, phenytoin, cyclosporin, vinblastine, valproate and tacrolimus, may be associated with elevations in serum levels of these other drugs. Rhabdomyolysis, co-incident with the co-administration of clarithromycin, and HMG-CoA reductase inhibitors, such as lovastatin and simvastatin have been reported.

The administration of clarithromycin to patients who are receiving theophylline has been associated with an increase in serum theophylline levels and potential theophylline toxicity.

The use of clarithromycin in patients receiving warfarin may result in potentiation of the effects of warfarin. Prothrombin time should be frequently monitored in these patients. The effects of digoxin may be potentiated with concomitant administration of clarithromycin. Monitoring of serum digoxin levels should be considered.

Clarithromycin may potentiate the effects of carbamazepine due to a reduction in the rate of excretion.

Simultaneous oral administration of clarithromycin tablets and zidovudine to HIV infected adult patients may result in decreased steady-state zidovudine levels. This can be largely avoided by staggering the doses of clarithromycin and zidovudine by 1-2 hours. No such reaction has been reported in children.

Ritonavir increases the area under the curve (AUC), C_{max} and C_{min} of clarithromycin when administered concurrently. Because of the large therapeutic window for clarithromycin, no dosage reduction should be necessary in patients with normal renal function. However, for patients with renal impairment, the following dosage adjustments should be considered: For patients with CL_{CR} 30 to 60 ml/min the dose of clarithromycin should be reduced by 50%. For patients with CL_{CR} <30ml/min the dose of clarithromycin should be decreased by 75%. Doses of clarithromycin greater than 1g/day should not be coadministered with ritonavir.

At the dosages recommended, there is no clinically significant interaction between clarithromycin and lansoprazole. Increased plasma concentrations of clarithromycin may occur when it is co-administered with Maalox or ranitidine. No adjustment to the dosage is necessary.

There have been postmarketed reports of Torsade de Pointes occurring with the concurrent use of clarithromycin and quinidine or disopyramide. Levels of these medications should be monitored during clarithromycin therapy.

Patients should be advised not to take alcohol during metronidazole therapy because of the possibility of a disulfiram-like reaction.

Some potentiation of anticoagulant therapy has been reported when metronidazole has been used with the warfarin type oral anticoagulants. Dosage of the latter may require reducing. Prothrombin times should be monitored. There is no interaction with heparin.

Antiepileptics interact with the metabolism of metronidazole. Patients receiving phenobarbitone metabolise metronidazole at a much greater rate than normally, reducing the half-life to approximately 3 hours. Metronidazole inhibits the metabolism of phenytoin.

Metronidazole interacts with the metabolism of cytotoxics – it inhibits the metabolism of fluorouracil, thus causing increased toxicity.

Cimetidine inhibits the metabolism of metronidazole.

Lithium retention accompanied by evidence of possible renal damage has been reported in patients treated simultaneously with lithium and metronidazole. Lithium treatment should be tapered or withdrawn before administering metronidazole. Plasma concentration of lithium, creatinine and electrolytes should be monitored in patients under treatment with lithium while they receive metronidazole.

4.6 Pregnancy and lactation

There is insufficient experience to recommend the use of lansoprazole in pregnancy. Animal studies do not reveal any teratogenic effect. Reproduction studies indicate slightly reduced litter survival and weights in rats and rabbits given very high doses of lansoprazole.

The safety of clarithromycin during pregnancy and breast feeding of infants has not been established. Some animal studies with clarithromycin have suggested an embryotoxic effect, but only at dose levels which are clearly toxic to mothers.

There is inadequate evidence of safety of metronidazole in pregnancy. Metronidazole should not therefore be given during pregnancy or during lactation unless the physician considers it essential.

HeliMet therapy should be avoided during pregnancy.

Lansoprazole and clarithromycin have been found in human breast milk and/or in the milk of lactating animals.

A significant amount of metronidazole is found in breast milk and therefore breast-feeding should be avoided after a large significant amount. It may give a bitter taste to the milk.

HeliMet therapy should be avoided during breast feeding unless the clinical benefit is considered to outweigh the risk.

4.7 Effects on ability to drive and use machines

As dizziness or drowsiness has been reported with metronidazole, but very rarely, patients should be warned to take care when driving or operating machinery.

4.8 Undesirable effects

Lansoprazole is well-tolerated, with adverse events generally being mild and transient. The most commonly reported adverse events are headache, dizziness, fatigue and malaise. Gastrointestinal effects include diarrhoea, constipation, abdominal pain, nausea, vomiting, flatulence and dry or sore mouth or throat. As with other PPIs, very rarely, cases of colitis have been reported. In severe and/or protracted cases of diarrhoea, discontinuation of therapy should be considered. In the majority of cases symptoms resolve on discontinuation of therapy. Alterations in liver function test values and, rarely, jaundice or hepatitis, have been reported. Dermatological reactions include skin rashes, urticaria and pruritus. These generally resolve on discontinuation of drug therapy. Serious dermatological reactions are rare but there have been occasional reports of Stevens-Johnson syndrome, toxic epidermal necrolysis and erythematous or bullous rashes including erythema multiforme. Cases of hair thinning and photosensitivity have also been reported. Other hypersensitivity reactions include angioedema, wheezing, and very rarely, anaphylaxis. Cases of interstitial nephritis have been reported which have sometimes resulted in renal failure. Haematological effects (thrombocytopenia, agranulocytosis, eosinophilia, leucopenia and pancytopenia) have occurred rarely. Bruising, purpura and petechiae have also been reported. Other reactions include arthralgia, myalgia, depression, peripheral oedema and, rarely, paraesthesia, blurred vision, taste disturbances, vertigo, confusion and hallucinations. Gynaecomastia and impotence have been reported rarely.

Clarithromycin is generally well tolerated. Side effects reported include nausea, dyspepsia, diarrhoea, vomiting, abdominal pain and paraesthesia. Stomatitis, glossitis, oral monilia and tongue discolouration have been reported. Other side-effects include headache, arthralgia, myalgia and allergic reactions ranging from urticaria and mild skin eruptions and angioedema to anaphylaxis have been reported. There have been reports of Stevens-Johnson syndrome/toxic epidermal necrolysis with orally administered clarithromycin. Reports of alteration of the sense of smell, usually in conjunction with taste perversion, have also been received. There have been reports of tooth discolouration in patients treated with clarithromycin. Tooth discolouration is usually reversible with professional dental cleaning. There have been reports of transient central nervous system side-effects including dizziness, vertigo, anxiety, insomnia, bad dreams, tinnitus, confusion, disorientation, hallucinations, psychosis and depersonalisation. There have been reports of hearing loss with clarithromycin which is usually reversible on withdrawal of therapy. Pseudomembranous colitis has been reported rarely with clarithromycin, and may range in severity from mild to life threatening. There have been rare reports of hypoglycaemia, some of which have occurred in patients on concomitant oral hypoglycaemic agents or insulin.

There have been rare reports of uveitis reported mainly in patients treated with concomitant rifabutin, most of these were reversible. Isolated cases of leucopenia and thrombocytopenia have been reported. As with other macrolides, hepatic dysfunction (which is usually reversible) including altered liver function tests, hepatitis and cholestasis with or without jaundice, has been reported. Dysfunction may be severe and very rarely fatal hepatic failure has been reported. Cases of increased serum creatinine, interstitial nephritis, renal failure, pancreatitis and convulsions have been reported rarely. As with other macrolides, QT prolongation, ventricular tachycardia and Torsade de Points have been reported rarely with clarithromycin.

Metronidazole is generally well-tolerated. Nausea, vomiting and gastro-intestinal disturbances, drowsiness, headache, rashes, leucopenia, darkening of urine, peripheral neuropathy in prolonged treatment, dizziness, ataxia, transient epileptiform seizures have been reported with high doses. Unpleasant taste in the mouth, furred tongue, urticaria and angiodema occur occasionally. Anaphylaxis may occur rarely. Skin rashes, pruritus, incoordination of movement, myalgia and arthralgia have been reported but very rarely.

Abnormal liver function tests, cholestatic hepatitis and jaundice which may be reversed upon drug withdrawal, have been reported with metronidazole usage.

Following treatment with metronidazole there have been reports of bone marrow depression disorders such as agranulocytosis, neutropenia, thrombocytopenia and pancytopenia which may be reversed on drug withdrawal, although fatalities have been reported.

Metronidazole may be associated with erythema multiforme which may be reversed on drug withdrawal.

4.9 Overdose

There is no information on the effect of overdosage with lansoprazole. However, it has been given at doses up to 120mg/day without significant adverse effects. Symptomatic and supportive therapy should be given as appropriate.

Reports indicate that the ingestion of large amounts of clarithromycin can be expected to produce gastro-intestinal symptoms. One patient who had a history of bipolar disorder ingested 8 grams of clarithromycin and showed altered mental status, paranoid behaviour, hypokalemia and hypoxemia. Adverse reactions accompanying overdosage should be treated by gastric lavage and supportive measures. As with other macrolides, clarithromycin serum levels are not expected to be appreciably affected by haemodialysis or peritoneal dialysis.

Overdose with metronidazole results in severe gastro-intestinal disturbances. Following overdose, patients should be observed for evidence of neuropathy.

There is no specific treatment for gross overdosage of metronidazole.

5. PHARMACOLOGICAL PROPERTIES

5.1 Pharmacodynamic properties

Lansoprazole is a proton pump inhibitor, it specifically inhibits the H^+/K^+ ATPase (proton pump) of the parietal cell in the stomach, the terminal step in acid production. By reducing gastric acidity, lansoprazole creates an environment in which clarithromycin and metronidazole can be effective against *H. pylori*.

Clarithromycin is a semi-synthetic derivative of erythromycin A and highly potent against a wide variety of aerobic and anaerobic gram-positive and gram-negative organisms.

Metronidazole is an antimicrobial agent with high activity against anaerobic bacteria and protozoa.

H. pylori is associated with acid peptic disease including duodenal and gastric ulceration in which about 95% and 80% of patients respectively are infected with the bacterium. Clinical studies using various different *H. pylori* eradication regimens have shown that eradication of *H. pylori* prevents ulcer recurrence. *H. pylori* is also implicated as a major contributory factor in the development of gastritis and ulcer recurrence in such patients. Recent evidence further suggests a causative link between *H. pylori* and gastric carcinoma.

Most available clinical experience from controlled randomised clinical trials indicate that lansoprazole 30 mg twice daily in combination with clarithromycin 500 mg twice daily and metronidazole 400 mg twice daily for one week achieve 90% *H. pylori* eradication rates in patients with gastro-duodenal ulcers. As would be expected, significantly lower eradication rates were observed in patients with baseline metronidazole-resistant *H. pylori* isolates. Hence, local information on the prevalence of resistance and local therapeutic guidelines should be taken into account in the choice of an appropriate combination regimen for *H. pylori* eradication therapy. In patients with persistent infection, potential development of secondary resistance (in patients with primary susceptible strains) to an antibacterial agent should be taken into account in the considerations for a new retreatment regimen.

The prevalence of metronidazole-resistant *H.pylori* strains has been described to be 30-50% in Western Europe. The prevalence of resistant strains to clarithromycin is significantly below that.

5.2 Pharmacokinetic properties

The plasma protein binding of lansoprazole is 97%. Following absorption, lansoprazole is extensively metabolised and is excreted by both the renal and biliary route. A study with ^{14}C-labelled lansoprazole indicated that up to 50% of the dose was excreted in the urine. Lansoprazole is metabolised substantially by the liver.

Clarithromycin penetrates the gastric mucus. Clarithromycin is 80% bound to plasma proteins at therapeutic levels. At 500mg b.i.d., urinary excretion is approximately 36%. The microbiologically active metabolite 14-hydroxyclarithromycin is the major urinary metabolite and accounts for 10-15% of the dose. Most of the remainder of the dose is eliminated in the faeces, primarily via the bile. 5-10% of the parent drug is recovered from the faeces.

Metronidazole is rapidly and almost completely absorbed on administration of Metronidazole Tablets. Peak plasma concentrations occur after 20 minutes to 3 hours. The elimination half-life is 7-8 hours.

5.3 Preclinical safety data

Gastric tumours have been observed in life-long studies with lansoprazole in rats. An increased incidence of spontaneous retinal atrophy has been observed in life-long studies with lansoprazole in rats. These lesions which are common to albino laboratory rats have not been observed in monkeys or dogs or life-long studies in mice. They are considered to be rat specific. No such treatment related changes have been observed in patients treated continuously for long periods.

In acute mouse and rat studies with clarithromycin, the median lethal dose was greater than the highest feasible dose for administration (5g/kg). In repeated dose studies, toxicity was related to dose, duration of treatment and species. Dogs were more sensitive than primates or rats. The major clinical signs at toxic doses included emesis, weakness, reduced food consumption and weight gain, salivation, dehydration and hyperactivity. In all species the liver was the primary target organ at toxic doses. Hepatotoxicity was detectable by early elevations of liver function tests. Discontinuation of clarithromycin generally resulted in a return to or toward normal results. Other tissues less commonly affected included the stomach, thymus and other lymphoid tissues and the kidneys. At near therapeutic doses, conjunctival injection and lacrimation occurred only in dogs. At a massive dose of 400mg/kg/day, some dogs and monkeys developed corneal opacities and/or oedema.

Fertility and reproduction studies with clarithromycin in rats have shown no adverse events. Teratogenicity studies with clarithromycin in rats (Wistar (p.o.) and Sprague-Dawley (p.o. and i.v.)), New Zealand White rabbits and cynomolgous monkeys failed to demonstrate any teratogenicity from clarithromycin. However, a further similar study in Sprague-Dawley rats indicated a low (6%) incidence of cardiovascular abnormalities which appeared to be due to spontaneous expression of genetic changes. Two mouse studies revealed a variable incidence (3-30%) of cleft palate and embryonic loss was seen in monkeys but only at dose levels which were clearly toxic to the mothers.

Metronidazole has been used for many years without proof of any relevant acute toxicity, chronic toxicity, mutagenic or carcinogenic potential or toxicity in reproduction.

6. PHARMACEUTICAL PARTICULARS

6.1 List of excipients

Zoton Capsules: Enteric Coated Granules: Magnesium carbonate, sugar spheres, sucrose, maize starch, low substituted hydroxypropyl cellulose, hydroxypropylcellulose, methacrylic acid-ethyl acrylate co-polymer (1:1) dispersion 30 per cent, talc, macrogol 8000, titanium dioxide, polysorbate 80 and colloidal anhydrous silica.

Capsule Shells: Gelatin, shellac, lecithin, simethicone, and colours: iron oxide black (E172), titanium dioxide (E171), erythrosine (E127), indigo carmine (E132).

Klaricid 500 Tablets: Croscarmellose sodium, cellulose microcrystalline, silicon dioxide, povidone, stearic acid, magnesium stearate, talc, hypromellose, hydroxypropylcellulose, propylene glycol, sorbitan monooleate, titanium dioxide, sorbic acid, vanillin, quinoline yellow (E104).

Metronidazole Tablets: Lactose, maize starch, povidone, colloidal silica anhydrous and magnesium stearate.

6.2 Incompatibilities

Not applicable.

6.3 Shelf life

The recommended shelf life is 36 months.

6.4 Special precautions for storage

Do not store above 25°C. Store in the original package. Keep containers in the outer carton.

6.5 Nature and contents of container

14 Zoton Capsules 30 mg, 14 Klaricid 500 tablets and 14 Metronidazole Tablets 400 mg in a blister patient pack. The blisters are packaged in a carton with a pack insert.

Blister material: PVC 300μm/PVdC 60gsm/Aluminium foil 20μm.

6.6 Instructions for use and handling

Not applicable

7. MARKETING AUTHORISATION HOLDER

John Wyeth and Brother Ltd.
Trading as Wyeth Laboratories
Huntercombe Lane South
Taplow, Maidenhead
Berkshire
SL6 0PH

8. MARKETING AUTHORISATION NUMBER(S)

PL 00011/0253

9. DATE OF FIRST AUTHORISATION/RENEWAL OF THE AUTHORISATION

14 August 2001

10. DATE OF REVISION OF THE TEXT

8 November 2004

Helixate NexGen 1000 IU

(ZLB Behring UK Limited)

1. NAME OF THE MEDICINAL PRODUCT

Helixate NexGen 1000 IU Powder and solvent for solution for injection.

2. QUALITATIVE AND QUANTITATIVE COMPOSITION

Recombinant Coagulation factor VIII, 1000 IU/vial.

INN: octocog alfa.

Recombinant Coagulation factor VIII is produced from genetically engineered baby hamster kidney cells containing the human factor VIII gene.

Solvent: water for injections.

The product reconstituted with the accompanying 2.5 ml of water for injections contains approximately 400 IU octocog alfa/ml.

The potency (IU) is determined using the one-stage clotting assay against the FDA Mega standard which was calibrated against WHO standard in IU.

The specific activity is approximately 4000 IU/mg protein.

For excipients, see 6.1.

3. PHARMACEUTICAL FORM

Powder and solvent for solution for injection.

4. CLINICAL PARTICULARS

4.1 Therapeutic indications

Treatment and prophylaxis of bleeding in patients with haemophilia A (congenital factor VIII deficiency).

This preparation does not contain von Willebrand factor and is therefore not indicated in von Willebrand's disease.

4.2 Posology and method of administration

Treatment should be initiated under the supervision of a physician experienced in the treatment of haemophilia.

Posology

The number of units of factor VIII administered is expressed in International Units (IU), which are related to the current WHO standard for factor VIII products. Factor VIII activity in plasma is expressed either as a percentage (relative to normal human plasma) or in International Units (relative to the International Standard for factor VIII in plasma). One International Unit (IU) of factor VIII activity is equivalent to that quantity of factor VIII in one ml of normal human plasma. The calculation of the required dosage of factor VIII is based on the empirical finding that 1 International Unit (IU) factor VIII per kg body weight raises the plasma factor VIII activity by 1.5% to 2.5% of normal activity. The required dosage is determined using the following formulae:

I. Required IU = body weight (kg) × desired factor VIII rise (% of normal) × 0.5

II. $\text{Expected factor VIII rise (\% of normal)} = \dfrac{2 \times \text{administered IU}}{\text{body weight (kg)}}$

The dosage and duration of the substitution therapy must be individualised according to the patient's needs (weight, severity of disorder of the haemostatic function, the site and extent of the bleeding, the titre of inhibitors, and the factor VIII level desired).

The following table provides a guide for factor VIII minimum blood levels. In the case of the haemorrhagic events listed, the factor VIII activity should not fall below the given level (in % of normal) in the corresponding period:

Degree of haemorrhage/ Type of surgical procedure	Factor VIII level required (%) (IU/dl)	Frequency of doses (hours)/ Duration of therapy (days)
Haemorrhage		
Early haemarthrosis, muscle bleed or oral bleed	20 - 40	Repeat every 12 to 24 hours. At least 1 day, until the bleeding episode as indicated by pain is resolved or healing is achieved.

More extensive haemarthrosis, muscle bleed or haematoma	30 - 60	Repeat infusion every 12 - 24 hours for 3 - 4 days or more until pain and disability are resolved.
Life threatening bleeds such as intracranial bleed, throat bleed, severe abdominal bleed	60 - 100	Repeat infusion every 8 to 24 hours until threat is resolved
Surgery *Minor* including tooth extraction	30 - 60	Every 24 hours, at least 1 day, until healing is achieved.
Major	80 - 100 (pre- and postoperative)	Repeat infusion every 8 - 24 hours until adequate wound healing, then therapy for at least another 7 days to maintain a factor VIII activity of 30% to 60%

The amount to be administered and the frequency of administration should always be adapted according to the clinical effectiveness in the individual case. Under certain circumstances larger amounts than those calculated may be required, especially in the case of the initial dose.

During the course of treatment, appropriate determination of factor VIII levels is advised in order to guide the dose to be administered and the frequency at which to repeat the infusions. In the case of major surgical interventions in particular, precise monitoring of the substitution therapy by means of coagulation analysis (plasma factor VIII activity) is indispensable. Individual patients may vary in their response to factor VIII, achieving different levels of *in vivo* recovery and demonstrating different half-lives.

For scheduled prophylaxis against bleeds in patients with severe haemophilia A, doses of 20 to 60 IU of Helixate NexGen per kg body weight should be given at intervals of 2 to 3 days. In some cases, especially in younger patients, shorter dosage intervals or higher doses may be necessary. Data have been obtained in 61 children under 6 years of age.

Patients with inhibitors

Patients should be monitored for the development of factor VIII inhibitors. If the expected plasma factor VIII activity levels are not attained, or if bleeding is not controlled with an appropriate dose, an assay should be performed to determine if a factor VIII inhibitor is present. If the inhibitor is present at levels less than 10 Bethesda Units (BU) per ml, administration of additional recombinant coagulation factor VIII may neutralise the inhibitor and permit continued clinically effective therapy with Helixate NexGen. However, in the presence of an inhibitor the doses required are variable and must be adjusted according to clinical response and monitoring of plasma factor VIII activity. In patients with inhibitor titres above 10 BU or with high anamnestic response, the use of (activated) prothrombin complex concentrate (PCC) or recombinant activated factor VII (rFVIIa) preparations has to be considered. These therapies should be directed by physicians with experience in the care of patients with haemophilia.

Administration

Dissolve the preparation as described in 6.6.

Helixate NexGen should be injected intravenously over several minutes. The rate of administration should be determined by the patient's comfort level (maximal rate of infusion: 2 ml/min).

4.3 Contraindications

Known hypersensitivity to the active substance, to mouse or hamster protein or to any of the excipients.

4.4 Special warnings and special precautions for use

Patients should be made aware that the potential occurrence of chest tightness, dizziness, mild hypotension and nausea during infusion can constitute an early warning for hypersensitivity and anaphylactic reactions. Symptomatic treatment and therapy for hypersensitivity should be instituted as appropriate. If allergic or anaphylactic reactions occur, the injection/infusion should be stopped immediately. In case of shock, the current medical standards for shock treatment should be observed.

The formation of neutralising antibodies (inhibitors) to factor VIII is a known complication in the management of individuals with haemophilia A. These inhibitors are invariably IgG immunoglobulins directed against the factor VIII procoagulant activity, which are quantified in Modified Bethesda Units (BU) per ml of plasma. The risk of developing inhibitors is correlated to the exposure to anti-haemophilic factor VIII, this risk being highest within the first 20 exposure days. Rarely, inhibitors may develop after the first 100 exposure days. Patients treated with recombinant coagulation factor VIII should be carefully monitored for the development of inhibitors by appropriate clinical observations and laboratory tests. See also 4.8 Undesirable effects.

4.5 Interaction with other medicinal products and other forms of Interaction

No interactions of Helixate NexGen with other medicinal products are known.

4.6 Pregnancy and lactation

Animal reproduction studies have not been conducted with Helixate NexGen.

Based on the rare occurrence of haemophilia A in women, experience regarding the use of Helixate NexGen during pregnancy and breast-feeding is not available. Therefore, Helixate NexGen should be used during pregnancy and lactation only if clearly indicated.

4.7 Effects on ability to drive and use machines

No effects on the ability to drive or to use machines have been observed.

4.8 Undesirable effects

After administration of Helixate NexGen mild to moderate adverse events were observed in rare cases. These included rash/pruritus, local reactions at the injection site (e.g. burning, transient erythema), hypersensitivity reactions (e.g. dizziness, nausea, chest pain/malaise, mildly reduced blood pressure), unusual taste in the mouth and fever. Furthermore, the possibility of an anaphylactic shock cannot be completely excluded.

The formation of neutralising antibodies to factor VIII (inhibitors) is a known complication in the management of individuals with haemophilia A. In studies with recombinant factor VIII preparations, development of inhibitors is predominantly observed in previously untreated haemophiliacs. Patients should be carefully monitored for the development of inhibitors by appropriate clinical observations and laboratory tests.

In clinical trials 9 out of 60 (15%) previously untreated and minimally treated patients treated with Helixate NexGen developed inhibitors: Overall 6 out of 60 (10%) with a titre above 10 BU and 3 out of 60 (5%) with a titre below 10 BU. The median number of exposure days at the time of inhibitor detection in these patients were 9 days (range 3 - 18 days).

During studies, no patient developed clinically relevant antibody titres against the trace amounts of mouse protein and hamster protein present in the preparation. However, the possibility of allergic reactions to constituents, e.g. trace amounts of mouse and hamster protein in the preparation exists in certain predisposed patients (see 4.3 and 4.4).

4.9 Overdose

No symptoms of overdose with recombinant coagulation factor VIII have been reported.

5. PHARMACOLOGICAL PROPERTIES

5.1 Pharmacodynamic properties

Pharmacotherapeutic group: blood coagulation factor VIII, ATC-Code B02B D02.

The factor VIII/von Willebrand factor (vWF) complex consists of two molecules (factor VIII and vWF) with different physiological functions. When infused into a haemophiliac patient, factor VIII binds to vWF in the patient's circulation. Activated factor VIII acts as a cofactor for activated factor IX, accelerating the conversion of factor X to activated factor X. Activated factor X converts prothrombin into thrombin. Thrombin then converts fibrinogen into fibrin and a clot can be formed. Haemophilia A is a sex-linked hereditary disorder of blood coagulation due to decreased levels of factor VIII:C and results in profuse bleeding into joints, muscles or internal organs, either spontaneously or as a results of accidental or surgical trauma. By replacement therapy the plasma levels of factor VIII are increased, thereby enabling a temporary correction of the factor deficiency and correction of the bleeding tendencies.

Determination of activated partial thromboplastin time (aPTT) is a conventional *in vitro* assay method for biological activity of factor VIII. The aPTT is prolonged in all haemophiliacs. The degree and duration of aPTT normalisation observed after administration of Helixate NexGen is similar to that achieved with plasma-derived factor VIII.

5.2 Pharmacokinetic properties

The analysis of all recorded *in vivo* recoveries in previously treated patients demonstrated a mean rise of 2 % per IU/kg body weight for Helixate NexGen. This result is similar to the reported values for factor VIII derived from human plasma.

After administration of Helixate NexGen, peak factor VIII activity decreased by a two-phase exponential decay with a mean terminal half-life of about 15 hours. This is similar to that of plasma-derived factor VIII which has a mean terminal half-life of approx. 13 hours. Additional pharmacokinetic parameters for Helixate NexGen are: mean residence time [MRT (0-48)] of about 22 hours and clearance of about 160 ml/h.

5.3 Preclinical safety data

Even doses several fold higher than the recommended clinical dose (related to body weight) failed to demonstrate any acute or subacute toxic effects for Helixate NexGen in laboratory animals (mouse, rat, rabbit, and dog).

Specific studies with repeated administration such as reproduction toxicity, chronic toxicity, and carcinogenicity were not performed with octocog alfa due to the immune response to heterologous proteins in all non-human mammalian species.

No studies were performed on the mutagenic potential of Helixate NexGen, since no mutagenic potential could be detected *in vitro* or *in vivo* for the predecessor product of Helixate NexGen.

6. PHARMACEUTICAL PARTICULARS

6.1 List of excipients

Powder

Glycine

Sodium chloride

Calcium chloride

Histidine

Polysorbate 80

Sucrose

Solvent

Water for injections

6.2 Incompatibilities

This medicinal product must not be mixed with other medicinal products or solvents.

Only the provided administration sets can be used because treatment failure can occur as a consequence of human coagulation factor VIII adsorption to the internal surfaces of some infusion equipment.

6.3 Shelf life

23 months

Chemical and physical in-use stability has been demonstrated for 4 hours at 25°C.

From a microbiological point of view, unless the method of reconstitution precludes the risk of microbial contamination, the product should be used immediately.

If not used immediately, in-use storage times and conditions are the responsibility of the user.

6.4 Special precautions for storage

Store in a refrigerator (2°C – 8°C). Do not freeze. Keep the vials in the outer carton in order to protect from light.

The product when kept in its outer carton may be stored at ambient room temperature (up to 25°C) for a limited period of 2 months. In this case, the product expires at the end of this 2-month period; the new expiry date must be noted on the top of the outer carton.

Do not refrigerate after reconstitution. For single use only. Any unused solution must be discarded.

6.5 Nature and contents of container

Each package of Helixate NexGen contains:

- one vial with powder (10 ml clear glass type 1 vial with latex-free grey bromobutyl rubber blend stopper and aluminium seal)
- one vial with solvent (10 ml clear glass type 2 vial with latex-free grey chlorobutyl rubber blend stopper and aluminium seal)
- an additional package with:

- 1 transfer device
- 1 filter needle
- 1 venipuncture set
- 1 plastic syringe (5 ml)
- two sterile alcohol swabs for single use

6.6 Instructions for use and handling

Detailed instructions for preparation and administration are contained in the package leaflet provided with Helixate NexGen.

Helixate NexGen powder should only be reconstituted with the supplied solvent (2.5 ml water for injections) using the supplied sterile transfer device. Gently rotate the vial until all powder is dissolved. Do not use Helixate NexGen if you notice visible particulate matter or turbidity.

After reconstitution, the solution is drawn through the sterile filter needle into the sterile disposable syringe (both supplied).

Any unused product or waste material should be disposed of in accordance with local requirements.

7. MARKETING AUTHORISATION HOLDER

Bayer AG

D-51368 Leverkusen

Germany

8. MARKETING AUTHORISATION NUMBER(S)

EU/1/00/144/003

9. DATE OF FIRST AUTHORISATION/RENEWAL OF THE AUTHORISATION

4 August 2000

10. DATE OF REVISION OF THE TEXT

26 November 2004

Helixate NexGen 250 IU

(ZLB Behring UK Limited)

1. NAME OF THE MEDICINAL PRODUCT

Helixate NexGen 250 IU Powder and solvent for solution for injection.

2. QUALITATIVE AND QUANTITATIVE COMPOSITION

Recombinant Coagulation factor VIII, 250 IU/vial.

INN: octocog alfa.

Recombinant Coagulation factor VIII is produced from genetically engineered baby hamster kidney cells containing the human factor VIII gene.

Solvent: water for injections.

The product reconstituted with the accompanying 2.5 ml of water for injections contains approximately 100 IU octocog alfa/ml.

The potency (IU) is determined using the one-stage clotting assay against the FDA Mega standard which was calibrated against WHO standard in IU.

The specific activity is approximately 4000 IU/mg protein.

For excipients, see 6.1.

3. PHARMACEUTICAL FORM

Powder and solvent for solution for injection.

4. CLINICAL PARTICULARS

4.1 Therapeutic indications

Treatment and prophylaxis of bleeding in patients with haemophilia A (congenital factor VIII deficiency).

This preparation does not contain von Willebrand factor and is therefore not indicated in von Willebrand's disease.

4.2 Posology and method of administration

Treatment should be initiated under the supervision of a physician experienced in the treatment of haemophilia.

Posology

The number of units of factor VIII administered is expressed in International Units (IU), which are related to the current WHO standard for factor VIII products. Factor VIII activity in plasma is expressed either as a percentage (relative to normal human plasma) or in International Units (relative to the International Standard for factor VIII in plasma). One International Unit (IU) of factor VIII activity is equivalent to that quantity of factor VIII in one ml of normal human plasma. The calculation of the required dosage of factor VIII is based on the empirical finding that 1 International Unit (IU) factor VIII per kg body weight raises the plasma factor VIII activity by 1.5% to 2.5% of normal activity. The required dosage is determined using the following formulae:

I. Required IU = body weight (kg) $\times$ desired factor VIII rise (% of normal) $\times$ 0.5

II. Expected factor VIII rise (% of normal) = $\frac{2 \times \text{administered IU}}{\text{body weight (kg)}}$

The dosage and duration of the substitution therapy must be individualised according to the patient's needs (weight, severity of disorder of the haemostatic function, the site and extent of the bleeding, the titre of inhibitors, and the factor VIII level desired).

The following table provides a guide for factor VIII minimum blood levels. In the case of the haemorrhagic events listed, the factor VIII activity should not fall below the given level (in % of normal) in the corresponding period:

Degree of haemorrhage/ Type of surgical procedure	Factor VIII level required (%) (IU/dl)	Frequency of doses (hours)/ Duration of therapy (days)
Haemorrhage		
Early haemarthrosis, muscle bleed or oral bleed	20 - 40	Repeat every 12 to 24 hours. At least 1 day, until the bleeding episode as indicated by pain is resolved or healing is achieved.
More extensive haemarthrosis, muscle bleed or haematoma	30 - 60	Repeat infusion every 12 - 24 hours for 3 - 4 days or more until pain and disability are resolved.
Life threatening bleeds such as intracranial bleed, throat bleed, severe abdominal bleed	60 - 100	Repeat infusion every 8 to 24 hours until threat is resolved
Surgery		
Minor including tooth extraction	30 - 60	Every 24 hours, at least 1 day, until healing is achieved.
Major	80 - 100 (pre- and postoperative)	Repeat infusion every 8 - 24 hours until adequate wound healing, then therapy for at least another 7 days to maintain a factor VIII activity of 30% to 60%

The amount to be administered and the frequency of administration should always be adapted according to the clinical effectiveness in the individual case. Under certain circumstances larger amounts than those calculated may be required, especially in the case of the initial dose.

During the course of treatment, appropriate determination of factor VIII levels is advised in order to guide the dose to be administered and the frequency at which to repeat the infusions. In the case of major surgical interventions in particular, precise monitoring of the substitution therapy by means of coagulation analysis (plasma factor VIII activity) is indispensable. Individual patients may vary in their response to factor VIII, achieving different levels of *in vivo* recovery and demonstrating different half-lives.

For scheduled prophylaxis against bleeds in patients with severe haemophilia A, doses of 20 to 60 IU of Helixate NexGen per kg body weight should be given at intervals of 2 to 3 days. In some cases, especially in younger patients, shorter dosage intervals or higher doses may be necessary. Data have been obtained in 61 children under 6 years of age.

Patients with inhibitors

Patients should be monitored for the development of factor VIII inhibitors. If the expected plasma factor VIII activity levels are not attained, or if bleeding is not controlled with an appropriate dose, an assay should be performed to determine if a factor VIII inhibitor is present. If the inhibitor is present at levels less than 10 Bethesda Units (BU) per ml, administration of additional recombinant coagulation factor VIII may neutralise the inhibitor and permit continued clinically effective therapy with Helixate NexGen. However, in the presence of an inhibitor the doses required are variable and must be adjusted according to clinical response and monitoring of plasma factor VIII activity. In patients with inhibitor titres above 10 BU or with high anamnestic response, the use of (activated) prothrombin complex concentrate (PCC) or recombinant activated factor VII (rFVIIa) preparations has to be considered. These therapies should be directed by physicians with experience in the care of patients with haemophilia.

Administration

Dissolve the preparation as described in 6.6.

Helixate NexGen should be injected intravenously over several minutes. The rate of administration should be determined by the patient's comfort level (maximal rate of infusion: 2 ml/min).

4.3 Contraindications

Known hypersensitivity to the active substance, to mouse or hamster protein or to any of the excipients.

4.4 Special warnings and special precautions for use

Patients should be made aware that the potential occurrence of chest tightness, dizziness, mild hypotension and nausea during infusion can constitute an early warning for hypersensitivity and anaphylactic reactions. Symptomatic treatment and therapy for hypersensitivity should be instituted as appropriate. If allergic or anaphylactic reactions occur, the injection/infusion should be stopped immediately. In case of shock, the current medical standards for shock treatment should be observed.

The formation of neutralising antibodies (inhibitors) to factor VIII is a known complication in the management of individuals with haemophilia A. These inhibitors are invariably IgG immunoglobulins directed against the factor VIII procoagulant activity, which are quantified in Modified Bethesda Units (BU) per ml of plasma. The risk of developing inhibitors is correlated to the exposure to anti-haemophilic factor VIII, this risk being highest within the first 20 exposure days. Rarely, inhibitors may develop after the first 100 exposure days. Patients treated with recombinant coagulation factor VIII should be carefully monitored for the development of inhibitors by appropriate clinical observations and laboratory tests. See also 4.8 Undesirable effects.

4.5 Interaction with other medicinal products and other forms of Interaction

No interactions of Helixate NexGen with other medicinal products are known.

4.6 Pregnancy and lactation

Animal reproduction studies have not been conducted with Helixate NexGen.

Based on the rare occurrence of haemophilia A in women, experience regarding the use of Helixate NexGen during pregnancy and breast-feeding is not available. Therefore, Helixate NexGen should be used during pregnancy and lactation only if clearly indicated.

4.7 Effects on ability to drive and use machines

No effects on the ability to drive or to use machines have been observed.

4.8 Undesirable effects

After administration of Helixate NexGen mild to moderate adverse events were observed in rare cases. These included rash/pruritus, local reactions at the injection site (e.g. burning, transient erythema), hypersensitivity reactions (e.g. dizziness, nausea, chest pain/malaise, mildly reduced blood pressure), unusual taste in the mouth and fever. Furthermore, the possibility of an anaphylactic shock cannot be completely excluded.

The formation of neutralising antibodies to factor VIII (inhibitors) is a known complication in the management of individuals with haemophilia A. In studies with recombinant factor VIII preparations, development of inhibitors is predominantly observed in previously untreated haemophiliacs. Patients should be carefully monitored for the development of inhibitors by appropriate clinical observations and laboratory tests.

In clinical trials 9 out of 60 (15%) previously untreated and minimally treated patients treated with Helixate NexGen developed inhibitors: Overall 6 out of 60 (10%) with a titre above 10 BU and 3 out of 60 (5%) with a titre below 10 BU. The median number of exposure days at the time of inhibitor detection in these patients were 9 days (range 3 - 18 days).

During studies, no patient developed clinically relevant antibody titres against the trace amounts of mouse protein and hamster protein present in the preparation. However, the possibility of allergic reactions to constituents, e.g. trace amounts of mouse and hamster protein in the preparation exists in certain predisposed patients (see 4.3 and 4.4).

4.9 Overdose

No symptoms of overdose with recombinant coagulation factor VIII have been reported.

5. PHARMACOLOGICAL PROPERTIES

5.1 Pharmacodynamic properties

Pharmacotherapeutic group: blood coagulation factor VIII, ATC-Code B02B D02.

The factor VIII/von Willebrand factor (vWF) complex consists of two molecules (factor VIII and vWF) with different physiological functions. When infused into a haemophiliac patient, factor VIII binds to vWF in the patient's circulation. Activated factor VIII acts as a cofactor for activated factor IX, accelerating the conversion of factor X to activated factor X. Activated factor X converts prothrombin into thrombin. Thrombin then converts fibrinogen into fibrin and a clot can be formed. Haemophilia A is a sex-linked hereditary disorder of blood coagulation due to decreased levels of factor VIII:C and results in profuse bleeding into joints, muscles or internal organs, either spontaneously or as a results of accidental or surgical trauma. By replacement therapy the plasma levels of factor VIII are increased, thereby enabling a temporary correction of the factor deficiency and correction of the bleeding tendencies.

Determination of activated partial thromboplastin time (aPTT) is a conventional *in vitro* assay method for biological activity of factor VIII. The aPTT is prolonged in all haemophiliacs. The degree and duration of aPTT normalisation observed after administration of Helixate NexGen is similar to that achieved with plasma-derived factor VIII.

5.2 Pharmacokinetic properties

The analysis of all recorded *in vivo* recoveries in previously treated patients demonstrated a mean rise of 2 % per IU/kg body weight for Helixate NexGen. This result is similar to the reported values for factor VIII derived from human plasma.

After administration of Helixate NexGen, peak factor VIII activity decreased by a two-phase exponential decay with a mean terminal half-life of about 15 hours. This is similar to that of plasma-derived factor VIII which has a mean terminal half-life of approx. 13 hours. Additional pharmacokinetic parameters for Helixate NexGen are: mean residence time [MRT (0-48)] of about 22 hours and clearance of about 160 ml/h.

5.3 Preclinical safety data

Even doses several fold higher than the recommended clinical dose (related to body weight) failed to demonstrate any acute or subacute toxic effects for Helixate NexGen in laboratory animals (mouse, rat, rabbit, and dog).

Specific studies with repeated administration such as reproduction toxicity, chronic toxicity, and carcinogenicity were not performed with octocog alfa due to the immune response to heterologous proteins in all non-human mammalian species.

No studies were performed on the mutagenic potential of Helixate NexGen, since no mutagenic potential could be detected *in vitro* or *in vivo* for the predecessor product of Helixate NexGen.

6. PHARMACEUTICAL PARTICULARS

6.1 List of excipients

Powder

Glycine

Sodium chloride

Calcium chloride

Histidine

Polysorbate 80

Sucrose

Solvent

Water for injections

6.2 Incompatibilities

This medicinal product must not be mixed with other medicinal products or solvents.

Only the provided administration sets can be used because treatment failure can occur as a consequence of human coagulation factor VIII adsorption to the internal surfaces of some infusion equipment.

6.3 Shelf life

23 months

Chemical and physical in-use stability has been demonstrated for 4 hours at 25°C.

From a microbiological point of view, unless the method of reconstitution precludes the risk of microbial contamination, the product should be used immediately.

If not used immediately, in-use storage times and conditions are the responsibility of the user.

6.4 Special precautions for storage

Store in a refrigerator (2°C – 8°C). Do not freeze. Keep the vials in the outer carton in order to protect from light.

The product when kept in its outer carton may be stored at ambient room temperature (up to 25°C) for a limited period of 2 months. In this case, the product expires at the end of this 2-month period; the new expiry date must be noted on the top of the outer carton.

Do not refrigerate after reconstitution. For single use only. Any unused solution must be discarded.

6.5 Nature and contents of container

Each package of Helixate NexGen contains:

- one vial with powder (10 ml clear glass type 1 vial with latex-free grey bromobutyl rubber blend stopper and aluminium seal)
- one vial with solvent (10 ml clear glass type 2 vial with latex-free grey chlorobutyl rubber blend stopper and aluminium seal)
- an additional package with:

- 1 transfer device
- 1 filter needle
- 1 venipuncture set
- 1 plastic syringe (5 ml)
- two sterile alcohol swabs for single use

6.6 Instructions for use and handling

Detailed instructions for preparation and administration are contained in the package leaflet provided with Helixate NexGen.

Helixate NexGen powder should only be reconstituted with the supplied solvent (2.5 ml water for injections) using the supplied sterile transfer device. Gently rotate the vial until all powder is dissolved. Do not use Helixate NexGen if you notice visible particulate matter or turbidity.

After reconstitution, the solution is drawn through the sterile filter needle into the sterile disposable syringe (both supplied).

Any unused product or waste material should be disposed of in accordance with local requirements.

7. MARKETING AUTHORISATION HOLDER

Bayer AG

D-51368 Leverkusen

Germany

8. MARKETING AUTHORISATION NUMBER(S)

EU/1/00/144/001

9. DATE OF FIRST AUTHORISATION/RENEWAL OF THE AUTHORISATION

4 August 2000

10. DATE OF REVISION OF THE TEXT

26 November 2004

Helixate NexGen 500 IU

(ZLB Behring UK Limited)

1. NAME OF THE MEDICINAL PRODUCT

Helixate NexGen 500 IU Powder and solvent for solution for injection.

2. QUALITATIVE AND QUANTITATIVE COMPOSITION

Recombinant Coagulation factor VIII, 500 IU/vial.

INN: octocog alfa.

Recombinant Coagulation factor VIII is produced from genetically engineered baby hamster kidney cells containing the human factor VIII gene.

Solvent: water for injections.

The product reconstituted with the accompanying 2.5 ml of water for injections contains approximately 200 IU octocog alfa/ml.

The potency (IU) is determined using the one-stage clotting assay against the FDA Mega standard which was calibrated against WHO standard in IU.

The specific activity is approximately 4000 IU/mg protein.

For excipients, see 6.1.

3. PHARMACEUTICAL FORM

Powder and solvent for solution for injection.

4. CLINICAL PARTICULARS

4.1 Therapeutic indications

Treatment and prophylaxis of bleeding in patients with haemophilia A (congenital factor VIII deficiency).

This preparation does not contain von Willebrand factor and is therefore not indicated in von Willebrand's disease.

4.2 Posology and method of administration

Treatment should be initiated under the supervision of a physician experienced in the treatment of haemophilia.

Posology

The number of units of factor VIII administered is expressed in International Units (IU), which are related to the current WHO standard for factor VIII products. Factor VIII activity in plasma is expressed either as a percentage (relative to normal human plasma) or in International Units (relative to the International Standard for factor VIII in plasma). One International Unit (IU) of factor VIII activity is equivalent to that quantity of factor VIII in one ml of normal human plasma. The calculation of the required dosage of factor VIII is based on the empirical finding that 1 International Unit (IU) factor VIII per kg body weight raises the plasma factor VIII activity by 1.5% to 2.5% of normal activity. The required dosage is determined using the following formulae:

I. Required IU = body weight (kg) $\times$ desired factor VIII rise (% of normal) $\times$ 0.5

II. $\text{Expected factor VIII rise (\% of normal)} = \dfrac{2 \times \text{administered IU}}{\text{body weight (kg)}}$

The dosage and duration of the substitution therapy must be individualised according to the patient's needs (weight, severity of disorder of the haemostatic function, the site and extent of the bleeding, the titre of inhibitors, and the factor VIII level desired).

The following table provides a guide for factor VIII minimum blood levels. In the case of the haemorrhagic events listed, the factor VIII activity should not fall below the given level (in % of normal) in the corresponding period:

Degree of haemorrhage/ Type of surgical procedure	Factor VIII level required (%) (IU/dl)	Frequency of doses (hours)/ Duration of therapy (days)
Haemorrhage Early haemarthrosis, muscle bleed or oral bleed	20 - 40	Repeat every 12 to 24 hours. At least 1 day, until the bleeding episode as indicated by pain is resolved or healing is achieved.
More extensive haemarthrosis, muscle bleed or haematoma	30 - 60	Repeat infusion every 12 - 24 hours for 3 - 4 days or more until pain and disability are resolved.
Life threatening bleeds such as intracranial bleed, throat bleed, severe abdominal bleed	60 - 100	Repeat infusion every 8 to 24 hours until threat is resolved
Surgery *Minor* including tooth extraction	30 - 60	Every 24 hours, at least 1 day, until healing is achieved.
Major	80 - 100 (pre- and postoperative)	Repeat infusion every 8 - 24 hours until adequate wound healing, then therapy for at least another 7 days to maintain a factor VIII activity of 30% to 60%

The amount to be administered and the frequency of administration should always be adapted according to the clinical effectiveness in the individual case. Under certain circumstances larger amounts than those calculated may be required, especially in the case of the initial dose.

During the course of treatment, appropriate determination of factor VIII levels is advised in order to guide the dose to be administered and the frequency at which to repeat the infusions. In the case of major surgical interventions in particular, precise monitoring of the substitution therapy by means of coagulation analysis (plasma factor VIII activity) is indispensable. Individual patients may vary in their response to factor VIII, achieving different levels of *in vivo* recovery and demonstrating different half-lives.

For scheduled prophylaxis against bleeds in patients with severe haemophilia A, doses of 20 to 60 IU of Helixate NexGen per kg body weight should be given at intervals of 2 to 3 days. In some cases, especially in younger patients, shorter dosage intervals or higher doses may be necessary. Data have been obtained in 61 children under 6 years of age.

Patients with inhibitors

Patients should be monitored for the development of factor VIII inhibitors. If the expected plasma factor VIII activity levels are not attained, or if bleeding is not controlled with an appropriate dose, an assay should be performed to determine if a factor VIII inhibitor is present. If the inhibitor is present at levels less than 10 Bethesda Units (BU) per ml, administration of additional recombinant coagulation factor VIII may neutralise the inhibitor and permit continued clinically effective therapy with Helixate NexGen. However, in the presence of an inhibitor the doses required are variable and must be adjusted according to clinical response and monitoring of plasma factor VIII activity. In patients with inhibitor titres above 10 BU or with high anamnestic response, the use of (activated) prothrombin complex concentrate (PCC) or recombinant activated factor VII (rFVIIa) preparations has to be considered. These therapies should be directed by physicians with experience in the care of patients with haemophilia.

Administration

Dissolve the preparation as described in 6.6.

Helixate NexGen should be injected intravenously over several minutes. The rate of administration should be determined by the patient's comfort level (maximal rate of infusion: 2 ml/min).

4.3 Contraindications

Known hypersensitivity to the active substance, to mouse or hamster protein or to any of the excipients.

4.4 Special warnings and special precautions for use

Patients should be made aware that the potential occurrence of chest tightness, dizziness, mild hypotension and nausea during infusion can constitute an early warning for hypersensitivity and anaphylactic reactions. Symptomatic treatment and therapy for hypersensitivity should be instituted as appropriate. If allergic or anaphylactic reactions occur, the injection/infusion should be stopped immediately. In case of shock, the current medical standards for shock treatment should be observed.

The formation of neutralising antibodies (inhibitors) to factor VIII is a known complication in the management of individuals with haemophilia A. These inhibitors are invariably IgG immunoglobulins directed against the factor VIII procoagulant activity, which are quantified in Modified Bethesda Units (BU) per ml of plasma. The risk of developing inhibitors is correlated to the exposure to anti-haemophilic factor VIII, this risk being highest within the first 20 exposure days. Rarely, inhibitors may develop after the first 100 exposure days. Patients treated with recombinant coagulation factor VIII should be carefully monitored for the development of inhibitors by appropriate clinical observations and laboratory tests. See also 4.8 Undesirable effects.

4.5 Interaction with other medicinal products and other forms of Interaction

No interactions of Helixate NexGen with other medicinal products are known.

4.6 Pregnancy and lactation

Animal reproduction studies have not been conducted with Helixate NexGen.

Based on the rare occurrence of haemophilia A in women, experience regarding the use of Helixate NexGen during pregnancy and breast-feeding is not available. Therefore, Helixate NexGen should be used during pregnancy and lactation only if clearly indicated.

4.7 Effects on ability to drive and use machines

No effects on the ability to drive or to use machines have been observed.

4.8 Undesirable effects

After administration of Helixate NexGen mild to moderate adverse events were observed in rare cases. These included rash/pruritus, local reactions at the injection site (e.g. burning, transient erythema), hypersensitivity reactions (e.g. dizziness, nausea, chest pain/malaise, mildly reduced blood pressure), unusual taste in the mouth and fever. Furthermore, the possibility of an anaphylactic shock cannot be completely excluded.

The formation of neutralising antibodies to factor VIII (inhibitors) is a known complication in the management of individuals with haemophilia A. In studies with recombinant factor VIII preparations, development of inhibitors is predominantly observed in previously untreated haemophiliacs. Patients should be carefully monitored for the development of inhibitors by appropriate clinical observations and laboratory tests.

In clinical trials 9 out of 60 (15%) previously untreated and minimally treated patients treated with Helixate NexGen developed inhibitors: Overall 6 out of 60 (10%) with a titre above 10 BU and 3 out of 60 (5%) with a titre below 10 BU. The median number of exposure days at the time of inhibitor detection in these patients were 9 days (range 3 - 18 days).

During studies, no patient developed clinically relevant antibody titres against the trace amounts of mouse protein and hamster protein present in the preparation. However, the possibility of allergic reactions to constituents, e.g. trace amounts of mouse and hamster protein in the preparation exists in certain predisposed patients (see 4.3 and 4.4).

4.9 Overdose

No symptoms of overdose with recombinant coagulation factor VIII have been reported.

5. PHARMACOLOGICAL PROPERTIES

5.1 Pharmacodynamic properties

Pharmacotherapeutic group: blood coagulation factor VIII, ATC-Code B02B D02.

The factor VIII/von Willebrand factor (vWF) complex consists of two molecules (factor VIII and vWF) with different physiological functions. When infused into a haemophiliac patient, factor VIII binds to vWF in the patient's circulation. Activated factor VIII acts as a cofactor for activated factor IX, accelerating the conversion of factor X to activated factor X. Activated factor X converts prothrombin into thrombin. Thrombin then converts fibrinogen into fibrin and a clot can be formed. Haemophilia A is a sex-linked hereditary disorder of blood coagulation due to decreased levels of factor VIII:C and results in profuse bleeding into joints, muscles or internal organs, either spontaneously or as a results of accidental or surgical trauma. By replacement therapy the plasma levels of factor VIII are increased, thereby enabling a temporary correction of the factor deficiency and correction of the bleeding tendencies.

Determination of activated partial thromboplastin time (aPTT) is a conventional *in vitro* assay method for biological activity of factor VIII. The aPTT is prolonged in all haemophiliacs. The degree and duration of aPTT normalisation observed after administration of Helixate NexGen is similar to that achieved with plasma-derived factor VIII.

5.2 Pharmacokinetic properties

The analysis of all recorded *in vivo* recoveries in previously treated patients demonstrated a mean rise of 2 % per IU/kg body weight for Helixate NexGen. This result is similar to the reported values for factor VIII derived from human plasma.

After administration of Helixate NexGen, peak factor VIII activity decreased by a two-phase exponential decay with a mean terminal half-life of about 15 hours. This is similar to that of plasma-derived factor VIII which has a mean terminal half-life of approx. 13 hours. Additional pharmacokinetic parameters for Helixate NexGen are: mean residence time [MRT (0-48)] of about 22 hours and clearance of about 160 ml/h.

5.3 Preclinical safety data

Even doses several fold higher than the recommended clinical dose (related to body weight) failed to demonstrate any acute or subacute toxic effects for Helixate NexGen in laboratory animals (mouse, rat, rabbit, and dog).

Specific studies with repeated administration such as reproduction toxicity, chronic toxicity, and carcinogenicity were not performed with octocog alfa due to the immune response to heterologous proteins in all non-human mammalian species.

No studies were performed on the mutagenic potential of Helixate NexGen, since no mutagenic potential could be detected *in vitro* or *in vivo* for the predecessor product of Helixate NexGen.

6. PHARMACEUTICAL PARTICULARS

6.1 List of excipients

Powder

Glycine

Sodium chloride

Calcium chloride

Histidine

Polysorbate 80

Sucrose

Solvent

Water for injections

6.2 Incompatibilities

This medicinal product must not be mixed with other medicinal products or solvents.

Only the provided administration sets can be used because treatment failure can occur as a consequence of human coagulation factor VIII adsorption to the internal surfaces of some infusion equipment.

6.3 Shelf life

23 months.

Chemical and physical in-use stability has been demonstrated for 4 hours at 25°C.

From a microbiological point of view, unless the method of reconstitution precludes the risk of microbial contamination, the product should be used immediately.

If not used immediately, in-use storage times and conditions are the responsibility of the user.

6.4 Special precautions for storage

Store in a refrigerator (2°C – 8°C). Do not freeze. Keep the vials in the outer carton in order to protect from light.

The product when kept in its outer carton may be stored at ambient room temperature (up to 25°C) for a limited period of 2 months. In this case, the product expires at the end of this 2-month period; the new expiry date must be noted on the top of the outer carton.

Do not refrigerate after reconstitution. For single use only. Any unused solution must be discarded.

6.5 Nature and contents of container

Each package of Helixate NexGen contains:

• one vial with powder (10 ml clear glass type 1 vial with latex-free grey bromobutyl rubber blend stopper and aluminium seal)

• one vial with solvent (10 ml clear glass type 2 vial with latex-free grey chlorobutyl rubber blend stopper and aluminium seal)

• an additional package with:

- 1 transfer device
- 1 filter needle
- 1 venipuncture set
- 1 plastic syringe (5 ml)
- two sterile alcohol swabs for single use

6.6 Instructions for use and handling

Detailed instructions for preparation and administration are contained in the package leaflet provided with Helixate NexGen.

Helixate NexGen powder should only be reconstituted with the supplied solvent (2.5 ml water for injections) using the supplied sterile transfer device. Gently rotate the vial until all powder is dissolved. Do not use Helixate NexGen if you notice visible particulate matter or turbidity.

After reconstitution, the solution is drawn through the sterile filter needle into the sterile disposable syringe (both supplied).

Any unused product or waste material should be disposed of in accordance with local requirements.

7. MARKETING AUTHORISATION HOLDER

Bayer AG

D-51368 Leverkusen

Germany

8. MARKETING AUTHORISATION NUMBER(S)

EU/1/00/144/002

9. DATE OF FIRST AUTHORISATION/RENEWAL OF THE AUTHORISATION

4 August 2000

10. DATE OF REVISION OF THE TEXT

26 November 2004

Hemabate Sterile Solution

(Pharmacia Limited)

1. NAME OF THE MEDICINAL PRODUCT

Hemabate Sterile Solution

2. QUALITATIVE AND QUANTITATIVE COMPOSITION

Each 1 ml contains carboprost tromethamine equivalent to carboprost 250 micrograms.

3. PHARMACEUTICAL FORM

Colourless, sterile, aqueous solution for intramuscular injection.

4. CLINICAL PARTICULARS

4.1 Therapeutic indications

Treatment of post-partum haemorrhage due to uterine atony and refractory to conventional methods of treatment with oxytocic agents and ergometrine used either alone or in combination.

Conventional therapy should usually consist of 0.5-1 mg ergometrine with up to 50 units of oxytocin infused intravenously over periods of time from 20 minutes to 12 hours. The dosage and duration of administration should reflect the seriousness of the clinical situation.

4.2 Posology and method of administration

Parenteral drug products should be inspected visually for particulate matter and discoloration prior to administration whenever solution and container permit.

An initial dose of 250 micrograms (1.0 ml) of Hemabate should be administered as a deep intramuscular injection.

If necessary, further doses of 250 micrograms may be administered at intervals of approximately 1.5 hours. In severe cases the interval between doses may be reduced at the discretion of the attending physician, but it should not be less than 15 minutes. The total dose of Hemabate should not exceed 2 mg (8 doses).

Elderly: Not applicable

Children: Not applicable

4.3 Contraindications

Hemabate should not be used where the patient is sensitive to carboprost tromethamine or any of the excipients.

Hemabate is not recommended in the following circumstances:

1. Acute pelvic inflammatory disease.

2. Patients with known cardiac, pulmonary, renal or hepatic disease.

4.4 Special warnings and special precautions for use

Warnings

This preparation should not be used for induction of labour.

Hemabate, as with other potent oxytocic agents, should be used only with strict adherence to recommended dosages. Hemabate should be used by medically trained personnel and is available only to hospitals and clinics with specialised obstetric units where 24 hour resident medical cover is provided.

Hemabate must not be given intravenously.

Very rare cases of cardiovascular collapse have been reported following the use of prostaglandins. This should always be considered when using Hemabate.

Precautions

Hemabate should be used with caution in patients with a history of glaucoma or raised intra-ocular pressure, asthma, hypertension or hypotension, cardiovascular disease, renal disease, hepatic disease, anaemia, jaundice, diabetes or epilepsy.

Animal studies lasting several weeks at high doses have shown that prostaglandins of the E and F series can induce proliferation of bone. Such effects have also been noted in newborn infants who have received prostaglandin E_1 during prolonged treatment. There is no evidence that short-term administration of Hemabate can cause similar bone effects.

Decreases in maternal arterial oxygen content have been observed in patients treated with carboprost tromethamine. A causal relationship to carboprost tromethamine has not been established, however, it is recommended that patients with pre-existing cardio-pulmonary problems receiving Hemabate are monitored during treatment and given additional oxygen if necessary.

4.5 Interaction with other medicinal products and other forms of Interaction

Prostaglandins may potentiate the effect of oxytocin

4.6 Pregnancy and lactation

Hemabate is contra-indicated in pregnancy.

In the unlikely event of a mother breastfeeding her baby whilst receiving Hemabate, no adverse effects to the nursing infant would be anticipated.

4.7 Effects on ability to drive and use machines

Not applicable

4.8 Undesirable effects

The adverse effects of Hemabate are generally transient and reversible when therapy ends.

The most frequent side-effects observed with the use of Hemabate are related to its contractile effect on smooth muscle. Thus nausea, vomiting and diarrhoea have been reported as commonly encountered. The incidence of vomiting and diarrhoea may be decreased by pre-treatment and concomitant use during treatment of anti-emetic and antidiarrhoeal agents.

Hyperthermia and flushing have been observed after intramuscular Hemabate, but if not complicated by endometritis, the temperature will usually return to normal within several hours of the last injection.

Asthma and wheezing have been noted with Hemabate treatment.

Less frequent, but potentially more serious adverse effects are elevated blood pressure, dyspnoea and pulmonary oedema. Other less serious adverse effects noted include chills, headache, diaphoresis, dizziness and injection site erythema and pain.

4.9 Overdose

Treatment of overdosage must be symptomatic at this time, as clinical studies with prostaglandin antagonists have not progressed to the point where recommendations may be made.

If evidence of excessive side-effects appears, the frequency of administration should be decreased or administration discontinued.

5. PHARMACOLOGICAL PROPERTIES

5.1 Pharmacodynamic properties

Carboprost is a synthetic 15-methyl analogue of dinoprost (prostaglandin F2 alpha). It is a uterine stimulant with a more prolonged action than dinoprost and when used in post-partum haemorrhage, it stimulates the uterus to contract in a manner similar to that normally observed in the uterus following delivery. The resulting myometrial contractions provide haemostasis at the site of placentation and hence prevent further blood loss. Whether or not this action results from a direct effect on the myometrium has not been determined with certainty at this time. The fundamental actions of the prostaglandins include inhibition or stimulation of smooth muscle contraction and inhibition of the release of noradrenaline or modulation of its effects at neuroeffector sites. They affect the uterus, the cardiovascular system, the gastro-intestinal system, the nervous system, the urinary system and metabolic processes.

5.2 Pharmacokinetic properties
The presence of the methyl group delays inactivation by enzymic dehydrogenation.

Peak plasma levels vary depending on the route of administration. In the Rhesus monkey after a single i.m. injection of 20-30 micrograms of 15-methyl PGF2 alpha peak levels of 0.4-5 nanograms/ml resulted at 30-60 minutes, declining to baseline levels 6-8 hours after injection. In pregnant women, an i.m. injection of 100-400 micrograms resulted in peak plasma levels of 1-1.6 nanograms/ml 20-30 minutes after injection. Levels declined to 0.2-0.4 nanograms/ml after 3 hours. When i.m. doses of 250 micrograms were given every two hours, pre-injection plasma levels stabilised after four injections at 1.2 nanograms/ml.

After administration of 2.5 mg 15-methyl PGF2 alpha intra-amniotically to 5 subjects, plasma levels were from 100-580 picograms/ml during the first 15 hours after administration. In three subjects the levels were low and fairly constant, while the two other had higher, but more variable levels.

6. PHARMACEUTICAL PARTICULARS
6.1 List of excipients
Benzyl alcohol

Sodium chloride

Tromethamine

Sodium hydroxide

Hydrochloric acid

Water for injections

6.2 Incompatibilities
None known

6.3 Shelf life
Ampoules: 48 months

Vial: 24 months

6.4 Special precautions for storage
The ampoules must be stored in a refrigerator at 2-8°C.

The vial must be stored in a refrigerator at 0-6°C

6.5 Nature and contents of container
Ampoule: Type 1 glass ampoule containing 1 ml solution, packed in cartons of two or ten ampoules.

Vial: Type 1 glass with butyl rubber closure, containing 10 ml solution, packed individually in a carton.

6.6 Instructions for use and handling
Parenteral drug products should be inspected visually for particulate matter and discoloration prior to administration whenever solution and container permit.

7. MARKETING AUTHORISATION HOLDER
Pharmacia Limited

Davy Avenue

Milton Keynes

MK5 8PH

UK

8. MARKETING AUTHORISATION NUMBER(S)
PL 0032/0152

9. DATE OF FIRST AUTHORISATION/RENEWAL OF THE AUTHORISATION
16 August 1990/23 February 1996

10. DATE OF REVISION OF THE TEXT
October 2001

Legal Category
POM.

Heminevrin Capsules

(AstraZeneca UK Limited)

1. NAME OF THE MEDICINAL PRODUCT
Heminevrin Capsules.

2. QUALITATIVE AND QUANTITATIVE COMPOSITION
Clomethiazole 192mg (as clomethiazole edisilate).

For excipients, see 6.1

3. PHARMACEUTICAL FORM
Capsule, soft.

4. CLINICAL PARTICULARS
4.1 Therapeutic indications
Heminevrin is a short acting hypnotic and sedative with anticonvulsant effect. It is used for the: management of restlessness and agitation in the elderly, short term treatment of severe insomnia in the elderly and treatment of alcohol withdrawal symptoms where close hospital supervision is also provided.

4.2 Posology and method of administration
For oral use.

Management of restlessness and agitation in the elderly: one capsule three times daily.

Severe insomnia in the elderly: 1 - 2 capsules before going to bed. The lower dose should be tried first. As with all psychotropic drugs, treatment should be kept to a minimum, reviewed regularly and discontinued as soon as possible.

Alcohol withdrawal states: Heminevrin is not a specific 'cure' for alcoholism. Alcohol withdrawal should be treated in hospital or, in exceptional circumstances, on an outpatient basis by specialist units when the daily dosage of Heminevrin must be monitored closely by community health staff. The dosage should be adjusted to patient response. The patient should be sedated but rousable. A suggested regimen is:

Initial dose: 2 to 4 capsules, if necessary repeated after some hours.

Day 1, first 24 hours: 9 to 12 capsules, divided into 3 or 4 doses.

Day 2: 6 to 8 capsules, divided into 3 or 4 doses.

Day 3: 4 to 6 capsules, divided into 3 or 4 doses.

Days 4 to 6: A gradual reduction in dosage until the final dose.

Administration for more than nine (9) days is not recommended.

4.3 Contraindications
Known sensitivity to clomethiazole. Acute pulmonary insufficiency.

4.4 Special warnings and special precautions for use
Heminevrin should be used cautiously in patients with chronic pulmonary insufficiency. Heminevrin may potentiate or be potentiated by centrally acting depressant drugs including alcohol and benzodiazepines. Fatal cardiorespiratory collapse has been reported when clomethiazole was combined with other CNS depressant drugs. When used concomitantly dosage should be appropriately reduced.

Hypoxia, resulting from, for example, cardiac and/or respiratory insufficiency, can manifest itself as an acute confusional state. Recognition and specific treatment of the cause is essential in such patients and in such cases sedatives/hypnotics should be avoided.

Moderate liver disorders associated with alcoholism do not preclude the use of clomethiazole, though an associated increase in systemic availability of oral doses and delayed elimination of the drug may require reduced dosage. Great caution should be observed in patients with gross liver damage and decreased liver function, particularly as sedation can mask the onset of liver coma.

Caution should be observed in patients with chronic renal disease.

Caution must be exercised in prescribing for individuals known to be addiction prone or for those whose histories suggest they may increase the dose on their own initiative since clomethiazole is not free from the risk of producing psychological and/or physical dependence. After prolonged administration of high doses, physical dependence has been reported with withdrawal symptoms such as convulsions, tremors, and organic psychosis. These reports have mainly been associated with indiscriminate prescribing to outpatient alcoholics and Heminevrin should not be prescribed to patients who continue to drink or abuse alcohol.

Alcoholism: Alcohol combined with clomethiazole particularly in alcoholics with cirrhosis can lead to fatal respiratory depression even with short term use. It should not therefore be prescribed for alcoholics who continue to drink alcoholic beverages.

Elderly: Caution is advised as there may be increased bioavailability and delayed elimination of clomethiazole.

Children: Oral Heminevrin is not recommended for use in children.

One capsule of Heminevrin contains 30mg of sorbitol. When taken according to the dosage recommendations each dose supplies up to 120mg of sorbitol. Unsuitable in hereditary fructose intolerance. Can cause stomach upset and diarrhoea.

4.5 Interaction with other medicinal products and other forms of Interaction
A combination of clomethiazole and diazoxide should be avoided as an adverse neonatal reaction suspected to be due to the maternal administration of this combination has been reported.

The combination of propranolol and clomethiazole has produced profound bradycardia in one patient possibly due to increased bioavailability of propranolol.

There is evidence to indicate that the metabolism of clomethiazole is inhibited by cimetidine, thus the co-administration of these drugs may lead to increased blood/plasma levels of clomethiazole.

When clomethiazole was administered by intravenous infusion in combination with carbamazepine, the clearance of clomethiazole increased by 30%, resulting in decreased plasma concentrations to the same extent. This interaction has not been studied after oral administration of clomethiazole. However, co-administration of carbamazepine and oral clomethiazole could result in both decreased bioavailability and increased clearance. Higher doses of clomethiazole could therefore be needed to obtain an effect when co-administered with carbamazepine or another potent inducer of the CYP3A4 enzyme.

4.6 Pregnancy and lactation
Do not use in pregnancy especially during the first and last trimesters, unless there are compelling reasons. There is no evidence of safety in human pregnancy, nor is there evidence from animal studies that it is entirely free from hazard.

Clomethiazole is excreted into the breast milk. The effect of even small quantities of sedative/hypnotic and anticonvulsant drugs on the infant brain is not established.

Clomethiazole should only be used in nursing mothers where the physician considers that the benefit outweighs the possible hazard to the infant.

4.7 Effects on ability to drive and use machines
As with all centrally acting depressant drugs, the driving of vehicles and the operating of machinery are to be avoided when under treatment.

4.8 Undesirable effects
The most common side-effect is nasal congestion and irritation, which may occur 15 to 20 minutes after drug ingestion. Conjunctival irritation has also been noted in some cases. Occasionally, these symptoms may be severe and may be associated with severe headache. This is commonest with the initial dose following which it decreases in severity with subsequent doses. Increased nasopharyngeal/bronchial secretions can occur.

Rash and urticaria have been reported. In rare cases, bullous skin eruptions have been reported.

Gastrointestinal disturbances have been reported.

Reversible increases of transaminases or bilirubin have been reported.

In rare cases anaphylactic reactions have occurred.

When Heminevrin has been given at higher than recommended doses for other than recommended indications over prolonged periods of time, physical dependence, tolerance and withdrawal reactions have been reported.

Great caution is required in prescribing Heminevrin for patients with a history of chronic alcoholism, drug abuse or marked personality disorder.

When used as a night-time hypnotic, hangover effects in the elderly may occur but are uncommon due to the short half-life.

Excessive sedation may occur, especially with higher doses or when given to the elderly for daytime sedation. Paradoxical excitement or confusion may occur rarely.

4.9 Overdose
The main effects to be expected with overdose of Heminevrin are: coma, respiratory depression, hypotension and hypothermia.

Hypothermia is thought to be due to a direct central effect as well as a result of lying unconscious for several hours. In addition, patients have increased secretion in the upper airways, which in one series was associated with a high incidence of pneumonia. The effects of overdosage are not usually severe in patients with no evidence of alcoholic liver disease, but they may be exacerbated when clomethiazole is taken in combination with alcohol and/or CNS depressant drugs, particularly those that are metabolised by the liver. There is no specific antidote to clomethiazole. Treatment of overdosage should therefore be carried out on a symptomatic basis, applying similar principles to those used in the treatment of barbiturate overdosage.

Charcoal column haemoperfusion is not and cannot be expected to be effective in treating clomethiazole poisoning.

5. PHARMACOLOGICAL PROPERTIES
5.1 Pharmacodynamic properties
Clomethiazole is pharmacologically distinct from both the benzodiazepines and the barbiturates

Clomethiazole has sedative, muscle relaxant and anticonvulsant properties. It is used for hypnosis in elderly and institutionalised patients, for preanaesthetic sedation and especially in the management of withdrawal from ethanol. Given alone its effects on respiration are slight and the therapeutic index high.

5.2 Pharmacokinetic properties
Clomethiazole has a short half-life, low oral bioavailability, high plasma clearance and shows no evidence of accumulation or altered pharmacokinetics after repeated dosage. It is excreted in urine after extensive metabolism in the liver. The rate of elimination is decreased by about 30% in liver cirrhosis.

5.3 Preclinical safety data
Extensive clinical use and experience with clomethiazole has provided a well established safety profile for this drug.

6. PHARMACEUTICAL PARTICULARS
6.1 List of excipients
Coconut oil fractionated, Gelatin, Glycerol, Sorbitol, Mannitol, Non hydrogenated Starch Hydrolysate, Titanium Dioxide, Brown Iron Oxide Paste (E172).

6.2 Incompatibilities
Not applicable.

6.3 Shelf life
Amber glass bottles: 36 months.

Aluminium foil blister packs: 24 months

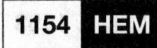

6.4 Special precautions for storage
Do not store above 25°C.

Store in the original container.

6.5 Nature and contents of container
Amber glass bottle with either a screw cap or clic-loc cap containing 60 or 100 capsules.

Transparent plastic bag in a cardboard outer for bulk packaging of 20,000 capsules.

Aluminium foil blister packs each containing 10 capsules.

6.6 Instructions for use and handling
The capsules should remain in the container in which they are supplied.

The capsules should be swallowed whole.

7. MARKETING AUTHORISATION HOLDER
AstraZeneca UK Ltd.,

600 Capability Green,

Luton,

LU1 3LU,

UK.

8. MARKETING AUTHORISATION NUMBER(S)
PL 17901/0126

9. DATE OF FIRST AUTHORISATION/RENEWAL OF THE AUTHORISATION
18th March 2002 / 7th March 2003

10. DATE OF REVISION OF THE TEXT
2nd February 2004

Heminevrin Syrup

(AstraZeneca UK Limited)

1. NAME OF THE MEDICINAL PRODUCT
Heminevrin Syrup.

2. QUALITATIVE AND QUANTITATIVE COMPOSITION
Clomethiazole 50mg/ml (as clomethiazole edisilate).

For excipients, see 6.1

3. PHARMACEUTICAL FORM
Syrup.

4. CLINICAL PARTICULARS

4.1 Therapeutic indications
Heminevrin is a short acting hypnotic and sedative with anticonvulsant effect. It is used for the: management of restlessness and agitation in the elderly, short term treatment of severe insomnia in the elderly and treatment of alcohol withdrawal symptoms where close hospital supervision is also provided.

4.2 Posology and method of administration
For oral use

Management of restlessness and agitation in the elderly: 5ml of syrup three times daily.

Severe insomnia in the elderly: 5 - 10ml of the syrup before going to bed. The lower dose should be tried first. As with all psychotropic drugs, treatment should be kept to a minimum, reviewed regularly and discontinued as soon as possible.

Alcohol withdrawal states: Heminevrin is not a specific 'cure' for alcoholism. Alcohol withdrawal should be treated in hospital or, in exceptional circumstances, on an out-patient basis by specialist units when the daily dosage of Heminevrin must be monitored closely by community health staff. The dosage should be adjusted to patient response. The patient should be sedated but rousable. A suggested regimen is:

Initial dose: 10 to 20ml, if necessary repeated after some hours.

Day 1, first 24 hours: 45 to 60ml, divided into 3 or 4 doses.

Day 2: 30 to 40ml, divided into 3 or 4 doses.

Day 3: 20 to 30ml, divided into 3 or 4 doses.

Days 4 to 6: A gradual reduction in dosage until the final dose.

Administration for more than nine (9) days is not recommended.

4.3 Contraindications
Known sensitivity to clomethiazole. Acute pulmonary insufficiency.

4.4 Special warnings and special precautions for use
Heminevrin should be used cautiously in patients with chronic pulmonary insufficiency. Heminevrin may potentiate or be potentiated by centrally acting depressant drugs including alcohol and benzodiazepines. Fatal cardiorespiratory collapse has been reported when clomethiazole was combined with other CNS depressant drugs. When used concomitantly dosage should be appropriately reduced.

Hypoxia, resulting from, for example, cardiac and/or respiratory insufficiency, can manifest itself as an acute confusional state. Recognition and specific treatment of the cause is essential in such patients and in such cases sedatives/hypnotics should be avoided.

Moderate liver disorders associated with alcoholism do not preclude the use of clomethiazole, though an associated increase in systemic availability of oral doses and delayed elimination of the drug may require reduced dosage. Great caution should be observed in patients with gross liver damage and decreased liver function, particularly as sedation can mask the onset of liver coma.

Caution should be observed in patients with chronic renal disease.

Caution must be exercised in prescribing for individuals known to be addiction prone or for those whose histories suggest they may increase the dose on their own initiative since clomethiazole is not free from the risk of producing psychological and/or physical dependence. After prolonged administration of high doses, physical dependence has been reported with withdrawal symptoms such as convulsions, tremors, and organic psychosis. These reports have mainly been associated with indiscriminate prescribing to outpatient alcoholics and Heminevrin should not be prescribed to patients who continue to drink or abuse alcohol.

Alcoholism: Alcohol combined with clomethiazole particularly in alcoholics with cirrhosis can lead to fatal respiratory depression even with short term use. It should not therefore be prescribed for alcoholics who continue to drink alcoholic beverages.

Elderly: Caution is advised as there may be increased bioavailability and delayed elimination of clomethiazole.

Children: Oral Heminevrin is not recommended for use in children.

Heminevrin syrup contains 0.13 vol % of ethanol. Each dose contains up to 20 mg of alcohol. Harmful for those suffering from liver disease, alcoholism, epilepsy, brain injury or disease, as well as for pregnant women and children. May modify or increase the effect of other medicines.

One ml of Heminevrin syrup contains 350 mg of sorbitol. When taken according to the dosage recommendations each dose supplies up to 7 g of sorbitol. Unsuitable in hereditary fructose intolerance. Can cause stomach upset and diarrhoea.

4.5 Interaction with other medicinal products and other forms of Interaction
A combination of clomethiazole and diazoxide should be avoided as an adverse neonatal reaction suspected to be due to the maternal administration of this combination has been reported.

The combination of propranolol and clomethiazole has produced profound bradycardia in one patient possibly due to increased bioavailability of propranolol.

There is evidence to indicate that the metabolism of clomethiazole is inhibited by cimetidine, thus the co-administration of these drugs may lead to increased blood/plasma levels of clomethiazole.

When clomethiazole was administered by intravenous infusion in combination with carbamazepine, the clearance of clomethiazole increased by 30%, resulting in decreased plasma concentrations to the same extent. This interaction has not been studied after oral administration of clomethiazole. However, co-administration of carbamazepine and oral clomethiazole could result in both decreased bioavailability and increased clearance. Higher doses of clomethiazole could therefore be needed to obtain an effect when co-administered with carbamazepine or another potent inducer of the CYP3A4 enzyme.

4.6 Pregnancy and lactation
Do not use in pregnancy especially during the first and last trimesters, unless there are compelling reasons. There is no evidence of safety in human pregnancy, nor is there evidence from animal studies that it is entirely free from hazard.

Clomethiazole is excreted into the breast milk. The effect of even small quantities of sedative/hypnotic and anticonvulsant drugs on the infant brain is not established.

Clomethiazole should only be used in nursing mothers where the physician considers that the benefit outweighs the possible hazard to the infant.

4.7 Effects on ability to drive and use machines
As with all centrally acting depressant drugs, the driving of vehicles and the operating of machinery are to be avoided when under treatment.

4.8 Undesirable effects
The most common side-effect is nasal congestion and irritation, which may occur 15 to 20 minutes after drug ingestion. Conjunctival irritation has also been noted in some cases. Occasionally, these symptoms may be severe and may be associated with severe headache. This is commonest with the initial dose following which it decreases in severity with subsequent doses. Increased nasopharyngeal/bronchial secretions can occur.

Rash and urticaria have been reported. In rare cases, bullous skin eruptions have been reported.

Gastrointestinal disturbances have been reported.

Reversible increases of transaminases or bilirubin have been reported.

In rare cases anaphylactic reactions have occurred.

When Heminevrin has been given at higher than recommended doses for other than recommended indications over prolonged periods of time, physical dependence, tolerance and withdrawal reactions have been reported.

Great caution is required in prescribing Heminevrin for patients with a history of chronic alcoholism, drug abuse or marked personality disorder.

When used as a night-time hypnotic, hangover effects in the elderly may occur but are uncommon due to the short half-life.

Excessive sedation may occur, especially with higher doses or when given to the elderly for daytime sedation. Paradoxical excitement or confusion may occur rarely.

4.9 Overdose
The main effects to be expected with overdose of Heminevrin are: coma, respiratory depression, hypotension and hypothermia.

Hypothermia is thought to be due to a direct central effect as well as a result of lying unconscious for several hours. In addition, patients have increased secretion in the upper airways, which in one series was associated with a high incidence of pneumonia. The effects of overdosage are not usually severe in patients with no evidence of alcoholic liver disease, but they may be exacerbated when clomethiazole is taken in combination with alcohol and/or CNS depressant drugs, particularly those that are metabolised by the liver. There is no specific antidote to clomethiazole. Treatment of overdosage should therefore be carried out on a symptomatic basis, applying similar principles to those used in the treatment of barbiturate overdosage.

Charcoal column haemoperfusion is not and cannot be expected to be effective in treating clomethiazole poisoning.

5. PHARMACOLOGICAL PROPERTIES

5.1 Pharmacodynamic properties
Clomethiazole is pharmacologically distinct from both the benzodiazepines and the barbiturates

Clomethiazole has sedative, muscle relaxant and anticonvulsant properties. It is used for hypnosis in elderly and institutionalised patients, for preanaesthetic sedation and especially in the management of withdrawal from ethanol. Given alone its effects on respiration are slight and the therapeutic index high.

5.2 Pharmacokinetic properties
Clomethiazole has a short half-life, low oral bioavailability, high plasma clearance and shows no evidence of accumulation or altered pharmacokinetics after repeated dosage. It is excreted in urine after extensive metabolism in the liver. The rate of elimination is decreased by about 30% in liver cirrhosis.

5.3 Preclinical safety data
Extensive clinical use and experience with clomethiazole has provided a well established safety profile for this drug.

6. PHARMACEUTICAL PARTICULARS

6.1 List of excipients
Sorbitol 70%, Cineole, Menthol, Ethanol 99.5% vol, Sodium hydroxide, Purified water.

6.2 Incompatibilities
Not applicable.

6.3 Shelf life
3 years.

6.4 Special precautions for storage
Store at 2-8°C (refrigerate). Do not freeze.

6.5 Nature and contents of container
300ml soda-glass bottle with a white polypropylene cap.

6.6 Instructions for use and handling
Not Applicable

7. MARKETING AUTHORISATION HOLDER
AstraZeneca UK Ltd.,

600 Capability Green,

Luton, LU1 3LU, UK.

8. MARKETING AUTHORISATION NUMBER(S)
PL 17901/0127

9. DATE OF FIRST AUTHORISATION/RENEWAL OF THE AUTHORISATION
18th March 2002 / 7th March 2003

10. DATE OF REVISION OF THE TEXT
16th January 2004

Hepatyrix

(GlaxoSmithKline UK)

1. NAME OF THE MEDICINAL PRODUCT
Hepatyrix

Hepatitis A (inactivated, adsorbed) and Typhoid Polysaccharide vaccine.

Suspension for injection

2. QUALITATIVE AND QUANTITATIVE COMPOSITION
1 dose (1 ml) contains:

Inactivated Hepatitis A virus (HM175 strain)* 1440 ELISA Units

Vi polysaccharide of Salmonella typhi (Ty2 strain) 25 micrograms

adsorbed on aluminium hydroxide (adjuvant) Total: 0.5 milligrams Al^{3+}

* propagated on MRC-5 human diploid cells

For excipients, see 6.1.

3. PHARMACEUTICAL FORM
Suspension for injection.

Slightly opaque white suspension.

4. CLINICAL PARTICULARS

4.1 Therapeutic indications
Active immunisation against hepatitis A virus infection and typhoid fever for adults and adolescents 15 years of age and older.

Hepatyrix should be given in accordance with official recommendations.

4.2 Posology and method of administration
Posology
Primary vaccination

A single dose of 1.0 ml is recommended for both adults and adolescents aged 15 years and older.

The vaccine should be given at least two weeks prior to risk of exposure to typhoid and hepatitis A (see section 5.1 for immunogenicity data).

Booster vaccination

In order to provide long term protection against infection caused by hepatitis A virus, a booster dose of an inactivated hepatitis A vaccine is recommended at any time between 6 and 12 months after a single dose of Hepatyrix.

Hepatyrix may also be given as a single dose of 1.0 ml for booster vaccination between 6 and 12 months following primary immunisation with an inactivated hepatitis A vaccine to subjects who also require protection against typhoid fever.

Subjects who remain at risk of typhoid fever should be revaccinated using a single dose of Vi polysaccharide vaccine every 3 years, unless it is also appropriate to administer a booster of hepatitis A vaccine, in which case Hepatyrix may be used.

As Hepatyrix has not been studied in subjects under 15 years of age, it is not recommended for use in this age group.

Method of Administration

Hepatyrix is for intramuscular administration in the deltoid region.

The vaccine should not be administered in the gluteal region.

Hepatyrix should under no circumstances be administered intravascularly.

Hepatyrix should not be administered subcutaneously/ intradermally since administration by these routes may result in a suboptimal response to the vaccine.

In exceptional circumstances, Hepatyrix may be administered subcutaneously to subjects with thrombocytopenia or bleeding disorders since bleeding may occur following an intramuscular administration to these subjects. Firm pressure should be applied to the injection site (without rubbing) for at least two minutes after the injection.

4.3 Contraindications
Hepatyrix should not be administered to subjects who have had a hypersensitivity reaction to a previous dose of Hepatyrix or a dose of either of the monovalent vaccines Havrix™ and Typherix™.

Hepatyrix should not be administered to subjects who are known to be hypersensitive to any component of the vaccine.

Hepatyrix contains traces of neomycin. The vaccine should not be used in subjects with known hypersensitivity to neomycin.

As with other vaccines, the administration of Hepatyrix should be postponed in subjects suffering from acute severe febrile illness. The presence of a minor infection, however, is not a contra-indication for vaccination.

4.4 Special warnings and special precautions for use
As with all injectable vaccines, appropriate medical treatment and supervision should always be readily available in case of a rare anaphylactic event following the administration of the vaccine.

In subjects with an impaired immune system, adequate anti-HAV and anti-Vi antibody titres may not be obtained after a single dose of Hepatyrix and such patients may therefore require administration of additional doses of vaccine. If possible, vaccination should be delayed until the completion of any immunosuppressive treatment. Subjects with chronic immunodeficiency such as HIV infection may be vaccinated if the underlying immunodeficiency allows the induction of an antibody response, even if limited.

It is possible that subjects may be in the incubation period of a hepatitis A infection at the time of vaccination. It is not known whether Hepatyrix will prevent clinically apparent hepatitis A infections in such cases.

Hepatyrix will not prevent infection caused by other hepatitis-causing agents such as hepatitis B virus, hepatitis C virus, hepatitis E virus or other pathogens known to infect the liver.

Hepatyrix protects only against typhoid fever caused by *Salmonella enterica serotype Typhi*. Protection is not conferred against paratyphoid fever or infections with any other serotypes of *S. enterica*.

As with any vaccine, a protective immune response may not be elicited in all vaccinees.

4.5 Interaction with other medicinal products and other forms of Interaction
Hepatyrix must not be mixed with any other vaccine in the same syringe.

If Hepatyrix is to be given at the same time as (an)other injectable vaccine(s), the vaccines should always be administered at different injection sites.

Hepatyrix contains purified inactivated hepatitis A antigen and purified Vi capsular polysaccharide. Although concomitant use with other inactivated vaccines has not specifically been studied, it is anticipated that no interaction will be observed.

Concomitant administration of yellow fever vaccine with Hepatyrix has not been specifically assessed. However, based on data obtained from the concomitant administration of various monovalent vaccines (purified Vi polysaccharide typhoid vaccine or inactivated hepatitis A vaccine) with yellow fever vaccine, no interference with the immune responses to any of these antigens would be expected.

The effect of concomitant administration of immunoglobulins on the immunogenicity of Hepatyrix has not been assessed. Therefore, interference with the immune response cannot be ruled out.

4.6 Pregnancy and lactation
Pregnancy

Adequate human data on use during pregnancy and adequate animal reproduction studies are not available. Hepatyrix should only be used after careful consideration of the risk-benefit relationship.

Lactation

Adequate data on the administration of Hepatyrix to women who are breast-feeding their infants are not available. Hepatyrix should be used during breast-feeding only when clearly needed.

4.7 Effects on ability to drive and use machines
Some of the effects mentioned under section 4.8 "Undesirable effects" may affect the ability to drive or operate machinery.

4.8 Undesirable effects
In controlled clinical studies, the most commonly reported reactions after administration of Hepatyrix were those at the site of injection. All local and general symptoms resolved without any sequelae.

Frequencies are reported as:

Very common: $\geqslant$ 10%

Common: $\geqslant$ 1% and $<$ 10%

Uncommon: $\geqslant$ 0.1% and $<$ 1%

Rare: $\geqslant$ 0.01% and $<$ 0.1%

Very rare: $<$ 0.01%

Application site:

Very common: pain, erythema

Common: swelling

Systemic adverse events with at least a suspected causal relationship to vaccination are listed below:

Body as a whole:

Common: malaise, headache, general aches, fever

Gastro-intestinal system:

Common: nausea

Skin and appendages:

Common: itching

During postmarketing surveillance, the following undesirable events have been reported in temporal association with Hepatyrix vaccination:

Body as a whole:

Very rare: allergic reactions, including anaphylaxis and anaphylactoid reactions

Cardiovascular general:

Very rare: syncope

Skin and appendages:

Very rare: skin rashes

In controlled clinical studies with the GlaxoSmithKline monovalent hepatitis A vaccine, systemic adverse events such as vomiting and loss of appetite have been reported.

During postmarketing surveillance, the following undesirable effects have been reported very rarely with the GlaxoSmithKline monovalent hepatitis A vaccine: convulsions, arthralgia, myalgia, neurological manifestations, including transverse myelitis, Guillain-Barre syndrome and neuralgic amyotrophy.

4.9 Overdose
No case of overdose has been reported.

5. PHARMACOLOGICAL PROPERTIES
Pharmaco-therapeutic group: Bacterial and viral vaccines combined, ATC code JO7C (combined)/P03 (typhoid)/C02 (Hepatitis A)

5.1 Pharmacodynamic properties
Hepatyrix confers immunity against typhoid fever and HAV infection by inducing specific anti-Vi and anti-HAV antibodies.

In clinical studies involving 462 subjects of 15-50 years of age, seropositivity rates for anti-HAV and anti-Vi antibodies were 89.8% and 97.5% respectively two weeks after primary immunisation. At month 1, seropositivity rates for anti-HAV and anti-Vi antibodies were 99.0% and 95.7% respectively.

In a clinical study where a group of 99 subjects received a booster dose of hepatitis A vaccine 12 months following the initial dose of Hepatyrix, all subjects were seropositive for anti-HAV antibodies one month later (i.e. at month 13).

When Hepatyrix was given 12 months following primary vaccination with the hepatitis A vaccine in a cohort of 97 subjects, the seropositivity rates for anti-Vi and anti-HAV antibodies were 88.2% and 100% respectively one month later (i.e. at month 13).

In a long term clinical study, the persistence of antibodies has been evaluated in 118 subjects up to 36 months after vaccination with Hepatyrix and a booster dose of Havrix™ 1440 administered six months later. At month 36, 53% were still seropositive with respect to anti-Vi antibody and 100% for anti-HAV antibodies. These seropositivity rates are similar to those seen in subjects in other clinical trials who were followed up for a similar period after vaccination with either of the licensed monovalent Vi polysaccharide vaccines or a licensed hepatitis A vaccine.

With respect to the hepatitis A component, based on data generated after administration of a booster dose of a monovalent hepatitis A vaccine between six and twelve months following the initial dose of the monovalent hepatitis A vaccine, it is predicted that anti-HAV antibodies persist for many years (at least 10 years).

5.2 Pharmacokinetic properties
Evaluation of pharmacokinetic properties is not required for vaccines.

5.3 Preclinical safety data
Preclinical data reveal no special hazard for humans based on general safety studies.

6. PHARMACEUTICAL PARTICULARS

6.1 List of excipients
Sodium chloride

2-phenoxyethanol (preservative)

Water for injections.

For adjuvants, see section 2.

6.2 Incompatibilities
This vaccine must not be mixed with other medicinal products.

6.3 Shelf life
2 years.

6.4 Special precautions for storage
Store at 2°C – 8°C (in a refrigerator).

Store in the original package in order to protect from light.

Do not freeze. Discard if vaccine has been frozen.

6.5 Nature and contents of container
1 ml of suspension in prefilled syringe (type I glass) with a plunger stopper (butyl rubber) with or without needles. Packs of 1 and 10 (with needles). Packs of 1, 10, 20 and 50 (without needles).

Not all packs may be marketed.

6.6 Instructions for use and handling
The vaccine's normal appearance is a cloudy white suspension, which may sediment during storage. Shake the container well to distribute the suspension uniformly before administering the vaccine.

The vaccine should be inspected visually for extraneous particulate matter and/or discolouration prior to administration. Any unused vaccine or waste material should be disposed of safely in accordance with local regulations.

Administrative Data

7. MARKETING AUTHORISATION HOLDER
SmithKline Beecham plc

Trading as:

GlaxoSmithKline UK,

Stockley Park West,

Uxbridge,

Middlesex, UB11 1BT8.

8. MARKETING AUTHORISATION NUMBER(S)
PL10592/0136

9. DATE OF FIRST AUTHORISATION/RENEWAL OF THE AUTHORISATION
22 June 2004

10. DATE OF REVISION OF THE TEXT
October 2004

11. Legal Status
POM

Hepsal injection 10 iu/ml

(Wockhardt UK Ltd)

1. NAME OF THE MEDICINAL PRODUCT
Hepsal 10 I.U./ml

2. QUALITATIVE AND QUANTITATIVE COMPOSITION
Heparin sodium (mucous) 10 I.U./ml

For excipients see 6.1

3. PHARMACEUTICAL FORM
Solution for injection

A colourless or straw coloured liquid, free from turbidity, and from matter that deposits on standing.

4. CLINICAL PARTICULARS
4.1 Therapeutic indications
Heparin is an anticoagulant and acts by potentiating the naturally occurring inhibitors of thrombin and factor X (Xa).

Hepsal is indicated in any clinical circumstances in which it is desired to maintain the patency of indwelling catheters/ cannulae, attendant lines or heparin locks.

4.2 Posology and method of administration
Hepsal is not recommended for systemic use.

For cleaning indwelling cannulae.

Material to be used as a cannula flush (5ml; 50 units) every four hours or as required.

4.3 Contraindications
The very rare occurrence of established hypersensitivity to heparin is the only contraindication to Hepsal.

4.4 Special warnings and special precautions for use
Caution should be exercised in patients with known hypersensitivity to low molecular weight heparins.

Rigorous aseptic technique should be observed at all times in its use.

Platelet counts should be measured in patients receiving heparin flushes for longer than seven days (or earlier in patients with previous exposure to heparin). In those who develop thrombocytopenia or paradoxical thrombosis, heparin should immediately be eliminated from all flushes and ports.

Repeated flushing of a catheter device with heparin may result in a systemic anticoagulant effect.

4.5 Interaction with other medicinal products and other forms of Interaction
When an indwelling device is used for repeated withdrawal of blood samples for laboratory analyses and the presence of heparin or saline is likely to interfere with or alter results of the desired blood tests, the in situ heparin flush solution should be cleared from the device by aspirating and discarding a volume of solution equivalent to that of the indwelling venipuncture device before the desired blood sample is taken.

4.6 Pregnancy and lactation
The safety of Hepsal in pregnancy is not established, but the dose of heparin involved would not be expected to constitute a hazard.

Heparin does not appear in breast milk.

4.7 Effects on ability to drive and use machines
None stated.

4.8 Undesirable effects
Used as directed, it is extremely unlikely that the low levels of heparin reaching the blood will have any systemic effect. However, there have been rare reports of immune-mediated thrombocytopenia and thrombosis in patients receiving heparin flushes (see also Section 4.4, Special Warnings and Precautions for Use).

Hypersensitivity reactions to heparin are rare. They include urticaria, conjunctivitis, rhinitis, asthma, cyanosis, tachypnoea, feeling of oppression, fever, chills, angioneurotic oedema and anaphylactic shock.

4.9 Overdose
None stated

5. PHARMACOLOGICAL PROPERTIES
5.1 Pharmacodynamic properties
Hepsal, containing only 50 I.U. of sodium heparin per ampoule (5ml), is used for flushing indwelling cannulae. This is unlikely to produce blood levels of heparin having any systemic effect.

5.2 Pharmacokinetic properties
None stated

5.3 Preclinical safety data
There are no pre-clinical data of relevance to the prescriber which are additional to those already included in other sections.

6. PHARMACEUTICAL PARTICULARS
6.1 List of excipients
Sodium chloride

Water for injections

Hydrochloric acid 3M

Sodium hydroxide 3M

6.2 Incompatibilities
Heparin and reteplase are incompatible when combined in solution.

If reteplase and heparin are to be given through the same line this, together with any Y-lines, must be thoroughly flushed with a 0.9% saline or a 5% glucose solution prior to and following the reteplase injection.

6.3 Shelf life
Unopened – 36 months

From a microbiological point of view, unless the method of opening precludes the risk of microbial contamination, the product should be used immediately.

If not used immediately, in-use storage times and conditions are the responsibility of the user.

6.4 Special precautions for storage
Do not store above 25°C

Store in the original package

6.5 Nature and contents of container
5ml clear glass ampoules. Carton contains 10 ampoules.

6.6 Instructions for use and handling
Not applicable

Administrative Data
7. MARKETING AUTHORISATION HOLDER
CP Pharmaceuticals Ltd

Ash Road North

Wrexham

LL13 9UF

UK.

8. MARKETING AUTHORISATION NUMBER(S)
4543/0228

9. DATE OF FIRST AUTHORISATION/RENEWAL OF THE AUTHORISATION
Date of first authorisation - 5 July 1991

Date of renewal – 28 September 2000

10. DATE OF REVISION OF THE TEXT
August 2001

Hepsera 10 mg tablets

(Gilead Sciences International Limited)

1. NAME OF THE MEDICINAL PRODUCT
Hepsera 10 mg tablets ▼

2. QUALITATIVE AND QUANTITATIVE COMPOSITION
Each tablet contains 10 mg adefovir dipivoxil equivalent to 5.45 mg adefovir.

For excipients, see 6.1.

3. PHARMACEUTICAL FORM
Tablet.

White to off-white, round, flat-faced, bevelled-edge tablets, debossed with "GILEAD" and "10" on one side and a stylised shape of a liver on the other side.

4. CLINICAL PARTICULARS
4.1 Therapeutic indications
Hepsera is indicated for the treatment of chronic hepatitis B in adults with:

• compensated liver disease with evidence of active viral replication, persistently elevated serum alanine aminotransferase (ALT) levels and histological evidence of active liver inflammation and fibrosis

• decompensated liver disease.

4.2 Posology and method of administration
Therapy should be initiated by a physician experienced in the management of chronic hepatitis B.

Adults: The recommended dose of Hepsera is 10 mg (one tablet) once daily taken orally with or without food.

Higher doses must not be administered.

The optimum duration of treatment is unknown. The relationship between treatment response and long-term outcomes such as hepatocellular carcinoma or decompensated cirrhosis is not known.

Patients should be monitored every six months for hepatitis B biochemical, virological and serological markers.

Treatment discontinuation may be considered as follows:

In HBeAg positive patients, treatment should be administered at least until HBeAg seroconversion (HBeAg and HBV DNA loss with HBeAb detection on 2 consecutive serum samples at least 3 months apart) or until HBsAg seroconversion or in case of evidence of loss of efficacy (see 4.4).

In HBeAg negative (pre-core mutant) patients, treatment should be administered at least until HBsAg seroconversion or in case of evidence of loss of efficacy (see 4.4).

In patients with decompensated liver disease or cirrhosis, treatment cessation is not recommended (see 4.4).

Children and adolescents: The safety and efficacy of Hepsera in patients under the age of 18 years have not been established. Hepsera should not be administered to children or adolescents.

Elderly: No data are available to support a dose recommendation for patients over the age of 65 years (see 4.4).

Renal insufficiency: Adefovir is eliminated by renal excretion, therefore adjustments of the dosing interval are required in patients with a creatinine clearance < 50 ml/min, as detailed below. The recommended dosing frequency according to renal function must not be exceeded (see 4.4 and 5.2). The proposed dose interval modification is based on extrapolation of limited data in patients with end stage renal disease (ESRD) and may not be optimal. The safety and effectiveness of these dosing interval adjustment guidelines have not been clinically evaluated. Therefore, clinical response to treatment and renal function should be closely monitored in these patients (see 4.4).

(see Table 1 below)

No dosing recommendations are available for non-haemodialysed patients with creatinine clearance < 10 ml/min.

Hepatic impairment: No dose adjustment is required in patients with hepatic impairment (see 5.2).

4.3 Contraindications
• Hypersensitivity to the active substance or to any of the excipients.

4.4 Special warnings and special precautions for use
Renal function: Treatment with adefovir dipivoxil may result in renal impairment. While the overall risk of renal impairment in patients with adequate renal function is low, this is of special importance in patients at risk of, or having underlying renal dysfunction and in patients receiving medicinal products that may affect renal function.

Adefovir is excreted renally, by a combination of glomerular filtration and active tubular secretion, therefore adjustments to the dosing interval of 10 mg adefovir dipivoxil are recommended in patients with creatinine clearance < 50 ml/min (see 4.2).

Apart from ibuprofen, lamivudine, paracetamol and trimethoprim/sulfamethoxazole, the effect of co-administration of 10 mg adefovir dipivoxil with medicinal products that are excreted renally or other medicinal products known to affect renal function has not been evaluated (e.g. intravenous aminoglycosides, amphotericin B, foscarnet, pentamidine, vancomycin, or medicinal products which are secreted by the same renal transporter, human Organic Anion Transporter 1 (hOAT1), such as cidofovir or tenofovir disoproxil fumarate). In healthy volunteers, a single dose of adefovir dipivoxil given with tenofovir disoproxil fumarate does not result in a relevant drug-drug interaction with regard to pharmacokinetics. However, the clinical safety, including potential renal effects of the co-administration of adefovir dipivoxil and tenofovir disoproxil fumarate is unknown. Such co-administration is only advisable if the patient is closely monitored.

Co-administration of 10 mg adefovir dipivoxil with medicinal products that are eliminated by active tubular secretion may lead to an increase in serum concentrations of either adefovir or a co-administered medicinal product due to competition for this elimination pathway (see 4.5).

Patients with normal renal function should be monitored for changes in serum creatinine every 3 months and creatinine clearance calculated.

Caution is advised in patients with creatinine clearance < 50 ml/min and in patients receiving medicinal products that may effect renal function. The renal function of these patients should be closely monitored with a frequency tailored to the individual patient's medical condition.

Patients with creatinine clearance below 10 ml/min have not been studied (see 4.2). These patients should be closely monitored for possible adverse reactions and to ensure efficacy is maintained.

Table 1

	Creatinine Clearance (ml/min)*		Haemodialysis Patients
	20-49	10-19	
Recommended Dosing Interval	Every 48 hours	Every 72 hours	Every 7 days following dialysis**

* Calculated using ideal body weight

** After 12 hours cumulative dialysis or three dialysis sessions, each of four hours duration

Patients with ESRD managed with other forms of dialysis such as ambulatory peritoneal dialysis have not been studied.

Hepatic function: Spontaneous exacerbations in chronic hepatitis B are relatively common and are characterised by transient increases in serum ALT. After initiating antiviral therapy, serum ALT may increase in some patients as serum HBV DNA levels decline. In patients with compensated liver disease, these increases in serum ALT are generally not accompanied by an increase in serum bilirubin concentrations or hepatic decompensation (see 4.8). Patients with cirrhosis may be at a higher risk for hepatic decompensation following hepatitis exacerbation, and therefore should be monitored closely during therapy.

Patients should be closely monitored for several months after stopping treatment as exacerbations of hepatitis have occurred after discontinuation of 10 mg adefovir dipivoxil. These exacerbations occurred in the absence of HBeAg seroconversion and presented as serum ALT elevations and increases in serum HBV DNA. Elevations in serum ALT that occurred in patients treated with 10 mg adefovir dipivoxil were not accompanied by clinical and laboratory changes associated with liver decompensation. Although most events appear to have been self-limiting or resolved with re-initiation of treatment, severe hepatitis flares, including fatalities, have been reported in some cases. The relationship of exacerbation of hepatitis to discontinuation of adefovir dipivoxil is unknown. Patients should be closely monitored after stopping treatment. Most post-treatment exacerbations of hepatitis were seen within 12 weeks of discontinuation of 10 mg adefovir dipivoxil. In patients with decompensated liver disease or cirrhosis, treatment cessation is not recommended.

Lactic acidosis and severe hepatomegaly with steatosis: Occurrences of lactic acidosis (in the absence of hypoxaemia), sometimes fatal, usually associated with severe hepatomegaly and hepatic steatosis, have been reported with the use of nucleoside analogues. As adefovir is structurally related to nucleoside analogues, this risk cannot be excluded. Treatment with nucleoside analogues should be discontinued when rapidly elevating aminotransferase levels, progressive hepatomegaly or metabolic/lactic acidosis of unknown aetiology occur. Benign digestive symptoms, such as nausea, vomiting and abdominal pain, might be indicative of lactic acidosis development. Severe cases, sometimes with fatal outcome, were associated with pancreatitis, liver failure/hepatic steatosis, renal failure and higher levels of serum lactate. Caution should be exercised when prescribing nucleoside analogues to any patient (particularly obese women) with hepatomegaly, hepatitis or other known risk factors for liver disease. These patients should be followed closely.

To differentiate between elevations in transaminases due to response to treatment and increases potentially related to lactic acidosis, physicians should ensure that changes in ALT are associated with improvements in other laboratory markers of chronic hepatitis B.

Co-infection with hepatitis C or D: There are no data on the efficacy of adefovir dipivoxil in patients co-infected with hepatitis C or hepatitis D.

Co-infection with HIV: Limited data are available on the safety and efficacy of 10 mg adefovir dipivoxil in patients with chronic hepatitis B, co-infected with HIV. To date there is no evidence that daily dosing with 10 mg adefovir dipivoxil results in emergence of adefovir-associated resistance mutations in the HIV reverse transcriptase. Nonetheless, there is a potential risk of selection of HIV strains resistant to adefovir with possible cross-resistance to other antiviral medicinal products.

As far as possible, treatment of hepatitis B by adefovir dipivoxil in an HIV co-infected patient should be reserved for patients whose HIV RNA is controlled. Treatment with 10 mg adefovir dipivoxil has not been shown to be effective against HIV replication and therefore should not be used to control HIV infection.

Elderly: The clinical experience in patients > 65 years of age is very limited. Caution should be exercised when prescribing adefovir dipivoxil to the elderly, keeping in mind the greater frequency of decreased renal or cardiac function in these patients, and the increase in concomitant diseases or concomitant use of other medicinal products in the elderly.

General: Patients should be advised that therapy with adefovir dipivoxil has not been proven to reduce the risk of transmission of hepatitis B virus to others and therefore appropriate precautions should still be taken.

4.5 Interaction with other medicinal products and other forms of Interaction

The potential for CYP450 mediated interactions involving adefovir with other medicinal products is low, based on the results of *in vitro* experiments in which adefovir did not influence any of the common CYP isoforms known to be involved in human drug metabolism and based on the known elimination pathway of adefovir.

Concomitant administration of 10 mg adefovir dipivoxil and 100 mg lamivudine did not alter the pharmacokinetic profile of either medicinal product.

Adefovir did not alter the pharmacokinetics of trimethoprim/sulfamethoxazole, paracetamol, ibuprofen and tenofovir disoproxil fumarate, four medicinal products that also undergo or may affect tubular secretion.

The pharmacokinetics of adefovir were unaltered when 10 mg adefovir dipivoxil was co-administered with trimethoprim/sulfamethoxazole, paracetamol or tenofovir disoproxil fumarate (see 4.4).

Concomitant administration of 10 mg adefovir dipivoxil and 800 mg ibuprofen 3 times daily resulted in increases in AUC and C_{max} of adefovir of 23 % and 33 %, respectively. These increases are considered to be due to higher bioavailability rather than a reduction in renal clearance and are not considered clinically relevant.

Adefovir is excreted renally, by a combination of glomerular filtration and active tubular secretion. Apart from ibuprofen, lamivudine, paracetamol, trimethoprim/sulfamethoxazole and tenofovir disoproxil fumarate the effect of co-administration of 10 mg adefovir dipivoxil with medicinal products that are excreted renally, or other medicinal products known to affect renal function has not been evaluated. Co-administration of 10 mg adefovir dipivoxil with other medicinal products that are eliminated by tubular secretion or alter tubular function may increase serum concentrations of either adefovir or the co-administered medicinal product (see 4.4).

At doses of adefovir dipivoxil 6- to 12-fold higher than the 10 mg dose recommended for the treatment of chronic hepatitis B, there were no interactions with zidovudine, nelfinavir, nevirapine, indinavir, efavirenz, delavirdine, or lamivudine. Concomitant administration of 60 mg adefovir dipivoxil with saquinavir soft capsules resulted in an increase in adefovir AUC (20 %) and concomitant administration with didanosine buffered tablets resulted in an increase in didanosine AUC (29 %). Neither of these increases in systemic exposure were considered clinically significant.

No data on the concomitant use with other medicinal products (including interferon) are available.

4.6 Pregnancy and lactation

Pregnancy: There are no adequate data on the use of adefovir dipivoxil in pregnant women.

Studies in animals administered adefovir intravenously have shown reproductive toxicity (see 5.3). Studies in orally dosed animals do not indicate teratogenic or foetotoxic effects.

Adefovir dipivoxil should be used during pregnancy only if the potential benefit justifies the potential risk to the foetus.

There are no data on the effect of adefovir dipivoxil on transmission of HBV from mother to infant. Therefore, the standard recommended procedures for immunisation of infants should be followed to prevent neonatal acquisition of HBV.

Given that the potential risks to developing human foetuses are unknown, it is recommended that women of child-bearing potential treated with adefovir dipivoxil use effective contraception.

Lactation: It is not known whether adefovir is excreted in human milk. Mothers should be instructed not to breast-feed if they are taking adefovir dipivoxil tablets.

4.7 Effects on ability to drive and use machines

No studies on the effects on the ability to drive and use machines have been performed.

4.8 Undesirable effects

Experience in patients with compensated liver disease: Assessment of adverse reactions is based on two placebo-controlled studies in which 522 patients with chronic hepatitis B and compensated liver disease received double-blind treatment with 10 mg adefovir dipivoxil (n=294) or placebo (n=228) for 48 weeks. With extended therapy 492 of these 522 patients were treated with 10 mg adefovir dipivoxil for up to 109 weeks, with a median duration of treatment of 49 weeks.

The adverse reactions considered at least possibly related to treatment in the first 48 weeks of treatment are listed below, by body system organ class, and absolute frequency. Frequencies are defined as very common ($> 1/10$) or common ($> 1/100$, $< 1/10$).

Gastrointestinal:

Common ($> 1/100$, $< 1/10$): nausea, flatulence, diarrhoea, dyspepsia.

Body as a whole:

Very common ($> 1/10$): asthenia.

Common ($> 1/100$, $< 1/10$): abdominal pain, headache.

There was no clinically relevant difference in laboratory abnormalities observed in these studies in the 10 mg adefovir dipivoxil and placebo-treated groups with the exception of hepatic transaminase elevations, which occurred more frequently in the placebo-treated group. With extended treatment, mild to moderate increases in serum creatinine were observed uncommonly ($< 1/100$) in patients with chronic hepatitis B and compensated liver disease treated with 10 mg adefovir dipivoxil for a median of 49 weeks and a maximum of 109 weeks. These increases in serum creatinine resolved, one with continuation of adefovir dipivoxil therapy and one following discontinuation of therapy. Clinical and laboratory evidence of exacerbations of hepatitis have occurred after discontinuation of treatment with 10 mg adefovir dipivoxil (see 4.4).

Experience in patients pre- and post-transplantation with lamivudine-resistant HBV: Pre- (n=128) and post-liver transplantation patients (n=196) with chronic hepatitis B and lamivudine-resistant HBV were treated in an open-label study with 10 mg adefovir dipivoxil once daily, for up to 129 weeks, with a median time on treatment of 19 and 56 weeks, respectively. The adverse reactions considered at least possibly related to treatment are listed below, by body system organ class, and absolute frequency. Frequencies are defined as very common ($> 1/10$) or common ($> 1/100$, $< 1/10$).

Gastrointestinal:

Common ($> 1/100$, $< 1/10$): nausea, flatulence, diarrhoea, dyspepsia.

Body as a whole:

Common ($> 1/100$, $< 1/10$): asthenia, abdominal pain, headache.

Urogenital system:

Very common ($> 1/10$): increases in creatinine.

Common ($> 1/100$, $< 1/10$): renal insufficiency and renal failure.

Changes in serum creatinine were observed very commonly. These changes were seen in patients with multiple risk factors for changes in renal function, including concomitant use of cyclosporin and tacrolimus, and were generally mild to moderate in severity, although some cases of renal failure have been reported.

Experience post-marketing: In addition to adverse drug reaction reports from clinical trials the following possible adverse reactions have also been identified during post-approval use of adefovir dipivoxil.

Skin and subcutaneous tissue disorders:

Rash, pruritus.

4.9 Overdose

Administration of 500 mg adefovir dipivoxil daily for 2 weeks and 250 mg daily for 12 weeks has been associated with the gastrointestinal disorders listed above and additionally vomiting and anorexia.

If overdose occurs, the patient must be monitored for evidence of toxicity, and standard supportive treatment applied as necessary.

Adefovir can be removed by haemodialysis; the median haemodialysis clearance of adefovir is 104 ml/min. The elimination of adefovir by peritoneal dialysis has not been studied.

5. PHARMACOLOGICAL PROPERTIES

5.1 Pharmacodynamic properties

Pharmacotherapeutic group: Antiviral for systemic use, ATC code: J05AF08.

Adefovir dipivoxil is an oral prodrug of adefovir, an acyclic nucleotide phosphonate analogue of adenosine monophosphate, which is actively transported into mammalian cells where it is converted by host enzymes to adefovir diphosphate. Adefovir diphosphate inhibits viral polymerases by competing for direct binding with the natural substrate (deoxyadenosine triphosphate) and, after incorporation into viral DNA, causes DNA chain termination. Adefovir diphosphate selectively inhibits HBV DNA polymerases at concentrations 12-, 700-, and 10-fold lower than those needed to inhibit human DNA polymerases α, β, and γ, respectively. Adefovir diphosphate has an intracellular half-life of 12 to 36 hours in activated and resting lymphocytes.

Adefovir is active against hepadnaviruses *in vitro*, including all common forms of lamivudine-resistant HBV (rtL180M, rtM204I, rtM204V, rtL180M/rtM204V), famciclovir-associated mutations (rtV173L, rtP177L, rtL180M, rtT184S or rtV207I) and hepatitis B immunoglobulin escape mutations (rtT128N and rtW153Q), and in *in vivo* animal models of hepadnavirus replication.

Clinical experience: The demonstration of the benefit of adefovir dipivoxil is based on histological, virological, biochemical, and serological responses in adults with:

- HBeAg positive and HBeAg negative chronic hepatitis B with compensated liver disease.
- clinical evidence of lamivudine-resistant HBV with either compensated or decompensated liver disease, including patients pre- and post-liver transplantation or co-infected with HIV. In the majority of these studies adefovir dipivoxil 10 mg was added to ongoing lamivudine treatment in patients failing lamivudine therapy. The optimal therapeutic management of patients with lamivudine-resistant HBV has not yet been established. It is therefore unknown whether adefovir dipivoxil should be added to ongoing lamivudine treatment or whether patients should be treated with adefovir dipivoxil alone.

In these clinical studies patients had active viral replication (HBV DNA $\geqslant$ 100,000 copies/ml) and elevated ALT levels ($\geqslant 1.2 \times$ Upper Limit of Normal (ULN)).

Experience in patients with compensated liver disease: In two placebo-controlled studies (total n=522) in HBeAg positive or in HBeAg negative chronic hepatitis B patients with compensated liver disease, significantly more patients ($p < 0.001$) in the 10 mg adefovir dipivoxil groups (53 and 64 %, respectively) had histological improvement from baseline at week 48 than in the placebo groups (25 and 33 %). Improvement was defined as a reduction from baseline of two points or more in the Knodell necro-inflammatory score with no concurrent worsening in the Knodell fibrosis score. Histological improvement was seen regardless of baseline demographic and hepatitis B characteristics, including prior interferon-alpha therapy. High baseline ALT levels (⩾ 2 × ULN) and Knodell Histology Activity Index (HAI) scores (⩾ 10) and low HBV DNA (< 7.6 $\log_{10}$ copies/ml) were associated with greater histological improvement. Blinded, ranked assessments of both necro-inflammatory activity and fibrosis at baseline and week 48, demonstrated that patients treated with 10 mg adefovir dipivoxil had improved necro-inflammatory and fibrosis scores relative to placebo-treated patients.

Assessment of the change in fibrosis after 48 weeks treatment using the Knodell scores confirms that patients treated with adefovir dipivoxil 10 mg had more regression and less progression of fibrosis than patients treated with placebo.

In the two studies mentioned above, treatment with 10 mg adefovir dipivoxil was associated with significant reductions in serum HBV DNA (3.52 and 3.91 $\log_{10}$ copies/ml, respectively, *versus* 0.55 and 1.35 $\log_{10}$ copies/ml), increased proportion of patients with normalisation of ALT (48 and 72 % *versus* 16 and 29 %) or increased proportion of patients with serum HBV DNA below the limits of quantification (< 400 copies/ml Roche Amplicor Monitor PCR assay) (21 and 51 % *versus* 0 %) when compared with placebo. In the study in HBeAg positive patients, HBeAg seroconversion (12 %) and HBeAg loss (24 %) was observed significantly more frequently in patients receiving 10 mg adefovir dipivoxil than in patients receiving placebo (6 % and 11 %, respectively) after 48 weeks of treatment.

In the HBeAg negative study patients on adefovir dipivoxil (0-48 weeks) were re-randomised in a blinded-manner to continue on adefovir dipivoxil or receive placebo for an additional 48 weeks. At week 96, patients continuing on adefovir dipivoxil 10 mg had sustained suppression of serum HBV with maintenance of the reduction seen at week 48. In over two thirds of patients suppression of serum HBV DNA was associated with normalisation of ALT levels. In most patients who stopped treatment with adefovir dipivoxil, serum HBV DNA and ALT levels returned towards baseline.

Treatment with adefovir dipivoxil resulted in improvement in the liver fibrosis from baseline to 96 weeks therapy when analysed using the Ishak score (median change: Δ= -1). No differences in the median fibrosis score were seen between groups using the Knodell fibrosis score.

In the HBeAg positive study, treatment beyond 48 weeks resulted in further reductions in serum HBV DNA levels and increases in the proportion of patients with ALT normalisation, HBeAg loss and seroconversion.

Experience in patients pre- and post-transplantation with lamivudine-resistant HBV: In a clinical study in 324 chronic hepatitis B patients with lamivudine-resistant HBV (pre-liver transplantation (n=128) and post-liver transplantation (n=196)), treatment with 10 mg adefovir dipivoxil resulted in a median reduction in serum HBV DNA of 4.1 and 4.3 $\log_{10}$ copies/ml, respectively, at week 48. Treatment with 10 mg adefovir dipivoxil showed similar efficacy regardless of the patterns of lamivudine-resistant HBV DNA polymerase mutations at baseline. Improvements or stabilisation were seen in Child-Pugh-Turcotte score. Normalisation of ALT, albumin, bilirubin and prothrombin time was seen at week 48. The clinical significance of these findings as they relate to histological improvement is not known.

Experience in patients with compensated liver disease and lamivudine-resistant HBV: In a double-blind comparative study in chronic hepatitis B patients with lamivudine-resistant HBV (n=58), there was no median reduction in HBV DNA from baseline after 48 weeks of treatment with lamivudine. Forty-eight weeks of treatment with adefovir dipivoxil 10 mg alone or in combination with lamivudine resulted in a similar significant decrease in median serum HBV DNA levels from baseline (4.04 $\log_{10}$ copies/ml and 3.59 $\log_{10}$ copies/ml, respectively). The clinical significance of these observed changes in HBV DNA has not been established.

Experience in patients with decompensated liver disease and lamivudine-resistant HBV: In 40 HBeAg positive or HBeAg negative patients with lamivudine-resistant HBV and decompensated liver disease receiving treatment with 100 mg lamivudine, addition of 10 mg adefovir dipivoxil treatment for 52 weeks resulted in a median reduction in HBV DNA of 4.6 $\log_{10}$ copies/ml. Improvement in liver function was also seen after one year of therapy.

Experience in patients with HIV co-infection and lamivudine-resistant HBV: In an open-label investigator study in 35 chronic hepatitis B patients with lamivudine-resistant HBV and co-infected with HIV, continued treatment with 10 mg adefovir dipivoxil resulted in progressive reductions in serum HBV DNA levels and ALT levels throughout the course of treatment up to 144 weeks.

Clinical resistance: In several clinical studies (HBeAg positive, HBeAg negative, pre- and post-liver transplantation with lamivudine resistant HBV and lamivudine resistant HBV co-infected with HIV patients), genotypic and phenotypic analyses were conducted on HBV isolates from 379 of a total of 629 patients, treated with adefovir dipivoxil for 48 weeks. No HBV DNA polymerase mutations associated with resistance to adefovir were identified when patients were genotyped at baseline and at week 48. After 96, 144 and 192 weeks of treatment with adefovir dipivoxil, resistance surveillance was performed for 293, 221 and 67 patients, respectively. Two novel conserved site mutations were identified in the HBV polymerase gene (rtN236T and rtA181V), which conferred clinical resistance to adefovir dipivoxil. The cumulative probabilities of developing these adefovir-associated resistance mutations in all patients treated with adefovir dipivoxil were 0 % at 48 weeks and approximately 2 %, 7 % and 15 % after 96, 144 and 192 weeks, respectively. These cumulative probabilities combine results in patients receiving adefovir dipivoxil as monotherapy and in combination with lamivudine. The currently available data both *in vitro* and in patients suggest that HBV expressing the adefovir-associated resistance mutation rtN236T is susceptible to lamivudine. Preliminary data, both *in vitro* and in patients, suggest the adefovir-associated resistance mutation rtA181V may confer a reduced susceptibility to lamivudine.

Table 2

Renal Function Group	Unimpaired	Mild	Moderate	Severe
Baseline Creatinine Clearance (ml/min)	**> 80 (n=7)**	**50-80 (n=8)**	**30-49 (n=7)**	**10-29 (n=10)**
C_{max} (ng/ml)	17.8±3.2	22.4±4.0	28.5±8.6	51.6±10.3
$AUC_{0-\infty}$ (ng·h/ml)	201±40.8	266±55.7	455±176	1240±629
CL/F (ml/min)	469±99.0	356±85.6	237±118	91.7±51.3
CL_{renal}(ml/min)	231±48.9	148±39.3	83.9±27.5	37.0±18.4

5.2 Pharmacokinetic properties

Absorption: Adefovir dipivoxil is a dipivaloyloxymethyl ester prodrug of the active substance adefovir. The oral bioavailability of adefovir from 10 mg adefovir dipivoxil is 59 %. Following oral administration of a single dose of 10 mg adefovir dipivoxil to chronic hepatitis B patients, the median (range) peak serum concentration (C_{max}) was achieved after 1.75 h (0.58-4.0 h). Median C_{max} and $AUC_{0-\infty}$ values were 16.70 (9.66-30.56) ng/ml and 204.40 (109.75-356.05) ng·h/ml, respectively. Systemic exposure to adefovir was not affected when 10 mg adefovir dipivoxil was taken with a high fat meal. The t_{max} was delayed by two hours.

Distribution: Preclinical studies show that after oral administration of adefovir dipivoxil, adefovir is distributed to most tissues with the highest concentrations occurring in kidney, liver and intestinal tissues. *In vitro* binding of adefovir to human plasma or human serum proteins is ⩽ 4 %, over the adefovir concentration range of 0.1 to 25 μg/ml. The volume of distribution at steady-state following intravenous administration of 1.0 or 3.0 mg/kg/day is 392±75 and 352±9 ml/kg, respectively.

Biotransformation: Following oral administration, adefovir dipivoxil is rapidly converted to adefovir. At concentrations substantially higher > 4,000-fold) than those observed *in vivo*, adefovir did not inhibit any of the following human CYP450 isoforms, CYP1A2, CYP2D6, CYP2C9, CYP2C19, CYP3A4. Based on the results of these *in vitro* experiments and the known elimination pathway of adefovir, the potential for CYP450 mediated interactions involving adefovir with other medicinal products is low.

Elimination: Adefovir is excreted renally by a combination of glomerular filtration and active tubular secretion. The median (min-max) renal clearance of adefovir in subjects with normal renal function (Cl_{cr}> 80 ml/min) is 211 ml/min (172-316 ml/min), approximately twice calculated creatinine clearance (Cockroft-Gault method). After repeated administration of 10 mg adefovir dipivoxil, 45 % of the dose is recovered as adefovir in the urine over 24 hours. Plasma adefovir concentrations declined in a biexponential manner with a median terminal elimination half-life of 7.22 h (4.72-10.70 h).

Linearity/non-linearity: The pharmacokinetics of adefovir are proportional to dose when given as adefovir dipivoxil over the dose range of 10 to 60 mg. Repeated dosing of adefovir dipivoxil 10 mg daily did not influence the pharmacokinetics of adefovir.

Gender, age and ethnicity: The pharmacokinetics of adefovir were similar in male and female patients. Pharmacokinetic studies have not been conducted in children or in the elderly. Pharmacokinetic studies were principally conducted in Caucasian patients. The available data do not appear to indicate any difference in pharmacokinetics with regard to race.

Renal impairment: The mean (± SD) pharmacokinetic parameters of adefovir following administration of a single dose of 10 mg adefovir dipivoxil to patients with varying degrees of renal impairment are described in the table below:

(see Table 2 above)

A four-hour period of haemodialysis removed approximately 35 % of the adefovir dose. The effect of peritoneal dialysis on adefovir removal has not been evaluated.

It is recommended that the dosing interval of 10 mg adefovir dipivoxil is modified in patients with creatinine clearance < 50 ml/min or in patients who already have ESRD and require dialysis (see 4.2).

Pharmacokinetics of adefovir have not been studied in patients with creatinine clearance < 10 ml/min and in patients with ESRD managed by other forms of dialysis (e.g. ambulatory peritoneal dialysis) (see 4.4).

Hepatic impairment: Pharmacokinetic properties were similar in patients with moderate and severe hepatic impairment compared to healthy volunteers (see 4.2).

5.3 Preclinical safety data

The primary dose-limiting toxic effect associated with administration of adefovir dipivoxil in animals (mice, rats and monkeys) was renal tubular nephropathy characterised by histological alterations and/or increases in blood urea nitrogen and serum creatinine. Nephrotoxicity was observed in animals at systemic exposures at least 3-10 times higher than those achieved in humans at the recommended therapeutic dose of 10 mg/day.

No effects on male or female fertility, or reproductive performance, occurred in rats and there was no embryotoxicity or teratogenicity in rats or rabbits administered adefovir dipivoxil orally.

When adefovir was administered intravenously to pregnant rats at doses associated with notable maternal toxicity (systemic exposure 38 times that achieved in humans at the therapeutic dose) embryotoxicity and an increased incidence of foetal malformations (anasarca, depressed eye bulge, umbilical hernia and kinked tail) were observed. No adverse effects on development were seen at systemic exposures approximately 12 times that achieved in humans at the therapeutic dose.

Adefovir dipivoxil was mutagenic in the *in vitro* mouse lymphoma cell assay (with or without metabolic activation), but was not clastogenic in the *in vivo* mouse micronucleus assay.

Adefovir was not mutagenic in microbial mutagenicity assays involving *Salmonella typhimurium* (Ames) and *Escherichia coli* in the presence and absence of metabolic activation. Adefovir induced chromosomal aberrations in the *in vitro* human peripheral blood lymphocyte assay without metabolic activation.

In long-term carcinogenicity studies in rats and mice with adefovir dipivoxil, no treatment-related increase in tumour incidence was found in mice or rats (systemic exposures approximately 10 and 4 times those achieved in humans at the therapeutic dose of 10 mg/day, respectively).

6. PHARMACEUTICAL PARTICULARS

6.1 List of excipients

Pregelatinised starch

Croscarmellose sodium

Lactose monohydrate

Talc

Magnesium stearate

6.2 Incompatibilities

Not applicable.

6.3 Shelf life

2 years.

6.4 Special precautions for storage

Do not store above 30°C. Store in original container.

6.5 Nature and contents of container

Hepsera is supplied in high-density polyethylene (HDPE) bottles with a child-resistant closure. Each bottle contains 30 tablets, silica gel desiccant and fibre packing material.

6.6 Instructions for use and handling

No special requirements.

7. MARKETING AUTHORISATION HOLDER

Gilead Sciences International Limited

Cambridge

CB1 6GT

United Kingdom

8. MARKETING AUTHORISATION NUMBER(S)

EU/1/03/251/001

9. DATE OF FIRST AUTHORISATION/RENEWAL OF THE AUTHORISATION

06 March 2003

10. DATE OF REVISION OF THE TEXT

13/09/05

Herceptin

(Roche Products Limited)

1. NAME OF THE MEDICINAL PRODUCT
Herceptin▼ 150 mg

Powder for concentrate for solution for infusion

2. QUALITATIVE AND QUANTITATIVE COMPOSITION
1 vial contains 150 mg of trastuzumab, a humanised IgG1 monoclonal antibody manufactured from a mammalian cell line (Chinese hamster ovary, CHO) by continuous perfusion. Reconstituted Herceptin solution contains 21 mg/ml of trastuzumab.

For excipients, see section 6.1.

3. PHARMACEUTICAL FORM
Powder for concentrate for solution for infusion.

Herceptin is a white to pale yellow lyophilised powder.

4. CLINICAL PARTICULARS

4.1 Therapeutic indications
Herceptin is indicated for the treatment of patients with metastatic breast cancer whose tumours overexpress HER2:

a) as monotherapy for the treatment of those patients who have received at least two chemotherapy regimens for their metastatic disease. Prior chemotherapy must have included at least an anthracycline and a taxane unless patients are unsuitable for these treatments. Hormone receptor positive patients must also have failed hormonal therapy, unless patients are unsuitable for these treatments.

b) in combination with paclitaxel for the treatment of those patients who have not received chemotherapy for their metastatic disease and for whom an anthracycline is not suitable.

c) in combination with docetaxel for the treatment of those patients who have not received chemotherapy for their metastatic disease.

Herceptin should only be used in patients whose tumours have either HER2 overexpression or HER2 gene amplification as determined by an accurate and validated assay (see 4.4 and 5.1).

4.2 Posology and method of administration
HER2 testing is mandatory prior to initiation of Herceptin therapy (see 4.4 and 5.1). Herceptin treatment should only be initiated by a physician experienced in the administration of cytotoxic chemotherapy (see 4.4).

The following loading and subsequent doses are recommended for monotherapy and in combination with paclitaxel or docetaxel.

Loading dose

The recommended initial loading dose of Herceptin is 4 mg/kg body weight.

Subsequent doses

The recommended weekly dose of Herceptin is 2 mg/kg body weight, beginning one week after the loading dose.

Method of administration

Herceptin is administered as a 90-minute intravenous infusion. Patients should be observed for at least six hours after the start of the first infusion and for two hours after the start of the subsequent infusions for symptoms like fever and chills or other infusion-related symptoms (see 4.4 and 4.8). Interruption of the infusion may help control such symptoms. The infusion may be resumed when symptoms abate.

If the initial loading dose was well tolerated, the subsequent doses can be administered as a 30-minute infusion. Emergency equipment must be available.

Do not administer as an intravenous push or bolus.

For instructions for use and handling refer to 6.6.

Administration in combination with Paclitaxel or docetaxel

In the pivotal trials, paclitaxel or docetaxel was administered the day following the first dose of Herceptin (for dose, see the Summary of Product Characteristics for paclitaxel or docetaxel) and immediately after the subsequent doses of Herceptin if the preceding dose of Herceptin was well tolerated.

Duration of treatment

Herceptin should be administered until progression of disease.

Dose reduction

No reductions in the dose of Herceptin were made during clinical trials. Patients may continue Herceptin therapy during periods of reversible, chemotherapy-induced myelosuppression but they should be monitored carefully for complications of neutropenia during this time. Refer to the Summary of Product Characteristics for paclitaxel or docetaxel for information on dose reduction or delays.

Special patient populations

Clinical data show that the disposition of Herceptin is not altered based on age or serum creatinine (see 5.2). In clinical trials, elderly patients did not receive reduced doses of Herceptin. Dedicated pharmacokinetic studies in the elderly and those with renal or hepatic impairment have not been carried out. However in a population pharmacokinetic analysis, age and renal impairment were not shown to affect trastuzumab disposition.

Paediatric use

The safety and efficacy of Herceptin in patients under the age of 18 years have not been established.

4.3 Contraindications
Patients with known hypersensitivity to trastuzumab, murine proteins, or to any of the excipients.

Patients with severe dyspnoea at rest due to complications of advanced malignancy or requiring supplementary oxygen therapy.

4.4 Special warnings and special precautions for use
HER2 testing must be performed in a specialised laboratory which can ensure adequate validation of the testing procedures (see 5.1).

The use of Herceptin is associated with cardiotoxicity. All candidates for treatment should undergo careful cardiac monitoring (see "*cardiotoxicity*" section below). The risk of cardiotoxicity is greatest when Herceptin is used in combination with anthracyclines. Therefore Herceptin and anthracyclines should not be used currently in combination except in a well-controlled clinical trial setting with cardiac monitoring. Patients who have previously received anthracyclines are also at risk of cardiotoxicity with Herceptin treatment, although the risk is lower than with concurrent use of Herceptin and anthracyclines.

Because the half-life of Herceptin is approximately 28.5 days (95 % confidence interval, 25.5 – 32.8 days), Herceptin may persist in the circulation for up to 24 weeks after stopping Herceptin treatment. Patients who receive anthracyclines after stopping Herceptin may possibly be at increased risk of cardiotoxicity. If possible, physicians should avoid anthracycline-based therapy for up to 24 weeks after stopping Herceptin. If anthracyclines are used, the patient's cardiac function should be monitored carefully (see "*cardiotoxicity*" section below). Serious adverse reactions including infusion reactions, hypersensitivity, allergic-like reactions and pulmonary events have been observed in patients receiving Herceptin therapy. Patients who are experiencing dyspnoea at rest due to complications of advanced malignancy and comorbidities may be at increased risk of a fatal infusion reaction. These severe reactions were usually associated with the first infusion of Herceptin and generally occurred during or immediately following the infusion. For some patients, symptoms progressively worsened and led to further pulmonary complications. Initial improvement followed by clinical deterioration and delayed reactions with rapid clinical deterioration have also been reported. Fatalities have occurred within hours and up to one week following infusion. On very rare occasions, patients have experienced the onset of infusion symptoms or pulmonary symptoms more than six hours after the start of the Herceptin infusion. Patients should be warned of the possibility of such a late onset and should be instructed to contact their physician if these symptoms occur.

Infusion reactions, allergic-like reactions and hypersensitivity

Serious adverse reactions to Herceptin infusion that have been reported infrequently include dyspnoea, hypotension, wheezing, hypertension, bronchospasm, supraventricular tachyarrythmia, reduced oxygen saturation, anaphylaxis, respiratory distress, urticaria and angioedema (see 4.8). The majority of these events occur during or within 2.5 hours of the start of the first infusion. Should an infusion reaction occur the Herceptin infusion should be discontinued and the patient monitored until resolution of any observed symptoms (see 4.2). The majority of patients experienced resolution of symptoms and subsequently received further infusions of Herceptin. Serious reactions have been treated successfully with supportive therapy such as oxygen, beta-agonists, and corticosteroids. In rare cases, these reactions are associated with a clinical course culminating in a fatal outcome. Patients who are experiencing dyspnoea at rest due to complications of advanced malignancy and comorbidities may be at increased risk of a fatal infusion reaction. Therefore, these patients should not be treated with Herceptin (see 4.3).

Pulmonary events

Severe pulmonary events have been reported rarely with the use of Herceptin in the post-marketing setting (see 4.8). These rare events have occasionally been fatal. In addition, rare cases of pulmonary infiltrates, acute respiratory distress syndrome, pneumonia, pneumonitis, pleural effusion, respiratory distress, acute pulmonary oedema and respiratory insufficiency have been reported. These events may occur as part of an infusion-related reaction or with a delayed onset. Patients who are experiencing dyspnoea at rest due to complications of advanced malignancy and comorbidities may be at increased risk of pulmonary events. Therefore, these patients should not be treated with Herceptin (see 4.3).

Cardiotoxicity

Heart failure (New York Heart Association [NYHA] class II-IV) has been observed in patients receiving Herceptin therapy alone or in combination with paclitaxel or docetaxel, particularly following anthracycline (doxorubicin or epirubicin)–containing chemotherapy. This may be moderate to severe and has been associated with death (see 4.8).

All candidates for treatment with Herceptin, but especially those with prior anthracycline and cyclophosphamide (AC) exposure, should undergo baseline cardiac assessment including history and physical examination, ECG, echocardiogram, and/or MUGA scan. A careful risk-benefit assessment should be made before deciding to treat with Herceptin. Cardiac function should be further monitored during treatment (e.g. every three months). Monitoring may help to identify patients who develop cardiac dysfunction. Patients who develop asymptomatic cardiac dysfunction may benefit from more frequent monitoring (e.g. every 6-8 weeks). If patients have a continued decrease in left ventricular function, but remain asymptomatic, the physician should consider discontinuing therapy if no clinical benefit of Herceptin therapy has been seen. Caution should be exercised in treating patients with symptomatic heart failure, a history of hypertension or documented coronary artery disease.

If symptomatic cardiac failure develops during Herceptin therapy, it should be treated with the standard medications for this purpose. Discontinuation of Herceptin therapy should be strongly considered in patients who develop clinically significant heart failure unless the benefits for an individual patient are deemed to outweigh the risks.

The safety of continuation or resumption of Herceptin in patients who experience cardiotoxicity has not been prospectively studied. However, most patients who developed heart failure in the pivotal trials improved with standard medical treatment. This included diuretics, cardiac glycosides, and/or angiotensin-converting enzyme inhibitors. The majority of patients with cardiac symptoms and evidence of a clinical benefit of Herceptin treatment continued on weekly therapy with Herceptin without additional clinical cardiac events.

4.5 Interaction with other medicinal products and other forms of Interaction
Drug interaction studies have not been performed with Herceptin in humans. A risk for interactions with concomitant medication cannot be excluded.

4.6 Pregnancy and lactation
Pregnancy

Reproduction studies have been conducted in cynomolgus monkeys at doses up to 25 times that of the weekly human maintenance dose of 2 mg/kg Herceptin and have revealed no evidence of impaired fertility or harm to the foetus. Placental transfer of trastuzumab during the early (Days 20–50 of gestation) and late (Days 120–150 of gestation) foetal development period was observed. It is not known whether Herceptin can cause foetal harm when administered to a pregnant woman or whether it can affect reproductive capacity. As animal reproduction studies are not always predictive of human response, Herceptin should be avoided during pregnancy unless the potential benefit for the mother outweighs the potential risk to the foetus.

In the postmarketing setting, cases of oligohydramnios have been reported in pregnant women receiving Herceptin.

Lactation

A study conducted in lactating cynomolgus monkeys at doses 25 times that of the weekly human maintenance dose of 2 mg/kg Herceptin demonstrated that trastuzumab is secreted in the milk. The presence of trastuzumab in the serum of infant monkeys was not associated with any adverse effects on their growth or development from birth to 1 month of age. It is not known whether trastuzumab is secreted in human milk. As human IgG1 is secreted into human milk, and the potential for harm to the infant is unknown, women should not breast-feed during Herceptin therapy and for 6 months after the last dose of Herceptin.

4.7 Effects on ability to drive and use machines
No studies on the effects on the ability to drive and to use machines have been performed. Patients experiencing infusion-related symptoms should be advised not to drive and use machines until symptoms abate.

4.8 Undesirable effects
The adverse event data reflect the clinical trial and post marketing experience of using Herceptin at the recommended dose regimen, either alone or in combination with paclitaxel.

Patients received Herceptin as monotherapy or in combination with paclitaxel in the two pivotal clinical trials. The most common adverse reactions are infusion-related symptoms, such as fever and chills, usually following the first infusion of Herceptin.

Adverse reactions attributed to Herceptin in ≥ 10 % of patients in the two pivotal clinical trials were the following:

Body as a Whole:	abdominal pain, asthenia, chest pain, chills, fever, headache, pain
Digestive:	diarrhoea, nausea, vomiting
Musculoskeletal:	arthralgia, myalgia
Skin and appendages:	rash

Adverse reactions attributed to Herceptin in > 1 % and < 10 % of patients in the two pivotal clinical trials were the following:

Body as a Whole:	influenza-like illness, back pain, infection, neck pain, malaise, hypersensitivity reaction, mastitis, weight loss
Cardiovascular:	vasodilation, supraventricular tachyarrythmia, hypotension, heart failure, cardiomyopathy, palpitation
Digestive:	anorexia, constipation, dyspepsia, liver tenderness, dry mouth, rectal disorder (haemorrhoids)
Blood and lymphatic:	leucopenia, ecchymosis
Metabolic:	peripheral oedema, oedema
Musculoskeletal:	bone pain, leg cramps, arthritis
Nervous:	dizziness, paraesthesia, somnolence, hypertonia, peripheral neuropathy, tremor
Psychiatric disorders:	anxiety, depression, insomnia
Respiratory:	asthma, cough increased, dyspnoea, epistaxis, lung disorders, pharyngitis, rhinitis, sinusitis
Urogenital:	urinary tract infection
Skin and appendages:	pruritus, sweating, nail disorder, dry skin, alopecia, acne, maculopapular rash
Special senses:	taste perversion

In a further randomised clinical trial (M77001), patients with metastatic breast cancer received docetaxel, with or without Herceptin. The following table displays adverse events which were reported in ⩾ 10% of patients, by study treatment:

(see Table 1)

There was an increased incidence of SAEs (40% vs. 31%) and Grade 4 AEs (34% vs. 23%) in the combination arm compared to docetaxel monotherapy.

Serious Adverse Reactions

At least one case of the following serious adverse reactions has occurred in at least one patient treated with Herceptin alone or in combination with chemotherapy in clinical trials or has been reported during post marketing experience:

Body as a Whole:	hypersensitivity reaction, anaphylaxis and anaphylactic shock, angioedema, ataxia, sepsis, chills and fever, asthenia, fever, rigor, headache, paresis, chest pain, fatigue, infusion-related symptoms, peripheral oedema, bone pain, coma, meningitis, cerebral oedema, thinking abnormal, progression of neoplasia
Cardiovascular:	cardiomyopathy, congestive heart failure, increased congestive heart failure, decreased ejection fraction, hypotension, pericardial effusion, bradycardia, cerebrovascular disorder, cardiac failure, cardiogenic shock, pericarditis
Digestive:	Hepatocellular damage, liver tenderness, diarrhoea, nausea and vomiting, pancreatitis, hepatic failure, jaundice
Blood and Lymphatic:	leukaemia, febrile neutropenia, neutropenia, thrombocytopenia, anaemia, hypoprothrombinemia
Metabolic:	hyperkalaemia
Musculoskeletal:	myalgia
Nervous:	paraneoplastic cerebellar degeneration
Renal:	membranous glomerulonephritis, glomerulonephropathy, renal failure
Respiratory:	bronchospasm, respiratory distress, acute pulmonary oedema, respiratory insufficiency, dyspnoea, hypoxia, laryngeal oedema, acute respiratory distress, acute respiratory distress syndrome, Cheyne-Stokes breathing, pulmonary infiltrates, pneumonia, pneumonitis, pulmonary fibrosis.
Skin and appendages:	rash, dermatitis, urticaria
Special Senses:	papilloedema, abnormal lacrimation, retinal haemorrhage, deafness

Infusion-Related Symptoms

During the first infusion of Herceptin chills and/or fever are observed commonly in patients. Other signs and/or symptoms may include nausea, hypertension, vomiting, pain, rigors, headache, cough, dizziness, rash, and asthenia. These symptoms are usually mild to moderate in severity, and occur infrequently with subsequent Herceptin infu-

Table 1

Body System	Adverse Event	Herceptin plus docetaxel N = 92 (%)	docetaxel N = 94 (%)
General disorders and administration site conditions	asthenia	45	41
	oedema peripheral	40	35
	fatigue	24	21
	mucosal inflammation	23	22
	pyrexia	29	15
	pain	12	9
	lethargy	7	11
	chest pain	11	5
	influenza like illness	12	2
	rigors	11	1
Skin and subcutaneous tissue disorders	alopecia	67	54
	nail disorder	17	21
	rash	24	12
	erythema	23	11
Gastrointestinal disorders	nausea	43	41
	diarrhoea	43	36
	vomiting	29	22
	constipation	27	23
	stomatitis	20	14
	abdominal pain	12	12
	dyspepsia	14	5
Nervous system disorders	paraesthesia	32	21
	headache	21	18
	dysgeusia	14	12
	hypoaesthesia	11	5
Blood and lymphatic system disorders	febrile neutropenia[1] / neutropenic sepsis	23	17
Musculoskeletal and connective tissue disorders	myalgia	27	26
	arthralgia	27	20
	pain in extremity	16	16
	back pain	10	14
	bone pain	14	6
Respiratory, thoracic and mediastinal disorders	cough	13	16
	dyspnoea	14	15
	pharyngolaryngeal pain	16	9
	epistaxis	18	5
	rhinorrhoea	12	1
Infections and infestations	nasopharyngitis	15	6
Eye disorders	lacrimation increased	21	10
	conjunctivitis	12	7
Vascular disorders	lymphoedema	11	6
Metabolism and nutrition disorders	anorexia	22	13
Investigations	weight increased	15	6
Psychiatric disorders	insomnia	11	4
Injury, poisoning and procedural complications	nail toxicity	11	7

[1] These numbers include patients with preferred terms of 'febrile neutropenia', 'neutropenic sepsis' or 'neutropenia' that was associated with fever (and antibiotic use). See also section 4.8

Table 05

	Herceptin plus paclitaxel N=91	paclitaxel N=95	Herceptin N=213
Symptomatic heart failure	8, 8.8 % [3.9-16.6]	4, 4.2 % [1.2-10.4]	18, 8.5 % 5.1-13.0]
Cardiac diagnosis other than heart failure	4, 4.4 % [1.2-10.9]	7, 7.4 % [3.0-14.6]	7, 3.3 % [1.3-6.7]

sions. These symptoms can be treated with an analgesic/antipyretic such as meperidine or paracetamol, or an antihistamine such as diphenhydramine (see 4.2). Some adverse reactions to Herceptin infusion including dyspnoea, hypotension, wheezing, bronchospasm, supraventricular tachyarrythmia, reduced oxygen saturation and respiratory distress can be serious and potentially fatal (see 4.4).

Allergic-like and hypersensitivity reactions

Allergic reactions, anaphylaxis and anaphylactic shock, urticaria and angioedema occurring during the first infusion of Herceptin, have been reported rarely. Over a third of these patients had a negative re-challenge and continued to receive Herceptin. Some of these reactions can be serious and potentially fatal (see 4.4).

Serious pulmonary events

Single cases of pulmonary infiltrates, pneumonia, pulmonary fibrosis, pleural effusion, respiratory distress, acute pulmonary oedema, acute respiratory distress syndrome (ARDS) and respiratory insufficiency have been reported rarely. These events have been reported rarely with fatal outcome (see 4.4).

Cardiac toxicity

Reduced ejection fraction and signs and symptoms of heart failure, such as dyspnoea, orthopnoea, increased cough, pulmonary oedema, and S_3 gallop, have been observed in patients treated with Herceptin. (see 4.4).

The incidence of cardiac adverse events from retrospective analysis of data from the combination therapy study (Herceptin plus paclitaxel versus paclitaxel alone) and the Herceptin monotherapy study is shown in the following table:

Cardiac Adverse Event Incidence; n,% [95 %-confidence limits]

(see Table 2 above)

The incidence of symptomatic congestive heart failure in the study of Herceptin plus docetaxel versus docetaxel alone (M77001), is shown in the following table:

	Herceptin plus docetaxel N = 92	docetaxel N = 94
Symptomatic heart failure	2 (2.2%)	0%

In this study, all patients had a baseline cardiac ejection fraction of greater than 50%. In the Herceptin plus docetaxel arm, 64% had received a prior anthracycline compared with 55% in the docetaxel alone arm.

Haematological toxicity

Haematological toxicity was infrequent following the administration of Herceptin as a single agent, WHO Grade 3 leucopenia, thrombocytopenia and anaemia occurring in < 1 % of patients. No WHO Grade 4 toxicities were observed.

There was an increase in WHO Grade 3 or 4 haematological toxicity in patients treated with the combination of Herceptin and paclitaxel compared with patients receiving paclitaxel alone (34 % versus 21 %). Haematological toxicity was also increased in patients receiving Herceptin and docetaxel, compared with docetaxel alone (32% grade 3/4 neutropenia versus 22%, using NCI-CTC criteria). Note that this is likely to be an underestimate since docetaxel alone at a dose of 100mg/m^2 is known to result in neutropenia in 97% of patients, 76% grade 4, based on nadir blood counts. The incidence of febrile neutropenia/neutropenic sepsis was also increased in patients treated with Herceptin plus docetaxel (23% versus 17% for patients treated with docetaxel alone).

Hepatic and renal toxicity

WHO Grade 3 or 4 hepatic toxicity was observed in 12 % of patients following administration of Herceptin as single agent. This toxicity was associated with progression of disease in the liver in 60 % of these patients. WHO Grade 3 or 4 hepatic toxicity was less frequently observed among patients receiving Herceptin and paclitaxel than among patients receiving paclitaxel (7 % compared with 15 %). No WHO Grade 3 or 4 renal toxicity was observed in patients treated with Herceptin.

Diarrhoea

Of patients treated with Herceptin as a single agent, 27 % experienced diarrhoea. An increase in the incidence of diarrhoea, primarily mild to moderate in severity, has also been observed in patients receiving Herceptin in combination with paclitaxel or docetaxel compared with patients receiving paclitaxel or docetaxel alone.

Infection

An increased incidence of infections, primarily mild upper respiratory infections of minor clinical significance or catheter infections, has been observed primarily in patients treated with Herceptin plus paclitaxel or docetaxel compared with patients receiving paclitaxel or docetaxel alone.

4.9 Overdose

There is no experience with overdosage in human clinical trials. Single doses of Herceptin alone greater than 10 mg/kg have not been administered in the clinical trials. Doses up to this level were well tolerated.

5. PHARMACOLOGICAL PROPERTIES

5.1 Pharmacodynamic properties

Pharmacotherapeutic group: Antineoplastic agents, ATC code: L01XC03

Trastuzumab is a recombinant humanised IgG1 monoclonal antibody against the human epidermal growth factor receptor 2 (HER2). Overexpression of HER2 is observed in 20 %-30 % of primary breast cancers. Studies indicate that patients whose tumours overexpress HER2 have a shortened disease-free survival compared to patients whose tumours do not overexpress HER2. The extracellular domain of the receptor (ECD, p105) can be shed into the blood stream and measured in serum samples.

Trastuzumab has been shown, in both *in vitro* assays and in animals, to inhibit the proliferation of human tumour cells that overexpress HER2. Additionally, trastuzumab is a potent mediator of antibody-dependent cell-mediated cytotoxicity (ADCC). *In vitro*, trastuzumab-mediated ADCC has been shown to be preferentially exerted on HER2 overexpressing cancer cells compared with cancer cells that do not overexpress HER2.

Detection of HER2 overexpression or HER2 gene amplification

Herceptin should only be used in patients whose tumours have HER2 overexpression or HER2 gene amplification. HER2 overexpression should be detected using an immunohistochemistry (IHC)-based assessment of fixed tumour blocks (see 4.4). HER2 gene amplification should be detected using fluorescence in situ hybridisation (FISH) or chromogenic in situ hybridisation (CISH) of fixed tumour blocks. Patients are eligible for Herceptin treatment if they show strong HER2 overexpression as described by a 3+ score by IHC or a positive FISH or CISH result.

To ensure accurate and reproducible results, the testing must be performed in a specialised laboratory, which can ensure validation of the testing procedures.

The recommended scoring system to evaluate the IHC staining patterns is as follows:

Staining Intensity Score	Staining pattern	HER2 Overexpression Assessment
0	No staining is observed or membrane staining is observed in < 10 % of the tumour cells	Negative
1+	A faint/barely perceptible membrane staining is detected in > 10 % of the tumour cells. The cells are only stained in part of their membrane.	Negative
2+	A weak to moderate complete membrane staining is detected in > 10 % of the tumour cells.	Weak to moderate overexpression
3+	A moderate to strong complete membrane staining is detected in > 10 % of the tumour cells.	Moderate to strong overexpression

In general, FISH is considered positive if the ratio of the HER2 gene copy number per tumour cell to the chromosome 17 copy number is greater than or equal to 2, or if there are more than 4 copies of the HER2 gene per tumour cell if no chromosome 17 control is used.

In general, CISH is considered positive if there are more than 5 copies of the HER2 gene per nucleus in greater than 50% of tumour cells.

For full instructions on assay performance and interpretation please refer to the package inserts of validated FISH and CISH assays.

For any other method that may be used for the assessment of HER2 protein or gene expression, the analyses should only be performed by laboratories that provide adequate state-of-the-art performance of validated methods. Such methods must clearly be precise and accurate enough to demonstrate overexpression of HER2 and must be able to distinguish between moderate (congruent with 2+) and strong (congruent with 3+) overexpression of HER2.

Clinical Data

Herceptin has been used in clinical trials as monotherapy for patients with metastatic breast cancer who have tumours that overexpress HER2 and who have failed one or more chemotherapy regimens for their metastatic disease (Herceptin alone).

Herceptin has also been used in combination with paclitaxel or docetaxel for the treatment of patients who have not received chemotherapy for their metastatic disease. Patients who had previously received anthracycline-based adjuvant chemotherapy were treated with paclitaxel (175 mg/m^2 infused over 3 hours) with or without Herceptin. In the pivotal trial of docetaxel (100 mg/m^2 infused over 1 hour) with or without Herceptin, 60% of the patients had received prior anthracycline-based adjuvant chemotherapy. Patients were treated with Herceptin until progression of disease.

The efficacy of Herceptin in combination with paclitaxel in patients who did not receive prior adjuvant anthracyclines has not been studied. However, Herceptin plus docetaxel was efficacious in patients whether or not they had received prior adjuvant anthracyclines.

The test method for HER2 overexpression used to determine eligibility of patients in the pivotal Herceptin monotherapy and Herceptin plus paclitaxel clinical trials employed immunohistochemical staining for HER2 of fixed material from breast tumours using the murine monoclonal antibodies CB11 and 4D5. These tissues were fixed in formalin or Bouin's fixative. This investigative clinical trial assay performed in a central laboratory utilised a 0 to 3+ scale. Patients classified as staining 2+ or 3+ were included, while those staining 0 or 1+ were excluded. Greater than 70 % of patients enrolled exhibited 3+ overexpression. The data suggest that beneficial effects were greater among those patients with higher levels of overexpression of HER2 (3+).

The main test method used to determine HER2 positivity in the pivotal trial of docetaxel, with or without Herceptin, was immunohistochemistry. A minority of patients were tested using fluorescence *in-situ* hybridisation (FISH). In this trial, 87% of patients entered had disease that was IHC3+, and 95% of patients entered had disease that was IHC3+ and/or FISH-positive.

Efficacy

The efficacy results from the monotherapy and combination therapy studies are summarised in the following table:

(see Table 3 on next page)

Immunogenicity

Nine hundred and three patients treated with Herceptin, alone or in combination with chemotherapy, have been evaluated for antibody production. Human anti-trastuzumab antibodies were detected in one patient, who had no allergic manifestations.

Sites of progression

After Herceptin and paclitaxel therapy for metastatic breast cancer in patients in the pivotal trial the following sites of disease progression were found:

(see Table 4 on next page)

The frequency of progression in the liver was significantly reduced in patients treated with the combination of Herceptin and paclitaxel. More patients treated with Herceptin and paclitaxel progressed in the central nervous system than those treated with paclitaxel alone.

5.2 Pharmacokinetic properties

The pharmacokinetics of trastuzumab have been studied in breast cancer patients with metastatic disease. Short duration intravenous infusions of 10, 50, 100, 250, and 500 mg trastuzumab once weekly in patients demonstrated dose-dependent pharmacokinetics. Drug interaction studies have not been performed with Herceptin.

Half-life

Using the recommended dose, the half-life is approximately 28.5 days (95 % confidence interval, 25.5 –32.8 days). The washout period is up to 24 weeks (95 % confidence interval, 18-24 weeks)

Steady State and Peak Concentration

Steady state pharmacokinetics should be reached by approximately 20 weeks (95 % confidence interval, 18 – 24 weeks). The estimated mean AUC was 578 mg day/L and the estimated mean peak and trough concentrations were 110 mg/L and 66 mg/L, respectively.

Table 3

Parameter	Monotherapy	Combination Therapy			
	Herceptin[1] N=172	Herceptin plus paclitaxel[2] N=68	Paclitaxel[2] N=77	Herceptin plus docetaxel[3] N=92	Docetaxel[3] N=94
Response rate (95%CI)	18% (13 - 25)	49% (36 - 61)	17% (9 - 27)	61% (50-71)	34% (25-45)
Median duration of response (months) (95%CI)	9.1 (5.6-10.3)	8.3 (7.3-8.8)	4.6 (3.7-7.4)	11.7 (9.3 – 15.0)	5.7 (4.6 -7.6)
Median TTP (months) (95%CI)	3.2 (2.6-3.5)	7.1 (6.2-12.0)	3.0 (2.0-4.4)	11.7 (9.2 -13.5)	6.1 (5.4 -7.2)
Median Survival (months) (95%CI)	16.4 (12.3-ne)	24.8 (18.6-33.7)	17.9 (11.2-23.8)	31.2 (27.3-40.8)	22.74 (19.1-30.8)

TTP = time to progression; "ne" indicates that it could not be estimated or it was not yet reached.

1. Study H0649g: IHC3+ patient subset
2. Study H0648g: IHC3+ patient subset
3. Study M77001: Full analysis set (intent-to-treat)

Table 4

Site*	Herceptin plus paclitaxel (N=87) %	paclitaxel (N=92) %	p-value
Any site	**70.1**	**95.7**	-
Abdomen	0	0	-
Bone	17.2	16.3	0.986
Chest	5.7	13.0	0.250
Liver	21.8	45.7	**0.004**
Lung	16.1	18.5	0.915
Dist. Node	3.4	6.5	0.643
Mediastinum	4.6	2.2	0.667
CNS	12.6	6.5	0.377
Other	4.6	9.8	0.410

*Patients may have had multiple sites of disease progression

Clearance

Clearance decreased with increased dose level. In clinical trials where a loading dose of 4 mg/kg trastuzumab followed by a subsequent weekly dose of 2 mg/kg was used, the mean clearance was 0.225L/day.

The effects of patient characteristics (such as age or serum creatinine) on the disposition of trastuzumab have been evaluated. The data suggest that the disposition of trastuzumab is not altered in any of these groups of patients (see 4.2), however, studies were not specifically designed to investigate the impact of renal impairment upon pharmacokinetics.

Volume of Distribution

In all clinical studies, volume of distribution approximated serum volume, 2.95 L.

Circulating Shed Antigen

Detectable concentrations of the circulating extracellular domain of the HER2 receptor (shed antigen) are found in the serum of some patients with HER2 overexpressing breast cancers. Determination of shed antigen in baseline serum samples revealed that 64 % (286/447) of patients had detectable shed antigen, which ranged as high as 1880 ng/ml (median = 11 ng/ml). Patients with higher baseline shed antigen levels were more likely to have lower serum trough concentrations of trastuzumab. However, with weekly dosing, most patients with elevated shed antigen levels achieved target serum concentrations of trastuzumab by week 6 and no significant relationship has been observed between baseline shed antigen and clinical response.

5.3 Preclinical safety data

There was no evidence of acute or multiple dose-related toxicity in studies of up to 6 months, or reproductive toxicity in teratology, female fertility or late gestational toxicity/placental transfer studies. Herceptin is not genotoxic. A study of trehalose, a major formulation excipient did not reveal any toxicities.

No long-term animal studies have been performed to establish the carcinogenic potential of Herceptin, or to determine its effects on fertility in males.

6. PHARMACEUTICAL PARTICULARS

6.1 List of excipients

L-histidine hydrochloride

L-histidine

α,α-trehalose dihydrate

polysorbate 20

6.2 Incompatibilities

Do not dilute with glucose solutions since these cause aggregation of the protein.

Herceptin should not be mixed or diluted with other products except those mentioned under section 6.6.

6.3 Shelf life

3 years

After reconstitution with sterile water for injections the reconstituted solution is physically and chemically stable for 48 hours at 2°C – 8°C. Any remaining reconstituted solution should be discarded.

Solutions of Herceptin for infusion are physically and chemically stable in polyvinylchloride or polyethylene bags containing 0.9 % sodium chloride for 24 hours at temperatures not exceeding 30°C.

From a microbiological point of view, the reconstituted solution and Herceptin infusion solution should be used immediately. The product is not intended to be stored after reconstitution and dilution unless this has taken place under controlled and validated aseptic conditions. If not used immediately, in-use storage times and conditions are the responsibility of the user.

6.4 Special precautions for storage

Store in a refrigerator (2°C – 8°C)

Do not freeze the reconstituted solution.

6.5 Nature and contents of container

Herceptin vial:

One 15 ml clear glass type I vial with butyl rubber stopper laminated with a fluoro-resin film.

Each carton contains one vial.

6.6 Instructions for use and handling

Preparation for Administration

Appropriate aseptic technique should be used. Each vial of Herceptin is reconstituted with 7.2 ml of sterile water for injections (not supplied). Use of other reconstitution solvents should be avoided.

This yields a 7.4 ml solution for single-dose use, containing approximately 21 mg/ml trastuzumab, at a pH of approximately 6.0. A volume overage of 4 % ensures that the labelled dose of 150 mg can be withdrawn from each vial.

Herceptin should be carefully handled during reconstitution. Causing excessive foaming during reconstitution or shaking the reconstituted Herceptin may result in problems with the amount of Herceptin that can be withdrawn from the vial.

Instructions for Reconstitution:

1) Using a sterile syringe, slowly inject 7.2 ml of sterile water for injections in the vial containing the lyophilised Herceptin, directing the stream into the lyophilised cake.

2) Swirl vial gently to aid reconstitution. DO NOT SHAKE!

Slight foaming of the product upon reconstitution is not unusual. Allow the vial to stand undisturbed for approximately 5 minutes. The reconstituted Herceptin results in a colourless to pale yellow transparent solution and should be essentially free of visible particulates.

Determine the volume of the solution required based on a loading dose of 4 mg trastuzumab/kg body weight, or a subsequent weekly dose of 2 mg trastuzumab/kg body weight:

$$\textbf{Volume}\ (\text{ml}) = \frac{\textbf{Body weight}\ (\text{kg}) \times \textbf{dose}\ (\textbf{4}\text{mg/kg for loading or }\textbf{2}\text{mg/kg for maintenance})}{\textbf{21}\ (\text{mg/ml, concentration of reconstituted solution})}$$

The appropriate amount of solution should be withdrawn from the vial and added to an infusion bag containing 250 ml of 0.9 % sodium chloride solution. Do not use with glucose-containing solutions (see 6.2). The bag should be gently inverted to mix the solution in order to avoid foaming. Parenteral solutions should be inspected visually for particulates and discoloration prior to administration. Once the infusion is prepared it should be administered immediately. If diluted aseptically, it may be stored for 24 hours (do not store above 30°C).

No incompatibilities between Herceptin and polyvinylchloride or polyethylene bags have been observed.

7. MARKETING AUTHORISATION HOLDER

Roche Registration Limited

40 Broadwater Road

Welwyn Garden City

Hertfordshire, AL7 3AY

United Kingdom

8. MARKETING AUTHORISATION NUMBER(S)

EU/1/00/145/001

9. DATE OF FIRST AUTHORISATION/RENEWAL OF THE AUTHORISATION

8 September 2005

10. DATE OF REVISION OF THE TEXT

28 June 2005

LEGAL STATUS

POM

Herpid

(Astellas Pharma Limited)

1. NAME OF THE MEDICINAL PRODUCT

Herpid.

2. QUALITATIVE AND QUANTITATIVE COMPOSITION

A clear, colourless solution containing idoxuridine BP 5% in dimethyl sulphoxide.

3. PHARMACEUTICAL FORM

Topical Solution.

4. CLINICAL PARTICULARS

4.1 Therapeutic indications

Cutaneous herpes simplex and herpes zoster (shingles).

4.2 Posology and method of administration

Administration: Herpid should be painted on the lesions and their erythematous bases four times daily for four days.

Adults and children over 12 years:

Treatment should start as soon as the condition has been diagnosed, ideally within two or three days after the rash appears. Good results are less likely if treatment is not started within seven days.

Children under 12 years:

The use of Herpid in children with malignant disease might be justified but, although not a contra-indication, its use in children under the age of 12 years is not recommended.

No specific information on the use of this product in the elderly is available. Clinical trials have included patients over 65 years and no adverse reactions specific to this age group have been reported.

4.3 Contraindications
Known hypersensitivity to either idoxuridine or dimethyl sulphoxide.

Dermographia.

4.4 Special warnings and special precautions for use
Herpid in the eye causes stinging: treat by washing out with water.

4.5 Interaction with other medicinal products and other forms of Interaction
Since the solvent in Herpid can increase the absorption of many substances it is important that no other topical medication be used on the same areas of skin treated with Herpid.

4.6 Pregnancy and lactation
Animal studies have shown idoxuridine to be teratogenic. Consequently, Herpid should not be prescribed for women who are pregnant or at risk of becoming pregnant. In a small number of cases of women who used Herpid inadvertently in early pregnancy and who were followed to term, the infant was normal in each case.

4.7 Effects on ability to drive and use machines
None.

4.8 Undesirable effects
Patients often experience stinging when applying Herpid and a distinctive taste during a course of treatment; both effects are transient.

Skin reactions have occasionally been reported.

Over-usage of the solution may lead to maceration of the skin.

4.9 Overdose
There is no clinical evidence of overdosage. Standard supportive measures should be adopted.

5. PHARMACOLOGICAL PROPERTIES

5.1 Pharmacodynamic properties
Idoxuridine is an antiviral agent which acts by blocking the uptake of thymidine into the deoxyribonucleic acid (DNA) of the virus and inhibits replication of viruses such as adenovirus, cytomegalovirus, herpes simplex (herpes virus hominus), varicella zoster or herpes zoster (herpes virus varicella) and vaccinia. It has no action against latent forms of the virus. It does not inhibit RNA viruses such as influenza virus or poliovirus.

5.2 Pharmacokinetic properties
The idoxuridine is dissolved in dimethyl sulphoxide which penetrates the skin and carries the antiviral agent to the deeper levels of the epidermis where the virus is replicating.

Idoxuridine is rapidly metabolised in the body to iodouracil, uracil and iodine which are rapidly excreted in the urine.

5.3 Preclinical safety data

6. PHARMACEUTICAL PARTICULARS

6.1 List of excipients
Dimethyl sulphoxide.

6.2 Incompatibilities
None stated.

6.3 Shelf life
2 years.

6.4 Special precautions for storage
Herpid should be stored in its box below 25°C. Do not refrigerate as the contents of the bottle may solidify. If crystals do form, allow to redissolve before use by warming the bottle gently (in the palm of the hand) until the solution is clear. Because the solution is hygroscopic, any remaining after completion of treatment should be discarded.

6.5 Nature and contents of container
5 ml bottle with brush (OP):

Bottle: Type III amber glass

Cap liner: high density natural polyethylene

Brush stem: low density natural polyethylene

6.6 Instructions for use and handling
Instructions for use:

1) Carefully unscrew the white cap and discard.

Replace it with the black cap and brush.

2) Apply the liquid sparingly with the brush 4 times a day to the affected area of skin.

It is important to treat only the affected areas.

3) Wash your hands thoroughly after using Herpid.

4) Do not continue a course of treatment on one area of the skin for more than four days.

5) Discard any solution remaining in the bottle as soon as the treatment period is complete.

Herpid can damage some synthetic materials (e.g. artificial silk and Terylene) and printed cotton fabrics. Contact between Herpid and these materials should therefore be avoided.

7. MARKETING AUTHORISATION HOLDER
Yamanouchi Pharma Limited

Yamanouchi House

Pyrford Road

West Byfleet

Surrey

KT14 6RA

8. MARKETING AUTHORISATION NUMBER(S)
PL 00166/0177

9. DATE OF FIRST AUTHORISATION/RENEWAL OF THE AUTHORISATION
Date of first authorisation 13.03.74

Date of latest renewal 17.01.01

10. DATE OF REVISION OF THE TEXT
Partial revision January 2001

Hexopal 500mg Tablets

(Genus Pharmaceuticals)

1. NAME OF THE MEDICINAL PRODUCT
Hexopal Tablets 500mg / Inositol Nicotinate Tablets BP 500mg.

2. QUALITATIVE AND QUANTITATIVE COMPOSITION
Inositol Nicotinate BP 500mg.

3. PHARMACEUTICAL FORM
Tablet.

4. CLINICAL PARTICULARS

4.1 Therapeutic indications
Hexopal is indicated for the symptomatic relief of severe intermittent claudication and Raynaud's phenomenon.

4.2 Posology and method of administration
For oral administration.

Adults (including the elderly): The usual dose is 3g daily (i.e. 2 tablets three times a day). The dose may be increased to 4g daily if necessary.

Children: Not recommended.

4.3 Contraindications
Use in patients who have suffered a recent myocardial infarction or are in the acute phase of a cerebrovascular accident.

Use in patients hypersensitive to the active ingredient.

4.4 Special warnings and special precautions for use
This product should be used with caution in the presence of cerebrovascular insufficiency or unstable angina.

4.5 Interaction with other medicinal products and other forms of Interaction
None.

4.6 Pregnancy and lactation
There is no evidence of the safety of Hexopal in human pregnancy nor is there adequate evidence from animal work that it is free from hazard. The use of Hexopal in pregnancy should therefore be avoided unless there is no safer alternative.

4.7 Effects on ability to drive and use machines
None.

4.8 Undesirable effects
Side effects are uncommon, but may include flushing, dizziness, headache, nausea, vomiting, syncope, paraesthesia, rash, oedema, and postural hypotension.

4.9 Overdose
Despite extensive clinical experience in Britain since 1959, no case of poisoning or overdosage with Hexopal has been reported. In an emergency, it is suggested that the stomach be emptied by gastric lavage and the patient be treated symptomatically.

5. PHARMACOLOGICAL PROPERTIES

5.1 Pharmacodynamic properties
The mode of action of inositol nicotinate in Raynaud's phenomenon and in intermittent claudication remains to be determined. Inositol nicotinate does not appear to produce general peripheral vasodilation.

5.2 Pharmacokinetic properties
Radiolabelled tracer studies indicate that with orally administered inositol nicotinate very low concentrations of nicotinic acid are found in the plasma. These levels appear to be maintained for approximately 24 hours.

5.3 Preclinical safety data
There are no preclinical safety data of relevance to the prescriber which are additional to that already included in other sections of the SPC.

6. PHARMACEUTICAL PARTICULARS

6.1 List of excipients
Pregelatinised starch, Maize starch, Purified talc, Magnesium stearate, Stearic acid, Sodium lauryl sulphate.

6.2 Incompatibilities
None.

6.3 Shelf life
60 months.

6.4 Special precautions for storage
Store below 25°C.

6.5 Nature and contents of container
Amber glass bottle with wadless polypropylene screws caps.

Pack size: 100 and 500 tablets.

200μm white opaque PVC/20μm aluminium blister pack.

Pack size: 100 tablets.

6.6 Instructions for use and handling
None.

7. MARKETING AUTHORISATION HOLDER
Genus Pharmaceuticals Limited (*trading as Genus Pharmaceuticals*)

Benham Valence

Newbury

Berkshire

RG20 8LU

United Kingdom

8. MARKETING AUTHORISATION NUMBER(S)
PL 06831/0147

9. DATE OF FIRST AUTHORISATION/RENEWAL OF THE AUTHORISATION
10th May 2005

10. DATE OF REVISION OF THE TEXT

Hexopal Forte 750mg Tablets / Inositol Nicotinate 750mg Tablets

(Genus Pharmaceuticals)

1. NAME OF THE MEDICINAL PRODUCT
Hexopal Forte Tablets / Inositol Nicotinate Tablets

2. QUALITATIVE AND QUANTITATIVE COMPOSITION
Each tablet contains Inositol Nicotinate BP 750 mg.

3. PHARMACEUTICAL FORM
Tablets

4. CLINICAL PARTICULARS

4.1 Therapeutic indications
Hexopal is indicated for the symptomatic relief of severe intermittent claudication and Raynauds phenomenon.

4.2 Posology and method of administration
Adults: The usual dose is 3g daily (two Hexopal Forte Tablets twice daily). The dose of Hexopal may be increased up to 4g daily if necessary.

Oral administration.

4.3 Contraindications
Use in patients who have suffered a recent myocardial infarction or are in the acute phase of a cerebrovascular accident.

Use in patients hypersensitive to the active ingredient.

4.4 Special warnings and special precautions for use
This product should be used with caution in the presence of cerebrovascular insufficiency or unstable angina.

4.5 Interaction with other medicinal products and other forms of Interaction
None.

4.6 Pregnancy and lactation
There is no evidence of the safety of Hexopal in human pregnancy nor is there any evidence from animal work that it is free from hazard. The use of Hexopal in pregnancy should therefore be avoided unless there is no safer alternative.

4.7 Effects on ability to drive and use machines
None.

4.8 Undesirable effects
Side effects are uncommon, but may include flushing, dizziness, headache, nausea, vomiting, syncope, paraesthesia, rash, oedema, and postural hypotension.

4.9 Overdose
Despite extensive clinical experience in Britain since 1959, no case of poisoning or overdosage with Hexopal has been reported. In an emergency, it is suggested that the stomach be emptied by gastric lavage and the patient be treated symptomatically.

5. PHARMACOLOGICAL PROPERTIES

5.1 Pharmacodynamic properties
In addition to a vasodilator effect, thought to be due to the slow release of nicotinic acid, Hexopal has been reported to reduce fibrinogen and blood viscosity and to have a beneficial effect on the fibrinolytic system and on blood lipids.

5.2 Pharmacokinetic properties
Radiolabelled tracer studies indicate that with orally administered inositol nicotinate very low concentrations of

nicotinic acid are found in the plasma. These levels appear to be maintained for approximately 24 hours.

5.3 Preclinical safety data

None.

6. PHARMACEUTICAL PARTICULARS

6.1 List of excipients

Pregelatinised starch, Talc, Magnesium stearate, Maize starch, Stearic acid, Sodium lauryl sulphate.

6.2 Incompatibilities

None.

6.3 Shelf life

60 months.

6.4 Special precautions for storage

The product should be stored below 25°C.

6.5 Nature and contents of container

Amber glass bottles containing 100, 250 and 500 tablets.

250μm clear PVC/20μm aluminium blister pack containing 112 tablets.

Not all pack sizes may be marketed.

6.6 Instructions for use and handling

No special requirements.

7. MARKETING AUTHORISATION HOLDER

Genus Pharmaceuticals Limited (*trading as Genus Pharmaceuticals*)

Benham Valence

Newbury

Berkshire

RG20 8LU

United Kingdom

8. MARKETING AUTHORISATION NUMBER(S)

PL 06831/0148

9. DATE OF FIRST AUTHORISATION/RENEWAL OF THE AUTHORISATION

10th May 2005

10. DATE OF REVISION OF THE TEXT

Hiberix

(GlaxoSmithKline UK)

1. NAME OF THE MEDICINAL PRODUCT

Hiberix Vaccine

Haemophilus influenzae type b (Hib) vaccine.

2. QUALITATIVE AND QUANTITATIVE COMPOSITION

Hiberix is a lyophilised vaccine of purified polyribosyl-ribitol-phosphate capsular polysaccharide (PRP) of Hib, covalently bound to tetanus toxoid.

The Hib polysaccharide is prepared from Hib, strain 20,752 and after activation with cyanogen bromide and derivatisation with adipic hydrazide spacer is coupled to tetanus toxoid via carbodiimide condensation. After purification the conjugate is lyophilised in the presence of lactose as a stabiliser.

Hiberix meets the World Health Organisation requirements for manufacture of biological substances of Hib conjugated vaccines.

Each 0.5 ml dose of the vaccine contains 10 micrograms of purified capsular polysaccharide of Hib covalently bound to approximately 30 micrograms tetanus toxoid.

3. PHARMACEUTICAL FORM

Hib vaccine (lyophilised) for reconstitution.

4. CLINICAL PARTICULARS

4.1 Therapeutic indications

Active immunisation against invasive disease caused by *Haemophilus influenzae* type b.

4.2 Posology and method of administration

Posology

Primary series

Under 13 months of age:

Three 0.5ml doses, with an interval of at least four weeks between doses, the first dose to be given not earlier than two months of age.

Hiberix can also be mixed with 'Infanrix', 'DTP Vaccine Behring' or 'Trivax-AD' immediately prior to administration (see Section 6.6 Instructions for Use/Handling).

13 months of age and over:

A single 0.5ml dose.

Booster

Following completion of a primary series in which one or more of the three doses consisted of Hiberix mixed with Infanrix, an additional (fourth) dose of Hib conjugate vaccine should be administered.

Children who were primed with Hiberix may be boosted with Hiberix or with another Hib conjugate vaccine. Similarly, Hiberix may be used to boost children who were primed with other Hib conjugate vaccines.

The timing of the Hib conjugate booster dose should be in accordance with official recommendations (see also section 5.1 Pharmacodynamic properties).

Method of administration

Intramuscular injection. (For patients with thrombocytopenia or bleeding disorders the injection should be given subcutaneously, see Section 4.4).

4.3 Contraindications

Hiberix should not be administered to subjects with known hypersensitivity to any component of the vaccine, or to subjects that have shown any signs of hypersensitivity after previous administration of Hib vaccines.

As with other vaccines, the administration of Hiberix should be postponed in subjects suffering from acute severe febrile illness. The presence of a minor non-febrile infection, however, is not a contra-indication to vaccination.

4.4 Special warnings and special precautions for use

It is good clinical practice that immunisation should be preceded by a review of the medical history (especially with regard to previous immunisation and possible occurrence of undesirable events) and a clinical examination.

As with all vaccinations, appropriate medical treatment should be available for injection should an anaphylactic reaction occur. Recipients of the vaccine should remain under observation until they have been seen to be in good health and not to be experiencing an immediate adverse reaction. It is not possible to specify an exact length of time.

Hiberix should be administered with caution to subjects with thrombocytopenia or a bleeding disorder since bleeding may occur following an intramuscular administration to these subjects. In these subjects Hiberix may be administered by deep subcutaneous injection, see Section 4.2.

Human Immunodeficiency Virus (HIV) infection is not considered as a contra-indication for Hiberix.

Although limited immune response to the tetanus toxoid component may occur, vaccination with Hiberix alone does not substitute for routine tetanus vaccination.

Excretion of capsular polysaccharide antigen in the urine has been described following receipt of the Hib vaccine and therefore antigen detection may not have a diagnostic value in suspected Hib disease within one to two weeks of vaccination.

Hiberix does not protect against disease caused by other types of *Haemophilus influenzae* nor against meningitis caused by other organisms.

Hiberix should under no circumstances be administered intravascularly.

4.5 Interaction with other medicinal products and other forms of Interaction

Hiberix can be administered either simultaneously or at any time before or after a different inactivated or live vaccine.

Different injectable vaccines should be administered at different injection sites, with the exception of Hiberix and either 'Infanrix', 'DTP Vaccine Behring' or 'Trivax-AD' which can be mixed (see section 6.6 for reconstitution instructions.).

As with other vaccines it may be expected that in patients receiving immunosuppressive therapy or patients with immunodeficiency, an adequate response may not be achieved.

4.6 Pregnancy and lactation

No reproductive studies have been conducted in animals since vaccination against Hib in adults is uncommon. There is no accurate information on the safety of this vaccine in pregnancy therefore this vaccine should not be used in pregnancy or during lactation.

4.7 Effects on ability to drive and use machines

There is no information available on the effect of Hiberix on driving and use of machines.

4.8 Undesirable effects

Clinical trials

Primary vaccination

Clinical trials involved the administration of over 1200 doses of Hiberix to infants from 2 months of age as primary vaccination. The occurrence of undesirable effects was actively monitored for approximately one month after vaccination. In all studies, Hiberix was administered concomitantly with a DTP (whole cell or acellular pertussis) vaccine.

Local reactions, particularly mild erythema, pain and mild swelling at the site of injection, are the most frequently observed adverse events, occurring after approximately 17% of all doses. They are commonly seen during the 48 hours following vaccination and normally resolve spontaneously. General symptoms that occur in the first 48 hours are usually mild and resolve spontaneously.

Adverse events considered as being at least possibly related to vaccination have been categorised by frequency. No increase in the incidence or severity of these events was seen with subsequent doses of the primary vaccination series.

Frequencies are reported as:

Very common: ⩾ 10%

Common: ⩾ 1% and < 10%

Uncommon: ⩾ 0.1% and < 1%

Rare: ⩾ 0.01% and < 0.1%

Very rare: < 0.01%

Application site

very common: redness

common: pain, swelling

Autonomic nervous system

uncommon: sweating increased

Body as a whole

very common: fever (rectal temperature ⩾ 38°C), unusual crying

Gastro-intestinal symptoms

very common: loss of appetite

common: vomiting, diarrhoea

Platelet bleeding and clotting

uncommon: purpura

Psychiatric

very common: restlessness

common: nervousness

uncommon: emotional lability, insomnia

Booster vaccination

Clinical trials involved the administration of over 1800 doses of Hiberix to children in the second year of life as a booster dose. In all studies, Hiberix was administered concomitantly with a DTP (whole cell or acellular pertussis) vaccine.

As has been reported with other vaccines, increases in the incidences of local reactions were observed after booster vaccination with Hiberix compared with the primary course; these reactions occurred after approximately 44% of all booster doses.

Adverse events considered as being at least possibly related to vaccination have been categorised by frequency (as above).

Application site

very common: pain, redness, swelling

uncommon: injections site mass

Body as a whole

very common: fever (rectal temperature ⩾ 38°C), unusual crying

uncommon: fatigue

Central and peripheral nervous system:

uncommon: gait abnormal

Gastro-intestinal symptoms

very common: loss of appetite

common: diarrhoea, vomiting

Platelet bleeding and clotting

uncommon: purpura

Psychiatric

very common: restlessness, somnolence, nervousness

uncommon: emotional lability

Resistance mechanism

uncommon: upper respiratory tract infection, otitis media

Skin and appendages:

uncommon: rash, urticaria, rash erythematous

Post-marketing surveillance

Adverse events similar to those observed in the clinical trials have been reported during post-marketing surveillance. Other, less frequent events and their reported incidences were:

Body as a whole

very rare: allergic reactions (including anaphylactoid reactions)

Central and peripheral nervous system:

very rare: collapse or shock-like state (hypotonic-hyporesponsiveness episode; HHE)

4.9 Overdose

Not applicable.

5. PHARMACOLOGICAL PROPERTIES

5.1 Pharmacodynamic properties

When Hiberix was given as a separate injection to various DTP vaccines at various primary schedules, an anti-PRP titre of ⩾ 0.15 micrograms/ml (the level generally considered as protective against Hib disease) was obtained in ⩾ 95% of infants one month after the third dose.

The percentages of infants with anti-PRP titres ⩾ 0.15 micrograms/ml following vaccination with Hiberix as a mix with the vaccines listed in section 4.5 were not different from those obtained with Hiberix when given as a separate injection. However, the geometric mean titres of anti-PRP in infants administered Hiberix as a mix with Infanrix as a three-dose primary course were approximately one-third of those seen in infants who received Hiberix as a separate injection.

Administration of a booster dose of Hiberix during the second year of life resulted in anti-PRP titres ⩾ 1.0 micrograms/ml in almost all vaccinated children, irrespective of the vaccine(s) that were used for primary immunisation.

5.2 Pharmacokinetic properties
Evaluation of pharmacokinetic properties is not required for vaccines.

5.3 Preclinical safety data
Not applicable.

6. PHARMACEUTICAL PARTICULARS

6.1 List of excipients
Vaccine: Lactose

Diluent: when provided contains Sodium Chloride, Water for Injections (as Sterile Saline Solution (0.9%))

6.2 Incompatibilities
Hiberix can be mixed in the same syringe with the vaccines mentioned (in section 4.5). No other vaccines should be mixed in the same syringe as Hiberix unless specified by the manufacturer.

6.3 Shelf life
The shelf-life of the Hiberix vaccine is three years when stored unopened and unmixed at 2°C to 8°C. The expiry date printed on the outer carton should be adhered to strictly.

6.4 Special precautions for storage
Store between 2°C and 8°C. Protect from light.

6.5 Nature and contents of container
Powder for reconstitution

Hiberix is supplied as a white pellet in a vial (Type I neutral glass) with stoppers (bromobutyl rubber) and overcaps with flip-off tops (aluminium), containing one dose.

Solvent for reconstitution

The diluent (Sterile Saline Solution (0.9%)), when provided, is a clear and colourless liquid in a glass ampoule or vial (PL 00002/0194) or pre-filled syringe (PL 00002/0236). The pre-filled syringe (Type I glass) contains 0.5 ml, with a plunger stopper (rubber butyl).

The green, 38mm, 21-gauge needle has been provided for reconstitution of the Hiberix vaccine.

The blue, 25mm, 23-gauge needle has been provided for administration of the Hiberix vaccine. This vaccine needs to be injected to the appropriate depth in order for it to be effective. Choose the most appropriate needle for your patient to ensure the vaccine reaches the correct tissue as specified in section 4.2 (Posology and Method of Administration). If the needle supplied for administration is not appropriate for your patient, a different needle can be used.

6.6 Instructions for use and handling
The reconstituted Hiberix vaccine should be inspected visually for any foreign particulate matter and/or variation of physical aspect prior to administration. In the event of either being observed, discard the vaccine.

The vaccine must be reconstituted by adding the entire contents of the ampoule, vial or syringe of diluent, when provided, to the vial containing the pellet. After the addition of the diluent, the mixture should be well shaken until the pellet is completely dissolved in the diluent.

Inject the entire contents of the vial.

After reconstitution, Hiberix should be injected promptly (within one hour). Any unused reconstituted vaccine should be discarded.

Full reconstitution instructions:

1. Attach the 38mm, 21-gauge (green) needle to a pre-filled syringe of diluent and inject the entire contents of the syringe into the Hib vial.

2. With the needle still inserted, shake the Hib vial vigorously and examine for complete dissolution.

3. Withdraw the entire mixture back into the syringe.

4. Replace the 21-gauge (green) needle with an appropriate size needle for injection, and administer the vaccine. Administer the vaccine by intramuscular injection.

5. After reconstitution, Hiberix should be injected immediately or at least within one hour.

6. If the vaccine is not administered immediately, shake the solution vigorously again before injection.

7. Any unused reconstituted vaccine should be discarded.

For mixing with DTP vaccines
Alternatively Hiberix can also be mixed with 'Infanrix', 'DTP Vaccine Behring' or 'Trivax-AD' immediately prior to administration as follows:

1. Attach a 38mm, 21-gauge (green) needle to the syringe (where DTP vaccine is supplied in a vial, first draw up the DTP vaccine suspension in to a syringe)

2. Inject the contents of the syringe of DTP vaccine suspension into the Hiberix vial.

3. With the needle still inserted, shake the Hiberix vial vigorously and examine for complete dissolution, i.e. a whitish liquid of uniform appearance should be formed.

4. Withdraw the entire mixture back into the syringe.

5. Replace the 38 mm, 21-gauge (green) needle with an appropriate size needle for injection, and administer the vaccine. The blue, 25mm, 23-gauge needle has been provided for administration of the Hiberix vaccine. This vaccine needs to be injected to the appropriate depth in order for it to be effective. Choose the most appropriate needle for your patient to ensure the vaccine reaches the correct tissue as specified in section 4.2 (Posology and Method of Administration). If the needle supplied for administration is not appropriate for your patient, a different needle can be used.

6. After reconstitution, the vaccine should be injected immediately or at least within one hour.

7. If the vaccine is not administered immediately, shake the solution vigorously again before injection.

8. Any unused reconstituted vaccine should be discarded.

Administrative Data

7. MARKETING AUTHORISATION HOLDER
SmithKline Beecham plc

Brentford

Middlesex

TW8 9GS

Trading as:

GlaxoSmithKline UK

Stockley Park West

Uxbridge

Middlesex UB11 1BT

8. MARKETING AUTHORISATION NUMBER(S)
PL 10592/0120

9. DATE OF FIRST AUTHORISATION/RENEWAL OF THE AUTHORISATION
3 September 1999

10. DATE OF REVISION OF THE TEXT
01 April 2004

11. Legal Status
POM

Hiprex Tablets

(3M Health Care Limited)

1. NAME OF THE MEDICINAL PRODUCT
Hiprex 1g Tablets

2. QUALITATIVE AND QUANTITATIVE COMPOSITION
Each Hiprex tablet contains methenamine hippurate 1 g.

For excipients see 6.1.

3. PHARMACEUTICAL FORM
White, oblong tablet with breakline marked HX on one side and 3M on the other.

4. CLINICAL PARTICULARS

4.1 Therapeutic indications
Hiprex is indicated in the prophylaxis and treatment of urinary tract infections:

1. As maintenance therapy after successful initial treatment of acute infections with antibiotics.

2. As long-term therapy in the prevention of recurrent cystitis.

3. To suppress urinary infection in patients with indwelling catheters and to reduce the incidence of catheter blockage.

4. To provide prophylaxis against the introduction of infection into the urinary tract during instrumental procedures.

5. Asymptomatic bacteriuria.

4.2 Posology and method of administration
Adults: 1g twice daily.

In patients with catheters the dosage may be increased to 1g three times daily.

Children under 6 years: Not recommended.

Children: 6-12 years: 500mg twice daily.

Elderly: No special dosage recommendations.

The tablets may be halved, or they can be crushed and taken with a drink of milk or fruit juice if the patient prefers.

4.3 Contraindications
Hepatic dysfunction, renal parenchymal infection, severe dehydration, metabolic acidosis, or severe renal failure (creatinine clearance or GFR<10 ml/min.). Hiprex may be used where mild (20-50 ml/min.) to moderate (10-20 ml/min.) renal insufficiency is present. (If the GFR is not available the serum creatinine concentration can be used as a guide.).

Hiprex should not be administered concurrently with sulphonamides because of the possibility of crystalluria, or with alkalising agents, such as a mixture of potassium citrate.

4.4 Special warnings and special precautions for use
None.

4.5 Interaction with other medicinal products and other forms of Interaction
Methenamine hippurate should not be given/administered concurrently with sulphonamides because of the possibility of crystalluria, or with alkalising agents such as potassium citrate. Concurrent use with acetazolamide should be avoided as the desired effect of hexamine will be lost.

4.6 Pregnancy and lactation
There is inadequate evidence of safety of the drug in human pregnancy but it has been in wide use for many years without apparent ill consequence, animal studies having shown no hazard.

Methenamine is excreted in breast milk but the quantities will be insignificant to the infant. Mothers can therefore breast feed their infants.

4.7 Effects on ability to drive and use machines
None.

4.8 Undesirable effects
Occasionally rashes, pruritis, gastric irritation, irritation of the bladder, may occur.

All side effects are reversible on the withdrawal of the drug.

4.9 Overdose
Vomiting and haematuria may occur. These can be treated by the use of an anti-emetic and drinking copious quantities of water respectively. Bladder symptoms can be treated by the consumption of copious quantities of water and 2-3 teaspoonfuls of bicarbonate of soda.

5. PHARMACOLOGICAL PROPERTIES

5.1 Pharmacodynamic properties
Pharmacotherapeutic group G04A A01

Hiprex is a urinary antibacterial agent with a wide antibacterial spectrum covering both gram-positive and gram-negative organisms. Urinary antibacterial activity can be shown within 30 minutes of administration.

The chemical structure of methenamine hippurate is such that a two-fold antibacterial action is obtained:

1. The slow release of the bactericidal formaldehyde, from the methenamine part, in the urine; acid pH is necessary for this reaction to occur. It is obtained and maintained there by the presence of hippuric acid.

2. The bacteriostatic effect of hippuric acid itself on urinary tract pathogens.

5.2 Pharmacokinetic properties
Methenamine hippurate is readily absorbed from the gastro-intestinal tract and excreted via the kidney.

Plasma concentrations of methenamine hippurate reach maximum 1-2 hours after a single dose and then decline with a half-life of about 4 hours. Methenamine recovered in the urine corresponds to about 80% of the dose given per 12 hours.

5.3 Preclinical safety data
Not applicable

6. PHARMACEUTICAL PARTICULARS

6.1 List of excipients
Magnesium Stearate

Povidone

Colloidal anhydrous silica

6.2 Incompatibilities
Not applicable.

6.3 Shelf life
5 years

6.4 Special precautions for storage
Do not store above 30°C. Keep bottle tightly closed.

6.5 Nature and contents of container
Glass bottles of 60 tablets

6.6 Instructions for use and handling
None

7. MARKETING AUTHORISATION HOLDER
3M Health Care Limited

3M House

Morley Street

Loughborough

Leics

LE11 1EP

8. MARKETING AUTHORISATION NUMBER(S)
PL 00068/5003R

9. DATE OF FIRST AUTHORISATION/RENEWAL OF THE AUTHORISATION
12 October 1989/29 March 1996

10. DATE OF REVISION OF THE TEXT
May 2001

Hormonin

(Shire Pharmaceuticals Limited)

1. NAME OF THE MEDICINAL PRODUCT
Hormonin®

2. QUALITATIVE AND QUANTITATIVE COMPOSITION
Per tablet:

Estrone 1.4 mg

Estradiol 0.6 mg

Estriol 0.27mg

3. PHARMACEUTICAL FORM
Tablets

4. CLINICAL PARTICULARS

4.1 Therapeutic indications

Hormone replacement therapy (HRT) for estrogen deficiency symptoms in peri- and post-menopausal women.

Prevention of osteoporosis in postmenopausal women at high risk of future fractures who are intolerant of, or contraindicated for, other medicinal products approved for the prevention of osteoporosis (see Section 4.4).

The experience of treating women older than 65 years is limited.

4.2 Posology and method of administration

Hormonin is an estrogen-only product which may be given to women with or without a uterus.

Hormonin may be given continuous sequentially or cyclically (three weeks out of four).

Continuous sequential therapy: 1-2 tablets should be taken daily without a break in therapy.

Cyclical therapy: Hormonin 1-2 tablets should be taken cyclically (three weeks on followed by one week off).

In women with an intact uterus the addition of an adequate dose and duration of progestogen (for 12-14 days) in each 28 day cycle is recommended to reduce the risk to the endometrium. Only progestogens approved for addition to estrogen treatment should be recommended e.g. Provera, Micronor HRT.

Unless there is a previous diagnosis of endometriosis, it is not normally recommended to add a progestogen in hysterectomised women.

For initiation and continuation of treatment of postmenopausal symptoms, the lowest effective dose for the shortest duration (see Section 4.4) should be used.

Starting Treatment

Therapy with Hormonin may be initiated with one tablet daily. This may be increased to 2 tablets daily if symptoms are not fully controlled.

In women who are not taking HRT and are not menstruating regularly, or women transferring from a continuous combined HRT product, treatment may be started on any convenient day.

If the patient is menstruating regularly, therapy can be started within the first five days of bleeding.

In women transferring from a sequential HRT regimen, treatment should begin on the day following the end of the previous 28 day cycle. In women transferring from a cyclical HRT regimen, treatment should begin within five days following the end of the previous 28 day cycle.

In hysterectomised women, treatment should be started on any convenient day.

Missed Tablet

If a tablet is missed it should be taken within 12 hours of when normally taken, otherwise the tablet should be discarded, and the usual tablet should be taken the following day.

If one extra tablet is taken inadvertently, the usual tablet should still be taken the following day.

Missing a dose may increase the likelihood of breakthrough bleeding and spotting.

4.3 Contraindications

- Known, past or suspected breast cancer
- Known or suspected estrogen-dependent malignant tumours (e.g. endometrial cancer)
- Undiagnosed genital bleeding
- Untreated endometrial hyperplasia
- Previous idiopathic or current venous thromboembolism (deep venous thrombosis, pulmonary embolism)
- Active or recent arterial thromboembolic disease (e.g. angina, myocardial infarction)
- Acute liver disease, or a recent history of liver disease as long as liver function tests have failed to return to normal
- Known hypersensitivity to the active substances or to any of the excipients
- Porphyria

4.4 Special warnings and special precautions for use

For the treatment of postmenopausal symptoms, HRT should only be initiated for symptoms that adversely affect quality of life. In all cases, a careful appraisal of the risks and benefits should be undertaken at least annually and HRT should only be continued as long as the benefit outweighs the risk.

Medical examination/follow up

Before initiating or reinstituting HRT, a complete personal and family medical history should be taken. Physical (including pelvic and breast) examination should be guided by this and by the contraindications and warnings for use. During treatment, periodic check-ups are recommended of a frequency and nature adapted to the individual woman. Women should be advised what changes in their breast should be reported to their doctor or nurse (see 'Breast cancer' below). Investigations, including mammography, should be carried out in accordance with currently accepted screening practices, modified to the clinical needs of the individual.

Conditions which need supervision

If any of the following conditions are present, have occurred previously, and/or have been aggravated during pregnancy or previous hormone treatment, the patient should be closely supervised. It should be taken into account that these conditions may recur or be aggravated during treatment with Hormonin, in particular:

- Leiomyoma (uterine fibroids) or endometriosis
- A history of, or risk factors for, thromboembolic disorders (see below)
- Risk factors for estrogen dependent tumours, e.g. first degree heredity for breast cancer
- Hypertension
- Liver disorders (e.g. liver adenoma)
- Diabetes mellitus with or without vascular involvement (see Other Conditions below)
- Cholelithiasis
- Migraine or (severe) headache
- Systemic lupus erythematosus
- A history of endometrial hyperplasia (see below)
- Epilepsy
- Asthma
- Otosclerosis

Reasons for immediate withdrawal of therapy

Therapy should be discontinued in case a contraindication is discovered and in the following situations:

- Jaundice or deterioration in liver function
- Significant increase in blood pressure
- New onset of migraine-type headache
- Pregnancy

Breast cancer

A randomised placebo-controlled trial, the Women's Health Initiative study (WHI), and epidemiological studies, including the Million Women Study (MWS), have reported an increased risk of breast cancer in women taking estrogens, estrogen-progestogen combinations, or tibolone for HRT for several years (see Section 4.8). For all HRT, an excess risk becomes apparent within a few years of use and increases with duration of intake of HRT but returns to baseline within a few (at most five) years after stopping treatment.

In the MWS, the relative risk of breast cancer with conjugated equine estrogens (CEE) or estradiol (E2) was greater when a progestogen was added, either sequentially or continuously, and regardless of type of progestogen. There was no evidence of a difference in risk between the different routes of administration.

In the WHI study, the continuous combined conjugated estrogen and medroxyprogesterone acetate (CEE + MPA) product used was associated with breast cancers that were slightly larger in size and more frequently had local lymph node metastases compared to placebo.

HRT, especially estrogen-progestogen combined treatment, increases the density of mammographic images, which may adversely affect the radiological detection of breast cancer.

Endometrial hyperplasia and cancer

The risk of endometrial hyperplasia and carcinoma is increased when estrogens are administered alone for prolonged periods (see Section 4.8). The addition of a progestogen for at least 12 days per cycle in non-hysterectomised women greatly reduces this risk.

Break-through bleeding and spotting may occur during the first months of treatment. If break-through bleeding or spotting appears after some time on therapy, or continues after treatment has been discontinued, the reason should be investigated, which may include endometrial biopsy to exclude endometrial malignancy.

Unopposed estrogen stimulation may lead to premalignant or malignant transformation in the residual foci of endometriosis. Therefore, the addition of progestogens to estrogen replacement therapy should be considered in women who have undergone hysterectomy because of endometriosis, if they are known to have residual endometriosis.

Ovarian Cancer

Long-term (at least 5 to 10 years) use of estrogen-only HRT products in hysterectomised women has been associated with an increased risk of ovarian cancer in some epidemiological studies. It is uncertain whether long-term use of combined HRT confers a different risk than estrogen-only products.

Venous thromboembolism

HRT is associated with a higher relative risk of developing venous thromboembolism (VTE), i.e. deep vein thrombosis or pulmonary embolism. One randomised controlled trial and epidemiological studies found a two- to threefold higher risk for users compared with non-users. For non-users, it is estimated that the number of cases of VTE that will occur over a 5 year period is about 3 per 1000 women aged 50-59 years and 8 per 1000 women aged 60-69 years. It is estimated that in healthy women who use HRT for 5 years, the number of additional cases of VTE over a 5 year period will be between 2 and 6 (best estimate = 4) per 1000 women aged 50-59 years and between 5 and 15 (best estimate = 9) per 1000 women aged 60-69 years. The occurrence of such an event is more likely in the first year of HRT than later.

Generally recognised risk factors for VTE include a personal history or family history, severe obesity (BM $>30kg/m^2$) and systemic lupus erythematosus (SLE). There is no consensus about the possible role of varicose veins in VTE.

Patients with a history of VTE or known thrombophilic states have an increased risk of VTE. HRT may add to this risk. Personal or strong family history of thromboembolism or recurrent spontaneous abortion should be investigated in order to exclude a thrombophilic predisposition. Until a thorough evaluation of thrombophilic factors has been made or anticoagulant treatment initiated, use of HRT in such patients should be viewed as contraindicated. Those women already on anticoagulant treatment require careful consideration of the benefit-risk of use of HRT.

The risk of VTE may be temporarily increased with prolonged immobilisation, major trauma or major surgery. As in all postoperative patients, scrupulous attention should be given to prophylactic measures to prevent VTE following surgery. When prolonged immobilisation is liable to follow elective surgery, particularly abdominal or orthopaedic surgery to the lower limbs, consideration should be given to temporarily stopping HRT 4 to 6 weeks earlier, if possible. Treatment should not be restarted until the woman is completely mobilised.

If VTE develops after initiating therapy, the drug should be discontinued. Patients should be told to contact their doctor immediately when they are aware of a potential thromboembolic symptom (e.g. painful swelling of a leg, sudden pain in the chest, dyspnoea).

Coronary artery disease (CAD)

There is no evidence from randomised controlled trials of cardiovascular benefit with continuous combined conjugated estrogens and medroxyprogesterone acetate. Two large clinical trials (WHI and HERS i.e. Heart and Estrogen/progestin Replacement Study) showed a possible increased risk of cardiovascular morbidity in the first year of use and no overall benefit. For other HRT products there are only limited data from randomised controlled trials examining effects in cardiovascular morbidity or mortality. Therefore, it is uncertain whether these findings also extend to other HRT products.

Stroke

One large randomised clinical trial (WHI trial) found, as a secondary outcome, an increased risk of ischaemic stroke in healthy women during treatment with continuous combined conjugated estrogens and MPA. For women who do not use HRT, it is estimated that the number of cases of stroke that will occur over a 5 year period is about 3 per 1000 women aged 50–59 years and 11 per 1000 women aged 60–69 years. It is estimated that for women who use conjugated estrogens and MPA for 5 years, the number of additional cases will be between 0 and 3 (best estimate = 1) per 1000 users aged 50–59 years and between 1 and 9 (best estimate = 4) per 1000 users aged 60–69 years. It is unknown whether the increased risk also extends to other HRT products.

Other conditions

Estrogens may cause fluid retention, and therefore patients with cardiac or renal dysfunction should be carefully observed. Patients with terminal renal insufficiency should be closely observed, since it is expected that the level of circulating active ingredients in Hormonin is increased.

Women with pre-existing hypertriglyceridemia should be followed closely during estrogen replacement or HRT, since rare cases of large increases of plasma triglycerides leading to pancreatitis have been reported with estrogen therapy in this condition.

Estrogens increase thyroid binding globulin (TBG), leading to increased circulating total thyroid hormone, as measured by protein-bound iodine (PBI), T4 levels (by column or by radio-immunoassay) or T3 levels (by radio-immunoassay). T3 resin uptake is decreased, reflecting the elevated TBG. Free T4 and free T3 concentrations are unaltered. Other binding proteins may be elevated in serum, i.e. corticoid binding globulin (CBG), sex-hormone-binding globulin (SHBG) leading to increased circulating corticosteroids and sex steroids, respectively. Free or biological active hormone concentrations are unchanged. Other plasma proteins may be increased (angiotensinogen/renin substrate, alpha-1-antitrypsin, ceruloplasmin).

There is no conclusive evidence for improvement of cognitive function. There is some evidence from the WHI trial of increased risk of probable dementia in women who start using continuous combined CEE and MPA after the age of 65. It is unknown whether the findings apply to younger post-menopausal women or other HRT products.

Glucose tolerance may be lowered and Hormonin may, therefore, increase the need for insulin or other anti-diabetic drugs in diabetics.

Hormonin is not an oral contraceptive. Non-hormonal contraception should be used if required.

Patients with rare hereditary problems of galactose intolerance, the Lapp lactase deficiency or glucose-galactose malabsoprtion should not take this medicine.

4.5 Interaction with other medicinal products and other forms of Interaction

The metabolism of estrogens may be increased by concomitant use of substances known to induce drug-metabolising enzymes, specifically cytochrome P450 enzymes, such as anticonvulsants (e.g. phenobarbital, phenytoin, carbamazepine) and anti-infectives (e.g. rifampicin, rifabutin, nevirapine, efavirenz).

Ritonavir and nelfinavir, although known as strong inhibitors, by contrast exhibit inducing properties when used concomitantly with steroid hormones. Herbal preparations containing St John's wort (Hypericum perforatum) may induce the metabolism of estrogens.

Clinically, an increased metabolism of estrogens may lead to decreased effect and changes in the uterine bleeding profile.

4.6 Pregnancy and lactation

Hormonin is not indicated during pregnancy. If pregnancy occurs during medication with Hormonin, treatment should be withdrawn immediately.

The results of most epidemiological studies to date relevant to inadvertent foetal exposure to estrogens indicate no teratogenic or foetotoxic effects.

Hormonin is not indicated during lactation.

4.7 Effects on ability to drive and use machines

None known.

4.8 Undesirable effects

From clinical trial data, approximately 42% of patients have experienced adverse reactions. These are mainly dose dependent and due to the pharmacological effects of the medicinal product.

The most commonly reported undesirable effects for Hormonin and other estrogen treatments are detailed in the following table.

System organ class	Undesirable effect
Cardiac disorders	Myocardial infarction
Endocrine disorders	Hirsutism
Eye disorders	Corneal discomfort (with contact lenses) Visual disturbance
Gastrointestinal disorders	Abdominal pain Dyspepsia Nausea Upper abdominal pain Vomiting
General disorders & administration site conditions	Fatigue
Hepatobiliary disorders	Cholelithiasis Cholestatic jaundice
Infections and infestations	Candidal infections
Investigations	Abnormal liver function tests Decreased glucose tolerance Raised blood pressure Weight fluctuation Weight gain
Musculoskeletal & connective tissue disorders	Back pain Muscle cramps
Nervous system disorders	Dizziness Headache Migraine Probable dementia Stroke Vertigo
Psychiatric disorders	Irritability Mood swings
Renal & urinary disorders	Fluid retention Sodium retention Urge incontinence
Reproductive system & breast disorders	Benign breast neoplasm Breast discharge Breast enlargement Breast pain Breast tenderness Dysmenorrhoea Endometrial cancer Endometrial hyperplasia Endometrial neoplasia Increase in size of uterine fibroids Intermenstrual bleeding Irregular menstruation Menorrhagia Ovarian cyst Pre-menstrual syndrome Vaginal discharge
Respiratory, thoracic & mediastinal system disorders	Dyspnoea
Skin & subcutaneous tissue disorders	Alopecia Chloasma Dry skin Erythema multiform Erythema nodosum Rash Vascular purpura
Vascular disorders	Hot flushes Hypertension Phlebitis Thromboembolism Thrombosis

Breast cancer

According to evidence from a large number of epidemiological studies and one randomised placebo-controlled trial, the WHI, the overall risk of breast cancer increases with increasing duration of HRT use in current or recent HRT users.

For *estrogen-only* HRT, estimates of relative risk (RR) from a reanalysis of original data from 51 epidemiological studies (in which >80% of HRT use was estrogen-only HRT) and from the epidemiological MWS are similar at 1.35 (95%CI 1.21-1.49) and 1.30 (95%CI 1.21-1.40), respectively.

For *estrogen plus progestogen* combined HRT, several epidemiological studies have reported an overall higher risk for breast cancer than with estrogens alone.

The MWS reported that, compared to never users, the use of various types of estrogen-progestogen combined HRT was associated with a higher risk of breast cancer (RR = 2.00, 95%CI 1.88-2.12) than use of estrogens alone (RR = 1.30, 95%CI 1.21-1.40) or use of tibolone (RR = 1.45, 95%CI 1.25-1.68).

The WHI trial reported a risk estimate of 1.24 (95%CI 1.01-1.54) after 5.6 years of use of estrogen-progestogen combined HRT (CEE + MPA) in all users compared with placebo.

The absolute risks calculated from the MWS and the WHI trial are presented below:

The MWS has estimated, from the known average incidence of breast cancer in developed countries, that:

• For women not using HRT, about 32 in every 1000 are expected to have breast cancer diagnosed between the ages of 50 and 64 years

• For 1000 current or recent users of HRT, the number of *additional* cases during the corresponding period will be

o For users of *estrogen-only* replacement therapy

§ Between 0 and 3 (best estimate = 1.5) for 5 years' use

§ Between 3 and 7 (best estimate = 5) for 10 years' use

o For users of estrogen plus progestogen combined HRT

§ Between 5 and 7 (best estimate = 6) for 5 years' use

§ Between 18 and 20 (best estimate = 19) for 10 years' use

The WHI trial estimated that after 5.6 years of follow-up of women between the ages of 50 and 79 years, an *additional* 8 cases of invasive breast cancer would be due to *estrogen-progestogen combined* HRT (CEE + MPA) per 10,000 women years. According to calculations from the trial data, it is estimated that:

• For 1000 women in the placebo group

o About 16 cases of invasive breast cancer would be diagnosed in 5 years

• For 1000 women who used estrogen-progestogen combined HRT (CEE + MPA), the number of *additional* cases would be

o Between 0 and 9 (best estimate = 4) for 5 years' use

The number of additional cases of breast cancer in women who use HRT is broadly similar for women who start HRT irrespective of age at start of use (between the ages of 45-65) (see Section 4.4).

Endometrial cancer

In women with an intact uterus, the risk of endometrial hyperplasia and endometrial cancer increases with increasing duration of use of unopposed estrogens. According to data from epidemiological studies, the best estimate of the risk is that for women not using HRT, about 5 in every 1000 are expected to have endometrial cancer diagnosed between the ages of 50 and 65. Depending on the duration of treatment and estrogen dose, the reported increase in endometrial cancer risk among unopposed estrogen users varies from 2- to 12-fold greater compared with non-users. Adding a progestogen to estrogen-only therapy greatly reduces this increased risk.

4.9 Overdose

Ingestion of large doses of estrogen containing oral contraceptives by young children have often been reported and show that acute serious ill effects do not occur. Overdosage of estrogen may cause nausea and withdrawal bleeding in females.

5. PHARMACOLOGICAL PROPERTIES

5.1 Pharmacodynamic properties

The active ingredients, synthetic 17β-estradiol, estriol and estrone are chemically and biologically identical to endogenous human estrogens. They substitute for the loss of estrogen production in menopausal women and alleviate menopausal symptoms.

The three natural hormone estrogens vary considerably in their potency. Estradiol is the most potent and estrone and estriol notably weaker. Pharmacologically, estriol occupies a unique position in that it has a shallow dose response curve and quickly reaches a plateau where substantially increased doses produce no increase in activity. It binds to its receptor site in competition with estradiol.

Estrogens prevent bone loss following menopause or ovariectomy. Estrogen deficiency at menopause is associated with an increasing bone turnover and decline in bone mass. The effect of estrogens on the bone mineral density is dose-dependent. Protection appears to be effective for as long as treatment is continued. After discontinuation of HRT, bone mass is lost at a rate similar to that in untreated women.

Evidence from the WHI trial and meta-analysed trials shows that current use of HRT, alone or in combination with a progestogen – given to predominately healthy women – reduces the risk of hip, vertebral, and other osteoporotic fractures. HRT may also prevent fractures in women with low bone density and/or established osteoporosis, but the evidence is limited.

5.2 Pharmacokinetic properties

The natural estrogens are generally quickly and well absorbed from the gastro-intestinal tract, there being little difference between estrone, estradiol and estriol. Estrogens are inactivated in the liver. A proportion of absorbed estrogen is excreted in the bile and then reabsorbed from the intestine. In the liver estradiol is readily oxidised to estrone and both estradiol and estrone are converted by hydration to estriol. Metabolites of estrogens are mainly excreted in the urine as conjugates of glucuronic and sulphuric acid.

Following administration of Hormonin, physiological estrogen concentrations are achieved at different rates. The maximum plasma levels and the time to reach the peak in the plasma level varied between subjects and was; estrone 750-2116 pmol/litre, 0.5-6.0 hours; estradiol 246-813 pmol/litre, 1-8 hours; estriol 173-241 pmol/litre, 5-12 hours. Following steady state conditions after cessation of Hormonin therapy, estrogen levels remained in the premenopausal range for approximately 48 hours.

5.3 Preclinical safety data

None stated.

6. PHARMACEUTICAL PARTICULARS

6.1 List of excipients

Sunset yellow

Amaranth

Lactose

Potato starch

Magnesium stearate

Methyl alcohol

Chloroform

6.2 Incompatibilities

None.

6.3 Shelf life

36 months

6.4 Special precautions for storage

Store in the original package. Do not store above 25°C.

6.5 Nature and contents of container

Blister packs of 84 tablets.

6.6 Instructions for use and handling

No special conditions.

7. MARKETING AUTHORISATION HOLDER

G. W. Carnrick Company Limited,
Greytown House,
221-227 High Street,
Orpington,
Kent BR6 ONZ
United Kingdom

8. MARKETING AUTHORISATION NUMBER(S)

PL 00271/5000R

9. DATE OF FIRST AUTHORISATION/RENEWAL OF THE AUTHORISATION

8 July 1988

10. DATE OF REVISION OF THE TEXT

July 2004

LEGAL CATEGORY

POM

HRF 100 Microgram

(Intrapharm Laboratories Ltd)

1. NAME OF THE MEDICINAL PRODUCT

HRF 100 microgram.

2. QUALITATIVE AND QUANTITATIVE COMPOSITION

Each vital contains 100 micrograms of Gonadorelin as Gonadorelin Hydrochloride BP.

3. PHARMACEUTICAL FORM

Powder and solvent for solution for injection.

4. CLINICAL PARTICULARS

4.1 Therapeutic indications

HRF as a single injection is indicated for evaluating the functional capacity and response of the gonadotropes of the anterior pituitary. The LH/FSH-RH response is used in testing patients with suspected gonadotropes deficiency, whether due to the hypothalamus alone or in combination with anterior pituitary failure. HRF is also indicated for evaluating residual gonadotropic function of the pituitary following removal of a pituitary tumour or surgery and/or irradiation.

The HRF test complements the clinical assessment of patients with a variety of endocrine disorders involving the hypothalamic-pituitary axis. In cases where there is a normal response, it indicates the presence of functional pituitary gonadotropes. The single injection test does not determine the patho-physiological cause for the subnormal response and does not measure pituitary gonadotropic reserve.

4.2 Posology and method of administration

Route of administration

For subcutaneous and intravenous administration.

Adults and elderly

100 micrograms, subcutaneously or intravenously. In females for whom the phrase of the menstrual cycle can be established, the test should be performed in early follicular phase (days 1 – 7).

Children

Do not use in children under one year of age as diluent contains 2% benzyl alcohol.

Test Methodology

To determine the status of the gonadotropin secretory capacity of the anterior pituitary, a test procedure requiring seven venous blood samples for LH/FSH-RH is recommended.

Procedure:

1. Venous blood samples should be drawn at -15minutes and immediately prior to HRF administration. The LH/FSH-RH baseline is obtained by averaging the LH/FSH-RH values of the two samples.

2. Administer a bolus of HRF subcutaneously or intravenously.

3. Draw venous blood samples at 15, 30, 45, 60 and 120 minutes after administration.

4. Blood samples should be handles as recommended by the laboratory that will determine the LH/FSH-RH content. It must be emphasized that the reliability of the test is directly related to the inter-assay and intra-assay reliability of the laboratory performing the assay.

Interpretation of Test Result: Interpretation of the LH/FSH-RH response to HRF requires an understanding of the hypothalamic-pituitary physiology, knowledge of the clinical status of the individual patient, and familiarity with the normal ranges and the standards used in the laboratory performing the LH/FSH-RH assays.

Curves provided represent the LH/FSH-RH response curves after administration in normal subjects. The normal LH/FSH-RH response curves were established between the 10th percentile (B line) and the 90th percentile (A line) of all LH/FSH-RH responses in normal subjects analysed from the results of clinical studies.

Individual patient responses should be plotted on the appropriate curve. A subnormal response in patients is defined as three or more LH/FSH-RH values which fall below the B line of the normal LH/FSH-RH response curve.

In cases where there is a blunted or boarderline response, the HRF test should be repeated.

The HRF test complements the clinical assessment of patients with a variety of endocrine disorders involving the hypothalamic-pituitary axis. In cases where there is a normal response, it indicates the presence of functional pituitary gonadotropes. The single injection test does not determine the patho-physiological cause for the subnormal response and does not measure pituitary gonadotropic reserve.

4.3 Contraindications

Hypersensitivity to HRF or and of the components. Known or suspected pregnancy. Do not use in children under one year of age as diluent contains 2% benzyl alcohol.

4.4 Special warnings and special precautions for use

Although allergic and hypersensitivity reactions have been observed with other polypeptide hormones, to date no such reactions have been encountered following the administration of a single 100 micrograms dose of HRF used for diagnostic purposes. Rare instances of hypersensitivity reactions have been reported. Therefore, patients treated by intermittent pulsatile therapy in whom re-administration is considered, particularly by the intravenous route, should be carefully observed. Administration during the follicular phase of a normal cycle may result in premature ovulation and appropriate measures are advised to prevent an unwanted pregnancy in these circumstances.

4.5 Interaction with other medicinal products and other forms of Interaction

The HRF test should be conducted in the absence of other drugs which directly affect the pituitary secretion of the gonadotropins. These would include a variety of preparations which contain androgens, oestrogens, progestins, or glucocorticoids. The gonadotropin levels may be transiently elevated by spironolactone, minimally elevated by levodopa, and suppressed by oral contraceptives and digoxin. The response to HRF may be blunted by phenothiazines and dopamine anyagonists which cause a rise in prolactin.

4.6 Pregnancy and lactation

HRF should not be administered to pregnant or nursing mothers.

4.7 Effects on ability to drive and use machines

None known.

4.8 Undesirable effects

Systemic complaints such as headaches, nausea, lightheadedness, abdominal discomfort and flushing have been reported rarely following administration of HRF. Local swelling, occasionally with pain and pruritus at the injection site may occur if HRF is administered subcutaneously. Local and generalized skin rash have been noted after chronic subcutaneous administration.

Thrombophlebitis with septicaemia, mild and severe, has been reported in isolated cases at the site of intravenous injection. Rare instances of hypersensitivity reaction (bronchospasm, tachycardia, flushing, urticaria, swelling, itching and redness of face, eyelids and lips, induration at injection site) have been reported following multiple-does administration of large doses. Antibody formation has also been reported rarely after chronic administration of large doses.

4.9 Overdose

HRF has been administered parenterally in doses up to 3 mg bd for 28 days without signs of symptoms of overdosage. In cases of overdosage or Idiosyncrasy, symptomatic treatment should be administered as required.

5. PHARMACOLOGICAL PROPERTIES

5.1 Pharmacodynamic properties

Gonadorelin stimulates the synthesis of follicle stimulating hormone and luteinising hormone in the anterior lobe of the pituitary as well as their release.

5.2 Pharmacokinetic properties

Gonadorelin is rapidly hydrolysed in plasma and excreted in urine with a half life of about 4 minutes.

5.3 Preclinical safety data

Not applicable.

6. PHARMACEUTICAL PARTICULARS

6.1 List of excipients

Lactose monohydrate USP

Solvent:

Benzyl alcohol BP

Water for injection BP

6.2 Incompatibilities

HRF should not be mixed with any other substance.

6.3 Shelf life

Unopened: 48 months

After reconstitution: 24 hours

6.4 Special precautions for storage

Store below 25°C

6.5 Nature and contents of container

HRF is supplied in a USP Type 1 clear glass vial with grey butyl rubber stopper and aluminium collar. The sterile solvent is 5 ml water for injections with 2% benzyl alcohol supplied in a Ph. Eur Type 1 clear glass ampoule.

6.6 Instructions for use and handling

Preparation for single injection administration: Reconstitute 100 micrograms vial with 1.0 ml of the accompanying sterile solvent of 2% benzyl alcohol. Prepare solution immediately before use. After reconstruction, refrigerate and use within 1 day. Discard unused reconstituted solution and solvent.

Administrative Data

7. MARKETING AUTHORISATION HOLDER

Intrapharm Laboratories Limited

60 Boughton Lane

Maidstone

Kent

ME15 9QS

United Kingdom

8. MARKETING AUTHORISATION NUMBER(S)

PL 17509/0005

9. DATE OF FIRST AUTHORISATION/RENEWAL OF THE AUTHORISATION

25 May 2001

10. DATE OF REVISION OF THE TEXT

Humalog 100U/ml, solution for injection in vial, 100U/ml, 100U/ml solution for injection in Cartridge and Pen 100U/ml, solution for injection

(Eli Lilly and Company Limited)

1. NAME OF THE MEDICINAL PRODUCT

Humalog* 100U/ml, solution for injection in vial.

Humalog 100U/ml, solution for injection in cartridge.

Humalog Pen 100U/ml, solution for injection.

2. QUALITATIVE AND QUANTITATIVE COMPOSITION

One ml contains 100U (equivalent to 3.5mg) insulin lispro (recombinant DNA origin produced in *E. coli*).

3ml cartridge: Each container includes 3ml equivalent to 300U insulin lispro.

Vial: Each container includes 10ml equivalent to 1000U insulin lispro.

Humalog Pen 3ml: Each container includes 3ml equivalent to 300U insulin lispro.

For excipients, see section 6.1.

3. PHARMACEUTICAL FORM

Solution for injection. Humalog and Humalog Pen is a sterile, clear, colourless, aqueous solution.

4. CLINICAL PARTICULARS

4.1 Therapeutic indications

For the treatment of adults and children with diabetes mellitus who require insulin for the maintenance of normal glucose homeostasis. Humalog or Humalog Pen is also indicated for the initial stabilisation of diabetes mellitus.

4.2 Posology and method of administration

The dosage should be determined by the physician, according to the requirement of the patient.

Humalog may be given shortly before meals. When necessary, Humalog can be given soon after meals.

Humalog preparations should be given by subcutaneous injection or by continuous subcutaneous infusion pump (see section 6.6), and may, although not recommended, also be given by intramuscular injection. If necessary, Humalog may also be administered intravenously, for example, for the control of blood glucose levels during ketoacidosis, acute illnesses, or during intraoperative and postoperative periods.

Subcutaneous administration should be in the upper arms, thighs, buttocks, or abdomen. Use of injection sites should be rotated so that the same site is not used more than approximately once a month.

When administered subcutaneously, care should be taken when injecting Humalog or Humalog Pen to ensure that a blood vessel has not been entered. After injection, the site of injection should not be massaged. Patients must be educated to use the proper injection techniques.

Humalog or Humalog Pen takes effect rapidly and has a shorter duration of activity (2 to 5 hours) given subcutaneously as compared with soluble insulin. This rapid onset of activity allows a Humalog injection (or in the case of administration by continuous subcutaneous infusion, a Humalog bolus) to be given very close to mealtime. The time course of action of any insulin may vary considerably in different individuals or at different times in the same individual. The faster onset of action compared to soluble human insulin is maintained regardless of injection site. As with all insulin preparations, the duration of action of Humalog or Humalog Pen is dependent on dose, site of injection, blood supply, temperature, and physical activity.

Humalog can be used in conjunction with a longer-acting human insulin or oral sulphonylurea agents, on the advice of a physician.

4.3 Contraindications

Hypoglycaemia.

Hypersensitivity to insulin lispro or to any of the excipients.

4.4 Special warnings and special precautions for use

Transferring a patient to another type or brand of insulin should be done under strict medical supervision. Changes in strength, brand (manufacturer), type (soluble, isophane, lente, etc), species (animal, human, human insulin analogue), and/or method of manufacture (recombinant DNA versus animal-source insulin) may result in the need for a change in dosage.

Vials: The shorter-acting Humalog should be drawn into the syringe first, to prevent contamination of the vial by the longer-acting insulin. Mixing of the insulins ahead of time or just before the injection should be on advice of the physician. However, a consistent routine must be followed.

Conditions which may make the early warning symptoms of hypoglycaemia different or less pronounced include long duration of diabetes, intensified insulin therapy, diabetic nerve disease, or medications such as beta-blockers.

A few patients who have experienced hypoglycaemic reactions after transfer from animal-source insulin to human insulin have reported that the early warning symptoms of hypoglycaemia were less pronounced or different from those experienced with their previous insulin. Uncorrected hypoglycaemic or hyperglycaemic reactions can cause loss of consciousness, coma, or death.

The use of dosages which are inadequate or discontinuation of treatment, especially in insulin-dependent diabetics, may lead to hyperglycaemia and diabetic ketoacidosis; conditions which are potentially lethal.

Insulin requirements may be reduced in the presence of renal impairment. Insulin requirements may be reduced in patients with hepatic impairment due to reduced capacity for gluconeogenesis and reduced insulin breakdown; however, in patients with chronic hepatic impairment, an increase in insulin resistance may lead to increased insulin requirements.

Insulin requirements may be increased during illness or emotional disturbances.

Adjustment of dosage may also be necessary if patients undertake increased physical activity or change their usual diet. Exercise taken immediately after a meal may increase the risk of hypoglycaemia. A consequence of the pharmacodynamics of rapid-acting insulin analogues is that if hypoglycaemia occurs, it may occur earlier after an injection when compared with soluble human insulin.

If the 40U/ml vial is the product normally prescribed, do not take insulin from a 100U/ml cartridge using a 40U/ml syringe.

Humalog should only be used in children in preference to soluble insulin when a fast action of insulin might be beneficial. For example, in the timing of the injection in relation to meals.

4.5 Interaction with other medicinal products and other forms of Interaction

Insulin requirements may be increased by medicinal products with hyperglycaemic activity, such as oral contraceptives, corticosteroids, or thyroid replacement therapy, danazol, beta$_2$ stimulants (such as ritodrine, salbutamol, terbutaline).

Insulin requirements may be reduced in the presence of medicinal products with hypoglycaemic activity, such as oral hypoglycaemics, salicylates (for example, acetylsalicylic acid), sulpha antibiotics, certain antidepressants (monoamine oxidase inhibitors), certain angiotensin converting enzyme inhibitors (captopril, enalapril), beta-blockers, octreotide, or alcohol.

The physician should be consulted when using other medications in addition to Humalog or Humalog Pen.

4.6 Pregnancy and lactation

Data on a large number of exposed pregnancies do not indicate any adverse effect of insulin lispro on pregnancy or on the health of the foetus/newborn.

It is essential to maintain good control of the insulin-treated (insulin-dependent or gestational diabetes) patient throughout pregnancy. Insulin requirements usually fall during the first trimester and increase during the second and third trimesters. Patients with diabetes should be advised to inform their doctor if they are pregnant or are contemplating pregnancy. Careful monitoring of glucose control, as well as general health, is essential in pregnant patients with diabetes.

Patients with diabetes who are lactating may require adjustments in insulin dose, diet, or both.

4.7 Effects on ability to drive and use machines

The patient's ability to concentrate and react may be impaired as a result of hypoglycaemia. This may constitute a risk in situations where these abilities are of special importance (eg, driving a car or operating machinery).

Patients should be advised to take precautions to avoid hypoglycaemia whilst driving, this is particularly important in those who have reduced or absent awareness of the warning signs of hypoglycaemia or have frequent episodes of hypoglycaemia. The advisability of driving should be considered in these circumstances.

4.8 Undesirable effects

Hypoglycaemia is the most frequent undesirable effect of insulin therapy that a patient with diabetes may suffer. Severe hypoglycaemia may lead to loss of consciousness, and in extreme cases, death.

Local allergy in patients occasionally occurs as redness, swelling, and itching at the site of insulin injection. This condition usually resolves in a few days to a few weeks. In some instances, this condition may be related to factors other than insulin, such as irritants in the skin cleansing agent or poor injection technique. Systemic allergy, less common but potentially more serious, is a generalised allergy to insulin. It may cause a rash over the whole body, shortness of breath, wheezing, reduction in blood pressure, fast pulse, or sweating. Severe cases of generalised allergy may be life-threatening.

Lipodystrophy may occur at the injection site.

4.9 Overdose

Insulins have no specific overdose definitions because serum glucose concentrations are a result of complex interactions between insulin levels, glucose availability, and other metabolic processes. Hypoglycaemia may occur as a result of an excess of insulin activity relative to food intake and energy expenditure.

Hypoglycaemia may be associated with listlessness, confusion, palpitations, headache, sweating, and vomiting.

Mild hypoglycaemic episodes will respond to oral administration of glucose or other sugar or saccharated products.

Correction of moderately severe hypoglycaemia can be accomplished by intramuscular or subcutaneous administration of glucagon, followed by oral carbohydrate when the patient recovers sufficiently. Patients who fail to respond to glucagon must be given glucose solution intravenously.

If the patient is comatose, glucagon should be administered intramuscularly or subcutaneously. However, glucose solution must be given intravenously if glucagon is not available or if the patient fails to respond to glucagon. The patient should be given a meal as soon as consciousness is recovered.

Sustained carbohydrate intake and observation may be necessary because hypoglycaemia may recur after apparent clinical recovery.

5. PHARMACOLOGICAL PROPERTIES

5.1 Pharmacodynamic properties

Pharmacotherapeutic group: Fast-acting human insulin analogue. ATC code: A10A B04.

The primary activity of insulin lispro is the regulation of glucose metabolism.

In addition, insulins have several anabolic and anti-catabolic actions on a variety of different tissues. Within muscle tissue this includes increasing glycogen, fatty acid, glycerol and protein synthesis, and amino acid uptake, while decreasing glycogenolysis, gluconeogenesis, ketogenesis, lipolysis, protein catabolism, and amino acid output.

Insulin lispro has a rapid onset of action (approximately 15 minutes), thus allowing it to be given closer to a meal (within zero to 15 minutes of the meal) when compared to soluble insulin (30 to 45 minutes before). Insulin lispro takes effect rapidly and has a shorter duration of activity (2 to 5 hours) when compared to soluble insulin.

Clinical trials in patients with Type 1 and Type 2 diabetes have demonstrated reduced postprandial hyperglycaemia with insulin lispro compared to soluble human insulin. For fast-acting insulins, any patient also on a basal insulin must optimise dosage of both insulins to obtain improved glucose control across the whole day.

As with all insulin preparations, the time course of insulin lispro action may vary in different individuals or at different times in the same individual and is dependent on dose, site of injection, blood supply, temperature, and physical activity. The typical activity profile following subcutaneous injection is illustrated below.

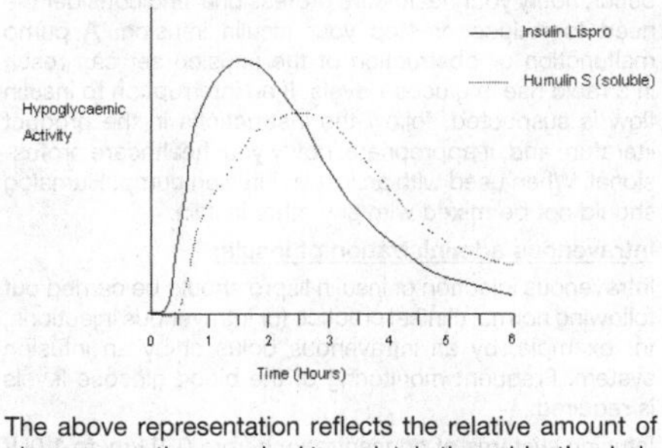

The above representation reflects the relative amount of glucose over time required to maintain the subject's whole blood glucose concentrations near fasting levels and is an indicator of the effect of these insulins on glucose metabolism over time.

Clinical trials have been performed in children (61 patients aged 2 to 11) and children and adolescents (481 patients aged 9 to 19 years), comparing insulin lispro to human soluble insulin. The pharmacodynamic profile of insulin lispro in children is similar to that seen in adults.

When used in subcutaneous infusion pumps, treatment with insulin lispro has been shown to result in lower glycosylated haemoglobin levels compared to soluble insulin. In a double-blind, crossover study, the reduction in glycosylated haemoglobin levels after 12 weeks dosing was 0.37 percentage points with insulin lispro, compared to 0.03 percentage points for soluble insulin ($P = 0.004$).

In patients with Type 2 diabetes on maximum doses of sulphonylurea agents, studies have shown that the addition of insulin lispro significantly reduces HbA_{1c} compared to sulphonylurea alone. The reduction of HbA_{1c} would also be expected with other insulin products, eg, soluble or isophane insulins.

Clinical trials in patients with Type 1 and Type 2 diabetes have demonstrated a reduced number of episodes of nocturnal hypoglycaemia with insulin lispro compared to soluble human insulin. In some studies, reduction of nocturnal hypoglycaemia was associated with increased episodes of daytime hypoglycaemia.

The glucodynamic response to insulin lispro is not affected by renal or hepatic function impairment. Glucodynamic differences between insulin lispro and soluble human insulin, as measured during a glucose clamp procedure, were maintained over a wide range of renal function.

Insulin lispro has been shown to be equipotent to human insulin on a molar basis but its effect is more rapid and of a shorter duration.

5.2 Pharmacokinetic properties

The pharmacokinetics of insulin lispro reflect a compound that is rapidly absorbed and achieves peak blood levels 30 to 70 minutes following subcutaneous injection. When considering the clinical relevance of these kinetics, it is more appropriate to examine the glucose utilisation curves (as discussed in section 5.1).

Insulin lispro maintains more rapid absorption when compared to soluble human insulin in patients with renal impairment. In patients with Type 2 diabetes, over a wide range of renal function, the pharmacokinetic differences between insulin lispro and soluble human insulin were generally maintained and shown to be independent of renal function. Insulin lispro maintains more rapid absorption and elimination when compared to soluble human insulin in patients with hepatic impairment.

5.3 Preclinical safety data

In *in vitro* tests, including binding to insulin receptor sites and effects on growing cells, insulin lispro behaved in a manner that closely resembled human insulin. Studies also demonstrate that the dissociation of binding to the insulin receptor of insulin lispro is equivalent to human insulin. Acute, one-month and twelve-month toxicology studies produced no significant toxicity findings.

Insulin lispro did not induce fertility impairment, embryotoxicity, or teratogenicity in animal studies.

6. PHARMACEUTICAL PARTICULARS

6.1 List of excipients

m-cresol (3.15mg/ml), glycerol, dibasic sodium phosphate.$7H_2O$, zinc oxide, water for injections. Hydrochloric acid and sodium hydroxide may be used to adjust pH to 7.0-7.8.

6.2 Incompatibilities

Humalog or Humalog Pen preparations should not be mixed with animal insulin preparations. This medicinal product must not be mixed with another medicinal product except those mentioned in section 6.6.

6.3 Shelf life

Two years. After insertion of the cartridge in a pen, or the first use of the vial or prefilled pen, the solution should be used within 28 days when stored below +30°C.

6.4 Special precautions for storage

Store at 2°C-8°C (in a refrigerator). Do not freeze. Do not expose to excessive heat or direct sunlight. Once in use, vials, cartridges, or Humalog Pens may be used for up to 28 days.

6.5 Nature and contents of container

Vials: The solution is contained in Type I flint glass vials, sealed with butyl or halobutyl stoppers, and secured with aluminium seals. Dimeticone or silicone emulsion may be used to treat the vial stoppers.

Cartridges/Humalog Pens: The solution is contained in Type I flint glass cartridges, sealed with butyl or halobutyl disc seals and plunger heads, and are secured with aluminium seals. Dimeticone or silicone emulsion may be used to treat the cartridge plunger and/or the glass cartridge. *Humalog Pens:* The 3ml cartridges are sealed in a disposable pen injector. Needles are not included.

Not all packs may be marketed in every country.

1 × 10ml Humalog vial.

5 × 3ml Humalog cartridges for a 3ml pen.

5 × 3ml Humalog Pens.

6.6 Instructions for use and handling

Humalog vials

The vial is to be used in conjunction with an appropriate syringe (100U markings).

a) Preparing a dose

Inspect the Humalog solution. It should be clear and colourless. Do not use Humalog if it appears cloudy, thickened, or slightly coloured, or if solid particles are visible.

1. Wash your hands.

2. If using a new vial, flip off the plastic protective cap, but **do not** remove the stopper.

3. If the therapeutic regimen requires the injection of basal insulin and Humalog at the same time, the two can be mixed in the syringe. If mixing insulins, refer to the instructions for mixing that follow in section b).

4. Draw air into the syringe equal to the prescribed Humalog dose. Wipe the top of the vial with an alcohol swab. Put the needle through the rubber top of the Humalog vial and inject the air into the vial.

5. Turn the vial and syringe upside down. Hold the vial and syringe firmly in one hand.

6. Making sure the tip of the needle is in the Humalog, withdraw the correct dose into the syringe.

7. Before removing the needle from the vial, check the syringe for air bubbles that reduce the amount of Humalog in it. If bubbles are present, hold the syringe straight up and

tap its side until the bubbles float to the top. Push them out with the plunger and withdraw the correct dose.

8. Remove the needle from the vial and lay the syringe down so that the needle does not touch anything.

b) Mixing Humalog with longer-acting human insulins

1. Humalog should be mixed with longer-acting human insulins only on the advice of a doctor.

2. Draw air into the syringe equal to the amount of longer-acting insulin being taken. Insert the needle into the longer-acting insulin vial and inject the air. Withdraw the needle.

3. Now inject air into the Humalog vial in the same manner, but **do not** withdraw the needle.

4. Turn the vial and syringe upside down.

5. Making sure the tip of the needle is in the Humalog, withdraw the correct dose of Humalog into the syringe.

6. Before removing the needle from the vial, check the syringe for air bubbles that reduce the amount of Humalog in it. If bubbles are present, hold the syringe straight up and tap its side until the bubbles float to the top. Push them out with the plunger and withdraw the correct dose.

7. Remove the needle from the vial of Humalog and insert it into the vial of the longer-acting insulin. Turn the vial and syringe upside down. Hold the vial and syringe firmly in one hand and shake gently. Making sure the tip of the needle is in the insulin, withdraw the dose of longer-acting insulin.

8. Withdraw the needle and lay the syringe down so that the needle does not touch anything.

c) Injecting a dose

1. Choose a site for injection.

2. Clean the skin as instructed.

3. Stabilise the skin by spreading it or pinching up a large area. Insert the needle and inject as instructed.

4. Pull the needle out and apply gentle pressure over the injection site for several seconds. Do not rub the area.

5. Dispose of the syringe and needle safely.

6. Use of the injection sites should be rotated so that the same is not used more than approximately once a month.

d) Mixing insulins

Do not mix insulin in vials with insulin in cartridges.

Humalog cartridges

Humalog cartridges are to be used with a CE marked pen as recommended in the information provided by the device manufacturer.

a) Preparing a dose

Inspect the Humalog solution. It should be clear and colourless. Do not use Humalog if it appears cloudy, thickened, or slightly coloured, or if solid particles are visible.

The following is a general description. The manufacturer's instructions with each individual pen must be followed for loading the cartridge, attaching the needle, and administering the insulin injection.

b) Injecting a dose

1. Wash your hands.

2. Choose a site for injection.

3. Clean the skin as instructed.

4. Remove outer needle cap.

5. Stabilise the skin by spreading it or pinching up a large area. Insert the needle as instructed.

6. Press the knob.

7. Pull the needle out and apply gentle pressure over the injection site for several seconds. Do not rub the area.

8. Using the outer needle cap, unscrew the needle and dispose of it safely.

9. Use of injection sites should be rotated so that the same site is not used more than approximately once a month.

c) Mixing insulins

Do not mix insulin in vials with insulin in cartridges.

Humalog Pens

a) Preparing a dose

1. Inspect the Humalog Pen solution.

It should be clear and colourless. Do not use Humalog Pen if it appears cloudy, thickened, or slightly coloured, or if solid particles are visible.

2. Put on the needle.

Wipe the rubber seal with alcohol. Remove the paper tab from the capped needle. Screw the capped needle clockwise onto the pen until it is tight. Hold the pen with needle pointing up and remove the outer needle cap and inner needle cover.

3. Priming the pen (check insulin flow).

(a) The arrow should be visible in the dose window. If the arrow is not present, turn the dose knob clockwise until the arrow appears and notch is felt or visually aligned.

(b) Pull dose knob out (in direction of the arrow) until a '0' appears in the dose window. A dose cannot be dialled until the dose knob is pulled out.

(c) Turn dose knob clockwise until a '2' appears in the dose window.

(d) Hold the pen with needle pointing up and tap the clear cartridge holder gently with your finger so any air bubbles collect near the top. Depress the injection button fully until you feel or hear a click. You should see a drop of insulin at the tip of the needle. If insulin does not appear, repeat the procedure until insulin appears.

(e) Always prime the pen (check the insulin flow) before each injection. Failure to prime the pen may result in an inaccurate dose.

4. Setting the dose.

(a) Turn the dose knob clockwise until the arrow appears in the dose window and a notch is felt or visually aligned.

(b) Pull the dose knob out (in the direction of the arrow) until a '0' appears in the dose window. A dose cannot be dialled until the dose knob is pulled out.

(c) Turn the dose knob clockwise until the dose appears in the dose window. If too high a dose is dialled, turn the dose knob backward (anti-clockwise) until the correct dose appears in the window. A dose greater than the number of units remaining in the cartridge cannot be dialled.

b) Injecting a dose

1. Wash your hands.

2. Choose a site for injection.

3. Clean the skin as instructed.

4. Remove outer needle cap.

5. Stabilise the skin by spreading it or pinching up a large area. Insert the needle as instructed.

6. Press the injection button down with the thumb (until you hear or feel a click); wait 5 seconds.

7. Pull the needle out and apply gentle pressure over the injection site for several seconds. Do not rub the area.

8. Immediately after an injection, use the outer needle cap to unscrew the needle. Remove the needle from the pen. This will ensure sterility, and prevent leakage, re-entry of air, and potential needle clogs. Do not reuse the needle. Dispose of the needle in a responsible manner. Needles and pens must not be shared.

The prefilled pen can be used until it is empty. Please properly discard or recycle.

9. Replace the cap on the pen.

10. Use of injection sites should be rotated so that the same site is not used more than approximately once a month.

11. The injection button should be fully depressed before using the pen again.

c) Mixing insulins

Do not mix insulin in vials with insulin in cartridges.

Use of Humalog in an insulin infusion pump

Minimed and Disetronic insulin infusion pumps may be used to infuse insulin lispro. Read and follow the instructions that accompany the infusion pump. Use the correct reservoir and catheter for the pump. Change the infusion set every 48 hours. Use aseptic technique when inserting the infusion set. In the event of a hypoglycaemic episode, the infusion should be stopped until the episode is resolved. If repeated or severe low blood glucose levels occur, notify your healthcare professional and consider the need to reduce or stop your insulin infusion. A pump malfunction or obstruction of the infusion set can result in a rapid rise in glucose levels. If an interruption to insulin flow is suspected, follow the instructions in the product literature and, if appropriate, notify your healthcare professional. When used with an insulin infusion pump, Humalog should not be mixed with any other insulin.

Intravenous administration of insulin

Intravenous injection of insulin lispro should be carried out following normal clinical practice for intravenous injections, for example, by an intravenous bolus or by an infusion system. Frequent monitoring of the blood glucose levels is required.

Infusion systems at concentrations from 0.1U/ml to 1.0U/ml insulin lispro in 0.9% sodium chloride or 5% dextrose are stable at room temperature for 48 hours. It is recommended that the system is primed before starting the infusion to the patient.

7. MARKETING AUTHORISATION HOLDER

Eli Lilly Nederland BV, Grootslag 1-5, 3991 RA Houten, The Netherlands.

8. MARKETING AUTHORISATION NUMBER(S)

Vial:	EU/1/96/007/002
3ml cartridge:	EU/1/96/007/004
Humalog Pen 3ml:	EU/1/96/007/015

9. DATE OF FIRST AUTHORISATION/RENEWAL OF THE AUTHORISATION

EMEA approval date:	Vial:	30 April 1996/April 2001
	3ml cartridge:	26 March 1997/April 2001
	Humalog Pen 3ml:	16 June 1997/April 2001
EMEA renewal date:	Vial:	April 2001
	3ml cartridge:	April 2001
	Humalog Pen 3ml:	April 2001

10. DATE OF REVISION OF THE TEXT

November 2003

LEGAL CATEGORY

POM (United Kingdom)

For further information in the United Kingdom contact:

Eli Lilly and Company Limited
Lilly House, Priestley Road
Basingstoke, Hampshire, RG24 9NL
Telephone: Basingstoke (01256) 315 999

For further information in the Republic of Ireland contact:

Eli Lilly and Company (Ireland) Limited
Hyde House, 65 Adelaide Road
Dublin 2, Republic of Ireland
Telephone: Dublin (01) 661 4377

*HUMALOG (insulin lispro) is a trademark of Eli Lilly and Company.

HLG21M

Humalog Mix25 100U/ml suspension for injection in cartridge,100U/ml Pen suspension for injection/Humalog Mix50 100U/ml Pen, suspension for injection

(Eli Lilly and Company Limited)

1. NAME OF THE MEDICINAL PRODUCT

Humalog Mix25* 100U/ml suspension for injection in cartridge.

Humalog Mix25 100U/ml Pen, suspension for injection.

Humalog Mix50* 100U/ml Pen, suspension for injection.

2. QUALITATIVE AND QUANTITATIVE COMPOSITION

One ml contains 100U (equivalent to 3.5mg) insulin lispro (recombinant DNA origin produced in *E. coli*). Each container includes 3ml equivalent to 300U insulin lispro.

Humalog Mix25 consists of 25% insulin lispro solution and 75% insulin lispro protamine suspension.

Humalog Mix50 consists of 50% insulin lispro solution and 50% insulin lispro protamine suspension.

For excipients, see section 6.1.

3. PHARMACEUTICAL FORM

Suspension for injection. Humalog Mix25 and Humalog Mix50 are white, sterile suspensions.

4. CLINICAL PARTICULARS

4.1 Therapeutic indications

Humalog Mix25 or Humalog Mix50 is indicated for the treatment of patients with diabetes mellitus who require insulin for the maintenance of normal glucose homeostasis.

4.2 Posology and method of administration

The dosage should be determined by the physician, according to the requirement of the patient.

Humalog Mix25 or Humalog Mix50 may be given shortly before meals. When necessary, Humalog Mix25 or Humalog Mix50 can be given soon after meals. Humalog Mix25 or Humalog Mix50 should only be given by subcutaneous injection. Under no circumstances should Humalog Mix25 or Humalog Mix50 be given intravenously.

Subcutaneous administration should be in the upper arms, thighs, buttocks, or abdomen. Use of injection sites should be rotated so that the same site is not used more than approximately once a month.

When administered subcutaneously, care should be taken when injecting Humalog Mix25 or Humalog Mix50 to ensure that a blood vessel has not been entered. After injection, the site of injection should not be massaged. Patients must be educated to use the proper injection techniques.

The rapid onset and early peak of activity of Humalog itself is observed following the subcutaneous administration of Humalog Mix25 or Humalog Mix50. This allows Humalog Mix25 or Humalog Mix50 to be given very close to mealtime. The duration of action of the insulin lispro protamine suspension (NPL) component of Humalog Mix25 or Humalog Mix50 is similar to that of a basal insulin (NPH [isophane]).

The time course of action of any insulin may vary considerably in different individuals or at different times in the same individual. As with all insulin preparations, the duration of action of Humalog Mix25 or Humalog Mix50 is dependent on dose, site of injection, blood supply, temperature, and physical activity.

4.3 Contraindications

Hypoglycaemia.

Hypersensitivity to insulin lispro or to any of the excipients.

4.4 Special warnings and special precautions for use

Under no circumstances should Humalog Mix25 or Humalog Mix50 be given intravenously.

Transferring a patient to another type or brand of insulin should be done under strict medical supervision. Changes in strength, brand (manufacturer), type (soluble, NPH, lente, etc), species (animal, human, human insulin analogue), and/or method of manufacture (recombinant DNA versus animal-source insulin) may result in the need for a change in dosage.

Conditions which may make the early warning symptoms of hypoglycaemia different or less pronounced include long duration of diabetes, intensified insulin therapy, diabetic nerve disease, or medications such as beta-blockers.

A few patients who have experienced hypoglycaemic reactions after transfer from animal-source insulin to human insulin have reported that the early warning symptoms of hypoglycaemia were less pronounced or different from those experienced with their previous insulin. Uncorrected hypoglycaemic or hyperglycaemic reactions can cause loss of consciousness, coma, or death.

The use of dosages which are inadequate or discontinuation of treatment, especially in insulin-dependent diabetics, may lead to hyperglycaemia and diabetic ketoacidosis; conditions which are potentially lethal.

Insulin requirements may be reduced in the presence of renal impairment. Insulin requirements may be reduced in patients with hepatic impairment due to reduced capacity for gluconeogenesis and reduced insulin breakdown; however, in patients with chronic hepatic impairment, an increase in insulin resistance may lead to increased insulin requirements.

Insulin requirements may be increased during illness or emotional disturbances.

Adjustment of dosage may also be necessary if patients undertake increased physical activity or change their usual diet. Exercise taken immediately after a meal may increase the risk of hypoglycaemia.

Administration of insulin lispro to children below 12 years of age should be considered only in case of an expected benefit when compared to soluble insulin.

4.5 Interaction with other medicinal products and other forms of Interaction

Insulin requirements may be increased by substances with hyperglycaemic activity, such as oral contraceptives, corticosteroids, or thyroid replacement therapy, danazol, $beta_2$ stimulants (such as ritodrine, salbutamol, terbutaline).

Insulin requirements may be reduced in the presence of substances with hypoglycaemic activity, such as oral hypoglycaemics, salicylates (for example, acetylsalicylic acid), sulpha antibiotics, certain antidepressants (monoamine oxidase inhibitors), certain angiotensin converting enzyme inhibitors (captopril, enalapril), beta-blockers, octreotide, or alcohol.

Mixing Humalog Mix25 or Humalog Mix50 with other insulins has not been studied.

The physician should be consulted when using other medications in addition to Humalog Mix25 or Humalog Mix50.

4.6 Pregnancy and lactation

Data on a large number of exposed pregnancies do not indicate any adverse effect of insulin lispro on pregnancy or on the health of the foetus/newborn.

It is essential to maintain good control of the insulin-treated (insulin-dependent or gestational diabetes) patient throughout pregnancy. Insulin requirements usually fall during the first trimester and increase during the second and third trimesters. Patients with diabetes should be advised to inform their doctor if they are pregnant or are contemplating pregnancy. Careful monitoring of glucose control, as well as general health, is essential in pregnant patients with diabetes.

Patients with diabetes who are lactating may require adjustments in insulin dose, diet, or both.

4.7 Effects on ability to drive and use machines

The patient's ability to concentrate and react may be impaired as a result of hypoglycaemia. This may constitute a risk in situations where these abilities are of special importance (eg, driving a car or operating machinery).

Patients should be advised to take precautions to avoid hypoglycaemia whilst driving, this is particularly important in those who have reduced or absent awareness of the warning signs of hypoglycaemia or have frequent episodes of hypoglycaemia. The advisability of driving should be considered in these circumstances.

4.8 Undesirable effects

Hypoglycaemia is the most frequent undesirable effect of insulin therapy that a patient with diabetes may suffer. Severe hypoglycaemia may lead to loss of consciousness, and in extreme cases, death.

Local allergy in patients occasionally occurs as redness, swelling, and itching at the site of insulin injection. This condition usually resolves in a few days to a few weeks. In some instances, this condition may be related to factors other than insulin, such as irritants in the skin cleansing agent or poor injection technique. Systemic allergy, less common but potentially more serious, is a generalised allergy to insulin. It may cause a rash over the whole body, shortness of breath, wheezing, reduction in blood pressure, fast pulse, or sweating. Severe cases of generalised allergy may be life-threatening.

Lipodystrophy may occur at the injection site.

4.9 Overdose

Insulins have no specific overdose definitions because serum glucose concentrations are a result of complex interactions between insulin levels, glucose availability, and other metabolic processes. Hypoglycaemia may occur as a result of an excess of insulin activity relative to food intake and energy expenditure.

Hypoglycaemia may be associated with listlessness, confusion, palpitations, headache, sweating, and vomiting.

Mild hypoglycaemic episodes will respond to oral administration of glucose or other sugar or saccharated products.

Correction of moderately severe hypoglycaemia can be accomplished by intramuscular or subcutaneous administration of glucagon, followed by oral carbohydrate when the patient recovers sufficiently. Patients who fail to respond to glucagon must be given glucose solution intravenously.

If the patient is comatose, glucagon should be administered intramuscularly or subcutaneously. However, glucose solution must be given intravenously if glucagon is not available or if the patient fails to respond to glucagon. The patient should be given a meal as soon as consciousness is recovered.

Sustained carbohydrate intake and observation may be necessary because hypoglycaemia may recur after apparent clinical recovery.

5. PHARMACOLOGICAL PROPERTIES

5.1 Pharmacodynamic properties

Pharmacotherapeutic group: Humalog Mix25 and Humalog Mix50 are premixed suspensions consisting of insulin lispro (fast acting human insulin analogue) and insulin lispro protamine suspension (intermediate acting human insulin analogue). ATC code: A10A D04.

The primary activity of insulin lispro is the regulation of glucose metabolism.

In addition, insulins have several anabolic and anti-catabolic actions on a variety of different tissues. Within muscle tissue this includes increasing glycogen, fatty acid, glycerol and protein synthesis, and amino acid uptake, while decreasing glycogenolysis, gluconeogenesis, ketogenesis, lipolysis, protein catabolism, and amino acid output.

Insulin lispro has a rapid onset of action (approximately 15 minutes), thus allowing it to be given closer to a meal (within zero to 15 minutes of the meal) when compared to soluble insulin (30 to 45 minutes before). The rapid onset and early peak of activity of insulin lispro is observed following the subcutaneous administration of Humalog Mix25 or Humalog Mix50. NPL has an activity profile that is very similar to that of a basal insulin (NPH) over a period of approximately 15 hours.

Clinical trials in patients with Type 1 and Type 2 diabetes have demonstrated reduced postprandial hyperglycaemia with Humalog Mix25 compared to human insulin mixture 30/70. In one clinical study there was a small (0.38mmol/l) increase in blood glucose levels at night (3 AM).

In the figures below the pharmacodynamics of Humalog Mix25, Humalog Mix50, and NPL are illustrated.

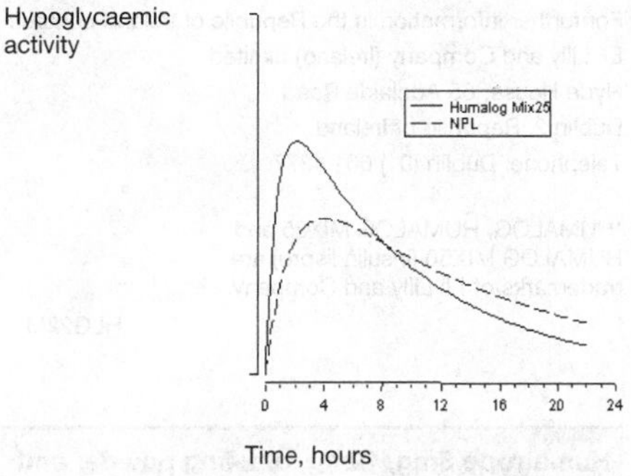

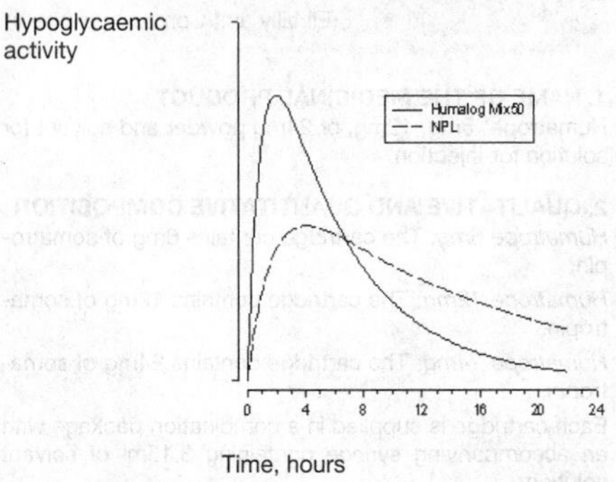

The above representations reflect the relative amount of glucose over time required to maintain the subject's whole blood glucose concentrations near fasting levels and is an indicator of the effect of these insulins on glucose metabolism over time.

The glucodynamic response to insulin lispro is not affected by renal or hepatic function impairment. Glucodynamic differences between insulin lispro and soluble human insulin, as measured during a glucose clamp procedure, were maintained over a wide range of renal function.

Insulin lispro has been shown to be equipotent to human insulin on a molar basis but its effect is more rapid and of a shorter duration.

5.2 Pharmacokinetic properties

The pharmacokinetics of insulin lispro reflect a compound that is rapidly absorbed and achieves peak blood levels 30 to 70 minutes following subcutaneous injection. The pharmacokinetics of insulin lispro protamine suspension are consistent with those of an intermediate acting insulin, such as NPH. The pharmacokinetics of Humalog Mix25 or Humalog Mix50 are representative of the individual pharmacokinetic properties of the two components. When considering the clinical relevance of these kinetics, it is more appropriate to examine the glucose utilisation curves (as discussed in section 5.1).

Insulin lispro maintains more rapid absorption when compared to soluble human insulin in patients with renal impairment. In patients with Type 2 diabetes, over a wide range of renal function, the pharmacokinetic differences between insulin lispro and soluble human insulin were generally maintained and shown to be independent of renal function. Insulin lispro maintains more rapid absorption and elimination when compared to soluble human insulin in patients with hepatic impairment.

5.3 Preclinical safety data

In *in vitro* tests, including binding to insulin receptor sites and effects on growing cells, insulin lispro behaved in a manner that closely resembled human insulin. Studies also demonstrate that the dissociation of binding to the insulin receptor of insulin lispro is equivalent to human insulin. Acute, one-month and twelve-month toxicology studies produced no significant toxicity findings.

Insulin lispro did not induce fertility impairment, embryotoxicity, or teratogenicity in animal studies.

6. PHARMACEUTICAL PARTICULARS

6.1 List of excipients

Each Humalog Mix25 cartridge contains the following excipients:

Protamine sulphate, *m*-cresol (1.76mg/ml), phenol (0.80mg/ml), glycerol, dibasic sodium phosphate.$7H_2O$, zinc oxide, water for injections. Hydrochloric acid and sodium hydroxide may be used to adjust pH to 7.0-7.8.

Each Humalog Mix50 cartridge contains the following excipients:

Protamine sulphate, *m*-cresol (2.20mg/ml), phenol (1.00mg/ml), glycerol, dibasic sodium phosphate.$7H_2O$, zinc oxide, water for injections. Hydrochloric acid and sodium hydroxide may be used to adjust pH to 7.0-7.8.

6.2 Incompatibilities

Mixing Humalog Mix25 or Humalog Mix50 with other insulins has not been studied. In the absence of compatibility studies, this medicinal product must not be mixed with another medicinal product.

6.3 Shelf life

Two years.

After first use of the prefilled Pen, the suspension should be used within 28 days, when stored below +30°C.

After insertion of the cartridge in a pen, the suspension should be used within 28 days, when stored below +30°C.

6.4 Special precautions for storage

Store at 2°C-8°C. (In a refrigerator.)

Do not freeze. Do not expose to excessive heat or direct sunlight.

Once in use, cartridges and Pens (prefilled) may be used for up to 28 days.

6.5 Nature and contents of container

Humalog Mix25 100U/ml suspension for injection in cartridge

The suspension is contained in Type I flint glass cartridges, sealed with butyl or halobutyl disc seals and plunger heads, and secured with aluminium seals. Dimeticone or silicone emulsion may have been used to treat the cartridge plunger and/or the glass cartridge.

5 × 3ml Humalog Mix25 cartridges for a 3ml pen.

Humalog Mix25 or Humalog Mix50 100U/ml Pen, suspension for injection

The suspension is contained in Type I flint glass cartridges, sealed with halobutyl disc seals and plunger heads, and secured with aluminium seals. Dimeticone or silicone emulsion may have been used to treat the cartridge plunger and/or the glass cartridge. The 3ml cartridges are sealed in a disposable pen injector, called the 'Pen'. Needles are not included.

5 × 3ml Humalog Mix25 100U/ml Pens.

5 × 3ml Humalog Mix50 100U/ml Pens.

6.6 Instructions for use and handling

Humalog Mix25 100U/ml suspension for injection in cartridge

Humalog Mix25 cartridges are to be used with a CE marked pen as recommended in the information provided by the device manufacturer.

(a) **Cartridge - Preparing a dose**

Cartridges containing Humalog Mix25 should be rotated in the palms of the hands ten times and inverted 180° ten times immediately before use to resuspend the insulin until it appears uniformly cloudy or milky. If not, repeat the above procedure until contents are mixed. Cartridges contain a small glass bead to assist mixing. Do not shake vigorously as this may cause frothing, which may interfere with the correct measurement of the dose.

The cartridges should be examined frequently and should not be used if clumps of material are present or if solid white particles stick to the bottom or wall of the cartridge, giving a frosted appearance.

Humalog Mix25 cartridges are not designed to allow any other insulin to be mixed in the cartridge. Cartridges are not designed to be refilled.

The following is a general description. The manufacturer's instructions with each individual pen must be followed for loading the cartridge, attaching the needle, and administering the insulin injection.

(b) Cartridge - Injecting a dose

1. Wash your hands.
2. Choose a site for injection.
3. Clean the skin as instructed.
4. Remove outer needle cap.
5. Stabilise the skin by spreading it or pinching up a large area. Insert the needle as instructed.
6. Press the knob.
7. Pull the needle out and apply gentle pressure over the injection site for several seconds. Do not rub the area.
8. Using the outer needle cap, unscrew the needle and dispose of it safely.
9. Use of injection sites should be rotated so that the same site is not used more than approximately once a month.

Humalog Mix25 or Humalog Mix50 100U/ml Pen, suspension for injection

(a) Pen (prefilled) - Preparing a dose

1. Inspect the Humalog Mix25 or Humalog Mix50 100U/ml Pen.

The Pen should be rotated in the palms of the hands ten times and inverted 180° ten times immediately before use to resuspend the insulin until it appears uniformly cloudy or milky. If not, repeat the above procedure until contents are mixed. Cartridges contain a small glass bead to assist mixing. Do not shake vigorously as this may cause frothing, which may interfere with the correct measurement of the dose.

The cartridges should be examined frequently and should not be used if clumps of material are present or if solid white particles stick to the bottom or wall of the cartridge, giving a frosted appearance.

2. Put on the needle.

Wipe the rubber seal with alcohol. Remove the paper tab from the capped needle. Screw the capped needle clockwise onto the Pen until it is tight. Hold the Pen with needle pointing up and remove the outer needle cap and inner needle cover.

3. Priming the Pen (check insulin flow).

(a) The arrow should be visible in the dose window. If the arrow is not present, turn the dose knob clockwise until the arrow appears and notch is felt or visually aligned.

(b) Pull dose knob out (in direction of the arrow) until a '0' appears in the dose window. A dose cannot be dialled until the dose knob is pulled out.

(c) Turn dose knob clockwise until a '2' appears in the dose window.

(d) Hold the Pen with needle pointing up and tap the clear cartridge holder gently with your finger so any air bubbles collect near the top. Depress the injection button fully until you feel or hear a click. You should see a drop of insulin at the tip of the needle. If insulin does not appear, repeat the procedure until insulin appears.

(e) Always prime the Pen (check the insulin flow) before each injection. Failure to prime the Pen may result in an inaccurate dose.

4. Setting the dose.

(a) Turn the dose knob clockwise until the arrow appears in the dose window and a notch is felt or visually aligned.

(b) Pull the dose knob out (in the direction of the arrow) until a '0' appears in the dose window. A dose cannot be dialled until the dose knob is pulled out.

(c) Turn the dose knob clockwise until the dose appears in the dose window. If too high a dose is dialled, turn the dose knob backward (anti-clockwise) until the correct dose appears in the window. A dose greater than the number of units remaining in the cartridge cannot be dialled.

(b) Pen (prefilled) - Injecting a dose

1. Wash your hands.
2. Choose a site for injection.
3. Clean the skin as instructed.
4. Remove outer needle cap.
5. Stabilise the skin by spreading it or pinching up a large area. Insert the needle as instructed.
6. Press the injection button down with the thumb (until you hear or feel a click); wait 5 seconds.
7. Pull the needle out and apply gentle pressure over the injection site for several seconds. Do not rub the area.
8. Immediately after an injection, use the outer needle cap to unscrew the needle. Remove the needle from the Pen. This will ensure sterility, and prevent leakage, re-entry of air, and potential needle clogs. Do not reuse the needle. Dispose of the needle in a responsible manner. Needles and pens must not be shared.

The prefilled Pen can be used until it is empty. Please properly discard or recycle.

9. Replace the cap on the Pen.
10. Use of injection sites should be rotated so that the same site is not used more than approximately once a month.
11. The injection button should be fully depressed before using the Pen again.

(c) Mixing insulins

Do not mix insulin in vials with insulin in cartridges.

7. MARKETING AUTHORISATION HOLDER

Eli Lilly Nederland BV, Grootslag 1-5, 3991 RA Houten, The Netherlands.

8. MARKETING AUTHORISATION NUMBER(S)

Humalog Mix25 100U/ml suspension for injection in cartridge:	EU/1/96/007/008
Humalog Mix25 100U/ml Pen, suspension for injection:	EU/1/96/007/016
Humalog Mix50 100U/ml Pen, suspension for injection:	EU/1/96/007/017

9. DATE OF FIRST AUTHORISATION/RENEWAL OF THE AUTHORISATION

19 November 1998/April 2001

10. DATE OF REVISION OF THE TEXT

November 2003

LEGAL CATEGORY

POM (United Kingdom)

For further information in the United Kingdom contact:

Eli Lilly and Company Limited
Lilly House, Priestley Road
Basingstoke, Hampshire, RG24 9NL
Telephone: Basingstoke (01256) 315 999

For further information in the Republic of Ireland contact:

Eli Lilly and Company (Ireland) Limited
Hyde House, 65 Adelaide Road
Dublin 2, Republic of Ireland
Telephone: Dublin (01) 661 4377

*HUMALOG, HUMALOG MIX25 and HUMALOG MIX50 (insulin lispro) are trademarks of Eli Lilly and Company.

HLG22M

Humatrope 6mg, 12mg, or 24mg powder and solvent for solution for injection

(Eli Lilly and Company Limited)

1. NAME OF THE MEDICINAL PRODUCT

Humatrope* 6mg, 12mg, or 24mg powder and solvent for solution for injection.

2. QUALITATIVE AND QUANTITATIVE COMPOSITION

Humatrope 6mg: The cartridge contains 6mg of somatropin.

Humatrope 12mg: The cartridge contains 12mg of somatropin.

Humatrope 24mg: The cartridge contains 24mg of somatropin.

Each cartridge is supplied in a combination package with an accompanying syringe containing 3.15ml of solvent solution.

Somatropin is produced by recombinant DNA technology in *Escherichia coli*.

For excipients, see section 6.1.

3. PHARMACEUTICAL FORM

Powder and solvent for solution for injection.

Somatropin is a white or almost white powder. The solvent is a clear solution.

4. CLINICAL PARTICULARS

4.1 Therapeutic indications

Paediatric Patients

Humatrope is indicated for the long-term treatment of children who have growth failure due to an inadequate secretion of normal endogenous growth hormone.

Humatrope is also indicated for the treatment of short stature in children with Turner's syndrome, confirmed by chromosome analysis.

Humatrope is also indicated for the treatment of growth retardation in prepubertal children with chronic renal insufficiency.

Adult Patients

Humatrope is indicated for replacement therapy in adults with pronounced growth hormone deficiency.

Patients with severe growth hormone deficiency in adulthood are defined as patients with known hypothalamic-pituitary pathology and at least one known deficiency of a pituitary hormone not being prolactin. These patients should undergo a single dynamic test in order to diagnose or exclude a growth deficiency. In patients with childhood onset isolated GH deficiency (no evidence of hypothalamic-pituitary disease or cranial irradiation), two dynamic tests should be recommended, except for those having low IGF-I concentrations (<2 SDS), who may be considered for one test. The cut-off point of the dynamic test should be strict.

4.2 Posology and method of administration

Humatrope in cartridges is administered by subcutaneous injection after reconstitution.

The dosage and administration schedule should be personalised for each individual; however, for

Growth Hormone Deficient Paediatric Patients

The recommended dosage is 0.025-0.035mg/kg of body weight per day by subcutaneous or intramuscular injection. This is the equivalent to approximately 0.7-1.0mg/m^2 body surface area per day.

Growth Hormone Deficient Adult Patients

The recommended starting dose is 0.15-0.30mg/day. A lower starting dose may be necessary in older and obese patients.

This dose should be gradually increased according to individual patient requirements based on the clinical response and serum IGF-I concentrations. Total daily dose usually does not exceed 1mg. IGF-I concentrations should be maintained below the upper limit of the age-specific normal range.

The minimum effective dose should be used, and dose requirements may decline with increasing age.

The dosage of somatropin should be decreased in cases of persistent oedema or severe paraesthesia, in order to avoid the development of carpal tunnel syndrome.

Patients With Turner's Syndrome

The recommended dosage is 0.045-0.050mg/kg of body weight per day, given as a subcutaneous injection, to be administered preferably in the evening. This is equivalent to approximately 1.4mg/m^2 per day.

Prepubertal Paediatric Patients With Chronic Renal Insufficiency

The recommended dosage is 0.045-0.050mg/kg of body weight per day, given as a subcutaneous injection.

The subcutaneous injection sites should be varied in order to avoid lipo-atrophy.

4.3 Contraindications

Humatrope should not be used when there is any evidence of activity of a tumour. Intracranial lesions must be inactive and antitumour therapy complete prior to the institution of growth hormone therapy. Humatrope should be discontinued if there is evidence of tumour growth.

Humatrope should not be reconstituted with the supplied solvent for patients with a known sensitivity to either metacresol or glycerol.

Humatrope should not be used for growth promotion in children with closed epiphyses.

Growth hormone should not be initiated to treat patients with acute critical illness due to complications following open heart or abdominal surgery, multiple accidental trauma, or to patients having acute respiratory failure (see section 4.4).

4.4 Special warnings and special precautions for use

Previous paediatric subjects who had been treated with growth hormone during childhood, until final height was attained, should be re-evaluated for growth hormone deficiency after epiphyseal closure before replacement therapy is commenced at the doses recommended for adults.

Diagnosis and therapy with Humatrope should be initiated and monitored by physicians who are appropriately qualified and experienced in the diagnosis and management of patients with growth hormone deficiency.

There is, so far, no evidence to suspect that growth hormone replacement influences the recurrence rate or regrowth of intracranial neoplasms, but standard clinical practice requires regular pituitary imaging in patients with a history of pituitary pathology. A baseline scan is recommended in these patients before instituting growth hormone replacement therapy.

In cases of severe or recurrent headache, visual problems, nausea, and/or vomiting, a fundoscopy for papilloedema is recommended. If papilloedema is confirmed, a diagnosis of benign intracranial hypertension should be considered and, if appropriate, the growth hormone treatment should be discontinued.

At present, there is insufficient evidence to guide clinical decision making in patients with resolved intracranial hypertension. If growth hormone treatment is restarted, careful monitoring for symptoms of intracranial hypertension is necessary.

Patients with endocrine disorders, including growth hormone deficiency, may develop slipped capital epiphyses more frequently. Any child with the onset of a limp during growth hormone therapy should be evaluated.

Growth hormone increases the extrathyroidal conversion of T4 to T3 and may, as such, unmask incipient hypothyroidism. Monitoring of thyroid function should therefore be conducted in all patients. In patients with hypopituitarism, standard replacement therapy must be closely monitored when somatropin therapy is administered.

For paediatric patients, the treatment should be continued until the end of the growth has been reached. It is advisable not to exceed the recommended dosage in view of the potential risks of acromegaly, hyperglycaemia, and glucosuria.

Before instituting treatment with somatropin for growth retardation secondary to chronic renal insufficiency, patients should have been followed for one year to verify growth disturbance. Conservative treatment for renal insufficiency (which include control of acidosis, hyperparathyroidism, and nutritional status for one year prior to the treatment) should have been established and should be maintained during treatment. Treatment with somatropin should be discontinued at the time of renal transplantation.

After intramuscular injection, hypoglycaemia may appear. Therefore, the recommended dosage should be accurately checked in case of intramuscular injection.

The effects of growth hormone on recovery were studied in two placebo-controlled clinical trials involving 522 adult patients who were critically ill due to complications following open heart or abdominal surgery, multiple accidental trauma, or who were having acute respiratory failure. Mortality was higher (41.9% versus 19.3%) among growth hormone-treated patients (doses 5.3-8mg/day) compared to those receiving placebo. The safety of continuing growth hormone in patients receiving replacement doses for approved indications who concurrently develop these illnesses has not been established. Therefore, the potential benefit of treatment continuation in patients having acute critical illnesses should be weighed against the potential risk.

In order to reach the defined treatment goal, men may need lower growth hormone doses than women. Oral oestrogen administration increases the dose requirements in women. An increasing sensitivity to growth hormone (expressed as change in IGF-I per growth hormone dose) over time may be observed, particularly in men. The accuracy of the growth hormone dose should therefore be controlled every 6 months.

Subjects with diabetes mellitus should be carefully monitored during treatment with Humatrope. An adjustment of the insulin dose may be required.

Experience with patients above 60 years is lacking.

Experience with prolonged treatment in adults is lacking.

4.5 Interaction with other medicinal products and other forms of Interaction

Because human growth hormone may induce a state of insulin resistance, patients should be monitored for evidence of glucose intolerance.

Excessive glucocorticoid therapy will inhibit the growth-promoting effect of human growth hormone. Patients with co-existing ACTH deficiency should have their glucocorticoid replacement dose carefully adjusted to avoid an inhibitory effect on growth.

In women on oral oestrogen replacement, a higher dose of growth hormone may be required to achieve the treatment goal (see section 4.4).

4.6 Pregnancy and lactation

Animal reproduction studies have not been conducted with Humatrope. It is not known whether Humatrope can cause foetal harm when administered to a pregnant woman or can affect reproduction capacity. Humatrope should be given to a pregnant woman only if clearly needed.

There have been no studies conducted with Humatrope in nursing mothers. It is not known whether this drug is excreted in human milk. Because many drugs are excreted in human milk, caution should be exercised when Humatrope is administered to a nursing woman.

4.7 Effects on ability to drive and use machines

Humatrope has no known effect on ability to drive or use machines.

4.8 Undesirable effects

The following table of undesirable effects and frequencies is based on clinical trial and post-marketing spontaneous reports.

Immune System Disorders Hypersensitivity to solvent (metacresol/glycerol): 1%-10%.
Endocrine Disorders Hypothyroidism: 1%-10%.
Reproductive System and Breast Disorders Gynaecomastia: <0.01% paediatrics; 0.1%-1% adults.
Metabolism and Nutrition Disorders Mild hyperglycaemia: 1% paediatrics; 1%-10% adults. Insulin resistance.
Nervous System Disorders Benign intracranial hypertension: 0.01%-0.1%. Headache: >10% adults. Insomnia: <0.01% paediatrics; 1%-10% adults. Paraesthesia: 0.01%-0.1% paediatrics; >10% adults.
Vascular Disorders Hypertension: <0.01% paediatrics; 1%-10% adults.
Musculoskeletal, Connective Tissue, and Bone Disorders Localised muscle pain (myalgia): 1%-10% adults. Joint pain and disorder (arthralgia): >10% adults.
General Disorders and Administration Site Conditions Weakness: 0.1%-1%. Injection site pain (reaction): 1%-10%. Oedema (local and generalised): 1%-10% paediatrics; 10% adults.
Investigations Glucosuria: <0.01% paediatrics; 0.01%-0.1% adults.

Paediatric Patients

In clinical trials with growth hormone deficient patients, approximately 2% of the patients developed antibodies to growth hormone. In trials in Turner's syndrome, where higher doses were used, up to 8% of patients developed antibodies to growth hormone. The binding capacity of these antibodies was low and growth rate was not affected adversely. Testing for antibodies to growth hormone should be carried out in any patient who fails to respond to therapy.

A mild and transient oedema was observed early during the course of treatment.

Leukaemia has been reported in a small number of children who have been treated with growth hormone. However, there is no evidence that leukaemia incidence is increased in growth hormone recipients without predisposing factors.

Adult Patients

In patients with adult onset growth hormone deficiency, oedema, muscle pain, and joint pain and disorder were reported early in therapy and tended to be transient.

Adult patients treated with growth hormone, following diagnosis of growth hormone deficiency in childhood, reported side-effects less frequently than those with adult onset growth hormone deficiency.

4.9 Overdose

Acute overdose could lead initially to hypoglycaemia and subsequently to hyperglycaemia. Long-term overdosage could result in signs and symptoms of acromegaly consistent with the known effects of excess human growth hormone.

5. PHARMACOLOGICAL PROPERTIES

5.1 Pharmacodynamic properties

Pharmacotherapeutic group: H01A C01.

Somatropin is a polypeptide hormone of recombinant DNA origin. It has 191 amino acid residues and a molecular weight of 22,125 daltons. The amino acid sequence of the product is identical to that of human growth hormone of pituitary origin. It is synthesised in a strain of *Escherichia coli* that has been modified by the addition of the gene for human growth hormone.

The biological effects of Humatrope are equivalent to human growth hormone of pituitary origin.

The most prominent effect of Humatrope is that it stimulates the growth plates of long bones. Additionally, it promotes cellular protein synthesis and nitrogen retention.

Humatrope stimulates lipid metabolism; it increases plasma fatty acids and HDL-cholesterols, and decreases total plasma cholesterol.

Humatrope therapy has a beneficial effect on body composition in growth hormone deficient patients, in that body fat stores are reduced and lean body mass is increased. Long-term therapy in growth hormone deficient patients increases bone mineral density.

Humatrope may induce insulin resistance. Large doses of human growth hormone may impair glucose tolerance.

The data available from clinical trials so far, in patients with Turner's syndrome, indicate that, while some patients may not respond to this therapy, an increase over predicted height has been observed, the average being 3.3 ± 3.9cm.

5.2 Pharmacokinetic properties

The bioavailability of Humatrope is the same whether presented in vials or cartridges. A dose of 100μg/kg to adult male volunteers will give a peak serum level (C_{max}) of about 55ng/ml, a half-life ($t_{1/2}$) of nearly four hours, and maximal absorption (AUC [0 to ∞]) of about 475ng/hr/ml.

5.3 Preclinical safety data

Humatrope is human growth hormone produced by recombinant technology. No serious events have been reported in subchronic toxicology studies. Long-term animal studies for carcinogenicity and impairment of fertility with this human growth hormone (Humatrope) have not been performed. There has been no evidence to date of Humatrope-induced mutagenicity.

6. PHARMACEUTICAL PARTICULARS

6.1 List of excipients

Cartridges: Mannitol, glycine, dibasic sodium phosphate, phosphoric acid, and sodium hydroxide.

Solvent syringes: Glycerol, metacresol, water for injections, hydrochloric acid, and sodium hydroxide.

6.2 Incompatibilities

There are no known incompatibilities with Humatrope.

6.3 Shelf life

Before reconstitution: 3 years.

After reconstitution: The product may be stored for a maximum of 28 days at 2°C-8°C. Daily room temperature exposure should not exceed 30 minutes.

6.4 Special precautions for storage

Store at 2°C-8°C (in a refrigerator). Do not freeze.

6.5 Nature and contents of container

Powder and solvent cartridges and syringes are of Type I glass.

Humatrope is available in the following pack sizes:

Humatrope 6mg: 1 cartridge with powder and 1 syringe with 3.15ml of solvent solution. Packs of 1, 5, and 10.

Humatrope 12mg: 1 cartridge with powder and 1 syringe with 3.15ml of solvent solution. Packs of 1, 5, and 10.

Humatrope 24mg: 1 cartridge with powder and 1 syringe with 3.15ml of solvent solution. Packs of 1, 5, and 10.

Not all pack sizes may be marketed.

6.6 Instructions for use and handling

Reconstitution: Each cartridge of Humatrope should be reconstituted using the accompanying solvent syringe and the solvent connector. To reconstitute, attach the solvent connector to the cartridge and then inject the entire contents of the pre-filled solvent syringe into the cartridge. The solvent connector automatically aims the stream of liquid against the glass wall of the cartridge. Following reconstitution, the cartridge should be gently rocked back and forth until the contents are completely dissolved. DO NOT SHAKE. The resulting solution should be clear, without particulate matter. If the solution is cloudy or contains particulate matter, the contents MUST NOT be injected.

Humatrope cartridges can be used in conjunction with compatible CE marked pen injection systems. The manufacturer's instructions with each individual pen must be followed for loading the cartridge, attaching the needle, and administering the Humatrope injection.

The solvent connector is for single use only. Discard it after use. A sterile needle should be used for each administration of Humatrope.

7. MARKETING AUTHORISATION HOLDER

Eli Lilly and Company Limited

Kingsclere Road

Basingstoke

RG21 6XA

Trading style:

Lilly Industries Limited

Dista Products Limited

Greenfield Pharmaceuticals

8. MARKETING AUTHORISATION NUMBER(S)

Cartridges 6mg:	PL 0006/0297
Cartridges 12mg:	PL 0006/0298
Cartridges 24mg:	PL 0006/0299
Diluent (6mg):	PL 0006/0254
Diluent (12 and 24mg):	PL 0006/0300

9. DATE OF FIRST AUTHORISATION/RENEWAL OF THE AUTHORISATION

22 November 2001

10. DATE OF REVISION OF THE TEXT

14 February 2002

LEGAL CATEGORY

POM

*HUMATROPE (somatropin) is a trademark of Eli Lilly and Company.

HT15M

Humira 40 mg Solution for Injection in Pre-filled Syringe

(Abbott Laboratories Limited)

1. NAME OF THE MEDICINAL PRODUCT

Humira▼ 40 mg solution for injection in pre-filled syringe

2. QUALITATIVE AND QUANTITATIVE COMPOSITION

Each 0.8 ml single dose pre-filled syringe contains 40 mg of adalimumab.

Adalimumab is a recombinant human monoclonal antibody expressed in Chinese Hamster Ovary cells.

For excipients, see section 6.1.

3. PHARMACEUTICAL FORM

Solution for injection in pre-filled syringe.

4. CLINICAL PARTICULARS

4.1 Therapeutic indications

Rheumatoid arthritis

Humira in combination with methotrexate, is indicated for:

the treatment of moderate to severe, active rheumatoid arthritis in adult patients when the response to disease-modifying anti-rheumatic drugs including methotrexate has been inadequate.

the treatment of severe, active and progressive rheumatoid arthritis in adults not previously treated with methotrexate.

Humira can be given as monotherapy in case of intolerance to methotrexate or when continued treatment with methotrexate is inappropriate.

Humira has been shown to reduce the rate of progression of joint damage as measured by X-ray and to improve physical function, when given in combination with methotrexate.

Psoriatic arthritis

Humira is indicated for the treatment of active and progressive psoriatic arthritis in adults when the response to previous disease-modifying anti rheumatic drug therapy has been inadequate.

4.2 Posology and method of administration

Humira treatment should be initiated and supervised by specialist physicians experienced in the diagnosis and treatment of rheumatoid arthritis. Patients treated with Humira should be given the special alert card.

After proper training in injection technique, patients may self-inject with Humira if their physician determines that it is appropriate and with medical follow-up as necessary.

Rheumatoid Arthritis

Adults

The recommended dose of Humira for adult patients with rheumatoid arthritis is 40 mg adalimumab administered every other week as a single dose via subcutaneous injection. Methotrexate should be continued during treatment with Humira.

Glucocorticoids, salicylates, nonsteroidal anti-inflammatory drugs, or analgesics can be continued during treatment with Humira. Regarding combination with disease modifying anti-rheumatic drugs other than methotrexate see sections 4.4 and 5.1.

In monotherapy, some patients who experience a decrease in their response to Humira may benefit from an increase in dose intensity to 40 mg adalimumab every week.

Available data suggest that the clinical response is usually achieved within 12 weeks of treatment. Continued therapy should be carefully reconsidered in a patient not responding within this time period.

Psoriatic arthritis

The recommended dose of Humira for patients with psoriatic arthritis is 40 mg adalimumab administered every other week as a single dose via subcutaneous injection.

Elderly patients

No dose adjustment is required.

Children and adolescents

Humira has not been studied in this patient population. Therefore, use of Humira cannot be recommended in patients aged below 18 years until further data become available.

Impaired renal and/or hepatic function

Humira has not been studied in these patient populations. No dose recommendations can be made.

4.3 Contraindications

Hypersensitivity to the active substance or to any of the excipients.

Active tuberculosis or other severe infections such as sepsis, and opportunistic infections (see section 4.4).

Moderate to severe heart failure (NYHA class III/IV) (see section 4.4).

4.4 Special warnings and special precautions for use

Infections

Patients must be monitored closely for infections including tuberculosis, before, during and after treatment with Humira. Because the elimination of adalimumab may take up to five months, monitoring should be continued throughout this period.

Treatment with Humira should not be initiated in patients with active infections including chronic or localized infections until infections are controlled.

Patients who develop a new infection while undergoing treatment with Humira should be monitored closely. Administration of Humira should be discontinued if a patient develops a new serious infection until infections are controlled. Physicians should exercise caution when considering the use of Humira in patients with a history of recurring infection or with underlying conditions which may predispose patients to infections.

Serious infections, sepsis, tuberculosis and other opportunistic infections, including fatalities, have been reported with Humira.

Before initiation of therapy with Humira, all patients must be evaluated for both active or inactive (latent) tuberculosis infection. This evaluation should include a detailed medical history with a personal history of tuberculosis or possible previous exposure to patients with active tuberculosis and previous and/or current immunosuppressive therapy. Appropriate screening tests, i.e. tuberculin skin test and chest X-ray, should be performed in all patients (local recommendations may apply). It is recommended that the conduct of these tests should be recorded in the patient alert card. Prescribers are reminded of the risk of false negative tuberculin skin test results, especially in patients who are severely ill or immunocompromised.

If active tuberculosis is diagnosed, Humira therapy must not be initiated (see section 4.3).

If latent tuberculosis is diagnosed, appropriate anti-tuberculosis prophylaxis in accordance with local recommendations must be initiated before starting treatment with Humira. In this situation, the benefit/risk balance of therapy with Humira should be very carefully considered.

Patients should be instructed to seek medical advice if signs/symptoms (eg, persistent cough, wasting/weight loss, low grade fever) suggestive of a tuberculosis infection occur during or after therapy with Humira.

Neurological events

TNF-antagonists including Humira have been associated in rare cases with exacerbation of clinical symptoms and/ or radiographic evidence of demyelinating disease. Prescribers should exercise caution in considering the use of Humira in patients with pre-existing or recent-onset central nervous system demyelinating disorders.

Allergic reactions

Serious allergic adverse reactions have not been reported with subcutaneous administration of Humira during clinical trials. Non-serious allergic reactions associated with Humira were uncommon during clinical trials. In postmarketing, serious allergic reactions including anaphylaxis have been reported very rarely following Humira administration. If an anaphylactic reaction or other serious allergic reaction occurs, administration of Humira should be discontinued immediately and appropriate therapy initiated.

Immunosuppression

In a study of 64 patients with rheumatoid arthritis that were treated with Humira, there was no evidence of depression of delayed-type hypersensitivity, depression of immunoglobulin levels, or change in enumeration of effector T-and B cells and NK-cells, monocyte/macrophages, and neutrophils.

Malignancies and lymphoproliferative disorders

In the controlled portions of clinical trials of TNF-antagonists, more cases of lymphoma have been observed among patients receiving a TNF-antagonist compared with control patients. However, the occurrence was rare, and the follow up period of placebo patients was shorter than for patients receiving TNF-antagonist therapy. Furthermore, there is an increased background lymphoma risk in rheumatoid arthritis patients with long-standing, highly active, inflammatory disease, which complicates the risk estimation. With the current knowledge, a possible risk for the development of lymphomas or other malignancies in patients treated with a TNF-antagonist cannot be excluded.

No studies have been conducted that include patients with a history of malignancy or that continue treatment in patients who develop malignancy while receiving Humira. Thus additional caution should be exercised in considering Humira treatment of these patients (see section 4.8).

Vaccinations

Sixty-one patients with rheumatoid arthritis were given pneumococcal vaccinations against a background of Humira and methotrexate therapy. Most patients receiving Humira were able to mount effective B-cell immune responses to pneumococcal polysaccharide vaccine. Since no data are available, concurrent administration of live vaccines and Humira is not recommended.

Congestive heart failure

In a clinical trial with another TNF antagonist worsening congestive heart failure and increased mortality due to congestive heart failure have been observed. Cases of worsening congestive heart failure have also been reported in patients receiving Humira. Humira should be used with caution in patients with mild heart failure (NYHA class I/II). Humira is contraindicated in moderate or severe heart failure (see section 4.3). Treatment with Humira must be discontinued in patients who develop new or worsening symptoms of congestive heart failure.

Autoimmune processes

Treatment with Humira may result in the formation of autoimmune antibodies. The impact of long-term treatment with Humira on the development of autoimmune diseases is unknown.

Concurrent administration of TNF-alpha antagonists and anakinra

Serious infections were seen in clinical studies with concurrent use of anakinra and another TNF-antagonist, etanercept, with no added clinical benefit compared to etanercept alone. Because of the nature of the adverse events seen with the combination of etanercept and anakinra therapy, similar toxicities may also result from the combination of anakinra and other TNF-antagonists. Therefore, the combination of adalimumab and anakinra is not recommended.

Surgery

There is limited safety experience of surgical procedures in patients treated with Humira. The long half-life of adalimumab should be taken into consideration if a surgical procedure is planned. A patient who requires surgery while on Humira should be closely monitored for infections, and appropriate actions should be taken. There is limited safety experience in patients undergoing arthroplasty while receiving Humira.

4.5 Interaction with other medicinal products and other forms of Interaction

Humira has been studied both in rheumatoid arthritis patients taking Humira as monotherapy and those taking concomitant methotrexate. Antibody formation was low (< 1%) when Humira was given together with methotrexate in comparison with use as monotherapy. Administration of Humira without methotrexate resulted in increased formation of antibodies and increased clearance of adalimumab (see section 5.1).

There is no experience with the efficacy and safety in patients previously treated with other TNF-antagonists.

4.6 Pregnancy and lactation

For adalimumab, there is no experience in pregnant women.

In a developmental toxicity study conducted in monkeys, there was no indication of maternal toxicity, embryotoxicity or teratogenicity. Preclinical data on postnatal toxicity and fertility effects of adalimumab are not available (see section 5.3).

Due to its inhibition of TNFα, adalimumab administered during pregnancy could affect normal immune responses in the newborn. Administration of adalimumab is not recommended during pregnancy. Women of childbearing potential are strongly recommended to use adequate contraception to prevent pregnancy and continue its use for at least five months after the last Humira treatment.

Use during lactation

It is not known whether adalimumab is excreted in human milk or absorbed systemically after ingestion.

However, because human immunoglobulins are excreted in milk, women must not breast-feed for at least five months after the last Humira treatment.

4.7 Effects on ability to drive and use machines

No studies on the effects on the ability to drive and use machines have been performed.

4.8 Undesirable effects

Clinical Trials

Rheumatoid Arthritis

Humira was studied in 2334 rheumatoid arthritis patients in placebo-controlled trials and in long term follow-up studies, including 2073 patients exposed for six months and 1497 patients exposed for greater than one year. The data in the table is based on the adequate and well-controlled studies I, II, III and IV (see section 5.1) involving 1380 patients receiving adalimumab during the placebo-controlled period by randomised treatment. The population had a mean age of 54.5 years, 77% were female, 91% were Caucasian and had moderate to severely active rheumatoid arthritis. Most patients received 40 mg Humira every other week.

The proportion of patients who discontinued treatment due to adverse events during the double-blind, placebo controlled portion of Studies I, II, III and IV was 6.6% for patients taking Humira and 4.2% for placebo-treated patients.

Adverse events at least possibly causally-related to adalimumab, both clinical and laboratory, are displayed by system organ class and frequency (very common > 1/10; common > 1/100 ≤ 1/10; uncommon > 1/1000 ≤ 1/100) in Table 1 below.

(see Table 1 on next page)

Injection site reactions

In placebo-controlled trials, 20% of patients treated with Humira developed injection site reactions (erythema and/ or itching, haemorrhage, pain or swelling), compared to 14% of patients receiving placebo. Injection site reactions generally did not necessitate discontinuation of the medicinal product.

Table 1 Undesirable Effects in Clinical Studies I-IV

Body system	Frequency	Adverse events
Neoplasia	Uncommon	Skin benign neoplasm
Haemic and Lymphatic system	Common	Decreased haemoglobin
	Uncommon	Granulocytopenia, coagulation time increased, antinuclear antibody present, eukopenia, lymphadenopathy, lymphocytosis, platelet count decreased, purpura
Metabolic and Nutritional Disorders	Common	Hypercholesterolaemia,
	Uncommon	Hypercholesterolaemia, alkaline phosphatase increased, BUN increased, hyperuricaemia, peripheral oedema, weight gain, creatine phosphokinase increased, healing abnormal, hypokalaemia, lactic dehydrogenase increased
Psychiatric Disorders	Uncommon	Depression, somnolence, insomnia, agitation
Nervous System	Common	Headache, dizziness
	Uncommon	Paresthaesia, vertigo, hypeasthesia, neuralgia, tremor
Special senses	Uncommon	Conjunctivitis, eye disorder*, otitis media, taste perversion, abnormal vision, blurred vision, dry eye, ear disorder*, eye pain
Cardiovascular System	Uncommon	Hypertension, vasodilatation, chest pain, migraine
Haemorrhage	Uncommon	Ecchymosis
Respiratory System	Common	Upper respiratory infection, rhinitis, sinusitis, bronchitis, cough increased, pneumonia
	Uncommon	Pharyngitis, dyspnoea, lung disorder*, asthma
Digestive System	Common	Nausea, diarrhoea, sore throat
	Uncommon	Liver function test abnormal, SGPT increased, SGOT increased, mouth ulceration, oesophagitis, vomiting, dyspepsia, constipation, gastrointestinal pain, tooth disorder*, gastritis, gastroenteritis, tongue disorder*, oral moniliasis, aphthous stomatitis, dysphagia, stomatitis, ulcerative stomatitis
Skin and Appendage	Common	Rash, pruritis, herpes simplex
	Uncommon	Skin disorder*, herpes zoster, maculopapular rash, nail disorder*, dry skin, sweating increased, alopecia, fungal dermatitis, urticaria, skin nodule, skin ulcer, eczema, subcutaneous haematoma
Musculo-skeletal System	Uncommon	Arthralgia, muscle cramps, myalgia, joint disorder, synovitis, tendon disorder*
Urogenital System	Common	Urinary tract infection
	Uncommon	Vaginal moniliasis, haematuria, cystitis, menorrhagia, proteinuria, increased urinary frequency
Body as a whole	Common	Laboratory test abnormal, asthenia, clinical flare reaction, flu syndrome, abdominal pain, infection
	Uncommon	Fever, mucous membrane disorder*, pain in extremity, face odema, back pain, cellulitis, chills, sepsis, surgery
Injection Site Reaction	Very common	Injection site pain
	Common	Injection site reaction, injection site Haemorrhage, injection site eruption
Hypersensitivity, general	Uncommon	Allergic reaction

* (not otherwise specified)

Infections

In placebo-controlled trials, the rate of infection was 1 per patient year in the Humira treated patients and 0.9 per patient year in the placebo-treated patients. The incidence of serious infections was 0.04 per patient year in Humira treated patients and 0.02 per patient year in placebo-treated patients. The infections consisted primarily of upper respiratory tract infections, bronchitis and urinary tract infections. Most patients continued on Humira after the infection resolved.

Malignancies and lymphoproliferative disorders

In the 4 pivotal trials, 21 malignancies were reported in 1380 Humira treated patients observed for 785 patient-years, and 2 malignancies were reported in 690 placebo treated patients observed for 362 patient-years. This included 2 lymphomas in the Humira treated patients and no lymphomas in the placebo treated patients.

In controlled trials and in open label extension studies, a total of 80 malignancies were observed in 2468 rheumatoid arthritis patients treated in clinical trials for a mean of 24 months (4870 patient years of therapy). This included 32 non-melanoma skin cancers. The expected rates of non melanoma skin cancers cannot be reliably estimated. Forty-eight other malignancies were observed and overall rates and incidences of malignancies in these patients was similar to that expected for an age and gender matched population. Among these other malignancies, 10 lymphomas were observed.

In post-marketing experience from January 2003 to June 2004, with an estimated exposure of 40100 patient-years, a total of 70 malignancies, including 13 lymphomas, have been reported, predominately in patients with rheumatoid arthritis (see section 4.4).

Autoantibodies

Patients had serum samples tested for autoantibodies at multiple time points. In the adequate and well-controlled trials, 12.6% of patients treated with Humira and 7.3% of placebo-treated patients that had negative baseline antinuclear antibody titres reported positive titres at week 24. One patient out of 2334 treated with Humira developed clinical signs suggestive of new-onset lupus-like syndrome. The patient improved following discontinuation of therapy. No patients developed lupus nephritis or central nervous system symptoms.

Information from further rheumatoid arthritis clinical trials

Humira has been studied in 542 patients with early rheumatoid arthritis (disease duration less than 3 years) who were methotrexate naïve (Study V). In the methotrexate monotherapy group, 3.9% of subjects had ALT values 3 × ULN, compared with 2.9% in Humira monotherapy and 8.6% in the combination arm (methotrexate plus Humira).

Psoriatic arthritis

Humira has been studied in 395 patients with psoriatic arthritis. Elevations in ALT were more common in these patients compared with patients in rheumatoid arthritis clinical studies.

Additional Adverse Reactions from Postmarketing Surveillance or Phase IV Clinical Trials

Anaphylaxis has been reported very rarely.

Cutaneous vasculitis has been reported rarely.

4.9 Overdose

No dose-limiting toxicity was observed during clinical trials. The highest dose level evaluated has been multiple intravenous doses of 10 mg/kg.

5. PHARMACOLOGICAL PROPERTIES

5.1 Pharmacodynamic properties

Pharmacotherapeutic group: Selective immunosuppressive agents. ATC code: L04AA17

Mechanism of action

Adalimumab binds specifically to TNF and neutralizes the biological function of TNF by blocking its interaction with the p55 and p75 cell surface TNF receptors.

Adalimumab also modulates biological responses that are induced or regulated by TNF, including changes in the levels of adhesion molecules responsible for leukocyte migration (ELAM-1, VCAM-1, and ICAM-1 with an IC_{50} of 1-2 X 10^{-10} M).

Pharmacodynamic effects

After treatment with Humira, a rapid decrease in levels of acute phase reactants of inflammation (C reactive protein (CRP) and erythrocyte sedimentation rate (ESR)) and serum cytokines (IL-6) was observed compared to baseline in patients with rheumatoid arthritis. Serum levels of matrix metalloproteinases (MMP-1 and MMP-3) that produce tissue remodelling responsible for cartilage destruction were also decreased after Humira administration. Patients treated with Humira usually experienced improvement in haematological signs of chronic inflammation.

Clinical trials

Rheumatoid arthritis

Humira was evaluated in over 3000 patients in all rheumatoid arthritis clinical trials. Some patients were treated for greater than 36 months duration. The efficacy and safety of Humira for the treatment of rheumatoid arthritis were assessed in five randomised, double-blind and well-controlled studies.

Study I evaluated 271 patients with moderately to severely active rheumatoid arthritis who were ≥ 18 years old, had failed therapy with at least one disease-modifying, anti rheumatic drugs and had insufficient efficacy with methotrexate at doses of 12.5 to 25 mg (10 mg if methotrexate-intolerant) every week and whose methotrexate dose remained constant at 10 to 25 mg every week. Doses of 20, 40 or 80 mg of Humira or placebo were given every other week for 24 weeks.

Study II evaluated 544 patients with moderately to severely active rheumatoid arthritis who were ≥ 18 years old and had failed therapy with at least one disease-modifying, anti-rheumatic drug. Doses of 20 or 40 mg of Humira were given by subcutaneous injection every other week with placebo on alternative weeks or every week for 26 weeks; placebo was given every week for the same duration. No other disease-modifying anti-rheumatic drugs were allowed.

Study III evaluated 619 patients with moderately to severely active rheumatoid arthritis who were ≥ 18 years old, had insufficient efficacy to methotrexate at doses of 12.5 to 25 mg (10 mg if methotrexate-intolerant) every week and whose methotrexate dose remained constant at 12.5 to 25 mg every week. There were three groups in this study. The first received placebo injections every week for 52 weeks. The second received 20 mg of Humira every week for 52 weeks. The third group received 40 mg of Humira every other week with placebo injections on alternate weeks. Thereafter, patients enrolled in an open-label extension phase in which 40 mg of Humira was administered every other week.

Table 2 ACR Responses in Placebo-Controlled Trials (Percent of Patients)

Response	Study I[a*]		Study II[a*]		Study III[a*]	
	Placebo/MTX[c] =60	Humira[b]/ MTX[c] n=63	Placebo n=110	Humira[b] n=113	Placebo/ MTX[c] n=200	Humira[b] MTX[c] n=207
ACR 20						
6 months	13.3%	65.1%	19.1%	46.0%	29.5%	63.3%
12 months	NA	NA	NA	NA	24.0%	58.9%
ACR 50						
6 months	6.7%	52.4%	8.2%	22.1%	9.5%	39.1%
12 months	NA	NA	NA	NA	9.5 %	41.5 %
ACR 70						
6 months	3.3%	23.8%	1.8%	12.4%	2.5%	20.8%
12 months	NA	NA	NA	NA	4.5%	23.2%

[a]Study I at 24 weeks, Study II at 26 weeks, and Study III at 24 and 52 weeks

[b]40mg Humira administered every other week

[c]MTX = methotrexate

*$p<0.01$, Humira versus placebo

Table 3 ACR Responses in Study V (percent of patients)

Response	MTX n=257	Humira n=274	Humira/MTX n=268	p-value[a]	p-value[b]	p-value[c]
ACR 20						
Week 52	62.6%	54.4%	72.8%	0.013	<0.001	0.043
Week 104	56.0%	49.3%	69.4%	0.002	<0.001	0.140
ACR 50						
Week 52	45.9%	41.2%	61.6%	<0.001	<0.001	0.317
Week 104	42.8%	36.9%	59.0%	<0.001	<0.001	0.162
ACR 70						
Week 52	27.2%	25.9%	45.5%	<0.001	<0.001	0.656
Week 104	28.4%	28.1%	46.6%	<0.001	<0.001	0.864

a. p-value is from the pairwise comparison of methotrexate monotherapy and Humira/methotrexate combination therapy using the Mann-Whitney U test.

b. p-value is from the pairwise comparison of Humira monotherapy and Humira/methotrexate combination therapy using the Mann-Whitney U test

c. p-value is from the pairwise comparison of Humira monotherapy and methotrexate monotherapy using the Mann-Whitney U test

Table 4 Radiographic Mean Changes Over 12 Months in Study III

	Placebo/MTX[a]	HUMIRA/MTX 40 mg every other week	Placebo/MTX-HUMIRA/MTX (95% Confidence Interval[b])	P-value
Total Sharp score	2.7	0.1	2.6 (1.4, 3.8)	<0.001[c]
Erosion score	1.6	0.0	1.6 (0.9, 2.2)	<0.001
JSN[d] score	1.0	0.1	0.9 (0.3, 1.4)	0.002

[a]methotrexate

[b]95% confidence intervals for the differences in change scores between methotrexate and Humira.

[c]Based on rank analysis

[d]Joint Space Narrowing

Study IV primarily assessed safety in 636 patients with moderately to severely active rheumatoid arthritis who were ⩾ 18 years old. Patients were permitted to be either disease-modifying, anti-rheumatic drug-naïve or to remain on their pre-existing rheumatologic therapy provided that therapy was stable for a minimum of 28 days. These therapies include methotrexate, leflunomide, hydroxychloroquine, sulfasalazine and/or gold salts. Patients were randomised to 40 mg of Humira or placebo every other week for 24 weeks.

Study V evaluated 799 methotrexate-naïve, adult patients with moderate to severely active early rheumatoid arthritis (mean disease duration less than 9 months). This study evaluated the efficacy of Humira 40 mg every other week/methotrexate combination therapy, Humira 40 mg every other week monotherapy and methotrexate monotherapy in reducing the signs and symptoms and rate of progression of joint damage in rheumatoid arthritis for 104 weeks.

The primary end point in Studies I, II and III and the secondary endpoint in Study IV was the percent of patients who achieved an ACR 20 response at week 24 or 26. The primary endpoint in Study V was the percent of patients who achieved an ACR 50 response at week 52. Study III and V had an additional primary endpoint at 52 weeks of retardation of disease progression (as detected by X-ray results). Study III also had a primary endpoint of changes in quality of life.

ACR response

The percent of Humira-treated patients achieving ACR 20, 50 and 70 responses was consistent across trials I, II and III. The results for the 40 mg every other week dose are summarized in Table 2.

(see Table 2 above)

In Studies I-IV, all individual components of the ACR response criteria (number of tender and swollen joints, physician and patient assessment of disease activity and pain, disability index (HAQ) scores and CRP (mg/dl) values) improved at 24 or 26 weeks compared to placebo. In Study III, these improvements were maintained throughout 52 weeks. In addition, ACR response rates were maintained in the majority of patients followed in the open-label extension phase to week 104.

In Study IV, the ACR 20 response of patients treated with Humira plus standard of care was statistically significantly better than patients treated with placebo plus standard of care ($p<0.001$).

In Studies I-IV, Humira-treated patients achieved statistically significant ACR 20 and 50 responses compared to placebo as early as one to two weeks after initiation of treatment.

In Study V with early rheumatoid arthritis patients who were methotrexate naïve, combination therapy with Humira and methotrexate led to faster and significantly greater ACR responses than methotrexate monotherapy and Humira monotherapy at week 52 and responses were sustained at week 104 (see Table 3).

(see Table 3)

At week 52, 42.9% of patients who received Humira/methotrexate combination therapy achieved clinical remission (DAS28 < 2.6) compared to 20.6% of patients receiving methotrexate monotherapy and 23.4% of patients receiving Humira monotherapy. Humira/methotrexate combination therapy was clinically and statistically superior to methotrexate ($p<0.001$) and Humira monotherapy ($p<0.001$) in achieving a low disease state in patients with recently diagnosed moderate to severe rheumatoid arthritis. The response for the two monotherapy arms was similar ($p=0.447$).

Radiographic response

In Study III, where Humira treated patients had a mean duration of rheumatoid arthritis of approximately 11 years, structural joint damage was assessed radiographically and expressed as change in modified total Sharp score and its components, the erosion score and joint space narrowing score. Humira/methotrexate patients demonstrated significantly less radiographic progression than patients receiving methotrexate alone at 6 and 12 months. Data from the open-label extension phase indicate that the reduction in rate of progression of structural damage is maintained through 104 weeks.

(see Table 4)

In Study V, structural joint damage was assessed radiographically and expressed as change in modified total Sharp score (see Table 5).

(see Table 5 on next page)

Following 52 weeks and 104 weeks of treatment, the percentage of patients without progression (change from baseline in modified total Sharp score ⩽ 0.5) was significantly higher with Humira/methotrexate combination therapy (63.8% and 61.2% respectively) compared to methotrexate monotherapy (37.4% and 33.5% respectively, $p<0.001$) and Humira monotherapy (50.7%, $p<0.002$ and 44.5%, $p<0.001$ respectively).

Quality of life and physical function

Health-related quality of life and physical function was assessed using the disability index of the Health Assessment Questionnaire (HAQ) in all the four original adequate and well-controlled trials, which was a pre-specified primary endpoint at week 52 in Study III. All doses/schedules of Humira in the four original studies showed statistically significantly greater improvement in the disability index of the HAQ from baseline to Month 6 compared to placebo and in Study III the same was seen at week 52. Results from the Short Form Health Survey (SF 36) for all doses/schedules of Humira in all four studies support these findings, with statistically significant physical component summary (PCS) scores, as well as statistically significant pain and vitality domain scores for the 40 mg every other week dose. A statistically significant decrease in fatigue as measured by functional assessment of chronic illness therapy (FACIT) scores was seen in all three studies in which it was assessed (Studies I, III, IV).

In Study III, improvement in physical function and quality of life was maintained through week 104 of open-label treatment.

In Study V, the improvement in the HAQ disability index and the physical component of the SF 36 showed greater improvement ($p<0.001$) for Humira/methotrexate combination therapy versus methotrexate monotherapy and Humira monotherapy at week 52, which was maintained through week 104.

Immunogenicity

Patients in Studies I, II and III were tested at multiple timepoints for antibodies to adalimumab during the 6 to 12 month period. In the pivotal trials, anti-adalimumab antibodies were identified in 58/1053 (5.5%) patients treated with adalimumab, compared to 2/370 (0.5%) on placebo. In patients not given concomitant methotrexate, the incidence was 12.4%, compared to 0.6% when adalimumab was used as add-on to methotrexate.

Table 5 Radiographic Mean Changes at Week 52 in Study V

	MTX n=257 (95% confidence interval)	Humira n=274 (95% confidence interval)	Humira/MTX n=268 (95% confidence interval)	p-value[a]	p-value[b]	p-value[c]
Total Sharp score	5.7 (4.2-7.3)	3.0 (1.7-4.3)	1.3 (0.5-2.1)	<0.001	0.0020	<0.001
Erosion score	3.7 (2.7-4.7)	1.7 (1.0-2.4)	0.8(0.4-1.2)	<0.001	0.0082	<0.001
JSN score	2.0 (1.2-2.8)	1.3 (0.5-2.1)	0.5 (0-1.0)	<0.001	0.0037	0.151

a. p-value is from the pairwise comparison of methotrexate monotherapy and Humira/methotrexate combination therapy using the Mann-Whitney U test.

b. p-value is from the pairwise comparison of Humira monotherapy and Humira/methotrexate combination therapy using the Mann-Whitney U test

c. p-value is from the pairwise comparison of Humira monotherapy and methotrexate monotherapy using the Mann-Whitney U test

Table 6 ACR Response in Placebo-Controlled Psoriatic Arthritis Studies (Percent of Patients)

Response	Study VI Placebo n=162	Study VI Humira n=151	Study VII Placebo n=49	Study VII Humira n=51
ACR 20				
Week 12	14%	58% [a]	16%	39%[b]
Week 24	15%	57% [a]	N/A	N/A
ACR 50				
Week 12	4%	36% [a]	2%	25%[a]
Week 24	6%	39% [a]	N/A	N/A
ACR 70				
Week 12	1%	20% [a]	0%	14% [b]
Week 24	1%	23% [a]	N/A	N/A

a $p<0.001$ for all comparisons between Humira and placebo

b $p<0.05$ for all comparisons between Humira and placebo

N/A not applicable

Because immunogenicity analyses are product-specific, comparison of antibody rates with those from other products is not appropriate.

Psoriatic arthritis

Humira, 40 mg every other week, was studied in patients with moderately to severely active psoriatic arthritis in two placebo-controlled studies, Studies VI and VII. Study VI with 24 week duration, treated 313 adult patients who had an inadequate response to non-steroidal anti-inflammatory drug therapy and of these, approximately 50% were taking methotrexate. Study VII with 12 week duration, treated 100 patients who had an inadequate response to DMARD therapy.

There is insufficient evidence of the efficacy of Humira in patients with ankylosing spondylitis-like psoriatic arthropathy due to the small number of patients studied.

(see Table 6 above)

ACR responses in Study VI were similar with and without concomitant methotrexate therapy.

Humira treated patients demonstrated improvement in physical function as assessed by HAQ and Short Form Health Survey (SF 36), from base-line to week 24.

5.2 Pharmacokinetic properties

After subcutaneous administration of a single 40 mg dose, absorption and distribution of adalimumab was slow, with peak serum concentrations being reached about 5 days after administration. The average absolute bioavailability of adalimumab estimated from three studies following a single 40 mg subcutaneous dose was 64%. After single intravenous doses ranging from 0.25 to 10 mg/kg, concentrations were dose proportional. After doses of 0.5 mg/kg (~40 mg), clearances ranged from 11 to 15 ml/hour, the distribution volume (V_{ss}) ranged from 5 to 6 litres and the mean terminal phase half-life was approximately two weeks. Adalimumab concentrations in the synovial fluid from several rheumatoid arthritis patients ranged from 31-96% of those in serum.

Following subcutaneous administration of 40 mg of Humira every other week the mean steady-state trough concentrations were approximately 5 μg/ml (without concomitant methotrexate) and 8 to 9 μg/ml (with concomitant methotrexate), respectively. The serum adalimumab trough levels at steady-state increased roughly proportionally with dose following 20, 40 and 80 mg every other week and every week subcutaneous dosing.

Population pharmacokinetic analyses with data from over 1300 patients revealed a trend toward higher apparent clearance of adalimumab with increasing body weight. After adjustment for weight differences, gender and age appeared to have a minimal effect on adalimumab clearance. The serum levels of free adalimumab (not bound to anti-adalimumab antibodies, AAA) were observed to be lower in patients with measurable AAA. Humira has not been studied in children or in patients with hepatic or renal impairment.

5.3 Preclinical safety data

Preclinical data reveal no special hazard for humans based on studies of single dose toxicity, repeated dose toxicity, and genotoxicity.

An embryo-foetal developmental toxicity/perinatal developmental study has been performed in cynomologous monkeys at 0, 30 and 100 mg/kg (9-17 monkeys / group) and has revealed no evidence of harm to the foetuses due to adalimumab. Carcinogenicity studies, and standard assessment of fertility and postnatal toxicity, were not performed with adalimumab due to the lack of appropriate models for an antibody with limited cross-reactivity to rodent TNF and the development of neutralizing antibodies in rodents.

6. PHARMACEUTICAL PARTICULARS

6.1 List of excipients

Mannitol

Citric acid monohydrate

Sodium citrate

Sodium dihydrogen phosphate dihydrate

Disodium phosphate dihydrate

Sodium chloride

Polysorbate 80

Sodium hydroxide

Water for injections

6.2 Incompatibilities

In the absence of compatibility studies, this medicinal product must not be mixed with other medicinal products.

6.3 Shelf life

18 months

6.4 Special precautions for storage

Store in a refrigerator (2°C – 8°C). Keep the vial in the outer carton. Do not freeze.

6.5 Nature and contents of container

Humira 40 mg solution for injection in single-use pre-filled syringe (type I glass) for patient use:

Packs of 2 pre-filled syringes (0.8 ml sterile solution), each with 1 alcohol pad, in a blister.

6.6 Instructions for use and handling

Any unused product or waste material should be disposed of in accordance with local requirements.

7. MARKETING AUTHORISATION HOLDER

Abbott Laboratories Ltd.

Queenborough

Kent ME11 5EL

United Kingdom

8. MARKETING AUTHORISATION NUMBER(S)

2 pre-filled syringes: EU/1/03/256/003

9. DATE OF FIRST AUTHORISATION/RENEWAL OF THE AUTHORISATION

8 September 2003

10. DATE OF REVISION OF THE TEXT

8 August 2005

Humulin Vials, Cartridges and Pens

(Eli Lilly and Company Limited)

1. NAME OF THE MEDICINAL PRODUCT

Humulin* S (Soluble) 100IU/ml solution for injection in vial

(Soluble insulin injection)

Humulin S (Soluble) 100IU/ml solution for injection in cartridge

(Soluble insulin injection)

Humulin I (Isophane) 100IU/ml suspension for injection in vial

(Isophane insulin injection)

Humulin I (Isophane) 100IU/ml suspension for injection in cartridge

(Isophane insulin injection)

Humulin I Pen (Isophane) 100IU/ml suspension for injection

(Isophane insulin injection)

Humulin M3 (Mixture 3) 100IU/ml suspension for injection in vial

(Biphasic isophane insulin injection - 30% soluble insulin/70% isophane insulin)

Humulin M3 (Mixture 3) 100IU/ml suspension for injection in cartridge

(Biphasic isophane insulin injection - 30% soluble insulin/70% isophane insulin)

Humulin M3 Pen (Mixture 3) 100IU/ml suspension for injection

(Biphasic isophane insulin injection - 30% soluble insulin/70% isophane insulin)

2. QUALITATIVE AND QUANTITATIVE COMPOSITION

1ml contains 100IU human insulin (produced in *E. coli* by recombinant DNA technology).

One vial contains 10ml equivalent to 1000IU.

One cartridge contains 3ml equivalent to 300IU.

One prefilled pen contains 3ml equivalent to 300IU.

For excipients, see section 6.1.

3. PHARMACEUTICAL FORM

A solution or suspension for injection filled into:

A. Cartridges administered via either

i) A reusable device.

A 3ml cartridge to be used with a CE marked pen, as recommended in the information provided by the device manufacturer.

or

ii) A non-reusable device.

A prefilled/disposable pen injector containing a 3.0ml cartridge. Humulin Pens deliver up to 60 units per dose in single unit increments.

B. Vials

A 10ml vial to be used in conjunction with an appropriate syringe (100IU/ml markings).

Humulin S is a sterile, clear, colourless, aqueous solution of human insulin, adjusted to a pH range of 7.0 to 7.8.

Humulin S is a rapidly acting insulin preparation.

Humulin I is a sterile suspension of a white, crystalline precipitate of isophane human insulin in an isotonic phosphate buffer adjusted to a pH range of 6.9 to 7.5.

Humulin I is an intermediate acting insulin preparation.

Humulin M3 is a sterile suspension of human insulin in the proportion of 30% soluble insulin to 70% isophane insulin, adjusted to a pH range of 6.9 to 7.5.

Humulin M3 is an intermediate acting insulin preparation.

4. CLINICAL PARTICULARS

4.1 Therapeutic indications

For the treatment of patients with diabetes mellitus who require insulin for the maintenance of glucose homeostasis. Humulin is also indicated for the initial control of diabetes mellitus and diabetes mellitus in pregnancy.

4.2 Posology and method of administration

The dosage should be determined by the physician, according to the requirement of the patient.

Humulin S should be given by subcutaneous injection but may, although not recommended, also be given by intramuscular injection. It may also be administered intravenously.

Humulin I and Humulin M3 in vials and cartridge presentations should be given by subcutaneous injection but may, although not recommended, also be given by intramuscular injection. These formulations should not be administered intravenously.

Subcutaneous administration should be in the upper arms, thighs, buttocks, or abdomen. Use of injection sites should be rotated so that the same site is not used more than approximately once a month.

Care should be taken when injecting any Humulin insulin preparations to ensure that a blood vessel has not been entered. After any insulin injection, the injection site should not be massaged. Patients must be educated to use proper injection techniques.

Humulin I may be administered in combination with Humulin S. (See section 6.6 for *'Mixing of insulins'*.)

The Humulin M3 formulation is a ready-made defined mixture of Humulin S and Humulin I insulin, designed to avoid the need for the patient to mix insulin preparations. A patient's treatment regimen should be based on their individual metabolic requirements.

4.3 Contraindications

Hypoglycaemia.

Hypersensitivity to Humulin or to the formulation excipients, unless used as part of a desensitisation programme.

Under no circumstances should any Humulin formulation, other than Humulin S, be given intravenously.

4.4 Special warnings and special precautions for use

Transferring a patient to another type or brand of insulin should be done under strict medical supervision. Changes in strength, brand (manufacturer), type (soluble, isophane, lente, etc), species (animal, human, human insulin analogue), and/or method of manufacture (recombinant DNA versus animal-source insulin) may result in the need for a change in dosage.

Some patients taking human insulin may require a change in dosage from that used with animal-source insulins. If an adjustment is needed, it may occur with the first dose or during the first several weeks or months.

A few patients who experienced hypoglycaemic reactions after transfer to human insulin have reported that the early warning symptoms were less pronounced or different from those experienced with their previous animal insulin. Patients whose blood glucose is greatly improved, eg, by intensified insulin therapy, may lose some or all of the warning symptoms of hypoglycaemia and should be advised accordingly. Other conditions which may make the early warning symptoms of hypoglycaemia different or less pronounced include long duration of diabetes, diabetic nerve disease, or medications such as beta-blockers. Uncorrected hypoglycaemic and hyperglycaemic reactions can cause loss of consciousness, coma, or death.

The use of dosages which are inadequate, or discontinuation of treatment, especially in insulin-dependent diabetics, may lead to hyperglycaemia and diabetic ketoacidosis, conditions which are potentially lethal.

Treatment with human insulin may cause formation of antibodies, but titres of antibodies are lower than those to purified animal insulin.

Insulin requirements may change significantly in diseases of the adrenal, pituitary, or thyroid glands, and in the presence of renal or hepatic impairment.

Insulin requirements may be increased during illness or emotional disturbances.

Adjustment of insulin dosage may also be necessary if patients change their level of physical activity or change their usual diet.

4.5 Interaction with other medicinal products and other forms of Interaction

Some medicinal products are known to interact with glucose metabolism. The physician should take possible interactions into account and ask patients about their other medications in addition to human insulin.

Insulin requirements may be increased by substances with hyperglycaemic activity, such as glucocorticoids, thyroid hormones, growth hormone, danazol, beta$_2$-sympathomimetics (such as ritodrine, salbutamol, terbutaline), thiazides.

Insulin requirements may be reduced in the presence of substances with hypoglycaemic activity, such as oral hypoglycaemics (OHA), salicylates (for example, acetylsalicylic acid), certain antidepressants (monoamine oxidase inhibitors), certain angiotensin converting enzyme (ACE) inhibitors (captopril, enalapril), non-selective beta-blocking agents, and alcohol.

Somatostatin analogues (octreotide, lanreotide) may both decrease and increase insulin requirements.

4.6 Pregnancy and lactation

It is essential to maintain good control of the insulin-treated (insulin-dependent or gestational diabetes) patient throughout pregnancy. Insulin requirements usually fall during the first trimester and increase during the second and third trimesters. Patients with diabetes should be advised to inform their doctors if they are pregnant or are contemplating pregnancy.

Careful monitoring of glucose control, as well as general health, is essential in pregnant patients with diabetes.

Diabetic patients who are lactating may require adjustments in insulin dose and/or diet.

4.7 Effects on ability to drive and use machines

The patient's ability to concentrate and react may be impaired as a result of hypoglycaemia. This may constitute a risk in situations where these abilities are of special importance (eg, driving a car or operating machinery).

Patients should be advised to take precautions to avoid hypoglycaemia whilst driving, this is particularly important in those who have reduced or absent awareness of the warning signs of hypoglycaemia or have frequent episodes of hypoglycaemia. The advisability of driving should be considered in these circumstances.

4.8 Undesirable effects

Hypoglycaemia is the most frequent undesirable effect of insulin therapy that a patient with diabetes may suffer. Severe hypoglycaemia may lead to loss of consciousness, and in extreme cases, death.

Local allergy in patients occurs as redness, swelling, and itching at the site of insulin injection. This condition usually resolves in a few days to a few weeks. In some instances, this condition may be related to factors other than insulin, such as irritants in the skin cleansing agent or poor injection technique.

Systemic allergy, less common but potentially more serious, is a generalised allergy to insulin. It may cause rash over the whole body, shortness of breath, wheezing, reduction in blood pressure, fast pulse, or sweating. Severe cases of generalised allergy may be life-threatening. In the rare event of a severe allergy to Humulin, treatment is required immediately. A change of insulin or desensitisation may be required.

Lipodystrophy may occur at the injection site.

4.9 Overdose

Insulin has no specific overdose definitions, because serum glucose concentrations are a result of complex interactions between insulin levels, glucose availability, and other metabolic processes. Hypoglycaemia may occur as a result of an excess of insulin relative to food intake and energy expenditure.

Hypoglycaemia may be associated with listlessness, confusion, palpitations, headache, sweating, and vomiting.

Mild hypoglycaemic episodes will respond to oral administration of glucose or sugar products.

Correction of moderately severe hypoglycaemia can be accomplished by intramuscular or subcutaneous administration of glucagon, followed by oral carbohydrate when the patient recovers sufficiently. Patients who fail to respond to glucagon must be given glucose solution intravenously.

If the patient is comatose, glucagon should be administered intramuscularly or subcutaneously. However, glucose solution must be given intravenously if glucagon is not available or if the patient fails to respond to glucagon. The patient should be given a meal as soon as consciousness is recovered.

5. PHARMACOLOGICAL PROPERTIES

5.1 Pharmacodynamic properties

Pharmacotherapeutic group:

Humulin S:	A10A B01
Humulin I:	A10A C01
Humulin M3:	A10A D01

The prime activity of insulin is the regulation of glucose metabolism.

In addition, insulin has several anabolic and anti-catabolic actions on a variety of different tissues. Within muscle tissue this includes increasing glycogen, fatty acid, glycerol and protein synthesis, and amino acid uptake, while decreasing glycogenolysis, gluconeogenesis, ketogenesis, lipolysis, protein catabolism, and amino acid output.

The typical activity profile (glucose utilisation curve) following subcutaneous injection is illustrated below by the heavy line. Variations that a patient may experience in timing and/or intensity of insulin activity are illustrated by the shaded area. Individual variability will depend on factors such as size of dose, site of injection temperature, and physical activity of the patient.

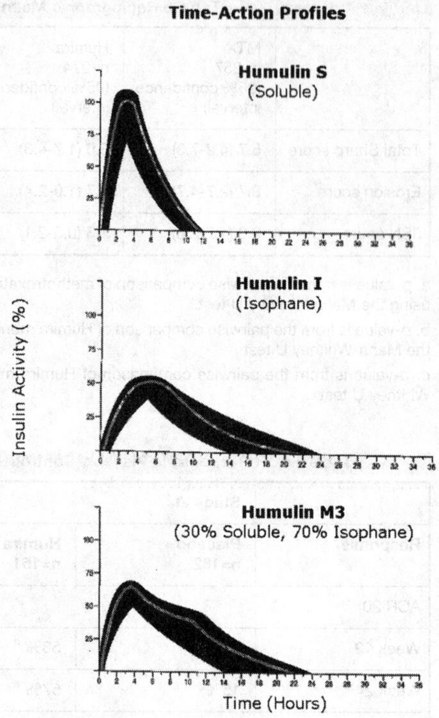

5.2 Pharmacokinetic properties

The pharmacokinetics of insulin do not reflect the metabolic action of that hormone. Therefore, it is more appropriate to examine glucose utilisation curves (as discussed above) when considering the activity of insulin.

5.3 Preclinical safety data

Humulin is human insulin produced by recombinant technology. No serious events have been reported in subchronic toxicology studies. Human insulin was not mutagenic in a series of *in vitro* and *in vivo* genetic toxicity assays.

6. PHARMACEUTICAL PARTICULARS

6.1 List of excipients

For Humulin S preparations:

Each vial or cartridge will contain human insulin (recombinant DNA origin) and the following excipients:

m-cresol

Glycerol

Water for injections

The following may be used to adjust pH:

Hydrochloric acid and/or

Sodium hydroxide

For Humulin I and Humulin M3 preparations:

Each vial, cartridge, or prefilled pen will contain human insulin (recombinant DNA origin) and the following excipients:

m-cresol

Glycerol

Phenol

Protamine sulphate

Dibasic sodium phosphate

Zinc oxide

Water for injections

The following may be used to adjust pH:

Hydrochloric acid and/or

Sodium hydroxide

6.2 Incompatibilities

Humulin preparations should not be mixed with insulins produced by other manufacturers or with animal insulin preparations.

6.3 Shelf life

The shelf-life for Humulin S, Humulin I, and Humulin M3 presentations is two years.

The in-use shelf-life for all Humulin vials, all Humulin 3.0ml cartridges, and the prefilled pens is 28 days.

6.4 Special precautions for storage

Store at 2°C-8°C (in a refrigerator).

Do not freeze. Do not expose to excessive heat or direct sunlight.

Keep the container in the outer carton.

Once in use, the vials, cartridges, and prefilled pens may be used for up to 28 days. Do not use beyond this period.

When in use, the vials, cartridges, and prefilled pens should not be stored above 30°C.

6.5 Nature and contents of container

Humulin vials: The product is filled in vials that comply with the requirements of the PhEur for Type I flint glass, stoppered with rubber closures, and sealed with aluminium seals combined with a plastic 'flip top'.

1 × 10ml vial

Humulin cartridges and prefilled pens: The product is filled in cartridges that comply with the requirements of the PhEur for Type I flint glass, and sealed with rubber closures consisting of a plunger head at the bottom and a disk seal at the top of the cartridge.

5 × 3ml cartridges

5 × 3ml pens

6.6 Instructions for use and handling

a) Preparing a dose

Vials or cartridges containing Humulin S formulation do not require resuspension and should only be used if they are clear, colourless, with no solid particles visible and if they are of water-like appearance.

Vials containing Humulin I or Humulin M3 formulations should be rotated several times in the palms of the hands before use to completely resuspend the insulin, until it appears uniformly cloudy or milky. If not, repeat the above procedure until contents are mixed. Cartridges or the Humulin Pens, containing Humulin I or Humulin M3 formulations, should be rolled in the palms of the hands ten-times and inverted 180° ten-times immediately before use to resuspend the insulin until it appears uniformly cloudy or milky. If not, repeat the above procedure until contents are mixed. Cartridges contain a small glass bead to assist mixing. Do not shake vigorously as this may cause frothing, which may interfere with the correct measurement of the dose.

The vials and cartridges should be examined frequently and should not be used if clumps of material are present or if solid white particles stick to the bottom or wall of the vial or cartridge, giving a frosted appearance.

The cartridges are not designed to allow any other insulin to be mixed in the cartridge. Cartridges are not designed to be refilled.

Mixing of insulins: The shorter acting insulin should be drawn into the syringe first, to prevent contamination of the vial or cartridge by the longer acting preparation. It is advisable to inject directly after mixing. However, if a delay is necessary, a consistent routine must be followed.

Alternatively, a separate syringe or separate cartridges can be used for administration of the correct amount of Humulin S and Humulin I.

Vials

Prepare your syringe prior to injection, as directed by your doctor or diabetic nurse.

Use an insulin syringe marked for the strength of insulin being administered.

Cartridges and prefilled pens

Reusable devices

The manufacturer's instructions with each individual pen must be followed for loading the cartridge, attaching the needle, and administering the insulin injection.

Non-reusable pens

Follow the instructions with Humulin Pens for attaching the needle and administering the insulin injection.

For Humulin Pens, a needle must always be attached before priming, dialling, and injecting an insulin dose. Humulin Pens should always be primed before each injection. Failure to prime Humulin Pens may result in an inaccurate dose.

b) Injecting a dose

Inject the correct dose of insulin, as directed by your doctor or diabetic nurse. Use of the injection sites should be rotated so that the same is not used more than approximately once a month.

Each pack contains a patient information leaflet with instructions on how tc inject insulin.

c) Disposal of used containers and needles

Do not reuse needles. Dispose of the needle in a responsible manner. Needles and pens must not be shared. Vials, cartridges, and Humulin Pens can be used until empty, then properly discard.

7. MARKETING AUTHORISATION HOLDER

Eli Lilly and Company Limited

Kingsclere Road

Basingstoke

Hampshire

RG21 6XA

8. MARKETING AUTHORISATION NUMBER(S)

Humulin S vial:	PL 0006/0216
Humulin I vial:	PL 0006/0228
Humulin M3 vial:	PL 0006/0233
Humulin S cartridge:	PL 0006/0242
Humulin I cartridge:	PL 0006/0257
Humulin M3 cartridge:	PL 0006/0260
Humulin I Pen:	PL 0006/0338
Humulin M3 Pen:	PL 0006/0341

9. DATE OF FIRST AUTHORISATION/RENEWAL OF THE AUTHORISATION

Humulin S vial:	Date of first authorisation:	16 February 1987
	Date of last renewal of the authorisation:	25 April 2001
Humulin I vial:	Date of first authorisation:	16 February 1987
	Date of last renewal of the authorisation:	25 April 2001
Humulin M3 vial:	Date of first authorisation:	28 April 1987
	Date of last renewal of the authorisation:	25 April 2001
Humulin S cartridge:	Date of first authorisation:	15 August 1994
	Date of last renewal of the authorisation:	25 April 2001
Humulin I cartridge:	Date of first authorisation:	15 August 1994
	Date of last renewal of the authorisation:	25 April 2001
Humulin M3 cartridge:	Date of first authorisation:	16 November 1990
	Date of last renewal of the authorisation:	25 April 2001
Humulin I Pen:	Date of first authorisation:	19 September 1997
	Date of last renewal of the authorisation:	19 September 2002
Humulin M3 Pen:	Date of first authorisation:	19 September 1997
	Date of last renewal of the authorisation:	19 September 2002

10. DATE OF REVISION OF THE TEXT

28 April 2004

LEGAL CATEGORY

POM

*HUMULIN (human insulin [prb]) is a trademark of Eli Lilly and Company.

HU17M

Hyalase (Hyaluronidase)

(Wockhardt UK Ltd)

1. NAME OF THE MEDICINAL PRODUCT

Hyalase® (Hyaluronidase for Injection BP).

2. QUALITATIVE AND QUANTITATIVE COMPOSITION

Each ampoule contains 1500 international units of Hyaluronidase for Injection BP (ovine).

3. PHARMACEUTICAL FORM

1ml neutral glass ampoule containing a white, sterile, freeze-dried powder of the enzyme hyaluronidase for subcutaneous and intramuscular injection.

4. CLINICAL PARTICULARS

4.1 Therapeutic indications

Hyalase® can be used to enhance permeation of subcutaneous or intramuscular injections, local anaesthetics and subcutaneous infusions and to promote resorption of excess fluids and blood in the tissues.

4.2 Posology and method of administration

Adults, children and the elderly:

With subcutaneous infusion (hypodermoclysis): 1500iu of Hyalase® dissolved in 1ml of water for injections or normal saline injected into the site, before the infusion is set up, or injected into the tubing of the infusion set, about 2cm back from the needle, at the start of the infusion. 1500iu is sufficient for administration of 500-1000ml of most fluids. Refer to Section 4.4 for information on solutions for hypodermoclysis. Care should be taken in young children and the elderly to control the speed and total volume of fluid administered and to avoid over-hydration, especially in renal impairment.

With subcutaneous or intramuscular injections: 1500iu of Hyalase® dissolved directly in the solution to be injected.

With local anaesthetics: 1500iu Hyalase® is mixed with the quantity of local anaesthetic solution to be used. In ophthalmology, 15iu of Hyalase® per ml is recommended.

Extravasation: Where dispersal rather than localisation is indicated, 1500iu of Hyalase® in 1ml water for injections or normal saline infiltrated into the affected area as soon as possible after the extravasation is noted.

Haematoma: 1500iu of Hyalase® dissolved in 1ml water for injections or normal saline infiltrated into the affected area.

Immediately before use dissolve the freeze-dried powder in approximately 1ml of water for injections or directly in the solution with which Hyalase® is to be combined.

4.3 Contraindications

Hypersensitivity to hyaluronidase

Not to be used to reduce the swelling of bites or stings or at sites where infection or malignancy is present. Not to be used for anaesthetic procedures in cases of unexplained premature labour.

4.4 Special warnings and special precautions for use

Do not apply directly to the cornea.

Not to be used for intravenous injections.

Solutions for subcutaneous administration should be isotonic with extracellular fluid. Hyalase® is physically compatible with the commonly used infusion fluids. Use in hypodermoclysis has been reported with 0.9% sodium chloride, 0.18% sodium chloride with 4% glucose, 0.45% sodium chloride with 2.5% glucose and 5% glucose.

Potassium 34mmol/litre has been administered in isotonic glucose or saline.

Electrolyte-free fluids are less preferable than those containing electrolytes and should not be given too rapidly. Hyalase® has also been mixed with morphine, diamorphine, hydromorphone, chlorpromazine, metoclopramide, promazine, dexamethasone, local anaesthetics and adrenaline (see 6.2. Incompatibilities).

4.5 Interaction with other medicinal products and other forms of Interaction

None stated.

4.6 Pregnancy and lactation

It is not known whether the drug enters breast milk although it is unlikely to harm the breast-fed infant. Caution should be exercised in administering it to nursing mothers.

There is no evidence on the drug's safety in human pregnancy nor is there evidence from animal work that it is free from hazard. Avoid use in pregnancy unless there is no safer alternative.

4.7 Effects on ability to drive and use machines

None known.

4.8 Undesirable effects

Oedema has been reported in association with hypodermoclysis. Severe allergic reactions including anaphylaxis have been reported rarely. Local irritation, infection, bleeding and bruising occur rarely.

4.9 Overdose

No cases of overdose appear to have been reported.

5. PHARMACOLOGICAL PROPERTIES

5.1 Pharmacodynamic properties

Hyaluronidase is an enzyme that has a temporary and reversible depolymerising effect on the polysaccharide hyaluronic acid, which is present in the intercellular matrix of connective tissue.

5.2 Pharmacokinetic properties

Not applicable

5.3 Preclinical safety data

There are no additional pre-clinical data of relevance to the prescriber.

6. PHARMACEUTICAL PARTICULARS

6.1 List of excipients

Water for Injections BP removed during the freeze drying process.

6.2 Incompatibilities

Physical incompatibility has been reported with heparin and adrenaline, although in clinical practice very low concentrations of adrenaline are combined with hyaluronidase without problems. Frusemide, the benzodiazepines and phenytoin have been found to be incompatible with hyaluronidase.

6.3 Shelf life

Three years from date of manufacture.

6.4 Special precautions for storage

Do not store above 25°C.

6.5 Nature and contents of container

1ml neutral glass ampoule containing a plug of white freeze-dried powder.

6.6 Instructions for use and handling

The solution should be used immediately after preparation.

Administrative Data

7. MARKETING AUTHORISATION HOLDER

CP Pharmaceuticals Ltd

Ash Road North

Wrexham

LL13 9UF

8. MARKETING AUTHORISATION NUMBER(S)

PL 4543/0337

9. DATE OF FIRST AUTHORISATION/RENEWAL OF THE AUTHORISATION

N/A

10. DATE OF REVISION OF THE TEXT

January 2002

Hyalgan

(Shire Pharmaceuticals Limited)

1. NAME OF THE MEDICINAL PRODUCT
HYALGAN®

2. QUALITATIVE AND QUANTITATIVE COMPOSITION
Each pre-filled syringe contains 20mg/2ml of hyaluronic acid sodium salt (Hyalectin®).

3. PHARMACEUTICAL FORM
Hyalgan is a sterile solution for intra-articular injection for single use only.

4. CLINICAL PARTICULARS

4.1 Therapeutic indications
For the sustained relief of pain in osteoarthritis of the knee.

4.2 Posology and method of administration
Adults (including the elderly)

The contents of one pre-filled syringe (20mg/2ml) to be injected into the affected joint once a week to a total of five injections, using a standard technique. No adjustment of dose is required in elderly patients.

This can be repeated at not less than 6 monthly intervals.

Children
At present there is not enough evidence to recommend a dosage regimen for use in children.

4.3 Contraindications
Hyalectin, the active principle in Hyalgan, is of avian origin. Do not administer to patients with known hypersensitivity to any ingredient of the product or to avian proteins.

Intra-articular injections are contraindicated in cases of infections or skin diseases in the area of the injection site.

4.4 Special warnings and special precautions for use
Remove joint effusion, if present, before injecting Hyalgan.

Patients should be carefully examined prior to administration to determine signs of acute inflammation and the physician should evaluate whether Hyalgan treatment should be initiated when objective signs of inflammation are present.

As with any invasive joint procedure, it is recommended that care be taken not to overburden the joint immediately following the intra-articular injection.

Use only if the solution is clear.

See also item 6.6.

4.5 Interaction with other medicinal products and other forms of Interaction
Since there is limited experience available, Hyalgan should not be administered simultaneously or mixed with other intra-articular injections.

Do not use concomitantly with disinfectants containing quaternary ammonium salts because hyaluronic acid can precipitate in their presence.

4.6 Pregnancy and lactation
No embryotoxicity or teratogenicity has been observed in animal studies. However, there is no experience of the use of Hyalgan in pregnant women and therefore the expected benefit to the mother should be weighed against any potential risk to the foetus.

If Hyalgan is prescribed to a woman of child bearing potential, she should be advised to contact her physician regarding discontinuance of the product if she intends to become, or suspects that she is, pregnant.

Although it is not expected that Hyalgan would be present in human milk, because many drugs are excreted by this route, caution should be exercised when Hyalgan is administered to a nursing mother and the expected benefit to the mother should be weighed against any potential risk to the neonate.

4.7 Effects on ability to drive and use machines
Hyalgan is not expected to have any effect on the patient's ability to drive or operate machinery.

4.8 Undesirable effects
Pain, swelling, effusion, heat and redness may rarely occur at the injection site. Such symptoms are benign, short lived, without sequelae and disappear spontaneously within a few days by resting the affected joint applying ice locally.

Systemic allergic reactions due to individual hypersensitivity have been rarely recorded. Isolated cases of an anaphylactic-like reaction have been reported in post-marketing experience and they had favourable outcomes. No case of anaphylactic-like reactions has been reported during clinical trials. Allergic-type signs and symptoms such as rash, pruritus, and urticaria are also very rare.

In a 495-patient US multicentre placebo- and naproxen-controlled clinical study, the following adverse events occurred with a frequency greater than 5% in the Hyalgan group (versus placebo): headache 18% (17%), rash 7% (9%), ecchymosis 7% (6%) and pruritus 7% (4%). As these events occurred with equal frequency in the placebo group, there is no proven causality in respect of Hyalgan.

4.9 Overdose
Overdosage is unlikely given the route of administration and the single use pack of the drug. No case of overdosage has been reported to date.

5. PHARMACOLOGICAL PROPERTIES

5.1 Pharmacodynamic properties
Hyalgan is a sterile, non-pyrogenic, viscous, aqueous buffered solution of a defined high molecular weight fraction of highly purified hyaluronic acid sodium salt (Hyalectin). Hyaluronic acid is an important component of the body's extracellular matrix and is present in a particularly high concentration in cartilage and synovial fluid. Endogenous hyaluronic acid provides viscosity and elasticity to synovial fluid, which is fundamental for its lubricating and shock absorbing properties, and it is essential for the correct structure of proteoglycans in articular cartilage. In osteoarthritis there is an insufficient amount of, and a change in the quality of, hyaluronic acid in synovial fluid and cartilage. The intra-articular administration of hyaluronic acid into arthritic joints with degenerating cartilage surfaces and pathologically altered synovial fluid improved joint functions. The observed beneficial effects of exogenous hyaluronic acid may be related to its interactions with various components of the synovial cavity (synoviocytes and chondrocytes).

In controlled clinical studies, treatment cycles with Hyalgan have been shown to ameliorate the symptoms of osteoarthritis for up to 6 months following the end of treatment.

5.2 Pharmacokinetic properties
Hyaluronic acid sodium salt (Hyalectin) administered intra-articularly is eliminated from the synovial fluid within 2 to 3 days. Pharmacokinetic studies have shown that it is quickly distributed to the synovial membrane. The highest concentrations of labelled hyaluronic acid have been detected in the synovial fluid and the articular capsule, followed by, in decreasing order, the synovial membrane, the ligaments and the adjacent muscle.

Hyaluronic acid in synovial fluid has been shown to be not significantly metabolised. Animal studies have shown that some degradation occurs in the tissue surrounding the joints, but the major site for metabolism is the liver and excretion is mainly through the kidneys.

5.3 Preclinical safety data
Hyalectin (hyaluronic acid sodium salt) was tested in a standard range of toxicological tests, including mutagenicity and reproductive toxicity studies, and produced negative results throughout.

6. PHARMACEUTICAL PARTICULARS

6.1 List of excipients
Sodium chloride, disodium hydrogen phosphate dodecahydrate, sodium dihydrogen phosphate dihydrate, water for injections.

6.2 Incompatibilities
There are currently insufficient data to support the compatibility of Hyalgan with other drugs administered intra-articularly. Therefore the mixing or simultaneous administration with other intra-articular drugs is not recommended.

6.3 Shelf life
Hyalgan pre-filled syringes have a shelf life of 36 months when in their original package.

Hyalgan should not be used after the expiry date, printed on the package.

6.4 Special precautions for storage
Do not use Hyalgan if package is opened or damaged. Store in original packaging (protected from light) below 25°C. DO NOT FREEZE.

6.5 Nature and contents of container
Sterile, colourless, Type 1 borosilicate glass syringes with rubber stoppers on which polypropylene plunger rods are tightened up, containing 2ml of Hyalgan solution, supplied in packs of 1 pre-filled syringe.

6.6 Instructions for use and handling
Hyalgan is for intra-articular injection and is supplied as a single-use, ready to use, sterile solution in a 2ml pre-filled syringe, and must not be diluted. The contents of the vial and syringe are sterile and must be used immediately once the container has been opened.

Intra-articular injection of Hyalgan should be made using precise, anatomical localisation into the joint cavity of the knee to be treated. The injection site in the knee is determined by that location which is easier to reach. Usually a lateral approach can be followed, but in some cases a medial approach is preferable. Strict aseptic precautions should be observed during the administration. The solution in the pre-filled syringe is ready for use and requires only a sterile disposable needle. To ensure sterility the injection site must be carefully cleansed with antiseptic. Care should be taken to expel any trapped air bubbles from the syringe containing Hyalgan prior to administration.

Joint effusion, if present, should be aspirated by arthrocentesis prior to injection of Hyalgan. The arthrocentesis should be made using a 20 gauge needle and the joint should be aspirated to almost dryness, but not to a degree that would compromise the accuracy of the subsequent Hyalgan injection. An appropriate examination of the joint fluid present should be carried out to exclude bacterial infection, prior to injection.

The intra-articular injection of Hyalgan can be given using the same needle as used for the arthrocentesis by simply detaching the aspirating syringe and attaching the syringe containing the Hyalgan. To make sure the needle is correctly positioned, some synovial fluid should be aspirated prior to the slow injection of Hyalgan. If the patient experiences pain during injection, the procedure may need to be stopped.

For the first 48 hours after the injection, the patient should be advised to rest the treated knee with as little exercise as possible, avoiding any strenuous or prolonged activity. Subsequently, they may gradually return to their normal level of activity.

Discard any unused Hyalgan.

7. MARKETING AUTHORISATION HOLDER
Fidia Farmaceutici S.p.A.

Via Ponte della Fabbrica 3/A

35031 Abano Terme (Padova)

Italy

8. MARKETING AUTHORISATION NUMBER(S)
PL 04530/0004

9. DATE OF FIRST AUTHORISATION/RENEWAL OF THE AUTHORISATION
14 January 1998

10. DATE OF REVISION OF THE TEXT
September 2002

LEGAL CATEGORY
POM

Hycamtin

(Merck Pharmaceuticals)

1. NAME OF THE MEDICINAL PRODUCT
HYCAMTIN 1 mg and 4 mg powder for concentrate for solution for infusion.

2. QUALITATIVE AND QUANTITATIVE COMPOSITION
Each 1 mg vial contains 1 mg topotecan as topotecan hydrochloride, with a 10% overage of fill.

Each 4 mg vial contains 4 mg topotecan as topotecan hydrochloride.

For excipients, see 6.1.

3. PHARMACEUTICAL FORM
Powder for concentrate for solution for infusion.

4. CLINICAL PARTICULARS

4.1 Therapeutic indications
Topotecan is indicated for the treatment of patients with metastatic carcinoma of the ovary after failure of first-line or subsequent therapy.

4.2 Posology and method of administration
The use of topotecan should be confined to units specialised in the administration of cytotoxic chemotherapy and should only be administered under the supervision of a physician experienced in the use of chemotherapy.

Initial Dose

The recommended dose of topotecan is 1.5 mg/m^2 body surface area/day administered by intravenous infusion over 30 minutes daily for 5 consecutive days with a 3 week interval between the start of each course. If well tolerated, treatment may continue until disease progression (see sections 4.8 Undesirable effects and 5.1 Pharmacodynamic properties).

Prior to administration of the first course of topotecan, patients must have a baseline neutrophil count of $\geqslant 1.5 \times 10^9$/l, and a platelet count of $\geqslant 100 \times 10^9$/l.

Routine pre-medication for non-haematological adverse events is not required with topotecan. Topotecan must be reconstituted and further diluted before use (see section 6.6 Instructions for use and handling, and disposal).

Subsequent Doses

Topotecan should not be re-administered unless the neutrophil count is $\geqslant 1 \times 10^9$/l, the platelet count is $\geqslant 100 \times 10^9$/l, and the haemoglobin level is $\geqslant$9 g/dl (after transfusion if necessary).

Patients who experience severe neutropenia (neutrophil count $< 0.5 \times 10^9$/l) for 7 days or more, or severe neutropenia associated with fever or infection, or who have had treatment delayed due to neutropenia, should be treated as follows:

either

be given a reduced dose i.e. 1.25 mg/m^2/day (or subsequently down to 1.0 mg/m^2/day if necessary)

or

be given G-CSF prophylactically in subsequent courses to maintain dose intensity, starting from day 6 of the course (the day after completion of topotecan administration). If neutropenia is not adequately managed with G-CSF administration, doses should be reduced.

Doses should be similarly reduced if the platelet count falls below 25×10^9/l. In clinical trials, topotecan was discontinued if the dose had been reduced to 1.0 mg/m^2 and a further dose reduction was required to manage adverse effects.

Dosage in Renally Impaired Patients

Insufficient data are available to make a recommendation for patients with a creatinine clearance < 20 ml/min. Limited data indicate that the dose should be reduced in patients with moderate renal impairment. The recommended dose in patients with creatinine clearance between 20 and 39 ml/min is 0.75 mg/m^2 /day.

4.3 Contraindications

Topotecan is contra-indicated in patients who:

- have a history of severe hypersensitivity to topotecan or to any of the excipients
- are pregnant or breast feeding (see section 4.6 Pregnancy and lactation)
- already have severe bone marrow depression prior to starting first course, as evidenced by baseline neutrophils < 1.5×10^9/l and/or a platelet count of $\leqslant 100 \times 10^9$/l.

4.4 Special warnings and special precautions for use

Haematological toxicity is dose-related and full blood count including platelets should be monitored regularly.

As expected, patients with poor performance status have a lower response rate and an increased incidence of complications such as fever and infection.

There is no experience of the use of topotecan in patients with severely impaired renal function (creatinine clearance < 20 ml/min) or severely impaired hepatic function (serum bilirubin $\geqslant$ 10 mg/dl) due to cirrhosis. Topotecan is not recommended to be used in these patient groups.

A small number of hepatically impaired patients (serum bilirubin between 1.5 and 10 mg/dl) were able to tolerate 1.5 mg/m^2 for five days every three weeks although a reduction in topotecan clearance was observed. There are insufficient data available to make a dose recommendation for this patient group.

4.5 Interaction with other medicinal products and other forms of Interaction

No *in vivo* human pharmacokinetic interaction studies have been performed.

Topotecan does not inhibit human P450 enzymes (see Section 5.2 Pharmacokinetic properties). In a population study, the co-administration of granisetron, ondansetron, morphine or corticosteroids did not appear to have a significant effect on the pharmacokinetics of total topotecan (active and inactive form).

In combining topotecan with other chemotherapy agents, reduction of the doses of each drug is required to improve tolerability. However, in combining with platinum agents, there is a distinct sequence-dependent interaction depending on whether the platinum agent is given on day 1 or 5 of the topotecan dosing. If either cisplatin or carboplatin is given on day 1 of the topotecan dosing, a lower dose of each agent must be given to improve tolerability compared to the dose of each agent which can be given if the platinum agent is given on day 5 of the topotecan dosing.

4.6 Pregnancy and lactation

Pregnancy

Topotecan is contraindicated during pregnancy. Topotecan has been shown to cause embryo-foetal lethality and malformations in preclinical studies. Women should be advised to avoid becoming pregnant during therapy with topotecan and to inform the treating physician immediately should this occur.

Lactation

Topotecan is contra-indicated during breast-feeding. Although it is not known whether topotecan is excreted in human breast milk, breast-feeding should be discontinued at the start of therapy.

4.7 Effects on ability to drive and use machines

Caution should be observed when driving or operating machinery if fatigue and asthenia persist.

4.8 Undesirable effects

Introduction

In dose-finding trials, the dose limiting toxicity was found to be haematological. Toxicity was predictable and reversible. There were no signs of cumulative haematological or non-haematological toxicity in an analysis of data derived from 523 patients with recurrent ovarian carcinoma, where 152 patients received more than 6 cycles of treatment and 46 patients received more than 10 cycles.

Adverse reactions are listed below, by system organ class and absolute frequency.

Frequencies are defined as: very common (> 1/10); common (> 1/100, < 1/10); uncommon (> 1/1,000, < 1/100); rare (> 1/10,000, < 1/1,000); very rare (< 1/10,000), including isolated reports.

Blood and lymphatic system disorders

Very Common: neutropenia*, thrombocytopenia*, anaemia*.

Immune system disorders

Rare: anaphylactic reaction, hypersensitivity reaction, angioedema, urticaria, rash.

Metabolism and nutrition disorders

Uncommon: anorexia.

Gastrointestinal disorders

Very common: nausea*, vomiting*, diarrhoea*, constipation, mucositis*.

Common: abdominal pain.

Hepato-biliary disorders

Uncommon: hyperbilirubinaemia.

Skin and subcutaneous tissue disorders

Very common: alopecia*.

Common: pruritis.

General disorders and administration site conditions

Very common: asthenia*, fatigue*.

Uncommon: malaise.

Rare: extravasation*.

** see detailed section below*

Haematological

Neutropenia: Severe (neutrophil count < 0.5×10^9/l) during course 1 was seen in 60% of the patients and with duration $\geqslant$ 7 days in 20% and overall in 79% of patients (42% of courses). In association with severe neutropenia, fever or infection occurred in 16% of patients during course 1 and overall in 21% of patients (7% of courses).

Median time to onset of severe neutropenia was 9 days and the median duration was 7 days. Severe neutropenia lasted beyond 7 days in 13% of courses overall. Among all patients treated in clinical studies (including both those with severe neutropenia and those who did not develop severe neutropenia), 13% (5% of courses) developed fever and 27% (10% of courses) developed infection. In addition, 5% of all patients treated (1% of courses) developed sepsis.

Thrombocytopenia: Severe (platelets less than 25×10^9/l) in 23% of patients (9% of courses); moderate (platelets between 25.0 and 49.9×10^9/l) in 20% of patients (13% of courses). Median time to onset of severe thrombocytopenia was Day 14 and the median duration was 5 days. Platelet transfusions were given in 4% of courses.

Significant sequelae associated with thrombocytopenia were rare.

Anaemia: Moderate to severe (Hb $\leqslant$ 7.9 g/dl) in 36% of patients (15% of courses).

Red cell transfusions were given in 54% of patients (23% of courses).

Non-haematological

In clinical trials of 445 ovarian cancer patients, frequently reported non-haematological effects were gastrointestinal such as nausea (68%), vomiting (44%), and diarrhoea (26%), constipation (14%) and mucositis (28.5%). Severe (grade 3 or 4) nausea, vomiting, diarrhoea and mucositis incidence was 6, 4, 3 and 2.5% respectively.

Mild abdominal pain was also reported amongst 8% of patients.

Fatigue was observed in approximately one third and asthenia in about one fifth of patients whilst receiving topotecan. Severe (grade 3 or 4) fatigue and asthenia incidence was 4% and 2% respectively.

Total or pronounced alopecia was observed in 42% of patients and partial alopecia in 17% of patients.

Other severe events occurring in $\geqslant$ 1% patients that were recorded as related or possibly related to topotecan treatment were anorexia (1%), malaise (1%) and hyperbilirubinaemia (1%).

Hypersensitivity reactions including rash, urticaria, angioedema and anaphylactic reactions have been reported rarely. In clinical trials, rash was reported in 12.4% of patients and pruritis in 2.7% of patients.

Extravasation has been reported rarely. Reactions have been mild and have not generally required specific therapy.

4.9 Overdose

There is no known antidote for topotecan overdosage. The primary complications of overdosage are anticipated to be bone marrow suppression and mucositis.

5. PHARMACOLOGICAL PROPERTIES

5.1 Pharmacodynamic properties

Pharmaco-therapeutic group: Antineoplastic and immunomodulating agent:

ATC-code: L01X X17.

The anti-tumour activity of topotecan involves the inhibition of topoisomerase-I, an enzyme intimately involved in DNA replication as it relieves the torsional strain introduced ahead of the moving replication fork. Topotecan inhibits topoisomerase-I by stabilising the covalent complex of enzyme and strand-cleaved DNA which is an intermediate of the catalytic mechanism. The cellular sequela of inhibition of topoisomerase-I by topotecan is the induction of protein-associated DNA single-strand breaks.

In a comparative study of topotecan and paclitaxel in patients previously treated for ovarian carcinoma with platinum based chemotherapy (n = 112 and 114, respectively), the response rate (95% CI) was 20.5% (13, 28) versus 14% (8, 20) and median time to progression 19 weeks versus 15 weeks (hazard ratio 0.7 [0.6, 1.0]), for topotecan and paclitaxel, respectively. Median overall survival was 62 weeks for topotecan versus 53 weeks for paclitaxel (hazard ratio 0.9 [0.6, 1.3]).

The response rate in the whole ovarian carcinoma programme (n = 392, all previously treated with cisplatin or cisplatin and paclitaxel) was 16%. The median time to response in clinical trials was 7.6-11.6 weeks. In patients refractory to, or relapsing within 3 months after cisplatin therapy (n = 186), the response rate was 10%. These data should be evaluated in the context of the overall safety profile of the drug, in particular to the important haematological toxicity (see section 4.8 Undesirable effects).

A supplementary retrospective analysis was conducted on data from 523 patients with relapsed ovarian cancer. Altogether, 87 complete and partial responses were observed, with 13 of these occurring during cycles 5 and 6 and 3 occurring thereafter. For patients administered more than 6 cycles of therapy, 91% completed the study as planned or were treated until disease progression with only 3% withdrawn for adverse events.

5.2 Pharmacokinetic properties

Following intravenous administration of topotecan at doses of 0.5 to 1.5 mg/m^2 as a 30 minute infusion daily for five days, topotecan demonstrated a high plasma clearance of 62 L/h (SD 22), corresponding to approximately 2/3 of liver blood flow. Topotecan also had a high volume of distribution, about 132 L, (SD 57) and a relatively short half-life of 2-3 hours. Comparison of pharmacokinetic parameters did not suggest any change in pharmacokinetics over the 5 days of dosing. Area under the curve increased approximately in proportion to the increase in dose. The binding of topotecan to plasma proteins was low (35%) and distribution between blood cells and plasma was fairly homogeneous.

In a population study, a number of factors including age, weight and ascites had no significant effect on clearance of total topotecan (active and inactive form).

The elimination of topotecan has only been partly investigated in man. A major route of clearance of topotecan was by hydrolysis of the lactone ring to form the ring-opened hydroxy acid. *In vitro* data using human liver microsomes indicate the formulation of small amounts of N-demethylated topotecan. In man, as in animal species, a significant proportion of the dose (generally 20-60%) was excreted in the urine as topotecan or the open ring form. In vitro, topotecan did not inhibit human P450 enzymes CYP1A2, CYP2A6, CYP2C8/9, CYP2C19, CYP2D6, CYP2E, CYP3A, or CYP4A nor did it inhibit the human cytosolic enzymes dihydropyrimidine or xanthine oxidase.

Plasma clearance in patients with hepatic impairment (serum bilirubin between 1.5 and 10 mg/dl) decreased to about 67% when compared with a control group of patients.

Topotecan half-life was increased by about 30% but no clear change in volume of distribution was observed. Plasma clearance of total topotecan (active and inactive form) in patients with hepatic impairment only decreased by about 10% compared with the control group of patients.

Plasma clearance in patients with renal impairment (creatinine clearance 41-60 ml/min.) decreased to about 67% compared with control patients. Volume of distribution was slightly decreased and thus half-life only increased by 14%. In patients with moderate renal impairment topotecan plasma clearance was reduced to 34% of the value in control patients. Mean half-life increased from 1.9 hours to 4.9 hours.

5.3 Preclinical safety data

Resulting from its mechanism of action, topotecan is genotoxic to mammalian cells (mouse lymphoma cells and human lymphocytes) *in vitro* and mouse bone marrow cells *in vivo*. Topotecan was also shown to cause embryo-foetal lethality when given to rats and rabbits. The carcinogenic potential of topotecan has not been studied.

6. PHARMACEUTICAL PARTICULARS

6.1 List of excipients

Tartaric acid (E334)

Mannitol (E421)

Hydrochloric acid (E507)

Sodium hydroxide

6.2 Incompatibilities

None known.

6.3 Shelf life

Vials

3 years.

Reconstituted and diluted solutions

The product should be used immediately after reconstitution as it contains no antibacterial preservative. If reconstitution and dilution is performed under strict aseptic conditions (e.g. an LAF bench) the product should be used (infusion completed) within 12 hours at room temperature or 24 hours if stored at 2-8°C after the first puncture of the vial.

6.4 Special precautions for storage

Keep the container in the outer carton in order to protect from light.

6.5 Nature and contents of container

HYCAMTIN 1 mg is supplied in 3 ml type I flint glass vials, together with 13 mm grey butyl rubber stoppers and 13 mm aluminium seals with plastic flip-off caps.

HYCAMTIN 1 mg is available in cartons containing 1 vial.

HYCAMTIN 4 mg is supplied in 5 ml type I flint glass vials, together with 20 mm grey butyl rubber stoppers and 20 mm aluminium seals with plastic flip-off caps.

HYCAMTIN 4 mg is available in cartons containing 1 vial.

6.6 Instructions for use and handling

HYCAMTIN 1 mg vials must be reconstituted with 1.1 ml water for injections. Since HYCAMTIN contains a 10% overage, the reconstituted solutions provide 1 mg per ml of topotecan. Further dilution of the appropriate volume of the reconstituted solution with either 0.9% w/v sodium chloride intravenous infusion or 5% w/v glucose intravenous infusion is required to a final concentration of between 25 and 50 microgram/ml.

HYCAMTIN 4 mg vials must be reconstituted with 4 ml water for injections. The reconstituted solutions provide 1 mg per ml of topotecan. Further dilution of the appropriate volume of the reconstituted solution with either 0.9% w/v sodium chloride intravenous infusion or 5% w/v glucose intravenous infusion is required to a final concentration of between 25 and 50 microgram/ml.

The normal procedures for proper handling and disposal of anticancer drugs should be adopted, namely:

- Personnel should be trained to reconstitute the drug.
- Pregnant staff should be excluded from working with this drug.
- Personnel handling this drug during reconstitution should wear protective clothing including mask, goggles and gloves.
- All items for administration or cleaning, including gloves, should be placed in high risk, waste disposal bags for high-temperature incineration. Liquid waste may be flushed with large amounts of water.
- Accidental contact with the skin or eyes should be treated immediately with copious amounts of water.

7. MARKETING AUTHORISATION HOLDER

SmithKline Beecham plc, 980 Great West Road, Brentford, Middlesex, TW8 9GS, United Kingdom.

8. MARKETING AUTHORISATION NUMBER(S)

1 mg vials:

1 vial: EU/1/96/027/005

4 mg vials:

1 vial: EU/1/96/027/003

9. DATE OF FIRST AUTHORISATION/RENEWAL OF THE AUTHORISATION

Date of renewal 12-11-2001 pursuant to a Commission Decision of 04-02-2002

10. DATE OF REVISION OF THE TEXT

30-07-2002

Hydrea Capsules 500mg

(E. R. Squibb & Sons Limited)

1. NAME OF THE MEDICINAL PRODUCT

Hydrea Capsules 500mg

2. QUALITATIVE AND QUANTITATIVE COMPOSITION

Pink, opaque capsule body with green, opaque cap, printed in black with 'BMS 303' containing 500 mg of hydroxycarbamide.

3. PHARMACEUTICAL FORM

Hard Gelatin Capsule

4. CLINICAL PARTICULARS

4.1 Therapeutic indications

The treatment of chronic myeloid leukaemia.

The treatment of cancer of the cervix in conjunction with radiotherapy.

4.2 Posology and method of administration

Adults

Treatment regimens can be continuous or intermittent. The continuous regimen is particularly suitable for chronic myeloid leukaemia, while the intermittent regimen, with its diminished effect on the bone marrow, is more satisfactory for the management of cancer of the cervix.

Hydrea should be started 7 days before concurrent irradiation therapy. If Hydrea is used concomitantly with radiotherapy, adjustment of radiation dosage is not usually necessary.

An adequate trial period for determining the antineoplastic effect of Hydrea is six weeks. Where there is a significant clinical response therapy may be continued indefinitely, provided that the patient is kept under adequate observation and shows no unusual or severe reactions. Therapy should be interrupted if the white cell count drops below $2.5x10^9$L or the platelet count below $100x10^9$/L.

Continuous therapy:

Hydrea 20-30mg/kg should be given daily in single doses. Dosage should be based on the patient's actual or ideal weight, whichever is the less. Therapy should be monitored by repeat blood counts.

Intermittent therapy:

Hydrea 80mg/kg in single doses should be given every third day. Using the intermittent regimes the likelihood of WBC depression is diminished, but if low counts are produced, 1 or more doses of Hydrea should be omitted.

Concurrent use of Hydrea with other myelosuppressive agents may require adjustments of dosages.

Children

Because of the rarity of these conditions in children, dosage regimens have not been established.

Elderly

Elderly patients may be more sensitive to the effects of hydroxycarbamide, and may require a lower dosage regimen.

NB: If the patient prefers, or is unable to swallow capsules, the contents of the capsules may be emptied into a glass of water and taken immediately. The contents of capsules should not be inhaled or allowed to come into contact with the skin or mucous membranes. Spillages must be wiped immediately.

4.3 Contraindications

Marked leucopenia (<2.5wbcx10^9/L), thrombocytopenia ($<$ $100x10^9$/L), or severe anaemia and those who have previously shown hypersensitivity to Hydrea.

4.4 Special warnings and special precautions for use

The complete status of the blood, including bone marrow examination, if indicated, as well as kidney function and liver function should be determined prior to, and repeatedly during, treatment. The determination of haemoglobin level, total leukocyte counts, and platelet counts should be performed at least once a week throughout the course of hydroxycarbamide therapy. If WBC falls below $2.5x10^9$/L or platelet count to $<100x10^9$/L, therapy should be interrupted. Counts should be rechecked after 3 days and treatment resumed when they rise significantly towards normal.

Severe anaemia must be corrected with whole blood replacement before initiating therapy with hydroxycarbamide. If, during treatment, anaemia occurs, correct without interrupting Hydrea therapy. Erythrocytic abnormalities; megaloblastic erythropoiesis, which is self-limiting, is often seen early in the course of hydroxycarbamide therapy. The morphologic change resembles pernicious anaemia, but is not related to vitamin B_{12} or folic acid deficiency. Hydroxycarbamide may also delay plasma iron clearance and reduce the rate of iron utilisation by erythrocytes but it does not appear to alter the red blood cell survival time.

Hydroxycarbamide should be used with caution in patients with marked renal dysfunction.

Hydroxycarbamide is not licensed for use in combination with antiretroviral agents for HIV disease and it may cause treatment failure and toxicities (in some cases fatal) in HIV patients (see section 4.5).

In patients receiving long-term therapy with hydroxycarbamide for myeloproliferative disorders, such as polycythemia, secondary leukaemia has been reported. It is unknown whether this leukaemogenic effect is secondary to hydroxycarbamide or associated with the patient's underlying disease.

The possibility of an increase in serum uric acid, resulting in the development of gout or, at worst, uric acid nephropathy, should be borne in mind in patients treated with hydroxycarbamide, especially when used with other cytotoxic agents. It is therefore important to monitor uric acid levels regularly and maintain a high fluid intake during treatment.

4.5 Interaction with other medicinal products and other forms of Interaction

The myelosuppressive activity may be potentiated by previous or concomitant radiotherapy or cytotoxic therapy. Fatal and non-fatal pancreatitis has occurred in HIV-infected patients during therapy with hydroxycarbamide and didanosine, with or without stavudine. Hepatotoxicity and hepatic failure resulting in death were reported during post-marketing surveillance in HIV-infected patients treated with hydroxycarbamide and other antiretroviral agents. Fatal hepatic events were reported most often in patients treated with the combination of hydroxycarbamide, didanosine and stavudine. Peripheral neuropathy, which was severe in some cases, has been reported in HIV-infected patients receiving hydroxycarbamide in combination with antiretroviral agents, including didanosine, with or without stavudine. (see section 4.4).

4.6 Pregnancy and lactation

Drugs which affect DNA synthesis, such as hydroxycarbamide, may be potent mutagenic agents. The physician should carefully consider this possibility before administering this drug to male or female patients who may contemplate conception. Since Hydrea is a cytotoxic agent it has produced a teratogenic effect in some animal species.

In rats and dogs, high doses of hydroxycarbamide reduced sperm production. Hydroxycarbamide is excreted in human breast milk.

Hydrea should not normally be administered to patients who are pregnant, or to mothers who are breast feeding, unless the potential benefits outweigh the possible hazards.

When appropriate both male and female patients should be counselled concerning the use of contraceptive measures before and during treatment with Hydrea.

4.7 Effects on ability to drive and use machines

Not applicable.

4.8 Undesirable effects

Bone-marrow suppression is the major toxic effect of Hydrea, while leucopenia, thrombocytopenia and anaemia may occur in that order. Other side-effects are generally rare, but the following have been reported; anorexia, nausea, vomiting, diarrhoea, constipation, headache, drowsiness, dizziness, stomatitis, alopecia, skin rash, melaena, abdominal pain, disorientations, pulmonary oedema, hallucinations, convulsions, potentiation of the erythema caused by irradiation, skin ulceration, dysuria and impairment of renal tubular function accompanied by elevation in serum uric acid, blood urea nitrogen, and creatinine levels. Fever, chills, malaise, asthenia and elevation of hepatic enzymes have been reported. Acute pulmonary reactions consisting of diffuse pulmonary infiltrates/fibrosis, and dyspnoea have been rarely reported. Skin cancer has also been rarely reported.

Cases of pancreatitis and hepatotoxicity (some with fatal outcomes) and severe peripheral neuropathy have been observed in HIV patients when hydroxycarbamide was administered with antiretroviral agents (see sections 4.4 and 4.5).

In some patients, hyperpigmentation, erythema, atrophy of skin and nails, scaling, violet papules and alopecia have been observed following several years of long-term daily maintenance therapy with hydroxycarbamide.

4.9 Overdose

Immediate treatment consists of gastric lavage, followed by supportive therapy for the cardiorespiratory systems if required. In the long term, careful monitoring of the haemopoietic system is essential and, if necessary, blood should be transfused.

Acute mucocutaneous toxicity has been reported in patients receiving hydroxycarbamide at a dosage several times greater than that recommended. Soreness, violet erythema, oedema on palms and foot soles followed by scaling of hands and feet, intense generalised hyperpigmentation of skin, and severe acute stomatitis were observed.

5. PHARMACOLOGICAL PROPERTIES

5.1 Pharmacodynamic properties

Hydroxycarbamide is an orally active antineoplastic agent. Although the mechanism of action has not yet been clearly defined, hydroxycarbamide appears to act by interfering with synthesis of DNA.

5.2 Pharmacokinetic properties

After oral administration hydroxycarbamide is readily absorbed from the gastrointestinal tract. Peak plasma concentrations are reached in 2 hours; by 24 hours the serum concentrations are virtually zero. Approximately 80% of an oral or intravenous dose of 7 to 30 mg/kg may be recovered from the urine within 12 hours. Hydroxycarbamide crosses the blood-brain barrier. Hydroxycarbamide is well distributed throughout the body.

5.3 Preclinical safety data

No further relevant data.

6. PHARMACEUTICAL PARTICULARS

6.1 List of excipients

Citric acid, erythrosine, gelatin, indigotine, lactose, magnesium stearate, sodium laurilsulfate, sodium phosphate, titanium dioxide, yellow iron oxide, opacode S-1-8100 HV black, purified water.

6.2 Incompatibilities

None known

6.3 Shelf life

Blisters - 24 months

6.4 Special precautions for storage

Do not store above 25°C. Keep tightly closed.

6.5 Nature and contents of container

100 capsules may be packaged in any of the following: PVC/PVDC blisters or PVC/aluminium blisters.

6.6 Instructions for use and handling

Procedures for proper handling and disposal of anticancer drugs should be considered.

7. MARKETING AUTHORISATION HOLDER

E.R. Squibb & Sons Limited

Uxbridge Business Park

Sanderson Road

Uxbridge

Middlesex

UB8 1DH

8. MARKETING AUTHORISATION NUMBER(S)

PL 0034/5044R

9. DATE OF FIRST AUTHORISATION/RENEWAL OF THE AUTHORISATION
29 May 1986 / 17 December 2002

10. DATE OF REVISION OF THE TEXT
June 2005

Hydrocortistab Injection 25 mg/ml

(Sovereign Medical)

1. NAME OF THE MEDICINAL PRODUCT
Hydrocortistab Injection or Hydrocortisone Acetate Injection BP 25 mg/ml

2. QUALITATIVE AND QUANTITATIVE COMPOSITION
Hydrocortisone Acetate Ph Eur 2.5% w/v (25 mg/ml)

3. PHARMACEUTICAL FORM
Suspension for injection.

4. CLINICAL PARTICULARS
4.1 Therapeutic indications
Hydrocortistab Injection is indicated for the local treatment, by intra-articular or periarticular injection, of arthritic conditions such as rheumatoid arthritis and osteoarthritis when few joints are involved. It is also suitable for the symptomatic treatment, by local injection, of certain non-articular inflammatory conditions such as inflamed tendon sheaths and bursae.

Hydrocortistab Injection is not suitable for the production of systemic effects.

4.2 Posology and method of administration
For intra-articular or periarticular injection. Hydrocortistab Injection may also be injected into non-articular tissues (e.g. tendon sheaths/bursae).

Adults: 5-50 mg, depending on the size of the joint.

Children: 5-30 mg daily in divided doses.

Elderly: Steroids should be used cautiously in the elderly, since adverse effects are enhanced in old age.

No more than three joints should be treated in one day. The injection may be repeated at intervals of about three weeks.

4.3 Contraindications
Hydrocortistab Injection is contra-indicated in patients with known hypersensitivity to any of the ingredients, and in patients with systemic infections, unless specific anti-infective therapy is employed.

Intra-articular and periarticular injections of Hydrocortistab Injection are contra-indicated when the joint or surrounding tissues are infected. The presence of infection also precludes injection into tendon sheaths and bursae. Hydrocortistab Injection must not be injected directly into tendons, nor should it be injected into spinal or other non-diarthrodial joints.

4.4 Special warnings and special precautions for use
Since joints and tissues injected with corticosteroids have an increased susceptibility to infection, local injections of Hydrocortistab should be carried out with full aseptic precautions.

Caution is necessary when prescribing corticosteroids in patients with the following conditions:

(a) Previous history of tuberculosis or characteristic appearance on chest X-ray. The emergence of active tuberculosis can, however, be prevented by the prophylactic use of antituberculous therapy.

(b) Diabetes mellitus (or a family history of diabetes).

(c) Osteoporosis (postmenopausal females are particularly at risk).

(d) Hypertension.

(e) History of severe affective disorders (especially previous history of steroid psychosis).

(f) Glaucoma (or a family history of glaucoma).

(g) Previous steroid myopathy.

(h) Peptic ulceration.

(i) Epilepsy.

(j) Vaccination with live vaccines.

Use in children:

Corticosteroids cause growth retardation in infancy, childhood and adolescence. Treatment should be limited to the minimum dosage for the shortest possible time, in order to minimise suppression of the hypothalamo-pituitary-adrenal axis and growth retardation.

Use in the elderly:

Treatment of elderly patients, particularly if long-term, should be planned bearing in mind the more serious consequences of the common side effects of corticosteroids in old age, especially osteoporosis, diabetes, hypertension, susceptibility to infection and thinning of the skin.

4.5 Interaction with other medicinal products and other forms of Interaction
The effectiveness of anticoagulants may be increased or decreased with concurrent corticosteroid therapy.

Serum levels of salicylates may increase considerably if corticosteroid therapy is withdrawn, possibly causing intoxication. Since both salicylates and corticosteroids are ulcerogenic, it is possible that there will be an increased rate of gastrointestinal ulceration.

The actions of hypoglycaemic drugs will be antagonised by the hyperglycaemic actions of corticosteroids.

Since amphotericin, diuretics (acetazolamide, loop diuretics and thiazides) and corticosteroids have potassium-depleting effects, signs of hypokalaemia should be looked for during their concurrent use.

There is a small amount of evidence that the simultaneous use of corticosteroids and methotrexate may cause increased methotrexate toxicity and possibly death, although this combination of drugs has been used very successfully.

The therapeutic effects of corticosteroids may be reduced by certain barbiturates (particularly when given at high doses), phenytoin and rifampicin.

The concurrent use of corticosteroids with antacids, cimetidine or theophylline appears to have no effect on the therapeutic use of either drug.

4.6 Pregnancy and lactation
There is evidence of harmful effects in pregnancy in animals.

There is inadequate evidence of safety in human pregnancy and there may be a very small risk of cleft palate and intra-uterine growth retardation in the foetus.

Trace amounts of hydrocortisone have been measured in breast milk but it is doubtful if these amounts are clinically significant. However, in lactation, continuous therapy with high doses could possibly affect the child's adrenal function. Monitor carefully.

The decision to use Hydrocortistab Injection during pregnancy and lactation must be made by weighing up the relative risks associated with the use of the drug against the potential benefits in maternal disease.

4.7 Effects on ability to drive and use machines
No adverse effects known.

4.8 Undesirable effects
With intra-articular or other local injections, the principal side effect encountered is a temporary local exacerbation with increased pain and swelling. This normally subsides after a few hours.

In certain circumstances, particularly after high or prolonged local dosage, corticosteroids can be absorbed in amounts sufficient to produce systemic effects.

The following side effects may be associated with the long-term systemic use of corticosteroids.

Gastrointestinal:

Dyspepsia, peptic ulceration with perforation and haemorrhage, abdominal distension, oesophageal ulceration, oesophageal candidiasis, acute pancreatitis.

Musculoskeletal:

Proximal myopathy, osteoporosis, vertebral and long bone fractures, avascular osteonecrosis, tendon rupture.

Fluid and electrolyte disturbance:

Sodium and water retention, hypertension, hypokalaemic alkalosis.

Dermatological:

Impaired healing, skin atrophy, bruising, striae, acne, telangiectasia.

Endocrine/metabolic:

Suppression of the hypothalamo-pituitary-adrenal axis, growth suppression in childhood and adolescence, menstrual irregularity and amenorrhoea. Cushingoid facies, hirsutism, weight gain, impaired carbohydrate tolerance with increased requirement for antidiabetic therapy, negative nitrogen balance.

Neuropsychiatric:

Euphoria, psychological dependence, depression, insomnia. Intracranial hypertension in children. Aggravation of schizophrenia.

Ophthalmic:

Increased intra-ocular pressure, glaucoma, papilloedema, cataracts, corneal or scleral thinning, exacerbation of ophthalmic viral disease.

General:

Opportunistic infection, recurrence of dormant tuberculosis, leucocytosis, hypersensitivity, thromboembolism, increased appetite, nausea, malaise.

Withdrawal symptoms and signs:

Fever, myalgia, arthralgia, adrenal insufficiency.

4.9 Overdose
Overdosage is unlikely with Hydrocortistab Injection but there is no specific antidote available. Treatment should be symptomatic.

5. PHARMACOLOGICAL PROPERTIES
5.1 Pharmacodynamic properties
Hydrocortisone has both glucocorticoid and mineralocorticoid activity.

5.2 Pharmacokinetic properties
Absorption following intra-articular or soft tissue injection is slow. Systemic absorption occurs slowly after local, intra-articular injection. Hydrocortisone is more than 90% bound to plasma proteins. Hydrocortisone is metabolised in the liver and most body tissues to hydrogenated and degraded forms, such as tetrahydrocortisone and tetrahydrocortisol. These are excreted in the urine, mainly conjugated as glucuronides, together with a very small proportion of unchanged hydrocortisone.

5.3 Preclinical safety data
There is no pre-clinical data of relevance to a prescriber which is additional to that already included in other sections of the SmPC.

6. PHARMACEUTICAL PARTICULARS
6.1 List of excipients
Water for injections, benzyl alcohol, sodium chloride for injections, sodium carboxymethylcellulose (Blanose 7M8SF), polysorbate 80 (Tween 80), with sodium hydroxide and/or hydrochloric acid as pH adjusters.

6.2 Incompatibilities
Not applicable.

6.3 Shelf life
36 months.

6.4 Special precautions for storage
Store at 15-25°C. Do not freeze. Protect from light.

6.5 Nature and contents of container
Glass ampoules. Pack size: 10 × 1 ml ampoules.

6.6 Instructions for use and handling
Shake the ampoule well before use. Do not freeze.

7. MARKETING AUTHORISATION HOLDER
Waymade PLC *trading as* Sovereign Medical
Sovereign House
Miles Gray Road
Basildon
Essex
SS14 3FR

8. MARKETING AUTHORISATION NUMBER(S)
PL 06464/0700

9. DATE OF FIRST AUTHORISATION/RENEWAL OF THE AUTHORISATION
11/01/1999

10. DATE OF REVISION OF THE TEXT
July 2004

Hydrocortone Tablets

(Merck Sharp & Dohme Limited)

1. NAME OF THE MEDICINAL PRODUCT
HYDROCORTONE® 10 mg Tablets
HYDROCORTONE® 20 mg Tablets

2. QUALITATIVE AND QUANTITATIVE COMPOSITION
10 mg tablet: 10 mg hydrocortisone

20 mg tablet: 20 mg hydrocortisone

3. PHARMACEUTICAL FORM
Tablets

10 mg tablets: white, quarter-scored tablets, marked 'MSD 619'.

20 mg tablets: white, half-scored tablets, marked 'MSD 625'.

4. CLINICAL PARTICULARS
4.1 Therapeutic indications
Corticosteroid.

For use as replacement therapy in primary, secondary, or acute adrenocortical insufficiency.

Pre-operatively, and during serious trauma or illness in patients with known adrenal insufficiency or doubtful adrenocortical reserve.

4.2 Posology and method of administration
Dosage must be individualised according to the response of the individual patient. The lowest possible dosage should be used.

Patients should be observed closely for signs that might require dosage adjustment, including changes in clinical status resulting from remissions or exacerbations of the disease, individual drug responsiveness, and the effect of stress (e.g. surgery, infection, trauma). During stress it may be necessary to increase the dosage temporarily.

To avoid hypoadrenalism and/or a relapse of the underlying disease, it may be necessary to withdraw the drug gradually (see 4.4 'Special warnings and special precautions for use').

In chronic adrenocortical insufficiency, a dosage of 20 to 30 mg a day is usually recommended, sometimes together with 4-6 g of sodium chloride or 50-300 micrograms of fludrocortisone daily. When immediate support is mandatory, one of the soluble adrenocortical hormone preparations (e.g. dexamethasone sodium phosphate), which may be effective within minutes after parenteral administration, can be life-saving.

Use in children: In chronic adrenocortical insufficiency, the dosage should be approximately 0.4 to 0.8 mg/kg/day in two or three divided doses, adjusted to the needs of the individual child.

Use in the elderly: Treatment of elderly patients, particularly if long term, should be planned bearing in mind the more serious consequences of the common side effects of corticosteroids in old age, especially osteoporosis, diabetes, hypertension, susceptibility to infection and thinning of the skin.

4.3 Contraindications

Systemic fungal infections. Hypersensitivity to any component of this product.

4.4 Special warnings and special precautions for use

Patients should carry 'steroid treatment' cards, which give clear guidance on the precautions to be taken to minimise risk and which provide details of prescriber, drug, dosage, and the duration of treatment.

The lowest possible dosage of corticosteroids should be used and when reduction in dosage is possible, the reduction should be gradual.

Corticosteroids may exacerbate systemic fungal infections and therefore should not be used in the presence of such infections unless they are needed to control life-threatening drug reactions due to amphotericin. Moreover, there have been cases reported in which concomitant use of amphotericin and hydrocortisone was followed by cardiac enlargement and congestive failure.

Literature reports suggest an apparent association between use of corticosteroids and left ventricular free wall rupture after a recent myocardial infarction; therefore, therapy with corticosteroids should be used with great caution in these patients.

Average and large dosages of hydrocortisone or cortisone can cause elevation of blood pressure, salt and water retention, and increase excretion of potassium. These effects are less likely to occur with the synthetic derivatives except when used in large doses. Dietary salt restriction and potassium supplementation may be necessary. All corticosteroids increase calcium excretion.

A report shows that the use of corticosteroids in cerebral malaria is associated with a prolonged coma and an increased incidence of pneumonia and gastro-intestinal bleeding.

Drug-induced secondary adrenocortical insufficiency may result from too rapid a withdrawal of corticosteroids and may be minimised by gradual reduction of dosage. This type of relative insufficiency may persist for months after discontinuation of therapy; therefore, in any situation of stress occurring during that period, corticosteroid therapy should be reinstated. If the patient is receiving steroids already, the dosage may have to be increased. Since mineralocorticoid secretion may be impaired, salt and/or a mineralocorticoid should be administered concurrently (see 4.5 'Interaction with other medicaments and other forms of interaction').

Stopping corticosteroid, after prolonged therapy may cause withdrawal symptoms, including fever, myalgia, arthralgia and malaise. In patients who have received more than physiological doses of systemic corticosteroids (approximately 30 mg hydrocortisone) for greater than three weeks, withdrawal should not be abrupt. How dose reduction should be carried out depends largely on whether the disease is likely to relapse as the dose of systemic corticosteroids is reduced. Clinical assessment of disease activity may be needed during withdrawal. If the disease is unlikely to relapse on withdrawal of systemic corticosteroids but there is uncertainty about hypothalamic-pituitary adrenal (HPA) suppression, the dose of systemic corticosteroid ***may*** be reduced rapidly to physiological doses. Once a daily dose of 30 mg hydrocortisone is reached, dose reduction should be slower to allow the HPA-axis to recover.

Abrupt withdrawal of systemic corticosteroid treatment, which has continued up to three weeks is appropriate if it is considered that the disease is unlikely to relapse. Abrupt withdrawal of doses of up to 160 mg hydrocortisone for three weeks is unlikely to lead to clinically relevant HPA-axis suppression, in the majority of patients. In the following patient groups, gradual withdrawal of systemic corticosteroid therapy should be ***considered*** even after courses lasting three weeks or less:

- Patients who have had repeated courses of systemic corticosteroids, particularly if taken for greater than three weeks,
- when a short course has been prescribed within one year of cessation of long-term therapy (months or years),
- patients who may have reasons for adrenocortical insufficiency other than exogenous corticosteroid therapy,
- patients receiving doses of systemic corticosteroid greater than 160 mg hydrocortisone,
- patients repeatedly taking doses in the evening.

If corticosteroids are indicated in patients with latent tuberculosis or tuberculin reactivity, close observation is necessary as reactivation may occur. During prolonged corticosteroid therapy, these patients should receive prophylactic chemotherapy.

The use of 'Hydrocortone' Tablets in active tuberculosis should be restricted to those cases of fulminating or disseminated tuberculosis.

Corticosteroids should be used with caution in renal insufficiency, hypertension, diabetes or in those with a family history of diabetes, congestive heart failure, osteoporosis, previous steroid myopathy, glaucoma (or family history of glaucoma), myasthenia gravis, non-specific ulcerative colitis, diverticulitis, fresh intestinal anastomoses, active or latent peptic ulcer. Signs of peritoneal irritation following gastro-intestinal perforation in patients receiving large doses of corticosteroids may be minimal or absent.

Fat embolism has been reported as a possible complication of hypercortisonism.

There is an enhanced effect of corticosteroids in patients with hypothyroidism and in those with cirrhosis.

Corticosteroids may mask some signs of infection, and new infections may appear during their use. There may be decreased resistance and inability to localise infection in patients on corticosteroids. Corticosteroids may affect the nitrobluetetrazolium test for bacterial infection and produce false negative results.

Corticosteroids may activate latent amoebiasis or strongyloidiasis or exacerbate active disease. Therefore, it is recommended that latent or active amoebiasis and strongyloidiasis be excluded before initiating corticosteroid therapy in any patient at risk of or with symptoms suggestive of either condition.

Prolonged use of corticosteroids may produce posterior subcapsular cataracts, glaucoma with possible damage to the optic nerves, and may enhance the establishment of secondary ocular infections due to fungi or viruses.

Corticosteroids should be used cautiously in patients with ocular herpes simplex because of possible corneal perforation.

Corticosteroids may increase or decrease motility and number of spermatozoa.

Children: Corticosteroids cause growth retardation in infancy, childhood and adolescence. Treatment should be limited to the minimum dosage in order to minimise suppression of the hypothalamo-pituitary-adrenal axis and growth retardation.

Growth and development of infants and children on prolonged corticosteroid therapy should be carefully monitored.

4.5 Interaction with other medicinal products and other forms of Interaction

Aspirin should be used cautiously in conjunction with corticosteroids in hypoprothrombinaemia.

Phenytoin, ephedrine, rifabutin, carbamazepine, barbiturates, rifampicin and aminoglutethimide may enhance the metabolic clearance of corticosteroids, resulting in decreased blood levels and lessened physiological activity, thus requiring adjustment in corticosteroid dosage.

The prothrombin time should be checked frequently in patients who are receiving corticosteroids and coumarin anticoagulants at the same time because of reports of altered response to these anticoagulants. Studies have shown that the usual effect produced by adding corticosteroids is inhibition of response to coumarins, although there have been some conflicting reports of potentiation not substantiated by studies.

Ketoconazole alone can inhibit adrenal corticosteroid synthesis and may cause adrenal insufficiency during corticosteroid withdraw (see 4.4 'Special warnings and special precautions for use').

When corticosteroids are administered concomitantly with potassium-depleting diuretics, patients should be observed closely for development of hypokalaemia.

Moreover, corticosteroids may affect the nitroblue tetrazolium test for bacterial infaction and produce false negative results.

4.6 Pregnancy and lactation

The ability of corticosteroids to cross the placenta varies between individual drugs, however, hydrocortisone readily crosses the placenta.

Administration of corticosteroids to pregnant animals can cause abnormalities of foetal development including cleft palate, intra-uterine growth retardation and effects on brain growth and development. There is no evidence that corticosteroids result in an increased incidence of congenital abnormalities, such as cleft palate/lip in man. However, when administered for prolonged periods or repeatedly during pregnancy, corticosteroids may increase the risk of intra-uterine growth retardation. Hypoadrenalism may, in theory, occur in the neonate following prenatal exposure to corticosteroids but usually resolves spontaneously following birth and is rarely clinically important. As with all drugs, corticosteroids should only be prescribed when the benefits to the mother and child outweigh the risks. When corticosteroids are essential however, patients with normal pregnancies may be treated as though they were in the non-gravid state.

Use in breast-feeding mothers: Corticosteroids are excreted in breast milk, although no data are available for hydrocortisone. Infants of mothers taking high doses of systemic corticosteroids for prolonged periods may have a degree of adrenal suppression.

4.7 Effects on ability to drive and use machines

Hydrocortisone may cause vertigo, visual field loss and muscle wasting and weakness. If affected, patients should not drive or operate machinery (see section 4.8 'Undesirable effects').

4.8 Undesirable effects

Fluid and electrolyte disturbances: Sodium retention, fluid retention, congestive heart failure in susceptible patients, potassium loss, hypokalaemic alkalosis, hypertension, increased calcium excretion.

Musculoskeletal effects: Muscle weakness, steroid myopathy, loss of muscle mass, osteoporosis (especially in post-menopausal females), vertebral compression fractures, aseptic necrosis of femoral and humeral heads, pathological fracture of long bones, tendon rupture.

Gastro-intestinal: Peptic ulcer with possible perforation and haemorrhage, perforation of the small and large bowel particularly in patients with inflammatory bowel disease, pancreatitis, abdominal distension, ulcerative oesophagitis, dyspepsia, oesophageal candidiasis.

Dermatological: Impaired wound healing, thin fragile skin, petechiae, and ecchymoses, erythema, striae, telangiectasia, acne, increased sweating, may suppress reactions to skin tests, other cutaneous reactions such as allergic dermatitis, urticaria, angioneurotic oedema.

Neurological: Convulsions, increased intracranial pressure with papilloedema (pseudotumour cerebri) usually after treatment, vertigo, headache, psychic disturbances.

Endocrine: Menstrual irregularities, amenorrhoea, development of Cushingoid state, suppression of growth in children, secondary adrenocortical and pituitary unresponsiveness (particularly in times of stress, as in trauma, surgery, or illness), decreased carbohydrate tolerance, manifestations of latent diabetes mellitus, hyperglycemia, increased requirements for insulin or oral hypoglycaemic agents in diabetes, hirsutism.

Ophthalmic: Posterior subcapsular cataracts, increased intra-ocular pressure, papilloedema, corneal or scleral thinning, exacerbation of ophthalmic viral disease, glaucoma, exophthalmos.

Metabolic: Negative nitrogen balance due to protein catabolism.

Cardiovascular: Myocardial rupture following recent myocardial infarction (see 4.4 'Special warnings and special precautions for use').

Other: Hypersensitivity, leucocytosis, thrombo-embolism, weight gain, increased appetite, nausea, malaise.

4.9 Overdose

Reports of acute toxicity and/or deaths following overdosage with glucocorticoids are rare. No antidote is available. Treatment is probably not indicated for reactions due to chronic poisoning unless the patient has a condition that would render him unusually susceptible to ill effects from corticosteroids. In this case, symptomatic treatment should be instituted as necessary.

Anaphylactic and hypersensitivity reactions may be treated with adrenaline, positive-pressure artificial respiration and aminophylline. The patient should be kept warm and quiet.

The biological half-life of hydrocortisone is about 100 minutes.

5. PHARMACOLOGICAL PROPERTIES

5.1 Pharmacodynamic properties

Hydrocortisone is a glucocorticoid. Glucocorticoids are adrenocortical steroids, both naturally-occurring and synthetic, which are readily absorbed from the gastro-intestinal tract.

Hydrocortisone is believed to be the principal corticosteroid secreted by the adrenal cortex. Naturally-occurring glucocorticosteroids (hydrocortisone and cortisone), which also have salt-retaining properties, are used as replacement therapy in adrenocortical deficiency states. They are also used for their potent anti-inflammatory effects in disorders of many organ systems. Glucocorticoids cause profound and varied metabolic effects. In addition they modify the body's immune responses to diverse stimuli.

5.2 Pharmacokinetic properties

Hydrocortisone is readily absorbed from the gastro-intestinal tract and 90% or more of the drug is reversibly bound to protein.

The binding is accounted for by two protein fractions. One, corticosteroid-binding globulin is a glycoprotein; the other is albumin.

Hydrocortisone is metabolised in the liver and most body tissues to hydrogenated and degraded forms such as tetrahydrocortisone and tetrahydrocortisol which are excreted in the urine, mainly conjugated as glucuronides, together with a very small proportion of unchanged hydrocortisone.

5.3 Preclinical safety data

No relevant data.

6. PHARMACEUTICAL PARTICULARS

6.1 List of excipients

Lactose

Magnesium stearate

Maize starch

6.2 Incompatibilities
None known.

6.3 Shelf life
36 months.

6.4 Special precautions for storage
Do not store above 25°C. Keep in original package, protected from light.

6.5 Nature and contents of container
PVC/aluminium blister containing 30 tablets.

6.6 Instructions for use and handling
None.

7. MARKETING AUTHORISATION HOLDER
Merck Sharp & Dohme Limited
Hertford Road
Hoddesdon
Hertfordshire
EN11 9BU
UK

8. MARKETING AUTHORISATION NUMBER(S)
10 mg tablets: PL 0025/5053
20 mg tablets: PL 0025/5054

9. DATE OF FIRST AUTHORISATION/RENEWAL OF THE AUTHORISATION
10 mg tablets: 23 February 1989 / 27 November 1995
20 mg tablets: 23 February 1989 / 13 December 1995

10. DATE OF REVISION OF THE TEXT
March 2004

LEGAL CATEGORY
POM.

® denotes registered trademark of Merck & Co., Inc., Whitehouse Station, NJ, USA.

SPC.HCT.03.UK.0954

Hydroxyurea medac 500 mg capsule, hard

(medac GmbH)

1. NAME OF THE MEDICINAL PRODUCT
Hydroxycarbamide medac 500 mg capsule, hard

2. QUALITATIVE AND QUANTITATIVE COMPOSITION
One capsule contains 500 mg hydroxycarbamide.

For excipients, see 6.1.

3. PHARMACEUTICAL FORM
Capsule, hard

White capsules.

4. CLINICAL PARTICULARS

4.1 Therapeutic indications
Treatment of patients with chronic myeloid leukaemia (CML) in the chronic or accelerated phase of the disease.

Treatment of patients with essential thrombocythemia or polycythemia vera with a high risk for thrombo-embolic complications.

4.2 Posology and method of administration
Therapy should only be conducted by a physician experienced in oncology or haematology. Doses are based on real or ideal bodyweight of the patient, whichever is the less.

In CML hydroxycarbamide is usually given at an initial dose of 40 mg/kg daily dependent on the white cell count. The dose is reduced by 50% (20 mg/kg daily) when the white cell count is dropped below 20 × 10^9/l. The dose is then adjusted individually to keep the white cell count at 5-10 × 10^9/l. Hydroxycarbamide dose should be reduced if white cell counts fall below 5 × 10^9/l and increased if white cell counts >10 × 10^9/l are observed.

If white cell count falls below 2.5 × 10^9/l, or the platelet count below 100 × 10^9/l, therapy should be interrupted until the counts rise significantly towards normal.

An adequate trial period for determining the antineoplastic effect of Hydroxycarbamide medac is six weeks. Therapy should be interrupted indefinitely, if there is a significant progress of the disease. If there is a significant clinical response therapy may be continued indefinitely.

In essential thrombocythemia hydroxycarbamide is usually given at starting doses of 15 mg/kg/day with dose adjustment to maintain a platelet count below 600 × 10^9 /l without lowering the white blood cell count below 4 × 10^9/l.

In polycythemia vera hydroxycarbamide should be started at a dosage of 15-20 mg/kg/day. Hydroxycarbamide dose should be adjusted individually to maintain the hematocrit below 45% and platelet count below 400 × 10^9/l. In most patients this can be achieved with hydroxycarbamide given continuously at average daily doses of 500 to 1000 mg.

If hematocrit and platelet count can be sufficiently controlled therapy should be continued indefinitely.

Children:

Because of the rarity of these conditions in children, dosage regimens have not been established.

Elderly:

Elderly patients may be more sensitive to the effects of hydroxycarbamide, and may require a lower dosage regimen.

Dosage in conditions of impaired renal and/or liver function:

There are no data available. Dose recommendation cannot be given to patients with impaired renal and/or liver function (see 4.4 Special warnings and precautions for use).

The capsules should be swallowed whole and not allowed to disintegrate within the mouth.

4.3 Contraindications
Hydroxycarbamide medac is contraindicated in severe bone marrow depression, leucocytopenia (<2,5 × 10^9 leukocytes/l), thrombocytopenia (< 100 × 10^9 platelets/l) or severe anaemia.

Hydroxycarbamide medac is contraindicated in patients with hypersensitivity to hydroxycarbamide or to any of the excipients. Therapy should be discontinued if hypersensitivity to Hydroxycarbamide medac occurs.

4.4 Special warnings and special precautions for use
Hydroxycarbamide can cause bone marrow depression with leucopenia as first and most often occurring sign of this depression. Thrombocytopenia and anaemia occur less frequently and are rare without preceding leucopenia. Complete blood counts including determination of haemoglobin level, total leukocyte differentiation counts, and platelet counts should be performed regularly also after the individual optimal dose has been established. The control interval should be individualised, but is normally once a week. If white cell count falls below 2.5 × 10^9/l, or the platelet count below 100 × 10^9/l, therapy should be interrupted until the counts rise significantly towards normal. (See 4.2 Posology and method of administration).

In case of anaemia before or during ongoing treatment red blood cells may be replaced when needed. Megaloblastic erythropoiesis, which is self limiting, is often seen early in the course of hydroxycarbamide therapy. The morphologic change resembles pernicious anaemia, but is not related to vitamin B_{12} or folic acid deficiency.

During therapy with Hydroxycarbamide medac frequent monitoring of blood counts should be conducted as well as monitoring of hepatic and renal function. In patients with impaired renal and/or liver function the experience is limited. Therefore special care should be taken in the treatment of these patients, especially at the beginning of therapy.

Patients should be instructed to drink abundantly.

In patients receiving long-term treatment with hydroxycarbamide for myeloproliferative disorders, such as polycythemia vera and thrombocythemia, secondary leukemia may develop. To what extent this relates to the underlying disease or to treatment with hydroxycarbamide is presently unknown.

The monitoring of skin changes is advisable during hydroxycarbamide treatment as in single cases squamous cell carcinoma of the skin was reported.

Hydroxycarbamide can induce painful leg ulcers which are usually difficult to treat and require cessation of therapy. Discontinuation of hydroxycarbamide usually leads to slow resolution of the ulcers over some weeks.

Hydroxycarbamide should be administered with caution to patients who receive concomitant or have received previous therapy with other antineoplastic drugs or irradiation, since adverse reactions can occur more frequently and more severe than those reported with the use of hydroxycarbamide, other antineoplastic drugs or irradiation alone. These effects primarily include bone marrow depression, gastric irritation, and mucositis.

An exacerbation of erythema caused by previous or simultaneous irradiation may occur.

The combination of hydroxycarbamide and nucleoside reverse transcriptase inhibitors (NRTI) may enhance the risk of side effects of NRTI, see also section 4.5, Interaction with other medicinal products and other forms of interaction.

Hydroxycarbamide may be genotoxic. Therefore, men under therapy are advised to use safe contraceptive measures during and for at least 3 months after therapy. They should be informed about the possibility of sperm conservation before the start of therapy.

Hydroxycarbamide medac should not be administered to patients who are pregnant or to mothers who are breast feeding, unless the benefits outweigh the possible hazards (see 4.6 Pregnancy and lactation).

Hydroxycarbamide medac should not be administered to patients with rare hereditary problems of galactose intolerance, the Lapp lactase deficiency or glucose-galactose malabsorption.

4.5 Interaction with other medicinal products and other forms of Interaction
Hydroxycarbamide should be administered with caution to patients who receive concomitant or have received previous therapy with other antineoplastic drugs or irradiation, since adverse reactions can occur more frequently and more severe than those reported with the use of hydroxycarbamide, other antineoplastic drugs or irradiation alone. These effects primarily include bone marrow depression, gastric irritation, and mucositis.

An exacerbation of erythema caused by previous or simultaneous irradiation may occur.

In-vitro studies have demonstrated hydroxycarbamidés ability to enhance the cytotoxicity of both ara-C and the fluoropyrimidines. Whether this interaction leads clinically to a co-operative toxicity or to the necessity of adjusting the doses is unclear.

Hydroxycarbamide may enhance the antiretroviral activity of nucleoside reverse transcriptase inhibitors like didanosine and stavudine. Hydroxycarbamide inhibits HIV DNA synthesis and HIV replication by decreasing the amount of intracellular deoxynucleotides. Hydroxycarbamide may also enhance the potential side effects of nucleoside reverse transcriptase inhibitors such as pancreatitis and peripheral neuropathy.

4.6 Pregnancy and lactation
Pregnancy

Hydroxycarbamide may be a potent mutagenic agent. Animal experiments with hydroxycarbamide indicated an increased incidence of congenital defects (see 5.3 Preclinical safety data). Hydroxycarbamide should not be administered to patients who are pregnant unless the benefits outweigh the possible hazards. Women of child-bearing potential have to take contraceptive precautions before the start of and during treatment with hydroxycarbamide.

If pregnancy still occurs during treatment the possibility of genetic consultation should be used. Hydroxycarbamide crosses the placenta.

Lactation:

As hydroxycarbamide passes into breast-milk, breast-feeding has to be interrupted before the start of treatment.

Fertility:

Hydroxycarbamide may be genotoxic, therefore, if a patient intends to become pregnant after a therapy with hydroxycarbamide a genetic consultation is recommended.

Men under therapy are advised to use safe contraceptive measures during and for at least 3 months after therapy. They should be informed about the possibility of sperm conservation before the start of therapy.

4.7 Effects on ability to drive and use machines
Ability to react may be impaired during treatment with Hydroxycarbamide medac. This should be borne in mind when heightened attention is required, e.g for driving and using machines.

4.8 Undesirable effects
Bone marrow depression is the dose limiting toxicity. Gastrointestinal side effects are common but require rarely dose reduction or cessation of treatment.

Common (> 1/100, < 1/10)

Blood: Bone marrow depression, leucopenia, megaloblastosis.

Gastrointestinal: Diarrhoea, constipation.

Uncommon > 1/1,000, < 1/100)

Blood: Thrombocytopenia, anaemia

Body as a whole: Nausea, vomiting, anorexia, stomatitis. Drug fever, chills, malaise.

Skin: Maculopapular rash, facial erythema, acral erythema.

Liver: Elevation of liver enzymes, bilirubin.

Urogenital: Transient impairment of the renal tubular function accompanied by elevation in serum uric acid, urea and creatinine.

Rare: > 1/10,000, < 1/1,000)

Body as a whole: Hypersensitive reactions

Skin: Alopecia.

Respiratory: Acute pulmonary reactions consisting of diffuse pulmonary infiltrates, fever and dyspnoe, allergic alveolitits.

Urogenital: Dysuria.

Neurological: Rare neurological disturbances including headache, dizziness, disorientation, hallucinations.

Very rare(< 1/10,000)

Skin: Dermatomyositis-like skin changes, Hyperpigmentation or atrophy of skin and nails, cutaneous ulcers (especially leg ulcers), Pruritus, actinic keratosis, skin cancer (squamous cell cancer, basal cell carcinoma), violet papules, desquamation.

Urogenital: renal impairment.

In the therapy with hydroxycarbamide megaloblastosis may occur which does not respond to treatment with folic acid or B_{12}.

The bone-marrow suppression subsides, however, when therapy is discontinued.

Severe gastric distress (nausea, emesis, anorexia) resulting from combined hydroxycarbamide and irradiation therapy may usually be controlled by temporarily discontinuing hydroxycarbamide administration.

Hydroxycarbamide may aggravate the inflammation of mucous membranes secondary to irradiation. It can cause a recall of erythema and hyperpigmentation in previously irradiated tissues. Erythema, atrophy of skin and nails, desquamation, violet papules, alopecia, dermatomyositis-like skin changes, actinic keratosis, skin cancer (squamous cell cancer, basal cell carcinoma), cutaneous ulcers (especially leg ulcers), pruritus and hyperpigmentation of skin and nails have been observed in isolated cases partly after years of long-term daily maintenance therapy with hydroxycarbamide.

High doses may cause moderate drowsiness.

Rare neurological disturbances including headache, dizziness, disorientation, hallucinations, and convulsions have been reported.

In rare cases dysuria or renal impairment, hypersensitive reactions.

In individual cases allergic alveolitis.

In patients receiving long-term treatment with hydroxycarbamide for myeloproliferative disorders, such as polycythemia vera and thrombocythemia, secondary leukemia may develop. To what extent this relates to the underlying disease or to treatment with hydroxycarbamide is presently unknown.

Hydroxycarbamide can reduce plasma iron clearance and iron utilisation by erythrocytes. However, it does not appear to alter the red blood cell survival time.

4.9 Overdose

Acute mucocutaneous symptoms have been observed in patients receiving hydroxycarbamide dosages several times the recommended dose. Soreness, violet erythema, oedema on palms and soles followed by scaling of hands and feet, severe generalised hyperpigmentation of the skin, and stomatitis have also been observed.

Immediate treatment consists of gastric lavage, followed by supportive care and monitoring of the haematopoetic system.

5. PHARMACOLOGICAL PROPERTIES

5.1 Pharmacodynamic properties

Pharmacotherapeutic group: Other antineoplastic agents

ATC-code: L01XX05

The exact mechanism of action of hydroxycarbamide is unknown. The most important effect of hydroxycarbamide appears to be blocking of the ribonucleotide reductase system resulting in inhibition of DNA synthesis. Cellular resistance is usually caused by increased ribonucleotide reductase levels as a result of gene amplification.

5.2 Pharmacokinetic properties

The pharmacokinetic information is limited. Hydroxycarbamide is well absorbed and the oral bioavailability is complete. After oral administration maximum plasma concentrations are reached within 0.5 to 2 hours. Hydroxycarbamide is eliminated partly via renal excretion. The contribution of this route of elimination to the total elimination of hydroxycarbamide is unclear since the fractions of the given dose recovered in urine ranged from 9 to 95 %. Metabolism of hydroxycarbamide has not been thoroughly studied in humans.

Hydroxycarbamide crosses the blood-brain barrier.

5.3 Preclinical safety data

Repeated dose toxicity

Bone marrow damages, lymphoid atrophy in the spleen and degenerative changes in the epithelium of the small and large intestines are toxic effects which have been observed in animal studies. The potential risk for similar effects in humans must be considered.

Reproduction toxicity

Teratogenicity of hydroxycarbamide was demonstrated in many species, including rat, mouse and rabbit. The large variety of teratogenic effects were ranging from death of a large proportion of embryos to limb deformities, neural defects and even behavioural effects.

Additionally, hydroxycarbamide affected spermatogenesis and sperm motility of mice after repeated administration.

Genotoxicity

Hydroxycarbamide showed genotoxic properties in conventional testing systems.

Carcinogenicity

The preclinical information on the carcinogenic potential of hydroxycarbamide is meagre. A 12 months study on mice where the occurrence of lung tumours was studied did not show any carcinogenic potential in hydroxycarbamide.

6. PHARMACEUTICAL PARTICULARS

6.1 List of excipients

Capsule content:

calcium citrate, disodium citrate, magnesium stearate, lactose monohydrate

Capsule shell:

titanium dioxide (E 171), gelatin

6.2 Incompatibilities

Not applicable.

6.3 Shelf life

4 years

6.4 Special precautions for storage

No special precautions for storage.

6.5 Nature and contents of container

The capsules are packed in blisters made of Al/PVDC and PVC/PVDC opacified with titanium dioxide.

Available pack sizes: 50 and 100 capsules.

6.6 Instructions for use and handling

Procedures for proper handling and disposal of anticancer drugs should be considered.

7. MARKETING AUTHORISATION HOLDER

medac

Gesellschaft für klinische Spezialpräparate mbH

Fehlandtstraβe 3

20354 Hamburg

Germany

8. MARKETING AUTHORISATION NUMBER(S)

PL 11587/0019

9. DATE OF FIRST AUTHORISATION/RENEWAL OF THE AUTHORISATION

23 May 2001/9 January 2004

10. DATE OF REVISION OF THE TEXT

24 March 2005

Hygroton Tablets 50mg

(Alliance Pharmaceuticals)

1. NAME OF THE MEDICINAL PRODUCT

Hygroton® Tablets 50mg

2. QUALITATIVE AND QUANTITATIVE COMPOSITION

Chlortalidone PhEur 50mg.

3. PHARMACEUTICAL FORM

Pale yellow, round, flat tablets with bevelled edges, impressed Geigy on one side with a breakline, and the letters Z/A on the other side.

4. CLINICAL PARTICULARS

4.1 Therapeutic indications

Treatment of arterial hypertension, essential or nephrogenic or isolated systolic. Treatment of stable, chronic heart failure of mild to moderate degree (New York Heart Association, NYHA: functional class II or III).

Oedema of specific origin

• Ascites due to cirrhosis of the liver in stable patients under close control.

• Oedema due to nephrotic syndrome.

Diabetes Insipidus.

4.2 Posology and method of administration

The dosage of Hygroton should be individually titrated to give the lowest effective dose; this is particularly important in the elderly. Hygroton should be taken orally, preferably as a single daily dose at breakfast time.

Adults:

Hypertension

The recommended starting dose is 25mg/day. This is sufficient to produce the maximum hypotensive effect in most patients. If the decrease in blood pressure proves inadequate with 25mg/day, then the dose can be increased to 50mg/day. If a further reduction in blood pressure is required, additional hypertensive therapy may be added to the dosage regime.

Stable, chronic heart failure (NYHA: functional class II /III):

The recommended starting dose is 25 to 50mg/day, in severe cases it may be increased up to 100 to 200mg/day. The usual maintenance dose is the lowest effective dose, eg 25 to 50mg/day either daily or every other day. If the response proves inadequate, digitalis or an ACE inhibitor, or both, may be added. (See Section 4.4 "Special warnings and precautions for use").

Oedema of specific origin (see Section 4.1 "Therapeutic indications")

The lowest effective dose is to be identified by titration and administered over limited periods only. It is recommended that doses should not exceed 50mg/day.

Diabetes insipidus:

Initially 100mg twice daily but reducing where possible to a daily maintenance dose of 50mg.

Children:

The lowest effective dose should also be used in children. For example, an initial dose of 0.5 to 1mg/kg/48hours and a maximum dose of 1.7mg/kg/48hours have been used.

Elderly patients and patients with renal impairment:

The lowest effective dose of Hygroton is also recommended for patients with mild renal insufficiency and for elderly patients (see Section 5.2 "Pharmacokinetic properties").

In elderly patients, the elimination of chlortalidone is slower than in healthy young adults, although absorption is the same. Therefore, a reduction in the recommended adult dosage may be needed. Close medical observation is indicated when treating patients of advanced age with chlortalidone.

Hygroton and the thiazide diuretics lose their diuretic effect when the creatinine clearance is < 30ml/min.

4.3 Contraindications

Known hypersensitivity to chlortalidone or any of the excipients. Anuria, severe hepatic or renal failure (creatinine clearance < 30ml/min), hypersensitivity to chlortalidone and other sulphonamide derivatives, refractory hypokalaemia, hyponatraemia and hypercalcaemia, symptomatic hyperuricaemia (history of gout or uric acid calculi), hypertension during pregnancy, untreated Addison's disease and concomitant lithium therapy.

4.4 Special warnings and special precautions for use

Warnings:

Hygroton should be used with caution in patients with impaired hepatic function or progressive liver disease since minor changes in the fluid and electrolyte balance due to thiazide diuretics may precipitate hepatic coma, especially in patients with liver cirrhosis (see Section 4.3 "Contra-indications").

Hygroton should also be used with caution in patients with severe renal disease. Thiazides may precipitate azotaemia in such patients, and the effects of repeated administration may be cumulative.

Precautions:

Electrolytes:

Treatment with thiazide diuretics has been associated with electrolyte disturbances such as hypokalaemia, hypomagnesaemia, hyperglycaemia and hyponatraemia. Since the excretion of electrolytes is increased, a very strict low-salt diet should be avoided.

Hypokalaemia can sensitise the heart or exaggerate its response to the toxic effects of digitalis.

Like all thiazide diuretics, kaluresis induced by Hygroton is dose dependent and varies in extent from one subject to another. With 25 to 50mg/day, the decrease in serum potassium concentrations averages 0.5mmol/l. Periodic serum electrolyte determinations should be carried out, particularly in digitalised patients.

If necessary, Hygroton may be combined with oral potassium supplements or a potassium-sparing diuretic (eg triamterene).

If hypokalaemia is accompanied by clinical signs (eg muscular weakness, paresis and ECG alteration), Hygroton should be discontinued.

Combined treatment consisting of Hygroton and a potassium salt or a potassium-sparing diuretic should be avoided in patients also receiving ACE inhibitors.

Monitoring of serum electrolytes is particularly indicated in the elderly, in patients with ascites due to liver cirrhosis, and in patients with oedema due to nephrotic syndrome. There have been isolated reports of hyponatraemia with neurological symptoms (eg nausea, debility, progressive disorientation and apathy) following thiazide treatment.

For nephrotic syndrome, Hygroton should be used only under close control in normokalaemic patients with no signs of volume depletion.

Metabolic effects:

Hygroton may raise the serum uric acid level, but attacks of gout are uncommon during chronic treatment.

As with the use of other thiazide diuretics, glucose intolerance may occur; this is manifest as hyperglycaemia and glycosuria. Hygroton may very seldom aggravate or precipitate diabetes mellitus; this is usually reversible on stopping therapy.

Small and partly reversible increases in plasma concentrations of total cholesterol, triglycerides, or low-density lipoprotein cholesterol were reported in patients during long-term treatment with thiazides and thiazide-like diuretics. The clinical relevance of these findings is a matter for debate.

Hygroton should not be used as a first-line drug for long-term treatment in patients with overt diabetes mellitus or in subjects receiving therapy for hypercholesterolaemia (diet or combined).

As with all antihypertensive agents, a cautious dosage schedule is indicated in patients with severe coronary or cerebral arteriosclerosis.

Other effects:

The antihypertensive effect of ACE inhibitors is potentiated by agents that increase plasma renin activity (diuretics). It is recommended that the diuretic be reduced in dosage or withdrawn for 2 to 3 days and/or that the ACE inhibitor therapy be started with a low initial dose of the ACE inhibitor. Patients should be monitored for several hours after the first dose.

4.5 Interaction with other medicinal products and other forms of Interaction

Diuretics potentiate the action of curare derivatives and antihypertensive drugs (e.g. guanethidine, methyldopa, β-blockers, vasodilators, calcium antagonists and ACE inhibitors).

The hypokalaemic effect of diuretics may be potentiated by corticosteroids, ACTH, β_2 – agonists, amphotericin and carbenoxolone.

It may prove necessary to adjust the dosage of insulin and oral anti-diabetic agents.

Thiazide-induced hypokalaemia or hypomagnesaemia may favour the occurrence of digitalis-induced cardiac arrhythmias (see Section 4.4 "Special warnings and precautions for use").

Concomitant administration of certain non-steroidal anti-inflammatory drugs (e.g. indometacin) may reduce the diuretic and antihypertensive activity of Hygroton; there have been isolated reports of a deterioration in renal function in predisposed patients.

The bioavailability of thiazide-type diuretics may be increased by anticholinergic agents (eg atropine, biperiden), apparently due to a decrease in gastrointestinal motility and stomach-emptying rate.

Absorption of thiazide diuretics is impaired in the presence of anionic exchange resins such as colestyramine. A decrease in the pharmacological effect may be expected.

Concurrent administration of thiazide diuretics may increase the incidence of hypersensitivity reactions to allopurinol, increase the risk of adverse effects caused by amantadine, enhance the hyperglycaemic effect of diazoxide, and reduce renal excretion of cytotoxic agents (eg cyclophosphamide, methotrexate) and potentiate their myelosuppressive effects.

The pharmacological effects of both calcium salts and vitamin D may be increased to clinically significant levels if given with thiazide diuretics. The resultant hypercalcaemia is usually transient but may be persistent and symptomatic (weakness, fatigue, anorexia) in patients with hyperparathyroidism.

Concomitant treatment with cyclosporin may increase the risk of hyperuricaemia and gout-type complications.

Thiazide and related diuretics can cause a rapid rise in serum lithium levels as the renal clearance of lithium is reduced by these compounds.

4.6 Pregnancy and lactation

Diuretics are best avoided for the management of oedema or hypertension in pregnancy as their use may be associated with hypovolaemia, increased blood viscosity and reduced placental perfusion. There have been reports of foetal bone marrow depression, thrombocytopenia, and foetal and neonatal jaundice associated with the use of thiazide diuretics.

Chlortalidone passes into the breast milk; mothers taking Hygroton should refrain from breast-feeding their infants.

4.7 Effects on ability to drive and use machines

Patients should be warned of the potential hazards of driving or operating machinery if they experience side effects such as dizziness.

4.8 Undesirable effects

Frequency estimate: very rare $<0.01\%$, rare $\leqslant 0.01\%$ to $\leqslant 0.1\%$;uncommon $\leqslant 0.1\%$ to $<1\%$; common $\leqslant 1\%$ to $<10\%$; very common $\geqslant 10\%$.

Electrolytes and metabolic disorders:

Very common: mainly at higher doses, hypokalaemia, hyperuricaemia, and rise in blood lipids.

Common: hyponatraemia, hypomagnesaemia and hyperglycaemia.

Uncommon: gout.

Rare: hypercalcaemia, glycosuria, worsening of diabetic metabolic state.

Very rare: hypochloraemic alkalosis.

Skin:

Common: urticaria and other forms of skin rash.

Rare: photosensitisation.

Liver:

Rare: intrahepatic cholestasis or jaundice.

Cardiovascular system:

Common: postural hypotension.

Rare: cardiac arrhythmias.

Central nervous system:

Common: Dizziness.

Rare: paraesthesia, headache.

Gastro-intestinal tract:

Common: loss of appetite and minor gastrointestinal distress.

Rare: mild nausea and vomiting, gastric pain, constipation and diarrhoea.

Very rare: pancreatitis.

Blood:

Rare: Thrombocytopenia, leucopenia, agranulocytosis and eosinophilia.

Other effects:

Common: impotence

Rare: Idiosyncratic pulmonary oedema (respiratory disorders), allergic interstitial nephritis.

4.9 Overdose

Signs and symptoms: In poisoning due to an overdosage the following signs and symptoms may occur: dizziness, nausea, somnolence, hypovolaemia, hypotension and electrolyte disturbances associated with cardiac arrhythmias and muscle spasms.

Treatment: There is no specific antidote to Hygroton. Gastric lavage, emesis or activated charcoal should be employed to reduce absorption. Blood pressure and fluid and electrolyte balance should be monitored and appropriate corrective measures taken. Intravenous fluid and electrolyte replacement may be indicated.

5. PHARMACOLOGICAL PROPERTIES

5.1 Pharmacodynamic properties

Chlortalidone is a benzothiadiazine (thiazide)-related diuretic with a long duration of action.

Thiazide and thiazide-like diuretics act primarily on the distal renal tubule (early convoluted part), inhibiting NaCl reabsorption (by antagonising the Na^+Cl cotransporter) and promoting Ca^{++} reabsorption (by an unknown mechanism). The enhanced delivery of Na^+ and water to the cortical collection tubule and/or the increased flow rate leads to increased secretion and excretion of K^+ and H^+.

In persons with normal renal function, diuresis is induced after the administration of 12.5mg Hygroton. The resulting increase in urinary excretion of sodium and chloride and the less prominent increase in urinary potassium are dose dependent and occur both in normal and in oedematous patients. The diuretic effect sets in after 2 to 3 hours, reaches its maximum after 4 to 24 hours, and may persist for 2 to 3 days.

Thiazide-induced diuresis initially leads to decreases in plasma volume, cardiac output, and systemic blood pressure. The renin-angiotensin-aldosterone system may possibly become activated.

In hypertensive individuals, chlortalidone gently reduces blood pressure. On continued administration, the hypotensive effect is maintained, probably due to the fall in peripheral resistance; cardiac output returns to pretreatment values, plasma volume remains somewhat reduced and plasma renin activity may be elevated.

On chronic administration, the antihypertensive effect of Hygroton is dose dependent between 12.5 and 50mg/day. Raising the dose above 50mg increases metabolic complications and is rarely of therapeutic benefit.

As with other diuretics, when Hygroton is given as monotherapy, blood pressure control is achieved in about half of patients with mild to moderate hypertension. In general, elderly and black patients are found to respond well to diuretics given as primary therapy. Randomised clinical trials in the elderly have shown that treatment of hypertension or predominant systolic hypertension in older persons with low-dose thiazide diuretics, including chlortalidone, reduces cerebrovascular (stroke), coronary heart and total cardiovascular morbidity and mortality.

Combined treatment with other antihypertensives potentiates the blood-pressure lowering effects. In the large proportion of patients failing to respond adequately to monotherapy, a further decrease in blood pressure can thus be achieved.

In renal diabetes insipidus, Hygroton paradoxically reduces polyuria. The mechanism of action has not been elucidated.

5.2 Pharmacokinetic properties

Absorption and plasma concentration

The bioavailability of an oral dose of 50mg Hygroton is approximately 64%, peak blood concentrations being attained after 8 to 12 hours. For doses of 25 and 50mg, C_{max} values average 1.5μg/ml (4.4μmol/L) and 3.2μg/ml (9.4μmol/L) respectively. For doses up to 100mg there is a proportional increase in AUC. On repeated daily doses of 50mg, mean steady-state blood concentrations of 7.2μg/ml (21.2μmol/L), measured at the end of the 24 hour dosage interval, are reached after 1 to 2 weeks.

Distribution

In blood, only a small fraction of chlortalidone is free, due to extensive accumulation in erythrocytes and binding to plasma proteins. Owing to the large degree of high affinity binding to the carbonic anhydrase of erythrocytes, only some 1.4% of the total amount of chlortalidone in whole blood was found in plasma at steady state during treatment with 50mg doses. *In vitro*, plasma protein binding of chlortalidone is about 76% and the major binding protein is albumin.

Chlortalidone crosses the placental barrier and passes into the breast milk. In mothers treated with 50mg chlortalidone daily before and after delivery, chlortalidone levels in fetal whole blood are about 15% of those found in maternal blood. Chlortalidone concentrations in amniotic fluid and in the maternal milk are approximately 4% of the corresponding maternal blood level.

Metabolism

Metabolism and hepatic excretion into bile constitute a minor pathway of elimination. Within 120 hours, about 70% of the dose is excreted in the urine and the faeces, mainly in unchanged form.

Elimination

Chlortalidone is eliminated from whole blood and plasma with an elimination half-life averaging 50 hours. The elimination half-life is unaltered after chronic administration. The major part of an absorbed dose of chlortalidone is excreted by the kidneys, with a mean renal clearance of 60ml/min.

Special patient groups

Renal dysfunction does not alter the pharmacokinetics of chlortalidone, the rate-limiting factor in the elimination of the drug from blood or plasma being most probably the affinity of the drug to the carbonic anhydrase of erythrocytes.

No dosage adjustment is needed in patients with impaired renal function.

In elderly patients, the elimination of chlortalidone is slower than in healthy young adults, although absorption is the same. Therefore, close medical observation is indicated when treating patients of advanced age with chlortalidone.

5.3 Preclinical safety data

There are no pre-clinical data of relevance to the prescriber which are additional to those already included in other sections of the Summary of Product Characteristics.

6. PHARMACEUTICAL PARTICULARS

6.1 List of excipients

Microcrystalline cellulose, silicon dioxide, maize starch, magnesium stearate, sodium carboxymethyl cellulose, yellow iron oxide (E172).

6.2 Incompatibilities

None known.

6.3 Shelf life

Five years.

6.4 Special precautions for storage

None.

6.5 Nature and contents of container

Aluminium/PVC blister packs of 28 tablets.

6.6 Instructions for use and handling

None

Administrative Data

7. MARKETING AUTHORISATION HOLDER

Alliance Pharmaceuticals Ltd

Avonbridge House

Bath Road

Chippenham

Wiltshire

SN15 2BB

8. MARKETING AUTHORISATION NUMBER(S)

PL16853/0007

9. DATE OF FIRST AUTHORISATION/RENEWAL OF THE AUTHORISATION

25 June 1998

10. DATE OF REVISION OF THE TEXT

February 2004

11. Legal status

POM

Alliance, Alliance Pharmaceuticals and associated devices are registered Trademarks of Alliance Pharmaceuticals Ltd.

Hyoscine Hydrobromide 400 micrograms Solution for Injection

(Wockhardt UK Ltd)

1. NAME OF THE MEDICINAL PRODUCT

Hyoscine Hydrobromide 400 micrograms Solution for Injection

2. QUALITATIVE AND QUANTITATIVE COMPOSITION

Each 1ml ampoule contains 400 micrograms of hyoscine hydrobromide.

For excipients, see 6.1.

3. PHARMACEUTICAL FORM

Solution for Injection.

A clear colourless solution, practically free from particles.

4. CLINICAL PARTICULARS

4.1 Therapeutic indications

Due to its anticholinergic activity, hyoscine injection is used as a preoperative medication to control bronchial, nasal, pharyngeal and salivary secretions, to prevent bronchospasm and laryngospasm and to block cardiac vagal inhibiting reflexes during induction of anaesthesia and intubation.

4.2 Posology and method of administration

Dosage

Adults

For pre-medication a dose of 200 to 600 micrograms is given by the subcutaneous or intramuscular route 30 to 60 minutes before induction of anaesthesia.

The injection may if required also be given by the intravenous route for acute use.

Children

A dose of 15 micrograms/kg is recommended in children.

Elderly

Hyoscine is not recommended for use in the elderly.

4.3 Contraindications
Hypersensitivity to hyoscine. Narrow angle glaucoma.

4.4 Special warnings and special precautions for use
Caution is necessary in treating patients with cardiovascular disease, gastrointestinal obstruction, paralytic ileus, prostatic enlargement, Down's Syndrome, myasthenia gravis, renal or hepatic impairment.

Because hyoscine may cause drowsiness, patients must not drive or operate machinery. Patients should avoid alcohol.

Heat prostration can occur at high ambient temperatures, due to decreased sweating.

4.5 Interaction with other medicinal products and other forms of Interaction
The antimuscarinic side-effects can be increased by concomitant administration of disopyramide, tricyclic and MAOI drugs, antihistamines, phenothiazines, amantadine and alcohol. Reduced effect of sub-lingual nitrates.

4.6 Pregnancy and lactation
Use of hyoscine during pregnancy may cause respiratory depression in the neonate, and should only be given during pregnancy when the potential benefit clearly outweighs the foetal hazard.

4.7 Effects on ability to drive and use machines
Because hyoscine may cause drowsiness, patients must not drive or operate machinery.

4.8 Undesirable effects
The most common side effects are drowsiness, dry mouth, dizziness, blurred vision and difficulty with micturition. Other reported effects include bradycardia, idiosyncratic reactions and mental confusion or excitement.

4.9 Overdose
Symptoms of overdose may include dilated pupils, tachycardia, rapid respiration, hyperpyrexia, restlessness, excitement, delirium and hallucinations. In the unlikely event of overdosage, supportive therapy should be implemented. Physostigmine by slow intravenous injection in a dose of 1 to 4mg has been used to reverse the anticholinergic effects, but this drug is rapidly metabolised. Neostigmine by slow intravenous injection in a dose of 0.5 to 2 mg antagonises only the peripheral effects. Diazepam may be given to control excitement.

5. PHARMACOLOGICAL PROPERTIES

5.1 Pharmacodynamic properties
Hyoscine is an anticholinergic drug which inhibits the muscarinic actions of acetylcholine at post-ganglionic parasympathetic neuroeffector sites including smooth muscle, secretory glands and CNS sites. Small doses effectively inhibit salivary and bronchial secretions and sweating and provide a degree of amnesia. Hyoscine is a more powerful suppressor of salivation than atropine and usually slows rather than increases heart rate.

5.2 Pharmacokinetic properties
Hyoscine is rapidly absorbed following IV or IM injection and is reversibly bound to plasma protein. Hyoscine is reported to cross the placenta and blood brain barrier. Hyoscine is almost completely metabolised by the liver and excreted in the urine. In one study in man, 3.4% of a single dose, administered by subcutaneous injection was excreted unchanged in urine within 72 hours.

5.3 Preclinical safety data
None stated

6. PHARMACEUTICAL PARTICULARS

6.1 List of excipients
Hydrobromic acid (47%)

Sodium hydroxide

Water for injections

6.2 Incompatibilities
None stated

6.3 Shelf life
24 months

6.4 Special precautions for storage
Do not store above 25°C

Store in the original container.

6.5 Nature and contents of container
1ml neutral glass (Type I) ampoules in packs of 5 or 10.

6.6 Instructions for use and handling
None stated.

Administrative Data

7. MARKETING AUTHORISATION HOLDER
CP Pharmaceuticals Ltd

Ash Road North

Wrexham

LL13 9UF

UK

8. MARKETING AUTHORISATION NUMBER(S)
PL 4543/0454

9. DATE OF FIRST AUTHORISATION/RENEWAL OF THE AUTHORISATION
30 June 2005

10. DATE OF REVISION OF THE TEXT

Hyoscine Hydrobromide 600 micrograms/ml Solution for Injection

(Wockhardt UK Ltd)

1. NAME OF THE MEDICINAL PRODUCT
Hyoscine Hydrobromide 600 micrograms/ml Solution for Injection

2. QUALITATIVE AND QUANTITATIVE COMPOSITION
Each 1ml ampoule contains 600 micrograms of hyoscine hydrobromide.

For excipients, see 6.1.

3. PHARMACEUTICAL FORM
Solution for Injection.

A clear colourless solution, practically free from particles.

4. CLINICAL PARTICULARS

4.1 Therapeutic indications
Due to its anticholinergic activity, hyoscine injection is used as a preoperative medication to control bronchial, nasal, pharyngeal and salivary secretions, to prevent bronchospasm and laryngospasm and to block cardiac vagal inhibiting reflexes during induction of anaesthesia and intubation.

4.2 Posology and method of administration
Dosage

Adults

For pre-medication a dose of 200 to 600 micrograms is given by the subcutaneous or intramuscular route 30 to 60 minutes before induction of anaesthesia.

The injection may if required also be given by the intravenous route for acute use.

Children

A dose of 15 micrograms/kg is recommended in children.

Elderly

Hyoscine is not recommended for use in the elderly.

4.3 Contraindications
Hypersensitivity to hyoscine. Narrow angle glaucoma.

4.4 Special warnings and special precautions for use
Caution is necessary in treating patients with cardiovascular disease, gastrointestinal obstruction, paralytic ileus, prostatic enlargement, Down's Syndrome, myasthenia gravis, renal or hepatic impairment.

Because hyoscine may cause drowsiness, patients must not drive or operate machinery. Patients should avoid alcohol.

Heat prostration can occur at high ambient temperatures, due to decreased sweating.

4.5 Interaction with other medicinal products and other forms of Interaction
The antimuscarinic side-effects can be increased by concomitant administration of disopyramide, tricyclic and MAOI drugs, antihistamines, phenothiazines, amantadine and alcohol. Reduced effect of sub-lingual nitrates.

4.6 Pregnancy and lactation
Use of hyoscine during pregnancy may cause respiratory depression in the neonate, and should only be given during pregnancy when the potential benefit clearly outweighs the foetal hazard.

4.7 Effects on ability to drive and use machines
Because hyoscine may cause drowsiness, patients must not drive or operate machinery.

4.8 Undesirable effects
The most common side effects are drowsiness, dry mouth, dizziness, blurred vision and difficulty with micturition. Other reported effects include bradycardia, idiosyncratic reactions and mental confusion or excitement.

4.9 Overdose
Symptoms of overdose may include dilated pupils, tachycardia, rapid respiration, hyperpyrexia, restlessness, excitement, delirium and hallucinations. In the unlikely event of overdosage, supportive therapy should be implemented. Physostigmine by slow intravenous injection in a dose of 1 to 4mg has been used to reverse the anticholinergic effects, but this drug is rapidly metabolised. Neostigmine by slow intravenous injection in a dose of 0.5 to 2 mg antagonises only the peripheral effects. Diazepam may be given to control excitement.

5. PHARMACOLOGICAL PROPERTIES

5.1 Pharmacodynamic properties
Hyoscine is an anticholinergic drug which inhibits the muscarinic actions of acetylcholine at post-ganglionic parasympathetic neuroeffector sites including smooth muscle, secretory glands and CNS sites. Small doses effectively inhibit salivary and bronchial secretions and sweating and provide a degree of amnesia. Hyoscine is a more powerful suppressor of salivation than atropine and usually slows rather than increases heart rate.

5.2 Pharmacokinetic properties
Hyoscine is rapidly absorbed following IV or IM injection and is reversibly bound to plasma protein. Hyoscine is reported to cross the placenta and blood brain barrier. Hyoscine is almost completely metabolised by the liver and excreted in the urine. In one study in man, 3.4% of a single dose, administered by subcutaneous injection was excreted unchanged in urine within 72 hours.

5.3 Preclinical safety data
None stated

6. PHARMACEUTICAL PARTICULARS

6.1 List of excipients
Hydrobromic acid (47%)

Sodium hydroxide

Water for injections

6.2 Incompatibilities
None stated

6.3 Shelf life
24 months

6.4 Special precautions for storage
Do not store above 25°C

Store in the original container.

6.5 Nature and contents of container
1ml neutral glass (Type I) ampoules in packs of 5 or 10.

6.6 Instructions for use and handling
None stated.

Administrative Data

7. MARKETING AUTHORISATION HOLDER
CP Pharmaceuticals Ltd

Ash Road North

Wrexham

LL13 9UF

UK

8. MARKETING AUTHORISATION NUMBER(S)
PL 4543/0455

9. DATE OF FIRST AUTHORISATION/RENEWAL OF THE AUTHORISATION
30 June 2005

10. DATE OF REVISION OF THE TEXT

Hyoscine Injection BP 400mcg/ml

(UCB Pharma Limited)

1. NAME OF THE MEDICINAL PRODUCT
Hyoscine Injection BP 400mcg/ml

2. QUALITATIVE AND QUANTITATIVE COMPOSITION
Hyoscine hydrobromide EP 0.04% w/v

For excipients, see 6.1

3. PHARMACEUTICAL FORM
Solution for Injection

4. CLINICAL PARTICULARS

4.1 Therapeutic indications
Due to its anticholinergic activity, hyoscine injection is used as a preoperative medication to control bronchial, nasal pharyngeal and salivary secretions, to prevent bronchospasms and laryngospasm and to block cardiac vagal inhibiting reflexes during induction of anaesthesia and intubation.

4.2 Posology and method of administration
Adults: For pre-medication a dose of 200 to 600 micrograms is given by the subcutaneous or intramuscular route 30 to 60 minutes before induction of anaesthesia.

The injection may if required also be given by the intravenous route for acute use.

Children: A dose of 15mcg/kg is recommended in children.

Elderly: Hyoscine is not recommended for use in the elderly.

4.3 Contraindications
Porphyria; hypersensitivity to hyoscine; narrow angle glaucoma.

4.4 Special warnings and special precautions for use
Caution is necessary in treating patients with cardiovascular disease, gastrointestinal obstruction, paralytic ileus, prostatic enlargement, Down's Syndrome, myasthenia gravis, renal or hepatic impairment.

Because hyoscine may cause drowsiness, patients must not drive or operate machinery. Patients should avoid alcohol.

Heat prostration can occur, at high ambient temperatures due to decreased sweating.

There have been rare reports of an increase in frequency of seizures in epileptic patients.

4.5 Interaction with other medicinal products and other forms of Interaction
The antimuscarinic side-effect can be increased by concomitant administration of disopyramide, tricyclic and

MAOI drugs, antihistamines, phenothiazines, amantadine and alcohol. Reduced effect of sub-lingual nitrates.

4.6 Pregnancy and lactation

Use of hyoscine during pregnancy may cause respiratory depression in the neonate, and should only be given during pregnancy when the potential benefit clearly outweighs the foetal hazard.

4.7 Effects on ability to drive and use machines

Because hyoscine may cause drowsiness, patients must not drive or operate machinery.

4.8 Undesirable effects

The most common side effects are drowsiness, dry mouth, dizziness, blurred vision and difficulty with micturition. Other reported effects include bradycardia, idiosyncratic reactions and mental confusion or excitement.

4.9 Overdose

Symptoms of overdose may include dilated pupils, tachycardia, rapid respiration, hyperpyrexia, restlessness, excitement, delirium and hallucinations. In the unlikely event of overdosage, supportive therapy should be implemented. Physostigmine by slow intravenous injection in a dose of 1 to 4mg has been used to reverse the anticholinergic effects, but this drug is rapidly metabolised. Neostigmine by slow intravenous injection in a dose of 0.5 to 2 mg antagonises only the peripheral effects. Diazepam may be given to control excitement.

5. PHARMACOLOGICAL PROPERTIES

5.1 Pharmacodynamic properties

Hyoscine is an anticholinergic drug which inhibits the muscarinic actions of acetylcholine at post ganglionic parasympathetic neuroeffector sites including smooth muscle, secretary glands and CNS sites. Small doses effectively inhibit salivary and bronchial secretions and sweating and provide a degree of amnesia. Hyoscine is a more powerful suppressor of salivation than atropine and usually slows rather than increases heart rate.

5.2 Pharmacokinetic properties

Hyoscine is rapidly absorbed following IV or IM injection and is reversibly bound to plasma protein. Hyoscine is reported to cross the placenta and blood brain barrier. Hyoscine is almost completely metabolised by the liver and excreted in the urine. In one study in man, 3.4% of a single dose, administered by subcutaneous injection was excreted unchanged in urine within 72 hours.

5.3 Preclinical safety data

None stated.

6. PHARMACEUTICAL PARTICULARS

6.1 List of excipients

Hydrobromic acid

Sodium hydroxide

Water for Injections

6.2 Incompatibilities

None stated.

6.3 Shelf life

36 months.

6.4 Special precautions for storage

Store below 25°C and protect from light.

6.5 Nature and contents of container

1ml neutral glass (Type I) ampoules in packs of 5 or 10.

Not all pack sizes may be marketed.

6.6 Instructions for use and handling

None stated.

7. MARKETING AUTHORISATION HOLDER

UCB Pharma Limited

208 Bath Road

Slough

Berkshire

SL1 3WE

UK

8. MARKETING AUTHORISATION NUMBER(S)

PL 00039/5677R

9. DATE OF FIRST AUTHORISATION/RENEWAL OF THE AUTHORISATION

Granted: 5 June 1987

Renewed: 17 June 1993

10 November 1998

10. DATE OF REVISION OF THE TEXT

June 2005

11. Legal Category

POM

Hypnomidate

(Janssen-Cilag Ltd)

1. NAME OF THE MEDICINAL PRODUCT

Hypnomidate®

2. QUALITATIVE AND QUANTITATIVE COMPOSITION

Each ml of Hypnomidate contains etomidate 2 mg.

3. PHARMACEUTICAL FORM

Injection.

4. CLINICAL PARTICULARS

4.1 Therapeutic indications

Hypnomidate is an intravenous induction agent of anaesthesia.

4.2 Posology and method of administration

For intravenous administration.

Adults and children:

A dose of 0.3 mg/kg given intravenously at induction of anaesthesia, gives sleep lasting from 6 to 10 minutes.

Elderly:

A dose of 0.15-0.2 mg/kg bodyweight should be given and the dose should be further adjusted according to effects.

Since Hypnomidate has no analgesic action, appropriate analgesics should be used in procedures involving painful stimuli.

Do not exceed a total dose of 30 ml (3 ampoules).

Hypnomidate should only be given by slow intravenous injection.

Hypnomidate may be diluted with sodium chloride infusion BP or dextrose infusion BP but it is not compatible with compound sodium lactate infusion BP (Hartmann's solution). Combinations with pancuronium bromide may show a very slight opalescence; for this reason the two should not be mixed together.

4.3 Contraindications

Hypnomidate is contra-indicated in patients with known hypersensitivity to etomidate.

4.4 Special warnings and special precautions for use

Warnings: In patients with liver cirrhosis, or in those who have already received neuroleptic, opiate or sedative agents, the dose of etomidate should be reduced.

When Hypnomidate is used, resuscitation equipment should be readily available to manage apnoea. In cases of adrenocortical gland dysfunction and during very long surgical procedures, a prophylactic cortisol supplement may be required (for example 50 to 100 mg hydrocortisone).

Reduced serum cortisol levels, unresponsive to ACTH injections, have been reported in some patients during induction of anaesthesia but particularly during maintenance of anaesthesia with etomidate; for this reason etomidate should not be used for maintenance. However, when etomidate is used for induction, the post-operative rise in serum cortisol which has been observed after thiopentone induction is delayed for approximately 3-6 hours.

Hypnomidate should not be administered to patients with evidence or suggestion of reduced adrenal cortical function.

Convulsions may occur in unpremedicated patients.

Precautions: Hypnomidate by injection should be given slowly.

4.5 Interaction with other medicinal products and other forms of Interaction

Sedative drugs potentiate the hypnotic effect of Hypnomidate.

Hypnomidate is pharmacologically compatible with the muscle relaxants, premedicant drugs and inhalation anaesthetics in current clinical use.

4.6 Pregnancy and lactation

Hypnomidate has no primary effect on fertility, nor primary embryotoxic or teratogenic effects. At maternally toxic doses in rats, decreased survival was noted. Safety in human pregnancy has not been established. As with other drugs, the possible risks should be weighed against the potential benefits before the drug is administered during pregnancy. Hypnomidate may cross the placental barrier during obstetric anaesthesia.

Lactation: It is not known whether etomidate is excreted in human milk. However, caution should be exercised when Hypnomidate is administered to a nursing mother.

4.7 Effects on ability to drive and use machines

Not applicable, but no effects likely. After very short surgical procedures (up to 15 minutes) the patient regains normal alertness 30 to 60 minutes after waking. After long operations, normal alertness is regained after 4 to 24 hours, depending on the duration of the operation.

4.8 Undesirable effects

The use of narcotic analgesics or diazepam as premedication and during surgery will reduce the uncontrolled spontaneous muscle movements shown by some patients after Hypnomidate administration.

Pain can occur after injection into the small veins of the dorsum of the hand. Use of larger veins or an intravenous application of a small dose of fentanyl 1-2 minutes before induction reduces pain on injection. In a small number of patients, thrombophlebitis has been reported.

Nausea and/or vomiting may occur although these are mainly as a result of concurrent use of opiates. Coughing, hiccough and/or shivering may also be experienced. Allergic reactions, including rare cases of bronchospasm and anaphylactoid reactions, have been reported. Rare cases of laryngospasm, cardiac arrhythmias and convulsions have also been reported.

A slight and transient drop in blood pressure may occur due to a reduction of the peripheral vascular resistance. In vulnerable patients, special care should be exercised to minimise this effect.

Respiratory depression and apnoea may occur.

4.9 Overdose

Overdosing is likely to result in prolonged anaesthesia with the possibility of respiratory depression and even arrest. Hypotension has also been observed. General supportive measures and close observation are recommended. In addition, administration of 50 -100 mg hydrocortisone (not ACTH) may be required for depression of cortisol secretion.

5. PHARMACOLOGICAL PROPERTIES

5.1 Pharmacodynamic properties

Etomidate is a short acting intravenous hypnotic with a broad safety margin. It is characterised by extremely slight effects on cardiac function and circulation and is rapidly inactivated by enzyme metabolism so that it does not give rise to a hangover effect. It does not release histamine, and has no effect on liver function. *In vitro* studies have shown etomidate to be an inhibitor of microsomal enzymes. Limited *in vivo* studies have demonstrated only minimal inhibition of hepatic metabolism.

5.2 Pharmacokinetic properties

After injection, etomidate is rapidly distributed to other body tissues. Plasma concentrations decrease rapidly for about 30 minutes and then more slowly; traces are still detectable after 6 hours. Metabolites, chiefly of hydrolysis, are more slowly excreted.

Etomidate is extensively (about 76%) bound to plasma proteins; metabolites are less extensively bound.

About 75% of a dose is excreted in the urine in 24 hours.

5.3 Preclinical safety data

No relevant information other than that contained elsewhere in the Summary of Product Characteristics.

6. PHARMACEUTICAL PARTICULARS

6.1 List of excipients

Propylene glycol

Water for injections

1N sodium hydroxide*

1N hydrochloric acid*

* for occasional pH adjustment only

6.2 Incompatibilities

Combinations with pancuronium bromide may show a very slight opalescence; for this reason the two should not be mixed together.

6.3 Shelf life

5 years.

6.4 Special precautions for storage

Store at room temperature.

6.5 Nature and contents of container

Colourless glass ampoule, PhEur Type I, containing 10 ml Hypnomidate, in packs of 5 ampoules.

6.6 Instructions for use and handling

None stated.

Administrative Data

7. MARKETING AUTHORISATION HOLDER

Janssen-Cilag Limited

Saunderton

High Wycombe

Buckinghamshire

HP14 4HJ

UK

8. MARKETING AUTHORISATION NUMBER(S)

PL 0242/0019

9. DATE OF FIRST AUTHORISATION/RENEWAL OF THE AUTHORISATION

27 October 1978/20 March 1999

10. DATE OF REVISION OF THE TEXT

May 2002

Legal category POM

Hypnovel 10mg/2ml

(Roche Products Limited)

1. NAME OF THE MEDICINAL PRODUCT

Hypnovel Ampoules 10mg/2ml

2. QUALITATIVE AND QUANTITATIVE COMPOSITION

Active ingredient: midazolam as hydrochloride.

Ampoules 10mg/2ml; for i.v., i.m. and rectal administration.

For excipients, see *6.1*.

3. PHARMACEUTICAL FORM

Solution for injection.

4. CLINICAL PARTICULARS

4.1 Therapeutic indications

Hypnovel is a short-acting sleep-inducing drug that is indicated:

In adults

- ***Conscious sedation*** before and during diagnostic or therapeutic procedures with or without local anaesthesia.
- ***Anaesthesia***
  - Premedication before induction of anaesthesia.
  - Induction of anaesthesia.
  - As an induction agent or as a sedative component in combined anaesthesia.
- ***Sedation in intensive care units***

In children

- ***Conscious sedation*** before and during diagnostic or therapeutic procedures with or without local anaesthesia.
- ***Anaesthesia***
  - Premedication before induction of anaesthesia.
- ***Sedation in intensive care units***

4.2 Posology and method of administration

STANDARD DOSAGE

Midazolam is a potent sedative agent that requires titration and slow administration. Titration is strongly recommended to safely obtain the desired level of sedation according to the clinical need, physical status, age and concomitant medication. In adults over 60 years, debilitated or chronically ill patients and paediatric patients, dose should be determined with caution and risk factors related to each patient should be taken into account. Standard dosages are provided in the table below. Additional details are provided in the text following the table.

(see Table 1)

Conscious sedation dosage

For conscious sedation prior to diagnostic or surgical intervention, midazolam is administered i.v. The dose must be individualised and titrated, and should not be administered by rapid or single bolus injection. The onset of sedation may vary individually depending on the physical status of the patient and the detailed circumstances of dosing (e.g. speed of administration, amount of dose). If necessary, subsequent doses may be administered according to the individual need. The onset of action is about 2 minutes after the injection. Maximum effect is obtained in about 5 to 10 minutes.

Adults

The i.v. injection of midazolam should be given slowly at a rate of approximately 1mg in 30 seconds. In adults below the age of 60 the initial dose is 2 to 2.5mg given 5 to10 minutes before the beginning of the procedure. Further doses of 1mg may be given as necessary. Mean total doses have been found to range from 3.5 to 7.5mg. A total dose greater than 5mg is usually not necessary. In adults over 60 years of age, debilitated or chronically ill patients, start by administering a dose of 0.5 to 1mg. Further doses of 0.5 to 1mg may be given as necessary. A total dose greater than 3.5mg is usually not necessary.

Children

I.V. administration: midazolam should be titrated slowly to the desired clinical effect. The initial dose of midazolam should be administered over 2 to 3 minutes. One must wait an additional 2 to 5 minutes to fully evaluate the sedative effect before initiating a procedure or repeating a dose. If further sedation is necessary, continue to titrate with small increments until the appropriate level of sedation is achieved. Infants and young children less than 5 years of age may require substantially higher doses (mg/kg) than older children and adolescents.

- Paediatric patients less than 6 months of age: paediatric patients less than 6 months of age are particularly vulnerable to airway obstruction and hypoventilation. For this reason, the use in conscious sedation in children less than 6 months of age is not recommended.
- Paediatric patients 6 months to 5 years of age: initial dose 0.05 to 0.1mg/kg. A total dose up to 0.6mg/kg may be necessary to reach the desired endpoint, but the total dose should not exceed 6mg. Prolonged sedation and risk of hypoventilation may be associated with the higher doses.
- Paediatric patients 6 to 12 years of age: initial dose 0.025 to 0.05mg/kg. A total dose of up to 0.4mg/kg to a maximum of 10mg may be necessary. Prolonged sedation and risk of hypoventilation may be associated with the higher doses.
- Paediatric patients 12 to 16 years of age: should be dosed as adults.

Rectal administration: the total dose of midazolam usually ranges from 0.3 to 0.5mg/kg. Rectal administration of the ampoule solution is performed by means of a plastic applicator fixed on the end of the syringe. If the volume to be administered is too small, water may be added up to a total volume of 10ml. Total dose should be administered at once and repeated rectal administration avoided.

The use in children less than 6 months of age is not recommended, as available data in this population are limited.

I.M. administration: the doses used range between 0.05 and 0.15mg/kg. A total dose greater than 10.0mg is usually not necessary. This route should only be used in exceptional cases. Rectal administration should be preferred as i.m. injection is painful.

In children less than 15kg of body weight, midazolam solutions with concentrations higher than 1mg/ml are not recommended. Higher concentrations should be diluted to 1mg/ml.

ANAESTHESIA DOSAGE

Premedication

Premedication with midazolam given shortly before a procedure produces sedation (induction of sleepiness or drowsiness and relief of apprehension) and pre-operative impairment of memory. Midazolam can also be administered in combination with anticholinergics. For this indication midazolam should be administered i.m., deep into a large muscle mass 20 to 60 minutes before induction of anaesthesia, or preferably via the rectal route in children (see below). Adequate observation of the patient after administration of premedication is mandatory as inter-individual sensitivity varies and symptoms of overdose may occur.

Adults

For pre-operative sedation and to impair memory of pre-operative events, the recommended dose for adults of ASA Physical Status I & II and below 60 years is 0.07 to 0.1mg/kg administered i.m. The dose must be reduced and individualised when midazolam is administered to adults over 60 years of age, debilitated, or chronically ill patients. A dose of 0.025 to 0.05mg/kg administered i.m. is recommended. The usual dose is 2 to 3mg.

Children

Rectal administration: The total dose of midazolam, usually ranging from 0.3 to 0.5mg/kg should be administered 15 to 30 minutes before induction of anaesthesia. Rectal administration of the ampoule solution is performed by means of a plastic applicator fixed on the end of the syringe. If the volume to be administered is too small, water may be added up to a total volume of 10ml.

I.M. administration: As i.m. injection is painful, this route should only be used in exceptional cases. Rectal administration should be preferred. However, a dose range from 0.08 to 0.2mg/kg of midazolam administered i.m. has been shown to be effective and safe. In children between ages 1 and 15 years, proportionally higher doses are required than in adults in relation to body-weight.

The use in children less than 6 months of age is not recommended as available data are limited.

In children less than 15kg of body weight, midazolam solutions with concentrations higher than 1mg/ml are not recommended. Higher concentrations should be diluted to 1mg/ml.

Induction

Adults

If midazolam is used for induction of anaesthesia before other anaesthetic agents have been administered, the individual response is variable. The dose should be titrated to the desired effect according to the patient's age and clinical status. When midazolam is used before or in combination with other i.v. or inhalation agents for induction of anaesthesia, the initial dose of each agent should be significantly reduced. The desired level of anaesthesia is reached by stepwise titration. The i.v. induction dose of midazolam should be given slowly in increments. Each increment of not more than 5mg should be injected over 20 to 30 seconds allowing 2 minutes between successive increments.

- In adults below the age of 60 years, an i.v. dose of 0.15 to 0.2mg/kg will usually suffice. In non-premedicated adults below the age of 60 the dose may be higher (0.3 to 0.35mg/kg i.v.). If needed to complete induction, increments of approximately 25% of the patient's initial dose may be used. Induction may instead be completed with inhalational anaesthetics. In resistant cases, a total dose of up to 0.6mg/kg may be used for induction, but such larger doses may prolong recovery.
- In adults over 60 years of age, debilitated or chronically ill patients, the dose is 0.1 to 0.2mg/kg administered i.v. Non-premedicated adults over 60 years of age usually require more midazolam for induction; an initial dose of 0.15 to 0.3mg/kg is recommended. Non-premedicated patients with severe systemic disease or other debilitation usually require less midazolam for induction. An initial dose of 0.15 to 0.25mg/kg will usually suffice.

Sedative component in combined anaesthesia

Adults

Midazolam can be given as a sedative component in combined anaesthesia by either further intermittent small i.v. doses (range between 0.03 and 0.1mg/kg) or continuous infusion of i.v. midazolam (range between 0.03 and 0.1mg/kg/h) typically in combination with analgesics. The dose and the intervals between doses vary according to the patient's individual reaction.

In adults over 60 years of age, debilitated or chronically ill patients, lower maintenance doses will be required.

Sedation in intensive care units

The desired level of sedation is reached by stepwise titration of midazolam followed by either continuous infusion or intermittent bolus, according to the clinical need, physical status, age and concomitant medication (see *4.5 Interaction with other medicinal products and other forms of interaction*).

Adults

I.V. loading dose: 0.03 to 0.3mg/kg should be given slowly in increments. Each increment of 1 to 2.5mg should be injected over 20 to 30 seconds allowing 2 minutes between successive increments. In hypovolaemic, vasoconstricted, or hypothermic patients the loading dose should be reduced or omitted. When midazolam is given with potent analgesics, the latter should be administered first so that

Table 1

Indication	Adults < 60 y	Adults ≥ 60 y / debilitated or chronically ill	Children
Conscious sedation	***i.v.*** Initial dose: 2 - 2.5mg Titration doses: 1mg Total dose: 3.5 - 7.5mg	***i.v*** Initial dose: 0.5 - 1mg Titration doses: 0.5 - 1mg Total dose: < 3.5mg	***i.v. in patients 6 months - 5 years*** Initial dose: 0.05 - 0.1mg/kg Total dose: < 6mg ***i.v. in patients 6-12 years*** Initial dose: 0.025 - 0.05mg/kg Total dose: < 10mg ***rectal> 6 months*** 0.3 - 0.5mg/kg ***i.m. 1 - 15 years*** 0.05 - 0.15mg/kg
Anaesthesia premedication	***i.m.*** 0.07 - 0.1mg/kg	***i.m.*** 0.025 - 0.05mg/kg	***rectal > 6 months*** 0.3 - 0.5mg/kg ***i.m. 1 - 15 years*** 0.08 - 0.2mg/kg
Anaesthesia induction	***i.v.*** 0.15 - 0.2mg/kg (0.3 -0.35 without premedication)	***i.v.*** 0.1 - 0.2mg/kg (0.15 -0.3 without premedication)	
Sedative component in combined anaesthesia	***i.v.*** intermittent doses of 0.03 - 0.1mg/kg or continuous infusion of 0.03-0.1mg/kg/h	***i.v.*** lower doses than recommended for adults < 60 years	
Sedation in ICU	***i.v.*** Loading dose: 0.03 - 0.3mg/kg in increments of 1 - 2.5mg Maintenance dose: 0.03 - 0.2mg/kg/h		***i.v. in neonates < 32 weeks gestational age*** 0.03mg/kg/h ***i.v in neonates > 32 weeks and children up to 6 months*** 0.06mg/kg/h ***i.v. in patients> 6 months of age*** Loading dose: 0.05 - 0.2mg/kg Maintenance dose: 0.06 - 0.12mg/kg/h

the sedative effects of midazolam can be safely titrated on top of any sedation caused by the analgesic.

I.V. maintenance dose: doses can range from 0.03 to 0.2mg/kg/h. In hypovolaemic, vasoconstricted, or hypothermic patients the maintenance dose should be reduced. The level of sedation should be assessed regularly. With long-term sedation, tolerance may develop and the dose may have to be increased.

Children over 6 months of age

In intubated and ventilated paediatric patients, a loading dose of 0.05 to 0.2mg/kg i.v. should be administered slowly over at least 2 to 3 minutes to establish the desired clinical effect. Midazolam should not be administered as a rapid intravenous dose. The loading dose is followed by a continuous i.v. infusion at 0.06 to 0.12mg/kg/h (1 to 2μg/kg/min). The rate of infusion can be increased or decreased (generally by 25% of the initial or subsequent infusion rate) as required, or supplemental i.v. doses of midazolam can be administered to increase or maintain the desired effect.

When initiating an infusion with midazolam in haemodynamically compromised patients, the usual loading dose should be titrated in small increments and the patient monitored for haemodynamic instability, e.g., hypotension. These patients are also vulnerable to the respiratory depressant effects of midazolam and require careful monitoring of respiratory rate and oxygen saturation.

Neonates and children up to 6 months of age

Midazolam should be given as a continuous i.v. infusion, starting at 0.03mg/kg/h (0.5μg/kg/min) in neonates with a gestational age $<$ 32 weeks or 0.06mg/kg/h (1μg/kg/min) in neonates with a gestational age $>$ 32 weeks and children up to 6 months.

Intravenous loading doses is not recommended in premature infants, neonates and children up to 6 months, rather the infusion may be run more rapidly for the first several hours to establish therapeutic plasma levels. The rate of infusion should be carefully and frequently reassessed, particularly after the first 24 hours so as to administer the lowest possible effective dose and reduce the potential for drug accumulation.

Careful monitoring of respiratory rate and oxygen saturation is required.

In premature infants, neonates and children less than 15 kg of body weight, midazolam solutions with concentrations higher than 1mg/ml are not recommended. Higher concentrations should be diluted to 1mg/ml.

4.3 Contraindications

Use of this drug in patients with known hypersensitivity to benzodiazepines or to any component of the product.

Use of this drug for conscious sedation in patients with severe respiratory failure or acute respiratory depression.

4.4 Special warnings and special precautions for use

Midazolam should be used only when age- and size-appropriate resuscitation facilities are available, as i.v. administration of midazolam may depress myocardial contractility and cause apnoea. Severe cardiorespiratory adverse events have occurred on rare occasions. These have included respiratory depression, apnoea, respiratory arrest and/or cardiac arrest. Such life-threatening incidents are more likely to occur when the injection is given too rapidly or when a high dosage is administered. Paediatric patients less than 6 months of age are particularly vulnerable to airway obstruction and hypoventilation, therefore titration with small increments to clinical effect and careful respiratory rate and oxygen saturation monitoring are essential.

When midazolam is used for premedication, adequate observation of the patient after administration is mandatory as inter-individual sensitivity varies and symptoms of overdose may occur.

Special caution should be exercised when administering midazolam to high-risk patients:

- adults over 60 years of age
- chronically ill or debilitated patients, e.g.
- patients with chronic respiratory insufficiency
- patients with chronic renal failure, impaired hepatic function or with impaired cardiac function
- paediatric patients specially those with cardiovascular instability.

These high-risk patients require lower dosages (see *4.2 Posology and method of administration*) and should be continuously monitored for early signs of alterations of vital functions.

Benzodiazepines should be used with caution in patients with a history of alcohol or drug abuse.

As with any substance with CNS depressant and/or muscle-relaxant properties, particular care should be taken when administering midazolam to a patient with myasthenia gravis.

Tolerance

Some loss of efficacy has been reported when midazolam was used as long-term sedation in intensive care units (ICU).

Dependence

When midazolam is used in long-term sedation in ICU, it should be borne in mind that physical dependence on midazolam may develop. The risk of dependence increases with dose and duration of treatment.

Withdrawal symptoms

During prolonged treatment with midazolam in ICU, physical dependence may develop. Therefore, abrupt termination of the treatment will be accompanied by withdrawal symptoms. The following symptoms may occur: headaches, muscle pain, anxiety, tension, restlessness, confusion, irritability, rebound insomnia, mood changes, hallucinations and convulsions. Since the risk of withdrawal symptoms is greater after abrupt discontinuation of treatment, it is recommended to decrease doses gradually.

Amnesia

Midazolam causes anterograde amnesia (frequently this effect is very desirable in situations such as before and during surgical and diagnostic procedures), the duration of which is directly related to the administered dose. Prolonged amnesia can present problems in outpatients, who are scheduled for discharge following intervention. After receiving midazolam parenterally, patients should be discharged from hospital or consulting room only if accompanied by an attendant.

Paradoxical reactions

Paradoxical reactions such as agitation, involuntary movements (including tonic/clonic convulsions and muscle tremor), hyperactivity, hostility, rage reaction, aggressiveness, paroxysmal excitement and assault, have been reported to occur with midazolam. These reactions may occur with high doses and/or when the injection is given rapidly. The highest incidence to such reactions has been reported among children and the elderly.

Delayed elimination of midazolam

Midazolam elimination may be altered in patients receiving compounds that inhibit or induce CYP3A4 (see 4.5 *Interaction with other medicaments and other forms of interaction*).

Midazolam elimination may also be delayed in patients with liver dysfunction, low cardiac output and in neonates (see *5.2 Pharmacokinetics in special populations*).

Preterm infants and neonates

Due to an increased risk of apnoea, extreme caution is advised when sedating pre-term and former pre-term patients. Careful monitoring of respiratory rate and oxygen saturation is required.

Rapid injection should be avoided in the neonatal population.

Neonates have reduced and/or immature organ function and are also vulnerable to profound and/or prolonged respiratory effects of midazolam.

Adverse haemodynamic events have been reported in paediatric patients with cardiovascular instability; rapid intravenous administration should be avoided in this population.

4.5 Interaction with other medicinal products and other forms of Interaction

The metabolism of midazolam is almost exclusively mediated by the isoenzyme CYP3A4 of the cytochrome P450 (CYP450). CYP3A4 inhibitors (see *4.4 Special warnings and precautions for use*) and inducers, but also other active substances (see below), may lead to drug-drug interactions with midazolam.

Since midazolam undergoes significant first pass effect, parenteral midazolam would theoretically be less affected by metabolic interactions and clinical relevant consequences should be limited.

- Itraconazole, fluconazole and ketoconazole

Co-administration of oral midazolam and some azole antifungals (itraconazole, fluconazole, ketokonazole) increased markedly midazolam plasma levels and prolonged its elimination half-life, leading to major impairment of psychosedative tests. Elimination half-lives were increased from 3 to 8 hours approximately.

When a single bolus dose of midazolam was given for short-term sedation, the effect of midazolam was not enhanced or prolonged to a clinically significant degree by itraconazole, and dosage reduction is therefore not required. However, administration of high doses or long-term infusions of midazolam to patients receiving itraconazole, fluconazole or ketoconazole, e.g. during intensive care treatment, may result in long-lasting hypnotic effects, possible delayed recovery, and possible respiratory depression, thus requiring dose adjustments.

- Verapamil and diltiazem

No *in vivo* interaction studies are available with intravenous midazolam and verapamil or diltiazem.

However, as expected, oral midazolam pharmacokinetics varied in a clinically significant way when combined to these calcium channel blockers, notably with almost a doubling of half-life value and peak plasma level, resulting in a strongly reduced performance in co-ordination and cognitive function tests while producing profound sedation. When oral midazolam is used, dosage adjustment is usually recommended. Although no clinically significant interaction is expected with midazolam used for short-term sedation, caution should be exercised if intravenous midazolam is concomitantly given with verapamil or diltiazem.

- Macrolide Antibiotics: Erythromycin and clarithromycin

Co-administration of oral midazolam and erythromycin or clarithromycin significantly increased the AUC of midazolam about four fold and more than doubled the elimination half-life of midazolam, depending on the study. Marked changes in psychomotor tests were observed and it is advised to adjust doses of midazolam, if given orally, due to significantly delayed recovery.

When a single bolus dose of midazolam was given for short-term sedation, the effect of midazolam was not enhanced or prolonged to a clinically significant degree by erythromycin, although a significant decrease in plasma clearance was recorded. Caution should be exercised if intravenous midazolam is concomitantly given with erythromycin or clarithromycin. No clinical significant interaction has been shown with midazolam and other macrolide antibiotics.

- Cimetidine and ranitidine

Co-administration of cimetidine (at doses equal or higher than 800mg/day) and intravenous midazolam slightly increased the steady-state plasma concentration of midazolam, which could possibly lead to a delayed recovery, whereas co-administration of ranitidine had no effect. Cimetidine and ranitidine did not affect oral midazolam pharmacokinetics. These data indicate that intravenous midazolam can be administered at usual doses of cimetidine (i.e. 400mg/day) and ranitidine without dosage adjustment.

- Saquinavir

Co-administration of a single intravenous dose of 0.05mg/kg midazolam after 3 or 5 days of saquinavir dosing (1200mg t.i.d) to 12 healthy volunteers decreased the midazolam clearance by 56% and increased the elimination half-life from 4.1 to 9.5 h. Only the subjective effects to midazolam (visual analogue scales with the item "overall drug effect") were intensified by saquinavir.

Therefore, a single bolus dose of intravenous midazolam can be given in combination with saquinavir. Nevertheless, during a prolonged midazolam infusion, a total dose reduction is recommended to avoid delayed recovery (see *4.4 Special warnings and precautions for use*).

- Other protease inhibitors: ritonavir, indinavir, nelfinavir and amprenavir

No *in vivo* interaction studies are available with intravenous midazolam and other protease inhibitors. Considering that saquinavir has the weakest CYP3A4 inhibitory potency among all protease inhibitors, midazolam should be systematically reduced during prolonged infusion when administered in combination with protease inhibitors other than saquinavir.

- CNS depressants

Other sedative drugs may potentiate midazolam effects.

The pharmacological classes of CNS depressants include opiates (when they are used as analgesics, antitussives or substitutive treatments), antipsychotics, other benzodiazepines used as anxiolytics or hypnotics, phenobarbital, sedative antidepressants, antihistaminics and centrally acting antihypertensive drugs.

Additional sedation should be taken into account when midazolam is combined with other sedative drugs.

Moreover, additional increase of respiratory depression should be particularly monitored in case of concomitant treatment with opiates, phenobarbital or benzodiazepines.

Alcohol may markedly enhance the sedative effect of midazolam. Alcohol intake should be strongly avoided in case of midazolam administration.

Other interactions

The i.v. administration of midazolam decreases the minimum alveolar concentration (MAC) of inhalation anaesthetics required for general anaesthesia.

4.6 Pregnancy and lactation

Insufficient data are available on midazolam to assess its safety during pregnancy. Animal studies do not indicate a teratogenic effect, but foetotoxicity was observed as with other benzodiazepines. No data on exposed pregnancies are available for the first two trimesters of pregnancy.

The administration of high doses of midazolam in the last trimester of pregnancy, during labour or when used as an induction agent of anaesthesia for caesarean section has been reported to produce maternal or foetal adverse effects (inhalation risk in mother, irregularities in the foetal heart rate, hypotonia, poor sucking, hypothermia and respiratory depression in the neonate).

Moreover, infants born from mothers who received benzodiazepines chronically during the latter stage of pregnancy may have developed physical dependence and may be at some risk of developing withdrawal symptoms in the post-natal period.

Consequently, midazolam should not be used during pregnancy unless clearly necessary. It is preferable to avoid using it for caesarean.

The risk for neonate should be taken into account in case of administration of midazolam for any surgery near the term.

Midazolam passes in low quantities into breast milk. Nursing mothers should be advised to discontinue breast-feeding for 24 hours following administration of midazolam.

4.7 Effects on ability to drive and use machines

Sedation, amnesia, impaired attention and impaired muscular function may adversely affect the ability to drive or use machines. Prior to receiving midazolam, the patient should be warned not to drive a vehicle or operate a machine until completely recovered. The physician should decide when these activities may be resumed. It is recommended that the patient is accompanied when returning home after discharge.

4.8 Undesirable effects

The following undesirable effects have been reported (very rarely) to occur when midazolam is injected:

Skin and appendages disorders: skin rash, urticarial reaction, pruritus.

Central and peripheral nervous system and psychiatric disorders: drowsiness and prolonged sedation, reduced alertness, confusion, euphoria, hallucinations, fatigue, headache, dizziness, ataxia, post-operative sedation, anterograde amnesia, the duration of which is directly related to the administered dose. Anterograde amnesia may still be present at the end of the procedure and in isolated cases prolonged amnesia has been reported.

Paradoxical reactions such as agitation, involuntary movements (including tonic/clonic movements and muscle tremor), hyperactivity, hostility, rage reaction, aggressiveness, paroxysmal excitement and assault, have been reported, particularly among children and the elderly.

Convulsions have been reported more frequently in premature infants and neonates.

Use of midazolam - even in therapeutic doses - may lead to the development of physical dependence after prolonged i.v. administration, abrupt discontinuation may be accompanied by withdrawal symptoms including withdrawal convulsions.

Gastrointestinal system disorders: nausea, vomiting, hiccough, constipation, dry mouth.

Cardiorespiratory disorders: severe cardiorespiratory adverse events: respiratory depression, apnoea, respiratory arrest and/or cardiac arrest, hypotension, heart rate changes, vasodilating effects, dyspnoea, laryngospasm.

Life-threatening incidents are more likely to occur in adults over 60 years of age and those with pre-existing respiratory insufficiency or impaired cardiac function, particularly when the injection is given too rapidly or when a high dosage is administered (see *4.4 Special warnings and precautions for use*).

Body-as-a-whole – general disorders: generalised hypersensitivity reactions: skin reactions, cardiovascular reactions, bronchospasm, anaphylactic shock.

Application site disorders: erythema and pain on injection site, thrombophlebitis, thrombosis.

4.9 Overdose

Symptoms

The symptoms of overdose are mainly an intensification of the pharmacological effects; drowsiness, mental confusion, lethargy and muscle relaxation or paradoxical excitation. More serious symptoms would be areflexia, hypotension, cardiorespiratory depression, apnoea and coma.

Treatment

In most cases monitoring of vital functions is only required. In the management of overdose special attention should be paid to the respiratory and cardiovascular functions in intensive care unit. The benzodiazepine antagonist flumazenil is indicated in case of severe intoxication accompanied with coma or respiratory depression. Caution should be observed in the use of flumazenil in case of mixed drug overdosage and in patients with epilepsy already treated with benzodiazepines. Flumazenil should not be used in patients treated with tricyclic antidepressant drugs, epileptogenic drugs, or patients with ECG abnormalities (QRS or QT prolongation).

5. PHARMACOLOGICAL PROPERTIES

5.1 Pharmacodynamic properties

Pharmacotherapeutic group:

Hypnotics and sedatives: benzodiazepine derivatives, ATC code: N05CD08.

Midazolam is a derivative of the imidazobenzodiazepine group. The free base is a lipophilic substance with low solubility in water.

The basic nitrogen in position 2 of the imidazobenzodiazepine ring system enables the active ingredient of midazolam to form water-soluble salts with acids. These produce a stable and well tolerated injection solution.

The pharmacological action of midazolam is characterised by short duration because of rapid metabolic transformation. Midazolam has a sedative and sleep-inducing effect of pronounced intensity. It also exerts an anxiolytic, an anticonvulsant and a muscle-relaxant effect.

After i.m. or i.v. administration anterograde amnesia of short duration occurs (the patient does not remember events that occurred during the maximal activity of the compound).

5.2 Pharmacokinetic properties

Absorption after i.m. injection

Absorption of midazolam from the muscle tissue is rapid and complete. Maximum plasma concentrations are reached within 30 minutes. The absolute bioavailability after i.m. injection is over 90%.

Absorption after rectal administration

After rectal administration midazolam is absorbed quickly. Maximum plasma concentration is reached in about 30 minutes. The absolute bioavailability is about 50%.

Distribution

When midazolam is injected i.v., the plasma concentration-time curve shows one or two distinct phases of distribution. The volume of distribution at steady state is 0.7 - 1.2 l/kg. 96 - 98% of midazolam is bound to plasma proteins. The major fraction of plasma protein binding is due to albumin. There is a slow and insignificant passage of midazolam into the cerebrospinal fluid. In humans, midazolam has been shown to cross the placenta slowly and to enter foetal circulation. Small quantities of midazolam are found in human milk.

Metabolism

Midazolam is almost entirely eliminated by biotransformation. The fraction of the dose extracted by the liver has been estimated to be 30 - 60%. Midazolam is hydroxylated by the cytochrome P4503A4 isozyme and the major urinary and plasma metabolite is alpha-hydroxymidazolam. Plasma concentrations of alpha-hydroxymidazolam are 12% of those of the parent compound. Alpha-hydroxymidazolam is pharmacologically active, but contributes only minimally (about 10%) to the effects of intravenous midazolam.

Elimination

In healthy volunteers, the elimination half-life of midazolam is between 1.5 - 2.5 hours. Plasma clearance is in the range of 300 - 500ml/min. Midazolam is excreted mainly by renal route (60 - 80% of the injected dose) and recovered as glucuroconjugated alpha-hydroxymidazolam. Less than 1% of the dose is recovered in urine as unchanged drug. The elimination half-life of alpha-hydroxy-midazolam is shorter than 1 hour. When midazolam is given by i.v. infusion, its elimination kinetics do not differ from those following bolus injection.

Pharmacokinetics in special populations

Elderly

In adults over 60 years of age, the elimination half-life may be prolonged up to four times.

Children

The rate of rectal absorption in children is similar to that in adults but the bioavailability is lower (5 - 18%). The elimination half-life after i.v. and rectal administration is shorter in children 3 - 10 years old (1 - 1.5) as compared with that in adults. The difference is consistent with an increased metabolic clearance in children.

Neonates

In neonates the elimination half-life is on average 6 - 12 hours, probably due to liver immaturity and the clearance is reduced (see *4.4 Special warnings and precautions for use*).

Obese

The mean half-life is greater in obese than in non-obese patients (5.9 vs 2.3 hours). This is due to an increase of approximately 50% in the volume of distribution corrected for total body weight. The clearance is not significantly different in obese and non-obese patients.

Patients with hepatic impairment

The elimination half-life in cirrhotic patients may be longer and the clearance smaller as compared to those in healthy volunteers (see *4.4 Special warnings and precautions for use*).

Patients with renal impairment

The elimination half-life in patients with chronic renal failure is similar to that in healthy volunteers.

Critically ill patients

The elimination half-life of midazolam is prolonged up to six times in the critically ill.

Patients with cardiac insufficiency

The elimination half-life is longer in patients with congestive heart failure compared with that in healthy subjects (see *4.4 Special warnings and precautions for use*).

5.3 Preclinical safety data

There are no preclinical data of relevance to the prescriber which are additional to that already included in other sections of the SPC.

6. PHARMACEUTICAL PARTICULARS

6.1 List of excipients

Sodium chloride, hydrochloric acid, sodium hydroxide, water for injection.

6.2 Incompatibilities

Admixture with Hartmann's solution is not recommended, as the potency of midazolam decreases.

6.3 Shelf life

60 months.

6.4 Special precautions for storage

None.

6.5 Nature and contents of container

Clear glass 2ml ampoules.

6.6 Instructions for use and handling

Hypnovel ampoule solution is stable, both physically and chemically, for up to 24 hours at room temperature when mixed with 500ml infusion fluids containing Dextrose 4% with Sodium Chloride 0.18%, Dextrose 5% or Sodium Chloride 0.9%.

There is no evidence of the adsorption of midazolam onto the plastic of infusion apparatus or syringes.

7. MARKETING AUTHORISATION HOLDER

Roche Products Limited, PO Box 8, Welwyn Garden City, Hertfordshire, AL7 3AY.

8. MARKETING AUTHORISATION NUMBER(S)

PL 0031/0126

9. DATE OF FIRST AUTHORISATION/RENEWAL OF THE AUTHORISATION

8 December 1982/22 April 1998

10. DATE OF REVISION OF THE TEXT

September 2002

Hypnovel is a registered trade mark

P999689/103

Hypnovel Ampoules 10mg/5ml

(Roche Products Limited)

1. NAME OF THE MEDICINAL PRODUCT

Hypnovel Ampoules 10mg/5ml

2. QUALITATIVE AND QUANTITATIVE COMPOSITION

Active ingredient: midazolam as hydrochloride.

Ampoules 10mg/5ml for i.v., i.m. and rectal administration.

For excipients, see *6.1*.

3. PHARMACEUTICAL FORM

Solution for injection.

4. CLINICAL PARTICULARS

4.1 Therapeutic indications

Hypnovel is a short-acting sleep-inducing drug that is indicated:

In adults

- ***Conscious sedation*** before and during diagnostic or therapeutic procedures with or without local anaesthesia.
- ***Anaesthesia***

– Premedication before induction of anaesthesia.

– Induction of anaesthesia.

– As an induction agent or as a sedative component in combined anaesthesia.

- ***Sedation in intensive care units***

In children

- ***Conscious sedation*** before and during diagnostic or therapeutic procedures with or without local anaesthesia.
- ***Anaesthesia***

– Premedication before induction of anaesthesia.

- ***Sedation in intensive care units***

4.2 Posology and method of administration

STANDARD DOSAGE

Midazolam is a potent sedative agent that requires titration and slow administration. Titration is strongly recommended to safely obtain the desired level of sedation according to the clinical need, physical status, age and concomitant medication. In adults over 60 years, debilitated or chronically ill patients and paediatric patients, dose should be determined with caution and risk factors related to each patient should be taken into account. Standard dosages are provided in the table below. Additional details are provided in the text following the table.

(see Table 1 on next page)

Conscious sedation dosage

For conscious sedation prior to diagnostic or surgical intervention, midazolam is administered i.v. The dose must be individualised and titrated, and should not be administered by rapid or single bolus injection. The onset of sedation may vary individually depending on the physical status of the patient and the detailed circumstances of dosing (e.g. speed of administration, amount of dose). If necessary, subsequent doses may be administered according to the individual need. The onset of action is about 2 minutes after the injection. Maximum effect is obtained in about 5 to 10 minutes.

Adults

The i.v. injection of midazolam should be given slowly at a rate of approximately 1mg in 30 seconds. In adults below the age of 60 the initial dose is 2 to 2.5mg given 5 to10 minutes before the beginning of the procedure. Further doses of 1mg may be given as necessary. Mean total

Table 1

Indication	**Adults < 60 y**	**Adults ≥ 60 y / debilitated or chronically ill**	**Children**
Conscious sedation	***i.v.*** Initial dose: 2 - 2.5mg Titration doses: 1mg Total dose: 3.5 - 7.5mg	***i.v*** Initial dose: 0.5 - 1mg Titration doses: 0.5 - 1mg Total dose: < 3.5mg	***i.v. in patients 6 months - 5 years*** Initial dose: 0.05 - 0.1mg/kg Total dose: < 6mg ***i.v.in patients 6-12 years*** Initial dose: 0.025 - 0.05mg/kg Total dose: < 10mg ***rectal >6 months*** 0.3 - 0.5mg/kg ***i.m. 1 - 15 years*** 0.05 - 0.15mg/kg
Anaesthesia premedication	***i.m.*** 0.07 - 0.1mg/kg	***i.m.*** 0.025 - 0.05mg/kg	***rectal >6 months*** 0.3 - 0.5mg/kg ***i.m. 1 - 15 years*** 0.08 - 0.2mg/kg
Anaesthesia induction	***i.v.*** 0.15 - 0.2mg/kg (0.3 -0.35 without premedication)	***i.v.*** 0.1 - 0.2mg/kg (0.15 -0.3 without premedication)	
Sedative component in combined anaesthesia	***i.v.*** intermittent doses of 0.03 - 0.1mg/kg or continuous infusion of 0.03 -0.1mg/kg/h	***i.v.*** lower doses than recommended for adults < 60 years	
Sedation in ICU	***i.v.*** Loading dose: 0.03 - 0.3mg/kg in increments of 1 - 2.5mg Maintenance dose: 0.03 - 0.2mg/kg/h		***i.v. in neonates <32 weeks gestational age*** 0.03mg/kg/h ***i.v in neonates >32 weeks and children up to 6 months*** 0.06mg/kg/h ***i.v. in patients >6 months of age*** Loading dose: 0.05 - 0.2mg/kg Maintenance dose: 0.06 - 0.12mg/kg/h

doses have been found to range from 3.5 to 7.5mg. A total dose greater than 5mg is usually not necessary. In adults over 60 years of age, debilitated or chronically ill patients, start by administering a dose of 0.5 to 1mg. Further doses of 0.5 to 1mg may be given as necessary. A total dose greater than 3.5mg is usually not necessary.

Children

I.V. administration: midazolam should be titrated slowly to the desired clinical effect. The initial dose of midazolam should be administered over 2 to 3 minutes. One must wait an additional 2 to 5 minutes to fully evaluate the sedative effect before initiating a procedure or repeating a dose. If further sedation is necessary, continue to titrate with small increments until the appropriate level of sedation is achieved. Infants and young children less than 5 years of age may require substantially higher doses (mg/kg) than older children and adolescents.

• Paediatric patients less than 6 months of age: paediatric patients less than 6 months of age are particularly vulnerable to airway obstruction and hypoventilation. For this reason, the use in conscious sedation in children less than 6 months of age is not recommended.

• Paediatric patients 6 months to 5 years of age: initial dose 0.05 to 0.1mg/kg. A total dose up to 0.6mg/kg may be necessary to reach the desired endpoint, but the total dose should not exceed 6mg. Prolonged sedation and risk of hypoventilation may be associated with the higher doses.

• Paediatric patients 6 to 12 years of age: initial dose 0.025 to 0.05mg/kg. A total dose of up to 0.4mg/kg to a maximum of 10mg may be necessary. Prolonged sedation and risk of hypoventilation may be associated with the higher doses.

• Paediatric patients 12 to 16 years of age: should be dosed as adults.

Rectal administration: the total dose of midazolam usually ranges from 0.3 to 0.5mg/kg. Rectal administration of the ampoule solution is performed by means of a plastic applicator fixed on the end of the syringe. If the volume to be administered is too small, water may be added up to a total volume of 10ml. Total dose should be administered at once and repeated rectal administration avoided.

The use in children less than 6 months of age is not recommended, as available data in this population are limited.

I.M. administration: the doses used range between 0.05 and 0.15mg/kg. A total dose greater than 10.0mg is usually not necessary. This route should only be used in exceptional cases. Rectal administration should be preferred as i.m. injection is painful.

In children less than 15kg of body weight, midazolam solutions with concentrations higher than 1mg/ml are not recommended. Higher concentrations should be diluted to 1mg/ml.

ANAESTHESIA DOSAGE

Premedication

Premedication with midazolam given shortly before a procedure produces sedation (induction of sleepiness or drowsiness and relief of apprehension) and pre-operative impairment of memory. Midazolam can also be administered in combination with anticholinergics. For this indication midazolam should be administered i.m., deep into a large muscle mass 20 to 60 minutes before induction of anaesthesia, or preferably via the rectal route in children (see below). Adequate observation of the patient after administration of premedication is mandatory as inter-individual sensitivity varies and symptoms of overdose may occur.

Adults

For pre-operative sedation and to impair memory of pre-operative events, the recommended dose for adults of ASA Physical Status I & II and below 60 years is 0.07 to 0.1mg/kg administered i.m. The dose must be reduced and individualised when midazolam is administered to adults over 60 years of age, debilitated, or chronically ill patients. A dose of 0.025 to 0.05mg/kg administered i.m. is recommended. The usual dose is 2 to 3mg.

Children

Rectal administration: The total dose of midazolam, usually ranging from 0.3 to 0.5mg/kg should be administered 15 to 30 minutes before induction of anaesthesia. Rectal administration of the ampoule solution is performed by means of a plastic applicator fixed on the end of the syringe. If the volume to be administered is too small, water may be added up to a total volume of 10ml.

I.M. administration: As i.m. injection is painful, this route should only be used in exceptional cases. Rectal administration should be preferred. However, a dose range from 0.08 to 0.2mg/kg of midazolam administered i.m. has been shown to be effective and safe. In children between ages 1 and 15 years, proportionally higher doses are required than in adults in relation to body-weight.

The use in children less than 6 months of age is not recommended as available data are limited.

In children less than 15kg of body weight, midazolam solutions with concentrations higher than 1mg/ml are not recommended. Higher concentrations should be diluted to 1mg/ml.

Induction

Adults

If midazolam is used for induction of anaesthesia before other anaesthetic agents have been administered, the individual response is variable. The dose should be titrated to the desired effect according to the patient's age and clinical status. When midazolam is used before or in combination with other i.v. or inhalation agents for induction of anaesthesia, the initial dose of each agent should be significantly reduced. The desired level of anaesthesia is reached by stepwise titration. The i.v. induction dose of midazolam should be given slowly in increments. Each increment of not more than 5mg should be injected over 20 to 30 seconds allowing 2 minutes between successive increments.

• In adults below the age of 60 years, an i.v. dose of 0.15 to 0.2mg/kg will usually suffice. In non-premedicated adults below the age of 60 the dose may be higher (0.3 to 0.35mg/kg i.v.). If needed to complete induction, increments of approximately 25% of the patient's initial dose may be used. Induction may instead be completed with inhalational anaesthetics. In resistant cases, a total dose of up to 0.6mg/kg may be used for induction, but such larger doses may prolong recovery.

• In adults over 60 years of age, debilitated or chronically ill patients, the dose is 0.1 to 0.2mg/kg administered i.v. Non-premedicated adults over 60 years of age usually require more midazolam for induction; an initial dose of 0.15 to 0.3mg/kg is recommended. Non-premedicated patients with severe systemic disease or other debilitation usually require less midazolam for induction. An initial dose of 0.15 to 0.25mg/kg will usually suffice.

Sedative component in combined anaesthesia

Adults

Midazolam can be given as a sedative component in combined anaesthesia by either further intermittent small i.v. doses (range between 0.03 and 0.1mg/kg) or continuous infusion of i.v. midazolam (range between 0.03 and 0.1mg/kg/h) typically in combination with analgesics. The dose and the intervals between doses vary according to the patient's individual reaction.

In adults over 60 years of age, debilitated or chronically ill patients, lower maintenance doses will be required.

Sedation in intensive care units

The desired level of sedation is reached by stepwise titration of midazolam followed by either continuous infusion or intermittent bolus, according to the clinical need, physical status, age and concomitant medication (see *4.5 Interaction with other medicinal products and other forms of interaction*).

Adults

I.V. loading dose: 0.03 to 0.3mg/kg should be given slowly in increments. Each increment of 1 to 2.5mg should be injected over 20 to 30 seconds allowing 2 minutes between successive increments. In hypovolaemic, vasoconstricted, or hypothermic patients the loading dose should be reduced or omitted. When midazolam is given with potent analgesics, the latter should be administered first so that the sedative effects of midazolam can be safely titrated on top of any sedation caused by the analgesic.

I.V. maintenance dose: doses can range from 0.03 to 0.2mg/kg/h. In hypovolaemic, vasoconstricted, or hypothermic patients the maintenance dose should be reduced. The level of sedation should be assessed regularly. With long-term sedation, tolerance may develop and the dose may have to be increased.

Children over 6 months of age

In intubated and ventilated paediatric patients, a loading dose of 0.05 to 0.2mg/kg i.v. should be administered slowly over at least 2 to 3 minutes to establish the desired clinical effect. Midazolam should not be administered as a rapid intravenous dose. The loading dose is followed by a continuous i.v. infusion at 0.06 to 0.12mg/kg/h (1 to 2μg/kg/min). The rate of infusion can be increased or decreased (generally by 25% of the initial or subsequent infusion rate) as required, or supplemental i.v. doses of midazolam can be administered to increase or maintain the desired effect.

When initiating an infusion with midazolam in haemodynamically compromised patients, the usual loading dose should be titrated in small increments and the patient monitored for haemodynamic instability, e.g., hypotension. These patients are also vulnerable to the respiratory depressant effects of midazolam and require careful monitoring of respiratory rate and oxygen saturation.

Neonates and children up to 6 months of age

Midazolam should be given as a continuous i.v. infusion, starting at 0.03mg/kg/h (0.5μg/kg/min) in neonates with a gestational age < 32 weeks or 0.06mg/kg/h (1μg/kg/min) in neonates with a gestational age > 32 weeks and children up to 6 months.

Intravenous loading doses is not recommended in premature infants, neonates and children up to 6 months, rather the infusion may be run more rapidly for the first several hours to establish therapeutic plasma levels. The rate of infusion should be carefully and frequently reassessed, particularly after the first 24 hours so as to administer the lowest possible effective dose and reduce the potential for drug accumulation.

Careful monitoring of respiratory rate and oxygen saturation is required.

In premature infants, neonates and children less than 15 kg of body weight, midazolam solutions with concentrations higher than 1mg/ml are not recommended. Higher concentrations should be diluted to 1mg/ml.

4.3 Contraindications

Use of this drug in patients with known hypersensitivity to benzodiazepines or to any component of the product.

Use of this drug for conscious sedation in patients with severe respiratory failure or acute respiratory depression.

4.4 Special warnings and special precautions for use

Midazolam should be used only when age- and size-appropriate resuscitation facilities are available, as i.v. administration of midazolam may depress myocardial contractility and cause apnoea. Severe cardiorespiratory adverse events have occurred on rare occasions. These have included respiratory depression, apnoea, respiratory arrest and/or cardiac arrest. Such life-threatening incidents are more likely to occur when the injection is given too rapidly or when a high dosage is administered. Paediatric patients less than 6 months of age are particularly vulnerable to airway obstruction and hypoventilation, therefore titration with small increments to clinical effect and careful respiratory rate and oxygen saturation monitoring are essential.

When midazolam is used for premedication, adequate observation of the patient after administration is mandatory as inter-individual sensitivity varies and symptoms of overdose may occur.

Special caution should be exercised when administering midazolam to high-risk patients:

– adults over 60 years of age

– chronically ill or debilitated patients, e.g.

– patients with chronic respiratory insufficiency

– patients with chronic renal failure, impaired hepatic function or with impaired cardiac function

– paediatric patients specially those with cardiovascular instability.

These high-risk patients require lower dosages (see *4.2 Posology and method of administration*) and should be continuously monitored for early signs of alterations of vital functions.

Benzodiazepines should be used with caution in patients with a history of alcohol or drug abuse.

As with any substance with CNS depressant and/or muscle-relaxant properties, particular care should be taken when administering midazolam to a patient with myasthenia gravis.

Tolerance

Some loss of efficacy has been reported when midazolam was used as long-term sedation in intensive care units (ICU).

Dependence

When midazolam is used in long-term sedation in ICU, it should be borne in mind that physical dependence on midazolam may develop. The risk of dependence increases with dose and duration of treatment.

Withdrawal symptoms

During prolonged treatment with midazolam in ICU, physical dependence may develop. Therefore, abrupt termination of the treatment will be accompanied by withdrawal symptoms. The following symptoms may occur: headaches, muscle pain, anxiety, tension, restlessness, confusion, irritability, rebound insomnia, mood changes, hallucinations and convulsions. Since the risk of withdrawal symptoms is greater after abrupt discontinuation of treatment, it is recommended to decrease doses gradually.

Amnesia

Midazolam causes anterograde amnesia (frequently this effect is very desirable in situations such as before and during surgical and diagnostic procedures), the duration of which is directly related to the administered dose. Prolonged amnesia can present problems in outpatients, who are scheduled for discharge following intervention. After receiving midazolam parenterally, patients should be discharged from hospital or consulting room only if accompanied by an attendant.

Paradoxical reactions

Paradoxical reactions such as agitation, involuntary movements (including tonic/clonic convulsions and muscle tremor), hyperactivity, hostility, rage reaction, aggressiveness, paroxysmal excitement and assault, have been reported to occur with midazolam. These reactions may occur with high doses and/or when the injection is given rapidly. The highest incidence to such reactions has been reported among children and the elderly.

Delayed elimination of midazolam

Midazolam elimination may be altered in patients receiving compounds that inhibit or induce CYP3A4 (see 4.5 *Interaction with other medicaments and other forms of interaction*).

Midazolam elimination may also be delayed in patients with liver dysfunction, low cardiac output and in neonates (see *5.2 Pharmacokinetics in special populations*).

Preterm infants and neonates

Due to an increased risk of apnoea, extreme caution is advised when sedating pre-term and former pre-term patients. Careful monitoring of respiratory rate and oxygen saturation is required.

Rapid injection should be avoided in the neonatal population.

Neonates have reduced and/or immature organ function and are also vulnerable to profound and/or prolonged respiratory effects of midazolam.

Adverse haemodynamic events have been reported in paediatric patients with cardiovascular instability; rapid intravenous administration should be avoided in this population.

4.5 Interaction with other medicinal products and other forms of Interaction

The metabolism of midazolam is almost exclusively mediated by the isoenzyme CYP3A4 of the cytochrome P450 (CYP450). CYP3A4 inhibitors (see *4.4 Special warnings and precautions for use*) and inducers, but also other active substances (see below), may lead to drug-drug interactions with midazolam.

Since midazolam undergoes significant first pass effect, parenteral midazolam would theoretically be less affected by metabolic interactions and clinical relevant consequences should be limited.

• Itraconazole, fluconazole and ketoconazole

Co-administration of oral midazolam and some azole antifungals (itraconazole, fluconazole, ketokonazole) increased markedly midazolam plasma levels and prolonged its elimination half-life, leading to major impairment of psychosedative tests. Elimination half-lives were increased from 3 to 8 hours approximately.

When a single bolus dose of midazolam was given for short-term sedation, the effect of midazolam was not enhanced or prolonged to a clinically significant degree by itraconazole, and dosage reduction is therefore not required. However, administration of high doses or long-term infusions of midazolam to patients receiving itraconazole, fluconazole or ketoconazole, e.g. during intensive care treatment, may result in long-lasting hypnotic effects, possible delayed recovery, and possible respiratory depression, thus requiring dose adjustments.

• Verapamil and diltiazem

No *in vivo* interaction studies are available with intravenous midazolam and verapamil or diltiazem.

However, as expected, oral midazolam pharmacokinetics varied in a clinically significant way when combined to these calcium channel blockers, notably with almost a doubling of half-life value and peak plasma level, resulting in a strongly reduced performance in co-ordination and cognitive function tests while producing profound sedation. When oral midazolam is used, dosage adjustment is usually recommended. Although no clinically significant interaction is expected with midazolam used for short-term sedation, caution should be exercised if intravenous midazolam is concomitantly given with verapamil or diltiazem.

• Macrolide Antibiotics: Erythromycin and clarithromycin

Co-administration of oral midazolam and erythromycin or clarithromycin significantly increased the AUC of midazolam about four fold and more than doubled the elimination half-life of midazolam, depending on the study. Marked changes in psychomotor tests were observed and it is advised to adjust doses of midazolam, if given orally, due to significantly delayed recovery.

When a single bolus dose of midazolam was given for short-term sedation, the effect of midazolam was not enhanced or prolonged to a clinically significant degree by erythromycin, although a significant decrease in plasma clearance was recorded. Caution should be exercised if intravenous midazolam is concomitantly given with erythromycin or clarithromycin. No clinical significant interaction has been shown with midazolam and other macrolide antibiotics.

• Cimetidine and ranitidine

Co-administration of cimetidine (at doses equal or higher than 800mg/day) and intravenous midazolam slightly increased the steady-state plasma concentration of midazolam, which could possibly lead to a delayed recovery, whereas co-administration of ranitidine had no effect. Cimetidine and ranitidine did not affect oral midazolam pharmacokinetics. These data indicate that intravenous midazolam can be administered at usual doses of cimetidine (i.e. 400mg/day) and ranitidine without dosage adjustment.

• Saquinavir

Co-administration of a single intravenous dose of 0.05mg/kg midazolam after 3 or 5 days of saquinavir dosing (1200mg t.i.d) to 12 healthy volunteers decreased the midazolam clearance by 56% and increased the elimination half-life from 4.1 to 9.5 h. Only the subjective effects to midazolam (visual analogue scales with the item "overall drug effect") were intensified by saquinavir.

Therefore, a single bolus dose of intravenous midazolam can be given in combination with saquinavir. Nevertheless, during a prolonged midazolam infusion, a total dose reduction is recommended to avoid delayed recovery (see *4.4 Special warnings and precautions for use*).

• Other protease inhibitors: ritonavir, indinavir, nelfinavir and amprenavir

No *in vivo* interaction studies are available with intravenous midazolam and other protease inhibitors. Considering that saquinavir has the weakest CYP3A4 inhibitory potency among all protease inhibitors, midazolam should be systematically reduced during prolonged infusion when administered in combination with protease inhibitors other than saquinavir.

• CNS depressants

Other sedative drugs may potentiate midazolam effects.

The pharmacological classes of CNS depressants include opiates (when they are used as analgesics, antitussives or substitutive treatments), antipsychotics, other benzodiazepines used as anxiolytics or hypnotics, phenobarbital, sedative antidepressants, antihistaminics and centrally acting antihypertensive drugs.

Additional sedation should be taken into account when midazolam is combined with other sedative drugs.

Moreover, additional increase of respiratory depression should be particularly monitored in case of concomitant treatment with opiates, phenobarbital or benzodiazepines.

Alcohol may markedly enhance the sedative effect of midazolam. Alcohol intake should be strongly avoided in case of midazolam administration.

Other interactions

The i.v. administration of midazolam decreases the minimum alveolar concentration (MAC) of inhalation anaesthetics required for general anaesthesia.

4.6 Pregnancy and lactation

Insufficient data are available on midazolam to assess its safety during pregnancy. Animal studies do not indicate a teratogenic effect, but foetotoxicity was observed as with other benzodiazepines. No data on exposed pregnancies are available for the first two trimesters of pregnancy.

The administration of high doses of midazolam in the last trimester of pregnancy, during labour or when used as an induction agent of anaesthesia for caesarean section has been reported to produce maternal or foetal adverse effects (inhalation risk in mother, irregularities in the foetal heart rate, hypotonia, poor sucking, hypothermia and respiratory depression in the neonate).

Moreover, infants born from mothers who received benzodiazepines chronically during the latter stage of pregnancy may have developed physical dependence and may be at some risk of developing withdrawal symptoms in the postnatal period.

Consequently, midazolam should not be used during pregnancy unless clearly necessary. It is preferable to avoid using it for caesarean.

The risk for neonate should be taken into account in case of administration of midazolam for any surgery near the term.

Midazolam passes in low quantities into breast milk. Nursing mothers should be advised to discontinue breastfeeding for 24 hours following administration of midazolam.

4.7 Effects on ability to drive and use machines

Sedation, amnesia, impaired attention and impaired muscular function may adversely affect the ability to drive or use machines. Prior to receiving midazolam, the patient should be warned not to drive a vehicle or operate a machine until completely recovered. The physician should decide when these activities may be resumed. It is recommended that the patient is accompanied when returning home after discharge.

4.8 Undesirable effects

The following undesirable effects have been reported (very rarely) to occur when midazolam is injected:

Skin and appendages disorders: skin rash, urticarial reaction, pruritus.

Central and peripheral nervous system and psychiatric disorders: drowsiness and prolonged sedation, reduced alertness, confusion, euphoria, hallucinations, fatigue, headache, dizziness, ataxia, post-operative sedation, anterograde amnesia, the duration of which is directly related to the administered dose. Anterograde amnesia may still be present at the end of the procedure and in isolated cases prolonged amnesia has been reported.

Paradoxical reactions such as agitation, involuntary movements (including tonic/clonic movements and muscle tremor), hyperactivity, hostility, rage reaction, aggressiveness, paroxysmal excitement and assault, have been reported, particularly among children and the elderly.

Convulsions have been reported more frequently in premature infants and neonates.

Use of midazolam - even in therapeutic doses - may lead to the development of physical dependence after prolonged i.v. administration, abrupt discontinuation may be accompanied by withdrawal symptoms including withdrawal convulsions.

Gastrointestinal system disorders: nausea, vomiting, hiccough, constipation, dry mouth.

Cardiorespiratory disorders: severe cardiorespiratory adverse events: respiratory depression, apnoea, respiratory arrest and/or cardiac arrest, hypotension, heart rate changes, vasodilating effects, dyspnoea, laryngospasm.

Life-threatening incidents are more likely to occur in adults over 60 years of age and those with pre-existing respiratory insufficiency or impaired cardiac function, particularly when the injection is given too rapidly or when a high dosage is administered (see *4.4 Special warnings and precautions for use*).

Body-as-a-whole – general disorders: generalised hypersensitivity reactions: skin reactions, cardiovascular reactions, bronchospasm, anaphylactic shock.

Application site disorders: erythema and pain on injection site, thrombophlebitis, thrombosis.

4.9 Overdose

Symptoms

The symptoms of overdose are mainly an intensification of the pharmacological effects; drowsiness, mental confusion, lethargy and muscle relaxation or paradoxical excitation. More serious symptoms would be areflexia, hypotension, cardiorespiratory depression, apnoea and coma.

Treatment

In most cases monitoring of vital functions is only required. In the management of overdose special attention should be paid to the respiratory and cardiovascular functions in intensive care unit. The benzodiazepine antagonist flumazenil is indicated in case of severe intoxication accompanied with coma or respiratory depression. Caution should be observed in the use of flumazenil in case of mixed drug overdosage and in patients with epilepsy already treated with benzodiazepines. Flumazenil should not be used in patients treated with tricyclic antidepressant drugs, epileptogenic drugs, or patients with ECG abnormalities (QRS or QT prolongation).

5. PHARMACOLOGICAL PROPERTIES

5.1 Pharmacodynamic properties

Pharmacotherapeutic group:

Hypnotics and sedatives: benzodiazepine derivatives, ATC code: N05CD08.

Midazolam is a derivative of the imidazobenzodiazepine group. The free base is a lipophilic substance with low solubility in water.

The basic nitrogen in position 2 of the imidazobenzodiazepine ring system enables the active ingredient of midazolam to form water-soluble salts with acids. These produce a stable and well tolerated injection solution.

The pharmacological action of midazolam is characterised by short duration because of rapid metabolic transformation. Midazolam has a sedative and sleep-inducing effect of pronounced intensity. It also exerts an anxiolytic, an anticonvulsant and a muscle-relaxant effect.

After i.m. or i.v. administration anterograde amnesia of short duration occurs (the patient does not remember events that occurred during the maximal activity of the compound).

5.2 Pharmacokinetic properties

Absorption after i.m. injection

Absorption of midazolam from the muscle tissue is rapid and complete. Maximum plasma concentrations are reached within 30 minutes. The absolute bioavailability after i.m. injection is over 90%.

Absorption after rectal administration

After rectal administration midazolam is absorbed quickly. Maximum plasma concentration is reached in about 30 minutes. The absolute bioavailability is about 50%.

Distribution

When midazolam is injected i.v., the plasma concentration-time curve shows one or two distinct phases of distribution. The volume of distribution at steady state is 0.7 - 1.2 l/kg. 96 - 98% of midazolam is bound to plasma proteins. The major fraction of plasma protein binding is due to albumin. There is a slow and insignificant passage of midazolam into the cerebrospinal fluid. In humans, midazolam has been shown to cross the placenta slowly and to enter foetal circulation. Small quantities of midazolam are found in human milk.

Metabolism

Midazolam is almost entirely eliminated by biotransformation. The fraction of the dose extracted by the liver has been estimated to be 30 - 60%. Midazolam is hydroxylated by the cytochrome P4503A4 isozyme and the major urinary and plasma metabolite is alpha-hydroxymidazolam. Plasma concentrations of alpha-hydroxymidazolam are 12% of those of the parent compound. Alpha-hydroxymidazolam is pharmacologically active, but contributes only minimally (about 10%) to the effects of intravenous midazolam.

Elimination

In healthy volunteers, the elimination half-life of midazolam is between 1.5 - 2.5 hours. Plasma clearance is in the range of 300 - 500ml/min. Midazolam is excreted mainly by renal route (60 - 80% of the injected dose) and recovered as glucuroconjugated alpha-hydroxymidazolam. Less than 1% of the dose is recovered in urine as unchanged drug. The elimination half-life of alpha-hydroxy-midazolam is shorter than 1 hour. When midazolam is given by i.v. infusion, its elimination kinetics do not differ from those following bolus injection.

Pharmacokinetics in special populations

Elderly

In adults over 60 years of age, the elimination half-life may be prolonged up to four times.

Children

The rate of rectal absorption in children is similar to that in adults but the bioavailability is lower (5 - 18%). The elimination half-life after i.v. and rectal administration is shorter in children 3 - 10 years old (1 - 1.5) as compared with that in adults. The difference is consistent with an increased metabolic clearance in children.

Neonates

In neonates the elimination half-life is on average 6 - 12 hours, probably due to liver immaturity and the clearance is reduced (see *4.4 Special warnings and precautions for use*).

Obese

The mean half-life is greater in obese than in non-obese patients (5.9 vs 2.3 hours). This is due to an increase of approximately 50% in the volume of distribution corrected for total body weight. The clearance is not significantly different in obese and non-obese patients.

Patients with hepatic impairment

The elimination half-life in cirrhotic patients may be longer and the clearance smaller as compared to those in healthy volunteers (see *4.4 Special warnings and precautions for use*).

Patients with renal impairment

The elimination half-life in patients with chronic renal failure is similar to that in healthy volunteers.

Critically ill patients

The elimination half-life of midazolam is prolonged up to six times in the critically ill.

Patients with cardiac insufficiency

The elimination half-life is longer in patients with congestive heart failure compared with that in healthy subjects (see *4.4 Special warnings and precautions for use*).

5.3 Preclinical safety data

There are no preclinical data of relevance to the prescriber which are additional to that already included in other sections of the SPC.

6. PHARMACEUTICAL PARTICULARS

6.1 List of excipients

Sodium Chloride	Ph. Eur.
Hydrochloric Acid	Ph. Eur.
IM Sodium Hydroxide Solution	Ph. Eur.
Water for Injections	Ph. Eur.

6.2 Incompatibilities

Admixture with Hartmann's solution is not recommended as the potency of midazolam decreases.

6.3 Shelf life

5 years.

6.4 Special precautions for storage

There are no special storage precautions.

6.5 Nature and contents of container

Type I Ph. Eur. 5ml colourless glass ampoules, in packs of 10.

6.6 Instructions for use and handling

Hypnovel ampoule solution is stable, both physically and chemically, for up to 24 hours at room temperature when mixed with 500ml infusion fluids containing Dextrose 4% with Sodium Chloride 0.18%, Dextrose 5% or Sodium Chloride 0.9%.

There is no evidence of the absorption of midazolam on to the plastic of infusion apparatus or syringes.

7. MARKETING AUTHORISATION HOLDER

Roche Products Limited, 40 Broadwater Road, Welwyn Garden City, Hertfordshire, AL7 3AY.

8. MARKETING AUTHORISATION NUMBER(S)

PL 00031/0189

9. DATE OF FIRST AUTHORISATION/RENEWAL OF THE AUTHORISATION

15 November 1984/15 November 1994/24 March 2000

10. DATE OF REVISION OF THE TEXT

September 2002

Hypnovel is a registered trade mark

P999690/103

Hypovase Tablets

(Pfizer Limited)

1. NAME OF THE MEDICINAL PRODUCT

HYPOVASE(TM) TABLETS

2. QUALITATIVE AND QUANTITATIVE COMPOSITION

500microgram tablets: prazosin hydrochloride Ph Eur equivalent to 500micrograms prazosin base, based on potency of 93.1% base activity.

1mg tablets: prazosin hydrochloride Ph Eur equivalent to 1mg prazosin based on a potency of 93.1% base activity.

2mg tablets: prazosin hydrochloride Ph Eur equivalent to 2mg prazosin based on a potency of 93.1% base activity.

3. PHARMACEUTICAL FORM

Tablets

4. CLINICAL PARTICULARS

4.1 Therapeutic indications

Hypertension: Hypovase is indicated in the treatment of all grades of essential (primary) hypertension and of all grades of secondary hypertension of varied aetiology. It can be used as the intial and sole agent or it may be employed in a treatment regimen in conjunction with a diuretic and/or other antihypertensive drug as needed for proper patient response.

Congestive heart failure: Hypovase may be used alone or added to the therapeutic regimen in those patients with congestive heart failure who are resistant or refractory to conventional therapy with diuretics and/or cardiac glycosides.

Raynaud's phenomenon and Raynaud's disease: Hypovase is indicated for the symptomatic treatment of patients with Raynaud's phenomenon and Raynaud's disease.

Benign prostatic hyperplasia: Hypovase is indicated as an adjunct in the symptomatic treatment of urinary obstruction caused by benign prostatic hyperplasia. It may therefore be of value in patients awaiting prostatic surgery.

4.2 Posology and method of administration

Hypovase tablets are for oral administration only.

Hypertension: The dosage range is from 500 micrograms - 20mg daily. It is recommended that therapy be initiated at the lowest dose, 500 micrograms, twice or three times daily for three to seven days, with the starting dose administered in the evening. This dose should be increased to 1mg twice or three times daily for a further three to seven days. Thereafter, the daily dose should be increased gradually as determined by the patient's response to the blood pressure lowering effect. Most patients are likely to be maintained on a dosage regimen of Hypovase alone of up to 15mg daily in divided doses. Maximum recommended daily dosage: 20mg in divided doses.

The b.d. starter pack is available for the convenience of prescribers to initiate treatment up to 2mg twice daily.

Patients receiving other antihypertensive therapy but with inadequate control: The dosage of the other drug should be reduced to a maintenance level and Hypovase initiated at 500 micrograms in the evening, then continuing with 500 micrograms twice or three times daily. Subsequent dosage increases should be made gradually depending upon the patient's response.

There is evidence that adding Hypovase to angiotensin converting enzyme inhibitor, beta-adrenergic antagonist or calcium antagonist therapy may bring about a substantial reduction in blood pressure. Therefore, the low initial dosage regimen is recommended.

Congestive cardiac failure: The recommended starting dose is 500 micrograms two, three or four times daily, increasing to 4mg in divided doses. Dosage should be adjusted according to the patient's clinical response, based on careful monitoring of cardiopulmonary signs and symptoms, and when indicated, haemodynamic studies. Dosage may be adjusted as often as every two to three days in patients under close medical supervision. In severely ill, decompensated patients, rapid dosage adjustment over one to two days may be indicated and is best done when haemodynamic monitoring is available. In clinical studies the therapeutic dosages ranged from 4mg to 20mg daily in divided doses. Adjustment of dosage may be required in the course of Hypovase therapy in some patients to maintain optimal clinical improvement.

Usual daily maintenance dosage: 4mg to 20mg in divided doses.

Raynaud's phenomenon and Raynaud's disease: The recommended starting dosage is 500 micrograms twice daily given for a period of three to seven days and should be adjusted according to the patient's clinical response. Usual maintenance dosage is 1mg or 2mg twice daily.

Benign prostatic hyperplasia: The recommended dosage is 500 micrograms twice daily for a period of 3 to 7 days, with the initial dose administered in the evening. The dosage should then be adjusted according to clinical response. The usual maintenance dosage is 2mg twice daily. This dose should not be exceeded unless the patient requires Hypovase as antihypertensive therapy. Patients with benign prostatic hyperplasia receiving hypertensive therapy, should be administered Hypovase only under the supervision of the practitioner responsible for treating the patient's hypertension.

Patients with moderate to severe grades of renal impairment

Evidence to date shows that Hypovase does not further compromise renal function when used in patients with renal impairment. As some patients in this category have responded to small doses of Hypovase, it is recommended that therapy be initiated at 500 micrograms daily and that dosage increases be instituted cautiously.

Patients with hepatic dysfunction: No information is available on the use of Hypovase in this patient group, however, since Hypovase normally undergoes substantial first pass metabolism and subsequent metabolism and excretion by the liver, it is recommended that therapy be initiated at 500 micrograms daily and that dosage increases be instituted cautiously.

Use in children: Hypovase is not recommended for the treatment of children under the age of 12 years since safe conditions for its use have not been established.

Use in the elderly: Since the elderly may be more susceptible to hypotension, therapy should be initiated with the lowest possible dose.

4.3 Contraindications
Hypovase is contraindicated in patients with known sensitivity to Hypovase, other quinazolines, prazosin or any of the excipients.

4.4 Special warnings and special precautions for use
In patients with benign prostatic hyperplasia: Hypovase is not recommended for patients with a history of micturition syncope.

Hypovase decreases peripheral vascular resistance and since many patients with this disorder are elderly, careful monitoring of blood pressure during initial administration and during adjustment of dosage is recommended. The possibility of postural hypotension, or rarely, loss of consciousness, as reported in other patient groups should be borne in mind. Close observation is especially recommended. For patients taking medications that are known to lower blood pressure, Hypovase may augment the efficacy of antihypertensive therapy, consequently, close observation is especially recommended for patients taking medications that are known to lower blood pressure. Hypovase should not normally be administered to patients already receiving another alpha-1-antagonist.

In patients with congestive cardiac failure: Hypovase is not recommended in the treatment of congestive cardiac failure due to mechanical obstruction such as aortic valve stenosis, mitral valve stenosis, pulmonary embolism and restrictive pericardial disease. Adequate data are not yet available to establish efficacy in patients with heart failure due to recent myocardial infarction.

When Hypovase is initially administered to patients with congestive cardiac failure who have undergone vigorous diuretic or other vasodilator treatment, particularly in higher than the recommended starting dose, the resultant decrease in left ventricular filling pressure may be associated with a significant fall in cardiac output and systemic blood pressure. In such patients, observance of the recommended starting dose of Hypovase followed by gradual dosage increase is particularly important.

The clinical efficacy of Hypovase in congestive cardiac failure has been reported to diminish after several months of treatment, in a proportion of patients. In these patients there is usually evidence of weight gain or peripheral oedema indicating fluid retention. Since spontaneous deterioration may occur in such severely ill patients, a causal relationship to prazosin therapy has not been established. Thus, as with all patients with congestive cardiac failure, careful adjustment of diuretic dosage according to the patient's clinical condition is required to prevent excessive fluid retention and consequent relief of symptoms.

In those patients without evidence of fluid retention, when clinical improvement has diminished, an increase in the dosage of Hypovase will usually restore clinical efficacy.

In patients with hypertension: A very small percentage of patients may respond in an abrupt and exaggerated manner to the initial dose of Hypovase. Postural hypotension evidenced by dizziness and weakness, or rarely loss of consciousness, has been reported, particularly with the commencement of therapy, but this effect is readily avoided by initiating treatment with a low dose of Hypovase and with small increases in dosage during the first one to two weeks of therapy. The effect when observed is not related to the severity of hypertension, is self-limiting and in most patients does not recur after the initial period of therapy or during subsequent titration steps.

Raynaud's phenomenon and Raynaud's disease: Because Hypovase decreases peripheral vascular resistance, careful monitoring of blood pressure during initial administration and during subsequent dosage increments of Hypovase is suggested. Close observation is especially recommended for patients already taking medications that are known to lower blood pressure.

4.5 Interaction with other medicinal products and other forms of Interaction
Hypovase has been administered without any adverse drug interaction in clinical experience to date with the following:

Cardiac glycosides: digitalis and digoxin.

Hypoglycaemic agents: insulin, chlorpropamide, phenformin, tolazamide and tolbutamide.

Tranquillizers and sedatives: chlordiazepoxide, diazepam and phenobarbital.

Agents for treatment of gout: allopurinol, colchicine and probenecid.

Anti-arrhythmic agents: procainamide and quinidine.

Analgesic, antipyretic and anti-inflammatory agents: dextropropoxyphene, aspirin, indomethacinand phenylbutazone.

There is evidence that adding Hypovase to beta-adrenergic antagonist or calcium antagonist therapy may produce a substantial reduction in blood pressure. Therefore the low initial dosage regimen is recommended.

Drug/Laboratory Test Interactions: False positive results may occur in screening tests for phaeochromocytoma urinary vanillylmandelic acid (VMA) and methoxyhydroxyphenyl glycol (MHPG) metabolites of norepinephrine (noradrenaline) in patients who are being treated with Hypovase.

4.6 Pregnancy and lactation
Although no teratogenic effects were seen in animal testing, the safety of Hypovase during pregnancy has not yet been established. The use of Hypovase and a beta-blocker for the control of severe hypertension in 44 pregnant women revealed no drug-related foetal abnormalities or adverse effects. Therapy with Hypovase was continued for as long as 14 weeks.

Hypovase has also been used alone or in combination with other hypotensive agents in severe hypertension of pregnancy. No foetal or neonatal abnormalities have been reported with the use of Hypovase.

Studies to date are inadequate to establish the safety of Hypovase in pregnancy, accordingly, it should be used only when, in the opinion of the physician, potential benefit outweighs potential risk. Hypovase has been shown to be excreted in small amounts in human milk. Caution should be exercised when Hypovase is administered to nursing mothers.

4.7 Effects on ability to drive and use machines
When instituting therapy with any effective antihypertensive agent, the patient should be advised on how to avoid symptoms resulting from postural hypotension and what measures to take should they develop. The patient should be cautioned to avoid situations where injury could result should dizziness or weakness occur during the initiation of Hypovase therapy (i.e. driving or operating machinery).

4.8 Undesirable effects
The following side-effects have been associated with Hypovase therapy:

MedDRA System Organ Class	Frequency	**Undesirable effects**
Immune System Disorders	Rare	Allergic reaction
Psychiatric Disorders	Common	Depression, nervousness
	Uncommon	Insomnia
	Rare	Hallucinations
Nervous System Disorders	Common	Dizziness, drowsiness, headache, faintness, syncope
	Uncommon	Paraesthesia
	Rare	Worsening of pre-existing narcolepsy
Eye Disorders	Common	Blurred vision
	Uncommon	Eye pain, reddened sclera
Ear and Labyrinth Disorders	Common	Vertigo
	Uncommon	Tinnitus
Cardiac Disorders	Common	Palpitations
	Uncommon	Angina pectoris, tachycardia,
	Rare	Bradycardia
Vascular Disorders	Rare	Flushing, orthostatic hypotension, vasculitis
Respiratory, Thoracic and Mediastinal Disorders	Common	Dyspnoea, nasal congestion
	Uncommon	Epistaxis
Gastrointestinal Disorders	Common	Constipation, diarrhoea, dry mouth, nausea, vomiting
	Uncommon	Abdominal discomfort and/ or pain
	Rare	Pancreatitis
Hepato-biliary Disorders	Rare	Liver function abnormalities
Skin and Subcutaneous Tissue Disorders	Common	Rash
	Uncommon	Diaphoresis, pruritis, urticaria
	Rare	Alopecia, lichen planus
Musculoskeletal and Connective Tissue Disorders	Uncommon	Arthralgia
Renal and Urinary Disorders	Common	Urinary frequency
	Rare	Incontinence
Reproductive System and Breast Disorders	Uncommon	Impotence
	Rare	Gynaecomastia, priapism
General Disorders and Administration Site Conditions	Common	Oedema, lack of energy, weakness
	Rare	Fever, pain
Investigations	Rare	Positive ANA titer

The frequency of side-effects observed in patients being managed for left ventricular failure with Hypovase when used in conjunction with cardiac glycosides and diuretics is shown below:

MedDRA System Organ Class	Frequency	Undesirable effects
Nervous System Disorders	Common	Dizziness
	Uncommon	Headache
	Rare	Drowsiness
Eye Disorders	Common	Blurred vision
Cardiac Disorders	Rare	Palpitations
Vascular Disorders	Common	Postural hypotension
Respiratory, Thoracic and Mediastinal Disorders	Rare	Nasal congestion
Gastrointestinal Disorders	Common	Dry mouth, nausea
	Uncommon	Diarrhoea
Reproductive System and Breast Disorders	Common	Impotence
General Disorders and Administration Site Conditions	Rare	Oedema

In most instances these occurrences have been mild to moderate in severity and have resolved with continued therapy or have been tolerated with no decrease in drug dosage.

4.9 Overdose
Should over-dosage lead to hypotension, support of the cardiovascular system is of first importance. Restoration of blood pressure and normalization of heart rate may be accomplished by keeping the patient in the supine position. If this measure is inadequate, shock should first be treated with volume expanders. If necessary vasopressors including angiotensin should then be used. Renal function should be monitored and supported as needed. Laboratory data indicate Hypovase is not dialysable because it is protein bound.

5. PHARMACOLOGICAL PROPERTIES

5.1 Pharmacodynamic properties

Hypovase causes a decrease in total peripheral vascular resistance through selective inhibition of postsynaptic alpha-1-adrenoreceptors in vascular smooth muscle. The results of forearm plethysmographic studies in humans demonstrate that the resultant peripheral vasodilatation is a balanced effect on both resistance vessels (arterioles) and capacitance vessels (veins).

In hypertensive patients, blood pressure is lowered in both the supine and standing positions; this effect is more pronounced on the diastolic blood pressure. Tolerance to the antihypertensive effect has not been observed in long-term clinical use; relatively little tachycardia or change in renin levels has been noted. Rebound elevation of blood pressure does not occur following abrupt cessation of Hypovase therapy.

The therapeutic efficacy of Hypovase in patients with congestive heart failure is ascribed to a reduction in left ventricular filling pressure, reduction in cardiac impedance and an augmentation of cardiac output. The use of Hypovase in congestive heart failure does not provoke a reflex tachycardia and blood pressure reduction is minimal in normotensive patients.

Hypovase has been found to successfully reduce the severity of the signs, symptoms, frequency and duration of attacks, in patients with Raynaud's disease.

In low dosage, antagonism of alpha-1-receptors on prostatic and urethral smooth muscle has been shown to improve the urinary pressure profile in men and to improve symptoms of benign prostatic hypertrophy.

Clinical studies have shown that Hypovase therapy is not associated with adverse changes in the serum lipid profile.

5.2 Pharmacokinetic properties

Following oral administration in normal volunteers and hypertensive patients plasma concentrations of prazosin reach a peak in one to two hours with a plasma half-life of two to three hours. Pharmacokinetic data in a limited number of patients with congestive heart failure, most of whom showed evidence of hepatic congestion, indicates that peak plasma concentrations are reached in 2.5 hours and plasma half life is approximately 7 hours. Hypovase is highly bound to plasma protein. Studies indicate that Hypovase is extensively metabolised, primarily by demethylation and conjugation, and excreted mainly via bile and faeces.

Renal blood flow and glomerular filtration rate are not impaired by long term oral administration and thus Hypovase can be used with safety in hypertensive patients with impaired renal function.

6. PHARMACEUTICAL PARTICULARS

6.1 List of excipients

Calcium phosphate dibasic anhydrous

Maize starch

Microcrystalline cellulose

Magnesium stearate

Sodium lauryl sulphate

Additionally, the 1mg tablet contains sunset yellow (E110).

6.2 Incompatibilities

None stated.

6.3 Shelf life

36 months

6.4 Special precautions for storage

Store below 30°C.

6.5 Nature and contents of container

b.d. starter pack, for the convenience of patients initiating Hypovase therapy, containing 8 × 500 microgram Hypovase tablets and 32 × 1mg Hypovase tablets.

Hypovase 500 microgram: Original packs of 56 tablets, (in blister strips of 4 × 14 tablets).

Hypovase 1mg: Original packs of 56 tablets, (in blister strips of 4 × 14 tablets).

Hypovase 2mg: Original packs of 56 tablets, (in blister strips of 4 × 14 tablets).

The two week b.d. starter pack has the following instructions to the patient:

Step 1 (500 microgram tablets) - evening day 1 to morning day 5

Step 2 (1mg tablets) - evening day 5 to morning day 9

Step 3 (2 × 1mg tablets) - evening day 9 to morning day 15

Your doctor will wish you to follow further dosage instructions beyond Step 3, and you should follow those instructions or see your doctor before the end of Step 3.

The tablets (500microgram and 1mg) are carefully packed in sequence, in blister strips to ensure correct usage.

6.6 Instructions for use and handling

None stated.

7. MARKETING AUTHORISATION HOLDER

Pfizer Limited

Ramsgate Road

Sandwich

Kent, CT13 9NJ

United Kingdom

8. MARKETING AUTHORISATION NUMBER(S)

PL 00057/0149R

PL 00057/0106R

PL 00057/0107R

9. DATE OF FIRST AUTHORISATION/RENEWAL OF THE AUTHORISATION

5 January 1994 / 22 November 2004

10. DATE OF REVISION OF THE TEXT

December 2004

11. LEGAL CATEGORY

POM

Ref: HY4_1 UK

Hypurin Bovine Isophane Cartridges

(Wockhardt UK Ltd)

1. NAME OF THE MEDICINAL PRODUCT

Hypurin® Bovine Isophane

2. QUALITATIVE AND QUANTITATIVE COMPOSITION

Crystalline Insulin Ph Eur (Bovine) 100 IU/ml.

Isophane Insulin Injection Ph Eur (Bovine)

For excipients, see 6.1

3. PHARMACEUTICAL FORM

Suspension for injection.

A white suspension

4. CLINICAL PARTICULARS

4.1 Therapeutic indications

The treatment of insulin dependent diabetes mellitus.

May be used for diabetics requiring a depot insulin of medium duration. Where a more rapid, intense onset is desirable it may be mixed with Hypurin Neutral.

4.2 Posology and method of administration

To be determined by the physician according to the needs of the patient.

Usually administered subcutaneously but where necessary it may be given intramuscularly in which case onset is more rapid and overall duration shorter. It should not be given intravenously. Onset of action occurs within 2 hours after subcutaneous injection with an overall duration of 18-24 hours. Maximum effect is exerted between 6-12 hours.

4.3 Contraindications

Hypoglycaemia.

4.4 Special warnings and special precautions for use

In no circumstances must Hypurin® Bovine Isophane be given intravenously.

Blood or urinary glucose concentrations should be monitored and the urine tested for ketones by patients on insulin therapy.

Patients transferred to Hypurin® Bovine insulins from other commercially available preparations may require dosage adjustments. Patients whose blood glucose control is greatly improved, e.g. by intensified insulin therapy, may lose some or all of the warning symptoms of hypoglycaemia and should be advised accordingly.

Insulin requirements may increase during illness (this includes infection and accidental and surgical trauma), puberty or emotional upset.

Insulin requirements may decrease with liver disease, disease of the adrenal, pituitary or thyroid glands and coeliac disease. In patients with severe renal impairment, insulin requirements may fall and dosage reduction may be necessary. The compensatory response to hypoglycaemia may also be impaired.

Insulin requirements are usually reduced but occasionally increased during periods of increased activity.

4.5 Interaction with other medicinal products and other forms of Interaction

Insulin requirements may increase during concurrent administration of drugs associated with hyperglycaemic activity e.g. oral contraceptives, chloropromazine, thyroid hormone replacement therapy, thiazide diuretics, sympathomimetic agents and corticosteroids.

Insulin requirements may decrease during concomitant use of drugs with hypoglycaemic activity, e.g salicylates, anabolic steroids, monoamine oxidase inhibitors, NSAIDS, ACE inhibitors and octreotide. Drugs which may decrease or increase insulin requirements include alcohol, cyclophosphamide, isoniazid and beta blockers (which may also mask some of the warning signs of insulin-induced hypoglycaemia). Nifedipine may occasionally impair glucose tolerance.

4.6 Pregnancy and lactation

A decreased requirement for insulin may be observed in the early stages of pregnancy. However, in the second and third trimesters, insulin requirements may increase. Insulin requirements should therefore be assessed frequently by an experienced diabetic physician. Diabetic patients who are breast-feeding may require adjustments in their insulin dose.

4.7 Effects on ability to drive and use machines

The patient's ability to concentrate and react may be impaired as a result of hypoglycaemia. This may constitute a risk in situations where these abilities are of special importance (e.g. driving a car or operating machinery).

Patients should be advised to take precautions to avoid hypoglycaemia whilst driving, this is particularly important in those who have reduced or absent awareness of the warning signs of hypoglycaemia or have frequent episodes of hypoglycaemia. The advisability of driving should be considered in these circumstances.

4.8 Undesirable effects

Lipodystrophy (atrophy or hypertrophy of the fat tissue) or oedema may occur at the injection site. Severe, generalised oedema is a rare adverse effect of insulin treatment occurring most often at the initiation of therapy. Insulin hypersensitivity can occur with animal insulins, but appears less likely with purified insulins and there is minimal evidence that such effects occur with Hypurin insulins.

Allergic reactions to phenol and m-cresol contained as preservative and to zinc and protamine may occur.

4.9 Overdose

a) Symptoms

Overdosage causes hypoglycaemia. Symptoms include weakness, sweating, trembling, nervousness, excitement and irritability which, if untreated, will lead to collapse and coma.

b) Treatment

Mild hypoglycaemia will respond to oral administration of glucose or sugar and rest.

Moderately severe hypoglycaemia can be treated by intramuscular or subcutaneous injection of glucagon followed by oral carbohydrate when the patient is sufficiently recovered.

For patients who are comatose or who have failed to respond to glucagon injection an intravenous injection of strong Dextrose Injection BP should be given.

5. PHARMACOLOGICAL PROPERTIES

5.1 Pharmacodynamic properties

ATC Code – A10A A

Insulin output from the pancreas of a healthy person is about 50 units per day, which is sufficient to maintain the fasting blood sugar concentration in the range 0.8 ± 0.2mg/ml. In diabetes mellitus, the blood sugar rises in an uncontrolled manner. Parenterally administered insulin causes a fall in blood sugar concentration and increased storage of glycogen in the liver. In the diabetic it raises the respiratory quotient after a carbohydrate meal and prevents the formation of ketone bodies. The rise in blood sugar concentration caused by adrenaline and corticosteroids, glucagon and posterior pituitary extract is reversed by insulin.

5.2 Pharmacokinetic properties

Insulin is rapidly absorbed from subcutaneous tissue or muscle following injection.

Insulin is metabolised mainly in the liver and a small amount is excreted in the urine.

The plasma half life is 4 to 5 minutes. The half life after subcutaneous injection is about 4 hours and after intramuscular injection about 2 hours.

5.3 Preclinical safety data

There are no preclinical data of relevance to the prescriber which are additional to that already included in other sections.

6. PHARMACEUTICAL PARTICULARS

6.1 List of excipients

Protamine sulphate

Zinc chloride

m-Cresol

Phenol

Sodium phosphate

Glycerol

Water for injections

6.2 Incompatibilities

None

6.3 Shelf life

36 months.

Following injection of the first dose the product should be used within 28 days. Discard any unused material after this time.

6.4 Special precautions for storage

Store at 2°C - 8°C.

Do not freeze.

Cartridges in use must not be stored in a refrigerator.

Chemical and physical in-use stability has been demonstrated for 28 days at 25°C.

From a microbiological point of view the opening carries a risk of microbial contamination and aseptic handling is a necessity.

In use storage times and conditions are the responsibility of the user.

6.5 Nature and contents of container
1.5ml neutral glass cartridge sealed with a bromobutyl rubber bung and metal closure in packs of five.

3ml neutral glass cartridge sealed with a bromobutyl rubber bung and metal closure in packs of five.

6.6 Instructions for use and handling
Prior to insertion in the pen, the cartridge of Hypurin® Bovine Isophane should be shaken vigorously up and down, with a "bell ringing" action at least ten times. Before each injection the pen should be inverted at least ten times to mix the insulin again.

The cartridge must not be used if the contents have been frozen or it contains lumps that do not disperse on mixing.

Administrative Data

7. MARKETING AUTHORISATION HOLDER
CP Pharmaceuticals Ltd

Ash Road North

Wrexham

LL13 9UF

8. MARKETING AUTHORISATION NUMBER(S)
PL 04543/0367

9. DATE OF FIRST AUTHORISATION/RENEWAL OF THE AUTHORISATION
N/A

10. DATE OF REVISION OF THE TEXT
July 2002

Hypurin Bovine Isophane Vials

(Wockhardt UK Ltd)

1. NAME OF THE MEDICINAL PRODUCT
Hypurin® Bovine Isophane

2. QUALITATIVE AND QUANTITATIVE COMPOSITION
Crystalline Insulin Ph Eur (Bovine) 100 IU/ml.

Isophane Insulin Injection Ph Eur (Bovine)

For excipients, see 6.1

3. PHARMACEUTICAL FORM
Suspension for injection.

A white suspension

4. CLINICAL PARTICULARS

4.1 Therapeutic indications
The treatment of insulin dependent diabetes mellitus.

May be used for diabetics requiring a depot insulin of medium duration. Where a more rapid, intense onset is desirable it may be mixed with Hypurin Neutral.

4.2 Posology and method of administration
Usually administered subcutaneously but where necessary it may be given intramuscularly in which case onset is more rapid and overall duration shorter. It should not be given intravenously. Onset of action occurs within 2 hours after subcutaneous injection with an overall duration of 18-24 hours. Maximum effect is exerted between 6-12 hours.

4.3 Contraindications
Hypoglycaemia.

4.4 Special warnings and special precautions for use
In no circumstances must Hypurin® Bovine Isophane be given intravenously.

Blood or urinary glucose concentrations should be monitored and the urine tested for ketones by patients on insulin therapy.

Patients transferred to Hypurin® Bovine insulins from other commercially available preparations may require dosage adjustments. Patients whose blood glucose control is greatly improved, e.g. by intensified insulin therapy, may lose some or all of the warning symptoms of hypoglycaemia and should be advised accordingly.

Insulin requirements may increase during illness (this includes infection and accidental and surgical trauma), puberty or emotional upset.

Insulin requirements may decrease with liver disease, disease of the adrenal, pituitary or thyroid glands and coeliac disease. In patients with severe renal impairment, insulin requirements may fall and dosage reduction may be necessary. The compensatory response to hypoglycaemia may also be impaired.

Insulin requirements are usually reduced but occasionally increased during periods of increased activity.

4.5 Interaction with other medicinal products and other forms of Interaction
Insulin requirements may increase during concurrent administration of drugs associated with hyperglycaemic activity e.g. oral contraceptives, chloropromazine, thyroid hormone replacement therapy, thiazide diuretics, sympathomimetic agents and corticosteroids.

Insulin requirements may decrease during concomitant use of drugs with hypoglycaemic activity, e.g salicylates, anabolic steroids, monoamine oxidase inhibitors, NSAIDS, ACE inhibitors and octreotide. Drugs which may decrease or increase insulin requirements include alcohol, cyclophosphamide, isoniazid and beta blockers (which may also mask some of the warning signs of insulin-induced hypoglycaemia). Nifedipine may occasionally impair glucose tolerance.

4.6 Pregnancy and lactation
A decreased requirement for insulin may be observed in the early stages of pregnancy. However, in the second and third trimesters, insulin requirements may increase. Insulin requirements should therefore be assessed frequently by an experienced diabetic physician. Diabetic patients who are breast-feeding may require adjustments in their insulin dose.

4.7 Effects on ability to drive and use machines
The patient's ability to concentrate and react may be impaired as a result of hypoglycaemia. This may constitute a risk in situations where these abilities are of special importance (e.g. driving a car or operating machinery).

Patients should be advised to take precautions to avoid hypoglycaemia whilst driving, this is particularly important in those who have reduced or absent awareness of the warning signs of hypoglycaemia or have frequent episodes of hypoglycaemia. The advisability of driving should be considered in these circumstances.

4.8 Undesirable effects
Lipodystrophy (atrophy or hypertrophy of the fat tissue) or oedema may occur at the injection site. Severe, generalised oedema is a rare adverse effect of insulin treatment occurring most often at the initiation of therapy. Insulin hypersensitivity can occur with animal insulins, but appears less likely with purified insulins and there is minimal evidence that such effects occur with Hypurin insulins.

Allergic reactions to phenol and m-cresol contained as preservative and to zinc and protamine may occur.

4.9 Overdose
a) Symptoms

Overdosage causes hypoglycaemia. Symptoms include weakness, sweating, trembling, nervousness, excitement and irritability which, if untreated, will lead to collapse and coma.

b) Treatment

Mild hypoglycaemia will respond to oral administration of glucose or sugar and rest.

Moderately severe hypoglycaemia can be treated by intramuscular or subcutaneous injection of glucagon followed by oral carbohydrate when the patient is sufficiently recovered.

For patients who are comatose or who have failed to respond to glucagon injection an intravenous injection of strong Dextrose Injection BP should be given.

5. PHARMACOLOGICAL PROPERTIES

5.1 Pharmacodynamic properties
ATC Code – A10A A

Insulin output from the pancreas of a healthy person is about 50 units per day, which is sufficient to maintain the fasting blood sugar concentration in the range 0.8 ± 0.2mg/ml. In diabetes mellitus, the blood sugar rises in an uncontrolled manner. Parenterally administered insulin causes a fall in blood sugar concentration and increased storage of glycogen in the liver. In the diabetic it raises the respiratory quotient after a carbohydrate meal and prevents the formation of ketone bodies. The rise in blood sugar concentration caused by adrenaline and corticosteroids, glucagon and posterior pituitary extract is reversed by insulin.

5.2 Pharmacokinetic properties
Insulin is rapidly absorbed from subcutaneous tissue or muscle following injection.

Insulin is metabolised mainly in the liver and a small amount is excreted in the urine.

The plasma half life is 4 to 5 minutes. The half life after subcutaneous injection is about 4 hours and after intramuscular injection about 2 hours.

5.3 Preclinical safety data
There are no preclinical data of relevance to the prescriber which are additional to those already included in other sections.

6. PHARMACEUTICAL PARTICULARS

6.1 List of excipients
Protamine sulphate

Zinc chloride

m-Cresol

Phenol

Sodium phosphate

Glycerol

Water for injections

6.2 Incompatibilities
None

6.3 Shelf life
36 months.

Following injection of the first dose the product should be used within 28 days. Discard any unused material after this time.

6.4 Special precautions for storage
Store at 2°C - 8°C.

Do not freeze.

Chemical and physical in-use stability has been demonstrated for 28 days at 25°C

From a microbiological point of view the opening carries a risk of microbial contamination and aseptic handling is a necessity.

In use storage times and conditions are the responsibility of the user.

6.5 Nature and contents of container
10ml neutral glass vial sealed with a rubber bung and metal closure.

6.6 Instructions for use and handling
The vial must not be used if the contents have been frozen or it contains lumps that do not disperse on mixing.

Prior to use the vial of Hypurin® Bovine Isophane should be rolled gently between the palms or inverted several times.

Hypurin® Bovine Isophane may be mixed with Hypurin® Bovine Neutral in the syringe, in which case Hypurin® Bovine Neutral should be the first dose to be withdrawn. The injection should then be made immediately upon withdrawal of the contents.

The use of each vial should be restricted to a single patient.

Administrative Data

7. MARKETING AUTHORISATION HOLDER
CP Pharmaceuticals Ltd

Ash Road North

Wrexham LL13 9UF

8. MARKETING AUTHORISATION NUMBER(S)
PL 4543/0196

9. DATE OF FIRST AUTHORISATION/RENEWAL OF THE AUTHORISATION
21 October 1986

10. DATE OF REVISION OF THE TEXT
November 2001

Hypurin Bovine Lente

(Wockhardt UK Ltd)

1. NAME OF THE MEDICINAL PRODUCT
Hypurin® Bovine Lente 100 IU/ml injection

2. QUALITATIVE AND QUANTITATIVE COMPOSITION
Crystalline Insulin Ph Eur (Bovine) 100 IU/ml.

Insulin Zinc Suspension (Mixed) Ph Eur (Bovine)

For excipients, see 6.1

3. PHARMACEUTICAL FORM
Suspension for injection.

A white suspension

4. CLINICAL PARTICULARS

4.1 Therapeutic indications
The treatment of insulin dependent diabetes mellitus.

Hypurin® Bovine Lente may be used for diabetics requiring a depot insulin of medium to extended duration.

4.2 Posology and method of administration
To be determined by the physician according to the needs of the patient.

Administered subcutaneously. It is not recommended for intramuscular use and should not be given intravenously. Onset of action occurs approximately 2 hours after subcutaneous injection with an overall duration extending up to 30 hours. Maximum effect is exerted between 8-12 hours.

Prior to use, the vial of Hypurin® Bovine Lente should be rolled gently between the palms or inverted several times.

4.3 Contraindications
Hypoglycaemia.

Known hypersensitivity to any of the constituents.

4.4 Special warnings and special precautions for use
In no circumstances must Hypurin® Bovine Lente be given intravenously.

Blood or urinary glucose concentrations should be monitored and the urine tested for ketones by patients on insulin therapy.

Patients transferred to Hypurin® Bovine insulins from other commercially available preparations may require dosage adjustments. Patients whose blood glucose control is greatly improved, e.g. by intensified insulin therapy, may lose some or all of the warning symptoms of hypoglycaemia and should be advised accordingly.

Insulin requirements may increase during illness (this includes infection and accidental and surgical trauma), puberty or emotional upset.

Insulin requirements may decrease with liver disease, disease of the adrenal, pituitary or thyroid glands and coeliac disease. In patients with severe renal impairment, insulin requirements may fall and dosage reduction may be necessary. The compensatory response to hypoglycaemia may also be impaired.

Insulin requirements are usually reduced but occasionally increased during periods of increased activity.

4.5 Interaction with other medicinal products and other forms of Interaction

Insulin requirements may increase during concurrent administration of drugs associated with hyperglycaemic activity e.g. oral contraceptives, chloropromazine, thyroid hormone replacement therapy, thiazide diuretics, sympathomimetic agents and corticosteroids.

Insulin requirements may decrease during concomitant use of drugs with hypoglycaemic activity, e.g salicylates, anabolic steroids, monoamine oxidase inhibitors, NSAIDS, ACE inhibitors and octreotide. Drugs which may decrease or increase insulin requirements include alcohol, cyclophosphamide, isoniazid and beta blockers (which may also mask some of the warning signs of insulin-induced hypoglycaemia). Nifedipine may occasionally impair glucose intolerance.

4.6 Pregnancy and lactation

A decreased requirement for insulin may be observed in the early stages of pregnancy. However, in the second and third trimesters, insulin requirements may increase. Insulin requirements should therefore be assessed frequently by an experienced diabetic physician. Diabetic patients who are breast-feeding may require adjustments in their insulin dose.

4.7 Effects on ability to drive and use machines

The patient's ability to concentrate and react may be impaired as a result of hypoglycaemia. This may constitute a risk in situations where these abilities are of special importance (e.g. driving a car or operating machinery).

Patients should be advised to take precautions to avoid hypoglycaemia whilst driving, this is particularly important in those who have reduced or absent awareness of the warning signs of hypoglycaemia or have frequent episodes of hypoglycaemia. The advisability of driving should be considered in these circumstances.

4.8 Undesirable effects

Lipodystrophy (atrophy or hypertrophy of the fat tissue) or oedema may occur at the injection site. Severe, generalised oedema is a rare adverse effect of insulin treatment occurring most often at the initiation of therapy. Insulin hypersensitivity can occur with animal insulins, but appears less likely with purified insulins and there is minimal evidence that such effects occur with Hypurin insulins.

Allergic reactions to phenol and m-cresol contained as preservative and to zinc and protamine may occur.

4.9 Overdose

a) Symptoms

Overdosage causes hypoglycaemia. Symptoms include weakness, sweating, trembling, nervousness, excitement and irritability which, if untreated, will lead to collapse and coma.

b) Treatment

Mild hypoglycaemia will respond to oral administration of glucose or sugar and rest.

Moderately severe hypoglycaemia can be treated by intramuscular or subcutaneous injection of glucagon followed by oral carbohydrate when the patient is sufficiently recovered.

For patients who are comatose or who have failed to respond to glucagon injection an intravenous injection of strong Dextrose Injection BP should be given.

5. PHARMACOLOGICAL PROPERTIES

5.1 Pharmacodynamic properties

ATC Code – A10A A

Insulin output from the pancreas of a healthy person is about 50 units per day, which is sufficient to maintain the fasting blood sugar concentration in the range 0.8 ± 0.2mg/ml. In diabetes mellitus, the blood sugar rises in an uncontrolled manner. Parenterally administered insulin causes a fall in blood sugar concentration and increased storage of glycogen in the liver. In the diabetic it raises the respiratory quotient after a carbohydrate meal and prevents the formation of ketone bodies. The rise in blood sugar concentration caused by adrenaline and corticosteroids, glucagon and posterior pituitary extract is reversed by insulin.

5.2 Pharmacokinetic properties

Insulin is rapidly absorbed from subcutaneous tissue following injection.

Insulin is metabolised mainly in the liver and a small amount is excreted in the urine.

The plasma half-life is 4 to 5 minutes. The half-life after subcutaneous injection is about 4 hours.

5.3 Preclinical safety data

There are no preclinical data of relevance to the prescriber which are additional to those already included in other sections.

6. PHARMACEUTICAL PARTICULARS

6.1 List of excipients

Sodium chloride

Sodium acetate

Methylparahydroxybenzoate

Zinc oxide

Water for injections

Hydrochloric acid

Sodium hydroxide

6.2 Incompatibilities

Not applicable

6.3 Shelf life

Three years.

Following injection of the first dose the product should be used within 28 days. Discard any unused material after this time.

6.4 Special precautions for storage

Store at 2°C - 8°C.

Do not freeze.

Chemical and physical in-use stability has been demonstrated for 28 days at 25°C.

From a microbiological point of view the opening carries a risk of microbial contamination and aseptic handling is a necessity.

In use storage times and conditions are the responsibility of the user.

6.5 Nature and contents of container

10ml Type I glass vial sealed with a rubber bung and metal closure.

6.6 Instructions for use and handling

The vial must not be used if the contents have been frozen or it contains lumps that do not disperse on mixing.

Prior to use the vial of Hypurin® Bovine Lente should be rolled gently between the palms or inverted several times. Hypurin® Bovine Lente may be mixed with bovine neutral insulin in the syringe, in which case the bovine neutral insulin should be the first dose to be withdrawn. The injection should then be made immediately upon withdrawal of the contents.

The use of each vial should be restricted to a single patient.

Administrative Data

7. MARKETING AUTHORISATION HOLDER

CP Pharmaceuticals Ltd

Ash Road North

Wrexham LL13 9UF

United Kingdom

8. MARKETING AUTHORISATION NUMBER(S)

PL 04543/0214

9. DATE OF FIRST AUTHORISATION/RENEWAL OF THE AUTHORISATION

28th October 1987

10. DATE OF REVISION OF THE TEXT

17 February 2002

Hypurin Bovine Neutral Cartridges

(Wockhardt UK Ltd)

1. NAME OF THE MEDICINAL PRODUCT

Hypurin® Bovine Neutral

2. QUALITATIVE AND QUANTITATIVE COMPOSITION

Crystalline Insulin Ph Eur (Bovine) 100IU/ml.

Neutral Insulin Injection Ph Eur (Bovine)

For excipients, see 6.1

3. PHARMACEUTICAL FORM

Solution for injection

A clear, colourless solution

4. CLINICAL PARTICULARS

4.1 Therapeutic indications

The treatment of insulin dependent diabetes mellitus.

May be used for diabetics who require an insulin of prompt onset and short duration. It is a suitable preparation for admixture with longer acting insulins. It is particularly useful where intermittent, short term or emergency therapy is required, during initial stabilisation and in the treatment of labile diabetes.

4.2 Posology and method of administration

To be determined by the physician according to the needs of the patient.

Usually administered subcutaneously but where necessary it may be given intramuscularly or intravenously. After subcutaneous injection onset of action occurs within 30-60 minutes with an overall duration of 6-8 hours. Maximum effect is exerted over the mid-range.

4.3 Contraindications

Hypoglycaemia.

4.4 Special warnings and special precautions for use

Blood or urinary glucose concentrations should be monitored and the urine tested for ketones by patients on insulin therapy.

Patients transferred to Hypurin® Bovine insulins from other commercially available preparations may require dosage adjustments. Patients whose blood glucose control is greatly improved, e.g. by intensified insulin therapy, may lose some or all of the warning symptoms of hypoglycaemia and should be advised accordingly.

Insulin requirements may increase during illness (this includes infection and accidental and surgical trauma), puberty or emotional upset.

Insulin requirements may decrease with liver disease, disease of the adrenal, pituitary or thyroid glands and coeliac disease. In patients with severe renal impairment, insulin requirements may fall and dosage reduction may be necessary. The compensatory response to hypoglycaemia may also be impaired.

Insulin requirements are usually reduced but occasionally increased during periods of increased activity.

4.5 Interaction with other medicinal products and other forms of Interaction

Insulin requirements may increase during concurrent administration of drugs associated with hyperglycaemic activity e.g. oral contraceptives, chloropromazine, thyroid hormone replacement therapy, thiazide diuretics, sympathomimetic agents and corticosteroids.

Insulin requirements may decrease during concomitant use of drugs with hypoglycaemic activity, e.g salicylates, anabolic steroids, monoamine oxidase inhibitors, NSAIDS, ACE inhibitors and octreotide. Drugs which may decrease or increase insulin requirements include alcohol, cyclophosphamide, isoniazid and beta blockers (which may also mask some of the warning signs of insulin-induced hypoglycaemia). Nifedipine may occasionally impair glucose tolerance.

4.6 Pregnancy and lactation

A decreased requirement for insulin may be observed in the early stages of pregnancy. However, in the second and third trimesters, insulin requirements may increase. Insulin requirements should therefore be assessed frequently by an experienced diabetic physician. Diabetic patients who are breast-feeding may require adjustments in their insulin dose.

4.7 Effects on ability to drive and use machines

The patient's ability to concentrate and react may be impaired as a result of hypoglycaemia. This may constitute a risk in situations where these abilities are of special importance (e.g. driving a car or operating machinery).

Patients should be advised to take precautions to avoid hypoglycaemia whilst driving, this is particularly important in those who have reduced or absent awareness of the warning signs of hypoglycaemia or have frequent episodes of hypoglycaemia. The advisability of driving should be considered in these circumstances.

4.8 Undesirable effects

Lipodystrophy (atrophy or hypertrophy of the fat tissue) or oedema may occur at the injection site. Severe, generalised oedema is a rare adverse effect of insulin treatment occurring most often at the initiation of therapy. Insulin hypersensitivity can occur with animal insulins, but appears less likely with purified insulins and there is minimal evidence that such effects occur with Hypurin insulins.

Allergic reactions to phenol and m-cresol contained as preservative and to zinc and protamine may occur.

4.9 Overdose

a) Symptoms

Overdosage causes hypoglycaemia. Symptoms include weakness, sweating, trembling, nervousness, excitement and irritability which, if untreated, will lead to collapse and coma.

b) Treatment

Mild hypoglycaemia will respond to oral administration of glucose or sugar and rest.

Moderately severe hypoglycaemia can be treated by intramuscular or subcutaneous injection of glucagon followed by oral carbohydrate when the patient is sufficiently recovered.

For patients who are comatose or who have failed to respond to glucagon injection an intravenous injection of strong Dextrose Injection BP should be given.

5. PHARMACOLOGICAL PROPERTIES

5.1 Pharmacodynamic properties

ATC Code – A10A A

Insulin output from the pancreas of a healthy person is about 50 units per day, which is sufficient to maintain the fasting blood sugar concentration in the range 0.8 ± 0.2mg/ml. In diabetes mellitus, the blood sugar rises in an uncontrolled manner. Parenterally administered insulin causes a fall in blood sugar concentration and increased storage of glycogen in the liver. In the diabetic it raises the respiratory quotient after a carbohydrate meal and prevents the formation of ketone bodies. The rise in blood sugar concentration caused by adrenaline and corticosteroids, glucagon and posterior pituitary extract is reversed by insulin.

5.2 Pharmacokinetic properties
Insulin is rapidly absorbed from subcutaneous tissue or muscle following injection.

Insulin is metabolised mainly in the liver and a small amount is excreted in the urine.

The plasma half life is 4 to 5 minutes. The half life after subcutaneous injection is about 4 hours and after intramuscular injection about 2 hours.

5.3 Preclinical safety data
There are no preclinical data of relevance to the prescriber which are additional to that already included in other sections.

6. PHARMACEUTICAL PARTICULARS

6.1 List of excipients
m-Cresol

Phenol

Sodium phosphate

Glycerol

Water for injections

6.2 Incompatibilities
None

6.3 Shelf life
36 months.

Following injection of the first dose the product should be used within 28 days. Discard any unused material after this time.

6.4 Special precautions for storage
Store at 2°C - 8°C.

Do not freeze.

Cartridges in use must not be stored in a refrigerator.

Chemical and physical in-use stability has been demonstrated for 28 days at 25°C.

From a microbiological point of view the opening carries a risk of microbial contamination and aseptic handling is a necessity.

In use storage times and conditions are the responsibility of the user.

6.5 Nature and contents of container
1.5ml neutral glass cartridge sealed with a bromobutyl rubber bung and metal closure in packs of five.

3ml neutral glass cartridge sealed with a bromobutyl rubber bung and metal closure in packs of five.

6.6 Instructions for use and handling
The cartridge must not be used if the contents have been frozen or it contains lumps that do not disperse on mixing.

Administrative Data

7. MARKETING AUTHORISATION HOLDER
CP Pharmaceuticals Ltd

Ash Road North

Wrexham

LL13 9UF

8. MARKETING AUTHORISATION NUMBER(S)
PL 04543/0366

9. DATE OF FIRST AUTHORISATION/RENEWAL OF THE AUTHORISATION
N/A

10. DATE OF REVISION OF THE TEXT
July 2002

Hypurin Bovine Neutral Vials

(Wockhardt UK Ltd)

1. NAME OF THE MEDICINAL PRODUCT
Hypurin® Bovine Neutral

2. QUALITATIVE AND QUANTITATIVE COMPOSITION
Crystalline Insulin Ph Eur (Bovine) 100IU/ml.

Neutral Insulin Injection Ph Eur (Bovine)

For excipients, see 6.1

3. PHARMACEUTICAL FORM
Solution for injection

A clear, colourless solution

4. CLINICAL PARTICULARS

4.1 Therapeutic indications
The treatment of insulin dependent diabetes mellitus.

May be used for diabetics who require an insulin of prompt onset and short duration. It is a suitable preparation for admixture with longer acting insulins. It is particularly useful where intermittent, short term or emergency therapy is required, during initial stabilisation and in the treatment of labile diabetes.

4.2 Posology and method of administration
To be determined by the physician according to the needs of the patient.

Usually administered subcutaneously but where necessary it may be given intramuscularly or intravenously. After subcutaneous injection onset of action occurs within 30-60 minutes with an overall duration of 6-8 hours. Maximum effect is exerted over the mid-range.

4.3 Contraindications
Hypoglycaemia.

4.4 Special warnings and special precautions for use
Blood or urinary glucose concentrations should be monitored and the urine tested for ketones by patients on insulin therapy.

Patients transferred to Hypurin® Bovine insulins from other commercially available preparations may require dosage adjustments. Patients whose blood glucose control is greatly improved, e.g. by intensified insulin therapy, may lose some or all of the warning symptoms of hypoglycaemia and should be advised accordingly.

Insulin requirements may increase during illness (this includes infection and accidental and surgical trauma), puberty or emotional upset.

Insulin requirements may decrease with liver disease, disease of the adrenal, pituitary or thyroid glands and coeliac disease. In patients with severe renal impairment, insulin requirements may fall and dosage reduction may be necessary. The compensatory response to hypoglycaemia may also be impaired.

Insulin requirements are usually reduced but occasionally increased during periods of increased activity.

4.5 Interaction with other medicinal products and other forms of Interaction
Insulin requirements may increase during concurrent administration of drugs associated with hyperglycaemic activity e.g. oral contraceptives, chloropromazine, thyroid hormone replacement therapy, thiazide diuretics, sympathomimetic agents and corticosteroids.

Insulin requirements may decrease during concomitant use of drugs with hypoglycaemic activity, e.g salicylates, anabolic steroids, monoamine oxidase inhibitors, NSAIDS, ACE inhibitors and octreotide. Drugs which may decrease or increase insulin requirements include alcohol, cyclophosphamide, isoniazid and beta blockers (which may also mask some of the warning signs of insulin-induced hypoglycaemia). Nifedipine may occasionally impair glucose tolerance.

4.6 Pregnancy and lactation
A decreased requirement for insulin may be observed in the early stages of pregnancy. However, in the second and third trimesters, insulin requirements may increase. Insulin requirements should therefore be assessed frequently by an experienced diabetic physician. Diabetic patients who are breast-feeding may require adjustments in their insulin dose.

4.7 Effects on ability to drive and use machines
The patient's ability to concentrate and react may be impaired as a result of hypoglycaemia. This may constitute a risk in situations where these abilities are of special importance (e.g. driving a car or operating machinery).

Patients should be advised to take precautions to avoid hypoglycaemia whilst driving, this is particularly important in those who have reduced or absent awareness of the warning signs of hypoglycaemia or have frequent episodes of hypoglycaemia. The advisability of driving should be considered in these circumstances.

4.8 Undesirable effects
Lipodystrophy (atrophy or hypertrophy of the fat tissue) or oedema may occur at the injection site. Severe, generalised oedema is a rare adverse effect of insulin treatment occuring most often at the initiation of therapy. Insulin hypersensitivity can occur with animal insulins, but appears less likely with purified insulins and there is minimal evidence that such effects occur with Hypurin insulins.

Allergic reactions to phenol and m-cresol contained as preservative and to zinc and protamine may occur.

4.9 Overdose

a) Symptoms

Overdosage causes hypoglycaemia. Symptoms include weakness, sweating, trembling, nervousness, excitement and irritability which, if untreated, will lead to collapse and coma.

b) Treatment

Mild hypoglycaemia will respond to oral administration of glucose or sugar and rest.

Moderately severe hypoglycaemia can be treated by intramuscular or subcutaneous injection of glucagon followed by oral carbohydrate when the patient is sufficiently recovered.

For patients who are comatose or who have failed to respond to glucagon injection an intravenous injection of strong Dextrose Injection BP should be given.

5. PHARMACOLOGICAL PROPERTIES

5.1 Pharmacodynamic properties

ATC Code – A10A A

Insulin output from the pancreas of a healthy person is about 50 units per day, which is sufficient to maintain the fasting blood sugar concentration in the range 0.8 ± 0.2mg/ml. In diabetes mellitus, the blood sugar rises in an uncontrolled manner. Parenterally administered insulin causes a fall in blood sugar concentration and increased storage of glycogen in the liver. In the diabetic it raises the respiratory quotient after a carbohydrate meal and prevents the formation of ketone bodies. The rise in blood sugar concentration caused by adrenaline and corticosteroids, glucagon and posterior pituitary extract is reversed by insulin.

5.2 Pharmacokinetic properties
Insulin is rapidly absorbed from subcutaneous tissue or muscle following injection.

Insulin is metabolised mainly in the liver and a small amount is excreted in the urine.

The plasma half life is 4 to 5 minutes. The half life after subcutaneous injection is about 4 hours and after intramuscular injection about 2 hours.

5.3 Preclinical safety data
There are no preclinical data of relevance to the prescriber which are additional to those already included in other sections.

6. PHARMACEUTICAL PARTICULARS

6.1 List of excipients
m-Cresol

Phenol

Sodium phosphate

Glycerol

Water for injections

6.2 Incompatibilities
None

6.3 Shelf life
36 months.

Following injection of the first dose the product should be used within 28 days. Discard any unused material after this time.

6.4 Special precautions for storage
Store at 2°C - 8°C.

Do not freeze.

Chemical and physical in-use stability has been demonstrated for 28 days at 25°C.

From a microbiological point of view the opening carries a risk of microbial contamination and aseptic handling is a necessity.

In use storage times and conditions are the responsibility of the user.

6.5 Nature and contents of container
10ml neutral glass vial sealed with a rubber bung and metal closure.

6.6 Instructions for use and handling
The vial must not be used if the contents have been frozen or it contains lumps that do not disperse on mixing.

Hypurin® Bovine Isophane and Hypurin® Bovine Lente may be mixed with Hypurin® Bovine Neutral in the syringe, in which case Hypurin® Bovine Neutral should be the first dose to be withdrawn. The injection should then be made immediately upon withdrawal of the contents.

Hypurin® Bovine Neutral and Hypurin® Bovine Protamine Zinc should not be mixed together.

The use of each vial should be restricted to a single patient.

Administrative Data

7. MARKETING AUTHORISATION HOLDER
CP Pharmaceuticals Ltd

Ash Road North

Wrexham LL13 9UF

8. MARKETING AUTHORISATION NUMBER(S)
PL 4543/0203

9. DATE OF FIRST AUTHORISATION/RENEWAL OF THE AUTHORISATION
4 November 1986

10. DATE OF REVISION OF THE TEXT
November 2001

Hypurin Bovine Protamine Zinc

(Wockhardt UK Ltd)

1. NAME OF THE MEDICINAL PRODUCT
Hypurin® Bovine Protamine Zinc

2. QUALITATIVE AND QUANTITATIVE COMPOSITION
Crystalline Insulin Ph Eur (Bovine) 100 IU/ml.

Protamine Zinc Insulin Injection BP (Bovine)

For excipients, see 6.1

3. PHARMACEUTICAL FORM
Suspension for injection.

A white suspension

4. CLINICAL PARTICULARS

4.1 Therapeutic indications
The treatment of insulin dependent diabetes mellitus.

May be used for diabetics requiring a depot insulin of extended duration. It is characteristically slow in onset and is commonly used in conjunction with Hypurin Neutral.

4.2 Posology and method of administration

Administered subcutaneously. It is not recommended for intramuscular use and should not be given intravenously. Onset of action occurs after 4-6 hours with an overall duration of 24-36 hours. Maximum effect is exerted between 10-20 hours.

4.3 Contraindications

Hypoglycaemia.

4.4 Special warnings and special precautions for use

In no circumstances must Hypurin® Bovine Protamine Zinc be given intravenously.

Blood or urinary glucose concentrations should be monitored and the urine tested for ketones by patients on insulin therapy.

Patients transferred to Hypurin® Bovine insulins from other commercially available preparations may require dosage adjustments. Patients whose blood glucose control is greatly improved, e.g. by intensified insulin therapy, may lose some or all of the warning symptoms of hypoglycaemia and should be advised accordingly.

Insulin requirements may increase during illness (this includes infection and accidental and surgical trauma), puberty or emotional upset.

Insulin requirements may decrease with liver disease, disease of the adrenal, pituitary or thyroid glands and coeliac disease. In patients with severe renal impairment, insulin requirements may fall and dosage reduction may be necessary. The compensatory response to hypoglycaemia may also be impaired.

Insulin requirements are usually reduced but occasionally increased during periods of increased activity.

4.5 Interaction with other medicinal products and other forms of Interaction

Insulin requirements may increase during concurrent administration of drugs associated with hyperglycaemic activity e.g. oral contraceptives, chloropromazine, thyroid hormone replacement therapy, thiazide diuretics, sympathomimetic agents and corticosteroids.

Insulin requirements may decrease during concomitant use of drugs with hypoglycaemic activity, e.g salicylates, anabolic steroids, monoamine oxidase inhibitors, NSAIDS, ACE inhibitors and octreotide. Drugs which may decrease or increase insulin requirements include alcohol, cyclophosphamide, isoniazid and beta blockers (which may also mask some of the warning signs of insulin-induced hypoglycaemia). Nifedipine may occasionally impair glucose tolerance.

4.6 Pregnancy and lactation

A decreased requirement for insulin may be observed in the early stages of pregnancy. However, in the second and third trimesters, insulin requirements may increase. Insulin requirements should therefore be assessed frequently by an experienced diabetic physician. Diabetic patients who are breast-feeding may require adjustments in their insulin dose.

4.7 Effects on ability to drive and use machines

The patient's ability to concentrate and react may be impaired as a result of hypoglycaemia. This may constitute a risk in situations where these abilities are of special importance (e.g. driving a car or operating machinery).

Patients should be advised to take precautions to avoid hypoglycaemia whilst driving, this is particularly important in those who have reduced or absent awareness of the warning signs of hypoglycaemia or have frequent episodes of hypoglycaemia. The advisability of driving should be considered in these circumstances.

4.8 Undesirable effects

Lipodystrophy (atrophy or hypertrophy of the fat tissue) or oedema may occur at the injection site. Severe, generalised oedema is a rare adverse effect of insulin treatment occurring most often at the initiation of therapy. Insulin hypersensitivity can occur with animal insulins, but appears less likely with purified insulins and there is minimal evidence that such effects occur with Hypurin insulins.

Allergic reactions to phenol and m-cresol contained as preservative and to zinc and protamine may occur.

4.9 Overdose

a) Symptoms

Overdosage causes hypoglycaemia. Symptoms include weakness, sweating, trembling, nervousness, excitement and irritability which, if untreated, will lead to collapse and coma.

b) Treatment

Mild hypoglycaemia will respond to oral administration of glucose or sugar and rest.

Moderately severe hypoglycaemia can be treated by intramuscular or subcutaneous injection of glucagon followed by oral carbohydrate when the patient is sufficiently recovered.

For patients who are comatose or who have failed to respond to glucagon injection an intravenous injection of strong Dextrose Injection BP should be given.

5. PHARMACOLOGICAL PROPERTIES

5.1 Pharmacodynamic properties

ATC Code – A10A A

Insulin output from the pancreas of a healthy person is about 50 units per day, which is sufficient to maintain the fasting blood sugar concentration in the range 0.8 ± 0.2mg/ml. In diabetes mellitus, the blood sugar rises in an uncontrolled manner. Parenterally administered insulin causes a fall in blood sugar concentration and increased storage of glycogen in the liver. In the diabetic it raises the respiratory quotient after a carbohydrate meal and prevents the formation of ketone bodies. The rise in blood sugar concentration caused by adrenaline and corticosteroids, glucagon and posterior pituitary extract is reversed by insulin.

5.2 Pharmacokinetic properties

Insulin is rapidly absorbed from subcutaneous tissue or muscle following injection.

Insulin is metabolised mainly in the liver and a small amount is excreted in the urine.

The plasma half life is 4 to 5 minutes. The half life after subcutaneous injection is about 4 hours and after intramuscular injection about 2 hours.

5.3 Preclinical safety data

There are no preclinical data of relevance to the prescriber which are additional to those already included in other sections.

6. PHARMACEUTICAL PARTICULARS

6.1 List of excipients

Protamine sulphate

Zinc chloride

Glycerol

Sodium phosphate

Phenol

Water for injections.

6.2 Incompatibilities

None

6.3 Shelf life

36 months.

Following injection of the first dose the product should be used within 28 days. Discard any unused material after this time.

6.4 Special precautions for storage

Store at 2°C - 8°C.

Do not freeze.

Chemical and physical in-use stability has been demonstrated for 28 days at 25°C.

From a microbiological point of view the opening carries a risk of microbial contamination and aseptic handling is a necessity.

In use storage times and conditions are the responsibility of the user.

6.5 Nature and contents of container

10ml neutral glass vial sealed with a rubber bung and metal closure.

6.6 Instructions for use and handling

The vial must not be used if the contents have been frozen or it contains lumps that do not disperse on mixing.

Prior to use the vial of Hypurin® Bovine Protamine Zinc should be rolled gently between the palms or inverted several times.

Hypurin® Bovine Neutral and Hypurin® Bovine Protamine Zinc should not be mixed together.

The use of each vial should be restricted to a single patient.

Administrative Data

7. MARKETING AUTHORISATION HOLDER

CP Pharmaceuticals Ltd

Ash Road North

Wrexham LL13 9UF

8. MARKETING AUTHORISATION NUMBER(S)

PL 4543/0199

9. DATE OF FIRST AUTHORISATION/RENEWAL OF THE AUTHORISATION

N/A

10. DATE OF REVISION OF THE TEXT

November 2001

Hypurin Porcine 30/70 Mix Cartridges

(Wockhardt UK Ltd)

1. NAME OF THE MEDICINAL PRODUCT

Hypurin® Porcine 30/70 Mix

2. QUALITATIVE AND QUANTITATIVE COMPOSITION

Crystalline Insulin Ph Eur (Porcine) 100 IU/ml.

Biphasic Isophane Insulin Injection Ph Eur 100 iu/ml (Porcine)

For excipients see 6.1.

3. PHARMACEUTICAL FORM

Suspension for injection.

A white suspension

4. CLINICAL PARTICULARS

4.1 Therapeutic indications

The treatment of insulin dependent diabetes mellitus.

May be used for diabetics requiring a depot insulin of intermediate duration.

4.2 Posology and method of administration

To be determined by the physician according to the needs of the patient.

Usually administered subcutaneously but where necessary it may be given intramuscularly in which case onset is more rapid and overall duration shorter. It should not be given intravenously. Onset of action occurs within 2 hours after subcutaneous injection with an overall duration up to 24 hours. Maximum effect is exerted between 4-12 hours.

4.3 Contraindications

Hypoglycaemia.

4.4 Special warnings and special precautions for use

In no circumstances must Hypurin® Porcine 30/70 Mix be given intravenously.

Blood or urinary glucose concentrations should be monitored and the urine tested for ketones by patients on insulin therapy.

Patients transferred to Hypurin® Porcine insulins from other commercially available preparations may require dosage adjustments. Patients whose blood glucose control is greatly improved, e.g. by intensified insulin therapy, may lose some or all of the warning symptoms of hypoglycaemia and should be advised accordingly.

Insulin requirements may increase during illness (this includes infection and accidental and surgical trauma), puberty or emotional upset.

Insulin requirements may decrease with liver disease, disease of the adrenal, pituitary or thyroid glands and coeliac disease. In patients with severe renal impairment, insulin requirements may fall and dosage reduction may be necessary. The compensatory response to hypoglycaemia may also be impaired.

Insulin requirements are usually reduced but occasionally increased during periods of increased activity.

4.5 Interaction with other medicinal products and other forms of Interaction

Insulin requirements may increase during concurrent administration of drugs associated with hyperglycaemic activity e.g. oral contraceptives, chloropromazine, thyroid hormone replacement therapy, thiazide diuretics, sympathomimetic agents and corticosteroids.

Insulin requirements may decrease during concomitant use of drugs with hypoglycaemic activity, e.g salicylates, anabolic steroids, monoamine oxidase inhibitors, NSAIDS, ACE inhibitors and octreotide. Drugs which may decrease or increase insulin requirements include alcohol, cyclophosphamide, isoniazid and beta blockers (which may also mask some of the warning signs of insulin-induced hypoglycaemia). Nifedipine may occasionally impair glucose tolerance.

4.6 Pregnancy and lactation

A decreased requirement for insulin may be observed in the early stages of pregnancy. However, in the second and third trimesters, insulin requirements may increase. Insulin requirements should therefore be assessed frequently by an experienced diabetic physician. Diabetic patients who are breast-feeding may require adjustments in their insulin dose.

4.7 Effects on ability to drive and use machines

The patient's ability to concentrate and react may be impaired as a result of hypoglycaemia. This may constitute a risk in situations where these abilities are of special importance (e.g. driving a car or operating machinery).

Patients should be advised to take precautions to avoid hypoglycaemia whilst driving, this is particularly important in those who have reduced or absent awareness of the warning signs of hypoglycaemia or have frequent episodes of hypoglycaemia. The advisability of driving should be considered in these circumstances.

4.8 Undesirable effects

Lipodystrophy (atrophy or hypertrophy of the fat tissue) or oedema may occur at the injection site. Severe, generalised oedema is a rare adverse effect of insulin treatment occurring most often at the initiation of therapy. Insulin hypersensitivity can occur with animal insulins, but appears less likely with purified insulins and there is minimal evidence that such effects occur with Hypurin insulins.

Allergic reactions to phenol and m-cresol contained as preservative and to zinc and protamine may occur.

4.9 Overdose

a) Symptoms

Overdosage causes hypoglycaemia. Symptoms include weakness, sweating, trembling, nervousness, excitement and irritability which, if untreated, will lead to collapse and coma.

b) Treatment

Mild hypoglycaemia will respond to oral administration of glucose or sugar and rest.

Moderately severe hypoglycaemia can be treated by intramuscular or subcutaneous injection of glucagon followed by oral carbohydrate when the patient is sufficiently recovered.

For patients who are comatose or who have failed to respond to glucagon injection an intravenous injection of strong Dextrose Injection BP should be given.

5. PHARMACOLOGICAL PROPERTIES

5.1 Pharmacodynamic properties

ATC Code – A10A A

Insulin output from the pancreas of a healthy person is about 50 units per day, which is sufficient to maintain the fasting blood sugar concentration in the range 0.8 ! 0.2mg/ml. In diabetes mellitus, the blood sugar rises in an uncontrolled manner. Parenterally administered insulin causes a fall in blood sugar concentration and increased storage of glycogen in the liver. In the diabetic it raises the respiratory quotient after a carbohydrate meal and prevents the formation of ketone bodies. The rise in blood sugar concentration caused by adrenaline and corticosteroids, glucagon and posterior pituitary extract is reversed by insulin.

5.2 Pharmacokinetic properties

Insulin is rapidly absorbed from subcutaneous tissue or muscle following injection.

Insulin is metabolised mainly in the liver and a small amount is excreted in the urine.

The plasma half-life is four to five minutes. The half-life after subcutaneous injection is about four hours and after intramuscular injection about two hours.

5.3 Preclinical safety data

There are no preclinical data of relevance to the prescriber that are additional to that already included in other sections.

6. PHARMACEUTICAL PARTICULARS

6.1 List of excipients

Protamine sulphate

Zinc chloride

m-Cresol

Phenol

Sodium phosphate

Glycerol

Water for injections

6.2 Incompatibilities

None

6.3 Shelf life

36 months.

Following injection of the first dose the product should be used within 28 days. Discard any unused material after this time.

6.4 Special precautions for storage

Store at 2°C - 8°C.

Do not freeze.

Cartridges in use must not be stored in a refrigerator.

Chemical and physical in-use stability has been demonstrated for 28 days at 25°C.

From a microbiological point of view the opening carries a risk of microbial contamination and aseptic handling is a necessity.

In use storage times and conditions are the responsibility of the user.

6.5 Nature and contents of container

1.5ml neutral glass cartridge sealed with a bromobutyl rubber bung and metal closure in packs of five.

3ml neutral glass cartridge sealed with a bromobutyl rubber bung and metal closure in packs of five.

6.6 Instructions for use and handling

Prior to insertion in the pen the cartridge of Hypurin® Porcine 30/70 Mix should be shaken vigorously up and down, with a "bell ringing" action, at least ten times.

Immediately before each injection the pen should be inverted at least ten times to mix the insulin again.

The cartridge must not be used if the contents have been frozen or it contains lumps that do not disperse on mixing.

Administrative Data

7. MARKETING AUTHORISATION HOLDER

CP Pharmaceuticals Ltd

Ash Road North

Wrexham

LL13 9UF

8. MARKETING AUTHORISATION NUMBER(S)

PL 04543/0375

9. DATE OF FIRST AUTHORISATION/RENEWAL OF THE AUTHORISATION

N/A

10. DATE OF REVISION OF THE TEXT

July 2002

Hypurin Porcine 30/70 Mix Vials

(Wockhardt UK Ltd)

1. NAME OF THE MEDICINAL PRODUCT

Hypurin® Porcine 30/70 Mix

2. QUALITATIVE AND QUANTITATIVE COMPOSITION

Crystalline Insulin Ph Eur (Porcine) 100 IU/ml.

Biphasic Isophane Insulin Injection Ph Eur 100 iu/ml (Porcine)

For excipients see 6.1.

3. PHARMACEUTICAL FORM

Suspension for injection.

A white suspension

4. CLINICAL PARTICULARS

4.1 Therapeutic indications

The treatment of insulin dependent diabetes mellitus.

May be used for diabetics requiring a depot insulin of intermediate duration.

4.2 Posology and method of administration

To be determined by the physician according to the needs of the patient.

Usually administered subcutaneously but where necessary it may be given intramuscularly in which case onset is more rapid and overall duration shorter. It should not be given intravenously. Onset of action occurs within 2 hours after subcutaneous injection with an overall duration up to 24 hours. Maximum effect is exerted between 4-12 hours.

4.3 Contraindications

Hypoglycaemia.

4.4 Special warnings and special precautions for use

In no circumstances must Hypurin® Porcine 30/70 Mix be given intravenously.

Blood or urinary glucose concentrations should be monitored and the urine tested for ketones by patients on insulin therapy.

Patients transferred to Hypurin® Porcine insulins from other commercially available preparations may require dosage adjustments. Patients whose blood glucose control is greatly improved, e.g. by intensified insulin therapy, may lose some or all of the warning symptoms of hypoglycaemia and should be advised accordingly.

Insulin requirements may increase during illness (this includes infection and accidental and surgical trauma), puberty or emotional upset.

Insulin requirements may decrease with liver disease, disease of the adrenal, pituitary or thyroid glands and coeliac disease. In patients with severe renal impairment, insulin requirements may fall and dosage reduction may be necessary. The compensatory response to hypoglycaemia may also be impaired.

Insulin requirements are usually reduced but occasionally increased during periods of increased activity.

4.5 Interaction with other medicinal products and other forms of Interaction

Insulin requirements may increase during concurrent administration of drugs associated with hyperglycaemic activity e.g. oral contraceptives, chloropromazine, thyroid hormone replacement therapy, thiazide diuretics, sympathomimetic agents and corticosteroids.

Insulin requirements may decrease during concomitant use of drugs with hypoglycaemic activity, e.g salicylates, anabolic steroids, monoamine oxidase inhibitors, NSAIDS, ACE inhibitors and octreotide. Drugs which may decrease or increase insulin requirements include alcohol, cyclophosphamide, isoniazid and beta blockers (which may also mask some of the warning signs of insulin-induced hypoglycaemia). Nifedipine may occasionally impair glucose tolerance.

4.6 Pregnancy and lactation

A decreased requirement for insulin may be observed in the early stages of pregnancy. However, in the second and third trimesters, insulin requirements may increase. Insulin requirements should therefore be assessed frequently by an experienced diabetic physician. Diabetic patients who are breast-feeding may require adjustments in their insulin dose.

4.7 Effects on ability to drive and use machines

The patient's ability to concentrate and react may be impaired as a result of hypoglycaemia. This may constitute a risk in situations where these abilities are of special importance (e.g. driving a car or operating machinery).

Patients should be advised to take precautions to avoid hypoglycaemia whilst driving, this is particularly important in those who have reduced or absent awareness of the warning signs of hypoglycaemia or have frequent episodes of hypoglycaemia. The advisability of driving should be considered in these circumstances.

4.8 Undesirable effects

Lipodystrophy (atrophy or hypertrophy of the fat tissue) or oedema may occur at the injection site. Severe, generalised oedema is a rare adverse effect of insulin treatment occurring most often at the initiation of therapy. Insulin hypersensitivity can occur with animal insulins, but appears less likely with purified insulins and there is minimal evidence that such effects occur with Hypurin insulins.

Allergic reactions to phenol and m-cresol contained as preservative and to zinc and protamine may occur.

4.9 Overdose

a) Symptoms

Overdosage causes hypoglycaemia. Symptoms include weakness, sweating, trembling, nervousness, excitement and irritability which, if untreated, will lead to collapse and coma.

b) Treatment

Mild hypoglycaemia will respond to oral administration of glucose or sugar and rest.

Moderately severe hypoglycaemia can be treated by intramuscular or subcutaneous injection of glucagon followed by oral carbohydrate when the patient is sufficiently recovered.

For patients who are comatose or who have failed to respond to glucagon injection an intravenous injection of strong Dextrose Injection BP should be given.

5. PHARMACOLOGICAL PROPERTIES

5.1 Pharmacodynamic properties

ATC Code – A10A A

Insulin output from the pancreas of a healthy person is about 50 units per day, which is sufficient to maintain the fasting blood sugar concentration in the range 0.8 ! 0.2mg/ml. In diabetes mellitus, the blood sugar rises in an uncontrolled manner. Parenterally administered insulin causes a fall in blood sugar concentration and increased storage of glycogen in the liver. In the diabetic it raises the respiratory quotient after a carbohydrate meal and prevents the formation of ketone bodies. The rise in blood sugar concentration caused by adrenaline and corticosteroids, glucagon and posterior pituitary extract is reversed by insulin.

5.2 Pharmacokinetic properties

Insulin is rapidly absorbed from subcutaneous tissue or muscle following injection.

Insulin is metabolised mainly in the liver and a small amount is excreted in the urine.

The plasma half-life is 4 to 5 minutes. The half-life after subcutaneous injection is about 4 hours and after intramuscular injection about 2 hours.

5.3 Preclinical safety data

There are no preclinical data of relevance to the prescriber that are additional to that already included in other sections.

6. PHARMACEUTICAL PARTICULARS

6.1 List of excipients

Protamine sulphate

Zinc chloride

m-Cresol,

Phenol

Sodium phosphate

Glycerol

Water for injections

6.2 Incompatibilities

None

6.3 Shelf life

36 months.

Following withdrawal of the first dose the product should be used within 28 days. Discard any unused material.

6.4 Special precautions for storage

Store at 2°C - 8°C.

Do not freeze.

Chemical and physical in-use stability has been demonstrated for 28 days at 25°C.

From a microbiological point of view the opening carries a risk of microbial contamination and aseptic handling is a necessity.

In use storage times and conditions are the responsibility of the user.

6.5 Nature and contents of container

10ml neutral glass vial sealed with a rubber bung and metal closure.

6.6 Instructions for use and handling

Prior to use the vial should be gently rolled between the palms or inverted several times.

The vial must not be used if the contents have been frozen or it contains lumps that do not disperse on mixing.

The injection should be made immediately upon withdrawal of the contents.

The use of each vial should be restricted to a single patient.

Administrative Data

7. MARKETING AUTHORISATION HOLDER

CP Pharmaceuticals Ltd

Ash Road North

Wrexham

LL13 9UF

8. MARKETING AUTHORISATION NUMBER(S)

PL 04543/0372

9. DATE OF FIRST AUTHORISATION/RENEWAL OF THE AUTHORISATION

12 February 1997

10. DATE OF REVISION OF THE TEXT

November 2001

Hypurin Porcine Isophane Cartridges

(Wockhardt UK Ltd)

1. NAME OF THE MEDICINAL PRODUCT

Hypurin® Porcine Isophane

2. QUALITATIVE AND QUANTITATIVE COMPOSITION

Crystalline Insulin Ph Eur (Porcine) 100 IU/ml.

Isophane Insulin Injection Ph Eur (Porcine)

For excipients, see 6.1

3. PHARMACEUTICAL FORM

Suspension for injection.

A white suspension

4. CLINICAL PARTICULARS

4.1 Therapeutic indications

The treatment of insulin dependent diabetes mellitus.

May be used for diabetics requiring a depot insulin of medium duration. Where a more rapid, intense onset is desirable it may be mixed with Hypurin® Porcine Neutral.

4.2 Posology and method of administration

To be determined by the physician according to the needs of the patient.

Usually administered subcutaneously but where necessary it may be given intramuscularly in which case onset is more rapid and overall duration shorter. It should not be given intravenously. Onset of action occurs within 2 hours after subcutaneous injection with an overall duration of 18-24 hours. Maximum effect is exerted between 6-12 hours.

4.3 Contraindications

Hypoglycaemia.

4.4 Special warnings and special precautions for use

In no circumstances must Hypurin® Porcine Isophane be given intravenously.

Blood or urinary glucose concentrations should be monitored and the urine tested for ketones by patients on insulin therapy.

Patients transferred to Hypurin® Porcine insulins from other commercially available preparations may require dosage adjustments. Patients whose blood glucose control is greatly improved, e.g. by intensified insulin therapy, may lose some or all of the warning symptoms of hypoglycaemia and should be advised accordingly.

Insulin requirements may increase during illness (this includes infection and accidental and surgical trauma), puberty or emotional upset.

Insulin requirements may decrease with liver disease, disease of the adrenal, pituitary or thyroid glands and coeliac disease. In patients with severe renal impairment, insulin requirements may fall and dosage reduction may be necessary. The compensatory response to hypoglycaemia may also be impaired.

Insulin requirements are usually reduced but occasionally increased during periods of increased activity.

4.5 Interaction with other medicinal products and other forms of Interaction

Insulin requirements may increase during concurrent administration of drugs associated with hyperglycaemic activity e.g. oral contraceptives, chloropromazine, thyroid hormone replacement therapy, thiazide diuretics, sympathomimetic agents and corticosteroids.

Insulin requirements may decrease during concomitant use of drugs with hypoglycaemic activity, e.g salicylates, anabolic steroids, monoamine oxidase inhibitors, NSAIDS, ACE inhibitors and octreotide. Drugs which may decrease or increase insulin requirements include alcohol, cyclophosphamide, isoniazid and beta blockers (which may also mask some of the warning signs of insulin-induced hypoglycaemia). Nifedipine may occasionally impair glucose tolerance.

4.6 Pregnancy and lactation

A decreased requirement for insulin may be observed in the early stages of pregnancy. However, in the second and third trimesters, insulin requirements may increase. Insulin requirements should therefore be assessed frequently by an experienced diabetic physician. Diabetic patients who are breast-feeding may require adjustments in their insulin dose.

4.7 Effects on ability to drive and use machines

The patient's ability to concentrate and react may be impaired as a result of hypoglycaemia. This may constitute a risk in situations where these abilities are of special importance (e.g. driving a car or operating machinery).

Patients should be advised to take precautions to avoid hypoglycaemia whilst driving, this is particularly important in those who have reduced or absent awareness of the warning signs of hypoglycaemia or have frequent episodes of hypoglycaemia. The advisability of driving should be considered in these circumstances.

4.8 Undesirable effects

Lipodystrophy (atrophy or hypertrophy of the fat tissue) or oedema may occur at the injection site. Severe, generalised oedema is a rare adverse effect of insulin treatment occurring most often at the initiation of therapy. Insulin hypersensitivity can occur with animal insulins, but appears less likely with purified insulins and there is minimal evidence that such effects occur with Hypurin insulins.

Allergic reactions to phenol and m-cresol contained as preservative and to zinc and protamine may occur.

4.9 Overdose

a) Symptoms

Overdosage causes hypoglycaemia. Symptoms include weakness, sweating, trembling, nervousness, excitement and irritability which, if untreated, will lead to collapse and coma.

b) Treatment

Mild hypoglycaemia will respond to oral administration of glucose or sugar and rest.

Moderately severe hypoglycaemia can be treated by intramuscular or subcutaneous injection of glucagon followed by oral carbohydrate when the patient is sufficiently recovered.

For patients who are comatose or who have failed to respond to glucagon injection an intravenous injection of strong Dextrose Injection BP should be given.

5. PHARMACOLOGICAL PROPERTIES

5.1 Pharmacodynamic properties

ATC Code – A10A A

Insulin output from the pancreas of a healthy person is about 50 units per day, which is sufficient to maintain the fasting blood sugar concentration in the range 0.8 ! 0.2mg/ml. In diabetes mellitus, the blood sugar rises in an uncontrolled manner. Parenterally administered insulin causes a fall in blood sugar concentration and increased storage of glycogen in the liver. In the diabetic it raises the respiratory quotient after a carbohydrate meal and prevents the formation of ketone bodies. The rise in blood sugar concentration caused by adrenaline and corticosteroids, glucagon and posterior pituitary extract is reversed by insulin.

5.2 Pharmacokinetic properties

Insulin is rapidly absorbed from subcutaneous tissue or muscle following injection.

Insulin is metabolised mainly in the liver and a small amount is excreted in the urine.

The plasma half-life is four to five minutes. The half-life after subcutaneous injection is about four hours and after intramuscular injection about two hours.

5.3 Preclinical safety data

There are no preclinical data of relevance to the prescriber that are additional to that already included in other sections.

6. PHARMACEUTICAL PARTICULARS

6.1 List of excipients

Protamine sulphate

Zinc chloride

m-Cresol

Phenol

Sodium phosphate

Glycerol

Water for injections

6.2 Incompatibilities

None

6.3 Shelf life

36 months.

Following injection of the first dose the product should be used within 28 days. Discard any unused material after this time.

6.4 Special precautions for storage

Store at 2°C - 8°C.

Do not freeze.

Cartridges in use must not be stored in a refrigerator.

Chemical and physical in-use stability has been demonstrated for 28 days at 25°C.

From a microbiological point of view the opening carries a risk of microbial contamination and aseptic handling is a necessity.

In use storage times and conditions are the responsibility of the user.

6.5 Nature and contents of container

1.5ml neutral glass cartridge sealed with a bromobutyl rubber bung and metal closure in packs of five.

3ml neutral glass cartridge sealed with a bromobutyl rubber bung and metal closure in packs of five.

6.6 Instructions for use and handling

Prior to insertion in the pen the cartridge of Hypurin® Porcine Isophane should be shaken vigorously up and down, with a "bell ringing" action, at least ten times.

Immediately before each injection the pen should be inverted at least ten times to mix the insulin again.

The cartridge must not be used if the contents have been frozen or it contains lumps that do not disperse on mixing.

Administrative Data

7. MARKETING AUTHORISATION HOLDER

CP Pharmaceuticals Ltd

Ash Road North

Wrexham

LL13 9UF

8. MARKETING AUTHORISATION NUMBER(S)

PL 04543/0374

9. DATE OF FIRST AUTHORISATION/RENEWAL OF THE AUTHORISATION

N/A

10. DATE OF REVISION OF THE TEXT

July 2002

Hypurin Porcine Isophane Vials

(Wockhardt UK Ltd)

1. NAME OF THE MEDICINAL PRODUCT

Hypurin® Porcine Isophane

2. QUALITATIVE AND QUANTITATIVE COMPOSITION

Crystalline Insulin Ph Eur (Porcine) 100 IU/ml.

Isophane Insulin Injection Ph Eur (Porcine)

For excipients, see 6.1

3. PHARMACEUTICAL FORM

Suspension for injection.

A white suspension

4. CLINICAL PARTICULARS

4.1 Therapeutic indications

The treatment of insulin dependent diabetes mellitus.

May be used for diabetics requiring a depot insulin of medium duration. Where a more rapid, intense onset is desirable it may be mixed with Hypurin Neutral.

4.2 Posology and method of administration

To be determined by the physician according to the needs of the patient.

Usually administered subcutaneously but where necessary it may be given intramuscularly in which case onset is more rapid and overall duration shorter. It should not be given intravenously. Onset of action occurs within 2 hours after subcutaneous injection with an overall duration of 18-24 hours. Maximum effect is exerted between 6-12 hours.

4.3 Contraindications

Hypoglycaemia.

4.4 Special warnings and special precautions for use

In no circumstances must Hypurin® Porcine Isophane be given intravenously.

Blood or urinary glucose concentrations should be monitored and the urine tested for ketones by patients on insulin therapy.

Patients transferred to Hypurin® Porcine insulins from other commercially available preparations may require dosage adjustments. Patients whose blood glucose control is greatly improved, e.g. by intensified insulin therapy, may lose some or all of the warning symptoms of hypoglycaemia and should be advised accordingly.

Insulin requirements may increase during illness (this includes infection and accidental and surgical trauma), puberty or emotional upset.

Insulin requirements may decrease with liver disease, disease of the adrenal, pituitary or thyroid glands and coeliac disease. In patients with severe renal impairment, insulin requirements may fall and dosage reduction may be necessary. The compensatory response to hypoglycaemia may also be impaired.

Insulin requirements are usually reduced but occasionally increased during periods of increased activity.

4.5 Interaction with other medicinal products and other forms of Interaction

Insulin requirements may increase during concurrent administration of drugs associated with hyperglycaemic activity e.g. oral contraceptives, chloropromazine, thyroid hormone replacement therapy, thiazide diuretics, sympathomimetic agents and corticosteroids.

Insulin requirements may decrease during concomitant use of drugs with hypoglycaemic activity, e.g salicylates, anabolic steroids, monoamine oxidase inhibitors, NSAIDS, ACE inhibitors and octreotide. Drugs which may decrease or increase insulin requirements include alcohol, cyclophosphamide, isoniazid and beta blockers (which may also mask some of the warning signs of insulin-induced hypoglycaemia). Nifedipine may occasionally impair glucose tolerance.

4.6 Pregnancy and lactation

A decreased requirement for insulin may be observed in the early stages of pregnancy. However, in the second and third trimesters, insulin requirements may increase. Insulin requirements should therefore be assessed frequently by an experienced diabetic physician. Diabetic patients who are breast-feeding may require adjustments in their insulin dose.

4.7 Effects on ability to drive and use machines

The patient's ability to concentrate and react may be impaired as a result of hypoglycaemia. This may constitute a risk in situations where these abilities are of special importance (e.g. driving a car or operating machinery).

Patients should be advised to take precautions to avoid hypoglycaemia whilst driving, this is particularly important in those who have reduced or absent awareness of the warning signs of hypoglycaemia or have frequent episodes of hypoglycaemia. The advisability of driving should be considered in these circumstances.

4.8 Undesirable effects

Lipodystrophy (atrophy or hypertrophy of the fat tissue) or oedema may occur at the injection site. Severe, generalised oedema is a rare adverse effect of insulin treatment occurring most often at the initiation of therapy. Insulin hypersensitivity can occur with animal insulins, but appears less likely with purified insulins and there is minimal evidence that such effects occur with Hypurin insulins.

Allergic reactions to phenol and m-cresol contained as preservative and to zinc and protamine may occur.

4.9 Overdose

a) Symptoms

Overdosage causes hypoglycaemia. Symptoms include weakness, sweating, trembling, nervousness, excitement and irritability which, if untreated, will lead to collapse and coma.

b) Treatment

Mild hypoglycaemia will respond to oral administration of glucose or sugar and rest.

Moderately severe hypoglycaemia can be treated by intramuscular or subcutaneous injection of glucagon followed by oral carbohydrate when the patient is sufficiently recovered.

For patients who are comatose or who have failed to respond to glucagon injection an intravenous injection of strong Dextrose Injection BP should be given.

5. PHARMACOLOGICAL PROPERTIES

5.1 Pharmacodynamic properties

ATC Code – A10A A

Insulin output from the pancreas of a healthy person is about 50 units per day, which is sufficient to maintain the fasting blood sugar concentration in the range 0.8 ! 0.2mg/ml. In diabetes mellitus, the blood sugar rises in an uncontrolled manner. Parenterally administered insulin causes a fall in blood sugar concentration and increased storage of glycogen in the liver. In the diabetic it raises the respiratory quotient after a carbohydrate meal and prevents the formation of ketone bodies. The rise in blood sugar concentration caused by adrenaline and corticosteroids, glucagon and posterior pituitary extract is reversed by insulin.

5.2 Pharmacokinetic properties

Insulin is rapidly absorbed from subcutaneous tissue or muscle following injection.

Insulin is metabolised mainly in the liver and a small amount is excreted in the urine.

The plasma half-life is 4 to 5 minutes. The half-life after subcutaneous injection is about 4 hours and after intramuscular injection about 2 hours.

5.3 Preclinical safety data

There are no preclinical data of relevance to the prescriber that are additional to that already included in other sections.

6. PHARMACEUTICAL PARTICULARS

6.1 List of excipients

Protamine sulphate

Zinc chloride

m-Cresol

Phenol

Sodium phosphate

Glycerol

Water for injections

6.2 Incompatibilities

None

6.3 Shelf life

36 months.

Following withdrawal of the first dose the product should be used within 28 days. Discard any unused material.

6.4 Special precautions for storage

Store at 2°C - 8°C.

Do not freeze.

Chemical and physical in-use stability has been demonstrated for 28 days at 25°C.

From a microbiological point of view the opening carries a risk of microbial contamination and aseptic handling is a necessity.

In use storage times and conditions are the responsibility of the user.

6.5 Nature and contents of container

10ml neutral glass vial sealed with a rubber bung and metal closure.

6.6 Instructions for use and handling

Prior to use the vial should be gently rolled between the palms or inverted several times.

The vial must not be used if the contents have been frozen or it contains lumps that do not disperse on mixing.

Hypurin® Porcine Isophane may be mixed with Hypurin® Porcine Neutral in the syringe, in which case Hypurin® Porcine Neutral should be the first dose to be withdrawn.

The injection should then be made immediately upon withdrawal of the contents.

The use of each vial should be restricted to a single patient.

Administrative Data

7. MARKETING AUTHORISATION HOLDER

CP Pharmaceuticals Ltd

Ash Road North

Wrexham

LL13 9UF

8. MARKETING AUTHORISATION NUMBER(S)

PL 04543/0371

9. DATE OF FIRST AUTHORISATION/RENEWAL OF THE AUTHORISATION

12 February 1997

10. DATE OF REVISION OF THE TEXT

November 2001

Hypurin Porcine Neutral Cartridges

(Wockhardt UK Ltd)

1. NAME OF THE MEDICINAL PRODUCT

Hypurin® Porcine Neutral

2. QUALITATIVE AND QUANTITATIVE COMPOSITION

Crystalline Insulin Ph Eur (Porcine) 100IU/ml.

Neutral Insulin Injection Ph Eur (Porcine)

For excipients, see 6.1

3. PHARMACEUTICAL FORM

Solution for injection

A clear, colourless solution

4. CLINICAL PARTICULARS

4.1 Therapeutic indications

The treatment of insulin dependent diabetes mellitus.

May be used for diabetics who require an insulin of prompt onset and short duration. It is a suitable preparation for admixture with longer acting insulins. It is particularly useful where intermittent, short term or emergency therapy is required, during initial stabilisation and in the treatment of labile diabetes.

4.2 Posology and method of administration

To be determined by the physician according to the needs of the patient.

Usually administered subcutaneously but where necessary it may be given intramuscularly or intravenously. After subcutaneous injection onset of action occurs within 30-60 minutes with an overall duration of 6-8 hours. Maximum effect is exerted over the mid-range.

4.3 Contraindications

Hypoglycaemia.

4.4 Special warnings and special precautions for use

Blood or urinary glucose concentrations should be monitored and the urine tested for ketones by patients on insulin therapy.

Patients transferred to Hypurin® Porcine insulins from other commercially available preparations may require dosage adjustments. Patients whose blood glucose control is greatly improved, e.g. by intensified insulin therapy, may lose some or all of the warning symptoms of hypoglycaemia and should be advised accordingly.

Insulin requirements may increase during illness (this includes infection and accidental and surgical trauma), puberty or emotional upset.

Insulin requirements may decrease with liver disease, disease of the adrenal, pituitary or thyroid glands and coeliac disease. In patients with severe renal impairment, insulin requirements may fall and dosage reduction may be necessary. The compensatory response to hypoglycaemia may also be impaired.

Insulin requirements are usually reduced but occasionally increased during periods of increased activity.

4.5 Interaction with other medicinal products and other forms of Interaction

Insulin requirements may increase during concurrent administration of drugs associated with hyperglycaemic activity e.g. oral contraceptives, chloropromazine, thyroid hormone replacement therapy, thiazide diuretics, sympathomimetic agents and corticosteroids.

Insulin requirements may decrease during concomitant use of drugs with hypoglycaemic activity, e.g salicylates, anabolic steroids, monoamine oxidase inhibitors, NSAIDS, ACE inhibitors and octreotide. Drugs which may decrease or increase insulin requirements include alcohol, cyclophosphamide, isoniazid and beta blockers (which may also mask some of the warning signs of insulin-induced hypoglycaemia). Nifedipine may occasionally impair glucose tolerance.

4.6 Pregnancy and lactation

A decreased requirement for insulin may be observed in the early stages of pregnancy. However, in the second and third trimesters, insulin requirements may increase. Insulin requirements should therefore be assessed frequently by an experienced diabetic physician. Diabetic patients who are breast-feeding may require adjustments in their insulin dose.

4.7 Effects on ability to drive and use machines

The patient's ability to concentrate and react may be impaired as a result of hypoglycaemia. This may constitute a risk in situations where these abilities are of special importance (e.g. driving a car or operating machinery).

Patients should be advised to take precautions to avoid hypoglycaemia whilst driving, this is particularly important in those who have reduced or absent awareness of the warning signs of hypoglycaemia or have frequent episodes of hypoglycaemia. The advisability of driving should be considered in these circumstances.

4.8 Undesirable effects

Lipodystrophy (atrophy or hypertrophy of the fat tissue) or oedema may occur at the injection site. Severe, generalised oedema is a rare adverse effect of insulin treatment occurring most often at the initiation of therapy. Insulin hypersensitivity can occur with animal insulins, but appears less likely with purified insulins and there is minimal evidence that such effects occur with Hypurin insulins.

Allergic reactions to phenol and m-cresol contained as preservative and to zinc and protamine may occur.

4.9 Overdose

a) Symptoms

Overdosage causes hypoglycaemia. Symptoms include weakness, sweating, trembling, nervousness, excitement and irritability which, if untreated, will lead to collapse and coma.

b) Treatment

Mild hypoglycaemia will respond to oral administration of glucose or sugar and rest.

Moderately severe hypoglycaemia can be treated by intramuscular or subcutaneous injection of glucagon followed by oral carbohydrate when the patient is sufficiently recovered.

For patients who are comatose or who have failed to respond to glucagon injection an intravenous injection of strong Dextrose Injection BP should be given.

5. PHARMACOLOGICAL PROPERTIES

5.1 Pharmacodynamic properties

ATC Code – A10A A

Insulin output from the pancreas of a healthy person is about 50 units per day, which is sufficient to maintain the fasting blood sugar concentration in the range 0.8 ! 0.2mg/ml. In diabetes mellitus, the blood sugar rises in an uncontrolled manner. Parenterally administered insulin causes a fall in blood sugar concentration and increased storage of glycogen in the liver. In the diabetic it raises the respiratory quotient after a carbohydrate meal and prevents the formation of ketone bodies. The rise in blood sugar concentration caused by adrenaline and corticosteroids, glucagon and posterior pituitary extract is reversed by insulin.

5.2 Pharmacokinetic properties

Insulin is rapidly absorbed from subcutaneous tissue or muscle following injection.

Insulin is metabolised mainly in the liver and a small amount is excreted in the urine.

The plasma half-life is four to five minutes. The half-life after subcutaneous injection is about four hours and after intramuscular injection about two hours.

5.3 Preclinical safety data

There are no preclinical data of relevance to the prescriber that are additional to that already included in other sections.

6. PHARMACEUTICAL PARTICULARS

6.1 List of excipients

m-Cresol

Phenol

Sodium phosphate

Glycerol

Water for injections

6.2 Incompatibilities

None

6.3 Shelf life

36 months.

Following injection of the first dose the product should be used within 28 days. Discard any unused material after this time.

6.4 Special precautions for storage
Store at 2°C - 8°C.

Do not freeze.

Cartridges in use must not be stored in a refrigerator.

Chemical and physical in-use stability has been demonstrated for 28 days at 25°C.

From a microbiological point of view the opening carries a risk of microbial contamination and aseptic handling is a necessity.

In use storage times and conditions are the responsibility of the user.

6.5 Nature and contents of container
1.5ml neutral glass cartridge sealed with a bromobutyl rubber bung and metal closure in packs of five.

3ml neutral glass cartridge sealed with a bromobutyl rubber bung and metal closure in packs of five.

6.6 Instructions for use and handling
The cartridge must not be used if the contents have been frozen or it contains lumps that do not disperse on mixing.

Administrative Data

7. MARKETING AUTHORISATION HOLDER
CP Pharmaceuticals Ltd

Ash Road North

Wrexham

LL13 9UF

8. MARKETING AUTHORISATION NUMBER(S)
PL 04543/0373

9. DATE OF FIRST AUTHORISATION/RENEWAL OF THE AUTHORISATION
N/A

10. DATE OF REVISION OF THE TEXT
July 2002

Hypurin Porcine Neutral Vials

(Wockhardt UK Ltd)

1. NAME OF THE MEDICINAL PRODUCT
Hypurin® Porcine Neutral

2. QUALITATIVE AND QUANTITATIVE COMPOSITION
Crystalline Insulin Ph Eur (Porcine) 100IU/ml.

Neutral Insulin Injection Ph Eur (Porcine)

For excipients, see 6.1

3. PHARMACEUTICAL FORM
Solution for injection

A clear, colourless solution

4. CLINICAL PARTICULARS
4.1 Therapeutic indications
The treatment of insulin dependent diabetes mellitus.

May be used for diabetics who require an insulin of prompt onset and short duration. It is a suitable preparation for admixture with longer acting insulins. It is particularly useful where intermittent, short term or emergency therapy is required, during initial stabilisation and in the treatment of labile diabetes.

4.2 Posology and method of administration
To be determined by the physician according to the needs of the patient.

Usually administered subcutaneously but where necessary it may be given intramuscularly or intravenously. After subcutaneous injection onset of action occurs within 30-60 minutes with an overall duration of 6-8 hours. Maximum effect is exerted over the mid-range.

4.3 Contraindications
Hypoglycaemia.

4.4 Special warnings and special precautions for use
Blood or urinary glucose concentrations should be monitored and the urine tested for ketones by patients on insulin therapy.

Patients transferred to Hypurin® Porcine insulins from other commercially available preparations may require dosage adjustments. Patients whose blood glucose control is greatly improved, e.g. by intensified insulin therapy, may lose some or all of the warning symptoms of hypoglycaemia and should be advised accordingly.

Insulin requirements may increase during illness (this includes infection and accidental and surgical trauma), puberty or emotional upset.

Insulin requirements may decrease with liver disease, disease of the adrenal, pituitary or thyroid glands and coeliac disease. In patients with severe renal impairment, insulin requirements may fall and dosage reduction may be necessary. The compensatory response to hypoglycaemia may also be impaired.

Insulin requirements are usually reduced but occasionally increased during periods of increased activity.

4.5 Interaction with other medicinal products and other forms of Interaction
Insulin requirements may increase during concurrent administration of drugs associated with hyperglycaemic activity e.g. oral contraceptives, chloropromazine, thyroid hormone replacement therapy, thiazide diuretics, sympathomimetic agents and corticosteroids.

Insulin requirements may decrease during concomitant use of drugs with hypoglycaemic activity, e.g salicylates, anabolic steroids, monoamine oxidase inhibitors, NSAIDS, ACE inhibitors and octreotide. Drugs which may decrease or increase insulin requirements include alcohol, cyclophosphamide, isoniazid and beta blockers (which may also mask some of the warning signs of insulin-induced hypoglycaemia). Nifedipine may occasionally impair glucose tolerance.

4.6 Pregnancy and lactation
A decreased requirement for insulin may be observed in the early stages of pregnancy. However, in the second and third trimesters, insulin requirements may increase. Insulin requirements should therefore be assessed frequently by an experienced diabetic physician. Diabetic patients who are breast-feeding may require adjustments in their insulin dose.

4.7 Effects on ability to drive and use machines
The patient's ability to concentrate and react may be impaired as a result of hypoglycaemia. This may constitute a risk in situations where these abilities are of special importance (e.g. driving a car or operating machinery).

Patients should be advised to take precautions to avoid hypoglycaemia whilst driving, this is particularly important in those who have reduced or absent awareness of the warning signs of hypoglycaemia or have frequent episodes of hypoglycaemia. The advisability of driving should be considered in these circumstances.

4.8 Undesirable effects
Lipodystrophy (atrophy or hypertrophy of the fat tissue) or oedema may occur at the injection site. Severe, generalised oedema is a rare adverse effect of insulin treatment occuring most often at the initiation of therapy. Insulin hypersensitivity can occur with animal insulins, but appears less likely with purified insulins and there is minimal evidence that such effects occur with Hypurin insulins.

Allergic reactions to phenol and m-cresol contained as preservative and to zinc and protamine may occur.

4.9 Overdose
a) Symptoms

Overdosage causes hypoglycaemia. Symptoms include weakness, sweating, trembling, nervousness, excitement and irritability which, if untreated, will lead to collapse and coma.

b) Treatment

Mild hypoglycaemia will respond to oral administration of glucose or sugar and rest.

Moderately severe hypoglycaemia can be treated by intramuscular or subcutaneous injection of glucagon followed by oral carbohydrate when the patient is sufficiently recovered.

For patients who are comatose or who have failed to respond to glucagon injection an intravenous injection of strong Dextrose Injection BP should be given.

5. PHARMACOLOGICAL PROPERTIES
5.1 Pharmacodynamic properties
ATC Code – A10A A

Insulin output from the pancreas of a healthy person is about 50 units per day, which is sufficient to maintain the fasting blood sugar concentration in the range 0.8 ! 0.2mg/ml. In diabetes mellitus, the blood sugar rises in an uncontrolled manner. Parenterally administered insulin causes a fall in blood sugar concentration and increased storage of glycogen in the liver. In the diabetic it raises the respiratory quotient after a carbohydrate meal and prevents the formation of ketone bodies. The rise in blood sugar concentration caused by adrenaline and corticosteroids, glucagon and posterior pituitary extract is reversed by insulin.

5.2 Pharmacokinetic properties
Insulin is rapidly absorbed from subcutaneous tissue or muscle following injection.

Insulin is metabolised mainly in the liver and a small amount is excreted in the urine.

The plasma half-life is 4 to 5 minutes. The half-life after subcutaneous injection is about 4 hours and after intramuscular injection about 2 hours.

5.3 Preclinical safety data
There are no preclinical data of relevance to the prescriber that are additional to that already included in other sections.

6. PHARMACEUTICAL PARTICULARS
6.1 List of excipients
m-Cresol

Phenol

Sodium phosphate

Glycerol

Water for injections

6.2 Incompatibilities
None

6.3 Shelf life
36 months.

Following withdrawal of the first dose the product should be used within 28 days. Discard any unused material.

6.4 Special precautions for storage
Store at 2°C - 8°C.

Do not freeze.

Chemical and physical in-use stability has been demonstrated for 28 days at 25°C.

From a microbiological point of view the opening carries a risk of microbial contamination and aseptic handling is a necessity.

In use storage times and conditions are the responsibility of the user.

6.5 Nature and contents of container
10ml neutral glass vial sealed with a rubber bung and metal closure.

6.6 Instructions for use and handling
The vial must not be used if the contents have been frozen or it contains lumps that do not disperse on mixing.

Hypurin® Porcine Isophane may be mixed with Hypurin® Porcine Neutral in the syringe, in which case Hypurin® Porcine Neutral should be the first dose to be withdrawn.

The injections should be made immediately upon withdrawal of the contents.

The use of each vial should be restricted to a single patient.

Administrative Data

7. MARKETING AUTHORISATION HOLDER
CP Pharmaceuticals Ltd

Ash Road North

Wrexham

LL13 9UF

8. MARKETING AUTHORISATION NUMBER(S)
PL 04543/0370

9. DATE OF FIRST AUTHORISATION/RENEWAL OF THE AUTHORISATION
12 February 1997

10. DATE OF REVISION OF THE TEXT
November 2001

Hytrin 1, 2, 5 & 10 mg Tablets

(Abbott Laboratories Limited)

1. NAME OF THE MEDICINAL PRODUCT
Hytrin 1mg Tablets, Hytrin 2mg Tablets, Hytrin 5mg Tablets, Hytrin 10mg Tablets.

2. QUALITATIVE AND QUANTITATIVE COMPOSITION

Tablet	Active	mg/Tablet
Hytrin 1mg	Terazosin as monohydrochloride dihydrate	1.0
Hytrin 2mg	Terazosin as monohydrochloride dihydrate	2.0
Hytrin 5mg	Terazosin as monohydrochloride dihydrate	5.0
Hytrin 10mg	Terazosin as monohydrochloride dihydrate	10.0

3. PHARMACEUTICAL FORM
Tablet.

4. CLINICAL PARTICULARS
4.1 Therapeutic indications
Orally administered Hytrin is indicated in the treatment of mild to moderate hypertension. It may be used in combination with thiazide diuretics and/or other antihypertensive drugs or as sole therapy where other agents are inappropriate or ineffective. The hypotensive effect is most pronounced on the diastolic pressure. Although the exact mechanism of the hypotensive action of terazosin is not established, the relaxation of peripheral blood vessels appears to be produced mainly by competitive antagonism of post-synaptic alpha$_1$ - adrenoceptors. Hytrin usually produces an initial gradual decrease in blood pressure followed by a sustained antihypertensive action.

Orally administered Hytrin is also indicated as a therapy for the symptomatic treatment of urinary obstruction caused by benign prostatic hyperplasia (BPH). Terazosin is a selective post synaptic alpha-1-adrenoreceptor antagonist. Antagonism of alpha-1-receptors on prostatic and urethral smooth muscle has been shown to improve urinary tract flow and relieve the urinary obstruction caused by BPH.

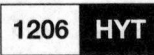

4.2 Posology and method of administration

a) Hypertension

Adults:

Initial dose: 1 mg before bedtime is the starting dose for all patients and should not be exceeded. Compliance with this initial dosage recommendation should be strictly observed to minimise potential for acute first-dose hypotensive episodes.

Subsequent doses: The single daily dosage may be increased by approximately doubling the dosage at weekly intervals to achieve the desired blood pressure response. The usual maintenance dose is 2mg to 10mg once daily. Doses over 20mg rarely improve efficacy and doses over 40mg have not been studied.

b) BPH

Adults Only: The dose of terazosin should be adjusted according to the patient's response. The following is a guide to administration:

Initial dose: 1 mg before bedtime is the starting dose for all patients and should not be exceeded. Strict compliance with this recommendation should be observed to minimise acute first-dose hypotensive episodes.

Subsequent dose: The dose may be increased by approximately doubling at weekly or bi-weekly intervals to achieve the desired reduction in symptoms. The maintenance dose is usually 5 to 10mg once daily. Improvements in symptoms have been detected as early as two weeks after starting treatment with terazosin.

At present there are insufficient data to suggest additional symptomatic relief with doses above 10mg once daily.

Treatment should be initiated using the Hytrin BPH Starter Pack and response to treatment reviewed at four weeks. Transient side effects may occur at each titration step. If any side effects persist, consideration should be given to reducing the dose.

Use in renal insufficiency: Pharmacokinetic studies indicate that patients with impaired renal function need no alteration in the recommended dosages.

Use in Children: Use in children for BPH is not applicable.

Use in the Elderly: Pharmacokinetic studies in the elderly indicate that no alteration in dosage recommendation is required.

Postural Hypotension: Postural hypotension has been reported to occur in patients receiving terazosin for the symptomatic treatment of urinary obstruction caused by BPH. In these cases, the incidence of postural hypotensive events was greater in patients aged 65 years and over (5.6%) than those aged less than 65 years (2.6%).

Use with thiazide diuretics and other antihypertensive agents: When adding a thiazide diuretic or another antihypertensive agent to a patient's regimen the dose of Hytrin should be reduced and retitration carried out if necessary. Caution should be observed when Hytrin is administered with thiazides or other antihypertensive agents as hypotension may develop.

4.3 Contraindications

Terazosin is contraindicated in patients known to be hypersensitive to alpha-adrenoreceptor antagonists.

4.4 Special warnings and special precautions for use

As with other alpha adrenoreceptor antagonists, terazosin is not recommended in patients with a history of micturition syncope.

In clinical trials, the incidence of postural hypotension was greater in patients who received terazosin for BPH than in patients who received terazosin for hypertension. In this indication the incidence of postural hypotensive events was greater in patients aged 65 years and over (5.6%) than those aged less than 65 years (2.6%).

If administration is discontinued for more than several days, therapy should be re-instituted using the initial dosing regimen.

4.5 Interaction with other medicinal products and other forms of Interaction

In patients receiving terazosin for BPH, plus ACE inhibitors or diuretics, the proportion reporting dizziness or related side effects was greater than in the total population of terazosin treated patients from clinical trials.

Caution should be observed when terazosin is administered with other antihypertensive agents, to avoid the possibility of significant hypotension. When adding terazosin to a diuretic or other antihypertensive agent, dosage reduction and retitration may be necessary.

Terazosin has been given without interaction with analgesics/anti-inflammatories, cardiac glycosides, hypoglycaemics, antiarrhythmics, anxiolytics/sedatives, antibacterials, hormones/steroids and drugs used for gout.

4.6 Pregnancy and lactation

Although no teratogenic effects were seen in animal testing, the safety during pregnancy and lactation has not yet been established. Hytrin should not be used therefore in pregnancy unless the potential benefit outweighs the risk.

4.7 Effects on ability to drive and use machines

Dizziness, light-headedness or drowsiness may occur with the initial dose or in association with missed doses and subsequent reinitiation of Hytrin therapy. Patients should be cautioned about these possible adverse events and the circumstances in which they may occur and advised to avoid driving or hazardous tasks for approximately the first 12 hours after the initial dose or when the dose is increased.

4.8 Undesirable effects

Hytrin, in common with other alpha-adrenoreceptor antagonists, may cause syncope. Syncopal episodes have occurred within 30 to 90 minutes of the initial dose of the drug. Syncope has occasionally occurred in association with rapid dosage increases or the introduction of another antihypertensive agent.

In clinical studies in hypertension, the incidence of syncopal episodes was approximately one percent. In most cases, this was believed to be due to an excessive postural hypotensive effect although occasionally the syncopal episode has been preceded by a bout of tachycardia with heart rates of 120 to 160 beats per minute.

If syncope occurs the patient should be placed in a recumbent position and given supportive treatment as necessary.

Dizziness, light-headedness or fainting may occur when standing up quickly from a lying or sitting position. Patients should be advised of this possibility and instructed to lie down if these symptoms appear and then sit for a few minutes before standing to prevent re-occurrence.

These adverse effects are self limiting and, in most cases, do not recur after the initial period of therapy or during subsequent titration.

Adverse events reported with terazosin: The most common events were asthenia, palpitations, nausea, peripheral oedema, dizziness, somnolence, nasal congestion/rhinitis and blurred vision/amblyopia.

In addition, the following have been reported: back pain; headache; tachycardia; postural hypotension; syncope; oedema; weight gain; pain in extremities; decreased libido; depression; nervousness; paraesthesia; vertigo; dyspnoea; sinusitis and impotence.

Additional adverse reactions reported in clinical trials or reported during marketing experience but not clearly associated with the use of terazosin include the following: chest pain; facial oedema; fever; abdominal pain; neck pain; shoulder pain; vasodilation; arrhythmia; constipation; diarrhoea; dry mouth; dyspepsia; flatulence; vomiting; gout; arthralgia; arthritis; joint disorders; myalgia; anxiety; insomnia; bronchitis; epistaxis; flu symptoms; pharyngitis; rhinitis; cold symptoms; pruritis; rash; increased cough; sweating; abnormal vision; conjunctivitis; tinnitus; urinary frequency; urinary tract infection and urinary incontinence primarily reported in post-menopausal women.

At least two cases of severe anaphylactoid reactions have been reported with the administration of terazosin.

Post marketing experience: Thrombocytopenia and priapism have been reported. Atrial fibrillation has been reported, however a cause and effect relationship has not been established.

Laboratory tests: Small but statistically significant decreases in haematocrit, haemoglobin, white blood cells, total protein and albumin were observed in controlled clinical trials. These laboratory findings suggest the possibility of haemodilution. Treatment with terazosin for up to 24 months had no significant effect on prostate specific antigen (PSA) levels.

4.9 Overdose

Should administration of terazosin lead to acute hypotension, cardiovascular support is of first importance. Restoration of blood pressure and normalisation of heart rate may be accomplished by keeping the patient in a supine position. If this measure is inadequate, shock should first be treated with volume expanders and, if necessary, vasopressors could then be used. Renal function should be monitored and general supportive measures applied as required. Dialysis may not be of benefit since laboratory data indicate that terazosin is highly protein bound.

5. PHARMACOLOGICAL PROPERTIES

5.1 Pharmacodynamic properties

Although the exact mechanism of the hypotensive action is not established, the relaxation of peripheral blood vessels appears to be produced mainly by competitive antagonism of post-synaptic alpha-adrenoceptors. Hytrin usually produces an initial gradual decrease in blood pressure followed by a sustained antihypertensive action.

Clinical experience indicates that a 2-5% decrease in total cholesterol plasma concentration and a 3-7% decrease in the combined LDL_c + $VLDL_c$ fraction plasma concentration from pretreatment values are associated with the administration of therapeutic doses of terazosin.

In clinical trials, plasma concentrates of total cholesterol and combined low density and very low density lipoproteins were found to be slightly reduced following Hytrin administration. Additionally, the increase in total cholesterol seen with other hypertensive agents did not occur when these were used in combination with Hytrin.

Studies suggest that alpha-1-adrenoreceptor antagonism is useful in improving the urodynamics in patients with chronic bladder obstruction such as in benign prostatic hyperplasia (BPH).

The symptoms of BPH are caused mainly by the presence of an enlarged prostate and by the increased smooth muscle tone of the bladder outlet and prostate, which is regulated by alpha-1-adrenergic receptors.

In in-vitro experiments, terazosin has been shown to antagonise phenylephrine-induced contractions of human prostatic tissue. In clinical trials terazosin has been shown to improve the urodynamics and symptomatology in patients with BPH.

5.2 Pharmacokinetic properties

The plasma concentration of the parent drug is a maximum 1 hour post administration and declines with a half-life of approximately 12 hours. Food has little or no effect on bioavailability. Approximately 40% of the administered dose is eliminated in the urine and 60% in the faeces. The drug is highly bound to plasma proteins.

5.3 Preclinical safety data

Carcinogenicity: terazosin has been shown to produce benign adrenal medullary tumours in male rats when administered in very high doses over a long period of time. No such findings were seen in female rats or in a similar study in mice. The relevance of these findings with respect to the clinical use of the drug in man is unknown.

6. PHARMACEUTICAL PARTICULARS

6.1 List of excipients

Lactose, maize starch, purified talc, magnesium stearate and purified water.

In addition: Hytrin 2mg tablets contains dye yellow (quinoline yellow, E104); Hytrin 5mg tablets contain dye (iron oxide burnt sienna, E172); Hytrin 10mg tablets contain dye blue (FD&C No. 2 lake).

6.2 Incompatibilities

None known.

6.3 Shelf life

36 months.

6.4 Special precautions for storage

None.

6.5 Nature and contents of container

Tablets in a blister pack. The 1mg tablets are only available as part of two starter packs. The hypertension starter pack consists of 7 × 1mg, 21 × 2mg and the BPH starter pack consists of 7 × 1mg, 14 × 2mg and 7 × 5mg tablets. The 2mg and 5mg tablets are also supplied in packs of 28 tablets. The 10mg tablets are supplied in packs of 28 tablets. The blisters, of PVC/PVdC, are heat sealed with 20 micron hard tempered aluminium foil and packaged in a carton with a pack insert.

6.6 Instructions for use and handling

Not applicable.

7. MARKETING AUTHORISATION HOLDER

Abbott Laboratories Limited, Queenborough, Kent, ME11 5EL.

8. MARKETING AUTHORISATION NUMBER(S)

Hytrin 1mg Tablets - PL 0037/0159

Hytrin 2mg Tablets - PL 0037/0160

Hytrin 5mg Tablets - PL 0037/0161

Hytrin 10mg Tablets - PL 0037/0162

9. DATE OF FIRST AUTHORISATION/RENEWAL OF THE AUTHORISATION

20/05/98

10. DATE OF REVISION OF THE TEXT

October 2000

Ibugel

(Dermal Laboratories Limited)

1. NAME OF THE MEDICINAL PRODUCT

IBUGEL™

2. QUALITATIVE AND QUANTITATIVE COMPOSITION

Ibuprofen 5.0% w/w.

3. PHARMACEUTICAL FORM

Non-greasy, fragrance-free, clear, aqueous-alcoholic gel.

4. CLINICAL PARTICULARS

4.1 Therapeutic indications

For the topical treatment of backache, rheumatic and muscular pain, sprains, strains and neuralgia. Ibugel is also indicated for symptomatic relief of pain due to non-serious arthritic conditions.

4.2 Posology and method of administration

Apply the gel to the affected areas, up to three times daily, or as directed by the physician. On each occasion apply only enough gel to thinly cover the affected area, and gently massage well into the skin, until completely absorbed. Do not use excessively. Hands should be washed immediately after use (unless treating them). Treatment should not normally continue for more than a few weeks, unless recommended to do so by a doctor.

The same dosage and dosage schedule applies to all age groups, although Ibugel is not normally recommended for use on children under the age of 12 years, unless instructed by their doctor.

4.3 Contraindications

Not to be used in cases of sensitivity to any of the ingredients, particularly if asthmatic or suffer from allergic disease, and have previously shown hypersensitivity to aspirin, ibuprofen or related painkillers. Not to be used on broken skin.

4.4 Special warnings and special precautions for use

Seek medical advice if symptoms worsen or persist. Oral NSAIDs, including ibuprofen, can sometimes be associated with renal impairment, aggravation of active peptic ulcers, and can induce allergic bronchial reactions in susceptible asthmatic patients. Although the systemic absorption of topically applied ibuprofen is less than for oral dosage forms, these complications can occur in rare cases. For these reasons, patients with an active peptic ulcer, a history of kidney problems, asthma or intolerance to aspirin or ibuprofen taken orally should seek medical advice before using Ibugel. Keep Ibugel away from the eyes and mucous membranes. For external use only.

The label will include statements to the following effect:

If symptoms persist, consult your doctor or pharmacist. Do not use if sensitive to any of the ingredients, particularly if asthmatic, suffer from rhinitis or urticaria and have previously shown hypersensitivity to aspirin, ibuprofen or related painkillers. Consult your doctor before use if you are taking aspirin or other pain-killers.

4.5 Interaction with other medicinal products and other forms of Interaction

Non-steroidal anti-inflammatory drugs may interact with blood pressure lowering drugs, although the chance of this occurring with a topically administered preparation is extremely remote. Concurrent aspirin or other NSAIDS may result in an increased incidence of adverse reactions.

4.6 Pregnancy and lactation

Do not use during pregnancy or lactation.

4.7 Effects on ability to drive and use machines

None known.

4.8 Undesirable effects

Very rarely, susceptible patients may experience the following side effects with ibuprofen, but these are extremely uncommon when ibuprofen is administered topically. If they occur, treatment should be discontinued:-

Hypersensitivity: hypersensitivity reactions have been reported following treatment with ibuprofen. These may consist of (a) non-specific allergic reactions and anaphylaxis, (b) respiratory tract reactivity comprising asthma, aggravated asthma, bronchospasm, or dyspnoea, or (c) assorted skin disorders, including rashes of various types, pruritus, urticaria, purpura, angioedema and, less commonly, bullous dermatoses (including epidermal necrolysis and erythema multiforme).

Renal: renal impairment can occur in patients with a history of kidney problems.

Gastrointestinal: side effects such as abdominal pain and dyspepsia have been reported.

4.9 Overdose

Not applicable. Any overdose with a topical presentation of ibuprofen is extremely unlikely.

5. PHARMACOLOGICAL PROPERTIES

5.1 Pharmacodynamic properties

Ibugel is a topical preparation which has anti-inflammatory and analgesic properties. It contains the active ingredient, ibuprofen, which exerts its effects directly in inflamed tissues underlying the site of application, mainly by inhibiting prostaglandin biosynthesis.

Because it is formulated in an aqueous/alcoholic gel, Ibugel also exerts a soothing and cooling effect when applied to the affected area.

5.2 Pharmacokinetic properties

Specially formulated for external application, the active ingredient penetrates through the skin rapidly and extensively, achieving high, therapeutically relevant local concentrations in underlying soft tissues, joints and synovial fluid, whilst producing plasma levels that are unlikely to be sufficient to cause any systemic side-effects, other than in rare individuals who are hypersensitive to ibuprofen.

Furthermore, there do not appear to be any appreciable differences between the oral and topical routes of administration regarding metabolism or excretion of ibuprofen.

5.3 Preclinical safety data

Published information on subchronic toxicity studies confirms that topically applied ibuprofen is well tolerated both locally and by the gastro-intestinal tract. Any local erythema is only mild and no signs of mucosal lesions or ulcerogenic effects have been determined in the gastro-intestinal tract.

In the course of assessing mucosal tolerance, topical ibuprofen has been found to cause acute, but reversible, irritant reactions in the eyes and mucous membranes.

6. PHARMACEUTICAL PARTICULARS

6.1 List of excipients

IMS; Carbomer; Propylene Glycol; Diethylamine; Purified Water.

6.2 Incompatibilities

None known.

6.3 Shelf life

36 months.

6.4 Special precautions for storage

Do not store above 25°C.

6.5 Nature and contents of container

100 g collapsible aluminium tube, fitted with a screw cap. This is supplied as an original pack (OP).

6.6 Instructions for use and handling

Not applicable.

7. MARKETING AUTHORISATION HOLDER

Dermal Laboratories
Tatmore Place, Gosmore
Hitchin, Herts SG4 7QR, UK.

8. MARKETING AUTHORISATION NUMBER(S)

0173/0050.

9. DATE OF FIRST AUTHORISATION/RENEWAL OF THE AUTHORISATION

2 September 2002.

10. DATE OF REVISION OF THE TEXT

April 2002.

Ibugel Forte 10%

(Dermal Laboratories Limited)

1. NAME OF THE MEDICINAL PRODUCT

IBUGEL™ FORTE 10%

2. QUALITATIVE AND QUANTITATIVE COMPOSITION

Ibuprofen 10.0% w/w.

3. PHARMACEUTICAL FORM

Aqueous-alcoholic, non-greasy, fragrance-free, clear or slightly hazy gel.

4. CLINICAL PARTICULARS

4.1 Therapeutic indications

For the topical treatment of rheumatic and muscular pain, sprains, strains, backache and neuralgia. Ibugel Forte 10% is also indicated for symptomatic relief of pain due to non-serious arthritic conditions.

4.2 Posology and method of administration

2 to 5 cm gel (50 to 125 mg ibuprofen) is to be applied to the affected area up to three times daily, or as directed by the physician. The gel should be massaged well into the skin until completely absorbed, and hands washed after use unless being treated.

Treatment should not normally continue for more than a few weeks, unless recommended to do so by a doctor.

The same dosage and dosage schedule applies to all age groups, although Ibugel Forte 10% is not normally recommended for use on children under the age of 12 years, unless instructed by the physician.

4.3 Contraindications

Not to be used if allergic to any of the ingredients, or in cases of hypersensitivity to aspirin, ibuprofen or related painkillers (including when taken by mouth), especially where associated with a history of asthma, rhinitis or urticaria. Not to be used on broken or damaged skin.

4.4 Special warnings and special precautions for use

To be kept away from the eyes and mucous membranes. Oral NSAIDs, including ibuprofen, can sometimes be associated with renal impairment, aggravation of active peptic ulcers, and can induce allergic bronchial reactions in susceptible asthmatic patients. Although the systemic absorption of topically applied ibuprofen is less than for oral dosage forms, these complications can occur in rare cases. For these reasons, caution should be exercised before prescribing Ibugel Forte 10% for patients with an active peptic ulcer, a history of kidney problems, asthma or intolerance to aspirin or ibuprofen taken orally. Patients should seek medical advice if symptoms worsen or persist.

4.5 Interaction with other medicinal products and other forms of Interaction

Non-steroidal anti-inflammatory drugs may interact with blood pressure lowering drugs, although the chance of this occurring with a topically administered preparation is extremely remote. Where aspirin or other NSAID tablets are taken concurrently, it is important to bear in mind that these may increase the incidence of undesirable effects.

4.6 Pregnancy and lactation

Not to be used during pregnancy or lactation. Although no teratogenic effects have been demonstrated, ibuprofen should be avoided during pregnancy. The onset of labour may be delayed, and the duration of labour increased. Ibuprofen appears in breast milk in very low concentrations, but is unlikely to affect breast fed infants adversely.

4.7 Effects on ability to drive and use machines

None known.

4.8 Undesirable effects

Very rarely, susceptible patients may experience the following side effects with ibuprofen, but these are extremely uncommon when ibuprofen is administered topically. If they occur, treatment should be discontinued:-

Hypersensitivity: hypersensitivity reactions have been reported following treatment with ibuprofen. These may consist of (a) non-specific allergic reactions and anaphylaxis, (b) respiratory tract reactivity comprising asthma, aggravated asthma, bronchospasm, or dyspnoea, or (c) assorted skin disorders, including rashes of various types, pruritus, urticaria, purpura, angioedema and, less commonly, bullous dermatoses (including epidermal necrolysis and erythema multiforme).

Renal: renal impairment can occur in patients with a history of kidney problems.

Gastrointestinal: side effects such as abdominal pain and dyspepsia have been reported.

4.9 Overdose

Not applicable. Any overdose with a topical presentation of ibuprofen is extremely unlikely. Symptoms of severe ibuprofen overdosage (eg following accidental oral ingestion) include headache, vomiting, drowsiness and hypotension. Correction of severe electrolyte abnormalities should be considered.

5. PHARMACOLOGICAL PROPERTIES

5.1 Pharmacodynamic properties

Ibugel Forte 10% is a topical preparation which has anti-inflammatory and analgesic properties. It contains the active ingredient, ibuprofen, which exerts its effects directly in inflamed tissues underlying the site of application, mainly by inhibiting prostaglandin biosynthesis.

Because it is formulated in an aqueous/alcoholic gel, Ibugel Forte 10% also exerts a soothing and cooling effect when applied to the affected area.

5.2 Pharmacokinetic properties

Specially formulated for external application, the active ingredient penetrates through the skin rapidly and extensively, achieving high, therapeutically relevant local concentrations in underlying soft tissues, joints and synovial fluid, whilst producing plasma levels that are unlikely to be sufficient to cause any systemic side effects, other than in rare individuals who are hypersensitive to ibuprofen. Furthermore, there do not appear to be any appreciable differences between the oral and topical routes of administration regarding metabolism or excretion of ibuprofen.

5.3 Preclinical safety data

Published information on subchronic toxicity studies confirms that topically applied ibuprofen is well tolerated both locally and by the gastro-intestinal tract. Any local erythema is only mild and no signs of mucosal lesions or ulcerogenic effects have been determined in the gastro-intestinal tract.

In the course of assessing mucosal tolerance, topical ibuprofen has been found to cause acute, but reversible, irritant reactions in the eyes and mucous membranes.

6. PHARMACEUTICAL PARTICULARS

6.1 List of excipients
IMS; Carbomers; Diethylamine; Purified Water.

6.2 Incompatibilities
None known.

6.3 Shelf life
36 months.

6.4 Special precautions for storage
Do not store above 25°C.

6.5 Nature and contents of container
100 g collapsible aluminium tube, fitted with a screw cap. This is supplied as an original pack (OP).

6.6 Instructions for use and handling
Not applicable.

7. MARKETING AUTHORISATION HOLDER
Dermal Laboratories
Tatmore Place, Gosmore
Hitchin, Herts SG4 7QR, UK.

8. MARKETING AUTHORISATION NUMBER(S)
0173/0175.

9. DATE OF FIRST AUTHORISATION/RENEWAL OF THE AUTHORISATION
3 March 2000.

10. DATE OF REVISION OF THE TEXT
October 2002.

Ibumousse

(Dermal Laboratories Limited)

1. NAME OF THE MEDICINAL PRODUCT
IBUMOUSSE™

2. QUALITATIVE AND QUANTITATIVE COMPOSITION
Ibuprofen 5.0% w/w.

3. PHARMACEUTICAL FORM
Non-greasy, fragrance-free, white aqueous cutaneous foam.

4. CLINICAL PARTICULARS

4.1 Therapeutic indications
For backache, rheumatic and muscular pain, and neuralgia. Ibumousse is also indicated for symptomatic relief of pain due to non-serious arthritic conditions.

4.2 Posology and method of administration
Shake container before use. Hold container upright, then press nozzle to dispense the mousse into the palm of your hand. Gently massage the mousse into and around the affected areas until absorbed. The exact amount to be applied will vary, depending on the extent and severity of the condition, but it should normally be sufficient to apply 1 to 2 g (1 to 2 golf-ball sized quantities of mousse dispensed into the palm of the hand). This amount may be repeated 3 to 4 times daily, unless otherwise directed by the doctor.

Treatment should not normally continue for more than a few weeks, unless recommended by a doctor.

The same dosage and dosage schedule applies to all age groups, although the mousse is not normally recommended for children under 12 years, unless instructed by their doctor.

4.3 Contraindications
Not to be used if allergic to any of the ingredients, or in cases of hypersensitivity to aspirin, ibuprofen or related painkillers (including when taken by mouth), especially where associated with a history of asthma, rhinitis or urticaria.

Not to be used on broken or damaged skin, or where there is infection or other skin disease.

4.4 Special warnings and special precautions for use
This product is flammable. Do not spray near flames, burning cigarettes, electric heaters or similar objects.

Keep away from the eyes and mucous membranes.

Oral NSAIDs, including ibuprofen, can sometimes be associated with renal impairment or aggravation of active peptic ulcers, and they can induce allergic bronchial reactions in susceptible asthmatic patients. Although systemic absorption of topically applied ibuprofen is much less than for oral dosage forms, these complications can still occur in rare cases. For these reasons, patients with asthma, an active peptic ulcer or a history of kidney problems, should seek medical advice before using the mousse, as should patients already taking other painkillers.

Patients should seek medical advice if symptoms worsen or persist.

For external use only.

Wash hands after use unless treating them.

Do not use excessively.

The label will include statements to the following effect:

Do not exceed the stated dose. Not recommended for children under 12 years without medical advice. For external use only. Not to be used during pregnancy or breast-feeding. Do not use if you are allergic to any of the ingredients or have experienced problems with aspirin, ibuprofen or related painkillers (including when taken by mouth). If symptoms persist consult your doctor or pharmacist. Keep out of the reach of children. Patients with asthma, an active peptic ulcer or a history of kidney problems should consult their doctor before use, as should patients already taking aspirin or other painkillers.

4.5 Interaction with other medicinal products and other forms of Interaction
Non-steroidal anti-inflammatory drugs may interact with blood pressure lowering drugs, although the chance of this occurring with a topically administered preparation is extremely remote. Concurrent aspirin or other NSAIDs may result in an increased incidence of undesirable effects.

4.6 Pregnancy and lactation
Not to be used during pregnancy or lactation. Although no teratogenic effects have been demonstrated, ibuprofen should be avoided during pregnancy. The onset of labour may be delayed, and the duration of labour increased. Ibuprofen appears in breast milk in very low concentrations, but is unlikely to affect breast-fed infants adversely.

4.7 Effects on ability to drive and use machines
None known.

4.8 Undesirable effects
The cooling effect of the mousse may result in a temporary paling of the skin. Very rarely, susceptible patients may experience the following side effects with ibuprofen, but these are extremely uncommon when ibuprofen is administered topically. If they occur, treatment should be discontinued:-

Hypersensitivity: hypersensitivity reactions have been reported following treatment with ibuprofen. These may consist of (a) non-specific allergic reactions and anaphylaxis, (b) respiratory tract reactivity comprising asthma, aggravated asthma, bronchospasm, or dyspnoea, or (c) assorted skin disorders, including rashes of various types, pruritus, urticaria, purpura, angioedema and, less commonly, bullous dermatoses (including epidermal necrolysis and erythema multiforme).

Renal: renal impairment can occur in patients with a history of kidney problems.

Gastrointestinal: side effects such as abdominal pain and dyspepsia have been reported.

4.9 Overdose
Any overdose with a topical presentation of ibuprofen is extremely unlikely.

Symptoms of severe ibuprofen overdosage (eg following accidental oral ingestion) include headache, vomiting, drowsiness and hypotension. Correction of severe electrolyte abnormalities should be considered.

5. PHARMACOLOGICAL PROPERTIES

5.1 Pharmacodynamic properties
The mousse is for topical application. Ibuprofen is a phenylpropionic acid derivative with analgesic and anti-inflammatory properties. It exerts its effects directly in inflamed tissues underlying the site of application, mainly by inhibiting prostaglandin biosynthesis.

Because it is formulated in an aqueous mousse, the preparation also exerts a soothing and cooling effect when applied to the affected area.

5.2 Pharmacokinetic properties
Ibumousse has been designed for external application. The formulation delivers the active ingredient through the skin rapidly and extensively, achieving high, therapeutically relevant local concentrations in underlying soft tissues, joints and the synovial fluid, whilst producing plasma levels that are unlikely to be sufficient to cause any systemic side-effects, other than in rare individuals who are hypersensitive to ibuprofen.

There do not appear to be any appreciable differences between the oral and topical routes of administration regarding metabolism or excretion of ibuprofen.

5.3 Preclinical safety data
No relevant information additional to that contained elsewhere in the SPC.

6. PHARMACEUTICAL PARTICULARS

6.1 List of excipients
Propylene Glycol; Carbomer; Phenoxyethanol; Diethylamine; Butane 40; Purified Water.

(The ozone-friendly aerosol propellent is a blend of C_2 - H_5 hydrocarbons consisting primarily of propane, iso-butane and n-butane).

6.2 Incompatibilities
None known.

6.3 Shelf life
48 months.

6.4 Special precautions for storage
Do not store above 25°C. Keep upright and away from direct heat or sunlight. Do not expose pressurised container to temperatures higher than 50°C. Do not pierce or burn container, even when empty.

6.5 Nature and contents of container
Aluminium pressurised container incorporating a spray valve and cap containing 125 g of product. This is supplied as an original pack (OP).

6.6 Instructions for use and handling
Not applicable.

7. MARKETING AUTHORISATION HOLDER
Dermal Laboratories
Tatmore Place, Gosmore
Hitchin, Herts SG4 7QR, UK.

8. MARKETING AUTHORISATION NUMBER(S)
0173/0169.

9. DATE OF FIRST AUTHORISATION/RENEWAL OF THE AUTHORISATION
26 August 1998.

10. DATE OF REVISION OF THE TEXT
October 2002.

Ibuspray

(Dermal Laboratories Limited)

1. NAME OF THE MEDICINAL PRODUCT
IBUSPRAY™

2. QUALITATIVE AND QUANTITATIVE COMPOSITION
Ibuprofen 5.0% w/w.

3. PHARMACEUTICAL FORM
Cutaneous spray solution.

Clear, colourless, fragrance-free, aqueous-alcoholic topical spray.

4. CLINICAL PARTICULARS

4.1 Therapeutic indications
For the topical treatment of backache, rheumatic and muscular pain, sprains, strains, and neuralgia. Ibuspray is also indicated for symptomatic relief of pain due to non-serious arthritic conditions.

4.2 Posology and method of administration
Hold the bottle upright or upside down and spray approximately 4 inches to 6 inches away from the skin. After every 2 to 3 sprays, gently massage the preparation into the skin, spreading the product over a wide area around the affected site. The exact amount to be applied will vary, depending on the extent and severity of the condition, but it should normally be sufficient to apply 5 to 10 sprays (1 to 2 ml). This amount may be repeated three to four times daily, or more often if required. Do not use excessively. Hands should be washed after use, unless treating them.

Treatment should not normally continue for more than a few weeks, unless recommended to do so by a doctor.

The same dosage and dosage schedule applies to all age groups, although Ibuspray is not normally recommended for use on children below the age of 12 years unless instructed by their doctor.

4.3 Contraindications
Not to be used in cases of sensitivity to any of the ingredients, particularly if asthmatic or suffer from rhinitis or urticaria, and have previously shown hypersensitivity to aspirin or ibuprofen or related painkillers. Not to be used on broken skin.

4.4 Special warnings and special precautions for use
This product is flammable. Do not spray near flames, electric heaters or similar objects. Seek medical advice if symptoms worsen or persist. Oral NSAIDs, including ibuprofen, can sometimes be associated with renal impairment, aggravation of active peptic ulcers, and can induce allergic bronchial reactions in susceptible asthmatic patients. Although the systemic absorption of topically applied ibuprofen is much less than from oral dosage forms, these complications can occur in rare cases. For these reasons, patients with an active peptic ulcer, a history of kidney problems, asthma or intolerance to aspirin or ibuprofen should seek medical advice before using Ibuspray.

Keep away from the eyes and mucous membranes. For external use only.

The label will include statements to the following effect:

If symptoms persist, consult your doctor or pharmacist.

Do not use if sensitive to any of the ingredients, particularly if asthmatic, suffer from rhinitis or urticaria and have previously shown hypersensitivity to aspirin, ibuprofen or related painkillers.

Consult your doctor before use if you are taking aspirin or other painkillers.

4.5 Interaction with other medicinal products and other forms of Interaction
Non-steroidal anti-inflammatory drugs may interact with blood pressure lowering drugs, although the chance of this occurring with a topically administered preparation is extremely remote. Concurrent aspirin or other NSAIDs may result in an increased incidence of undesirable effects.

4.6 Pregnancy and lactation
Do not use during pregnancy or lactation.

4.7 Effects on ability to drive and use machines
None known.

4.8 Undesirable effects
Very rarely, susceptible patients may experience the following side effects with ibuprofen, but these are extremely uncommon when ibuprofen is administered topically. If they occur, treatment should be discontinued:-

Hypersensitivity: hypersensitivity reactions have been reported following treatment with ibuprofen. These may consist of (a) non-specific allergic reactions and anaphylaxis, (b) respiratory tract reactivity comprising asthma, aggravated asthma, bronchospasm, or dyspnoea, or (c) assorted skin disorders, including rashes of various types, pruritus, urticaria, purpura, angioedema and, less commonly, bullous dermatoses (including epidermal necrolysis and erythema multiforme).

Renal: renal impairment can occur in patients with a history of kidney problems.

Gastrointestinal: side effects such as abdominal pain and dyspepsia have been reported.

4.9 Overdose
Not applicable. Any overdose with a topical presentation of ibuprofen is unlikely.

5. PHARMACOLOGICAL PROPERTIES

5.1 Pharmacodynamic properties
Ibuspray is a topical preparation which has anti-inflammatory and analgesic properties. It contains the active ingredient, ibuprofen, which exerts its effects directly in inflamed tissues underlying the site of application, mainly by inhibiting prostaglandin biosynthesis. Because it is formulated in an evaporative aqueous/alcoholic solution, Ibuspray also exerts a soothing and cooling effect when applied to the affected area.

5.2 Pharmacokinetic properties
Specially formulated for external application, the active ingredient penetrates through the skin rapidly and extensively, achieving high, therapeutically relevant local concentrations in underlying soft tissues, joints and synovial fluid, whilst producing plasma levels that are unlikely to be sufficient to cause any systemic side effects, other than in rare individuals who are hypersensitive to ibuprofen. Furthermore, there do not appear to be any appreciable differences between the oral and topical routes of administration regarding metabolism or excretion of ibuprofen.

5.3 Preclinical safety data
No relevant information additional to that contained elsewhere in the SPC.

6. PHARMACEUTICAL PARTICULARS

6.1 List of excipients
IMS; Macrogol 300; Cetomacrogol 1000; Purified Water.

6.2 Incompatibilities
None known.

6.3 Shelf life
36 months.

6.4 Special precautions for storage
Do not store above 25°C.

6.5 Nature and contents of container
100 ml plastic bottle incorporating a controlled dose spray pump dispenser and overcap. This is supplied as an original pack (OP).

6.6 Instructions for use and handling
Not applicable.

7. MARKETING AUTHORISATION HOLDER
Dermal Laboratories

Tatmore Place, Gosmore

Hitchin, Herts SG4 7QR, UK.

8. MARKETING AUTHORISATION NUMBER(S)
0173/0150.

9. DATE OF FIRST AUTHORISATION/RENEWAL OF THE AUTHORISATION
27 January 2000.

10. DATE OF REVISION OF THE TEXT
September 2004.

Icthaband

(Medlock Medical Ltd)

1. NAME OF THE MEDICINAL PRODUCT
Icthaband.

2. QUALITATIVE AND QUANTITATIVE COMPOSITION
Zinc Oxide BP 15% w/w; Ichthammol BP 2% w/w.

3. PHARMACEUTICAL FORM
Open wove bleached cotton bandage impregnated with the paste formulation.

4. CLINICAL PARTICULARS

4.1 Therapeutic indications
Icthaband may be used for the following conditions: subacute eczematous conditions; chronic eczema, where tar is not tolerated; subacute gravitational eczema and all other forms of leg eczema; varicose and gravitational ulcers, in conjunction with a compression bandage, when a protective barrier to thin and fragile skin is required.

4.2 Posology and method of administration
For topical use. Adults, the elderly, and children: Frequency of dressing changes is at the discretion of the responsible physician. There are no differences in use between adults, children and the elderly.

4.3 Contraindications
Hypersensitivity to any ingredient of the paste, and acute eczematous lesions.

4.4 Special warnings and special precautions for use
Avoid use on grossly macerated skin. The skin of leg ulcers is easily sensitised to topical medicaments including preservatives. Sensitisation should be suspected in patients particularly where there is deterioration of the ulcer or surrounding skin. Such patients should be referred for special diagnosis including patch testing. One of the functions of occlusive bandages is to increase absorption. Care should be taken, therefore, if it is decided to apply topical steroid preparations under these bandages as their absorption may be significantly increased.

4.5 Interaction with other medicinal products and other forms of Interaction
None stated.

4.6 Pregnancy and lactation
No special precautions required.

4.7 Effects on ability to drive and use machines
Not applicable.

4.8 Undesirable effects
Not applicable.

4.9 Overdose
Not applicable.

5. PHARMACOLOGICAL PROPERTIES

5.1 Pharmacodynamic properties
The product is a paste bandage with the active constituent presented in a glycerine, modified starch and castor oil based paste spread onto a cotton bandage. Zinc Oxide as a zinc salt has astringent properties and has been shown to play a role in wound healing. Ichthammol has an antipruritic action and has slight bacteriostatic properties. These substances are well established in use, but only the subject of brief references in recent literature and pharmacopoeias (e.g. Martindale). Much of the therapeutic action of paste bandages is attributable to the bandaging technique, the physical support and protection provided and to the maintenance of moist wound healing conditions.

5.2 Pharmacokinetic properties
The pharmacokinetics of the active ingredient are those relevant to topical application of the substances through whole or broken skin. Contemporary literature describes the biochemical properties but with the exception of the zinc salts does directly relate these properties to the disease states being treated. Zinc compounds are the subject of current re-appraisal for their role in wound healing.

5.3 Preclinical safety data
None stated.

6. PHARMACEUTICAL PARTICULARS

6.1 List of excipients
Propyl hydroxybenzoate; modified starch; citric acid; glycerine; castor oil; purified water; open wove cotton bandage.

6.2 Incompatibilities
None stated.

6.3 Shelf life
Thirty months.

6.4 Special precautions for storage
Store in a dry place not exceeding 25°C.

6.5 Nature and contents of container
Bandages are wrapped individually in waxed paper or polythene film and then placed in a nylon/foil/polythene laminate bag in a cardboard carton, or a sealed polythene bag in a cardboard carton. 12 cartons are packed per corrugated cardboard outer.

6.6 Instructions for use and handling
None.

7. MARKETING AUTHORISATION HOLDER
Seton Healthcare Group plc, Tubiton House, Oldham, OL1 3HS.

8. MARKETING AUTHORISATION NUMBER(S)
PL 0223/5001R.

9. DATE OF FIRST AUTHORISATION/RENEWAL OF THE AUTHORISATION
27th July 1990 / 17th July 2003.

10. DATE OF REVISION OF THE TEXT
July 2003.

Idrolax 10g

(SCHWARZ PHARMA Limited)

1. NAME OF THE MEDICINAL PRODUCT
IDROLAX 10g

2. QUALITATIVE AND QUANTITATIVE COMPOSITION
Macrogol 4000 10.000 g

Excipients: see 6.1.

3. PHARMACEUTICAL FORM
Powder for oral solution in sachet.

Single dose sachet containing an almost white powder with an odour and taste of orange grapefruit.

4. CLINICAL PARTICULARS

4.1 Therapeutic indications
Symptomatic treatment of constipation in adults and children aged 8 years and above.

An organic disorder should have been ruled out before initiation of treatment. IDROLAX 10g should remain a temporary adjuvant treatment to appropriate lifestyle and dietary management of constipation, with a maximum 3-months treatment course in children. If symptoms persist despite associated dietary measures, an underlying cause should be suspected and treated.

4.2 Posology and method of administration
1 to 2 sachets per day, preferably taken as a single dose in the morning. Each sachet should be dissolved in a glass of water.

The effect of IDROLAX becomes apparent within 24 to 48 hours after its administration.

In children, treatment should not exceed 3 months. Treatment-induced restoration of bowel movements will be maintained by lifestyle and dietary measures.

4.3 Contraindications
- severe inflammatory bowel disease (such as ulcerative colitis, Crohn's disease) or toxic megacolon, associated with symptomatic stenosis,
- perforation or risk of perforation,
- ileus or suspicion of intestinal obstruction,
- painful abdominal syndromes of indeterminate cause,
- known hypersensitivity to IDROLAX or to one of the components.

4.4 Special warnings and special precautions for use
Warning

Safety data in children were obtained in patients aged 6 months to 3 years.

The treatment of constipation with any medicinal product is only an adjuvant to a healthy lifestyle and diet, for example:
- increased intake of liquids and dietary fibre,
- appropriate physical activity and rehabilitation of the bowel reflex.

Due to the presence of sorbitol (traces), this medicine is contraindicated in persons who are intolerant to fructose.

Precautions for use

This medicinal product contains polyethylene glycol.

Very rare cases of hypersensitivity reactions (rash, urticaria, oedema) have been reported with drugs containing polyethylene glycol. Exceptional cases of anaphylactic shock have been reported.

IDROLAX does not contain a significant quantity of sugar or polyol and can be prescribed to diabetic patients or patients on a galactose-free diet

4.5 Interaction with other medicinal products and other forms of Interaction
Not applicable

4.6 Pregnancy and lactation
Pregnancy

Macrogol 4000 was not teratogenic in rats or rabbits

There are no adequate data from use of IDROLAX in pregnant women

Therefore caution should be exercised when prescribing IDROLAX to pregnant women.

Lactation

There are no data on the excretion of macrogol 4000 in breast milk. As macrogol 4000 is not significantly absorbed, IDROLAX may be administrated during lactation.

4.7 Effects on ability to drive and use machines
None

4.8 Undesirable effects
Adults:

Undesirable effects reported during clinical trials with the following frequencies have always been minor and transitory and have mainly concerned the gastrointestinal system:

- common (≥1/100, <1/10): abdominal distension and/or pain, nausea, diarrhoea,

- uncommon (≥1/1000, <1/100): vomiting, and the more common consequence of the diarrhoea: urgency to defecate and faecal incontinence.

Children:

Undesirable effects reported during clinical trials are of the same nature as for adults.

Excessive doses may cause diarrhoea, which generally disappears when the dosage is reduced or treatment temporarily interrupted.

Additional information from post-marketing surveillance included very rare (<1/10000) cases of hypersensitivity reactions: pruritus, urticaria, rash, face oedema, Quincke oedema and isolated cases of anaphylactic shock have been reported.

4.9 Overdose

Leads to diarrhoea which disappears when treatment is temporarily interrupted or the dosage is reduced.

Cases of aspiration have been reported when extensive volumes of polyethylene glycol and electrolytes were administered with nasogastric tube. Neurologically impaired children who have oromotor dysfunction are particularly at risk of aspiration.

5. PHARMACOLOGICAL PROPERTIES

5.1 Pharmacodynamic properties

OSMOTIC LAXATIVE

A: gastrointestinal tract and metabolism

ATC code: A06AD15

High molecular weight (4000) macrogols are long linear polymers which retain water molecules by means of hydrogen bonds. When administered by the oral route, they lead to an increase in volume of intestinal fluids.

The volume of unabsorbed intestinal fluid accounts for the laxative properties of the solution.

5.2 Pharmacokinetic properties

The pharmacokinetic data confirm that macrogol 4000 undergoes neither gastrointestinal resorption nor biotransformation following oral ingestion.

5.3 Preclinical safety data

Toxicological studies in different species of animals did not reveal any signs of systemic or local gastrointestinal toxicity of macrogol 4000. Macrogol 4000 had no teratogenic, mutagenic, nor carcinogenic effect. Potential drug interactions studies performed in rats on some NSAIDs, anticoagulants, gastric antisecretory agents, or on a hypoglycaemic sulfamide showed that IDROLAX did not interfere with gastrointestinal absorption of these compounds.

6. PHARMACEUTICAL PARTICULARS

6.1 List of excipients

Saccharin sodium (E954), orange-grapefruit flavour**

** Composition of the orange-grapefruit flavour:

Orange and grapefruit oils, concentrated orange juice, citral, acetaldehyde, linalol, ethyl butyrate, alpha terpineol, octanal, beta gamma hexenol, maltodextrine, gum arabic, sorbitol.

6.2 Incompatibilities

Not applicable

6.3 Shelf life

5 years

6.4 Special precautions for storage

No special precaution for storage

6.5 Nature and contents of container

(Paper / Aluminium / PE) sachet.

10.167 g single dose sachets contained in a box of 10, 20, 50 sachets

Not all pack sizes may be marketed

6.6 Instructions for use and handling

None

7. MARKETING AUTHORISATION HOLDER

SCHWARZ PHARMA Limited

East Street

Chesham

Buckinghamshire

HP5 1DG

England

8. MARKETING AUTHORISATION NUMBER(S)

04438/0062

9. DATE OF FIRST AUTHORISATION/RENEWAL OF THE AUTHORISATION

January 2002

10. DATE OF REVISION OF THE TEXT

March 2004

Code IDR 2856

Ikorel Tablets

(sanofi-aventis)

1. NAME OF THE MEDICINAL PRODUCT

Ikorel™ Tablets 10mg and 20mg

2. QUALITATIVE AND QUANTITATIVE COMPOSITION

Nicorandil 10mg or 20mg

3. PHARMACEUTICAL FORM

Tablets, off-white, round, with faceted edges, scored on one side and bearing the inscription IK10 (10mg) or IK20 (20mg).

4. CLINICAL PARTICULARS

4.1 Therapeutic indications

Ikorel tablets are indicated for the following:

• The prevention and long term treatment of chronic stable angina pectoris

• A reduction in the risk of acute coronary syndromes in patients with chronic stable angina and at least one of the following risk factors:

Previous MI

Previous CABG

CHD on angiography **or** a positive exercise test together with one of the following: LVH on ECG, left ventricular dysfunction, Age ≥ 65, diabetes mellitus (type I or II excluding those on sulphonylureas, see section 5.1), hypertension or documented vascular disease

4.2 Posology and method of administration

Route of administration: oral.

Adults: The recommended starting dose is 10mg nicorandil twice daily, although 5mg twice daily may be employed in patients particularly susceptible to headache. Subsequently the dosage should be titrated upward depending on the clinical response. The usual therapeutic dosage is in the range 10 to 20mg nicorandil twice daily, although up to 30mg twice daily may be employed if necessary.

Elderly: There is no special requirement for dosage reduction in elderly patients. As with all medicines, the lowest effective dosage should be used.

Children: A paediatric dosage has not been established and use of nicorandil is not recommended.

4.3 Contraindications

Ikorel is contraindicated in patients with cardiogenic shock, left ventricular failure with low filling pressures and in hypotension. It is also contraindicated in patients who have demonstrated an idiosyncratic response or hypersensitivity to nicorandil. Due to the risk of severe hypotension, the concomitant use of Ikorel and phosphodiesterase 5 inhibitors (e.g. sildenafil, tadalafil, vardenafil) is contraindicated.

4.4 Special warnings and special precautions for use

The use of nicorandil should be avoided in patients with depleted blood volume, low systolic blood pressure, acute pulmonary oedema or acute myocardial infarction with acute left ventricular failure and low filling pressures.

Therapeutic doses of nicorandil may lower the blood pressure of hypertensive patients and therefore nicorandil, as with other antianginal agents, should be used with care when prescribed with antihypertensive drugs.

Alternative therapy should be considered if persistent aphtosis or severe mouth ulceration occurs.

4.5 Interaction with other medicinal products and other forms of Interaction

No pharmacological or pharmacokinetic interactions have been observed in humans or animals with beta-blockers, digoxin, rifampicin, cimetidine, nicoumalone, a calcium antagonist or a combination of digoxin and frusemide. Nevertheless, there is the possibility that nicorandil may potentiate the hypotensive effects of other vasodilators, tricyclic antidepressants or alcohol.

As the hypotensive effects of nitrates or nitric oxide donors are potentiated by phosphodiesterase 5 inhibitors, the concomitant use of Ikorel and phosphodiesterase 5 inhibitors is contraindicated.

4.6 Pregnancy and lactation

Pregnancy: Animal studies have not revealed any harmful effect of nicorandil on the foetus although there is no experience in humans. It should not be used in pregnant patients unless there is no safer alternative.

Lactation: As it is not known whether nicorandil is excreted in human milk, breastfeeding should be avoided by lactating patients who require therapy.

4.7 Effects on ability to drive and use machines

Patients should be warned not to drive or operate machinery until it is established that their performance is unimpaired by nicorandil.

4.8 Undesirable effects

The most frequent effect to be anticipated is headache, usually of a transitory nature, especially when treatment is initiated.

Cutaneous vasodilation with flushing is less frequent. Nausea, vomiting dizziness and a feeling of weakness have been reported occasionally. Myalgia and different types of rash have been reported rarely.

There have been very rare reports of angioedema and hepatic function abnormalities.

Hypotension may occur at high therapeutic doses. An increase in heart rate may occur at high doses.

Rare cases of persistent aphtosis or mouth ulcers which were occasionally severe have been reported. These resolved following treatment discontinuation.

4.9 Overdose

Acute overdosage is likely to be associated with peripheral vasodilation, decreased blood pressure and reflex tachycardia. Cardiac function should be monitored and general supportive measures employed. If necessary, circulating plasma volume should be increased by infusion of suitable fluid. In life-threatening situations, administration of vasopressors should be considered. There is no experience of massive overdosage in humans, although the LD_{50} in dogs is in the range 62.5 to 125 mg/kg and in rodents it is in the order of 1200 mg/kg.

5. PHARMACOLOGICAL PROPERTIES

5.1 Pharmacodynamic properties

Nicorandil provides a dual mode of action leading to relaxation of vascular smooth muscle. A potassium channel opening action provides arterial vasodilation, thus reducing afterload, while the nitrate component promotes venous relaxation and a reduction in preload. Nicorandil has a direct effect on coronary arteries without leading to a steal phenomenon. The overall action improves blood flow to post-stenotic regions and the oxygen balance in the myocardium.

A reduction of coronary heart disease complications has been shown in patients suffering from angina pectoris who were treated with nicorandil in the IONA study.

The study was a randomised, double blind, placebo controlled, cardiovascular endpoint study carried out in 5126 patients to determine if Nicorandil could reduce the frequency of coronary events in men and women with chronic stable angina and standard anti anginal treatment at high risk of cardiovascular events defined by either: 1) previous myocardial infarction, or 2) coronary artery bypass grafting, or 3) coronary artery disease confirmed by angiography, or a positive exercise test in the previous two years, together with one of the following: left ventricular hypertrophy on the ECG, left ventricular ejection fraction ≤ 45%, or an end diastolic dimension of >55 mm, age ≥ 65, diabetes (either type 1 or type 2), hypertension, peripheral vascular disease, or cerebrovascular disease. Patients were excluded from the study if they were receiving a sulphonylurea as it was felt these patients may not benefit; (sulphonylurea agents have the potential to close potassium channels and may thus antagonise some of the effects of nicorandil). Study follow up for endpoint analysis was between 12 and 36 months with a mean of 1.6 years.

The primary endpoint of coronary heart disease (CHD) death, non-fatal myocardial infarction, or unplanned hospital admission for cardiac chest pain, occurred in 13.1% of patients treated with nicorandil compared with 15.5% of patients receiving placebo (hazard ratio 0.83, p=0.014). The rate of acute coronary syndrome (CHD death, non fatal MI or unstable angina) was 6.1% in patients treated with nicorandil compared with 7.6% in patients receiving placebo (hazard ratio 0.79, p=0.028). All cardiovascular events were significantly less in the nicorandil than placebo group 14.7% vs 17.0% (hazard ratio 0.86 p=0.027). The validity of these findings was confirmed by re-analysing the primary endpoint using all cause rather than cardiovascular mortality (nicorandil 14.9% compared with placebo 17.3%, hazard ratio 0.85, p=0.021). The study was not expressly powered to, nor did it detect any statistically significant reduction in any individual component endpoints.

5.2 Pharmacokinetic properties

Nicorandil is well absorbed with no significant first-pass metabolism. Maximum plasma concentrations are achieved in 30 to 60 minutes and are directly related to the dosage. Metabolism is mainly by denitration of the molecule into the nicotinamide pathway with less than 20% of an administered dose being excreted in the urine. The main phase of elimination has a half-life of about 1 hour. Nicorandil is only slightly bound to plasma proteins.

No clinically relevant modifications in the pharmacokinetic profile have been seen in the elderly or in patients with liver disease or chronic renal failure.

5.3 Preclinical safety data

There are no preclinical data of relevance to the prescriber which are additional to that included in other sections of the SPC.

6. PHARMACEUTICAL PARTICULARS

6.1 List of excipients

Maize starch, croscarmellose sodium, stearic acid and mannitol.

6.2 Incompatibilities

None stated.

6.3 Shelf life

18 months.

Each blister strip should be used within 30 days of opening.

6.4 Special precautions for storage
Store in a dry place below 25°C.

6.5 Nature and contents of container
Ikorel tablets 10mg and 20mg are presented in soft tempered aluminium foil/PVC blister strips of 10 tablets, in which each tablet is linked to a silica gel capsule dessicant.

The blister strips are packaged in cartons of 60 tablets.

6.6 Instructions for use and handling
None stated.

7. MARKETING AUTHORISATION HOLDER
May and Baker Ltd
T/A Aventis Pharma, or Rhône-Poulenc Rorer
50 Kings Hill Avenue
Kings Hill
West Malling
Kent ME19 4AH

8. MARKETING AUTHORISATION NUMBER(S)
Ikorel tablets 10mg: PL 00012/0229
Ikorel tablets 20mg: PL 00012/0230

9. DATE OF FIRST AUTHORISATION/RENEWAL OF THE AUTHORISATION
26 October 1999

10. DATE OF REVISION OF THE TEXT
June 2004

11 LEGAL CLASSIFICATION
POM

Imdur Tablets 60mg

(AstraZeneca UK Limited)

1. NAME OF THE MEDICINAL PRODUCT
Imdur ® Tablets 60mg.

2. QUALITATIVE AND QUANTITATIVE COMPOSITION
Isosorbide mononitrate 60mg
For excipients, see Section 6.1.

3. PHARMACEUTICAL FORM
Extended release film coated tablet (Durules®)

4. CLINICAL PARTICULARS

4.1 Therapeutic indications
Prophylactic treatment of angina pectoris.

4.2 Posology and method of administration

Dosage

Adults:
Imdur 60mg (one tablet) once daily given in the morning. The dose may be increased to 120mg (two tablets) daily, both to be taken once daily in the morning. The dose can be titrated to minimise the possibility of headache, by initiating treatment with 30mg (half a tablet) for the first 2-4 days.

Administration:
Imdur Tablets must not be chewed or crushed. They should be swallowed whole with half a glass of water.

Children
The safety and efficacy of Imdur in children has not been established.

Elderly
No evidence of a need for routine dosage adjustment in the elderly has been found, but special care may be needed in those with increased susceptibility to hypotension or marked hepatic or renal insufficiency.

The core of the tablet is insoluble in the digestive juices but disintegrates into small particles when all active substance has been released. Very occasionally the matrix may pass through the gastrointestinal tract without disintegrating and be found visible in the stool, but all active substance has been released.

4.3 Contraindications
Hypersensitivity to any of the components. Constrictive cardiomyopathy and pericarditis, aortic stenosis, cardiac tamponade, mitral stenosis and severe anaemia.

Sildenafil has been shown to potentiate the hypotensive effects of nitrates, and its co-administration with nitrates or nitric oxide donors is therefore contraindicated.

Severe cerebrovascular insufficiency or hypotension are relative contraindications to the use of Imdur.

4.4 Special warnings and special precautions for use
Imdur is not indicated for relief of acute angina attacks; in the event of an acute attack, sublingual or buccal glyceryl trinitrate tablets should be used.

4.5 Interaction with other medicinal products and other forms of Interaction
The hypotensive effect of nitrates are potentiated by concurrent administration of sildenafil.

4.6 Pregnancy and lactation
The safety and efficacy of Imdur during pregnancy or lactation has not been established.

4.7 Effects on ability to drive and use machines
None known.

4.8 Undesirable effects
Most of the adverse reactions are pharmacodynamically mediated and dose dependent. Headache may occur when treatment is initiated, but usually disappears after 1-2 weeks of treatment. The dose can be titrated to minimise the possibility of headache, by initiating treatment with 30mg. Hypotension, with symptoms such as dizziness and nausea, has occasionally been reported. These symptoms generally disappear during continued treatment. Rash and pruritus have been reported rarely. Myalgia has been reported very rarely.

4.9 Overdose

Symptoms
Pulsing headache. More serious symptoms are excitation, flushing, cold perspiration, nausea, vomiting, vertigo, syncope, tachycardia and a fall in blood pressure.

Management
Induction of emesis, activated charcoal. In case of pronounced hypotension the patient should first be placed in the supine position with legs raised. If necessary fluids should be administered intravenously.

5. PHARMACOLOGICAL PROPERTIES

5.1 Pharmacodynamic properties
Pharmacotherapeutic group: Vasodilators used in cardiovascular disease (organic nitrates). ATC Code: C01D A.

The principal pharmacological action of isosorbide mononitrate, an active metabolite of isosorbide dinitrate, is relaxation of vascular smooth muscle, producing vasodilation of both arteries and veins with the latter effect predominating. The effect of the treatment is dependent on the dose. Low plasma concentrations lead to venous dilatation, resulting in peripheral pooling of blood, decreased venous return and reduction in left ventricular end-diastolic pressure (preload). High plasma concentrations also dilate the arteries reducing systemic vascular resistance and arterial pressure leading to a reduction in cardiac afterload. Isosorbide mononitrate may also have a direct dilatory effect on the coronary arteries. By reducing the end diastolic pressure and volume, the preparation lowers the intramural pressure, thereby leading to an improvement in the subendocardial blood flow.

The net effect when administering isosorbide mononitrate is therefore a reduced workload of the heart and an improved oxygen supply/demand balance in the myocardium.

5.2 Pharmacokinetic properties
Isosorbide mononitrate is completely absorbed and is not subject to first pass metabolism by the liver. This reduces the intra- and inter-individual variations in plasma levels and leads to predictable and reproducible clinical effects.

The elimination half-life of isosorbide mononitrate is around 5 hours. The plasma protein binding is less than 5%. The volume of distribution for isosorbide mononitrate is about 0.6 l/kg and total clearance around 115 ml/minute. Elimination is primarily by denitration and conjugation in the liver. The metabolites are excreted mainly via the kidneys. Only about 2% of the dose given is excreted intact via the kidneys.

Impaired liver or kidney function have no major influence on the pharmacokinetic properties.

Imdur is an extended release formulation (Durules). The active substance is released independently of pH, over a 10-hour period. Compared to ordinary tablets the absorption phase is prolonged and the duration of effect is extended.

The extent of bioavailability of Imdur is about 90% compared to immediate release tablets. Absorption is not significantly affected by food intake and there is no accumulation during steady state. Imdur exhibits dose proportional kinetics up to 120mg. After repeated peroral administration with 60mg once daily, maximal plasma concentration (around 3000 nmol/l) is achieved after around 4 hours. The plasma concentration then gradually falls to under 500 nmol/l at the end of the dosage interval (24 hours after dose intake). The tablets are divisible.

In placebo-controlled studies, Imdur once daily has been shown to effectively control angina pectoris both in terms of exercise capacity and symptoms, and also in reducing signs of myocardial ischaemia. The duration of the effect is at least 12 h, at this point the plasma concentration is at the same level as at around 1 hour after dose intake (around 1300 nmol/l).

Imdur is effective as monotherapy as well as in combination with chronic -blocker therapy.

The clinical effects of nitrates may be attenuated during repeated administration owing to high and/or even plasma levels. This can be avoided by allowing low plasma levels for a certain period of the dosage interval. Imdur, when administered once daily in the morning, produces a plasma profile of high levels during the day and low levels during the night. With Imdur 60mg or 120mg once daily no development of tolerance with respect to antianginal effect has been observed. Rebound phenomenon between doses as described with intermittent nitrate patch therapy has not been seen with Imdur.

5.3 Preclinical safety data
The accessible data indicate that isosorbide mononitrate has expected pharmacodynamic properties of an organic nitrate ester, has simple pharmacokinetic properties, and is devoid of toxic, mutagenic or oncogenic effects.

6. PHARMACEUTICAL PARTICULARS

6.1 List of excipients
Aluminium silicate, paraffin special, hydroxypropylcellulose LF, magnesium stearate, colloidal anhydrous silica, hypromellose 6cps, macrogol 6000, titanium dioxide E171 and iron oxide yellow E172.

6.2 Incompatibilities
Not applicable for extended release products.

6.3 Shelf life
Glass bottle: 3 years
Blister pack: 3 years

6.4 Special precautions for storage
Store below 30°C.

6.5 Nature and contents of container
Amber glass bottles with a LD-polyethylene cap in a pack of 100 tablets.

Press-through package of thermoformed PVC, in packs of 7, 14, 28 and 98 tablets.

6.6 Instructions for use and handling
Do not crush or chew tablets. The tablets should be taken with half a glass of water.

7. MARKETING AUTHORISATION HOLDER
AstraZeneca UK Ltd.,
600 Capability Green,
Luton, LU1 3LU, UK.

8. MARKETING AUTHORISATION NUMBER(S)
PL 17901/0129

9. DATE OF FIRST AUTHORISATION/RENEWAL OF THE AUTHORISATION
18th May 2004

10. DATE OF REVISION OF THE TEXT
15th December 2004

Imigran 10mg and 20mg Nasal Spray

(GlaxoSmithKline UK)

1. NAME OF THE MEDICINAL PRODUCT
Imigran® 10mg Nasal Spray.
Imigran® 20mg Nasal Spray.

2. QUALITATIVE AND QUANTITATIVE COMPOSITION
Imigran 10mg Nasal Spray: Unit dose spray device for intranasal administration. The device delivers 10mg of sumatriptan in 0.1ml of an aqueous buffered solution.

Imigran 20mg Nasal Spray: Unit dose spray device for intranasal administration. The device delivers 20mg of sumatriptan in 0.1ml of an aqueous buffered solution.

For excipients see 6.1. List of Excipients

3. PHARMACEUTICAL FORM
Nasal Spray, solution.

Clear pale yellow to dark yellow liquid, in glass vials in a single dose nasal spray device.

4. CLINICAL PARTICULARS

4.1 Therapeutic indications
Imigran Nasal Spray is indicated for the acute treatment of migraine attacks with or without aura.

4.2 Posology and method of administration
Imigran Nasal Spray should not be used prophylactically.

Imigran is recommended as monotherapy for the acute treatment of a migraine attack and should not be given concomitantly with ergotamine or derivatives of ergotamine (including methysergide) (see Section 4.3 Contraindications).

It is advisable that Imigran be given as early as possible after the onset of a migraine headache. It is equally effective at whatever stage of the attack it is administered.

Adults (18 years of age and over)
The optimal dose of Imigran Nasal Spray is 20mg for administration into one nostril. Although, due to inter/intra patient variability of both the migraine attacks and the absorption of sumatriptan, 10mg may be effective in some patients.

If a patient does not respond to the first dose of Imigran, a second dose should not be taken for the same attack. However the attack can be treated with paracetamol, aspirin or non-steroidal anti-inflammatory drugs. Imigran may be taken for subsequent attacks.

If the patient has responded to the first dose, but the symptoms recur a second dose may be given in the next 24 hours, provided that there is a minimum interval of two hours between the two doses.

No more than two Imigran 20mg Nasal Sprays to be used in any 24 hour period.

Adolescents (12-17 years of age)

Use of sumatriptan in adolescents should be on the recommendation of a specialist or physician who has significant experience in treating migraine, taking into account local guidance.

The recommended dose of Imigran Nasal Spray is 10mg for administration into one nostril.

If a patient does not respond to the first dose of Imigran, a second dose should not be taken for the same attack. In these cases the attack can be treated with paracetamol, aspirin or non-steroidal anti-inflammatory drugs.

Imigran may be taken for subsequent attacks.

If the patient has responded to the first dose but the symptoms recur, a second dose may be given in the following 24 hours, provided that there is a minimum interval of 2 hours between the two doses.

No more than two doses of Imigran 10mg Nasal Spray should be taken in any 24-hour period.

Children (under 12 years of age)

The safety and effectiveness of Imigran Nasal Spray in children has not yet been established.

Elderly (over 65)

There is no experience of the use of Imigran Nasal Spray in patients over 65. The kinetics in elderly patients have not been sufficiently studied. Therefore the use of sumatriptan is not recommended until further data are available.

4.3 Contraindications

Hypersensitivity to any component of the preparation.

Sumatriptan should not be given to patients who have had myocardial infarction or have ischaemic heart disease, coronary vasospasm (Prinzmetal's angina), peripheral vascular disease or patients who have symptoms or signs consistent with ischaemic heart disease.

Sumatriptan should not be administered to patients with a history of cerebrovascular accident (CVA) or transient ischaemic attack (TIA).

Sumatriptan should not be administered to patients with severe hepatic impairment.

The use of sumatriptan in patients with moderate and severe hypertension and mild uncontrolled hypertension is contraindicated.

The concomitant administration of ergotamine, or derivatives of ergotamine (including methysergide) is contra-indicated (See Section 4.5 Interactions With Other Medicinal Products).

Concurrent administration of monoamine oxidase inhibitors (MAOIs) and sumatriptan is contraindicated.

Imigran must not be used within two weeks of discontinuation of therapy with monoamine oxidase inhibitors.

4.4 Special warnings and special precautions for use

Imigran Nasal Spray should only be used where there is a clear diagnosis of migraine.

Sumatriptan is not indicated for use in the management of hemiplegic, basilar or ophthalmoplegic migraine.

As with other acute migraine therapies, before treating headaches in patients not previously diagnosed as migraineurs, and in migraineurs who present with atypical symptoms, care should be taken to exclude other potentially serious neurological conditions.

It should be noted that migraineurs may be at increased risk of certain cerebrovascular events (eg. CVA, TIA).

Following administration, sumatriptan can be associated with transient symptoms including chest pain and tightness which may be intense and involve the throat (see Section 4.8 Undesirable effects). Where such symptoms are thought to indicate ischaemic heart disease, no further doses of sumatriptan should be given and appropriate evaluation should be carried out.

Sumatriptan should not be given to patients with risk factors for ischaemic heart disease without prior cardiovascular evaluation (See Section 4.3. Contraindications). Special consideration should be given to postmenopausal women and males over 40 with these risk factors. These evaluations however, may not identify every patient who has cardiac disease and, in very rare cases, serious cardiac events have occurred in patients without underlying cardiovascular disease.

There have been rare postmarketing reports describing patients with weakness, hyper-reflexia, and incoordination following the use of a selective serotonin reuptake inhibitor (SSRI) and sumatriptan. If concomitant treatment with sumatriptan and an SSRI is clinically warranted, appropriate observation of the patient is advised.

Sumatriptan should be administered with caution to patients with conditions which may affect significantly the absorption, metabolism or excretion of the drug, eg. impaired hepatic or renal function.

Sumatriptan should be used with caution in patients with a history of seizures or other risk factors which lower the seizure threshold, as seizures have been reported in association with sumatriptan (see section 4.8).

Patients with known hypersensitivity to sulphonamides may exhibit an allergic reaction following administration of sumatriptan. Reactions may range from cutaneous hypersensitivity to anaphylaxis.

Undesirable effects may be more common during concomitant use of triptans and herbal preparations containing St John's Wort (Hypericum perforatum).

As with other acute migraine treatments, chronic daily headache/exacerbation of headache have been reported with overuse of sumatriptan, which may necessitate a drug withdrawal.

The recommended dose of Imigran should not be exceeded.

4.5 Interaction with other medicinal products and other forms of Interaction

There is no evidence of interactions with propranolol, flunarizine, pizotifen or alcohol.

There are limited data on an interaction with ergotamine containing preparations. The increased risk of coronary vasospasm is a theoretical possibility and concomitant administration is contra-indicated.

The period of time that should elapse between the use of sumatriptan and ergotamine containing preparations is not known. This will also depend on the doses and type of ergotamine containing products used. The effects may be additive. It is advised to wait at least 24 hours following the use of ergotamine containing preparations before administering sumatriptan. Conversely it is advised to wait at least six hours following use of sumatriptan before administering an ergotamine containing product. (see Section 4.3 Contra-indications)

An interaction may occur between sumatriptan and MAOIs and concomitant administration is contraindicated (see Section 4.3 Contraindications). Rarely an interaction may occur between sumatriptan and SSRIs.

4.6 Pregnancy and lactation

Post-marketing data from the use of sumatriptan during the first trimester in over 1,000 women are available. Although these data contain insufficient information to draw definitive conclusions, they do not point to an increased risk of congenital defects. Experience with the use of sumatriptan in the second and third trimester is limited.

Evaluation of experimental animal studies does not indicate direct teratogenic effects or harmful effects on peri- and postnatal development. However, embryofoetal viability might be affected in the rabbit (see section 5.3 Preclinical Safety Data). Administration of sumatriptan should only be considered if the expected benefit to the mother is greater than any possible risk to the foetus.

It has been demonstrated that following subcutaneous administration sumatriptan is secreted into breast milk. Infant exposure can be minimised by avoiding breast feeding for 24 hours after treatment.

4.7 Effects on ability to drive and use machines

No data are available. Drowsiness may occur as a result of migraine or its treatment with sumatriptan. This may influence the ability to drive and to operate machinery.

4.8 Undesirable effects

Adverse events are listed below by system organ class and frequency. Frequencies are defined as: very common >1/10), common >1/100, <1/10), uncommon >1/1000, <1/100), rare >1/10,000, <1/1000) and very rare (<1/10,000) including isolated reports. The most frequently reported side effect following the use of Imigran Nasal Spray is its taste.

Clinical Trial Data

Nervous System Disorders

Common: Tingling, dizziness, drowsiness.

Vascular disorders

Common: Transient increases in blood pressure arising soon after treatment. Flushing.

Respiratory, Thoracic and Mediastinal Disorders

Common: Following administration of sumatriptan nasal spray mild, transient irritation or burning sensation in the nose or throat or epistaxis have been reported.

Gastrointestinal

Common: Nausea and vomiting occurred in some patients but it is if this related to sumatriptan or the underlying condition.

Musculoskeletal, connective tissue and bone disorders

Common: Sensations of heaviness (usually transient and may be intense and can affect any part of the body including the chest and throat).

General Disorders and Administration Site Conditions

Common: Pain, sensations of heat, pressure or tightness (these events are usually transient and may be intense and can affect any part of the body including the chest and throat).

Common: Feelings of weakness, fatigue (both events are mostly mild to moderate in intensity and transient).

Investigations

Very rare: Minor disturbances in liver function tests have occasionally been observed.

Post-Marketing Data

Immune System Disorders

Very rare: Hypersensitivity reactions ranging from cutaneous hypersensitivity to rare cases of anaphylaxis.

Nervous System Disorders

Very rare: Seizures, although some have occurred in patients with either a history of seizures or concurrent conditions predisposing to seizures there are also reports in patients where no such predisposing factors are apparent.

Nystagmus, scotoma.

Eye disorders

Very rare: Flickering, diplopia, reduced vision. Loss of vision including reports of permanent defects. However, visual disorders may also occur during a migraine attack itself.

Cardiac disorders

Very rare: Bradycardia, tachycardia, palpitations, cardiac arrhythmias, transient ischaemic ECG changes, coronary artery vasospasm, myocardial infarction (see Contraindications, Special Warnings and Precautions for Use).

Vascular disorders

Very rare: Hypotension, Raynaud's phenomenon.

Gastrointestinal

Very rare: Ischaemic colitis.

Musculoskeletal, connective tissue and bone disorders

Very rare: Neck stiffness.

4.9 Overdose

Single doses, of sumatriptan, up to 40mg intranasally and in excess of 16mg subcutaneously and 400mg orally have not been associated with side effects other than those mentioned.

In clinical studies volunteers have received 20mg of sumatriptan by the intranasal route three times a day for a period of 4 days without significant adverse effects.

If overdosage occurs, the patient should be monitored for at least ten hours and standard supportive treatment applied as required. It is unknown what effect haemodialysis or peritoneal dialysis has on the plasma concentrations of sumatriptan.

5. PHARMACOLOGICAL PROPERTIES

5.1 Pharmacodynamic properties

Pharmacotherapeutic group:- Selective $5HT_1$ receptor agonists. ATC code: N02CC01

Sumatriptan has been demonstrated to be a selective vascular 5-hydroxytryptamine-1-($5HT_{1d}$) receptor agonist with no effect at other 5HT receptor (5HT2-$5HT_7$) subtypes. The vascular $5HT_{1d}$ receptor is found predominantly in cranial blood vessels and mediates vasoconstriction. In animals sumatriptan selectively constricts the carotid arterial circulation, the carotid arterial circulation supplies blood to the extracranial and intracranial tissues such as the meninges and dilatation and/or oedema formation in these vessels is thought to be the underlying mechanism of migraine in man. In addition, evidence from animal studies suggests that sumatriptan inhibits trigeminal nerve activity. Both these actions (cranial vasoconstriction and inhibition of trigeminal nerve activity) may contribute to the anti-migraine action of sumatriptan in humans.

Clinical response begins 15 minutes following a 20mg dose given by intra-nasal administration.

Because of its route of administration Imigran nasal spray may be particularly suitable for patients who suffer with nausea and vomiting during an attack.

The magnitude of the treatment effect is smaller in adolescents as compared with adults. This might be due to a much higher placebo response observed in adolescents compared with adults. The reason for the high placebo response remains unclear.

5.2 Pharmacokinetic properties

After intranasal administration, sumatriptan is rapidly absorbed, median times to maximum plasma concentrations being 1.5 (range: 0.25-3) hours in adults and 2 (range: 0.5-3) hours in adolescents. After a 20mg dose, the mean maximum concentration is 13ng/mL. Mean intranasal bioavailability, relative to subcutaneous administration is about 16%, partly due to pre-systemic metabolism.

Following oral administration, presystemic clearance is reduced in patients with hepatic impairment resulting in increased plasma levels of sumatriptan, a similar increase would be expected following intranasal administration.

Plasma protein binding is low (14-21%), the mean volume of distribution is 170 litres. The elimination half-life is approximately 2 hours. The mean total plasma clearance is approximately 1160ml/min and the mean renal plasma clearance is approximately 260ml/min.

A pharmacokinetic study in adolescent subjects (12-17 years) indicated that the mean maximum plasma concentration was 13.9ng/mL and mean elimination half-life was approximately 2 hours following a 20mg intranasal dose. Population pharmacokinetic modelling indicated that clearance and volume of distribution both increase with body size in the adolescent population resulting in higher exposure in lower bodyweight adolescents.

Non-renal clearance accounts for about 80% of the total clearance. Sumatriptan is eliminated primarily by oxidative metabolism mediated by monoamine oxidase A. The major metabolite, the indole acetic acid analogue of sumatriptan is mainly excreted in urine, where it is present as a free acid and the glucuronide conjugate. It has no known 5HT1 or 5HT2 activity. Minor metabolites have not been identified. The pharmacokinetics of intra-nasal sumatriptan do not appear to be significantly affected by migraine attacks.

The kinetics in the elderly have been insufficiently studied to justify a statement on possible differences in kinetics between elderly and young volunteers.

5.3 Preclinical safety data

In studies carried out to test for local and ocular irritancy, following administration of sumatriptan nasal spray, there was no nasal irritancy seen in laboratory animals and no ocular irritancy observed when the spray was applied directly to the eyes of rabbits.

In a rat fertility study a reduction in success of insemination was seen at exposures sufficiently in excess of the maximum human exposure. In rabbits embryolethality, without marked teratogenic defects, was seen. The relevance for humans of these findings is unknown.

Sumatriptan was devoid of genotoxic and carcinogenic activity in in-vitro systems and animal studies.

6. PHARMACEUTICAL PARTICULARS

6.1 List of excipients

Potassium Dihydrogen Phosphate

Dibasic Sodium Phosphate anhydrous

Sulphuric Acid

Sodium Hydroxide

Purified Water

6.2 Incompatibilities

Not applicable

6.3 Shelf life

3 years.

6.4 Special precautions for storage

Do not store above 30°C. Do not freeze.

Imigran Nasal Spray should be kept in the sealed blister, preferably in the box, to protect from light.

6.5 Nature and contents of container

The container consists of a type I Ph.Eur. glass vial with rubber stopper and applicator.

Imigran 10mg Nasal Spray: unit dose spray device containing 0.1ml solution.

Pack contains 1, 2, 4, 6, 12, or 18 sprays.

Imigran 20mg Nasal Spray: unit dose spray device containing 0.1ml solution.

Pack contains 1, 2, 4, 6, 12, or 18 sprays.

Not all pack sizes may be marketed.

6.6 Instructions for use and handling

No special requirements.

Administrative Data

7. MARKETING AUTHORISATION HOLDER

Glaxo Wellcome UK Ltd

Trading as

GlaxoSmithKline UK

Stockley Park West

Uxbridge

Middlesex

UB11 1BT.

8. MARKETING AUTHORISATION NUMBER(S)

Imigran 10mg Nasal Spray: PL 10949/0260

Imigran 20mg Nasal Spray: PL 10949/0261

9. DATE OF FIRST AUTHORISATION/RENEWAL OF THE AUTHORISATION

Renewal: 29 March 2001

10. DATE OF REVISION OF THE TEXT

08 July 2004

11. Legal Status

POM

Imigran Injection, Subject

(GlaxoSmithKline UK)

1. NAME OF THE MEDICINAL PRODUCT

Imigran Injection

Imigran Subject

2. QUALITATIVE AND QUANTITATIVE COMPOSITION

Each pre-filled syringe contains 6mg of sumatriptan base, as the succinate salt, in an isotonic solution of 0.5ml.

3. PHARMACEUTICAL FORM

Pre-filled syringes for use in conjunction with an auto injector for subcutaneous injection.

4. CLINICAL PARTICULARS

4.1 Therapeutic indications

Subcutaneous Injection is indicated for the acute relief of migraine attacks, with or without aura, and for the acute treatment of cluster headache. Imigran should only be used where there is a clear diagnosis of migraine or cluster headache.

4.2 Posology and method of administration

Imigran should not be used prophylactically.

It is recommended to start the treatment at the first sign of a migraine headache or associated symptoms such as nausea, vomiting or photophobia. It is equally effective at whatever stage of the attack it is administered. Imigran Injection should be injected subcutaneously using an autoinjector. Patients should be advised to observe strictly the instruction leaflet for the Imigran auto-injector especially regarding the safe disposal of syringes and needles.

Migraine:

Adult: The recommended adult dose of Imigran is a single 6mg subcutaneous injection. Patients who do not respond to this dose should not take a second dose of Imigran for the same attack. Imigran may be taken for subsequent attacks. Patients who respond initially but whose migraine returns may take a further dose at any time in the next 24 hours provided that one hour has elapsed since the first dose.

The maximum dose in 24 hours is two 6mg injections (12mg).

Imigran is recommended as monotherapy for the acute treatment of migraine and should not be given concomitantly with other acute migraine therapies. If a patient fails to respond to a single dose of Imigran there are no reasons, either on theoretical grounds or from limited clinical experience, to withhold products containing aspirin or non-steroidal anti-inflammatory drugs or paracetamol for further treatment of the attack.

Cluster headache:

Adult:

The recommended adult dose is a single 6mg subcutaneous injection for each cluster attack. The maximum dose in 24 hours is two 6mg injections (12mg) with a minimum interval of one hour between the two doses.

Children (under 18 years of age):

The safety and effectiveness of Imigran in children has not yet been established.

Elderly (over 65):

Experience of the use of Imigran in patients aged over 65 years is limited. The pharmacokinetics do not differ significantly from a younger population but, until further clinical data are available, the use of Sumatriptan in patients aged over 65 years is not recommended.

4.3 Contraindications

Hypersensitivity to any component of the preparation.

Sumatriptan should not be given to patients who have had myocardial infarction or have ischaemic heart disease, coronary vasospasm (Prinzmetal's angina), peripheral vascular disease or patients who have symptoms or signs consistent with ischaemic heart disease.

Sumatriptan should not be administered to patients with a history of cerebovascular accident (CVA) or transient ischaemic attack (TIA).

Sumatriptan should not be administered to patients with severe hepatic impairment.

The use of sumatriptan in patients with moderate and severe hypertension and mild uncontrolled hypertension is contraindicated.

The concomitant administration of ergotamine or derivatives of ergotamine (including methysergide) is contraindicated. (See interactions)

Concurrent administration of monoamine oxidase inhibitors and sumatriptan is contraindicated.

Imigran Injection must not be used within two weeks of discontinuation of therapy with monoamine oxidase inhibitors.

4.4 Special warnings and special precautions for use

Warnings: Imigran should only be used where there is a clear diagnosis of migraine or cluster headache.

Sumatriptan is not indicated for use in the management of hemiplegic, basilar or opthalmoplegic migraine.

The recommended doses of Sumatriptan should not be exceeded.

Imigran Injection should not be given intravenously because of its potential to cause vasospasm. The vasospasm may result in arrhythmias, ischaemic ECG changes or myocardial infarction.

Before treating headaches in patients not previously diagnosed as migraineurs, and in migraineurs who present with atypical symptoms, care should be taken to exclude other potentially serious neurological conditions. It should be noted that migraineurs may be at risk of certain cerebrovascular events (e.g. cerebrovascular accident, transient ischaemic attack).

Following administration, sumatriptan can be associated with transient symptoms including chest pain and tightness which may be intense and involve the throat. Where such symptoms are thought to indicate ischaemic heart disease, no further doses of sumatriptan should be given and appropriate evaluation should be carried out.

Sumatriptan should not be given to patients with risk factors for ischaemic heart disease without prior cardiovascular evaluation (See Section 4.3 Contraindications). Special consideration should be given to postmenopausal women and males over 40 with these risk factors. These evaluations however, may not identify every patient who has cardiac disease and, in very rare cases, serious cardiac events have occurred in patients without underlying cardiovascular disease.

If the patient experiences symptoms which are severe or persistent or are consistent with angina, further doses should not be taken until appropriate investigations have been carried out to check for the possibility of ischaemic changes.

Precautions: Sumatriptan should be administered with caution to patients with controlled hypertension as transient increases in blood pressure and peripheral vascular resistance have been observed in a small proportion of patients.

There have been rare post-marketing reports describing patients with weakness, hyper-reflexia, and in coordination following the use of a selective serotonin reuptake inhibitor (SSRI) and sumatriptan. If concomitant treatment with sumatriptan and an SSRI is clinically warranted, appropriate observation of the patient is advised.

Sumatriptan should be administered with caution to patients with conditions which may affect significantly the absorption, metabolism or excretion of the drug e.g. impaired hepatic or renal function.

Patients with known hypersensitivity to sulphonamides may exhibit an allergic reaction following administration of Sumatriptan. Reactions may range from cutaneous hypersensitivity to anaphylaxis.

Evidence of cross- sensitivity is limited, however, caution should be exercised before using sumatriptan in these patients.

Undesirable effects may be more common during concomitant use of triptans and herbal preparations containing St John's Wort (*Hypericum perforatum*).

4.5 Interaction with other medicinal products and other forms of Interaction

Studies in healthy subjects show that Imigran does not interact with propranolol, flunarizine, pizotifen or alcohol. Sumatriptan has the potential to interact with MAOIs, ergotamine and derivatives of ergotamine. (See also Contraindications).

Rarely an interaction may occur between sumatriptan and SSRI's. (See special warnings and special precautions for use).

Prolonged vasospastic reactions have been reported with ergotamine. As these effects may be additive, 24 hours should elapse before sumatriptan can be taken following any ergotamine-containing preparation. Conversely, ergotamine-containing preparations should not be taken until 6 hours have elapsed following sumatriptan administration.

4.6 Pregnancy and lactation

Post-marketing data from the use of sumatriptan during the first trimester in over 1,000 women are available. Although these data contain insufficient information to draw definitive conclusions, they do not point to an increased risk of congenital defects. Experience with the use of sumatriptan in the second and third trimester is limited.

Evaluation of experimental animal studies does not indicate direct teratogenic effects or harmful effects on peri- and postnatal development. However, embryofoetal viability might be affected in the rabbit (see section 5.3). Administration of sumatriptan should only be considered if the expected benefit to the mother is greater than any possible risk to the foetus.

It has been demonstrated that following subcutaneous administration sumatriptan is excreted into breast milk. Infant exposure can be minimised by avoiding breast feeding for 24 hours after treatment.

4.7 Effects on ability to drive and use machines

Drowsiness may occur as a result of migraine or its treatment with Sumatriptan. Caution is recommended in patients performing skilled tasks, e.g., driving or operating machinery.

4.8 Undesirable effects

General: The most common side effect associated with treatment with Imigran administered subcutaneously is transient pain at the site of injection. Stinging/burning, erythema, bruising and bleeding at the injection site have also been reported.

These symptoms are usually transient and may be intense and can affect any part of the body including the chest and throat: pain, sensations of tingling, heat, heaviness, pressure or tightness.

The following symptoms are mild to moderate in intensity and transient: flushing, dizziness and feelings of weakness.

Fatigue and drowsiness have been reported.

Cardiovascular: Hypotension, bradycardia, tachycardia, palpitations. Transient increases in blood pressure arising soon after treatment have been recorded. In extremely rare cases, serious coronary events have been reported which have included cardiac arrhythmias, ischaemic ECG changes, coronary artery vasospasm or myocardial infarction.

There have also been rare reports of Raynaud's phenomenon and ischaemic colitis.

Gastrointestinal: Nausea and vomiting occurred in some patients but the relationship to Imigran is not clear.

CNS: There have been rare reports of seizures following use of sumatriptan. Although some have occurred in patients with either a history of seizures or concurrent conditions predisposing to seizures there are also reports in patients where no such predisposing factors are apparent.

Eye Disorders: Patients treated with Imigran rarely exhibit visual disorders like flickering and diplopia. Additionally, cases of nystagmus, scotoma and reduced vision have been observed. Very rarely, loss of vision has occurred, which is usually transient. However, visual disorders may also occur during a migraine attack itself.

Hypersensitivity/skin: Hypersensitivity reactions ranging from cutaneous hypersensitivity to, in rare cases, anaphylaxis.

Laboratory Values: Minor disturbances in liver function tests have occasionally been observed.

4.9 Overdose

There have been some reports of overdosage with Imigran Injection. Patients have received single injections of up to 12mg subcutaneously without significant adverse effects. Doses in excess of 16mg subcutaneously were not associated with side effects other than those mentioned.

If overdosage with Imigran occurs, the patient should be monitored for at least ten hours and standard supportive treatment applied as required.

It is unknown what effect haemodialysis or peritoneal dialysis has on the plasma concentrations of Imigran.

5. PHARMACOLOGICAL PROPERTIES

5.1 Pharmacodynamic properties

Pharmacotherapeutic group: Analgesics: Selective 5-HT_1 receptor agonists.

ATC Code: N02CC01

Sumatriptan has been demonstrated to be a specific and selective 5-hydroxytryptamine (5-HT_{1D}) receptor agonist with no effect on other 5-HT receptor (5-HT_2-5-HT_7) subtypes. The vascular 5-HT_{1D} receptor is found predominantly in cranial blood vessels and mediates vasoconstriction. In animals, sumatriptan selectively constricts the carotid arterial circulation but does not alter cerebral blood flow. The carotid arterial circulation supplies blood to the extracranial and intracranial tissues, such as the meninges and dilatation and/or oedema formation in these vessels is thought to be the underlying mechanism of migraine in man. In addition, experimental evidence from animal studies suggests that sumatriptan inhibits trigeminal nerve activity. Both these actions (cranial vasoconstriction and inhibition of trigeminal nerve activity) may contribute to the anti-migraine action of sumatriptan in humans.

Sumatriptan remains effective in treating menstrual migraine i.e. migraine without aura that occurs between 3 days prior and up to 5 days post onset of menstruation. Sumatriptan should be taken as soon as possible in an attack.

Clinical response begins 10 to 15 minutes following a 6mg subcutaneous injection.

Because of its route of administration Imigran Injection may be particularly suitable for patients who suffer with nausea and vomiting during an attack.

5.2 Pharmacokinetic properties

Following subcutaneous injection, sumatriptan has a high mean bioavailability (96%) with peak serum concentrations occurring in 25 minutes. Average peak serum concentration after a 6mg subcutaneous dose is 72ng/ml. The elimination phase half life is approximately two hours.

Plasma protein binding is low (14 to 21%), mean volume of distribution is 170 litres. Mean total plasma clearance is approximately 1160ml/min and the mean renal plasma clearance is approximately 260ml/min. Non-renal clearance accounts for about 80% of the total clearance. Sumatriptan is eliminated primarily by oxidative metabolism mediated by monoamine oxidase A.

The major metabolite, the indole acetic acid analogue of sumatriptan, is mainly excreted in the urine where it is present as a free acid and the glucuronide conjugate. It has no known 5-HT_1 or 5-HT_2 activity. Minor metabolites have not been identified.

In a pilot study no significant differences were found in the pharmacokinetic parameters between the elderly and young healthy volunteers.

5.3 Preclinical safety data

Sumatriptan was devoid of genotoxic and carcinogenic activity in *in-vitro* systems and animal studies.

In a rat fertility study oral doses of sumatriptan resulting in plasma levels approximately 150 times those seen in man after a 6 mg subcutaneous dose were associated with a reduction in the success of insemination.

This effect did not occur during a subcutaneous study where maximum plasma levels achieved approximately 100 times those in man by the subcutaneous route.

In rabbits embryolethality, without marked teratogenic defects, was seen. The relevance for humans of these findings is unknown.

6. PHARMACEUTICAL PARTICULARS

6.1 List of excipients

Sodium Chloride

Water for Injection

6.2 Incompatibilities

None Reported

6.3 Shelf life

Two years when stored below 30°C and protected from light

6.4 Special precautions for storage

Imigran Injection should be stored below 30°C and protected from light.

6.5 Nature and contents of container

Treatment pack: 2 pre-filled syringes (in cases) plus an auto-injector, in a plastic tray within a carton.

Refill pack: 2 pre-filled syringes (in cases) in a carton or 6 pre-filled syringes(ie three cases each containing 2 prefilled syringes).

6.6 Instructions for use and handling

None stated.

Administrative Data

7. MARKETING AUTHORISATION HOLDER

Glaxo Wellcome UK Limited Trading as GlaxoSmithKline UK

Stockley Park West

Uxbridge

Middlesex, UB11 1BT

8. MARKETING AUTHORISATION NUMBER(S)

PL 10949/0113

9. DATE OF FIRST AUTHORISATION/RENEWAL OF THE AUTHORISATION

11 July 2002

10. DATE OF REVISION OF THE TEXT

19 September 2003

11. Legal Category

POM

Imigran Radis 100mg Tablets

(GlaxoSmithKline UK)

1. NAME OF THE MEDICINAL PRODUCT

Imigran Radis 100mg Tablets

2. QUALITATIVE AND QUANTITATIVE COMPOSITION

100mg sumatriptan base as the succinate salt.

3. PHARMACEUTICAL FORM

Film-coated Tablet

White film-coated, triangular shaped, biconvex tablets debossed with 'GS YE7' on one face and '100' on the other.

4. CLINICAL PARTICULARS

4.1 Therapeutic indications

Imigran Radis tablets are indicated for the acute relief of migraine attacks, with or without aura. Imigran should only be used where there is a clear diagnosis of migraine.

4.2 Posology and method of administration

Adults

Imigran Radis is indicated for the acute intermittent treatment of migraine. It should not be used prophylactically.

It is advisable that Imigran be given as early as possible after the onset of migraine attack but it is equally effective at whatever stage of the attack it is administered.

The recommended dose of oral Imigran is a single 50mg tablet. Some patients may require 100mg. If the patient has responded to the first dose but the symptoms recur a second dose may be given in the next 24 hours provided that there is a minimum interval of two hours between the two doses and no more than 300mg is taken in any 24 hour period.

Patients who do not respond to the prescribed dose of Imigran Radis should not take a second dose for the same attack. Imigran Radis may be taken for subsequent attacks.

Imigran Radis is recommended as monotherapy for the acute treatment of migraine and should not be given concomitantly with other acute migraine therapies. If a patient fails to respond to a single dose of Imigran Radis there are no reasons, either on theoretical grounds or from limited clinical experience, to withhold products containing aspirin or non-steroidal anti-inflammatory drugs for further treatment of the attack.

The tablets should be swallowed whole with water.

Children (under 18 years of age)

The safety and effectiveness of Imigran Radis in children has not yet been established

Elderly (Over 65)

Experience of the use of Imigran Radis in patients aged over 65 years is limited. The pharmacokinetics do not differ significantly from a younger population but until further clinical data are available, the use of Imigran Radis in patients aged over 65 years is not recommended

4.3 Contraindications

Hypersensitivity to any component of the preparation.

Sumatriptan should not be given to patients who have had myocardial infarction or have ischaemic heart disease, coronary vasospasm (Prinzmetal's angina), peripheral vascular disease or patients who have symptoms or sign consistent with ischaemic heart disease.

Sumatriptan should not be administered to patients with a history of cerebrovascular accident (CVA) or transient ischaemic attack (TIA).

Sumatriptan should not be administered to patients with severe hepatic impairment.

The use of sumatriptan in patients with moderate and severe hypertension and mild uncontrolled hypertension is contraindicated.

The concomitant administration of ergotamine or derivatives of ergotamine (including methysergide) is contraindicated. (See interactions)

Concurrent administration of monoamine oxidase inhibitors and sumatriptan is contraindicated. Sumatriptan must not be used within two weeks of discontinuation of therapy with monoamine oxidase inhibitors.

4.4 Special warnings and special precautions for use

Imigran Radis should only be used where there is a clear diagnosis of migraine

Sumatriptan is not indicated for use in the management of hemiplegic, basilar or ophthalmoplegic migraine.

The recommended doses of sumatriptan should not be exceeded. As with other migraine therapies, before treating headaches in patients not previously diagnosed as migraineurs, and in migraineurs who present atypical symptoms, care should be taken to exclude other potentially serious neurological conditions.

It should be noted that migraineurs may be at risk of certain cerebrovascular events (e.g. cerebrovascular accident, transient ischaemic attack).

Following administration, sumatriptan can be associated with transient symptoms including chest pain and tightness which may be intense and involve the throat (See Side effects). Where such symptoms are thought to indicate ischaemic heart disease, no further doses of sumatriptan should be given and appropriate evaluation should be carried out.

Sumatriptan should not be given to patients with risk factors for ischaemic heart disease without prior cardiovascular evaluation (See Section 4.3 Contraindications). Special consideration should be given to postmenopausal women and males over 40 with these risk factors. These evaluations however, may not identify every patient who has cardiac disease and, in very rare cases, serious cardiac events have occurred in patients without underlying cardiovascular disease.

Sumatriptan should be administered with caution to patients with controlled hypertension as transient increases in blood pressure and peripheral vascular resistance have been observed in a small proportion of patients.

There have been rare post-marketing reports describing patients with weakness, hyper-reflexia, and incoordination following the use of a selective serotonin reuptake inhibitor (SSRI) and sumatriptan. If concomitant treatment with sumatriptan and an SSRI is clinically warranted, appropriate observation of the patient is advised.

Sumatriptan should be administered with caution to patients with conditions which may affect significantly the absorption, metabolism or excretion of drugs, e.g. impaired hepatic or renal function. A 50mg dose should be considered in patients with hepatic impairment.

Sumatriptan should be used with caution in patients with a history of seizures or other risk factors which lower the seizure threshold, as seizures have been reported in association with sumatriptan (see section 4.8).

Patients with known hypersensitivity to sulphonamides may exhibit an allergic reaction following administration of sumatriptan. Reactions may range from cutaneous hypersensitivity to anaphylaxis. Evidence of cross-sensitivity is limited, however, caution should be exercised before using sumatriptan in these patients.

Undesirable effects may be more common during concomitant use of triptans and herbal preparations containing St John's Wort (Hypericum perforatum).

As with other acute migraine treatments, chronic daily headache/exacerbation of headache have been reported with overuse of sumatriptan, which may necessitate a drug withdrawal.

4.5 Interaction with other medicinal products and other forms of Interaction

Studies in healthy subjects show that sumatriptan does not interact with propranolol, flunarizine, pizotifen or alcohol. Sumatriptan has the potential to interact with MAOIs, ergotamine and derivatives of ergotamine. The increased risk of coronary vasospasm is a theoretical possibility and concomitant administration is contra-indicated. (see also contraindications).

Prolonged vasospastic reactions have been reported with ergotamine. As these effects may be additive, 24 hours should elapse before sumatriptan can be taken following any ergotamine-containing preparation. Conversely, ergotamine-containing preparations should not be taken until 6 hours have elapsed following sumatriptan administration.

Rarely, an interaction may occur between sumatriptan and SSRI's (see Special Warnings and special Precautions for Use).

4.6 Pregnancy and lactation

Post-marketing data from the use of sumatriptan during the first trimester in over 1,000 women are available. Although these data contain insufficient information to draw definitive conclusions, they do not point to an increased risk of congenital defects. Experience with the use of sumatriptan in the second and third trimester is limited.

Evaluation of experimental animal studies does not indicate direct teratogenic effects or harmful effects on peri- and postnatal development. However, embryofoetal viability might be affected in the rabbit (see section 5.3). Administration of sumatriptan should only be considered if the expected benefit to the mother is greater than any possible risk to the foetus.

It has been demonstrated that following subcutaneous administration, sumatriptan is excreted into breast milk. Infant exposure can be minimised by avoiding breast feeding for 24 hours after treatment.

4.7 Effects on ability to drive and use machines

Drowsiness may occur as a result of migraine or its treatment with sumatriptan. Caution is recommended in patients performing skilled tasks, e.g. driving or operating machinery

4.8 Undesirable effects

General

The following symptoms are usually transient and may be intense and can affect any part of the body including the chest and throat; pain, sensations of tingling, heat, heaviness, pressure or tightness. The following symptoms are mild to moderate in intensity and transient: flushing, dizziness and feelings of weakness.

Fatigue and drowsiness have been reported.

Cardiovascular

Hypotension, bradycardia, tachycardia, palpitations.

Transient increases in blood pressure arising soon after treatment have been recorded. In extremely rare cases, serious coronary events have been reported which have included cardiac arrhythmias, ischaemic ECG changes, coronary artery vasospasm or myocardial infarction. (see contraindications and Precautions and Warnings).

There have also been rare reports of Raynaud's phenomenon and ischaemic colitis.

Gastrointestinal

Nausea and vomiting occurred in some patients but the relationship to sumatriptan is not clear.

CNS

There have been rare reports of seizures following use of sumatriptan. Although some have occurred in patients with either a history of seizures or concurrent conditions predisposing to seizures there are also reports in patients where no such predisposing factors are apparent.

Eye Disorders

Patients treated with Imigran rarely exhibit visual disorders like flickering and diplopia. Additionally, cases of nystagmus, scotoma and reduced vision have been observed. Very rarely, loss of vision has occurred, which is usually transient. However, visual disorders may also occur during a migraine attack itself.

Hypersensitivity/skin

Hypersensitivity reactions ranging from cutaneous hypersensitivity to, in rare cases, anaphylaxis.

Laboratory values

Minor disturbances in liver function tests have occasionally been observed.

4.9 Overdose

There have been some reports of overdosage with Imigran Tablets. Doses in excess of 400mg orally were not associated with side effects other than those mentioned.

If overdosage occurs, the patient should be monitored for at least ten hours and standard supportive treatment applied as required.

It is unknown what effect haemodialysis or peritoneal dialysis has on the plasma concentrations of Imigran

5. PHARMACOLOGICAL PROPERTIES

5.1 Pharmacodynamic properties

Pharmacotherapeutic group: Analgesics: Selective 5-HT_1 receptor agonists.

ATC code: N02CC01

Sumatriptan has been demonstrated to be a specific and selective 5-Hydroxytryptamine$_1$ ($5HT_{1D}$) receptor agonist with no effect on other 5HT receptor ($5\text{-}HT_2\text{-}5\text{-}HT_7$) subtypes. The vascular 5-HT_{1D} receptor is found predominantly in cranial blood vessels and mediates vasoconstriction. In animals, sumatriptan selectively constricts the carotid arterial circulation but does not alter cerebral blood flow. The carotid arterial circulation supplies blood to the extracranial and intracranial tissues such as the meninges and dilatation of and/or oedema formation in these vessels is thought to be the underlying mechanism of migraine in man.

In addition, evidence from animal studies suggests that sumatriptan inhibits trigeminal nerve activity. Both these actions (cranial vasoconstriction and inhibition of trigeminal nerve activity) may contribute to the anti-migraine action of sumatriptan in humans.

Sumatriptan remains effective in treating menstrual migraine i.e. migraine without aura that occurs between 3 days prior and up to 5 days post onset of menstruation. Sumatriptan should be taken as soon as possible in an attack.

Clinical response begins around 30 minutes following a 100mg oral dose.

Although the recommended dose of oral sumatriptan is 50mg, migraine attacks vary in severity both within and between patients. Doses of 25-100mg have shown greater efficacy than placebo in clinical trials, but 25mg is statistically significantly less effective than 50 and 100mg.

5.2 Pharmacokinetic properties

Following oral administration, sumatriptan is rapidly absorbed, 70% of maximum concentration occurring at 45 minutes. After 100mg dose, the maximum plasma concentration is 54ng/ml. Mean absolute oral bioavailability is 14% partly due to presystemic metabolism and partly due to incomplete absorption. The elimination phase half-life is approximately 2 hours, although there is an indication of a longer terminal phase. Plasma protein binding is low (14-21%), mean volume of distribution is 170 litres. Mean total plasma clearance is approximately 1160ml/min and the mean renal plasma clearance is approximately 260ml/min. Non-renal clearance accounts for about 80% of the total clearance. Sumatriptan is eliminated primarily by oxidative metabolism mediated by monoamine oxidase A. The major metabolite, the indole acetic acid analogue of Sumatriptan is mainly excreted in the urine, where it is present as a free acid and the glucuronide conjugate. It has no known $5HT_1$ or $5HT_2$ activity. Minor metabolites have not been identified. The pharmacokinetics of oral Sumatriptan do not appear to be significantly affected by migraine attacks.

In a pilot study, no significant differences were found in the pharmacokinetic parameters between the elderly and young healthy volunteers.

5.3 Preclinical safety data

Sumatriptan was devoid of genotoxic and carcinogenic activity in *in-vitro* systems and animal studies.

In a rat fertility study oral doses of sumatriptan resulting in plasma levels approximately 200 times those seen in man after a 100 mg oral dose were associated with a reduction in the success of insemination.

This effect did not occur during a subcutaneous study where maximum plasma levels achieved approximately 150 times those in man by the oral route.

In rabbits embryolethality, without marked teratogenic defects, was seen. The relevance for humans of these findings is unknown.

6. PHARMACEUTICAL PARTICULARS

6.1 List of excipients

Calcium Hydrogen Phosphate, Anhydrous

Microcrystalline Cellulose

Sodium Hydrogen Carbonate

Croscarmellose Sodium

Magnesium Stearate

Hypromellose

Titanium Dioxide

Glycerol Triacetate

6.2 Incompatibilities

None stated.

6.3 Shelf life

36 months

6.4 Special precautions for storage

Do not store above 30°C

6.5 Nature and contents of container

Aluminium double foil blister packs in a cardboard carton, containing either 2, 4, 6,12 or 18 tablets.

Not all pack sizes may be marketed.

6.6 Instructions for use and handling

None stated

Administrative Data

7. MARKETING AUTHORISATION HOLDER

GlaxoSmithKline UK Ltd.

Stockley Park West

Uxbridge

Middlesex. UB11 1BT

8. MARKETING AUTHORISATION NUMBER(S)

PL 19494/0014

9. DATE OF FIRST AUTHORISATION/RENEWAL OF THE AUTHORISATION

8th June 2004

10. DATE OF REVISION OF THE TEXT

07 December 2004

11. Legal Status

POM

Imigran Radis 50mg Tablets

(GlaxoSmithKline UK)

1. NAME OF THE MEDICINAL PRODUCT

Imigran Radis 50mg Tablets

2. QUALITATIVE AND QUANTITATIVE COMPOSITION

50mg sumatriptan base as the succinate salt.

3. PHARMACEUTICAL FORM

Film-coated Tablet

Pink film-coated, triangular shaped, biconvex tablets debossed with 'GS 1YM' on one face and '50' on the other.

4. CLINICAL PARTICULARS

4.1 Therapeutic indications

Imigran Radis tablets are indicated for the acute relief of migraine attacks, with or without aura. Imigran should only be used where there is a clear diagnosis of migraine.

4.2 Posology and method of administration

Adults

Imigran Radis is indicated for the acute intermittent treatment of migraine. It should not be used prophylactically.

It is advisable that Imigran be given as early as possible after the onset of migraine attack but it is equally effective at whatever stage of the attack it is administered.

The recommended dose of oral Imigran is a single 50mg tablet. Some patients may require 100mg. If the patient has responded to the first dose but the symptoms recur a second dose may be given in the next 24 hours provided that there is a minimum interval of two hours between the two doses and no more than 300mg is taken in any 24 hour period.

Patients who do not respond to the prescribed dose of Imigran Radis should not take a second dose for the same attack. Imigran Radis may be taken for subsequent attacks.

Imigran Radis is recommended as monotherapy for the acute treatment of migraine and should not be given concomitantly with other acute migraine therapies. If a patient fails to respond to a single dose of Imigran Radis there are no reasons, either on theoretical grounds or from limited clinical experience, to withhold products containing aspirin or non-steroidal anti-inflammatory drugs for further treatment of the attack.

The tablets should be swallowed whole with water.

Children (under 18 years of age)

The safety and effectiveness of Imigran Radis in children has not yet been established

Elderly (Over 65)

Experience of the use of Imigran Radis in patients aged over 65 years is limited. The pharmacokinetics do not differ significantly from a younger population but until further clinical data are available, the use of Imigran Radis in patients aged over 65 years is not recommended

4.3 Contraindications

Hypersensitivity to any component of the preparation.

Sumatriptan should not be given to patients who have had myocardial infarction or have ischaemic heart disease, coronary vasospasm (Prinzmetal's angina), peripheral vascular disease or patients who have symptoms or sign consistent with ischaemic heart disease.

Sumatriptan should not be administered to patients with a history of cerebovascular accident (CVA) or transient ischaemic attack (TIA).

Sumatriptan should not be administered to patients with severe hepatic impairment.

The use of sumatriptan in patients with moderate and severe hypertension and mild uncontrolled hypertension is contraindicated.

The concomitant administration of ergotamine or derivatives of ergotamine (including methysergide) is contraindicated. (See interactions)

Concurrent administration of monoamine oxidase inhibitors and sumatriptan is contraindicated. Sumatriptan must not be used within two weeks of discontinuation of therapy with monoamine oxidase inhibitors.

4.4 Special warnings and special precautions for use

Imigran Radis should only be used where there is a clear diagnosis of migraine

Sumatriptan is not indicated for use in the management of hemiplegic, basilar or ophthalmoplegic migraine.

The recommended doses of sumatriptan should not be exceeded. As with other migraine therapies, before treating headaches in patients not previously diagnosed as migraineurs, and in migraineurs who present atypical symptoms, care should be taken to exclude other potentially serious neurological conditions.

It should be noted that migraineurs may be at risk of certain cerebrovascular events (e.g. cerebrovascular accident, transient ischaemic attack).

Following administration, sumatriptan can be associated with transient symptoms including chest pain and tightness which may be intense and involve the throat (See Side effects). Where such symptoms are thought to indicate ischaemic heart disease, no further doses of sumatriptan should be given and appropriate evaluation should be carried out.

Sumatriptan should not be given to patients with risk factors for ischaemic heart disease without prior cardiovascular evaluation (See Section 4.3 Contraindications). Special consideration should be given to postmenopausal women and males over 40 with these risk factors. These evaluations however, may not identify every patient who has cardiac disease and, in very rare cases, serious cardiac events have occurred in patients without underlying cardiovascular disease.

Sumatriptan should be administered with caution to patients with controlled hypertension as transient increases in blood pressure and peripheral vascular resistance have been observed in a small proportion of patients.

There have been rare post-marketing reports describing patients with weakness, hyper-reflexia, and incoordination following the use of a selective serotonin reuptake inhibitor (SSRI) and sumatriptan. If concomitant treatment with sumatriptan and an SSRI is clinically warranted, appropriate observation of the patient is advised.

Sumatriptan should be administered with caution to patients with conditions which may affect significantly the absorption, metabolism or excretion of drugs, e.g. impaired hepatic or renal function. A 50mg dose should be considered in patients with hepatic impairment.

Sumatriptan should be used with caution in patients with a history of seizures or other risk factors which lower the seizure threshold, as seizures have been reported in association with sumatriptan (see section 4.8).

Patients with known hypersensitivity to sulphonamides may exhibit an allergic reaction following administration of sumatriptan. Reactions may range from cutaneous hypersensitivity to anaphylaxis. Evidence of cross-sensitivity is limited, however, caution should be exercised before using sumatriptan in these patients.

Undesirable effects may be more common during concomitant use of triptans and herbal preparations containing St John's Wort (*Hypericum perforatum*).

As with other acute migraine treatments, chronic daily headache/exacerbation of headache have been reported with overuse of sumatriptan, which may necessitate a drug withdrawal.

4.5 Interaction with other medicinal products and other forms of Interaction

Studies in healthy subjects show that sumatriptan does not interact with propranolol, flunarizine, pizotifen or alcohol. Sumatriptan has the potential to interact with MAOIs, ergotamine and derivatives of ergotamine. The increased risk of coronary vasospasm is a theoretical possibility and concomitant administration is contra-indicated. (see also contraindications).

Prolonged vasospastic reactions have been reported with ergotamine. As these effects may be additive, 24 hours should elapse before sumatriptan can be taken following any ergotamine-containing preparation. Conversely, ergotamine-containing preparations should not be taken until 6 hours have elapsed following sumatriptan administration.

Rarely, an interaction may occur between sumatriptan and SSRI's (see Special Warnings and special Precautions for Use).

4.6 Pregnancy and lactation

Post-marketing data from the use of sumatriptan during the first trimester in over 1,000 women are available. Although these data contain insufficient information to draw definitive conclusions, they do not point to an increased risk of congenital defects. Experience with the use of sumatriptan in the second and third trimester is limited.

Evaluation of experimental animal studies does not indicate direct teratogenic effects or harmful effects on peri- and postnatal development. However, embryofoetal viability might be affected in the rabbit (see section 5.3). Administration of sumatriptan should only be considered if the expected benefit to the mother is greater than any possible risk to the foetus.

It has been demonstrated that following subcutaneous administration, sumatriptan is excreted into breast milk. Infant exposure can be minimised by avoiding breast feeding for 24 hours after treatment.

4.7 Effects on ability to drive and use machines

Drowsiness may occur as a result of migraine or its treatment with sumatriptan. Caution is recommended in patients performing skilled tasks, e.g. driving or operating machinery

4.8 Undesirable effects

General

The following symptoms are usually transient and may be intense and can affect any part of the body including the chest and throat; pain, sensations of tingling, heat, heaviness, pressure or tightness. The following symptoms are mild to moderate in intensity and transient: flushing, dizziness and feelings of weakness.

Fatigue and drowsiness have been reported.

Cardiovascular

Hypotension, bradycardia, tachycardia, palpitations.

Transient increases in blood pressure arising soon after treatment have been recorded. In extremely rare cases, serious coronary events have been reported which have included cardiac arrhythmias, ischaemic ECG changes, coronary artery vasospasm or myocardial infarction. (see contraindications and Precautions and Warnings).

There have also been rare reports of Raynaud's phenomenon and ischaemic colitis.

Gastrointestinal

Nausea and vomiting occurred in some patients but the relationship to sumatriptan is not clear.

CNS

There have been rare reports of seizures following use of sumatriptan. Although some have occurred in patients with either a history of seizures or concurrent conditions predisposing to seizures there are also reports in patients where no such predisposing factors are apparent.

Eye Disorders

Patients treated with Imigran rarely exhibit visual disorders like flickering and diplopia. Additionally, cases of nystagmus, scotoma and reduced vision have been observed. Very rarely, loss of vision has occurred, which is usually transient. However, visual disorders may also occur during a migraine attack itself.

Hypersensitivity/skin

Hypersensitivity reactions ranging from cutaneous hypersensitivity to, in rare cases, anaphylaxis.

Laboratory values

Minor disturbances in liver function tests have occasionally been observed.

4.9 Overdose

There have been some reports of overdosage with Imigran Tablets. Doses in excess of 400mg orally were not associated with side effects other than those mentioned.

If overdosage occurs, the patient should be monitored for at least ten hours and standard supportive treatment applied as required.

It is unknown what effect haemodialysis or peritoneal dialysis has on the plasma concentrations of Imigran

5. PHARMACOLOGICAL PROPERTIES

5.1 Pharmacodynamic properties

Pharmacotherapeutic group: Analgesics: Selective $5\text{-}HT_1$ receptor agonists.

ATC code: N02CC01

Sumatriptan has been demonstrated to be a specific and selective 5-Hydroxytryptamine$_1$ ($5HT_{1D}$) receptor agonist with no effect on other 5HT receptor ($5\text{-}HT_2\text{-}5\text{-}HT_7$) subtypes. The vascular $5\text{-}HT_{1D}$ receptor is found predominantly in cranial blood vessels and mediates vasoconstriction. In animals, sumatriptan selectively constricts the carotid arterial circulation but does not alter cerebral blood flow. The carotid arterial circulation supplies blood to the extracranial and intracranial tissues such as the meninges and dilatation of and/or oedema formation in these vessels is thought to be the underlying mechanism of migraine in man.

In addition, evidence from animal studies suggests that sumatriptan inhibits trigeminal nerve activity. Both these actions (cranial vasoconstriction and inhibition of trigeminal nerve activity) may contribute to the anti-migraine action of sumatriptan in humans.

Sumatriptan remains effective in treating menstrual migraine i.e. migraine without aura that occurs between 3 days prior and up to 5 days post onset of menstruation. Sumatriptan should be taken as soon as possible in an attack.

Clinical response begins around 30 minutes following a 100mg oral dose.

Although the recommended dose of oral sumatriptan is 50mg, migraine attacks vary in severity both within and between patients. Doses of 25-100mg have shown greater efficacy than placebo in clinical trials, but 25mg is statistically significantly less effective than 50 and 100mg.

5.2 Pharmacokinetic properties

Following oral administration, sumatriptan is rapidly absorbed, 70% of maximum concentration occurring at 45 minutes. After 100mg dose, the maximum plasma concentration is 54ng/ml. Mean absolute oral bioavailability is 14% partly due to presystemic metabolism and partly due to incomplete absorption. The elimination phase half-life is approximately 2 hours, although there is an indication of a longer terminal phase. Plasma protein binding is low (14-21%), mean volume of distribution is 170 litres. Mean total plasma clearance is approximately 1160ml/min and the mean renal plasma clearance is approximately 260ml/min. Non-renal clearance accounts for about 80% of the total clearance. Sumatriptan is eliminated primarily by oxidative metabolism mediated by monoamine oxidase A. The major metabolite, the indole acetic acid analogue of Sumatriptan is mainly excreted in the urine, where it is present as a free acid and the glucuronide conjugate. It has no known $5HT_1$ or $5HT_2$ activity. Minor metabolites have not been identified. The pharmacokinetics of oral Sumatriptan do not appear to be significantly affected by migraine attacks.

In a pilot study, no significant differences were found in the pharmacokinetic parameters between the elderly and young healthy volunteers.

5.3 Preclinical safety data

Sumatriptan was devoid of genotoxic and carcinogenic activity in *in-vitro* systems and animal studies.

In a rat fertility study oral doses of sumatriptan resulting in plasma levels approximately 200 times those seen in man after a 100 mg oral dose were associated with a reduction in the success of insemination.

This effect did not occur during a subcutaneous study where maximum plasma levels achieved approximately 150 times those in man by the oral route.

In rabbits embryolethality, without marked teratogenic defects, was seen. The relevance for humans of these findings is unknown.

6. PHARMACEUTICAL PARTICULARS

6.1 List of excipients

Calcium Hydrogen Phosphate, Anhydrous

Microcrystalline Cellulose

Sodium Hydrogen Carbonate

Croscarmellose Sodium

Magnesium Stearate

Hypromellose

Titanium Dioxide

Glycerol Triacetate

Iron Oxide Red

6.2 Incompatibilities

None stated.

6.3 Shelf life

36 months

6.4 Special precautions for storage

Do not store above 30°C

6.5 Nature and contents of container

Aluminium double foil blister packs in a cardboard carton, containing either 2, 4, 6, 12 or 18 tablets.

Not all pack sizes may be marketed.

6.6 Instructions for use and handling

None stated

Administrative Data

7. MARKETING AUTHORISATION HOLDER

GlaxoSmithKline UK Ltd.

Stockley Park West

Uxbridge

Middlesex. UB11 1BT

8. MARKETING AUTHORISATION NUMBER(S)

PL 19494/0013

9. DATE OF FIRST AUTHORISATION/RENEWAL OF THE AUTHORISATION

8th June 2004

10. DATE OF REVISION OF THE TEXT

07 December 2004

11. Legal Status

POM

Imigran Tablets 50mg Imigran Tablets 100mg

(GlaxoSmithKline UK)

1. NAME OF THE MEDICINAL PRODUCT

Imigran Tablets 50mg

Imigran Tablets 100mg

2. QUALITATIVE AND QUANTITATIVE COMPOSITION

50mg sumatriptan base as the succinate salt.

100mg sumatriptan base as the succinate salt.

3. PHARMACEUTICAL FORM

Tablet

4. CLINICAL PARTICULARS

4.1 Therapeutic indications

Imigran tablets are indicated for the acute relief of migraine attacks, with or without aura. Imigran should only be used where there is a clear diagnosis of migraine.

4.2 Posology and method of administration

Adults

Imigran is indicated for the acute intermittent treatment of migraine. It should not be used prophylactically.

It is advisable that Imigran be given as early as possible after the onset of migraine attack but it is equally effective at whatever stage of the attack it is administered.

The recommended dose of oral Imigran is a single 50mg tablet. Some patients may require 100mg. If the patient has responded to the first dose but the symptoms recur a second dose may be given in the next 24 hours provided that there is a minimum interval of two hours between the two doses and no more than 300mg is taken in any 24 hour period.

Patients who do not respond to the prescribed dose of Imigran should not take a second dose for the same attack. Imigran may be taken for subsequent attacks.

Imigran is recommended as monotherapy for the acute treatment of migraine and should not be given concomitantly with other acute migraine therapies. If a patient fails to respond to a single dose of Imigran there are no reasons, either on theoretical grounds or from limited clinical experience, to withhold products containing aspirin or non-steroidal anti-inflammatory drugs for further treatment of the attack.

The tablets should be swallowed whole with water.

Children (under 18 years of age)

The safety and effectiveness of Imigran in children has not yet been established

Elderly (Over 65)

Experience of the use of Imigran in patients aged over 65 years is limited. The pharmacokinetics do not differ significantly from a younger population but until further clinical data are available, the use of Imigran in patients aged over 65 years is not recommended

4.3 Contraindications

Hypersensitivity to any component of the preparation.

Sumatriptan should not be given to patients who have had myocardial infarction or have ischaemic heart disease, coronary vasospasm (Prinzmetal's angina), peripheral vascular disease or patients who have symptoms or sign consistent with ischaemic heart disease.

Sumatriptan should not be administered to patients with a history of cerebovascular accident (CVA) or transient ischaemic attack (TIA).

Sumatriptan should not be administered to patients with severe hepatic impairment.

The use of sumatriptan in patients with moderate and severe hypertension and mild uncontrolled hypertension is contraindicated.

The concomitant administration of ergotamine or derivatives of ergotamine (including methysergide) is contraindicated. (See interactions)

Concurrent administration of monoamine oxidase inhibitors and sumatriptan is contraindicated.

Imigran Tablets must not be used within two weeks of discontinuation of therapy with monoamine oxidase inhibitors.

4.4 Special warnings and special precautions for use

Imigran should only be used where there is a clear diagnosis of migraine

Sumatriptan is not indicated for use in the management of hemiplegic, basilar or ophthalmoplegic migraine.

The recommended doses of sumatriptan should not be exceeded. As with other migraine therapies, before treating headaches in patients not previously diagnosed as migraineurs, and in migraineurs who present atypical symptoms, care should be taken to exclude other potentially serious neurological conditions.

It should be noted that migraineurs may be at risk of certain cerebrovascular events (e.g. cerebrovascular accident, transient ischaemic attack).

Following administration, sumatriptan can be associated with transient symptoms including chest pain and tightness which may be intense and involve the throat (See Side effects). Where such symptoms are thought to indicate ischaemic heart disease, no further doses of sumatriptan should be given and appropriate evaluation should be carried out.

Sumatriptan should not be given to patients with risk factors for ischaemic heart disease without prior cardiovascular evaluation (See Section 4.3 Contraindications). Special consideration should be given to postmenopausal women and males over 40 with these risk factors. These evaluations however, may not identify every patient who has cardiac disease and, in very rare cases, serious cardiac events have occurred in patients without underlying cardiovascular disease.

Sumatriptan should be administered with caution to patients with controlled hypertension as transient increases in blood pressure and peripheral vascular resistance have been observed in a small proportion of patients.

There have been rare post-marketing reports describing patients with weakness, hyper-reflexia, and incoordination following the use of a selective serotonin reuptake inhibitor (SSRI) and sumatriptan. If concomitant treatment with sumatriptan and an SSRI is clinically warranted, appropriate observation of the patient is advised.

Sumatriptan should be administered with caution to patients with conditions which may affect significantly the absorption, metabolism or excretion of drugs, e.g. impaired hepatic or renal function. A 50mg dose should be considered in patients with hepatic impairment.

Patients with known hypersensitivity to sulphonamides may exhibit an allergic reaction following administration of sumatriptan. Reactions may range from cutaneous hypersensitivity to anaphylaxis. Evidence of cross-sensitivity is limited, however, caution should be exercised before using sumatriptan in these patients.

Undesirable effects may be more common during concomitant use of triptans and herbal preparations containing St John's Wort (*Hypericum perforatum*).

4.5 Interaction with other medicinal products and other forms of Interaction

Studies in healthy subjects show that sumatriptan does not interact with propranolol, flunarizine, pizotifen or alcohol. Sumatriptan has the potential to interact with MAOIs, ergotamine and derivatives of ergotamine. The increased risk of coronary vasospasm is a theoretical possibility and concomitant administration is contra-indicated. (see also contraindications).

Prolonged vasospastic reactions have been reported with ergotamine. As these effects may be additive, 24 hours should elapse before sumatriptan can be taken following any ergotamine-containing preparation. Conversely, ergotamine-containing preparations should not be taken until 6 hours have elapsed following sumatriptan administration.

Rarely, an interaction may occur between sumatriptan and SSRI's (see Special Warnings and special Precautions for Use).

4.6 Pregnancy and lactation

Post-marketing data from the use of sumatriptan during the first trimester in over 1,000 women are available. Although these data contain insufficient information to draw definitive conclusions, they do not point to an increased risk of congenital defects. Experience with the use of sumatriptan in the second and third trimester is limited.

Evaluation of experimental animal studies does not indicate direct teratogenic effects or harmful effects on peri- and postnatal development. However, embryofoetal viability might be affected in the rabbit (see section 5.3). Administration of sumatriptan should only be considered if the expected benefit to the mother is greater than any possible risk to the foetus.

It has been demonstrated that following subcutaneous administration, sumatriptan is excreted into breast milk. Infant exposure can be minimised by avoiding breast feeding for 24 hours after treatment.

4.7 Effects on ability to drive and use machines

Drowsiness may occur as a result of migraine or its treatment with sumatriptan. Caution is recommended in patients performing skilled tasks, e.g. driving or operating machinery

4.8 Undesirable effects

General

The following symptoms are usually transient and may be intense and can affect any part of the body including the chest and throat; pain, sensations of tingling, heat, heaviness, pressure or tightness. The following symptoms are mild to moderate in intensity and transient: flushing, dizziness and feelings of weakness.

Fatigue and drowsiness have been reported.

Cardiovascular

Hypotension, bradycardia, tachycardia, palpitations.

Transient increases in blood pressure arising soon after treatment have been recorded. In extremely rare cases, serious coronary events have been reported which have included cardiac arrhythmias, ischaemic ECG changes, coronary artery vasospasm or myocardial infarction. (see contraindications and Precautions and Warnings).

There have also been rare reports of Raynaud's phenomenon and ischaemic colitis.

Gastrointestinal

Nausea and vomiting occurred in some patients but the relationship to sumatriptan is not clear.

CNS

There have been rare reports of seizures following use of sumatriptan. Although some have occurred in patients with either a history of seizures or concurrent conditions predisposing to seizures there are also reports in patients where no such predisposing factors are apparent.

Eye Disorders

Patients treated with Imigran rarely exhibit visual disorders like flickering and diplopia. Additionally, cases of nystagmus, scotoma and reduced vision have been observed. Very rarely, loss of vision has occurred, which is usually transient. However, visual disorders may also occur during a migraine attack itself.

Hypersensitivity/skin

Hypersensitivity reactions ranging from cutaneous hypersensitivity to, in rare cases, anaphylaxis.

Laboratory values

Minor disturbances in liver function tests have occasionally been observed.

4.9 Overdose

There have been some reports of overdosage with Imigran Tablets. Doses in excess of 400mg orally were not associated with side effects other than those mentioned.

If overdosage occurs, the patient should be monitored for at least ten hours and standard supportive treatment applied as required.

It is unknown what effect haemodialysis or peritoneal dialysis has on the plasma concentrations of Imigran

5. PHARMACOLOGICAL PROPERTIES

5.1 Pharmacodynamic properties

Pharmacotherapeutic group: Analgesics: Selective 5-HT_1 receptor agonists.

ATC code: N02CC01

Sumatriptan has been demonstrated to be a specific and selective 5-Hydroxytryptamine$_1$ ($5HT_{1D}$) receptor agonist with no effect on other 5HT receptor ($5\text{-}HT_2\text{-}5\text{-}HT_7$) subtypes. The vascular 5-HT_{1D} receptor is found predominantly in cranial blood vessels and mediates vasoconstriction. In animals, sumatriptan selectively constricts the carotid arterial circulation but does not alter cerebral blood flow. The carotid arterial circulation supplies blood to the extracranial and intracranial tissues such as the meninges and dilatation of and/or oedema formation in these vessels is thought to be the underlying mechanism of migraine in man.

In addition, evidence from animal studies suggests that sumatriptan inhibits trigeminal nerve activity. Both these actions (cranial vasoconstriction and inhibition of trigeminal nerve activity) may contribute to the anti-migraine action of sumatriptan in humans.

Sumatriptan remains effective in treating menstrual migraine i.e. migraine without aura that occurs between 3 days prior and up to 5 days post onset of menstruation. Sumatriptan should be taken as soon as possible in an attack.

Clinical response begins around 30 minutes following a 100mg oral dose.

Although the recommended dose of oral sumatriptan is 50mg, migraine attacks vary in severity both within and between patients. Doses of 25-100mg have shown greater efficacy than placebo in clinical trials, but 25mg is statistically significantly less effective than 50 and 100mg.

5.2 Pharmacokinetic properties

Following oral administration, sumatriptan is rapidly absorbed, 70% of maximum concentration occurring at 45 minutes. After 100mg dose, the maximum plasma concentration is 54ng/ml. Mean absolute oral bioavailability is 14% partly due to presystemic metabolism and partly due to incomplete absorption. The elimination phase half-life is approximately 2 hours, although there is an indication of a longer terminal phase. Plasma protein binding is low (14-21%), mean volume of distribution is 170 litres. Mean total plasma clearance is approximately 1160ml/min and the mean renal plasma clearance is approximately 260ml/min. Non-renal clearance accounts for about 80% of the total clearance. Sumatriptan is eliminated primarily by oxidative metabolism mediated by monoamine oxidase A. The major metabolite, the indole acetic acid analogue of Sumatriptan is mainly excreted in the urine, where it is present as a free acid and the glucuronide conjugate. It has no known $5HT_1$ or $5HT_2$ activity. Minor metabolites have not been identified. The pharmacokinetics of oral Sumatriptan do not appear to be significantly affected by migraine attacks.

In a pilot study, no significant differences were found in the pharmacokinetic parameters between the elderly and young healthy volunteers.

5.3 Preclinical safety data

Sumatriptan was devoid of genotoxic and carcinogenic activity in *in-vitro* systems and animal studies.

In a rat fertility study oral doses of sumatriptan resulting in plasma levels approximately 200 times those seen in man after a 100 mg oral dose were associated with a reduction in the success of insemination.

This effect did not occur during a subcutaneous study where maximum plasma levels achieved approximately 150 times those in man by the oral route.

In rabbits embryolethality, without marked teratogenic defects, was seen. The relevance for humans of these findings is unknown.

6. PHARMACEUTICAL PARTICULARS

6.1 List of excipients

Imigran 50mg Tablets: Lactose, microcrystalline cellulose, croscarmellose sodium, magnesium stearate, methylhydroxypropylcellulose, titanium dioxide, triacetin and iron oxide.

Imigran 100mg Tablets: Lactose, microcrystalline cellulose, croscarmellose sodium, magnesium stearate, methylhydroxypropylcellulose and opaspray white.

6.2 Incompatibilities

None stated.

6.3 Shelf life

Imigran 50mg Tablets: 36 months

Imigran 100mg Tablets: 48 months

6.4 Special precautions for storage

Store below 30°C

6.5 Nature and contents of container

Imigran 50mg Tablets: Aluminium double foil blister packs in a cardboard carton, containing either 2, 3, 6, 12, 18 or 24 tablets.

Imigran 100mg Tablets: Aluminium double foil blister packs in a cardboard carton, containing either 2, 3, 6 or12 tablets.

6.6 Instructions for use and handling

None stated

Administrative Data

7. MARKETING AUTHORISATION HOLDER

Glaxo Wellcome UK Ltd., trading as GlaxoSmithKline UK.

Stockley Park West

Uxbridge

Middlesex. UB11 1BT

8. MARKETING AUTHORISATION NUMBER(S)

Imigran 50mg Tablets: PL 10949/0222

Imigran 100mg Tablets: PL 10949/0231

9. DATE OF FIRST AUTHORISATION/RENEWAL OF THE AUTHORISATION

Imigran 50mg Tablets: 21 June 2000

Imigran 100mg Tablets: 09 February 2003

10. DATE OF REVISION OF THE TEXT

19 September 2003

11. Legal Status

POM

ImmuCyst 81mg

(Cambridge Laboratories)

1. NAME OF THE MEDICINAL PRODUCT

Trade Name: ImmuCyst® 81 mg

Proper name: BCG Immunotherapy

2. QUALITATIVE AND QUANTITATIVE COMPOSITION

The product is presented as a lyophilisate, which is a white powder. This is reconstituted in sterile preservative-free normal saline.

ImmuCyst® 81 mg is freeze-dried preparation made from a culture of the Connaught strain of Bacillus of Calmette and Guérin (BCG), which is an attenuated strain of living bovine tubercle bacillus, *Mycobacterium bovis*. The bacilli are lyophilised (freeze-dried) and are viable upon reconstitution. The product contains no preservative.

Lyophilisate	Content per Vial
BCG	81 mg (dry weight)
(Bacillus of Calmette and Guérin)	1.8 to 15.9 $\times 10^8$ Colony Forming Units (CFU) throughout the shelf life
Monosodium glutamate	150 mg (5% w/v prior to lyophilisation)

3. PHARMACEUTICAL FORM

ImmuCyst® 81 mg is supplied as a lyophilisate, for intravesicular use.

4. CLINICAL PARTICULARS

4.1 Therapeutic indications

ImmuCyst® 81 mg is indicated for intravesicular use in the treatment and prophylaxis of primary or recurrent carcinoma *in situ* (CIS) of the urinary bladder, and for the prophylaxis following transurethral resection (TUR) of primary or recurrent stage Ta and/or T1 papillary tumours, or any combination thereof, regardless of antecedent intravesicular treatment.

4.2 Posology and method of administration

Adults

One dose of ImmuCyst® 81 mg consists of the intravesicular instillation of 81 mg (dry weight) BCG. This dose is prepared by reconstituting the vial containing freeze-dried BCG with preservative-free normal saline. The vial of reconstituted BCG is diluted in 50 ml of sterile, preservative-free saline, to a total of 53 ml instillation volume (see instructions for use and handling).

A urethral catheter is inserted into the bladder under aseptic conditions, the bladder is drained, and then 53 ml suspension of ImmuCyst® 81 mg is instilled slowly by gravity, following which the catheter is withdrawn.

The patient retains the suspension for as long as possible for up to two hours. During the first 15 minutes following instillation, the patient should lie prone. Thereafter, the patient is allowed to be up. At the end of 2 hours, all patients should void in a seated position for environmental safety reasons. Patients should be instructed to maintain adequate hydration.

Clinical trials carried out with ImmuCyst® 81 mg included a percutaneous inoculation with each intravesicular dose. A 0.5 ml portion of the 53 ml intravesical dose of ImmuCyst® 81 mg was administered percutaneously (e.g., on inner, upper thigh). Some studies have suggested that there is no additional benefit of administering BCG systemically. If severe reactions occur, such as ulceration at the site of regional lymphadenitis, the percutaneous treatment should be discontinued.

Treatment Schedule

Intravesicular treatment of the urinary bladder should begin 10 to 14 days after biopsy of TUR, and consists of induction and maintenance treatments.

The induction treatment consists of one intravesicular instillation of ImmuCyst® 81mg each week for 6 weeks. After a 6 week pause, one intravesical instillation should be given once each week for 1-3 weeks. Clinical studies have demonstrated that 3 weekly instillations significantly increase the complete response rate from 73% to 87% at 6 months, compared with no additional treatment given at 3 months. Three weekly instillations should definitely be given to patients who still have evidence of bladder cancer.

Based on clinical studies performed with ImmuCyst® 81 mg, maintenance therapy following induction is highly recommended. This consists of one dose given each week for 1 to 3 weeks at 6 months following the initial dose, and then every 6 months thereafter until 36 months.

Children

Safety and effectiveness in children have not been established.

4.3 Contraindications

ImmuCyst® 81 mg is contraindicated for patients:

- who have had a TUR or traumatic bladder catheterisation (associated with hematuria) in the previous 10 days,
- who are immunosuppressed as a result of malignancies or receiving immunosuppressive therapies, including irradiation, antimetabolites, alkylating agents, cytotoxic drugs, or who are otherwise immunocompromised (including HIV-infected individuals),
- with active tuberculosis, because of the danger of exacerbation or of concomitant systemic BCG infection,
- with current or previous evidence of a systemic BCG infection,
- with fever, unless the cause of the fever has been determined and evaluated, and
- with bacterial urinary tract infection, until all the infection has resolved.

4.4 Special warnings and special precautions for use

Contains viable attenuated mycobacteria. Handle as infectious.

ImmuCyst® 81 mg should not be handled by persons with immune deficiency.

It is recommended that intravesicular ImmuCyst® 81 mg not be administered any sooner than 10 days following TUR. Given the specialised nature of BCG intravesical treatment, ImmuCyst® 81 mg should be administered under the supervision of a qualified physician, such as a urologist, experienced in the use of anti-cancer agents.

Care must be taken during administration of intravesicular ImmuCyst® 81 mg not to introduce contaminants into the urinary tract nor to traumatise unduly the urinary mucosa. If the physician believes that the bladder catheterisation has been traumatic (e.g. associated with bleeding), then ImmuCyst® 81 mg should not be administered and there must be a treatment delay of at least 10 days. Subsequent treatment should be resumed as if no interruption in the schedule had occurred.

Intravesicular treatment with ImmuCyst® 81 mg may induce a sensitivity to tuberculin purified protein derivative (PPD) which could complicate future interpretations of skin test reactions to tuberculin in the diagnosis of suspected mycobacterial infections. Determination of a patient's reactivity to tuberculin prior to administration of ImmuCyst® 81 mg may therefore be desirable.

For patients with small bladder capacity, increased risk of bladder contracture should be considered in decisions to treat with ImmuCyst® 81 mg.

If a bacterial urinary tract infection (UTI) occurs during the course of ImmuCyst® 81mg treatment, ImmuCyst® 81 mg instillation should be withheld until complete resolution of the bacterial UTI for two reasons: (1) the combination of a UTI and BCG- induced cystitis may lead to more severe adverse effects on the genitourinary tract, and (2) BCG bacilli are sensitive to a wide variety of antibiotics; antimicrobial administration may therefore diminish the efficacy of ImmuCyst® 81 mg.

Patients undergoing antimicrobial therapy for other infections should be evaluated to assess whether the therapy might diminish the efficacy of ImmuCyst® 81 mg.

BCG infection of aneurysms and prosthetic devices (including arterial grafts, cardiac devices, and artificial joints) have been reported following intravesicular administration of BCG. The risk of these ectopic BCG infections has not been determined, but is considered to be very small. The benefits of BCG therapy must carefully be weighed against the possibility of an ectopic BCG infection in patients with pre-existing arterial aneurysms or prosthetic devices of any kind.

4.5 Interaction with other medicinal products and other forms of Interaction

Patients must be advised that drug combinations containing bone marrow depressants and/or immunosuppressants and/or radiation may impair the response to ImmuCyst® 81 mg and/or increase the risk of disseminated BCG infection. For patients with a condition that may in future require mandatory immunosuppression (e.g. awaiting an organ transplant, myasthenia gravis), the decision to treat with ImmuCyst® 81 mg should be considered carefully.

4.6 Pregnancy and lactation

Animal reproduction studies have not been conducted with ImmuCyst® 81 mg. It is also not known whether ImmuCyst® 81 mg can cause fetal harm when administered to a pregnant woman or can affect reproduction capacity. ImmuCyst® 81 mg should be given to a pregnant woman only if clearly needed.

A nursing woman with a systemic BCG infection could infect her infant.

It is not known whether this drug is excreted in human milk. Therefore, caution should be exercised when ImmuCyst® 81 mg is administered to a nursing woman.

4.7 Effects on ability to drive and use machines

There are no indications that ability to drive and use machines is impaired.

4.8 Undesirable effects

Administration of intravesicular ImmuCyst® 81 mg causes an inflammatory response in the bladder and has been frequently associated with transient fever, haematuria, urinary frequency and dysuria. Such reactions may to some degree be taken as evidence that BCG is evoking the desired response, but patients should be carefully monitored for serious adverse events. Serious adverse events have occurred in <1% of ImmuCyst® 81 mg recipients.

Local:

The most common local reactions are transient dysuria and urinary frequency. During the induction course, these reactions occurred on at least one occasion in 26% and 14% of patients, respectively. This rose to 46% and 34% respectively, among patients during maintenance therapy. Gross hematuria has occurred among 11-19% of ImmuCyst® 81 mg recipients, while more serious genitourinary adverse events have occurred in <0.5% of recipients. Infrequent associations include bacterial UTI, bladder contracture, symptomatic granulomatous prostatitis, epididymo-orchitis, urethral obstruction, and renal abscess.

Systemic:

Transient fever of <38.5° C of < 48 hours duration has occurred among 17% of ImmuCyst® 81 mg recipients during induction and among 31% during maintenance.

Skin rash, arthralgia, and migratory arthritis are rare, and are considered to be strictly allergic reactions.

Ocular symptoms (including uveitis, conjunctivitis, iritis, keratitis, and granulomatous choreoretinitis) alone, or in combination with joint symptoms (arthritis or arthralgia), urinary symptoms and/or skin rash, have been reported following administration of intravesicular BCG. The risk seems to be elevated among patients who are positive for HLA-B27.

BCG Infection

Systemic BCG infection is a serious side effect of ImmuCyst® 81 mg administration and fatalities have occurred.

BCG infection may be more common after traumatic bladder catheterisation or bladder perforation. BCG treatment should be delayed in such patients until mucosal damage has healed.

Treatment should be delayed for 10-14 days after TUR or biopsy of bladder lesions.

All patients receiving the product should be carefully monitored and advised to report all incidences of fever and other events outside the urinary tract. Fever lasting over 24 hours and any unusual event should be investigated to exclude another cause and to try and isolate organisms. Blood cultures and samples from affected sites should be cultured for BCG.

The infection may manifest as pneumonitis, hepatitis and/or cytopenia after a period of fever and malaise.

Fever lasting more than 48 hours for which there is no explanation and any other unexplained reactions should be treated with antituberculous therapy, following the regular treatment schedules for tuberculosis.

ImmuCyst® 81 mg is sensitive to Isoniazid, Rifampicin and Ethambutol.

No further treatment with BCG should be given.

Treatment of undesirable effects:

Table 1 summarises the recommended treatment of adverse events.

Irritative bladder side effects associated with ImmuCyst® 81 mg administration can be managed symptomatically with propantheline bromide. Paracetamol may be administered for symptomatic relief of transient fever or irritative bladder symptoms.

BCG organisms, including the Connaught strain, are susceptible to all currently used anti-tuberculosis drugs with the exception of pyrazinamide. Accordingly, for more serious reactions other than a systemic BCG infection (e.g., severe urinary tract adverse events or allergic reaction), Isoniazid with or without Rifampicin should be administered for 3-6 months.

If a systemic BCG infection occurs, an Infectious Diseases consultation should be sought. ImmuCyst® 81 mg should be permanently discontinued, and triple anti-tuberculosis therapy should be initiated promptly and continued for 6 months. Commonly, this will comprise Isoniazid (300 mg daily), Rifampicin (600 mg daily), and Ethambutol (1000 mg daily). In the presence of signs of septic shock as a manifestation of a systemic BCG infection, the addition of short-term corticosteroids (e.g. Prednisolone, 40 mg daily) has been shown to be beneficial, and should be considered.

If a systemic BCG infection has occurred, a report should be submitted to both the manufacturer and the appropriate health authorities. The report should include details of the treatment history with ImmuCyst® 81 mg, the symptoms and signs of the BCG infection, the treatment administered for the reaction, and the response to this treatment.

Patients must be advised to check with their doctor as soon as possible if there is an increase in their existing symptoms, or if their symptoms persist even after receiving a number of treatments, or if any of the following symptoms develop.

More common: Blood in the urine; painful or frequent urination lasting $>$ 2 days; nausea and vomiting; fever and chill lasting $>$ 24 hours.

Rare: Cough; skin rash; high or persistent fever; joint pains; jaundice; eye complaints.

Table 1

Recommended Treatment of Adverse Events Associated with ImmuCyst® 81 mg

Symptom, Sign or Syndrome	Treatment
Irritative bladder symptoms $<$ 48 hours duration	Symptomatic treatment.
Irritative bladder symptoms $\geq$48 hours duration	Symptomatic treatment; postpone next ImmuCyst® 81 mg treatment until complete resolution. If complete resolution has not occurred within one week, administer Isoniazid (INH), 300 mg daily until complete resolution.
Concomitant bacterial UTI	Postpone next ImmuCyst® 81 mg treatment until completion of antimicrobial therapy and negative urine culture.
Other genitourinary tract adverse events: symptomatic granulomatous prostatitis, epididymo-orchitis, urethral obstruction or renal abscess.	Discontinue ImmuCyst® 81 mg. Administer INH, 300 mg daily and Rifampicin, 600 mg daily for 3-6 months.
Fever $<$38.5° C of $<$48 hours duration.	Symptomatic treatment with Paracetamol
Skin rash, arthralgia, or migratory arthritis.	Anti-histamines or non-steroidal anti-inflammatories. If no response, discontinue ImmuCyst® 81 mg and administer INH 300 mg daily for 3 months. Consider administration of Prednisolone.
Systemic BCG infection without signs of septic shock.	Discontinue ImmuCyst® 81 mg. Seek an Infectious Disease consultation. Administer triple-drug anti-tuberculosis therapy for 6 months.
Systemic BCG infection with signs of septic shock.	As for immediately above. Consider addition of short-term high-dose systemic corticosteroids.
Ocular complaints	Consult Ophthalmologist for specific treatment

4.9 Overdose

In case of overdose, patients should be monitored closely, and any adverse events should be treated according to the recommendations in "Treatment of undesirable effects", above.

5. PHARMACOLOGICAL PROPERTIES

5.1 Pharmacodynamic properties

ATC Code: LO3AX

ImmuCyst® 81 mg promotes a local acute inflammatory and immunological reaction, and sub-acute granulomatous reaction with macrophage and lymphocyte infiltration in the urothelium and lamina propria of the urinary bladder.

5.2 Pharmacokinetic properties

ImmuCyst® 81 mg has been administered intravesically with concomitant percutaneous administration. Acid-fast bacteria have been observed in the urine. Cultures and strains for acid-fast bacilli at other sites have usually been negative even in the cases of suspected systemic BCG infection. However, traumatic catheterisation or treatment following extensive tumour resection or bladder perforation could result in systemic BCG infection.

5.3 Preclinical safety data

ImmuCyst® 81 mg administered intravesically induced no serious systemic toxicity in studies in guinea pigs and monkeys. Studies in animals suggest that there is a possibility of a potential for allergenicity to the product.

No animal reproduction studies have been performed. Studies on mutagenicity and carcinogenicity have also not been performed.

6. PHARMACEUTICAL PARTICULARS

6.1 List of excipients

Monosodium glutamate

6.2 Incompatibilities

BCG bacilli are sensitive to a wide variety of antibiotics. Antimicrobial administration may therefore diminish the efficacy of ImmuCyst® 81 mg. Patients undergoing antimicrobial therapy for infections should be evaluated to assess whether the therapy might diminish the efficacy of ImmuCyst® 81 mg.

ImmuCyst® 81 mg is contraindicated in persons receiving immunosuppressive therapies, including irradiation, antimetabolites, alkylating agents or cytotoxic drugs because of risk of disseminated BCG infection.

6.3 Shelf life

Twenty-four months from the date of initiation of the viability (potency:viable count) test when stored between 2° and 8°C.

6.4 Special precautions for storage

ImmuCyst® 81 mg should be kept in a refrigerator at a temperature between 2° and 8°C. it should not be used after the expiration date marked on the vial.

At no time should the freeze-dried or reconstituted ImmuCyst® 81 mg be exposed to sunlight, direct or indirect. Exposure to artificial light should be kept to a minimum.

6.5 Nature and contents of container

The lyophilisate is contained in a 5 ml type 1 amber glass vial sealed with a grey butyl silicone stopper and held closed with an aluminium seal with a blue flip-off plastic top.

6.6 Instructions for use and handling

Reconstitution of Freeze-Dried Product and Withdrawal from Rubber-Stoppered Vial

DO NOT REMOVE THE RUBBER STOPPERS FROM THE VIALS. HANDLE AS INFECTIOUS MATERIAL

Reconstitute and dilute immediately prior to use, using aseptic technique in a low traffic, high airflow area (e.g., in a biocontainment cabinet). Persons handling product should wear gloves. If and when the product is handled outside of a biocontainment cabinet, persons handling the product should also wear a mask and eye protection.

ImmuCyst® 81 mg should not be handled by persons with an immune deficiency.

ImmuCyst® 81 mg is to be reconstituted only with sterile preservative-free normal saline to ensure proper dispersion of the organisms.

Using a 5 ml sterile syringe and needle, draw up 3ml of saline from an ampoule.

Prepare the surface of the ImmuCyst® 81 mg vial using a suitable antiseptic and using a 5 ml syringe containing 3ml of saline, pierce the stopper of the vial. Holding the vial upright pull the plunger of the syringe back to the 5 ml marking on the barrel. This will create a mild vacuum in the vial. Release the plunger and allow the vacuum to pull the saline from the syringe into the vial. After all the saline has passed into the freeze-dried material, remove the needle and syringe.

Shake the vial gently.

Two options for intravesicular administration are possible:

Option 1:

Further dilute the reconstituted material from the vial (1 dose) in an additional 50 ml of sterile preservative-free normal saline to a final volume of 53 ml intravesicular instillation (and 0.5 ml of the 53 ml for percutaneous inoculation, if administered).

The reconstituted product is then transferred to a bladder syringe.

Option 2:

The entire contents from the reconstituted vial is added to a saline bladder irrigation bag.

The product should be used immediately after reconstitution. In the event of a delay between reconstitution and administration, the reconstituted and diluted suspension may be stored, protected from light, for up to 8 hours at room temperature (up to 25° C). Any reconstituted product, which exhibits flocculation or clumping that cannot be dispersed with gentle shaking should not be used.

At no time should the reconstituted product be exposed to sunlight, direct or indirect. Exposure to artificial light should be kept to a minimum.

Special Instructions

After use, unused product, packaging, and all equipment and materials used for instillation should be sterilised or disposed of properly as with any other biohazardous waste.

Urine voided over 6 hours following ImmuCyst® 81 mg instillation should be disinfected with an equal volume of 5% hypochlorite solution (undiluted household bleach) and allowed to stand for 15 minutes before flushing.

Administrative Data

7. MARKETING AUTHORISATION HOLDER

Cambridge Laboratories Limited

Deltic House,

Kingfisher Way, Silverlink Business Park,

Wallsend, Tyne and Wear

NE28 9NX, United Kingdom

8. MARKETING AUTHORISATION NUMBER(S)

PL 12070/0024

9. DATE OF FIRST AUTHORISATION/RENEWAL OF THE AUTHORISATION

19 September 2001

10. DATE OF REVISION OF THE TEXT

March 2004

Immukin

(Boehringer Ingelheim Limited)

1. NAME OF THE MEDICINAL PRODUCT

Immukin® Solution for Injection 2×10^6 IU (0.1mg)

2. QUALITATIVE AND QUANTITATIVE COMPOSITION

Immukin contains 2×10^6 IU (0.1 mg) recombinant human interferon gamma-1b per vial. Interferon gamma 1-b is produced in an E. coli expression system.

For excipients, see 6.1.

3. PHARMACEUTICAL FORM

Solution for injection.

A clear, colourless solution.

4. CLINICAL PARTICULARS

4.1 Therapeutic indications

Immukin is indicated for the reduction of the frequency of serious infections in patients with chronic granulomatous disease (CGD) (see section 4.4).

Immukin is indicated for the reduction in frequency of serious infections in patients with severe, malignant osteopetrosis (see also section 5.1).

4.2 Posology and method of administration

Immukin is for subcutaneous use. The recommended dosage of Immukin for the treatment of patients with CGD or severe, malignant osteopetrosis is 50 mcg/m^2 for patients whose body surface area is greater than 0.5 m^2, and 1.5 mcg/kg/dose for patients whose body surface area is equal to or less than 0.5 m^2. The actually drawn volume has to be controlled before injection. Injections should be administered subcutaneously preferably in the evening three times weekly (for example, Monday, Wednesday, Friday). The optimum sites of injection are the right and the left deltoid and anterior thigh. Immukin can be administered by a physician, nurse, family member or patient when trained in the administration of subcutaneous injections.

Although the most beneficial dose of Immukin is not known yet higher doses are not recommended. Safety and efficacy has not been established for Immukin given in doses greater or less than the recommended dose of 50 mcg/m^2. If severe reactions occur, the dosage should be modified (50% reduction) or therapy should be discontinued until the adverse reaction abates.

Safety and effectiveness in children under the age of 6 months have not been established in patients with CGD, but have been established in patients with severe, malignant osteopetrosis.

4.3 Contraindications

Immukin is contra-indicated in patients who develop or have known acute hypersensitivity to interferon gamma or known hypersensitivity to closely related interferons or to any of the excipients.

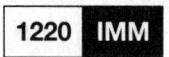

4.4 Special warnings and special precautions for use

The use of Immukin does not exclude the need for any additional antimicrobial coverage that might be required for the management of CGD. In the pivotal clinical efficacy study, the overwhelming majority of the patients were receiving prophylactic antimicrobial therapy (see section 5.1).

Patients with pre-existing cardiac disease may experience an acute, self-limited exacerbation of their cardiac condition at doses of 250mcg/m^2/day or higher as observed in early clinical trials, although no direct cardiotoxic effect has been demonstrated.

Caution should be exercised when treating patients with known seizure disorders and/or compromised central nervous system function.

Patients with serious liver disease and patients with severe renal insufficiency should be treated with caution since the possibility of interferon gamma-1b accumulation exists in those patients.

Simultaneous administration of interferon gamma-1b with other heterologous serum protein preparations or immunological preparations (e.g. vaccines) should be avoided because of the risk for unexpected amplified immune response.

In addition to tests normally required for monitoring patients with CGD or severe, malignant osteopetrosis, patients should have performed the following tests before beginning Immukin therapy and at appropriate periods during treatment: haematologic tests, including complete blood counts, differential and platelet counts; blood chemistries, including renal and liver function tests; urinalysis.

Interferon gamma 1b is an exogenous protein, which may lead to the occurrence of antibodies during the course of treatment. Up to now Immukin administered to CGD or severe, malignant osteopetrosis patients in the recommended dose does not seem to be associated with significant risk for the induction of neutralising antibodies to interferon gamma-1b.

Based on the information available, it cannot be excluded that the presence of higher levels of interferon gamma may impair male and female fertility.

4.5 Interaction with other medicinal products and other forms of Interaction

Immukin does not reduce the efficacy of antibiotics or glucocorticoids in CGD or severe, malignant osteopetrosis patients.

Drug interactions seen with Immukin are similar to those seen with other interferons in animal experiments.

It is theoretically possible that hepatotoxic and/or nephrotoxic drugs might have effects on the clearance of Immukin. Also the effects of anti-inflammatory drugs, NSAIDs, theophylline, immunosuppressive and cytostatic drugs on the acute cellular effects of Immukin and its therapeutic effects in CGD or severe, malignant osteopetrosis patients when such drugs are used concomitantly in chronic conditions are not known.

Immukin potentially can prolong the half-lives of simultaneously administered drugs, which are metabolised by the cytochrome P-450 system.

Concurrent use of drugs having neurotoxic (including effects on the central nervous system); haemotoxic or cardiotoxic effects may increase the toxicity of interferons in these systems.

4.6 Pregnancy and lactation

Pregnancy

There are no data on the use of interferon gamma during pregnancy. Higher levels of endogenous interferon gamma were found in women with recurrent first trimester miscarriage compared to women with normal pregnancy. There is no evidence of any clinical relevance for Immukin. In animal studies, reproductive toxicity was observed (see section 5.3). Immukin should not be used during pregnancy unless vitally indicated.

Lactation

It is not known whether interferon gamma is excreted in human milk. Because of the lack of data on neonatal effects, breast feeding is not recommended.

4.7 Effects on ability to drive and use machines

Even when given at the recommended dosage of 50mcg/m^2 by subcutaneous injection, Immukin may affect reactions such that the ability to drive a vehicle or to operate machinery is impaired. This effect may be enhanced by alcohol.

4.8 Undesirable effects

a) General Description

The clinical and laboratory toxicity associated with multiple-dose Immukin therapy is dose-, and schedule-dependent.

The most common adverse events are flu-like symptoms characterised by fever, headache, chills, myalgia or fatigue.

b) Table of Adverse Reactions

System Organ Class	
MedDRA Term	**Frequency**[1]
Psychiatric disorders	
Confusion	Rare[2]
Nervous system disorders	
Headache	Very common
Gastro-intestinal disorders	
Nausea	Common
Vomiting	Common
Skin and subcutaneous tissue disorders	
Rash	Very common
Musculoskeletal, connective tissue and bone disorders	
Myalgia	Common
Arthralgia	Common
Systemic lupus erythematosus	Rare[2]
General disorders and administration	
Fever	Very common
Chills	Very common
Injection site pain	Very common
Fatigue	Common
Investigations	
Autoantibody response	Rare[2]

[1]very common > 1/10; common > 1/100, < 1/10; rare > 1/10,000, < 1/1,000 according to frequency

[2]It has been assumed that these events have a reporting frequency of less than 1/1,000 and, therefore, they have been systematically classified "rare".

c) Information Characterising Individual Serious and/or Frequently Occurring Adverse Reactions

The flu-like symptoms may decrease in severity as treatment continues. Some of these symptoms can be minimised by bedtime administration. Acetaminophen (paracetamol) may also be used to ameliorate these effects. Vomiting, nausea, arthralgia and injection site tenderness have been reported in some patients.

Transient cutaneous rashes, e.g. dermatitis, maculopapular rash, pustular and vesicular eruptions, and erythema at injection site have occurred in some patients following injection but have rarely necessitated treatment interruption.

In some patients treated with gamma interferon an increased production of autoantibodies, including the development of systemic lupus erythematosus, has been observed.

Isolated cases of confusion, which may have been triggered by the administration of Immukin, have been reported in some patients with diseases involving CNS other than CGD or severe, malignant osteopetrosis.

4.9 Overdose

Immukin has been administered at higher doses (>100 mcg/m^2) to patients with advanced malignancies by the intravenous or intramuscular route.

Central nervous system adverse reactions including decreased mental status, gait disturbance and dizziness have been observed, particularly in cancer patients receiving doses greater than 100mcg/m^2/day. These abnormalities were reversible within a few days upon dose reduction or discontinuation of therapy.

Blood disorders, including reversible neutropenia and thrombocytopenia as well as the onset of increased hepatic enzymes and of triglycerides, have also been observed.

Patients with pre-existing cardiac disease, may experience an acute, self-limited exacerbation of their cardiac condition at doses of 250 mcg/m^2/day or higher, as observed in early clinical trials, although no direct cardiotoxic effect has been demonstrated.

5. PHARMACOLOGICAL PROPERTIES

5.1 Pharmacodynamic properties

Pharmacotherapeutic group: Immunostimulants, Cytokines and immunomodulators, ATC code: L03A B03

Interferons are a family of functionally related proteins synthesised by eukaryotic cells in response to viruses and a variety of neutral and synthetic stimuli. The real mechanism of action of interferon gamma-1b in CGD is still unknown. Findings related to superoxide anion production remain unequivocal. However, it is presumed that interferon-gamma increases macrophage cytotoxicity by enhancing the respiratory burst via generation of toxic oxygen metabolites capable of mediating the killing of intracellular micro-organisms. It increases HLA-DR expression on macrophages and augments Fc receptor expression, which results in increased antibody-dependent cell-mediated cytotoxicity.

In a placebo-controlled clinical trial in 128 patients with CGD, Immukin was shown to reduce the frequency of serious infections during the trial period of 12 months by 77% in patients treated with Immukin compared to 30% in the placebo group (p=0.0006). The overwhelming majority of these patients were also receiving prophylactic antimicrobial therapy.

In severe, malignant osteopetrosis (inherited disorder characterised by an osteoclast defect leading to bone overgrowth and deficient phagocyte oxidative metabolism), a treatment-related enhancement of superoxide production by phagocytes was observed in situ.

In a controlled, randomised study in 16 patients with severe, malignant osteopetrosis, Immukin in combination with calcitriol was shown to reduce the frequency of serious infections versus calcitriol alone. In an analysis which combined data from two clinical studies, 19 out of 24 patients treated with Immukin in combination with or without calcitriol for at least 6 months had reduced trabecular bone volume compared to baseline. The clinical relevance of this observed decrease in Immukin treated patients versus a control group could not be established.

5.2 Pharmacokinetic properties

Immukin is rapidly cleared after intravenous administration and slowly and well absorbed after intramuscular or subcutaneous administration.

With the recommended dosage regimen of subcutaneous administration of 0.05 mg/m^2 Immukin, the mean elimination half-lives were 4.9 hours and the mean residence time was 2.5 hours. Time to reach maximum plasma concentration ranged from 4 to 14 hours with a mean of 8 hours.

Interferon gamma was not detected in the urine of healthy male subjects following administration of 100 mcg/m^2 by the intramuscular or subcutaneous injection.

5.3 Preclinical safety data

Although difficult to interpret, due to species restrictions, pre-clinical data reveal no special hazard to humans based on studies of acute toxicity, repeated dose toxicity, mutagenicity, local tolerance and skin sensitisation.

An increased incidence of abortion has been observed in pregnant non-human primates which received the drug in doses manifold higher than that recommended for human use.

6. PHARMACEUTICAL PARTICULARS

6.1 List of excipients

D-Mannitol

Disodium succinate hexahydrate

Polysorbate 20

Succinic acid

Water for injections

6.2 Incompatibilities

In the absence of compatibility studies, this medicinal product must not be mixed with other medicinal products.

6.3 Shelf life

18 months.

6.4 Special precautions for storage

Store at 2°C – 8°C (in a refrigerator)

Do not freeze

Immukin is for single use only.

The formulation does not contain a preservative. Once opened, the content of a vial should be used immediately. The unused portion of any vial should be discarded.

6.5 Nature and contents of container

3ml sterilised glass vials (Type I borosilicate glass), which are stoppered with sterile grey butyl rubber stoppers with aluminium/polypropylene flip-off type caps.

Pack sizes: 1,3,5,6 and 12 vial(s) in one folding box. Not all pack sizes may be marketed.

6.6 Instructions for use and handling

Vials of Immukin must not be shaken vigorously.

Parenteral drug products should be inspected visually for particulate matter and discolouration prior to administration.

7. MARKETING AUTHORISATION HOLDER

Boehringer Ingelheim Limited

Ellesfield Avenue

Bracknell

Berkshire

RG12 8YS

United Kingdom

8. MARKETING AUTHORISATION NUMBER(S)

PL 00015/0154

9. DATE OF FIRST AUTHORISATION/RENEWAL OF THE AUTHORISATION

7 October 1992 / 9th April 1998/ 29th September 2002

10. DATE OF REVISION OF THE TEXT

June 2004

11. Legal category

POM

I2/UK/SPC/5

Imodium Capsules & Syrup

(Janssen-Cilag Ltd)

1. NAME OF THE MEDICINAL PRODUCT
Imodium® Capsules.
[Diareze *(when marketed by Boots under OLS)*]
Imodium® Syrup.

2. QUALITATIVE AND QUANTITATIVE COMPOSITION
Capsules: Loperamide hydrochloride 2 mg.

Syrup: Loperamide hydrochloride 0.2 mg/ml.

3. PHARMACEUTICAL FORM
Capsules and syrup for oral administration.

4. CLINICAL PARTICULARS
4.1 Therapeutic indications
Capsules:

POM: For the symptomatic treatment of acute diarrhoea of any aetiology including acute exacerbations of chronic diarrhoea for periods of up to 5 days in adults and children over 8 years. For the symptomatic treatment of chronic diarrhoea in adults.

P and GSL: For the symptomatic treatment of acute diarrhoea in adults and children aged 12 years and over.

P: For the symptomatic treatment of acute episodes of diarrhoea associated with Irritable Bowel Syndrome in adults following initial diagnosis by a doctor.

Syrup:

POM Classification: For the symptomatic treatment of acute diarrhoea of any aetiology including acute exacerbations of chronic diarrhoea for periods of up to 5 days in adults and children over 4 years. For the symptomatic treatment of chronic diarrhoea in adults.

P Classification: For the symptomatic treatment of acute diarrhoea in adults and children aged 12 years and over.

4.2 Posology and method of administration
Acute diarrhoea

GSL

Adults and children

over 12: 2 capsules initially followed by 1 capsule after every loose stool.

The maximum daily dose should not exceed 6 capsules.

P and POM

Adults and children

over 12: Two capsules or four 5 ml spoonfuls initially, followed by one capsule or two 5 ml spoonfuls after each loose stool. The usual dose is 3-4 capsules a day. The total daily dose should not exceed 8 capsules or sixteen spoonfuls.

POM

Children: The following doses should not be exceeded.

Children

9 to 12 years: One capsule or two 5 ml spoonfuls four times daily until diarrhoea is controlled (up to 5 days).

Children 4 - 8 years: Use syrup: One 5 ml spoonful three or four times daily with the duration limited to 3 days.

Not recommended for children under 4 years of age.

Further investigation into the cause of the diarrhoea should be considered if there is no improvement within two days of starting treatment with Imodium.

Chronic Diarrhoea (POM)

Adults: Patients may need widely differing amounts of Imodium. The starting dose should be between two and four capsules, or four and eight 5 ml spoonfuls per day in divided doses, depending on severity. If required this dose can be adjusted up to a maximum of eight capsules or sixteen 5 ml spoonfuls daily.

Having established the patient's daily maintenance dose, Imodium may be administered on a twice daily regimen. Tolerance has not been observed and therefore subsequent dosage adjustment should be unnecessary.

Symptomatic treatment of acute episodes of diarrhoea associated with Irritable Bowel Syndrome in adults (P)

Two capsules to be taken initially. The usual dose is between 2 and 4 capsules per day in divided doses, depending on severity. If required, this dose can be adjusted according to result, up to a maximum of 8 capsules daily.

USE IN ELDERLY

No dose adjustment is required for the elderly.

RENAL IMPAIRMENT

No dose adjustment is required for patients with renal impairment.

HEPATIC IMPAIRMENT

Although no pharmacokinetic data are available in patients with hepatic impairment, Imodium should be used with caution in such patients because of reduced first pass metabolism. (see 4.4 Special warnings and special precautions for use).

Method of administration

Oral use.

4.3 Contraindications
Imodium is contraindicated in:

- patients with a known hypersensitivity to loperamide hydrochloride or to any of the excipients.
- children less than 4 years of age.
- when inhibition of peristalsis is to be avoided due to the possible risk of significant sequelae including ileus, megacolon and toxic megacolon, in particular:

- when ileus or constipation are present or when abdominal distension develops, particularly in severely dehydrated children,

- in patients with acute ulcerative colitis,

- in patients with bacterial enterocolitis caused by invasive organisms including Salmonella, Shigella, and Campylobacter,

- in patients with pseudomembranous colitis associated with the use of broad-spectrum antibiotics.

Imodium should not be used alone in acute dysentery, which is characterised by blood in stools and elevated body temperatures.

GSL - not for use when inflammatory bowel disease is present.

4.4 Special warnings and special precautions for use
In patients with diarrhoea, especially young children, fluid and electrolyte depletion may occur. Use of Imodium does not preclude the administration of appropriate fluid and electrolyte replacement therapy.

Since persistent diarrhoea can be an indicator of potentially more serious conditions, Imodium should not be used for prolonged periods until the underlying cause of the diarrhoea has been investigated.

Imodium must be used with caution when the hepatic function necessary for the drug's metabolism is defective (eg in cases of severe hepatic disturbance), as this might result in a relative overdose leading to CNS toxicity.

Patients with AIDS treated with Imodium for diarrhoea should have therapy stopped at the earliest signs of abdominal distension. There have been isolated reports of toxic megacolon in AIDS patients with infectious colitis from both viral and bacterial pathogens treated with loperamide hydrochloride.

Also for P use only

If symptoms persist for more than 24 hours, consult your doctor.

If you are taking Imodium to control episodes of diarrhoea associated with Irritable Bowel Syndrome diagnosed by your doctor, you should return to him/her if the pattern of your symptoms changes. You should also return to your doctor if your episodes of acute symptoms continue for more than two weeks or there is a need for continuous treatment of more than two weeks.

Also for GSL use only

The first line of treatment in acute diarrhoea is the prevention or treatment of fluid and electrolyte depletion. This is of particular importance in frail and elderly patients with acute diarrhoea.

If symptoms persist for more than 24 hours, consult your doctor.

4.5 Interaction with other medicinal products and other forms of Interaction
Non-clinical data have shown that loperamide is a P-glycoprotein substrate. Concomitant administration of loperamide (16 mg single dose) with quinidine, or ritonavir, which are both P-glycoprotein inhibitors, resulted in a 2 to 3-fold increase in loperamide plasma levels. The clinical relevance of this pharmacokinetic interaction with P-glycoprotein inhibitors, when loperamide is given at recommended dosages (2 mg, up to 16 mg maximum daily dose), is unknown.

4.6 Pregnancy and lactation
Safety in human pregnancy has not been established although studies in animals have not demonstrated any teratogenic effects. As with other drugs, it is not advisable to administer Imodium in pregnancy. Small amounts of loperamide may appear in human breast milk. Therefore, Imodium is not recommended during breast-feeding.

Women who are pregnant or breast feeding infants should therefore be advised to consult their doctor for appropriate treatment.

4.7 Effects on ability to drive and use machines
Tiredness, dizziness, or drowsiness may occur when diarrhoea is treated with Imodium. If affected, do not drive or operate machinery.

4.8 Undesirable effects
In clinical trials, constipation and dizziness have been reported with greater frequency in loperamide hydrochloride treated patients than placebo treated patients.

The following adverse events have also been reported with use of loperamide hydrochloride:

Skin and Appendages

Very rare: rash, urticaria and pruritus.

Isolated occurrences of angioedema, and bullous eruptions including Stevens-Johnson Syndrome, erythema multiforme, and toxic epidermal necrolysis.

Body as a whole, general

Very rare: isolated occurrences of allergic reactions and in some cases severe hypersensitivity reactions including anaphylactic shock and anaphylactoid reactions.

Gastrointestinal System Disorders

Very rare: abdominal pain, ileus, abdominal distension, nausea, constipation, vomiting, megacolon including toxic megacolon, flatulence, and dyspepsia.

Genitourinary

Very rare: isolated reports of urinary retention.

Psychiatric

Very rare: drowsiness

Central and Peripheral Nervous System

Very rare: dizziness

A number of the adverse events reported during the clinical investigations and post-marketing experience with loperamide are frequent symptoms of the underlying diarrhoeal syndrome (abdominal pain/discomfort, nausea, vomiting, dry mouth, tiredness, drowsiness, dizziness, constipation, and flatulence). These symptoms are often difficult to distinguish from undesirable drug effects.

4.9 Overdose
In case of overdose the following effects may be observed: constipation, urinary retention, ileus and neurological symptoms (miosis, muscular hypertonia, somnolence and bradypnoea). If intoxication is suspected, naloxone may be given as an antidote. Since the duration of action of loperamide is longer than that of naloxone, the patient should be kept under constant observation for at least 48 hours in order to detect any possible depression of the central nervous system. Children, and patients with hepatic dysfunction, may be more sensitive to CNS effects. Gastric lavage, or induced emesis and or enema or laxatives may be recommended.

5. PHARMACOLOGICAL PROPERTIES
5.1 Pharmacodynamic properties
Loperamide binds to the opiate receptor in the gut wall, reducing propulsive peristalsis and increasing intestinal transit time. Loperamide increases the tone of the anal sphincter.

In a double blind randomised clinical trial in 56 patients with acute diarrhoea receiving loperamide, onset of anti-diarrhoeal action was observed within one hour following a single 4 mg dose. Clinical comparisons with other antidiarrhoeal drugs confirmed this exceptionally rapid onset of action of loperamide.

5.2 Pharmacokinetic properties
The half-life of loperamide in man is 10.8 hours with a range of 9-14 hours. Studies on distribution in rats show high affinity for the gut wall with preference for binding to the receptors in the longitudinal muscle layer. Loperamide is well absorbed from the gut, but is almost completely extracted and metabolised by the liver where it is conjugated and excreted via the bile. Due to its high affinity for the gut wall and its high first pass metabolism, very little loperamide reaches the systemic circulation.

5.3 Preclinical safety data
No relevant information additional to that contained elsewhere in the Summary of Product Characteristics.

6. PHARMACEUTICAL PARTICULARS
6.1 List of excipients
Capsules:

Lactose

Maize starch

Talc

Magnesium stearate

Capsule cap:

Titanium dioxide

Yellow ferric oxide

Indigotindisulphonate sodium

Gelatin

Capsule body:

Titanium dioxide

Black ferrous oxide

Indigotindisulphonate sodium

Erythrosin

Gelatin

Syrup:

Glycerol

Sodium saccharin

Methyl parahydroxybenzoate

Propyl parahydroxybenzoate

Cochineal Red A

Raspberry Flavour

Red Currant Flavour

Alcohol

Citric acid monohydrate

Purified water

6.2 Incompatibilities
Not applicable.

6.3 Shelf life
Capsules: 60 months.

Syrup: 60 months.

6.4 Special precautions for storage
Capsules: None.

Syrup: None.

6.5 Nature and contents of container
Capsules:

Blister packs consisting of aluminium foil, hermetalu and polyvinyl chloride genotherm glass clear.

The blister strips are packed in cardboard cartons to contain 2, 6, 8, 12, 18 or 30 capsules.

OR

Tubs of capsules containing 250 capsules.

Syrup:

Amber glass bottle with either a pilfer-proof aluminium screw cap coated on the inside with PVC or a child resistant polypropylene screw cap lined inside with an LDPE insert and a 5 ml or 10 ml polypropylene measuring cup.

Imodium syrup in bottle sizes of 100 mls.

6.6 Instructions for use and handling
Not applicable.

7. MARKETING AUTHORISATION HOLDER
Janssen-Cilag Ltd.

Saunderton

High Wycombe

Bucks

HP14 4HJ

UK

8. MARKETING AUTHORISATION NUMBER(S)
Capsules PL 0242/0028

Syrup PL 0242/0040

9. DATE OF FIRST AUTHORISATION/RENEWAL OF THE AUTHORISATION
Capsules: Date of Renewal of Authorisation: 18 June 2001

Syrup: Date of Renewal of Authorisation: 20 December 1996

10. DATE OF REVISION OF THE TEXT
Capsules: 6 July 2004

Syrup: 6 July 2004

Legal category Capsules: POM/P/GSL

Syrup: POM/P

Implanon 68mg implant for subdermal use

(Organon Laboratories Limited)

1. NAME OF THE MEDICINAL PRODUCT
Implanon®, 68mg implant for subdermal use.

2. QUALITATIVE AND QUANTITATIVE COMPOSITION
One implant contains 68mg of etonogestrel; the release rate is 60-70 μg/day in week 5-6 and has decreased to approximately 35-45 μg/day at the end of the first year, to approximately 30-40 μg/day at the end of the second year and to approximately 25-30 μg/day at the end of the third year.

For excipients see section 6.1

3. PHARMACEUTICAL FORM
Implant for subdermal use.

(Non-biodegradable white to off-white flexible rod).

4. CLINICAL PARTICULARS

4.1 Therapeutic indications
Contraception.

Safety and efficacy have been established in women between 18 and 40 years of age.

4.2 Posology and method of administration
4.2.1 HOW TO USE IMPLANON

Pregnancy should be excluded before insertion of Implanon.

Prior to inserting Implanon it is strongly recommended to carefully read the instructions for insertion and removal of the implant in section 4.2.2 ''How to insert Implanon'' and section 4.2.4 ''How to remove Implanon''.

Implanon is a long-acting contraceptive. One implant is inserted subdermally. The user should be informed that she can request the removal of Implanon at any time but the implant should not be left in place more than three years. Only a physician who is familiar with the removal technique should perform, on request or at the end of the 3 years of use, the removal of Implanon. After the removal of the implant, immediate insertion of another implant will result in continued contraceptive protection.

To ensure uncomplicated removal it is necessary that Implanon is inserted correctly, directly under the skin. The risk of complications is small if the provided instructions are followed.

Some cases have been reported in which the implant was not inserted correctly or was not inserted at all. Incidentally, this has resulted in an unintended pregnancy. The occurrence of such incidents can be minimised when the instructions for insertion (section 4.2.2 ''How to insert Implanon'') are strictly followed. The presence of the implant should be verified by palpation directly after insertion. In case the implant cannot be palpated or when the presence of the implant is doubtful, other methods must be applied to confirm its presence (see paragraph 4.2.2 ''How to insert Implanon''). Until the presence of Implanon has been verified a contraceptive barrier method must be used.

It is strongly recommended that physicians, prior to practicing the insertion of Implanon, participate in training sessions organised by Organon. Physicians who have little experience with subdermal insertion are advised to acquire the correct technique under supervision of a more experienced colleague. Additional information and more detailed instructions concerning the insertion and removal of Implanon will be sent on request free of charge (Organon Laboratories Ltd, Telephone 01223 432700).

The Implanon package contains a USER CARD intended for the user, and an adhesive label intended for the physician's user record. The USER CARD records the batch number of the provided implant, and helps to memorise the date of insertion, the arm of insertion, the name of the doctor and / or the hospital, and the intended day of removal. The adhesive label records the batch number and date of insertion.

4.2.2 HOW TO INSERT IMPLANON
(see Table 1 below)

4.2.3 WHEN TO INSERT IMPLANON
No preceding hormonal contraceptive use

Implanon should be inserted between Day 1-5, but at the latest on Day 5 of the woman's natural cycle (Day 1 is the first day of her menstrual bleeding).

Changing from a combined oral contraceptive (COC)

Implanon should be inserted preferably on the day after the last active tablet (the last tablet containing the active substances) of her previous COC, but at the latest on the day following the usual tablet-free interval or following the last placebo tablet of her previous COC.

Changing from a progestagen-only-method (minipill, injectable, a different implant)

Implanon may be inserted any day when the woman is switching from a minipill (from another implant on the day of its removal, from an injectable when the next injection would be due).

Following first-trimester abortion

Implanon should be inserted immediately.

Table 1 HOW TO INSERT IMPLANON

- Insertion of Implanon should be performed under aseptic conditions, and only by a physician who is familiar with the procedure.
- Insertion of Implanon is performed with the specially designed applicator. The use of this applicator differs substantially from that of a classical syringe. A drawing of a dismantled applicator and its individual components (e.g. cannula, obturator and needle with double-angled bevel) is shown in this leaflet to clarify their specific functions.
- The procedure used for insertion of Implanon **is opposite to giving an injection.** When inserting Implanon the **obturator** must remain fixed while the **cannula** (needle) is retracted from the arm. For normal injections the **plunger** is pushed and the **body** of the syringe remains fixed.
- Allow the subject to lie on her back with her non-dominant arm (the arm, which the woman does not use for writing) turned outwards and bent at the elbow.
- Implanon should be inserted at the inner side of the upper arm (non-dominant arm) about 6-8 cm above the elbow crease in the groove between the biceps and the triceps (sulcus bicipitalis medialis).
- Mark the insertion site.
- Clean the insertion site with a disinfectant.
- Anaesthetise with an anaesthetic spray, or with 2 ml of lidocaine (1%) applied just under the skin along the 'insertion canal'.
- Remove the sterile disposable applicator carrying Implanon from its blister and remove the needle shield.
- Always hold the applicator in the upward position (i.e. with the needle pointed upwards) until the time of insertion. This is to prevent the implant from dropping out.
- Visually verify the presence of the implant inside the metal part of the cannula (the needle). The implant can be seen as a white tip inside the needle. If the implant protrudes from the needle, return it to its original position by tapping against the plastic part of the cannula. Keep the needle and the implant sterile. If contamination occurs, a new package with a new sterile applicator must be used.

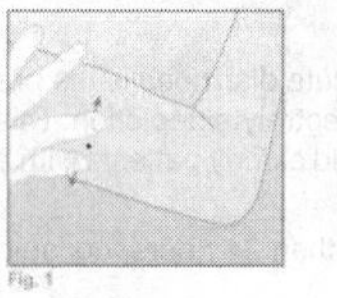
Fig. 1

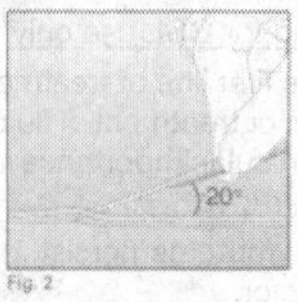

Fig. 2

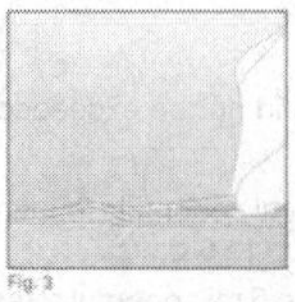
Fig. 3

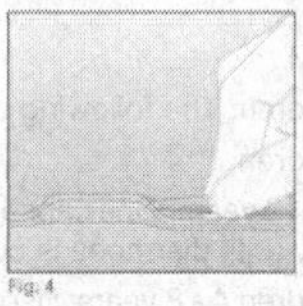
Fig. 4

- Stretch the skin around the insertion site with thumb and index finger (Figure 1).
- Insert only the tip of the needle, slightly angled (~ 20°) (Figure 2).
- Release the skin.
- Lower the applicator to a horizontal position (Figure 3).
- Lift the skin with the tip of the needle, but keep the needle in the subdermal connective tissue (Figure 4).
- Gently insert, while lifting the skin, the needle to its full length without using force.
- Keep the applicator parallel to the surface of the skin.
- **When the implant is placed too deeply the removal can be hampered later on.**

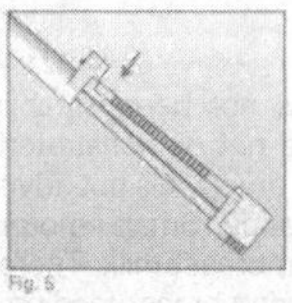
Fig. 5

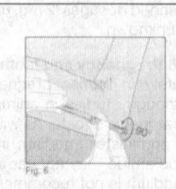

Fig. 6

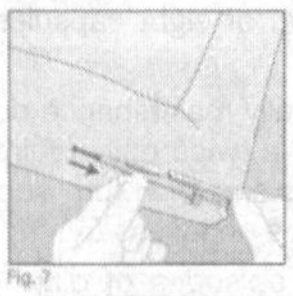
Fig. 7

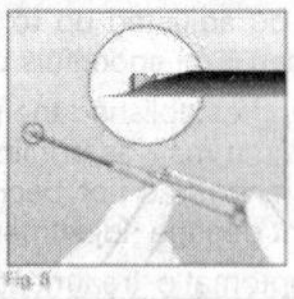
Fig. 8

- Break the seal of the applicator (Figure 5).
- Turn the **obturator** 90° (Figure 6).
- Fix the obturator with one hand against the arm and with the other hand slowly retract the **cannula** (needle) out of the arm (Figure 7).
- **Never push against the obturator.**
- Check the needle for the absence of the implant. After retraction of the cannula, the grooved tip of the obturator should be visible (Figure 8).
- **Always verify the presence of the implant by palpation.**
- In case the implant can not be palpated or when the presence of the implant is doubtful, other methods must be applied to confirm its presence. Suitable methods to locate the implant are first of all ultrasound (USS) and secondly magnetic resonance imaging (MRI). Prior to the application of USS or MRI for the localisation of Implanon it is recommended to consult Organon for instructions. In case these imaging methods fail, it is advised to verify the presence of the implant by measuring the etonogestrel level in a blood sample of the subject. In this case Organon will also provide the appropriate procedure.
- **Until the presence of Implanon has been confirmed a contraceptive barrier method must be used.**
- Apply sterile gauze with a pressure bandage to prevent bruising.
- Fill out the User Card and hand it over to the subject to facilitate removal of the implant later on.
- The applicator is for single use only and must be adequately disposed of, in accordance with local regulations for the handling of biohazardous waste.

Following childbirth or a second-trimester abortion

For breastfeeding women see "Use during pregnancy and lactation" (4.6)

Implanon should be inserted on day 21-28 after delivery or second-trimester abortion. When the implant is inserted later, the woman should be advised to additionally use a barrier method on the first 7 days after the insertion. However, if intercourse has already occurred, pregnancy should be excluded or the woman's first natural period should be awaited before the actual insertion of the implant.

4.2.4 HOW TO REMOVE IMPLANON

(see Table 2)

4.3 Contraindications

- Active venous thromboembolic disorder.
- Progestagen-dependent tumours.
- Presence or history of severe hepatic disease as long as liver function values have not returned to normal.
- Undiagnosed vaginal bleeding.
- Hypersensitivity to the active substance or to any of the excipients of Implanon.

4.4 Special warnings and special precautions for use

4.4.1 WARNINGS

If any of the conditions / risk factors mentioned below is present, the benefits of progestagen use should be weighed against the possible risks for each individual woman and discussed with the woman before she decides to start with Implanon. In the event of aggravation, exacerbation or first appearance of any of these conditions, the woman should contact her physician. The physician should then decide on whether the use of Implanon should be discontinued.

- The risk for breast cancer increases in general with increasing age. During the use of oral contraceptives (OCs) the risk of having breast cancer diagnosed is slightly increased. This increased risk disappears gradually within 10 years after discontinuation of OC use and is not related to the duration of use, but to the age of the woman when using the OC. The expected number of cases diagnosed per 10,000 women who use combined OCs (up to 10 years after stopping) relative to never users over the same period have been calculated for the respective age groups to be: 4.5/4 (16-19 years), 17.5/16 (20-24 years), 48.7/44 (25-29 years), 110/100 (30-34 years), 180/160 (35-39 years) and 260/230 (40-44 years). The risk in users of contraceptive methods, which only contain progestagens, is possibly of similar magnitude as that associated with combined OCs. However, for these methods, the evidence is less conclusive. Compared to the risk of getting breast cancer ever in life, the increased risk associated with OCs is low. The cases of breast cancer diagnosed in OC users tend to be less advanced than in those who have not used OCs. The increased risk observed in OC users may be due to an earlier diagnosis, biological effects of the OC or a combination of both. Since a biological effect of hormones cannot be excluded, an individual benefit/risk assessment should be made in women with pre-existing breast cancer and in women in whom breast cancer is diagnosed while using Implanon.
- Epidemiological investigations have associated the use of combined OCs with an increased incidence of venous thromboembolism (VTE, deep venous thrombosis and pulmonary embolism). Although the clinical relevance of this finding for etonogestrel (the biologically active metabolite of desogestrel) used as a contraceptive in the absence of an estrogenic component is unknown, Implanon should be removed in the event of a thrombosis. Removal of Implanon should also be considered in case of long-term immobilisation due to surgery or illness. Women with a history of thrombo-embolic disorders should be made aware of the possibility of a recurrence.
- If a sustained hypertension develops during the use of Implanon, or if a significant increase in blood pressure does not adequately respond to antihypertensive therapy, the use of Implanon should be discontinued.
- When acute or chronic disturbances of liver function occur the woman should be referred to a specialist for examination and advice.
- The use of progestagen-containing contraceptives may have an effect on peripheral insulin resistance and glucose tolerance. Therefore, diabetic women should be carefully monitored during the first months of Implanonuse.
- Chloasma may occasionally occur, especially in women with a history of chloasma gravidarum. Women with a tendency to chloasma should avoid exposure to the sun or ultraviolet radiation whilst using Implanon.
- The contraceptive effect of Implanon is related to the plasma levels of etonogestrel, which are inversely related to body weight, and decrease with time after insertion. The clinical experience with Implanon in heavier women in the third year of use is limited. Therefore it can not be excluded that the contraceptive effect in these women during the third year of use may be lower than for women of normal weight. Clinicians may therefore consider earlier replacement of the implant in heavier women.
- Expulsion may occur if the implant is inserted not according to the instructions given in section 4.2.2 "How to insert Implanon".

Table 2 HOW TO REMOVE IMPLANON

- Removal of Implanon should only be performed by a physician who is familiar with the removal technique.

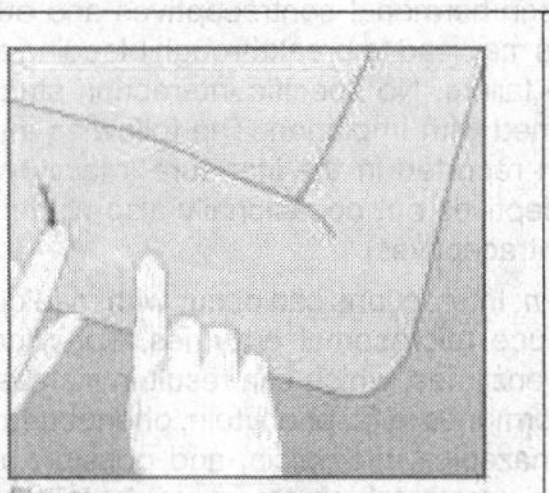

Fig. a

- The precise location of the implant is indicated on the USER CARD
- Locate the implant by palpation and mark the distal end. In case that Implanon cannot be palpated it is strongly advised to locate the implant by either ultrasound (USS) or magnetic resonance imaging (MRI). Prior to the application of USS and MRI for the localisation of Implanon it is recommended to consult Organon for the proper instructions (Figure a).
- A non-palpable implant should always first be localised by USS (or MRI) and subsequently be removed under the guidance of USS.
- Wash the area and apply a disinfectant

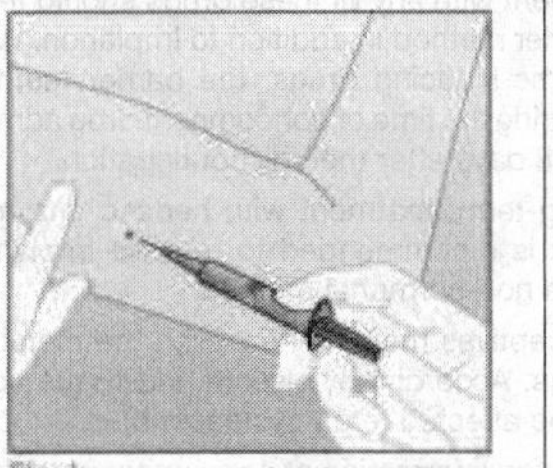

Fig. b

- Anaesthetise the arm with 0.5-1 ml lidocaine (1%) at the site of incision, which is just below the distal end of the implant. Note: Apply the anaesthetic **under** the implant. Application **above** the implant makes the skin swell, which may cause difficulties in locating the implant (Figure b).

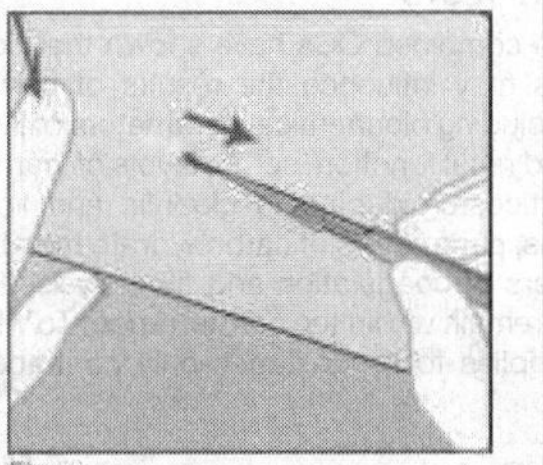

Fig. c

- Make an incision of 2 mm in length in the longitudinal direction of the arm at the distal end of the implant (Figure c).

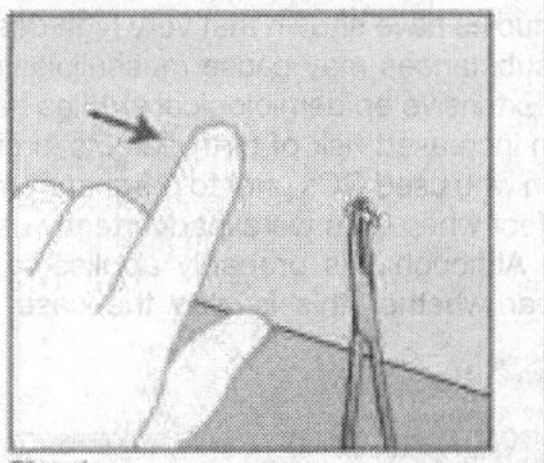

Fig. d

- Gently push the implant towards the incision until the tip is visible. Grasp the implant with forceps (preferably 'mosquito' forceps) and remove it (Figure d).

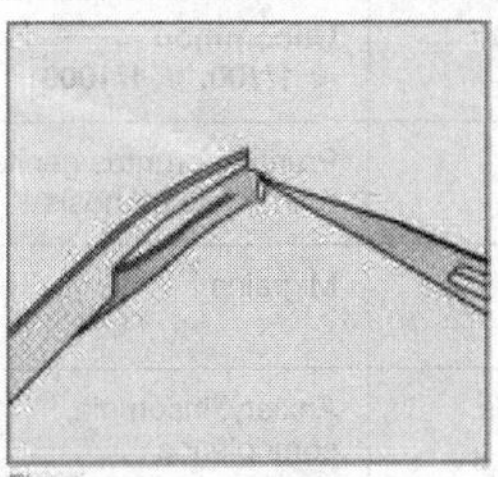

Fig. e

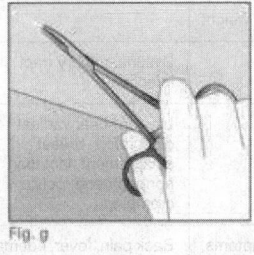

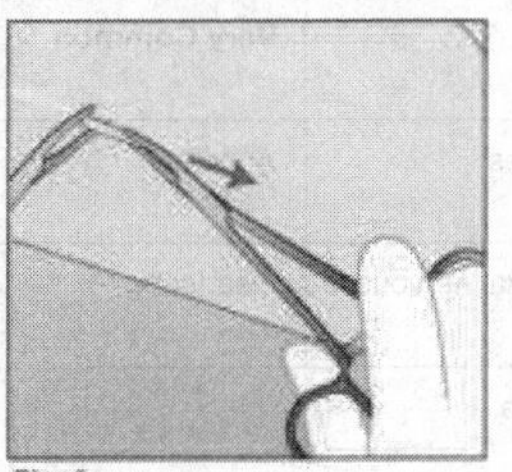

Fig. f

- If the implant is encapsulated, an incision into the tissue sheath should be made and the implant then removed with forceps (Figures e and f).

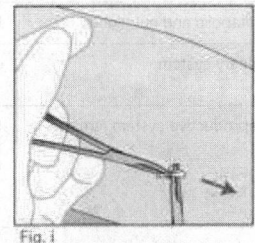

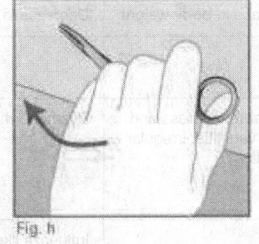

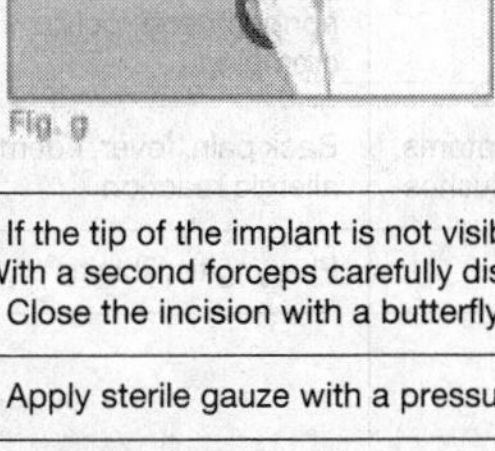

Fig. g

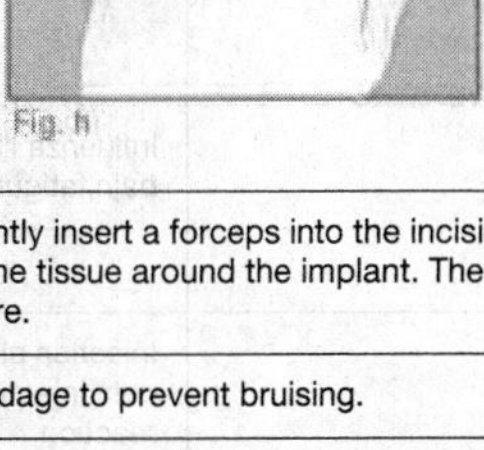

Fig. h

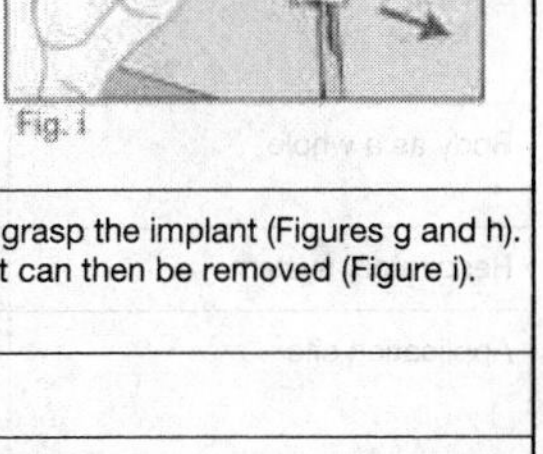

Fig. i

- If the tip of the implant is not visible, gently insert a forceps into the incision and grasp the implant (Figures g and h). With a second forceps carefully dissect the tissue around the implant. The implant can then be removed (Figure i).
- Close the incision with a butterfly closure.

- Apply sterile gauze with a pressure bandage to prevent bruising.

- There have been occasional reports of displacement of the implant; usually this involves minor movement relative to the original position. This may somewhat complicate removal.

• With all low-dose hormonal contraceptives, follicular development occurs and occasionally the follicle may continue to grow beyond the size it would attain in a normal cycle. Generally, these enlarged follicles disappear spontaneously. Often, they are asymptomatic; in some cases they are associated with mild abdominal pain. They rarely require surgical intervention.

• The protection with traditional progestagen-only contraceptives against ectopic pregnancies is not as good as with combined OCs, which has been associated with the frequent occurrence of ovulations during the use of these methods. Despite the fact that Implanon consistently inhibits ovulation, ectopic pregnancy should be taken into account in the differential diagnosis if the woman gets amenorrhoea or abdominal pain.

• The following conditions have been reported both during pregnancy and during sex steroid use, but an association with the use of progestagens has not been established: jaundice and/or pruritus related to cholestasis; gallstone formation; porphyria; systemic lupus erythematosis; haemolytic uraemic syndrome; Sydenham's chorea; herpes gestationis; otosclerosis-related hearing loss.

4.4.2 MEDICAL EXAMINATION/CONSULTATION

Prior to the initiation or reinstitution of Implanon a complete medical history (including family medical history) should be taken and pregnancy should be excluded. Blood pressure should be measured and a physical examination should be performed, guided by the contraindications (Section 4.3) and warnings (Section 4.4.1). It is recommended that the woman returns for a medical check-up three months after insertion of Implanon. During this check-up, the blood pressure should be measured and an enquiry should be made after any questions, complaints or the occurrence of undesirable effects. The frequency and nature of further periodic checks should be adapted to the individual woman, guided by clinical judgment.

Women should be advised that Implanon does not protect against HIV (AIDS) and other sexually transmitted diseases.

4.4.3 REDUCED EFFICACY

The efficacy of Implanon may be reduced when concomitant medication is used (See "Interactions" (4.5.1)).

4.4.4 CHANGES IN THE VAGINAL BLEEDING PATTERN

During the use of Implanon, vaginal bleeding may become more frequent or of longer duration in most women. In other women bleeding may become incidental or be totally absent (approximately in 1 out of 5 women). Information, counselling and the use of a bleeding diary can improve the woman's acceptance of a bleeding pattern. Evaluation of vaginal bleeding should be done on an ad hoc basis and may include an examination to exclude gynaecological pathology or pregnancy.

4.5 Interaction with other medicinal products and other forms of Interaction

4.5.1 INTERACTIONS

Interactions between hormonal contraceptives and other medicinal products may lead to breakthrough bleeding and / or contraceptive failure. No specific interaction studies have been performed with Implanon. The following interactions have been reported in the literature (mainly with combined contraceptives but occasionally also with progestogen-only contraceptives).

Hepatic metabolism: Interactions can occur with medicinal products that induce microsomal enzymes, specifically cytochrome P450 enzymes, which can result in increased clearance of sex hormones (e.g., phenytoin, phenobarbital, primidone, carbamazepine, rifampicin, and possibly also oxcarbazepine, topiramate, felbamate, ritonavir, nelfinavir, griseofulvin and the herbal remedy St. John's wort).

Women on treatment with any of these drugs should temporarily use a barrier method in addition to Implanon. With microsomal enzyme-inducing drugs, the barrier method should be used during the time of concomitant drug administration and for 28 days after their discontinuation.

In women on long-term treatment with hepatic enzyme-inducing drugs, it is recommended to remove Implanon and to prescribe a non-hormonal method.

Hormonal contraceptives may interfere with the metabolism of other drugs. Accordingly, plasma and tissue concentrations may be affected (e.g., cyclosporin).

Note: The prescribing information of concomitant medications should be consulted to identify potential interactions.

4.5.2 LABORATORY TESTS

Data obtained with combined OCs have shown that contraceptive steroids may influence the results of certain laboratory tests, including biochemical parameters of liver, thyroid, adrenal and renal function, serum levels of (carrier) proteins, e.g., corticosteroid binding globulin and lipid/lipoprotein fractions, parameters of carbohydrate metabolism and parameters of coagulation and fibrinolysis. The changes generally remain within the normal range. To what extent this also applies to progestagen-only contraceptives is not known.

4.6 Pregnancy and lactation

Implanon is not indicated during pregnancy. If pregnancy occurs during use of Implanon, the implant should be removed. Animal studies have shown that very high doses of progestagenic substances may cause masculinisation of female fetuses. Extensive epidemiological studies have revealed neither an increased risk of birth defects in children born to women who used OCs prior to pregnancy, nor of a teratogenic effect when OCs were inadvertently used during pregnancy. Although this probably applies to all OCs, it is not clear whether this is also the case for Implanon.

Pharmacovigilance data with various desogestrel-containing combined OCs (etonogestrel is a metabolite of desogestrel) also do not indicate an increased risk.

Implanon does not influence the production or the quality (protein, lactose or fat concentrations) of breast milk. However, small amounts of etonogestrel are excreted in breast milk. Based on daily milk ingestion of 150 ml/kg, the mean daily infant etonogestrel dose calculated after one month of etonogestrel release is approximately 27 ng/kg/day. This corresponds to approximately 2.2% of the weight-adjusted maternal daily dose and to approximately 0.2% of the estimated absolute maternal daily dose. Subsequently the milk etonogestrel concentration decreases with time during the lactation period.

Limited long-term data are available on 38 children, whose mothers started using Implanon during the 4th to 8th week postpartum. They were breast-fed for a mean duration of 14 months and followed-up to 36 months of age. Evaluation of growth, and physical and psychomotor development did not indicate any differences in comparison to nursing infants whose mothers used an IUD (n=33). Nevertheless, development and growth of the child should be carefully followed. Based on the available data, Implanon may be used during lactation.

4.7 Effects on ability to drive and use machines

On the basis of the pharmacodynamic profile, Implanon is expected to have no or negligible influence on the ability to drive or use machines.

4.8 Undesirable effects

Possibly related undesirable effects in the clinical trials with Implanon have been listed in the Table below.

(see Table 3)

In rare cases, a clinically relevant rise in blood pressure has been observed during the use of Implanon. Insertion or removal of Implanon may cause some bruising, slight local irritation, pain or itching. Occasionally fibrosis at the injection site may occur or a scar may be formed.

A number of undesirable effects have been reported in women using oral contraceptives, which are discussed in more detail in Section 4.4 "Special warnings and precautions for use." These include: venous thromboembolic disorders, arterial thromboembolic disorders, hypertension, hormone-dependent tumours (e.g. liver tumours, breast cancer) and chloasma.

4.9 Overdose

An implant should always be removed before inserting a new one. There are no data available on overdose with etonogestrel. There have been no reports of serious deleterious effects from an overdose of contraceptives in general.

5. PHARMACOLOGICAL PROPERTIES

5.1 Pharmacodynamic properties

(PHARMACOTHERAPEUTIC GROUP: PROGESTAGENS, ATC-classification G03AC08)

Implanon is a non-biodegradable, etonogestrel-containing implant for subdermal use. Etonogestrel is the biologically active metabolite of desogestrel, a progestagen widely used in OCs. It is structurally derived from 19-nortestosterone and binds with high affinity to progesterone receptors in the target organs. The contraceptive effect of Implanon is primarily achieved by inhibition of ovulation. Ovulations were not observed in the first two years of use and only rarely in the third year. Besides inhibition of ovulation, Implanon also causes changes in the cervical mucus, which hinders the passage of spermatozoa. Clinical trials were conducted in women between 18 and 40 years Although no direct comparison was made, the contraceptive efficacy appeared to be at least comparable with that known for combined oral contraceptives. The high degree of protection against pregnancy is obtained among other reasons because, in contrast to OCs, the contraceptive action of Implanon is not dependent on the regular intake of tablets. The contraceptive action of Implanon is reversible, which is apparent from the rapid return of the normal menstrual cycle after removal of the implant. Although Implanon inhibits ovulation, ovarian activity is not completely suppressed. Mean estradiol concentrations remain above the level seen in the early-follicular phase. In a two-year study, in which the bone mineral density in 44 Implanon users has been compared with that in a control group of 29 IUD-users no adverse effects on bone mass have been observed. During the use of Implanon no clinically relevant effects on lipid metabolism have been observed. The use of progestagen-containing contraceptives may have an effect on insulin resistance and glucose tolerance. In clinical trials it has further been shown that Implanon users often have a less painful menstrual bleeding.

5.2 Pharmacokinetic properties

ABSORPTION

After the insertion of Implanon, etonogestrel is rapidly absorbed into the circulation. Ovulation-inhibiting concentrations are reached within 1 day. Maximum serum concentrations (between 472 and 1270 pg/ml) are reached within 1 to 13 days. The release rate of the implant decreases with time. As a result serum concentrations decline rapidly over the first few months. By the end of the first year a mean concentration of approximately 200 pg/ml (range 150-261 pg/ml) is measured, which slowly

Table 3

Body system	Frequency of adverse reactions		
	Very Common > 1/10	**Common < 1/10 ⩾ 1/100**	**Uncommon < 1/100, ⩾ 1/1000**
Skin and appendages	Acne	Alopecia	Pruritus, pruritus genital, rash, hypertrichosis
Central and peripheral nervous system	Headache	Dizziness	Migraine
Psychiatric disorders		Depressive moods, emotional lability, nervousness, libido changes, appetite decreased	Anxiety, insomnia, somnolence
Gastro-intestinal system		Abdominal pain, nausea, flatulence	Diarrhoea, vomiting, constipation
Metabolic and nutritional	Increase in body weight	Decrease in body weight	
Urinary system			Dysuria, urinary tract infection
Reproductive system female	Breast tenderness and pain, vaginitis, irregular bleeding	Dysmenorrhoea	Leukorrhoea, vaginal discomfort, breast enlargement, lactation nonpeurperal, pelvic cramping
Body as a whole		Influenza like symptoms, pain,fatigue, hot flushes	Back pain, fever, edema, allergic reaction
Respiratory system			Pharyngitis,Rhinitis
Application site		Injection site pain,injection site reaction	
Musculoskeletal system			Arthralgia,myalgia, skeletal pain

decreases to 156 pg/ml (range 111-202 pg/ml) by the end of the third year. The variations observed in serum concentrations can be partly attributed to differences in body weight.

DISTRIBUTION

Etonogestrel is for 95.5-99% bound to serum proteins, predominantly to albumin and to a lesser extent to sex hormone binding globulin. The central and total volume of distribution are 27 l and 220 l, respectively, and hardly change during the use of Implanon.

METABOLISM

Etonogestrel undergoes hydroxylation and reduction. Metabolites are conjugated to sulfates and glucuronides. Animal studies show that enterohepatic circulation probably does not contribute to the progestagenic activity of etonogestrel.

ELIMINATION

After intravenous administration of etonogestrel, the mean elimination half-life is approximately 25 hours and the serum clearance is approximately 7.5 l/hour. Both clearance and elimination-half-life remain constant during the treatment period. The excretion of etonogestrel and its metabolites, either as free steroids or as conjugates, is with urine and faeces (ratio 1.5:1). After oral intake of desogestrel by lactating women, the active metabolite etonogestrel is excreted in breast milk with a milk/serum ratio of 0.37-0.55. In lactating women using Implanon, the mean transfer of etonogestrel to the infant is approximately 2.2% of the maternal etonogestrel daily dose (values normalised per kg bodyweight). Concentrations show a gradual and statistically significant decrease over the time.

5.3 Preclinical safety data

Toxicological studies did not reveal any effects other than those, which can be explained on the basis of the hormonal properties of etonogestrel, regardless of the route of administration.

6. PHARMACEUTICAL PARTICULARS

6.1 List of excipients

Implant

Core: Ethylene vinylacetate copolymer (28% vinyl acetate).

Skin: Ethylene vinylacetate copolymer (14% vinyl acetate).

6.2 Incompatibilities

Not applicable

6.3 Shelf life

5 years

Implanon should not be inserted after the expiry date as indicated on the primary package.

6.4 Special precautions for storage

Store in the original package in order to protect from light.

6.5 Nature and contents of container

The pack contains one implant (4 cm in length and 2 mm in diameter) in the cannula of a disposable sterile applicator. The applicator consists of acrylonitrile-butadiene-styrene body with a stainless steel needle and a polypropylene shield. The applicator containing the implant is packed in a blister pack made of transparent polyethyleneterephtalate glycol sealed with coated paper.

6.6 Instructions for use and handling

See Section 4.2 (Posology and Method of Administration).

The applicator is for single use only.

7. MARKETING AUTHORISATION HOLDER

ORGANON LABORATORIES LTD, CAMBRIDGE SCIENCE PARK, MILTON ROAD, CAMBRIDGE, CB4 0FL, UK

8. MARKETING AUTHORISATION NUMBER(S)

PL 0065/0161

9. DATE OF FIRST AUTHORISATION/RENEWAL OF THE AUTHORISATION

9 June 1999 / 11 December 2003

10. DATE OF REVISION OF THE TEXT

December 2004

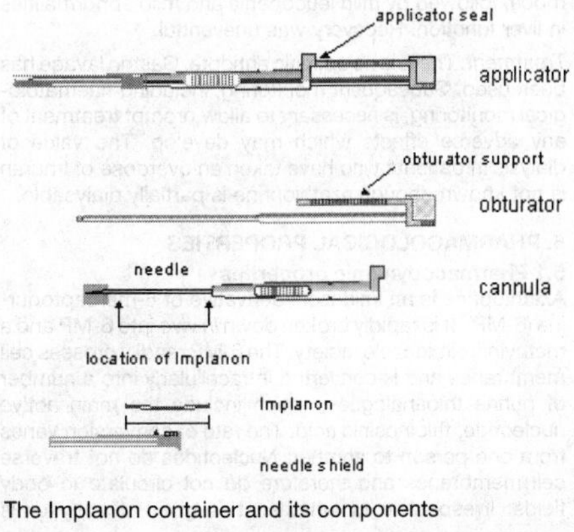

The Implanon container and its components

Imuran Injection

(GlaxoSmithKline UK)

1. NAME OF THE MEDICINAL PRODUCT

Imuran Injection.

2. QUALITATIVE AND QUANTITATIVE COMPOSITION

Azathioprine EP 50 mg/vial.

3. PHARMACEUTICAL FORM

Injection.

4. CLINICAL PARTICULARS

4.1 Therapeutic indications

Imuran is used as an immunosuppressant antimetabolite either alone or, more commonly, in combination with other agents (usually corticosteroids) and procedures which influence the immune response. Therapeutic effect may be evident only after weeks or months and can include a steroid-sparing effect, thereby reducing the toxicity associated with high dosage and prolonged usage of corticosteroids.

Imuran, in combination with corticosteroids and/or other immunosuppressive agents and procedures, is indicated to enhance the survival of organ transplants, such as renal transplants, cardiac transplants, and hepatic transplants, and to reduce the corticosteroid requirement of renal transplant recipients.

Imuran, either alone or more usually in combination with corticosteroids and/or other drugs and procedures, has been used with clinical benefit (which may include reduction of dosage or discontinuation of corticosteroids) in a proportion of patients suffering from the following:

severe rheumatoid arthritis;

systemic lupus erythematosus;

dermatomyositis and polymyositis;

auto-immune chronic active hepatitis;

pemphigus vulgaris;

polyarteritis nodosa;

auto-immune haemolytic anaemia;

chronic refractory idiopathic thrombocytopenic purpura.

4.2 Posology and method of administration

Imuran Injection should be used ONLY when the oral route is impractical, and should be discontinued as soon as oral therapy is tolerated. It must be administered only by the intravenous route.

Specialist medical literature should be consulted for guidance as to clinical experience in particular conditions.

Dosage in transplantation - adults and children

Depending on the immunosuppressive regimen employed, a dosage of up to 5 mg/kg bodyweight/day may be given on the first day of therapy, either orally or intravenously.

Maintenance dosage should range from 1 to 4 mg/kg bodyweight/day and must be adjusted according to clinical requirements and haematological tolerance.

Evidence indicates that Imuran therapy should be maintained indefinitely, even if only low doses are necessary, because of the risk of graft rejection.

Dosage in other conditions - adults and children

In general, starting dosage is from 1 to 3 mg/kg bodyweight/day, and should be adjusted, within these limits, depending on the clinical response (which may not be evident for weeks or months) and haematological tolerance.

When therapeutic response is evident, consideration should be given to reducing the maintenance dosage to the lowest level compatible with the maintenance of that response. If no improvement occurs in the patient's condition within 3 months, consideration should be given to withdrawing Imuran.

The maintenance dosage required may range from less than 1 mg/kg bodyweight/day to 3 mg/kg bodyweight/day, depending on the clinical condition being treated and the individual patient response, including haematological tolerance.

In patients with renal and/or hepatic insufficiency, dosages should be given at the lower end of the normal range (see Special Precautions for Use for further details).

Use in the elderly (see Renal and/or hepatic insufficiency)

There is a limited experience of the administration of Imuran to elderly patients. Although the available data do not provide evidence that the incidence of side effects among elderly patients is higher than that among other patients treated with Imuran, it is recommended that the dosages used should be at the lower end of the range.

Particular care should be taken to monitor haematological response and to reduce the maintenance dosage to the minimum required for clinical response.

Reconstitution and dilution of Imuran Injection

Precautions should always be taken when handling Imuran Injection (see section 6.6 Instructions for Use/Handling).

No antimicrobial preservative is included. Therefore reconstitution and dilution must be carried out under full aseptic conditions, preferably immediately before use. Any unused solution should be discarded.

The contents of each vial should be reconstituted by the addition of 5 ml to 15 ml of Water for Injections BP. The reconstituted solution is stable for up to 5 days when stored between 5°C and 25°C.

When diluted on the basis of 5 ml of reconstituted solution to a volume of between 20 ml and 200 ml of one of the following infusion solutions, Imuran is stable for up to 24 hours at room temperature (15°C to 25°C):

Sodium Chloride Intravenous Infusion BP (0.45% w/v and 0.9% w/v)

Sodium Chloride (0.18% w/v) and Glucose (4.0% w/v) Intravenous Infusion BP.

Should any visible turbidity or crystallisation appear in the reconstituted or diluted solution the preparation must be discarded.

Imuran Injection should ONLY be reconstituted with the recommended volume of Water for Injections BP and should be diluted as specified above. Imuran Injection should not be mixed with other drugs or fluids, except those specified above, before administration.

Administration of Imuran Injection

Imuran Injection, when reconstituted as directed, is a very irritant solution with a pH of 10 to 12.

When the reconstituted solution is diluted as directed above, the pH of the resulting solution may be expected to be within the range pH 8.0 to 9.5 (the greater the dilution, the lower the pH).

Where dilution is not practicable, the reconstituted solution should be injected slowly over a period of not less than one minute and followed immediately by not less than 50 ml of one of the recommended infusion solutions.

Care must be taken to avoid perivenous injection, which may produce tissue damage.

4.3 Contraindications

Imuran is contra-indicated in patients known to be hypersensitive to azathioprine. Hypersensitivity to 6-mercaptopurine (6-MP) should alert the prescriber to probable hypersensitivity to Imuran.

Imuran therapy should not be initiated in patients who may be pregnant, or who are likely to become pregnant without careful assessment of risk versus benefit (see section 4.4 Special Warnings and Precautions for Use & section 4.6 Pregnancy and Lactation).

4.4 Special warnings and special precautions for use

Monitoring

There are potential hazards in the use of Imuran. It should be prescribed only if the patient can be adequately monitored for toxic effects throughout the duration of therapy.

It is suggested that during the first 8 weeks of therapy, complete blood counts, including platelets, should be performed weekly or more frequently if high dosage is used or if severe renal and/or hepatic disorder is present. The blood count frequency may be reduced later in therapy, but it is suggested that complete blood counts are repeated monthly, or at least at intervals of not longer than 3 months.

Patients receiving Imuran should be instructed to report immediately any evidence of infection, unexpected bruising or bleeding or other manifestations of bone marrow depression.

There are individuals with an inherited deficiency of the enzyme thiopurine methyltransferase (TPMT) who may be unusually sensitive to the myelosuppressive effect of azathioprine and prone to developing rapid bone marrow depression following the initiation of treatment with Imuran. This problem could be exacerbated by co-administration with drugs that inhibit TPMT, such as olsalazine, mesalazine or sulphasalazine.

Renal and/or hepatic insufficiency

It has been suggested that the toxicity of Imuran may be enhanced in the presence of renal insufficiency, but controlled studies have not supported this suggestion. Nevertheless, it is recommended that the dosages used should be at the lower end of the normal range and that haematological response should be carefully monitored. Dosage should be further reduced if haematological toxicity occurs.

Caution is necessary during the administration of Imuran to patients with hepatic dysfunction, and regular complete blood counts and liver function tests should be undertaken. In such patients the metabolism of Imuran may be impaired, and the dosage of Imuran should therefore be reduced if hepatic or haematological toxicity occurs.

Limited evidence suggests that Imuran is not beneficial to patients with hypoxanthine-guanine-phosphoribosyltransferase deficiency (Lesch-Nyhan syndrome). Therefore, given the abnormal metabolism in these patients, it is not prudent to recommend that these patients should receive Imuran.

Mutagenicity

Chromosomal abnormalities have been demonstrated in both male and female patients treated with Imuran. It is difficult to assess the role of Imuran in the development of these abnormalities.

Effects on fertility

Relief of chronic renal insufficiency by renal transplantation involving the administration of Imuran has been accompanied by increased fertility in both male and female transplant recipients.

Carcinogenicity (see also section 4.8 Undesirable Effects)

Patients receiving immunosuppressive therapy are at an increased risk of developing lymphomas and other malignancies, notably skin cancers. The risk appears to be related to the intensity and duration of immunosuppression rather than to the use of any specific agent. It has been reported that reduction or discontinuation of immunosuppression may cause lymphomas to regress.

Patients receiving multiple immunosuppressive agents may be at risk of over-immunosuppression, therefore such therapy should be maintained at the lowest effective level.

As is usual for patients with increased risk for skin cancer, exposure to sunlight and UV light should be limited by wearing protective clothing and using a sunscreen with a high protection factor.

4.5 Interaction with other medicinal products and other forms of Interaction

Allopurinol/ oxipurinol/ thiopurinol

Xanthine oxidase activity is inhibited by allopurinol, oxipurinol and thiopurinol which results in reduced conversion of biologically active 6-thioinosinic acid to biologically inactive 6-thiouric acid. When allopurinol, oxipurinol and/or thiopurinol are given concomitantly with 6-mercaptopurine or azathioprine, the dose of 6-mercaptopurine and azathioprine should be reduced to one-quarter of the original dose.

Neuromuscular blocking agents

Imuran can potentiate the neuromuscular blockade produced by depolarising agents such as succinylcholine and can reduce the blockade produced by non-depolarising agents such as tubocurarine. There is considerable variation in the potency of this interaction.

Warfarin

Inhibition of the anticoagulant effect of warfarin, when administered with azathioprine, has been reported.

Cytostatic/myelosuppressive agents

Where possible, concomitant administration of cytostatic drugs, or drugs which may have a myelosuppressive effect, such as penicillamine, should be avoided. There are conflicting clinical reports of interactions, resulting in serious haematological abnormalities, between Imuran and co-trimoxazole.

There has been a case report suggesting that haematological abnormalities may develop due to the concomitant administration of Imuran and captopril.

It has been suggested that cimetidine and indomethacin may have myelosuppressive effects, which may be enhanced by concomitant administration of Imuran.

Other interactions

As there is *in vitro* evidence that aminosalicylate derivatives (eg. olsalazine, mesalazine or sulphasalazine) inhibit the TPMT enzyme, they should be administered with caution to patients receiving concurrent Imuran therapy (see section 4.4 Special Warnings and Special Precautions for Use).

Frusemide has been shown to impair the metabolism of azathioprine by human hepatic tissue *in vitro*. The clinical significance is unknown.

Vaccines

The immunosuppressive activity of Imuran could result in an atypical and potentially deleterious response to live vaccines and so the administration of live vaccines to patients receiving Imuran therapy is contra-indicated on theoretical grounds.

A diminished response to killed vaccines is likely and such a response to hepatitis B vaccine has been observed among patients treated with a combination of azathioprine and corticosteroids.

A small clinical study has indicated that standard therapeutic doses of Imuran do not deleteriously affect the response to polyvalent pneumococcal vaccine, as assessed on the basis of mean anti-capsular specific antibody concentration.

4.6 Pregnancy and lactation

Teratogenicity

Studies in pregnant rats, mice and rabbits using azathioprine in dosages from 5 to 15 mg/kg body weight/day over the period of organogenesis have shown varying degrees of foetal abnormalities. Teratogenicity was evident in rabbits at 10 mg/kg body weight/day.

Evidence of the teratogenicity of Imuran in man is equivocal. As with all cytotoxic chemotherapy, adequate contraceptive precautions should be advised when either partner is receiving Imuran.

Mutagenicity

Chromosomal abnormalities, which disappear with time, have been demonstrated in lymphocytes from the offspring of patients treated with Imuran. Except in extremely rare cases, no overt physical evidence of abnormality has been observed in the offspring of patients treated with Imuran. Azathioprine and long-wave ultraviolet light have been shown to have a synergistic clastogenic effect in patients treated with azathioprine for a range of disorders.

Use in Pregnancy and Lactation

Imuran should not be given to patients who are pregnant or likely to become pregnant without careful assessment of risk versus benefit.

There have been reports of premature birth and low birth weight following maternal exposure to azathioprine, particularly in combination with corticosteroids. There have also been reports of spontaneous abortion following either maternal or paternal exposure.

Azathioprine and/or its metabolites have been found in low concentrations in foetal blood and amniotic fluid after maternal administration of azathioprine.

Leucopenia and/or thrombocytopenia have been reported in a proportion of neonates whose mothers took azathioprine throughout their pregnancies. Extra care in haematological monitoring is advised during pregnancy.

Lactation

6-Mercaptopurine has been identified in the colostrum and breast-milk of women receiving azathioprine treatment.

4.7 Effects on ability to drive and use machines

None known.

4.8 Undesirable effects

For this product there is no modern clinical documentation that can be used as support for determining the frequency of undesirable effects. Undesirable effects may vary in their incidence depending on the indication. The following convention has been utilised for the classification of frequency: Very common, $\geqslant$ 1/10; common, $\geqslant$ 1/100 and $<$ 1/10; uncommon, $\geqslant$ 1/1000 and $<$ 1/100; rare, $\geqslant$ 1/10000 and $<$ 1/1000; very rare, $<$ 1/10000.

Infection and infestations

Transplant patients receiving Imuran in combination with other immunosuppressants.

Very common:	Viral, fungal, and bacterial infections.

Other indications.

Uncommon:	Viral, fungal and bacterial infections.

Patients receiving Imuran alone, or in combination with other immunosupressants, particularly corticosteroids, have shown increased susceptibility to viral, fungal and bacterial infections.

<u>Neoplasms benign and malignant (including cysts and polyps).</u>

Rare:	Neoplasms including lymphomas, skin cancers, acute myloid leukaemia and myelodysplasia (see also section 4.4 Special Warnings and Special Precautions for Use).

The risk of developing lymphomas and other malignancies, notably skin cancer is increased in patients who receive immunosuppressive drugs, particularly in transplant recipients receiving aggressive treatment and such therapy should be maintained at the lowest effective levels. The increased risk of developing lymphomas in immunosuppressed rheumatoid arthritis patients compared with the general population appears to be related at least in part to the disease itself.

There have been rare reports of acute myeloid leukaemia and myelodysplasia (some in association with chromosomal abnormalities).

<u>Blood and lymphatic system disorders</u>

Very common:	Depression of bone marrow function; leucopenia.
Common:	Thrombocytopenia.
Uncommon:	Anaemia.
Rare:	Agranulocytosis, pancytopenia, aplastic anaemia, megaloblastic anaemia, erythriod hypoplasia.

Imuran may be associated with a dose-related, generally reversible, depression of bone marrow function, most frequently expressed as leucopenia, but also sometimes as anaemia and thrombocytopenia, and rarely as agranulocytosis, pancytopenia and aplastic anaemia. These occur particularly in patients predisposed to myelotoxicity, such as those with TPMP deficiency and renal or hepatic insufficiency and in patients failing to reduce the dose of Imuran when receiving concurrent allopurinol therapy.

Reversible, dose-related increases in mean corpuscular volume and red cell haemoglobin content have occurred in association with Imuran therapy. Megaloblastic bone marrow changes have also been observed but severe megaloblastic anaemia and erythroid hypoplasia are rare.

<u>Respiratory, thorasic and mediastinal disorders</u>

Very rare:	Reversible pneumonitis.

Reversible pneumonitis has been described very rarely.

<u>Gastrointestinal disorders</u>

Uncommon:	Pancreatitis.
Rare:	Colitis, diverticulitis and bowel perforation reported in transplant population, severe diarrhoea in inflammatory bowel disease population.

Serious complications, including colitis, diverticulitis and bowel perforation, have been described in transplant recipients receiving immunosuppressive therapy. However, the aetiology is not clearly established and high-dose corticosteroids may be implicated. Severe diarrhoea, recurring on re-challenge, has been reported in patients treated with Imuran for inflammatory bowel disease. The possibility that exacerbation of symptoms might be drug-related should be borne in mind when treating such patients.

Pancreatitis has been reported in a small percentage of patients on Imuran therapy, particularly in renal transplant patients and those diagnosed as having inflammatory bowel disease. There are difficulties in relating the pancreatitis to the administration of one particular drug, although re-challenge has confirmed an association with Imuran on occasions.

<u>Hepato-biliary disorders</u>

Uncommon:	Cholestasis and degeneration of liver function tests.
Rare:	Life-threatening hepatic damage.

Cholestasis and deterioration of liver function have occasionally been reported in association with Imuran therapy and are usually reversible on withdrawal of therapy. This may be associated with symptoms of a hypersensitivity reaction (see Hypersensitivity reactions).

Rare, but life-threatening hepatic damage associated with chronic administration of azathioprine has been described, primarily in transplant patients. Histological findings include sinusoidal dilatation, peliosis hepatis, veno-occlusive disease and nodular regenerative hyperplasia. In some cases withdrawal of azathioprine has resulted in either a temporary or permanent improvement in liver histology and symptoms.

<u>Skin and subcutaneous tissue disorders</u>

Rare:	Alopecia

Hair loss has been described on a number of occasions in patients receiving azathioprine and other immunosuppressive agents. In many instances the condition resolved spontaneously despite continuing therapy. The relationship between alopecia and azathioprine treatment is uncertain.

<u>Immune system disorders</u>

Uncommon:	Hypersensitivity reactions

Several different clinical syndromes, which appear to be idiosyncratic manifestations of hypersensitivity, have been described occasionally following administration of Imuran. Clinical features include general malaise, dizziness, nausea, vomiting, diarrhoea, fever, rigors, exanthema, rash, vasculitis, myalgia, arthralgia, hypotension, renal dysfunction, hepatic dysfunction and cholestasis (see Hepato-biliary disorders).

In many cases, re-challenge has confirmed an association with Imuran.

Immediate withdrawal of azathioprine and institution of circulatory support where appropriate have led to recovery in the majority of cases.

Other marked underlying pathology has contributed to the very rare deaths reported.

Following a hypersensitivity reaction to Imuran, the necessity for continued administration of Imuran should be carefully considered on an individual basis.

4.9 Overdose

Symptoms and signs: Unexplained infection, ulceration of the throat, bruising and bleeding are the main signs of overdosage with Imuran and result from bone marrow depression which may be maximal after 9 to 14 days. These signs are more likely to be manifest following chronic overdosage, rather than after a single acute overdose. There has been a report of a patient who ingested a single overdose of 7.5 g of azathioprine. The immediate toxic effects of this overdose were nausea, vomiting and diarrhoea, followed by mild leucopenia and mild abnormalities in liver function. Recovery was uneventful.

Treatment: There is no specific antidote. Gastric lavage has been used. Subsequent monitoring, including haematological monitoring, is necessary to allow prompt treatment of any adverse effects which may develop. The value of dialysis in patients who have taken an overdose of Imuran is not known, though azathioprine is partially dialysable.

5. PHARMACOLOGICAL PROPERTIES

5.1 Pharmacodynamic properties

Azathioprine is an imidazole derivative of 6-mercaptopurine (6-MP). It is rapidly broken down *in vivo* into 6-MP and a methylnitroimidazole moiety. The 6-MP readily crosses cell membranes and is converted intracellularly into a number of purine thioanalogues, which include the main active nucleotide, thioinosinic acid. The rate of conversion varies from one person to another. Nucleotides do not traverse cell membranes and therefore do not circulate in body fluids. Irrespective of whether it is given directly or is derived *in vivo* from azathioprine, 6-MP is eliminated mainly as the inactive oxidised metabolite thiouric acid. This oxidation is brought about by xanthine oxidase, an enzyme that is inhibited by allopurinol. The activity of the methylnitroimidazole moiety has not been defined clearly. However, in several systems it appears to modify the activity of azathioprine as compared with that of 6-MP. Determination of plasma concentrations of azathioprine or 6-MP have no prognostic values as regards effectiveness or toxicity of these compounds.

Mode of action: While the precise modes of action remain to be elucidated, some suggested mechanisms include:

1. the release of 6-MP which acts as a purine antimetabolite.
2. the possible blockade of -SH groups by alkylation.
3. the inhibition of many pathways in nucleic acid biosynthesis, hence preventing proliferation of cells involved in determination and amplification of the immune response.
4. damage to deoxyribonucleic acid (DNA) through incorporation of purine thio-analogues.

Because of these mechanisms, the therapeutic effect of Imuran may be evident only after several weeks or months of treatment.

Imuran appears to be well absorbed from the upper gastro-intestinal tract.

Studies in mice with [^{35}S]-azathioprine showed no unusually large concentration in any particular tissue, and there was very little [^{35}S]-label found in brain.

Plasma levels of azathioprine and 6-MP do not correlate well with the therapeutic efficacy or toxicity of Imuran.

5.2 Pharmacokinetic properties

Azathioprine is well absorbed following oral administration. After oral administration of [^{35}S]-azathioprine, the maximum plasma radioactivity occurs at 1-2 hours and decays with a half-life of 4-6 hours. This is not an estimate of the half-life of azathioprine itself, but reflects the elimination from plasma of azathioprine and the [^{35}S]-containing metabolites of the drug. As a consequence of the rapid and extensive metabolism of azathioprine, only a fraction of the radioactivity measured in plasma is comprised of unmetabolised drug. Studies in which the plasma concentration of azathioprine and 6-MP have been determined, following intravenous administration of azathioprine, have estimated the mean plasma $T_{1/2}$ for azathioprine to be in the range of 6-28 minutes and the mean plasma $T_{1/2}$ for 6-MP to be in the range 38-114 minutes.

Azathioprine is principally excreted as 6-thiouric uric acid in the urine. 1-methyl-4-nitro-5-thioimidazole has also been detected in urine as a minor excretory product. This would indicate that, rather than azathioprine being exclusive cleaved by nucleophilic attack at the 5-position of the nitroimidazole ring to generate 6-MP and 1-methyl-4-nitro-5-(S-glutathionyl)imidazole. A small proportion of the drug may be cleaved between the sulphur-atom and the purine ring. Only a small amount of the dose of azathioprine administered is excreted unmetabolised in the urine.

5.3 Preclinical safety data

No additional data of clinical relevance to the prescriber.

6. PHARMACEUTICAL PARTICULARS

6.1 List of excipients

Sodium hydroxide pellets* BP 7.2 mg

Sodium hydroxide pellets* to adjust pH

Water for Injections EP

*In the form of a 1M solution in water for injections.

6.2 Incompatibilities

Imuran Injection should ONLY be reconstituted with the recommended volume of Water for Injections BP and should be diluted as specified above. Imuran Injection should not be mixed with other drugs or fluids, except those specified above, before administration.

6.3 Shelf life

3 years unopened

5 days when reconstituted with 5 ml to 15 ml water for injections and stored at 5 to 25°C.

1 day for 5 ml of the reconstituted injection further diluted with between 20 ml and 200 ml of an appropriate infusion solution and stored at 15°C to 25°C.

6.4 Special precautions for storage

Store below 25°C

Keep dry

Protect from light

6.5 Nature and contents of container

Neutral glass vials with synthetic butyl rubber closures and aluminium collars. Each vial contains the equivalent of 50 mg azathioprine.

6.6 Instructions for use and handling

Health professionals who handle Imuran Injection should follow guidelines for the handling of cytotoxic drugs according to prevailing local recommendations and/or regulations (e.g., the Royal Pharmaceutical Society of Great Britain Working Party Report on the Handling of Cytotoxic Drugs, 1983).

Administrative Data

7. MARKETING AUTHORISATION HOLDER

The Wellcome Foundation Limited
Glaxo Wellcome House
Berkeley Avenue
Greenford
Middlesex
UB6 0NN
Trading as
GlaxoSmithKline UK
Stockley Park West
Uxbridge
Middlesex UB11 1BT

8. MARKETING AUTHORISATION NUMBER(S)

PL0003/5043R

9. DATE OF FIRST AUTHORISATION/RENEWAL OF THE AUTHORISATION

11 February 1997

10. DATE OF REVISION OF THE TEXT

2 April 2003

11. Legal Status

POM

Imuran Tablets 25mg

(GlaxoSmithKline UK)

1. NAME OF THE MEDICINAL PRODUCT

Imuran tablets 25 mg

2. QUALITATIVE AND QUANTITATIVE COMPOSITION

Orange, round, biconvex, film-coated tablets, impressed 'GX EL5' and containing 25 mg Azathioprine BP in each tablet.

3. PHARMACEUTICAL FORM

Tablet.

4. CLINICAL PARTICULARS

4.1 Therapeutic indications

Imuran tablets are used as an immunosuppressant antimetabolite either alone or, more commonly, in combination with other agents (usually corticosteroids) and procedures which influence the immune response. Therapeutic effect may be evident only after weeks or months and can include a steroid-sparing effect, thereby reducing the toxicity associated with high dosage and prolonged usage of corticosteroids.

Imuran, in combination with corticosteroids and/or other immunosuppressive agents and procedures, is indicated to enhance the survival of organ transplants, such as renal transplants, cardiac transplants, and hepatic transplants; and to reduce the corticosteroid requirements of renal transplant recipients.

Imuran, either alone or more usually in combination with corticosteroids and/or other drugs and procedures, has been used with clinical benefit (which may include reduction of dosage or discontinuation of corticosteroids) in a proportion of patients suffering from the following:

severe rheumatoid arthritis;

systemic lupus erythematosus;

dermatomyositis and polymyositis;

auto-immune chronic active hepatitis;

pemphigus vulgaris;

polyarteritis nodosa;

auto-immune haemolytic anaemia;

chronic refractory idiopathic thrombocytopenic purpura.

4.2 Posology and method of administration

Transplantation - adults and children

Depending on the immunosuppressive regimen employed, a dosage of up to 5 mg/kg body weight/day may be given on the first day of therapy, either orally or intravenously.

Maintenance dosage should range from 1 to 4 mg/kg body weight/day and must be adjusted according to clinical requirements and haematological tolerance.

Evidence indicates that Imuran therapy should be maintained indefinitely, even if only low doses are necessary, because of the risk of graft rejection.

Dosage in other conditions - adults and children

In general, starting dosage is from 1 to 3 mg/kg body weight/day, and should be adjusted, within these limits, depending on the clinical response (which may not be evident for weeks or months) and haematological tolerance.

When therapeutic response is evident, consideration should be given to reducing the maintenance dosage to the lowest level compatible with the maintenance of that response. If no improvement occurs in the patient's condition within 3 months, consideration should be given to withdrawing Imuran.

The maintenance dosage required may range from less than 1 mg/kg body weight/day to 3 mg/kg body weight/day, depending on the clinical condition being treated and the individual patient response, including haematological tolerance.

In patients with renal and/or hepatic insufficiency, dosages should be given at the lower end of the normal range (see Special Warnings and Precautions for Use for further details).

Use in the elderly (see Renal and/or hepatic insufficiency)

There is limited experience of the administration of Imuran to elderly patients. Although the available data do not provide evidence that the incidence of side effects among elderly patients is higher than that among other patients treated with Imuran, it is recommended that the dosages used should be at the lower end of the range.

Particular care should be taken to monitor haematological response and to reduce the maintenance dosage to the minimum required for clinical response.

4.3 Contraindications

Imuran is contra-indicated in patients known to be hypersensitive to azathioprine. Hypersensitivity to 6-mercaptopurine (6-MP) should alert the prescriber to probable hypersensitivity to Imuran.

Imuran therapy should not be initiated in patients who may be pregnant, or who are likely to become pregnant without careful assessment of risk versus benefit (see Special Warnings and Precautions for Use & Pregnancy and Lactation).

4.4 Special warnings and special precautions for use

Monitoring

There are potential hazards in the use of Imuran. It should be prescribed only if the patient can be adequately monitored for toxic effects throughout the duration of therapy.

It is suggested that during the first 8 weeks of therapy, complete blood counts, including platelets, should be performed weekly or more frequently if high dosage is used or if severe renal and/or hepatic disorder is present. The blood count frequency may be reduced later in therapy, but it is suggested that complete blood counts are repeated monthly, or at least at intervals of not longer than 3 months.

Patients receiving Imuran should be instructed to report immediately any evidence of infection, unexpected bruising or bleeding or other manifestations of bone marrow depression.

There are individuals with an inherited deficiency of the enzyme thiopurine methyltransferase (TPMT) who may be unusually sensitive to the myelosuppressive effect of azathioprine and prone to developing rapid bone marrow depression following the initiation of treatment with Imuran. This problem could be exacerbated by co-administration with drugs that inhibit TPMT, such as olsalazine, mesalazine or sulphasalazine.

Renal and/or hepatic insufficiency

It has been suggested that the toxicity of Imuran may be enhanced in the presence of renal insufficiency, but controlled studies have not supported this suggestion. Nevertheless, it is recommended that the dosages used should be at the lower end of the normal range and that haematological response should be carefully monitored. Dosage should be further reduced if haematological toxicity occurs.

Caution is necessary during the administration of Imuran to patients with hepatic dysfunction, and regular complete blood counts and liver function tests should be undertaken. In such patients the metabolism of Imuran may be impaired, and the dosage of Imuran should therefore be reduced if hepatic or haematological toxicity occurs.

Limited evidence suggests that Imuran is not beneficial to patients with hypoxanthine-guanine-phosphoribosyltransferase deficiency (Lesch-Nyhan syndrome). Therefore, given the abnormal metabolism in these patients, it is not prudent to recommend that these patients should receive Imuran.

Mutagenicity

Chromosomal abnormalities have been demonstrated in both male and female patients treated with Imuran. It is difficult to assess the role of Imuran in the development of these abnormalities.

Effects on fertility

Relief of chronic renal insufficiency by renal transplantation involving the administration of Imuran has been accompanied by increased fertility in both male and female transplant recipients.

Carcinogenicity (see also section 4.8 Undesirable Effects)

Patients receiving immunosuppressive therapy are at an increased risk of developing lymphomas and other malignancies, notably skin cancers. The risk appears to be related to the intensity and duration of immunosuppression rather than to the use of any specific agent. It has been reported that reduction or discontinuation of immunosuppression may cause lymphomas to regress.

Patients receiving multiple immunosuppressive agents may be at risk of over-immunosuppression, therefore such therapy should be maintained at the lowest effective level.

As is usual for patients with increased risk for skin cancer, exposure to sunlight and UV light should be limited by wearing protective clothing and using a sunscreen with a high protection factor.

4.5 Interaction with other medicinal products and other forms of Interaction

Allopurinol/ oxipurinol/ thiopurinol

Xanthine oxidase activity is inhibited by allopurinol, oxipurinol and thiopurinol which results in reduced conversion of biologically active 6-thioinosinic acid to biologically inactive 6-thiouric acid. When allopurinol, oxipurinol and/or thiopurinol are given concomitantly with 6-mercaptopurine or azathioprine, the dose of 6-mercaptopurine and azathioprine should be reduced to one-quarter of the original dose.

Neuromuscular blocking agents

Imuran can potentiate the neuromuscular blockade produced by depolarising agents such as succinylcholine and can reduce the blockade produced by non-depolarising agents such as tubocurarine. There is considerable variation in the potency of this interaction.

Warfarin

Inhibition of the anticoagulant effect of warfarin, when administered with azathioprine, has been reported.

Cytostatic/myelosuppressive agents

Where possible, concomitant administration of cytostatic drugs, or drugs which may have a myelosuppressive effect, such as penicillamine, should be avoided. There are conflicting clinical reports of interactions, resulting in serious haematological abnormalities, between Imuran and co-trimoxazole.

There has been a case report suggesting that haematological abnormalities may develop due to the concomitant administration of Imuran and captopril.

It has been suggested that cimetidine and indomethacin may have myelosuppressive effects, which may be enhanced by concomitant administration of Imuran.

Other interactions

As there is *in vitro* evidence that aminosalicylate derivatives (eg. olsalazine, mesalazine or sulphasalazine) inhibit the TPMT enzyme, they should be administered with caution to patients receiving concurrent Imuran therapy (see Special Warnings and Special Precautions for Use).

Frusemide has been shown to impair the metabolism of azathioprine by human hepatic tissue *in vitro*. The clinical significance is unknown.

Vaccines

The immunosuppressive activity of Imuran could result in an atypical and potentially deleterious response to live vaccines and so the administration of live vaccines to patients receiving Imuran therapy is contra-indicated on theoretical grounds.

A diminished response to killed vaccines is likely and such a response to hepatitis B vaccine has been observed among patients treated with a combination of azathioprine and corticosteroids.

A small clinical study has indicated that standard therapeutic doses of Imuran do not deleteriously affect the response to polyvalent pneumococcal vaccine, as assessed on the basis of mean anti-capsular specific antibody concentration.

4.6 Pregnancy and lactation

Teratogenicity

Studies in pregnant rats, mice and rabbits using azathioprine in dosages from 5 to 15 mg/kg body weight/day over the period of organogenesis have shown varying degrees of foetal abnormalities. Teratogenicity was evident in rabbits at 10 mg/kg body weight/day.

Evidence of the teratogenicity of Imuran in man is equivocal. As with all cytotoxic chemotherapy, adequate contraceptive precautions should be advised when either partner is receiving Imuran.

Mutagenicity

Chromosomal abnormalities, which disappear with time, have been demonstrated in lymphocytes from the offspring of patients treated with Imuran. Except in extremely rare cases, no overt physical evidence of abnormality has been observed in the offspring of patients treated with Imuran. Azathioprine and long-wave ultraviolet light have been shown to have a synergistic clastogenic effect in patients treated with azathioprine for a range of disorders.

Use in Pregnancy and Lactation

Imuran should not be given to patients who are pregnant or likely to become pregnant without careful assessment of risk versus benefit.

There have been reports of premature birth and low birth weight following maternal exposure to azathioprine, particularly in combination with corticosteroids. There have also been reports of spontaneous abortion following either maternal or paternal exposure.

Azathioprine and/or its metabolites have been found in low concentrations in foetal blood and amniotic fluid after maternal administration of azathioprine.

Leucopenia and/or thrombocytopenia have been reported in a proportion of neonates whose mothers took azathioprine throughout their pregnancies. Extra care in haematological monitoring is advised during pregnancy.

Lactation

6-Mercaptopurine has been identified in the colostrum and breast-milk of women receiving azathioprine treatment.

4.7 Effects on ability to drive and use machines

None known.

4.8 Undesirable effects

For this product there is no modern clinical documentation that can be used as support for determining the frequency of undesirable effects. Undesirable effects may vary in their incidence depending on the indication. The following convention has been utilised for the classification of frequency: Very common, ≥ 1/10; common, ≥ 1/100 and < 1/1000; uncommon, ≥ 1/1000 and < 1/100; rare, ≥ 1/10000 and < 1/1000; very rare, < 1/10000.

Infection and infestations

Transplant patients receiving Imuran in combination with other immunosuppressants.

Very common:	Viral, fungal and bacterial infections.

Other indications.

Uncommon:	Viral, fungal and bacterial infections.

Patients receiving Imuran alone, or in combination with other immunosupressants, particularly corticosteroids, have shown increased susceptibility to viral, fungal and bacterial infections.

Neoplasms benign and malignant (including cysts and polyps)

Rare: Neoplasms including lymphomas, skin cancers, acute myeloid leukaemia and myelodysplasia (see also section 4.4 Special Warnings and Special Precautions for Use)

The risk of developing lymphomas and other malignancies, notably skin cancers is increased in patients who receive immunosuppressive drugs, particularly in transplant recipients receiving aggressive treatment and such therapy should be maintained at the lowest effective levels. The increased risk of developing lymphomas in immunosuppressed rheumatoid arthritis patients compared with the general population appears to be related at least in part to the disease itself.

There have been rare reports of acute myeloid leukaemia and myelodysplasia (some in association with chromasomal abnormalities)

Blood and lymphatic system disorders

Very common:	Depression of bone marrow function; leucopenia.
Common:	Thrombocytopenia.
Uncommon:	Anaemia.
Rare:	Agranulocytosis, pancytopenia, aplastic anaemia, megaloblastic anaemia, erythriod hypoplasia.

Imuran may be associated with a dose-related, generally reversible, depression of bone marrow function, most frequently expressed as leucopenia, but also sometimes as anaemia and thrombocytopenia, and rarely as agranulocytosis, pancytopenia and aplastic anaemia. These occur particularly in patients predisposed to myelotoxicity, such as those with TPMP deficiency and renal or hepatic insufficiency and in patients failing to reduce the dose of Imuran when receiving concurrent allopurinol therapy.

Reversible, dose-related increases in mean corpuscular volume and red cell haemoglobin content have occurred in association with Imuran therapy. Megaloblastic bone marrow changes have also been observed but severe megaloblastic anaemia and erythroid hypoplasia is rare.

Respiratory, thorasic and mediastinal disorders

Very rare:	Reversible pneumonitis.

Reversible pneumonitis has been described very rarely.

Gastrointestinal disorders

Uncommon:	Pancreatitis.
Rare:	Colitis, diverticulitis and bowel perforation reported in transplant population, severe diarrhoea in inflammatory bowel disease population.

A minority of patients experience nausea when first given Imuran. This appears to be relieved by administering the tablets after meals.

Serious complications, including colitis, diverticulitis and bowel perforation, have been described in transplant recipients receiving immunosuppressive therapy. However, the aetiology is not clearly established and high-dose corticosteroids may be implicated. Severe diarrhoea, recurring on re-challenge, has been reported in patients treated with Imuran for inflammatory bowel disease. The possibility that exacerbation of symptoms might be drug-related should be borne in mind when treating such patients.

Pancreatitis has been reported in a small percentage of patients on Imuran therapy, particularly in renal transplant patients and those diagnosed as having inflammatory bowel disease. There are difficulties in relating the pancreatitis to the administration of one particular drug, although re-challenge has confirmed an association with Imuran on occasions.

Hepato-biliary disorders

Uncommon:	Cholestasis and degeneration of liver function tests.
Rare:	Life-threatening hepatic damage.

Cholestasis and deterioration of liver function have occasionally been reported in association with Imuran therapy and are usually reversible on withdrawal of therapy. This may be associated with symptoms of a hypersensitivity reaction (see Hypersensitivity reactions).

Rare, but life-threatening hepatic damage associated with chronic administration of azathioprine has been described primarily in transplant patients. Histological findings include sinusoidal dilatation, peliosis hepatis, veno-occlusive disease and nodular regenerative hyperplasia. In some cases withdrawal of azathioprine has resulted in either a temporary or permanent improvement in liver histology and symptoms.

Skin and subcutaneous tissue disorders

Rare:	Alopecia

Hair loss has been described on a number of occasions in patients receiving azathioprine and other immunosuppressive agents. In many instances the condition resolved spontaneously despite continuing therapy. The relationship between alopecia and azathioprine treatment is uncertain.

Immune system disorders

Uncommon:	Hypersensitivity reactions

Several different clinical syndromes, which appear to be idiosyncratic manifestations of hypersensitivity, have been described occasionally following administration of Imuran. Clinical features include general malaise, dizziness, nausea, vomiting, diarrhoea, fever, rigors, exanthema, rash, vasculitis, myalgia, arthralgia, hypotension, renal dysfunction, hepatic dysfunction and cholestasis (see Hepato-biliary disorders).

In many cases, re-challenge has confirmed an association with Imuran.

Immediate withdrawal of azathioprine and institution of circulatory support where appropriate have led to recovery in the majority of cases.

Other marked underlying pathology has contributed to the very rare deaths reported.

Following a hypersensitivity reaction to Imuran, the necessity for continued administration of Imuran should be carefully considered on an individual basis.

4.9 Overdose

Symptoms and signs

Unexplained infection, ulceration of the throat, bruising and bleeding are the main signs of overdosage with Imuran and result from bone marrow depression which may be maximal after 9 to 14 days. These signs are more likely to be manifest following chronic overdosage, rather than after a single acute overdose. There has been a report of a patient who ingested a single overdose of 7.5 g of azathioprine. The immediate toxic effects of this overdose were nausea, vomiting and diarrhoea, followed by mild leucopenia and mild abnormalities in liver function. Recovery was uneventful.

Treatment

There is no specific antidote. Gastric lavage has been used. Subsequent monitoring, including haematological monitoring, is necessary to allow prompt treatment of any adverse effects which may develop. The value of dialysis in patients who have taken an overdose of Imuran is not known, though azathioprine is partially dialysable.

5. PHARMACOLOGICAL PROPERTIES

5.1 Pharmacodynamic properties

Azathioprine is an imidazole derivative of 6-mercaptopurine (6-MP). It is rapidly broken down *in vivo* into 6-MP and a methylnitroimidazole moiety. The 6-MP readily crosses cell membranes and is converted intracellularly into a number of purine thioanalogues, which include the main active nucleotide, thioinosinic acid. The rate of conversion varies from one person to another. Nucleotides do not traverse cell membranes and therefore do not circulate in body fluids. Irrespective of whether it is given directly or is derived *in vivo* from azathioprine, 6-MP is eliminated mainly as the inactive oxidised metabolite thiouric acid. This oxidation is brought about by xanthine oxidase, an enzyme that is inhibited by allopurinol. The activity of the methylnitroimidazole moiety has not been defined clearly. However, in several systems it appears to modify the activity of azathioprine as compared with that of 6-MP. Determination of plasma concentrations of azathioprine or 6-MP have no prognostic values as regards effectiveness or toxicity of these compounds.

While the precise modes of action remain to be elucidated, some suggested mechanisms include:

1. the release of 6-MP which acts as a purine antimetabolite.

2. the possible blockade of -SH groups by alkylation.

3. the inhibition of many pathways in nucleic acid biosynthesis, hence preventing proliferation of cells involved in determination and amplification of the immune response.

4. damage to deoxyribonucleic acid (DNA) through incorporation of purine thio-analogues.

Because of these mechanisms, the therapeutic effect of Imuran may be evident only after several weeks or months of treatment.

Imuran appears to be well absorbed from the upper gastrointestinal tract.

Studies in mice with [^{35}S]-azathioprine showed no unusually large concentration in any particular tissue, and there was very little [^{35}S]-label found in brain.

Plasma levels of azathioprine and 6-MP do not correlate well with the therapeutic efficacy or toxicity of Imuran.

5.2 Pharmacokinetic properties

Azathioprine is well absorbed following oral administration. After oral administration of [^{35}S]-azathioprine, the maximum plasma radioactivity occurs at 1-2 hours and decays with a half-life of 4-6 hours. This is not an estimate of the half-life of azathioprine itself, but reflects the elimination from plasma of azathioprine and the [^{35}S]-containing metabolites of the drug. As a consequence of the rapid and extensive metabolism of azathioprine, only a fraction of the radioactivity measured in plasma is comprised of unmetabolised drug. Studies in which the plasma concentration of azathioprine and 6-MP have been determined following intravenous administration of azathioprine have estimated the mean plasma $T^1/_2$ for azathioprine to be in the range of 6-28 minutes and the mean plasma $T^1/_2$ for 6-MP to be in the range 38-114 minutes after i.v. administration of the drug.

Azathioprine is principally excreted as 6-thiouric uric acid in the urine. 1-methyl-4-nitro-5-thioimidazole has also been detected in urine as a minor excretory product. This would indicate that, rather than azathioprine being exclusive cleaved by nucleophilic attack at the 5-position of the nitroimidazole ring to generate 6-MP and 1-methyl-4-nitro-5-(S-glutathionyl)imidazole. A small proportion of the drug may be cleaved between the S atom and the purine ring. Only a small amount of the dose of azathioprine administered is excreted unmetabolised in the urine.

5.3 Preclinical safety data

No additional data of clinical relevance to the prescriber.

6. PHARMACEUTICAL PARTICULARS

6.1 List of excipients

Lactose, pregelatinised starch, maize starch, stearic acid, magnesium sterate, methylhydroxylpropyl cellulose, polyethylene glycol 400, titanium dioxide (E171), iron oxide, yellow (E172), iron oxide, red (E172), industrial methylated spirit, purified water.

6.2 Incompatibilities

None known.

6.3 Shelf life

5 years.

6.4 Special precautions for storage

Store below 25°C. Protect from light.

6.5 Nature and contents of container

Blister strips in a pack.

Pack sizes: 28, 30, 56, 60 and 100 tablets.

6.6 Instructions for use and handling

Health professionals who handle Imuran Injection should follow guidelines for the handling of cytotoxic drugs (for example, the Royal Pharmaceutical Society of Great Britain Working Party Report on the Handling of Cytotoxic Drugs, 1983).

Provided that the film-coating is intact, there is no risk in handling film-coated Imuran Tablets. Imuran Tablets should not be divided and, provided the coating is intact, no additional precautions are required when handling them.

Administrative Data

7. MARKETING AUTHORISATION HOLDER

The Wellcome Foundation

Berkeley Avenue

Greenford

Middlesex

UB6 0NN

8. MARKETING AUTHORISATION NUMBER(S)

PL0003/0225

9. DATE OF FIRST AUTHORISATION/RENEWAL OF THE AUTHORISATION

20 March 1992

10. DATE OF REVISION OF THE TEXT

31st May 2003

11. Legal Status

POM

Imuran Tablets 50mg

(GlaxoSmithKline UK)

1. NAME OF THE MEDICINAL PRODUCT

Imuran tablets 50 mg

2. QUALITATIVE AND QUANTITATIVE COMPOSITION

Yellow, round, biconvex, scored, film-coated tablets, impressed 'GX CH1' and containing 50 mg Azathioprine BP in each tablet.

3. PHARMACEUTICAL FORM

Tablet.

4. CLINICAL PARTICULARS

4.1 Therapeutic indications

Imuran tablets are used as an immunosuppressant antimetabolite either alone or, more commonly, in combination with other agents (usually corticosteroids) and procedures which influence the immune response. Therapeutic effect may be evident only after weeks or months and can include a steroid-sparing effect, thereby reducing the toxicity associated with high dosage and prolonged usage of corticosteroids.

Imuran, in combination with corticosteroids and/or other immunosuppressive agents and procedures, is indicated to enhance the survival of organ transplants, such as renal transplants, cardiac transplants, and hepatic transplants; and to reduce the corticosteroid requirements of renal transplant recipients.

Imuran, either alone or more usually in combination with corticosteroids and/or other drugs and procedures, has been used with clinical benefit (which may include reduction of dosage or discontinuation of corticosteroids) in a proportion of patients suffering from the following:

severe rheumatoid arthritis;

systemic lupus erythematosus;

dermatomyositis and polymyositis;

auto-immune chronic active hepatitis;

pemphigus vulgaris;

polyarteritis nodosa;

auto-immune haemolytic anaemia;

chronic refractory idiopathic thrombocytopenic purpura.

4.2 Posology and method of administration

<u>Transplantation - adults and children</u>

Depending on the immunosuppressive regimen employed, a dosage of up to 5 mg/kg body weight/day may be given on the first day of therapy, either orally or intravenously.

Maintenance dosage should range from 1 to 4 mg/kg body weight/day and must be adjusted according to clinical requirements and haematological tolerance.

Evidence indicates that Imuran therapy should be maintained indefinitely, even if only low doses are necessary, because of the risk of graft rejection.

<u>Dosage in other conditions - adults and children</u>

In general, starting dosage is from 1 to 3 mg/kg body weight/day, and should be adjusted, within these limits, depending on the clinical response (which may not be evident for weeks or months) and haematological tolerance.

When therapeutic response is evident, consideration should be given to reducing the maintenance dosage to the lowest level compatible with the maintenance of that response. If no improvement occurs in the patient's condition within 3 months, consideration should be given to withdrawing Imuran.

The maintenance dosage required may range from less than 1 mg/kg body weight/day to 3 mg/kg body weight/day, depending on the clinical condition being treated and the individual patient response, including haematological tolerance.

In patients with renal and/or hepatic insufficiency, dosages should be given at the lower end of the normal range (see Special Warnings and Precautions for Use for further details).

<u>Use in the elderly</u> (see Renal and/or hepatic insufficiency)

There is limited experience of the administration of Imuran to elderly patients. Although the available data do not provide evidence that the incidence of side effects among elderly patients is higher than that among other patients treated with Imuran, it is recommended that the dosages used should be at the lower end of the range.

Particular care should be taken to monitor haematological response and to reduce the maintenance dosage to the minimum required for clinical response.

4.3 Contraindications

Imuran is contra-indicated in patients known to be hypersensitive to azathioprine. Hypersensitivity to 6-mercaptopurine (6-MP) should alert the prescriber to probable hypersensitivity to Imuran.

Imuran therapy should not be initiated in patients who may be pregnant, or who are likely to become pregnant without careful assessment of risk versus benefit (see Special Warnings and Precautions for Use & Pregnancy and Lactation).

4.4 Special warnings and special precautions for use

Monitoring

There are potential hazards in the use of Imuran. It should be prescribed only if the patient can be adequately monitored for toxic effects throughout the duration of therapy.

It is suggested that during the first 8 weeks of therapy, complete blood counts, including platelets, should be performed weekly or more frequently if high dosage is used or if severe renal and/or hepatic disorder is present. The blood count frequency may be reduced later in therapy, but it is suggested that complete blood counts are repeated monthly, or at least at intervals of not longer than 3 months.

Patients receiving Imuran should be instructed to report immediately any evidence of infection, unexpected bruising or bleeding or other manifestations of bone marrow depression.

There are individuals with an inherited deficiency of the enzyme thiopurine methyltransferase (TPMT) who may be unusually sensitive to the myelosuppressive effect of azathioprine and prone to developing rapid bone marrow depression following the initiation of treatment with Imuran. This problem could be exacerbated by co-administration with drugs that inhibit TPMT, such as olsalazine, mesalazine or sulphasalazine.

Renal and/or hepatic insufficiency

It has been suggested that the toxicity of Imuran may be enhanced in the presence of renal insufficiency, but controlled studies have not supported this suggestion. Nevertheless, it is recommended that the dosages used should be at the lower end of the normal range and that haematological response should be carefully monitored. Dosage should be further reduced if haematological toxicity occurs.

Caution is necessary during the administration of Imuran to patients with hepatic dysfunction, and regular complete blood counts and liver function tests should be undertaken. In such patients the metabolism of Imuran may be impaired, and the dosage of Imuran should therefore be reduced if hepatic or haematological toxicity occurs.

Limited evidence suggests that Imuran is not beneficial to patients with hypoxanthine-guanine-phosphoribosyltransferase deficiency (Lesch-Nyhan syndrome). Therefore, given the abnormal metabolism in these patients, it is not prudent to recommend that these patients should receive Imuran.

Mutagenicity

Chromosomal abnormalities have been demonstrated in both male and female patients treated with Imuran. It is difficult to assess the role of Imuran in the development of these abnormalities.

Effects on fertility

Relief of chronic renal insufficiency by renal transplantation involving the administration of Imuran has been accompanied by increased fertility in both male and female transplant recipients.

Carcinogenicity (see also section 4.8 Undesirable Effects)

Patients receiving immunosuppressive therapy are at an increased risk of developing lymphomas and other malignancies, notably skin cancers. The risk appears to be related to the intensity and duration of immunosuppression rather than to the use of any specific agent. It has been reported that reduction or discontinuation of immunosuppression may cause lymphomas to regress.

Patients receiving multiple immunosuppressive agents may be at risk of over-immunosuppression, therefore such therapy should be maintained at the lowest effective level.

As is usual for patients with increased risk for skin cancer, exposure to sunlight and UV light should be limited by wearing protective clothing and using a sunscreen with a high protection factor.

4.5 Interaction with other medicinal products and other forms of Interaction

Allopurinol/ oxipurinol/ thiopurinol

Xanthine oxidase activity is inhibited by allopurinol, oxipurinol and thiopurinol which results in reduced conversion of biologically active 6-thioinosinic acid to biologically inactive 6-thiouric acid. When allopurinol, oxipurinol and/or thiopurinol are given concomitantly with 6-mercaptopurine or azathioprine, the dose of 6-mercaptopurine and azathioprine should be reduced to one-quarter of the original dose.

Neuromuscular blocking agents

Imuran can potentiate the neuromuscular blockade produced by depolarising agents such as succinylcholine and can reduce the blockade produced by non-depolarising agents such as tubocurarine. There is considerable variation in the potency of this interaction.

Warfarin

Inhibition of the anticoagulant effect of warfarin, when administered with azathioprine, has been reported.

Cytostatic/myelosuppressive agents

Where possible, concomitant administration of cytostatic drugs, or drugs which may have a myelosuppressive effect, such as penicillamine, should be avoided. There are conflicting clinical reports of interactions, resulting in serious haematological abnormalities, between Imuran and co-trimoxazole.

There has been a case report suggesting that haematological abnormalities may develop due to the concomitant administration of Imuran and captopril.

It has been suggested that cimetidine and indomethacin may have myelosuppressive effects, which may be enhanced by concomitant administration of Imuran.

Other interactions

As there is *in vitro* evidence that aminosalicylate derivatives (eg. olsalazine, mesalazine or sulphasalazine) inhibit the TPMT enzyme, they should be administered with caution to patients receiving concurrent Imuran therapy (see Special Warnings and Special Precautions for Use).

Frusemide has been shown to impair the metabolism of azathioprine by human hepatic tissue *in vitro*. The clinical significance is unknown.

Vaccines

The immunosuppressive activity of Imuran could result in an atypical and potentially deleterious response to live vaccines and so the administration of live vaccines to patients receiving Imuran therapy is contra-indicated on theoretical grounds.

A diminished response to killed vaccines is likely and such a response to hepatitis B vaccine has been observed among patients treated with a combination of azathioprine and corticosteroids.

A small clinical study has indicated that standard therapeutic doses of Imuran do not deleteriously affect the response to polyvalent pneumococcal vaccine, as assessed on the basis of mean anti-capsular specific antibody concentration.

4.6 Pregnancy and lactation

Teratogenicity

Studies in pregnant rats, mice and rabbits using azathioprine in dosages from 5 to 15 mg/kg body weight/day over the period of organogenesis have shown varying degrees of foetal abnormalities. Teratogenicity was evident in rabbits at 10 mg/kg body weight/day.

Evidence of the teratogenicity of Imuran in man is equivocal. As with all cytotoxic chemotherapy, adequate contraceptive precautions should be advised when either partner is receiving Imuran.

Mutagenicity

Chromosomal abnormalities, which disappear with time, have been demonstrated in lymphocytes from the offspring of patients treated with Imuran. Except in extremely rare cases, no overt physical evidence of abnormality has been observed in the offspring of patients treated with Imuran. Azathioprine and long-wave ultraviolet light have been shown to have a synergistic clastogenic effect in patients treated with azathioprine for a range of disorders.

Use in Pregnancy and Lactation

Imuran should not be given to patients who are pregnant or likely to become pregnant without careful assessment of risk versus benefit.

There have been reports of premature birth and low birth weight following maternal exposure to azathioprine, particularly in combination with corticosteroids. There have also been reports of spontaneous abortion following either maternal or paternal exposure.

Azathioprine and/or its metabolites have been found in low concentrations in foetal blood and amniotic fluid after maternal administration of azathioprine.

Leucopenia and/or thrombocytopenia have been reported in a proportion of neonates whose mothers took azathioprine throughout their pregnancies. Extra care in haematological monitoring is advised during pregnancy.

Lactation

6-Mercaptopurine has been identified in the colostrum and breast-milk of women receiving azathioprine treatment.

4.7 Effects on ability to drive and use machines

None known.

4.8 Undesirable effects

For this product there is no modern clinical documentation that can be used as support for determining the frequency of undesirable effects. Undesirable effects may vary in their incidence depending on the indication. The following convention has been utilised for the classification of frequency: Very common, ≥ 1/10; common, ≥ 1/100 and < 1/10; uncommon, ≥ 1/1000 and < 1/100; rare, ≥ 1/10000 and < 1/1000; very rare, < 1/10000.

<u>Infection and infestations</u>

Transplant patients receiving Imuran in combination with other immunosuppressants.

Very common:	Viral, fungal, and bacterial infections.

Other indications.

Uncommon:	Viral, fungal and bacterial infections.

Patients receiving Imuran alone, or in combination with other immunosuppressants, particularly corticosteroids, have shown increased susceptibility to viral, fungal and bacterial infections.

<u>Neoplasms benign and malignant (including cysts and polyps)</u>

Rare:	Neoplasms including lymphomas, skin cancers, acute myloid leukaemia and myelodysplasia (see also section 4.4 Special Warnings and Special Precautions for Use).

The risk of developing lymphomas and other malignancies, notably skin cancers is increased in patients who receive immunosuppressive drugs, particularly in transplant recipients receiving aggressive treatment and such therapy should be maintained at the lowest effective levels. The increased risk of developing lymphomas in immunosuppressed rheumatoid arthritis patients compared with the general population appears to be related at least in part to the disease itself.

There have been rare reports of acute myeloid leukaemia and myelodysplasia (some in association with chromasomal abnormalities).

<u>Blood and lymphatic system disorders</u>

Very common:	Depression of bone marrow function; leucopenia.
Common:	Thrombocytopenia.
Uncommon:	Anaemia.
Rare:	Agranulocytosis, pancytopenia, aplastic anaemia, megaloblastic anaemia, erythriod hypoplasia.

Imuran may be associated with a dose-related, generally reversible, depression of bone marrow function, most frequently expressed as leucopenia, but also sometimes as anaemia and thrombocytopenia, and rarely as agranulocytosis, pancytopenia and aplastic anaemia. These occur particularly in patients predisposed to myelotoxicity, such as those with TPMP deficiency and renal or hepatic insufficiency and in patients failing to reduce the dose of Imuran when receiving concurrent allopurinol therapy.

Reversible, dose-related increases in mean corpuscular volume and red cell haemoglobin content have occurred in association with Imuran therapy. Megaloblastic bone marrow changes have also been observed but severe megaloblastic anaemia and erythroid hypoplasia are rare.

Respiratory, thorasic and mediastinal disorders

Very rare:	Reversible pneumonitis.

Reversible pneumonitis has been described very rarely.

<u>Gastrointestinal disorders</u>

Uncommon:	Pancreatitis.
Rare:	Colitis, diverticulitis and bowel perforation reported in transplant population, severe diarrhoea in inflammatory bowel disease population.

A minority of patients experience nausea when first given Imuran. This appears to be relieved by administering the tablets after meals.

Serious complications, including colitis, diverticulitis and bowel perforation, have been described in transplant recipients receiving immunosuppressive therapy. However, the aetiology is not clearly established and high-dose corticosteroids may be implicated. Severe diarrhoea, recurring on re-challenge, has been reported in patients treated with Imuran for inflammatory bowel disease. The possibility that exacerbation of symptoms might be drug-related should be borne in mind when treating such patients.

Pancreatitis has been reported in a small percentage of patients on Imuran therapy, particularly in renal transplant patients and those diagnosed as having inflammatory bowel disease. There are difficulties in relating the pancreatitis to the administration of one particular drug, although re-challenge has confirmed an association with Imuran on occasions.

<u>Hepato-biliary disorders</u>

Uncommon:	Cholestasis and degeneration of liver function tests.
Rare:	Life-threatening hepatic damage.

Cholestasis and deterioration of liver function have occasionally been reported in association with Imuran therapy and are usually reversible on withdrawal of therapy. This may be associated with symptoms of a hypersensitivity reaction (see Hypersensitivity reactions).

Rare, but life-threatening hepatic damage associated with chronic administration of azathioprine has been described primarily in transplant patients. Histological findings include sinusoidal dilatation, peliosis hepatis, veno-occlusive disease and nodular regenerative hyperplasia. In some cases withdrawal of azathioprine has resulted in either a temporary or permanent improvement in liver histology and symptoms.

Skin and subcutaneous tissue disorders

Rare:	Alopecia

Hair loss has been described on a number of occasions in patients receiving azathioprine and other immunosuppressive agents. In many instances the condition resolved spontaneously despite continuing therapy. The relationship between alopecia and azathioprine treatment is uncertain.

<u>Immune system disorders</u>

Uncommon:	Hypersensitivity reactions

Several different clinical syndromes, which appear to be idiosyncratic manifestations of hypersensitivity, have been described occasionally following administration of Imuran. Clinical features include general malaise, dizziness, nausea, vomiting, diarrhoea, fever, rigors, exanthema, rash, vasculitis, myalgia, arthralgia, hypotension, renal dysfunction, hepatic dysfunction and cholestasis (see Hepato-biliary disorders).

In many cases, re-challenge has confirmed an association with Imuran.

Immediate withdrawal of azathioprine and institution of circulatory support where appropriate have led to recovery in the majority of cases.

Other marked underlying pathology has contributed to the very rare deaths reported.

Following a hypersensitivity reaction to Imuran, the necessity for continued administration of Imuran should be carefully considered on an individual basis.

4.9 Overdose

Symptoms and signs

Unexplained infection, ulceration of the throat, bruising and bleeding are the main signs of overdosage with Imuran and result from bone marrow depression which may be maximal after 9 to 14 days. These signs are more likely to be manifest following chronic overdosage, rather than after a single acute overdose. There has been a report of a patient who ingested a single overdose of 7.5 g of azathioprine. The immediate toxic effects of this overdose were nausea, vomiting and diarrhoea, followed by mild leucopenia and mild abnormalities in liver function. Recovery was uneventful.

Treatment

There is no specific antidote. Gastric lavage has been used. Subsequent monitoring, including haematological monitoring, is necessary to allow prompt treatment of any adverse effects which may develop. The value of dialysis in patients who have taken an overdose of Imuran is not known, though azathioprine is partially dialysable.

5. PHARMACOLOGICAL PROPERTIES

5.1 Pharmacodynamic properties

Azathioprine is an imidazole derivative of 6-mercaptopurine (6-MP). It is rapidly broken down *in vivo* into 6-MP and a methylnitroimidazole moiety. The 6-MP readily crosses cell membranes and is converted intracellularly into a number of purine thioanalogues, which include the main active nucleotide, thioinosinic acid. The rate of conversion varies from one person to another. Nucleotides do not traverse cell membranes and therefore do not circulate in body fluids. Irrespective of whether it is given directly or is derived *in vivo* from azathioprine, 6-MP is eliminated mainly as the inactive oxidised metabolite thiouric acid. This oxidation is brought about by xanthine oxidase, an enzyme that is inhibited by allopurinol. The activity of the methylnitroimidazole moiety has not been defined clearly. However, in several systems it appears to modify the activity of azathioprine as compared with that of 6-MP. Determination of plasma concentrations of azathioprine or 6-MP have no prognostic values as regards effectiveness or toxicity of these compounds.

While the precise modes of action remain to be elucidated, some suggested mechanisms include:

1. the release of 6-MP which acts as a purine antimetabolite.
2. the possible blockade of -SH groups by alkylation.
3. the inhibition of many pathways in nucleic acid biosynthesis, hence preventing proliferation of cells involved in determination and amplification of the immune response.
4. damage to deoxyribonucleic acid (DNA) through incorporation of purine thio-analogues.

Because of these mechanisms, the therapeutic effect of Imuran may be evident only after several weeks or months of treatment.

Imuran appears to be well absorbed from the upper gastrointestinal tract.

Studies in mice with $[^{35}S]$-azathioprine showed no unusually large concentration in any particular tissue, and there was very little $[^{35}S]$-label found in brain.

Plasma levels of azathioprine and 6-MP do not correlate well with the therapeutic efficacy or toxicity of Imuran.

5.2 Pharmacokinetic properties

Azathioprine is well absorbed following oral administration. After oral administration of $[^{35}S]$-azathioprine, the maximum plasma radioactivity occurs at 1-2 hours and decays with a half-life of 4-6 hours. This is not an estimate of the half-life of azathioprine itself, but reflects the elimination from plasma of azathioprine and the $[^{35}S]$-containing metabolites of the drug. As a consequence of the rapid and extensive metabolism of azathioprine, only a fraction of the radioactivity measured in plasma is comprised of unmetabolised drug. Studies in which the plasma concentration of azathioprine and 6-MP have been determined following intravenous administration of azathioprine have estimated the mean plasma $T^{1}/_{2}$ for azathioprine to be in the range of 6-28 minutes and the mean plasma $T^{1}/_{2}$ for 6-MP to be in the range 38-114 minutes after i.v. administration of the drug.

Azathioprine is principally excreted as 6-thiouric acid in the urine. 1-methyl-4-nitro-5-thioimidazole has also been detected in urine as a minor excretory product. This would indicate that, rather than azathioprine being exclusive cleaved by nucleophilic attack at the 5-position of the nitroimidazole ring to generate 6-MP and 1-methyl-4-nitro-5-(S-glutathionyl)imidazole. A small proportion of the drug may be cleaved between the sulphur-atom and the purine ring. Only a small amount of the dose of azathioprine administered is excreted unmetabolised in the urine.

5.3 Preclinical safety data
No additional data of clinical relevance to the prescriber.

6. PHARMACEUTICAL PARTICULARS

6.1 List of excipients
Lactose, pregelatinised starch, maize starch, stearic acid, magnesium sterate, purified water, methylhydroxylpropyl cellulose, polyethylene glycol 400.

6.2 Incompatibilities
None known.

6.3 Shelf life
5 years.

6.4 Special precautions for storage
Store below 25°C. Protect from light.

6.5 Nature and contents of container
Blister strips in a pack.

Pack sizes: 28, 30, 56, 60, 100 and 1000 tablets.

6.6 Instructions for use and handling
Health professionals who handle Imuran Injection should follow guidelines for the handling of cytotoxic drugs (for example, the Royal Pharmaceutical Society of Great Britain Working Party Report on the Handling of Cytotoxic Drugs, 1983).

Provided that the film-coating is intact, there is no risk in handling film-coated Imuran Tablets. Imuran Tablets should not be divided and, provided the coating is intact, no additional precautions are required when handling them.

Administrative Data

7. MARKETING AUTHORISATION HOLDER
The Wellcome Foundation

Berkeley Avenue

Greenford

Middlesex

UB6 ONN

8. MARKETING AUTHORISATION NUMBER(S)
PL0003/0226

9. DATE OF FIRST AUTHORISATION/RENEWAL OF THE AUTHORISATION
20 March 1992

10. DATE OF REVISION OF THE TEXT
30 May 2003

11. Legal Status
POM

Inactivated Influenza Vaccine (Split Virion) BP

(Sanofi Pasteur MSD)

1. NAME OF THE MEDICINAL PRODUCT
Inactivated Influenza Vaccine (Split Virion) BP, suspension for injection in prefilled syringe

2. QUALITATIVE AND QUANTITATIVE COMPOSITION
Split influenza virus* inactivated containing antigens equivalent to:

A/New Caledonia/20/99 (H_1N_1) – like strain

(A/New Caledonia/20/99(IVR-116)) .... 15 micrograms**

A/Califonia/7/2004 (H_3N_2) – like strain

(A/New York/55/2004 (NYMC X-157)) ..... 15 micrograms**

B/Shanghai/361/2002 – like strain

(B/Jiangsu/10/2003)................................. 15 micrograms**

per one 0.5 mL dose

* propagated in eggs

** haemagglutinin

This vaccine complies with the WHO recommendation (northern hemisphere) and EU decision for the "2005/2006" season.

For excipients, see section 6.1

3. PHARMACEUTICAL FORM
Suspension for injection in prefilled syringe.

4. CLINICAL PARTICULARS

4.1 Therapeutic indications
Prophylaxis of influenza especially in those who run an increased risk of associated complications.

4.2 Posology and method of administration
POSOLOGY

Adults and children from 36 months: one 0.5 mL dose.

Children from 6 months to 35 months: clinical data are limited. Dosages of 0.25 mL or 0.5 mL have been used.

For children who have not previously been vaccinated, a second dose should be given after an interval of at least 4 weeks.

METHOD OF ADMINISTRATION

Immunisation should be carried out by intramuscular or deep subcutaneous injection.

4.3 Contraindications
Hypersensitivity to the active substances, to any of the excipients, to eggs, chicken protein, neomycin, formaldehyde and octoxinol 9.

Immunisation shall be postponed in patients with febrile illness or acute infection.

4.4 Special warnings and special precautions for use
As with all injectable vaccines, appropriate medical treatment and supervision should always be readily available in case of a rare anaphylactic event following the administration of the vaccine.

Inactivated Influenza Vaccine (Split Virion) BP should under no circumstances be administered intravascularly.

Antibody response in patients with endogenous or iatrogenic immunosuppression may be insufficient.

4.5 Interaction with other medicinal products and other forms of Interaction
Inactivated Influenza Vaccine (Split Virion) BP may be given at the same time as other vaccines. Immunisation should be carried out on separate limbs. It should be noted that the adverse reactions may be intensified.

The immunological response may be diminished if the patient is undergoing immunosuppressant treatment.

Following influenza vaccination, false positive results in serology tests using the ELISA method to detect antibodies against HIV1, hepatitis C and especially HTLV1 have been observed. The Western Blot technique disproves the results. The transient false positive reactions could be due to IgM response by the vaccine.

4.6 Pregnancy and lactation
Limited data from vaccinations in women do not indicate that the adverse foetal and maternal outcomes were attributable to the vaccine. The use of this vaccine may be considered from the second trimester of pregnancy. For pregnant women with medical conditions that increase their risk of complications from influenza, administration of the vaccine is recommended, irrespective of their stage of pregnancy.

Inactivated Influenza Vaccine (Split Virion) BP may be used during lactation.

4.7 Effects on ability to drive and use machines
The vaccine is unlikely to produce an effect on the ability to drive and use machines.

4.8 Undesirable effects
Adverse reactions from clinical trials:

The safety of trivalent inactivated influenza vaccines is assessed in open label, uncontrolled clinical trials performed as annual update requirement, including at least 50 adults aged 18 - 60 years of age and at least 50 elderly aged 60 years or older. Safety evaluation is performed during the first 3 days following vaccination.

Undesirable effects reported are listed according to the following frequency.

Adverse events from clinical trials:

<u>Common (>1/100, <1/10):</u>

Local reaction: redness, swelling, pain, ecchymosis, induration

Systemic reactions: fever, malaise, shivering, fatigue, headache, sweating, myalgia, arthralgia.

These reactions usually disappear within 1 - 2 days without treatment.

From post-marketing surveillance additionally, the following adverse events have been reported:

Uncommon (>1/1,000, <1/100):

Generalised skin reactions including pruritus, urticaria or non-specific rash.

Rare (>1/10,000, <1/1,000):

Neuralgia, paraesthesia, convulsions, transient thrombocytopenia.

Allergic reactions, in rare cases leading to shock, have been reported.

Very rare (<1/10,000):

Vasculitis with transient renal involvement.

Neurological disorders, such as encephalomyelitis, neuritis and Guillain-Barré syndrome.

4.9 Overdose
Overdosage is unlikely to have any untoward effect.

5. PHARMACOLOGICAL PROPERTIES

5.1 Pharmacodynamic properties
Pharmacotherapeutic group: INFLUENZA VACCINE

ATC code: J: ANTI-INFECTIOUS

Seroprotection is generally obtained within 2 to 3 weeks. The duration of postvaccinal immunity to homologous strains or to strains closely related to the vaccine strains varies but is usually 6-12 months.

5.2 Pharmacokinetic properties
Not applicable.

5.3 Preclinical safety data
Not applicable.

6. PHARMACEUTICAL PARTICULARS

6.1 List of excipients
Buffer solution:

Sodium chloride

Potassium chloride

Disodium phosphate dihydrate

Potassium dihydrogen phosphate

Water for injections.

6.2 Incompatibilities
In the absence of compatibility studies, this vaccine must not be mixed with other injection fluids.

6.3 Shelf life
1 year.

6.4 Special precautions for storage
The product should be stored at +2°C to +8°C (in a refrigerator). Do not freeze. Protect from light.

6.5 Nature and contents of container
0.5 mL of suspension in prefilled syringe (type I glass) with attached needle equipped with an elastomer plunger stopper (chlorobromobutyl) - pack of 1 or 10.

0.5 mL of suspension in prefilled syringe (type I glass) without attached needle, equipped with an elastomer plunger stopper (chlorobromobutyl) and a tip cap (chlorobromobutyl) – pack of 1 or 10.

6.6 Instructions for use and handling
The vaccine should be allowed to reach room temperature before use.

Shake before use.

For children, when one dose of 0.25 mL is indicated, push the plunger exactly to the edge of the mark so that the half of the volume should be eliminated. The remaining volume should be injected.

7. MARKETING AUTHORISATION HOLDER
Sanofi Pasteur MSD Limited

Mallards Reach

Bridge Avenue

Maidenhead

Berkshire

SL6 1QP

8. MARKETING AUTHORISATION NUMBER(S)
PL 6745/0095

9. DATE OF FIRST AUTHORISATION/RENEWAL OF THE AUTHORISATION
20th March 1998 / 30th December 2002

10. DATE OF REVISION OF THE TEXT
June 2005

Inactivated Influenza Vaccine (Split Virion) For Paediatric Use

(Sanofi Pasteur MSD)

1. NAME OF THE MEDICINAL PRODUCT
Inactivated Influenza Vaccine (Split Virion) for Paediatric use, suspension for injection in prefilled syringe.

2. QUALITATIVE AND QUANTITATIVE COMPOSITION
Split influenza virus*, inactivated containing antigens equivalent to:

A/New Caledonia/20/99 (H_1N_1) - like strain

(A/New Caledonia/20/99 (IVR-116)) .... 7.5 micrograms**

A/Califonia/7/2004 (H_3N_2) – like strain

(A/New York/55/2004 (NYMC X-157)).............. 7.5 micrograms**

B/Shanghai/361/2002 – like strain

(B/Jiangsu/10/2003)... 7.5 micrograms**

per one 0.25 mL dose

* propagated in eggs

** haemagglutinin

The vaccine complies with the WHO recommendation (Northern hemisphere) and the EU decision for the 2005/2006 season.

For excipients, see section 6.1.

3. PHARMACEUTICAL FORM
Suspension for injection in pre-filled syringe.

4. CLINICAL PARTICULARS

4.1 Therapeutic indications
Prophylaxis of influenza, especially in children from 6 to 35 months who run an increased risk of associated complications.

4.2 Posology and method of administration
Posology

Children from 6 to 35 months: one dose of 0.25 mL.

For children who have not previously been vaccinated, a second dose should be given after an interval of at least 4 weeks.

Method of administration

Immunisation should be carried out by intramuscular or deep subcutaneous injection.

4.3 Contraindications
Hypersensitivity to the active substances, to any of the excipients, to eggs, chicken proteins, neomycin, formaldehyde, and octoxinol 9.

Immunisation shall be postponed in patients with febrile illness or acute infection.

4.4 Special warnings and special precautions for use
As with all injectable vaccines, appropriate medical treatment and supervision should always be readily available in case of a rare anaphylactic event following the administration of the vaccine.

Inactivated Influenza Vaccine (Split Virion) for Paediatric use should under no circumstances be administered intravascularly.

Antibody response in children with endogenous or iatrogenic immunosuppression may be insufficient.

4.5 Interaction with other medicinal products and other forms of Interaction
Inactivated Influenza Vaccine (Split Virion) for Paediatric use may be given at the same time as other vaccines. Immunisation should be carried out on separate limbs. It should be noted that the adverse reactions may be intensified.

The immunological response may be diminished if the child is undergoing immunosuppressant treatment.

Following influenza vaccination, false positive results in serology tests using the ELISA method to detect antibodies against HIV1, Hepatitis C and especially HTLV1 have been observed. The Western Blot technique disproves the results. The transient false positive reactions could be due to IgM response by the vaccine.

4.6 Pregnancy and lactation
Not applicable.

4.7 Effects on ability to drive and use machines
Not applicable.

4.8 Undesirable effects
Adverse reactions from clinical trials:

The safety of trivalent inactivated influenza vaccines is assessed in open label, uncontrolled clinical trials performed as annual update requirement, including at least 50 adults aged 18 – 60 years of age and at least 50 elderly aged 60 years or older. Safety evaluation is performed during the first 3 days following vaccination.

Undesirable effects reported are listed according to the following frequency.

Adverse events from clinical trials:

Common (> 1/100, < 1/10):

Local reactions: redness, swelling, pain, ecchymosis, induration;

Systemic reactions: fever, malaise, shivering, fatigue, headache, sweating, myalgia, arthralgia.

These reactions usually disappear within 1 - 2 days without treatment.

From post-marketing surveillance additionally, the following adverse events have been reported:

Uncommon (>1/1,000, <1/100):

Generalised skin reactions including pruritus, urticaria or non-specific rash.

Rare (>1/10,000, <1/1,000):

Neuralgia, paraesthesia, convulsions, transient thrombocytopenia.

Allergic reactions, in rare cases leading to shock, have been reported.

Very rare (<1/10,000):

Vasculitis with transient renal involvement.

neurological disorders such as encephalomyelitis, neuritis and Guillain-Barré syndrome.

4.9 Overdose
Overdosage is unlikely to have any untoward effect.

5. PHARMACOLOGICAL PROPERTIES

5.1 Pharmacodynamic properties
Pharmacotherapeutic group: INFLUENZA VACCINE

ATC Code: J: ANTI-INFECTIOUS

Seroprotection is generally obtained within 2 to 3 weeks. The duration of post vaccinal immunity to homologous strains or to strains closely related to the vaccine strains varies but is usually 6 to 12 months.

5.2 Pharmacokinetic properties
Not applicable.

5.3 Preclinical safety data
Not applicable.

6. PHARMACEUTICAL PARTICULARS

6.1 List of excipients
Buffer solution:

- Sodium chloride
- Potassium chloride
- Disodium phosphate dihydrate
- Potassium dihydrogen phosphate
- Water for injections.

6.2 Incompatibilities
In the absence of compatibility studies, this vaccine must not be mixed with other injection fluids.

6.3 Shelf life
1 year.

6.4 Special precautions for storage
Store at +2 to +8°C (in a refrigerator) and protect from light. Do not freeze. Protect from light.

6.5 Nature and contents of container
0.25 mL of suspension in prefilled syringe (type I glass), equipped with an elastomer plunger stopper (chlorobromobutyl) – pack of 1.

0.25 mL of suspension in prefilled syringe (type I glass) without attached needle, equipped with an elastomer plunger stopper (chlorobromobutyl) and a tip cap (chlorobromobutyl) – pack of 1.

6.6 Instructions for use and handling
The vaccine should be allowed to reach room temperature before use.

Shake before use.

7. MARKETING AUTHORISATION HOLDER
Sanofi Pasteur MSD Limited

Mallards Reach

Bridge Avenue

Maidenhead

Berkshire

SL6 1QP

8. MARKETING AUTHORISATION NUMBER(S)
PL 06745/0105

9. DATE OF FIRST AUTHORISATION/RENEWAL OF THE AUTHORISATION
30th December 2002

10. DATE OF REVISION OF THE TEXT
June 2005

Inderal Injection

(AstraZeneca UK Limited)

1. NAME OF THE MEDICINAL PRODUCT
Inderal Injection.

2. QUALITATIVE AND QUANTITATIVE COMPOSITION
Propranolol Hydrochloride Ph. Eur. 0.1% w/v.

3. PHARMACEUTICAL FORM
Solution for intravenous injection.

4. CLINICAL PARTICULARS

4.1 Therapeutic indications
The emergency treatment of cardiac dysrhythmias and thyrotoxic crisis.

4.2 Posology and method of administration
For intravenous injection.

Adults

The initial dose of Inderal is 1 mg (1 ml) injected over 1 minute. This may be repeated at 2-minute intervals until a response is observed or to a maximum dose of 10 mg in conscious patients or 5 mg in patients under anaesthesia.

Elderly

Evidence concerning the relation between blood level and age is conflicting. Inderal should be used to treat the elderly with caution. It is suggested that treatment should start with the lowest dose. The optimum dose should be individually determined according to clinical response.

Children

Dysrhythmias, thyrotoxicosis

Dosage should be individually determined and the following is only a guide:

Intravenous: 0.025 to 0.05 mg/kg injected slowly under ECG control and repeated 3 or 4 times daily as required.

Fallot's tetralogy

The value of Inderal in this condition is confined mainly to the relief of right-ventricular outflow tract shut-down. It is also useful for treatment of associated dysrhythmias and angina. Dosage should be individually determined and the following is only a guide:

Intravenous: Up to 0.1 mg/kg injected slowly under ECG control, repeated 3 or 4 times daily as required.

4.3 Contraindications
Inderal must not be used if there is a history of bronchial asthma or bronchospasm. The product label and patient information leaflets state the following warnings:

Label: "Do not use Inderal if the patient has a history of asthma or wheezing".

Patient Information Leaflet: "If you have ever had asthma or wheezing, you should not be given Inderal injection. Talk to your doctor".

Bronchospasm can usually be reversed by $beta_2$- agonist bronchodilators such as salbutamol. Large doses of the $beta_2$- agonist bronchodilator may be required to overcome the beta-blockade produced by propranolol and the dose should be titrated according to the clinical response; both intravenous and inhalational administration should be considered. The use of intravenous aminophylline and/or the use of ipratropium (given by nebuliser) may also be considered. Glucagon (1 to 2 mg given intravenously) has also been reported to produce a bronchodilator effect in asthmatic patients. Oxygen or artificial ventilation may be required in severe cases.

Inderal as with other beta-adrenoceptor blocking drugs must not be used in patients with any of the following conditions: known hypersensitivity to the substance; bradycardia; cardiogenic shock; hypotension; metabolic acidosis; after prolonged fasting; severe peripheral arterial circulatory disturbances; second or third degree heart block; sick sinus syndrome; untreated phaeochromocytoma; uncontrolled heart failure or Prinzmetal's angina.

Inderal must not be used in patients prone to hypoglycaemia, i.e., patients after prolonged fasting or patients with restricted counter-regulatory reserves. Patients with restricted counter regulatory reserves may have reduced autonomic and hormonal responses to hypoglycaemia which includes glycogenolysis, gluconeogenesis and /or impaired modulation of insulin secretion. Patients at risk for an inadequate response to hypoglycaemia includes individuals with malnutrition, prolonged fasting, starvation, chronic liver disease, diabetes and concomitant use of drugs which block the full response to catecholamines.

4.4 Special warnings and special precautions for use
Inderal as with other beta-adrenoceptor blocking drugs:

- although contraindicated in uncontrolled heart failure (see Section 4.3), may be used in patients whose signs of heart failure have been controlled. Caution must be exercised in patients whose cardiac reserve is poor.

Should not be used in combination with calcium channel blockers with negative inotropic effects (e.g. verapamil, diltiazem), as it can lead to an exaggeration of these effects particularly in patients with impaired ventricular function and/or SA or AV conduction abnormalities. This may result in severe hypotension, bradycardia and cardiac failure. Neither the beta-blocker nor the calcium channel blocker should be administered intravenously within 48 hours of discontinuing the other.

- although contraindicated in severe peripheral arterial circulatory disturbances (see Section 4.3), may also aggravate less severe peripheral arterial circulatory disturbances.

- due to its negative effect on conduction time, caution must be exercised if it is given to patients with first degree heart block.

- may block/modify the signs and symptoms of the hypoglycaemia (especially tachycardia). Inderal occasionally causes hypoglycaemia, even in non-diabetic patients, e.g., neonates, infants, children (Inderal is not recommended for use in children – see section 4.2), elderly patients, patients on haemodialysis or patients suffering from chronic liver disease and patients suffering from overdose. Severe hypoglycaemia associated with Inderal has rarely presented with seizures and/or coma in isolated patients. Caution must be exercised in the concurrent use of Inderal and hypoglycaemic therapy in diabetic patients. Inderal may prolong the hypoglycaemic response to insulin. (see section 4.3).

- may mask the signs of thyrotoxicosis.

- should not be used in untreated phaeochromocytoma. However, in patients with phaeochromocytoma, an alpha-blocker may be given concomitantly.

- will reduce heart rate as a result of its pharmacological action. In the rare instances when a treated patient develops symptoms which may be attributable to a slow heart rate, the dose may be reduced.

- may cause a more severe reaction to a variety of allergens when given to patients with a history of anaphylactic reaction to such allergens. Such patients may be unresponsive to the usual doses of adrenaline used to treat the allergic reactions.

Abrupt withdrawal of beta-blockers is to be avoided. The dosage should be withdrawn gradually over a period of 7 to 14 days. Patients should be followed during withdrawal especially those with ischaemic heart disease.

When a patient is scheduled for surgery and a decision is made to discontinue beta-blocker therapy, this should be done at least 24 hours prior to the procedure. The risk/benefit of stopping beta blockade should be made for each patient.

Since the half-life may be increased in patients with significant hepatic or renal impairment, caution must be exercised when starting treatment and selecting the initial dose.

Inderal must be used with caution in patients with decompensated cirrhosis (see section 4.2).

In patients with portal hypertension, liver function may deteriorate and hepatic encephalopathy may develop. There have been reports suggesting that treatment with propranolol may increase the risk of developing hepatic encephalopathy (see section 4.2).

Interference with laboratory tests. Inderal has been reported to interfere with the estimation of serum bilirubin by the diazo method and with the determination of catecholamines by methods using fluorescence.

4.5 Interaction with other medicinal products and other forms of Interaction

Inderal modifies the tachycardia of hypoglycaemia. Caution must be exercised in the concurrent use of Inderal and hypoglycaemic therapy in diabetic patients. Inderal may prolong the hypoglycaemic response to insulin.

Caution must be exercised in prescribing a beta-adrenoceptor blocking drug with Class I antiarrhythmic agents such as disopyramide.

Digitalis glycosides in association with beta-adrenoceptor blocking drugs may increase atrioventricular conduction time.

Combined use of beta-adrenoceptor blocking drugs and calcium channel blockers with negative inotropic effects (eg, verapamil, diltiazem) can lead to an exaggeration of these effects particularly in patients with impaired ventricular function and/or SA or AV conduction abnormalities. This may result in severe hypotension, bradycardia and cardiac failure. Neither the beta-adrenoceptor blocking drug nor the calcium channel blocker should be administered intravenously within 48 hours of discontinuing the other.

Concomitant therapy with dihydropyridines calcium channel blockers eg, nifedipine, may increase the risk of hypotension, and cardiac failure may occur in patients with latent cardiac insufficiency.

Concomitant use of sympathomimetic agents eg, adrenaline, may counteract the effect of beta-adrenoceptor blocking drugs. Caution must be exercised in the parenteral administration of preparations containing adrenaline to patients taking beta-adrenoceptor blocking drugs as, in rare cases, vasoconstriction, hypertension and bradycardia may result.

Administration of Inderal during infusion of lignocaine may increase the plasma concentration of lignocaine by approximately 30%. Patients already receiving Inderal tend to have higher lignocaine levels than controls. The combination should be avoided.

Concomitant use of cimetidine or hydralazine will increase, whereas concomitant use of alcohol will decrease, the plasma levels of propranolol.

Beta-adrenoceptor blocking drugs may exacerbate the rebound hypertension which can follow the withdrawal of clonidine. If the two drugs are co-administered, the beta-adrenoceptor blocking drug should be withdrawn several days before discontinuing clonidine. If replacing clonidine by beta-adrenoceptor blocking drug therapy, the introduction of beta-adrenoceptor blocking drugs should be delayed for several days after clonidine administration has stopped.

Caution must be exercised if ergotamine, dihydroergotamine or related compounds are given in combination with Inderal since vasospastic reactions have been reported in a few patients.

Concomitant use of prostaglandin synthetase inhibiting drugs eg, ibuprofen and indomethacin, may decrease the hypotensive effects of Inderal.

Concomitant administration of Inderal and chlorpromazine may result in an increase in plasma levels of both drugs. This may lead to an enhanced antipsychotic effect for chlorpromazine and an increased antihypertensive effect for Inderal.

Caution must be exercised when using anaesthetic agents with Inderal. The anaesthetist should be informed and the choice of anaesthetic should be an agent with as little negative inotropic activity as possible. Use of beta-adrenoceptor blocking drugs with anaesthetic drugs may result in attenuation of the reflex tachycardia and increase the risk of hypotension. Anaesthetic agents causing myocardial depression are best avoided.

Pharmacokinetic studies have shown that the following agents may interact with propranolol due to effects on enzyme systems in the liver which metabolise propranolol and these agents: quinidine, propafenone, rifampicin, theophylline, warfarin, thioridazine and dihydropyridine calcium channel blockers such as nifedipine, nisoldipine, nicardipine, isradipine and lacidipine. Owing to the fact that blood concentrations of either agent may be affected dosage adjustments may be needed according to clinical judgement. (See also the interaction above concerning the concomitant therapy with dihydropyridine calcium channel blockers).

4.6 Pregnancy and lactation

Pregnancy

As with all drugs Inderal should not be given during pregnancy unless its use is essential. There is no evidence of teratogenicity with Inderal. However beta-adrenoceptor blocking drugs reduce placental perfusion, which may result in intra-uterine foetal death, immature and premature deliveries. In addition, adverse effects (especially hypoglycaemia and bradycardia in the neonate and bradycardia in the foetus) may occur. There is an increased risk of cardiac and pulmonary complications in the neonate in the postnatal period.

Lactation

Most beta-adrenoceptor blocking drugs, particularly lipophilic compounds, will pass into breast milk although to a variable extent. Breast feeding is therefore not recommended following administration of these compounds.

4.7 Effects on ability to drive and use machines

Use is unlikely to result in any impairment of the ability of patients to drive or operate machinery. However it should be taken into account that occasionally dizziness or fatigue may occur.

4.8 Undesirable effects

Inderal is usually well tolerated. In clinical studies the undesired events reported are usually attributable to the pharmacological actions of propranolol.

The following undesired events, listed by body system, have been reported.

Cardiovascular: bradycardia; heart failure deterioration; postural hypotension which may be associated with syncope; cold cyanotic extremities. In susceptible patients: precipitation of heart block; exacerbation of intermittent claudication; Raynaud's phenomenon.

CNS: confusion; dizziness; mood changes; nightmares; psychoses and hallucinations; sleep disturbances.

Endocrine: Hypoglycaemia in neonates, infants, children (Inderal is not recommended for use in children – see section 4.2), elderly patients, patients on haemodialysis, patients on concomitant antidiabetic therapy, patients with prolonged fasting and patients with chronic liver disease has been reported (see section 4.3, 4.4 and 4.5).

Gastrointestinal: gastrointestinal disturbance.

Haematological: purpura; thrombocytopenia.

Integumentary: alopecia; dry eyes; psoriasiform skin reactions; exacerbation of psoriasis; skin rashes.

Neurological: paraesthesia.

Respiratory: bronchospasm may occur in patients with bronchial asthma or a history of asthmatic complaints, sometimes with fatal outcome (see Section 4.3).

Special senses: visual disturbances.

Others: fatigue and/or lassitude (often transient); an increase in ANA (Antinuclear Antibodies) has been observed, however the clinical relevance of this is not clear; isolated reports of myasthenia gravis like syndrome or exacerbation of myasthenia gravis have been reported in patients administered propranolol.

Discontinuance of the drug should be considered if, according to clinical judgement, the well-being of the patient is adversely affected by any of the above reactions. Cessation of therapy with a beta-adrenoceptor blocking drug should be gradual. In the rare event of intolerance, manifested as bradycardia and hypotension, the drug should be withdrawn and, if necessary, treatment for overdosage instituted.

4.9 Overdose

The symptoms of overdosage may include bradycardia, hypotension, acute cardiac insufficiency and bronchospasm.

General treatment should include: close supervision, treatment in an intensive care ward, the use of gastric lavage, activated charcoal and a laxative to prevent absorption of any drug still present in the gastrointestinal tract, the use of plasma or plasma substitutes to treat hypotension and shock.

Excessive bradycardia can be countered with atropine 1 to 2 mg intravenously and/or a cardiac pacemaker. If necessary, this may be followed by a bolus dose of glucagon 10 mg intravenously. If required, this may be repeated or followed by an intravenous infusion of glucagon 1 to 10 mg/hour depending on response. If no response to glucagon occurs or if glucagon is unavailable, a beta-adrenoceptor stimulant such as dobutamine 2.5 to 10 microgram/kg/minute by intravenous infusion may be given. Dobutamine, because of its positive inotropic effect, could also be used to treat hypotension and acute cardiac insufficiency. It is likely that these doses would be inadequate to reverse the cardiac effects of beta-adrenoceptor blockade if a large overdose has been taken. The dose of dobutamine should therefore be increased if necessary to achieve the required response according to the clinical condition of the patient.

5. PHARMACOLOGICAL PROPERTIES

5.1 Pharmacodynamic properties

Inderal is a competitive antagonist at both the beta$_1$- and beta$_2$ adrenoceptors. It has no agonist activity at the beta-adrenoceptor, but has membrane stabilising activity at concentrations exceeding 1 to 3 mg/litre, though such concentrations are rarely achieved during oral therapy. Competitive beta-adrenoceptor blockade has been demonstrated in man by a parallel shift to the right in the dose-heart rate response curve to beta agonists such as isoprenaline.

Propranolol as with other beta-adrenoceptor blocking drugs, has negative inotropic effects, and is therefore contraindicated in uncontrolled heart failure.

Inderal is a racemic mixture and the active form is the S (-) isomer of propranolol. With the exception of inhibition of the conversion of thyroxine to triiodothyronine, it is unlikely that any additional ancillary properties possessed by R (+) propranolol, in comparison with the racemic mixture, will give rise to different therapeutic effects.

Inderal is effective and well tolerated in most ethnic populations, although the response may be less in black patients.

5.2 Pharmacokinetic properties

Following intravenous administration the plasma half-life of propranolol is about 2 hours and the ratio of metabolites to parent drug in the blood is lower than after oral administration. In particular 4-hydroxypropranolol is not present after intravenous administration. Propranolol is completely absorbed after oral administration and peak plasma concentrations occur 1 to 2 hours after dosing in fasting patients. The liver removes up to 90% of an oral dose with an elimination half-life of 3 to 6 hours. Propranolol is widely and rapidly distributed throughout the body with highest levels occurring in the lungs, liver, kidney, brain and heart. Propranolol is highly protein bound (80 to 95%).

5.3 Preclinical safety data

Propranolol is a drug on which extensive clinical experience has been obtained. Relevant information for the prescriber is provided elsewhere in this Summary of Product Characteristics.

6. PHARMACEUTICAL PARTICULARS

6.1 List of excipients

Citric acid (anhydrous) Ph. Eur.
Water for injections Ph. Eur.

6.2 Incompatibilities

None known.

6.3 Shelf life

5 years.

6.4 Special precautions for storage

Store below 30°C, protected from light

6.5 Nature and contents of container

Ampoule containing 1 ml.

6.6 Instructions for use and handling

None stated.

7. MARKETING AUTHORISATION HOLDER

AstraZeneca UK Limited,
600 Capability Green,
Luton, LU1 3LU, UK.

8. MARKETING AUTHORISATION NUMBER(S)

PL 17901/0018

9. DATE OF FIRST AUTHORISATION/RENEWAL OF THE AUTHORISATION

11th June 2000 / 4th June 2003

10. DATE OF REVISION OF THE TEXT

4th June 2003

Inderal LA 160mg

(AstraZeneca UK Limited)

1. NAME OF THE MEDICINAL PRODUCT

Inderal LA 160mg.

2. QUALITATIVE AND QUANTITATIVE COMPOSITION

Propranolol hydrochloride Ph Eur 160 mg

3. PHARMACEUTICAL FORM

Pink/lavender prolonged release capsules, marked Inderal LA in white

4. CLINICAL PARTICULARS

4.1 Therapeutic indications

a) Control of hypertension

b) Management of angina

c) Prophylaxis of migraine

d) Management of essential tremor

e) Management of anxiety

f) Adjunctive management of thyrotoxicosis

g) Prophylaxis of upper gastro-intestinal bleeding in patients with portal hypertension and oesophageal varices

4.2 Posology and method of administration

For oral administration.

Adults

Hypertension: The usual starting dose is one 160 mg Inderal LA capsule daily, taken either morning or evening. An adequate response is seen in most patients at this dosage. If necessary, it can be increased in 80 mg Half-Inderal LA increments until an adequate response is achieved. A further reduction in blood pressure can be obtained if a diuretic or other antihypertensive agent is given in addition to Inderal LA and Half-Inderal LA.

Angina, anxiety, essential tremor, thyrotoxicosis and the prophylaxis of migraine: One Half-Inderal LA capsule daily, taken either morning or evening, may be sufficient to provide adequate control in many patients. If necessary the dose may be increased to one Inderal LA capsule per day and an additional Half-Inderal LA increment may be given.

Portal hypertension: Dosage should be titrated to achieve approximately 25% reduction in resting heart rate. Dosing should begin with one 80 mg Half-Inderal LA capsule daily, increasing to one 160 mg Inderal LA capsule daily depending on heart rate response. Further 80 mg Half-Inderal LA increments may be added up to a maximum dose of 320 mg once daily.

Patients who are already established on equivalent daily doses of Inderal tablets should be transferred to the equivalent doses of Half-Inderal LA or Inderal LA daily, taken either morning or evening.

Children

Inderal LA and Half-Inderal LA are not intended for use in children.

Elderly Patients

Evidence concerning the relation between blood level and age is conflicting. It is suggested that treatment should start with one Half-Inderal LA capsule once daily. The dose may be increased to one Inderal LA capsule daily or higher as appropriate.

4.3 Contraindications

Inderal LA and Half-Inderal LA must not be used if there is a history of bronchial asthma or bronchospasm. The product label states the following warning: "Do not take Inderal LA if you have a history of asthma or wheezing". A similar warning appears in the Patient Information Leaflet.

Bronchospasm can usually be reversed by $beta_2$- agonist bronchodilators such as salbutamol. Large doses of the $beta_2$- agonist bronchodilator may be required to overcome the beta-blockade produced by propranolol and the dose should be titrated according to the clinical response; both intravenous and inhalational administration should be considered. The use of intravenous aminophylline and/or the use of ipratropium (given by nebuliser) may also be considered. Glucagon (1 to 2 mg given intravenously) has also been reported to produce a bronchodilator effect in asthmatic patients. Oxygen or artificial ventilation may be required in severe cases.

Inderal LA and Half-Inderal LA, as with other beta-adrenoceptor blocking drugs, must not be used in patients with any of the following conditions: known hypersensitivity to the substance, bradycardia, cardiogenic shock, hypotension, metabolic acidosis, after prolonged fasting, severe peripheral arterial circulatory disturbances, second or third degree heart block, sick sinus syndrome, untreated phaeochromocytoma, uncontrolled heart failure or Prinzmetal's angina.

Inderal LA and Half-Inderal LA must not be used in patients prone to hypoglycaemia, i.e., patients after prolonged fasting or patients with restricted counter-regulatory reserves.

4.4 Special warnings and special precautions for use

Inderal LA and Half-Inderal LA as with other beta-adrenoceptor blocking drugs:

- although contra-indicated in uncontrolled heart failure (see Section 4.3) may be used in patients whose signs of heart failure have been controlled. Caution must be exercised in patients whose cardiac reserve is poor.
- should not be used in combination with calcium channel blockers with negative inotropic effects (e.g. verapamil, diltiazem), as it can lead to an exaggeration of these effects particularly in patients with impaired ventricular function and/or SA or AV conduction abnormalities. This may result in severe hypotension, bradycardia and cardiac failure. Neither the beta-blocker nor the calcium channel blocker should be administered intravenously within 48 hours of discontinuing the other.
- should not be used in patients with Prinzmetal's angina and beta-1 selective agents should be used with care. (see section 4.3).
- although contra-indicated in severe peripheral arterial circulatory disturbances (see Section 4.3) may also aggravate less severe peripheral arterial circulatory disturbances.
- due to its negative effect on conduction time, caution must be exercised if it is given to patients with first degree heart block.
- may block/modify the signs and symptoms of the hypoglycaemia (especially tachycardia). Inderal LA and Half-Inderal LA occasionally causes hypoglycaemia, even in non-diabetic patients, e.g., neonates, infants, children, elderly patients, patients on haemodialysis or patients suffering from chronic liver disease and patients suffering from overdose. Severe hypoglycaemia associated with Inderal LA and Half-Inderal LA has rarely presented with seizures and/or coma in isolated patients. Caution must be exercised in the concurrent use of Inderal LA and Half-Inderal LA and hypoglycaemic therapy in diabetic patients. Inderal LA and Half-Inderal LA may prolong the hypoglycaemic response to insulin. (see section 4.3).
- may mask the signs of thyrotoxicosis.
- should not be used in untreated phaeochromocytoma. However, in patients with phaeochromocytoma, an alpha-blocker may be given concomitantly.
- should be used to treat the elderly with caution starting with a lower dose. (see section 4.2).
- will reduce heart rate as a result of its pharmacological action. In the rare instances when a treated patient develops symptoms that may be attributable to a slow heart rate, the dose may be reduced.
- may cause a more severe reaction to a variety of allergens, when given to patients with a history of anaphylactic reaction to such allergens. Such patients may be unresponsive to the usual doses of adrenaline used to treat the allergic reactions.

Abrupt withdrawal of beta-blockers is to be avoided. The dosage should be withdrawn gradually over a period of 7 to 14 days. An equivalent dosage of another beta-blocker may be substituted during the withdrawal period to facilitate a reduction in dosage below Inderal LA 80mg. Patients should be followed during withdrawal especially those with ischaemic heart disease.

When a patient is scheduled for surgery and a decision is made to discontinue beta-blocker therapy, this should be done at least 24 hours prior to the procedure. The risk/benefit of stopping beta blockade should be made for each patient.

Since the half-life may be increased in patients with significant hepatic or renal impairment, caution must be exercised when starting treatment and selecting the initial dose.

Inderal LA and Half-Inderal LA must be used with caution in patients with decompensated cirrhosis. (see section 4.2)

In patients with portal hypertension, liver function may deteriorate and hepatic encephalopathy may develop. There have been reports suggesting that treatment with propranolol may increase the risk of developing hepatic encephalopathy (see section 4.2).

Interference with laboratory tests: Inderal LA and Half-Inderal LA have been reported to interfere with the estimation of serum bilirubin by the diazo method and with the determination of catecholamines by methods using fluorescence.

4.5 Interaction with other medicinal products and other forms of Interaction

Inderal LA and Half-Inderal LA modify the tachycardia of hypoglycaemia. Caution must be exercised in the concurrent use of Inderal LA or Half-Inderal LA and hypoglycaemic therapy in diabetic patients. Propranolol may prolong the hypoglycaemic response to insulin.(see section 4.3 and 4.4).

Caution must be exercised when prescribing a beta-adrenoceptor blocking drug with Class 1 antiarrhythmic agents such as disopyramide.

Digitalis glycosides, in association with beta-adrenoceptor blocking drugs, may increase atrio-ventricular conduction time.

Combined use of beta-adrenoceptor blocking drugs and calcium channel blockers with negative inotropic effects eg, verapamil, diltiazem, can lead to an exaggeration of these effects, particularly in patients with impaired ventricular function and/or sino-atrial or atrio-ventricular conduction abnormalities. This may result in severe hypotension, bradycardia and cardiac failure. Neither the beta-adrenoceptor blocking drug nor the calcium channel blocker should be administered intravenously within 48 hours of discontinuing the other.

Concomitant therapy with dihydropyridine calcium channel blockers eg, nifedipine, may increase the risk of hypotension, and cardiac failure may occur in patients with latent cardiac insufficiency.

Concomitant use of sympathomimetic agents, eg, adrenaline, may counteract the effect of beta-adrenoceptor blocking drugs. Caution must be exercised in the parenteral administration of preparations containing adrenaline to patients taking beta-adrenoceptor blocking drugs as, in rare cases, vasoconstriction, hypertension and bradycardia may result.

Administration of propranolol during infusion of lignocaine may increase the plasma concentration of lignocaine by approximately 30%. Patients already receiving propranolol tend to have higher lignocaine levels than controls. The combination should be avoided.

Concomitant use of cimetidine will increase, whereas concomitant use of alcohol will decrease, the plasma levels of propranolol.

Beta-adrenoceptor blocking drugs may exacerbate the rebound hypertension, which can follow the withdrawal of clonidine. If the two drugs are co-administered, the beta-adrenoceptor blocking drug should be withdrawn several days before discontinuing clonidine. If replacing clonidine by beta-adrenoceptor blocking drug therapy, the introduction of beta-adrenoceptor blocking drugs should be delayed for several days after clonidine administration has stopped.

Caution must be exercised if ergotamine, dihydroergotamine or related compounds are given in combination with propranolol since vasospastic reactions have been reported in a few patients.

Concomitant use of prostaglandin synthetase inhibiting drugs, eg, ibuprofen or indomethacin, may decrease the hypotensive effects of propranolol.

Concomitant administration of propranolol and chlorpromazine may result in an increase in plasma levels of both drugs. This may lead to an enhanced antipsychotic effect for chlorpromazine and an increased antihypertensive effect for propranolol.

Caution must be exercised when using anaesthetic agents with Inderal LA and Half-Inderal LA. The anaesthetist should be informed and the choice of anaesthetic should be the agent with as little negative inotropic activity as possible. Use of beta-adrenoceptor blocking drugs with anaesthetic drugs may result in attenuation of the reflex tachycardia and increase the risk of hypotension. Anaesthetic agents causing myocardial depression are best avoided.

Pharmacokinetic studies have shown that the following agents may interact with propranolol due to effects on enzyme systems in the liver which metabolise propranolol and these agents: quinidine, propafenone, rifampicin, theophylline, warfarin, thioridazine and dihydropyridine calcium channel blockers such as nifedipine, nisoldipine, nicardipine, isradipine and lacidipine. Owing to the fact that blood concentrations of either agent may be affected, dosage adjustments may be needed according to clinical judgement. (See also the interaction above concerning concomitant therapy with dihydropyridine calcium channel blockers).

4.6 Pregnancy and lactation

Pregnancy: As with all drugs, Inderal LA and Half-Inderal LA should not be given during pregnancy unless their use is essential. There is no evidence of teratogenicity with Inderal. However beta-adrenoceptor blocking drugs reduce placental perfusion, which may result in intra-uterine foetal death, immature and premature deliveries. In addition, adverse effects (especially hypoglycaemia and bradycardia in the neonate and bradycardia in the foetus) may occur. There is an increased risk of cardiac and pulmonary complications in the neonate in the post-natal period.

Lactation: Most beta-adrenoceptor blocking drugs, particularly lipophilic compounds, will pass into breast milk although to a variable extent. Breast feeding is therefore not recommended following administration of these compounds.

4.7 Effects on ability to drive and use machines

The use of Inderal LA or Half-Inderal LA is unlikely to result in any impairment of the ability of patients to drive or operate machinery. However, it should be taken into account that occasionally dizziness or fatigue may occur.

4.8 Undesirable effects

Inderal LA and Half-Inderal LA are usually well tolerated. In clinical studies, the undesired events reported are usually attributable to the pharmacological actions of propranolol.

The following undesired events, listed by body system, have been reported.

Cardiovascular: bradycardia, heart failure deterioration, postural hypotension which may be associated with syncope, cold cyanotic extremities. In susceptible patients: precipitation of heart block, exacerbation of intermittent claudication, Raynaud's phenomenon.

CNS: confusion, dizziness, mood changes, nightmares, psychoses and hallucinations, sleep disturbances.

Endocrine: Hypoglycaemia in neonates, infants, children, elderly patients, patients on haemodialysis, patients on concomitant antidiabetic therapy, patients with prolonged fasting and patients with chronic liver disease has been reported (see section 4.3, 4.4 and 4.5).

Gastrointestinal: gastrointestinal disturbance.

Haematological: purpura, thrombocytopenia.

Integumentary: alopecia, dry eyes, psoriasiform skin reactions, exacerbation of psoriasis, skin rashes.

Neurological: paraesthesia.

Respiratory: bronchospasm may occur in patients with bronchial asthma or a history of asthmatic complaints, sometimes with fatal outcome (see Section 4.3).

Special senses: visual disturbances.

Others: fatigue and/or lassitude (often transient), an increase in ANA (antinuclear antibodies) has been observed, however the clinical relevance of this is not clear; isolated reports of myasthenia gravis like syndrome or exacerbation of myasthenia gravis have been reported in patients administered propranolol.

Discontinuance of the drug should be considered if, according to clinical judgement, the well-being of the patient is adversely affected by any of the above reactions. Cessation of therapy with a beta-adrenoceptor blocking drug should be gradual. In the rare event of intolerance manifested as bradycardia and hypotension, the drug should be withdrawn and, if necessary, treatment for overdosage instituted.

4.9 Overdose

The symptoms of overdosage may include bradycardia, hypotension, acute cardiac insufficiency and bronchospasm.

General treatment should include: close supervision, treatment in an intensive care ward, the use of gastric lavage, activated charcoal and a laxative to prevent absorption of any drug still present in the gastrointestinal tract, the use of plasma or plasma substitutes to treat hypotension and shock.

Excessive bradycardia can be countered with atropine 1 to 2 mg intravenously and/or a cardiac pacemaker. If necessary, this may be followed by a bolus dose of glucagon 10 mg intravenously. If required, this may be repeated or followed by an intravenous infusion of glucagon 1 to 10 mg/hour depending on response. If no response to glucagon occurs or if glucagon is unavailable, a beta-adrenoceptor stimulant such as dobutamine 2.5 to 10 microgram/kg/minute by intravenous infusion may be given. Dobutamine, because of its positive inotropic effect, could also be used to treat hypotension and acute cardiac insufficiency. It is likely that these doses would be inadequate to reverse the cardiac effects of beta-blockade if a large overdose has been taken. The dose of dobutamine should therefore be increased if necessary to achieve the required response according to the clinical condition of the patient.

5. PHARMACOLOGICAL PROPERTIES

5.1 Pharmacodynamic properties

Propranolol is a competitive antagonist at both $beta_1$ and $beta_2$-adrenoceptors. It has no agonist activity at the beta-adrenoceptor, but has membrane stabilising activity at concentrations exceeding 1 to 3 mg/litre, though such concentrations are rarely achieved during oral therapy. Competitive beta-adrenoceptor blockade has been demonstrated in man by a parallel shift to the right in the dose-heart rate response curve to beta-agonists such as isoprenaline.

Propranolol, as with other beta-adrenoceptor blocking drugs, has negative inotropic effects, and is therefore contra-indicated in uncontrolled heart failure.

Propranolol is a racemic mixture and the active form is the S (-) isomer. With the exception of inhibition of the conversion of thyroxine to triiodothyronine it is unlikely that any additional ancillary properties possessed by R (+) propranolol, in comparison with the racemic mixture will give rise to different therapeutic effects.

Propranolol is effective and well tolerated in most ethnic populations, although the response may be less in black patients.

The sustained release preparation of propranolol maintains a higher degree of $beta_1$-blockade 24 hours after dosing compared with conventional propranolol.

5.2 Pharmacokinetic properties

Propranolol is completely absorbed after oral administration and peak plasma concentrations occur 1-2 hours after dosing in fasting patients. Following oral dosing with the sustained release preparation of propranolol, the blood profile is flatter than after conventional Inderal but the half-life is increased to between 10 and 20 hours. The liver removes up to 90% of an oral dose with an elimination half-life of 3 to 6 hours. Propranolol is widely and rapidly distributed throughout the body with highest levels occurring in the lungs, liver, kidney, brain and heart. Propranolol is highly protein bound (80 to 95%).

5.3 Preclinical safety data

Propranolol is a drug on which extensive clinical experience has been obtained. Relevant information for the prescriber is provided elsewhere in this Summary of Product Characteristics.

6. PHARMACEUTICAL PARTICULARS

6.1 List of excipients

Erythrosine (E127)

Ethyl cellulose

Gelatin

Glycerol

Iron oxide, red (E172)

Iron oxide, black (E172)

Methylhydroxypropylcellulose

Microcrystalline cellulose

Titanium dioxide (E171)

6.2 Incompatibilities

None known.

6.3 Shelf life

5 years.

6.4 Special precautions for storage

Store below 30°C, protected from light and moisture.

6.5 Nature and contents of container

Patient calendar pack of 28 capsules.

6.6 Instructions for use and handling

Use as directed by the prescriber.

Administrative Data

7. MARKETING AUTHORISATION HOLDER

AstraZeneca UK Limited

600 Capability Green

Luton

LU1 3LU

UK

8. MARKETING AUTHORISATION NUMBER(S)

PL 17901/0019

9. DATE OF FIRST AUTHORISATION/RENEWAL OF THE AUTHORISATION

11th June 2000

10. DATE OF REVISION OF THE TEXT

25th October 2001

Inderal Tablets 10mg, 40mg & 80mg

(AstraZeneca UK Limited)

1. NAME OF THE MEDICINAL PRODUCT

Inderal Tablets 10 mg.

Inderal Tablets 40 mg.

Inderal Tablets 80 mg.

2. QUALITATIVE AND QUANTITATIVE COMPOSITION

Propranolol Hydrochloride Ph. Eur. 10 mg.

Propranolol Hydrochloride Ph. Eur. 40 mg.

Propranolol Hydrochloride Ph. Eur. 80 mg.

3. PHARMACEUTICAL FORM

Round pink film coated tablets.

4. CLINICAL PARTICULARS

4.1 Therapeutic indications

a) the control of hypertension;

b) the management of angina pectoris;

c) long term management against re-infarction after recovery from acute myocardial infarction;

d) the control of most forms of cardiac dysrhythmias;

e) the prophylaxis of migraine;

f) the management of essential tremor;

g) relief of situational anxiety and generalised anxiety symptoms, particularly those of somatic type;

h) prophylaxis of upper gastrointestinal bleeding in patients with portal hypertension and oesophageal varices;

i) the adjunctive management of thyrotoxicosis and thyrotoxic crisis;

j) management of hypertrophic obstructive cardiomyopathy;

k) management of phaeochromocytoma peri-operatively (with an alpha-blocker).

4.2 Posology and method of administration

For oral administration

Adults

Hypertension

A starting dose of 80 mg twice a day may be increased at weekly intervals according to response. The usual dose range is 160 to 320 mg per day. With concurrent diuretic or other antihypertensive drugs a further reduction of blood pressure is obtained.

Angina, migraine and essential tremor

A starting dose of 40 mg two or three times daily may be increased by the same amount at weekly intervals according to patient response. An adequate response in migraine and essential tremor is usually seen in the range 80 to 160 mg/day and in angina in the range 120 to 240 mg/day.

Situational and generalised anxiety

A dose of 40 mg daily may provide short term relief of acute situational anxiety. Generalised anxiety, requiring longer term therapy, usually responds adequately to 40 mg twice daily which, in individual cases, may be increased to 40 mg three times daily. Treatment should be continued according to response. Patients should be reviewed after 6 to 12 months treatment.

Dysrhythmias, anxiety tachycardia, hypertrophic obstructive cardiomyopathy and thyrotoxicosis

A dosage range of 10 to 40 mg three or four times a day usually achieves the required response.

Post myocardial infarction

Treatment should start between days 5 and 21 after myocardial infarction, with an initial dose of 40 mg four times a day for 2 or 3 days. In order to improve compliance the total daily dosage may thereafter be given as 80 mg twice a day.

Portal hypertension

Dosage should be titrated to achieve approximately 25% reduction in resting heart rate. Dosage should begin with 40 mg twice daily, increasing to 80 mg twice daily depending on heart rate response. If necessary, the dose may be increased incrementally to a maximum of 160 mg twice daily.

Phaeochromocytoma

(Used only with an alpha-receptor blocking drug).

Pre-operative: 60 mg daily for 3 days is recommended. Non-operable malignant cases: 30 mg daily.

Elderly

Evidence concerning the relation between blood level and age is conflicting. Inderal should be used to treat the elderly with caution. It is suggested that treatment should start with the lowest dose. The optimum dose should be individually determined according to clinical response.

Children

Dysrhythmias, phaeochromocytoma, thyrotoxicosis

Dosage should be individually determined and the following is only a guide:

Oral: 0.25 to 0.5 mg/kg three or four times daily as required.

Migraine

Oral: Under the age of 12: 20 mg two or three times daily. Over the age of 12: The adult dose.

Fallot's tetralogy

The value of Inderal in this condition is confined mainly to the relief of right-ventricular outflow tract shut-down. It is also useful for treatment of associated dysrhythmias and angina. Dosage should be individually determined and the following is only a guide:

Oral: Up to 1 mg/kg repeated three or four times daily as required.

4.3 Contraindications

Inderal must not be used if there is a history of bronchial asthma or bronchospasm. The product label states the following warning: "Do not take Inderal if you have a history of asthma or wheezing". A similar warning appears in the patient information leaflet.

Bronchospasm can usually be reversed by $beta_2$- agonist bronchodilators such as salbutamol. Large doses of the $beta_2$- agonist bronchodilator may be required to overcome the beta-blockade produced by propranolol and the dose should be titrated according to the clinical response; both intravenous and inhalational administration should be considered. The use of intravenous aminophylline and/or the use of ipratropium (given by nebuliser) may also be considered. Glucagon (1 to 2 mg given intravenously) has also been reported to produce a bronchodilator effect in asthmatic patients. Oxygen or artificial ventilation may be required in severe cases.

Inderal as with other beta-adrenoceptor blocking drugs must not be used in patients with any of the following conditions: known hypersensitivity to the substance; bradycardia; cardiogenic shock; hypotension; metabolic acidosis; after prolonged fasting; severe peripheral arterial circulatory disturbances; second or third degree heart block; sick sinus syndrome; untreated phaeochromocytoma; uncontrolled heart failure or Prinzmetal's angina.

Inderal must not be used in patients prone to hypoglycaemia, i.e., patients after prolonged fasting or patients with restricted counter-regulatory reserves. Patients with restricted counter regulatory reserves may have reduced autonomic and hormonal responses to hypoglycaemia which includes glycogenolysis, gluconeogenesis and /or impaired modulation of insulin secretion. Patients at risk for an inadequate response to hypoglycaemia includes individuals with malnutrition, prolonged fasting, starvation, chronic liver disease, diabetes and concomitant use of drugs which block the full response to catecholamines.

4.4 Special warnings and special precautions for use

Inderal as with other beta-adrenoceptor blocking drugs:

- although contraindicated in uncontrolled heart failure (see Section 4.3), may be used in patients whose signs of heart failure have been controlled. Caution must be exercised in patients whose cardiac reserve is poor.

- should not be used in combination with calcium channel blockers with negative inotropic effects (e.g. verapamil, diltiazem), as it can lead to an exaggeration of these effects particularly in patients with impaired ventricular function and/or SA or AV conduction abnormalities. This may result in severe hypotension, bradycardia and cardiac failure. Neither the beta-blocker nor the calcium channel blocker should be administered intravenously within 48 hours of discontinuing the other.

- although contraindicated in severe peripheral arterial circulatory disturbances (see section 4.3), may also aggravate less severe peripheral arterial circulatory disturbances

- due to its negative effect on conduction time, caution must be exercised if it is given to patients with first degree heart block.

- may block/modify the signs and symptoms of the hypoglycaemia (especially tachycardia). Inderal occasionally causes hypoglycaemia, even in non-diabetic patients, e.g., neonates, infants, children (Inderal is not recommended for use in children – see section 4.2), elderly patients, patients on haemodialysis or patients suffering from chronic liver disease and patients suffering from overdose. Severe hypoglycaemia associated with Inderal has rarely presented with seizures and/or coma in isolated patients. Caution must be exercised in the concurrent use of Inderal and hypoglycaemic therapy in diabetic patients. Inderal may prolong the hypoglycaemic response to insulin. (see section 4.3).

- may mask the signs of thyrotoxicosis.

- should not be used in untreated phaeochromocytoma. However, in patients with phaeochromocytoma, an alpha-blocker may be given concomitantly.

- will reduce heart rate as a result of its pharmacological action. In the rare instances when a treated patient develops symptoms which may be attributable to a slow heart rate, the dose may be reduced.

- may cause a more severe reaction to a variety of allergens when given to patients with a history of anaphylactic reaction to such allergens. Such patients may be unresponsive to the usual doses of adrenaline used to treat the allergic reactions.

Abrupt withdrawal of beta-blockers is to be avoided. The dosage should be withdrawn gradually over a period of 7 to 14 days. Patients should be followed during withdrawal especially those with ischaemic heart disease.

When a patient is scheduled for surgery and a decision is made to discontinue beta-blocker therapy, this should be done at least 24 hours prior to the procedure. The risk/benefit of stopping beta blockade should be made for each patient

Since the half-life may be increased in patients with significant hepatic or renal impairment, caution must be exercised when starting treatment and selecting the initial dose.

Inderal must be used with caution in patients with decompensated cirrhosis (see section 4.2).

In patients with portal hypertension, liver function may deteriorate and hepatic encephalopathy may develop. There have been reports suggesting that treatment with propranolol may increase the risk of developing hepatic encephalopathy (see section 4.2).

Interference with laboratory tests: Inderal has been reported to interfere with the estimation of serum bilirubin by the diazo method and with the determination of catecholamines by methods using fluorescence.

4.5 Interaction with other medicinal products and other forms of Interaction

Inderal modifies the tachycardia of hypoglycaemia. Caution must be exercised in the concurrent use of Inderal and hypoglycaemic therapy in diabetic patients. Inderal may prolong the hypoglycaemic response to insulin.

Caution must be exercised in prescribing a beta-adrenoceptor blocking drug with Class I antiarrhythmic agents such as disopyramide.

Digitalis glycosides in association with beta-adrenoceptor blocking drugs may increase atrioventricular conduction time.

Combined use of beta-adrenoceptor blocking drugs and calcium channel blockers with negative inotropic effects (eg, verapamil, diltiazem) can lead to an exaggeration of these effects particularly in patients with impaired ventricular function and/or SA or AV conduction abnormalities. This may result in severe hypotension, bradycardia and cardiac failure. Neither the beta-adrenoceptor blocking drug nor the calcium channel blocker should be administered intravenously within 48 hours of discontinuing the other.

Concomitant therapy with dihydropyridine calcium channel blockers eg, nifedipine, may increase the risk of hypotension, and cardiac failure may occur in patients with latent cardiac insufficiency.

Concomitant use of sympathomimetic agents eg, adrenaline, may counteract the effect of beta-adrenoceptor blocking drugs. Caution must be exercised in the parenteral administration of preparations containing adrenaline to patients taking beta-adrenoceptor blocking drugs as, in rare cases, vasoconstriction, hypertension and bradycardia may result.

Administration of Inderal during infusion of lignocaine may increase the plasma concentration of lignocaine by approximately 30%. Patients already receiving Inderal tend to have higher lignocaine levels than controls. The combination should be avoided.

Concomitant use of cimetidine or hydralazine will increase, whereas concomitant use of alcohol will decrease, the plasma levels of propranolol.

Beta-adrenoceptor blocking drugs may exacerbate the rebound hypertension which can follow the withdrawal of clonidine. If the two drugs are co-administered, the beta-adrenoceptor blocking drug should be withdrawn several days before discontinuing clonidine. If replacing clonidine by beta-adrenoceptor blocking drug therapy, the introduction of beta-adrenoceptor blocking drugs should be delayed for several days after clonidine administration has stopped.

Caution must be exercised if ergotamine, dihydroergotamine or related compounds are given in combination with Inderal since vasospastic reactions have been reported in a few patients.

Concomitant use of prostaglandin synthetase inhibiting drugs e.g., ibuprofen and indomethacin, may decrease the hypotensive effects of Inderal.

Concomitant administration of Inderal and chlorpromazine may result in an increase in plasma levels of both drugs. This may lead to an enhanced antipsychotic effect for chlorpromazine and an increased antihypertensive effect for Inderal.

Caution must be exercised when using anaesthetic agents with Inderal. The anaesthetist should be informed and the choice of anaesthetic should be an agent with as little negative inotropic activity as possible. Use of beta-adrenoceptor blocking drugs with anaesthetic drugs may result in attenuation of the reflex tachycardia and increase the risk of hypotension. Anaesthetic agents causing myocardial depression are best avoided.

Pharmacokinetic studies have shown that the following agents may interact with propranolol due to effects on enzyme systems in the liver which metabolise propranolol and these agents: quinidine, propafenone, rifampicin, theophylline, warfarin, thioridazine and dihydropyridine calcium channel blockers such as nifedipine, nisoldipine, nicardipine, isradipine, and lacidipine. Owing to the fact that blood concentrations of either agent may be affected, dosage adjustments may be needed according to clinical judgement. (See also the interaction above concerning the concomitant therapy with dihydropyridine calcium channel blockers).

4.6 Pregnancy and lactation

Pregnancy

As with all drugs Inderal should not be given during pregnancy unless its use is essential. There is no evidence of teratogenicity with Inderal. However beta-adrenoceptor blocking drugs reduce placental perfusion, which may result in intra-uterine foetal death, immature and premature deliveries. In addition, adverse effects (especially hypoglycaemia and bradycardia in the neonate and bradycardia in the foetus) may occur. There is an increased risk of cardiac and pulmonary complications in the neonate in the post-natal period.

Lactation

Most beta-adrenoceptor blocking drugs, particularly lipophilic compounds, will pass into breast milk although to a variable extent. Breast feeding is therefore not recommended following administration of these compounds.

4.7 Effects on ability to drive and use machines

Use is unlikely to result in any impairment of the ability of patients to drive or operate machinery. However it should be taken into account that occasionally dizziness or fatigue may occur.

4.8 Undesirable effects

Inderal is usually well tolerated. In clinical studies the undesired events reported are usually attributable to the pharmacological actions of propranolol.

The following undesired events, listed by body system, have been reported.

Cardiovascular: bradycardia; heart failure deterioration; postural hypotension which may be associated with syncope; cold cyanoticextremities. In susceptible patients: precipitation of heart block; exacerbation of intermittent claudication; Raynaud's phenomenon.

CNS: confusion; dizziness; mood changes; nightmares; psychoses and hallucinations; sleep disturbances.

Endocrine: hypoglycaemia in neonates, infants, children (Inderal is not recommended for use in children – see section 4.2), elderly patients, patients on haemodialysis, patients on concomitant antidiabetic therapy, patients with prolonged fasting and patients with chronic liver disease has been reported (see section 4.3, 4.4 and 4.5).

Gastrointestinal: gastrointestinal disturbance.

Haematological: purpura; thrombocytopenia.

Integumentary: alopecia; dry eyes; psoriasiform skin reactions; exacerbation of psoriasis; skin rashes.

Neurological: paraesthesia.

Respiratory: bronchospasm may occur in patients with bronchial asthma or a history of asthmatic complaints, sometimes with fatal outcome (see Section 4.3).

Special senses: visual disturbances.

Others: fatigue and/or lassitude (often transient); an increase in ANA (Antinuclear Antibodies) has been observed, however the clinical relevance of this is not clear; isolated reports of myasthenia gravis like syndrome or exacerbation of myasthenia gravis have been reported in patients administered propranolol.

Discontinuance of the drug should be considered if, according to clinical judgement, the well-being of the patient is adversely affected by any of the above reactions. Cessation of therapy with a beta-adrenoceptor blocking drug should be gradual. In the rare event of intolerance, manifested as bradycardia and hypotension, the drug should be withdrawn and, if necessary, treatment for overdosage instituted.

4.9 Overdose

The symptoms of overdosage may include bradycardia, hypotension, acute cardiac insufficiency and bronchospasm.

General treatment should include: close supervision, treatment in an intensive care ward, the use of gastric lavage, activated charcoal and a laxative to prevent absorption of any drug still present in the gastrointestinal tract, the use of plasma or plasma substitutes to treat hypotension and shock.

Excessive bradycardia can be countered with atropine 1 to 2 mg intravenously and/or a cardiac pacemaker. If necessary, this may be followed by a bolus dose of glucagon 10 mg intravenously. If required, this may be repeated or followed by an intravenous infusion of glucagon 1 to 10 mg/hour depending on response. If no response to glucagon occurs or if glucagon is unavailable, a beta-adrenoceptor stimulant such as dobutamine 2.5 to10microgram/kg/minute by intravenous infusion may be given. Dobutamine, because of its positive inotropic effect, could also be used to treat hypotension and acute cardiac insufficiency. It is likely that these doses would be inadequate to reverse the cardiac effects of beta-adrenoceptor blockade if a large overdose has been taken. The dose of dobutamine should therefore be increased if necessary to achieve the required response according to the clinical condition of the patient.

5. PHARMACOLOGICAL PROPERTIES

5.1 Pharmacodynamic properties

Inderal is a competitive antagonist at both the beta$_1$- and beta$_2$ adrenoceptors. It has no agonist activity at the beta-adrenoceptor, but has membrane stabilising activity at concentrations exceeding 1 to 3 mg/litre, though such concentrations are rarely achieved during oral therapy. Competitive beta-adrenoceptor blockade has been demonstrated in man by a parallel shift to the right in the dose-heart rate response curve to beta agonists such as isoprenaline.

Propranolol as with other beta-adrenoceptor blocking drugs, has negative inotropic effects, and is therefore contraindicated in uncontrolled heart failure.

Inderal is a racemic mixture and the active form is the S (-) isomer of propranolol. With the exception of inhibition of the conversion of thyroxine to triiodothyronine, it is unlikely that any additional ancillary properties possessed by R (+) propranolol, in comparison with the racemic mixture, will give rise to different therapeutic effects.

Inderal is effective and well tolerated in most ethnic populations, although the response may be less in black patients.

5.2 Pharmacokinetic properties

Following intravenous administration the plasma half-life of propranolol is about 2 hours and the ratio of metabolites to parent drug in the blood is lower than after oral administration. In particular 4-hydroxypropranolol is not present after intravenous administration. Propranolol is completely absorbed after oral administration and peak plasma concentrations occur 1 to 2 hours after dosing in fasting patients. The liver removes up to 90% of an oral dose with an elimination half-life of 3 to 6 hours. Propranolol is widely and rapidly distributed throughout the body with highest levels occurring in the lungs, liver, kidney, brain and heart. Propranolol is highly protein bound (80 to 95%).

5.3 Preclinical safety data

Propranolol is a drug on which extensive clinical experience has been obtained. Relevant information for the prescriber is provided elsewhere in this Summary of Product Characteristics.

6. PHARMACEUTICAL PARTICULARS

6.1 List of excipients

10 mg, 40 mg and 80 mg:

Calcium Carboxymethyl
Cellulose USNF
Carmine BPC (E120)
Gelatin Ph. Eur.
Glycerol Ph. Eur.
Lactose Ph. Eur.
Light Magnesium Carbonate Ph.
Eur.
Magnesium Stearate Ph. Eur.
Methylhydroxypropylcellulose
Ph. Eur.
Titanium Dioxide Ph. Eur. (E171)

6.2 Incompatibilities

None known.

6.3 Shelf life

5 years.

6.4 Special precautions for storage

Store below 30°C, protected from light and moisture.

6.5 Nature and contents of container

10 mg & 40 mg: HDPE bottles of 100 tablets.

80 mg: HDPE bottles of 60 tablets.

6.6 Instructions for use and handling

None stated.

7. MARKETING AUTHORISATION HOLDER

AstraZeneca UK Ltd

600 Capability Green,

Luton, LU1 3LU, UK.

8. MARKETING AUTHORISATION NUMBER(S)

10 mg PL 17901/0021

40 mg PL 17901/0022

80 mg PL 17901/0023

9. DATE OF FIRST AUTHORISATION/RENEWAL OF THE AUTHORISATION

10 mg: 11th June 2000 / 4th June 2003

40 mg: 11th June 2000 / 4th June 2003

80 mg: 11th June 2000 / 4th June 2003

10. DATE OF REVISION OF THE TEXT

4th June 2003

Indivina

(Orion Pharma (UK) Limited)

1. NAME OF THE MEDICINAL PRODUCT

Indivina 1 mg/2.5 mg tablets

Indivina 1 mg/5 mg tablets

Indivina 2 mg/5 mg tablets

2. QUALITATIVE AND QUANTITATIVE COMPOSITION

One Indivina 1 mg/2.5 mg tablet contains:

Estradiol valerate 1 mg

Medroxyprogesterone acetate 2.5 mg

One Indivina 1 mg/5 mg tablet contains:

Estradiol valerate 1 mg

Medroxyprogesterone acetate 5 mg

One Indivina 2 mg/5 mg tablet contains:

Estradiol valerate 2 mg

Medroxyprogesterone acetate 5 mg

For excipients, see 6.1.

3. PHARMACEUTICAL FORM

Tablet. White, round, bevelled-edge, diameter 7 mm, flat tablets with a code on one side with 1+2,5, 1+5, and 2+5, respectively.

4. CLINICAL PARTICULARS

4.1 Therapeutic indications

Hormone replacement therapy (HRT) for estrogen deficiency symptoms in women with an intact uterus more than three years after menopause.

Prevention of osteoporosis in postmenopausal women at high risk of future fractures who are intolerant of, or contraindicated for, other medicinal products approved for the prevention of osteoporosis.

The experience of treating women older than 65 years is limited.

4.2 Posology and method of administration

Indivina is a continuous combined HRT regimen in which estrogen and progestagen are given every day without interruption.

Dosage: One tablet each day orally without a tablet-free interval. Tablet should be taken approximately at the same time of the day.

Treatment is recommended to be initiated with Indivina 1 mg/2.5 mg tablet. Depending on the clinical response to treatment, the dosage can then be adjusted to individual needs.

Medroxyprogesterone acetate (MPA) 2.5 mg is usually sufficient to prevent breakthrough bleeding. If breakthrough bleeding occurs and persists, and endometrial abnormality has been ruled out, the dose can be increased to 5 mg (Indivina 1mg/5 mg tablet).

If 1 mg of estradiol valerate (E_2V) is not sufficient to alleviate estrogen deficiency symptoms, the dose can be increased to 2 mg (Indivina 2 mg/5 mg tablet).

In women with amenorrhea and not taking HRT or women who switch from another continuous combined HRT product, treatment with Indivina may be started on any day. Women who switch from cyclic HRT regimen should start Indivina treatment one week after completion of the cycle.

The effect of estrogen on bone mineral density is dose dependent and therefore the effect of 1 mg E_2V may be less than with 2 mg (see section 5.1).

If the patient has forgotten to take one tablet, the forgotten tablet is to be discarded. Forgetting a dose may increase the likelihood of breakthrough bleeding and spotting.

For initiation and continuation of treatment of postmenopausal symptoms, the lowest effective dose for the shortest duration (see also Section 4.4) should be used.

4.3 Contraindications

Known, past or suspected breast cancer

Known or suspected estrogen-dependent malignant tumours (e.g. endometrial cancer)

Undiagnosed genital bleeding

Untreated endometrial hyperplasia

Previous idiopathic or current venous thromboembolism [deep venous thrombosis (DVT), pulmonary embolism]

Active or recent arterial thromboembolic disease (e.g. angina, myocardial infarction)

Acute liver disease or a history of liver disease as long as liver function tests have failed to return to normal

Known hypersensitivity to the active substances or to any of the excipients

Porphyria.

4.4 Special warnings and special precautions for use

For the treatment of postmenopausal symptoms, HRT should only be initiated for symptoms that adversely affect quality of life. In all cases, a careful appraisal of the risks and benefits should be undertaken at least annually and HRT should only be continued as long as the benefit outweighs the risk.

Medical examination/follow-up

Before initiating or reinstituting HRT, a complete personal and family medical history should be taken. Physical (including pelvic and breast) examination should be guided by this and by the contraindications and warnings for use.

During treatment, periodic check-ups are recommended of a frequency and nature adapted to the individual woman. Women should be advised what changes in their breasts should be reported to their doctor or nurse (see 'Breast cancer' below). Investigations, including mammography, should be carried out in accordance with currently accepted screening practices, modified to the clinical needs of the individual.

Conditions which need supervision

If any of the following conditions are present, have occurred previously and/or have been aggravated during pregnancy or previous hormone treatment, the patient should be closely supervised. It should be taken into account that these conditions may recur or be aggravated during treatment with Indivina, in particular:

Leiomyoma (uterine fibroids) or endometriosis

A history of or risk factors for thromboembolic disorders (see below)

Risk factors for estrogen dependent tumours, e.g. 1st degree heredity for breast cancer

Hypertension

Liver disorders (e.g. liver adenoma)

Diabetes mellitus with or without vascular involvement

Cholelithiasis

Migraine or (severe) headache

Systemic lupus erythematosus

A history of endometrial hyperplasia (see below)

Epilepsy

Asthma

Otosclerosis

Reasons for immediate withdrawal of therapy:

Therapy should be discontinued in case a contra-indication is discovered and in the following situations:

Jaundice or deterioration of liver function

Significant increase in blood pressure

New onset of migraine-type headache

Pregnancy

Endometrial hyperplasia

The risk of endometrial hyperplasia and carcinoma is increased when estrogens are administered alone for prolonged periods (see section 4.8). The addition of a progestagen for at least 12 days per cycle (for cyclic or sequential products) or every day (for combination products like Indivina) in non-hysterectomised women greatly reduces this risk.

Break-through bleeding and spotting may occur during the first months of treatment. If break-through bleeding or spotting appears after some time of therapy, or continues after treatment has been discontinued, the reason should be investigated, which may include endometrial biopsy to excluded endometrial malignancy.

Breast cancer

A randomised placebo-controlled trial, the Women's Health Initiative study (WHI), and epidemiological studies, including the Million Women Study (MWS), have reported an increased risk of breast cancer in women taking estrogens, estrogen-progestagen combinations or tibolone for HRT for several years (see section 4.8). For all HRT, an excess risk becomes apparent within a few years of use and increases with duration of intake but returns to baseline within a few (at most five) years after stopping treatment.

In the MWS, the relative risk of breast cancer with conjugated equine estrogens (CEE) or estradiol (E2) was greater when a progestagen was added, either sequentially or continuously, and regardless of type of progestagen. There was no evidence of a difference in risk between the different routes of administration.

In the WHI study, the continuous combined conjugated equine estrogen and medroxyprogesterone acetate (CEE + MPA) product used was associated with breast cancers that were slightly larger in size and more frequently had local lymph node metastases compared to placebo.

HRT, especially estrogen-progestagen combined treatment, increases the density of mammographic images which may adversely affect the radiological detection of breast cancer.

Venous thromboembolism

HRT is associated with a higher relative risk of developing venous thromboembolism (VTE), i.e. deep vein thrombosis or pulmonary embolism. One randomised controlled trial and epidemiological studies found a two- to threefold higher risk for users compared with non-users. For non-users it is estimated that the number of cases of VTE that will occur over a 5 year period is about 3 per 1000 women aged 50-59 years and 8 per 1000 women aged between 60-69 years. It is estimated that in healthy women who use HRT for 5 years, the number of additional cases of VTE over a 5 year period will be between 2 and 6 (best estimate = 4) per 1000 women aged 50-59 years and between 5 and 15 (best estimate = 9) per 1000 women aged 60-69 years. The occurrence of such an event is more likely in the first year of HRT than later.

Generally recognised risk factors for VTE include a personal history or family history, severe obesity (BMI > 30 kg/m²) and systemic lupus erythematosus (SLE). There is no consensus about the possible role of varicose veins in VTE.

Patients with a history of VTE or known thrombophilic states have an increased risk of VTE. HRT may add to this risk. Personal or strong family history of thromboembolism or recurrent spontaneous abortion should be investigated in order to exclude a thrombophilic predisposition. Until a thorough evaluation of thrombophilic factors has been made or anticoagulant treatment initiated, use of HRT in such patients should be viewed as contraindicated. Those women already on anticoagulant treatment require careful consideration of the benefit-risk of use of HRT.

The risk of VTE may be temporarily increased with prolonged immobilisation, major trauma or major surgery. As in all postoperative patients, scrupulous attention should be given to prophylactic measures to prevent VTE following surgery. Where prolonged immobilisation is liable to follow elective surgery, particularly abdominal or orthopaedic surgery to the lower limbs, consideration should be given to temporarily stopping HRT 4 to 6 weeks earlier, if possible. Treatment should not be restarted until the woman is completely mobilised.

If VTE develops after initiating therapy, the drug should be discontinued. Patients should be told to contact their doctors immediately when they are aware of a potential thromboembolic symptom (e.g., painful swelling of a leg, sudden pain in the chest, dyspnea).

Coronary artery disease (CAD)

There is no evidence from randomised controlled trials of cardiovascular benefit with continuous combined conjugated estrogens and medroxyprogesterone acetate (MPA). Two large clinical trials (WHI and HERS i.e. Heart and Estrogen/progestin Replacement Study) showed a possible increased risk of cardiovascular morbidity in the first year of use and no overall benefit. For other HRT products there are only limited data from randomised controlled trials examining effects in cardiovascular morbidity and mortality. Therefore, it is uncertain whether these findings also extend to other HRT products.

Stroke

One large randomised clinical trial (WHI-trial) found, as a secondary outcome, an increased risk of ischaemic stroke in healthy women during treatment with continuous combined conjugated estrogens and MPA. For women who do not use HRT, it is estimated that the number of cases of stroke that will occur over a 5 year period is about 3 per 1000 women aged 50-59 years and 11 per 1000 women aged 60-69 years. It is estimated that for women who use conjugated estrogens and MPA for 5 years, the number of additional cases will be between 0 and 3 (best estimate = 1) per 1000 users aged 50-59 years and between 1 and 9 (best estimate = 4) per 1000 users aged 60-69 years. It is unknown whether the increased risk also extends to other HRT products.

Ovarian cancer

Long-term (at least 5-10 years) use of estrogen-only HRT products in hysterectomised women has been associated with an increased risk of ovarian cancer in some epidemiological studies. It is uncertain whether long-term use of combined HRT confers a different risk than estrogen-only products.

Other conditions

Estrogens may cause fluid retention and, therefore, patients with cardiac or renal dysfunction should be carefully observed. Patients with terminal renal insufficiency should be closely observed, since it is expected that the level of circulating active ingredients of Indivina is increased.

Women with pre-existing hypertriglyceridaemia should be followed closely during HRT, since rare cases of large increases of plasma triglycerides leading to pancreatitis have been reported with estrogen therapy in this condition.

Estrogens increase thyroid binding globulin (TBG), leading to increased circulating total thyroid hormone, as measured by protein-bound iodine (PBI), T4 levels (by column or by radio-immunoassay) or T3 levels (by radio-immunoassay). T3 resin uptake is decreased, reflecting the elevated TBG. Free T4 and free T3 concentrations are unaltered. Other binding proteins may be elevated in serum, i.e. corticoid binding globulin (CBG), sex-hormone-binding globulin (SHBG) leading to increased circulating corticosteroids and sex steroids, respectively. Free

Table 1

Organ group	Common >1/100)	Uncommon>1/1,000, <1/100	Rare >1/10,000; <1/1,000)
Gastrointestinal	Nausea, abdominal pain	Dyspepsia, vomiting, flatulence, gallbladder disease/gall stones	
Skin			Alopecia, hirsutism, rash, itching
CNS	Headache	Dizziness, migraine	
Urogenital	Uterine bleeding, increase in size of uterine fibroids	Vaginal candidiasis	
Cardiovascular		Increase in blood pressure	Venous thromboembolism
Miscellaneous	Weight increase/ decrease, oedema, breast tenderness, breast enlargement, changes in mood including anxiety and depressive mood, changes in libido	Leg cramps	

or biological active hormone concentrations are unchanged. Other plasma proteins may be increased (angiotensinogen/ennin substrate, alpha-1-antitrypsin, ceruloplasmin).

There is no conclusive evidence for improvement of cognitive function. There is some evidence from the WHI trial of increased risk of probable dementia in women who start using continuous combined CEE and MPA after the age of 65. It is unknown whether the findings apply to younger post-menopausal women or other HRT products.

Patients with rare hereditary problems of galactose intolerance, the Lapp lactase deficiency or glucose-galactose malabsorption should not take this medicine.

4.5 Interaction with other medicinal products and other forms of Interaction

The metabolism of estrogens and progestagens may be increased by concomitant use of substances known to induce drug-metabolising enzymes, specifically cytochrome P450 enzymes, such as anticonvulsants (e.g. phenobarbital, phenytoin, carbamazepine) and anti-infectives (e.g. rifampicin, rifabutin, nevirapine, efavirenz).

Ritonavir and nelfinavir, although known as strong inhibitors, by contrast exhibit inducing properties when used concomitantly with steroid hormones. Herbal preparations containing St John's wort (*Hypericum perforatum*) may induce the metabolism of estrogens and progestagens.

Clinically, an increased metabolism of estrogens and progestagens may lead to decreased effect and changes in the uterine bleeding profile.

4.6 Pregnancy and lactation

Pregnancy

Indivina is not indicated during pregnancy. If pregnancy occurs during medication with Indivina, treatment should be withdrawn immediately. Data on limited number of exposed pregnancies indicate adverse effects of medroxyprogesterone acetate on sexual differentiation of the foetus. Studies in animals have shown reproductive toxicity (see section 5.3). The potential risk for humans is unknown.

The results of most epidemiological studies to date relevant to inadvertent foetal exposure to combinations of estrogens and progestagen indicate no teratogenic or foetotoxic effect.

Lactation

Indivina is not indicated during lactation.

4.7 Effects on ability to drive and use machines

No effects on ability to drive and use machines have been observed.

4.8 Undesirable effects

The most frequently reported undesirable effect during Indivina treatment in clinical trials was breast tenderness, which occurred in 10.6% of users.

Undesirable effects according to system organ class associated with Indivinatreatment are presented in the table below.

(see Table 1 above)

Breast cancer

According to evidence from a large number of epidemiological studies and one randomised placebo-controlled trial, the Women's Health Initiative (WHI), the overall risk of breast cancer increases with increasing duration of HRT use in current or recent HRT users.

For estrogen-only HRT, estimates of relative risk (RR) from a reanalysis of original data from 51 epidemiological studies (in which >80% of HRT use was estrogen-only HRT) and from the epidemiological Million Women Study (MWS) are similar at 1.35 (95% CI 1.21 – 1.49) and 1.30 (95% CI 1.21 – 1.40), respectively.

For oestrogen plus progestagen combined HRT, several epidemiological studies have reported an overall higher risk for breast cancer than with estrogens alone.

The MWS reported that, compared to never users, the use of various types of estrogen-progestagen combined HRT was associated with a higher risk of breast cancer (RR = 2.00, 95%CI: 1.88 – 2.12) than use of estrogens alone (RR = 1.30, 95%CI: 1.21 – 1.40) or use of tibolone (RR = 1.45; 95%CI 1.25-1.68).

The WHI trial reported a risk estimate of 1.24 (95%CI 1.01 – 1.54) after 5.6 years of use of estrogen-progestagen combined HRT (CEE + MPA) in all users compared with placebo.

The absolute risks calculated from the MWS and the WHI trial are presented below:

The MWS has estimated, from the known average incidence of breast cancer in developed countries, that:

For women not using HRT, about 32 in every 1000 are expected to have breast cancer diagnosed between the ages of 50 and 64 years.

For 1000 current or recent users of HRT, the number of additional cases during the corresponding period will be

For users of estrogen-only replacement therapy

- between 0 and 3 (best estimate = 1.5) for 5 years' use
- between 3 and 7 (best estimate = 5) for 10 years' use

For users of estrogen plus progestagen combined HRT,

- between 5 and 7 (best estimate = 6) for 5 years' use
- between 18 and 20 (best estimate = 19) for 10 years' use.

The WHI trial estimated that after 5.6 years of follow-up of women between the ages of 50 and 79 years, an additional 8 cases of invasive breast cancer would be due to estrogen- progestagen combined HRT (CEE + MPA) per 10,000 women years.

According to calculations from the trial data, it is estimated that:

For 1000 women in the placebo group,

- about 16 cases of invasive breast cancer would be diagnosed in 5 years.

For 1000 women who used estrogen + progestagen combined HRT (CEE + MPA), the number of additional cases would be

- between 0 and 9 (best estimate = 4) for 5 years' use.

The number of additional cases of breast cancer in women who use HRT is broadly similar for women who start HRT irrespective of age at start of use (between the ages of 45-65) (see section 4.4).'

Endometrial cancer

In women with an intact uterus, the risk of endometrial hyperplasia and endometrial cancer increases with increasing duration of use of unopposed estrogens. According to data from epidemiological studies, the best estimate of the risk is that for women not using HRT about 5 in every 1000 are expected to have endometrial cancer diagnosed between the ages of 50 and 65. Depending on the duration of treatment and estrogen dose, the reported increase in endometrial cancer risk among unopposed estrogen users varies from 2- to 12-fold greater compared with non-users. Adding a progestagen to estrogen-only therapy greatly reduces this increased risk.

Other adverse reactions have been reported in association with estrogen/progestagen treatment:

Estrogen-dependent neoplasms benign and malignant, e.g. endometrial cancer.

Venous thromboembolism, i.e. deep leg or pelvic venous thrombosis and pulmonary embolism, is more frequent among HRT users than among non-users. For further information see sections 4.3 and 4.4.

Myocardial infarction and stroke.

Gall bladder disease.

Skin and subcutaneous disorders: chloasma, erythema multiforme, erythema nodosum, vascular purpura.

Probable dementia (see section 4.4).

4.9 Overdose

Estrogen overdose may cause nausea, headache and uterine bleeding. Numerous reports on high doses of estrogen-containing oral contraceptives ingested by young children indicate that serious harmful effects do not occur. Treatment of estrogen overdose is symptomatic. High doses of medroxyprogesterone acetate (MPA) used for cancer treatment have not resulted in serious undesirable effects.

5. PHARMACOLOGICAL PROPERTIES

5.1 Pharmacodynamic properties

Pharmacotherapeutic group: Progestagens and estrogens, fixed combinations; ATC code: G03FA12.

The active form of estradiol valerate, synthetic 17β-estradiol is chemically and biologically identical to endogenous human estradiol. It substitutes for the loss of estrogen production in menopausal women, and alleviates menopausal symptoms.

Estrogens prevent bone loss following menopause or ovariectomy.

Medroxyprogesterone acetate is a derivative of the natural progesterone, 17-alpha-hydroxy-6-methylprogesterone. Medroxyprogesterone acetate binds to progestin-specific receptors and acts on the endometrium to convert the status of the endometrium from proliferative to secretory.

As estrogens promote the growth of the endometrium, unopposed estrogens increase the risk of endometrial hyperplasia and cancer. The addition of medroxyprogesterone acetate greatly reduces the estrogen-induced risk of endometrial hyperplasia in non-hysterectomised women.

Clinical trial information

Relief of estrogen deficiency symptoms and bleeding patterns

Relief of menopausal symptoms was achieved during the first few weeks of treatment.

Bleeding and/or spotting appeared in 41% of the women receiving 1 mg estradiol valerate and 51% of women receiving 2 mg estradiol valerate during the first three months of treatment and in 9% of the women receiving 1 mg estradiol valerate and in 20% of women receiving 2 mg estradiol valerate during 10-12 months of treatment.

Amenorrhoea was seen in 91% of women receiving 1 mg estradiol valerate and in 80% of women receiving 2 mg estradiol valerate after 10-12 months of treatment.

Prevention of osteoporosis

Estrogen deficiency at menopause is associated with an increasing bone turnover and decline in bone mass. The effect of estrogens on bone mineral density (BMD) is dose dependent. Protection appears to be effective for as long as treatment is continued. After discontinuation of HRT, bone mass is lost at a rate similar to that in untreated women.

Evidence from the WHI trial and meta-analysed trials shows that current use of HRT, alone or in combination with a progestagen – given to predominantly healthy women – reduces the risk of hip, vertebral, and other osteoporotic fractures. HRT may also prevent fractures in women with low bone density and/or established osteoporosis, but the evidence for that is limited.

After 4 years of treatment with Indivina combinations containing the 1 mg dose, the increase in lumbar spine bone mineral density (BMD) was6.2 ± 0.5% (mean ± SE). The percentage of women who gained BMD in lumbar zone during treatment was 86.6%.

Indivina combinations containing the 1 mg dose also had an effect on hip BMD. The increase after 4 years was 2.9 ± 0.4% (mean ± SE) at femoral neck. The percentage of women who gained BMD in hip zone during treatment was 80.4%.

After 4 years of treatment with Indivina combinations containing the 2 mg dose, the increase in lumbar spine BMD was 7.4 ± 0.4% (mean ± SE). The percentage of women who gained BMD in lumbar zone during treatment was 95.8%.

Indivina combinations containing the 2 mg dose also had an effect on hip BMD. The increase after 4 years was 2.9 ± 0.4% (mean ± SE) at femoral neck. The percentage of women who gained BMD in hip zone during treatment was 72.3%.

5.2 Pharmacokinetic properties

Following oral administration estradiol valerate is absorbed from the gastrointestinal tract and rapidly hydrolysed to estradiol by esterases. In postmenopausal women aged 50-65 years the maximum concentration of estradiol in serum (C_{max}) was reached within 4 to 6 hours after multiple dosing of 1 mg or 2 mg estradiol valerate. After 1 mg dose C_{max} was about 166 pmol/l, trough concentration (C_{min}) about 101 pmol/l and average concentration ($C_{average}$) about 123 pmol/l. For 2 mg dose C_{max} was 308 pmol/l, C_{min} 171 pmol/l and $C_{average}$ 228 pmol/l. Comparable estradiol concentrations were observed in women over 65 years.

Circulating estradiol is bound to plasma proteins, mainly to sex hormone binding globulin (SHBG) and serum albumin. Estradiol undergoes extensive biotransformation. Its metabolites are excreted in the urine as glucuronide and sulphate conjugates together with a small proportion of unchanged estradiol. Besides urinary excretion, estrogen metabolites undergo an enterohepatic circulation. Only a small amount of a dose is excreted in the faeces.

The absorption of medroxyprogesterone acetate after oral administration is low due to low solubility and there is large individual variation. Medroxyprogesterone acetate undergoes virtually no first-pass metabolism. After multiple dosing of 2.5 mg or 5 mg medroxyprogesterone acetate to women aged 50-65 years, maximum concentration in serum was reached in less than 2 hours. After 2.5 mg dose C_{max} was about 0.37 ng/ml, C_{min} about 0.05 ng/ml and $C_{average}$ about 0.11 ng/ml. After 5 mg dose C_{max} was about 0.64 ng/ml, C_{min} about 0.12 ng/ml and $C_{average}$ about 0.21 ng/ml. Comparable medroxyprogesterone acetate concentrations were observed in women over 65 years.

Medroxyprogesterone acetate is over 90% bound to plasma proteins, mainly to albumin. The elimination half-life of oral medroxyprogesterone acetate is approximately 24 hours. Medroxyprogesterone acetate is extensively metabolised by hepatic hydroxylation and conjugation and excreted in the urine and the bile. Metabolism is poorly documented and the pharmacological activity of the metabolites is not known.

5.3 Preclinical safety data

Animal studies with estradiol and medroxyprogesterone acetate have shown expected estrogenic and gestagenic effect. Both compounds induced adverse effects in reproductive toxicity studies. Chiefly, estradiol showed embryotoxic effects and induced feminisation of male foetuses. Medroxyprogesterone showed embryotoxic effects and induced anti-androgenic effects in male foetuses and masculinization in female foetuses. The relevance of these data for human exposure is unknown (see section 4.6). Concerning other preclinical effects, the toxicity profiles of estradiol valerate and medroxyprogesterone acetate are well known and reveal no particular human health risks beyond those discussed in other sections of the SPC and which generally apply to hormone replacement therapy.

6. PHARMACEUTICAL PARTICULARS

6.1 List of excipients

Lactose monohydrate, maize starch, elatine, magnesium stearate.

6.2 Incompatibilities

Not applicable.

6.3 Shelf life

3 years.

6.4 Special precautions for storage

Do not store above 30 °C. Store in the original package in order to protect from moisture.

6.5 Nature and contents of container

28 tablets in PVC/PVDC/Aluminium blister. Pack of 1x28 tablets and 3x28 tablets

6.6 Instructions for use and handling

No special requirements.

7. MARKETING AUTHORISATION HOLDER

Orion Corporation

Orionintie 1

FI-02200 Espoo

Finland

8. MARKETING AUTHORISATION NUMBER(S)

Indivina 1 mg/2.5 mg: 15396

Indivina 1 mg/5 mg: 15397

Indivina 2 mg/5 mg: 15399

9. DATE OF FIRST AUTHORISATION/RENEWAL OF THE AUTHORISATION

Date of first authorisation: 10 December 1999

Date of last renewal: 10 December 2004

10. DATE OF REVISION OF THE TEXT

18 February 2005

Indocid PDA

(Merck Sharp & Dohme Limited)

1. NAME OF THE MEDICINAL PRODUCT

INDOCID® PDA

2. QUALITATIVE AND QUANTITATIVE COMPOSITION

'Indocid' PDA contains indometacin sodium trihydrate equivalent to 1.0 mg indometacin.

3. PHARMACEUTICAL FORM

'Indocid' PDA is available in vials containing a sterile, off-white to yellow lyophilised powder for solution for injection, of indometacin sodium trihydrate.

4. CLINICAL PARTICULARS

4.1 Therapeutic indications

'Indocid' PDA is indicated for the closure of patent ductus arteriosus in premature babies.

4.2 Posology and method of administration

For intravenous use only.

A course of therapy is defined as three intravenous doses of 'Indocid' PDA given at 12- to 24-hour intervals, with careful attention to urinary output.

If anuria or marked oliguria (urinary output of 0.6 ml/kg/hour) is evident at the time of the scheduled second or third dose, 'Indocid' PDA must not be given until laboratory studies indicate that renal function has returned to normal.

Dosage recommendations depend closely on the age of the infant:

	Dosage (mg/kg)		
Age at 1st dose	*1st*	*2nd*	*3rd*
Less than 48 hours	0.2	0.1	0.1
2-7 days	0.2	0.2	0.2
Over 7 days	0.2	0.25	0.25

If the ductus arteriosus is closed or significantly reduced in size 48 hours after the first course of therapy, no further treatment is necessary. If the ductus arteriosus reopens, a second course of therapy may be given.

If the condition is unchanged after the second course of therapy, surgery may then be necessary. If severe adverse reactions occur, stop the treatment.

4.3 Contraindications

'Indocid' PDA is contra-indicated in infants with established or suspected untreated infection; infants who are bleeding, especially with active intracranial haemorrhage or gastro-intestinal bleeding; infants with congenital heart disease in whom patency of the ductus arteriosus is necessary for satisfactory pulmonary or systemic blood flow (e.g. pulmonary atresia, severe tetralogy of Fallot, severe coarctation of the aorta); infants with thrombocytopenia; infants with coagulation defects; infants with known or suspected necrotising enterocolitis; infants with significant impairment of renal function.

4.4 Special warnings and special precautions for use

General: 'Indocid' may mask the usual signs and symptoms of infection. The drug must therefore be used cautiously in the presence of existing controlled infection.

Because severe hepatic reactions have been reported in adults on prolonged therapy with oral indometacin, 'Indocid' PDA should be discontinued if signs and symptoms consistent with liver disease develop in the neonate.

'Indocid' PDA may inhibit platelet aggregation. Premature babies should be observed for signs of bleeding.

'Indocid' PDA should be administered carefully to avoid extravasation and resultant irritation to tissues.

Gastro-intestinal effects

Clinical results indicate that major gastro-intestinal bleeding was no more common in those babies receiving indometacin than those receiving placebo. However, minor gastro-intestinal bleeding (i.e. chemical detection of blood in the stool) was more common in infants treated with indometacin. Severe gastro-intestinal effects have been reported in adults treated for prolonged periods with oral indometacin.

CNS reactions

Prematurity *per se* is associated with an increased incidence of spontaneous intraventricular haemorrhage. Because indometacin may inhibit platelet aggregation, the potential for intraventricular bleeding may be increased.

Renal effects

'Indocid' PDA may cause significant reduction in urine output (50% or more) with elevated blood urea and creatinine, and reduced GFR and creatinine clearance. In most babies, these effects are transient and disappear when therapy with 'Indocid' PDA is stopped. However, because adequate renal function can depend on renal prostaglandin synthesis, 'Indocid' PDA may precipitate renal insufficiency including acute renal failure. This is most likely in babies with conditions such as extracellular volume depletion from any cause, congestive heart failure, sepsis, or hepatic dysfunction or who are undergoing therapy with nephrotoxic drugs which may affect renal function.

Whenever a significant suppression of urine volume occurs with treatment, treatment with 'Indocid' PDA must stop until urine output returns to normal.

'Indocid' PDA may suppress water excretion in premature babies to a greater extent than the excretion of sodium. This may result in hyponatraemia. Renal function and plasma electrolytes should be monitored.

4.5 Interaction with other medicinal products and other forms of Interaction

The half-life of digitalis in premature babies with patent ductus arteriosus and with cardiac failure is often prolonged by indometacin. When both drugs are used concomitantly, frequent monitoring of ECG and serum digitalis may help prevention or early detection of digitalis toxicity.

In a study of premature infants treated with 'Indocid' PDA and also receiving gentamicin or amikacin, both peak and trough levels of these aminoglycosides were significantly elevated.

'Indocid' may reduce the diuretic effect of furosemide.

4.6 Pregnancy and lactation

Not applicable.

4.7 Effects on ability to drive and use machines

Not applicable.

4.8 Undesirable effects

Haemorrhagic: gross or microscopic bleeding into the gastro-intestinal tract; oozing from the skin after needle puncture; pulmonary haemorrhage; and disseminated intravascular coagulopathy.

Renal: renal dysfunction including one or more of the following: reduced urinary output; reduced urine sodium, chloride or potassium, urine osmolality, free water clearance, or glomerular filtration rate; uraemia; transient oliguria; and hypercreatinaemia.

Gastro-intestinal: vomiting; abdominal distension; melaena; transient ileus; and localised perforations of the small and/or large intestine, necrotising enterocolitis.

Metabolic: hypersensitivity; hyponatraemia; elevated plasma potassium; elevated blood urea; hypoglycaemia.

Cardiovascular: pulmonary hypertension, intracranial bleeding.

Coagulation: decreased platelet aggregation.

General: weight gain (fluid retention); and exacerbation of infection.

Causal relationship unknown

Although the following reactions have been reported in babies, a definite causal relationship has not been established.

Cardiovascular: bradycardia.

Respiratory: apnoea; exacerbation of pre-existing pulmonary infection.

Haematological: disseminated intravascular coagulation.

Metabolic: acidosis, alkalosis.

Ophthalmic: retrolental fibroplasia.

4.9 Overdose

It is recommended that 'Indocid' PDA should be administered only in a neonatal intensive-care unit.

Dosage is critical. The following signs and symptoms have occurred in individuals (not necessarily in premature infants) following an overdose of oral indometacin: nausea, vomiting, intense headache, dizziness, mental confusion, disorientation, lethargy, paraesthesiae, numbness, and convulsions. There are no specific measures to treat acute overdosage with 'Indocid' PDA. The patient should be monitored for several days because gastro-intestinal ulceration and haemorrhage have been reported as adverse reactions of indometacin. Any complications occurring in the gastro-intestinal, renal and central nervous systems should be treated symptomatically and supportively.

Plasma half-life of intravenous indometacin was inversely variable to the post-natal age and weight of the baby. In one study, a mean plasma half-life in babies less than a week old averaged 20 hours, while older babies showed a 12-hour average. Grouping the same babies by weight, the mean plasma half-life seen in babies under 1,000 g was 21 hours, in heavier babies the half-life was reduced to an average of 15 hours.

5. PHARMACOLOGICAL PROPERTIES

5.1 Pharmacodynamic properties

Although the exact mechanism of action through which indometacin causes closure of patent ductus arteriosus is not known, it is believed to be through inhibition of prostaglandin synthesis. Indometacin has been shown to be a potent inhibitor of prostaglandin synthesis, both *in vitro* and *in vivo*. In human newborns with certain congenital heart malformations, PGE 1 dilates the ductus arteriosus. In foetal and newborn lambs, E type prostaglandins have also been shown to maintain the patency of the ductus; as in human newborns, indometacin causes its constriction.

Studies in healthy young animals and in premature infants with patent ductus arteriosus indicated that, after the first dose of intravenous indometacin, there was a transient reduction in cerebral blood flow velocity and cerebral blood flow. Similar decreases in mesenteric blood flow and velocity have been observed. The clinical significance of these effects have not been established.

5.2 Pharmacokinetic properties

The disposition of indometacin following intravenous administration in preterm neonates with patent ductus arteriosus has not been extensively evaluated. Even though the plasma half-life of indometacin was variable among premature infants, it was shown to vary inversely with post-natal age and weight. In one study of 28 evaluable infants, the plasma half-life in those infants less than 7 days old averaged 20 hours, and in infants older than 7 days, the mean plasma half-life was 12 hours. Grouping the infants by weight, the mean plasma half-life in those weighing less than 1,000 g was 21 hours, and in those weighing more than 1,000 g was 15 hours.

5.3 Preclinical safety data

No relevant information.

6. PHARMACEUTICAL PARTICULARS

6.1 List of excipients

Water for injection.

6.2 Incompatibilities

None reported.

6.3 Shelf life

36 months.

6.4 Special precautions for storage

Do not store above 25°C. Keep in outer carton. Intravenous solution should be prepared just prior to use and any unused portion remaining in the opened vial should be discarded.

When reconstituted, 'Indocid' PDA is acceptable for use only when clear and free from particulate matter.

Further dilution with intravenous infusion solutions is not recommended. 'Indocid' PDA is not buffered, and reconstitution at pH levels below 6 may cause precipitation of insoluble indometacin.

6.5 Nature and contents of container

Available in cartons of three Type I glass vials each containing 1 mg.

6.6 Instructions for use and handling

The solution should be prepared only with 1 to 2 ml 0.9% Sodium Chloride Injection BP or Water for Injections Ph Eur. Preparations containing dextrose must not be used.

Preservatives should be carefully avoided at every stage because of the risk of toxicity in the newborn; any unused portion remaining in the opened vial should be discarded.

A fresh solution should be prepared just prior to each administration according to the dilution table below:

Amount of diluent used for each vial	Concentration achieved
1 ml 2 ml	0.1 mg/0.1 ml 0.05 mg/0.1 ml

While the optimal rate of injection has not been established, published literature suggests an infusion rate over 20-30 minutes.

Further dilution with intravenous infusion solutions is not recommended.

7. MARKETING AUTHORISATION HOLDER

Merck Sharp & Dohme Limited

Hertford Road, Hoddesdon, Hertfordshire EN11 9BU, UK

8. MARKETING AUTHORISATION NUMBER(S)

PL 0025/0201

9. DATE OF FIRST AUTHORISATION/RENEWAL OF THE AUTHORISATION

14 January 1986/13 May 1997

10. DATE OF REVISION OF THE TEXT

July 2004.

LEGAL CATEGORY

POM

® denotes registered trademark of Merck & Co., Inc., Whitehouse Station, NJ, USA.

MSD (logo)

Merck Sharp & Dohme Limited

Hertford Road, Hoddesdon, Hertfordshire EN11 9BU, UK.

SPC.IDC.04.UK.2005

InductOs 12mg

(Wyeth Pharmaceuticals)

1. NAME OF THE MEDICINAL PRODUCT

InductOs 12 mg ▼

Kit for implant

2. QUALITATIVE AND QUANTITATIVE COMPOSITION

One vial contains 12 mg dibotermin alfa*. After reconstitution, InductOs contains 1.5 mg/ml dibotermin alfa.

*dibotermin alfa (recombinant human Bone Morphogenetic Protein-2; rhBMP-2) is a human protein derived from a recombinant Chinese Hamster Ovary (CHO) cell line.

For excipients, see 6.1.

3. PHARMACEUTICAL FORM

Kit for implant.

The kit consists of dibotermin alfa powder for solution, a solvent (water for injections), and a matrix.

4. CLINICAL PARTICULARS

4.1 Therapeutic indications

InductOs is indicated for single-level (L_4 – S_1) anterior lumbar spine fusion as a substitute for autogenous bone graft in adults with degenerative disc disease who have had at least 6 months of non-operative treatment for this condition.

InductOs is indicated for the treatment of acute tibia fractures in adults, as an adjunct to standard care using open fracture reduction and intramedullary nail fixation.

See also section 5.1.

4.2 Posology and method of administration

InductOs should be used by an appropriately qualified surgeon.

InductOs is prepared immediately prior to use from a kit containing all necessary components. Once prepared, InductOs contains dibotermin alfa at a concentration of 1.5 mg/ml (12 mg per kit).

InductOs should not be used in concentrations higher than 1.5 mg/ml (see 4.9 Overdosage).

There is very limited experience of the efficacy and safety of the medicinal product in the elderly (>65 years of age).

The safety and effectiveness of InductOs have not been established in pediatric patients (see also 4.3 Contraindications).

Product preparation

In the non-sterile field

1. Using sterile technique, place one syringe, one needle and the matrix inner package in the sterile field.

2. Disinfect the stoppers of the dibotermin alfa and solvent vials.

3. Using the remaining syringe and needle from the kit, reconstitute the dibotermin alfa vial with 8.4 ml of solvent. Slowly inject the solvent into the vial containing the lyophilised dibotermin alfa. Swirl the vial gently to aid reconstitution. Do not shake. Discard syringe and needle after use.

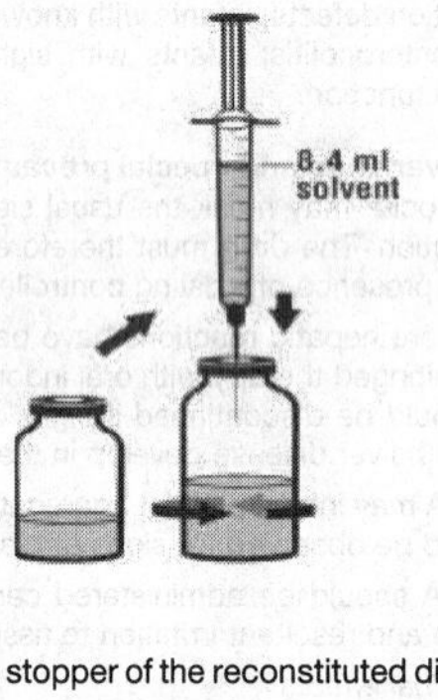

4. Disinfect the stopper of the reconstituted dibotermin alfa vial.

In the sterile field

5. Peel open the interior package of the matrix and leave the matrix in its tray.

6. Using aseptic transfer technique and the syringe and needle from step 1, withdraw 8 ml of the reconstituted dibotermin alfa solution from the vial in the non-sterile field holding up the inverted vial to facilitate withdrawal.

7. Leaving the matrix in its tray, UNIFORMLY distribute the dibotermin alfa solution on the matrix following the pattern in the figure below.

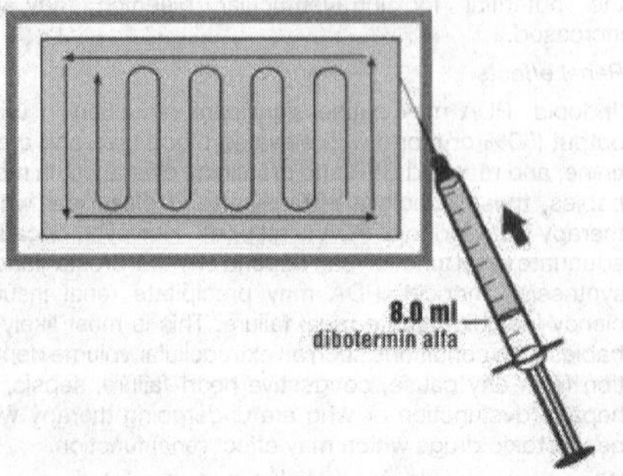

8. Wait a MINIMUM of 15 minutes before using the prepared InductOs product. The product must be used within 2 hours after preparation.

To prevent overloading the matrix, it is important to reconstitute the dibotermin alfa and to wet the entire sponge as described above.

9. Follow instructions relevant to the planned surgery – anterior lumbar spine fusion or acute tibia fracture repair.

Instructions for use in anterior lumbar spine fusion surgery

InductOs should not be used alone for this indication, but must be used with the LT-CAGE Lumbar Tapered Fusion Device.

Pre-Implantation

Cut the wetted matrix of InductOs into 6 equal (approximately 2.5 × 5 cm) pieces. During cutting and handling, avoid excessive fluid loss from InductOs. Do not squeeze.

The number of pieces of InductOs required is determined by the size of the LT-CAGE Lumbar Tapered Fusion Device being used. Using the table below, identify the number of 2.5 × 5 cm pieces of InductOs required for the size of LT-CAGE Lumbar Tapered Fusion Device.

LT-CAGE Lumbar Tapered Fusion Device size (lead diameter × length)	Number of 2.5 × 5 cm pieces of InductOs per LT-CAGE Lumbar Tapered Fusion Device
14 mm × 20 mm	1
14 mm × 23 mm	1
16 mm × 20 mm	1
16 mm × 23 mm	2
16 mm × 26 mm	2
18 mm × 23 mm	2
18 mm × 26 mm	2

Implantation

Using forceps to avoid excessive squeezing, carefully roll the required number of InductOs pieces for each LT-CAGE device and insert each roll into the matching LT-CAGE Lumbar Tapered Fusion Device, as shown in the figure below.

For instructions of implantation of the LT-CAGE Lumbar Tapered Fusion Device, please refer to the package insert for the LT-CAGE device.

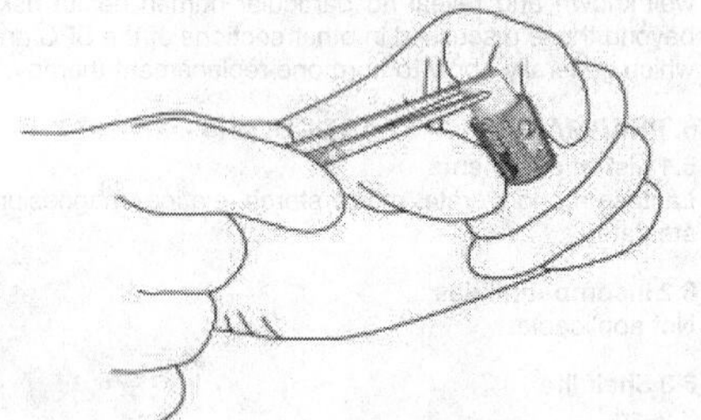

Post-Implantation

Once InductOs and the LT-CAGE device are implanted, do not irrigate the wound region.

If a surgical drain is required, place the drain remote from the implantation site or, preferably, one layer superficial to the implantation site.

Instructions for use in acute tibia fractures

Pre-Implantation

Achieve definitive fracture reduction, fixation, and hemostasis prior to InductOs implantation.

InductOs does not provide mechanical stability and should not be used to fill spaces in the presence of compressive forces.

Fold or cut InductOs as needed prior to implantation. During handling, avoid excessive fluid loss from InductOs. Do not squeeze. If the surgical setting requires that only a portion of the product is needed, first prepare the entire InductOs product (following steps 1-8 above), and then cut the product to the desired size and discard the unused portion.

Implantation

InductOs is implanted after the completion of standard fracture and wound management, i.e. at the time of soft-tissue closure. The number of InductOs kits to use and the volume of InductOs to be implanted are determined by the fracture anatomy and the ability to close the wound without overly packing or compressing the product. Generally, each fracture site is treated with the contents of one kit. The maximum dosage of InductOs is limited to 2 kits. To the extent possible, the accessible surface area of the fracture (fracture lines and defects) should be covered with InductOs. Place InductOs so that it bridges the fracture region and makes good contact with the major proximal and distal fragments. It is not necessary to overlay the contents of multiple kits to achieve the desired effect.

During implantation, use forceps to handle InductOs to avoid excessive loss of fluid.

InductOs may be placed into a void (loosely packed), folded, rolled, or wrapped, as the geometry of the fracture requires. Do not squeeze.

Post-Implantation

Once InductOs is implanted, do not irrigate the wound.

If a surgical drain is required, place the drain remote from the implantation site or, preferably, one layer superficial to the implantation site.

In order to achieve maximum potential efficacy, it is important to achieve complete soft-tissue coverage of InductOs following its implantation.

4.3 Contraindications

InductOs is contraindicated for patients with:

– A known hypersensitivity to dibotermin alfa, bovine Type I collagen or to any of the other excipients of the medicinal product

– Skeletal immaturity

– Any active malignancy or patient undergoing treatment for a malignancy

– Pregnancy

– An active infection at the operative site

– Persistent compartment syndrome or neurovascular residua of compartment syndrome

– Pathological fractures such as those observed in (but not limited to) Paget's disease or in metastatic bone

4.4 Special warnings and special precautions for use

InductOs can cause initial resorption of surrounding trabecular bone. Therefore, in the absence of clinical data, the product should not be used for direct applications to trabecular bone when transient bone resorption may create a risk of bone fragility. When InductOs was used with the LT-CAGE device (as instructed in Section 4.2 of this SmPC) in clinical trials for anterior lumbar spine fusion, the frequency and severity of resorption of bone as evidenced by radiolucencies and/or device migration was similar to that observed for patients treated with autogenous bone graft.

There are no data on the efficacy and safety of the product in concomitant use with bone graft.

In the absence of any experience, the repeated use of the medicinal product is not recommended.

The safety and efficacy of the use of InductOs in patients with known autoimmune disease, including rheumatoid arthritis, systemic lupus erythematosus, scleroderma, Sjögren's syndrome and dermatomyositis/polymyositis have not been established.

The safety and efficacy of InductOs have not been demonstrated in patients with metabolic bone diseases.

No studies have been performed in patients with hepatic or renal impairment.

Use of InductOs may cause heterotopic ossification in the surrounding tissues, which can result in complications. Exuberant bone formation at the site of implantation and ectopic bone formation have been observed.

Commonly, both dibotermin alfa and bovine Type I collagen have been found to elicit immune responses in patients.

Anti-dibotermin alfa antibodies: In anterior lumbar spine fusion studies, 0.7% of patients receiving InductOs developed antibodies vs 0.8% of patients receiving autogenous bone graft. In acute tibia fracture studies, 4.4% of patients receiving InductOs developed antibodies vs 0.6% in the control group.

Anti-bovine Type I collagen antibodies: In anterior lumbar spine fusion studies, 19% of patients receiving InductOs developed antibodies to bovine Type I collagen vs. 13% of patients receiving autogenous bone graft. In acute tibia fracture studies,15.7% of patients receiving InductOs developed antibodies to bovine Type I collagen vs. 11.8% of control patients. In either of the 2 indications, no patients who tested positive for anti-bovine Type I collagen antibodies developed antibodies to human Type I collagen.

Although no clear association with clinical outcome or undesirable effects could be observed in clinical studies, the possibility of developing neutralising antibodies or hypersensitivity-type reactions cannot be excluded. Special consideration of risks and benefits should be given for patients who have previously received injectable collagen (see also 4.3 Contraindications). The possibility of an immune response to the product should be evaluated in cases where an undesirable effect with immunological background is suspected.

Failure to follow the Instructions for Use for InductOs may compromise its effectiveness.

Localised oedema associated with the use of InductOs has been reported in patients undergoing cervical spine surgery. The oedema was delayed in onset and, in some cases, severe enough to result in airway compromise. The safety and efficacy of InductOs in cervical spine surgery have not been established and InductOs should not be used in this condition.

Special warnings and special precautions for use specific to anterior lumbar spine fusion

The safety and efficacy of InductOs used with spinal implants other than the LT-CAGE device, implanted at locations other than L_4-S_1 in the lower lumbar spine, or used in surgical techniques other than anterior open or anterior laparoscopic approaches have not been established. When degenerative disc disease was treated by a posterior lumbar interbody fusion procedure with cylindrical threaded cages and dibotermin alfa, posterior bone formation was observed in some instances.

Special warnings and special precautions for use specific to acute tibia fractures

InductOs is intended for use in patients with the following:

– adequate fracture reduction and stabilization to ensure mechanical stability

– adequate neurovascular status (e.g. absence of compartment syndrome, low risk of amputation)

– adequate hemostasis (providing a relatively dry implantation site)

– absence of large segmental defect repair of long bones, in which significant soft tissue compression can occur

The implant may only be administered to the fracture site under adequate vision and with utmost care (see also 4.2 Posology and method of administration).

Efficacy information in tibia fracture is available only from controlled clinical trials in which open tibial fractures were treated using intramedullary nail fixation (see section 5.1 Pharmacodynamic properties).

InductOs does not provide mechanical stability and should not be used to fill space in the presence of compressive forces. Long-bone fracture and soft-tissue management procedures should be based on standard practice, including control of infection.

4.5 Interaction with other medicinal products and other forms of Interaction

No metabolism studies have been carried out. As dibotermin alfa is a protein and has not been identified in the general circulation, it is an unlikely candidate for pharmacokinetic drug-drug interactions.

Information from clinical studies in acute tibia fractures, indicated that the use of InductOs in patients receiving glucocorticoids was not associated with any apparent adverse effect. In preclinical studies, concurrent administration of glucocorticoids depressed bone repair (measured as a % change from control), but the effects of InductOs were not altered.

In acute tibia fracture clinical trials, more InductOs patients receiving concomitant NSAIDs for 14 consecutive days experienced mild or moderate adverse events related to wound healing (e.g. wound drainage) than InductOs patients not taking NSAIDs. Although patient outcome was not affected, an interaction between NSAIDs and InductOs cannot be excluded.

4.6 Pregnancy and lactation

Pregnancy

The safety and effectiveness of InductOs have not been established in pregnant women.

Animal studies have shown reproductive toxicity (see section 5.3). The potential risk for humans is unknown.

Due to the unknown risks to the fetus associated with the potential development of neutralising antibodies to dibotermin alfa, InductOs is contraindicated in pregnancy (see sections 4.3 and 4.4).

Lactation

It is not known if dibotermin alfa is excreted in human milk. The safety and effectiveness of InductOs have not been established in nursing mothers. Caution should be exercised when prescribing to nursing mothers.

4.7 Effects on ability to drive and use machines

No studies have been performed, but since InductOs has no systemic effect, it is not likely to interfere with the ability to drive or use machinery.

4.8 Undesirable effects

Over 1490 patients have been evaluated in clinical studies, of which more than 955 received InductOs treatment. In the long bone fracture studies, over 418 patients received InductOs. In the anterior lumber spine fusion studies, over 288 patients received InductOs.

There have been post-marketing reports of localised oedema in patients undergoing cervical spine surgery associated with the use of InductOs. The oedema was delayed in onset and, in some cases, severe enough to result in airway compromise (see Section 4.4, Special warnings and special precautions for use).

Undesirable effects specific to use in anterior lumbar spine fusion

The undesirable effects observed in anterior lumbar spine fusion patients were generally representative of the morbidity associated with spine fusion using autogenous bone graft taken from the iliac crest. Very common (>10%) undesirable effects: accidental injury, neuralgia, back pain and bone disorder, were similar in both control and InductOs treatment groups.

Undesirable effects specific to use in acute tibia fractures

The undesirable effects observed in long bone fracture patients were generally representative of the morbidity associated with either orthopaedic trauma or the surgical procedure. The incidence of frequent (>10%) undesirable effects was similar in both control and InductOs treatment groups, with two exceptions: pain and infection (both specific to the fractured limb) were observed more frequently in the control group than in the InductOs treatment group. Common (1% to 10% incidence) undesirable effects were observed with equal incidence in control and InductOs treatment groups, with four exceptions: Increased amylasemia (without overt signs of pancreatitis in InductOs treated patients), headache, tachycardia, and hypomagnesemia were observed significantly more frequently in the InductOs treatment group than in the control group.

4.9 Overdose

Use of InductOs in concentrations or amounts greater than those recommended in 4.2 Posology and method of administration have been associated with reports of localised oedema in patients undergoing cervical spine surgery (see Section 4.4 Special warnings and special precautions for use).

5. PHARMACOLOGICAL PROPERTIES

5.1 Pharmacodynamic properties

Pharmacotherapeutic group: Bone Morphogenetic Proteins, ATC code: M05BC01

Dibotermin alfa is an osteoinductive protein that results in the induction of new bone tissue at the site of implantation. Dibotermin alfa binds to receptors on the surface of mesenchymal cells and causes cells to differentiate into cartilage- and bone-forming cells. The differentiated cells form trabecular bone as the matrix is degraded, with vascular invasion evident at the same time. The bone formation process develops from the outside of the implant towards the center until the entire InductOs implant is replaced by trabecular bone.

Remodeling of the surrounding trabecular bone occurs in a manner that is consistent with the biomechanical forces placed on it. Placement of InductOs into trabecular bone resulted in transient resorption of the bone surrounding the implant, followed by replacement with new, more dense bone. The ability of InductOs to support bone remodeling may be responsible for the biological and biomechanical integration of the new bone induced by InductOs with that of the surrounding bone. Radiographic, biomechanical, and histologic evaluation of the induced bone indicates that it functions biologically and biomechanically as native bone. Furthermore, preclinical studies have indicated that the bone induced by InductOs, if fractured, can repair itself in a manner indistinguishable from native bone.

Preclinical studies have suggested that bone formation initiated by InductOs is a self-limiting process, forming a well-defined volume of bone. This self-limitation is likely due to the loss of dibotermin alfa from the implant site, as well as the presence of BMP inhibitors in the surrounding tissues. In addition, several preclinical studies indicate that there is a negative feedback mechanism at the molecular level that limits bone induction by BMPs.

Clinical pharmacology studies demonstrate that the matrix alone is not osteoinductive and is no longer present in biopsies taken as early as 16 weeks post-implantation.

Pharmacodynamic information specific to anterior lumbar spine fusion studies

The efficacy and safety of InductOs were demonstrated in a randomised, controlled, multicenter, non-inferiority study of 279 patients aged 19 – 78 years undergoing an open anterior lumbar interbody fusion procedure. Patients had received at least six months of non-operative treatment prior to treatment with InductOs for anterior lumbar spine fusion. Patients were randomised to receive the LT-CAGE Lumbar Tapered Fusion Device filled with either InductOs or autogenous bone graft taken from the iliac crest.

At 24 months post-operation, InductOs was demonstrated to be statistically non-inferior to autogenous bone graft. The success rate for radiologically determined fusion was 94.4% versus 88.9% (95% two-sided CI of the difference: -1.53, 12.46) for InductOs and autogenous bone graft, respectively. For pain and disability (Oswestry score), the success rate was 72.9% versus 72.5% (95% two-sided CI of the difference: -11.2, 12.0). A single, multi-component endpoint, known as overall success was the primary variable of the study. Overall success consists of the following primary efficacy and safety considerations:

1. Radiographically demonstrated fusion
2. Oswestry pain/disability improvement
3. Maintenance or improvement in neurological status
4. No Grade 3 or 4 adverse event classified as implant-associated or implant-/surgical procedure associated
5. No additional surgical procedure performed that was classified as a "failure"

At 24 months post-operation, the overall success rate was 57.5% versus 55.8% (95% two-sided CI of the difference: -10.72, 14.01) for InductOs and autogenous bone graft, respectively.

An additional, non-comparative study of 134 patients who received anterior lumbar interbody fusion procedures via a laparoscopic surgical technique yielded similar success rates of 92.9%, 85.6% and 90.3% for fusion, pain and disability, and neurological status, respectively. The study confirmed the applicability of anterior lumbar spine fusion using InductOs via laparoscopic surgical implantation techniques.

Pharmacodynamic information specific to acute tibia fracture studies

The efficacy of InductOs was demonstrated in a multinational, randomized, controlled, single-blind study of 450 patients (age range 18 to 87 years; 81% male) with open tibial shaft fractures requiring surgical management. Patients received (in a 1:1:1 ratio) standard care (control group) consisting of intramedullary (IM) nail fixation and routine soft tissue management, standard care plus InductOs 0.75 mg/ml, or standard care plus InductOs 1.5 mg/ml. Patients were followed for 12 months after soft-tissue closure.

In the acute tibia fracture pivotal trial, InductOs increased the probability of fracture healing; patients treated with InductOs 1.5 mg/ml had a 44% reduced risk for treatment failure (secondary intervention to promote fracture healing) compared with patients in the standard-care group (RR = 0.56; 95% CI = 0.40 to 0.78). These results were independently corroborated by a radiology panel blinded to treatment. The number of secondary and subsequent interventions was significantly reduced for the InductOs patients, particularly with regard to more invasive interventions such as bone graft and exchange nailing (P=0.0326).

In the subgroup of patients who received reamed IM nail fixation, InductOs was not observed to reduce the rate of secondary intervention. However, statistically significant differences in favour of InductOs were observed for some of the secondary efficacy variables (i.e. acceleration of the rate of fracture and soft tissue healing, and reduction of the rate of hardware failure).

The proportion of patients healed after treatment with InductOs 1.5 mg/ml was significantly higher at all visits from 10 weeks to 12 months post-operative, suggesting accelerated fracture healing.

InductOs 1.5 mg/ml was significantly effective (compared to standard care) in patients both with or without a history of smoking.

Severity of fractures:Treatment with InductOs 1.5 mg/ml was significantly effective in all fracture classes, including severe Gustilo IIIB fractures (52% reduced risk of secondary interventions as compared to standard-care patients). Moreover, patients with Gustilo III fractures treated with InductOs 1.5 mg/ml had significantly less infections of the limb studied.

The proportion of patients with healed soft-tissue wounds was significantly higher at the 6-week post-treatment visit in the InductOs 1.5 mg/ml group compared with the standard-care group (83% vs. 65%; P=0.0010). The proportion of patients with hardware failure (locking screws bent or broken) was significantly lower in the InductOs 1.5 mg/ml group as compared to standard-care group (11% vs. 22%; P=0.0174).

5.2 Pharmacokinetic properties

InductOs is active at the site of implantation. In two exploratory studies, pre- and post-surgery serum samples were collected from a few long-bone fracture patients. Dibotermin alfa was not detectable in serum.

In animal studies (rats) using InductOs containing radiolabelled dibotermin alfa, the mean residence time at the site of implantation was 4-8 days. Peak levels of circulating dibotermin alfa (0.1% of the implanted dose) were observed within 6 hours following implantation. When injected intravenously, the terminal half-life of dibotermin alfa was 16 minutes in rats and 6.7 minutes in cynomolgus monkeys. It is concluded therefore that at the site of implantation dibotermin alfa is slowly released from the matrix and rapidly cleared when taken up into the systemic circulation.

5.3 Preclinical safety data

Preclinical data reveal no special hazard for humans on conventional studies of pharmacology, acute and repeat exposure toxicity.

Animal studies do not indicate direct or indirect harmful effects with respect to pregnancy, maternal toxicity, embryolethality, or fetotoxicity. However, in reproductive toxicity studies in rats, where dibotermin alfa was administered intravenously to maximize systemic exposure, increased fetal weight and increased fetal ossification was observed and a treatment related effect could not be ruled out. The potential effects of anti-dibotermin antibodies have not been investigated.

InductOs has not been tested for *in vivo* carcinogenicity. Dibotermin alfa has demonstrated variable effects on human tumour cell lines *in vitro*. Although the available *in vitro* data suggest a low potential for promotion of tumour growth, the use of InductOs is contraindicated in patients with an active malignancy or in patients undergoing treatment for a malignancy (see also section 4.3 Contraindications).

InductOs has been studied in a canine spinal implantation model. InductOs was implanted directly onto the exposed dura following a laminectomy. Although narrowing of the neuroforamen and stenosis was observed, no mineralization of the dura, no spinal cord stenosis, and no neurological deficits subsequent to the application of InductOs were observed. The significance of these data for humans is not known.

6. PHARMACEUTICAL PARTICULARS

6.1 List of excipients

Powder for solution:

Sucrose, Glycine, Glutamic acid, Sodium chloride, Polysorbate 80, Sodium hydroxide

Solvent: Water for injections

Matrix: Bovine Type I collagen.

6.2 Incompatibilities

InductOs must not be mixed with other medicinal products.

6.3 Shelf life

3 years

6.4 Special precautions for storage

Store at 15°C to 30°C. Store in the original package.

6.5 Nature and contents of container

Each kit of InductOs is provided with one vial delivering 12 mg sterile dibotermin alfa, one 10 ml vial of solvent for dibotermin alfa, one sterile matrix (7.5 × 10 cm), 2 sterile 10 ml syringes and 2 sterile needles.

The container-closure system for dibotermin alfa consists of a 20 ml vial constructed of Type I glass, stoppered with a bromobutyl rubber closure sealed with an aluminum flip-off seal and plastic cap.

The container-closure system for the solvent (water for injections) consists of a 10 ml vial constructed of Type I glass, stoppered with a bromobutyl rubber closure sealed with an aluminum flip-off seal and plastic cap.

The packaging for the sterile matrix consists of a blister package formed from polyvinyl chloride (PVC) sealed with a Tyvek lid.

The sterile 10 ml disposable syringes are manufactured of polypropylene with a rubber piston. The sterile precision needles are manufactured of stainless steel.

6.6 Instructions for use and handling

Dibotermin alfa must be used only with the accompanying solvent and matrix provided in the InductOs kit. See also section 4.2 Posology and method of administration.

7. MARKETING AUTHORISATION HOLDER

Wyeth Europa Ltd.
Huntercombe Lane South
Taplow, Maidenhead
Berkshire, SL6 0PH
United Kingdom

8. MARKETING AUTHORISATION NUMBER(S)

EU/1/02/226/001

9. DATE OF FIRST AUTHORISATION/RENEWAL OF THE AUTHORISATION

9 September 2002

10. DATE OF REVISION OF THE TEXT

March 2005

INEGY Tablets

(MSD-SP LTD)

1. NAME OF THE MEDICINAL PRODUCT

INEGY® ▼ 10 mg/20 mg, 10 mg/40 mg, or 10 mg/80 mg Tablets

2. QUALITATIVE AND QUANTITATIVE COMPOSITION

Each tablet contains 10 mg ezetimibe and 20, 40 or 80 mg of simvastatin.

For excipients, see section 6.1.

3. PHARMACEUTICAL FORM

Tablet.

White to off-white capsule-shaped tablets with code "311", "312", "313", or "315" on one side.

4. CLINICAL PARTICULARS

4.1 Therapeutic indications

Hypercholesterolaemia

INEGY is indicated as adjunctive therapy to diet for use in patients with primary (heterozygous familial and non-familial) hypercholesterolaemia or mixed hyperlipidaemia where use of a combination product is appropriate:

- patients not appropriately controlled with a statin alone
- patients already treated with a statin and ezetimibe

INEGY contains ezetimibe and simvastatin. Simvastatin (20-40 mg) has been shown to reduce the frequency of cardiovascular events (see section 5.1). Studies to demonstrate the efficacy of INEGY or ezetimibe in the prevention of complications of atherosclerosis have not been completed.

Homozygous Familial Hypercholesterolaemia (HoFH)

INEGY is indicated as adjunctive therapy to diet for use in patients with HoFH. Patients may also receive adjunctive treatments (e.g., low-density lipoprotein [LDL] apheresis).

4.2 Posology and method of administration

Hypercholesterolaemia

The patient should be on an appropriate lipid-lowering diet and should continue on this diet during treatment with INEGY.

Route of administration is oral. The dosage range of INEGY is 10/10 mg/day through 10/80 mg/day in the evening. All dosages may not be available in all member states. The typical dose is 10/20 mg/day or 10/40 mg/day given as a single dose in the evening. The 10/80 mg dose is only recommended in patients with severe hypercholesterolaemia and high risk for cardiovascular complications. The patient's low-density lipoprotein cholesterol (LDL-C) level, coronary heart disease risk status, and response to current cholesterol-lowering therapy should be considered when starting therapy or adjusting the dose.

The dose of INEGY should be individualised based on the known efficacy of the various dose strengths of INEGY (see section 5.1, Table 1) and the response to the current cholesterol-lowering therapy. Adjustments of dosage, if required, should be made at intervals of not less than 4 weeks. INEGY can be administered with or without food. So far, comparative studies with INEGY are limited to simvastatin and atorvastatin.

Homozygous Familial Hypercholesterolaemia

The recommended dosage for patients with homozygous familial hypercholesterolaemia is INEGY 10/40 mg/day or 10/80 mg/day in the evening. INEGY may be used as an adjunct to other lipid-lowering treatments (e.g., LDL apheresis) in these patients or if such treatments are unavailable.

Coadministration with other medicines

Dosing of INEGY should occur either ≥2 hours before or ≥4 hours after administration of a bile acid sequestrant.

In patients taking amiodaroneor verapamil concomitantly with INEGY, the dose of INEGY should not exceed 10/20 mg/day (see sections 4.4 and 4.5).

In patients taking ciclosporin, danazol or lipid-lowering doses (≥1 g/day) of niacin concomitantly with INEGY, the dose of INEGY should not exceed 10/10 mg/day (see sections 4.4 and 4.5).

Use in the Elderly

No dosage adjustment is required for elderly patients (see section 5.2).

Use in Children and adolescents

Efficacy and safety of use in children have not been established. Therefore, INEGY is not recommended for paediatric use (see section 5.2).

Use in Hepatic Impairment

No dosage adjustment is required in patients with mild hepatic insufficiency (Child Pugh score 5 to 6). Treatment with INEGY is not recommended in patients with moderate (Child Pugh score 7 to 9) or severe (Child Pugh score >9) liver dysfunction. (See sections 4.4 and 5.2.)

Use in Renal Impairment

No modification of dosage should be necessary in patients with moderate renal insufficiency. If treatment in patients with severe renal insufficiency (creatinine clearance ≤30 ml/min) is deemed necessary, dosages above 10/10 mg/day should be implemented cautiously (see section 5.2).

4.3 Contraindications

Hypersensitivity to ezetimibe, simvastatin, or to any of the excipients.

Pregnancy and lactation (see section 4.6).

Active liver disease or unexplained persistent elevations in serum transaminases.

Concomitant administration of potent CYP3A4 inhibitors (e.g., itraconazole, ketoconazole, erythromycin, clarithromycin, telithromycin, HIV protease inhibitors and nefazodone) (see sections 4.4 and 4.5).

4.4 Special warnings and special precautions for use

Myopathy/Rhabdomyolysis

In post-marketing experience with ezetimibe, cases of myopathy and rhabdomyolysis have been reported. Most patients who developed rhabdomyolysis were taking a statin concomitantly with ezetimibe. However, rhabdomyolysis has been reported very rarely with ezetimibe monotherapy and very rarely with the addition of ezetimibe to other agents known to be associated with increased risk of rhabdomyolysis.

INEGY contains simvastatin. Simvastatin, like other inhibitors of HMG-CoA reductase, occasionally causes myopathy manifested as muscle pain, tenderness or weakness with creatine kinase (CK) above 10X the upper limit of normal (ULN). Myopathy sometimes takes the form of rhabdomyolysis with or without acute renal failure secondary to myoglobinuria, and very rare fatalities have occurred. The risk of myopathy is increased by high levels of HMG-CoA reductase inhibitory activity in plasma.

The risk of myopathy/rhabdomyolysis is dose related for simvastatin. The incidence in clinical trials, in which patients were carefully monitored and some interacting drugs were excluded, has been approximately 0.03% at 20 mg, 0.08% at 40 mg, and 0.4% at 80 mg simvastatin.

Creatine Kinase measurement

Creatine Kinase (CK) should not be measured following strenuous exercise or in the presence of any plausible alternative cause of CK increase as this makes value interpretation difficult. If CK levels are significantly elevated at baseline (> 5 X ULN), levels should be re-measured within 5 to 7 days later to confirm the results.

Before the treatment

All patients starting therapy with INEGY, or whose dose of INEGY is being increased, should be advised of the risk of myopathy and told to report promptly any unexplained muscle pain, tenderness or weakness.

Caution should be exercised in patients with pre-disposing factors for rhabdomyolysis. In order to establish a reference baseline value, a CK level should be measured before starting treatment in the following situations:

- Elderly (age >70 years)
- Renal impairment
- Uncontrolled hypothyroidism
- Personal or familial history of hereditary muscular disorders
- Previous history of muscular toxicity with a statin or fibrate
- Alcohol abuse.

In such situations, the risk of treatment should be considered in relation to possible benefit, and clinical monitoring is recommended. If a patient has previously experienced a muscle disorder on a fibrate or a statin, treatment with any statin-containing product (such as INEGY) should only be initiated with caution. If CK levels are significantly elevated at baseline (>5 X ULN), treatment should not be started.

Whilst on treatment

If muscle pain, weakness or cramps occur whilst a patient is receiving treatment with INEGY, their CK levels should be measured. If these levels are found, in the absence of strenuous exercise, to be significantly elevated (>5 X ULN), treatment should be stopped. If muscular symptoms are severe and cause daily discomfort, even if CK levels are <5 X ULN, treatment discontinuation may be considered. If myopathy is suspected for any other reason, treatment should be discontinued.

If symptoms resolve and CK levels return to normal, then re-introduction of INEGY or introduction of another statin-containing product may be considered at the lowest dose and with close monitoring.

Therapy with INEGY should be temporarily stopped a few days prior to elective major surgery and when any major medical or surgical condition supervenes.

Measures to reduce the risk of myopathy caused by medicinal product interactions (see also section 4.5)

The risk of myopathy and rhabdomyolysis is significantly increased by concomitant use of INEGY with potent inhibitors of CYP3A4 (such as itraconazole, ketoconazole, erythromycin, clarithromycin, telithromycin, HIV protease inhibitors, nefazodone), as well as ciclosporin, danazol and gemfibrozil (see section 4.2).

Due to the simvastatin component of INEGY, the risk of myopathy and rhabdomyolysis is also increased by concomitant use of other fibrates, lipid-lowering doses (≥1 g/day) of niacin or by concomitant use of amiodarone or verapamil with higher doses of INEGY (see sections 4.2 and 4.5). There is also a slight increase in risk when diltiazem is used with INEGY 10 mg/80 mg.

Consequently, regarding CYP3A4 inhibitors, the use of INEGY concomitantly with itraconazole, ketoconazole, HIV protease inhibitors, erythromycin, clarithromycin, telithromycin, and nefazodone is contraindicated (see sections 4.3 and 4.5). If treatment with itraconazole, ketoconazole, erythromycin, clarithromycin or telithromycin is unavoidable, therapy with INEGY must be suspended during the course of treatment. Moreover, caution should be exercised when combining INEGY with certain other less potent CYP3A4 inhibitors: ciclosporin, verapamil, diltiazem (see sections 4.2 and 4.5). Concomitant intake of grapefruit juice and INEGY should be avoided.

The dose of INEGY should not exceed 10/10 mg daily in patients receiving concomitant medication with ciclosporin, danazol or lipid-lowering doses (≥ 1 g/day) of niacin. The combined use of INEGY with fibrates should be avoided. The benefits of the combined use of INEGY 10 mg/10 mg daily with ciclosporin, danazol or niacin should be carefully weighed against the potential risks of these combinations. (See sections 4.2 and 4.5.)

The combined use of INEGY at doses higher than 10/20 mg daily with amiodarone or verapamil should be avoided unless the clinical benefit is likely to outweigh the increased risk of myopathy (see sections 4.2 and 4.5).

Liver Enzymes

In controlled coadministration trials in patients receiving ezetimibe with simvastatin, consecutive transaminase elevations (≥3 X ULN) have been observed (see section 4.8).

It is recommended that liver function tests be performed before treatment with INEGY begins and thereafter when clinically indicated. Patients titrated to the 10/80-mg dose should receive an additional test prior to titration, 3 months after titration to the 10/80-mg dose, and periodically thereafter (e.g., semiannually) for the first year of treatment. Special attention should be paid to patients who develop elevated serum transaminase levels, and in these patients, measurements should be repeated promptly and then performed more frequently. If the transaminase levels show evidence of progression, particularly if they rise to 3 X ULN and are persistent, the drug should be discontinued.

INEGY should be used with caution in patients who consume substantial quantities of alcohol.

Hepatic Insufficiency

Due to the unknown effects of the increased exposure to ezetimibe in patients with moderate or severe hepatic insufficiency, INEGY is not recommended (see section 5.2).

Fibrates

The safety and efficacy of ezetimibe administered with fibrates have not been established; therefore, coadministration of INEGY and fibrates is not recommended (see section 4.5).

Ciclosporin

Caution should be exercised when initiating INEGY in the setting of ciclosporin. Ciclosporin concentrations should be monitored in patients receiving INEGY and ciclosporin (see section 4.5).

Warfarin

If INEGY is added to warfarin or another coumarin anticoagulant, the International Normalised Ratio (INR) should be appropriately monitored (see section 4.5).

Excipient

Patients with rare hereditary problems of galactose intolerance, the Lapp lactase deficiency or glucose-galactose malabsorption should not take this medicine.

4.5 Interaction with other medicinal products and other forms of interaction

Pharmacodynamic interactions

Interactions with lipid-lowering medicinal products that can cause myopathy when given alone

The risk of myopathy, including rhabdomyolysis, is increased during concomitant administration of simvastatin with fibrates and niacin (nicotinic acid) (≥1 g/day). Additionally, there is a pharmacokinetic interaction of simvastatin with gemfibrozil resulting in increased simvastatin plasma levels (see below *Pharmacokinetic interactions*).

Fibrates may increase cholesterol excretion into the bile, leading to cholelithiasis. In a preclinical study in dogs, ezetimibe increased cholesterol in the gallbladder bile (see section 5.3). Although the relevance of this preclinical finding to humans is unknown, coadministration of INEGY with fibrates is not recommended until use in patients is studied (see section 4.4).

Pharmacokinetic interactions

Effects of other medicinal products on INEGY

Ezetimibe

Antacids: Concomitant antacid administration decreased the rate of absorption of ezetimibe but had no effect on the bioavailability of ezetimibe. This decreased rate of absorption is not considered clinically significant.

Colestyramine: Concomitant colestyramine administration decreased the mean area under the curve (AUC) of total ezetimibe (ezetimibe + ezetimibe glucuronide) approximately 55%. The incremental LDL-C reduction due to adding INEGY to colestyramine may be lessened by this interaction (see section 4.2).

Ciclosporin: In a study of eight post-renal transplant patients with creatinine clearance of >50 ml/min on a stable dose of ciclosporin, a single 10-mg dose of ezetimibe resulted in a 3.4-fold (range 2.3- to 7.9-fold) increase in the mean AUC for total ezetimibe compared to a healthy control population, receiving ezetimibe alone, from another study (n=17). In a different study, a renal transplant patient with severe renal insufficiency who was receiving ciclosporin and multiple other medications, demonstrated a 12-fold greater exposure to total ezetimibe compared to concurrent controls receiving ezetimibe alone. In a two-period crossover study in twelve healthy subjects, daily administration of 20 mg ezetimibe for 8 days with a single 100-mg dose of ciclosporin on Day 7 resulted in a mean 15% increase in ciclosporin AUC (range 10% decrease to 51% increase) compared to a single 100-mg dose of ciclosporin alone. A controlled study on the effect of coadministered ezetimibe on ciclosporin exposure in renal transplant patients has not been conducted. Caution should be exercised when initiating INEGY in the setting of ciclosporin. Ciclosporin concentrations should be monitored in patients receiving INEGY and ciclosporin (see section 4.4).

Fibrates: Concomitant fenofibrate or gemfibrozil administration increased total ezetimibe concentrations approximately 1.5- and 1.7-fold, respectively. Although these increases are not considered clinically significant, coadministration of INEGY with fibrates is not recommended until use in patients is studied (see section 4.4).

Simvastatin

Simvastatin is a substrate of cytochrome P450 3A4. Potent inhibitors of cytochrome P450 3A4 increase the risk of myopathy and rhabdomyolysis by increasing the concentration of HMG-CoA reductase inhibitory activity in plasma during simvastatin therapy. Such inhibitors include itraconazole, ketoconazole, erythromycin, clarithromycin, telithromycin, HIV protease inhibitors, and nefazodone. Concomitant administration of itraconazole resulted in a more than 10-fold increase in exposure to simvastatin acid (the active beta-hydroxyacid metabolite). Telithromycin caused an 11-fold increase in exposure to simvastatin acid.

Therefore, combination with itraconazole, ketoconazole, HIV protease inhibitors, erythromycin, clarithromycin, telithromycin, and nefazodone is contraindicated. If treatment with itraconazole, ketoconazole, erythromycin, clarithromycin or telithromycin is unavoidable, therapy with INEGY must be suspended during the course of treatment. Caution should be exercised when combining INEGY with certain other less potent CYP3A4 inhibitors: ciclosporin, verapamil, diltiazem (see sections 4.2 and 4.4).

Ciclosporin: The risk of myopathy/rhabdomyolysis is increased by concomitant administration of ciclosporin particularly with higher doses of INEGY (see sections 4.2 and 4.4). Therefore, the dose of INEGY should not exceed 10/10 mg daily in patients receiving concomitant medication with ciclosporin. Although the mechanism is not fully understood, ciclosporin increases the AUC of simvastatin acid, presumably due, in part, to inhibition of CYP3A4.

Danazol: The risk of myopathy and rhabdomyolysis is increased by concomitant administration of danazol with higher doses of INEGY (see section 4.2 and section 4.4).

Gemfibrozil: Gemfibrozil increases the AUC of simvastatin acid by 1.9-fold, possibly due to inhibition of the glucuronidation pathway.

Amiodarone and verapamil: The risk of myopathy and rhabdomyolysis is increased by concomitant administration of amiodarone or verapamil with higher doses of simvastatin (see section 4.4). In an ongoing clinical trial, myopathy has been reported in 6% of patients receiving simvastatin 80 mg and amiodarone.

An analysis of the available clinical trials showed an approximately 1% incidence of myopathy in patients receiving simvastatin 40 mg or 80 mg and verapamil. In a pharmacokinetic study, concomitant administration of simvastatin with verapamil resulted in 2.3-fold increase in exposure of simvastatin acid, presumably due, in part, to inhibition of CYP3A4. Therefore, the dose of INEGY should not exceed 10/20 mg daily in patients receiving concomitant medication with amiodarone or verapamil, unless the clinical benefit is likely to outweigh the increased risk of myopathy and rhabdomyolysis.

Diltiazem: An analysis of the available clinical trials showed a 1% incidence of myopathy in patients receiving simvastatin 80 mg and diltiazem. The risk of myopathy in patients taking simvastatin 40 mg was not increased by concomitant diltiazem(see section 4.4). In a pharmacokinetic study, concomitant administration of diltiazem with simvastatin caused a 2.7-fold increase in exposure of simvastatin acid, presumably due to inhibition of CYP3A4. Therefore, the dose of INEGY should not exceed 10/40 mg daily in patients receiving concomitant medication with diltiazem, unless the clinical benefit is likely to outweigh the increased risk of myopathy and rhabdomyolysis.

Grapefruit juice: Grapefruit juice inhibits cytochrome P450 3A4. Concomitant intake of large quantities (over 1 litre daily) of grapefruit juice and simvastatin resulted in a 7-fold increase in exposure to simvastatin acid. Intake of 240 ml of grapefruit juice in the morning and administration of simvastatin in the evening also resulted in a 1.9-fold increase. Intake of grapefruit juice during treatment with INEGY should therefore be avoided.

Effects of INEGY on the pharmacokinetics of other medicinal products

Ezetimibe

In preclinical studies, it has been shown that ezetimibe does not induce cytochrome P450 drug metabolising enzymes. No clinically significant pharmacokinetic interactions have been observed between ezetimibe and drugs known to be metabolised by cytochromes P450 1A2, 2D6, 2C8, 2C9, and 3A4, or N-acetyltransferase.

Warfarin

Concomitant administration of ezetimibe (10 mg once daily) had no significant effect on bioavailability of warfarin and prothrombin time in a study of twelve healthy adult males. However, there have been post-marketing reports of increased International Normalised Ratio (INR) in patients who had ezetimibe added to warfarin. If INEGY is added to warfarin or another coumarin anticoagulant, INR should be appropriately monitored. (see section 4.4).

Simvastatin

Simvastatin does not have an inhibitory effect on cytochrome P450 3A4. Therefore, simvastatin is not expected to affect plasma concentrations of substances metabolised via cytochrome P450 3A4.

Oral anticoagulants: In two clinical studies, one in normal volunteers and the other in hypercholesterolaemic patients, simvastatin 20-40 mg/day modestly potentiated the effect of coumarin anticoagulants: the prothrombin time, reported as International Normalised Ratio (INR), increased from a baseline of 1.7 to 1.8 and from 2.6 to 3.4 in the volunteer and patient studies, respectively. Very rare cases of elevated INR have been reported. In patients taking coumarin anticoagulants, prothrombin time should be determined before starting INEGY and frequently enough during early therapy to ensure that no significant alteration of prothrombin time occurs. Once a stable prothrombin time has been documented, prothrombin times can be monitored at the intervals usually recommended for patients on coumarin anticoagulants. If the dose of INEGY is changed or discontinued, the same procedure should be repeated. Simvastatin therapy has not been associated with bleeding or with changes in prothrombin time in patients not taking anticoagulants.

4.6 Pregnancy and lactation

Pregnancy:

Atherosclerosis is a chronic process, and ordinarily discontinuation of lipid-lowering drugs during pregnancy should have little impact on the long-term risk associated with primary hypercholesterolaemia.

INEGY

INEGY is contraindicated during pregnancy. No clinical data are available on the use of INEGY during pregnancy. Animal studies on combination therapy have demonstrated reproduction toxicity. (See section 5.3.)

Simvastatin

The safety of simvastatin in pregnant women has not been established. No controlled clinical trials with simvastatin have been conducted in pregnant women. Rare reports of congenital anomalies following intrauterine exposure to HMG-CoA reductase inhibitors have been received. However, in an analysis of approximately 200 prospectively followed pregnancies exposed during the first trimester to simvastatin or another closely related HMG-CoA reductase inhibitor, the incidence of congenital anomalies was comparable to that seen in the general population. This number of pregnancies was statistically sufficient to exclude a 2.5-fold or greater increase in congenital anomalies over the background incidence.

Although there is no evidence that the incidence of congenital anomalies in offspring of patients taking simvastatin or another closely related HMG-CoA reductase inhibitor differs from that observed in the general population, maternal treatment with simvastatin may reduce the foetal levels of mevalonate which is a precursor of cholesterol biosynthesis. For this reason, INEGY should not be used in women who are pregnant, trying to become pregnant or suspect they are pregnant. Treatment with INEGY should be suspended for the duration of pregnancy or until it has been determined that the woman is not pregnant. (See section 4.3.)

Ezetimibe

No clinical data are available on the use of ezetimibe during pregnancy.

Lactation:

INEGY is contraindicated during lactation. Studies on rats have shown that ezetimibe is excreted into breast milk. It is not known if the active components of INEGY are secreted into human breast milk. (See section 4.3.)

4.7 Effects on ability to drive and use machines

No studies of the effects on the ability to drive and use of machines have been performed. However, when driving vehicles or operating machines, it should be taken into account that dizziness has been reported.

4.8 Undesirable effects

INEGY (or coadministration of ezetimibe and simvastatin equivalent to INEGY) has been evaluated for safety in more than 3,800 patients in clinical trials.

The frequencies of adverse events are ranked according to the following: Very common (⩾ 1/10), Common (⩾ 1/100, < 1/10), Uncommon (⩾ 1/1000), < 1/100), Rare (⩾ 1/10,000, < 1/1000), Very rare (< 1/10,000) including isolated reports.

INEGY

Nervous system disorders:

Common: headache

Gastro-intestinal disorders:

Common: flatulence

Musculoskeletal, connective tissue, and bone disorders:

Common: myalgia

Laboratory Values

In coadministration trials, the incidence of clinically important elevations in serum transaminases (ALT and/or AST ⩾3 X ULN, consecutive) was 1.7% for patients treated with INEGY. These elevations were generally asymptomatic, not associated with cholestasis, and returned to baseline after discontinuation of therapy or with continued treatment. (See section 4.4.)

Clinically important elevations of CK (⩾10 X ULN) were seen in 0.2% of the patients treated with INEGY.

Post-marketing Experience

The adverse reactions reported for INEGY are consistent with those previously reported with ezetimibe and/or simvastatin.

Additional information on individual components: in addition to the adverse reactions listed above for the combination product, other undesirable effects previously reported during clinical studies or post-marketing use with one of the individual components may be potential undesirable effects with INEGY.

Ezetimibe

Blood and lymphatic system disorders:

Very rare: thrombocytopaenia

Gastro-intestinal disorders:

Common: abdominal pain, diarrhoea

Rare: nausea

Very rare: pancreatitis

Hepto-biliary disorders:

Rare: hepatitis

Very rare: cholelithiasis, cholecystitis

Skin and subcutaneous tissue disorders:

Rare: hypersensitivity reactions, including rash and very rarely, angio-oedema

Musculoskeletal, connective tissue disorders:

Very rare: myopathy/rhabdomyolysis (see section 4.4)

General disorders and administration site conditions:

Common: fatigue

Laboratory values

Rare: increased transaminases; increased CK

In clinical trials, CPK > 10 X ULN was reported for 4 of 1674 (0.2%) patients administered ezetimibe alone vs 1 of 786 (0.1%) patients administered placebo, and for 1 of 917 (0.1%) patients coadministered ezetimibe and a statin vs 4 of 929 (0.4%) patients administered a statin alone. There was no excess of myopathy or rhabdomyolysis associated with ezetimibe compared with the relevant control arm (placebo or statin alone). (See section 4.4).

Simvastatin

Blood and lymphatic system disorders:

Rare: anaemia

Nervous system disorders:

Rare: dizziness, paresthaesia, peripheral neuropathy

Gastro-intestinal disorders:

Rare: constipation, abdominal pain, dyspepsia, diarrhoea, nausea, vomiting, pancreatitis

Hepato-biliary disorders:

Rare: hepatitis/jaundice

Skin and subcutaneous tissue disorders:

Rare: rash, pruritus, alopecia

Musculoskeletal, connective tissue and bone disorders:

Rare: myopathy, rhabdomyolysis (see section 4.4), muscle cramps

General disorders and administration site conditions:

Rare: aesthenia

An apparent hypersensitivity syndrome has been reported rarely which has included some of the following features: angio-oedema, lupus-like syndrome, polymyalgia rheumatica, dermatomyositis, vasculitis, thrombocytopaenia, eosinophilia, red blood cell sedimentation rate increased, arthritis and arthralgia, urticaria, photosensitivity reaction, pyrexia, flushing, dyspnoea and malaise.

Laboratory Values

Rare: increases in γ-glutamyl transpeptidase, elevated alkaline phosphatase.

4.9 Overdose

INEGY

In the event of an overdose, symptomatic and supportive measures should be employed. Coadministration of ezetimibe (1000 mg/kg) and simvastatin (1000 mg/kg) was well-tolerated in acute, oral toxicity studies in mice and rats. No clinical signs of toxicity were observed in these animals. The estimated oral LD_{50} for both species was ezetimibe ⩾1000 mg/kg/simvastatin ⩾1000 mg/kg.

Ezetimibe

In clinical studies, administration of ezetimibe, 50 mg/day to 15 healthy subjects for up to 14 days, or 40 mg/day to 18 patients with primary hypercholesterolaemia for up to 56 days, was generally well tolerated. A few cases of overdosage have been reported; most have not been associated with adverse experiences. Reported adverse experiences have not been serious. In animals, no toxicity was observed after single oral doses of 5000 mg/kg of ezetimibe in rats and mice and 3000 mg/kg in dogs.

Simvastatin

A few cases of overdosage have been reported; the maximum dose taken was 3.6 g. All patients recovered without sequelae.

5. PHARMACOLOGICAL PROPERTIES

5.1 Pharmacodynamic properties

Pharmacotherapeutic group: Other cholesterol and triglyceride reducers, ATC code: C10AX

INEGY (ezetimibe/simvastatin) is a lipid-lowering product that selectively inhibits the intestinal absorption of cholesterol and related plant sterols and inhibits the endogenous synthesis of cholesterol.

Mechanism of action:

INEGY

Plasma cholesterol is derived from intestinal absorption and endogenous synthesis. INEGY contains ezetimibe and simvastatin, two lipid-lowering compounds with complementary mechanisms of action. INEGY reduces elevated total cholesterol (total-C), LDL-C, apolipoprotein B (Apo B), triglycerides (TG), and non-high-density lipoprotein cholesterol (non-HDL-C), and increases high-density lipoprotein cholesterol (HDL-C) through dual inhibition of cholesterol absorption and synthesis.

Ezetimibe

Ezetimibe inhibits the intestinal absorption of cholesterol. Ezetimibe is orally active and has a mechanism of action that differs from other classes of cholesterol-reducing compounds (e.g., statins, bile acid sequestrants [resins], fibric acid derivatives, and plant stanols).

Ezetimibe localises at the brush border of the small intestine and inhibits the absorption of cholesterol, leading to a decrease in the delivery of intestinal cholesterol to the liver; statins reduce cholesterol synthesis in the liver and together these distinct mechanisms provide complementary cholesterol reduction. The molecular mechanism of action is not fully understood. In a 2-week clinical study in 18 hypercholesterolaemic patients, ezetimibe inhibited intestinal cholesterol absorption by 54%, compared with placebo.

A series of preclinical studies was performed to determine the selectivity of ezetimibe for inhibiting cholesterol absorption. Ezetimibe inhibited the absorption of [^{14}C]-cholesterol with no effect on the absorption of triglycerides, fatty acids, bile acids, progesterone, ethinyl estradiol, or fat soluble vitamins A and D.

Simvastatin

After oral ingestion, simvastatin, which is an inactive lactone, is hydrolysed in the liver to the corresponding active β-hydroxyacid form which has a potent activity in inhibiting HMG-CoA reductase (3 hydroxy - 3 methylglutaryl CoA reductase). This enzyme catalyses the conversion of HMG-CoA to mevalonate, an early and rate-limiting step in the biosynthesis of cholesterol.

Simvastatin has been shown to reduce both normal and elevated LDL-C concentrations. LDL is formed from very-low-density protein (VLDL) and is catabolised predominantly by the high affinity LDL receptor. The mechanism of the LDL-lowering effect of simvastatin may involve both reduction of VLDL-cholesterol (VLDL-C) concentration and induction of the LDL receptor, leading to reduced production and increased catabolism of LDL-C. Apolipoprotein B also falls substantially during treatment with simvastatin. In addition, simvastatin moderately increases HDL-C and reduces plasma TG. As a result of these changes, the ratios of total- to HDL-C and LDL- to HDL-C are reduced.

CLINICAL TRIALS

In controlled clinical studies, INEGY significantly reduced total-C, LDL-C, Apo B, TG, and non-HDL-C, and increased HDL-C in patients with hypercholesterolaemia.

Primary Hypercholesterolaemia

In a double-blind, placebo-controlled, 8-week study, 240 patients with hypercholesterolaemia already receiving simvastatin monotherapy and not at National Cholesterol Education Program (NCEP) LDL-C goal (2.6 to 4.1 mmol/l [100 to 160 mg/dl], depending on baseline characteristics) were randomised to receive either ezetimibe 10 mg or placebo in addition to their on-going simvastatin therapy. Among simvastatin-treated patients not at LDL-C goal at baseline (~80%), significantly more patients randomised to ezetimibe coadministered with simvastatin achieved their LDL-C goal at study endpoint compared to patients randomised to placebo coadministered with simvastatin, 76% and 21.5%, respectively. The corresponding LDL-C reductions for ezetimibe or placebo coadministered with simvastatin were also significantly different (27% or 3%, respectively). In addition, ezetimibe coadministered with simvastatin significantly decreased total-C, Apo B, and TG compared with placebo coadministered with simvastatin.

In a multicentre, double-blind, 24-week trial, 214 patients with type 2 diabetes mellitus treated with thiazolidinediones (rosiglitazone or pioglitazone) for a minimum of 3 months and simvastatin 20 mg for a minimum of 6 weeks with a mean LDL-C of 2.4 mmol/L (93 mg/dl), were randomised to receive either simvastatin 40 mg or the coadministered active ingredients equivalent to INEGY 10 mg/20 mg. INEGY 10 mg/20 mg was significantly more effective than doubling the dose of simvastatin to 40 mg in further reducing LDL-C (-21% and 0%, respectively), total-C (-14% and -1%, respectively), Apo B (-14% and -2%, respectively), and non-HDL-C (-20% and -2%, respectively) beyond the reductions observed with simvastatin 20 mg. Results for HDL-C and TG between the two treatment groups were not significantly different. Results were not affected by type of thiazolidinedione treatment.

The efficacy of the different dose-strengths of INEGY (10/10 to 10/80 mg/day) was demonstrated in a multicentre, double-blind, placebo-controlled 12-week trial that included all available doses of INEGY and all relevant doses of simvastatin. When patients receiving all doses of INEGY were compared to those receiving all doses of simvastatin, INEGY significantly lowered total-C, LDL-C, and TG (see Table 1) as well as Apo B (-42% and -29%, respectively), non-HDL-C (-49% and -34%, respectively) and C-reactive protein (-33% and -9%, respectively). The effects of INEGY on HDL-C were similar to the effects seen with simvastatin. Further analysis showed INEGY significantly increased HDL-C compared with placebo.

Table 1

Response to INEGY in Patients with Primary Hypercholesterolemia

(Mean[a] % Change from Untreated Baseline[b])

(see Table 1 on next page)

In a similarly designed study, results for all lipid parameters were generally consistent. In a pooled analysis of these two studies, the lipid response to INEGY was similar in patients with TG levels greater than or less than 200 mg/dl.

Table 1 Response to INEGY in Patients with Primary Hypercholesterolemia (Mean[a] % Change from Untreated Baseline[b])

Treatment (Daily Dose)	N	Total-C	LDL-C	HDL-C	TG[a]
Pooled data (All INEGY doses)[c]	353	-38	-53	+8	-28
Pooled data (All simvastatin doses)[c]	349	-26	-38	+8	-15
Ezetimibe10 mg	92	-14	-20	+7	-13
Placebo	93	+2	+3	+2	-2
INEGY by dose					
10/10	87	-32	-46	+9	-21
10/20	86	-37	-51	+8	-31
10/40	89	-39	-55	+9	-32
10/80	91	-43	-61	+6	-28
Simvastatin by dose					
10 mg	81	-21	-31	+5	-4
20 mg	90	-24	-35	+6	-14
40 mg	91	-29	-42	+8	-19
80 mg	87	-32	-46	+11	-26

[a] For triglycerides, median % change from baseline

[b] Baseline - on no lipid-lowering drug

[c] INEGY doses pooled (10/10-10/80) significantly reduced total-C, LDL-C, and TG, compared to simvastatin, and significantly increased HDL-C compared to placebo.

INEGY contains simvastatin. In two large placebo-controlled clinical trials, the Scandinavian Simvastatin Survival Study (20-40 mg; N=4,444 patients) and the Heart Protection Study (40 mg; N=20,536 patients), the effects of treatment with simvastatin were assessed in patients at high risk of coronary events because of existing coronary heart disease, diabetes, peripheral vessel disease, history of stroke or other cerebrovascular disease. Simvastatin was proven to reduce: the risk of total mortality by reducing CHD deaths; the risk of non-fatal myocardial infarction and stroke; and the need for coronary and non-coronary revascularisation procedures.

Studies to demonstrate the efficacy of INEGY in the prevention of complications of atherosclerosis have not been completed.

Homozygous Familial Hypercholesterolaemia (HoFH)

A double-blind, randomised, 12-week study was performed in patients with a clinical and/or genotypic diagnosis of HoFH. Data were analysed from a subgroup of patients (n=14) receiving simvastatin 40 mg at baseline. Increasing the dose of simvastatin from 40 to 80 mg (n=5) produced a reduction of LDL-C of 13% from baseline on simvastatin 40 mg. Coadministered ezetimibe and simvastatin equivalent to INEGY (10 mg/40 mg and 10 mg/80 mg pooled, n=9), produced a reduction of LDL-C of 23% from baseline on simvastatin 40 mg. In those patients coadministered ezetimibe and simvastatin equivalent to INEGY (10 mg/80 mg, n=5), a reduction of LDL-C of 29% from baseline on simvastatin 40 mg was produced.

5.2 Pharmacokinetic properties

No clinically significant pharmacokinetic interaction was seen when ezetimibe was coadministered with simvastatin.

Absorption:

INEGY

INEGY is bioequivalent to coadministered ezetimibe and simvastatin.

Ezetimibe

After oral administration, ezetimibe is rapidly absorbed and extensively conjugated to a pharmacologically active phenolic glucuronide (ezetimibe-glucuronide). Mean maximum plasma concentrations (C_{max}) occur within 1 to 2 hours for ezetimibe-glucuronide and 4 to 12 hours for ezetimibe. The absolute bioavailability of ezetimibe cannot be determined as the compound is virtually insoluble in aqueous media suitable for injection.

Concomitant food administration (high fat or non-fat meals) had no effect on the oral bioavailability of ezetimibe when administered as 10-mg tablets.

Simvastatin

The availability of the active β-hydroxyacid to the systemic circulation following an oral dose of simvastatin was found to be less than 5% of the dose, consistent with extensive hepatic first-pass extraction. The major metabolites of simvastatin present in human plasma are the β-hydroxyacid and four additional active metabolites.

Relative to the fasting state, the plasma profiles of both active and total inhibitors were not affected when simvastatin was administered immediately before a test meal.

Distribution:

Ezetimibe

Ezetimibe and ezetimibe-glucuronide are bound 99.7% and 88 to 92% to human plasma proteins, respectively.

Simvastatin

Both simvastatin and the β-hydroxyacid are bound to human plasma proteins (95%).

The pharmacokinetics of single and multiple doses of simvastatin showed that no accumulation of drug occurred after multiple dosing. In all of the above pharmacokinetic studies, the maximum plasma concentration of inhibitors occurred 1.3 to 2.4 hours post-dose.

Biotransformation:

Ezetimibe

Ezetimibe is metabolised primarily in the small intestine and liver via glucuronide conjugation (a phase II reaction) with subsequent biliary excretion. Minimal oxidative metabolism (a phase I reaction) has been observed in all species evaluated. Ezetimibe and ezetimibe-glucuronide are the major drug-derived compounds detected in plasma, constituting approximately 10 to 20% and 80 to 90% of the total drug in plasma, respectively. Both ezetimibe and ezetimibe-glucuronide are slowly eliminated from plasma with evidence of significant enterohepatic recycling. The half-life for ezetimibe and ezetimibe-glucuronide is approximately 22 hours.

Simvastatin

Simvastatin is an inactive lactone which is readily hydrolyzed *in vivo* to the corresponding β-hydroxyacid, a potent inhibitor of HMG-CoA reductase. Hydrolysis takes place mainly in the liver; the rate of hydrolysis in human plasma is very slow.

In man simvastatin is well absorbed and undergoes extensive hepatic first-pass extraction. The extraction in the liver is dependent on the hepatic blood flow. The liver is its primary site of action, with subsequent excretion of drug equivalents in the bile. Consequently, availability of active drug to the systemic circulation is low.

Following an intravenous injection of the β-hydroxyacid metabolite, its half-life averaged 1.9 hours.

Elimination:

Ezetimibe

Following oral administration of ^{14}C-ezetimibe (20 mg) to human subjects, total ezetimibe accounted for approximately 93% of the total radioactivity in plasma. Approximately 78% and 11% of the administered radioactivity were recovered in the faeces and urine, respectively, over a 10-day collection period. After 48 hours, there were no detectable levels of radioactivity in the plasma.

Simvastatin

Following an oral dose of radioactive simvastatin to man, 13% of the radioactivity was excreted in the urine and 60% in the faeces within 96 hours. The amount recovered in the faeces represents absorbed drug equivalents excreted in bile as well as unabsorbed drug. Following an intravenous injection of the β-hydroxyacid metabolite, an average of only 0.3% of the IV dose was excreted in urine as inhibitors.

Special Populations:

Paediatric Patients

The absorption and metabolism of ezetimibe are similar between children and adolescents (10 to 18 years) and adults. Based on total ezetimibe, there are no pharmacokinetic differences between adolescents and adults. Pharmacokinetic data in the paediatric population $<$10 years of age are not available. Clinical experience in paediatric and adolescent patients (ages 9 to 17) has been limited to patients with HoFH or sitosterolaemia. (See section 4.2.)

Geriatric Patients

Plasma concentrations for total ezetimibe are about 2-fold higher in the elderly ($\geqslant$65 years) than in the young (18 to 45 years). LDL-C reduction and safety profile are comparable between elderly and younger subjects treated with ezetimibe. (See section 4.2.)

Hepatic Insufficiency

After a single 10-mg dose of ezetimibe, the mean AUC for total ezetimibe was increased approximately 1.7-fold in patients with mild hepatic insufficiency (Child Pugh score 5 or 6), compared to healthy subjects. In a 14-day, multiple-dose study (10 mg daily) in patients with moderate hepatic insufficiency (Child Pugh score 7 to 9), the mean AUC for total ezetimibe was increased approximately 4-fold on Day 1 and Day 14 compared to healthy subjects. No dosage adjustment is necessary for patients with mild hepatic insufficiency. Due to the unknown effects of the increased exposure to ezetimibe in patients with moderate or severe (Child Pugh score $>$9) hepatic insufficiency, ezetimibe is not recommended in these patients (see sections 4.2 and 4.4).

Renal Insufficiency

Ezetimibe

After a single 10-mg dose of ezetimibe in patients with severe renal disease (n=8; mean CrCl $\leqslant$30 ml/min), the mean AUC for total ezetimibe was increased approximately 1.5-fold, compared to healthy subjects (n=9). (See section 4.2.)

An additional patient in this study (post-renal transplant and receiving multiple medications, including ciclosporin) had a 12-fold greater exposure to total ezetimibe.

Simvastatin

In a study of patients with severe renal insufficiency (creatinine clearance $<$30 ml/min), the plasma concentrations of total inhibitors after a single dose of a related HMG-CoA reductase inhibitor were approximately two-fold higher than those in healthy volunteers.

Gender

Plasma concentrations for total ezetimibe are slightly higher (approximately 20%) in women than in men. LDL-C reduction and safety profile are comparable between men and women treated with ezetimibe.

5.3 Preclinical safety data

INEGY

In coadministration studies with ezetimibe and simvastatin, the toxic effects observed were essentially those typically associated with statins. Some of the toxic effects were more pronounced than observed during treatment with statins alone. This is attributed to pharmacokinetic and/or pharmacodynamic interactions following coadministration. No such interactions occurred in the clinical studies. Myopathies occurred in rats only after exposure to doses that were several times higher than the human therapeutic dose (approximately 20 times the AUC level for simvastatin and 1800 times the AUC level for the active metabolite). There was no evidence that coadministration of ezetimibe affected the myotoxic potential of simvastatin.

The coadministration of ezetimibe and simvastatin was not teratogenic in rats. In pregnant rabbits a small number of skeletal deformities (fused caudal vertebrae, reduced number of caudal vertebrae) were observed.

In a series of *in vivo* and *in vitro* assays, ezetimibe, given alone or coadministered with simvastatin, exhibited no genotoxic potential.

Ezetimibe

Animal studies on the chronic toxicity of ezetimibe identified no target organs for toxic effects. In dogs treated for four weeks with ezetimibe ($\geqslant$0.03 mg/kg/day) the cholesterol concentration in the cystic bile was increased by a factor of 2.5 to 3.5. However, in a one-year study on dogs given doses of up to 300 mg/kg/day no increased incidence of cholelithiasis or other hepatobiliary effects were observed. The significance of these data for humans is not known. A lithogenic risk associated with the therapeutic use of ezetimibe cannot be ruled out.

Long-term carcinogenicity tests on ezetimibe were negative.

Ezetimibe had no effect on the fertility of male or female rats, nor was it found to be teratogenic in rats or rabbits, nor did it affect prenatal or postnatal development. Ezetimibe crossed the placental barrier in pregnant rats and rabbits given multiple doses of 1000 mg/kg/day.

Simvastatin

Based on conventional animal studies regarding pharmacodynamics, repeated dose toxicity, genotoxicity and carcinogenicity, there are no other risks for the patient than may be expected on account of the pharmacological mechanism. At maximally tolerated doses in both the rat and the rabbit, simvastatin produced no foetal malformations, and had no effects on fertility, reproductive function or neonatal development.

6. PHARMACEUTICAL PARTICULARS

6.1 List of excipients

Butylated hydroxyanisole

Citric acid monohydrate

Croscarmellose sodium

Hypromellose

Lactose monohydrate

Magnesium stearate

Microcrystalline cellulose

Propyl gallate

6.2 Incompatibilities
Not applicable.

6.3 Shelf life
24 months.

6.4 Special precautions for storage
Do not store above 30°C.

Blisters: Store in the original package.

Bottles: Keep bottles tightly closed.

6.5 Nature and contents of container
INEGY 10 mg/20 mg, and 10 mg/40 mg

White HDPE bottles with foil induction seals, white child-resistant polypropylene closure, and silica gel desiccant, containing 100 tablets.

INEGY 10 mg/20 mg, 10 mg/40 mg, and 10 mg/80 mg

Push-through blisters of opaque polychlorotrifluoroethylene/PVC sealed to vinyl coated aluminum in packs of 7, 10, 14, 28, 30, 50, 56, 98, 100, or 300 tablets.

Unit dose push-through blisters of opaque polychlorotrifluoroethylene/PVC sealed to vinyl coated aluminum in packs of 30, 50, 100, or 300 tablets.

Not all pack sizes may be marketed.

6.6 Instructions for use and handling
No special requirements.

7. MARKETING AUTHORISATION HOLDER
MSD-SP Ltd
Hertford Road
Hoddesdon
Hertfordshire
EN11 9BU
United Kingdom

8. MARKETING AUTHORISATION NUMBER(S)
INEGY 10 mg/20 mg Tablets PL 19945/0008

INEGY 10 mg/40 mg Tablets PL 19945/0009

INEGY 10 mg/80 mg Tablets PL 19945/0010

9. DATE OF FIRST AUTHORISATION/RENEWAL OF THE AUTHORISATION
18 November 2004

10. DATE OF REVISION OF THE TEXT
July 2005

LEGAL CATEGORY
POM

® denotes registered trademark of MSP Singapore Company, LLC

INEGY SPC.VYT.04.UK-IRL.2124 II-005

Infacol

(Forest Laboratories UK Limited)

1. NAME OF THE MEDICINAL PRODUCT
INFACOL

2. QUALITATIVE AND QUANTITATIVE COMPOSITION
Simethicone USP 40mg/ml

3. PHARMACEUTICAL FORM
Oral suspension

4. CLINICAL PARTICULARS

4.1 Therapeutic indications
An antiflatulent for the relief of griping pain, colic or wind due to swallowed air.

4.2 Posology and method of administration
For adults and elderly:

Not applicable.

For infants:

20mg (0.5ml) administered before each feed. If necessary this may be increased to 40mg (1ml). Treatment with Infacol may provide a progressive improvement in symptoms over several days.

4.3 Contraindications
None stated

4.4 Special warnings and special precautions for use
If symptoms persist, seek medical advice.

4.5 Interaction with other medicinal products and other forms of Interaction
None stated

4.6 Pregnancy and lactation
Not applicable

4.7 Effects on ability to drive and use machines
Not applicable

4.8 Undesirable effects
None stated

4.9 Overdose
In the event of deliberate or accidental overdosage, treat symptoms on appearance.

5. PHARMACOLOGICAL PROPERTIES

5.1 Pharmacodynamic properties
Physiologically the active ingredient is a chemically inert, non-systemic gastric defoaming agent that works by altering the elasticity of interfaces of mucus-embedded bubbles in the gastrointestinal tract.

The gas bubbles are thus broken down or coalesced and in this form gas is more easily eliminated through eructation or passing flatus.

5.2 Pharmacokinetic properties
Simethicone is not absorbed from the gastrointestinal tract.

5.3 Preclinical safety data
There are no preclinical data of relevance to the prescriber which are additional to that already included in other sections of the SPC.

6. PHARMACEUTICAL PARTICULARS

6.1 List of excipients
Saccharin Sodium

Hydroxypropyl Methylcellulose

Orange flavour

Methyl Paraben

Propyl Paraben

Purified Water

6.2 Incompatibilities
None stated.

6.3 Shelf life
2 years

6.4 Special precautions for storage
Store at room temperature (below 25°C).

6.5 Nature and contents of container
High-density polyethylene bottle fitted with a low-density polyethylene dropper and evoprene teat containing 50ml of liquid.

6.6 Instructions for use and handling
Not stated.

7. MARKETING AUTHORISATION HOLDER
Forest Laboratories UK Limited

Bourne Road

Bexley

Kent DA5 1NX

8. MARKETING AUTHORISATION NUMBER(S)
PL 0108/0100

9. DATE OF FIRST AUTHORISATION/RENEWAL OF THE AUTHORISATION
29th October 1986 / 20 January 1997

10. DATE OF REVISION OF THE TEXT
July 1996

11. Legal Category
GSL

Infanrix

(GlaxoSmithKline UK)

1. NAME OF THE MEDICINAL PRODUCT
Infanrix®▼

Diphtheria-tetanus-acellular pertussis vaccine (DTPa)

2. QUALITATIVE AND QUANTITATIVE COMPOSITION
Infanrix contains diphtheria toxoid, tetanus toxoid and three purified pertussis antigens [pertussis toxoid (PT), filamentous haemagglutinin (FHA) and pertactin (69 kilo-Dalton outer membrane protein)] adsorbed on to aluminium salts.

The diphtheria and tetanus toxins obtained from cultures of *Corynebacterium diphtheriae* and *Clostridium tetani* are detoxified and purified. The acellular pertussis vaccine components (PT, FHA and pertactin) are prepared by growing phase I *Bordetella pertussis* from which the PT and FHA and pertactin are extracted, purified and detoxified.

The diphtheria toxoid, tetanus toxoid and acellular pertussis vaccine components are adsorbed on aluminium salts. The final vaccine is formulated in saline and contains 2-phenoxyethanol as preservative.

Infanrix meets the World Health Organisation requirements for manufacture of biological substances and for diphtheria and tetanus vaccines. No substances of human origin are used in its manufacture.

A 0.5 ml dose of the vaccine contains not less than 30 International Units (IU) of diphtheria toxoid, 40 IU of tetanus toxoid, 25 μg of PT, 25 μg of FHA and 8 μg of pertactin.

3. PHARMACEUTICAL FORM
Turbid suspension for deep intramuscular injection.

4. CLINICAL PARTICULARS

4.1 Therapeutic indications
Infanrix is indicated for active primary immunisation against diphtheria, tetanus and pertussis from 2 months of age.

Infanrix is also indicated as a booster dose for children who have previously been immunised with 3 doses of either DTPa or DTPw vaccine according to the national policy in effect at the time.

4.2 Posology and method of administration

Posology

Primary series

Children (up to and including 6 years of age):

Three 0.5 ml doses of the vaccine by deep intramuscular injection, with an interval of at least four weeks between doses, the first dose to be given not earlier than two months of age.

Infanrix can be mixed with Hiberix for use in primary immunisation. If these two vaccines are mixed the reconstitution should be done immediately prior to administration (see Section 6.6 Instructions for Use/Handling).

Booster

After completion of the primary series, booster doses of DTP should be given in accordance with official recommendations.

Following completion of a primary series in which one or more of the three doses consisted of Infanrix mixed with Hiberix, an additional (fourth) dose of Hib conjugate vaccine (Hiberix or another monovalent Hib conjugate vaccine) should be administered. The timing of the Hib conjugate booster dose should be in accordance with official recommendations (see also section 5.1).

Method of administration

Deep intramuscular injection.

4.3 Contraindications
As with other vaccines, the administration of Infanrix should be postponed in subjects suffering from acute severe febrile illness. The presence of a minor infection, however, is not a contra-indication.

Infanrix is contraindicated if the child has experienced an encephalopathy of unknown aetiology, occurring within 7 days following previous vaccination with pertussis containing vaccine. In these circumstances the vaccination course should be continued with diphtheria and tetanus vaccine.

Infanrix should not be administered to subjects with known hypersensitivity to any component of the vaccine or to subjects having shown signs of hypersensitivity after previous administration of Infanrix, diphtheria and tetanus vaccine or DTPw.

4.4 Special warnings and special precautions for use
It is good clinical practice that immunisation should be preceded by a review of the medical history (especially with regard to previous immunisation and possible occurrence of undesirable events) and a clinical examination.

If any of the following events occur in temporal relation to receipt of DTPa or DTPw, the decision to give subsequent doses of vaccine containing the pertussis component should be carefully considered. There may be circumstances, such as a high incidence of pertussis, when the potential benefits outweigh possible risks, particularly since these events are not associated with permanent sequelae.

The following events were previously considered contra-indications for DTPw and can now be considered to be general precautions:

Temperature of $\geqslant$ 40.5 C within 48 hours of vaccination, not due to another identifiable cause.

Collapse or shock-like state (hypotonic-hyporesponsive episode) within 48 hours of vaccination.

Persistent, inconsolable crying lasting $\geqslant$ 3 hours, occurring within 48 hours of vaccination.

Convulsions with or without fever, occurring within 3 days of vaccination.

A history of febrile convulsions and a family history of convulsive fits do not constitute contra-indications.

HIV infection is not considered as a contra-indication.

As with all vaccinations, a solution of 1:1000 adrenaline should be available for injection should an anaphylactic reaction occur. Recipients of the vaccine should remain under observation until they have been seen to be in good health and not to be experiencing an immediate adverse reaction. It is not possible to specify an exact length of time.

As for all diphtheria, tetanus and pertussis vaccines, the vaccine should be given by deep intramuscular injection.

Infanrix should be administered with caution to subjects with thrombocytopenia or bleeding disorders since bleeding may occur following an intramuscular administration to these subjects. Following injection, firm pressure should be applied to the site (without rubbing) for at least two minutes.

Infanrix should under no circumstances be administered intravenously.

Do not administer by intradermal injection.

4.5 Interaction with other medicinal products and other forms of Interaction

Infanrix can be administered in any temporal relationship with other childhood vaccines.

Different injectable vaccines should always be administered at different injection sites with the exception of Infanrix and Hiberix which can be mixed (see Sections 5.1 and 6.6).

In patients receiving immunosuppressive therapy or patients with immunodeficiency an adequate immunologic response may not be achieved.

4.6 Pregnancy and lactation

As Infanrix is not intended for use in adults, information on the safety of the vaccine when used during pregnancy or lactation is not available.

4.7 Effects on ability to drive and use machines

Not applicable.

4.8 Undesirable effects

These are usually mild and confined to the first 48 hours after vaccination. The commonest local symptoms are likely to be mild soreness, erythema, swelling and induration at the injection site. Some children will experience a mild fever. Less common symptoms that may be observed are: unusual crying, vomiting, diarrhoea, eating or drinking less than usual, sleeping less than usual/restlessness and sleeping more than usual/drowsiness.

The following symptoms have been very rarely reported: fatigue, malaise, headache, arthralgia, myalgia, urticaria, allergic reactions including anaphylactoid reactions. Extremely rare cases of collapse or shock-like state (hypotonic-hyporesponsiveness episode) and convulsions within 2 to 3 days of vaccination have been reported. All the subjects recovered totally and spontaneously without sequelae.

4.9 Overdose

Not applicable.

5. PHARMACOLOGICAL PROPERTIES

5.1 Pharmacodynamic properties

Immune response of Infanrix primary immunisation

One month after a three-dose primary vaccination course in the first 6 months of life more than 99% of infants vaccinated with Infanrix had antibody titres of more than 0.1 IU/ml to both diphtheria and tetanus.

The vaccine contains PT, FHA and pertactin, antigens which are considered to play an important role in protection against pertussis disease. In clinical studies, the vaccine response to these pertussis antigens was more than 95%.

Immune response of Infanrix booster immunisation

Following administration of an Infanrix booster in the second year of life (13-24 months) all Infanrix primed infants had antibody titres of more than 0.1 IU/ml to both diphtheria and tetanus.

The booster response to the pertussis antigens was seen in more than 96% of these children.

Protective efficacy of Infanrix

The protective efficacy of Infanrix against WHO-defined typical pertussis (⩾ 21 days of paroxysmal cough with laboratory confirmation) was demonstrated in:

- a prospective blinded household contact study performed in Germany (3, 4, 5 months schedule).

Based on data collected from secondary contacts in households where there was an index case with typical pertussis, the protective efficacy of the vaccine was 88.7%. Protection against laboratory confirmed mild disease, defined as 14 days or more of cough of any type was 73% and 67% when defined as 7 days or more of cough of any type.

- an NIH sponsored efficacy study performed in Italy (2, 4, 6 months schedule).

The vaccine efficacy was found to be 84%. When the definition of pertussis was expanded to include clinically milder cases with respect to type and duration of cough, the efficacy of Infanrix was calculated to be 71% against > 7 days of any cough and 73% against > 14 days of any cough.

Immune response to Hiberix when administered as a mix with Infanrix

In the majority of studies that have been conducted with different primary immunisation schedules in infants, an anti-PRP titre of ⩾ 0.15 micrograms/ml (the level generally considered as protective against Hib disease) was obtained in ⩾ 95% of infants at one month after the third dose. However, the geometric mean titres of anti-PRP in infants administered the vaccines as a mix for the three-dose primary course were approximately one-third those seen in infants who received Hiberix as a separate injection.

The responses to DT and Pa components were not reduced as a result of mixing Infanrix with Hiberix.

Administration of a booster dose of Hiberix (see section 4.2) during the second year of life to children who had received a primary vaccination course of Hiberix as a mix with Infanrix resulted in anti-PRP titres ⩾ 1.0 micrograms/ml in almost all vaccinated children.

5.2 Pharmacokinetic properties

Evaluation of pharmacokinetic properties is not required for vaccines.

5.3 Preclinical safety data

Appropriate safety tests are performed.

6. PHARMACEUTICAL PARTICULARS

6.1 List of excipients

Aluminium salts, 2-phenoxyethanol, sodium chloride, Water for Injection.

6.2 Incompatibilities

Infanrix can be used to reconstitute Hiberix (see sections 4.5 and 6.6). No other vaccines should be mixed in the same syringe as Infanrix unless specified by the manufacturer.

6.3 Shelf life

The expiry date of the vaccine is indicated on the label and packaging.

When stored between 2°C and 8°C, the shelf-life is 36 months.

6.4 Special precautions for storage

Infanrix should be stored at 2°C to 8°C and protected from light.

Do not freeze. Discard if the vaccine has been frozen.

6.5 Nature and contents of container

Infanrix is presented as 0.5 ml single dose presentation in either 3 ml glass vials or 1 ml glass prefilled syringes.

The vials and prefilled syringes are made of neutral glass type I, which conforms to European Pharmacopoeia Requirements. Vials are closed with grey butyl rubber stoppers and flip-off caps. Syringes are presented with or without needles. Syringes without needles are fitted with grey butyl rubber tip caps. Syringes with needles are fitted with grey butyl rubber shields. Plunger stoppers are grey butyl rubber.

6.6 Instructions for use and handling

Upon storage a white deposit and clear supernatant is observed.

The vaccine should be well shaken in order to obtain a homogenous turbid suspension and inspected visually for any foreign particulate matter and/or variation of physical aspect prior to administration. In the event of either being observed, discard the vaccine.

For mixing with Hiberix

The DTPa vaccine can be used to reconstitute Hiberix by adding the entire contents of the container of the DTPa vaccine to the Hiberix vial containing the pellet. After the addition of the DTPa vaccine to the pellet, the mixture should be well shaken. The reconstituted vaccine must not be injected until the pellet has completely dissolved. After reconstitution, the vaccine should be injected promptly. The full reconstitution instructions are:

1. Attach a green needle to the syringe (where DTPa vaccine is supplied in a vial, first draw up the DTPa vaccine suspension in to a syringe)

2. Inject the contents of the syringe of DTPa vaccine suspension into the Hib vial.

3. With the needle still inserted, shake the Hib vial vigorously and examine for complete dissolution.

4. Withdraw the entire mixture back into the syringe.

5. Replace the green needle with a smaller orange needle and administer the vaccine by intramuscular injection.

6. If the vaccine is not administered immediately, shake the solution vigorously again before injection.

Administrative Data

7. MARKETING AUTHORISATION HOLDER

SmithKline Beecham plc
Great West Road, Brentford, Middlesex TW8 9GS
Trading as:
GlaxoSmithKline UK
Stockley Park West
Uxbridge
Middlesex UB11 1BT

8. MARKETING AUTHORISATION NUMBER(S)

PL 10592/0075

9. DATE OF FIRST AUTHORISATION/RENEWAL OF THE AUTHORISATION

13 April 1999

10. DATE OF REVISION OF THE TEXT

27 March 2003

11. Legal Status

POM

Infanrix IPV

(GlaxoSmithKline UK)

1. NAME OF THE MEDICINAL PRODUCT

Infanrix-IPV▼, suspension for injection in pre-filled syringe

Diphtheria, tetanus, pertussis (acellular, component) and poliomyelitis (inactivated) vaccine (adsorbed)

2. QUALITATIVE AND QUANTITATIVE COMPOSITION

One dose (0.5 ml) contains

Diphtheria toxoid* ⩾ 30 IU

Tetanus toxoid* ⩾ 40 IU

Bordetella pertussis antigens

Toxoid* 25 micrograms

Filamentous Haemagglutinin* 25 micrograms

Pertactin* 8 micrograms

Inactivated poliovirus type 1** 40 DU***

Inactivated poliovirus type 2** 8 DU***

Inactivated poliovirus type 3** 32 DU***

* adsorbed on aluminium oxide hydrated 0.5 mg

** propagated in VERO cells

*** DU: D antigen units

For excipients, see section 6.1.

3. PHARMACEUTICAL FORM

Suspension for injection in pre-filled syringe.

4. CLINICAL PARTICULARS

4.1 Therapeutic indications

This vaccine is indicated for booster vaccination against diphtheria, tetanus, pertussis, and poliomyelitis diseases in individuals from 16 months to 13 years of age inclusive.

The administration of Infanrix-IPV should be based on official recommendations.

4.2 Posology and method of administration

Posology

A single dose of 0.5 ml should be administered.

Infanrix-IPV may be administered to subjects who have previously received whole cell or acellular pertussis-containing vaccines, and oral live attenuated or injected inactivated poliomyelitis vaccines. (See also sections 4.8 and 5.1).

Method of administration

The vaccine is for intramuscular injection, usually into the deltoid muscle. However, the anterolateral thigh may be used in very young subjects if preferred.

Do not administer intravascularly.

4.3 Contraindications

Hypersensitivity reaction after previous administration of diphtheria, tetanus, pertussis or polio vaccines.

Known hypersensitivity to any component of the vaccine (see 6.1) or to neomycin, polymyxin B or formaldehyde (which may be present in the vaccine as trace residues of manufacture).

Infanrix-IPV should not be administered to subjects who experienced neurological complications (for convulsions or hypotonic-hyporesponsive episodes, see section 4.4) following previous immunisation with any of the antigens in the vaccine.

Infanrix-IPV should not be administered to subjects who experienced an encephalopathy of unknown aetiology, occurring within 7 days following previous vaccination with a pertussis containing vaccine.

As with other vaccines, administration of Infanrix-IPV should be postponed in subjects suffering from an acute severe febrile illness. The presence of a minor infection is not a contra-indication.

4.4 Special warnings and special precautions for use

As with all injectable vaccines, appropriate medical treatment and supervision should always be readily available in case of a rare anaphylactic event following the administration of the vaccine.

Vaccination should be preceded by a review of the medical history (especially with regard to previous vaccination and possible occurrence of undesirable events) and a clinical examination. A family history of convulsions or a family history of Sudden Infant Death Syndrome (SIDS) does not constitute a contra-indication.

If any of the following events are known to have occurred in temporal relation to receipt of pertussis-containing vaccine, the decision to give further doses of pertussis-containing vaccines should be carefully considered:

- temperature of ⩾ 40.0°C within 48 hours, not due to another identifiable cause,

- collapse or shock-like state (hypotonic-hyporesponsiveness episode) within 48 hours of vaccination,

- persistent, inconsolable crying lasting ⩾ 3 hours, occurring within 48 hours of vaccination,

- convulsions with or without fever, occurring within 3 days of vaccination.

There may be circumstances, such as a high incidence of pertussis, when the potential benefits outweigh possible risks.

Infanrix-IPV should be administered with caution to subjects with thrombocytopenia or a bleeding disorder since bleeding may occur following an intramuscular administration to these subjects.

HIV infection is not considered as a contra-indication. The expected immunological response may not be obtained after vaccination of immunosuppressed patients.

For children under immunosuppressive treatment (corticosteroid therapy, antimitotic chemotherapy, etc.), it is recommended to postpone vaccination until the end of treatment.

Infanrix-IPV should under no circumstances be administered intravascularly.

4.5 Interaction with other medicinal products and other forms of Interaction

Infanrix-IPV has been administered concomitantly with measles-mumps-rubella vaccine or Hib vaccine in clinical trials. The data available do not suggest any clinically relevant interference in the antibody response to each of the individual antigens.

Interaction studies have not been carried out with other vaccines, biological products or therapeutic medications. However, in accordance with commonly accepted immunisation guidelines, since Infanrix-IPV is an inactivated product, there is no theoretical reason why it should not be administered concomitantly with other vaccines or immunoglobulins at separate sites.

As with other vaccines it may be expected that in patients receiving immunosuppressive therapy or patients with immunodeficiency, a protective immune response to one or more antigens in the vaccine may not be achieved.

4.6 Pregnancy and lactation

It is anticipated that Infanrix-IPV would only rarely be administered to subjects of child-bearing potential. Adequate human data on the use of Infanrix-IPV during pregnancy and lactation are not available and animal studies on reproductive toxicity have not been conducted. Consequently the use of this combined vaccine is not recommended during pregnancy. It is preferable to avoid the use of this vaccine during lactation.

4.7 Effects on ability to drive and use machines

It is anticipated that Infanrix-IPV would only rarely be administered to subjects who would be driving or using machines. However, somnolence, commonly reported after vaccination, may temporarily affect the ability to drive and use machines.

4.8 Undesirable effects

The safety of Infanrix-IPV has been evaluated in 2030 subjects in clinical studies. All vaccinees had previously received either 3 or 4 doses of a combined diphtheria, tetanus and pertussis vaccine. These vaccines contained either whole cell (Pw) or acellular (Pa) pertussis components as follows:

-736 children aged 15-26 months had previously been given 3 doses of DTP –37 had received DTPw, 699 had received DTPa,

– 593 children aged 4-7 years had previously been given either 3 or 4 doses of DTP – 128 had received 3 doses of DTPw, 211 had received 3 doses of DTPa, 73 had received 4 doses of DTPw, 181 had received 4 doses of DTPa

– 701 children aged 10-14 years had received 4 doses of DTPw

All had received a full primary course of either IPV or OPVVaccinees aged 10-14 years had also received an additional dose of diphtheria, tetanus and polio antigens at approximately 5-6 years.

Booster doses of DTPa-containing vaccines may be more reactogenic in children who have been previously primed with acellular pertussis-containing vaccines.

Adverse reactions reported during these studies were mostly reported within 48 hours following vaccination, were of mild to moderate severity and resolved spontaneously.

Very common (⩾ 10%):

Local reactions: pain, redness and swelling at the injection site*

General symptoms: fever, headache, malaise, somnolence, irritability, loss of appetite, restlessness, unusual crying

Common (⩾ 1% and < 10%):

Nausea, vomiting, diarrhoea, asthenia.

Uncommon (⩾ 0.1% and < 1%)

Lymphadenopathy, rash, insomnia, rhinitis, coughing, urinary incontinence, abdominal pain, back pain

Rare (⩾ 0.01% and < 0.1%)

Pruritis, earache, pharyngitis, eye pain

* Information on extensive swelling of the injected limb (defined as swelling with a diameter > 50mm, noticeable diffuse swelling or noticeable increase of limb circumference) occurring after Infanrix-IPV was actively solicited in two clinical trials. When Infanrix-IPV was administered as either a fourth dose or a fifth dose of DTPa to children 4-6 years of age, extensive injection site swelling was reported with incidences of 13% and 25% respectively. The most frequent reactions were large, localised swelling (diameter > 50mm) occurring around the injection site. A smaller percentage of children (3% and 6% respectively) experienced diffuse swelling of the injected limb, sometimes involving the adjacent joint. In general, these reactions began within 48 hours of vaccination and spontaneously resolved over an average of 4 days without sequelae.

Allergic reactions, including urticaria, rash and anaphylactoid reactions have been reported very rarely during post-marketing surveillance.

4.9 Overdose

No case of overdose has been reported.

5. PHARMACOLOGICAL PROPERTIES

Vaccine against diphtheria, tetanus, pertussis and poliomyelitis

ATC code: J07 CA02

5.1 Pharmacodynamic properties

The immune response after booster vaccination with Infanrix-IPV was evaluated in 917 vaccinees. The immune response observed was independent of the number of doses and type of vaccines administered previously (DTPw or DTPa, OPV or IPV) as shown in the tables below.

One month after vaccination of children aged 15 to 26 months, the immune responses were the following:

(see Table 1 opposite)

One month after vaccination of children aged 4-7 years, the immune responses were the following:

(see Table 2 opposite)

One month after vaccination of children/adolescents aged 10-13 years, the immune responses were the following:

Antigen	Previous vaccination history/schedule (N subjects)	4 doses of DTPw+IPV at 2, 3, 4 + 16-18 months + 1 dose of DT-IPV at 5-6 years (N = 53)
Diphtheria	% vaccinees with titres ⩾ 0.1 IU/ml by ELISA*	100
Tetanus	% vaccinees with titres ⩾ 0.1 IU/ml by ELISA*	100
Pertussis	% vaccinees with titres ⩾ 5 EL.U/ml by ELISA	100
Pertussis toxoid		100
Pertactin		100
Polio	% vaccinees with titres ⩾ 8 by neutralisation*	
type 1		100
type 2		100
type 3		100

* These levels are considered to be protective

After vaccination, ⩾ 99% of all subjects had protective antibody levels against diphtheria, tetanus and the three poliovirus types.

No serological correlate of protection has been defined for the pertussis antigens. The antibody titres to the three pertussis components were in all cases higher than those

Table 1

Antigen	Previous vaccination history/schedule (N subjects)	3 doses of DTPw + IPV 2, 3, 4 months (N = 37)	3 doses of DTPa + IPV 2, 3, 4 / 2, 4, 6 / 3, 4, 5 or 3, 4.5, 6 months (N = 252)
Diphtheria	% vaccinees with titres ⩾ 0.1 IU/ml by ELISA*	100	99.6
Tetanus	% vaccinees with titres ⩾ 0.1 IU/ml by ELISA*	100	100
Pertussis	% vaccinees with titres ⩾ 5 EL.U/ml by ELISA		
Pertussis toxoid		100	100
Filamentous haemagglutinin		100	100
Pertactin		100	100
Polio	% vaccinees with titres ⩾ 8 by neutralisation*		
type 1		100	100
type 2		100	100
type 3		100	100

* These levels are considered to be protective

Table 2

Antigen	Previous vaccination history/schedule(N subjects)	3 doses of DTPw + IPV 3, 5, 11 months (N = 128)	3 doses of DTPa + IPV or OPV 3, 5, 11-12 months(N=208)	4 doses of DTPw + IPV 2, 3, 4 + 16-18 months (N = 73)	4 doses of DTPa + IPV or OPV 2, 4, 6 + 18 months (N = 166)
Diphtheria	% vaccinees with titres ⩾ 0.1 IU/ml by ELISA*	100	99.0	100	100
Tetanus	% vaccinees with titres ⩾ 0.1 IU/ml by ELISA*	100	100	100	100
Pertussis	% vaccinees with titres ⩾ 5 EL.U/ml by ELISA				
Pertussis toxoid		98.3	100	95.5	99.4
Filamentous haemagglutinin		100	100	100	100
Pertactin		100	100	100	100
Polio	% vaccinees with titres ⩾ 8 by neutralisation*				
type 1		100	100	100	100
type 2		100	100	100	100
type 3		100	99.5	100	100

* These levels are considered to be protective

observed after primary vaccination with the paediatric acellular pertussis combination vaccine (DTPa, *Infanrix*™), for which efficacy has been demonstrated in a household contact efficacy study. Based on these comparisons, it can therefore be anticipated that Infanrix-IPV would provide protection against pertussis, although the degree and duration of protection afforded by the vaccine are undetermined.

5.2 Pharmacokinetic properties
Not applicable.

5.3 Preclinical safety data
Not applicable

6. PHARMACEUTICAL PARTICULARS

6.1 List of excipients
Phenoxyethanol

Sodium chloride

Medium 199 (containing principally amino acids, mineral salts, vitamins)

Water for injections

6.2 Incompatibilities
In the absence of compatibility studies, this medicinal product must not be mixed with other medicinal products.

6.3 Shelf life
3 years.

6.4 Special precautions for storage
Store at 2°C - 8°C (in a refrigerator).

Do not freeze.

Store in the original package, in order to protect from light.

6.5 Nature and contents of container
0.5 ml of suspension for injection in pre-filled syringe (glass) with plunger stopper (butyl) - pack sizes of 1 or 20.

6.6 Instructions for use and handling
Upon storage, a white deposit and clear supernatant may be observed. This does not constitute a sign of deterioration.

The syringe should be well shaken in order to obtain a homogeneous turbid white suspension.

The suspension should be inspected visually for any foreign particulate matter and/or abnormal physical appearance. In the event of either being observed, discard the vaccine.

Any unused product or waste material should be disposed of in accordance with local requirements.

Administrative Data

7. MARKETING AUTHORISATION HOLDER
SmithKline Beecham plc

Trading as:

GlaxoSmithKline UK

Stockley Park West, Uxbridge

Middlesex UB11 1BT

8. MARKETING AUTHORISATION NUMBER(S)
PL10592/0209

9. DATE OF FIRST AUTHORISATION/RENEWAL OF THE AUTHORISATION
4th June 2004

10. DATE OF REVISION OF THE TEXT
19 August 2004

Infanrix-Hib Prefilled Syringe/ Vial

(GlaxoSmithKline UK)

1. NAME OF THE MEDICINAL PRODUCT
Infanrix® _ Hib ▼

Infanrix-Hib powder (vial) and suspension (in a pre-filled syringe) for suspension for injection.

Diphtheria, tetanus, acellular pertussis (DTPa) and conjugated *Haemophilus influenzae* type b vaccine (Hib)

2. QUALITATIVE AND QUANTITATIVE COMPOSITION
After reconstitution, 1 dose (0.5ml) contains:

Diphtheria toxoid* not less than 30 IU

Tetanus toxoid* not less than 40 IU

Pertussis antigens

Pertussis toxoid* 25 micrograms

Filamentous haemagglutinin* 25 micrograms

Pertactin 8 micrograms

Haemophilus influenzae type b polysaccharide 10 micrograms

conjugated to tetanus toxoid 20-40 micrograms

*adsorbed on aluminium oxide hydrated Total: 0.95 milligrams

For excipients, see 6.1

3. PHARMACEUTICAL FORM
Powder (vial) and suspension (in a pre-filled syringe) for suspension for injection

The diphtheria, tetanus and acellular pertussis (DTPa) is a turbid white suspension.

The lyophilised *Haemophilus influenzae* type b (Hib) component is a white powder

4. CLINICAL PARTICULARS

4.1 Therapeutic indications
'Infanrix-Hib' is indicated for active primary immunisation against diphtheria, tetanus, pertussis (DTP) and invasive disease caused by Hib from 2 months of age.

4.2 Posology and method of administration
Posology
Primary series
Infants: Three 0.5 ml doses of the vaccine by deep intramuscular injection, with an interval of at least four weeks between doses, the first dose to be given not earlier than two months of age.

Booster
Following completion of a primary series in which one or more of the three doses consisted of Infanrix-Hib, an additional (fourth) dose of Hib conjugate vaccine (Hiberix or another monovalent Hib conjugate vaccine) should be administered. The timing of the Hib conjugate booster dose should be in accordance with official recommendations (see also section 5.1 Pharmacodynamic properties).

Booster doses of DTP should also be given in accordance with official recommendations.

Method of administration
The reconstituted vaccine is for deep intramuscular injection.

4.3 Contraindications
'Infanrix-Hib' should not be administered to subjects with known hypersensitivity to any component of the vaccine or to subjects having shown signs of hypersensitivity after previous administration of diphtheria, tetanus, pertussis or Hib vaccines.

As with other vaccines, the administration of 'Infanrix-Hib' should be postponed in subjects suffering from acute severe febrile illness. The presence of a minor infection, however, is not a contra-indication.

'Infanrix-Hib' is contraindicated if the child has experienced an encephalopathy of unknown aetiology, occurring within 7 days following previous vaccination with pertussis containing vaccine. In these circumstances the vaccination course should be continued with diphtheria, tetanus and Hib vaccines.

4.4 Special warnings and special precautions for use
It is good clinical practice that immunisation should be preceded by a review of the medical history (especially with regard to previous immunisation and possible occurrence of undesirable events) and a clinical examination.

If any of the following events occur in temporal relation to receipt of DTP-containing vaccines, the decision to give subsequent doses of vaccine containing the pertussis component should be carefully considered. There may be circumstances, such as a high incidence of pertussis, when the potential benefits outweigh possible risks, particularly since these events are not associated with permanent sequelae.

The following events were previously considered contra-indications for DTPw and can now be considered to be general precautions:

- Temperature of ⩾ 40.5°C within 48 hours of vaccination, not due to another identifiable cause.
- Collapse or shock-like state (hypotonic-hyporesponsive episode) within 48 hours of vaccination.
- Persistent, inconsolable crying lasting ⩾ 3 hours, occurring within 48 hours of vaccination.
- Convulsions with or without fever, occurring within three days of vaccination.

A history of febrile convulsions and a family history of convulsive fits do not constitute contra-indications.

HIV infection is not considered as a contra-indication.

As with all vaccinations, a solution of 1:1000 adrenaline (epinephrine) should be available for injection should an anaphylactic reaction occur. Recipients of the vaccine should remain under observation until they have been seen to be in good health and not to be experiencing an immediate adverse reaction. It is not possible to specify an exact length of time.

'Infanrix-Hib' should be administered with caution to subjects with thrombocytopenia or bleeding disorders since bleeding may occur following an intramuscular administration to these subjects.

Excretion of capsular polysaccharide antigen in the urine has been described following receipt of Hib vaccines and therefore antigen detection may not have a diagnostic value in suspected Hib disease within 1 to 2 weeks of vaccination.

'Infanrix-Hib' does not protect against diseases due to other types of *H. influenzae* nor against meningitis caused by other organisms.

'Infanrix-Hib' should under no circumstances be administered intravenously.

Do not administer by intradermal injection.

4.5 Interaction with other medicinal products and other forms of Interaction
'Infanrix-Hib' can be administered either simultaneously or at any time before or after a different inactivated or live vaccine. Different injectable vaccines should always be administered at different injection sites.

As with other vaccines, it may be expected that in patients receiving immunosuppressive therapy or patients with immunodeficiency an adequate immunologic response may not be achieved.

4.6 Pregnancy and lactation
As 'Infanrix-Hib' is not intended for use in adults, adequate human data on use during pregnancy or lactation and adequate animal reproduction studies are not available.

4.7 Effects on ability to drive and use machines
Not applicable.

4.8 Undesirable effects
The following undesirable effects have been reported in temporal relation to DTPa/Hib. In many instances the causal relationship to the vaccine has not been established.

Very common:

Local reactions: pain, redness, swelling and induration at the injection site.

Systemic reactions: fever, unusual crying, sleepiness, restlessness, diarrhoea, loss of appetite, vomiting.

Common:

Coughing, rhinitis, bronchitis, upper respiratory tract infection, viral infections, otitis media, conjunctivitis, gastroenteritis.

Very rare:

Fatigue, malaise, headache, arthralgia, myalgia, urticaria, allergic reactions, collapse or shock-like state (hypotonic-hyporesponsiveness episode) and convulsions within 2 to 3 days of vaccination.

Anaphylactoid reactions have been reported infrequently with other DTPa containing vaccines.

4.9 Overdose
Not applicable.

5. PHARMACOLOGICAL PROPERTIES

5.1 Pharmacodynamic properties
DTPa component:

One month after the primary vaccination course more than 99.6% of infants vaccinated with 'Infanrix-Hib' had antibody titres of ⩾ 0.1 IU/ml to tetanus and diphtheria. The mean vaccine response to the pertussis antigens (PT, FHA, pertactin) was 97.7%.

The protective efficacy of 'Infanrix' against WHO-defined typical pertussis (⩾ 21 days of paroxysmal cough with laboratory confirmation) was demonstrated in:

- a prospective blinded household contact study performed in Germany (3, 4, 5 months schedule).

Based on data collected from secondary contacts in households where there was an index case with typical pertussis, the protective efficacy of the vaccine was 88.7%. Protection against laboratory confirmed mild disease, defined as 14 days or more of cough of any type was 73% and 67% when defined as 7 days or more of cough of any type.

- an NIH sponsored efficacy study performed in Italy (2, 4, 6 months schedule).

The vaccine efficacy was found to be 84%. When the definition of pertussis was expanded to include clinically milder cases with respect to type and duration of cough, the efficacy of 'Infanrix' was calculated to be 71% against >7 days of any cough and 73% against >14 days of any cough.

Hib component:

In the majority of studies that have been conducted with different primary immunisation schedules in infants, an anti-PRP titre of ⩾0.15 micrograms/ml (the level generally accepted as protective against Hib disease) was obtained in ⩾ 95% of infants at one month after the third dose. However, the geometric mean titres of anti-PRP of infants administered Infanrix-Hib for the three-dose primary course were approximately one-third those seen in infants who received Hiberix as a separate injection.

Administration of a booster dose of Hiberix (see section 4.2) during the second year of life to infants who had received a primary vaccination course of Infanrix-Hib resulted in anti-PRP titres of ⩾ 1.0 micrograms/ml in almost all vaccinated children.

5.2 Pharmacokinetic properties
Evaluation of pharmacokinetic properties is not required for vaccines.

5.3 Preclinical safety data
Not applicable.

6. PHARMACEUTICAL PARTICULARS

6.1 List of excipients
Lyophilised Hib vaccine

Lactose

DTPa vaccine

Aluminium salts

2-phenoxyethanol

Sodium chloride

Water for Injections

6.2 Incompatibilities
'Infanrix-Hib' should not be mixed with other vaccines in the same syringe, unless specified by the manufacturer.

6.3 Shelf life
36 months.

After reconstitution, immediate use is recommended.

The carton and ALL its contents should be discarded on reaching the outer carton expiry date.

6.4 Special precautions for storage
Store between +2°C to +8°C in a refrigerator Do not freeze

Store in the original package, in order to protect from light.

6.5 Nature and contents of container
Powder in vial (Type 1 glass) closed with butyl stopper.

Suspension for injection in pre-filled syringe (Type 1 glass, 1.0ml) with butyl plunger stoppers

Pack sizes of 10 vials of powder and 10 pre-filled syringes of suspension with separate needles

6.6 Instructions for use and handling
Upon storage of the DTPa suspension, a white deposit and clear supernatant is observed. The syringe should be well shaken to obtain a homogenous turbid white suspension. The DTPa suspension and reconstituted vaccine should be inspected visually for any foreign particulate matter prior to administration. If foreign particulates are observed, discard the vaccine.

The vaccine is reconstituted by adding the **entire contents** of the prefilled syringe of DTPa suspension to the vial containing the Hib powder. The mixture should then be well shaken until the powder has completely dissolved. After reconstitution, Infanrix-Hib should be injected immediately or at least within one hour. The full reconstitution instructions are:

1. Attach a 21G (gauge size) needle to a pre-filled syringe of DTPa suspension and inject the entire contents of the syringe into the Hib vial.

2. With the needle still inserted, shake the Hib vial vigorously and examine for complete dissolution. (The reconstituted, combined vaccine will appear more turbid than the DTPa suspension alone and may contain minute air bubbles. This appearance is normal).

3 Withdraw the entire mixture back into the syringe.

4. Replace the 21G needle with an appropriate size needle for injection, and administer the vaccine.

5. If the vaccine is not administered immediately, shake the solution vigorously again before injection.

6. Any unused reconstituted vaccine should be discarded.

Administrative Data

7. MARKETING AUTHORISATION HOLDER
SmithKline Beecham plc

Great West Road, Brentford, Middlesex TW8 9GS

Trading as:

SmithKline Beecham Pharmaceuticals or GlaxoSmithKline UK, at

Stockley Park West

Uxbridge

Middlesex UB11 1BT

8. MARKETING AUTHORISATION NUMBER(S)
PL 10592/0163

9. DATE OF FIRST AUTHORISATION/RENEWAL OF THE AUTHORISATION
14/01/2002

10. DATE OF REVISION OF THE TEXT
27 March 2003

11. Legal Status
POM

Infanrix is a registered trade mark.

Inflexal V

(Sanofi Pasteur MSD)

1. NAME OF THE MEDICINAL PRODUCT
INFLEXAL V

Suspension for injection

Influenza vaccine (surface antigen, inactivated, virosome) 2005/2006 season

2. QUALITATIVE AND QUANTITATIVE COMPOSITION
Influenza virus surface antigen, inactivated, virosome, containing antigens*:

A/California/7/2004 (H3N2)
(A/New York/55/2004 NYMC X-157) ......15 micrograms **

A/New Caledonia/20/99 (H1N1)
(A/New Caledonia/20/99 IVR-116)..........15 micrograms **

B/Shanghai/361/2002
(B/Jiangsu/10/2003)...............................15 micrograms **

per 0,5 ml dose

* propagated in hen's eggs

** haemagglutinin

Inflexal V is an inactivated influenza vaccine formulated with virosomes as carrier/adjuvant system, composed of highly purified surface antigens of strain A and B of the influenza virus propagated in fertilized hen's eggs.

This vaccine complies with the WHO recommendations (northern hemisphere) and EU decision for the 2005/2006 season.

For excipients see 6.1

3. PHARMACEUTICAL FORM
Suspension for injection.

4. CLINICAL PARTICULARS

4.1 Therapeutic indications
Prophylaxis of influenza, especially in those who run an increased risk of associated complications.

4.2 Posology and method of administration
Adults and children from 36 months: 0.5 ml.

Children from 6 months to 35 months: Clinical data are limited. Dosages of 0.25 or 0.5 ml have been used.

For children who have not previously been vaccinated, a second dose should be given after an interval of at least 4 weeks.

Immunisation should be carried out by intramuscular or deep subcutaneous injection.

4.3 Contraindications
Hypersensitivity to the active substances, to any of the excipients, to eggs, to chicken proteins, to polymyxin B or to neomycin.

Immunisation should be postponed in patients with febrile illness or acute infection.

4.4 Special warnings and special precautions for use
As with all injectable vaccines, appropriate medical treatment and supervision should always be readily available in case of a rare anaphylactic event following the administration of the vaccine.

The vaccine (Inflexal V) should under no circumstances be administered intravascularly.

Antibody response in patients with endogenous or iatrogenic immunosuppression may be insufficient.

4.5 Interaction with other medicinal products and other forms of Interaction
The vaccine (Inflexal V) may be given at the same time as other vaccines. Immunisations should be administered into separate limbs. It should be noted that the adverse reactions may be intensified.

The immunological response may be diminished if the patient is undergoing imunosuppressant treatment.

Following influenza vaccination, false-positive serology test results may be obtained by the ELISA method for antibody to HIV-1, hepatitis C virus and, especially, HTLV-1. In such cases, the Western blot method is negative. These transitory false-positive results may be due to IgM production in response to the vaccine.

4.6 Pregnancy and lactation
Limited data from vaccinations in pregnant women do not indicate that adverse foetal and maternal outcomes were attributable to the vaccine. The use of this vaccine may be considered from the second trimester of pregnancy. For pregnant women with medical conditions that increase their risk of complications from influenza, administration of the vaccine is recommended, irrespective of their stage of pregnancy.

The vaccine (Inflexal V) may be used during lactation.

4.7 Effects on ability to drive and use machines
The vaccine is unlikely to produce an effect on the ability to drive and use machines.

4.8 Undesirable effects
Adverse reactions from clinical trials:

The safety of trivalent inactivated influenza vaccines is assessed in open label, uncontrolled clinical trials performed as annual update requirement, including at least 50 adults aged 18 – 60 years of age and at least 50 elderly aged 60 years or older. Safety evaluation is performed during the first 3 days following vaccination.

Undesirable effects reported are listed according to the following frequency.

Adverse events from clinical trials:

Common (>1/100, <1/10):

Local reactions: redness, swelling, pain, ecchymosis, induration.

Systemic reactions: Fever, malaise, shivering, fatigue, headache, sweating, myalgia, arthralgia.

These reactions usually disappear within 1-2 days without treatment.

From Post-marketing surveillance additionally, the following adverse events have been reported:

Uncommon (>1/1,000, <1/100):

Generalised skin reactions including pruritus, urticaria or non-specific rash.

Rare (>1/10,000, <1/1,000):

Neuralgia, paraesthesia, convulsions, transient thrombocytopenia.

Allergic reactions, in rare cases leading to shock, have been reported.

Very rare (<1/10,000):

Vasculitis with transient renal involvement.

Neurological disorders, such as encephalomyelitis, neuritis and Guillain Barré syndrome.

4.9 Overdose
Overdosage is unlikely to have any untoward effect.

5. PHARMACOLOGICAL PROPERTIES

5.1 Pharmacodynamic properties
Seroprotection is generally obtained within 2 to 3 weeks. The duration of postvaccinal immunity to homologous strains or to strains closely related to the vaccine strains varies but is usually 6-12 months.

5.2 Pharmacokinetic properties
Not applicable.

5.3 Preclinical safety data
Not applicable.

6. PHARMACEUTICAL PARTICULARS

6.1 List of excipients
Sodium chloride, disodium phosphate dihydrate, potassium dihydrogen phosphate, lecithin, water for injections.

6.2 Incompatibilities
In the absence of compatibility studies, Inflexal V must not be mixed with other medicinal products.

6.3 Shelf life
1 year.

6.4 Special precautions for storage
Store in a refrigerator (2°C to 8°C)

Do not freeze: the vaccine must not be used if it is inadvertently frozen.

Protect from the light.

6.5 Nature and contents of container
0.5 ml of suspension in pre-filled syringe (type I glass) – pack of 1 or 10.

6.6 Instructions for use and handling
The vaccine should be allowed to reach room temperature before use.

Shake before use.

When a dose of 0.25 ml is indicated, the prefilled syringe should be held in upright position and half of the volume should be eliminated. The remaining volume should be injected.

7. MARKETING AUTHORISATION HOLDER
ISTITUTO SIEROTERAPICO BERNA S.r.l.

Via Bellinzona 39

I-22100 COMO

Italy

8. MARKETING AUTHORISATION NUMBER(S)
PL 15747/0004

9. DATE OF FIRST AUTHORISATION/RENEWAL OF THE AUTHORISATION
15 February 2002

10. DATE OF REVISION OF THE TEXT
June 2005

Influvac Sub-Unit

(Solvay Healthcare Limited)

1. NAME OF THE MEDICINAL PRODUCT
Influvac® Sub-unit, suspension for injection (influenza vaccine, surface antigen, inactivated)

2. QUALITATIVE AND QUANTITATIVE COMPOSITION
Influenza virus surface antigens (haemagglutinin and neuraminidase)* of strains:

A/California/7/2004 (H_3N_2)-like strain - (A/New York/55/2004 NYMC X-157 reass.) 15 micrograms**

A/New Caledonia/20/99 (H_1N_1)-like strain - (A/New Caledonia/20/99 IVR-116 reass.) 15 micrograms

B/Shanghai/361/2002-like strain - (B/Jiangsu/10/2003) 15 micrograms

per 0.5 ml dose.

* propagated in hens' eggs

** haemagglutinin

This vaccine complies with the WHO recommendation (northern hemisphere), and the decision of the EU for the 2005/2006 season.

For excipients, see 6.1.

3. PHARMACEUTICAL FORM

Suspension for injection in pre-filled syringes.

4. CLINICAL PARTICULARS

4.1 Therapeutic indications

Prophylaxis of influenza, especially in those who run an increased risk of associated complications.

4.2 Posology and method of administration

Adults and children from 36 months: 0.5 ml.

Children from 6 months to 35 months: Clinical data are limited; doses of 0.25 ml or 0.5 ml have been used.

For children who have not previously been vaccinated, a second dose should be given after an interval of at least 4 weeks.

Immunisation should be carried out by intramuscular or deep subcutaneous injection.

4.3 Contraindications

Hypersensitivity to the active substances, to any of the excipients and to eggs, chicken protein, formaldehyde, cetyltrimethylammonium bromide, polysorbate 80, or gentamicin.

Immunisation shall be postponed in patients with febrile illness or acute infection.

4.4 Special warnings and special precautions for use

As with all injectable vaccines, appropriate medical treatment and supervision should always be readily available in case of a rare anaphylactic event following the administration of the vaccine.

Influvac should under no circumstances be administered intravascularly.

Antibody response in patients with endogenous or iatrogenic immunosuppression may be insufficient.

4.5 Interaction with other medicinal products and other forms of Interaction

Influvac may be given at the same time as other vaccines. Immunisation should be carried out on separate limbs. It should be noted that the adverse reactions may be intensified.

The immunological response may be diminished if the patient is undergoing immunosuppressant treatment.

Following influenza vaccination, false positive results in serology tests using the ELISA method to detect antibodies against HIV1, Hepatitis C and especially HTLV1 have been observed. The Western Blot technique disproves the results. The transient false positive reactions could be due to the IgM response by the vaccine.

4.6 Pregnancy and lactation

Limited data from vaccinations in pregnant women do not indicate that adverse fetal and maternal outcomes were attributable to the vaccine. The use of this vaccine may be considered from the second trimester of pregnancy. For pregnant women with medical conditions that increase their risk of complications from influenza, administration of the vaccine is recommended, irrespective of their stage of pregnancy.

Influvac may be used during lactation.

4.7 Effects on ability to drive and use machines

Influvac is unlikely to produce an effect on the ability to drive and use machines.

4.8 Undesirable effects

Adverse events from clinical trials:

The safety of trivalent inactivated influenza vaccines is assessed in open label, uncontrolled clinical trials performed as annual update requirement, including at least 50 adults aged 18-60 and at least 50 elderly subjects aged 60 or older. Safety evaluation is performed during the first 3 days following vaccination.

Undesirable effects reported are listed according to the following frequency:

Adverse events from clinical trials:

Common >1/100, <1/10)

Local reactions: redness, swelling, pain, ecchymosis, induration.

Systemic reactions: fever, malaise, shivering, fatigue, headache, sweating, myalgia, arthralgia. These reactions usually disappear within 1-2 days without treatment.

From post-marketing surveillance additionally, the following adverse events have been reported:

Uncommon >1/1,000, <1/100)

Generalised skin reactions including pruritus, urticaria or non-specific rash.

Rare >1/10,000, <1/1,000)

Neuralgia, paraesthesia, convulsions, transient thrombocytopenia.

Allergic reactions, in rare cases leading to shock, have been reported.

Very rare (<1/10,000)

Vasculitis with transient renal involvement. Neurological disorders, such as encephalomyelitis, neuritis and Guillain Barré syndrome.

4.9 Overdose

Overdosage is unlikely to have any untoward effect.

5. PHARMACOLOGICAL PROPERTIES

5.1 Pharmacodynamic properties

Seroprotection is generally obtained within 2 to 3 weeks. The duration of postvaccinal immunity to homologous strains or to strains closely related to the vaccine strains varies but is usually 6-12 months.

5.2 Pharmacokinetic properties

Not applicable.

5.3 Preclinical safety data

Not applicable.

6. PHARMACEUTICAL PARTICULARS

6.1 List of excipients

Potassium chloride, potassium dihydrogen phosphate, disodium phosphate dihydrate, sodium chloride, calcium chloride, magnesium chloride hexahydrate and water for injections.

6.2 Incompatibilities

In the absence of compatibility studies, this medicinal product must not be mixed with other medicinal products.

6.3 Shelf life

1 year.

6.4 Special precautions for storage

Influvac should be stored at +2°C to +8°C (in a refrigerator). Do not freeze. Protect from light.

6.5 Nature and contents of container

0.5 ml suspension for injection in pre-filled syringe (glass, type 1), pack of 1 or 10.

Not all pack sizes may be marketed.

6.6 Instructions for use and handling

Influvac should be allowed to reach room temperature before use. Shake before use.

For administration of a 0.25 ml dose from a syringe, push the front side of the plunger exactly to the edge of the hub (the knurled polypropylene ring); a reproducible volume of vaccine remains in the syringe, suitable for administration.

7. MARKETING AUTHORISATION HOLDER

Solvay Healthcare Limited

Mansbridge Road

West End

Southampton

SO18 3JD

8. MARKETING AUTHORISATION NUMBER(S)

PL 00512/0156

9. DATE OF FIRST AUTHORISATION/RENEWAL OF THE AUTHORISATION

17 March 1998

10. DATE OF REVISION OF THE TEXT

22 August 2005

Legal category

POM

Infukoll 6% solution for infusion

(Beacon Pharmaceuticals)

1. NAME OF THE MEDICINAL PRODUCT

Infukoll® 6 % solution for infusion

2. QUALITATIVE AND QUANTITATIVE COMPOSITION

1000 ml contains:

Poly (O-2-hydroxyethyl)starch 60.0 g

(Molar substitution 0.45-0.55)

(Average molecular weight: 200 000 Da)

Sodium chloride 9.00 g

Na^+ 154 mmol

Cl^- 154 mmol

Theoretical osmolarity 309 mosmol/l

pH 5.0-7.0

For excipients, see 6.1.

3. PHARMACEUTICAL FORM

Solution for infusion

Clear, colourless, aqueous solution

4. CLINICAL PARTICULARS

4.1 Therapeutic indications

Treatment and prevention of hypovolaemia and shock.

Normovolaemic haemodilution.

4.2 Posology and method of administration

HES must be administered intravenously.

Total dosage, duration and rate of infusion will depend upon the amount of blood lost and/or the haemodynamic status and general clinical condition of the patient. Dosage will need to be adjusted as necessary by monitoring the usual circulatory parameters e.g. blood pressure.

The risk of circulatory overload by too rapid rate of infusion or inappropriately large doses must be borne in mind.

Due to the risk for occurrence of an anaphylactic reaction, the first 10 ml - 20 ml of Infukoll® 6 % should be infused slowly and under careful observation of the patient.

Maximum infusion rate:

The maximum rate of infusion should be adjusted to the clinical situation.

Patients with acute haemorrhagic shock: Up to 20 ml/kg bodyweight/hour (equivalent to 0.33 ml/kg BW/min).

In life-threatening situations: 500 ml as a rapid infusion (under pressure). The rates of infusion selected for perioperative indications and for burns and septic shock patients will usually be lower.

Maximum daily dosage:

A maximum daily dosage of 2 g/kg bodyweight/day of hydroxyethyl starch (HES) should not be exceeded. This corresponds to 33 ml/kg bodyweight/day of the 6 % solution (approximately 2,500 ml/day in a person of 75 kg).

Experience of treatment of more than 1-2 days is limited. In cases of longer treatment the daily doses have generally been lower. An increasing risk of undesirable effects with high cumulative doses (see section 4.8) should be considered.

Children:

There are no data concerning usage of Infukoll® 6 % in children.

Administration to children should only be managed after careful benefit/risk assessment.

Further information:

Patients with primarily interstitial fluid losses must firstly be treated with crystalloids. After infusion of HES controls of serum electrolytes and fluid balance are required. Electrolytes must be administered as required. In all patients adequate fluid supply is essential. Renal function must be monitored during treatment (control of serum creatinine).

Because of the possibility of allergic (anaphylactic/anaphylactoid) reactions, appropriate monitoring of patients is necessary.(See section 4.4)

4.3 Contraindications

Known hypersensitivity to hydroxyethyl starch Hypervolaemia Hyper-hydration (e.g. water intoxication) Hyperchloraemia (or hypernatriaemia) Congestive cardiac failure

- Pulmonary oedema Renal failure, with oliguria and anuria Cerebral haemorrhage Severe blood coagulation disorders
- Severe hepatic impairment

4.4 Special warnings and special precautions for use

Particular caution should be exercised and the dosage adjusted as appropriate in patients who have impaired renal clearance since this is the principal way in which Infukoll® 6 % is eliminated. In these patients especially, adequate fluid supply is essential. Renal function, including serum creatinine, must be monitored both before and during treatment.

Monitoring of the serum electrolytes and fluid balance is necessary.

Circulatory overload: The possibility of circulatory overload should be considered. Caution should be exercised in patients at risk of pulmonary oedema and/or congestive cardiac failure; and severely impaired renal function.

Because of the possibility of allergic (anaphylactic/anaphylactoid) reactions, appropriate monitoring of patients is necessary. (See section 4.4)

In case of an allergic reaction, the infusion must be stopped immediately and appropriate treatment given.

Like all colloidal plasma substitutes, Infukoll® 6 % produces coagulation factor dilution. In particular, there is a change in Factor VIII activity, which is, however, temporary and reversible, and, in the absence of other blood coagulation disorders, has no clinical significance. Infukoll® 6 % should be used with caution in patients with preexisting blood coagulation disorders, impaired hepatic function or haemorrhagic diathesis.

Haematocrit may be decreased and plasma proteins diluted by infusion of large volumes of Infukoll® 6 %. Administration of packed red cells, fresh frozen plasma, platelets or full blood should also be considered if excessive dilution occurs.

Samples for blood group determination must be obtained before HES administration because the product may interfere with the tests and cause false positive answers for irregular agglutinins.

Elevated serum alpha amylase concentrations about three times the upper limit of normal may be observed temporarily following administration of HES solutions which may interfere with the diagnosis of pancreatitis. This elevated alpha amylase activity is due to the formation of an enzyme-substrate complex of amylase and HES subject to slow renal elimination and therefore must not be considered diagnostic of impaired pancreatic function. (See sections 4.8 and 5.2).

4.5 Interaction with other medicinal products and other forms of Interaction

Concomitant use of heparin or oral anticoagulants may increase coagulation time.

4.6 Pregnancy and lactation

For Infukoll® 6 % no clinical data on exposed pregnancies are available. No reproductive toxicological studies in animals with Infukoll® 6 % have been performed, but studies with similar hydroxyethyl starch products have caused vaginal bleeding and embryolethality during repeated treatment of test animals. Harmful embryo effects may occur with HES associated anaphylactic reactions in the pregnant mother. Infukoll® 6 % should only be used during pregnancy when the potential effects outweigh the potential risks to the embryo.

There is as yet no experience with usage of this product in nursing mothers.

4.7 Effects on ability to drive and use machines

Not applicable.

4.8 Undesirable effects

Medical products containing hydroxyethyl starch may in rare cases cause anaphylactic reactions of varying degrees of severity.

In the event of an allergic reaction, the infusion must be stopped immediately and appropriate measures to manage the reaction in response to its intensity must be taken. (See section 4.4)

Administration of hydroxyethyl starch may result in dose dependent coagulation disturbances. A transient fall in Factor VIII levels may be seen followed by a prolonged coagulation time. This lacks clinical relevance in the majority of patients. Haematocrit value may be decreased and plasma proteins diluted by infusion of large volumes of Infukoll® 6 %. (See section 4.4)

The concentration of serum α-amylase may increase during the infusion of hydroxyethyl starch. This elevated α-amylase is due to the formation of an enzyme-substrate complex of amylase and hydroxyethyl starch subject to slow renal elimination and must not be considered diagnostic of pancreatitis.

Itching is a known adverse event after long-term administration of high doses of hydroxyethyl starch. This itching may not appear until weeks after the last infusion and may persist for months.

4.9 Overdose

The main risk of an acute overdose would be volume overload. In this case infusion must be stopped immediately and if necessary diuretics should be administered.

5. PHARMACOLOGICAL PROPERTIES

5.1 Pharmacodynamic properties

Pharmacotherapeutic group: Blood substitute and plasma proteins. ATC code: B 05 AA 07.

Infukoll® 6 % is a colloidal plasma volume substitute containing 6 % hydroxyethyl starch (HES) in isotonic saline (0.9 % sodium chloride). The average molecular weight (Mw) of the colloid is 200,000 Da and the molar substitution (MS) 0.45- 0.55, meaning that HES on average contains approximately 5 hydroxyethylgroups per 10 glucose units.

Infukoll® 6 % is iso-oncotic, i.e., the increase in plasma volume is approximately 100% of the infused volume.

The duration of the plasma volume effect depends primarily on the level of molecular substitution and to a lesser extent on the average molecular weight. Intravascular hydrolysis of the hydroxyethyl starch polymers continually releases smaller molecules, which, in turn, are oncotically active before being eliminated via the kidneys.

Infusion of Infukoll® 6 % lowers haematocrit and plasma viscosity.

After infusion of Infukoll® 6 % to hypovolaemic patients the blood volume increasing effect is in general maintained for 3 to 6 hours.

5.2 Pharmacokinetic properties

Hydroxyethyl starch is a mixture of several different substances with different degree of substitution and molecular weight. The elimination depends on molecular weight and degree of substitution. Molecules smaller than the renal threshold (60 000 Da – 70 000 Da) are eliminated via glomerular filtration. Larger molecules are degraded by α-amylase and are thereafter eliminated renally. The rate of degradation decreases with increased degree of substitution. The initial half-life in serum is approximately 6 hours. Approximately 50 % of a given dose is excreted into urine within 24 hours.

5.3 Preclinical safety data

No toxicological animal studies have been conducted with Infukoll® 6 %. Publications of toxicological evaluations of animal studies conducted with repeated hypervolaemic treatment with similar hydroxyethyl starch products have shown bleeding and histiocytosis (accumulation of foam-like histiocytes/macrophages) in several organs including gained weight of the liver, kidneys and the spleen. Infiltration of fat and vacuolation of organs and increasing plasma ASAT and ALAT have been reported. Possible explanations of some of these effects are blood dilution, increased circulatory load and uptake and accumulation of starch in phagocyting cells.

Similar hydroxyethyl starch products have been reported to not being geno-toxic during standard testing. Repro-toxicological studies of similar hydroxyethyl starch products have not shown any signs of teratogenicity. However, vaginal bleeding and embryolethal effects have been observed after evaluation of repeated treatment of test animals.

6. PHARMACEUTICAL PARTICULARS

6.1 List of excipients

Water for injections

6.2 Incompatibilities

In the absence of incompatibility studies this medicinal product must not be mixed with other medicinal products.

6.3 Shelf life

Bottles 3 years

Bags 2 years

6.4 Special precautions for storage

Do not freeze.

6.5 Nature and contents of container

Infukoll® 6 % is available in the following containers and pack sizes:

Bottle (type II-glass) with stopper (bromobutyl rubber) 10 × 500 ml

Bags (plastic polypropylene) with stopper (chlorobutyl rubber) and outer bag (polypropen)

10 × 500 ml

6.6 Instructions for use and handling

Use immediately after first opening and discard any unused product.

Use clear solutions from intact containers.

7. MARKETING AUTHORISATION HOLDER

Serumwerk Bernburg AG

Hallesche Landstrasse 105 b

06406 Bernburg

Germany

8. MARKETING AUTHORISATION NUMBER(S)

PL 20631/0001

9. DATE OF FIRST AUTHORISATION/RENEWAL OF THE AUTHORISATION

22 March 2004

10. DATE OF REVISION OF THE TEXT

Innohep 10,000 IU/ml and Innohep Syringe 10,000 IU/ml

(Leo Laboratories Limited)

1. NAME OF THE MEDICINAL PRODUCT

INNOHEP® 10,000 IU/ML AND **INNOHEP®** SYRINGE 10,000 IU/ML.

2. QUALITATIVE AND QUANTITATIVE COMPOSITION

Tinzaparin sodium 10,000 anti-Factor Xa IU/ml.

3. PHARMACEUTICAL FORM

Solution for Injection.

4. CLINICAL PARTICULARS

4.1 Therapeutic indications

For the prevention of thromboembolic events, including deep vein thrombosis in patients undergoing general and orthopaedic surgery.

For the prevention of clotting in the extracorporeal circuit during haemodialysis in patients with chronic renal insufficiency.

4.2 Posology and method of administration

For prevention of thromboembolic events:

Administration is by subcutaneous injection.

Adults at low to moderate risk, e.g. patients undergoing general surgery:

3,500 anti-Factor Xa IU two hours before surgery and then once daily for 7 to 10 days post-operatively.

Adults at high risk, e.g. patients undergoing orthopaedic surgery:

In this high risk group the recommended dose is either a fixed dose of 4,500 anti-Factor Xa IU given 12 hours before surgery followed by a once daily dose, or 50 anti-Factor Xa IU/kilogram body weight 2 hours before surgery followed by a once daily dose for 7 to 10 days post-operatively.

For haemodialysis:

The dose of Innohep should be given into the arterial side of the dialyser or intravenously. The dialyser can be primed by flushing with 500-1000ml isotonic sodium chloride (9mg/ml) containing 5,000 anti-Factor Xa IU Innohep per litre.

Patients with chronic renal insufficiency:

a) Short-term haemodialysis (up to 4 hours)

A bolus dose of 2,000 - 2,500 anti-Factor Xa IU into the arterial side of the dialyser (or intravenously).

b) Long-term haemodialysis (more than 4 hours)

A bolus dose of 2,500 anti-Factor Xa IU into the arterial side of the dialyser (or intravenously) followed by 750 anti-Factor Xa IU/hour infused into the extracorporeal circuit.

Dosage adjustment

The bolus Innohep dose may be adjusted (increased or decreased) by 250 - 500 anti-Factor Xa IU until a satisfactory response is obtained.

Additional Innohep (500 - 1,000 anti-Factor Xa IU) may be given if concentrated red cells or blood transfusions (which may increase the likelihood of clotting in the dialyser) are given during dialysis or additional treatment beyond the normal dialysis duration is employed.

Dose monitoring

Determination of plasma anti-Factor Xa may be used to monitor the Innohep dose during haemodialysis. Plasma anti-Factor Xa, one hour after dosing should be within the range 0.4 - 0.5 IU/ml.

Use in the elderly

No dose modifications are necessary.

Use in children

There is no experience of use in children.

4.3 Contraindications

Known hypersensitivity to constituents. Generalised haemorrhagic tendency, uncontrolled severe hypertension, active peptic ulcer, septic endocarditis. Thrombocytopenia in patients with a positive *in vitro* aggregation test in the presence of tinzaparin.

In patients receiving heparin for treatment rather than prophylaxis, locoregional anaesthesia in elective surgical procedures is contra-indicated because the use of heparin may be very rarely associated with epidural or spinal haematoma resulting in prolonged or permanent paralysis.

4.4 Special warnings and special precautions for use

Care should be taken when Innohep is administered to patients with severe liver or kidney insufficiency who are undergoing general or orthopaedic surgery. Care should also be taken when Innohep is administered to patients with severe liver insufficiency during haemodialysis. In such cases a dose reduction should be considered.

Innohep should not be administered by intramuscular injection due to the risk of haematoma.

Care should be taken when Innohep is administered to patients who have recently suffered from cerebral haemorrhage, trauma and/or had recent surgery to the central nervous system.

Innohep should be used with caution in patients with hypersensitivity to heparin or to other low molecular weight heparins.

Heparin can suppress adrenal secretion of aldosterone leading to hyperkalaemia, particularly in patients such as those with diabetes mellitus, chronic renal failure, pre-existing metabolic acidosis, a raised plasma potassium or taking potassium-sparing drugs. The risk of hyperkalaemia appears to increase with duration of therapy but is usually reversible. Plasma potassium should be measured in patients at risk before starting heparin therapy and monitored regularly thereafter particularly if treatment is prolonged beyond about 7 days.

In patients undergoing peridural or spinal anaesthesia or spinal puncture, the prophylactic use of heparin may be very rarely associated with epidural or spinal haematoma resulting in prolonged or permanent paralysis. The risk is increased by the use of a peridural or spinal catheter for anaesthesia, by the concomitant use of drugs affecting haemostasis such as non-steroidal anti-inflammatory drugs (NSAIDs), platelet inhibitors or anticoagulants, and by traumatic or repeated puncture.

In decision making on the interval between the last administration of heparin at prophylactic doses and the placement or removal of a peridural or spinal catheter, the product characteristics and the patient profile should be taken into account. Subsequent dose should not take place before at least four hours have elapsed. Re-administration should be delayed until the surgical procedure is completed.

Should a physician decide to administer anti-coagulation in the context of peridural or spinal anaesthesia, extreme vigilance and frequent monitoring must be exercised to detect any signs and symptoms of neurologic impairment, such as back pain, sensory and motor deficits and bowel or bladder dysfunction. Patients should be instructed to inform immediately a nurse or a clinician if they experience any of these.

As there is a risk of antibody-mediated heparin-induced thrombocytopenia, platelet counts should be measured in patients receiving heparin treatment for longer than 5 days and the treatment should be stopped immediately in those who develop thrombocytopenia.

Prosthetic Heart Valves:

There have been no adequate studies to assess the safe and effective use of tinzaparin sodium in preventing valve thrombosis in patients with prosthetic heart valves; therefore no dosage recommendations can be given. High doses of tinzaparin sodium (175 IU/kg) may not be sufficient prophylaxis to prevent valve thrombosis in patients with prosthetic heart valves. The use of tinzaparin sodium cannot be recommended for this purpose.

4.5 Interaction with other medicinal products and other forms of Interaction
Any drug which affects platelet function or aggregation or blood coagulation, e.g. salicylates, non-steroidal anti-inflammatory drugs, vitamin K antagonists (such as warfarin) and dextran should be used with caution in patients receiving Innohep.

Innohep does not appear to interact with other drugs used widely in chronic renal failure, including vitamin B supplements, aluminium hydroxide, calcium supplements, alfacalcidol, ranitidine, vitamin C supplements, ferrous sulphate, folic acid, nifedipine, erythropoietin and azatadine.

4.6 Pregnancy and lactation
No transplacental passage of Innohep was found (assessed by anti-Factor Xa and anti-Factor IIa activity) in patients given a dose of 35 to 40 anti-Factor Xa IU/kg in the second trimester of pregnancy. In rabbits, no transplacental passage of anti-Factor Xa or anti-Factor IIa activity was observed after doses of 1750 anti-Factor Xa IU/kg. Toxicological studies in rats have shown no embryotoxic or teratogenic effects, although a lower birthweight was found.

Although these animal studies show no hazard, as a precaution Innohep should not be used in pregnancy unless no safer alternative is available.

It is not known whether Innohep is excreted in breast milk. However, patients are advised to stop breast-feeding while receiving Innohep.

Prosthetic Heart Valves:

Therapeutic failures and maternal death have been reported in pregnant women with prosthetic heart valves on full anti-coagulant doses of low molecular weight heparins. In the absence of clear dosing, efficacy and safety information in this circumstance, tinzaparin sodium is not recommended for use in pregnant women with prosthetic heart valves

4.7 Effects on ability to drive and use machines
No adverse effects to be expected.

4.8 Undesirable effects
Skin rashes and minor bruising at the site of injection have occurred occasionally. Systemic allergic reactions have been reported extremely rarely.

Innohep, like heparin, has been shown to increase the risk of haemorrhage. However, at the recommended dose this risk is low. As with heparin, thrombocytopenia may occur rarely.

As for heparin, a transient increase in aminotransferase levels is frequently seen. Cessation of treatment is not usually required.

Heparin products can cause hypoaldosteronism which may result in an increase in plasma potassium. Rarely, clinically significant hyperkalaemia may occur particularly in patients with chronic renal failure and diabetes mellitus (see Special Warnings and Precautions for Use).

Very rare cases of epidural and spinal haematoma have been reported in patients receiving heparin for prophylaxis undergoing spinal or epidural anaesthesia or spinal puncture. For further information, see Section 4.4, Special Warnings and Precautions for Use.

Skin necrosis has been reported. If this occurs treatment must be withdrawn immediately.

Priapism has been reported rarely.

Valve thrombosis in patients with prosthetic heart valves have been reported rarely in patients receiving low molecular weight heparins, usually associated with inadequate dosing (see Special warnings and precautions for use).

4.9 Overdose
Overdose of Innohep may be complicated by haemorrhage. With recommended dosages there should be no need for an antidote but in the event of accidental administration of an overdose, the effect of Innohep can be reversed by intravenous administration of 1% protamine sulphate solution.

The dose of protamine sulphate required for neutralisation should be accurately determined by titrating with the patient's plasma. As a rule, 1mg of protamine sulphate neutralises the effect of 100 anti-Factor Xa IU tinzaparin. The anti-Factor Xa activity of tinzaparin is only partially neutralised by protamine sulphate and the anti-Factor Xa and anti-Factor IIa (APTT) activities are seen to return 3 hours after its reversal.

It is recommended that protamine sulphate (1mg/100 anti-Factor Xa IU of tinzaparin) should be given as intermittent injections or continuous infusion. Potential side-effects of protamine sulphate must be considered and patients carefully observed.

Transfusion of fresh plasma may be used, if necessary. Plasma anti-Factor Xa and anti-Factor IIa activity should be measured during the management of overdose situations.

5. PHARMACOLOGICAL PROPERTIES

5.1 Pharmacodynamic properties
Innohep is an antithrombotic agent. It potentiates the inhibition of several activated coagulation factors, especially Factor Xa, its activity being mediated via antithrombin III.

5.2 Pharmacokinetic properties
The pharmacokinetics/pharmacodynamic activity of Innohep is monitored by anti-Factor Xa activity.

Innohep has a bioavailability of around 90% following a subcutaneous injection. The absorption half-life is 200 minutes, peak plasma activity being observed after 4 to 6 hours. The elimination half-life is about 90 minutes.

The half-life of Innohep in patients with renal insufficiency given a bolus intravenous dose of 2,500 anti-Factor Xa IU is about 2.5 hours.

There is a linear dose response relationship between plasma activity and the dose administered.

5.3 Preclinical safety data
There are no preclinical data of relevance to the prescriber which are additional to that already included in other sections of the SPC.

6. PHARMACEUTICAL PARTICULARS

6.1 List of excipients
Innohep 10,000 IU/ml: Benzyl alcohol, Sodium acetate, Sodium hydroxide, Water for Injections.

Innohep Syringe 10,000 IU/ml: Sodium acetate, Water for Injections. As pH adjuster: sodium hydroxide.

6.2 Incompatibilities
Innohep should not be mixed with any other injection.

6.3 Shelf life
2 years.

6.4 Special precautions for storage
Do not store above 25°C.

6.5 Nature and contents of container
Innohep 10,000 IU/ml: 2ml glass vial containing 10,000 anti-Factor Xa IU/ml in packs of 10 vials.

Innohep Syringe 10,000 IU/ml: A prefilled unit dose syringe containing:

2,500 anti-Factor Xa IU in 0.25ml

3,500 anti-Factor Xa IU in 0.35ml

4,500 anti-Factor Xa IU in 0.45ml

in packs of 10 syringes.

6.6 Instructions for use and handling
Innohep 10,000 IU/ml: The vial should be discarded 14 days after first use.

Innohep Syringe 10,000 IU/ml: Contains no preservative, any portion of the contents not used at once should be discarded with the syringe.

7. MARKETING AUTHORISATION HOLDER
LEO Laboratories Limited

Longwick Road

Princes Risborough

Bucks HP27 9RR

8. MARKETING AUTHORISATION NUMBER(S)
Innohep 10,000 IU/ml: PL 00043/0205.

Innohep Syringe 10,000 IU/ml: PL 00043/0204.

9. DATE OF FIRST AUTHORISATION/RENEWAL OF THE AUTHORISATION
Innohep 10,000 IU/ml: 30 September 1998.

Innohep Syringe 10,000 IU/ml: 20 November 1997.

10. DATE OF REVISION OF THE TEXT
March 2004.

LEGAL CATEGORY
POM

Innohep 20,000 IU/ml and Innohep syringe 20,000 IU/ml

(Leo Laboratories Limited)

1. NAME OF THE MEDICINAL PRODUCT
INNOHEP® 20,000 IU/ML AND **INNOHEP**® SYRINGE 20,000 IU/ML

2. QUALITATIVE AND QUANTITATIVE COMPOSITION
Tinzaparin sodium 20,000 anti-Factor Xa IU/ml

3. PHARMACEUTICAL FORM
Solution for Injection

4. CLINICAL PARTICULARS

4.1 Therapeutic indications
Treatment of deep-vein thrombosis and of pulmonary embolus.

4.2 Posology and method of administration
Administration is by subcutaneous injection only.

Adults: 175 anti-Factor Xa IU/kg bodyweight once daily, for at least 6 days and until adequate oral anti-coagulation is established. There is no need to monitor the anticoagulant activity of Innohep.

Use in the elderly: No dose modifications are necessary.

Use in children: There is no experience of use in children.

4.3 Contraindications
Known hypersensitivity to constituents. Generalised haemorrhagic tendency, uncontrolled severe hypertension, active peptic ulcer, septic endocarditis. Thrombocytopenia in patients with a positive *in vitro* aggregation test in the presence of tinzaparin.

In patients receiving heparin for treatment rather than prophylaxis, locoregional anaesthesia in elective surgical procedures is contra-indicated because the use of heparin may be very rarely associated with epidural or spinal haematoma resulting in prolonged or permanent paralysis.

4.4 Special warnings and special precautions for use
Care should be taken when Innohep is administered to patients with severe liver or kidney insufficiency. In such cases a dose reduction should be considered.

Innohep should not be administered by intramuscular injection due to the risk of haematoma.

Innohep should be used with caution in patients with a history of asthma due to the presence of sodium bisulphite.

Care should be taken when Innohep is administered to patients who have recently suffered from cerebral haemorrhage, trauma and/or had recent surgery to the central nervous system.

Innohep should be used with caution in patients with hypersensitivity to heparin or to other low molecular weight heparins.

For some patients with pulmonary embolism (e.g. those with severe haemodynamic instability) alternative treatment, such as surgery or thrombolysis may be indicated.

Heparin can suppress adrenal secretion of aldosterone leading to hyperkalaemia, particularly in patients such as those with diabetes mellitus, chronic renal failure, pre-existing metabolic acidosis, a raised plasma potassium or taking potassium sparing drugs. The risk of hyperkalaemia appears to increase with duration of therapy but is usually reversible. Plasma potassium should be measured in patients at risk before starting heparin therapy and monitored regularly thereafter particularly if treatment is prolonged beyond about 7 days.

In patients undergoing peridural or spinal anaesthesia or spinal puncture, the prophylactic use of heparin may be very rarely associated with epidural or spinal haematoma resulting in prolonged or permanent paralysis. The risk is increased by the use of a peridural or spinal catheter for anaesthesia, by the concomitant use of drugs affecting haemostasis such as non-steroidal anti-inflammatory drugs (NSAIDs), platelet inhibitors or anticoagulants, and by traumatic or repeated puncture.

In decision making on the interval between the last administration of heparin at prophylactic doses and the placement or removal of a peridural or spinal catheter, the product characteristics and the patient profile should be taken into account. Subsequent dose should not take place before at least four hours have elapsed. Re-administration should be delayed until the surgical procedure is completed.

Should a physician decide to administer anti-coagulation in the context of peridural or spinal anaesthesia, extreme vigilance and frequent monitoring must be exercised to detect any signs and symptoms of neurologic impairment, such as back pain, sensory and motor deficits and bowel or bladder dysfunction. Patients should be instructed to inform immediately a nurse or a clinician if they experience any of these.

As there is a risk of antibody-mediated heparin-induced thrombocytopenia, platelet counts should be measured in patients receiving heparin treatment for longer than 5 days and the treatment should be stopped immediately in those who develop thrombocytopenia.

Prosthetic Heart Valves:

There have been no adequate studies to assess the safe and effective use of tinzaparin sodium in preventing valve thrombosis in patients with prosthetic heart valves; therefore no dosage recommendations can be given. High doses of tinzaparin sodium (175 IU/kg) may not be sufficient prophylaxis to prevent valve thrombosis in patients with prosthetic heart valves. The use of tinzaparin sodium cannot be recommended for this purpose.

4.5 Interaction with other medicinal products and other forms of Interaction
Any drug which affects platelet function or aggregation or blood coagulation, e.g. salicylates, non-steroidal anti-inflammatory drugs, vitamin K antagonists (such as warfarin) and dextran, should be used with caution in patients receiving Innohep.

4.6 Pregnancy and lactation
No transplacental passage of Innohep was found (assessed by anti-Factor Xa and anti-Factor IIa activity) in patients given a dose of 35-40 anti-Factor Xa IU/kg in the second trimester of pregnancy. In rabbits, no transplacental passage of anti-Factor Xa or anti-Factor IIa activity was observed after doses of 1750 anti-Factor Xa IU/kg. Toxicological studies in rats have shown no embryotoxic or teratogenic effects, although a lower birthweight was found.

Although these animal studies show no hazard, as a precaution Innohep should not be used in pregnancy unless no safer alternative is available.

It is not known whether Innohep is excreted in breast milk. However, patients are advised to stop breast-feeding while receiving Innohep.

Prosthetic Heart Valves:
Therapeutic failures and maternal death have been reported in pregnant women with prosthetic heart valves on full anti-coagulant doses of low molecular weight heparins. In the absence of clear dosing, efficacy and safety information in this circumstance, tinzaparin sodium is not recommended for use in pregnant women with prosthetic heart valves.

4.7 Effects on ability to drive and use machines
No adverse effects to be expected.

4.8 Undesirable effects
Skin rashes and minor bruising at the site of injection have occurred occasionally. Systemic allergic reactions have been reported extremely rarely.

Innohep, like heparin, has been shown to increase the risk of haemorrhage. However, at the recommended dose this risk is low. As with heparin, thrombocytopenia may occur rarely.

As for heparin, a transient increase in aminotransferase levels is frequently seen. Cessation of treatment is not usually required.

Heparin products can cause hypoaldosteronism which may result in an increase in plasma potassium. Rarely, clinically significant hyperkalaemia may occur particularly in patients with chronic renal failure and diabetes mellitus (see Special Warnings and Precautions for Use).

Very rare cases of epidural and spinal haematoma have been reported in patients receiving heparin for prophylaxis undergoing spinal or epidural anaesthesia or spinal puncture. For further information, see Section 4.4, Special Warnings and Precautions for Use.

Skin necrosis has been reported. If this occurs treatment must be withdrawn immediately.

Priapism has been reported rarely.

Valve thrombosis in patients with prosthetic heart valves have been reported rarely in patients receiving low molecular weight heparins, usually associated with inadequate dosing (see Special warnings and precautions for use).

4.9 Overdose
Overdose of Innohep may be complicated by haemorrhage. With recommended dosages there should be no need for an antidote but in the event of accidental administration of an overdose, the effect of Innohep can be reversed by intravenous administration of 1% protamine sulphate solution.

The dose of protamine sulphate required for neutralisation should be accurately determined by titrating with the patient's plasma. As a rule, 1mg of protamine sulphate neutralises the effect of 100 anti-Factor Xa IU tinzaparin. The anti-Factor Xa activity of tinzaparin is only partially neutralised by protamine sulphate and the anti-Factor Xa and anti-Factor IIa (APTT) activities are seen to return 3 hours after its reversal.

It is recommended that protamine sulphate (1mg/100 anti-Factor Xa IU of tinzaparin) should be given as intermittent injections or continuous infusion. Potential side-effects of protamine sulphate must be considered and patients carefully observed.

Transfusion of fresh plasma may be used, if necessary. Plasma anti-Factor Xa and anti-Factor IIa activity should be measured during the management of overdose situations.

5. PHARMACOLOGICAL PROPERTIES

5.1 Pharmacodynamic properties
Innohep is an antithrombotic agent. It potentiates the inhibition of several activated coagulation factors, especially Factor Xa, its activity being mediated via antithrombin III.

5.2 Pharmacokinetic properties
The pharmacokinetics/pharmacodynamic activity of Innohep is monitored by anti-Factor Xa activity. Following subcutaneous injection of Innohep, anti-Factor Xa activity reaches a maximum at 4-6 hours (peak anti-Factor Xa activity, after administration of 175 anti-Factor Xa IU/kg bodyweight once daily, is approximately 0.5-1.0 IU/ml). Detectable anti-Factor Xa activity persists for 24 hours.

5.3 Preclinical safety data
There are no preclinical data of relevance to the prescriber which are additional to that already included in other sections of the SPC.

6. PHARMACEUTICAL PARTICULARS

6.1 List of excipients
Innohep 20,000IU/ml - Sodium metabisulphite, Benzyl alcohol, Sodium hydroxide, Water for Injections.

Innohep Syringe 20,000IU/ml - Sodium metabisulphite, Sodium hydroxide, Water for Injections.

6.2 Incompatibilities
Innohep should be given by subcutaneous injection only. It should not be mixed with any other injection.

6.3 Shelf life
2 years.

6.4 Special precautions for storage
Do not store above 25°C.

6.5 Nature and contents of container
Innohep 20,000 IU/ml - A 2ml glass vial containing 20,000 anti-Factor Xa IU/ml in packs of 1 vial.

Innohep Syringe 20,000 IU/ml - A prefilled variable dose graduated syringe containing: 0.5ml (10,000 anti-Factor Xa IU), 0.7ml (14,000 anti-Factor Xa IU), 0.9ml (18,000 anti-Factor Xa IU) in packs of 2 and 6 syringes.

6.6 Instructions for use and handling
Innohep 20,000 IU/ml - The vial should be discarded 14 days after first use.

Innohep Syringe 20,000 IU/ml - Contains no bactericide, any portion of the contents not used at once should be discarded together with the syringe.

7. MARKETING AUTHORISATION HOLDER
LEO Laboratories Limited

Longwick Road

Princes Risborough

Bucks HP27 9RR

8. MARKETING AUTHORISATION NUMBER(S)
Innohep 20,000 IU/ml - PL 0043/0192

Innohep Syringe 20,000 IU/ml - PL 0043/0197

9. DATE OF FIRST AUTHORISATION/RENEWAL OF THE AUTHORISATION
Innohep 20,000 IU/ml - 18 October 1994

Innohep Syringe 20,000 IU/ml - 3 October 1996

10. DATE OF REVISION OF THE TEXT
March 2004

LEGAL CATEGORY
POM

Innovace Tablets

(Merck Sharp & Dohme Limited)

1. NAME OF THE MEDICINAL PRODUCT
INNOVACE® 2.5 mg Tablets

INNOVACE® 5 mg Tablets

INNOVACE® 10 mg Tablets

INNOVACE® 20 mg Tablets

2. QUALITATIVE AND QUANTITATIVE COMPOSITION
Each tablet contains 2.5 mg, 5 mg, 10 mg or 20 mg of enalapril maleate.

For excipients, see section 6.1.

3. PHARMACEUTICAL FORM
Tablets.

'Innovace' 2.5 mg Tablets are white, round, biconvex tablets one side embossed 'MSD 14', the other plain.

'Innovace' 5 mg Tablets are white rounded, triangle-shaped tablets one side scored the other embossed 'MSD 712'.

'Innovace' 10 mg Tablets are rust-red coloured, rounded, triangle-shaped tablets one side embossed 'MSD 713' the other side scored.

'Innovace' 20 mg Tablets are peach-coloured, rounded, triangle-shaped tablets one side embossed 'MSD 714', the other side scored.

4. CLINICAL PARTICULARS

4.1 Therapeutic indications
- Treatment of hypertension
- Treatment of symptomatic heart failure
- Prevention of symptomatic heart failure in patients with asymptomatic left ventricular dysfunction (ejection fraction ⩽35%).

(See Section 5.1 'Pharmacodynamic properties'.)

4.2 Posology and method of administration
The absorption of 'Innovace' is not affected by food.

The dose should be individualised according to patient profile (see 4.4 'Special warnings and special precautions for use') and blood pressure response.

Hypertension
The initial dose is 5 to maximally 20 mg, depending on the degree of hypertension and the condition of the patient (see below). 'Innovace' is given once daily. In mild hypertension, the recommended initial dose is 5 to 10 mg. Patients with a strongly activated renin-angiotensin-aldosterone system, (e.g. renovascular hypertension, salt and/or volume depletion, cardiac decompensation, or severe hypertension) may experience an excessive blood pressure fall following the initial dose. A starting dose of 5 mg or lower is recommended in such patients and the initiation of treatment should take place under medical supervision.

Prior treatment with high dose diuretics may result in volume depletion and a risk of hypotension when initiating therapy with enalapril. A starting dose of 5 mg or lower is recommended in such patients. If possible, diuretic therapy should be discontinued for 2-3 days prior to initiation of therapy with 'Innovace'. Renal function and serum potassium should be monitored.

The usual maintenance dose is 20 mg daily. The maximum maintenance dose is 40 mg daily.

Heart failure/asymptomatic left ventricular dysfunction
In the management of symptomatic heart failure 'Innovace' is used in addition to diuretics and, where appropriate, digitalis or beta-blockers. The initial dose of 'Innovace' in patients with symptomatic heart failure or asymptomatic left ventricular dysfunction is 2.5 mg, and it should be administered under close medical supervision to determine the initial effect on the blood pressure. In the absence of, or after effective management of, symptomatic hypotension following initiation of therapy with 'Innovace' in heart failure, the dose should be increased gradually to the usual maintenance dose of 20 mg, given in a single dose or two divided doses, as tolerated by the patient. This dose titration is recommended to be performed over a 2 to 4 week period. The maximum dose is 40 mg daily given in two divided doses.

Suggested dosage titration of 'Innovace' in patients with heart failure/asymptomatic left ventricular dysfunction

Week	Dose mg/day
Week 1	**Days 1 to 3:** 2.5 mg/day* in a single dose **Days 4 to 7:** 5 mg/day in two divided doses
Week 2	10 mg/day in a single dose or in two divided doses
Weeks 3 and 4	20 mg/day in a single dose or in two divided doses

*Special precautions should be followed in patients with impaired renal function or taking diuretics (See 4.4 'Special warnings and special precautions for use').

Blood pressure and renal function should be monitored closely both before and after starting treatment with 'Innovace' (see 4.4 'Special warnings and special precautions for use') because hypotension and (more rarely) consequent renal failure have been reported. In patients treated with diuretics, the dose should be reduced if possible before beginning treatment with 'Innovace'. The appearance of hypotension after the initial dose of 'Innovace' does not imply that hypotension will recur during chronic therapy with 'Innovace' and does not preclude continued use of the drug. Serum potassium and renal function also should be monitored.

Dosage in renal insufficiency
Generally, the intervals between the administration of enalapril should be prolonged and/or the dosage reduced.

Creatinine clearance (CrCL) mL/min	Initial dose mg/day
30 < CrCL < 80 ml/min.	5 - 10 mg
10 < CrCL ⩽ 30 ml/min.	2.5 mg
CrCL ⩽ 10 ml/min.	2.5 mg on dialysis days*

* See 4.4 'Special warnings and special precautions for use' - *Haemodialysis Patients*.

Enalaprilat is dialysable. Dosage on non-dialysis days should be adjusted depending on the blood pressure response.

Use in elderly
The dose should be in line with the renal function of the elderly patient (see 4.4 'Special warnings and special precautions for use', *Renal function impairment*).

Use in paediatrics
There is limited clinical trial experience of the use of 'Innovace' in hypertensive paediatric patients (see 4.4 'Special warnings and special precautions for use', 5.1 'Pharmacodynamic properties' and 5.2 'Pharmacokinetic properties').

For patients who can swallow tablets, the dose should be individualised according to patient profile and blood pressure response. The recommended initial dose is 2.5 mg in patients 20 to <50 kg and 5 mg in patients ⩾50 kg. 'Innovace' is given once daily. The dosage should be adjusted according to the needs of the patient to a maximum of 20 mg daily in patients 20 to <50 kg and 40 mg in patients ⩾50 kg. (See 4.4 'Special warnings and special precautions for use').

'Innovace' is not recommended in neonates and in paediatric patients with glomerular filtration rate <30 ml/min/1.73 m^2, as no data are available.

4.3 Contraindications
- Hypersensitivity to enalapril, to any of the excipients or any other ACE inhibitor
- History of angioedema associated with previous ACE-inhibitor therapy
- Hereditary or idiopathic angioedema
- Second and third trimesters of pregnancy (see 4.6 'Pregnancy and lactation').

4.4 Special warnings and special precautions for use

Symptomatic hypotension

Symptomatic hypotension is rarely seen in uncomplicated hypertensive patients. In hypertensive patients receiving 'Innovace', symptomatic hypotension is more likely to occur if the patient has been volume depleted, e.g. by diuretic therapy, dietary salt restriction, dialysis, diarrhoea or vomiting (see 4.5 'Interaction with other medicinal products and other forms of interaction' and 4.8 'Undesirable effects'). In patients with heart failure, with or without associated renal insufficiency, symptomatic hypotension has been observed. This is most likely to occur in those patients with more severe degrees of heart failure, as reflected by the use of high doses of loop diuretics, hyponatraemia or functional renal impairment. In these patients, therapy should be started under medical supervision and the patients should be followed closely whenever the dose of 'Innovace' and/or diuretic is adjusted. Similar considerations may apply to patients with ischaemic heart or cerebrovascular disease in whom an excessive fall in blood pressure could result in a myocardial infarction or cerebrovascular accident.

If hypotension occurs, the patient should be placed in the supine position and, if necessary, should receive an intravenous infusion of normal saline. A transient hypotensive response is not a contra-indication to further doses, which can be given usually without difficulty once the blood pressure has increased after volume expansion.

In some patients with heart failure who have normal or low blood pressure, additional lowering of systemic blood pressure may occur with 'Innovace'. This effect is anticipated, and usually is not a reason to discontinue treatment. If hypotension becomes symptomatic, a reduction of dose and/or discontinuation of the diuretic and/or 'Innovace' may be necessary.

Aortic or mitral valve stenosis/hypertrophic cardiomyopathy

As with all vasodilators, ACE inhibitors should be given with caution in patients with left ventricular valvular and outflow tract obstruction and avoided in cases of cardiogenic shock and haemodynamically significant obstruction.

Renal function impairment

In cases of renal impairment (creatinine clearance <80 ml/min) the initial enalapril dosage should be adjusted according to the patient's creatinine clearance (see 4.2 'Posology and method of administration') and then as a function of the patient's response to treatment. Routine monitoring of potassium and creatinine are part of normal medical practice for these patients.

Renal failure has been reported in association with enalapril and has been mainly in patients with severe heart failure or underlying renal disease, including renal artery stenosis. If recognised promptly and treated appropriately, renal failure when associated with therapy with enalapril is usually reversible.

Some hypertensive patients, with no apparent pre-existing renal disease have developed increases in blood urea and creatinine when enalapril has been given concurrently with a diuretic. Dosage reduction of enalapril and/or discontinuation of the diuretic may be required. This situation should raise the possibility of underlying renal artery stenosis (see 4.4 'Special warnings and special precautions for use', *Renovascular hypertension*).

Renovascular hypertension

There is an increased risk of hypotension and renal insufficiency when patients with bilateral renal artery stenosis or stenosis of the artery to a single functioning kidney are treated with ACE inhibitors. Loss of renal function may occur with only mild changes in serum creatinine. In these patients, therapy should be initiated under close medical supervision with low doses, careful titration, and monitoring of renal function.

Kidney transplantation

There is no experience regarding the administration of 'Innovace' in patients with a recent kidney transplantation. Treatment with 'Innovace' is therefore not recommended.

Hepatic failure

Rarely, ACE inhibitors have been associated with a syndrome that starts with cholestatic jaundice and progresses to fulminant hepatic necrosis and (sometimes) death. The mechanism of this syndrome is not understood. Patients receiving ACE inhibitors who develop jaundice or marked elevations of hepatic enzymes should discontinue the ACE inhibitor and receive appropriate medical follow-up.

Neutropenia/Agranulocytosis

Neutropenia/agranulocytosis, thrombocytopenia and anaemia have been reported in patients receiving ACE inhibitors. In patients with normal renal function and no other complicating factors, neutropenia occurs rarely. Enalapril should be used with extreme caution in patients with collagen vascular disease, immunosuppressant therapy, treatment with allopurinol or procainamide, or a combination of these complicating factors, especially if there is pre-existing impaired renal function. Some of these patients developed serious infections which in a few instances did not respond to intensive antibiotic therapy. If enalapril is used in such patients, periodic monitoring of white blood cell counts is advised and patients should be instructed to report any sign of infection.

Hypersensitivity/Angioneurotic oedema

Angioneurotic oedema of the face, extremities, lips, tongue, glottis and/or larynx has been reported in patients treated with angiotensin-converting enzyme inhibitors, including 'Innovace'. This may occur at any time during treatment. In such cases, 'Innovace' should be discontinued promptly and appropriate monitoring should be instituted to ensure complete resolution of symptoms prior to dismissing the patient. In those instances where swelling has been confined to the face and lips the condition generally resolved without treatment, although antihistamines have been useful in relieving symptoms.

Angioneurotic oedema associated with laryngeal oedema may be fatal. Where there is involvement of the tongue, glottis or larynx, likely to cause airway obstruction, appropriate therapy, which may include subcutaneous epinephrine solution 1:1000 (0.3 ml to 0.5 ml) and/or measures to ensure a patent airway, should be administered promptly.

Black patients receiving ACE inhibitors have been reported to have a higher incidence of angioedema compared to non-blacks.

Patients with a history of angioedema unrelated to ACE-inhibitor therapy may be at increased risk of angioedema while receiving an ACE inhibitor. (Also see 4.3 'Contra-indications').

Anaphylactoid reactions during hymenoptera desensitisation

Rarely, patients receiving ACE inhibitors during desensitisation with hymenoptera venom have experienced life-threatening anaphylactoid reactions. These reactions were avoided by temporarily withholding ACE-inhibitor therapy prior to each desensitisation.

Anaphylactoid reactions during LDL Apheresis

Rarely, patients receiving ACE inhibitors during low density lipoprotein LDL apheresis with dextran sulfate have experienced life-threatening anaphylactoid reactions. These reactions were avoided by temporarily withholding ACE-inhibitor therapy prior to each apheresis.

Haemodialysis patients

Anaphylactoid reactions have been reported in patients dialysed with high-flux membranes (e.g. AN 69) and treated concomitantly with an ACE inhibitor. In these patients, consideration should be given to using a different type of dialysis membrane or a different class of antihypertensive agent.

Diabetic patients

In diabetic patients treated with oral antidiabetic agents or insulin, glycaemic control should be closely monitored during the first month of treatment with an ACE inhibitor. (See 4.5 'Interaction with other medicinal products and other forms of interaction', *Antidiabetics*.)

Cough

Cough has been reported with the use of ACE inhibitors. Characteristically, the cough is non-productive, persistent and resolves after discontinuation of therapy. ACE inhibitor-induced cough should be considered as part of the differential diagnosis of cough.

Surgery/Anaesthesia

In patients undergoing major surgery or during anaesthesia with agents that produce hypotension, enalapril blocks angiotensin II formation secondary to compensatory renin release. If hypotension occurs and is considered to be due to this mechanism, it can be corrected by volume expansion.

Hyperkalaemia

Elevations in serum potassium have been observed in some patients treated with ACE inhibitors, including enalapril. Patients at risk for the development of hyperkalaemia include those with renal insufficiency, diabetes mellitus, or those using concomitant potassium-sparing diuretics, potassium supplements or potassium-containing salt substitutes; or those patients taking other drugs associated with increases in serum potassium, (e.g. heparin). If concomitant use of the above mentioned agents is deemed appropriate, regular monitoring of serum potassium is recommended.

Lithium

The combination of lithium and enalapril is generally not recommended (see 4.5 'Interaction with other medicinal products and other forms of interaction').

Lactose

'Innovace' contains less than 200 mg of lactose per tablet.

Paediatric use

There is limited efficacy and safety experience in hypertensive children >6 years old, but no experience in other indications. Limited pharmacokinetic data are available in children above 2 months of age. (Also see 4.2 'Posology and method of administration', 5.1 'Pharmacodynamic properties', and 5.2 'Pharmacokinetic properties'.) 'Innovace' is not recommended in children in other indications than hypertension.

'Innovace' is not recommended in neonates and in paediatric patients with glomerular filtration rate <30 ml/min/1.73 m^2, as no data are available. (See 4.2 'Posology and method of administration'.)

Pregnancy and lactation

Enalapril should not be used during the first trimester of pregnancy. 'Innovace' is contra-indicated in the second and third trimesters of pregnancy (see 4.3 'Contra-indications'). When pregnancy is detected, enalapril treatment should be discontinued as soon as possible (see 4.6 'Pregnancy and lactation').

Use of enalapril is not recommended during breast feeding.

Ethnic differences

As with other angiotensin-converting enzyme inhibitors, enalapril is apparently less effective in lowering blood pressure in black people than in non-blacks, possibly because of a higher prevalence of low-renin states in the black hypertensive population.

4.5 Interaction with other medicinal products and other forms of Interaction

Potassium-sparing diuretics or potassium supplements

ACE inhibitors attenuate diuretic-induced potassium loss. Potassium-sparing diuretics (e.g. spironolactone, triamterene or amiloride), potassium supplements, or potassium-containing salt substitutes may lead to significant increases in serum potassium. If concomitant use is indicated because of demonstrated hypokalaemia they should be used with caution and with frequent monitoring of serum potassium (see 4.4 'Special warnings and special precautions for use').

Diuretics (thiazide or loop diuretics)

Prior treatment with high dose diuretics may result in volume depletion and a risk of hypotension when initiating therapy with enalapril (see 4.4 'Special warnings and special precautions for use'). The hypotensive effects can be reduced by discontinuation of the diuretic, by increasing volume or salt intake or by initiating therapy with a low dose of enalapril.

Other antihypertensive agents

Concomitant use of these agents may increase the hypotensive effects of enalapril. Concomitant use with nitroglycerine and other nitrates, or other vasodilators, may further reduce blood pressure.

Lithium

Reversible increases in serum lithium concentrations and toxicity have been reported during concomitant administration of lithium with ACE inhibitors. Concomitant use of thiazide diuretics may further increase lithium levels and enhance the risk of lithium toxicity with ACE inhibitors. Use of enalapril with lithium is not recommended, but if the combination proves necessary, careful monitoring of serum lithium levels should be performed (see 4.4 'Special warnings and special precautions for use').

Tricyclic antidepressants/Antipsychotics/Anaesthetics/Narcotics

Concomitant use of certain anaesthetic medicinal products, tricyclic antidepressants and antipsychotics with ACE inhibitors may result in further reduction of blood pressure (see 4.4 'Special warnings and special precautions for use').

Non-Steroidal Anti-Inflammatory Drugs (NSAIDs)

Chronic administration of NSAIDs may reduce the antihypertensive effect of an ACE inhibitor.

NSAIDs and ACE inhibitors exert an additive effect on the increase in serum potassium, and may result in a deterioration of renal function. These effects are usually reversible. Rarely, acute renal failure may occur, especially in patients with compromised renal function such as the elderly or dehydrated.

Sympathomimetics

Sympathomimetics may reduce the antihypertensive effects of ACE inhibitors.

Antidiabetics

Epidemiological studies have suggested that concomitant administration of ACE inhibitors and antidiabetic medicines (insulins, oral hypoglycaemic agents) may cause an increased blood-glucose-lowering effect with risk of hypoglycaemia. This phenomenon appeared to be more likely to occur during the first weeks of combined treatment and in patients with renal impairment.

Alcohol

Alcohol enhances the hypotensive effect of ACE inhibitors.

Acetyl salicylic acid, thrombolytics and β-blockers

Enalapril can be safely administered concomitantly with acetyl salicylic acid (at cardiologic doses), thrombolytics and β-blockers.

4.6 Pregnancy and lactation

Pregnancy

Enalapril should not be used during the first trimester of pregnancy. When a pregnancy is planned or confirmed the switch to an alternative treatment should be initiated as soon as possible. Controlled studies with ACE inhibitors have not been done in humans, but a limited number of cases with first trimester exposure have not appeared to manifest malformations consistent with human foetotoxicity as described below.

Enalapril is contra-indicated during the second and third trimesters of pregnancy.

Prolonged enalapril exposure during the second and third trimesters is known to induce human foetotoxicity (decreased renal function, oligohydramnios, skull ossification retardation) and neonatal toxicity (renal failure, hypotension, hyperkalaemia). (See also 5.3 'Preclinical safety data').

Should exposure to enalapril have occurred from the second trimester of pregnancy, ultrasound check of renal function and skull is recommended.

Infants whose mothers have taken 'Innovace' should be closely observed for hypotension, oliguria and hyperkalaemia. Enalapril, which crosses the placenta, has been removed from the neonatal circulation by peritoneal dialysis with some clinical benefit, and theoretically may be removed by exchange transfusion.

Lactation

Enalapril and enalaprilat are excreted in breast milk, but their effect on the nursing infant has not been determined. Consequently, use of enalapril is not recommended if breast feeding.

4.7 Effects on ability to drive and use machines

When driving vehicles or operating machines it should be taken into account that occasionally dizziness or weariness may occur.

4.8 Undesirable effects

Undesirable effects reported for enalapril include:

[Very common >1/10); Common >1/100, <1/10); Uncommon >1/1,000), <1/100); Rare >1/10,000, <1/1,000); Very rare (<1/10,000), including isolated reports.]

Blood and the lymphatic system disorders:

Uncommon: anaemia (including aplastic and haemolytic).

Rare: neutropenia, decreases in haemoglobin, decreases in haematocrit, thrombocytopenia, agranulocytosis, bone marrow depression, pancytopenia, lymphadenopathy, autoimmune diseases.

Metabolism and nutrition disorders:

Uncommon: hypoglycaemia (see 4.4 'Special warnings and special precautions for use,' *Diabetic patients*).

Nervous system and psychiatric disorders:

Common: headache, depression.

Uncommon: confusion, somnolence, insomnia, nervousness, paraesthesia, vertigo

Rare: dream abnormality, sleep disorders.

Eye disorders:

Very common: blurred vision.

Cardiac and vascular disorders:

Very common: dizziness.

Common: hypotension (including orthostatic hypotension), syncope, myocardial infarction or cerebrovascular accident, possibly secondary to excessive hypotension in high-risk patients (see 4.4 'Special warnings and special precautions for use'), chest pain, rhythm disturbances, angina pectoris, tachycardia.

Uncommon: orthostatic hypotension, palpitations.

Rare: Raynaud's phenomenon.

Respiratory, thoracic and mediastinal disorders:

Very common: cough.

Common: dyspnoea.

Uncommon: rhinorrhoea, sore throat and hoarseness, bronchospasm/asthma.

Rare: pulmonary infiltrates, rhinitis, allergic alveolitis/eosinophilic pneumonia.

Gastro-intestinal disorders:

Very common: nausea.

Common: diarrhoea, abdominal pain, taste alteration.

Uncommon: ileus, pancreatitis, vomiting, dyspepsia, constipation, anorexia, gastric irritations, dry mouth, peptic ulcer.

Rare: stomatitis/aphthous ulcerations, glossitis.

Very rare: intestinal angioedema

Hepatobiliary disorders:

Rare: hepatic failure, hepatitis – either hepatocellular or cholestatic, hepatitis including necrosis, cholestasis (including jaundice).

Skin and subcutaneous tissue disorders:

Common: rash, hypersensitivity/angioneurotic oedema: angioneurotic oedema of the face, extremities, lips, tongue, glottis and/or larynx has been reported (see 4.4 'Special warnings and special precautions for use').

Uncommon: diaphoresis, pruritus, urticaria, alopecia.

Rare: erythema multiforme, Stevens-Johnson syndrome, exfoliative dermatitis, toxic epidermal necrolysis, pemphigus, erythroderma.

A symptom complex has been reported which may include some or all of the following: fever, serositis, vasculitis, myalgia/myositis, arthralgia/arthritis, a positive ANA, elevated ESR, eosinophilia, and leukocytosis. Rash, photosensitivity or other dermatologic manifestations may occur.

Renal and urinary disorders:

Uncommon: renal dysfunction, renal failure, proteinuria.

Rare: oliguria.

Reproductive system and breast disorders:

Uncommon: impotence.

Rare: gynecomastia.

General disorders and administration site conditions:

Very common: asthenia.

Common: fatigue.

Uncommon: muscle cramps, flushing, tinnitus, malaise, fever.

Investigations:

Common: hyperkalaemia, increases in serum creatinine.

Uncommon: increases in blood urea, hyponatraemia.

Rare: elevations of liver enzymes, elevations of serum bilirubin.

4.9 Overdose

Limited data are available for overdosage in humans. The most prominent features of overdosage reported to date are marked hypotension, beginning some six hours after ingestion of tablets, concomitant with blockade of the renin-angiotensin system, and stupor. Symptoms associated with overdosage of ACE inhibitors may include circulatory shock, electrolyte disturbances, renal failure, hyperventilation, tachycardia, palpitations, bradycardia, dizziness, anxiety, and cough. Serum enalaprilat levels 100- and 200-fold higher than usually seen after therapeutic doses have been reported after ingestion of 300 mg and 440 mg of enalapril, respectively.

The recommended treatment of overdosage is intravenous infusion of normal saline solution. If hypotension occurs, the patient should be placed in the shock position. If available, treatment with angiotensin II infusion and/or intravenous catecholamines may also be considered. If ingestion is recent, take measures aimed at eliminating enalapril maleate (e.g. emesis, gastric lavage, administration of absorbents, and sodium sulfate). Enalaprilat may be removed from the general circulation by haemodialysis. (See 4.4 'Special warnings and special precautions for use', *Haemodialysis patients*). Pacemaker therapy is indicated for therapy-resistant bradycardia. Vital signs, serum electrolytes and creatinine concentrations should be monitored continuously.

5. PHARMACOLOGICAL PROPERTIES

5.1 Pharmacodynamic properties

Pharmacotherapeutic group: Angiotensin-converting enzyme inhibitors, ATC Code: C09A A02

'Innovace' (enalapril maleate) is the maleate salt of enalapril, a derivative of two amino-acids, L-alanine and L-proline. Angiotensin converting enzyme (ACE) is a peptidyl dipeptidase which catalyses the conversion of angiotensin I to the pressor substance angiotensin II. After absorption, enalapril is hydrolysed to enalaprilat, which inhibits ACE. Inhibition of ACE results in decreased plasma angiotensin II, which leads to increased plasma renin activity (due to removal of negative feedback of renin release), and decreased aldosterone secretion.

ACE is identical to kininase II. Thus 'Innovace' may also block the degradation of bradykinin, a potent vasodepressor peptide. However, the role that this plays in the therapeutic effects of 'Innovace' remains to be elucidated.

While the mechanism through which 'Innovace' lowers blood pressure is believed to be primarily suppression of the renin-angiotensin-aldosterone system, 'Innovace' is antihypertensive even in patients with low-renin hypertension.

Administration of 'Innovace' to patients with hypertension results in a reduction of both supine and standing blood pressure without a significant increase in heart rate.

Symptomatic postural hypotension is infrequent. In some patients the development of optimal blood pressure reduction may require several weeks of therapy. Abrupt withdrawal of 'Innovace' has not been associated with rapid increase in blood pressure.

Effective inhibition of ACE activity usually occurs 2 to 4 hours after oral administration of an individual dose of enalapril. Onset of antihypertensive activity was usually seen at one hour, with peak reduction of blood pressure achieved by 4 to 6 hours after administration. The duration of effect is dose-related. However, at recommended doses, antihypertensive and haemodynamic effects have been shown to be maintained for at least 24 hours.

In haemodynamic studies in patients with essential hypertension, blood pressure reduction was accompanied by a reduction in peripheral arterial resistance with an increase in cardiac output and little or no change in heart rate. Following administration of 'Innovace' there was an increase in renal blood flow; glomerular filtration rate was unchanged. There was no evidence of sodium or water retention. However, in patients with low pre-treatment glomerular filtration rates, the rates were usually increased.

In short-term clinical studies in diabetic and non-diabetic patients with renal disease, decreases in albuminuria and urinary excretion of IgG and total urinary protein were seen after the administration of enalapril.

When given together with thiazide-type diuretics, the blood pressure-lowering effects of 'Innovace' are at least additive. 'Innovace' may reduce or prevent the development of thiazide-induced hypokalaemia.

In patients with heart failure on therapy with digitalis and diuretics, treatment with oral or injection 'Innovace' was associated with decreases in peripheral resistance and blood pressure. Cardiac output increased, while heart rate (usually elevated in patients with heart failure) decreased. Pulmonary capillary wedge pressure was also reduced. Exercise tolerance and severity of heart failure, as measured by New York Heart Association criteria, improved. These actions continued during chronic therapy.

In patients with mild to moderate heart failure, enalapril retarded progressive cardiac dilatation/enlargement and failure, as evidenced by reduced left ventricular end diastolic and systolic volumes and improved ejection fraction.

A multicentre, randomised, double-blind, placebo-controlled trial (SOLVD Prevention trial) examined a population with asymptomatic left ventricular dysfunction (LVEF<35%). 4228 patients were randomised to receive either placebo (n=2117) or enalapril (n=2111). In the placebo group, 818 patients had heart failure or died (38.6%) as compared with 630 in the enalapril group (29.8%) (risk reduction: 29%; 95% CI; 21 - 36%; p<0.001). 518 patients in the placebo group (24.5%) and 434 in the enalapril group (20.6%) died or were hospitalised for new or worsening heart failure (risk reduction 20%; 95% CI; 9-30%; p<0.001).

A multicentre, randomised, double-blind, placebo-controlled trial (SOLVD treatment trial) examined a population with symptomatic congestive heart failure due to systolic dysfunction (ejection fraction <35%). 2569 patients receiving conventional treatment for heart failure were randomly assigned to receive either placebo (n=1284) or enalapril (n=1285). There were 510 deaths in the placebo group (39.7%) as compared with 452 in the enalapril group (35.2%) (reduction in risk, 16%; 95% CI, 5 - 26%; p=0.0036). There were 461 cardiovascular deaths in the placebo group as compared with 399 in the enalapril group (risk reduction 18%, 95% CI, 6 - 28%, p<0.002), mainly due to a decrease of deaths due to progressive heart failure (251 in the placebo group vs 209 in the enalapril group, risk reduction 22%, 95% CI, 6 - 35%). Fewer patients died or were hospitalised for worsening heart failure (736 in the placebo group and 613 in the enalapril group; risk reduction, 26%; 95% CI, 18 - 34%; p<0.0001). Overall in SOLVD study, in patients with left ventricular dysfunction, 'Innovace' reduced the risk of myocardial infarction by 23% (95% CI, 11 – 34%; p<0.001) and reduced the risk of hospitalisation for unstable angina pectoris by 20% (95% CI, 9 – 29%; p<0.001).

There is limited experience of the use in hypertensive paediatric patients >6 years. In a clinical study involving 110 hypertensive paediatric patients 6 to 16 years of age with a body weight ≥20 kg and a glomerular filtration rate >30 ml/min/1.73 m^2, patients who weighed <50 kg received either 0.625, 2.5 or 20 mg of enalapril daily and patients who weighed ≥50 kg received either 1.25, 5 or 40 mg of enalapril daily. Enalapril administration once daily lowered trough blood pressure in a dose-dependent manner. The dose-dependent antihypertensive efficacy of enalapril was consistent across all subgroups (age, Tanner stage, gender, race). However, the lowest doses studied, 0.625 mg and 1.25 mg, corresponding to an average of 0.02 mg/kg once daily, did not appear to offer consistent antihypertensive efficacy. The maximum dose studied was 0.58 mg/kg (up to 40 mg) once daily. The adverse experience profile for paediatric patients is not different from that seen in adult patients.

5.2 Pharmacokinetic properties

Absorption

Oral enalapril is rapidly absorbed, with peak serum concentrations of enalapril occurring within one hour. Based on urinary recovery, the extent of absorption of enalapril from oral enalapril tablet is approximately 60%. The absorption of oral enalapril is not influenced by the presence of food in the gastro-intestinal tract.

Following absorption, oral enalapril is rapidly and extensively hydrolysed to enalaprilat, a potent angiotensin-converting enzyme inhibitor. Peak serum concentrations of enalaprilat occur about 4 hours after an oral dose of enalapril tablet. The effective half-life for accumulation of enalaprilat following multiple doses of oral enalapril is 11 hours. In subjects with normal renal function, steady-state serum concentrations of enalaprilat were reached after 4 days of treatment.

Distribution

Over the range of concentrations which are therapeutically relevant, enalaprilat binding to human plasma proteins does not exceed 60%.

Biotransformation

Except for conversion to enalaprilat, there is no evidence for significant metabolism of enalapril.

Elimination

Excretion of enalaprilat is primarily renal. The principal components in urine are enalaprilat, accounting for about 40% of the dose, and intact enalapril (about 20%).

Renal impairment

The exposure of enalapril and enalaprilat is increased in patients with renal insufficiency. In patients with mild to moderate renal insufficiency (creatinine clearance 40-60 ml/min) steady state AUC of enalaprilat was approximately two-fold higher than in patients with normal renal function after administration of 5 mg once daily. In severe renal impairment (creatinine clearance ≤30 ml/min), AUC was increased approximately 8-fold. The effective half-life of enalaprilat following multiple doses of enalapril maleate is prolonged at this level of renal insufficiency and time to steady state is delayed. (See 4.2 'Posology and method of administration'). Enalaprilat may be removed from the general circulation by haemodialysis. The dialysis clearance is 62 ml/min.

Children and adolescents

A multiple dose pharmacokinetic study was conducted in 40 hypertensive male and female paediatric patients aged 2 months to ≤16 years following daily oral administration of 0.07 to 0.14 mg/kg enalapril maleate. There were no major differences in the pharmacokinetics of enalaprilat in children compared with historic data in adults. The data indicate an increase in AUC (normalised to dose per body weight) with increased age; however, an increase in AUC is not observed when data are normalised by body surface area. At steady state, the mean effective half-life for accumulation of enalaprilat was 14 hours.

5.3 Preclinical safety data

Preclinical data reveal no special hazard for humans based on conventional studies of safety pharmacology, repeated dose toxicity, genotoxicity and carcinogenic potential. Reproductive toxicity studies suggest that enalapril has no effects on fertility and reproductive performance in rats, and is not teratogenic. In a study in which female rats were dosed prior to mating through gestation, an increased incidence of rat pup deaths occurred during lactation. The compound has been shown to cross the placenta and is secreted in milk. Angiotensin-converting enzyme inhibitors, as a class, have been shown to be foetotoxic (causing injury and/or death to the foetus) when given in the second or third trimester.

6. PHARMACEUTICAL PARTICULARS

6.1 List of excipients

Lactose monohydrate

Magnesium stearate E572

Maize starch

Pregelatinised maize starch

Sodium bicarbonate E500

In addition the red 10 mg tablets contain red iron oxide E172 and the peach-coloured 20 mg tablets contain red iron oxide E172 and yellow iron oxide E172.

6.2 Incompatibilities

Not applicable

6.3 Shelf life

2.5 mg, 5 mg, and 10 mg: 3 years

20 mg: 2 years

6.4 Special precautions for storage

Do not store above 25°C. Store in the original package.

6.5 Nature and contents of container

'Innovace' tablets are available in aluminium foil blisters containing 28 tablets.

6.6 Instructions for use and handling

No special requirements

7. MARKETING AUTHORISATION HOLDER

Merck Sharp & Dohme Limited

Hertford Road, Hoddesdon, Hertfordshire, EN11 9BU, UK.

8. MARKETING AUTHORISATION NUMBER(S)

2.5 mg Tablet: PL0025/0220

5 mg Tablet: PL0025/0194

10 mg Tablet: PL0025/0195

20 mg Tablet: PL0025/0196

9. DATE OF FIRST AUTHORISATION/RENEWAL OF THE AUTHORISATION

2.5 mg tablets PL 0025/0220 first licensed 17 April 1986

2.5 mg tablets PL 0025/0220 last renewed 30 October 2003.

5 mg tablets PL 0025/0194 first licensed 6 December 1984.

5 mg tablets PL 0025/0194 last renewed 30 October 2003.

10 mg tablets PL 0025/0195 first licensed 6 December 1984

10 mg tablets PL 0025/0195 last renewed 30 October 2003.

20 mg tablets PL 0025/0196 first licensed 6 December 1984

20 mg tablets PL 0025/0196 last renewed 30 October 2003.

10. DATE OF REVISION OF THE TEXT

July 2004

® denotes registered trademark of Merck & Co., Inc., Whitehouse Station, NJ, USA.

Merck Sharp & Dohme Limited

Hertford Road, Hoddesdon, Hertfordshire, EN11 9BU, UK

SPC.RNT.04.UK.1062

Innozide Tablets

(Merck Sharp & Dohme Limited)

1. NAME OF THE MEDICINAL PRODUCT

INNOZIDE®

2. QUALITATIVE AND QUANTITATIVE COMPOSITION

Each tablet of 'Innozide' contains 20 mg enalapril maleate and 12.5 mg hydrochlorothiazide.

3. PHARMACEUTICAL FORM

'Innozide' is supplied as round, fluted, yellow tablets with 'MSD 718' on one side and scored on the other.

4. CLINICAL PARTICULARS

4.1 Therapeutic indications

'Innozide' is indicated for the treatment of mild to moderate hypertension in patients who have been stabilised on the individual components given in the same proportions.

4.2 Posology and method of administration

The dosage of 'Innozide' should be determined primarily by the experience with the enalapril maleate component.

Adults

Essential hypertension

The usual dosage is one tablet, taken once daily. If necessary, the dosage may be increased to two tablets, taken once daily.

Prior diuretic therapy: symptomatic hypotension may occur following the initial dose of 'Innozide'; this is more likely in patients who are volume and/or salt depleted as a result of prior diuretic therapy. The diuretic therapy should be discontinued for 2-3 days prior to initiation of therapy with 'Innozide'.

Dosage in renal insufficiency

Thiazides may not be appropriate diuretics for use in patients with renal impairment and are ineffective at creatinine clearance values of 30 ml/min or below (i.e. moderate or severe renal insufficiency).

In patients with creatinine clearance of >30 and <80 ml/min, 'Innozide' should be used only after titration of the individual components.

Use in the elderly

In clinical studies the efficacy and tolerability of enalapril maleate and hydrochlorothiazide, administered concomitantly, were similar in both elderly and younger hypertensive patients.

Paediatric use

Safety and effectiveness in children have not been established.

Route of administration: Oral.

4.3 Contraindications

'Innozide' is contra-indicated in patients with anuria.

'Innozide' is contra-indicated in patients who are hypersensitive to any component of this product and in patients with a history of angioneurotic oedema relating to previous treatment with an angiotensin-converting enzyme (ACE) inhibitor and in patients with hereditary or idiopathic angioedema.

'Innozide' is contra-indicated in patients who are hypersensitive to other sulphonamide-derived drugs.

'Innozide' is contra-indicated in patients with stenosis of the renal arteries.

'Innozide' is contra-indicated in pregnancy and lactation (see section 4.6 'Pregnancy and lactation').

4.4 Special warnings and special precautions for use

Hypotension and electrolyte/fluid imbalance: as with all antihypertensive therapy, symptomatic hypotension may occur in some patients. This was rarely seen in uncomplicated hypertensive patients but is more likely in the presence of fluid or electrolyte imbalance, e.g. volume depletion, hyponatraemia, hypochloraemic alkalosis, hypomagnesaemia or hypokalaemia which may occur from prior diuretic therapy, dietary salt restriction, dialysis, or during intercurrent diarrhoea or vomiting. Periodic determination of serum electrolytes should be performed at appropriate intervals in such patients.

Particular consideration should be given when therapy is administered to patients with ischaemic heart or cerebrovascular disease because an excessive fall in blood pressure could result in a myocardial infarction or cerebrovascular accident.

If hypotension occurs, the patient should be placed in the supine position and, if necessary, should receive an intravenous infusion of normal saline. A transient hypotensive response is not a contra-indication to further doses. Following restoration of effective blood volume and pressure, reinstitution of therapy at reduced dosage may be possible; or either of the components may be used appropriately alone.

Aortic stenosis/hypertrophic cardiomyopathy: As with all vasodilators, ACE inhibitors should be given with caution to patients with obstruction in the outflow tract of the left ventricle.

Kalaemia modifications: the combination of enalapril and a low-dose diuretic cannot exclude the possibility of hyperkalaemia to occur.

Renal function impairment: thiazides may not be appropriate diuretics for use in patients with renal impairment and are ineffective at creatinine clearance values of 30 ml/min or below (i.e. moderate or severe renal insufficiency).

'Innozide' should not be administered to patients with renal insufficiency (creatinine clearance ≤80 ml/min) until titration of the individual components has shown the need for the doses present in the combination tablet.

Some hypertensive patients with no apparent pre-existing renal disease have developed usually minor and transient increases in blood urea and serum creatinine when enalapril maleate has been given concomitantly with a diuretic. If this occurs during therapy with 'Innozide', the combination should be discontinued. Reinstitution of therapy at reduced dosage may be possible, or either of the components may be used appropriately alone.

In some patients, with bilateral renal artery stenosis or stenosis in the artery to a solitary kidney, increases in blood urea and serum creatinine, reversible upon discontinuation of therapy, have been seen with angiotensin-converting enzyme (ACE) inhibitors (see section 4.3 'Contra-indications').

Haemodialysis patients: a high incidence of anaphylactoid reactions, facial swelling, flushing, hypotension and dyspnoea, has been reported in patients dialysed with high-flux membranes and treated concomitantly with an ACE inhibitor. This combination should therefore be avoided. It is recommended that an alternative membrane or an alternative antihypertensive medicine be used.

Anaphylactic reactions during LDL apheresis: rarely, patients receiving ACE inhibitors during low-density lipoprotein (LDL) apheresis with dextran sulphate have experienced life-threatening anaphylactoid reactions. These reactions were avoided by temporarily withholding ACE-inhibitor therapy prior to each apheresis.

Hepatic disease: thiazides should be used with caution in patients with impaired hepatic function or progressive liver disease, since minor alterations of fluid and electrolyte balance may precipitate hepatic coma.

Surgery/anaesthesia: in patients undergoing major surgery or during anaesthesia with agents that produce hypotension, enalaprilat blocks angiotensin-II formation secondary to compensatory renin release. If hypotension occurs and is considered to be due to this mechanism, it can be corrected by volume expansion.

Metabolic and endocrine effects: thiazide therapy may impair glucose tolerance. Dosage adjustment of antidiabetic agents, including insulin, may be required.

Thiazides may decrease urinary calcium excretion and may cause intermittent and slight elevation of serum calcium. Marked hypercalcaemia may be evidence of hidden hyperparathyroidism. Thiazides should be discontinued before carrying out tests for parathyroid function.

Increases in cholesterol and triglyceride levels may be associated with thiazide diuretic therapy; however, at the 12.5 mg dose contained in 'Innozide', minimal or no effect was reported.

Thiazide therapy may precipitate hyperuricaemia and/or gout in certain patients. However, enalapril may increase urinary uric acid and thus may attenuate the hyperuricaemic effect of hydrochlorothiazide.

Hypersensitivity/angioneurotic oedema: angioneurotic oedema of the face, extremities, lips, tongue, glottis and/or larynx has been reported rarely in patients treated with angiotensin-converting enzyme inhibitors, including enalapril maleate. This may occur at any time during treatment. In such cases, enalapril maleate should be discontinued promptly and appropriate monitoring should be carried out to ensure complete resolution of symptoms before discharging the patient.

In those instances where swelling has been confined to the face and lips the condition generally resolved without treatment, although antihistamines have been useful in relieving symptoms.

Angioneurotic oedema associated with laryngeal oedema may be fatal. Where there is involvement of the tongue, glottis or larynx, likely to cause airway obstruction, appropriate therapy which may include subcutaneous adrenaline solution 1:1000 (0.3 ml to 0.5 ml) and/or measures to ensure a patent airway, should be administered promptly.

Black patients receiving ACE inhibitors have been reported to have a higher incidence of angioedema compared to patients of other racial origin.

Patients with a history of angioneurotic oedema unrelated to ACE-inhibitor therapy may be at increased risk of angioneurotic oedema while receiving an ACE inhibitor. (See also: section 4.3 'Contra-indications').

In patients receiving thiazides, sensitivity reactions may occur with or without a history of allergy or bronchial asthma. Exacerbation or activation of systemic lupus erythematosus has been reported with the use of thiazides.

Anaphylactoid reactions during Hymenoptera desensitisation: rarely, patients receiving ACE inhibitors during desensitisation with hymenoptera venom (e.g. Bee or Wasp venom) have experienced life-threatening anaphylactoid reactions. These reactions were avoided by temporarily withholding ACE-inhibitor therapy prior to each desensitisation.

Cough: cough has been reported with the use of ACE inhibitors. Characteristically, the cough is non-productive, persistent and resolves after discontinuation of therapy. ACE-inhibitor-induced cough should be considered as part of the differential diagnosis of cough.

4.5 Interaction with other medicinal products and other forms of Interaction

Serum potassium:

The potassium-losing effect of thiazide diuretics is usually attenuated by the effect of enalapril maleate. Serum potassium usually remains within normal limits, although in clinical trials with enalapril maleate hyperkalaemia did occur in a few cases.

The use of potassium supplements, potassium-sparing agents or potassium-containing salt substitutes, particularly in patients with impaired renal function, may lead to a significant increase in serum potassium. If concomitant use of 'Innozide' and any of these agents is deemed appropriate, they should be used with caution and with frequent monitoring of serum potassium.

Lithium:

Diuretic agents and ACE-Inhibitors reduce the renal clearance of lithium and add a high risk of lithium toxicity; concomitant use is not recommended. Refer to the prescribing information for lithium preparations before use of such preparations.

Non-depolarising muscle relaxants:

Thiazides may increase the responsiveness to tubocurarine.

Narcotic drugs/antispsychotics:

Postural hypotension may occur with ACE inhibitors. Concomitant administration of thiazide diuretics with barbiturates, narcotics or phenothiazine may result in potentiation of orthostatic hypotension.

Antihypertensive agents:

The combination of enalapril maleate with beta-adrenergic blocking agents, methyldopa, or calcium entry blockers has been shown to improve the efficacy of lowering the blood pressure.

Ganglionic-blocking agents or adrenergic-blocking agents, combined with enalapril, should only be administered under careful observation of the patient.

Allopurinol, cytostatic or immunosuppressive agents, systemic corticosteroids or procainamide:

Concomitant administration with ACE inhibitors may lead to an increased risk for leucopenia.

Corticosteroids, ACTH: may result in intensified electrolyte depletion, particularly hypokalaemia with thiazide diuretics.

Cyclosporin: increase the risk of hyperkalaemia with ACE inhibitors.

Non-steroidal anti-inflammatory drugs:

The administration of a non-steroidal anti-inflammatory agent may reduce the antihypertensive effect of an ACE inhibitor. However, in a clinical pharmacology study, indomethacin or sulindac was administered to hypertensive patients receiving 'Innovace' and there was no evidence of a blunting of the antihypertensive action of 'Innovace'. Furthermore, it has been described that NSAIDS and ACE inhibitors exert an additive effect on the increase in serum potassium., whereas renal function may decrease. These effects are in principle reversible, and occur especially in patients with compromised renal function.

In some patients, the administration of NSAIDS can reduce the diuretic, natriuretic, and antihypertensive effects of diuretics.

Antacids: induce decreased bioavailability of ACE inhibitors.

Sympathomimetics: may reduce the antihypertensive effects of ACE inhibitors; patients should be carefully monitored to confirm that the desired effect is being obtained.

Alcohol:

Alcohol enhances the hypotensive effect with ACE inhibitors. Alcohol may interact with thiazide diuretic to produce potentiation of orthostatic hypotension.

Antidiabetic drugs (oral hypoglycaemic agents and insulin):

Epidemiological studies have suggested that concomitant administration of ACE inhibitors and antidiabetic medicines may cause an increased blood-glucose-lowering effect with risk of hypoglycaemia. This phenomenon appeared to be more likely to occur during the first weeks of combined treatment and in patients with renal impairment. Long-term controlled clinical trials with enalapril have not confirmed these findings and do not preclude the use of enalapril in diabetic patients. It is advised, however, that these patients be monitored

The use of antidiabetic drugs and thiazide diuretics may require dosage adjustment of the antidiabetic drug.

Cholestyramine and colestipol resins:

Absorption of hydrochlorothiazide is impaired in the presence of anionic exchange resins. Single doses of either cholestyramine or colestipol resins bind the hydrochlorothiazide and reduce its absorption from the gastrointestinal tract by up to 85 and 43 percent respectively.

Pressor amines (e.g. adrenaline): possible decreased response to pressor amines but not sufficient to preclude their use.

4.6 Pregnancy and lactation

'Innozide' is contra-indicated in pregnancy. ACE inhibitors have been shown to be fetotoxic in rabbits during middle and late pregnancy. Effects of exposure of the foetus to ACE inhibitors during the first trimester of human pregnancy are unknown. Foetal exposure during the second and third trimesters of pregnancy has been associated with foetal and neonatal morbidity and mortality. ACE inhibitors in human pregnancy have been associated with oligohydramnios. Hypotension and renal failure have occurred in the new-born.

Breast-feeding mothers: Enalapril, enalaprilat and thiazides appear in human milk. If use of 'Innozide' is deemed essential, breast-feeding should stop.

4.7 Effects on ability to drive and use machines

There are no data to suggest that 'Innozide' affects the ability to drive or use machines. When driving vehicles or operating machines it should be taken into account that occasionally dizziness or weariness may occur.

4.8 Undesirable effects

'Innozide' is usually well tolerated. In clinical studies, side effects have usually been mild and transient, and in most instances have not required interruption of therapy.

The most common clinical side effects were dizziness and fatigue, which generally responded to dosage reduction and seldom required discontinuation of therapy.

Other side effects (1-2%) were: muscle cramps, nausea, asthenia, orthostatic effects including hypotension, headache, cough, and impotence.

Less common side effects which occurred either during controlled trials or during marketed use include:

Cardiovascular: syncope, non-orthostatic hypotension, palpitation, tachycardia, chest pain.

Gastro-intestinal: pancreatitis, diarrhoea, vomiting, dyspepsia, abdominal pain, flatulence, constipation.

Nervous system/psychiatric: insomnia, somnolence, paraesthesia, vertigo, nervousness.

Respiratory: dyspnoea.

Skin: Stevens-Johnson syndrome, rash, pruritus, diaphoresis.

Other: renal dysfunction, renal failure, decreased libido, dry mouth, gout, tinnitus, arthralgia.

A symptom complex has been reported which may include some or all of the following: fever, serositis, vasculitis, myalgia/myositis, arthralgia/arthritis, a positive ANA, elevated ESR, eosinophilia and leucocytosis. Rash, photosensitivity or other dermatological manifestations may occur.

Hypersensitivity/angioneurotic oedema: Angioneurotic oedema of the face, extremities, lips, tongue, glottis and/or larynx has been reported rarely (see section 4.4 'Special warnings and precautions for use'). In very rare cases intestinal angioedema has been reported with angiotensin-converting enzyme inhibitors including enalapril.

Side effects due to individual components

Additional side effects that have been seen with one of the individual components and may be potential side effects with 'Innozide' are the following:

Enalapril maleate: Ileus, hepatic failure, hepatitis - either hepatocellular or cholestatic, jaundice, depression, confusion, dream abnormality, pulmonary infiltrates, bronchospasm/asthma, sore throat and hoarseness, rhythm disturbances, angina pectoris, myocardial infarction or cerebrovascular accident, possibly secondary to excessive hypotension in high-risk patients, Raynaud's phenomenon, rhinorrhoea, photosensitivity, alopecia, flushing, taste alteration, anorexia, blurred vision, urticaria, stomatitis, glossitis, oliguria, toxic epidermal necrolysis, erythema multiforme, exfoliative dermatitis, pemphigus.

Hydrochlorothiazide: Anorexia, gastric irritation, jaundice (intrahepatic cholestatic jaundice), sialoadenitis, xanthopsia, leucopenia, agranulocytosis, thrombocytopenia, aplastic anaemia, haemolytic anaemia, purpura, photosensitivity, fever, urticaria, necrotising angiitis (vasculitis), respiratory distress (including pneumonitis and pulmonary oedema), interstitial nephritis, anaphylactic reaction, toxic epidermal necrolysis, glycosuria, electrolyte imbalance including hyponatraemia, restlessness, muscle spasm, transient blurred vision.

Laboratory test findings: Clinically important changes in standard laboratory parameters were rarely associated with administration of 'Innozide'. Occasional hyperglycaemia, hyperuricaemia and hyper- or hypokalaemia have been noted. Increases in blood urea and serum creatinine, and elevations of liver enzymes and/or serum bilirubin have been seen. Decreases in haemoglobin and haematocrit have been reported in hypertensive patients treated with 'Innozide'. These are usually reversible upon discontinuation of 'Innozide'.

Decreases in platelets and white-cell count, and rare cases of neutropenia, thrombocytopenia and bone-marrow depression have been reported, but a causal relationship to 'Innozide' has not been established.

Hyponatraemia has occurred with enalapril and may be a potential finding with 'Innozide'.

4.9 Overdose

No specific information is available on the treatment of overdosage with 'Innozide'. Treatment is symptomatic and supportive. Therapy with 'Innozide' should be discontinued and the patient observed closely. Suggested measures include induction of emesis and/or gastric lavage, and correction of dehydration, electrolyte imbalance and hypotension by established procedures.

Enalapril maleate

The most prominent feature of overdosage reported to date is marked hypotension, beginning some six hours after ingestion of tablets, concomitant with blockade of the renin-angiotensin-aldosterone system, and stupor. Serum enalaprilat levels 100 times and 200 times higher than usually seen after therapeutic doses have been reported after ingestion of 300 mg and 440 mg of enalapril maleate respectively.

The recommended treatment of overdosage is intravenous infusion of normal saline solution. If available angiotensin II infusion may be beneficial. Enalaprilat may be removed from the general circulation by haemodialysis (see section 4.4 'Special warnings and special precautions for use': haemodialysis patients).

Hydrochlorothiazide

The most common signs and symptoms observed are those caused by electrolyte depletion (hypokalaemia, hypochloraemia, hyponatraemia) and dehydration resulting from excessive diuresis. If digitalis has also been administered, hypokalaemia may accentuate cardiac arrhythmias.

5. PHARMACOLOGICAL PROPERTIES

5.1 Pharmacodynamic properties

Pharmacotherapeutic group: enalapril and diuretics, ATC code C09 BA02.

Enalapril maleate

Angiotensin-converting enzyme (ACE) is a peptidyl dipeptidase which catalyses the conversion of angiotensin I to the pressor substance angiotensin II. After absorption, enalapril is hydrolysed to enalaprilat, which inhibits ACE, which leads to increased plasma renin activity (due to removal of negative feedback on renin release), and decreased aldosterone secretion.

ACE is identical to kininase II. Thus enalapril may also block the degradation of bradykinin, a potential vasodepressor peptide. However, the role that this plays in the therapeutic effects of enalapril remains to be elucidated. While the mechanism through which enalapril lowers blood pressure is believed to be primarily suppression of the renin-angiotensin-aldosterone system, which plays a major role in the regulation of blood pressure, enalapril is antihypertensive even in patients with low-renin hypertension.

Enalapril maleate - hydrochlorothiazide

Hydrochlorothiazide is a diuretic and antihypertensive agent which increases plasma renin activity. Although enalapril alone is antihypertensive even in patients with low-renin hypertension, concomitant administration of hydrochlorothiazide in these patients leads to greater reduction of blood pressure.

5.2 Pharmacokinetic properties

Absorption

Oral enalapril maleate is rapidly absorbed, with peak serum concentrations of enalapril occurring within one hour. Based on urinary recovery, the extent of absorption of enalapril from oral enalapril maleate is approximately 60%. Following absorption, oral enalapril is rapidly and extensively hydrolysed to enalaprilat, a potent angiotensin-converting enzyme inhibitor. Peak serum concentrations of enalaprilat occur 3 to 4 hours after an oral dose of enalapril maleate. The principal components in urine are enalaprilat, accounting for about 40% of the dose, and intact enalapril. Except for conversion to enalaprilat, there is no evidence of significant metabolism of enalapril. The serum concentration profile of enalaprilat exhibits a prolonged terminal phase, apparently associated with binding to ACE. In subjects with normal renal function, steady state serum concentrations of enalaprilat were achieved by the fourth day of administration of enalapril maleate. The absorption of oral enalapril maleate is not influenced by the presence of food in the gastro-intestinal tract. The extent of absorption and hydrolysis of enalapril are similar for the various doses in the recommended therapeutic range.

Distribution

Studies in dogs indicate that enalapril crosses the blood-brain barrier poorly, if at all; enalaprilat does not enter the brain. Enalapril crosses the placental barrier. Hydrochlorothiazide crosses the placental but not the blood-brain barrier.

Biotransformation

Except for conversion to enalaprilat, there is no evidence for significant metabolism of enalapril. Hydrochlorothiazide is not metabolised but is eliminated rapidly by the kidney.

Elimination

Excretion of enalapril is primarily renal. The principal components in urine are enalaprilat, accounting for about 40%

of the dose, and intact enalapril. The effective half-life for accumulation of enalaprilat following multiple doses of oral enalapril maleate is 11 hours. When plasma levels of hydrochlorothiazide have been followed for at least 24 hours, the plasma half-life has been observed to vary between 5.6 and 14.8 hours. Hydrochlorothiazide is not metabolised but is eliminated rapidly by the kidney. At least 61% of the oral dose is eliminated unchanged within 24 hours.

Characteristics in patients

Enalaprilat may be removed from the general circulation by haemodialysis.

5.3 Preclinical safety data

No relevant information.

6. PHARMACEUTICAL PARTICULARS

6.1 List of excipients

Sodium hydrogen carbonate E500, lactose, maize starch, yellow ferric oxide E172, pregelatinised starch, and magnesium stearate E572.

6.2 Incompatibilities

None

6.3 Shelf life

36 months.

6.4 Special precautions for storage

Do not store above 25°C. Store in the original container.

6.5 Nature and contents of container

PVC/nylon/aluminium blister calendar packs containing 28 tablets.

6.6 Instructions for use and handling

None.

7. MARKETING AUTHORISATION HOLDER

Merck Sharp & Dohme Limited

Hertford Road, Hoddesdon, Hertfordshire EN11 9BU, UK

8. MARKETING AUTHORISATION NUMBER(S)

PL 0025/0249

9. DATE OF FIRST AUTHORISATION/RENEWAL OF THE AUTHORISATION

First authorised: 8 May 1991.

Last renewed: 10 November 1999.

10. DATE OF REVISION OF THE TEXT

Revision approved: April 2004.

SPC.CRN.03.UK.0973 F.T. 14 May 2004

Inspra 25mg & 50 mg film-coated tablets

(Pfizer Limited)

1. NAME OF THE MEDICINAL PRODUCT

INSPRA®▼ 25 mg film-coated tablets.

INSPRA®▼ 50 mg film-coated tablets.

2. QUALITATIVE AND QUANTITATIVE COMPOSITION

Each tablet contains 25 mg of eplerenone.

Each tablet contains 50 mg of eplerenone.

For excipients see section 6.1.

3. PHARMACEUTICAL FORM

Film-coated tablet.

25 mg tablet: yellow tablet with stylized "Pfizer" on one side of tablet, "NSR" over "25" on the other side of tablet.

50 mg tablet: yellow tablet with stylized "Pfizer" on one side of tablet, "NSR" over "50" on the other side of tablet.

4. CLINICAL PARTICULARS

4.1 Therapeutic indications

Eplerenone is indicated, in addition to standard therapy including beta-blockers, to reduce the risk of cardiovascular mortality and morbidity in stable patients with left ventricular dysfunction (LVEF ≤ 40 %) and clinical evidence of heart failure after recent myocardial infarction.

4.2 Posology and method of administration

For the individual adjustment of dose, the strengths of 25 mg and 50 mg are available.

The recommended maintenance dose of eplerenone is 50 mg once daily (OD). Treatment should be initiated at 25 mg once daily and titrated to the target dose of 50 mg once daily preferably within 4 weeks, taking into account the serum potassium level (see Table 1). Eplerenone therapy should usually be started within 3-14 days after an acute myocardial infarction.

Patients with a serum potassium of > 5.0 mmol/L should not be started on eplerenone (see section 4.3).

Serum potassium should be measured before initiating eplerenone therapy, within the first week and at one month after the start of treatment or dose adjustment. Serum potassium should be assessed as needed periodically thereafter.

After initiation, the dose should be adjusted based on the serum potassium level as shown in Table 1.

Table 1: Dose adjustment table after initiation

Serum potassium (mmol/L)	Action	Dose adjustment
< 5.0	Increase	25 mg EOD* to 25 mg OD 25 mg OD to 50 mg OD
5.0 - 5.4	Maintain	No dose adjustment
5.5 - 5.9	Decrease	50 mg OD to 25 mg OD 25 mg OD to 25 mg EOD* 25 mg EOD* to withhold
≥ 6.0	Withhold	N/A

* EOD: Every Other Day

Following withholding eplerenone due to serum potassium ≥ 6.0 mmol/L, eplerenone can be re-started at a dose of 25 mg every other day when potassium levels have fallen below 5.0 mmol/L.

Children and adolescents

There are no data to recommend the use of eplerenone in the paediatric population, and therefore, use in this age group is not recommended.

Elderly

No initial dose adjustment is required in the elderly. Due to an age-related decline in renal function, the risk of hyperkalaemia is increased in elderly patients. This risk may be further increased when co-morbidity associated with increased systemic exposure is also present, in particular mild-to-moderate hepatic impairment. Periodic monitoring of serum potassium is recommended (see section 4.4).

Renal impairment

No initial dose adjustment is required in patients with mild renal impairment. Periodic monitoring of serum potassium is recommended (see section 4.4).

Eplerenone is not dialysable.

Hepatic impairment

No initial dosage adjustment is necessary for patients with mild-to-moderate hepatic impairment. Due to an increased systemic exposure to eplerenone in patients with mild-to-moderate hepatic impairment, frequent and regular monitoring of serum potassium is recommended in these patients, especially when elderly (see section 4.4).

Concomitant treatment

In case of concomitant treatment with mild to moderate CYP3A4 inhibitors, e.g. amiodarone, diltiazem and verapamil, a starting dose of 25 mg OD may be initiated. Dosing should not exceed 25 mg OD (see section 4.5).

Eplerenone may be administered with or without food (see section 5.2).

4.3 Contraindications

- Hypersensitivity to eplerenone or any of the excipients (see section 6.1).
- Patients with serum potassium level > 5.0 mmol/L at initiation
- Patients with moderate to severe renal insufficiency (creatinine clearance < 50 mL/min)
- Patients with severe hepatic insufficiency (Child-Pugh Class C)
- Patients receiving potassium-sparing diuretics, potassium-supplements or strong inhibitors of CYP 3A4 (e.g. itraconazole, ketoconazole, ritonavir, nelfinavir, clarithromycin, telithromycin and nefazodone) (see section 4.5).

4.4 Special warnings and special precautions for use

Hyperkalaemia: Consistent with its mechanism of action, hyperkalaemia may occur with eplerenone. Serum potassium levels should be monitored in all patients at initiation of treatment and with a change in dosage. Thereafter, periodic monitoring is recommended especially in patients at risk for the development of hyperkalaemia, such as (elderly) patients with renal insufficiency (see section 4.2) and patients with diabetes. The use of potassium supplements after initiation of eplerenone therapy is not recommended, due to an increased risk of hyperkalaemia. Dose reduction of eplerenone has been shown to decrease serum potassium levels. In one study, the addition of hydrochlorothiazide to eplerenone therapy has been shown to offset increases in serum potassium.

Impaired renal function: Potassium levels should be monitored regularly in patients with impaired renal function, including diabetic microalbuminuria. The risk of hyperkalaemia increases with decreasing renal function. While the data from EPHESUS in patients with type 2 diabetes and microalbuminuria is limited, an increased occurrence of hyperkalaemia was observed in this small number of patients. Therefore, these patients should be treated with caution. Eplerenone is not removed by haemodialysis.

Impaired hepatic function: No elevations of serum potassium above 5.5 mmol/L were observed in patients with mild to moderate hepatic impairment (Child Pugh class A and B). Electrolyte levels should be monitored in patients with mild to moderate hepatic impairment. The use of eplerenone in patients with severe hepatic impairment has not been evaluated and its use is therefore contra-indicated (see section 4.3).

CYP3A4 inducers: Co-administration of eplerenone with strong CYP3A4 inducers is not recommended (see section 4.5).

Lithium, cyclosporin, tacrolimus should be avoided during treatment with eplerenone (see section 4.5).

Lactose: The tablets contain lactose and should not be administered in patients with rare hereditary problems of galactose intolerance, the Lapp lactase deficiency or glucose-galactose malabsorption.

4.5 Interaction with other medicinal products and other forms of Interaction

Pharmacodynamic interactions

Potassium-sparing diuretics and potassium supplements: Due to increased risk of hyperkalaemia, eplerenone should not be administered to patients receiving potassium-sparing diuretics and potassium supplements (see section 4.3). Potassium-sparing diuretics may potentiate the effect of anti-hypertensive agents and other diuretics.

Lithium: Drug interaction studies of eplerenone have not been conducted with lithium. However, lithium toxicity has been reported in patients receiving lithium concomitantly with diuretics and ACE inhibitors (see section 4.4). Co-administration of eplerenone and lithium should be avoided. If this combination appears necessary, lithium plasma concentrations should be monitored (see section 4.4).

Cyclosporin, tacrolimus: Cyclosporin and tacrolimus may lead to impaired renal function and increase the risk of hyperkalaemia. The concomitant use of eplerenone and cyclosporin or tacrolimus should be avoided. If needed, close monitoring of serum potassium and renal function are recommended when cyclosporin and tacrolimus are to be administered during treatment with eplerenone (see section 4.4).

Non-steroidal anti-inflammatory drugs (NSAIDs): Treatment with NSAIDs may lead to acute renal failure by acting directly on glomerular filtration, especially in at-risk patients (elderly and/or dehydrated patients). Patients receiving eplerenone and NSAIDs should be adequately hydrated and be monitored for renal function prior to initiating treatment.

Trimethoprim: The concomitant administration of trimethoprim with eplerenone increases the risk of hyperkalaemia. Monitoring of serum potassium and renal function should be made, particularly in patients with renal impairment and in the elderly.

ACE inhibitors, angiotensin-II receptors antagonists (AIIA): Eplerenone and ACE inhibitors or angiotensin-II receptors antagonists should be co-administered with caution. Combining eplerenone with these drugs may increase risk of hyperkalaemia in patients at risk for impaired renal function, eg the elderly. A close monitoring of serum potassium and renal function is recommended.

Alpha 1 blockers (eg prazosin, alfuzosine): When alpha-1-blockers are combined with eplerenone, there is the potential for increased hypotensive effect and/or postural hypotension. Clinical monitoring for postural hypotension is recommended during alpha-1-blocker co-administration.

Tricyclic anti-depressants, neuroleptics, amifostine, baclofene: Co-administration of these drugs with eplerenone may potentially increase antihypertensive effects and risk of postural hypotension.

Glucocorticoids, tetracosactide: Co-administration of these drugs with eplerenone may potentially decrease antihypertensive effects (sodium and fluid retention).

Pharmacokinetic interactions

In vitro studies indicate that eplerenone is not an inhibitor of CYP1A2, CYP2C19, CYP2C9, CYP2D6 or CYP3A4 isozymes. Eplerenone is not a substrate or an inhibitor of P-Glycoprotein.

Digoxin: Systemic exposure (AUC) to digoxin increases by 16% (90% CI: 4% - 30%) when co-administered with eplerenone. Caution is warranted when digoxin is dosed near the upper limit of therapeutic range.

Warfarin: No clinically significant pharmacokinetic interactions have been observed with warfarin. Caution is warranted when warfarin is dosed near the upper limit of therapeutic range.

CYP3A4 substrates: Results of pharmacokinetic studies with CYP3A4 probe-substrates, i.e. midazolam and cisapride, showed no significant pharmacokinetic interactions when these drugs were co-administered with eplerenone.

CYP3A4 inhibitors:

- Strong CYP3A4 inhibitors: Significant pharmacokinetic interactions may occur when eplerenone is co-acministered with drugs that inhibit the CYP3A4 enzyme. A strong inhibitor of CYP3A4 (ketoconazole 200 mg BID) led to a 441% increase in AUC of eplerenone (see section 4.3). The concomitant use of eplerenone with strong CYP3A4 inhibitors such as ketoconazole, itraconazole, ritonavir, nelfinavir, clarithromycin, telithromycin and nefazadone, is contra-indicated (see section 4.3).
- Mild to moderate CYP3A4 inhibitors: Co-administration with erythromycin, saquinavir, amiodarone, diltiazem,

verapamil, and fluconazole have led to significant pharmacokinetic interactions with rank order increases in AUC ranging from 98% to 187%. Eplerenone dosing should therefore not exceed 25 mg when mild to moderate inhibitors of CYP3A4 are co-administered with eplerenone (see section 4.2).

CYP3A4 inducers: Co-administration of St John's Wort (a strong CYP3A4 inducer) with eplerenone caused a 30 % decrease in eplerenone AUC. A more pronounced decrease in eplerenone AUC may occur with stronger CYP3A4 inducers such as rifampicin. Due to the risk of decreased eplerenone efficacy, the concomitant use of strong CYP3A4 inducers (rifampicin, carbamazepine, phenytoin, phenobarbital, St John's Wort) with eplerenone is not recommended (see section 4.4).

Antacids: Based on the results of a pharmacokinetic clinical study, no significant interaction is expected when antacids are co-administered with eplerenone.

4.6 Pregnancy and lactation
Pregnancy: There are no adequate data on the use of eplerenone in pregnant women. Animal studies did not indicate direct or indirect adverse effects with respect to pregnancy, embryofoetal development, parturition and postnatal development (see section 5.3). Caution should be exercised prescribing eplerenone to pregnant women.

Lactation: It is unknown if eplerenone is excreted in human breast milk after oral administration. However, preclinical data show that eplerenone and/or metabolites are present in rat breast milk and that rat pups exposed by this route developed normally. Because of the unknown potential for adverse effects on the breast fed infant, a decision should be made whether to discontinue breast-feeding or discontinue the drug, taking into account the importance of the drug to the mother.

4.7 Effects on ability to drive and use machines
No studies on the effect of eplerenone on the ability to drive or use machines have been performed. Eplerenone does not cause drowsiness or impairment of cognitive function but when driving vehicles or operating machines it should be taken into account that dizziness may occur during treatment.

4.8 Undesirable effects
In the eplerenone post-acute myocardial infarction heart failure efficacy and survival study (EPHESUS), the overall incidence of adverse events reported with eplerenone (78.9%) was similar to placebo (79.5%). The discontinuation rate due to adverse events in these studies was 4.4% for patients receiving eplerenone and for 4.3% patients receiving placebo.

Adverse events reported below are taken from EPHESUS and are those with suspected relationship to treatment and in excess of placebo, or are serious and significantly in excess of placebo. Adverse events are listed by body system and absolute frequency. Frequencies are defined as: common > 1/100, < 1/10; uncommon > 1/1000, < 1/100.

Blood and lymphatic system disorders
Uncommon: eosinophilia

Metabolism and nutrition disorders
Common: hyperkalaemia
Uncommon: dehydration, hypercholesterolaemia, hypertriglyceridaemia, hyponatraemia

Psychiatric disorders
Uncommon: insomnia

Nervous system disorders
Common: dizziness
Uncommon: headache

Cardiac disorders
Uncommon: atrial fibrillation, myocardial infarction, left cardiac failure

Vascular disorders
Common: hypotension
Uncommon: postural hypotension, arterial leg thrombosis

Respiratory, thoracic and mediastinal disorders
Uncommon: pharyngitis

Gastrointestinal disorders
Common: diarrhoea, nausea
Uncommon: flatulence, vomiting

Skin and subcutaneous tissue disorders
Uncommon: pruritus, increased sweating

Musculoskeletal and connective tissue disorders
Uncommon: back pain, leg cramps

Renal and urinary disorders
Common: abnormal renal function

General disorders and administration site conditions
Uncommon: asthenia, malaise

Investigations
Uncommon: increased BUN, creatinine increase

Infections and infestations
Uncommon: pyelonephritis

In EPHESUS, there were numerically more cases of stroke in the elderly group (≥ 75 years old). There was however no statistical significant difference between the occurrence of stroke in the eplerenone (30) vs placebo (22) groups.

4.9 Overdose
No cases of human overdosage with eplerenone have been reported. The most likely manifestation of human overdosage would be anticipated to be hypotension or hyperkalaemia. Eplerenone cannot be removed by haemodialysis. Eplerenone has been shown to bind extensively to charcoal. If symptomatic hypotension should occur, supportive treatment should be initiated. If hyperkalaemia develops, standard treatment should be initiated.

5. PHARMACOLOGICAL PROPERTIES

5.1 Pharmacodynamic properties
Pharmacotherapeutic group: aldosterone antagonists, ATC code: C03DA04

Eplerenone has relative selectivity in binding to recombinant human mineralocorticoid receptors compared to its binding to recombinant human glucocorticoid, progesterone and androgen receptors. Eplerenone prevents the binding of aldosterone, a key hormone in the renin-angiotensin-aldosterone-system (RAAS), which is involved in the regulation of blood pressure and the pathophysiology of cardiovascular disease.

Eplerenone has been shown to produce sustained increases in plasma renin and serum aldosterone, consistent with inhibition of the negative regulatory feedback of aldosterone on renin secretion. The resulting increased plasma renin activity and aldosterone circulating levels do not overcome the effects of eplerenone.

In dose-ranging studies of chronic heart failure (NYHA classification II-IV), the addition of eplerenone to standard therapy resulted in expected dose-dependent increases in aldosterone. Similarly, in a cardiorenal substudy of EPHESUS, therapy with eplerenone led to a significant increase in aldosterone. These results confirm the blockade of the mineralocorticoid receptor in these populations.

Eplerenone was studied in the eplerenone post-acute myocardial infarction heart failure efficacy and survival study (EPHESUS). EPHESUS was a double-blind, placebo-controlled study, of 3 year duration, in 6632 patients with acute myocardial infarction (MI), left ventricular dysfunction (as measured by left ventricular ejection fraction [LVEF] ≤40%), and clinical signs of heart failure. Within 3-14 days (median 7 days) after an acute MI, patients received eplerenone or placebo in addition to standard therapies at an initial dose of 25 mg once daily and titrated to the target dose of 50 mg once daily after 4 weeks if serum potassium was < 5.0 mmol/L. During the study patients received standard care including acetylsalicylic acid (92%), ACE inhibitors (90%), β-blockers (83%), nitrates (72%), loop diuretics (66%), or HMG CoA reductase inhibitors (60%).

In EPHESUS, the co-primary endpoints were all-cause mortality and the combined endpoint of CV death or CV hospitalisation; 14.4 % of patients assigned to eplerenone and 16.7 % of patients assigned to placebo died (all causes), while 26.7 % of patients assigned to eplerenone and 30.0 % assigned to placebo met the combined endpoint of CV death or hospitalisation. Thus, in EPHESUS, eplerenone reduced the risk of death from any cause by 15% (RR 0.85; 95% CI, 0.75-0.96; p= 0.008) compared to placebo, primarily by reducing cardiovascular (CV) mortality. The risk of CV death or CV hospitalisation was reduced by 13% with eplerenone (RR 0.87; 95% CI, 0.79-0.95; p=0.002). The absolute risk reductions for the endpoints of all cause mortality and CV mortality/hospitalisation were 2.3 and 3.3%, respectively. Clinical efficacy was primarily demonstrated when eplerenone therapy was initiated in patients aged < 75 years old. The benefits of therapy in those patients over the age of 75 are unclear. NYHA functional classification improved or remained stable for a statistically significantly greater proportion of patients receiving eplerenone compared to placebo. The incidence of hyperkalaemia was 3.4 % in the eplerenone group vs 2.0 % in the placebo group ($p < 0.001$). The incidence of hypokalaemia was 0.5 % in the eplerenone group vs 1.5 % in the placebo group ($p < 0.001$).

No consistent effects of eplerenone on heart rate, QRS duration, or PR or QT interval were observed in 147 normal subjects evaluated for electrocardiographic changes during pharmacokinetic studies.

5.2 Pharmacokinetic properties
Absorption and Distribution:

The absolute bioavailability of eplerenone is unknown. Maximum plasma concentrations are reached after about 2 hours. Both peak plasma levels (C_{max}) and area under the curve (AUC) are dose proportional for doses of 10 to 100 mg and less than proportional at doses above 100 mg. Steady state is reached within 2 days. Absorption is not affected by food.

The plasma protein binding of eplerenone is about 50% and is primarily bound to alpha 1-acid glycoproteins. The apparent volume of distribution at steady state is estimated at 50 (±7) L. Eplerenone does not preferentially bind to red blood cells.

Metabolism and Excretion:

Eplerenone metabolism is primarily mediated via CYP3A4. No active metabolites of eplerenone have been identified in human plasma.

Less than 5% of an eplerenone dose is recovered as unchanged drug in the urine and faeces. Following a single oral dose of radiolabeled drug, approximately 32% of the dose was excreted in the faeces and approximately 67% was excreted in the urine. The elimination half-life of eplerenone is approximately 3 to 5 hours. The apparent plasma clearance is approximately 10 L/hr.

Special Populations

Age, Gender, and Race: The pharmacokinetics of eplerenone at a dose of 100 mg once daily have been investigated in the elderly (≥65 years), in males and females, and in blacks. The pharmacokinetics of eplerenone did not differ significantly between males and females. At steady state, elderly subjects had increases in C_{max} (22%) and AUC (45%) compared with younger subjects (18 to 45 years). At steady state, C_{max} was 19% lower and AUC was 26% lower in blacks. (see section 4.2.)

Renal Insufficiency: The pharmacokinetics of eplerenone were evaluated in patients with varying degrees of renal insufficiency and in patients undergoing haemodialysis. Compared with control subjects, steady-state AUC and C_{max} were increased by 38% and 24%, respectively, in patients with severe renal impairment and were decreased by 26% and 3%, respectively, in patients undergoing haemodialysis. No correlation was observed between plasma clearance of eplerenone and creatinine clearance. Eplerenone is not removed by haemodialysis (see section 4.4.).

Hepatic Insufficiency: The pharmacokinetics of eplerenone 400 mg have been investigated in patients with moderate (Child-Pugh Class B) hepatic impairment and compared with normal subjects. Steady-state C_{max} and AUC of eplerenone were increased by 3.6% and 42%, respectively (see section 4.2). Since the use of eplerenone has not been investigated in patients with severe hepatic impairment, eplerenone is contra-indicated in this patients' group (see section 4.3).

Heart Failure: The pharmacokinetics of eplerenone 50 mg were evaluated in patients with heart failure (NYHA classification II-IV). Compared with healthy subjects matched according to age, weight and gender, steady state AUC and Cmax in heart failure patients were 38% and 30% higher, respectively. Consistent with these results, a population pharmacokinetic analysis of eplerenone based on a subset of patients from EPHESUS indicates that clearance of eplerenone in patients with heart failure was similar to that in healthy elderly subjects.

5.3 Preclinical safety data
Preclinical studies on safety pharmacology, genotoxicity, carcinogenic potential and toxicity to reproduction revealed no special hazard for humans.

In repeated dose toxicity studies, prostate atrophy was observed in rats and dogs at exposure levels slightly above clinical exposure levels. The prostatic changes were not associated with adverse functional consequences. The clinical relevance of these findings is unknown.

6. PHARMACEUTICAL PARTICULARS

6.1 List of excipients
Tablet core:

Lactose monohydrate
Microcrystalline cellulose (E460i)
Croscarmellose sodium (E466)
Hypromellose (E464)
Sodium laurilsulfate
Talc (E553b)
Magnesium stearate (E470b)

Tablet coating:

Opadry yellow:
Hypromellose (E464)
Titanium dioxide (E171)
Macrogol 400
Polysorbate 80 (E433)
Iron oxide yellow (E172)
Iron oxide red (E172)

6.2 Incompatibilities
Not applicable.

6.3 Shelf life
3 years.

6.4 Special precautions for storage
No special precautions for storage.

6.5 Nature and contents of container
Opaque PVC/Al blisters containing 10, 20, 28, 30, 50, 90 100 or 200 tablets

Opaque PVC/Al perforated unit dose blisters containing 20 × 1, 30 × 1, 50 × 1, 90 × 1, 100 × 1 or 200 × 1 (10 packs of 20 × 1) tablets

Not all pack sizes may be marketed.

6.6 Instructions for use and handling
No special requirements.

7. MARKETING AUTHORISATION HOLDER
Pfizer Limited
Ramsgate Road
Sandwich
Kent
CT13 9NJ
United Kingdom

8. MARKETING AUTHORISATION NUMBER(S)
Inspra® ▼ 25 mg film-coated tablets: PL 00057/0615
Inspra ® ▼50 mg film-coated tablets: PL 00057/0616

9. DATE OF FIRST AUTHORISATION/RENEWAL OF THE AUTHORISATION
21st September 2004

10. DATE OF REVISION OF THE TEXT
18th July 2005

11. LEGAL CATEGORY
POM
Company Reference IN2_0

Insulatard Insulatard 100 IU/ml, Insulatard Penfill 100 IU/ml, Insulatard NovoLet 100 IU/ml, Insulatard InnoLet 100 IU/ml, Insulatard FlexPen 100 IU/ml

(Novo Nordisk Limited)

1. NAME OF THE MEDICINAL PRODUCT
Insulatard 100 IU/ml
Suspension for injection in a vial
Insulatard Penfill 100 IU/ml
Suspension for injection in a cartridge
Insulatard NovoLet 100 IU/ml
Suspension for injection in a pre-filled pen
Insulatard InnoLet 100 IU/ml
Suspension for injection in a pre-filled pen
Insulatard FlexPen 100 IU/ml
Suspension for injection in a pre-filled pen

2. QUALITATIVE AND QUANTITATIVE COMPOSITION
Insulin human, rDNA (produced by recombinant DNA technology in *Saccharomyces cerevisiae*).

1 ml contains 100 IU of insulin human

1 vial contains 10 ml equivalent to 1000 IU

1 cartridge contains 3 ml equivalent to 300 IU

1 pre-filled pen contains 3 ml equivalent to 300 IU

One IU (International Unit) corresponds to 0.035 mg of anhydrous human insulin.

Insulatard is a suspension of isophane (NPH) insulin.

For excipients, see Section 6.1 List of excipients.

3. PHARMACEUTICAL FORM
Suspension for injection in a vial.
Suspension for injection in cartridge.
Suspension for injection in a pre-filled pen.
Insulatard is a cloudy, white, aqueous suspension.

4. CLINICAL PARTICULARS

4.1 Therapeutic indications
Treatment of diabetes mellitus.

4.2 Posology and method of administration
Insulatard is a long-acting insulin.

Dosage

Dosage is individual and determined in accordance with the needs of the patient. The individual insulin requirement is usually between 0.3 and 1.0 IU/kg/day. The daily insulin requirement may be higher in patients with insulin resistance (e.g. during puberty or due to obesity) and lower in patients with residual, endogenous insulin production.

The physician determines whether one or several daily injections are necessary. Insulatard may be used alone or mixed with fast-acting insulin. In intensive insulin therapy the suspension may be used as basal insulin (evening and/or morning injection) with fast-acting insulin given at meals.

In patients with diabetes mellitus optimised glycaemic control delays the onset of late diabetic complications. Close blood glucose monitoring is recommended.

Dosage adjustment

Concomitant illness, especially infections and feverish conditions, usually increases the patient's insulin requirement.

Renal or hepatic impairment may reduce insulin requirement.

Adjustment of dosage may also be necessary if patients change physical activity or their usual diet.

Dosage adjustment may be necessary when transferring patients from one insulin preparation to another (see section 4.4 Special warnings and special precautions for use).

Administration

For subcutaneous use.

Insulatard is usually administered subcutaneously in the thigh. If convenient, the abdominal wall, the gluteal region or the deltoid region may also be used.

Subcutaneous injection into the thigh results in a slower and less variable absorption compared to the other injection sites.

Injection into a lifted skin fold minimises the risk of unintended intramuscular injection.

Keep the needle under the skin for at least 6 seconds to make sure the entire dose is injected.

Injection sites should be rotated within an anatomic region in order to avoid lipodystrophy.

Insulin suspensions are never to be administered intravenously.

Insulatard is accompanied by a package leaflet with detailed instruction for use to be followed.

The vials are for use with insulin syringes with a corresponding unit scale. When two types of insulin are mixed, draw the amount of fast-acting insulin first, followed by the amount of long-acting insulin.

The cartridges are designed to be used with Novo Nordisk delivery systems (durable devices for repeated use) and NovoFine needles. Detailed instruction accompanying the delivery system must be followed.

Insulatard NovoLet is designed to be used with NovoFine needles.

NovoLet delivers 2-78 units in increments of 2 units.

Insulatard InnoLet is designed to be used with NovoFine short cap needles of 8 mm or shorter in length. The needle box is marked with an **S.**

InnoLet delivers 1-50 units in increments of 1 unit.

Insulatard FlexPen is designed to be used with NovoFine short cap needles of 8 mm or shorter in length. The needle box is marked with an **S.**

FlexPen delivers 1-60 units in increments of 1 unit.

The pens should be primed before injection so that the dose selector returns to zero and a drop of insulin appears at the needle tip.

The dose is set by turning the selector, which returns to zero during the injection.

4.3 Contraindications
Hypoglycaemia

Hypersensitivity to human insulin or to any of the excipients (see section 6.1 List of excipients).

4.4 Special warnings and special precautions for use
Inadequate dosage or discontinuation of treatment, especially in type 1 diabetes, may lead to **hyperglycaemia**.

Usually the first symptoms of hyperglycaemia set in gradually, over a period of hours or days. They include thirst, increased frequency of urination, nausea, vomiting, drowsiness, flushed dry skin, dry mouth, loss of appetite as well as acetone odour of breath.

In type 1 diabetes, untreated hyperglycaemic events eventually lead to diabetic ketoacidosis, which is potentially lethal.

Hypoglycaemia may occur if the insulin dose is too high in relation to the insulin requirement (see sections 4.8 and 4.9).

Omission of a meal or unplanned, strenuous physical exercise may lead to hypoglycaemia.

Patients whose blood glucose control is greatly improved e.g. by intensified insulin therapy, may experience a change in their usual warning symptoms of hypoglycaemia and should be advised accordingly.

Usual warning symptoms may disappear in patients with long-standing diabetes.

Transferring a patient to another type or brand of insulin should be done under strict medical supervision. Changes in strength, brand (manufacturer), type (fast-, dual-, long-acting insulin etc.), origin (animal, human or analogue insulin) and/or method of manufacture (recombinant DNA versus animal source insulin) may result in a need for a change in dosage.

If an adjustment is needed when switching the patients to Insulatard, it may occur with the first dose or during the first several weeks or months.

A few patients who have experienced hypoglycaemic reactions after transfer from animal source insulin have reported that early warning symptoms of hypoglycaemia were less pronounced or different from those experienced with their previous insulin.

Before travelling between different time zones, the patient should be advised to consult the doctor, since this may mean that the patient has to take insulin and meals at different times.

Insulin suspensions are not to be used in insulin infusion pumps.

Insulatard contains metacresol, which may cause allergic reactions.

4.5 Interaction with other medicinal products and other forms of Interaction
A number of medicinal products are known to interact with glucose metabolism. The physician must therefore take possible interactions into account and should always ask their patients about any medicinal products they take.

The following substances may reduce insulin requirement:
Oral hypoglycaemic agents (OHA), monoamine oxidase inhibitors (MAOI), non-selective beta-blocking agents, angiotensin converting enzyme (ACE) inhibitors, salicylates and alcohol.

The following substances may increase insulin requirement:
Thiazides, glucocorticoids, thyroid hormones and beta-sympathomimetics, growth hormone and danazol.

Beta-blocking agents may mask the symptoms of hypoglycaemia and delay recovery from hypoglycaemia.

Octreotide/lanreotide may both decrease and increase insulin requirement.

Alcohol may intensify and prolong the hypoglycaemic effect of insulin.

4.6 Pregnancy and lactation
There are no restrictions on treatment of diabetes with insulin during pregnancy, as insulin does not pass the placental barrier.

Both hypoglycaemia and hyperglycaemia, which can occur in inadequately controlled diabetes therapy, increase the risk of malformations and death *in utero*. Intensified control in the treatment of pregnant women with diabetes is therefore recommended throughout pregnancy and when contemplating pregnancy.

Insulin requirements usually fall in the first trimester and increase subsequently during the second and third trimesters.

After delivery, insulin requirements return rapidly to pre-pregnancy values.

Insulin treatment of the nursing mother presents no risk to the baby. However, the Insulatard dosage may need to be adjusted.

4.7 Effects on ability to drive and use machines
The patient's ability to concentrate and react may be impaired as a result of hypoglycaemia. This may constitute a risk in situations where these abilities are of special importance (e.g. driving a car or operating machinery).

Patients should be advised to take precautions to avoid hypoglycaemia whilst driving. This is particularly important in those who have reduced or absent awareness of the warning signs of hypoglycaemia or have frequent episodes of hypoglycaemia. The advisability of driving should be considered in these circumstances.

4.8 Undesirable effects
As for other insulin products, hypoglycaemia, in general is the most frequently occurring undesirable effect. It may occur if the insulin dose is too high in relation to the insulin requirement. In clinical trials and during marketed use the frequency varies with patient population and dose regimens. Therefore, no specific frequency can be presented. Severe hypoglycaemia may lead to unconsciousness and/or convulsions and may result in temporary or permanent impairment of brain function or even death.

Frequencies of adverse drug reactions from clinical trials, that are considered related to Insulatard are listed below. The frequencies are defined as: Uncommon $> 1/1000$, $< 1/100$). Isolated spontaneous cases are presented as very rare defined as $< 1/10,000$.

Immune system disorders

Uncommon – Urticaria, rash

Very rare – Anaphylactic reactions

Symptoms of generalized hypersensitivity may include generalized skin rash, itching, sweating, gastrointestinal upset, angioneurotic oedema, difficulties in breathing, palpitation, reduction in blood pressure and fainting/loss of consciousness. Generalised hypersensitivity reactions are potentially life threatening.

Nervous system disorders

Very rare – Peripheral neuropathy

Fast improvement in blood glucose control may be associated with a condition termed "acute painful neuropathy", which is usually reversible.

Eye disorders

Very rare – Refraction disorders

Refraction anomalies may occur upon initiation of insulin therapy. These symptoms are usually of transitory nature.

Uncommon – Diabetic retinopathy

Long-term improved glycaemic control decreases the risk of progression of diabetic retinopathy. However, intensification of insulin therapy with abrupt improvement in glycaemic control may be associated with temporary worsening of diabetic retinopathy.

Skin and subcutaneous tissue disorders

Uncommon – Lipodystrophy

Lipodystrophy may occur at the injection site as a consequence of failure to rotate injection sites within an area.

General disorders and administration site conditions

Uncommon – Injection site reactions

Injection site reactions (redness, swelling, itching, pain and haematoma at the injection site) may occur during treatment with insulin. Most reactions are transitory and disappear during continued treatment.

Uncommon – Oedema

Oedema may occur upon initiation of insulin therapy. These symptoms are usually of transitory nature.

4.9 Overdose

A specific overdose of insulin cannot be defined. However, hypoglycaemia may develop over sequential stages:

• Mild hypoglycaemic episodes can be treated by oral administration of glucose or sugary products. It is therefore recommended that the diabetic patients carry some sugar lumps, sweets, biscuits or sugary fruit juice.

• Severe hypoglycaemic episodes, where the patient has become unconscious, can be treated by glucagon (0.5 to 1 mg) given intramuscularly or subcutaneously by a person who has received appropriate instruction, or by glucose given intravenously by a medical professional. Glucose must also be given intravenously, if the patient does not respond to glucagon within 10 to 15 minutes.

Upon regaining consciousness, administration of oral carbohydrate is recommended for the patient in order to prevent relapse.

5. PHARMACOLOGICAL PROPERTIES

5.1 Pharmacodynamic properties

Pharmacotherapeutic group: Insulins and analogues, intermediate-acting, insulin human. ATC code: A10A C01.

The blood glucose lowering effect of insulin is due to the facilitated uptake of glucose following binding of insulin to receptors on muscle and fat cells and to the simultaneous inhibition of glucose output from the liver.

Insulatard is a long-acting insulin.

Onset of action is within 1½ hours, reaches a maximum effect within 4-12 hours and the entire time of duration is approximately 24 hours.

5.2 Pharmacokinetic properties

Insulin in the blood stream has a half-life of a few minutes. Consequently, the time-action profile of an insulin preparation is determined solely by its absorption characteristics.

This process is influenced by several factors (e.g. insulin dosage, injection route and site, thickness of subcutaneous fat, type of diabetes). The pharmacokinetics of insulins is therefore affected by significant intra- and inter-individual variation.

Absorption

The maximum plasma concentration of the insulin is reached within 2-18 hours after subcutaneous administration.

Distribution

No profound binding to plasma proteins, except circulating insulin antibodies (if present) has been observed.

Metabolism

Human insulin is reported to be degraded by insulin protease or insulin-degrading enzymes and possibly protein disulfide isomerase. A number of cleavage (hydrolysis) sites on the human insulin molecule have been proposed; none of the metabolites formed following the cleavage are active.

Elimination

The terminal half-life is determined by the rate of absorption from the subcutaneous tissue. The terminal half-life ($t_{½}$) is therefore a measure of the absorption rather than of the elimination *per se* of insulin from plasma (insulin in the blood stream has a $t_{½}$ of a few minutes). Trials have indicated a $t_{½}$ of about 5-10 hours.

5.3 Preclinical safety data

Preclinical data reveal no special hazard for humans based on conventional studies of safety pharmacology, repeated dose toxicity, genotoxicity, carcinogenic potential, toxicity to reproduction.

6. PHARMACEUTICAL PARTICULARS

6.1 List of excipients

Zinc chloride

Glycerol

Metacresol

Phenol

Disodium phosphate dihydrate

Sodium hydroxide or/and hydrochloric acid (for pH adjustment)

Protamine sulphate

Water for injections

6.2 Incompatibilities

Insulin suspensions should not be added to infusion fluids.

6.3 Shelf life

30 months.

After first opening: 6 weeks.

6.4 Special precautions for storage

Store in a refrigerator (2°C - 8°C).

Do not freeze.

Insulatard:

Keep the vial in the outer carton in order to protect from light.

During use: do not refrigerate. Do not store above 25°C.

Insulatard Penfill:

Keep the cartridge in the outer carton in order to protect from light.

During use: do not refrigerate. Do not store above 30°C.

Insulatard NovoLet, Insulatard InnoLet and Insulatard FlexPen:

During use: do not refrigerate. Do not store above 30°C.

Keep the pen cap on in order to protect the insulin from light.

Protect from excessive heat and sunlight.

6.5 Nature and contents of container

Glass vial (type 1) closed with a bromobutyl/polyisoprene rubber stopper and a protective tamper-proof plastic cap.

Pack size: 1 vial × 10 ml.

Glass cartridge (type 1) with a bromobutyl rubber plunger and a bromobutyl/polyisoprene rubber stopper. The cartridge contains a glass ball to facilitate the re-suspension.

Pack size: 5 cartridges × 3 ml.

Pre-filled pen (multidose disposable pen) comprising a pen injector with a cartridge (3 ml). The cartridge is made of glass (type 1), containing a bromobutyl rubber plunger and a bromobutyl/polyisoprene rubber stopper. The cartridge contains a glass ball to facilitate the re-suspension. The pen injector is made of plastic.

Pack size: 5 pre-filled pens × 3 ml.

6.6 Instructions for use and handling

Cartridges and pens should only be used in combination with products that are compatible with them and allow the cartridge and pen to function safely and effectively.

Insulatard Penfill, Insulatard NovoLet, Insulatard InnoLet and Insulatard FlexPen are for single person use only. The container must not be refilled.

Insulin preparations, which have been frozen, must not be used.

Insulin suspensions should not be used if they do not appear uniformly white and cloudy after re-suspension.

7. MARKETING AUTHORISATION HOLDER

Novo Nordisk A/S

Novo Allé

DK-2880 Bagsværd

Denmark

8. MARKETING AUTHORISATION NUMBER(S)

Insulatard 100 IU/ml EU/1/02/233/003

Insulatard Penfill 100 IU/ml EU/1/02/233/006

Insulatard NovoLet 100 IU/ml EU/1/02/233/008

Insulatard InnoLet 100 IU/ml EU/1/02/233/011

Insulatard FlexPen 100 IU/ml EU/1/02/233/014

9. DATE OF FIRST AUTHORISATION/RENEWAL OF THE AUTHORISATION

October 2002

10. DATE OF REVISION OF THE TEXT

2 August 2004

Legal Status

POM

Insuman Basal 100 IU/ml

(sanofi-aventis)

1. NAME OF THE MEDICINAL PRODUCT

Insuman ® Basal 100 IU/ml suspension for injection in a vial ▼

Insuman ® Basal 100 IU/ml suspension for injection in a cartridge ▼

Insuman ® Basal 100 IU/ml OptiSet® suspension for injection ▼

2. QUALITATIVE AND QUANTITATIVE COMPOSITION

Insuman Basal is an isophane insulin suspension.

Each ml of Insuman Basal contains 100 IU of the active substance insulin human.

Each vial contains 5 ml, equal to 500 IU insulin.

Each cartridge contains 3 ml, equal to 300 IU insulin.

Insuman Basal OptiSet is a pre-filled disposable pen containing Insuman Basal.

Each pen contains 3 ml, equivalent to 300 IU insulin.

One IU (International Unit) corresponds to 0.035 mg of anhydrous human insulin.

The human insulin in Insuman Basal is produced by recombinant DNA technology using K 12 strains of *Escherichia coli*.

For the excipients, see 6.1.

3. PHARMACEUTICAL FORM

Suspension for injection in a vial, cartridge or pre-filled disposable pen.

4. CLINICAL PARTICULARS

4.1 Therapeutic indications

Diabetes mellitus where treatment with insulin is required.

4.2 Posology and method of administration

The desired blood glucose levels, the insulin preparations to be used and the insulin dosage (doses and timings) must be determined individually and adjusted to suit the patient's diet, physical activity and life-style.

Daily doses and timing of administration

There are no fixed rules for insulin dosage. However, the average insulin requirement is often 0.5 to 1.0 IU per kg body weight per day. The basal metabolic requirement is 40% to 60% of the total daily requirement.

Insuman Basal is injected subcutaneously 45 to 60 minutes before a meal.

Insuman Basal OptiSet delivers insulin in increments of 2 IU up to a maximum single dose of 40 IU.

Transfer to Insuman Basal

Dosage adjustment may be necessary when transferring patients from one insulin preparation to another. This applies, for example, when transferring from:

• an animal insulin (especially a bovine insulin) to human insulin,

• one human insulin preparation to another.

• a regimen with only regular insulin to one with a longer-acting insulin.

The need to adjust (e.g. reduce) the dose may become evident immediately after transfer. Alternatively, it may emerge gradually over a period of several weeks.

Following transfer from an animal insulin to human insulin, dosage reduction may be required in particular in patients who:

• were previously already controlled on rather low blood glucose levels.

• have a tendency to hypoglycaemia.

• previously required high insulin doses due to the presence of insulin antibodies.

Close metabolic monitoring is recommended during the transition and in the initial weeks thereafter. In patients who require high insulin doses because of the presence of insulin antibodies, transfer under medical supervision in a hospital or similar setting must be considered.

Secondary dose adjustment

Improved metabolic control may result in increased insulin sensitivity, leading to a reduced insulin requirement. Dose adjustment may also be required, for example, if:

• the patient's weight changes,

• the patient's life-style changes,

• other circumstances arise that may promote an increased susceptibility to hypo- or hyperglycaemia (see section 4.4).

Use in specific patient groups

In patients with hepatic or renal impairment as well as in the elderly, insulin requirements may be diminished (see section 4.4).

Administration

Vials: Insuman Basal contains 100 IU of insulin per ml suspension. Only syringes designed for this strength of insulin (100 IU per ml) are to be used. The syringes must not contain any other medicinal product or residue (e.g. traces of heparin).

Cartridges: Insuman Basal in cartridges has been developed for use in the OptiPen® series. For further details on handling, see section 6.6.

OptiSet: Insuman Basal OptiSet is a pre-filled disposable pen. For handling of the pen, see section 6.6.

Insuman Basal is administered subcutaneously. Insuman Basal must never be injected intravenously.

Insulin absorption and hence the blood glucose lowering effect of a dose may vary from one injection area to another (e.g. the abdominal wall compared with the thigh). Injection sites within an injection area must be rotated from one injection to the next.

Mixing of insulins

Insuman Basal vials or cartridges may be mixed with all Aventis Pharma human insulins, but NOT with those designed specifically for use in insulin pumps. Insuman Basal must also NOT be mixed with insulins of animal origin or with insulin analogues.

Insuman Basal OptiSet must not be mixed with any other insulins or with insulin analogues.

4.3 Contraindications

Hypersensitivity to the active substance or to any of the excipients (see section 6.1).

Insuman Basal must not be administered intravenously and must not be used in infusion pumps or external or implanted insulin pumps.

4.4 Special warnings and special precautions for use

Patients hypersensitive to Insuman Basal for whom no better tolerated preparation is available must only continue treatment under close medical supervision and – where necessary – in conjunction with anti-allergic treatment.

In patients with an allergy to animal insulin intradermal skin testing is recommended prior to a transfer to Insuman

Basal, since they may experience immunological cross-reactions.

In patients with renal impairment, insulin requirements may be diminished due to reduced insulin metabolism. In the elderly, progressive deterioration of renal function may lead to a steady decrease in insulin requirements.

In patients with severe hepatic impairment, insulin requirements may be diminished due to reduced capacity for gluconeogenesis and reduced insulin metabolism.

In case of insufficient glucose control or a tendency to hyper- or hypoglycaemic episodes, the patient's adherence to the prescribed treatment regimen, injection sites and proper injection technique and all other relevant factors must be reviewed before dose adjustment is considered.

Hypoglycaemia

Hypoglycaemia may occur if the insulin dose is too high in relation to the insulin requirement.

Particular caution should be exercised, and intensified blood glucose monitoring is advisable in patients in whom hypoglycaemic episodes might be of particular clinical relevance, such as in patients with significant stenoses of the coronary arteries or of the blood vessels supplying the brain (risk of cardiac or cerebral complications of hypoglycaemia) as well as in patients with proliferative retinopathy, particularly if not treated with photocoagulation (risk of transient amaurosis following hypoglycaemia).

Patients should be aware of circumstances where the warning symptoms of hypoglycaemia are diminished. The warning symptoms of hypoglycaemia may be changed, be less pronounced or absent in certain risk groups. These include patients:

- in whom glycaemic control has been markedly improved,
- in whom hypoglycaemia develops gradually,
- who are in elderly,
- in whom an autonomic neuropathy is present,
- with a long history of diabetes,
- suffering from a psychiatric illness,
- receiving concurrent treatment with certain other medicinal products (see section 4.5).

Such situations may result in severe hypoglycaemia (and possibly loss of consciousness) prior to the patients awareness of hypoglycaemia.

If normal or decreased values for glycated haemoglobin are noted, the possibility of recurrent, unrecognised (especially nocturnal) episodes of hypoglycaemia must be considered.

Adherence of the patient to the dosage and dietary regimen, correct insulin administration and awareness of hypoglycaemia symptoms are essential to reduce the risk of hypoglycaemia. Factors increasing the susceptibility to hypoglycaemia require particularly close monitoring and may necessitate dose adjustment. These include:

- change in the injection area,
- improved insulin sensitivity(e.g. by removal of stress factors.),
- unaccustomed, increased or prolonged physical activity,
- intercurrent illness (eg. vomiting, diarrhoea.),
- inadequate food intake,
- missed meals,
- alcohol consumption,
- certain uncompensated endocrine disorders (e.g. in hypothyroidism and in anterior pituitary or adrenocortical insufficiency),
- concomitant treatment with certain other medicinal products.

Intercurrent illnesses

Intercurrent illness requires intensified metabolic monitoring. In many cases, urine tests for ketones are indicated, and often it is necessary to adjust the insulin dose. The insulin requirement is often increased. Patients with type I diabetes must continue to consume at least a small amount of carbohydrates on a regular basis, even if they are able to eat only little or no food, or are vomiting etc. and they must never omit insulin entirely.

4.5 Interaction with other medicinal products and other forms of Interaction

A number of substances affect glucose metabolism and may require dose adjustment of human insulin.

Substances that may enhance the blood –glucose-lowering effect and increase susceptibility to hypoglycaemia include oral antidiabetic agents, ACE inhibitors, disopyramide, fibrates, fluoxetine, MAO inhibitors, pentoxifylline, propoxyphene, salicylates and sulfonamide antibiotics.

Substances that may reduce the blood –glucose- lowering effect include corticosteroids, danazol, diazoxide, diuretics, glucagon, isoniazid, oestrogens and progestogens; phenothiazines derivatives, somatropin, sympathomimetic agents (e.g. epinephrine (adrenaline), salbutamol, terbutaline) and thyroid hormones.

Beta-blockers, clonidine, lithium salts or alcohol may either potentiate or weaken the blood-glucose-lowering effect of insulin. Pentamidine may cause hypoglycaemia which may sometimes be followed by hyperglycaemia.

In addition, under the influence of sympatholytic medicinal products such as beta-blockers, clonidine, guanethidine and reserpine, the signs of adrenergic counter-regulation may be reduced or absent.

4.6 Pregnancy and lactation

There is no experience with the use of Insuman Basal in pregnant women.

Insulin does not cross the placental barrier.

It is essential for patients with pre-existing or gestational diabetes to maintain good metabolic control throughout pregnancy. Insulin requirements may decrease during the first trimester and generally increase during the second and third trimesters. Immediately after delivery, insulin requirements decline rapidly (increased risk of hypoglycaemia). Careful monitoring of glucose control is essential.

There are no restrictions on the use of Insuman Basal in breast-feeding women. Lactating women may require adjustments in insulin dose and diet.

4.7 Effects on ability to drive and use machines

The patient's ability to concentrate and react may be impaired as a result of hypoglycaemia or hyperglycaemia or, for example, as a result of visual impairment.

This may constitute a risk in situations where these abilities are of special importance (e.g. driving a car or operating machinery).

Patients should be advised to take precautions to avoid hypoglycaemia whilst driving. This is particularly important in those who have reduced or absent awareness of the warning symptoms of hypoglycaemia or have frequent episodes of hypoglycaemia. It should be considered whether it is advisable to drive or operate machinery in these circumstances.

4.8 Undesirable effects

Hypoglycaemia

Hypoglycaemia, in general the most frequent undesirable effect of insulin therapy, may occur if the insulin dose is too high in relation to the insulin requirement. Severe hypoglycaemic attacks, especially if recurrent, may lead to neurological damage. Prolonged or severe hypoglycaemic episodes may be life-threatening.

In many patients, the signs and symptoms of neuroglycopenia are preceded by signs of adrenergic counter-regulation. Generally, the greater and more rapid the decline in blood glucose, the more marked is the phenomenon of counter-regulation and its symptoms.

Eyes

A marked change in glycaemic control may cause temporary visual impairment, due to temporary alteration in the turgidity and hence the refractive index of the lens.

Long-term improved glycaemic control decreases the risk of progression of diabetic retinopathy. However, intensification of insulin therapy with abrupt improvement in glycaemic control may be associated with temporary worsening of diabetic retinopathy. In patients with proliferative retinopathy, particularly if not treated with photocoagulation, severe hypoglycaemic episodes may result in transient amaurosis.

Lipodystrophy

As with any insulin therapy, lipodystrophy may occur at the injection site and delay local insulin absorption. Continuous rotation of the injection site within the given injection area may help to reduce or prevent these reactions.

Injection site and allergic reactions

In rare cases mild reactions at the injection site may occur. Such reactions include redness, pain, itching, hives, swelling, or inflammation. Most minor reactions to insulins at the injection site usually resolve in a few days to a few weeks.

Immediate-type allergic reactions to insulin are very rare. Such reactions to insulin or the excipients may, for example, be associated with generalised skin reactions, angiooedema, bronchospasm, hypotension and shock, and may be life-threatening.

Other reactions

Insulin administration may cause insulin antibodies to form. In rare cases, the presence of such insulin antibodies may necessitate adjustment of the insulin dose in order to correct a tendency to hyperglycaemia or hypoglycaemia.

Insulin may cause sodium retention and oedema, particularly if previously poor metabolic control is improved by intensified insulin therapy.

4.9 Overdose

Symptoms

Insulin overdose may lead to severe and sometimes long-term and life-threatening hypoglycaemia.

Management

Mild episodes of hypoglycaemia can usually be treated with oral carbohydrates. Adjustments in dosage of the medicinal product, meal patterns, or physical activity may be needed.

More severe episodes with coma, seizure, or neurologic impairment may be treated with intramuscular/subcutaneous glucagon or concentrated intravenous glucose. Sustained carbohydrate intake and observation may be necessary because hypoglycaemia may recur after apparent clinical recovery.

5. PHARMACOLOGICAL PROPERTIES

5.1 Pharmacodynamic properties

Pharmaco-therapeutic group: Antidiabetic agent. Insulins and analogues, intermediate-acting.

ATC Code: A10AC01.

Mode of action

Insulin:

- lowers blood glucose and promotes anabolic effects as well as decreasing catabolic effects.
- increases the transport of glucose into cells as well as the formation of glycogen in the muscles and the liver, and improves pyruvate utilisation. It inhibits glycogenolysis and gluconeogenesis.
- increases lipogenesis in the liver and adipose tissue and inhibits lipolysis.
- promotes the uptake of amino acids into cells and promotes protein synthesis.
- enhances the uptake of potassium into cells.

Pharmacodynamic characteristics

Insuman Basal (an isophane insulin suspension) is an insulin with gradual onset and long duration of action. Following subcutaneous injection, onset of action is within 60 minutes, the phase of maximum action is between 3 and 4 hours after injection and the duration of action is 11 to 20 hours.

5.2 Pharmacokinetic properties

In healthy subjects, the serum half-life of insulin is approximately 4 to 6 minutes. It is longer in patients with severe renal insufficiency. However, it must be noted that the pharmacokinetics of insulin do not reflect its metabolic action.

5.3 Preclinical safety data

The acute toxicity was studied following subcutaneous administration in rats. No evidence of toxic effects was found. Studies of pharmacodynamic effects following subcutaneous administration in rabbits and dogs revealed the expected hypoglycaemic reactions.

6. PHARMACEUTICAL PARTICULARS

6.1 List of excipients

Protamine sulphate, m-cresol, phenol, zinc chloride, sodium dihydrogen phosphate dihydrate, glycerol, sodium hydroxide, hydrochloric acid, water for injections.

6.2 Incompatibilities

As with all insulin preparations, Insuman Basal must not be mixed with solutions containing reducing agents such as thioles and sulfites. It must also be remembered that insulin protamine crystals dissolve in an acid pH range.

Concerning mixing and incompatibility with other insulins see section 4.2.

Care must be taken to ensure that no alcohol or other disinfectants enter the insulin suspension.

6.3 Shelf life

2 years.

Vials: Once in use, the vial may be used for up to four weeks. It is recommended that the date of the first withdrawal from the vial be noted on the label.

Cartridges: Once in use, the cartridges may be kept for up to four weeks. This applies irrespective of whether the cartridges are immediately put into the pen or are first carried as a spare for a while.

OptiSet: Once in use the OptiSet pens may be kept for up to four weeks. This applies irrespective of whether the pens are immediately used or are first carried as a spare for a while.

6.4 Special precautions for storage

Store at 2°C - 8°C. Keep the container in the outer carton. Do not freeze. Ensure that the container is not directly touching the freezer compartment or freezer packs.

Vials: Once in use, do not store above 25°C, and protect from direct heat or light.

Cartridges: Once in use do not store above 25°C and protect from direct heat or light. When in use (in the pen), do not store in a refrigerator.

OptiSet: Once in use, do not store above 25°C and protect from direct heat or light. When in use, do not store in a refrigerator.

6.5 Nature and contents of container

Vials

5 ml type I colourless glass vial with flanged aluminium cap, chlorobutyl rubber,(type I,) stopper and tear-off polypropylene lid.

Each vial contains 5 ml suspension (500 IU insulin human). Pack of 1 vial is available.

Cartridges

3.0 ml, type I colourless, glass cartridge with bromobutyl rubber (type I), plunger and flanged aluminium cap with bromobutyl rubber (type I) stopper.

Each cartridge contains 3 balls (stainless steel).

Each cartridge contains 3 ml suspension (300 IU insulin human). Pack of 5 cartridges is available.

OptiSet

Disposable pen filled with 3 ml, type I colourless glass cartridge with bromobutyl rubber (type I) plunger and flanged aluminium cap with bromobutyl rubber (type I) stopper

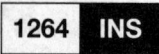

Each cartridge contains 3 balls (stainless steel).

Each cartridge contains 3 ml suspension (300 IU insulin human). The cartridges are sealed in a disposable pen injector. Needles are not included in the pack. Pack of 5 pens is available.

6.6 Instructions for use and handling

Vials

Before withdrawing insulin from the vial for the first time, remove the plastic protective cap.

Immediately before withdrawal from the vial into the syringe, the insulin must be re-suspended. This is best done by rolling the vial at an oblique angle between the palms of the hands. Do not shake the vial vigorously as this may lead to changes in the suspension (giving the vial a frosted appearance; see below) and cause frothing. Froth may interfere with the correct measurement of the dose.

After resuspension, the fluid must have a uniformly milky appearance. Insuman Basal must not be used if this cannot be achieved, i.e. if the suspension remains clear, for example, or if clumps, particles or flocculation appear in the insulin or stick to the wall or bottom of the vial. These changes sometimes give the vial a frosted appearance. In such cases, a new vial yielding a uniform suspension must be used. It is also necessary to change to a new vial if the insulin requirement changes substantially.

Mixing of insulins

If two different insulins have to be drawn into one single syringe, it is recommended that the shorter-acting insulin be drawn first to prevent contamination of the vial by the longer-acting preparation. It is advisable to inject immediately after mixing. Insulins of different concentration (e.g. 100 IU per ml and 40 IU per ml) must not be mixed.

Cartridges

Before insertion into the pen, Insuman Basal must be kept at room temperature for 1 to 2 hours and then resuspended to check the contents. This is best done by gently tilting the cartridge back and forth (at least ten times). Each cartridge contains three small metal balls to facilitate quick and thorough mixing of the contents.

Later on, when the cartridge has been inserted into the pen, the insulin must be resuspended again prior to each injection. This is best done by gently tilting the pen back and forth (at least ten times).

After resuspension, the fluid must have a uniformly milky appearance. Insuman Basal must not be used if this cannot be achieved, i.e. if the suspension remains clear, for example, or if clumps, particles or flocculation appear in the insulin or stick to the wall or bottom of the cartridge. These changes sometimes give the cartridge a frosted appearance. In such cases, a new cartridge yielding a uniform suspension must be used. It is also necessary to change to a new cartridge if the insulin requirement changes substantially.

Air bubbles must be removed from the cartridge before injection (see instructions for using the pen).

The instructions for using the pen must be followed carefully. Empty cartridges must not be refilled.

Insuman Basal cartridges are not designed to allow any other insulin to be mixed in the cartridge.

If the pen malfunctions, the suspension may be drawn from the cartridge into a syringe (suitable for an insulin with 100 IU/ml) and injected.

OptiSet

Before first use, Insuman Basal OptiSet must be kept at room temperature for 1 to 2 hours and then resuspended to check the contents. This is best done by gently tilting the cartridge back and forth (at least ten times). Each cartridge contains three small metal balls to facilitate quick and thorough mixing of the contents. Later on, the insulin must be resuspended again prior to each injection.

After resuspension, the fluid must have a uniformly milky appearance. Insuman Basal OptiSet must not be used if this cannot be achieved, i.e. if the suspension remains clear, for example, or if clumps, particles or flocculation appear in the insulin or stick to the wall or bottom of the cartridge. These changes sometimes give the cartridge a frosted appearance.

In such cases, a new pen yielding a uniform suspension must be used. It is also necessary to change to a new pen if the insulin requirement changes substantially.

Air bubbles must be removed from the cartridge before injection. The instructions for using the pen must be followed carefully (see below). Empty pens must never be reused and must be properly discarded.

To prevent the possible transmission of disease, each pen must be used by one patient only.

The insulin pen must not be dropped or subjected to impact (otherwise, the insulin cartridge in the transparent insulin reservoir may break and the pen will not work). If this happens, a new pen must be used.

A new needle must be affixed prior to each injection. The following needles may be used in conjunction with the OptiSet: Needles designed for the OptiSet or those for which the needle manufacturer has demonstrated suitability for use in OptiSet. The needle is removed after the injection and the pen is stored without the needle. The needle must also be removed before disposal of the pen. Needles must not be reused.

Handling of the pen

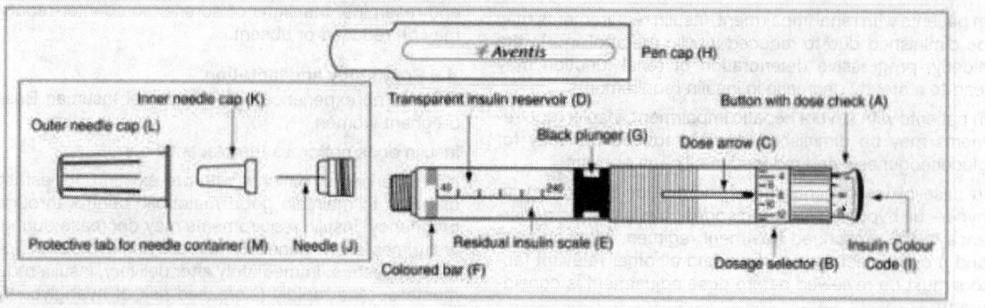

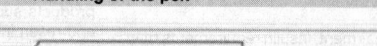

Schematic diagram of the pen

(see Handling of the pen above)

PREPARATION OF THE PEN

(a) Before using your pen for the first time, remove the pen cap (H).

(b) Take a new needle. Use needles designed for the OptiSet or those needles for which the needle manufacturer has demonstrated that they can be used with the OptiSet pre-filled pen. Remove the protective tab (M) from the needle container and affix the needle (J) together with the outer needle cap (L) onto the pen. As you do this, hold the pen firmly by the transparent insulin reservoir (D) (Figure 1).

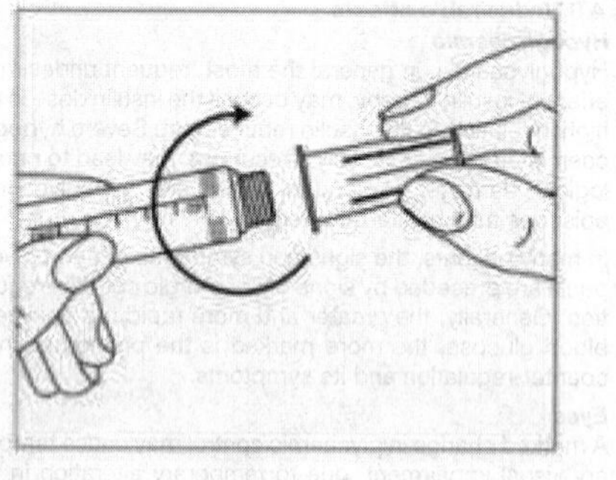

Figure 1

MAKE SURE THAT YOU AFFIX THE NEEDLE CAREFULLY. IMPRECISE AFFIXING (E.G. AT A SLANT) MAY LEAD TO BREAKAGE OF THE NEEDLE OR LEAKAGE OF THE INJECTION SYSTEM, RESULTING IN IMPRECISE DOSING.

FUNCTION TEST PRIOR TO FIRST INJECTION

(a) Check to ensure that the dose arrow (C) is pointing to the number 8 (Figure 2).

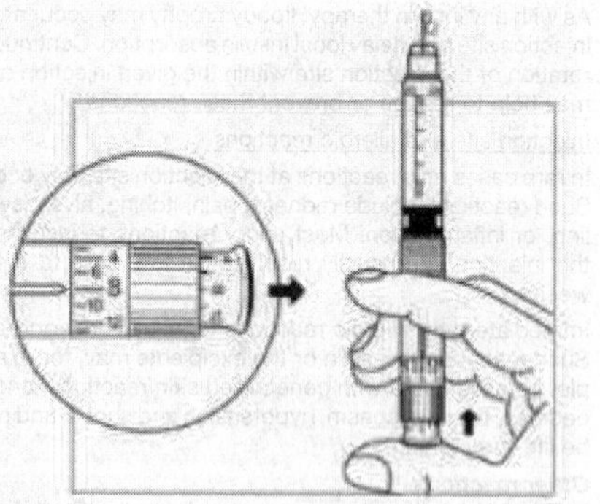

Figure 2

(b) Pull out button (A) as far as it will go, remove the inner and outer needle caps (K+L) and hold the pen with the needle pointing upwards.

(c) With the needle still pointing upwards, press button (A) fully home. Insulin must appear at the tip of the needle; this indicates that your pen is primed for injection. The amount of insulin seen at the needle tip is just the excess from the pen (generally less than 8 units). If no insulin appears, check to ensure that your pen is working properly (follow steps a-c under "Removal of air bubbles/In-use function test") and repeat until a drop of insulin is seen at the needle tip.

REMOVAL OF AIR BUBBLES/IN-USE FUNCTION TEST

Small amounts of air may be present in the needle and insulin reservoir during normal use. You must remove this air. (Small persistent air bubbles in the insulin reservoir do not interfere with the correct dosage.)

If your pen has not been used for several days, you should also check that it is working properly and repeat steps a-c given below, after affixing a new needle.

(a) Set the dose arrow to 2 by turning the dosage selector (B). (The dosage selector (B) may be turned in either direction.) Now pull button (A) out as far as it will go. Remove the inner and outer needle caps (K+L) (Figure 3a).

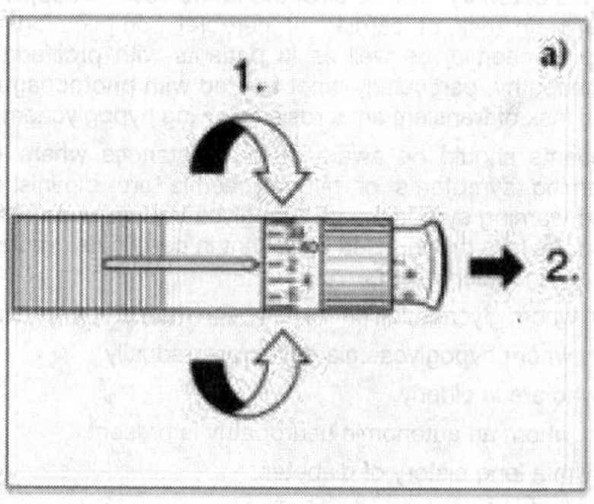

Figure 3a

(b) Hold the pen with the needle pointing upwards and tap the insulin reservoir (D) gently with the finger so that any air bubbles rise up towards the needle (Figure 3b).

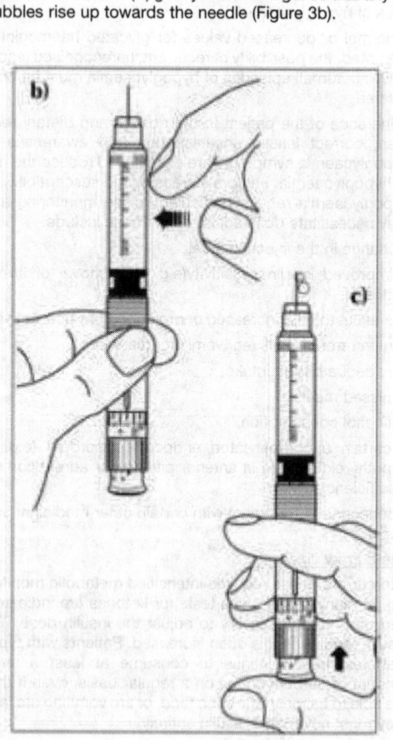

Figure 3b/c

(c) Press button (A) fully home. If insulin appears at the needle tip, then your pen is working properly (Figure 3c).

If no insulin appears at the needle tip, repeat steps a-c until you see an insulin drop at the needle tip.

If no insulin appears at the tip of the needle even after steps a-c have been repeated several times, the needle may be clogged. Please change the needle.

SETTING AND INJECTING THE FIRST INSULIN DOSE

(a) To ensure that the insulin suspension is uniformly mixed, gently tilt the pen back and forth (at least ten times) (see also above). Set the required dose by turning the dosage selector (B) in either direction until the dose arrow (C) is pointing to the dose you require (Figure 4a). (The dosage selector lets you set the dose in steps of 2 units.)

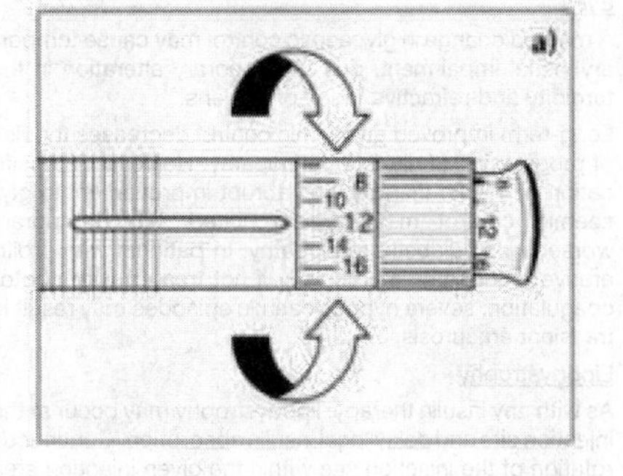

Figure 4a

(b) Once you have set your dose, load it by pulling button (A) out as far as it will go (Figure 4b).

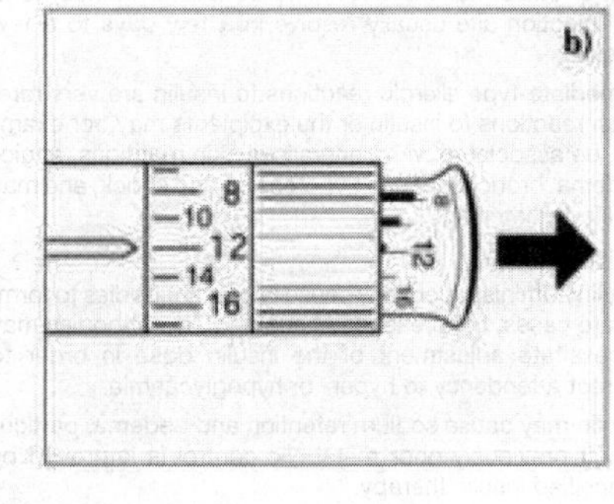

Figure 4b

The button allows you to check the dose: When the button is pulled out, the last thick bar visible indicates the dose that has been loaded (the example in Figure 4b shows the button pulled out and a loaded dose of 12 IU insulin).

(c) Injection: Insert the needle into the skin and press the button completely home (Figure 4c). Allow the needle to remain in the skin for at least 10 seconds (count to 10 slowly). Keep the button pressed down until you have taken the needle out of the skin. This ensures that you have injected the full insulin dose.

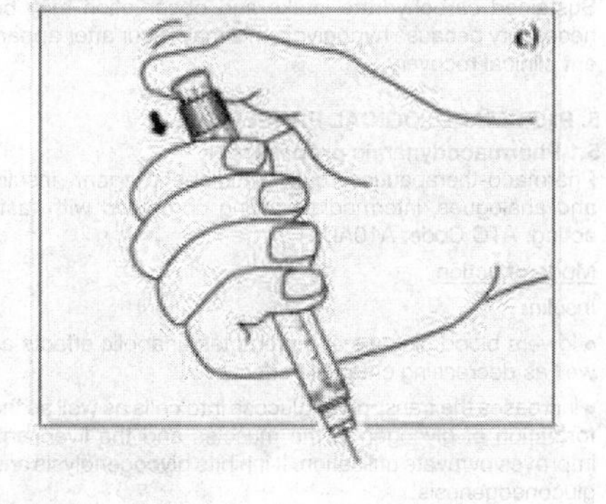

Figure 4c

REMOVING THE NEEDLE

Remove the needle after each injection and discard it. This will prevent contamination as well as leakage, re-entry of air and potential needle clogs. Needles must not be reused.

(a) Hold the pen firmly by the transparent insulin reservoir (D). Replace the inner needle cap (K) onto the needle (J) to avoid injuries. Unscrew the needle by turning the needle hub (that part of the needle not protected by the cap) anticlockwise (Figure 5). Dispose of the used needle safely.

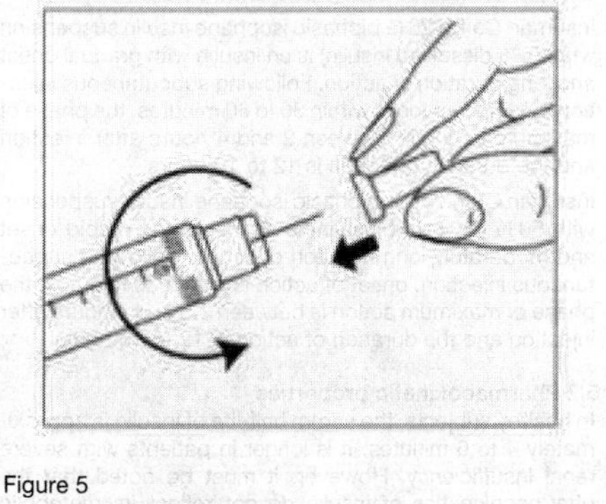

Figure 5

(b) Now replace the pen cap (H) on the pen.

SUBSEQUENT INJECTIONS

(a) Affix a new needle for each injection. To ensure that the insulin suspension is uniformly mixed, gently tilt the pen back and forth (at least ten times) (see also above).

(b) If the same dose is required every time, then the dose arrow can be left pointing at the same position on the dosage selector (B). To deliver an injection, you need only pull the button out as far as it will go, then pushing it home.

(c) If you need to change the dose, please follow precisely the steps described under "Setting and injecting the first insulin dose" above.

Note:

The residual insulin scale (E) on the transparent insulin reservoir (D) shows you whether the volume remaining is sufficient for your next injection.

The residual insulin scale (E) is intended solely to enable you to estimate the remaining insulin volume in the pen. This scale must not be used to set the insulin dose.

If the black plunger (G) is at the 40 mark at the beginning of the coloured bar (F), then the insulin volume remaining is approx. 40 IU. The end of the coloured bar indicates that the pen still contains approx. 20 IU insulin. If the plunger has already advanced beyond the end of the coloured bar, then less than 20 IU remain in the pen (Figure 6a).

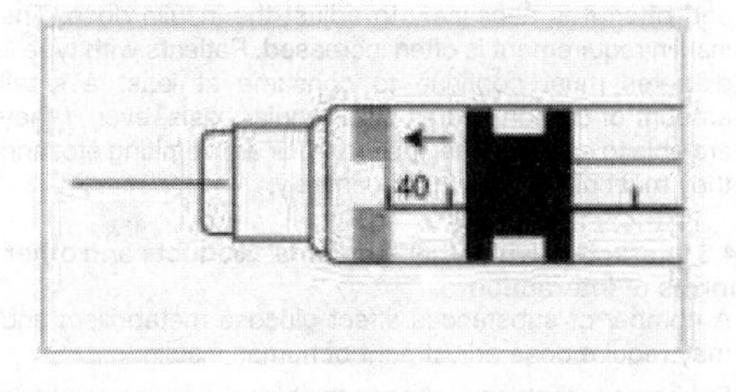

Figure 6a

Button (A) enables you to make a further check: it can only be pulled out as far as the stop indicating the amount of insulin remaining in the reservoir.

Example:

If you have set the dose arrow (C) to 20 IU and button (A) can only be pulled out to the stop for 12 IU, then only 12 IU insulin can be injected with this pen (Figure 6b).

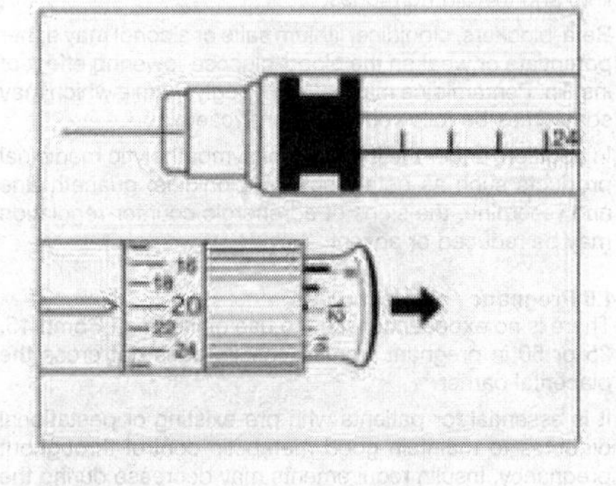

Figure 6b

In this example, either the other 8 IU will have to be injected using a new pen, or the entire 20 IU dose will have to be injected using a new pen.

General Note

The insulin in the OptiSet is distinguished by the international Insulin Colour Code on the button (I) and the coloured bar (F) on the insulin reservoir.

7. MARKETING AUTHORISATION HOLDER

Aventis Pharma Deutschland GmbH

D-65926 Frankfurt am Main

Germany

8. MARKETING AUTHORISATION NUMBER(S)

1 vial of 5 ml: EU/1/97/030/033

5 cartridges of 3 ml: EU/1/97/030/035

5 OptiSet pens of 3 ml: EU/1/97/030/071

9. DATE OF FIRST AUTHORISATION/RENEWAL OF THE AUTHORISATION

Vial: 11 November 1998 / 22 March 2002

Cartridge: 18 February 1999 / 22 March 2002

OptiSet: 20 March 2000 / 22 March 2002

10. DATE OF REVISION OF THE TEXT

14/06/2001

11. Legal Category

POM

Insuman Comb 15, 25 and 50 (100 IU/ml)

(sanofi-aventis)

1. NAME OF THE MEDICINAL PRODUCT

Insuman® Comb 15 100 IU/ml OptiSet® suspension for injection ▼

Insuman® Comb 25 100 IU/ml suspension for injection in a vial ▼

Insuman® Comb 25 100 IU/ml suspension for injection in a cartridge ▼

Insuman® Comb 25 100 IU/ml OptiSet® suspension for injection ▼

Insuman® Comb 50 100 IU/ml suspension for injection in a cartridge ▼

Insuman® Comb 50 100 IU/ml OptiSet® suspension for injection ▼

2. QUALITATIVE AND QUANTITATIVE COMPOSITION

Insuman Comb 15 is a biphasic isophane insulin suspension consisting of 15% dissolved insulin and 85% crystalline protamine insulin.

Insuman Comb 25 is a biphasic isophane insulin suspension consisting of 25% dissolved insulin and 75% crystalline protamine insulin.

Insuman Comb 50 is a biphasic isophane insulin suspension consisting of 50% dissolved insulin and 50% crystalline protamine insulin.

Each ml of Insuman Comb 15, 25 or 50 contains 100 IU of the active substance insulin human.

Each vial contains 5 ml, equivalent to 500 IU insulin.

Each cartridge contains 3 ml, equivalent to 300 IU insulin.

Insuman Comb 15, 25 or 50 OptiSet is a pre-filled disposable pen. Each pen contains 3 ml, equivalent to 300 IU insulin.

One IU (International Unit) corresponds to 0.035 mg of anhydrous human insulin.

The human insulin in Insuman Comb 15, 25 or 50 is produced by recombinant DNA technology using K 12 strains of *Escherichia coli*.

For excipients, see section 6.1.

3. PHARMACEUTICAL FORM

Suspension for injection in a vial, cartridge or pre-filled disposable pen.

4. CLINICAL PARTICULARS

4.1 Therapeutic indications

Diabetes mellitus where treatment with insulin is required.

4.2 Posology and method of administration

The desired blood glucose levels, the insulin preparations to be used and the insulin dosage (doses and timings) must be determined individually and adjusted to suit the patient's diet, physical activity and life-style.

Daily doses and timing of administration

There are no fixed rules for insulin dosage. However, the average insulin requirement is often 0.5 to 1.0 IU per kg body weight per day. The basal metabolic requirement is 40% to 60% of the total daily requirement.

Insuman Comb 15 and 25 are injected subcutaneously 30 to 45 minutes before a meal.

Insuman Comb 50 is injected subcutaneously 20 to 30 minutes before a meal.

Insuman Comb 15, 25 or 50 OptiSet delivers insulin in increments of 2 IU up to a maximum single dose of 40 IU.

Transfer to Insuman Comb 15, 25 or 50

Dosage adjustment may be necessary when transferring patients from one insulin preparation to another. This applies, for example, when transferring from:

- an animal insulin (especially a bovine insulin) to human insulin,
- one human insulin preparation to another,
- a regimen with only regular insulin to one with a longer-acting insulin.

The need to adjust (e.g. reduce) the dose may become evident immediately after transfer. Alternatively, it may emerge gradually over a period of several weeks.

Following transfer from an animal insulin to human insulin, dosage reduction may be required in particular in patients who

- were previously already controlled on rather low blood glucose levels,
- have a tendency to hypoglycaemia,
- previously required high insulin doses due to the presence of insulin antibodies.

Close metabolic monitoring is recommended during the transition and in the initial weeks thereafter. In patients who require high insulin doses because of the presence of insulin antibodies, transfer under medical supervision in a hospital or similar setting must be considered.

Secondary dose adjustment

Improved metabolic control may result in increased insulin sensitivity, leading to a reduced insulin requirement. Dose adjustment may also be required, for example, if

- the patient's weight changes,

- the patient's life-style changes,

- other circumstances arise that may promote an increased susceptibility to hypo- or hyperglycaemia (see section 4.4).

Use in specific patient groups

In patients with hepatic or renal impairment as well as in the elderly, insulin requirements may be diminished (see section 4.4).

Administration

Vial: Insuman Comb 25 contains 100 IU of insulin per ml suspension. Only syringes designed for this strength of insulin (100 IU per ml) are to be used. The syringes must not contain any other medicinal product or residue (e.g. traces of heparin).

Cartridges: Insuman Comb 25 or 50 in cartridges has been developed for use in the OptiPen® series. For further details on handling, see section 6.6.

OptiSet: Insuman Comb 15, 25 or 50 OptiSet is a pre-filled disposable pen. For handling of the pen, see section 6.6.

Insuman Comb 15, 25 or 50 is administered subcutaneously. Insuman Comb 15, 25 or 50 must never be injected intravenously.

Insulin absorption and hence the blood glucose lowering effect of a dose may vary from one injection area to another (e.g. the abdominal wall compared with the thigh). Injection sites within an injection area must be rotated from one injection to the next.

Mixing of insulins

Insuman Comb 25 or 50 vials or cartridges may be mixed with all Aventis Pharma human insulins, but NOT with those designed specifically for use in insulin pumps. Insuman Comb 15, 25 or 50 must also NOT be mixed with insulins of animal origin or with insulin analogues.

Insuman Comb 15, 25 or 50 OptiSet must not be mixed with any other insulin or with insulin analogues.

4.3 Contraindications

Hypersensitivity to the active substance or to any of the excipients (see section 6.1).

Insuman Comb 15, 25 or 50 must not be administered intravenously and must not be used in infusion pumps or external or implanted insulin pumps.

4.4 Special warnings and special precautions for use

Patients hypersensitive to Insuman Comb 15, 25 or 50 for whom no better tolerated preparation is available must only continue treatment under close medical supervision and – where necessary – in conjunction with anti-allergic treatment.

In patients with an allergy to animal insulin intradermal skin testing is recommended prior to a transfer to Insuman Comb 15, 25 or 50, since they may experience immunological cross-reactions.

In patients with renal impairment, insulin requirements may be diminished due to reduced insulin metabolism. In the elderly, progressive deterioration of renal function may lead to a steady decrease in insulin requirements.

In patients with severe hepatic impairment, insulin requirements may be diminished due to reduced capacity for gluconeogenesis and reduced insulin metabolism.

In case of insufficient glucose control or a tendency to hyper- or hypoglycaemic episodes, the patient's adherence to the prescribed treatment regimen, injection sites and proper injection technique and all other relevant factors must be reviewed before dose adjustment is considered.

Hypoglycaemia

Hypoglycaemia may occur if the insulin dose is too high in relation to the insulin requirement.

Particular caution should be exercised, and intensified blood glucose monitoring is advisable in patients in whom hypoglycaemic episodes might be of particular clinical relevance, such as in patients with significant stenoses of the coronary arteries or of the blood vessels supplying the brain (risk of cardiac or cerebral complications of hypoglycaemia) as well as in patients with proliferative retinopathy, particularly if not treated with photocoagulation (risk of transient amaurosis following hypoglycaemia).

Patients should be aware of circumstances where warning symptoms of hypoglycaemia are diminished. The warning symptoms of hypoglycaemia may be changed, be less pronounced or be absent in certain risk groups. These include patients:

- in whom glycaemic control is markedly improved,
- in whom hypoglycaemia develops gradually,
- who are elderly,
- in whom an autonomic neuropathy is present,
- with a long history of diabetes,
- suffering from a psychiatric illness,
- receiving concurrent treatment with certain other medicinal products (see section 4.5).

Such situations may result in severe hypoglycaemia (and possibly loss of consciousness) prior to the patient's awareness of hypoglycaemia.

If normal or decreased values for glycated haemoglobin are noted, the possibility of recurrent, unrecognised (especially nocturnal) episodes of hypoglycaemia must be considered.

Adherence of the patient to the dosage and dietary regimen, correct insulin administration and awareness of hypoglycaemia symptoms are essential to reduce the risk of hypoglycaemia. Factors increasing the susceptibility to hypoglycaemia require particularly close monitoring and may necessitate dose adjustment. These include:

- change in the injection area,
- improved insulin sensitivity (by, e.g., removal of stress factors),
- unaccustomed, increased or prolonged physical activity,
- intercurrent illness (e.g. vomiting, diarrhoea),
- inadequate food intake,
- missed meals,
- alcohol consumption,
- certain uncompensated endocrine disorders (e.g. in hypothyroidism and in anterior pituitary or adrenocortical insufficiency),
- concomitant treatment with certain other medicinal products.

Intercurrent illness

Intercurrent illness requires intensified metabolic monitoring. In many cases, urine tests for ketones are indicated, and often it is necessary to adjust the insulin dose. The insulin requirement is often increased. Patients with type 1 diabetes must continue to consume at least a small amount of carbohydrates on a regular basis, even if they are able to eat only little or no food, or are vomiting etc. and they must never omit insulin entirely.

4.5 Interaction with other medicinal products and other forms of Interaction

A number of substances affect glucose metabolism and may require dose adjustment of human insulin.

Substances that may enhance the blood-glucose-lowering effect and increase susceptibility to hypoglycaemia include oral antidiabetic agents, ACE inhibitors, disopyramide, fibrates, fluoxetine, MAO inhibitors, pentoxifylline, propoxyphene, salicylates and sulphonamide antibiotics.

Substances that may reduce the blood-glucose-lowering effect include corticosteroids, danazol, diazoxide, diuretics, glucagon, isoniazid, oestrogens and progestogens, phenothiazine derivatives, somatropin, sympathomimetic agents (e.g. epinephrine [adrenaline], salbutamol, terbutaline) and thyroid hormones.

Beta-blockers, clonidine, lithium salts or alcohol may either potentiate or weaken the blood-glucose-lowering effect of insulin. Pentamidine may cause hypoglycaemia which may sometimes be followed by hyperglycaemia.

In addition, under the influence of sympatholytic medicinal products such as beta-blockers, clonidine, guanethidine and reserpine, the signs of adrenergic counter-regulation may be reduced or absent.

4.6 Pregnancy and lactation

There is no experience with the use of Insuman Comb 15, 25 or 50 in pregnant women. Insulin does not cross the placental barrier.

It is essential for patients with pre-existing or gestational diabetes to maintain good metabolic control throughout pregnancy. Insulin requirements may decrease during the first trimester and generally increase during the second and third trimesters. Immediately after delivery, insulin requirements decline rapidly (increased risk of hypoglycaemia). Careful monitoring of glucose control is essential.

There are no restrictions on the use of Insuman Comb 15, 25 or 50 in breast-feeding women. Lactating women may require adjustments in insulin dose and diet.

4.7 Effects on ability to drive and use machines

The patient's ability to concentrate and react may be impaired as a result of hypoglycaemia or hyperglycaemia or, for example, as a result of visual impairment. This may constitute a risk in situations where these abilities are of special importance (e.g. driving a car or operating machinery).

Patients should be advised to take precautions to avoid hypoglycaemia whilst driving. This is particularly important in those who have reduced or absent awareness of the warning symptoms of hypoglycaemia or have frequent episodes of hypoglycaemia. It should be considered whether it is advisable to drive or operate machinery in these circumstances.

4.8 Undesirable effects

Hypoglycaemia

Hypoglycaemia, in general the most frequent undesirable effect of insulin therapy, may occur if the insulin dose is too high in relation to the insulin requirement. Severe hypoglycaemic attacks, especially if recurrent, may lead to neurological damage. Prolonged or severe hypoglycaemic episodes may be life-threatening.

In many patients, the signs and symptoms of neuroglycopenia are preceded by signs of adrenergic counter-regulation. Generally, the greater and more rapid the decline in blood glucose, the more marked is the phenomenon of counter-regulation and its symptoms.

Eyes

A marked change in glycaemic control may cause temporary visual impairment, due to temporary alteration in the turgidity and refractive index of the lens.

Long-term improved glycaemic control decreases the risk of progression of diabetic retinopathy. However, intensification of insulin therapy with abrupt improvement in glycaemic control may be associated with temporary worsening of diabetic retinopathy. In patients with proliferative retinopathy, particularly if not treated with photocoagulation, severe hypoglycaemic episodes may result in transient amaurosis.

Lipodystrophy

As with any insulin therapy, lipodystrophy may occur at the injection site and delay local insulin absorption. Continuous rotation of the injection site within the given injection area may help to reduce or prevent these reactions.

Injection site and allergic reactions

In rare cases mild reactions at the injection site may occur. Such reactions include redness, pain, itching, hives, swelling, or inflammation. Most minor reactions to insulins at the injection site usually resolve in a few days to a few weeks.

Immediate-type allergic reactions to insulin are very rare. Such reactions to insulin or the excipients may, for example, be associated with generalised skin reactions, angiooedema, bronchospasm, hypotension and shock, and may be life-threatening.

Other reactions

Insulin administration may cause insulin antibodies to form. In rare cases, the presence of such insulin antibodies may necessitate adjustment of the insulin dose in order to correct a tendency to hyper- or hypoglycaemia.

Insulin may cause sodium retention and oedema, particularly if previously poor metabolic control is improved by intensified insulin therapy.

4.9 Overdose

Symptoms

Insulin overdose may lead to severe and sometimes long-term and life-threatening hypoglycaemia.

Management

Mild episodes of hypoglycaemia can usually be treated with oral carbohydrates. Adjustments in dosage of the medicinal product, meal patterns, or physical activity may be needed.

More severe episodes with coma, seizure, or neurologic impairment may be treated with intramuscular/subcutaneous glucagon or concentrated intravenous glucose. Sustained carbohydrate intake and observation may be necessary because hypoglycaemia may recur after apparent clinical recovery.

5. PHARMACOLOGICAL PROPERTIES

5.1 Pharmacodynamic properties

Pharmaco-therapeutic group: Antidiabetic agent. Insulin and analogues, intermediate-acting combined with fast-acting. ATC Code: A10AD01,

Mode of action

Insulin:

- lowers blood glucose and promotes anabolic effects as well as decreasing catabolic effects.
- increases the transport of glucose into cells as well as the formation of glycogen in the muscles and the liver, and improves pyruvate utilisation. It inhibits glycogenolysis and gluconeogenesis.
- increases lipogenesis in the liver and adipose tissue and inhibits lipolysis.
- promotes the uptake of amino acids into cells and promotes protein synthesis.
- enhances the uptake of potassium into cells.

Pharmacodynamic characteristics

Insuman Comb 15 (a biphasic isophane insulin suspension with 15% dissolved insulin) is an insulin with gradual onset and long duration of action. Following subcutaneous injection, onset of action is within 30 to 60 minutes, the phase of maximum action is between 2 and 4 hours after injection and the duration of action is 11 to 20 hours.

Insuman Comb 25 (a biphasic isophane insulin suspension with 25% dissolved insulin) is an insulin with gradual onset and long duration of action. Following subcutaneous injection, onset of action is within 30 to 60 minutes, the phase of maximum action is between 2 and 4 hours after injection and the duration of action is 12 to 19 hours.

Insuman Comb 50 (a biphasic isophane insulin suspension with 50% dissolved insulin) is an insulin with rapid onset and moderately long duration of action. Following subcutaneous injection, onset of action is within 30 minutes, the phase of maximum action is between 1.5 and 4 hours after injection and the duration of action is 12 to 16 hours.

5.2 Pharmacokinetic properties

In healthy subjects, the serum half-life of insulin is approximately 4 to 6 minutes. It is longer in patients with severe renal insufficiency. However, it must be noted that the pharmacokinetics of insulin do not reflect its metabolic action.

5.3 Preclinical safety data

The acute toxicity was studied following subcutaneous administration in rats. No evidence of toxic effects was found. Studies of pharmacodynamic effects following subcutaneous administration in rabbits and dogs revealed the expected hypoglycaemic reactions.

6. PHARMACEUTICAL PARTICULARS

6.1 List of excipients

Protamine sulphate, m-cresol, phenol, zinc chloride, sodium dihydrogen phosphate dihydrate, glycerol, sodium hydroxide, hydrochloric acid, water for injections.

6.2 Incompatibilities

As with all insulin preparations, Insuman Comb 15, 25 or 50 must not be mixed with solutions containing reducing agents such as thioles and sulfites.

It must also be remembered that:

- insulin protamine crystals dissolve in an acid pH range.
- the soluble insulin part precipitates out at a pH of approximately 4.5 to 6.5.

Concerning mixing and incompatibility with other insulins see section 4.2. Care must be taken to ensure that no alcohol or other disinfectants enter the insulin suspension.

6.3 Shelf life

2 years.

Vial: Once in use, the vial may be used for up to four weeks. It is recommended that the date of the first withdrawal from the vial be noted on the label.

Cartridges: Once in use, the cartridges may be kept for up to four weeks. This applies irrespective of whether the cartridges are immediately put into the pen or are first carried as a spare for a while.

OptiSet: Once in use the pens may be kept for up to four weeks. This applies irrespective of whether the pens are immediately used or are first carried as a spare for a while.

6.4 Special precautions for storage

Store at 2°C to 8°C. Keep the container in the original carton. Do not freeze. Ensure that the container is not directly touching the freezer compartment or freezer packs.

Vials: Once in use, do not store above 25°C, and protect from direct heat and light.

Cartridges: Once in use, do not store above 25°C and protect from direct heat and light. When in use (in the pen) do not store in a refrigerator.

OptiSet: Once in use, do not store above 25°C and protect from direct heat and light. When in use, do not store in a refrigerator.

6.5 Nature and contents of container

Vial

5 ml, type 1 colourless glass vial with flanged aluminium cap, chlorobutyl rubber (type 1) stopper and tear-off polypropylene lid.

Each vial contains 5 ml suspension (500 IU insulin human). Packs of 1 vial are available.

Cartridge

3 ml, type 1 colourless glass cartridge with bromobutyl rubber (type 1) plunger and flanged aluminium cap with bromobutyl rubber (type 1) stopper.

Each cartridge contains 3 balls (stainless steel).

Each cartridge contains 3 ml suspension (300 IU insulin human). Packs of 5 cartridges are available.

OptiSet

Disposable pen filled with 3 ml, type 1 colourless glass cartridge with bromobutyl rubber (type 1) plunger and flanged aluminium cap with bromobutyl rubber (type 1) stopper.

Each cartridge contains 3 balls (stainless steel).

Each cartridge contains 3 ml suspension (300 IU insulin human). The cartridges are sealed in a disposable pen injector. Needles are not included in the pack. Packs of 5 pens are available.

6.6 Instructions for use and handling

Vial

Before withdrawing insulin from the vial for the first time, remove the plastic protective cap.

Immediately before withdrawal from the vial into the syringe, the insulin must be re-suspended. This is best done by rolling the vial at an oblique angle between the palms of the hands.

Do not shake the vial vigorously as this may lead to changes in the suspension (giving the vial a frosted appearance; see below) and cause frothing. Froth may interfere with the correct measurement of the dose.

After resuspension, the fluid must have a uniformly milky appearance. Insuman Comb 25 vial must not be used if this cannot be achieved, i.e. if the suspension remains clear, for example, or if clumps, particles or flocculation appear in the insulin or stick to the wall or bottom of the vial. These changes sometimes give the vial a frosted appearance. In such cases, a new vial yielding a uniform suspension must be used. It is also necessary to change to a new vial if the insulin requirement changes substantially.

Mixing of insulins

If two different insulins have to be drawn into one single syringe, it is recommended that the shorter-acting insulin be drawn first to prevent contamination of the vial by the longer-acting preparation. It is advisable to inject immediately after mixing. Insulins of different concentration (e.g. 100 IU per ml and 40 IU per ml) must not be mixed.

Cartridge

Before insertion into the pen, Insuman Comb 25 or 50 cartridge must be stored at room temperature for 1 to 2 hours and then resuspended to check the contents. This is best done by gently tilting the cartridge back and forth(at least ten times). Each cartridge contains three small metal balls to facilitate quick and thorough mixing of the contents.

Later on, when the cartridge has been inserted into the pen, the insulin must be resuspended again prior to each injection. This is best done by gently tilting the pen back and forth (at least ten times).

After resuspension, the fluid must have a uniformly milky appearance. Insuman Comb 25 or 50 cartridge must not be used if this cannot be achieved, i.e. if the suspension remains clear, for example, or if clumps, particles or flocculation appear in the insulin or stick to the wall or bottom of the cartridge. These changes sometimes give the cartridge a frosted appearance. In such cases, a new cartridge yielding a uniform suspension must be used. It is also necessary to change to a new cartridge if the insulin requirement changes substantially.

Air bubbles must be removed from the cartridge before injection (see instructions for using the pen).

The instructions for using the pen must be followed carefully. Empty cartridges must not be refilled.

Insuman Comb 25 or 50 cartridges are not designed to allow any other insulin to be mixed in the cartridge.

If the pen malfunctions, the suspension may be drawn from the cartridge into a syringe (suitable for an insulin with 100 IU/ml) and injected.

OptiSet

Before first use, Insuman Comb OptiSet must be stored at room temperature for 1 to 2 hours and then resuspended to check the contents. This is best done by gently tilting the pen back and forth (at least ten times). Each cartridge contains three small metal balls to facilitate quick and thorough mixing of the contents. Later on, the insulin must be resuspended again prior to each injection.

After resuspension, the fluid must have a uniformly milky appearance. Insuman Comb 15, 25 or 50 OptiSet must not be used if this cannot be achieved, i.e. if the suspension remains clear, for example, or if clumps, particles or flocculation appear in the insulin or stick to the wall or bottom of the cartridge. These changes sometimes give the cartridge a frosted appearance.

In such cases, a new pen yielding a uniform suspension must be used. It is also necessary to change to a new pen if the insulin requirement changes substantially.

Air bubbles must be removed from the cartridge before injection. The instructions for using the pen must be followed carefully (see below). Empty pens must never be reused and must be properly discarded.

To prevent the possible transmission of disease, each pen must be used by one patient only.

The insulin pen must not be dropped or subjected to impact (otherwise, the insulin cartridge in the transparent insulin reservoir may break and the pen will not work). If this happens, a new pen must be used.

A new needle must be affixed prior to each injection. The following needles may be used in conjunction with the OptiSet: Needles designed for the OptiSet or those for which the needle manufacturer has demonstrated suitability for use in OptiSet. The needle is removed after the injection and the pen is stored without the needle. The needle must also be removed before disposal of the pen. Needles must not be reused.

(see Handling of the pen below)

PREPARATION OF THE PEN

(a) Before using your pen for the first time, remove the pen cap (H).

(b) Take a new needle. Use needles designed for the OptiSet or those needles for which the needle manufacturer has demonstrated that they can be used with the OptiSet pre-filled pen. Remove the protective tab (M) from the needle container and affix the needle (J) together with the outer needle cap (L) onto the pen. As you do this, hold the pen firmly by the transparent insulin reservoir (D) (Figure 1).

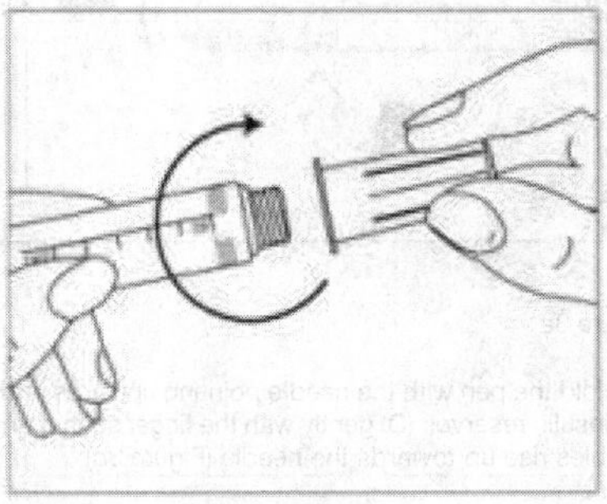

Figure 1

Make sure that you affix the needle carefully. Imprecise affixing (e.g. at a slant) may lead to breakage of the needle or leakage of the injection system, resulting in imprecise dosing.

FUNCTION TEST PRIOR TO FIRST INJECTION

(a) Check to ensure that the dose arrow (C) is pointing to the number 8 (Figure 2).

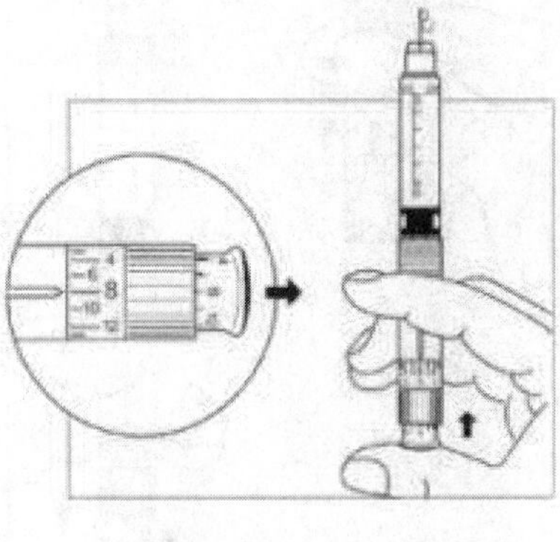

Figure 2

(b) Pull out button (A) as far as it will go, remove the inner and outer needle caps (K+L) and hold the pen with the needle pointing upwards.

(c) With the needle still pointing upwards, press button (A) fully home. Insulin must appear at the tip of the needle; this indicates that your pen is primed for injection. The amount of insulin seen at the needle tip is just the excess from the pen (generally less than 8 units). If no insulin appears, check to ensure that your pen is working properly (follow steps a-c under "Removal of air bubbles/In-use function test") and repeat until a drop of insulin is seen at the needle tip.

Removal of air bubbles/In-use function test Small amounts of air may be present in the needle and insulin reservoir during normal use. You must remove this air. (Small persistent air bubbles in the insulin reservoir do not interfere with the correct dosage.) If your pen has not been used for several days, you should also check that it is working properly and repeat steps a-c given below, after affixing a new needle.

(a) Set the dose arrow to 2 by turning the dosage selector (B). (The dosage selector (B) may be turned in either direction.) Now pull button (A) out as far as it will go. Remove the inner and outer needle caps (K+L) (Figure 3a).

Handling of the pen

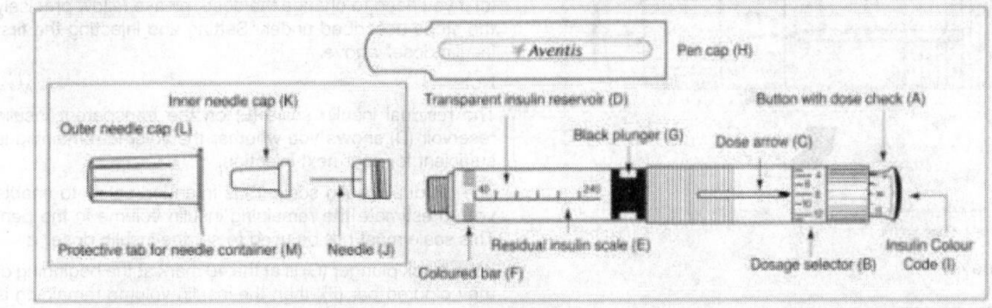

Schematic diagram of the pen

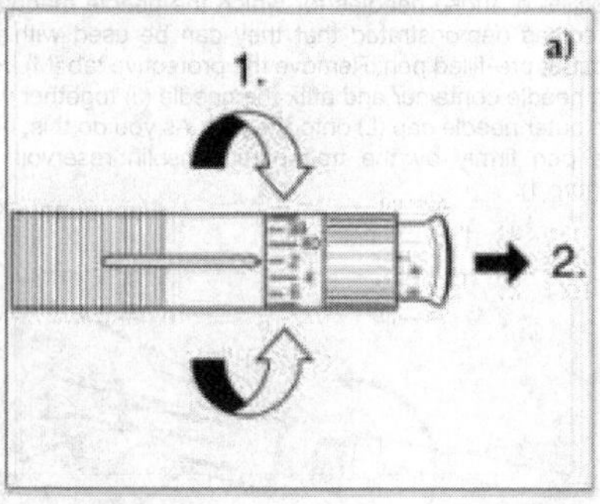

Figure 3a

(b) Hold the pen with the needle pointing upwards and tap the insulin reservoir (D) gently with the finger so that any air bubbles rise up towards the needle (Figure 3b).

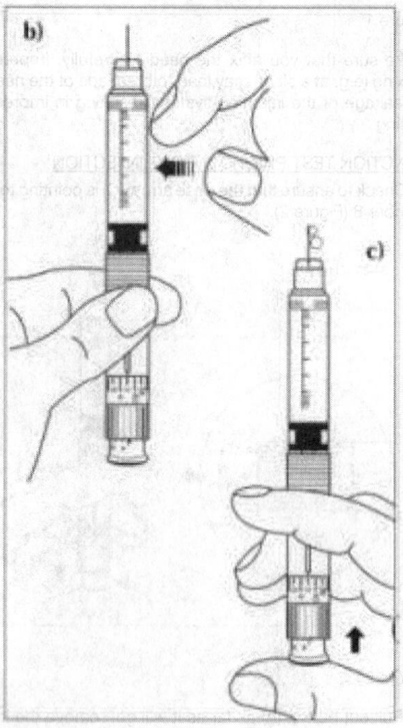

Figure 3b/c

(c) Press button (A) fully home. If insulin appears at the needle tip, then your pen is working properly (Figure 3c).

If no insulin appears at the needle tip, repeat steps a-c until you see an insulin drop at the needle tip.

If no insulin appears at the tip of the needle even after steps a-c have been repeated several times, the needle may be clogged. Please change the needle.

SETTING AND INJECTING THE FIRST INSULIN DOSE

(a) To ensure that the insulin suspension is uniformly mixed, gently tilt the pen back and forth (at least ten times) (see also above). Set the required dose by turning the dosage selector (B) in either direction until the dose arrow (C) is pointing to the dose you require (Figure 4a). (The dosage selector lets you set the dose in steps of 2 units.)

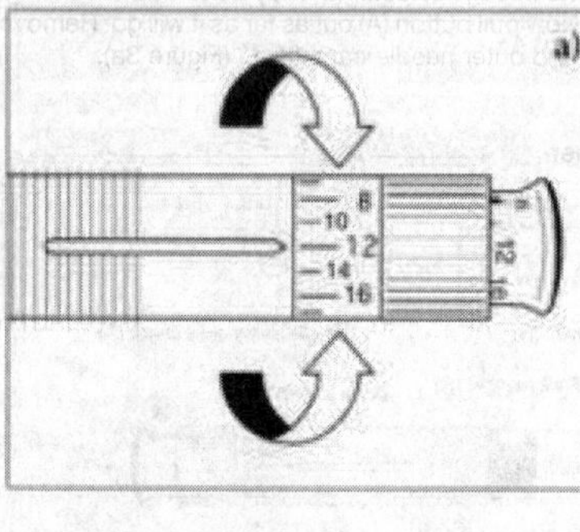

Figure 4a

(b) Once you have set your dose, load it by pulling button (A) out as far as it will go (Figure 4b).

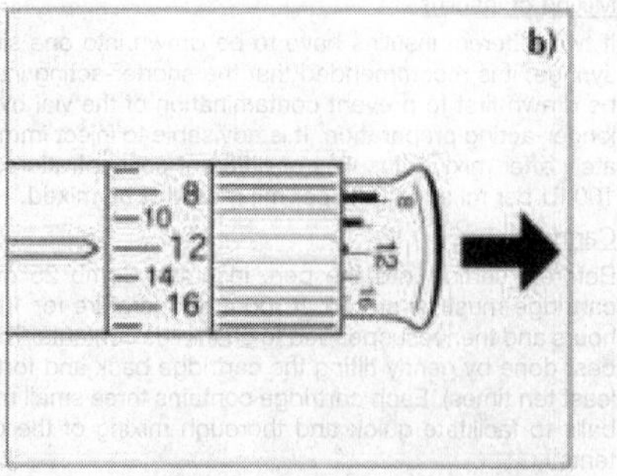

Figure 4b

The button allows you to check the dose: When the button is pulled out, the last thick bar visible indicates the dose that has been loaded (the example in Figure 4b shows the button pulled out and a loaded dose of 12 IU insulin).

(c) Injection: Insert the needle into the skin and press the button completely home (Figure 4c). Allow the needle to remain in the skin for at least 10 seconds (count to 10 slowly). Keep the button pressed down until you have taken the needle out of the skin. This ensures that you have injected the full insulin dose.

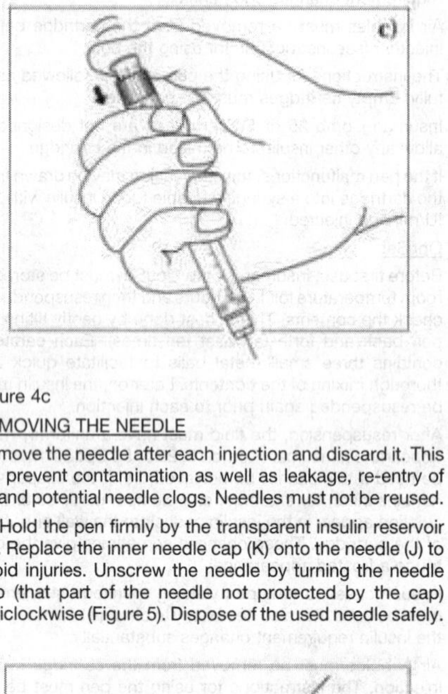

Figure 4c

REMOVING THE NEEDLE

Remove the needle after each injection and discard it. This will prevent contamination as well as leakage, re-entry of air and potential needle clogs. Needles must not be reused.

(a) Hold the pen firmly by the transparent insulin reservoir (D). Replace the inner needle cap (K) onto the needle (J) to avoid injuries. Unscrew the needle by turning the needle hub (that part of the needle not protected by the cap) anticlockwise (Figure 5). Dispose of the used needle safely.

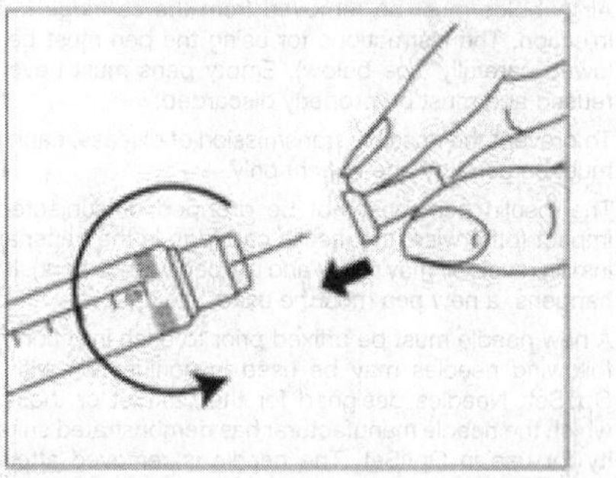

Figure 5

(b) Now replace the pen cap (H) on the pen.

SUBSEQUENT INJECTIONS

(a) Affix a new needle for each injection. To ensure that the insulin suspension is uniformly mixed, gently tilt the pen back and forth (at least ten times) (see also above).

(b) If the same dose is required every time, then the dose arrow can be left pointing at the same position on the dosage selector (B). To deliver an injection, you need only pull the button out as far as it will go, then pushing it home.

(c) If you need to change the dose, please follow precisely the steps described under "Setting and injecting the first insulin dose" above.

Note:

The residual insulin scale (E) on the transparent insulin reservoir (D) shows you whether the volume remaining is sufficient for your next injection.

The residual insulin scale (E) is intended solely to enable you to estimate the remaining insulin volume in the pen. This scale must not be used to set the insulin dose.

If the black plunger (G) is at the 40 mark at the beginning of the coloured bar (F), then the insulin volume remaining is approx. 40 IU. The end of the coloured bar indicates that the pen still contains approx. 20 IU insulin. If the plunger has already advanced beyond the end of the coloured bar, then less than 20 IU remain in the pen (Figure 6a).

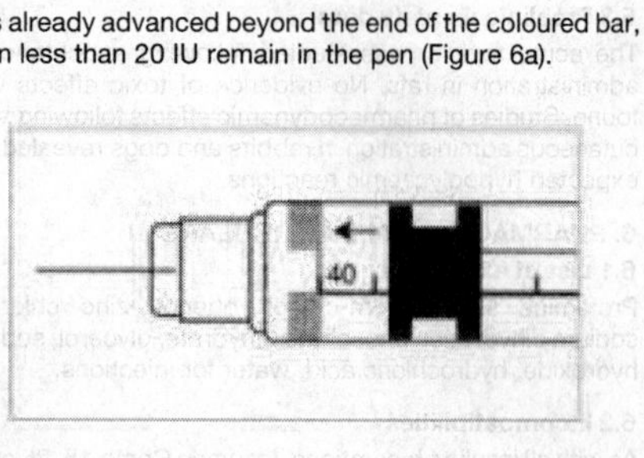

Figure 6a

Button (A) enables you to make a further check: it can only be pulled out as far as the stop indicating the amount of insulin remaining in the reservoir.

Example:

If you have set the dose arrow (C) to 20 IU and button (A) can only be pulled out to the stop for 12 IU, then only 12 IU insulin can be injected with this pen (Figure 6b).

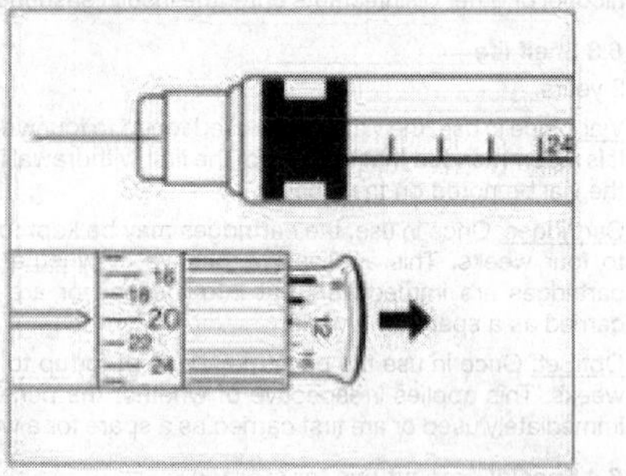

Figure 6b

In this example, either the other 8 IU will have to be injected using a new pen, or the entire 20 IU dose will have to be injected using a new pen.

General Note

The insulin in this pen is distinguished by the International Insulin Colour Code on the button (I) and the coloured bar (F) on the insulin reservoir.

7. MARKETING AUTHORISATION HOLDER

Aventis Pharma Deutschland GmbH

D-65926 Frankfurt am Main

Germany

8. MARKETING AUTHORISATION NUMBER(S)

Insuman Comb 25 100 IU/ml	1 vial of 5 ml:	EU/1/97/030/043
	5 cartridges of 3 ml:	EU/1/97/030/045

Insuman Comb 50 100 IU/ml	5 cartridges of 3 ml:	EU/1/97/030/050

Insuman Comb 15 100 IU/ml OptiSet: 5 OptiSet pens of 3 ml: EU/1/97/030/075
Insuman Comb 25 100 IU/ml OptiSet: 5 OptiSet pens of 3 ml: EU/1/97/030/079
Insuman Comb 50 100 IU/ml OptiSet: 5 OptiSet pens of 3 ml: EU/1/97/030/083

9. DATE OF FIRST AUTHORISATION/RENEWAL OF THE AUTHORISATION

Vial: 11 November 1998 / 22 March 2002

Cartridges: 18 February 1999 / 22 March 2002

OptiSet: 20 March 2000 / 22 March 2002

10. DATE OF REVISION OF THE TEXT

14.06.2001

11. Legal Category

POM

Insuman Rapid (100 IU/ml)

(sanofi-aventis)

1. NAME OF THE MEDICINAL PRODUCT

Insuman® Rapid 100 IU/ml solution for injection in a cartridge ▼

Insuman® Rapid 100 IU/ml OptiSet® solution for injection ▼

2. QUALITATIVE AND QUANTITATIVE COMPOSITION

Insuman Rapid is a neutral insulin solution (regular insulin).

Each ml of Insuman Rapid contains 100 IU of the active substance insulin human.

Each cartridge contains 3 ml, equivalent to 300 IU insulin.

Insuman Rapid OptiSet is a pre-filled disposable pen. Each pen contains 3 ml, equivalent to 300 IU insulin.

One IU (International Unit) corresponds to 0.035 mg of anhydrous human insulin.

The human insulin in Insuman Rapid is produced by recombinant DNA technology using K 12 strains of *Escherichia coli*.

For excipients, see section 6.1.

3. PHARMACEUTICAL FORM

Solution for injection in a cartridge or pre-filled disposable pen.

4. CLINICAL PARTICULARS

4.1 Therapeutic indications

Diabetes mellitus where treatment with insulin is required.

Insuman Rapid cartridges are also suitable for the treatment of hyperglycaemic coma and ketoacidosis, as well as for achieving pre-, intra- and post-operative stabilisation in patients with diabetes mellitus

4.2 Posology and method of administration

The desired blood glucose levels, the insulin preparations to be used and the insulin dosage (doses and timings) must be determined individually and adjusted to suit the patient's diet, physical activity and life-style.

Daily doses and timing of administration

There are no fixed rules for insulin dosage. However, the average insulin requirement is often 0.5 to 1.0 IU per kg body weight per day. The basal metabolic requirement is 40% to 60% of the total daily requirement. Insuman Rapid is injected subcutaneously 15 to 20 minutes before a meal.

Insuman Rapid OptiSet delivers insulin in increments of 2 IU up to a maximum single dose of 40 IU.

In the treatment of severe hyperglycaemia or ketoacidosis in particular, insulin administration is part of a complex therapeutic regimen which includes measures to protect patients from possible severe complications of a relatively rapid lowering of blood glucose. This regimen requires close monitoring (metabolic status, acid-base and electrolyte status, vital parameters etc.) in an intensive care unit or similar setting.

Transfer to Insuman Rapid

Dosage adjustment may be necessary when transferring patients from one insulin preparation to another. This applies, for example, when transferring from:

- an animal insulin (especially a bovine insulin) to human insulin,
- one human insulin preparation to another,
- a regimen with only regular insulin to one with a longer-acting insulin.

The need to adjust (e.g. reduce) the dose may become evident immediately after transfer. Alternatively, it may emerge gradually over a period of several weeks.

Following transfer from an animal insulin to human insulin, dosage reduction may be required in particular in patients who

- were previously already controlled on rather low blood glucose levels,
- have a tendency to hypoglycaemia,
- previously required high insulin doses due to the presence of insulin antibodies.

Close metabolic monitoring is recommended during the transition and in the initial weeks thereafter. In patients who require high insulin doses because of the presence of insulin antibodies, transfer under medical supervision in a hospital or similar setting must be considered.

Secondary dose adjustment

Improved metabolic control may result in increased insulin sensitivity, leading to a reduced insulin requirement. Dose adjustment may also be required, for example, if

- the patient's weight changes,
- the patient's life-style changes,
- other circumstances arise that may promote an increased susceptibility to hypo- or hyperglycaemia (see section 4.4).

Use in specific patient groups

In patients with hepatic or renal impairment as well as in the elderly, insulin requirements may be diminished (see section 4.4).

Administration

Cartridges: Insuman Rapid in cartridges has been developed for use in the OptiPen® series. For further details on handling, see section 6.6.

OptiSet: Insuman Rapid OptiSet is a pre-filled disposable pen. For handling of the OptiSet pen, see section 6.6.

Insuman Rapid is administered subcutaneously.

Insulin absorption and hence the blood glucose lowering effect of a dose may vary from one injection area to another (e.g. the abdominal wall compared with the thigh). Injection sites within an injection area must be rotated from one injection to the next.

Insuman Rapid cartridges may also be administered intravenously. Intravenous insulin therapy must generally take place in an intensive care unit or under comparable monitoring and treatment conditions (see "Daily doses and timing of administration").

Mixing of insulins

Insuman Rapid cartridges may be mixed with all Aventis Pharma human insulins, but NOT with those designed specifically for use in insulin pumps. Insuman Rapid must also NOT be mixed with insulins of animal origin or with insulin analogues.

Insuman Rapid OptiSet must not be mixed with any other insulin or with insulin analogues.

4.3 Contraindications

Hypersensitivity to the active substance or to any of the excipients (see section 6.1).

Insuman Rapid must not be used in external or implanted insulin pumps or in peristaltic pumps with silicone tubing.

4.4 Special warnings and special precautions for use

Patients hypersensitive to Insuman Rapid for whom no better tolerated preparation is available must only continue treatment under close medical supervision and – where necessary – in conjunction with anti-allergic treatment.

In patients with an allergy to animal insulin intradermal skin testing is recommended prior to a transfer to Insuman Rapid, since they may experience immunological cross-reactions.

In patients with renal impairment, insulin requirements may be diminished due to reduced insulin metabolism. In the elderly, progressive deterioration of renal function may lead to a steady decrease in insulin requirements.

In patients with severe hepatic impairment, insulin requirements may be diminished due to reduced capacity for gluconeogenesis and reduced insulin metabolism.

In case of insufficient glucose control or a tendency to hyper- or hypoglycaemic episodes, the patient's adherence to the prescribed treatment regimen, injection sites and proper injection technique and all other relevant factors must be reviewed before dose adjustment is considered.

Hypoglycaemia

Hypoglycaemia may occur if the insulin dose is too high in relation to the insulin requirement.

Particular caution should be exercised, and intensified blood glucose monitoring is advisable in patients in whom hypoglycaemic episodes might be of particular clinical relevance, such as in patients with significant stenoses of the coronary arteries or of the blood vessels supplying the brain (risk of cardiac or cerebral complications of hypoglycaemia) as well as in patients with proliferative retinopathy, particularly if not treated with photocoagulation (risk of transient amaurosis following hypoglycaemia).

Patients should be aware of circumstances where warning symptoms of hypoglycaemia are diminished. The warning symptoms of hypoglycaemia may be changed, be less pronounced or be absent in certain risk groups. These include patients:

- in whom glycaemic control is markedly improved,
- in whom hypoglycaemia develops gradually,
- who are elderly,
- in whom an autonomic neuropathy is present,
- with a long history of diabetes,
- suffering from a psychiatric illness,
- receiving concurrent treatment with certain other medicinal products (see section 4.5).

Such situations may result in severe hypoglycaemia (and possibly loss of consciousness) prior to the patient's awareness of hypoglycaemia.

If normal or decreased values for glycated haemoglobin are noted, the possibility of recurrent, unrecognised (especially nocturnal) episodes of hypoglycaemia must be considered.

Adherence of the patient to the dosage and dietary regimen, correct insulin administration and awareness of hypoglycaemia symptoms are essential to reduce the risk of hypoglycaemia. Factors increasing the susceptibility to hypoglycaemia require particularly close monitoring and may necessitate dose adjustment. These include:

- change in the injection area,
- improved insulin sensitivity (by, e.g., removal of stress factors),
- unaccustomed, increased or prolonged physical activity,
- intercurrent illness (e.g. vomiting, diarrhoea),
- inadequate food intake,
- missed meals,
- alcohol consumption,
- certain uncompensated endocrine disorders (e.g. in hypothyroidism and in anterior pituitary or adrenocortical insufficiency),
- concomitant treatment with certain other medicinal products.

Intercurrent illness

Intercurrent illness requires intensified metabolic monitoring. In many cases, urine tests for ketones are indicated, and often it is necessary to adjust the insulin dose. The insulin requirement is often increased. Patients with type 1 diabetes must continue to consume at least a small amount of carbohydrates on a regular basis, even if they are able to eat only little or no food, or are vomiting etc. and they must never omit insulin entirely.

4.5 Interaction with other medicinal products and other forms of Interaction

A number of substances affect glucose metabolism and may require dose adjustment of human insulin.

Substances that may enhance the blood-glucose-lowering effect and increase susceptibility to hypoglycaemia include oral antidiabetic agents, ACE inhibitors, disopyramide, fibrates, fluoxetine, MAO inhibitors, pentoxifylline, propoxyphene, salicylates and sulphonamide antibiotics.

Substances that may reduce the blood-glucose-lowering effect include corticosteroids, danazol, diazoxide, diuretics, glucagon, isoniazid, oestrogens and progestogens, phenothiazine derivatives, somatropin, sympathomimetic agents (e.g. epinephrine [adrenaline], salbutamol, terbutaline) and thyroid hormones.

Beta-blockers, clonidine, lithium salts or alcohol may either potentiate or weaken the blood-glucose-lowering effect of insulin. Pentamidine may cause hypoglycaemia which may sometimes be followed by hyperglycaemia.

In addition, under the influence of sympatholytic medicinal products such as beta-blockers, clonidine, guanethidine and reserpine, the signs of adrenergic counter-regulation may be reduced or absent.

4.6 Pregnancy and lactation

There is no experience with the use of Insuman Rapid in pregnant women. Insulin does not cross the placental barrier.

It is essential for patients with pre-existing or gestational diabetes to maintain good metabolic control throughout pregnancy. Insulin requirements may decrease during the first trimester and generally increase during the second and third trimesters. Immediately after delivery, insulin requirements decline rapidly (increased risk of hypoglycaemia). Careful monitoring of glucose control is essential.

There are no restrictions on the use of Insuman Rapid in breast-feeding women. Lactating women may require adjustments in insulin dose and diet.

4.7 Effects on ability to drive and use machines

The patient's ability to concentrate and react may be impaired as a result of hypoglycaemia or hyperglycaemia or, for example, as a result of visual impairment. This may constitute a risk in situations where these abilities are of special importance (e.g. driving a car or operating machinery).

Patients should be advised to take precautions to avoid hypoglycaemia whilst driving. This is particularly important in those who have reduced or absent awareness of the warning symptoms of hypoglycaemia or have frequent episodes of hypoglycaemia. It should be considered whether it is advisable to drive or operate machinery in these circumstances.

4.8 Undesirable effects

Hypoglycaemia

Hypoglycaemia, in general the most frequent undesirable effect of insulin therapy, may occur if the insulin dose is too high in relation to the insulin requirement. Severe hypoglycaemic attacks, especially if recurrent, may lead to neurological damage. Prolonged or severe hypoglycaemic episodes may be life-threatening.

In many patients, the signs and symptoms of neuroglycopenia are preceded by signs of adrenergic counter-regulation. Generally, the greater and more rapid the decline in blood glucose, the more marked is the phenomenon of counter-regulation and its symptoms.

Eyes

A marked change in glycaemic control may cause temporary visual impairment, due to temporary alteration in the turgidity and refractive index of the lens.

Long-term improved glycaemic control decreases the risk of progression of diabetic retinopathy. However, intensification of insulin therapy with abrupt improvement in glycaemic control may be associated with temporary worsening of diabetic retinopathy. In patients with proliferative retinopathy, particularly if not treated with photocoagulation, severe hypoglycaemic episodes may result in transient amaurosis.

Lipodystrophy

As with any insulin therapy, lipodystrophy may occur at the injection site and delay local insulin absorption. Continuous rotation of the injection site within the given injection area may help to reduce or prevent these reactions.

Injection site and allergic reactions

In rare cases mild reactions at the injection site may occur. Such reactions include redness, pain, itching, hives, swelling, or inflammation. Most minor reactions to insulins at the injection site usually resolve in a few days to a few weeks.

Immediate-type allergic reactions to insulin are very rare. Such reactions to insulin or the excipients may, for example, be associated with generalised skin reactions, angio-oedema, bronchospasm, hypotension and shock, and may be life-threatening.

Other reactions

Insulin administration may cause insulin antibodies to form. In rare cases, the presence of such insulin antibodies may necessitate adjustment of the insulin dose in order to correct a tendency to hyper- or hypoglycaemia.

Insulin may cause sodium retention and oedema, particularly if previously poor metabolic control is improved by intensified insulin therapy.

4.9 Overdose

Symptoms

Insulin overdose may lead to severe and sometimes long-term and life-threatening hypoglycaemia.

Management

Mild episodes of hypoglycaemia can usually be treated with oral carbohydrates. Adjustments in dosage of the medicinal product, meal patterns, or physical activity may be needed.

More severe episodes with coma, seizure, or neurologic impairment may be treated with intramuscular/subcutaneous glucagon or concentrated intravenous glucose. Sustained carbohydrate intake and observation may be necessary because hypoglycaemia may recur after apparent clinical recovery.

5. PHARMACOLOGICAL PROPERTIES

5.1 Pharmacodynamic properties

Pharmaco-therapeutic group: Antidiabetic agent. Insulins and analogues, fast-acting.

ATC Code: A10AB01,

Mode of action

Insulin:

- lowers blood glucose and promotes anabolic effects as well as decreasing catabolic effects.
- increases the transport of glucose into cells as well as the formation of glycogen in the muscles and the liver, and improves pyruvate utilisation. It inhibits glycogenolysis and gluconeogenesis.
- increases lipogenesis in the liver and adipose tissue and inhibits lipolysis.
- promotes the uptake of amino acids into cells and promotes protein synthesis.
- enhances the uptake of potassium into cells.

Pharmacodynamic characteristics

Insuman Rapid is an insulin with rapid onset and short duration of action. Following subcutaneous injection, onset of action is within 30 minutes, the phase of maximum action is between 1 and 4 hours after injection and the duration of action is 7 to 9 hours.

5.2 Pharmacokinetic properties

In healthy subjects, the serum half-life of insulin is approximately 4 to 6 minutes. It is longer in patients with severe renal insufficiency. However, it must be noted that the pharmacokinetics of insulin do not reflect its metabolic action.

5.3 Preclinical safety data

The acute toxicity was studied following subcutaneous administration in rats. No evidence of toxic effects was found. Local tolerability studies following subcutaneous and intramuscular administration in rabbits gave no remarkable findings. Studies of pharmacodynamic effects following subcutaneous administration in rabbits and dogs revealed the expected hypoglycaemic reactions.

6. PHARMACEUTICAL PARTICULARS

6.1 List of excipients

M-cresol, sodium dihydrogen phosphate dihydrate, glycerol, sodium hydroxide, hydrochloric acid, water for injections.

6.2 Incompatibilities

As with all insulin preparations, Insuman Rapid must not be mixed with solutions containing reducing agents such as thioles and sulfites. It must also be remembered that neutral regular insulin precipitates out at a pH of approximately 4.5 to 6.5.

Concerning mixing and incompatibility with other insulins see section 4.2.

Care must be taken to ensure that no alcohol or other disinfectants enter the insulin solution.

6.3 Shelf life

2 years.

Cartridges: Once in use, the cartridges may be kept for up to four weeks. This applies irrespective of whether the cartridges are immediately put into the pen or are first carried as a spare for a while.

OptiSet: Once in use the pens may be kept for up to four weeks. This applies irrespective of whether the pens are immediately used or are first carried as a spare for a while.

6.4 Special precautions for storage

Store at 2°C to 8°C. Keep the container in the outer carton. Do not freeze. Ensure that the container is not directly touching the freezer compartment or freezer packs.

Cartridges: Once in use, do not store above 25°C, and protect from direct heat and light. When in use (in the pen), do not store in a refrigerator.

OptiSet pens: Once in use, do not store above 25°C, and protect from direct heat and light. When in use (in the pen), do not store in a refrigerator.

6.5 Nature and contents of container

Cartridges

3 ml, type 1 colourless glass cartridge with bromobutyl rubber (type 1) plunger and flanged aluminium cap with bromobutyl rubber (type 1) stopper.

Each cartridge contains 3 ml solution (300 IU insulin human). Pack of 5 cartridges are available.

OptiSet

Disposable pen filled with a 3 ml, type 1 colourless glass cartridge with bromobutyl rubber (type 1) plunger and flanged aluminium cap with bromobutyl rubber (type 1) stopper.

Each cartridge contains 3 ml solution (300 IU insulin human). The cartridges are sealed in a disposable pen injector. Needles are not included in the pack. Pack of 5 pens are available.

6.6 Instructions for use and handling

Mixing of insulins

If two different insulins have to be drawn into one single syringe, it is recommended that the shorter-acting insulin be drawn first to prevent contamination of the vial by the longer-acting preparation. It is advisable to inject immediately after mixing.

Insulins of different concentration (e.g. 100 IU per ml and 40 IU per ml) must not be mixed.

Cartridges

Before insertion into the pen, Insuman Rapid must be stored at room temperature for 1 to 2 hours.

Insuman Rapid must only be used if the solution is clear, colourless, with no solid particles visible, and if it is of a water-like consistency.

Air bubbles must be removed from the cartridge before injection (see instructions for using the pen).

The instructions for using the pen must be followed carefully. Empty cartridges must not be refilled.

Insuman Rapid cartridges are not designed to allow any other insulin to be mixed in the cartridge. If the pen malfunctions, the solution may be drawn from the cartridge into a syringe (suitable for an insulin with 100 IU/ml) and injected.

OptiSet

Before first use, Insuman Rapid OptiSet must be stored at room temperature for 1 to 2 hours. Insuman Rapid must only be used if the solution is clear, colourless, with no solid particles visible, and if it is of a water-like consistency.

Air bubbles must be removed from the cartridge before injection.

The instructions for using the pen must be followed carefully (see below). Empty pens must never be reused and must be properly discarded.

To prevent the possible transmission of disease, each pen must be used by one patient only.

The insulin pen must not be dropped or subjected to impact (otherwise, the insulin cartridge in the transparent insulin reservoir may break and the pen will not work). If this happens, a new pen must be used.

A new needle must be affixed prior to each injection. The following needles may be used in conjunction with the OptiSet: Needles designed for the OptiSet or those for which the needle manufacturer has demonstrated suitability for use in OptiSet. The needle is removed after the injection and the pen is stored without the needle. The needle must also be removed before disposal of the pen. Needles must not be reused.

(see Handling of the pen below)

PREPARATION OF THE PEN

(a) Before using your pen for the first time, remove the pen cap (H).

(b) Take a new needle. Use needles designed for the OptiSet or those needles for which the needle manufacturer has demonstrated that they can be used with the OptiSet pre-filled pen. Remove the protective tab (M) from the needle container and affix the needle (J) together with the outer needle cap (L) onto the pen. As you do this, hold the pen firmly by the transparent insulin reservoir (D) (Figure 1).

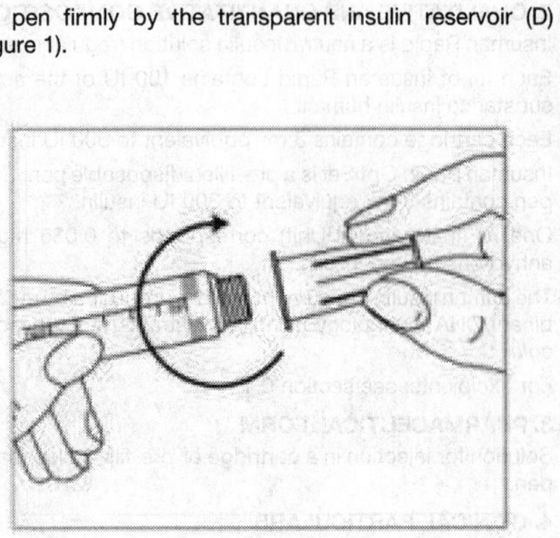

Figure 1

Make sure that you affix the needle carefully. Imprecise affixing (e.g. at a slant) may lead to breakage of the needle or leakage of the injection system, resulting in imprecise dosing.

FUNCTION TEST PRIOR TO FIRST INJECTION

(a) Check to ensure that the dose arrow (C) is pointing to the number 8 (Figure 2).

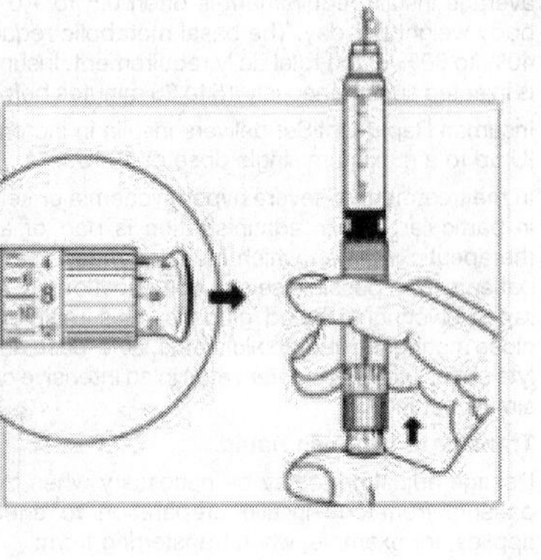

Figure 2

(b) Pull out button (A) as far as it will go, remove the inner and outer needle caps (K+L) and hold the pen with the needle pointing upwards.

(c) With the needle still pointing upwards, press button (A) fully home. Insulin must appear at the tip of the needle; this indicates that your pen is primed for injection. The amount of insulin seen at the needle tip is just the excess from the pen (generally less than 8 units). If no insulin appears, check to ensure that your pen is working properly (follow steps a-c under "Removal of air bubbles/In-use function test") and repeat until a drop of insulin is seen at the needle tip.

REMOVAL OF AIR BUBBLES/IN-USE FUNCTION TEST

Small amounts of air may be present in the needle and insulin reservoir during normal use. You must remove this air. (Small persistent air bubbles in the insulin reservoir do not interfere with the correct dosage.)

If your pen has not been used for several days, you should also check that it is working properly and repeat steps a-c given below, after affixing a new needle.

(a) Set the dose arrow to 2 by turning the dosage selector (B). (The dosage selector (B) may be turned in either direction.) Now pull button (A) out as far as it will go. Remove the inner and outer needle caps (K+L) (Figure 3a).

Handling of the pen

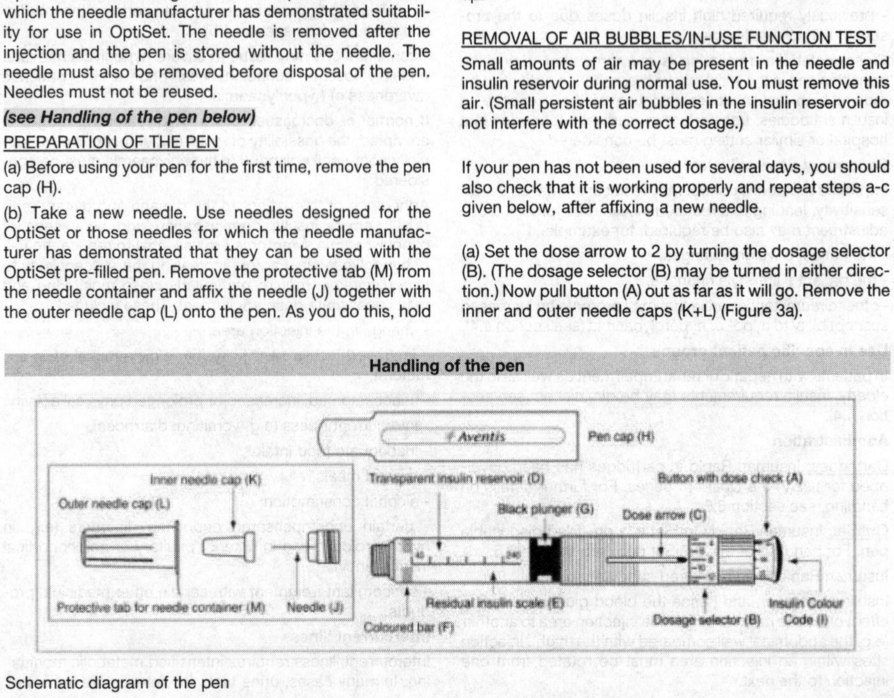

Schematic diagram of the pen

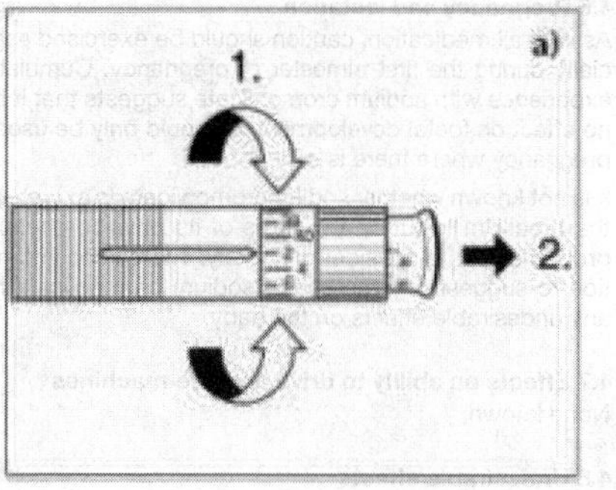

Figure 3a

(b) Hold the pen with the needle pointing upwards and tap the insulin reservoir (D) gently with the finger so that any air bubbles rise up towards the needle (Figure 3b).

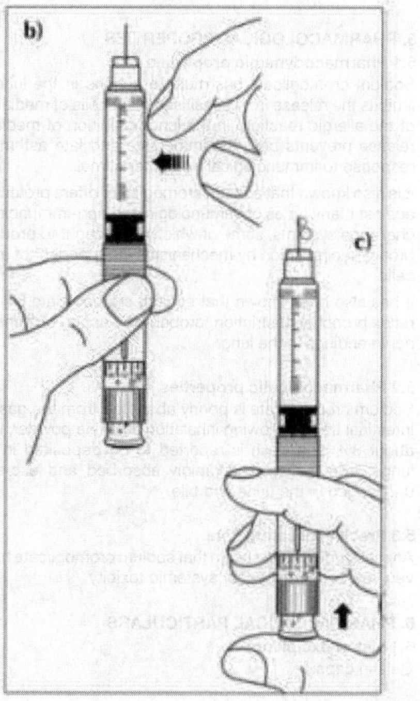

Figure 3b/c

(c) Press button (A) fully home. If insulin appears at the needle tip, then your pen is working properly (Figure 3c).

If no insulin appears at the needle tip, repeat steps a-c until you see an insulin drop at the needle tip.

If no insulin appears at the tip of the needle even after steps a-c have been repeated several times, the needle may be clogged. Please change the needle.

<u>SETTING AND INJECTING THE FIRST INSULIN DOSE</u>

(a) Set the required dose by turning the dosage selector (B) in either direction until the dose arrow (C) is pointing to the dose you require (Figure 4a). (The dosage selector lets you set the dose in steps of 2 units.)

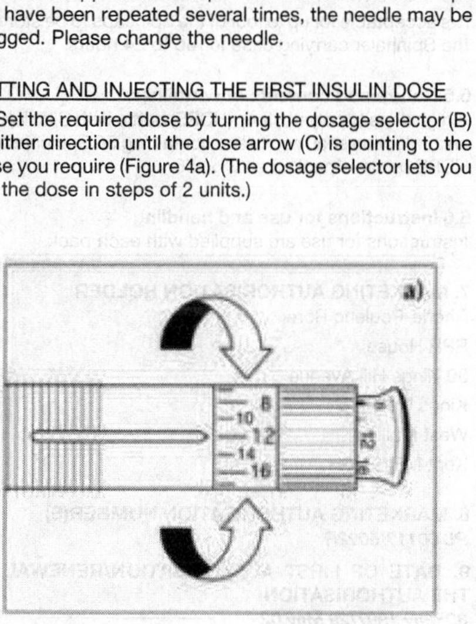

Figure 4a

(b) Once you have set your dose, load it by pulling button (A) out as far as it will go (Figure 4b).

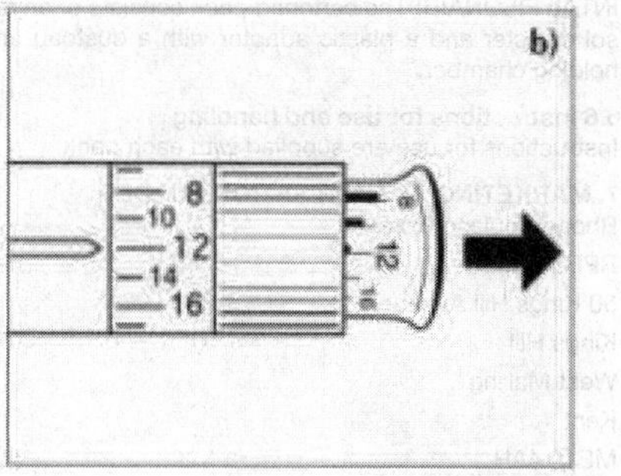

Figure 4b

The button allows you to check the dose: When the button is pulled out, the last thick bar visible indicates the dose that has been loaded (the example in Figure 4b shows the button pulled out and a loaded dose of 12 IU insulin).

(c) Injection: Insert the needle into the skin and press the button completely home (Figure 4c). Allow the needle to remain in the skin for at least 10 seconds (count to 10 slowly). Keep the button pressed down until you have taken the needle out of the skin. This ensures that you have injected the full insulin dose.

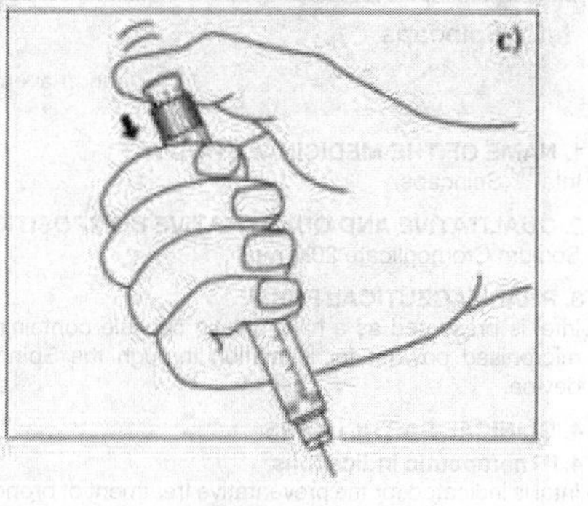

Figure 4c

<u>REMOVING THE NEEDLE</u>

Remove the needle after each injection and discard it. This will prevent contamination as well as leakage, re-entry of air and potential needle clogs. Needles must not be reused.

(a) Hold the pen firmly by the transparent insulin reservoir (D). Replace the inner needle cap (K) onto the needle (J) to avoid injuries. Unscrew the needle by turning the needle hub (that part of the needle not protected by the cap) counterclockwise (Figure 5). Dispose of the used needle safely.

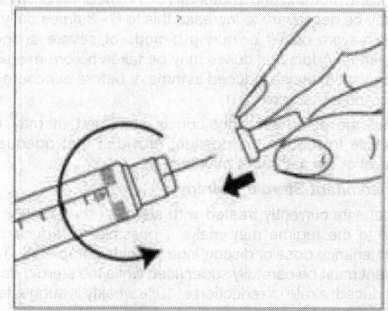

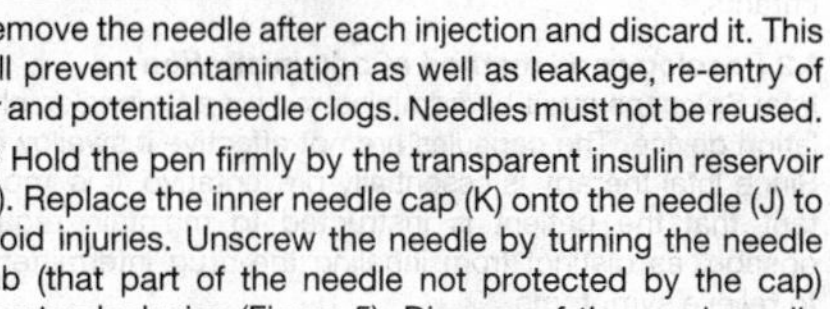

Figure 5

(b) Now replace the pen cap (H) on the pen.

<u>SUBSEQUENT INJECTIONS</u>

(a) Affix a new needle for each injection.

(b) If the same dose is required every time, then the dose arrow can be left pointing at the same position on the dosage selector (B). To deliver an injection, you need only pull the button out as far as it will go, then pushing it home.

(c) If you need to change the dose, please follow precisely the steps described under "Setting and injecting the first insulin dose" above.

Note:

The residual insulin scale (E) on the transparent insulin reservoir (D) shows you whether the volume remaining is sufficient for your next injection.

The residual insulin scale (E) is intended solely to enable you to estimate the remaining insulin volume in the pen. This scale must not be used to set the insulin dose.

If the black plunger (G) is at the 40 mark at the beginning of the coloured bar (F), then the insulin volume remaining is approx. 40 IU. The end of the coloured bar indicates that the pen still contains approx. 20 IU insulin. If the plunger has already advanced beyond the end of the coloured bar, then less than 20 IU remain in the pen (Figure 6a).

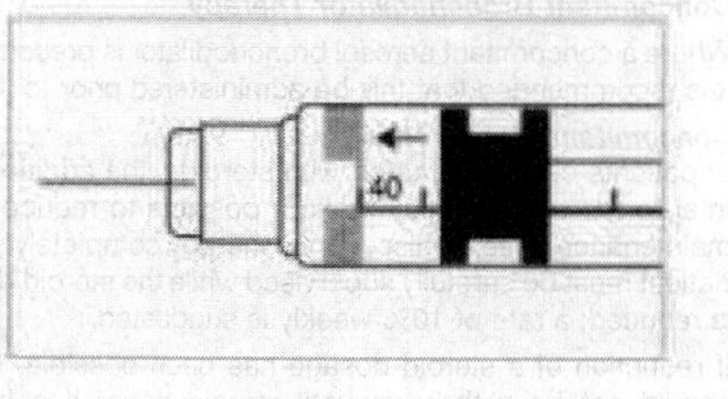

Figure 6a

Button (A) enables you to make a further check: it can only be pulled out as far as the stop indicating the amount of insulin remaining in the reservoir.

Example:

If you have set the dose arrow (C) to 20 IU and button (A) can only be pulled out to the stop for 12 IU, then only 12 IU insulin can be injected with this pen (Figure 6b).

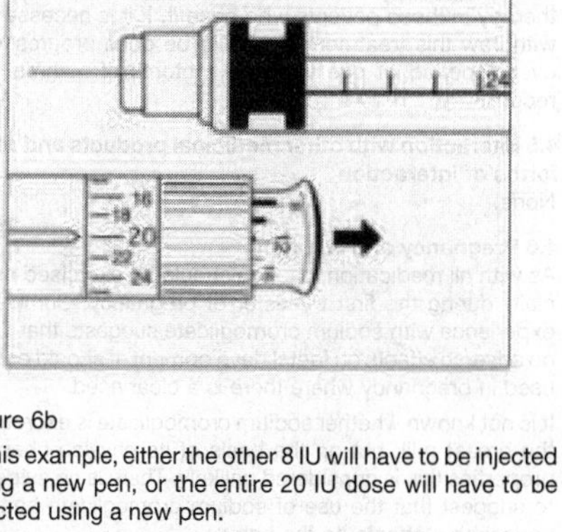

Figure 6b

In this example, either the other 8 IU will have to be injected using a new pen, or the entire 20 IU dose will have to be injected using a new pen.

General Note

The insulin in this pen is distinguished by the International Insulin Colour Code on the button (I) and the coloured bar (F) on the insulin reservoir.

7. MARKETING AUTHORISATION HOLDER

Aventis Pharma Deutschland GmbH

D-65926 Frankfurt am Main

Germany

8. MARKETING AUTHORISATION NUMBER(S)

5 cartridges of 3 ml: EU/1/97/030/030

5 OptiSet pens of 3 ml: EU/1/97/030/067

9. DATE OF FIRST AUTHORISATION/RENEWAL OF THE AUTHORISATION

Cartridge: 18 February 1999 / 22 March 2002

OptiSet: 20 March 2000 / 22 March 2002

10. DATE OF REVISION OF THE TEXT

14.06.2001

11. Legal Category

POM

Intal Fisonair

(sanofi-aventis)

1. NAME OF THE MEDICINAL PRODUCT

Intal™ Fisonair

2. QUALITATIVE AND QUANTITATIVE COMPOSITION

The active component per actuation of Intal is: sodium cromoglicate 5.0 mg

3. PHARMACEUTICAL FORM

Intal is presented as a metered dose pressurised aerosol containing sodium cromoglicate as a suspension in chlorofluorocarbon propellants, for inhalation.

4. CLINICAL PARTICULARS

4.1 Therapeutic indications

Intal is indicated for the preventative treatment of bronchial asthma, in adults and children.

4.2 Posology and method of administration

Adults and Children

The initial dose is two inhalations of the aerosol four times daily. Once adequate control of symptoms has been achieved it may be possible to reduce to a maintenance dose of one inhalation four times daily. However, the dose may be increased to two inhalations six or eight times daily in more severe cases or during periods of severe antigen challenge. An additional dose before exercise may also be taken.

Elderly

No current evidence for alteration of the recommended adult dose.

Concomitant Bronchodilator Therapy

Where a concomitant aerosol bronchodilator is prescribed it is recommended that this be administered prior to Intal.

Concomitant Steroid Therapy

In patients currently treated with steroids, the addition of Intal to the regimen may make it possible to reduce the maintenance dose, or discontinue therapy completely. The patient must be carefully supervised while the steroid dose is reduced; a rate of 10% weekly is suggested.

If reduction of a steroid dosage has been possible, Intal should not be withdrawn until steroid cover has been reinstituted.

4.3 Contraindications

Intal is contraindicated in patients with known hypersensitivity to sodium cromoglicate, sorbitan trioleate or aerosol propellants.

4.4 Special warnings and special precautions for use

Intal must not be used for relief of an acute attack of bronchospasm.

Withdrawal of Intal therapy

Since the therapy is prophylactic, it is important to continue therapy in those patients who benefit. If it is necessary to withdraw this treatment, it should be done progressively over a period of one week. Symptoms of asthma may recur.

4.5 Interaction with other medicinal products and other forms of Interaction

None.

4.6 Pregnancy and lactation

As with all medication, caution should be exercised especially during the first trimester of pregnancy. Cumulative experience with sodium cromoglicate suggests that it has no adverse effects on foetal development. It should only be used in pregnancy where there is a clear need.

It is not known whether sodium cromoglicate is excreted in the breast milk but on the basis of its physico-chemical properties this is considered unlikely. There is no evidence to suggest that the use of sodium cromoglicate has any undesirable effects on the baby.

4.7 Effects on ability to drive and use machines

None.

4.8 Undesirable effects

Mild throat irritation, coughing and transient bronchospasm may occur. Very rarely severe bronchospasm associated with a marked fall in pulmonary function has been reported. In such cases treatment should be stopped and should not be reintroduced.

4.9 Overdose

No action other than medical supervision should be necessary.

5. PHARMACOLOGICAL PROPERTIES

5.1 Pharmacodynamic properties

Sodium cromoglicate has multiple actions in the lung. It inhibits the release from sensitised mast cells of mediators of the allergic reaction. In the lung, this inhibition of mediator release prevents both the immediate and late asthmatic response to immunological stimuli.

It is also known that sodium cromoglicate offers protection against many types of immunologic and non-immunologic challenge systems, some of which are thought to produce bronchoconstriction by mechanisms independent of mast cells.

It has also been shown that sodium cromoglicate inhibits reflex bronchoconstriction, probably by acting on sensory nerve endings in the lung.

5.2 Pharmacokinetic properties

Sodium cromoglicate is poorly absorbed from the gastrointestinal tract. Following inhalation as a fine powder, about 8% of a dose is reported to be deposited in the lungs, from where it is rapidly absorbed and excreted unchanged in the urine and bile.

5.3 Preclinical safety data

Animal studies have shown that sodium cromoglicate has a very low order of local or systemic toxicity.

6. PHARMACEUTICAL PARTICULARS

6.1 List of excipients

Sorbitan Trioleate, propellant mixture of Dichlorotetrafluoroethane (Propellant 114) and Dichlorodifluoromethane (propellant 12).

6.2 Incompatibilities

None known.

6.3 Shelf life

36 months.

6.4 Special precautions for storage

Store below 30°C, not in a refrigerator.

The aerosol canister is pressurised and should be protected from direct sunlight, heat and frost and must not be punctured or burnt, even when empty.

6.5 Nature and contents of container

The aluminium can is fitted with a metering valve which delivers 112 actuations each containing 5 mg of sodium cromoglicate.

INTAL FISONAIR: The cartoned pack consists of an aerosol canister and a plastic adaptor with a dustcap and a holding chamber.

6.6 Instructions for use and handling

Instructions for use are supplied with each pack.

7. MARKETING AUTHORISATION HOLDER

Rhone Poulenc Rorer

RPR House

50 Kings Hill Avenue

Kings Hill

West Malling

Kent

ME19 4AH

8. MARKETING AUTHORISATION NUMBER(S)

PL 00113/0109

9. DATE OF FIRST AUTHORISATION/RENEWAL OF THE AUTHORISATION

9 April 1997

10. DATE OF REVISION OF THE TEXT

August 2004

11. Legal Category

POM

Intal Spincaps

(sanofi-aventis)

1. NAME OF THE MEDICINAL PRODUCT

Intal™ Spincaps.

2. QUALITATIVE AND QUANTITATIVE COMPOSITION

Sodium Cromoglicate 20.0 mg.

3. PHARMACEUTICAL FORM

Intal is presented as a hard gelatin capsule containing a micronised powder for inhalation through the Spinhaler device.

4. CLINICAL PARTICULARS

4.1 Therapeutic indications

Intal is indicated for the preventative treatment of bronchial asthma, in adults and children, which may be due to allergy, exercise, cold air, or chemical and occupational irritants.

4.2 Posology and method of administration

Intal Spincaps must be administered via a Spinhaler inhalation device. The capsules are not effective if swallowed. Since Intal therapy is essentially preventative, it is important that the patient is instructed to maintain regular dosage, as distinct from inhaling the drug intermittently to relieve symptoms.

Adults (including the elderly) and children:

The normal dose is one Spincap four times daily, i.e. one night and morning and at intervals of 3 - 6 hours in between. It may be necessary to increase this to 6 - 8 times daily in more severe cases or during periods of severe antigen challenge. Additional doses may be taken before exertion to prevent exercise induced asthma or before exposure to other trigger factors.

When the asthmatic condition is stabilised, it may be possible to reduce the dosage, provided that adequate control of the asthma is maintained.

Concomitant Steroid Therapy:

In patients currently treated with steroids, the addition of Intal to the regime may make it possible to reduce the maintenance dose or discontinue steroids completely. The patient must be carefully supervised while the steroid dose is reduced; a rate of reduction of 10% weekly is suggested.

An increase in steroid dosage may be necessary if symptoms increase, and at times of infection, severe antigen challenge or stress.

If reduction of steroid dosage has been possible, Intal should not be withdrawn until steroid cover has been re-instituted.

Concomitant Bronchodilator Therapy:

If bronchodilators are used concomitantly, patients may find that the frequency of bronchodilator usage can be reduced as their asthma is stabilised with Intal.

4.3 Contraindications

Intal is contraindicated in patients with known sensitivity to sodium cromoglicate.

4.4 Special warnings and special precautions for use

Intal must not be used for relief of an acute attack of bronchospasm.

Withdrawal of Intal therapy:

Since sodium cromoglicate acts prophylactically, it is important to continue treatment in those patients who benefit. If it is necessary to withdraw Intal, this should be done progressively over a period of one week. Symptoms of asthma may recur.

4.5 Interaction with other medicinal products and other forms of Interaction

None known.

4.6 Pregnancy and lactation

As with all medication, caution should be exercised especially during the first trimester of pregnancy. Cumulative experience with sodium cromoglicate suggests that it has no effect on foetal development. It should only be used in pregnancy where there is a clear need.

It is not known whether sodiumcromoglicate is excreted in the breast milk but on the basis of its physico-chemical properties this is considered unlikely. There is no information to suggest that the use of sodium cromoglicate has any undesirable effects on the baby.

4.7 Effects on ability to drive and use machines

None known.

4.8 Undesirable effects

Mild throat irritation, coughing and transient bronchospasm may occur. Very rarely severe bronchospasm associated with a marked fall in pulmonary function has been reported. In such cases treatment should be stopped and should not be reintroduced.

4.9 Overdose

No action other than medical supervision should be necessary.

5. PHARMACOLOGICAL PROPERTIES

5.1 Pharmacodynamic properties

Sodium cromoglicate has multiple actions in the lung. It inhibits the release from sensitised mast cells of mediators of the allergic reaction. In the lung, inhibition of mediator release prevents both the immediate and late asthmatic response to immunological and other stimuli.

It is also known that sodium cromoglicate offers protection against many types of immunologic and non-immunologic challenge systems, some of which are thought to produce bronchoconstriction by mechanisms independent of mast cells.

It has also been shown that sodium cromoglicate inhibits reflex bronchoconstriction, probably by acting on sensory nerve endings in the lung.

5.2 Pharmacokinetic properties

Sodium cromoglicate is poorly absorbed from the gastrointestinal tract. Following inhalation as a fine powder, only about 8% of a dose is reported to be deposited in the lungs, from where it is rapidly absorbed and excreted unchanged in the urine and bile.

5.3 Preclinical safety data

Animal studies have shown that sodium cromoglicate has a very low order of local or systemic toxicity.

6. PHARMACEUTICAL PARTICULARS

6.1 List of excipients

Gelatin capsule.

6.2 Incompatibilities

None known.

6.3 Shelf life

60 months

6.4 Special precautions for storage

Store in a cool, dry place, protect from light. Intal Spincaps can be adversely affected by moisture ingress. To prevent possible deterioration of this product, it is essential that the cartridges are kept in their containers at all times.

It is acceptable for up to four of the Spincaps to be stored in the Spinhaler carrying case for up to 24 hours.

6.5 Nature and contents of container

A high density polyethylene (HDPE) bottle with Clicklok cap and induction seal membrane containing 56 Spincaps. The HDPE bottle is packed as 2 × 56.

6.6 Instructions for use and handling

Instructions for use are supplied with each pack.

7. MARKETING AUTHORISATION HOLDER

Rhône-Poulenc Rorer

RPR House

50 Kings Hill Avenue

Kings Hill

West Malling

Kent ME19 4AH

8. MARKETING AUTHORISATION NUMBER(S)

PL 00113/5022R

9. DATE OF FIRST AUTHORISATION/RENEWAL OF THE AUTHORISATION

30 May 1997/29 May 02

10. DATE OF REVISION OF THE TEXT

December 2004

11 LEGAL CATEGORY

POM

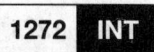

Integrilin 2mg solution for injection, 0.75mg solution for infusion

(GlaxoSmithKline UK)

1. NAME OF THE MEDICINAL PRODUCT
Integrilin 2 mg/ml, solution for injection

Integrilin 0.75 mg/ml, solution for infusion

2. QUALITATIVE AND QUANTITATIVE COMPOSITION
Integrilin solution for injection contains 2 mg/ml of eptifibatide.

Integrilin solution for infusion contains 0.75 mg/ml of eptifibatide.

For excipients, see section 6.1.

3. PHARMACEUTICAL FORM
Solution for infusion and solution for infusion

Both are clear, colourless solutions

4. CLINICAL PARTICULARS
4.1 Therapeutic indications
Integrilin is intended for use with acetylsalicylic acid and unfractionated heparin.

Integrilin is indicated for the prevention of early myocardial infarction in patients presenting with unstable angina or non-Q-wave myocardial infarction with the last episode of chest pain occurring within 24 hours and with ECG changes and/or elevated cardiac enzymes.

Patients most likely to benefit from Integrilin treatment are those at high risk of developing myocardial infarction within the first 3-4 days after onset of acute angina symptoms including for instance those that are likely to undergo an early PTCA (Percutaneous Transluminal Coronary Angioplasty) (see section 5.1).

4.2 Posology and method of administration
This product is for hospital use only, by specialist physicians experienced in the management of acute coronary syndromes.

Integrilin solution for infusion must be used in conjunction with Integrilin solution for injection.

Adults (⩾ 18 years of age) presenting with unstable angina or non-Q-wave myocardial infarction: The recommended dosage is an intravenous bolus of 180 microgram/kg administered as soon as possible following diagnosis, followed by a continuous infusion of 2.0 microgram/kg/min for up to 72 hours, until initiation of coronary artery bypass graft (CABG) surgery, or until discharge from the hospital (whichever occurs first). If Percutaneous Coronary Intervention (PCI) is performed during Integrilin therapy, continue the infusion for 20-24 hours post-PCI for an overall maximum duration of therapy of 96 hours.

Emergency or semi-elective surgery

If the patient requires emergency or urgent cardiac surgery during the course of Integrilin therapy, terminate the infusion immediately. If the patient requires semi-elective surgery, stop the Integrilin infusion at an appropriate time to allow time for platelet function to return towards normal.

Hepatic impairment
Experience in patients with hepatic impairment is very limited. Administer with caution to patients with hepatic impairment in whom coagulation could be affected (see section 4.3, prothrombin time).

Renal impairment
In patients presenting with UA/NQMI (Unstable Angina and non-Q-wave Myocardial Infarction), who may or may not require PCI Integrilin may be administered at the standard dose to patients with mild to moderate renal impairment (serum creatinine between 175 – 350 micromols/l). Experience in patients with more severe renal impairment is limited.

Pediatric use
Safety and efficacy in children and adolescents less than 18 years of age have not been established. Therefore, use in patients less than 18 years old is not recommended.

4.3 Contraindications
Integrilin must not be used to treat patients with:

– evidence of gastrointestinal bleeding, gross genitourinary bleeding or other active abnormal bleeding within the previous 30 days of treatment;

– history of stroke within 30 days or any history of haemorrhagic stroke;

– known history of intracranial disease (neoplasm, arteriovenous malformation, aneurysm);

– major surgery or severe trauma within past 6 weeks;

– a history of bleeding diathesis;

– thrombocytopaenia (< 100,000 cells/mm^3);

– prothrombin time > 1.2 times control, or International Normalized Ratio (INR) ⩾ 2.0;

– severe hypertension (systolic blood pressure > 200 mm Hg or diastolic blood pressure > 110 mm Hg on antihypertensive therapy);

– creatinine clearance < 30 ml/min or severe renal failure;

– clinically significant hepatic impairment;

– concomitant or planned administration of another parenteral GP IIb/IIIa inhibitor;

– hypersensitivity to the active substance or to any of the excipients.

4.4 Special warnings and special precautions for use
Bleeding
Integrilin is an antithrombotic agent that acts by inhibition of platelet aggregation; therefore the patient must be observed carefully for indications of bleeding during treatment (see section 4.8). Women, the elderly and patients with low body weight may have an increased risk of bleeding. Monitor these patients closely with regard to bleeding.

Bleeding is most common at the arterial access site in patients undergoing percutaneous arterial procedures. All potential bleeding sites, e.g., catheter insertion sites; arterial, venous, or needle puncture sites; cutdown sites; gastrointestinal and genitourinary tracts must be observed carefully. Other potential bleeding sites such as central and peripheral nervous system and retroperitoneal sites, must be carefully considered too.

Because Integrilin inhibits platelet aggregation, caution must be employed when it is used with other medicinal products that affect haemostasis, including ticlopidine, clopidogrel, thrombolytics, oral anticoagulants, dextran solutions (see section 6.2), adenosine, sulfinpyrazone, prostacyclin, non-steroidal anti-inflammatory agents, or dypyridamole (see section 4.5).

There is no experience with Integrilin and low molecular weight heparins.

There is limited therapeutic experience with Integrilin in patients for whom thrombolytic therapy is generally indicated (e.g., acute transmural myocardial infarction with new pathological Q-waves or elevated ST-segments or left bundle branch block in the ECG). Consequently the use of Integrilin is not recommended in these circumstances.

Stop the Integrilin infusion immediately if circumstances arise that necessitate thrombolytic therapy or if the patient must undergo an emergency CABG surgery or requires an intraortic balloon pump.

If serious bleeding occurs that is not controllable with pressure, immediately stop the Integrilin infusion and any unfractionated heparin that is given concomitantly.

Arterial procedures
During treatment with eptifibatide there is a significant increase in bleeding rates, especially in the femoral artery area, where the catheter sheath is introduced. Take care to ensure that only the anterior wall of the femoral artery is punctured. Arterial sheaths may be removed when coagulation has returned to normal (e.g., when activated clotting time [ACT] is less than 180 seconds (usually 2-6 hours after discontinuation of heparin). After removal of the introducer sheath, careful haemostasis must be ensured under close observation.

Thrombocytopaenia
Integrilin inhibits platelet aggregation, but does not appear to affect the viability of platelets. As demonstrated in clinical trials, the incidence of thrombocytopaenia was low, and similar in patients treated with Integrilin or placebo. Thrombocytopaenia, including acute profound thrombocytopaenia, has been observed with Integrilin administration (see section 4.8). Platelet counts should be monitored prior to treatment, within 6 hours of administration, and at least once daily thereafter while on therapy and immediately at clinical signs of unexpected bleeding tendency. If the patient experiences a confirmed platelet decrease to < 100,000/mm^3, discontinue Integrilin and unfractionated heparin and monitor and treat the patient appropriately. The decision to use platelet transfusions should be based upon clinical judgment on an individual basis. In patients with previous thrombocytopaenia from other parenteral GP IIb/IIIa inhibitors, there are no data with the use of Integrilin, and thus these patients require close monitoring as noted above.

Heparin administration
Heparin administration is recommended unless a contraindication (such as a history of thrombocytopaenia associated with use of heparin) is present.

UA/NQMI: For a patient who weighs ⩾ 70 kg, it is recommended that a bolus dose of 5,000 units is given, followed by a constant intravenous infusion of 1,000 units/hr. If the patient weighs < 70 kg, a bolus dose of 60 units/kg is recommended, followed by an infusion of 12 units/kg/hr. The activated partial thromboplastin time (aPTT) must be monitored in order to maintain a value between 50 and 70 seconds, above 70 seconds there may be an increased risk of bleeding.

If PCI is to be performed in the setting of UA/NQMI, monitor the activated clotting time (ACT) to maintain a value between 300-350 seconds. Stop heparin administration if the ACT exceeds 300 seconds; do not administer until the ACT falls below 300 seconds.

Monitoring of laboratory values
Before infusion of Integrilin, the following laboratory tests are recommended before treatment to identify pre-existing haemostatic abnormalities: prothrombin time (PT) and aPTT, serum creatinine, platelet count, haemoglobin and haematocrit levels. Haemoglobin, haematocrit, and platelet count are to be monitored as well within 6 hours after start of therapy and at least once daily thereafter while on therapy (or more often if there is evidence of a marked decrease). If the platelet count falls below 100,000/mm^3, further platelet counts are required to rule out pseudothrombocytopaenia. Discontinue unfractionated heparin. In patients undergoing PCI, measure the ACT also.

Patients must be monitored for bleeding and treated if necessary (see section 4.9).

Immunogenicity
Immunogenic response or antibodies against Integrilin have been observed in isolated cases in naïve patients or in rare cases of patients re-exposed to Integrilin. Only limited experience exists for readministration of Integrilin. If treatment with Integrilin is repeated, no diminished therapeutic response is expected.

4.5 Interaction with other medicinal products and other forms of Interaction
Integrilin did not appear to increase the risk of major and minor bleeding associated with concomitant use of warfarin and dipyridamole. Integrilin-treated patients who had a prothrombin time (PT) > 14.5 seconds and received warfarin concomitantly did not appear to be at an increased risk of bleeding.

Data are limited on the use of Integrilin in patients receiving thrombolytic agents. There was no consistent evidence that Integrilin increased the risk of major or minor bleeding associated with tissue plasminogen activator in either a PCI or an acute myocardial infarction study; however, Integrilin appeared to increase the risk of bleeding when administered with streptokinase in an acute myocardial infarction study.

In an acute myocardial infarction study involving 181 patients, Integrilin (in regimens up to a bolus injection of 180 microgram/kg, followed by an infusion up to 2 microgram/kg/min for up to 72 hours) was administered concomitantly with streptokinase (1.5 million units over 60 minutes). At the highest infusion rates (1.3 microgram/kg/min and 2.0 microgram/kg/min) studied, Integrilin was associated with an increased incidence of bleeding and transfusions compared to the incidence seen when streptokinase was given alone.

4.6 Pregnancy and lactation
There are no adequate data from the use of Integrilin in pregnant women.

Animal studies are insufficient with respect to effects on pregnancy, embryonal/foetal development, parturition or postnatal development (see section 5.3). The potential risk for humans is unknown.

Integrilin should not be used during pregnancy unless clearly necessary.

It is not known whether Integrilin is excreted in human milk. Interruption of breast-feeding during the treatment period is recommended.

4.7 Effects on ability to drive and use machines
Integrilin is intended for use in hospitalised patients. There are no data in patients treated with Integrilin outside the hospital setting.

4.8 Undesirable effects
The majority of undesirable effects experienced by patients treated with Integrilin were generally related to bleeding, or to cardiovascular events that occur frequently in this patient population.

At the recommended therapeutic dose, as administered in the PURSUIT trial involving nearly 11,000 patients, bleeding was the most common complication encountered during Integrilin therapy. Administration of Integrilin is associated with an increase in major and minor bleeding, as classified by the criteria of the Thrombolysis in Myocardial Infarction (TIMI) study group.

Bleeding
Minor bleeding was a very common (> 1/10) complication of Integrilin administration (13.1 % Integrilin vs 7.6 % placebo). Minor bleeding was defined as spontaneous gross haematuria, spontaneous haematemesis, observed blood loss with a haemoglobin decrease of more than 3 g/dl, or more than 4 g/dl in the absence of an observed bleeding site. Bleeding events were more frequent in patients receiving concurrent heparin while undergoing PCI, when ACT exceeded 350 seconds (see section 4.4, heparin use).

Major bleeding was also very common (> 1/10) and reported more frequently in patients treated with Integrilin than with placebo, i.e., 10.8 % vs 9.3 %, respectively. Major bleeding was defined as either an intracranial haemorrhage or a decrease in haemoglobin concentrations of more than 5 g/dl (see table 1).

The incidence of severe or life-threatening bleeding events with Integrilin was common (> 1/100, < 1/10); 1.9 % vs 1.1 % with placebo. Integrilin treatment increased the need for blood transfusions modestly (11.8 % vs 9.3 %, placebo).

In the subgroup of patients undergoing PCI, major bleeding was observed commonly, in 9.7 % of Integrilin-treated patients vs 4.6 % of placebo-treated patients.

Other undesirable effects
Overall, in the same trial, serious non-bleeding adverse events were reported at a similar rate in patients treated with Integrilin and those treated with placebo.

Commonly (> 1/100, < 1/10) reported events (occurring in ⩾ 2 % across all groups) in PURSUIT were events related to the underlying disease, such as atrial fibrillation, hypotension, congestive heart failure, cardiac arrest and shock.

Adverse events reported within 30 days of initiation of Integrilin treatment in PURSUIT are reported in Table 1 below. Patients with unstable angina/non-Q wave myocardial infarction (NQMI) [PURSUIT trial] received an IV bolus of 180 microgram/kg followed by continuous infusion of 2.0 microgram/kg/min for up to 72 hours (96 hours if PCI performed).

Table 1. Reported Adverse Events in PURSUIT at 30 Days*

Very common (> 1/10), Common (> 1/100, < 1/10), Uncommon (> 1/1,000, < 1/100), Rare (> 1/10,000, < 1/1,000), Very rare (< 1/10,000)

Adverse Event	Placebo (N=4,696)	Eptifibatide (N=4,679)
Major Bleeding very common	9.3 %	10.8 %
Type or Location of Major Bleeding		
Femoral Artery Access	1.3	2.7
CABG-related	6.7	6.5
Genitourinary	0.3	0.8
Gastrointestinal	0.4	1.5
Retroperitoneal	0.04	0.2
Oral/Oropharyngeal	0.2	1.6
Haemoglobin/Haematocrit decrease	1.5	1.4
Intracranial	0.06	0.1
Minor Bleeding very common	7.6 %	13.1 %
Type or Location of Minor Bleeding		
Femoral Artery Access	1.3	3.3
CABG-related	2.7	2.8
Genitourinary	1.6	3.9
Gastrointestinal	0.8	2.8
Oral/Oropharyngeal	0.3	3.0
Haemoglobin/Haematocrit decrease	1.4	1.4
Any Non-Bleeding Adverse Event	18.7 %	19.0 %
Cardiac disorders common		
Atrial Fibrillation	6.4	6.3
Congestive Heart Failure	5.5	5.1
Cardiac Arrest	2.7	2.3
Atrioventricular Block	1.3	1.5
Ventricular Fibrillation	1.4	1.3
Ventricular Tachycardia	1.1	1.1
Vascular disorder common		
Hypotension	6.2	6.9
Shock	2.5	2.6
Phlebitis	1.5	1.4
Blood and lymphatic system disorders uncommon		
Thrombocytopaenia	< 0.1	0.2
Nervous system disorders uncommon		
Cerebral ischaemia	0.5	0.4

*Causality has not been determined for all adverse events.

Table 2 (below) depicts the incidence of bleeding by TIMI criteria and by invasive cardiac procedures in the PURSUIT trial.

(see Table 2 on next page)

The most common bleeding complications were associated with cardiac invasive procedures (CABG-related or at femoral artery access site). Major bleeding was infrequent in the PURSUIT trial in the large majority of patients who did not undergo CABG within 30 days of enrollment.

Adverse events reported in the ESPRIT trial are listed in Table 3.

Table 3. Reported Adverse Events in ESPRIT *

Very common (> 1/10), Common (> 1/100, < 1/10), Uncommon (> 1/1,000, < 1/100), Rare (> 1/10,000, < 1/1,000), Very rare (< 1/10,000)

Adverse Event	Placebo (N=1,024)	Integrilin (N=1,040)
Major Bleeding common	**(4) 0.4 %**	**(13) 1.3 %**
Type or Location of Major Bleeding		
Femoral Artery Access	0.1	0.8
Genitourinary	0.0	0.1
Retroperitoneal	0.0	0.3
Intracranial	0.1	0.2
Hematemesis	0.0	0.1
Hematuria	0.0	0.1
Other	0.2	0.4
Minor Bleeding common	**(18) 1.8 %**	**(29) 2.8 %**
Type or Location of Minor Bleeding		
Femoral Artery Access	0.9	1.0
Gastrointestinal	0.2	0.1
Hematemesis	0.4	0.6
Hematuria	0.9	1.4
Other	0.2	0.5
Any Non-Bleeding Adverse Event common	**(35) 3.4 %**	**(34) 3.3 %**
Cardiac disorders		
uncommon Atrial Fibrillation	0.3	0.3
Heart Failure	0.5	0.0
Cardiac Arrest	0.4	0.3
Atrioventricular Block	0.1	0.0
Ventricular Fibrillation	0.0	0.1
Ventricular Tachycardia	0.1	0.1
Vascular disorders		
Hypotension	0.2	0.0
Blood and lymphatic system disorders		
uncommon Thrombocytopaenia	0.0	0.2
Nervous sytem disorders		
uncommon Cerebral ischaemia	0.1	0.2

*Causality has not been determined for all adverse events. Bleeding events were reported at 48 hours and non bleeding events are reported at 30 days.

Post-marketing experience:

Blood and lymphatic system disorders

Very rare: fatal bleeding (the majority involved central and peripheral nervous system disorders: cerebral or intracranial haemorrhages); acute profound thrombocytopaenia, haematoma, anaemia.

Immune system disorders

Very rare: anaphylactic reactions.

Skin and subcutaneous tissue disorders

Very rare: rash, application site disorders such as urticaria.

Laboratory values

Changes during Integrilin treatment result from its known pharmacological action, i.e., inhibition of platelet aggregation. Thus, changes in laboratory parameters associated with bleeding (e.g., bleeding time) are common and expected. No apparent differences were observed between patients treated with Integrilin or with placebo in values for liver function (SGOT/AST, SGPT/ALT, bilirubin, alkaline phosphatase) or renal function (serum creatinine, blood urea nitrogen).

4.9 Overdose

The experience in humans with overdosage of Integrilin is extremely limited. There was no indication of severe adverse events associated with administration of accidental large bolus doses, rapid infusion reported as overdose or large cumulative doses. In the PURSUIT trial, there were 9 patients who received bolus and/or infusion doses more than double that specified in the protocol, or who were identified by the investigator as having received an overdose. There was no excessive bleeding in any of these patients, although one patient undergoing CABG surgery was reported as having had a moderate bleed. Specifically, no patients experienced an intracranial bleed.

Potentially, an overdose of Integrilin could result in bleeding. Because of its short half-life and rapid clearance, the activity of Integrilin may be halted readily by discontinuing the infusion. Thus, although Integrilin can be dialysed, the need for dialysis is unlikely.

5. PHARMACOLOGICAL PROPERTIES

5.1 Pharmacodynamic properties

Pharmacotherapeutic group: Antithrombotic agent (platelet aggregation inhibitor excl. heparin), ATC code: B01A C16

Eptifibatide, a synthetic cyclic heptapeptide containing six amino acids, including one cysteine amide and one mercaptopropionyl (desamino cysteinyl) residue, is an inhibitor of platelet aggregation and belongs to the class of RGD (arginine-glycine-aspartate)-mimetics.

Eptifibatide reversibly inhibits platelet aggregation by preventing the binding of fibrinogen, von Willebrand factor and other adhesive ligands to the glycoprotein (GP)IIb/IIIa receptors.

Eptifibatide inhibits platelet aggregation in a dose- and concentration-dependent manner as demonstrated by *ex vivo* platelet aggregation using adenosine diphosphate (ADP) and other agonists to induce platelet aggregation. The effect of eptifibatide is observed immediately after administration of a 180 microgram/kg intravenous bolus. When followed by a 2.0 microgram/kg/min continuous infusion, this regimen produces a > 80 % inhibition of ADP-induced *ex vivo* platelet aggregation, at physiologic calcium concentrations, in more than 80 % of patients.

Platelet inhibition was readily reversed, with a return of platelet function towards baseline (> 50 % platelet aggregation) 4 hours after stopping a continuous infusion of 2.0 microgram/kg/min. Measurements of ADP-induced *ex vivo* platelet aggregation at physiologic calcium concentrations (D-phenylalanyl-L-prolyl-L-arginine chloromethyl ketone [PPACK] anticoagulant) in patients presenting with unstable angina and Non Q-Wave Myocardial Infarction showed a concentration-dependent inhibition with an IC_{50} (50 % inhibitory concentration) of approximately 550 ng/ml and an IC_{80} (80 % inhibitory concentration) of approximately 1,100 ng/ml.

PURSUIT trial

The pivotal clinical trial for Unstable Angina (UA)/Non-Q Wave Myocardial Infarction (NQMI) was PURSUIT. This study was a 726-center, 27-country, double-blind, randomised, placebo-controlled study in 10,948 patients presenting with UA or NQMI. Patients could be enrolled only if they had experienced cardiac ischemia at rest (≥ 10 minutes) within the previous 24 hours and had:

- either ST-segment changes: ST depression > 0.5 mm of less than 30 minutes or persistent ST elevation > 0.5 mm not requiring reperfusion therapy or thrombolytic agents, T-wave inversion (> 1 mm),
- or increased CK-MB.

Patients were randomised to either placebo, Integrilin 180 microgram/kg bolus followed by a 2.0 microgram/kg/min infusion (180/2.0), or Integrilin 180 microgram/kg bolus followed by a 1.3 microgram/kg/min infusion (180/1.3).

The infusion was continued until hospital discharge, until the time of coronary artery bypass grafting (CABG) or for up to 72 hours, whichever occurred first. If PCI was performed, the Integrilin infusion was continued for 24 hours after the procedure, allowing for a duration of infusion up to 96 hours.

The 180/1.3 arm was stopped after an interim analysis, as prespecified in the protocol, when the two active-treatment arms appeared to have a similar incidence of bleeding.

Patients were managed according to the usual standards of the investigational site; frequencies of angiography, PCI and CABG therefore differed widely from site to site and

Table 2 Bleeding (TIMI Criteria) by Procedures in the PURSUIT Trial

	Major		Minor	
	Placebo n (%)	**Eptifibatide n (%)**	**Placebo n (%)**	**Eptifibatide n (%)**
Patients	**4,577**	**4,604**	**4,577**	**4,604**
Overall Incidence of Bleeding	425 (9.3 %)	498 (10.8 %)	347 (7.6 %)	604 (13.1 %)
Breakdown by Procedure: CABG	375 (8.2 %)	377 (8.2 %)	157 (3.4 %)	156 (3.4 %)
Angioplasty without CABG	27 (0.6 %)	64 (1.4 %)	102 (2.2 %)	197 (4.3 %)
Angiography without angioplasty or CABG	11 (0.2 %)	29 (0.6 %)	36 (0.8 %)	102 (2.2 %)
Medical Therapy Only	12 (0.3 %)	28 (0.6 %)	52 (1.1 %)	149 (3.2 %)

Denominators are based on the total number of patients whose TIMI classification was resolved.

Table 4 Incidence of Death/CEC-Assessed MI («Treated as Randomised» Population)

Time	Placebo	Integrilin	p-Value
30 days	743/4,697 (15.8 %)	667/4,680 (14.3 %)	0.034[a]

a: Pearson's chi-square test of difference between placebo and Integrilin.

from country to country. Of the patients in PURSUIT, 13 % were managed with PCI during Integrilin infusion, of whom approximately 50 % received intracoronary stents; 87 % were managed medically (without PCI during Integrilin infusion).

The vast majority of patients received acetylsalicylic acid (75-325 mg once daily).

Unfractionated heparin was administered intravenously or subcutaneously at the physician's discretion, most commonly as an intravenous bolus of 5,000 U followed by a continuous infusion of 1,000 U/h. A target aPTT of 50-70 seconds was recommended. A total of 1,250 patients underwent PCI within 72 hours after randomisation, in which case they received intravenous unfractionated heparin to maintain an activated clotting time (ACT) of 300-350 seconds.

The primary endpoint of the study was the occurrence of death from any cause or new myocardial infarction (MI) (evaluated by a blinded Clinical Events Committee) within 30 days of randomisation. The component MI could be defined as asymptomatic with enzymatic elevation of CK-MB or new Q wave.

Compared to placebo, Integrilin administered as 180/2.0 significantly reduced the incidence of the primary endpoint events (table 4): this represents around 15 events avoided for 1,000 patients treated:

(see Table 4 above)

Results on the primary endpoint were principally attributed to the occurrence of myocardial infarction.

The reduction in the incidence of endpoint events in patients receiving Integrilin appeared early during treatment (within the first 72-96 hours) and this reduction was maintained through 6 months, without any significant effect on mortality.

Patients most likely to benefit from Integrilin treatment are those at high risk of developing myocardial infarction within the first 3-4 days after onset of acute angina.

According to epidemiological findings, a higher incidence of cardiovascular events has been associated with certain indicators, for instance:

- age
- elevated heart rate or blood pressure
- persistent or recurrent ischemic cardiac pain
- marked ECG changes (in particular ST-segment abnormalities)
- raised cardiac enzymes or markers (e.g. CK-MB, troponins) and
- heart failure

ESPRIT trial

ESPRIT (Enhanced Suppression of the Platelet IIb/IIIa Receptor with Integrilin Therapy) was a double-blind, randomised, placebo-controlled trial (n= 2,064) for nonurgent PCI with intracoronary stenting.

All patients received routine standard of care and were randomised to either placebo or Integrilin (2 bolus doses of 180 microgram/kg and a continuous infusion until discharge from hospital or a maximum of 18-24 hours).

The first bolus and the infusion were started simultaneously, immediately before the PCI procedure and were followed by a second bolus 10 minutes after the first. The rate of infusion was 2.0 microgram/kg/min for patients with serum creatinine $\leqslant$ 175 micromols/l or 1.0 microgram/kg/min for serum creatinine > 175 up to 350 micromols/l.

In the Integrilin arm of the trial, virtually all patients received aspirin (99.7 %), and 98.1 % received a thienopyridine, (clopidogrel in 95.4 % and ticlopidine in 2.7 %). On the day of PCI, prior to catheterization, 53.2 % received a thienopyridine (clopidogrel 52.7 %; ticlopidine 0.5 %) – mostly as a loading dose (300 mg or more). The placebo arm was comparable (aspirin 99.7 %, clopidogrel 95.9 %, ticlopidin 2.6 %).

The ESPRIT trial used a simplified regimen of heparin during PCI that consisted of an initial bolus of 60 units/kg, with a target ACT of 200 - 300 seconds. The primary endpoint of the trial was death (D), MI, urgent target vessel revascularisation (UTVR), and acute antithrombotic rescue with GP IIb/IIIa inhibitor therapy (RT) within 48 hours of randomisation.

MI was identified per the CK-MB core laboratory criteria. For this diagnosis, within 24 hours after the index PCI procedure, there had to be at least two CK-MB values $\geqslant 3 \times$ the upper limit of normal; thus, validation by the CEC was not required. MI could also be reported following CEC adjudication of an investigator report.

The primary endpoint analysis [quadruple composite of death, MI, urgent target vessel revascularisation (UTVR) and thrombolytic bail-out (TBO) at 48 hours] showed a 37 % relative and 3.9 % absolute reduction in the eptifibatide group (6.6 % events versus 10.5 %, p = 0.0015). Results on the primary endpoint were mainly attributed to the reduction of enzymatic MI occurrence, identified as the occurrence of early elevation of cardiac enzymes after PCI (80 out of 92 MIs in the placebo group vs. 47 out of 56 MIs in the eptifibitide group). The clinical relevance of such enzymatic MIs is still controversial.

Similar results were also obtained for the 2 secondary endpoints assessed at 30 days: a triple composite of death, MI and UTVR, and the more robust combination of death and MI.

The reduction in the incidence of endpoint events in patients receiving eptifibatide appeared early during treatment. There was no increased benefit thereafter, up to 1 year.

Prolongation of bleeding time

Administration of Integrilin by intravenous bolus and infusion causes up to a 5-fold increase in bleeding time. This increase is readily reversible upon discontinuation of the infusion with bleeding times returning towards baseline inapproximately 6 (2-8) hours. When administered alone, Integrilin has no measurable effect on prothrombin time (PT) or activated partial thromboplastin time (aPTT).

5.2 Pharmacokinetic properties

The pharmacokinetics of eptifibatide are linear and dose proportional for bolus doses ranging from 90 to 250 microgram/kg and infusion rates from 0.5 to 3.0 microgram/kg/min. For a 2.0 microgram/kg/min infusion, mean steady-state plasma eptifibatide concentrations range from 1.5 to 2.2 microgram/ml in patients with coronary artery disease. These plasma concentrations are achieved rapidly when the infusion is preceded by a 180 microgram/kg bolus. The extent of eptifibatide binding to human plasma protein is about 25 %. In the same population, plasma elimination half-life is approximately 2.5 hours, plasma clearance 55 to 80 ml/kg/hr and volume of distribution of approximately 185 to 260 ml/kg. In healthy subjects, renal excretion accounted for approximately 50 % of total body clearance; approximately 50 % of the amount cleared is excreted unchanged.

No formal pharmacokinetic interaction studies have been conducted. However, in a population pharmacokinetic study there was no evidence of a pharmacokinetic interaction between Integrilin and the following concomitant medicinal products: amlodipine, atenolol, atropine, captopril, cefazolin, diazepam, digoxin, diltiazem, diphenhydramine, enalapril, fentanyl, furosemide, heparin, lidocaine, lisinopril, metoprolol, midazolam, morphine, nitrates, nifedipine, and warfarin.

5.3 Preclinical safety data

Toxicology studies conducted with eptifibatide include single and repeated dose studies in the rat, rabbit and monkey, reproduction studies in the rat and rabbit, *in vitro* and *in vivo* genetic toxicity studies, and irritation, hypersensitivity and antigenicity studies. No unexpected toxic effects for an agent with this pharmacologic profile were observed and findings were predictive of clinical experience, with bleeding effects being the principal adverse event. No genotoxic effects were observed with eptifibatide.

Teratology studies have been performed by continuous intravenous infusion of eptifibatide in pregnant rats at total daily doses of up to 72 mg/kg/day (about 4 times the recommended maximum daily human dose on a body surface area basis) and in pregnant rabbits at total daily doses of up to 36 mg/kg/day (about 4 times the recommended maximum daily human dose on a body surface area basis). These studies revealed no evidence of impaired fertility or harm to the foetus due to eptifibatide. Reproduction studies in animal species where eptifibatide shows a similar pharmacologic activity as in humans are not available. Consequently these studies are not suitable to evaluate the toxicity of eptifibatide on reproductive function (see section 4.6).

The carcinogenic potential of eptifibatide has not been evaluated in long-term studies.

6. PHARMACEUTICAL PARTICULARS

6.1 List of excipients

- citric acid monohydrate
- sodium hydroxide
- water for injections

6.2 Incompatibilities

Integrilin is not compatible with furosemide.

There are no data on the use of Integrilin in combination with Dextran.

In the absence of compatibility studies, Integrilin must not be mixed with other medicinal products except those mentioned in 6.6.

6.3 Shelf life

3 years

6.4 Special precautions for storage

Store in a refrigerator (2°C - 8°C). Keep the vial in the outer carton.

6.5 Nature and contents of container

Integrilin 2 mg/ml, solution for injection: One 10 ml Type I glass vial, closed with a butyl rubber stopper and sealed with a crimped aluminium seal.

Integrilin 0.75 mg/ml, solution for infusion: One 100 ml Type I glass vial, closed with a butyl rubber stopper and sealed with a crimped aluminium seal

6.6 Instructions for use and handling

Physical and chemical compatibility testing indicate that Integrilin may be administered through an intravenous line with atropine sulfate, dobutamine, heparin, lidocaine, meperidine, metoprolol, midazolam, morphine, nitroglycerin, tissue plasminogen activator, or verapamil. Integrilin is compatible with 0.9 % sodium chloride solution for infusion and with Dextrose 5 % in Normosol R, in the presence or absence of potassium chloride.

Before using, inspect the vial contents. Do not use if particulate matter or discoloration is present. Protection of Integrilin solution from light is not necessary during administration. Discard any unused material after opening.

7. MARKETING AUTHORISATION HOLDER

Glaxo Group Ltd

Greenford

Middlesex

UB6 0NN

United Kingdom

8. MARKETING AUTHORISATION NUMBER(S)

Integrilin 2 mg/ml, solution for injection: EU/1/99/109/002

Integrilin 0.75 mg/ml, solution for infusion: EU/1/99/109/001

9. DATE OF FIRST AUTHORISATION/RENEWAL OF THE AUTHORISATION

1 July 1999

10. DATE OF REVISION OF THE TEXT

4 January 2005

11 Legal Status

POM

IntronA 18,30 and 60 million IU solution for injection, multidose pen

(Schering-Plough Ltd)

1. NAME OF THE MEDICINAL PRODUCT

IntronA 18, 30 or 60 million IU solution for injection, multidose pen

2. QUALITATIVE AND QUANTITATIVE COMPOSITION

One cartridge contains 18, 30 or 60 million IU of recombinant interferon alfa-2b* in 1.2 ml.

*produced in *E.coli* by recombinant DNA technology.

One ml contains 15, 25 or 50 million IU of interferon alfa-2b.

IntronA 18 million IU solution for injection, multidose pen

The pen is designed to deliver its contents of 18 million IU in doses ranging from 1.5 to 6 million IU. The pen will deliver a maximum of 12 doses of 1.5 million IU over a period not to exceed 4 weeks.

IntronA 30 million IU solution for injection, multidose pen

The pen is designed to deliver its contents of 30 million IU in doses ranging from 2.5 to 10 million IU. The pen will deliver a maximum of 12 doses of 2.5 million IU over a period not to exceed 4 weeks.

IntronA 60 million IU solution for injection, multidose pen

The pen is designed to deliver its contents of 60 million IU in doses ranging from 5 to 20 million IU. The pen will deliver a maximum of 12 doses of 5 million IU over a period not to exceed 4 weeks.

For excipients, see section 6.1.

3. PHARMACEUTICAL FORM

Solution for injection

Solution is clear and colourless.

4. CLINICAL PARTICULARS

4.1 Therapeutic indications

Chronic Hepatitis B: Treatment of adult patients with chronic hepatitis B associated with evidence of hepatitis B viral replication (presence of HBV-DNA and HBeAg), elevated ALT and histologically proven active liver inflammation and/or fibrosis.

Chronic Hepatitis C:

Adult patients:

IntronA is indicated for the treatment of adult patients with chronic hepatitis C who have elevated transaminases without liver decompensation and who are positive for serum HCV-RNA or anti-HCV (see section **4.4**).

The best way to use IntronA in this indication is in combination with ribavirin.

Chidren and adolescents:

IntronA is intended for use, in a combination regimen with ribavirin, for the treatment of children and adolescents 3 years of age and older, who have chronic hepatitis C, not previously treated, without liver decompensation, and who are positive for serum HCV-RNA. The decision to treat should be made on a case by case basis, taking into account any evidence of disease progression such as hepatic inflammation and fibrosis, as well as prognostic factors for response, HCV genotype and viral load. The expected benefit of treatment should be weighed against the safety findings observed for paediatric subjects in the clinical trials (see sections **4.4**, **4.8** and **5.1**).

Hairy Cell Leukaemia: Treatment of patients with hairy cell leukaemia.

Chronic Myelogenous Leukaemia:

Monotherapy: Treatment of adult patients with Philadelphia chromosome or bcr/abl translocation positive chronic myelogenous leukaemia.

Clinical experience indicates that a haematological and cytogenetic major/minor response is obtainable in the majority of patients treated. A major cytogenetic response is defined by < 34 % Ph+ leukaemic cells in the bone marrow, whereas a minor response is ⩾ 34 %, but < 90 % Ph+ cells in the marrow.

Combination therapy: The combination of interferon alfa-2b and cytarabine (Ara-C) administered during the first 12 months of treatment has been demonstrated to significantly increase the rate of major cytogenetic responses and to significantly prolong the overall survival at three years when compared to interferon alfa-2b monotherapy.

Multiple Myeloma: As maintenance therapy in patients who have achieved objective remission (more than 50 % reduction in myeloma protein) following initial induction chemotherapy.

Current clinical experience indicates that maintenance therapy with interferon alfa-2b prolongs the plateau phase; however, effects on overall survival have not been conclusively demonstrated.

Follicular Lymphoma: Treatment of high tumour burden follicular lymphoma as adjunct to appropriate combination induction chemotherapy such as a CHOP-like regimen. High tumour burden is defined as having at least one of the following: bulky tumour mass (> 7 cm), involvement of three or more nodal sites (each > 3 cm), systemic symptoms (weight loss > 10 %, fever > 38°C for more than 8 days, or nocturnal sweats), splenomegaly beyond the umbilicus, major organ obstruction or compression syndrome, orbital or epidural involvement, serous effusion, or leukaemia.

Carcinoid Tumour: Treatment of carcinoid tumours with lymph node or liver metastases and with "carcinoid syndrome".

Malignant Melanoma: As adjuvant therapy in patients who are free of disease after surgery but are at high risk of systemic recurrence, e.g., patients with primary or recurrent (clinical or pathological) lymph node involvement.

4.2 Posology and method of administration

Multidose presentations must be for individual patient use only.

Not all dosage forms and strengths are appropriate for some indications. Please make sure to select an appropriate dosage form and strength.

Treatment must be initiated by a physician experienced in the management of the disease.

If adverse events develop during the course of treatment with IntronA for any indication, modify the dosage or discontinue therapy temporarily until the adverse events abate. If persistent or recurrent intolerance develops following adequate dosage adjustment, or disease progresses, discontinue treatment with IntronA. At the discretion of the physician, the patient may self-administer the dose for maintenance dosage regimens administered subcutaneously.

Chronic Hepatitis B: The recommended dosage is in the range 5 to 10 million IU administered subcutaneously three times a week (every other day) for a period of 4 to 6 months.

The administered dose should be reduced by 50 % in case of occurrence of haematological disorders (white blood cells < 1,500/mm^3, granulocytes < 1,000/mm^3, thrombocytes < 100,000/mm^3). Treatment should be discontinued in case of severe leukopaenia (< 1,200/mm^3), severe neutropaenia (< 750/mm^3) or severe thrombocytopaenia (< 70,000/mm^3).

For all patients, if no improvement on serum HBV-DNA is observed after 3 to 4 months of treatment (at the maximum tolerated dose), discontinue IntronA therapy.

Chronic Hepatitis C: IntronA is administered subcutaneously at a dose of 3 million IU three times a week (every other day) to adult patients, whether administered as monotherapy or in combination with ribavirin.

Children 3 years of age or older and adolescents: Interferon alfa-2b 3 MIU/m^2 is administered subcutaneously 3 times a week (every other day) in combination with ribavirin capsules or oral solution administered orally in two divided doses daily with food (morning and evening).

(See ribavirin capsule SPC for dose of ribavirin capsules and dosage modification guidelines for combination therapy. For paediatric patients who weigh < 47 kg or cannot swallow capsules, see ribavirin oral solution SPC).

Relapse patients (adults):

IntronA is given in combination with ribavirin.

Based on the results of clinical trials, in which data are available for 6 months of treatment, it is recommended that patients be treated with IntronA in combination with ribavirin for 6 months.

Naïve patients:

Adults: The efficacy of IntronA is enhanced when given in combination with ribavirin. IntronA should be given alone mainly in case of intolerance or contraindication to ribavirin.

IntronA in combination with ribavirin:

Based on the results of clinical trials, in which data are available for 12 months of treatment, it is recommended that patients be treated with IntronA in combination with ribavirin for at least 6 months.

Treatment should be continued for another 6-month period (i.e., a total of 12 months) in patients who exhibit negative HCV-RNA at month 6, and with viral genotype 1 (as determined in a pre-treatment sample) and high pre-treatment viral load.

Other negative prognostic factors (age > 40 years, male gender, bridging fibrosis) should be taken into account in order to extend therapy to 12 months.

During clinical trials, patients who failed to show a virologic response after 6 months of treatment (HCV-RNA below lower limit of detection) did not become sustained virologic responders (HCV-RNA below lower limit of detection six months after withdrawal of treatment).

IntronA alone:

The optimal duration of therapy with IntronA alone is not yet fully established, but a therapy of between 12 and 18 months is advised.

It is recommended that patients be treated with IntronA alone for at least 3 to 4 months, at which point HCV-RNA status should be determined. Treatment should be continued in patients who exhibit negative HCV-RNA.

Children and adolescents: The efficacy and safety of IntronA in combination with ribavirin has been studied in children and adolescents who have not been previously treated for chronic hepatitis C.

Genotype 1: The recommended duration of treatment is one year. Patients who fail to achieve virological response at 12 weeks are highly unlikely to become sustained virological responders (negative predictive value 96 %). Virological response is defined as absence of detectable HCV-RNA at Week 12. Treatment should be discontinued in these patients.

Genotype 2/3: The recommended duration of treatment is 24 weeks.

Virological responses after 1 year of treatment and 6 months of follow-up were 36 % for genotype 1 and 81 % for genotype 2/3/4.

Hairy Cell Leukaemia: The recommended dosage is 2 million IU/m^2 administered subcutaneously three times a week (every other day) for both splenectomised and non-splenectomised patients. For most patients with Hairy Cell Leukaemia, normalisation of one or more haematological variables occurs within one to two months of IntronA treatment. Improvement in all three haematological variables (granulocyte count, platelet count and haemoglobin level) may require six months or more. This regimen must be maintained unless the disease progresses rapidly or severe intolerance is manifested.

Chronic Myelogenous Leukaemia: The recommended dosage of IntronA is 4 to 5 million IU/m^2 administered daily subcutaneously. Some patients have been shown to benefit from IntronA 5 million IU/m^2 administered daily subcutaneously in association with cytarabine (Ara-C) 20 mg/m^2 administered daily subcutaneously for 10 days per month (up to a maximum daily dose of 40 mg). When the white blood cell count is controlled, administer the maximum tolerated dose of IntronA (4 to 5 million IU/m^2 daily) to maintain haematological remission.

IntronA treatment must be discontinued after 8 to 12 weeks of treatment if at least a partial haematological remission or a clinically meaningful cytoreduction has not been achieved.

Multiple Myeloma: Maintenance therapy: In patients who are in the plateau phase (more than 50 % reduction of myeloma protein) following initial induction chemotherapy, interferon alfa-2b may be administered as monotherapy, subcutaneously, at a dose of 3 million IU/m^2 three times a week (every other day).

Follicular Lymphoma: Adjunctively with chemotherapy, interferon alfa-2b may be administered subcutaneously, at a dose of 5 million IU three times a week (every other day) for a duration of 18 months. CHOP-like regimens are advised, but clinical experience is available only with CHVP (combination of cyclophosphamide, doxorubicin, teniposide and prednisolone).

Carcinoid Tumour: The usual dose is 5 million IU (3 to 9 million IU) administered subcutaneously three times a week (every other day). Patients with advanced disease may require a daily dose of 5 million IU. The treatment is to be temporarily discontinued during and after surgery. Therapy may continue for as long as the patient responds to interferon alfa-2b treatment.

Malignant Melanoma: As induction therapy, interferon alfa-2b is administered intravenously at a dose of 20 million IU/m^2 daily for five days a week for a four-week period; the calculated interferon alfa-2b dose is added to 0.9 % sodium chloride solution and administered as a 20-minute infusion (see section **6.6**). As maintenance treatment, the recommended dose is 10 million IU/m^2 administered subcutaneously three days a week (every other day) for 48 weeks.

If severe adverse events develop during interferon alfa-2b treatment, particularly if granulocytes decrease to < 500/mm^3 or ALT/AST rises to > 5 × upper limit of normal, discontinue treatment temporarily until the adverse event abates. Interferon alfa-2b treatment is to be restarted at 50 % of the previous dose. If intolerance persists after dose adjustment or if granulocytes decrease to < 250/mm^3 or ALT/AST rises to > 10 × upper limit of normal, discontinue interferon alfa-2b therapy.

Although the optimal (minimum) dose for full clinical benefit is unknown, patients must be treated at the recommended dose, with dose reduction for toxicity as described.

4.3 Contraindications

- Hypersensitivity to the active substance or to any of the excipients

- A history of severe pre-existing cardiac disease, e.g., uncontrolled congestive heart failure, recent myocardial infarction, severe arrhythmic disorders

- Severe renal or hepatic dysfunction; including that caused by metastases

- Epilepsy and/or compromised central nervous system (CNS) function (see section **4.4**)

- Chronic hepatitis with decompensated cirrhosis of the liver

- Chronic hepatitis in patients who are being or have been treated recently with immunosuppressive agents excluding short term corticosteroid withdrawal

- Autoimmune hepatitis; or history of autoimmune disease; immunosuppressed transplant recipients

- Pre-existing thyroid disease unless it can be controlled with conventional treatment

Children and adolescents:

- Existence of, or history of severe psychiatric condition, particularly severe depression, suicidal ideation or suicide attempt.

Combination therapy with ribavirin: Also see ribavirin labelling if interferon alfa-2b is to be administered in combination with ribavirin in patients with chronic hepatitis C.

4.4 Special warnings and special precautions for use

For all patients:

Acute hypersensitivity reactions (e.g., urticaria, angioedema, bronchoconstriction, anaphylaxis) to interferon alfa-2b have been observed rarely during IntronA therapy. If such a reaction develops, discontinue the medication and institute appropriate medical therapy. Transient rashes do not necessitate interruption of treatment.

Moderate to severe adverse experiences may require modification of the patient's dosage regimen, or in some cases, termination of IntronA therapy. Any patient developing liver function abnormalities during treatment with IntronA must be monitored closely and treatment discontinued if signs and symptoms progress.

Hypotension may occur during IntronA therapy or up to two days post-therapy and may require supportive treatment.

Adequate hydration must be maintained in patients undergoing IntronA therapy since hypotension related to fluid depletion has been seen in some patients. Fluid replacement may be necessary.

While fever may be associated with the flu-like syndrome reported commonly during interferon therapy, other causes of persistent fever must be ruled out.

IntronA must be used cautiously in patients with debilitating medical conditions, such as those with a history of pulmonary disease (e.g., chronic obstructive pulmonary disease) or diabetes mellitus prone to ketoacidosis. Caution must be observed also in patients with coagulation disorders (e.g., thrombophlebitis, pulmonary embolism) or severe myelosuppression.

Pulmonary infiltrates, pneumonitis, and pneumonia, occasionally resulting in fatality, have been observed rarely in interferon alpha treated patients, including those treated with IntronA. The aetiology has not been defined. These symptoms have been reported more frequently when shosaikoto, a Chinese herbal medicine, is administered concomitantly with interferon alpha (see section **4.5**). Any patient developing fever, cough, dyspnea or other respiratory symptoms must have a chest X-ray taken. If the chest X-ray shows pulmonary infiltrates or there is evidence of pulmonary function impairment, the patient is to be monitored closely, and, if appropriate, discontinue interferon alpha. While this has been reported more often in patients with chronic hepatitis C treated with interferon alpha, it has also been reported in patients with oncologic diseases treated with interferon alpha. Prompt discontinuation of interferon alpha administration and treatment with corticosteroids appear to be associated with resolution of pulmonary adverse events.

Ocular adverse events (see section **4.8**) including retinal haemorrhages, cotton wool spots, and retinal artery or vein obstruction have been reported in rare instances after treatment with alpha interferons. All patients should have a baseline eye examination. Any patient complaining of changes in visual acuity or visual fields, or reporting other ophthalmologic symptoms during treatment with IntronA, must have a prompt and complete eye examination. Periodic visual examinations during IntronA therapy are recommended particularly in patients with disorders that may be associated with retinopathy, such as diabetes mellitus or hypertension. Discontinuation of IntronA should be considered in patients who develop new or worsening ophthalmological disorders.

Psychiatric and central nervous system (CNS): Severe CNS effects, particularly depression, suicidal ideation and attempted suicide have been observed in some patients during IntronA therapy, and in the follow-up period. Among children and adolescents treated with IntronA in combination with ribavirin, suicidal ideation or attempts were reported more frequently compared to adult patients (2.4 % vs 1 %) during treatment and during the 6-month follow-up after treatment. As in adult patients, children and adolescents experienced other psychiatric adverse events (e.g., depression, emotional lability, and somnolence). Other CNS effects including aggressive behaviour (sometimes directed against others), confusion and alterations of mental status have been observed with alpha interferons. If patients develop psychiatric or CNS problems, including clinical depression, it is recommended that the patient be carefully monitored by the prescribing physicians during treatment and in the follow-up period. If such symptoms appear, the potential seriousness of these undesirable effects must be borne in mind by the prescribing physician. If psychiatric symptoms persist or worsen, or suicidal ideation is identified, it is recommended that treatment with IntronA be discontinued, and the patient followed, with psychiatric intervention, as appropriate.

Patients with existence of or history of severe psychiatric conditions:

If treatment with interferon alfa-2b is judged necessary in adult patients with existence or history of severe psychiatric conditions, this should only be initiated after having ensured appropriate individualised diagnostic and therapeutic management of the psychiatric condition. The use of interferon alfa-2b in children and adolescents with existence of or history of severe psychiatric conditions is contraindicated (see section **4.3**).

More significant obtundation and coma, including cases of encephalopathy, have been observed in some patients, usually elderly, treated at higher doses. While these effects are generally reversible, in a few patients full resolution took up to three weeks. Very rarely, seizures have occurred with high doses of IntronA.

Adult patients with a history of congestive heart failure, myocardial infarction and/or previous or current arrhythmic disorders, who require IntronA therapy, must be closely monitored. It is recommended that those patients who have pre-existing cardiac abnormalities and/or are in advanced stages of cancer have electrocardiograms taken prior to and during the course of treatment. Cardiac arrhythmias (primarily supraventricular) usually respond to conventional therapy but may require discontinuation of IntronA therapy. There are no data in children or adolescents with a history of cardiac disease.

Hypertriglyceridemia and aggravation of hypertriglyceridemia, sometimes severe, have been observed. Monitoring of lipid levels is, therefore, recommended.

Due to reports of interferon alpha exacerbating pre-existing psoriatic disease and sarcoidosis, use of IntronA in patients with psoriasis or sarcoidosis is recommended only if the potential benefit justifies the potential risk.

Preliminary data indicates that interferon alpha therapy may be associated with an increased rate of kidney graft rejection. Liver graft rejection has also been reported.

The development of auto-antibodies and autoimmune disorders has been reported during treatment with alpha interferons. Patients predisposed to the development of autoimmune disorders may be at increased risk. Patients with signs or symptoms compatible with autoimmune disorders should be evaluated carefully, and the benefit-risk of continued interferon therapy should be reassessed (see also section **4.4 Chronic hepatitis C, Monotherapy** (thyroid abnormalities) and section **4.8**).

Discontinue treatment with IntronA in patients with chronic hepatitis who develop prolongation of coagulation markers which might indicate liver decompensation.

Chronic HepatitisC:

Combination therapy with ribavirin: Also see ribavirin labelling if IntronA is to be administered in combination with ribavirin in patients with chronic hepatitis C.

All patients in the chronic hepatitis C studies had a liver biopsy before inclusion, but in certain cases (i.e. patients with genotype 2 and 3), treatment may be possible without histological confirmation. Current treatment guidelines should be consulted as to whether a liver biopsy is needed prior to commencing treatment.

Monotherapy: Infrequently, adult patients treated for chronic hepatitis C with IntronA developed thyroid abnormalities, either hypothyroidism or hyperthyroidism. In clinical trials using IntronA therapy, 2.8 % patients overall developed thyroid abnormalities. The abnormalities were controlled by conventional therapy for thyroid dysfunction. The mechanism by which IntronA may alter thyroid status is unknown. Prior to initiation of IntronA therapy for the treatment of chronic hepatitis C, evaluate serum thyroid-stimulating hormone (TSH) levels. Any thyroid abnormality detected at that time must be treated with conventional therapy. IntronA treatment may be initiated if TSH levels can be maintained in the normal range by medication. Determine TSH levels if, during the course of IntronA therapy, a patient develops symptoms consistent with possible thyroid dysfunction. In the presence of thyroid dysfunction, IntronA treatment may be continued if TSH levels can be maintained in the normal range by medication. Discontinuation of IntronA therapy has not reversed thyroid dysfunction occurring during treatment (also see Children and adolescents, Thyroid monitoring).

Supplemental monitoring specific for children and adolescents

Thyroid Monitoring: Approximately 12 % of children treated with interferon alfa-2b and ribavirin developed increase in TSH. Another 4 % had a transient decrease below the lower limit of normal. Prior to initiation of IntronA therapy, TSH levels must be evaluated and any thyroid abnormality detected at that time must be treated with conventional therapy. IntronA therapy may be initiated if TSH levels can be maintained in the normal range by medication. Thyroid dysfunction during treatment with interferon alfa-2b and ribavirin has been observed. If thyroid abnormalities are detected, the patient's thyroid status should be evaluated and treated as clinically appropriate. Children and adolescents should be monitored every 3 months for evidence of thyroid dysfunction (e.g. TSH).

Growth and Development: During a 1-year course of therapy there was a decrease in the rate of linear growth (mean percentile decrease of 9 %) and a decrease in the rate of weight gain (mean percentile decrease of 13 %). A general reversal of these trends was noted during the 6 months follow-up post treatment. However, based on interim data from a long-term follow-up study, 12 (14 %) of 84 children had a > 15 percentile decrease in rate of linear growth, of whom 5 (6 %) children had a > 30 percentile decrease despite being off treatment for more than 1 year. There are no data on long term effects on growth and development and on sexual maturation.

HCV/HIV Coinfection: Patients co-infected with HIV and receiving Highly Active Anti-Retroviral Therapy (HAART) may be at increased risk of developing lactic acidosis. Caution should be used when adding IntronA and ribavirin to HAART therapy (see ribavirin SPC).

Co-infected patients with advanced cirrhosis receiving HAART may be at increased risk of hepatic decompensation and death. Adding treatment with alfa interferons alone or in combination with ribavirin may increase the risk in this patient subset.

Concomitant chemotherapy:

Administration of IntronA in combination with other chemotherapeutic agents (e.g., Ara-C, cyclophosphamide, doxorubicin, teniposide) may lead to increased risk of toxicity (severity and duration), which may be life-threatening or fatal as a result of the concomitantly administered medicinal product. The most commonly reported potentially life-threatening or fatal adverse events include mucositis, diarrhoea, neutropaenia, renal impairment, and electrolyte disturbance. Because of the risk of increased toxicity, careful adjustments of doses are required for IntronA and for the concomitant chemotherapeutic agents (see section **4.5**).

Laboratory Tests:

Standard haematological tests and blood chemistries (complete blood count and differential, platelet count, electrolytes, liver enzymes, serum protein, serum bilirubin and serum creatinine) are to be conducted in all patients prior to and periodically during systemic treatment with IntronA.

During treatment for hepatitis B or C the recommended testing schedule is at weeks 1, 2, 4, 8, 12, 16, and every other month, thereafter, throughout treatment. If ALT flares during IntronA therapy to greater than or equal to 2 times baseline, IntronA therapy may be continued unless signs and symptoms of liver failure are observed. During ALT flare, liver function tests: ALT, prothrombin time, alkaline phosphatase, albumin and bilirubin must be monitored at two-week intervals.

In patients treated for malignant melanoma, liver function and white blood cell (WBC) count and differential must be monitored weekly during the induction phase of therapy and monthly during the maintenance phase of therapy.

Effect on fertility: Interferon may impair fertility (see section **4.6** and section **5.3**).

4.5 Interaction with other medicinal products and other forms of Interaction

Narcotics, hypnotics or sedatives must be administered with caution when used concomitantly with IntronA.

Interactions between IntronA and other medicinal products have not been fully evaluated. Caution must be exercised when administering IntronA in combination with other potentially myelosuppressive agents.

Interferons may affect the oxidative metabolic process. This must be considered during concomitant therapy with medicinal products metabolised by this route, such as the xanthine derivatives theophylline or aminophylline. During concomitant therapy with xanthine agents, serum theophylline levels must be monitored and dosage adjusted if necessary.

Pulmonary infiltrates, pneumonitis, and pneumonia, occasionally resulting in fatality, have been observed rarely in interferon alpha treated patients, including those treated with IntronA. The aetiology has not been defined. These symptoms have been reported more frequently when shosaikoto, a Chinese herbal medicine, is administered concomitantly with interferon alpha (see section **4.4**).

Administration of IntronA in combination with other chemotherapeutic agents (e.g., Ara-C, cyclophosphamide, doxorubicin, teniposide) may lead to increased risk of toxicity (severity and duration) (see section **4.4**).

(Also see ribavirin labelling if IntronA is to be administered in combination with ribavirin in patients with chronic hepatitis C).

4.6 Pregnancy and lactation

Women of childbearing potential have to use effective contraception during treatment. IntronA must be used with caution in fertile men. Decreased serum estradiol and progesterone concentrations have been reported in women treated with human leukocyte interferon.

There are no adequate data from the use of interferon alfa-2b in pregnant women. Studies in animals have shown reproductive toxicity (see section **5.3**). The potential risk for humans is unknown. IntronA is to be used during pregnancy only if the potential benefit justifies the potential risk to the foetus.

It is not known whether the components of this medicinal product are excreted in human milk. Because of the potential for adverse events from IntronA in nursing infants, a decision must be made whether to discontinue nursing or to discontinue the medicinal product, taking into account the importance of the treatment to the mother.

Combination therapy with ribavirin: Ribavirin causes serious birth defects when administered during pregnancy. IntronA in combination with ribavirin is contraindicated (see ribavirin SPC). Females of childbearing potential have to use effective contraception during treatment and for 4 months after treatment.

4.7 Effects on ability to drive and use machines

Patients are to be advised that they may develop fatigue, somnolence, or confusion during treatment with IntronA, and therefore it is recommended that they avoid driving or operating machinery.

4.8 Undesirable effects

See ribavirin labelling for ribavirin-related undesirable effects if IntronA is to be administered in combination with ribavirin in patients with chronic hepatitis C.

In clinical trials conducted in a broad range of indications and at a wide range of doses (from 6 MIU/m^2/week in hairy cell leukaemia up to 100 MIU/m^2/week in melanoma), the most commonly reported undesirable effects were fever, fatigue, headache and myalgia. Fever and fatigue were often reversible within 72 hours of interruption or cessation of treatment.

The safety profile shown here was determined from 4 clinical trials in hepatitis C in which patients were treated with IntronA alone or in combination with ribavirin for one year. All patients in these trials received 3 MIU of IntronA three times a week. The percentage of patients reporting (treatment related) undesirable effects ⩾ 10 % is presented in **Table 1** as a range to capture the incidences reported in individual treatment groups among these clinical trials in naïve patients treated for one year. Severity was generally mild to moderate.

Table 1. Undesirable effects reported very commonly in any of the clinical trials in naïve patients treated for one year with monotherapy or combination therapy, Very common (> 1/10) (CIOMS III)

Body System	IntronA n=806	IntronA + Rebetol n=1,010
Infections and infestations		
Infection viral	0-7 %	3-10 %
Metabolism and nutrition disorders		
Weight decrease	6-11 %	9-19 %
Psychiatric disorders		
Depression	16-36 %	25-34 %
Irritability	13-27 %	18-34 %
Insomnia	21-28 %	33-41 %
Anxiety	8-12 %	8-16 %
Concentration impaired	8-14 %	9-21 %
Emotional lability	5-8 %	5-11 %
Nervous system disorders		
Headache	51-64 %	48-64 %
Respiratory, thoracic and mediastinal disorders		
Pharyngitis	3-7 %	7-13 %
Coughing	3-7 %	8-11 %
Dyspnoea	2-9 %	10-22 %
Gastrointestinal disorders		
Nausea/Vomiting	18-31 %/ 3-10 %	25-44 %/ 6-10 %
Anorexia	14-19 %	19-26 %
Diarrhoea	12-22 %	13-18 %
Abdominal pain	9-17 %	9-14 %
Skin and subcutaneous tissue disorders		
Alopecia	22-31 %	26-32 %
Pruritus	6-9 %	18-27 %
Skin dry	5-8 %	10-21 %
Rash	5-7 %	15-24 %
Musculoskeletal and connective tissue disorders		
Myalgia	41-61 %	30-62 %
Arthralgia	25-31 %	21-29 %
Musculoskeletal pain	15-20 %	11-20 %
General disorders and administration site conditions		
Injection site inflammation	9-16 %	6-17 %
Injection site reaction	5-8 %	3-36 %
Fatigue	42-70 %	43-68 %
Rigors	15-39 %	19-41 %
Fever	29-39 %	29-41 %
Flu-like symptoms	19-37 %	18-29 %
Asthenia	9-30 %	9-30 %
Dizziness	8-18 %	10-22 %

Table 2. Undesirable effects reported commonly in clinical trials of 483 patients treated with IntronA + Ribavirin
(IntronA 3 MIU 3 times a week, ribavirin > 10.6 mg/kg for one year) Common (> 1/100, < 1/10) (CIOMS III)

Body System	IntronA + Rebetol
Infections and infestations 1-5 %	Herpes simplex (resistance)
Blood and lymphatic system disorders 5-10 %:	Leukopaenia
1-5 %:	Thrombocytopaenia, lymphadenopathy, lymphopenia
Endocrine disorders 1-5 %:	Hyperthyroidism, hypothyroidism
Metabolism and nutrition disorders 1-5 %:	Hyperuricemia, hypocalcemia, thirst
Psychiatric disorders 5-10 %:	Agitation, nervousness
1-5 %:	Sleep disorder, somnolence, libido decreased
Nervous system disorders 5-10 %	Mouth dry, sweating increased
1-5 %:	Hypoesthesia, vertigo, confusion, parasthesia, tremor, migraine, flushing, lacrimal gland disorder
Eye disorders 5-10 %:	Vision blurred
1-5 %:	Conjunctivitis, eye pain, vision abnormal
Ear and labyrinth disorders 1-5 %:	Tinnitus
Cardiac disorders 1-5 %:	Palpitation, tachycardia
Vascular disorders 1-5 %:	Hypertension
Respiratory, thoracic and mediastinal disorders 1-5 %:	Bronchitis, cough nonproductive, epistaxis, nasal congestion, respiratory disorder, rhinitis, rhinorrhea, sinusitis
Gastrointestinal disorders 5-10 %:	Dyspepsia, stomatitis
1-5 %:	Constipation, dehydration, gingivitis, glossitis, loose stools, stomatitis ulcerative, taste perversion
Hepatobiliary disorders 1-5 %:	Hepatomegaly
Skin and subcutaneous tissue disorders 1-5 %:	Eczema, psoriasis (new or aggravated), rash erythematous, rash maculopapular, skin disorder, erythema
Musculoskeletal and connective tissue disorders 1-5 %:	Arthritis
Renal and urinary disorders 1-5 %:	Micturition frequency
Reproductive system and breast disorders 1-5 %:	Amenorrhea, breast pain, dysmenorrhea, menorrhagia, menstrual disorder, vaginal disorder
General disorders and administration site conditions 5-10 %:	Malaise, chest pain
1-5 %:	Injection site pain, right upper quadrant pain

These undesirable effects have also been reported with IntronA alone.

The undesirable effects seen with hepatitis C are representative of those reported when IntronA is administered in other indications, with some anticipated dose-related increases in incidence. For example, in a trial of high-dose adjuvant IntronA treatment in patients with melanoma, incidences of fatigue, fever, myalgia, neutropaenia/anaemia, anorexia, nausea and vomiting, diarrhoea, chills, flu-like symptoms, depression, alopecia, altered taste, and dizziness were greater than in the hepatitis C trials. Severity also increased with high dose therapy (WHO Grade 3 and 4, in 66 % and 14 % of patients, respectively), in comparison with the mild to moderate severity usually associated with lower doses. Undesirable effects were usually managed by dose adjustment.

Additional adverse events were reported rarely (> 1/10,000, < 1/1,000) or very rarely (< 1/10,000) during clinical trials in other indications or following the marketing of interferon alfa-2b:

Immune system disorders:

very rarely: sarcoidosis or exacerbation of sarcoidosis

Endocrine disorders:

very rarely: diabetes, aggravated diabetes

Metabolism and nutrition disorders:

very rarely: hyperglycaemia, hypertriglyceridaemia

Psychiatric disorders:

rarely: suicide ideation

very rarely: aggressive behaviour (sometimes directed against others), suicide attempts, suicide, psychosis, including hallucinations

Nervous system disorders:

very rarely: impaired consciousness, neuropathy, polyneuropathy, seizure, encephalopathy, cerebrovascular ischaemia, cerebrovascular haemorrhage

Eye disorders:

rarely: retinal haemorrhages, retinopathies (including macular oedema), cotton-wool spots, retinal artery or vein obstruction, loss of visual acuity or visual field, optic neuritis and papilloedema

Ear and labyrinth disorders:

very rarely: hearing disorder, hearing loss

Cardiac disorders:

very rarely: cardiac ischaemia and myocardial infarction

Vascular disorders:

very rarely: hypotension; peripheral ischaemia

Respiratory, thoracic and mediastinal disorders:

rarely: pneumonia

very rarely: pulmonary infiltrates, pneumonitis

Gastrointestinal:

very rarely: pancreatitis; increased appetite; gingival bleeding; colitis, mainly ulcerative and ischemic

Hepatobiliary disorders:

very rarely: hepatotoxicity, including fatality

Skin and subcutaneous tissue disorders:

very rarely: face oedema, erythema multiforme, Stevens Johnson syndrome, toxic epidermal necrolysis, injection site necrosis

Musculoskeletal and connective tissue disorders:

very rarely: rhabdomyolysis, sometimes serious; leg cramps; back pain; myositis

Renal and urinary disorders:

very rarely: nephrotic syndrome, renal insufficiency, renal failure

Very rarely IntronA used alone or in combination with ribavirin may be associated with aplastic anaemia.

Cardiovascular (CVS) adverse events, particularly arrhythmia, appeared to be correlated mostly with pre-existing CVS disease and prior therapy with cardiotoxic agents (see section **4.4**). Cardiomyopathy, that may be reversible upon discontinuation of interferon alpha, has been reported rarely in patients without prior evidence of cardiac disease.

A wide variety of autoimmune and immune-mediated disorders have been reported with alpha interferons including thyroid disorders, systemic lupus erythematosus, rheumatoid arthritis (new or aggravated), idiopathic and thrombotic thrombocytopenic purpura, vasculitis, neuropathies including mononeuropathies (see also section **4.4**).

Clinically significant laboratory abnormalities, most frequently occurring at doses greater than 10 million IU daily, include reduction in granulocyte and white blood cell counts; decreases in haemoglobin level and platelet count; increases in alkaline phosphatase, LDH, serum creatinine and serum urea nitrogen levels. Increase in serum ALT/AST (SGPT/SGOT) levels have been noted as an abnormality in some non-hepatitis subjects and also in some patients with chronic hepatitis B coincident with clearance of viral DNAp.

Children and adolescents – Chronic Hepatitis C

In clinical trials of 118 children or adolescents 3 to 16 years of age, 6 % discontinued therapy due to adverse events. In general, the adverse event profile in the limited paediatric population studied was similar to that observed in adults, although there is a paediatric specific concern regarding

Table 3 Undesirable effects very commonly and commonly reported in paediatric clinical trials ($\geqslant$ 1 % of patients treated with IntronA + ribavirin) Very common (> 1/10) - Common (> 1/100, < 1/10)

Body system	$\geqslant$ 10%	5 % - < 10 %	1 % - < 5 %
Infection and infestations	Viral infection		Tooth abscess, bacterial infection, fungal infection, herpes simplex, otitis media
Neoplasms benign, malignant and unspecified (including cysts and polyps)			Neoplasm (unspecified),
Blood and lymphatic system disorders	Anaemia, neutropenia		Bruise, thrombocytopaenia, lymphadenopathy
Endocrine disorders	Hypothyroidism		Hyperthyroidism, virilism,
Metabolism and nutrition disorders			Hypertriglyceridemia, hyperuricemia
Psychiatric disorders	Depression, emotional lability, insomnia, irritability	Agitation, somnolence	Aggressive reaction, anxiety, apathy, increased appetite, behavior disorder, concentration impaired, abnormal dreaming, nervousness, sleep disorder, somnambulism, suicidal ideation
Nervous system disorders	Headache, dizziness	Tremor	Confusion, hyperkinesia, dysphonia, paresthaesia, hyperaesthesia, hypoaesthesia
Eye disorders			Conjunctivitis, eye pain, abnormal vision, lacrimal gland disorder
Vascular disorders		Pallor	Raynaud's disease
Respiratory, thoracic and mediastinal disorders	Pharyngitis	Epistaxis	Coughing, dyspnoea, nasal congestion, nasal irritation, pulmonary infection, rhinorrhea, sneezing, tachypnea
Gastrointestinal disorders	Abdominal pain, anorexia, diarrhoea, nausea, vomiting		Constipation, dyspepsia, gastroenteritis, gastroesophogeal reflux, gastrointestinal disorder, glossitis, loose stools, mouth ulceration, rectal disorder, stomatitis, stomatitis ulcerative, toothache, tooth disorder
Hepatobiliary disorders			Hepatic function abnormal
Skin and subcutaneous tissue disorders	Alopecia, rash	Pruritus	Acne, eczema, skin laceration, nail disorder, dry skin, photosensitivity reaction, maculopapular rash, skin discolouration, skin disorder, erythema, sweating increased
Musculoskeletal and connective tissue disorders	Arthralgia, musculoskeletal pain, myalgia		
Renal and urinary disorders			Enuresis, micturition disorder, urinary tract infection, urinary incontinence
Reproductive system and breast disorders			Female: amenorrhea, menorrhagia, menstrual disorder, vaginal disorder, vaginitis Male: testicular pain
General disorders and administration site conditions	Injection site reaction, injection site inflammation, fatigue, fever, rigors, influenza-like symptoms, malaise, growth rate decrease (height and/or weight decrease for age)	Injection site pain	Asthenia, flushing, oedema, chest pain, right upper quadrant pain

growth inhibition as decrease in height (mean percentile decrease of growth velocity of 9 %) and weight (mean percentile decrease of 13 %) percentile were observed during treatment (see section **4.4**). Furthermore, suicidal ideation or attempts were reported more frequently compared to adult patients (2.4 % vs 1 %) during treatment and during the 6 month follow-up after treatment. As in adult patients, children and adolescents also experienced other psychiatric adverse events (e.g., depression, emotional lability, and somnolence) (see section **4.4**). In addition, injection site disorders, fever, anorexia, vomiting, and emotional lability occurred more frequently in children and adolescents compared to adult patients. Dose modifications were required in 30 % of patients, most commonly for anaemia and neutropaenia.

Undesirable effects reported in paediatric clinical trials, and not previously reported at an incidence $\geqslant$ 1 % in adults, are shown in **Table 3**. All effects reported at a $\geqslant$ 10 % incidence in paediatric trials were previously reported in adults (**Table 2**) and are not repeated in the paediatric table.

(see Table 3 on next page)

4.9 Overdose

No case of overdose has been reported that has led to acute clinical manifestations. However, as for any pharmacologically active compound, symptomatic treatment with frequent monitoring of vital signs and close observation of the patient is indicated.

5. PHARMACOLOGICAL PROPERTIES

5.1 Pharmacodynamic properties

Pharmacotherapeutic group: Immunostimulants, cytokines and immunomodulators, interferons, interferon alfa-2b, ATC code: L03A B05

IntronA is a sterile, stable, formulation of highly purified interferon alfa-2b produced by recombinant DNA techniques. Recombinant interferon alfa-2b is a water-soluble protein with a molecular weight of approximately 19,300 daltons. It is obtained from a clone of E. coli, which harbours a genetically engineered plasmid hybrid encompassing an interferon alfa-2b gene from human leukocytes.

The activity of IntronA is expressed in terms of IU, with 1 mg of recombinant interferon alfa-2b protein corresponding to 2.6 $\times$ 10^8 IU. International Units are determined by comparison of the activity of the recombinant interferon alfa-2b with the activity of the international reference preparation of human leukocyte interferon established by the World Health Organisation.

The interferons are a family of small protein molecules with molecular weights of approximately 15,000 to 21,000 daltons. They are produced and secreted by cells in response to viral infections or various synthetic and biological inducers. Three major classes of interferons have been identified: alpha, beta and gamma. These three main classes are themselves not homogeneous and may contain several different molecular species of interferon. More than 14 genetically distinct human alpha interferons have been identified. IntronA has been classified as recombinant interferon alfa-2b.

Interferons exert their cellular activities by binding to specific membrane receptors on the cell surface. Human interferon receptors, as isolated from human lymphoblastoid (Daudi) cells, appear to be highly asymmetric proteins. They exhibit selectivity for human but not murine interferons, suggesting species specificity. Studies with other interferons have demonstrated species specificity. However, certain monkey species, eg, rhesus monkeys, are susceptible to pharmacodynamic stimulation upon exposure to human type 1 interferons.

The results of several studies suggest that, once bound to the cell membrane, interferon initiates a complex sequence of intracellular events that include the induction of certain enzymes. It is thought that this process, at least in part, is responsible for the various cellular responses to interferon, including inhibition of virus replication in virus-infected cells, suppression of cell proliferation and such immunomodulating activities as enhancement of the phagocytic activity of macrophages and augmentation of the specific cytotoxicity of lymphocytes for target cells. Any or all of these activities may contribute to interferon's therapeutic effects.

Recombinant interferon alfa-2b has exhibited antiproliferative effects in studies employing both animal and human cell culture systems as well as human tumour xenografts in animals. It has demonstrated significant immunomodulatory activity *in vitro*.

Recombinant interferon alfa-2b also inhibits viral replication *in vitro* and *in vivo*. Although the exact antiviral mode of action of recombinant interferon alfa-2b is unknown, it appears to alter the host cell metabolism. This action inhibits viral replication or if replication occurs, the progeny virions are unable to leave the cell.

Chronic hepatitis B:

Current clinical experience in patients who remain on interferon alfa-2b for 4 to 6 months indicates that therapy can produce clearance of serum HBV-DNA. An improvement in liver histology has been observed. In adult patients with loss of HBeAg and HBV-DNA, a significant reduction in morbidity and mortality has been observed.

Interferon alfa-2b (6 MIU/m^2 3 times a week for 6 months) has been given to children with chronic active hepatitis B. Because of a methodological flaw, efficacy could not be demonstrated. Moreover children treated with interferon alfa-2b experienced a reduced rate of growth and some cases of depression were observed.

Chronic hepatitis C:

In adult patients receiving interferon in combination with ribavirin, the achieved sustained response rate is 47 %. Superior efficacy has been demonstrated with the combination of pegylated interferon with ribavirin (sustained response rate of 61 % achieved in a study performed in naïve patients with a ribavirin dose > 10.6 mg/kg, $p < 0.01$).

Adult patients: IntronA alone or in combination with ribavirin has been studied in 4 randomised Phase III clinical trials in 2,552 interferon-naïve patients with chronic hepatitis C. The trials compared the efficacy of IntronA used

Table 4 Sustained virologic response rates with IntronA + ribavirin (one year of treatment) by genotype and viral load

HCV Genotype	I N=503 C95-132/I95-143	I/R N=505 C95-132/I95-143	I/R N=505 C/I98-580
All Genotypes	**16 %**	**41 %**	**47 %**
Genotype 1	9 %	29 %	33 %
Genotype 1 ⩽ 2 million copies/ml	25 %	33 %	45 %
Genotype 1 > 2 million copies/ml	3 %	27 %	29 %
Genotype 2/3	31 %	65 %	79 %

I IntronA (3 MIU 3 times a week)

I/R IntronA (3 MIU 3 times a week) + ribavirin (1,000/1,200 mg/day)

alone or in combination with ribavirin. Efficacy was defined as sustained virologic response, 6 months after the end of treatment. Eligible patients for these trials had chronic hepatitis C confirmed by a positive HCV-RNA polymerase chain reaction assay (PCR) (> 100 copies/ml), a liver biopsy consistent with a histologic diagnosis of chronic hepatitis with no other cause for the chronic hepatitis, and abnormal serum ALT.

IntronA was administered at a dose of 3 MIU 3 times a week as monotherapy or in combination with ribavirin. The majority of patients in these clinical trials were treated for one year. All patients were followed for an additional 6 months after the end of treatment for the determination of sustained virologic response. Sustained virologic response rates for treatment groups treated for one year with IntronA alone or in combination with ribavirin (from two studies) are shown in **Table 4**.

Co-administration of IntronA with ribavirin increased the efficacy of IntronA by at least two fold for the treatment of chronic heptatitis C in naïve patients. HCV genotype and baseline virus load are prognostic factors which are known to affect response rates. The increased response rate to the combination of IntronA + ribavirin, compared with IntronA alone, is maintained across all subgroups. The relative benefit of combination therapy with IntronA + ribavirin is particularly significant in the most difficult to treat subgroup of patients (genotype 1 and high virus load) (**Table 4**).

Response rates in these trials were increased with compliance. Regardless of genotype, patients who received IntronA in combination with ribavirin and received ⩾ 80 % of their treatment had a higher sustained response 6 months after 1 year of treatment than those who took < 80 % of their treatment (56 % vs. 32 % in trial C/I98-580). ***(see Table 4)***

Relapse patients: A total of 345 interferon alpha relapse patients were treated in two clinical trials with IntronA monotherapy or in combination with ribavirin. In these patients, the addition of ribavirin to IntronA increased by as much as 10-fold the efficacy of IntronA used alone in the treatment of chronic hepatitis C (48.6 % vs. 4.7 %). This enhancement in efficacy included loss of serum HCV (< 100 copies/ml by PCR), improvement in hepatic inflammation, and normalisation of ALT, and was sustained when measured 6 months after the end of treatment.

Clinical trials in paediatric patients with chronic hepatitis C:

Children and adolescents 3 to 16 years of age with compensated chronic hepatitis C and detectable HCV-RNA (assessed by a central laboratory using a research-based RT-PCR assay) were enrolled in two multicentre trials and received IntronA 3 MIU/m^2 3 times a week plus ribavirin 15 mg/kg per day for 1 year followed by 6 months follow-up after-treatment. A total of 118 patients were enrolled: 57 % male, 80 % Caucasian, and 78 % genotype 1, 64 % ⩽ 12 years of age. The population enrolled mainly consisted in children with mild to moderate hepatitis C. Sustained virological response rates in children and adolescents were similar to those in adults. Due to the lack of data in children with severe progression of the disease, and the potential for undesirable effects, the benefit/risk of the combination of ribavirin and interferon alfa-2b needs to be carefully considered in this population (see sections **4.1**, **4.4** and **4.8**).

Study results are summarized in **Table 5**.

Table 5. Virological response in previously untreated paediatric patients

	IntronA 3 MIU/m^2 3 times a week **+ ribavirin 15 mg/kg/day**
Overall Response[1] (n=118)	54 (46 %)*
Genotype 1 (n=92)	33 (36 %)*
Genotype 2/3/4 (n=26)	21 (81 %)*

*Number (%) of patients

1. Defined as HCV-RNA below limit of detection using a research based RT-PCR assay at end of treatment and during follow-up period

5.2 Pharmacokinetic properties

The pharmacokinetics of IntronA were studied in healthy volunteers following single 5 million IU/m^2 and 10 million IU doses administered subcutaneously, at 5 million IU/m^2 administered intramuscularly and as a 30-minute intravenous infusion. The mean serum interferon concentrations following subcutaneous and intramuscular injections were comparable. C_{max} occurred three to 12 hours after the lower dose and six to eight hours after the higher dose. The elimination half-lives of interferon injections were approximately two to three hours, and six to seven hours, respectively. Serum levels were below the detection limit 16 and 24 hours, respectively, post-injection. Both subcutaneous and intramuscular administration resulted in bioavailabilities greater than 100 %.

After intravenous administration, serum interferon levels peaked (135 to 273 IU/ml) by the end of the infusion, then declined at a slightly more rapid rate than after subcutaneous or intramuscular administration of medicinal product, becoming undetectable four hours after the infusion. The elimination half-life was approximately two hours.

Urine levels of interferon were below the detection limit following each of the three routes of administration.

Children and adolescents: Multiple-dose pharmacokinetic properties for IntronA injection and ribavirin capsules in children and adolescents with chronic hepatitis C, between 5 and 16 years of age, are summarized in **Table 6**. The pharmacokinetics of IntronA and ribavirin (dose-normalized) are similar in adults and children or adolescents.

Table 6. Mean (% CV) multiple-dose pharmacokinetic parameters for IntronA and ribavirin capsules when administered to children or adolescents with chronic hepatitis C

Parameter	**Ribavirin** 15 mg/kg/day as 2 divided doses (n = 17)	IntronA 3 MIU/m^2 3 times a week (n = 54)
T_{max} (hr)	1.9 (83)	5.9 (36)
C_{max} (ng/ml)	3,275 (25)	51 (48)
AUC*	29,774 (26)	622 (48)
Apparent clearance l/hr/kg	0.27 (27)	Not done

*AUC_{12} (ng.hr/ml) for ribavirin; AUC_{0-24} (IU.hr/ml) for IntronA

Interferon neutralising factor assays were performed on serum samples of patients who received IntronA in Schering-Plough monitored clinical trials. Interferon neutralising factors are antibodies which neutralise the antiviral activity of interferon. The clinical incidence of neutralising factors developing in cancer patients treated systemically is 2.9 % and in chronic hepatitis patients is 6.2 %. The detectable titres are low in almost all cases and have not been regularly associated with loss of response or any other autoimmune phenomenon. In patients with hepatitis, no loss of response was observed apparently due to the low titres.

5.3 Preclinical safety data

Although interferon is generally recognised as being species specific, toxicity studies in animals were conducted. Injections of human recombinant interferon alfa-2b for up to three months have shown no evidence of toxicity in mice, rats, and rabbits. Daily dosing of cynomolgus monkeys with 20 × 10^6 IU/kg/day for 3 months caused no remarkable toxicity. Toxicity was demonstrated in monkeys given 100 × 10^6 IU/kg/day for 3 months.

In studies of interferon use in non-human primates, abnormalities of the menstrual cycle have been observed (see section **4.4**).

Results of animal reproduction studies indicate that recombinant interferon alfa-2b was not teratogenic in rats or rabbits, nor did it adversely affect pregnancy, foetal development or reproductive capacity in offspring of treated rats. Interferon alfa-2b has been shown to have abortifacient effects in *Macaca mulatta* (rhesus monkeys) at 90 and 180 times the recommended intramuscular or subcutaneous dose of 2 million IU/m^2. Abortion was observed in all dose groups (7.5 million, 15 million and 30 million IU/kg), and was statistically significant versus control at the mid- and high-dose groups (corresponding to 90 and 180 times the recommended intramuscular or subcutaneous dose of 2 million IU/m^2). High doses of other forms of interferons alpha and beta are known to produce dose-related anovulatory and abortifacient effects in rhesus monkeys.

Mutagenicity studies with interferon alfa-2b revealed no adverse events.

No studies have been conducted in juvenile animals to examine the effects of treatment on growth, development, sexual maturation, and behaviour.

6. PHARMACEUTICAL PARTICULARS

6.1 List of excipients

Sodium phosphate dibasic, sodium phosphate monobasic, edetate disodium, sodium chloride, m-cresol, polysorbate 80, water for injections q.s. Deliverable volume from pen = 1.2 ml (an overfill is included for proper dispensing from the pen delivery system).

6.2 Incompatibilities

This medicinal product must not be mixed with other medicinal products except those mentioned in section 6.6.

6.3 Shelf life

15 months

Chemical and physical in-use stability has been demonstrated for 27 days at 2°C – 8°C.

From a microbiological point of view, once opened, the product may be stored for a maximum of 27 days at 2°C – 8°C. Other in-use storage times and conditions are the responsibility of the user.

6.4 Special precautions for storage

Store in a refrigerator (2°C – 8°C). Do not freeze.

6.5 Nature and contents of container

The solution is contained in a 1.5 ml cartridge, type I flint glass. The cartridge is sealed at one end with an aluminium cap containing a bromobutyl rubber liner and at the other end by a bromobutyl rubber plunger.

IntronA 18 million IU solution for injection, multidose pen

The pen is designed to deliver its contents of 18 million IU in doses ranging from 1.5 to 6 million IU. The pen will deliver a maximum of 12 doses of 1.5 million IU over a period not to exceed 4 weeks.

IntronA 30 million IU solution for injection, multidose pen

The pen is designed to deliver its contents of 30 million IU in doses ranging from 2.5 to 10 million IU. The pen will deliver a maximum of 12 doses of 2.5 million IU over a period not to exceed 4 weeks.

IntronA 60 million IU solution for injection, multidose pen

The pen is designed to deliver its contents of 60 million IU in doses ranging from 5 to 20 million IU. The pen will deliver a maximum of 12 doses of 5 million IU over a period not to exceed 4 weeks.

- 1 pen, 12 injection needles and 12 cleansing swabs
- 2 pens, 24 injection needles and 24 cleansing swabs
- 8 pens, 96 injection needles and 96 cleansing swabs

Not all pack sizes may be marketed.

6.6 Instructions for use and handling

Not all dosage forms and strengths are appropriate for some indications. Please make sure to select an appropriate dosage form and strength (see section **4.2**).

IntronA, solution for injection, multidose pen is injected subcutaneously after attaching an injection needle and dialing the prescribed dose.

Remove the pen from the refrigerator approximately 30 minutes before administration to allow the injectable solution to reach room temperature (not more than 25°C).

Detailed instructions for the use of the product is provided with the package leaflet.

Each pen is intended for a maximum four-week use period and must then be discarded. A new injection needle must be used for each dose. After each use, the injection needle must be discarded safely and the pen must be returned immediately to the refrigerator. A maximum of 48 hours (two days) of exposure to 25°C is permitted over the four-week use period to cover accidental delays in returning the pen to the refrigerator.

Sufficient needles and swabs are provided to use the IntronA pen for administering the smallest measurable doses. Instruct the patient that any extra needles and swabs that remain after the final dose has been taken from the pen, must be discarded appropriately and safely.

As for all parenteral medicinal products, inspect the reconstituted solution visually for particulate matter and discoloration prior to administration. The reconstituted solution should be clear and colourless.

7. MARKETING AUTHORISATION HOLDER

SP Europe

73, rue de Stalle

B-1180 Bruxelles

Belgium

8. MARKETING AUTHORISATION NUMBER(S)

IntronA 18 million IU solution for injection, multidose pen: EU/1/99/127/031-033

IntronA 30 million IU solution for injection, multidose pen: EU/1/99/127/034-036

IntronA 60 million IU solution for injection, multidose pen: EU/1/99/127/037-039

9. DATE OF FIRST AUTHORISATION/RENEWAL OF THE AUTHORISATION

Date of first authorisation: 9 March 2000

Date of last renewal: 23 May 2005

10. DATE OF REVISION OF THE TEXT

23 May 2005

Legal Category

Prescription Only Medicine

IntronA-Pen/05-05/7

IntronA 10miu Powder and 25miu Multidose Solution

(Schering-Plough Ltd)

1. NAME OF THE MEDICINAL PRODUCT

IntronA 10 million IU/ml powder and solvent for solution for injection or infusion

IntronA 25 million IU/2.5 ml solution for injection or infusion

2. QUALITATIVE AND QUANTITATIVE COMPOSITION

IntronA 10 million IU/ml powder and solvent for solution for injection or infusion:

After reconstitution, 1 ml contains:

Interferon alfa-2b* 10 million IU

*produced in *E.coli* by recombinant DNA technology.

One vial of powder contains 10 million IU of interferon alfa-2b.

IntronA 25 million IU/2.5ml solution for injection or infusion:

One vial of IntronA solution for injection or infusion, multiple dose vial, contains 25 million IU of recombinant interferon alfa-2b* in 2.5 ml of solution.

*produced in *E.coli* by recombinant DNA technology.

One ml of solution contains 10 million IU of interferon alfa-2b.

For excipients, see section 6.1.

3. PHARMACEUTICAL FORM

IntronA 10 million IU/ml powder and solvent for solution for injection or infusion:

Powder and solvent for solution for injection or infusion

The white to cream coloured powder is contained in a 2 ml glass vial and the clear and colourless solvent is presented in a 2 ml glass ampoule.

IntronA 25 million IU/2.5ml solution for injection or infusion:

Solution for injection or infusion

Solution is clear and colourless.

4. CLINICAL PARTICULARS

4.1 Therapeutic indications

Chronic Hepatitis B: Treatment of adult patients with chronic hepatitis B associated with evidence of hepatitis B viral replication (presence of HBV-DNA and HBeAg), elevated ALT and histologically proven active liver inflammation and/or fibrosis.

Chronic Hepatitis C:

Adult patients:

IntronA is indicated for the treatment of adult patients with chronic hepatitis C who have elevated transaminases without liver decompensation and who are positive for serum HCV-RNA or anti-HCV (see section **4.4**).

The best way to use IntronA in this indication is in combination with ribavirin.

Chidren and adolescents:

IntronA is intended for use, in a combination regimen with ribavirin, for the treatment of children and adolescents 3 years of age and older, who have chronic hepatitis C, not previously treated, without liver decompensation, and who are positive for serum HCV-RNA. The decision to treat should be made on a case by case basis, taking into account any evidence of disease progression such as hepatic inflammation and fibrosis, as well as prognostic factors for response, HCV genotype and viral load. The expected benefit of treatment should be weighed against the safety findings observed for paediatric subjects in the clinical trials (see sections **4.4**, **4.8** and **5.1**).

Hairy Cell Leukaemia: Treatment of patients with hairy cell leukaemia.

Chronic Myelogenous Leukaemia:

Monotherapy: Treatment of adult patients with Philadelphia chromosome or bcr/abl translocation positive chronic myelogenous leukaemia.

Clinical experience indicates that a haematological and cytogenetic major/minor response is obtainable in the majority of patients treated. A major cytogenetic response is defined by < 34 % Ph+ leukaemic cells in the bone marrow, whereas a minor response is $\geqslant 34$ %, but < 90 % Ph+ cells in the marrow.

Combination therapy: The combination of interferon alfa-2b and cytarabine (Ara-C) administered during the first 12 months of treatment has been demonstrated to significantly increase the rate of major cytogenetic responses and to significantly prolong the overall survival at three years when compared to interferon alfa-2b monotherapy.

Multiple Myeloma: As maintenance therapy in patients who have achieved objective remission (more than 50 % reduction in myeloma protein) following initial induction chemotherapy.

Current clinical experience indicates that maintenance therapy with interferon alfa-2b prolongs the plateau phase; however, effects on overall survival have not been conclusively demonstrated.

Follicular Lymphoma: Treatment of high tumour burden follicular lymphoma as adjunct to appropriate combination induction chemotherapy such as a CHOP-like regimen. High tumour burden is defined as having at least one of the following: bulky tumour mass ($>$ 7 cm), involvement of three or more nodal sites (each $>$ 3 cm), systemic symptoms (weight loss $>$ 10 %, fever $>$ 38°C for more than 8 days, or nocturnal sweats), splenomegaly beyond the umbilicus, major organ obstruction or compression syndrome, orbital or epidural involvement, serous effusion, or leukaemia.

Carcinoid Tumour: Treatment of carcinoid tumours with lymph node or liver metastases and with "carcinoid syndrome".

Malignant Melanoma: As adjuvant therapy in patients who are free of disease after surgery but are at high risk of systemic recurrence, e.g., patients with primary or recurrent (clinical or pathological) lymph node involvement.

4.2 Posology and method of administration

IntronA may be administered using either glass or plastic disposable injection syringes.

Not all dosage forms and strengths are appropriate for some indications. Please make sure to select an appropriate dosage form and strength.

Treatment must be initiated by a physician experienced in the management of the disease.

If adverse events develop during the course of treatment with IntronA for any indication, modify the dosage or discontinue therapy temporarily until the adverse events abate. If persistent or recurrent intolerance develops following adequate dosage adjustment, or disease progresses, discontinue treatment with IntronA. At the discretion of the physician, the patient may self-administer the dose for maintenance dosage regimens administered subcutaneously.

Chronic Hepatitis B: The recommended dosage is in the range 5 to 10 million IU administered subcutaneously three times a week (every other day) for a period of 4 to 6 months.

The administered dose should be reduced by 50 % in case of occurrence of haematological disorders (white blood cells $< 1{,}500/mm^3$, granulocytes $< 1{,}000/mm^3$, thrombocytes $< 100{,}000/mm^3$). Treatment should be discontinued in case of severe leukopaenia ($< 1{,}200/mm^3$), severe neutropaenia ($< 750/mm^3$) or severe thrombocytopaenia ($< 70{,}000/mm^3$).

For all patients, if no improvement on serum HBV-DNA is observed after 3 to 4 months of treatment (at the maximum tolerated dose), discontinue IntronA therapy.

Chronic Hepatitis C: IntronA is administered subcutaneously at a dose of 3 million IU three times a week (every other day) to adult patients, whether administered as monotherapy or in combination with ribavirin.

Children 3 years of age or older and adolescents: Interferon alfa-2b 3 MIU/m^2 is administered subcutaneously 3 times a week (every other day) in combination with ribavirin capsules or oral solution administered orally in two divided doses daily with food (morning and evening).

(See ribavirin capsule SPC for dose of ribavirin capsules and dosage modification guidelines for combination therapy. For paediatric patients who weigh $<$ 47 kg or cannot swallow capsules, see ribavirin oral solution SPC).

Relapse patients (adults):

IntronA is given in combination with ribavirin.

Based on the results of clinical trials, in which data are available for 6 months of treatment, it is recommended that patients be treated with IntronA in combination with ribavirin for 6 months.

Naïve patients:

Adults: The efficacy of IntronA is enhanced when given in combination with ribavirin. IntronA should be given alone mainly in case of intolerance or contraindication to ribavirin.

IntronA in combination with ribavirin:

Based on the results of clinical trials, in which data are available for 12 months of treatment, it is recommended that patients be treated with IntronA in combination with ribavirin for at least 6 months.

Treatment should be continued for another 6-month period (i.e., a total of 12 months) in patients who exhibit negative HCV-RNA at month 6, and with viral genotype 1 (as determined in a pre-treatment sample) and high pre-treatment viral load.

Other negative prognostic factors (age $>$ 40 years, male gender, bridging fibrosis) should be taken into account in order to extend therapy to 12 months.

During clinical trials, patients who failed to show a virologic response after 6 months of treatment (HCV-RNA below lower limit of detection) did not become sustained virologic responders (HCV-RNA below lower limit of detection six months after withdrawal of treatment).

IntronA alone:

The optimal duration of therapy with IntronA alone is not yet fully established, but a therapy of between 12 and 18 months is advised.

It is recommended that patients be treated with IntronA alone for at least 3 to 4 months, at which point HCV-RNA status should be determined. Treatment should be continued in patients who exhibit negative HCV-RNA.

Children and adolescents: The efficacy and safety of IntronA in combination with ribavirin has been studied in children and adolescents who have not been previously treated for chronic hepatitis C.

Genotype 1: The recommended duration of treatment is one year. Patients who fail to achieve virological response at 12 weeks are highly unlikely to become sustained virological responders (negative predictive value 96 %). Virological response is defined as absence of detectable HCV-RNA at Week 12. Treatment should be discontinued in these patients.

Genotype 2/3: The recommended duration of treatment is 24 weeks.

Virological responses after 1 year of treatment and 6 months of follow-up were 36 % for genotype 1 and 81 % for genotype 2/3/4.

Hairy Cell Leukaemia: The recommended dosage is 2 million IU/m^2 administered subcutaneously three times a week (every other day) for both splenectomised and non-splenectomised patients. For most patients with Hairy Cell Leukaemia, normalisation of one or more haematological variables occurs within one to two months of IntronA treatment. Improvement in all three haematological variables (granulocyte count, platelet count and haemoglobin level) may require six months or more. This regimen must be maintained unless the disease progresses rapidly or severe intolerance is manifested.

Chronic Myelogenous Leukaemia: The recommended dosage of IntronA is 4 to 5 million IU/m^2 administered daily subcutaneously. Some patients have been shown to benefit from IntronA 5 million IU/m^2 administered daily subcutaneously in association with cytarabine (Ara-C) 20 mg/m^2 administered daily subcutaneously for 10 days per month (up to a maximum daily dose of 40 mg). When the white blood cell count is controlled, administer the maximum tolerated dose of IntronA (4 to 5 million IU/m^2 daily) to maintain haematological remission.

IntronA treatment must be discontinued after 8 to 12 weeks of treatment if at least a partial haematological remission or a clinically meaningful cytoreduction has not been achieved.

Multiple Myeloma: Maintenance therapy: In patients who are in the plateau phase (more than 50 % reduction of myeloma protein) following initial induction chemotherapy, interferon alfa-2b may be administered as monotherapy, subcutaneously, at a dose of 3 million IU/m^2 three times a week (every other day).

Follicular Lymphoma: Adjunctively with chemotherapy, interferon alfa-2b may be administered subcutaneously, at a dose of 5 million IU three times a week (every other day) for a duration of 18 months. CHOP-like regimens are advised, but clinical experience is available only with CHVP (combination of cyclophosphamide, doxorubicin, teniposide and prednisolone).

Carcinoid Tumour: The usual dose is 5 million IU (3 to 9 million IU) administered subcutaneously three times a week (every other day). Patients with advanced disease may require a daily dose of 5 million IU. The treatment is to be temporarily discontinued during and after surgery. Therapy may continue for as long as the patient responds to interferon alfa-2b treatment.

Malignant Melanoma: As induction therapy, interferon alfa-2b is administered intravenously at a dose of 20 million IU/m^2 daily for five days a week for a four-week period; the calculated interferon alfa-2b dose is added to 0.9 % sodium chloride solution and administered as a 20-minute infusion (see section **6.6**). As maintenance treatment, the recommended dose is 10 million IU/m^2 administered subcutaneously three days a week (every other day) for 48 weeks.

If severe adverse events develop during interferon alfa-2b treatment, particularly if granulocytes decrease to $< 500/mm^3$ or ALT/AST rises to $> 5 \times$ upper limit of normal, discontinue treatment temporarily until the adverse event abates. Interferon alfa-2b treatment is to be restarted at 50 % of the previous dose. If intolerance persists after dose adjustment or if granulocytes decrease to $< 250/mm^3$ or ALT/AST rises to $> 10 \times$ upper limit of normal, discontinue interferon alfa-2b therapy.

Although the optimal (minimum) dose for full clinical benefit is unknown, patients must be treated at the recommended dose, with dose reduction for toxicity as described.

4.3 Contraindications

- Hypersensitivity to the active substance or to any of the excipients

- A history of severe pre-existing cardiac disease, e.g., uncontrolled congestive heart failure, recent myocardial infarction, severe arrhythmic disorders

- Severe renal or hepatic dysfunction; including that caused by metastases

- Epilepsy and/or compromised central nervous system (CNS) function (see section **4.4**)

- Chronic hepatitis with decompensated cirrhosis of the liver

- Chronic hepatitis in patients who are being or have been treated recently with immunosuppressive agents excluding short term corticosteroid withdrawal

- Autoimmune hepatitis; or history of autoimmune disease; immunosuppressed transplant recipients

- Pre-existing thyroid disease unless it can be controlled with conventional treatment

Children and adolescents:

- Existence of, or history of severe psychiatric condition, particularly severe depression, suicidal ideation or suicide attempt.

Combination therapy with ribavirin: Also see ribavirin labelling if interferon alfa-2b is to be administered in combination with ribavirin in patients with chronic hepatitis C.

4.4 Special warnings and special precautions for use
For all patients:

Acute hypersensitivity reactions (e.g., urticaria, angioedema, bronchoconstriction, anaphylaxis) to interferon alfa-2b have been observed rarely during IntronA therapy. If such a reaction develops, discontinue the medication and institute appropriate medical therapy. Transient rashes do not necessitate interruption of treatment.

Moderate to severe adverse experiences may require modification of the patient's dosage regimen, or in some cases, termination of IntronA therapy. Any patient developing liver function abnormalities during treatment with IntronA must be monitored closely and treatment discontinued if signs and symptoms progress.

Hypotension may occur during IntronA therapy or up to two days post-therapy and may require supportive treatment.

Adequate hydration must be maintained in patients undergoing IntronA therapy since hypotension related to fluid depletion has been seen in some patients. Fluid replacement may be necessary.

While fever may be associated with the flu-like syndrome reported commonly during interferon therapy, other causes of persistent fever must be ruled out.

IntronA must be used cautiously in patients with debilitating medical conditions, such as those with a history of pulmonary disease (e.g., chronic obstructive pulmonary disease) or diabetes mellitus prone to ketoacidosis. Caution must be observed also in patients with coagulation disorders (e.g., thrombophlebitis, pulmonary embolism) or severe myelosuppression.

Pulmonary infiltrates, pneumonitis, and pneumonia, occasionally resulting in fatality, have been observed rarely in interferon alpha treated patients, including those treated with IntronA. The aetiology has not been defined. These symptoms have been reported more frequently when shosaikoto, a Chinese herbal medicine, is administered concomitantly with interferon alpha (see section **4.5**). Any patient developing fever, cough, dyspnea or other respiratory symptoms must have a chest X-ray taken. If the chest X-ray shows pulmonary infiltrates or there is evidence of pulmonary function impairment, the patient is to be monitored closely, and, if appropriate, discontinue interferon alpha. While this has been reported more often in patients with chronic hepatitis C treated with interferon alpha, it has also been reported in patients with oncologic diseases treated with interferon alpha. Prompt discontinuation of interferon alpha administration and treatment with corticosteroids appear to be associated with resolution of pulmonary adverse events.

Ocular adverse events (see section **4.8**) including retinal haemorrhages, cotton wool spots, and retinal artery or vein obstruction have been reported in rare instances after treatment with alpha interferons. All patients should have a baseline eye examination. Any patient complaining of changes in visual acuity or visual fields, or reporting other ophthalmologic symptoms during treatment with IntronA, must have a prompt and complete eye examination. Periodic visual examinations during IntronA therapy are recommended particularly in patients with disorders that may be associated with retinopathy, such as diabetes mellitus or hypertension. Discontinuation of IntronA should be considered in patients who develop new or worsening ophthalmological disorders.

Psychiatric and central nervous system (CNS): Severe CNS effects, particularly depression, suicidal ideation and attempted suicide have been observed in some patients during IntronA therapy, and in the follow-up period. Among children and adolescents treated with IntronA in combination with ribavirin, suicidal ideation or attempts were reported more frequently compared to adult patients (2.4 % vs 1 %) during treatment and during the 6-month follow-up after treatment. As in adult patients, children and adolescents experienced other psychiatric adverse events (e.g., depression, emotional lability, and somnolence). Other CNS effects including aggressive behaviour (sometimes directed against others), confusion and alterations of mental status have been observed with alpha interferons. If patients develop psychiatric or CNS problems, including clinical depression, it is recommended that the patient be carefully monitored by the prescribing physicians during treatment and in the follow-up period. If such symptoms appear, the potential seriousness of these undesirable effects must be borne in mind by the prescribing physician. If psychiatric symptoms persist or worsen, or suicidal ideation is identified, it is recommended that treatment with IntronA be discontinued, and the patient followed, with psychiatric intervention, as appropriate.

Patients with existence of or history of severe psychiatric conditions:

If treatment with interferon alfa-2b is judged necessary in adult patients with existence or history of severe psychiatric conditions, this should only be initiated after having ensured appropriate individualised diagnostic and therapeutic management of the psychiatric condition. The use of interferon alfa-2b in children and adolescents with existence of or history of severe psychiatric conditions is contraindicated (see section **4.3**).

More significant obtundation and coma, including cases of encephalopathy, have been observed in some patients, usually elderly, treated at higher doses. While these effects are generally reversible, in a few patients full resolution took up to three weeks. Very rarely, seizures have occurred with high doses of IntronA.

Adult patients with a history of congestive heart failure, myocardial infarction and/or previous or current arrhythmic disorders, who require IntronA therapy, must be closely monitored. It is recommended that those patients who have pre-existing cardiac abnormalities and/or are in advanced stages of cancer have electrocardiograms taken prior to and during the course of treatment. Cardiac arrhythmias (primarily supraventricular) usually respond to conventional therapy but may require discontinuation of IntronA therapy. There are no data in children or adolescents with a history of cardiac disease.

Hypertriglyceridemia and aggravation of hypertriglyceridemia, sometimes severe, have been observed. Monitoring of lipid levels is, therefore, recommended.

Due to reports of interferon alpha exacerbating pre-existing psoriatic disease and sarcoidosis, use of IntronA in patients with psoriasis or sarcoidosis is recommended only if the potential benefit justifies the potential risk.

Preliminary data indicates that interferon alpha therapy may be associated with an increased rate of kidney graft rejection. Liver graft rejection has also been reported.

The development of auto-antibodies and autoimmune disorders has been reported during treatment with alpha interferons. Patients predisposed to the development of autoimmune disorders may be at increased risk. Patients with signs or symptoms compatible with autoimmune disorders should be evaluated carefully, and the benefit-risk of continued interferon therapy should be reassessed (see also section **4.4 Chronic hepatitis C, Monotherapy** (thyroid abnormalities) and section **4.8**).

Discontinue treatment with IntronA in patients with chronic hepatitis who develop prolongation of coagulation markers which might indicate liver decompensation.

Appropriate vaccination (hepatitis A and B) should be considered for patients in regular/repeated receipt of human plasma-derived albumin.

Standard measures to prevent infections resulting from the use of medicinal products prepared from human blood or plasma include selection of donors, screening of individual donations and plasma pools for specific markers of infection and the inclusion of effective manufacturing steps for the inactivation/removal of viruses. Despite this, when medicinal products prepared from human blood or plasma are administered, the possibility of transmitting infective agents cannot be totally excluded. This also applies to unknown or emerging viruses and other pathogens.

There are no reports of virus transmissions with albumin manufactured to European Pharmacopoeia specifications by established processes.

It is strongly recommended that every time that IntronA is administered to a patient, the name and batch number of the product are recorded in order to maintain a link between the patient and the batch of the product.

Chronic HepatitisC:

Combination therapy with ribavirin: Also see ribavirin labelling if IntronA is to be administered in combination with ribavirin in patients with chronic hepatitis C.

All patients in the chronic hepatitis C studies had a liver biopsy before inclusion, but in certain cases (i.e. patients with genotype 2 and 3), treatment may be possible without histological confirmation. Current treatment guidelines should be consulted as to whether a liver biopsy is needed prior to commencing treatment.

Monotherapy: Infrequently, adult patients treated for chronic hepatitis C with IntronA developed thyroid abnormalities, either hypothyroidism or hyperthyroidism. In clinical trials using IntronA therapy, 2.8 % patients overall developed thyroid abnormalities. The abnormalities were controlled by conventional therapy for thyroid dysfunction. The mechanism by which IntronA may alter thyroid status is unknown. Prior to initiation of IntronA therapy for the treatment of chronic hepatitis C, evaluate serum thyroid-stimulating hormone (TSH) levels. Any thyroid abnormality detected at that time must be treated with conventional therapy. IntronA treatment may be initiated if TSH levels can be maintained in the normal range by medication. Determine TSH levels if, during the course of IntronA therapy, a patient develops symptoms consistent with possible thyroid dysfunction. In the presence of thyroid dysfunction, IntronA treatment may be continued if TSH levels can be maintained in the normal range by medication. Discontinuation of IntronA therapy has not reversed thyroid dysfunction occurring during treatment (also see Children and adolescents, Thyroid monitoring).

Supplemental monitoring specific for children and adolescents

Thyroid Monitoring: Approximately 12 % of children treated with interferon alfa-2b and ribavirin developed increase in TSH. Another 4 % had a transient decrease below the lower limit of normal. Prior to initiation of IntronA therapy, TSH levels must be evaluated and any thyroid abnormality detected at that time must be treated with conventional therapy. IntronA therapy may be initiated if TSH levels can be maintained in the normal range by medication. Thyroid dysfunction during treatment with interferon alfa-2b and ribavirin has been observed. If thyroid abnormalities are detected, the patient's thyroid status should be evaluated and treated as clinically appropriate. Children and adolescents should be monitored every 3 months for evidence of thyroid dysfunction (e.g. TSH).

Growth and Development: During a 1-year course of therapy there was a decrease in the rate of linear growth (mean percentile decrease of 9 %) and a decrease in the rate of weight gain (mean percentile decrease of 13 %). A general reversal of these trends was noted during the 6 months follow-up post treatment. However, based on interim data from a long-term follow-up study, 12 (14 %) of 84 children had a > 15 percentile decrease in rate of linear growth, of whom 5 (6 %) children had a > 30 percentile decrease despite being off treatment for more than 1 year. There are no data on long term effects on growth and development and on sexual maturation.

HCV/HIV Coinfection: Patients co-infected with HIV and receiving Highly Active Anti-Retroviral Therapy (HAART) may be at increased risk of developing lactic acidosis. Caution should be used when adding IntronA and ribavirin to HAART therapy (see ribavirin SPC).

Co-infected patients with advanced cirrhosis receiving HAART may be at increased risk of hepatic decompensation and death. Adding treatment with alfa interferons alone or in combination with ribavirin may increase the risk in this patient subset.

Concomitant chemotherapy:

Administration of IntronA in combination with other chemotherapeutic agents (e.g., Ara-C, cyclophosphamide, doxorubicin, teniposide) may lead to increased risk of toxicity (severity and duration), which may be life-threatening or fatal as a result of the concomitantly administered medicinal product. The most commonly reported potentially life-threatening or fatal adverse events include mucositis, diarrhoea, neutropaenia, renal impairment, and electrolyte disturbance. Because of the risk of increased toxicity, careful adjustments of doses are required for IntronA and for the concomitant chemotherapeutic agents (see section **4.5**).

Laboratory Tests:

Standard haematological tests and blood chemistries (complete blood count and differential, platelet count, electrolytes, liver enzymes, serum protein, serum bilirubin and serum creatinine) are to be conducted in all patients prior to and periodically during systemic treatment with IntronA.

During treatment for hepatitis B or C the recommended testing schedule is at weeks 1, 2, 4, 8, 12, 16, and every other month, thereafter, throughout treatment. If ALT flares during IntronA therapy to greater than or equal to 2 times baseline, IntronA therapy may be continued unless signs and symptoms of liver failure are observed. During ALT flare, liver function tests: ALT, prothrombin time, alkaline phosphatase, albumin and bilirubin must be monitored at two-week intervals.

In patients treated for malignant melanoma, liver function and white blood cell (WBC) count and differential must be monitored weekly during the induction phase of therapy and monthly during the maintenance phase of therapy.

Effect on fertility: Interferon may impair fertility (see section **4.6** and section **5.3**).

4.5 Interaction with other medicinal products and other forms of Interaction

Narcotics, hypnotics or sedatives must be administered with caution when used concomitantly with IntronA.

Interactions between IntronA and other medicinal products have not been fully evaluated. Caution must be exercised when administering IntronA in combination with other potentially myelosuppressive agents.

Interferons may affect the oxidative metabolic process. This must be considered during concomitant therapy with medicinal products metabolised by this route, such as the xanthine derivatives theophylline or aminophylline. During concomitant therapy with xanthine agents, serum theophylline levels must be monitored and dosage adjusted if necessary.

Pulmonary infiltrates, pneumonitis, and pneumonia, occasionally resulting in fatality, have been observed rarely in interferon alpha treated patients, including those treated with IntronA. The aetiology has not been defined. These symptoms have been reported more frequently when shosaikoto, a Chinese herbal medicine, is administered concomitantly with interferon alpha (see section **4.4**).

Administration of IntronA in combination with other chemotherapeutic agents (e.g., Ara-C, cyclophosphamide, doxorubicin, teniposide) may lead to increased risk of toxicity (severity and duration) (see section **4.4**).

(Also see ribavirin labelling if IntronA is to be administered in combination with ribavirin in patients with chronic hepatitis C).

4.6 Pregnancy and lactation

Women of childbearing potential have to use effective contraception during treatment. IntronA must be used with caution in fertile men. Decreased serum estradiol and progesterone concentrations have been reported in women treated with human leukocyte interferon.

There are no adequate data from the use of interferon alfa-2b in pregnant women. Studies in animals have shown reproductive toxicity (see section **5.3**). The potential risk for humans is unknown. IntronA is to be used during pregnancy only if the potential benefit justifies the potential risk to the foetus.

It is not known whether the components of this medicinal product are excreted in human milk. Because of the potential for adverse events from IntronA in nursing infants, a decision must be made whether to discontinue nursing or to discontinue the medicinal product, taking into account the importance of the treatment to the mother.

Combination therapy with ribavirin: Ribavirin causes serious birth defects when administered during pregnancy. IntronA in combination with ribavirin is contraindicated (see ribavirin SPC). Females of childbearing potential have to use effective contraception during treatment and for 4 months after treatment.

4.7 Effects on ability to drive and use machines

Patients are to be advised that they may develop fatigue, somnolence, or confusion during treatment with IntronA, and therefore it is recommended that they avoid driving or operating machinery.

4.8 Undesirable effects

See ribavirin labelling for ribavirin-related undesirable effects if IntronA is to be administered in combination with ribavirin in patients with chronic hepatitis C.

In clinical trials conducted in a broad range of indications and at a wide range of doses (from 6 MIU/m^2/week in hairy cell leukaemia up to 100 MIU/m^2/week in melanoma), the most commonly reported undesirable effects were fever, fatigue, headache and myalgia. Fever and fatigue were often reversible within 72 hours of interruption or cessation of treatment.

The safety profile shown here was determined from 4 clinical trials in hepatitis C in which patients were treated with IntronA alone or in combination with ribavirin for one year. All patients in these trials received 3 MIU of IntronA three times a week. The percentage of patients reporting (treatment related) undesirable effects ≥ 10 % is presented in **Table 1** as a range to capture the incidences reported in individual treatment groups among these clinical trials in naïve patients treated for one year. Severity was generally mild to moderate.

Table 1. Undesirable effects reported very commonly in any of the clinical trials in naïve patients treated for one year with monotherapy or combination therapy, Very common (>1/10) (CIOMS III)

Body System	IntronA n=806	IntronA + Rebetol n=1,010
Infections and infestations		
Infection viral	0-7 %	3-10 %
Metabolism and nutrition disorders		
Weight decrease	6-11 %	9-19 %
Psychiatric disorders		
Depression	16-36 %	25-34 %
Irritability	13-27 %	18-34 %
Insomnia	21-28 %	33-41 %
Anxiety	8-12 %	8-16 %
Concentration impaired	8-14 %	9-21 %
Emotional lability	5-8 %	5-11 %
Nervous system disorders		
Headache	51-64 %	48-64 %
Respiratory, thoracic and mediastinal disorders		
Pharyngitis	3-7 %	7-13 %
Coughing	3-7 %	8-11 %
Dyspnoea	2-9 %	10-22 %
Gastrointestinal disorders		
Nausea/Vomiting	18-31 %/ 3-10 %	25-44 %/ 6-10 %
Anorexia	14-19 %	19-26 %
Diarrhoea	12-22 %	13-18 %
Abdominal pain	9-17 %	9-14 %
Skin and subcutaneous tissue disorders		
Alopecia	22-31 %	26-32 %
Pruritus	6-9 %	18-27 %
Skin dry	5-8 %	10-21 %
Rash	5-7 %	15-24 %
Musculoskeletal and connective tissue disorders		
Myalgia	41-61 %	30-62 %
Arthralgia	25-31 %	21-29 %
Musculoskeletal pain	15-20 %	11-20 %
General disorders and administration site conditions		
Injection site inflammation	9-16 %	6-17 %
Injection site reaction	5-8 %	3-36 %
Fatigue	42-70 %	43-68 %
Rigors	15-39 %	19-41 %
Fever	29-39 %	29-41 %
Flu-like symptoms	19-37 %	18-29 %
Asthenia	9-30 %	9-30 %
Dizziness	8-18 %	10-22 %

Table 2. Undesirable effects reported commonly in clinical trials of 483 patients treated with IntronA + Ribavirin
(IntronA 3 MIU 3 times a week, ribavirin >10.6 mg/kg for one year) Common (>1/100, <1/10) (CIOMS III)

Body System	IntronA + Rebetol
Infections and infestations 1-5 %	Herpes simplex (resistance)
Blood and lymphatic system disorders 5-10 %: 1-5 %:	Leukopaenia Thrombocytopaenia, lymphadenopathy, lymphopenia
Endocrine disorders 1-5 %:	Hyperthyroidism, hypothyroidism
Metabolism and nutrition disorders 1-5 %:	Hyperuricemia, hypocalcemia, thirst
Psychiatric disorders 5-10 %: 1-5 %:	Agitation, nervousness Sleep disorder, somnolence, libido decreased
Nervous system disorders 5-10 % 1-5 %:	Mouth dry, sweating increased Hypoesthesia, vertigo, confusion, parasthesia, tremor, migraine, flushing, lacrimal gland disorder
Eye disorders 5-10 %: 1-5 %:	Vision blurred Conjunctivitis, eye pain, vision abnormal
Ear and labyrinth disorders 1-5 %:	Tinnitus
Cardiac disorders 1-5 %:	Palpitation, tachycardia
Vascular disorders 1-5 %:	Hypertension
Respiratory, thoracic and mediastinal disorders 1-5 %:	Bronchitis, cough nonproductive, epistaxis, nasal congestion, respiratory disorder, rhinitis, rhinorrhea, sinusitis
Gastrointestinal disorders 5-10 %: 1-5 %:	Dyspepsia, stomatitis Constipation, dehydration, gingivitis, glossitis, loose stools, stomatitis ulcerative, taste perversion
Hepatobiliary disorders 1-5 %:	Hepatomegaly
Skin and subcutaneous tissue disorders 1-5 %:	Eczema, psoriasis (new or aggravated), rash erythematous, rash maculopapular, skin disorder, erythema
Musculoskeletal and connective tissue disorders 1-5 %:	Arthritis
Renal and urinary disorders 1-5 %:	Micturition frequency
Reproductive system and breast disorders 1-5 %:	Amenorrhea, breast pain, dysmenorrhea, menorrhagia, menstrual disorder, vaginal disorder
General disorders and administration site conditions 5-10 %: 1-5 %:	Malaise, chest pain Injection site pain, right upper quadrant pain

These undesirable effects have also been reported with IntronA alone.

The undesirable effects seen with hepatitis C are representative of those reported when IntronA is administered in other indications, with some anticipated dose-related increases in incidence. For example, in a trial of high-dose adjuvant IntronA treatment in patients with melanoma, incidences of fatigue, fever, myalgia, neutropaenia/anaemia, anorexia, nausea and vomiting, diarrhoea, chills, flu-like symptoms, depression, alopecia, altered taste, and dizziness were greater than in the hepatitis C trials. Severity also increased with high dose therapy (WHO Grade 3 and 4, in 66 % and 14 % of patients, respectively), in comparison with the mild to moderate severity usually associated with lower doses. Undesirable effects were usually managed by dose adjustment.

Additional adverse events were reported rarely (> 1/10,000, < 1/1,000) or very rarely (< 1/10,000) during clinical trials in other indications or following the marketing of interferon alfa-2b:

Immune system disorders:

very rarely: sarcoidosis or exacerbation of sarcoidosis

Endocrine disorders:

very rarely: diabetes, aggravated diabetes

Metabolism and nutrition disorders:

very rarely: hyperglycaemia, hypertriglyceridaemia

Psychiatric disorders:

rarely: suicide ideation

very rarely: aggressive behaviour (sometimes directed against others), suicide attempts, suicide, psychosis, including hallucinations

Nervous system disorders:

very rarely: impaired consciousness, neuropathy, polyneuropathy, seizure, encephalopathy, cerebrovascular ischaemia, cerebrovascular haemorrhage

Eye disorders:

rarely: retinal haemorrhages, retinopathies (including macular oedema), cotton-wool spots, retinal artery or vein obstruction, loss of visual acuity or visual field, optic neuritis and papilloedema

Ear and labyrinth disorders:

very rarely: hearing disorder, hearing loss

Cardiac disorders:

very rarely: cardiac ischaemia and myocardial infarction

Vascular disorders:

very rarely: hypotension; peripheral ischaemia

Respiratory, thoracic and mediastinal disorders:

rarely: pneumonia

very rarely: pulmonary infiltrates, pneumonitis

Gastrointestinal:

very rarely: pancreatitis; increased appetite; gingival bleeding; colitis, mainly ulcerative and ischemic

Hepatobiliary disorders:

very rarely: hepatotoxicity, including fatality

Skin and subcutaneous tissue disorders:

very rarely: face oedema, erythema multiforme, Stevens Johnson syndrome, toxic epidermal necrolysis, injection site necrosis

Musculoskeletal and connective tissue disorders:

very rarely: rhabdomyolysis, sometimes serious; leg cramps; back pain; myositis

Renal and urinary disorders:

very rarely: nephrotic syndrome, renal insufficiency, renal failure

Very rarely IntronA used alone or in combination with ribavirin may be associated with aplastic anaemia.

Cardiovascular (CVS) adverse events, particularly arrhythmia, appeared to be correlated mostly with pre-existing CVS disease and prior therapy with cardiotoxic agents (see section **4.4**). Cardiomyopathy, that may be reversible upon discontinuation of interferon alpha, has been reported rarely in patients without prior evidence of cardiac disease.

A wide variety of autoimmune and immune-mediated disorders have been reported with alpha interferons including thyroid disorders, systemic lupus erythematosus, rheumatoid arthritis (new or aggravated), idiopathic and thrombotic thrombocytopenic purpura, vasculitis, neuropathies including mononeuropathies (see also section **4.4**).

Clinically significant laboratory abnormalities, most frequently occurring at doses greater than 10 million IU daily, include reduction in granulocyte and white blood cell counts; decreases in haemoglobin level and platelet count; increases in alkaline phosphatase, LDH, serum creatinine and serum urea nitrogen levels. Increase in serum ALT/AST (SGPT/SGOT) levels have been noted as an abnormality in some non-hepatitis subjects and also in some patients with chronic hepatitis B coincident with clearance of viral DNAp.

For safety with respect to transmissible agents, see section **4.4.**

Children and adolescents – Chronic Hepatitis C

In clinical trials of 118 children or adolescents 3 to 16 years of age, 6 % discontinued therapy due to adverse events. In general, the adverse event profile in the limited paediatric population studied was similar to that observed in adults, although there is a paediatric specific concern regarding growth inhibition as decrease in height (mean percentile decrease of growth velocity of 9 %) and weight (mean percentile decrease of 13 %) percentile were observed during treatment (see section **4.4**). Furthermore, suicidal ideation or attempts were reported more frequently compared to adult patients (2.4 % vs 1 %) during treatment and during the 6 month follow-up after treatment. As in adult patients, children and adolescents also experienced other psychiatric adverse events (e.g., depression, emotional lability, and somnolence) (see section **4.4**). In addition, injection site disorders, fever, anorexia, vomiting, and emotional lability occurred more frequently in children and adolescents compared to adult patients. Dose modifications were required in 30 % of patients, most commonly for anaemia and neutropaenia.

Undesirable effects reported in paediatric clinical trials, and not previously reported at an incidence ⩾ 1 % in adults, are shown in **Table 3**. All effects reported at a ⩾ 10 % incidence in paediatric trials were previously reported in adults (**Table 2**) and are not repeated in the paediatric table.

(see Table 3)

Table 3 Undesirable effects very commonly and commonly reported in paediatric clinical trials (⩾ 1 % of patients treated with IntronA + ribavirin) Very common (>1/10) - Common (>1/100, <1/10)

Body system	⩾ 10%	5 % - < 10 %	1 % - < 5 %
Infection and infestations	Viral infection		Tooth abscess, bacterial infection, fungal infection, herpes simplex, otitis media
Neoplasms benign, malignant and unspecified (including cysts and polyps)			Neoplasm (unspecified),
Blood and lymphatic system disorders	Anaemia, neutropenia		Bruise, thrombocytopaenia, lymphadenopathy
Endocrine disorders	Hypothyroidism		Hyperthyroidism, virilism,
Metabolism and nutrition disorders			Hypertriglyceridemia, hyperuricemia
Psychiatric disorders	Depression, emotional lability, insomnia, irritability	Agitation, somnolence	Aggressive reaction, anxiety, apathy, increased appetite, behavior disorder, concentration impaired, abnormal dreaming, nervousness, sleep disorder, somnambulism, suicidal ideation
Nervous system disorders	Headache, dizziness	Tremor	Confusion, hyperkinesia, dysphonia, paresthaesia, hyperaesthesia, hypoaesthesia
Eye disorders			Conjunctivitis, eye pain, abnormal vision, lacrimal gland disorder
Vascular disorders		Pallor	Raynaud's disease
Respiratory, thoracic and mediastinal disorders	Pharyngitis	Epistaxis	Coughing, dyspnoea, nasal congestion, nasal irritation, pulmonary infection, rhinorrhea, sneezing, tachypnea
Gastrointestinal disorders	Abdominal pain, anorexia, diarrhoea, nausea, vomiting		Constipation, dyspepsia, gastroenteritis, gastroesophogeal reflux, gastrointestinal disorder, glossitis, loose stools, mouth ulceration, rectal disorder, stomatitis, stomatitis ulcerative, toothache, tooth disorder
Hepatobiliary disorders			Hepatic function abnormal
Skin and subcutaneous tissue disorders	Alopecia, rash	Pruritus	Acne, eczema, skin laceration, nail disorder, dry skin, photosensitivity reaction, maculopapular rash, skin discolouration, skin disorder, erythema, sweating increased
Musculoskeletal and connective tissue disorders	Arthralgia, musculoskeletal pain, myalgia		
Renal and urinary disorders			Enuresis, micturition disorder, urinary tract infection, urinary incontinence
Reproductive system and breast disorders			Female: amenorrhea, menorrhagia, menstrual disorder, vaginal disorder, vaginitis Male: testicular pain
General disorders and administration site conditions	Injection site reaction, injection site inflammation, fatigue, fever, rigors, influenza-like symptoms, malaise, growth rate decrease (height and/or weight decrease for age)	Injection site pain	Asthenia, flushing, oedema, chest pain, right upper quadrant pain

4.9 Overdose

No case of overdose has been reported that has led to acute clinical manifestations. However, as for any pharmacologically active compound, symptomatic treatment with frequent monitoring of vital signs and close observation of the patient is indicated.

5. PHARMACOLOGICAL PROPERTIES

5.1 Pharmacodynamic properties

Pharmacotherapeutic group: Immunostimulants, cytokines and immunomodulators, interferons, interferon alfa-2b, ATC code: L03A B05

IntronA is a sterile, stable, formulation of highly purified interferon alfa-2b produced by recombinant DNA techniques. Recombinant interferon alfa-2b is a water-soluble protein with a molecular weight of approximately 19,300 daltons. It is obtained from a clone of E. coli, which harbours a genetically engineered plasmid hybrid encompassing an interferon alfa-2b gene from human leukocytes.

The activity of IntronA is expressed in terms of IU, with 1 mg of recombinant interferon alfa-2b protein corresponding to

Table 4 Sustained virologic response rates with IntronA + ribavirin (one year of treatment) by genotype and viral load

HCV Genotype	I N=503 C95-132/I95-143	I/R N=505 C95-132/I95-143	I/R N=505 C/I98-580
All Genotypes	**16 %**	**41 %**	**47 %**
Genotype 1	9 %	29 %	33 %
Genotype 1 ⩽ 2 million copies/ml	25 %	33 %	45 %
Genotype 1 > 2 million copies/ml	3 %	27 %	29 %
Genotype 2/3	31 %	65 %	79 %

I IntronA (3 MIU 3 times a week)

I/R IntronA (3 MIU 3 times a week) + ribavirin (1,000/1,200 mg/day)

2.6×10^8 IU. International Units are determined by comparison of the activity of the recombinant interferon alfa-2b with the activity of the international reference preparation of human leukocyte interferon established by the World Health Organisation.

The interferons are a family of small protein molecules with molecular weights of approximately 15,000 to 21,000 daltons. They are produced and secreted by cells in response to viral infections or various synthetic and biological inducers. Three major classes of interferons have been identified: alpha, beta and gamma. These three main classes are themselves not homogeneous and may contain several different molecular species of interferon. More than 14 genetically distinct human alpha interferons have been identified. IntronA has been classified as recombinant interferon alfa-2b.

Interferons exert their cellular activities by binding to specific membrane receptors on the cell surface. Human interferon receptors, as isolated from human lymphoblastoid (Daudi) cells, appear to be highly asymmetric proteins. They exhibit selectivity for human but not murine interferons, suggesting species specificity. Studies with other interferons have demonstrated species specificity. However, certain monkey species, eg, rhesus monkeys, are susceptible to pharmacodynamic stimulation upon exposure to human type 1 interferons.

The results of several studies suggest that, once bound to the cell membrane, interferon initiates a complex sequence of intracellular events that include the induction of certain enzymes. It is thought that this process, at least in part, is responsible for the various cellular responses to interferon, including inhibition of virus replication in virus-infected cells, suppression of cell proliferation and such immunomodulating activities as enhancement of the phagocytic activity of macrophages and augmentation of the specific cytotoxicity of lymphocytes for target cells. Any or all of these activities may contribute to interferon's therapeutic effects.

Recombinant interferon alfa-2b has exhibited antiproliferative effects in studies employing both animal and human cell culture systems as well as human tumour xenografts in animals. It has demonstrated significant immunomodulatory activity *in vitro*.

Recombinant interferon alfa-2b also inhibits viral replication *in vitro* and *in vivo*. Although the exact antiviral mode of action of recombinant interferon alfa-2b is unknown, it appears to alter the host cell metabolism. This action inhibits viral replication or if replication occurs, the progeny virions are unable to leave the cell.

Chronic hepatitis B:

Current clinical experience in patients who remain on interferon alfa-2b for 4 to 6 months indicates that therapy can produce clearance of serum HBV-DNA. An improvement in liver histology has been observed. In adult patients with loss of HBeAg and HBV-DNA, a significant reduction in morbidity and mortality has been observed.

Interferon alfa-2b (6 MIU/m^2 3 times a week for 6 months) has been given to children with chronic active hepatitis B. Because of a methodological flaw, efficacy could not be demonstrated. Moreover children treated with interferon alfa-2b experienced a reduced rate of growth and some cases of depression were observed.

Chronic hepatitis C:

In adult patients receiving interferon in combination with ribavirin, the achieved sustained response rate is 47 %. Superior efficacy has been demonstrated with the combination of pegylated interferon with ribavirin (sustained response rate of 61 % achieved in a study performed in naïve patients with a ribavirin dose > 10.6 mg/kg, p < 0.01).

Adult patients: IntronA alone or in combination with ribavirin has been studied in 4 randomised Phase III clinical trials in 2,552 interferon-naïve patients with chronic hepatitis C. The trials compared the efficacy of IntronA used alone or in combination with ribavirin. Efficacy was defined as sustained virologic response, 6 months after the end of treatment. Eligible patients for these trials had chronic hepatitis C confirmed by a positive HCV-RNA polymerase chain reaction assay (PCR) (> 100 copies/ml), a liver biopsy consistent with a histologic diagnosis of chronic hepatitis with no other cause for the chronic hepatitis, and abnormal serum ALT.

IntronA was administered at a dose of 3 MIU 3 times a week as monotherapy or in combination with ribavirin. The majority of patients in these clinical trials were treated for one year. All patients were followed for an additional 6 months after the end of treatment for the determination of sustained virologic response. Sustained virologic response rates for treatment groups treated for one year with IntronA alone or in combination with ribavirin (from two studies) are shown in **Table 4**.

Co-administration of IntronA with ribavirin increased the efficacy of IntronA by at least two fold for the treatment of chronic heptatitis C in naïve patients. HCV genotype and baseline virus load are prognostic factors which are known to affect response rates. The increased response rate to the combination of IntronA + ribavirin, compared with IntronA alone, is maintained across all subgroups. The relative benefit of combination therapy with IntronA + ribavirin is particularly significant in the most difficult to treat subgroup of patients (genotype 1 and high virus load) (**Table 4**).

Response rates in these trials were increased with compliance. Regardless of genotype, patients who received IntronA in combination with ribavirin and received ⩾ 80 % of their treatment had a higher sustained response 6 months after 1 year of treatment than those who took < 80 % of their treatment (56 % vs. 32 % in trial C/I98-580).

(see Table 4 above)

Relapse patients: A total of 345 interferon alpha relapse patients were treated in two clinical trials with IntronA monotherapy or in combination with ribavirin. In these patients, the addition of ribavirin to IntronA increased by as much as 10-fold the efficacy of IntronA used alone in the treatment of chronic hepatitis C (48.6 % vs. 4.7 %). This enhancement in efficacy included loss of serum HCV (< 100 copies/ml by PCR), improvement in hepatic inflammation, and normalisation of ALT, and was sustained when measured 6 months after the end of treatment.

Clinical trials in paediatric patients with chronic hepatitis C:

Children and adolescents 3 to 16 years of age with compensated chronic hepatitis C and detectable HCV-RNA (assessed by a central laboratory using a research-based RT-PCR assay) were enrolled in two multicentre trials and received IntronA 3 MIU/m^2 3 times a week plus ribavirin 15 mg/kg per day for 1 year followed by 6 months follow-up after-treatment. A total of 118 patients were enrolled: 57 % male, 80 % Caucasian, and 78 % genotype 1, 64 % ⩽ 12 years of age. The population enrolled mainly consisted in children with mild to moderate hepatitis C. Sustained virological response rates in children and adolescents were similar to those in adults. Due to the lack of data in children with severe progression of the disease, and the potential for undesirable effects, the benefit/risk of the combination of ribavirin and interferon alfa-2b needs to be carefully considered in this population (see sections **4.1**, **4.4** and **4.8**).

Study results are summarized in **Table 5**.

Table 5. Virological response in previously untreated paediatric patients

	IntronA 3 MIU/m^2 3 times a week **+ ribavirin 15 mg/kg/day**
Overall Response[1] (n=118)	54 (46 %)*
Genotype 1 (n=92)	33 (36 %)*
Genotype 2/3/4 (n=26)	21 (81 %)*

*Number (%) of patients

1. Defined as HCV-RNA below limit of detection using a research based RT-PCR assay at end of treatment and during follow-up period

5.2 Pharmacokinetic properties

The pharmacokinetics of IntronA were studied in healthy volunteers following single 5 million IU/m^2 and 10 million IU doses administered subcutaneously, at 5 million IU/m^2 administered intramuscularly and as a 30-minute intravenous infusion. The mean serum interferon concentrations following subcutaneous and intramuscular injections were comparable. C_{max} occurred three to 12 hours after the lower dose and six to eight hours after the higher dose. The elimination half-lives of interferon injections were approximately two to three hours, and six to seven hours, respectively. Serum levels were below the detection limit 16 and 24 hours, respectively, post-injection. Both subcutaneous and intramuscular administration resulted in bioavailabilities greater than 100 %.

After intravenous administration, serum interferon levels peaked (135 to 273 IU/ml) by the end of the infusion, then declined at a slightly more rapid rate than after subcutaneous or intramuscular administration of medicinal product, becoming undetectable four hours after the infusion. The elimination half-life was approximately two hours.

Urine levels of interferon were below the detection limit following each of the three routes of administration.

Children and adolescents: Multiple-dose pharmacokinetic properties for IntronA injection and ribavirin capsules in children and adolescents with chronic hepatitis C, between 5 and 16 years of age, are summarized in **Table 6**. The pharmacokinetics of IntronA and ribavirin (dose-normalized) are similar in adults and children or adolescents.

Table 6. Mean (% CV) multiple-dose pharmacokinetic parameters for IntronA and ribavirin capsules when administered to children or adolescents with chronic hepatitis C

Parameter	**Ribavirin** 15 mg/kg/day as 2 divided doses (n = 17)	**IntronA** 3 MIU/m^2 3 times a week (n = 54)
T_{max} (hr)	1.9 (83)	5.9 (36)
C_{max} (ng/ml)	3,275 (25)	51 (48)
AUC*	29,774 (26)	622 (48)
Apparent clearance l/hr/kg	0.27 (27)	Not done

*AUC_{12} (ng.hr/ml) for ribavirin; AUC_{0-24} (IU.hr/ml) for IntronA

Interferon neutralising factor assays were performed on serum samples of patients who received IntronA in Schering-Plough monitored clinical trials. Interferon neutralising factors are antibodies which neutralise the antiviral activity of interferon. The clinical incidence of neutralising factors developing in cancer patients treated systemically is 2.9 % and in chronic hepatitis patients is 6.2 %. The detectable titres are low in almost all cases and have not been regularly associated with loss of response or any other autoimmune phenomenon. In patients with hepatitis, no loss of response was observed apparently due to the low titres.

5.3 Preclinical safety data

Although interferon is generally recognised as being species specific, toxicity studies in animals were conducted. Injections of human recombinant interferon alfa-2b for up to three months have shown no evidence of toxicity in mice, rats, and rabbits. Daily dosing of cynomolgus monkeys with 20×10^6 IU/kg/day for 3 months caused no remarkable toxicity. Toxicity was demonstrated in monkeys given 100×10^6 IU/kg/day for 3 months.

In studies of interferon use in non-human primates, abnormalities of the menstrual cycle have been observed (see section **4.4**).

Results of animal reproduction studies indicate that recombinant interferon alfa-2b was not teratogenic in rats or rabbits, nor did it adversely affect pregnancy, foetal development or reproductive capacity in offspring of treated rats. Interferon alfa-2b has been shown to have abortifacient effects in *Macaca mulatta* (rhesus monkeys) at 90 and 180 times the recommended intramuscular or subcutaneous dose of 2 million IU/m^2. Abortion was observed in all dose groups (7.5 million, 15 million and 30 million IU/kg), and was statistically significant versus control at the mid- and high-dose groups (corresponding to 90 and 180 times the recommended intramuscular or subcutaneous dose of 2 million IU/m^2). High doses of other forms of interferons alpha and beta are known to produce dose-related anovulatory and abortifacient effects in rhesus monkeys.

Mutagenicity studies with interferon alfa-2b revealed no adverse events.

No studies have been conducted in juvenile animals to examine the effects of treatment on growth, development, sexual maturation, and behaviour.

6. PHARMACEUTICAL PARTICULARS

6.1 List of excipients

IntronA 10 million IU/ml powder and solvent for solution for injection or infusion:

Glycine, sodium phosphate dibasic, sodium phosphate monobasic and albumin solution human.

Solvent: water for injections

IntronA 25 million IU/2.5ml solution for injection or infusion:

Sodium phosphate dibasic, sodium phosphate monobasic, edetate disodium, sodium chloride, m-cresol, polysorbate 80 and water for injections.

6.2 Incompatibilities

This medicinal product must not be mixed with other medicinal products except those mentioned in section 6.6.

6.3 Shelf life

IntronA 10 million IU/ml powder and solvent for solution for injection or infusion:

3 years

After reconstitution: Chemical and physical in-use stability has been demonstrated for 24 hours at 25°C.

From a microbiological point of view, the product is to be used immediately. If not used immediately, in-use storage times and conditions prior to use are the responsibility of the user and would normally not be longer than 24 hours at 2°C - 8°C.

IntronA 25 million IU/2.5ml solution for injection or infusion:

2 years

After first opening the container: Chemical and physical in-use stability has been demonstrated for 28 days at 2°C – 8°C.

From a microbiological point of view, once opened, the product may be stored for a maximum of 28 days at 2°C – 8°C. Other in-use storage times and conditions are the responsibility of the user.

6.4 Special precautions for storage

IntronA 10 million IU/ml powder and solvent for solution for injection or infusion:

Store in a refrigerator (2°C – 8°C). Do not freeze. For the purpose of transport and/or to facilitate ambulatory use the non-reconstituted product can be kept at or below 25°C for a period up to four weeks before use. If the product is not reconstituted during the four-week period, it cannot be put back in the refrigerator for a new storage period and is to be discarded.

IntronA 25 million IU/2.5ml solution for injection or infusion:

Store in a refrigerator (2°C – 8°C). Do not freeze. For the purpose of transport, the solution can be kept at or below 25°C for a period up to seven days before use. IntronA can be put back in the refrigerator at any time during this seven-day period. If the product is not used during the seven-day period, it cannot be put back in the refrigerator for a new storage period and is to be discarded.

6.5 Nature and contents of container

IntronA 10 million IU/ml powder and solvent for solution for injection or infusion:

The powder is contained in a 2 ml vial, type I flint glass, with a butyl rubber stopper in an aluminium flip-off seal with a polypropylene bonnet. The solvent is presented in a 2 ml ampoule, type I flint glass.

- 1 vial of powder for solution for injection or infusion, 1 ampoule of water for injections, 1 injection syringe, 2 injection needles and 1 cleansing swab

- 6 vials of powder for solution for injection or infusion, 6 ampoules of water for injections

- 10 vials of powder for solution for injection or infusion, 10 ampoules of water for injections, 10 injection syringes, 20 injection needles and 10 cleansing swabs

IntronA 25 million IU/2.5ml solution for injection or infusion:

The solution is contained in a 5 ml vial, type I flint glass, with a halobutyl rubber stopper in an aluminium flip-off seal with a polypropylene bonnet.

- 1 vial

- 1 vial, 6 injection syringes, 6 injection needles and 12 cleansing swabs

- 2 vials,

- 2 vials, 12 injection syringes, 12 injection needles and 24 cleansing swabs

- 12 vials

- 12 vials, 72 injection syringes, 72 injection needles and 144 cleansing swabs

Not all pack sizes may be marketed.

6.6 Instructions for use and handling

Not all dosage forms and strengths are appropriate for some indications. Please make sure to select an appropriate dosage form and strength (see section **4.2**).

IntronA 10 million IU/ml powder and solvent for solution for injection or infusion:

Reconstitution of IntronA, powder for solution for injection or infusion, for parenteral administration: IntronA is supplied as a powder at strengths of 1 million IU/ml for single-dose use. Vials must be reconstituted with 1 ml of water for injections. The reconstituted solutions are isotonic for parenteral administration.

Using a sterilised injection syringe and injection needle, inject 1 ml water for injections into the vial of IntronA. Agitate gently to facilitate complete dissolution of the powder. The appropriate dose can then be withdrawn with a sterile injection syringe and injected.

As for all parenteral medicinal products, inspect the reconstituted solution visually for particulate matter and discoloration prior to administration. The reconstituted solution should be clear and colourless.

Detailed instructions for the subcutaneous use of the product are provided with the package leaflet.

Preparation of IntronA for intravenous infusion: The infusion must be prepared immediately prior to use. The lyophilised powder form of IntronA is to be reconstituted by adding 1 ml of water for injections to the vial. The calculated amount of interferon for the appropriate dose then is withdrawn from the vial(s), added to 100 ml of 0.9 % sodium chloride solution and administered over 20 minutes. Final concentration of interferon in sodium chloride solution must not be less than 1×10^5 IU/ml.

NO OTHER MEDICINAL PRODUCT CAN BE INFUSED CONCOMITANTLY WITH INTRONA.

Any unused product must be discarded after withdrawal of the dose.

IntronA 25 million IU/2.5ml solution for injection or infusion:

IntronA solution for injection or infusion, may be injected directly after withdrawal of the appropriate doses from the vial with a sterile injection syringe.

Detailed instructions for the subcutaneous use of the product are provided with the package leaflet.

Preparation of IntronA for intravenous infusion: The infusion is to be prepared immediately prior to use. Any size vial may be used to measure the required dose; however, final concentration of interferon in sodium chloride solution must be not less than 0.3 million IU/ml. The appropriate dose of IntronA is withdrawn from the vial(s), added to 50 ml of 0.9 % sodium chloride solution in a PVC bag or glass bottle for intravenous use and administered over 20 minutes.

NO OTHER MEDICINAL PRODUCT CAN BE INFUSED CONCOMITANTLY WITH INTRONA.

As with all parenteral medicinal products, prior to administration inspect IntronA, solution for injection or infusion, visually for particulate matter and discolouration. The solution should be clear and colourless.

7. MARKETING AUTHORISATION HOLDER

SP Europe

73, rue de Stalle

B-1180 Bruxelles

Belgium

8. MARKETING AUTHORISATION NUMBER(S)

IntronA 10 million IU/ml powder and solvent for solution for injection or infusion: EU/1/99/127/006-008

IntronA 25 million IU/2.5ml solution for injection or infusion: EU/1/99/127/027-030; 043-044

9. DATE OF FIRST AUTHORISATION/RENEWAL OF THE AUTHORISATION

Date of first authorisation: 9 March 2000

Date of last renewal: 23 May 2005

10. DATE OF REVISION OF THE TEXT

23 May 2005

Legal Category

Prescription Only Medicine

IntronA/6-05/7

INVANZ 1g powder for concentrate for solution for infusion

(Merck Sharp & Dohme Limited)

1. NAME OF THE MEDICINAL PRODUCT

INVANZ▼ 1 g powder for concentrate for solution for infusion.

2. QUALITATIVE AND QUANTITATIVE COMPOSITION

Each vial contains 1.0 g ertapenem equivalent to 1.046 g ertapenem sodium.

For excipients, see section 6.1.

3. PHARMACEUTICAL FORM

Powder for concentrate for solution for infusion. White to off-white powder.

4. CLINICAL PARTICULARS

4.1 Therapeutic indications

Treatment of the following infections when caused by bacteria known or very likely to be susceptible to ertapenem and when parenteral therapy is required (see section 4.4 and section 5.1):

- Intra-abdominal infections
- Community acquired pneumonia
- Acute gynaecological infections

Consideration should be given to official guidance on the appropriate use of antibacterial agents.

4.2 Posology and method of administration

Adults and adolescents (13 to 17 years of age): The dose of INVANZ is 1 gram (g) given once a day by the intravenous route.

Children (3 months to 12 years of age): The dose of INVANZ is 15 mg/kg given twice daily (not to exceed 1 g/day) by the intravenous route. INVANZ is not recommended in children under 3 months of age, as no data are available (see section 4.4).

Intravenous administration: INVANZ should be infused over a period of 30 minutes.

The usual duration of therapy with INVANZ is 3 to 14 days but may vary depending on the type and severity of infection and causative pathogen(s). When clinically indicated, a switch to an appropriate oral antibacterial agent may be implemented if clinical improvement has been observed.

Renal insufficiency:

INVANZ may be used for the treatment of infections in adult patients with renal insufficiency. In patients whose creatinine clearance is > 30 ml/min/1.73 m², no dosage adjustment is necessary. There are inadequate data on the safety and efficacy of ertapenem in patients with advanced renal insufficiency to support a dose recommendation. Therefore, ertapenem should not be used in these patients. (See section 5.2.) There are no data in children and adolescents with renal insufficiency.

Patients on haemodialysis:

There are inadequate data on the safety and efficacy of ertapenem in patients on haemodialysis to support a dose recommendation. Therefore, ertapenem should not be used in these patients.

Hepatic insufficiency:

No dosage adjustment is recommended in patients with impaired hepatic function (see section 5.2).

Elderly:

The recommended dose of INVANZ should be administered, except in cases of advanced renal insufficiency (see *Renal insufficiency*).

4.3 Contraindications

- Hypersensitivity to ertapenem or to any of the excipients
- Hypersensitivity to any other carbapenem antibacterial agent
- Severe hypersensitivity (e.g. anaphylactic reaction, severe skin reaction) to any other type of beta-lactam antibacterial agent (e.g. penicillins or cephalosporins).

4.4 Special warnings and special precautions for use

Serious and occasionally fatal hypersensitivity (anaphylactic) reactions have been reported in patients receiving therapy with beta-lactams. These reactions are more likely to occur in individuals with a history of sensitivity to multiple allergens. Before initiating therapy with ertapenem, careful inquiry should be made concerning previous hypersensitivity reactions to penicillins, cephalosporins, other beta-lactams and other allergens (see section 4.3). If an allergic reaction to ertapenem occurs, discontinue the therapy immediately. **Serious anaphylactic reactions require immediate emergency treatment.**

As with other antibiotics, prolonged use of ertapenem may result in overgrowth of non-susceptible organisms. Repeated evaluation of the patient's condition is essential. If superinfection occurs during therapy, appropriate measures should be taken.

Antibiotic-associated colitis and pseudomembranous colitis have been reported with nearly all antibacterial agents, including ertapenem, and may range in severity from mild to life-threatening. Therefore, it is important to consider this diagnosis in patients who present with diarrhoea subsequent to the administration of antibacterial agents. Discontinuation of therapy with INVANZ and the administration of specific treatment for *Clostridium difficile* should be considered. Medicinal products that inhibit peristalsis should not be given.

The efficacy of INVANZ in the treatment of community acquired pneumonia due to penicillin-resistant *Streptococcus pneumoniae* has not been established. There is relatively little experience with ertapenem in children less than two years of age. In this age group, particular care should be taken to establish the susceptibility of the infecting organism(s) to ertapenem. No data are available in children under 3 months of age.

Experience in the use of ertapenem in the treatment of severe infections is limited. In clinical studies for the treatment of community-acquired pneumonia, in adults, 25 % of evaluable patients treated with ertapenem had severe disease (defined as pneumonia severity index > III). In a clinical study for the treatment of acute gynaecologic infections, in adults, 26 % of evaluable patients treated with ertapenem had severe disease (defined as temperature ⩾ 39°C and/or bacteraemia); ten patients had bacteraemia. Of evaluable patients treated with ertapenem in a clinical study for the treatment of intra-abdominal infections, in adults, 30 % had generalised peritonitis and 39 % had infections involving sites other than the appendix including the stomach, duodenum, small bowel, colon, and gallbladder; there were limited numbers of evaluable patients who were enrolled with APACHE II scores $\geq$ 15 and efficacy in these patients has not been established.

4.5 Interaction with other medicinal products and other forms of Interaction

Interactions caused by inhibition of P-glycoprotein-mediated clearance or CYP-mediated clearance of medicinal products are unlikely (see section 5.2).

Penem and carbapenem antibacterial agents may decrease the serum levels of valproic acid. Monitoring of serum levels of valproic acid should be considered if ertapenem is to be co-administered with valproic acid.

4.6 Pregnancy and lactation

Adequate and well-controlled studies have not been performed in pregnant women. Animal studies do not indicate direct or indirect harmful effects with respect to pregnancy, embryo-foetal development, parturition or post-natal development. However, ertapenem should not be used during pregnancy unless the potential benefit outweighs the possible risk to the foetus.

Ertapenem is excreted in human milk. Because of the potential for adverse effects on the infant, mothers should not breast-feed their infants while receiving ertapenem.

4.7 Effects on ability to drive and use machines

Dizziness and somnolence can occur (see section 4.8), which may affect some patients' ability to drive and/or operate machinery.

4.8 Undesirable effects

Adults 18 years of age and older:

The total number of patients treated with ertapenem in clinical studies was over 1,900 of which over 1,850 received a 1 g dose of ertapenem. Adverse reactions (i.e. considered by the investigator to be possibly, probably, or definitely related to the medicinal product) were reported in approximately 20 % of patients treated with ertapenem. Treatment was discontinued due to adverse reactions in 1.3 % of patients.

For patients who received only INVANZ, the most common adverse reactions reported during therapy plus follow-up for 14 days after treatment was stopped were: diarrhoea (4.8 %), infused vein complication (4.5 %) and nausea (2.8 %).

For patients who received only INVANZ, the following adverse reactions were reported during therapy plus follow-up for 14 days after treatment was stopped:

Common = $\geq$ 1/100, $<$ 1/10; Uncommon = $>$ 1/1,000, $<$ 1/100; Rare = $>$ 1/10,000, $<$ 1/1,000

Infections and infestations:

Uncommon: Oral candidiasis

Blood and the lymphatic disorders:

Rare: Neutropenia, thrombocytopenia

Metabolism and nutrition disorders:

Uncommon: Anorexia

Rare: Hypoglycaemia

Nervous system disorders:

Common: Headache

Uncommon: Dizziness, somnolence, insomnia, confusion, seizure

Rare: Agitation, anxiety, depression, tremor

Cardiac disorders:

Rare: Arrhythmia, tachycardia

Vascular disorders:

Common: Phlebitis/thrombophlebitis

Uncommon: Hypotension

Rare: Haemorrhage, increased blood pressure

Respiratory, thoracic and mediastinal disorders:

Uncommon: Dyspnoea, pharyngeal discomfort

Rare: Nasal congestion, cough, epistaxis, pneumonia, rales/rhonchi, wheezing

Gastrointestinal disorders:

Common: Diarrhoea, nausea, vomiting

Uncommon: Constipation, pseudomembranous enterocolitis, acid regurgitation, dry mouth, dyspepsia

Rare: Dysphagia, faecal incontinence

Hepato-biliary disorders:

Rare: Cholecystitis, jaundice, liver disorder

Skin and subcutaneous tissue disorders:

Common: Rash, pruritus

Uncommon: Erythema

Rare: Dermatitis, dermatomycosis, desquamation, post-operative wound infection

Musculoskeletal, connective tissue and bone disorders:

Rare: Muscle cramp, shoulder pain

Renal and urinary disorders:

Rare: Urinary tract infection, renal insufficiency, acute renal insufficiency

Reproductive system and breast disorders:

Uncommon: Vaginitis

Rare: Abortion, genital bleeding

General disorders and administration site conditions:

Common Infused vein complication

Uncommon: Extravasation, abdominal pain, candidiasis, asthenia/fatigue, fungal infection, fever, oedema/swelling, chest pain, taste perversion

Rare: Allergy, injection-site induration, malaise, pelvic peritonitis, scleral disorder, syncope

Children and adolescents (3 months to 17 years of age):

The total number of patients treated with ertapenem in clinical studies was 384. The overall safety profile is comparable to that in adult patients. Adverse reactions (i.e. considered by the investigator to be possibly, probably, or definitely related to the medicinal product) were reported in approximately 20.8 % of patients treated with ertapenem. Treatment was discontinued due to adverse reactions in 0.5 % of patients.

For patients who received only INVANZ, the most common adverse reactions reported during therapy plus follow-up for 14 days after treatment was stopped were: diarrhoea (5.2 %) and infusion site pain (6.1 %).

For patients who received only INVANZ, the following adverse reactions were reported during therapy plus follow-up for 14 days after treatment was stopped:

Nervous system disorders:

Uncommon: Headache

Vascular disorders:

Uncommon: Hot flush, hypertension, petechiae

Gastro-intestinal disorders:

Common: Diarrhoea

Uncommon: Faeces discoloured, melaena

Skin and subcutaneous tissue disorders:

Common: Diaper dermatitis

Uncommon: Erythema, rash

General disorders and administration site conditions:

Common: Infusion site pain

Uncommon: Infusion site burning, infusion site pruritus, infusion site erythema, injection site erythema, infusion site warmth

Post-marketing experience:

The following post-marketing adverse experiences have been reported:

Immune system: anaphylaxis including anaphylactoid reactions (very rare)

Nervous system disorders: hallucinations (very rare)

Laboratory test findings: for adult patients who received only INVANZ, the most frequently reported laboratory abnormalities and their respective incidence rates during therapy plus follow-up for 14 days after treatment was stopped were: elevations in ALT (4.6 %), AST (4.6 %), alkaline phosphatase (3.8 %) and platelet count (3.0 %). For children and adolescents (3 months to 17 years of age) who received only INVANZ, the most frequently reported laboratory abnormalities and their respective incidence rates during therapy plus follow-up for 14 days after treatment was stopped were: decreases in neutrophil count (3.0 %), and elevations in ALT (2.9 %) and AST (2.8 %).

For patients who received only INVANZ, the following laboratory abnormalities were reported during therapy plus follow-up 14 days after treatment was stopped:

Common = $\geq$ 1/100, $<$ 1/10; Uncommon = $>$ 1/1,000, $<$ 1/100; Rare = $>$ 1/10,000, $<$ 1/1,000

Investigations:

Adults 18 years of age and older:

Chemistry:

Common: Elevations in ALT, AST, alkaline phosphatase

Uncommon: Increases in total serum bilirubin, direct serum bilirubin, indirect serum bilirubin, serum creatinine, serum urea, serum glucose

Rare: Decreases in serum bicarbonate, serum creatinine, and serum potassium; increases in serum LDH, serum phosphorus, serum potassium

Haematology:

Common: Elevation in platelet count

Uncommon: Decreases in white blood cells, platelet count, segmented neutrophils, haemoglobin and haematocrit; increases in eosinophils, activated partial thromboplastin time, segmented neutrophils, and white blood cells

Rare: Decrease in lymphocytes; increases in band neutrophils, lymphocytes, metamyelocytes, monocytes, myelocytes; atypical lymphocytes

Urinalysis:

Uncommon: Increases in urine bacteria, urine white blood cells, urine epithelial cells, and urine red blood cells; urine yeast present

Rare: Increase in urobilinogen

Miscellaneous:

Uncommon: Positive *Clostridium difficile* toxin

Children and adolescents (3 months to 17 years of age):

Chemistry:

Common: Elevations in ALT and AST

Haematology:

Common: Decreases in neutrophil count

Uncommon: Increases in platelet count, activated partial thromboplastin time, prothrombin time, decreases in haemoglobin

4.9 Overdose

No specific information is available on the treatment of overdose with ertapenem. Overdosing of ertapenem is unlikely. Intravenous administration of ertapenem at a 3 g daily dose for 8 days to healthy adult volunteers did not result in significant toxicity. In clinical studies in adults inadvertent administration of up to 3 g in a day did not result in clinically important adverse reactions. In paediatric clinical studies, a single IV dose of 40 mg/kg up to a maximum of 2 g did not result in toxicity.

However, in the event of an overdose, treatment with INVANZ should be discontinued and general supportive treatment given until renal elimination takes place.

Ertapenem can be removed to some extent by haemodialysis (see section 5.2); however, no information is available on the use of haemodialysis to treat overdose.

5. PHARMACOLOGICAL PROPERTIES

5.1 Pharmacodynamic properties

Pharmacotherapeutic group: carbapenems, ATC code: J01D H03

Mechanism of action

Ertapenem inhibits bacterial cell wall synthesis following attachment to penicillin binding proteins (PBPs). In *Escherichia coli*, affinity is strongest to PBPs 2 and 3.

Microbiological Susceptibility

The NCCLS MIC breakpoints are as follows:

- *Enterobacteriaceae and staphylococci: S $\leq$ 2 mg/l and R $\geq$ 8 mg/l*
- *S. Pneumoniae: S $\leq$ 1 mg/l and R $\geq$ 4 mg/l*
- *Streptococcus species (beta-haemolytic only): S $\leq$ 1 mg/l*
- *Haemophilus species: S $\leq$ 0.5 mg/l*
- *Anaerobes: S $\leq$ 4 mg/l and R $\geq$ 16 mg/l*

(NB: the breakpoint values for staphylococci and S. pneumoniae are applicable only to methicillin-susceptible staphylococci and penicillin-susceptible pneumococci, respectively)

The prescribers are informed that local MIC breakpoints, if available, should be consulted.

The prevalence of acquired resistance may vary geographically and with time for selected species and local information on resistance is desirable, particularly when treating severe infections. Localised clusters of infections due to carbapenem-resistant organisms have been reported in the European Union. The information below gives only approximate guidance on the probability as to whether the micro-organism will be susceptible to ertapenem or not.

Pathogen	European range of observed resistance
Susceptible:	
Gram-positive aerobes:	
Methicillin-susceptible staphylococci (including *Staphylococcus aureus*)*	0 - 5 %
*Streptococcus agalactiae**	
*Streptococcus pneumoniae**†	
Streptococcus pyogenes	
Gram-negative aerobes:	
Citrobacter freundii	
Enterobacter aerogenes	0 - 20 %
Enterobacter cloacae	
*Escherichia coli**	
*Haemophilus influenzae**	
Haemophilus parainfluenzae	
Klebsiella oxytoca	
*Klebsiella pneumoniae**	
*Moraxella catarrhalis**	
Morganella morganii	
Proteus mirabilis	
Proteus vulgaris	
Serratia marcescens	
Anaerobes:	
Bacteroides fragilis and species in the *B. fragilis* Group*	
Clostridium species (excluding *C. difficile*)*	
Eubacterium species*	
Fusobacterium species*	
Peptostreptococcus species*	
*Porphyromonas asaccharolytica**	
Prevotella species*	
Resistant:	
Gram-positive aerobes:	
Corynebacterium jeikeium	
Methicillin-resistant staphylococci (including *Staphylococcus aureus*)	
Enterococci including *Enterococcus faecalis* and *Enterococcus faecium*	

Gram-negative aerobes:
Aeromonas species
Acinetobacter species
Burkholderia cepacia
Pseudomonas aeruginosa
Stenotrophomonas maltophilia

Anaerobes:
Lactobacillus species

Others:
Chlamydia species
Mycoplasma species
Rickettsia species
Legionella species

* Clinical efficacy has been demonstrated for susceptible isolates in the approved clinical indications.

† The efficacy of INVANZ in the treatment of community acquired pneumonia due to penicillin-resistant *Streptococcus pneumoniae* has not been established.

Resistance

For species considered susceptible to ertapenem, resistance was uncommon in surveillance studies in Europe. In resistant isolates, resistance to other antibacterial agents of the carbapenem class was seen in some but not all isolates. Ertapenem is effectively stable to hydrolysis by most classes of beta-lactamases, including penicillinases, cephalosporinases and extended spectrum beta-lactamases, but not metallo-beta-lactamases.

The mechanism of action of ertapenem differs from that of other classes of antibiotics, such as quinolones, aminoglycosides, macrolides and tetracyclines. There is no target-based cross-resistance between ertapenem and these substances. However, micro-organisms may exhibit resistance to more than one class of antibacterial agents when the mechanism is, or includes, impermeability to some compounds and/or an efflux pump.

Efficacy in paediatric studies

Ertapenem was evaluated primarily for paediatric safety and secondarily for efficacy in randomised comparative, multicentre studies in patients 3 months to 17 years of age with community acquired pneumonia (CAP), urinary tract infections (UTI), skin and soft tissue infections (SSTI), intra-abdominal infections (IAI) and acute pelvic infections (API).

The proportion of patients with a favourable clinical response assessment at post-treatment visit in the clinical MITT population is shown below:

(see Table 1 below)

5.2 Pharmacokinetic properties

Plasma concentrations

Average plasma concentrations of ertapenem following a single 30 minute intravenous infusion of a 1 g dose in healthy young adults (25 to 45 years of age) were 155 micrograms/ml (C_{max}) at 0.5 hour post-dose (end of infusion), 9 micrograms/ml at 12 hour post-dose, and 1 microgram/ml at 24 hour post-dose.

Area under the plasma concentration curve (AUC) of ertapenem in adults increases nearly dose-proportionally over the 0.5 to 2 g dose range.

There is no accumulation of ertapenem in adults following multiple intravenous doses ranging from 0.5 to 2 g daily.

Average plasma concentrations of ertapenem following a single 30 minute intravenous infusion of a 15 mg/kg (up to a maximum dose of 1 g) dose in patients 3 to 23 months of age were 103.8 micrograms/ml (C_{max}) at 0.5 hour postdose (end of infusion), 13.5 micrograms/ml at 6 hour post-dose, and 2.5 micrograms/ml at 12 hour post-dose.

Average plasma concentrations of ertapenem following a single 30 minute intravenous infusion of a 15 mg/kg (up to a maximum dose of 1 g) dose in patients 2 to 12 years of age were 113.2 micrograms/ml (C_{max}) at 0.5 hour postdose (end of infusion), 12.8 micrograms/ml at 6 hour post-dose, and 3.0 micrograms/ml at 12 hour post-dose.

Average plasma concentrations of ertapenem following a single 30 minute intravenous infusion of a 20 mg/kg (up to a maximum dose of 1 g) dose in patients 13 to 17 years of age were 170.4 micrograms/ml (C_{max}) at 0.5 hour post-dose (end of infusion), 7.0 micrograms/ml at 12 hour post-dose, and 1.1 microgram/ml at 24 hour post-dose.

Average plasma concentrations of ertapenem following a single 30 minute intravenous infusion of a 1 g dose in three patients 13 to 17 years of age were 155.9 micrograms/ml (C_{max}) at 0.5 hour post-dose (end of infusion), and 6.2 micrograms/ml at 12 hour post-dose.

Distribution

Ertapenem is highly bound to human plasma proteins. In healthy young adults (25 to 45 years of age), the protein binding of ertapenem decreases, as plasma concentrations increase, from approximately 95 % bound at an approximate plasma concentration of < 50 micrograms/ml to approximately 92 % bound at an approximate plasma concentration of 155 micrograms/ml (average concentration achieved at the end of infusion following 1 g intravenously).

The volume of distribution (V_{dss}) of ertapenem in adults is approximately 8 litres (0.11 litre/kg) and approximately 0.2 litre/kg in paediatric patients 3 months to 12 years of age and approximately 0.16 litre/kg in paediatric patients 13 to 17 years of age.

Concentrations of ertapenem achieved in adult skin blister fluid at each sampling point on the third day of 1 g once daily intravenous doses showed a ratio of AUC in skin blister fluid: AUC in plasma of 0.61.

In-vitro studies indicate that the effect of ertapenem on the plasma protein binding of highly protein bound medicinal products (warfarin, ethinyl estradiol, and norethindrone) was small. The change in binding was < 12 % at peak plasma ertapenem concentration following a 1 g dose. *In vivo*, probenecid (500 mg every 6 hours) decreased the bound fraction of ertapenem in plasma at the end of infusion in subjects administered a single 1 g intravenous dose from approximately 91 % to approximately 87 %. The effects of this change are anticipated to be transient. A clinically significant interaction due to ertapenem displacing another medicinal product or another medicinal product displacing ertapenem is unlikely.

In-vitro studies indicate that ertapenem does not inhibit P-glycoprotein-mediated transport of digoxin or vinblastine and that ertapenem is not a substrate for P-glycoprotein-mediated transport.

Metabolism

In healthy young adults (23 to 49 years of age), after intravenous infusion of radiolabelled 1 g ertapenem, the plasma radioactivity consists predominantly (94 %) of ertapenem. The major metabolite of ertapenem is the ring-opened derivative formed by dehydropeptidase-I-mediated hydrolysis of the beta-lactam ring.

In-vitro studies in human liver microsomes indicate that ertapenem does not inhibit metabolism mediated by any of the six major CYP isoforms: 1A2, 2C9, 2C19, 2D6, 2E1 and 3A4.

Elimination

Following administration of a 1 g radiolabelled intravenous dose of ertapenem to healthy young adults (23 to 49 years of age), approximately 80 % is recovered in urine and 10 % in faeces. Of the 80 % recovered in urine, approximately 38 % is excreted as unchanged ertapenem and approximately 37 % as the ring-opened metabolite.

In healthy young adults (18 to 49 years of age) and patients 13 to 17 years of age given a 1 g intravenous dose, the mean plasma half-life is approximately 4 hours. The mean plasma half-life in children 3 months to 12 years of age is approximately 2.5 hours. Average concentrations of ertapenem in urine exceed 984 micrograms/ml during the period 0 to 2 hours post-dose and exceed 52 micrograms/ml during the period 12 to 24 hours post-administration.

Special populations

Gender

The plasma concentrations of ertapenem are comparable in men and women.

Elderly

Plasma concentrations following a 1 g and 2 g intravenous dose of ertapenem are slightly higher (approximately 39 % and 22 %, respectively) in healthy elderly adults (≥ 65 years) relative to young adults (< 65 years). In the absence of advanced renal insufficiency, no dosage adjustment is necessary in elderly patients.

Paediatric patients

Plasma concentrations of ertapenem are comparable in paediatric patients 13 to 17 years of age and adults following a 1 g once daily intravenous dose.

Following the 20 mg/kg dose (up to a maximum dose of 1 g), the pharmacokinetic parameter values in patients 13 to 17 years of age were generally comparable to those in healthy young adults. To provide an estimate of the pharmacokinetic data if all patients in this age group were to receive a 1 g dose, the pharmacokinetic data were calculated adjusting for a 1 g dose, assuming linearity. A comparison of results show that a 1 g once daily dose of ertapenem achieves a pharmacokinetic profile in patients 13 to 17 years of age comparable to that of adults. The ratios (13 to 17 years/adults) for AUC, the end of infusion concentration and the concentration at the midpoint of the dosing interval were 0.99, 1.20, and 0.84, respectively.

Plasma concentrations at the midpoint of the dosing interval following a single 15 mg/kg intravenous dose of ertapenem in patients 3 months to 12 years of age are comparable to plasma concentrations at the midpoint of the dosing interval following a 1 g once daily intravenous dose in adults (see Plasma concentrations). The plasma clearance (ml/min/kg) of ertapenem in patients 3 months to 12 years of age is approximately 2-fold higher as compared to that in adults. At the 15 mg/kg dose, the AUC value and plasma concentrations at the midpoint of the dosing interval in patients 3 months to 12 years of age were comparable to those in young healthy adults receiving a 1 g intravenous dose of ertapenem.

Hepatic insufficiency

The pharmacokinetics of ertapenem in patients with hepatic insufficiency have not been established. Due to the limited extent of hepatic metabolism of ertapenem, its pharmacokinetics are not expected to be affected by hepatic impairment. Therefore, no dosage adjustment is recommended in patients with hepatic impairment.

Renal insufficiency

Following a single 1 g intravenous dose of ertapenem in adults, AUCs of total ertapenem (bound and unbound) and of unbound ertapenem are similar in patients with mild renal insufficiency (Cl_{cr} 60 to 90 ml/min/1.73 m^2) compared with healthy subjects (ages 25 to 82 years). AUCs of total ertapenem and of unbound ertapenem are increased in patients with moderate renal insufficiency (Cl_{cr} 31 to 59 ml/min/1.73 m^2) approximately 1.5-fold and 1.8-fold, respectively, compared with healthy subjects. AUCs of total ertapenem and of unbound ertapenem are increased in patients with advanced renal insufficiency (Cl_{cr} 5 to 30 ml/min/1.73 m^2) approximately 2.6-fold and 3.4-fold, respectively, compared with healthy subjects. AUCs of total ertapenem and of unbound ertapenem are increased in patients who require haemodialysis approximately 2.9-fold and 6.0-fold, respectively, between dialysis sessions,

Table 1

Disease Stratum†	Age Stratum	Ertapenem		Ceftriaxone	
		n/m	%	n/m	%
CAP	3 to 23 months	31/35	88.6	13/13	100.0
	2 to 12 years	55/57	96.5	16/17	94.1
	13 to 17 years	3/3	100.0	3/3	100.0
UTI‡	3 to 23 months	27/31	87.1	11/11	100.0
	2 to 12 years	38/45	84.4	15/16	93.8
	13 to 17 years	4/4	100.0	2/2	100.0
SSTI‡	3 to 23 months	24/30	80.0	6/6	100.0
	2 to 12 years	47/50	94.0	19/19	100.0
	13 to 17 years	7/8	87.5	2/2	100.0

Disease Stratum	Age Stratum	Ertapenem		Ticarcillin/clavulanate	
		n/m	%	n/m	%
IAI	2 to 12 years	28/34	82.4	7/9	77.8
	13 to 17 years	15/16	93.8	4/6	66.7
API	13 to 17 years	25/25	100.0	8/8	100.0

† This includes 13 patients in the ertapenem group (1 UTI, 3 SSTI, 7 CAP and 2 IAI), 3 patients in the ceftriaxone group (1 SSTI, 2 CAP), and 1 patient with IAI in the ticarcillin/clavulanate group with secondary bacteraemia at entry into the study.

‡ This includes 8 patients in the ertapenem group (7 SSTI and 1 UTI) and none in the comparator group with methicillin resistant *Staphylococcus aureus*.

compared with healthy subjects. Following a single 1 g intravenous dose given immediately prior to a haemodialysis session, approximately 30 % of the dose is recovered in the dialysate. There are no data in paediatric patients with renal insufficiency.

There are inadequate data on the safety and efficacy of ertapenem in patients with advanced renal insufficiency and patients who require haemodialysis to support a dose recommendation. Therefore, ertapenem should not be used in these patients.

5.3 Preclinical safety data

Preclinical data reveal no special hazard for humans based on conventional studies of safety, pharmacology, repeated-dose toxicity, genotoxicity and toxicity in reproduction. Decreased neutrophil counts, however, occurred in rats that received high doses of ertapenem, which was not considered a significant safety issue.

Long-term studies in animals to evaluate the carcinogenic potential of ertapenem have not been performed.

6. PHARMACEUTICAL PARTICULARS

6.1 List of excipients

Sodium bicarbonate (E500).

Sodium hydroxide (E524) to adjust pH to 7.5

The sodium content is approximately 137 mg (approximately 6.0 mEq).

6.2 Incompatibilities

Do not use solvents or infusion fluids containing dextrose for reconstitution or administration of ertapenem sodium.

In the absence of compatibility studies, this medicinal product must not be mixed with other medicinal products.

6.3 Shelf life

2 years.

6.4 Special precautions for storage

Do not store above 25°C.

After reconstitution:

Reconstituted solutions and solutions for infusion: reconstituted solutions should be diluted in sodium chloride 9 mg/ml (0.9 %) solution immediately after preparation (see section 6.6). Diluted solutions should be used immediately. If not used immediately, in use storage times are the responsibility of the user. Diluted solutions (approximately 20 mg/ml ertapenem) are physically and chemically stable for 6 hours at room temperature (25°C) or for 24 hours at 2 to 8°C (in a refrigerator). Solutions should be used within 4 hours of their removal from the refrigerator.

Do not freeze solutions of INVANZ.

6.5 Nature and contents of container

20 ml Type I glass vials with a grey butyl stopper and a white plastic cap on a coloured aluminium band seal.

Supplied in packs of 1 vial or 10 vials.

Not all pack sizes may be marketed.

6.6 Instructions for use and handling

For single use only.

Preparation for intravenous administration:

INVANZ must be reconstituted and then diluted prior to administration.

Adults and adolescents (13 to 17 years of age):

1. **Reconstitution**:

Reconstitute the contents of a 1 g vial of INVANZ with 10 ml of water for injection or sodium chloride 9 mg/ml (0.9 %) solution to yield a reconstituted solution of approximately 100 mg/ml. Shake well to dissolve. (See section 6.4)

2. **Dilution**:

For a 50 ml bag of diluent: For a 1 g dose, immediately transfer contents of the reconstituted vial to a 50 ml bag of sodium chloride 9 mg/ml (0.9 %) solution; or

For a 50 ml vial of diluent: For a 1 g dose, withdraw 10 ml from a 50 ml vial of sodium chloride 9 mg/ml (0.9 %) solution and discard. Transfer the contents of the reconstituted 1 g vial of INVANZ to the 50 ml vial of sodium chloride 9 mg/ml (0.9 %) solution.

3. **Infusion**:

Infuse over a period of 30 minutes.

Children (3 months to 12 years of age):

1. **Reconstitution**:

Reconstitute the contents of a 1 g vial of INVANZ with 10 ml of water for injection or sodium chloride 9 mg/ml (0.9 %) solution to yield a reconstituted solution of approximately 100 mg/ml. Shake well to dissolve. (See section 6.4.)

2. **Dilution**:

For a bag of diluent: Transfer a volume equal to 15 mg/kg of body weight (not to exceed 1 g/day) to a bag of sodium chloride 9 mg/ml (0.9 %) solution for a final concentration of 20 mg/ml or less; or

For a vial of diluent: Transfer a volume equal to 15 mg/kg of body weight (not to exceed 1 g/day) to a vial of sodium chloride 9 mg/ml (0.9 %) solution for a final concentration of 20 mg/ml or less.

3. **Infusion**:

Infuse over a period of 30 minutes.

Compatibility of INVANZ with intravenous solutions containing heparin sodium and potassium chloride has been demonstrated.

The reconstituted solutions should be inspected visually for particulate matter and discoloration prior to administration, whenever the container permits. Solutions of INVANZ range from colourless to pale yellow. Variations of colour within this range do not affect potency.

Any unused solution should be discarded.

7. MARKETING AUTHORISATION HOLDER

Merck Sharp & Dohme Limited
Hertford Road, Hoddesdon
Hertfordshire EN11 9BU
United Kingdom

8. MARKETING AUTHORISATION NUMBER(S)

EU/1/02/216/001

EU/1/02/216/002

9. DATE OF FIRST AUTHORISATION/RENEWAL OF THE AUTHORISATION

18 April 2002

10. DATE OF REVISION OF THE TEXT

07 July 2005

SPC.IVZ.05.UK/IRL.2223

Invirase

(Roche Products Limited)

1. NAME OF THE MEDICINAL PRODUCT

INVIRASE 200 mg hard capsules.

2. QUALITATIVE AND QUANTITATIVE COMPOSITION

One capsule of Invirase contains saquinavir mesylate corresponding to 200 mg saquinavir. For excipients, see section 6.1.

3. PHARMACEUTICAL FORM

Hard capsule.

4. CLINICAL PARTICULARS

4.1 Therapeutic indications

Invirase is indicated for the treatment of HIV-1 infected adult patients. Invirase should only be given in combination with ritonavir and other antiretroviral medicinal products (see section 4.2).

4.2 Posology and method of administration

Therapy with Invirase should be initiated by a physician experienced in the management of HIV infection.

Adults and adolescents over the age of 16 years

In combination with ritonavir

The recommended dose of Invirase is 1000 mg (5 × 200 mg capsules) two times daily with ritonavir 100 mg two times daily in combination with other antiretroviral agents.

Invirase capsules should be swallowed whole and taken at the same time as ritonavir within 2 hours following a meal (see section 5.2).

In combination with other protease inhibitors (PIs) and non-nucleoside reverse transcriptase inhibitors

Dose reduction may be required when Invirase/ritonavir is administered with some other HIV protease inhibitors (e.g. nelfinavir, indinavir and delavirdine), since these drugs may increase saquinavir plasma levels (see section 4.5).

Renal and hepatic impairment

No dosage adjustment is necessary for patients with mild to moderate renal or mild hepatic impairment. Caution should be exercised in patients with severe renal or moderate hepatic impairment. Invirase/ritonavir is contraindicated in patients with severe hepatic impairment. (see sections 4.3 and 4.4).

Paediatric and elderly patients

There is only limited information on the safety and efficacy of saquinavir in HIV infected patients younger than 16 years and in adults over 60 years. Due to the significantly lower saquinavir plasma levels in children compared to adults, Invirase should not be used as the sole PI in children (see section 4.4).

For further information on special patient groups refer to section 4.4 and for pharmacokinetic interactions see sections 4.5. and 5.2.

4.3 Contraindications

Invirase/ritonavir is contraindicated in patients with hypersensitivity to saquinavir, ritonavir or any of the excipients contained in the capsules.

Invirase/ritonavir should not be given together with other drugs which may interact and result in potentially life threatening side effects. Drugs which should not be given with Invirase/ritonavir include terfenadine, astemizole, pimozide, cisapride, amiodarone, propafenone and flecainide (potential for life threatening cardiac arrhythmia), midazolam, triazolam (potential for prolonged or increased sedation, respiratory depression), simvastatin, lovastatin (increased risk of myopathy including rhabdomyolysis), ergot alkaloids (e.g. ergotamine, dihydroergotamine, ergonovine, and methylergonovine) (potential for acute ergot toxicity) and rifampicin (risk of severe hepatocellular toxicity) (see section 4.5).

Invirase/ritonavir is contraindicated in patients with severe hepatic impairment (see section 4.4).

4.4 Special warnings and special precautions for use

Considerations when initiating Invirase therapy: Invirase should not be given as the sole protease inhibitor. Invirase should only be given in combination with ritonavir (see section 4.2).

Patients should be informed that saquinavir is not a cure for HIV infection and that they may continue to acquire illnesses associated with advanced HIV infection, including opportunistic infections. Patients should also be advised that they might experience undesirable effects associated with co-administered medications.

Liver disease: The safety and efficacy of saquinavir has not been established in patients with significant underlying liver disorders. Invirase/ritonavir is contraindicated in patients with severe hepatic impairment (see section 4.3). Patients with chronic hepatitis B or C and treated with combination antiretroviral therapy are at an increased risk for severe and potentially fatal hepatic adverse events. In case of concomitant antiviral therapy for hepatitis B or C, please refer also to the relevant product information for these medicinal products.

Patients with pre-existing liver dysfunction including chronic active hepatitis have an increased frequency of liver function abnormalities during combination antiretroviral therapy and should be monitored according to standard practice. If there is evidence of worsening liver disease in such patients, interruption or discontinuation of treatment must be considered.

In cases of mild hepatic impairment no initial dosage adjustment is necessary at the recommended dose. The use of Invirase in combination with ritonavir in patients with moderate hepatic impairment has not been studied. In the absence of such studies, caution should be exercised, as increases in saquinavir levels and/or increases in liver enzymes may occur.

There have been reports of exacerbation of chronic liver dysfunction, including portal hypertension, in patients with underlying hepatitis B or C, cirrhosis and other underlying liver abnormalities.

Renal impairment: Renal clearance is only a minor elimination pathway, the principal route of metabolism and excretion for saquinavir being via the liver. Therefore, no initial dose adjustment is necessary for patients with renal impairment. However, patients with severe renal impairment have not been studied and caution should be exercised when prescribing saquinavir in this population.

Patients with chronic diarrhoea or malabsorption: Only limited information on the safety and efficacy of saquinavir is available for patients suffering from chronic diarrhoea or malabsorption. It is unknown whether patients with such conditions could receive subtherapeutic drug levels.

Young and elderly patients: The safety and efficacy of saquinavir in HIV-infected patients younger than 16 years have not been established. Limited information is available in children treated with Fortovase and none for children treated with Invirase as the sole protease inhibitor. Due to the significantly lower saquinavir plasma levels in children compared with adults, neither Invirase nor Fortovase should be used as the sole protease inhibitor in children. When Fortovase (50 mg/kg bid) is co-administered with nelfinavir or ritonavir in children, saquinavir exposures are greatly increased and, when combined with ritonavir, may provide saquinavir exposures up to 2-fold greater than those achieved with Fortovase 1200 mg tid in adults. Only limited experience is available in patients older than 60 years.

Lactose intolerance: Invirase 200 mg capsules contain lactose. Patients with rare hereditary problems of galactose intolerance, the Lapp lactase deficiency or glucose-galactose malabsorption should not take this medicine.

Use during pregnancy and lactation: See section 4.6.

Patients with haemophilia: There have been reports of increased bleeding, including spontaneous skin haematomas and haemarthroses, in haemophiliac patients type A and B treated with protease inhibitors. In some patients additional factor VIII was given. In more than a half of the reported cases, treatment with protease inhibitors was continued or reintroduced if treatment had been discontinued. A causal relationship has been evoked, although the mechanism of action has not been elucidated. Haemophiliac patients should therefore be made aware of the possibility of increased bleeding.

Diabetes mellitus and hyperglycaemia: New onset diabetes mellitus, hyperglycaemia or exacerbation of existing diabetes mellitus has been reported in patients receiving protease inhibitors. In some of these patients, the hyperglycaemia was severe and in some cases was also associated with ketoacidosis. Many patients had confounding medical conditions, some of which required therapy with agents that have been associated with the development of diabetes mellitus or hyperglycaemia.

Lipodystrophy: Combination antiretroviral therapy has been associated with the redistribution of body fat (lipodystrophy) in HIV infected patients. The long-term consequences of these events are currently unknown. Knowledge about the mechanism is incomplete. A connection between visceral lipomatosis and PIs and lipoatrophy and Nucleoside Reverse Transcriptase Inhibitors

(NRTIs) has been hypothesised. A higher risk of lipodystrophy has been associated with individual factors such as older age, and with drug related factors such as longer duration of antiretroviral treatment and associated metabolic disturbances. Clinical examination should include evaluation for physical signs of fat redistribution. Consideration should be given to the measurement of fasting serum lipids and blood glucose. Lipid disorders should be managed as clinically appropriate (see section 4.8.).

Immune Reactivation Syndrome: In HIV-infected patients with severe immune deficiency at the time of institution of combination antiretroviral therapy (CART), an inflammatory reaction to asymptomatic or residual opportunistic pathogens may arise and cause serious clinical conditions, or aggravation of symptoms. Typically, such reactions have been observed within the first few weeks or months of initiation of CART. Relevant examples are cytomegalovirus retinitis, generalised and/or focal mycobacterial infections, and Pneumocystis carinii pneumonia. Any inflammatory symptoms should be evaluated and treatment instituted when necessary.

Interaction with ritonavir: The recommended dose of Invirase and ritonavir is 1000 mg Invirase plus 100 mg ritonavir bid. Higher doses of ritonavir have been shown to be associated with an increased incidence of adverse events. Co-administration of saquinavir and ritonavir has led to severe adverse events, mainly diabetic ketoacidosis and liver disorders, especially in patients with pre-existing liver disease.

Interaction with HMG-CoA reductase inhibitors: Caution must be exercised if Invirase/ritonavir is used concurrently with atorvastatin, which is metabolised to a lesser extent by CYP3A4. In this situation a reduced dose of atorvastatin should be considered. If treatment with a HMG-CoA reductase inhibitor is indicated, pravastatin or fluvastatin is recommended (see section 4.5).

Oral contraceptives: Because concentration of ethinyl estradiol may be decreased when co-administered with Invirase/ritonavir, alternative or additional contraceptive measures should be used when estrogen-based oral contraceptives are co-administered (see section 4.5).

Glucocorticoids: Concomitant use of boosted saquinavir and fluticasone or other glucocorticoids that are metabolised by CYP3A4 is not recommended unless the potential benefit of treatment outweighs the risk of systemic corticosteroid effects, including Cushing's syndrome and adrenal suppression (see section 4.5).

4.5 Interaction with other medicinal products and other forms of Interaction

Most drug interaction studies with saquinavir have been completed with unboosted Invirase and Fortovase. A limited number of studies have been completed with ritonavir boosted Invirase/Fortovase.

Observations from drug interaction studies done with unboosted saquinavir might not be representative of the effects seen with saquinavir/ritonavir therapy. Furthermore, results seen with Fortovase may not predict the magnitude of these interactions with Invirase and vice versa.

The metabolism of saquinavir is mediated by cytochrome P450, with the specific isoenzyme CYP3A4 responsible for 90% of the hepatic metabolism. Additionally, *in vitro* studies have shown that saquinavir is a substrate and an inhibitor for P-glycoprotein (P-gp). Therefore, drugs that either share this metabolic pathway or modify CYP3A4 and/or P-gp activity (see "*Other potential interactions*") may modify the pharmacokinetics of saquinavir. Similarly, saquinavir might also modify the pharmacokinetics of other drugs that are substrates for CYP3A4 or P-gp.

Ritonavir can affect the pharmacokinetics of other drugs because it is a potent inhibitor of CYP3A4 and P-gp. Therefore, when saquinavir is co-administered with ritonavir, consideration should be given to the potential effects of ritonavir on other drugs (see the Summary of Product Characteristics for Norvir).

Antiretroviral agents

Nucleoside reverse transcriptase inhibitors (NRTIs):

Zalcitabine and/or zidovudine: ***Saquinavir:*** Concomitant use of Invirase with zalcitabine and/or zidovudine has been studied in adults. Absorption, distribution and elimination of each of the drugs are unchanged when they are used together. ***Saquinavir/ritonavir:*** No pharmacokinetic interaction studies have been completed with these agents given in combination with saquinavir/ritonavir. However, for zalcitabine an interaction is unlikely as this product has differential routes of metabolism and excretion and is unlikely to affect absorption of saquinavir/ritonavir. For zidovudine given 200mg q8h a 25% decrease in AUC of zidovudine was reported when combined with ritonavir (300mg q6h), whereas the pharmacokinetics of ritonavir was not affected by zidovudine. No dose modification of zidovudine is warranted when zidovudine is co-administered with ritonavir.

Didanosine: ***Saquinavir/ritonavir:*** The effects of a single dose of didanosine 400 mg on the pharmacokinetics of saquinavir in eight healthy subjects who received Fortovase/ritonavir 1600/100 mg QD for 2 weeks was investigated. Didanosine decreased saquinavir AUC and C_{max} approximately 30 % and 25 %, respectively, and had essentially no effect on C_{min} of saquinavir. These changes are of doubtful clinical significance.

Non-nucleoside reverse transcriptase inhibitors (NNRTIs):

Delavirdine: ***Saquinavir:*** Co-administration of delavirdine with Invirase resulted in a 348% increase in saquinavir plasma AUC. Currently there are limited safety and no efficacy data available from the use of this combination. In a small, preliminary study, hepatocellular enzyme elevations occurred in 13% of subjects during the first several weeks of the delavirdine and saquinavir combination (6% Grade 3 or 4). Hepatocellular changes should be monitored frequently if this combination is prescribed. ***Saquinavir/ritonavir:*** The interaction between Invirase/ritonavir and delavirdine has not been evaluated.

Efavirenz: ***Saquinavir:*** Co-administration of efavirenz (600 mg) and Fortovase (1200 mg tid) to 12 healthy volunteers decreased saquinavir AUC by 62% and C_{max} by 50%. The concentrations of efavirenz were also decreased by about 10%, but this was not suggested to be clinically significant. Because of these results, saquinavir should only be given in combination with efavirenz if the saquinavir blood levels are increased by the addition of other antiretroviral agents such as ritonavir. ***Saquinavir/ritonavir:*** No clinically relevant alterations of either saquinavir or efavirenz concentrations were noted in a study in twenty-four healthy subjects who received Fortovase/ritonavir/efavirenz 1600/200/600 mg QD. Two additional studies in HIV patients investigated the effect of concomitant administration of efavirenz with either a twice-daily boosted regimen (Invirase/ritonavir 1000/100 mg BID) (n=32) or a once-daily boosted regimen (Fortovase/ritonavir 1200/100 mg QD) (n=35). No clinically significant alterations of either saquinavir or efavirenz concentrations were noted in either study.

Nevirapine: ***Saquinavir:*** Co-administration of nevirapine and Invirase resulted in a 24% decrease in plasma saquinavir AUC and no change to nevirapine AUC. The decrease is not thought to be clinically relevant and no dose adjustments of Invirase or nevirapine are recommended. ***Saquinavir/ritonavir:*** The interaction between Invirase/ritonavir and nevirapine has not been evaluated.

HIV protease inhibitors (PIs):

Indinavir: ***Saquinavir:*** Co-administration of indinavir (800 mg tid) and single doses of Invirase (600 mg) or Fortovase (800 or 1200 mg) in six healthy volunteers each resulted in 4.6 – 7.2 fold increases in plasma saquinavir AUC_{0-24}. Indinavir plasma levels remained unchanged. Currently, no safety and efficacy data are available from the use of this combination. Appropriate doses of the combination have not been established. ***Saquinavir/ritonavir:*** The administration of low dose ritonavir increases the concentrations of indinavir, which may result in nephrolithiasis.

Nelfinavir: ***Saquinavir:*** Concomitant administration of a single 1200 mg dose of Fortovase on the fourth day of multiple nelfinavir dosing (750 mg tid) to 14 HIV infected patients resulted in saquinavir AUC and C_{max} values which were 392% and 179% higher than those seen with saquinavir alone. Concomitant administration of a single 750 mg dose of nelfinavir on the fourth day of multiple Fortovase dosing (1200 mg tid) to the same patients resulted in nelfinavir AUC values which were 18% higher than those seen with nelfinavir alone, while C_{max} values remained unchanged. Quadruple therapy, including Fortovase and nelfinavir in addition to two nucleoside reverse transcriptase inhibitors gave a more durable response (prolongation of time to virological relapse) than triple therapy with either single protease inhibitor. The regimens were generally well tolerated. However, concomitant administration of nelfinavir and Fortovase resulted in a moderate increase in the incidence of diarrhoea. ***Saquinavir/ritonavir:*** The interaction between Invirase/ritonavir and nelfinavir has not been evaluated.

Ritonavir: Saquinavir has been shown not to alter the pharmacokinetics of ritonavir following single or multiple doses in healthy volunteers. Ritonavir extensively inhibits the metabolism of saquinavir resulting in greatly increased saquinavir plasma concentrations. Saquinavir steady-state AUC_{0-24} and C_{max} values obtained from 10 patients, who received Invirase 600 mg tid, were 2598 ng·h/ml and 197 ng/ml, respectively. Invirase, given at a dose of 1000 mg bid in combination with ritonavir 100 mg bid resulted in steady-state saquinavir plasma concentration as follows (N=24): AUC_{0-24} of 29214 ng·h/ml, C_{max} of 2623 ng/ml, and C_{min} of 371 ng/ml.

In HIV-infected patients, Invirase or Fortovase in combination with ritonavir at doses of 1000/100 mg bid provide saquinavir systemic exposure over a 24 hour period similar to or greater than those achieved with Fortovase 1200 mg tid (see section 5.2).

HIV fusion inhibitor:

Enfuvirtide: ***Saquinavir/ritonavir:*** No clinically significant interaction was noted from a study in 12 HIV patients who received enfuvirtide concomitantly with Fortovase/ritonavir 1000/100 mg BID.

Other medicinal products

Antiarrhythmics:

Bepridil, systemic lidocaine, quinidine: Concentrations of these products may be increased when co-administered with Invirase/ritonavir. Caution is warranted and therapeutic concentration monitoring, if available, is recommended if these antiarrhythmics are given with Invirase/ritonavir.

Amiodarone, flecainide and propafenone: Concentrations of these drugs may be increased when co-administered with Invirase/ritonavir. Due to a potential for life threatening cardiac arrhythmia, amiodarone, flecainide and propafenone are contra-indicated with Invirase/ritonavir (see section 4.3).

Anticoagulant:

Warfarin: Concentrations of warfarin may be affected. It is recommended that INR (international normalised ratio) be monitored.

Anticonvulsants:

Carbamazepine, phenobarbital, phenytoin: These products will induce CYP3A4 and may decrease saquinavir concentrations if Invirase is taken without ritonavir. The interaction between Invirase/ritonavir and these products has not been evaluated.

Antidepressants:

Tricyclic antidepressants (e.g. amitriptyline, imipramine): Invirase/ritonavir may increase the concentrations of tricyclic antidepressants. Therapeutic concentration monitoring is recommended for tricyclic antidepressants when co-administered with Invirase/ritonavir.

Nefazodone: Will inhibit CYP3A4 and may increase saquinavir concentrations. If nefazodone is taken concomitantly with saquinavir, monitoring for saquinavir toxicity is recommended. The interaction between Invirase/ritonavir and nefazodone has not been evaluated.

Antihistamines:

Terfenadine, astemizole: Co-administration of terfenadine and Fortovase leads to an increase in plasma terfenadine exposure (AUC) associated with a prolongation of QTc intervals. Hence, terfenadine is contraindicated in patients receiving saquinavir or saquinavir/ritonavir. As similar interactions are likely, saquinavir or saquinavir/ritonavir should not be administered with astemizole (see section 4.3).

Anti-infectives:

Clarithromycin: ***Saquinavir:*** Concomitant administration of clarithromycin (500 mg bid) and Fortovase (1200 mg tid) to 12 healthy volunteers resulted in steady-state saquinavir AUC and C_{max} values which were 177% and 187% higher than those seen with saquinavir alone. Clarithromycin AUC and C_{max} values were approximately 40% higher than those seen with clarithromycin alone. No dose adjustment is required when the two drugs are co-administered for a limited time at the doses studied. ***Saquinavir/ritonavir:*** The interaction between Invirase/ritonavir and clarithromycin has not been evaluated.

Erythromycin: ***Saquinavir:*** Concomitant administration of erythromycin (250 mg qid) and Fortovase (1200 mg tid) to 22 HIV-infected patients resulted in steady-state saquinavir AUC and C_{max} values which were 99% and 106% higher than those seen with saquinavir alone. No dose adjustment is required when the two drugs are co-administered. ***Saquinavir/ritonavir:*** The interaction between Invirase/ritonavir and erythromycin has not been evaluated.

Streptogramin antibiotics such as quinupristin/dalfopristin: Will inhibit CYP3A4 and may increase saquinavir concentrations. If these products are taken concomitantly with saquinavir, monitoring for saquinavir toxicity is recommended. The interaction between Invirase/ritonavir and quinupristin/dalfopristin has not been evaluated.

Antifungals:

Ketoconazole: ***Saquinavir:*** Concomitant use of ketoconazole (200 mg once daily) and Invirase (600 mg three times daily) to 12 healthy volunteers led to an increase in saquinavir AUC by about 160% at steady state (day 6 of treatment) with no increase in the elimination half-life or any change in the absorption rate. Ketoconazole pharmacokinetics were not affected by co-administration with saquinavir at a dose of 600 mg tid. No dose adjustment for either drug is required when the two drugs are co-administered at the doses studied. ***Saquinavir/ritonavir:*** The interaction between Invirase/ritonavir and ketoconazole has not been evaluated.

Itraconazole: ***Saquinavir:*** Like ketoconazole, itraconazole is a moderately potent inhibitor of the CYP3A4 isoenzyme and an interaction of similar magnitude is possible. If itraconazole is taken concomitantly with saquinavir, monitoring for saquinavir toxicity is recommended. ***Saquinavir/ritonavir:*** The interaction between Invirase/ritonavir and itraconazole has not been evaluated.

Fluconazole/miconazole: No specific drug interaction studies with either of these products have been performed.

Antimycobacterials:

Rifampicin: ***Saquinavir:*** Rifampicin (600 mg once daily) was shown to decrease plasma concentrations of saquinavir by 80%. Since this may result in sub-therapeutic concentrations of saquinavir, rifampicin should not be administered concomitantly with Invirase. ***Saquinavir/ritonavir:*** In a study investigating the interaction of rifampicin 600 mg once daily and Invirase 1000 mg/ritonavir 100 mg given twice daily, 11 of 17 (65%) healthy volunteers developed severe hepatocellular toxicity with transaminase elevations up to > 20-fold the upper limit of normal after 1 to 5 days of co-administration. Therefore, rifampicin is contraindicated in patients taking ritonavir boosted Invirase as part of an ART regimen (see section 4.3).

Rifabutin: ***Saquinavir:*** Rifabutin reduces saquinavir plasma concentrations by 40%. Rifabutin and Invirase should not be co-administered. ***Saquinavir/ritonavir:*** Concomitant administration of rifabutin with Invirase/ritonavir 400 mg/400 mg had no clinical significant effect on saquinavir exposure in 24 HIV patients.

Benzodiazepines:

Midazolam: ***Saquinavir:*** Co-administration of a single oral dose of midazolam (7.5 mg) after 3 or 5 days of Fortovase (1200 mg tid) to 12 healthy volunteers in a double-blind cross-over study, increased midazolam C_{max} to 235% and AUC to 514% of control. Saquinavir increased the elimination half-life of oral midazolam from 4.3 to 10.9 hours and the absolute bioavailability from 41 to 90%. Volunteers experienced impairment in psychomotor skills and an increase in sedative effects. Consequently the dose of oral midazolam should be greatly reduced when given with saquinavir and the combination should be used with caution. When combined with intravenous midazolam (0.05 mg/kg), saquinavir decreased the clearance of midazolam by 56% and increased its elimination half-life from 4.1 to 9.5 hours, however, only the subjective feeling to the drug effects was increased. Therefore, bolus doses of intravenous midazolam can be given in combination with Fortovase. During prolonged midazolam infusion, a total dose reduction of 50% is recommended. ***Saquinavir/ritonavir:*** The interaction between Invirase/ritonavir and midazolam has not been evaluated. Midazolam is contraindicated with Invirase/ritonavir due to the risk of potential for prolonged or increased sedation and respiratory depression (see section 4.3).

Alprazolam, clorazepate, diazepam, flurazepam: Concentrations of these products may be increased when co-administered with Invirase/ritonavir. Careful monitoring of patients with regard to sedative effects is warranted, a decrease in the dose of the benzodiazepine may be required.

Triazolam: Concentrations of triazolam may be increased when co-administered with Invirase/ritonavir. Triazolam is contra-indicated with Invirase/ritonavir, due to the risk of potential for prolonged or increased sedation and respiratory depression (see section 4.3).

Calcium channel blockers:

Felodipine, nifedipine, nicardipine, diltiazem, nimodipine, verapamil, amlodipine, nisoldipine, isradipine: Concentrations of these products may be increased when co-administered with Invirase/ritonavir. Caution is warranted and clinical monitoring of patients is recommended.

Corticosteroids:

Dexamethasone: Will induce CYP3A4 and may decrease saquinavir concentrations. Use with caution, saquinavir may be less effective in patients taking these products concomitantly. The interaction between Invirase/ritonavir and dexamethasone has not been evaluated.

Fluticasone propionate (interaction with ritonavir): In a clinical study where ritonavir 100 mg capsules bid were co-administered with 50μg intranasal fluticasone propionate (4 times daily) for 7 days in healthy subjects, the fluticasone propionate plasma levels increased significantly, whereas the intrinsic cortisol levels decreased by approximately 86 % (90 % confidence interval 82-89 %). Greater effects may be expected when fluticasone propionate is inhaled. Systemic corticosteroid effects including Cushing's syndrome and adrenal suppression have been reported in patients receiving ritonavir and inhaled or intranasally administered fluticasone propionate; this could also occur with other corticosteroids metabolised via the P450 3A pathway e.g. busesonide. Consequently, concomitant administration of boosted saquinavir and these glucocorticoids is not recommended unless the potential benefit of treatment outweighs the risk of systemic corticosteroid effects (see section 4.4). A dose reduction of the glucocorticoid should be considered with close monitoring of local and systemic effects or a switch to a glucocorticoid, which is not a substrate for CYP3A4 (e.g. beclomethasone). Moreover, in case of withdrawal of glucocorticoids progressive dose reduction may have to be performed over a longer period. The effects of high fluticasone systemic exposure on ritonavir plasma levels is yet unknown.

Histamine H_2-receptor antagonist:

Ranitidine: ***Saquinavir:*** There was an increase in exposure of saquinavir when Invirase was dosed in the presence of both ranitidine and food, relative to Invirase dosed with food alone. This resulted in AUC values of saquinavir, which were 67% higher. This increase is not thought to be clinically relevant and no dose adjustment of saquinavir is recommended. ***Saquinavir/ritonavir:*** The interaction between Invirase/ritonavir and ranitidine has not been evaluated.

HMG-CoA reductase inhibitors:

Pravastatin, fluvastatin: Are not metabolised by CYP3A4, and interactions are not expected with protease inhibitors including ritonavir. If treatment with a HMG-CoA reductase inhibitor is indicated, either pravastatin or fluvastatin are the products recommended.

Simvastatin, lovastatin: Are highly dependent on CYP3A4 metabolism, and plasma concentrations are markedly increased when co-administered with Invirase/ritonavir. Increased concentrations of these products have been associated with rhabdomyolysis and these products are contraindicated for use with Invirase/ritonavir (see section 4.3).

Atorvastatin: Is less dependent on CYP3A4 for metabolism. When used with Invirase/ritonavir, the lowest possible dose of atorvastatin should be administered and the patient carefully monitored for signs/symptoms of myopathy (muscle weakness, muscle pain, rising plasma creatinine kinase levels).

Immunosuppressants:

Cyclosporin, tacrolimus, rapamycin: Concentrations of these products may be increased when co-administered with Invirase/ritonavir. Therapeutic concentration monitoring is recommended for immunosuppressant agents when co-administered with Invirase/ritonavir.

Narcotic analgesic:

Methadone: Concentration of methadone may be decreased when co-administered with Invirase/ritonavir. Dosage of methadone may need to be increased.

Neuroleptics:

Pimozide: Concentrations of pimozide may be increased when co-administered with Invirase/ritonavir. Due to a potential for life threatening cardiac arrhythmias, Invirase/ritonavir is contra-indicated in combination with pimozide (see section 4.3).

Oral contraceptives:

Ethinyl estradiol: Concentration of ethinyl estradiol may be decreased when co-administered with Invirase/ritonavir. Alternative or additional contraceptive measures should be used when estrogen-based oral contraceptives are co-administered.

Phosphodiesterase type 5 (PDE5) inhibitors:

Sildenafil: The co-administration of Fortovase at steady state (1200 mg tid) with sildenafil (100 mg single dose), a substrate of CYP3A4, resulted in a 140% increase in sildenafil C_{max} and a 210% increase in sildenafil AUC. Sildenafil had no effect on saquinavir pharmacokinetics. Use sildenafil with caution at reduced doses of no more than 25 mg every 48 hours with increased monitoring of adverse events when administered concomitantly with Invirase/ritonavir.

Vardenafil: Concentrations of vardenafil may be increased when co-administered with Invirase/ritonavir. Use vardenafil with caution at reduced doses of no more than 2.5 mg every 72 hours with increased monitoring of adverse events when administered concomitantly with Invirase/ritonavir.

Tadalafil: Concentrations of tadalafil may be increased when co-administered with Invirase/ritonavir. Use tadalafil with caution at reduced doses of no more than 10 mg every 72 hours with increased monitoring of adverse events when administered concomitantly with Invirase/ritonavir.

Others:

Ergot alkaloids (e.g. ergotamine, dihydroergotamine, ergonovine, and methylergonovine):

Invirase/ritonavir may increase ergot alkaloids exposure and consequently increase the potential for acute ergot toxicity. Thus, the concomitant use of Invirase/ritonavir, and ergot alkaloids is contra-indicated (see section 4.3).

Grapefruit juice: ***Saquinavir:*** Co-administration of Invirase and grapefruit juice as single administration in healthy volunteers results in a 50% and 100% increase in exposure to saquinavir for normal and double strength grapefruit juice, respectively. This increase is not thought to be clinically relevant and no dose adjustment of Invirase is recommended. ***Saquinavir/ritonavir:*** The interaction between Invirase/ritonavir and grapefruit juice has not been evaluated.

Garlic capsules: ***Saquinavir:*** Concomitant administration of garlic capsules (dose approx. equivalent to two 4 g cloves of garlic daily) and saquinavir (Fortovase) 1200 mg tid to nine healthy volunteers resulted in a decrease of saquinavir AUC by 51% and a decrease of the mean trough levels at 8 hours post dose by 49%. Saquinavir mean C_{max} levels decreased by 54%. Therefore, patients on saquinavir treatment must not take garlic capsules due to the risk of decreased plasma concentrations and loss of virological response and possible resistance to one or more components of the antiretroviral regimen. ***Saquinavir/ritonavir:*** The interaction between Invirase/ritonavir and garlic capsules has not been evaluated.

St. John's wort *(Hypericum perforatum)*: ***Saquinavir:*** Plasma levels of saquinavir can be reduced by concomitant use of the herbal preparation St. John's wort *(Hypericum perforatum)*. This is due to induction of drug metabolising enzymes and/or transport proteins by St. John's wort. Herbal preparations containing St. John's wort must not be used concomitantly with Invirase. If a patient is already taking St. John's wort, stop St. John's wort, check viral levels and if possible saquinavir levels. Saquinavir levels may increase on stopping St. John's wort, and the dose of saquinavir may need adjusting. The inducing effect of St. John's wort may persist for at least 2 weeks after cessation of treatment. ***Saquinavir/ritonavir:*** The interaction between Invirase/ritonavir and St. John's wort has not been evaluated.

Other potential interactions

Drugs that are substrates of CYP3A4:

Although specific studies have not been performed, co-administration of Invirase/ritonavir with drugs that are mainly metabolised by CYP3A4 pathway (e.g. dapsone, disopyramide, quinine, fentanyl, and alfentanyl) may result in elevated plasma concentrations of these drugs. Therefore these combinations should be given with caution.

Drugs that are substrates of P-glycoprotein:

Concomitant use of Invirase/ritonavir and drugs that are substrates of P-glycoprotein (P-gp) (e.g. digoxin) may lead to elevated plasma concentrations of these drugs, hence monitoring for toxicity is recommended.

Drugs reducing gastrointestinal transit time:

It is unknown, whether drugs which reduce the gastrointestinal transit time (e.g. metoclopramide) could lead to lower saquinavir plasma concentrations.

4.6 Pregnancy and lactation

Pregnancy: Evaluation of experimental animal studies does not indicate direct or indirect harmful effects with respect to the development of the embryo or foetus, the course of gestation and peri- and post-natal development. Clinical experience in pregnant women is limited: Congenital malformations, birth defects and other disorders (without a congenital malformation) have been reported rarely in pregnant women who had received saquinavir in combination with other antiretroviral agents. However, so far the available data are insufficient and do not identify specific risks for the unborn child. Saquinavir should be used during pregnancy only if the potential benefit justifies the potential risk to the foetus (see section 5.3).

Lactation: There are no laboratory animal or human data available on secretion of saquinavir in breast milk. The potential for adverse reactions to saquinavir in nursing infants cannot be assessed, and therefore, breast-feeding should be discontinued prior to receiving saquinavir. It is recommended that HIV-infected women do not breast feed their infants under any circumstances in order to avoid transmission of HIV.

4.7 Effects on ability to drive and use machines

It is not known whether saquinavir has an effect on the ability to drive and to use machines.

4.8 Undesirable effects

Undesirable effects from clinical trials with unboosted Invirase

The most frequently reported adverse events among patients receiving Invirase as monotherapy 600 mg tid in clinical trials (excluding those toxicities known to be associated with zidovudine and/or zalcitabine when used in combinations) were diarrhoea, abdominal discomfort and nausea.

Adverse events from a pivotal study (n = 327) which included a treatment arm with saquinavir used as single drug (600 mg tid) are listed below. Adverse events (mild, moderate and severe) with an incidence > 2% considered by the investigator at least remotely related to saquinavir are summarised in Table 1:

Table 1: Incidences of undesirable effects in clinical trials, considered at least remotely related to treatment with Invirase with mild, moderate and severe intensity, occurring in > 2% of patients.

(Very common (⩾ 10%); common (⩾ 1% and < 10%))

Body System **Frequency of event**	**Adverse Events**
Nervous system disorders	
Common	Headache, peripheral neuropathy, numbness extremities, paraesthesia, dizziness
Gastrointestinal disorders	
Very common	Diarrhoea, nausea
Common	Buccal mucosa ulceration, abdominal discomfort, vomiting, abdominal pain, flatulence
Skin and subcutaneous tissue disorders	
Common	Rash, pruritus
Musculoskeletal, connective tissue and bone disorders	
Common	Pain
General disorders and administration site conditions	
Common	Fatigue, asthenia, fever

Invirase does not alter or add to the toxicity profile of zalcitabine and/or zidovudine, when given in combination.

At least possibly related serious adverse reactions reported from clinical trials where Invirase was used as the sole protease inhibitor

Serious adverse reactions, at least possibly related to the use of saquinavir, reported from clinical trials with a frequency of less than 2% and not mentioned above, are listed below. These adverse reactions are from a database of over 6000 patients; of whom more than 100 had been on saquinavir therapy for over 2 years. Patients received saquinavir either as monotherapy or in combination with a wide variety of other antiretroviral drugs (nucleoside analogues, non-nucleoside reverse transcriptase inhibitors and protease inhibitors).

Confusion, ataxia and weakness, acute myeloblastic leukaemia, haemolytic anaemia, attempted suicide, Stevens-Johnson syndrome, severe cutaneous reaction associated with increased liver function tests, thrombocytopenia and intracranial haemorrhage, exacerbation of chronic liver disease with Grade 4 elevated liver function test, jaundice, ascites, drug fever, bullous skin eruption and polyarthritis, nephrolithiasis, pancreatitis, intestinal obstruction, portal hypertension, and peripheral vasoconstriction.

Adverse events that occurred in clinical trials with Fortovase are given for completeness.

Undesirable effects from clinical trials with unboosted Fortovase (saquinavir soft capsule)

The safety of Fortovase was studied in more than 500 patients who received the drug either alone or in combination with other antiretroviral agents. The majority of adverse events were of mild intensity. The most frequently reported adverse events among patients receiving Fortovase were diarrhoea, nausea, abdominal discomfort and dyspepsia.

Clinical adverse events of at least moderate intensity which occurred in greater than or equal to 2% of patients in an open label safety study (NV15182) and in a double blind study comparing Fortovase and Invirase (NV15355) are summarised in Table 2.

Table 2: Incidences of undesirable effects* in clinical trials, considered related to treatment with Fortovase of at least moderate intensity, occurring in ⩾ 2% of patients.

(Very common (⩾ 10%); common (⩾ 1% and < 10%))

Body System **Frequency of event**	**Adverse Events**
Psychiatric disorders	
Common	Depression, insomnia, anxiety, libido disorder
Nervous system disorders	
Common	Headaches
Gastrointestinal disorders	
Very common	Diarrhoea, nausea
Common	Abdominal discomfort, dyspepsia, flatulence, vomiting, abdominal pain, constipation
Skin and subcutaneous tissue disorders	
Common	Verruca
Musculoskeletal, connective tissue and bone disorders	
Common	Pain
General disorders and administration site conditions	
Common	Fatigue, appetite decreased, chest pain
Special senses disorders	
Common	Taste alteration

*Includes adverse events at least possibly related to study drug or of unknown intensity and/or relationship to treatment (corresponding to ACTG Grade 3 and 4).

At least possibly related serious undesirable effects reported from clinical trials where Fortovase was used as the sole protease inhibitor:

Serious adverse reactions at least possibly related to the use of Fortovase reported from clinical trials with a frequency of less than 2% are:

Nephrolithiasis; pancreatitis; thrombocytopenia; erythema; dehydration; eructation; abdominal distension.

Fortovase does not alter the pattern, frequency or severity of known major toxicities associated with nucleoside analogues. For comprehensive dose adjustment recommendations and drug-associated adverse reactions for other drugs used in combination, physicians should refer to the Summary of Product Characteristics for each of these medicinal products.

Undesirable effects from clinical trials with boosted Fortovase

The safety of Fortovase (1000 mg bid) when used in combination with low dose ritonavir (100 mg bid) for at least 48 weeks was studied in 148 patients. The most frequently reported adverse reactions among patients receiving this boosted protease inhibitor regimen as part of their antiretroviral therapy were nausea, diarrhoea, fatigue, vomiting, flatulence, and abdominal pain.

Adverse reactions of grade 3 and 4 severity that were considered to be at least possibly related to Fortovase, or which were of unknown causality or severity, and which occurred at a frequency of at least 2% in the pivotal study (n=148) were nausea (4.1%), vomiting (2%), anaemia (2%) and fatigue (2%).

Laboratory abnormalities with Invirase

The most common marked laboratory abnormalities seen during treatment with saquinavir containing regimens (as the sole protease inhibitor or in combination with low dose ritonavir) in clinical trials were isolated CPK increase, glucose decrease, glucose increase, raised transaminase values and neutropenia.

Laboratory abnormalities with Fortovase

Marked clinical laboratory abnormalities (change from grade 0 to grade 3 or 4, or change from grade 1 to grade 4) reported in greater than 2% of patients treated with 1200 mg tid in the open label safety study included decreased glucose (6.4%), increased CPK (7.8%), increased gamma glutamyltransferase (5.7%), increased ALT (5.7%), increased AST (4.1%), increased potassium (2.7%) and neutropenia (2.9%).

The following additional marked clinical laboratory abnormalities have been reported following treatment with Fortovase as the sole protease inhibitor (saquinavir) containing regimens: calcium (high/low), phosphate (low), bilirubin (high), amylase (high), potassium (low), sodium (low/high), haemoglobin (low), platelets (low), alkaline phosphatase (high), glucose (high), triglyceride (high).

In the safety study there was a 27%-33% incidence of greater than or equal to 1 grade shifts in ALT and AST during the 48 week study period. 46% of these were single abnormal values. Only 3%-4% of patients had greater than or equal to 3 grade shifts in transaminase levels and less than 0.5% of patients had to discontinue the study for increased liver function tests.

Marked laboratory abnormalities (Grade 1- 4) that have been observed with Fortovase in combination with ritonavir (at 48 weeks) included low haemoglobin (4%), WBC (3%), platelets (11%), and lymphocyte counts (5%), and high amylase (2%), creatinine (2%), bilirubin (7%), AST (19%), ALT (26%), cholesterol (27%), LDL-cholesterol (62%), and triglyceride (32%) levels.

Post-marketing experience with Invirase and Fortovase

Serious and non-serious adverse events from post-marketing spontaneous reports (where Fortovase and Invirase were taken as the sole protease inhibitor or in combination with ritonavir), not mentioned previously in section 4.8, for which a causal relationship to saquinavir cannot be excluded, are summarised below (rare: ⩾ 0.01% and < 0.1%; very rare: < 0.01%):

- Infections and infestations: Hepatitis (rare).
- Immune system disorders: Allergic reactions (very rare).
- Nervous system disorders: Somnolence (very rare), seizures (rare).
- Renal and urinary disorders: Abnormal renal function (very rare).
- Metabolism and nutrition disorders:

- Diabetes mellitus or hyperglycaemia, sometimes associated with ketoacidosis (rare) (see section 4.4).

- Lipodystrophy: Combination antiretroviral therapy has been associated with redistribution of body fat (lipodystrophy) in HIV infected patients including the loss of peripheral and facial subcutaneous fat, increased intra-abdominal and visceral fat, breast hypertrophy and dorsicervical fat accumulation (buffalo hump) (rare).

- Combination antiretroviral therapy has been associated with metabolic abnormalities such as hypertriglyceridaemia, hypercholesterolaemia, insulin resistance, hyperglycaemia and hyperlactataemia (very rare; see section 4.4.).

- Vascular disorders: There have been reports of increased bleeding, including spontaneous skin haematomas and haemarthroses, in haemophilic patients type A and B treated with protease inhibitors (rare) (see section 4.4).
- Musculoskeletal, connective tissue and bone disorders: Increased CPK, myalgia, myositis and rarely, rhabdomyolysis have been reported with protease inhibitors, particularly in combination with nucleoside analogues (rare).
- In HIV-infected patients with severe immune deficiency at the time of initiation of combination antiretroviral therapy (CART), an inflammatory reaction to asymptomatic or residual opportunistic infections may arise (see section 4.4).

4.9 Overdose

There are two reports of patients who had overdoses with Invirase. One patient exceeded the recommended daily dose of saquinavir and took 8000 mg at once. The patient was treated with induction of emesis within two hours after ingestion of the overdose. The patient did not experience any sequelae. The second patient ingested 2.4 g of Invirase in combination with 600 mg of ritonavir and experienced pain in the throat that lasted for 6 hours and then resolved. In an exploratory small study, oral dosing with saquinavir at 3600 mg per day has not shown increased toxicity through the first 16 weeks of treatment.

Two cases of Fortovase overdosage have been received (1 case with unknown amount of Fortovase, second case 3.6 g to 4 g at once). No adverse events were reported in any of the cases.

5. PHARMACOLOGICAL PROPERTIES

5.1 Pharmacodynamic properties

Pharmaco-therapeutic group: Antiviral agent, ATC code J05A E01

Mechanism of action: The HIV protease carries out specific cleavages of viral precursor proteins as virions bud from infected cells. This is an essential step in the creation of fully formed, infectious virus particles. These viral precursor proteins contain a type of cleavage site which is recognised only by HIV and closely related viral proteases. Saquinavir is a mimetic of such cleavage sites and fits closely into the HIV-1 and HIV-2 protease active sites, acting as a reversible and selective inhibitor. Saquinavir has approximately 50,000-fold greater affinity for HIV protease than for human proteases. In *in vitro* antiviral assays saquinavir blocks the formation of infectious virus, and hence the spread of infection to naïve cells.

Antiviral activity in vitro: Unlike nucleoside analogues (zidovudine, etc.), saquinavir acts directly on its viral target enzyme. It does not require metabolic activation. This extends its potential effectiveness into resting cells. Saquinavir is active at nanomolar concentrations in lymphoblastoid and monocytic lines and in primary cultures of lymphocytes and monocytes infected with laboratory strains or clinical isolates of HIV-1. Experiments in cell culture show that saquinavir produces an additive to synergistic antiviral effect against HIV-1 in double and triple combination with various reverse transcriptase inhibitors (including zidovudine, zalcitabine, didanosine, lamivudine, stavudine and nevirapine) without enhanced cytotoxicity, and clear synergy in double combination with lopinavir.

Pharmacodynamic effects: The effects of saquinavir in combination with zalcitabine and zidovudine on biological markers (CD4 cell counts and plasma RNA) were evaluated in HIV-1 infected patients.

Clinical studies performed with Invirase

In a study (NV14256) with zidovudine pre-treated patients (CD4 ⩾ 50 ⩽ 300 cells/mm^3), the combination of Invirase plus zalcitabine compared to zalcitabine monotherapy prolonged the time to first AIDS-defining illness or death. In this study, the combination therapy reduced the risk of a patient having an AIDS-defining illness or dying by 53%. For death alone the combination of Invirase plus zalcitabine reduced the risk by 72%. This corresponds to a reduction in the rate of an AIDS-defining illness or death from 29.4% to 16.0% over 18 months. Similarly for death alone, the rate was reduced from 8.6% to 4.1% over 18 months. In the three treatment groups, median treatment duration was 11 to 13 months and median follow-up has been 17 months.

In this study the median CD4 cell count at baseline over all treatment arms was 156 to 176 cells/mm^3. The average change from baseline over 16 weeks (median DAVG16) for saquinavir plus zalcitabine was +26 cells/mm^3 for the CD4 cell count and -0.6 $\log_{10}$ RNA copies/ml of plasma for viral load. The peak mean increase in the CD4 cell count was 47 cells/mm^3 at week 16. The peak mean reduction in viral load was 0.7 $\log_{10}$ RNA copies/ml of plasma at week 12.

Study SV14604 is a randomised, multi-centre, double blind phase III parallel study of zidovudine + zalcitabine, vs. saquinavir + zidovudine, vs. saquinavir + zidovudine + zalcitabine, in untreated/minimally treated HIV infected patients. A fourth treatment arm of zidovudine monotherapy was discontinued; patients originally on zidovudine monotherapy were switched to saquinavir + zidovudine + zalcitabine, constituting a "delayed" triple therapy group.

A total of 3485 patients was treated and had follow up data available (the intent to treat population). Median baseline CD4 across the 3 arms was 199-204 cells/mm^3, and median baseline HIV RNA was 5.0 - 5.1 $\log_{10}$ copies/ml. Median duration of study drug treatment was approximately 14 months and the median duration of follow up for AIDS defining events and deaths approximately 17 months.

Progression to first AIDS defining event or death was significantly decreased for patients on saquinavir + zidovudine + zalcitabine with 76 first AIDS defining events/deaths compared to 142 events on zidovudine + zalcitabine (p = 0.0001). An exploratory comparison of initial saquinavir + zidovudine + zalcitabine compared to the delayed triple therapy group showed superiority of initial triple therapy including saquinavir with 76 AIDS defining events or deaths on initial triple therapy vs. 116 on the initial zidovudine monotherapy-delayed triple therapy regimen (p = 0.001).

Patients receiving triple therapy had greater increases in CD4 count, with a 71 cells/mm^3 median peak increase from baseline compared to a 40 cells/mm^3 median peak increase on zidovudine + zalcitabine. Similarly, reductions in HIV RNA were greater on triple therapy with a -1.5 $\log_{10}$

copies/ml median peak change from baseline compared to a -1.1 log_{10} copies/ml median peak change on zidovudine + zalcitabine. For both CD4 and HIV RNA, comparisons over 48 weeks between the triple therapy arm and zidovudine + zalcitabine reached statistical significance (p = 0.0001).

Clinical study performed with Fortovase and Invirase

Study NV15355 is an open-label, randomised, parallel study comparing Fortovase (n = 90) and Invirase (n = 81) in combination with two nucleoside reverse transcriptase inhibitors of choice in treatment-naïve patients. Mean baseline CD4 cell count was 429 cells/mm^3 and mean baseline plasma HIV-RNA was 4.8 log_{10} copies/ml. After 16 weeks of treatment, there was a mean viral load suppression of -2.0 log_{10} copies/ml in the Fortovase containing arm compared to -1.6 log_{10} copies/ml in the Invirase containing arm. The magnitude of the reduction in viral load was limited by the sensitivity of the assay used, especially in the Fortovase arm in which 80% of patients had viral loads below the limit of quantification (< 400 copies/ml) at 16 weeks compared to 43% of patients on Invirase (p = 0.001). At 16 weeks, the increases in CD4 cell counts were 97 and 115 cells/mm^3 for the Fortovase and Invirase arms, respectively.

Clinical studies performed with Fortovase

In the MaxCmin 1 study, the safety and efficacy of Fortovase/ritonavir 1000/100 mg bid plus 2 NRTIs/Non-Nucleoside Reverse Transcriptase Inhibitors (NNRTIs) was compared to indinavir/ritonavir 800/100 mg bid plus 2 NRTIs/NNRTIs in over 300 (both protease inhibitor treatment naïve and experienced) subjects. Median baseline CD4 cell count was 272 cells/mm^3, and median baseline plasma HIV-RNA was 4.0 log_{10} copies/ml in the saquinavir/ritonavir arm. Median baseline CD4 cell count was 280 cells/mm^3, and median baseline plasma HIV-RNA was 3.9 log_{10} copies/ml in the indinavir/ritonavir arm. At 48 weeks, the median increases in CD4 cell counts were 85 and 73 cells/mm^3 for the saquinavir and indinavir arms, respectively. For the intent to treat analysis (switch = failure) at week 48, the proportion of patients in the saquinavir containing arm with viral load below the limit of detection (< 400 copies/ml) was 69% (N=102) compared with 53% (N=84) in the indinavir containing arm. The combination of saquinavir and ritonavir exhibited a superior virological activity compared with the indinavir and ritonavir arm when switch from the assigned treatment was counted as virological failure. This was to be expected as a higher proportion of subjects in the indinavir/ritonavir arm (40%) than in the saquinavir/ritonavir arm (27%, p=0.01) switched from the randomised treatment. In addition patients randomised to indinavir/ritonavir had an increased risk of treatment-limiting adverse events, and adverse events of grade 3 and/or 4 (41% in the indinavir/ritonavir arm versus 24% in the saquinavir/ritonavir arm; p=0.002).

In the MaxCmin2 study, the safety and efficacy of Fortovase/ritonavir 1000/100 mg bid plus 2 NRTIs/NNRTIs was compared with lopinavir/ritonavir 400/100 mg bid plus 2 NRTIs/NNRTIs in 324 (both protease inhibitor treatment naïve and experienced) subjects. Values for median baseline CD4 count and median baseline plasma HIV RNA were 241 cells/mm^3 and 4.4 log_{10} copies/ml in the saquinavir/ritonavir arm, and 239 cells/mm^3 and 4.6 log_{10} copies/ml in the lopinavir/ritonavir arm, respectively. None of the subjects in the lopinavir/ritonavir arm had been exposed to lopinavir prior to randomisation whereas 16 of the subjects in the saquinavir/ritonavir arm had previously been exposed to saquinavir.

In the primary efficacy analysis, incidence of virological failure, including all subjects that took at least one dose of the study medication (ITT/exposed population), 29 failures were observed in the lopinavir/ritonavir arm and 53 failures in the saquinavir/ritonavir arm (hazard ratio: 0.5; 95 % C.I. 0.3 – 0.8). At 48 weeks, the proportion of subjects with HIV RNA below the limit of detection (< 50 copies/ml) was 53% (N=161) for the saquinavir arm versus 60% (N=163) for the lopinavir arm in the intent-to-treat, switch equals failure analysis, and 74% (N=114) for the saquinavir arm versus 70% (N=141) for the lopinavir arm in the on-treatment analysis (p = ns for both comparisons). The combination of saquinavir and ritonavir exhibited comparable virological activity with the lopinavir and ritonavir arm when switch from the assigned treatment was counted as virological failure. Over 48 weeks a similar immunological response was seen in both arms with median increases in CD4 count of 106 cells/mm^3 for the lopinavir/ritonavir arm, and 110 cells/mm^3 for the saquinavir/ritonavir arm. More subjects in the saquinavir/ritonavir arm (30 %) than in the lopinavir/ritonavir arm (14 %) prematurely discontinued the assigned treatment (p = 0.001). The primary reasons for premature discontinuation were non-fatal adverse events and subject's choice. No difference in the incidence of adverse events of grade 3 and/or 4 was seen between the two arms.

Potential for resistance and cross-resistance to saquinavir:

Resistance: The objective of antiretroviral therapy is to suppress viral replication to below the limits of quantification. Incomplete viral suppression may lead to the development of drug resistance to one or more components of the regimen. Drug resistance is measured as the change in viral susceptibility to drug in culture (="phenotypic resistance") or in protease amino acid sequence (="genotypic resistance").

Two primary mutations in the viral protease (L90M and G48V, the former predominating and the combination rare even with saquinavir monotherapy) are found in post-treatment resistant isolates. The G48V and L90M mutations give modest (typically less than 10-fold) reductions in susceptibility to saquinavir. In one study, 24 clinical isolates containing G48V and/or L90M after therapy with Invirase used as a single protease inhibitor showed a geometric mean reduction of susceptibility (increase in IC_{50}) of 7.3-fold relative to baseline virus (range 1.2 to 97-fold). In another study, 32 saquinavir-naïve patients, of whom 26 were resistant to ritonavir and/or indinavir, were treated with Invirase 1000 mg in combination with ritonavir 100 mg both two times daily, efavirenz and nucleoside analogues. 19/32 were sensitive to saquinavir at baseline. HIV RNA levels below 50 copies/ml were achieved at week 24 for 58% of those patients carrying saquinavir-sensitive virus and for 25% of those carrying virus with reduced (> 10 fold) sensitivity to saquinavir.

Secondary mutations (e.g. L10I/V, K20R, M36I/L, A71T, V82X) may accompany or precede the primary resistance mutations and give rise to greater reductions in susceptibility to saquinavir.

The overall incidence of protease genotypic resistance to saquinavir observed in a cohort of 51 antiretroviral naïve subjects after a mean of 46 weeks (range 15 to 50 weeks) treatment with Fortovase 1200 mg tid in combination with 2 NRTIs was 4%.

Cross-resistance: Resistance mutations selected by one drug can in principle also result in reduced susceptibility to other drugs, particularly those in the same drug class. When this occurs it is termed cross-resistance.

Cross- resistance can result in weakened virological response to drug therapy. The application of data from phenotypic and/or genotypic resistance testing following incomplete viral suppression or virological failure can improve the response to subsequent treatments.

Cross-resistance between saquinavir and reverse transcriptase inhibitors: Cross-resistance between saquinavir and reverse transcriptase inhibitors is unlikely because of their different enzyme targets. HIV isolates resistant to zidovudine are sensitive to saquinavir, and conversely, HIV isolates resistant to saquinavir are sensitive to zidovudine.

Cross-resistance to other protease inhibitors: In a study of virus isolates from four clinical trials with Invirase as the sole protease inhibitor, 22 virus isolates were identified as being resistant to saquinavir following treatment for 24 - 147 weeks. Susceptibility of each isolate was assessed to indinavir, ritonavir, nelfinavir and amprenavir. Of the isolates, 6/22 did not show cross-resistance to the other inhibitors, while 4/22 showed broad cross-resistance. The remaining 12/22 retained activity against at least one other protease inhibitor.

Cross-resistance with lopinavir is as yet undetermined in clinical isolates, although laboratory strains with substitutions at residues 10, 84 and 90 or 10, 48, 82 and 90 did not show significant reduction in susceptibility to lopinavir.

Cross-resistance from other protease inhibitors: Subjects with high level resistance to other protease inhibitors do not necessarily show cross-resistance to saquinavir. Studies of molecular clones containing resistance mutations associated with ritonavir, nelfinavir or amprenavir showed significant resistance to these individual protease inhibitors, but not in all cases to saquinavir. In a clinical study of individuals pre-treated with indinavir or ritonavir, 81% showed reduced susceptibility to indinavir and 59% to ritonavir at baseline. Of these, 40% showed reduced (> 10 fold) susceptibility to saquinavir at baseline. Following 24 weeks of therapy with Invirase 1000 mg in combination with ritonavir both 100 mg two times daily, efavirenz and nucleoside analogues, the median decrease in plasma HIV-RNA was 0.9 log_{10} copies/ml for patients with phenotypic resistance to saquinavir versus 1.52 log_{10} copies/ml for those without resistance (p=0.03). The median number of resistance mutations in the protease gene in individuals with phenotypic resistance to saquinavir was 5.5 (range 4 - 8), whereas it was 3 (range 0-6) in those sensitive to saquinavir (p=0.0003). However, extensive treatment of subjects with protease inhibitors after failure can lead to broad cross-resistance in a complex, dynamic process.

Hypersusceptibility to mutant virus: Some virus isolates with reduced susceptibility to other protease inhibitors can have enhanced susceptibility (hypersusceptibility) to inhibition with saquinavir, for example viruses containing the D30N substitution after nelfinavir therapy and viruses, carrying complex substitutions patterns including I50V. Many viruses with substitutions at residue 82, commonly selected by indinavir or ritonavir therapy, either retain, or show enhanced susceptibility to saquinavir. The clinical significance of hypersusceptibility to saquinavir has not been established.

5.2 Pharmacokinetic properties

Absorption and bioavailability in adults and effect of food: In healthy volunteers the extent of absorption (as reflected by AUC) after a 600 mg oral dose of saquinavir was increased from 24 ng·h/ml (CV 33%), under fasting conditions, to 161 ng·h/ml (CV35%) when saquinavir was given following a heavy breakfast (48 g protein, 60 g carbohydrate, 57 g fat; 1006 kcal).

The presence of food also increased the time taken to achieve maximum concentration from 2.4 hours to 3.8 hours and substantially increased the mean maximum plasma concentrations (C_{max}) from 3.0 ng/ml to 35.5 ng/ml. The effect of food has been shown to persist for up to 2 hours. Therefore, Invirase should be taken within 2 hours after a meal.

Absolute bioavailability averaged 4% (CV 73%, range: 1% to 9%) in 8 healthy volunteers who received a single 600 mg dose (3 × 200 mg) of Invirase following a heavy breakfast. The low bioavailability is thought to be due to a combination of incomplete absorption and extensive first-pass metabolism. Gastric pH has been shown to be only a minor component in the large increase in bioavailability seen when given with food.

After multiple oral doses (25 – 600 mg tid) in the presence of food, the increase in exposure

(50-fold) was greater than directly proportional to the increase in dose (24-fold). Following multiple dosing (600 mg tid) in HIV-infected patients (n = 29), the steady state area under the plasma concentration versus time curve (AUC) was 2.5 times (95% CI 1.6 to 3.8) higher than that observed after a single dose.

In one study, HIV-infected patients were given saquinavir 600 mg tid after a meal or a substantial snack. AUC and maximum plasma concentration (C_{max}) values were about twice those observed in healthy volunteers receiving the same treatment regimen.

In HIV-infected patients, Invirase or Fortovase in combination with ritonavir at doses of 1000/100 mg bid provides saquinavir systemic exposures over a 24-hour period similar to or greater than those achieved with Fortovase 1200 mg tid (see Table 3). The pharmacokinetics of saquinavir are stable during long-term treatment. Studies with saquinavir in combination with ritonavir have been performed with food only. No data are available for the intake of ritonavir boosted saquinavir in the fasting state.

Table 3: Mean (%CV) AUC, C_{max} and C_{min} of saquinavir in patients following multiple dosing of Invirase, Fortovase, Invirase/ritonavir, and Fortovase/ritonavir

(see Table 3)

Effective therapy in treatment naïve patients is associated with a C_{min} of approximately 50 ng/ml and an AUC_{0-24} of about 20,000 (ng·h/ml). Effective therapy in treatment experienced patients is associated with a C_{min} of approximately 100 ng/ml and an AUC_{0-24} of about 20,000 (ng·h/ml).

In vitro studies have shown that saquinavir is a substrate for P-glycoprotein (P-gp).

Distribution in adults: Saquinavir partitions extensively into the tissues. The mean steady-state volume of distribution following intravenous administration of a 12 mg dose of saquinavir was 700 l (CV 39%). It has been shown that

Table 3 Mean (%CV) AUC, C_{max} and C_{min} of saquinavir in patients following multiple dosing of Invirase, Fortovase, Invirase/ritonavir, and Fortovase/ritonavir

Treatment	N	AUCτ (ng·h/ml)	AUC_{0-24} (ng·h/ml)	C_{max} (ng/ml)	C_{min} (ng/ml)
Invirase 600 mg tid	10	866 (62)	2,598	197 (75)	75 (82)
Fortovase 1200 mg tid	31	7,249 (85)	21,747	2,181 (74)	216 (84)
Fortovase 1000 mg bid plus ritonavir 100 mg bid*	24	19,085 (13,943-26,124)	38,170	3,344 (2,478-4,513)	433 (301-622)
Invirase 1000 mg bid plus ritonavir 100 mg bid*	24	14,607 (10,218-20,882)	29,214	2,623 (1,894-3,631)	371 (245-561)

τ = dosing interval, i.e. 8 hour for tid and 12 h for bid dosing.

C_{min} = the observed plasma concentration at the end of the dose interval.

* results are mean (95% CI).

saquinavir is approximately 97% bound to plasma proteins up to 30 μg/ml. In two patients receiving Invirase 600 mg tid, cerebrospinal fluid concentrations of saquinavir were negligible when compared to concentrations from matching plasma samples.

Metabolism and elimination in adults: *In vitro* studies using human liver microsomes have shown that the metabolism of saquinavir is cytochrome P450 mediated with the specific isoenzyme, CYP3A4, responsible for more than 90% of the hepatic metabolism. Based on *in vitro* studies, saquinavir is rapidly metabolised to a range of mono- and di-hydroxylated inactive compounds. In a mass balance study using 600 mg 14C-saquinavir (n = 8), 88% and 1% of the orally administered radioactivity, was recovered in faeces and urine, respectively, within 4 days of dosing. In an additional four subjects administered 10.5 mg 14C-saquinavir intravenously, 81% and 3% of the intravenously administered radioactivity was recovered in faeces and urine, respectively, within 4 days of dosing. 13% of circulating saquinavir in plasma was present as unchanged drug after oral administration and the remainder as metabolites. Following intravenous administration 66% of circulating saquinavir was present as unchanged drug and the remainder as metabolites, suggesting that saquinavir undergoes extensive first pass metabolism. *In vitro* experiments have shown that the hepatic metabolism of saquinavir becomes saturable at concentrations above 2 μg/ml.

Systemic clearance of saquinavir was high, 1.14 l/h/kg (CV 12%), slightly above the hepatic plasma flow, and constant after intravenous doses of 6, 36 and 72 mg. The mean residence time of saquinavir was 7 hours (n = 8).

Effect of gender following treatment with Invirase/ritonavir: A gender difference was observed with females showing higher saquinavir exposure than males (AUC on average 56 % higher and C_{max} on average 26 % higher) in the bioequivalence study comparing Invirase 500 mg film coated tablets with Invirase 200 mg hard capsules both in combination with ritonavir. There was no evidence that age and body-weight explained the gender difference in this study. Limited data from controlled clinical studies with the approved dosage regimen do not indicate a major difference in the efficacy and safety profile between men and women.

5.3 Preclinical safety data

Acute and chronic toxicity: Saquinavir was well tolerated in oral acute and chronic toxicity studies in mice, rats, dogs and marmosets at dose levels that gave maximum plasma exposures (AUC values) approximately 1.5, 1.0, 4 to 9-and 3 fold greater, respectively, than those achieved in humans at the recommended dose.

Mutagenesis: Studies with and without metabolic activation (as appropriate) have shown that saquinavir has no mutagenic or genotoxic activity.

Carcinogenesis: There was no evidence of carcinogenic activity after the administration of saquinavir mesylate for 96 to 104 weeks to rats (maximum dose 1000 mg/kg/day) and mice (maximum dose 2500 mg/kg/day). The plasma exposures (AUC values) in the respective species were up to 60% of those obtained in humans at the recommended clinical dose of Fortovase (saquinavir soft capsule) or equivalent to them.

Reproductive toxicity: (see section 4.6). Fertility and reproductive performance were not affected in rats at plasma exposures (AUC values) approximately 50% of those achieved in humans at the recommended dose.

Reproduction studies conducted with saquinavir in rats have shown no embryotoxicity or teratogenicity at plasma exposures (AUC values) approximately 50% of those achieved in humans at the recommended dose or in rabbits at plasma exposures approximately 40% of those achieved at the recommended clinical dose. Distribution studies in these species showed that placental transfer of saquinavir is low (less than 5% of maternal plasma concentrations).

Studies in rats indicated that exposure to saquinavir from late pregnancy through lactation at plasma concentrations (AUC values) approximately 50% of those achieved in humans at the recommended dose had no effect on the survival, growth and development of offspring to weaning.

6. PHARMACEUTICAL PARTICULARS

6.1 List of excipients

Capsule filling: lactose (anhydrous), microcrystalline cellulose, povidone, sodium starch glycollate, talc, magnesium stearate.

Capsule shell: gelatine, iron oxide black, red and yellow (E172), indigocarmine (E132), titanium dioxide (E171).

Printing ink: titanium dioxide (E 171), shellac, soya lecithin, polydimethylsiloxane.

Capsule appearance: light brown and green, opaque; marking "ROCHE" and the code "0245" on each half of the capsule shell.

6.2 Incompatibilities

Not applicable.

6.3 Shelf life

3 years.

6.4 Special precautions for storage

Store in the closed original container.

6.5 Nature and contents of container

Container: Amber glass bottles with plastic screw cap containing 270 capsules of Invirase.

6.6 Instructions for use and handling

Not applicable.

7. MARKETING AUTHORISATION HOLDER

Roche Registration Limited

40 Broadwater Road

Welwyn Garden City

Hertfordshire, AL7 3AY

United Kingdom

8. MARKETING AUTHORISATION NUMBER(S)

EU/1/96/026/001

9. DATE OF FIRST AUTHORISATION/RENEWAL OF THE AUTHORISATION

04 October 1996 / 12 November 2001

10. DATE OF REVISION OF THE TEXT

31 August 2005

LEGAL STATUS

POM

Invirase is a registered trade mark.

Invirase 500mg Film-Coated Tablets

(Roche Products Limited)

1. NAME OF THE MEDICINAL PRODUCT

INVIRASE® 500 mg film-coated tablet.

2. QUALITATIVE AND QUANTITATIVE COMPOSITION

One film-coated tablet contains 500 mg of saquinavir as saquinavir mesylate. For excipients, see section 6.1.

3. PHARMACEUTICAL FORM

Film-coated tablet.

Light orange to greyish or brownish orange film-coated tablet of oval cylindrical biconvex shape with the marking "SQV 500" on the one side and "ROCHE" on the other side.

4. CLINICAL PARTICULARS

4.1 Therapeutic indications

Invirase is indicated for the treatment of HIV-1 infected adult patients. Invirase should only be given in combination with ritonavir and other antiretroviral medicinal products (see section 4.2).

4.2 Posology and method of administration

Therapy with Invirase should be initiated by a physician experienced in the management of HIV infection.

Adults and adolescents over the age of 16 years

In combination with ritonavir

The recommended dose of Invirase is 1000 mg (2 × 500 mg film-coated tablets) two times daily with ritonavir 100 mg two times daily in combination with other antiretroviral agents.

Invirase film-coated tablets should be taken at the same time as ritonavir within 2 hours following a meal (see section 5.2).

In combination with other protease inhibitors (PIs) and non-nucleoside reverse transcriptase inhibitors

Dose reduction may be required when Invirase/ritonavir is administered with some other HIV protease inhibitors (e.g. nelfinavir, indinavir and delavirdine), since these medicinal products may increase saquinavir plasma levels (see section 4.5).

Renal and hepatic impairment

No dosage adjustment is necessary for patients with mild to moderate renal or mild hepatic impairment. Caution should be exercised in patients with severe renal or moderate hepatic impairment. Invirase/ritonavir is contraindicated in patients with severe hepatic impairment. (see sections 4.3 and 4.4).

Paediatric and elderly patients

There is only limited information on the safety and efficacy of saquinavir in HIV infected patients younger than 16 years and in adults over 60 years. Due to the significantly lower saquinavir plasma levels in children compared to adults, Invirase should not be used as the sole PI in children (see section 4.4).

For further information on special patient groups refer to section 4.4 and for pharmacokinetic interactions see sections 4.5. and 5.2.

4.3 Contraindications

Invirase/ritonavir is contraindicated in patients with hypersensitivity to saquinavir, ritonavir or any of the excipients contained in the film-coated tablet.

Invirase/ritonavir should not be given together with other medicinal products which may interact and result in potentially life threatening side effects. Medicinal products which should not be given with Invirase/ritonavir include terfenadine, astemizole, pimozide, cisapride, amiodarone, propafenone and flecainide (potential for life threatening cardiac arrhythmia), midazolam, triazolam (potential for prolonged or increased sedation, respiratory depression), simvastatin, lovastatin (increased risk of myopathy including rhabdomyolysis), ergot alkaloids (e.g. ergotamine, dihydroergotamine, ergonovine, and methylergonovine) (potential for acute ergot toxicity) and rifampicin (risk of severe hepatocellular toxicity) (see section 4.5).

Invirase/ritonavir is contraindicated in patients with severe hepatic impairment (see section 4.4).

4.4 Special warnings and special precautions for use

Considerations when initiating Invirase therapy: Invirase should not be given as the sole protease inhibitor. Invirase should only be given in combination with ritonavir (see section 4.2).

Patients should be informed that saquinavir is not a cure for HIV infection and that they may continue to acquire illnesses associated with advanced HIV infection, including opportunistic infections. Patients should also be advised that they might experience undesirable effects associated with co-administered medications.

Liver disease: The safety and efficacy of saquinavir has not been established in patients with significant underlying liver disorders. Invirase/ritonavir is contraindicated in patients with severe hepatic impairment (see section 4.3). Patients with chronic hepatitis B or C and treated with combination antiretroviral therapy are at an increased risk for severe and potentially fatal hepatic adverse events. In case of concomitant antiviral therapy for hepatitis B or C, please refer also to the relevant product information for these medicinal products.

Patients with pre-existing liver dysfunction including chronic active hepatitis have an increased frequency of liver function abnormalities during combination antiretroviral therapy and should be monitored according to standard practice. If there is evidence of worsening liver disease in such patients, interruption or discontinuation of treatment must be considered.

In cases of mild hepatic impairment no initial dosage adjustment is necessary at the recommended dose. The use of Invirase in combination with ritonavir in patients with moderate hepatic impairment has not been studied. In the absence of such studies, caution should be exercised, as increases in saquinavir levels and/or increases in liver enzymes may occur.

There have been reports of exacerbation of chronic liver dysfunction, including portal hypertension, in patients with underlying hepatitis B or C, cirrhosis and other underlying liver abnormalities.

Renal impairment: Renal clearance is only a minor elimination pathway, the principal route of metabolism and excretion for saquinavir being via the liver. Therefore, no initial dose adjustment is necessary for patients with renal impairment. However, patients with severe renal impairment have not been studied and caution should be exercised when prescribing saquinavir in this population.

Patients with chronic diarrhoea or malabsorption: Only limited information on the safety and efficacy of saquinavir is available for patients suffering from chronic diarrhoea or malabsorption. It is unknown whether patients with such conditions could receive subtherapeutic saquinavir levels.

Young and elderly patients: The safety and efficacy of saquinavir in HIV-infected patients younger than 16 years have not been established. Limited information is available in children treated with Fortovase and none for children treated with Invirase as the sole protease inhibitor. Due to the significantly lower saquinavir plasma levels in children compared with adults, neither Invirase nor Fortovase should be used as the sole protease inhibitor in children. When Fortovase (50 mg/kg twice daily) is co-administered with nelfinavir or ritonavir in children, saquinavir exposures are greatly increased and, when combined with ritonavir, may provide saquinavir exposures up to 2-fold greater than those achieved with Fortovase 1200 mg three times daily in adults. Only limited experience is available in patients older than 60 years. For patients in whom the 500 mg film-coated tablet is not suitable, Invirase is also available in the form of 200 mg hard capsules.

Lactose intolerance: Invirase 500 mg film-coated tablets contain lactose. Patients with rare hereditary problems of galactose intolerance, the Lapp lactase deficiency or glucose-galactose malabsorption should not take this medicine.

Use during pregnancy and lactation: See section 4.6.

Patients with haemophilia: There have been reports of increased bleeding, including spontaneous skin haematomas and haemarthroses, in haemophiliac patients type A and B treated with protease inhibitors. In some patients additional factor VIII was given. In more than a half of the reported cases, treatment with protease inhibitors was continued or reintroduced if treatment had been discontinued. A causal relationship has been evoked, although the mechanism of action has not been elucidated. Haemophiliac patients should therefore be made aware of the possibility of increased bleeding.

Diabetes mellitus and hyperglycaemia: New onset diabetes mellitus, hyperglycaemia or exacerbation of existing diabetes mellitus has been reported in patients receiving protease inhibitors. In some of these patients, the hyperglycaemia was severe and in some cases was also associated with ketoacidosis. Many patients had confounding medical conditions, some of which required therapy with agents that have been associated with the development of diabetes mellitus or hyperglycaemia.

Lipodystrophy: Combination antiretroviral therapy has been associated with the redistribution of body fat (lipodystrophy) in HIV infected patients. The long-term consequences of these events are currently unknown. Knowledge about the mechanism is incomplete. A connection between visceral lipomatosis and PIs and lipoatrophy and Nucleoside Reverse Transcriptase Inhibitors (NRTIs) has been hypothesised. A higher risk of lipodystrophy has been associated with individual factors such as older age, and with drug related factors such as longer duration of antiretroviral treatment and associated metabolic disturbances. Clinical examination should include evaluation for physical signs of fat redistribution. Consideration should be given to the measurement of fasting serum lipids and blood glucose. Lipid disorders should be managed as clinically appropriate (see section 4.8.).

Immune Reactivation Syndrome: In HIV-infected patients with severe immune deficiency at the time of institution of combination antiretroviral therapy (CART), an inflammatory reaction to asymptomatic or residual opportunistic pathogens may arise and cause serious clinical conditions, or aggravation of symptoms. Typically, such reactions have been observed within the first few weeks or months of initiation of CART. Relevant examples are cytomegalovirus retinitis, generalised and/or focal mycobacterial infections, and Pneumocystis carinii pneumonia. Any inflammatory symptoms should be evaluated and treatment instituted when necessary.

Interaction with ritonavir: The recommended dose of Invirase and ritonavir is 1000 mg Invirase plus 100 mg ritonavir twice daily. Higher doses of ritonavir have been shown to be associated with an increased incidence of adverse events. Co-administration of saquinavir and ritonavir has led to severe adverse events, mainly diabetic ketoacidosis and liver disorders, especially in patients with pre-existing liver disease.

Interaction with HMG-CoA reductase inhibitors: Caution must be exercised if Invirase/ritonavir is used concurrently with atorvastatin, which is metabolised to a lesser extent by CYP3A4. In this situation a reduced dose of atorvastatin should be considered. If treatment with a HMG-CoA reductase inhibitor is indicated, pravastatin or fluvastatin is recommended (see section 4.5).

Oral contraceptives: Because concentration of ethinyl oestradiol may be decreased when co-administered with Invirase/ritonavir, alternative or additional contraceptive measures should be used when oestrogen-based oral contraceptives are co-administered (see section 4.5).

Glucocorticoids: Concomitant use of boosted saquinavir and fluticasone or other glucocorticoids that are metabolized by CYP3A4 is not recommended unless the potential benefit of treatment outweighs the risk of systemic corticosteroid effects, including Cushing's syndrome and adrenal suppression (see section 4.5).

4.5 Interaction with other medicinal products and other forms of Interaction

Most drug interaction studies with saquinavir have been completed with unboosted Invirase and Fortovase. A limited number of studies have been completed with ritonavir boosted Invirase/Fortovase.

Observations from drug interaction studies done with unboosted saquinavir might not be representative of the effects seen with saquinavir/ritonavir therapy. Furthermore, results seen with Fortovase may not predict the magnitude of these interactions with Invirase and vice versa.

The metabolism of saquinavir is mediated by cytochrome P450, with the specific isoenzyme, CYP3A4, responsible for 90 % of the hepatic metabolism. Additionally, *in vitro* studies have shown that saquinavir is a substrate and an inhibitor for P-glycoprotein (P-gp). Therefore, medicinal products that either share this metabolic pathway or modify CYP3A4 and/or P-gp activity (see "*Other potential interactions*") may modify the pharmacokinetics of saquinavir. Similarly, saquinavir might also modify the pharmacokinetics of other medicinal products that are substrates for CYP3A4 or P-gp.

Ritonavir can affect the pharmacokinetics of other medicinal products because it is a potent inhibitor of CYP3A4 and P-gp. Therefore, when saquinavir is co-administered with ritonavir, consideration should be given to the potential effects of ritonavir on other medicinal products (see the Summary of Product Characteristics for Norvir).

Antiretroviral agents

Nucleoside reverse transcriptase inhibitors (NRTIs):

Zalcitabine and/or zidovudine: ***Saquinavir:*** Concomitant use of Invirase with zalcitabine and/or zidovudine has been studied in adults. Absorption, distribution and elimination of each of the medicinal products are unchanged when they are used together. ***Saquinavir/ritonavir:*** No pharmacokinetic interaction studies have been completed with these agents given in combination with saquinavir/ritonavir. However, for zalcitabine an interaction is unlikely as this medicinal product has differential routes of metabolism and excretion and is unlikely to affect absorption of saquinavir/ritonavir. For zidovudine given 200 mg every 8 hours a 25 % decrease in AUC of zidovudine was reported when combined with ritonavir (300 mg every 6 hours), whereas the pharmacokinetics of ritonavir was not affected by zidovudine. No dose modification of zidovudine is warranted when zidovudine is co-administered with ritonavir.

Didanosine: ***Saquinavir/ritonavir:*** The effects of a single dose of didanosine 400 mg on the pharmacokinetics of saquinavir in eight healthy subjects who received Fortovase/ritonavir 1600/100 mg once daily for 2 weeks was investigated. Didanosine decreased saquinavir AUC and C_{max} approximately 30 % and 25 %, respectively, and had essentially no effect on C_{min} of saquinavir. These changes are of doubtful clinical significance.

Non-nucleoside reverse transcriptase inhibitors (NNRTIs):

Delavirdine: ***Saquinavir:*** Co-administration of delavirdine with Invirase resulted in a 348 % increase in saquinavir plasma AUC. Currently there are limited safety and no efficacy data available from the use of this combination. In a small, preliminary study, hepatocellular enzyme elevations occurred in 13 % of subjects during the first several weeks of the delavirdine and saquinavir combination (6 % Grade 3 or 4). Hepatocellular changes should be monitored frequently if this combination is prescribed. ***Saquinavir/ritonavir:*** The interaction between Invirase/ritonavir and delavirdine has not been evaluated.

Efavirenz: ***Saquinavir:*** Co-administration of efavirenz (600 mg) and Fortovase (1200 mg three times daily) to 12 healthy volunteers decreased saquinavir AUC by 62 % and C_{max} by 50 %. The concentrations of efavirenz were also decreased by about 10 %, but this was not suggested to be clinically significant. Because of these results, saquinavir should only be given in combination with efavirenz if the saquinavir blood levels are increased by the addition of other antiretroviral agents such as ritonavir. ***Saquinavir/Ritonavir:*** No clinically relevant alterations of either saquinavir or efavirenz concentrations were noted in a study in twenty-four healthy subjects who received Fortovase/ritonavir/efavirenz 1600/200/600 mg once daily. Two additional studies in HIV patients investigated the effect of concomitant administration of efavirenz with either a twice-daily boosted regimen (Invirase/ritonavir 1000/100 mg twice daily) (n=32) or a once-daily boosted regimen (Fortovase/ritonavir 1200/100 mg once daily) (n=35). No clinically significant alterations of either saquinavir or efavirenz concentrations were noted in either study.

Nevirapine: ***Saquinavir:*** Co-administration of nevirapine and Invirase resulted in a 24 % decrease in plasma saquinavir AUC and no change to nevirapine AUC. The decrease is not thought to be clinically relevant and no dose adjustments of Invirase or nevirapine are recommended. ***Saquinavir/ritonavir:*** The interaction between Invirase/ritonavir and nevirapine has not been evaluated.

HIV protease inhibitors (PIs):

Indinavir: ***Saquinavir:*** Co-administration of indinavir (800 mg three times daily) and single doses of Invirase (600 mg) or Fortovase (800 or 1200 mg) in six healthy volunteers each resulted in 4.6 – 7.2 fold increases in plasma saquinavir AUC_{0-24}. Indinavir plasma levels remained unchanged. Currently, no safety and efficacy data are available from the use of this combination. Appropriate doses of the combination have not been established. ***Saquinavir/ritonavir:*** The administration of low dose ritonavir increases the concentrations of indinavir, which may result in nephrolithiasis.

Nelfinavir: ***Saquinavir:*** Concomitant administration of a single 1200 mg dose of Fortovase on the fourth day of multiple nelfinavir dosing (750 mg three times daily) to 14 HIV infected patients resulted in saquinavir AUC and C_{max} values which were 392 % and 179 % higher than those seen with saquinavir alone. Concomitant administration of a single 750 mg dose of nelfinavir on the fourth day of multiple Fortovase dosing (1200 mg three times daily) to the same patients resulted in nelfinavir AUC values which were 18 % higher than those seen with nelfinavir alone, while C_{max} values remained unchanged. Quadruple therapy, including Fortovase and nelfinavir in addition to two nucleoside reverse transcriptase inhibitors gave a more durable response (prolongation of time to virological relapse) than triple therapy with either single protease inhibitor. The regimens were generally well tolerated. However, concomitant administration of nelfinavir and Fortovase resulted in a moderate increase in the incidence of diarrhoea. ***Saquinavir/ritonavir:*** The interaction between Invirase/ritonavir and nelfinavir has not been evaluated.

Ritonavir: Saquinavir has been shown not to alter the pharmacokinetics of ritonavir following single or multiple doses in healthy volunteers. Ritonavir extensively inhibits the metabolism of saquinavir resulting in greatly increased saquinavir plasma concentrations. Saquinavir steady-state AUC_{0-24} and C_{max} values obtained from 10 patients, who received Invirase 600 mg three times daily, were 2598 ng·h/ml and 197 ng/ml, respectively. Invirase, given at a dose of 1000 mg twice daily in combination with ritonavir 100 mg twice daily resulted in steady-state saquinavir plasma concentration as follows (N=24): AUC_{0-24} of 29214 ng·h/ml, C_{max} of 2623 ng/ml, and C_{min} of 371 ng/ml.

In HIV-infected patients, Invirase or Fortovase in combination with ritonavir at doses of 1000/100 mg twice daily provide saquinavir systemic exposure over a 24 hour period similar to or greater than those achieved with Fortovase 1200 mg three times daily (see section 5.2).

HIV fusion inhibitor:

Enfuvirtide: ***Saquinavir/ritonavir:*** No clinically significant interaction was noted from a study in 12 HIV patients who received enfuvirtide concomitantly with Fortovase/ritonavir 1000/100 mg twice daily.

Other medicinal products

Antiarrhythmics:

Bepridil, systemic lidocaine, quinidine: Concentrations of these medicinal products may be increased when co-administered with Invirase/ritonavir. Caution is warranted and therapeutic concentration monitoring, if available, is recommended if these antiarrhythmics are given with Invirase/ritonavir.

Amiodarone, flecainide and propafenone: Concentrations of these medicinal products may be increased when co-administered with Invirase/ritonavir. Due to a potential for life threatening cardiac arrhythmia, amiodarone, flecainide and propafenone are contraindicated with Invirase/ritonavir (see section 4.3).

Anticoagulant:

Warfarin: Concentrations of warfarin may be affected. It is recommended that INR (international normalised ratio) be monitored.

Anticonvulsants:

Carbamazepine, phenobarbital, phenytoin: These medicinal products will induce CYP3A4 and may decrease saquinavir concentrations if Invirase is taken without ritonavir. The interaction between Invirase/ritonavir and these medicinal products has not been evaluated.

Antidepressants:

Tricyclic antidepressants (e.g. amitriptyline, imipramine): Invirase/ritonavir may increase the concentrations of tricyclic antidepressants. Therapeutic concentration monitoring is recommended for tricyclic antidepressants when co-administered with Invirase/ritonavir.

Nefazodone: Will inhibit CYP3A4 and may increase saquinavir concentrations. If nefazodone is taken concomitantly with saquinavir, monitoring for saquinavir toxicity is recommended. The interaction between Invirase/ritonavir and nefazodone has not been evaluated.

Antihistamines:

Terfenadine, astemizole: Co-administration of terfenadine and Fortovase leads to an increase in plasma terfenadine exposure (AUC) associated with a prolongation of QTc intervals. Hence, terfenadine is contraindicated in patients receiving saquinavir or saquinavir/ritonavir. As similar interactions are likely, saquinavir or saquinavir/ritonavir should not be administered with astemizole (see section 4.3).

Anti-infectives:

Clarithromycin: ***Saquinavir:*** Concomitant administration of clarithromycin (500 mg twice daily) and Fortovase (1200 mg three times daily) to 12 healthy volunteers resulted in steady-state saquinavir AUC and C_{max} values which were 177 % and 187 % higher than those seen with saquinavir alone. Clarithromycin AUC and C_{max} values were approximately 40 % higher than those seen with clarithromycin alone. No dose adjustment is required when the two medicinal products are co-administered for a limited time at the doses studied. ***Saquinavir/ritonavir:*** The interaction between Invirase/ritonavir and clarithromycin has not been evaluated.

Erythromycin: ***Saquinavir:*** Concomitant administration of erythromycin (250 mg four times daily) and Fortovase (1200 mg three times daily) to 22 HIV-infected patients resulted in steady-state saquinavir AUC and C_{max} values which were 99 % and 106 % higher than those seen with saquinavir alone. No dose adjustment is required when the two medicinal products are co-administered. ***Saquinavir/ritonavir:*** The interaction between Invirase/ritonavir and erythromycin has not been evaluated.

Streptogramin antibiotics such as quinupristin/dalfopristin: Will inhibit CYP3A4 and may increase saquinavir concentrations. If these medicinal products are taken concomitantly with saquinavir, monitoring for saquinavir toxicity is recommended. The interaction between Invirase/ritonavir and quinupristin/dalfopristin has not been evaluated.

Antifungals:

Ketoconazole: ***Saquinavir:*** Concomitant use of ketoconazole (200 mg once daily) and Invirase (600 mg three times daily) to 12 healthy volunteers led to an increase in saquinavir AUC by about 160 % at steady state (day 6 of treatment) with no increase in the elimination half-life or any change in the absorption rate. Ketoconazole pharmacokinetics were not affected by co-administration with saquinavir at a dose of 600 mg three times daily. No dose adjustment for either medicinal product is required when the two medicinal products are co-administered at the doses studied. ***Saquinavir/ritonavir:*** The interaction between Invirase/ritonavir and ketoconazole has not been evaluated.

Itraconazole: ***Saquinavir:*** Like ketoconazole, itraconazole is a moderately potent inhibitor of the CYP3A4 isoenzyme and an interaction of similar magnitude is possible. If itraconazole is taken concomitantly with saquinavir, monitoring for saquinavir toxicity is recommended. ***Saquinavir/ritonavir:*** The interaction between Invirase/ritonavir and itraconazole has not been evaluated.

Fluconazole/miconazole: No specific drug interaction studies with either of these medicinal products have been performed.

Antimycobacterials:

Rifampicin: ***Saquinavir:*** Rifampicin (600 mg once daily) was shown to decrease plasma concentrations of saquinavir by 80 %. Since this may result in sub-therapeutic concentrations of saquinavir, rifampicin should not be administered concomitantly with Invirase. ***Saquinavir/ritonavir:*** In a study investigating the interaction of rifampicin 600 mg once daily and Invirase 1000 mg/ritonavir 100 mg given twice daily, 11 of 17 (65%) healthy volunteers developed severe hepatocellular toxicity with transaminase elevations up to > 20-fold the upper limit of normal after 1 to 5 days of co-administration. Therefore, rifampicin is contraindicated in patients taking ritonavir boosted Invirase as part of an ART regimen (see section 4.3).

Rifabutin: ***Saquinavir:*** Rifabutin reduces saquinavir plasma concentrations by 40 %. Rifabutin and Invirase should not be co-administered. ***Saquinavir/ritonavir:*** Concomitant administration of rifabutin with Invirase/ritonavir 400 mg/400 mg had no clinical significant effect on saquinavir exposure in 24 HIV patients.

Benzodiazepines:

Midazolam: ***Saquinavir:*** Co-administration of a single oral dose of midazolam (7.5 mg) after 3 or 5 days of Fortovase (1200 mg three times daily) to 12 healthy volunteers in a double-blind cross-over study, increased midazolam C_{max} to 235 % and AUC to 514 % of control. Saquinavir increased the elimination half-life of oral midazolam from 4.3 to 10.9 hours and the absolute bioavailability from 41 to 90 %. Volunteers experienced impairment in psychomotor skills and an increase in sedative effects. Consequently the dose of oral midazolam should be greatly reduced when given with saquinavir and the combination should be used with caution. When combined with intravenous midazolam (0.05 mg/kg), saquinavir decreased the clearance of midazolam by 56 % and increased its elimination half-life from 4.1 to 9.5 hours, however, only the subjective feeling to the midazolam effects was increased. Therefore, bolus doses of intravenous midazolam can be given in combination with Fortovase. During prolonged midazolam infusion, a total dose reduction of 50 % is recommended. ***Saquinavir/ritonavir:*** The interaction between Invirase/ritonavir and midazolam has not been evaluated. Midazolam is contraindicated with Invirase/ritonavir due to the risk of potential for prolonged or increased sedation and respiratory depression (see section 4.3).

Alprazolam, clorazepate, diazepam, flurazepam: Concentrations of these medicinal products may be increased when co-administered with Invirase/ritonavir. Careful monitoring of patients with regard to sedative effects is warranted, a decrease in the dose of the benzodiazepine may be required.

Triazolam: Concentrations of triazolam may be increased when co-administered with Invirase/ritonavir. Triazolam is contraindicated with Invirase/ritonavir, due to the risk of potential for prolonged or increased sedation and respiratory depression (see section 4.3).

Calcium channel blockers:

Felodipine, nifedipine, nicardipine, diltiazem, nimodipine, verapamil, amlodipine, nisoldipine, isradipine: Concentrations of these medicinal products may be increased when co-administered with Invirase/ritonavir. Caution is warranted and clinical monitoring of patients is recommended.

Corticosteroids:

Dexamethasone: Will induce CYP3A4 and may decrease saquinavir concentrations. Use with caution, saquinavir may be less effective in patients taking these medicinal products concomitantly. The interaction between Invirase/ritonavir and dexamethasone has not been evaluated.

Fluticasone propionate (interaction with ritonavir): In a clinical study where ritonavir 100 mg capsules bid were co-administered with 50 μg intranasal fluticasone propionate (4 times daily) for 7 days in healthy volunteers, the fluticasone propionate plasma levels increased significantly, whereas the intrinsic cortisol levels decreased by approximately 86 % (90 % confidence interval 82-89 %). Greater effects may be expected when fluticasone propionate is inhaled. Systemic corticosteroid effects including Cushing's syndrome and adrenal suppression have been reported in patients receiving ritonavir and inhaled or intranasally administered fluticasone propionate; this could also occur with other corticosteroids metabolised via the P450 3A pathway e.g. budesonide. Consequently, concomitant administration of boosted saquinavir and these glucocorticoids is not recommended unless the potential benefit of treatment outweighs the risk of systemic corticosteroid effects (see section 4.4). A dose reduction of the glucocorticoid should be considered with close monitoring of local and systemic effects or a switch to a glucocorticoid, which is not a substrate for CYP3A4 (e.g. beclomethasone). Moreover, in case of withdrawal of glucocorticoids progressive dose reduction may have to be performed over a longer period. The effects of high fluticasone systemic exposure on ritonavir plasma levels is yet unknown.

Histamine H_2-receptor antagonist:

Ranitidine: ***Saquinavir:*** There was an increase in exposure of saquinavir when Invirase was dosed in the presence of both ranitidine and food, relative to Invirase dosed with food alone. This resulted in AUC values of saquinavir, which were 67 % higher. This increase is not thought to be clinically relevant and no dose adjustment of saquinavir is recommended. ***Saquinavir/ritonavir:*** The interaction between Invirase/ritonavir and ranitidine has not been evaluated.

HMG-CoA reductase inhibitors:

Pravastatin, fluvastatin: Are not metabolised by CYP3A4, and interactions are not expected with protease inhibitors including ritonavir. If treatment with a HMG-CoA reductase inhibitor is indicated, either pravastatin or fluvastatin are the products recommended.

Simvastatin, lovastatin: Are highly dependent on CYP3A4 metabolism and plasma concentrations are markedly increased when co-administered with Invirase/ritonavir. Increased concentrations of these medicinal products have been associated with rhabdomyolysis and these medicinal products are contraindicated for use with Invirase/ritonavir (see section 4.3).

Atorvastatin: Is less dependent on CYP3A4 for metabolism. When used with Invirase/ritonavir, the lowest possible dose of atorvastatin should be administered and the patient carefully monitored for signs/symptoms of myopathy (muscle weakness, muscle pain, rising plasma creatinine kinase levels).

Immunosuppressants:

Cyclosporin, tacrolimus, rapamycin: Concentrations of these medicinal products may be increased when co-administered with Invirase/ritonavir. Therapeutic concentration monitoring is recommended for immunosuppressant agents when co-administered with Invirase/ritonavir.

Narcotic analgesic:

Methadone: Concentration of methadone may be decreased when co-administered with Invirase/ritonavir. Dosage of methadone may need to be increased.

Neuroleptics:

Pimozide: Concentrations of pimozide may be increased when co-administered with Invirase/ritonavir. Due to a potential for life threatening cardiac arrhythmias, Invirase/ritonavir is contraindicated in combination with pimozide (see section 4.3).

Oral contraceptives:

Ethinyl oestradiol: Concentration of ethinyl oestradiol may be decreased when co-administered with Invirase/ritonavir. Alternative or additional contraceptive measures should be used when oestrogen-based oral contraceptives are co-administered.

Phosphodiesterase type 5 (PDE5) inhibitors:

Sildenafil: The co-administration of Fortovase at steady state (1200 mg three times daily) with sildenafil (100 mg single dose), a substrate of CYP3A4, resulted in a 140 % increase in sildenafil C_{max} and a 210 % increase in sildenafil AUC. Sildenafil had no effect on saquinavir pharmacokinetics. Use sildenafil with caution at reduced doses of no more than 25 mg every 48 hours with increased monitoring of adverse events when administered concomitantly with Invirase/ritonavir.

Vardenafil: Concentrations of vardenafil may be increased when co-administered with Invirase/ritonavir. Use vardenafil with caution at reduced doses of no more than 2.5 mg every 72 hours with increased monitoring of adverse events when administered concomitantly with Invirase/ritonavir.

Tadalafil: Concentrations of tadalafil may be increased when co-administered with Invirase/ritonavir. Use tadalafil with caution at reduced doses of no more than 10 mg every 72 hours with increased monitoring of adverse events when administered concomitantly with Invirase/ritonavir.

Others:

Ergot alkaloids (e.g. ergotamine, dihydroergotamine, ergonovine, and methylergonovine):

Invirase/ritonavir may increase ergot alkaloids exposure and consequently increase the potential for acute ergot toxicity. Thus, the concomitant use of Invirase/ritonavir, and ergot alkaloids is contra-indicated (see section 4.3).

Grapefruit juice: ***Saquinavir:*** Co-administration of Invirase and grapefruit juice as single administration in healthy volunteers results in a 50 % and 100 % increase in exposure to saquinavir for normal and double strength grapefruit juice, respectively. This increase is not thought to be clinically relevant and no dose adjustment of Invirase is recommended. ***Saquinavir/ritonavir:*** The interaction between Invirase/ritonavir and grapefruit juice has not been evaluated.

Garlic capsules: ***Saquinavir:*** Concomitant administration of garlic capsules (dose approx. equivalent to two 4 g cloves of garlic daily) and saquinavir (Fortovase) 1200 mg three times daily to nine healthy volunteers resulted in a decrease of saquinavir AUC by 51 % and a decrease of the mean trough levels at 8 hours post dose by 49 %. Saquinavir mean C_{max} levels decreased by 54 %. Therefore, patients on saquinavir treatment must not take garlic capsules due to the risk of decreased plasma concentrations and loss of virological response and possible resistance to one or more components of the antiretroviral regimen. ***Saquinavir/ritonavir:*** The interaction between Invirase/ritonavir and garlic capsules has not been evaluated.

St. John's wort *(Hypericum perforatum)*: ***Saquinavir:*** Plasma levels of saquinavir can be reduced by concomitant use of the herbal preparation St. John's wort *(Hypericum perforatum)*. This is due to induction of drug metabolising enzymes and/or transport proteins by St. John's wort. Herbal preparations containing St. John's wort must not be used concomitantly with Invirase. If a patient is already taking St. John's wort, stop St. John's wort, check viral levels and if possible saquinavir levels. Saquinavir levels may increase on stopping St. John's wort, and the dose of saquinavir may need adjusting. The inducing effect of St. John's wort may persist for at least 2 weeks after cessation of treatment. ***Saquinavir/ritonavir:*** The interaction between Invirase/ritonavir and St. John's wort has not been evaluated.

Other potential interactions

Medicinal products that are substrates of CYP3A4:

Although specific studies have not been performed, co-administration of Invirase/ritonavir with medicinal products that are mainly metabolised by CYP3A4 pathway (e.g. dapsone, disopyramide, quinine, fentanyl, and alfentanyl) may result in elevated plasma concentrations of these medicinal products. Therefore these combinations should be given with caution.

Medicinal products that are substrates of P-glycoprotein:

Concomitant use of Invirase/ritonavir and medicinal products that are substrates of P-glycoprotein (P-gp) (e.g. digoxin) may lead to elevated plasma concentrations of these medicinal products, hence monitoring for toxicity is recommended.

Medicinal products reducing gastrointestinal transit time:

It is unknown, whether medicinal products which reduce the gastrointestinal transit time (e.g. metoclopramide) could lead to lower saquinavir plasma concentrations.

4.6 Pregnancy and lactation

Pregnancy: Evaluation of experimental animal studies does not indicate direct or indirect harmful effects with respect to the development of the embryo or foetus, the course of gestation and peri- and post-natal development. Clinical experience in pregnant women is limited: congenital malformations, birth defects and other disorders (without a congenital malformation) have been reported rarely in pregnant women who had received saquinavir in combination with other antiretroviral agents. However, so far the available data are insufficient and do not identify specific risks for the unborn child. Saquinavir should be used during pregnancy only if the potential benefit justifies the potential risk to the foetus (see section 5.3).

Lactation: There are no laboratory animal or human data available on secretion of saquinavir in breast milk. The potential for adverse reactions to saquinavir in nursing infants cannot be assessed, and therefore, breast-feeding should be discontinued prior to receiving saquinavir. It is recommended that HIV-infected women do not breast feed their infants under any circumstances in order to avoid transmission of HIV.

4.7 Effects on ability to drive and use machines

It is not known whether saquinavir has an effect on the ability to drive and to use machines.

4.8 Undesirable effects

Undesirable effects from clinical trials with unboosted Invirase

The most frequently reported adverse reactions among patients receiving Invirase as monotherapy 600 mg three times daily (in the form of Invirase 200 mg hard capsules) in clinical trials (excluding those toxicities known to be associated with zidovudine and/or zalcitabine when used in combinations) were diarrhoea, abdominal discomfort and nausea.

Adverse reactions from a pivotal study (n = 327) which included a treatment arm with saquinavir used as single medicinal product (600 mg three times daily) are listed below. Adverse reactions (mild, moderate and severe) with an incidence > 2 % considered by the investigator at least remotely related to saquinavir are summarised in Table 1:

Table 1: Incidences of undesirable effects in clinical trials, considered at least remotely related to treatment with Invirase with mild, moderate and severe intensity, occurring in > 2 % of patients.

(Very common (⩾ 10 %); common (⩾ 1 % and < 10 %))

Body System Frequency of Reaction	**Adverse Reactions**
Nervous system disorders	
Common	Headache, peripheral neuropathy, numbness extremities, paraesthesia, dizziness
Gastrointestinal disorders	
Very common	Diarrhoea, nausea
Common	Buccal mucosa ulceration, abdominal discomfort, vomiting, abdominal pain, flatulence

Skin and subcutaneous tissue disorders	
Common	Rash, pruritus
Musculoskeletal, connective tissue and bone disorders	
Common	Pain
General disorders and administration site conditions	
Common	Fatigue, asthenia, fever

Invirase does not alter or add to the toxicity profile of zalcitabine and/or zidovudine, when given in combination.

At least possibly related serious adverse reactions reported from clinical trials where Invirase was used as the sole protease inhibitor:

Serious adverse reactions, at least possibly related to the use of saquinavir, reported from clinical trials with a frequency of less than 2 % and not mentioned above, are listed below. These adverse reactions are from a database of over 6000 patients, of whom more than 100 had been on saquinavir therapy for over 2 years. Patients received saquinavir either as monotherapy or in combination with a wide variety of other antiretroviral medicinal products (nucleoside analogues, non-nucleoside reverse transcriptase inhibitors and protease inhibitors).

Confusion, ataxia and weakness, acute myeloblastic leukaemia, haemolytic anaemia, attempted suicide, Stevens-Johnson syndrome, severe cutaneous reaction associated with increased liver function tests, thrombocytopenia and intracranial haemorrhage, exacerbation of chronic liver disease with Grade 4 elevated liver function test, jaundice, ascites, drug fever, bullous skin eruption and polyarthritis, nephrolithiasis, pancreatitis, intestinal obstruction, portal hypertension, and peripheral vasoconstriction.

Adverse reactions that occurred in clinical trials with Fortovase are given for completeness.

Undesirable effects from clinical trials with unboosted Fortovase (saquinavir soft capsule)

The safety of Fortovase was studied in more than 500 patients who received the medicinal product either alone or in combination with other antiretroviral agents. The majority of adverse reactions were of mild intensity. The most frequently reported adverse reactions among patients receiving Fortovase were diarrhoea, nausea, abdominal discomfort and dyspepsia.

Clinical adverse reactions of at least moderate intensity which occurred in greater than or equal to 2 % of patients in an open label safety study (NV15182) and in a double blind study comparing Fortovase and Invirase (NV15355) are summarised in Table 2.

Table 2: Incidences of undesirable effects* in clinical trials, considered related to treatment with Fortovase of at least moderate intensity, occurring in ⩾ 2 % of patients.

(Very common (⩾ 10 %); common (⩾ 1 % and < 10 %))

Body System Frequency of reactions	**Adverse Reactions**
Psychiatric disorders	
Common	Depression, insomnia, anxiety, libido disorder
Nervous system disorders	
Common	Headaches
Gastrointestinal disorders	
Very common	Diarrhoea, nausea
Common	Abdominal discomfort, dyspepsia, flatulence, vomiting, abdominal pain, constipation
Skin and subcutaneous tissue disorders	
Common	Verruca
Musculoskeletal, connective tissue and bone disorders	
Common	Pain
General disorders and administration site conditions	
Common	Fatigue, appetite decreased, chest pain
Special senses disorders	
Common	Taste alteration

*Includes adverse reactions at least possibly related to study medication or of unknown intensity and/or relationship to treatment (corresponding to ACTG Grade 3 and 4).

At least possibly related serious undesirable effects reported from clinical trials where Fortovase was used as the sole protease inhibitor:

Serious adverse reactions at least possibly related to the use of Fortovase reported from clinical trials with a frequency of less than 2 % are:

Nephrolithiasis; pancreatitis; thrombocytopenia; erythema; dehydration; eructation; abdominal distension.

Fortovase does not alter the pattern, frequency or severity of known major toxicities associated with nucleoside analogues. For comprehensive dose adjustment recommendations and drug-associated adverse reactions for other medicinal products used in combination, physicians should refer to the Summary of Product Characteristics for each of these medicinal products.

Undesirable effects from clinical trials with boosted Fortovase

The safety of Fortovase (1000 mg twice daily) when used in combination with low dose ritonavir (100 mg twice daily) for at least 48 weeks was studied in 148 patients. The most frequently reported adverse reactions among patients receiving this boosted protease inhibitor regimen as part of their antiretroviral therapy were nausea, diarrhoea, fatigue, vomiting, flatulence, and abdominal pain.

Adverse reactions of grade 3 and 4 severity that were considered to be at least possibly related to Fortovase, or which were of unknown causality or severity, and which occurred at a frequency of at least 2 % in the pivotal study (n=148) were nausea (4.1 %), vomiting (2 %), anaemia (2 %) and fatigue (2 %).

Laboratory abnormalities with Invirase

The most common marked laboratory abnormalities seen during treatment with saquinavir containing regimens (as the sole protease inhibitor or in combination with low dose ritonavir) in clinical trials were isolated CPK increase, glucose decrease, glucose increase, raised transaminase values and neutropenia.

Laboratory abnormalities with Fortovase

Marked clinical laboratory abnormalities (change from grade 0 to grade 3 or 4, or change from grade 1 to grade 4) reported in greater than 2 % of patients treated with 1200 mg three times daily in the open label safety study included decreased glucose (6.4 %), increased CPK (7.8 %), increased gamma glutamyltransferase (5.7 %), increased ALT (5.7 %), increased AST (4.1 %), increased potassium (2.7 %) and neutropenia (2.9 %).

The following additional marked clinical laboratory abnormalities have been reported following treatment with Fortovase as the sole protease inhibitor (saquinavir) containing regimens: calcium (high/low), phosphate (low), bilirubin (high), amylase (high), potassium (low), sodium (low/high), haemoglobin (low), platelets (low), alkaline phosphatase (high), glucose (high), triglyceride (high).

In the safety study there was a 27 %-33 % incidence of greater than or equal to 1 grade shifts in ALT and AST during the 48 week study period. 46 % of these were single abnormal values. Only 3 % - 4 % of patients had greater than or equal to 3 grade shifts in transaminase levels and less than 0.5 % of patients had to discontinue the study for increased liver function tests.

Marked laboratory abnormalities (Grade 1 - 4) that have been observed with Fortovase in combination with ritonavir (at 48 weeks) included low haemoglobin (4 %), WBC (3 %), platelets (11 %), and lymphocyte counts (5 %), and high amylase (2 %), creatinine (2 %), bilirubin (7 %), AST (19 %), ALT (26 %), cholesterol (27 %), LDL-cholesterol (62 %), and triglyceride (32 %) levels.

Post-marketing experience with Invirase and Fortovase

Serious and non-serious adverse reactions from post-marketing spontaneous reports (where Fortovase and Invirase were taken as the sole protease inhibitor or in combination with ritonavir), not mentioned previously in section 4.8, for which a causal relationship to saquinavir cannot be excluded, are summarised below (rare: ⩾ 0.01 % and < 0.1 %; very rare: < 0.01 %):

- Infections and infestations: Hepatitis (rare).
- Immune system disorders: Allergic reactions (very rare).
- Nervous system disorders: Somnolence (very rare), seizures (rare).
- Renal and urinary disorders: Abnormal renal function (very rare).
- Metabolism and nutrition disorders:

- Diabetes mellitus or hyperglycaemia, sometimes associated with ketoacidosis (rare) (see section 4.4).

- Lipodystrophy: Combination antiretroviral therapy has been associated with redistribution of body fat (lipodystrophy) in HIV infected patients including the loss of peripheral and facial subcutaneous fat, increased intra-abdominal and visceral fat, breast hypertrophy and dorsicervical fat accumulation (buffalo hump) (rare).

- Combination antiretroviral therapy has been associated with metabolic abnormalities such as hypertriglyceridaemia, hypercholesterolaemia, insulin resistance, hyperglycaemia and hyperlactataemia (very rare; see section 4.4.).

- Vascular disorders: There have been reports of increased bleeding, including spontaneous skin haematomas and haemarthroses, in haemophilic patients type A and B treated with protease inhibitors (rare) (see section 4.4).
- Musculoskeletal, connective tissue and bone disorders: Increased CPK, myalgia, myositis and rarely, rhabdomyolysis have been reported with protease inhibitors, particularly in combination with nucleoside analogues (rare).
- In HIV-infected patients with severe immune deficiency at the time of initiation of combination antiretroviral therapy (CART), an inflammatory reaction to asymptomatic or residual opportunistic infections may arise (see section 4.4).

4.9 Overdose

There are two reports of patients who had overdoses with Invirase. One patient exceeded the recommended daily dose of saquinavir and took 8000 mg at once. The patient was treated with induction of emesis within two hours after ingestion of the overdose. The patient did not experience any sequelae. The second patient ingested 2.4 g of Invirase in combination with 600 mg of ritonavir and experienced pain in the throat that lasted for 6 hours and then resolved. In an exploratory small study, oral dosing with saquinavir at 3600 mg per day has not shown increased toxicity through the first 16 weeks of treatment.

Two cases of Fortovase overdosage have been received (1 case with unknown amount of Fortovase, second case 3.6 g to 4 g at once). No adverse events were reported in any of the cases.

5. PHARMACOLOGICAL PROPERTIES

5.1 Pharmacodynamic properties

Pharmaco-therapeutic group: Antiviral agent, ATC code J05A E01

Mechanism of action: The HIV protease carries out specific cleavages of viral precursor proteins as virions bud from infected cells. This is an essential step in the creation of fully formed, infectious virus particles. These viral precursor proteins contain a type of cleavage site which is recognised only by HIV and closely related viral proteases. Saquinavir is a mimetic of such cleavage sites and fits closely into the HIV-1 and HIV-2 protease active sites, acting as a reversible and selective inhibitor. Saquinavir has approximately 50,000-fold greater affinity for HIV protease than for human proteases. In *in vitro* antiviral assays saquinavir blocks the formation of infectious virus, and hence the spread of infection to naïve cells.

Antiviral activity in vitro: Unlike nucleoside analogues (zidovudine, etc.), saquinavir acts directly on its viral target enzyme. It does not require metabolic activation. This extends its potential effectiveness into resting cells. Saquinavir is active at nanomolar concentrations in lymphoblastoid and monocytic lines and in primary cultures of lymphocytes and monocytes infected with laboratory strains or clinical isolates of HIV-1. Experiments in cell culture show that saquinavir produces an additive to synergistic antiviral effect against HIV-1 in double and triple combination with various reverse transcriptase inhibitors (including zidovudine, zalcitabine, didanosine, lamivudine, stavudine and nevirapine) without enhanced cytotoxicity, and clear synergy in double combination with lopinavir.

Pharmacodynamic effects: The effects of saquinavir in combination with zalcitabine and zidovudine on biological markers (CD4 cell counts and plasma RNA) were evaluated in HIV-1 infected patients.

Clinical studies performed with Invirase (saquinavir mesylate)

In a study (NV14256) with zidovudine pre-treated patients (CD4 ⩾ 50 ⩽ 300 cells/mm^3), the combination of Invirase plus zalcitabine compared to zalcitabine monotherapy prolonged the time to first AIDS-defining illness or death. In this study, the combination therapy reduced the risk of a patient having an AIDS-defining illness or dying by 53 %. For death alone the combination of Invirase plus zalcitabine reduced the risk by 72 %. This corresponds to a reduction in the rate of an AIDS-defining illness or death from 29.4 % to 16.0 % over 18 months. Similarly for death alone, the rate was reduced from 8.6 % to 4.1 % over 18 months. In the three treatment groups, median treatment duration was 11 to 13 months and median follow-up has been 17 months.

In this study the median CD4 cell count at baseline over all treatment arms was 156 to 176 cells/mm^3. The average change from baseline over 16 weeks (median DAVG16) for saquinavir plus zalcitabine was +26 cells/mm^3 for the CD4 cell count and -0.6 $\log_{10}$ RNA copies/ml of plasma for viral load. The peak mean increase in the CD4 cell count was 47 cells/mm^3 at week 16. The peak mean reduction in viral load was 0.7 $\log_{10}$ RNA copies/ml of plasma at week 12.

Study SV14604 is a randomised, multi-centre, double blind phase III parallel study of zidovudine + zalcitabine, vs. saquinavir + zidovudine, vs. saquinavir + zidovudine + zalcitabine, in untreated/minimally treated HIV infected patients. A fourth treatment arm of zidovudine monotherapy was discontinued; patients originally on zidovudine monotherapy were switched to saquinavir + zidovudine + zalcitabine, constituting a "delayed" triple therapy group.

A total of 3485 patients was treated and had followed up data available (the intent to treat population). Median baseline CD4 across the 3 arms was 199-204 cells/mm^3, and median baseline HIV RNA was 5.0 - 5.1 $\log_{10}$ copies/ml. Median duration of study treatment was approximately 14 months and the median duration of follow up for AIDS defining events and deaths approximately 17 months.

Progression to first AIDS defining event or death was significantly decreased for patients on saquinavir + zidovudine + zalcitabine with 76 first AIDS defining events/deaths compared to 142 events on zidovudine + zalcitabine (p = 0.0001). An exploratory comparison of initial saquinavir + zidovudine + zalcitabine compared to the delayed triple therapy group showed superiority of initial triple therapy including saquinavir with 76 AIDS defining events or deaths on initial triple therapy vs. 116 on the initial zidovudine monotherapy-delayed triple therapy regimen (p = 0.001).

Patients receiving triple therapy had greater increases in CD4 count, with a 71 cells/mm^3 median peak increase from baseline compared to a 40 cells/mm^3 median peak increase on zidovudine + zalcitabine. Similarly, reductions in HIV RNA were greater on triple therapy with a -1.5 log_{10} copies/ml median peak change from baseline compared to a -1.1 log_{10} copies/ml median peak change on zidovudine + zalcitabine. For both CD4 and HIV RNA, comparisons over 48 weeks between the triple therapy arm and zidovudine + zalcitabine reached statistical significance (p = 0.0001).

Clinical study performed with Fortovase (saquinavir) and Invirase (saquinavir mesylate)

Study NV15355 is an open-label, randomised, parallel study comparing Fortovase (n = 90) and Invirase (n = 81) in combination with two nucleoside reverse transcriptase inhibitors of choice in treatment-naïve patients. Mean baseline CD4 cell count was 429 cells/mm^3 and mean baseline plasma HIV-RNA was 4.8 log_{10} copies/ml. After 16 weeks of treatment, there was a mean viral load suppression of -2.0 log_{10} copies/ml in the Fortovase containing arm compared to -1.6 log_{10} copies/ml in the Invirase containing arm. The magnitude of the reduction in viral load was limited by the sensitivity of the assay used, especially in the Fortovase arm in which 80 % of patients had viral loads below the limit of quantification (< 400 copies/ml) at 16 weeks compared to 43 % of patients on Invirase (p = 0.001). At 16 weeks, the increases in CD4 cell counts were 97 and 115 cells/mm^3 for the Fortovase and Invirase arms, respectively.

Clinical studies performed with Fortovase (saquinavir)

In the MaxCmin 1 study, the safety and efficacy of Fortovase/ritonavir 1000/100 mg twice daily plus 2 NRTIs/Non-Nucleoside Reverse Transcriptase Inhibitors (NNRTIs) was compared to indinavir/ritonavir 800/100 mg twice daily plus 2 NRTIs/NNRTIs in over 300 (both protease inhibitor treatment naïve and experienced) subjects. Median baseline CD4 cell count was 272 cells/mm^3, and median baseline plasma HIV-RNA was 4.0 log_{10} copies/ml in the saquinavir/ritonavir arm. Median baseline CD4 cell count was 280 cells/mm^3, and median baseline plasma HIV-RNA was 3.9 log_{10} copies/ml in the indinavir/ritonavir arm. At 48 weeks, the median increases in CD4 cell counts were 85 and 73 cells/mm^3 for the saquinavir and indinavir arms, respectively. For the intent to treat analysis (switch = failure) at week 48, the proportion of patients in the saquinavir containing arm with viral load below the limit of detection (< 400 copies/ml) was 69 % (N=102) compared with 53 % (N=84) in the indinavir containing arm. The combination of saquinavir and ritonavir exhibited a superior virological activity compared with the indinavir and ritonavir arm when switch from the assigned treatment was counted as virological failure. This was to be expected as a higher proportion of subjects in the indinavir/ritonavir arm (40 %) than in the saquinavir/ritonavir arm (27 %, p=0.01) switched from the randomised treatment. In addition patients randomised to indinavir/ritonavir had an increased risk of treatment-limiting adverse events and adverse events of grade 3 and/or 4 (41 % in the indinavir/ritonavir arm versus 24 % in the saquinavir/ritonavir arm; p=0.002).

In the MaxCmin2 study, the safety and efficacy of Fortovase/ritonavir 1000/100 mg twice daily plus 2 NRTIs/NNRTIs was compared with lopinavir/ritonavir 400/100 mg twice daily plus 2 NRTIs/NNRTIs in 324 (both protease inhibitor treatment naïve and experienced) subjects. Values for median baseline CD4 count and median baseline plasma HIV RNA were 241 cells/mm^3 and 4.4 log_{10} copies/ml in the saquinavir/ritonavir arm, and 239 cells/mm^3 and 4.6 log_{10} copies/ml in the lopinavir/ritonavir arm, respectively. None of the subjects in the lopinavir/ritonavir arm had been exposed to lopinavir prior to randomisation whereas 16 of the subjects in the saquinavir/ritonavir arm had previously been exposed to saquinavir.

In the primary efficacy analysis, incidence of virological failure, including all subjects that took at least one dose of the study medication (ITT/exposed population), 29 failures were observed in the lopinavir/ritonavir arm and 53 failures in the saquinavir/ritonavir arm (hazard ratio: 0.5; 95 % C.I. 0.3 – 0.8). At 48 weeks, the proportion of subjects with HIV RNA below the limit of detection (< 50 copies/ml) was 53 % (N=161) for the saquinavir arm versus 60 % (N=163) for the lopinavir arm in the intent-to-treat, switch equals failure analysis, and 74 % (N=114) for the saquinavir arm versus 70 % (N=141) for the lopinavir arm in the on-treatment analysis (p = ns for both comparisons). The combination of saquinavir and ritonavir exhibited comparable virological activity with the lopinavir and ritonavir arm when switch from the assigned treatment was counted as virological failure. Over 48 weeks a similar immunological response was seen in both arms with median increases in CD4 count of 106 cells/mm^3 for the lopinavir/ritonavir arm, and 110 cells/mm^3 for the saquinavir/ritonavir arm. More subjects in the saquinavir/ritonavir arm (30 %) than in the lopinavir/ritonavir arm (14 %) prematurely discontinued the assigned treatment (p = 0.001). The primary reasons for premature discontinuation were non-fatal adverse events and subject's choice. No difference in the incidence of adverse events of grade 3 and/or 4 was seen between the two arms.

Potential for resistance and cross-resistance to saquinavir:

Resistance: The objective of antiretroviral therapy is to suppress viral replication to below the limits of quantification. Incomplete viral suppression may lead to the development of drug resistance to one or more components of the regimen. Drug resistance is measured as the change in viral susceptibility to drug in culture (="phenotypic resistance") or in protease amino acid sequence (="genotypic resistance").

Two primary mutations in the viral protease (L90M and G48V, the former predominating and the combination rare even with saquinavir monotherapy) are found in post-treatment resistant isolates. The G48V and L90M mutations give modest (typically less than 10-fold) reductions in susceptibility to saquinavir. In one study, 24 clinical isolates containing G48V and/or L90M after therapy with Invirase used as a single protease inhibitor showed a geometric mean reduction of susceptibility (increase in IC_{50}) of 7.3-fold relative to baseline virus (range 1.2 to 97-fold). In another study, 32 saquinavir-naïve patients, of whom 26 were resistant to ritonavir and/or indinavir, were treated with Invirase 1000 mg in combination with ritonavir 100 mg both two times daily, efavirenz and nucleoside analogues. 19/32 were sensitive to saquinavir at baseline. HIV RNA levels below 50 copies/ml were achieved at week 24 for 58 % of those patients carrying saquinavir-sensitive virus and for 25 % of those carrying virus with reduced (> 10 fold) sensitivity to saquinavir.

Secondary mutations (e.g. L10I/V, K20R, M36I/L, A71T, V82X) may accompany or precede the primary resistance mutations and give rise to greater reductions in susceptibility to saquinavir.

The overall incidence of protease genotypic resistance to saquinavir observed in a cohort of 51 antiretroviral naïve subjects after a mean of 46 weeks (range 15 to 50 weeks) treatment with Fortovase 1200 mg three times daily in combination with 2 NRTIs was 4 %.

Cross-resistance: Resistance mutations selected by one drug can in principle also result in reduced susceptibility to other drugs, particularly those in the same drug class. When this occurs it is termed cross-resistance.

Cross-resistance can result in weakened virological response to drug therapy. The application of data from phenotypic and/or genotypic resistance testing following incomplete viral suppression or virological failure can improve the response to subsequent treatments.

Cross-resistance between saquinavir and reverse transcriptase inhibitors: Cross-resistance between saquinavir and reverse transcriptase inhibitors is unlikely because of their different enzyme targets. HIV isolates resistant to zidovudine are sensitive to saquinavir, and conversely HIV isolates resistant to saquinavir are sensitive to zidovudine.

Cross-resistance to other protease inhibitors: In a study of virus isolates from four clinical trials with Invirase as the sole protease inhibitor, 22 virus isolates were identified as being resistant to saquinavir following treatment for 24 - 147 weeks. Susceptibility of each isolate was assessed to indinavir, ritonavir, nelfinavir and amprenavir. Of the isolates, 6/22 did not show cross-resistance to the other inhibitors, while 4/22 showed broad cross-resistance. The remaining 12/22 retained activity against at least one other protease inhibitor.

Cross-resistance with lopinavir is as yet undetermined in clinical isolates, although laboratory strains with substitutions at residues 10, 84 and 90 or 10, 48, 82 and 90 did not show significant reduction in susceptibility to lopinavir.

Cross-resistance from other protease inhibitors: Subjects with high level resistance to other protease inhibitors do not necessarily show cross-resistance to saquinavir. Studies of molecular clones containing resistance mutations associated with ritonavir, nelfinavir or amprenavir showed significant resistance to these individual protease inhibitors, but not in all cases to saquinavir. In a clinical study of individuals pre-treated with indinavir or ritonavir, 81 % showed reduced susceptibility to indinavir and 59 % to ritonavir at baseline. Of these, 40 % showed reduced (> 10 fold) susceptibility to saquinavir at baseline. Following 24 weeks of therapy with Invirase 1000 mg in combination with ritonavir both 100 mg two times daily, efavirenz and nucleoside analogues, the median decrease in plasma HIV-RNA was 0.9 log_{10} copies/ml for patients with phenotypic resistance to saquinavir versus 1.52 log_{10} copies/ml for those without resistance (p=0.03). The median number of resistance mutations in the protease gene in individuals with phenotypic resistance to saquinavir was 5.5 (range 4 - 8), whereas it was 3 (range 0-6) in those sensitive to saquinavir (p=0.0003). However, extensive treatment of subjects with protease inhibitors after failure can lead to broad cross-resistance in a complex, dynamic process.

Hypersusceptibility to mutant virus: Some virus isolates with reduced susceptibility to other protease inhibitors can have enhanced susceptibility (hypersusceptibility) to inhibition with saquinavir, for example viruses containing the D30N substitution after nelfinavir therapy and viruses, carrying complex substitutions patterns including I50V. Many viruses with substitutions at residue 82, commonly selected by indinavir or ritonavir therapy, either retain, or show enhanced susceptibility to saquinavir. The clinical significance of hypersusceptibility to saquinavir has not been established.

5.2 Pharmacokinetic properties

Absorption and bioavailability in adults and effect of food: In healthy volunteers the extent of absorption (as reflected by AUC) after a 600 mg oral dose of saquinavir was increased from 24 ng·h/ml (CV 33 %), under fasting conditions, to 161 ng·h/ml (CV35 %) when saquinavir was given following a heavy breakfast (48 g protein, 60 g carbohydrate, 57 g fat; 1006 kcal).

The presence of food also increased the time taken to achieve maximum concentration from 2.4 hours to 3.8 hours and substantially increased the mean maximum plasma concentrations (C_{max}) from 3.0 ng/ml to 35.5 ng/ml. The effect of food has been shown to persist for up to 2 hours. Therefore, Invirase should be taken within 2 hours after a meal.

Absolute bioavailability averaged 4 % (CV 73 %, range: 1 % to 9 %) in 8 healthy volunteers who received a single 600 mg dose (3 × 200 mg hard capsule) of Invirase following a heavy breakfast. The low bioavailability is thought to be due to a combination of incomplete absorption and extensive first-pass metabolism. Gastric pH has been shown to be only a minor component in the large increase in bioavailability seen when given with food.

After multiple oral doses (25 – 600 mg three times daily) in the presence of food, the increase in exposure (50-fold) was greater than directly proportional to the increase in dose (24-fold). Following multiple dosing (600 mg three times daily, in the form of Invirase 200 mg hard capsules) in HIV-infected patients (n = 29), the steady state area under the plasma concentration versus time curve (AUC) was 2.5 times (95 % CI 1.6 to 3.8) higher than that observed after a single dose.

In one study, HIV-infected patients were given saquinavir 600 mg three times daily after a meal or a substantial snack. AUC and maximum plasma concentration (C_{max})

Table 3 Mean (%CV) AUC, C_{max} and C_{min} of saquinavir in patients following multiple dosing of Invirase, Fortovase, Invirase/ritonavir, and Fortovase/ritonavir

Treatment	N	AUCτ (ng·h/ml)	AUC_{0-24} (ng·h/ml)	C_{max} (ng/ml)	C_{min} (ng/ml)
Invirase (hard capsule) 600 mg tid	10	866 (62)	2,598	197 (75)	75 (82)
Fortovase (soft capsule) 1200 mg tid	31	7,249 (85)	21,747	2,181 (74)	216 (84)
Fortovase (soft capsule) 1000 mg bid plus ritonavir 100 mg bid*	24	19,085 (13,943-26,124)	38,170	3,344 (2,478-4,513)	433 (301-622)
Invirase(hard capsule) 1000 mg bid plus ritonavir 100 mg bid*	24	14,607 (10,218-20,882)	29,214	2,623 (1,894-3,631)	371 (245-561)

τ = dosing interval, i.e. 8 hour for tid and 12 h for bid dosing.

C_{min} = the observed plasma concentration at the end of the dose interval.

* results are mean (95 % CI).

values were about twice those observed in healthy volunteers receiving the same treatment regimen.

In HIV-infected patients, Invirase or Fortovase in combination with ritonavir at doses of 1000/100 mg twice daily (bid) provides saquinavir systemic exposures over a 24-hour period similar to or greater than those achieved with Fortovase 1200 mg three times daily (tid) (see Table 3). The pharmacokinetics of saquinavir are stable during long-term treatment. Studies with saquinavir in combination with ritonavir have been performed with food only. No data are available for the intake of ritonavir boosted saquinavir in the fasting state.

Table 3: Mean (%CV) AUC, C_{max} and C_{min} of saquinavir in patients following multiple dosing of Invirase, Fortovase, Invirase/ritonavir, and Fortovase/ritonavir

(see Table 3 on previous page)

Bioequivalence of Invirase 500 mg film-coated tablets (FCT) and Invirase 200 mg hard capsules (HC) was demonstrated in 94 healthy male and female volunteers who received either 1000 mg (2 × 500 mg) Invirase FCT or (5 × 200 mg) Invirase HC under fed conditions in combination with 100 mg ritonavir twice daily. Mean exposure ratios were estimated to be 1.10 for $AUC_{0-\infty}$ and 1.19 for C_{max} of saquinavir with corresponding 90 % confidence intervals of 1.04-1.16 and 1.14-1.25, respectively.

Effective therapy in treatment naïve patients is associated with a C_{min} of approximately 50 ng/ml and an AUC_{0-24} of about 20,000 ng·h/ml. Effective therapy in treatment experienced patients is associated with a C_{min} of approximately 100 ng/ml and an AUC_{0-24} of about 20,000 ng·h/ml.

In vitro studies have shown that saquinavir is a substrate for P-glycoprotein (P-gp).

Distribution in adults: Saquinavir partitions extensively into the tissues. The mean steady-state volume of distribution following intravenous administration of a 12 mg dose of saquinavir was 700 l (CV 39 %). It has been shown that saquinavir is approximately 97 % bound to plasma proteins up to 30 μg/ml. In two patients receiving Invirase 600 mg three times daily, cerebrospinal fluid concentrations of saquinavir were negligible when compared to concentrations from matching plasma samples.

Metabolism and elimination in adults: *In vitro* studies using human liver microsomes have shown that the metabolism of saquinavir is cytochrome P450 mediated with the specific isoenzyme, CYP3A4, responsible for more than 90 % of the hepatic metabolism. Based on *in vitro* studies, saquinavir is rapidly metabolised to a range of mono- and di-hydroxylated inactive compounds. In a mass balance study using 600 mg 14C-saquinavir (n = 8), 88 % and 1 % of the orally administered radioactivity, was recovered in faeces and urine, respectively, within 4 days of dosing. In an additional four subjects administered 10.5 mg 14C-saquinavir intravenously, 81 % and 3 % of the intravenously administered radioactivity was recovered in faeces and urine, respectively, within 4 days of dosing. 13 % of circulating saquinavir in plasma was present as unchanged compound after oral administration and the remainder as metabolites. Following intravenous administration 66 % of circulating saquinavir was present as unchanged compound and the remainder as metabolites, suggesting that saquinavir undergoes extensive first pass metabolism. *In vitro* experiments have shown that the hepatic metabolism of saquinavir becomes saturable at concentrations above 2 μg/ml.

Systemic clearance of saquinavir was high, 1.14 l/h/kg (CV 12 %), slightly above the hepatic plasma flow, and constant after intravenous doses of 6, 36 and 72 mg. The mean residence time of saquinavir was 7 hours (n = 8).

Effect of gender following treatment with Invirase/ritonavir: A gender difference was observed with females showing higher saquinavir exposure than males (AUC on average 56 % higher and C_{max} on average 26 % higher) in the bioequivalence study comparing Invirase 500 mg film coated tablets with Invirase 200 mg hard capsules both in combination with ritonavir. There was no evidence that age and body-weight explained the gender difference in this study. Limited data from controlled clinical studies with the approved dosage regimen do not indicate a major difference in the efficacy and safety profile between men and women.

5.3 Preclinical safety data

Acute and chronic toxicity: Saquinavir was well tolerated in oral acute and chronic toxicity studies in mice, rats, dogs and marmosets at dose levels that gave maximum plasma exposures (AUC values) approximately 1.5, 1.0, 4 to 9-and 3 fold greater, respectively, than those achieved in humans at the recommended dose.

Mutagenesis: Studies with and without metabolic activation (as appropriate) have shown that saquinavir has no mutagenic or genotoxic activity.

Carcinogenesis: There was no evidence of carcinogenic activity after the administration of saquinavir mesylate for 96 to 104 weeks to rats (maximum dose 1000 mg/kg/day) and mice (maximum dose 2500 mg/kg/day). The plasma exposures (AUC values) in the respective species were up to 60 % of those obtained in humans at the recommended clinical dose of Fortovase (saquinavir soft capsule) or equivalent to them.

Reproductive toxicity: (see section 4.6). Fertility and reproductive performance were not affected in rats at plasma exposures (AUC values) approximately 50 % of those achieved in humans at the recommended dose.

Reproduction studies conducted with saquinavir in rats have shown no embryotoxicity or teratogenicity at plasma exposures (AUC values) approximately 50 % of those achieved in humans at the recommended dose or in rabbits at plasma exposures approximately 40 % of those achieved at the recommended clinical dose. Distribution studies in these species showed that placental transfer of saquinavir is low (less than 5 % of maternal plasma concentrations).

Studies in rats indicated that exposure to saquinavir from late pregnancy through lactation at plasma concentrations (AUC values) approximately 50 % of those achieved in humans at the recommended dose had no effect on the survival, growth and development of offspring to weaning.

6. PHARMACEUTICAL PARTICULARS

6.1 List of excipients

Tablet core:

Microcrystalline cellulose

Croscarmellose sodium

Povidone

Lactose (monohydrate)

Magnesium stearate

Tablet coat:

Hypromellose

Titanium dioxide (E 171)

Talc

Glycerol triacetate

Iron oxide yellow and red (E172)

6.2 Incompatibilities

Not applicable.

6.3 Shelf life

2 years.

6.4 Special precautions for storage

This medicinal product does not require any special storage conditions.

6.5 Nature and contents of container

Plastic bottles (HDPE) containing 120 tablets.

6.6 Instructions for use and handling

No special requirements.

7. MARKETING AUTHORISATION HOLDER

Roche Registration Limited

40 Broadwater Road

Welwyn Garden City

Hertfordshire, AL7 3AY

United Kingdom

8. MARKETING AUTHORISATION NUMBER(S)

EU/1/96/026/002

9. DATE OF FIRST AUTHORISATION/RENEWAL OF THE AUTHORISATION

May 2005

10. DATE OF REVISION OF THE TEXT

31 August 2005

LEGAL STATUS

POM

Invirase is a registered trade mark

Invivac

(Solvay Healthcare Limited)

1. NAME OF THE MEDICINAL PRODUCT

Invivac ® 2005/2006, suspension for injection

Influenza vaccine (surface antigen, inactivated, virosome).

2. QUALITATIVE AND QUANTITATIVE COMPOSITION

Influenza virus surface antigens (haemagglutinin and neuraminidase)* of strains:

A/California/7/2004 (H_3N_2)-like strain - (A/New York/55/2004 NYMC X-157 reass.)	15 micrograms**
A/New Caledonia/20/99 (H_1N_1)-like strain - (A/New Caledonia/20/99 IVR-116 reass.)	15 micrograms
B/Shanghai/361/2002-like strain - (B/Jiangsu/10/2003)	15 micrograms

per 0.5 ml dose.

* propagated in hens' eggs

** haemagglutinin

This vaccine complies with the WHO recommendation (northern hemisphere), and

the decision of the EU for the 2005/2006 season.

For excipients see 6.1.

3. PHARMACEUTICAL FORM

Suspension for injection.

4. CLINICAL PARTICULARS

4.1 Therapeutic indications

Prophylaxis of influenza in adults and the elderly, especially in those who run an increased risk of associated complications.

4.2 Posology and method of administration

Adults: 0.5 ml.

Immunisation should be carried out by intramuscular or deep subcutaneous injection.

Children: the clinical data available are too limited to vaccinate children with Invivac.

4.3 Contraindications

Hypersensitivity to the active substances, to any of the excipients and to eggs, chicken protein or gentamicin.

Immunisation shall be postponed in patients with febrile illness or acute infection.

4.4 Special warnings and special precautions for use

As with all injectable vaccines, appropriate medical treatment and supervision should always be readily available in case of a rare anaphylactic event following the administration of the vaccine.

Invivac should under no circumstances be administered intravascularly.

Antibody response in patients with endogenous or iatrogenic immunosuppression may be insufficient.

4.5 Interaction with other medicinal products and other forms of Interaction

Invivac may be given at the same time as other vaccines. Immunisation should be carried out on separate limbs. It should be noted that the adverse reactions may be intensified.

The immunological response may be diminished if the patient is undergoing immunosuppressant treatment.

Following influenza vaccination, false positive results in serology tests using the ELISA method to detect antibodies against HIV1, Hepatitis C and especially HTLV1 have been observed. The Western Blot technique disproves the results. The transient false positive reactions could be due to the IgM response by the vaccine.

4.6 Pregnancy and lactation

Limited data from vaccinations in pregnant women do not indicate that adverse foetal and maternal outcomes were attributable to the vaccine. The use of this vaccine may be considered from the second trimester of pregnancy. For pregnant women with medical conditions that increase their risk of complications from influenza, administration of the vaccine is recommended, irrespective of their stage of pregnancy.

Invivac may be used during lactation.

4.7 Effects on ability to drive and use machines

Invivac is unlikely to produce an effect on the ability to drive and use machines.

4.8 Undesirable effects

Adverse events from clinical trials:

The safety of trivalent inactivated influenza vaccines is assessed in open label, uncontrolled clinical trials performed as annual update requirement, including at least 50 adults aged 18-60 and at least 50 elderly subjects aged 60 or older. Safety evaluation is performed during the first 3 days following vaccination.

Undesirable effects reported are listed according to the following frequency.

Adverse events from clinical trials:

Common >1/100, <1/10)

Local reactions: redness, swelling, pain, ecchymosis, induration.

Systemic reactions: fever, malaise, shivering, fatigue, headache, sweating, myalgia, arthralgia. These reactions usually disappear within 1-2 days without treatment.

From post-marketing surveillance additionally, the following adverse events have been reported:

Uncommon >1/1,000, <1/100)

Generalised skin reactions including pruritus, urticaria or non-specific rash.

Rare >1/10,000, <1/1,000)

Neuralgia, paraesthesia, convulsions, transient thrombocytopenia.

Allergic reactions, in rare cases leading to shock, have been reported.

Very rare (<1/10,000)

Vasculitis with transient renal involvement.

Neurological disorders, such as encephalomyelitis, neuritis and Guillain Barré syndrome.

4.9 Overdose

Overdosage is unlikely to have any untoward effect.

5. PHARMACOLOGICAL PROPERTIES

5.1 Pharmacodynamic properties

Seroprotection is generally obtained within 2 to 3 weeks. The duration of post-vaccinal immunity to homologous strains or to strains closely related to the vaccine strains varies but is usually 6 to 12 months.

5.2 Pharmacokinetic properties
Not applicable.

5.3 Preclinical safety data
Not applicable.

6. PHARMACEUTICAL PARTICULARS

6.1 List of excipients
Sodium chloride

Disodium phosphate dihydrate

Potassium dihydrogen phosphate

Lecithin

Water for injections

6.2 Incompatibilities
In the absence of compatibility studies, this medicinal product must not be mixed with other medicinal products.

6.3 Shelf life
1 year.

6.4 Special precautions for storage
Store in a refrigerator (+2°C to +8°C). Do not freeze. Protect from light.

6.5 Nature and contents of container
0.5 ml suspension for injection in prefilled syringe (glass, type I), pack of 1 or 10.

6.6 Instructions for use and handling
Invivac should be allowed to reach room temperature before use. Shake gently before use.

7. MARKETING AUTHORISATION HOLDER
Solvay Healthcare Limited

Mansbridge Road

West End

Southampton

SO18 3JD

8. MARKETING AUTHORISATION NUMBER(S)
PL 0512/0186

9. DATE OF FIRST AUTHORISATION/RENEWAL OF THE AUTHORISATION
July 2004

10. DATE OF REVISION OF THE TEXT
23 August 2005

Legal category
POM

Ismelin ampoules 10mg/ml

(Amdipharm)

1. NAME OF THE MEDICINAL PRODUCT
Ismelin Ampoules 10mg/ml

2. QUALITATIVE AND QUANTITATIVE COMPOSITION
Guanethidine monosulphate Ph.Eur. 10mg/ml

3. PHARMACEUTICAL FORM
A colourless solution in a clear glass 1 ml ampoule, for intramuscular administration.

4. CLINICAL PARTICULARS

4.1 Therapeutic indications
Control of hypertensive crises, and to obtain more rapid blood pressure control.

4.2 Posology and method of administration
Adults:

Ismelin should be given by intramuscular injection. One injection of 10 to 20mg will generally cause a fall in blood pressure within 30 minutes which reaches a maximum in one to two hours and is maintained for four to six hours. If a further dose of 10 to 20mg is deemed necessary, then three hours should be allowed to elapse between doses.

In hypertensive patients with moderate renal insufficiency, the intervals between dosing should be extended or the dosage reduced to avoid accumulation as the drug is renally excreted. (For patients with renal failure, see Section 4.3, "Contra-indications").

Children: Not recommended.

Elderly: Clinical evidence would indicate that no special dosage regime is necessary, but concurrent coronary or cerebral insufficiency should be taken into account.

4.3 Contraindications
Cases of phaeochromocytoma and patients previously treated with monoamine oxidase inhibitors (see Section 4.5, "Interactions with other medicaments and other forms of interaction"); in such cases, Ismelin may lead to the release of large quantities of catecholamines, which may cause a hypertensive crisis.

Patients with known hypersensitivity to guanethidine and related derivatives. Heart failure due to causes other than hypertension. Renal failure (creatinine clearance 10 to 40ml/min).

4.4 Special warnings and special precautions for use
Heat and physical exertion may increase the antihypertensive effect of Ismelin.

Ismelin should be used with caution in patients with moderate renal insufficiency (creatinine clearance 41 to 65ml/min), or with coronary and/or cerebral arteriosclerosis; abrupt lowering of blood pressure should be avoided. Caution should be exercised in asthmatic patients or in patients with a history of gastro-intestinal ulceration.

The concurrent administration of guanethidine and β-blockers may provoke severe bradycardia.

When patients have to undergo surgery, it is recommended that treatment with Ismelin be withdrawn a few days before the operation. To avoid excessive bradycardia during anaesthesia, it is advisable to premedicate with larger than usual doses of atropine.

After prolonged treatment with Ismelin, latent heart failure may develop. This is due to salt and water retention, and mild negative inotropic and chronotropic effects. Concomitant administration of diuretics can readily correct this condition.

If patients develop fever, the dose of Ismelin should be lowered.

4.5 Interaction with other medicinal products and other forms of Interaction
Monoamine oxidase inhibitors should be withdrawn at least fourteen days before starting treatment with Ismelin (See Section 4.3, "Contra-indications").

Concurrent administration of Ismelin with anti-arrhythmic agents and digitalis may lead to sinus bradycardia.

The anti-hypertensive action of Ismelin may be enhanced by other anti-hypertensive agents such as reserpine, methyldopa, vasodilators (especially minoxidil), calcium antagonists, β-blockers, ACE inhibitors and alcohol.

The anti-hypertensive action of Ismelin may be reduced by chlorpromazine, phenothiazine derivatives, tricyclic antidepressants and related anti-psychotic drugs, and oral contraceptives. Consequently if larger doses of Ismelin are prescribed, care must be taken upon the withdrawal of any of the drugs listed, as severe hypotension may ensue if the dose of Ismelin is not adjusted in advance.

After prolonged treatment with Ismelin, it may be necessary to adjust the dosage of insulin or oral anti-diabetic drugs.

Patients on Ismelin may become hypersensitive to adrenaline, amphetamines or other sympathomimetic agents. Therefore caution should be exercised when taking or using preparations containing these drugs.

4.6 Pregnancy and lactation
No foetal toxicity or fertility studies have been carried out in animals. Therefore the drug should only be used if there is no safer alternative. However, in particular, it should not be used during the first trimester of pregnancy nor within at least two weeks prior to the birth or during labour since it may induce paralytic ileus in the newborn infant.

In mothers receiving Ismelin in therapeutic doses, the active substance passes into the breast milk, but in quantities so small that no undesirable effects on the infant are to be expected.

4.7 Effects on ability to drive and use machines
Patients should be warned of the potential hazards of driving or operating machinery if they experience side effects such as dizziness, blurred vision or drowsiness.

4.8 Undesirable effects
Side effects are often an indication of excessive dosage. The following effects may occur:

Central nervous system: Particularly at the start of treatment: dizziness, tiredness, lethargy, paraesthesia and headache. Occasional: blurred vision and depression. Rare: myalgia and muscular tremor.

Cardiovascular system: Postural hypotension (which may be associated with cerebral or myocardial ischaemia in severe cases) especially when getting up in the morning or after physical exertion, sick-sinus syndrome, oedema, exacerbation of intermittent claudication and bradycardia. Occasional: heart failure. Rare: angina pectoris.

Gastro-intestinal tract: Diarrhoea and gaseous distension. Occasional: vomiting, nausea and dry mouth. Rare: swelling of parotid glands.

Respiratory tract: Nasal congestion. Rare: asthma.

Urogenital system: Raised BUN levels or uraemia in patients with latent or manifest renal failure, and ejaculation disturbances.

Skin and hair: Occasional: dermatitis. Rare: hair loss.

Blood: Isolated reports of anaemia, leucopenia, and/or thrombocytopenia.

4.9 Overdose
Symptoms: may include postural hypotension which may cause syncope, sinus bradycardia (although tachycardia has been observed), tiredness, dizziness, blurring of vision, muscular weakness, nausea, vomiting, severe diarrhoea and oliguria.

Treatment: Postural hypotension may be overcome by keeping the patient recumbent, or by instituting fluid and electrolyte replacement, and if necessary, by cautious administration of pressor agents (see Section 4.5, "Interactions with other medicaments and other forms of interaction"). Sinus bradycardia can be treated with atropine, and diarrhoea with an anticholinergic agent.

5. PHARMACOLOGICAL PROPERTIES

5.1 Pharmacodynamic properties
Ismelin is a peripheral sympathetic blocking drug which lowers blood pressure by depleting and inhibiting reformation of noradrenaline in postganglionic nerve endings. Guanethidine, being highly polar, does not cross the blood-brain barrier and is unlikely therefore to exert any effect on the central nervous system. In addition, guanethidine has no effect on the parasympathetic nervous system.

5.2 Pharmacokinetic properties
Guanethidine may be excreted more slowly in those patients with moderate to severely compromised renal function, therefore the potential for accumulation of the drug will be higher.

5.3 Preclinical safety data
There are no pre-clinical data of relevance to the prescriber which are additional to those already included in other sections of the Summary of Product Characteristics.

6. PHARMACEUTICAL PARTICULARS

6.1 List of excipients
Sodium chloride, sulphuric acid and water for injections.

6.2 Incompatibilities
None known.

6.3 Shelf life
5 years.

6.4 Special precautions for storage
None.

6.5 Nature and contents of container
Clear glass type I, 1 ml ampoules containing 10mg/ml: Boxes of 5.

6.6 Instructions for use and handling
None.

7. MARKETING AUTHORISATION HOLDER
Amdipharm Plc

Regency House

Miles Gray Road

Basildon

Essex

SS14 3AF

United Kingdom

8. MARKETING AUTHORISATION NUMBER(S)
PL 20072/0027

9. DATE OF FIRST AUTHORISATION/RENEWAL OF THE AUTHORISATION
18th April 2005

10. DATE OF REVISION OF THE TEXT

LEGAL STATUS
POM

Ismo 10

(Roche Products Limited)

1. NAME OF THE MEDICINAL PRODUCT
Ismo 10

2. QUALITATIVE AND QUANTITATIVE COMPOSITION
10mg isosorbide-5-mononitrate.

3. PHARMACEUTICAL FORM
Tablet for oral use.

Each tablet is marked Ismo on one face and 10 on the reverse.

4. CLINICAL PARTICULARS

4.1 Therapeutic indications
Ismo products are indicated for use in the treatment and prophylaxis of angina pectoris and as adjunctive therapy in congestive heart failure which does not respond adequately to cardiac glycosides and/or diuretics.

4.2 Posology and method of administration
Route of administration

Oral.

Adults

The recommended dosage is from 20 to 120mg isosorbide-5-mononitrate daily in divided doses. The majority of patients will require a dosage in the range of 40 to 60mg daily in divided doses. The tablets should be taken with fluid and swallowed whole without chewing.

The lowest effective dose should be used.

For patients who have not previously received prophylactic nitrate therapy it is recommended that the Ismo Starter Pack be employed. This provides an initial dosage of 10mg isosorbide-5-mononitrate (1 tablet) daily for 2 days followed by a dosage of 20mg daily (1 tablet morning and evening) for a further 3 days. Subsequently the daily dosage may be increased to the normal prophylactic level using the Ismo 20 tablets also included in the Starter Pack. Patients already accustomed to chronic nitrate therapy normally may be transferred directly to a therapeutic dose of Ismo.

For those previously treated with isosorbide dinitrate in conventional form the dosage of Ismo should be the same initially. Ismo is effectively twice as potent as sustained release forms of isosorbide dinitrate and patients transferred from such treatment should receive Ismo at half the previous dosage.

Therapy should not be discontinued suddenly. Both dosage and frequency should be tapered gradually (see Section 4.4)

Elderly

There is no evidence to suggest an adjustment of dose is necessary. However, caution may be required in elderly patients who are known to be susceptible to the effects of hypotensive medication.

Children

The safety and efficacy of Ismo in children has not been established.

Renal and hepatic impairment

No dosage reduction is necessary.

4.3 Contraindications

Ismo tablets are contraindicated in patients with a known hypersensitivity to isosorbide-5-mononitrate or isosorbide dinitrate, in cases of marked low blood pressure (BP ⩽ 90mm Hg systolic), circulatory collapse, shock, cardiogenic shock and acute myocardial infarction with low left ventricular filling pressure, hypertrophic obstructive cardiomyopathy, constrictive pericarditis, cardiac tamponade, aortic/mitral valve stenosis, severe anaemia, closed-angle glaucoma and conditions associated with raised intracerebral pressure e.g. following head trauma and cerebral haemorrhage.

Sildenafil has been shown to potentiate the hypotensive effects of nitrates (see Section 4.8), and its co-administration with nitrates or nitric oxide donors is therefore contraindicated.

4.4 Special warnings and special precautions for use

Ismo is not indicated for relief of an acute attack, sublingual or buccal glyceryl trinitrate tablets or spray should be used.

The lowest effective dose should be used (see Section 4.2)

Since a rebound phenomenon cannot be excluded, therapy with isosorbide-5-mononitrate should be terminated gradually rather than stopping abruptly (see Section 4.2).

Caution should be exercised in patients suffering from hypothyroidism, malnutrition, severe renal or hepatic impairment, hypothermia and recent history of myocardial infarction.

Hypotension induced by nitrates may be accompanied by paradoxical bradycardia and increased angina.

Severe postural hypotension with light-headedness and dizziness is frequently observed after the consumption of alcohol.

Ismo 10 tablets contain 74 mg lactose and are unsuitable for patients with lactase insufficiency, galactosaemia or glucose/galactose malabsorption syndrome.

4.5 Interaction with other medicinal products and other forms of Interaction

The hypotensive effects of other drugs such as alprostadil, aldesleukin and angiotensin II receptor antagonists may be potentiated. In particular, the hypotensive effects of nitrates are potentiated by concurrent co-administration of phosphodiesterase type-5 inhibitors e.g. sildenafil (see Section 4.3).

4.6 Pregnancy and lactation

There is inadequate evidence of safety of isosorbide-5-mononitrate in human pregnancy although nitrates have been in wide use for many years without ill consequence, animal studies having shown no adverse effects on the foetus. There is no information on excretion of isosorbide-5-mononitrate in breast milk. Use in pregnancy and lactation is not recommended unless considered essential by the patient's physician.

4.7 Effects on ability to drive and use machines

In theory, the ability to drive or to operate machinery may be impaired in patients experiencing hypotensive side effects such as dizziness or blurred vision.

4.8 Undesirable effects

Central nervous system:

– frequently, particularly at the start of treatment, a transient "nitrate headache" may occur which normally subsides after some days of continued treatment.

– occasionally, particularly when first used, slight states of dizziness or feeling of weakness may occur which normally improve during treatment.

Cardiovascular system:

– occasionally, especially at the beginning of treatment, hypotension (including postural hypotension), tachycardia or flushing, which normally improves on continuation of therapy.

– rarely, collapse, in some instances accompanied by bradyarrhythmias and syncope.

– in rare cases where there is a significant drop in blood pressure the symptoms of angina pectoris may be intensified.

– administration of isosorbide-5-nitrate may produce transient hypoxaemia as a result of redistribution of blood flow with a relative increase in perfusion of poorly ventilated areas of the lung. This may cause ischaemia in patients with coronary heart disease.

Gastro-intestinal system:

– occasionally, especially when first used, gastro-intestinal symptoms, e.g. nausea and/or vomiting may occur.

Haematological:

– formation of methaemoglobin might occur, in particular in susceptible patients such as those with methaemoglobin reductase deficiency.

Skin:

– rarely allergic skin reactions (e.g. exfoliative dermatitis).

4.9 Overdose

Symptoms: Nausea, vomiting, restlessness, warm flushed skin, blurred vision, headache, fainting, tachycardia, hypotension and palpitations. A rise in intracranial pressure with confusion and neurological deficits can sometimes occur.

Management: Consider oral activated charcoal if ingestion of a potentially toxic amount has occurred within 1 hour. Observe for at least 12 hours after the overdose. Monitor blood pressure and pulse. Correct hypotension by raising the foot of the bed and/or by expanding the intravascular volume. Other measures as indicated by the patient's clinical condition. If severe hypotension persists despite the above measures consider use of inotropes such as dopamine or dobutamine.

5. PHARMACOLOGICAL PROPERTIES

5.1 Pharmacodynamic properties

Ismo provides long-term nitrate treatment of angina pectoris and heart failure in a form with complete biological availability due to lack of any significant hepatic first-pass metabolism. This provides consistently uniform blood levels of drug substance and a predictable clinical response. The onset of activity occurs within 20 minutes, and, depending on dosage, is maintained for up to 10 hours.

Beta-blocking drugs have a different pharmacological action in angina and may have a complementary effect when co-administered with Ismo.

The main effect of isosorbide-5-mononitrate is to produce a marked venous vasodilation without a significant effect on the systemic arteries. The venous dilation leads to an accumulation of blood in the capacitance vessels resulting in a reduction of venous return to the heart. This results in a reduction of the ventricular diastolic volume, which produces a reduction in intramural tension (afterload) as well as reductions of filling pressures and pulmonary capillary pressure (preload) and as a result, a reduction in myocardial oxygen requirements from which arises the antianginal effect.

5.2 Pharmacokinetic properties

Isosorbide-5-mononitrate displays 100% bioavailability on oral administration. Consequently, serum levels are predictable, isosorbide-5-mononitrate is rapidly absorbed - peak serum concentrations occuring 1 hour after oral administration. Elimination half life is approximately 5 hours.

The drug is eliminated solely by the liver and therefore can be used in renal insufficiency.

5.3 Preclinical safety data

No special findings.

6. PHARMACEUTICAL PARTICULARS

6.1 List of excipients

Ismo 10 tablets also contain lactose, colloidal silicon dioxide and magnesium stearate.

6.2 Incompatibilities

Not applicable.

6.3 Shelf life

60 months.

6.4 Special precautions for storage

No special storage or handling precautions apply although it is recommended that Ismo products be kept in a cool, dry place in accordance with good pharmaceutical practice.

6.5 Nature and contents of container

Ismo Starter Pack: 8 tablets of Ismo 10 and 60 tablets of Ismo 20 in calendarised blister strips.

Ismo 10 - packs of 100 tablets.

6.6 Instructions for use and handling

No special instructions.

7. MARKETING AUTHORISATION HOLDER

Roche Products Limited, 40 Broadwater Road, Welwyn Garden City, Hertfordshire, AL7 3AY.

8. MARKETING AUTHORISATION NUMBER(S)

PL 00031/0526

9. DATE OF FIRST AUTHORISATION/RENEWAL OF THE AUTHORISATION

1 April 1999

10. DATE OF REVISION OF THE TEXT

17 May 2005

11. LEGAL CATEGORY

P

Ismo is a registered trade mark

Item Code

Ismo 20

(Roche Products Limited)

1. NAME OF THE MEDICINAL PRODUCT

Ismo 20

2. QUALITATIVE AND QUANTITATIVE COMPOSITION

In terms of the active ingredients:

Ismo 20: 20mg isosorbide-5-mononitrate.

3. PHARMACEUTICAL FORM

Tablets for oral administration.

Ismo tablets are white, circular, uncoated and contain isosorbide-5-mononitrate. Lactose is present in the formulation.

Ismo 20 tablets: Marked with a score line and BM 3B on both faces.

4. CLINICAL PARTICULARS

4.1 Therapeutic indications

Ismo products are indicated for use in the treatment and prophylaxis of angina pectoris and as adjunctive therapy in congestive heart failure which does not respond adequately to cardiac glycosides and/or diuretics.

4.2 Posology and method of administration

Route of administration

Oral.

Adults

The recommended dosage is from 20 to 120mg isosorbide-5-mononitrate daily in divided doses. The majority of patients will require a dosage in the range of 40 to 60mg daily in divided doses. The tablets should be taken with fluid and swallowed whole without chewing.

The lowest effective dose should be used.

For patients who have not previously received prophylactic nitrate therapy it is recommended that the Ismo Starter Pack be employed. This provides an initial dosage of 10mg isosorbide-5-mononitrate (1 tablet) daily for 2 days followed by a dosage of 20mg daily (1 tablet morning and evening) for a further 3 days. Subsequently the daily dosage may be increased to the normal prophylactic level using the Ismo 20 tablets also included in the Starter Pack. Patients already accustomed to chronic nitrate therapy normally may be transferred directly to a therapeutic dose of Ismo.

For those previously treated with isosorbide dinitrate in conventional form the dosage of Ismo should be the same initially. Ismo is effectively twice as potent as sustained release forms of isosorbide dinitrate and patients transferred from such treatment should receive Ismo at half the previous dosage.

Therapy should not be discontinued suddenly. Both dosage and frequency should be tapered gradually (see Section 4.4)

Elderly

There is no evidence to suggest an adjustment of dose is necessary. However, caution may be required in elderly patients who are known to be susceptible to the effects of hypotensive medication.

Children

The safety and efficacy of Ismo in children has not been established.

Renal and hepatic impairment

No dosage reduction is necessary.

4.3 Contraindications

Ismo tablets are contraindicated in patients with a known hypersensitivity to isosorbide-5-mononitrate or isosorbide dinitrate, in cases of marked low blood pressure (BP ⩽ 90mm Hg systolic), circulatory collapse, shock, cardiogenic shock and acute myocardial infarction with low left ventricular filling pressure, hypertrophic obstructive cardiomyopathy, constrictive pericarditis, cardiac tamponade, aortic/mitral valve stenosis, severe anaemia, closed-angle glaucoma and conditions associated with raised intracerebral pressure e.g. following head trauma and cerebral haemorrhage.

Sildenafil has been shown to potentiate the hypotensive effects of nitrates (see Section 4.8), and its co-administration with nitrates or nitric oxide donors is therefore contraindicated.

4.4 Special warnings and special precautions for use

Ismo is not indicated for relief of an acute attack, sublingual or buccal glyceryl trinitrate tablets or spray should be used.

The lowest effective dose should be used (see Section 4.2).

Since a rebound phenomenon cannot be excluded, therapy with isosorbide-5-mononitrate should be terminated gradually rather than stopping abruptly (see Section 4.2).

Caution should be exercised in patients suffering from hypothyroidism, malnutrition, severe renal or hepatic impairment, hypothermia and recent history of myocardial infarction.

Hypotension induced by nitrates may be accompanied by paradoxical bradycardia and increased angina.

Severe postural hypotension with light-headedness and dizziness is frequently observed after the consumption of alcohol.

Ismo 20 tablets contain 148 mg lactose and are unsuitable for patients with lactase insufficiency, galactosaemia or glucose/galactose malabsorption syndrome.

4.5 Interaction with other medicinal products and other forms of Interaction

The hypotensive effects of other drugs such as alprostadil, aldesleukin and angiotensin II receptor antagonists may be potentiated. In particular, the hypotensive effects of nitrates are potentiated by concurrent co-administration of phosphodiesterase type-5 inhibitors e.g. sildenafil (see Section 4.3).

4.6 Pregnancy and lactation

There is inadequate evidence of safety of isosorbide-5-mononitrate in human pregnancy although nitrates have been in wide use for many years without ill consequence, animal studies having shown no adverse effects on the foetus. There is no information on excretion of isosorbide-5-mononitrate in breast milk. Use in pregnancy and lactation is not recommended unless considered essential by the patient's physician.

4.7 Effects on ability to drive and use machines

In theory, the ability to drive or to operate machinery may be impaired in patients experiencing hypotensive side effects such as dizziness or blurred vision.

4.8 Undesirable effects

Central nervous system:

– frequently, particularly at the start of treatment, a transient "nitrate headache" may occur which normally subsides after some days of continued treatment.

– occasionally, particularly when first used, slight states of dizziness or feeling of weakness may occur which normally improve during treatment.

Cardiovascular system:

– occasionally, especially at the beginning of treatment, hypotension (including postural hypotension), tachycardia or flushing, which normally improves on continuation of therapy.

– rarely, collapse, in some instances accompanied by bradyarrhythmias and syncope.

– in rare cases where there is a significant drop in blood pressure the symptoms of angina pectoris may be intensified.

– administration of isosorbide-5-nitrate may produce transient hypoxaemia as a result of redistribution of blood flow with a relative increase in perfusion of poorly ventilated areas of the lung. This may cause ischaemia in patients with coronary heart disease.

Gastro-intestinal system:

– occasionally, especially when first used, gastro-intestinal symptoms, e.g. nausea and/or vomiting may occur.

Haematological:

– formation of methaemoglobin might occur, in particular in susceptible patients such as those with methaemoglobin reductase deficiency.

Skin:

– rarely allergic skin reactions (e.g. exfoliative dermatitis).

4.9 Overdose

Symptoms: Nausea, vomiting, restlessness, warm flushed skin, blurred vision, headache, fainting, tachycardia, hypotension and palpitations. A rise in intracranial pressure with confusion and neurological deficits can sometimes occur.

Management: Consider oral activated charcoal if ingestion of a potentially toxic amount has occurred within 1 hour. Observe for at least 12 hours after the overdose. Monitor blood pressure and pulse. Correct hypotension by raising the foot of the bed and/or by expanding the intravascular volume. Other measures as indicated by the patient's clinical condition. If severe hypotension persists despite the above measures consider use of inotropes such as dopamine or dobutamine.

5. PHARMACOLOGICAL PROPERTIES

5.1 Pharmacodynamic properties

The main effect of isosorbide-5-mononitrate is to produce a marked venous vasodilation without a significant effect on the systemic arteries. The venous dilation leads to an accumulation of blood in the capacitance vessels resulting in a reduction of venous return to the heart. This results in a reduction of the ventricular diastolic volume, which produces a reduction in intramural tension (afterload) as well as reductions of filling pressures (preload) and as a result, a reduction in myocardial oxygen requirements from which arises the antianginal effect.

5.2 Pharmacokinetic properties

Isosorbide-5-mononitrate displays 100% bioavailability on oral administration. Consequently, serum levels are predictable, isosorbide-5-mononitrate is rapidly absorbed - peak serum concentrations occuring 1 hour after oral administration. Elimination half life is approximately 5 hours.

The drug is eliminated solely by the liver and therefore can be used in renal insufficiency.

5.3 Preclinical safety data

No special findings.

6. PHARMACEUTICAL PARTICULARS

6.1 List of excipients

Ismo 20 tablets also contain anhydrous lactose, colloidal silicon dioxide and magnesium stearate.

6.2 Incompatibilities

Not applicable.

6.3 Shelf life

5 years.

6.4 Special precautions for storage

None.

6.5 Nature and contents of container

Ismo Starter Pack: 8 tablets of Ismo 10 and 56 or 60 tablets of Ismo 20 in calendarised blister strips.

Ismo 20: Packs of 56, 60 and 100 tablets in blister strips or 100, 250 or 500 tablets in Securitainers.

6.6 Instructions for use and handling

No special instructions.

7. MARKETING AUTHORISATION HOLDER

Roche Products Limited, 40 Broadwater Road, Welwyn Garden City, Hertfordshire, AL7 3AY.

8. MARKETING AUTHORISATION NUMBER(S)

PL 00031/0527

9. DATE OF FIRST AUTHORISATION/RENEWAL OF THE AUTHORISATION

1 April 1999

10. DATE OF REVISION OF THE TEXT

March 2005

11. LEGAL CATEGORY

P

Ismo is a registered trade mark

Item Code

Ismo 40

(Roche Products Limited)

1. NAME OF THE MEDICINAL PRODUCT

Ismo 40

2. QUALITATIVE AND QUANTITATIVE COMPOSITION

In terms of the active ingredients:

Ismo 40: 40mg isosorbide-5-mononitrate.

3. PHARMACEUTICAL FORM

Tablets for oral administration.

Ismo tablets are white, circular, uncoated and contain isosorbide-5-mononitrate. Lactose is present in the formulation.

Ismo 40 tablets: marked Ismo on one face with a score line and 40 on the reverse.

4. CLINICAL PARTICULARS

4.1 Therapeutic indications

Ismo products are indicated for use in the treatment and prophylaxis of angina pectoris and as adjunctive therapy in congestive heart failure which does not respond adequately to cardiac glycosides and/or diuretics.

4.2 Posology and method of administration

Route of administration

Oral.

Adults

The recommended dosage is from 20 to 120mg isosorbide-5-mononitrate daily in divided doses. The majority of patients will require a dosage in the range of 40 to 60mg daily in divided doses. The tablets should be taken with fluid and swallowed whole without chewing.

The lowest effective dose should be used.

For those previously treated with isosorbide dinitrate in conventional form the dosage of Ismo should be the same initially. Ismo is effectively twice as potent as sustained release forms of isosorbide dinitrate and patients transferred from such treatment should receive Ismo at half the previous dosage.

Therapy should not be discontinued suddenly. Both dosage and frequency should be tapered gradually (see Section 4.4)

Elderly

There is no evidence to suggest an adjustment of dose is necessary. However, caution may be required in elderly patients who are known to be susceptible to the effects of hypotensive medication.

Children

The safety and efficacy of Ismo in children has not been established.

Renal and hepatic impairment

No dosage reduction is necessary.

4.3 Contraindications

Ismo tablets are contraindicated in patients with a known hypersensitivity to isosorbide-5-mononitrate or isosorbide dinitrate, in cases of marked low blood pressure (BP ⩽ 90mm Hg systolic), circulatory collapse, shock, cardiogenic shock and acute myocardial infarction with low left ventricular filling pressure, hypertrophic obstructive cardiomyopathy, constrictive pericarditis, cardiac tamponade, aortic/mitral valve stenosis, severe anaemia, closed-angle glaucoma and conditions associated with raised intracerebral pressure e.g. following head trauma and cerebral haemorrhage.

Sildenafil has been shown to potentiate the hypotensive effects of nitrates (see Section 4.8), and its co-administration with nitrates or nitric oxide donors is therefore contraindicated.

4.4 Special warnings and special precautions for use

Ismo is not indicated for relief of an acute attack, sublingual or buccal glyceryl trinitrate tablets or spray should be used.

The lowest effective dose should be used (see Section 4.2).

Since a rebound phenomenon cannot be excluded, therapy with isosorbide-5-mononitrate should be terminated gradually rather than stopping abruptly (see Section 4.2).

Caution should be exercised in patients suffering from hypothyroidism, malnutrition, severe renal or hepatic impairment, hypothermia and recent history of myocardial infarction.

Hypotension induced by nitrates may be accompanied by paradoxical bradycardia and increased angina.

Severe postural hypotension with light-headedness and dizziness is frequently observed after the consumption of alcohol.

Ismo 40 tablets contain 296 mg lactose and are unsuitable for patients with lactase insufficiency, galactosaemia or glucose/galactose malabsorption syndrome.

4.5 Interaction with other medicinal products and other forms of Interaction

The hypotensive effects of other drugs such as alprostadil, aldesleukin and angiotensin II receptor antagonists may be potentiated. In particular, the hypotensive effects of nitrates are potentiated by concurrent co-administration of phosphodiesterase type-5 inhibitors e.g. sildenafil (see Section 4.3).

4.6 Pregnancy and lactation

There is inadequate evidence of safety of isosorbide-5-mononitrate in human pregnancy although nitrates have been in wide use for many years without ill consequence, animal studies having shown no adverse effects on the foetus. There is no information on excretion of isosorbide-5-mononitrate in breast milk. Use in pregnancy and lactation is not recommended unless considered essential by the patient's physician.

4.7 Effects on ability to drive and use machines

In theory, the ability to drive or to operate machinery may be impaired in patients experiencing hypotensive side effects such as dizziness or blurred vision.

4.8 Undesirable effects

Central nervous system:

– frequently, particularly at the start of treatment, a transient "nitrate headache" may occur which normally subsides after some days of continued treatment.

– occasionally, particularly when first used, slight states of dizziness or feeling of weakness may occur which normally improve during treatment.

Cardiovascular system:

– occasionally, especially at the beginning of treatment, hypotension (including postural hypotension), tachycardia or flushing, which normally improves on continuation of therapy.

– rarely, collapse, in some instances accompanied by bradyarrhythmias and syncope.

– in rare cases where there is a significant drop in blood pressure the symptoms of angina pectoris may be intensified.

– administration of isosorbide-5-nitrate may produce transient hypoxaemia as a result of redistribution of blood flow with a relative increase in perfusion of poorly ventilated areas of the lung. This may cause ischaemia in patients with coronary heart disease.

Gastro-intestinal system:

– occasionally, especially when first used, gastro-intestinal symptoms, e.g. nausea and/or vomiting may occur.

Haematological:

– formation of methaemoglobin might occur, in particular in susceptible patients such as those with methaemoglobin reductase deficiency.

Skin:

– rarely allergic skin reactions (e.g. exfoliative dermatitis).

4.9 Overdose

Symptoms: Nausea, vomiting, restlessness, warm flushed skin, blurred vision, headache, fainting, tachycardia, hypotension and palpitations. A rise in intracranial pressure with confusion and neurological deficits can sometimes occur.

Management: Consider oral activated charcoal if ingestion of a potentially toxic amount has occurred within 1 hour. Observe for at least 12 hours after the overdose. Monitor blood pressure and pulse. Correct hypotension by raising the foot of the bed and/or by expanding the intravascular volume. Other measures as indicated by the patient's clinical condition. If severe hypotension persists despite the above measures consider use of inotropes such as dopamine or dobutamine.

5. PHARMACOLOGICAL PROPERTIES

5.1 Pharmacodynamic properties

The main effect of isosorbide-5-mononitrate is to produce a marked venous vasodilation without a significant effect on the systemic arteries. The venous dilation leads to an accumulation of blood in the capacitance vessels resulting in a reduction of venous return to the heart. This results in a reduction of the ventricular diastolic volume, which produces a reduction in intramural tension (afterload) as well as reductions of filling (preload) and as a result, a reduction in myocardial oxygen requirements from which arises the antianginal effect.

5.2 Pharmacokinetic properties

Isosorbide-5-mononitrate displays 100% bioavailability on oral administration. Consequently, serum levels are predictable, isosorbide-5-mononitrate is rapidly absorbed - peak serum concentrations occuring 1 hour after oral administration. Elimination half life is approximately 5 hours.

The drug is eliminated solely by the liver and therefore can be used in renal insufficiency.

5.3 Preclinical safety data

No special findings.

6. PHARMACEUTICAL PARTICULARS

6.1 List of excipients

Ismo 40 tablets also contain anhydrous lactose, colloidal silicon dioxide and magnesium stearate.

6.2 Incompatibilities

Not applicable.

6.3 Shelf life

5 years.

6.4 Special precautions for storage

None.

6.5 Nature and contents of container

Ismo 40: packs of 60 and 100 tablets in blister strips or 100 in Securitainers.

6.6 Instructions for use and handling

No special instructions.

7. MARKETING AUTHORISATION HOLDER

Roche Products Limited, 40 Broadwater Road, Welwyn Garden City, Hertfordshire, AL7 3AY.

8. MARKETING AUTHORISATION NUMBER(S)

PL 00031/0528

9. DATE OF FIRST AUTHORISATION/RENEWAL OF THE AUTHORISATION

1 April 1999

10. DATE OF REVISION OF THE TEXT

March 2005

11. LEGAL CATEGORY

P

Ismo is a registered trade mark

Item Code

Ismo Retard

(Roche Products Limited)

1. NAME OF THE MEDICINAL PRODUCT

Ismo Retard®.

2. QUALITATIVE AND QUANTITATIVE COMPOSITION

40mg isosorbide-5-mononitrate.

3. PHARMACEUTICAL FORM

Circular, white sugar coated tablets for oral administration.

4. CLINICAL PARTICULARS

4.1 Therapeutic indications

Ismo Retard is indicated for the prophylaxis of angina pectoris.

4.2 Posology and method of administration

Route of administration

Oral.

Dosage

Ismo Retard has been developed to provide a convenient, once daily dosage form of isosorbide mononitrate. It is designed to achieve therapeutic blood concentrations within 30 minutes which persist up to 17 hours. A nitrate free interval of up to 7 hours makes the development of anti-anginal tolerance during chronic therapy unlikely.

The tablets should be taken with fluid and swallowed whole without chewing.

Adults

One tablet daily to be taken in the morning.

Elderly

There is no evidence to suggest an adjustment of dose is necessary. However, caution may be required in elderly patients who are known to be susceptible to the effects of hypotensive medication.

Children

The safety and efficacy of Ismo in children has not been established.

Renal and hepatic impairment

No dosage reduction is necessary.

4.3 Contraindications

Ismo Retard is contra-indicated in patients with a known hypersensitivity to isosorbide mononitrate or isosorbide dinitrate, in cases of marked low blood pressure (BP ⩽ 90mm Hg systolic), circulatory collapse, shock, cardiogenic shock and acute myocardial infarction with low left ventricular filling pressure.

Sildenafil has been shown to potentiate the hypotensive effects of nitrates, and its co-administration with nitrates or nitric oxide donors is therefore contra-indicated.

4.4 Special warnings and special precautions for use

Ismo Retard is not indicated for relief of acute anginal attacks. In the event of an acute attack, sublingual or buccal glyceryl trinitrate tablets or spray should be used.

Patients who have not previously received nitrates may initially be started with a low dose which should be gradually increased before introducing Ismo Retard.

In the case of acute myocardial infarction, Ismo Retard should be continued only under strict medical supervision; reduction of the systolic blood pressure to below 90mm Hg should be avoided.

Ismo Retard should be used with caution in the presence of hypertrophic obstructive cardiomyopathy, constrictive pericarditis, cardiac tamponade, aortic and/or mitral stenosis, orthostatic disorders of circulatory regulation and increased intracranial pressure.

Since a rebound phenomenon cannot be excluded, therapy with isosorbide mononitrate should be terminated gradually rather than stopping abruptly.

4.5 Interaction with other medicinal products and other forms of Interaction

The hypotensive effects of other drugs may be potentiated. In particular, the hypotensive effects of nitrates are potentiated by concurrent administration of sildenafil.

4.6 Pregnancy and lactation

There is inadequate evidence of safety of isosorbide-5-mononitrate in human pregnancy although nitrates have been in wide use for many years without ill consequence, animal studies having shown no adverse effects on the foetus. There is no information on excretion of isosorbide-5-mononitrate in breast milk. Use in pregnancy and lactation is not recommended unless considered essential by the patient's physician.

4.7 Effects on ability to drive and use machines

In theory, the ability to drive or to operate machinery may be impaired in patients experiencing hypotensive side effects.

4.8 Undesirable effects

Central nervous system:

– frequently, particularly at the start of treatment, a transient "nitrate headache" may occur which normally subsides after some days of continued treatment.

– occasionally, particularly when first used, slight states of dizziness or feeling of weakness may occur which normally improve during treatment.

Cardiovascular system:

– occasionally, especially at the beginning of treatment, hypotension (including postural hypotension), tachycardia or flushing, which normally improves on continuation of therapy.

– rarely, collapse, in some instances accompanied by bradyarrhythmias and syncope.

– in rare cases where there is a significant drop in blood pressure the symptoms of angina pectoris may be intensified.

– administration of isosorbide-5-nitrate may produce transient hypoxaemia as a result of redistribution of blood flow with a relative increase in perfusion of poorly ventilated areas of the lung. This may cause ischaemia in patients with coronary heart disease.

Gastro-intestinal system:

– occasionally, especially when first used, gastro-intestinal symptoms, e.g. nausea and/or vomiting may occur.

Haematological:

– formation of methaemoglobin might occur, in particular in susceptible patients such as those with methaemoglobin reductase deficiency.

Skin:

– rarely allergic skin reactions (i.e. exfoliative dermatitis).

4.9 Overdose

Symptoms and signs: In the event of overdosage the main sign is liable to be hypotension.

Treatment: The stomach should be aspirated to remove any remaining tablets. The patient should be placed in a supine position with the legs elevated to promote venous return. Symptomatic and supportive treatment e.g. plasma expanders and, if necessary, the careful use of vasopressor agents to counterbalance the hypotensive effects may be necessary. Methaemoglobinaemia will normally respond to methylene blue infusion.

5. PHARMACOLOGICAL PROPERTIES

5.1 Pharmacodynamic properties

The main effect of isosorbide-5-mononitrate is to produce a marked venous vasodilation without a significant effect on the systemic arteries. The venous dilation leads to an accumulation of blood in the capacitance vessels resulting in a reduction of venous return to the heart. This results in a reduction of the ventricular diastolic volume, which produces a reduction in intramural tension (afterload) as well as reductions of filling pressures and pulmonary capillary pressure (preload) and as a result, a reduction in myocardial oxygen requirements from which arises the antianginal effect.

Beta-blocking drugs have a different pharmacological action in angina and may have a complementary effect when co-administered with Ismo Retard.

5.2 Pharmacokinetic properties

Isosorbide-5-mononitrate rapidly and completely absorbed following oral administration. Elimination is by hepatic metabolism to inactive metabolites. The elimination half life is slightly more than 4 hours.

Ismo Retard releases isosorbide-5-mononitrate over several hours. Therapeutic serum levels are present within 30 minutes of a dose. Peak serum concentrations occur between 3 and 4 hours post administration. Pharmacologically active serum concentrations are maintained for up to 17 hours. Simulation studies indicate that accumulation will not occur in hepatically normal patients.

The drug is eliminated solely by the liver and therefore can be used in renal insufficiency.

Anti-anginal tolerance is unlikely to occur during chronic use as the dosage regime provides up to 7 hours daily when isosorbide-5-mononitrate serum concentration is below pharmacologically active values.

5.3 Preclinical safety data

No special findings.

6. PHARMACEUTICAL PARTICULARS

6.1 List of excipients

Ismo Retard also contains lactose, montanic acid/ethanediol ester, povidone, colloidal silicone dioxide and magnesium stearate. The tablets are covered by a sugar coating which contains polymethacrylic acid esters, talc, sucrose, kaolin, polyethyleneglycol, titanium dioxide, povidone, glucose and montanic acid/ethanediol ester. No azo dyes are used as colouring substances. (The sugar content of each tablet is less than 36mg).

6.2 Incompatibilities

Not applicable.

6.3 Shelf life

3 years.

6.4 Special precautions for storage

Store at or below 25°C.

6.5 Nature and contents of container

Packs of 30 tablets in blister strips.

6.6 Instructions for use and handling

No special instructions.

7. MARKETING AUTHORISATION HOLDER

Roche Products Limited, 40 Broadwater Road, Welwyn Garden City, Hertfordshire, AL7 3AY.

8. MARKETING AUTHORISATION NUMBER(S)

0031/0529

9. DATE OF FIRST AUTHORISATION/RENEWAL OF THE AUTHORISATION

1 April 1999

10. DATE OF REVISION OF THE TEXT

June 2001

11. LEGAL STATUS

P

Ismo is a registered trade mark

P999657/102

Isocarboxazid Tablets 10mg

(Cambridge Laboratories)

1. NAME OF THE MEDICINAL PRODUCT

Isocarboxazid Tablets 10mg

2. QUALITATIVE AND QUANTITATIVE COMPOSITION

Each tablet contains 10mg Isocarboxazid.

3. PHARMACEUTICAL FORM
Tablets

4. CLINICAL PARTICULARS
4.1 Therapeutic indications
For the treatment of the symptoms of depressive illness.

4.2 Posology and method of administration
Isocarboxazid Tablets are for oral administration.

Adults
A daily dose of 30mg, in single or divided doses, should be given until improvement is obtained. The maximal effect is only observed after a period varying from 1 - 4 weeks. If no improvement has been seen by 4 weeks, doses up to 60mg may be tried, according to the patient's tolerance, for no longer than 4 - 6 weeks, provided the patient is closely monitored because of the increased risk of adverse reactions occurring.

Once the optimal effect is achieved, the dose should be reduced to the lowest possible amount sufficient to maintain the improvement. Clinical experience has shown this to be usually 10 - 20mg daily but up to 40mg daily may be required in some cases.

The elderly
The elderly are more likely to experience adverse reactions such as agitation, confusion and postural hypotension. Half the normal maintenance dose may be sufficient to produce a satisfactory clinical response.

Children
Isocarboxazid Tablets are not indicated for paediatric use.

4.3 Contraindications
Isocarboxazid is contra-indicated in patients with any impairment of hepatic function, cerebrovascular disorders or severe cardiovascular disease, and in those with actual or suspected phaeochromocytoma.

4.4 Special warnings and special precautions for use
Some monoamine oxidase inhibitors have occasionally caused hepatic complications and jaundice in patients, therefore regular monitoring of liver function should be carried out during Isocarboxazid therapy. If there is any evidence of a hepatotoxic reaction, the drug should be withdrawn immediately.

The drug should be used cautiously in patients with impaired renal function, to prevent accumulation taking place, and also in the elderly or debilitated and those with cardiovascular disease, diabetes or blood dyscrasias.

In restless or agitated patients, Isocarboxazid may precipitate states of excessive excitement. Isocarboxazid appears to have varying effects in epileptic patients; while some have a decrease in frequency of seizures, others have more seizures.

4.5 Interaction with other medicinal products and other forms of Interaction
Like other monoamine oxidase inhibitors, Isocarboxazid potentiates the action of a number of drugs and foods. Patients being treated with a monoamine oxidase inhibitor should not receive indirectly-acting sympathomimetic agents such as amphetamines, metaraminol, fenfluramine or similar anorectic agents, ephedrine or phenylpropanolamine (contained in many proprietary 'cold-cure' medications), dopamine or levodopa. Patients should also be warned to avoid foodstuffs and beverages with a high tyramine content: mature cheeses (including processed cheeses), hydrolysed yeast or meat extracts, alcoholic beverages, particularly heavy red wines such as Chianti, non-alcoholic beers, lagers and wines, and other foods which are not fresh and are fermented, pickled, 'hung', 'matured' or otherwise subject to protein degradation before consumption. Broad bean pods (which contain levodopa) and banana skins may also present a hazard. In extreme cases interactions may result in severe hypertensive episodes. Isocarboxazid should therefore be discontinued immediately upon the occurrence of palpitations or frequent headaches.

Pethidine should not be given to patients receiving monoamine oxidase inhibitors as serious, potentially fatal reactions, including central excitation, muscle rigidity, hyperpyrexia, circulatory collapse, respiratory depression and coma, can result. Such reactions are less likely with morphine, but experience of the interaction of Isocarboxazid with narcotic analgesics other than pethidine is limited and extreme caution is therefore necessary when administering morphine to patients undergoing therapy with Isocarboxazid.

Isocarboxazid should not be administered together with other monoamine oxidase inhibitors or most tricyclic antidepressants (clomipramine, desipramine, imipramine, butriptyline, nortriptyline or protriptyline). Although there is no proof that combined therapy will be effective, refractory cases of depression may be treated with Isocarboxazid in combination with amitriptyline or trimipramine, provided appropriate care is taken. Hypotensive and other adverse reactions are likely to be increased.

An interval of 1 - 2 weeks should be allowed after treatment with Isocarboxazid before the administration of antidepressants with a different mode of action or any other drug which may interact. A similar interval is recommended before administration of Isocarboxazid when another antidepressant has been used; in the case of drugs with a very long half-life (such as fluoxetine), it may be advisable to extend this interval.

Isocarboxazid should be discontinued for at least 2 weeks prior to elective surgery requiring general anaesthesia. The anaesthetist should be warned that a patient is being treated with Isocarboxazid, in the event of emergency surgery being necessary. Concurrent administration of Isocarboxazid with other central nervous system depressants (especially barbiturates and phenothiazines), stimulants, local anaesthetics, ganglion-blocking agents and other hypotensives (including methyl-dopa and reserpine), diuretics, vasopressors, anticholinergic drugs and hypoglycaemic agents may lead to potentiation of their effects. This should be borne in mind if dentistry, surgery or a change in treatment of a patient becomes necessary during treatment with Isocarboxazid.

All patients taking Isocarboxazid should be warned against self-medication with proprietary 'cold-cure' preparations and nasal decongestants and advised of the dietary restrictions listed under 'warnings'.

With Isocarboxazid, as with other drugs acting on the central nervous system, patients should be instructed to avoid alcohol while under treatment, since the individual response cannot be foreseen.

4.6 Pregnancy and lactation
Do not use in pregnancy, especially during the first and last trimesters, unless there are compelling reasons. There is no evidence as to drug safety in human pregnancy, nor is there evidence from animal work that it is free from hazard. In addition, the effect of psychotropic drugs on the fine brain structure of the foetus is unknown. Since there is no information on the secretion of the drug into breast milk, Isocarboxazid is contra-indicated during lactation.

4.7 Effects on ability to drive and use machines
Like all medicaments of this type, Isocarboxazid may modify patients' reactions (driving ability, operation of machinery etc.) to a varying extent, depending on dosage and individual susceptibility.

4.8 Undesirable effects
In general, Isocarboxazid is well tolerated by the majority of patients. Side-effects, if they occur, are those common to the group of monoamine oxidase inhibitors.

The most frequently reported have been orthostatic hypotension, associated in some patients with disturbances in cardiac rhythm, peripheral oedema, complaints of dizziness, dryness of the mouth, nausea and vomiting, constipation, blurred vision, insomnia, drowsiness, weakness and fatigue. These side-effects can usually be controlled by dosage reduction.

There have been infrequent reports of mild headaches, sweating, paraesthesiae, peripheral neuritis, hyperreflexia, agitation, overactivity, muscle tremor, confusion and other behavioural changes, difficulty in micturition, impairment of erection and ejaculation, and skin rashes. Although rare, blood dyscrasias (purpura, granulocytopenia) have been reported. Response to Isocarboxazid may be accompanied by increased appetite and weight gain.

4.9 Overdose
The primary symptoms of overdosage include dizziness, ataxia and irritability. In acute cases, hypotension or hypertension, tachycardia, pyrexia, psychotic manifestations, convulsions, respiratory depression and coma may occur and continue for 8 - 14 days before recovery.

Gastric lavage should be performed soon after ingestion and intensive supportive therapy carried out. Sympathomimetic agents should not be given to treat hypotension but plasma expanders may be used in severe cases. Hypertensive crises may be treated by pentolinium or phentolamine, severe shock with hydrocortisone. Diazepam may be used to control convulsions or severe excitement. Dialysis is of value in eliminating the drug in severe cases.

5. PHARMACOLOGICAL PROPERTIES
5.1 Pharmacodynamic properties
Isocarboxazid is a monoamine oxidase inhibitor, effective in small doses. Its antidepressant action is thought to be related to its effect on physiological amines such as serotonin and noradrenaline, and this effect is cumulative and persistent.

5.2 Pharmacokinetic properties
Isocarboxazid is readily absorbed after oral administration. Most of the drug-related material is excreted as metabolites in the urine.

5.3 Preclinical safety data
There are no pre-clinical data of relevance to the prescriber which are additional to that already included in other sections of the SPC.

6. PHARMACEUTICAL PARTICULARS
6.1 List of excipients
Lactose
Starch
Talc
Magnesium stearate
Gelatin
Iron oxide yellow E172
Iron Oxide red E172

6.2 Incompatibilities
None known.

6.3 Shelf life
Three years.

6.4 Special precautions for storage
The recommended maximum storage temperature is 25°C.

Isocarboxazid Tablets should be stored in well-closed containers.

6.5 Nature and contents of container
HDPE bottles with snap closures, containing 56 tablets.

6.6 Instructions for use and handling
None.

7. MARKETING AUTHORISATION HOLDER
Cambridge Laboratories Limited
Deltic House
Kingfisher Way
Silverlink Business Park
Wallsend
Tyne & Wear
NE28 9NX

8. MARKETING AUTHORISATION NUMBER(S)
PL 12070/0003

9. DATE OF FIRST AUTHORISATION/RENEWAL OF THE AUTHORISATION
21 April 1992

10. DATE OF REVISION OF THE TEXT
March 2000

Isoflurane

(Abbott Laboratories Limited)

1. NAME OF THE MEDICINAL PRODUCT
Isoflurane or Forane

2. QUALITATIVE AND QUANTITATIVE COMPOSITION
Isoflurane 99.9% w/w

3. PHARMACEUTICAL FORM
Isoflurane is an inhalation anaesthetic with a mildly pungent ethereal odour. No additive or stabiliser present.

4. CLINICAL PARTICULARS
4.1 Therapeutic indications
Isoflurane is indicated as a general anaesthetic by inhalation.

4.2 Posology and method of administration
Vaporisers specially calibrated for isoflurane should be used so that the concentration of anaesthetic delivered can be accurately controlled.

MAC values for isoflurane vary with age. The table below indicates average MAC values for different age groups.

Age	Average MAC Value In Oxygen
0-1 month	1.6%
1-6 months	1.87%
6-12 months	1.8%
1-5 years	1.6%
mid twenties	1.28%
mid forties	1.15%
mid sixties	1.05%

Premedication:
Drugs used for premedication should be selected for the individual patient bearing in mind the respiratory depressant effect of isoflurane. The use of anticholinergic drugs is a matter of choice, but may be advisable for inhalation induction in paediatrics.

Induction:
A short-acting barbiturate or other intravenous induction agent is usually administered followed by inhalation of the isoflurane mixture. Alternatively, isoflurane with oxygen or with an oxygen/nitrous oxide mixture may be used.

It is recommended that induction with isoflurane be initiated at a concentration of 0.5%. Concentrations of 1.5 to 3.0% usually produce surgical anaesthesia in 7 to 10 minutes.

Maintenance:
Surgical levels of anaesthesia may be maintained with 1.0-2.5% Isoflurane in oxygen/nitrous oxide mixtures. An additional 0.5-1.0% isoflurane may be required when given with oxygen alone.

For caesarean section, 0.5-0.75% isoflurane in a mixture of oxygen/nitrous oxide is suitable to maintain anaesthesia for this procedure.

Arterial pressure levels during maintenance tend to be inversely related to alveolor isoflurane concentrations in the absence of other complicating factors. Excessive falls in blood pressure may be due to depth of anaesthesia and in these circumstances, should be corrected by reducing the inspired isoflurane concentration.

Elderly: As with other agents, lesser concentrations of isoflurane are normally required to maintain surgical anaesthesia in elderly patients. See above for MAC values related to age.

4.3 Contraindications
Isoflurane is contra-indicated in patients with known sensitivity to isoflurane or other halogenated anaesthetics. It is also contraindicated in patients with known or suspected genetic susceptibility to malignant hyperpyrexia.

4.4 Special warnings and special precautions for use
Since levels of anaesthesia may be altered quickly and easily with isoflurane, only vaporisers which deliver a predictable output with reasonable accuracy, or techniques during which inspired or expired concentrations can be monitored, should be used. The degree of hypotension and respiratory depression may provide some indication of anaesthetic depth.

Reports demonstrate that isoflurane can produce hepatic injury ranging from mild transient increase in liver enzymes to fatal hepatic necrosis in very rare instances.

As with other halogenated agents, isoflurane must be used with caution in patients with increased intracranial pressure. In such cases hyperventilation may be necessary.

Isoflurane has been reported to interact with dry carbon dioxide absorbents to form carbon monoxide. In order to minimise the risk of formation of carbon monoxide in rebreathing circuits and the possibility of elevated carboxyhaemoglobin levels, carbon dioxide absorbent should not be allowed to dry out.

4.5 Interaction with other medicinal products and other forms of Interaction
The actions of non-depolarising relaxants are markedly potentiated with isoflurane, therefore, when administered with isoflurane, dosage adjustments of these agents should be made.

4.6 Pregnancy and lactation
Reproduction studies have been carried out on animals after repeated exposures to anaesthetic concentrations of isoflurane. Studies in the rat demonstrated no effect on the fertility, pregnancy or delivery or on the viability of offspring. No evidence of teratogenicity was revealed. Comparable experiments in rabbits produced similar negative results. The relevance of these studies to the human is not known. As there is insufficient experience in the use of isoflurane in pregnant women safety in human pregnancy has not been established. Blood losses comparable with those found following anaesthesia with other inhalation agents have been recorded with isoflurane in patients undergoing induced abortion. Adequate data have not been developed to establish the safety of isoflurane in obstetric anaesthesia other than for caesarean section.

4.7 Effects on ability to drive and use machines
Not applicable.

4.8 Undesirable effects
Arrhythmias have been occasionally reported.

Elevation of the white blood cell count has been observed, even in the absence of surgical stress.

Minimally raised levels of serum inorganic fluoride occur during and after isoflurane anaesthesia, due to biodegradation of the agent. It is unlikely that the low levels of serum inorganic fluoride observed (mean 4.4 μmol/l in one study) could cause renal toxicity, as these are well below the proposed threshold levels for kidney toxicity.

Undesirable effects during recovery (shivering, nausea and vomiting) are minor in nature and comparable in incidence with those found with other anaesthetics.

Malignant hyperthermia has been reported.

Reports demonstrate that isoflurane can produce hepatic injury ranging from mild transient increase of liver enzymes to fatal hepatic necrosis in very rare instances.

4.9 Overdose
As with other halogenated anaesthetics, hypotension and respiratory depression have been observed. Close monitoring of blood pressure and respiration is recommended. Supportive measures may be necessary to correct hypotension and respiratory depression resulting from excessively deep levels of anaesthesia.

5. PHARMACOLOGICAL PROPERTIES

5.1 Pharmacodynamic properties
Induction and particularly recovery are rapid. Although slight pungency may limit the rate of induction, excessive salivation and tracheo-bronchial secretions are not stimulated. Pharyngeal and laryngeal reflexes are diminished quickly. Levels of anaesthesia change rapidly with isoflurane. Heart rhythm remains stable. Spontaneous respiration becomes depressed as depth of anaesthesia increases and should be closely monitored.

During induction there is a decrease in blood pressure which returns towards normal with surgical stimulation.

Blood pressure tends to fall during maintenance in direct relation to depth of anaesthesia, due to peripheral vasodilation, but cardiac rhythm remains stable. With controlled respiration and normal $PaCO_2$, cardiac output tends to be maintained despite increasing depth of anaesthesia, primarily through a rise in heart rate. With spontaneous respiration, the resulting hypercapnia may increase heart rate and cardiac output above awake levels.

Cerebral blood flow remains unchanged during light isoflurane anaesthesia but tends to rise at deeper levels. Increases in cerebrospinal fluid pressure may be prevented or reversed by hyperventilating the patient before or during anaesthesia. Electro-encephalographic changes and convulsion are extremely rare with isoflurane.

Isoflurane appears to sensitise the myocardium to adrenaline to an even lesser extent than Enflurane. Limited data suggest that subcutaneous infiltration of up to 50ml of 1:200,000 solution adrenaline does not induce ventricular arrhythmias, in patients anaesthetised with isoflurane.

Muscular relaxation may be adequate for some intra-abdominal operations at normal levels of anaesthesia, but should greater relaxation be required small doses of intravenous muscle relaxants may be used. All commonly used muscle relaxants are markedly potentiated by isoflurane, the effect being most profound with non-depolarising agents. Neostigmine reverses the effects of non-depolarising muscle relaxants but has no effect on the relaxant properties of isoflurane itself. All commonly used muscle relaxants are compatible with isoflurane.

Isoflurane may be used for the induction and maintenance of general anaesthesia. Adequate data are not available to establish its place in pregnancy or obstetric anaesthesia other than for caesarean section.

Relatively little metabolism of isoflurane occurs in the human body. In the post operative period only 0.17% of the isoflurane taken up can be recovered as urinary metabolites. Peak serum inorganic fluoride values usually average less than 5μmol/litre and occur about four hours after anaesthesia, returning to normal within 24 hours. No signs of renal injury have been reported after isoflurane administration.

5.2 Pharmacokinetic properties
MAC (Minimum Alveolar Concentration in man):

Age	100% Oxygen	70% N_2O
26 ± 4	1.28	0.56
44 ± 7	1.15	0.50
64 ± 5	1.05	0.37

5.3 Preclinical safety data
None stated.

6. PHARMACEUTICAL PARTICULARS

6.1 List of excipients
None.

6.2 Incompatibilities
Isoflurane has been reported to interact with dry carbon dioxide absorbents to form carbon monoxide. In order to minimise the risk of formation of carbon monoxide in rebreathing circuits and the possibility of elevated carboxyhaemoglobin levels, carbon dioxide absorbents should not be allowed to dry out. (See also section 4.4).

6.3 Shelf life
The recommended shelf life is 5 years.

6.4 Special precautions for storage
Store below 25°C. Keep container well closed.

6.5 Nature and contents of container
100 ml and 250 ml glass bottles.

6.6 Instructions for use and handling
Vaporisers specially calibrated for isoflurane should be used so that the concentration of anaesthetic delivered can be accurately controlled.

It is recommended that vapour from this and other inhalation agents be efficiently extracted from the area of use.

7. MARKETING AUTHORISATION HOLDER
Abbott Laboratories Limited
Queenborough
Kent
ME11 5EL

8. MARKETING AUTHORISATION NUMBER(S)
PL 00037/0115

9. DATE OF FIRST AUTHORISATION/RENEWAL OF THE AUTHORISATION
23 March 1983/17 July 2001

10. DATE OF REVISION OF THE TEXT
February 2000

Isoket 0.05%

(SCHWARZ PHARMA Limited)

1. NAME OF THE MEDICINAL PRODUCT
ISOKET 0.05 %

2. QUALITATIVE AND QUANTITATIVE COMPOSITION
Isosorbide dinitrate 500 micrograms (0.05% w/v) 5mg/10ml
For excipients, See 6.1

3. PHARMACEUTICAL FORM
Sterile colourless solution for intravenous infusion.

4. CLINICAL PARTICULARS

4.1 Therapeutic indications
1. Intravenous

Isoket is indicated in the treatment of unresponsive left ventricular failure secondary to acute myocardial infarction, unresponsive left ventricular failure of various aetiology and severe to unstable angina pectoris.

2. Intra-coronary

Isoket is indicated during percutaneous transluminal coronary angioplasty to facilitate prolongation of balloon inflation and to prevent or relieve coronary spasm.

4.2 Posology and method of administration
Adults, including the elderly

Intravenous route
Isoket 0.05% is intended for intravenous administration by slow infusion via a syringe pump.

A dose of between 2mg and 12mg per hour is usually satisfactory. However, dosages up to 20mg per hour may be required. In all cases the dose administered should be adjusted to the patient response.

Intra-coronary Route
Isoket 0.05% 10ml prefilled syringes may be used for direct administration (through a catheter by means of an adaptor, if necessary) during percutaneous transluminal coronary angioplasty.

The usual dose is 1mg given as a bolus injection prior to balloon inflation. Further doses may be given not exceeding 5mg within a 30 minute period.

Children
The safety and efficacy of Isoket has not yet been established in children.

4.3 Contraindications
These are common to all nitrates: known hypersensitivity to nitrates, marked anaemia, cerebral haemorrhage, head trauma, hypovolaemia, and severe hypotension. Use in circulatory collapse or low filling pressure is also contraindicated. Isoket should not be used in the treatment of cardiogenic shock, unless some means of maintaining an adequate diastolic pressure is undertaken.

Sildenafil has been shown to potentiate the hypotensive effects of nitrates, and its co-administration with nitrates or nitric oxide donors is therefore contraindicated.

4.4 Special warnings and special precautions for use
Isoket should be used with caution in patients who are suffering from hypothyroidism, malnutrition, severe liver or renal disease or hypothermia. Close attention to pulse and blood pressure is necessary during the administration of Isoket infusions.

4.5 Interaction with other medicinal products and other forms of Interaction
Concurrent intake of drugs with blood pressure lowering properties e.g. beta-blockers, calcium antagonists, vasodilators etc. and/or alcohol may potentiate the hypotensive effect of Isoket.

The hypotensive effect of nitrates is potentiated by concurrent administration of sildenafil (Viagra®). This might also occur with neuroleptics and tricyclic antidepressants.

4.6 Pregnancy and lactation
No data have been reported which would indicate the possibility of adverse effects resulting from the use of isosorbide dinitrate in pregnancy. Safety in pregnancy, however, has not been established. Isosorbide dinitrate should only be used in pregnancy and during lactation if, in the opinion of the physician, the possible benefits of treatment outweigh the possible hazards.

4.7 Effects on ability to drive and use machines
None known.

4.8 Undesirable effects
In common with other nitrates, headaches, nausea and tachycardia may occur during administration. Whilst sharp falls in systemic arterial pressure can give rise to symptoms of cerebral flow deficiency and decreased coronary perfusion, clinical experience with Isoket has shown that this is not normally a problem.

4.9 Overdose
General supportive therapy is recommended.

5. PHARMACOLOGICAL PROPERTIES
ATC Code: C02D A 08 Vasodilators used in cardiac diseases.

5.1 Pharmacodynamic properties
Isosorbide dinitrate is an organic nitrate, which in common with other cardioactive nitrates, is a vasodilator. It produces decreased left and right ventricular end-diastolic pressures to a greater extent than the decrease in systemic arterial pressure, thereby reducing afterload and especially the preload of the heart.

Isosorbide dinitrate influences the oxygen supply to ischaemic myocardium by causing the redistribution of blood flow along collateral channels and from epicardial to endocardial regions by selective dilatation of large epicardial vessels.

It reduces the requirement of the myocardium for oxygen by increasing venous capacitance, causing a pooling of blood in peripheral veins, thereby reducing ventricular volume and heart wall distension.

5.2 Pharmacokinetic properties
Isosorbide dinitrate (ISDN) is eliminated from plasma with a short half-life (about 0.7h). The metabolic degradation of ISDN occurs via denitration and glucuronidation, like all organic nitrates. The rate of formation of the metabolites has been calculated for isosorbide-5-mononitrate (IS-5-MN) with $0.57h^{-1}$ followed by isosorbide-2-mononitrate (IS-2-MN) with $0.27h^{-1}$and isosorbide (IS) with $0.16h^{-1}$, IS-5-MN and IS-2-MN are the primary metabolites, which are also pharmacologically active. IS-5-MN is metabolised to isosorbide 5-mononitrate-2-glucuronide (IS-5-MN-2-GLU). The half-life of this metabolite (about 2.5h) is shorter than that of IS-5-MN (about 5.1h). The half-life of ISDN is the shortest of all and that of IS-2-MN (about 3.2h) lies in between.

5.3 Preclinical safety data
None stated.

6. PHARMACEUTICAL PARTICULARS

6.1 List of excipients
Sodium chloride

Water for injection

Hydrochloric acid for pH adjustment

Sodium hydroxide for pH adjustment

6.2 Incompatibilities
Isoket contains isosorbide dinitrate in isotonic saline and is compatible with commonly employed infusion fluids, no incompatibilities have so far been demonstrated.

Isoket is compatible with glass infusion bottles and infusion packs made from polyethylene. Isoket may be infused slowly using a syringe pump with glass or plastic syringe. The use of PVC giving sets and containers should be avoided since significant losses of the active ingredient by adsorption can occur.

6.3 Shelf life
50ml glass bottles (glass type 1): 5 years as packaged for sale.

50ml glass bottles (glass type 2): 2 years as packaged for sale.

Admixtures are stable for approximately 24 hours at room temperature in the recommended containers.

Open ampoules or bottles should be used immediately and any unused drug discarded.

Prefilled glass syringes: 3 years

6.4 Special precautions for storage
There are no special precautions for storage of the product as packaged for sale.

6.5 Nature and contents of container
50ml glass bottles (glass type 1 or 2) with a laminated rubber stopper. The stopper consists of butyl rubber. The inner side of the stopper, coming into contact with the product is laminated with a film, consisting of a copolymer of tetrafluorethylene, ethylene and a fluorine containing vinyl monomer.

10ml prefilled glass syringes with rubber plunger, stopper and cap and polystyrene plunger rod.

6.6 Instructions for use and handling
None

7. MARKETING AUTHORISATION HOLDER
SCHWARZ PHARMA Limited

Schwarz House

East Street

Chesham

Bucks

HP5 1DG

England

8. MARKETING AUTHORISATION NUMBER(S)
PL 04438/0017

9. DATE OF FIRST AUTHORISATION/RENEWAL OF THE AUTHORISATION
October 2003

10. DATE OF REVISION OF THE TEXT
September 2003

Isoket 0.1%

(SCHWARZ PHARMA Limited)

1. NAME OF THE MEDICINAL PRODUCT
Isoket 0.1%

2. QUALITATIVE AND QUANTITATIVE COMPOSITION
Isosorbide dinitrate 0.1% w/v.

3. PHARMACEUTICAL FORM
Sterile colourless solution for intravenous infusion.

4. CLINICAL PARTICULARS

4.1 Therapeutic indications
1. Intravenous

Isoket is indicated in the treatment of unresponsive left ventricular failure secondary to acute myocardial infarction, unresponsive left ventricular failure of various aetiology and severe or unstable angina pectoris.

2. Intra-coronary

Isoket is indicated during percutaneous transluminal coronary angioplasty to facilitate prolongation of balloon inflation and to prevent or relieve coronary spasm.

4.2 Posology and method of administration
Dosage: Adults, including the elderly

Intravenous route

A dose of between 2mg and 12mg per hour is usually satisfactory. However, dosages up to 20mg per hour administered should be adjusted to the patient response.

Intra-coronary Route

The usual dose is 1mg given as a bolus injection prior to balloon inflation. Further doses maybe given not exceeding 5mg within a 30 minute period.

Children

The safety and efficacy of Isoket has not yet been established in children.

Administration

Isoket is a concentrated solution and must be diluted prior use. The diluted solution should never be injected directly in the form of a bolus except via the intra-coronary route prior to balloon inflation. A dilution of 50% is advocated for intracoronary administration.

Isoket can be administered as an intravenous admixture with a suitable vehicle such as sodium chloride injection BP or dextrose injection BP.

Prepared Isoket admixtures should be given by intravenous infusion or with the aid of a syringe pump incorporating a glass or rigid plastic syringe. During administration the patients blood pressure and pulse should be closely monitored.

4.3 Contraindications
These are common to all nitrates; known hypersensitivity to nitrates, marked anaemia, cerebral haemorrhage, head trauma, hypovolaemia, and severe hypotension. Use in circulatory collapse or low filling pressure is also contraindicated. Isoket should not be used in the treatment of cardiogenic shock, unless some means of maintaining an adequate diastolic pressure is undertaken.

Sildenafil has been shown to potentiate the hypotensive effects of nitrates, and its co-administration with nitrates or nitric oxide donors is therefore contraindicated.

4.4 Special warnings and special precautions for use
Isoket should be used with caution in patients who are suffering from hypothyroidism, malnutrition, severe liver or renal disease or hypothermia. Close attention to pulse and blood pressure is necessary during the administration of Isoket infusions.

4.5 Interaction with other medicinal products and other forms of Interaction
Concurrent intake of drugs with blood pressure lowering properties e.g. beta-blockers, calcium antagonists, vasodilators etc. and or/alcohol may potentiate the hypotensive effect of Isoket 0.1%.

The hypotensive effect of nitrates is potentiated by concurrent administration of sildenafil (Viagra®). This might also occur with neuroleptics and tricyclic antidepressants.

4.6 Pregnancy and lactation
No data have been reported which would indicate the possibility of adverse effects resulting from the use of isosorbide dinitrate in pregnancy. Safety in pregnancy, however, has not been established. Isosorbide dinitrate should only be used in pregnancy and during lactation if, in the opinion of the physician, the possible benefits of treatment outweigh the possible hazards.

4.7 Effects on ability to drive and use machines
None known.

4.8 Undesirable effects
In common with other nitrates, headaches, nausea and tachycardia may occur during administration. Whilst sharp falls in systemic arterial pressure can give rise to symptoms of cerebral flow deficiency and decreased coronary perfusion, clinical experience with Isoket has shown that this is not normally a problem.

4.9 Overdose
General supportive therapy.

5. PHARMACOLOGICAL PROPERTIES

5.1 Pharmacodynamic properties
ATC Code: CO1D A08 Vasodilators used in cardiac diseases – organic nitrates.

Isosorbide dinitrate is an organic nitrate, which in common with other cardioactive nitrates, is a vasodilator. It produces decreased left and right ventricular end-diastolic pressures to a greater extent than the decrease in systemic arterial pressure, thereby reducing afterload and especially the preload of the heart.

Isosorbide dinitrate influences the oxygen supply to ischaemic myocardium by causing the redistribution of blood flow along collateral channels and from epicardial to endocardial regions by selective dilatation of large epicardial vessels.

It reduces the requirement of the myocardium for oxygen by increasing venous capacitance, causing a pooling of blood in peripheral veins, thereby reducing ventricular volume and heart wall distension.

5.2 Pharmacokinetic properties
Isosorbide dinitrate (ISDN) is eliminated from plasma with a short half-life (about 0.7h). The metabolic degradation of ISDN occurs via denitration and glucuronidation, like all organic nitrates. The rate of formation of the metabolites has been calculated for isosorbide-5-mononitrate (IS-5-MN) with $0.27\ h^{-1}$, and isosorbide (IS) with $0.16\ h^{-1}$. IS-5-MN and IS-2-MN are the primary metabolites which are also pharmacologically active. IS-5-MN is metabolised to isosorbide 5-mononitrate-2-glucuronide (IS-5-MN-2-GLU). The half-life of this metabolite (about 2.5h) is shorter than that of IS-5-MN (about 5.1h). The half-life of ISDN is the shortest of all and that of IS-2-MN (about 3.2h) lies in between.

5.3 Preclinical safety data
None stated.

6. PHARMACEUTICAL PARTICULARS

6.1 List of excipients
Sodium chloride

Water for injection

Sodium hydroxide 1N

Hydrochloric acid solution 2N

6.2 Incompatibilities
Isoket contains isosorbide dinitrate in isotonic saline and is compatible with commonly employed infusion fluids, no incompatibilities have so far been demonstrated.

Isoket is compatible with glass infusion bottles and infusion packs made from polyethylene. Isoket may be infused slowly using a syringe pump with glass or plastic syringe. The use of PVC giving sets and containers should be avoided since significant losses of the active ingredient by adsorption can occur.

6.3 Shelf life
5 years, as packaged for sale.

Admixtures are stable for approximately 24 hours at room temperature in the recommended containers.

Open ampoules or bottles should be used immediately and any unused drug discarded.

6.4 Special precautions for storage
There are no special precautions for storage of the product as packaged for sale.

6.5 Nature and contents of container
10ml glass ampoules and 50ml, 100ml glass vials.

Clear, Type I glass vials sealed with a grey stopper and a red flip-off aluminium cap, containing 50ml or 100ml of concentrate. The bottle is packed in a cardboard carton containing a Sterifix Minispike to aid withdrawal of the product from the bottle.

6.6 Instructions for use and handling
Example of admixture preparation

To obtain a dose of 6 mg per hour, add 50 ml of Isoket 0.1% to 450 ml of a suitable vehicle, under aseptic conditions. The resultant admixture (500ml) contains 100 μg/ml (1mg/10ml) isosorbide dinitrate. An infusion rate of 60ml per hour (equivalent to 60 paediatric microdrops per minute or 20 standard drops per minute) will deliver the required dose of 6mg per hour.

Should it be necessary to reduce fluid intake, 100ml of Isoket 0.1% may be diluted to 500ml using a suitable vehicle. The resultant solution now contains 200 μg/ml (2mg/10ml) isosorbide dinitrate. An infusion rate of 30ml per hour (equivalent to 30 paediatric microdrops per minute or 10 standard drops per minute), will deliver the required dose of 6 mg per hour.

A dilution of 50% is advocated to produce a solution containing 0.5 mg/ml where fluid intake is strictly limited.

7. MARKETING AUTHORISATION HOLDER
SCHWARZ PHARMA Limited

Schwarz House

East Street

Chesham

Bucks HP5 1DG

England

8. MARKETING AUTHORISATION NUMBER(S)
PL 04438/0001

9. DATE OF FIRST AUTHORISATION/RENEWAL OF THE AUTHORISATION
10 February 2002

10. DATE OF REVISION OF THE TEXT
19th March 2003

Isoket Retard 20

(SCHWARZ PHARMA Limited)

1. NAME OF THE MEDICINAL PRODUCT
ISOKET RETARD 20 TABLETS

2. QUALITATIVE AND QUANTITATIVE COMPOSITION
Each tablet contains isosorbide dinitrate 20mg in a prolonged release formulation.

For excipients see 6.1.

3. PHARMACEUTICAL FORM
Prolonged release tablets.

White with break score, marked IR 20 on the upper side and with SCHWARZ PHARMA on the reverse side.

4. CLINICAL PARTICULARS
4.1 Therapeutic indications
For the prophylaxis and treatment of angina pectoris.

4.2 Posology and method of administration
For oral administration.

Adults: One tablet to be taken twice daily without chewing and with a sufficient amount of fluid. The second dose should be given 6 to 8 hours after the first. For patients with higher nitrate requirements the dose may be increased to one tablet three times daily; the last dose should be taken around 6pm.

Elderly: Clinical experience has not necessitated alternative advice for use in elderly patients.

Children: The safety and efficacy of Isoket Retard has yet to be established.

4.3 Contraindications
This product should not be given to patients with a known sensitivity to nitrates (or any other ingredient in this product), very low blood pressure, acute myocardial infarction with low filling pressure, marked anaemia, head trauma, cerebral haemorrhage, acute circulatory failure, severe hypotension or hypovolaemia.

Phosphodiesterase inhibitors (e.g. Sildenafil) have been shown to potentiate the hypotensive effects of nitrates, and their co-administration with nitrates or nitric oxide donors is therefore contraindicated.

4.4 Special warnings and special precautions for use
These tablets should be used with caution in patients who are suffering from hypothyroidism, hypothermia, malnutrition, severe liver disease or renal disease.

Symptoms of circulatory collapse may arise after the first dose, particularly in patients with labile circulation.

This product may give rise to symptoms of postural hypotension and sycope in some patients.

These tablets should be used with particular caution and under medical supervison in the following:

Hypertrophic obstructive cardiomyopathy (HOCM), constrictive pericarditis, cardiac tamponade, low cardiac filling pressures, aortic/mitral valve stenosis, and diseases associated with raised intracranial pressure.

Treatment with these tablets must not be interrupted or stopped to take phosphodiestearase inhibitors due to the increased risk of inducing an attack of angina pectoris.

If these tablets are not taken as indicated with the appropriate dosing interval (see section 4.2) tolerance to the medication could develop.

4.5 Interaction with other medicinal products and other forms of Interaction
Concurrent intake of drugs with blood pressure lowering properties e.g. beta blockers, calcium antagonists, vasodilators etc. and/or alcohol may potentiate the hypotensive effect of the tablets. Symptoms of circulatory collapse can arise in patients already taking ACE inhibitors.

The hypotensive effect of nitrates is potentiated by concurrent administration of phosphodiesterase inhibitors (eg. sildenafil). This might also occur with neuroleptics and tricyclic antidepressants.

Reports suggest that when administered concomitantly, nitrates may increase the blood level of dihydroergotamine and its hypertensive effect.

4.6 Pregnancy and lactation
This product should not be used during pregnancy or lactation unless considered essential by the physician.

4.7 Effects on ability to drive and use machines
Headaches, tiredness and dizziness may occur. These may affect the ability to drive and operate machinery. Patients should not drive or operate machinery if their ability is impaired.

4.8 Undesirable effects
A very common (> 10% of patients) adverse reaction to these tablets is headache. The incidence of headache diminishes gradually with time and continued use,

At start of therapy or when the dosage is increased, hypotension and/or light-headedness on standing are observed commonly (i.e. in 1-10% of patients.) These symptoms may be associated with dizziness, drowsiness, reflex tachycardia, and a feeling of weakness.

Infrequently (i.e in less than 1% of patients), nausea, vomiting, flush and allergic skin reaction (e.g. rash), which may be sometimes severe may infrequently occur. In isolated cases exfoliative dermatitis may occur. Very rarely, Stevens-Johnson-Syndrome or angiodema may occur.

Severe hypotensive responses have been reported for organic nitrates and include nausea, vomiting, restlessness, pallor and excessive perspiration. Uncommonly collapse may occur (sometimes accompanied by bradyarrhythmia and syncope). Uncommonly severe hypotension may lead to enhanced angina symptoms.

A few reports on heartburn most likely due to a nitrate-induced sphincter relaxation have been recorded.

During treatment with these tablets, a temporary hypoxaemia may occur due to a relative redistribution of the blood flow in hypoventilated alveolar areas. Particularly in patients with coronary artery disease this may lead to a myocardial hypoxia.

4.9 Overdose
Clinical Features:

- Fall of blood pressure ⩽ 90mmHg, paleness, sweating, weak pulse, tachycardia, light-headedness on standing, headache, weakness, dizziness, nausea and vomiting
- During isosorbide monintrate biotransformation nitrite ions are released, which may include methaemoglobinaemia and cyanosis with subsequent tachypnoea, anxiety, loss of consciousness and cardiac arrest. It can not be excluded that an overdose of isosorbide dinitrate may cause this adverse reaction.
- In very high doses the intracranial pressure may be increased. This might lead to cerebral symptoms.

Supportive measures

- Stop intake of the drug
- General procedures in the event of nitrate-related hypotension:

- Patient should be kept horizontal with the head lowered and legs raised

- Supply oxygen

- Expand plasma volume

- For specific shock treatment admit patient to intensive care unit

Specific Procedures:

- Raising the blood pressure if the blood pressure is very low
- Treatment of methaeglobinaemia

- Reduction therapy of choice with vitamin C, methylene-blue, or toluidine-blue

- Administer oxygen (if necessary)

- Initiate artificial ventilation

- Hemodialysis (if necessary)

- Resuscitation measures:

In case of signs of respiratory and circulatory arrest, initiate resuscitation measures immediately.

5. PHARMACOLOGICAL PROPERTIES
5.1 Pharmacodynamic properties
ATC Code: C01D A08 (Organic nitrates)

Isosorbide dinitrate causes a relaxation of vascular smooth muscle thereby inducing a vasodilation.

Both peripheral arteries and veins are relaxed by isosorbide dinitrate. The latter effect promotes venous pooling of blood and decreases venous return to the heart, thereby reducing ventricular end-diastolic pressure and volume (preload).

The action on arterial, and at higher dosages arteriolar vessels, reduce the systemic vascular resistance (afterload). This in turn reduces the cardiac work.

The effects on both preload and afterload lead subsequently to a reduced oxygen consumption of the heart.

Furthermore, isosorbide dinitrate causes redistribution of blood flow to the subendocardial regions of the heart when the coronary circulation is partially occluded by arteriosclerotic lesions. This last effect is likely to be due to a selective dilation of large coronary vessels. Nitrate-induced dilation of collateral arteries can improve the perfusion of poststenotic myocardium. Nitrates also dilate eccentric stenoses as they can counteract possible constricting factors acting on the residual arch of compliant smooth muscle at the site of the coronary narrowing. Furthermore, coronary spasms can be relaxed by nitrates.

Nitrates were shown to improve resting and exercise haemodynamics in patients suffering from congestive heart failure. In this beneficial effect several mechansims including an improvement of valvular regurgitation (due to the lessening of ventricular dilation) and the reduction of myocardial oxygen demand are involved.

By decreasing the oxygen demand and increasing the oxygen supply, the area of myocardial damage is reduced. Therefore, isosorbide dinitrate may be useful in selected patients who suffered a myocardial infarction.

Effects on other organ systems include a relaxation of the bronchial muscle, the muscles of the gastrointestinal, the biliary and the urinary tract. Relaxation of the uterine smooth muscles is reported as well.

Mechanism of action:

Like all organic nitrates, isosorbide dinitrate acts as a donor of nitric oxide (NO). NO causes a relaxation of vascular smooth muscle via the stimulation of guanylyl cyclase and the subsequent increase of intracellular cyclic guanosine monophosphate (cGMP) concentration. A cGMP-dependent protein kinase is thus stimulated, with resultant alteration of the phosphorylation of various proteins in the smooth muscle cell. This eventually leads to the dephosphorylation of the light chain of myosin and the lowering of contractility

5.2 Pharmacokinetic properties
After administration of one tablet of Isoket Retard 20 at least two peak concentrations of ISDN occurred in the plasma. The initial peak (mean 1.9 ng/ml, range 1.0 to 3.4 ng/ml) occurred during 0.5 to 2 hours and then the mean plasma concentrations declined to 1.3 ng/ml at 3 hours. The concentration then increased again to reach a major peak level (mean 6.2 ng/ml range 1.6 to 12.3 ng/ml) during 4 to 6 hours after dosing. Plasma concentrations of ISDN have been measured after administration of increasing doses in the range 20 to 100mg as Isoket Retard 20 tablets. Means of peak concentrations of 4.2 ng/ml, 13.1 ng/ml, 20.7 ng/ml, 36.8 ng/ml and 34.9 ng/ml were measured after doses of 20mg, 40mg, 60mg, 80mg and 100mg respectively.

Gastrointestinal absorption is slower than absorption through the oral mucosa. The first pass effect is higher when given orally. Isosorbide dinitrate is metabolized to isosorbide 2-mononitrate with a half life of 2.01h (±0.4h) to 2.5h and isosorbide 5-mononitrate with a half-life of 4.6h (±0.8h). Both metabolites are pharmocologically active.

The relative bioavailability of Isoket Retard in comparison to the non-sustained-release tablet amounts to more than 80% after oral use.

5.3 Preclinical safety data
None stated.

6. PHARMACEUTICAL PARTICULARS
6.1 List of excipients
Lactose monohydrate

Talc

Polyvinyl acetate

Magnesium stearate

Potato starch

6.2 Incompatibilities
None known.

6.3 Shelf life
5 years.

6.4 Special precautions for storage
None

6.5 Nature and contents of container
Cartons of blister strips of polypropylene (PP) and aluminium or of PP/PP

Pack sizes: 56 and 84 tablets.

6.6 Instructions for use and handling
None

7. MARKETING AUTHORISATION HOLDER
SCHWARZ PHARMA Limited

Schwarz House

East Street

Chesham

Bucks HP5 1DG

England

8. MARKETING AUTHORISATION NUMBER(S)
PL 04438/0004

9. DATE OF FIRST AUTHORISATION/RENEWAL OF THE AUTHORISATION
27 August 2001

10. DATE OF REVISION OF THE TEXT
March 2005

Legal Category

P

Isoket Retard 40

(SCHWARZ PHARMA Limited)

1. NAME OF THE MEDICINAL PRODUCT
ISOKET RETARD 40 TABLETS

2. QUALITATIVE AND QUANTITATIVE COMPOSITION
Each tablet contains isosorbide dinitrate 40 mg in a prolonged release formulation.

For excipients see 6.1

3. PHARMACEUTICAL FORM
Prolonged release tablets.

White with break score, marked IR 40 on the upper side and with SCHWARZ PHARMA on the reverse side.

4. CLINICAL PARTICULARS
4.1 Therapeutic indications
For the prophylaxis and treatment of angina pectoris.

4.2 Posology and method of administration
For oral administration.

Adults: One tablet to be taken once daily without chewing and with a sufficient amount of fluid. For patients with higher nitrate requirements the dose may be increased to one tablet twice daily; the second dose should be given 6 to 8 hours after the first.

Elderly: Clinical experience has not necessitated alternative advice for use in elderly patients.

Children: The safety and efficacy of Isoket Retard has yet to be established.

4.3 Contraindications
This product should not be given to patients with a known sensitivity to nitrates (or any other ingredient in this product), very low blood pressure, acute myocardial infarction with low filling pressure, marked anaemia, head trauma, cerebral haemorrhage, acute circulatory failure, severe hypotension or hypovolaemia.

Phosphodiesterase inhibitors (e.g. Sildenafil) have been shown to potentiate the hypotensive effects of nitrates, and their co-administration with nitrates or nitric oxide donors is therefore contraindicated.

4.4 Special warnings and special precautions for use
These tablets should be used with caution in patients who are suffering from hypothyroidism, hypothermia, malnutrition, severe liver disease or renal disease.

Symptoms of circulatory collapse may arise after the first dose, particularly in patients with labile circulation.

This product may give rise to symptoms of postural hypotension and sycope in some patients.

These tablets should be used with particular caution and under medical supervison in the following:

Hypertrophic obstructive cardiomyopathy (HOCM), constrictive pericarditis, cardiac tamponade, low cardiac filling pressures, aortic/mitral valve stenosis, and diseases associated with raised intracranial pressure.

Treatment with these tablets must not be interrupted or stopped to take phosphodiesterase inhibitors due to the increased risk of inducing an attack of angina pectoris.

If these tablets are not taken as indicated with the appropriate dosing interval (see section 4.2) tolerance to the medication could develop.

4.5 Interaction with other medicinal products and other forms of Interaction
Concurrent intake of drugs with blood pressure lowering properties e.g. beta blockers, calcium antagonists, vasodilators etc. and/or alcohol may potentiate the hypotensive effect of the tablets. Symptoms of circulatory collapse can arise in patients already taking ACE inhibitors.

The hypotensive effect of nitrates is potentiated by concurrent administration of phosphodiesterase inhibitors (e.g. sildenafil). This might also occur with neuroleptics and tricyclic antidepressants.

Reports suggest that when administered concomitantly, nitrates may increase the blood level of dihydroergotamine and its hypertensive effect.

4.6 Pregnancy and lactation
This product should not be used during pregnancy or lactation unless considered essential by the physician.

4.7 Effects on ability to drive and use machines
Headaches, tiredness and dizziness may occur. These may affect the ability to drive and operate machinery. Patients should not drive or operate machinery if their ability is impaired.

4.8 Undesirable effects
A very common (> 10% of patients) adverse reaction to these tablets is headache. The incidence of headache diminishes gradually with time and continued use.

At start of therapy or when the dosage is increased, hypotension and/or light-headedness on standing are observed commonly (i.e. in 1-10% of patients.) These symptoms may be associated with dizziness, drowsiness, reflex tachycardia, and a feeling of weakness.

Infrequently (i.e. in less than 1% of patients), nausea, vomiting, flush and allergic skin reaction (e.g. rash), which may be sometimes severe may infrequently occur. In isolated cases exfoliative dermatitis may occur. Very rarely, Stevens-Johnson-Syndrome or angiodema may occur.

Severe hypotensive responses have been reported for organic nitrates and include nausea, vomiting, restlessness, pallor and excessive perspiration. Uncommonly collapse may occur (sometimes accompanied by bradyarrhythmia and syncope). Uncommonly severe hypotension may lead to enhanced angina symptoms.

A few reports on heartburn most likely due to a nitrate-induced sphincter relaxation have been recorded.

During treatment with these tablets, a temporary hypoxaemia may occur due to a relative redistribution of the blood flow in hypoventilated alveolar areas. Particularly in patients with coronary artery disease this may lead to a myocardial hypoxia.

4.9 Overdose
Clinical Features:

- Fall of blood pressure ≤ 90mm Hg, paleness, sweating, weak pulse, tachycardia, light-headedness on standing, headache, weakness, dizziness, nausea and vomiting
- During isosorbide monintrate biotransformation nitrite ions are released, which may include methaemoglobinaemia and cyanosis with subsequent tachypnoea, anxiety, loss of consciousness and cardiac arrest. It can not be excluded that an overdose of isosorbide dinitrate may cause this adverse reaction.
- In very high doses the intracranial pressure may be increased. This might lead to cerebral symptoms.

Supportive measures

- Stop intake of the drug
- General procedures in the event of nitrate-related hypotension:

- Patient should be kept horizontal with the head lowered and legs raised
- Supply oxygen
- Expand plasma volume
- For specific shock treatment admit patient to intensive care unit

Specific Procedures:

- Raising the blood pressure if the blood pressure is very low
- Treatment of methaeglobinaemia

- Reduction therapy of choice with vitamin C, methylene-blue, or toluidine-blue
- Administer oxygen (if necessary)
- Initiate artificial ventilation
- Hemodialysis (of necessary)

- Resuscitation measures:

In case of signs of respiratory and circulatory arrest, initiate resuscitation measures immediately.

5. PHARMACOLOGICAL PROPERTIES
5.1 Pharmacodynamic properties
ATC Code: C01D A08 (Organic nitrates)

Isosorbide dinitrate causes a relaxation of vascular smooth muscle thereby inducing a vasodilation.

Both peripheral arteries and veins are relaxed by isosorbide dinitrate. The latter effect promotes venous pooling of blood and decreases venous return to the heart, thereby reducing ventricular end-diastolic pressure and volume (preload).

The action on arterial, and at higher dosages arteriolar vessels, reduce the systemic vascular resistance (afterload). This in turn reduces the cardiac work.

The effects on both preload and afterload lead subsequently to a reduced oxygen consumption of the heart.

Furthermore, isosorbide dinitrate causes redistribution of blood flow to the subendocardial regions of the heart when the coronary circulation is partially occluded by arteriosclerotic lesions. This last effect is likely to be due to a selective dilation of large coronary vessels. Nitrate-induced dilation of collateral arteries can improve the perfusion of poststenotic myocardium. Nitrates also dilate eccentric stenoses as they can counteract possible constricting factors acting on the residual arch of compliant smooth muscle at the site of the coronary narrowing. Furthermore, coronary spasms can be relaxed by nitrates.

Nitrates were shown to improve resting and exercise haemodynamics in patients suffering from congestive heart failure. In this beneficial effect several mechansims including an improvement of valvular regurgitation (due to the lessening of ventricular dilation) and the reduction of myocardial oxygen demand are involved.

By decreasing the oxygen demand and increasing the oxygen supply, the area of myocardial damage is reduced. Therefore, isosorbide dinitrate may be useful in selected patients who suffered a myocardial infarction.

Effects on other organ systems include a relaxation of the bronchial muscle, the muscles of the gastrointestinal, the biliary and the urinary tract. Relaxation of the uterine smooth muscles is reported as well.

Mechanism of action:

Like all organic nitrates, isosorbide dinitrate acts as a donor of nitric oxide (NO). NO causes a relaxation of vascular smooth muscle via the stimulation of guanylyl cyclase and the subsequent increase of intracellular cyclic guanosine monophosphate (cGMP) concentration. A cGMP-dependent protein kinase is thus stimulated, with resultant alteration of the phosphorylation of various proteins in the smooth muscle cell. This eventually leads to the dephosphorylation of the light chain of myosin and the lowering of contractility

5.2 Pharmacokinetic properties
After administration of one tablet of Isoket Retard 40 mean peak plasma concentrations of ISDN (8.0 ± 12 ng/ml) at 7.7 ± 2.9 hours and IS-5N (190 ± 33 ng/ml) at 8.7 ± 2.1 hours. The terminal half life of IS-5N which was least affected by the absorption process was 5.4 hours ± 0.5 sd.

Gastrointestinal absorption is slower than absorption through the oral mucosa. The first pass effect is higher when given orally. Isosorbide dinitrate is metabolized to isosorbide 2-mononitrate with a half-life of 2.01 h (±0.4 h) to 2.5 h and isosorbide 5-mononitrate with a half-life of 4.6 h (± 8 h). Both metabolites are pharmacologically active.

The relative bioavailability of Isoket Retard in comparison to the non-sustained-release tablet amounts to more than 80% after oral use.

5.3 Preclinical safety data
None stated.

6. PHARMACEUTICAL PARTICULARS
6.1 List of excipients
Lactose monohydrate

Talc

Polyvinyl acetate

Magnesium stearate

Potato starch

6.2 Incompatibilities
None known.

6.3 Shelf life
5 years.

6.4 Special precautions for storage
None

6.5 Nature and contents of container
Cartons of blister strips of polypropylene (PP) and aluminium or of PP/PP

Pack sizes 56 and 84 tablets.

6.6 Instructions for use and handling
None

7. MARKETING AUTHORISATION HOLDER
SCHWARZ PHARMA Limited

Schwarz House

East Street

Chesham

Bucks HP5 1DG

England

8. MARKETING AUTHORISATION NUMBER(S)
PL 04438/0002

9. DATE OF FIRST AUTHORISATION/RENEWAL OF THE AUTHORISATION
17 September 2002

10. DATE OF REVISION OF THE TEXT
March 2005

Legal Category

P

Isoniazid Ampoules 50mg/2ml

(Cambridge Laboratories)

1. NAME OF THE MEDICINAL PRODUCT
Isoniazid Ampoules 50 mg/2 ml.

2. QUALITATIVE AND QUANTITATIVE COMPOSITION
Each ampoule contains 50 mg Isoniazid BP in 2 ml of solution.

3. PHARMACEUTICAL FORM
Ampoules

4. CLINICAL PARTICULARS
4.1 Therapeutic indications
For all forms of pulmonary and extra-pulmonary tuberculosis.

4.2 Posology and method of administration
Isoniazid ampoules are for intramuscular, intravenous, intrapleural, or intrathecal injection.

<u>Adults and children</u>

The usual intramuscular or intravenous dose for adults is 200 to 300 mg as a single daily dose, for children 100 to 300 mg daily (10 - 20 mg/kg), but doses much larger than these are sometimes given, especially in conditions such as tuberculous meningitis. It is recommended to give an intravenous dose slowly as an undiluted bolus injection, although other methods may be employed.

<u>Neonates</u>

The recommended intravenous or intramuscular dose for neonates is 3-5 mg/kg with a maximum of 10 mg/kg daily. Isoniazid may be present in the milk of lactating mothers.

<u>The elderly</u>

No dosage reduction is necessary in the elderly.

<u>Intrapleural use</u>

50 to 250 mg may be instilled intrapleurally after aspiration of pus, the dosage of oral isoniazid on that day being correspondingly reduced. The ampoule solution is also used for the local treatment of tuberculous ulcers, for irrigation of fistulae, etc.

<u>Intrathecal use:</u>

It should be noted that CSF concentrations of isoniazid are approximately 90% of plasma concentrations. Where intrathecal use is required, 25 - 50 mg daily has been given to adults and 10 - 20 mg daily for children, according to age.

It is usual to give Isoniazid together with other antituberculous therapy, as determined by current practice and/or sensitivity testing.

It is recommended that pyridoxine 10 - 50mg daily be given during Isoniazid therapy to minimise adverse reactions, especially in malnourished patients and those predisposed to neuropathy (eg. diabetics and alcoholics).

4.3 Contraindications
Isoniazid should not be given to patients with a history of sensitivity to isoniazid.

4.4 Special warnings and special precautions for use
Use in renal and hepatic impairment: no dosage reduction of Isoniazid is necessary when given to patients with mild renal failure. Patients with severe renal failure (glomerular filtration rate of less than 10 ml/minute) and slow acetylator status might require a dose reduction of about 100mg to maintain trough plasma levels at less than 1 mcg/ml. The possible risks of administration of Isoniazid to patients with pre-existing non-tuberculous hepatic disease should be balanced against the benefits expected from treating tuberculosis.

Care is also required in chronic alcoholism and when prescribing isoniazid for patients with pre-existing hepatitis. Convulsions and psychotic reactions have occurred, especially in patients with a previous history of these conditions. These manifestations usually subside rapidly when the drug is withdrawn. Isoniazid should therefore be given with caution to patients with convulsive disorders and should be avoided in those with manic or hypomanic psychoses.

Isoniazid is metabolised by acetylation, which is subject to genetic variation. The 'slow acetylators' may be more susceptible to drug-induced peripheral neuropathy. However, dose adjustment is not normally required.

4.5 Interaction with other medicinal products and other forms of Interaction
Isoniazid may inhibit the metabolism of phenytoin, primidone and carbamazepine. Plasma levels of these drugs should be monitored if concurrent therapy with Isoniazid is necessary. See also statement under 4.8 regarding Rifampicin.

4.6 Pregnancy and lactation
While Isoniazid is generally regarded to be safe in pregnancy, there is a possibility of an increased risk of foetal malformations occurring when Isoniazid is given in early pregnancy. If pregnancy cannot be excluded possible risks should be balanced against therapeutic benefits. Isoniazid is excreted in breast milk at concentrations equivalent to those found in maternal plasma, ie. 6-12 mcg/ml. this could result in an infant ingesting up to 2 mg/kg/day.

4.7 Effects on ability to drive and use machines
None known.

4.8 Undesirable effects
Isoniazid is generally well tolerated. Side-effects have been reported mainly in association with high doses or in slow acetylators who develop higher blood levels of the drug. Fever, peripheral neuropathy (preventable with pyridoxine), optic neuritis and atrophy, allergic skin conditions (including erythema multiforme), and rarely lupoid syndrome, pellagra, purpura and haematological reactions have occurred during isoniazid therapy. Hyperglycaemia and gynaeco-mastia have been reported with isoniazid treatment. Isoniazid, especially if given with rifampicin, may induce abnormalities in liver function, particularly in patients with pre-existing liver disorders, in the elderly, the very young and the malnourished. Monthly review is suggested to detect and limit the severity of this side-effect by stopping treatment if plasma transaminases exceed three times the upper limit of normal. There is conflicting opinion as to the relationship of this side-effect to acetylator status.

4.9 Overdose
In severe poisoning the main risk is of epileptiform convulsions. In addition any of the side-effects listed above may occur together with metabolic acidosis and hyperglycaemia. Treatment should be directed to the control of convulsions and large doses of pyridoxine may limit the occurrence of other adverse effects. Metabolic acidosis may require sodium bicarbonate infusion. The drug is removed by dialysis.

5. PHARMACOLOGICAL PROPERTIES
5.1 Pharmacodynamic properties
Isoniazid is a highly active tuberculostatic drug, and at high concentrations it is bactericidal to mycobacterium tuberculosis, possibly acting by interference with the synthesis of mycolic acid (a constituent of the bacterial cell wall).

5.2 Pharmacokinetic properties
Isoniazid is not appreciably protein-bound and diffuses readily throughout the body. It affects intracellular as well as extracellular bacilli. The primary metabolic route involves acetylation the rate of which is determined genetically.

5.3 Preclinical safety data
There are no pre-clinical data of relevance to the prescriber which are additional to that already included in other sections of the SPC.

6. PHARMACEUTICAL PARTICULARS
6.1 List of excipients
Hydrochloric Acid
Water for Injections BP

6.2 Incompatibilities
None known.

6.3 Shelf life
Three years.

6.4 Special precautions for storage
The recommended maximum storage temperature is 25°C.
Protect from light.

6.5 Nature and contents of container
Colourless glass ampoules coded with dark red and orange colour rings, each containing 2 ml of solution, in packs of 10 ampoules.

6.6 Instructions for use and handling
None.

Administrative Data
7. MARKETING AUTHORISATION HOLDER
Cambridge Laboratories Limited
Deltic House
Kingfisher Way
Silverlink Business Park
Wallsend
Tyne & Wear
NE28 9NX

8. MARKETING AUTHORISATION NUMBER(S)
PL 12070/0005

9. DATE OF FIRST AUTHORISATION/RENEWAL OF THE AUTHORISATION
30 July 1997

10. DATE OF REVISION OF THE TEXT
April 2002

Isoniazid Tablets BP 100mg

(Celltech Manufacturing Services Limited)

1. NAME OF THE MEDICINAL PRODUCT
Isoniazid Tablets BP 100mg

2. QUALITATIVE AND QUANTITATIVE COMPOSITION
Isoniazid BP 100mg

3. PHARMACEUTICAL FORM
White biconvex uncoated tablets embossed 100 152 on one face and EVANS on the obverse.

4. CLINICAL PARTICULARS
4.1 Therapeutic indications
Isoniazid is indicated in the treatment of all forms of pulmonary and extra-pulmonary tuberculosis.

4.2 Posology and method of administration
As directed by the medical practitioner.

Recommended dosage

Patients should be given the following single daily dose and preferably on an empty stomach, i.e. at least 30 minutes before a meal or 2 hours after a meal.

Adults

The usual dose of isoniazid in tuberculosis is 4 to 5mg per kilogram body-weight daily given by mouth in single or divided doses to a maximum of 300mg daily. Up to 10mg per kilogram body-weight daily may be given particularly during the first 1 to 2 weeks of treatment of tuberculous meningitis. A dose of 15mg per kg has been given twice weekly in intermittent treatment regimens; slow-release preparations of isoniazid have also been used in such regimens, especially in patients who are rapid acetylators of isoniazid.

Elderly

No dosage reduction is necessary in the elderly, but caution should be exercised in such patients, in view of the possible decrease of the excretory function of the kidney and of the liver.

Children

The usual daily doses for children are 10 to 20mg per kilogram body-weight daily in single or divided doses.

An effective level of isoniazid in the cerebrospinal fluid usually follows oral administration.

4.3 Contraindications
Patients who are known to be hypersensitive to isoniazid or drug-induced liver disease.

4.4 Special warnings and special precautions for use
All patients should have baseline liver function tests performed and repeated at regular intervals during treatment. If serum AST rises to more than three times normal, or there is any increase in bilirubin, treatment should be withdrawn. Special precautions are required in patients with impaired liver function. Any deterioration in liver function in these patients is an indication for stopping treatment.

Care should be taken in giving isoniazid to patients suffering from convulsive disorders, chronic alcoholism or impaired kidney function.

4.5 Interaction with other medicinal products and other forms of Interaction
Isoniazid should not be given to patients who have experience severe adverse reactions includingdrug-induced liver disease. Care should be taken in giving isoniazid to patients suffering from convulsive disorders, diabetes mellitus, chronic alcoholism, or impaired liver or kidney function or to patients taking other potentially hepatoxic agents. If symptoms of hepatitis such as malaise, fatigue, anorexia, and nausea develop isoniazid should be discontinued immediately.

When isoniazid is given to patients who inactivate it slowly or to patients receiving PAS concurrently, tissue concentrations may be enhanced, and adverse effects are more likely to appear. There may be an increased risk of liver damage in patients receiving rifampicin and isoniazid but liver enzymes are raised only transiently.

Isoniazid enhances the effect of phenytoin and may also inhibit the metabolism of primadone; there may be increased toxicity when used with disulfiram.

Patients may require additional treatment with pyridoxine.

There may be an increased risk of distal sensory neuropathy when isoniazid is used in patients taking stavudine (d4T).

4.6 Pregnancy and lactation
There are no well controlled studies in pregnant women. Therefore, isoniazid should only be used in pregnant women or in women of child-bearing potential only of the potential benefit justifies the potential risk to the foetus. When administered to nursing mother, breast-fed infants should be monitored for possible signs of isoniazid toxicity.

4.7 Effects on ability to drive and use machines
No specific statement, but unlikely to effect the ability to drive or use machinery.

4.8 Undesirable effects
Patients may experience **fever**, nausea, vomiting and other gastro-intestinal effects. Many of the adverse effects of isoniazid are related to hypersensitivity or to the use of large doses; patients who are slow inactivators may experience a greater incidence of toxicity.

Peripheral neuropathy, constipation, difficulty in starting urination, dryness of the mouth, and sometimes vertigo and hyperreflexia may be troublesome with doses of 10mg per kg body weight. Convulsions, optic neuritis, systemic lupus erythematosus, lupus-like syndrome, gynaecomastiaand psychotic reactions have been reported. Liver damage has occurred especially over the age of 35; it may be serious and sometimes fatal with the development of necrosis. Blood disorders include haemolytic and aplastic anaemia and agranulocytosis.

Various skin reactions including erythema multiforme, have occurred as have hyperglycaemia and acidosis. Pellagra may be related to an isoniazid-induced pyridoxine deficiency which affects the conversion of tryptophan to nicotinic acid. Although isoniazid usually has a mood elevating effect, mental disturbances, ranging from minor personality changes to major mental derangement have been reported; these are usually reversed on withdrawal of the drug.

Withdrawal symptoms, which may occur on the cessation of the treatment, include headache, insomnia, excessive dreaming, irritability and nervousness.

4.9 Overdose
Treatment of overdosage consists of gastric lavage following intubation and the control of convulsions by anti-convulsants given intravenously as well as the intravenous injection of large doses of pyridoxine. Any acidosis is corrected with sodium bicarbonate. Forced diuresis may be tried and haemodialysis or peritoneal dialysis has been used.

5. PHARMACOLOGICAL PROPERTIES
5.1 Pharmacodynamic properties
Isoniazid has no significant antibacterial action against any micro-organisms except the mycobacteria; against mycobacterium tuberculosis it is bacteriostatic in extremely low concentrations.

Isoniazid is used mainly in the treatment of pulmonary tuberculosis but it appears to be effective also in the treatment of extrapulmonary lesions, including meningitis and genito-urinary disease.

5.2 Pharmacokinetic properties
Absorption

Readily and completely absorbed after oral administration.

Distribution

Readily diffuses into all tissues and fluids including the cerebrospinal fluid. Isoniazid is retained in the skin and in infected tissue; it crosses the placenta and is secreted in the milk of lactating mothers.

Protein binding

Isoniazid does not appear to be bound in the blood.

Half-life

Plasma elimination half-life, in rapid acetylators about 1.2 hours and in slow acetylators about 3.5 hours.

Metabolic reactions

Acetylation, hydrolysis and glycine conjugation, hydrazone formation, and n-methylation; acetylation is polymorphic and two groups of acetylators have been identified, rapid and slow acetylators. The rate of hydrolysis is more rapid in the rapid acetylators than in the slow ones. The metabolites formed include acetyl isoniazid, isonicotinic acid, isonicotinuric acid, isonicotinoylhydrazones of pyruvic and glutaric acids, and n-methylisoniazid.

Excretion

Over 90% of a dose is excreted in the urine in 24 hours, most being excreted in the first 12 hours, 4-32% is unchanged, but no more than 10% of a dose is excreted in the faeces.

5.3 Preclinical safety data

Not applicable since isoniazid tablets have been used in clinical practice for many years and its effects in man are well known.

6. PHARMACEUTICAL PARTICULARS

6.1 List of excipients

Lactose 170 Mesh BP

Maize Starch BP

Microcrystalline Cellulose BP

Alginic Acid BPC

Magnesium Stearate BP

Purified Water BP

6.2 Incompatibilities

None.

6.3 Shelf life

36 months.

6.4 Special precautions for storage

Store below 25°C.

6.5 Nature and contents of container

Pigmented polypropylene container fitted with a tamper-evident closure containing 7, 14, 21, 28, 30, 50, 56, 60, 84, 90, 100, 112, 120 or 250 tablets. Not all pack sizes may be marketed.

6.6 Instructions for use and handling

No special precautions are required.

Administrative Data

7. MARKETING AUTHORISATION HOLDER

Celltech Manufacturing Services Limited

Vale of Bardsley

Ashton-under-Lyne

Lancashire

OL7 9RR, UK

8. MARKETING AUTHORISATION NUMBER(S)

PL 18816/0011

9. DATE OF FIRST AUTHORISATION/RENEWAL OF THE AUTHORISATION

7 October 2001

10. DATE OF REVISION OF THE TEXT

November 2001

POM

Isoniazid Tablets BP 50mg

(Celltech Manufacturing Services Limited)

1. NAME OF THE MEDICINAL PRODUCT

Isoniazid Tablets BP 50mg

2. QUALITATIVE AND QUANTITATIVE COMPOSITION

Isoniazid BP 50mg

3. PHARMACEUTICAL FORM

White biconvex uncoated tablets embossed 50 151 on one face and EVANS on the obverse.

4. CLINICAL PARTICULARS

4.1 Therapeutic indications

Isoniazid is indicated in the treatment of all forms of pulmonary and extra-pulmonary tuberculosis.

4.2 Posology and method of administration

As directed by the medical practitioner.

Recommended dosage

Patients should be given the following single daily dose and preferably on an empty stomach, i.e. at least 30 minutes before a meal or 2 hours after a meal.

Adults

The usual dose of isoniazid in tuberculosis is 4 to 5mg per kilogram body-weight daily given by mouth in single or divided doses to a maximum of 300mg daily. Up to 10mg per kilogram body-weight daily may be given particularly during the first 1 to 2 weeks of treatment of tuberculous meningitis. A dose of 15mg per kg has been given twice weekly in intermittent treatment regimens; slow-release preparations of isoniazid have also been used in such regimens, especially in patients who are rapid acetylators of isoniazid.

Elderly

No dosage reduction is necessary in the elderly, but caution should be exercised in such patients, in view of the possible decrease of the excretory function of the kidney and of the liver.

Children

The usual daily doses for children are 10 to 20mg per kilogram body-weight daily in single or divided doses.

An effective level of isoniazid in the cerebrospinal fluid usually follows oral administration.

4.3 Contraindications

Patients who are known to be hypersensitive to isoniazid or drug-induced liver disease.

4.4 Special warnings and special precautions for use

All patients should have baseline liver function tests performed and repeated at regular intervals during treatment. If serum AST rises to more than three times normal, or there is any increase in bilirubin, treatment should be withdrawn. Special precautions are required in patients with impaired liver function. Any deterioration in liver function in these patients is an indication for stopping treatment.

Care should be taken in giving isoniazid to patients suffering from convulsive disorders, chronic alcoholism or impaired kidney function.

4.5 Interaction with other medicinal products and other forms of Interaction

Isoniazid should not be given to patients who have experience severe adverse reactions including drug-induced liver disease. Care should be taken in giving isoniazid to patients suffering from convulsive disorders, diabetes mellitus, chronic alcoholism, or impaired liver or kidney function or to patients taking other potentially hepatoxic agents. If symptoms of hepatitis such as malaise, fatigue, anorexia, and nausea develop isoniazid should be discontinued immediately.

When isoniazid is given to patients who inactivate it slowly or to patients receiving PAS concurrently, tissue concentrations may be enhanced, and adverse effects are more likely to appear. There may be an increased risk of liver damage in patients receiving rifampicin and isoniazid but liver enzymes are raised only transiently.

Isoniazid enhances the effect of phenytoin and may also inhibit the metabolism of primadone; there may be increased toxicity when used with disulfiram.

Patients may require additional treatment with pyridoxine.

There may be an increased risk of distal sensory neuropathy when isoniazid is used in patients taking stavudine (d4T).

4.6 Pregnancy and lactation

There are no well controlled studies in pregnant women. Therefore, isoniazid should only be used in pregnant women or in women of child-bearing potential only of the potential benefit justifies the potential risk to the foetus. When administered to nursing mother, breast-fed infants should be monitored for possible signs of isoniazid toxicity.

4.7 Effects on ability to drive and use machines

No specific statement, but unlikely to effect the ability to drive or use machinery.

4.8 Undesirable effects

Patients may experience fever, nausea, vomiting and other gastro-intestinal effects. Many of the adverse effects of isoniazid are related to hypersensitivity or to the use of large doses; patients who are slow inactivators may experience a greater incidence of toxicity.

Peripheral neuropathy, constipation, difficulty in starting urination, dryness of the mouth, and sometimes vertigo and hyperreflexia may be troublesome with doses of 10mg per kg body weight. Convulsions, optic neuritis, systemic lupus erythematosus, lupus-like syndrome, gynaecomastiaand psychotic reactions have been reported. Liver damage has occurred especially over the age of 35; it may be serious and sometimes fatal with the development of necrosis. Blood disorders include haemolytic and aplastic anaemia and agranulocytosis.

Various skin reactions including erythema multiforme, have occurred as have hyperglycaemia and acidosis. Pellagra may be related to an isoniazid-induced pyridoxine deficiency which affects the conversion of tryptophan to nicotinic acid. Although isoniazid usually has a mood elevating effect, mental disturbances, ranging from minor personality changes to major mental derangement have been reported; these are usually reversed on withdrawal of the drug.

Withdrawal symptoms, which may occur on the cessation of the treatment, include headache, insomnia, excessive dreaming, irritability and nervousness.

4.9 Overdose

Treatment of overdosage consists of gastric lavage following intubation and the control of convulsions by anti-convulsants given intravenously as well as the intravenous injection of large doses of pyridoxine. Any acidosis is corrected with sodium bicarbonate. Forced diuresis may be tried and haemodialysis or peritoneal dialysis has been used.

5. PHARMACOLOGICAL PROPERTIES

5.1 Pharmacodynamic properties

Isoniazid has no significant antibacterial action against any micro-organisms except the mycobacteria; against mycobacterium tuberculosis it is bacteriostatic in extremely low concentrations.

Isoniazid is used mainly in the treatment of pulmonary tuberculosis but it appears to be effective also in the treatment of extrapulmonary lesions, including meningitis and genito-urinary disease.

5.2 Pharmacokinetic properties

Absorption

Readily and completely absorbed after oral administration.

Distribution

Readily diffuses into all tissues and fluids including the cerebrospinal fluid. Isoniazid is retained in the skin and in infected tissue; it crosses the placenta and is secreted in the milk of lactating mothers.

Protein binding

Isoniazid does not appear to be bound in the blood.

Half-life

Plasma elimination half-life, in rapid acetylators about 1.2 hours and in slow acetylators about 3.5 hours.

Metabolic reactions

Acetylation, hydrolysis and glycine conjugation, hydrazone formation, and n-methylation; acetylation is polymorphic and two groups of acetylators have been identified, rapid and slow acetylators. The rate of hydrolysis is more rapid in the rapid acetylators than in the slow ones. The metabolites formed include acetyl isoniazid, isonicotinic acid, isonicotinuric acid, isonicotinoylhydrazones of pyruvic and glutaric acids, and n-methylisoniazid.

Excretion

Over 90% of a dose is excreted in the urine in 24 hours, most being excreted in the first 12 hours, 4-32% is unchanged, but no more than 10% of a dose is excreted in the faeces.

5.3 Preclinical safety data

Not applicable since isoniazid tablets have been used in clinical practice for many years and its effects in man are well known.

6. PHARMACEUTICAL PARTICULARS

6.1 List of excipients

Lactose 170 Mesh BP

Maize Starch BP

Microcrystalline Cellulose BP

Alginic Acid BPC

Magnesium Stearate BP

Purified Water BP

6.2 Incompatibilities

None.

6.3 Shelf life

36 months.

6.4 Special precautions for storage

Store below 25°C.

6.5 Nature and contents of container

Pigmented polypropylene container fitted with a tamper-evident closure containing 7, 14, 21, 28, 30, 50, 56, 60, 84, 90, 100, 112, 120 or 250 tablets. Not all pack sizes may be marketed.

6.6 Instructions for use and handling

No special precautions are required.

Administrative Data

7. MARKETING AUTHORISATION HOLDER

Celltech Manufacturing Services Limited

Vale of Bardsley

Ashton-under-Lyne

Lancashire

OL7 9RR, UK

8. MARKETING AUTHORISATION NUMBER(S)

PL 18816/0010

9. DATE OF FIRST AUTHORISATION/RENEWAL OF THE AUTHORISATION

7 October 2001

10. DATE OF REVISION OF THE TEXT

November 2001

POM

Isotard XL

(Strakan Pharmaceuticals Ltd)

1. NAME OF THE MEDICINAL PRODUCT

Isotard 25XL, 40XL, 50XL and 60XL Tablets

2. QUALITATIVE AND QUANTITATIVE COMPOSITION

Isosorbide-5-mononitrate 25mg

Isosorbide-5-mononitrate 40mg

Isosorbide-5-mononitrate 50mg

Isosorbide-5-mononitrate 60mg

International non-proprietary name (INN): Isosorbide mononitrate.

Isosorbide mononitrate is also referred to as ISMN.

Chemical name: 1,4:3,6 dianhydro-D-glucitol-5-mononitrate.

3. PHARMACEUTICAL FORM

Tablets (modified release).

4. CLINICAL PARTICULARS

4.1 Therapeutic indications

Prophylactic treatment of angina pectoris.

4.2 Posology and method of administration

Adults

One tablet, once daily given in the morning. The dose may be increased to two tablets, the whole dose to be given together (dose range 25 to 120 mg).

For Isotard 60XL only, the dose can be titrated to minimise the possibility of headache by initiating treatment with half a tablet (30 mg) for the first two to four days.

The tablets should not be chewed or crushed and should be swallowed with half a glass of fluid.

Children

The safety and efficacy of Isotard XL ISMN modified release tablets has not been established.

Elderly

No need for routine dosage adjustment in the elderly has been found, but special care may be needed in those with increased susceptibility to hypotension or marked hepatic or renal insufficiency.

The lowest effective dose should be used.

Attenuation of effect has occurred in some patients being treated with prolonged release preparations. In such patients intermittent therapy may be more appropriate (see Section 4.4).

Therapy should not be discontinued suddenly. Both dosage and frequency should be tapered gradually (see Section 4.4).

4.3 Contraindications

Hypertrophic obstructive cardiomyopathy, constrictive pericarditis, cardiac tamponade, aortic/mitral valve stenosis, severe anaemia, closed-angle glaucoma, conditions associated with raised intracerebral pressure e.g. following head trauma, cerebral haemorrhage. Acute myocardial infarction with low filling pressures, acute circulatory failure (shock, vascular collapse) or very low blood pressure. Phosphodiesterase type-5 inhibitors e.g. sildenafil, tadalafil and vardenafil have been shown to potentiate the hypotensive effects of nitrates, and their co-administration with nitrates or nitric oxide donors is therefore contraindicated (see section 4.5). Isotard XL should not be given to patients with a known sensitivity to nitrates.

4.4 Special warnings and special precautions for use

Isotard XL ISMN modified release tablets are not indicated for relief of acute anginal attacks. In the event of an acute attack, sublingual or buccal glyceryl trinitrate tablets should be used.

Isotard XL ISMN should be used with caution in patients who have a recent history of myocardial infarction, or who are suffering from hypothyroidism, hypothermia, malnutrition and severe liver or renal disease.

The lowest effective dose should be used.

Attenuation of effect has occurred in some patients being treated with prolonged release preparations. In such patients intermittent therapy may be more appropriate (see Section 4.2).

Therapy should not be discontinued suddenly. Both dosage and frequency should be tapered gradually (see Section 4.2).

Hypotension induced by nitrates may be accompanied by paradoxical bradycardia and increased angina.

Severe postural hypotension with light-headedness and dizziness is frequently observed after the consumption of alcohol.

4.5 Interaction with other medicinal products and other forms of Interaction

Alprostadil, aldesleukin, angiotensin II receptor antagonists.

This product may potentiate some of the effects of alcohol and the action of hypotensive agents. The hypotensive effects of nitrates are potentiated by concurrent administration of phosphodiesterase type-5 inhibitors e.g. sildenafil (see section 4.3).

4.6 Pregnancy and lactation

No data have been reported which would indicate the possibility of adverse effects resulting from the use of isosorbide mononitrate in pregnancy. Safety in pregnancy, however, has not been established. It is not known whether nitrates are excreted in human milk and therefore caution should be exercised when administered to nursing women.

Isosorbide mononitrate should only be used in pregnancy and during lactation if, in the opinion of the physician, the possible benefits of treatment outweigh the possible hazards.

4.7 Effects on ability to drive and use machines

The patient should be warned not to drive or operate machinery if hypotension, blurred vision or dizziness occurs.

4.8 Undesirable effects

Throbbing headache may occur when treatment is initiated, but usually disappears after 1–2 weeks of treatment. Hypotension with symptoms such as dizziness, nausea and fatigue has occasionally been reported. Infrequently, flushing and allergic rashes can occur. These symptoms generally disappear during long-term treatment.

Tachycardia and paroxysmal bradycardia have been reported.

4.9 Overdose

Symptoms: Nausea, vomiting, restlessness, warm flushed skin, blurred vision, headache, fainting, tachycardia, hypotension and palpitations. A rise in intracranial pressure with confusion and neurological deficits can sometimes occur.

Management: Consider oral activated charcoal if ingestion of a potentially toxic amount has occurred within 1 hour. Observe for at least 12 hours after the overdose. Monitor blood pressure and pulse. Correct hypotension by raising the foot of the bed and/or by expanding the intravascular volume. Other measures as indicated by the patient's clinical condition. If severe hypotension persists despite the above measures consider use of inotropes such as dopamine or dobutamine.

5. PHARMACOLOGICAL PROPERTIES

5.1 Pharmacodynamic properties

Organic nitrates (including GTN, ISDN, and ISMN) are potent relaxers of smooth muscle. They have a powerful effect on vascular smooth muscle with less effect on bronchiolar, gastrointestinal, ureteral and uterine smooth muscle. Low concentrations dilate both arteries and veins. Venous dilatation pools blood in the periphery leading to a decrease in venous return, central blood volume, and ventricular filling volumes and pressures. Cardiac output may remain unchanged or it may decline as a result of the decrease in venous return. Arterial blood pressure usually declines secondary to a decrease in cardiac output or arteriolar vasodilatation, or both. A modest reflex increase in heart rate results from the decrease in arterial blood pressure. Nitrates can dilate epicardial coronary arteries including atherosclerotic stenoses.

The cellular mechanism of nitrate-induced smooth muscle relaxation has become apparent in recent years. Nitrates enter the smooth muscle cell and are cleaved to inorganic nitrate and eventually to nitric oxide. This cleavage requires the presence of sulphydryl groups, which apparently come from the amino acid cysteine. Nitric oxide undergoes further reduction to nitrosothiol by further interaction with sulphydryl groups. Nitrosothiol activates guanylate cyclase in the vascular smooth muscle cells, thereby generating cyclic guanosine monophosphate (cGMP). It is this latter compound, cGMP, that produces smooth muscle relaxation by accelerating the release of calcium from these cells.

5.2 Pharmacokinetic properties

Absorption

Isosorbide-5-mononitrate is readily absorbed from the gastro-intestinal tract.

Distribution

Following oral administration of conventional tablets, peak plasma levels are reached in about 1 hour. Unlike isosorbide dinitrate, ISMN does not undergo first-pass hepatic metabolism and bioavailability is 100%. ISMN has a volume of distribution of about 40 litres and is not significantly protein bound.

Elimination

ISMN is metabolised to inactive metabolites including isosorbide and isosorbide glucuronide. The pharmacokinetics are unaffected by the presence of heart failure, renal or hepatic insufficiency. Only 20% of ISMN is excreted unchanged in the urine. An elimination half life of about 4-5 hours has been reported.

5.3 Preclinical safety data

Not applicable.

6. PHARMACEUTICAL PARTICULARS

6.1 List of excipients

Stearic acid

Carnauba wax

Hydroxypropylmethylcellulose

Lactose

Magnesium stearate

Talc

Purified siliceous earth

Polyethylene glycol 4000

E171

E172.

6.2 Incompatibilities

None known.

6.3 Shelf life

36 months

6.4 Special precautions for storage

Do not store above 25°C. Store in the original package. Keep container in the outer carton

6.5 Nature and contents of container

The tablets are packed in blisters which consist of 250μm PVC with a 25μm PVdC coating which is sealed to 25μm thick aluminium foil with 20μm PVdC sealing lacquer. The tablets are packaged in boxes of 28 tablets.

Isotard 25XL, 40XL and 50XL tablets are round, biconvex, cream coloured tablets marked IM25, 40 or 50 on one side, as appropriate. The Isotard 60XL tablets, only, are oval, cream coloured tablets scored on both sides but with '6 (score) 0' on one side.

6.6 Instructions for use and handling

The tablets should be swallowed whole with half a glass of water. They must not be chewed or crushed.

Administrative Data

7. MARKETING AUTHORISATION HOLDER

Strakan Limited

Buckholm Mill

Galashiels

TD1 2HB

UK

8. MARKETING AUTHORISATION NUMBER(S)

Isotard 25XL: PL 16508/0018

Isotard 40XL: PL 16508/0020

Isotard 50XL: PL 16508/0021

Isotard 60XL: PL 16508/0022

9. DATE OF FIRST AUTHORISATION/RENEWAL OF THE AUTHORISATION

08 April 2002

10. DATE OF REVISION OF THE TEXT

7 October 2004

11. Legal Category

P

Isotretinoin 20mg capsules

(Beacon Pharmaceuticals)

1. NAME OF THE MEDICINAL PRODUCT

Isotretinoin 20mg Capsules

2. QUALITATIVE AND QUANTITATIVE COMPOSITION

Each capsule contains 20mg isotretinoin

For excipients, see section 6.1

3. PHARMACEUTICAL FORM

Soft capsules.

Red/orange soft gelatin capsules marked 'P20'.

4. CLINICAL PARTICULARS

4.1 Therapeutic indications

Isotretinoin capsules are indicated for the treatment of severe forms of acne (such as nodular or conglobate acne or acne at risk of permanent scarring), resistant to adequate courses of standard therapy with systemic antibacterials and topical therapy.

4.2 Posology and method of administration

Isotretinoin should only be prescribed by or under the supervision of physicians with expertise in the use of systemic retinoids for the treatment of severe acne and a full understanding of the risks of isotretinoin therapy and monitoring requirements.

The capsules should be taken with food once or twice daily.

<u>Adults including adolescents and the elderly:</u>

Isotretinoin therapy should be started at a dose of 0.5 mg/kg daily. The therapeutic response to isotretinoin and some of the adverse effects are dose-related and vary between patients. This necessitates individual dosage adjustment during therapy. For most patients, the dose ranges from 0.5-1.0 mg/kg per day.

Long-term remission and relapse rates are more closely related to the total dose administered than to either duration of treatment or daily dose. It has been shown that no substantial additional benefit is to be expected beyond a cumulative treatment dose of 120-150 mg/kg. The duration of treatment will depend on the individual daily dose. A treatment course of 16-24 weeks is normally sufficient to achieve remission.

In the majority of patients, complete clearing of the acne is obtained with a single treatment course. In the event of a definite relapse a further course of isotretinoin therapy may be considered using the same daily dose and cumulative treatment dose. As further improvement of the acne can be observed up to 8 weeks after discontinuation of treatment, a further course of treatment should not be considered until at least this period has elapsed.

Patients with severe renal insufficiency

In patients with severe renal insufficiency treatment should be started at a lower dose (e.g. 10 mg/day). The dose should then be increased up to 1 mg/kg/day or until the patient is receiving the maximum tolerated dose (see section 4.4 "Special warnings and special precautions for use").

Children

Isotretinoin is not indicated for the treatment of prepubertal acne and is not recommended in patients less than 12 years of age.

Patients with intolerance

In patients who show severe intolerance to the recommended dose, treatment may be continued at a lower dose with the consequences of a longer therapy duration and a higher risk of relapse. In order to achieve the maximum possible efficacy in these patients the dose should normally be continued at the highest tolerated dose.

4.3 Contraindications

Isotretinoin is contraindicated in women who are pregnant or breastfeeding.

(see section 4.6 "Pregnancy and lactation").

Isotretinoin is contraindicated in women of childbearing potential unless all of the conditions of the Pregnancy Prevention Programme are met (see section 4.4 "Special warnings and special precautions for use").

Isotretinoin is also contraindicated in patients

With hepatic insufficiency

With excessively elevated blood lipid values

With hypervitaminosis A

With hypersensitivity to isotretinoin or to any of the excipients (the medicine contains hydrogenated soya-bean oil and refined soya-bean oil).

Receiving concomitant treatment with tetracyclines (see section 4.5 "Interaction with other medicinal products and other forms of interactions")

4.4 Special warnings and special precautions for use

Pregnancy Prevention Programme

This medicinal product is TERATOGENIC

Isotretinoin is contraindicated in women of childbearing potential unless all of the following conditions of the Pregnancy Prevention Programme are met:

She has severe acne (such as nodular or conglobate acne or acne at risk of permanent scarring) resistant to adequate courses of standard therapy with systemic antibacterials and topical therapy (see section 4.1 "Therapeutic indications").

She understands the teratogenic risk.

She understands the need for rigorous follow-up, on a monthly basis.

She understands and accepts the need for effective contraception, without interruption, 1 month before starting treatment, throughout the duration of treatment and 1 month after the end of treatment. At least one and preferably two complementary forms of contraception including a barrier method should be used.

Even if she has amenorrhea she must follow all of the advice on effective contraception.

She should be capable of complying with effective contraceptive measures.

She is informed and understands the potential consequences of pregnancy and the need to rapidly consult if there is a risk of pregnancy.

She understands the need and accepts to undergo pregnancy testing before, during and 5 weeks after the end of treatment.

She has acknowledged that she has understood the hazards and necessary precautions associated with the use of isotretinoin.

These conditions also concern women who are not currently sexually active unless the prescriber considers that there are compelling reasons to indicate that there is no risk of pregnancy.

The prescriber must ensure that:

The patient complies with the conditions for pregnancy prevention as listed above, including confirmation that she has an adequate level of understanding.

The patient has acknowledged the aforementioned conditions.

The patient has used at least one and preferably two methods of effective contraception including a barrier method for at least 1 month prior to starting treatment and is continuing to use effective contraception throughout the treatment period and for at least 1 month after cessation of treatment.

Negative pregnancy test results have been obtained before, during and 5 weeks after the end of treatment. The dates and results of pregnancy tests should be documented.

Contraception

Female patients must be provided with comprehensive information on pregnancy prevention and should be referred for contraceptive advice if they are not using effective contraception.

As a minimum requirement, female patients at potential risk of pregnancy must use at least one effective method of contraception. Preferably the patient should use two complementary forms of contraception including a barrier method. Contraception should be continued for at least 1 month after stopping treatment with isotretinoin, even in patients with amenorrhea.

Pregnancy testing

According to local practice, medically supervised pregnancy tests with a minimum sensitivity of 25mIU/mL are recommended to be performed in the first 3 days of the menstrual cycle, as follows.

Prior to starting therapy:

In order to exclude the possibility of pregnancy prior to starting contraception, it is recommended that an initial medically supervised pregnancy test should be performed and its date and result recorded. In patients without regular menses, the timing of this pregnancy test should reflect the sexual activity of the patient and should be undertaken approximately 3 weeks after the patient last had unprotected sexual intercourse. The prescriber should educate the patient about contraception.

A medically supervised pregnancy test should also be performed during the consultation when isotretinoin is prescribed or in the 3 days prior to the visit to the prescriber, and should have been delayed until the patient had been using effective contraception for at least 1 month. This test should ensure the patient is not pregnant when she starts treatment with isotretinoin.

Follow-up visits

Follow-up visits should be arranged at 28 day intervals. The need for repeated medically supervised pregnancy tests every month should be determined according to local practice including consideration of the patient's sexual activity and recent menstrual history (abnormal menses, missed periods or amenorrhea). Where indicated, follow-up pregnancy tests should be performed on the day of the prescribing visit or in the 3 days prior to the visit to the prescriber.

End of treatment

Five weeks after stopping treatment, women should undergo a final pregnancy test to exclude pregnancy.

Prescribing and dispensing restrictions

Prescriptions of isotretinoin for women of childbearing potential should be limited to 30 days of treatment and continuation of treatment requires a new prescription. Ideally, pregnancy testing, issuing a prescription and dispensing of isotretinoin should occur on the same day. Dispensing of isotretinoin should be completed within a maximum of 7 days of the prescription.

Male patients

The available data suggest that the level of maternal exposure from the semen of the patients receiving isotretinoin is not of sufficient magnitude to be associated with the teratogenic effects of isotretinoin.

Male patients should be reminded that they must not share their medication with anyone, particularly not females.

Additional precautions

Patients should be instructed never to give this medicinal product to another person and to return any unused capsules to their pharmacist at the end of treatment.

Patients should not donate blood during therapy and for 1 month following discontinuation of isotretinoin because of the potential risk to the foetus of a pregnant transfusion recipient.

Educational material

In order to assist prescribers, pharmacists and patients in avoiding foetal exposure to isotretinoin the Marketing Authorisation Holder will provide educational material to reinforce the warnings about the teratogenicity of isotretinoin, to provide advice on contraception before therapy is started and to provide guidance on the need for pregnancy testing.

Full patient information about the teratogenic risk and the strict pregnancy prevention measures as specified in the Pregnancy Prevention Programme should be given by the physician to all patients, both male and female.

Psychiatric disorders

Depression, psychotic symptoms and, rarely, suicide attempts and suicide have been reported in patients treated with isotretinoin (see section 4.8 "Undesirable effects"). Particular care needs to be taken in patients with a history of depression and all patients should be monitored for signs of depression and referred for appropriate treatment if necessary. However, discontinuation of isotretinoin may be insufficient to alleviate symptoms and therefore further psychiatric or psychological evaluation may be necessary.

Skin and subcutaneous tissues disorders

Acute exacerbation of acne is occasionally seen during the initial period but this subsides with continued treatment, usually within 7-10 days, and usually does not require dose adjustment.

Exposure to intense sunlight or to UV rays should be avoided. Where necessary a sun-protection product with a high protection factor of at least SPF 15 should be used.

Aggressive chemical dermabrasion and cutaneous laser treatment should be avoided in patients on isotretinoin for a period of 5-6 months after the end of the treatment because of the risk of hypertrophic scarring in atypical areas and more rarely post inflammatory hyper or hypo-pigmentation in treated areas. Wax depilation should be avoided in patients on isotretinoin for at least a period of 6 months after treatment because of the risk of epidermal stripping.

Concurrent administration of isotretinoin with topical keratolytic or exfoliative anti-acne agents should be avoided as local irritation may increase.

Patients should be advised to use a skin moisturising ointment or cream and a lip balm from the start of treatment as isotretinoin is likely to cause dryness of the skin and lips.

Eye disorders

Dry eyes, corneal opacities, decreased night vision and keratitis usually resolve after discontinuation of therapy. Dry eyes can be helped by the application of a lubricating eye ointment or by the application of tear replacement therapy. Intolerance to contact lenses may occur which may necessitate the patient to wear glasses during treatment.

Decreased night vision has also been reported and the onset in some patients was sudden (see section 4.7 "Effects on ability to drive and to use machines"). Patients experiencing visual difficulties should be referred for an expert ophthalmological opinion. Withdrawal of isotretinoin may be necessary.

Musculo-skeletal and connective tissue disorders

Myalgia, arthralgia and increased serum creatine phosphokinase values have been reported in patients receiving isotretinoin, particularly in those undertaking vigorous physical activity (see section 4.8 "Undesirable effects").

Bone changes including premature epiphyseal closure, hyperostosis, and calcification of tendons and ligaments have occurred after several years of administration at very high doses for treating disorders of keratinisation. The dose levels, duration of treatment and total cumulative dose in these patients generally far exceeded those recommended for the treatment of acne.

Benign intracranial hypertension

Cases of benign intracranial hypertension have been reported, some of which involved concomitant use of tetracyclines (see sections 4.3 "Contraindications" and 4.5 "Interactions with other medicinal products and other forms of interaction"). Signs and symptoms of benign intracranial hypertension include headache, nausea and vomiting, visual disturbances and papilloedema. Patients who develop benign intracranial hypertension should discontinue isotretinoin immediately.

Hepatobiliary disorders

Liver enzymes should be checked before treatment, 1 month after the start of treatment, and subsequently at 3 monthly intervals unless more frequent monitoring is clinically indicated. Transient and reversible increases in liver transaminases have been reported. In many cases these changes have been within the normal range and values have returned to baseline levels during treatment. However, in the event of persistent clinically relevant elevation of transaminase levels, reduction of the dose or discontinuation of treatment should be considered.

Renal insufficiency

Renal insufficiency and renal failure do not affect the pharmacokinetics of isotretinoin. Therefore, isotretinoin can be given to patients with renal insufficiency. However, it is recommended that patients are started on a low dose and titrated up to the maximum tolerated dose (see section 4.2 "Posology and Method of Administration").

Lipid Metabolism

Serum lipids (fasting values) should be checked before treatment, 1 month after the start of treatment, and subsequently at 3 monthly intervals unless more frequent monitoring is clinically indicated. Elevated serum lipid values usually return to normal on reduction of the dose or discontinuation of treatment and may also respond to dietary measures.

Isotretinoin has been associated with an increase in plasma triglyceride levels. Isotretinoin should be discontinued if hypertriglyceridaemia cannot be controlled at an acceptable level or if symptoms of pancreatitis occur (see section 4.8 "Undesirable effects"). Levels in excess of 800mg/dL or 9mmol/L are sometimes associated with acute pancreatitis, which may be fatal.

Gastrointestinal disorders

Isotretinoin has been associated with inflammatory bowel disease (inlcuding regional ileitis) in patients without a prior history of intestinal disorders. Patients experiencing severe (haemorrhagic) diarrhoea should discontinue isotretinoin immediately. Patients with rare hereditary problems of fructose intolerance should not take this medicine.

Allergic reactions

Anaphylactic reactions have been rarely reported, in some cases after previous topical exposure to retinoids. Allergic cutaneous reactions are reported infrequently. Serious cases of allergic vasculitis, often with purpura (bruises and red patches) of the extremities and extracutaneous involvement have been reported. Severe allergic reactions necessitate interruption of therapy and careful monitoring.

High Risk Patients

In patients with diabetes, obesity, alcoholism or a lipid metabolism disorder undergoing treatment with isotretinoin, more frequent checks of serum values for lipids and/or blood glucose may be necessary. Elevated fasting blood sugars have been reported, and new cases of diabetes have been diagnosed during isotretinoin therapy.

4.5 Interaction with other medicinal products and other forms of Interaction

Patients should not take vitamin A as concurrent medication due to the risk of developing hypervitaminosis A.

Cases of benign intracranial hypertension (pseudotumor cerebri) have been reported with concomitant use of isotretinoin and tetracyclines. Therefore, concomitant treatment with tetracyclines must be avoided (see section 4.3 "Contraindications" and section 4.4 "Special warnings and special precautions for use").

4.6 Pregnancy and lactation

Pregnancy is an absolute contraindication to treatment with isotretinoin (see section 4.3 "Contraindications"). If pregnancy does occur in spite of these precautions during treatment with isotretinoin or in the month following, there is a great risk of very severe and serious malformation of the foetus.

The foetal malformations associated with exposure to isotretinoin include central nervous system abnormalities (hydrocephalus, cerebellar malformation/abnormalities, microcephaly), facial dysmorphia, cleft palate, external ear abnormalities (absence of external ear, small or absent external auditory canals), eye abnormalities (microphthalmia), cardiovascular abnormalities (conotruncal malformations such as tetralogy of Fallot, transposition of great vessels, septal defects), thymus gland abnormality and parathyroid gland abnormalities. There is also an increased incidence of spontaneous abortion.

If pregnancy occurs in a woman treated with isotretinoin, treatment must be stopped and the patient should be referred to a physician specialised or experienced in teratology for evaluation and advice.

Lactation:

Isotretinoin is highly lipophilic, therefore the passage of isotretinoin into human milk is very likely. Due to the potential for adverse effects in the mother and exposed child, the use of isotretinoin is contraindicated in nursing mothers.

4.7 Effects on ability to drive and use machines

A number of cases of decreased night vision have occurred during isotretinoin therapy and in rare instances have persisted after therapy (see section 4.4 "Special warnings and special precautions for use" and section 4.8 "Undesirable effects"). Because the onset in some patients was sudden, patients should be advised of this potential problem and warned to be cautious when driving or operating machines.

4.8 Undesirable effects

The following symptoms are the most commonly reported undesirable effects with isotretinoin: dryness of the mucosa e.g. of the lips, cheilitis, the nasal mucosa, epistaxis, and the eyes, conjunctivitis, dryness of the skin. Some of the side effects associated with the use of isotretinoin are dose-related. The side effects are generally reversible after altering the dose or discontinuation of treatment, however some may persist after treatment has stopped.

(see Table 1)

4.9 Overdose

Isotretinoin is a derivative of vitamin A. Although the acute toxicity of isotretinoin is low, signs of hypervitaminosis A could appear in cases of accidental overdose. Manifestations of acute vitamin A toxicity include severe headache, nausea or vomiting, drowsiness, irritability and pruritus. Signs and symptoms of accidental or deliberate overdosage with isotretinoin would probably be similar. These symptoms would be expected to be reversible and to subside without the need for treatment.

5. PHARMACOLOGICAL PROPERTIES

5.1 Pharmacodynamic properties

Pharmacotherapeutic group: anti-acne preparations for systemic use

ATC code: D10BA01

Mechanism of action

Isotretinoin is a stereoisomer of all-trans retinoic acid (tretinoin). The exact mechanism of action of isotretinoin has not yet been elucidated in detail, but it has been established that the improvement observed in the clinical picture of severe acne is associated with suppression of sebaceous gland activity and a histologically demonstrated reduction in the size of the sebaceous glands. Furthermore, a dermal anti-inflammatory effect of isotretinoin has been established.

Efficacy

Hypercornification of the epithelial lining of the pilosebaceous unit leads to shedding of comeocytes into the duct and blockage by keratin and excess sebum. This is followed by formation of a comedone and, eventually, inflam-

Table 1

Infections:	
Very Rare (≤1/10 000)	Gram positive (mucocutaneous) bacterial infection
Blood and lymphatic system disorders:	
Very common (≥1/10)	Anaemia, Red blood cell sedimentation rate increased, Thrombocytopenia, Thrombocytosis
Common (≥1/100, <1/10)	Neutropenia
Very Rare (≤1/10000)	Lymphadenopathy
Immune system disorders:	
Rare (≥l/10000, <l/1000)	Allergic skin reaction, Anaphylactic reactions, Hypersensitivity
Metabolism and nutrition disorders:	
Very Rare (≤1/10000)	Diabetes mellitus, Hyperuricaemia
Psychiatric disorders:	
Rare (≥l/10000, <l/1000)	Depression
Very Rare (≤1/10000)	Abnormal behaviour. Psychotic disorder. Suicide attempt, Suicide
Nervous system disorders:	
Common (≥1/100, <1/10)	Headache
Very Rare (≤1/10 000)	Benign intracranial hypertension. Convulsions, Drowsiness
Eye disorders:	
Very common (≥1/10)	Blepharitis, Conjunctivitis, Dry eye. Eye irritation
Very Rare (≤1/10000)	Blurred vision, Cataract, Colour blindness (colour vision deficiencies). Contact lens intolerance, Corneal opacity, Decreased night vision, Keratitis, Papilloedema (as sign of benign intracranial hypertension). Photophobia
Ear and labyrinth disorders:	
Very Rare (≤1/10 000)	Hearing impaired
Vascular disorders:	
Very Rare (≤1/10000)	Vasculitis (for example Wegener's granulomatosis, allergic vasculitis)
Respiratory, thoracic and mediastinal disorders:	
Common (≥1/100, <1/10)	Epistaxis, Nasal dryness, Nasopharyngitis
Very Rare (≤1/10000)	Bronchospasm (particularly in patients with asthma), Hoarseness
Gastrointestinal disorders:	
Very Rare (≤1/10000)	Colitis, Ileitis, Dry throat, Gastrointestinal haemorrhage, haemorrhagic diarrhoea and inflammatory bowel disease, Nausea, Pancreatitis (see section 4.4 "Special warnings and special precautions for use")
Hepatobiliary disorders	
Very common (≥1/10)	Transaminase increased (see section 4.4 "Special warnings and special precautions for use")
Very Rare (≤1/10000)	Hepatitis
Skin and subcutaneous tissues disorders:	
Very common (≥1/10)	Cheilitis, Dermatitis, Dry skin. Localised exfoliation, Pruritus, Rash erythematous, Skin fragility (risk of frictional trauma)
Rare (≥l/10000, <l/1000)	Alopecia
Very Rare (≤1/10 000)	Acne fulminans. Acne aggravated (acne flare). Erythema (facial). Exanthema, Hair disorders, Hirsutism, Nail dystrophy, Paronychia, Photosensitivity reaction, Pyogenic granuloma. Skin hyperpigmentation, Sweating increased
Musculo-skeletal and connective tissue disorders:	
Very common (≥1/10)	Arthralgia, Myalgia, Back pain (particularly adolescent patients) bone density, Tendonitis
Very Rare (≤1/10 000)	Arthritis, Calcinosis (calcification of ligaments and tendons), Epiphyses premature fusion, Exostosis, (hyperostosis). Reduced bone density, Tendonitis
Renal and urinary disorders	
Very Rare (≤1/10 000)	Glomerulonephritis
General disorders and administration site conditions:	
Very Rare (≤1/10 000)	Granulation tissue (increased formation of). Malaise
Investigations:	
Very common (≥1/10)	Blood triglycerides increased, High density lipoprotein decreased
Common (≥1/100, <1/10)	Blood cholesterol increased. Blood glucose increased, Haematuria, Proteinuria
Very Rare (≤1/10000)	Blood creatine phosphokinase increased

The incidence of the adverse events was calculated from pooled clinical trial data involving 824 patients and from post-marketing data.

matory lesions. Isotretinoin inhibits proliferation of sebocytes and appears to act in acne by re-setting the orderly program of differentiation. Sebum is a major substrate for the growth of Propionibacterium acnes so that reduced sebum production inhibits bacterial colonisation of the duct.

5.2 Pharmacokinetic properties

Absorption

The absorption of isotretinoin from the gastro-intestinal tract is variable and dose-linear over the therapeutic range. The absolute bioavailability of isotretinoin has not been determined, since the compound is not available as an intravenous preparation for human use, but extrapolation from dog studies would suggest a fairly low and variable systemic bioavailability. When isotretinoin is taken with food, the bioavailability is doubled relative to fasting conditions.

Distribution

Isotretinoin is extensively bound to plasma proteins, mainly albumin (99.9%). The volume of distribution of isotretinoin in man has not been determined since isotretinoin is not available as an intravenous preparation for human use. In humans little information is available on the distribution of isotretinoin into tissue. Concentrations of isotretinoin in the epidermis are only half of those in serum. Plasma concentrations of isotretinoin are about 1.7 times those of whole blood due to poor penetration of isotretinoin into red blood cells.

Metabolism

After oral administration of isotretinoin, three major metabolites have been identified in plasma: 4-oxo-isotretinoin, tretinoin, (all-trans retinoic acid), and 4-oxo-tretinoin. These metabolites have shown biological activity in several in vitro tests. 4-oxo-isotretinoin has been shown in a clinical study to be a significant contributor to the activity of isotretinoin (reduction in sebum excretion rate despite no effect on plasma levels of isotretinoin and tretinoin). Other minor metabolites includes glucuronide conjugates. The major metabolite is 4-oxo-isotretinoin with plasma concentrations at steady state, that are 2.5 times higher than those of the parent compound.

Isotretinoin and tretinoin (all-trans retinoic acid) are reversibly metabolised (interconverted), and the metabolism of tretinoin is therefore linked with that of isotretinoin. It has been estimated that 20-30% of an isotretinoin dose is metabolised by isomerisation.

Enterohepatic circulation may play a significant role in the pharmacokinetics of isotretinoin in man. In vitro metabolism studies have demonstrated that several CYP enzymes are involved in the metabolism of isotretinoin to 4-oxo-isotretinoin and tretinoin. No single isoform appears to have a predominant role. Isotretinoin and its metabolites do not significantly affect CYP activity.

Elimination

After oral administration of radiolabelled isotretinoin approximately equal fractions of the dose were recovered in urine and faeces. Following oral administration of isotretinoin, the terminal elimination half-life of unchanged drug in patients with acne has a mean value of 19 hours. The terminal elimination half-life of 4-oxo-isotretinoin is longer, with a mean value of 29 hours.

Isotretinoin is a physiological retinoid and endogenous retinoid concentrations are reached within approximately two weeks following the end of isotretinoin therapy.

Pharmacokinetics in special populations

Since isotretinoin is contraindicated in patients with hepatic impairment, limited information on the kinetics of isotretinoin is available in this patient population. Renal failure does not significantly reduce the plasma clearance of isotretinoin or 4-oxo-isotretinoin.

5.3 Preclinical safety data

Acute toxicity

The acute oral toxicity of isotretinoin was determined in various animal species. LD50 is approximately 2000 mg/kg in rabbits, approximately 3000 mg/kg in mice, and over 4000 mg/kg in rats.

Chronic toxicity

A long-term study in rats over 2 years (isotretinoin dosage 2, 8 and 32 mg/kg/d) produced evidence of partial hair loss and elevated plasma triglycerides in the higher dose groups. The side effect spectrum of isotretinoin in the rodent thus closely resembles that of vitamin A, but does not include the massive tissue and organ calcifications observed with vitamin A in the rat. The liver cell changes observed with vitamin A did not occur with isotretinoin.

All observed side effects of hypervitaminosis A syndrome were spontaneously reversible after withdrawal of isotretinoin. Even experimental animals in a poor general state had largely recovered within 1-2 weeks.

Teratogenicity

Like other vitamin A derivatives, isotretinoin has been shown in animal experiments to be teratogenic and embryotoxic.

Due to the teratogenic potential of isotretinoin there are therapeutic consequences for the administration to women of a childbearing age (see section 4.3 "Contraindications", section 4.4 "Special warnings and special precautions for use" and section 4.6 "Pregnancy and lactation").

Fertility

Isotretinoin, in therapeutic dosages, does not affect the number, motility and morphology of sperm and does not jeopardise the formation and development of the embryo on the part of the men taking isotretinoin.

Mutagenicity

Isotretinoin has not been shown to be mutagenic nor carcinogenic in in vitro or in vivo animal tests respectively.

6. PHARMACEUTICAL PARTICULARS

6.1 List of excipients

Capsule contents:

refined soya-bean oil

yellow beeswax

hydrogenated soya-bean oil

partially hydrogenated vegetable oil.

Capsule shell:

Gelatin

Glycerol

titanium dioxide E171

ferrous oxide red E172

ferrous oxide yellow E172

Printing ink:

Brilliant Blue FCF Dye

sorbitol

maltitol

phosphatidylcholine

lysophosphatidylcholine.

6.2 Incompatibilities

Not applicable

6.3 Shelf life

Two years

6.4 Special precautions for storage

Do not store above 25°C. Store in the original container.

6.5 Nature and contents of container

PVC/PE/PVdC aluminium blisters in cardboard carton containing 56 capsules

6.6 Instructions for use and handling

Not applicable

7. MARKETING AUTHORISATION HOLDER

Beacon Pharmaceuticals Ltd.

85, High Street

Tunbridge Wells

Kent TN1 1YG

8. MARKETING AUTHORISATION NUMBER(S)

PL 18157/0007

9. DATE OF FIRST AUTHORISATION/RENEWAL OF THE AUTHORISATION

18th October 2004

10. DATE OF REVISION OF THE TEXT

10th June 2005

Isotretinoin 5mg capsules

(Beacon Pharmaceuticals)

1. NAME OF THE MEDICINAL PRODUCT

Isotretinoin 5mg Capsules

2. QUALITATIVE AND QUANTITATIVE COMPOSITION

Each capsule contains 5mg isotretinoin

For excipients, see section 6.1

3. PHARMACEUTICAL FORM

Soft capsules.

Red/orange soft gelatin capsules marked 'P5'

4. CLINICAL PARTICULARS

4.1 Therapeutic indications

Isotretinoin capsules are indicated for the treatment of severe forms of acne (such as nodular or conglobate acne or acne at risk of permanent scarring), resistant to adequate courses of standard therapy with systemic antibacterials and topical therapy.

4.2 Posology and method of administration

Isotretinoin should only be prescribed by or under the supervision of physicians with expertise in the use of systemic retinoids for the treatment of severe acne and a full understanding of the risks of isotretinoin therapy and monitoring requirements.

The capsules should be taken with food once or twice daily.

Adults including adolescents and the elderly:

Isotretinoin therapy should be started at a dose of 0.5 mg/kg daily. The therapeutic response to isotretinoin and some of the adverse effects are dose-related and vary between patients. This necessitates individual dosage adjustment during therapy. For most patients, the dose ranges from 0.5-1.0 mg/kg per day.

Long-term remission and relapse rates are more closely related to the total dose administered than to either duration of treatment or daily dose. It has been shown that no substantial additional benefit is to be expected beyond a cumulative treatment dose of 120-150 mg/kg. The duration of treatment will depend on the individual daily dose. A treatment course of 16-24 weeks is normally sufficient to achieve remission.

In the majority of patients, complete clearing of the acne is obtained with a single treatment course. In the event of a definite relapse a further course of isotretinoin therapy may be considered using the same daily dose and cumulative treatment dose. As further improvement of the acne can be observed up to 8 weeks after discontinuation of treatment, a further course of treatment should not be considered until at least this period has elapsed.

Patients with severe renal insufficiency

In patients with severe renal insufficiency treatment should be started at a lower dose (e.g.10 mg/day). The dose should then be increased up to 1 mg/kg/day or until the patient is receiving the maximum tolerated dose (see section 4.4 "Special warnings and special precautions for use").

Children

Isotretinoin is not indicated for the treatment of prepubertal acne and is not recommended in patients less than 12 years of age.

Patients with intolerance

In patients who show severe intolerance to the recommended dose, treatment may be continued at a lower dose with the consequences of a longer therapy duration and a higher risk of relapse. In order to achieve the maximum possible efficacy in these patients the dose should normally be continued at the highest tolerated dose.

4.3 Contraindications

Isotretinoin is contraindicated in women who are pregnant or breastfeeding.

(see section 4.6 "Pregnancy and lactation").

Isotretinoin is contraindicated in women of childbearing potential unless all of the conditions of the Pregnancy Prevention Programme are met (see section 4.4 "Special warnings and special precautions for use").

Isotretinoin is also contraindicated in patients

With hepatic insufficiency

With excessively elevated blood lipid values

With hypervitaminosis A

With hypersensitivity to isotretinoin or to any of the excipients (the medicine contains hydrogenated soya-bean oil and refined soya-bean oil).

Receiving concomitant treatment with tetracyclines (see section 4.5 "Interaction with other medicinal products and other forms of interactions")

4.4 Special warnings and special precautions for use

Pregnancy Prevention Programme

This medicinal product is TERATOGENIC

Isotretinoin is contraindicated in women of childbearing potential unless all of the following conditions of the Pregnancy Prevention Programme are met:

She has severe acne (such as nodular or conglobate acne or acne at risk of permanent scarring) resistant to adequate courses of standard therapy with systemic antibacterials and topical therapy (see section 4.1 "Therapeutic indications").

She understands the teratogenic risk.

She understands the need for rigorous follow-up, on a monthly basis.

She understands and accepts the need for effective contraception, without interruption, 1 month before starting treatment, throughout the duration of treatment and 1 month after the end of treatment. At least one and preferably two complementary forms of contraception including a barrier method should be used.

Even if she has amenorrhea she must follow all of the advice on effective contraception.

She should be capable of complying with effective contraceptive measures.

She is informed and understands the potential consequences of pregnancy and the need to rapidly consult if there is a risk of pregnancy.

She understands the need and accepts to undergo pregnancy testing before, during and 5 weeks after the end of treatment.

She has acknowledged that she has understood the hazards and necessary precautions associated with the use of isotretinoin.

These conditions also concern women who are not currently sexually active unless the prescriber considers that there are compelling reasons to indicate that there is no risk of pregnancy.

The prescriber must ensure that:

The patient complies with the conditions for pregnancy prevention as listed above, including confirmation that she has an adequate level of understanding.

The patient has acknowledged the aforementioned conditions.

The patient has used at least one and preferably two methods of effective contraception including a barrier method for at least 1 month prior to starting treatment and is continuing to use effective contraception throughout the treatment period and for at least 1 month after cessation of treatment.

Negative pregnancy test results have been obtained before, during and 5 weeks after the end of treatment. The dates and results of pregnancy tests should be documented.

Contraception

Female patients must be provided with comprehensive information on pregnancy prevention and should be referred for contraceptive advice if they are not using effective contraception.

As a minimum requirement, female patients at potential risk of pregnancy must use at least one effective method of contraception. Preferably the patient should use two complementary forms of contraception including a barrier method. Contraception should be continued for at least 1 month after stopping treatment with isotretinoin, even in patients with amenorrhea.

Pregnancy testing

According to local practice, medically supervised pregnancy tests with a minimum sensitivity of 25mIU/mL are recommended to be performed in the first 3 days of the menstrual cycle, as follows.

Prior to starting therapy:

In order to exclude the possibility of pregnancy prior to starting contraception, it is recommended that an initial medically supervised pregnancy test should be performed and its date and result recorded. In patients without regular menses, the timing of this pregnancy test should reflect the sexual activity of the patient and should be undertaken approximately 3 weeks after the patient last had unprotected sexual intercourse. The prescriber should educate the patient about contraception.

A medically supervised pregnancy test should also be performed during the consultation when isotretinoin is prescribed or in the 3 days prior to the visit to the prescriber, and should have been delayed until the patient had been using effective contraception for at least 1 month. This test should ensure the patient is not pregnant when she starts treatment with isotretinoin.

Follow-up visits

Follow-up visits should be arranged at 28 day intervals. The need for repeated medically supervised pregnancy tests every month should be determined according to local practice including consideration of the patient's sexual activity and recent menstrual history (abnormal menses, missed periods or amenorrhea). Where indicated, follow-up pregnancy tests should be performed on the day of the prescribing visit or in the 3 days prior to the visit to the prescriber.

End of treatment

Five weeks after stopping treatment, women should undergo a final pregnancy test to exclude pregnancy.

Prescribing and dispensing restrictions

Prescriptions of isotretinoin for women of childbearing potential should be limited to 30 days of treatment and continuation of treatment requires a new prescription. Ideally, pregnancy testing, issuing a prescription and dispensing of isotretinoin should occur on the same day. Dispensing of isotretinoin should be completed within a maximum of 7 days of the prescription.

Male patients

The available data suggest that the level of maternal exposure from the semen of the patients receiving isotretinoin is not of sufficient magnitude to be associated with the teratogenic effects of isotretinoin.

Male patients should be reminded that they must not share their medication with anyone, particularly not females.

Additional precautions

Patients should be instructed never to give this medicinal product to another person and to return any unused capsules to their pharmacist at the end of treatment.

Patients should not donate blood during therapy and for 1 month following discontinuation of isotretinoin because of the potential risk to the foetus of a pregnant transfusion recipient.

Educational material

In order to assist prescribers, pharmacists and patients in avoiding foetal exposure to isotretinoin the Marketing Authorisation Holder will provide educational material to reinforce the warnings about the teratogenicity of isotretinoin, to provide advice on contraception before therapy is started and to provide guidance on the need for pregnancy testing.

Full patient information about the teratogenic risk and the strict pregnancy prevention measures as specified in the Pregnancy Prevention Programme should be given by the physician to all patients, both male and female.

Psychiatric disorders

Depression, psychotic symptoms and, rarely, suicide attempts and suicide have been reported in patients treated with isotretinoin (see section 4.8 "Undesirable effects"). Particular care needs to be taken in patients with a history of depression and all patients should be monitored for signs of depression and referred for appropriate treatment if necessary. However, discontinuation of isotretinoin may be insufficient to alleviate symptoms and therefore further psychiatric or psychological evaluation may be necessary.

Skin and subcutaneous tissues disorders

Acute exacerbation of acne is occasionally seen during the initial period but this subsides with continued treatment, usually within 7-10 days, and usually does not require dose adjustment.

Exposure to intense sunlight or to UV rays should be avoided. Where necessary a sun-protection product with a high protection factor of at least SPF 15 should be used.

Aggressive chemical dermabrasion and cutaneous laser treatment should be avoided in patients on isotretinoin for a period of 5-6 months after the end of the treatment because of the risk of hypertrophic scarring in atypical areas and more rarely post inflammatory hyper or hypopigmentation in treated areas. Wax depilation should be avoided in patients on isotretinoin for at least a period of 6 months after treatment because of the risk of epidermal stripping.

Concurrent administration of isotretinoin with topical keratolytic or exfoliative anti-acne agents should be avoided as local irritation may increase.

Patients should be advised to use a skin moisturising ointment or cream and a lip balm from the start of treatment as isotretinoin is likely to cause dryness of the skin and lips.

Eye disorders

Dry eyes, corneal opacities, decreased night vision and keratitis usually resolve after discontinuation of therapy. Dry eyes can be helped by the application of a lubricating eye ointment or by the application of tear replacement therapy. Intolerance to contact lenses may occur which may necessitate the patient to wear glasses during treatment.

Decreased night vision has also been reported and the onset in some patients was sudden (see section 4.7 "Effects on ability to drive and to use machines"). Patients experiencing visual difficulties should be referred for an expert ophthalmological opinion. Withdrawal of isotretinoin may be necessary.

Musculo-skeletal and connective tissue disorders

Myalgia, arthralgia and increased serum creatine phosphokinase values have been reported in patients receiving isotretinoin, particularly in those undertaking vigorous physical activity (see section 4.8 "Undesirable effects").

Bone changes including premature epiphyseal closure, hyperostosis, and calcification of tendons and ligaments have occurred after several years of administration at very high doses for treating disorders of keratinisation. The dose levels, duration of treatment and total cumulative dose in these patients generally far exceeded those recommended for the treatment of acne.

Benign intracranial hypertension

Cases of benign intracranial hypertension have been reported, some of which involved concomitant use of tetracyclines (see sections 4.3 "Contraindications" and 4.5 "Interactions with other medicinal products and other forms of interaction"). Signs and symptoms of benign intracranial hypertension include headache, nausea and vomiting, visual disturbances and papilloedema. Patients who develop benign intracranial hypertension should discontinue isotretinoin immediately.

Hepatobiliary disorders

Liver enzymes should be checked before treatment, 1 month after the start of treatment, and subsequently at 3 monthly intervals unless more frequent monitoring is clinically indicated. Transient and reversible increases in liver transaminases have been reported. In many cases these changes have been within the normal range and values have returned to baseline levels during treatment. However, in the event of persistent clinically relevant elevation of transaminase levels, reduction of the dose or discontinuation of treatment should be considered.

Renal insufficiency

Renal insufficiency and renal failure do not affect the pharmacokinetics of isotretinoin. Therefore, isotretinoin can be given to patients with renal insufficiency. However, it is recommended that patients are started on a low dose and titrated up to the maximum tolerated dose (see section 4.2 "Posology and Method of Administration").

Lipid Metabolism

Serum lipids (fasting values) should be checked before treatment, 1 month after the start of treatment, and subsequently at 3 monthly intervals unless more frequent monitoring is clinically indicated. Elevated serum lipid values usually return to normal on reduction of the dose or discontinuation of treatment and may also respond to dietary measures.

Isotretinoin has been associated with an increase in plasma triglyceride levels. Isotretinoin should be discontinued if hypertriglyceridaemia cannot be controlled at an acceptable level or if symptoms of pancreatitis occur (see section 4.8 "Undesirable effects"). Levels in excess of 800mg/dL or 9mmol/L are sometimes associated with acute pancreatitis, which may be fatal.

Gastrointestinal disorders

Isotretinoin has been associated with inflammatory bowel disease (inlcuding regional ileitis) in patients without a prior history of intestinal disorders. Patients experiencing severe (haemorrhagic) diarrhoea should discontinue isotretinoin immediately. Patients with rare hereditary problems of fructose intolerance should not take this medicine.

Allergic reactions

Anaphylactic reactions have been rarely reported, in some cases after previous topical exposure to retinoids. Allergic cutaneous reactions are reported infrequently. Serious cases of allergic vasculitis, often with purpura (bruises and red patches) of the extremities and extracutaneous involvement have been reported. Severe allergic reactions necessitate interruption of therapy and careful monitoring.

High Risk Patients

In patients with diabetes, obesity, alcoholism or a lipid metabolism disorder undergoing treatment with isotretinoin, more frequent checks of serum values for lipids and/or blood glucose may be necessary. Elevated fasting blood sugars have been reported, and new cases of diabetes have been diagnosed during isotretinoin therapy.

4.5 Interaction with other medicinal products and other forms of Interaction

Patients should not take vitamin A as concurrent medication due to the risk of developing hypervitaminosis A.

Cases of benign intracranial hypertension (pseudotumor cerebri) have been reported with concomitant use of isotretinoin and tetracyclines. Therefore, concomitant treatment with tetracyclines must be avoided (see section 4.3 "Contraindications" and section 4.4 "Special warnings and special precautions for use").

4.6 Pregnancy and lactation

Pregnancy is an absolute contraindication to treatment with isotretinoin (see section 4.3 "Contraindications"). If pregnancy does occur in spite of these precautions during treatment with isotretinoin or in the month following, there is a great risk of very severe and serious malformation of the foetus.

The foetal malformations associated with exposure to isotretinoin include central nervous system abnormalities (hydrocephalus, cerebellar malformation/abnormalities, microcephaly), facial dysmorphia, cleft palate, external ear abnormalities (absence of external ear, small or absent external auditory canals), eye abnormalities (microphthalmia), cardiovascular abnormalities (conotruncal malformations such as tetralogy of Fallot, transposition of great vessels, septal defects), thymus gland abnormality and parathyroid gland abnormalities. There is also an increased incidence of spontaneous abortion.

If pregnancy occurs in a woman treated with isotretinoin, treatment must be stopped and the patient should be referred to a physician specialised or experienced in teratology for evaluation and advice.

Lactation:

Isotretinoin is highly lipophilic, therefore the passage of isotretinoin into human milk is very likely. Due to the potential for adverse effects in the mother and exposed child, the use of isotretinoin is contraindicated in nursing mothers.

4.7 Effects on ability to drive and use machines

A number of cases of decreased night vision have occurred during isotretinoin therapy and in rare instances have persisted after therapy (see section 4.4 "Special warnings and special precautions for use" and section 4.8 "Undesirable effects"). Because the onset in some patients was sudden, patients should be advised of this potential problem and warned to be cautious when driving or operating machines.

4.8 Undesirable effects

The following symptoms are the most commonly reported undesirable effects with isotretinoin:dryness of the mucosa e.g. of the lips, cheilitis, the nasal mucosa, epistaxis, and the eyes, conjunctivitis, dryness of the skin. Some of the side effects associated with the use of isotretinoin are dose-related. The side effects are generally reversible after altering the dose or discontinuation of treatment, however some may persist after treatment has stopped.

(see Table 1 on next page)

4.9 Overdose

Isotretinoin is a derivative of vitamin A. Although the acute toxicity of isotretinoin is low, signs of hypervitaminosis A could appear in cases of accidental overdose. Manifestations of acute vitamin A toxicity include severe headache, nausea or vomiting, drowsiness, irritability and pruritus. Signs and symptoms of accidental or deliberate overdosage with isotretinoin would probably be similar. These symptoms would be expected to be reversible and to subside without the need for treatment.

5. PHARMACOLOGICAL PROPERTIES

5.1 Pharmacodynamic properties

Pharmacotherapeutic group: anti-acne preparations for systemic use

ATC code: D10BA01

Table 1

Infections:	
Very Rare (≤1/10 000)	Gram positive (mucocutaneous) bacterial infection
Blood and lymphatic system disorders:	
Very common (≥1/10)	Anaemia, Red blood cell sedimentation rate increased, Thrombocytopenia, Thrombocytosis
Common (≥1/100, <1/10)	Neutropenia
Very Rare (≤1/10000)	Lymphadenopathy
Immune system disorders:	
Rare (≥1/10 000, <1/1000)	Allergic skin reaction, Anaphylactic reactions, Hypersensitivity
Metabolism and nutrition disorders:	
Very Rare (≤1/10000)	Diabetes mellitus, Hyperuricaemia
Psychiatric disorders:	
Rare (≤1/10 000, <1/1000)	Depression
Very Rare (≤1/10000)	Abnormal behaviour. Psychotic disorder. Suicide attempt, Suicide
Nervous system disorders:	
Common (≥1/100, <1/10)	Headache
Very Rare (≤1/10 000)	Benign intracranial hypertension. Convulsions, Drowsiness
Eye disorders:	
Very common (≥1/10)	Blepharitis, Conjunctivitis, Dry eye. Eye irritation
Very Rare (≤1/10000)	Blurred vision, Cataract, Colour blindness (colour vision deficiencies). Contact lens intolerance, Corneal opacity, Decreased night vision, Keratitis, Papilloedema (as sign of benign intracranial hypertension). Photophobia
Ear and labyrinth disorders:	
Very Rare (≤1/10 000)	Hearing impaired
Vascular disorders:	
Very Rare (≤1/10000)	Vasculitis (for example Wegener's granulomatosis, allergic vasculitis)
Respiratory, thoracic and mediastinal disorders:	
Common (≥1/100, <1/10)	Epistaxis, Nasal dryness, Nasopharyngitis
Very Rare (≤1/10000)	Bronchospasm (particularly in patients with asthma), Hoarseness
Gastrointestinal disorders:	
Very Rare (≤1/10000)	Colitis, Ileitis, Dry throat, Gastrointestinal haemorrhage, haemorrhagic diarrhoea and inflammatory bowel disease, Nausea, Pancreatitis (see section 4.4 "Special warnings and special precautions for use")
Hepatobiliary disorders	
Very common (≥1/10)	Transaminase increased (see section 4.4 "Special warnings and special precautions for use")
Very Rare (≤1/10000)	Hepatitis
Skin and subcutaneous tissues disorders:	
Very common (≥1/10)	Cheilitis, Dermatitis, Dry skin. Localised exfoliation, Pruritus, Rash erythematous, Skin fragility (risk of frictional trauma)
Rare(≥1/10000,<1/1000)	Alopecia
Very Rare (≤1/10 000)	Acne fulminans. Acne aggravated (acne flare). Erythema (facial). Exanthema, Hair disorders, Hirsutism, Nail dystrophy, Paronychia, Photosensitivity reaction, Pyogenic granuloma. Skin hyperpigmentation, Sweating increased
Musculo-skeletal and connective tissue disorders:	
Very common (≥1/10)	Arthralgia, Myalgia, Back pain (particularly adolescent patients) bone density, Tendonitis
Very Rare (≤1/10 000)	Arthritis, Calcinosis (calcification of ligaments and tendons), Epiphyses premature fusion, Exostosis, (hyperostosis). Reduced bone density, Tendonitis
Renal and urinary disorders	
Very Rare (≤1/10 000)	Glomerulonephritis
General disorders and administration site conditions:	
Very Rare (≤1/10 000)	Granulation tissue (increased formation of). Malaise
Investigations:	
Very common (≥1/10)	Blood triglycerides increased, High density lipoprotein decreased
Common (≥1/100, <1/10)	Blood cholesterol increased. Blood glucose increased, Haematuria, Proteinuria
Very Rare (≤1/10000)	Blood creatine phosphokinase increased

The incidence of the adverse events was calculated from pooled clinical trial data involving 824 patients and from post-marketing data.

Mechanism of action

Isotretinoin is a stereoisomer of all-trans retinoic acid (tretinoin). The exact mechanism of action of isotretinoin has not yet been elucidated in detail, but it has been established that the improvement observed in the clinical picture of severe acne is associated with suppression of sebaceous gland activity and a histologically demonstrated reduction in the size of the sebaceous glands. Furthermore, a dermal anti-inflammatory effect of isotretinoin has been established.

Efficacy

Hypercornification of the epithelial lining of the pilosebaceous unit leads to shedding of comeocytes into the duct and blockage by keratin and excess sebum. This is followed by formation of a comedone and, eventually, inflammatory lesions. Isotretinoin inhibits proliferation of sebocytes and appears to act in acne by re-setting the orderly program of differentiation. Sebum is a major substrate for the growth of Propionibacterium acnes so that reduced sebum production inhibits bacterial colonisation of the duct.

5.2 Pharmacokinetic properties

Absorption

The absorption of isotretinoin from the gastro-intestinal tract is variable and dose-linear over the therapeutic range. The absolute bioavailability of isotretinoin has not been determined, since the compound is not available as an intravenous preparation for human use, but extrapolation from dog studies would suggest a fairly low and variable systemic bioavailability. When isotretinoin is taken with food, the bioavailability is doubled relative to fasting conditions.

Distribution

Isotretinoin is extensively bound to plasma proteins, mainly albumin (99.9%). The volume of distribution of isotretinoin in man has not been determined since isotretinoin is not available as an intravenous preparation for human use. In humans little information is available on the distribution of isotretinoin into tissue. Concentrations of isotretinoin in the epidermis are only half of those in serum. Plasma concentrations of isotretinoin are about 1.7 times those of whole blood due to poor penetration of isotretinoin into red blood cells.

Metabolism

After oral administration of isotretinoin, three major metabolites have been identified in plasma: 4-oxo-isotretinoin, tretinoin, (all-trans retinoic acid), and 4-oxo-tretinoin. These metabolites have shown biological activity in several in vitro tests. 4-oxo-isotretinoin has been shown in a clinical study to be a significant contributor to the activity of isotretinoin (reduction in sebum excretion rate despite no effect on plasma levels of isotretinoin and tretinoin). Other minor metabolites includes glucuronide conjugates. The major metabolite is 4-oxo-isotretinoin with plasma concentrations at steady state, that are 2.5 times higher than those of the parent compound.

Isotretinoin and tretinoin (all-trans retinoic acid) are reversibly metabolised (interconverted), and the metabolism of tretinoin is therefore linked with that of isotretinoin. It has been estimated that 20-30% of an isotretinoin dose is metabolised by isomerisation.

Enterohepatic circulation may play a significant role in the pharmacokinetics of isotretinoin in man. In vitro metabolism studies have demonstrated that several CYP enzymes are involved in the metabolism of isotretinoin to 4-oxo-isotretinoin and tretinoin. No single isoform appears to have a predominant role. Isotretinoin and its metabolites do not significantly affect CYP activity.

Elimination

After oral administration of radiolabelled isotretinoin approximately equal fractions of the dose were recovered in urine and faeces. Following oral administration of isotretinoin, the terminal elimination half-life of unchanged drug in patients with acne has a mean value of 19 hours. The terminal elimination half-life of 4-oxo-isotretinoin is longer, with a mean value of 29 hours.

Isotretinoin is a physiological retinoid and endogenous retinoid concentrations are reached within approximately two weeks following the end of isotretinoin therapy.

Pharmacokinetics in special populations

Since isotretinoin is contraindicated in patients with hepatic impairment, limited information on the kinetics of isotretinoin is available in this patient population. Renal failure does not significantly reduce the plasma clearance of isotretinoin or 4-oxo-isotretinoin.

5.3 Preclinical safety data

Acute toxicity

The acute oral toxicity of isotretinoin was determined in various animal species. LD50 is approximately 2000 mg/kg in rabbits, approximately 3000 mg/kg in mice, and over 4000 mg/kg in rats.

Chronic toxicity

A long-term study in rats over 2 years (isotretinoin dosage 2, 8 and 32 mg/kg/d) produced evidence of partial hair loss and elevated plasma triglycerides in the higher dose groups. The side effect spectrum of isotretinoin in the rodent thus closely resembles that of vitamin A, but does not include the massive tissue and organ calcifications observed with vitamin A in the rat. The liver cell changes observed with vitamin A did not occur with isotretinoin.

All observed side effects of hypervitaminosis A syndrome were spontaneously reversible after withdrawal of isotretinoin. Even experimental animals in a poor general state had largely recovered within 1-2 weeks.

Teratogenicity

Like other vitamin A derivatives, isotretinoin has been shown in animal experiments to be teratogenic and embryotoxic.

Due to the teratogenic potential of isotretinoin there are therapeutic consequences for the administration to women of a childbearing age (see section 4.3 "Contraindications", section 4.4 "Special warnings and special precautions for use" and section 4.6 "Pregnancy and lactation").

Fertility

Isotretinoin, in therapeutic dosages, does not affect the number, motility and morphology of sperm and does not jeopardise the formation and development of the embryo on the part of the men taking isotretinoin.

Mutagenicity

Isotretinoin has not been shown to be mutagenic nor carcinogenic in in vitro or in vivo animal tests respectively.

6. PHARMACEUTICAL PARTICULARS

6.1 List of excipients

Capsule contents:

refined soya-bean oil

yellow beeswax

hydrogenated soya-bean oil

partially hydrogenated vegetable oil.

Capsule shell:

Gelatin

Glycerol

titanium dioxide E171

ferrous oxide red E172

ferrous oxide yellow E172

Printing ink:

Brilliant Blue FCF Dye

sorbitol

maltitol

phosphatidylcholine

lysophosphatidylcholine.

6.2 Incompatibilities

Not applicable

6.3 Shelf life

Two years

6.4 Special precautions for storage

Do not store above 25°C. Store in the original container.

6.5 Nature and contents of container

PVC/PE/PVdC aluminium blisters in cardboard carton containing 56 capsules

6.6 Instructions for use and handling

Not applicable

7. MARKETING AUTHORISATION HOLDER

Beacon Pharmaceuticals Ltd.

85, High Street

Tunbridge Wells

Kent TN1 1YG

8. MARKETING AUTHORISATION NUMBER(S)

PL 18157/0005

9. DATE OF FIRST AUTHORISATION/RENEWAL OF THE AUTHORISATION

18th October 2004

10. DATE OF REVISION OF THE TEXT

10th June 2005

Isotrex Gel

(Stiefel Laboratories (UK) Limited)

1. NAME OF THE MEDICINAL PRODUCT

Isotrex Gel

2. QUALITATIVE AND QUANTITATIVE COMPOSITION

Isotretinoin 0.05% w/w

For excipients, see 6.1

3. PHARMACEUTICAL FORM

Gel for topical application

4. CLINICAL PARTICULARS

4.1 Therapeutic indications

Isotrex Gel is intended for use in the treatment of mild to moderate inflammatory and non-flammatory acne vulgaris.

4.2 Posology and method of administration

Apply Isotrex Gel sparingly over the whole affected area once or twice daily.

Patients should be advised that 6-8 weeks of treatment may be required before a therapeutic effect is observed.

The safety and efficacy of Isotrex Gel has not been established in children since acne vulgaris rarely presents in this age group.

There are no specific recommendations for use in the elderly. Acne vulgaris does not present in the elderly.

4.3 Contraindications

Isotrex Gel should not be used in patients with known hypersensitivity to any of the ingredients.

4.4 Special warnings and special precautions for use

Contact with the eyes, mouth and mucous membranes and with abraded or eczematous skin should be avoided. Care should be taken not to let the medication accumulate in skin fold areas and in the angles of the nose.

Application to sensitive areas of skin, such as the neck, should be made with caution.

Although tretinoin has not been shown to initiate or promote carcinogenesis in humans, tretinoin applied topically to albino hairless mice had resulted in a dose-related acceleration in ultraviolet-B radiation induced cutaneous tumours. The same author also observed the opposite effect in another study of low, non-irritating concentrations of tretinoin. The significance of these findings as related to man is unknown; however, caution should be observed in patients with a personal or family history of cutaneous epithelioma. Exposure to sunlight of areas treated with Isotrex Gel should be avoided or minimised. When exposure to strong sunlight cannot be avoided a sunscreen product and protective clothing should be used. Patients with sunburn should not use Isotrex Gel due to the possibility of increased sensitivity to sunlight. The use of sunlamps should be avoided during treatment.

4.5 Interaction with other medicinal products and other forms of Interaction

Concomitant topical medication should be used with caution during therapy with Isotrex Gel. Particular caution should be exercised when using preparations containing a peeling agent (for example Benzoyl Peroxide) or abrasive cleansers.

4.6 Pregnancy and lactation

Category B1.

There is inadequate evidence of the safety of topically applied isotretinoin in human pregnancy.

Isotretinoin has been associated with teratogenicity in humans when administered systemically. Reproduction studies conducted in rabbits using Isotrex Gel applied topically at up to 60 times the human dose have, however, revealed no harm to the foetus. The use of Isotrex gel should be avoided during pregnancy.

Use during lactation

Percutaneous absorption of isotretinoin from Isotrex Gel is negligible. It is not known, however, whether isotretinoin is excreted in human milk. Isotrex Gel should not be used during lactation.

4.7 Effects on ability to drive and use machines

Not applicable; the product is a topical preparation which acts locally at the site of application.

4.8 Undesirable effects

In normal use, Isotrex Gel may cause stinging, burning or irritation; erythema and peeling at the site of application may occur.

If undue irritation occurs, treatment should be interrupted temporarily and resumed once the reaction subsides. If irritation persists, treatment should be discontinued. Reactions will normally resolve on discontinuation of therapy.

4.9 Overdose

Acute overdosage of Isotrex Gel has not been reported to date. Accidental ingestion of Isotrex Gel resulting in overdosage of isotretinoin could be expected to induce symptoms of hypervitaminosis A. These include severe headaches, nausea or vomiting, drowsiness, irritability and pruritus.

5. PHARMACOLOGICAL PROPERTIES

5.1 Pharmacodynamic properties

Isotretinoin is structurally and pharmacologically related to Vitamin A which regulates epithelial cell growth and differentiation.

The pharmacological action of isotretinoin remains to be fully elucidated. When used systemically it suppresses sebaceous gland activity and reduces sebum production; it also affects comedogenesis, suppresses *Propionibacterium acnes* and reduces inflammation.

When applied topically, the mode of action of isotretinoin may be comparable with its stereoisomer, tretinoin. Tretinoin stimulates mitosis in the epidermis and reduces intercellular cohesion in the stratum corneum; it contests the hyperkeratosis characteristic of acne vulgaris and aids desquamation, preventing the formation of lesions. Tretinoin also mediates an increased production of less cohesive epidermal sebaceous cells, this appears to promote the initial expulsion and subsequent prevention of comedones.

5.2 Pharmacokinetic properties

Percutaneous absorption of isotretinoin from the gel is negligible. After applying 30g per day of isotretinoin 0.05% gel to acne of the face, chest and back for 30 days, HPLC assays for isotretinoin and tretinoin demonstrated non-detectable levels in the plasma samples (0.02μg/ml). Applying ^{14}C isotretinoin in a cream base on the healthy skim of human volunteers resulted in only 0.03% of the topically applied dose being recovered through estimating the radioactivity of blood, urine and faecal samples

5.3 Preclinical safety data

Not applicable. The relevant information is given in Section 4.

6. PHARMACEUTICAL PARTICULARS

6.1 List of excipients

Butylated Hydroxytoluene; Hydroxypropylcellulose; Ethanol

6.2 Incompatibilities

Not applicable.

6.3 Shelf life

a) For the product as packaged for sale

3 years

b) After first opening the container

Two months

6.4 Special precautions for storage

Store below 25°C

6.5 Nature and contents of container

Aluminium tube of 30g fitted with a screw cap.

6.6 Instructions for use and handling

There are no special instructions for use or handling of Isotrex Gel.

7. MARKETING AUTHORISATION HOLDER

Stiefel Laboratories (UK) Ltd

Holtspur Lane,

Wooburn Green,

High Wycombe,

Bucks HP10 0AU

8. MARKETING AUTHORISATION NUMBER(S)

PL 0174/0073

9. DATE OF FIRST AUTHORISATION/RENEWAL OF THE AUTHORISATION

January 1992

10. DATE OF REVISION OF THE TEXT

April 1997

Isotrexin Gel

(Stiefel Laboratories (UK) Limited)

1. NAME OF THE MEDICINAL PRODUCT

Isotrexin Gel

2. QUALITATIVE AND QUANTITATIVE COMPOSITION

Active Ingredients:

Isotretinoin 0.05% w/w

Erythromycin 2.00% w/w

1 g Gel contains:

Isotretinoin 0.5mg

Erythromycin 20.0mg

For excipients, see 6.1.

3. PHARMACEUTICAL FORM

Gel.

A pale yellow soft gel.

4. CLINICAL PARTICULARS

4.1 Therapeutic indications

Isotrexin is indicated for the topical treatment of moderate acne.

4.2 Posology and method of administration

Adults

Apply Isotrexin sparingly over the entire affected area once or twice daily, preferably after cleaning the skin.

Patients should be advised that, in some cases, six to eight weeks of treatment may be required before the full therapeutic effect is observed.

Patients should wash their hands after application of Isotrexin Gel.

The patient should be advised to avoid over-saturation with Isotrexin to the extent that excess medication could run into their eyes, and angles of the nose or other areas where treatment is not intended. Patients should be advised that if Isotrexin is applied excessively, no more rapid or better results would be obtained and marked redness, peeling or discomfort may occur. Should this occur accidentally or through over enthusiastic use application should be discontinued for a few days.

Use in children

Not established for prepubescent children, in whom acne vulgaris rarely presents.

Use in elderly

No specific recommendations as acne vulgaris does not present in the elderly.

4.3 Contraindications
Isotrexin should not be used in patients with known hypersensitivity to any of the ingredients.

Isotrexin should not be used in patients with acute eczema, rosacea and perioral dermatitis.

Isotrexin is contraindicated in pregnancy and lactation.

4.4 Special warnings and special precautions for use
Contact with the mouth, eyes and mucous membranes and with abraded or eczematous skin should be avoided. Application to sensitive areas of skin, such as the neck, should be made with caution. As Isotrexin may cause increased sensitivity to sunlight, deliberate or prolonged exposure to sunlight or sunlamps should be avoided or minimised. In case of "sunburn" reaction the treatment should be temporarily interrupted.

When exposure to sunlight cannot be avoided use of sunscreen products providing adequate UVB and UVA protection and protective clothing over treated areas is recommended. Following prolonged use of a peeling agent it is advisable to "rest" a patient's skin until the effects of the peeling subside before starting to use Isotrexin. When Isotrexin and peeling agents are alternated, irritancy or dermatitis may result and the frequency of application may have to be reduced.

4.5 Interaction with other medicinal products and other forms of Interaction
Concomitant topical antibiotics, medicated or abrasive soaps and cleaners, soaps and cosmetics that have a strong drying effect, and products with high concentrations of alcohol and/or astringents, should be used with caution as a cumulative irritant effect may occur. Particular caution should be exercised when using preparations containing a peeling agent (for example benzoyl peroxide.)

4.6 Pregnancy and lactation
The safety of Isotrexin for use in human pregnancy has not been established (see section 5.3).

Isotretinoin has been associated with teratogenicity in humans when administered systemically. Isotrexin is contraindicated in pregnant women and those intending to conceive. Treatment should be discontinued for one cycle prior to intended conception.

Use during lactation

Percutaneous absorption of isotretinoin from Isotrexin is negligible. However, as it is not known if isotretinoin is excreted into maternal milk, Isotrexin must not be used during lactation.

4.7 Effects on ability to drive and use machines
None.

4.8 Undesirable effects
Isotrexin may cause stinging, burning or irritation; erythema and peeling at the site of application may occur. These local effects usually subside with continued treatment. If undue irritation occurs, treatment should be interrupted temporarily and resumed once the reaction subsides. If irritation persists, treatment should be discontinued. Reactions will usually resolve on discontinuation of therapy.

Heightened susceptibility to either sunlight or other sources of UVB light has been reported (See 4.4).

Long-term use of erythromycin-containing preparations may rarely trigger gram-negative folliculitis. In this case the product should be withdrawn and therapy continued with an antibiotic-free monopreparation.

4.9 Overdose
Acute overdose of Isotrexin has not been reported to date. The isotretinoin and erythromycin components are not expected to cause problems on ingestion of the topical gel.

Excessive application of Isotrexin does not improve the results of treatment and may induce marked irritation e.g. erythema, peeling, pruritis etc.

5. PHARMACOLOGICAL PROPERTIES
5.1 Pharmacodynamic properties
ATC Code: D10A X30

Isotretinoin is structurally and pharmacologically related to vitamin A, which regulates epithelial cell growth and differentiation. The pharmacological action of isotretinoin has not been fully determined. When used systemically, it suppresses sebaceous gland activity and reduces sebum production; it also affects comedogenesis, inhibits follicular keratinisation, suppresses *Propionibacterium acnes* and reduces inflammation. It is thought that topically applied isotretinoin stimulates mitosis in the epidermis and reduces intercellular cohesion in the stratum corneum; contests the hyperkeratosis characteristic of acne vulgaris and aids desquamation, preventing the formation of lesions. It is also thought that it mediates an increased production of less cohesive epidermal sebaceous cells. This appears to promote the initial expulsion and subsequent prevention of comedones.

Studies in animal models have shown similar activity when isotretinoin is applied topically. Inhibition of sebum production by topical isotretinoin has been demonstrated in the ears and flank organs of the Syrian hamster. Application of isotretinoin to the ear for 15 days led to a 50% reduction in sebaceous gland size, and application to the flank organ resulted in a 40% reduction. Topical application of isotretinoin has also been shown to have an effect on the epidermal differentiation of rhino mouse skin. Reduction in the size of the utriculi or superficial cysts leading to normal looking follicles was a predominant feature of isotretinoin treatment and has been used to quantify the antikeratinising effects of isotretinoin.

Isotretinoin has topical anti-inflammatory actions. Topically applied isotretinoin inhibits leukotriene-B_4-induced migration of polymorphonuclear leukocytes, which accounts for topical isotretinoin's anti-inflammatory action. A significant inhibition was produced by topically applied isotretinoin but only a weak inhibition by topical tretinoin. This may account for the reduced rebound effect seen with topical isotretinoin when compared with topical tretinoin.

Erythromycin is a macrolide antibiotic which acts by interfering with bacterial protein synthesis by reversibly binding to ribosomal subunits, thereby inhibiting translocation of aminoacyl transfer-RNA and inhibiting polypeptide synthesis. In the treatment of acne, it is effective through reduction in the population of *Propionibacterium acnes* and through prevention of release of inflammatory mediators by the bacteria. Resistance of *P. acnes* to topical erythromycin can occur, but evidence exists that the combination of erythromycin and isotretinoin in Isotrexin is effective against erythromycin-resistant strains of *P. acnes*.

Isotrexin is effective in treating both inflammatory and non-inflammatory lesions. The isotretinoin component treats the comedonal phase of the disease. The erythromycin component is effective in the treatment of moderate inflammatory acne vulgaris.

5.2 Pharmacokinetic properties
Percutaneous absorption of isotretinoin and erythromycin from Isotrexin is negligible. In a maximised study of the topical absorption of the two components from Isotrexin in patients suffering from widespread acne, isotretinoin levels were shown to be only slightly raised from baseline levels (isotretinoin is normally present in plasma). Levels remained below 5 ng/ml, and were not increased in the presence of erythromycin when compared to topical isotretinoin alone. The levels of erythromycin were not detectable.

Under conditions of normal use in patients with acne, percutaneous absorption of the active components was negligible.

5.3 Preclinical safety data
Isotretinoin and erythromycin, the active ingredients in Isotrexin, are well-established pharmacopoeial substances which are regularly used in the topical and systemic treatment of acne vulgaris. Preclinical safety studies have not been conducted on Isotrexin, as an extensive range of toxicological studies has been conducted on isotretinoin and erythromycin as well as their respective topical formulations. A human patch test for irritation has shown the combination to be comparable to the application of either component alone, with an acceptably low potential for irritation.

Isotretinoin has been associated with teratogenicity in humans when administered systemically. However, reproduction studies conducted in rabbits using topical isotretinoin applied at up to 10 times the human therapeutic dose have revealed no harm to the foetus.

6. PHARMACEUTICAL PARTICULARS
6.1 List of excipients
Hydroxypropylcellulose,

Butylated Hydroxytoluene (BHT)

Anhydrous Ethanol

6.2 Incompatibilities
Not applicable.

6.3 Shelf life
2 years

6.4 Special precautions for storage
Do not store above 25°C.

6.5 Nature and contents of container
Internally lacquered membrane-sealed aluminium tubes fitted with a polypropylene screw-cap, packed into a carton. Pack size: 30g.

6.6 Instructions for use and handling
See section 4.2.

7. MARKETING AUTHORISATION HOLDER
Stiefel Laboratories (UK) Ltd

Holtspur Lane,

Wooburn Green,

High Wycombe,

Bucks HP10 0AU

8. MARKETING AUTHORISATION NUMBER(S)
PL 0174/0200

9. DATE OF FIRST AUTHORISATION/RENEWAL OF THE AUTHORISATION
26 March 1997 / 26 March 2002

10. DATE OF REVISION OF THE TEXT
May 2002

Isovorin
(Wyeth Pharmaceuticals)

1. NAME OF THE MEDICINAL PRODUCT
ISOVORIN*▼ Solution for Injection

2. QUALITATIVE AND QUANTITATIVE COMPOSITION
Calcium levofolinate (INN: calcium levofolinate) equivalent to 1.00% w/v (10mg/ml) of levoleucovorin (levofolinic acid).

The product is presented as vials containing 25mg, 50mg or 175mg of levofolinic acid (as calcium levofolinate) in 2.5ml, 5ml or 17.5ml of solution respectively.

3. PHARMACEUTICAL FORM
Solution for injection.

4. CLINICAL PARTICULARS
4.1 Therapeutic indications
4.1.1 Calcium Levofolinate Rescue
Calcium levofolinate is used to diminish the toxicity and counteract the action of folic acid antagonists such as methotrexate in cytotoxic therapy. This procedure is known as Calcium Levofolinate Rescue.

4.1.2 Advanced Colorectal Cancer - Enhancement of 5-Fluorouracil (5-FU) Cytotoxicity
Calcium levofolinate increases the thymine depleting effects of 5-FU resulting in enhanced cytotoxic activity. Combination regimens of 5-fluorouracil and levofolinate give greater efficacy compared to 5-FU given alone.

4.2 Posology and method of administration
For single use only.

4.2.1 Calcium Levofolinate Rescue
Adults, Children and the Elderly:

Calcium Levofolinate Rescue therapy should commence 24 hours after the beginning of methotrexate infusion. Dosage regimes vary depending upon the dose of methotrexate administered. In general, the calcium levofolinate should be administered at a dose of 7.5mg (approximately 5mg/m^2) every 6 hours for 10 doses by intramuscular injection, bolus intravenous injection or intravenous infusion, (refer to 4.2.2 for information concerning use of calcium levofolinate with infusion fluids). **Do not administer calcium levofolinate intrathecally.**

Where overdose of methotrexate is suspected, the dose of calcium levofolinate should be at least 50% of the offending dose of methotrexate and should be administered in the first hour. In the case of intravenous administration, no more than 160mg of calcium levofolinate should be injected per minute due to the calcium content of the solution.

In addition to calcium levofolinate administration, measures to ensure the prompt excretion of methotrexate are important as part of Calcium Levofolinate Rescue therapy. These measures include:

a. Alkalinisation of urine so that the urinary pH is greater than 7.0 before methotrexate infusion (to increase solubility of methotrexate and its metabolites).

b. Maintenance of urine output of 1800-2000 cc/m^2/24 hr by increased oral or intravenous fluids on days 2, 3 and 4 following methotrexate therapy.

c. Plasma methotrexate concentration, BUN and creatinine should be measured on days 2, 3 and 4.

These measures must be continued until the plasma methotrexate level is less than 10^{-7} molar (0.1μM).

Delayed methotrexate excretion may be seen in some patients. This may be caused by a third space accumulation (as seen in ascites or pleural effusion for example), renal insufficiency or inadequate hydration. Under such circumstances, higher doses of calcium levofolinate or prolonged administration may be indicated. Dosage and administration guidelines for these patients are given in Table 1. Patients who experience delayed early methotrexate elimination are likely to develop reversible renal failure.

(see Table 1 on next page)

4.2.2 Colorectal Cancer: Enhancement of 5-FU Cytotoxicity
Adults and the Elderly:

Administration: The 175mg in 17.5ml vial of Calcium Levofolinate Solution for Injection should be used to administer the high doses of calcium levofolinate required in combination regimens.

When used in combination regimens with 5-FU, calcium levofolinate should only be given by the intravenous route. The agents should not be mixed together. Each vial of calcium levofolinate 175mg contains 0.7mEq (0.35mmol) of calcium per vial and it is recommended that the solution is administered over not less than 3 minutes.

For intravenous infusion, the 175mg in 17.5ml Solution for Injection may be diluted with any of the following infusion fluids before use: Sodium Chloride 0.9%; Glucose 5%; Glucose 10%; Glucose 10% and Sodium Chloride 0.9% Injection; Compound Sodium Lactate Injection.

Calcium levofolinate should not be mixed together with 5-FU in the same infusion and, because of the risk of degradation, the giving set should be protected from light.

TABLE 1 Dosage and Administration Guidelines for Calcium Levofolinate Rescue

Clinical Situation	Laboratory Findings	Levofolinate Dosage and Duration
Normal Methotrexate Elimination	Serum methotrexate level approximately 10μM at 24 hours after administration, 1μM at 48 hours and less than 0.2μM at 72 hours.	7.5mg IM or IV every 6 hours for 60 hours (10 doses starting at 24 hours after start of methotrexate infusion).
Delayed Late Methotrexate Elimination	Serum methotrexate level remaining above 0.2μM at 72 hours, and more than 0.05μM at 96 hours after administration.	Continue 7.5mg IM or IV every 6 hours, until methotrexate level is less than 0.05μM.
Delayed Early Methotrexate Elimination and/or Evidence of Acute Renal Injury	Serum methotrexate level of 50μM or more at 24 hours or 5μM or more at 48 hours after administration, OR; a 100% or greater increase in serum creatinine level at 24 hours after methotrexate administration.	75mg IV every 3 hours, until methotrexate level is less than 1μM; then 7.5mg IV every 3 hours until methotrexate level is less than 0.05μM.

Dosage: Based on the available clinical evidence, the following regimen is effective in advanced colorectal carcinoma:

Calcium levofolinate given at a dose of 100mg/m^2 by slow intravenous injection, followed immediately by 5-FU at an initial dose of 370mg/m^2 by intravenous injection. The injection of levofolinate should not be given more rapidly than over 3 minutes because of the calcium content of the solution. This treatment is repeated daily for 5 consecutive days. Subsequent courses may be given after a treatment-free interval of 21-28 days.

For the above regimen, modification of the 5-FU dosage and the treatment-free interval may be necessary depending on patient condition, clinical response and dose limiting toxicity. A reduction of calcium levofolinate dosage is not required. The number of repeat cycles used is at the discretion of the clinician.

On the basis of the available data, no specific dosage modifications are recommended in the use of the combination regimen with 5-FU in the elderly. However, particular care should be taken when treating elderly or debilitated patients as these patients are at increased risk of severe toxicity with this therapy (See 'Warnings and Precautions').

Children:

There are no data available on the use of this combination in children.

4.3 Contraindications

Calcium levofolinate should not be used for the treatment of pernicious anaemia or other megaloblastic anaemias where vitamin B_{12} is deficient.

4.4 Special warnings and special precautions for use

Calcium levofolinate should only be used with methotrexate or 5-FU under the direct supervision of a clinician experienced in the use of cancer chemotherapeutic agents. When calcium levofolinate has been administered intrathecally, following intrathecal overdose of methotrexate, a death has been reported.

4.5 Interaction with other medicinal products and other forms of Interaction

Calcium levofolinate should not be given simultaneously with an anti-neoplastic folic acid antagonist, (e.g. methotrexate), to modify or abort clinical toxicity, as the therapeutic effect of the antagonist may be nullified. Concomitant calcium levofolinate will not however inhibit the antibacterial activity of other folic acid antagonists such as trimethoprim and pyrimethamine.

Folinates given in large amounts may counteract the antiepileptic effect of phenobarbitone, phenytoin and primidone and increase the frequency of seizures in susceptible patients.

Seizures and/or syncope have been reported rarely in cancer patients receiving leucovorin, usually in association with fluoropyrimidine administration and most commonly in those with CNS metastases or other predisposing factors; however a causal relationship has not been established.

4.6 Pregnancy and lactation

Reproduction studies have been performed in rats and rabbits at doses of at least 50 times the human dose. These studies have revealed no evidence of harm to the foetus due to calcium levofolinate. There are, however, no adequate and well controlled studies in pregnant women. Because animal reproduction studies are not always predictive of human response, calcium levofolinate should only be used in pregnant women if the potential benefit justifies the potential risk to the foetus.

It is not known whether calcium levofolinate is excreted in human milk. Because many drugs are excreted in human milk, caution should be exercised when calcium levofolinate is administered to a nursing mother.

4.7 Effects on ability to drive and use machines

None.

4.8 Undesirable effects

Adverse reactions to calcium levofolinate are rare but occasional pyrexial reactions and anaphylactoid/anaphylactic reactions (including shock) have been reported following parenteral administration.

In the combination regimen with 5-FU, the toxicity profile of 5-FU is enhanced by calcium levofolinate. The most common manifestations are leucopenia, mucositis, stomatitis and/or diarrhoea which may be dose limiting. When calcium levofolinate and 5-FU are used in the treatment of colorectal cancer, the 5-FU dosage must be reduced more in cases of toxicity than when 5-FU is used alone. Toxicities observed in patients treated with the combination are qualitatively similar to those observed in patients treated with 5-FU alone. Gastrointestinal toxicities are observed more commonly and may be more severe or even life threatening. In severe cases, treatment is the withdrawal of 5-FU and calcium levofolinate and provision of supportive intravenous therapy. Elderly or debilitated patients are at a greater risk of severe toxicity with this therapy.

4.9 Overdose

There have been no reported sequelae in patients who have received significantly more calcium levofolinate than the recommended dosage. There is no specific antidote. In cases of overdose, patients should be given appropriate supportive care. Should overdose of the combination of 5-FU with calcium levofolinate occur, the overdose instructions for 5-FU should be followed.

5. PHARMACOLOGICAL PROPERTIES

5.1 Pharmacodynamic properties

Levofolinate is the pharmacologically active isomer of 5-formyltetrahydrofolic acid. Levofolinate does not require reduction by the enzyme dihydrofolate reductase in order to participate in reactions utilising folates as a source of "one carbon" moieties. Levofolinate is actively and passively transported across cell membranes.

Administration of levofolinate can "rescue" normal cells and thereby prevent toxicity of folic acid antagonists such as methotrexate which act by inhibiting dihydrofolate reductase.

Levofolinate can enhance the therapeutic and toxic effects of fluoropyrimidines used in cancer therapy such as 5-fluorouracil. 5-fluorouracil is metabolised to 5-fluoro-2'-deoxyuridine-5'-monophosphate (FDUMP), which binds to and inhibits thymidylate synthase. Levofolinate is readily converted to another reduced folate, 5, 10-methylenetetrahydrofolate, which acts to stabilise the binding of FDUMP to thymidylate synthase and thereby enhances the inhibition of this enzyme.

Levofolinate is also effective in the treatment of megaloblastic anaemias due to folate deficiencies.

5.2 Pharmacokinetic properties

When levofolinate is injected intravenously it is 100% bioavailable.

The pharmacokinetics of levofolinate after intravenous administration of a 15mg dose were studied in healthy male volunteers. After rapid intravenous administration, serum total tetrahydrofolate (total-THF) concentrations reached a mean peak of 1722ng/ml. Serum levo-5-methyl-THF concentrations reached a mean peak of 275ng/ml and the mean time to peak concentration was 0.9 hours. The mean half-life for total-THF and levo-5-methyl-THF was 5.1 and 6.8 hours respectively.

The distribution and plasma levels of levofolinate following intramuscular administration have not been established.

The distribution in tissue and body fluids and protein binding have not been determined.

In vivo, levofolinate is converted to levo-5-methyltetrahydrofolic acid (levo-5-methyl-THF), the primary circulating form of active reduced folate. Levofolinate and levo-5-methyl-THF are polyglutamated intracellularly by the enzyme folylpolyglutamate synthetase. Folylpolyglutamates are active and participate in biochemical pathways that require reduced folate.

Levofolinate and levo-5-methyl-THF are excreted renally.

Due to the inherent lack of levofolinate toxicity, the influence of impaired renal or hepatic function on levofolinate disposition was not evaluated.

5.3 Preclinical safety data

The pre-clinical data raises no concerns for the clinical uses indicated.

6. PHARMACEUTICAL PARTICULARS

6.1 List of excipients

Sodium Chloride, Water for Injection, Hydrochloric Acid, Sodium Hydroxide

6.2 Incompatibilities

Calcium levofolinate should not be mixed together with 5-FU in the same intravenous injection or infusion.

6.3 Shelf life

24 months.

6.4 Special precautions for storage

Store ISOVORIN Solution for Injection under refrigerated conditions (2 - 8°C) in original containers. Protect from light.

Discard any unused products.

When ISOVORIN Solution for Injection is diluted with the recommended infusion fluids, the resulting solutions are intended for immediate use but may be stored for up to 24 hours under refrigerated conditions (2 - 8°C). Because of the risk of degradation, reconstituted solutions should be protected from light prior to use if necessary.

6.5 Nature and contents of container

Type I amber glass vials each containing the equivalent of 25mg, 50mg or 175mg of calcium levofolinate in 2.5ml, 5ml or 17.5ml of solution respectively. Isovorin is packed in boxes of 1 vial.

6.6 Instructions for use and handling

See sections 4.2 and 6.4.

7. MARKETING AUTHORISATION HOLDER

John Wyeth and Brother Limited trading as Wyeth Laboratories

Huntercombe Lane South

Taplow, Maidenhead

Berkshire

SL6 OPH

8. MARKETING AUTHORISATION NUMBER(S)

PL 0011/0235

9. DATE OF FIRST AUTHORISATION/RENEWAL OF THE AUTHORISATION

12/6/1998

10. DATE OF REVISION OF THE TEXT

July 2002

* Registered Trademark

Istin

(Pfizer Limited)

1. NAME OF THE MEDICINAL PRODUCT

ISTIN™

2. QUALITATIVE AND QUANTITATIVE COMPOSITION

Active Ingredient: amlodipine

The tablets contain amlodipine besilate (equivalent to 5mg and 10mg amlodipine)

3. PHARMACEUTICAL FORM

Tablet for oral administration

5mg tablets coded "ITN5" on one side and "PFIZER" on the other

10mg tablets coded "ITN10" on one side and "PFIZER" on the other

4. CLINICAL PARTICULARS

4.1 Therapeutic indications

Hypertension

Prophylaxis of chronic stable angina pectoris

Prinzmetal's (variant) angina when diagnosed by a cardiologist

In hypertensive patients, Istin has been used in combination with a thiazide diuretic, alpha blocker, beta-adrenoceptor blocking agent, or an angiotensin converting enzyme inhibitor. For angina, Istin may be used as monotherapy or in combination with other antianginal drugs in patients with angina that is refractory to nitrates and/or adequate doses of beta blockers.

Istin is well tolerated in patients with heart failure and a history of hypertension or ischaemic heart disease.

4.2 Posology and method of administration

In adults: For both hypertension and angina the usual initial dose is 5mg Istin once daily which may be increased to a maximum dose of 10mg depending on the individual patient's response.

No dose adjustment of Istin is required upon concomitant administration of thiazide diuretics, beta blockers, and angiotensin-converting enzyme inhibitors.

Use in children: Not recommended.

Use in the elderly: Istin, used at similar doses in elderly or younger patients, is equally well tolerated. Therefore normal dosage regimens are recommended.

Patients with hepatic impairment: See section 4.4 Special warnings and precautions for use.

Patients with renal impairment: Changes in amlodipine plasma concentrations are not correlated with degree of renal impairment, therefore the normal dosage is recommended. Amlodipine is not dialysable.

4.3 Contraindications

Istin is contra-indicated in patients with a known sensitivity to dihydropyridines, amlodipine or any of the excipients.

Istin should not be used in cardiogenic shock, clinically significant aortic stenosis, unstable angina (excluding Prinzmetal's angina).

Pregnancy and lactation

4.4 Special warnings and special precautions for use

Use in patients with Heart Failure: In a long-term, placebo controlled study (PRAISE-2) of Istin in patients with NYHA III and IV heart failure of nonischaemic aetiology, amlodipine was associated with increased reports of pulmonary oedema despite no significant difference in the incidence of worsening heart failure as compared to placebo. See section 5.1 "Pharmacodynamic Properties".

Use in patients with impaired hepatic function: As with all calcium antagonists, amlodipine's half-life is prolonged in patients with impaired liver function and dosage recommendations have not been established. The drug should therefore be administered with caution in these patients.

There are no data to support the use of Istin alone, during or within one month of a myocardial infarction.

The safety and efficacy of Istin in hypertensive crisis has not been established.

4.5 Interaction with other medicinal products and other forms of Interaction

Istin has been safely administered with thiazide diuretics, alpha-blockers, beta-blockers, angiotensin-converting enzyme inhibitors, long-acting nitrates, sublingual glyceryl trinitrate, non-steroidal anti-inflammatory drugs, antibiotics, and oral hypoglycaemic drugs.

In vitro data from studies with human plasma, indicate that amlodipine has no effect on protein binding of digoxin, phenytoin, warfarin or indomethacin.

Special Studies: Effect of other agents on amlodipine

Cimetidine: Co-administration of Istin with cimetidine did not alter the pharmacokinetics of Istin.

Grapefruit Juice: Co-administration of 240ml of grapefruit juice with a single oral dose of Istin 10mg in 20 healthy volunteers had no significant effect on the pharmacokinetics of Istin.

Sildenafil: When Istin and sildenafil were used in combination, each agent independently exerted its own blood pressure lowering effect.

Special Studies: Effect of amlodipine on other agents

Atorvastatin: Co-administration of multiple 10mg doses of Istin with 80mg of atorvastatin resulted in no significant change in the steady state pharmacokinetic parameters of atorvastatin.

Digoxin: Co-administration of Istin with digoxin did not change serum digoxin levels or digoxin renal clearance in normal volunteers.

Warfarin: In healthy male volunteers, the co-administration of Istin does not significantly alter the effect of warfarin on prothrombin response time. Co-administration of Istin with warfarin did not change the warfarin prothrombin response time.

Cyclosporin: Pharmacokinetic studies with cyclosporin have demonstrated that Istin does not significantly alter the pharmacokinetics of cyclosporin.

Drug/Laboratory test Interactions: None known.

4.6 Pregnancy and lactation

Although some dihydropyridine compounds have been found to be teratogenic in animals, data in the rat and rabbit for amlodipine provide no evidence for a teratogenic effect. There is, however, no clinical experience with the preparation in pregnancy or lactation. Accordingly, Istin should not be administered during pregnancy, or lactation, or to women of childbearing potential unless effective contraception is used.

4.7 Effects on ability to drive and use machines

Clinical experience with Istin indicates that therapy is unlikely to impair a patient's ability to drive or use machinery.

4.8 Undesirable effects

Adverse events that have been reported in amlodipine trials are categorised below, according to system organ class and frequency. Frequencies are defined as: very common (>10%); common (>1%, <10%); uncommon (>0.1%, <1%); rare (>0.01%, <0.1%) and very rare (<0.01%).

(see Table 1)

Table 1

Blood and the Lymphatic System Disorders	thrombocytopenia	Very Rare
Immune System Disorders	allergic reaction	Very Rare
Metabolism and Nutrition Disorders	hyperglycaemia	Very Rare
Psychiatric Disorders	insomnia, mood changes	Uncommon
Nervous System Disorders	somnolence, dizziness, headache	Common
	tremor, taste perversion, syncope, hypoaesthesia, paraesthesia	Uncommon
	peripheral neuropathy	Very Rare
Eye Disorders	visual disturbances	Uncommon
Ear and Labyrinth Disorders	tinnitus	Uncommon
Cardiac Disorders	palpitations	Common
	myocardial infarction, arrhythmia, ventricular tachycardia and atrial fibrillation)	Very Rare
Vascular Disorders	flushing	Common
	hypotension	Uncommon
	vasculitis	Very Rare
Respiratory, Thoracic and Mediastinal Disorders	dyspnoea, rhinitis	Uncommon
	coughing	Very Rare
Gastrointestinal Disorders	abdominal pain, nausea	Common
	vomiting, dyspepsia, altered bowel habits, dry mouth	Uncommon
	pancreatitis, gastritis, gingival hyperplasia	Very Rare
Hepato-biliary Disorders	hepatitis, jaundice and hepatic enzyme elevations (mostly consistent with cholestasis)	Very Rare
Skin and Subcutaneous Tissue Disorders	alopecia, purpura, skin discolouration, increased sweating, pruritus, rash	Uncommon
	angioedema, erythema multiforme, urticaria	Very Rare
Musculoskeletal and Connective Tissue Disorders	arthralgia, myalgia, muscle cramps, back pain	Uncommon
Renal and Urinary Disorders	micturition disorder, nocturia, increased urinary frequency	Uncommon
Reproductive System and Breast Disorders	impotence, gynaecomastia	Uncommon
General Disorders and Administration Site Conditions	oedema, fatigue	Common
	chest pain, asthenia, pain, malaise	Uncommon
Investigations	weight increase, weight decrease	Uncommon

4.9 Overdose

Available data suggest that gross overdosage could result in excessive peripheral vasodilatation and possibly reflex tachycardia. Marked and probably prolonged systemic hypotension up to and including shock with fatal outcome have been reported.

Administration of activated charcoal to healthy volunteers immediately or up to two hours after ingestion of amlodipine 10mg has been shown to significantly decrease amlodipine absorption. Gastric lavage may be worthwhile in some cases. Clinically significant hypotension due to Istin overdosage calls for active cardiovascular support including frequent monitoring of cardiac and respiratory function, elevation of extremities, and attention to circulating fluid volume and urine output. A vasoconstrictor may be helpful in restoring vascular tone and blood pressure, provided that there is no contraindication to its use. Intravenous calcium gluconate may be beneficial in reversing the effects of calcium channel blockade. Since Istin is highly protein-bound, dialysis is not likely to be of benefit.

5. PHARMACOLOGICAL PROPERTIES

5.1 Pharmacodynamic properties

Istin is a calcium ion influx inhibitor of the dihydropyridine group (slow channel blocker or calcium ion antagonist) and inhibits the transmembrane influx of calcium ions into cardiac and vascular smooth muscle.

The mechanism of the antihypertensive action of Istin is due to a direct relaxant effect on vascular smooth muscle. The precise mechanism by which Istin relieves angina has not been fully determined but Istin reduces total ischaemic burden by the following two actions.

1) Istin dilates peripheral arterioles and thus, reduces the total peripheral resistance (afterload) against which the heart works. Since the heart rate remains stable, this unloading of the heart reduces myocardial energy consumption and oxygen requirements.

2) The mechanism of action of Istin also probably involves dilatation of the main coronary arteries and coronary arterioles, both in normal and ischaemic regions. This dilatation increases myocardial oxygen delivery in patients with coronary artery spasm (Prinzmetal's or variant angina).

In patients with hypertension, once daily dosing provides clinically significant reductions of blood pressure in both the supine and standing positions throughout the 24 hour interval. Due to the slow onset of action, acute hypotension is not a feature of Istin administration.

In patients with angina, once daily administration of Istin increases total exercise time, time to angina onset, and time to 1mm ST segment depression, and decreases both angina attack frequency and glyceryl trinitrate tablet consumption.

Istin has not been associated with any adverse metabolic effects or changes in plasma lipids and is suitable for use in patients with asthma, diabetes, and gout.

Use in Patients with Heart Failure: Haemodynamic studies and exercise based controlled clinical trials in NYHA Class II-IV heart failure patients have shown that Istin did not lead to clinical deterioration as measured by exercise tolerance, left ventricular ejection fraction and clinical symptomatology.

A placebo controlled study (PRAISE) designed to evaluate patients in NYHA Class III-IV heart failure receiving digoxin, diuretics and ACE inhibitors has shown that Istin did not lead to an increase in risk of mortality or combined mortality and morbidity with heart failure.

In a follow-up, long term, placebo controlled study (PRAISE-2) of Istin in patients with NYHA III and IV heart failure without clinical symptoms or objective findings suggestive or underlying ischaemic disease, on stable doses of ACE inhibitors, digitalis, and diuretics, Istin had no effect on total cardiovascular mortality. In this same population Istin was associated with increased reports of pulmonary oedema despite no significant difference in the incidence of worsening heart failure as compared to placebo.

A randomized double-blind morbidity-mortality study called the Antihypertensive and Lipid-Lowering Treatment to Prevent Heart Attack Trial (ALLHAT) was performed to compare newer drug therapies: amlodipine 2.5-10 mg/d (calcium channel blocker) or lisinopril 10-40 mg/d (ACE-inhibitor) as first-line therapies to that of the thiazide-diuretic, chlorthalidone 12.5-25 mg/d in mild to moderate hypertension."

A total of 33,357 hypertensive patients aged 55 or older were randomized and followed for a mean of 4.9 years. The patients had at least one additional CHD risk factor, including: previous myocardial infarction or stroke > 6 months prior to enrollment) or documentation of other atherosclerotic CVD (overall 51.5%), type 2 diabetes (36.1%), HDL-C < 35 mg/dL (11.6%), left ventricular hypertrophy diagnosed by electrocardiogram or echocardiography (20.9%), current cigarette smoking (21.9%).

The primary endpoint was a composite of fatal CHD or non-fatal myocardial infarction. There was no significant difference in the primary endpoint between amlodipine-based therapy and chlorthalidone-based therapy: RR 0.98 95% CI(0.90-1.07) p=0.65. Among Secondary Endpoints, the incidence of heart failure (component of a composite combined cardiovascular endpoint) was significantly higher in the amlodipine group as compared to the chlorthalidone group (10.2% % vs 7.7%, RR 1.38, 95% CI [1.25-1.52] p<0.001). However, there was no significant difference in all-cause mortality between amlodipine-based therapy and chlorthalidone-based therapy. RR 0.96 95% CI [0.89-1.02] p=0.20.

In a study involving 268 children aged 6-17 years with predominantly secondary hypertension, comparison of a 2.5mg dose, and 5.0mg dose of amlodipine with placebo, showed that both doses reduced Systolic Blood Pressure significantly more than placebo. The difference between the two doses was not statistically significant.

The long-term effects of amlodipine on growth, puberty and general development have not been studied. The long-term efficacy of amlodipine on therapy in childhood to reduce cardiovascular morbidity and mortality in adulthood have also not been established.

5.2 Pharmacokinetic properties

Absorption, distribution, plasma protein binding: After oral administration of therapeutic doses, amlodipine is well absorbed with peak blood levels between 6-12 hours post dose. Absolute bioavailability has been estimated to be between 64 and 80%. The volume of distribution is approximately 21 l/kg. *In vitro* studies have shown that approximately 97.5% of circulating amlodipine is bound to plasma proteins.

Biotransformation/elimination: The terminal plasma elimination half-life is about 35-50 hours and is consistent with once daily dosing. Amlodipine is extensively metabolised by the liver to inactive metabolites with 10% of the parent compound and 60% of metabolites excreted in the urine.

Use in the elderly: The time to reach peak plasma concentrations of amlodipine is similar in elderly and younger subjects. Amlodipine clearance tends to be decreased with resulting increases in AUC and elimination half-life in elderly patients. Increases in AUC and elimination half-life in patients with congestive heart failure were as expected for the patient age group studied.

5.3 Preclinical safety data

None

6. PHARMACEUTICAL PARTICULARS

6.1 List of excipients

Microcrystalline cellulose, E460

Dibasic calcium phosphate anhydrous

Sodium starch glycollate

Magnesium stearate, E572

6.2 Incompatibilities

Not applicable

6.3 Shelf life

4 years

6.4 Special precautions for storage

Do not store above 25°C

6.5 Nature and contents of container

Istin is available as:

Calendar packs of 28 tablets. Aluminium/PVC blister strips, 14 tablets/strip, 2 strips in a carton box.

6.6 Instructions for use and handling

No special requirements

7. MARKETING AUTHORISATION HOLDER

Pfizer Limited

Ramsgate Road

Sandwich

Kent

CT13 9NJ

United Kingdom

8. MARKETING AUTHORISATION NUMBER(S)

Istin Tablets 5mg PL 00057/0297

Istin Tablets 10mg PL 00057/0298

9. DATE OF FIRST AUTHORISATION/RENEWAL OF THE AUTHORISATION

30 January 1995 / 25 April 2001

10. DATE OF REVISION OF THE TEXT

15th April 2005

11. LEGAL CATEGORY

POM

Ref: IS 8_0

Junior Meltus Dry Coughs with Congestion

(SSL International plc)

1. NAME OF THE MEDICINAL PRODUCT

Junior Meltus Dry Coughs with Congestion

2. QUALITATIVE AND QUANTITATIVE COMPOSITION

Dextromethorphan Hydrobromide BP 3.5mg/5ml; Pseudoephedrine Hydrochloride BP 10.0mg/5ml.

3. PHARMACEUTICAL FORM

Oral solution.

4. CLINICAL PARTICULARS

4.1 Therapeutic indications

An oral solution for the symptomatic relief of unproductive coughs accompanied by congestion of the upper respiratory tract.

4.2 Posology and method of administration

To be given four times a day. Do not repeat dosage more frequently than every four hours. Children 6-12 years: Two 5ml spoonfuls. Children 2-5 years: One 5ml spoonful. Adults, the elderly and children over 12 years are recommended to take Adult Meltus Dry Coughs with Congestion. Not to be given to children under two years of age.

4.3 Contraindications

Junior Meltus Dry Coughs with Congestion is contraindicated in patients with a known hypersensitivity to pseudoephedrine or dextromethorphan. Contraindicated in persons under treatment with monoamine oxidase inhibitors or within 2 weeks of stopping such treatment. Contraindicated in patients with severe hypertension or severe coronary artery disease. Junior Meltus Dry Coughs with Congestion should not be administered to patients where the cough is associated with asthma or where the cough is accompanied by excessive secretions. Dextromethorphan, in common with other centrally acting antitussive agents, should not be given to patients in or at risk of developing respiratory failure. Although pseudoephedrine has virtually no pressor effect in patients with normal blood pressure, Junior Meltus Dry Coughs with Congestion should be used with caution in patients taking antihypertensive agents, tricyclic antidepressants, other sympathomimetic agents, such as decongestants, appetite suppressants and amphetamine-like psychostimulants. The effects of a single dose of Junior Meltus Dry Coughs with Congestion on the blood pressure of these patients should be observed before recommending repeated or unsupervised treatment. As with other sympathomimetic agents, caution should be exercised in patients with uncontrolled diabetes, hyperthyroidism, elevated intraocular pressure and prostatic enlargement.

4.4 Special warnings and special precautions for use

Keep out of the reach of children. Do not exceed the stated dose. If currently taking any other medicine, consult with a doctor or pharmacist before taking this product. If symptoms persist, consult your doctor.

4.5 Interaction with other medicinal products and other forms of Interaction

Concomitant use of Junior Meltus Dry Coughs with Congestion with sympathomimetic agents such as decongestants, tricyclic antidepressants, appetite suppressants and amphetamine-like psychostimulants, or with monoamine oxidase inhibitors which interfere with the catabolism of sympathomimetic amines, may occasionally cause a rise in blood pressure. Because of its pseudoephedrine content, the effect of antihypertensive agents which modify sympathetic activity may be partially reversed by Junior Meltus Dry Coughs with Congestion. The antibacterial agent, furazolidine, is known to cause a dose-related inhibition of monoamine oxidase and although there are no reports of a hypertensive crisis having occurred, it should not be administered concurrently with Junior Meltus Dry Coughs with Congestion. The product may potentiate the effects of alcohol and other central nervous system depressants.

4.6 Pregnancy and lactation

Not applicable.

4.7 Effects on ability to drive and use machines

Not applicable.

4.8 Undesirable effects

In some patients, pseudoephedrine may occasionally cause insomnia. Rarely, sleep disturbance and hallucinations have been reported. Fixed drug eruption due to pseudoephedrine, taking the form of erythematous nummular patches, has been reported as a rare event. Side-effects attributed to dextromethorphan are uncommon; occasionally dizziness, nausea, vomiting or gastrointestinal disturbance may occur.

4.9 Overdose

The effects of acute toxicity from Junior Meltus Dry Coughs with Congestion may include nystagmus, hypertension, irritability, restlessness, tremor, palpitations, visual and auditory hallucinations, convulsions, respiratory depression, difficulty with micturition, nausea and vomiting. Gastric lavage and supportive measures for respiration and circulation should be performed if indicated. Convulsions should be controlled with an anticonvulsant. Catheterisation of the bladder may be necessary. If desired, the elimination of pseudoephedrine can be accelerated by acid diuresis or by dialysis. Naloxone has been used successfully as a specific antagonist to dextromethorphan toxicity in a child.

5. PHARMACOLOGICAL PROPERTIES

5.1 Pharmacodynamic properties

Cough suppressant; decongestant.

5.2 Pharmacokinetic properties

Not applicable.

5.3 Preclinical safety data

None stated.

6. PHARMACEUTICAL PARTICULARS

6.1 List of excipients

Sorbitol Syrup (Non Crystallising) BP; Menthol BP; Chloroform BP; Loganberry Flavour 500195E; Methylhydroxybenzoate BP; Propylhydroxybenzoate BP; Alcohol 96% BP; Glycerin BP; Sodium Saccharin BP; Sodium Cyclamate 1968 BP; Carmellose Sodium BP; Water.

6.2 Incompatibilities

None known.

6.3 Shelf life

36 months unopened.

6.4 Special precautions for storage

Store below 25°C and avoid prolonged storage at 5°C or below.

6.5 Nature and contents of container

Amber glass bottle with tamper evident cap with fitted polycone liner packed in an outer carton. Bottle contains 100ml of product.

6.6 Instructions for use and handling

None stated.

7. MARKETING AUTHORISATION HOLDER

Cupal Limited

Tubiton House

Oldham

OL1 3HS

8. MARKETING AUTHORISATION NUMBER(S)

PL 0338/0070.

9. DATE OF FIRST AUTHORISATION/RENEWAL OF THE AUTHORISATION

11th October 1991 / 12th June 2003

10. DATE OF REVISION OF THE TEXT

June 2003

Kaletra Oral Solution

(Abbott Laboratories Limited)

1. NAME OF THE MEDICINAL PRODUCT

Kaletra oral solution

2. QUALITATIVE AND QUANTITATIVE COMPOSITION

Each 5 ml of Kaletra oral solution contains 400 mg of lopinavir co-formulated with 100 mg of ritonavir as a pharmacokinetic enhancer.

For excipients, see section 6.1.

3. PHARMACEUTICAL FORM

Oral solution

The solution is light yellow to golden.

4. CLINICAL PARTICULARS

4.1 Therapeutic indications

Kaletra is indicated for the treatment of HIV-1 infected adults and children above the age of 2 years, in combination with other antiretroviral agents.

Most experience with Kaletra is derived from the use of the product in antiretroviral therapy naïve patients. Data in heavily pretreated protease inhibitor experienced patients are limited. There are limited data on salvage therapy on patients who have failed therapy with Kaletra.

The choice of Kaletra to treat protease inhibitor experienced HIV-1 infected patients should be based on individual viral resistance testing and treatment history of patients (see sections 4.4 and 5.1).

4.2 Posology and method of administration

Kaletra should be prescribed by physicians who are experienced in the treatment of HIV infection.

Adult and adolescent use: the recommended dosage of Kaletra is 5 ml of oral solution (400/100 mg) twice daily taken with food.

Paediatric use (2 years of age and above): the recommended dosage of Kaletra is 230/57.5 mg/m^2 twice daily taken with food, up to a maximum dose of 400/100 mg twice daily. The 230/57.5 mg/m^2 dosage might be insufficient in some children when co-administered with nevirapine or efavirenz. An increase of the dose of Kaletra to 300/75 mg/m^2 should be considered in these patients. Dose should be administered using a calibrated oral dosing syringe.

The oral solution is the recommended option for the most accurate dosing in children based on body surface area. However, if it is judged necessary to resort to soft capsules in children, they should be used with particular caution since they are associated with less precise dosing capabilities. Therefore, children receiving soft capsules might have higher exposure (with the risk of increased toxicity) or suboptinal exposure (with the risk of insufficient efficacy). Consequently when dosing children with soft capsules, therapeutic drug monitoring may be a useful tool to ensure appropriate lopinavir exposure in an individual patient.

Paediatric Dosing Guidelines for the dose 230/57.5 mg/m^2

Body Surface Area* (m^2)	Twice Daily Oral Solution Dose (dose in mg)	Twice Daily Soft Capsule Dose (dose in mg)
0.25	0.7 ml (57.5/14.4 mg)	NA
0.40	1.2 ml (96/24 mg)	1 soft capsule (133.3/33.3 mg)
0.50	1.4 ml (115/28.8 mg)	1 soft capsule (133.3/33.3 mg)
0.75	2.2 ml (172.5/43.1 mg)	1 soft capsule (133.3/33.3 mg)
0.80	2.3 ml (184/46 mg)	2 soft capsules (266.6/66.6 mg)
1.00	2.9 ml (230/57.5 mg)	2 soft capsules (266.6/66.6 mg)
1.25	3.6 ml (287.5/71.9 mg)	2 soft capsules (266.6/66.6 mg)
1.3	3.7 ml (299/74.8 mg)	2 soft capsules (266.6/66.6 mg)
1.4	4.0 ml (322/80.5 mg)	3 soft capsules (400/100 mg)
1.5	4.3 ml (345/86.3 mg)	3 soft capsules (400/100 mg)
1.75	5 ml (402.5/100.6 mg)	3 soft capsules (400/100 mg)

* Body surface area can be calculated with the following equation

BSA (m^2) = $\sqrt{}$ (Height (cm) X Weight (kg) / 3600)

Children less than 2 years of age: Kaletra is not recommended for use in children less than 2 years of age because of limited safety and efficacy data. Paediatric patients should switch from Kaletra oral solution to soft capsules as soon as they are able to swallow the capsule formulation (see section 4.4).

Hepatic impairment: In HIV-infected patients with mild to moderate hepatic impairment, an increase of approximately 30% in lopinavir exposure has been observed but is not expected to be of clinical relevance. (see section 5.2). No data are available in patients with severe hepatic impairment. Kaletra should not be given to these patients (see section 4.3).

Renal impairment: No dose adjustment is necessary in patients with renal impairment. Caution is warranted when Kaletra is used in patients with severe renal impairment (see section 4.4).

4.3 Contraindications

Patients with known hypersensitivity to lopinavir, ritonavir or any of the excipients.

Patients with severe hepatic insufficiency.

Kaletra contains lopinavir and ritonavir, both of which are inhibitors of the P450 isoform CYP3A. Kaletra should not be co-administered with medicinal products that are highly dependent on CYP3A for clearance and for which elevated plasma concentrations are associated with serious and/or life threatening events. These medicinal products include astemizole, terfenadine, midazolam, triazolam, cisapride, pimozide, amiodarone, ergot alkaloids (e.g. ergotamine, dihydroergotamine and ergonovine and methylergonovine).

Herbal preparations containing St John's wort (*Hypericum perforatum)* must not be used while taking lopinavir and ritonavir due to the risk of decreased plasma concentrations and reduced clinical effects of lopinavir and ritonavir. (see section 4.5).

Kaletra oral solution is contraindicated in children below the age of 2 years, pregnant women, patients with hepatic or renal failure and patients treated with disulfiram or metronidazole due to the potential risk of toxicity from the excipient propylene glycol (see section 4.4).

Rifampicin should not be used in combination with Kaletra because co-administration may cause large decreases in lopinavir concentrations which may in turn significantly decrease the lopinavir therapeutic effect (see section 4.5).

4.4 Special warnings and special precautions for use

Patients with coexisting conditions

Liver disease: the safety and efficacy of Kaletra has not been established in patients with significant underlying liver disorders. Kaletra is contraindicated in patients with severe liver impairment (see section 4.3). Patients with chronic hepatitis B or C and treated with combination antiretroviral therapy are at an increased risk for severe and potentially fatal hepatic adverse events. In case of concomitant antiviral therapy for hepatitis B or C, please refer to the relevant product information for these medicinal products.

Patients with pre-existing liver dysfunction including chronic hepatitis have an increased frequency of liver function abnormalities during combination antiretroviral therapy and should be monitored according to standard practice. If there is evidence of worsening liver disease in such patients, interruption or discontinuation of treatment should be considered.

Renal disease: since the renal clearance of lopinavir and ritonavir is negligible, increased plasma concentrations are not expected in patients with renal impairment. Because lopinavir and ritonavir are highly protein bound, it is unlikely that they will be significantly removed by haemodialysis or peritoneal dialysis.

Haemophilia: there have been reports of increased bleeding, including spontaneous skin haematomas and haemarthrosis in patients with haemophilia type A and B treated with protease inhibitors. In some patients additional factor VIII was given. In more than half of the reported cases, treatment with protease inhibitors was continued or reintroduced if treatment had been discontinued. A causal relationship had been evoked, although the mechanism of action had not been elucidated. Haemophiliac patients should therefore be made aware of the possibility of increased bleeding.

Lipid elevations

Treatment with Kaletra has resulted in increases, sometimes marked, in the concentration of total cholesterol and triglycerides. Triglyceride and cholesterol testing is to be performed prior to initiating Kaletra therapy and at periodic intervals during therapy. Particular caution should be paid to patients with high values at baseline and with history of lipid disorders. Lipid disorders are to be managed as clinically appropriate (see also section 4.5 for additional information on potential interactions with HMG-CoA reductase inhibitors).

Pancreatitis

Cases of pancreatitis have been reported in patients receiving Kaletra, including those who developed hypertriglyceridaemia. In most of these cases patients have had a prior history of pancreatitis and/or concurrent therapy with other medicinal products associated with pancreatitis. Marked triglyceride elevation is a risk factor for development of pancreatitis. Patients with advanced HIV disease may be at risk of elevated triglycerides and pancreatitis.

Pancreatitis should be considered if clinical symptoms (nausea, vomiting, abdominal pain) or abnormalities in laboratory values (such as increased serum lipase or amylase values) suggestive of pancreatitis should occur. Patients who exhibit these signs or symptoms should be evaluated and Kaletra therapy should be suspended if a diagnosis of pancreatitis is made (see section 4.8).

Hyperglycaemia

New onset diabetes mellitus, hyperglycaemia or exacerbation of existing diabetes mellitus has been reported in patients receiving protease inhibitors. In some of these the hyperglycaemia was severe and in some cases also associated with ketoacidosis. Many patients had confounding medical conditions some of which required therapy with agents that have been associated with the development of diabetes mellitus or hyperglycaemia.

Fat redistribution & metabolic disorders

Combination antiretroviral therapy has been associated with redistribution of body fat (lipodystrophy) in HIV patients. The long-term consequences of these events are currently unknown. Knowledge about the mechanism is incomplete. A connection between visceral lipomatosis and protease inhibitors (PIs) and lipoatrophy and nucleoside reverse transcriptase inhibitors (NRTIs) has been hypothesised. A higher risk of lipodystrophy has been associated with individual factors such as older age, and with drug related factors such as longer duration of antiretroviral treatment and associated metabolic disturbances. Clinical examination should include evaluation for physical signs of fat redistribution. Consideration should be given to measurement of fasting serum lipids and blood glucose. Lipid disorders should be managed as clinically appropriate (see section 4.8).

Immune Reactivation Syndrome

In HIV-infected patients with severe immune deficiency at the time of institution of combination antiretroviral therapy (CART), an inflammatory reaction to asymtomatic or residual opportunistic pathogens may arise and cause serious clinical conditions, or aggravation of symptoms. Typically, such reactions have been observed within the first few weeks or months of initiation of CART. Relevant examples are cytomegalovirus retinitis, generalised and/or focal mycobacterial infections, and Pneumocystis carinii pneumonia. Any inflammatory symptoms should be evaluated and treatment instituted when necessary.

Interactions with medicinal products

Kaletra contains lopinavir and ritonavir, both of which are inhibitors of the P450 isoform CYP3A. Kaletra is likely to increase plasma concentrations of medicinal products that are primarily metabolised by CYP3A. These increases of plasma concentrations of co-administered medicinal products could increase or prolong their therapeutic effect and adverse events (see sections 4.3 and 4.5).

Particular caution must be used when prescribing sildenafil in patients receiving Kaletra. Co-administration of Kaletra with sildenafil is expected to substantially increase sildenafil concentrations and may result in an increase in sildenafil-associated adverse events including hypotension, syncope, visual changes and prolonged erection (see section 4.5).

The HMG-CoA reductase inhibitors simvastatin and lovastatin are highly dependent on CYP3A for metabolism, thus concomitant use of Kaletra with simvastatin or lovastatin is not recommended due to an increased risk of myopathy including rhabdomyolysis. Caution must also be exercised and reduced doses should be considered if Kaletra is used concurrently with atorvastatin, which is metabolised to a lesser extent by CYP3A4. If treatment with an HMG-CoA reductase inhibitor is indicated, pravastatin or fluvastatin is recommended (see section 4.5).

Particular caution must be used when prescribing Kaletra and medicinal products known to induce QT interval prolongation such as: chlorpheniramine, quinidine, erythromycin, clarithromycin. Indeed, Kaletra could increase concentrations of the co-administered medicinal products and this may result in an increase of their associated cardiac adverse events. Cardiac events have been reported with Kaletra in preclinical studies; therefore, the potential cardiac effects of Kaletra cannot be currently ruled out (see sections 4.8 and 5.3).

Rifampicin should not be used in combination with Kaletra because this may cause large decreases in lopinavir concentrations which may in turn significantly decrease the lopinavir therapeutic effect (see sections 4.3 and 4.5).

Oral Contraceptives: since levels of ethinyl oestradiol may be decreased alternative or additional contraceptive measures are to be used when oestrogen-based oral contraceptives are co-administered (see section 4.5).

Other

Patients taking the oral solution, particularly those with renal impairment or with decreased ability to metabolise propylene glycol (e.g. those of Asian origin), should be monitored for adverse reactions potentially related to propylene glycol toxicity (i.e. seizures, stupor, tachycardia, hyperosmolarity, lactic acidosis, renal toxicity, haemolysis) (see section 4.3).

Kaletra is not a cure for HIV infection or AIDS. It does not reduce the risk of passing HIV to others through sexual contact or blood contamination. Appropriate precautions should be taken. People taking Kaletra may still develop infections or other illnesses associated with HIV disease and AIDS.

There are limited data on salvage therapy on patients who have failed with Kaletra. There are ongoing studies to further establish the usefulness of potential salvage therapy regimens (e.g. amprenavir or saquinavir). There are currently limited data on the use of Kaletra in protease inhibitor-experienced patients.

Besides propylene glycol as described above, Kaletra oral solution contains alcohol (42% v/v) which is potentially harmful for those suffering from liver disease, alcoholism, epilepsy, brain injury or disease as well as for pregnant women and children. It may modify or increase the effects of other medicines. Kaletra oral solution contains up to 0.8 g of fructose per dose when taken according to the dosage recommendations. This may be unsuitable in hereditary fructose intolerance. Kaletra oral solution contains up to 0.3 g of glycerol per dose. Only at high inadvertent doses, it can cause headache and gastrointestinal upset. Furthermore, polyoxol 40 hydrogenated castor oil and potassium present in Kaletra oral solution may cause only at high inadvertent doses gastrointestinal upset. Patients on a low potassium diet should be cautioned.

Concomitant use of ritonavir (including low-dose) and fluticasone propionate significantly increased fluticasone propionate plasma concentrations and reduced serum cortisol concentrations in a clinical study. Concomitant use of ritonavir (including low-dose) and fluticasone is therefore not recommended unless the potential benefit of treatment outweighs the risk of systemic corticosteroid effects. Systemic corticosteroid effects including Cushing's syndrome and adrenal suppression have been reported when ritonavir has been co-administered with inhaled or intranasal administered fluticasone propionate (see section 4.5).

4.5 Interaction with other medicinal products and other forms of Interaction

Kaletra contains lopinavir and ritonavir, both of which are inhibitors of the P450 isoform CYP3A *in vitro*. Co-administration of Kaletra and medicinal products primarily metabolised by CYP3A may result in increased plasma concentrations of the other medicinal product, which could increase or prolong its therapeutic and adverse effects. Kaletra does not inhibit CYP2D6, CYP2C9, CYP2C19, CYP2E1, CYP2B6 or CYP1A2 at clinically relevant concentrations (see section 4.3).

Kaletra has been shown *in vivo* to induce its own metabolism and to increase the biotransformation of some medicinal products metabolised by cytochrome P450 enzymes and by glucuronidation. This may result in lowered plasma concentrations and potential decrease of efficacy of co-administered medicinal products.

Medicinal products that are contraindicated specifically due to the expected magnitude of interaction and potential for serious adverse events are listed in section 4.3.

Antiretroviral agents

Nucleoside reverse transcriptase inhibitors (NRTIs):

Stavudine and Lamivudine: no change in the pharmacokinetics of lopinavir was observed when Kaletra was given alone or in combination with stavudine and lamivudine in clinical studies.

Didanosine: it is recommended that didanosine be administered on an empty stomach; therefore, didanosine is to be given one hour before or two hours after Kaletra (given with food). The gastroresistant formulation of didanosine should be administered at least two hours after a meal.

Zidovudine and Abacavir: Kaletra induces glucuronidation, therefore Kaletra has the potential to reduce zidovudine and abacavir plasma concentrations. The clinical significance of this potential interaction is unknown.

Non-nucleoside reverse transcriptase inhibitors (NNRTIs):

Nevirapine: no change in the pharmacokinetics of lopinavir was apparent in healthy volunteers during nevirapine and Kaletra co-administration. Results from a study in HIV-positive paediatric patients revealed a decrease in lopinavir concentrations during nevirapine co-administration. The effect of nevirapine in HIV-positive adults is expected to be similar to that in paediatric patients and lopinavir concentrations may be decreased. The clinical significance of the pharmacokinetic interaction is unknown. No formal recommendation could be drawn on dosage adjustment when Kaletra is used in combination with nevirapine. However, based on clinical experience, Kaletra dose increase to 533/133 mg twice daily (~6.5 ml) may be considered when co-administered with nevirapine, particularly for patients in whom reduced lopinavir susceptibility is likely.

Efavirenz: when used in combination with efavirenz and two nucleoside reverse transcriptase inhibitors in multiple protease inhibitor-experienced patients, increasing the dose of Kaletra 33.3% from 400/100 mg (3 capsules) twice daily to 533/133 mg (4 capsules) twice daily yielded similar lopinavir plasma concentrations as compared to historical data of Kaletra 400/100 mg (3 capsules) twice daily.

Dosage increase of Kaletra from 400/100 mg (5 ml) twice daily to 533/133 mg (~6.5 ml) twice daily should be considered when co-administered with efavirenz. Caution is warranted since this dosage adjustment might be insufficient in some patients.

Co-administration with other HIV protease inhibitors (PIs):

Kaletra (400/100 mg twice daily) has been studied in combination with reduced doses of amprenavir, indinavir, nelfinavir and saquinavir in steady-state controlled healthy volunteer studies relative to clinical doses of each HIV protease inhibitor in the absence of ritonavir. Comparisons to published pharmacokinetic data with ritonavir-enhanced amprenavir and saquinavir regimens are also described. Additionally, the effect of additional ritonavir on the pharmacokinetics of lopinavir are discussed. Note that the historical comparisons to ritonavir-enhanced protease inhibitor regimens should be interpreted with caution (see details of combinations below). Appropriate doses of HIV-protease inhibitors in combination with Kaletra with respect to safety and efficacy have not been established. Therefore, the concomitant administration of Kaletra with PIs requires close monitoring.

Amprenavir: the concomitant use of Kaletra with amprenavir 750 mg twice daily, resulted in an increase in amprenavir AUC by 70% and of C_{min} by 4.6-fold, relative to amprenavir 1200 mg twice daily alone. On the other hand, the AUC of lopinavir decreases by 38%. A dose increase of Kaletra may be necessary but may further affect concentrations of amprenavir.

Combined with Kaletra, amprenavir concentrations were lower (approximately 30%) relative to boosted amprenavir (amprenavir 600 mg/ritonavir 100 mg) twice daily alone.

Indinavir: indinavir 600 mg twice daily in combination with Kaletra produces similar indinavir AUC, higher C_{min} (by 3.5-fold) and lower C_{max} relative to indinavir 800 mg three times daily alone. Furthermore, concentrations of lopinavir do not appear to be affected when both drugs, Kaletra and indinivir, are combined, based on historical comparison with Kaletra alone.

Nelfinavir: administration of nelfinavir 1000 mg twice daily in combination with Kaletra produces a similar nelfinavir C_{max} and AUC and higher C_{min} relative to nelfinavir 1250 mg twice daily alone. Additionally, concentrations of the active M8 metabolite of nelfinavir were increased.

On the other hand, lopinavir AUC was decreased by 27% during nelfinavir co-administration with Kaletra. A dose increase of Kaletra may be necessary but may further affect concentrations of nelfinavir and its active metabolite. Higher doses of Kaletra have not been studied.

Saquinavir: saquinavir 800 mg twice daily co-administered with Kaletra produces an increase of saquinavir AUC by 9.6-fold relative to saquinavir 1200 mg three times daily given alone.

Saquinavir 800 mg twice daily co-administered with Kaletra resulted in an increase of saquinavir AUC by approximately 30% relative to saquinavir/ritonavir 1000/100 mg twice daily, and produces similar exposure to those reported after saquinavir/ritonavir 400/400 mg twice daily.

When saquinavir 1200 mg twice daily was combined with Kaletra, no further increase of concentrations was noted. Furthermore, concentrations of lopinavir do not appear to be affected when both drugs, Kaletra and saquinavir, are combined, based on historical comparison with Kaletra alone.

Ritonavir: Kaletra co-administered with an additional 100 mg ritonavir twice daily resulted in an increase of lopinavir AUC and C_{min} of 33% and 64%, respectively, as compared to Kaletra alone.

Other medicinal products:

Antiarrhythmics: (bepridil, systemic lidocaine and quinidine): concentrations may be increased when co-administered with Kaletra. Caution is warranted and therapeutic concentration monitoring is recommended when available.

Anticoagulants: warfarin concentrations may be affected when co-administered with Kaletra. It is recommended that INR (international normalised ratio) be monitored.

Anticonvulsants: (phenobarbital, phenytoin, carbamazepine): will induce CYP3A4 and may decrease lopinavir concentrations.

Dihydropyridine calcium channel blockers: (e.g. felodipine, nifedipine, nicardipine): may have their serum concentrations increased by Kaletra.

Disulfiram, metronidazole: Kaletra oral solution contains alcohol which can produce disulfiram-like reactions when co-administered with disulfiram or other medicinal products that produce this reaction.

HMG-CoA reductase inhibitors: HMG-CoA reductase inhibitors which are highly dependent on CYP3A4 metabolism, such as lovastatin and simvastatin, are expected to have markedly increased plasma concentrations when co-administered with Kaletra. Since increased concentrations of HMG-CoA reductase inhibitors may cause myopathy, including rhabdomyolysis, the combination of these medicinal products with Kaletra is not recommended. Atorvastatin is less dependent on CYP3A for metabolism. When atorvastatin was given concurrently with Kaletra, a mean 4.7-fold and 5.9-fold increase in atorvastatin C_{max} and AUC, respectively, was observed. When used with Kaletra, the lowest possible dose of atorvastatin should be administered. Results from an interaction study with Kaletra and pravastatin reveal no clinically significant interaction. The metabolism of pravastatin and fluvastatin is not dependent on CYP3A4, and interactions are not expected with Kaletra. If treatment with a HMG-CoA reductase inhibitor is indicated, pravastatin or fluvastatin is recommended.

Dexamethasone: may induce CYP3A4 and may decrease lopinavir concentrations.

Sildenafil: co-administration of sildenafil 100 mg single dose with ritonavir 500 mg twice daily at steady-state resulted in a 1000% increase in sildenafil plasma AUC. On the basis of these data, concomitant use of sildenafil with Kaletra is not recommended and in no case should the starting dose of sildenafil exceed 25 mg within 48 hours (see section 4.4).

Cyclosporin, sirolimus (rapamycin) and tacrolimus: concentrations may be increased when co-administered with Kaletra. More frequent therapeutic concentration monitoring is recommended until plasma levels of these products have been stabilised.

Ketoconazole and itraconazole: may have serum concentrations increased by Kaletra. High doses of ketoconazole and itraconazole > 200 mg/day) are not recommended.

Clarithromycin: moderate increases in clarithromycin AUC are expected when co-administered with Kaletra. For patients with renal or hepatic impairment dose reduction of clarithromycin should be considered (see section 4.4).

Methadone: Kaletra was demonstrated to lower plasma concentrations of methadone. Monitoring plasma concentrations of methadone is recommended.

Oral Contraceptives: since levels of ethinyl oestradiol may be decreased alternative or additional contraceptive measures are to be used when oestrogen-based oral contraceptives are co-administered.

Rifabutin: when rifabutin and Kaletra were co-administered for 10 days, rifabutin (parent drug and active 25-O-desacetyl metabolite) C_{max} and AUC were increased by 3.5- and 5.7-fold, respectively. On the basis of these data, a rifabutin dose reduction of 75% (i.e. 150 mg every other day or 3 times per week) is recommended when administered with Kaletra. Further reduction may be necessary.

Rifampicin: due to large decreases in lopinavir concentrations, rifampicin should not be used in combination with Kaletra (see sections 4.3 and 4.4).

St John's wort: serum levels of lopinavir and ritonavir can be reduced by concomitant use of the herbal preparation St John's wort (*Hypericum perforatum).* This is due to the induction of drug metabolising enzymes by St John's wort. Herbal preparations containing St John's wort should therefore not be combined with lopinavir and ritonavir. If a patient is already taking St John's wort, stop St John's wort and if possible check viral levels. Lopinavir and ritonavir levels may increase on stopping St John's wort. The dose of Kaletra may need adjusting. The inducing effect may persist for at least 2 weeks after cessation of treatment with St John's wort (see section 4.3).

Fluticasone propionate: in a clinical study where ritonavir 100 mg capsules twice daily were co – administered with 50 μg intranasal fluticasone propionate (4 times daily) for seven days in healthy subjects, the fluticasone propionate plasma levels increased significantly, whereas the intrinsic cortisol levels decreased by approximately 86% (90% confidence interval 82 – 89%). Greater effects may be expected when fluticasone propionate is inhaled. Systemic corticosteroid effects including Cushing's syndrome and adrenal suppression have been reported when ritonavir has been co – administered with inhaled or intranasally administered fluticasone propionate; this could also occur with other corticosteroids eg budesonide. Consequently, concomitant administration of Kaletra (including low dose of ritonavir) and inhaled or intranasally administered glucocorticoids is not recommended unless the potential benefit of treatment outweighs the risk of systemic corticosteroid effects. A dose reduction of the glucocorticoid should be considered with close monitoring. Moreover, in case of withdrawal of glucocorticoids progressive dose reduction may have to be performed over a longer period.

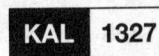

Table 1 Undesirable Effects in Clinical Studies in Adult Patients

Infections and infestations	Uncommon	Otitis media, bronchitis, sinusitis, furunculosis, bacterial infection, viral infection
Neoplasms benign, malignant and unspecified	Uncommon	Skin benign neoplasm, cyst
Blood and lymphatic system Disorders	Uncommon	Anaemia, leucopenia and lymphadenopathy
Endocrine disorders	Uncommon	Hypogonadism male, Cushing syndrome, hypothyroidism
Metabolic and nutritional disorders	Uncommon	Avitaminosis, dehydration, oedema, increased appetite, lactic acidosis, obesity, anorexia, diabetes mellitus, hyperglycaemia, hypocholesteremia
Psychiatric disorders	Common	Insomnia
	Uncommon	Abnormal dreams, agitation, anxiety, confusion, depression, dyskinesia, emotional lability, decreased libido, nervousness, abnormal thinking
Nervous system disorders	Common	Headache
	Uncommon	Dizziness, amnesia, ataxia, encephalopathy, facial paralysis, hypertonia, neuropathy, paresthesia, peripheral neuritis, somnolence, tremor, taste perversion, migraine, amnesia, extrapyramidal syndrome
Eye disorders	Uncommon	Abnormal vision, eye disorder
Ear and labyrinth disorders	Uncommon	Tinnitus
Cardiac disorders	Uncommon	Palpitation, lung oedema, myocardial infarct[1]
Vascular disorders	Uncommon	Hypertension, thrombophlebitis, vasculitis, varicose vein, deep thrombophlebitis, vascular disorder
Respiratory, thoracic and mediastinal disorders	Uncommon	Dyspnea, rhinitis, cough increased
Gastrointestinal disorders	Very common	Diarrhoea
	Common	Nausea, vomiting, abdominal pain, abnormal stools, dyspepsia, flatulence, gastrointestinal disorder
	Uncommon	Abdomen enlarged, constipation, dry mouth, dysphagia, enterocolitis, eructation, oesophagitis, faecal incontinence, gastritis, gastroenteritis, haemorrhagic colitis, mouth ulcerations, pancreatitis[2], sialadenitis, stomatitis, ulcerative stomatitis, periodontitis
Hepatobiliary disorders	Uncommon	Cholecystitis, hepatitis, hepatomegaly, liver fatty deposit, liver tenderness
Skin and subcutaneous tissue disorders	Common	Rash, lipodystrophy
	Uncommon	Alopecia, dry skin, eczema, exfoliative dermatitis, maculopapular rash, nail disorder, pruritis, seborrhea, skin discoloration, skin ulcer, face oedema, acne, sweating, skin striae
Musculoskeletal and connective tissue disorders	Uncommon	Arthralgia, arthrosis, myalgia, back pain, joint disorder
Renal and urinary disorders	Uncommon	Kidney calculus, urine abnormality, albuminuria, hypercalcinuria, hyperuricemia
Reproductive system and breast disorders	Uncommon	Abnormal ejaculation, breast enlargement, gynecomastia, impotence, menorrhagia
General disorders and administration site conditions	Common	Asthenia
	Uncommon	Chest pain, chest pain substernal, chills, fever, flu syndrome, malaise, pain, peripheral oedema, drug interaction
Investigations	Very common (Grade 3 or 4)	Increased triglycerides, increased total cholesterol, increased GGT
	Common (Grade 3 or 4)	Increased glucose, increased amylase, increased SGOT/AST, increased SGPT/ALT, liver function tests abnormal
	Uncommon	Decreased glucose tolerance, weight gain, weight loss, increased bilirubin, hormone level altered, lab test abnormal

[1] This event had a fatal outcome.

[2] See section 4.4: pancreatitis and lipids

The effects of high fluticasone systemic exposure on ritonavir plasma levels is yet unknown (see section 4.4).

Based on known metabolic profiles, clinically significant interactions are not expected between Kaletra and fluvastatin, dapsone, trimethoprim/sulfamethoxazole, azithromycin or fluconazole.

4.6 Pregnancy and lactation

There are no data from the use of Kaletra in pregnant women. Studies in animals have shown reproductive toxicity (see section 5.3). The potential risk for humans is unknown. Kaletra should not be used during pregnancy unless clearly necessary.

Studies in rats revealed that lopinavir is excreted in the milk. It is not known whether this medicinal product is excreted in human milk. HIV-infected women must not breast-feed their infants under any circumstances to avoid transmission of HIV.

4.7 Effects on ability to drive and use machines

No studies on the effects on the ability to drive a car and use machines have been performed.

Kaletra oral solution contains approximately 42% v/v alcohol.

4.8 Undesirable effects

The safety of Kaletra has been investigated in 612 patients in Phase II/III clinical trials, of which 442 have received a dose of 400/100 mg (3 capsules) twice daily. In some studies, Kaletra was used in combination with efavirenz or nevirapine.

The most common adverse event associated with Kaletra therapy was diarrhoea and was generally of mild to moderate severity. Discontinuation due to adverse reactions was 4.5% (naïve patients) and 9% (experienced patients) over a 48 week period.

It is important to note that cases of pancreatitis have been reported in patients receiving Kaletra, including those who developed hypertriglyceridaemia. Furthermore, rare increases in PR interval have been reported during Kaletra therapy (see section 4.4: sections pancreatitis and lipid elevations).

Increased CPK, myalgia, myositis, and rarely, rhabdomyolysis have been reported with protease inhibitors, particularly in combination with nucleoside reverse transcriptase inhibitors.

Combination antiretroviral therapy has been associated with redistribution of body fat (lipodystrophy) in HIV patients including the loss of peripheral and facial subcutaneous fat, increased intra-abdominal and visceral fat, breast hypertrophy and dorsocervical fat accumulation (buffalo hump).

Combination antiretroviral therapy has been associated with metabolic abnormalities such as hypertriglyceridaemia, hypercholesterolaemia, insulin resistance, hyperglycaemia and hyperlactataemia (see section 4.4).

In HIV-infected patients with severe immune deficiency at the time of initiation of combination antiretroviral therapy (CART), an inflammatory reaction to asymptomatic or residual opportunistic infections may arise (see section 4.4).

Adult patients

Adverse events:

The following adverse reactions of moderate to severe intensity with possible or probable relationship to Kaletra have been reported. The adverse reactions are displayed by system organ class. Within the system organ class adverse reactions are listed by frequency, using the following groupings: very common >1/10, common > 1/100, < 1/10, uncommon > 1/1000, < 1/100.

(see Table 1 opposite)

Paediatric patients

In children 2 years of age and older, the nature of the safety profile is similar to that seen in adults.

Undesirable Effects in Clinical Studies in Paediatric Patients

Infections and infestations	Common	Viral infection
Nervous system disorders	Common	Taste perversion
Gastrointestinal disorders	Common	Constipation, vomiting, pancreatitis*
Hepatobiliary disorders	Common	Hepatomegaly
Skin and subcutaneous tissue disorders	Common	Rash, dry skin
General disorders and administration site conditions	Common	Fever

Investigations	Common (Grade 3 or 4)	Increased activated partial thromboplastin time, decreased haemoglobin, decreased platelets, increased sodium, increased potassium, increased calcium, increased bilirubin, increased SGPT/ALT, increased SGOT/AST, increased total cholesterol, increased amylase, increased uric acid, decreased sodium, decreased potassium, decreased calcium, decreased neutrophils

*see section 4.4: pancreatitis and lipids

Post marketing experience

Hepatitis, and rarely jaundice, have been reported in patients on Kaletra therapy in the presence or absence of identifiable risk factors for hepatitis.

4.9 Overdose

To date, there is limited human experience of acute overdose with Kaletra.

The adverse clinical signs observed in dogs included salivation, emesis and diarrhoea/abnormal stool. The signs of toxicity observed in mice, rats or dogs included decreased activity, ataxia, emaciation, dehydration and tremors.

There is no specific antidote for overdose with Kaletra. Treatment of overdose with Kaletra is to consist of general supportive measures including monitoring of vital signs and observation of the clinical status of the patient. If indicated, elimination of unabsorbed active substance is to be achieved by emesis or gastric lavage. Administration of activated charcoal may also be used to aid in removal of unabsorbed active substance. Since Kaletra is highly protein bound, dialysis is unlikely to be beneficial in significant removal of the active substance.

5. PHARMACOLOGICAL PROPERTIES

5.1 Pharmacodynamic properties

Pharmaco-therapeutic group: antiviral for systemic use, ATC code: J05AE06

Mechanism of action: Lopinavir provides the antiviral activity of Kaletra. Lopinavir is an inhibitor of the HIV-1 and HIV-2 proteases. Inhibition of HIV protease prevents cleavage of the *gag-pol* polyprotein resulting in the production of immature, non-infectious virus.

Antiviral activity in vitro: the *in vitro* antiviral activity of lopinavir against laboratory and clinical HIV strains was evaluated in acutely infected lymphoblastic cell lines and peripheral blood lymphocytes, respectively. In the absence of human serum, the mean EC_{50} of lopinavir against five different HIV-1 laboratory strains was 19 nM. In the absence and presence of 50% human serum, the mean EC_{50} of lopinavir against HIV-1_{IIIB} in MT4 cells was 17 nM and 102 nM, respectively. In the absence of human serum, the mean EC_{50}- of lopinavir was 6.5 nM against several HIV-1 clinical isolates.

Resistance

HIV-1 isolates with reduced susceptibility to lopinavir have been selected *in vitro*. HIV-1 has been passaged *in vitro* with lopinavir alone and with lopinavir plus ritonavir at concentration ratios representing the range of plasma concentration ratios observed during Kaletra therapy. Genotypic and phenotypic analysis of viruses selected in these passages suggest that the presence of ritonavir, at these concentration ratios, does not measurably influence the selection of lopinavir-resistant viruses. Overall, the *in vitro* characterisation of phenotypic cross-resistance between lopinavir and other protease inhibitors suggest that decreased susceptibility to lopinavir correlated closely with decreased susceptibility to ritonavir and indinavir, but did not correlate closely with decreased susceptibility to amprenavir, saquinavir, and nelfinavir.

Genotypic correlates of reduced phenotypic susceptibility to lopinavir in viruses selected by other protease inhibitors. The *in vitro* antiviral activity of lopinavir against 112 clinical isolates taken from patients failing therapy with one or more protease inhibitors was assessed. Within this panel, the following mutations in HIV protease were associated with reduced *in vitro* susceptibility to lopinavir: L10F/I/R/V, K20M/R, L24I, M46I/L, F53L, I54L/T/V, L63P, A71I/L/T/V, V82A/F/T, I84V and L90M. The median EC_{50} of lopinavir against isolates with 0 – 3, 4 – 5, 6 – 7 and 8 – 10 mutations at the above amino acid positions was 0.8, 2.7 13.5 and 44.0-fold higher than the EC_{50} against wild type HIV, respectively. The 16 viruses that displayed > 20-fold change in susceptibility all contained mutations at positions 10, 54, 63 plus 82 and/or 84. In addition, they contained a median of 3 mutations at amino acid positions 20, 24, 46, 53, 71 and 90.

Antiviral activity of Kaletra in patients failing protease inhibitor therapy: the clinical relevance of reduced *in vitro* susceptibility to lopinavir has been examined by assessing the virologic response to Kaletra therapy, with respect to baseline viral genotype and phenotype, in 56 patients previous failing therapy with multiple protease inhibitors. The EC_{50} of lopinavir against the 56 baseline viral isolates ranged from 0.6 to 96-fold higher than the EC_{50} against wild type HIV. After 48 weeks of treatment with Kaletra, efavirenz and nucleoside reverse transcriptase inhibitors, plasma HIV RNA $\leqslant$ 400 copies/ml was observed in 93% (25/27), 73% (11/15), and 25% (2/8) of patients with < 10-fold, 10 to 40-fold, and > 40-fold reduced susceptibility to lopinavir at baseline, respectively. In addition, virologic response was observed in 91% (21/23), 71% (15/21) and 33% (2/6) patients with 0 – 5, 6 – 7, and 8 – 10 mutations of the above mutations in HIV protease associated with reduced *in vitro* susceptibility to lopinavir. Since these patients had not previously been exposed to either Kaletra or efavirenz, part of the response may be attributed to the antiviral activity of efavirenz, particularly in patients harbouring highly lopinavir resistant virus. The study did not contain a control arm of patients not receiving Kaletra.

Selection of viral resistance during Kaletra therapy: in Phase II studies of 227 antiretroviral treatment naïve and protease inhibitor experienced patients, isolates from four patients with quantifiable > 400 copies/ml) viral load following treatment with Kaletra for $\geqslant$ 12 weeks displayed significantly reduced susceptibility to lopinavir compared to the corresponding baseline viral isolates. The mean EC_{50} of lopinavir against the four baseline isolates was 2.8-fold (range: 0.7 to 5.2-fold) higher than the EC_{50} against wild type HIV, and each of the four baseline isolates contained four or more mutations in HIV protease associated with resistance to protease inhibitors. Following treatment of the four patients with Kaletra, the mean EC_{50} of lopinavir increased to 55-fold (range: 9.4 to 99-fold) compared to wild type HIV, and 2 – 3 additional mutations at amino acids 10, 24, 33, 46, 54, 63, 71 and/or 82 were observed.

In a Phase II (M97-720) through 204 weeks of treatment, genotypic analysis of viral isolates was successfully conducted in 11 of 16 patients with confirmed HIV RNA above 400 copies/ml revealed no primary or active site mutations in protease (amino acids at positions 8, 30, 32, 36, 47, 48, 50, 82, 84 and 90) or protease inhibitor phenotypic resistance.

Cross-resistance: at this stage of development, little information is available on the cross-resistance of viruses selected during therapy with Kaletra. Isolates from 4 patients previously treated with one or more protease inhibitors that developed increased lopinavir phenotypic resistance during Kaletra therapy either remained or developed cross-resistance to ritonavir, indinavir, and nelfinavir. All rebound viruses either remained fully sensitive or demonstrated modestly reduced susceptibility to amprenavir (up to 8.6-fold concurrent with 99-fold resistance to lopinavir). The rebound isolates from the two patients with no prior saquinavir treatment remained fully sensitive to saquinavir.

Clinical pharmacodynamic data

The effects of Kaletra (in combination with other antiretroviral agents) on biological markers (plasma HIV RNA levels and CD_4 counts) have been investigated in a controlled study of Kaletra of 48 weeks duration, and in additional studies of Kaletra of 204 weeks duration.

Adult Use

Patients without prior antiretroviral therapy

Study M98-863 is a randomised, double-blind trial of 653 antiretroviral treatment naïve patients investigating Kaletra (400/100 mg twice daily) compared to nelfinavir (750 mg three times daily) plus nucleoside reverse transcriptase inhibitors. By intent to treat analysis where patients with missing values are considered virologic failures, the proportion of patients at 48 weeks with HIV RNA < 400 copies/ml in the Kaletra arm was 75% and 63% in the nelfinavir arm. Mean baseline CD_4 cell count was 259 cells/mm^3 (range: 2 to 949 cells/mm^3) and mean baseline plasma HIV-1 RNA was 4.9 log_{10} copies/ml (range: 2.6 to 6.8 log_{10} copies/ml). Through 48 weeks of therapy, the proportion of patients in the Kaletra arm with plasma RNA < 50 copies/ml was 67% and 52% in the nelfinavir arm. The mean increase from baseline in CD_4 cell count was 207 cells/mm^3 in the Kaletra arm and 195 cells/mm^3 in the nelfinavir arm. Through 48 weeks of therapy, a statistically significantly higher proportion of patients in the Kaletra arm had HIV RNA < 50 copies/ml compared to the nelfinavir arm.

Sustained virological response to Kaletra (in combination with lamivudine and stavudine) has been also observed in a small Phase II study (M97-720) through 204 weeks of treatment. Through 204 weeks of treatment, the proportion of patients with HIV RNA < 400 (< 50) copies/ml was 71% (70%) [n=100 including 40 patients having received the recommended dose of Kaletra for the entire 204 weeks], and the corresponding mean increase in CD_4 cell count was 440 cells/mm^3. Twenty-eight patients (28%) discontinued the study, including nine (9%) discontinuations due to adverse events and one (1%) death.

Patients with prior antiretroviral therapy

Study M97-765 is a randomised, double-blind trial evaluating Kaletra at two dose levels (400/100 mg and 400/200 mg, both twice daily) plus nevirapine (200 mg twice daily) and two nucleoside reverse transcriptase inhibitors in 70 single protease inhibitor experienced, non-nucleoside reverse transcriptase inhibitor naïve patients. Median baseline CD_4 cell count was 349 cells/mm^3 (range 72 to 807 cells/mm^3) and median baseline plasma HIV-1 RNA was 4.0 log_{10} copies/ml (range 2.9 to 5.8 log_{10} copies/ml). By intent-to-treat analysis where patients with missing values are considered virologic failures, the proportion of patients with HIV RNA < 400 (< 50) copies/ml at 24 weeks was 75% (58%) and the mean increase from baseline in CD_4 cell count was 174 cells/mm^3 for the 36 patients receiving the 400/100 mg dose of Kaletra.

M98-957 is a randomised, open-label study evaluating Kaletra treatment at two dose levels (400/100 mg and 533/133 mg, both twice daily) plus efavirenz (600 mg once daily) and nucleoside reverse transcriptase inhibitors in 57 multiple protease inhibitor experienced, non-nucleoside reverse transcriptase inhibitor naïve patients. Between week 24 and 48, patients randomised to a dose of 400/100 mg were converted to a dose of 533/133 mg. Median baseline CD_4 cell count was 220 cells/mm^3 (range13 to 1030 cells/mm^3). By intent-to-treat analysis of both dose groups combined (n=57), where patients with missing values are considered virologic failures, the proportion of patients with HIV RNA < 400 copies/ml at 48 weeks was 65% and the mean increase from baseline CD_4 cell count was 94 cells/mm^3.

Paediatric Use

M98-940 is an open-label study of a liquid formulation of Kaletra in 100 antiretroviral naïve (44%) and experienced (56%) paediatric patients. All patients were non-nucleoside reverse transcriptase inhibitor naïve. Patients were randomised to either 230 mg lopinavir/57.5 mg ritonavir per m^2 or 300 mg lopinavir/75 mg ritonavir per m^2. Naïve patients also received nucleoside reverse transcriptase inhibitors. Experienced patients received nevirapine plus up to two nucleoside reverse transcriptase inhibitors. Safety, efficacy and pharmacokinetic profiles of the two dose regimens were assessed after 3 weeks of therapy in each patient. Subsequently, all patients were continued on the 300/75 mg per m^2 dose. Patients had a mean age of 5 years (range 6 months to 12 years) with 14 patients less than 2 years old and 6 patients one year or less. Mean baseline CD_4 cell count was 838 cells/mm^3 and mean baseline plasma HIV-1 RNA was 4.7 log_{10} copies/ml. Through 48 weeks of therapy, the proportion of patients with HIV RNA < 400 copies/ml was 84% for antiretroviral naïve patients and 75% for antiretroviral experienced patients and the mean increase from baseline in CD_4 cell count were 404 cells/mm^3 and 284 cells/mm^3 respectively.

5.2 Pharmacokinetic properties

The pharmacokinetic properties of lopinavir co-administered with ritonavir have been evaluated in healthy adult volunteers and in HIV-infected patients; no substantial differences were observed between the two groups. Lopinavir is essentially completely metabolised by CYP3A. Ritonavir inhibits the metabolism of lopinavir, thereby increasing the plasma levels of lopinavir. Across studies, administration of Kaletra 400/100 mg twice daily yields mean steady-state lopinavir plasma concentrations 15 to 20-fold higher than those of ritonavir in HIV-infected patients. The plasma levels of ritonavir are less than 7% of those obtained after the ritonavir dose of 600 mg twice daily. The *in vitro* antiviral EC_{50} of lopinavir is approximately 10-fold lower than that of ritonavir. Therefore, the antiviral activity of Kaletra is due to lopinavir.

Absorption: multiple dosing with 400/100 mg Kaletra twice daily for 3 to 4 weeks and without meal restriction produced a mean ± SD lopinavir peak plasma concentration (C_{max}) of 9.6 ± 4.4 μg/ml, occurring approximately 4 hours after administration. The mean steady-state trough concentration prior to the morning dose was 5.5 ± 4.0 μg/ml. Lopinavir AUC over a 12 hour dosing interval averaged 82.8 ± 44.5 μg•h/ml. The absolute bioavailability of lopinavir coformulated with ritonavir in humans has not been established.

Effects of food on oral absorption: Kaletra soft capsules and liquid have been shown to be bioequivalent under nonfasting conditions (moderate fat meal). Administration of a single 400/100 mg dose of Kaletra soft capsules with a moderate fat meal (500 – 682 kcal, 22.7 –25.1% from fat) was associated with a mean increase of 48% and 23% in lopinavir AUC and C_{max}, respectively, relative to fasting. For Kaletra oral solution, the corresponding increases in lopinavir AUC and C_{max} were 80% and 54%, respectively. Administration of Kaletra with a high fat meal (872 kcal, 55.8% from fat) increased lopinavir AUC and C_{max} by 96% and 43%, respectively, for soft capsules, and 130% and 56%, respectively, for oral solution. To enhance bioavailability and minimise variability Kaletra is to be taken with food.

Distribution: at steady state, lopinavir is approximately 98 – 99% bound to serum proteins. Lopinavir binds to both alpha-1-acid glycoprotein (AAG) and albumin, however, it has a higher affinity for AAG. At steady state, lopinavir protein binding remains constant over the range of observed concentrations after 400/100 mg Kaletra twice daily, and is similar between healthy volunteers and HIV-positive patients.

Metabolism: *in vitro* experiments with human hepatic microsomes indicate that lopinavir primarily undergoes oxidative metabolism. Lopinavir is extensively metabolised by the hepatic cytochrome P450 system, almost exclusively by isozyme CYP3A. Ritonavir is a potent CYP3A inhibitor which inhibits the metabolism of lopinavir and therefore, increases plasma levels of lopinavir. A ^{14}C-lopinavir study in humans showed that 89% of the plasma radioactivity after a single 400/100 mg Kaletra dose was due to parent drug. At least 13 lopinavir oxidative metabolites have been identified in man. The 4-oxo and 4-hydroxymetabolite epimeric pair are the major metabolites with antiviral activity, but comprise only minute amounts of total plasma radioactivity. Ritonavir has been shown to induce metabolic enzymes, resulting in the induction of its own metabolism, and likely the induction of lopinavir metabolism. Pre-dose lopinavir concentrations decline with time during multiple dosing, stabilising after approximately 10 days to 2 weeks.

Elimination: after a 400/100 mg ^{14}C-lopinavir/ritonavir dose, approximately 10.4 ± 2.3% and 82.6 ± 2.5% of an administered dose of ^{14}C-lopinavir can be accounted for in urine and faeces, respectively. Unchanged lopinavir accounted for approximately 2.2% and 19.8% of the administered dose in urine and faeces, respectively. After multiple dosing, less than 3% of the lopinavir dose is excreted unchanged in the urine. The effective (peak to trough) half-life of lopinavir over a 12 hour dosing interval averaged 5 – 6 hours, and the apparent oral clearance (CL/F) of lopinavir is 6 to 7 l/h.

Special Populations

Paediatrics:

There are limited pharmacokinetic data in children below 2 years of age. The pharmacokinetics of Kaletra 300/75 mg/m^2 twice daily and 230/57.5 mg/m^2 twice daily have been studied in a total of 53 paediatric patients, ranging in age from 6 months to 12 years. The lopinavir mean steady-state AUC, C_{max}, and C_{min} were 72.6 ± 31.1 μg•h/ml, 8.2 ± 2.9 μg/ml and 3.4 ± 2.1 μg/ml, respectively after Kaletra 230/57.5 mg/m^2 twice daily without nevirapine (n=12), and were 85.8 ± 36.9 μg•h/ml, 10.0 ± 3.3 μg/ml and 3.6 ± 3.5 μg/ml, respectively after 300/75 mg/m^2 twice daily with nevirapine (n=12). The 230/57.5 mg/m^2 twice daily regimen without nevirapine and the 300/75 mg/m^2 twice daily regimen with nevirapine provided lopinavir plasma concentrations similar to those obtained in adult patients receiving the 400/100 mg twice daily regimen without nevirapine. Kaletra soft capsules and Kaletra oral solution are bioequivalent under nonfasting conditions.

Gender, Race and Age:

Kaletra pharmacokinetics have not been studied in the elderly. No age or gender related pharmacokinetic differences have been observed in adult patients. Pharmacokinetic differences due to race have not been identified.

Renal Insufficiency:

Kaletra pharmacokinetics have not been studied in patients with renal insufficiency; however, since the renal clearance of lopinavir is negligible, a decrease in total body clearance is not expected in patients with renal insufficiency.

Hepatic Insufficiency:

The steady state pharmacokinetic parameters of lopinavir in HIV-infected patients with mild to moderate hepatic impairment were compared with those of HIV-infected patients with normal hepatic function in a multiple dose study with lopinavir/ritonavir 400/100 mg twice daily. A limited increase in total lopinavir concentrations of approximately 30% has been observed which is not expected to be of clinical relevance (see section 4.2).

5.3 Preclinical safety data

Repeat-dose toxicity studies in rodents and dogs identified major target organs as the liver, kidney, thyroid, spleen and circulating red blood cells. Hepatic changes indicated cellular swelling with focal degeneration. While exposure eliciting these changes were comparable to or below human clinical exposure, dosages in animals were over 6-fold the recommended clinical dose. Mild renal tubular degeneration was confined to mice exposed with at least twice the recommended human exposure; the kidney was unaffected in rats and dogs. Reduced serum thyroxine led to an increased release of TSH with resultant follicular cell hypertrophy in the thyroid glands of rats. These changes were reversible with withdrawal of the active substance and were absent in mice and dogs. Coombs-negative anisocytosis and poikilocytosis were observed in rats, but not in mice or dogs. Enlarged spleens with histiocytosis were seen in rats but not other species. Serum cholesterol was elevated in rodents but not dogs, while triglycerides were elevated only in mice.

During *in vitro* studies, cloned human cardiac potassium channels (HERG) were inhibited by 30% at the highest concentrations of lopinavir/ritonavir tested, corresponding to a lopinavir exposure 7-fold total and 15-fold free peak plasma levels achieved in humans at the maximum recommended therapeutic dose. In contrast, similar concentrations of lopinavir/ritonavir demonstrated no repolarisation delay in the canine cardiac Purkinje fibres. Lower concentrations of lopinavir/ritonavir did not produce significant potassium (HERG) current blockade. Tissue distribution studies conducted in the rat did not suggest significant cardiac retention of the drug; 72-hour AUC in heart was approximately 50% of measured plasma AUC. Therefore, it is reasonable to expect that cardiac lopinavir levels would not be significantly higher than plasma levels.

In dogs, prominent U waves on the electrocardiogram have been observed associated with prolonged PR interval and bradycardia. These effects have been assumed to be caused by electrolyte disturbance.

The clinical relevance of these preclinical data is unknown, however, the potential cardiac effects of this product in humans cannot be ruled out (see also sections 4.4 and 4.8).

In rats, embryofoetotoxicity (pregnancy loss, decreased foetal viability, decreased foetal body weights, increased frequency of skeletal variations) and postnatal developmental toxicity (decreased survival of pups) was observed at maternally toxic dosages. The systemic exposure to lopinavir/ritonavir at the maternal and developmental toxic dosages was lower than the intended therapeutic exposure in humans.

Long-term carcinogenicity studies of lopinavir/ritonavir in mice revealed a nongenotoxic, mitogenic induction of liver tumours, generally considered to have little relevance to human risk. Carcinogenicity studies in rats revealed no tumourigenic findings. Lopinavir/ritonavir was not found to be mutagenic or clastogenic in a battery of *in vitro* and *in vivo* assays including the Ames bacterial reverse mutation assay, the mouse lymphoma assay, the mouse micronucleus test and chromosomal aberration assays in human lymphocytes.

6. PHARMACEUTICAL PARTICULARS

6.1 List of excipients

Oral solution contains:

Alcohol (42% v/v),

high fructose corn syrup,

propylene glycol,

purified water,

glycerol,

povidone,

Magnasweet-110 flavour (mixture of monoammonium glycyrrhizinate and glycerol),

vanilla flavour (containing p-hydroxybenzoic acid, p-hydroxybenzaldehyde, vanillic acid, vanillin, heliotrope, ethyl vanillin),

polyoxyl 40 hydrogenated castor oil,

cotton candy flavour (containing ethyl maltol, ethyl vanillin, acetoin, dihydrocoumarin, propylene glycol),

acesulfame potassium,

saccharin sodium,

sodium chloride,

peppermint oil,

sodium citrate,

citric acid,

menthol.

6.2 Incompatibilities

Not applicable.

6.3 Shelf life

2 years.

6.4 Special precautions for storage

Store Kaletra oral solution in a refrigerator (2°C - 8°C).

In use storage: If kept outside of the refrigerator, do not store above 25°C and discard any unused contents after 42 days (6 weeks). It is advised to write the date of removal from the refrigerator on the package.

Avoid exposure to excessive heat.

6.5 Nature and contents of container

Amber coloured multiple-dose polyethylene terephthalate (PET) bottles in a 60 ml size. Each pack contains 5 bottles of 60 ml (300 ml). The pack also contains 5 × 5 ml syringes with 0.1 ml graduations from 0 to 5 ml (400/100 mg).

6.6 Instructions for use and handling

No special requirements.

7. MARKETING AUTHORISATION HOLDER

Abbott Laboratories Limited

Queenborough

Kent ME11 5EL

United Kingdom

8. MARKETING AUTHORISATION NUMBER(S)

EU/1/01/172/003

9. DATE OF FIRST AUTHORISATION/RENEWAL OF THE AUTHORISATION

20 March 2001

10. DATE OF REVISION OF THE TEXT

12 January 2005

Kaletra Soft Capsules

(Abbott Laboratories Limited)

1. NAME OF THE MEDICINAL PRODUCT

Kaletra soft capsules

2. QUALITATIVE AND QUANTITATIVE COMPOSITION

Each Kaletra soft capsule contains 133.3 mg of lopinavir co-formulated with 33.3 mg of ritonavir as a pharmacokinetic enhancer.

For excipients, see section 6.1.

3. PHARMACEUTICAL FORM

Soft capsules

The capsules are orange with a black ink imprint of [Abbott logo] and "PK".

4. CLINICAL PARTICULARS

4.1 Therapeutic indications

Kaletra is indicated for the treatment of HIV-1 infected adults and children above the age of 2 years, in combination with other antiretroviral agents.

Most experience with Kaletra is derived from the use of the product in antiretroviral therapy naïve patients. Data in heavily pretreated protease inhibitor experienced patients are limited. There are limited data on salvage therapy on patients who have failed therapy with Kaletra.

The choice of Kaletra to treat protease inhibitor experienced HIV-1 infected patients should be based on individual viral resistance testing and treatment history of patients (see sections 4.4 and 5.1).

4.2 Posology and method of administration

Kaletra should be prescribed by physicians who are experienced in the treatment of HIV infection.

Adult and adolescent use: the recommended dosage of Kaletra is three capsules twice daily taken with food. Oral solution is available to patients with difficulty swallowing.

Paediatric use (2 years of age and above): the oral solution is the recommended option for the most accurate dosing in children based on body surface area* (please refer to the Kaletra oral solution Summary of Product Characteristics). However, if it is judged necessary to resort to soft capsules in children, they should be used with particular caution since they are associated with less precise dosing capabilities. Therefore, children receiving soft capsules might have higher exposure (with the risk of increased toxicity) or sub optimal exposure (with the risk of insuffcient efficacy). Consequently when dosing children with soft capsules, therapeutic drug monitoring may be a useful tool to ensure appropriate lopinavir exposure in an individual patient.

Paediatric Dosing Guidelines with Soft Capsules

Body Surface Area* (m^2)	Twice Daily Dose (dose in mg)
0.40 – 0.75	1 soft capsule (133.3/33.3 mg)
0.80 – 1.3	2 soft capsules (266.6/66.6 mg)
1.4 – 1.75	3 soft capsules (400/100 mg)

* Body surface area can be calculated with the following equation

BSA (m^2) = $\sqrt{}$ (Height (cm) X Weight (kg) / 3600)

Children less than 2 years of age: Kaletra is not recommended for use in children less than 2 years of age because of limited safety and efficacy data.

Hepatic impairment: In HIV-infected patients with mild to moderate hepatic impairment, an increase of approximately 30% in lopinavir exposure has been observed but is not expected to be of clinical relevance. (see section 5.2). No data are available in patients with severe hepatic impairment. Kaletra should not be given to these patients (see section 4.3).

Renal impairment: no dose adjustment is necessary in patients with renal impairment. Caution is warranted when Kaletra is used in patients with severe renal impairment (see section 4.4).

4.3 Contraindications

Patients with known hypersensitivity to lopinavir, ritonavir or any of the excipients.

Patients with severe hepatic insufficiency.

Kaletra contains lopinavir and ritonavir, both of which are inhibitors of the P450 isoform CYP3A. Kaletra should not be co-administered with medicinal products that are highly dependent on CYP3A for clearance and for which elevated plasma concentrations are associated with serious and/or life threatening events. These medicinal products include astemizole, terfenadine, midazolam, triazolam, cisapride, pimozide, amiodarone, ergot alkaloids (e.g. ergotamine, dihydroergotamine, ergonovine and methylergonovine).

Herbal preparations containing St John's wort (*Hypericum perforatum)* must not be used while taking lopinavir and ritonavir due to the risk of decreased plasma concentrations and reduced clinical effects of lopinavir and ritonavir. (see section 4.5).

Rifampicin should not be used in combination with Kaletra because co-administration may cause large decreases in lopinavir concentrations which may in turn significantly decrease the lopinavir therapeutic effect (see section 4.5).

4.4 Special warnings and special precautions for use

Patients with coexisting conditions

Liver disease: the safety and efficacy of Kaletra has not been established in patients with significant underlying liver disorders. Kaletra is contraindicated in patients with severe liver impairment (see section 4.3). Patients with chronic hepatitis B or C and treated with combination antiretroviral therapy are at an increased risk for severe and potentially fatal hepatic adverse events. In case of concomitant antiviral therapy for hepatitis B or C, please refer to the relevant product information for these medicinal products.

Patients with pre-existing liver dysfunction including chronic hepatitis have an increased frequency of liver function abnormalities during combination antiretroviral therapy and should be monitored according to standard practice. If there is evidence of worsening liver disease in such patients, interruption or discontinuation of treatment should be considered.

Renal disease: since the renal clearance of lopinavir and ritonavir is negligible, increased plasma concentrations are not expected in patients with renal impairment. Because lopinavir and ritonavir are highly protein bound, it is unlikely that they will be significantly removed by haemodialysis or peritoneal dialysis.

Haemophilia: there have been reports of increased bleeding, including spontaneous skin haematomas and haemarthrosis in patients with haemophilia type A and B treated with protease inhibitors. In some patients additional factor VIII was given. In more than half of the reported cases, treatment with protease inhibitors was continued or reintroduced if treatment had been discontinued. A causal relationship had been evoked, although the mechanism of action had not been elucidated. Haemophiliac patients should therefore be made aware of the possibility of increased bleeding.

Lipid elevations

Treatment with Kaletra has resulted in increases, sometimes marked, in the concentration of total cholesterol and triglycerides. Triglyceride and cholesterol testing is to be performed prior to initiating Kaletra therapy and at periodic intervals during therapy. Particular caution should be paid to patients with high values at baseline and with history of lipid disorders. Lipid disorders are to be managed as clinically appropriate (see also section 4.5 for additional information on potential interactions with HMG-CoA reductase inhibitors).

Pancreatitis

Cases of pancreatitis have been reported in patients receiving Kaletra, including those who developed hypertriglyceridaemia. In most of these cases patients have had a prior history of pancreatitis and/or concurrent therapy with other medicinal products associated with pancreatitis. Marked triglyceride elevation is a risk factor for development of pancreatitis. Patients with advanced HIV disease may be at risk of elevated triglycerides and pancreatitis

Pancreatitis should be considered if clinical symptoms (nausea, vomiting, abdominal pain) or abnormalities in laboratory values (such as increased serum lipase or amylase values) suggestive of pancreatitis should occur. Patients who exhibit these signs or symptoms should be evaluated and Kaletra therapy should be suspended if a diagnosis of pancreatitis is made (see section 4.8).

Hyperglycaemia

New onset diabetes mellitus, hyperglycaemia or exacerbation of existing diabetes mellitus has been reported in patients receiving protease inhibitors. In some of these the hyperglycaemia was severe and in some cases also associated with ketoacidosis. Many patients had confounding medical conditions some of which required therapy with agents that have been associated with the development of diabetes mellitus or hyperglycaemia.

Fat redistribution & metabolic disorders

Combination antiretroviral therapy has been associated with redistribution of body fat (lipodystrophy) in HIV patients. The long-term consequences of these events are currently unknown. Knowledge about the mechanism is incomplete. A connection between visceral lipomatosis and protease inhibitors (PIs) and lipoatrophy and nucleoside reverse transcriptase inhibitors (NRTIs) has been hypothesised. A higher risk of lipodystrophy has been associated with individual factors such as older age, and with drug related factors such as longer duration of antiretroviral treatment and associated metabolic disturbances. Clinical examination should include evaluation for physical signs of fat redistribution. Consideration should be given to measurement of fasting serum lipids and blood glucose. Lipid disorders should be managed as clinically appropriate (see section 4.8).

Immune Reactivation Syndrome

In HIV-infected patients with severe immune deficiency at the time of institution of combination antiretroviral therapy (CART), an inflammatory reaction to asymtomatic or residual opportunistic pathogens may arise and cause serious clinical conditions, or aggravation of symptoms. Typically, such reactions have been observed within the first few weeks or months of initiation of CART. Relevant examples are cytomegalovirus retinitis, generalised and/or focal mycobacterial infections, and Pneumocystis carinii pneumonia. Any inflammatory symptoms should be evaluated and treatment instituted when necessary.

Interactions with medicinal products

Kaletra contains lopinavir and ritonavir, both of which are inhibitors of the P450 isoform CYP3A. Kaletra is likely to increase plasma concentrations of medicinal products that are primarily metabolised by CYP3A. These increases of plasma concentrations of co-administered medicinal products could increase or prolong their therapeutic effect and adverse events (see sections 4.3 and 4.5).

Particular caution must be used when prescribing sildenafil in patients receiving Kaletra. Co-administration of Kaletra with sildenafil is expected to substantially increase sildenafil concentrations and may result in an increase in sildenafil-associated adverse events including hypotension, syncope, visual changes and prolonged erection (see section 4.5).

The HMG-CoA reductase inhibitors simvastatin and lovastatin are highly dependent on CYP3A for metabolism, thus concomitant use of Kaletra with simvastatin or lovastatin is not recommended due to an increased risk of myopathy including rhabdomyolysis. Caution must also be exercised and reduced doses should be considered if Kaletra is used concurrently with atorvastatin, which is metabolised to a lesser extent by CYP3A4. If treatment with a HMG-CoA reductase inhibitor is indicated, pravastatin or fluvastatin is recommended (see section 4.5).

Particular caution must be used when prescribing Kaletra and medicinal products known to induce QT interval prolongation such as: chlorpheniramine, quinidine, erythromycin, clarithromycin. Indeed, Kaletra could increase concentrations of the co-administered medicinal products and this may result in an increase of their associated cardiac adverse events. Cardiac events have been reported with Kaletra in preclinical studies; therefore, the potential cardiac effects of Kaletra cannot be currently ruled out (see sections 4.8 and 5.3).

Rifampicin should not be used in combination with Kaletra because this may cause large decreases in lopinavir concentrations which may in turn significantly decrease the lopinavir therapeutic effect (see sections 4.3 and 4.5).

Oral Contraceptives: since levels of ethinyl oestradiol may be decreased alternative or additional contraceptive measures are to be used when oestrogen-based oral contraceptives are co-administered (see section 4.5).

Other

Kaletra is not recommended for use in children less than 2 years of age because of limited efficacy and safety data.

Kaletra is not a cure for HIV infection or AIDS. It does not reduce the risk of passing HIV to others through sexual contact or blood contamination. Appropriate precautions should be taken. People taking Kaletra may still develop infections or other illnesses associated with HIV disease and AIDS.

There are limited data on salvage therapy on patients who have failed with Kaletra. There are ongoing studies to further establish the usefulness of potential salvage therapy regimens (e.g. amprenavir or saquinavir). There are currently limited data on the use of Kaletra in protease inhibitor-experienced patients.

Kaletra soft capsules contain sunset yellow [E110] as an excipient, which can cause allergic-type reaction. Allergy is more common in those people who are allergic to aspirin.

Concomitant use of ritonavir (including low-dose) and fluticasone propionate significantly increased fluticasone propionate plasma concentrations and reduced serum cortisol concentrations in a clinical study. Concomitant use of ritonavir (including low-dose) and fluticasone is therefore not recommended unless the potential benefit of treatment outweighs the risk of systemic corticosteroid effects. Systemic corticosteroid effects including Cushing's syndrome and adrenal suppression have been reported when ritonavir has been co-administered with inhaled or intranasal administered fluticasone propionate (see section 4.5).

4.5 Interaction with other medicinal products and other forms of Interaction

Kaletra contains lopinavir and ritonavir, both of which are inhibitors of the P450 isoform CYP3A *in vitro*. Co-administration of Kaletra and medicinal products primarily metabolised by CYP3A may result in increased plasma concentrations of the other medicinal product, which could increase or prolong its therapeutic and adverse effects. Kaletra does not inhibit CYP2D6, CYP2C9, CYP2C19, CYP2E1, CYP2B6 or CYP1A2 at clinically relevant concentrations (see section 4.3).

Kaletra has been shown *in vivo* to induce its own metabolism and to increase the biotransformation of some medicinal products metabolised by cytochrome P450 enzymes and by glucuronidation. This may result in lowered plasma concentrations and potential decrease of efficacy of co-administered medicinal products.

Medicinal products that are contraindicated specifically due to the expected magnitude of interaction and potential for serious adverse events are listed in section 4.3.

Antiretroviral agents

Nucleoside reverse transcriptase inhibitors (NRTIs):

Stavudine and Lamivudine: no change in the pharmacokinetics of lopinavir was observed when Kaletra was given alone or in combination with stavudine and lamivudine in clinical studies.

Didanosine: it is recommended that didanosine be administered on an empty stomach; therefore, didanosine is to be given one hour before or two hours after Kaletra (given with food). The gastroresistant formulation of didanosine should be administered at least two hours after a meal.

Zidovudine and Abacavir: Kaletra induces glucuronidation, therefore Kaletra has the potential to reduce zidovudine and abacavir plasma concentrations. The clinical significance of this potential interaction is unknown.

Non-nucleoside reverse transcriptase inhibitors (NNRTIs):

Nevirapine: no change in the pharmacokinetics of lopinavir was apparent in healthy volunteers during nevirapine and Kaletra co-administration. Results from a study in HIV-positive paediatric patients revealed a decrease in lopinavir concentrations during nevirapine co-administration. The effect of nevirapine in HIV-positive adults is expected to be similar to that in paediatric patients and lopinavir concentrations may be decreased. The clinical significance of the pharmacokinetic interaction is unknown. No formal recommendation could be drawn on dosage adjustment when Kaletra is used in combination with nevirapine. However, based on clinical experience, Kaletra dose increase to 533/133 mg (4 capsules) twice daily may be considered when co-administered with nevirapine, particularly for patients in whom reduced lopinavir susceptibility is likely.

Efavirenz: when used in combination with efavirenz and two nucleoside reverse transcriptase inhibitors in multiple protease inhibitor-experienced patients, increasing the dose of Kaletra 33.3% from 400/100 mg (3 capsules) twice daily to 533/133 mg (4 capsules) twice daily yielded similar lopinavir plasma concentrations as compared to historical data of Kaletra 400/100 mg (3 capsules) twice daily.

Dosage increase of Kaletra from 400/100 mg (3 capsules) twice daily to 533/133 mg (4 capsules) twice daily should be considered when co-administered with efavirenz. Caution is warranted since this dosage adjustment might be insufficient in some patients.

Co-administration with other HIV protease inhibitors (PIs):

Kaletra (400/100 mg twice daily) has been studied in combination with reduced doses of amprenavir, indinavir, nelfinavir and saquinavir in steady-state controlled healthy volunteer studies relative to clinical doses of each HIV protease inhibitor in the absence of ritonavir. Comparisons to published pharmacokinetic data with ritonavir-enhanced amprenavir and saquinavir regimens are also described. Additionally, the effect of additional ritonavir on the pharmacokinetics of lopinavir are discussed. Note that the historical comparisons to ritonavir-enhanced protease inhibitor regimens should be interpreted with caution (see details of combinations below). Appropriate doses of HIV-protease inhibitors in combination with Kaletra with respect to safety and efficacy have not been established. Therefore, the concomitant administration of Kaletra with PIs requires close monitoring.

Amprenavir: the concomitant use of Kaletra with amprenavir 750 mg twice daily, resulted in an increase in amprenavir AUC by 70% and of C_{min} by 4.6-fold, relative to amprenavir 1200 mg twice daily alone. On the other hand, the AUC of lopinavir decreases by 38%. A dose increase of Kaletra may be necessary but may further affect concentrations of amprenavir.

Combined with Kaletra, amprenavir concentrations were lower (approximately 30%) relative to boosted amprenavir (amprenavir 600 mg/ritonavir 100 mg) twice daily alone.

Indinavir: indinavir 600 mg twice daily in combination with Kaletra produces similar indinavir AUC, higher C_{min} (by 3.5-fold) and lower C_{max} relative to indinavir 800 mg three times daily alone. Furthermore, concentrations of lopinavir do not appear to be affected when both drugs, Kaletra and indinivir, are combined, based on historical comparison with Kaletra alone.

Nelfinavir: administration of nelfinavir 1000 mg twice daily in combination with Kaletra produces a similar nelfinavir C_{max} and AUC and higher C_{min} relative to nelfinavir 1250 mg twice daily alone. Additionally, concentrations of the active M8 metabolite of nelfinavir were increased.

On the other hand, lopinavir AUC was decreased by 27% during nelfinavir co-administration with Kaletra. A dose increase of Kaletra may be necessary but may further affect concentrations of nelfinavir and its active metabolite. Higher doses of Kaletra have not been studied.

Saquinavir: saquinavir 800 mg twice daily co-administered with Kaletra produces an increase of saquinavir AUC by 9.6-fold relative to saquinavir 1200 mg three times daily given alone.

Saquinavir 800 mg twice daily co-administered with Kaletra resulted in an increase of saquinavir AUC by approximately 30% relative to saquinavir/ritonavir 1000/100 mg twice daily, and produces similar exposure to those reported after saquinavir/ritonavir 400/400 mg twice daily.

When saquinavir 1200 mg twice daily was combined with Kaletra, no further increase of concentrations was noted. Furthermore, concentrations of lopinavir do not appear to be affected when both drugs, Kaletra and saquinavir, are combined, based on historical comparison with Kaletra alone.

Ritonavir: Kaletra co-administered with an additional 100 mg ritonavir twice daily resulted in an increase of lopinavir AUC and C_{min} of 33% and 64%, respectively, as compared to Kaletra alone.

Other medicinal products:

Antiarrhythmics: (bepridil, systemic lidocaine and quinidine): concentrations may be increased when co-administered with Kaletra. Caution is warranted and therapeutic concentration monitoring is recommended when available.

Anticoagulants: warfarin concentrations may be affected when co-administered with Kaletra. It is recommended that INR (international normalised ratio) be monitored.

Anticonvulsants: (phenobarbital, phenytoin, carbamazepine): will induce CYP3A4 and may decrease lopinavir concentrations.

Dihydropyridine calcium channel blockers: (e.g. felodipine, nifedipine, nicardipine): may have their serum concentrations increased by Kaletra.

HMG-CoA reductase inhibitors: HMG-CoA reductase inhibitors which are highly dependent on CYP3A4 metabolism, such as lovastatin and simvastatin, are expected to have markedly increased plasma concentrations when co-administered with Kaletra. Since increased concentrations of HMG-CoA reductase inhibitors may cause myopathy, including rhabdomyolysis, the combination of these medicinal products with Kaletra is not recommended. Atorvastatin is less dependent on CYP3A for metabolism. When atorvastatin was given concurrently with Kaletra, a mean 4.7-fold and 5.9-fold increase in atorvastatin C_{max} and AUC, respectively, was observed. When used with Kaletra, the lowest possible dose of atorvastatin should be administered. Results from an interaction study with Kaletra and pravastatin reveal no clinically significant interaction. The metabolism of pravastatin and fluvastatin is not dependent on CYP3A4, and interactions are not expected with Kaletra. If treatment with a HMG-CoA reductase inhibitor is indicated, pravastatin or fluvastatin is recommended.

Dexamethasone: may induce CYP3A4 and may decrease lopinavir concentrations.

Sildenafil: co-administration of sildenafil 100 mg single dose with ritonavir 500 mg twice daily at steady-state resulted in a 1000% increase in sildenafil plasma AUC. On the basis of these data, concomitant use of sildenafil with Kaletra is not recommended and in no case should the starting dose of sildenafil exceed 25 mg within 48 hours (see section 4.4).

Cyclosporin, sirolimus (rapamycin) and tacrolimus: concentrations may be increased when co-administered with Kaletra. More frequent therapeutic concentration monitoring is recommended until plasma levels of these products have been stabilised.

Ketoconazole and itraconazole: may have serum concentrations increased by Kaletra. High doses of ketoconazole and itraconazole > 200 mg/day) are not recommended.

Clarithromycin: moderate increases in clarithromycin AUC are expected when co-administered with Kaletra. For patients with renal or hepatic impairment dose reduction of clarithromycin should be considered (see section 4.4).

Methadone: Kaletra was demonstrated to lower plasma concentrations of methadone. Monitoring plasma concentrations of methadone is recommended.

Oral Contraceptives: since levels of ethinyl oestradiol may be decreased alternative or additional contraceptive measures are to be used when oestrogen-based oral contraceptives are co-administered.

Rifabutin: when rifabutin and Kaletra were co-administered for 10 days, rifabutin (parent drug and active 25-O-desacetyl metabolite) C_{max} and AUC were increased by 3.5- and 5.7-fold, respectively. On the basis of these data, a rifabutin dose reduction of 75% (i.e. 150 mg every other day or 3 times per week) is recommended when administered with Kaletra. Further reduction may be necessary.

Rifampicin: due to large decreases in lopinavir concentrations, rifampicin should not be used in combination with Kaletra (see sections 4.3 and 4.4).

St John's wort: serum levels of lopinavir and ritonavir can be reduced by concomitant use of the herbal preparation St John's wort (*Hypericum perforatum).* This is due to the induction of drug metabolising enzymes by St John's wort. Herbal preparations containing St John's wort should therefore not be combined with lopinavir and ritonavir. If a patient is already taking St John's wort, stop St John's wort and if possible check viral levels. Lopinavir and ritonavir levels may increase on stopping St John's wort. The dose of Kaletra may need adjusting. The inducing effect may persist for at least 2 weeks after cessation of treatment with St John's wort (see section 4.3).

Fluticasone propionate: in a clinical study where ritonavir 100 mg capsules twice daily were co – administered with 50 μg intranasal fluticasone propionate (4 times daily) for seven days in healthy subjects, the fluticasone propionate plasma levels increased significantly, whereas the intrinsic cortisol levels decreased by approximately 86% (90% confidence interval 82 – 89%). Greater effects may be expected when fluticasone propionate is inhaled. Systemic corticosteroid effects including Cushing's syndrome and

Table 1 Undesirable Effects in Clinical Studies in Adult Patients

Infections and infestations	Uncommon	Otitis media, bronchitis, sinusitis, furunculosis, bacterial infection, viral infection
Neoplasms benign, malignant and unspecified	Uncommon	Skin benign neoplasm, cyst
Blood and lymphatic system Disorders	Uncommon	Anaemia, leucopenia and lymphadenopathy
Endocrine disorders	Uncommon	Hypogonadism male, Cushing syndrome, hypothyroidism
Metabolic and nutritional disorders	Uncommon	Avitaminosis, dehydration, oedema, increased appetite, lactic acidosis, obesity, anorexia, diabetes mellitus, hyperglycaemia, hypocholesteremia
Psychiatric disorders	Common	Insomnia
	Uncommon	Abnormal dreams, agitation, anxiety, confusion, depression, dyskinesia, emotional lability, decreased libido, nervousness, abnormal thinking
Nervous system disorders	Common	Headache
	Uncommon	Dizziness, amnesia, ataxia, encephalopathy, facial paralysis, hypertonia, neuropathy, paresthesia, peripheral neuritis, somnolence, tremor, taste perversion, migraine, amnesia, extrapyramidal syndrome
Eye disorders	Uncommon	Abnormal vision, eye disorder
Ear and labyrinth disorders	Uncommon	Tinnitus
Cardiac disorders	Uncommon	Palpitation, lung oedema, myocardial infarct[1]
Vascular disorders	Uncommon	Hypertension, thrombophlebitis, vasculitis, varicose vein, deep thrombophlebitis, vascular disorder
Respiratory, thoracic and mediastinal disorders	Uncommon	Dyspnea, rhinitis, cough increased
Gastrointestinal disorders	Very common	Diarrhoea
	Common	Nausea, vomiting, abdominal pain, abnormal stools, dyspepsia, flatulence, gastrointestinal disorder
	Uncommon	Abdomen enlarged, constipation, dry mouth, dysphagia, enterocolitis, eructation, oesophagitis, faecal incontinence, gastritis, gastroenteritis, haemorrhagic colitis, mouth ulcerations, pancreatitis[2], sialadenitis, stomatitis, ulcerative stomatitis, periodontitis
Hepatobiliary disorders	Uncommon	Cholecystitis, hepatitis, hepatomegaly, liver fatty deposit, liver tenderness
Skin and subcutaneous tissue disorders	Common	Rash, lipodystrophy
	Uncommon	Alopecia, dry skin, eczema, exfoliative dermatitis, maculopapular rash, nail disorder, pruritis, seborrhea, skin discoloration, skin ulcer, face oedema, acne, sweating, skin striae
Musculoskeletal and connective tissue disorders	Uncommon	Arthralgia, arthrosis, myalgia, back pain, joint disorder
Renal and urinary disorders	Uncommon	Kidney calculus, urine abnormality, albuminuria, hypercalcinuria, hyperuricemia
Reproductive system and breast disorders	Uncommon	Abnormal ejaculation, breast enlargement, gynecomastia, impotence, menorrhagia
General disorders and administration site conditions	Common	Asthenia
	Uncommon	Chest pain, chest pain substernal, chills, fever, flu syndrome, malaise, pain, peripheral oedema, drug interaction
Investigations	Very common (Grade 3 or 4)	Increased triglycerides, increased total cholesterol, increased GGT
	Common (Grade 3 or 4)	Increased glucose, increased amylase, increased SGOT/AST, increased SGPT/ALT, liver function tests abnormal
	Uncommon	Decreased glucose tolerance, weight gain, weight loss, increased bilirubin, hormone level altered, lab test abnormal

[1] This event had a fatal outcome.

[2] See section 4.4: pancreatitis and lipids

adrenal suppression have been reported when ritonavir has been co – administered with inhaled or intranasally administered fluticasone propionate; this could also occur with other corticosteroids eg budesonide. Consequently, concomitant administration of Kaletra (including low dose of ritonavir) and inhaled or intranasally administered glucocorticoids is not recommended unless the potential benefit of treatment outweighs the risk of systemic corticosteroid effects. A dose reduction of the glucocorticoid should be considered with close monitoring. Moreover, in case of withdrawal of glucocorticoids progressive dose reduction may have to be performed over a longer period. The effects of high fluticasone systemic exposure on ritonavir plasma levels is yet unknown (see section 4.4).

Based on known metabolic profiles, clinically significant interactions are not expected between Kaletra and fluvastatin, dapsone, trimethoprim/sulfamethoxazole, azithromycin or fluconazole.

4.6 Pregnancy and lactation

There are no data from the use of Kaletra in pregnant women. Studies in animals have shown reproductive toxicity (see section 5.3). The potential risk for humans is unknown. Kaletra should not be used during pregnancy unless clearly necessary.

Studies in rats revealed that lopinavir is excreted in the milk. It is not known whether this medicinal product is excreted in human milk. HIV infected women must not breast-feed their infants under any circumstances to avoid transmission of HIV.

4.7 Effects on ability to drive and use machines

No studies on the effects on the ability to drive a car and use machines have been performed.

4.8 Undesirable effects

The safety of Kaletra has been investigated in 612 patients in Phase II/III clinical trials, of which 442 have received a dose of 400/100 mg (3 capsules) twice daily. In some studies, Kaletra was used in combination with efavirenz or nevirapine.

The most common adverse event associated with Kaletra therapy was diarrhoea and was generally of mild to moderate severity. Discontinuation due to adverse reactions was 4.5% (naïve patients) and 9% (experienced patients) over a 48 week period.

It is important to note that cases of pancreatitis have been reported in patients receiving Kaletra, including those who developed hypertriglyceridaemia. Furthermore, rare increases in PR interval have been reported during Kaletra therapy (see section 4.4: sections pancreatitis and lipid elevations).

Increased CPK, myalgia, myositis, and rarely, rhabdomyolysis have been reported with protease inhibitors, particularly in combination with nucleoside reverse transcriptase inhibitors.

Combination antiretroviral therapy has been associated with redistribution of body fat (lipodystrophy) in HIV patients including the loss of peripheral and facial subcutaneous fat, increased intra-abdominal and visceral fat, breast hypertrophy and dorsocervical fat accumulation (buffalo hump).

Combination antiretroviral therapy has been associated with metabolic abnormalities such as hypertriglyceridaemia, hypercholesterolaemia, insulin resistance, hyperglycaemia and hyperlactataemia (see section 4.4).

In HIV-infected patients with severe immune deficiency at the time of initiation of combination antiretroviral therapy (CART), an inflammatory reaction to asymptomatic or residual opportunistic infections may arise (see section 4.4).

Adult patients

Adverse events:

The following adverse reactions of moderate to severe intensity with possible or probable relationship to Kaletra have been reported. The adverse reactions are displayed by system organ class. Within the system organ class adverse reactions are listed by frequency, using the following groupings: very common >1/10, common > 1/100, < 1/10, uncommon > 1/1000, < 1/100.

(see Table 1 on previous page)

Paediatric patients

In children 2 years of age and older, the nature of the safety profile is similar to that seen in adults.

Undesirable Effects in Clinical Studies in Paediatric Patients		
Infections and infestations	Common	Viral infection
Nervous system disorders	Common	Taste perversion
Gastrointestinal disorders	Common	Constipation, vomiting, pancreatitis*
Hepatobiliary disorders	Common	Hepatomegaly
Skin and subcutaneous tissue disorders	Common	Rash, dry skin
General disorders and administration site conditions	Common	Fever
Investigations	Common (Grade 3 or 4)	Increased activated partial thromboplastin time, decreased haemoglobin, decreased platelets, increased sodium, increased potassium, increased calcium, increased bilirubin, increased SGPT/ALT, increased SGOT/AST, increased total cholesterol, increased amylase, increased uric acid, decreased sodium, decreased potassium, decreased calcium, decreased neutrophils

*see section 4.4: pancreatitis and lipids

Post marketing experience

Hepatitis, and rarely jaundice, have been reported in patients on Kaletra therapy in the presence or absence of identifiable risk factors for hepatitis.

4.9 Overdose

To date, there is limited human experience of acute overdose with Kaletra.

The adverse clinical signs observed in dogs included salivation, emesis and diarrhoea/abnormal stool. The signs of toxicity observed in mice, rats or dogs included decreased activity, ataxia, emaciation, dehydration and tremors.

There is no specific antidote for overdose with Kaletra. Treatment of overdose with Kaletra is to consist of general supportive measures including monitoring of vital signs and observation of the clinical status of the patient. If indicated, elimination of unabsorbed active substance is to be achieved by emesis or gastric lavage. Administration of activated charcoal may also be used to aid in removal of unabsorbed active substance. Since Kaletra is highly protein bound, dialysis is unlikely to be beneficial in significant removal of the active substance.

5. PHARMACOLOGICAL PROPERTIES

5.1 Pharmacodynamic properties

Pharmaco-therapeutic group: antiviral for systemic use, ATC code: J05AE06

Mechanism of action: Lopinavir provides the antiviral activity of Kaletra. Lopinavir is an inhibitor of the HIV-1 and HIV-2 proteases. Inhibition of HIV protease prevents cleavage of the *gag-pol* polyprotein resulting in the production of immature, non-infectious virus.

Antiviral activity in vitro: the *in vitro* antiviral activity of lopinavir against laboratory and clinical HIV strains was evaluated in acutely infected lymphoblastic cell lines and peripheral blood lymphocytes, respectively. In the absence of human serum, the mean EC_{50} of lopinavir against five different HIV-1 laboratory strains was 19 nM. In the absence and presence of 50% human serum, the mean EC_{50} of lopinavir against HIV-1_{IIIB} in MT4 cells was 17 nM and 102 nM, respectively. In the absence of human serum, the mean EC_{50}- of lopinavir was 6.5 nM against several HIV-1 clinical isolates.

Resistance

HIV-1 isolates with reduced susceptibility to lopinavir have been selected *in vitro*. HIV-1 has been passaged *in vitro* with lopinavir alone and with lopinavir plus ritonavir at concentration ratios representing the range of plasma concentration ratios observed during Kaletra therapy. Genotypic and phenotypic analysis of viruses selected in these passages suggest that the presence of ritonavir, at these concentration ratios, does not measurably influence the selection of lopinavir-resistant viruses. Overall, the *in vitro* characterisation of phenotypic cross-resistance between lopinavir and other protease inhibitors suggest that decreased susceptibility to lopinavir correlated closely with decreased susceptibility to ritonavir and indinavir, but did not correlate closely with decreased susceptibility to amprenavir, saquinavir, and nelfinavir.

Genotypic correlates of reduced phenotypic susceptibility to lopinavir in viruses selected by other protease inhibitors. The *in vitro* antiviral activity of lopinavir against 112 clinical isolates taken from patients failing therapy with one or more protease inhibitors was assessed. Within this panel, the following mutations in HIV protease were associated with reduced *in vitro* susceptibility to lopinavir: L10F/I/R/V, K20M/R, L24I, M46I/L, F53L, I54L/T/V, L63P, A71I/L/T/V, V82A/F/T, I84V and L90M. The median EC_{50} of lopinavir against isolates with 0 – 3, 4 – 5, 6 – 7 and 8 – 10 mutations at the above amino acid positions was 0.8, 2.7 13.5 and 44.0-fold higher than the EC_{50} against wild type HIV, respectively. The 16 viruses that displayed > 20-fold change in susceptibility all contained mutations at positions 10, 54, 63 plus 82 and/or 84. In addition, they contained a median of 3 mutations at amino acid positions 20, 24, 46, 53, 71 and 90.

Antiviral activity of Kaletra in patients failing protease inhibitor therapy: the clinical relevance of reduced *in vitro* susceptibility to lopinavir has been examined by assessing the virologic response to Kaletra therapy, with respect to baseline viral genotype and phenotype, in 56 patients previous failing therapy with multiple protease inhibitors. The EC_{50} of lopinavir against the 56 baseline viral isolates ranged from 0.6 to 96-fold higher than the EC_{50} against wild type HIV. After 48 weeks of treatment with Kaletra, efavirenz and nucleoside reverse transcriptase inhibitors, plasma HIV RNA ⩽ 400 copies/ml was observed in 93% (25/27), 73% (11/15), and 25% (2/8) of patients with < 10-fold, 10 to 40-fold, and > 40-fold reduced susceptibility to lopinavir at baseline, respectively. In addition, virologic response was observed in 91% (21/23), 71% (15/21) and 33% (2/6) patients with 0 – 5, 6 – 7, and 8 – 10 mutations of the above mutations in HIV protease associated with reduced *in vitro* susceptibility to lopinavir. Since these patients had not previously been exposed to either Kaletra or efavirenz, part of the response may be attributed to the antiviral activity of efavirenz, particularly in patients harbouring highly lopinavir resistant virus. The study did not contain a control arm of patients not receiving Kaletra.

Selection of viral resistance during Kaletra therapy: in Phase II studies of 227 antiretroviral treatment naïve and protease inhibitor experienced patients, isolates from four patients with quantifiable > 400 copies/ml) viral load following treatment with Kaletra for ⩾ 12 weeks displayed significantly reduced susceptibility to lopinavir compared to the corresponding baseline viral isolates. The mean EC_{50} of lopinavir against the four baseline isolates was 2.8 fold (range: 0.7 to 5.2 fold) higher than the EC_{50} against wild type HIV, and each of the four baseline isolates contained four or more mutations in HIV protease associated with resistance to protease inhibitors. Following treatment of the four patients with Kaletra, the mean EC_{50} of lopinavir increased to 55-fold (range: 9.4 to 99-fold) compared to wild type HIV, and 2 – 3 additional mutations at amino acids 10, 24, 33, 46, 54, 63, 71 and/or 82 were observed.

In a Phase II study (M97-720) through 204 weeks of treatment, genotypic analysis of viral isolates was successfully conducted in 11 of 16 patients with confirmed HIV RNA above 400 copies/ml revealed no primary or active site mutations in protease (amino acids at positions 8, 30, 32, 36, 47, 48, 50, 82, 84 and 90) or protease inhibitor phenotypic resistance.

Cross-resistance: at this stage of development, little information is available on the cross-resistance of viruses selected during therapy with Kaletra. Isolates from 4 patients previously treated with one or more protease inhibitors that developed increased lopinavir phenotypic resistance during Kaletra therapy either remained or developed cross-resistance to ritonavir, indinavir, and nelfinavir. All rebound viruses either remained fully sensitive or demonstrated modestly reduced susceptibility to amprenavir (up to 8.6-fold concurrent with 99-fold resistance to lopinavir). The rebound isolates from the two patients with no prior saquinavir treatment remained fully sensitive to saquinavir.

Clinical pharmacodynamic data

The effects of Kaletra (in combination with other antiretroviral agents) on biological markers (plasma HIV RNA levels and CD_4 counts) have been investigated in a controlled study of Kaletra of 48 weeks duration, and in additional studies of Kaletra of 204 weeks duration.

Adult Use

Patients without prior antiretroviral therapy

Study M98-863 is a randomised, double-blind trial of 653 antiretroviral treatment naïve patients investigating Kaletra (400/100 mg twice daily) compared to nelfinavir (750 mg three times daily) plus nucleoside reverse transcriptase inhibitors. By intent to treat analysis where patients with missing values are considered virologic failures, the proportion of patients at 48 weeks with HIV RNA < 400 copies/ml in the Kaletra arm was 75% and 63% in the nelfinavir arm. Mean baseline CD_4 cell count was 259 cells/mm^3 (range: 2 to 949 cells/ mm^3) and mean baseline plasma HIV-1 RNA was 4.9 log_{10} copies/ml (range: 2.6 to 6.8 log_{10} copies/ml). Through 48 weeks of therapy, the proportion of patients in the Kaletra arm with plasma RNA < 50 copies/ml was 67% and 52% in the nelfinavir arm. The mean increase from baseline in CD_4 cell count was 207 cells/mm^3 in the Kaletra arm and 195 cells/mm^3 in the nelfinavir arm. Through 48 weeks of therapy, a statistically significantly higher proportion of patients in the Kaletra arm had HIV RNA < 50 copies/ml compared to the nelfinavir arm.

Sustained virological response to Kaletra (in combination with lamivudine and stavudine) has been also observed in a small Phase II study (M97-720) through 204 weeks of treatment. Through 204 weeks of treatment, the proportion of patients with HIV RNA < 400 (< 50) copies/ml was 71% (70%) [n=100 including 40 patients having received the recommended dose of Kaletra for the entire 204 weeks], and the corresponding mean increase in CD_4 cell count was 440 cells/mm^3. Twenty-eight patients (28%) discontinued the study, including nine (9%) discontinuations due to adverse events and one (1%) death.

Patients with prior antiretroviral therapy

Study M97-765 is a randomised, double-blind trial evaluating Kaletra at two dose levels (400/100 mg and 400/200 mg, both twice daily) plus nevirapine (200 mg twice daily) and two nucleoside reverse transcriptase inhibitors in 70 single protease inhibitor experienced, non-nucleoside reverse transcriptase inhibitor naïve patients. Median baseline CD_4 cell count was 349 cells/mm^3 (range 72 to 807 cells/mm^3) and median baseline plasma HIV-1 RNA was 4.0 $\log_{10}$ copies/ml (range 2.9 to 5.8 $\log_{10}$ copies/ml). By intent to treat analysis where patients with missing values are considered virologic failures, the proportion of patients with HIV RNA < 400 (< 50) copies/ml at 24 weeks was 75% (58%) and the mean increase from baseline in CD_4 cell count was 174 cells/mm^3 for the 36 patients receiving the 400/100 mg dose of Kaletra.

M98-957 is a randomised, open-label study evaluating Kaletra treatment at two dose levels (400/100 mg and 533/133 mg, both twice daily) plus efavirenz (600 mg once daily) and nucleoside reverse transcriptase inhibitors in 57 multiple protease inhibitor experienced, non-nucleoside reverse transcriptase inhibitor naïve patients. Between week 24 and 48, patients randomised to a dose of 400/100 mg were converted to a dose of 533/133 mg. Median baseline CD_4 cell count was 220 cells/mm^3 (range 13 to 1030 cells/mm^3). By intent-to-treat analysis of both dose groups combined (n=57), where patients with missing values are considered virologic failures, the proportion of patients with HIV RNA < 400 copies/ml at 48 weeks was 65% and the mean increase from baseline CD_4 cell count was 94 cells/mm^3.

Paediatric Use

M98-940 is an open-label study of a liquid formulation of Kaletra in 100 antiretroviral naïve (44%) and experienced (56%) paediatric patients. All patients were non-nucleoside reverse transcriptase inhibitor naïve. Patients were randomised to either 230 mg lopinavir/57.5 mg ritonavir per m^2 or 300 mg lopinavir/75 mg ritonavir per m^2. Naïve patients also received nucleoside reverse transcriptase inhibitors. Experienced patients received nevirapine plus up to two nucleoside reverse transcriptase inhibitors. Safety, efficacy and pharmacokinetic profiles of the two dose regimens were assessed after 3 weeks of therapy in each patient. Subsequently, all patients were continued on the 300/75 mg per m^2 dose. Patients had a mean age of 5 years (range 6 months to 12 years) with 14 patients less than 2 years old and 6 patients one year or less. Mean baseline CD_4 cell count was 838 cells/mm^3 and mean baseline plasma HIV-1 RNA was 4.7 $\log_{10}$ copies/ml. Through 48 weeks of therapy, the proportion of patients with HIV RNA < 400 copies/ml was 84% for antiretroviral naïve patients and 75% for antiretroviral experienced patients and the mean increases from baseline in CD_4 cell count were 404 cells/mm^3 and 284 cells/mm^3 respectively.

5.2 Pharmacokinetic properties

The pharmacokinetic properties of lopinavir co-administered with ritonavir have been evaluated in healthy adult volunteers and in HIV-infected patients; no substantial differences were observed between the two groups. Lopinavir is essentially completely metabolised by CYP3A. Ritonavir inhibits the metabolism of lopinavir, thereby increasing the plasma levels of lopinavir. Across studies, administration of Kaletra 400/100 mg twice daily yields mean steady-state lopinavir plasma concentrations 15 to 20-fold higher than those of ritonavir in HIV-infected patients. The plasma levels of ritonavir are less than 7% of those obtained after the ritonavir dose of 600 mg twice daily. The *in vitro* antiviral EC_{50} of lopinavir is approximately 10-fold lower than that of ritonavir. Therefore, the antiviral activity of Kaletra is due to lopinavir.

Absorption: multiple dosing with 400/100 mg Kaletra twice daily for 3 to 4 weeks and without meal restriction produced a mean ± SD lopinavir peak plasma concentration (C_{max}) of 9.6 ± 4.4 μg/ml, occurring approximately 4 hours after administration. The mean steady-state trough concentration prior to the morning dose was 5.5 ± 4.0 μg/ml. Lopinavir AUC over a 12 hour dosing interval averaged 82.8 ± 44.5 μg•h/ml. The absolute bioavailability of lopinavir coformulated with ritonavir in humans has not been established.

Effects of food on oral absorption: Kaletra soft capsules and liquid have been shown to be bioequivalent under nonfasting conditions (moderate fat meal). Administration of a single 400/100 mg dose of Kaletra soft capsules with a moderate fat meal (500 – 682 kcal, 22.7 –25.1% from fat) was associated with a mean increase of 48% and 23% in lopinavir AUC and C_{max}, respectively, relative to fasting. For Kaletra oral solution, the corresponding increases in lopinavir AUC and C_{max} were 80% and 54%, respectively. Administration of Kaletra with a high fat meal (872 kcal, 55.8% from fat) increased lopinavir AUC and C_{max} by 96% and 43%, respectively, for soft capsules, and 130% and 56%, respectively, for oral solution. To enhance bioavailability and minimise variability Kaletra is to be taken with food.

Distribution: at steady state, lopinavir is approximately 98 – 99% bound to serum proteins. Lopinavir binds to both alpha-1-acid glycoprotein (AAG) and albumin, however, it has a higher affinity for AAG. At steady state, lopinavir protein binding remains constant over the range of observed concentrations after 400/100 mg Kaletra twice daily, and is similar between healthy volunteers and HIV-positive patients.

Metabolism: *in vitro* experiments with human hepatic microsomes indicate that lopinavir primarily undergoes oxidative metabolism. Lopinavir is extensively metabolised by the hepatic cytochrome P450 system, almost exclusively by isozyme CYP3A. Ritonavir is a potent CYP3A inhibitor which inhibits the metabolism of lopinavir and therefore, increases plasma levels of lopinavir. A ^{14}C-lopinavir study in humans showed that 89% of the plasma radioactivity after a single 400/100 mg Kaletra dose was due to parent drug. At least 13 lopinavir oxidative metabolites have been identified in man. The 4-oxo and 4-hydroxymetabolite epimeric pair are the major metabolites with antiviral activity, but comprise only minute amounts of total plasma radioactivity. Ritonavir has been shown to induce metabolic enzymes, resulting in the induction of its own metabolism, and likely the induction of lopinavir metabolism. Pre-dose lopinavir concentrations decline with time during multiple dosing, stabilising after approximately 10 days to 2 weeks.

Elimination: after a 400/100 mg ^{14}C-lopinavir/ritonavir dose, approximately 10.4 ± 2.3% and 82.6 ± 2.5% of an administered dose of ^{14}C-lopinavir can be accounted for in urine and faeces, respectively. Unchanged lopinavir accounted for approximately 2.2% and 19.8% of the administered dose in urine and faeces, respectively. After multiple dosing, less than 3% of the lopinavir dose is excreted unchanged in the urine. The effective (peak to trough) half-life of lopinavir over a 12 hour dosing interval averaged 5 – 6 hours, and the apparent oral clearance (CL/F) of lopinavir is 6 to 7 l/h.

Special Populations

Paediatrics:

There are limited pharmacokinetic data in children below 2 years of age. The pharmacokinetics of Kaletra 300/75 mg/m^2 twice daily and 230/57.5 mg/m^2 twice daily have been studied in a total of 53 paediatric patients, ranging in age from 6 months to 12 years. The lopinavir mean steady-state AUC, C_{max}, and C_{min} were 72.6 ± 31.1 μg•h/ml, 8.2 ± 2.9 μg/ml and 3.4 ± 2.1 μg/ml, respectively after Kaletra 230/57.5 mg/m^2 twice daily without nevirapine (n=12), and were 85.8 ± 36.9 μg•h/ml, 10.0 ± 3.3 μg/ml and 3.6 ± 3.5 μg/ml, respectively after 300/75 mg/m^2 twice daily with nevirapine (n=12). The 230/57.5 mg/m^2 twice daily regimen without nevirapine and the 300/75 mg/m^2 twice daily regimen with nevirapine provided lopinavir plasma concentrations similar to those obtained in adult patients receiving the 400/100 mg twice daily regimen without nevirapine. Kaletra soft capsules and Kaletra oral solution are bioequivalent under nonfasting conditions.

Gender, Race and Age:

Kaletra pharmacokinetics have not been studied in the elderly. No age or gender related pharmacokinetic differences have been observed in adult patients. Pharmacokinetic differences due to race have not been identified.

Renal Insufficiency:

Kaletra pharmacokinetics have not been studied in patients with renal insufficiency; however, since the renal clearance of lopinavir is negligible, a decrease in total body clearance is not expected in patients with renal insufficiency.

Hepatic Insufficiency:

The steady state pharmacokinetic parameters of lopinavir in HIV-infected patients with mild to moderate hepatic impairment were compared with those of HIV-infected patients with normal hepatic function in a multiple dose study with lopinavir/ritonavir 400/100 mg twice daily. A limited increase in total lopinavir concentrations of approximately 30% has been observed which is not expected to be of clinical relevance (see section 4.2).

5.3 Preclinical safety data

Repeat-dose toxicity studies in rodents and dogs identified major target organs as the liver, kidney, thyroid, spleen and circulating red blood cells. Hepatic changes indicated cellular swelling with focal degeneration. While exposure eliciting these changes were comparable to or below human clinical exposure, dosages in animals were over 6-fold the recommended clinical dose. Mild renal tubular degeneration was confined to mice exposed with at least twice the recommended human exposure; the kidney was unaffected in rats and dogs. Reduced serum thyroxine led to an increased release of TSH with resultant follicular cell hypertrophy in the thyroid glands of rats. These changes were reversible with withdrawal of the active substance and were absent in mice and dogs. Coombs-negative anisocytosis and poikilocytosis were observed in rats, but not in mice or dogs. Enlarged spleens with histiocytosis were seen in rats but not other species. Serum cholesterol was elevated in rodents but not dogs, while triglycerides were elevated only in mice.

During *in vitro* studies, cloned human cardiac potassium channels (HERG) were inhibited by 30% at the highest concentrations of lopinavir/ritonavir tested, corresponding to a lopinavir exposure 7-fold total and 15-fold free peak plasma levels achieved in humans at the maximum recommended therapeutic dose. In contrast, similar concentrations of lopinavir/ritonavir demonstrated no repolarisation delay in the canine cardiac Purkinje fibres. Lower concentrations of lopinavir/ritonavir did not produce significant potassium (HERG) current blockade. Tissue distribution studies conducted in the rat did not suggest significant cardiac retention of the drug; 72-hour AUC in heart was approximately 50% of measured plasma AUC. Therefore, it is reasonable to expect that cardiac lopinavir levels would not be significantly higher than plasma levels.

In dogs, prominent U waves on the electrocardiogram have been observed associated with prolonged PR interval and bradycardia. These effects have been assumed to be caused by electrolyte disturbance.

The clinical relevance of these preclinical data is unknown, however, the potential cardiac effects of this product in humans cannot be ruled out (see also sections 4.4 and 4.8).

In rats, embryofoetotoxicity (pregnancy loss, decreased foetal viability, decreased foetal body weights, increased frequency of skeletal variations) and postnatal developmental toxicity (decreased survival of pups) was observed at maternally toxic dosages. The systemic exposure to lopinavir/ritonavir at the maternal and developmental toxic dosages was lower than the intended therapeutic exposure in humans.

Long-term carcinogenicity studies of lopinavir/ritonavir in mice revealed a nongenotoxic, mitogenic induction of liver tumours, generally considered to have little relevance to human risk. Carcinogenicity studies in rats revealed no tumourigenic findings. Lopinavir/ritonavir was not found to be mutagenic or clastogenic in a battery of *in vitro* and *in vivo* assays including the Ames bacterial reverse mutation assay, the mouse lymphoma assay, the mouse micronucleus test and chromosomal aberration assays in human lymphocytes.

6. PHARMACEUTICAL PARTICULARS

6.1 List of excipients

Capsule contents:

oleic acid,

propylene glycol,

polyoxyl 35 castor oil,

purified water

Capsule shell:

gelatine,

anhydrized liquid sorbitol (mixture of sorbitol, sorbitol anhydrides and mannitol),

glycerol,

titanium dioxide (E171),

sunset yellow (E110)

medium-chain triglycerides,

lecithin

Black ink containing:

propylene glycol,

black iron oxide (E172),

polyvinyl acetate phthalate,

polyethylene glycol 400,

ammonium hydroxide

6.2 Incompatibilities

Not applicable.

6.3 Shelf life

2 years.

6.4 Special precautions for storage

Store Kaletra soft capsules in a refrigerator (2°C- 8°C).

In use storage: If kept outside of the refrigerator, do not store above 25°C and discard any unused contents after 42 days (6 weeks). It is advised to write the date of removal from the refrigerator on the package.

Avoid exposure to excessive heat.

6.5 Nature and contents of container

High density polyethylene (HDPE) bottles closed with polypropylene caps. Each bottle contains 90 capsules. Each pack contains 2 bottles (180 capsules).

Blisters consisting of PVC/fluoropolymer foil. Each carton contains 6 foil blisters each containing 6 capsules (36 capsules). Each pack contains 5 cartons (180 capsules).

6.6 Instructions for use and handling

No special requirements.

7. MARKETING AUTHORISATION HOLDER

Abbott Laboratories Limited

Queenborough

Kent ME11 5EL

United Kingdom

8. MARKETING AUTHORISATION NUMBER(S)

EU/1/01/172/001

EU/1/01/172/002

9. DATE OF FIRST AUTHORISATION/RENEWAL OF THE AUTHORISATION

20 March 2001

10. DATE OF REVISION OF THE TEXT

12 January 2005

Kaodene

(Sovereign Medical)

1. NAME OF THE MEDICINAL PRODUCT
Kaodene.

2. QUALITATIVE AND QUANTITATIVE COMPOSITION

Codeine Phosphate fine cryst	EP	0.1% w/v
Irradiated Light Kaolin	BP	30.0% w/v

3. PHARMACEUTICAL FORM
Suspension.

4. CLINICAL PARTICULARS

4.1 Therapeutic indications
For the symptomatic relief of simple diarrhoea.

4.2 Posology and method of administration
Adults, elderly and children over 12 years: 20ml, three or four times a day.

Children aged 5 to 12 years: 10ml three or four times a day.

Children under 5 years: Not recommended.

For oral administration.

4.3 Contraindications
Kaodene is contraindicated in patients with pseudomembraneous colitis, diverticular disease, or respiratory depression.

4.4 Special warnings and special precautions for use
Kaodene should be used with caution in patients with ulcerative colitis and impaired liver or kidney function. The long term administration of Kaodene, particularly in the elderly, is not recommended. It cannot be used as a substitute for rehydration therapy.

Keep all medicines out of the reach of children.

This medicines should not be taken in pregnancy without consulting your doctor.

Warning. May cause drowsiness. If affected do not drive or operate machinery. Avoid alcoholic drink. Do not exceed the stated dose.

If diarrhoea is severe and persists for more than 24 hours, consult your doctor.

4.5 Interaction with other medicinal products and other forms of Interaction
Kaodene may interfere with the absorption of some drugs from the gastrointestinal tract including certain antibiotics and digoxin. The depressant effects of codeine are enhanced by alcohol. May interact with monoamine oxidase inhibitors. Administration of Kaodene may interfere with laboratory estimations of serum amylase and certain liver function tests.

4.6 Pregnancy and lactation
The safety of Kaodene during pregnancy has not been established and therefore use of the product during this period should be avoided, unless under medical supervision. In limited studies codeine appears in the breast milk in very low concentrations and is unlikely to affect the breast fed infant adversely.

4.7 Effects on ability to drive and use machines
May cause drowsiness and therefore may influence the ability to drive and operate machinery.

4.8 Undesirable effects
Occasionally may cause drowsiness, nausea, vomiting and constipation.

4.9 Overdose
Symptoms of overdosage include the adverse effects given under (4.8.) above. In addition large overdoses may produce respiratory depression, hypotension, circulatory failure and deepening coma. Initial treatment includes emptying the stomach by aspiration and lavage. Intensive supportive therapy may be required to correct respiratory failure and shock. In addition the narcotic antagonist naloxone hydrochloride, may be used to counteract very rapidly the severe respiratory depression and coma. A dose in adults of 0.4-2mg is given intravenously or intramuscularly, repeated at intervals of 2-3 minutes if necessary up to 10mg. In children, doses of naloxone of 5-10 micrograms/kg bodyweight may be given intravenously or intramuscularly.

5. PHARMACOLOGICAL PROPERTIES

5.1 Pharmacodynamic properties
Codeine phosphate is a narcotic analgesic which reduces intestinal motility.

Light kaolin is adsorbent and when given orally adsorbs toxic and other substances from the gastrointestinal tract and increases the bulk of the faeces.

5.2 Pharmacokinetic properties
Kaolin is not absorbed from the gastrointestinal tract. Codeine phosphate is absorbed from the gastrointestinal tract, peak levels being achieved in about one hour. Codeine is metabolised by O-and N-demethylation in the liver to morphine and norcodeine. Codeine and its metabolites are excreted almost entirely by the kidney, mainly as conjugates of glucuronic acid.

The plasma half-life of codeine is between 3 and 4 hours.

5.3 Preclinical safety data
None stated.

6. PHARMACEUTICAL PARTICULARS

6.1 List of excipients
Methyl hydroxybenzoate

Propyl hydroxybenzoate

Sodium saccharin recryst (76% saccharin)

Xanthan gum

Blanose sodium carboxymethyl cellulose 7MF

Vanilla essence H96 Rayner

Anise Oil

Peppermint oil

Chloroform

Purified water

6.2 Incompatibilities
Not applicable.

6.3 Shelf life
Unopened shelf-life is 36 months for all pack sizes.

6.4 Special precautions for storage
None stated.

6.5 Nature and contents of container

Pack 1 - a 50ml amber winchester bottle with a screw-neck and a polypropylene wadless cap.

Pack 2 - a 250ml amber winchester bottle with a screw-neck and a polypropylene wadless cap.

Pack 3 - a 300ml amber glass bottle with a roll on pilfer-proof cap with a triseal liner.

6.6 Instructions for use and handling
None stated.

7. MARKETING AUTHORISATION HOLDER
Waymade PLC

Trading as Sovereign Medical

Sovereign House

Miles Gray Road

Basildon

Essex

SS14 3FR

8. MARKETING AUTHORISATION NUMBER(S)
PL 06464/0708

9. DATE OF FIRST AUTHORISATION/RENEWAL OF THE AUTHORISATION
11 January 1999

10. DATE OF REVISION OF THE TEXT
None stated.

Keflex tablets, Capsules and Granules

(Flynn Pharma Ltd)

1. NAME OF THE MEDICINAL PRODUCT
Keflex* tablets.

Keflex capsules.

Keflex Granules for Oral Suspension BP.

2. QUALITATIVE AND QUANTITATIVE COMPOSITION
Each tablet contains, as the active ingredient, cefalexin monohydrate equivalent to 250mg or 500mg of cefalexin base.

Each capsule contains, as the active ingredient, cefalexin monohydrate equivalent to 250mg or 500mg of cefalexin base.

Each bottle, when prepared as directed, contains, as the active ingredient, cefalexin monohydrate equivalent to 125mg/5ml or 250mg/5ml of cefalexin base.

3. PHARMACEUTICAL FORM
Tablets 250mg: 9.5mm diameter, peach, marked 'GP3'.

Tablets 500mg: Pillow-shaped, 16mm long, scored, peach, marked 'GP4'.

Capsules 250mg: Green and white, coded 'GP1'.

Capsules 500mg: Pale green and dark green, coded 'GP2'.

Granules for oral suspension 125mg: White granules.

Granules for oral suspension 250mg: White granules.

4. CLINICAL PARTICULARS

4.1 Therapeutic indications
Cefalexin is a semi-synthetic cephalosporin antibiotic for oral administration.

Cefalexin is indicated in the treatment of the following infections due to susceptible micro-organisms:

Respiratory tract infections

Otitis media

Skin and soft tissue infections

Bone and joint infections

Genito-urinary tract infections, including acute prostatitis

Dental infections

4.2 Posology and method of administration
Cefalexin is administered orally.

The bottle is first inverted and tapped to loosen the powder then a total of 60ml water in two portions is added, shaking after each addition until suspended. If dilution is unavoidable, Syrup BP should be used after the suspension has been prepared as described. Shake well before use.

Adults: The adult dosage ranges from 1-4g daily in divided doses; most infections will respond to a dosage of 500mg every 8 hours. For skin and soft tissue infections, streptococcal pharyngitis, and mild, uncomplicated urinary tract infections, the usual dosage is 250mg every 6 hours, or 500mg every 12 hours.

For more severe infections or those caused by less susceptible organisms, larger doses may be needed. If daily doses of cefalexin greater than 4g are required, parenteral cephalosporins, in appropriate doses, should be considered.

The elderly and patients with impaired renal function: As for adults. Reduce dosage if renal function is markedly impaired (see section 4.4).

Children: The usual recommended daily dosage for children is 25-50mg/kg (10-20mg/lb) in divided doses. For skin and soft tissue infections, streptococcal pharyngitis, and mild, uncomplicated urinary tract infections, the total daily dose may be divided and administered every 12 hours. For most infections the following schedule is suggested:

Children under 5 years: 125mg every 8 hours.

Children 5 years and over: 250mg every 8 hours.

In severe infections, the dosage may be doubled. In the therapy of otitis media, clinical studies have shown that a dosage of 75 to 100mg/kg/day in 4 divided doses is required.

In the treatment of beta-haemolytic streptococcal infections, a therapeutic dose should be administered for at least 10 days.

4.3 Contraindications
Cefalexin is contra-indicated in patients with known allergy to the cephalosporin group of antibiotics.

4.4 Special warnings and special precautions for use
Before instituting therapy with cefalexin, every effort should be made to determine whether the patient has had previous hypersensitivity reactions to the cephalosporins, penicillins, or other drugs. Cefalexin should be given cautiously to penicillin-sensitive patients. There is some clinical and laboratory evidence of partial cross-allergenicity of the penicillins and cephalosporins. Patients have had severe reactions (including anaphylaxis) to both drugs.

Pseudomembranous colitis has been reported with virtually all broad-spectrum antibiotics, including macrolides, semi-synthetic penicillins, and cephalosporins. It is important, therefore, to consider its diagnosis in patients who develop diarrhoea in association with the use of antibiotics. Such colitis may range in severity from mild to life-threatening. Mild cases of pseudomembranous colitis usually respond to drug discontinuance alone. In moderate to severe cases, appropriate measures should be taken.

If an allergic reaction to cefalexin occurs, the drug should be discontinued and the patient treated with the appropriate agents.

Prolonged use of cefalexin may result in the overgrowth of non-susceptible organisms. Careful observation of the patient is essential. If superinfection occurs during therapy, appropriate measures should be taken.

Cefalexin should be administered with caution in the presence of markedly impaired renal function. Careful clinical and laboratory studies should be made because safe dosage may be lower than that usually recommended.

Positive direct Coombs' tests have been reported during treatment with the cephalosporin antibiotics. In haematological studies, or in transfusion cross-matching procedures when antiglobulin tests are performed on the minor side, or in Coombs' testing of newborns whose mothers have received cephalosporin antibiotics before parturition, it should be recognised that a positive Coombs' test may be due to the drug.

A false positive reaction for glucose in the urine may occur with Benedict's or Fehling's solutions, or with copper sulphate test tablets.

4.5 Interaction with other medicinal products and other forms of Interaction
As with other beta-lactam drugs, renal excretion of cefalexin is inhibited by probenecid.

In a single study of 12 healthy subjects given single 500mg doses of cefalexin and metformin, plasma metformin C_{max} and AUC increased by an average of 34% and 24%, respectively, and metformin renal clearance decreased by an average of 14%. No side-effects were reported in the 12 healthy subjects in this study. No information is available about the interaction of cefalexin and metformin following multiple dose administration. The clinical significance of this study is unclear, particularly as no cases of "lactic acidosis" have been reported in association with concomitant metformin and cefalexin treatment.

4.6 Pregnancy and lactation

Usage in pregnancy: Although laboratory and clinical studies have shown no evidence of teratogenicity, caution should be exercised when prescribing for the pregnant patient.

Usage in nursing mothers: The excretion of cefalexin in human breast milk increased up to 4 hours following a 500mg dose. The drug reached a maximum level of 4 micrograms/ml, then decreased gradually and had disappeared 8 hours after administration. Caution should be exercised when cefalexin is administered to a nursing woman.

4.7 Effects on ability to drive and use machines

None known.

4.8 Undesirable effects

Gastro-intestinal: Symptoms of pseudomembranous colitis may appear either during or after antibiotic treatment. Nausea and vomiting have been reported rarely. The most frequent side-effect has been diarrhoea. It was very rarely severe enough to warrant cessation of therapy. Dyspepsia and abdominal pain have also occurred. As with some penicillins and some other cephalosporins, transient hepatitis and cholestatic jaundice have been reported rarely.

Hypersensitivity: Allergic reactions have been observed in the form of rash, urticaria, angioedema, and, rarely, erythema multiforme, Stevens-Johnson syndrome, and toxic epidermal necrolysis. These reactions usually subsided upon discontinuation of the drug, although in some cases supportive therapy may be necessary. Anaphylaxis has also been reported.

Haemic and lymphatic system: Eosinophilia, neutropenia, thrombocytopenia, and haemolytic anaemia have been reported.

Other: These have included genital and anal pruritus, genital candidiasis, vaginitis and vaginal discharge, dizziness, fatigue, headache, agitation, confusion, hallucinations, arthralgia, arthritis, and joint disorder. Reversible interstitial nephritis has been reported rarely. Slight elevations in AST and ALT have been reported.

4.9 Overdose

Symptoms of oral overdose may include nausea, vomiting, epigastric distress, diarrhoea, and haematuria.

In the event of severe overdosage, general supportive care is recommended, including close clinical and laboratory monitoring of haematological, renal, and hepatic functions, and coagulation status until the patient is stable. Forced diuresis, peritoneal dialysis, haemodialysis, or charcoal haemoperfusion have not been established as beneficial for an overdose of cefalexin. It would be extremely unlikely that one of these procedures would be indicated.

Unless 5 to 10 times the normal total daily dose has been ingested, gastro-intestinal decontamination should not be necessary.

There have been reports of haematuria, without impairment of renal function, in children accidentally ingesting more than 3.5g of cefalexin in a day. Treatment has been supportive (fluids) and no sequelae have been reported.

5. PHARMACOLOGICAL PROPERTIES

5.1 Pharmacodynamic properties

In vitro tests demonstrate that cephalosporins are bactericidal because of their inhibition of cell-wall synthesis.

Cefalexin is active against the following organisms *in vitro:*

Beta-haemolytic streptococci

Staphylococci, including coagulase-positive, coagulase-negative, and penicillinase-producing strains

Streptococcus pneumoniae

Escherichia coli

Proteus mirabilis

Klebsiella species

Haemophilus influenzae

Branhamella catarrhalis

Most strains of enterococci (*Streptococcus faecalis*) and a few strains of staphylococci are resistant to cefalexin. It is not active against most strains of *Enterobacter* species, *Morganella morganii*, and *Pr. vulgaris*. It has no activity against *Pseudomonas* or *Herellea* species or *Acinetobacter calcoaceticus*. Penicillin-resistant *Streptococcus pneumoniae* is usually cross-resistant to beta-lactam antibiotics. When tested by *in vitro* methods, staphylococci exhibit cross-resistance between cefalexin and methicillin-type antibiotics.

5.2 Pharmacokinetic properties

Cefalexin is acid stable and may be given without regard to meals. It is rapidly absorbed after oral administration. Following doses of 250mg, 500mg, and 1g, average peak serum levels of approximately 9, 18, and 32mg/l, respectively, were obtained at 1 hour. Measurable levels were present 6 hours after administration. Cefalexin is excreted in the urine by glomerular filtration and tubular secretion. Studies showed that over 90% of the drug was excreted unchanged in the urine within 8 hours. During this period, peak urine concentrations following the 250mg, 500mg, and 1g doses were approximately 1,000, 2,200, and 5,000mg/l, respectively.

Cefalexin is almost completely absorbed from the gastro-intestinal tract, and 75-100% is rapidly excreted in active form in the urine. Absorption is slightly reduced if the drug is administered with food. The half-life is approximately 60 minutes in patients with normal renal function. Haemodialysis and peritoneal dialysis will remove cefalexin from the blood.

Peak blood levels are achieved one hour after administration, and therapeutic levels are maintained for 6-8 hours. Approximately 80% of the active drug is excreted in the urine within 6 hours. No accumulation is seen with dosages above the therapeutic maximum of 4g/day.

The half-life may be increased in neonates due to their renal immaturity, but there is no accumulation when given at up to 50mg/kg/day.

5.3 Preclinical safety data

The daily oral administration of cefalexin to rats in doses of 250 or 500mg/kg prior to and during pregnancy, or to rats and mice during the period of organogenesis only, had no adverse effect on fertility, foetal viability, foetal weight, or litter size.

Cefalexin showed no enhanced toxicity in weanling and newborn rats as compared with adult animals.

The oral LD_{50} of cefalexin in rats is 5,000mg/kg.

6. PHARMACEUTICAL PARTICULARS

6.1 List of excipients

The tablets contain the following excipients:

Sodium starch glycollate type A

Pregelatinised maize starch (250mg tablet only)

Starch dry-flow (250mg tablet only)

Stearic acid (250mg tablet only)

Maize starch (250mg tablet only)

Magnesium stearate

Povidone (500mg tablet only)

Methylhydroxypropylcellulose

Glycerol

Talc

Titanium dioxide

Iron oxide yellow

Iron oxide red

The capsules contain the following excipients:

Cellulose with sodium carboxymethylcellulose

Dimeticone

Magnesium stearate

Patent blue V

Quinoline yellow

Titanium dioxide

Gelatin

The granules contain the following excipients:

Sucrose

Imitation guarana flavour

Allura red AC

Sodium lauryl sulphate

Methylcellulose 15

Dimeticone

Xanthan gum

Pregelatinised starch

6.2 Incompatibilities

None known.

6.3 Shelf life

Tablets or capsules: When stored appropriately, 3 years.

Suspension: When stored appropriately,

Unreconstituted product: 2 years (Keflex suspension 125mg/5ml).

3 years (Keflex suspension 250mg/5ml).

Bottles of reconstituted product: 10 days.

6.4 Special precautions for storage

Tablets or capsules: Do not store above 30°C. Keep containers tightly closed.

Suspension: Do not store granules above 25°C.

After mixing, Keflex suspensions should be stored in a cool place (6°C-15°C) or in a refrigerator (2°C-8°C) and be used within 10 days. Where dilution is unavoidable, Syrup BP should be used after the suspension has been prepared according to the manufacturer's instructions.

6.5 Nature and contents of container

Tablets: The products are filled into HDPE bottles of 100 tablets, or blister strips of 28 tablets consisting of UPVC with aluminium foil backing. Additionally, the 500mg product may be packed into blisters of 21 tablets.

Capsules: The products are filled into HDPE bottles of 100 capsules, or blister strips of 28 capsules consisting of UPVC with aluminium foil backing. Additionally, the 500mg product may be packed into blisters of 21 capsules.

Suspension: The product is filled into 100ml HDPE bottles with screw caps.

6.6 Instructions for use and handling

For oral use.

Suspension: First invert the bottle and tap to loosen the powder then add a total of 60ml water in two portions, shaking after each addition until suspended. The solution is red. If dilution is unavoidable, Syrup BP should be used after the suspension has been prepared as described. Shake well before use.

7. MARKETING AUTHORISATION HOLDER

Flynn Pharma Limited

Alton House

4 Herbert Street

Dublin

Ireland

8. MARKETING AUTHORISATION NUMBER(S)

Tablets: PL13621/0020 (250mg)

PL13621/0022 (500mg)

Capsules: PL13621/0025 (250mg)

PL13621/0021 (500mg)

Suspension: PL13621/0023 (125mg/5ml)

PL13621/0023 (250mg/5ml)

9. DATE OF FIRST AUTHORISATION/RENEWAL OF THE AUTHORISATION

Tablets: Date of first authorisation: 30 April 1985 (250mg)

30 April 1985 (500mg)

Date of last renewal of authorisation: August 2001 (250mg)

13 August 2001 (500mg)

Capsules: Date of first authorisation: 30 September 1985 (250mg)

30 April 1985 (500mg)

Date of last renewal of authorisation: 13 August 2001 (250mg)

13 August 2001 (500mg)

Suspension: Date of first authorisation: 14 March 1985

Date of last renewal of authorisation: 14 June 2001

10. DATE OF REVISION OF THE TEXT

September 2005

LEGAL CATEGORY

POM

*KEFLEX (cefalexin) is a trademark of Eli Lilly and Company. KFL7M

Kemadrin Tablets 5 mg

(GlaxoSmithKline UK)

1. NAME OF THE MEDICINAL PRODUCT

Kemadrin Tablets 5mg

2. QUALITATIVE AND QUANTITATIVE COMPOSITION

Procyclidine Hydrochloride BP 5mg per tablet

3. PHARMACEUTICAL FORM

Tablet

4. CLINICAL PARTICULARS

4.1 Therapeutic indications

Kemadrin is indicated for the treatment and symptomatic relief of all forms of Parkinson's disease e.g. idiopathic (paralysis agitans), postencephalitic and arteriosclerotic disease.

Kemadrin is also indicated for the control of extrapyramidal symptoms induced by neuroleptic drugs including pseudo-parkinsonism, acute dystonic reactions and akathisia.

4.2 Posology and method of administration

The variation in optimum dosage from one patient to another should be taken into consideration by the physician.

Dosage in adults:-

Parkinson's disease:-

Treatment is usually started at 2.5mg procyclidine three times per day, increasing by 2.5 to 5mg per day at intervals of two or three days until the optimum clinical response is achieved.

The usual maintenance dose to achieve optimal response is 15 to 30 mg procyclidine per day.

Addition of a fourth dose before retiring has been seen to be beneficial in some patients. Doses up to 60mg procyclidine have been well tolerated, and at the discretion of the attending physician dosing to this level may be appropriate.

In general younger patients or those with postencephalitic parkinsonism may require higher doses for a therapeutic response than older patients and those with arteriosclerotic parkinsonism.

Kemadrin may be combined with levodopa or amantadine in patients who are inadequately controlled on a single agent.

Neuroleptic-induced extrapyramidal symptoms:-

Treatment is usually initiated at 2.5mg procyclidine three times per day increasing by 2.5mg daily until symptoms are relieved.

The effective maintenance dose is usually 10 to 30mg procyclidine per day.

After a period of 3 to 4 months of therapy, KEMADRIN should be withdrawn and the patient observed to see whether the neuroleptic-induced extra-pyramidal symptoms recur.

If this is the case KEMADRIN should be reintroduced to avoid debilitating extra-pyramidal symptoms. Cessation of treatment periodically is to be recommended even in patients who appear to require the drug for longer periods.

Dosage in children:-

The use of Kemadrin in this age group is not recommended.

Dosage in the Elderly:-

Elderly patients may be more susceptible than younger adults to the anticholinergic effects of Kemadrin and a reduced dosage may be required (See Special Warnings and Special Precautions for Use).

Administration:-

Pharmacokinetic studies have indicated that the mean plasma elimination half life of Kemadrin is sufficient to allow twice daily administration orally or intravenously, if more convenient.

Oral administration may be better tolerated if associated with a meal.

4.3 Contraindications

Kemadrin is contra-indicated in individuals with known hypersensitivity to any component of the preparation, untreated urinary retention, closed angle glaucoma and gastro-intestinal obstruction.

4.4 Special warnings and special precautions for use

As with all anticholinergics the benefit/risk ratio should be assessed when prescribing Kemadrin in patients with existing angle-closure (narrow angle) glaucoma or those considered to be predisposed to glaucoma. Cautious prescribing is also indicated in patients predisposed to obstructive disease of the gastro-intestinal tract and those with urinary symptoms associated with prostatic hypertrophy.

In a proportion of patients undergoing neuroleptic treatment, tardive dysknesias will occur. While anticholinergic agents do not cause this syndrome, when given in combination with neuroleptics they may exacerbate the symptoms of tardive dyskinesia or reduce the threshold at which these symptoms appear in predisposed patients. In such individuals subsequent adjustment of neuroleptic therapy or reduction in anticholinergic treatment should be considered.

Patients with mental disorders occasionally experience a precipitation of a psychotic episode when procyclidine is administered for the treatment of the extrapyramidal side effects of neuroleptics.

Elderly patients, especially those on high doses of anticholinergics may be more susceptible to the adverse events associated with such therapy (See ADVERSE EVENTS). Specifically, the elderly patient may be particularly vulnerable to Central Nervous System disturbances such as confusion, impairment of cognitive function and memory, disorientation and hallucinations. These effects are usually reversible on reduction or discontinuation of anticholinergic therapy.

There is no specific information available concerning the use of procyclidine hydrochloride in patients with impaired renal or hepatic function. However, since procyclidine is metabolised in the liver and excreted via the urine care should be exercised when administering procyclidine to patients with impairment of renal or hepatic function.

Kemadrin should not be withdrawn abruptly as rebound parkinsonian symptoms may occur.

Abuse

Kemadrin, along with other anticholinergic drugs, has the potential to be abused. Although the cases of abuse are rare, physicians should exercise caution in prescribing Kemadrin to patients with symptoms that may not be genuine.

4.5 Interaction with other medicinal products and other forms of Interaction

Monoamine oxidase inhibitors or drugs with anticholinergic properties, such as amantadine, memantine, antihistamines, phenothiazines, tricyclic and related antidepressants, clozapine, disopyramide and nefopam may increase the anticholinergic action of procyclidine.

The use of drugs with cholinergic properties, such as tacrine, may reduce the therapeutic response to Kemadrin. Furthermore, drugs with anticholinergic properties may antagonise the effect of parasympathomimetic agents.

The concomitant use of procyclidine with some neuroleptics for the treatment of extrapyramidal symptoms has been associated with a reduction in neuroleptic plasma concentrations. However this reduction is unlikely to be associated with a significant reduction in clinical effect.

Drugs with anticholinergic properties may decrease salivation causing dry mouth and, in theory, may reduce the absorption and therefore the therapeutic effect of sublingual or buccal nitrate tablets.

Anticholinergics, including procyclidine, may reduce the efficacy of levodopa by increasing gastric emptying time, resulting in enhanced gastric degradation.

The effect of anticholinergics such as procyclidine may antagonise the gastrointestinal effects of cisapride, domperidone and metoclopramide.

Procyclidine may potentiate the vagolytic effects of quinidine.

Anticholinergics may reduce the absorption of ketoconazole.

Exposure to high environmental temperature and humidity in association with a phenothiazine/anticholinergic drug regimen has rarely resulted in hyperpyrexia.

Daily administration of paroxetine increases significantly the plasma levels of procyclidine. If anticholinergic effects are seen, the dose of procyclidine should be reduced

4.6 Pregnancy and lactation

Pregnancy:-

The safety of using Kemadrin during pregnancy has not been established. However, extensive clinical use has not given any evidence that it in any way compromises the normal course of pregnancy. Nevertheless, as with all drugs, use should be considered only when the expected clinical benefit of treatment for the mother outweighs any possible risk to the developing foetus.

Lactation:-

No information is available on the passage of procyclidine into human breast milk following administration of Kemadrin.

4.7 Effects on ability to drive and use machines

Adverse events of a neurological character such as blurred vision, dizziness, confusion and disorientation have been reported with procyclidine. Therefore, if affected, patients should be advised not to drive or operate machinery.

4.8 Undesirable effects

The main side effects are those to be expected from any anticholinergic agent. Dry mouth, blurring of vision, constipation, urinary retention are most commonly recorded. Nausea, vomiting, gingivitis, nervousness and rash have occasionally been reported.

The unwanted anticholinergic effects are easily reversed by reducing the dosage.

With high doses of procyclidine dizziness, mental confusion, impaired cognition and memory, disorientation, anxiety, agitation and hallucinations may occur.

Rarely the development of psychotic-like symptoms have been reported in association with procyclidine.

4.9 Overdose

Symptoms & Signs:

Reports of overdosage are relatively rare and no fatalities are known. Symptoms of overdosage are agitation, restlessness and confusion with severe sleeplessness lasting up to 24 hours or more. Visual and auditory hallucinations have been reported. Most subjects are euphoric but the occasional patient may be anxious and aggressive. The pupils are widely dilated and unreactive to light.

In recorded cases, the disorientation has lasted 1 to 4 days and ended in a recuperative sleep.

Tachycardia has also been reported in association with cases of Kemadrin overdose.

Treatment:

If procyclidine has been ingested within the previous hour or two (or possibly longer in view of its likely effects on gastric motility) then gastric lavage is probably indicated. Other active measures such as the use of cholinergic agents or haemodialysis are extremely unlikely to be of clinical value although if convulsions occur they should be controlled by injections of diazepam.

5. PHARMACOLOGICAL PROPERTIES

5.1 Pharmacodynamic properties

Procyclidine is a synthetic anticholinergic agent which blocks the excitatory effects of acetylcholine at the muscarinic receptor.

Idiopathic Parkinson's disease is thought to result from degeneration of neurones in the substantia nigra whose axons project and inhibit cells in the corpus striatum. Blockade by neuroleptic drugs of the dopamine released by these terminals produces a similar clinical picture. The cell bodies in the corpus striatum also receive cholinergic innervation which is excitatory.

Relief of the Parkinsonian syndrome can be achieved, either by potentiation of the dopaminergic system or blockade of the cholinergic input by anticholinergics. It is by a central action of this latter type by which procyclidine exerts its effect.

Procyclidine is particularly effective in the alleviation of rigidity. Tremor, akinesia, speech and writing difficulties, gait, sialorrhoea and drooling, sweating, oculogyric crises and depressed mood are also beneficially influenced.

5.2 Pharmacokinetic properties

Procyclidine is adequately absorbed from the gastro-intestinal tract with a bioavailability of 75% and disappears rapidly from the tissues. The relatively low clearance of 68ml/min represents a predominantly metabolic change with a small first pass effect. The mean plasma elimination half-life after both oral and intravenous administration is approximately 12 hours.

No detailed information is available on the metabolic fate of procyclidine but very little of the parent compound is excreted in the urine unchanged. When given orally about one fifth of the dose is known to be metabolised in the liver, principally by cytochrome P450 and then conjugated with glucuronic acid. This conjugate has been detected in the urine.

5.3 Preclinical safety data

Fertility:-

A three generation study in rats dosed at 40 mg/kg/day via the diet before and during pregnancy showed only that the number of viable pups was slightly decreased from the second mating. No other parameters were affected.

Teratogenicity:-

No teratogenic effects were seen in rats dosed subcutaneously with 10, 30 or 100 mg/kg/day on days 8 to 16 of pregnancy. Maternal bodyweight gain was reduced at doses of 30 or 100 mg/kg/day, and a 10% reduction in foetal weight was seen at 100 mg/kg/day

Mutagenicity:-

No data is available regarding the mutagenic potential of procyclidine hydrochloride.

Carcinogenicity:-

There is no data on the carcinogenic potential of procyclidine hydrochloride.

6. PHARMACEUTICAL PARTICULARS

6.1 List of excipients

Lactose

Sodium Starch Glycollate

Povidone

Magnesium Stearate

6.2 Incompatibilities

None

6.3 Shelf life

5 years

6.4 Special precautions for storage

Store below 25°C

6.5 Nature and contents of container

Amber glass bottles with low density polyethylene snap fit closures.

Polypropylene containers with polyethylene snap-fit lids.

Round enamelled tins with lever lids.

6.6 Instructions for use and handling

See posology and method of administration.

Administrative Data

7. MARKETING AUTHORISATION HOLDER

The Wellcome Foundation

Glaxo Wellcome House

Berkeley Avenue

Greenford

Middlesex

UB6 ONN

Trading as

GlaxoSmithKline UK

Stockley Park West

Uxbridge

Middlesex UB11 1BT

8. MARKETING AUTHORISATION NUMBER(S)

PL 00003/5255R

9. DATE OF FIRST AUTHORISATION/RENEWAL OF THE AUTHORISATION

29th January 2001

10. DATE OF REVISION OF THE TEXT

21 February 2005

11 Legal Status

POM

Kemicetine Succinate Injection

(Pharmacia Limited)

1. NAME OF THE MEDICINAL PRODUCT

Kemicetine Succinate Injection or Chloramphenicol Sodium Succinate 1.377g Injection

2. QUALITATIVE AND QUANTITATIVE COMPOSITION

Chloramphenicol sodium succinate (BP) 1.377 g

– equivalent to laevorotatory chloramphenicol 1.0 g

3. PHARMACEUTICAL FORM

Freeze dried powder for injection.

4. CLINICAL PARTICULARS

4.1 Therapeutic indications

Kemicetine (chloramphenicol) is a broad-spectrum antibiotic and is active against many gram-negative organisms, *Spirillae* and *Rickettsia*. Kemicetine should not be used for trivial infections due to the possibility of severe blood dyscrasias, which may prove fatal.

Table 1

Concentration	Solution strength	Volume of diluent to be added	Total volume after dilution
40%	400 mg/ml	1.7 ml	2.5 ml
25%	250 mg/ml	3.2 ml	4.0 ml
20%	200 mg/ml	4.2 ml	5.0 ml

Kemicetine succinate is indicated for typhoid, meningitis caused by *H. influenzae* and other serious infections caused by bacteria susceptible to chloramphenicol. It is also indicated wherever chloramphenicol is deemed the antibiotic of choice and oral administration is not possible, or where higher than usual blood concentrations are required.

4.2 Posology and method of administration

To be given by i.v. or i.m. injection.

In order to ensure rapid attainment of high blood levels, Kemicetine succinate is best administered by i.v. injection. Where this is not possible, however, intramuscular administration may be used, although it should be borne in mind that absorption may be slow and unpredictable.

The injection should be reconstituted with Water for Injections, Sodium Chloride Injection, or Dextrose Injection 5 %. The following dilution table may be useful for the administration of a proportion of the contents of a vial:

(see Table 1 above)

The dose administered and the concentration used is dependent on the severity of the infection. The recommended standard dosage is as follows:

Adults: The equivalent of 1 g of chloramphenicol every 6-8 hours.

Elderly: The usual adult dosage should be given subject to normal hepatic and renal function.

Children: The equivalent of 50 mg/kg chloramphenicol according to body weight, daily in divided doses every 6 hours (this dose should not be exceeded). The patient should be carefully observed for signs of toxicity.

Neonates and Premature Infants: 25 mg/kg in divided doses.

Only 10% or lower concentrations to be used. The 10% solution can be prepared by extracting 5ml of the 20% solution and adding 5ml of diluent (Water for Injections, Sodium Chloride Injection or Dextrose Injection 5%) under aseptic conditions.

The 10 % solution should be given by intravenous injection over a period of about a minute, or in a larger volume of fluid, by slow intravenous infusion. The concurrent administration of i.v. Kemicetine succinate with topical treatment has been found to be very effective in the treatment of osteomyelitic foci, abscesses, empyema and skin and urinary infections.

In exceptional cases, such as patients with septicaemia or meningitis, dosage schedule up to 100 mg/kg/day may be prescribed. However, these high doses should be decreased as soon as clinically indicated. To prevent relapses treatment should be continued after the temperature has returned to normal for 4 days in rickettsial diseases and for 8 – 10 days in typhoid fever.

4.3 Contraindications

Kemicetine succinate is contra-indicated in patients with a previous history of sensitivity and/or toxic reaction to chloramphenicol.

4.4 Special warnings and special precautions for use

Kemicetine is to be administered only under the direction of a medical practitioner.

Chloramphenicol may cause severe bone marrow depression which may lead to agranulocytosis, thrombocytopenic purpura or aplastic anaemia. These effects of the haemopoietic system are usually associated with a high dose, prolonged administration, or repeated courses, but they may occur at relatively low doses.

Chloramphenicol should not be used in the treatment of any infection for which a less toxic antibiotic is available. It is also advisable to perform blood tests in the case of prolonged or repeated administration. Evidence of any detrimental effect on blood elements is an indication to discontinue therapy immediately.

The dosage of chloramphenicol should be reduced in patients with impairment of hepatic or renal function.

Because of its toxic nature it is important to monitor serum levels of this antibiotic particularly in new-born and premature infants, in the elderly, in patients with renal or hepatic disease and in those receiving other drugs with which chloramphenicol may interact.

4.5 Interaction with other medicinal products and other forms of Interaction

Chloramphenicol has been shown to interact with, and enhance the effects of coumarin anticoagulants, some hypoglycaemic agents (e.g. tolbutamide) and phenytoin. When given concurrently, a dose reduction of these agents may be necessary.

Plasma concentrations of chloramphenicol may be reduced with concomitant usage of phenobarbitone and rifampicin.

4.6 Pregnancy and lactation

The use of chloramphenicol is contra-indicated in pregnancy and whilst breastfeeding.

4.7 Effects on ability to drive and use machines

None stated.

4.8 Undesirable effects

The following may become apparent after chloramphenicol treatment: dryness of the mouth, nausea and vomiting, diarrhoea, urticaria, optic neuritis with blurring or temporary loss of vision, peripheral neuritis, headache and depression.

Superinfection by fungi e.g. *C. albicans* in the gastro-intestinal tract or vagina, may also occur due to the disturbance of normal bacterial flora.

Chloramphenicol may also impede the development of immunity and should therefore not be given during active immunisation.

The "Grey syndrome" may occur after administration in patients with immature hepatic metabolic capacity, i.e. infants and neonates, usually in those treated with doses substantially in excess of those recommended.

4.9 Overdose

General supportive therapy.

5. PHARMACOLOGICAL PROPERTIES

5.1 Pharmacodynamic properties

After administration chloramphenicol is rapidly released from chloramphenicol sodium succinate. Chloramphenicol is active against many gram-positive and gram negative organisms, *Spirillae* and *Rickettsia*. It acts b interfering with bacterial protein synthesis. Chloramphenicol is widely distributed in body tissues and fluids and enters the cerebrospinal fluid.

Chloramphenicol sodium succinate, free chloramphenicol and metabolites are excreted in the urine.

5.2 Pharmacokinetic properties

After intravenous administration of chloramphenicol succinate every 6 hours elimination half-lives were 4.03 hours for chloramphenicol and 2.65 hours for chloramphenicol succinate. After intravenous chloramphenicol sodium succinate, steady state peak concentrations were reached on average 18.0 minutes after cessation of the infusion.

In infants and children aged 3 days to 16 years the apparent half-life was extremely variable ranging from 1.7 to 12.0 hours.

5.3 Preclinical safety data

None stated.

6. PHARMACEUTICAL PARTICULARS

6.1 List of excipients

There are no excipients.

6.2 Incompatibilities

None stated.

6.3 Shelf life

48 months.

6.4 Special precautions for storage

Do not store above 25 °C.

Keep container in the outer carton.

6.5 Nature and contents of container

Type IIIcolourless glass vials with grey chlorobutyl rubber bung and aluminium seal. Pack size: 1, 20 or 25 vials.

6.6 Instructions for use and handling

To be reconstituted with Water for Injection, Sodium Chloride Injection or Dextrose Injection 5%.

Administrative Data

7. MARKETING AUTHORISATION HOLDER

Pharmacia Limited

Davy Avenue

Milton Keynes

MK5 8PH

Buckinghamshire

United Kingdom

8. MARKETING AUTHORISATION NUMBER(S)

PL 00032/0341

9. DATE OF FIRST AUTHORISATION/RENEWAL OF THE AUTHORISATION

13th September 2002

10. DATE OF REVISION OF THE TEXT

March 2004

Company Reference: KM1_4

Kenalog Intra-articular / Intramuscular Injection

(E. R. Squibb & Sons Limited)

1. NAME OF THE MEDICINAL PRODUCT

Kenalog Intra-articular / Intramuscular Injection

2. QUALITATIVE AND QUANTITATIVE COMPOSITION

Kenalog Intra-articular / Intramuscular Injection contains triamcinolone acetonide 40mg per ml of sterile suspension.

3. PHARMACEUTICAL FORM

Sterile aqueous suspension for injection.

4. CLINICAL PARTICULARS

4.1 Therapeutic indications

Intra-articular use: for alleviating the joint pain, swelling and stiffness associated with rheumatoid arthritis and osteoarthrosis, with an inflammatory component; also for bursitis, epicondylitis, and tenosynovitis.

Intramuscular use: Where sustained systemic corticosteroid treatment is required: *Allergic states*, e.g. bronchial asthma, seasonal or perennial allergic rhinitis. In seasonal allergies, patients who do not respond to conventional therapy may achieve a remission of symptoms over the entire period with a single intramuscular injection (see Dosage); *Endocrine disorders*, e.g. primary or secondary adrenocortical insufficiency. *Collagen disorders*, e.g. during an exacerbation of maintenance therapy of selected cases of SLE or acute rheumatic carditis; *Dermatological diseases*, e.g. pemphigus, severe dermatitis and Stevens Johnson Syndrome; *Rheumatic, Gastrointestinal or Respiratory disorders* - as an adjunctive, short-term therapy; *Haematological disorders*, e.g. acquired (autoimmune) haemolytic anaemia; *Neoplastic diseases*, e.g. palliative management of leukaemia and lymphomas; *Renal disease*, such as acute interstitial nephritis, minimal change nephrotic syndrome or lupus nephritis.

4.2 Posology and method of administration

Kenalog is for Intra-articular/Intramuscular injection. The safety and efficacy of administration by other routes has yet to be established. Strict aseptic precautions should be observed. Since the duration of effect is variable, subsequent doses should be given when symptoms recur and not at set intervals.

Intra-Articular Injection: For intra-articular administration or injection into tendon sheaths and bursae, the dose of Kenalog Injection may vary from 5mg to 10mg (0.125 - 0.25ml) for smaller joints and up to 40mg (1.0ml) for larger joints, depending on the specific disease entity being treated. Single injections into several sites for multiple joint involvement, up to a total of 80mg, have been given without undue reactions.

It is recommended that, when injections are given into the sheaths of short tendons, Adcortyl Injection (triamcinolone acetonide 10mg/ml) should be used. (See under Precautions, re Achilles tendon).

Intramuscular Injection: To avoid the danger of subcutaneous fat atrophy, it is important to ensure that deep intramuscular injection is given into the gluteal site. The deltoid should not be used. Alternate sides should be used for subsequent injections.

Adults and Children over 12 Years: The suggested initial dose is 40mg (1.0ml) injected deeply into the upper, outer quadrant of the gluteal muscle. Subsequent dosage depends on the patient's response and period of relief. Patients with hay fever or pollen asthma who do not respond to conventional therapy may obtain a remission of symptoms lasting throughout the pollen season after a single dose of 40-100mg given when allergic symptoms appear. (See Warnings and Precautions.)

Elderly: Treatment of elderly patients, particularly if long term, should be planned bearing in mind the more serious consequences of the common side effects of corticosteroids in old age, especially osteoporosis, diabetes, hypertension, susceptibility to infection and thinning of the skin. Close clinical supervision is required to avoid life-threatening reactions.

Children from 6-12 Years of Age: The suggested initial dose of 40mg (1.0ml injected deeply into the gluteal muscle should be scaled according to the severity of symptoms and the age and weight of the child. Kenalog is not recommended for children under six years. Growth and development of children on prolonged corticosteroid therapy should be carefully observed. Caution should be used in the event of exposure to chickenpox, measles or other communicable diseases. (See 4.4 Special Warnings and Special Precautions for Use.)

Triamcinolone withdrawal: In patients who have received more than physiological doses of Kenalog (more than one injection during a three week period), withdrawal should not be abrupt. The dose should be reduced and the dosage interval increased until a dose of not more than 40mg and a dosage interval of at least three weeks have been achieved as the dose of systemic corticosteroid is reduced. Clinical assessment of disease activity may be needed.

Abrupt withdrawal of short term systemic corticosteroid treatment is appropriate if it is considered that the disease is unlikely to relapse. A single dose, which is not repeated within a three week period, is unlikely to lead to clinically relevant hpa-axis suppression in the majority of patients. However, in the following patient groups, gradual withdrawal of systemic corticosteroid therapy should always be considered:

- Patients who have had repeated courses of systemic corticosteroids.
- When a course of Kenalog has been prescribed within one year of cessation of long-term therapy (months or years).
- Patients who may have reasons for adrenocortical insufficiency other than exogenous corticosteroid therapy.

4.3 Contraindications

Hypersensitivity to any of the ingredients.

Systemic infections unless specific anti-infective therapy is employed.

Administration by intravenous or intrathecal injection.

4.4 Special warnings and special precautions for use

Warnings

(Intra-Articular Injection):

Corticosteroids should not be injected into unstable joints.

Patients should be specifically warned to avoid over-use of joints in which symptomatic benefit has been obtained. Severe joint destruction with necrosis of bone may occur if repeated intra-articular injections are given over a long period of time. Care should be taken if injections are given into tendon sheaths to avoid injection into the tendon itself. Repeated injection into inflamed tendons should be avoided as it has been shown to cause tendon rupture.

Due to the absence of a true tendon sheath, the Achilles tendon should not be injected with depot corticosteroids.

(Intramuscular Injection):

During prolonged therapy a liberal protein intake is essential to counteract the tendency to gradual weight loss sometimes associated with negative nitrogen balance and wasting of skeletal muscle.

Precautions:

Intra-articular injection should not be carried out in the presence of active infection in or near joints. The preparation should not be used to alleviate joint pain arising from infectious states such as gonococcal or tubercular arthritis.

Undesirable effects may be minimised using the lowest effective dose for the minimum period, and by administering the daily requirement, whenever possible, as a single morning dose on alternate days. Frequent patient review is required to titrate the dose appropriately against disease activity. (See dosage section).

Adrenal cortical atrophy develops during prolonged therapy and may persist for years after stopping treatment. Withdrawal of corticosteroids after prolonged therapy must, therefore, always be gradual to avoid acute adrenal insufficiency and should be tapered off over weeks or months according to the dose and duration of treatment. During prolonged therapy any intercurrent illness, trauma or surgical procedure will require a temporary increase in dosage. If corticosteroids have been stopped following prolonged therapy they may need to be reintroduced temporarily.

Patients should carry steroid treatment cards which give clear guidance on the precautions to be taken to minimise risk and which provide details of prescriber, drug, dosage and the duration of treatment.

Suppression of the inflammatory response and immune function increases the susceptibility to infections and their severity. The clinical presentation may often be atypical and serious infections such as septicaemia and tuberculosis may be masked and may reach an advanced stage before being recognised.

Chickenpox and measles are of particular concern since these normally minor illnesses may be fatal in immunosuppressed patients.

Unless they have had chickenpox, patients receiving parenteral corticosteroids for purposes other than replacement should be regarded as being *at risk of severe chickenpox.* Manifestations of fulminant illness include pneumonia, hepatitis and disseminated intravascular coagulation; rash is not necessarily a prominent feature. Passive immunisation with varicella zoster immunoglobulin (VZIG) is needed by exposed non- immune patients who are receiving systemic corticosteroids or who have used them within the previous 3 months; varicella-zoster immunoglobulin should preferably be given within 3 days of exposure and not later than 10 days. Confirmed chickenpox warrants specialist care and urgent treatment. Corticosteroids should not be stopped and the dose may need to be increased.

Patients should be advised to avoid exposure to measles and to seek medical advice without delay if exposure occurs. Prophylaxis with normal immunoglobulin may be needed.

During corticosteroid therapy antibody response will be reduced and therefore affect the patient's response to vaccines. Live vaccines should not be administered.

Special Precautions:

Particular care is required when considering use of systemic corticosteroids in patients with the following conditions and frequent patient monitoring is necessary.

Recent intestinal anastomoses, diverticulitis, thrombophlebitis, existing or previous history of severe affective disorders (especially previous steroid psychosis), exanthematous disease, chronic nephritis, or renal insufficiency, metastatic carcinoma, osteoporosis (post-menopausal females are particularly at risk); in patients with an active peptic ulcer (or a history of peptic ulcer). Myasthenia gravis. Latent or healed tuberculosis; in the presence of local or systemic viral infection, systemic fungal infections or in active infections not controlled by antibiotics. In acute psychoses; in acute glomerulonephritis. Hypertension; congestive heart failure; glaucoma (or a family history of glaucoma), previous steroid myopathy or epilepsy. Liver failure.

Corticosteroid effects may be enhanced in patients with hypothyroidism or cirrhosis and decreased in hyperthyroid patients.

Diabetes may be aggravated, necessitating a higher insulin dosage. Latent diabetes mellitus may be precipitated.

Menstrual irregularities may occur, and this possibility should be mentioned to female patients.

Rare instances of anaphylactoid reactions have occurred in patients receiving corticosteroids, especially when a patient has a history of drug allergies.

All corticosteroids increase calcium excretion

Aspirin should be used cautiously in conjunction with corticosteroids in patients with hypoprothrombinaemia.

Use in Children:

Kenalog is not recommended for children under six years. Corticosteroids cause dose-related growth retardation in infancy, childhood and adolescence which may be irreversible, therefore growth and development of children on prolonged corticosteroid therapy should be carefully observed.

Use in Elderly:

The common adverse effects of systemic corticosteroids may be associated with more serious consequences in old age, especially osteoporosis, hypertension, hypokalaemia, diabetes, susceptibility to infection and thinning of the skin. Close clinical supervision is required to avoid life-threatening reactions.

4.5 Interaction with other medicinal products and other forms of Interaction

Amphotericin B injection and potassium-depleting agents: Patients should be observed for hypokalaemia.

Anticholinesterases: Effects of anticholinesterase agent may be antagonised.

Anticoagulants, oral: Corticosteroids may potentiate or decrease anticoagulant action. Patients receiving oral anticoagulants and corticosteroids should therefore be closely monitored.

Antidiabetics: Corticosteroids may increase blood glucose; diabetic control should be monitored, especially when corticosteroids are initiated, discontinued, or changed in dosage.

Antihypertensives, including diuretics: Corticosteroids antagonise the effects of antihypertensives and diuretics. The hypokalaemic effect of diuretics, including acetazolamide, is enhanced.

Anti-tubercular drugs: Isoniazid serum concentrations may be decreased.

Cyclosporin: Monitor for evidence of increased toxicity of cyclosporin when the two are used concurrently.

Digitalis glycosides: Co-administration may enhance the possibility of digitalis toxicity.

Oestrogens, including oral contraceptives: Corticosteroid half-life and concentration may be increased and clearance decreased.

Hepatic Enzyme Inducers (e.g. barbiturates, phenytoin, carbamazepine, rifampicin, primidone, aminoglutethimide): There may be increased metabolic clearance of Kenalog. Patients should be carefully observed for possible diminished effect of steroid, and the dosage should be adjusted accordingly.

Human growth hormone: The growth-promoting effect may be inhibited.

Ketoconazole: Corticosteroid clearance may be decreased, resulting in increased effects.

Nondepolarising muscle relaxants: Corticosteroids may decrease or enhance the neuromuscular blocking action.

Nonsteroidal anti-inflammatory agents (NSAIDS): Corticosteroids may increase the incidence and/or severity of GI bleeding and ulceration associated with NSAIDS. Also, corticosteroids can reduce serum salicylate levels and therefore decrease their effectiveness. Conversely, discontinuing corticosteroids during high-dose salicylate therapy may result in salicylate toxicity. Aspirin should be used cautiously in conjunction with corticosteroids in patients with hypoprothrombinaemia.

Thyroid drugs: Metabolic clearance of adrenocorticoids is decreased in hypothyroid patients and increased in hyperthyroid patients. Changes in thyroid status of the patient may necessitate adjustment in adrenocorticoid dosage.

Vaccines: Neurological complications and lack of antibody response may occur when patients taking corticosteroids are vaccinated. (See 4.4 Special Warnings and Special Precautions for Use.)

4.6 Pregnancy and lactation

The ability of corticosteroids to cross the placenta varies between individual drugs, however triamcinolone does cross the placenta.

Administration of corticosteroids to pregnant animals can cause abnormalities of foetal development including cleft palate, intra-uterine growth retardation and effects on brain growth and development. There is no evidence that corticosteroids result in an increased incidence of congenital abnormalities, such as cleft palate / lip in man. However, when administered for prolonged periods or repeatedly during pregnancy, corticosteroids may increase the risk of intra-uterine growth retardation. Hypoadrenalism may, in theory, occur in the neonate following prenatal exposure to corticosteroids but usually resolves spontaneously following birth and is rarely clinically important.

As with all drugs, corticosteroids should only be prescribed when the benefits to the mother and child outweigh the risks. When corticosteroids are essential, however, patients with normal pregnancies may be treated as though they were in the non-gravid state.

Lactation

Corticosteroids may pass into breast milk, although no data are available for triamcinolone. Infants of mothers taking high doses of systemic corticosteroids for prolonged periods may have a degree of adrenal suppression.

4.7 Effects on ability to drive and use machines

None known.

4.8 Undesirable effects

Where adverse reactions occur they are usually reversible on cessation of therapy. The incidence of predictable side-effects, including hypothalamic-pituitary-adrenal suppression correlate with the relative potency of the drug, dosage, timing of administration and duration of treatment. (See Warnings and Precautions).

Absorption of triamcinolone following injection by the intra-articular route is rare. However, patients should be watched closely for the following adverse reactions which may be associated with any corticosteroid therapy:

Anti-inflammatory and immunosuppressive effects: Increased susceptibility and severity of infections with suppression of clinical symptoms and signs, opportunistic infections, recurrence of dormant tuberculosis. (See Warnings and Precautions).

Fluid and electrolyte disturbances: sodium retention, fluid retention, congestive heart failure in susceptible patients, potassium loss, cardiac arrhythmias or ECG changes due to potassium deficiency, hypokalaemic alkalosis, increased calcium excretion and hypertension.

Musculoskeletal: muscle weakness, fatigue, steroid myopathy, loss of muscle mass, osteoporosis, avascular osteonecrosis, vertebral compression fractures, delayed healing of fractures, aseptic necrosis of femoral and humeral heads, pathological fractures of long bones and spontaneous fractures, tendon rupture.

Hypersensitivity: Anaphylactic reactions, angiodema, rash, pruritus and urticaria, particularly where there is a history of drug allergies.

Dermatological: impaired wound healing, thin fragile skin, petechiae and ecchymoses, facial erythema, increased sweating, purpura, striae, hirsutism, acneiform eruptions, lupus erythematous-like lesions and suppressed reactions to skin tests.

Gastrointestinal: dyspepsia, peptic ulcer with possible subsequent perforation and haemorrhage, pancreatitis, abdominal distension and ulcerative oesophagitis, candidiasis.

Neurological: euphoria, psychological dependence, depression, insomnia, convulsions, increased intracranial pressure with papilloedema (pseudo-tumour cerebri) usually after treatment, vertigo, headache, neuritis or paraesthesias and aggravation of pre-existing psychiatric conditions and epilepsy.

Endocrine: menstrual irregularities and amenorrhoea; development of the Cushingoid state; suppression of growth in childhood and adolescence; secondary adrenocortical and pituitary unresponsiveness, particularly in times of stress (e.g. trauma, surgery or illness); decreased carbohydrate tolerance; manifestations of latent diabetes mellitus and increased requirements for insulin or oral hypoglycaemic agents in diabetes, weight gain. Negative protein and calcium balance. Increased appetite.

Ophthalmic: posterior subcapsular cataracts, increased intraocular pressure, glaucoma, exophthalmos, papilloedema, corneal or scleral thinning, exacerbation of ophthalmic viral or fungal diseases.

Others: necrotising angiitis, thrombophlebitis, thromboembolism, leucocytosis, insomnia and syncopal episodes.

Withdrawal Symptoms and Signs:

On withdrawal, fever, myalgia, arthralgia, rhinitis, conjunctivitis, painful itchy skin nodules and weight loss may occur. Too rapid a reduction in dose following prolonged treatment can lead to acute adrenal insufficiency, hypotension and death. (See Warnings and Precautions.)

Intra-Articular Injection:

Reactions following intra-articular administration have been rare. In a few instances, transient flushing and dizziness have occurred. Local symptoms such as post-injection flare, transient pain, irritation, sterile abscesses, hyper- or hypo-pigmentation, Charcot-like arthropathy and occasional increase in joint discomfort may occur. Local fat atrophy may occur if the injection is not given into the joint space, but is temporary and disappears within a few weeks to months.

Intramuscular Injection:

Severe pain has been reported following intramuscular administration. Sterile abscesses, cutaneous and subcutaneous atrophy, hyperpigmentation, hypopigmentation and Charcot-like arthropathy have also occurred.

4.9 Overdose

Not applicable.

5. PHARMACOLOGICAL PROPERTIES

5.1 Pharmacodynamic properties

Triamcinolone acetonide is a synthetic glucocorticoid with marked anti-inflammatory and anti-allergic actions.

Intra-Articular Injection: Following local injection, relief of pain and swelling and greater freedom of movement are usually obtained within a few hours.

Intramuscular Injection: Provides an extended duration of therapeutic effect and fewer side effects of the kind associated with oral corticosteroid therapy, particularly gastro-intestinal reactions such as peptic ulceration. Studies indicate that, following a single intramuscular dose of 80mg triamcinolone acetonide, adrenal suppression occurs within 24 - 48 hours and then gradually returns to normal, usually in approximately three weeks. This finding correlates closely with the extended duration of therapeutic action of triamcinolone acetonide.

5.2 Pharmacokinetic properties

Triamcinolone acetonide may be absorbed into the systemic circulation from synovial spaces. However clinically significant systemic levels after intra-articular injection are unlikely to occur except perhaps following treatment of large joints with high doses. Systemic effects do not ordinarily occur with intra-articular injections when the proper techniques of administration and the recommended dosage regimens are observed.

Triamcinolone acetonide is absorbed slowly, though almost completely, following depot administration by deep intramuscular injection; biologically active levels are achieved systemically for prolonged periods (weeks to months). In common with other corticosteroids, triamcinolone is metabolised largely hepatically but also by the kidney and is excreted in urine. The main metabolic route is 6-beta-hydroxylation; no significant hydrolytic cleavage of the acetonide occurs.

In view of the hepatic metabolism and renal excretion of triamcinolone acetonide, functional impairments of the liver or kidney may affect the pharmacokinetics of the drug.

5.3 Preclinical safety data

See 4.6 Pregnancy and Lactation.

6. PHARMACEUTICAL PARTICULARS

6.1 List of excipients

Benzyl alcohol, polysorbate 80, carmellose sodium, sodium chloride, water.

6.2 Incompatibilities

The injection should not be physically mixed with other medicinal products.

6.3 Shelf life

36 months

6.4 Special precautions for storage

Do not store above 25°C. Do not freeze. Store in an upright position.

6.5 Nature and contents of container

Carton containing glass ampoules 5 × 1ml or individually cartoned 1ml and 2ml syringes.

6.6 Instructions for use and handling

No special handling instructions.

7. MARKETING AUTHORISATION HOLDER

E.R. Squibb & Sons Ltd.

Uxbridge Business Park

Sanderson Road

Uxbridge

Middlesex

UB8 1DH

8. MARKETING AUTHORISATION NUMBER(S)

PL 0034/5045R

9. DATE OF FIRST AUTHORISATION/RENEWAL OF THE AUTHORISATION

10 July 1986

10. DATE OF REVISION OF THE TEXT

June 2005

Kentera 3.9 mg/24 hours, transdermal patch

(UCB Pharma Limited)

1. NAME OF THE MEDICINAL PRODUCT

▼Kentera 3.9 mg / 24 hours, transdermal patch

2. QUALITATIVE AND QUANTITATIVE COMPOSITION

Each transdermal patch contains 36 mg of oxybutynin. The area of the patch is 39 cm^2, releasing a nominal 3.9 mg of oxybutynin per 24 hours.

For excipients, see section 6.1.

3. PHARMACEUTICAL FORM

Transdermal patch.

4. CLINICAL PARTICULARS

4.1 Therapeutic indications

Symptomatic treatment of urge incontinence and/or increased urinary frequency and urgency as may occur in patients with unstable bladder.

4.2 Posology and method of administration

The patch should be applied to dry, intact skin on the abdomen, hip, or buttock immediately after removal from the protective sachet. A new application site should be selected with each new patch to avoid reapplication to the same site within 7 days.

The recommended dose is one 3.9 mg transdermal patch applied twice weekly (every 3 to 4 days).

No studies have been performed in children or adolescents, therefore Kentera is not recommended for use in children or adolescents.

4.3 Contraindications

Hypersensitivity to the active substance or to any other excipients of the transdermal patch.

Kentera is contraindicated in patients with urinary retention, severe gastro-intestinal condition, myasthenia gravis or narrow-angle glaucoma and in patients who are at risk for these conditions.

4.4 Special warnings and special precautions for use

Kentera should be used with caution in patients with hepatic or renal impairment. The use of Kentera in patients with hepatic impairment should be carefully monitored. Other causes of frequent urination (heart failure or renal disease) should be assessed before treatment with Kentera. If urinary tract infection is present, an appropriate antibacterial therapy should be started.

Urinary Retention: Anticholinergic products should be administered with caution to patients with clinically significant bladder outflow obstruction because of the risk of urinary retention.

Because anticholinergic agents such as oxybutynin may produce drowsiness, somnolence, or blurred vision, patients should be advised to exercise caution. Patients should be informed that alcohol may enhance the drowsiness caused by anticholinergic agents such as oxybutynin.

Kentera should be used with caution in elderly patients, who may be more sensitive to the effects of centrally acting anticholinergics and exhibit differences in pharmacokinetics.

Oral administration of oxybutynin may warrant the following cautionary statements, but these events were not observed during clinical trials with Kentera:

Gastrointestinal Disorders: Anticholinergic medicinal products may decrease gastrointestinal motility and should be used with caution in patients with gastrointestinal obstructive disorders because of the risk of gastric retention. Also in conditions such as ulcerative colitis, and intestinal atony. Anticholinergic medicinal products should be used with caution in patients who have hiatus hernia/gastro-oesophageal reflux and/or who are concurrently taking medicinal products (such as bisphosphonates) that can cause or exacerbate oesophagitis.

Anticholinergic medicinal products should be used with caution in patients who have autonomic neuropathy, cognitive impairment or Parkinson's disease.

Patients should be informed that heat prostration (fever and heat stroke due to decreased sweating) can occur when anticholinergics such as oxybutynin are used in a hot environment.

Oxybutynin may exacerbate the symptoms of hyperthyroidism, coronary heart disease, congestive heart failure, cardiac arrhythmias, tachycardia, hypertension and prostatic hypertrophy.

Oxybutynin may lead to suppressed salivary secretions which could result in dental caries, parodontosis or oral candidiasis.

4.5 Interaction with other medicinal products and other forms of Interaction

The concomitant use of oxybutynin with other anticholinergic medicinal products or with other agents that compete for CYP3A4 enzyme metabolism may increase the frequency or severity of dry mouth, constipation, and drowsiness.

Anticholinergic agents may potentially alter the absorption of some concomitantly administered drugs due to anticholinergic effects on gastrointestinal motility. As oxybutynin is metabolised by cytochrome P 450 isoenzyme CYP 3A4, interactions with drugs that inhibit this isoenzyme cannot be ruled out. This should be borne in mind when using azole antifungals (e.g. ketoconazole) or macrolide antibiotics (e.g. erythromycin) concurrently with oxybutynin.

The anticholinergic activity of oxybutynin is increased by concurrent use of other anticholinergics or drugs with anticholinergic activity, such as amantadine and other anticholinergic antiparkinsonian drugs (e.g. biperiden, levodopa), antihistamines, antipsychotics (e.g. phenothiazines, butyrophenones, clozapine), quinidine, tricyclic antidepressants, atropine and related compounds like atropinic antispasmodics, dipyridamole.

Oxybutynin may antagonise prokinetic therapies.

4.6 Pregnancy and lactation

Pregnancy

There are no adequate data on the use of oxybutynin transdermal patch in pregnant women.

Studies in animals have shown minor reproductive toxicity (see section 5.3). Kentera should not to be used during pregnancy unless clearly necessary

Lactation

When oxybutynin is used during lactation, a small amount is excreted in the mother's milk. Breast feeding while using oxybutynin is therefore not recommended.

4.7 Effects on ability to drive and use machines

Oxybutynin may cause drowsiness, blurred vision, dizziness and fatigue, therefore caution is recommended when driving or operating machines.

4.8 Undesirable effects

The most commonly reported adverse drug reactions were application site reaction (Kentera 23.1 %, placebo 7.6%). Other adverse drug reactions reported were dry mouth (Kentera 8.6%, placebo 5.2%), constipation (Kentera 3.9%, placebo 2%), diarrhoea (Kentera 3.2%, placebo 2%), headache (Kentera 3.0%, placebo 2.4%), dizziness (Kentera 2.3%, placebo 1.2%), and blurred vision (Kentera 2.3%, placebo 0.89%).

Undesirable effects known to be associated with anticholinergic therapy, but not observed with Kentera during clinical studies are anorexia, vomiting, reflux oesophagitis, decreased sweating, heat stroke, decreased lacrimation, mydriasis, tachycardia, arrhythmia, disorientation, poor ability to concentrate, fatigue, nightmares, restlessness, convulsion, intraocular hypertension and induction of glaucoma, confusion, anxiety, paranoia, hallucinations, photosensitivity, erectile dysfunction.

Reported Adverse Drug Reactions and rate of occurrence:

(see Table 1 on next page)

4.9 Overdose

Plasma concentration of oxybutynin declines within 1 to 2 hours after removal of transdermal system(s). Patients should be monitored until symptoms resolve. Overdosage with oxybutynin has been associated with anticholinergic effects including CNS excitation, flushing, fever, dehydration, cardiac arrhythmia, vomiting, and urinary retention. Ingestion of 100 mg oral oxybutynin chloride in association with alcohol has been reported in a 13 year old boy who experienced memory loss, and in a 34 year old woman who developed stupor, followed by disorientation and agitation on awakening, dilated pupils, dry skin, cardiac arrhythmia, and retention of urine. Both patients recovered fully with symptomatic treatment.

No cases of overdose have been reported with Kentera.

5. PHARMACOLOGICAL PROPERTIES

5.1 Pharmacodynamic properties

Pharmacotherapeutic group: urinary antispasmodic, ATC code: G04B D04.

Mechanism of action: *oxybutynin acts as a competitive antagonist of acetylcholine at post-ganglionic muscarinic receptors, resulting in relaxation of bladder smooth muscle.*

Pharmacodynamic effects:

In patients with overactive bladder, characterised by detrusor muscle instability or hyperreflexia, cystometric studies have demonstrated that oxybutynin increases maximum urinary bladder capacity and increases the volume to first detrusor contraction. Oxybutynin thus decreases urinary urgency and the frequency of both incontinence episodes and voluntary urination.

Oxybutynin is a racemic (50:50) mixture of R- and S-isomers. Antimuscarinic activity resides predominantly in the R-isomer. The R-isomer of oxybutynin shows greater selectivity for the M_1 and M_3 muscarinic subtypes (predominant in bladder detrusor muscle and parotid gland) compared to the M_2 subtype (predominant in cardiac tissue). The active metabolite, N-desethyloxybutynin, has pharmacological activity on the human detrusor muscle that is similar to that of oxybutynin *in vitro* studies, but has a greater binding affinity for parotid tissue than oxybutynin. The free base form of oxybutynin is pharmacologically equivalent to oxybutynin hydrochloride.

Table 1 Reported Adverse Drug Reactions and rate of occurrence

Application site reactions		
All application site reactions	23.1%	Very common
- Application site pruritis	14.3 %	very common
- Application site erythema	5.7 %	common
- Application site reaction	3.5 %	common
- Application site rash	3.0 %	common
Infections and infestations:		
Urinary Tract	1.2 %	common
Upper Respiratory Tract	0.2 %	uncommon
Fungal	0.2 %	uncommon
Eye disorders		
Vision abnormalities	2.3 %	common
Ear and labyrinth disorders		
Dizziness	2.3%	common
Cardiac Disorders		
Palpitations	0.3 %	uncommon
Vascular disorders		
Hot flushes	0.3 %	uncommon
Urticaria	0.4%	uncommon
Gastrointestinal disorders		
Dry Mouth	8.6 %	common
Constipation	3.9 %	common
Diarrhoea	3.2 %	common
Nausea	2.1 %	common
Abdominal Pain	1.2 %	common
Dyspepsia	0.4%	uncommon
Abdominal Discomfort	0.5%	uncommon
Musculoskeletal disorders		
Back Pain	0.8 %	uncommon
Renal and urinary disorders		
Urinary retention	0.3 %	uncommon
Dysuria	0.9 %	uncommon
General disorders		
Headache	3.0 %	common
Somnolence	1.2 %	common
Rhinitis	0.5 %	uncommon
Injury		
Inflicted Injury	0.3 %	uncommon

Clinical efficacy:

A total of 957 patients with urge urinary incontinence were evaluated in three controlled studies comparing Kentera to either placebo, oral oxybutynin and/or tolterodine long acting capsules. Reductions in weekly incontinence episodes, urinary frequency, and urinary void volume were evaluated. Kentera led to consistent improvements in overactive bladder symptoms compared with placebo.

5.2 Pharmacokinetic properties

Absorption

Kentera has a concentration of oxybutynin sufficient to maintain continuous transport over the 3 to 4 day dosing interval. Oxybutynin is transported across intact skin and into the systemic circulation by passive diffusion across the stratum corneum. Following the application of Kentera, oxybutynin plasma concentration increases for approximately 24 to 48 hours, reaching average maximum concentrations of 3 to 4ng/ml. Steady-state conditions are reached during the second application of the transdermal patch. Thereafter, steady concentrations are maintained for up to 96 hours. The difference in AUC and Cmax of oxybutynin and the active metabolite N-desethyloxybutynin following transdermal administration of Kentera on either the abdomen, buttocks or hip is not clinically relevant.

Distribution

Oxybutynin is widely distributed in body tissues following systemic absorption. The volume of distribution was estimated to be 193 l after intravenous administration of 5 mg oxybutynin hydrochloride.

Metabolism

Oxybutynin administered orally is metabolised primarily by the cytochrome P450 enzyme systems, particularly CYP3A4, found mostly in the liver and gut wall. Metabolites include phenylcyclohexylglycolic acid, which is pharmacologically inactive, and N-desethyloxybutynin, which is pharmacologically active. Transdermal administration of oxybutynin bypasses the first-pass gastrointestinal and hepatic metabolism, reducing the formation of the N-desethyl metabolite.

Excretion

Oxybutynin is extensively metabolised by the liver, see above with less than 0.1% of the administered dose excreted unchanged in the urine. Also, less than 0.1% of the administered dose is excreted as the metabolite N-desethyloxybutynin.

5.3 Preclinical safety data

Pre-clinical data reveal no special hazard for humans based on studies for acute toxicology, repeat dose toxicity, genotoxicity, carcinogenic potential and local toxicity. At a concentration of 0.4 mg/kg/day oxybutynin administered subcutaneously, the occurrence of organ anomalies is significantly increased, but is observed only in the presence of maternal toxicity. Kentera delivers approximately 0.08 mg/kg/day. However, in the absence of understanding the association between maternal toxicity and developmental effect, the relevance to human safety cannot be addressed. In the subcutaneous fertility study in rats, while no effects were reported in males, in females, fertility was impaired and a NOAEL (no observed adverse effect level) of 5 mg/kg was identified.

6. PHARMACEUTICAL PARTICULARS

6.1 List of excipients

The transdermal patch is composed of three layers: a backing film, an adhesive/drug layer and a release liner. The backing film provides the matrix system with occlusivity and physical integrity and protects the adhesive/drug layer. The adhesive/drug layer contains oxybutynin and glycerol triacetate. The release liner is two overlapped siliconised polyester strips that are peeled off and discarded by the patient prior to applying the patch.

Backing Film:

Polyethylene/ethyl vinyl acetate (PET/EVA), clear

Middle layer:

Glycerol Triacetate

Acrylic Copolymer Adhesive Solution containing 2-ethylhexyl acrylate N-vinyl pyrrolidone and hexamethyleneglycol dimethacrylate polymer domains

Release Liner:

Siliconised Polyester

6.2 Incompatibilities

Not applicable.

6.3 Shelf life

2 years.

6.4 Special precautions for storage

Store in the original package. Do not refrigerate. Do not freeze.

6.5 Nature and contents of container

The transdermal patches are individually contained in LDPE/paper laminate sachets and supplied in Patient Calendar Boxes of 8 or 24 patches.

6.6 Instructions for use and handling

Apply immediately upon removal from the protective sachet. After use the patch still contains substantial quantities of active ingredients. Remaining active ingredients of the patch may have harmful effects if reaching the aquatic environment. Hence, after removal, the used patch should be folded in half, adhesive side inwards so that the release membrane is not exposed, placed in the original sachet and then discarded safely out of reach of children. Any used or unused patches should be discarded according to local requirements or returned to the pharmacy. Used patches should not be flushed down the toilet nor placed in liquid waste disposal systems.

Activities that may lead to excessive sweating, or exposure to water or extreme temperature may contribute to adhesion problems. Do not expose the patch to the sun.

7. MARKETING AUTHORISATION HOLDER

Nicobrand Limited

189 Castleroe Road

Coleraine

Northern Ireland

BT51 3RP

8. MARKETING AUTHORISATION NUMBER(S)

EU/1/03/270/001

EU/1/03/270/002

EU/1/03/270/003

9. DATE OF FIRST AUTHORISATION/RENEWAL OF THE AUTHORISATION

15/06/2004

10. DATE OF REVISION OF THE TEXT

Keppra Tablets and Solution

(UCB Pharma Limited)

1. NAME OF THE MEDICINAL PRODUCT

▼Keppra 250 mg film-coated tablets.

▼Keppra 500 mg film-coated tablets.

▼Keppra 750 mg film-coated tablets.

▼Keppra 1000 mg film-coated tablets.

▼Keppra 100 mg/ml, oral solution.

2. QUALITATIVE AND QUANTITATIVE COMPOSITION

Tablets:

Each film-coated tablet contains 250 mg levetiracetam, 500 mg levetiracetam, 750 mg levetiracetam or 1000 mg levetiracetam.

Oral solution:

Each ml contains 100 mg levetiracetam.

For excipients, see section 6.1.

3. PHARMACEUTICAL FORM

Film-coated tablets:

Blue, oblong and debossed with the code "ucb 250" on one side. Yellow, oblong and debossed with the code "ucb 500" on one side. Orange, oblong and debossed with the code "ucb 750" on one side.

White, oblong and debossed with the code "ucb 1000" on one side.

Oral solution:

Clear liquid.

4. CLINICAL PARTICULARS

4.1 Therapeutic indications

Keppra is indicated as adjunctive therapy in the treatment of partial onset seizures with or without secondary generalisation in adults and children from 4 years of age with epilepsy.

4.2 Posology and method of administration

Tablets:

The film-coated tablets must be taken orally, swallowed with a sufficient quantity of liquid and may be taken with or without food. The daily dose is administered in two equally divided doses.

Oral solution:

The oral solution should be diluted in a glass of water and may be taken with or without food. A graduated oral syringe and instruction for use in the package leaflet are provided with this medicine. The daily dose is administered in 2 equally divided doses.

Adults (≥ 18 years) and adolescents (12 to 17 years) of 50 kg or more

The initial therapeutic dose is 500 mg twice daily. This dose can be started on the first day of treatment.

Depending upon the clinical response and tolerability, the daily dose can be increased up to 1,500 mg twice daily. Dose changes can be made in 500 mg twice daily increments or decrements every two to four weeks.

Elderly (65 years and older)

Adjustment of the dose is recommended in elderly patients with compromised renal function (see "Patients with renal impairment" below).

Children aged 4 to 11 years and adolescents (12 to 17 years) of less than 50 kg

The initial therapeutic dose is 10 mg/kg twice daily.

Depending upon the clinical response and tolerability, the dose can be increased up to 30 mg/kg twice daily. Dose changes should not exceed increments or decrements of 10 mg/kg twice daily every two weeks. The lowest effective dose should be used.

Dosage in children 50 kg or greater is the same as in adults.

The physician should prescribe the most appropriate pharmaceutical form and strength according to weight and dose.

Dosage recommendations for children and adolescents:

Weight	Starting dose: 10 mg/kg twice daily	Maximum dose: 30 mg/kg twice daily
15 kg (1)	150 mg twice daily	450 mg twice daily
20 kg (1)	200 mg twice daily	600 mg twice daily
25 kg	250 mg twice daily	750 mg twice daily
From 50 kg (2)	500 mg twice daily	1500 mg twice daily

(1) Children 20 kg or less should preferably start the treatment with Keppra 100 mg/ml oral solution.

(2) Dosage in children and adolescents 50 kg or more is the same as in adults.

The graduated oral syringe contains up to 1,000 mg levetiracetam (corresponding to 10 ml) with a graduation every 25 mg (corresponding to 0.25 ml).

Infants and children less than 4 years

There are insufficient data to recommend the use of levetiracetam in children under 4 years of age.

Patients with renal impairment

The daily dose must be individualised according to renal function.

For adult patients, refer to the following table and adjust the dose as indicated. To use this dosing table, an estimate of the patient's creatinine clearance (CLcr) in ml/min is needed. The CLcr in ml/min may be estimated from serum creatinine (mg/dl) determination using the following formula:

$$CLcr = \frac{[140\text{-age (years)}] \times \text{weight (kg)}}{72 \times \text{serum creatinine (mg/dl)}} \quad (\times 0.85 \text{ for women})$$

Dosing adjustment for adult patients with impaired renal function

Group	Creatinine clearance (ml/min)	Dosage and frequency
Normal	> 80	500 to 1,500 mg twice daily
Mild	50-79	500 to 1,000 mg twice daily
Moderate	30-49	250 to 750 mg twice daily
Severe	< 30	250 to 500 mg twice daily
End-stage renal disease patients Undergoing dialysis (1)		500 to 1,000 mg once daily (2)

(1) A 750 mg loading dose is recommended on the first day of treatment with levetiracetam.

(2) Following dialysis, a 250 to 500 mg supplemental dose is recommended.

For children with renal impairment, levetiracetam dose needs to be adjusted based on the renal function as levetiracetam clearance is related to renal function. This recommendation is based on a study in adult renally impaired patients.

Patients with hepatic impairment

No dose adjustment is needed in patients with mild to moderate hepatic impairment. In patients with severe hepatic impairment, the creatinine clearance may underestimate the renal insufficiency. Therefore a 50 % reduction of the daily maintenance dose is recommended when the creatinine clearance is < 70 ml/min.

4.3 Contraindications

Hypersensitivity to levetiracetam or other pyrrolidone derivatives or any of the excipients.

4.4 Special warnings and special precautions for use

In accordance with current clinical practice, if Keppra has to be discontinued it is recommended to withdraw it gradually (*e.g.* in adults: 500 mg twice daily decrements every two to four weeks; in children: dose decrease should not exceed decrements of 10 mg/kg twice daily every two weeks).

In a study reflecting clinical practice, the concomitant antiepileptic medication could be withdrawn in a limited number of patients who responded to levetiracetam adjunctive therapy (36 adult patients out of 69).

Available data in children did not suggest impact on growth and puberty. However, long term effects on learning, intelligence, growth, endocrine function, puberty and childbearing potential in children remain unknown.

An increase in seizure frequency of more than 25 % was reported in 14 % of levetiracetam treated adult and paediatric patients, whereas it was reported in 26 % and 21 % of placebo treated adult and paediatric patients, respectively.

The administration of Keppra to patients with renal impairment may require dose adjustment. In patients with severely impaired hepatic function, assessment of renal function is recommended before dose selection (see section 4.2 "Posology").

Keppra 100 mg/ml oral solution includes methyl parahydroxybenzoate (E218) and propyl parahydroxybenzoate (E216) which may cause allergic reactions (possibly delayed).

It also includes maltitol; patients with rare hereditary problems of fructose intolerance should not take this medicine.

4.5 Interaction with other medicinal products and other forms of Interaction

Pre-marketing data from clinical studies conducted in adults indicate that Keppra did not influence the serum concentrations of existing antiepileptic medicinal products (phenytoin, carbamazepine, valproic acid, phenobarbital, lamotrigine, gabapentin and primidone) and that these antiepileptic medicinal products did not influence the pharmacokinetics of Keppra.

Consistent with formal pharmacokinetic studies in adults, there has been no clear evidence of clinically significant medicinal product interactions in paediatric patients receiving up to 60 mg/kg/day levetiracetam.

A retrospective assessment of pharmacokinetic interactions in children and adolescents with epilepsy (4 to 17 years) confirmed that adjunctive therapy with levetiracetam did not influence the steady-state serum concentrations of concomitantly administered carbamazepine and valproate. However, data suggested that enzyme-inducing antiepileptic medicinal products increase levetiracetam clearance by 22 %. Dosage adjustment is not required.

Probenecid (500 mg four times daily), a renal tubular secretion blocking agent, has been shown to inhibit the renal clearance of the primary metabolite but not of levetiracetam. Nevertheless, the concentration of this metabolite remains low. It is expected that other drugs excreted by active tubular secretion could also reduce the renal clearance of the metabolite. The effect of levetiracetam on probenecid was not studied and the effect of levetiracetam on other actively secreted drugs, *e.g.* NSAIDs, sulfonamides and methotrexate, is unknown.

Levetiracetam 1,000 mg daily did not influence the pharmacokinetics of oral contraceptives (ethinyl-estradiol and levonorgestrel); endocrine parameters (luteinizing hormone and progesterone) were not modified. Levetiracetam 2,000 mg daily did not influence the pharmacokinetics of digoxin and warfarin; prothrombin times were not modified. Co-administration with digoxin, oral contraceptives and warfarin did not influence the pharmacokinetics of levetiracetam.

No data on the influence of antacids on the absorption of levetiracetam are available.

The extent of absorption of levetiracetam was not altered by food, but the rate of absorption was slightly reduced.

No data on the interaction of levetiracetam with alcohol are available.

4.6 Pregnancy and lactation

There are no adequate data from the use of Keppra in pregnant women. Studies in animals have shown reproductive toxicity (see section 5.3). The potential risk for human is unknown.

Keppra should not be used during pregnancy unless clearly necessary. Discontinuation of antiepileptic treatments may result in disease worsening, harmful to the mother and the foetus.

Levetiracetam is excreted in human breast milk. Therefore, breast-feeding is not recommended.

4.7 Effects on ability to drive and use machines

No studies on the effects on the ability to drive and use machines have been performed.

Due to possible different individual sensitivity, some patients might experience somnolence or other central nervous system related symptoms, at the beginning of treatment or following a dose increase. Therefore, caution is recommended in those patients when performing skilled tasks, *e.g.* driving vehicles or operating machinery.

4.8 Undesirable effects

Pooled safety data from clinical studies showed that 46.4 % and 42.2 % of the patients experienced undesirable effects in the Keppra and placebo groups, respectively, and that 2.4 % and 2.0 % of the patients experienced serious undesirable effects in the Keppra and placebo groups, respectively. The most commonly reported undesirable effects were somnolence, asthenia and dizziness. In the pooled safety analysis, there was no clear dose-response relationship but incidence and severity of the central nervous system related undesirable effects decreased over time.

A study conducted in paediatric patients (4 to 16 years) showed that 55.4 % of the patients in the Keppra group and 40.2 % of the patients in the placebo group experienced undesirable effects. Serious undesirable effects were experienced in 0.0 % of the patients in the Keppra group and 1.0 % of the patients in the placebo group. The most commonly reported undesirable effects were somnolence, hostility, nervousness, emotional lability, agitation, anorexia, asthenia and headache in the paediatric population. Safety results in paediatric patients were consistent with the safety profile of levetiracetam in adults except for behavioural and psychiatric adverse events which were more common in children than in adults (38.6% versus 18.6%). However, the relative risk was similar in children as compared to adults.

Undesirable effects reported in clinical studies (adults and children) or from post-marketing experience are listed in the following table per System Organ Class and per frequency. For clinical trials, the frequency is defined as follows: very common: > 10 %; common: > 1 - 10 %; uncommon: > 0.1 % - 1 %; rare: 0.01 % - 0.1 %; very rare: < 0.01 %, including isolated reports. Data from post-marketing experience are insufficient to support an estimate of their incidence in the population to be treated.

- General disorders and administration site conditions

Very common: asthenia

- Nervous system disorders

Very common: somnolence

Common: amnesia, ataxia, convulsion, dizziness, headache, hyperkinesia, tremor

- Psychiatric disorders

Common: agitation, depression, emotional lability, hostility, insomnia, nervousness, personality disorders, thinking abnormal

Post-marketing experience: abnormal behaviour, aggression, anger, anxiety, confusion, hallucination, irritability, psychotic disorder, suicide, suicide attempt and suicidal ideation

- Gastrointestinal disorders

Common: diarrhoea, dyspepsia, nausea, vomiting

- Metabolism and nutrition disorders

Common: anorexia. The risk of anorexia is higher when topiramate is coadministered with levetiracetam.

- Ear and labyrinth disorders

Common: vertigo

- Eye disorders

Common: diplopia

- Injury, poisoning and procedural complications

Common: accidental injury

- Infections and infestations

Common: infection

- Respiratory, thoracic and mediastinal disorders

Common: cough increased

- Skin and subcutaneous tissue disorders

Common: rash

Post-marketing experience: alopecia: in several cases, recovery was observed when Keppra was discontinued.

- Blood and lymphatic system disorders

Post-marketing experience: leukopenia, neutropenia, pancytopenia, thrombocytopenia

4.9 Overdose

Symptoms

Somnolence, agitation, aggression, depressed level of consciousness, respiratory depression and coma were observed with Keppra overdoses.

Management of overdose

After an acute overdose, the stomach may be emptied by gastric lavage or by induction of emesis. There is no specific antidote for levetiracetam. Treatment of an overdose will be symptomatic and may include haemodialysis. The dialyser extraction efficiency is 60 % for levetiracetam and 74 % for the primary metabolite.

5. PHARMACOLOGICAL PROPERTIES

5.1 Pharmacodynamic properties

Pharmacotherapeutic group: antiepileptics, ATC code: N03AX14.

The active substance, levetiracetam, is a pyrrolidone derivative (S-enantiomer of α-ethyl-2-oxo-1-pyrrolidine acetamide), chemically unrelated to existing antiepileptic active substances.

Mechanism of action

The mechanism of action of levetiracetam still remains to be fully elucidated but appears to be different from the mechanisms of current antiepileptic medicinal products. *In vitro* and *in vivo* experiments suggest that levetiracetam does not alter basic cell characteristics and normal neurotransmission.

In vitro studies show that levetiracetam affects intranueronal Ca^{2+} levels by partial inhibition of N-type CA^{2+} currents and by reducing the release of Ca^{2+} from intraneuronal stores. In addition it partially reverses the reductions in GABA- and glycine-gated currents induced by zinc and β-carbolines. Further more, levetiracetam has been shown in *in vitro* studies to bind to a specific site in rodent brain tissue. This binding site is the synaptic vesicle protein 2A, believed to be involved in vesicle fusion and neurotransmitter exocytosis. Levetiracetam and related analogs show a rank order of affinity for binding to the synaptic vesicle protein 2A which correlates with the potency of their anti-seizure protection in the mouse audiogenic model of epilepsy. This finding suggests the interaction between levetiracetam and the synaptic vesicle protein 2A seems to contribute to the antiepileptic mechanism of action of the drug.

Pharmacodynamic effects

Levetiracetam induces seizure protection in a broad range of animal models of partial and primarily generalised seizures without having a pro-convulsant effect. The primary metabolite is inactive.

In man, an activity in both partial and generalised epilepsy conditions (epileptiform discharge/photoparoxysmal response) has confirmed the broad spectrum of the preclinical pharmacological profile.

5.2 Pharmacokinetic properties

Levetiracetam is a highly soluble and permeable compound. The pharmacokinetic profile is linear with low intra- and inter-subject variability. There is no modification of the clearance after repeated administration. There is no evidence for any relevant gender, race or circadian variability. The pharmacokinetic profile is comparable in healthy volunteers and in patients with epilepsy.

Due to its complete and linear absorption, plasma levels can be predicted from the oral dose of levetiracetam expressed as mg/kg bodyweight. Therefore there is no need for plasma level monitoring of levetiracetam.

A significant correlation between saliva and plasma concentrations has been shown in adults and children (ratio of saliva/plasma concentrations ranged from 1 to 1.7 for oral tablet formulation and after 4 hours post-dose for oral solution formulation).

Adults and adolescents

Absorption

Levetiracetam is rapidly absorbed after oral administration. Oral absolute bioavailability is close to 100 %.

Peak plasma concentrations (C_{max}) are achieved at 1.3 hours after dosing. Steady-state is achieved after two days of a twice daily administration schedule.

Peak concentrations (C_{max}) are typically 31 and 43 μg/ml following a single 1,000 mg dose and repeated 1,000 mg twice daily dose, respectively.

The extent of absorption is dose-independent and is not altered by food.

Distribution

No tissue distribution data are available in humans.

Neither levetiracetam nor its primary metabolite are significantly bound to plasma proteins (< 10 %).

The volume of distribution of levetiracetam is approximately 0.5 to 0.7 l/kg, a value close to the total body water volume.

Biotransformation

Levetiracetam is not extensively metabolised in humans. The major metabolic pathway (24 % of the dose) is an enzymatic hydrolysis of the acetamide group. Production of the primary metabolite, ucb L057, is not supported by liver cytochrome P_{450} isoforms. Hydrolysis of the acetamide group was measurable in a large number of tissues including blood cells. The metabolite ucb L057 is pharmacologically inactive.

Two minor metabolites were also identified. One was obtained by hydroxylation of the pyrrolidone ring (1.6 % of the dose) and the other one by opening of the pyrrolidone ring (0.9 % of the dose).

Other unidentified components accounted only for 0.6 % of the dose.

No enantiomeric interconversion was evidenced *in vivo* for either levetiracetam nor its primary metabolite.

In vitro, levetiracetam and its primary metabolite have been shown not to inhibit the major human liver cytochrome P_{450} isoforms (CYP3A4, 2A6, 2C8/9/10, 2C19, 2D6, 2E1 and 1A2), glucuronyl transferase (UGT1*6, UGT1*1 and UGT [PL6.2]) and epoxide hydroxylase activities. In addition, levetiracetam does not affect the *in vitro* glucuronidation of valproic acid.

In human hepatocytes in culture, levetiracetam did not cause enzyme induction. Therefore, the interaction of Keppra with other substances, or *vice versa,* is unlikely.

Elimination

The plasma half-life in adults was 7±1 hours and did not vary either with dose, route of administration or repeated administration. The mean total body clearance was 0.96 ml/min/kg.

The major route of excretion was via urine, accounting for a mean 95 % of the dose (approximately 93 % of the dose was excreted within 48 hours). Excretion *via* faeces accounted for only 0.3 % of the dose.

The cumulative urinary excretion of levetiracetam and its primary metabolite accounted for 66 % and 24 % of the dose, respectively during the first 48 hours.

The renal clearance of levetiracetam and ucb L057 is 0.6 and 4.2 ml/min/kg respectively indicating that levetiracetam is excreted by glomerular filtration with subsequent tubular reabsorption and that the primary metabolite is also excreted by active tubular secretion in addition to glomerular filtration. Levetiracetam elimination is correlated to creatinine clearance.

Elderly

In the elderly, the half-life is increased by about 40 % (10 to 11 hours). This is related to the decrease in renal function in this population (see section 4.2 "Posology").

Children (4 to 12 years)

Following single dose administration (20 mg/kg) to epileptic children (6 to 12 years), the half-life of levetiracetam was 6.0 hours. The apparent body weight adjusted clearance was approximately 30 % higher than in epileptic adults.

Following repeated oral dose administration (20 to 60 mg/kg/day) to epileptic children (4 to 12 years), levetiracetam was rapidly absorbed. Peak plasma concentration was observed 0.5 to 1.0 hour after dosing. Linear and dose proportional increases were observed for peak plasma concentrations and area under the curve. The elimination half-life was approximately 5 hours. The apparent body clearance was 1.1 ml/min/kg.

Infants and children (1 month to 4 years)

Following single dose administration (20 mg/kg) of a 100 mg/ml oral solution to epileptic children (1 month to 4 years), levetiracetam was rapidly absorbed and peak plasma concentrations were observed approximately 1 hour after dosing. The pharmacokinetic results indicated that half-life was shorter (5.3 h) than for adults (7.2 h) and apparent clearance was faster (1.5 ml/min/kg) than for adults (0.96 ml/min/kg).

Renal impairment

The apparent body clearance of both levetiracetam and of its primary metabolite is correlated to the creatinine clearance. It is therefore recommended to adjust the maintenance daily dose of Keppra, based on creatinine clearance in patients with moderate and severe renal impairment (see section 4.2 "Posology").

In anuric end-stage renal disease subjects the half-life was approximately 25 and 3.1 hours during interdialytic and intradialytic periods, respectively.

The fractional removal of levetiracetam was 51 % during a typical 4-hour dialysis session.

Hepatic impairment

In subjects with mild and moderate hepatic impairment, there was no relevant modification of the clearance of levetiracetam. In most subjects with severe hepatic impairment, the clearance of levetiracetam was reduced by more than 50 % due to a concomitant renal impairment (see section 4.2 "Posology").

5.3 Preclinical safety data

Preclinical data reveal no special hazard for humans based on conventional studies of safety pharmacology, genotoxicity and carcinogenicity. Although no evidence for carcinogenicity was seen, the potential carcinogenicity has not been fully evaluated due to some shortcomings in the studies performed.

Adverse effects not observed in clinical studies but seen in the rat and to a lesser extent in the mouse at exposure levels similar to human exposure levels and with possible relevance for clinical use were liver changes, indicating an adaptive response such as increased weight and centrilobular hypertrophy, fatty infiltration and increased liver enzymes in plasma.

In reproductive toxicity studies in the rat, levetiracetam induced developmental toxicity (increase in skeletal variations/minor anomalies, retarded growth, increased pup mortality) at exposure levels similar to or greater than the human exposure. In the rabbit foetal effects (embryonic death, increased skeletal anomalies, and increased malformations) were observed in the presence of maternal toxicity. The systemic exposure at the observed no effect level in the rabbit was about 4 to 5 times the human exposure.

Neonatal and juvenile animal studies in rats and dogs demonstrated that there were no adverse effects seen in any of the standard developmental or maturation endpoints at doses up to 1800 mg/kg/day corresponding to 30 times the maximum recommended human dose.

6. PHARMACEUTICAL PARTICULARS

6.1 List of excipients

Keppra 250 mg, Keppra 500 mg, Keppra 750 mg, Keppra 1000 mg film coated tablets

Core: Sodium croscarmellose, Macrogol 6000, colloidal anhydrous silica, magnesium stearate.

Keppra 250 mg:

Film-coating: Opadry 85F20694: Polyvinyl alcohol-part.hydrolyzed, Titanium dioxide (E171), Macrogol 3350, Talc, Indigo carmine aluminium lake (E132).

Keppra 500 mg:

Film-coating: Opadry 85F32004: Polyvinyl alcohol-part.hydrolyzed, Titanium dioxide (E171), Macrogol 3350, Talc, Iron oxide yellow (E172).

Keppra 750 mg:

Film-coating: Opadry 85F23452:Polyvinyl alcohol-part.hydrolyzed, Titanium dioxide (E171)

Macrogol 3350, Talc, sunset yellow FCF aluminium lake (E110), Iron oxide red (E172).

Keppra 1000 mg

Film-coating: Opadry 85F18422: Polyvinyl alcohol-part.hydrolyzed, Titanium dioxide (E171)

Macrogol 3350, Talc.

Keppra 100 mg/ml, oral solution

Sodium citrate, citric acid monohydrate, methyl parahydroxybenzoate (E 218), propyl parahydroxybenzoate (E 216), ammonium glycyrrhizate, glycerol (E 422), maltitol (E 965), acesulfame potassium (E 950), grape flavour, purified water.

6.2 Incompatibilities

Not applicable.

6.3 Shelf life

Tablets:

3 years.

Oral solution:

2 years

6.4 Special precautions for storage

Tablets:

No special precautions for storage.

Oral solution:

Store in original container.

6.5 Nature and contents of container

Keppra 250 mg, Keppra 500mg, Keppra 750mg, Keppra 1000 mg film-coated tablets are packaged in aluminium/PVC blisters placed into cardboard boxes containing 20, 30, 50, 60 and 100 film-coated tablets.

Keppra 100 mg/ml, oral solution is packaged in a 300 ml amber glass bottle (type III) with a white child resistant closure (polypropylene) in a cardboard box also containing a graduated oral syringe (polyethylene, polystyrene) and a patient information leaflet.

Not all pack sizes may be marketed.

6.6 Instructions for use and handling

No special requirements.

7. MARKETING AUTHORISATION HOLDER

UCB S.A.

Allée de la Recherche 60

B-1070 Bruxelles

Belgium

8. MARKETING AUTHORISATION NUMBER(S)

Keppra 250 mg × 60 tablets: EU/1/00/146/004.

Keppra 500 mg × 60 tablets: EU/1/00/146/010.

Keppra 750 mg × 60 tablets EU/1/00/146/017.

Keppra 1000 mg × 60 tablets: EU/1/00/146/024.

Keppra 300 ml oral solution: EU/1/00/146/027.

9. DATE OF FIRST AUTHORISATION/RENEWAL OF THE AUTHORISATION

Tablets:

29 September 2000/08 July 2005

Oral solution:

03 March 2004/08 July 2005

10. DATE OF REVISION OF THE TEXT

September 2005

11. Legal Category

POM

Keral

(A. Menarini Pharma U.K. S.R.L.)

1. NAME OF THE MEDICINAL PRODUCT

KERAL 25 mg film-coated tablets

2. QUALITATIVE AND QUANTITATIVE COMPOSITION

Each tablet contains: Dexketoprofen trometamol 36.9mg corresponding to dexketoprofen (INN) 25 mg.

For excipients, see 6.1

3. PHARMACEUTICAL FORM

Film coated tablets.

Keral 25mg: white, round, scored film-coated tablets

4. CLINICAL PARTICULARS

4.1 Therapeutic indications

Symptomatic treatment of pain of mild to moderate intensity, such as musculo-skeletal pain, dysmenorrhoea, dental pain.

4.2 Posology and method of administration

General population:

According to the nature and severity of pain, the recommended dosage is generally 12.5 mg every 4-6 hours or 25 mg every 8 hours. The total daily dose should not exceed 75 mg. KERAL tablets are not intended for long term use and the treatment must be limited to the symptomatic period.

Concomitant administration with food delays the absorption rate of the drug (see Pharmacokinetic Properties), thus in case of acute pain it is recommended that administration is at least 30 minutes before meals.

Elderly:

In elderly patients it is recommended to start the therapy at the lower end of the dosage range (50 mg total daily dose). The dosage may be increased to that recommended for the general population only after good general tolerance has been ascertained.

Hepatic dysfunction:

Patients with mild to moderate hepatic dysfunction should start therapy at reduced doses (50 mg total daily dose) and be closely monitored. KERAL tablets should not be used in patients with severe hepatic dysfunction.

Renal dysfunction:

The initial dosage should be reduced to 50 mg total daily dose in patients with mildly impaired renal function. KERAL tablets should not be used in patients with moderate to severe renal dysfunction.

Children:

KERAL tablets has not been studied in children. Therefore, safety and efficacy have not been established and the product should not be used in children.

4.3 Contraindications

KERAL tablets must not be administered in the following cases:

- patients previously sensitive to dexketoprofen, to any other NSAID, or to any of the excipients of the product.
- patients in whom substances with a similar action (e.g. aspirin, or other NSAIDs) precipitate attacks of asthma, bronchospasm, acute rhinitis, or cause nasal polyps, urticaria or angioneurotic oedema.
- patients with active or suspected gastrointestinal ulcer or history of gastrointestinal ulcer or chronic dyspepsia.
- patients who have gastrointestinal bleeding or other active bleedings or bleeding disorders.
- patients with Crohn's disease or ulcerative colitis.
- patients with a history of bronchial asthma.
- patients with severe heart failure.
- patients with moderate to severe renal dysfunction.
- patients with severely impaired hepatic function.
- patients with haemorrhagic diathesis and other coagulation disorders, or patients receiving anticoagulant therapy.
- during pregnancy and lactation period.

4.4 Special warnings and special precautions for use

The safe use in children has not been established.

Administer with caution in patients with a history of allergic conditions.

As with all NSAIDs, any history of oesophagitis, gastritis and/or peptic ulcer must be sought in order to ensure their total cure before starting treatment with dexketoprofen.

Patients with gastrointestinal symptoms or history of gastrointestinal disease should be monitored for digestive disturbances, especially gastrointestinal bleeding. In the rare instances where gastrointestinal bleeding or ulceration occurs in patients receiving dexketoprofen trometamol, treatment should be immediately discontinued.

As with all NSAIDs, it can increase plasma urea nitrogen and creatinine. As with other inhibitors of prostaglandin synthesis, it can be associated with adverse effects on the renal system which can lead to glomerular nephritis, interstitial nephritis, renal papillary necrosis, nephrotic syndrome and acute renal failure.

As with other NSAIDs, it can cause transient small increases in some liver parameters, and also significant increases in SGOT and SGPT. In case of a relevant increase in such parameters, therapy must be discontinued.

KERAL tablets should be administered with caution to patients suffering from haematopoietic disorders, systemic lupus erythematosus or mixed connective tissue disease.

As other NSAIDs, dexketoprofen can mask the symptoms of infectious diseases.

Caution should be exercised in patients with impairment of hepatic, renal or cardiac functions as well as in patients with other conditions predisposing to fluid retention. In these patients, the use of NSAIDs may result in deterioration of renal function and fluid retention. Caution is also required in patients receiving diuretic therapy or those who are likely to be hypovolaemic as there is an increased risk of nephrotoxicity.

Caution should be exercised in the treatment of elderly patients who are generally more prone to adverse reactions. The consequences, e.g. gastrointestinal bleeding and/or perforation are dose-dependent, often more serious and may occur without warning symptoms or previous history, at any time during treatment. Elderly patients are more likely to be suffering from impaired renal cardiovascular or hepatic function.

4.5 Interaction with other medicinal products and other forms of Interaction

The following interactions apply to non-steroidal antiinflammatory drugs (NSAIDs) in general:

Inadvisable combinations:

- Other NSAIDs, including high doses of salicylates (⩾ 3 g/day): administration of several NSAIDs together may increase the risk of gastrointestinal ulcers and bleeding, via a synergistic effect.
- Oral anticoagulants, parenteral heparin and ticlopidine: increased risk of bleeding, via inhibition of platelet function and damage to the gastrointestinal mucosa.
- Lithium (described with several NSAIDs): NSAIDs increase blood lithium levels, which may reach toxic values (decreased renal excretion of lithium). This parameter therefore requires monitoring during the initiation, adjustment and withdrawal of treatment with dexketoprofen.
- Methotrexate, used at high doses of 15 mg/week or more: increased haematological toxicity of methotrexate via a decrease in its renal clearance by antiinflammatory agents in general.
- Hydantoines and sulphonamides: the toxic effects of these substances may be increased.

Combinations requiring precautions:

- Diuretics, angiotensin converting enzyme inhibitors: treatment with NSAIDs is associated with a risk of acute renal failure in dehydrated patients (decreased glomerular filtration via decreased renal prostaglandin synthesis). Treatment with a NSAID may decrease their antihypertensive effect. In case of combined prescription of dexketoprofen and a diuretic, it is essential to ensure that the patient is adequately hydrated and to monitor renal function at the start of the treatment.
- Methotrexate, used at low doses, less than 15 mg/week: increased haematological toxicity of methotrexate via a decrease in its renal clearance by antiinflammatory agents in general. Weekly monitoring of blood count during the first weeks of the combination. Increased surveillance in the presence of even mildly impaired renal function, as well as in the elderly.
- Pentoxyfilline: increased risk of bleeding. Increase clinical monitoring and check bleeding time more often.
- Zidovudine: risk of increased red cell line toxicity via action on reticulocytes, with severe anaemia occurring one week after the NSAID is started. Check CBC and reticulocyte count one to two weeks after starting treatment with the NSAID.
- Sulfonylureas: NSAIDs can increase the hypoglycaemic effect of sulfonylureas by displacement from plasma protein binding sites.

Associations needing to be taken into account:

- Beta-blockers: treatment with a NSAID may decrease their antihypertensive effect via inhibition of prostaglandin synthesis.
- Cyclosporin and tacrolimus: nephrotoxicity may be enhanced by NSAIDs via renal prostaglandin mediated effects. During combination therapy, renal function has to be measured.
- Thrombolytics: increased risk of bleeding.
- Probenecid: plasma concentrations of dexketoprofen may be increased; this interaction can be due to an inhibitory mechanism at the site of renal tubular secretion and of glucuronoconjugation and requires adjustment of the dose of dexketoprofen.
- Cardiac Glycosides: NSAIDS may increase plasma glycoside concentration.
- Mifepristone: Because of a theoretical risk that prostaglandin synthetase inhibitors may alter the efficacy of mifepristone, NSAIDS should not be used for 8-12 days after mifepristone administration.
- Quinolone antibiotics: Animal data indicate that high doses of quinolones incombination with NSAIDS can increase the risk of developing convulsions.

4.6 Pregnancy and lactation

KERAL tablets should not be administered during pregnancy and lactation.

Insufficient information is available to assess the safety of the use of KERAL tablets during pregnancy.

In animal studies foetal effects were found at high doses, probably resulting from the inhibitory effects of dexketoprofen on prostaglandin synthesis.

NSAIDs may block uterine contractions and delay delivery. They may induce intrauterine constriction or closure of the ductus arteriosus leading to neonatal pulmonary hypertension and respiratory insufficiency. NSAIDs may depress foetal platelet function and inhibit foetal renal function, resulting in oligohydramniosis and neonatal anuria.

It is not known whether dexketoprofen is excreted in human milk.

4.7 Effects on ability to drive and use machines

KERAL can cause minor or moderate effects on the ability to drive or use machines due to the possibility of dizziness or drowsiness occurring.

4.8 Undesirable effects

The adverse reactions reported as at least possibly related with dexketoprofen trometamol in clinical trials, as well as the adverse reactions reported after the marketing of KERAL tablets are tabulated below, classified by system organ class and ordered by frequency:

(see Table 1 on next page)

The following undesirable effects may appear because they have been observed with other non-steroidal antiinflammatory drugs and may be associated with prostaglandin synthesis inhibitors: aseptic meningitis, which might predominantly occur in patients with systemic lupus erythematosus or mixed connective tissue disease; and haematological reactions (purpura, aplastic and haemolytic anaemia, and rarely agranulocytosis and medullar hypoplasia).

4.9 Overdose

In case of accidental or excessive intake, immediately institute symptomatic therapy and perform gastric lavage if required.

Dexketoprofen trometamol may be removed by dialysis.

5. PHARMACOLOGICAL PROPERTIES

5.1 Pharmacodynamic properties

Dexketoprofen trometamol is the tromethamine salt of S-(+)-2-(3-benzoylphenyl)propionic acid, an analgesic, antiinflammatory and antipyretic drug, which belongs to the non-steroidal anti-inflammatory group of drugs (M01AE).

The mechanism of action of non-steroidal antiinflammatory drugs is related to the reduction of prostaglandin synthesis by the inhibition of cyclooxygenase pathway. Specifically, there is an inhibition of the transformation of arachidonic

Table 1

SYSTEM ORGAN CLASS	Common (1-10%)	Uncommon (0.1-1%)	Rare (0.01-0.1%)	Very rare / Isolated reports (<0.01%)
Blood and the lymphatic system disorders				Neutropenia Thrombocytopenia
Psychiatric disorders		sleep disorders, anxiety		
Nervous system disorders		headache, dizziness, vertigo	paraesthesia	
Eye disorders				blurred vision
Ear and labirynth disorders				Tinnitus
Cardiac disorders		Palpitations		tachycardia
Vascular disorders			hypertension, peripheral oedema	Hypotension
Respiratory, thoracic and mediastinal disorders			bradypnoea	bronchospasm, dyspnoea
Gastrointestinal disorders	Nausea and/or Vomiting, abdominal pain, diarrhoea, dyspepsia.	gastritis, constipation, dry mouth, flatulence	peptic ulceration, haemorrhage or perforation (see section 4.4), anorexia	pancreatic damage
Hepatobiliary disorders			hepatic enzymes increased	hepatic damage
Skin and subcutaneous tissue disorders		Skin rash	urticaria, acne, sweating increased	severe mucocutaneous skin reactions (Steven Johnson, Lyell syndromes), angioedema, dermatological reactions, photosensitivity reactions, pruritus
Renal and urinary disorders			polyuria	renal damage (nephritis or nephrotic syndrome)
Reproductive system and breast disorders			female: menstrual disorders; male: prostatic disorders	
General disorders and administration site conditions		Fatigue, hot flushes, pain, asthenia, rigors, malaise	back pain, syncope	anaphylaxis, facial oedema.

acid into cyclic endoperoxides, PGG_2 and PGH_2, which produce prostaglandins PGE_1, PGE_2, $PGF_{2\alpha}$ and PGD_2 and also prostacyclin PGI_2 and thromboxanes (TxA_2 and TxB_2). Furthermore, the inhibition of the synthesis of prostaglandins could affect other inflammation mediators such as kinins, causing an indirect action which would be additional to the direct action.

Dexketoprofen has been demonstrated to be an inhibitor for COX-1 and COX-2 activities in experimental animals and humans.

Clinical studies performed on several pain models demonstrated effective analgesic activity of dexketoprofen trometamol. The onset of the analgesic activity was obtained in some studies at30 minutes post-administration. The analgesic effect persists for 4 to 6 hours.

5.2 Pharmacokinetic properties

After oral administration of dexketoprofen trometamol to humans, the Cmax is reached at 30 min (range 15 to 60 min).

The distribution half-life and elimination half-life values of dexketoprofen trometamol are 0.35 and 1.65 hours, respectively. As with other drugs with a high plasma protein binding (99%), its volume of distribution has a mean value below 0.25 l/kg. The main elimination route for dexketoprofen is glucuronide conjugation followed by renal excretion.

After administration of dexketoprofen trometamol only the S-(+) enantiomer is obtained in urine, demonstrating that no conversion to the R-(-) enantiomer occurs in humans.

In multiple-dose pharmacokinetic studies, it was observed that the AUC after the last administration is not different from that obtained following a single dose, indicating that no drug accumulation occurs.

When administered concomitantly with food, the AUC does not change, however the Cmax of dexketoprofen trometamol decreases and its absorption rate is delayed (increased tmax).

5.3 Preclinical safety data

Preclinical data revealed no special hazard for humans based on conventional studies of safety pharmacology, repeated dose toxicity, genotoxicity, toxicity to reproduction and immunopharmacology. The chronic toxicity studies carried out in mice and monkeys gave a No Observed Adverse Effect Level (NOAEL) of 3 mg/kg/day. The main adverse effect observed at high doses was gastrointestinal erosions and ulcers that developed dose-dependently.

6. PHARMACEUTICAL PARTICULARS

6.1 List of excipients

Maize starch, microcrystalline cellulose, sodium starch glycollate, glycerol palmitostearate,

hypromellose, titanium dioxide, propylene glycol, macrogol 6000.

6.2 Incompatibilities

Not applicable

6.3 Shelf life

2 years.

6.4 Special precautions for storage

Do not store above 30°C; keep the blister packs in the outer carton in order to protect from light.

6.5 Nature and contents of container

Tablets are provided in blister packs (PVC-aluminium blister) 4,10, 20, 30, 40, 50 or 500 film-coated tablets/pack.

(Not all pack sizes may be marketed.)

6.6 Instructions for use and handling

No special requirements.

7. MARKETING AUTHORISATION HOLDER

MENARINI INTERNATIONAL OPERATIONS LUXEMBOURG, S.A.

1, Avenue de la Gare

L-1611-Luxembourg.

8. MARKETING AUTHORISATION NUMBER(S)

PL 16239/0007

9. DATE OF FIRST AUTHORISATION/RENEWAL OF THE AUTHORISATION

25 April 2001

10.

10. DATE OF REVISION OF THE TEXT

March 2001

Keri Therapeutic Lotion

(Bristol-Myers Pharmaceuticals)

1. NAME OF THE MEDICINAL PRODUCT

Keri Therapeutic Lotion

2. QUALITATIVE AND QUANTITATIVE COMPOSITION

Mineral Oil 16%.

3. PHARMACEUTICAL FORM

Lotion.

4. CLINICAL PARTICULARS

4.1 Therapeutic indications

Keri Therapeutic Lotion has emollient properties. It is indicated for the symptomatic treatment of dermatitis, eczema, ichthyosis, nappy rash, protection of raw and abraded skin areas, pruritus and related conditions where dry scaly skin is a problem It is also indicated as an emollient before bathing for dry/eczematous skin, to alleviate drying effects.

4.2 Posology and method of administration

Topical Administration

Adults and Children:

Keri Therapeutic Lotion should be gently massaged into the skin three times daily or as often as required.

Elderly:

No dosage adjustment is necessary.

4.3 Contraindications

Keri Therapeutic Lotion contains lanolin oil and is therefore contraindicated in those patients allergic to this ingredient.

4.4 Special warnings and special precautions for use

None known.

4.5 Interaction with other medicinal products and other forms of Interaction

None known.

4.6 Pregnancy and lactation

No special precautions.

4.7 Effects on ability to drive and use machines

Not applicable

4.8 Undesirable effects

None known.

4.9 Overdose

Not applicable.

5. PHARMACOLOGICAL PROPERTIES

5.1 Pharmacodynamic properties

Mineral oil has emollient properties. Keri lotion lubrication helps hydrate the skin. It relieves itching, helps maintain a normal moisture balance and supplements the protective action of skin lipids.

5.2 Pharmacokinetic properties

Not applicable for this type of product.

5.3 Preclinical safety data

Nothing of relevance to the prescriber.

6. PHARMACEUTICAL PARTICULARS

6.1 List of excipients

Carbomer 934, glyceryl monostearate, lanolin oil, laureth 4, methylparaben, perfume, PEG-4 dilaurate, polyethylene glycol 40 stearate, propylparaben, propylene glycol, quaternium 15, sodium dioctyl sulphosuccinate, triethanolamine, water.

6.2 Incompatibilities

None known.

6.3 Shelf life

36 months.

6.4 Special precautions for storage

Store at room temperature (below 25°C)

6.5 Nature and contents of container

HDPE opaque white bottle with either a polypropylene pump or a polypropylene disc cap closure (Pack sizes of 190 or 380 ml).

6.6 Instructions for use and handling

Not applicable to this product.

7. MARKETING AUTHORISATION HOLDER
Bristol-Myers Squibb Holdings Ltd

T/A Bristol-Myers Pharmaceuticals or Westwood Pharmaceuticals Ltd

Uxbridge Business Park

Sanderson Road,

Uxbridge

Middlesex

UB8 1DH

8. MARKETING AUTHORISATION NUMBER(S)
PL 0125/0152

9. DATE OF FIRST AUTHORISATION/RENEWAL OF THE AUTHORISATION
18th October 1992 / 17th October 1997

10. DATE OF REVISION OF THE TEXT
22 July 2005

Ketalar Injection

(Pfizer Limited)

1. NAME OF THE MEDICINAL PRODUCT
KetalarTM Injection 10 mg/ml, 50 mg/ml, 100 mg/ml

2. QUALITATIVE AND QUANTITATIVE COMPOSITION
Each 1 ml of solution contains:

Ketalar Injection 10 mg/ml: ketamine hydrochloride Ph Eur equivalent to 10 mg ketamine base per ml.

Ketalar Injection 50 mg/ml: ketamine hydrochloride Ph Eur equivalent to 50 mg ketamine base per ml.

Ketalar Injection 100mg/ml: ketamine hydrochloride Ph Eur equivalent to 100 mg ketamine base per ml.

3. PHARMACEUTICAL FORM
A clear solution for injection.

4. CLINICAL PARTICULARS

4.1 Therapeutic indications
Ketalar is recommended:

As the sole anaesthetic agent for diagnostic and surgical procedures. When used by intravenous or intramuscular injection, Ketalar is best suited for short procedures. With additional doses, or by intravenous infusion, Ketalar can be used for longer procedures. If skeletal muscle relaxation is desired, a muscle relaxant should be used and respiration should be supported.

For the induction of anaesthesia prior to the administration of other general anaesthetic agents.

To supplement other anaesthetic agents.

Specific areas of application or types of procedures:

When the intramuscular route of administration is preferred.

Debridement, painful dressings, and skin grafting in burned patients, as well as other superficial surgical procedures.

Neurodiagnostic procedures such as pneumoencephalograms, ventriculograms, myelograms, and lumbar punctures.

Diagnostic and operative procedures of the eye, ear, nose, and mouth, including dental extractions.

Note: Eye movements may persist during ophthalmological procedures.

Anaesthesia in poor-risk patients with depression of vital functions or where depression of vital functions must be avoided, if at all possible.

Orthopaedic procedures such as closed reductions, manipulations, femoral pinning, amputations, and biopsies.

Sigmoidoscopy and minor surgery of the anus and rectum, circumcision and pilonidal sinus.

Cardiac catheterization procedures.

Caesarian section; as an induction agent in the absence of elevated blood pressure.

Anaesthesia in the asthmatic patient, either to minimise the risks of an attack of bronchospasm developing, or in the presence of bronchospasm where anaesthesia cannot be delayed.

4.2 Posology and method of administration
For intravenous infusion, intravenous injection or intramuscular injection.

NOTE: All doses are given in terms of ketamine base

Adults, elderly (over 65 years) and children:

For surgery in elderly patients ketamine has been shown to be suitable either alone or supplemented with other anaesthetic agents.

Preoperative preparations
Ketalar has been safely used alone when the stomach was not empty. However, since the need for supplemental agents and muscle relaxants cannot be predicted, when preparing for elective surgery it is advisable that nothing be given by mouth for at least six hours prior to anaesthesia.

Atropine, hyoscine, or another drying agent should be given at an appropriate interval prior to induction.

Midazolam, diazepam, lorazepam, or flunitrazepam used as a premedicant or as an adjunct to ketamine, have been effective in reducing the incidence of emergence reactions.

Onset and duration
As with other general anaesthetic agents, the individual response to Ketalar is somewhat varied depending on the dose, route of administration, age of patient, and concomitant use of other agents, so that dosage recommendation cannot be absolutely fixed. The dose should be titrated against the patient's requirements.

Because of rapid induction following intravenous injection, the patient should be in a supported position during administration. An intravenous dose of 2 mg/kg of bodyweight usually produces surgical anaesthesia within 30 seconds after injection and the anaesthetic effect usually lasts 5 to 10 minutes. An intramuscular dose of 10 mg/kg of bodyweight usually produces surgical anaesthesia within 3 to 4 minutes following injection and the anaesthetic effect usually lasts 12 to 25 minutes. Return to consciousness is gradual.

A. Ketalar as the sole anaesthetic agent

Intravenous Infusion
The use of Ketalar by continuous infusion enables the dose to be titrated more closely, thereby reducing the amount of drug administered compared with intermittent administration. This results in a shorter recovery time and better stability of vital signs.

A solution containing 1 mg/ml of ketamine in dextrose 5% or sodium chloride 0.9% is suitable for administration by infusion.

Induction
An infusion corresponding to 0.5 – 2 mg/kg as total induction dose.

Maintenance of anaesthesia
Anaesthesia may be maintained using a microdrip infusion of 10 - 45 microgram/kg/min (approximately 1 – 3 mg/min).

The rate of infusion will depend on the patient's reaction and response to anaesthesia. The dosage required may be reduced when a long acting neuromuscular blocking agent is used.

Intermittent Injection

Induction
Intravenous Route

The initial dose of Ketalar administered intravenously may range from 1 mg/kg to 4.5mg/kg (in terms of ketamine base). The average amount required to produce 5 to 10 minutes of surgical anaesthesia has been 2.0 mg/kg. It is recommended that intravenous administration be accomplished slowly (over a period of 60 seconds). More rapid administration may result in respiratory depression and enhanced pressor response.

Note: the 100 mg/ml concentration of ketamine should not be injected intravenously without proper dilution. It is recommended that the drug be diluted with an equal volume of either sterile water for injection, normal saline, or 5% dextrose in water.

Intramuscular Route
The initial dose of Ketalar administered intramuscularly may range from 6.5 to 13 mg/kg (in terms of ketamine base). A low initial intramuscular dose of 4 mg/kg has been used in diagnostic manoeuvres and procedures not involving intensely painful stimuli. A dose of 10 mg/kg will usually produce 12 to 25 minutes of surgical anaesthesia.

Maintenance of anaesthesia
Lightening of anaesthesia may be indicated by nystagmus, movements in response to stimulation, and vocalization. Anaesthesia is maintained by the administration of additional doses of Ketalar by either the intravenous or intramuscular route.

Each additional dose is from ½ to the full induction dose recommended above for the route selected for maintenance, regardless of the route used for induction.

The larger the total amount of Ketalar administered, the longer will be the time to complete recovery.

Purposeless and tonic-clonic movements of extremities may occur during the course of anaesthesia. These movements do not imply a light plane and are not indicative of the need for additional doses of the anaesthetic.

B. Ketalar as induction agent prior to the use of other general anaesthetics
Induction is accomplished by a full intravenous or intramuscular dose of Ketalar as defined above. If Ketalar has been administered intravenously and the principal anaesthetic is slow-acting, a second dose of Ketalar may be required 5 to 8 minutes following the initial dose. If Ketalar has been administered intramuscularly and the principal anaesthetic is rapid-acting, administration of the principal anaesthetic may be delayed up to 15 minutes following the injection of Ketalar.

C. Ketalar as supplement to anaesthetic agents
Ketalar is clinically compatible with the commonly used general and local anaesthetic agents when an adequate respiratory exchange is maintained. The dose of Ketalar for use in conjunction with other anaesthetic agents is usually in the same range as the dosage stated above; however, the use of another anaesthetic agent may allow a reduction in the dose of Ketalar.

D. Management of patients in recovery
Following the procedure the patient should be observed but left undisturbed. This does not preclude the monitoring of vital signs. If, during the recovery, the patient shows any indication of emergence delirium, consideration may be given to the use of diazepam (5 to 10 mg I.V. in an adult). A hypnotic dose of a thiobarbiturate (50 to 100 mg I.V.) may be used to terminate severe emergence reactions. If any one of these agents is employed, the patient may experience a longer recovery period.

4.3 Contraindications
Ketalar is contra-indicated in persons in whom an elevation of blood pressure would constitute a serious hazard (see Undesirable effects) and in those who have shown hypersensitivity to the drug. Ketalar should not be used in patients with eclampsia or pre-eclampsia, severe coronary or myocardial disease, cerebrovascular accident or cerebral trauma.

4.4 Special warnings and special precautions for use
To be used only in hospitals by or under the supervision of experienced medically qualified anaesthetists except under emergency conditions.

As with any general anaesthetic agent, resuscitative equipment should be available and ready for use.

Emergence delirium phenomena may occur during the recovery period. The incidence of these reactions may be reduced if verbal and tactile stimulation of the patient is minimised during the recovery period. This does not preclude the monitoring of vital signs.

Because pharyngeal and laryngeal reflexes usually remain active, mechanical stimulation of the pharynx should be avoided unless muscle relaxants, with proper attention to respiration, are used.

Although aspiration of contrast medium has been reported during Ketalar anaesthesia under experimental conditions (Taylor, P A and Towey, R M, Brit. Med. J. 1971, 2: 688), in clinical practice aspiration is seldom a problem.

Cardiac function should be continually monitored during the procedure in patients found to have hypertension or cardiac decompensation.

Since an increase in cerebrospinal fluid pressure has been reported during Ketalar anaesthesia, Ketalar should be used with special caution in patients with preanaesthetic elevated cerebrospinal fluid pressure.

Respiratory depression may occur with overdosage of Ketalar, in which case supportive ventilation should be employed. Mechanical support of respiration is preferred to the administration of analeptics.

The intravenous dose should be administered over a period of 60 seconds. More rapid administration may result in transient respiratory depression or apnoea and enhanced pressor response.

In surgical procedures involving visceral pain pathways, Ketalar should be supplemented with an agent which obtunds visceral pain.

Use with caution in the chronic alcoholic and the acutely alcohol-intoxicated patient.

When Ketalar is used on an outpatient basis, the patient should not be released until recovery from anaesthesia is complete and then should be accompanied by a responsible adult.

Ketalar has been reported as being a drug of abuse. If used on a daily basis for a few weeks, dependence and tolerance may develop, particularly in individuals with a history of drug abuse and dependence. Therefore the use of Ketalar should be closely supervised and it should be prescribed and administered with caution.

4.5 Interaction with other medicinal products and other forms of Interaction
Prolonged recovery time may occur if barbiturates and/or narcotics are used concurrently with Ketalar.

Ketalar is chemically incompatible with barbiturates and diazepam because of precipitate formation. Therefore, these should not be mixed in the same syringe or infusion fluid.

4.6 Pregnancy and lactation
Ketalar crosses the placenta. This should be borne in mind during operative obstetric procedures in pregnancy. With the exception of administration during surgery for abdominal delivery or vaginal delivery, no controlled clinical studies in pregnancy have been conducted. The safe use in pregnancy, and in lactation, has not been established and such use is not recommended.

4.7 Effects on ability to drive and use machines
Patients should be cautioned that driving a car, operating hazardous machinery or engaging in hazardous activities should not be undertaken for 24 hours or more after anaesthesia.

4.8 Undesirable effects

Cardiovascular
Temporary elevation of blood pressure and pulse rate is frequently observed following administration of ketamine hydrochloride. However, hypotension and bradycardia have been reported. Arrhythmias have also occurred. The median peak rise of blood pressure has ranged from 20 to 25 per cent of preanaesthetic values. Depending on the condition of the patient, this elevation of blood pressure

may be considered an adverse reaction or a beneficial effect.

Respiratory
Depression of respiration or apnoea may occur following over rapid intravenous administration or high doses of ketamine hydrochloride. Laryngospasm and other forms of airway obstruction have occurred during ketamine hydrochloride anaesthesia.

Ocular
Diplopia and nystagmus may occur following ketamine hydrochloride administration. A slight elevation in intraocular pressure may also occur.

Psychological
Reports suggest that ketamine produces a variety of symptoms including, but not limited to, flashbacks, hallucinations, dysphoria, anxiety, insomnia or disorientation. During recovery from anaesthesia the patient may experience emergence delirium, characterised by vivid dreams (pleasant or unpleasant), with or without psychomotor activity, manifested by confusion and irrational behaviour. The fact that these reactions are observed less often in the young (15 years of age or less) makes Ketalar especially useful in paediatric anaesthesia. These reactions are also less frequent in the elderly (over 65 years of age) patient. The incidence of emergence reactions is reduced as experience with the drug is gained. No residual psychological effects are known to have resulted from the use of Ketalar.

Neurological
In some patients, enhanced skeletal muscle tone may be manifested by tonic and clonic movements sometimes resembling seizures. These movements do not imply a light plane of anaesthesia and are not indicative of a need for additional doses of the anaesthetic.

Gastro-intestinal
Anorexia, nausea, and vomiting have been observed; however, these are uncommon and are not usually severe. The great majority of patients are able to take liquids by mouth shortly after regaining consciousness.

Hypersensitivity reactions
There have been a number of reported cases of anaphylaxis.

Local pain and exanthema at the injection site have infrequently been reported. Transient erythema and/or morbilliform rash have also been reported. Increased salivation leading to respiratory difficulties may occur unless an antisialogogue is used.

4.9 Overdose
Respiratory depression can result from an overdosage of ketamine hydrochloride. Supportive ventilation should be employed. Mechanical support of respiration that will maintain adequate blood oxygen saturation and carbon dioxide elimination is preferred to administration of analeptics.

Ketalar has a wide margin of safety; several instances of unintentional administration of overdoses of Ketalar (up to 10 times that usually required) have been followed by prolonged but complete recovery.

5. PHARMACOLOGICAL PROPERTIES
5.1 Pharmacodynamic properties
Ketamine is a rapidly acting general anaesthetic for intravenous or intramuscular use with a distinct pharmacological action. Ketamine hydrochloride produces dissociative anaesthesia characterised by catalepsy, amnesia, and marked analgesia which may persist into the recovery period. Pharyngeal-laryngeal reflexes remain normal and skeletal muscle tone may be normal or can be enhanced to varying degrees. Mild cardiac and respiratory stimulation and occasionally respiratory depression occur.

5.2 Pharmacokinetic properties
Ketamine is rapidly distributed into perfused tissues including brain and placenta. Animal studies have shown ketamine to be highly concentrated in body fat, liver and lung. Biotransformation takes place in liver. Termination of anaesthetic is partly by redistribution from brain to other tissues and partly by metabolism. Elimination half-life is approximately 2-3 hours, and excretion renal, mostly as conjugated metabolites.

5.3 Preclinical safety data
Preclinical safety data does not add anything of further significance to the prescriber.

6. PHARMACEUTICAL PARTICULARS
6.1 List of excipients
Ketalar Injection 10 mg/ml: sodium chloride, benzethonium chloride, water for injection

Ketalar Injection 50 mg/ml: benzethonium chloride, water for injection

Ketalar Injection 100 mg/ml: benzethonium chloride, water for injection

6.2 Incompatibilities
Ketalar is chemically incompatible with barbiturates and diazepam because of precipitate formation. Therefore, these should not be mixed in the same syringe or infusion fluid.

6.3 Shelf life
3 years

6.4 Special precautions for storage
Store at a temperature not exceeding 25°C. Protect from light. Do not freeze. Discard any unused product at the end of each operating session.

After dilution the solutions should be used immediately.

6.5 Nature and contents of container
Ketalar Injection 10 mg/ml: 20 ml white neutral glass vial with rubber closure and aluminium flip-off cap containing 10 mg ketamine base per ml.

Ketalar Injection 50 mg/ml: 12 ml vials containing 10 ml of solution as 50 mg ketamine base per ml.

Ketalar Injection 100 mg/ml: 12 ml vials containing 10 ml of solution as 100 mg ketamine base per ml.

6.6 Instructions for use and handling
See Section 6.2 Incompatibilities.

7. MARKETING AUTHORISATION HOLDER
Pfizer Limited, Sandwich, Kent CT13 9NJ, United Kingdom

8. MARKETING AUTHORISATION NUMBER(S)
PL 00057/0529, PL 00057/0530, PL 00057/0531

9. DATE OF FIRST AUTHORISATION/RENEWAL OF THE AUTHORISATION
1st July 2003

10. DATE OF REVISION OF THE TEXT
August 2003

Company Reference: KE 2_1 UK

Ketek 400mg Tablets

(sanofi-aventis)

1. NAME OF THE MEDICINAL PRODUCT
Ketek 400 mg film-coated tablets. ▼

2. QUALITATIVE AND QUANTITATIVE COMPOSITION
Each film-coated tablet of Ketek contains 400 mg of telithromycin as active substance.

For excipients, see 6.1.

3. PHARMACEUTICAL FORM
Film-coated tablet.

Light orange, oblong, biconvex tablet, imprinted with H3647 on one side and 400 on the other.

4. CLINICAL PARTICULARS
4.1 Therapeutic indications
When prescribing Ketek, consideration should be given to official guidance on the appropriate use of antibacterial agents (See also sections 4.4 and 5.1).

Ketek is indicated for the treatment of the following infections:

-In patients of 18 years and older:

- Community-acquired pneumonia, mild or moderate (see section 4.4).
- Acute exacerbation of chronic bronchitis,
- Acute sinusitis
- Tonsillitis/pharyngitis caused by Group A *beta streptococci,* as an alternative when beta lactam antibiotics are not appropriate.

-In patients of 12 to 18 years old:

- Tonsillitis/pharyngitis caused by Group A *beta streptococci*, as an alternative when beta lactam antibiotics are not appropriate.

4.2 Posology and method of administration
The recommended dose is 800 mg once a day i.e. two 400 mg tablets once a day. The tablets should be swallowed whole with a sufficient amount of water. The tablets may be taken with or without food.

In patients of 18 years and older, according to the indication, the treatment regimen will be:

- Community-acquired pneumonia: 800 mg once a day for 7 to 10 days,
- Acute exacerbation of chronic bronchitis: 800 mg once a day for 5 days,
- Acute sinusitis: 800 mg once a day for 5 days,
- Tonsillitis/pharyngitis caused by Group A *beta streptococci:* 800 mg once a day for 5 days.

In patients of 12 to 18 years old, the treatment regimen will be:

- Tonsillitis/pharyngitis caused by Group A *beta streptococci:* 800 mg once a day for 5 days.

In the elderly:

No dosage adjustment is required in elderly patients based on age alone.

In children:

The safety and efficacy of Ketek in patient populations less than 12 years old have not yet been established.

Impaired renal function:

No dosage adjustment is necessary in patients with mild or moderate renal impairment. In the presence of severe renal impairment (creatinine clearance <30ml/min) with or without co-existing hepatic impairment, the dose should be halved.

In haemodialysed patients, the tablets should be given after the dialysis session on dialysis days.

Impaired hepatic function:

No dosage adjustment is necessary in patients with mild, moderate, or severe hepatic impairment, unless renal function is severely impaired.

4.3 Contraindications
Hypersensitivity to telithromycin, to any of the macrolide antibacterial agents, or to any of the excipients.

Concomitant administration of Ketek and any of the following substances is contraindicated: cisapride, ergot alkaloid derivatives (such as ergotamine and dihydroergotamine), pimozide, astemizole and terfenadine (see section 4.5).

Ketek should not be used concomitantly with simvastatin, atorvastatin and lovastastin. Treatment with these agents should be interrupted during Ketek treatment (see section 4.5).

Ketek is contraindicated in patients with a history of congenital or a family history of long QT syndrome (if not excluded by ECG) and in patients with known acquired QT interval prolongation.

4.4 Special warnings and special precautions for use
As with macrolides, due to a potential to increase QT, Ketek should be used with care in patients with coronary heart disease, a history of ventricular arrhythmias, uncorrected hypokalaemia and or hypomagnesaemia, bradycardia (<50 bpm), or during concomitant administration of Ketek with QT prolonging agents or potent CYP 3A4 inhibitors such as protease inhibitors and ketoconazole.

As with nearly all antibacterial agents, diarrhoea, particularly if severe, persistent and /or bloody, during or after treatment with Ketek may be caused by *pseudomembranous colitis*. If *pseudomembranous colitis* is suspected, the treatment must be stopped immediately and patients should be treated with supportive measures and/or specific therapy.

Exacerbation of myasthenia gravis has been reported in patients with myasthenia gravis treated with telithromycin. This usually occurred within one to three hours after intake of first dose of telithromycin.

Reports have included potentially life threatening acute respiratory failure with a rapid onset in myasthenic patients treated for respiratory tract infections with telithromycin. Telithromycin is not recommended in patients with myasthenia gravis unless other therapeutic alternatives are not available.

Patients with myasthenia gravis taking telithromycin should be advised to immediately seek medical attention if they experience exacerbation of their symptoms. Ketek must then be discontinued and supportive care administered as medically indicated (see section 4.8).

Due to limited experience, Ketek should be used with caution in patients with liver impairment (see section 5.2).

Ketek should not be used during and 2 weeks after treatment with CYP3A4 inducers (such as rifampicin, phenytoin, carbamazepine, phenobarbital, St John's wort). Concomitant treatment with these drugs is likely to result in subtherapeutic levels of telithromycin and therefore encompass a risk of treatment failure (see section 4.5 *Effect of other medicinal products on Ketek*).

Ketek is an inhibitor of CYP3A4 and should only be used under specific circumstances during treatment with other medicinal products that are metabolised by CYP3A4.

In areas with a high incidence of erythromycin A resistance, it is especially important to take into consideration the evolution of the pattern of susceptibility to telithromycin and other antibiotics.

In community acquired pneumonia, efficacy has been demonstrated in a limited number of patients with risk factors such as pneumococcal bacteraemia or age higher than 65 years.

Experience of treatment of infections caused by penicillin/ or erythromycin resistant *S. pneumoniae* is limited, but so far, clinical efficacy and eradication rates have been similar compared with the treatment of susceptible *S. pneumoniae*. Caution should be taken when *S. aureus* is the suspected pathogen and there is a likelihood of erythromycin resistance based on local epidemiology.

L. pneumophila is highly susceptible to telithromycin *in vitro*, however, the clinical experience of the treatment of pneumonia caused by *legionella* is limited.

As for macrolides, *H. influenzae* is classified as intermediately susceptible. This should be taken into account when treating infections caused by *H. influenzae.*

This medicine contains lactose. Patients with rare hereditary problems of galactose intolerance, the Lapp lactase deficiency or glucose-galactose malabsorption should not take this medicine.

4.5 Interaction with other medicinal products and other forms of Interaction
Effect of Ketek on other medicinal product
Telithromycin is an inhibitor of CYP3A4 and a weak inhibitor of CYP2D6. In vivo studies with simvastatin, midazolam and cisapride have demonstrated a potent inhibition of

intestinal CYP3A4 and a moderate inhibition of hepatic CYP3A4. The degree of inhibition with different CYP3A4 substrates is difficult to predict. Hence, Ketek should not be used during treatment with medicinal products that are CYP3A4 substrates, unless plasma concentrations of the CYP3A4 substrate, efficacy or adverse events can be closely monitored. Alternatively, interruption in the treatment with the CYP3A4 substrate should be made during treatment with Ketek.

Medicinal products with a potential to prolong QT interval

Ketek is expected to increase the plasma levels of cisapride, pimozide, astemizole and terfenadine. This could result in QT prolongation and cardiac arrhythmias including ventricular tachycardia, ventricular fibrillation and torsades de pointes. Concomitant administration of Ketek and any of these medicinal products is contraindicated (see section 4.3).

Caution is warranted when Ketek is administered to patients taking other medicinal products with the potential to prolong QT (see section 4.4).

Ergot alkaloid derivatives (such as ergotamine and dihydroergotamine)

By extrapolation from erythromycin A and josamycin, concomitant medication of Ketek and alkaloid derivatives could lead to severe vasoconstriction ("ergotism") with possibly necrosis of the extremities The combination is contraindicated (see section 4.3).

Statins

When simvastatin was coadministered with Ketek, there was a 5.3 fold increase in simvastatin C_{max}, an 8.9 fold increase in simvastatin AUC, a 15-fold increase in simvastatin acid C_{max} and an 11-fold increase in simvastatine acid AUC. In vivo interaction studies with other statins have not been performed, but Ketek may produce a similar interaction with lovastatin and atorvastatin, a lesser interaction with cerivastatin and little or no interaction with pravastatin and fluvastatin. Ketek should not be used concomitantly with simvastatin, atorvastastin and lovastatin. Treatment with these agents should be interrupted during Ketek treatment. Cerivastatin should be used with caution and patients should be carefully monitored for signs and symptoms of myopathy.

Benzodiazepins

When midazolam was coadministered with Ketek, midazolam AUC was increased 2.2-fold after intravenous administration of midazolam and 6.1-fold after oral administration. The midazolam half-life was increased about 2.5-fold. Oral administration of midazolam concomitantly with Ketek should be avoided. Intravenous dosage of midazolam should be adjusted as necessary and monitoring of the patient be undertaken. The same precautions should also apply to the other benzodiazepins which are metabolized by CYP3A4, (especially triazolam but also to a lesser extent alprazolam). For those benzodiazepins which are not metabolized by CYP3A4 (temazepam, nitrazepam, lorazepam) an interaction with Ketek is unlikely.

Cyclosporin, tacrolimus, sirolimus

Due to its CYP3A4 inhibitory potential, telithromycin can increase blood concentrations of these CYP34A4 substrates. Thus, when initiating telithromycin in patients already receiving any of theses immunosuppressive agents, cyclosporin, tacrolimus or sirolimus levels must be carefully monitored and their doses decreased as necessary. When telithromycin is discontinued, cyclosporin, tacrolimus or sirolimus levels must be again carefully monitored and their dose increased as necessary.

Metoprolol

When metoprolol (a CYP2D6 substrate) was coadministered with Ketek, metropolol Cmax and AUC were increased by approximately 38%, however, there was no effect on the elimination half-life of metoprolol. The increase exposure to metoprolol may be of clinical importance in patients with heart failure treated with metoprolol. In these patients, co-administration of Ketek and metoprolol, a CYP2D6 substrate, should be considered with caution.

Digoxin

Ketek has been shown to increase the plasma concentrations of digoxin. The plasma trough levels, C_{max}, AUC and renal clearance were increased by 20 %, 73 %, 37 % and 27% respectively, in healthy volunteers. There were no significant changes in ECG parameters and no signs of digoxin toxicity were observed. Nevertheless, monitoring of serum digoxin level should be considered during concomitant administration of digoxin and Ketek.

Theophylline

There is no clinically relevant pharmacokinetic interaction of Ketek and theophylline administered as extended release formulation. However, the co-administration of both medicinal products should be separated by one hour in order to avoid possible digestive side effects such as nausea and vomiting.

Warfarin

Ketek has no clinically relevant pharmacokinetic or pharmacodynamic interaction with warfarin after single dose administration. However, a pharmacodynamic interaction after multiple dose administration cannot be ruled out.

There is no pharmacodynamic or clinically relevant pharmacokinetic interaction with low-dose triphasic oral contraceptives in healthy subjects.

Effect of other medicinal products on Ketek

During concomitant administration of rifampicin and telithromycin in repeated doses, C_{max} and AUC of telithromycin were on average decreased by 79% and 86% respectively. Therefore, concomitant administration of CYP3A4 inducers (such as rifampicin, phenytoin, carbamazepine, phenobarbital, St John's wort) is likely to result in subtherapeutic levels of telithromycin and loss of effect. The induction gradually decreases during 2 weeks after cessation of treatment with CYP3A4 inducers. Ketek should not be used during and 2 weeks after treatment with CYP3A4 inducers.

Interaction studies with itraconazole and ketoconazole, two CYP3A4 inhibitors, showed that maximum plasma concentrations of telithromycin were increased respectively by 1.22 and 1.51 fold and AUC by respectively 1.54 fold and 2.0 fold. These changes in the pharmacokinetics of telithromycin do not necessitate dosage adjustment as telithromycin exposure remains within a well tolerated range. The effect of ritonavir on telithromycin has not been studied and could lead to larger increase in telithromycin exposure. The combination should be used with caution.

Ranitidine (taken 1 hour before Ketek) and antacid containing aluminium and magnesium hydroxide has no clinically relevant influence on telithromycin pharmacokinetics.

4.6 Pregnancy and lactation

Pregnancy

There are no adequate data from the use of Ketek in pregnant women. Studies in animals have shown reproductive toxicity (see section 5.3). The potential risk for humans is unknown. Ketek should not be used during pregnancy unless clearly necessary.

Lactation

Telithromycin is excreted in the milk of lactating animals, at concentrations about 5 times those of maternal plasma. Corresponding data for humans is not available. Ketek should not be used by breast-feeding women.

4.7 Effects on ability to drive and use machines

Ketek may cause undesirable effects such as visual disturbances which may reduce the capacity for the completion of certain tasks (see section 4.8). Patients should be informed of the potential for these undesirable effects that they may occur as early as the first dose of medication, and if they experience these symptoms, consideration should be given not to drive or operate machinery.

4.8 Undesirable effects

In 2461 patients treated by Ketek in phase III clinical trials, the following undesirable effects possibly or probably related to telithromycin have been reported. This is shown below.

(see Table 1 below)

Cases of rapid onset of exacerbation of myasthenia gravis have been reported (see section 4.4).

In addition, the following undesirable effects have been reported in sporadic cases: *pseudomembranous colitis*, erythema multiforme, parosmia,, muscle cramps.

Visual disturbances (<1%) associated with the use of KETEK, including blurred vision, difficulty focusing and diplopia, were mostly mild to moderate. They typically occurred within a few hours after the first or second dose, recurred upon subsequent dosing, lasted several hours and were fully reversible either during therapy or following the end of treatment. These events have not been associated with signs of ocular abnormality.

In clinical trials the effect on QTc was small (mean of approximately 1 msec). In comparative trials, similar effects to those observed with clarithromycin were seen with an on-therapy ΔQTc >30 msec in 7.6% and 7.0% of cases, respectively. No patient in either group developed a ΔQTc >60 msec. There were no reports of TdP or other serious ventricular arrhythmias or related syncope in the clinical program and no subgroups at risk were identified.

4.9 Overdose

In the event of acute overdose the stomach should be emptied. The patients should be carefully observed and given symptomatic and supportive treatment. Adequate hydration should be maintained. Blood electrolytes (especially potassium) must be controlled. Due to the potential for the prolongation of the QT interval and increased risk of arrhythmia, ECG monitoring must take place

5. PHARMACOLOGICAL PROPERTIES

5.1 Pharmacodynamic properties

Pharmacotherapeutic group: antibacterial for systemic use, ATC Code: J01.

Telithromycin is a semisynthetic derivative of erythromycin A belonging to the ketolides, a class of antibacterial agents related to macrolides.

Mode of action

Telithromycin inhibits protein synthesis by acting at the ribosome level.

The affinity of telithromycin for the 50S bacterial subunit of ribosome is 10 fold higher than that of erythromycin A when the strain is susceptible to erythromycin A. Against erythromycin A resistant strains, due to an MLS_B mechanism of resistance, telithromycin shows a more than 20 fold affinity compared to erythromycin A in the 50S bacterial subunit.

Telithromycin interferes with the ribosome translation at the 23S ribosomal RNA level, where it interacts with domain V and II. Furthermore, telithromycin is able to block the formation of the 50S and 30S ribosomal subunits.

Table 1

Organ systems	Very common side effects ≥ 10 % of patients	Common side effects 1 to 10 % of patients	Uncommon side effects 0.1 to 1 % of patients	Rare side effects 0.01 to 0.1 % of patients	Very rare side effects < 0.01 % of patients
Gastro-intestinal disorders	Diarrhoea	1. Nausea, vomiting, gastrointestinal pain, flatulence	Constipation, anorexia, oral moniliasis, stomatitis		
Hepato-biliary disorders		Increase in liver enzymes (AST, ALT, alkaline phosphatase)		Cholestatic jaundice	Hepatitis
Nervous system disorders		Dizziness, headache	Somnolence, insomnia, nervousness	Paraesthesia	
Blood and the lymphatic system disorders			Eosinophilia		
Eye and sensory organs disorders		Disturbance of taste	Blurred vision	Diplopia	
Reproductive system disorders		Vaginal moniliasis			
Skin disorders			Rash, urticaria, pruritus	Eczema	Angioneurotic oedema, anaphylactic reactions including anaphylactic shock
Cardiovascular disorders			Flush Palpitations	Atrial arrhythmia, hypotension, bradycardia	

Breakpoints

The recommended MIC breakpoints for telithromycin, separating susceptible organisms from intermediately susceptible organisms and intermediately susceptible organisms from resistant organisms, are: susceptible ≤0.5 mg/l, resistant >2mg/l.

Antibacterial spectrum

The prevalence of resistance may vary geographically and with time for selected species and local information on resistance is desirable, particularly when treating severe infections. This information provides only an approximate guidance on probabilities as to whether microorganisms will be susceptible to telithromycin. Where resistance patterns for particular species are known to vary within the European Union, this is shown below.

	Category with European range of resistance where this is known to vary
Susceptible Aerobic Gram-positive bacteria	
Streptococcus pneumoniae penicillin G susceptible or resistant and erythromycin A susceptible or resistant*	<1 %
*Streptococcus pyogenes**	1 – 22%
Streptococcus agalactiae	
Viridans group streptococci	
Lancefield group C and G (β haemolytic) *streptococci*	
Staphylococcus aureus erythromycin A susceptible* or resistant by inducible MLS_B mechanism	
Aerobic Gram- negative bacteria *Moraxella catarrhalis**	
Other *Legionella spp* *Legionella pneumophila* *Chlamydia pneumoniae** *Chlamydia psittaci* *Mycoplasma pneumoniae**	
Intermediately susceptible Haemophilus influenzae* *Haemophilus parainfluenzae*	
Resistant	
Staphylococcus aureus erythromycin A resistant by constitutive mechanism* * *Enterobacteriaceae* *Pseudomonas* *Acinetobacter*	

*** Clinical efficacy has been demonstrated for susceptible isolates in the approved clinical indications.**

* * Among MRSA the rate of MLSBc resistant strains is more than 80%.

Resistance

Telithromycin does not induce MLS_B resistance in vitro to *S. aureus*, *S. pneumoniae*, and *S. pyogenes*, an attribute related to its 3 keto function. Development of in vitro resistance to telithromycin due to spontaneous mutation is rare. The majority of MRSA are resistant to erythromycin A by a constitutive MLS_B mechanism.

In vitro results have shown that telithromycin is affected by the erythromycin ermB or mefA related resistance mechanisms but to lesser extent than erythromycin. While exposure to telithromycin did select for pneumococcal mutants with increased MICs, the MICs remained within the proposed susceptibility range.

For *S. pneumoniae*, there is no cross-resistance between telithromycin and other antibacterial classes.

For *S. pyogenes*, cross-resistance occurs for high-level erythromycin A resistant strains.

Effect on oral and faecal flora

In a comparative study in healthy human volunteers, telithromycin 800 mg daily and clarithromycin 500 mg twice daily for 10 days showed a similar and reversible reduction of oral and faecal flora. However, in contrast to clarithromycin, no resistant strains of alpha streptococci emerged in saliva on treatment with telithromycin.

5.2 Pharmacokinetic properties

Absorption

Following oral administration, telithromycin is fairly rapidly absorbed. A mean maximum plasma concentration of about 2 mg/l is reached within 1-3 hour after dose with once-daily dosing of telithromycin 800 mg. The absolute bioavailability is about 57 % after a single dose of 800 mg. The rate and extent of absorption is unaffected by food intake, and thus Ketek tablets can be given without regard to food.

Mean steady-state trough plasma concentrations of between 0.04 and 0.07 mg/l are reached within 3 to 4 days with once-daily dosing of telithromycin 800 mg. At steady-state AUC is approximately 1.5 fold increased compared to the single dose.

Mean peak and trough plasma concentrations at steady state in patients were 2.9±1.6 mg/l (range 0.02-7.6 mg/l) and 0.2±0.2 mg/l (range 0.010 to 1.29 mg/l), during a therapeutic 800 mg once-daily dose regimen.

Distribution

The in vitro protein binding is approximately 60 % to 70 %. Telithromycin is widely distributed throughout the body. The volume of distribution is 2.9±1.0 l/kg. Rapid distribution of telithromycin into tissues results in significantly higher telithromycin concentrations in most target tissues than in plasma. The maximum total tissue concentration in epithelial lining fluid, alveolar macrophages, bronchial mucosa, tonsils and sinus tissue were 14.9±11.4 mg/l, 318.1±231 mg/l, 3.88±1.87 mg/kg, 3.95±0.53 mg/kg and 6.96±1.58 mg/kg, respectively. The total tissue concentration 24 h after dose in epithelial lining fluid, alveolar macrophages, bronchial mucosa, tonsils and sinus tissue were 0.84±0.65 mg/l, 162±96 mg/l, 0.78±0.39 mg/kg, 0.72±0.29 mg/kg and 1.58±1.68 mg/kg, respectively. The mean maximum white blood cell concentration of telithromycin was 83±25 mg/l.

Metabolism

Telithromycin is metabolized primarily by the liver. After oral administration, two-thirds of the dose is eliminated as metabolites and one-third unchanged. The main circulating compound in plasma is telithromycin. Its principal circulating metabolite represents approximately 13 % of telithromycin AUC, and has little antimicrobial activity compared with the parent medicinal product. Other metabolites were detected in plasma, urine and faeces and represent less or equal than 3 % of plasma AUC.

Telithromycin is metabolized both by CYP450 isoenzymes and non-CYP enzymes. The major CYP450 enzyme involved in the metabolism of telithromycin is CYP3A4. Telithromycin is an inhibitor of CYP3A4 and CYP2D6, but has no or limited effect on CYP1A, 2A6, 2B6, 2C8, 2C9, 2C19 and 2E1.

Elimination

After oral administration of radiolabelled telithromycin, 76 % of the radioactivity was recovered from faeces, and 17 % from the urine. Approximately one-third of telithromycin was eliminated unchanged; 20 % in faeces and 12 % in urine. Telithromycin displays moderate non-linear pharmacokinetics. The non-renal clearance is decreased as the dose is increased. The total clearance (mean ±SD) is approximately 58±5 l/h after an intravenous administration with renal clearance accounting for about 22 % of this. Telithromycin displays a tri-exponential decay from plasma, with a rapid distribution half-life of 0.17 h. The main elimination half-life of telithromycin is 2-3 h and the terminal, less important, half-life is about 10 h at the dose 800 mg once daily.

Special populations

Renal impairment

The effect of renal impairment was evaluated after single dose administration.

In patients with mild to severe renal impairment, mean C_{max} and AUC values increased by an average of 37-38 % and 41-52 %, respectively, compared to normal healthy subjects. The inter-individual variability was increased in patients with renal impairment, but plasma exposure remained in the well tolerated range. The effect of dialysis on the elimination of telithromycin has not been assessed.

Hepatic impairment

The effect of hepatic impairment was evaluated after single dose administration. AUC of telithromycin was not affected but C_{max} decreased 20 %, trough concentration increased two fold and half-lives increased 20 to 40 % in patients with mild to severe hepatic insufficiency. The effect of hepatic impairment on the pharmacokinetics after multiple dose administration cannot be predicted from these data. Ketek should be used with caution in patients with hepatic impairment.

Elderly subjects: In subjects over 65 (median 75 years), the maximum plasma concentration and AUC of telithromycin were increased approximately 2 fold compared with those achieved in young healthy adults. These changes in pharmacokinetics do not necessitate dosage adjustment.

Paediatric patients: The pharmacokinetics of telithromycin in paediatric population less than 12 years old have not yet been studied. Limited data, obtained in paediatric patients 13 to 17 years of age, showed that telithromycin concentrations in this age group were similar to the concentrations in patients 18 to 40 years of age.

Gender

The pharmacokinetics of telithromycin are similar between males and females.

5.3 Preclinical safety data

Repeated dose toxicity studies of 1, 3 and 6 months duration with telithromycin conducted in rat, dog and monkey showed that the liver was the principal target for toxicity with elevations of liver enzymes, and histological evidence of damage. These effects showed a tendency to regress after cessation of treatment. Plasma exposures based on free fraction of drug, at the no observed adverse effect levels ranged from 1.6 to 13 times the expected clinical exposure.

Phospholipidosis (intracellular phospholipid accumulation) affecting a number of organs and tissues (e.g., liver, kidney, lung, thymus, spleen, gall bladder, mesenteric lymph nodes, GI-tract) has been observed in rats and dogs administered telithromycin at repeated doses of 150 mg/kg/day or more for 1 month and 20 mg/kg/day or more for 3-6 months. This administration corresponds to free drug systemic exposure levels of at least 9 times the expected levels in human after 1 month and less than the expected level in humans after 6 months, respectively. There was evidence of reversibility upon cessation of treatment. The significance of these findings for humans is unknown.

In similarity to some macrolides, telithromycin caused a prolongation of QTc in dogs and on action potential duration in rabbit Purkinje fibers in vitro. Effects were evident at plasma levels of free drug 8 to 13 times the expected clinical level. Hypokalaemia and quinidine had additive/supra-additive effects in vitro while potentiation was evident with sotalol. Telithromycin, but not its major human metabolites, had inhibitory activity on HERG and Kv1.5 channels.

Reproduction toxicity studies showed reduced gamete maturation in rat and adverse effects on fertilization. At high doses embryotoxicity was apparent and an increase in incomplete ossification and in skeletal anomalies was seen. Studies in rats and rabbits were inconclusive with respect to potential for teratogenicity, there was equivocal evidence of adverse effects on foetal development at high doses.

Telithromycin, and its principal human metabolites, were negative in tests on genotoxic potential *in vitro* and *in vivo*. No carcinogenicity studies have been conducted with telithromycin.

6. PHARMACEUTICAL PARTICULARS

6.1 List of excipients

Tablet core:

Maize starch

Microcrystalline cellulose

Povidone K25

Croscarmellose sodium

Magnesium stearate

Lactose monohydrate

Tablet coating:

Talc

Macrogol 8000

Hypromellose 6 cp

Titanium dioxide E171

Yellow iron oxide E172

Red iron oxide E172

6.2 Incompatibilities

Not applicable.

6.3 Shelf life

3 years.

6.4 Special precautions for storage

No special precautions for storage.

6.5 Nature and contents of container

Opaque PVC/Aluminium blisters.

Two tablets are contained in each blister cavity.

Available as packs of 10 tablets.

6.6 Instructions for use and handling

No special requirements.

7. MARKETING AUTHORISATION HOLDER

Aventis Pharma S.A.

20, Avenue Raymond Aron

F-92160 ANTONY

France

8. MARKETING AUTHORISATION NUMBER(S)

EU/1/01/191/001 – 10 tablet pack

9. DATE OF FIRST AUTHORISATION/RENEWAL OF THE AUTHORISATION

9th July 2001

10. DATE OF REVISION OF THE TEXT

27th January 2004

Ketovite Liquid

(Paines & Byrne Limited)

1. NAME OF THE MEDICINAL PRODUCT
Ketovite Liquid.

2. QUALITATIVE AND QUANTITATIVE COMPOSITION
Vitamin A as palmitate (1.7 × 10^6 units/g) HSE 2500 units
Vitamin D_2 (ergocalciferol) BP 400 units
Cyanocobalamin BP 12.5 microgram
Choline chloride HSE 150.0 mg

3. PHARMACEUTICAL FORM
Oral emulsion.

4. CLINICAL PARTICULARS
4.1 Therapeutic indications
As a sugar-free therapeutic supplement for the prevention of vitamin deficiency in conditions such as galactosaemia, disaccharide intolerance, phenylketonuria and other disorders of carbohydrate or amino acid metabolism, as well as in patients who are on restricted, specialised or synthetic diets.

In order to achieve complete vitamin supplementation Ketovite Liquid should be used in conjunction with Ketovite Tablets.

4.2 Posology and method of administration
For adults, children and the elderly: 5 ml daily, by oral administration.

4.3 Contraindications
Hypersensitivity to the product. Hypercalcaemia.

4.4 Special warnings and special precautions for use
The recommended dose should not be exceeded without medical advice. No other vitamin supplement containing Vitamins A and D should be taken with Ketovite Liquid except under medical supervision. Warning: do not exceed the stated dose.

4.5 Interaction with other medicinal products and other forms of Interaction
Absorption of some vitamins in this preparation may be reduced in conditions of fat malabsorption or with the concurrent use of neomycin, cholestyramine, liquid paraffin, aminoglycosides, aminosalicylic acid, anticonvulsants, biguanides, chloramphenicol, cimetidine, colchicine, potassium salts and methyl-dopa. Serum B_{12} concentrations may be decreased by concurrent administration of oral contraceptives.

4.6 Pregnancy and lactation
Caution should be used in pregnancy as excessive doses of Vitamin A may be teratogenic, especially when taken in the first trimester.

Large doses of Vitamin D in lactating mothers may cause hypercalcaemia in infants.

4.7 Effects on ability to drive and use machines
None known.

4.8 Undesirable effects
None, in the absence of overdosage.

4.9 Overdose
Symptoms of overdosage may include anorexia, nausea, vomiting, rough dry skin, polyuria, thirst, loss of hair, painful bones and joints as well as raised plasma and urine calcium and phosphate concentration.

No emergency procedure or antidote is applicable and symptoms are rapidly reduced upon withdrawal of the preparation.

5. PHARMACOLOGICAL PROPERTIES
5.1 Pharmacodynamic properties
The product is a multivitamin supplemental product.

5.2 Pharmacokinetic properties
The pharmacokinetics of the active substances would not differ from that of the same substance when derived naturally from oral foodstuffs.

5.3 Preclinical safety data
No relevant pre-clinical data has been generated.

6. PHARMACEUTICAL PARTICULARS
6.1 List of excipients
Methyl cellulose (methocel E4M) HSE
Saccharin BP
Methyl hydroxybenzoate BP
Polysorbate 80 BP
Ascorbic acid BP
DL α tocopherol HSE
Terpeneless orange oil BP
Ammonia solution 0.88m HSE
Deionised water HSE

6.2 Incompatibilities
None known.

6.3 Shelf life
24 months.

6.4 Special precautions for storage
Store at 2-8°C.

6.5 Nature and contents of container
Amber glass bottle with plastic screw cap. Pack sizes 100,150 & 140

6.6 Instructions for use and handling
Not applicable.

Administrative Data
7. MARKETING AUTHORISATION HOLDER
Paines and Byrne Ltd
Yamanouchi House
Pyrford Road
West Byfleet
Surrey
KT14 6RA

8. MARKETING AUTHORISATION NUMBER(S)
Product Licence 0051/5080R

9. DATE OF FIRST AUTHORISATION/RENEWAL OF THE AUTHORISATION
First authorisation granted 30 January 1990
Renewal granted 29th June 2000.

10. DATE OF REVISION OF THE TEXT
5th September 2000

Ketovite Tablets

(Paines & Byrne Limited)

1. NAME OF THE MEDICINAL PRODUCT
Ketovite Tablets.

2. QUALITATIVE AND QUANTITATIVE COMPOSITION
Thiamine hydrochloride BP 1.0 mg
Riboflavin BP 1.0 mg
Pyridoxine hydrochloride 0.33 mg
Nicotinamide BP 3.3 mg
Calcium pantothenate PhEur 1.16 mg
Ascorbic acid BP 16.6 mg
Acetomenaphthone BP 1973 0.5 mg
Alpha-tocopheryl acetate BP 5.0 mg
Inositol NF XII 50.0 mg
Biotin USP 0.17 mg
Folic acid BP 0.25 mg

3. PHARMACEUTICAL FORM
Tablet

4. CLINICAL PARTICULARS
4.1 Therapeutic indications
As a therapeutic supplement for the prevention of vitamin deficiency in conditions such as galactosaemia, disaccharide intolerance, phenylketonuria and other disorders of carbohydrate or amino acid metabolism, as well as in patients who are on restricted, specialised or synthetic diets.

In order to achieve complete vitamin supplementation Ketovite Tablets should be used in conjunction with Ketovite Liquid.

4.2 Posology and method of administration
For Adults, Children and the Elderly: One tablet three times a day, by oral administration.

4.3 Contraindications
Hypersensitivity to the product.

4.4 Special warnings and special precautions for use
None stated.

4.5 Interaction with other medicinal products and other forms of Interaction
Pyridoxine may increase the peripheral metabolism of levodopa reducing therapeutic efficacy in patients with Parkinson's disease.

4.6 Pregnancy and lactation
The recommended dose should not be exceeded without medical advice.

4.7 Effects on ability to drive and use machines
None.

4.8 Undesirable effects
None stated.

4.9 Overdose
Large overdoses of water-soluble vitamins are readily excreted in the urine. No emergency procedure or antidote is applicable and any symptoms are rapidly reduced upon withdrawal of the preparation.

5. PHARMACOLOGICAL PROPERTIES
5.1 Pharmacodynamic properties
Multivitamin preparation.

5.2 Pharmacokinetic properties
In normal circumstances the active constituents are obtained by the same route of administration (oral) from food.

5.3 Preclinical safety data
No relevant pre-clinical data has been generated.

6. PHARMACEUTICAL PARTICULARS
6.1 List of excipients
Heavy magnesium carbonate
Magnesium stearate
Magnesium trisilicate
Stearic acid
Methylcellulose
Colloidal silicon dioxide

6.2 Incompatibilities
None.

6.3 Shelf life
Two years.

6.4 Special precautions for storage
Store at 2-8°C.

6.5 Nature and contents of container
Securitainers containing 84, 90, 100 or 500 tablets.

6.6 Instructions for use and handling
None.

Administrative Data
7. MARKETING AUTHORISATION HOLDER
Paines and Byrne Ltd
Yamanouchi House
Pyrford Road
West Byfleet
Surrey KT14 6RA
United Kingdom

8. MARKETING AUTHORISATION NUMBER(S)
0051/5079R

9. DATE OF FIRST AUTHORISATION/RENEWAL OF THE AUTHORISATION
27 March 1987; renewed 21 January 2005

10. DATE OF REVISION OF THE TEXT
Date of partial revision = 2nd October 2003.

11. Legal Category
POM.

Kinidin Durules

(AstraZeneca UK Limited)

1. NAME OF THE MEDICINAL PRODUCT
Kinidin® Durules®.

2. QUALITATIVE AND QUANTITATIVE COMPOSITION
Each tablet contains 250mg quinidine bisulphate (hydrate) equivalent to quinidine sulphate BP 200mg.

3. PHARMACEUTICAL FORM
Film coated white to off-white oval tablet in an extended - release formulation (Durules).

4. CLINICAL PARTICULARS
4.1 Therapeutic indications
Maintenance of sinus rhythm following cardioversion of atrial fibrillation. Suppression of supraventricular and ventricular tachyarrhythmias.

4.2 Posology and method of administration
Initiation of treatment, as with other antiarrhythmic agents used to treat life-threatening ventricular arrhythmias, should be carried out in hospital.

An initial test dose of one tablet should be given to detect hypersensitivity.

Dosage is adjusted according to individual patient requirements. The quinidine dose should preferably be established by determination of the serum concentration after about one week of treatment. The therapeutic plasma concentration range is 1-6mg/L (3-18μmol/L). The QT-time should be checked before and during treatment. The normal dose is 2-5 tablets (0.4-1.0g) morning and evening. The normal dose for maintenance treatment after conversion of atrial fibrillation is 3 tablets (0.6g) morning and evening.

Concomitant food intake may increase the tolerability.

Kinidin Durules must not be chewed or crushed. They should be swallowed whole with half a glass of water.

4.3 Contraindications
Kinidin Durules are contra-indicated in patients with known hypersensitivity to quinidine, a history of quinidine induced thrombocytopenia or complete heart block.

Quinidine should be used with extreme caution in patients with incomplete atrio-ventricular block, uncompensated cardiac failure, digitalis toxicity, myocarditis, severe myocardial damage or myasthenia gravis.

The use of Kinidin Durules is contra-indicated in pregnancy.

4.4 Special warnings and special precautions for use
The patient should be observed after the first dose with special attention to hypersensitivity reactions. Quinidine should be administered with caution to patients with prolonged AV-conduction, sustained cardiac decompensation, cardiogenic shock, hypotension, bradycardia or disturbed potassium balance.

Caution is indicated in combined therapy with other class I antiarrhythmic drugs, β-blockers and digitalis glycosides (see further interaction with digoxin and digitoxin). Myocarditis or severe myocardial damage also requires caution.

Heart failure and hypokalaemia should be corrected before quinidine treatment is started. In patients treated with digoxin, the digoxin dosage should be halved if quinidine is given in addition.

Like other antiarrhythmic drugs quinidine may worsen arrhythmias.

At toxic quinidine concentrations, and in some patients even at therapeutic levels, the QT-interval may be considerably prolonged, which increases the risk of ventricular tachycardia, often of the torsades de pointes type and in some cases also ventricular fibrillation.

Kinidin Durules should be used with caution in the presence of obstructive changes in the digestive tract, oesophagus, when there is a potential risk of oesophageal complications.

4.5 Interaction with other medicinal products and other forms of Interaction

Digoxin: The plasma concentration of digoxin increases (may be doubled) when quinidine is given in addition. This is due to reduced renal clearance and a reduced distribution volume of digoxin. When quinidine is administered, the dose of digoxin should be halved and the plasma concentration of digoxin checked.

This recommendation is based on the assumption that the digoxin concentration is within the therapeutic range when quinidine treatment is started.

Digitoxin: The interaction between digitoxin and quinidine is a controversial issue. Several studies indicate, however, that quinidine increases the plasma concentration of digitoxin.

Cimetidine: Cimetidine decreases the clearance of quinidine, thereby increasing the plasma level.

Coumarin derivates: Quinidine may enhance the anticoagulant effect of coumarin derivatives.

Rifampicin, barbituric acid derivatives and phenytoin: These drugs increase the metabolism of quinidine, thereby reducing the plasma concentration to sub-therapeutic levels if the normal dosage is maintained.

Verapamil, amiodarone and nifedipine: Concomitant administration of verapamil or amiodarone can produce clinically important increases in serum quinidine concentrations. Conversely, simultaneous administration of nifedipine has been reported to significantly reduce plasma quinidine levels.

Appropriate quinidine dose changes and ECG monitoring should be carried out when these drugs are added or discontinued. During quinidine therapy 30-50% change in quinidine dosage may be required in order to avoid systemic toxicity or lack of efficacy.

Desipramine and imipramine: Quinidine inhibits the metabolism of desipramine and imipramine in rapid hydroxylators resulting in increased plasma concentrations. In addition they have additive antiarrhythmic properties. The combination should be avoided.

Procainamide: One case-report indicates that the plasma concentration of procainamide and its main metabolite N-acetyl-procainamide may increase significantly if quinidine is given simultaneously.

Metoprolol: In rapid hydroxylators quinidine may inhibit the metabolism of metoprolol resulting in increased plasma concentrations of metoprolol.

4.6 Pregnancy and lactation

The use of Kinidin Durules is contra-indicated in pregnancy.

Quinidine is excreted in breast milk but is unlikely to cause effects at therapeutic doses.

4.7 Effects on ability to drive and use machines

None known.

4.8 Undesirable effects

Gastrointestinal adverse reactions are frequent and occur in approximately 30% of the patients.

Gastrointestinal: Diarrhoea, nausea and vomiting.

Central and peripheral nervous system: Rarely signs of cinchonism e.g. tinnitus, blurred vision, headache and dizziness.

Cardiovascular: Arrhythmias such as ventricular tachycardia, mostly of the torsades de pointes type or ventricular fibrillation. Rarely hypotension and bradycardia, which may lead to cardiac arrest.

Hypersensitivity reactions: Rarely urticaria, skin rash and fever. In isolated cases hepatitis, thrombocytopenia, pancytopenia, agranulocytosis, photosensitisation, lupus erythematosus-like syndrome, myalgia and arthralgia.

4.9 Overdose

Poisoning due to an overdose of Kinidin Durules may lead to widening of the QRS complex and prolongation of the QT interval, atrioventricular block, sinoatrial block or arrest, asystole, paroxysmal ventricular tachycardia, flutter or fibrillation, myocardial depression, severe hypotension and cardiac arrest. Cinchonism, nausea, vomiting, drowsiness and sometimes convulsions also occur. Metabolic acidosis and hypokalaemia may complicate severe poisoning.

Treatment should include close monitoring of cardiovascular, respiratory and renal function, electrolytes and continuous ECG monitoring. Further absorption may be prevented by induction of vomiting or gastric lavage, or administration of activated charcoal if ingestion is recent. Cardiovascular complications should be treated symptomatically, which may require the use of sympathomimetic agents (e.g. noradrenaline, metaraminol), or inotropic agents (e.g. dopamine, dobutamine). Temporary pacing may be required for AV block. Glucagon may be used to treat hypotension, and intravenous sodium bicarbonate to correct acidosis and intravenous diazepam for convulsions.

Quinidine and its metabolites cannot be removed effectively by peritoneal or haemodialysis, or charcoal column haemoperfusion but repeated oral administration of activated charcoal may enhance elimination. Forced acid diuresis is not recommended.

As Kinidin Durules is an extended release formulation, treatment of overdosage may be required for a longer period.

5. PHARMACOLOGICAL PROPERTIES

5.1 Pharmacodynamic properties

Quinidine reduces the excitability, automaticity and conduction velocity in the atrium, AV node and ventricle and increases the duration of the action potential and the effective refractory period. These effects are closely related to the blockade of the "fast sodium channels" in the cell membranes, resulting in a reduced rate of the rise of action potential and thus a slower conduction and reduced automaticity in the purkinje fibres. The effect is considerably diminished when the extracellular potassium concentration is reduced and enhanced when it is increased.

The direct electrophysiological effects are modified by a relatively pronounced anticholinergic effect dominating particularly at lower plasma concentrations.

5.2 Pharmacokinetic properties

Oral bioavailabilty of quinidine is 70%–80%, the absorption is not influenced by concomitant intake of food. Plasma protein binding is 70%–95%. Half life in the elimination phase is approximately 6 hours and the dose is almost entirely excreted in the urine, 10%–20% as unchanged drug. Alkaline urine prolongs the elimination time.

The Durules formulation provides gradual release of active substance, thereby reducing the plasma concentration peaks. The absorption phase is prolonged compared to ordinary tablets and a more constant and prolonged effect is achieved, reducing the number of doses needed per day. The peak serum concentration is reached 4 hours after intake of Kinidin Durules.

5.3 Preclinical safety data

Quinidine bisulphate is an established active ingredient.

6. PHARMACEUTICAL PARTICULARS

6.1 List of excipients

Hydoxypropyl methylcellulose, Polyethylene glycol, Paraffin, Polyvinyl chloride, Polyvinyl acetate, Magnesium stearate and Colour (E171)

6.2 Incompatibilities

None Known.

6.3 Shelf life

Glass bottle - 60 months

Securitainer - 24 months

Press-through packages - 60 months.

6.4 Special precautions for storage

Glass bottle - store below 30°C

Securitainer - store below 30°C

PVC press-through packs - store below 25°C

6.5 Nature and contents of container

Glass bottle 100 or 250 tablets

Securitainer 100 or 250 tablets

Press-through packages of thermoformed PVC (10 tablets per strip) 100 tablets

6.6 Instructions for use and handling

None.

7. MARKETING AUTHORISATION HOLDER

AstraZeneca UK Ltd.,
600 Capability Green,
Luton, LU1 3LU, UK.

8. MARKETING AUTHORISATION NUMBER(S)

PL 17901/0131

9. DATE OF FIRST AUTHORISATION/RENEWAL OF THE AUTHORISATION

11th June 2002

10. DATE OF REVISION OF THE TEXT

11th June 2002

Kivexa film-coated tablets

(GlaxoSmithKline UK)

1. NAME OF THE MEDICINAL PRODUCT

Kivexa▼ film-coated tablets

2. QUALITATIVE AND QUANTITATIVE COMPOSITION

Each film-coated tablet contains 600 mg of abacavir (as sulfate) and 300 mg lamivudine.

For excipients see section 6.1.

3. PHARMACEUTICAL FORM

Film-coated tablet.

Orange, film-coated, modified capsule shaped tablets, debossed with GS FC2 on one side.

4. CLINICAL PARTICULARS

4.1 Therapeutic indications

Kivexa is a fixed-dose combination of two nucleoside analogues (abacavir and lamivudine). It is indicated in antiretroviral combination therapy for the treatment of Human Immunodeficiency Virus (HIV) infection in adults and adolescents from 12 years of age.

The demonstration of the benefit of the combination abacavir/lamivudine as a once daily regimen in antiretroviral therapy, is mainly based on results of one study performed in primarily asymptomatic treatment-naïve adult patients (see sections 4.4 and 5.1).

4.2 Posology and method of administration

Therapy should be prescribed by a physician experienced in the management of HIV infection.

The recommended dose of Kivexa in adults and adolescents is one tablet once daily.

Kivexa should not be administered to adults or adolescents who weigh less than 40 kg because it is a fixed-dose tablet that cannot be dose reduced.

Kivexa can be taken with or without food.

Kivexa is a fixed-dose tablet and should not be prescribed for patients requiring dosage adjustments. Separate preparations of abacavir or lamivudine are available in cases where discontinuation or dose adjustment of one of the active substances is indicated. In these cases the physician should refer to the individual product information for these medicinal products.

Renal impairment: Kivexa is not recommended for use in patients with a creatinine clearance < 50 ml/min (see section 5.2).

Hepatic impairment: No data are available in patients with moderate hepatic impairment, therefore the use of Kivexa is not recommended unless judged necessary. In patients with mild and moderate hepatic impairment close monitoring is required, and if feasible, monitoring of abacavir plasma levels is recommended (see sections 4.4 and 5.2). Kivexa is contraindicated in patients with severe hepatic impairment (see section 4.3).

Elderly: No pharmacokinetic data are currently available in patients over 65 years of age. Special care is advised in this age group due to age associated changes such as the decrease in renal function and alteration of haematological parameters.

Children: Kivexa is not recommended for treatment of children less than 12 years of age as the necessary dose adjustment cannot be made.

4.3 Contraindications

Kivexa is contraindicated in patients with known hypersensitivity to abacavir or lamivudine or to any of the excipients. See BOXED INFORMATION ON ABACAVIR HYPERSENSITIVITY REACTIONS in section 4.4 and section 4.8.

Patients with severe hepatic impairment.

4.4 Special warnings and special precautions for use

The special warnings and precautions relevant to abacavir and lamivudine are included in this section. There are no additional precautions and warnings relevant to Kivexa.

(see Table 1 on next page)

Lactic acidosis: lactic acidosis, usually associated with hepatomegaly and hepatic steatosis, has been reported with the use of nucleoside analogues. Early symptoms (symptomatic hyperlactatemia) include benign digestive symptoms (nausea, vomiting and abdominal pain), non-specific malaise, loss of appetite, weight loss, respiratory symptoms (rapid and/or deep breathing) or neurological symptoms (including motor weakness).

Lactic acidosis has a high mortality and may be associated with pancreatitis, liver failure, or renal failure.

Lactic acidosis generally occurred after a few or several months of treatment.

Treatment with nucleoside analogues should be discontinued in the setting of symptomatic hyperlactatemia and metabolic/lactic acidosis, progressive hepatomegaly, or rapidly elevating aminotransferase levels.

Caution should be exercised when administering nucleoside analogues to any patient (particularly obese women) with hepatomegaly, hepatitis or other known risk factors for liver disease and hepatic steatosis (including certain medicinal products and alcohol). Patients co-infected with

Table 1

Hypersensitivity Reaction

(see also section 4.8)

In clinical studies approximately 5% of subjects receiving abacavir develop a hypersensitivity reaction. Some of these cases were life-threatening and resulted in a fatal outcome despite taking precautions.

- **Description**

Hypersensitivity reactions are characterised by the appearance of symptoms indicating multi-organ system involvement. Almost all hypersensitivity reactions will have fever and/or rash as part of the syndrome.

Other signs and symptoms may include respiratory signs and symptoms such as dyspnoea, sore throat, cough, and abnormal chest x-ray findings (predominantly infiltrates, which can be localised), gastrointestinal symptoms, such as nausea, vomiting, diarrhoea, or abdominal pain, **and may lead to misdiagnosis of hypersensitivity as respiratory disease (pneumonia, bronchitis, pharyngitis), or gastroenteritis.**
Other frequently observed signs or symptoms of the hypersensitivity reaction may include lethargy or malaise and musculoskeletal symptoms (myalgia, rarely myolysis, arthralgia).

The symptoms related to this hypersensitivity reaction worsen with continued therapy and can be life- threatening. These symptoms usually resolve upon discontinuation of abacavir.

- **Management**

Hypersensitivity reaction symptoms usually appear within the first six weeks of initiation of treatment with abacavir, although these reactions **may occur at any time during therapy**. Patients should be monitored closely, especially during the first two months of treatment with abacavir, with consultation every two weeks.

Patients who are diagnosed with a hypersensitivity reaction whilst on therapy **MUST discontinue Kivexa immediately.**

Kivexa, or any other medicinal product containing abacavir (Ziagen or Trizivir), MUST NEVER be restarted in patients who have stopped therapy due to a hypersensitivity reaction.
Restarting abacavir following a hypersensitivity reaction results in a prompt return of symptoms within hours. This recurrence is usually more severe than on initial presentation, and may include life-threatening hypotension and death.

To avoid a delay in diagnosis and minimise the risk of a life-threatening hypersensitivity reaction, Kivexa must be permanently discontinued if hypersensitivity cannot be ruled out, even when other diagnoses are possible (respiratory diseases, flu-like illness, gastroenteritis or reactions to other medicinal products).

Special care is needed for those patients simultaneously starting treatment with Kivexa and other medicinal products known to induce skin toxicity (such as non-nucleoside reverse transcriptase inhibitors - NNRTIs). This is because it is currently difficult to differentiate between rashes induced by these products and abacavir related hypersensitivity reactions.

- **Management after an interruption of Kivexa therapy**

If therapy with Kivexa has been discontinued for any reason and restarting therapy is under consideration, the reason for discontinuation must be established to assess whether the patient had any symptoms of a hypersensitivity reaction. **If a hypersensitivity reaction cannot be ruled out, Kivexa or any other medicinal product containing abacavir (Ziagen or Trizivir) must not be restarted.**

Hypersensitivity reactions with rapid onset, including life-threatening reactions have occurred after restarting abacavir in patients who had only one of the key symptoms of hypersensitivity (skin rash, fever, gastrointestinal, respiratory or constitutional symptoms such as lethargy and malaise) prior to stopping abacavir. The most common isolated symptom of a hypersensitivity reaction was a skin rash. Moreover, on very rare occasions hypersensitivity reactions have been reported in patients who have restarted therapy, and who had no preceding symptoms of a hypersensitivity reaction.
In both cases if a decision is made to restart abacavir this must be done in a setting where medical assistance is readily available.

- **Essential patient information**

***Prescribers* must ensure that patients are fully informed regarding the following information on the hypersensitivity reaction:**
- Patients must be made aware of the possibility of a hypersensitivity reaction to abacavir that may result in a life-threatening reaction or death.

- Patients developing signs or symptoms possibly linked with a hypersensitivity reaction **MUST CONTACT their doctor IMMEDIATELY.**

- Patients who are hypersensitive to abacavir should be reminded that they must never take Kivexa or any other medicinal product containing abacavir (Ziagen or Trizivir) again.

- In order to avoid restarting abacavir, patients who have experienced a hypersensitivity reaction should dispose of their remaining Kivexa tablets in their possession in accordance with the local requirements, and ask their doctor or pharmacist for advice.

- Patients who have stopped Kivexa for any reason, and particularly due to possible adverse reactions or illness, must be advised to contact their doctor before restarting.

- Patients should be advised of the importance of taking Kivexa regularly.

- Each patient should be reminded to read the Package Leaflet included in the Kivexa package.

- They should be reminded of the importance of removing the Alert Card included in the package, and keeping it with them at all times.

hepatitis C and treated with alpha interferon and ribavirin may constitute a special risk.

Patients at increased risk should be followed closely.

Lipodystrophy: combination antiretroviral therapy has been associated with the redistribution of body fat (lipodystrophy) in HIV patients. The long-term consequences of these events are currently unknown. Knowledge about the mechanism is incomplete. A connection between visceral lipomatosis and protease inhibitors (PIs) and lipoatrophy and nucleoside reverse transcriptase inhibitors (NRTIs) has been hypothesised. A higher risk of lipodystrophy has been associated with individual factors such as older age, and with drug related factors such as longer duration of antiretroviral treatment and associated metabolic disturbances. Clinical examination should include evaluation for physical signs of fat redistribution. Consideration should be given to the measurement of fasting serum lipids and blood glucose. Lipid disorders should be managed as clinically appropriate (see section 4.8).

Pancreatitis: pancreatitis has been reported, but a causal relationship to lamivudine and abacavir is uncertain.

Clinical studies: the benefit of the combination of abacavir and lamivudine as a once daily regimen is mainly based on a study performed in combination with efavirenz, in antiretroviral-naïve adults patients (see section 5.1).

Triple nucleoside therapy: There have been reports of a high rate of virological failure, and of emergence of resistance at an early stage when abacavir and lamivudine were combined with tenofovir disoproxil fumarate as a once daily regimen.

Liver disease: if lamivudine is being used concomitantly for the treatment of HIV and HBV, additional information relating to the use of lamivudine in the treatment of hepatitis B infection is available in the Zeffix SPC.

The safety and efficacy of Kivexa has not been established in patients with significant underlying liver disorders. Kivexa is contraindicated in patients with severe hepatic impairment (see section 4.3).

Patients with chronic hepatitis B or C and treated with combination antiretroviral therapy are at an increased risk of severe and potentially fatal hepatic adverse events. In case of concomitant antiviral therapy for hepatitis B or C, please refer also to the relevant product information for these medicinal products.

If Kivexa is discontinued in patients co-infected with hepatitis B virus, periodic monitoring of both liver function tests and markers of HBV replication is recommended, as withdrawal of lamivudine may result in an acute exacerbation of hepatitis (see Zeffix SPC).

Patients with pre-existing liver dysfunction, including chronic active hepatitis have an increased frequency of liver function abnormalities during combination antiretroviral therapy, and should be monitored according to standard practice. If there is evidence of worsening liver disease in such patients, interruption or discontinuation of treatment must be considered.

Mitochondrial dysfunction: nucleoside and nucleotide analogues have been demonstrated *in vitro* and *in vivo* to cause a variable degree of mitochondrial damage. There have been reports of mitochondrial dysfunction in HIV-negative infants exposed *in utero* and/or post-natally to nucleoside analogues. The main adverse events reported are haematological disorders (anaemia, neutropenia), metabolic disorders (hyperlactatemia, hyperlipasemia). These events are often transitory. Some late-onset neurological disorders have been reported (hypertonia, convulsion, abnormal behaviour). Whether the neurological disorders are transient or permanent is currently unknown. Any child exposed *in utero* to nucleoside and nucleotide analogues, even HIV-negative children, should have clinical and laboratory follow-up and should be fully investigated for possible mitochondrial dysfunction in case of relevant signs or symptoms. These findings do not affect current national recommendations to use antiretroviral therapy in pregnant women to prevent vertical transmission of HIV.

Immune Reactivation Syndrome: in HIV-infected patients with severe immune deficiency at the time of institution of combination antiretroviral therapy (CART), an inflammatory reaction to asymptomatic or residual opportunistic pathogens may arise and cause serious clinical conditions, or aggravation of symptoms. Typically, such reactions have been observed within the first few weeks or months of initiation of CART. Relevant examples are cytomegalovirus retinitis, generalised and/or focal mycobacterial infections, and *Pneumocystis carinii* pneumonia. Any inflammatory symptoms should be evaluated and treatment instituted when necessary.

Excipients: Kivexa contains the azo colouring agent sunset yellow, which may cause allergic reactions.

Opportunistic infections: patients should be advised that Kivexa or any other antiretroviral therapy does not cure HIV infection and that they may still develop opportunistic infections and other complications of HIV infection. Therefore patients should remain under close clinical observation by physicians experienced in the treatment of these associated HIV diseases.

Transmission of HIV: patients should be advised that current antiretroviral therapy, including Kivexa, has not been proven to prevent the risk of transmission of HIV to others through sexual contact or blood contamination. Appropriate precautions should continue to be taken.

4.5 Interaction with other medicinal products and other forms of Interaction

Kivexa contains abacavir and lamivudine, therefore any interactions identified for these individually are relevant to Kivexa. Clinical studies have shown that there are no clinically significant interactions between abacavir and lamivudine.

Abacavir and lamivudine are not significantly metabolised by cytochrome P_{450} enzymes (such as CYP 3A4, CYP 2C9 or CYP 2D6) nor do they inhibit or induce this enzyme system. Therefore, there is little potential for interactions with antiretroviral protease inhibitors, non-nucleosides and other medicinal products metabolised by major P_{450} enzymes. The interactions listed below should not be considered exhaustive but are representative of the classes of medicinal products where caution should be exercised.

Interactions relevant to abacavir

Potent enzymatic inducers such as rifampicin, phenobarbital and phenytoin may via their action on

Table 2

Abacavir hypersensitivity

(see also section 4.4)

In clinical studies, approximately 5 % of subjects receiving abacavir developed a hypersensitivity reaction. In clinical studies with abacavir 600 mg once daily the reported rate of hypersensitivity remained within the range recorded for abacavir 300 mg twice daily.

Some of these hypersensitivity reactions were life-threatening and resulted in fatal outcome despite taking precautions. This reaction is characterised by the appearance of symptoms indicating multi-organ/body-system involvement.

Almost all patients developing hypersensitivity reactions will have fever and/or rash (usually maculopapular or urticarial) as part of the syndrome, however reactions have occurred without rash or fever.

The signs and symptoms of this hypersensitivity reaction are listed below. These have been identified either from clinical studies or post marketing surveillance. Those reported **in at least 10% of patients** with a hypersensitivity reaction are in bold text.

Skin	**Rash** (usually maculopapular or urticarial)
Gastrointestinal tract	**Nausea, vomiting, diarrhoea, abdominal pain**, mouth ulceration
Respiratory tract	**Dyspnoea, cough**, sore throat, adult respiratory distress syndrome, respiratory failure
Miscellaneous	**Fever, lethargy, malaise**, oedema, lymphadenopathy, hypotension, conjunctivitis, anaphylaxis
Neurological/Psychiatry	**Headache**, paraesthesia
Haematological	Lymphopenia
Liver/pancreas	**Elevated liver function tests**, hepatitis, hepatic failure
Musculoskeletal	**Myalgia**, rarely myolysis, arthralgia, elevated creatine phosphokinase
Urology	Elevated creatinine, renal failure

Some patients with hypersensitivity reactions were initially thought to have gastroenteritis, respiratory disease (pneumonia, bronchitis, pharyngitis) or a flu-like illness. This delay in diagnosis of hypersensitivity has resulted in abacavir being continued or re-introduced, leading to more severe hypersensitivity reactions or death. Therefore, the diagnosis of hypersensitivity reaction should be carefully considered for patients presenting with symptoms of these diseases.

Symptoms usually appeared within the first six weeks (median time to onset 11 days) of initiation of treatment with abacavir, although these reactions may occur at any time during therapy. Close medical supervision is necessary during the first two months, with consultations every two weeks.

It is likely that intermittent therapy may increase the risk of developing sensitisation and therefore occurrence of clinically significant hypersensitivity reactions. Consequently, patients should be advised of the importance of taking Kivexa regularly.

Restarting abacavir following a hypersensitivity reaction results in a prompt return of symptoms within hours. This recurrence of the hypersensitivity reaction was usually more severe than on initial presentation, and may include life-threatening hypotension and death. **Patients who develop this hypersensitivity reaction must discontinue Kivexa and must never be rechallenged with Kivexa, or any other medicinal product containing abacavir (Ziagen or Trizivir).**

To avoid a delay in diagnosis and minimise the risk of a life-threatening hypersensitivity reaction, abacavir must be permanently discontinued if hypersensitivity cannot be ruled out, even when other diagnoses are possible (respiratory diseases, flu-like illness, gastroenteritis or reactions to other medicinal products).

Hypersensitivity reactions with rapid onset, including life-threatening reactions have occurred after restarting abacavir in patients who had only one of the key symptoms of hypersensitivity (skin rash, fever, gastrointestinal, respiratory or constitutional symptoms such as lethargy and malaise) prior to stopping abacavir. The most common isolated symptom of a hypersensitivity reaction was a skin rash. Moreover, on very rare occasions hypersensitivity reactions have been reported in patients who have restarted therapy and who had <u>no preceding symptoms</u> of a hypersensitivity reaction. In both cases, if a decision is made to restart abacavir this must be done in a setting where medical assistance is readily available.

Each patient must be warned about this hypersensitivity reaction to abacavir.

UDP-glucuronyltransferases slightly decrease the plasma concentrations of abacavir.

The metabolism of abacavir is altered by concomitant consumption of ethanol resulting in an increase in AUC of abacavir of about 41%. These findings are not considered clinically significant. Abacavir has no effect on the metabolism of ethanol.

Retinoid compounds are eliminated via alcohol dehydrogenase. Interaction with abacavir is possible but has not been studied.

In a pharmacokinetic study, coadministration of 600 mg abacavir twice daily with methadone showed a 35% reduction in abacavir C_{max} and a 1 hour delay in t_{max}, but the AUC was unchanged. The changes in abacavir pharmacokinetics are not considered clinically relevant. In this study, abacavir increased the mean methadone systemic clearance by 22%. The induction of metabolizing enzymes cannot therefore be excluded. Patients being treated with methadone and abacavir should be monitored for evidence of withdrawal symptoms indicating under dosing, as occasionally methadone re-titration may be required.

<u>Interactions relevant to lamivudine</u>

The likelihood of metabolic interactions with lamivudine is low due to limited metabolism and plasma protein binding, and almost complete renal clearance. The possibility of interactions with other medicinal products administered concurrently with Kivexa should be considered, particularly when the main route of elimination is active renal secretion, especially via the cationic transport system e.g. trimethoprim. Other medicinal products (e.g. ranitidine, cimetidine) are eliminated only in part by this mechanism and were shown not to interact with lamivudine. The nucleoside analogues (e.g. zidovudine and didanosine) are not metabolised by this mechanism and are unlikely to interact with lamivudine.

Administration of trimethoprim/sulfamethoxazole 160 mg/800 mg results in a 40% increase in lamivudine exposure, because of the trimethoprim component. However, unless the patient has renal impairment, no dosage adjustment of lamivudine is necessary (see section 4.2). The pharmacokinetics of trimethoprim or sulfamethoxazole are not affected. When concomitant administration with co-trimoxazole is warranted, patients should be monitored clinically. Co-administration of Kivexa with high doses of co-trimoxazole for the treatment of *Pneumocystis carinii* pneumonia (PCP) and toxoplasmosis should be avoided.

Co-administration of lamivudine with intravenous ganciclovir or foscarnet is not recommended until further information is available.

Lamivudine may inhibit the intracellular phosphorylation of zalcitabine when the two medicinal products are used concurrently. Kivexa is therefore not recommended to be used in combination with zalcitabine.

4.6 Pregnancy and lactation

<u>Pregnancy</u>

Kivexa is not recommended during pregnancy. The safety of abacavir and lamivudine in human pregnancy has not been established. Studies with abacavir and lamivudine in animals have shown reproductive toxicity (see section 5.3).

<u>Lactation</u>

It is recommended that HIV-infected women do not breast-feed their infants under any circumstances in order to avoid transmission of HIV. Lamivudine is excreted in human milk at similar concentrations to those found in serum. It is expected that abacavir will also be secreted into human milk, although this has not been confirmed. It is therefore recommended that mothers do not breast-feed their babies while receiving treatment with Kivexa.

4.7 Effects on ability to drive and use machines

No studies on the effects on ability to drive and use machines have been performed. The clinical status of the patient and the adverse event profile of Kivexa should be borne in mind when considering the patient's ability to drive or operate machinery.

4.8 Undesirable effects

The adverse reactions reported for Kivexa were consistent with the known safety profiles of abacavir and lamivudine when given as separate medicinal products. For many of these adverse reactions it is unclear whether they are related to the active substance, the wide range of other medicinal products used in the management of HIV infection, or whether they are a result of the underlying disease process.

(see Table 2 opposite)

Many of the adverse reactions listed in the table below occur commonly (nausea, vomiting, diarrhoea, fever, lethargy, rash) in patients with abacavir hypersensitivity. Therefore, patients with any of these symptoms should be carefully evaluated for the presence of this hypersensitivity reaction. If Kivexa has been discontinued in patients due to experiencing any one of these symptoms and a decision is made to restart a medicinal product containing abacavir, this must be done in a setting where medical assistance is readily available (see section 4.4). Very rarely cases of erythema multiforme, Stevens-Johnson syndrome or toxic epidermal necrolysis have been reported where abacavir hypersensitivity could not be ruled out. In such cases medicinal products containing abacavir should be permanently discontinued.

The adverse reactions considered at least possibly related to abacavir or lamivudine are listed by body system, organ class and absolute frequency. Frequencies are defined as very common > 1/10), common > 1/100, < 1/10), uncommon > 1/1000, < 1/100), rare > 1/10,000, < 1/1000), very rare (< 1/10,000).

Body system	**Abacavir**	**Lamivudine**
Blood and lymphatic systems disorders		*Uncommon:* Neutropenia and anaemia (both occasionally severe), thrombocytopenia *Very rare:* Pure red cell aplasia
Immune system disorders	*Common:* hypersensitivity	
Metabolism and nutrition disorders	*Common:* anorexia	
Nervous system disorders	*Common:* headache	*Common:* Headache, insomnia. *Very rare:* Cases of peripheral neuropathy (or paraesthesia) have been reported
Respiratory, thoracic and mediastinal disorders		*Common:* Cough, nasal symptoms
Gastrointestinal disorders	*Common:* nausea, vomiting, diarrhoea *Rare:* pancreatitis has been reported, but a causal relationship to abacavir treatment is uncertain	*Common:* Nausea, vomiting, abdominal pain or cramps, diarrhoea *Rare:* Rises in serum amylase. Cases of pancreatitis have been reported

Hepatobiliary disorders		*Uncommon:* Transient rises in liver enzymes (AST, ALT), *Rare:* Hepatitis
Skin and subcutaneous tissue disorders	*Common:* rash (without systemic symptoms) *Very rare:* erythema multiforme, Stevens-Johnson syndrome and toxic epidermal necrolysis	*Common:* Rash, alopecia
Musculoskeletal and connective tissue disorders		*Common:* Arthralgia, muscle disorders *Rare:* Rhabdomyolysis
General disorders and administration site conditions	*Common:* fever, lethargy, fatigue.	*Common:* fatigue, malaise, fever.

Cases of lactic acidosis, sometimes fatal, usually associated with severe hepatomegaly and hepatic steatosis, have been reported with the use of nucleoside analogues (see section 4.4).

Combination antiretroviral therapy has been associated with redistribution of body fat (lipodystrophy) in HIV patients including the loss of peripheral and facial subcutaneous fat, increased intra-abdominal and visceral fat, breast hypertrophy and dorsocervical fat accumulation (buffalo hump).

Combination antiretroviral therapy has been associated with metabolic abnormalities such as hypertriglyceridaemia, hypercholesterolaemia, insulin resistance, hyperglycaemia and hyperlactataemia (see section 4.4).

In HIV-infected patients with severe immune deficiency at the time of initiation of combination antiretroviral therapy, an inflammatory reaction to asymptomatic or residual opportunistic infections may arise (see section 4.4).

4.9 Overdose

No specific symptoms or signs have been identified following acute overdose with abacavir or lamivudine, apart from those listed as undesirable effects.

If overdose occurs the patient should be monitored for evidence of toxicity (see section 4.8), and standard supportive treatment applied as necessary. Since lamivudine is dialysable, continuous haemodialysis could be used in the treatment of overdose, although this has not been studied. It is not known whether abacavir can be removed by peritoneal dialysis or haemodialysis.

5. PHARMACOLOGICAL PROPERTIES

5.1 Pharmacodynamic properties

Pharmacotherapeutic group, nucleoside reverse transcriptase inhibitors (NRTIs), ATC code: J05A F30

Mechanism of action and resistance

Abacavir and lamivudine are NRTIs, and are potent selective inhibitors of HIV-1 and HIV-2. Both abacavir and lamivudine are metabolised sequentially by intracellular kinases to the respective 5'-triphosphate (TP) which are the active moieties. Lamivudine-TP and carbovir-TP (the active triphosphate form of abacavir) are substrates for and competitive inhibitors of HIV reverse transcriptase (RT). However, their main antiviral activity is through incorporation of the monophosphate form into the viral DNA chain, resulting in chain termination. Abacavir and lamivudine triphosphates show significantly less affinity for host cell DNA polymerases.

Lamivudine has been shown to be highly synergistic with zidovudine, inhibiting the replication of HIV in cell culture. Abacavir shows synergy *in vitro* in combination with amprenavir, nevirapine and zidovudine. It has been shown to be additive in combination with didanosine, stavudine and lamivudine.

HIV-1 resistance to lamivudine involves the development of a M184V amino acid change close to the active site of the viral RT. This variant arises both *in vitro* and in HIV-1 infected patients treated with lamivudine-containing antiretroviral therapy.

Abacavir-resistant isolates of HIV-1 have been selected *in vitro* and are associated with specific genotypic changes in the reverse transcriptase (RT) codon region (codons M184V, K65R, L74V and Y115F). Viral resistance to abacavir develops relatively slowly *in vitro* and *in vivo*, requiring multiple mutations to reach an eight-fold increase in IC_{50} over wild-type virus, which may be a clinically relevant level. Isolates resistant to abacavir may also show reduced sensitivity to lamivudine, zalcitabine, tenofovir, emtricitabine and/or didanosine, but remain sensitive to zidovudine and stavudine.

Cross-resistance between abacavir or lamivudine and antiretrovirals from other classes e.g. PIs or NNRTIs is unlikely. Reduced susceptibility to abacavir has been demonstrated in clinical isolates of patients with uncontrolled viral replication, who have been pre-treated with and are resistant to other nucleoside inhibitors.

Clinical isolates with three or more mutations associated with NRTIs are unlikely to be susceptible to abacavir. Cross-resistance conferred by the M184V RT is limited within the nucleoside inhibitor class of antiretroviral agents. Zidovudine, stavudine, abacavir and tenofovir maintain their antiretroviral activities against lamivudine-resistant HIV-1. Abacavir maintains its antiretroviral activities against lamivudine-resistant HIV-1 harbouring only the M184V mutation.

Clinical experience

Therapy-naïve patients

The combination of abacavir and lamivudine as a once daily regimen is supported by a 48 weeks multi-centre, double-blind, controlled study (CNA30021) of 770 HIV-infected, therapy-naïve adults. These were primarily asymptomatic HIV infected patients (CDC stage A). They were randomised to receive either abacavir (ABC) 600 mg once daily or 300 mg twice daily, in combination with lamivudine 300 mg once daily and efavirenz 600 mg once daily. The results are summarised in the table below:

Virological Response Based on Plasma HIV-1 RNA < 50 copies/ml at Week 48

ITT-Exposed Population

Treatment regimen	ABC once/day (N = 384)	ABC twice/day (N = 386)
Virological response	253/384 (66%)	261/386 (68%)

Similar clinical success (point estimate for treatment difference: -1.7, 95% CI –8.4, 4.9) was observed for both regimens. From these results, it can be concluded with 95% confidence that the true difference is no greater than 8.4% in favour of the twice daily regimen. This potential difference is sufficiently small to draw an overall conclusion of non-inferiority of abacavir once daily over abacavir twice daily.

There was a low, similar overall incidence of virologic failure (viral load > 50 copies/ml) in both the once and twice daily treatment groups (10% and 8% respectively). In the small sample size for genotypic analysis, there was a trend toward a higher rate of NRTI-associated mutations in the once daily versus the twice daily abacavir regimens. No firm conclusion could be drawn due to the limited data derived from this study. Long term data with abacavir used as a once daily regimen (beyond 48 weeks) are currently limited.

Therapy-experienced patients

In study CAL30001, 182 treatment-experienced patients with virologic failure were randomised to receive either Kivexa or abacavir 300 mg twice daily plus lamivudine 300 mg once daily, both in combination with tenofovir and a PI or an NNRTI for 48 weeks. Preliminary data at 24 weeks indicate that the Kivexa group was non-inferior to the abacavir twice daily group, based on similar reductions in HIV-1 RNA as measured by average area under the curve minus baseline (AAUCMB, -1.6 versus -1.87 respectively, 95% CI -0.06, 0.37). Proportions with HIV-1 RNA < 50 copies/ml (56% versus 47%) and < 400 copies/ml (65% versus 63%) were also similar in each group. However, as there were only moderately experienced patients included in this study with an imbalance in baseline viral load and treatment discontinuations between the arms, these results should be interpreted with caution.

In study ESS30008, 260 patients with virologic suppression on a first line therapy regimen containing abacavir 300 mg plus lamivudine 150 mg, both given twice daily and a PI or NNRTI, were randomised to continue this regimen or switch to Kivexa plus a PI or NNRTI for 48 weeks. Preliminary data at 24 weeks indicate that the Kivexa group was associated with a similar virologic outcome (non-inferior) compared to the abacavir plus lamivudine group, based on proportions of subjects with HIV-1 RNA < 50 copies/ml (91% and 86% respectively, 95% CI -11.1, 1.9).

5.2 Pharmacokinetic properties

The fixed-dose combination tablet of abacavir/lamivudine (FDC) has been shown to be bioequivalent to lamivudine and abacavir administered separately. This was demonstrated in a single dose, 3-way crossover bioequivalence study of FDC (fasted) versus 2 × 300 mg abacavir tablets plus 2 × 150 mg lamivudine tablets (fasted) versus FDC administered with a high fat meal, in healthy volunteers (n = 30). In the fasted state there was no significant difference in the extent of absorption, as measured by the area under the plasma concentration-time curve (AUC) and maximal peak concentration (C_{max}), of each component. There was also no clinically significant food effect observed between administration of FDC in the fasted or fed state. These results indicate that FDC can be taken with or without food. The pharmacokinetic properties of lamivudine and abacavir are described below.

Absorption

Abacavir and lamivudine are rapidly and well absorbed from the gastro-intestinal tract following oral administration. The absolute bioavailability of oral abacavir and lamivudine in adults is about 83% and 80-85% respectively. The mean time to maximal serum concentrations (t_{max}) is about 1.5 hours and 1.0 hour for abacavir and lamivudine, respectively. Following a single dose of 600 mg of abacavir, the mean (CV) C_{max} is 4.26 μg/ml (28%) and the mean (CV) AUC_{∞} is 11.95 μg.h/ml (21%). Following multiple-dose oral administration of lamivudine 300 mg once daily for seven days, the mean (CV) steady-state C_{max} is 2.04 μg/ml (26%) and the mean (CV) AUC_{24} is 8.87 μg.h/ml (21%).

Distribution

Intravenous studies with abacavir and lamivudine showed that the mean apparent volume of distribution is 0.8 and 1.3 l/kg respectively. Plasma protein binding studies *in vitro* indicate that abacavir binds only low to moderately (~49%) to human plasma proteins at therapeutic concentrations. Lamivudine exhibits linear pharmacokinetics over the therapeutic dose range and displays limited plasma protein binding *in vitro* (< 36%). This indicates a low likelihood for interactions with other medicinal products through plasma protein binding displacement.

Data show that abacavir and lamivudine penetrate the central nervous system (CNS) and reach the cerebrospinal fluid (CSF). Studies with abacavir demonstrate a CSF to plasma AUC ratio of between 30 to 44%. The observed values of the peak concentrations are 9 fold greater than the IC_{50} of abacavir of 0.08 μg/ml or 0.26 μM when abacavir is given at 600 mg twice daily. The mean ratio of CSF/serum lamivudine concentrations 2-4 hours after oral administration was approximately 12%. The true extent of CNS penetration of lamivudine and its relationship with any clinical efficacy is unknown.

Metabolism

Abacavir is primarily metabolised by the liver with approximately 2% of the administered dose being renally excreted, as unchanged compound. The primary pathways of metabolism in man are by alcohol dehydrogenase and by glucuronidation to produce the 5'-carboxylic acid and 5'-glucuronide which account for about 66% of the administered dose. These metabolites are excreted in the urine.

Metabolism of lamivudine is a minor route of elimination. Lamivudine is predominately cleared by renal excretion of unchanged lamivudine. The likelihood of metabolic drug interactions with lamivudine is low due to the small extent of hepatic metabolism (5-10%).

Elimination

The mean half-life of abacavir is about 1.5 hours. Following multiple oral doses of abacavir 300 mg twice a day there is no significant accumulation of abacavir. Elimination of abacavir is via hepatic metabolism with subsequent excretion of metabolites primarily in the urine. The metabolites and unchanged abacavir account for about 83% of the administered abacavir dose in the urine. The remainder is eliminated in the faeces.

The observed lamivudine half-life of elimination is 5 to 7 hours. The mean systemic clearance of lamivudine is approximately 0.32 l/h/kg, predominantly by renal clearance > 70%) via the organic cationic transport system. Studies in patients with renal impairment show lamivudine elimination is affected by renal dysfunction. Dose reduction is required for patients with creatinine clearance < 50 ml/min (see section 4.2).

Intracellular pharmacokinetics

In a study of 20 HIV-infected patients receiving abacavir 300 mg twice daily, with only one 300 mg dose taken prior to the 24 hour sampling period, the geometric mean terminal carbovir-TP intracellular half-life at steady-state was 20.6 hours, compared to the geometric mean abacavir plasma half-life in this study of 2.6 hours. Similar intracellular kinetics are expected from abacavir 600 mg once daily. For patients receiving lamivudine 300 mg once daily, the terminal intracellular half-life of lamivudine-TP was prolonged to 16-19 hours, compared to the plasma lamivudine half-life of 5-7 hours. These data support the use of lamivudine 300 mg and abacavir 600 mg once daily for the treatment of HIV-infected patients. Additionally, the efficacy of this combination given once daily has been demonstrated in a pivotal clinical study (CNA30021- See Clinical experience).

Special populations

Hepatically impaired: There are no data available on the use of Kivexa in hepatically impaired patients. Pharmacokinetic data has been obtained for abacavir and lamivudine alone.

Abacavir is metabolised primarily by the liver. The pharmacokinetics of abacavir have been studied in patients with mild hepatic impairment (Child-Pugh score 5-6) receiving a single 600 mg dose. The results showed that there was a mean increase of 1.89 fold [1.32; 2.70] in the abacavir AUC, and 1.58 [1.22; 2.04] fold in the elimination half-life. No recommendation on dosage reduction is possible in patients with mild hepatic impairment due to substantial variability of abacavir exposure.

Data obtained in patients with moderate to severe hepatic impairment show that lamivudine pharmacokinetics are not significantly affected by hepatic dysfunction.

Renally impaired: Pharmacokinetic data have been obtained for lamivudine and abacavir alone. Abacavir is primarily metabolised by the liver with approximately 2% of abacavir excreted unchanged in the urine. The pharmacokinetics of abacavir in patients with end-stage renal disease is similar to patients with normal renal function. Studies with lamivudine show that plasma concentrations (AUC) are increased in patients with renal dysfunction due to decreased clearance. Dose reduction is required for patients with creatinine clearance of < 50 ml/min.

Elderly: No pharmacokinetic data are available in patients over 65 years of age.

5.3 Preclinical safety data

There are no data available on the effects of the combination of abacavir and lamivudine in animals.

Mutagenicity and carcinogenicity

Neither abacavir nor lamivudine were mutagenic in bacterial tests, but like many nucleoside analogues they show activity in the *in vitro* mammalian tests such as the mouse lymphoma assay. This is consistent with the known activity of other nucleoside analogues.

Lamivudine has not shown any genotoxic activity in the *in vivo* studies at doses that gave plasma concentrations up to 30-40 times higher than clinical plasma concentrations. Abacavir has a weak potential to cause chromosomal damage both *in vitro* and *in vivo* at high tested concentrations.

The carcinogenic potential of a combination of abacavir and lamivudine has not been tested. In long-term oral carcinogenicity studies in rats and mice, lamivudine did not show any carcinogenic potential. Carcinogenicity studies with orally administered abacavir in mice and rats showed an increase in the incidence of malignant and non-malignant tumours. Malignant tumours occurred in the preputial gland of males and the clitoral gland of females of both species, and in rats in the thyroid gland of males and in the liver, urinary bladder, lymph nodes and the subcutis of females.

The majority of these tumours occurred at the highest abacavir dose of 330 mg/kg/day in mice and 600 mg/kg/day in rats. The exception was the preputial gland tumour which occurred at a dose of 110 mg/kg in mice. The systemic exposure at the no effect level in mice and rats was equivalent to 3 and 7 times the human systemic exposure during therapy. While the carcinogenic potential in humans is unknown, these data suggest that a carcinogenic risk to humans is outweighed by the potential clinical benefit.

Repeat-dose toxicity

In toxicology studies abacavir was shown to increase liver weights in rats and monkeys. The clinical relevance of this is unknown. There is no evidence from clinical studies that abacavir is hepatotoxic. Additionally, autoinduction of abacavir metabolism or induction of the metabolism of other medicinal products hepatically metabolised has not been observed in man.

Mild myocardial degeneration in the heart of mice and rats was observed following administration of abacavir for two years. The systemic exposures were equivalent to 7 to 24 times the expected systemic exposure in humans. The clinical relevance of this finding has not been determined.

Reproductive toxicology

In reproductive toxicity studies in animals, lamivudine and abacavir were shown to cross the placenta.

Lamivudine was not teratogenic in animal studies but there were indications of an increase in early embryonic deaths in rabbits at relatively low systemic exposures, comparable to those achieved in humans. A similar effect was not seen in rats even at very high systemic exposure.

Abacavir demonstrated toxicity to the developing embryo and foetus in rats, but not in rabbits. These findings included decreased foetal body weight, foetal oedema, and an increase in skeletal variations/malformations, early intra-uterine deaths and still births. No conclusion can be drawn with regard to the teratogenic potential of abacavir because of this embryo-foetal toxicity.

A fertility study in rats has shown that abacavir and lamivudine had no effect on male or female fertility.

6. PHARMACEUTICAL PARTICULARS

6.1 List of excipients

Core:

magnesium stearate

microcrystalline cellulose

sodium starch glycollate.

Coating:

Opadry Orange YS-1-13065-A containing:

hypromellose

titanium dioxide (E171)

macrogol 400, polysorbate 80

sunset yellow aluminium lake (E110).

6.2 Incompatibilities

Not applicable.

6.3 Shelf life

3 years.

6.4 Special precautions for storage

Do not store above 30°C.

6.5 Nature and contents of container

30 tablets in opaque white (PVC/PVDC/Aluminium) blister packs and white (HDPE) bottles with child-resistant closure.

6.6 Instructions for use and handling

No special requirements.

Administrative Data

7. MARKETING AUTHORISATION HOLDER

Glaxo Group Ltd

Greenford

Middlesex UB6 0NN

United Kingdom

8. MARKETING AUTHORISATION NUMBER(S)

EU\1\04\298\001

EU\1\04\298\002

9. DATE OF FIRST AUTHORISATION/RENEWAL OF THE AUTHORISATION

17 December 2004

10. DATE OF REVISION OF THE TEXT

Klaricid 250mg Tablets

(Abbott Laboratories Limited)

1. NAME OF THE MEDICINAL PRODUCT

Klaricid **or Clarithromycin 250 mg Tablets**

2. QUALITATIVE AND QUANTITATIVE COMPOSITION

Active: Clarithromycin 250 mg/tablet

3. PHARMACEUTICAL FORM

A yellow, ovaloid film-coated tablet containing 250 mg of clarithromycin.

4. CLINICAL PARTICULARS

4.1 Therapeutic indications

Clarithromycin is indicated for treatment of infections caused by susceptible organisms. Indications include:

Lower respiratory tract infections for example, acute and chronic bronchitis, and pneumonia.

Upper respiratory tract infections for example, sinusitis and pharyngitis.

Clarithromycin is appropriate for initial therapy in community acquired respiratory infections and has been shown to be active *in vitro* against common and atypical respiratory pathogens as listed in the microbiology section.

Clarithromycin is also indicated in skin and soft tissue infections of mild to moderate severity.

Clarithromycin in the presence of acid suppression effected by omeprazole or lansoprazole is also indicated for the eradication of *H. pylori* in patients with duodenal ulcers. See Dosage and Administration section.

Clarithromycin is usually active against the following organisms in vitro:

Gram-positive Bacteria: *Staphylococcus aureus* (methicillin susceptible); *Streptococcus pyogenes* (Group A beta-hemolytic streptococci); alpha-hemolytic streptococci (viridans group); *Streptococcus (Diplococcus) pneumoniae; Streptococcus agalactiae; Listeria monocytogenes*.

Gram-negative Bacteria: *Haemophilus influenzae; Haemophilus parainfluenzae; Moraxella (Branhamella) catarrhalis; Neisseria gonorrhoeae; Legionella pneumophila; Bordetella pertussis; Helicobacter pylori; Campylobacter jejuni.*

Mycoplasma: *Mycoplasma pneumoniae; Ureaplasma urealyticum.*

Other Organisms: *Chlamydia trachomatis; Mycobacterium avium; Mycobacterium leprae.*

Anaerobes: Macrolide-*susceptible Bacteroides fragilis; Clostridium perfringens*; Peptococcus species; Peptostreptococcus species; *Propionibacterium acnes*.

Clarithromycin has bactericidal activity against several bacterial strains. The organisms include *Haemophilus influenzae; Streptococcus pneumoniae; Streptococcus pyogenes; Streptococcus agalactiae; Moraxella (Branhamella) catarrhalis; Neisseria gonorrhoeae; H. pylori* and Campylobacter spp.

The activity of clarithromycin against *H. pylori* is greater at neutral pH than at acid pH.

4.2 Posology and method of administration

Patients with respiratory tract/skin and soft tissue infections.

Adults: The usual dose is 250 mg twice daily for 7 days although this may be increased to 500mg twice daily for up to 14 days in severe infections.

Children older than 12 years: As for adults.

Children younger than 12 years: Use Clarithromycin Paediatric Suspension.

Eradication of *H. pylori* in patients with duodenal ulcers (Adults)

Triple Therapy (7 - 14 days)

Clarithromycin (500mg) twice daily and lansoprazole 30mg twice daily should be given with amoxycillin 1000mg twice daily for 7 - 14 days.

Triple Therapy (7 days)

Clarithromycin (500mg) twice daily and lansoprazole 30mg twice daily should be given with metronidazole 400mg twice daily for 7 days.

Triple Therapy (7 days)

Clarithromycin (500mg) twice daily and omeprazole 40mg daily should be given with amoxycillin 1000mg twice daily or metronidazole 400mg twice daily for 7 days.

Triple Therapy (10 days)

Clarithromycin (500mg) twice daily should be given with amoxycillin 1000mg twice daily and omeprazole 20mg daily for 10 days.

Dual Therapy (14 days)

The usual dose of Clarithromycin is 500 mg three times daily for 14 days. Clarithromycin should be administered with oral omeprazole 40 mg once daily. The pivotal study was conducted with omeprazole 40 mg once daily for 28 days. Supportive studies have been conducted with omeprazole 40 mg once daily for 14 days.

For further information on the dosage for omeprazole see the Astra data sheet.

Elderly: As for adults.

Renal impairment: Dosage adjustments are not usually required except in patients with severe renal impairment (creatinine clearance < 30 ml/min). If adjustment is necessary, the total daily dosage should be reduced by half, e.g. 250 mg once daily or 250 mg twice daily in more severe infections.

Clarithromycin may be given without regard to meals as food does not affect the extent of bioavailability.

4.3 Contraindications

Clarithromycin is contra-indicated in patients with known hypersensitivity to macrolide antibiotic drugs.

Clarithromycin and ergot derivatives should not be co-administered.

Concomitant administration of clarithromycin and any of the following drugs is contraindicated: cisapride, pimozide and terfenadine. Elevated cisapride, pimozide and terfenadine levels have been reported in patients receiving either of these drugs and clarithromycin concomitantly. This may result in QT prolongation and cardiac arrhythmias including ventricular tachycardia, ventricular fibrillation and Torsade de Pointes. Similar effects have been observed with concomitant administration of astemizole and other macrolides.

4.4 Special warnings and special precautions for use

Clarithromycin is principally excreted by the liver and kidney. Caution should be exercised in administering this antibiotic to patients with impaired hepatic or renal function.

Prolonged or repeated used of clarithromycin may result in an overgrowth of non-susceptible bacteria or fungi. If super-infection occurs, clarithromycin should be discontinued and appropriate therapy instituted.

H. pylori organisms may develop resistance to clarithromycin in a small number of patients.

4.5 Interaction with other medicinal products and other forms of Interaction

Clarithromycin has been shown not to interact with oral contraceptives.

As with other macrolide antibiotics the use of clarithromycin in patients concurrently taking drugs metabolised by the cytochrome P450 system (eg. warfarin, ergot alkaloids, triazolam, midazolam, disopyramide, lovastatin, rifabutin, phenytoin, cyclosporin and tacrolimus) may be associated with elevations in serum levels of these other drugs. Rhabdomyolysis, co-incident with the co- administration of clarithromycin, and HMG-CoA reductase inhibitors, such as lovastatin and simvastatin has been reported.

The administration of clarithromycin to patients who are receiving theophylline has been associated with an increase in serum theophylline levels and potential theophylline toxicity.

The use of clarithromycin in patients receiving warfarin may result in potentiation of the effects of warfarin. Prothrombin time should be frequently monitored in these patients. The effects of digoxin may be potentiated with concomitant administration of Klaricid **or Clarithromycin 250 mg Tablets**. Monitoring of serum digoxin levels should be considered.

Clarithromycin may potentiate the effects of carbamazepine due to a reduction in the rate of excretion.

Simultaneous oral administration of clarithromycin tablets and zidovudine to HIV infected adult patients may result in decreased steady-state zidovudine levels. This can be largely avoided by staggering the doses of Clarithromycin and zidovudine by 1 -2 hours. No such reaction has been reported in children.

Ritonavir increases the area under the curve (AUC), C_{max} and C_{min} of clarithromycin when administered concurrently. Because of the large therapeutic window for clarithromycin, no dosage reduction should be necessary in patients with normal renal function. However, for patients with renal impairment, the following dosage adjustments should be considered: For patients with CL_{CR} 30 to 60 ml/min the dose of clarithromycin should be reduced by 50%.

For patients with CL_{CR} <30ml/min the dose of clarithromycin should be decreased by 75%. Doses of clarithromycin greater than 1g/day should not be coadministered with ritonavir.

Although the plasma concentrations of clarithromycin and omeprazole may be increased when they are administered concurrently, no adjustment to the dosage is necessary. At the dosages recommended, there is no clinically significant interaction between clarithromycin and lansoprazole. Increased plasma concentrations of clarithromycin may also occur when it is co-administered with Maalox or ranitidine. No adjustment to the dosage is necessary.

4.6 Pregnancy and lactation

The safety of clarithromycin during pregnancy and breast feeding of infants has not been established. Clarithromycin should thus not be used during pregnancy or lactation unless the benefit is considered to outweigh the risk. Some animal studies have suggested an embryotoxic effect, but only at dose levels which are clearly toxic to mothers. Clarithromycin has been found in the milk of lactating animals and in human breast milk.

4.7 Effects on ability to drive and use machines

None known.

4.8 Undesirable effects

Clarithromycin is generally well tolerated. Side effects include nausea, dyspepsia, diarrhoea, vomiting, abdominal pain and paraesthesia. Stomatitis, glossitis, oral monilia and tongue discolouration have been reported. Other side-effects include headache, arthralgia, myalgia and allergic reactions ranging from urticaria, mild skin eruptions and angioedema to anaphylaxis and rarely Stevens-Johnson syndrome / toxic epidermal necrolysis.

Reports of alteration of the sense of smell, usually in conjunction with taste perversion have also been received. There have been reports of tooth discolouration in patients treated with clarithromycin. Tooth discolouration is usually reversible with professional dental cleaning.

There have been reports of transient central nervous system side-effects including dizziness, vertigo, anxiety, insomnia, bad dreams, tinnitus, confusion, disorientation, hallucinations, psychosis and depersonalisation. There have been reports of hearing loss with clarithromycin which is usually reversible on withdrawal of therapy. Pseudomembranous colitis has been reported rarely with clarithromycin, and may range in severity from mild to life threatening. There have been rare reports of hypoglycaemia, some of which have occurred in patients on concomitant oral hypoglycaemic agents or insulin. There have been very rare reports of uveitis mainly in patients treated with concomitant rifabutin, most of these were reversible. Isolated cases of leukopenia and thrombocytopenia have been reported.

As with other macrolides, hepatic dysfunction (which is usually reversible) including altered liver function tests, hepatitis and cholestasis with or without jaundice, has been reported. Dysfunction may be severe and very rarely fatal hepatic failure has been reported.

Cases of increased serum creatinine, interstitial nephritis, renal failure, pancreatitis and convulsions have been reported rarely.

As with other macrolides, QT prolongation, ventricular tachycardia and Torsade de Pointes have been rarely reported with clarithromycin.

4.9 Overdose

Reports indicate that the ingestion of large amounts of clarithromycin can be expected to produce gastro-intestinal symptoms. One patient who had a history of bipolar disorder ingested 8 grams of clarithromycin and showed altered mental status, paranoid behaviour, hypokalemia and hypoxemia. Adverse reactions accompanying overdosage should be treated by gastric lavage and supportive measures. As with other macrolides, clarithromycin serum levels are not expected to be appreciably affected by haemodialysis or peritoneal dialysis.

5. PHARMACOLOGICAL PROPERTIES

5.1 Pharmacodynamic properties

Clarithromycin is a semi-synthetic derivative of erythromycin A. It exerts its antibacterial action by binding to the 50s ribosomal sub-unit of susceptible bacteria and suppresses protein synthesis. It is highly potent against a wide variety of aerobic and anaerobic gram-positive and gram-negative organisms. The minimum inhibitory concentrations (MICs) of clarithromycin are generally two-fold lower than the MICs of erythromycin.

The 14-hydroxy metabolite of clarithromycin also has antimicrobial activity. The MICs of this metabolite are equal or two-fold higher than the MICs of the parent compound, except for *H. influenzae* where the 14-hydroxy metabolite is two-fold more active than the parent compound.

Clarithromycin is usually active against the following organisms in vitro:-

Gram-positive Bacteria: *Staphylococcus aureus* (methicillin susceptible); *Streptococcus pyogenes* (Group A beta-hemolytic streptococci); alpha-hemolytic streptococci (viridans group); *Streptococcus (Diplococcus) pneumoniae; Streptococcus agalactiae; Listeria monocytogenes*.

Gram-negative Bacteria: *Haemophilus influenzae; Haemophilus parainfluenzae; Moraxella (Branhamella) catarrhalis; Neisseria gonorrhoeae; Legionella pneumophila; Bordetella pertussis; Helicobacter pylori; Campylobacter jejuni.*

Mycoplasma: *Mycoplasma pneumoniae; Ureaplasma urealyticum*.

Other Organisms: *Chlamydia trachomatis; Mycobacterium avium; Mycobacterium leprae*.

Anaerobes: Macrolide-susceptible *Bacteroides fragilis; Clostridium perfringens*; Peptococcus species; Peptostreptococcus species; *Propionibacterium acnes*.

Clarithromycin has bactericidal activity against several bacterial strains. The organisms include *Haemophilus influenzae, Streptococcus pneumoniae, Streptococcus pyogenes, Streptococcus agalactiae, Moraxella (Branhamella) catarrhalis, Neisseria gonorrhoeae, H. pylori* and Campylobacter spp.

5.2 Pharmacokinetic properties

H. pylori is associated with acid peptic disease including duodenal ulcer and gastric ulcer in which about 95% and 80% of patients respectively are infected with the agent. *H. pylori* is also implicated as a major contribution factor in the development of gastric and ulcer recurrence in such patients.

Clarithromycin has been used in small numbers of patients in other treatment regimens. Possible kinetic interactions have not been fully investigated. These regimens include:

Clarithromycin plus tinidazole and omeprazole; clarithromycin plus tetracycline, bismuth subsalicylate and ranitidine; clarithromycin plus ranitidine alone.

Clinical studies using various different *H. pylori* eradication regimens have shown that eradication of *H. pylori* prevents ulcer recurrence.

Clarithromycin is rapidly and well absorbed from the gastro-intestinal tract after oral administration of Clarithromycin tablets. The microbiologically active metabolite 14-hydroxyclarithromycin is formed by first pass metabolism. Clarithromycin may be given without regard to meals as food does not affect the extent of bioavailability of Clarithromycin tablets. Food does slightly delay the onset of absorption of clarithromycin and formation of the 14-hydroxymetabolite. The pharmacokinetics of clarithromycin are non linear; however, steady-state is attained within 2 days of dosing. At 250 mg b.i.d. 15-20% of unchanged drug is excreted in the urine. With 500 mg b.i.d. daily dosing urinary excretion is greater (approximately 36%). The 14-hydroxyclarithromycin is the major urinary metabolite and accounts for 10-15% of the dose. Most of the remainder of the dose is eliminated in the faeces, primarily via the bile. 5-10% of the parent drug is recovered from the faeces.

When clarithromycin 500 mg is given three times daily, the clarithromycin plasma concentrations are increased with respect to the 500 mg twice daily dosage.

Clarithromycin provides tissue concentrations that are several times higher than the circulating drug levels. Increased levels have been found in both tonsillar and lung tissue. Clarithromycin is 80% bound to plasma proteins at therapeutic levels.

Clarithromycin also penetrates the gastric mucus. Levels of clarithromycin in gastric mucus and gastric tissue are higher when clarithromycin is co-administered with omeprazole than when clarithromycin is administered alone.

5.3 Preclinical safety data

In acute mouse and rat studies, the median lethal dose was greater than the highest feasible dose for administration (5g/kg).

In repeated dose studies, toxicity was related to dose, duration of treatment and species. Dogs were more sensitive than primates or rats. The major clinical signs at toxic doses included emesis, weakness, reduced food consumption and weight gain, salivation, dehydration and hyperactivity. In all species the liver was the primary target organ at toxic doses. Hepatotoxicity was detectable by early elevations of liver function tests. Discontinuation of the drug generally resulted in a return to or toward normal results. Other tissues less commonly affected included the stomach, thymus and other lymphoid tissues and the kidneys. At near therapeutic doses, conjunctival injection and lacrimation occurred only in dogs. At a massive dose of 400mg/kg/day, some dogs and monkeys developed corneal opacities and/or oedema.

Fertility and reproduction studies in rats have shown no adverse effects. Teratogenicity studies in rats (Wistar (p.o.) and Spraque-Dawley (p.o. and i.v.)), New Zealand White rabbits and cynomolgous monkeys failed to demonstrate any teratogenicity from clarithromycin. However, a further similar study in Sprague-Dawley rats indicated a low (6%) incidence of cardiovascular abnormalities which appeared to be due to spontaneous expression of genetic changes. Two mouse studies revealed a variable incidence (3-30%) of cleft palate and embryonic loss was seen in monkeys but only at dose levels which were clearly toxic to the mothers.

6. PHARMACEUTICAL PARTICULARS

6.1 List of excipients

Croscarmellose sodium, starch pregelatinised, cellulose microcrystalline, silica gel, povidone, stearic acid, magnesium stearate, talc, hypromellose, hydroxypropylcellulose, propylene glycol, sorbitan monooleate, titanium dioxide, sorbic acid, vanillin, quinoline yellow E104.

6.2 Incompatibilities

None known.

6.3 Shelf life

The recommended shelf life is 24 months.

6.4 Special precautions for storage

Protect from light. Store in a dry place.

6.5 Nature and contents of container

2/14/56 tablets in a blister original pack. The blisters are packaged in a carton with a pack insert.

6.6 Instructions for use and handling

Not applicable

7. MARKETING AUTHORISATION HOLDER

Abbott Laboratories Limited

Queenborough

Kent

ME11 5EL, UK

8. MARKETING AUTHORISATION NUMBER(S)

PL 0037/0211

9. DATE OF FIRST AUTHORISATION/RENEWAL OF THE AUTHORISATION

09/04/91

10. DATE OF REVISION OF THE TEXT

February 2005

Klaricid 500

(Abbott Laboratories Limited)

1. NAME OF THE MEDICINAL PRODUCT

Klaricid 500 or **Clarithromycin 500 mg Tablets**

2. QUALITATIVE AND QUANTITATIVE COMPOSITION

Active Clarithromycin 500 mg/tablet

3. PHARMACEUTICAL FORM

A yellow, ovaloid film-coated tablet containing 500 mg of clarithromycin.

4. CLINICAL PARTICULARS

4.1 Therapeutic indications

Clarithromycin is indicated for treatment of infections caused by susceptible organisms. Indications include:

Lower respiratory tract infections for example, acute and chronic bronchitis, and pneumonia.

Upper respiratory tract infections for example, sinusitis and pharyngitis.

Clarithromycin is appropriate for initial therapy in community acquired respiratory infections and has been shown to be active in vitro against common and atypical respiratory pathogens as listed in the microbiology section.

Clarithromycin is also indicated in skin and soft tissue infections of mild to moderate severity.

Clarithromycin in the presence of acid suppression effected by omeprazole or lansoprazole is also indicated for the eradication of *H. pylori* in patients with duodenal ulcers. See Dosage and Administration section.

Clarithromycin is usually active against the following organisms *in vitro*:

Gram-positive Bacteria: *Staphylococcus aureus* (methicillin susceptible); *Streptococcus pyogenes* (Group A beta-hemolytic streptococci), alpha-hemolytic streptococci (viridans group)*; Streptococcus (Diplococcus) pneumoniae; Streptococcus agalactiae; Listeria monocytogenes*.

Gram-negative Bacteria: *Haemophilus influenzae, Haemophilus parainfluenzae, Moraxella (Branhamella) catarrhalis, Neisseria gonorrhoeae; Legionella pneumophila, Bordetella pertussis, Helicobacter pylori; Campylobacter jejuni.*

Mycoplasma: *Mycoplasma pneumoniae; Ureaplasma urealyticum.*

Other Organisms: *Chlamydia trachomatis; Mycobacterium avium; Mycobacterium leprae; Mycobacterum kansasii; Mycobacterium chelonae; Mycobacterium fortuitum; Mycobacterium intracellulare.*

Anaerobes: Macrolide-susceptible *Bacteroides fragilis; Clostridium perfringens*; Peptococcus species; Peptostreptococcus species; *Propionibacterium acnes*.

Clarithromycin has bactericidal activity against several bacterial strains. The organisms include *Haemophilus influenzae, Streptococcus pneumoniae, Streptococcus pyogenes, Streptococcus agalactiae, Moraxella (Branhamella) catarrhalis, Neisseria gonorrhoeae, H. pylori* and Campylobacter spp.

The activity of clarithromycin against *H. pylori* is greater at neutral pH than at acid pH.

4.2 Posology and method of administration

Patients with respiratory tract/skin and soft tissue infections.

Adults: The usual dose is 250 mg twice daily for 7 days although this may be increased to 500mg twice daily for up to 14 days in severe infections.

Children older than 12 years: As for adults.

Children younger than 12 years: Use Clarithromycin Paediatric Suspension.

Eradication of *H. pylori* in patients with duodenal ulcers (Adults)

Triple Therapy (7 - 14 days)

Clarithromycin (500mg) twice daily and lansoprazole 30mg twice daily should be given with amoxycillin 1000mg twice daily for 7 - 14 days.

Triple Therapy (7 days)

Clarithromycin (500mg) twice daily and lansoprazole 30mg twice daily should be given with metronidazole 400mg twice daily for 7 days.

Triple Therapy (7 days)

Clarithromycin (500mg) twice daily and omeprazole 40mg daily should be given with amoxycillin 1000mg twice daily or metronidazole 400mg twice daily for 7 days.

Triple Therapy (10 days)

Clarithromycin (500mg) twice daily should be given with amoxycillin 1000mg twice daily and omeprazole 20mg daily for 10 days.

Dual Therapy (14 days)

The usual dose of Clarithromycin is 500 mg three times daily for 14 days. Clarithromycin should be administered with oral omeprazole 40 mg once daily. The pivotal study was conducted with omeprazole 40 mg once daily for 28 days. Supportive studies have been conducted with omeprazole 40 mg once daily for 14 days.

For further information on the dosage for omeprazole see the Astra data sheet.

Elderly: As for adults.

Renal impairment: Dosage adjustments are not usually required except in patients with severe renal impairment (creatinine clearance < 30 ml/min). If adjustment is necessary, the total daily dosage should be reduced by half, e.g. 250 mg once daily or 250 mg twice daily in more severe infections.

Clarithromycin may be given without regard to meals as food does not affect the extent of bioavailability.

4.3 Contraindications

Clarithromycin is contra-indicated in patients with known hypersensitivity to macrolide antibiotic drugs.

Clarithromycin and ergot derivatives should not be co-administered.

Concomitant administration of clarithromycin and any of the following drugs is contraindicated: cisapride, pimozide and terfenadine. Elevated cisapride, pimozide and terfenadine levels have been reported in patients receiving either of these drugs and clarithromycin concomitantly. This may result in QT prolongation and cardiac arrhythmias including ventricular tachycardia, ventricular fibrillation and Torsade de Pointes. Similar effects have been observed with concomitant administration of astemizole and other macrolides.

4.4 Special warnings and special precautions for use

Clarithromycin is principally excreted by the liver and kidney. Caution should be exercised in administering this antibiotic to patients with impaired hepatic or renal function.

Prolonged or repeated used of clarithromycin may result in an overgrowth of non-susceptible bacteria or fungi. If super-infection occurs, clarithromycin should be discontinued and appropriate therapy instituted.

H. pylori organisms may develop resistance to clarithromycin in a small number of patients.

4.5 Interaction with other medicinal products and other forms of Interaction

Clarithromycin has been shown not to interact with oral contraceptives.

As with other macrolide antibiotics the use of clarithromycin in patients concurrently taking drugs metabolised by the cytochrome P450 system (eg. warfarin, ergot alkaloids, triazolam, midazolam, disopyramide, lovastatin, rifabutin, phenytoin, cyclosporin and tacrolimus.) may be associated with elevations in serum levels of these other drugs. Rhabdomyolysis, co-incident with the co- administration of clarithromycin, and HMG-CoA reductase inhibitors, such as lovastatin and simvastatin has been reported.

The administration of clarithromycin to patients who are receiving theophylline has been associated with an increase in serum theophylline levels and potential theophylline toxicity.

The use of clarithromycin in patients receiving warfarin may result in potentiation of the effects of warfarin. Prothrombin time should be frequently monitored in these patients. The effects of digoxin may be potentiated with concomitant administration of Clarithromycin. Monitoring of serum digoxin levels should be considered.

Clarithromycin may potentiate the effects of carbamazepine due to a reduction in the rate of excretion.

Simultaneous oral administration of clarithromycin tablets and zidovudine to HIV infected adult patients may result in decreased steady-state zidovudine levels. This can be largely avoided by staggering the doses of Clarithromycin and zidovudine by 1 -2 hours. No such reaction has been reported in children.

Ritonavir increases the area under the curve (AUC), C_{max} and C_{min} of clarithromycin when administered concurrently. Because of the large therapeutic window for clarithromycin, no dosage reduction should be necessary in patients with normal renal function. However, for patients with renal impairment, the following dosage adjustments should be considered: For patients with CL_{CR} 30 to 60 ml/min the dose of clarithromycin should be reduced by 50%. For patients with CL_{CR} <30ml/min the dose of clarithromycin should be decreased by 75%. Doses of clarithromycin greater than 1g/day should not be coadministered with ritonavir.

Although the plasma concentrations of clarithromycin and omeprazole may be increased when they are administered concurrently, no adjustment to the dosage is necessary. At the dosages recommended, there is no clinically significant interaction between clarithromycin and lansoprazole. Increased plasma concentrations of clarithromycin may also occur when it is co-administered with Maalox or ranitidine. No adjustment to the dosage is necessary.

4.6 Pregnancy and lactation

The safety of clarithromycin during pregnancy and breast feeding of infants has not been established. Clarithromycin should thus not be used during pregnancy or lactation unless the benefit is considered to outweigh the risk. Some animal studies have suggested an embryotoxic effect, but only at dose levels which are clearly toxic to mothers. Clarithromycin has been found in the milk of lactating animals and in human breast milk.

4.7 Effects on ability to drive and use machines

None known.

4.8 Undesirable effects

Clarithromycin is generally well tolerated. Side effects include nausea, dyspepsia, diarrhoea, vomiting, abdominal pain and paraesthesia. Stomatitis, glossitis, oral monilia and tongue discolouration have been reported. Other side-effects include headache, arthralgia, myalgia and allergic reactions ranging from urticaria, mild skin eruptions and angioedema to anaphylaxis and rarely Stevens-Johnson syndrome / toxic epidermal necrolysis.

Reports of alteration of the sense of smell, usually in conjunction with taste perversion have also been received. There have been reports of tooth discolouration in patients treated with clarithromycin. Tooth discolouration is usually reversible with professional dental cleaning.

There have been reports of transient central nervous system side-effects including dizziness, vertigo, anxiety, insomnia, bad dreams, tinnitus, confusion, disorientation, hallucinations, psychosis and depersonalisation. There have been reports of hearing loss with clarithromycin which is usually reversible on withdrawal of therapy. Pseudomembranous colitis has been reported rarely with clarithromycin, and may range in severity from mild to life threatening. There have been rare reports of hypoglycaemia, some of which have occurred in patients on concomitant oral hypoglycaemic agents or insulin. There have been very rare reports of uveitis mainly in patients treated with concomitant rifabutin, most of these were reversible. Isolated cases of leukopenia andthrombocytopenia have been reported.

As with other macrolides, hepatic dysfunction (which is usually reversible) including altered liver function tests, hepatitis and cholestasis with or without jaundice, has been reported. Dysfunction may be severe and very rarely fatal hepatic failure has been reported.

Cases of increased serum creatinine, interstitial nephritis, renal failure, pancreatitis and convulsions have been reported rarely.

As with other macrolides, QT prolongation, ventricular tachycardia and Torsade de Pointes have been rarely reported with clarithromycin.

4.9 Overdose

Reports indicate that the ingestion of large amounts of clarithromycin can be expected to produce gastro-intestinal symptoms. One patient who had a history of bipolar disorder ingested 8 grams of clarithromycin and showed altered mental status, paranoid behaviour, hypokalemia and hypoxemia. Adverse reactions accompanying overdosage should be treated by gastric lavage and supportive measures. As with other macrolides, clarithromycin serum levels are not expected to be appreciably affected by haemodialysis or peritoneal dialysis.

5. PHARMACOLOGICAL PROPERTIES

5.1 Pharmacodynamic properties

Clarithromycin is a semi-synthetic derivative of erythromycin A. It exerts its antibacterial action by binding to the 50s ribosomal sub-unit of susceptible bacteria and suppresses protein synthesis. It is highly potent against a wide variety of aerobic and anaerobic gram-positive and gram-negative organisms. The minimum inhibitory concentrations (MICs) of clarithromycin are generally two-fold lower than the MICs of erythromycin.

The 14-hydroxy metabolite of clarithromycin also has antimicrobial activity. The MICs of this metabolite are equal or two-fold higher than the MICs of the parent compound, except for *H. influenzae* where the 14-hydroxy metabolite is two-fold more active than the parent compound.

Clarithromycin is usually active against the following organisms in vitro:-

Gram-positive Bacteria: *Staphylococcus aureus* (methicillin susceptible); *Streptococcus pyogenes* (Group A beta-hemolytic streptococci) alpha-hemolytic streptococci (viridans group); *Streptococcus (Diplococcus) pneumoniae; Streptococcus agalactiae; Listeria monocytogenes*.

Gram-negative Bacteria: *Haemophilus influenzae, Haemophilus parainfluenzae, Moraxella (Branhamella) catarrhalis, Neisseria gonorrhoeae; Legionella pneumophila, Bordetella pertussis, Helicobacter pylori; Campylobacter jejuni.*

Mycoplasma: *Mycoplasma pneumoniae; Ureaplasma urealyticum.*

Other Organisms: *Chlamydia trachomatis; Mycobacterium avium; Mycobacterium leprae; Mycobacterum kansasii; Mycobacterium chelonae; Mycobacterium fortuitum; Mycobacterium intracellulare*.

Anaerobes: Macrolide-susceptible *Bacteroides fragilis; Clostridium perfringens*; Peptococcus species; Peptostreptococcus species; *Propionibacterium acnes*.

Clarithromycin has bactericidal activity against several bacterial strains. The organisms include *Haemophilus influenzae, Streptococcus pneumoniae, Streptococcus pyogenes, Streptococcus agalactiae, Moraxella (Branhamella) catarrhalis, Neisseria gonorrhoeae, H. pylori* and Campylobacter spp.

5.2 Pharmacokinetic properties

H. pylori is associated with acid peptic disease including duodenal ulcer and gastric ulcer in which about 95% and 80% of patients respectively are infected with the agent. *H. pylori* is also implicated as a major contribution factor in the development of gastritis and ulcer recurrence in such patients.

Clarithromycin has been used in small numbers of patients in other treatment regimens. Possible kinetic interactions have not been fully investigated. These regimens include:

Clarithromycin plus tinidazole and omeprazole; clarithromycin plus tetracycline, bismuth subsalicylate and ranitidine; clarithromycin plus ranitidine alone.

Clinical studies using various different *H. pylori* eradication regimens have shown that eradication of *H. pylori* prevents ulcer recurrence.

Clarithromycin is rapidly and well absorbed from the gastro-intestinal tract after oral administration of Clarithromycin tablets. The microbiologically active metabolite 14-hydroxyclarithromycin is formed by first pass metabolism. Clarithromycin may be given without regard to meals as food does not affect the extent of bioavailability of Clarithromycin tablets. Food does slightly delay the onset of absorption of clarithromycin and formation of the 14-hydroxymetabolite. The pharmacokinetics of clarithromycin are non linear; however, steady-state is attained within 2 days of dosing. At 250 mg b.i.d. 15-20% of unchanged drug is excreted in the urine. With 500 mg b.i.d. daily dosing urinary excretion is greater (approximately 36%). The 14-hydroxyclarithromycin is the major urinary metabolite and accounts for 10-15% of the dose. Most of the remainder of the dose is eliminated in the faeces, primarily via the bile. 5-10% of the parent drug is recovered from the faeces.

When clarithromycin 500 mg is given three times daily, the clarithromycin plasma concentrations are increased with respect to the 500 mg twice daily dosage.

Clarithromycin provides tissue concentrations that are several times higher than the circulating drug levels. Increased levels have been found in both tonsillar and lung tissue. Clarithromycin is 80% bound to plasma proteins at therapeutic levels.

Clarithromycin also penetrates the gastric mucus. Levels of clarithromycin in gastric mucus and gastric tissue are higher when clarithromycin is co-administered with omeprazole than when clarithromycin is administered alone.

5.3 Preclinical safety data

In acute mouse and rat studies, the median lethal dose was greater than the highest feasible dose for administration (5g/kg).

In repeated dose studies, toxicity was related to dose, duration of treatment and species. Dogs were more sensitive than primates or rats. The major clinical signs at toxic doses included emesis, weakness, reduced food consumption and weight gain, salivation, dehydration and hyperactivity. In all species the liver was the primary target organ at toxic doses. Hepatotoxicity was detectable by early elevations of liver function tests. Discontinuation of the drug generally resulted in a return to or toward normal results. Other tissues less commonly affected included the stomach, thymus and other lymphoid tissues and the kidneys. At near therapeutic doses, conjunctival injection and lacrimation occurred only in dogs. At a massive dose of 400mg/kg/day, some dogs and monkeys developed corneal opacities and/or oedema.

Fertility and reproduction studies in rats have shown no adverse effects. Teratogenicity studies in rats (Wistar (p.o.) and Sprague-Dawley (p.o. and i.v.)), New Zealand White rabbits and cynomolgous monkeys failed to demonstrate any teratogenicity from clarithromycin. However, a further similar study in Sprague-Dawley rats indicated a low (6%) incidence of cardiovascular abnormalities which appeared to be due to spontaneous expression of genetic changes. Two mouse studies revealed a variable incidence (3-30%) of cleft palate and embryonic loss was seen in monkeys but only at dose levels which were clearly toxic to the mothers.

6. PHARMACEUTICAL PARTICULARS

6.1 List of excipients

Croscarmellose sodium, cellulose microcrystalline, silicon dioxide, povidone, stearic acid, magnesium stearate, talc, hypromellose, hydroxypropylcellulose, propylene glycol, sorbitan monooleate, titanium dioxide, sorbic acid, vanillin, quinoline yellow E104.

6.2 Incompatibilities

None known.

6.3 Shelf life

36 months.

6.4 Special precautions for storage

Store in a dry place, protected from light.

6.5 Nature and contents of container

Tablets in a 300μ PVC/60gsm PVdC/20μ Al foil blister pack. Pack sizes are 14,20,28,42,84,168 tablets in a carton with a patient leaflet.

Tablets in HDPE bottle with a patient leaflet. Pack sizes are 100,250,500,1000 tablets.

6.6 Instructions for use and handling

Not applicable

7. MARKETING AUTHORISATION HOLDER

Abbott Laboratories Limited
Queenborough
Kent
ME11 5EL,
England
United Kingdom

8. MARKETING AUTHORISATION NUMBER(S)

PL 0037/0254

9.

9. DATE OF FIRST AUTHORISATION/RENEWAL OF THE AUTHORISATION

24/03/94

10. DATE OF REVISION OF THE TEXT

February 2005

Klaricid IV

(Abbott Laboratories Limited)

1. NAME OF THE MEDICINAL PRODUCT

Klaricid IV **or Clarithromycin 500 mg/vial Powder for Solution for Injection**

2. QUALITATIVE AND QUANTITATIVE COMPOSITION

Active: Clarithromycin 500mg/vial

3. PHARMACEUTICAL FORM

Lyophilised powder for reconstitution to give a solution for IV administration.

4. CLINICAL PARTICULARS

4.1 Therapeutic indications

Klaricid IV **or Clarithromycin 500 mg/vial Powder for Solution for Injection** is indicated whenever parenteral therapy is required for treatment of infections caused by susceptible organisms in the following conditions;

- Lower respiratory tract infections for example, acute and chronic bronchitis, and pneumonia.
- Upper respiratory tract infections for example, sinusitis and pharyngitis.
- Skin and soft tissue infections.

4.2 Posology and method of administration

For intravenous administration only.

Intravenous therapy may be given for 2 to 5 days and should be changed to oral clarithromycin therapy when appropriate.

Adults: The recommended dosage of Klaricid IV **or Clarithromycin 500 mg/vial Powder for Solution for Injection** is 1.0 gram daily, divided into two 500mg doses, appropriately diluted as described below.

Children: At present, there are insufficient data to recommend a dosage regimen for routine use in children.

Elderly: As for adults.

Renal Impairment: In patients with renal impairment who have creatinine clearance less than 30ml/min, the dosage of clarithromycin should be reduced to one half of the normal recommended dose.

Recommended administration:

Klaricid IV **or Clarithromycin 500 mg/vial Powder for Solution for Injection** should be administered into one of the larger proximal veins as an IV infusion over 60 minutes, using a solution concentration of about 2mg/ml. Clarithromycin should not be given as a bolus or an intramuscular injection.

4.3 Contraindications

Klaricid IV **or Clarithromycin 500 mg/vial Powder for Solution for Injection** is contra-indicated in patients with known hypersensitivity to macrolide antibiotic drugs.

Clarithromycin and ergot derivatives should not be co-administered.

Concomitant administration of clarithromycin and any of the following drugs is contraindicated: cisapride, pimozide and terfenadine. Elevated cisapride, pimozide and terfenadine levels have been reported in patients receiving either of these drugs and clarithromycin concomitantly. This may result in QT prolongation and cardiac arrhythmias including ventricular tachycardia, ventricular fibrillation and Torsade de Pointes. Similar effects have been observed with concomitant administration of astemizole and other macrolides.

4.4 Special warnings and special precautions for use

Clarithromycin is principally excreted by the liver and kidney. Caution should be exercised in administering this antibiotic to patients with impaired hepatic and renal function.

Prolonged or repeated use of clarithromycin may result in an overgrowth of non-susceptible bacteria or fungi. If super-infection occurs, clarithromycin should be discontinued and appropriate therapy instituted.

4.5 Interaction with other medicinal products and other forms of Interaction

Clarithromycin has been shown not to interact with oral contraceptives.

As with other macrolide antibiotics the use of clarithromycin in patients concurrently taking drugs metabolised by the cytochrome p450 system (e.g. warfarin, ergot alkaloids, triazolam, midazolam, disopyramide, lovastatin, rifabutin, phenytoin, cyclosporin and tacrolimus) may be associated with elevations in serum levels of these other drugs. Rhabdomyolysis, co-incident with the co-administration of clarithromycin, and HMG-CoA reductase inhibitors, such as lovastatin and simvastatin has been reported.

The administration of Clarithromycin to patients who are receiving theophylline has been associated with increased serum theophylline levels and potential theophylline toxicity.

The use of Clarithromycin in patients receiving warfarin may result in a potentiation of the effects of warfarin. Prothrombin time should be frequently monitored in these patients. The effects of digoxin may be potentiated with concomitant administration of Clarithromycin. Monitoring of serum digoxin levels should be considered.

Clarithromycin may potentiate the effects of carbamazepine due to a reduction in the rate of excretion.

Simultaneous oral administration of clarithromycin tablets and zidovudine to HIV infected adults may result in decreased steady-state zidovudine concentrations. Since this interaction in adults is thought to be due to interference of clarithromycin with simultaneously administered oral zidovudine, this interaction should not be a problem when clarithromycin is administered intravenously. With oral clarithromycin, the interaction can be largely avoided by staggering the doses; see Summary of Product Characteristics for Clarithromycin tablets for further information. No similar reaction has been reported in children.

Ritonavir increases the area under the curve (AUC), C_{max} and C_{min} of clarithromycin when administered concurrently. Because of the large therapeutic window for clarithromycin, no dosage reduction should be necessary in patients with normal renal function. However, for patients with renal impairment, the following dosage adjustments should be considered: For patients with CL_{CR} 30 to 60ml/min the dose of clarithromycin should be decreased by 50%. For patients with CL_{CR} <30ml/min the dose of clarithromycin should be decreased by 75%. Doses of clarithromycin greater than 1g/day should not be coadministered with ritonavir.

4.6 Pregnancy and lactation

The safety of Clarithromycin during pregnancy and breast feeding of infants has not been established. Clarithromycin should thus not be used during pregnancy or lactation unless the benefit is considered to outweigh the risk. Some animal studies have suggested an embryotoxic effect but only at dose levels which are clearly toxic to mothers. Clarithromycin has been found in the milk of lactating animals and in human breast milk.

4.7 Effects on ability to drive and use machines

None reported.

4.8 Undesirable effects

The most frequently reported infusion-related adverse events in clinical studies were injection-site inflammation, tenderness, phlebitis and pain. The most common non-infusion related adverse event reported was taste perversion.

During clinical studies with oral Clarithromycin, the drug was generally well tolerated. Side-effects included nausea, vomiting, diarrhoea, dyspepsia and abdominal pain and paraesthesia. Stomatitis, glossitis and oral monilia have been reported. Other side-effects include headache, tooth and tongue discolouration, arthralgia, myalgia and allergic reactions ranging from urticaria, mild skin eruptions and angioedema to anaphylaxis and, rarely, Stevens-Johnson syndrome/ toxic epidermal necrolysis. Reports of alteration of the sense of smell, usually in conjunction with taste perversion have also been received. There have been reports of transient central nervous system side-effects including dizziness, vertigo, anxiety, insomnia, bad dreams, tinnitus, confusion, disorientation, hallucinations, psychosis, and depersonalisation. There have been reports of hearing loss with clarithromycin which is usually reversible upon withdrawal of therapy.

Pseudomembranous colitis has been reported rarely with clarithromycin, and may range in severity from mild to life threatening.

There have been rare reports of hypoglycaemia, some of which have occurred in patients on concomitant oral hypoglycaemic agents or insulin.

There have been very rare reports of uveitis mainly in patients treated with concomitant rifabutin, most of these were reversible.

Isolated cases of leukopenia and thrombocytopenia have been reported.

As with other macrolides, hepatic dysfunction (which is usually reversible) including altered liver function tests, hepatitis and cholestasis with or without jaundice, has been reported. Dysfunction may be severe and very rarely fatal hepatic failure has been reported.

Cases of increased serum creatinine, interstitial nephritis, renal failure, pancreatitis and convulsions have been reported rarely.

As with other macrolides, QT prolongation, ventricular tachycardia and Torsade de Pointes have been rarely reported with clarithromcyin.

4.9 Overdose

There is no experience of overdosage after IV administration of clarithromycin. However, reports indicate that the ingestion of large amounts of clarithromycin orally can be expected to produce gastro-intestinal symptoms. Adverse reactions accompanying overdosage should be treated by gastric lavage and supportive measures.

As with other macrolides, clarithromycin serum levels are not expected to be appreciably affected by haemodialysis or peritoneal dialysis.

One patient who had a history of bipolar disorder ingested 8 grams of clarithromycin and showed altered mental status, paranoid behaviour, hypokalaemia and hypoxaemia.

5. PHARMACOLOGICAL PROPERTIES

5.1 Pharmacodynamic properties

Clarithromycin is a semi-synthetic derivative of erythromycin A. It exerts its antibacterial action by binding to the 50s ribosomal sub-unit of susceptible bacteria and suppresses protein synthesis. Clarithromycin demonstrates excellent *in vitro* activity against standard strains of clinical isolates. It is highly potent against a wide variety of aerobic and anaerobic gram positive and negative organisms. The minimum inhibitory concentrations (MICs) of clarithromycin are generally two-fold lower than the MICs of erythromycin.

The 14-(R)-hydroxy metabolite of clarithromycin, formed in man by first pass metabolism also has anti-microbial activity. The MICs of this metabolite are equal to or two-fold higher than the MICs of the parent compound except for *H. influenzae* where the 14-hydroxy metabolite is two-fold more active than the parent compound.

Klaricid IV **or Clarithromycin 500 mg/vial Powder for Solution for Injection** is usually active against the following organisms in vitro:

Gram-positive Bacteria:*Staphylococcus aureus* (methicillin susceptible); *Streptococcus pyogenes* (Group A beta-haemolytic streptococci); alpha-haemolytic streptococcus (viridans group); *Streptococcus (Diplococcus) pneumoniae; Streptococcus agalactiae; Listeria monocytogenes.*

Gram-negative Bacteria:*Haemophilus influenzae, Haemophilus parainfluenzae, Moraxella (Branhamella) catarrhalis, Neisseria gonorrhoeae; Legionella pneumophila, Bordetella pertussis, Helicobacter pylori; Campylobacter jejuni.*

Mycoplasma:*Mycoplasma pneumoniae; Ureaplasma urealyticum.*

Other Organisms:*Chlamydia trachomatis; Mycobacterium avium; Mycobacterium leprae; Chlamydia pneumoniae.*

Anaerobes: Macrolide-susceptible *Bacteriodes fragilis; Clostridium perfringens*; Peptococcus species; Peptostreptococcus species; *Propionibacterium acnes.*

Clarithromycin has bactericidal activity against several bacterial strains. These organisms include *H. influenzae, Streptococcus pneumoniae, Streptococcus pyogenes, Streptococcus agalactiae, Morazella (Brahamella) catarrhalis, Neisseria gonorrhoeae, Helicobacter pylori* and Campylobacter spp.

The activity of clarithromycin against *H. pylori* is greater at neutral pH than at acid pH.

5.2 Pharmacokinetic properties

The microbiologically active metabolite 14-hydroxyclarithromycin is formed by first pass metabolism as indicated by lower bioavailability of the metabolite following IV administration. Following IV administration the blood levels of clarithromycin achieved are well in excess of the MIC $_{90}$s for the common pathogens and the levels of 14-hydroxy-clarithromycin exceed the necessary concentrations for important pathogens, e.g. *H. influenzae*.

The pharmacokinetics of clarithromycin and the 14-hydroxy metabolite are non-linear; steady state is achieved by day 3 of IV dosing. Following a single 500mg IV dose over 60 minutes, about 33% clarithromycin and 11% 14-hydroxyclarithromycin is excreted in the urine at 24 hours.

Klaricid IV **or Clarithromycin 500 mg/vial Powder for Solution for Injection** does not contain tartrazine or other azo dyes, lactose or gluten.

5.3 Preclinical safety data

There are no pre-clinical data of relevance to the prescriber which are additional to that already included in other sections of the SPC.

6. PHARMACEUTICAL PARTICULARS

6.1 List of excipients

Lactobionic acid and Sodium Hydroxide EP.

6.2 Incompatibilities

None known. However, Klaricid IV **or Clarithromycin 500 mg/vial Powder for Solution for Injection** should only be diluted with the diluents recommended.

6.3 Shelf life

48 months unopened.

24 hours (at 5°C - 25°C) once reconstituted in 10ml water for injections.

6 hours (at 25°C) or 24 hours at (5°C) once diluted in 250ml of appropriate diluent.

6.4 Special precautions for storage

Do not store above 30° C. Store in the original container.

6.5 Nature and contents of container

30ml Ph.Eur. Type I flint glass tubing vial with a 20mm grey halo-butyl lyophilisation stopper with flip-off capor 15ml Ph.Eur. flint glass tubing vial with a grey bromobutyl lyophilisation stopper with a flip-off cap. Vials are packed in units of 1,4 and 6. Pack size 500mg.

6.6 Instructions for use and handling

Klaricid IV **or Clarithromycin 500 mg/vial Powder for Solution for Injection** should be administered into one of the larger proximal veins as an IV infusion over 60 minutes, using a solution concentration of about 2mg/ml. Clarithromycin should not be given as a bolus or an intramuscular injection.

7. MARKETING AUTHORISATION HOLDER

Abbott Laboratories Limited

Queenborough

Kent

ME11 5EL.

8. MARKETING AUTHORISATION NUMBER(S)

PL 0037 / 0251

9. DATE OF FIRST AUTHORISATION/RENEWAL OF THE AUTHORISATION

22/09/93

10. DATE OF REVISION OF THE TEXT

February 2005

Klaricid Paediatric Suspension

(Abbott Laboratories Limited)

1. NAME OF THE MEDICINAL PRODUCT

Klaricid Paediatric Suspension **or Clarithromycin 125 mg/5ml Granules for Oral Suspension**

2. QUALITATIVE AND QUANTITATIVE COMPOSITION

Active	mg/5ml
Clarithromycin	125

3. PHARMACEUTICAL FORM

White to off - white granules for reconstitution.

4. CLINICAL PARTICULARS

4.1 Therapeutic indications

Klaricid Paediatric Suspension **or Clarithromycin 125 mg/5ml Granules for Oral Suspension** is indicated for the treatment of infections caused by susceptible organisms. Indications include:

Lower respiratory tract infections.

Upper respiratory tract infections.

Skin and skin structure infections.

Acute otitis media.

Klaricid Paediatric Suspension **or Clarithromycin 125 mg/5ml Granules for Oral Suspension** is usually active against the following organisms *in vitro*:

Gram-positive Bacteria:*Staphylococcus aureus* (methicillin susceptible); *Streptococcus pyogenes* (Group A beta-haemolytic streptococci); alpha-haemolytic streptococci (viridans group); *Streptococcus (Diplococcus) pneumoniae*; *Streptococcus agalactiae*; *Listeria monocytogenes*.

Gram-negative Bacteria: *Haemophilus influenzae*, *Haemophilus parainfluenzae*, *Moraxella (Branhamella) catarrhalis*, *Neisseria gonorrhoeae*; *Legionella pneumophila*, *Bordetella pertussis*, *Helicobacter pylori*; *Campylobacter jejuni*.

Mycoplasma: *Mycoplasma pneumoniae*; *Ureaplasma urealyticum*.

Other Organisms:*Chlamydia trachomatis*; *Mycobacterium avium*; *Mycobacterium leprae*; *Chlamydia pneumoniae*.

Anaerobes: Macrolide-susceptible *Bacteroides fragilis*; *Clostridium perfringens*; *Peptococcus* species; *Peptostreptococcus* species; *Propionibacterium acnes*.

Klaricid Paediatric Suspension **or Clarithromycin 125 mg/5ml Granules for Oral Suspension** has bactericidal activity against several bacterial strains. These organisms include *H. influenzae, Streptococcus pneumoniae, Streptococcus pyogenes, Streptococcus agalactiae, Moraxella (Branhamella) catarrhalis, Neisseria gonorrhoeae, Helicobacter pylori and Campylobacter* species.

The activity of clarithromycin against *H. pylori* is greater at neutral pH than at acid pH.

4.2 Posology and method of administration

Recommended doses and dosage schedules:

The usual duration of treatment is for 5 to 10 days depending on the pathogen involved and the severity of the condition. The recommended daily dosage of Klaricid Paediatric Suspension **or Clarithromycin 125 mg/5ml Granules for Oral Suspension** in children is given in the following table and is based on a 7.5mg/kg b.i.d. dosing regime. Doses up to 500mg b.i.d. have been used in the treatment of severe infections.

KLARICID PAEDIATRIC SUSPENSION **OR CLARITHROMYCIN 125 MG/5ML GRANULES FOR ORAL SUSPENSION**

DOSAGE IN CHILDREN

(see Table 1 below)

Preparation for use: 140ml bottle: 74ml of water should be added to the granules in the bottle and shaken to yield 140ml of reconstituted suspension. The concentration of clarithromycin in the reconstituted suspension is 125mg per 5ml.

100 ml bottle:

53ml of water should be added to the granules in the bottle and shaken to yield 100ml of reconstituted suspension. The concentration of clarithromycin in the reconstituted suspension is 125mg per 5ml.

70 ml bottle:

37ml of water should be added to the granules in the bottle and shaken to yield 70ml of reconstituted suspension. The concentration of clarithromycin in the reconstituted suspension is 125mg per 5ml.

50 ml bottle:

27ml of water should be added to the granules in the bottle and shaken to yield 50ml of reconstituted suspension. The concentration of clarithromycin in the reconstituted suspension is 125mg per 5ml.

Sachet: After cutting along the dotted line, empty contents of sachet into a glass, half fill the sachet with cold water. Add to glass and stir thoroughly before taking.

4.3 Contraindications

Klaricid Paediatric Suspension **or Clarithromycin 125 mg/5ml Granules for Oral Suspension** is contra-indicated in patients with known hypersensitivity to macrolide antibiotic drugs and other ingredients.

Klaricid Paediatric Suspension **or Clarithromycin 125 mg/5ml Granules for Oral Suspension** and ergot derivatives should not be co-administered.

Concomitant administration of clarithromycin and any of the following drugs is contraindicated: cisapride, pimozide and terfenadine. Elevated cisapride, pimozide and terfenadine levels have been reported in patients receiving either of these drugs and clarithromycin concomitantly. This may result in QT prolongation and cardiac arrhythmias including ventricular tachycardia, ventricular fibrillation and Torsade de Pointes. Similar effects have been observed with concomitant administration of astemizole and other macrolides.

4.4 Special warnings and special precautions for use

Clarithromycin is principally excreted by the liver and kidneys. This antibiotic should not be administered to paediatric patients with hepatic or renal failure.

Prolonged or repeated use of clarithromycin may result in an overgrowth of non-susceptible bacteria or fungi. If super-infection occurs, clarithromycin should be discontinued and appropriate therapy instituted.

4.5 Interaction with other medicinal products and other forms of Interaction

As with other macrolide antibiotics, the use of clarithromycin in patients concurrently taking drugs metabolised by the cytochrome P450 system (eg. warfarin, ergot alkaloids, triazolam, midazolam, disopyramide, lovastatin, rifabutin, phenytoin, cyclosporin and tacrolimus) may be associated with elevations in serum levels of these other drugs. Rhabdomyolysis, co-incident with the co- administration of clarithromycin, and HMG-CoA reductase inhibitors, such as lovastatin and simvastatin has been reported.

The administration of clarithromycin to patients who are receiving theophylline has been associated with an increase of serum theophylline levels and potential theophylline toxicity.

The use of Klaricid Paediatric Suspension **or Clarithromycin 125 mg/5ml Granules for Oral Suspension** in patients receiving digoxin, warfarin and carbamazepine may result in potentiation of their effects due to a reduction in the rate of excretion. Prothrombin time should be frequently monitored in patients receiving warfarin. Monitoring of serum digoxin levels should be considered.

Ritonavir increases the AUC (area under the curve) of clarithromycin when administered concurrently. Because of the large therapeutic window for clarithromycin, no dosage reduction should be necessary in patients with normal renal function. However, for patients with renal impairment, the following dosage adjustments should be considered: For patients with CL_{CR} 30 to 60 ml/min the dose of clarithromycin should be reduced by 50%. For patients with CL_{CR}<30ml/min the dose of clarithromycin should be decreased by 75%. Doses of clarithromycin greater than 1g/day should not be coadministered with ritonavir.

Simultaneous oral administration of clarithromycin tablets and zidovudine to HIV-infected adult patients may result in decreased steady-state zidovudine levels. To date, this interaction does not appear to occur in paediatric HIV-infected patients taking Klaricid Paediatric Suspension **or Clarithromycin 125 mg/5ml Granules for Oral Suspension** with zidovudine or dideoxyinosine.

4.6 Pregnancy and lactation

The safety of clarithromycin during pregnancy and breast feeding of infants has not been established. Some animal studies have suggested an embryotoxic effect but only at dose levels which are clearly toxic to mothers. Therefore, if a patient of post-pubertal age becomes pregnant, clarithromycin should not be used during pregnancy or lactation unless the benefit outweighs the risk. Clarithromycin has been found in the milk of lactating animals and in human breast milk.

4.7 Effects on ability to drive and use machines

None known.

4.8 Undesirable effects

Clarithromycin is generally well tolerated. Side effects reported include nausea, dyspepsia, diarrhoea, vomiting, abdominal pain and paraesthesia. Stomatitis, glossitis, oral monilia and tongue discolouration have been reported. Other side-effects include headache, arthralgia, myalgia and allergic reactions ranging from urticaria, mild skin eruptions and angioedema to anaphylaxis and rarely Stevens-Johnson syndrome / toxic epidermal necrolysis. Reports of alteration of the sense of smell, usually in conjunction with taste perversion have also been received. There have been reports of tooth discolouration in patients treated with clarithromycin. Tooth discolouration is usually reversible with professional dental cleaning. There have been reports of transient central nervous system side-effects including dizziness, vertigo, anxiety, insomnia, bad dreams, tinnitus, confusion, disorientation, hallucinations, psychosis and depersonalisation. There have been reports of hearing loss with clarithromycin which is usually reversible upon withdrawal of therapy. Pseudomembranous colitis has been reported rarely with clarithromycin, and may range in severity from mild to life threatening. There have been rare reports of hypoglycaemia, some of

Table 1 KLARICID PAEDIATRIC SUSPENSION OR CLARITHROMYCIN 125 MG/5ML GRANULES FOR ORAL SUSPENSION - DOSAGE IN CHILDREN

Dosage Based on Body Weight (kg)

Weight* (kg)	Approx Age (yrs)	Dosage (ml) bid	Dosage per 5ml teaspoonful twice daily
8-11	1 - 2	2.50	1/2
12-19	3 - 6	5.00	1.00
20-29	7 - 9	7.50	1 1/2
30-40	10 - 12	10.00	2.00

* Children < 8 kg should be dosed on a per kg basis (approx. 7.5 mg/kg bid)

which have occurred in patients on concomitant oral hypoglycaemic agents or insulin. There have been very rare reports of uveitis mainly in patients treated with concomitant rifabutin, most of these were reversible.

Isolated cases of leukopenia and thrombocytopenia have been reported. As with other macrolides, hepatic dysfunction (which is usually reversible) including altered liver function tests, hepatitis and cholestasis with or without jaundice, has been reported.

Dysfunction may be severe and very rarely fatal hepatic failure has been reported.

Cases of increased serum creatinine, interstitial nephritis, renal failure, pancreatitis and convulsions have been reported rarely.

As with other macrolides, QT prolongation, ventricular tachycardia and Torsade de Pointes have been rarely reported with clarithromycin.

4.9 Overdose

Reports indicate that the ingestion of large amounts of clarithromycin can be expected to produce gastro-intestinal symptoms. Adverse reactions accompanying overdosage should be treated by gastric lavage and general supportive measures. One patient who had a history of bipolar disorder ingested 8 grams of clarithromycin and showed altered mental status, paranoid behaviour, hypokalaemia and hypoxaemia. As with other macrolides, clarithromycin serum levels are not expected to be appreciably affected by haemodialysis or peritoneal dialysis.

5. PHARMACOLOGICAL PROPERTIES

5.1 Pharmacodynamic properties

Clarithromycin is a semi-synthetic derivative of erythromycin A. It exerts its anti-bacterial action by binding to the 50s ribosomal sub-unit of susceptible bacteria and suppresses protein synthesis. Clarithromycin demonstrates excellent *in-vitro* activity against standard strains of clinical isolates. It is highly potent against a wide variety of aerobic and anaerobic gram-positive and gram-negative organisms. The minimum inhibitory concentrations (MICs) of clarithromycin are generally two-fold lower than the MICs of erythromycin.

The 14-(R)-hydroxy metabolite of clarithromycin formed in man by first pass metabolism also has anti-microbial activity. The MICs of this metabolite are equal or two-fold higher than the MICs of the parent compound, except for H.influenzae where the 14-hydroxy metabolite is two-fold more active than the parent compound. Clarithromycin is also bactericidal against several bacterial strains.

Clarithromycin is usually active against the following organisms in vitro:-

Gram-positive Bacteria:*Staphylococcus aureus* (methicillin susceptible); *Streptococcus pyogenes* (Group A beta-haemolytic streptococci); alpha-haemolytic streptococci (viridans group); *Streptococcus (Diplococcus) pneumoniae*; *Streptococcus agalactiae*; *Listeria monocytogenes*.

Gram-negative Bacteria: *Haemophilus influenzae, Haemophilus parainfluenzae, Moraxella (Branhamella) catarrhalis, Neisseria gonorrhoeae; Legionella pneumophila, Bordetella pertussis, Helicobacter pylori; Campylobacter jejuni*.

Mycoplasma: *Mycoplasma pneumoniae; Ureaplasma urealyticum*.

Other Organisms:*Chlamydia trachomatis; Mycobacterium avium; Mycobacterium leprae; Chlamydia pneumoniae*.

Anaerobes: Macrolide-susceptible *Bacteroides fragilis*; *Clostridium perfringens*; *Peptococcus* species; *Peptostreptococcus* species; *Propionibacterium acnes*.

Clarithromycin also has bactericidal activity against several bacterial strains. These organisms include *H. influenzae, Streptococcus pneumoniae, Streptococcus pyogenes, Streptococcus agalactiae, Moraxella (Brahamella) catarrhalis, Neisseria gonorrhoeae, Helicobacter pylori* and *Campylobacter* species.

5.2 Pharmacokinetic properties

Clarithromycin is rapidly and well absorbed from the gastro-intestinal tract after oral administration. The microbiologically active 14(R)-hydroxyclarithromycin is formed by first pass metabolism. Clarithromycin, may be given without regard to meals as food does not affect the extent of bioavailability. Food does slightly delay the onset of absorption of clarithromycin and formation of the 14-hydroxy metabolite. Although the pharmacokinetics of clarithromycin are non linear, steady state is attained within 2 days of dosing. 14-Hydroxyclarithromycin is the major urinary metabolite and accounts for 10-15% of the dose. Most of the remainder of the dose is eliminated in the faeces, primarily via the bile. 5-10% of the parent drug is recovered from the faeces.

Clarithromycin provides tissue concentrations that are several times higher than circulating drug level. Increased levels of clarithromycin have been found in both tonsillar and lung tissue. Clarithromycin penetrates into the middle ear fluid at concentrations greater than in the serum. Clarithromycin is 80% bound to plasma proteins at therapeutic levels.

Klaricid Paediatric Suspension **or Clarithromycin 125 mg/5ml Granules for Oral Suspension** does not contain tartrazine or other azo dyes, lactose or gluten.

5.3 Preclinical safety data

The acute oral LD_{50} values for a clarithromycin suspension administered to 3-day old mice were 1290 mg/kg for males and 1230 mg/kg for females. The LD_{50} values in 3-day old rats were 1330 mg/kg for males and 1270 mg/kg for females. For comparison, the LD_{50} of orally-administered clarithromycin is about 2700 mg/kg for adult mice and about 3000 mg/kg for adult rats. These results are consistent with other antibiotics of the penicillin group, cephalosporin group and macrolide group in that the LD_{50} is generally lower in juvenile animals than in adults.

In both mice and rats, body weight was reduced or its increase suppressed and suckling behaviour and spontaneous movements were depressed for the first few days following drug administration. Necropsy of animals that died disclosed dark-reddish lungs in mice and about 25% of the rats; rats treated with 2197 mg/kg or more of a clarithromycin suspension were also noted to have a reddish - black substance in the intestines, probably because of bleeding. Deaths of these animals were considered due to debilitation resulting from depressed suckling behaviour or bleeding from the intestines.

Pre-weaning rats (5 days old) were administered a clarithromycin suspension formulation for two weeks at doses of 0, 15, 55 and 200 mg/kg/day. Animals from the 200 mg/kg/day group had decreased body-weight gains, decreased mean haemoglobin and haematocrit values, and increased mean relative kidney weights compared to animals from the control group. Treatment-related minimal to mild multifocal vacuolar degeneration of the intrahepatic bile duct epithelium and an increased incidence of nephritic lesions were also observed in animals from this treatment group. The "no-toxic effect" dosage for this study was 55 mg/kg/day.

An oral toxicity study was conducted in which immature rats were administered a clarithromycin suspension (granules for suspension) for 6 weeks at daily dosages of 0, 15, 50 and 150 mg base/kg/day. No deaths occurred and the only clinical sign observed was excessive salivation for some of the animals at the highest dosage from 1 to 2 hours after administration during the last 3 weeks of treatment. Rats from the 150 mg/kg dose group had lower mean body weights during the first three weeks, and were observed to have decreased mean serum albumin values and increased mean relative liver weight compared to the controls. No treatment-related gross or microscopic histopathological changes were found. A dosage of 150 mg/kg/day produced slight toxicity in the treated rats and the "no effect dosage" was considered to be 50 mg/kg/day.

Juvenile beagle dogs, 3 weeks of age, were treated orally daily for four weeks with 0, 30, 100, or 300 mg/kg of clarithromycin, followed by a 4-week recovery period. No deaths occurred and no changed in the general condition of the animals were observed. Necropsy revealed no abnormalities. Upon histological examination, fatty deposition of centrilobular hepatocytes and cell infiltration of portal areas were observed by light microscopy and an increase in hepatocellular fat droplets was noted by electron microscopy in the 300 mg/kg dose group. The toxic dose in juvenile beagle dogs was considered to be greater than 300 mg/kg and the "no effect dose" 100 mg/kg.

Fertility, Reproduction and Teratogenicity

Fertility and reproduction studies have shown daily dosages of 150-160 mg/kg/day to male and female rats caused no adverse effects on the oestrus cycle, fertility, parturition and number and viability of offspring. Two teratogenicity studies in both Wistar (p.o.) and Sprague-Dawley (p.o. and i.v.) rats, one study in New Zealand white rabbits and one study in cynomolgus monkeys failed to demonstrate any teratogenicity from clarithromycin.

6. PHARMACEUTICAL PARTICULARS

6.1 List of excipients

Carbopol 974P, povidone K90, water purified, hydroxypropylmethylcellulose

phthalate (HP-55), castor oil, acetone, ethanol, silicon dioxide, sucrose, xanthan gum, flavour - fruit punch, potassium sorbate, citric acid, titanium dioxide and maltodextrin

6.2 Incompatibilities

None known.

6.3 Shelf life

Bottles: The recommended shelf life is 36 months.

Once reconstituted, Klaricid Paediatric Suspension **or Clarithromycin 125 mg/5ml Granules for Oral Suspension** should be used within 14 days.

Sachets: The recommended shelf life is 18 months.

6.4 Special precautions for storage

Do not store above 25°C.

6.5 Nature and contents of container

Granules for reconstitution in a HDPE bottle. Pack sizes of 50, 70, 100 and 140ml are available.

Granules for reconstitution in paper/LDPE/Al foil/LDPE sachet. Packs of 2 sachets.

6.6 Instructions for use and handling

Not applicable

7. MARKETING AUTHORISATION HOLDER

Abbott Laboratories Limited
Queenborough
Kent, ME11 5EL

8. MARKETING AUTHORISATION NUMBER(S)

PL 0037/0264

9. DATE OF FIRST AUTHORISATION/RENEWAL OF THE AUTHORISATION

16 October 1995

10. DATE OF REVISION OF THE TEXT

February 2005

Klaricid Paediatric Suspension 250

(Abbott Laboratories Limited)

1. NAME OF THE MEDICINAL PRODUCT

Klaricid Paediatric Suspension 250mg/5ml **or Clarithromycin 250mg/5ml Granules for Oral Suspension**

2. QUALITATIVE AND QUANTITATIVE COMPOSITION

Active	mg/5ml
Clarithromycin	250

3. PHARMACEUTICAL FORM

White to off - white granules for oral suspension.

4. CLINICAL PARTICULARS

4.1 Therapeutic indications

Klaricid Paediatric Suspension 250mg/5ml **or Clarithromycin 250mg/5ml Granules for Oral Suspension** is indicated for the treatment of infections caused by susceptible organisms. Indications include:

Lower respiratory tract infections.

Upper respiratory tract infections.

Skin and skin structure infections.

Acute otitis media.

Klaricid Paediatric Suspension 250mg/5ml **or Clarithromycin 250mg/5ml Granules for Oral Suspension** is usually active against the following organisms *in vitro*:

Gram-positive Bacteria:*Staphylococcus aureus* (methicillin susceptible); *Streptococcus pyogenes* (Group A beta-haemolytic streptococci); alpha-haemolytic streptococci (viridans group); *Streptococcus (Diplococcus) pneumoniae*; *Streptococcus agalactiae*; *Listeria monocytogenes*.

Gram-negative Bacteria: *Haemophilus influenzae*; *Haemophilus parainfluenzae*; *Moraxella (Branhamella) catarrhalis*; *Neisseria gonorrhoeae*; *Legionella pneumophila*; *Bordetella pertussis*; *Helicobacter pylori*; *Campylobacter jejuni*.

Mycoplasma: *Mycoplasma pneumoniae*; *Ureaplasma urealyticum*.

Other Organisms:*Chlamydia trachomatis*; *Mycobacterium avium*; *Mycobacterium leprae*; *Chlamydia pneumoniae*.

Anaerobes: Macrolide-susceptible *Bacteroides fragilis*; *Clostridium perfringens*; Peptococcus species; Peptostreptococcus species; *Propionibacterium acnes*.

Klaricid Paediatric Suspension 250mg/5ml **or Clarithromycin 250mg/5ml Granules for Oral Suspension** has bactericidal activity against several bacterial strains. These organisms include *H. influenzae, Streptococcus pneumoniae, Streptococcus pyogenes, Streptococcus agalactiae, Moraxella (Branhamella) catarrhalis, Neisseria gonorrhoeae, Helicobacter pylori* and Campylobacter species.

The activity of clarithromycin against *H. pylori* is greater at neutral pH than at acid pH.

4.2 Posology and method of administration

Recommended doses and dosage schedules:

The usual duration of treatment is for 5 to 10 days depending on the pathogen involved and the severity of the condition. The recommended daily dosage of Klaricid Paediatric Suspension 250mg/5ml **or Clarithromycin 250mg/5ml Granules for Oral Suspension** in children is given in the following table and is based on a 7.5mg/kg twice a day dosage regimen. Doses up to 500mg twice a day have been used in the treatment of severe infections.

KLARICID PAEDIATRIC SUSPENSION 250MG/5ML **OR CLARITHROMYCIN 250MG/5ML GRANULES FOR ORAL SUSPENSION**

DOSAGE IN CHILDREN

(see Table 1 on next page)

Preparation for use: 140ml bottle: 74ml of water should be added to the granules in the bottle and shaken to yield 140ml of reconstituted suspension. The concentration of clarithromycin in the reconstituted suspension is 250mg per 5ml.

Table 1 KLARICID PAEDIATRIC SUSPENSION 250MG/5ML OR CLARITHROMYCIN 250MG/5ML GRANULES FOR ORAL SUSPENSION - DOSAGE IN CHILDREN

Dosage Based on Body Weight (kg)

Weight * (kg)	Approx Age (yrs)	Dosage twice a day (ml)	(mg)
8-11	1 - 2	1.25	62.50
12-19	3 - 6	2.5	125.00
20-29	7 - 9	3.75	187.50
30-40	10 - 12	5	250.00

* Children < 8 kg should be dosed on a per kg basis (approx. 7.5 mg/kg twice a day)

100 ml bottle:

53ml of water should be added to the granules in the bottle and shaken to yield 100ml of reconstituted suspension. The concentration of clarithromycin in the reconstituted suspension is 250mg per 5ml.

70 ml bottle:

37ml of water should be added to the granules in the bottle and shaken to yield 70ml of reconstituted suspension. The concentration of clarithromycin in the reconstituted suspension is 250mg per 5ml.

50 ml bottle:

27ml of water should be added to the granules in the bottle and shaken to yield 50ml of reconstituted suspension. The concentration of clarithromycin in the reconstituted suspension is 250mg per 5ml.

4.3 Contraindications

Klaricid Paediatric Suspension 250mg/5ml **or Clarithromycin 250mg/5ml Granules for Oral Suspension** is contra-indicated in patients with known hypersensitivity to macrolide antibiotic drugs and other ingredients.

Klaricid Paediatric Suspension 250mg/5ml **or Clarithromycin 250mg/5ml Granules for Oral Suspension** and ergot derivatives should not be co-administered.

Concomitant administration of clarithromycin and any of the following drugs is contraindicated: cisapride, pimozide and terfenadine. Elevated cisapride, pimozide and terfenadine levels have been reported in patients receiving either of these drugs and clarithromycin concomitantly. This may result in QT prolongation and cardiac arrhythmias including ventricular tachycardia, ventricular fibrillation and Torsade de Pointes. Similar effects have been observed with concomitant administration of astemizole and other macrolides.

4.4 Special warnings and special precautions for use

Clarithromycin is principally excreted by the liver and kidneys. This antibiotic should not be administered to paediatric patients with hepatic or renal failure.

Prolonged or repeated use of clarithromycin may result in an overgrowth of non-susceptible bacteria or fungi. If super-infection occurs, clarithromycin should be discontinued and appropriate therapy instituted.

4.5 Interaction with other medicinal products and other forms of Interaction

As with other macrolide antibiotics the use of clarithromycin in patients concurrently taking drugs metabolised by the cytochrome P450 system (eg. warfarin, ergot alkaloids, triazolam, midazolam, disopyramide, lovastatin, rifabutin, phenytoin, cyclosporin and tacrolimus) may be associated with elevations in serum levels of these other drugs. Rhabdomyolysis, co-incident with the co- administration of clarithromycin, and HMG-CoA reductase inhibitors, such as lovastatin and simvastatin has been reported.

The administration of clarithromycin to patients who are receiving theophylline has been associated with an increase of serum theophylline levels and potential theophylline toxicity.

The use of Klaricid Paediatric Suspension 250mg/5ml **or Clarithromycin 250mg/5ml Granules for Oral Suspension** in patients receiving digoxin, warfarin and carbamazepine may result in potentiation of their effects due to a reduction in the rate of excretion. Prothrombin time should be frequently monitored in patients receiving warfarin. Monitoring of serum digoxin levels should be considered.

Ritonavir increases the AUC (area under the curve) of clarithromycin when administered concurrently. Because of the large therapeutic window for clarithromycin, no dosage reduction should be necessary in patients with normal renal function. However, for patients with renal impairment, the following dosage adjustments should be considered: For patients with CL_{CR} 30 to 60 ml/min the dose of clarithromycin should be reduced by 50%. For patients with CL_{CR}<30ml/min the dose of clarithromycin should be decreased by 75%. Doses of clarithromycin greater than 1g/day should not be coadministered with ritonavir.

Simultaneous oral administration of clarithromycin tablets and zidovudine to HIV-infected adult patients may result in decreased steady-state zidovudine levels. To date, this interaction does not appear to occur in paediatric HIV-infected patients taking Klaricid Paediatric Suspension 250mg/5ml **or Clarithromycin 250mg/5ml Granules for Oral Suspension** with zidovudine or dideoxyinosine.

4.6 Pregnancy and lactation

The safety of clarithromycin during pregnancy and breast feeding of infants has not been established. Some animal studies have suggested an embryotoxic effect but only at dose levels which are clearly toxic to mothers. Therefore, if a patient of post-pubertal age becomes pregnant, clarithromycin should not be used during pregnancy or lactation unless the benefit outweighs the risk. Clarithromycin has been found in the milk of lactating animals and in human breast milk.

4.7 Effects on ability to drive and use machines

None known.

4.8 Undesirable effects

Clarithromycin is generally well tolerated. Side effects reported include nausea, dyspepsia, diarrhoea, vomiting and abdominal pain and paraesthesia. Stomatitis, glossitis and oral monilia and tongue discolouration have been reported. Other side-effects include headache, arthralgia, myalgia and allergic reactions ranging from urticaria, mild skin eruptions and angioedema to anaphylaxis and rarely Stevens-Johnson syndrome / toxic epidermal necrolysis.

Reports of alteration of the sense of smell, usually in conjunction with taste perversion have also been received. There have been reports of tooth discolouration in patients treated with clarithromycin. Tooth discolouration is usually reversible with professional dental cleaning.

There have been reports of transient central nervous system side-effects including dizziness, vertigo, anxiety, insomnia, bad dreams, tinnitus, confusion, disorientation, hallucinations, psychosis and depersonalisation. There have been reports of hearing loss with clarithromycin which is usually reversible upon withdrawal of therapy. Pseudomembranous colitis has been reported rarely with clarithromycin, and may range in severity from mild to life threatening. There have been rare reports of hypoglycaemia, some of which have occurred in patients on concomitant oral hypoglycaemic agents or insulin. There have been very rare reports of uveitis in patients treated with concomitant rifabutin, most of these were reversible. Isolated cases of leukopenia andthrombocytopenia have been reported.

As with other macrolides, hepatic dysfunction (which is usually reversible) including altered liver function tests, hepatitis and cholestasis with or without jaundice, has been reported. Dysfunction may be severe and very rarely fatal hepatic failure has been reported.

Cases of increased serum creatinine, interstitial nephritis, renal failure, pancreatitis and convulsions have been reported rarely.

As with other macrolides, QT prolongation, ventricular tachycardia and Torsade de Pointes have been rarely reported with clarithromycin.

4.9 Overdose

Reports indicate that the ingestion of large amounts of clarithromycin can be expected to produce gastro-intestinal symptoms. Adverse reactions accompanying overdosage should be treated by gastric lavage and general supportive measures. One patient who had a history of bipolar disorder ingested 8 grams of clarithromycin and showed altered mental status, paranoid behaviour, hypokalaemia and hypoxaemia. As with other macrolides, clarithromycin serum levels are not expected to be appreciably affected by haemodialysis or peritoneal dialysis.

5. PHARMACOLOGICAL PROPERTIES

5.1 Pharmacodynamic properties

Clarithromycin is a semi-synthetic derivative of erythromycin A. It exerts its anti-bacterial action by binding to the 50s ribosomal sub-unit of susceptible bacteria and suppresses protein synthesis. Clarithromycin demonstrates excellent *in-vitro* activity against standard strains of clinical isolates. It is highly potent against a wide variety of aerobic and anaerobic gram-positive and gram-negative organisms. The minimum inhibitory concentrations (MICs) of clarithromycin are generally two-fold lower than the MICs of erythromycin.

The 14-(R)-hydroxy metabolite of clarithromycin formed in man by first pass metabolism also has anti-microbial activity. The MICs of this metabolite are equal or two-fold higher than the MICs of the parent compound, except for *H.influenzae* where the 14-hydroxy metabolite is two-fold more active than the parent compound. Clarithromycin is also bactericidal against several bacterial strains.

Clarithromycin is usually active against the following organisms *in vitro*:-

Gram-positive Bacteria:*Staphylococcus aureus* (methicillin susceptible); *Streptococcus pyogenes* (Group A beta-haemolytic streptococci); alpha-haemolytic streptococci (viridans group); *Streptococcus (Diplococcus) pneumoniae*; *Streptococcus agalactiae*; *Listeria monocytogenes*.

Gram-negative Bacteria: *Haemophilus influenzae; Haemophilus parainfluenzae; Moraxella (Branhamella) catarrhalis; Neisseria gonorrhoeae; Legionella pneumophila; Bordetella pertussis; Helicobacter pylori; Campylobacter jejuni*.

Mycoplasma: *Mycoplasma pneumoniae; Ureaplasma urealyticum*.

Other Organisms:*Chlamydia trachomatis; Mycobacterium avium; Mycobacterium leprae; Chlamydia pneumoniae*.

Anaerobes: Macrolide-susceptible *Bacteroides fragilis*; *Clostridium perfringens*; Peptococcus species; Peptostreptococcus species; *Propionibacterium acnes*.

Clarithromycin also has bactericidal activity against several bacterial strains. These organisms include *H. influenzae, Streptococcus pneumoniae, Streptococcus pyogenes, Streptococcus agalactiae, Moraxella (Branhamella) catarrhalis, Neisseria gonorrhoeae, Helicobacter pylori* and Campylobacter species.

5.2 Pharmacokinetic properties

Clarithromycin is rapidly and well absorbed from the gastro-intestinal tract after oral administration. The microbiologically active 14(R)-hydroxyclarithromycin is formed by first pass metabolism. Clarithromycin may be given without regard to meals as food does not affect the extent of bioavailability. Food does slightly delay the onset of absorption of clarithromycin and formation of the 14-hydroxy metabolite. Although the pharmacokinetics of clarithromycin are non linear, steady state is attained within 2 days of dosing. 14-Hydroxyclarithromycin is the major urinary metabolite and accounts for 10-15% of the dose. Most of the remainder of the dose is eliminated in the faeces, primarily via the bile. 5-10% of the parent drug is recovered from the faeces.

Clarithromycin provides tissue concentrations that are several times higher than circulating drug level. Increased levels of clarithromycin have been found in both tonsillar and lung tissue. Clarithromycin penetrates into the middle ear fluid at concentrations greater than in the serum. Clarithromycin is 80% bound to plasma proteins at therapeutic levels.

Klaricid Paediatric Suspension 250mg/5ml **or Clarithromycin 250mg/5ml Granules for Oral Suspension** does not contain tartrazine or other azo dyes, lactose or gluten.

5.3 Preclinical safety data

In both mice and rats, body weight was reduced or its increase suppressed and suckling behaviour and spontaneous movements were depressed for the first few days following drug administration. Necropsy of animals that died disclosed dark-reddish lungs in mice and about 25% of the rats; rats treated with 2197 mg/kg or more of a clarithromycin suspension were also noted to have a reddish - black substance in the intestines, probably because of bleeding. Deaths of these animals were considered due to debilitation resulting from depressed suckling behaviour or bleeding from the intestines.

Pre-weaning rats (5 days old) were administered a clarithromycin suspension formulation for two weeks at doses of 0, 15, 55 and 200 mg/kg/day. Animals from the 200 mg/kg/day group had decreased body-weight gains, decreased mean haemoglobin and haematocrit values, and increased mean relative kidney weights compared to animals from the control group. Treatment-related minimal to mild multifocal vacuolar degeneration of the intrahepatic bile duct epithelium and an increased incidence of nephritic lesions were also observed in animals from this treatment group. The "no-toxic effect" dosage for this study was 55 mg/kg/day.

An oral toxicity study was conducted in which immature rats were administered a clarithromycin suspension (granules for suspension) for 6 weeks at daily dosages of 0, 15, 50 and 150 mg base/kg/day. No deaths occurred and the only clinical sign observed was excessive salivation for some of the animals at the highest dosage from 1 to 2 hours after administration during the last 3 weeks of treatment. Rats from the 150 mg/kg dose group had lower mean body weights during the first three weeks, and were observed to have decreased mean serum albumin values and increased mean relative liver weight compared to the controls. No treatment-related gross or microscopic histopathological changes were found. A dosage of 150 mg/kg/day produced slight toxicity in the treated rats and the "no effect dosage" was considered to be 50 mg/kg/day.

Juvenile beagle dogs, 3 weeks of age, were treated orally daily for four weeks with 0, 30, 100, or 300 mg/kg of clarithromycin, followed by a 4-week recovery period. No deaths occurred and no changes in the general condition of the animals were observed. Necropsy revealed no abnormalities. Upon histological examination, fatty deposition of centrilobular hepatocytes and cell infiltration of portal areas were observed by light microscopy and an increase in hepatocellular fat droplets was noted by electron microscopy in the 300 mg/kg dose group. The toxic dose in juvenile beagle dogs was considered to be greater than 300 mg/kg and the "no effect dose" 100 mg/kg.

Fertility, Reproduction and Teratogenicity

Fertility and reproduction studies have shown daily dosages of 150-160 mg/kg/day to male and female rats caused no adverse effects on the oestrus cycle, fertility, parturition and number and viability of offspring. Two teratogenicity studies in both Wistar (p.o.) and Sprague-Dawley (p.o. and i.v.) rats, one study in New Zealand white rabbits and one study in cynomolgus monkeys failed to demonstrate any teratogenicity from clarithromycin.

6. PHARMACEUTICAL PARTICULARS

6.1 List of excipients
Carbopol 974P, povidone K90, water purified, hypromellose phthalate (HP-55), castor oil, silicon dioxide, sucrose, xanthan gum, flavour - fruit punch, potassium sorbate, citric acid, titanium dioxide and maltodextrin.

6.2 Incompatibilities
None known.

6.3 Shelf life
The recommended shelf life of the dry granule is 24 months.

Once reconstituted, Klaricid Paediatric Suspension 250mg/5ml **or Clarithromycin 250mg/5ml Granules for Oral Suspension** should be used within 14 days.

6.4 Special precautions for storage
Do not store above 30°C. Do not refrigerate or freeze.

6.5 Nature and contents of container
Granules for reconstitution in a HDPE bottle. Pack sizes of 50, 70, 100 and 140ml are available.

6.6 Instructions for use and handling
Not applicable.

7. MARKETING AUTHORISATION HOLDER
Abbott Laboratories Limited

Queenborough

Kent

ME11 5EL

8. MARKETING AUTHORISATION NUMBER(S)
0037/0277

9. DATE OF FIRST AUTHORISATION/RENEWAL OF THE AUTHORISATION
19th May 1999

10. DATE OF REVISION OF THE TEXT
February 2005

Klaricid XL

(Abbott Laboratories Limited)

1. NAME OF THE MEDICINAL PRODUCT
Klaricid XL **or Clarithromycin 500 mg Modified Release Tablets**

2. QUALITATIVE AND QUANTITATIVE COMPOSITION
Active: Clarithromycin 500.00 mg/tablet

3. PHARMACEUTICAL FORM
A yellow, ovaloid tablet containing 500mg clarithromycin in a modified-release preparation.

4. CLINICAL PARTICULARS

4.1 Therapeutic indications
Klaricid XL **or Clarithromycin 500 mg Modified Release Tablets** is indicated for treatment of infections caused by susceptible organisms. Indications include:

Lower respiratory tract infections for example, acute and chronic bronchitis, and pneumonia.

Upper respiratory tract infections for example, sinusitis and pharyngitis.

Klaricid XL **or Clarithromycin 500 mg Modified Release Tablets** is also indicated in skin and soft tissue infections of mild to moderate severity, for example folliculitis, cellulitis and erysipelas.

4.2 Posology and method of administration
Adults: The usual recommended dosage of Klaricid XL **or Clarithromycin 500 mg Modified Release Tablets** in adults is one 500mg modified-release tablet daily to be taken with food.

In more severe infections, the dosage can be increased to two 500mg modified-release tablets daily. The usual duration of treatment is 7 to 14 days.

Children older than 12 years: As for adults.

Children younger than 12 years: Use Klaricid Paediatric Suspension **or Clarithromycin 125 mg/5ml Granules for Oral Suspension.**

Klaricid XL **or Clarithromycin 500 mg Modified Release Tablets** should not be used in patients with renal impairment (creatinine clearance less than 30 mL/min). Clarithromycin immediate release tablets may be used in this patient population. (See 4.3 Contra-indications).

4.3 Contraindications
Clarithromycin is contra-indicated in patients with known hypersensitivity to macrolide antibiotic drugs.

Clarithromycin and ergot derivatives should not be co-administered.

As the dose cannot be reduced from 500mg daily, Klaricid XL **or Clarithromycin 500 mg Modified Release Tablets** is contraindicated in patients with creatinine clearance less than 30 mL/min.

Concomitant administration of clarithromycin and any of the following drugs is contraindicated: cisapride, pimozide and terfenadine. Elevated cisapride, pimozide and terfenadine levels have been reported in patients receiving either of these drugs and clarithromycin concomitantly. This may result in QT prolongation and cardiac arrhythmias including ventricular fibrillation and torsade de pointes. Similar effects have been observed with concomitant administration of astemizole and other macrolides.

4.4 Special warnings and special precautions for use
Clarithromycin is principally excreted by the liver and kidney. Caution should be exercised in administering this antibiotic to patients with impaired hepatic and renal function.

Prolonged or repeated used of clarithromycin may result in an overgrowth of non-susceptible bacteria or fungi. If super-infection occurs, clarithromycin should be discontinued and appropriate therapy instituted.

4.5 Interaction with other medicinal products and other forms of Interaction
Clarithromycin has been shown not to interact with oral contraceptives.

As with other macrolide antibiotics the use of clarithromycin in patients concurrently taking drugs metabolised by the cytochrome P450 system (eg. warfarin, ergot alkaloids, triazolam, midazolam, disopyramide, lovastatin, rifabutin, phenytoin, cyclosporin and tacrolimus) may be associated with elevations in serum levels of these other drugs. Rhabdomyolysis, co-incident with the co- administration of clarithromycin, and HMG-CoA reductase inhibitors, such as lovastatin and simvastatin has been reported.

The administration of clarithromycin to patients who are receiving theophylline has been associated with an increase in serum theophylline levels and potential theophylline toxicity.

The use of clarithromycin in patients receiving warfarin may result in potentiation of the effects of warfarin. Prothrombin time should be frequently monitored in these patients.

The effects of digoxin may be potentiated with concomitant administration of clarithromycin. Monitoring of serum digoxin levels should be considered.

Clarithromycin may potentiate the effects of carbamazepine due to a reduction in the rate of excretion.

Interaction studies have not been conducted with Klaricid XL **or Clarithromycin 500 mg Modified Release Tablets** and zidovudine. If concomitant administration of clarithromycin and zidovudine is required, then an immediate release formulation of clarithromycin should be used.

Ritonavir increases the area under the curve (AUC), C_{max} and C_{min} of clarithromycin when administered concurrently. Because of the large therapeutic window for clarithromycin, no dosage reduction should be necessary in patients with normal renal function. However, for patients with renal impairment an immediate release form of clarithromycin should be used. Doses of clarithromycin greater than 1g/day should not be coadministered with ritonavir.

4.6 Pregnancy and lactation
The safety of clarithromycin during pregnancy and breast feeding of infants has not been established. Clarithromycin should thus not be used during pregnancy or lactation unless the benefit is considered to outweigh the risk. Some animal studies have suggested an embryotoxic effect, but only at dose levels which are clearly toxic to mothers. Clarithromycin has been found in the milk of lactating animals and in human breast milk.

4.7 Effects on ability to drive and use machines
The medicine is unlikely to produce an effect.

4.8 Undesirable effects
Clarithromycin is generally well tolerated. Side effects include nausea, dyspepsia, diarrhoea, vomiting, abdominal pain and paraesthesia. Stomatitis, glossitis, oral monilia and tongue discolouration have been reported. Other side-effects include headache, arthralgia, myalgia and allergic reactions ranging from urticaria, mild skin eruptions and angioedema to anaphylaxis and rarely Stevens-Johnson syndrome / toxic epidermal necrolysis.

Reports of alteration of the sense of smell, usually in conjunction with taste perversion have also been received. There have been reports of tooth discolouration in patients treated with clarithromycin. Tooth discolouration is usually reversible with professional dental cleaning.

There have been reports of transient central nervous system side-effects including dizziness, vertigo, anxiety, insomnia, bad dreams, tinnitus, confusion, disorientation, hallucinations, psychosis and depersonalisation. There have been reports of hearing loss with clarithromycin which is usually reversible on withdrawal of therapy. Pseudomembranous colitis has been reported rarely with clarithromycin, and may range in severity from mild to life threatening. There have been rare reports of hypoglycaemia, some of which have occurred in patients on concomitant oral hypoglycaemic agents or insulin. There have been very rare reports of uveitis mainly in patients treated with concomitant rifabutin, most of these were reversible. Isolated cases of leukopenia andthrombocytopenia have been reported.

As with other macrolides, hepatic dysfunction (which is usually reversible) including altered liver function tests, hepatitis and cholestasis with or without jaundice, has been reported. Dysfunction may be severe and very rarely fatal hepatic failure has been reported.

Cases of increased serum creatinine, interstitial nephritis, renal failure, pancreatitis and convulsions have been reported rarely.

As with other macrolides, QT prolongation, ventricular tachycardia and Torsade de Pointes have been rarely reported with clarithromycin.

4.9 Overdose
Reports indicate that the ingestion of large amounts of clarithromycin can be expected to produce gastro-intestinal symptoms. One patient who had a history of bipolar disorder ingested 8 grams of clarithromycin and showed altered mental status, paranoid behaviour, hypokalaemia and hypoxaemia. Adverse reactions accompanying overdosage should be treated by gastric lavage and supportive measures. As with other macrolides, clarithromycin serum levels are not expected to be appreciably affected by haemodialysis or peritoneal dialysis.

5. PHARMACOLOGICAL PROPERTIES

5.1 Pharmacodynamic properties
Clarithromycin is a semi-synthetic derivative of erythromycin A. It exerts its antibacterial action by binding to the 50s ribosomal sub-unit of susceptible bacteria and suppresses protein synthesis. It is highly potent against a wide variety of aerobic and anaerobic gram-positive and gram-negative organisms. The minimum inhibitory concentrations (MICs) of clarithromycin are generally two-fold lower than the MICs of erythromycin.

The 14-hydroxy metabolite of clarithromycin also has antimicrobial activity. The MICs of this metabolite are equal or two-fold higher than the MICs of the parent compound, except for *H. influenzae* where the 14-hydroxy metabolite is two-fold more active than the parent compound.

Clarithromycin is usually active against the following organisms in vitro:

Gram-positive Bacteria: *Staphylococcus aureus* (methicillin susceptible); *Streptococcus pyogenes* (Group A beta-hemolytic streptococci); alpha-hemolytic streptococci (viridans group); *Streptococcus (Diplococcus) pneumoniae; Streptococcus agalactiae; Listeria monocytogenes.*

Gram-negative Bacteria: *Haemophilus influenza; Haemophilus parainfluenza; Moraxella (Branhamella) catarrhalis; Neisseria gonorrhoeae; Legionella pneumophila; Bordetella pertussis; Campylobacter jejuni.*

Mycoplasma: *Mycoplasma pneumoniae; Ureaplasma urealyticum.*

Other Organisms: *Chlamydia trachomatis; Mycobacterium avium; Mycobacterium leprae; Mycobacterium kansasii; Mycobacterium chelonae; Mycobacterium fortuitum; Mycobacterium intracellularis; Chlamydia pneumoniae.*

Anaerobes: *Clostridium perfringens*; Peptococcus species; Peptostreptococcus species; *Propionibacterium acnes*.

Clarithromycin has bactericidal activity against several bacterial strains. The organisms include *Haemophilus influenzae; Streptococcus pneumoniae; Streptococcus pyogenes; Streptococcus agalactiae; Moraxella (Branhamella) catarrhalis; Neisseria gonorrhoeae* and Campylobacter spp.

5.2 Pharmacokinetic properties
The kinetics of orally administered modified-release clarithromycin have been studied in adult humans and compared with clarithromycin 250mg and 500mg immediate release tablets. The extent of absorption was found to be equivalent when equal total daily doses were administered. The absolute bioavailability is approximately 50%. Little or no unpredicted accumulation was found and the metabolic disposition did not change in any species following multiple dosing. Based upon the finding of equivalent absorption the following *in vitro* and *in vivo* data are applicable to the modified-release formulation.

In vitro: Results of in vitro studies showed that the protein binding of clarithromycin in human plasma averaged about 70 % at concentrations of 0.45 - 4.5μg/mL. A decrease in binding to 41% at 45.0μg/mL suggested that the binding sites might become saturated, but this only occurred at concentrations far in excess of therapeutic drug levels.

In vivo: Clarithromycin levels in all tissues, except the central nervous system, were several times higher than the circulating drug levels. The highest concentrations were found in the liver and lung tissue, where the tissue to plasma ratios reached 10 to 20.

The pharmacokinetic behaviour of clarithromycin is non-linear. In fed patients given 500mg clarithromycin modified-release daily, the peak steady state plasma concentration of clarithromycin and 14 hydroxy clarithromycin were 1.3 and 0.48μg/mL, respectively. When the dosage was increased to 1000mg daily, these steady-state values were 2.4μg/mL and 0.67μg/mL respectively. Elimination half-lives of the parent drug and metabolite were approximately 5.3 and 7.7 hours respectively. The apparent half-lives of both clarithromycin and its hydroxylated metabolite tended to be longer at higher doses.

Urinary excretion accounted for approximately 40% of the clarithromycin dose. Faecal elimination accounts for approximately 30%.

5.3 Preclinical safety data
In repeated dose studies, clarithromycin toxicity was related to dose and duration of treatment. The primary target organ was the liver in all species, with hepatic lesions seen after 14 days in dogs and monkeys. Systemic exposure levels associated with this toxicity are not known but toxic mg/kg doses were higher than the dose recommended for patient treatment.

No evidence of mutagenic potential of clarithromycin was seen during a range of in vitro and in vivo tests.

Fertility and reproduction studies in rats have shown no adverse effects. Teratogenicity studies in rats (Wistar (p.o.) and Sprague-Dawley (p.o. and i.v.)), New Zealand White rabbits and cynomolgous monkeys failed to demonstrate any teratogenicity from clarithromycin. However, a further similar study in Sprague-Dawley rats indicated a low (6%) incidence of cardiovascular abnormalities which appeared to be due to spontaneous expression of genetic changes. Two mouse studies revealed a variable incidence (3-30%) of cleft palate and in monkeys embryonic loss was seen but only at dose levels which were clearly toxic to the mothers.

No other toxicological findings considered to be of relevance to the dose level recommended for patient treatment have been reported.

6. PHARMACEUTICAL PARTICULARS

6.1 List of excipients
Citric acid anhydrous, sodium alginate, sodium calcium alginate, lactose, povidone K30, talc, stearic acid, magnesium stearate, methyl hydroxypropylcellulose 6cps, polyethylene glycol 400, polyethylene glycol 8000, titanium dioxide (E171), sorbic acid, quinoline yellow (dye) aluminium lake (E104).

6.2 Incompatibilities
None known.

6.3 Shelf life
The shelf-life is 18 months when stored in HDPE or glass bottles and 36 months when stored in PVC/PVdC blisters.

6.4 Special precautions for storage
Do not store above 30°C Store in the original package.

6.5 Nature and contents of container
1,4,5,6,7 or 14 tablets in a blister original pack or in bottles. The blisters, of PVC/PVdC, are heat sealed with 20 micron hard tempered aluminium foil and packaged in a cardboard carton with a pack insert. The bottles, of HDPE or glass, are packaged in a cardboard carton with a pack insert.

6.6 Instructions for use and handling
Not applicable.

7. MARKETING AUTHORISATION HOLDER
Abbott Laboratories Limited

Queenborough

Kent

ME11 5EL

8. MARKETING AUTHORISATION NUMBER(S)
PL00037/0275

9. DATE OF FIRST AUTHORISATION/RENEWAL OF THE AUTHORISATION
December 1996

10. DATE OF REVISION OF THE TEXT
February 2005

Klean-Prep

(Norgine Limited)

1. NAME OF THE MEDICINAL PRODUCT
KLEAN-PREP.

2. QUALITATIVE AND QUANTITATIVE COMPOSITION
Each sachet of KLEAN-PREP contains the following active ingredients:

Polyethylene Glycol 3350 USNF	59.000 g
Anhydrous Sodium Sulphate Ph Eur	5.685 g
Sodium Bicarbonate Ph Eur	1.685 g
Sodium Chloride	1.465 g
Potassium Chloride Ph Eur	0.7425 g

The content of electrolyte ions per sachet when made up to one litre of water is as follows:

Sodium	125 mM
Sulphate	40 mM
Chloride	35 mM
Bicarbonate	20 mM
Potassium	10 mM

3. PHARMACEUTICAL FORM
A whitish powder which, when dissolved in water, gives a clear, colourless solution for oral administration.

4. CLINICAL PARTICULARS

4.1 Therapeutic indications
For colonic lavage prior to diagnostic examination or surgical procedures requiring a clean colon, e.g. colonoscopy, barium enema or colonic resection.

4.2 Posology and method of administration
Adults: Each sachet should be dissolved in 1 litre of water. The usual dose is up to 4 sachets taken at a rate of 250 ml every 10 to 15 minutes until the total volume is consumed or rectal effluent is clear, or as directed by the physician.

The solutions from all 4 sachets should be drunk within 4 to 6 hours. Alternatively, administration may be divided, for example, taking 2 sachets during the evening before the examination, and the remaining 2 sachets on the morning of the examination.

If administration is by nasogastric tube, the usual rate should be 20 to 30 ml/minute.

Children: There is no recommended dosage for children.

Renal patients: No dosage adjustment need be made.

4.3 Contraindications
Use in patients with known or suspected gastrointestinal obstruction or perforation, ileus, gastric retention, acute intestinal or gastric ulceration, toxic colitis or toxic megacolon.

4.4 Special warnings and special precautions for use
No solid food should be eaten for at least 2 hours before taking

KLEAN-PREP. The product should only be administered with caution to patients with impaired gag reflex, reflux oesophagitis or those with diminished levels of consciousness and patients with ulcerative colitis.

Unconscious, semi-conscious patients or patients prone to aspiration or regurgitation should be observed during administration especially if this is via the nasogastric route.

4.5 Interaction with other medicinal products and other forms of Interaction
Oral medication taken within one hour of administration of KLEAN-PREP may be flushed from the gastro-intestinal tract and not absorbed.

4.6 Pregnancy and lactation
The preparation should only be used during pregnancy and lactation if considered essential by the physician. There is no experience of use during pregnancy. The purpose and mechanisms of use should be borne in mind if the physician is considering administration.

4.7 Effects on ability to drive and use machines
There is no known effect on the ability to drive and use machines.

4.8 Undesirable effects
Nausea, abdominal fullness and bloating may be experienced. Should distension or pain arise, the rate of administration should be slowed down or temporarily stopped until symptoms subside. Abdominal cramps, vomiting and anal irritation occur less frequently.

These effects normally subside rapidly. Urticaria and allergic reactions have been reported rarely.

4.9 Overdose
In case of gross accidental overdosage, where diarrhoea is severe, conservative measures are usually sufficient; generous amounts of fluid, especially fruit juices, should be given.

5. PHARMACOLOGICAL PROPERTIES

5.1 Pharmacodynamic properties
Polyethylene glycol 3350 exerts its effects by virtue of its osmotic effect in the gut, which induces a laxative effect. The electrolytes also present in the formulation ensure that there is virtually no net gain or loss of sodium, potassium or water, and thus no dehydration.

5.2 Pharmacokinetic properties
Polyethylene glycol 3350 is unchanged along the gut. It is virtually unabsorbed from the gastro-intestinal tract and has no known pharmacological activity. Any polyethylene glycol 3350 that is absorbed is excreted via the urine.

5.3 Preclinical safety data
Pre-clinical studies provide evidence that polyethylene glycol 3350 has no significant systemic toxicity potential.

6. PHARMACEUTICAL PARTICULARS

6.1 List of excipients
Vanilla flavour

Aspartame

6.2 Incompatibilities
None are known.

6.3 Shelf life

Sachets:	2 years
Solution:	24 hours

6.4 Special precautions for storage
Sachets: Store in a dry place below 25°C.

6.5 Nature and contents of container
Sachets containing 69gm white powder, in a box of 4 sachets.

6.6 Instructions for use and handling
The solution should be used within 24 hours.

7. MARKETING AUTHORISATION HOLDER
Norgine Limited

Chaplin House

Widewater Place

Moorhall Road

Harefield

UXBRIDGE

Middlesex UB9 6NS

United Kingdom

8. MARKETING AUTHORISATION NUMBER(S)
PL 00322/0068

9. DATE OF FIRST AUTHORISATION/RENEWAL OF THE AUTHORISATION
March 1997

10. DATE OF REVISION OF THE TEXT
March 2000

Legal Category: **P**

Kliofem

(Novo Nordisk Limited)

1. NAME OF THE MEDICINAL PRODUCT
Kliofem

2. QUALITATIVE AND QUANTITATIVE COMPOSITION

Active ingredients:	Estradiol 2 mg
	Norethisterone acetate 1 mg

The tablets also contain lactose and maize starch, but do not contain clinically significant amounts of gluten.

3. PHARMACEUTICAL FORM
Film-coated tablet for oral administration.

4. CLINICAL PARTICULARS

4.1 Therapeutic indications

4.1 Therapeutic Indications

1 The treatment of symptoms due to oestrogen deficiency.

2 Second line therapy for prevention of osteoporosis in postmenopausal women at high risk of future fractures who are intolerant of, or contraindicated for, other medicinal products approved for the prevention of osteoporosis.

Kliofem is for use in postmenopausal women with an intact uterus. In perimenopausal women treated with Kliofem the incidence of vaginal bleeding is unacceptably high and therefore therapy should not be initiated earlier than one year after the last natural menstrual period

4.2 Posology and method of administration
4.2.1 **Dosage**
Adults: Menopausal symptoms and prophylaxis of osteoporosis.

Kliofem is administered orally, without chewing, one tablet daily without interruption, preferably at the same time each day.

Prophylaxis of osteoporosis: Hormone replacement therapy (HRT) has been found to be effective in the prevention of osteoporosis especially when started soon after the menopause and used for 5 years and probably up to 10 years or more. Treatment should ideally start as soon as possible after the onset of the menopause and certainly within 2 to 3 years, but benefit may also be obtained even if treatment is started at a later date. Protection appears to be effective for as long as treatment is continued. However, data beyond 10 years are limited. A careful re-appraisal of the risk-benefit ratio should be undertaken before treating for longer than 5 to 10 years.

Not intended for children or males.

Use in the elderly: There are no special dosage requirements.

4.2.2 Administration
In women not previously treated with HRT, treatment may be started on any convenient day. In women transferred from sequential HRT, treatment should probably be started at the end of the scheduled bleed.

Before initiation of therapy it is recommended that the patient is fully informed of all likely benefits and potential risks.

Since progestogens are only administered to protect against hyperplastic changes of the endometrium patients without a uterus should be treated with an oestrogen-only-preparation.

4.3 Contraindications

1 Known, suspected, or past history of cancer of the breast.

2 Known or suspected oestrogen-dependent neoplasia. Vaginal bleeding of unknown aetiology.

3 Known or suspected pregnancy.

4 Active deep venous thrombosis, thromboembolic disorders, or a history of confirmed venous thromboembolism. See also Warnings and Precautions, number 4.

5 Acute or chronic liver disease or history of liver disease where the liver function tests have failed to return to normal.

6 Rotor's syndrome or Dubin-Johnson syndrome.

7 Severe cardiac or renal disease.

8 Allergy to one or more of the constituents.

4.4 Special warnings and special precautions for use

1 Assessment of each woman prior to taking hormone replacement therapy (and at regular intervals thereafter) should include a personal and family medical history. Physical examination should be guided by this and by the contraindications (section 4.3) and warnings (section 4.4) for this product. During assessment of each individual woman clinical examination of the breasts and pelvic examination should be performed where clinically indicated rather than as a routine procedure. Women should be encouraged to participate in the national breast cancer screening programme (mammography) and the national cervical cancer screening programme (cervical cytology) as appropriate for their age. Breast awareness should also be encouraged and women advised to report any changes in their breasts to their doctor or nurse.

2 Endometrial assessment should be carried out if indicated; this may be particularly relevant in patients who are, or who have been, previously treated with oestrogens unopposed by a progestogen. In the female there is an increased risk of endometrial hyperplasia and carcinoma associated with unopposed oestrogen administered long term (for more than one year). However, the appropriate addition of a progestogen to an oestrogen regimen lowers this additional risk.

During the first few months of Kliofem therapy, a high proportion of patients will experience bleeding or spotting. About half of women will become amenorrhoeic after 3-4 months' treatment with Kliofem. In a further group, bleeding or spotting may still occur infrequently but will remain acceptable. This means that after 3 months treatment the majority of women will derive benefit from Kliofem in terms of either having no bleeding at all or only light spotting. The patient should be asked to keep a diary of any spotting or bleeding that occurs during treatment with Kliofem.

If, at any time, bleeding or spotting is unacceptable, Kliofem should be discontinued; if all bleeding subsides completely within 3 weeks of stopping Kliofem, then no further investigation is needed.

Bleeding after a period of amenorrhoea or heavy bleeding after a period of light bleeding may indicate poor compliance or concurrent antibiotics use. However, any doubt as to the cause of bleeding is a reason for endometrial evaluation including some form of endometrial biopsy.

3 A reanalysis of original data from 51 epidemiological studies reported a small or moderate increase in the probability of having breast cancer *diagnosed* in women currently or recently using HRT. The findings may be due to biological effects of HRT, earlier diagnosis, or a combination of both. The relative risk increased with duration of treatment (by 2.3% per year of use) and returned to normal in the course of five years after cessation of HRT use. This is comparable to the increase in relative risk when natural menopause is delayed in the absence of HRT. Breast cancers diagnosed in current or recent users of HRT are more likely to be localised to the breast than those found in non-users. HRT use may not be associated with increased mortality from breast cancer.

Between the ages of 50 and 70, about 45 women in every 1000 not using HRT will have breast cancer diagnosed. It is estimated that among those who use HRT for 5 years starting at age 50, 2 extra cases of breast cancer will be detected by age 70 in every 1000 women. For those who use HRT for 10 years there will be 6 extra cases of breast cancer, and for 15 years use, 12 extra cases of breast cancer in every 1000 women during the 20 year period until age 70.

It is important that the increased risk of being diagnosed with breast cancer is discussed with the patient and weighed against the known benefits of HRT.

4 Certain diseases may be made worse by hormone replacement therapy and patients with these conditions should be closely monitored. These include otosclerosis, multiple sclerosis, systemic lupus erythematosus, porphyria, melanoma, epilepsy, migraine and asthma. In addition, pre-existing uterine fibroids may increase in size during oestrogen therapy and symptoms associated with endometriosis may be exacerbated.

5 Epidemiological studies have suggested that hormone replacement therapy (HRT) is associated with a higher relative risk of developing venous thromboembolism (VTE), i.e. deep vein thrombosis or pulmonary embolism. The studies find a 2-3 fold higher risk for users compared with non-users which for healthy women amounts to one extra case of VTE each year for every 5000 patients taking HRT.

Generally recognised risk factors for VTE include a personal or family history and severe obesity (Body Mass Index >30 kg/m5). In women with these factors the benefits of treatment with HRT need to be carefully weighed against risks. There is no consensus about the possible role of varicose veins in VTE.

The risk of VTE may be temporarily increased with prolonged immobilisation, major trauma or major surgery. In women on HRT scrupulous attention should be given to prophylactic measures to prevent VTE following surgery. Where prolonged immobilisation is liable to follow elective surgery, particularly abdominal or orthopaedic surgery to the lower limbs, consideration should be given to temporarily stopping HRT four weeks earlier, if possible.

If venous thromboembolism develops after initiating therapy the drug should be discontinued.

6 Oestrogens may cause fluid retention and, therefore, patients with cardiac or renal dysfunction should be carefully observed.

7 If jaundice, migraine-like headaches, visual disturbance, or a significant increase in blood pressure develop after initiating therapy, the medication should be discontinued while the cause is investigated.

8 Kliofem is not a contraceptive, neither will it restore fertility.

9 Most studies indicate that oestrogen replacement therapy has little effect on blood pressure and some indicate that oestrogen use may be associated with a small decrease in B.P. In addition, most studies on combined therapy, including Kliofem, indicate that the addition of a progestogen also has little effect on blood pressure. Rarely, idiosyncratic hypertension may occur.

However, when oestrogens are administered to hypertensive women, supervision is necessary and blood pressure should be monitored at regular intervals.

10 Diabetic patients should be carefully observed when initiating hormone replacement therapy, as worsening glucose tolerance may occur.

11 Changed oestrogen levels may affect certain endocrine and liver function tests.

12 It has been reported that there is an increase in the risk of surgically confirmed gall bladder disease in women receiving postmenopausal oestrogens.

4.5 Interaction with other medicinal products and other forms of Interaction

Drugs such as barbiturates, phenytoin, rifampicin and carbamazepine which induce the activity of microsomal drug metabolising enzymes may decrease the effectiveness of Kliofem.

4.6 Pregnancy and lactation

Kliofem is contra-indicated during pregnancy and lactation.

4.7 Effects on ability to drive and use machines

No effects known.

4.8 Undesirable effects

The following side effects have been reported with oestrogen/progestogen therapy:

1 Genitourinary system - breakthrough bleeding, spotting, change in menstrual flow, dysmenorrhoea, premenstrual-like syndrome, increase in size of uterine fibromyomata, vaginal candidiasis, change in cervical erosion and in degree of cervical secretion, cystitis-like syndrome.

2 Breasts - tenderness, enlargement, secretion.

3 Gastrointestinal - nausea, vomiting, abdominal cramps, bloating, cholestatic jaundice.

4 Skin - chloasma or melasma which may persist when drug is discontinued, erythema multiforme, erythema nodosum, haemorrhagic eruption, loss of scalp hair, hirsutism.

5 Eyes - steepening of corneal curvature, intolerance to contact lenses.

6 CNS - headaches, migraine, dizziness, mental depression, chorea.

7 Miscellaneous - increase or decrease in weight, reduced carbohydrate tolerance, aggravation of porphyria, oedema, change in libido, leg cramps.

4.9 Overdose

Overdosage may be manifested by nausea and vomiting. There is no specific antidote and treatment should be symptomatic.

5. PHARMACOLOGICAL PROPERTIES

5.1 Pharmacodynamic properties

The oestrogen component of Kliofem substitutes for the loss of endogenous oestrogen production in postmenopausal women, whilst the progestogen component counteracts hyperstimulation of the endometrium. A regular shedding of the endometrium is not induced by Kliofem. Studies based on measurement of bone mineral content have shown that Kliofem is effective in the prevention of progressive bone loss following the menopause.

5.2 Pharmacokinetic properties

The micronised oestradiol in Kliofem is rapidly and efficiently absorbed from the gastrointestinal tract, maximum plasma concentration being reached after 2-4 hours. Oestrogens are partly bound to plasma proteins. Oestradiol is oxidised to oestrone which, in turn, is hydrated to oestriol; both transformations take place mainly in the liver. Oestrogens are excreted into the bile and then undergo reabsorption from the intestine. During this entero-hepatic circulation, degradation of the oestrogens occur. They are excreted in the urine (90-95%) as biologically inactive glucuronide and sulphate conjugates or in the faeces (5-10%) mostly unconjugated.

Norethisterone acetate is rapidly absorbed and transformed to norethisterone, then metabolised and excreted as glucuronide and sulphate conjugates. About half the dose is recovered in the urine within 24 hours, the remainder being reduced to less than 1% of the dose within 5-6 days. Mean plasma half-life is 3-6 hours.

6. PHARMACEUTICAL PARTICULARS

6.1 List of excipients

Lactose monohydrate

Maize starch

Gelatin

Talc

Magnesium stearate

Methyl hydroxypropyl cellulose (E464)

Titanium dioxide (E171)

Iron oxide (E172)

Propylene glycol

Purified water

6.2 Incompatibilities

None known.

6.3 Shelf life

48 months.

6.4 Special precautions for storage

Store at room temperature (max 25°C); protect from light and moisture.

6.5 Nature and contents of container

Polypropylene/polystyrene calendar dial pack containing 28 tablets. Calendar dial packs (3 × 28 tablets) are contained within outer carton.

6.6 Instructions for use and handling

Each carton contains a patient information leaflet with instructions for use of the calendar dial pack.

7. MARKETING AUTHORISATION HOLDER

Novo Nordisk Limited

Broadfield Park, Brighton Road

Crawley, West Sussex, RH11 9RT

8. MARKETING AUTHORISATION NUMBER(S)

PL 3132/0080

9. DATE OF FIRST AUTHORISATION/RENEWAL OF THE AUTHORISATION

3 March 1995

10. DATE OF REVISION OF THE TEXT

February 1998, April 1999, April 2001, April 2002, December 2003

LEGAL CATEGORY

POM.

Kliovance

(Novo Nordisk Limited)

1. NAME OF THE MEDICINAL PRODUCT

Kliovance® film-coated tablets.

2. QUALITATIVE AND QUANTITATIVE COMPOSITION

Each film-coated tablet contains:

Estradiol anhydrous 1 mg (as estradiol hemihydrate) and norethisterone acetate 0.5 mg.

For excipients, see 6.1.

3. PHARMACEUTICAL FORM

Film-coated tablets.

White film-coated, round, biconvex tablets with a diameter of 6 mm. The tablets are engraved with NOVO 288 on one side and the APIS on the other.

4. CLINICAL PARTICULARS

4.1 Therapeutic indications

Hormone Replacement Therapy (HRT) for oestrogen deficiency symptoms in women more than one year after menopause.

Prevention of osteoporosis in postmenopausal women at high risk of future fractures who are intolerant of, or contra-indicated for, other medicinal products approved for the prevention of osteoporosis.

The experience of treating women older than 65 years is limited.

4.2 Posology and method of administration

Kliovance is a continuous-combined hormone replacement product intended for use in women with an intact uterus. One tablet should be taken orally once a day without interruption, preferably at the same time every day.

For initiation and continuation of treatment of postmenopausal symptoms, the lowest effective dose for the shortest duration (see also section 4.4) should be used.

A switch to a higher dose combination product could be indicated if the response after three months is insufficient for satisfactory symptom relief.

In women with amenorrhea and not taking HRT or women transferring from another continuous combined HRT product, treatment with Kliovance may be started on any convenient day. In women transferring from sequential HRT regimens, treatment should start as soon as their withdrawal bleeding has ended.

If the patient has forgotten to take one tablet, the forgotten tablet is to be discarded. Forgetting a dose may increase the likelihood of breakthrough bleeding and spotting.

4.3 Contraindications

- Known, past or suspected breast cancer
- Known or suspected oestrogen-dependent malignant tumours (e.g. endometrial cancer)
- Undiagnosed genital bleeding
- Untreated endometrial hyperplasia
- Previous idiopathic or current venous thromboembolism (deep venous thrombosis, pulmonary embolism)
- Active or recent arterial thromboembolic disease (e.g. angina, myocardial infarction)
- Acute liver disease, or a history of liver disease as long as liver function tests have failed to return to normal
- Known hypersensitivity to the active substances or to any of the excipients
- Porphyria

4.4 Special warnings and special precautions for use

For the treatment of postmenopausal symptoms, HRT should only be initiated for symptoms that adversely affect quality of life. In all cases, a careful appraisal of the risks and benefits should be undertaken at least annually and HRT should only be continued as long as the benefit outweighs the risk.

Medical examination/follow-up

Before initiating or reinstituting HRT, a complete personal and family medical history should be taken. Physical (including pelvic and breast) examination should be guided by this and by the contraindications and warnings for use. During treatment periodic check-ups are recommended of a frequency and nature adapted to the individual woman. Women should be advised what changes in their breasts should be reported to their doctor or nurse (see 'Breast cancer' below). Investigations, including mammography, should be carried out in accordance with currently accepted screening practices, modified to the clinical needs of the individual.

Conditions which need supervision

If any of the following conditions are present, have occurred previously and/or have been aggravated during pregnancy or previous hormone treatment, the patient should be closely supervised. It should be taken into account that these conditions may recur or be aggravated during treatment with Kliovance, in particular:

- Leiomyoma (uterine fibroids) or endometriosis
- A history of, or risk factors for, thromboembolic disorders (see below)
- Risk factors for oestrogen dependent tumours, e.g. 1st degree heredity for breast cancer
- Hypertension
- Liver disorders (e.g. liver adenoma)
- Diabetes mellitus with or without vascular involvement
- Cholelithiasis
- Migraine or (severe) headache
- Systemic lupus erythematosus
- A history of endometrial hyperlasia (see below)
- Epilepsy
- Asthma
- Otosclerosis

Reasons for immediate withdrawal of therapy

Therapy should be discontinued in case a contra-indication is discovered and in the following situations:

- Jaundice or deterioration in liver function
- Significant increase in blood pressure
- New onset of migraine-type headache
- Pregnancy

Endometrial hyperplasia

The risk of endometrial hyperplasia and carcinoma is increased when oestrogens are administered alone for prolonged periods (see section 4.8). The addition of a progestogen for at least 12 days per cycle in non-hysterectomised women greatly reduces this risk.

Breakthrough bleeding and spotting may occur during the first months of treatment. If breakthrough bleeding or spotting appears after some time on therapy, or continues after treatment has been discontinued, the reason should be investigated, which may include endometrial biopsy to exclude endometrial malignancy.

Breast cancer

A randomised placebo-controlled trial, the Women's Health Initiative study (WHI), and epidemiological studies, including the Million Women Study (MWS), have reported an increased risk of breast cancer in women taking oestrogens, oestrogen-progestogen combinations or tibolone for HRT for several years (see Section 4.8). For all HRT an excess risk becomes apparent within a few years of use and increases with duration of intake but returns to baseline within a few (at most five) years after stopping treatment.

In the MWS, the relative risk of breast cancer with conjugated equine oestrogens (CEE) or estradiol (E2) was greater when a progestogen was added, either sequentially or continuously, and regardless of type of progestogen. There was no evidence of a difference in the risk between the different routes of administration.

In the WHI study, the continuous combined conjugated equine oestrogen and medroxyprogesterone acetate (CEE + MPA) product used was associated with breast cancers that were slightly larger in size and more frequently had local lymph node metastases compared to placebo.

HRT, especially oetrogen-progestogen combined treatment, increases the density of mammographic images which may adversely affect the radiological detection of breast cancers.

Venous thromboembolism

HRT is associated with a higher relative risk of developing venous thromboembolism (VTE), i.e. deep vein thrombosis or pulmonary embolism. One randomised controlled trial and epidemiological studies found a two- to threefold higher risk for users compared with non-users. For non-users it is estimated that the number of cases of VTE that will occur over a 5 year period is about 3 per 1000 women aged 50-59 years and 8 per 1000 women aged between 60-69 years. It is estimated that in healthy women who use HRT for 5 years, the number of additional cases of VTE over a 5 year period will be between 2 and 6 (best estimate=4) per 1000 women aged 50-59 years and between 5 and 15 (best estimate=9) per 1000 women aged 60-69 years. The occurrence of such an event is more likely in the first year of HRT than later.

Generally recognised risk factors for VTE include a personal history or family history, severe obesity (Body Mass Index > 30 kg/m^2) and systemic lupus erythematosus (SLE). There is no consensus about the possible role of varicose veins in VTE.

Patients with a history of VTE or known thrombophilic states have an increased risk of VTE. HRT may add to this risk. Personal or strong family history of thromboembolism, or recurrent spontaneous abortion, should be investigated in order to exclude a thrombophilic predisposition. Until a thorough evaluation of thrombophilic factors has been made or anticoagulant treatment initiated, use of HRT in such patients should be viewed as contraindicated. Those women already on anticoagulant treatment require careful consideration of the benefit-risk of use of HRT.

The risk of VTE may be temporarily increased with prolonged immobilisation, major trauma or major surgery. As in all post-operative patients, scrupulous attention should be given to prophylactic measures to prevent VTE following surgery. Where prolonged immobilisation is liable to follow elective surgery, particularly abdominal or orthopaedic surgery to the lower limbs, consideration should be given to temporarily stopping HRT four to six weeks earlier, if possible. Treatment should not be restarted until the woman is completely mobilised.

If VTE develops after initiating therapy, the drug should be discontinued. Patients should be told to contact their doctors immediately when they are aware of a potential thromboembolic symptom (e.g. painful swelling of a leg, sudden pain in the chest, dyspnea).

Coronary artery disease (CAD)

There is no evidence from randomised controlled trials of cardiovascular benefit with continuous combined conjugated oestrogens and medroxyprogesterone acetate (MPA). Two large clinical trials (WHI and HERS i.e. Heart and Estrogen/progestin Replacement Study) showed a possible increased risk of cardiovascular morbidity in the first year of use and no overall benefit. For other HRT products there are only limited data from randomised controlled trials examining effects in cardiovascular morbidity or mortality. Therefore, it is uncertain whether these findings also extend to other HRT products.

Stroke

One large randomised clinical trial (WHI-trial) found, as a secondary outcome, an increased risk of ischaemic stroke in healthy women during treatment with continuous combined conjugated oestrogens and MPA. For women who do not use HRT, it is estimated that the number of cases of stroke that will occur over a 5 year period is about 3 per 1000 women aged 50-59 years and 11 per 1000 women aged 60-69 years. It is estimated that for women who use conjugated oestrogens and MPA for 5 years, the number of additional cases will be between 0 and 3 (best estimate=1) per 1000 users aged 50-59 years and between 1 and 9 (best estimate=4) per 1000 users aged 60-69 years. It is unknown whether the increased risk also extends to other HRT products.

Ovarian cancer

Long-term (at least 5-10 years) use of oestrogen-only HRT products in hysterectomised women has been associated with an increased risk of ovarian cancer in some epidemiological studies. It is uncertain whether long-term use of combined HRT confers a different risk than oestrogen-only products.

Other conditions

Oestrogens may cause fluid retention, and therefore patients with cardiac or renal dysfunction should be carefully observed. Patients with terminal renal insufficiency should be closely observed, since it is expected that the level of circulating active ingredients in Kliovance will increase.

Women with pre-existing hypertriglyceridemia should be followed closely during oestrogen replacement or hormone replacement therapy, since rare cases of large increases of plasma triglycerides leading to pancreatitis have been reported with oestrogen therapy in this condition.

Oestrogens increase thyroid binding globulin (TBG), leading to increased circulating total thyroid hormone, as measured by protein-bound iodine (PBI), T4 levels (by column or by radio-immunoassay) or T3 levels (by radio-immunoassay). T3 resin uptake is decreased, reflecting the elevated TBG. Free T4 and free T3 concentrations are unaltered. Other binding proteins may be elevated in serum, i.e. corticoid binding globulin (CBG), sex-hormone-binding globulin (SHBG) leading to increased circulating corticosteroids and sex steroids, respectively. Free or biological active hormone concentrations are unchanged. Other plasma proteins may be increased (angiotensinogen/renin substrate, alpha-I-antitrypsin, ceruloplasmin).

There is no conclusive evidence for improvement of cognitive function. There is some evidence from the WHI trial of increased risk of probable dementia in women who start using continuous combined CEE and MPA after the age of 65. It is unknown whether the findings apply to younger post-menopausal women or other HRT products.

4.5 Interaction with other medicinal products and other forms of Interaction

The metabolism of oestrogens and progestogens may be increased by concomitant use of substances known to induce drug-metabolising enzymes, specifically cytochrome P450 enzymes such as anticonvulsants (e.g. phenobarbital, phenytoin, carbamazepin) and anti-infectives (e.g. rifampicin, rifabutin, nevirapine, efavirenz).

Ritonavir and nelfinavir, although known as strong inhibitors, by contrast exhibit inducing properties when used concomitantly with steroid hormones. Herbal preparations containing St John's Wort (*Hypericum perforatum*) may induce the metabolism of oestrogens and progestogens.

Clinically, an increased metabolism of oestrogens and progestogens may lead to decreased effect and changes in the uterine bleeding profile.

Drugs that inhibit the activity of hepatic microsomal drug metabolizing enzymes e.g. ketoconazole, may increase circulating levels of the active substances in Kliovance.

4.6 Pregnancy and lactation

Kliovance is not indicated during pregnancy.

If pregnancy occurs during medication with Kliovance, treatment should be withdrawn immediately.

Data on a limited number of exposed pregnancies indicate adverse effects of norethisterone acetate on the foetus. At doses higher than normally used in OC and HRT formulations masculinisation of female foetuses was observed. The results of most epidemiological studies to date relevant to inadvertent foetal exposure to combinations of oestrogens and progestogens indicate no teratogenic or foetotoxic effect.

Lactation

Kliovance is not indicated during lactation.

4.7 Effects on ability to drive and use machines

No effects known.

4.8 Undesirable effects

The most frequently reported adverse events in the clinical trials with Kliovance were vaginal bleeding and breast pain/tenderness, reported in approximately 10% to 20% of patients. Vaginal bleeding usually occurred in the first months of treatment. Breast pain usually disappeared after a few months of therapy. All adverse events observed in the randomised clinical trials with a higher frequency in patients treated with Kliovance as compared to placebo and which on an overall judgement are possibly related to treatment are presented in the table below.

(see Table 1 on next page)

Breast cancer

According to evidence from a large number of epidemiological studies and one randomised placebo-controlled trial, the Women's Health Initiative (WHI), the overall risk of breast cancer increases with increasing duration of HRT use in current or recent HRT users.

For *oestrogen-only* HRT, estimates of relative risk (RR) from a reanalysis of original data from 51 epidemiological studies (in which >80% of HRT use was oestrogen-only

Table 1

System organ class	Very common >1/10	Common >1/100; <1/10	Uncommon >1/1,000; <1/100	Rare >1/10,000; <1/1,000
Infections and infestations		Genital candidiasis or vaginitis, see also "Reproductive system and breast disorders"		
Immune system disorders			Hypersensi-tivity, see also "Skin and subcutaneous tissue disorders"	
Metabolism and nutrition disorders		Fluid retention, see also "General disorders and administration site conditions"		
Psychiatric disorders		Depression or depression aggravated	Nervousness	
Nervous system disorders		Headache, migraine or migraine aggravated		
Vascular disorders			Thrombo phlebitis superficial	Deep venous tromboembolism Pulmonary embolism
Gastrointestinal disorders		Nausea	Abdominal pain, abdominal distension or abdominal discomfort Flatulence or bloating	
Skin and subcutaneous tissue disorders			Alopecia, hirsutism or acne Pruritus or urticaria	
Muscle-skeletal, connective tissue and bone disorders		Back pain	Leg cramps	
Reproductive system and breast disorders	Breast pain or breast tenderness Vaginal haemor- rhage	Breast oedema or breast enlargement Uterine fibroids aggravated or uterine fibroids re-occurrence or uterine fibroids		
General disorders and administration site conditions		Oedema peripheral	Drug ineffective	
Investigations		Weight increased		

HRT) and from the epidemiological Million Women Study (MWS) are similar at 1.35 (95% CI: 1.21-1.49) and 1.30 (95% CI: 1.21-1.40), respectively.

For *oestrogen plus progestogen* combined HRT, several epidemiological studies have reported an overall higher risk for breast cancer than with oestrogens alone.

The MWS reported that, compared to never users, the use of various types of oestrogen-progestogen combined HRT was associated with a higher risk of breast cancer (RR = 2.00, 95% CI: 1.88-2.12) than use of oestrogens alone (RR = 1.30, 95% CI: 1.21-1.40) or use of tibolone (RR = 1.45, 95% CI: 1.25-1.68).

The WHI trial reported a risk estimate of 1.24 (95% CI: 1.01-1.54) after 5.6 years of use of oestrogen-progestogen combined HRT (CEE + MPA) in all users compared with placebo.

The absolute risks calculated from the MWS and the WHI trial are presented below:

The MWS has estimated, from the known average incidence of breast cancer in developed countries, that:

- For women not using HRT, about 32 in every 1000 are expected to have breast cancer diagnosed between the ages of 50 and 64 years.
- For 1000 current or recent users of HRT, the number of *additional* cases during the corresponding period will be
- For users of *oestrogen-only* replacement therapy,

- between 0 and 3 (best estimate = 1.5) for 5 years' use

- between 3 and 7 (best estimate = 5) for 10 years' use.

- For users of *oestrogen plus progestogen* combined HRT,

- between 5 and 7 (best estimate = 6) for 5 years' use

- between 18 and 20 (best estimate = 19 for 10 years use.

The WHI trial estimated that after 5.6 years of follow-up of women between the ages of 50 and 79 years, an *additional* 8 cases of invasive breast cancer would be due to *oestrogen-progestogen combined* HRT (CEE + MPA) per 10,000 women years. According to calculations from the trial data, it is estimated that:

- For 1000 women in the placebo group,

- about 16 cases of invasive breast cancer would be diagnosed in 5 years.

- For 1000 women who used oestrogen + progestogen combined HRT (CEE + MPA), the number of additional cases would be

- between 0 an 9 (best estimate = 4) for 5 years' use.

The number of additional cases of breast cancer in women who use HRT is broadly similar for women who start HRT irrespective of age at start of use (between the ages of 45-65) (see section 4.4).

Endometrial cancer

In women with an intact uterus, the risk of endometrial hyperplasia and endometrial cancer increases with increasing duration of use of unopposed oestrogens. According to data from epidemiological studies, the best estimate of the risk is that for women not using HRT, about 5 in every 1000 are expected to have endometrial cancer diagnosed between the ages of 50 and 65. Depending on the duration of treatment and oestrogen dose, the reported increase in endometrial cancer risk among unopposed oestrogen users varies from 2- to 12-fold greater compared with non-users. Adding a progestogen to oestrogen-only therapy greatly reduces this increased risk.

Post marketing experience:

In addition to the above mentioned adverse drug reactions, those presented below have been spontaneously reported, and are by an overall judgement considered possibly related to Kliovance treatment. The reporting rate of these spontaneous adverse drug reactions is very rare (<1/10,000 patient years). Post-marketing experience is subject to underreporting especially with regard to trivial and well known adverse drug reactions. The presented frequencies should be interpreted in that light:

Neoplasms benign and malignant (incl. cysts and polyps): Endometrial cancer

Psychiatric disorders: Insomnia, anxiety, libido decreased, libido increased

Nervous system disorders: Dizziness

Eye disorders: Visual disturbances

Vascular disorders: Hypertension aggravated

Gastrointestinal disorders: Dyspepsia, vomiting

Hepatobilitary disorders: Gallbladder disease, cholelithiasis, cholelithiasis aggravated, cholelithiasis re-occurrence

Skin and subcutaneous tissue disorder: Seborrhoea, rash, angioneurotic oedema

Reproductive system and breast disorders: Hyperplasia endometrial, vulvovaginal pruritus

Investigations: Weight decreased, blood pressure increased

Other adverse reactions have been reported in association with oestrogen/progestogen treatment:

- Oestrogen-dependent neoplasms benign and malignant, e.g. endometrial cancer

- Venous thromboembolism, i.e. deep leg or pelvic venous thrombosis and pulmonary embolism, is more frequent among hormone replacement therapy users than among non-users. For further information, see section 4.3 Contra-indications and 4.4 Special warnings and precautions for use.

- Myocardial infarction and stroke

- Skin and subcutaneous disorders: chloasma, erythema multiforme, erythema nodosum, vascular purpura

- Probable dementia (see section 4.4).

4.9 Overdose

Overdose may be manifested by nausea and vomiting. Treatment should be symptomatic.

5. PHARMACOLOGICAL PROPERTIES

5.1 Pharmacodynamic properties

ATC code G03F A01

Oestrogen and progestogen for continuous combined hormone replacement therapy (HRT).

Oestradiol: The active ingredient, synthetic 17 beta-oestradiol, is chemically and biologically identical to endogenous human oestradiol. It substitutes for the loss of oestrogen production in menopausal women, and alleviates menopausal symptoms.

Oestrogens prevent bone loss following menopause or ovariectomy.

Norethisterone acetate: As oestrogens promote the growth of the endometrium, unopposed oestrogens increase the risk of endometrial hyperplasia and cancer. The addition of a progestogen greatly reduces the oestrogen-induced risk of endometrial hyperplasia in non-hysterectomised women.

In clinical trials with Kliovance, the addition of the norethisterone acetate component enhanced the vasomotor symptom relieving effect of 17beta-estradiol.

Relief of menopausal symptoms is achieved during the first few weeks of treatment.

Kliovance is a continuous combined HRT given with the intent of avoiding the regular withdrawal bleeding associated with cyclic or sequential HRT. Amenorrhoea (no bleeding and spotting) was seen in 90% of the women during months 9-12 of treatment. Bleeding and/or spotting appeared in 27% of the women during the first three months of treatment and in 10% during months 10-12 of treatment.

Oestrogen deficiency at menopause is associated with an increasing bone turnover and decline in bone mass. The effect of oestrogens on the bone mineral density is dose-dependent. Protection appears to be effective for as long as treatment is continued. After discontinuation of HRT, bone mass is lost at a rate similar to that in untreated women.

Evidence from the WHI trial and meta-analysed trials shows that current use of HRT, alone or in combination with a progestogen – given to predominantly healthy women – reduces the risk of hip, vertebral, and other osteoporotic fractures. HRT may also prevent fractures in women with low bone density and/or established osteoporosis, but the evidence for that is limited.

The effects of Kliovance on bone mineral density were examined in two 2-year, randomised, double-blind, placebo-controlled clinical trials in postmenopausal women (n=327 in one trial, including 47 on Kliovance and 48 on Kliofem (2 mg estradiol and 1 mg norethisterone acetate); and n=135 in the other trial including 46 on Kliovance). All women received calcium supplementation ranging from 500 to 1000 mg daily. Kliovance significantly prevented bone loss at the lumbar spine, total hip, distal radius and total body in comparison with calcium supplemented placebo-treated women. In early postmenopausal women (1 to 5 years since last menses), the percentage change from baseline in bone mineral density at lumbar spine, femoral neck and femoral trochanter in patients completing 2 years of treatment with Kliovance was 4.8 ± 0.6%, 1.6 ± 0.7% and 4.3 ± 0.7% (mean ± SEM), respectively, while with the higher dose combination containing 2 mg E_2 and 1 mg NETA (Kliofem) it was 5.4 ± 0.7%, 2.9 ± 0.8% and 5.0 ± 0.9%, respectively. The percentage of women who maintained or gained bone mineral density during treatment with Kliovance and Kliofem was 87% and 91%, respectively, after 2 years of treatment. In a study conducted in postmenopausal women with a mean age of 58 years, treatment with Kliovance for 2 years increased the bone mineral density at lumbar spine by 5.9 ± 0.9%, at total hip by 4.2 ± 1.0%, at distal radius by 2.1 ± 0.6%, and at total body by 3.7 ± 0.6%.

5.2 Pharmacokinetic properties

Following oral administration of 17 beta-estradiol in micronized form, rapid absorption from the gastrointestinal tract occurs. It undergoes extensive first-pass metabolism in the liver and other enteric organs and reaches a peak plasma concentration of approximately 35 pg/ml (range 21-52 pg/ml) within 5-8 hours. The half-life of 17beta-estradiol is about 12-14 hours. It circulates bound to SHBG (37%) and to albumin (61%), while only approximately 1-2% is unbound. Metabolism of 17 beta-estradiol, occurs mainly in the liver and gut but also in target organs, and involves the formation of less active or inactive metabolites, including oestrone, catecholoestrogens and several oestrogen sulphates and glucuronides. Oestrogens are excreted with the bile, where they are hydrolysed and reabsorbed (enterohepatic circulation), and mainly in urine in biologically inactive form.

After oral administration norethisterone acetate is rapidly absorbed and transformed to norethisterone (NET). It undergoes first-pass metabolism in the liver and other enteric organs and reaches a peak plasma concentration of approximately 3.9 ng/ml (range 1.4-6.8 ng/ml) within 0.5-1.5 hour. The terminal half-life of NET is about 8-11 hours. NET binds to SHBG (36%) and to albumin (61%). The most important metabolites are isomers of 5α-dihydro-NET and of tetrahydro-NET, which are excreted mainly in the urine as sulphate or glucuronide conjugates.

The pharmacokinetics in the elderly have not been studied.

5.3 Preclinical safety data

Acute toxicity of oestrogens is low. Because of marked differences between animal species and between animals and humans preclinical results possess a limited predictive value for the application of oestrogens in humans.

In experimental animals oestradiol or oestradiol valerate displayed an embryolethal effect already at relatively low doses; malformations of the urogenital tract and feminisation of male foetuses were observed.

Norethisterone, like other progestogens, caused virilisation of female foetuses in rats and monkeys. After high doses of norethisterone embryolethal effects were observed.

Preclinical data based on conventional studies of repeated dose toxicity, genotoxicity and carcinogenic potential revealed no particular human risks beyond those discussed in other sections of the SPC.

6. PHARMACEUTICAL PARTICULARS

6.1 List of excipients

Tablet core:

Lactose monohydrate

Maize starch

Copovidone

Talc

Magnesium stearate

Film-coating:

Hypromellose

Triacetin

Talc

6.2 Incompatibilities

Not applicable.

6.3 Shelf life

3 years.

6.4 Special precautions for storage

Do not store above 25°C. Do not refrigerate. Keep the container in the outer carton.

6.5 Nature and contents of container

The tablets are contained in calendar dial packs; each calendar dial pack contains 28 tablets.

Packs containing 3 calendar dial packs are available (3 × 28 tablets)

The calendar dial pack with 28 tablets consists of the following 3 parts:

- The base made of coloured non-transparent polypropylene
- The ring-shaped lid made of transparent polystyrene
- The centre-dial made of coloured non-transparent polystyrene

6.6 Instructions for use and handling

No special requirements.

7. MARKETING AUTHORISATION HOLDER

Novo Nordisk Limited

Broadfield Park

Brighton Road

Crawley, West Sussex

RH11 9RT

8. MARKETING AUTHORISATION NUMBER(S)

PL 03132/0125

9. DATE OF FIRST AUTHORISATION/RENEWAL OF THE AUTHORISATION

20 August 1998/20 August 2003

10. DATE OF REVISION OF THE TEXT

5 October 1999, 10 September 2002, 23 May 2003, 5 December 2003, 9 March 2004.

LEGAL CATEGORY

Prescription-only medicine (POM)

Kloref Tablets

(Alpharma Limited)

1. NAME OF THE MEDICINAL PRODUCT

KLOREF TABLETS

2. QUALITATIVE AND QUANTITATIVE COMPOSITION

Each tablet contains 740mg Betaine Hydrochloride BPC 1949, 455mg Potassium Bicarbonate BPC, 140mg Potassium Chloride PhEur and 50mg Potassium Benzoate USNF. Each tablet provides 6.7mmol of potassium (K^+) and 6.7mmol of chloride (Cl^-), equivalent to 500mg potassium chloride, when dissolved in water.

3. PHARMACEUTICAL FORM

White uncoated tablets.

4. CLINICAL PARTICULARS

4.1 Therapeutic indications

1) Kloref is indicated in all cases of potassium depletion resulting from prolonged or intensive diuretic therapy, an inadequate dietary potassium intake, and those receiving digitalis - here the elderly population are a special risk. A lack of cellular potassium in the latter can increase the toxic effect of digitalis.

2) Other indications are corticosteroid therapy, use of carbenoxolone sodium, advanced hepatic cirrhosis, chronic renal disease, Cushing's syndrome, diabetic ketosis, patients on a low salt diet and in conditions requiring potassium supplementation due to prolonged or chronic diarrhoea or vomiting.

4.2 Posology and method of administration

Posology

Each tablet should be fully dissolved in at least 100ml of cold or refrigerated water before drinking. The tablets themselves should not be swallowed.

Adults: In most cases 1-2 tablets three times daily (20-40mmol K^+ and Cl^-). A few patients may need considerably bigger doses.

Children and pregnant women: Treatment should only be initiated under close medical supervision in hospital, with frequent monitoring of serum electrolytes.

Elderly: The elderly also require monitoring of serum electrolytes.

Method of Administration

To be dissolved in water for oral administration.

4.3 Contraindications

Hyperchloraemia; renal tubular or metabolic acidosis.

4.4 Special warnings and special precautions for use

Cautious administration required in cases of chronic renal disease.

4.5 Interaction with other medicinal products and other forms of Interaction

None known.

4.6 Pregnancy and lactation

Potassium may be indicated as replacement therapy for pregnant women with low potassium levels such as those receiving diuretics. Serum levels should be closely monitored.

Administration of potassium during lactation is considered to be safe providing that maternal serum levels are maintained in the physiological range.

4.7 Effects on ability to drive and use machines

None known.

4.8 Undesirable effects

None known.

4.9 Overdose

Hyperkalaemia. Poisoning is usually minimal below 6.5mmol/l, moderate between 6.5-8mmol/l and severe above that level. The absolute toxicity is governed by both pH and associated sodium levels.

Hyperkalaemic symptoms and particularly the ECG effects, may be transiently controlled by calcium gluconate, administration of glucose or glucose and insulin, sodium bicarbonate or hypertonic sodium infusions, cation exchange resins or by haemodialysis and peritoneal dialysis. Caution should be exercised in patients who are digitalised and who may experience acute digitalis intoxication in the course of potassium removal.

5. PHARMACOLOGICAL PROPERTIES

5.1 Pharmacodynamic properties

Betaine hydrochloride has been given as a source of hydrochloride acid in the treatment of hypochlorhydria. A wide variety of betaine salts have been used in various countries, mainly for GI disturbances.

Potassium bicarbonate, potassium chloride and potassium benzoate are potassium supplements.

5.2 Pharmacokinetic properties

Potassium salts other than the phosphate, sulphate and tartrate are generally readily absorbed from the GI tract. Potassium is excreted mainly by the kidneys, it is secreted in the distal tubules which are also the site of sodium-potassium exchange. The capacity of the kidneys to conserve potassium is poor and urinary excretion of potassium continues even when there is severe depletion. Tubular secretion of potassium is influenced by several factors, including chloride ion concentration, hydrogen ion exchange, acid-base equilibrium, and adrenal hormones. Some potassium is excreted in the faeces and small amounts may also be excreted in saliva, sweat, bile and pancreatic juice.

5.3 Preclinical safety data

Not applicable.

6. PHARMACEUTICAL PARTICULARS

6.1 List of excipients

Also contains: polyvidone, docusate sodium, saccharin calcium, citric acid (E330), macrogol, lime flavour, lemon flavour.

6.2 Incompatibilities

None known.

6.3 Shelf life

Shelf-life

A three year shelf-life is claimed and our marketed products includes a three year expiry date.

Shelf-life after dilution/reconstitution

Not applicable.

Shelf-life after first opening

Not applicable.

6.4 Special precautions for storage

i) Prescription Packs: Store below 25°C in a dry place.

Dispense in original or other moisture-proof container.

CAUTION: Securely fasten lid immediately after use.

(ii) Hospital Packs: Store below 25°C in a dry place.

Dispense in a moisture-proof container.

CAUTION: Securely fasten bag and lid immediately after use.

6.5 Nature and contents of container

(i) Prescription Packs: The product containers are rigid injection moulded polypropylene or injection blow-moulded polyethylene containers with snap-on polyethylene lids. One 3g silica gel sachet - 50s; two 3g silica gel sachets - 100s.

(ii) Dispensing Packs: The product is contained in a black plastic bag with one 50g silica gel sachet, sealed with a metal twist and contained in a white polybucket.

Pack sizes: 7s, 14s, 21s, 28s, 50s, 56s, 60s, 84s, 100s, 1000s.

6.6 Instructions for use and handling

Not applicable.

Administrative Data

7. MARKETING AUTHORISATION HOLDER

Alpharma Limited (Trading styles: Alpharma, Cox Pharmaceuticals)

Whiddon Valley

BARNSTAPLE

N Devon EX32 8NS

8. MARKETING AUTHORISATION NUMBER(S)

PL 0142/0275

9. DATE OF FIRST AUTHORISATION/RENEWAL OF THE AUTHORISATION

April 1988; June 1993; September 1998

10. DATE OF REVISION OF THE TEXT

May 2003

Kogenate Bayer 250IU, 500IU & 1000IU (Bio-Set)

(Bayer plc)

1. NAME OF THE MEDICINAL PRODUCT

KOGENATE Bayer 250 IU Powder and solvent for solution for injection.

KOGENATE Bayer 500 IU Powder and solvent for solution for injection.

KOGENATE Bayer 1000 IU Powder and solvent for solution for injection.

2. QUALITATIVE AND QUANTITATIVE COMPOSITION

KOGENATE Bayer 250 IU - Recombinant coagulation Factor VIII, 250 IU/vial.

KOGENATE Bayer 500 IU – Recombinant coagulation Factor VIII, 500 IU/vial.

KOGENATE Bayer 1000 IU – Recombinant coagulation Factor VIII, 1000 IU/vial.

INN: octocog alfa.

Recombinant Coagulation Factor VIII is produced from genetically engineered baby hamster kidney cells containing the human factor VIII gene.

Solvent: water for injections.

KOGENATE Bayer 250 IU – The product reconstituted with the accompanying 2.5 ml of water for injections contains approximately 100 IU octocog alfa/ml.

KOGENATE Bayer 500 IU - The product reconstituted with the accompanying 2.5 ml of water for injections contains approximately 200 IU octocog alfa/ml.

KOGENATE Bayer 1000 IU - The product reconstituted with the accompanying 2.5 ml of water for injections contains approximately 400 IU octocog alfa/ml.

The potency (IU) is determined using the one-stage clotting assay against the FDA Mega standard which was calibrated against WHO standard in IU.

The specific activity is approximately 4000 IU/mg protein.

For excipients, see 6.1.

3. PHARMACEUTICAL FORM

Powder and solvent for solution for injection.

The powder is provided in a vial as a dry white to slightly yellow powder or cake.

The solvent is water for injections provided in a pre-filled syringe.

4. CLINICAL PARTICULARS

4.1 Therapeutic indications

Treatment and prophylaxis of bleeding in patients with haemophilia A (congenital factor VIII deficiency).

This preparation does not contain von Willebrand factor and is therefore not indicated in von Willebrand's disease.

4.2 Posology and method of administration

Treatment should be initiated under the supervision of a physician experienced in the treatment of haemophilia.

Posology

The number of units of factor VIII administered is expressed in International Units (IU), which are related to the current WHO standard for factor VIII products. Factor VIII activity in plasma is expressed either as a percentage (relative to normal human plasma) or in International Units (relative to the International Standard for factor VIII in plasma). One International Unit (IU) of factor VIII activity is equivalent to that quantity of factor VIII in one ml of normal human plasma. The calculation of the required dosage of factor VIII is based on the empirical finding that 1 International Unit (IU) factor VIII per kg body weight raises the plasma factor VIII activity by 1.5% to 2.5% of normal activity. The required dosage is determined using the following formulae:

I.	Required IU = body weight (kg) × desired factor VIII rise (% of normal) × 0.5	
II.	Expected factor VIII rise (% of normal) =	$\frac{2 \times \text{administered IU}}{\text{body weight (kg)}}$

The dosage and duration of the substitution therapy must be individualised according to the patient's needs (weight, severity of disorder of the haemostatic function, the site and extent of the bleeding, the titre of inhibitors, and the factor VIII level desired).

The following table provides a guide for factor VIII minimum blood levels. In the case of the haemorrhagic events listed, the factor VIII activity should not fall below the given level (in % of normal) in the corresponding period:

Degree of haemorrhage/ Type of surgical procedure	Factor VIII level required (%) (IU/dl)	Frequency of doses (hours)/ Duration of therapy (days)
Haemorrhage		
Early haemarthrosis, muscle bleed or oral bleed	20 - 40	Repeat every 12 to 24 hours. At least 1 day, until the bleeding episode as indicated by pain is resolved or healing is achieved.
More extensive haemarthrosis, muscle bleed or haematoma	30 - 60	Repeat infusion every 12 - 24 hours for 3 - 4 days or more until pain and disability are resolved.
Life threatening bleeds such as intracranial bleed, throat bleed, severe abdominal bleed	60 - 100	Repeat infusion every 8 to 24 hours until threat is resolved
Surgery		
Minor including tooth extraction	30 - 60	Every 24 hours, at least 1 day, until healing is achieved.
Major	80 - 100 (pre- and postoperative)	Repeat infusion every 8 - 24 hours until adequate wound healing, then therapy for at least another 7 days to maintain a factor VIII activity of 30% to 60%

The amount to be administered and the frequency of administration should always be adapted according to the clinical effectiveness in the individual case. Under certain circumstances larger amounts than those calculated may be required, especially in the case of the initial dose.

During the course of treatment, appropriate determination of factor VIII levels is advised in order to guide the dose to be administered and the frequency at which to repeat the infusions. In the case of major surgical interventions in particular, precise monitoring of the substitution therapy by means of coagulation analysis (plasma factor VIII activity) is indispensable. Individual patients may vary in their response to factor VIII, achieving different levels of *in vivo* recovery and demonstrating different half-lives.

For scheduled prophylaxis against bleeds in patients with severe haemophilia A, doses of 20 to 60 IU of KOGENATE Bayer per kg body weight should be given at intervals of 2 to 3 days. In some cases, especially in younger patients, shorter dosage intervals or higher doses may be necessary. Data have been obtained in 61 children under 6 years of age.

Patients with inhibitors

Patients should be monitored for the development of factor VIII inhibitors. If the expected plasma factor VIII activity levels are not attained, or if bleeding is not controlled with an appropriate dose, an assay should be performed to determine if a factor VIII inhibitor is present. If the inhibitor is present at levels less than 10 Bethesda Units (BU) per ml, administration of additional recombinant coagulation factor VIII may neutralise the inhibitor and permit continued clinically effective therapy with KOGENATE Bayer. However, in the presence of an inhibitor the doses required are variable and must be adjusted according to clinical response and monitoring of plasma factor VIII activity. In patients with inhibitor titres above 10 BU or with high anamnestic response, the use of (activated) prothrombin complex concentrate (PCC) or recombinant activated factor VII (rFVIIa) preparations has to be considered. These therapies should be directed by physicians with experience in the care of patients with haemophilia.

Administration

Reconstitute the preparation as described in 6.6.

KOGENATE Bayer should be injected intravenously over several minutes. The rate of administration should be determined by the patient's comfort level (maximal rate of injection: 2 ml/min).

4.3 Contraindications

Known hypersensitivity to the active substance, to mouse or hamster protein or to any of the excipients.

4.4 Special warnings and special precautions for use

Patients should be made aware that the potential occurrence of chest tightness, dizziness, mild hypotension and nausea during infusion can constitute an early warning for hypersensitivity and anaphylactic reactions. Symptomatic treatment and therapy for hypersensitivity should be instituted as appropriate. If allergic or anaphylactic reactions occur, the injection/infusion should be stopped immediately. In case of shock, the current medical standards for shock treatment should be observed.

The formation of neutralising antibodies (inhibitors) to factor VIII is a known complication in the management of individuals with haemophilia A. These inhibitors are invariably IgG immunoglobulins directed against the factor VIII procoagulant activity, which are quantified in Modified Bethesda Units (BU) per ml of plasma. The risk of developing inhibitors is correlated to the exposure to anti-haemophilic factor VIII, this risk being highest within the first 20 exposure days. Rarely, inhibitors may develop after the first 100 exposure days. Patients treated with recombinant coagulation factor VIII should be carefully monitored for the development of inhibitors by appropriate clinical observations and laboratory tests. See also 4.8 Undesirable effects.

4.5 Interaction with other medicinal products and other forms of Interaction

No interactions of KOGENATE Bayer with other medicinal products are known.

4.6 Pregnancy and lactation

Animal reproduction studies have not been conducted with KOGENATE Bayer.

Based on the rare occurrence of haemophilia A in women, experience regarding the use of KOGENATE Bayer during pregnancy and breast-feeding is not available. Therefore, KOGENATE Bayer should be used during pregnancy and lactation only if clearly indicated.

4.7 Effects on ability to drive and use machines

No effects on the ability to drive or to use machines have been observed.

4.8 Undesirable effects

After administration of KOGENATE Bayer mild to moderate adverse events were observed in rare cases. These included rash/pruritus, local reactions at the injection site (e.g. burning, transient erythema), hypersensitivity reactions (e.g. dizziness, nausea, chest pain/malaise, mildly reduced blood pressure), unusual taste in the mouth and fever. Furthermore, the possibility of an anaphylactic shock cannot be completely excluded.

The formation of neutralising antibodies to factor VIII (inhibitors) is a known complication in the management of individuals with haemophilia A. In studies with recombinant factor VIII preparations, development of inhibitors is predominantly observed in previously untreated haemophiliacs. Patients should be carefully monitored for the development of inhibitors by appropriate clinical observations and laboratory tests.

In clinical trials 9 out of 60 (15%) previously untreated and minimally treated patients treated with KOGENATE Bayer developed inhibitors: Overall 6 out of 60 (10%) with a titre above 10 BU and 3 out of 60 (5%) with a titre below 10 BU. The median number of exposure days at the time of inhibitor detection in these patients were 9 days (range 3 - 18 days).

During studies, no patient developed clinically relevant antibody titres against the trace amounts of mouse protein and hamster protein present in the preparation. However, the possibility of allergic reactions to constituents, e.g. trace amounts of mouse and hamster protein in the preparation exists in certain predisposed patients (see 4.3 and 4.4).

4.9 Overdose

No symptoms of overdose with recombinant coagulation factor VIII have been reported.

5. PHARMACOLOGICAL PROPERTIES

5.1 Pharmacodynamic properties

Pharmacotherapeutic group: blood coagulation factor VIII, ATC-Code B02B D02.

The factor VIII/von Willebrand factor (vWF) complex consists of two molecules (factor VIII and vWF) with different physiological functions. When infused into a haemophiliac patient, factor VIII binds to vWF in the patient's circulation. Activated factor VIII acts as a cofactor for activated factor IX, accelerating the conversion of factor X to activated factor X. Activated factor X converts prothrombin into thrombin. Thrombin then converts fibrinogen into fibrin and a clot can be formed. Haemophilia A is a sex-linked hereditary disorder of blood coagulation due to decreased levels of factor VIII:C and results in profuse bleeding into joints, muscles or internal organs, either spontaneously or as a results of accidental or surgical trauma. By replacement therapy the plasma levels of factor VIII are increased, thereby enabling a temporary correction of the factor deficiency and correction of the bleeding tendencies.

Determination of activated partial thromboplastin time (aPTT) is a conventional *in vitro* assay method for biological activity of factor VIII. The aPTT is prolonged in all haemophiliacs. The degree and duration of aPTT normalisation observed after administration of KOGENATE Bayer is similar to that achieved with plasma-derived factor VIII.

5.2 Pharmacokinetic properties

The analysis of all recorded *in vivo* recoveries in previously treated patients demonstrated a mean rise of 2 % per IU/kg body weight for KOGENATE Bayer. This result is similar to the reported values for factor VIII derived from human plasma.

After administration of KOGENATE Bayer, peak factor VIII activity decreased by a two-phase exponential decay with a mean terminal half-life of about 15 hours. This is similar to that of plasma-derived factor VIII which has a mean terminal half-life of approx. 13 hours. Additional pharmacokinetic parameters for KOGENATE Bayer are: mean residence time [MRT (0-48)] of about 22 hours and clearance of about 160 ml/h.

5.3 Preclinical safety data

Even doses several fold higher than the recommended clinical dose (related to body weight) failed to demonstrate any acute or subacute toxic effects for KOGENATE Bayer in laboratory animals (mouse, rat, rabbit, and dog).

Specific studies with repeated administration such as reproduction toxicity, chronic toxicity, and carcinogenicity were not performed with octocog alfa due to the immune response to heterologous proteins in all non-human mammalian species.

No studies were performed on the mutagenic potential of KOGENATE Bayer, since no mutagenic potential could be detected *in vitro* or *in vivo* for the predecessor product of KOGENATE Bayer.

6. PHARMACEUTICAL PARTICULARS

6.1 List of excipients

Powder

Glycine

Sodium chloride

Calcium chloride

Histidine

Polysorbate 80

Sucrose

Solvent

Water for injections

6.2 Incompatibilities

This medicinal product must not be mixed with other medicinal products or solvents.

Only the provided components (powder vial with Bio-Set device, pre-filled syringe containing solvent and venipuncture set) should be used for reconstitution and injection because treatment failure can occur as a consequence of human coagulation factor VIII adsorption to the internal surfaces of some infusion equipment.

6.3 Shelf life

23 months.

Chemical and physical in-use stability has been demonstrated for 4 hours at 25°C.

From a microbiological point of view, unless the method of reconstitution precludes the risk of microbial contamination, the product should be used immediately.

If not used immediately, in-use storage times and conditions are the responsibility of the user.

6.4 Special precautions for storage

Store in a refrigerator (2°C – 8°C). Do not freeze. Keep the vial and the pre-filled syringe in the outer carton in order to protect from light.

The product when kept in its outer carton may be stored at ambient room temperature (up to 25°C) for a limited period of 2 months. In this case, the product expires at the end of this 2-month period; the new expiry date must be noted on the outer carton.

Do not refrigerate after reconstitution. For single use only. Any unused solution must be discarded.

6.5 Nature and contents of container

Each package of KOGENATE Bayer contains:

• one vial plus Bio-Set device, containing powder (10 ml clear glass type 1 vial with latex-free grey bromobutyl rubber blend stopper plus transfer device with protective cap [Bio-Set])

• one pre-filled syringe with 2.5 ml solvent (clear glass cylinder type 2 with latex-free grey bromobutyl rubber blend stoppers)

• syringe plunger rod

• one venipuncture set

• two sterile alcohol swabs for single use

• two dry swabs

• two plasters

6.6 Instructions for use and handling

Detailed instructions for preparation and administration are contained in the package leaflet provided with KOGENATE Bayer.

KOGENATE Bayer powder should only be reconstituted with the supplied solvent (2.5 ml water for injections) in the prefilled syringe and the integrated transfer device (Bio-Set). Gently rotate the vial until all powder is dissolved. Do not use KOGENATE Bayer if you notice visible particulate matter or turbidity.

After reconstitution, the solution is drawn back into the syringe.

Use the provided venipuncture set for intravenous injection.

Any unused product or waste material should be disposed of in accordance with local requirements.

7. MARKETING AUTHORISATION HOLDER

Bayer AG

D-51368 Leverkusen

Germany

8. MARKETING AUTHORISATION NUMBER(S)

KOGENATE Bayer 250 IU – EU/1/00/143/004

KOGENATE Bayer 500 IU – EU/1/00/143/005

KOGENATE Bayer 1000 IU – EU/1/00/143/006

9. DATE OF FIRST AUTHORISATION/RENEWAL OF THE AUTHORISATION

21 September 2004

10. DATE OF REVISION OF THE TEXT

November 2004

LEGAL CATEGORY

POM

Distributed in the United Kingdom by:

Bayer plc

Pharmaceutical Division

Bayer House

Strawberry Hill

Newbury

Berkshire

RG14 1JA

Konakion MM

(Roche Products Limited)

1. NAME OF THE MEDICINAL PRODUCT

Konakion MM.

2. QUALITATIVE AND QUANTITATIVE COMPOSITION

Each Konakion MM Ampoule contains 10.0mg vitamin K_1 (phytomenadione) Ph. Eur in 1ml.

3. PHARMACEUTICAL FORM

Amber glass ampoules containing 10mg phytomenadione in 1ml. The ampoule solution is clear to slightly opalescent, pale yellow in colour and contains the active constituent in a mixed micelles vehicle of glycocholic acid and lecithin.

4. CLINICAL PARTICULARS

4.1 Therapeutic indications

Konakion MM is indicated as an antidote to anticoagulant drugs of the coumarin type in the treatment of haemorrhage or threatened haemorrhage, associated with a low blood level of prothrombin or factor VII.

4.2 Posology and method of administration

Adults:*As an antidote to anticoagulant drugs*

For potentially fatal and severe haemorrhages: Konakion MM therapy should be accompanied by a more immediate effective treatment such as transfusions of whole blood or blood clotting factors. The anticoagulant should be withdrawn and an intravenous injection of Konakion MM given slowly in a dose of 10 – 20mg. The prothrombin level should be estimated three hours later and, if the response has been inadequate, the dose should be repeated. Not more than 40mg of Konakion MM should be given intravenously in 24 hours. Coagulation profiles must be monitored on a daily basis until these have returned to acceptable levels; in severe cases more frequent monitoring is necessary and where there is no immediate efficacy, transfusion of whole blood or blood clotting factors should be used.

Less severe haemorrhage: Oral treatment with Konakion tablets may be used.

Elderly

Elderly patients tend to be more sensitive to reversal of anticoagulation with Konakion MM; dosage in this group should be at the lower end of the ranges recommended.

Instructions for infusion in adults

Konakion MM Ampoules are for intravenous injection and should be diluted with 55ml of 5% glucose before slowly infusing the product. The solution should be freshly prepared and protected from light. Konakion MM Ampoule solution should not be diluted or mixed with other injectables, but may be injected into the lower part of an infusion apparatus.

Children aged 1 to 18 years

It is advisable that a haematologist is consulted about appropriate investigation and treatment in any child in whom Konakion MM is being considered.

Likely indications for using vitamin K in children are limited and may include:

1. Children with disorders that interfere with absorption of vitamin K (chronic diarrhoea, cystic fibrosis, biliary atresia, hepatitis, coeliac disease).

2. Children with poor nutrition who are receiving broad spectrum antibiotics.

3. Liver disease.

4. Patients receiving anticoagulant therapy with warfarin in whom the INR is increased outside the therapeutic range and therefore are at risk of, or are bleeding, and those with an INR in the therapeutic range who are bleeding.

For patients on warfarin therapy, therapeutic intervention must take into consideration the reason for the child being on warfarin and whether or not anticoagulant therapy has to be continued (e.g. in a child with mechanical heart valve or repeated thromboembolic complications) as vitamin K administration is likely to interfere with anticoagulation with warfarin for 2 – 3 weeks.

It should be noted that the earliest effect seen with vitamin K treatment is at 4 – 6 hours and therefore in patients with severe haemorrhage replacement with coagulation factors may be indicated (discuss with haematologist).

Dose of vitamin K

There are few data available regarding use of Konakion MM in children over 1 year. There have been no dose ranging studies in children with haemorrhage. Suggested dosages based on clinical experience are as follows:

Haemorrhage in children: 2 – 5mg i.v.

Asymptomatic children at risk of bleeding: 1 – 5mg i.v.

Prothrombin levels should be measured 2 to 6 hours later and if the response has not been adequate, the dose may be repeated. Frequent monitoring of vitamin K dependent clotting factors is essential in these patients.

Children on warfarin therapy who need to remain anticoagulated are not included in the above dosage recommendations.

Neonates and babies

Konakion MM Paediatric should be used in these patients. (See separate prescribing information.)

4.3 Contraindications

Use in patients with a known hypersensitivity to any of the constituents.

4.4 Special warnings and special precautions for use

When treating patients with severely impaired liver function, it should be borne in mind that one Konakion MM Ampoule 10mg/1ml contains 54.6mg glycocholic acid and this may have a bilirubin displacing effect.

At the time of use, the ampoule contents should be clear. Following incorrect storage, the contents may become turbid or present a phase-separation. In this case the ampoule must no longer be used.

In potentially fatal and severe haemorrhage due to overdosage of coumarin anticoagulants, intravenous injections of Konakion MM must be administered slowly and not more than 40mg should be given during a period of 24 hours. Konakion MM therapy should be accompanied by a more immediate effective treatment such as transfusion of whole blood or blood clotting factors. When patients with prosthetic heart valves are given transfusions for the treatment of severe or potentially fatal haemorrhages, fresh frozen plasma should be used.

Large doses of Konakion MM (more than 40mg per day) should be avoided if it is intended to continue with anticoagulant therapy because there is no experience with doses above this maximum of 40mg per day and higher doses may give rise to unexpected adverse events. Clinical studies have shown a sufficient decrease in the prothrombin time with the recommended dosage. If haemorrhage is severe, a transfusion of fresh whole blood may be necessary whilst awaiting the effect of the vitamin K_1.

Vitamin K_1 is not an antidote to heparin.

4.5 Interaction with other medicinal products and other forms of Interaction

No significant interactions are known other than antagonism of coumarin anticoagulants.

4.6 Pregnancy and lactation

There is no specific evidence regarding the safety of Konakion MM in pregnancy but, as with most drugs, the administration during pregnancy should only occur if the benefits outweigh the risks.

4.7 Effects on ability to drive and use machines

None.

4.8 Undesirable effects

There are only few unconfirmed reports of the occurrence of possible anaphylactoid reactions after intravenous injection of Konakion MM. Very rarely, venous irritation or phlebitis has been reported in association with intravenous administration of Konakion mixed micelle solution. Injection site reactions have been reported after intramuscular injection of Konakion.

4.9 Overdose

Hypervitaminosis of vitamin K_1 is unknown.

5. PHARMACOLOGICAL PROPERTIES

5.1 Pharmacodynamic properties

Konakion MM is a synthetic preparation of vitamin K. The presence of vitamin K (i.e. vitamin K or substances with vitamin K activity) is essential for the formation within the body of prothrombin, factor VII, factor IX and factor X. Lack of vitamin K leads to an increased tendency to haemorrhage. When an antidote to an anticoagulant is necessary it is essential to use vitamin K_1 itself, as vitamin K analogues are much less effective.

In the mixed micelles solution, vitamin K_1 is solubilised by means of a physiological colloidal system, also found in the human body, consisting of lecithin and bile acid. Owing to the absence of organic solvents, the Konakion mixed micelles solution is well tolerated on intravenous administration.

5.2 Pharmacokinetic properties

In blood plasma, 90% of vitamin K_1 is bound to lipoproteins. Following an intramuscular dose of 10mg vitamin K, plasma concentrations of 10 – 20mcg/l are produced (normal range 0.4 – 1.2mcg/l). Systemic availability following intramuscular administration is about 50% and elimination half-life in plasma is approximately 1.5 – 3 hours.

5.3 Preclinical safety data

None applicable.

6. PHARMACEUTICAL PARTICULARS

6.1 List of excipients

Glycocholic acid HSE

Sodium hydroxide Ph. Eur

Lecithin (phospholipon 100) HSE

Hydrochloric acid Ph. Eur.

Water for injection Ph. Eur.

6.2 Incompatibilities

None.

6.3 Shelf life

The recommended shelf-life of Konakion MM Ampoules is 36 months.

6.4 Special precautions for storage

The recommended maximum storage temperature is 25°C. Do not use if the solution is turbid.

6.5 Nature and contents of container

Konakion MM is supplied in amber glass ampoules containing 10mg phytomenadione in 1ml. The ampoule solution is clear to slightly opalescent, pale yellow in colour and contains the active constituent in a mixed micelles vehicle of glycocholic acid and lecithin.

6.6 Instructions for use and handling

See section 4.2.

7. MARKETING AUTHORISATION HOLDER

Roche Products Limited, 40 Broadwater Road, Welwyn Garden City, Hertfordshire, AL7 3AY.

8. MARKETING AUTHORISATION NUMBER(S)

PL 0031/0254

9. DATE OF FIRST AUTHORISATION/RENEWAL OF THE AUTHORISATION

17 August 1993

10. DATE OF REVISION OF THE TEXT

November 2002

Konakion is a registered trade mark

Item Code

Konakion MM Paediatric

(Roche Products Limited)

1. NAME OF THE MEDICINAL PRODUCT

Konakion MM Paediatric.

2. QUALITATIVE AND QUANTITATIVE COMPOSITION

Each ampoule contains 2mg phytomenadione in 0.2ml.

3. PHARMACEUTICAL FORM

The ampoule solution is clear to slightly opalescent, pale yellow in colour and contains the active constituent in a mixed micelles vehicle of glycocholic acid and lecithin.

4. CLINICAL PARTICULARS

4.1 Therapeutic indications

Konakion MM is indicated for the prophylaxis and treatment of haemorrhagic disease of the newborn.

4.2 Posology and method of administration

Neonates and Babies

Prophylaxis

*Healthy neonates of 36 weeks gestation and older:*2mg orally at birth or soon after birth. This should be followed by a second dose of 2mg at 4 - 7 days.

*Preterm neonates of less than 36 weeks gestation weighing 2.5kg or greater, and term neonates at special risk:*1mg IM or IV at birth or soon after birth, the size and frequency of further doses depending on coagulation status.

*Preterm neonates of less than 36 weeks gestation weighing less than 2.5kg:*0.4mg/kg (equivalent to 0.04ml/kg) IM or IV at birth or soon after birth. This parenteral dose should not be exceeded (see *Special warnings and special precautions for use*). The frequency of further doses should depend on coagulation status.

Exclusively breast-fed babies: In addition to the doses at birth and at 4 - 7 days, a further 2mg oral dose should be given 1 month after birth. Further monthly 2mg oral doses until formula feeding is introduced have been advised, but no safety or efficacy data exist for these additional doses.

Therapy

Initially 1mg IV and further doses as required, depending on clinical picture and coagulation status. Konakion therapy may need to be accompanied by a more immediate effective treatment, such as transfusion of whole blood or blood clotting factors to compensate for severe blood loss and delayed response to vitamin K_1.

4.3 Contraindications

Use in patients with a known hypersensitivity to any of the constituents.

4.4 Special warnings and special precautions for use

At the time of use, the ampoule contents should be clear. Following incorrect storage, the contents may become turbid or present a phase-separation. In this case the ampoule must no longer be used.

For oral use: After breaking the ampoule open, 0.2ml of solution should be withdrawn into the oral dispenser until it reaches the mark on the dispenser (0.2ml = 2mg vitamin K). Drop the contents of the dispenser directly into the baby's mouth by pressing the plunger.

For parenteral use: Konakion MM paediatric should not be diluted or mixed with other parenteral medications, but may be injected into the lower part of an infusion set.

Parenteral administration to premature babies weighing less than 2.5kg may increase the risk for the development of kernicterus (bilirubin encephalopathy).

4.5 Interaction with other medicinal products and other forms of Interaction

No significant interactions are known other than antagonism of coumarin anticoagulants.

4.6 Pregnancy and lactation

Not applicable.

4.7 Effects on ability to drive and use machines

Not applicable.

4.8 Undesirable effects

There are only few unconfirmed reports on the occurrence of possible anaphylactoid reactions after IV injection of Konakion MM. Local irritation may occur at the injection site but is unlikely due to the small injection volume. Rarely, injection site reactions may occur which may be severe, including inflammation, atrophy and necrosis.

4.9 Overdose

No overdose effects are known.

5. PHARMACOLOGICAL PROPERTIES

5.1 Pharmacodynamic properties

Konakion MM is a preparation of synthetic phytomenadione (vitamin K_1). The presence of vitamin K_1 is essential for the formation within the body of prothrombin, factor VII, factor IX and factor X, and of the coagulation inhibitors, protein C and protein S.

Vitamin K_1 does not readily cross the placental barrier from mother to child and is poorly excreted in breast milk.

Lack of vitamin K_1 leads to an increased tendency to haemorrhagic disease in the newborn. Vitamin K_1 administration, which promotes synthesis of the above-mentioned coagulation factors by the liver, can reverse an abnormal coagulation status due to vitamin K_1 deficiency.

5.2 Pharmacokinetic properties

In the mixed micelle solution, vitamin K_1 is solubilised by means of a physiological colloidal system consisting of lecithin and a bile acid.

Vitamin K_1 is absorbed from the small intestine. Absorption is limited in the absence of bile.

Vitamin K_1 accumulates predominantly in the liver, is up to 90% bound to lipoproteins in the plasma and is stored in the body only for short periods of time.

Vitamin K_1 is transformed to more polar metabolites, such as phytomenadione-2,3-epoxide.

The half-life of vitamin K_1 in plasma is about 1.5 to 3 hours. Vitamin K_1 is excreted in bile and urine as the glucuronide and sulphate conjugates.

5.3 Preclinical safety data

None applicable.

6. PHARMACEUTICAL PARTICULARS

6.1 List of excipients

Glycocholic acid, lecithin, sodium hydroxide, hydrochloric acid and water.

6.2 Incompatibilities

See section 4.4.

6.3 Shelf life

3 years.

6.4 Special precautions for storage

Konakion MM Paediatric ampoule solution should be stored below 25°C and be protected from light. The solution should not be frozen. Do not use if the solution is turbid.

6.5 Nature and contents of container

Amber glass ampoules containing 2mg phytomenadione in 0.2ml. Plastic oral dispensers. Packs of 1, 5 or 10.

6.6 Instructions for use and handling

See section 4.4.

7. MARKETING AUTHORISATION HOLDER

Roche Products Limited, 40 Broadwater Road, Welwyn Garden City, Hertfordshire, AL7 3AY.

8. MARKETING AUTHORISATION NUMBER(S)

PL 0031/0346

9. DATE OF FIRST AUTHORISATION/RENEWAL OF THE AUTHORISATION

20 June 1996

10. DATE OF REVISION OF THE TEXT

August 1998

Konakion is a registered trade mark

P465032/1098

Konakion Neonatal Ampoules

(Roche Products Limited)

1. NAME OF THE MEDICINAL PRODUCT

Konakion Neonatal Ampoules

2. QUALITATIVE AND QUANTITATIVE COMPOSITION

Each Konakion Neonatal Ampoule contains 1mg vitamin K_1 (phytomenadione) Ph. Eur. in 0.5ml.

3. PHARMACEUTICAL FORM

Amber glass ampoules containing 1mg phytomenadione in 0.5ml. The ampoule solution is clear to opalescent, greenish-yellow in colour and contains a polyethoxylated castor oil as a non-ionic surfactant.

4. CLINICAL PARTICULARS

4.1 Therapeutic indications

Konakion Neonatal Ampoules are indicated for the *intramuscular* prophylaxis of haemorrhagic disease of healthy neonates of 36 weeks gestation and older.

For the prophylaxis of haemorrhage in pre-term neonates of less than 36 weeks gestation and term neonates at special risk, refer to Konakion MM Paediatric prescribing information.

For *oral* prophylaxis of haemorrhagic disease in healthy neonates of 36 weeks gestation and older, refer to Konakion MM Paediatric prescribing information.

For the treatment of the haemorrhagic disease of the newborn, refer to Konakion MM Paediatric prescribing information.

Konakion Neonatal Ampoules are used as an antidote to anticoagulant drugs of the coumarin type in infants and babies under 1 year. For use as an antidote to anticoagulant drugs of the coumarin type in adults and children (age 1 to 18 years), refer to Konakion MM Ampoules.

4.2 Posology and method of administration

Prophylaxis of healthy neonates of 36 weeks gestation and older:

1mg by intramuscular injection at birth or shortly after birth.

There have been no dose ranging studies performed to recommend a dose of Konakion Neonatal Ampoules used as an antidote to anticoagulant drugs of the coumarin type in infants and babies under 1 year. It is advisable that a haematologist is consulted about appropriate investigation and treatment in any infant or baby under 1 year in whom Konakion Neonatal Ampoules is being considered.

4.3 Contraindications

Use in patients with a known hypersensitivity to any of the constituents.

4.4 Special warnings and special precautions for use

Konakion Neonatal Ampoules contain a polyethoxylated castor oil as a non-ionic surfactant. In animal studies, polyethoxylated castor oil can produce severe anaphylactoid reactions associated with histamine release. There is strong circumstantial evidence that similar reactions occurring in patients may have been caused by polyethoxylated castor oil. Polyethoxylated castor oil, when given to patients over a period of several days, can also produce abnormal lipoprotein electrophoretic patterns, alterations in blood viscosity and erythrocyte aggregation.

4.5 Interaction with other medicinal products and other forms of Interaction

None known.

4.6 Pregnancy and lactation

Not applicable. Konakion Neonatal Ampoules are only recommended for use in neonates.

4.7 Effects on ability to drive and use machines

Not applicable. Konakion Neonatal Ampoules are only recommended for use in neonates.

4.8 Undesirable effects

Local irritation may occur at the injection site, but is unlikely in view of the small injection volume.

Konakion Neonatal Ampoules must not be administered by intravenous injection. After rapid intravenous administration of vitamin K_1 the following undesirable effects have been reported: flushing of the face, sweating, a sense of chest constriction, cyanosis and peripheral vascular collapse.

Repeated intramuscular injections of Konakion Neonatal Ampoules are not recommended. Repeated intramuscular injections of vitamin K_1 preparations, usually over prolonged periods in patients with hepatic disease have been reported to give rise to local cutaneous and subcutaneous changes.

4.9 Overdose

Hypervitaminosis of vitamin K_1 is unknown.

5. PHARMACOLOGICAL PROPERTIES

5.1 Pharmacodynamic properties

Konakion is a synthetic preparation of vitamin K_1. The presence of vitamin K (i.e. vitamin K_1 itself or substances with vitamin K activity) is essential for the formation within the body of prothrombin, factor VII, factor IX and factor X. Lack of vitamin K leads to increased tendency to haemorrhage. When an antidote to an anticoagulant is necessary it is essential to use vitamin K_1 itself, as vitamin K analogues are much less effective.

5.2 Pharmacokinetic properties
The fat-soluble vitamin compound phytomenadione (Vitamin K_1) requires the presence of bile for its absorption from the gastro-intestinal tract. Vitamin K accumulates mainly in the liver but is stored in the body only for short periods of time. Vitamin K does not appear to cross the placenta readily and it is poorly distributed into breast milk. Phytomenadione is rapidly metabolised to more polar metabolites and is excreted in bile and urine as glucuronide and sulphate conjugates.

5.3 Preclinical safety data
LD_{50} (i.v.) of Konakion MM (10mg/ml) in mice: 12.1 - 17.7ml/kg.

6. PHARMACEUTICAL PARTICULARS

6.1 List of excipients
Polyoxyl 35 castor oil USP

Propylene glycol Ph. Eur.

Phenol Ph. Eur.

Water for injections Ph. Eur.

6.2 Incompatibilities
None known.

6.3 Shelf life
The recommended shelf life of Konakion Ampoules is 60 months.

6.4 Special precautions for storage
Konakion Ampoule solution should be protected from light; it should not be allowed to freeze. The recommended maximum storage temperature for Konakion Ampoules is 30°C.

6.5 Nature and contents of container
Konakion is supplied in 1ml amber glass ampoules containing 0.6ml of solution.

6.6 Instructions for use and handling
Konakion Ampoule solution should not be diluted.

7. MARKETING AUTHORISATION HOLDER
Roche Products Limited, 40 Broadwater Road, Welwyn Garden City, Hertfordshire, AL7 3AY.

8. MARKETING AUTHORISATION NUMBER(S)
PL 0031/5023R

9. DATE OF FIRST AUTHORISATION/RENEWAL OF THE AUTHORISATION
3 July 1985

10. DATE OF REVISION OF THE TEXT
November 2000

Konakion is a registered trade mark

P465036/101

Konakion Tablets 10mg

(Roche Products Limited)

1. NAME OF THE MEDICINAL PRODUCT
Konakion Tablets 10mg

2. QUALITATIVE AND QUANTITATIVE COMPOSITION
Each Konakion Tablet contains 10mg phytomenadione (vitamin K_1).

For excipients, see 6.1.

3. PHARMACEUTICAL FORM
Round off-white sugar-coated tablets.

4. CLINICAL PARTICULARS

4.1 Therapeutic indications
Konakion is indicated in the treatment of haemorrhage or threatened haemorrhage associated with a low blood level of prothrombin or factor VII. The main indications are:

As an antidote to anticoagulant drugs of the coumarin type.

4.2 Posology and method of administration
Konakion tablets are for oral administration and should be chewed or allowed to dissolve slowly in the mouth.

Adults: As an antidote to anticoagulant drugs

For potentially fatal and severe haemorrhages: Konakion intravenous injection (see separate prescribing information).

Less severe haemorrhage: Konakion is given orally in doses of 10 - 20mg (1 to 2 tablets). The prothrombin level is estimated 8 to 12 hours later, and if the response has been inadequate, the dose should be repeated.

Lowering of prothrombin to dangerous level but no haemorrhage: A dose of 5 - 10mg Konakion orally may be given to bring the prothrombin level back to within safe limits. In such instances it is not usually necessary to discontinue the anticoagulant.

Adults: Other indications

Doses of 10 - 20mg as required.

Elderly

Elderly patients tend to be more sensitive to reversal of anticoagulation with Konakion; dosage in this group should be at the lower end of the ranges recommended.

Children

If, on the recommendation of a physician, a children's dosage is required, then it is suggested that 5 - 10mg be given.

4.3 Contraindications
Use in patients with a known hypersensitivity to any of the constituents.

4.4 Special warnings and special precautions for use
Large doses of Konakion should be avoided if it is intended to continue with anticoagulant therapy.

Vitamin K_1 is not an antidote to heparin.

Konakion tablets contain glucose, sucrose and lactose (skimmed milk powder). Patients with rare galactose intolerance, Lapp Lactase deficiency, fructose intolerance, glucose-galactose malabsorption or sucrase-isomaltase insufficiency should not take this medicine.

4.5 Interaction with other medicinal products and other forms of interaction
None known.

4.6 Pregnancy and lactation
There is no specific evidence regarding the safety of Konakion in pregnancy but, as with most drugs, the administration during pregnancy should only occur if the benefits outweigh the risks.

4.7 Effects on ability to drive and use machines
None known.

4.8 Undesirable effects
None known.

4.9 Overdose
Hypervitaminosis of vitamin K_1 is unknown.

5. PHARMACOLOGICAL PROPERTIES

5.1 Pharmacodynamic properties
Konakion is a synthetic preparation of vitamin K_1. The presence of vitamin K (i.e. vitamin K_1 itself or substances with vitamin K activity) is essential for the formation within the body of prothrombin, factor VII, factor IX and factor X. Lack of vitamin K leads to increased tendency to haemorrhage. When an antidote to an anticoagulant is necessary it is essential to use vitamin K_1 itself, as vitamin K analogues are much less effective.

5.2 Pharmacokinetic properties
The fat-soluble vitamin compound phytomenadione (Vitamin K_1) requires the presence of bile for its absorption from the gastro-intestinal tract. Vitamin K accumulates mainly in the liver but is stored in the body only for short periods of time. Vitamin K does not appear to cross the placenta readily and it is poorly distributed into breast milk. Phytomenadione is rapidly metabolised to more polar metabolites and is excreted in bile and urine as glucuronide and sulphate conjugates.

5.3 Preclinical safety data
None stated.

6. PHARMACEUTICAL PARTICULARS

6.1 List of excipients
Tablet core:

Silica, colloidal hydrated

Sucrose

Glucose, anhydrous

Skim Milk Powder

Cocoa

Theobroma oil

Carob Bean Gum

Glycerol

Tablet coat:

Sucrose

Rice Starch

Titanium Dioxide (E171)

Ethyl Vanillin

Acacia, Spray-Dried

Paraffin, Light Liquid

Paraffin, Hard

Talc

Carmellose sodium

6.2 Incompatibilities
Not applicable.

6.3 Shelf life
The recommended shelf life of Konakion Tablets is 5 years.

6.4 Special precautions for storage
Keep the bottle tightly closed. Store the bottle in the outer carton in order to protect from light.

6.5 Nature and contents of container
Konakion Tablets are supplied in white HDPE bottles with tamper evident snap-fit, containing 25 coated tablets or in amber glass bottles with HDPE closures and cotton-viscose pads, containing 10 coated tablets.

6.6 Instructions for use and handling
No special requirements.

7. MARKETING AUTHORISATION HOLDER
Roche Products Limited, 40 Broadwater Road, Welwyn Garden City, Hertfordshire AL7 3AY, England.

8. MARKETING AUTHORISATION NUMBER(S)
PL 0031/5022R

PA 50/51/1

9. DATE OF FIRST AUTHORISATION/RENEWAL OF THE AUTHORISATION
PL 0031/5022R: 31 May 1996

PA 50/51/1: 1 April 2003

10. DATE OF REVISION OF THE TEXT
March 2005

Konakion is a registered trade mark

Kytril Ampoules 1mg/1ml

(Roche Products Limited)

1. NAME OF THE MEDICINAL PRODUCT
Kytril Ampoules 1mg/1ml

2. QUALITATIVE AND QUANTITATIVE COMPOSITION
Each 1ml contains 1mg granisetron (as the hydrochloride). For excipients, see section *6.1*.

3. PHARMACEUTICAL FORM
A glass ampoule containing a sterile, clear colourless solution. The content allows withdrawal of 1ml.

Concentrate for solution for infusion or injection.

4. CLINICAL PARTICULARS

4.1 Therapeutic indications
Kytril is indicated for the prevention or treatment of nausea and vomiting induced by cytostatic therapy and for the prevention and treatment of post-operative nausea and vomiting.

4.2 Posology and method of administration
Cytostatic therapy

Children

Prevention: A single dose of 40μg/kg bodyweight (up to 3mg) should be administered as an intravenous infusion, diluted in 10 to 30ml infusion fluid and administered over five minutes. Administration should be completed prior to the start of cytostatic therapy.

Treatment: The same dose of Kytril as above should be used for treatment as prevention.

One additional dose of 40μg/kg bodyweight (up to 3mg) may be administered within a 24-hour period if required. This additional dose should be administered at least 10 minutes apart from the initial infusion.

Renally impaired

No special requirements apply.

Hepatically impaired

No special requirements apply.

Post-operative nausea and vomiting

Adults

For prevention in adults, a single dose of 1mg of Kytril should be diluted to 5ml and administered as a slow intravenous injection (over 30 seconds). Administration should be completed prior to induction of anaesthesia.

For the treatment of established post-operative nausea and vomiting in adults, a single dose of 1mg of Kytril should be diluted to 5ml and administered by slow intravenous injection (over 30 seconds).

Maximum dose and duration of treatment

Two doses (2mg) in one day.

Children

There is no experience in the use of Kytril in the prevention and treatment of post-operative nausea and vomiting in children. Kytril is not therefore recommended for the treatment of post-operative nausea and vomiting in this age group.

Elderly

As for adults.

Renally impaired

As for adults.

Hepatically impaired

As for adults.

4.3 Contraindications
Hypersensitivity to granisetron or related substances.

4.4 Special warnings and special precautions for use
As Kytril may reduce lower bowel motility, patients with signs of sub-acute intestinal obstruction should be monitored following administration of Kytril.

No special precautions are required for the elderly or renally or hepatically impaired patient.

4.5 Interaction with other medicinal products and other forms of Interaction
In studies in healthy subjects, no evidence of any interaction has been indicated between Kytril and cimetidine or lorazepam. No evidence of drug interactions has been observed in clinical studies conducted.

No specific interaction studies have been conducted in anaesthetised patients, but Kytril has been safely administered with commonly used anaesthetic and analgesic agents. In addition, *in vitro* human microsomal studies have shown that the cytochrome P450 sub-family 3A4 (involved in the metabolism of some of the main narcotic analgesic agents) is not modified by Kytril.

4.6 Pregnancy and lactation
Whilst animal studies have shown no teratogenic effects, there is no experience of Kytril in human pregnancy. Therefore Kytril should not be administered to women who are pregnant unless there are compelling clinical reasons. There are no data on the excretion of Kytril in breast milk. Breast feeding should therefore be discontinued during therapy.

4.7 Effects on ability to drive and use machines
There has been no evidence from human studies that Kytril has any adverse effect on alertness.

4.8 Undesirable effects
Kytril has been generally well tolerated in human studies. As reported with other drugs of this class, headache and constipation have been the most frequently noted adverse events but the majority have been mild or moderate in nature. Rare cases of hypersensitivity reaction, occasionally severe (e.g. anaphylaxis) have been reported. Other allergic reactions including minor skin rashes have also been reported. In clinical trials, transient increases in hepatic transaminases, generally within the normal range, have been seen.

4.9 Overdose
There is no specific antidote for Kytril. In the case of overdosage, symptomatic treatment should be given. One patient has received 30mg of Kytril intravenously. The patient reported a slight headache but no other sequelae were observed.

5. PHARMACOLOGICAL PROPERTIES

5.1 Pharmacodynamic properties
Kytril is a potent anti-emetic and highly selective antagonist of 5-hydroxytryptamine (5-HT_3) receptors. Radioligand binding studies have demonstrated that Kytril has negligible affinity for other receptor types including 5-HT and dopamine D_2 binding sites.

Kytril is effective intravenously, either prophylactically or by intervention, in abolishing the retching and vomiting evoked by administration of cytotoxic drugs or by whole body X-irradiation.

Kytril is effective, intravenously, in the prevention and treatment of post-operative nausea and vomiting.

5.2 Pharmacokinetic properties
General characteristics

Distribution

Kytril is extensively distributed, with a mean volume of distribution of approximately 3L/kg; plasma protein binding is approximately 65%.

Biotransformation

Biotransformation pathways involve N-demethylation and aromatic ring oxidation followed by conjugation.

Elimination

Clearance is predominantly by hepatic metabolism. Urinary excretion of unchanged Kytril averages 12% of dose whilst that of metabolites amounts to about 47% of dose. The remainder is excreted in faeces as metabolites. Mean plasma half-life in patients is approximately nine hours, with a wide inter-subject variability.

Characteristics in patients

The plasma concentration of Kytril is not clearly correlated with anti-emetic efficacy. Clinical benefit may be conferred even when Kytril is not detectable in plasma.

In elderly subjects after single intravenous doses, pharmacokinetic parameters were within the range found for non-elderly subjects. In patients with severe renal failure, data indicate that pharmacokinetic parameters after a single intravenous dose are generally similar to those in normal subjects. In patients with hepatic impairment due to neoplastic liver involvement, total plasma clearance of an intravenous dose was approximately halved compared to patients without hepatic involvement. Despite these changes, no dosage adjustment is necessary.

5.3 Preclinical safety data
Data from two-year carcinogenicity studies have shown an increase in hepatocellular carcinoma and/or adenoma in rats and mice of both sexes given 50mg/kg (rat dosage reduced to 25mg/kg/day at week 59). Increases in hepatocellular neoplasia were also detected at 5mg/kg in male rats. In both species, drug-induced effects (hepatocellular neoplasia) were not observed in the low-dose group (1mg/kg).

In several *in vitro* and *in vivo* assays, Kytril was shown to be non-genotoxic in mammalian cells.

6. PHARMACEUTICAL PARTICULARS

6.1 List of excipients
Sodium Chloride

Water for Injection

Citric acid, monohydrate

Hydrochloric acid

Sodium hydroxide

6.2 Incompatibilities
As a general precaution, Kytril should not be mixed in solution with other drugs. Prophylactic administration of Kytril should be completed prior to the start of cytostatic therapy or induction of anaesthesia.

6.3 Shelf life
Kytril ampoules have a shelf-life of three years.

Once opened 24 hours.

6.4 Special precautions for storage
Do not store above 30°C. Keep container in the outer carton. Do not freeze.

6.5 Nature and contents of container
Kytril is supplied in clear glass ampoules in packs of five, with an outer carton.

6.6 Instructions for use and handling
Preparing the infusion

Children: To prepare the dose of 40 μg/kg, the appropriate volume is withdrawn and diluted with infusion fluid to a total volume of 10 to 30ml. Any one of the following solutions may be used:

0.9% w/v Sodium Chloride Injection BP; 0.18% w/v Sodium Chloride and 4% w/v Glucose Injection BP; 5% w/v Glucose Injection BP; Hartmann's Solution for Injection BP; Sodium Lactate Injection BP; or 10% Mannitol Injection BP. No other diluents should be used.

Ideally, intravenous infusions of Kytril should be prepared at the time of administration. After dilution (see above), or when the container is opened for the first time, the shelf-life is 24 hours when stored at ambient temperature in normal indoor illumination protected from direct sunlight. It must not be used after 24 hours. If to be stored after preparation, Kytril infusions must be prepared under appropriate aseptic conditions.

Adults: to prepare a dose of 1mg, 1ml should be withdrawn from the ampoule and diluted to 5ml with 0.9% w/v Sodium Chloride Injection BP. No other diluent should be used.

7. MARKETING AUTHORISATION HOLDER
Roche Products Limited, 40 Broadwater Road, Welwyn Garden City, Hertfordshire, AL7 3AY.

8. MARKETING AUTHORISATION NUMBER(S)
PL 00031/0595

9. DATE OF FIRST AUTHORISATION/RENEWAL OF THE AUTHORISATION
23rd October 1995/23rd October 2000.

10. DATE OF REVISION OF THE TEXT
November 2003

11. LEGAL CATEGORY
POM

Kytril is a registered trade mark

P467059/1203

Kytril Infusion 3mg/3ml

(Roche Products Limited)

1. NAME OF THE MEDICINAL PRODUCT
Kytril Infusion 3mg/3ml.

2. QUALITATIVE AND QUANTITATIVE COMPOSITION
Each 3ml contains 3.0mg granisetron (as the hydrochloride).

For excipients, see *6.1*.

3. PHARMACEUTICAL FORM
An ampoule containing a sterile, clear, colourless or slightly straw-coloured solution equivalent to 1mg of granisetron per 1ml of solution. The content allows withdrawal of 3ml.

Concentrate for solution for infusion, or bolus injection.

4. CLINICAL PARTICULARS

4.1 Therapeutic indications
Kytril is indicated for the prevention or treatment of nausea and vomiting induced by cytostatic therapy.

4.2 Posology and method of administration
Adults

Kytril ampoules are for intravenous administration only.

3mg Kytril, which should be administered *either* in 15ml infusion fluid as an intravenous bolus over not less than 30 seconds *or* diluted in 20 to 50ml infusion fluid and administered over five minutes.

Prevention: In clinical trials, the majority of patients have required only a single dose of Kytril to control nausea and vomiting over 24 hours. Up to two additional doses of 3mg Kytril may be administered within a 24-hour period. There is clinical experience in patients receiving daily administration for up to five consecutive days in one course of therapy. Prophylactic administration of Kytril should be completed prior to the start of cytostatic therapy.

Treatment: The same dose of Kytril should be used for treatment as prevention. Additional doses should be administered at least 10 minutes apart.

Maximum daily dosage

Up to three doses of 3mg Kytril may be administered within a 24-hour period. The maximum dose of Kytril to be administered over 24 hours should not exceed 9mg.

Concomitant use of dexamethasone

The efficacy of Kytril may be enhanced by the addition of dexamethasone.

Children

Prevention: A single dose of 40 μg/kg body weight (up to 3mg) should be administered as an intravenous infusion, diluted in 10 to 30ml infusion fluid and administered over five minutes. Administration should be completed prior to the start of cytostatic therapy.

Treatment: The same dose of Kytril as above should be used for treatment as prevention.

One additional dose of 40 μg/kg body weight (up to 3mg) may be administered within a 24-hour period. This additional dose should be administered at least 10 minutes apart from the initial infusion.

Elderly

No special requirements apply to elderly patients.

Patients with renal or hepatic impairment

No special requirements apply to those patients with renal or hepatic impairment.

4.3 Contraindications
Hypersensitivity to granisetron, related substances or the excipients (see section *6.1*).

4.4 Special warnings and special precautions for use
As Kytril may reduce lower bowel motility, patients with signs of sub-acute intestinal obstruction should be monitored following administration of Kytril.

No special precautions are required for the elderly, renally or hepatically impaired patient.

4.5 Interaction with other medicinal products and other forms of Interaction
In studies in healthy subjects, no evidence of any interaction has been indicated between Kytril and cimetidine or lorazepam. No evidence of drug interactions has been observed in clinical studies conducted.

4.6 Pregnancy and lactation
Whilst animal studies have shown no teratogenic effects, there is no experience of Kytril in human pregnancy. Therefore Kytril should not be administered to women who are pregnant unless there are compelling clinical reasons. There are no data on the excretion of Kytril in breast milk. Breast feeding should therefore be discontinued during therapy.

4.7 Effects on ability to drive and use machines
There has been no evidence from human studies that Kytril has any adverse effect on alertness.

4.8 Undesirable effects
Kytril has been generally well tolerated in human studies. As reported with other drugs of this class, headache and constipation have been the most frequently noted adverse events but the majority have been mild or moderate in nature. Rare cases of hypersensitivity reaction, occasionally severe (e.g. anaphylaxis) have been reported. Other allergic reactions including minor skin rashes have also been reported. In clinical trials transient increases in hepatic transaminases, generally within the normal range, have been seen.

4.9 Overdose
There is no specific antidote for Kytril. In the case of overdosage, symptomatic treatment should be given. One patient has received 30mg of Kytril intravenously. The patient reported a slight headache but no other sequelae were observed.

5. PHARMACOLOGICAL PROPERTIES

5.1 Pharmacodynamic properties
Kytril is a potent anti-emetic and highly selective antagonist of 5-hydroxytryptamine (5-HT_3) receptors. Radioligand binding studies have demonstrated that Kytril has negligible affinity for other receptor types including 5-HT and dopamine D_2 binding sites.

Kytril is effective intravenously, either prophylactically or by intervention, in abolishing the retching and vomiting evoked by administration of cytotoxic drugs or by whole body X-irradiation.

5.2 Pharmacokinetic properties
General characteristics

Distribution

Kytril is extensively distributed, with a mean volume of distribution of approximately 3 L/kg; plasma protein binding is approximately 65%.

Biotransformation

Biotransformation pathways involve N-demethylation and aromatic ring oxidation followed by conjugation.

Elimination

Clearance is predominantly by hepatic metabolism. Urinary excretion of unchanged Kytril averages 12% of dose whilst that of metabolites amounts to about 47% of dose. The remainder is excreted in faeces as metabolites. Mean plasma half-life in patients is approximately nine hours, with a wide inter-subject variability.

Characteristics in patients

The plasma concentration of Kytril is not clearly correlated with anti-emetic efficacy. Clinical benefit may be conferred even when Kytril is not detectable in plasma.

In elderly subjects after single intravenous doses, pharmacokinetic parameters were within the range found for non-elderly subjects. In patients with severe renal failure, data indicate that pharmacokinetic parameters after a single intravenous dose are generally similar to those in normal subjects. In patients with hepatic impairment due to neoplastic liver involvement, total plasma clearance of an intravenous dose was approximately halved compared to patients without hepatic involvement. Despite these changes, no dosage adjustment is necessary.

5.3 Preclinical safety data

Data from two-year carcinogenicity studies have shown an increase in hepatocellular carcinoma and/or adenoma in rats and mice of both sexes given 50mg/kg (rat dosage reduced to 25mg/kg/day at week 59). Increases in hepatocellular neoplasia were also detected at 5mg/kg in male rats. In both species, drug-induced effects (hepatocellular neoplasia) were not observed in the low-dose group (1mg/kg).

In several *in vitro* and *in vivo* assays, Kytril was shown to be non-genotoxic in mammalian cells.

6. PHARMACEUTICAL PARTICULARS

6.1 List of excipients

Sodium Chloride

Water for Injection

Citric acid, monohydrate

Hydrochloric acid

Sodium hydroxide

6.2 Incompatibilities

As a general precaution, Kytril should not be mixed in solution with other drugs. Prophylactic administration of Kytril should be completed prior to the start of cytostatic therapy.

6.3 Shelf life

Kytril ampoules have a shelf-life of three years.

6.4 Special precautions for storage

Kytril ampoules should be stored protected from light. Do not freeze.

6.5 Nature and contents of container

Kytril is supplied in clear glass ampoules packaged in boxes of 5 or 10 ampoules.

6.6 Instructions for use and handling

Preparing the infusion

Adults: To prepare a dose of 3mg, 3ml is withdrawn from the ampoule and diluted either to 15ml with 0.9% w/v Sodium Chloride Injection BP (for bolus administration) or in infusion fluid to a total volume of 20 to 50ml in any of the following solutions: 0.9% w/v Sodium Chloride Injection BP; 0.18% w/v Sodium Chloride and 4% w/v Glucose Injection BP; 5% w/v Glucose Injection BP; Hartmann's Solution for Injection BP; Sodium Lactate Injection BP; or 10% Mannitol Injection BP (for infusion). No other diluents should be used.

Children: To prepare the dose of 40μg/kg the appropriate volume (up to 3ml) is withdrawn from the ampoule and diluted with infusion fluid (as for adults) to a total volume of 10 to 30ml.

Ideally, intravenous infusions of Kytril should be prepared at the time of administration. After dilution (see above) the shelf life is 24 hours when stored at ambient temperature in normal indoor illumination protected from direct sunlight. It must not be used after 24 hours. If to be stored after preparation, Kytril infusions must be prepared under appropriate aseptic conditions.

As a general precaution, Kytril should not be mixed in solution with other drugs.

7. MARKETING AUTHORISATION HOLDER

Roche Products Limited, 40 Broadwater Road, Welwyn Garden City, Hertfordshire, AL7 3AY.

8. MARKETING AUTHORISATION NUMBER(S)

PL 00031/0594

9. DATE OF FIRST AUTHORISATION/RENEWAL OF THE AUTHORISATION

15 October 2001

10. DATE OF REVISION OF THE TEXT

February 2004

11. Legal Category

POM

Kytril is a registered trade mark P467061/504

Kytril Tablets

(Roche Products Limited)

1. NAME OF THE MEDICINAL PRODUCT

Kytril Tablets 1mg and 2mg.

2. QUALITATIVE AND QUANTITATIVE COMPOSITION

Each tablet contains 1mg or 2mg granisetron (as hydrochloride).

For excipients, see section *6.1*.

3. PHARMACEUTICAL FORM

Film-coated Tablet.

White triangular film-coated tablets marked 'K1' or 'K2' on one side.

4. CLINICAL PARTICULARS

4.1 Therapeutic indications

Kytril tablets are indicated for the prevention of nausea and vomiting induced by cytostatic therapy.

4.2 Posology and method of administration

Adults

The dose of Kytril is 1mg twice a day or 2mg once a day during cytostatic therapy.

The first dose of Kytril should be administered within one hour before the start of cytostatic therapy.

Concomitant use of dexamethasone: The efficacy of Kytril may be enhanced by the addition of dexamethasone.

Maximum Dose and Duration of Treatment

Kytril is also available as ampoules for intravenous administration. The maximum dose of Kytril administered orally and/or intravenously over 24 hours should not exceed 9mg.

Children

There is insufficient evidence on which to base appropriate dosage regimens for children under

12 years old. Kytril Tablets are therefore not recommended in this age group.

Elderly

As for adults.

Renally Impaired

As for adults.

Hepatically Impaired

As for adults.

4.3 Contraindications

Hypersensitivity to granisetron, related substances, or the excipients (see section *6.1*).

4.4 Special warnings and special precautions for use

As Kytril may reduce lower bowel motility, patients with signs of sub-acute intestinal obstruction should be monitored following administration of Kytril.

4.5 Interaction with other medicinal products and other forms of Interaction

In studies in healthy subjects, no evidence of any interaction has been indicated between Kytril and cimetidine or lorazepam. No evidence of drug interactions has been observed in clinical studies.

4.6 Pregnancy and lactation

Whilst animal studies have shown no teratogenic effects, there is no experience of Kytril in human pregnancy. Therefore Kytril should not be administered to women who are pregnant unless there are compelling clinical reasons. There are no data on the excretion of Kytril in breast milk. Breast feeding should therefore be discontinued during therapy.

4.7 Effects on ability to drive and use machines

There has been no evidence from human studies that Kytril has any adverse effect on alertness.

4.8 Undesirable effects

Kytril has been generally well tolerated in human studies. As reported with other drugs of this class, headache and constipation have been the most frequently noted adverse events, but the majority have been mild or moderate in nature. Rare cases of hypersensitivity reaction, occasionally severe (e.g. anaphylaxis), have been reported. Other allergic reactions including minor skin rashes have also been reported. In clinical trials, transient increases in hepatic transaminases, generally within the normal range, have been seen.

4.9 Overdose

There is no specific antidote for Kytril. In the case of overdosage, symptomatic treatment should be given. One patient has received 30mg of Kytril intravenously. The patient reported a slight headache but no other sequelae were observed.

5. PHARMACOLOGICAL PROPERTIES

5.1 Pharmacodynamic properties

Kytril is a potent anti-emetic and highly selective antagonist of 5-hydroxytryptamine (5-HT_3) receptors. Radioligand binding studies have demonstrated that Kytril has negligible affinity for other receptor types including 5-HT and dopamine D_2 binding sites.

Kytril is effective orally prophylactically in abolishing the retching and vomiting evoked by cytostatic therapy.

5.2 Pharmacokinetic properties

General Characteristics

Absorption

Absorption of Kytril is rapid and complete, though oral bioavailability is reduced to about 60% as a result of first pass metabolism. Oral bioavailability is generally not influenced by food.

Distribution

Kytril is extensively distributed, with a mean volume of distribution of approximately 3 l/kg; plasma protein binding is approximately 65%.

Biotransformation

Biotransformation pathways involve N-demethylation and aromatic ring oxidation followed by conjugation.

Elimination

Clearance is predominantly by hepatic metabolism. Urinary excretion of unchanged Kytril averages 12% of dose whilst that of metabolites amounts to about 47% of dose. The remainder is excreted in faeces as metabolites. Mean plasma half-life in patients is approximately nine hours, with a wide inter-subject variability.

The pharmacokinetics of Kytril demonstrate no marked deviations from linear pharmacokinetics at oral doses up to 2.5-fold of the recommended clinical dose.

Characteristics in Patients

The plasma concentration of Kytril is not clearly correlated with anti-emetic efficacy. Clinical benefit may be conferred even when Kytril is not detectable in plasma.

In elderly subjects after single intravenous doses, pharmacokinetic parameters were within the range found for non-elderly subjects. In patients with severe renal failure, data indicate that pharmacokinetic parameters after a single intravenous dose are generally similar to those in normal subjects. In patients with hepatic impairment due to neoplastic liver involvement, total plasma clearance of an intravenous dose was approximately halved compared to patients without hepatic involvement. Despite these changes, no dosage adjustment is necessary.

5.3 Preclinical safety data

Data from two-year carcinogenicity studies have shown an increase in hepatocellular carcinoma and/or adenoma in rats and mice of both sexes given 50mg/kg (rat dosage reduced to 25mg/kg/day at week 59). Increases in hepatocellular neoplasia were also detected at 5mg/kg in male rats. In both species, drug-induced effects (hepatocellular neoplasia) were not observed in the low-dose group (1mg/kg).

In several *in vitro* and *in vivo* assays, Kytril was shown to be non-genotoxic in mammalian cells.

6. PHARMACEUTICAL PARTICULARS

6.1 List of excipients

Microcrystalline Cellulose (E460)

Sodium Starch Glycolate

Hypromellose (E464)Lactose monohydrate

Magnesium Stearate (E572)

***Film coat*:**

Hypromellose (E464)Titanium dioxide (E171)

Macrogol 400

Polysorbate 80 (E433)

6.2 Incompatibilities

None.

6.3 Shelf life

Kytril Tablets have a shelf-life of three years.

6.4 Special precautions for storage

None.

6.5 Nature and contents of container

Opaque PVC/aluminium foil blister packs packed in cartons containing 10 tablets (1mg) or 5 tablets (2mg).

6.6 Instructions for use and handling

None.

7. MARKETING AUTHORISATION HOLDER

Roche Products Limited, 40 Broadwater Road, Welwyn Garden City, Hertfordshire, AL7 3AY.

8. MARKETING AUTHORISATION NUMBER(S)

PL 00031/0591 (1mg)

PL 0031/0592 (2mg)

9. DATE OF FIRST AUTHORISATION/RENEWAL OF THE AUTHORISATION

15 September 2001

10. DATE OF REVISION OF THE TEXT

July 2004

11. Legal Category

POM

Kytril is a registered trade mark

Item code

Labiton Tonic

(Laboratories for Applied Biology Limited)

1. NAME OF THE MEDICINAL PRODUCT
Labiton

2. QUALITATIVE AND QUANTITATIVE COMPOSITION
Vitamin B1 0.375 mg/5ml

Alcohol (96%) 1.45 ml/5ml

Caffeine (total) 3.3 mg/5ml

Dried extract of Kola Nuts 3.025 mg/5ml

3. PHARMACEUTICAL FORM
Liquid for oral use.

4. CLINICAL PARTICULARS

4.1 Therapeutic indications
For use as a tonic for fatigue, anorexia and debility in convalescence after infections, such as influenza, and after operations.

4.2 Posology and method of administration
10 - 20 ml twice daily, before or after meals, with or without water.

Not intended for administration to children.

4.3 Contraindications
Where intake of alcohol is contraindicated, e.g., in cases of hepatitis.

Where there is hypersensitivity to any of the ingredients.

4.4 Special warnings and special precautions for use
The alcohol content should be born in mind.

4.5 Interaction with other medicinal products and other forms of Interaction
Alcohol may enhance the acute effect of drugs which depress the CNS.

4.6 Pregnancy and lactation
Not recommended for use in pregnant and breastfeeding women.

4.7 Effects on ability to drive and use machines
Car drivers taking tranquillisers should be made aware of the presence of alcohol and should be advised not to exceed the recommended dose.

4.8 Undesirable effects
With the correct dosage the ill effects of sensitivity to caffeine, such as tremors or palpitations, should not occur.

4.9 Overdose
Ill effects due to the alcohol content should predominate over those from the caffeine and will require appropriate treatment.

5. PHARMACOLOGICAL PROPERTIES

5.1 Pharmacodynamic properties
The pharmacology of all the active ingredients are well documented. See, e.g., Martindale.

Caffeine acts on the central nervous system, on muscle, including cardiac muscle, and on the kidney.

Vitamin B1 is fundamentally associated with carbohydrate metabolism. It is converted in the body to its pyrophosphate, which acts as a coenzyme.

Alcohol has a depressant action on the central nervous system, but by masking hesitancy, circumspection and self-criticism, in small doses it may appear to stimulate.

5.2 Pharmacokinetic properties
The pharmacokinetics of all the active ingredients are well documented. See, eg, Martindale.

Caffeine is readily absorbed from the gastrointestinal tract and is widely distributed to most body tissues. It is not stored to any appreciable amount in the body.

Alcohol is absorbed from the stomach and small intestine and is rapidly distributed throughout the body fluids. It is mainly metabolised in the liver to acetate.

Vitamin B1 is absorbed from the gastrointestinal tract and is widely distributed to most body tissues. It is not stored to any appreciable extent in the body.

5.3 Preclinical safety data
The product has been on the market for over 40 years with no problems reported.

6. PHARMACEUTICAL PARTICULARS

6.1 List of excipients
Sucrose 1.0 gm/5ml

x-tocopherol acetate 7.5mg/5ml

Cremophore RH 40 25mg/5ml

p-Aminobenzoic acid 2.0mg/5ml

Glycerophos. ac 20% 0.01ml/5ml

Caramel 5.0mg/5ml

6.2 Incompatibilities
Alcohol may enhance the acute effect of drugs which depress the CNS.

6.3 Shelf life
3 years. 6 months after opening.

6.4 Special precautions for storage
No special precautions

6.5 Nature and contents of container
Amber glass bottle containing 200 ml.

Amber glass bottle containing 1000ml.

6.6 Instructions for use and handling
No special instructions.

Administrative Data

7. MARKETING AUTHORISATION HOLDER
Laboratories for Applied Biology Ltd

91 Amhurst Park

London N 16 5 DR

8. MARKETING AUTHORISATION NUMBER(S)
PL 00118/5005R

9. DATE OF FIRST AUTHORISATION/RENEWAL OF THE AUTHORISATION
Date of Grant 23 June 1982

Renewed 17 June 2002

Expires 23 June 2007

10. DATE OF REVISION OF THE TEXT
20.09.99 Reduction of x-tocopherol acetate

24.04.02 Corrections to 4.3, 4.6, and 5.2

Lacri-lube

(Allergan Ltd)

1. NAME OF THE MEDICINAL PRODUCT
LACRI-LUBE® Eye ointment

REFRESH NIGHT TIME® Eye ointment

2. QUALITATIVE AND QUANTITATIVE COMPOSITION
No pharmacologically active ingredient is present.

For excipients, see 6.1.

3. PHARMACEUTICAL FORM
Eye ointment.

Smooth, homogeneous, off-white, preservative-free ointment.

4. CLINICAL PARTICULARS

4.1 Therapeutic indications
As adjunctive therapy to lubricate and protect the eye in conditions such as exposure keratitis, decreased corneal sensitivity, recurrent corneal erosions, keratitis sicca, ophthalmic and non-ophthalmic surgery.

4.2 Posology and method of administration
For topical ocular administration.

Pull lower eye lid down to form a pocket and apply small amount as required.

There is no variation in dosage for age.

4.3 Contraindications
Hypersensitivity to lanolin alcohols.

4.4 Special warnings and special precautions for use
To avoid contamination during use, do not touch the tube tip to any surface.

If irritation, pain, redness and changes in vision occur or worsen, treatment discontinuation should be considered and a re-evaluation of the patient's condition should be made.

Contact lenses should not be worn during instillation of the drug. After instillation there should be an interval of at least 30 minutes before reinsertion.

In circumstances where concomitant topical ocular medication is necessary, there should be an interval of at least 5 minutes between the two medications. LACRI-LUBE® / REFRESH NIGHT TIME® should always be the last medication instilled.

4.5 Interaction with other medicinal products and other forms of Interaction
No interactions have been observed with LACRI-LUBE® / REFRESH NIGHT TIME®. Since the constituents have a well-established medicinal use, no interactions are anticipated.

4.6 Pregnancy and lactation
The constituents of LACRI-LUBE® / REFRESH NIGHT TIME® have been used as pharmaceutical agents for many years with no untoward effects. No special precautions are therefore necessary for the use of LACRI-LUBE® / REFRESH NIGHT TIME® in pregnancy and lactation.

Women of child-bearing potential: suitable for use.

Fertility: no known implications.

4.7 Effects on ability to drive and use machines
May cause transient blurring of vision. Do not drive or use machinery unless vision is clear.

4.8 Undesirable effects
Local (ocular) effects:

Transient blurring of vision (typically lasting 1-15 minutes) may occur.

Rare $>1/10{,}000$, $<1/1{,}000$): irritation/stinging/burning sensation,

Very rare ($<1/10{,}000$): allergic reaction, pain, hyperaemia, and conjunctivitis.

Isolated reports of oedema, and pruritus.

4.9 Overdose
Accidental topical ocular overdosage will present no hazard, apart from a transient effect on vision (see 4.7).

5. PHARMACOLOGICAL PROPERTIES

5.1 Pharmacodynamic properties
Pharmacotherapeutic group (ATC code) = *S01X A* 20.

The ingredients of LACRI-LUBE® / REFRESH NIGHT TIME® are pharmacologically inert, bland oleaginous substances for lubrication and to maintain hydration of the ocular surfaces by occlusion.

5.2 Pharmacokinetic properties
Not applicable.

5.3 Preclinical safety data
No information.

6. PHARMACEUTICAL PARTICULARS

6.1 List of excipients
White soft paraffin (white petroleum jelly)

Mineral oil

Lanolin alcohols

6.2 Incompatibilities
None known.

6.3 Shelf life
Shelf life of the medicinal product as packaged for sale = 36 months.

Shelf life after first opening of container = 1 month.

6.4 Special precautions for storage
Do not store above 25°C.

6.5 Nature and contents of container
Container: 3.5 and 5.0g per tube

Collapsible metal tube; aluminium (99.7%) with melanine-epoxy resin internal coating or epoxyphenolic liner, or pig tin (98.8%).

Closure

Low density polyethylene; colorant: teknor apex PE-151 black.

Sealant

Darex cold seal (AD2311BLS)

Dispensing under medical prescription or sale from registered pharmacies.

6.6 Instructions for use and handling
Discard any unused product 1 month after first opening.

Administrative Data

7. MARKETING AUTHORISATION HOLDER
Allergan Ltd

Coronation Road

High Wycombe

Bucks. HP12 3SH

United Kingdom

8. MARKETING AUTHORISATION NUMBER(S)
PL 00426/0041

9. DATE OF FIRST AUTHORISATION/RENEWAL OF THE AUTHORISATION
23rd July 2003

10. DATE OF REVISION OF THE TEXT
23rd July 2003

Lacticare

(Stiefel Laboratories (UK) Limited)

1. NAME OF THE MEDICINAL PRODUCT
LactiCare

2. QUALITATIVE AND QUANTITATIVE COMPOSITION
Lactic acid 5% w/w, sodium pyrrolidone carboxylate 2.5% w/w

3. PHARMACEUTICAL FORM
Lotion for cutaneous use.

4. CLINICAL PARTICULARS

4.1 Therapeutic indications
LactiCare is indicated for the symptomatic relief of hyper-keratotic and other chronic dry skin conditions, and for dry skin conditions caused by low humidity or the use of detergents.

4.2 Posology and method of administration
Use as required on affected areas or as directed by a doctor.

4.3 Contraindications
None.

4.4 Special warnings and special precautions for use
Keep away from the eyes and mucous membranes. Should contact with the eyes occur, remove with water. Keep out of the reach of children.

4.5 Interaction with other medicinal products and other forms of Interaction
None.

4.6 Pregnancy and lactation
Although there is no experimental evidence to support the safety of the drug during pregnancy and lactation, no adverse effects have been reported.

4.7 Effects on ability to drive and use machines
None.

4.8 Undesirable effects
Occasionally a transient mild stinging sensation may occur. Should prolonged irritation develop when used on abraded or inflamed skin, discontinue use.

4.9 Overdose
Not applicable.

5. PHARMACOLOGICAL PROPERTIES

5.1 Pharmacodynamic properties
Both lactic acid and sodium pyrrolidone carboxylic acid are hygroscopic. They enhance the ability of the stratum corneum to retain water and counteract the tendency of the skin to dry out. Lactic acid also modulates epidermal keratinisation and increases skin extensibility.

5.2 Pharmacokinetic properties
Not applicable.

5.3 Preclinical safety data
There are no preclinical data of any relevance additional to that already included in other sections of the SmPC.

6. PHARMACEUTICAL PARTICULARS

6.1 List of excipients
Carbomer 940

Imidazolidinyl urea

Dehydroacetic acid

Sodium hydroxide

Polyethylene glycol ether complex

Glyceryl monostearate

Cetyl alcohol

Isopropyl palmitate

Light liquid paraffin

Myristyl lactate

Perfume Antaria 73/82

Purified water.

6.2 Incompatibilities
None.

6.3 Shelf life
a) For the product as packaged for sale - 3 years

b) After first opening the container - Comply with expiry date

6.4 Special precautions for storage
None.

6.5 Nature and contents of container
High density polyethylene bottles containing 150ml.

6.6 Instructions for use and handling
There are no special instructions for use or handling of LactiCare.

Administrative Data

7. MARKETING AUTHORISATION HOLDER
Stiefel Laboratories (UK) Ltd.

Holtspur Lane,

Wooburn Green,

High Wycombe,

Bucks. HP10 0AU

8. MARKETING AUTHORISATION NUMBER(S)
PL 0174/0038

9. DATE OF FIRST AUTHORISATION/RENEWAL OF THE AUTHORISATION
8th June 1979

10. DATE OF REVISION OF THE TEXT
September 2005.

Lactugal

(Intrapharm Laboratories Ltd)

1. NAME OF THE MEDICINAL PRODUCT
Lactugal.

2. QUALITATIVE AND QUANTITATIVE COMPOSITION
Active Ingredient:

Lactulose Solution BP 99.897 % v/v

(Equivalent to 62.0-74.0% w/v of Lactulose).

3. PHARMACEUTICAL FORM
Oral solution. Banana Flavour

4. CLINICAL PARTICULARS

4.1 Therapeutic indications
Constipation; Hepatic encephalopathy (Portal systemic encephalopathy).

4.2 Posology and method of administration
For oral administration.

Adults:

Constipation: 15ml once or twice daily.

Hepatic Encephalopathy: Initially 30-50ml three times daily, adjust dose to produce 2 or 3 soft stools daily.

Children:

1-5 years: 5ml twice daily.

5-10 years: l0ml twice daily.

Elderly:

The normal adult dosage is appropriate.

4.3 Contraindications
Lactugal is contra-indicated where there is evidence of gastro-intestinal obstruction and to patients with galactosaemia.

4.4 Special warnings and special precautions for use
There are no warnings or precautions for patients with any impaired organ function.

Lactulose should be used with caution in patients exhibiting lactose intolerance.

Due to the product's physiological mode of action it may take up to 48 hours before effects are obtained, however, the product does exhibit a 'carry over' effect which may enable the patient to reduce the dose gradually over a period of time.

Lactulose solution has a calorific value of approximately 19Kcals/5ml. As, however, only negligible amounts of lactulose are absorbed from the gastrointestinal tract the available calories will be much lower than this, and therefore, is unlikely to adversely affect diabetes.

4.5 Interaction with other medicinal products and other forms of Interaction
There are no known interactions with lactulose.

4.6 Pregnancy and lactation
Wide clinical experience in combination with data from animal production studies has not revealed any embryotoxic hazards to the foetus if used in the recommended dosage during pregnancy. If drug therapy is required during pregnancy or for lactating mothers, the use of this drug is acceptable.

4.7 Effects on ability to drive and use machines
There is no evidence to show that lactulose affects driving ability.

4.8 Undesirable effects
A normal dosage of lactulose may cause mild abdominal pain and flatulence which will disappear spontaneously after a few days. High doses may provoke nausea in some patients and this can be minimised by administration with water, fruit juice or meals.

4.9 Overdose
If clinically important electrolyte disturbances occur, suitable corrective measures should be taken.

5. PHARMACOLOGICAL PROPERTIES

5.1 Pharmacodynamic properties
Lactulose is a synthetic disaccharide which is metabolised by gastro-intestinal bacterial flora to low molecular weight acids (chiefly lactic and acetic acids). There is no endogenous metabolising enzyme in the human gut.

Its mode of action in constipation is as an osmotic agent producing soft stools.

A dual mode of action is proposed for the efficacy of lactulose in Portal System Encephalopathy, relating to the metabolism of ammonia and subsequent nitrogenous toxins. The reduction in gastro-intestinal pH results in a net entrapment of ammonia in the gut lumen. Lactulose has also been shown to alter ammonia metabolism by microbial flora.

5.2 Pharmacokinetic properties
Lactulose is absorbed from the gastro-intestinal tract to 0.4 - 2% and is excreted unchanged with the urine. There are no human lactulose disaccharide enzymes; metabolism of lactulose to lactic acid occurs via gastro-intestinal microbial flora only. Due to its poor bioavailability, plasma lactulose concentrations are negligible.

There are no known changes in kinetic properties in patients with organic diseases which may alter drug disposition.

5.3 Preclinical safety data
None stated.

6. PHARMACEUTICAL PARTICULARS

6.1 List of excipients
Banana Flavour Quinoline Yellow

(17.41.0042) (E 1 04)

6.2 Incompatibilities
There are no known incompatibilities.

6.3 Shelf life
36 months from the date of manufacture.

6.4 Special precautions for storage
Store at a temperature not exceeding 20°C. Do not freeze

6.5 Nature and contents of container
Amber glass winchesters with polypropylene caps as closures. Polyethylene containers with polypropylene caps as closures.

6.6 Instructions for use and handling
There are no special storage or handling instructions for this product.

Administrative Data

7. MARKETING AUTHORISATION HOLDER
Intrapharm Laboratories Ltd

Maidstone

Kent

ME15 9QS

United Kingdom

8. MARKETING AUTHORISATION NUMBER(S)
PL 17509/0011

9. DATE OF FIRST AUTHORISATION/RENEWAL OF THE AUTHORISATION
4 September 2003

10. DATE OF REVISION OF THE TEXT

Lactulose Solution

(Novartis Consumer Health)

1. NAME OF THE MEDICINAL PRODUCT
Lactulose Liquid EP

2. QUALITATIVE AND QUANTITATIVE COMPOSITION
Lactulose 67.0% w/v

3. PHARMACEUTICAL FORM
Oral Solution

4. CLINICAL PARTICULARS

4.1 Therapeutic indications
A. Chronic constipation.

B. Chronic portal systemic encephalopathy.

4.2 Posology and method of administration
Adults

Initially: 15-30ml daily for first 2-3 days (45ml may be given in obstinate cases).

Maintenance: 10-15ml daily or according to the need of the patient.

Children

Initially: 10-25ml daily for first 2-3 days.

Maintenance: 5-15ml daily or according to the need of the patient.

Dosage does not appear to be related to the age or weight of the child and should be adjusted to produce the required response.

Chronic portal systemic encephalopathy

Initially 30-50ml three times daily according to the requirements of the patient for adequate acidification of the colonic contents.

Use in the elderly

No evidence exists that elderly patients require different dosages or show different side-effects from younger patients.

4.3 Contraindications
In common with other preparations used for the treatment of constipation, Lactulose solution should not be used in patients with gastrointestinal obstruction. Lactulose solution should not be given to patients with galactosaemia or lactose intolerance.

4.4 Special warnings and special precautions for use
Prolonged use of Lactulose in children may contribute to the development of dental caries. Patients should be instructed to pay careful attention to dental hygiene.

4.5 Interaction with other medicinal products and other forms of Interaction
There are no known interactions involving Lactulose.

4.6 Pregnancy and lactation
Lactulose solution should be used with caution during the first trimester of pregnancy.

4.7 Effects on ability to drive and use machines
There is no evidence that Lactulose affects driving ability.

4.8 Undesirable effects
Side-effects rarely occur after the administration of Lactulose solution. Mild transient effects such as abdominal distension or cramps and flatulence, which subside after the initial stages of treatment, have occasionally been reported. High doses may provoke nausea in some patients.
This can be minimised by administration with water, fruit juice or with meals.

4.9 Overdose
No cases of intoxication due to deliberate or accidental overdosage with Lactulose solution have been reported to the company.

5. PHARMACOLOGICAL PROPERTIES
5.1 Pharmacodynamic properties
The active principle of Lactulose solution, lactulose, is neither broken down nor absorbed in the stomach and small intestine. In the colon it acts as a substrate for and promotes the growth of naturally occurring glycolytic micro-organisms, and is broken down to lactic acid. The pH of the intestinal contents is lowered, the growth of acidophilic flora is promoted and the putrefactive micro-organisms are suppressed. This reduces the formation of ammonia and amines and their absorption from the gut, thus leading to a fall in blood ammonia levels (responsible for hepatic encephalopathy). By normalising the intestinal flora Lactulose solution ensures the passage of normal stools, without excessive peristalsis.

5.2 Pharmacokinetic properties
Not appropriate.

5.3 Preclinical safety data
There are no preclinical data of relevance to the prescriber which are additional to those already included in other sections of the Summary of Product Characteristics.

6. PHARMACEUTICAL PARTICULARS
6.1 List of excipients
Other sugars (lactose, galactose, tagatose and other ketoses)
Purified water

6.2 Incompatibilities
Not applicable.

6.3 Shelf life
36 months.

6.4 Special precautions for storage
Do not store above 25°C.

6.5 Nature and contents of container
Amber glass bottles or plastic bottles containing 200 ml, 300 ml, 500 ml or 1 litre of Lactulose solution.

6.6 Instructions for use and handling
Not applicable.

Administrative Data
7. MARKETING AUTHORISATION HOLDER
Novartis Consumer Health UK Limited
Trading as Novartis Consumer Health
Wimblehurst Road
Horsham
West Sussex
RH12 5AB
UK

8. MARKETING AUTHORISATION NUMBER(S)
PL 00030/0175

9. DATE OF FIRST AUTHORISATION/RENEWAL OF THE AUTHORISATION
10 April 2000

10. DATE OF REVISION OF THE TEXT
November 2002

Legal category:
Pharmacy

Lamictal Combined Tablets

(GlaxoSmithKline UK)

1. NAME OF THE MEDICINAL PRODUCT
Lamictal Tablets 25mg
Lamictal Tablets 50mg
Lamictal Tablets 100mg
Lamictal Tablets 200mg
Lamictal Dispersible 2mg
Lamictal Dispersible 5mg
Lamictal Dispersible 25mg
Lamictal Dispersible 100mg

2. QUALITATIVE AND QUANTITATIVE COMPOSITION
Lamictal Tablets containing 25mg lamotrigine.
Lamictal Tablets containing 50mg lamotrigine.
Lamictal Tablets containing 100mg lamotrigine.
Lamictal Tablets containing 200mg lamotrigine.
Lamictal Dispersible 2 mg contain 2 mg lamotrigine.
Lamictal Dispersible 5 mg contain 5 mg lamotrigine.
Lamictal Dispersible 25 mg contain 25 mg lamotrigine.
Lamictal Dispersible 100 mg contain 100 mg lamotrigine.
For excipients see section 6.1.

3. PHARMACEUTICAL FORM
Lamictal Tablets 25mg are pale-yellow rounded-square tablets. They are multifaceted with '25' on one side and flat with "GSEC7" on the other.

Lamictal Tablets 50mg are pale-yellow rounded-square tablets. They are multifaceted with '50' on one side and flat with "GSEE1" on the other.

Lamictal Tablets 100mg are pale-yellow rounded-square tablets. They are multifaceted with '100' on one side and flat with "GSEE5" on the other.

Lamictal Tablets 200mg are pale-yellow rounded-square tablets. They are multifaceted with '200' on one side and flat with "GSEE7" on the other.

Lamictal Dispersible 2mg are white to off-white round tablets with a blackcurrant odour. One side has a bevelled edge and is engraved with LTG over the number 2. The other side is engraved with two overlapping super-ellipses at right angles.

Lamictal Dispersible 5mg are white elongated, biconvex, tablets with "5" on one side and "GSCL2" on the other.

Lamictal Dispersible 25mg are white, multifaceted, super elliptical tablets with "25" on one side and "GSCL5" on the other.

Lamictal Dispersible 100mg are white multifaceted, super elliptical tablets with "100" on one side and "GSCL7" on the other.

4. CLINICAL PARTICULARS
4.1 Therapeutic indications
Epilepsy: *Monotherapy in adults and children over 12 years of age:*

Simple partial seizures

Complex partial seizures

Secondarily generalised tonic-clonic seizures

Primary generalised tonic-clonic seizures

Monotherapy in children under 12 years of age is not recommended until such time as adequate information is made available from controlled trials in this particular target population.

Add-on therapy in adults and children over 2 years of age

Simple partial seizures

Complex partial seizures

Secondarily generalised tonic-clonic seizures

Primary generalised tonic-clonic seizures

Lamictal is also indicated for the treatment of seizures associated with Lennox-Gastaut Syndrome.

4.2 Posology and method of administration
Administration
Lamictal Tablets should be swallowed whole with a little water.

Lamictal Dispersible tablets may be chewed, dispersed in a small volume of water (at least enough to cover the whole tablet) or swallowed whole with a little water.

To ensure a therapeutic dose is maintained the weight of a child must be monitored and the dose reviewed as weight changes occur.

If a calculated dose of lamotrigine (e.g. for use in children and patients with hepatic impairment) does not equate to whole tablets the dose to be administered is that equal to the lower number of whole tablets.

When concomitant antiepileptic drugs are withdrawn to achieve Lamictal monotherapy or other antiepileptic drugs (AEDs) are added-on to treatment regimes containing Lamictal consideration should be given to the effect this may have on lamotrigine pharmacokinetics (see 4.5 Interaction with other Medicinal Products and other Forms of Interaction).

<u>Restarting Therapy</u>
Prescribers should assess the need for escalation to maintenance dose when restarting lamotrigine in patients who have discontinued lamotrigine for any reason, since the risk of serious rash is associated with high initial doses and exceeding the recommended dose escalation for lamotrigine (see section 4.4). The greater the interval of time since the previous dose, the more consideration should be given to escalation to the maintenance dose. When the interval since discontinuing lamotrigine exceeds five half-lives (see section 5.2), lamotrigine should generally be escalated to the maintenance dose according to the appropriate schedule, as though initiating therapy (see section 4.2).

Dosage in monotherapy
Adults and children over 12 years (see Table 1)

The initial Lamictal dose in monotherapy is 25mg once a day for two weeks, followed by 50mg once a day for two weeks. Thereafter, the dose should be increased by a maximum of 50mg-100mg every 1-2 weeks until the optimal response is achieved. The usual maintenance dose to achieve optimal response is 100 - 200mg/day given once a day or as two divided doses. Some patients have required 500mg/day of Lamictal to achieve the desired response.

The initial dose and subsequent dose escalation should not be exceeded to minimise the risk of rash (see Special Warnings and Special Precautions for Use).

Children aged 2 to 12 years

There is insufficient evidence available from appropriate studies in children, upon which to base dosage recommendations for monotherapy use in children under the age of 12 years (see Therapeutic Indications).

Dosage in add-on therapy
Adults and children over 12 years (see Table 1)

In patients taking valproate with / without any other antiepileptic drug (AED) the initial Lamictal dose is 25 mg every alternate day for two weeks, followed by 25 mg once a day for two weeks. Thereafter, the dose should be increased by a maximum of 25-50mg every 1-2 weeks until the optimal response is achieved. The usual maintenance dose to achieve optimal response is 100-200mg/day given once a day or in two divided doses.

In those patients taking enzyme inducing AED's with / without other AED's (except valproate) the initial Lamictal dose is 50 mg once a day for two weeks, followed by 100 mg/day given in two divided doses for two weeks. Thereafter, the dose should be increased by a maximum of 100mg every 1-2 weeks until the optimal response is achieved. The usual maintenance dose to achieve optimal response is 200-400mg/day given in two divided doses. Some patients have required 700 mg/day of Lamictal to achieve the desired response.

In patients taking AED's where the pharmacokinetic interaction with lamotrigine is currently not known, the dose escalation as recommended for lamotrigine with concurrent valproate should be used, thereafter, the dose should be increased until optimal response is achieved.

Table 1 Recommended treatment regimen for adults and children over 12 years of age

(see Table 1 on next page)

The initial dose and subsequent dose escalation should not be exceeded to minimise the risk of rash (see Special Warnings and Special Precautions for Use).

Children aged 2 to 12 years

In patients taking valproate with / without any other antiepileptic drug (AED), the initial Lamictal dose is 0.15 mg/kg bodyweight/day given once a day for two weeks, followed by 0.3 mg/kg/day given once a day for two weeks. Thereafter, the dose should be increased by a maximum of 0.3 mg/kg every 1-2 weeks until the optimal response is achieved. The usual maintenance dose to achieve optimal response is 1-5 mg/kg/day given once a day or in two divided doses.

In those patients taking enzyme inducing AED's with / without other AED's (except valproate) the initial Lamictal dose is 0.6 mg/kg bodyweight/day given in two divided doses for two weeks, followed by 1.2mg/kg/day for two weeks. Thereafter, the dose should be increased by a maximum of 1.2 mg/kg every 1-2 weeks until the optimal response is achieved. The usual maintenance dose to achieve optimal response is 5-15mg/kg/day given in two divided doses.

In patients taking AED's where the pharmacokinetic interaction with lamotrigine is currently not known, the dose escalation as recommended for lamotrigine with concurrent valproate should be used, thereafter, the dose should be increased until optimal response is achieved.

Table 2 Recommended treatment regimen of Lamictal for children aged 2-12 years on combined drug therapy (Total daily dose in mg/kg bodyweight/day)

(see Table 2 on next page)

The initial dose and subsequent dose escalation should not be exceeded to minimise the risk of rash (see Special Warnings and Special Precautions for Use).

It is likely that patients aged 2-6 years will require a maintenance dose at the higher end of the recommended range.

Children aged less than 2 years

There is insufficient information on the use of Lamictal in children aged less than 2 years.

Women and Hormonal Contraceptives (see sections 4.4 and 4.5)

(a) Starting lamotrigine in patients taking hormonal contraceptives

Dose escalation should follow the guidelines recommended in Table 1 above (see sections 4.4 and 4.5).

(b) Starting hormonal contraceptives in patients taking lamotrigine

For women NOT taking inducers of lamotrigine glucuronidation such as phenytoin, carbamazepine, phenobarbital, primidone or rifampicin, the maintenance dose of lamotrigine may need to be increased by as much as two-fold, according to clinical response (see sections 4.4 and 4.5). For women taking lamotrigine in addition to inducers of

Table 1 Recommended treatment regimen for adults and children over 12 years of age

Treatment regimen		Weeks 1 + 2	Weeks 3 + 4	Usual Maintenance Dose
Monotherapy		25 mg (once a day)	50 mg (once a day)	100 – 200 mg (once a day or two divided doses) To achieve maintenance, doses may be increased by 50 – 100 mg every one to two weeks
Add-on therapy with valproate regardless of any concomitant medications		12.5 mg (given 25 mg **on** alternate days)	25 mg (once a day)	100 – 200 mg (once a day or two divided doses) To achieve maintenance, doses may be increased by 25 – 50 mg every one to two weeks
Add-on therapy without valproate	This dosage regimen should be used with: phenytoin carbamazepine phenobarbital primidone or with other inducers of lamotrigine glucuronidation (see section 4.5).	50 mg (once a day)	100 mg (two divided doses)	200 – 400 mg (two divided doses) To achieve maintenance, doses may be increased by 100 mg every one to two weeks

Note: In patients taking AEDs where the pharmacokinetic interaction with lamotrigine is currently not known (see section 4.5), the treatment regimen as recommended for lamotrigine with concurrent valproate should be used, thereafter, the dose should be increased until optimal response is achieved.

Table 2 Recommended treatment regimen of Lamictal for children aged 2-12 years on combined drug therapy (Total daily dose in mg/kg bodyweight/day)

Treatment regimen		Weeks 1 + 2	Weeks 3 + 4	Usual Maintenance Dose
Add-on therapy with valproate regardless of any other concomitant medication		0.15 mg/kg* (once a day)	0.3 mg/kg (once a day)	0.3 mg/kg increments every one to two weeks to achieve a maintenance dose of 1 – 5 mg/kg (once a day or two divided doses).
Add-on therapy without valproate	This dosage regimen should be used with: phenytoin carbamazepine phenobarbital primidone or with other inducers of lamotrigine glucuronidation (see section 4.5).	0.6 mg/kg (two divided doses)	1.2 mg/kg (two divided doses)	1.2 mg/kg increments every one to two weeks to achieve a maintenance dose of 5 – 15 mg/kg (two divided doses).

Note: In patients taking AEDs where the pharmacokinetic interaction with lamotrigine is currently not known (see section 4.5), the treatment regimen as recommended for lamotrigine with concurrent valproate should be used, thereafter, the dose should be increased until optimal response is achieved.

* If the calculated daily dose in patients taking valproate is 1 to 2 mg, then 2 mg lamotrigine may be taken on alternate days for the first two weeks. If the calculated daily dose in patients taking valproate is less than 1 mg, then lamotrigine should not be administered.

lamotrigine glucoronidation, adjustment may not be necessary.

(c) Stopping hormonal contraceptives in patients taking lamotrigine

For women NOT taking inducers of lamotrigine glucoronidation the maintenance dose of lamotrigine may need to be decreased by as much as 50%, according to clinical response (see sections 4.4 and 4.5).

For women taking lamotrigine in addition to inducers of lamotrigine glucuronidation, adjustment may not be necessary.

Pregnancy and *post-partum*

Dose adjustment may be necessary during pregnancy and post-partum (see section 4.6).

Elderly

No dosage adjustment from recommended schedule is required. The pharmacokinetics of lamotrigine in this age group do not differ significantly from a non-elderly population.

Hepatic Impairment

Initial, escalation and maintenance doses should generally be reduced by approximately 50% in patients with moderate (Child-Pugh grade B) and 75% in severe (Child-Pugh grade C) hepatic impairment. Escalation and maintenance doses should be adjusted according to clinical response.

4.3 Contraindications

Lamictal is contraindicated in individuals with known hypersensitivity to lamotrigine.

4.4 Special warnings and special precautions for use

There have been reports of adverse skin reactions, which have generally occurred within the first 8 weeks after initiation of lamotrigine (Lamictal) treatment. The majority of rashes are mild and self limiting, however rarely, serious potentially life threatening skin rashes including Stevens Johnson syndrome (SJS) and toxic epidermal necrolysis (TEN) have been reported (see Undesirable Effects).

The approximate incidence of serious skin rashes reported as SJS in adults and children over the age of 12 is 1 in 1000. The risk in children under the age of 12 is higher than in adults. Available data from a number of studies suggest that the incidence of rashes associated with hospitalisation in children under the age of 12 is from 1 in 300 to 1 in 100 (see Undesirable Effects).

In children, the initial presentation of a rash can be mistaken for an infection; physicians should consider the possibility of a drug reaction in children that develop symptoms of rash and fever during the first eight weeks of therapy.

Additionally the overall risk of rash appears to be strongly associated with:-

- High initial doses of lamotrigine and exceeding the recommended dose escalation of lamotrigine therapy (see Posology and Method of Administration).
- Concomitant use of valproate (See Posology and Method of Administration).

All patients (adults and children) who develop a rash should be promptly evaluated and lamotrigine withdrawn immediately unless the rash is clearly not drug related. Lamotrigine should not be restarted in patients with previous hypersensitivity (see section 4.3).

Rash has also been reported as part of a hypersensitivity syndrome associated with a variable pattern of systemic symptoms including fever, lymphadenopathy, facial oedema and abnormalities of the blood and liver. The syndrome shows a wide spectrum of clinical severity and may, rarely, lead to disseminated intravascular coagulation (DIC) and multiorgan failure. It is important to note that early manifestations of hypersensitivity (e.g., fever, lymphadenopathy) may be present even though rash is not evident. Patients should be warned to seek immediate medical advice if signs and symptoms develop. If such signs and symptoms are present the patient should be evaluated immediately and Lamictal discontinued if an alternative aetiology cannot be established

Specialist contraceptive advice should be given to women who are of child-bearing age. Women of child-bearing age should be encouraged to use effective alternative non-hormonal methods of contraception.

Effects of hormonal contraceptives on lamotrigine efficacy:

Systemic lamotrigine concentrations are approximately halved during co-administration of oral contraceptives. This may result in reduced seizure control in women on a stable lamotrigine dose who start an oral contraceptive, or in adverse effects following withdrawal of an oral contraceptive. Dose adjustments of lamotrigine may be required (see sections 4.2 and 4.5).

The effects of co-administration of other hormonal contraceptives and hormone replacement therapy have not been studied; they may similarly affect lamotrigine pharmacokinetic parameters.

Effects of lamotrigine on hormonal contraceptive efficacy:

An interaction study demonstrated some loss of suppression of the hypothalamic-pituitary-ovarian axis when 300mg lamotrigine was co-administered with a combined oral contraceptive (see section 4.5). The impact of these changes on ovarian ovulatory activity is unknown. However, the possibility of decreased contraceptive efficacy cannot be excluded. Therefore, women should have a review of their contraception when starting lamotrigine, and the use of alternative non-hormonal methods of contraception should be encouraged. A hormonal contraceptive should only be used as the sole method of contraception if there is no other alternative. If the oral contraceptive pill is chosen as the sole method of contraception, women should be advised to promptly notify their physician if they experience changes in menstrual pattern (e.g. breakthrough bleeding) while taking Lamictal as this may be an indication of decreased contraceptive efficacy. Women taking Lamictal should notify their physician if they plan to start or stop use of oral contraceptives or other female hormonal preparations.

As with other AEDs, abrupt withdrawal of Lamictal may provoke rebound seizures. Unless safety concerns (for example rash) require an abrupt withdrawal, the dose of Lamictal should be gradually decreased over a period of 2 weeks.

During clinical experience with lamotrigine used as add-on therapy, there have been, rarely, deaths following rapidly progressive illnesses with status epilepticus, rhabdomyolysis, multiorgan dysfunction and disseminated intravascular coagulation (DIC). The contribution of lamotrigine to these events remains to be established.

Lamictal is a weak inhibitor of dihydrofolate reductase hence there is a possibility of interference with folate metabolism during long-term therapy. However, during prolonged human dosing, lamotrigine did not induce significant changes in the haemoglobin concentration, mean corpuscular volume, or serum or red blood cell folate concentrations up to 1 year or red blood cell folate concentrations for up to 5 years.

In single dose studies in subjects with end stage renal failure, plasma concentrations of lamotrigine were not significantly altered. However, accumulation of the glucuronide metabolite is to be expected; caution should therefore be exercised in treating patients with renal failure.

In patients with severe hepatic impairment (Child-Pugh grade C) it has been shown that initial and maintenance doses should be reduced by 75%. Caution should be exercised when dosing this severely hepatically impaired population.

4.5 Interaction with other medicinal products and other forms of Interaction

UDP-glucuronyl transferases have been identified as the enzymes responsible for metabolism of lamotrigine. There is no evidence that lamotrigine causes clinically significant induction or inhibition of hepatic oxidative drug-metabolising enzymes, and interactions between lamotrigine and drugs metabolised by cytochrome P450 enzymes are unlikely to occur. Lamotrigine may induce its own metabolism but the effect is modest and unlikely to have significant clinical consequences.

Table 3 Effects of other drugs on glucuronidation of lamotrigine

Drugs that significantly inhibit glucuronidation of lamotrigine	Drugs that significantly induce glucuronidation of lamotrigine
Valproate	Carbamazepine
	Phenytoin
	Primidone
	Phenobarbital
	Rifampicin
	Ethinylestradiol/ levonorgestrel combination*

* Other hormonal contraceptives and hormone replacement therapy have not been studied; they may similarly affect lamotrigine pharmacokinetic parameters.

Antiepileptic agents which induce drug-metabolising enzymes (such as phenytoin, carbamazepine, phenobarbital and primidone) enhance the metabolism of lamotrigine and may increase dose requirements.

Sodium valproate, which competes with lamotrigine for hepatic drug-metabolising enzymes, reduces the metabolism of lamotrigine and increases the mean half life of lamotrigine nearly two fold.

Although changes in the plasma concentrations of other antiepileptic drugs have been reported, controlled studies have shown no evidence that lamotrigine affects the plasma concentrations of concomitant antiepileptic drugs. Evidence from in vitro studies indicates that lamotrigine does not displace other antiepileptic drugs from protein binding sites.

There have been reports of central nervous system events including headache, nausea, blurred vision, dizziness, diplopia and ataxia in patients taking carbamazepine following the introduction of lamotrigine. These events usually resolve when the dose of carbamazepine is reduced.

Interactions involving Oral Contraceptives

Effect of oral contraceptives on lamotrigine:

Systemic lamotrigine concentrations are approximately halved during co-administration of oral contraceptives. This may result in reduced seizure control after the addition of an oral contraceptive, or adverse effects following withdrawal of an oral contraceptive. Dose adjustments of lamotrigine may be required (see section 4.2).

In a study of 16 female volunteers, 30 mcg ethinylestradiol/150 mcg levonorgestrel in a combined oral contraceptive pill caused an approximately two-fold increase in lamotrigine oral clearance, resulting in an average 52% and 39% reduction in lamotrigine AUC and Cmax, respectively. Serum lamotrigine concentrations gradually increased during the course of the week of inactive medication (e.g. "pill-free" week), with pre-dose concentrations at the end of the week of inactive medication being, on average, approximately two-fold higher than during co-therapy.

The effect of other hormonal contraceptive products or hormone replacement therapy has not been evaluated although the effect may be similar.

Effect of lamotrigine on oral contraceptives:

Co-administration of 300mg lamotrigine in a study of 16 female volunteers had no effect on the pharmacokinetics of the ethinylestradiol component of a combined oral contraceptive pill. A modest increase in oral clearance of the levonorgestrel component was observed, resulting in an average 19% and 12% reduction in levonorgestrel AUC and Cmax, respectively. Measurement of serum follicle-stimulating hormone (FSH), luteinising hormone (LH) and estradiol during the study indicated some loss of suppression of ovarian hormonal activity, although measurement of serum progesterone indicated that there was no hormonal evidence of ovulation in any of the 16 subjects. The impact of the modest increase in levonorgestrel clearance, and the changes in serum FSH and LH, on ovarian ovulatory activity is unknown (see section 4.4). Vaginal bleeding was reported by some volunteers (see section 4.4). The effects of doses of lamotrigine other than 300mg/day have not been studied and studies with other female hormonal preparations have not been conducted.

4.6 Pregnancy and lactation

Fertility

Administration of Lamictal did not impair fertility in animal reproductive studies.

There is no experience of the effect of Lamictal on human fertility.

Teratogenicity

Lamotrigine is a weak inhibitor of dihydrofolate reductase. There is a theoretical risk of human foetal malformations when the mother is treated with a folate inhibitor during pregnancy. However, reproductive toxicology studies with Lamotrigine in animals at doses in excess of the human therapeutic dosage showed no teratogenic effects.

Pregnancy

There are insufficient data available on the use of Lamotrigine in human pregnancy to evaluate its safety. Lamotrigine should not be used in pregnancy unless, in the opinion of the physician, the potential benefits of treatment to the mother outweigh any possible risks to the developing foetus.

Physiological changes during pregnancy may result in decreased lamotrigine levels. These changes in lamotrigine levels can occur from early in pregnancy and progress during pregnancy, then revert quickly after delivery. The dose of lamotrigine should not be increased routinely in pregnancy but should only be adjusted on clinical grounds. To maintain seizure control during pregnancy a dose increase may be needed, although other factors including vomiting should also be considered if seizure control deteriorates. *Post-partum* a dose decrease may be needed to avoid toxicity. Women on lamotrigine must be monitored closely during pregnancy and *post-partum*.

Lactation

There is limited information on the use of lamotrigine in lactation. Preliminary data indicate that it passes into breast milk in concentrations usually of the order of 40-60% of the serum concentration. In a small number of infants known to have been breastfed, the serum concentrations of lamotrigine reached levels at which pharmacological effects may occur. The potential benefits of breast feeding should be weighed against the potential risk of adverse effects occurring in the infant.

4.7 Effects on ability to drive and use machines

Two volunteer studies have demonstrated that the effect of lamotrigine on fine visual motor co-ordination, eye movements, body sway and subjective sedative effects did not differ from placebo.

In clinical trials with lamotrigine adverse events of a neurological character such as dizziness and diplopia have been reported. As there is individual variation in response to all antiepileptic drug therapy patients should consult their physician on the specific issues of driving and epilepsy.

4.8 Undesirable effects

In double-blind, add-on clinical trials, skin rashes occurred in up to 10% of patients taking lamotrigine and in 5% of patients taking placebo. The skin rashes led to the withdrawal of lamotrigine treatment in 2% of patients. The rash, usually maculopapular in appearance, generally appears within eight weeks of starting treatment and resolves on withdrawal of lamotrigine (see Special Warnings and Special Precautions for Use).

Rarely, serious potentially life threatening skin rashes, including Stevens Johnson syndrome and toxic epidermal necrolysis (Lyell Syndrome) have been reported. Although the majority recover on drug withdrawal, some patients experience irreversible scarring and there have been rare cases of associated death. (See Special Warnings and Special Precautions for Use)

The approximate incidence of serious skin rashes reported as SJS in adults and children over the age of 12 is 1 in 1000. The risk in children under the age of 12 is higher than in adults. Available data from a number of studies suggest that the incidence in children under the age of 12 requiring hospitalisation due to rash ranges from 1 in 300 to 1 in 100 (see Special Warnings and Special Precautions for Use).

In children, the initial presentation of a rash can be mistaken for an infection; physicians should consider the possibility of a drug reaction in children that develop symptoms of rash and fever during the first eight weeks of therapy.

Additionally the overall risk of rash appears to be strongly associated with:-

High initial doses of lamotrigine and exceeding the recommended dose escalation of lamotrigine therapy (see Posology and Method of Administration).

Concomitant use of valproate (See Posology and Method of Administration).

All patients (adults and children) who develop a rash should be promptly evaluated and lamotrigine withdrawn immediately unless the rash is clearly not drug related.

Rash has also been reported as part of a hypersensitivity syndrome associated with a variable pattern of systemic symptoms including fever, lymphadenopathy, facial oedema and abnormalities of the blood and liver. The syndrome shows a wide spectrum of clinical severity and may, rarely, lead to disseminated intravascular coagulation (DIC) and multiorgan failure. It is important to note that early manifestations of hypersensitivity (e.g., fever, lymphadenopathy) may be present even though rash is not evident. Patients should be warned to seek immediate medical advice if signs and symptoms develop. If such signs and symptoms are present the patient should be evaluated immediately and Lamictal discontinued if an alternative aetiology cannot be established

Adverse experiences reported during Lamictal monotherapy trials include headache, tiredness, rash, nausea, dizziness, drowsiness and insomnia.

Other adverse experiences have included diplopia, blurred vision, conjunctivitis, dizziness, drowsiness, headache, tiredness, gastrointestinal disturbance (including vomiting and diarrhoea), irritability/aggression, tremor, agitation, confusion and hallucinations. Very rarely, lupus-like reactions have been reported.

There have been reports of haematological abnormalities which may or may not be associated with the hypersensitivity syndrome. These have included neutropenia, leucopenia, anaemia, thrombocytopenia, pancytopenia, and very rarely aplastic anaemia and agranulocytosis.

Movement disorders such as tics, unsteadiness, ataxia, nystagmus and tremor have also been reported. There have been reports that Lamictal may worsen parkinsonian symptoms in patients with pre-existing Parkinson's disease, and isolated reports of extrapyramidal effects and choreoathetosis in patients with this underlying condition. Very rarely, increase in seizure frequency has been reported.

Elevations of liver function tests and rare reports of hepatic dysfunction, including hepatic failure, have been reported. Hepatic dysfunction usually occurs in association with hypersensitivity reactions but isolated cases have been reported without overt signs of hypersensitivity.

4.9 Overdose

Symptoms and signs

Acute ingestion of doses in excess of 10 – 20 times the maximum therapeutic dose has been reported. Overdose has resulted in symptoms including nystagmus, ataxia, impaired consciousness and coma.

Treatment

In the event of overdosage, the patient should be admitted to hospital and given appropriate supportive therapy. Gastric lavage should be performed if indicated.

5. PHARMACOLOGICAL PROPERTIES

5.1 Pharmacodynamic properties

Mode of action

The results of pharmacological studies suggest that lamotrigine is a use-dependent blocker of voltage gated sodium channels. It produces a use- and voltage-dependent block of sustained repetitive firing in cultured neurones and inhibits pathological release of glutamate (the amino acid which plays a key role in the generation of epileptic seizures), as well as inhibiting glutamate-evoked bursts of action potentials.

Pharmacodynamics

In tests designed to evaluate the central nervous system effects of drugs, the results obtained using doses of 240 mg lamotrigine administered to healthy volunteers did not differ from placebo, whereas both 1000 mg phenytoin and 10 mg diazepam each significantly impaired fine visual motor co-ordination and eye movements, increased body sway and produced subjective sedative effects.

In another study, single oral doses of 600mg carbamazepine significantly impaired fine visual motor co-ordination and eye movements, while increasing both body sway and heart rate, whereas results with lamotrigine at doses of 150mg and 300mg did not differ from placebo.

5.2 Pharmacokinetic properties

Lamotrigine is rapidly and completely absorbed from the gut with no significant first pass metabolism. Peak plasma concentrations occur approximately 2.5 hours after oral drug administration. Time to maximum concentration is slightly delayed after food but the extent of absorption is unaffected. The pharmacokinetics are linear up to 450mg, the highest single dose tested. There is considerable inter-individual variation in steady state maximum concentrations but within an individual concentrations vary very little.

Binding to plasma proteins is about 55%. It is very unlikely that displacement from plasma proteins would result in toxicity. The volume of distribution is 0.92 to 1.22 L/kg.

The mean steady state clearance in healthy adults is 39 ± 14 mL/min. Clearance of lamotrigine is primarily metabolic with subsequent elimination of glucuronide-conjugated material in urine. Less than 10% is excreted unchanged in the urine. Only about 2% of drug-related material is excreted in faeces. Clearance and half-life are independent of dose. The mean elimination half-life in healthy adults is 24 to 35 hours. UDP-glucuronyl transferases have been identified as the enzymes responsible for metabolism of lamotrigine. In a study of subjects with Gilbert's Syndrome, mean apparent clearance was reduced by 32% compared with normal controls but the values are within the range for the general population.

Lamotrigine induces its own metabolism to a modest extent depending on dose. However, there is no evidence that lamotrigine affects the pharmacokinetics of other AEDs and data suggest that interactions between lamotrigine and drugs metabolised by cytochrome P450 enzymes are unlikely to occur.

The half-life of lamotrigine is greatly affected by concomitant medication. Mean half-life is reduced to approximately 14 hours when given with enzyme-inducing drugs such as carbamazepine and phenytoin and is increased to a mean of approximately 70 hours when co-administered with sodium valproate alone. (see Posology and Method of Administration).

Clearance adjusted for bodyweight is higher in children aged 12 years and under than in adults with the highest values in children under five years. The half-life of lamotrigine is generally shorter in children than in adults with a mean value of approximately 7 hours when given with enzyme-inducing drugs such as carbamazepine and phenytoin and increasing to mean values of 45 to 50 hours when co-administered with sodium valproate alone (see Posology and Method of Administration).

The results of pharmacokinetic studies of lamotrigine in 12 healthy elderly volunteers aged 65 to 76 years and 12 young volunteers aged 26 to 38 years following a 150mg single dose revealed that average plasma clearance was about 37% lower in the elderly. However the mean clearance in the elderly (0.39 mL/min/kg) lies within the range of the mean clearance values (0.31 to 0.65 mL/min/kg) obtained in 9 studies with non-elderly adults after single doses of 30 to 450mg. A population pharmacokinetic analysis with both young and elderly subjects (including 12 elderly volunteers from the pharmacokinetic study and 13 elderly epilepsy patients enrolled in monotherapy clinical trials) indicated that the clearance of lamotrigine did not change to a clinically relevant extent. After single doses apparent clearance decreased by 12% from 35mL/min at age 20 to 31 mL/min at 70 years. The decrease after 48 weeks of treatment was 10% from 41 to 37mL/min between the young and elderly groups. To date there have been no specific studies of lamotrigine pharmacokinetics in elderly patients with epilepsy.

There is no experience of treatment with lamotrigine of patients with renal failure. Pharmacokinetic studies using single doses in subjects with renal failure indicate that lamotrigine pharmacokinetics are little affected but plasma concentrations of the major glucuronide metabolite increase almost eight-fold due to reduced renal clearance.

A single dose pharmacokinetic study was performed in 24 subjects with various degrees of hepatic impairment and 12 healthy subjects as controls. The median apparent clearance of lamotrigine was 0.31, 0.24, 0.10 mL/min/kg in patients with Grade A, B or C (Child-Pugh Classification) hepatic impairment respectively, compared to 0.34 mL/min/kg in the healthy controls. Reduced doses should generally be used in patients with Grade B or C hepatic impairment (see 4.2 Posology and Method of Administration)

5.3 Preclinical safety data

Mutagenicity

The results of a wide range of mutagenicity tests indicate that Lamictal does not present a genetic risk to man.

Carcinogenicity

Lamictal was not carcinogenic in long-term studies in the rat and the mouse.

6. PHARMACEUTICAL PARTICULARS

6.1 List of excipients

Lamictal Tablets
Lactose
Microcrystalline Cellulose
Povidone
Sodium Starch Glycollate
Iron Oxide Yellow (E172) EEC Requirements
Magnesium Stearate
Lamictal Dispersible Tablets
Calcium carbonate
Low substituted hydroxypropyl cellulose
Aluminium magnesium silicate
Sodium starch glycollate
Povidone K30
Saccharin sodium
Blackcurrant flavour
Magnesium stearate

6.2 Incompatibilities

Not applicable.

6.3 Shelf life

Lamictal Tablets 25mg	3 years.
Lamictal Tablets 50mg	3 years
Lamictal Tablets 100mg	3 years
Lamictal Tablets 200mg	3 years
Lamictal Dispersible 2mg	2 years
Lamictal Dispersible 5mg	3 years
Lamictal Dispersible 25mg	3 years
Lamictal Dispersible 100mg	3 years

6.4 Special precautions for storage

Lamictal Tablets 25mg	Store below 30°C. Keep dry.
Lamictal Tablets 50mg	Store below 30°C. Keep dry.
Lamictal Tablets 100mg	Store below 30°C. Keep dry.
Lamictal Tablets 200mg	Store below 30°C. Keep dry.
Lamictal Dispersible 2mg	No special precautions for storage
Lamictal Dispersible 5mg	Store below 30°C. Keep dry.
Lamictal Dispersible 25mg	Store below 30°C. Keep dry.
Lamictal Dispersible 100mg	Store below 30°C. Keep dry.

6.5 Nature and contents of container

Lamictal Tablets 25mg	PVC/Aluminium foil blister packs containing 21 or 42 tablets.
Lamictal Tablets 50mg	PVC/Aluminium foil blisters containing 42 tablets
Lamictal Tablets 100mg	PVC/Aluminium foil blisters containing 56 tablets
Lamictal Tablets 200mg	PVC /Aluminium foil blisters containing 56 tablets
Lamictal Dispersible 2mg	HDPE bottle containing 30 tablets
Lamictal Dispersible 5mg	PVC/Aluminium foil blisters containing 28 tablets
Lamictal Dispersible 25mg	PVC/Aluminium foil blisters containing 56 tablets
Lamictal Dispersible 100mg	PVC/Aluminium foil blisters containing 28 tablets

6.6 Instructions for use and handling

None

Administrative Data

7. MARKETING AUTHORISATION HOLDER

The Wellcome Foundation Ltd
Glaxo Wellcome House
Berkeley Avenue
Greenford
Middlesex UB6 0NN
Trading as
GlaxoSmithKline UK
Stockley Park West
Uxbridge
Middlesex UB11 1BT

8. MARKETING AUTHORISATION NUMBER(S)

Lamictal Tablets 25mg: PL 0003/0272
Lamictal Tablets 50mg: PL 0003/0273
Lamictal Tablets 100mg: PL 0003/0274
Lamictal Tablets 200mg: PL 0003/0297
Lamictal Dispersible 2mg: PL 0003/0375
Lamictal Dispersible 5mg: PL 0003/0346
Lamictal Dispersible 25mg: PL 0003/0347
Lamictal Dispersible 100mg: PL 0003/0348

9. DATE OF FIRST AUTHORISATION/RENEWAL OF THE AUTHORISATION

Lamictal Tablets 25mg: 27th August 1997
Lamictal Tablets 50mg: 27th August 1997
Lamictal Tablets 100mg: 27th August 1997
Lamictal Tablets 200mg: 6th September 1999
Lamictal Dispersible 2mg: 18th December 2000
Lamictal Dispersible 5mg: 6th September 1999
Lamictal Dispersible 25mg: 6th September 1999
Lamictal Dispersible 100mg: 6th September 1999

10. DATE OF REVISION OF THE TEXT

27th June 2005

11. Legal Status

POM

Lamisil Cream

(Novartis Pharmaceuticals UK Ltd)

1. NAME OF THE MEDICINAL PRODUCT

LAMISIL® Cream

2. QUALITATIVE AND QUANTITATIVE COMPOSITION

Terbinafine hydrochloride 1.0% w/w

3. PHARMACEUTICAL FORM

White, smooth or almost smooth glossy cream

4. CLINICAL PARTICULARS

4.1 Therapeutic indications

Fungal infections of the skin caused by *Trichophyton* (e.g. *T. Rubrum*, *T.Mentagrophytes*, *T. Verrucosum*, *T. Violaceum*), *Microsporum canis* and *Epidermophyton floccosum*.

Yeast infections of the skin, principally those caused by the genus *Candida* (eg. *C. albicans*).

Pityriasis (tinea) versicolor due to *Pityrosporum orbiculare* (also known as *Malassezia furfur*).

4.2 Posology and method of administration

LAMISIL can be applied once or twice daily. Cleanse and dry the affected areas thoroughly before application of LAMISIL. Apply the cream to the affected skin and surrounding area in a thin layer and rub in lightly. In the case of intertriginous infections (submammary, interdigital, intergluteal, inguinal) the application may be covered with a gauze strip, especially at night.

The likely durations of treatment are as follows:

Tinea corporis, cruris: 1 to 2 weeks
Tinea pedis: 1 week
Cutaneous candidiasis: 2 weeks
Pityriasis versicolor: 2 weeks

Relief of clinical symptoms usually occurs within a few days. Irregular use or premature discontinuation of treatment carries the risk of recurrence. If there are no signs of improvement after two weeks, the diagnosis should be verified.

<u>Children</u>

The experience with topical LAMISIL in children is still limited and its use cannot therefore be recommended.

<u>Use in the elderly</u>

There is no evidence to suggest that elderly patients require different dosages or experience side-effects different to those of younger patients.

<u>Method of administration</u>

Via the topical route.

4.3 Contraindications

Hypersensitivity to terbinafine or any of the excipients contained in the cream.

4.4 Special warnings and special precautions for use

LAMISIL Cream is for external use only. Contact with the eyes should be avoided.

4.5 Interaction with other medicinal products and other forms of Interaction

There are no known drug interactions with LAMISIL Cream.

4.6 Pregnancy and lactation

Foetal toxicity and fertility studies in animals suggest no adverse effects.

There is no clinical experience with LAMISIL Cream in pregnant women, therefore, unless the potential benefits outweigh any potential risks, LAMISIL Cream should not be administered during pregnancy.

Terbinafine is excreted in breast milk and therefore mothers should not receive LAMISIL whilst breast-feeding.

4.7 Effects on ability to drive and use machines

None known.

4.8 Undesirable effects

Redness, itching or stinging occasionally occur at the site of application; however, treatment rarely has to be discontinued for this reason. This must be distinguished from allergic reactions which are rare but require discontinuation.

4.9 Overdose

No case of ingestion of LAMISIL Cream has been reported to the company. However, if accidental ingestion of LAMISIL Cream occurs, an appropriate method of gastric emptying may be used if considered appropriate.

5. PHARMACOLOGICAL PROPERTIES

5.1 Pharmacodynamic properties

Terbinafine is an allylamine which has a broad spectrum of antifungal activity. At low concentrations terbinafine is fungicidal against dermatophytes, moulds and certain dimorphic fungi. The activity versus yeasts is fungicidal or fungistatic depending on the species.

Terbinafine interferes specifically with fungal sterol biosynthesis at an early step. This leads to a deficiency in ergosterol and to an intracellular accumulation of squalene, resulting in fungal cell death. Terbinafine acts by inhibition of squalene epoxidase in the fungal cell membrane.

The enzyme squalene epoxidase is not linked to the cytochrome P450 system. Terbinafine does not influence the metabolism of hormones or other drugs.

5.2 Pharmacokinetic properties

Less than 5% of the dose is absorbed after topical application to humans; systemic exposure is therefore very slight.

6. PHARMACEUTICAL PARTICULARS

6.1 List of excipients

Sodium hydroxide, benzyl alcohol, sorbitan monostearate, cetyl palmitate, cetyl alcohol, stearyl alcohol, polysorbate 60, isopropyl myristate, demineralised water.

6.2 Incompatibilities

None known.

6.3 Shelf life

Aluminium tube: 5 years.

6.4 Special precautions for storage

None.

6.5 Nature and contents of container

Aluminium tube with membrane, with an interior coating of phenol-epoxy based lacquer, closed with a polypropylene cap, containing 15g or 30g LAMISIL Cream.

6.6 Instructions for use and handling

Not applicable.

7. MARKETING AUTHORISATION HOLDER

Novartis Pharmaceuticals UK Ltd
Trading as Sandoz Pharmaceuticals
Frimley Business Park
Frimley
Camberley
Surrey
GU16 7SR

8. MARKETING AUTHORISATION NUMBER(S)

PL 0101/0305

9. DATE OF FIRST AUTHORISATION/RENEWAL OF THE AUTHORISATION

Date Present Licence Granted: 29/11/95

10. DATE OF REVISION OF THE TEXT

July 2000

Lamisil Tablets 250mg

(Novartis Pharmaceuticals UK Ltd)

1. NAME OF THE MEDICINAL PRODUCT

Lamisil® Tablets 250mg

2. QUALITATIVE AND QUANTITATIVE COMPOSITION

Each tablet contains 281.25mg terbinafine hydrochloride, equivalent to 250mg terbinafine.

3. PHARMACEUTICAL FORM

Tablets for oral administration.

Whitish to yellow tinged white, circular, biconvex tablets, scored and coded S T on one side.

4. CLINICAL PARTICULARS

4.1 Therapeutic indications

Fungal infections of the skin and nails caused by *Trichophyton* (eg. *T. rubrum*, *T.mentagrophytes*, *T. verrucosum*, *T. violaceum*), *Microsporum canis* and *Epidermophyton floccosum*.

1. Oral Lamisil is indicated in the treatment of ringworm (tinea corporis, tinea cruris and tinea pedis) where oral therapy is considered appropriate due to the site, severity or extent of the infection.

2. Oral Lamisil is indicated in the treatment of onychomycosis.

4.2 Posology and method of administration

Adults

250mg once daily.

The duration of treatment varies according to the indication and the severity of the infection.

Skin infections

Likely durations of treatment are as follows:

Tinea pedis (interdigital, plantar/moccasin type): 2 to 6 weeks

Tinea corporis: 4 weeks

Tinea cruris: 2 to 4 weeks

Onychomycosis

The duration of treatment for most patients is between 6 weeks and 3 months. Treatment periods of less than 3 months can be anticipated in patients with fingernail infection, toenail infection other than of the big toe, or patients of younger age. In the treatment of toenail infections, 3 months is usually sufficient although a few patients may require treatment of 6 months or longer. Poor nail outgrowth during the first weeks of treatment may enable identification of those patients in whom longer therapy is required.

Complete resolution of the signs and symptoms of infection may not occur until several weeks after mycological cure.

Children

A review of safety experience with oral Lamisil in children, which includes 314 patients involved in the UK Lamisil Post Marketing Surveillance study, has shown that the adverse event profile in children is similar to that seen in adults. No evidence of any new, unusual or more severe reactions to those seen in the adult population have been noted. However, as data is still limited its use is not recommended.

Use in the elderly

There is no evidence to suggest that elderly patients require different dosages or experience side-effects different to those of younger patients. The possibility of impairment of liver or kidney function should be considered in this age group (see Precautions).

Method of administration

Via the oral route.

4.3 Contraindications

Hypersensitivity to Lamisil

4.4 Special warnings and special precautions for use

Rarely, cases of cholestasis and hepatitis have been reported, these usually occur within two months of starting treatment. If a patient presents with signs or symptoms suggestive of liver dysfunction such as pruritis, unexplained persistent nausea, anorexia or tiredness, or jaundice, vomiting, fatigue, abdominal pain or dark urine, or pale stools, hepatic origin should be verified and Lamisil therapy should be discontinued (see 4.8 Undesirable effects).

Single dose pharmacokinetic studies in patients with pre-existing liver disease have shown that the clearance of Lamisil may be reduced by about 50%. The therapeutic use of Lamisil in patients with chronic or active liver disease has not been studied in prospective clinical trials, and therefore cannot be recommended.

Lamisil should be used with caution in patients with psoriasis, as very rare cases of exacerbation of psoriasis have been reported

Patients with impaired renal function (creatinine clearance less than 50ml/minute or serum creatinine of more than 300μmol/l) should receive half the normal dose.

4.5 Interaction with other medicinal products and other forms of Interaction

The plasma clearance of terbinafine may be accelerated by drugs which induce metabolism (such as rifampicin) and may be inhibited by drugs which inhibit cytochrome P450 (such as cimetidine). Where co-administration of such agents is necessary, the dosage of Lamisil may need to be adjusted accordingly.

In vitro studies have shown, that terbinafine inhibits the CYP2D6-mediated metabolism. This in vitro finding may be of clinical relevance for patients receiving compounds predominantly metabolised by this enzyme, such as tricyclic antidepressants (TCA's), *B*-blockers, selective serotonine reuptake inhibitors (SSRIs), and monoamine oxidase inhibitors (MAO-Is) Type B.

Other studies undertaken in vitro and in healthy volunteers suggest that terbinafine shows negligible potential to inhibit or induce the clearance of drugs that are metabolised via other cytochrome P450 enzymes (e.g. cyclosporin, tolbutamine, terfenadine, triazolam, oral contraceptives). However, some cases of menstrual disturbance (breakthrough bleeding and irregular cycle) have been reported in patients taking Lamisil concomitantly with oral contraceptives.

4.6 Pregnancy and lactation

Foetal toxicity and fertility studies in animals suggest no adverse effects.

There is no clinical experience with Lamisil in pregnant women, therefore, unless the potential benefits outweigh any potential risks, Lamisil should not be administered during pregnancy.

Terbinafine is excreted in breast milk and therefore mothers should not receive Lamisil treatment whilst breast-feeding.

4.7 Effects on ability to drive and use machines

None.

4.8 Undesirable effects

Frequency estimate: very common $\geqslant$ 10%, common $\geqslant$ 1% to < 10%, uncommon $\geqslant$ 0.1% to < 1%, rare $\geqslant$ 0.01% to < 0.1%, very rare < 0.01%.

Side effects are generally mild to moderate, and transient. The most common are gastrointestinal symptoms (dyspepsia, fullness, loss of appetite, nausea, mild abdominal pain, diarrhoea), allergic skin reactions (rash, urticaria) and headache. Musculo-skeletal disorders including arthralgia and myalgia have been reported. These may occur as part of a hypersensitivity reaction in association with allergic skin reactions.

Rare: cases of serious skin reactions (eg. Stevens-Johnson syndrome, toxic epidermal necrolysis, photosensitivity and angioneurotic oedema) have been reported. If progressive skin rash occurs, Lamisil treatment should be discontinued.

Uncommon: taste loss and taste disturbance have been reported in approximately 0.6% of patients treated with Lamisil. This usually resolves slowly on drug discontinuation. Very rare cases of prolonged taste disturbance have been reported, sometimes leading to a decrease of food intake and significant weight loss.

Rare: cases of serious hepatic dysfunction, including jaundice, cholestasis and hepatitis have been reported. If hepatic dysfunction develops, treatment with Lamisil should be discontinued (see also precautions).

Rare: paraesthesia, hypoaesthesia, dizziness, malaise and fatigue.

Very rare: haematological disorders such as neutropenia, thrombocytopenia and agranulocytosis.

Very rare: exacerbation of psoriasis has been reported very rarely (see section 4.4).

Very rare: psychiatric disturbances such as depression and anxiety.

Very rare: cases of vertigo.

Very rare: precipitation and exacerbation of cutaneous and systemic lupus erythematosus have been reported.

4.9 Overdose

A few cases of overdose (up to 5g) have been reported, giving rise to headache, nausea, epigastric pain and dizziness. The recommended treatment of overdosage consists in eliminating the drug, primarily by the administration of activated charcoal, and giving symptomatic supportive therapy if needed.

5. PHARMACOLOGICAL PROPERTIES

5.1 Pharmacodynamic properties

Terbinafine is an allylamine which has a broad spectrum of antifungal activity. At low concentrations terbinafine is fungicidal against dermatophytes, moulds and certain dimorphic fungi. The activity versus yeasts is fungicidal or fungistatic depending on the species.

Terbinafine interferes specifically with fungal sterol biosynthesis at an early step. This leads to a deficiency in ergosterol and to an intracellular accumulation of squalene, resulting in fungal cell death. Terbinafine acts by inhibition of squalene epoxidase in the fungal cell membrane.

The enzyme squalene epoxidase is not linked to the cytochrome P450 system. Terbinafine does not influence the metabolism of hormones or other drugs.

When given orally, the drug concentrates in skin at levels associated with fungicidal activity.

5.2 Pharmacokinetic properties

A single oral dose of 250mg terbinafine results in mean peak plasma concentrations of 0.97μg/ml within 2 hours after administration. The absorption half-life is 0.8 hours and the distribution half-life is 4.6 hours. Terbinafine binds strongly to plasma proteins. It rapidly diffuses through the dermis and concentrates in the lipophilic stratum corneum. Terbinafine is also secreted in sebum, thus achieving high concentrations in hair follicles, hair and sebum rich skins. There is also evidence that terbinafine is distributed into the nail plate within the first few weeks of commencing therapy. Biotransformation results in metabolites with no antifungal activity, which are excreted predominantly in the urine. The elimination half-life is 17 hours. There is no evidence of accumulation.

No age-dependent changes in pharmacokinetics have been observed but the elimination rate may be reduced in patients with renal or hepatic impairment, resulting in higher blood levels of terbinafine.

The bioavailability of Lamisil is unaffected by food.

5.3 Preclinical safety data

In long-term studies (up to 1 year) in rats and dogs no marked toxic effects were seen in either species up to oral doses of about 100mg/kg a day. At high oral doses, the liver and possibly also the kidneys were identified as potential target organs.

In a two-year oral carcinogenicity study in mice, no neoplastic or other abnormal findings attributable to treatment were made up to doses of 130 (males) and 156 (females) mg/kg a day. In a two-year oral carcinogenicity study in rats, an increased incidence of liver tumours was observed in males at the highest dosage level of 69mg/kg a day. The changes which may be associated with peroxisome proliferation have been shown to be species-specific since they were not seen in the carcinogenicity study in mice, dogs or monkeys.

During high-dose studies in monkeys, refractile irregularities were observed in the retina at the higher doses (non-toxic effect level 50mg/kg). These irregularities were associated with the presence of a terbinafine metabolite in ocular tissue and disappeared after drug discontinuation. They were not associated with histological changes.

A standard battery of *in vitro* and *in vivo* genotoxicity tests revealed no evidence of mutagenic or clastogenic potential.

No adverse effects on fertility or other reproduction parameters were observed in studies in rats or rabbits.

6. PHARMACEUTICAL PARTICULARS

6.1 List of excipients

Magnesium stearate, colloidal anhydrous silica, hydroxy propyl methylcellulose, sodium carboxy methyl starch, microcrystalline cellulose.

6.2 Incompatibilities

None known.

6.3 Shelf life

5 years.

6.4 Special precautions for storage

Protect from light. Store below 25°C

6.5 Nature and contents of container

PVC or PVC/PVDC blister pack, containing 14 or 28 tablets.

6.6 Instructions for use and handling

Not applicable.

7. MARKETING AUTHORISATION HOLDER

NOVARTIS PHARMACEUTICALS UK LIMITED

(Trading as Sandoz Pharmaceuticals)

Frimley Business Park

Frimley

Camberley

Surrey

GU16 7SR

8. MARKETING AUTHORISATION NUMBER(S)

PL 0101/0304

9. DATE OF FIRST AUTHORISATION/RENEWAL OF THE AUTHORISATION

01 November 2001

10. DATE OF REVISION OF THE TEXT

10 December 2004

LEGAL CATEGORY

POM

Lanoxin 125 Tablets

(GlaxoSmithKline UK)

1. NAME OF THE MEDICINAL PRODUCT

Lanoxin 125 Tablets

2. QUALITATIVE AND QUANTITATIVE COMPOSITION

Digoxin Ph Eur 0.125 mg/tablet

3. PHARMACEUTICAL FORM

Tablet

4. CLINICAL PARTICULARS

4.1 Therapeutic indications

Lanoxin is indicated in the management of chronic cardiac failure where the dominant problem is systolic dysfunction. Its therapeutic benefit is greatest in those patients with ventricular dilatation.

Lanoxin is specifically indicated where cardiac failure is accompanied by atrial fibrillation.

Lanoxin is indicated in the management of certain supraventricular arrhythmias, particularly chronic atrial flutter and fibrillation,.

4.2 Posology and method of administration

The dose of Lanoxin for each patient has to be tailored individually according to age, lean body weight and renal function. Suggested doses are intended only as an initial guide.

The difference in bioavailability between injectable Lanoxin and oral formulations must be considered when changing from one dosage form to another. For example, if patients are switched from oral to the i.v. formulation the dosage should be reduced by approximately 33 %.

Adults and children over 10 years:

Rapid Oral Loading: 750 to 1500 micrograms (0.75 to 1.5 mg) as a single dose.

Where there is less urgency, or greater risk of toxicity eg. in the elderly, the oral loading dose should be given in divided doses 6 hours apart, assessing clinical response before giving each additional dose. (See *Special Warnings and Precautions for Use*).

Slow Oral Loading: 250 to 750 micrograms (0.25 to 0.75 mg) should be given daily for 1 week followed by an appropriate maintenance dose. A clinical response should be seen within one week.

NOTE: The choice between slow and rapid oral loading depends on the clinical state of the patient and the urgency of the condition.

Maintenance: The maintenance dosage should be based upon the percentage of the peak body stores lost each day through elimination. The following formula has had wide clinical use:

$$\text{Maintenance Dose} = \text{Peak body stores} \times \frac{\%\ \text{daily loss}}{100}$$

Where:

Peak Body Stores = Loading Dose

% Daily Loss = 14 + Creatinine Clearance (C_{cr})/5.

C_{cr} is creatinine clearance corrected to 70 kg body weight or 1.73 m^2 body surface area. If only serum creatinine (S_{cr}) concentrations are available, a C_{cr} (Corrected to 70 kg body weight) may be estimated in men as

$$C_{cr} = \frac{(140 - \text{age})}{S_{cr}\ (\text{in mg/100 ml})}$$

NOTE: Where serum creatinine values are obtained in micromol/l these may be converted to mg/100 ml (mg %) as follows

$$S_{cr}\ (\text{mg/100 ml}) = \frac{S_{cr}\ (\text{micromol/L}) \times 113.12}{10{,}000} = \frac{S_{cr}\ (\text{micromol/L})}{88.4}$$

Where 113.12 is the molecular weight of creatinine.

For *women*, this result should be multiplied by 0.85.

NOTE: These formulae cannot be used for creatinine clearance in children.

In practice, this will mean that most patients will be maintained on 0.125 to 0.75 mg digoxin daily; however in those who show increased sensitivity to the adverse effects of digoxin, a dosage of 62.5 microgram (0.0625 mg) daily or less may suffice.

Neonates, infants and children up to 10 years of age (if cardiac glycosides have not been given in the preceding two weeks):

In the newborn, particularly in the premature infant, renal clearance of digoxin is diminished and suitable dose reductions must be observed, over and above general dosage instructions.

Beyond the immediate newborn period, children generally require proportionally larger doses than adults on the basis of body weight or body surface area, as indicated in the schedule below. Children over 10 years of age require adult dosages in proportion to their body weight.

Oral Loading Dose:

This should be administered in accordance with the following schedule:

Preterm neonates < 1.5 kg	25 microgram/kg over 24 hours
Preterm neonates 1.5 to 2.5 kg	30 microgram/kg over 24 hours
Term neonates to 2 years	45 microgram/kg over 24 hours
2 to 5 years	35 microgram/kg over 24 hours
5 to 10 years	25 microgram/kg over 24 hours

The loading dose should be administered in divided doses with approximately half the total dose given as the first dose and further fractions of the total dose given at intervals of 4 to 8 hours, assessing clinical response before giving each additional dose.

Maintenance:

The maintenance dose should be administered in accordance with the following schedule:

Preterm neonates:

daily dose = 20% of 24-hour loading dose (intravenous or oral)

Term neonates and children up to 10 years

daily dose = 25% of 24-hour loading dose (intravenous or oral)

These dosage schedules are meant as guidelines and careful clinical observation and monitoring of serum digoxin levels (see *Monitoring*) should be used as a basis for adjustment of dosage in these paediatric patients groups.

If cardiac glycosides have been given in the two weeks preceding commencement of Lanoxin therapy, it should be anticipated that optimum loading doses of Lanoxin will be less than those recommended above.

Use in the Elderly: The tendency to impaired renal function and low lean body mass in the elderly influences the pharmacokinetic of Lanoxin such that high serum digoxin levels and associated toxicity can occur quite readily, unless dosages of Lanoxin lower than those in non-elderly patients are used. Serum digoxin levels should be checked regularly and hypokalaemia avoided.

Dose recommendations in renal disorder or with diuretic therapy: See *Special Warnings and Precautions for Use*.

Monitoring: Serum concentrations of digoxin may be expressed in conventional units of nanogram/ml (ng/ml) or SI units of nanomol/L (nmol/L). To convert ng/ml to nmol/L, multiply ng/ml by 1.28.

The serum concentration of digoxin can be determined by radioimmunoassay. Blood should be taken 6 hours or more after the last dose of Lanoxin. There are no rigid guidelines as to the range of serum concentrations that are most efficacious but most patients will benefit, with little risk of toxic symptoms and signs developing, with digoxin concentrations from 0.8 ng/ml (1.02 nmol/L) to 2 ng/ml (2.56 nmol/L). Above this range, toxic symptoms and signs become more frequent and levels above 3 ng/ml (3.84 nmol/L) are quite likely to be toxic. However, in deciding whether a patients symptoms are due to digoxin, the patients clinical state together with the serum potassium level and thyroid function are important factors.

Other glycosides, including metabolites of digoxin, can interfere with the assays that are available and one should always be wary of values which do not seem commensurate with the clinical state of the patient.

4.3 Contraindications

Lanoxin is contra-indicated in intermittent complete heart block or second degree atrioventricular block, especially if there is a history of Stokes-Adams attacks.

Lanoxin is contra-indicated in arrhythmias caused by cardiac glycoside intoxication.

Lanoxin is contra-indicated in supraventricular arrhythmias associated with an accessory atrioventricular pathway, as in the Wolff-Parkinson-White syndrome, unless the electrophysiological characteristics of the accessory pathway and any possible deleterious effect of digoxin on these characteristics has been evaluated. If an accessory pathway is known or suspected to be present and there is no history of previous supraventricular arrhythmias, Lanoxin is similarly contra-indicated.

Lanoxin is contra-indicated in ventricular tachycardia or ventricular fibrillation.

Lanoxin is contra-indicated in Hypertrophic Obstructive Cardiomyopathy, unless there is concomitant atrial fibrillation and heart failure but even then caution should be exercised if Lanoxin is to be used.

Lanoxin is contra-indicated in patients known to be hypersensitive to digoxin or other digitalis glycosides.

4.4 Special warnings and special precautions for use

Arrhythmias may be precipitated by digoxin toxicity, some of which can resemble arrhythmias for which the drug could be advised. For example, atrial tachycardia with varying atrioventricular block requires care as clinically the rhythm resembles atrial fibrillation.

In some cases of sinoatrial disorder (ie. Sick Sinus Syndrome) digoxin may cause or exacerbate sinus bradycardia or cause sinoatrial block.

Determination of the serum digoxin concentration may be very helpful in making a decision to treat with further digoxin, but toxic doses of other glycosides may cross-react in the assay and wrongly suggest apparently satisfactory measurements. Observations during the temporary withholding of digoxin might be more appropriate.

In cases where cardiac glycosides have been taken in the preceding two weeks the recommendations for initial dosing of a patient should be reconsidered and a reduced dose is advised.

The dosing recommendations should be reconsidered if patients are elderly or there are other reasons for the renal clearance of digoxin being reduced. A reduction in both initial and maintenance doses should be considered.

Hypokalaemia sensitises the myocardium to the actions of cardiac glycosides.

Hypoxia, hypomagnesaemia and marked hypercalcaemia increase myocardial sensitivity to cardiac glycosides.

Administering Lanoxin to a patient with thyroid disease requires care. Initial and maintenance doses of Lanoxin should be reduced when thyroid function is subnormal. In hyperthyroidism there is relative digoxin resistance and the dose may have to be increased. During the course of treatment of thyrotoxicosis, dosage should be reduced as the thyrotoxicosis comes under control.

Patients with malabsorption syndrome or gastro-intestinal reconstructions may require larger doses of digoxin.

The risk of provoking dangerous arrhythmias with direct current cardioversion is greatly increased in the presence of digitalis toxicity and is in proportion to the cardioversion energy used.

For elective direct current cardioversion of a patient who is taking digoxin, the drug should be withheld for 24 hours before cardioversion is performed. In emergencies, such as cardiac arrest when attempting cardioversion the lowest effective energy should be applied. Direct current cardioversion is inappropriate in the treatment of arrhythmias though to be caused by cardiac glycosides.

Many beneficial effects of digoxin on arrhythmias result from a degree of atrioventricular conduction blockage. However, when incomplete atrioventricular block already exists the effects of a rapid progression in the block should be anticipated. In complete heart block the idioventricular escape rhythm may be suppressed.

The administration of digoxin in the period immediately following myocardial infarction is not contra-indicated. However, the use of inotropic drugs in some patients in this setting may result in undesirable increased in myocardial oxygen demand and ischaemia, and some retrospective follow-up studies have suggested digoxin to be associated with an increased risk of death. However, the possibility of arrhythmias arising in patients who may be hypokalaemic after myocardial infarction and are likely to be cardiologically unstable must be borne in mind. The limitations imposed thereafter on direct current cardioversion must also be remembered.

Digoxin improves exercise tolerance in patients with impaired left ventricular systolic dysfunction and normal sinus rhythm. This may or may not be associated with an improved haemodynamic profile. However, the benefit of patients with supraventricular arrhythmias is most evident at rest, less evident with exercise.

In patients receiving diuretics and an ACE inhibitor, or diuretics alone, the withdrawal of digoxin has been shown to result in clinical deterioration.

The use of therapeutic doses of digoxin may cause prolongation of the PR interval and depression of the ST segment on the electrocardiogram.

Digoxin may produce false positive ST-T changes on the electrocardiogram during exercise testing. These electrophysiologic effects reflect an expected effect of the drug and are not indicative of toxicity.

Patients receiving digoxin should have their serum electrolytes and renal function (serum creatinine concentration) assessed periodically; the frequency of assessments will depend on the clinical setting.

Although many patients with chronic congestive cardiac failure benefit from acute administration of digoxin. There are some in whom it does not lead to constant, marked or lasting haemodynamic improvement. It is therefore important to evaluate the response of each patient individually when Lanoxin is continued long-term.

Patients with severe respiratory disease may have an increased myocardial sensitivity to digitalis glycosides.

4.5 Interaction with other medicinal products and other forms of Interaction

These may arise from effects on the renal excretion, tissue binding, plasma protein binding, distribution within the body, gut absorptive capacity and sensitivity to Lanoxin. Consideration of the possibility of an interaction whenever concomitant therapy is contemplated is the best precaution and a check on serum digoxin concentration is recommended when any doubt exists.

Digoxin, in association with beta-adrenoceptor blocking drugs, may increase atrio-ventricular conduction time.

Agents causing hypokalaemia or intracellular potassium deficiency may cause increased sensitivity to Digoxin; they include diuretics, lithium salts, corticosteroids and carbenoxolone.

Patients receiving Digoxin are more susceptible to the effects of suxamethonium-exacerbation hyperkalaemia.

Calcium, particularly if administered rapidly by the intravenous route, may produce serious arrhythmias in digitalized patients.

Serum levels or digoxin may be ***increased*** by concomitant administration of the following:

Alprazolam, amiodarone, diphenoxylate with atropine, flecainide, gentamicin, indomethacin, itraconazole, prazosin, propafenone, quinidine, quinine, spironolactone, macrolide antibiotics (e.g neomycyn), tetracycline (and possibly other antibiotics), trimethoprim, and propantheline.

Serum levels of digoxin may be ***reduced*** by concomitant administration of the following:

Adrenaline, antacids, kaolin-pectin, some bulk laxatives and cholestyramine, acarbose, salbutamol, sulphasalazine, neomycin, rifampicin, some cytostatics, phenytoin, metoclopramide, penicillamine and the herbal remedy St John's wort (*Hypericum perforatum*).

Calcium channel blocking agents may either increase or cause no change in serum digoxin levels. Verapamil, felodipine and tiapamil increase serum digoxin levels. Nifedipine and diltiazem may increase or have no effect on serum digoxin levels. Isradipine causes no change in serum digoxin levels. Angiotensin converting enzyme (ACE) inhibitors may also increase or cause no change in serum digoxin concentrations.

Milrinone does not alter steady-state serum digoxin levels.

4.6 Pregnancy and lactation

No data are available on whether or not digoxin has teratogenic effects.

There is no information available on the effect of digoxin on human fertility.

The use of digoxin in pregnancy is not contra-indicated, although the dosage and control may be less predictable in pregnant than in non-pregnant women with some requiring an increased dosage of digoxin during pregnancy. As with all drugs, use should be considered only when the expected clinical benefit of treatment to the mother outweighs any possible risk to the developing foetus.

Despite extensive antenatal exposure to digitalis preparations, no significant adverse effects have been observed in the foetus or neonate when maternal serum digoxin concentrations are maintained within the normal range. Although it has been speculated that a direct effect of digoxin on the myometrium may result in relative prematurity and low birthweight, a contributing role of the underlying cardiac disease cannot be excluded. Maternally administered digoxin has been successfully used to treat foetal tachycardia and congestive heart failure.

Adverse foetal effects have been reported in mothers with digitalis toxicity.

Although digoxin is excreted in breast milk, the quantities are minute and breast feeding is not contra-indicated.

4.7 Effects on ability to drive and use machines

Since central nervous system and visual disturbances have been reported in patients receiving Lanoxin, patients should exercise caution before driving, using machinery or participating in dangerous activities.

4.8 Undesirable effects

In general, the adverse reactions of digoxin are dose-dependent and occur at doses higher than those needed to achieve a therapeutic effect.

Hence, adverse reactions are less common when digoxin is used within the recommended dose range or therapeutic serum concentration range and when there is careful attention to concurrent medications and conditions.

The side effects of digoxin in infants and children differ from those seen in adults in several respects.

In children, the use of digoxin may produce any type of arrhythmia. The most common are conduction disturbances or supraventricular tachyarrhythmias, such as atrial tachycardia (with or without block) and junctional (nodal) tachycardia. Ventricular arrhythmias are less common.

Sinus bradycardia may be a sign of impending digoxin intoxication, especially in infants, even in the absence of first-degree heart block. Any arrhythmia or alteration in cardiac conduction that develops in a child taking digoxin should be assumed to be caused by digoxin, until further evaluation proves otherwise.

Although digoxin may produce anorexia, nausea, vomiting, diarrhoea, and CNS disturbances in young patients, these are rarely the initial symptoms of overdose. Rather, the earliest and most frequent manifestation of excessive dosing with digoxin in infants and children is the appearance of cardiac arrhythmias, including sinus bradycardia.

Non-cardiac:

These are principally associated with overdosage but may occur from a temporarily high serum concentration due to rapid absorption. They include anorexia, nausea and vomiting and usually disappear within a few hours of taking the drug. Diarrhoea can also occur. It is inadvisable to rely on nausea as an early warning of excessive digoxin dosage.

Gynaecomastia can occur with long-term administration.

Weakness, dizziness, confusion, apathy, fatigue, malaise, headache, depression and even psychosis have been reported as adverse central nervous system effects.

Digoxin can produce visual disturbances (blurred or yellow vision).

Oral digoxin has also been associated with intestinal ischaemia and, rarely, with intestinal necrosis.

Skin rashes of urticarial or scarlatiniform character are rare reactions to digoxin and may be accompanied by pronounced eosinophilia.

Very rarely, digoxin can cause thrombocytopenia.

Cardiac:

Digoxin toxicity can cause various arrhythmias and conduction disturbances. Usually an early sign is the occurrence of ventricular premature contractions; they can proceed to bigeminy or even trigeminy. Atrial tachycardias, frequently an indication for digoxin may occur with excessive dosage of the drug. Atrial tachycardia with some degree of atrioventricular block is particularly characteristic, and the pulse rate may not necessarily be fast. (See also *Special Warnings and Precautions for Use*). Digoxin produces PR prolongation and ST segment depression which should not by themselves be considered digoxin toxicity. Cardiac toxicity can also occur at therapeutic doses in patients who have conditions which may alter their sensitivity to digoxin (see *Special Warnings and Special Precautions for Use*).

4.9 Overdose

For symptoms and signs see *Undesirable Effects*.

After recent ingestion, such as accidental or deliberate self-poisoning, the load available for absorption may be reduced by gastric lavage.

Patients with massive digitalis ingestion should receive large doses of activated charcoal to prevent absorption and bind digoxin in the gut during enteroenteric recirculation.

An overdose of digoxin of 10 to 15 mg in adults without heart disease and of 6 to 10 mg in children aged 1 to 3 years without heart disease appeared to be the dose resulting in death in half of the patients.

If more than 25 mg of digoxin was ingested by an adult without heart disease, death or progressive toxicity responsive only to digoxin-binding Fab antibody fragments (Digibind®) resulted. If more that 10 mg of digoxin was ingested by a child aged 1 to 3 years without heart disease, the outcome was uniformly fatal when Fab fragment treatment was not given.

If hypokalaemia is present, it should be corrected with potassium supplements either orally or intravenously depending on the urgency of the situation. In cases where a large amount of Lanoxin has been ingested hyperkalaemia may be present due to release of potassium from skeletal muscle. Before administering potassium in digoxin overdose the serum potassium level must be known.

Bradyarrhythmias may respond to atropine but temporary cardiac pacing may be required. Ventricular arrhythmias may respond to lignocaine or phenytoin.

Dialysis is not particularly effective in removing digoxin from the body in potentially life-threatening toxicity.

Rapid reversal of the complications that are associated with serious poisoning by digoxin, digitoxin and related glycosides has followed intravenous administration of digoxin-specific (ovine) antibody fragments (Fab) when other therapies have failed. Digibind® is the only specific treatment for digoxin toxicity and is very effective. For details consult the literature supplied with Digibind®.

5. PHARMACOLOGICAL PROPERTIES

5.1 Pharmacodynamic properties

Mode of Action:-

Digoxin increases contractility of the myocardium by direct activity. This effect is proportional to dose in the lower range and some effect is achieved with quite low dosing; it occurs even in normal myocardium although it is then entirely without physiological benefit. The primary action of digoxin is specifically to inhibit adenosine triphosphatase, and thus sodium-potassium (Na^+-K^+) exchange activity, the altered ionic distribution across the membrane resulting in an augmented calcium ion influx and thus an increase in the availability of calcium at the time of excitation-contraction coupling. The potency of digoxin may therefore appear considerably enhanced when the extracellular potassium concentration is low, with hyperkalaemia having the opposite effect.

Digoxin exerts the same fundamental effect of inhibition of the Na^+-K^+ exchange mechanism on cells of the autonomic nervous system, stimulating them to exert indirect cardiac activity. Increases in efferent vagal impulses result in reduced sympathetic tone and diminished impulse conduction rate through the atria and atrioventricular node. Thus, the major beneficial effect of digoxin is reduction of ventricular rate.

Indirect cardiac contractility changes also result from changes in venous compliance brought about by the altered autonomic activity and by direct venous stimulation. The interplay between direct and indirect activity governs the total circulatory response, which is not identical for all subjects. In the presence of certain supraventricular arrhythmias, the neurogenically mediated slowing of AV conduction is paramount.

The degree of neurohormonal activation occurring in patients with heart failure is associated with clinical deterioration and an increased risk of death. Digoxin reduces activation of both the sympathetic nervous system and the (renin-angiotensin) system independently of its inotropic actions, and may thus favourably influence survival. Whether this is achieved via direct sympathoinhibitory effects or by re-sensitising baroreflex mechanisms remains unclear.

5.2 Pharmacokinetic properties

Intravenous administration of a loading dose produces an appreciable pharmacological effect within 5 to 30 minutes; this reaches a maximum in 1 to 5 hours. Upon oral administration, digoxin is absorbed from the stomach and upper part of the small intestine. Absorption is delayed by taking a meal although the total amount absorbed is unchanged. Using the oral route the onset of effect occurs in 0.5 to 2 hours and reaches its maximum at 2 to 6 hours. The bioavailability of orally administered Lanoxin is approximately 63% in tablet form and 75% as paediatric elixir.

The initial distribution of digoxin from the central to the peripheral compartment generally lasts from 6 to 8 hours. This is followed by a more gradual decline in serum digoxin concentration, which is dependent upon digoxin elimination from the body. The volume of distribution is large (Vd_{ss} = 510 litres in healthy volunteers), indicating digoxin to be extensively bound to body tissues. The highest digoxin concentrations are seen in the heart, liver and kidney, that in the heart averaging 30- fold that in the systemic circulation. Although the concentration in skeletal muscle is far lower, this store cannot be overlooked since skeletal muscle represents 40% of total body weight. Of the small proportion of digoxin circulating in plasma, approximately 25% is bound to protein.

The major route of elimination is renal excretion of the unchanged drug.

Following intravenous administration to healthy volunteers, between 60 and 75% of a digoxin dose is recovered unchanged in the urine over a 6 day follow-up period. Total body clearance of digoxin has been shown to be directly related to renal function, and percent daily loss is thus a function of creatinine clearance, which in turn may be estimated from a stable serum creatinine. The total and renal clearances of digoxin have been found to be 193 ± 25 ml/min and 152 ± 24 mil/min in a healthy control population.

In a small percentage of individuals, orally administered digoxin is converted to cardioinactivate reduction products (digoxin reduction products or DRPs) by colonic bacteria in the gastrointestinal tract. In these subjects over 40% of the dose may be excreted as DRPs in the urine. Renal clearances of the two main metabolites, dihydrodigoxin and digoxygenin, have been found to be 79 ± 13 ml/min and 100 ± 26 ml/min respectively.

In the majority of cases however, the major route of digoxin elimination is renal excretion of the unchanged drug.

The terminal elimination half life of digoxin in patients with normal renal function is 30 to 40 hours. It is prolonged in patients with impaired renal function, and in anuric patients may be of the order of 100 hours.

In the newborn period, renal clearance of digoxin is diminished and suitable dosage adjustments must be observed. This is specially pronounced in the premature infant since renal clearance reflects maturation of renal function. Digoxin clearance has been found to be 65.6 ± 30 ml/min/1.73m^2 at 3 months, compared to only 32 ± 7 ml/min/1.73m^2 at 1 week. Beyond the immediate newborn period, children generally require proportionally larger doses than adults on the basis of body weight and body surface area.

Since most of the drug is bound to the tissues rather than circulating in the blood, digoxin is not effectively removed from the body during cardiopulmonary by-pass. Furthermore, only about 3% of a digoxin dose is removed from the body during five hours of haemodialysis.

5.3 Preclinical safety data

No data are available on whether or not digoxin has mutagenic or carcinogenic effects.

6. PHARMACEUTICAL PARTICULARS

6.1 List of excipients

Lactose Ph Eur

Starches Ph Eur

Hydrolysed Starch HSE

Magnesium Stearate Ph Eur

6.2 Incompatibilities

None known

6.3 Shelf life

60 months

6.4 Special precautions for storage

Store below 25°C

6.5 Nature and contents of container

Amber glass bottle with low density polyethylene snap-fit closure

Pack sizes: 28, 50, 500

Amber glass bottle with a clic-loc child resistant closure

Pack size: 56

6.6 Instructions for use and handling

Not applicable.

Adminsitrative Data

7. MARKETING AUTHORISATION HOLDER

The Wellcome Foundation Limited

Greenford

Middlesex

UB6 0NN

Trading as:
GlaxoSmithKline UK
Stockley Park West
Uxbridge
Middlesex UB11 1BT

8. MARKETING AUTHORISATION NUMBER(S)
PL 0003/0102R

9. DATE OF FIRST AUTHORISATION/RENEWAL OF THE AUTHORISATION
24.04.03

10. DATE OF REVISION OF THE TEXT
21 May 2003

11. Legal Status
POM

Lanoxin Injection

(GlaxoSmithKline UK)

1. NAME OF THE MEDICINAL PRODUCT
Lanoxin Injection.

2. QUALITATIVE AND QUANTITATIVE COMPOSITION
Digoxin 0.025 % w/v

3. PHARMACEUTICAL FORM
Solution for Injection.

4. CLINICAL PARTICULARS

4.1 Therapeutic indications
Lanoxin is indicated in the management of chronic cardiac failure where the dominant problem is systolic dysfunction. Its therapeutic benefit is greatest in those patients with ventricular dilatation.

Lanoxin is specifically indicated where cardiac failure is accompanied by atrial fibrillation.

Lanoxin is indicated in the management of certain supraventricular arrhythmias, particularly chronic atrial flutter and fibrillation.

4.2 Posology and method of administration
The dose of Lanoxin for each patient has to be tailored individually according to age, lean body weight and renal function. Suggested doses are intended only as an initial guide.

The difference in bioavailability between injectable Lanoxin and oral formulations must be considered when changing from one dosage form to another. For example, if patients are switched from oral to the i.v. formulation the dosage should be reduced by approximately 33 %.

Emergency Parenteral Loading (In patients who have not been given cardiac glycosides within the preceding two weeks): The loading of parenteral Lanoxin is 500 to 1000 micrograms (0.5 to 1.0 mg) depending on age, lean body weight and renal function.

The loading dose should be administered in divided doses with approximately half the total dose given as the first dose and further fractions of the total dose given at intervals of 4 to 8 hours, assessing clinical response before giving each additional dose. Each dose should be given by intravenous infusion (see *Dilution*) over 10 to 20 minutes.

Neonates, infants and children up to 10 years of age (if cardiac glycosides have not been given in the preceding two weeks):

In the newborn, particularly in the premature infant, renal clearance of digoxin is diminished and suitable dose reductions must be observed, over and above general dosage instructions.

Beyond the immediate newborn period, children generally require proportionally larger doses than adults on the basis of body weight or body surface area, as indicated in the schedule below. Children over 10 years of age require adult dosages in proportion to their body weight.

The *intravenous loading dose* in the above groups should be administered in accordance with the following schedule:

Preterm neonates < 1.5 kg	20 microgram/kg over 24 hours
Preterm neonates 1.5 kg to 2.5 kg	30 microgram/kg over 24 hours
Term neonates to 2 years	35 microgram/kg over 24 hours
2 to 5 years	35 microgram/kg over 24 hours
5 to 10 years	25 microgram/kg over 24 hours

The loading dose should be administered in divided doses with approximately half the total dose given as the first dose and further fractions of the total dose given at intervals of 4 to 8 hours, assessing clinical response before giving each additional dose. Each dose should be given by intravenous infusion (see *Dilution*) over 10 to 20 minutes.

Maintenance:

The maintenance dose should be administered in accordance with the following schedule:

Preterm neonates:

daily dose = 20% of 24-hour loading dose (intravenous or oral

Term neonates and children up to 10 years:

daily dose = 25% of 24-hour loading dose (intravenous or oral)

These dosage schedules are meant as guidelines and careful clinical observation and monitoring of serum digoxin levels (see *Monitoring*) should be used as a basis for adjustment of dosage in these paediatric patient groups.

If cardiac glycosides have been given in the two weeks preceding commencement of Lanoxin therapy, it should be anticipated that optimum loading doses of Lanoxin will be less than those recommended above.

Use in the elderly: The tendency to impaired renal function and low lean body mass in the elderly influences the pharmacokinetics of Lanoxin such that high serum digoxin levels and associated toxicity can occur quite readily, unless doses of Lanoxin lower than those in non-elderly patients are used. Serum digoxin levels should be checked regularly and hypokalaemia avoided.

Dose Recommendations in Renal Disorder or with Diuretic Therapy: See *Special Warnings and Precautions for use.*

Dilution: Lanoxin Injection can be administered undiluted or diluted with a 4-fold or greater volume of diluent. The use of less than a 4-fold volume of diluent could lead to precipitation of digoxin.

Lanoxin Injection, 250 micrograms/ml when diluted in the ratio of 1 to 250 (i.e. One 2 ml ampoule containing 500 micrograms added to 500 ml of infusion solution) is known to be compatible with the following infusion solutions:

Sodium Chloride Intravenous Infusion, BP, 0.9% w/v

Sodium Chloride (0.18% w/v) and Glucose (4% w/v) Intravenous Infusion, BP

Glucose Intravenous Infusion, BP, 5% w/v

Chemical in-use stability has been demonstrated for up to 96 hours at ambient temperature (20-25°C).

From a microbiological point of view, the product should be used immediately. If not used immediately, in-use storage times and conditions prior to use are the responsibility of the user and would normally not be longer than 24 hours at 2 to 8°C, unless reconstitution / dilution (etc) has taken place in controlled and validated aseptic conditions.

Any unused solution should be discarded.

Monitoring: Serum concentrations of digoxin may be expressed in conventional units of nanogram/ml (ng/ml) or SI Units of nanomol/L (nmol/L). To convert ng/ml to nmol/L, multiply ng/ml by 1.28.

The serum concentration of digoxin can be determined by radioimmunoassay. Blood should be taken 6 hours or more after the last dose of Lanoxin. There are no rigid guidelines as to the range of serum concentrations that are most efficacious but most patients will benefit, with little risk of toxic symptoms developing, with digoxin concentrations from 0.8 ng/ml (1.02 nmol/L) to 2.0 ng/ml (2.56 nmol/L). Above this range toxic symptoms and signs become more frequent and levels above 3.0 ng/ml (3.84 nmol/L) are quite likely to be toxic. However, in deciding whether a patient's symptoms are due to digoxin, the patient's clinical state together with the serum potassium level and thyroid function are important factors.

Other glycosides, including metabolites of digoxin, can interfere with the assays that are available and one should always be wary of values which do not seem commensurate with the clinical state of the patient.

4.3 Contraindications
Lanoxin is contra-indicated in intermittent complete heart block or second degree atrioventricular block, especially if there is a history of Stokes-Adams attacks.

Lanoxin is contra-indicated in arrhythmias caused by cardiac glycoside intoxication.

Lanoxin is contra-indicated in supraventricular arrhythmias associated with an accessory atrioventricular pathway, as in the Wolff-Parkinson-White syndrome unless the electrophysiological characteristics of the accessory pathway and any possible deleterious effect of digoxin on these characteristics has been evaluated. If an accessory pathway is known or suspected to be present and there is no history of previous supraventricular arrhythmias, Lanoxin is similarly contra-indicated.

Lanoxin is contra-indicated in ventricular tachycardia or ventricular fibrillation.

Lanoxin is contra-indicated in hypertrophic obstructive cardiomyopathy, unless there is concomitant atrial fibrillation and heart failure, but even then caution should be exercised if digoxin is to be used.

Lanoxin is contra-indicated in patients known to be hypersensitive to digoxin or other digitalis glycosides.

4.4 Special warnings and special precautions for use
Arrhythmias may be precipitated by digoxin toxicity, some of which can resemble arrhythmias for which the drug could be advised. For example, atrial tachycardia with varying atrioventricular block requires particular care as clinically the rhythm resembles atrial fibrillation.

In some cases of sinoatrial disorder (i.e. Sick Sinus Syndrome) digoxin may cause or exacerbate sinus bradycardia or cause sinoatrial block.

Determination of the serum digoxin concentration may be very helpful in making a decision to treat with further digoxin, but toxic doses of other glycosides may cross-react in the assay and wrongly suggest apparently satisfactory measurements. Observations during the temporary withholding of digoxin might be more appropriate.

In cases where cardiac glycosides have been taken in the preceding two weeks, the recommendations for initial dosing of a patient should be reconsidered and a reduced dose is advised.

The dosing recommendations should be reconsidered if patients are elderly or there are other reasons for the renal clearance of digoxin being reduced. A reduction in both initial and maintenance doses should be considered.

Hypokalaemia sensitises the myocardium to the actions of cardiac glycosides.

Hypoxia, hypomagnesaemia and marked hypercalcaemia increase myocardial sensitivity to cardiac glycosides.

Rapid intravenous injection can cause vasoconstriction producing hypertension and/or reduced coronary flow. A slow injection rate is therefore important in hypertensive heart failure and acute myocardial infarction.

Administering Lanoxin to a patient with thyroid disease requires care. Initial and maintenance doses of Lanoxin should be reduced when thyroid function is subnormal. In hyperthyroidism there is relative digoxin resistance and the dose may have to be increased. During the course of treatment of thyrotoxicosis, dosage should be reduced as the thyrotoxicosis comes under control.

Patients with malabsorption syndrome or gastro-intestinal reconstructions may require larger doses of digoxin.

The risk of provoking dangerous arrhythmias with direct current cardioversion is greatly increased in the presence of digitalis toxicity and is in proportion to the cardioversion energy used.

For elective direct current cardioversion of a patient who is taking digoxin, the drug should be withheld for 24 hours before cardioversion is performed. In emergencies, such as cardiac arrest, when attempting cardioversion the lowest effective energy should be applied. Direct current cardioversion is inappropriate in the treatment of arrhythmias thought to be caused by cardiac glycosides.

Many beneficial effects of digoxin on arrhythmias result from a degree of atrioventricular conduction blockade. However, when incomplete atrioventricular block already exists the effects of a rapid progression in the block should be anticipated. In complete heart block the idioventricular escape rhythm may be suppressed.

The administration of digoxin in the period immediately following myocardial infarction is not contra-indicated. However, the use of inotropic drugs in some patients in this setting may result in undesirable increases in myocardial oxygen demand and ischaemia, and some retrospective follow-up studies have suggested digoxin to be associated with an increased risk of death. However, the possibility of arrhythmias arising in patients who may be hypokalaemic after myocardial infarction and are likely to be cardiologically unstable must be borne in mind. The limitations imposed thereafter on direct current cardioversion must also be remembered.

Digoxin improves exercise tolerance in patients with impaired left ventricular systolic dysfunction and normal sinus rhythm. This may or may not be associated with an improved haemodynamic profile. However, the benefit of patients with supraventricular arrhythmias is most evident at rest, less evident with exercise.

In patients receiving diuretics and an ACE inhibitor, or diuretics alone, the withdrawal of digoxin has been shown to result in clinical deterioration.

The use of therapeutic doses of digoxin may cause prolongation of the PR interval and depression of the ST segment on the electrocardiogram.

Digoxin may produce false positive ST-T changes on the electrocardiogram during exercise testing. These electrophysiologic effects reflect an expected effect of the drug and are not indicative of toxicity.

Patients receiving digoxin should have their serum electrolytes and renal function (serum creatinine concentration) assessed periodically; the frequency of assessments will depend on the clinical setting.

Although many patients with chronic congestive cardiac failure benefit from acute administration of digoxin, there are some in whom it does not lead to constant, marked or lasting haemodynamic improvement. It is therefore important to evaluate the response of each patient individually when Lanoxin is continued long-term.

The intramuscular route is painful and is associated with muscle necrosis. This route cannot be recommended.

Patients with severe respiratory disease may have an increased myocardial sensitivity to digitalis glycosides.

The packs will carry the following statements:

Do not store above 25°C

Protect from light

For intravenous injection under medical supervision

Keep out of reach of children

4.5 Interaction with other medicinal products and other forms of Interaction

These may arise from effects on the renal excretion, tissue binding, plasma protein binding, distribution within the body, gut absorptive capacity and sensitivity to Lanoxin. Consideration of the possibility of an interaction whenever concomitant therapy is contemplated is the best precaution and a check on serum digoxin concentration is recommended when any doubt exists.

Digoxin, in association with beta-adrenoceptor blocking drugs, may increase atrio-ventricular conduction time.

Agents causing hypokalaemia or intracellular potassium deficiency may cause increased sensitivity to Digoxin; they include diuretics, lithium salts, corticosteroids and carbenoxolone.

Patients receiving Digoxin are more susceptible to the effects of suxamethonium-exacerbated hyperkalaemia.

Calcium, particularly if administered rapidly by the intravenous route, may produce serious arrhthmias in digitalized patients.

Serum levels of digoxin may be **increased** by concomitant administration of the following:

Alprazolam, amiodarone, diphenoxylate with atropine, flecainide, gentamicin, indomethacin, itraconazole, prazosin, propafenone, quinidine, quinine, spironolactone, macrolide antibiotics (e.g. neomycyn), tetracycline, trimethoprim, (and possibly other antibiotics), and propantheline.

Serum levels of digoxin may be **reduced** by concomitant administration of the following:

Adrenaline, antacids, kaolin-pectin, some bulk laxatives and cholestyramine, acarbose,, salbutamol, sulphasalazine, neomycin, rifampicin, some cytostatics, phenytoin, metoclopramide, penicillamine and the herbal remedy St John's wort (*Hypericum perforatum*).

Calcium channel blocking agents may either increase or cause no change in serum digoxin levels. Verapamil, felodipine and tiapamil increase serum digoxin levels. Nifedipine and diltiazem may increase or have no effect on serum digoxin levels. Isradipine causes no change in serum digoxin levels. Angiotensin converting enzyme (ACE) inhibitors may also increase or cause no change in serum digoxin concentrations.

Milrinone does not alter steady-state serum digoxin levels.

4.6 Pregnancy and lactation

No data are available on whether or not digoxin has teratogenic effects.

There is no information available on the effect of digoxin on human fertility.

The use of digoxin in pregnancy is not contra-indicated, although the dosage and control may be less predictable in pregnant than in non-pregnant women with some requiring an increased dosage of digoxin during pregnancy. As with all drugs, use should be considered only when the expected clinical benefit of treatment to the mother outweighs any possible risk to the developing foetus.

Despite extensive antenatal exposure to digitalis preparations, no significant adverse effects have been observed in the foetus or neonate when maternal serum digoxin concentrations are maintained within the normal range. Although it has been speculated that a direct effect of digoxin in the myometrium may result in relative prematurity and low birthweight, a contributing role of the underlying cardiac disease cannot be excluded. Maternally administered digoxin has been successfully used to treat foetal tachycardia and congestive heart failure.

Adverse foetal effects have been reported in mothers with digitalis toxicity.

Although digoxin is excreted in breast milk, the quantities are minute and breast feeding is not contra-indicated.

4.7 Effects on ability to drive and use machines

Since central nervous system and visual disturbances have been reported in patients receiving Lanoxin, patients should exercise caution before driving, using machinery or participating in dangerous activities.

4.8 Undesirable effects

In general, the adverse reactions of digoxin are dose-dependent and occur at doses higher than those needed to achieve a therapeutic effect. Hence, adverse reactions are less common when digoxin is used within the recommended dose range or therapeutic serum concentration range and when there is careful attention to concurrent medications and conditions.

The side effects of digoxin in infants and children differ from those seen in adults in several respects.

Although digoxin may produce anorexia, nausea, vomiting, diarrhoea, and CNS disturbances in young patients, these are rarely the initial symptoms of overdose. Rather, the earliest and most frequent manifestation of excessive dosing with digoxin in infants and children is the appearance of cardiac arrhythmias, including sinus bradycardia.

In children, the use of digoxin may produce any type of arrhythmia. The most common are conduction disturbances or supraventricular tachyarrhythmias, such as atrial tachycardia (with or without block) and junctional (nodal) tachycardia. Ventricular arrhythmias are less common.

Sinus bradycardia may be a sign of impending digoxin intoxication, especially in infants, even in the absence of first-degree heart block. Any arrhythmia or alteration in cardiac conduction that develops in a child taking digoxin should be assumed to be caused by digoxin, until further evaluation proves otherwise.

Non-cardiac:

These are principally associated with overdosage but may occur from a temporarily high serum concentration due to rapid absorption. They include anorexia, nausea and vomiting and usually disappear within a few hours of taking the drug. Diarrhoea can also occur. It is inadvisable to rely on nausea as an early warning of excessive digoxin dosage.

Gynaecomastia can occur with long-term administration.

Weakness, dizziness, confusion, apathy, fatigue, malaise, headache, depression and even psychosis have been reported as adverse central nervous system effects.

Digoxin can produce visual disturbances (blurred or yellow vision).

Oral digoxin has also been associated with intestinal ischaemia and, rarely, with intestinal necrosis.

Skin rashes of urticarial or scarlatiniform character are rare reactions to digoxin, and may be accompanied by pronounced eosinophilia.

Very rarely, digoxin can cause thrombocytopenia.

Cardiac:

Digoxin toxicity can cause various arrhythmias and conduction disturbances. Usually an early sign is the occurrence of ventricular premature contractions; they can proceed to bigeminy or even trigeminy. Atrial tachycardias, frequently an indication for digoxin, may nevertheless occur with excessive dosage of the drug. Atrial tachycardia with some degree of atrioventricular block is particularly characteristic, and the pulse rate may not necessarily be fast. (See also *Special Warnings and Precautions for Use*). Digoxin produces PR prolongation and ST segment depression which should not by themselves be considered digoxin toxicity. Cardiac toxicity can also occur at therapeutic doses in patients who have conditions which may alter their sensitivity to digoxin (see *Special Warnings and Precautions for Use*).

4.9 Overdose

For symptoms and signs see *Undesirable Effects.*

After recent ingestion, such as accidental or deliberate self-poisoning, the load available for absorption may be reduced by gastric lavage.

Patients with massive digitalis ingestion should receive large doses of activated charcoal to prevent absorption and bind digoxin in the gut during enteroenteric recirculation.

An overdosage of digoxin of 10 to 15 mg in adults without heart disease and of 6 to 10 mg in children aged 1 to 3 years without heart disease appeared to be the dose resulting in death in half of the patients.

If more than 25 mg of digoxin was ingested by an adult without heart disease, death or progressive toxicity responsive only to digoxin-binding Fab antibody fragments (Digibind®) resulted. If more than 10 mg of digoxin was ingested by a child aged 1 to 3 years without heart disease, the outcome was uniformly fatal when Fab fragment treatment was not given.

If hypokalaemia is present, it should be corrected with potassium supplements either orally or intravenously depending on the urgency of the situation. In cases where a large amount of Lanoxin has been ingested, hyperkalaemia may be present due to release of potassium from skeletal muscle. Before administering potassium in digoxin overdose the serum potassium level must be known.

Bradyarrhythmias may respond to atropine but temporary cardiac pacing may be required. Ventricular arrhythmias may respond to lignocaine or phenytoin.

Dialysis is not particularly effective in removing digoxin from the body in potentially life-threatening toxicity.

Rapid reversal of the complications that are associated with serious poisoning by digoxin, digitoxin and related glycosides has followed intravenous administration of digoxin-specific (ovine) antibody fragments (Fab) when other therapies have failed. Digibind® is the only specific treatment for digoxin toxicity and is very effective. For details consult the literature supplied with Digibind®.

5. PHARMACOLOGICAL PROPERTIES

5.1 Pharmacodynamic properties

Mode of Action:-

Digoxin increases contractility of the myocardium by direct activity. This effect is proportional to dose in the lower range and some effect is achieved with quite low dosing; it occurs even in normal myocardium although it is then entirely without physiological benefit. The primary action of digoxin is specifically to inhibit adenosine triphosphatase, and thus sodium-potassium (Na^+-K^+) exchange activity, the altered ionic distribution across the membrane resulting in an augmented calcium ion influx and thus an increase in the availability of calcium at the time of excitation-contraction coupling. The potency of digoxin may therefore appear considerably enhanced when the extracellular potassium concentration is low, with hyperkalaemia having the opposite effect.

Digoxin exerts the same fundamental effect of inhibition of the Na^+-K^+ exchange mechanism on cells of the autonomic nervous system, stimulating them to exert indirect cardiac activity. Increases in efferent vagal impulses result in reduced sympathetic tone and diminished impulse conduction rate through the atria and atrioventricular node. Thus, the major beneficial effect of digoxin is reduction of ventricular rate.

Indirect cardiac contractility changes also result from changes in venous compliance brought about by the altered autonomic activity and by direct venous stimulation. The interplay between direct and indirect activity governs the total circulatory response, which is not identical for all subjects. In the presence of certain supraventricular arrhythmias, the neurogenically mediated slowing of AV conduction is paramount.

The degree of neurohormonal activation occurring in patients with heart failure is associated with clinical deterioration and an increased risk of death. Digoxin reduces activation of both the sympathetic nervous system and the (renin-angiotensin) system independently of its inotropic actions, and may thus favourably influence survival. Whether this is achieved via direct sympathoinhibitory effects or by re-sensitising baroreflex mechanisms remains unclear.

5.2 Pharmacokinetic properties

Intravenous administration of a loading dose produces an appreciable pharmacological effect within 5 to 30 minutes; this reaches a maximum in 1 to 5 hours. Upon oral administration, digoxin is absorbed from the stomach and upper part of the small intestine. Absorption is delayed by taking a meal although the total amount absorbed is unchanged. Using the oral route the onset of effect occurs in 0.5 to 2 hours and reaches its maximum at 2 to 6 hours. The bioavailability of orally administered Lanoxin is approximately 63% in tablet form and 75% as paediatric elixir.

The initial distribution of digoxin from the central to the peripheral compartment generally lasts from 6 to 8 hours. This is followed by a more gradual decline in serum digoxin concentration, which is dependent upon digoxin elimination from the body. The volume of distribution is large (Vd_{ss} = 510 litres in healthy volunteers), indicating digoxin to be extensively bound to body tissues. The highest digoxin concentrations are seen in the heart, liver and kidney, that in the heart averaging 30- fold that in the systemic circulation. Although the concentration in skeletal muscle is far lower, this store cannot be overlooked since skeletal muscle represents 40% of total body weight. Of the small proportion of digoxin circulating in plasma, approximately 25% is bound to protein.

The major route of elimination is renal excretion of the unchanged drug.

Following intravenous administration to healthy volunteers, between 60 and 75% of a digoxin dose is recovered unchanged in the urine over a 6 day follow-up period. Total body clearance of digoxin has been shown to be directly related to renal function, and percent daily loss is thus a function of creatinine clearance, which in turn may be estimated from a stable serum creatinine. The total and renal clearances of digoxin have been found to be 193 ± 25 ml/min and 152 ± 24 mil/min in a healthy control population.

In a small percentage of individuals, orally administered digoxin is converted to cardioinactivate reduction products (digoxin reduction products or DRPs) by colonic bacteria in the gastrointestinal tract. In these subjects over 40% of the dose may be excreted as DRPs in the urine. Renal clearances of the two main metabolites, dihydrodigoxin and digoxygenin, have been found to be 79 ± 13 ml/min and 100 ± 26 ml/min respectively.

In the majority of cases however, the major route of digoxin elimination is renal excretion of the unchanged drug.

The terminal elimination half life of digoxin in patients with normal renal function is 30 to 40 hours. It is prolonged in patients with impaired renal function, and in anuric patients may be of the order of 100 hours.

In the newborn period, renal clearance of digoxin is diminished and suitable dosage adjustments must be observed. This is specially pronounced in the premature infant since renal clearance reflects maturation of renal function. Digoxin clearance has been found to be 65.6 ± 30 ml/min/1.73m² at 3 months, compared to only 32 ± 7 ml/min/1.73m² at 1 week. Beyond the immediate newborn period, children generally require proportionally larger doses than adults on the basis of body weight and body surface area.

Since most of the drug is bound to the tissues rather than circulating in the blood, digoxin is not effectively removed from the body during cardiopulmonary by-pass. Furthermore, only about 3% of a digoxin dose is removed from the body during five hours of haemodialysis.

5.3 Preclinical safety data
No data are available on whether or not digoxin has mutagenic or carcinogenic effects.

6. PHARMACEUTICAL PARTICULARS

6.1 List of excipients

Ethanol	10.4 v/v
Propylene Glycol	40.0 v/v
Citric Acid Monohydrate	0.075 w/v
Sodium phosphate anhydrous	0.179 w/v
or	
Sodium phosphate	0.45 w/v
Water for Injections	to 2 ml

6.2 Incompatibilities
None known.

6.3 Shelf life
5 years.

6.4 Special precautions for storage
Do not store above 25°C.

Store in the original container

6.5 Nature and contents of container
Neutral glass ampoules

6.6 Instructions for use and handling
(Ampoule instructions and diagram)

Lanoxin Injection can be administered undiluted or diluted with a 4-fold or greater volume of diluent. The use of less than a 4-fold volume of diluent could lead to precipitation of digoxin.

Lanoxin Injection, 250 micrograms/ml when diluted in the ratio of 1 to 250 (i.e. One 2 ml ampoule containing 500 micrograms added to 500 ml of infusion solution) is known to be compatible with the following infusion solutions:

Sodium Chloride Intravenous Infusion, BP, 0.9% w/v

Sodium Chloride (0.18% w/v) and Glucose (4% w/v) Intravenous Infusion, BP

Glucose Intravenous Infusion, BP, 5% w/v

Chemical in-use stability has been demonstrated for up to 96 hours at ambient temperature (20-25°C).

From a microbiological point of view, the product should be used immediately. If not used immediately, in-use storage times and conditions prior to use are the responsibility of the user and would normally not be longer than 24 hours at 2 to 8°C, unless reconstitution / dilution (etc) has taken place in controlled and validated aseptic conditions.

Any unused solution should be discarded.

Administrative Data

7. MARKETING AUTHORISATION HOLDER
The Wellcome Foundation Limited

Greenford

Middlesex

UB6 0NN

8. MARKETING AUTHORISATION NUMBER(S)
PL0003/5259R

9. DATE OF FIRST AUTHORISATION/RENEWAL OF THE AUTHORISATION
24.04.03

10. DATE OF REVISION OF THE TEXT
24 November 2003

11. Legal Status
POM

Lanoxin PG Elixir

(GlaxoSmithKline UK)

1. NAME OF THE MEDICINAL PRODUCT
Lanoxin PG Elixir

2. QUALITATIVE AND QUANTITATIVE COMPOSITION
Digoxin 0.005 % w/v

3. PHARMACEUTICAL FORM
Liquid

4. CLINICAL PARTICULARS

4.1 Therapeutic indications
Lanoxin is indicated in the management of chronic cardiac failure where the dominant problem is systolic dysfunction. Its therapeutic benefit is greatest in those patients with ventricular dilatation.

Lanoxin is specifically indicated where cardiac failure is accompanied by atrial fibrillation.

Lanoxin is indicated in the management of certain supraventricular arrhythmias, particularly chronic atrial flutter and fibrillation.

4.2 Posology and method of administration
The dose of Lanoxin for each patient has to be tailored individually according to age, lean body weight and renal function. Suggested doses are intended only as an initial guide.

The difference in bioavailability between injectable Lanoxin and oral formulations must be considered when changing from one dosage form to another. For example, if patients are switched from oral to the i.v. formulation the dosage should be reduced by approximately 33 %.

Lanoxin PG Elixir, 50 micrograms in 1 ml, is supplied with a graduated pipette and this should be used for measurement of all doses.

Adults and children over 10 years.

Rapid Oral Loading: 750 to 1500 micrograms (0.75 to 1.5 mg) as a single dose.

Where there is less urgency, or greater risk of toxicity (e.g. in the elderly), the oral loading dose should be given in divided doses 6 hours apart, assessing clinical response before giving each additional dose (see *Special Warnings and Precautions for Use*).

Slow Oral Loading: 250 to 750 micrograms (0.25 to 0.75 mg) should be given daily for 1 week followed by an appropriate maintenance dose. A clinical response should be seen within one week.

Note: The choice between slow and rapid oral loading depends on the clinical state of the patient and the urgency of the condition.

Maintenance: The maintenance dosage should be based upon the percentage of the peak body stores lost each day through elimination. The following formula has had wide clinical use:

$$\text{Maintenance Dose} = \text{Peak body stores} \times \frac{\%\ \text{daily loss}}{100}$$

Where:

Peak Body Stores = Loading Dose

% Daily Loss = 14 + Creatinine Clearance (C_{cr})/5.

C_{cr} is creatinine clearance corrected to 70 kg body weight or 1.73 m^2 body surface area. If only serum creatinine (S_{cr}) concentrations are available, a C_{cr} (corrected to 70 kg body weight) maybe estimated in men as:

$$C_{cr} = \frac{(140 - \text{age})}{S_{cr}\ (\text{in mg/100 ml})}$$

NOTE: Where serum creatinine values are obtained in micromol/L. These may be converted to mg/100 ml (mg %) as follows:

$$S_{cr}\ (\text{mg/100 ml}) = \frac{S_{cr}\ (\text{micromol/L}) \times 113.12}{10{,}000} = \frac{S_{cr}\ (\text{micromol/L})}{88.4}$$

Where 113.12 is the molecular weight of creatinine.

For women, this result should be multiplied by 0.85

NOTE: These formulae cannot be used for creatinine clearance in children.

In practice, this will mean that most patients will be maintained on 0.125 to 0.75 mg digoxin daily; however in those who show increased sensitivity to the adverse effects of digoxin, a dosage of 62.5 microgram (0.0625 mg) daily or less may suffice.

Neonates, infants and children up to 10 years of age (if cardiac glycosides have not been given in preceding two weeks):

In the newborn, particularly in the premature infant, renal clearance of digoxin is diminished and suitable dose reductions must be observed, over and above general dosage instructions.

Beyond the immediate newborn period, children generally require proportionally larger doses than adults on the basis of body weight or body surface area, as indicated in the schedule below. Children over 10 years of age require adult dosages in proportion to their body weight.

Oral Loading Dose:

This should be administered in accordance with the following schedule:-

Preterm neonates < 1.5 kg	25 microgram/kg over 24 hours
Preterm neonates 1.5 to 2.5 kg	30 microgram/kg over 24 hours
Term neonates to 2 years	45 microgram/kg over 24 hours
2 to 5 years	35 microgram/kg over 24 hours
5 to 10 years	25 microgram/kg over 24 hours

The loading dose should be administered in divided doses with approximately half the total dose given as the first dose and further fractions of the total dose given at intervals of 4 to 8 hours, assessing clinical response before giving each additional dose.

Maintenance:

The maintenance dose should be administered in accordance with the following schedule:

Preterm neonates:

daily dose = 20% of 24-hour loading dose (intravenous or oral)

Term neonates and children up to10 years:

daily dose = 25% of 24-hour loading dose (intravenous or oral)

These dosage schedules are meant as guidelines and careful clinical observation and monitoring of serum digoxin levels (see *Monitoring*) should be used as a basis for adjustment of dosage in these paediatric patient groups.

If cardiac glycosides have been given in the two weeks preceding commencement of Lanoxin therapy, it should be anticipated that optimum loading doses of Lanoxin will be less than those recommended above.

Use in the Elderly: The tendency to impaired renal function and low lean body mass in the elderly influences the pharmacokinetics of Lanoxin such that high serum digoxin levels and associated toxicity can occur quite readily, unless doses of Lanoxin lower than those in non-elderly patients are used. Serum digoxin levels should be checked regularly and hypokalaemia avoided.

Dose recommendations in renal disorder or with diuretic therapy: See *Special Warnings and Precautions for Use.*

Monitoring: Serum concentrations of digoxin may be expressed in conventional units of nanogram/ml (ng/ml) or SI units of nanomol/L (nmol/L). To convert ng/ml to nmol/L, multiply ng/ml by 1.28.

The serum concentration of digoxin can be determined by radioimmunoassay. Blood should be taken 6 hours or more after the last dose of Lanoxin. There are no rigid guidelines as to the range of serum concentrations that are most efficacious but most patients will benefit, with little risk of toxic symptoms and signs developing, with digoxin concentrations from 0.8 ng/ml (1.02 nmol/L) to 2 ng/ml (2.56 nmol/L). Above this range, toxic symptoms and signs become more frequent and levels above 3 ng/ml (3.84 nmol/L) are quite likely to be toxic. However, in deciding whether a patient's symptoms are due to digoxin, the patient's clinical state together with the serum potassium level and thyroid function are important factors.

Other glycosides, including metabolites of digoxin, can interfere with the assays that are available and one should always be wary of values which do not seem commensurate with the clinical state of the patient.

4.3 Contraindications
Lanoxin is contra-indicated in intermittent complete heart block or second degree atrioventricular block, especially if there is a history of Strokes-Adams attacks.

Lanoxin is contra-indicated in arrhythmias caused by cardiac glycoside intoxication.

Lanoxin is contra-indicated in supraventricular arrhythmias associated with an accessory atrioventricular pathway, as in the Wolff-Parkinson-White syndrome, unless the electrophysiological characteristics of the accessory pathway and any possible deleterious effect of digoxin on these characteristics has been evaluated. If an accessory pathway is known or suspected to be present and there is no history of previous supraventricular arrhythmias Lanoxin is similarly contra-indicated.

Lanoxin is contra-indicated in ventricular tachycardia or ventricular fibrillation.

Lanoxin is contra-indicated in hypertrophic obstructive cardiomyopathy, unless there is concomitant atrial fibrillation and heart failure but even then caution should be exercised if Lanoxin is to be used.

Lanoxin is contra-indicated in patients known to be hypersensitive to digoxin or other digitalis glycosides.

4.4 Special warnings and special precautions for use
Arrhythmias may be precipitated by digoxin toxicity, some of which can resemble arrhythmias for which the drug could be advised. For example, atrial tachycardia with varying atrioventricular block requires particular care as clinically the rhythm resembles atrial fibrillation.

In some cases of sinoatrial disorder (i.e. sick sinus syndrome) digoxin may cause or exacerbate sinus bradycardia or cause sinoatrial block.

Determination of the serum digoxin concentration may be very helpful in making a decision to treat with further digoxin, but toxic doses of other glycosides may cross-react in the assay and wrongly suggest apparently satisfactory measurements. Observations during the temporary withholding of digoxin may be more appropriate.

In cases where cardiac glycosides have been taken in the preceding two weeks the recommendations for initial dosing of a patient should be reconsidered and a reduced dose is advised.

The dosing recommendations should be reconsidered if patients are elderly or there are other reasons for the renal clearance of digoxin being reduced. A reduction in both initial and maintenance doses should be considered.

Hypokalaemia sensitises the myocardium to the actions of cardiac glycosides.

Hypoxia, hypomagnesaemia and marked hypercalcaemia increase myocardial sensitivity to cardiac glycosides.

Administering Lanoxin to a patient with thyroid disease requires care. Initial and maintenance doses of Lanoxin should be reduced when thyroid function is subnormal. In hyperthyroidism there is relative digoxin resistance and the dose may have to be increased. During the course of treatment of thyrotoxicosis, dosage should be reduced as the thyrotoxicosis comes under control.

Patients with malabsorption syndrome or gastro-intestinal reconstruction may require larger doses of digoxin.

The risk of provoking dangerous arrhythmias with direct current cardioversion is greatly increased in the presence of digitalis toxicity and is in proportion to the cardioversion energy used.

For elective direct current cardioversion of a patient who is taking digoxin, the drug should be withheld for 24 hours before cardioversion is performed. In emergencies, such as cardiac arrest, when attempting cardioversion the lowest effective energy should be applied.

Direct current cardioversion is inappropriate in the treatment of arrhythmias thought to be caused by cardiac glycosides.

Many beneficial effects of digoxin on arrhythmias result from a degree of atrioventricular conduction blockade. However, when incomplete atrioventricular block already exists, the effects of a rapid progression in the block should be anticipated. In complete heart block the idioventricular escape rhythm may be suppressed.

The administration of digoxin in the period immediately following myocardial infarction is not contra-indicated. However, the use of inotropic drugs in some patients in this setting may result in undesirable increases in myocardial oxygen demand and ischaemia, and some retrospective follow-up studies have suggested digoxin to be associated with an increased risk of death. However, the possibility of arrhythmias arising in patients who may be hypokalaemic after myocardial infarction and are likely to be cardiologicially unstable must be borne in mind. The limitations imposed thereafter on direct current cardioversion must also be remembered.

Digoxin improves exercise tolerance in patients with impaired left ventricular systolic dysfunction and normal sinus rhythm. This may or may not be associated with an improved haemodynamic profile. However, the benefit of digoxin in patients with supreaventricular arrythmias is most evident at rest, less evident with exercise.

In patients receiving diuretics and an ACE inhibitor, or diuretics alone, the withdrawal of digoxin has been shown to result in clinical deterioration.

The use of therapeutic doses of digoxin may cause prolongation of the PR interval and depression of the ST segment on the electrocardiogram.

Digoxin may produce false positive ST-T changes on the electrocardiogram during exercise testing. These electrophysiologic effects reflect an expected effect of the drug and are not indicative of toxicity.

Patients receiving digoxin should have their serum electrolytes and renal function (serum creatinine concentration) assessed periodically; the frequency of assessments will depend on the clinical setting.

Although many patients with chronic congestive cardiac failure benefit from acute administration of digoxin, there are some in whom it does not lead to constant, marked or lasting haemodynamic improvement. It is therefore important to evaluate the response of each patient individually when the Lanoxin is continued long-term.

Patients with severe respiratory diseases may have an increased myocardial sensitivity to digitalis glycosides.

4.5 Interaction with other medicinal products and other forms of Interaction

These may arise from effects on the renal excretion, tissue binding, plasma protein binding, distribution within the body, gut absorptive capacity and sensitivity to Lanoxin. Consideration of the possibility of an interaction whenever concomitant therapy is contemplated is the best precaution and a check on serum digoxin concentration is recommended when any doubt exists.

Digoxin, in association with beta-adrenoceptor blocking drugs, may increase atrio-ventricular conduction time.

Agents causing hypokalaemia or intracellular potassium deficiency may cause increased sensitivity to Digoxin; they include diuretics, lithium salts, corticosteroids and carbenoxolone.

Patients receiving Digoxin are more susceptible to the effects of suxamethonium-exacerbated hyperkalaemia.

Calcium, particularly if administered rapidly by the intravenous route, may produce serious arrhythmias in digitalized patients.

Serum levels of digoxin may be **increased** by concomitant administration of the following:

Amiodarone, flecainide, prazosin, propafenone, quinidine, spironolactone, macrolide antibiotics (e.g. neomycin), tetracycline, (and possibly other antibiotics), gentamicin, itraconazole, trimethoprim, quinine, alprazolam, diphenoxylate with atropine, indomethacin, and propantheline.

Serum levels of digoxin may be **reduced** by concomitant administration of the following:

Antacids, kaolin-pectin, some bulk laxatives, cholestyramine, acarbose, adrenaline, salbutamol, sulphasalazine, neomycin, rifampicin, some cytostatics, phenytoin, metoclopramide, penicillamine and the herbal remedy St John's wort (*Hypericum perforatum*).

Calcium channel blocking agents may either increase or cause no change in serum digoxin levels. Verapamil, felodipine and tiapamil increase serum digoxin levels. Nifedipine and diltiazem may increase or have no effect on serum digoxin levels. Isradipine causes no change in serum digoxin levels. Angiotensin converting enzyme (ACE) inhibitors may also increase or cause no change in serum digoxin concentrations.

Milrinone dose not alter steady-state serum digoxin levels.

4.6 Pregnancy and lactation

No data are available on whether or not digoxin has teratogenic effects.

There is no information available on the effect of digoxin on human fertility.

The use of digoxin in pregnancy is not contra-indicated, although the dosage may be less predictable in pregnant than in non-pregnant women with some requiring an increased dosage of digoxin during pregnancy. As with all drugs, use should be considered only when the expected clinical benefit of treatment to the mother outweighs any possible risk to the developing foetus.

Despite extensive antenatal exposure to digitalis preparations, no significatn adverse effects have been observed in the foetus or neonate when maternal serum digoxin concentrations are mantained withing the normal range. Although it has been speculated that a direct effect of digoxin n the myometrium may result in relative prematurity and low birthweight, a contributing role of the underlying cardiac disease cannot be excluded. Maternally administered digoxin has been successfully used to treat foetal tachycardia and congestive heart failure.

Adverse foetal effects have been reported in mothers with digitalis toxicity.

Although digoxin is excreted in breast milk, the quantities are minute and breast feeding is not contra-indicated.

4.7 Effects on ability to drive and use machines

Since central nervous system and visual disturbances have been reported in patients receiving Lanoxin, patients should exercise caution before driving, using machinery or participating in dangerous activities.

4.8 Undesirable effects

In general, the adverse reactions of digoxin are dose-dependent and occur at doses higher than those needed to achieve a therapeutic effect.

Hence, adverse reactions are less common when digoxin is used within the recommended dose range or therapeutic serum concentration range and when there is careful attention to concurrent medications and conditions.

The side effects of digoxin in infants and children differ from those seen in adults in several respects.

Although digoxin may produce anorexia, nausea, vomiting, diarrhoea, and CNS disturbances in young patients, these are rarely the initial symptoms of overdose. Rather, the earliest and most frequent manifestation of excessive dosing with digoxin in infants and children is the appearance of cardiac arrhythmias, including sinus bradycardia.

In children, the use of digoxin may produce any type of arrhythmia. The most common are conduction disturbances or supraventricular tachyarrhythmias, such as atrial tachycardia (with or without block) and junctional (nodal) tachycardia. Ventricular arrhythmias are less common.

Sinus bradycardia may be a sign of impending digoxin intoxication, especially in infants, even in the absence of first-degree heart block. Any arrhythmia or alteration in cardiac conduction that develops in a child taking digoxin should be assumed to be caused by digoxin, until further evaluation proves otherwise.

Non-cardiac:

These are principally associated with overdosage but may occur from a temporarily high serum concentration due to rapid absorption. They include anorexia, nausea and vomiting and usually disappear within a few hours of taking the drug. Diarrhoea can also occur. It is inadvisable to rely on nausea as an early warning of excessive digoxin dosage.

Gynaecomastia can occur with long-term administration.

Weakness, dizziness, confusion, apathy, fatigue, malaise, headache, depression and even psychosis have been reported as adverse central nervous system effects.

Digoxin can produce visual disturbances (blurred or yellow vision).

Oral digoxin has also been associated with intestinal ischaemia and, rarely, with intestinal necrosis.

Skin rashes of urticarial or scarlatiniform character are rare reactions to digoxin and may be accompanied by pronounced eosinophilia.

Very rarely, digoxin can cause thrombocytopenia.

Cardiac:

Digoxin toxicity can cause various arrhythmias and conduction disturbances, Usually an early sign is the occurrence of ventricular premature contractions; they can proceed to bigeminy or even trigeminy. Atrial tachycardias, frequently an indication for digoxin, may occur with excessive dosage of the drug. Atrial tachycardia with some degree of atrioventricular block is particularly characteristic, and the pulse rate may not necessarily be fast (also see *Special Warnings and Precautions for Use*). Digoxin produces PR prolongation and ST segment depression which should not by themselves be considered digoxin toxicity. Cardiac toxicity can also occur at therapeutic doses in patients who have conditions which may alter their sensitivity to digoxin (see *Special Warnings and Special Precautions for Use*).

4.9 Overdose

For symptoms and signs see *Undesirable Effects*.

After recent ingestion, such as accidental or deliberate self-poisoning, the load available for absorption may be reduced by gastric lavage.

Patients with massive digitalis ingestion should receive large doses of activated charcoal to prevent absorption and bind digoxin in the gut during enteroenteric recirculation.

An overdose of digoxin 10 to 15 mg in adults without heart disease and of 6 to 10 mg in children aged 1 to 3 years without heart disease appeared to be the dose resulting in death in half of the patients.

If more than 25 mg of digoxin was ingested by an adult without hear disease, death or progressive toxicity responsive only to digoxin-binding Fab antibody fragments (Digibind®) resulted. If more than 10mg of digoxin was ingested by a child aged 1 to 3 years without heart disease, the outcome was uniformly fatal when Fab fragment treatment was not given.

If hypokalaemia is present, it should be corrected with potassium supplements either orally or intravenously depending on the urgency of the situation. In cases where a large amount of Lanoxin has been ingested hyperkalaemia may be present due to release of potassium from skeletal muscle. Before administering potassium in digoxin overdose the serum potassium level must be known.

Bradyarrhythmias may respond to atropine but temporary cardiac pacing may be required. Ventricular arrhythmias may respond to lignocaine or phenytoin.

Dialysis is not particularly effective in removing digoxin from the body in potentially life-threatening toxicity.

Rapid reversal of the complications that are associated with serious poisoning by digoxin, digitoxin and related glycosides has followed intravenous administration of digoxin-specific (ovine) antibody fragments (Fab) when other therapies have failed. Digibind is the only specific treatment for digoxin toxicity and is very effective. For details consult the literature supplied with Digibind®.

5. PHARMACOLOGICAL PROPERTIES

5.1 Pharmacodynamic properties

Mode of Action:-

Digoxin increases contractility of the myocardium by direct activity. This effect is proportional to dose in the lower range and some effect is achieved with quite low dosing; it occurs even in normal myocardium although it is then entirely without physiological benefit. The primary action of digoxin is specifically to inhibit adenosine triphosphatase, and thus sodium-potassium (Na^+-K^+) exchange activity, the altered ionic distribution across the membrane resulting in an augmented calcium ion influx and thus an increase in the availability of calcium at the time of excitation-contraction coupling. The potency of digoxin may therefore appear considerably enhanced when the extracellular potassium concentration is low, with hyperkalaemia having the opposite effect.

Digoxin exerts the same fundamental effect of inhibition of the Na^+-K^+ exchange mechanism on cells of the autonomic nervous system, stimulating them to exert indirect cardiac activity. Increases in efferent vagal impulses result in reducted sympathetic tone and diminished impulse conduction rate through the atria and atrioventricular node. Thus, the major beneficial effect of digoxin is reduction of ventricular rate.

Indirect cardiac cotnractility changes also result from changes in venous comliance brought about by the altered autonomic activity and by direct venous stimulation. The interplay between direct and indirect activity governs the total circulatory response, which is not identical for all subjects. In the presence of certain supraventricular arrhythmias, the neurogenically mediated slowing of AV conduction is paramount.

The degree of neurohormonal activation occurring in patients with heart failure is associated with clinical deterioration and an increased risk of death. Digoxin reduces activation of both the sympathetic nervous system and the (renin-angiotensin) system independently of its inotropic actions, and may thus favourably influence survival. Whether this is achieved via direct sympathoinhibitory effects or by re-sensitizing baroreflex mechanisms remains unclear.

5.2 Pharmacokinetic properties

Intravenous administration of a loading dose produces an appreciable pharmacological effect within 5 to 30 minutes; this reaches a maximun in 1 to 5 hours. Upon oral administration, digoxin is absorbed from the stomach and upper part of the small intestine. Absorption is delayed byt taking a meal although the total amount absorbed is unchanged. Using the oral route the onset of effect occurs in 0.5 to 2 hours and reaches its maximun at 2 to 6 hours. The bioavailability of orally administered Lanoxin is approximately 63% in tablet form and 75% as paediatric elixir.

The initial distribution of digoxin from the central to the peripheral compartment generally lasts from 6 to 8 hours. This is followed by a more gradual decline in serum digoxin concentration, which is dependent upon digoxin elimination from the body. The volume of distribution is large (Vd_{ss} = 510 litres in healthy volunteers), indicating digoxin to be extensively bound to body tissues. The highest digoxin concentrations are seen in the heart, liver and kidney, that in the heart averaging 30- fold that in the systemic circulation. Although the concentration in skeletal muscle is far lower, this store cannot be overlooked since skeletal muscle represents 40% of total body weight. Of the small proportion of digoxin circulating in plasma, approximately 25% is bound to protein.

The major route of elimination is renal excretion of the unchanged drug.

Following intravenous administration to healthy volunteers, between 60 and 75% of a digoxin dose is recovered unchanged in the urine over a 6 day follow-up period. Total body clearance of digoxin has been shown to be directly related to renal function, and percent daily loss is thus a function of creatinine clearance, which in turn may be estimated from a stable serum creatinine. The total and renal clearances of digoxin have been found to be 193 ± 25 ml/min and 152 ± 24 mil/min in a healthy control population.

In a small percentage of individuals, orally administered digoxin is converted to cardioinactivate reduction products (digoxin reduction products or DRPs) by colonic bacteria in the gastrointestinal tract. In these subjects over 40% of the dose may be excreted as DRPs in the urine. Renal clearances of the two main metabolites, dihydrodigoxin and digoxygenin, have been found to be 79 ± 13 ml/min and 100 ± 26 ml/min respectively.

In the majority of cases however, the major route of digoxin elimination is renal excretion of the unchanged drug.

The terminal elimnation half life of digoxin in patients with normal renal function is 30 to 40 hours. It is prolonged in patients with impaired renal function, and in anuric patients may be of the order of 100 hours.

In the newborn period, renal clearance of digoxin is diminished and suitable dosage adjustments must be observed. This is specially pronounced in the premature infant since renal clearance reflects maturation of renal function. Digoxin clearance has been found to be 65.6 ± 30 ml/min/1.73m^2 at 3 months, compared to only 32 ± 7 ml/min/1.73m^2 at 1 week. Beyond the immediate newborn period, children generally require proportionally larger doses than adults on the basis of body weight and body surface area.

Since most of the drug is bound to the tissues rather than circulating in the blood, digoxin is not effectively removed from the body during cardiopulmonary by-pass. Furthermore, only abount 3% of a digoxin dose is removed from the body during five hours of haemodialysis.

5.3 Preclinical safety data
No data are available on whether or not digoxin has mutagenic or carcinogenic effects.

6. PHARMACEUTICAL PARTICULARS

6.1 List of excipients
Methyl Hydroxybenzoate Ph Eur

Sucrose Ph Eur*

Syrup BP*

Anhydrous Sodium Phosphate HSE

Citric Acid Monohydrate Ph Eur

Quinine Yellow HSE

Ethanol (96%) BP

Propylene Glycol Ph Eur

Lime Flavour No. 1 NA HSE

Purified Water Ph Eur

*These ingredients are alternatives.

6.2 Incompatibilities
None known.

6.3 Shelf life
36 months

6.4 Special precautions for storage
Store below 25°C.

6.5 Nature and contents of container
Amber glass bottle with a metal roll-on closure and a graduated polyethene dropper assembly plus cap.

Pack size: 60 ml

6.6 Instructions for use and handling
Do not dilute.

Administrative Data

7. MARKETING AUTHORISATION HOLDER
The Wellcome Foundation Limited

Greenford

Middlesex

UB6 0NN

Trading as:

GlaxoSmithKline UK

Stockley Park West

Uxbridge

Middlesex UB11 1BT

8. MARKETING AUTHORISATION NUMBER(S)
PL0003/5260R

9. DATE OF FIRST AUTHORISATION/RENEWAL OF THE AUTHORISATION
24.04.03

10. DATE OF REVISION OF THE TEXT
21 May 2003

11. Legal Status
POM

Lanoxin PG Tablets

(GlaxoSmithKline UK)

1. NAME OF THE MEDICINAL PRODUCT
Lanoxin PG Tablets

2. QUALITATIVE AND QUANTITATIVE COMPOSITION
Digoxin Ph Eur 0.0625 mg/tablet

3. PHARMACEUTICAL FORM
Tablet

4. CLINICAL PARTICULARS

4.1 Therapeutic indications
Lanoxin is indicated in the management of chronic cardiac failure where the dominant problem is systolic dysfunction Its therapeutic benefit is greatest in those patients with ventricular dilatation.

Lanoxin is specifically indicated where cardiac failure is accompanied by atrial fibrillation.

Lanoxin is indicated in the management of certain supraventricular arrhythmias, particularly chronic atrial flutter and fibrillation,.

4.2 Posology and method of administration
The dose of Lanoxin for each patient has to be tailored individually according to age, lean body weight and renal function. Suggested doses are intended only as an initial guide.

The difference in bioavailability between injectable Lanoxin and oral formulations must be considered when changing from one dosage form to another. For example, if patients are switched from oral to the i.v. formulation the dosage should be reduced by approximately 33 %.

Adults and children over 10 years:

Rapid Oral Loading: 750 to 1500 micrograms (0.75 to 1.5 mg) as a single dose.

Where there is less urgency, or greater risk of toxicity (e.g. in the elderly), the oral loading dose should be given in divided doses 6 hours apart, assessing clinical response before giving each additional dose (See *Special Warnings and Precautions for Use*).

Slow Oral Loading: 250 to 750 micrograms (0.25 to 0.75 mg) should be given daily for 1 week followed by an appropriate maintenance dose. A clinical response should be seen within one week.

NOTE:The choice between slow and rapid oral loading depends on the clinical state of the patient and the urgency of the condition.

Maintenance: The maintenance dosage should be based upon the percentage of the peak body stores lost each day through elimination. The following formula has had wide clinical use:

$$\text{Maintenance Dose} = \text{Peak body stores} \times \frac{\%\ \text{daily loss}}{100}$$

Where:

Peak Body Stores = Loading Dose

% Daily Loss = 14 + Creatinine Clearance (C_{cr})/5.

C_{cr} is creatinine clearance corrected to 70 kg body weight or 1.73 m^2 body surface area. If only serum creatinine (S_{cr}) concentrations are available, a C_{cr} (corrected to 70 kg body weight) may be estimated in men as

$$C_{cr} = \frac{(140 - \text{age})}{S_{cr}\ (\text{in mg/100 ml})}$$

NOTE: Where serum creatinine values are obtained in micromol/L these may be converted to mg/100 ml (mg %) as follows:

$$S_{cr}\ (\text{mg/100 ml}) = \frac{S_{cr}\ (\text{micromol/L}) \times 113.12}{10{,}000} = \frac{S_{cr}\ (\text{micromol/L})}{88.4}$$

Where 113.12 is the molecular weight of creatinine.

For women, this result should be multiplied by 0.85.

NOTE: These formulae cannot be used for creatinine clearance in children.

In practice, this will mean that most patients will be maintained on 0.125 to 0.75 mg digoxin daily; however in those who show increased sensitivity to the adverse effects of digoxin, a dosage of 62.5 microgram (0.0625 mg) daily or less may suffice.

Neonates, infants and children up to 10 years of age (if cardiac glycosides have not been given in the preceding two weeks):

In the newborn, particularly in the premature infant, renal clearance of digoxin is diminished and suitable dose reductions must be observed, over and above general dosage instructions.

Beyond the immediate newborn period, children generally require proportionally larger doses than adults on the basis of body weight or body surface area, as indicated in the schedule below. Children over 10 years of age require adult dosages in proportion to their body weight.

Oral loading dose:

This should be administered in accordance with the following schedule:

Preterm neonates < 1.5 kg	25 microgram/kg over 24 hours
Preterm neonates 1.5 kg to 2.5 kg	30 microgram/kg over 24 hours
Term neonates to 2 years	45 microgram/kg over 24 hours
2 to 5 years	35 microgram/kg over 24 hours
5 to 10 years	25 microgram/kg over 24 hours

The loading dose should be administered in divided doses with approximately half the total dose given as the first dose and further fractions of the total dose given at intervals of 4 to 8 hours, assessing clinical response before giving each additional dose.

Maintenance:

The maintenance dose should be administered in accordance with the following schedule:

Preterm neonates:

daily dose = 20% of 24-hour loading dose (intravenous or oral)

Term neonates and children up to 10 years:

daily dose = 25% of 24-hour loading dose (intravenous or oral)

These dosage schedules are meant as guidelines and careful clinical observation and monitoring of serum digoxin levels (see *Monitoring*) should be used as a basis for adjustment of dosage in these paediatric patient groups.

If cardiac glycosides have been given in the two weeks preceding commencement of Lanoxin therapy, it should be anticipated that optimum loading doses of Lanoxin will be less than those recommended above.

Use in the elderly: The tendency to impaired renal function and low lean body mass in the elderly influences the pharmacokinetics of Lanoxin such that high serum digoxin levels and associated toxicity can occur quite readily, unless doses of Lanoxin lower than those in non-elderly patients are used. Serum digoxin levels should be checked regularly and hypokalaemia avoided.

Dose Recommendations in Renal Disorder or with Diuretic Therapy: See *Special Warnings and Precautions for use.*

Monitoring: Serum concentrations of digoxin may be expressed in conventional units of nanogram/ml (ng/ml) or SI units of nanomol//L (nmol/L). To convert ng/ml to nmol/L, multiply ng/ml by 1.28.

The serum concentration of digoxin can be determined by radioimmunoassay. Blood should be taken 6 hours or more after the last dose of Lanoxin. There are no rigid guidelines as to the range of serum concentrations that are most efficacious but most patients will benefit, with little risk of toxic symptoms and signs developing, with digoxin concentrations from 0.8 ng/ml (1.02 nmol/L) to 2.0 ng/ml (2.56 nmol/L). Above this range toxic symptoms and signs become more frequent and levels above 3.0 ng/ml (3.84 nmol/L) are quite likely to be toxic. However, in deciding whether a patient's symptoms are due to digoxin, the patient's clinical state together with the serum potassium level and thyroid function are important factors.

Other glycosides, including metabolites of digoxin, can interfere with the assays that are available and one should always be wary of values which do not seem commensurate with the clinical state of the patient.

4.3 Contraindications
Lanoxin is contra-indicated in intermittent complete heart block or second degree atrioventricular block, especially if there is a history of Stokes-Adams attacks.

Lanoxin is contra-indicated in arrhythmias caused by cardiac glycoside intoxication.

Lanoxin is contra-indicated in supraventricular arrhythmias associated with an accessory atrioventricular pathway, as in the Wolff-Parkinson-White Syndrome, unless the electrophysiological characteristics of the accessory pathway and any possible deleterious effect of digoxin on these characteristics has been evaluated. If an accessory pathway is known or suspected to be present and there is no history of previous supraventricular arrhythmias, Lanoxin is similarly contra-indicated.

Lanoxin is contra-indicated in ventricular tachycardia or ventricular fibrillation.

Lanoxin is contra-indicated in hypertrophic obstructive cardiomyopathy, unless there is concomitant atrial fibrillation and heart failure but even then caution should be exercised if Lanoxin is to be used.

Lanoxin is contra-indicated in patients known to be hypersensitive to digoxin or other digitalis glycosides.

4.4 Special warnings and special precautions for use

Arrhythmias may be precipitated by digoxin toxicity, some of which can resemble arrhythmias for which the drug could be advised. For example, atrial tachycardia with varying atrioventricular block requires care, as clinically the rhythm resembles atrial fibrillation.

In some cases of sinoatrial disorder (i.e. Sick Sinus Syndrome) digoxin may cause or exacerbate sinus bradycardia or cause sinoatrial block.

Determination of the serum digoxin concentration may be very helpful in making a decision to treat with further digoxin, but toxic doses of other glycosides may cross-react in the assay and wrongly suggest apparently satisfactory measurements. Observations during the temporary withholding of digoxin might be more appropriate.

In cases where cardiac glycosides have been taken in the preceding two weeks, therecommendations for initial dosing of a patient should be reconsidered and a reduced dose is advised.

The dosing recommendations should be reconsidered if patients are elderly or there are other reasons for the renal clearance of digoxin being reduced. A reduction in both initial and maintenance doses should be considered.

Hypokalaemia sensitises the myocardium to the actions of cardiac glycosides.

Hypoxia, hypomagnesaemia and marked hypercalcaemia increase myocardial sensitivity to cardiac glycosides.

Administering Lanoxin to a patient with thyroid disease requires care. Initial and maintenance doses of Lanoxin should be reduced when thyroid function is subnormal. In hyperthyroidism there is relative digoxin resistance and the dose may have to be increased. During the course of treatment of thyrotoxicosis, dosage should be reduced as the thyrotoxicosis comes under control.

Patients with malabsorption syndrome or gastro-intestinal reconstructions may require larger doses of digoxin.

The risk of provoking dangerous arrhythmias with direct current cardioversion is greatly increased in the presence of digitalis toxicity and is in proportion to the cardioversion energy used.

For elective direct current cardioversion of a patient who is taking digoxin, the drug should be withheld for 24 hours before cardioversion is performed. In emergencies, such as cardiac arrest, when attempting cardioversion the lowest effective energy should be applied. Direct current cardioversion is inappropriate in the treatment of arrhythmias thought to be caused by cardiac glycosides.

Many beneficial effects of digoxin on arrhythmias result from a degree of atrioventricular conduction blockade. However, when incomplete atrioventricular block already exists the effects of a rapid progression in the block should be anticipated. In complete heart block the idioventricular escape rhythm may be suppressed.

The administration of digoxin in the period immediately following myocardial infarction is not contra-indicated. However, the use of inotropic drugs in some patients in this setting may result in undesirable increases in myocardial oxygen demand and ischaemia, and some retrospective follow-up studies have suggested digoxin to be associated with an increased risk of death. However, the possibility of arrhythmias arising in patients who may be hypokalaemic after myocardial infarction and are likely to be cardiologically unstable must be borne in mind. The limitations imposedthereafter on direct current cardioversion must also be remembered.

Digoxin improves exercise tolerance in patients with impaired left ventricular systolic dysfunction and normal sinus rhythm. This may or may not be associated with an improved haemodynamic profile. However, the benefit of digoxin in patients with supraventricular arrythmias is most evident at rest, less evident with exercise.

In patients receiving diuretics and an ACE inhibitor, or diuretics alone, the withdrawal of digoxin has been shown to result in clinical deterioration.

The use of therapeutic doses of digoxin may cause prolongation of the PR interval and depression of the ST segment on the electrocardiogram.

Digoxin may produce false positive ST-T changes on the electrocardiogram during exercise testing. These electrophysiologic effects reflect an expected effect of the drug and are not indicative of toxicity.

Patients receiving digoxin should have their serum electrolytes and renal function (serum creatinine concentration) assessed periodically; the frequency of assessments will depend on the clinical setting.

Although many patients with chronic congestive cardiac failure benefit from acute administration of digoxin, there are some in whom it does not lead to constant, marked or lasting haemodynamic improvement. It is therefore important to evaluate the response of each patient individually when Lanoxin is continued long-term.

Patients with severe respiratory disease may have an increased myocardial sensitivity to digitalis glycosides.

4.5 Interaction with other medicinal products and other forms of Interaction

These may arise from effects on the renal excretion, tissue binding, plasma protein binding, distribution within the body, gut absorptive capacity and sensitivity to Lanoxin. Consideration of the possibility of an interaction whenever concomitant therapy is contemplated is the best precaution and a check on serum digoxin concentration is recommended when any doubt exists.

Digoxin, in association with beta-adrenoceptor blocking drugs, may increase atrio-ventricular conduction time.

Agents causing hypokalaemia or intracellular potassium deficiency may cause increased sensitivity to Digoxin; they include diuretics, lithium salts, corticosteroids and carbenoxolone.

Patients receiving Digoxin are more susceptible to the effects of suxamethonium-exacerbated hyperkalaemia.

Calcium, particularly if administered rapidly by the intravenous route, may produce serious arrhythmias in digitalized patients.

Serum levels of digoxin may be ***increased*** by concomitant administration of the following:

Alprazolam, amiodarone, diphenoxylate with atropine, flecainide, gentamicin, indomethacin, itraconazole, prazosin, propafenone, quinidine, quinine, spironolactone, macrolide antibiotics (e.g. neomycin), tetracycline (and possibly other antibiotics), trimethoprim and propantheline.

Serum levels of digoxin may be ***reduced*** by concomitant administration of the following:

Adrenaline, antacids, kaolin-pectin, some bulk laxatives and cholestyramine, acarbose, salbutamol, sulphasalazine, neomycin, rifampicin, some cytostatics, phenytoin, metoclopramide, penicillamine and the herbal remedy St John's wort (*Hypericum perforatum*).

Calcium channel blocking agents may either increase or cause no change in serum digoxin levels. Verapamil, felodipine and tiapamil increase serum digoxin levels. Nifedipine and diltiazem may increase or have no effect on serum digoxin levels. Isradipine causes no change in serum digoxin levels. Angiotensin converting enzyme (ACE) inhibitors may also increase or cause no change in serum digoxin concentrations.

Milrinone does not alter steady-state serum digoxin levels.

4.6 Pregnancy and lactation

No data are available on whether or not digoxin has teratogenic effects.

There is no information available on the effect of digoxin on human fertility.

The use of digoxin in pregnancy is not contra-indicated, although the dosage and control may be less predictable in pregnant than in non-pregnant women with some requiring an increased dosage of digoxin during pregnancy. As with all drugs, use should be considered only when the expected clinical benefit of treatment to the mother outweighs any possible risk to the developing foetus.

Despite extensive antenatal exposure to digitalis preparations, no significant adverse effects have been observed in the foetus or neonate when maternal serum digoxin concentrations are maintained within the normal range. Although it has been speculated that a direct effect of digoxin on the myometrium may result in relative prematurity and low birthweight, a contributing role of the underlying cardiac disease cannot be excluded. Maternally administered digoxin has been successfully used to treat foetal tachycardia and congestive heart failure.

Adverse foetal effects have been reported in mothers with digitalis toxicity.

Although digoxin is excreted in breast milk, the quantities are minute and breast feeding is not contra-indicated.

4.7 Effects on ability to drive and use machines

Since central nervous system and visual disturbances have been reported in patients receiving Lanoxin, patients should exercise caution before driving, using machinery or participating in dangerous activities.

4.8 Undesirable effects

In general, the adverse reactions of digoxin are dose-dependent and occur at doses higher than those needed to achieve a therapeutic effect.

Hence, adverse reactions are less common when digoxin is used within the recommended dose range or therapeutic serum concentration range and when there is careful attention to concurrent medications and conditions.

The side effects of digoxin in infants and children differ from those seen in adults in several respects.

Although digoxin may produce anorexia, nausea, vomiting, diarrhoea, and CNS disturbances in young patients, these are rarely the initial symptoms of overdose. Rather, the earliest and most frequent manifestation of excessive dosing with digoxin in infants and children is the appearance of cardiac arrhythmias, including sinus bradycardia.

In children, the use of digoxin may produce any type of arrhythmia. The most common are conduction disturbances or supraventricular tachyarrhythmias, such as atrial tachycardia (with or without block) and junctional (nodal) tachycardia. Ventricular arrhythmias are less common.

Sinus bradycardia may be a sign of impending digoxin intoxication, especially in infants, even in the absence of first-degree heart block. Any arrhythmia or alteration in cardiac conduction that develops in a child taking digoxin should be assumed to be caused by digoxin, until further evaluation proves otherwise.

Non-cardiac:

These are principally associated with overdosage but may occur from a temporarily high serum concentration due to rapid absorption. They include anorexia, nausea and vomiting and usually disappear within a few hours of taking the drug. Diarrhoea can also occur. It is inadvisable to rely on nausea as an early warning of excessive digoxin dosage.

Gynaecomastia can occur with long-term administration.

Weakness, dizziness, confusion, apathy, fatigue, malaise, headache, depression and even psychosis have been reported as adverse central nervous system effects.

Digoxin can produce visual disturbances (blurred or yellow vision).

Oral digoxin has also been associated with intestinal ischaemia and, rarely, with intestinal necrosis.

Skin rashes of urticarial or scarlatiniform character are rare reactions to digoxin, and may be accompanied by pronounced eosinophilia.

Very rarely, digoxin can cause thrombocytopenia.

Cardiac:

Digoxin toxicity can cause various arrhythmias and conduction disturbances. Usually an early sign is the occurrence of ventricular premature contractions; they can proceed to bigeminy or even trigeminy. Atrial tachycardias, frequently an indication for digoxin, may occur with excessive dosage of the drug. Atrial tachycardia with some degree of atrioventricular block is particularly characteristic, and the pulse rate may not necessarily be fast. (See also *Special Warnings and Precautions for Use*). Digoxin produces PR prolongation and ST segment depression which should not by themselves be considered digoxin toxicity. Cardiac toxicity can also occur at therapeutic doses in patients who have conditions which may alter their sensitivity to digoxin (see *Special Warnings and Special Precautions for Use*).

4.9 Overdose

For symptoms and signs see *Undesirable Effects*,

After recent ingestion, such as accidental or deliberate self-poisoning, the load available for absorption may be reduced by gastric lavage.

Patients with massive digitalis ingestion should receive large doses of activated charcoal to prevent absorption and bind digoxin in the gut during enteroenteric recirculation.

An overdosage of digoxin of 10 to 15 mg in adults without heart disease and of 6 to 10 mg in children aged 1 to 3 years without heart disease appeared to be the dose resulting in death in half of the patients.

If more than 25 mg of digoxin was ingested by an adult without heart disease, death or progressive toxicity responsive only to digoxin-binding Fab antibody fragments (Digibind®) resulted. If more than 10 mg of digoxin was ingested by a child aged 1 to 3 years without heart disease, the outcome was uniformly fatal when Fab fragment treatment was not given.

If hypokalaemia is present, it should be corrected with potassium supplements either orally or intravenously depending on the urgency of the situation. In cases where a large amount of Lanoxin has been ingested, hyperkalaemia may be present due to release of potassium from skeletal muscle. Before administering potassium in digoxin overdose the serum potassium level must be known.

Bradyarrhythmias may respond to atropine but temporary cardiac pacing may be required. Ventricular arrhythmias may respond to lignocaine or phenytoin.

Dialysis is not particularly effective in removing digoxin from the body in potentially life-threatening toxicity.

Rapid reversal of the complications that are associated with serious poisoning by digoxin, digitoxin and related glycosides has followed intravenous administration of digoxin-specific (ovine) antibody fragments (Fab) when other therapies have failed. Digibind® is the only specific treatment for digoxin toxicity and is very effective. For details consult the literature supplied with Digibind®.

5. PHARMACOLOGICAL PROPERTIES

5.1 Pharmacodynamic properties

Mode of Action:-

Digoxin increases contractility of the myocardium by direct activity. This effect is proportional to dose in the lower range and some effect is achieved with quite low dosing; it occurs even in normal myocardium although it is then entirely without physiological benefit. The primary action of digoxin is specifically to inhibit adenosine triphosphatase, and thus sodium-potassium (Na^+-K^+) exchange activity, the altered ionic distribution across the membrane resulting in an augmented calcium ion influx and thus an increase in the availability of calcium at the time of excitation-contraction coupling. The potency of digoxin may therefore appear considerably enhanced when the extracellular potassium concentration is low, with hyperkalaemia having the opposite effect.

Digoxin exerts the same fundamental effect of inhibition of the Na^+-K^+ exchange mechanism on cells of the autonomic nervous system, stimulating them to exert indirect cardiac activity. Increases in efferent vagal impulses result in reduced sympathetic tone and diminished impulse conduction rate through the atria and atrioventricular node. Thus, the major beneficial effect of digoxin is reduction of ventricular rate.

Indirect cardiac contractility changes also result from changes in venous compliance brought about by the altered autonomic activity and by direct venous stimulation. The interplay between direct and indirect activity governs the total circulatory response, which is not identical for all subjects. In the presence of certain supraventricular arrhythmias, the neurogenically mediated slowing of AV conduction is paramount.

The degree of neurohormonal activation occurring in patients with heart failure is associated with clinical deterioration and an increased risk of death. Digoxin reduces activation of both the sympathetic nervous system and the (renin-angiotensin) system independently of its inotropic actions, and may thus favourably influence survival. Whether this is achieved via direct sympathoinhibitory effects or by re-sensitising baroreflex mechanisms remains unclear.

5.2 Pharmacokinetic properties

Intravenous administration of a loading dose produces an appreciable pharmacological effect within 5 to 30 minutes; this reaches a maximum in 1 to 5 hours. Upon oral administration, digoxin is absorbed from the stomach and upper part of the small intestine. Absorption is delayed by taking a meal although the total amount absorbed is unchanged. Using the oral route the onset of effect occurs in 0.5 to 2 hours and reaches its maximum at 2 to 6 hours. The bioavailability of orally administered Lanoxin is approximately 63% in tablet form and 75% as paediatric elixir.

The initial distribution of digoxin from the central to the peripheral compartment generally lasts from 6 to 8 hours. This is followed by a more gradual decline in serum digoxin concentration, which is dependent upon digoxin elimination from the body. The volume of distribution is large (Vd_{ss} = 510 litres in healthy volunteers), indicating digoxin to be extensively bound to body tissues. The highest digoxin concentrations are seen in the heart, liver and kidney, that in the heart averaging 30- fold that in the systemic circulation. Although the concentration in skeletal muscle is far lower, this store cannot be overlooked since skeletal muscle represents 40% of total body weight. Of the small proportion of digoxin circulating in plasma, approximately 25% is bound to protein.

The major route of elimination is renal excretion of the unchanged drug.

Following intravenous administration to healthy volunteers, between 60 and 75% of a digoxin dose is recovered unchanged in the urine over a 6 day follow-up period. Total body clearance of digoxin has been shown to be directly related to renal function, and percent daily loss is thus a function of creatinine clearance, which in turn may be estimated from a stable serum creatinine. The total and renal clearances of digoxin have been found to be 193 ± 25 ml/min and 152 ± 24 mil/min in a healthy control population.

In a small percentage of individuals, orally administered digoxin is converted to cardioinactivate reduction products (digoxin reduction products or DRPs) by colonic bacteria in the gastrointestinal tract. In these subjects over 40% of the dose may be excreted as DRPs in the urine. Renal clearances of the two main metabolites, dihydrodigoxin and digoxygenin, have been found to be 79 ± 13 ml/min and 100 ± 26 ml/min respectively.

In the majority of cases however, the major route of digoxin elimination is renal excretion of the unchanged drug.

The terminal elimination half life of digoxin in patients with normal renal function is 30 to 40 hours. It is prolonged in patients with impaired renal function, and in anuric patients may be of the order of 100 hours.

In the newborn period, renal clearance of digoxin is diminished and suitable dosage adjustments must be observed. This is specially pronounced in the premature infant since renal clearance reflects maturation of renal function. Digoxin clearance has been found to be 65.6 ± 30 ml/min/1.73m^2 at 3 months, compared to only 32 ± 7 ml/min/1.73m^2 at 1 week. Beyond the immediate newborn period, children generally require proportionally larger doses than adults on the basis of body weight and body surface area.

Since most of the drug is bound to the tissues rather than circulating in the blood, digoxin is not effectively removed from the body during cardiopulmonary by-pass. Furthermore, only about 3% of a digoxin dose is removed from the body during five hours of haemodialysis.

5.3 Preclinical safety data

No data are available on whether or not digoxin has mutagenic or carcinogenic effects.

6. PHARMACEUTICAL PARTICULARS

6.1 List of excipients

Lactose Ph Eur

Starches Ph Eur

Indigo Carmine HSE

Hydrolysed Starch HSE

Povidone BP

Magnesium Stearate Ph Eur

6.2 Incompatibilities

None known

6.3 Shelf life

60 months

6.4 Special precautions for storage

Store below 25°C

6.5 Nature and contents of container

Amber glass bottle with polyethylene snap fit closure

Pack sizes: 28, 50, 100, 500 tablets

15 ml amber glass bottle with a clic-loc child resistant closure

Pack size: 56 tablets

6.6 Instructions for use and handling

Not applicable

Administrative Data

7. MARKETING AUTHORISATION HOLDER

The Wellcome Foundation Limited

Greenford

Middlesex

UB6 0NN

Trading as:

GlaxoSmithKline UK

Stockley Park West

Uxbridge

Middlesex UB11 1BT

8. MARKETING AUTHORISATION NUMBER(S)

PL0003/0091R

9. DATE OF FIRST AUTHORISATION/RENEWAL OF THE AUTHORISATION

24.04.03

10. DATE OF REVISION OF THE TEXT

21 May 2003

11. Legal Status

POM

Lanoxin Tablets 0.25mg

(GlaxoSmithKline UK)

1. NAME OF THE MEDICINAL PRODUCT

Lanoxin Tablets 0.25 mg

2. QUALITATIVE AND QUANTITATIVE COMPOSITION

Digoxin Ph Eur 0.25 mg/tablet

3. PHARMACEUTICAL FORM

Tablet

4. CLINICAL PARTICULARS

4.1 Therapeutic indications

Lanoxin is indicated in the management of chronic cardiac failure where the dominant problem is systolic dysfunction. Its therapeutic benefit is greatest in those patients with ventricular dilatation.

Lanoxin is specifically indicated where cardiac failure is accompanied by atrial fibrillation.

Lanoxin is indicated in the management of certain supraventricular arrhythmias, particularly chronic atrial flutter and fibrillation.

4.2 Posology and method of administration

The dose of Lanoxin for each patient has to be tailored individually according to age, lean body weight and renal function. Suggested doses are intended only as an initial guide.

The difference in bioavailability between injectable Lanoxin and oral formulations must be considered when changing from one dosage form to another. For example, if patients are switched from oral to the i.v. formulation the dosage should be reduced by approximately 33 %.

Adults and children over 10 years:

Rapid Oral Loading: 750 to 1500 micrograms (0.75 to 1.5 mg) as a single dose.

Where there is less urgency, or greater risk of toxicity e.g. in the elderly, the oral loading dose should be given in divided doses 6 hours apart, assessing clinical response before giving each additional dose (*See Special Warnings and Precautions for Use*).

Slow Oral Loading: 250 to 750 micrograms (0.25 to 0.75 mg) should be given daily for 1 week followed by an appropriate maintenance dose. A clinical response should be seen within one week.

NOTE: The choice between slow and rapid oral loading depends on the clinical state of the patient and the urgency of the condition.

Maintenance: The maintenance dosage should be based upon the percentage of the peak body stores lost each day through elimination. The following formula has had wide clinical use:

$$\text{Maintenance Dose} = \text{Peak body stores} \times \frac{\%\text{ daily loss}}{100}$$

Where:

Peak Body Stores = Loading Dose

% Daily Loss = 14 + Creatinine Clearance (C_{cr})/5.

C_{cr} is creatinine clearance corrected to 70 kg body weight or 1.73 m^2 body surface area. If only serum creatinine (S_{cr}) concentrations are available, a C_{cr} (corrected to 70 kg body weight) may be estimated in men as

$$C_{cr} = \frac{(140 - age)}{S_{cr}\text{ (in mg/100 ml)}}$$

NOTE: Where serum creatinine values are obtained in micromol/L these may be converted to mg/100 ml (mg %) as follows:

$$S_{cr}\text{ (mg/100 ml)} = \frac{S_{cr}\text{ (micromol/L)} \times 113.12}{10{,}000}$$

$$= \frac{S_{cr}\text{ (micromol/L)}}{88.4}$$

Where 113.12 is the molecular weight of creatinine.

For *women*, this result should be multiplied by 0.85.

NOTE: These formulae cannot be used for creatinine clearance in children.

In practice, this will mean that most patients will be maintained on 0.125 to 0.75 mg digoxin daily; however in those who show increased sensitivity to the adverse effects of digoxin, a dosage of 62.5 microgram (0.0625 mg) daily or less may suffice.

Neonates, infants and children up to 10 years of age (if cardiac glycosides have not been given in the preceding two weeks):

In the newborn, particularly in the premature infant, renal clearance of digoxin is diminished and suitable dose reductions must be observed, over and above general dosage instructions.

Beyond the immediate newborn period, children generally require proportionally larger doses than adults on the basis of body weight or body surface area, as indicated in the schedule below. Children over 10 years of age require adult dosages in proportion to their body weight.

Oral loading dose:

This should be administered in accordance with the following schedule:

Preterm neonates < 1.5 kg	25 microgram/kg over 24 hours
Preterm neonates 1.5 kg to 2.5 kg	30 microgram/kg over 24 hours
Term neonates to 2 years	45 microgram/kg over 24 hours
2 to 5 years	35 microgram/kg over 24 hours
5 to 10 years	25 microgram/kg over 24 hours

The loading dose should be administered in divided doses with approximately half the total dose given as the first dose and further fractions of the total dose given at intervals of 4 to 8 hours, assessing clinical response before giving each additional dose.

Maintenance:

The maintenance dose should be administered in accordance with the following schedule:

Preterm neonates:

daily dose = 20% of 24-hour loading dose (intravenous or oral)

Term neonates and children up to 10 years:

daily dose = 25% of 24-hour loading dose (intravenous or oral)

These dosage schedules are meant as guidelines and careful clinical observation and monitoring of serum digoxin levels (see *Monitoring*) should be used as a basis for adjustment of dosage in these paediatric patient groups.

If cardiac glycosides have been given in the two weeks preceding commencement of Lanoxin therapy, it should be anticipated that optimum loading doses of Lanoxin will be less than those recommended above.

Use in the elderly: The tendency to impaired renal function and low lean body mass in the elderly influences the pharmacokinetics of Lanoxin such that high serum digoxin levels and associated toxicity can occur quite readily, unless doses of Lanoxin lower than those in non-elderly patients are used. Serum digoxin levels should be checked regularly and hypokalaemia avoided.

Dose Recommendations in Renal Disorder or with Diuretic Therapy: See *Special Warnings and Precautions for Use*.

Monitoring: Serum concentrations of digoxin may be expressed in conventional units of nanogram/ml (ng/ml) or SI Units of nanomol/L (nmol/L). To convert ng/ml to nmol/L, multiply ng/ml by 1.28.

The serum concentration of digoxin can be determined by radioimmunoassay. Blood should be taken 6 hours or more after the last dose of Lanoxin. There are no rigid guidelines as to the range of serum concentrations that are most efficacious but most patients will benefit, with little risk of toxic symptoms developing, with digoxin concentrations from 0.8 ng/ml (1.02 nmol/L) to 2.0 ng/ml (2.56 nmol/L). Above this range toxic symptoms and signs become more frequent and levels above 3.0 ng/ml (3.84 nmol/L) are quite likely to be toxic. However, in deciding whether a patient's symptoms are due to digoxin, the patient's clinical state together with the serum potassium level and thyroid function are important factors.

Other glycosides, including metabolites of digoxin, can interfere with the assays that are available and one should always be wary of values which do not seem commensurate with the clinical state of the patient.

4.3 Contraindications

Lanoxin is contra-indicated in intermittent complete heart block or second degree atrioventricular block, especially if there is a history of Stokes-Adams attacks.

Lanoxin is contra-indicated in arrhythmias caused by cardiac glycoside intoxication.

Lanoxin is contra-indicated in supraventricuar arrhythmias associated with an accessory atrioventricular pathway, as in the Wolff-Parkinson-White Syndrome, unless the electrophysiological characteristics of the accessory pathway and any possible deleterious effect of digoxin on these characteristics have been evaluated. If an accessory pathway is known or suspected to be present and there is no history of previous supraventricular arrhythmias, Lanoxin is similarly contra-indicated.

Lanoxin is contra-indicated in ventricular tachycardia or ventricular fibrillation.

Lanoxin is contra-indicated in hypertrophic obstructive cardiomyopathy, unless there is concomitant atrial fibrillation and heart failure but even then caution should be exercised if Lanoxin is to be used.

Lanoxin is contra-indicated in patients known to be hypersensitive to digoxin or other digitalis glycosides.

4.4 Special warnings and special precautions for use

Arrhythmias may be precipitated by digoxin toxicity, some of which can resemble arrhythmias for which the drug could be advised. For example, atrial tachycardia with varying atrioventricular block requires particular care as clinically the rhythm resembles atrial fibrillation.

In some cases of sinoatrial disorder (i.e. Sick Sinus Syndrome) digoxin may cause or exacerbate sinus bradycardia or cause sinoatrial block.

Determination of the serum digoxin concentration may be very helpful in making a decision to treat with further digoxin, but toxic doses of other glycosides may cross-react in the assay and wrongly suggest apparently satisfactory measurements. Observations during the temporary withholding of digoxin might be more appropriate.

In cases where cardiac glycosides have been taken in the preceding two weeks, the recommendations for initial dosing of a patient should be reconsidered and a reduced dose is advised.

The dosing recommendations should be reconsidered if patients are elderly or there are other reasons for the renal clearance of digoxin being reduced. A reduction in both initial and maintenance doses should be considered.

Hypokalaemia sensitises the myocardium to the actions of cardiac glycosides.

Hypoxia, hypomagnesaemia and marked hypercalcaemia increase myocardial sensitivity to cardiac glycosides.

Administering Lanoxin to a patient with thyroid disease requires care. Initial and maintenance doses of Lanoxin should be reduced when thyroid function is subnormal. In hyperthyroidism there is relative digoxin resistance and the dose may have to be increased. During the course of treatment of thyrotoxicosis, dosage should be reduced as the thyrotoxicosis comes under control.

Patients with malabsorption syndrome or gastro-intestinal reconstructions may require larger doses of digoxin.

The risk of provoking dangerous arrhythmias with direct current cardioversion is greatly increased in the presence of digitalis toxicity and is in proportion to the cardioversion energy used.

For elective direct current cardioversion of a patient who is taking digoxin, the drug should be withheld for 24 hours before cardioversion is performed. In emergencies, such as cardiac arrest, when attempting cardioversion the lowest effective energy should be applied. Direct current cardioversion is inappropriate in the treatment of arrhythmia thought to be caused by cardiac glycosides.

Many beneficial effects of digoxin on arrhythmias result from a degree of atrioventricular conduction blockade. However, when incomplete atrioventricular block already exists the effects of a rapid progression in the block should be anticipated. In complete heart block the idioventricular escape rhythm may be suppressed.

The administration of digoxin in the period immediately following myocardial infarction is not contra-indicated. However, the use of inotropic drugs in some patients in this setting may result in undesirable increases in myocardial oxygen demand and ischaemia, and some retrospective follow-up studies have suggested digoxin to be associated with an increased risk of death. However, the possibility of arrhythmias arising in patients who may be hypokalaemic after myocardial infarction and are likely to be cardiologically unstable must be borne in mind. The limitations imposed thereafter on direct current cardioversion must also be remembered.

Digoxin improves exercise tolerance in patients with impaired left ventricular systolic dysfunction and normal sinus rhythm. This may or may not be associated with an improved haemodynamic profile. However, the benefit of patients with supraventricular arrhythmias is most evident at rest, less evident with exercise.

In patients receiving diuretics and an ACE inhibitor, or diuretics alone, the withdrawal of digoxin has been shown to result in clinical deterioration.

The use of therapeutic doses of digoxin may cause prolongation of the PR interval and depression of the ST segment on the electrocardiogram.

Digoxin may produce false positive ST-T changes on the electrocardiogram during exercise testing. These electrophysiologic effects reflect an expected effect of the drug and are not indicative of toxicity.

Patients receiving digoxin should have their serum electrolytes and renal function (serum creatinine concentration) assessed periodically; the frequency of assessments will depend on the clinical setting.

Although many patients with chronic congestive cardiac failure benefit from acute administration of digoxin, there are some in whom it does not lead to constant, marked or lasting haemodynamic improvement. It is therefore important to evaluate the response of each patient individually when Lanoxin is continued long-term.

Patients with severe respiratory disease may have an increased myocardial sensitivity to digitalis glycosides.

4.5 Interaction with other medicinal products and other forms of Interaction

These may arise from effects on the renal excretion, tissue binding, plasma protein binding, distribution within the body, gut absorptive capacity and sensitivity to Lanoxin. Consideration of the possibility of an interaction whenever concomitant therapy is contemplated is the best precaution and a check on serum digoxin concentration is recommended when any doubt exists.

Digoxin, in association with beta-adrenoceptor blocking drugs, may increase atrio-ventricular conduction time.

Agents causing hypokalaemia or intracellular potassium deficiency may cause increased sensitivity to Digoxin; they include diuretics, lithium salts, corticosteroids and carbenoxolone.

Patients receiving Digoxin are more susceptible to the effects of suxamethonium-exacerbated hyperkalaemia.

Calcium, particularly if administered rapidly by the intravenous route, may produce serious arrhythmias in digitalized patients.

Serum levels of digoxin may be **increased** by concomitant administration of the following:

Alprazolam, amiodarone, diphenoxylate with atropine, flecainide, gentamicin, indomethacin, itraconazole, prazosin, propafenone, quinidine, quinine, spironolactone, macrolide antibiotics (e.g. neomycyn), tetracycline (and possibly other antibiotics), trimethoprimand propantheline.

Serum levels of digoxin may be **reduced** by concomitant administration of the following:

Adrenaline, antacids, kaolin-pectin, some bulk laxatives, cholestyramine, acarbose, salbutamol, sulphasalazine, neomycin, rifampicin, some cytostatics, phenytoin, metoclopramide, penicillamine and the herbal remedy St John's wort (*Hypericum perforatum*).

Calcium channel blocking agents may either increase or cause no change in serum digoxin levels. Verapamil, felodipine and tiapamil increase serum digoxin levels. Nifedipine and diltiazem may increase or have no effect on serum digoxin levels. Isradipine causes no change in serum digoxin levels. Angiotensin converting enzyme (ACE) inhibitors may also increase or cause no change in serum digoxin concentrations.

Milrinone does not alter steady-state serum digoxin levels.

4.6 Pregnancy and lactation

No data are available on whether or not digoxin has teratogenic effects.

There is no information available on the effect of digoxin on human fertility.

The use of digoxin in pregnancy is not contra-indicated, although the dosage and control may be less predictable in pregnant than in non-pregnant women with some requiring an increased dosage of digoxin during pregnancy. As with all drugs, use should be considered only when the expected clinical benefit of treatment to the mother outweighs any possible risk to the developing foetus.

Despite extensive antenatal exposure to digitalis preparations, no significant adverse effects have been observed in the foetus or neonate when maternal serum digoxin concentrations are maintained within the normal range. Although it has been speculated that a direct effect of digoxin on the myometrium may result in relative prematurity and low birthweight, a contributing role of the underlying cardiac disease cannot be excluded. Maternally administered digoxin has been successfully used to treat foetal tachycardia and congestive heart failure.

Adverse foetal effects have been reported in mothers with digitalis toxicity.

Although digoxin is excreted in breast milk, the quantities are minute and breast feeding is not contra-indicated.

4.7 Effects on ability to drive and use machines

Since central nervous system and visual disturbances have been reported in patients receiving Lanoxin, patients should exercise caution before driving, using machinery or participating in dangerous activities.

4.8 Undesirable effects

In general, the adverse reactions of digoxin are dose-dependent and occur at doses higher than those needed to achieve a therapeutic effect.

Hence, adverse reactions are less common when digoxin is used within the recommended dose range or therapeutic serum concentration range and when there is careful attention to concurrent medications and conditions.

The side effects of digoxin in infants and children differ from those seen in adults in several respects. In children, the use of digoxin may produce any type of arrhythmia. The most common are conduction disturbances or supraventricular tachyarrhythmias, such as atrial tachycardia (with or without block) and junctional (nodal) tachycardia. Ventricular arrhythmias are less common.

Sinus bradycardia may be a sign of impending digoxin intoxication, especially in infants, even in the absence of first-degree heart block. Any arrhythmia or alteration in cardiac conduction that develops in a child taking digoxin should be assumed to be caused by digoxin, until further evaluation proves otherwise.

Although digoxin may produce anorexia, nausea, vomiting, diarrhoea, and CNS disturbances in young patients, these are rarely the initial symptoms of overdose. Rather, the earliest and most frequent manifestation of excessive dosing with digoxin in infants and children is the appearance of cardiac arrhythmias, including sinus bradycardia.

Non-cardiac:

These are principally associated with overdosage but may occur from a temporarily high serum concentration due to rapid absorption. They include anorexia, nausea and vomiting and usually disappear within a few hours of taking the drug. Diarrhoea can also occur. It is inadvisable to rely on nausea as an early warning of excessive digoxin dosage.

Gynaecomastia can occur with long-term administration.

Weakness, dizziness, confusion, apathy, fatigue, malaise, headache, depression and even psychosis have been reported as adverse central nervous system effects.

Digoxin can produce visual disturbances (blurred or yellow vision).

Oral digoxin has also been associated with intestinal ischaemia and, rarely, with intestinal necrosis.

Skin rashes of urticarial or scarlatiniform character are rare reactions to digoxin, and may be accompanied by pronounced eosinophilia.

Very rarely, digoxin can cause thrombocytopenia.

Cardiac:

Digoxin toxicity can cause various arrhythmias and conduction disturbances. Usually an early sign is the occurrence of ventricular premature contractions; they can proceed to bigeminy or even trigeminy. Atrial tachycardias, frequently an indication for digoxin, may occur with excessive dosage of the drug. Atrial tachycardia with some degree of atrioventricular block is particularly characteristic, and the pulse rate may not necessarily be fast. (See also *Special Warnings and Precautions for Use*). Digoxin produces PR prolongation and ST segment depression which should not by themselves be considered digoxin toxicity. Cardiac toxicity can also occur at therapeutic doses in patients who have conditions which may alter their sensitivity to digoxin (see *Special Warnings and Special Precautions for Use*).

4.9 Overdose

For symptoms and signs see *Undesirable Effects*.

After recent ingestion, such as accidental or deliberate self-poisoning, the load available for absorption may be reduced by gastric lavage.

Patients with massive digitalis ingestion should receive large doses of activated charcoal to prevent absorption and bind digoxin in the gut during enteroenteric recirculation.

An overdosage of digoxin of 10 to 15 mg in adults without heart disease and of 6 to 10 mg in children aged 1 to 3 years without heart disease appeared to be the dose resulting in death in half of the patients. If more than 25 mg of digoxin was ingested by an adult without heart disease, death or progressive toxicity responsive only to digoxin-binding Fab antibody fragments (Digibind®) resulted. If more than 10 mg of digoxin was ingested by a child aged 1 to 3 years without heart disease, the outcome was uniformly fatal when Fab fragment treatment was not given.

If hypokalaemia is present, it should be corrected with potassium supplements either orally or intravenously depending on the urgency of the situation. In cases where a large amount of Lanoxin has been ingested, hyperkalaemia may be present due to release of potassium from skeletal muscle. Before administering potassium in digoxin overdose the serum potassium level must be known.

Bradyarrhythmias may respond to atropine but temporary cardiac pacing may be required. Ventricular arrhythmias may respond to lignocaine or phenytoin.

Dialysis is not particularly effective in removing digoxin from the body in potentially life-threatening toxicity.

Rapid reversal of the complications that are associated with serious poisoning by digoxin, digitoxin and related glycosides has followed intravenous administration of digoxin-specific (ovine) antibody fragments (Fab) when other therapies have failed. Digibind® is the only specific treatment for digoxin toxicity and is very effective. For details consult the literature supplied with Digibind®.

5. PHARMACOLOGICAL PROPERTIES

5.1 Pharmacodynamic properties

Mode of Action:-

Digoxin increases contractility of the myocardium by direct activity. This effect is proportional to dose in the lower range and some effect is achieved with quite low dosing; it occurs even in normal myocardium although it is then entirely without physiological benefit. The primary action of digoxin is specifically to inhibit adenosine triphosphatase, and thus sodium-potassium (Na^+-K^+) exchange activity, the altered ionic distribution across the membrane resulting in an augmented calcium ion influx and thus an increase in the availability of calcium at the time of excitation-contraction coupling. The potency of digoxin may therefore appear considerably enhanced when the extracellular potassium concentration is low, with hyperkalaemia having the opposite effect.

Digoxin exerts the same fundamental effect of inhibition of the Na^+-K^+ exchange mechanism on cells of the autonomic nervous system, stimulating them to exert indirect cardiac activity. Increases in efferent vagal impulses result in reduced sympathetic tone and diminished impulse conduction rate through the atria and atrioventricular node. Thus, the major beneficial effect of digoxin is reduction of ventricular rate.

Indirect cardiac contractility changes also result from changes in venous compliance brought about by the altered autonomic activity and by direct venous stimulation. The interplay between direct and indirect activity governs the total circulatory response, which is not identical for all subjects. In the presence of certain supraventricular arrhythmias, the neurogenically mediated slowing of AV conduction is paramount.

The degree of neurohormonal activation occurring in patients with heart failure is associated with clinical deterioration and an increased risk of death. Digoxin reduces activation of both the sympathetic nervous system and the (renin-angiotensin) system independently of its inotropic actions, and may thus favourably influence survival. Whether this is achieved via direct sympathoinhibitory effects or by re-sensitising baroreflex mechanisms remains unclear.

5.2 Pharmacokinetic properties

Intravenous administration of a loading dose produces an appreciable pharmacological effect within 5 to 30 minutes; this reaches a maximum in 1 to 5 hours. Upon oral administration, digoxin is absorbed from the stomach and upper part of the small intestine. Absorption is delayed by taking a meal although the total amount absorbed is unchanged. Using the oral route the onset of effect occurs in 0.5 to 2 hours and reaches its maximum at 2 to 6 hours. The bioavailability of orally administered Lanoxin is approximately 63% in tablet form and 75% as paediatric elixir.

The initial distribution of digoxin from the central to the peripheral compartment generally lasts from 6 to 8 hours. This is followed by a more gradual decline in serum digoxin concentration, which is dependent upon digoxin elimination from the body. The volume of distribution is large (Vd_{ss} = 510 litres in healthy volunteers), indicating digoxin to be extensively bound to body tissues. The highest digoxin concentrations are seen in the heart, liver and kidney, that in the heart averaging 30- fold that in the systemic circulation. Although the concentration in skeletal muscle is far lower, this store cannot be overlooked since skeletal muscle represents 40% of total body weight. Of the small proportion of digoxin circulating in plasma, approximately 25% is bound to protein.

The major route of elimination is renal excretion of the unchanged drug.

Following intravenous administration to healthy volunteers, between 60 and 75% of a digoxin dose is recovered unchanged in the urine over a 6 day follow-up period. Total body clearance of digoxin has been shown to be directly related to renal function, and percent daily loss is thus a function of creatinine clearance, which in turn may be estimated from a stable serum creatinine. The total and renal clearances of digoxin have been found to be 193 ± 25 ml/min and 152 ± 24 mil/min in a healthy control population.

In a small percentage of individuals, orally administered digoxin is converted to cardioinactivate reduction products (digoxin reduction products or DRPs) by colonic bacteria in the gastrointestinal tract. In these subjects over 40% of the dose may be excreted as DRPs in the urine. Renal clearances of the two main metabolites, dihydrodigoxin and digoxygenin, have been found to be 79 ± 13 ml/min and 100 ± 26 ml/min respectively.

In the majority of cases however, the major route of digoxin elimination is renal excretion of the unchanged drug.

The terminal elimination half life of digoxin in patients with normal renal function is 30 to 40 hours. It is prolonged in patients with impaired renal function, and in anuric patients may be of the order of 100 hours.

In the newborn period, renal clearance of digoxin is diminished and suitable dosage adjustments must be observed. This is specially pronounced in the premature infant since renal clearance reflects maturation of renal function. Digoxin clearance has been found to be 65.6 ± 30 ml/min/1.73m^2 at 3 months, compared to only 32 ± 7 ml/min/1.73m^2 at 1 week. Beyond the immediate newborn period, children generally require proportionally larger doses than adults on the basis of body weight and body surface area.

Since most of the drug is bound to the tissues rather than circulating in the blood, digoxin is not effectively removed from the body during cardiopulmonary by-pass. Furthermore, only about 3% of a digoxin dose is removed from the body during five hours of haemodialysis.

5.3 Preclinical safety data

No data are available on whether or not digoxin has mutagenic or carcinogenic effects.

6. PHARMACEUTICAL PARTICULARS

6.1 List of excipients

Lactose Ph Eur

Maize Starch Ph Eur

Hydrolysed Starch HSE

Magnesium Stearate Ph Eur

Rice Starch Ph Eur

6.2 Incompatibilities

None known

6.3 Shelf life

60 months

6.4 Special precautions for storage

Store below 25°C

6.5 Nature and contents of container

Amber glass bottle and low-density polyethene snap fit closures

Pack sizes: 28, 50, 500 tablets

15 ml amber glass bottle and a clic-loc child resistant closure

Pack size: 56 tablets

Polypropylene containers with polyethyene snap fit closures

Pack sizes: 1000, 5000 tablets

6.6 Instructions for use and handling

Not applicable

Administrative Data

7. MARKETING AUTHORISATION HOLDER

The Wellcome Foundation Limited

Greenford

Middlesex

UB6 0NN

Trading as:

GlaxoSmithKline UK

Stockley Park West

Uxbridge

Middlesex UB11 1BT

8. MARKETING AUTHORISATION NUMBER(S)

PL0003/0090R

9. DATE OF FIRST AUTHORISATION/RENEWAL OF THE AUTHORISATION

24.04.03

10. DATE OF REVISION OF THE TEXT

21 May 2003

11. Legal Status

POM

Lantus 100 IU/ml

(sanofi-aventis)

1. NAME OF THE MEDICINAL PRODUCT

Lantus® 100 IU/ml solution for injection in a vial▼

Lantus® 100 IU/ml solution for injection in a cartridge▼

Lantus® 100 IU/ml OptiSet® solution for injection▼

2. QUALITATIVE AND QUANTITATIVE COMPOSITION

Each ml of the solution for injection contains 3.64 mg of the active substance insulin glargine, corresponding to 100 IU human insulin.

Each vial contains 10 ml, equivalent to 1000 IU

Each cartridge contains 3 ml, equivalent to 300 IU.

Each OptiSet pen contains 3 ml, equivalent to 300 IU.

Insulin glargine is an insulin analogue produced by recombinant DNA technology using *Escherichia coli* (K 12 strains).

For excipients, see section 6.1.

3. PHARMACEUTICAL FORM

Solution for injection in a vial, cartridge or pre-filled disposable pen.

Lantus is a clear colourless solution.

4. CLINICAL PARTICULARS

4.1 Therapeutic indications

For the treatment of adults, adolescents and children of 6 years or above with diabetes mellitus, where treatment with insulin is required.

4.2 Posology and method of administration

Lantus contains insulin glargine, an insulin analogue with a prolonged duration of action. It should be administered once daily at any time, but at the same time each day.

Lantus OptiSet delivers insulin in increments of 2 IU up to a maximum single dose of 40 IU.

The dosage and timing of dose of Lantus should be individually adjusted. In patients with type 2 diabetes mellitus, Lantus can also be given together with orally active antidiabetic medicinal products.

Children

In children efficacy and safety of Lantus have only been demonstrated when given in the evening. Due to limited experience the efficacy and safety of Lantus have not been demonstrated in children below the age of 6 years.

Transition from other insulins to Lantus

When changing from a treatment regimen with an intermediate or long-acting insulin to a regimen with Lantus, a change of the dose of the basal insulin may be required and the concomitant antidiabetic treatment may need to be adjusted (dose and timing of additional regular insulins or fast-acting insulin analogues or the dose of oral antidiabetic agents).

To reduce the risk of nocturnal and early morning hypoglycaemia, patients who are changing their basal insulin regimen from a twice daily NPH insulin to a once daily regimen with Lantus should reduce their daily dose of basal insulin by 20-30% during the first weeks of treatment.

During the first weeks the reduction should, at least partially, be compensated by an increase in mealtime insulin, after this period the regimen should be adjusted individually.

As with other insulin analogues, patients with high insulin doses because of antibodies to human insulin may experience an improved insulin response with Lantus.

Close metabolic monitoring is recommended during the transition and in the initial weeks thereafter.

With improved metabolic control and resulting increase in insulin sensitivity a further adjustment in dosage regimen may become necessary. Dose adjustment may also be required, for example, if the patient's weight or life-style changes, changes of timing of insulin dose or other circumstances arise that increase susceptibility to hypo-or hyperglycaemia (see section 4.4).

Administration

Lantus is administered subcutaneously.

Lantus should not be administered intravenously. The prolonged duration of action of Lantus is dependent on its injection into subcutaneous tissue. Intravenous administration of the usual subcutaneous dose could result in severe hypoglycaemia.

There are no clinically relevant differences in serum insulin or glucose levels after abdominal, deltoid or thigh administration of Lantus. Injection sites must be rotated within a given injection area from one injection to the next.

Lantus must not be mixed with any other insulin or diluted. Mixing or diluting can change its time/action profile and mixing can cause precipitation.

For further details on handling, see section 6.6.

Due to limited experience the efficacy and safety of Lantus could not be assessed in the following groups of patients: patients with impaired liver function or patients with moderate/severe renal impairment (see 4.4).

4.3 Contraindications

Hypersensitivity to insulin glargine or to any of the excipients (see section 6.1).

4.4 Special warnings and special precautions for use

Lantus is not the insulin of choice for the treatment of diabetic ketoacidosis. Instead, regular insulin administered intravenously is recommended in such cases.

Safety and efficacy of Lantus has been established in adolescents and children of 6 years and above.

Due to limited experience the efficacy and safety of Lantus could not be assessed in children below 6 years of age, in patients with impaired liver function or in patients with moderate/severe renal impairment (see 4.2).

In patients with renal impairment, insulin requirements may be diminished due to reduced insulin metabolism. In the elderly, progressive deterioration of renal function may lead to a steady decrease in insulin requirements.

In patients with severe hepatic impairment, insulin requirements may be diminished due to reduced capacity for gluconeogenesis and reduced insulin metabolism.

In case of insufficient glucose control or a tendency to hyper- or hypoglycaemic episodes, the patient's adherence to the prescribed treatment regimen, injection sites and proper injection technique and all other relevant factors must be reviewed before dose adjustment is considered.

Hypoglycaemia

The time of occurrence of hypoglycaemia depends on the action profile of the insulins used and may, therefore, change when the treatment regimen is changed. Due to more sustained basal insulin supply with Lantus, less nocturnal but more early morning hypoglycaemia can be expected.

Particular caution should be exercised, and intensified blood glucose monitoring is advisable in patients in whom hypoglycaemic episodes might be of particular clinical relevance, such as in patients with significant stenoses of the coronary arteries or of the blood vessels supplying the brain (risk of cardiac or cerebral complications of hypoglycaemia) as well as in patients with proliferative retinopathy, particularly if not treated with photocoagulation (risk of transient amaurosis following hypoglycaemia).

Patients should be aware of circumstances where warning symptoms of hypoglycaemia are diminished. The warning symptoms of hypoglycaemia may be changed, be less pronounced or be absent in certain risk groups. These include patients:

- in whom glycaemic control is markedly improved,
- in whom hypoglycaemia develops gradually,
- who are elderly,
- after transfer from animal insulin to human insulin,
- in whom an autonomic neuropathy is present,
- with a long history of diabetes,
- suffering from a psychiatric illness,
- receiving concurrent treatment with certain other medicinal products (see section 4.5).

Such situations may result in severe hypoglycaemia (and possibly loss of consciousness) prior to the patient's awareness of hypoglycaemia.

The prolonged effect of subcutaneous insulin glargine may delay recovery from hypoglycaemia.

If normal or decreased values for glycated haemoglobin are noted, the possibility of recurrent, unrecognised (especially nocturnal) episodes of hypoglycaemia must be considered.

Adherence of the patient to the dosage and dietary regimen, correct insulin administration and awareness of hypoglycaemia symptoms are essential to reduce the risk of hypoglycaemia. Factors increasing the susceptibility to hypoglycaemia require particularly close monitoring and may necessitate dose adjustment. These include:

- change in the injection area,
- improved insulin sensitivity (by, e.g., removal of stress factors),
- unaccustomed, increased or prolonged physical activity,
- intercurrent illness (e.g. vomiting, diarrhoea),
- inadequate food intake,
- missed meals,
- alcohol consumption,
- certain uncompensated endocrine disorders, (e.g. in hypothyroidism and in anterior pituitary or adrenocortical insufficiency),
- concomitant treatment with certain other medicinal products.

Intercurrent illness

Intercurrent illness requires intensified metabolic monitoring. In many cases urine tests for ketones are indicated, and often it is necessary to adjust the insulin dose. The insulin requirement is often increased. Patients with type 1 diabetes must continue to consume at least a small amount of carbohydrates on a regular basis, even if they are able to eat only little or no food, or are vomiting etc. and they must never omit insulin entirely.

4.5 Interaction with other medicinal products and other forms of Interaction

A number of substances affect glucose metabolism and may require dose adjustment of insulin glargine.

Substances that may enhance the blood-glucose-lowering effect and increase susceptibility to hypoglycaemia include oral antidiabetic agents, ACE inhibitors, disopyramide, fibrates, fluoxetine, MAO inhibitors, pentoxifylline, propoxyphene, salicylates and sulphonamide antibiotics.

Substances that may reduce the blood-glucose-lowering effect include corticosteroids, danazol, diazoxide, diuretics, glucagon, isoniazid, oestrogens and progestogens, phenothiazine derivatives, somatropin, sympathomimetic agents (e.g. epinephrine [adrenaline], salbutamol, terbutaline), thyroid hormones, atypical antipsychotic medicinal products (e.g. clozapine and olanzapine) and protease inhibitors.

Beta-blockers, clonidine, lithium salts or alcohol may either potentiate or weaken the blood-glucose-lowering effect of insulin. Pentamidine may cause hypoglycaemia, which may sometimes be followed by hyperglycaemia.

In addition, under the influence of sympatholytic medicinal products such as beta-blockers, clonidine, guanethidine and reserpine, the signs of adrenergic counter-regulation may be reduced or absent.

4.6 Pregnancy and lactation

For insulin glargine, no clinical data on exposed pregnancies are available. Animal studies do not indicate direct or indirect harmful effects with respect to pregnancy, embryonal or foetal development, parturition or postnatal development (see also section 5.3).

Caution should be exercised when prescribing to pregnant women,

It is essential for patients with pre-existing or gestational diabetes to maintain good metabolic control throughout pregnancy. Insulin requirements may decrease during the first trimester and generally increase during the second and third trimesters. Immediately after delivery, insulin requirements decline rapidly (increased risk of hypoglycaemia). Careful monitoring of glucose control is essential.

Lactating women may require adjustments in insulin dose and diet.

4.7 Effects on ability to drive and use machines

The patient's ability to concentrate and react may be impaired as a result of hypoglycaemia or hyperglycaemia or, for example, as a result of visual impairment. This may constitute a risk in situations where these abilities are of special importance (e.g. driving a car or operating machinery).

Patients should be advised to take precautions to avoid hypoglycaemia whilst driving. This is particularly important in those who have reduced or absent awareness of the warning symptoms of hypoglycaemia or have frequent episodes of hypoglycaemia. It should be considered whether it is advisable to drive or operate machinery in these circumstances.

4.8 Undesirable effects

Hypoglycaemia

Hypoglycaemia, in general the most frequent undesirable effect of insulin therapy, may occur if the insulin dose is too high in relation to the insulin requirement. Severe hypoglycaemic attacks, especially if recurrent, may lead to neurological damage. Prolonged or severe hypoglycaemic episodes may be life-threatening.

In many patients, the signs and symptoms of neuroglycopenia are preceded by signs of adrenergic counter-regulation. Generally, the greater and more rapid the decline in blood glucose, the more marked is the phenomenon of counter-regulation and its symptoms.

Eyes

A marked change in glycaemic control may cause temporary visual impairment, due to temporary alteration in the turgidity and refractive index of the lens.

Long-term improved glycaemic control decreases the risk of progression of diabetic retinopathy. However, intensification of insulin therapy with abrupt improvement in glycaemic control may be associated with temporary worsening of diabetic retinopathy. In patients with proliferative retinopathy, particularly if not treated with photocoagulation, severe hypoglycaemic episodes may result in transient amaurosis.

Lipodystrophy

As with any insulin therapy, lipodystrophy may occur at the injection site and delay local insulin absorption. In clinical studies, in regimens which included Lantus, lipohypertrophy was observed in 1 to 2% of patients, whereas lipoatrophy was uncommon. Continuous rotation of the injection site within the given injection area may help to reduce or prevent these reactions.

Injection site and allergic reactions

In clinical studies, in regimens which included Lantus, reactions at the injection site were observed in 3 to 4% of patients. Such reactions include redness, pain, itching, hives, swelling, or inflammation. Most minor reactions to insulins at the injection site usually resolve in a few days to a few weeks.

Immediate-type allergic reactions to insulin are rare. Such reactions to insulin (including insulin glargine) or the excipients may, for example, be associated with generalised skin reactions, angio-oedema, bronchospasm, hypotension and shock, and may be life-threatening.

Other reactions

Insulin administration may cause insulin antibodies to form. In clinical studies, antibodies that cross-react with human insulin and insulin glargine were observed with the same frequency in both NPH and insulin glargine treatment groups. In rare cases, the presence of such insulin antibodies may necessitate adjustment of the insulin dose in order to correct a tendency to hyper- or hypoglycaemia.

Rarely, insulin may cause sodium retention and oedema, particularly if previously poor metabolic control is improved by intensified insulin therapy.

4.9 Overdose

Symptoms

Insulin overdose may lead to severe and sometimes long-term and life-threatening hypoglycaemia.

Management

Mild episodes of hypoglycaemia can usually be treated with oral carbohydrates. Adjustments in dosage of the medicinal product, meal patterns, or physical activity may be needed.

More severe episodes with coma, seizure, or neurologic impairment may be treated with intramuscular/subcutaneous glucagon or concentrated intravenous glucose. Sustained carbohydrate intake and observation may be necessary because hypoglycaemia may recur after apparent clinical recovery.

5. PHARMACOLOGICAL PROPERTIES

5.1 Pharmacodynamic properties

Pharmacotherapeutic group: Antidiabetic agent. Insulin and analogues, long-acting. ATC Code: A10A E04.

Insulin glargine is a human insulin analogue designed to have a low solubility at neutral pH. It is completely soluble at the acidic pH of the Lantus injection solution (pH 4). After injection into the subcutaneous tissue, the acidic solution is neutralised leading to formation of micro-precipitates from which small amounts of insulin glargine are continuously released, providing a smooth, peakless, predictable concentration/time profile with a prolonged duration of action.

Insulin receptor binding: Insulin glargine is very similar to human insulin with respect to insulin receptor binding kinetics. It can, therefore, be considered to mediate the same type of effect via the insulin receptor as insulin.

The primary activity of insulin, including insulin glargine, is regulation of glucose metabolism. Insulin and its analogues lower blood glucose levels by stimulating peripheral glucose uptake, especially by skeletal muscle and fat, and by inhibiting hepatic glucose production. Insulin inhibits lipolysis in the adipocyte, inhibits proteolysis and enhances protein synthesis.

In clinical pharmacology studies, intravenous insulin glargine and human insulin have been shown to be equipotent when given at the same doses. As with all insulins, the time course of action of insulin glargine may be affected by physical activity and other variables.

In euglycaemic clamp studies in healthy subjects or in patients with type 1 diabetes, the onset of action of subcutaneous insulin glargine was slower than with human NPH insulin, its effect profile was smooth and peakless, and the duration of its effect was prolonged.

The following graph shows the results from a study in patients:

(see Figure 1 on next page)

The longer duration of action of insulin glargine is directly related to its slower rate of absorption and supports once daily administration. The time course of action of insulin and insulin analogues such as insulin glargine may vary considerably in different individuals or within the same individual.

In a clinical study, symptoms of hypoglycaemia or counter-regulatory hormone responses were similar after intravenous insulin glargine and human insulin both in healthy volunteers and patients with type 1 diabetes.

5.2 Pharmacokinetic properties

In healthy subjects and diabetic patients, insulin serum concentrations indicated a slower and much more prolonged absorption and showed a lack of a peak after subcutaneous injection of insulin glargine in comparison to human NPH insulin. Concentrations were thus consistent with the time profile of the pharmacodynamic activity of insulin glargine. The graph above shows the activity profiles over time of insulin glargine and NPH insulin.

Insulin glargine injected once daily will reach steady state levels in 2-4 days after the first dose.

When given intravenously the elimination half-life of insulin glargine and human insulin were comparable.

In man, insulin glargine is partly degraded in the subcutaneous tissue at the carboxyl terminus of the Beta chain with formation of the active metabolites 21^A-Gly-insulin and 21^A-Gly-des-30^B-Thr-insulin. Unchanged insulin glargine and degradation products are also present in the plasma.

Figure 1

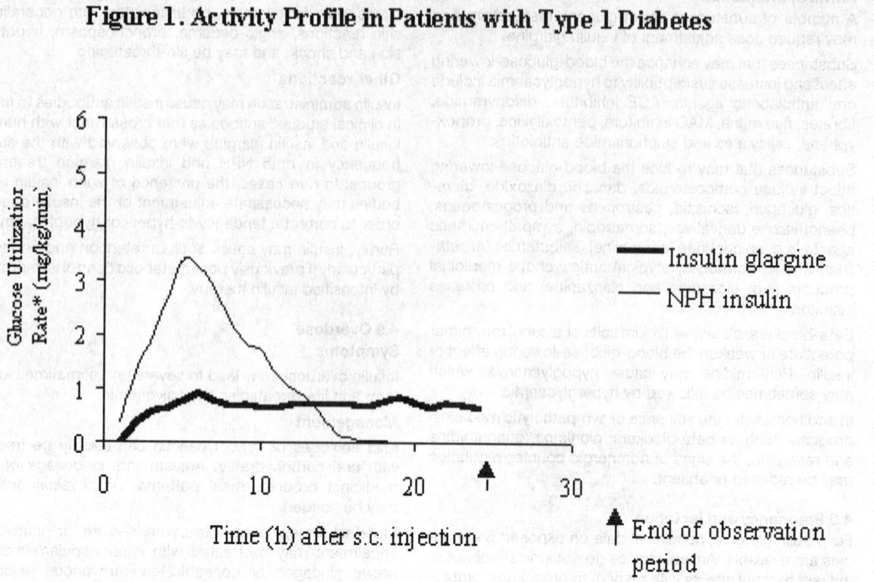

*determined as amount of glucose infused to maintain constant plasma glucose levels (hourly mean values)

In clinical studies, subgroup analyses based on age and gender did not indicate any difference in safety and efficacy in insulin glargine-treated patients compared to the entire study population.

5.3 Preclinical safety data

Preclinical data reveal no special hazard for humans based on conventional studies of safety pharmacology, repeated-dose toxicity, genotoxicity, carcinogenic potential and toxicity to reproduction.

6. PHARMACEUTICAL PARTICULARS

6.1 List of excipients

Zinc chloride, m-cresol, glycerol, hydrochloric acid, sodium hydroxide, water for injections.

6.2 Incompatibilities

Lantus must not be mixed with any other product. It is important to ensure that syringes do not contain traces of any other material.

6.3 Shelf life

2 years.

Vials or Cartridges Shelf-life after first opening: 4 weeks.

It is recommended that the date of first withdrawal from the vial be noted on the label.

OptiSet Pens Shelf-life for pens in use: 4 weeks

6.4 Special precautions for storage

Store at 2°C - 8°C (in a refrigerator).

Keep in the outer carton.

Do not freeze.

Ensure that the container/pen is not directly touching the freezer compartment or freezer packs.

Vial:	Once in use, do not store above 25°C and keep in the outer carton.
Cartridge:	Once in use, do not store above 25°C. The pen containing a cartridge must not be stored in the refrigerator.
OptiSet:	Once in use, do not store above 25°C. Pens in use must not be stored in the refrigerator

6.5 Nature and contents of container

Vial

10 ml, type 1 colourless glass vial with flanged aluminium cap, rubber (type 1, laminate of polyisoprene and bromobutyl) stopper and tear-off polypropylene lid. Each vial contains 10 ml solution (1000 IU insulin glargine). Packs of 1 vial are available.

Cartridge

3 ml, type 1 colourless glass cartridge with black bromobutyl rubber plunger and flanged aluminium cap with black bromobutyl rubber stopper. Each cartridge contains 3 ml solution (300 IU insulin glargine). Packs of 5 cartridges are available.

OptiSet

3 ml, type 1 colourless glass cartridge with black bromobutyl rubber plunger and flanged aluminium cap with black bromobutyl rubber stopper. Each cartridge contains 3 ml solution (300 IU insulin glargine). The cartridges are sealed in a disposable pen injector. Needles are not included in the pack.

Packs of 5 OptiSet pens are available.

6.6 Instructions for use and handling

Vial

Inspect the vial before use. It must only be used if the solution is clear, colourless, with no solid particles visible, and if it is of water-like consistency. Since Lantus is a solution, it does not require resuspension before use.

Cartridge

Before insertion into the pen, the cartridge must be stored at room temperature for 1 to 2 hours.

Inspect the cartridge before use. It must only be used if the solution is clear, colourless, with no solid particles visible, and if it is of water-like consistency. Since Lantus is a solution, it does not require resuspension before use.

Air bubbles must be removed from the cartridge before injection (see instructions for using the pen). Empty cartridges must not be refilled.

Optiset

Before first use, the pen must be stored at room temperature for 1 to 2 hours.

Inspect the cartridge before use. It must only be used if the solution is clear, colourless, with no solid particles visible, and if it is of water-like consistency. Since Lantus is a solution, it does not require resuspension before use.

Empty pens must never be reused and must be properly discarded.

To prevent the possible transmission of disease, each pen must be used by one patient only.

Handling of the pen

The Instructions for Use included in the Package Leaflet must be read carefully before using OptiSet.

(see Figure 2 below)

Important information for use of OptiSet:

Before each use, a new needle must be attached and a safety test must be performed. The dosage selector must never be turned after the injection button has been pulled out. If a problem occurs with OptiSet, the section "Troubleshooting" in the Instructions for Use should be referred to. If OptiSet is damaged or not working properly (due to mechanical defects) it has to be discarded and a new OptiSet has to be used.

- General Notes

- The injection button allows checking the actual loaded dose: The button should be pulled out. While holding it out, the last thick bar visible (only the top part can be seen) shows the amount of insulin loaded. If it is difficult to see, the pen may be held at an angle.

- The insulin pen must not be dropped or subjected to impact; otherwise, the insulin cartridge in the transparent insulin reservoir may break and the pen will not work. If this happens, a new pen must be used.

Step 1. Check the Insulin

After removing the pen cap, the label on the insulin reservoir should be checked to make sure it contains the correct insulin. The appearance of insulin should also be checked: the insulin solution must be clear, colourless, with no solid particles visible, and must have a water-like consistency.

Step 2. Attaching the needle

Only needles that have been approved for use with OptiSet should be used.

The needle should be carefully attached straight onto the pen.

Step 3. Safety test

Prior to each injection a safety test has to be performed.

For a new and unused OptiSet, the dose arrow should point to the number 8, as preset by the manufacturer.

Otherwise, the dosage selector should be turned until the dose arrow points to 2.

Then the injection button should be pulled out as far as it will go.

The outer and inner needle caps should be removed.

While holding the pen with the needle pointing upwards, the insulin reservoir should be tapped gently with the finger so that any air bubbles rise up towards the needle

Then the injection button should be pressed in completely.

If insulin has been expelled through the needle tip, then the pen and the needle are working properly.

If no insulin appears at the needle tip, step 3 should be repeated until insulin appears at the needle tip.

Step 4. Setting and loading the insulin dose

The dose can be set in steps of 2 units, from a minimum of 2 units to a maximum of 40 units. If a dose greater than 40 units is required, it should be given as two or more injections.

The dosage selector should be turned in either direction until the dose arrow points to the required dose.

The injection button should be pulled out as far as it will go in order to load the pen.

Step 5. Injecting the insulin dose

The patient should be informed on the injection technique by his health care professional.

The needle should be inserted into the skin.

The injection button should be pressed in completely. Then the injection button should be held down 10 seconds before withdrawing the needle. This ensures that the full dose of insulin has been injected.

Step 6. Removing the needle

The needle should be removed after each injection and discarded. This will prevent contamination as well as leakage, re-entry of air and potential needle blocks. Needles must not be reused.

The pen cap should be replaced on the pen.

Checking the reservoir for remaining insulin

The residual insulin scale on the transparent insulin reservoir shows approximately how much insulin remains in the OptiSet. This scale must not be used to set the insulin dose.

The actual loaded dose should be checked as per "General notes". In case, the patient is not sure whether enough insulin remains in the reservoir, the OptiSet should be discarded.

Example: If the dose arrow has been set to 30 units and injection button can only be pulled out to as far as 12 units,

Figure 2

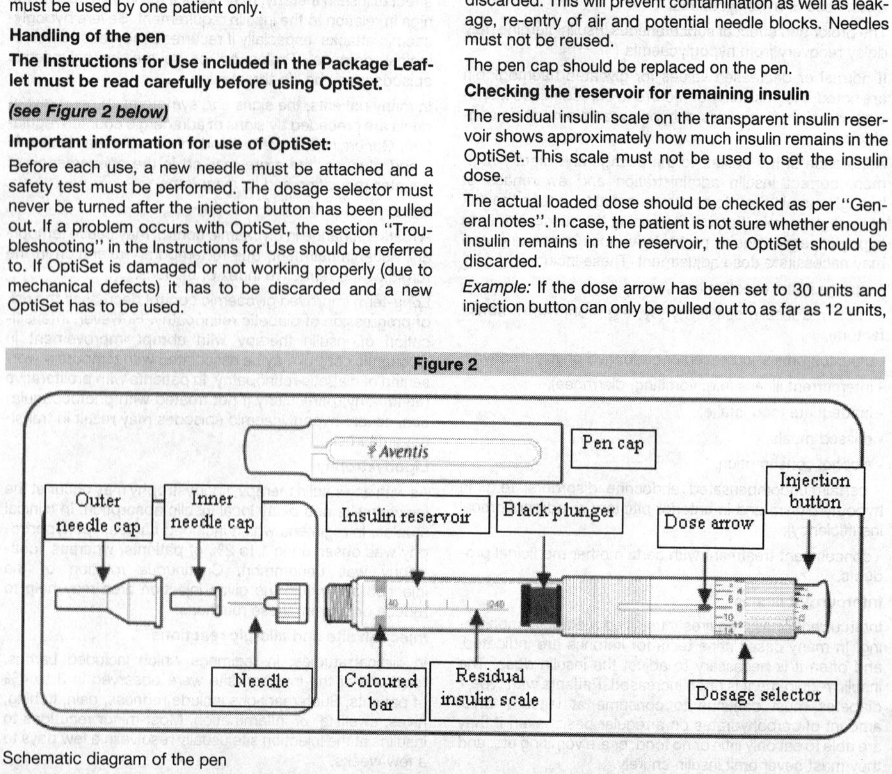

Schematic diagram of the pen

then only 12 units insulin can be injected with this pen. In this example, either the other 18 units will have to be injected using a new pen, or the entire 30 units dose will have to be injected using a new pen.

7. MARKETING AUTHORISATION HOLDER
Aventis Pharma Deutschland GmbH, D-65926 Frankfurt am Main, Germany.

8. MARKETING AUTHORISATION NUMBER(S)
EU/1/00/134/012 Lantus 100 IU/ml solution for injection in a 10 ml vial (1 vial/pack)

EU/1/00/134/006 Lantus 100 IU/ml solution for injection in a cartridge (5 cartridges/pack)

EU/1/00/134/010 Lantus 100 IU/ml OptiSet solution for injection (5 pens)

9. DATE OF FIRST AUTHORISATION/RENEWAL OF THE AUTHORISATION
Vials: 09 June 2000

Cartridges: 09 June 2000

OptiSet: 09 June 2000

10. DATE OF REVISION OF THE TEXT
September 2004

11. LEGAL CLASSIFICATION
POM

Lanvis Tablets

(GlaxoSmithKline UK)

1. NAME OF THE MEDICINAL PRODUCT
Lanvis Tablets

2. QUALITATIVE AND QUANTITATIVE COMPOSITION
40mg Tioguanine BP per tablet

3. PHARMACEUTICAL FORM
Tablet

4. CLINICAL PARTICULARS

4.1 Therapeutic indications
Lanvis is indicated primarily for the treatment of acute leukaemias especially acute myelogenous leukaemia and acute lymphoblastic leukaemia.

Lanvis is also used in the treatment of chronic granulocytic leukaemia.

4.2 Posology and method of administration
Route of administration: oral.

The exact dose and duration of administration will depend on the nature and dosage of other cytotoxic drugs given in conjunction with Lanvis.

Lanvis is variably absorbed following oral administration and plasma levels may be reduced following emesis or intake of food.

Lanvis can be used at various stages of treatment in short term cycles. However it is not recommended for use during maintenance therapy or similar long-term continuous treatments due to the high risk of liver toxicity (see Special Warnings and Precautions for Use and Undesirable Effects).

Adults

The usual dosage of Lanvis is between 100 and 200 mg/m^2 body surface area, per day.

Children

Similar dosages to those used in adults, with appropriate correction for body surface area, have been used.

Use in the elderly

There are no specific dosage recommendations in elderly patients (see dosage in renal or hepatic impairment).

Lanvis has been used in various combination chemotherapy schedules in elderly patients with acute leukaemia at equivalent doses to those used in younger patients.

Dosage in renal or hepatic impairment

Consideration should be given to reducing the dosage in patients with impaired hepatic or renal function.

4.3 Contraindications
In view of the seriousness of the indications there are no absolute contra-indications.

4.4 Special warnings and special precautions for use
Lanvis is an active cytotoxic agent for use only under the direction of physicians experienced in the administration of such agents.

Hepatic Effects

Lanvis is not recommended for maintenance therapy or similar long-term continuous treatments due to the high risk of liver toxicity associated with vascular endothelial damage (see Posology and Method of Administration and Undesirable Effects). This liver toxicity has been observed in a high proportion of children receiving Lanvis as part of maintenance therapy for acute lymphoblastic leukaemia and in other conditions associated with continuous use of tioguanine. This liver toxicity is particularly prevalent in males. Liver toxicity usually presents as the clinical syndrome of hepatic veno-occlusive disease (hyperbilirubinaemia, tender hepatomegaly, weight gain due to fluid retention and ascites) or with signs of portal hypertension (splenomegaly, thrombocytopenia and oesophageal varices). Histopathological features associated with this toxicity include hepatoportal sclerosis, nodular regenerative hyperplasia, peliosis hepatis and periportal fibrosis.

Lanvis therapy should be discontinued in patients with evidence of liver toxicity as reversal of signs and symptoms of liver toxicity have been reported upon withdrawal.

Monitoring

Patients must be carefully monitored during therapy including blood cell counts and weekly liver function tests. Early indications of liver toxicity are signs associated with portal hypertension such as thrombocytopenia out of proportion with neutropenia and splenomegaly. Elevations of liver enzymes have also been reported in association with liver toxicity but do not always occur.

Haematological Effects

Treatment with Lanvis causes bone marrow suppression leading to leucopenia and thrombocytopenia. Anaemia has been reported less frequently.

Bone marrow suppression is readily reversible if Lanvis is withdrawn early enough.

There are individuals with an inherited deficiency of the enzyme thiopurine methyltransferase (TPMT) who may be unusually sensitive to the myelosuppressive effect of Lanvis and prone to developing rapid bone marrow depression following the initiation of treatment with Lanvis. This problem could be exacerbated by coadministration with drugs that inhibit TPMT, such as olsalazine, mesalazine or sulphasalazine. Some laboratories offer testing for TPMT deficiency, although these tests have not been shown to identify all patients at risk of severe toxicity. Therefore close monitoring of blood counts is still necessary.

During remission indication in acute myelogenous leukaemia the patient may frequently have to survive a period of relative bone marrow aplasia and it is important that adequate supportive facilities are available.

Patients on myelosuppressive chemotherapy are particularly susceptible to a variety of infections.

During remission induction, particularly when rapid cell lysis is occurring, adequate precautions should be taken to avoid hyperuricaemia and/or hyperuricosuria and the risk of uric acid nephropathy.

Monitoring

During remission induction, full blood counts must be carried out frequently.

The leucocyte and platelet counts continue to fall after treatment is stopped, so at the first sign of an abnormally large fall in these counts, treatment should be temporarily discontinued.

In view of its action on cellular DNA, tioguanine is potentially mutagenic and carcinogenic.

It is recommended that the handling of Lanvis tablets follows the "Guidelines for the handling of cytotoxic drugs" issued by the Royal Pharmaceutical Society of Great Britain Working Party on the handling of cytotoxic drugs.

If halving of a tablet is required, care should be taken not to contaminate the hands or inhale the drug.

Lesch-Nyhan syndrome

Since the enzyme hypoxanthine guanine phosphoribosyl transferase is responsible for the conversion of Lanvis to its active metabolite, it is possible that patients deficient in this enzyme, such as those suffering from Lesch-Nyhan Syndrome, may be resistant to the drug. Resistance to azathioprine (Imuran*) which has one of the same active metabolites as Lanvis, has been demonstrated in two children with Lesch-Nyhan Syndrome.

4.5 Interaction with other medicinal products and other forms of Interaction
As there is *in vitro* evidence that aminosalicylate derivatives (eg. olsalazine, mesalazine or sulfasalazine) inhibit the TPMT enzyme, they should be administered with caution to patients receiving concurrent Lanvis therapy (see Special Warnings and Precautions for Use).

4.6 Pregnancy and lactation
Lanvis, like other cytotoxic agents is potentially teratogenic. There have been isolated cases where men, who have received combinations of cytotoxic agents including Lanvis, have fathered children with congenital abnormalities. Its use should be avoided whenever possible during pregnancy, particularly during the first trimester. In any individual case the potential hazard to the foetus must be balanced against the expected benefit to the mother.

As with all cytotoxic chemotherapy, adequate contraceptive precautions should be advised when either partner is receiving Lanvis.

There are no reports documenting the presence of Lanvis or its metabolites in maternal milk. It is suggested that mothers receiving Lanvis should not breast feed.

4.7 Effects on ability to drive and use machines
None known.

4.8 Undesirable effects
For this product there is a lack of modern clinical documentation which can be used as support for determining the frequency of undesirable effects. Lanvis is usually one component of combination chemotherapy and consequently it is not possible to ascribe the side effects unequivocally to this drug alone.

The following convention has been utilised for the classification of frequency of undesirable effects:- Very common $\geq$1/10 ($\geq$10%), Common $\geq$1/100 and <1/10 ($\geq$1% and <10%), Uncommon $\geq$1/1000 and <1/100 ($\geq$0.1% and <1%), Rare $\geq$1/10,000 and <1/1000 ($\geq$0.01% and <0.1%), Very rare <1/10,000 (<0.01%).

Blood and lymphatic system disorders

Very Common: Bone marrow suppression

Gastrointestinal disorders

Common: stomatitis, gastrointestinal intolerance

Rare: intestinal necrosis and perforation

Hepato-biliary disorders

Very Common: liver toxicity associated with vascular endothelial damage when Lanvis is used in maintenance or similar long term continuous therapy which is not recommended (see Dosage and Administration and Warnings and Precautions).

Usually presenting as the clinical syndrome of hepatic veno-occlusive disease (hyperbilirubinaemia, tender hepatomegaly, weight gain due to fluid retention and ascites) or signs and symptoms of portal hypertension (splenomegaly, thrombocytopenia and oesophageal varices). Elevation of liver transaminases, alkaline phosphatase and gamma glutamyl transferase and jaundice may also occur. Histopathalogical features associated with this toxicity include hepatoportal sclerosis, nodular regenerative hyperplasia, peliosis hepatis and periportal fibrosis.

Common: liver toxicity during short term cyclical therapy presenting as veno-occlusive disease.

Reversal of signs and symptoms of this liver toxicity has been reported upon withdrawal of short term or long term continuous therapy.

Rare: centrilobular hepatic necrosis has been reported in a few cases including patients receiving combination chemotherapy, oral contraceptives, high dose Lanvis and alcohol.

4.9 Overdose
The principal toxic effect is on the bone marrow and haematological toxicity is likely to be more profound with chronic overdosage than with a single ingestion of Lanvis. As there is no known antidote the blood picture should be closely monitored and general supportive measures, together with appropriate blood transfusion instituted if necessary.

5. PHARMACOLOGICAL PROPERTIES

5.1 Pharmacodynamic properties
Tioguanine is a sulphydryl analogue of guanine and behaves as a purine antimetabolite. It is activated to its nucleotide, thioguanylic acid. Tioguanine metabolites inhibit *de novo* purine synthesis and purine nucleotide interconversions. Tioguanine is also incorporated into nucleic acids and DNA (deoxyribonucleic acid) incorporation is claimed to contribute to the agent's cytotoxicity. Cross resistance usually exists between tioguanine and mercaptopurine, and it is not to be expected that patients resistant to one will respond to the other.

5.2 Pharmacokinetic properties
Tioguanine is extensively metabolised *in vivo*. There are two principal catabolic routes: methylation to 2-amino-6-methyl-thiopurine and deamination to 2-hydroxy-6-mercaptopurine, followed by oxidation to 6-thiouric acid.

Studies with radioactive tioguanine show that peak blood levels of total radioactivity are achieved about 8-10 hours after oral administration and decline slowly thereafter. Later studies using HPLC have shown 6-tioguanine to be the major thiopurine present for at least the first 8 hours after intravenous administration. Peak plasma concentrations of 61-118 nanomol (nmol)/ml are obtainable following intravenous administration of 1 to 1.2 g of 6-tioguanine/m^2 body surface area.

Plasma levels decay biexponentially with initial and terminal half-lives of 3 and 5.9 hours, respectively. Following oral administration of 100 mg/m2, peak levels as measured by HPLC occur at 2-4 hours and lie in the range of 0.03-0.94 micromolar (0.03-0.94 nmol/ml). Levels are reduced by concurrent food intake (as well as vomiting).

5.3 Preclinical safety data
There are no pre-clinical data of relevance to the prescriber which are additional to that already included in other sections of the SPC.

6. PHARMACEUTICAL PARTICULARS

6.1 List of excipients

Lactose	NF
Starch, potato	HSE
Acacia	NF
Stearic acid	NF
Magnesium stearate	NF
Purified water	USP

6.2 Incompatibilities
None known.

6.3 Shelf life
60 months (unopened).

6.4 Special precautions for storage
Store below 25°C

Keep dry

Protect from light

6.5 Nature and contents of container
Amber glass bottles with child-resistant polyethylene/polypropylene closures

Pack size 25

6.6 Instructions for use and handling
None

Administrative Data

7. MARKETING AUTHORISATION HOLDER
The Wellcome Foundation Limited

Glaxo Wellcome House

Berkeley Avenue

Greenford

Middlesex UB6 0NN

Trading as

GlaxoSmithKline UK

Stockley Park West

Uxbridge

Middlesex UB11 1BT

8. MARKETING AUTHORISATION NUMBER(S)
PL0003/0083

9. DATE OF FIRST AUTHORISATION/RENEWAL OF THE AUTHORISATION
29 October 1997

10. DATE OF REVISION OF THE TEXT
18th April 2005

Largactil Injection

(sanofi-aventis)

1. NAME OF THE MEDICINAL PRODUCT
Largactil Injection.

2. QUALITATIVE AND QUANTITATIVE COMPOSITION
2.5% w/v chlorpromazine hydrochloride.

3. PHARMACEUTICAL FORM
Sterile solution for injection.

4. CLINICAL PARTICULARS

4.1 Therapeutic indications
Largactil injection is a phenothiazine neuroleptic. It is indicated in the following conditions:

- Schizophrenia and other psychoses (especially paranoid) mania and hypomania.

- Anxiety, psychomotor agitation, excitement, violent or dangerously impulsive behaviour. Largactil is used as an adjunct in the short-term treatment of these conditions.

- Intractable hiccup.

- Nausea and vomiting of terminal illness (where other drugs have failed or are not available).

- Induction of hypothermia is facilitated by Largactil which prevents shivering and causes vasodilation.

- Childhood schizophrenia and autism.

4.2 Posology and method of administration
Route of administration: Deep intramuscular injection.

Oral route administration should be used wherever possible.

Parenteral formulations may be used in emergencies. They may only be administered by deep intramuscular injection. Largactil is too irritant to give subcutaneously. Repeated injections should be avoided if possible.

ADULTS: A single deep intramuscular injection of 25-50mg followed by oral therapy will suffice in many cases, but the intramuscular dose may be repeated if required at 6 to 8 hour intervals. As soon as possible oral administration should be substituted.

ELDERLY: Should be started on half or even quarter of the adult dosage.

Dosage of chlopromazine in schizophrenia, other psychoses, anxiety and agitation, childhood schizophrenias and autism:

(see Table 1)

Hiccup, induction of hypothermia to prevent shivering:

(see Table 2)

Nausea and vomiting of terminal illness:

(see Table 3)

4.3 Contraindications
Known hypersensitivity to chlorpromazine or to any of the excipients. Bone marrow depression.

4.4 Special warnings and special precautions for use
Largactil should be avoided in patients with liver or renal dysfunction, Parkinson's disease, hypothyroidism, cardiac failure, phaeochromocytoma, myasthenia gravis and prostate hypertrophy. It should be avoided in patients known to be hypersensitive to phenothiazines or with a history of narrow angle glaucoma or agranulocytosis. It should be used with caution in the elderly, particularly during very hot or cold weather (risk of hyper-, hypothermia). The elderly are particularly susceptible to postural hypotension.

Postural hypotension with tachycardia as well as local pain or nodule formation may occur after intramuscular administration. The patient should be kept supine and blood pressure monitored when receiving parenteral chlorpromazine. The elderly are particularly susceptible to postural hypotension.

Close monitoring is required in patients with epilepsy or a history of seizures, as phenothiazines may lower the seizure threshold.

As agranulocytosis has been reported, regular monitoring of the complete blood count is recommended. The occurrence of unexplained infections or fever may be evidence of blood dyscrasia (see section 4.8 below), and requires immediate haematological investigation.

It is imperative that treatment be discontinued in the event of unexplained fever, as this may be a sign of neuroleptic malignant syndrome (pallor, hyperthermia, autonomic dysfunction, altered consciousness, muscle rigidity). Signs of autonomic dysfunction, such as sweating and arterial instability, may precede the onset of hyperthermia and serve as early warning signs. Although neuroleptic malignant syndrome may be idiosyncratic in origin, dehydration and organic brain disease are predisposing factors.

Acute withdrawal symptoms, including nausea, vomiting and insomnia, have very rarely been reported following the abrupt cessation of high doses of neuroleptics. Relapse may also occur, and the emergence of extrapyramidal reactions has been reported. Therefore, gradual withdrawal is advisable.

In schizophrenia, the response to neuroleptic treatment may be delayed. If treatment is withdrawn, the recurrence of symptoms may not become apparent for some time.

As with other neuroleptics, cases of QT interval prolongation have been reported with chlorpromazine very rarely (see section 4.8, below). The risk-benefit should be fully assessed before Largactil treatment is commenced, and patients with predisposing factors for ventricular arrhythmias, (e.g. cardiac disease; metabolic abnormalities such as hypokalaemia, hypocalcaemia or hypomagnesaemia; starvation; alcohol abuse; concomitant therapy with other drugs known to prolong the QT interval) should be carefully monitored (biochemical status and ECG), particularly during the initial phase of treatment.

As with all antipsychotic drugs, Largactil should not be used alone where depression is predominant. However, it may be combined with antidepressant therapy to treat those conditions in which depression and psychosis coexist.

Because of the risk of photosensitisation, patients should be advised to avoid exposure to direct sunlight (see section 4.8).

In those frequently handling preparations of phenothiazines, the greatest care must be taken to avoid contact of the drug with the skin.

4.5 Interaction with other medicinal products and other forms of Interaction
Adrenaline must not be used in patients overdosed with Largactil.

The CNS depressant actions of Largactil and other neuroleptic agents may be intensified (additively) by alcohol, barbiturates and other sedatives. Respiratory depression may occur.

Anticholinergic drugs may reduce the antipsychotic effect of Largactil and the mild anticholinergic effect of Largactil may be enhanced by other anticholinergic drugs possibly leading to constipation, heat stroke, etc.

Some drugs interfere with absorption of neuroleptic agents: antacids, anti-Parkinson drugs and lithium.

Documented adverse clinically significant interactions occur with alcohol, guanethidine and hypoglycaemic agents.

Where treatment for neuroleptic-induced extrapyramidal symptoms is required, anticholinergic antiparkinsonian agents should be used in preference to levodopa, since neuroleptics antagonise the antiparkinsonian action of dopaminergics.

High doses of Largactil reduce the response to hypoglycaemic agents the dosage of which might have to be raised.

The hypotensive effect of most antihypertensive drugs especially alpha adrenoceptor blocking agents may be exaggerated by Largactil.

The action of some drugs may be opposed by Largactil; these include amphetamine, levodopa, clonidine, guanethidine, adrenaline.

Increases or decreases in the plasma concentrations of a number of drugs, e.g. propranolol, phenobarbitone have been observed but were not of clinical significance.

Simultaneous administration of desferrioxamine and prochlorperazine has been observed to induce a transient metabolic encephalopathy characterised by loss of consciousness for 48-72 hours. It is possible this may occur with Largactil since it shares many of the pharmacological properties of prochlorperazine.

There is an increased risk of arrhythmias when neuroleptics are used concurrently with drugs which prolong the QT interval, including certain antiarrhythmics, antidepressants, and other antipsychotics (see section 4.8, below).

Table 1 Dosage of chlopromazine in schizophrenia, other psychoses, anxiety and agitation, childhood schizophrenias and autism

Route	Adults	Children under 1 year	Children 1-5 years	Children 6-12 years	Elderly or debilitated patients
i.m.	For acute relief of symptoms 25-50 mg every 6-8 hours.	Do not use unless need is life saving.	0.5 mg/kg bodyweight every 6-8 hours. Dosage is not advised to exceed 40 mg daily.	0.5 mg/kg bodyweight every 6-8 hours. Dosage is not advised to exceed 75 mg daily.	Doses in the lower range for adults should be sufficient to control symptoms i.e. 25 mg 8 hourly.

Table 2 Hiccup, induction of hypothermia to prevent shivering

Indication	Route	Adults	Children under 1 year	Children 1-5 years	Children 6-12 years	Elderly or debilitated patients
Hiccups	i.m.	25-50 mg and if this fails 25-50 mg in 500-1000 ml sodium chloride injection by slow intravenous infusion.	No information available.			
Induction of hypothermia to prevent shivering	i.m.	25-50 mg every 6-8 hours.	Do not use.	Initial dose 0.5 to 1 mg/kg. Maintenance 0.5 mg/kg every 4-6 hours.	Initial dose 0.5 to 1 mg/kg. Maintenance 0.5 mg/kg every 4-6 hours.	No data available.

Table 3 Nausea and vomiting of terminal illness

Route	Adults	Children under 1 year	Children 1-5 years	Children 6-12 years	Elderly or debilitated patients
i.m.	25 mg initially then 25-50 mg every 3-4 hours until vomiting stops then drug to be taken orally.	Do not use unless need is life saving.	0.5 mg/kg 6-8 hourly. It is advised that maximum daily dosage should not exceed 40 mg.	0.5 mg/kg every 6-8 hours. It is advised that maximum daily dosage should not exceed 75 mg.	Not recommended.

There is an increased risk of agranulocytosis when neuroleptics are used concurrently with drugs with myelosuppressive potential, such as carbamazepine or certain antibiotics and cytotoxics.

In patients treated concurrently with neuroleptics and lithium, there have been rare reports of neurotoxicity.

4.6 Pregnancy and lactation

There is inadequate evidence of the safety of Largactil in human pregnancy. There is evidence of harmful effects in animals. Like other drugs it should be avoided in pregnancy unless the physician considers it essential. It may occasionally prolong labour and at such a time should be withheld until the cervix is dilated 3-4 cm. Possible adverse effects on the foetus include lethargy or paradoxical hyperexcitability, tremor and low Apgar score. Largactil may be excreted in milk, therefore breastfeeding should be suspended during treatment.

4.7 Effects on ability to drive and use machines

Patients should be warned about drowsiness during the early days of treatment and advised not to drive or operate machinery.

4.8 Undesirable effects

Generally, adverse reactions occur at low frequency; the most common reported adverse reactions are nervous system disorders.

Blood and lymphatic system disorders: A mild leucopaenia occurs in up to 30% of patients on prolonged high dosage. Agranulocytosis may occur rarely; it is not dose related.

Immune system disorders: Allergic phenomena such as angiodema, bronchospasm, and urticaria have occurred with phenothiazines but anaphylactic reactions have been exceedingly rare. In very rare cases, treatment with chlorpromazine may be associated with systemic lupus erythematosus.

Endocrine: Hyperprolactinaemia which may result in galactorrhoea, gynaecomastia, amenorrhoea and impotence.

Nervous system disorders: Acute dystonias or dyskenias, usually transitory are more common in children and young adults and usually occur within the first 4 days of treatment or after dosage increases.

Akathisia characteristically occurs after large initial doses.

Parkinsonism is more common in adults and the elderly. It usually develops after weeks or months of treatment. One or more of the following may be seen: tremor, rigidity, akinesia or other features of Parkinsonism. Commonly just tremor.

Tardive Dyskinesia: If this occurs it is usually, but not necessarily, after prolonged high dosage. It can even occur after treatment has been stopped. Dosage should therefore be kept low whenever possible.

Insomnia and agitation may occur.

Eye disorders: Ocular changes and the development of a metallic greyish-mauve coloration of exposed skin have been noted in some individuals, mainly females, who have received chlorpromazine continuously for long periods (four to eight years).

Cardiac disorders: Cardiac arrhythmia's including atrial arrythmia, A-V block, ventricular tachycardia and fibrillation have been reported during neuroleptic therapy, possibly related to dosage. Pre-existing cardiac disease, old age, hypokalaemia and concurrent tricyclic antidepressant may predispose. ECG changes, usually benign, including widened QT interval, ST depression, U-waves and T-wave changes (see section 4.4, above).

Vascular disorders: Hypotension, usually postural, commonly occurs. Elderly or volume depleted subjects are particularly susceptible: it is more likely to occur after intramuscular administration.

Gastrointestinal disorders: dry mouth may occur.

Respiratory, thoracic and mediastinal disorders: Respiratory depression is possible in susceptible patients. Nasal stuffiness may occur.

Hepato-biliary disorders: Jaundice, usually transient, occurs in a very small percentage of patients taking chlorpromazine. A premonitory sign may be a sudden onset of fever after one to three weeks of treatment followed by the development of jaundice. Chlorpromazine jaundice has the biochemical and other characteristics of obstructive (cholestatic) jaundice and is associated with obstructions of the canaliculi by bile thrombi; the frequent presence of an accompanying eosinophilia indicates the allergic nature of this phenomenon. Liver injury, sometimes fatal, has been reported rarely in patients treated with chlorpromazine. Treatment should be withheld on the development of jaundice (see section 4.4, above).

Skin and subcutaneous tissue disorders: Contact skin sensitisation may occur rarely in those frequently handling preparations of chlorpromazine (see section 4.4, above). Skin rashes of various kinds may also be seen in patients treated with the drug. Patients on high dosage may develop photosensitivity in sunny weather and should avoid exposure to direct sunlight.

Reproductive system and breast disorders: Priapism has been very rarely reported in patients treated with chlorpromazine.

General disorders and administration site conditions: Neuroleptic malignant syndrome (hyperthermia, rigidity, autonomic dysfunction and altered consciousness) may occur (see section 4.4, above).

4.9 Overdose

Toxicity and treatment of overdosage: Symptoms of chlorpromazine overdosage include drowsiness or loss of consciousness, hypotension, tachycardia, ECG changes, ventricular arrhythmia's and hypothermia. Severe extrapyramidal dyskinesias may occur.

If the patient is seen sufficiently soon (up to 6 hours) after ingestion of a toxic dose, gastric lavage may be attempted. Pharmacological induction of emesis is unlikely to be of any use. Activated charcoal should be given. There is no specific antidote. Treatment is supportive.

Generalised vasodilation may result in circulatory collapse; raising the patient's legs may suffice. In severe cases, volume expansion by intravenous fluids may be needed; infusion fluids should be warmed before administration in order not to aggravate hypothermia.

Positive inotropic agents such as dopamine may be tried if fluid replacement is insufficient to correct the circulatory collapse. Peripheral vasoconstriction agents are not generally recommended; avoid the use of adrenaline.

Ventricular or supraventricular tachy-arrhythmias usually respond to restoration of normal body temperature and correction of circulatory or metabolic disturbances. If persistent or life threatening, appropriate anti-arrhythmic therapy may be considered. Avoid lignocaine and, as far as possible, long acting anti-arrhythmic drugs.

Pronounced central nervous system depression requires airway maintenance or, in extreme circumstances, assisted respiration. Severe dystonic reactions usually respond to procyclidine (5-10mg) or orphenadrine (20-40mg) administered intramuscularly or intravenously. Convulsions should be treated with intravenous diazepam.

Neuroleptic malignant syndrome should be treated with cooling. Dantrolene sodium may be tried.

5. PHARMACOLOGICAL PROPERTIES

5.1 Pharmacodynamic properties

Largactil is a phenothiazine neuroleptic.

5.2 Pharmacokinetic properties

Chlorpromazine is rapidly absorbed and widely distributed in the body. It is metabolised in the liver and excreted in the urine and bile. Whilst plasma concentration of chlorpromazine itself rapidly declines excretion of chlorpromazine metabolites is very slow. The drug is highly bound to plasma protein. It readily diffuses across the placenta. Small quantities have been detected in milk from treated women. Children require smaller dosages per kg than adults.

5.3 Preclinical safety data

There are no preclinical data of relevance to the prescriber which are additional to that already included in other sections of the SPC.

6. PHARMACEUTICAL PARTICULARS

6.1 List of excipients

Sodium sulphite anhydrous BP (E221), Sodium citrate BP, Sodium metabisulphite powder BP (E223), Sodium chloride PhEur, Water for Injections.

6.2 Incompatibilities

Largactil injection solutions have a pH of 5.0-6.5; they are incompatible with benzylpenicillin potassium, pentobarbitone sodium and phenobarbitone sodium.

6.3 Shelf life

The shelf life of the Largactil Injection is 60 months.

6.4 Special precautions for storage

Largactil injection should be stored protected from light. Discoloured solution should not be used.

6.5 Nature and contents of container

Largactil Injection 2.5% w/v is supplied in boxes containing 10 × 1 ml or 10 × 2 ml in glass ampoules.

6.6 Instructions for use and handling

None.

7. MARKETING AUTHORISATION HOLDER

Hawgreen Limited
4, Priory Hall
Stillorgan Road
Stillorgan
Dublin
Eire

8. MARKETING AUTHORISATION NUMBER(S)

PL 17077/0011

9. DATE OF FIRST AUTHORISATION/RENEWAL OF THE AUTHORISATION

September 1998

10. DATE OF REVISION OF THE TEXT

March 2004

Legal Category: POM

Largactil Tablets, Syrup & Forte Suspension

(sanofi-aventis)

1. NAME OF THE MEDICINAL PRODUCT

Largactil Tablets 10mg
Largactil Tablets 25mg
Largactil Tablets 50mg
Largactil Tablets 100mg
Largactil Syrup
Largactil Forte Suspension

2. QUALITATIVE AND QUANTITATIVE COMPOSITION

Tablets: The active component of Largactil is chlorpromazine hydrochloride. Each tablet contains 10mg, 25mg, 50mg or 100mg chlorpromazine hydrochloride.

Syrup: 0.5% w/v chlorpromazine hydrochloride (25 mg chlorpromazine hydrochloride in 5 ml).

Forte Suspension: 2.9% w/v chlorpromazine embonate, equivalent to 100 mg/5 ml of chlorpromazine hydrochloride.

3. PHARMACEUTICAL FORM

Tablets: White to off-white circular, biconvex, film coated tablets: one face impressed LG/10, LG/25, LG/50 or LG/100 reverse face plain.

Syrup: A clear, bright golden-brown syrup.

Forte Suspension: An orange coloured suspension.

4. CLINICAL PARTICULARS

4.1 Therapeutic indications

Largactil is a phenothiazine neuroleptic. It is indicated in the following conditions:

- Schizophrenia and other psychoses (especially paranoid) mania and hypomania.

- Anxiety, psychomotor agitation, excitement, violent or dangerously impulsive behaviour. Largactil is used as an adjunct in the short-term treatment of these conditions.

- Intractable hiccup.

- Nausea and vomiting of terminal illness (where other drugs have failed or are not available).

- Childhood schizophrenia and autism.

4.2 Posology and method of administration

Oral route of administration should be used whenever possible. Patients unwilling to swallow tablets may be treated with suspension or syrup.

Dosage should be low to begin with and gradually increased under close supervision until the optimum dosage within the recommended range, for the individual is reached.

Individuals vary considerably and the optimum dose may be affected by the formulation used.

Dosage of chloropromazine in schizophrenia, other psychoses, anxiety and agitation, childhood schizophrenias and autism:

(see Table 1 on next page)

Hiccup:

(see Table 2 on next page)

Nausea and vomiting of terminal illness:

(see Table 3 on next page)

4.3 Contraindications

Known hypersensitivity to chlorpromazine or to any of the excipients. Bone marrow depression.

4.4 Special warnings and special precautions for use

Largactil should be avoided in patients with liver or renal dysfunction, Parkinson's disease, hypothyroidism, cardiac failure, phaeochromocytoma, myasthenia gravis and prostate hypertrophy. It should be avoided in patients known to be hypersensitive to phenothiazines or with a history of narrow angle glaucoma or agranulocytosis. It should be used with caution in the elderly, particularly during very hot or cold weather (risk of hyper-, hypothermia). The elderly are particularly susceptible to postural hypotension.

Close monitoring is required in patients with epilepsy or a history of seizures, as phenothiazines may lower the seizure threshold.

As agranulocytosis has been reported, regular monitoring of the complete blood count is recommended. The occurrence of unexplained infections or fever may be evidence of blood dyscrasia (see section 4.8 below), and requires immediate haematological investigation.

It is imperative that treatment be discontinued in the event of unexplained fever, as this may be a sign of neuroleptic malignant syndrome (pallor, hyperthermia, autonomic dysfunction, altered consciousness, muscle rigidity). Signs of autonomic dysfunction, such as sweating and arterial instability, may precede the onset of hyperthermia and serve as early warning signs. Although neuroleptic malignant syndrome may be idiosyncratic in origin, dehydration and organic brain disease are predisposing factors.

Acute withdrawal symptoms, including nausea, vomiting and insomnia, have very rarely been reported following the abrupt cessation of high doses of neuroleptics. Relapse may also occur, and the emergence of extrapyramidal

Table 1 Dosage of chlopromazine in schizophrenia, other psychoses, anxiety and agitation, childhood schizophrenias and autism

Route	Adults	Children under 1 year	Children 1-5 years	Children 6-12 years	Elderly or debilitated patients
Oral	Initially 25 mg t.d.s. or 75 mg at bedtime increasing by daily amounts of 25 mg to an effective maintenance dose. This is usually in the range 75 to 300 mg daily, but some patients may require up to 1 g daily.	Do not use unless need is life saving.	0.5 mg/kg bodyweight every 4-6 hours to a recommended dose of 40 mg daily.	1/3 to 1/2 the adult dose to a maximum recommended dose of 75 mg daily.	Start with 1/3 to 1/2 the usual adult dose with a more gradual increase in dosage.

Table 2 Hiccup

Route	Adults	Children under 1 year	Children 1-5 years	Children 6-12 years	Elderly or debilitated patients
Oral	25-50 mg t.d.s. or q.d.s.	No information available.			

Table 3 Nausea and vomiting of terminal illness

Route	Adults	Children under 1 year	Children 1-5 years	Children 6-12 years	Elderly or debilitated patients
Oral	10-25 mg every 4-6 hours	Do not use unless need is life saving.	0.5 mg/kg every 4-6 hours. Maximum daily dosage should not exceed 40 mg.	0.5 mg/kg every 4-6 hours. Maximum daily dosage should not exceed 75 mg.	Initially 1/3 to 1/2 the adult dose. The physician should then use his clinical judgement to obtain control.

reactions has been reported. Therefore, gradual withdrawal is advisable.

In schizophrenia, the response to neuroleptic treatment may be delayed. If treatment is withdrawn, the recurrence of symptoms may not become apparent for some time.

As with other neuroleptics, cases of QT interval prolongation have been reported with chlorpromazine very rarely (see section 4.8, below). The risk-benefit should be fully assessed before Largactil treatment is commenced, and patients with predisposing factors for ventricular arrhythmias, (e.g. cardiac disease; metabolic abnormalities such as hypokalaemia, hypocalcaemia or hypomagnesaemia; starvation; alcohol abuse; concomitant therapy with other drugs known to prolong the QT interval) should be carefully monitored (biochemical status and ECG), particularly during the initial phase of treatment.

As with all antipsychotic drugs, Largactil should not be used alone where depression is predominant. However, it may be combined with antidepressant therapy to treat those conditions in which depression and psychosis coexist.

Because of the risk of photosensitisation, patients should be advised to avoid exposure to direct sunlight (see section 4.8).

In those frequently handling preparations of phenothiazines, the greatest care must be taken to avoid contact of the drug with the skin.

4.5 Interaction with other medicinal products and other forms of Interaction

Adrenaline must not be used in patients overdosed with Largactil.

The CNS depressant actions of Largactil and other neuroleptic agents may be intensified (additively) by alcohol, barbiturates and other sedatives. Respiratory depression may occur.

Anticholinergic drugs may reduce the antipsychotic effect of Largactil and the mild anticholinergic effect of Largactil may be enhanced by other anticholinergic drugs possibly leading to constipation, heat stroke, etc.

Some drugs interfere with absorption of neuroleptic agents: antacids, anti-Parkinson drugs and lithium.

Documented adverse clinically significant interactions occur with alcohol, guanethidine and hypoglycaemic agents.

Where treatment for neuroleptic-induced extrapyramidal symptoms is required, anticholinergic antiparkinsonian agents should be used in preference to levodopa, since neuroleptics antagonise the antiparkinsonian action of dopaminergics.

High doses of Largactil reduce the response to hypoglycaemic agents the dosage of which might have to be raised.

The hypotensive effect of most antihypertensive drugs especially alpha adrenoceptor blocking agents may be exaggerated by Largactil.

The action of some drugs may be opposed by Largactil; these include amphetamine, levodopa, clonidine, guanethidine, adrenaline.

Increases or decreases in the plasma concentrations of a number of drugs, e.g. propranolol, phenobarbitone have been observed but were not of clinical significance.

Simultaneous administration of desferrioxamine and prochlorperazine has been observed to induce a transient metabolic encephalopathy characterised by loss of consciousness for 48-72 hours. It is possible this may occur with Largactil since it shares many of the pharmacological properties of prochlorperazine.

There is an increased risk of arrhythmias when neuroleptics are used concurrently with drugs which prolong the QT interval, including certain antiarrhythmics, antidepressants, and other antipsychotics (see section 4.8, below).

There is an increased risk of agranulocytosis when neuroleptics are used concurrently with drugs with myelosuppressive potential, such as carbamazepine or certain antibiotics and cytotoxics.

In patients treated concurrently with neuroleptics and lithium, there have been rare reports of neurotoxicity.

4.6 Pregnancy and lactation

There is inadequate evidence of the safety of Largactil in human pregnancy. There is evidence of harmful effects in animals. Like other drugs it should be avoided in pregnancy unless the physician considers it essential. It may occasionally prolong labour and at such time should be withheld It may be withheld until the cervix is dilated 3-4 cm. Possible adverse effects on the foetus include lethargy or paradoxical hyperexcitability, tremor and low Apgar score. Largactil may be excreted in milk, therefore breastfeeding should be suspended during treatment.

4.7 Effects on ability to drive and use machines

Patients should be warned about drowsiness during the early days of treatment and advised not to drive or operate machinery.

4.8 Undesirable effects

Generally, adverse reactions occur at low frequency; the most common reported adverse reactions are nervous system disorders.

Blood and lymphatic system disorders: A mild leucopaenia occurs in up to 30% of patients on prolonged high dosage. Agranulocytosis may occur rarely; it is not dose related.

Immune system disorders: Allergic phenomena such as angiodema, bronchospasm, and urticaria have occurred with phenothiazines but anaphylactic reactions have been exceedingly rare. In very rare cases, treatment with chlorpromazine may be associated with systemic lupus erythematosus.

Endocrine: Hyperprolactinaemia which may result in galactorrhoea, gynaecomastia, amenorrhoea and impotence.

Nervous system disorders: Acute dystonias or dyskenias, usually transitory are more common in children and young adults and usually occur within the first 4 days of treatment or after dosage increases.

Akathisia characteristically occurs after large initial doses.

Parkinsonism is more common in adults and the elderly. It usually develops after weeks or months of treatment. One or more of the following may be seen: tremor, rigidity, akinesia or other features of Parkinsonism. Commonly just tremor.

Tardive Dyskinesia: If this occurs it is usually, but not necessarily, after prolonged high dosage. It can even occur after treatment has been stopped. Dosage should therefore be kept low whenever possible.

Insomnia and agitation may occur.

Eye disorders: Ocular changes and the development of a metallic greyish-mauve coloration of exposed skin have been noted in some individuals, mainly females, who have received chlorpromazine continuously for long periods (four to eight years).

Cardiac disorders: Cardiac arrhythmia's including atrial arrythmia, A-V block, ventricular tachycardia and fibrillation have been reported during neuroleptic therapy, possibly related to dosage. Pre-existing cardiac disease, old age, hypokalaemia and concurrent tricyclic antidepressant may predispose. ECG changes, usually benign, including widened QT interval, ST depression, U-waves and T-wave changes (see section 4.4, above).

Vascular disorders: Hypotension, usually postural, commonly occurs. Elderly or volume depleted subjects are particularly susceptible: it is more likely to occur after intramuscular administration.

Gastrointestinal disorders: dry mouth may occur.

Respiratory, thoracic and mediastinal disorders: Respiratory depression is possible in susceptible patients. Nasal stuffiness may occur.

Hepato-biliary disorders: Jaundice, usually transient, occurs in a very small percentage of patients taking chlorpromazine. A premonitory sign may be a sudden onset of fever after one to three weeks of treatment followed by the development of jaundice. Chlorpromazine jaundice has the biochemical and other characteristics of obstructive (cholestatic) jaundice and is associated with obstructions of the canaliculi by bile thrombi; the frequent presence of an accompanying eosinophilia indicates the allergic nature of this phenomenon. Liver injury, sometimes fatal, has been reported rarely in patients treated with chlorpromazine. Treatment should be withheld on the development of jaundice (see section 4.4, above).

Skin and subcutaneous tissue disorders: Contact skin sensitisation may occur rarely in those frequently handling preparations of chlorpromazine (see section 4.4, above). Skin rashes of various kinds may also be seen in patients treated with the drug. Patients on high dosage may develop photosensitivity in sunny weather and should avoid exposure to direct sunlight.

Reproductive system and breast disorders: Priapism has been very rarely reported in patients treated with chlorpromazine.

General disorders and administration site conditions: Neuroleptic malignant syndrome (hyperthermia, rigidity, autonomic dysfunction and altered consciousness) may occur (see section 4.4, above).

4.9 Overdose

Toxicity and treatment of overdosage: Symptoms of chlorpromazine overdosage include drowsiness or loss of consciousness, hypotension, tachycardia, ECG changes, ventricular arrhythmia's and hypothermia. Severe extrapyramidal dyskinesias may occur.

If the patient is seen sufficiently soon (up to 6 hours) after ingestion of a toxic dose, gastric lavage may be attempted. Pharmacological induction of emesis is unlikely to be of any use. Activated charcoal should be given. There is no specific antidote. Treatment is supportive.

Generalised vasodilation may result in circulatory collapse; raising the patient's legs may suffice. In severe cases, volume expansion by intravenous fluids may be needed; infusion fluids should be warmed before administration in order not to aggravate hypothermia.

Positive inotropic agents such as dopamine may be tried if fluid replacement is insufficient to correct the circulatory collapse. Peripheral vasoconstriction agents are not generally recommended; avoid the use of adrenaline.

Ventricular or supraventricular tachy-arrhythmias usually respond to restoration of normal body temperature and correction of circulatory or metabolic disturbances. If persistent or life threatening, appropriate anti-arrhythmic therapy may be considered. Avoid lignocaine and, as far as possible, long acting anti-arrhythmic drugs.

Pronounced central nervous system depression requires airway maintenance or, in extreme circumstances, assisted respiration. Severe dystonic reactions usually respond to procyclidine (5-10mg) or orphenadrine (20-40mg) administered intramuscularly or intravenously. Convulsions should be treated with intravenous diazepam.

Neuroleptic malignant syndrome should be treated with cooling. Dantrolene sodium may be tried.

5. PHARMACOLOGICAL PROPERTIES

5.1 Pharmacodynamic properties

Largactil is a phenothiazine neuroleptic.

5.2 Pharmacokinetic properties

Chlorpromazine is rapidly absorbed and widely distributed in the body. It is metabolised in the liver and excreted in the urine and bile. Whilst plasma concentration of chlorpromazine itself rapidly declines excretion of chlorpromazine metabolites is very slow. The drug is highly bound to plasma protein. It readily diffuses across the placenta. Small quantities have been detected in milk from treated women. Children require smaller dosages per kg than adults.

5.3 Preclinical safety data

There is no preclinical data of relevance to the prescriber which are additional to that already included in other sections of the SPC.

6. PHARMACEUTICAL PARTICULARS

6.1 List of excipients

Tablets: Lactose BP, Maize starch BP, Aerosil 200 (E464), Magnesium sterate BP. Tablet coating: Pharmacoat 606, Polyethylene glycol 200, Demineralised water BP, White opaspray M-1-7111B, (Titanium Dioxide Ph Eur (E171), Hydroxypropylmethylcellulose Ph Eur (E464))

Syrup: Sucrose PhEur, Tween 20, Oil peppermint Chinese, Oil spearmint BP, Fruit cup 868 (Zimmerman), Citric acid anhydrous BP (E330), Sodium citrate gran. BP (E331), Ascorbic acid BP (E300), Sodium sulphite anhydrous BP (E221), Sodium metabisuphite powder BP (E223), Caramel H.T. (E150), Sodium benzoate BP (E211), Demineralised water.

Forte Suspension: Sorbitol solution 1973 BPC or Sorbitol powder BP (E420), Sodium benzoate BP (E211), Veegum RG, Citric acid anhydrous BP (E330), Sodium citrate gran.BP, Standacol sunset yellow dye (E110), Saccharin sodium BP, Oil orange terpeneless BP, Propylene glycol BP, Sodium alginate BPC (E401), Povidone K30 BP (E1201), Demineralised water BP

6.2 Incompatibilities

None stated.

6.3 Shelf life

Tablets: Shelf life is 36 months.

Syrup: The shelf life of the Largactil Syrup is 36 months. After opening for the first time the shelf life is 1 month. After dilution the shelf life is 14 days.

Forte Suspension: The shelf-life of the Largactil Forte Suspension is 36 months. After opening for the first time the shelf-life is 6 months. After dilution with Simple Syrup BP the shelf-life is 7 days.

6.4 Special precautions for storage

Tablets: Protect from light. Store below 30°C.

Syrup: Largactil Syrup should be stored protected from light, below 25°C.

Forte Suspension: Largactil Forte Suspension should be stored protected from light, below 25°C.

6.5 Nature and contents of container

Largactil Tablets are available in PVDC coated UPVC/aluminium foil blister of 56 tablets.

Largactil Syrup is supplied in type III glass bottles containing 100ml with either a rolled on pilfer proof aluminium cap and a PVDC emulsion coated wad or a HDPE/polypropylene child resistant cap with a tamper evident band.

Largactil Forte Suspension is supplied in amber glass bottles containing 100 ml.

6.6 Instructions for use and handling

None.

7. MARKETING AUTHORISATION HOLDER

Hawgreen Limited

4 Priory Hall

Stillorgan Road

Stillorgan

County Dublin

Ireland

8. MARKETING AUTHORISATION NUMBER(S)

10mg Tablets: PL 17077/0007

25mg Tablets: PL 17077/0008

50mg Tablets: PL 17077/0009

100mg Tablets: PL 17077/0010

Syrup: PL 17077/0012

Forte Suspension: PL17077/0013

9. DATE OF FIRST AUTHORISATION/RENEWAL OF THE AUTHORISATION

Tablets and Forte Suspension: 1 September 1998

Syrup: November 1998

10. DATE OF REVISION OF THE TEXT

Tablets and Syrup: March 2004

Forte Suspension: December 2003

11. LEGAL CLASSIFICATION

POM

Lariam

(Roche Products Limited)

1. NAME OF THE MEDICINAL PRODUCT

Lariam 250mg tablets

2. QUALITATIVE AND QUANTITATIVE COMPOSITION

Each tablet contains 250mg mefloquine (as 274.09mg mefloquine hydrochloride).

For excipients, see section *6.1*.

3. PHARMACEUTICAL FORM

Tablet. White to off-white cylindrical biplanar tablets, cross scored and imprinted with Roche on one face.

4. CLINICAL PARTICULARS

4.1 Therapeutic indications

Therapy and prophylaxis of malaria.

Therapy: Lariam is especially indicated for therapy of *P. falciparum* malaria in which the pathogen has become resistant to other antimalarial agents.

Following treatment of *P. vivax* malaria with Lariam, relapse prophylaxis with an 8-amino-quinoline derivative, for example primaquine, should be considered in order to eliminate parasites in the hepatic phase.

Prophylaxis: Malaria prophylaxis with Lariam is particularly recommended for travellers to malarious areas in which multiple resistant *P. falciparum* strains occur.

For current advice on geographical resistance patterns and appropriate chemoprophylaxis, current guidelines or the Malaria Reference Laboratory should be consulted, details of which can be found in the British National Formulary (BNF).

4.2 Posology and method of administration

Curative treatment

The recommended total therapeutic dose of mefloquine for non-immune patients is 20 – 25mg/kg. A lower total dose of 15mg/kg may suffice for partially immune individuals.

The recommended total therapeutic dosages of Lariam tablets relative to body weight and immune status are presented in the following table.*

	Non-immune patients	Partially immune patients
< 20kg **	¼ tablet / 2.5 – 3kg 1 tablet / 10 – 12 kg	¼ tablet / 4kg 1 tablet / 16kg
20 – 30kg	2 – 3 tablets	1 ¼ – 2 tablets
> 30 – 45kg	3 – 4 tablets	2 – 3 tablets
> 45 – 60kg	4 – 5 tablets	3 – 4 tablets
> 60kg ***	6 tablets	4 – 6 tablets

* Splitting the total curative dosage into 2 – 3 doses (e.g. 3 + 1, 3 + 2 or 3 + 2 + 1 tablets) taken 6 – 8 hours apart may reduce the occurrence or severity of adverse events.

** Experience with Lariam in infants less than 3 months old or weighing less than 5kg is limited.

*** There is no specific experience with total dosages of more than 6 tablets in very heavy patients.

A second full dose should be given to patients who vomit less than 30 minutes after receiving the drug. If vomiting occurs 30 – 60 minutes after a dose, an additional half-dose should be given.

If a full treatment course with Lariam does not lead to improvement within 48 – 72 hours, alternative treatments should be considered. When breakthrough malaria occurs during Lariam prophylaxis, physicians should carefully evaluate which antimalarial to use for therapy.

Lariam can be given for severe acute malaria after an initial course of intravenous quinine lasting at least 2 – 3 days. Interactions leading to adverse events can largely be prevented by allowing an interval of at least 12 hours after the last dose of quinine (see section *4.5 Interaction with other medicaments and other forms of interaction*).

In areas with multi-resistant malaria, initial treatment with artemisinin or a derivative, if available, followed by Lariam is also an option.

Malaria prophylaxis

Prophylaxis of malaria with Lariam should be initiated at least one week and up to 2 – 3 weeks before arrival in a malarious area. The stated dose to be given once weekly, always on the same day for a minimum of six weeks. Further doses at weekly intervals during, and for four weeks after visiting the malarious area. The following dosage schedule is given as a guide.

	Dosage
Adults and children of more than 45kg bodyweight	1 tablet
Children and adults weighing less than 45kg	
5 – 19kg	¼ tablet
20 – 30kg	½ tablet
31 – 45kg	¾ tablet

The maximum recommended duration of administration of Lariam is 12 months.

The tablets should be swallowed whole preferably after a meal with plenty of liquid.

Elderly

No specific adaptation of the usual adult dosage is required for elderly patients.

4.3 Contraindications

Prophylactic use in patients with severe impairment of liver function should be regarded for the time being as a contra-indication as no experience has been gained in such patients.

Patients with a history of psychiatric disturbances (including depression) or convulsions should not be prescribed Lariam prophylactically, as it may precipitate these conditions (see section *4.4 Special warnings and special precautions for use* and section *4.5 Interaction with other medicaments and other forms of interaction*).

Lariam should not be administered to patients with a known hypersensitivity to mefloquine or related compounds, e.g. quinine.

Because of the danger of a potentially fatal prolongation of the QTc interval, halofantrine must not be given simultaneously with or subsequent to Lariam. No data are available where Lariam was given after halofantrine.

4.4 Special warnings and special precautions for use

Women of childbearing potential travelling to malarious areas in which multiple resistant *P. falciparum* is found and who are receiving Lariam for the treatment and prophylaxis of malaria should take reliable contraceptive precautions for the entire duration of therapy and for three months after the last dose of Lariam (see section *4.6 Pregnancy and lactation*).

If psychiatric disturbances occur during prophylactic use, Lariam should be discontinued and an alternative prophylactic agent should be recommended (see section *4.3 Contra-indications*).

Experience with Lariam in infants less than 3 months old or weighing less than 5kg is limited.

There is no evidence that dose adjustment is necessary for patients with renal insufficiency. However, since clinical evidence in such patients is limited, caution should be exercised when using Lariam in patients with impaired renal function.

In patients with epilepsy, mefloquine may increase the risk of convulsions. Therefore in such cases, Lariam should be used only for curative treatment and only if compelling reasons exist (see section *4.3 Contra-indications* and section *4.5 Interaction with other medicaments and other forms of interaction*).

Lariam should be taken with caution in patients suffering from cardiac conduction disorders, since transient cardiac conduction alterations have been observed during curative and preventative use.

Patients should not disregard the possibility that re-infection or recrudescence may occur after effective antimalarial therapy.

Patients with rare hereditary problems of galactose intolerance, the Lapp lactose deficiency or glucose – galactose malabsorption should not take this medicine.

4.5 Interaction with other medicinal products and other forms of Interaction

Concomitant administration of Lariam and other related compounds (e.g. quinine, quinidine and chloroquine) may produce electrocardiographic abnormalities and increase the risk of convulsions. There is evidence that the use of halofantrine after mefloquine causes a significant lengthening of the QTc interval. Clinically significant QTc prolongation has not been found with mefloquine alone.

This appears to be the only clinically relevant interaction of this kind with Lariam, although theoretically co-administration of other drugs known to alter cardiac conduction (e.g. anti-arrhythmic or β-adrenergic blocking agents, calcium channel blockers, antihistamines or H_1-blocking agents, tricyclic antidepressants and phenothiazines) might also contribute to a prolongation of the QTc interval.

In patients taking an anticonvulsant (e.g. valproic acid, carbamazepine, phenobarbital or phenytoin), the concomitant use of Lariam may reduce seizure control by lowering the plasma levels of the anticonvulsant. Dosage adjustments of anti-seizure medication may be necessary in some cases (see section *4.3 Contra-indications* and section *4.4 Special warnings and special precautions for use*).

When Lariam is taken concurrently with oral live typhoid vaccines, attenuation of immunisation cannot be excluded. Vaccinations with oral attenuated live bacteria should therefore be completed at least 3 days before the first dose of Lariam.

No other drug interactions are known. Nevertheless, the effects of Lariam on travellers receiving co-medication, particularly those on anticoagulants or antidiabetics, should be checked before departure.

4.6 Pregnancy and lactation

There is too little clinical experience in humans to assess any possible damaging effects of Lariam during pregnancy. However, mefloquine is teratogenic when administered to rats and mice in early gestation. Therefore, Lariam should be used in pregnancy only if there are compelling medical reasons. In the absence of clinical experience, prophylactic use during pregnancy should be avoided as a matter of principle.

As mefloquine is secreted into the breast milk, nursing mothers should not breast-feed while taking Lariam.

4.7 Effects on ability to drive and use machines

Mefloquine can cause dizziness or disturbed sense of balance. It is consequently recommended not to drive or carry out tasks demanding fine co-ordination and spatial discrimination during treatment with mefloquine. Patients should avoid such tasks for at least 3 weeks following therapeutic use, as dizziness, a disturbed sense of balance or neuropsychiatric reactions have been reported up to three weeks after the use of Lariam.

Prophylactic use

Caution should be exercised with regard to driving, piloting aircraft and operating machines, as dizziness, a disturbed sense of balance or neuropsychiatric reactions have been reported during and up to three weeks after use of Lariam.

4.8 Undesirable effects

At the doses given for acute malaria, adverse reactions to Lariam may not be distinguishable from symptoms of the disease itself. The overall incidence of adverse events reported during mefloquine prophylaxis is comparable to that reported for other chemoprophylactic regimens. However, the profile of mefloquine adverse events is predominantly characterised by neuropsychological adverse events. Because of the long half-life of mefloquine, adverse reactions to Lariam may occur or persist for more than several weeks after the last dose.

Patients should be advised to obtain medical advice before the next weekly dose of Lariam, if any concerning or neuropsychiatric symptoms develop. Discontinuation of Lariam should be considered, particularly if neuropsychiatric reactions occur. The need for alternative antimalarial therapy or prophylaxis can then be evaluated.

Common adverse reactions

Nausea, vomiting, dizziness or vertigo, loss of balance, headache, somnolence, sleep disorders (insomnia, abnormal dreams), loose stools or diarrhoea and abdominal pain.

Uncommon adverse reactions

Psychiatric: Psychiatric reactions sometimes disabling and prolonged have been reported in association with Lariam. These include depression, mood changes, anxiety, confusion, hallucinations, panic attacks, restlessness, forgetfulness, psychosis and paranoia, emotional instability, aggression and agitation. There have been rare reports of suicidal ideation and suicide but no relationship to drug administration has been established.

Neurological: Convulsions, sensory and motor neuropathies (including paraesthesia), tremor, tinnitus and vestibular disorders, including hearing impairment, abnormal co-ordination, ataxia and visual disturbances.

Cardiovascular system: Circulatory disturbances (hypotension, hypertension, flushing, syncope), chest pain, tachycardia or palpitations, bradycardia, irregular pulse, extrasystoles and other transient cardiac conduction alterations.

Skin: Rash, exanthema, erythema, urticaria, pruritus, oedema, hair loss, erythema multiforme, Stevens-Johnson syndrome.

Musculo-skeletal system: Muscle weakness and muscle cramps, myalgia, arthralgia.

General symptoms: Asthenia, malaise, fatigue, fever, sweating, chills, loss of appetite, dyspepsia and dyspnoea.

Haematological: Leucopenia or leucocystosis, thrombocytopenia.

Laboratory abnormalities: Transient elevation of transaminases.

Very rare adverse reactions: AV-block and encephalopathy. There have also been rare reports of anaphylaxis in patients taking Lariam.

Studies *in vitro* and *in vivo* showed no haemolysis associated with G6PD deficiency.

4.9 Overdose

In cases of overdosage with Lariam, the symptoms mentioned under section *4.8* (*Undesirable effects*) may be more pronounced.

Countermeasures: Induce vomiting or perform gastric lavage as appropriate. Monitor cardiac function (if possible by ECG) and neuropsychiatric status for at least 24 hours. Provide symptomatic and intensive supportive treatment as required, particularly for cardiovascular disorders.

5. PHARMACOLOGICAL PROPERTIES

5.1 Pharmacodynamic properties

The effectiveness of Lariam in the therapy and prophylaxis of malaria is due essentially to destruction of the asexual forms of the malarial pathogens that affect humans (*Plasmodium falciparum, P. vivax, P. malariae, P. ovale*).

Lariam is also effective against malarial parasites resistant to other antimalarials such as chloroquine and other 4-aminoquinoline derivatives, proguanil, pyrimethamine and pyrimethamine-sulphonamide combinations. However, strains of *P. falciparum* resistant to mefloquine have been reported (e.g. in parts of Indochina). Cross-resistance between mefloquine and halofantrine has been observed.

In vitro and *in vivo* studies with mefloquine showed no haemolysis associated with glucose-6-phosphate dehydrogenase deficiency.

5.2 Pharmacokinetic properties

Absorption: The maximum plasma concentration is reached within 6 to 24 hours after a single oral dose of Lariam. The level in micrograms per litre is roughly equivalent to the dose in milligrams (for example approximately 1000μg/l after a single dose of 1000mg). The presence of food significantly enhances the rate and extent of absorption.

At a dose of 250mg once weekly, maximum steady state plasma concentrations of 1000 – 2000μg/l are reached after 7 – 10 weeks. The RBC concentration is almost twice as high as the plasma level. Plasma protein binding is about 98%. Clinical experience suggests a minimal suppressive plasma concentration of mefloquine in the order of 600μg/l.

Elimination: The average half-life of mefloquine in Europeans is 21 days. There is evidence that mefloquine is excreted mainly in the bile and faeces. In volunteers, urinary excretion of unchanged mefloquine and its main metabolite accounted for about 9% and 4% of the dose, respectively.

Special clinical situations: The pharmacokinetics of mefloquine may be altered in acute malaria. Pharmacokinetic differences have been observed between various ethnic populations. In practice however, these are of minor importance compared with the host immune status and sensitivity of the parasite.

Mefloquine crosses the placenta. Excretion into breast milk appears to be minimal.

5.3 Preclinical safety data

Mefloquine crosses the placenta and is teratogenic when administered to rats and mice in early gestation (see section *4.6 Pregnancy and lactation*).

6. PHARMACEUTICAL PARTICULARS

6.1 List of excipients

Microcrystalline cellulose

lactose

crospovidone

maize starch

ammonium-calcium alginate

poloxamer (polyoxyethylene-polyoxypropylene copolymer)

talc

magnesium stearate

6.2 Incompatibilities

Not applicable.

6.3 Shelf life

3 years.

6.4 Special precautions for storage

Store in the original package.

6.5 Nature and contents of container

Aluminium foil packs or aluminium/PVC blister packs containing 6 or 8 tablets.

Glass bottle with desiccant unit containing 100 tablets.

6.6 Instructions for use and handling

Not applicable.

7. MARKETING AUTHORISATION HOLDER

Roche Products Limited, 40 Broadwater Road, Welwyn Garden City, Hertfordshire, AL7 3AY.

8. MARKETING AUTHORISATION NUMBER(S)

PL 00031/0236

9. DATE OF FIRST AUTHORISATION/RENEWAL OF THE AUTHORISATION

5 October 1989/1 February 1999

10. DATE OF REVISION OF THE TEXT

February 2005

Lariam is a registered trade mark

Item Code

Lasilactone

(sanofi-aventis)

1. NAME OF THE MEDICINAL PRODUCT

Lasilactone

2. QUALITATIVE AND QUANTITATIVE COMPOSITION

Lasilactone contains 20mg Furosemide and 50mg Spironolactone.

3. PHARMACEUTICAL FORM

Capsule.

4. CLINICAL PARTICULARS

4.1 Therapeutic indications

Lasilactone contains a short-acting diuretic and a long-acting aldosterone antagonist. It is indicated in the treatment of resistant oedema where this is associated with secondary hyperaldosteronism; conditions include chronic congestive cardiac failure and hepatic cirrhosis.

Treatment with Lasilactone should be reserved for cases refractory to a diuretic alone at conventional doses.

This fixed ratio combination should only be used if titration with the component drugs separately indicates that this product is appropriate.

The use of Lasilactone in the management of essential hypertension should be restricted to patients with demonstrated hyperaldosteronism. It is recommended that in these patients also, this combination should only be used if titration with the component drugs separately indicates that this product is appropriate.

4.2 Posology and method of administration

For oral administration.

Adults: 1-4 capsules daily.

Children: The product is not suitable for use in children.

Elderly: Furosemide and Spironolactone may both be excreted more slowly in the elderly.

The capsules should be swallowed whole. They are best taken at breakfast and/or lunch with a generous amount of liquid (approx. 1 glass). An evening dose is not recommended, especially during initial treatment, because of the increased nocturnal output of urine to be expected in such cases.

4.3 Contraindications

Patients with hypovolaemia or dehydration (with or without accompanying hypotension). Patients with an impaired renal function and a creatinine clearance below 30ml/min per 1.73m^2 body surface area, acute renal failure, anuria, hepatorenal syndrome and hepatic encephalopathy, hyperkalaemia, severe hypokalaemia, severe hyponatraemia, Addison's diseaseor breast feeding women.

Hypersensitivity to furosemide, spironolactone, sulphonamides or sulphonamide derivatives, or any of the excipients of Lasilactone.

4.4 Special warnings and special precautions for use

Spironolactone may cause vocal changes. In determining whether to initiate treatment with Lasilactone, special attention must be given to this possibility in patients whose voice is particularly important for their work (e.g., actors, singers, teachers).

Urinary output must be secured. Patients with partial obstruction of urinary outflow, for example patients with prostatic hypertrophy or impairment of micturition have an increased risk of developing acute retention and require careful monitoring.

Where indicated, steps should be taken to correct hypotension or hypovolaemia before commencing therapy.

Particularly careful monitoring is necessary in:

- patients with hypotension.
- patients who are at risk from a pronounced fall in blood pressure.
- patients where latent diabetes may become manifest or the insulin requirements of diabetic patients may increase.
- patients with gout.
- patients with liver disease as hepatic coma may be precipitated in susceptible cases.
- patients with hypoproteinaemia, e.g. associated with nephrotic syndrome (the effect of furosemide may be weakened and its ototoxicity potentiated). Cautious dose titration is required.

Administration of Lasilactone should be avoided in the presence of a raised serum potassium. Concomitant administration of triamterene, amiloride, potassium supplements or non-steroidal anti-inflammatory drugs is not recommended as hyperkalaemia may result.

Caution should be observed in patients liable to electrolyte deficiency. Regular monitoring of serum sodium, potassium, creatinine and glucose is generally recommended during therapy; particularly close monitoring is required in patients at high risk of developing electrolyte imbalances or in case of significant additional fluid loss. Hypovolaemia or dehydration as well as any significant electrolyte and acid-base disturbances must be corrected. This may require temporary discontinuation of furosemide.

Frequent checks of the serum potassium level are necessary in patients with impaired renal function and a creatinine clearance below 60ml/min per 1.73m^2 body surface area as well as in cases where Lasilactone is taken in combination with certain other drugs which may lead to an increase in potassium levels.

4.5 Interaction with other medicinal products and other forms of Interaction

The dosage of concurrently administered cardiac glycosides or anti-hypertensive agents may require adjustment.

A marked fall in blood pressure and deterioration in renal function may be seen when ACE inhibitors are added to furosemide therapy. The dose of Lasilactone should be reduced, or the drug stopped, before initiating the ACE inhibitor or increasing the dose of an ACE inhibitor.

When Lasilactone is taken in combination with potassium salts, with drugs which reduce potassium excretion, with non-steroidal anti-inflammatory drugs or with ACE inhibitors, an increase in serum potassium concentration and hyperkalaemia may occur.

The toxic effects of nephrotoxic antibiotics may be potentiated by concurrent administration of potent diuretics such as furosemide.

Lasilactone and sucralfate must not be taken within a brief time span of each other because sucralfate decreases the absorption of furosemide from the intestine and so reduced its effect.

In common with other diuretics, serum lithium levels may be increased when lithium is given concomitantly with furosemide, resulting in increased lithium toxicity. Therefore, it is recommended that lithium levels are carefully monitored and where necessary the lithium dosage is adjusted in patients receiving this combination.

Certain non-steroidal anti-inflammatory agents (e.g.indometacin, acetylsalicylic acid) may attenuate the action of Lasilactone and may cause acute renal failure in cases of pre-existing hypovolaemia or dehydration.

Impairment of renal function may develop in patients receiving concurrent treatment with furosemide and high doses of certain cephalosporins.

Salicylate toxicity may be increased by Lasilactone. Furosemide may sometimes attenuate the effects of other drugs (e.g. the effects of antidiabetics and pressor amines) and sometimes potentiate them (e.g. the effects of salicylates, theophylline and curare-type muscle relaxants).

Lasilactone may potentiate the ototoxicity of aminoglycosides and other ototoxic drugs. Since this may lead to irreversible damage, these drugs must only be used with furosemide if there are compelling medical reasons.

There is a risk of ototoxic effects if cisplatin and furosemide are given concomitantly. In addition, nephrotoxicity of cisplatin may be enhanced if furosemide is not given in low doses (e.g. 40 mg in patients with normal renal function) and with positive fluid balance when used to achieve forced diuresis during cisplatin treatment.

Spironolactone may cause raised digoxin levels. Some electrolyte disturbances (e.g. hypokalaemia, hypomagnesaemia) may increase the toxicity of certain other drugs (e.g. digitalis preparations and drugs inducing QT interval prolongation syndrome).

Attenuation of the effect of furosemide may occur following concurrent administration of phenytoin.

Concomitant administration of carbamazepine or aminoglutethimide may increase the risk of hyponatraemia.

Corticosteroids administered concurrently may cause sodium retention.

Both spironolactone and carbenoloxone may impair the action of the other substance. In this regard, liquorice in larger amounts acts in a similar manner to carbenoxolone. Corticosteroids, carbenoxolone, liquorice, B_2 sympathomimetics in large amounts, prolonged use of laxatives, reboxetine and amphotericin may increase the risk of developing hypokalaemia.

Probenecid, methotrexate and other drugs which, like furosemide, undergo significant renal tubular secretion may reduce the effect of furosemide. Conversely, furosemide may decrease renal elimination of these drugs. In case of high-dose treatment (in particular, of both furosemide and the other drugs), this may lead to increased serum levels and an increased risk of adverse effects due to furosemide or the concomitant medication.

4.6 Pregnancy and lactation

Results of animal work, in general, show no hazardous effect of furosemide in pregnancy. There is clinical evidence of safety of the drug in the third trimester of human pregnancy; however, furosemide crosses the placental barrier.

Spironolactone or its metabolites may cross the placental barrier.

Lasilactone must not be used in pregnancy unless there are compelling medical reasons. Treatment during pregnancy requires monitoring of foetal growth.

Furosemide passes into breast milk and may inhibit lactation. Canrenone, a metabolite of spironolactone, appears in breast milk, Lasilactone must be avoided in nursing mothers.

4.7 Effects on ability to drive and use machines

Reduced mental alertness may impair the ability to drive or operate dangerous machinery. This applies especially at the commencement of treatment.

4.8 Undesirable effects

Furosemide is generally well tolerated.

Bone marrow depression has been reported as a rare complication and necessitates withdrawal of treatment.

Occasionally, thrombocytopenia may occur. In rare cases, leucopenia and, in isolated cases, agranulocytosis, aplastic anaemia or haemolytic anaemia may develop. Eosinophilia is rare.

Rarely, paraesthesiae may occur.

Serum calcium levels may be reduced; in very rare cases tetany has been observed. Nephrocalcinosis / Nephrolithiasis has been reported in premature infants.

Serum cholesterol and triglyceride levels may rise during furosemide treatment. During long-term therapy they will usually return to normal within six months.

Glucose tolerance may decrease with furosemide. In patients with diabetes mellitus this may lead to a deterioration of metabolic control; latent diabetes mellitus may become manifest.

Hearing disorders and tinnitus, although usually transitory, may occur in rare cases, particularly in patients with renal failure, hypoproteinaemia (e.g. in nephrotic syndrome) and/or when intravenous furosemide has been given too rapidly.

Furosemide may cause a reduction in blood pressure which, if pronounced may cause signs and symptoms such as impairment of concentration and reactions, light-headedness, sensations of pressure in the head, headache, dizziness, drowsiness, weakness, disorders of vision, dry mouth, orthostatic intolerance.

In isolated cases, intrahepatic cholestasis, an increase in liver transaminases or acute pancreatitis may develop.

The incidence of allergic reactions, such as skin rashes, photosensitivity, vasculitis, fever or interstitial nephritis, is very low, but when these occur treatment should be withdrawn. Skin and mucous membrane reactions may occasionally occur, e.g. itching, urticaria, other rashes or bullous lesions, erythema multiforme, exfoliative dermatitis, purpura.

As with other diuretics, electrolytes and water balance may be disturbed as a result of diuresis after prolonged therapy.

Furosemide leads to increased excretion of sodium and chloride and consequently water. In addition excretion of other electrolytes (in particular, calcium and magnesium) is increased. The two active ingredients exert opposing influences on potassium excretion. The serum potassium concentration may decrease, especially at the commencement of treatment (owing to the earlier onset of action of furosemide), although particularly as treatment is continued, the potassium concentration may increase (owing to the later onset of action of spironolactone), especially in patients with renal failure.

Symptomatic electrolyte disturbances and metabolic alkalosis may develop in the form of a gradually increasing electrolyte deficit or, e.g. where higher furosemide doses are administered to patients with normal renal function, acute severe electrolyte losses. Warning signs of electrolyte disturbances include increased thirst, headache, hypotension, confusion, muscle cramps, tetany, muscle weakness, disorders of cardiac rhythm and gastrointestinal symptoms. In the event of an irregular pulse, tiredness or muscle weakness (e.g., in the legs), particular consideration must be given to the possibility of hyperkalaemia. Pre-existing metabolic alkalosis (e.g. in decompensated cirrhosis of the liver) may be aggravated by furosemide treatment.

Disturbances in electrolyte balance, particularly if pronounced, must be corrected.

The diuretic action may lead to or contribute to hypovolaemia and dehydration, especially in elderly patients. To avert these, it is important to compensate any undesired losses of fluid (e.g., due to vomiting or diarrhoea, or to intense sweating). Severe fluid depletion may lead to haemoconcentration with a tendency for thromboses to develop.

Increased production of urine may provoke or aggravate complaints in patients with an obstruction of urinary outflow. Thus, acute retention of urine with possible secondary complications may occur for example, in patients with bladder-emptying disorders, prostatic hyperplasia or narrowing of the urethra.

If furosemide is administered to premature infants during the first weeks of life, it may increase the risk of persistence of patent ductus arteriosus.

Severe anaphylactic or anaphylactoid reactions (e.g. with shock) occur rarely.

Side-effects of a minor nature such as nausea, malaise or gastric upset (vomiting or diarrhoea) may occur but are not usually severe enough to necessitate withdrawal of treatment.

As with other diuretics, treatment with furosemide may lead to transitory increases in blood creatinine and urea levels. Serum levels of uric acid may increase and attacks of gout may occur.

Spironolactone has been reported to induce gastrointestinal intolerance. Stomach ulcers (sometimes with bleeding) have been reported rarely. Spironolactone may also cause drowsiness, headache, ataxia and mental confusion.

Because of its chemical similarity to the sex hormones, spironolactone may make the nipples more sensitive to touch. Dose dependent mastodynia and reversible gynaecomastia may occur in both sexes. Maculopapular or erythematous cutaneous eruptions have been reported rarely, as have mild androgenic manifestation such as hirsutism and menstrual irregularities. In men, potency may occasionally be impaired. Rarely, spironolactone may cause vocal changes in the form of hoarseness and (in women), deepening of the voice or (in men) increase in pitch. In some patients these vocal changes persist even after Lasilactone has been discontinued.

4.9 Overdose

The clinical picture in acute or chronic overdose depends primarily on the extent and consequences of electrolyte and fluid loss, e.g. hypovolaemia, dehydration, haemoconcentration, cardiac arrhythmias due to excessive diuresis. Symptoms of these disturbances include severe hypotension (progressing to shock), acute renal failure, thrombosis, delirious states, flaccid paralysis, apathy and confusion.

Treatment should therefore be aimed at fluid replacement and correction of the electrolyte imbalance. Together with the prevention and treatment of serious complications resulting from such disturbances and of other effects on the body (e.g., hyperkalaemia), this corrective action may necessitate general and specific intensive medical monitoring and therapeutic measures (e.g., to promote potassium elimination).

No specific antidote to furosemide is known. If ingestion has only just taken place, attempts may be made to limit further systemic absorption of the active ingredient by measures such as gastric lavage or those designated to reduce absorption (e.g. activated charcoal).

5. PHARMACOLOGICAL PROPERTIES

5.1 Pharmacodynamic properties

Furosemide: Furosemide is a diuretic acting on the Loop of Henle.

Spironolactone: Spironolactone is a competitive inhibitor of aldosterone.

5.2 Pharmacokinetic properties

Furosemide: Furosemide is a short-acting diuretic; diuresis usually commences within one hour and lasts for four to six hours.

Spironolactone: Spironolactone, a competitive inhibitor of aldosterone, increases sodium excretion whilst reducing potassium loss at the distal renal tubule. It has a slow and prolonged action, maximum response being usually attained after 2-3 days' treatment.

5.3 Preclinical safety data

Carcinogenicity: Spironolactone has been shown to produce tumours in rats when administered at high doses over a long period of time. The significance of these findings with respect to clinical use is not certain. However, the long-term use of spironolactone in young patients requires careful consideration of the benefits and the potential hazard involved.

6. PHARMACEUTICAL PARTICULARS

6.1 List of excipients

Lasilactone capsules contain microcrystalline cellulose, lactose, talc, magnesium stearate, sodium amylopectin glycolate, indigotin (FD&C Blue 2), titanium dioxide and gelatin.

6.2 Incompatibilities

None known.

6.3 Shelf life

Four years.

6.4 Special precautions for storage

Store at ambient temperature proteced from light.

6.5 Nature and contents of container

Blister pack containing 28 capsules.

6.6 Instructions for use and handling

Not applicable.

Administrative Data

7. MARKETING AUTHORISATION HOLDER

Hoechst Marion Roussel Limited

Broadwater Park

Denham

Uxbridge

Middlesex.

UB9 5HP.

8. MARKETING AUTHORISATION NUMBER(S)

PL 13402/0033

9. DATE OF FIRST AUTHORISATION/RENEWAL OF THE AUTHORISATION

31 December 1997.

10. DATE OF REVISION OF THE TEXT

November 2004

Lasix Injection 20mg/2ml

(sanofi-aventis)

1. NAME OF THE MEDICINAL PRODUCT

Lasix 20 mg /2 ml Injection

2. QUALITATIVE AND QUANTITATIVE COMPOSITION

Lasix 20 mg/2 ml Injection contains 20 mg Furosemide in 2 ml aqueous solution.

3. PHARMACEUTICAL FORM

Solution for injection.

4. CLINICAL PARTICULARS

4.1 Therapeutic indications

Lasix 20 mg/2 ml Injection is a diuretic indicated for use when a prompt and effective diuresis is required. The intravenous formulation is appropriate for use in emergencies or when oral therapy is precluded. Indications include cardiac, pulmonary, hepatic and renal oedema.

4.2 Posology and method of administration

Route of administration: intramuscular or intravenous

Intravenous furosemide must be injected or infused slowly; a rate of 4 mg per minute must not be exceeded. In patients with severe impairment of renal function (serum creatinine >5 mg/dl), it is recommended that an infusion rate of 2.5 mg per minute is not exceeded.

Intramuscular administration must be restricted to exceptional cases where neither oral nor intravenous administration are feasible. It must be noted that intramuscular injection is not suitable for the treatment of acute conditions such as pulmonary oedema.

To achieve optimum efficacy and suppress counter-regulation, a continuous furosemide infusion is generally to be preferred to repeated bolus injections. Where continuous furosemide infusion is not feasible for follow-up treatment after one or several acute bolus doses, a follow-up regimen with low doses given at short intervals (approx. 4 hours) is to be preferred to a regimen with higher bolus doses at longer intervals.

Doses of 20 to 50 mg intramuscularly or intravenously may be given initially. If larger doses are required, they should be given increasing by 20 mg increments and not given more often than every two hours. If doses greater than 50 mg are required it is recommended that they be given by slow intravenous infusion. The recommended maximum daily dose of furosemide administration is 1,500 mg.

Elderly: The dosage recommendations for adults apply, but in the elderly furosemide is generally eliminated more slowly. Dosage should be titrated until the required response is achieved.

Children: Parenteral doses for children range from 0.5 to 1.5 mg/kg body weight daily up to a maximum total daily dose of 20 mg.

4.3 Contraindications

Lasix 20 mg/2 ml Injection is contra-indicated in patients with hypovolaemia or dehydration, anuria or renal failure with anuria not responding to furosemide, renal failure as a result of poisoning by nephrotoxic or hepatotoxic agents or renal failure associated with hepatic coma, severe hypokalaemia, severe hyponatraemia, pre-comatose and comatose states associated with hepatic encephalopathy and breast feeding women.

Hypersensitivity to furosemide or any of the excipients of Lasix 20 mg/2 ml Injection. Patients allergic to sulphonamides may show cross-sensitivity to furosemide.

4.4 Special warnings and special precautions for use

Urinary output must be secured. Patients with partial obstruction of urinary outflow, for example patients with prostatic hypertrophy or impairment of micturition have an increased risk of developing acute retention and require careful monitoring.

Where indicated, steps should be taken to correct hypotension or hypovolaemia before commencing therapy.

Particularly careful monitoring is necessary in:

- patients with hypotension.
- patients who are at risk from a pronounced fall in blood pressure.
- patients where latent diabetes may become manifest or the insulin requirements of diabetic patients may increase.
- patients with gout
- patients with hepatorenal syndrome
- patients with hypoproteinaemia, e.g. associated with nephritic syndrome (the effect of furosemide may be weakened and its ototoxicity potentiated). Cautious dose titration is required.
- premature infants (possible development nephrocalcinosis nephrolithiasis; renal function must be monitored and renal ultrasonography performed).

Caution should be observed in patients liable to electrolyte deficiency. Regular monitoring of serum sodium, potassium and creatinine is generally recommended during furosemide therapy; particularly close monitoring is required in patients at high risk of developing electrolyte imbalances or in case of significant additional fluid loss. Hypovolaemia or dehydration as well as any significant electrolyte and acid-base disturbances must be corrected. This may require temporary discontinuation of furosemide.

4.5 Interaction with other medicinal products and other forms of Interaction

The dosage of concurrently administered cardiac glycosides or anti-hypertensive agents may require adjustment.

A marked fall in blood pressure and deterioration in renal function may be seen when ACE inhibitors are added to furosemide therapy. The dose of furosemide should be reduced for at least three days, or the drug stopped, before initiating the ACE inhibitor or increasing the dose of an ACE inhibitor.

The toxic effects of nephrotoxic antibiotics may be increased by concomitant administration of potent diuretics such as furosemide.

Impairment of renal function may develop in patients receiving treatment with furosemide and high doses of certain cephalosporins.

Oral furosemide and sucralfate must not be taken within 2 hours of each other because sucralfate decreases the absorption of furosemide from the intestine and so reduces its effect.

In common with other diuretics, serum lithium levels may be increased when lithium is given concomitantly with furosemide, resulting in increased lithium toxicity. Therefore, it is recommended that lithium levels are carefully monitored and where necessary the lithium dosage is adjusted in patients receiving this combination.

Certain non-steroidal anti-inflammatory agents (e.g. indometacin, acetylsalicylic acid) may attenuate the action of furosemide and may cause acute renal failure in cases of pre-existing hypovolaemia or dehydration. Salicylate toxicity may be increased by furosemide. Furosemide may sometimes attenuate the effects of other drugs (e.g. the effects of anti-diabetics and of pressor amines) and sometimes potentiate them (e.g. the effects of salicylates, theophylline and curare-type muscle relaxants).

Furosemide may potentiate the ototoxicity of aminoglycosides and other ototoxic drugs. Since this may lead to irreversible damage, these drugs must only be used with furosemide if there are compelling medical reasons.

There is a risk of ototoxic effects if cisplatin and furosemide are given concomitantly. In addition, nephrotoxicity of cisplatin may be enhanced if furosemide is not given in low doses (e.g. 40 mg in patients with normal renal function) and with positive fluid balance when used to achieve forced diuresis during cisplatin treatment.

Some electrolyte disturbances (e.g. hypokalaemia, hypomagnesaemia) may increase the toxicity of certain other drugs (e.g. digitalis preparations and drugs inducing QT interval prolongation syndrome).

Attenuation of the effect of furosemide may occur following concurrent administration of phenytoin.

Concomitant administration of carbamazepine or aminoglutethimide may increase the risk of hyponatraemia.

Corticosteroids administered concurrently may cause sodium retention.

Corticosteroids, carbenoxolone, liquorice, B_2 sympathomimetics in large amounts, prolonged use of laxatives, reboxetine and amphotericin may increase the risk of developing hypokalaemia.

Probenecid, methotrexate and other drugs which, like furosemide, undergo significant renal tubular secretion may reduce the effect of furosemide. Conversely, furosemide may decrease renal elimination of these drugs. In case of high-dose treatment (in particular, of both furosemide and the other drugs), this may lead to increased serum levels and an increased risk of adverse effects due to furosemide or the concomitant medication.

4.6 Pregnancy and lactation

Results of animal work, in general, show no hazardous effect of furosemide in pregnancy. There is clinical evidence of safety of the drug in the third trimester of human pregnancy; however, furosemide crosses the placental barrier. It must not be given during pregnancy unless there are compelling medical reasons. Treatment during pregnancy requires monitoring of fetal growth.

Furosemide passes into breast milk and may inhibit lactation. Women must not breast-feed if they are treated with furosemide.

4.7 Effects on ability to drive and use machines

Reduced mental alertness may impair ability to drive or operate dangerous machinery.

4.8 Undesirable effects

Lasix 20 mg/2 ml Injection is generally well tolerated.

Eosinophilia is rare.

Occasionally, thrombocytopenia may occur. In rare cases, leucopenia and, in isolated cases, agranulocytosis, aplastic anaemia or haemolytic anaemia may develop.

Bone marrow depression has been reported as a rare complication and necessitates withdrawal of treatment.

Rarely, paraesthesiae may occur.

Serum calcium levels may be reduced; in very rare cases tetany has been observed. Nephrocalcinosis / Nephrolithiasis has been reported in premature infants.

Serum cholesterol and triglyceride levels may rise during furosemide treatment. During long term therapy they will usually return to normal within six months.

Glucose tolerance may decrease with furosemide. In patients with diabetes mellitus this may lead to a deterioration of metabolic control; latent diabetes mellitus may become manifest.

Hearing disorders and tinnitus, although usually transitory, may occur in rare cases, particularly in patients with renal failure, hypoproteinaemia (e.g. in nephritic syndrome) and/ or when intravenous furosemide has been given too rapidly.

Furosemide may cause a reduction in blood pressure which, if pronounced may cause signs and symptoms such as impairment of concentration and reactions, light-headedness, sensations of pressure in the head, headache, dizziness, drowsiness, weakness, disorders of vision, dry mouth, orthostatic intolerance.

In isolated cases, intrahepatic cholestasis, an increase in liver transaminases or acute pancreatitis may develop.

The incidence of allergic reactions, such as skin rashes, photosensitivity, vasculitis, fever, interstitial nephritis or shock is very low, but when these occur treatment should be withdrawn. Skin and mucous membrane reactions may occasionally occur, e.g. itching, urticaria, other rashes or bullous lesions, erythema multiforme, exfoliative dermatitis, purpura.

As with other diuretics, electrolytes and water balance may be disturbed as a result of diuresis after prolonged therapy. Furosemide leads to increased excretion of sodium and chloride and consequently water. In addition excretion of other electrolytes (in particular potassium, calcium and magnesium) is increased. Symptomatic electrolyte disturbances and metabolic alkalosis may develop in the form of a gradually increasing electrolyte deficit or, e.g. where higher furosemide doses are administered to patients with normal renal function, acute severe electolyte losses. Warning signs of electrolyte disturbances include increased thirst, headache, hypotension, confusion, muscle cramps, tetany, muscle weakness, disorders of cardiac rhythm and gastrointestinal symptoms. Pre-existing metabolic alkalosis (e.g. in decompensated cirrhosis of the liver) may be aggravated by furosemide treatment.

The diuretic action of furosemide may lead to or contribute to hypovolaemia and dehydration, especially in elderly patients. Severe fluid depletion may lead to haemoconcentration with a tendency for thromboses to develop.

Increased production of urine may provoke or aggravate complaints in patients with an obstruction of urinary outflow. Thus, acute retention of urine with possible secondary complications may occur, for example, in patients with bladder-emptying disorders, prostatic hyperplasia or narrowing of the urethra.

If furosemide is administered to premature infants during the first weeks of life, it may increase the risk of persistence of patent ductus arteriosus.

Severe anaphylactic or anaphylactoid reactions (e.g. with shock) occur rarely.

Side-effects of a minor nature such as nausea, malaise or gastric upset (vomiting or diarrhoea) may occur but are not usually severe enough to necessitate withdrawal of treatment.

Following intramuscular injection, local reactions such as pain may occur.

As with other diuretics, treatment with furosemide may lead to transitory increases in blood creatinine and urea levels. Serum levels of uric acid may increase and attacks of gout may occur.

4.9 Overdose

The clinical picture in acute or chronic overdose depends primarily on the extent and consequences of electrolyte and fluid loss, e.g. hypovolaemia, dehydration, haemoconcentration, cardiac arrhythmias due to excessive diuresis. Symptoms of these disturbances include severe hypotension (progressing to shock), acute renal failure, thrombosis, delirious states, flaccid paralysis, apathy and confusion.

Treatment should therefore be aimed at fluid replacement and correction of the electrolyte imbalance. Together with the prevention and treatment of serious complications resulting from such disturbances and of other effects on the body, this corrective action may necessitate general and specific intensive medical monitoring and therapeutic measures.

No specific antidote to furosemide is known. If ingestion has only just taken place, attempts may be made to limit further systemic absorption of the active ingredient by measures such as gastric lavage or those designated to reduce absorption (e.g. activated charcoal).

5. PHARMACOLOGICAL PROPERTIES

5.1 Pharmacodynamic properties

The evidence from many experimental studies suggests that furosemide acts along the entire nephron with the exception of the distal exchange site. The main effect is on the ascending limb of the loop of Henle with a complex effect on renal circulation. Blood-flow is diverted from the juxta-medullary region to the outer cortex. The principle renal action of furosemide is to inhibit active chloride transport in the thick ascending limb. Re-absorption of sodium chloride from the nephron is reduced and a hypotonic or isotonic urine produced. It has been established that prostaglandin (PG) biosynthesis and the renin-angiotensin system are affected by furosemide administration and that furosemide alters the renal permeability of the glomerulus to serum proteins.

5.2 Pharmacokinetic properties

Furosemide is a weak carboxylic acid which exists mainly in the dissociated form in the gastrointestinal tract. Furosemide is rapidly but incompletely absorbed (60-70%) on oral administration and its effect is largely over within 4 hours. The optimal absorption site is the upper duodenum at pH 5.0. Regardless of route of administration 69-97% of activity from a radio-labelled dose is excreted in the first 4 hours after the drug is given. Furosemide is bound to plasma albumin and little biotransformation takes place. Furosemide is mainly eliminated via the kidneys (80-90%); a small fraction of the dose undergoes biliary elimination and 10-15% of the activity can be recovered from the faeces.

<u>In renal/ hepatic impairment</u>

Where liver disease is present, biliary elimination is reduced up to 50%. Renal impairment has little effect on the elimination rate of Lasix 20 mg/2 ml Injection, but less than 20% residual renal function increases the elimination time.

The elderly

The elimination of furosemide is delayed in the elderly where a certain degree of renal impairment is present.

New born

A sustained diuretic effect is seen in the newborn, possibly due to immature tubular function.

5.3 Preclinical safety data
Not applicable

6. PHARMACEUTICAL PARTICULARS

6.1 List of excipients
Sodium hydroxide BP, Sodium chloride BP, Water for Injection BP.

6.2 Incompatibilities
Furosemide may precipitate out of solution in fluids of low pH (e.g. dextrose solutions).

6.3 Shelf life
60 months

6.4 Special precautions for storage
Lasix 20 mg/2 ml Injection should be stored protected from light.

6.5 Nature and contents of container
Each pack contains 5x 2ml Lasix 20 mg/2 ml Injection in amber glass ampoules.

6.6 Instructions for use and handling
Lasix 20 mg/2 ml Injection solution should not be mixed with any other drugs in the injection bottle.

7. MARKETING AUTHORISATION HOLDER
Hoechst Marion Roussel Limited
Broadwater Park
Denham
Uxbridge
Middlesex, UB9 5HP
UK

8. MARKETING AUTHORISATION NUMBER(S)
PL13402/0035

9. DATE OF FIRST AUTHORISATION/RENEWAL OF THE AUTHORISATION
31 December 1997

10. DATE OF REVISION OF THE TEXT
December 2004

Legal Category: POM

Lasonil/Bruiseze

(Bayer plc)

1. NAME OF THE MEDICINAL PRODUCT
Lasonil (also available GSL as Bruiseze).

2. QUALITATIVE AND QUANTITATIVE COMPOSITION
100g of ointment contains Heparinoid 'Bayer' 5000 HDB-U (Heparinoid Bayer Units). This is equivalent to 0.8% w/w.

3. PHARMACEUTICAL FORM
Ointment.

4. CLINICAL PARTICULARS

4.1 Therapeutic indications
The relief of traumatic conditions: e.g. bruises, sprains and soft tissue injuries.

4.2 Posology and method of administration
Adults and Elderly:

The ointment should be applied thickly and gently massaged into the affected area two or three times daily.

Children:

No clinical studies have been performed in children up to the age of 12 years. However, there is documented use of this product in children and the safety profile is similar to that reported in adults.

For GSL use:

Not recommended in children under 6 years of age. Medical advice should be sought if no improvement is seen within 5 days of treatment.

4.3 Contraindications
The ointment is contraindicated for use in:

Patients with known hypersensitivity to any of the ingredients.

Patients taking oral anticoagulants (see Section 4.5 Interactions).

Senile purpura.

4.4 Special warnings and special precautions for use
Lasonil should be applied to unbroken skin only. It should not be applied to open or infected wounds or ulcers, mucous membranes and large areas of skin.

A physician should be consulted if the patient:

Experiences spontaneous bruising.

Is unable to weight-bear as a result of the injury.

Has extensive bruising of the lower limbs.

Suffers recurrent bruising or bruising in response to minor trauma.

First aid measures such as rest, ice, compression and elevation should be implemented before the ointment is applied.

4.5 Interaction with other medicinal products and other forms of Interaction
Concurrent use of this product with systemically administered anticoagulants may lead to further prolongation of prothrombin time.

4.6 Pregnancy and lactation
There is no evidence to suggest that Lasonil should not be used during pregnancy and lactation. However, it should be used with caution during the first trimester.

4.7 Effects on ability to drive and use machines
None.

4.8 Undesirable effects
Very rarely (<1/10,000) erythema and hypersensitivity reactions occur which subside when treatment with the ointment is stopped.

4.9 Overdose
In the unlikely event of Lasonil being taken orally, treat symptomatically.

5. PHARMACOLOGICAL PROPERTIES

5.1 Pharmacodynamic properties
Heparinoid has been shown to prolong blood-clotting time locally and has anti-inflammatory, thrombolytic and anti-exudatory activity.

5.2 Pharmacokinetic properties
Heparinoids have a half-life of 2-6 hours after intravenous administration. There is no definitive evidence to date that heparins or heparinoids are absorbed after oral administration.

The transdermal absorption under intact anatomical conditions is between 1% and 2%. The transdermal absorption of high-dose heparinoids has been demonstrated by detecting their anticoagulant activities in both intact and surface-modified skin preparations (skin without epidermis) from various animals and man. Topical effects are assessed by measuring the influence of the substances on oedemas and haematomas.

The recalcification time and the thrombin time in blood were significantly prolonged after topical application of a heparinoid ointment to human subjects. The anticoagulant effect was seen about 2 hours after application of the ointment. It reached a peak after 5 hours and remained detectable for 8 hours.

The absorption rate of radio-labelled heparinoid in guinea-pigs following depilation of the skin was over 33% after 10 hours.

5.3 Preclinical safety data
There are no pre-clinical data of relevance to the prescriber which are additional to the information included in other sections of the SPC.

6. PHARMACEUTICAL PARTICULARS

6.1 List of excipients
Lasonil contains the following excipients:

White petroleum jelly DAB

Wool Alcohols Ph.Eur

6.2 Incompatibilities
None known.

6.3 Shelf life
36 months.

6.4 Special precautions for storage
Do not store above 30°C.

6.5 Nature and contents of container
Aluminium tube with an inner protective layer and cardboard outer carton. Sizes available are 20g (GSL) and 40g (P).

6.6 Instructions for use and handling
Not applicable.

7. MARKETING AUTHORISATION HOLDER
Bayer plc
Bayer House
Strawberry Hill
Newbury
Berkshire RG14 1JA
Trading as Bayer plc, Consumer Care Division

8. MARKETING AUTHORISATION NUMBER(S)
PL 0010/0241

9. DATE OF FIRST AUTHORISATION/RENEWAL OF THE AUTHORISATION
Date of first authorisation: 4 October 1999.

10. DATE OF REVISION OF THE TEXT
August 2001

LEGAL CATEGORY

Lasonil	P
Bruiseze	GSL

Lasoride

(sanofi-aventis)

1. NAME OF THE MEDICINAL PRODUCT
LASORIDE ™

2. QUALITATIVE AND QUANTITATIVE COMPOSITION
In terms of the active ingredient

The active ingredient is Furosemide 40.0mg and amiloride hydrochloride equivalent to 5.0mg anhydrous amiloride hydrochloride.

3. PHARMACEUTICAL FORM
Tablets for oral administration.

4. CLINICAL PARTICULARS

4.1 Therapeutic indications
Lasoride is a potassium sparing diuretic which is indicated where a prompt diuresis is required. It is of particular value in conditions where potassium conservation is important: congestive cardiac failure, nephrosis, corticosteroid therapy, oestrogen therapy and for ascites associated with cirrhosis.

4.2 Posology and method of administration
Adults: One or two tablets to be taken in the morning.

Children: Not recommended for children under 18 years of age as safety and efficacy have not been established.

Elderly: The dosage should be adjusted according to the diuretic response; serum electrolytes and urea should be carefully monitored.

4.3 Contraindications
Hyperkalaemia (serum potassium >5.3mmol/litre), Addison's disease, acute renal failure, anuria, severe progressive renal disease, electrolyte imbalance, precomatose states associated with cirrhosis, concomitant potassium supplements or potassium sparing diuretics, known sensitivity to furosemide or amiloride.

Lasoride is contra-indicated in children under 18 years of age as safety in this age group has not been established.

4.4 Special warnings and special precautions for use
Lasoride should be discontinued before a glucose tolerance test.

Patients who are being treated with this preparation require regular supervision, with monitoring of fluid electrolyte states to avoid excessive loss of fluid.

Lasoride should be used with particular caution in elderly patients or those with potential obstruction of the urinary tract or disorders rendering electrolyte balance precarious.

4.5 Interaction with other medicinal products and other forms of Interaction
Lasoride may enhance the nephrotoxicity of cephalosporin antibacterials such as cephalothin, NSAID's or cisplatin, and enhance the ototoxicity of aminoglycoside antibacterials and other ototoxic drugs.

Concurrent use of other diuretics, reboxetine, sympathomimetic agents, corticosteroids, ampotericin and carbenoxolone may lead to an increased risk of hypokalaemia.

The diuretic effect of Lasoride may be reduced by concurrent use of phenytoin or NSAID's, notably indomethacin and ketorolac. Severe diuresis may occur if metolazone is administered concomitantly.

Hyperkalaemia may occur in patients receiving potassium salts, ACE Inhibitors, indometacin and possibly other NSAID's, ciclosporin or trilostane.

Potentially serious hypokalaemia may result from beta$_2$-adreno-receptor stimulant therapy. Particular caution is required with concomitant therapy with diuretics.

If other antihypertensives or drugs which can lead to a reduction in blood pressure are taken concurrently with Lasoride, a more pronounced fall in blood pressure must be anticipated. Profound first-dose hypotension may occur when ACE inhibitors are introduced to patients with heart failure who are already taking a high dose of a loop diuretic (e.g. furosemide 80mg daily or more). Temporary withdrawal of the loop diuretic reduces the risk, but may cause severe rebound pulmonary oedema. The ACE inhibitor should, therefore, be started at a very low dosage (e.g. captopril 6.25mg), with the patient recumbent and under close medical supervision and with facilities to treat profound hypotension. In these circumstances the patient should be admitted to hospital for initiation of therapy.

Lasoride may antagonise the effects of antidiabetic drugs and pressor amines and potentiate the effects of lithium and curare-type muscle relaxants.

Concomitant administration of carbamazepine or aminoglutethimide may increase the risk of hyponatraemia.

The dosage of concurrently administered cardiac glycosides may also require adjustment.

4.6 Pregnancy and lactation
The safety of Lasoride during pregnancy and lactation has not been established.

4.7 Effects on ability to drive and use machines
None stated.

4.8 Undesirable effects

Serum uric acid levels may rise during treatment with Lasoride and acute attacks of gout may be precipitated.

Malaise, dry mouth, gastric upset, nausea, vomiting, diarrhoea and constipation may occur.

If skin rashes or pruritus occur treatment should be withdrawn. Rare complications may include minor psychiatric disturbances, disturbances in liver function tests and ototoxicity. Bone marrow depression occasionally complicates treatment, necessitating withdrawal of the product. The haematopoietic state should be regularly monitored during treatment.

Hyponatraemia, hypochloraemia and raised blood urea nitrogen may occur during vigorous diuresis, especially in seriously ill patients. Careful monitoring of serum electrolytes and urea should therefore be undertaken in these patients. Hyperkalaemia has been observed in patients receiving amiloride hydrochloride.

As ACE inhibitors may elevate serum potassium levels, especially in the presence of renal impairment, combination with Lasoride is best avoided in elderly patients or in any others in whom renal function may be compromised. If use of the combination is deemed essential clinical condition and serum electrolytes must be continuously monitored.

Furosemidemay cause latent diabetes to become manifest. It may be necessary to increase the dose of hypoglycaemic agents in diabetic patients.

Patients with prostatic hypertrophy or impairment of micturition have an increased risk of developing acute urinary retention during diuretic therapy.

4.9 Overdose

Treatment of overdosage should be aimed at reversing dehydration and correcting electrolyte imbalance, particularly hyperkalaemia. Emesis should be induced or gastric lavage performed. Treatment should be symptomatic and supportive. If hyperkalaemia is seen, appropriate measures to reduce serum potassium must be instituted.

5. PHARMACOLOGICAL PROPERTIES

5.1 Pharmacodynamic properties

FUROSEMIDE:

Furosemide is a loop diuretic which acts primarily to inhibit electrolyte reabsorption in the thick ascending Loop of Henle. Excretion of sodium, potassium and chloride ions is increased and water excretion enhanced.

AMILORIDE:

Amiloride is a mild diuretic which moderately increases the excretion of sodium and chloride and reduces potassium excretion, and appears to act mainly on the distal renal tubules. It does not appear to act by inhibition of aldosterone and does not inhibit carbonic anhydrase. Amiloride adds to the natiuretic but diminishes the kaliuretic effect of other diuretics.

A combination of Furosemide and Amiloride is a diuretic which reduces the potassium loss of furosemidealone while avoiding the possible gastro-intestinal disturbances of potassium supplements.

5.2 Pharmacokinetic properties

FUROSEMIDE:

Approximately 65% of the dose is absorbed after oral administration. The plasma half-life is biphasic with a terminal elimination phase of about 1½ hours. Furosemideis up to 99% bound to plasma proteins and is mainly excreted in the urine, largely unchanged, but also excreted in the bile, non-renal elimination being considerably increased in renal failure. Furosemide crosses the placental barrier and is excreted in the milk.

AMILORIDE:

Approximately 50% of the dose is absorbed after oral administration and peak serum concentrations are achieved by about 3 - 4 hours. The serum half-life is estimated to be about 6 hours. Amiloride is not bound to plasma proteins. Amiloride is not metabolised and is excreted unchanged in the urine.

Pharmacokinetic studies have been completed on Lasoride.

FUROSEMIDE	AMILORIDE
Cp MAX = 1/14 μg/ml	Cp MAX = 13.42 ng/ml
SD = 0.67	SD = 5.74
Tmax = 3.0 hours	Tmax = 4.0 hours
AUC = 3.17μg/ml hr SD = ± 1.25	AUC = 154 ng/ml hr SD = ± 65.2

5.3 Preclinical safety data

No further information available

6. PHARMACEUTICAL PARTICULARS

6.1 List of excipients

Lasoride tablets contain the following excipients:

Lactose

Starch Maize

Microcrystalline Cellulose

Sodium Starch Glycollate

Sunset Yellow Dye (E110)

French Chalk Powdered

Colloidal Anhydrous Silica

Magnesium Stearate

6.2 Incompatibilities

None stated.

6.3 Shelf life

The shelf-life of Lasoride is 3 years.

6.4 Special precautions for storage

Store below 25°C in a dry place. Protect from light.

6.5 Nature and contents of container

Blister packs of 28 tablets.

6.6 Instructions for use and handling

None

Administrative Data

7. MARKETING AUTHORISATION HOLDER

Helios Healthcare Limited

11A Ferraidy Street

Peyki-Attikis

Greece

8. MARKETING AUTHORISATION NUMBER(S)

PL 17076/0001

9. DATE OF FIRST AUTHORISATION/RENEWAL OF THE AUTHORISATION

01 September 1998

10. DATE OF REVISION OF THE TEXT

November 2004

Legal Category: POM

Laxoberal & Dulco-Lax Liquid

(Boehringer Ingelheim Limited Self-Medication Division)

1. NAME OF THE MEDICINAL PRODUCT

LAXOBERAL Liquid*

DULCO-LAX Liquid**

* P ** GSL

2. QUALITATIVE AND QUANTITATIVE COMPOSITION

Each 5ml of liquid contains 5mg sodium picosulfate.

For excipients, see 6.1.

3. PHARMACEUTICAL FORM

Oral solution.

Golden orange coloured liquid, with a fruit-like odour and taste.

4. CLINICAL PARTICULARS

4.1 Therapeutic indications

Pharmacy only and GSL:

Short term relief of constipation

Pharmacy only:

For the management of constipation of any aetiology. For bowel clearance before surgery, childbirth or radiological investigations.

4.2 Posology and method of administration

For oral administration

Unless otherwise prescribed by the doctor, the following dosages are recommended:

Pharmacy only and GSL:

Adults and children over 10 years:

One to two 5 ml spoonfuls (5 - 10 mg) at night.

Pharmacy only:

Children under 10 years:

Not to be taken by children under 10 years without medical advice.

Children (4 - 10 years):

Half to one 5 ml spoonful (2.5 - 5 mg) at night.

Children under 4 years:

The recommended dosage is 250 micrograms per kilogram body weight.

In the management of constipation, once regularity has restarted dosage should be reduced and can usually be discontinued.

Diluent: Can be diluted with purified water.

4.3 Contraindications

Not to be used in patients with ileus, intestinal obstruction, acute surgical abdominal conditions like acute appendicitis, acute inflammatory bowel diseases, and in severe dehydration. Not to be used in patients with a known hypersensitivity to sodium picosulfate or any other component of the product.

4.4 Special warnings and special precautions for use

As with all laxatives, Laxoberal should not be taken on a continuous daily basis for long periods. Patients who need to take laxatives frequently should do so under medical supervision only and should have the cause of their constipation investigated.

Prolonged excessive use may lead to fluid and electrolyte imbalance and hypokalaemia, and may precipitate onset of rebound constipation.

Not to be taken by children under 10 years without medical advice.

4.5 Interaction with other medicinal products and other forms of Interaction

The concomitant use of diuretics or adreno-corticosteroids may increase the risk of electrolyte imbalance. However, this situation only arises if excessive doses are taken (See Overdose Section).

Concurrent administration of broad spectrum antibiotics may reduce the laxative action of this product.

4.6 Pregnancy and lactation

There are no reports of undesirable or damaging effects during pregnancy or to the foetus attributable to the use of this product. Nevertheless, medicines should not be used in pregnancy, especially the first trimester, unless the expected benefit is thought to outweigh any possible risk to the foetus.

Although the active ingredient is not known to be excreted in breast milk, use of this product during breast feeding is not recommended.

4.7 Effects on ability to drive and use machines

None stated.

4.8 Undesirable effects

Abdominal discomfort (including abdominal pain and cramps) and diarrhoea may occasionally occur.

Isolated cases of allergic reactions, including skin reactions and angio-oedema have been reported rarely in association with the administration of sodium picosulfate.

4.9 Overdose

Symptoms: If high doses are taken diarrhoea, abdominal cramps and a clinically significant loss of potassium and other electrolytes can occur. This may also lead to increased sensitivity to cardiac glycosides.

Furthermore, cases of colonic mucosal ischaemia have been reported in association with doses of Laxoberal considerably higher than those recommended for the routine management of constipation.

Laxatives in chronic overdosage are known to cause chronic diarrhoea, abdominal pain, hypokalaemia, secondary hyperaldosteronism and renal calculi. Renal tubular damage, metabolic alkalosis and muscle weakness secondary to hypokalaemia have also been described in association with chronic laxative abuse.

Therapy: Within a short time of ingestion, absorption can be minimised or prevented by inducing vomiting or by gastric lavage. Replacement of fluids and correction of electrolyte imbalance may be required. This is especially important in the elderly and the young. Administration of antispasmodics may be of some value.

5. PHARMACOLOGICAL PROPERTIES

5.1 Pharmacodynamic properties

Sodium picosulfate is a locally acting laxative from the triarylmethane group, which after bacterial cleavage in the colon, has the dual-action of stimulating the mucosa of both the large intestine causing peristalsis and of the rectum causing increased motility and a feeling of rectal fullness. The rectal effect may help to restore the "call to stool" although its clinical relevance remains to be established.

5.2 Pharmacokinetic properties

After oral ingestion, sodium picosulfate reaches the colon without any appreciable absorption. Therefore, enterohepatic circulation is avoided. By bacterial cleavage the active form, the free diphenol, is formed in the colon. Consequently, there is an onset of action between 6 - 12 hours, which is determined by the conversion of the drug substance to the active substance.

After administration, only small amounts of the drug are systemically available. Urinary excretion reflects low systemic burden after oral administration.

There is no relationship between the laxative effect and plasma levels of diphenol.

5.3 Preclinical safety data

There are no pre-clinical data of relevance to the prescriber which are additional to that already included in other sections of the SPC.

6. PHARMACEUTICAL PARTICULARS

6.1 List of excipients

Sodium Carboxymethylcellulose

Methyl p-Hydroxybenzoate

Propyl p-Hydroxybenzoate

Glycerol

Aroma Tutti Frutti (flavouring)

Saccharin Sodium

FD & C Yellow 6 (E110) (colouring)

Ethanol 96%

0.1 M Sodium Hydroxide

Purified Water

6.2 Incompatibilities

None stated

6.3 Shelf life

5 years

6.4 Special precautions for storage

Keep the container in the outer carton

6.5 Nature and contents of container
Amber glass bottles with aluminium ROPP caps.

Pack sizes of 30, 40, 50, 60, 90, and 500 ml.

Amber glass bottles with polypropylene tamper-evident closure with expanded polyethylene (coated with LDPE) liner.

Pack sizes of 100, 250 and 300 ml.

Not all pack sizes may be marketed.

6.6 Instructions for use and handling
Not applicable.

7. MARKETING AUTHORISATION HOLDER
Boehringer Ingelheim Limited

Ellesfield Avenue

Bracknell

Berkshire

RG12 8YS

Trading as Boehringer Ingelheim Self-Medication Division

8. MARKETING AUTHORISATION NUMBER(S)
PL 00015/0249

9. DATE OF FIRST AUTHORISATION/RENEWAL OF THE AUTHORISATION
1st April 1999

10. DATE OF REVISION OF THE TEXT
January 2004

11. Legal Category
90, 100, 250, 300, 500 ml: **P**

30, 40, 50, 60 ml: **GSL**

L1a/UK/SPC/15

Lederfolin Solution (Calcium Leucovorin Solution for Injection 350mg/vial)

(Wyeth Pharmaceuticals)

1. NAME OF THE MEDICINAL PRODUCT
Lederfolin 350mg/35ml Solution for Injection or Infusion

2. QUALITATIVE AND QUANTITATIVE COMPOSITION
Each vial of 35ml solution contains 10 mg/ml of folinic acid provided as calcium folinate

For excipients, see 6.1.

3. PHARMACEUTICAL FORM
Solution for Injection or Infusion

Clear, yellow solution

4. CLINICAL PARTICULARS

4.1 Therapeutic indications
Calcium folinate is indicated

- to diminish the toxicity and counteract the action of folic acid antagonists such as methotrexate in cytotoxic therapy and overdose in adults and children. In cytotoxic therapy, this procedure is commonly known as "Calcium Folinate Rescue"

- in combination with 5-fluorouracil in cytotoxic therapy.

4.2 Posology and method of administration
For intravenous and intramuscular administration only. In the case of intravenous administration, no more than 160 mg of calcium folinate should be injected per minute due to the calcium content of the solution.

For intravenous infusion, calcium folinate may be diluted with 0.9% sodium chloride solution or 5% glucose solution before use. Refer also to sections 6.3 and 6.6.

Calcium folinate rescue in methotrexate therapy:

Since the calcium folinate rescue dosage regimen depends heavily on the posology and method of the intermediate- or high-dose methotrexate administration, the methotrexate protocol will dictate the dosage regimen of calcium folinate rescue. Therefore, it is best to refer to the applied intermediate or high dose methotrexate protocol for posology and method of administration of calcium folinate.

The following guidelines may serve as an illustration of regimens used in adults, elderly and children:

Calcium folinate rescue has to be performed by parenteral administration in patients with malabsorption syndromes or other gastrointestinal disorders where enteral absorption is not assured. Dosages above 25-50 mg should be given parenterally due to saturable enteral absorption of calcium folinate.

Calcium folinate rescue is necessary when methotrexate is given at doses exceeding 500 mg/m^2 body surface and should be considered with doses of 100 mg – 500 mg/m^2 body surface.

Dosage and duration of calcium folinate rescue primarily depend on the type and dosage of methotrexate therapy, the occurrence of toxicity symptoms, and the individual excretion capacity for methotrexate. As a rule, the first dose of calcium folinate is 15 mg (6-12 mg/m^2) to be given 12-24 hours (24 hours at the latest) after the beginning of methotrexate infusion. The same dose is given every 6 hours throughout a period of 72 hours. After several parenteral doses treatment can be switched over to the oral form.

In addition to calcium folinate administration, measures to ensure the prompt excretion of methotrexate (maintenance of high urine output and alkalinisation of urine) are integral parts of the calcium folinate rescue treatment. Renal function should be monitored through daily measurements of serum creatinine.

Forty-eight hours after the start of the methotrexate infusion, the residual methotrexate-level should be measured. If the residual methotrexate-level is >0.5 μmol/l, calcium folinate dosages should be adapted according to the following table:

Residual methotrexate blood level 48 hours after the start of the methotrexate administration:	Additional calcium folinate to be administered every 6 hours for 48 hours or until levels of methotrexate are lower than 0.05 μmol/l:
$\geqslant$0.5 μmol/l	15 mg/m^2
$\geqslant$1.0 μmol/l	100 mg/m^2
$\geqslant$2.0 μmol/l	200 mg/m^2

In combination with 5-fluorouracil in cytotoxic therapy:

Different regimens and different dosages are used, without any dosage having been proven to be the optimal one.

The following regimens have been used in adults and elderly in the treatment of advanced or metastatic colorectal cancer and are given as examples. There are no data on the use of these combinations in children:

Bimonthly regimen: Calcium folinate 200 mg/m^2 by intravenous infusion over two hours, followed by bolus 400 mg/m^2 of 5-FU and 22-hour infusion of 5-FU (600 mg/m^2) for 2 consecutive days, every 2 weeks on days 1 and 2.

Weekly regimen: Calcium folinate 20 mg/m^2 by bolus i.v. injection or 200 to 500 mg/m^2 as i.v. infusion over a period of 2 hours plus 500 mg/m^2 5-fluorouracil as i.v. bolus injection in the middle or at the end of the calcium folinate infusion.

Monthly regimen: Calcium folinate 20 mg/m^2 by bolus i.v. injection or 200 to 500 mg/m^2 as i.v. infusion over a period of 2 hours immediately followed by 425 or 370 mg/m^2 5-fluorouracil as i.v. bolus injection during five consecutive days.

For the combination therapy with 5-fluorouracil, modification of the 5-fluorouracil dosage and the treatment-free interval may be necessary depending on patient condition, clinical response and dose limiting toxicity as stated in the product information of 5-fluorouracil. A reduction of calcium folinate dosage is not required.

The number of repeat cycles used is at the discretion of the clinician.

Antidote to the folic acid antagonists trimetrexate, trimethoprime, and pyrimethamine:

Trimetrexate toxicity:

• Prevention: Calcium folinate should be administered every day during treatment with trimetrexate and for 72 hours after the last dose of trimetrexate. Calcium folinate can be administered either by the intravenous route at a dose of 20 mg/m^2 for 5 to 10 minutes every 6 hours for a total daily dose of 80 mg/m^2, or by oral route with four doses of 20 mg/m^2 administered at equal time intervals. Daily doses of calcium folinate should be adjusted depending on the haematological toxicity of trimetrexate.

• Overdosage (possibly occurring with trimetrexate doses above 90 mg/m^2 without concomitant administration of calcium folinate): after stopping trimetrexate, calcium folinate 40 mg/m^2 IV every 6 hours for 3 days.

Trimethoprime toxicity:

• After stopping trimethoprime, 3-10 mg/day calcium folinate until recovery of a normal blood count.

Pyrimethamine toxicity:

• In case of high dose pyrimethamine or prolonged treatment with low doses, calcium folinate 5 to 50 mg/day should be simultaneously administered, based on the results of the peripheral blood counts.

4.3 Contraindications
• Known hypersensitivity to calcium folinate, or to any of the excipients.

• Pernicious anaemia or other anaemias due to vitamin B_{12} deficiency.

Regarding the use of calcium folinate with methotrexate or 5-fluorouracil during pregnancy and lactation, see section 4.6, "Pregnancy and Lactation" and the summaries of product characteristics for methotrexate- and 5-fluorouracil- containing medicinal products.

4.4 Special warnings and special precautions for use
Calcium folinate should only be given by intramuscular or intravenous injection and must not be administered intrathecally. When folinic acid has been administered intrathecally following intrathecal overdose of methotrexate, death has been reported.

General

Calcium folinate should be used with methotrexate or 5-fluorouracil only under the direct supervision of a clinician experienced in the use of cancer chemotherapeutic agents.

Calcium folinate treatment may mask pernicious anaemia and other anaemias resulting from vitamin B_{12} deficiency.

Many cytotoxic medicinal products – direct or indirect DNA synthesis inhibitors – lead to macrocytosis (hydroxycarbamide, cytarabine, mecaptopurine, thioguanine). Such macrocytosis should not be treated with folinic acid.

In epileptic patients treated with phenobarbital, phenytoine, primidone, and succinimides there is a risk to increase the frequency of seizures due to a decrease of plasma concentrations of anti-epileptic drugs. Clinical monitoring, possibly monitoring of the plasma concentrations and, if necessary, dose adaptation of the anti-epileptic drug during calcium folinate administration and after discontinuation is recommended (see also section 4.5 Interactions).

Calcium folinate/5-fluorouracil

Calcium folinate may enhance the toxicity risk of 5-fluorouracil, particularly in elderly or debilitated patients. The most common manifestations are leucopenia, mucositis, stomatitis and/or diarrhoea, which may be dose limiting. When calcium folinate and 5-fluorouracil are used in combination, the 5-fluorouracil dosage has to be reduced more in cases of toxicity than when 5-fluorouracil is used alone.

Combined 5-fluorouracil/calcium folinate treatment should neither be initiated nor maintained in patients with symptoms of gastrointestinal toxicity, regardless of the severity, until all of these symptoms have completely disappeared.

Because diarrhoea may be a sign of gastrointestinal toxicity, patients presenting with diarrhoea must be carefully monitored until the symptoms have disappeared completely, since a rapid clinical deterioration leading to death can occur. If diarrhoea and/or stomatitis occur, it is advisable to reduce the dose of 5-FU until symptoms have fully disappeared. Especially the elderly and patients with a low physical performance due to their illness are prone to these toxicities. Therefore, particular care should be taken when treating these patients.

In elderly patients and patients who have undergone preliminary radiotherapy, it is recommended to begin with a reduced dosage of 5-fluorouracil.

Calcium folinate must not be mixed with 5-fluorouracil in the same IV injection or infusion.

Calcium levels should be monitored in patients receiving combined 5-fluorouracil/calcium folinate treatment and calcium supplementation should be provided if calcium levels are low.

Calcium folinate/methotrexate

For specific details on reduction of methotrexate toxicity refer to the SPC of methotrexate.

Calcium folinate has no effect on non-haematological toxicities of methotrexate such as the nephrotoxicity resulting from methotrexate and/or metabolite precipitation in the kidney. Patients who experience delayed early methotrexate elimination are likely to develop reversible renal failure and all toxicities associated with methotrexate (please refer to the SPC for methotrexate). The presence of pre-existing- or methotrexate-induced renal insufficiency is potentially associated with delayed excretion of methotrexate and may increase the need for higher doses or more prolonged use of calcium folinate.

Excessive calcium folinate doses must be avoided since this might impair the antitumour activity of methotrexate, especially in CNS tumours where calcium folinate accumulates after repeated courses.

Resistance to methotrexate as a result of decreased membrane transport implies also resistance to folinic acid rescue as both medicinal products share the same transport system.

An accidental overdose with a folate antagonist, such as methotrexate, should be treated as a medical emergency. As the time interval between methotrexate administration and calcium folinate rescue increases, calcium folinate effectiveness in counteracting toxicity decreases.

The possibility that the patient is taking other medications that interact with methotrexate (eg, medications which may interfere with methotrexate elimination or binding to serum albumin) should always be considered when laboratory abnormalities or clinical toxicities are observed.

4.5 Interaction with other medicinal products and other forms of Interaction
When calcium folinate is given in conjunction with a folic acid antagonist (e.g. cotrimoxazole, pyrimethamine) the efficacy of the folic acid antagonist may either be reduced or completely neutralised.

Calcium folinate may diminish the effect of anti-epileptic substances: phenobarbital, primidone, phenytoine and succinimides, and may increase the frequency of seizures (a decrease of plasma levels of enzymatic inductor anticonvulsant drugs may be observed because the hepatic metabolism is increased as folates are one of the cofactors) (see also sections 4.4 and 4.8).

Concomitant administration of calcium folinate with 5-fluorouracil has been shown to enhance the efficacy and toxicity of 5-fluorouracil (see sections 4.2, 4.4 and 4.8).

4.6 Pregnancy and lactation

Pregnancy

There are no adequate and well-controlled clinical studies conducted in pregnant or breast-feeding women. No formal animal reproductive toxicity studies with calcium folinate have been conducted. There are no indications that folic acid induces harmful effects if administered during pregnancy.

During pregnancy, methotrexate should only be administered on strict indications, where the benefits of the drug to the mother should be weighed against possible hazards to the foetus. Should treatment with methotrexate or other folate antagonists take place despite pregnancy or lactation, there are no limitations as to the use of calcium folinate to diminish toxicity or counteract the effects.

5-fluorouracil use is generally contraindicated during pregnancy and contraindicated during breast-feeding; this applies also to the combined use of calcium folinate with 5-fluorouracil.

Please refer also to the summaries of product characteristics for methotrexate-, other folate antagonists and 5-fluorouracil- containing medicinal products.

Lactation

It is not known whether calcium folinate is excreted into human breast milk. Calcium folinate can be used during breast feeding when considered necessary according to the therapeutic indications.

4.7 Effects on ability to drive and use machines

There is no evidence that calcium folinate has an effect on the ability to drive or use machines.

4.8 Undesirable effects

Both therapeutic indications:

Immune system disorders

Very rare (<0.01%): allergic reactions, including anaphylactoid reactions and urticaria.

Psychiatric disorders

Rare (0.01-0.1%): insomnia, agitation and depression after high doses.

Gastrointestinal disorders

Rare (0.01-0.1%): gastrointestinal disorders after high doses.

Neurological disorders

Rare (0.01-0.1%): increase in the frequency of attacks in epileptics (see also section 4.5 Interactions..).

General disorders and administration site conditions

Uncommon (0.1-1%): fever has been observed after administration of calcium folinate as solution for injection.

Combination therapy with 5-fluorouracil:

Generally, the safety profile depends on the applied regimen of 5-fluorouracil due to enhancement of the 5-fluorouracil induced toxicities:

Monthly regimen:

Gastrointestinal disorders

Very common (>10%): vomiting and nausea

General disorders and administration site conditions

Very common (>10%): (severe) mucosal toxicity.

No enhancement of other 5-fluorouracil induced toxicities (e.g. neurotoxicity).

Weekly regimen:

Gastrointestinal disorders

Very common (>10%): diarrhoea with higher grades of toxicity, and dehydration, resulting in hospital admission for treatment and even death.

4.9 Overdose

There have been no reported sequelae in patients who have received significantly more calcium folinate than the recommended dosage. However, excessive amounts of calcium folinate may nullify the chemotherapeutic effect of folic acid antagonists.

Should overdosage of the combination of 5-fluorouracil and calcium folinate occur, the overdosage instructions for 5-FU should be followed.

5. PHARMACOLOGICAL PROPERTIES

5.1 Pharmacodynamic properties

Pharmacotherapeutic group: Detoxifying agents for antineoplastic treatment; ATC code: V03AF03

Calcium folinate is the calcium salt of 5-formyl tetrahydrofolic acid. It is an active metabolite of folinic acid and an essential coenzyme for nucleic acid synthesis in cytotoxic therapy.

Calcium folinate is frequently used to diminish the toxicity and counteract the action of folate antagonists, such as methotrexate. Calcium folinate and folate antagonists share the same membrane transport carrier and compete for transport into cells, stimulating folate antagonist efflux. It also protects cells from the effects of folate antagonist by repletion of the reduce folate pool. Calcium folinate serves as a pre-reduced source of H4 folate; it can therefore bypass folate antagonist blockage and provide a source for the various coenzyme forms of folic acid.

Calcium folinate is also frequently used in the biochemical modulation of fluoropyridine (5-FU) to enhance its cytotoxic activity. 5-FU inhibits thymidylate synthase (TS), a key enzyme involved in pyrimidine biosynthesis, and calcium folinate enhances TS inhibition by increasing the intracellular folate pool, thus stabilising the 5FU-TS complex and increasing activity.

Finally intravenous calcium folinate can be administered for the prevention and treatment of folate deficiency when it cannot be prevented or corrected by the administration of folic acid by the oral route. This may be the case during total parenteral nutrition and severe malabsorption disorders. It is also indicated for the treatment of megaloblastic anaemia due to folic acid deficiency, when oral administration is not feasible.

5.2 Pharmacokinetic properties

Absorption

Following intramuscular administration of the aqueous solution, systemic availability is comparable to an intravenous administration. However, lower peak serum levels (C_{max}) are achieved.

Metabolism

Calcium folinate is a racemate where the L-form (L-5-formyl-tetrahydrofolate, L-5-formyl-THF), is the active enantiomer.

The major metabolic product of folinic acid is 5-methyl-tetrahydrofolic acid (5-methyl-THF) which is predominantly produced in the liver and intestinal mucosa.

Distribution

The distribution volume of folinic acid is not known.

Peak serum levels of the parent substance (D/L-5-formyl-tetrahydrofolic acid, folinic acid) are reached 10 minutes after i.v. administration.

AUC for L-5-formyl-THF and 5-methyl-THF were 28.4±3.5 mg.min/l and 129±112 mg.min/l after a dose of 25 mg. The inactive D-isomer is present in higher concentration than L-5-formyl-tetrahydrofolate.

Elimination

The elimination half-life is 32 - 35 minutes for the active L-form and 352 - 485 minutes for the inactive D-form, respectively.

The total terminal half-life of the active metabolites is about 6 hours (after intravenous and intramuscular administration).

Excretion

80-90 % with the urine (5- and 10-formyl-tetrahydrofolates inactive metabolites), 5-8 % with the faeces.

5.3 Preclinical safety data

There are no preclinical data considered relevant to clinical safety beyond data included in other sections of the SPC.

6. PHARMACEUTICAL PARTICULARS

6.1 List of excipients

Sodium Chloride

Hydrochloric Acid

Sodium Hydroxide

Water for Injections

6.2 Incompatibilities

Incompatibilities have been reported between injectable forms of calcium folinate and injectable forms of droperidol, fluorouracil, foscarnet and methotrexate.

Droperidol

1. Droperidol 1.25 mg/0.5 ml with calcium folinate 5 mg/0.5 ml, immediate precipitation in direct admixture in syringe for 5 minutes at 25° C followed by 8 minutes of centrifugation.

2. Droperidol 2.5 mg/0.5 ml with calcium folinate 10 mg/0.5 ml, immediate precipitation when the drugs were injected sequentially into a Y-site without flushing the Y-side arm between injections.

Fluorouracil

Calcium folinate must not be mixed in the same infusion as 5-fluorouracil because a precipitate may form. Fluorouracil 50 mg/ml with calcium folinate 20 mg/ml, with or without dextrose 5% in water, has been shown to be incompatible when mixed in different amounts and stored at 4° C, 23° C, or 32° C in polyvinyl chloride containers.

Foscarnet

Foscarnet 24 mg/ml with calcium folinate 20 mg/ml formation of a cloudy yellow solution reported.

6.3 Shelf life

18 months

6.4 Special precautions for storage

Store at 2°C – 8°C (in a refrigerator).

Store in original container to protect from light

Chemical and physical in-use stability has been demonstrated for 24 hours at 2 – 8°C.

From a microbiological point of view, the product should be used immediately. If not used immediately, in-use storage times and conditions prior to use are the responsibility of the user and would normally not be longer than 24 hours at 2-8°C, unless dilution has taken place in controlled and validated aseptic conditions.

6.5 Nature and contents of container

35ml Type I amber glass vial with silicon treated butyl rubber stopper, aluminium seal and flip-off cap containing a clear, yellowish solution.

6.6 Instructions for use and handling

Prior to administration, calcium folinate should be inspected visually. The solution for injection or infusion should be a clear and yellowish solution. If cloudy in appearance or particles are observed, the solution should be discarded. Calcium folinate solution for injection or infusion is intended only for single use. Any unused portion of the solution should be disposed of in accordance with the local requirements.

7. MARKETING AUTHORISATION HOLDER

Cyanamid of Great Britain Limited

Fareham Road

Gosport

Hampshire PO13 0AS

UK

8. MARKETING AUTHORISATION NUMBER(S)

PL 00095/0274

9. DATE OF FIRST AUTHORISATION/RENEWAL OF THE AUTHORISATION

18 June 1993

10. DATE OF REVISION OF THE TEXT

March 2004

Lemsip Cold & Flu Lemon

(Reckitt Benckiser Healthcare (UK) Ltd)

1. NAME OF THE MEDICINAL PRODUCT

Lemsip Cold & Flu Lemon.

2. QUALITATIVE AND QUANTITATIVE COMPOSITION

Paracetamol, 650 mg/sachet, Ph Eur

Phenylephrine hydrochloride, *10 mg/sachet, Ph Eur

*Equivalent to phenylephrine base 8.21 mg.

3. PHARMACEUTICAL FORM

Oral powder.

4. CLINICAL PARTICULARS

4.1 Therapeutic indications

For the relief of the symptoms of colds and influenza, including the relief of aches and pains and nasal congestion, and lowering of temperature.

4.2 Posology and method of administration

Oral, after dissolution in water.

Adults and children 12 and over: Contents of one sachet dissolved by stirring in hot water and sweetened to taste.

The dose may be repeated every 4 to 6 hours as required.

No more than four doses should be taken in 24 hours.

There is no indication that dosage need be modified for the elderly.

Not to be given to children under 12.

4.3 Contraindications

Severe coronary heart disease, hypertension, hypersensitivity to paracetamol, phenylephrine or any other ingredient.

4.4 Special warnings and special precautions for use

Use with caution in patients with Raynaud's Phenomenon or diabetes. Each sachet contains approximately 2.6 g of carbohydrate. Due to its aspartame content this product should not be given to patients with phenylketonuria. Care is advised in the administration of paracetamol to patients with severe renal or severe hepatic impairment. The hazard of overdose is greater in those with non-cirrhotic alcoholic liver disease. Patients should be advised not to take other paracetamol-containing products concurrently.

Label warnings: Do not exceed the stated dose. Keep out of the reach of children. Contains paracetamol (panel). If symptoms persist consult your doctor. If you are pregnant or are being prescribed medicine by your doctor, seek his advice before taking this product. Total sugars 2.6 g. Contains aspartame. Do not take with any other paracetamol-containing products. Immediate medical advice should be sought in the event of an overdose, even if you feel well.

Leaflet: Immediate medical advice should be sought in the event of an overdose, even if you feel well, because of the risk of delayed, serious liver damage.

4.5 Interaction with other medicinal products and other forms of Interaction

Phenylephrine may adversely interact with other sympathomimetics, vasodilators and beta-blockers. Drugs which induce hepatic microsomal enzymes such as alcohol, barbiturates, monoamine oxidase inhibitors and tricyclic antidepressants, may increase the hepatotoxicity of paracetamol particularly after overdosage.

Not recommended for patients currently receiving or within two weeks of stopping therapy with monoamine oxidase inhibitors.

The speed of absorption of paracetamol may be increased by metoclopramide or domperidone and absorption reduced by cholestyramine.

The anticoagulant effect of warfarin and other coumarins may be enhanced by prolonged regular daily use of paracetamol with increased risk of bleeding; occasional doses have no significant effect.

4.6 Pregnancy and lactation

Due to the vasoconstrictive properties of phenylephrine the product should be used with caution in patients with a history of pre-eclampsia. Phenylephrine may reduce placental perfusion and the product should be used in pregnancy only if the benefits outweigh this risk. There is no information on use in lactation.

Epidemiological studies in human pregnancy have shown no ill effects due to paracetamol used in the recommended dosage, but patients should follow the advice of their doctor regarding its use. Paracetamol is excreted in breast milk, but not in a clinically significant amount. Available published data do not contraindicate breast feeding.

4.7 Effects on ability to drive and use machines

None known.

4.8 Undesirable effects

Adverse effects of paracetamol are rare, but hypersensitivity including skin rash may occur. There have been a few reports of blood dyscrasias including thrombocytopenia and agranulocytosis, but these were not necessarily causally related to paracetamol.

4.9 Overdose

Symptoms of paracetamol overdosage in the first 24 hours are pallor, nausea, vomiting, anorexia and abdominal pain. Liver damage may become apparent 12 to 48 hours after ingestion. Abnormalities of glucose metabolism and metabolic acidosis may occur. In severe poisoning, hepatic failure may progress to encephalopathy, coma and death. Acute renal failure with acute tubular necrosis may develop even in the absence of severe liver damage. Cardiac arrhythmias and pancreatitis have been reported. Liver damage is possible in adults who have taken 10 g or more of paracetamol. It is considered that excess quantities of a toxic metabolite (usually adequately detoxified by glutathione when normal doses of paracetamol are ingested) become irreversibly bound to liver tissue.

Immediate treatment is essential in the management of paracetamol overdose. Despite a lack of significant early symptoms, patients should be referred to hospital urgently for immediate medical attention and any patient who has ingested around 7.5 g or more of paracetamol in the preceding 4 hours should undergo gastric lavage. Administration of oral methionine or intravenous N-acetylcysteine, which may have a beneficial effect up to at least 48 hours after the overdose, may be required. General supportive measures must be available.

Features of severe overdosage of phenylephrine include haemodynamic changes and cardiovascular collapse with respiratory depression. Treatment includes early gastric lavage and symptomatic and supportive measures. Hypertensive effects may be treated with an i.v. alpha-receptor blocking agent.

5. PHARMACOLOGICAL PROPERTIES

5.1 Pharmacodynamic properties

Paracetamol

Paracetamol has both analgesic and antipyretic activity which is believed to be mediated principally through its inhibition of prostaglandin synthesis within the central nervous system.

Phenylephrine

Phenylephrine is a postsynaptic alpha-receptor agonist with low cardioselective beta-receptor affinity and minimal central stimulant activity. It is a recognised decongestant and acts by vasoconstriction to reduce oedema and nasal swelling.

5.2 Pharmacokinetic properties

Paracetamol

Paracetamol is absorbed rapidly and completely mainly from the small intestine producing peak plasma levels after 15-20 minutes following oral dosing. The systemic availability is subject to first-pass metabolism and varies with dose between 70% and 90%. The drug is rapidly and widely distributed throughout the body and is eliminated from plasma with a T½ of approximately 2 hours. The major metabolites are glucuronide and sulphate conjugates >80%) which are excreted in urine.

Phenylephrine

Phenylephrine is absorbed from the gastrointestinal tract, but has reduced bioavailability by the oral route due to first pass metabolism. It retains activity as a nasal decongestant when given orally, the drug distributing through the systemic circulation to the vascular bed of the nasal mucosa. When taken by mouth as a nasal decongestant phenylephrine is usually given at intervals of 4 to 6 hours.

5.3 Preclinical safety data

No preclinical findings of relevance have been reported.

6. PHARMACEUTICAL PARTICULARS

6.1 List of excipients

Caster sugar, pulverised sucrose, citric acid anhydrous, sodium citrate, lemon flavour no. 1, aspartame, ascorbic acid, saccharin sodium and curcumin WD.

6.2 Incompatibilities

None known.

6.3 Shelf life

Three years.

6.4 Special precautions for storage

Store below 25°C in a dry place.

6.5 Nature and contents of container

Heat-sealed laminate sachet of 41 gsm paper/10-12 gsm LD polyethylene/8-9 micron aluminium foil/18 gsm polyethylene. In a cardboard outer carton.

Pack size: 5, **7**, 10 and 16 sachets. (The pack sizes printed in bold are currently marketed).

6.6 Instructions for use and handling

Oral administration, after dissolution in hot water.

7. MARKETING AUTHORISATION HOLDER

Reckitt Benckiser Healthcare (UK) Limited, Dansom Lane, Hull, HU8 7DS.

8. MARKETING AUTHORISATION NUMBER(S)

PL 0063/0034.

9. DATE OF FIRST AUTHORISATION/RENEWAL OF THE AUTHORISATION

24th April, 1995.

10. DATE OF REVISION OF THE TEXT

September 2004.

Lemsip Max Cold & Flu Capsules

(Reckitt Benckiser Healthcare (UK) Ltd)

1. NAME OF THE MEDICINAL PRODUCT

Lemsip Max Cold & Flu Capsules.

2. QUALITATIVE AND QUANTITATIVE COMPOSITION

Paracetamol, 500 mg/capsule, Ph Eur

Caffeine anhydrous, 25 mg/capsule, Ph Eur

Phenylephrine hydrochloride, 6.1 mg/capsule, Ph Eur

3. PHARMACEUTICAL FORM

Red/yellow hard gelatine capsules.

4. CLINICAL PARTICULARS

4.1 Therapeutic indications

For the relief of symptoms associated with the common cold and influenza, including relief of aches and pains, sore throat, headache, fatigue and drowsiness, nasal congestion and lowering of temperature.

4.2 Posology and method of administration

Adults (over 12 years): Two capsules every 4 hours to a maximum of four doses in any 24 hours. Do not exceed eight capsules in any 24 hours.

Children 6-12 years: One capsule every 4 hours to a maximum of four doses in any 24 hours. Do not exceed four capsules in any 24 hours.

Swallow whole with water. Do not chew.

Not recommended for children under 6 years of age.

4.3 Contraindications

Paracetamol: Hypersensitivity to paracetamol or any of the other constituents.

Caffeine: Should be given with care to patients with a history of peptic ulcer.

Phenylephrine hydrochloride: Severe coronary heart disease and cardiovascular disorders. Hypertension. Hyperthyroidism. Contraindicated in patients currently receiving or within two weeks of stopping therapy with monoamine oxidase inhibitors.

4.4 Special warnings and special precautions for use

Care is advised in the administration of paracetamol to patients with severe renal or severe hepatic impairment. The hazard of overdose is greater in those with non-cirrhotic alcoholic liver disease.

Use with caution in patients with Raynaud's Phenomenon and diabetes mellitus.

Label: Immediate medical advice should be sought in the event of an overdose, even if you feel well.

Leaflet: Immediate medical advice should be sought in the event of an overdose, even if you feel well, because of the risk of delayed, serious liver damage.

Do not exceed the stated dose. Do not take with any other paracetamol-containing products. If symptoms persist consult your doctor. Keep out of the reach of children. If you are pregnant or are being prescribed medicine by your doctor, seek his advice before taking this product. Contains paracetamol (panel).

4.5 Interaction with other medicinal products and other forms of Interaction

The speed of absorption of paracetamol may be increased by metoclopramide or domperidone and absorption reduced by cholestyramine.

The anticoagulant effect of warfarin and other coumarins may be enhanced by prolonged regular daily use of paracetamol with increased risk of bleeding; occasional doses have no significant effect.

Phenylephrine may adversely interact with other sympathomimetics, vasodilators and beta-blockers. Drugs which induce hepatic microsomal enzymes, such as alcohol, barbiturates, monoamine oxidase inhibitors and tricyclic antidepressants, may increase the hepatotoxicity of paracetamol, particularly after overdosage. Contraindicated in patients currently receiving or within two weeks of stopping therapy with monoamine oxidase inhibitors because of a risk of hypertensive crisis.

4.6 Pregnancy and lactation

Epidemiological studies in human pregnancy have shown no ill effects due to paracetamol used in the recommended dosage, but patients should follow the advice of their doctor regarding its use.

Paracetamol is excreted in breast milk, but not in a clinically significant amount. Available published data do not contraindicate breastfeeding.

Caffeine: Taken during pregnancy it appears that the half-life of caffeine is prolonged. This is a possible contributing factor in hyperemesis gravidarum.

Phenylephrine hydrochloride: Due to the vasoconstrictive properties of phenylephrine the product should be used with caution in patients with a history of pre-eclampsia. Phenylephrine may reduce placental perfusion and the product should be used in pregnancy only if the benefits outweigh this risk. There is no information on use in lactation.

4.7 Effects on ability to drive and use machines

None known.

4.8 Undesirable effects

Adverse effects of paracetamol are rare, but hypersensitivity including skin rash may occur. There have been a few reports of blood dyscrasias including thrombocytopenia and agranulocytosis, but these were not necessarily causally related to paracetamol.

Phenylephrine hydrochloride: High blood pressure with headache, vomiting and rarely, palpitations. Also rare reports of allergic reactions.

Caffeine: If taken close to bedtime, may interfere with sleep.

4.9 Overdose

Paracetamol: Symptoms of paracetamol overdosage in the first 24 hours are pallor, nausea, vomiting, anorexia and abdominal pain. Liver damage may become apparent 12 to 48 hours after ingestion. Abnormalities of glucose metabolism and metabolic acidosis may occur. In severe poisoning, hepatic failure may progress to encephalopathy, coma and death. Acute renal failure with acute tubular necrosis may develop even in the absence of severe liver damage. Cardiac arrhythmias and pancreatitis have been reported. Liver damage is possible in adults who have taken 10 g or more of paracetamol. It is considered that excess quantities of a toxic metabolite (usually adequately detoxified by glutathione when normal doses of paracetamol are ingested) become irreversibly bound to liver tissue.

Immediate treatment is essential in the management of paracetamol overdose. Despite a lack of significant early symptoms, patients should be referred to hospital urgently for immediate medical attention and any patient who has ingested around 7.5 g or more of paracetamol in the preceding 4 hours should undergo gastric lavage. Administration of oral methionine or intravenous N-acetylcysteine, which may have a beneficial effect up to at least 48 hours after the overdose, may be required. General supportive measures must be available.

Caffeine: Symptoms - emesis and convulsions may occur. No specific antidote. However, treatment is usually fluid therapy. Fatal poisoning is rare. If symptoms become apparent or overdose is suspected, consult a doctor immediately.

Phenylephrine hydrochloride: Features of severe overdosage of phenylephrine include haemodynamic changes and cardiovascular collapse with respiratory depression. Treatment includes early gastric lavage and symptomatic and supportive measures. Hypertensive effects may be treated with an i.v. alpha-receptor blocking agent.

5. PHARMACOLOGICAL PROPERTIES

5.1 Pharmacodynamic properties

Paracetamol: Paracetamol has both analgesic and antipyretic activity which is believed to be mediated principally through its inhibition of prostaglandin synthesis within the central nervous system.

Caffeine: Caffeine is a central nervous system stimulant. It inhibits the enzyme phosphodiesterase and has an antagonistic effect at central adenosine receptors. Its action on the central nervous system is mainly on the higher centres and it produces a condition of wakefulness and increased mental activity.

Phenylephrine hydrochloride: Phenylephrine is a post-synaptic alpha-receptor agonist with low cardioselective beta-receptor affinity and minimal central stimulant activity. It is a recognised decongestant and acts by vasoconstriction to reduce oedema and nasal swelling.

5.2 Pharmacokinetic properties

Paracetamol: Paracetamol is absorbed rapidly and completely from the small intestine, producing peak plasma levels after 15-20 minutes following oral dosing. The systemic availability is subject to first-pass metabolism and varies with dose between 70% and 90%. The drug is rapidly and widely distributed throughout the body and is eliminated from plasma with a T½ of approximately 2 hours. The major metabolites are glucuronide and sulphate conjugates (>80%) which are excreted in urine.

Caffeine: Caffeine is absorbed readily after oral, rectal or parenteral administration, but absorption from the gastrointestinal tract may be erratic. There is little evidence of accumulation in any particular tissue. Caffeine passes readily into the central nervous system and into saliva. Concentrations have also been detected in breast milk. It is metabolised almost completely and is excreted in the urine as 1-methyluric acid, 1-methylxanthine and other metabolites with only about 1% unchanged.

Phenylephrine hydrochloride: Phenylephrine is absorbed from the gastrointestinal tract, but has reduced bioavailability by the oral route due to first-pass metabolism. It retains activity as a nasal decongestant when given orally, the drug distributing through the systemic circulation to the vascular bed of the nasal mucosa. When taken by mouth as a nasal decongestant phenylephrine is usually given at intervals of 4-6 hours.

5.3 Preclinical safety data

No preclinical findings of relevance have been reported.

6. PHARMACEUTICAL PARTICULARS

6.1 List of excipients

Starch, croscarmellose sodium, sodium lauryl sulphate, magnesium stearate, talc, gelatine, titanium dioxide (E171), quinoline yellow (E104), patent blue V (E131), erythrosin (E127), shellac, tartrazine (E102) and aluminium hydroxide.

6.2 Incompatibilities

None known.

6.3 Shelf life

Three years.

6.4 Special precautions for storage

Store up to 25°C.

6.5 Nature and contents of container

250 micron opaque uPVC blister with foil/paper laminate, 35 gsm paper/9 micron soft-temper foil and heat-seal coated, contained in an outer cardboard carton.

Pack sizes: 4, 6, 8, 12 and 16 capsules.

6.6 Instructions for use and handling

The capsules are to be taken orally, with water if preferred, and swallowed without being chewed.

7. MARKETING AUTHORISATION HOLDER

Reckitt Benckiser Healthcare (UK) Limited, Dansom Lane, Hull, HU8 7DS, East Yorkshire.

8. MARKETING AUTHORISATION NUMBER(S)

PL 0063/0104.

9. DATE OF FIRST AUTHORISATION/RENEWAL OF THE AUTHORISATION

9th October, 1998.

10. DATE OF REVISION OF THE TEXT

March 2005.

Lemsip Max Cold & Flu Direct Blackcurrant

(Reckitt Benckiser Healthcare (UK) Ltd)

1. NAME OF THE MEDICINAL PRODUCT

Lemsip Max Cold & Flu Direct Blackcurrant.

2. QUALITATIVE AND QUANTITATIVE COMPOSITION

Paracetamol, 1000.0 mg/sachet.

Phenylephrine hydrochloride, *12.2 mg/sachet.

*This is equivalent to 10 mg phenylephrine base.

For excipients, see Section 6.1.

3. PHARMACEUTICAL FORM

Oral powder.

A white to off-white unit-dose powder with the odour and flavour of blackcurrants.

4. CLINICAL PARTICULARS

4.1 Therapeutic indications

For relief of symptoms associated with the common cold and influenza, including the relief of aches and pains, sore throat, headache, nasal congestion and lowering of temperature.

4.2 Posology and method of administration

Oral administration.

Adults and children 12 and over: One single-dose container. The product is taken orally without water.

The dose may be repeated in 4 hours.

No more than four doses should be taken in 24 hours.

Not to be given to children under 12 without medical advice.

There is no indication that dosage need be modified in the elderly.

4.3 Contraindications

Severe coronary heart disease and cardiovascular disorders. Hypertension. Hyperthyroidism. Contraindicated in patients currently receiving or within two weeks of stopping therapy with monoamine oxidase inhibitors. Hypersensitivity to paracetamol, phenylephrine or any other ingredient.

4.4 Special warnings and special precautions for use

Use with caution in patients with Raynaud's phenomenon or diabetes mellitus. Care is advised in the administration of paracetamol to patients with severe renal or severe hepatic impairment. The hazard of overdose is greater in those with non-cirrhotic alcoholic liver disease. Patients should be advised not to take other paracetamol-containing products concurrently.

Label warnings: Do not exceed the stated dose. Keep out of the reach and sight of children. Contains paracetamol (panel). If symptoms persist consult your doctor. If you are pregnant or are being prescribed medicine by your doctor, seek his advice before taking this product.

Do not take with any other paracetamol-containing products. Immediate medical advice should be sought in the event of an overdose, even if you feel well.

Leaflet: Immediate medical advice should be sought in the event of an overdose, even if you feel well, because of the risk of delayed, serious liver damage.

4.5 Interaction with other medicinal products and other forms of Interaction

Phenylephrine may adversely interact with other sympathomimetics, vasodilators and beta-blockers. Drugs which induce hepatic microsomal enzymes, such as alcohol, barbiturates, monoamine oxidase inhibitors and tricyclic antidepressants, may increase the hepatotoxicity of paracetamol, particularly after overdosage. Contraindicated in patients currently receiving or within two weeks of stopping therapy with monoamine oxidase inhibitors because of a risk of hypertensive crisis.

The speed of absorption of paracetamol may be increased by metoclopramide or domperidone and absorption reduced by cholestyramine. The anticoagulant effect of warfarin and other coumarins may be enhanced by prolonged regular daily use of paracetamol with increased risk of bleeding; occasional doses have no significant effect.

4.6 Pregnancy and lactation

Due to the vasoconstrictive properties of phenylephrine the product should be used with caution in patients with a history of pre-eclampsia. Phenylephrine may reduce placental perfusion and the product should be used in pregnancy only if the benefits outweigh the risk. There is no information on use in lactation.

Epidemiological studies in human pregnancy have shown no ill-effects due to paracetamol used in the recommended dosage, but patients should follow the advice of their doctor regarding its use. Paracetamol is excreted in breast milk, but not in a clinically significant amount. Available published data do not contraindicate breast feeding.

4.7 Effects on ability to drive and use machines

None known.

4.8 Undesirable effects

Paracetamol: Adverse effects of paracetamol are rare, but hypersensitivity including skin rash may occur. There have been a few reports of blood dyscrasias including thrombocytopenia and agranulocytosis, but these were not necessarily causally related to paracetamol.

Phenylephrine hydrochloride: Rarely, high blood pressure with headache, vomiting and palpitations, which are only likely to occur with overdose. Also rare reports of allergic reactions.

4.9 Overdose

Symptoms of paracetamol overdosage in the first 24 hours are pallor, nausea, vomiting, anorexia and abdominal pain. Liver damage may become apparent 12 to 48 hours after ingestion. Abnormalities of glucose metabolism and metabolic acidosis may occur. In severe poisoning, hepatic failure may progress to encephalopathy, coma and death. Acute renal failure with acute tubular necrosis may develop even in the absence of severe liver damage. Cardiac arrhythmias and pancreatitis have been reported. Liver damage is possible in adults who have taken 10 g or more of paracetamol. It is considered that excess quantities of a toxic metabolite (usually adequately detoxified by glutathione when normal doses of paracetamol are ingested) become irreversibly bound to liver tissue.

Immediate treatment is essential in the management of paracetamol overdose. Despite a lack of significant early symptoms, patients should be referred to hospital urgently for immediate medical attention and any patient who has ingested around 7.5 g or more of paracetamol in the preceding 4 hours should undergo gastric lavage. Administration of oral methionine or intravenous N-acetylcysteine, which may have a beneficial effect up to at least 48 hours after the overdose, may be required. General supportive measures must be available.

Features of severe overdosage of phenylephrine include haemodynamic changes and cardiovascular collapse with respiratory depression. Treatment includes early gastric lavage and symptomatic and supportive measures. Hypertensive effects may be treated with an i.v. alpha-receptor blocking agent.

5. PHARMACOLOGICAL PROPERTIES

5.1 Pharmacodynamic properties

Paracetamol: Paracetamol has both analgesic and antipyretic activity which is believed to be mediated principally through its inhibition of prostaglandin synthesis within the central nervous system.

Phenylephrine: Phenylephrine is a post-synaptic alpha-receptor agonist with low cardioselective beta-receptor affinity and minimal central stimulant activity. It is a recognised decongestant and acts by vasoconstriction to reduce oedema and nasal swelling.

5.2 Pharmacokinetic properties

Paracetamol: Paracetamol is absorbed rapidly and completely mainly from the small intestine producing peak plasma levels after 15-20 minutes following oral dosing. The systemic availability is subject to first-pass metabolism and varies with dose between 70% and 90%. The drug is rapidly and widely distributed throughout the body and is eliminated from plasma with a T½ of approximately 2 hours. The major metabolites are glucuronide and sulphate conjugates (>80%) which are excreted in urine.

Phenylephrine: Phenylephrine is absorbed from the gastrointestinal tract, but has reduced bioavailability by the oral route due to first-pass metabolism. It retains activity as a nasal decongestant when given orally, the drug distributing through the systemic circulation to the vascular bed of nasal mucosa. When taken by mouth as a nasal decongestant phenylephrine is usually given at intervals of 4-6 hours.

5.3 Preclinical safety data

No preclinical findings of relevance have been reported.

6. PHARMACEUTICAL PARTICULARS

6.1 List of excipients

Ethyl cellulose, ascorbic acid, glyceryl tristearate, tartaric acid, sodium carbonate anhydrous, aspartame, blackcurrant flavour, sweet flavour and xylitol.

6.2 Incompatibilities

None known.

6.3 Shelf life

Two years.

6.4 Special precautions for storage

Do not store above 25°C and store in the original package.

6.5 Nature and contents of container

Polyethylene terephthalate/aluminium/ polyethylene sachets.

Pack size: 1, 8 and 10.

6.6 Instructions for use and handling

There are no special instructions for handling.

7. MARKETING AUTHORISATION HOLDER

Reckitt Benckiser Healthcare (UK) Limited, Dansom Lane, Hull, HU8 7DS, United Kingdom.

8. MARKETING AUTHORISATION NUMBER(S)

PL 00063/0115.

9. DATE OF FIRST AUTHORISATION/RENEWAL OF THE AUTHORISATION

19th July, 2002.

10. DATE OF REVISION OF THE TEXT

May 2003.

Lemsip Max Cold & Flu Direct Lemon

(Reckitt Benckiser Healthcare (UK) Ltd)

1. NAME OF THE MEDICINAL PRODUCT

Lemsip Max Cold & Flu Direct Lemon.

2. QUALITATIVE AND QUANTITATIVE COMPOSITION

Paracetamol, 1000.0 mg/sachet.

Phenylephrine hydrochloride, *12.2 mg/sachet.

*This is equivalent to 10 mg phenylephrine base.

For excipients, see Section 6.1.

3. PHARMACEUTICAL FORM

Oral powder.

A white to off-white unit-dose powder with the odour and flavour of lemons.

4. CLINICAL PARTICULARS

4.1 Therapeutic indications

For relief of symptoms associated with the common cold and influenza, including the relief of aches and pains, sore throat, headache, nasal congestion and lowering of temperature.

4.2 Posology and method of administration
Oral administration.

Adults and children 12 and over: One single-dose container. The product is taken orally without water.

The dose may be repeated in 4 hours.

No more than four doses should be taken in 24 hours.

Not to be given to children under 12 without medical advice.

There is no indication that dosage need be modified in the elderly.

4.3 Contraindications
Severe coronary heart disease and cardiovascular disorders. Hypertension. Hyperthyroidism. Contraindicated in patients currently receiving or within two weeks of stopping therapy with monoamine oxidase inhibitors. Hypersensitivity to paracetamol, phenylephrine or any other ingredient.

4.4 Special warnings and special precautions for use
Use with caution in patients with Raynaud's phenomenon or diabetes mellitus. Care is advised in the administration of paracetamol to patients with severe renal or severe hepatic impairment. The hazard of overdose is greater in those with non-cirrhotic alcoholic liver disease. Patients should be advised not to take other paracetamol-containing products concurrently.

Label warnings: Do not exceed the stated dose. Keep out of the reach and sight of children. Contains paracetamol (panel). If symptoms persist consult your doctor. If you are pregnant or are being prescribed medicine by your doctor, seek his advice before taking this product.

Do not take with any other paracetamol-containing products. Immediate medical advice should be sought in the event of an overdose, even if you feel well.

Leaflet: Immediate medical advice should be sought in the event of an overdose, even if you feel well, because of the risk of delayed, serious liver damage.

4.5 Interaction with other medicinal products and other forms of Interaction
Phenylephrine may adversely interact with other sympathomimetics, vasodilators and beta-blockers. Drugs which induce hepatic microsomal enzymes, such as alcohol, barbiturates, monoamine oxidase inhibitors and tricyclic antidepressants, may increase the hepatotoxicity of paracetamol, particularly after overdose. Contraindicated in patients currently receiving or within two weeks of stopping therapy with monoamine oxidase inhibitors because of a risk of hypertensive crisis.

The speed of absorption of paracetamol may be increased by metoclopramide or domperidone and absorption reduced by cholestyramine. The anticoagulant effect of warfarin and other coumarins may be enhanced by prolonged regular daily use of paracetamol with increased risk of bleeding; occasional doses have no significant effect.

4.6 Pregnancy and lactation
Due to the vasoconstrictive properties of phenylephrine the product should be used with caution in patients with a history of pre-eclampsia. Phenylephrine may reduce placental perfusion and the product should be used in pregnancy only if the benefits outweigh the risk. There is no information on use in lactation.

Epidemiological studies in human pregnancy have shown no ill-effects due to paracetamol used in the recommended dosage, but patients should follow the advice of their doctor regarding its use. Paracetamol is excreted in breast milk, but not in a clinically significant amount. Available published data do not contraindicate breast feeding.

4.7 Effects on ability to drive and use machines
None known.

4.8 Undesirable effects
Paracetamol: Adverse effects of paracetamol are rare, but hypersensitivity including skin rash may occur. There have been a few reports of blood dyscrasias including thrombocytopenia and agranulocytosis, but these were not necessarily causally related to paracetamol.

Phenylephrine hydrochloride: Rarely, high blood pressure with headache, vomiting and palpitations, which are only likely to occur with overdose. Also rare reports of allergic reactions.

4.9 Overdose
Symptoms of paracetamol overdosage in the first 24 hours are pallor, nausea, vomiting, anorexia and abdominal pain. Liver damage may become apparent 12 to 48 hours after ingestion. Abnormalities of glucose metabolism and metabolic acidosis may occur. In severe poisoning, hepatic failure may progress to encephalopathy, coma and death. Acute renal failure with acute tubular necrosis may develop even in the absence of severe liver damage. Cardiac arrhythmias and pancreatitis have been reported. Liver damage is possible in adults who have taken 10 g or more of paracetamol. It is considered that excess quantities of a toxic metabolite (usually adequately detoxified by glutathione when normal doses of paracetamol are ingested) become irreversibly bound to liver tissue.

Immediate treatment is essential in the management of paracetamol overdose. Despite a lack of significant early symptoms, patients should be referred to hospital urgently for immediate medical attention and any patient who has ingested around 7.5 g or more of paracetamol in the preceding 4 hours should undergo gastric lavage. Administration of oral methionine or intravenous N-acetylcysteine, which may have a beneficial effect up to at least 48 hours after the overdose, may be required. General supportive measures must be available.

Features of severe overdose of phenylephrine include haemodynamic changes and cardiovascular collapse with respiratory depression. Treatment includes early gastric lavage and symptomatic and supportive measures. Hypertensive effects may be treated with an i.v. alpha-receptor blocking agent.

5. PHARMACOLOGICAL PROPERTIES

5.1 Pharmacodynamic properties
Paracetamol: Paracetamol has both analgesic and antipyretic activity which is believed to be mediated principally through its inhibition of prostaglandin synthesis within the central nervous system.

Phenylephrine: Phenylephrine is a post-synaptic alpha-receptor agonist with low cardioselective beta-receptor affinity and minimal central stimulant activity. It is a recognised decongestant and acts by vasoconstriction to reduce oedema and nasal swelling.

5.2 Pharmacokinetic properties
Paracetamol: Paracetamol is absorbed rapidly and completely mainly from the small intestine producing peak plasma levels after 15-20 minutes following oral dosing. The systemic availability is subject to first-pass metabolism and varies with dose between 70% and 90%. The drug is rapidly and widely distributed throughout the body and is eliminated from plasma with a T½ of approximately 2 hours. The major metabolites are glucuronide and sulphate conjugates (>80%) which are excreted in urine.

Phenylephrine: Phenylephrine is absorbed from the gastrointestinal tract, but has reduced bioavailability by the oral route due to first-pass metabolism. It retains activity as a nasal decongestant when given orally, the drug distributing through the systemic circulation to the vascular bed of nasal mucosa. When taken by mouth as a nasal decongestant phenylephrine is usually given at intervals of 4-6 hours.

5.3 Preclinical safety data
No preclinical findings of relevance have been reported.

6. PHARMACEUTICAL PARTICULARS

6.1 List of excipients
Ethyl cellulose, ascorbic acid, glyceryl tristearate, tartaric acid, sodium carbonate anhydrous, aspartame, lemon flavour, sweet flavour and xylitol.

6.2 Incompatibilities
None known.

6.3 Shelf life
Two years.

6.4 Special precautions for storage
Do not store above 25°C and store in the original package.

6.5 Nature and contents of container
Polyethylene terephthalate/aluminium/ polyethylene sachets.

Pack size: 1, 8 and 10.

6.6 Instructions for use and handling
There are no special instructions for handling.

7. MARKETING AUTHORISATION HOLDER
Reckitt Benckiser Healthcare (UK) Limited, Dansom Lane, Hull, HU8 7DS, United Kingdom.

8. MARKETING AUTHORISATION NUMBER(S)
PL 00063/0114.

9. DATE OF FIRST AUTHORISATION/RENEWAL OF THE AUTHORISATION
19th July, 2002

10. DATE OF REVISION OF THE TEXT
May 2003.

Lemsip Max Cold & Flu Lemon

(Reckitt Benckiser Healthcare (UK) Ltd)

1. NAME OF THE MEDICINAL PRODUCT
Lemsip Max Cold & Flu Lemon.

2. QUALITATIVE AND QUANTITATIVE COMPOSITION
Paracetamol, 1000.00 mg/sachet, Ph Eur

Phenylephrine hydrochloride*, 12.20 mg/sachet, Ph Eur

*Equivalent to phenylephrine (base) 10.0 mg.

3. PHARMACEUTICAL FORM
Oral powder.

4. CLINICAL PARTICULARS

4.1 Therapeutic indications
For relief of the symptoms of colds and influenza, including the relief of aches and pains, sore throat, headache, nasal congestion and lowering of temperature.

4.2 Posology and method of administration
Oral administration after dissolution in water.

Adults and children over 12: One sachet dissolved by stirring in hot water and sweetened to taste.

The dose may be repeated in 4-6 hours.

No more than four doses should be taken in 24 hours.

Not to be given to children under 12 without medical advice.

There is no indication that dosage need be modified in the elderly.

4.3 Contraindications
Severe coronary heart disease. Hypertension. Hypersensitivity to paracetamol, phenylephrine or any other ingredient.

4.4 Special warnings and special precautions for use
Use with caution in patients with Raynaud's phenomenon or diabetes. Each sachet contains approximately 2.2 g of carbohydrate. Care is advised in the administration of paracetamol to patients with severe renal or severe hepatic impairment. The hazard of overdose is greater in those with non-cirrhotic alcoholic liver disease. Patients should be advised not to take other paracetamol-containing products concurrently.

Label warnings: Do not exceed the stated dose. Keep out of the reach of children. Contains paracetamol (panel). If symptoms persist, consult your doctor. If you are pregnant or are being prescribed medicine by your doctor, seek his advice before taking this product. Total sugars 2.2 g.

Do not take with any other paracetamol-containing products. Immediate medical advice should be sought in the event of an overdose, even if you feel well.

Leaflet: Immediate medical advice should be sought in the event of an overdose, even if you feel well, because of the risk of delayed, serious liver damage.

4.5 Interaction with other medicinal products and other forms of Interaction
Phenylephrine may adversely interact with other sympathomimetics, vasodilators and beta-blockers. Drugs which induce hepatic microsomal enzymes, such as alcohol, barbiturates, monoamine oxidase inhibitors and tricyclic antidepressants, may increase the hepatotoxicity of paracetamol, particularly after overdosage. Not recommended for patients currently receiving or within two weeks of stopping therapy with monoamine oxidase inhibitors.

The speed of absorption of paracetamol may be increased by metoclopramide or domperidone and absorption reduced by cholestyramine. The anticoagulant effect of warfarin and other coumarins may be enhanced by prolonged regular daily use of paracetamol with increased risk of bleeding; occasional doses have no significant effect.

4.6 Pregnancy and lactation
Due to the vasoconstrictive properties of phenylephrine the product should be used with caution in patients with a history of pre-eclampsia. Phenylephrine may reduce placental perfusion and the product should be used in pregnancy only if the benefits outweigh the risk. There is no information on use in lactation.

Epidemiological studies in human pregnancy have shown no ill-effects due to paracetamol used in the recommended dosage, but patients should follow the advice of their doctor regarding its use. Paracetamol is excreted in breastmilk, but not in a clinically significant amount. Available published data do not contraindicate breast feeding.

4.7 Effects on ability to drive and use machines
None known.

4.8 Undesirable effects
Adverse effects of paracetamol are rare, but hypersensitivity including skin rash may occur. There have been a few reports of blood dyscrasias including thrombocytopenia and agranulocytosis, but these were not necessarily causally related to paracetamol.

4.9 Overdose
Symptoms of paracetamol overdosage in the first 24 hours are pallor, nausea, vomiting, anorexia and abdominal pain. Liver damage may become apparent 12 to 48 hours after ingestion. Abnormalities of glucose metabolism and metabolic acidosis may occur. In severe poisoning, hepatic failure may progress to encephalopathy, coma and death. Acute renal failure with acute tubular necrosis may develop even in the absence of severe liver damage. Cardiac arrhythmias and pancreatitis have been reported. Liver damage is possible in adults who have taken 10 g or more of paracetamol. It is considered that excess quantities of a toxic metabolite (usually adequately detoxified by glutathione when normal doses of paracetamol are ingested) become irreversibly bound to liver tissue.

Immediate treatment is essential in the management of paracetamol overdose. Despite a lack of significant early symptoms, patients should be referred to hospital urgently for immediate medical attention and any patient who has ingested around 7.5 g or more of paracetamol in the preceding 4 hours should undergo gastric lavage. Administration of oral methionine or intravenous N-acetylcysteine, which may have a beneficial effect up to at least 48 hours after the overdose, may be required. General supportive measures must be available.

Features of severe overdosage of phenylephrine include haemodynamic changes and cardiovascular collapse with respiratory depression. Treatment includes early gastric lavage and symptomatic and supportive measures. Hypertensive effects may be treated with an i.v. alpha-receptor blocking agent.

5. PHARMACOLOGICAL PROPERTIES

5.1 Pharmacodynamic properties

Paracetamol: Paracetamol has both analgesic and antipyretic activity which is believed to be mediated principally through its inhibition of prostaglandin synthesis within the central nervous system.

Phenylephrine: Phenylephrine is a post-synaptic alpha-receptor agonist with low cardioselective beta-receptor affinity and minimal central stimulant activity. It is a recognised decongestant and acts by vasoconstriction to reduce oedema and nasal swelling.

5.2 Pharmacokinetic properties

Paracetamol: Paracetamol is absorbed rapidly and completely mainly from the small intestine producing peak plasma levels after 15-20 minutes following oral dosing. The systemic availability is subject to first-pass metabolism and varies with dose between 70% and 90%. The drug is rapidly and widely distributed throughout the body and is eliminated from plasma with a $T^{1}/_{2}$ of approximately 2 hours. The major metabolites are glucuronide and sulphate conjugates (>80%) which are excreted in urine.

Phenylephrine: Phenylephrine is absorbed from the gastrointestinal tract, but has reduced bioavailability by the oral route due to first-pass metabolism. It retains activity as a nasal decongestant when given orally, the drug distributing through the systemic circulation to the vascular bed of nasal mucosa. When taken by mouth as a nasal decongestant phenylephrine is usually given at intervals of 4-6 hours.

5.3 Preclinical safety data

No preclinical findings of relevance have been reported.

6. PHARMACEUTICAL PARTICULARS

6.1 List of excipients

Sodium citrate, citric acid, curcumin, lemon flavour, aspartame, saccharin sodium, pulverised sucrose, caster sugar and ascorbic acid.

6.2 Incompatibilities

None known.

6.3 Shelf life

Three years.

6.4 Special precautions for storage

Store below 25°C in a dry place.

6.5 Nature and contents of container

Heat-sealed sachet of paper/polyethylene/aluminium foil/polyethylene laminate in an outer cardboard carton.

Pack sizes: 1, 5, 7, 10 and 16 sachets.

6.6 Instructions for use and handling

Oral administration after dissolution in water.

7. MARKETING AUTHORISATION HOLDER

Reckitt Benckiser Healthcare (UK) Limited, Dansom Lane, Hull, HU8 7DS, East Yorkshire.

8. MARKETING AUTHORISATION NUMBER(S)

PL 0063/0069.

9. DATE OF FIRST AUTHORISATION/RENEWAL OF THE AUTHORISATION

24th April, 1995.

10. DATE OF REVISION OF THE TEXT

September 2004.

Lescol

(Novartis Pharmaceuticals UK Ltd)

1. NAME OF THE MEDICINAL PRODUCT

LESCOL® (fluvastatin* sodium) 20 mg and 40mg capsules.

*INN rec.

2. QUALITATIVE AND QUANTITATIVE COMPOSITION

One 20mg capsule contains 21.06 mg fluvastatin sodium corresponding to 20 mg fluvastatin free acid.

One 40mg capsule contains 42.12 mg fluvastatin sodium corresponding to 40 mg fluvastatin free acid.

For excipients, see Section 6.1.

3. PHARMACEUTICAL FORM

Capsule, hard

20-mg capsules are No. 3 size hard gelatine capsules with a strong reddish brown opaque cap with a Sandoz triangle imprinted in white, and a pale yellow opaque body with XU 20 mg imprinted in red.

40-mg capsules are No. 1 size hard gelatine capsules with a strong reddish brown opaque cap with a Sandoz triangle imprinted in white, and a moderate orange yellow body with XU 40 mg imprinted in red.

4. CLINICAL PARTICULARS

4.1 Therapeutic indications

LESCOL is indicated as an adjunct to diet for the reduction of elevated total-C, LDL-C, apo B and TG levels in patients with primary hypercholesterolaemia and mixed dyslipidaemia (Fredrickson types IIa and IIb).

LESCOL is also indicated to slow the progression of coronary atherosclerosis in patients with primary hypercholesterolaemia and concomitant coronary heart disease who do not adequately respond to dietary control.

LESCOL is also indicated in patients with coronary heart disease for the secondary prevention of coronary events after percutaneous coronary intervention, see Section 5.1.

4.2 Posology and method of administration

Prior to initiating LESCOL, secondary causes of hypercholesterolaemia should be excluded, and the patient placed on a standard cholesterol-lowering diet. Dietary therapy should be continued during treatment.

• Dose recommendations for lipid lowering effect

The recommended starting dose is 40 mg (1 capsule LESCOL 40 mg) once daily in the evening, although a dose of 20 mg fluvastatin (1 capsule LESCOL 20 mg) once daily may be adequate in mild cases. Most patients will require a dose of 20 mg to 40 mg once daily but the dose may be increased to 80 mg daily (1 tablet LESCOL XL 80 mg or 1 capsule LESCOL 40 mg twice daily), individualised according to baseline LDL-C levels and the recommended goal of therapy to be accomplished. The maximum recommended daily dose is 80 mg.

The maximum lipid-lowering effect with a given dose of the drug is achieved within 4 weeks. Doses should be adjusted according to the patient's response and dose adjustment made at intervals of 4 weeks or more. The therapeutic effect of LESCOL is maintained with prolonged administration.

For patients requiring a dose of 40 mg twice daily, a calendar pack of 56 LESCOL Capsules 40 mg is available containing morning and evening doses in marked blister strips.

LESCOL is efficacious in monotherapy or in combination with bile acid sequestrants. When LESCOL is used in combination with cholestyramine or other resins, it should be administered at least 4 hours after the resin to avoid a significant interaction due to binding of the drug to the resin. Minimal data exist to support the efficacy and safety of LESCOL in combination with nicotinic acid or fibrates (see Section 4.5 Interactions with other medicaments and other forms of interaction).

• Dose recommendations for slowing the progression of coronary atherosclerosis

In a study in patients with primary hypercholesterolaemia and concomitant coronary heart disease 40 mg daily slowed the progression of coronary atherosclerosis.

• Dose recommendations for the secondary prevention of coronary events after percutaneous coronary intervention

In patients with coronary heart disease after percutaneous coronary intervention, the dose is 80 mg daily.

Patients with impaired kidney function

Fluvastatin is cleared by the liver, with less than 6% of the administered dose excreted into the urine. The pharmacokinetics of fluvastatin remain unchanged in patients with mild to severe renal insufficiency (creatinine > 260 μmol/L). No dose adjustments are therefore necessary in these patients.

Patients with impaired liver function

LESCOL/LESCOL XL is contraindicated in patients with active liver disease, or unexplained, persistent elevations in serum transaminases (see 4.3 Contraindications and 4.4 Special warnings and special precautions for use).

USE IN THE ELDERLY

There is no evidence of reduced tolerability or altered dosage requirements in elderly patients.

USE IN CHILDREN

As there is no experience with the use of LESCOL in individuals less than 18 years of age, its use is contraindicated in this group.

4.3 Contraindications

Known hypersensitivity to any component of LESCOL.

Patients with active liver disease, hepatic impairment, or unexplained, persistent elevations in serum transaminases.

Individuals under 18 years of age.

4.4 Special warnings and special precautions for use

HMG-CoA reductase inhibitors, including LESCOL, are unlikely to be of benefit in patients with rare homozygous familial hypercholesterolaemia.

As with other lipid-lowering drugs, it is recommended that liver function tests be performed before the initiation of treatment and periodically thereafter in all patients. Should an increase in aspartate aminotransferase (AST) or alanine aminotransferase (ALT) exceed 3 times the upper limit of normal and persist, therapy should be discontinued. In very rare cases, possibly drug-related hepatitis was observed that resolved upon discontinuation of treatment.

Caution should be exercised when LESCOL is administered to patients with a history of liver disease or heavy alcohol ingestion.

Since fluvastatin is eliminated primarily via the biliary route and is subject to significant pre-systemic metabolism, the potential exists for drug accumulation in patients with hepatic insufficiency.

The use of fluvastatin in combination with glibenclamide should be avoided whenever possible (see Section 4.5 Interaction with other medicaments and other forms of interaction).

Skeletal muscle:

With LESCOL, myopathy has rarely been reported, whereas myositis and rhabdomyolysis have been reported very rarely. In patients with unexplained diffuse myalgias, muscle tenderness or muscle weakness, and/or marked elevation of creatine kinase (CK) values myopathy, myositis or rhabdomyolysis have to be considered. Patients should therefore be advised to report promptly unexplained muscle pain, muscle tenderness or muscle weakness, particularly if accompanied by malaise or fever.

Creatine kinase measurement:

There is no current evidence to require routine monitoring of plasma total creatine kinase or other muscle enzyme levels in asymptomatic patients on statins. If creatine kinase has to be measured it should not be done following strenuous exercise or in the presence of any plausible alternative cause of CK-increase as this makes the value interpretation difficult.

Before the treatment:

As with all other statins physicians should prescribe fluvastatin with caution in patients with pre-disposing factors for rhabdomyolysis and its complications. A creatine kinase level should be measured before starting fluvastatin treatment in the following situations:

- Renal impairment
- Hypothyroidism
- Personal or familial history of hereditary muscular disorders
- Previous history of muscular toxicity with a statin or fibrate
- Alcohol abuse
- In elderly (age > 70 years), the necessity of such measurement should be considered, according to the presence of other predisposing factors for rhabdomyolysis.

In such situations, the risk of treatment should be considered in relation to the possible benefit and clinical monitoring is recommended. If CK-levels are significantly elevated at baseline (> 5 × ULN), levels should be re-measured within 5 to 7 days later to confirm the results. If CK-levels are still significantly elevated (> 5 × ULN) at baseline, treatment should not be started.

Whilst on treatment:

If muscular symptoms like pain, weakness or cramps occur in patients receiving fluvastatin, their CK-levels should be measured. Treatment should be stopped, if these levels are found to be significantly elevated (> 5 × ULN).

If muscular symptoms are severe and cause daily discomfort, even if CK-levels are elevated to ≤ 5 × ULN, treatment discontinuation should be considered.

Should the symptoms resolve and CK-levels return to normal, then re-introduction of fluvastatin or another statin may be considered at the lowest dose and under close monitoring.

The risk of myopathy is known to be increased in patients receiving immunosuppressive drugs (including cyclosporin), fibrates, nicotinic acid or erythromycin together with other HMG-CoA reductase inhibitors. Minimal data exist to support the efficacy or safety of LESCOL in combination with nicotinic acid, its derivatives, fibrates or cyclosporin. LESCOL should be used with caution in patients receiving such concomitant medication (see Section 4.5).

4.5 Interaction with other medicinal products and other forms of Interaction

Fluvastatin is substantially metabolised by cytochrome P450 (CYP2C9). Other substrates or inhibitors of CYP2C9 administered concomitantly may therefore potentially result in increased plasma levels of fluvastatin, with a consequent increased risk of myopathy (see section 4.4).

Food - Although AUC and C_{max} were lowered and t_{max} prolonged when LESCOL was taken with food, there was no apparent difference in the lipid-lowering effects whether LESCOL was taken with food or not.

Cyclosporin - In an interaction study concomitant administration of fluvastatin and cyclosporin resulted in an increase in the bioavailability of fluvastatin by a factor of 1.9. The combination should be used with caution due to the theoretical potential for an increased risk of myopathy and/or rhabdomyolysis. No effect was seen on cyclosporin levels.

Fibric acid derivatives (fibrates) and nicotinic acid:

Bezafibrate - An interaction study between 20mg o.d. fluvastatin and 200mg t.d.s. bezafibrate showed that mean AUC and C_{max} values of fluvastatin were increased on average by about 50-60%. No effect was seen on bezafibrate pharmacokinetics. This combination should be used with caution, however, due to the increased risk of developing myopathy and/or rhabdomyolysis when HMG-CoA reductase inhibitors including fluvastatin have been combined with fibrates. Any patient complaining of myalgia should be carefully evaluated.

Gemfibrozil - In an interaction study the concomitant administration of fluvastatin and gemfibrozil had no effect on the pharmacokinetics of either drug. The combination should be used with caution however, due to reports of an increased risk of myopathy and/or rhabdomyolysis when other HMG-CoA reductase inhibitors have been combined with fibrates.

Ciprofibrate - Concomitant administration of fluvastatin and ciprofibrate has no effect on the bioavailability of fluvastatin. However, the combination should be used with caution due to reports of an increased risk of myopathy and/or rhabdomyolysis when ciprofibrate is used in combination with other HMG-CoA reductase inhibitors.

Nicotinic acid - Concomitant administration of fluvastatin and nicotinic acid has no effect on the bioavailability of fluvastatin. However, the combination should be used with caution due to reports of an increased risk of myopathy and/or rhabdomyolysis when nicotinic acid is used in combination with other HMG-CoA reductase inhibitors.

Erythromycin - There are reports of an increased risk of myopathy and/or rhabdomyolysis when other HMG-CoA reductase inhibitors have been combined with erythromycin. The results from an interaction study with a small number of healthy volunteers suggested that erythromycin and fluvastatin were not metabolised by the same isoenzyme, however caution should be exercised when these two drugs are given in combination in view of the interaction seen with other HMG-CoA reductase inhibitors.

Itraconazole - No interactions have been seen with itraconazole. Nevertheless patients should be closely monitored.

Antipyrine - Administration of LESCOL does not influence the metabolism and excretion of antipyrine. As antipyrine is a model for drugs metabolised by the microsomal hepatic enzyme systems, interactions with other drugs metabolised by these systems are not expected.

Propranolol - Concomitant administration of LESCOL with propranolol has no effect on the bioavailability of LESCOL.

Bile-acid sequestering agents - Administration of LESCOL 4 hours after cholestyramine results in a clinically significant additive effect compared with that achieved with either drug alone. LESCOL should be administered at least 4 hours after the resin (e.g. cholestyramine) to avoid a significant interaction due to drug binding to the resin.

Digoxin - Concomitant administration of LESCOL with digoxin has no effect on digoxin plasma concentrations.

Cimetidine/ranitidine/omeprazole - Concomitant administration of LESCOL with cimetidine, ranitidine or omeprazole results in an increase in the bioavailability of LESCOL, which, however, is of no clinical relevance.

Rifampicin - Administration of LESCOL to subjects pretreated with rifampicin resulted in a reduction of the bioavailability of LESCOL by about 50%. Although at present there is no clinical evidence that fluvastatin efficacy in lowering lipid levels is altered, for patients undertaking long-term rifampicin therapy (e.g. treatment of tuberculosis), appropriate adjustment of fluvastatin dosage may be warranted to ensure a satisfactory reduction in lipid levels.

Phenytoin - Co-administration of fluvastatin (40 mg b.i.d. for 5 days) increased the mean C_{max} of phenytoin by 5% whereas the mean AUC was increased by 22%. Patients on phenytoin should be carefully monitored when fluvastatin therapy is initiated or when the dose is increased. Fluvastatin mean AUC and Cmax values were also increased by 40% and 27% respectively. This combination should be used with caution due to the increased risk of developing phenytoin toxicity or myoptahy and/or rhabdomyolysis.

Warfarin and other coumarin derivatives - Co-administration of fluvastatin with warfarin may commonly cause significant increases in prothrombin time. This has resulted very rarely in serious haemorrhage. It is recommended that prothrombin times are monitored when fluvastatin therapy is initiated, discontinued or the dosage changed in patients receiving warfarin or other coumarin derivative.

Glibenclamide - An interaction study between fluvastatin 40mg b.i.d. and glibenclamide was done in diabetic patients stabilised on 5-20mg of glibenclamide. The AUC for glibenclamide increased on average by 1.7 times (range: 0.9 – 3.5), Cmax increased on average by 1.6 times (range: 0.9 -3.0) and the mean t1/2 of glibenclamide increased from 8.5 to 18.8 hours when taken with fluvastatin. In this study there were no significant changes in glucose levels but in view of the increases seen in glibenclamide levels there remains a potential for serious hypoglycaemia and this combination should be avoided whenever possible.

Other concomitant therapy - In clinical studies in which LESCOL was used concomitantly with angiotensin converting enzyme (ACE) inhibitors, beta-blockers, calcium channel blockers, salicylic acid, H_2-blockers and non-steroidal anti-inflammatory drugs (NSAIDs), no clinically significant adverse interactions occurred.

4.6 Pregnancy and lactation

Animal studies have indicated that fluvastatin is devoid of embryotoxic and teratogenic potential. However, since HMG-CoA reductase inhibitors decrease the synthesis of cholesterol and possibly of other biologically active substances derived from cholesterol, they may cause fetal harm when administered to pregnant women. Therefore, HMG-CoA reductase inhibitors are contraindicated during pregnancy and in women of childbearing potential not taking adequate contraceptive precautions. If a patient becomes pregnant while taking this class of drug, therapy should be discontinued. As small amounts of fluvastatin have been found in rat milk, LESCOL is contraindicated in nursing mothers.

4.7 Effects on ability to drive and use machines

No data exist on the effects of LESCOL on the ability to drive and use machines.

4.8 Undesirable effects

Frequency estimate: very rare < 0.01%; rare ⩽ 0.01% to < 0.1%; uncommon ⩽ 0.1% to < 1%; common ⩾ 1% to < 10%.

The most commonly reported adverse drug reactions are minor gastrointestinal symptoms, insomnia and headache.

Gastrointestinal tract:

Common: dyspepsia, abdominal pain and nausea.

Central and peripheral nervous system:

Common: headache and insomnia.

Very rare: paresthesia, dysesthesia, hypoesthesia and peripheral neuropathy also known to be associated with underlying hyperlipidemic disorders.

Hypersensitivity reactions:

Rare: rash and urticaria.

Very rare: other skin reactions (e.g. eczema, dermatitis and bullous exanthema), face, edema, angiodema, thrombocytopenia, vasculitis, lupus erythematosus-like reactions.

Musculoskeletal system:

(see section 4.4, skeletal muscle):

Rare: myalgia, muscle tenderness, muscle weakness and myopathy.

Very rare: myositis and rhabdomyolysis.

Liver:

(see section 4.4, skeletal muscle):

Very rare: hepatitis.

Biochemical abnormalities of liver function have been associated with HMG-CoA reductase inhibitors and other lipid-lowering agents. Confirmed elevations of transaminase levels to more than 3 times the upper limit of normal (ULN) developed in a small number of patients (less than or equal to 1%). Marked elevations of CK levels to more than 5 × ULN developed 0.3 - 1.0% of patients receiving licensed doses of fluvastatin in clinical trials.

4.9 Overdose

The experience with overdoses of LESCOL is very limited. Should an accidental overdosage occur, administration of activated charcoal is recommended. In the case of a very recent oral intake gastric lavage may be considered. Treatment should be symptomatic.

5. PHARMACOLOGICAL PROPERTIES

5.1 Pharmacodynamic properties

LESCOL, a fully synthetic cholesterol-lowering agent, is a competitive inhibitor of HMG-CoA reductase, which is responsible for the conversion of HMG-CoA to mevalonate, a precursor of sterols, including cholesterol. LESCOL exerts its main effect in the liver. The inhibition of cholesterol biosynthesis reduces the cholesterol in hepatic cells, which stimulates the synthesis of LDL receptors and thereby increases the uptake of LDL particles. The ultimate result of these mechanisms is a reduction of the plasma cholesterol concentration.

A variety of clinical studies has demonstrated that elevated levels of total cholesterol (total-C), LDL-C and apolipoprotein B (a membrane transport complex for LDL-C) promote human atherosclerosis. Similarly, decreased levels of high density lipoprotein cholesterol (HDL-C) and its transport complex, apolipoprotein A, are associated with the development of atherosclerosis. Epidemiologic investigations have established that cardiovascular morbidity and mortality vary directly with the level of total-C and LDL-C and inversely with the level of HDL-C. In multicentre clinical trials, those pharmacologic and/or non-pharmacologic interventions that simultaneously lowered LDL-C and increased HDL-C reduced the rate of cardiovascular events (both fatal and non-fatal myocardial infarctions). The overall cholesterol profile is improved with the principal effects being the reduction of total-C and LDL-C. LESCOL also produces a moderate reduction in triglycerides and a moderate increase in HDL-C.

In a pooled analysis of all placebo-controlled studies, patients with primary mixed dyslipidaemia (Type IIb) defined as baseline TG levels ⩾ 200 mg/dL, treatment with LESCOL in daily doses ranging from 20 mg to 80 mg (40 mg b.i.d.) demonstrated consistent and significant decreases in total-C, LDL-C, and apo-B, TG, and a modest increase in HDL-C.

In the Lescol Intervention Prevention Study (LIPS), the effect of fluvastatin on major adverse cardiac events (MACE) was assessed in patients with coronary heart disease who had first successful transcatheter therapy (TCT). The study included male and female patients (18-80 years old) and with baseline total cholesterol levels ranging from 3.5-7.0 mmol/L.

In this randomised, double-blind, placebo-controlled trial, a total of 1677 patients were recruited (844 in fluvastatin group and 833 in placebo group). The MACE was defined as cardiac death, non fatal MI and re-intervention (including CABG, repeat TCT, or TCT of a new lesion). The dose of fluvastatin used in this study was 80 mg daily over 4 years. Although the overall composite endpoint showed significant reduction in MACE (22%) compared to placebo (p=0.013), the individual components (cardiac death, non fatal MI and re-intervention) failed to reach statistical significance. There was however a trend in favour of fluvastatin. Therapy with fluvastatin reduced the risk of cardiac death and/or myocardial infarction by 31% (p=0.065).

5.2 Pharmacokinetic properties

LESCOL is a racemate of the two erythro enantiomers of which one exerts the pharmacological activity. LESCOL is absorbed rapidly and completely (98%) following oral administration to fasted volunteers. In a fed state, the drug is absorbed at a reduced rate. Fluvastatin exerts its main effect in the liver, which is also the main organ for its metabolism. The absolute bioavailability assessed from systemic blood concentrations is 24%. The apparent volume of distribution (V_zf) for the drug is 330 L. More than 98% of the circulating drug is bound to plasma proteins, and this binding is unaffected by drug concentration.

The major circulating blood components are fluvastatin and the pharmacologically inactive N-desisopropyl-propionic acid metabolite. The hydroxylated metabolites have pharmacological activity but do not circulate systemically.

The hepatic metabolic pathways of fluvastatin in humans have been characterised. There are multiple, alternative cytochrome P_{450} (CYP_{450}) pathways involved. However, the major pathway is mediated by CYP2C9 and this pathway is subject to potential interactions with other CYP2C9 substrates or inhibitors. In addition there are several minor pathways (e.g. CYP3A4).

Several detailed *in vitro* studies have addressed the inhibitory potential of fluvastatin on common CYP isoenzymes. Fluvastatin inhibited only the metabolism of compounds that are metabolized by CYP2C9.

Following administration of ^{3}H-fluvastatin to healthy volunteers, excretion of radioactivity is about 6% in the urine and 93% in the faeces, and fluvastatin accounts for less than 2% of the total radioactivity excreted. The plasma clearance (CL/f)for fluvastatin in man is calculated to be 1.8 ± 0.8 L/min. Steady-state plasma concentrations show no evidence of fluvastatin accumulation following administration of 40 mg daily. Following oral administration of 40 mg of LESCOL, the terminal disposition half-life for fluvastatin is 2.3 ± 0.9 hours.

Food: Although AUC and C_{max} were lowered and t_{max} prolonged when LESCOL was taken with food, there was no apparent difference in the lipid-lowering effect whether LESCOL was taken with food or not.

Plasma concentrations of fluvastatin do not vary as a function of either age or gender in the general population.

5.3 Preclinical safety data

The safety of fluvastatin was extensively investigated in toxicity studies in rats, dogs, monkeys, mice and hamsters. A variety of changes were identified that are common to HMG-CoA reductase inhibitors, *viz.* hyperplasia and hyperkeratosis of the rodent non-glandular stomach, cataracts in dogs, myopathy in rodents, mild liver changes in most laboratory animals with gall bladder changes in dog, monkey and hamster, thyroid weight increases in the rat and testicular degeneration in the hamster. Fluvastatin is devoid of the CNS vascular and degenerative changes recorded in dogs with other members of this class of compound.

A carcinogenicity study was performed in rats at dose levels of 6, 9 and 18 mg/kg a day (escalated to 24 mg/kg a day after 1 year) to establish a clear maximum tolerated dose. These treatment levels yielded plasma drug levels approximately 9, 13 and 26 to 35 times the mean human plasma drug concentration after a 40 mg oral dose. A low incidence of forestomach squamous papillomas and one carcinoma of the forestomach was observed at the 24 mg/kg a day dose level. In addition, an increased incidence of thyroid follicular cell adenomas and carcinomas was recorded in male rats treated with 18 to 24 mg/kg a day.

The forestomach neoplasms observed in rats and mice reflect chronic hyperplasia caused by direct contact exposure to fluvastatin rather than a genotoxic effect of the drug. The increased incidence of thyroid follicular cell neoplasms in male rats given fluvastatin appears to be consistent with species-specific findings with other HMG-CoA reductase inhibitors. In contrast to other HMG-CoA reductase inhibitors, no treatment-related increases in the incidences of hepatic adenomas or carcinomas were observed.

The carcinogenicity study conducted in mice at dose levels of 0.3, 15 and 30 mg/kg a day revealed, as in rats, a statistically significant increase in forestomach squamous cell papillomas in males and females at 30 mg/kg a day and in females at 15 mg/kg a day. These treatment levels yielded plasma drug levels approximately 0.2, 10 and 21 times the mean human plasma drug concentration after a 40-mg oral dose.

No evidence of mutagenicity was observed *in vitro*, with or without rat-liver metabolic activation, in the following studies: microbial mutagen tests using mutant strains of *Salmonella typhimurium* or *Escherichia coli*: malignant transformation assay in BALB/3T3 cells; unscheduled DNA synthesis in rat primary hepatocytes; chromosomal aberrations in V79 Chinese hamster cells; HGPRT V79 Chinese hamster cells. In addition, there was no evidence of mutagenicity *in vivo* in either a rat or mouse micronucleus test.

In a study in rats at dose levels in females of 0.6, 2 and 6 mg/kg a day and in males of 2, 10 and 20 mg/kg a day, fluvastatin had no adverse effects on the fertility or reproductive performance. Teratology studies in rats and rabbits showed maternal toxicity at high dose levels, but there was no evidence of embryotoxic or teratogenic potential. A study in which female rats were dosed at 12 and 24 mg/kg a day during late gestation until weaning of the pups resulted in maternal mortality at or near term and post partum accompanied by fetal and neonatal lethality. No effects on the pregnant females or fetuses occurred at the low dose level of 2 mg/kg a day.

A second study at levels of 2, 6, 12 and 24 mg/kg a day during late gestation and early lactation showed similar effects at 6 mg/kg a day and above caused by cardiotoxicity. In a third study, pregnant rats were administered 12 or 24 mg/kg a day during late gestation until weaning of pups with or without the presence of concurrent supplementation with mevalonic acid, a derivative of HMG-CoA that is essential for cholesterol biosynthesis. The concurrent administration of mevalonic acid completely prevented the cardiotoxicity and the maternal and neonatal mortality. Therefore, the maternal and neonatal lethality observed with fluvastatin reflects its exaggerated pharmacologic effect during pregnancy.

6. PHARMACEUTICAL PARTICULARS

6.1 List of excipients

Capsule content:

Magnesium stearate

Sodium hydrogen carbonate

Talc

Cellulose microcrystalline, fine powder

Cellulose microcrystalline, granular powder

Maize starch, physically modified

Calcium carbonate

Capsule shell:

Titanium dioxide E171

Iron oxide red E172

Iron oxide yellow E172

Gelatin

6.2 Incompatibilities

None

6.3 Shelf life

3 years.

6.4 Special precautions for storage

Do not store above 25°C.

6.5 Nature and contents of container

Alu/alu blister consisting of an aluminium coating foil and an aluminium covering foil.

HDPE bottle with a tight closure consisting of a polyethylene container (high density polyethylene, grey pigmented) and a closure.

The 20 mg capsules are contained in calendar packs of 28.

The 40mg capsules are contained in calendar packs of 28 capsules and available in calendar packs of 56 capsules for twice daily dosing.

6.6 Instructions for use and handling

None

7. MARKETING AUTHORISATION HOLDER

Novartis Pharmaceuticals UK Ltd

Trading as Sandoz Pharmaceuticals

Frimley Business Park

Frimley

Camberley

Surrey

GU16 7SR

8. MARKETING AUTHORISATION NUMBER(S)

20 mg capsules: PL 00101/0360

40mg capsules: PL 00101/0361

9. DATE OF FIRST AUTHORISATION/RENEWAL OF THE AUTHORISATION

23 August 1993.

10. DATE OF REVISION OF THE TEXT

16 February 2004

Legal category

POM

Lescol XL 80 mg Prolonged Release Tablets

(Novartis Pharmaceuticals UK Ltd)

1. NAME OF THE MEDICINAL PRODUCT

Lescol® XL 80 mg Prolonged Release Tablets.

2. QUALITATIVE AND QUANTITATIVE COMPOSITION

One prolonged release tablet containing 84.24 mg fluvastatin sodium corresponding to 80 mg fluvastatin free acid.

For excipients, see Section 6.1.

3. PHARMACEUTICAL FORM

Prolonged release tablet.

Lescol XL tablets are yellow, round, slightly biconvex with bevelled edges and are marked "LESCOL XL" on one side and "80" on the other.

4. CLINICAL PARTICULARS

4.1 Therapeutic indications

Lescol XL is indicated as an adjunct to diet for the reduction of elevated total cholesterol (total-C), low-density lipoprotein cholesterol (LDL-C), apolipoprotein B (apo B) and triglyceride (TG) levels and for the increase of high-density lipoprotein cholesterol (HDL-C) in patients with primary hypercholesterolaemia and mixed dyslipidaemia (Fredrickson Types IIa and IIb).

Lescol XL is also indicated to slow the progression of coronary atherosclerosis in patients with primary hypercholesterolaemia, including mild forms, and coronary heart disease who do not adequately respond to dietary control.

Lescol XL is also indicated in patients with coronary heart disease for the secondary prevention of coronary events after percutaneous coronary intervention, see Section 5.1.

4.2 Posology and method of administration

Prior to initiating Lescol XL, secondary causes of hypercholesterolaemia should be excluded, and the patient placed on a standard cholesterol-lowering diet. Dietary therapy should be continued during treatment.

Dose recommendations for lipid lowering effect

The recommended starting dose is 40 mg (1 capsule Lescol 40 mg) once daily although a dose of 20 mg fluvastatin (1 capsule Lescol 20 mg) once daily may be adequate in mild cases. Most patients will require a dose of 20 mg to 40 mg once daily but the dose may be increased to 80 mg (1 tablet Lescol XL 80mg) once daily, individualised according to baseline LDL-C levels and the recommended goal of therapy to be accomplished. The maximum recommended daily dose is 80 mg once daily.

Lescol XL can be administered as a single dose at any time of the day with or without food and must be swallowed whole with a glass of water. The maximum lipid-lowering effect with a given dose of the drug is achieved within 4 weeks. Doses should be adjusted according to the patient's response and dose adjustment made at intervals of 4 weeks or more. The therapeutic effect of Lescol XL is maintained with prolonged administration.

Lescol XL is efficacious in monotherapy or in combination with bile acid sequestrants. When Lescol XL is used in combination with cholestyramine or other resins, it should be administered at least 4 hours after the resin to avoid a significant interaction due to binding of the drug to the resin. Minimal data exist to support the efficacy and safety of Lescol XL in combination with nicotinic acid or fibrates (see Section 4.5 Interactions with other medicaments and other forms of interaction).

Dose recommendations for the secondary prevention of coronary events after percutaneous coronary intervention

In patients with coronary heart disease after percutaneous coronary intervention, the dose is 80 mg daily.

Patients with impaired kidney function

Fluvastatin is cleared by the liver, with less than 6% of the administered dose excreted into the urine. The pharmacokinetics of fluvastatin remain unchanged in patients with mild to severe renal insufficiency (creatinine > 260 μmol/L). No dose adjustments are therefore necessary in these patients.

Patients with impaired liver function

Lescol/Lescol XL is contraindicated in patients with active liver disease, or unexplained, persistent elevations in serum transaminases (see 4.3 Contraindications and 4.4 Special warnings and special precautions for use).

USE IN THE ELDERLY

There is no evidence of reduced tolerability or altered dosage requirements in elderly patients.

USE IN CHILDREN

As there is no experience with the use of Lescol XL in individuals less than 18 years of age, its use is contraindicated in this group.

4.3 Contraindications

Known hypersensitivity to any component of Lescol XL.

Patients with active liver disease, hepatic impairment, or unexplained, persistent elevations in serum transaminases.

Individuals under 18 years of age.

4.4 Special warnings and special precautions for use

HMG-CoA reductase inhibitors, including Lescol XL, are unlikely to be of benefit in patients with rare homozygous familial hypercholesterolaemia.

As with other lipid-lowering drugs, it is recommended that liver function tests be performed before the initiation of treatment and periodically thereafter in all patients. Should an increase in aspartate aminotransferase (AST) or alanine aminotransferase (ALT) exceed 3 times the upper limit of normal and persist, therapy should be discontinued. In very rare cases, possibly drug-related hepatitis was observed that resolved upon discontinuation of treatment.

Caution should be exercised when Lescol XL is administered to patients with a history of liver disease or heavy alcohol ingestion.

Since fluvastatin is eliminated primarily via the biliary route and is subject to significant pre-systemic metabolism, the potential exists for drug accumulation in patients with hepatic insufficiency.

The use of fluvastatin in combination with glibenclamide should be avoided whenever possible (see Section 4.5 Interactions with other medicaments and other forms of interaction).

Skeletal muscle

With Lescol XL, myopathy has rarely been reported, whereas myositis and rhabdomyolysis have been reported very rarely. In patients with unexplained diffuse myalgias, muscle tenderness or muscle weakness, and/or marked elevation of creatine kinase (CK) values, myopathy, myositis or rhabdomyolysis have to be considered. Patients should, therefore, be advised to report promptly unexplained muscle pain, muscle tenderness or muscle weakness, particularly if accompanied by malaise or fever.

Creatine kinase measurement

There is no current evidence to require routine monitoring of plasma total creatine kinase or other muscle enzyme levels in asymptomatic patients on statins. If creatine kinase has to be measured it should not be done following strenuous exercise or in the presence of any plausible alternative cause of CK-increase as this makes the value interpretation difficult.

Before the treatment

As with all other statins physicians should prescribe fluvastatin with caution in patients with pre-disposing factors for rhabdomyolysis and its complications. A creatine kinase level should be measured before starting fluvastatin treatment in the following situations:

- Renal impairment
- Hypothyroidism
- Personal or familial history of hereditary muscular disorders
- Previous history of muscular toxicity with a statin or fibrate
- Alcohol abuse
- In elderly (age > 70 years), the necessity of such measurement should be considered, according to the presence of other predisposing factors for rhabdomyolysis.

In such situations, the risk of treatment should be considered in relation to the possible benefit and clinical monitoring is recommended. If CK-levels are significantly elevated at baseline > 5 × ULN), levels should be re-measured within 5 to 7 days later to confirm the results. If CK-levels are still significantly elevated > 5 × ULN) at baseline, treatment should not be started.

Whilst on treatment

If muscular symptoms like pain, weakness or cramps occur in patients receiving fluvastatin, their CK-levels should be measured. Treatment should be stopped, if these levels are found to be significantly elevated (> 5 × ULN).

If muscular symptoms are severe and cause daily discomfort, even if CK-levels are elevated to ≤ 5 × ULN, treatment discontinuation should be considered.

Should the symptoms resolve and CK-levels return to normal, then re-introduction of fluvastatin or another statin may be considered at the lowest dose and under close monitoring.

The risk of myopathy is known to be increased in patients receiving immunosuppressive drugs (including cyclosporin), fibrates, nicotinic acid or erythromycin together with other HMG-CoA reductase inhibitors. Minimal data exist to support the efficacy or safety of Lescol XL in combination with nicotinic acid, its derivatives, fibrates or cyclosporin. Lescol XL should be used with caution in patients receiving such concomitant medication (see Section 4.5).

4.5 Interaction with other medicinal products and other forms of Interaction

Fluvastatin is substantially metabolised by cytochrome P450 (CYP2C9). Other substrates or inhibitors of CYP2C9 administered concomitantly may, therefore, potentially result in increased plasma levels of fluvastatin, with a consequent increased risk of myopathy (see section 4.4).

Food

Mean AUC and C_{max} were increased by 49% and 45% respectively and t_{max} prolonged when fluvastatin (Lescol XL) was taken with food, compared to fasting state. However, no clinically obvious differences in the lipid-lowering effects and safety are anticipated when Lescol XL is taken with or without food.

Cyclosporin

In an interaction study concomitant administration of fluvastatin and cyclosporin resulted in an increase in the bioavailability of fluvastatin by a factor of 1.9. The combination should be used with caution due to the theoretical potential for an increased risk of myopathy and/or rhabdomyolysis. No effect was seen on cyclosporin levels.

Fibric acid derivatives (fibrates) and nicotinic acid

Bezafibrate

An interaction study between 20 mg o.d. fluvastatin and 200 mg t.d.s. bezafibrate showed that mean AUC and C_{max} values of fluvastatin were increased on average by about 50-60%. No effect was seen on bezafibrate pharmacokinetics. This combination should be used with caution, however, due to the increased risk of developing myopathy and/or rhabdomyolysis when HMG-CoA reductase inhibitors including fluvastatin have been combined with fibrates. Any patient complaining of myalgia should be carefully evaluated.

Gemfibrozil

In an interaction study the concomitant administration of fluvastatin and gemfibrozil had no effect on the pharmacokinetics of either drug. The combination should be used with caution however, due to reports of an increased risk of myopathy and/or rhabdomyolysis when other HMG-CoA reductase inhibitors have been combined with fibrates.

Ciprofibrate

Concomitant administration of fluvastatin and ciprofibrate has no effect on the bioavailability of fluvastatin. However, the combination should be used with caution due to reports of an increased risk of myopathy and/or rhabdomyolysis when ciprofibrate is used in combination with other HMG-CoA reductase inhibitors.

Nicotinic acid

Concomitant administration of fluvastatin and nicotinic acid has no effect on the bioavailability of fluvastatin. However, the combination should be used with caution due to reports of an increased risk of myopathy and/or rhabdomyolysis when nicotinic acid is used in combination with other HMG-CoA reductase inhibitors.

Erythromycin

There are reports of an increased risk of myopathy and/or rhabdomyolysis when other HMG-CoA reductase inhibitors have been combined with erythromycin. The results from an interaction study with a small number of healthy volunteers suggested that erythromycin and fluvastatin were not metabolised by the same isoenzyme, however, caution should be exercised when these two drugs are given in combination in view of the interaction seen with other HMG-CoA reductase inhibitors.

Itraconazole

No interactions have been seen with itraconazole. Nevertheless, patients should be closely monitored.

Antipyrine

Administration of fluvastatin does not influence the metabolism and excretion of antipyrine. As antipyrine is a model for drugs metabolised by the microsomal hepatic enzyme systems, interactions with other drugs metabolised by these systems are not expected.

Propranolol

Concomitant administration of fluvastatin with propranolol has no effect on the bioavailability of fluvastatin.

Bile-acid sequestering agents

Administration of fluvastatin 4 hours after cholestyramine results in a clinically significant additive effect compared with that achieved with either drug alone. Lescol XL should be administered at least 4 hours after the resin (e.g. cholestyramine) to avoid a significant interaction due to drug binding to the resin.

Digoxin

Concomitant administration of fluvastatin with digoxin has no effect on digoxin plasma concentrations.

Cimetidine/ranitidine/omeprazole

Concomitant administration of fluvastatin with cimetidine, ranitidine or omeprazole results in an increase in the bioavailability of fluvastatin, which, however, is of no clinical relevance.

Rifampicin

Administration of fluvastatin to subjects pre-treated with rifampicin resulted in a reduction of the bioavailability of fluvastatin by about 50%. Although at present there is no clinical evidence that fluvastatin efficacy in lowering lipid levels is altered, for patients undertaking long-term rifampicin therapy (e.g. treatment of tuberculosis), appropriate adjustment of fluvastatin dosage may be warranted to ensure a satisfactory reduction in lipid levels.

Phenytoin

Co-administration of fluvastatin (40 mg b.i.d. for 5 days) increased the mean C_{max} of phenytoin by 5%, whereas the mean AUC was increased by 22%. Patients on phenytoin should be carefully monitored when fluvastatin therapy is initiated or when the dose is increased. Fluvastatin mean AUC and Cmax values were also increased by 40% and 27% respectively. This combination should be used with caution due to the increased risk of developing phenytoin toxicity or myopathy and/or rhabdomyolysis.

Warfarin and other coumarin derivatives

Co-administration of fluvastatin with warfarin may commonly cause significant increases in prothrombin time. This has resulted, very rarely, in serious haemorrhage. It is recommended that prothrombin times are monitored when fluvastatin therapy is initiated, discontinued or the dosage changed in patients receiving warfarin or other coumarin derivative.

Glibenclamide

An interaction study between fluvastatin 40 mg b.i.d. and glibenclamide was done in diabetic patients stabilised on 5-20 mg of glibenclamide. The AUC for glibenclamide increased on average by 1.7 times (range: 0.9 – 3.5), C_{max} increased on average by 1.6 times (range: 0.9 -3.0) and the mean $t_{1/2}$ of glibenclamide increased from 8.5 to 18.8 hours when taken with fluvastatin. In this study there were no significant changes in glucose levels, but in view of the increases seen in glibenclamide levels there remains a potential for serious hypoglycaemia and this combination should be avoided whenever possible.

Other concomitant therapy

In clinical studies in which fluvastatin was used concomitantly with angiotensin converting enzyme (ACE) inhibitors, beta-blockers, calcium channel blockers, salicylic acid, H_2-blockers and non-steroidal anti-inflammatory drugs (NSAIDs), no clinically significant adverse interactions occurred.

4.6 Pregnancy and lactation

Animal studies have indicated that fluvastatin is devoid of embryotoxic and teratogenic potential. However, since HMG-CoA reductase inhibitors decrease the synthesis of cholesterol and possibly of other biologically active substances derived from cholesterol, they may cause foetal harm when administered to pregnant women. Therefore, HMG-CoA reductase inhibitors are contraindicated during pregnancy and in women of childbearing potential not taking adequate contraceptive precautions. If a patient becomes pregnant while taking this class of drug, therapy should be discontinued. As small amounts of fluvastatin have been found in rat milk, Lescol XL is contraindicated in nursing mothers.

4.7 Effects on ability to drive and use machines

No data exist on the effects of Lescol XL on the ability to drive and use machines.

4.8 Undesirable effects

Frequency estimate:

very rare $< 0.01\%$

rare $\geqslant 0.01\%$ to $< 0.1\%$

uncommon $\geqslant 0.1\%$ to $< 1\%$

common $\geqslant 1\%$ to $< 10\%$.

The most commonly reported adverse drug reactions are minor gastrointestinal symptoms, insomnia and headache.

Gastrointestinal tract

Common: dyspepsia, abdominal pain and nausea.

Central and peripheral nervous system

Common: headache and insomnia.

Very rare: paresthesia, dysesthesia, hypoesthesia and peripheral neuropathy also known to be associated with underlying hyperlipidemic disorders.

Hypersensitivity reactions

Rare: rash and urticaria.

Very rare: other skin reactions (e.g. eczema, dermatitis and bullous exanthema), face oedema, angioedema, thrombocytopenia, vasculitis, lupus erythematosus-like reactions.

Musculoskeletal system (see section 4.4, skeletal muscle)

Rare: myalgia, muscle tenderness, muscle weakness and myopathy.

Very rare: myositis and rhabdomyolysis.

Liver (see section 4.4, skeletal muscle)

Very rare: hepatitis.

Confirmed elevations of transaminase levels to more than 3 times the upper limit of normal (ULN) developed in a small number of patients (less than or equal to 2%). Marked elevations of CK levels to more than 5 × ULN developed in 0.3-1.0% of patients receiving licensed doses of fluvastatin in clinical trials.

4.9 Overdose

In a placebo-controlled study including 40 hypercholesterolaemic patients, doses up to 320 mg/day (n=7 per dose group) administered as Lescol XL 80 mg tablets over two weeks were well tolerated.

The experience with overdoses of Lescol XL is very limited. Should an accidental overdosage occur, administration of activated charcoal is recommended. In the case of a very recent oral intake gastric lavage may be considered. Treatment should be symptomatic.

5. PHARMACOLOGICAL PROPERTIES

5.1 Pharmacodynamic properties

Fluvastatin, a fully synthetic cholesterol-lowering agent, is a competitive inhibitor of HMG-CoA reductase, which is responsible for the conversion of HMG-CoA to mevalonate, a precursor of sterols, including cholesterol. Lescol XL exerts its main effect in the liver. The inhibition of cholesterol biosynthesis reduces the cholesterol in hepatic cells, which stimulates the synthesis of LDL receptors and thereby increases the uptake of LDL particles. The ultimate result of these mechanisms is a reduction of the plasma cholesterol concentration.

A variety of clinical studies have demonstrated that elevated levels of total cholesterol (total-C), LDL-C and apolipoprotein B (a membrane transport complex for LDL-C) promote human atherosclerosis. Similarly, decreased levels of high density lipoprotein cholesterol (HDL-C) and its transport complex, apolipoprotein A, are associated with the development of atherosclerosis. Epidemiologic investigations have established that cardiovascular morbidity and mortality vary directly with the level of total-C and LDL-C and inversely with the level of HDL-C. In multicentre clinical trials, those pharmacologic and/or nonpharmacologic interventions that simultaneously lowered LDL-C and increased HDL-C reduced the rate of cardiovascular events (both fatal and non-fatal myocardial infarctions). The overall cholesterol profile is improved with the principal effects being the reduction of total-C and LDL-C. Lescol XL also produces a moderate reduction in triglycerides and a moderate increase in HDL-C. Therapeutic response is well established within 2 weeks, and maximum response is achieved within 4 weeks from treatment initiation and maintained during chronic therapy.

In the Lescol Intervention Prevention Study (LIPS), the effect of fluvastatin on major adverse cardiac events (MACE) was assessed in patients with coronary heart disease who had first successful transcatheter therapy (TCT). The study included male and female patients (18-80 years old) and with baseline total cholesterol levels ranging from 3.5-7.0 mmol/L.

In this randomised, double-blind, placebo-controlled trial, a total of 1677 patients were recruited (844 in fluvastatin group and 833 in placebo group). The MACE was defined as cardiac death, non fatal MI and re-intervention (including CABG, repeat TCT, or TCT of a new lesion). The dose of fluvastatin used in this study was 80 mg daily over 4 years. Although the overall composite endpoint showed significant reduction in MACE (22%) compared to placebo (p=0.013), the individual components (cardiac death, non fatal MI and re-intervention) failed to reach statistical significance. There was, however, a trend in favour of fluvastatin. Therapy with fluvastatin reduced the risk of cardiac death and/or myocardial infarction by 31% (p=0.065).

5.2 Pharmacokinetic properties

Lescol XL is a racemate of the two erythro enantiomers of which one exerts the pharmacological activity. Fluvastatin is absorbed rapidly and completely (98%) following oral administration to fasted volunteers. After oral administration of Lescol XL 80 and in comparison with the capsules, the absorption rate of fluvastatin is almost 60% slower while the mean residence time of fluvastatin is increased by approximately 4 hours. In a fed state, the drug is absorbed at a reduced rate. Fluvastatin exerts its main effect in the liver, which is also the main organ for its metabolism. The absolute bioavailability assessed from systemic blood concentrations is 24%. The apparent volume of distribution (V_zf) for the drug is 330 L. More than 98% of the circulating drug is bound to plasma proteins, and this binding is unaffected by drug concentration.

The major circulating blood components are fluvastatin and the pharmacologically inactive N-desisopropyl-propionic acid metabolite. The hydroxylated metabolites have pharmacological activity but do not circulate systemically.

The hepatic metabolic pathways of fluvastatin in humans have been characterised. There are multiple, alternative cytochrome P450 (CYP450) pathways involved. However, the major pathway is mediated by CYP2C9 and this pathway is subject to potential interactions with other CYP2C9 substrates or inhibitors. In addition there are several minor pathways (e.g. CYP3A4).

Several detailed *in vitro* studies have addressed the inhibitory potential of fluvastatin on common CYP isoenzymes. Fluvastatin inhibited only the metabolism of compounds that are metabolised by CYP2C9.

Following administration of ^3H-fluvastatin to healthy volunteers, excretion of radioactivity is about 6% in the urine and 93% in the faeces and fluvastatin accounts for less than 2% of the total radioactivity excreted. The plasma clearance (CL/f) for fluvastatin in man is calculated to be 1.8 ± 0.8 L/min. Steady-state plasma concentrations show no evidence of fluvastatin accumulation following administration of 80 mg daily. Following oral administration of 40 mg of LESCOL, the terminal disposition half-life for fluvastatin is 2.3 ± 0.9 hours.

Food

Mean AUC and C_{max} were increased by 49% and 45% respectively and t_{max} prolonged when fluvastatin (Lescol XL) was taken with food, compared to fasting state. However, no clinically obvious differences in the lipid-lowering effects and safety are anticipated when Lescol XL is taken with or without food.

Plasma concentrations of fluvastatin do not vary as a function of age. Mean AUC and C_{max} were increased by 36% and 44% respectively in females compared to males. However, no clinically obvious differences in the lipid-lowering effects of fluvastatin are anticipated between males and females.

5.3 Preclinical safety data

The safety of fluvastatin was extensively investigated in toxicity studies in rats, dogs, monkeys, mice and hamsters. A variety of changes were identified that are common to HMG-CoA reductase inhibitors, *viz.* hyperplasia and hyperkeratosis of the rodent non-glandular stomach, cataracts in dogs, myopathy in rodents, mild liver changes in most laboratory animals with gall bladder changes in dog, monkey and hamster, thyroid weight increases in the rat and testicular degeneration in the hamster. Fluvastatin is devoid of the CNS vascular and degenerative changes recorded in dogs with other members of this class of compound.

A carcinogenicity study was performed in rats at dose levels of 6, 9 and 18 mg/kg a day (escalated to 24 mg/kg a day after 1 year) to establish a clear maximum tolerated dose. These treatment levels yielded plasma drug levels approximately 9, 13 and 26 to 35 times the mean human plasma drug concentration after a 40 mg oral dose. A low incidence of forestomach squamous papillomas and one carcinoma of the forestomach was observed at the 24 mg/kg a day dose level. In addition, an increased incidence of thyroid follicular cell adenomas and carcinomas was recorded in male rats treated with 18 to 24 mg/kg a day.

The forestomach neoplasms observed in rats and mice reflect chronic hyperplasia caused by direct contact exposure to fluvastatin rather than a genotoxic effect of the drug. The increased incidence of thyroid follicular cell neoplasms in male rats given fluvastatin appears to be consistent with species-specific findings with other HMG-CoA reductase inhibitors. In contrast to other HMG-CoA reductase inhibitors, no treatment-related increases in the incidences of hepatic adenomas or carcinomas were observed.

The carcinogenicity study conducted in mice at dose levels of 0.3, 15 and 30 mg/kg a day revealed, as in rats, a statistically significant increase in forestomach squamous cell papillomas in males and females at 30 mg/kg a day and in females at 15 mg/kg a day. These treatment levels yielded plasma drug levels approximately 0.2, 10 and 21 times the mean human plasma drug concentration after a 40-mg oral dose.

No evidence of mutagenicity was observed *in vitro*, with or without rat-liver metabolic activation, in the following studies: microbial mutagen tests using mutant strains of *Salmonella typhimurium* or *Escherichia coli*; malignant transformation assay in BALB/3T3 cells; unscheduled DNA synthesis in rat primary hepatocytes; chromosomal aberrations in V79 Chinese hamster cells; HGPRT V79 Chinese hamster cells. In addition, there was no evidence of mutagenicity *in vivo* in either a rat or mouse micronucleus test.

In a study in rats at dose levels in females of 0.6, 2 and 6 mg/kg a day and in males of 2, 10 and 20 mg/kg a day, fluvastatin had no adverse effects on the fertility or reproductive performance. Teratology studies in rats and rabbits showed maternal toxicity at high dose levels, but there was no evidence of embryotoxic or teratogenic potential. A study in which female rats were dosed at 12 and 24 mg/kg a day during late gestation until weaning of the pups resulted in maternal mortality at, or near, term and post partum accompanied by feotal and neonatal lethality. No effects on the pregnant females or feotuses occurred at the low dose level of 2 mg/kg a day.

A second study at levels of 2, 6, 12 and 24 mg/kg a day during late gestation and early lactation showed similar effects at 6 mg/kg a day and above caused by cardiotoxicity. In a third study, pregnant rats were administered 12 or 24 mg/kg a day during late gestation until weaning of pups with or without the presence of concurrent supplementation with mevalonic acid, a derivative of HMG-CoA that is essential for cholesterol biosynthesis. The concurrent administration of mevalonic acid completely prevented the cardiotoxicity and the maternal and neonatal mortality. Therefore, the maternal and neonatal lethality observed with fluvastatin reflects its exaggerated pharmacologic effect during pregnancy.

6. PHARMACEUTICAL PARTICULARS

6.1 List of excipients

Cellulose microcrystalline

Hypromellose

Hydroxypropyl cellulose

Potassium hydrogen carbonate

Povidone

Magnesium stearate

Iron oxide yellow E172

Titanium dioxide E171

Macrogol 8000

6.2 Incompatibilities

None

6.3 Shelf life

Two years

6.4 Special precautions for storage

Do not store above 25°C. Store in the original package.

6.5 Nature and contents of container

Alu/Alu blister consisting of an aluminium coating foil and an aluminium covering foil. Lescol XL tablets come in packs of 28 tablets.

6.6 Instructions for use and handling

None

7. MARKETING AUTHORISATION HOLDER

Novartis Pharmaceuticals UK Ltd

Trading as Sandoz Pharmaceuticals

Frimley Business Park

Frimley

Camberley

Surrey

GU16 7SR

8. MARKETING AUTHORISATION NUMBER(S)

PL 00101/0587

9. DATE OF FIRST AUTHORISATION/RENEWAL OF THE AUTHORISATION

30 June 2004

10. DATE OF REVISION OF THE TEXT

15 September 2005

LEGAL CATEGORY

POM

Leukeran Tablets 2mg

(GlaxoSmithKline UK)

1. NAME OF THE MEDICINAL PRODUCT

Leukeran Tablets 2 mg

2. QUALITATIVE AND QUANTITATIVE COMPOSITION

Each tablet contains 2 mg of the active ingredient chlorambucil.

3. PHARMACEUTICAL FORM

Film-coated tablet

4. CLINICAL PARTICULARS

4.1 Therapeutic indications

Leukeran is indicated in the treatment of Hodgkin's disease, certain forms of non-Hodgkin's lymphoma, chronic lymphocytic leukaemia, and Waldenstrom's macroglobulinaemia.

4.2 Posology and method of administration

Adults:Hodgkin's Disease: Used as a single agent in the palliative treatment of advanced disease a typical dosage is 0.2 mg/kg/day for 4-8 weeks. Leukeran is usually included in combination therapy and a number of regimes have been used. Leukeran has been used as an alternative to nitrogen mustard with a reduction in toxicity but similar therapeutic results.

Non-Hodgkin's Lymphoma: Used as a single agent the usual dosage is 0.1-0.2 mg/kg/day for 4-8 weeks initially, maintenance therapy is then given either by a reduced daily dosage or intermittent courses of treatment. Leukeran is useful in the management of patients with advanced diffuse lymphocytic lymphoma and those who have relapsed after radiotherapy. There is no significant difference in the overall response rate obtained with chlorambucil as a single agent and combination chemotherapy in patients with advanced non-Hodgkin's lymphocytic lymphoma.

Chronic Lymphocytic Leukaemia: Treatment with Leukeran is usually started after the patient has developed symptoms or when there is evidence of impaired bone marrow function (but not bone marrow failure) as indicated by the peripheral blood count. Initially Leukeran is given at a dosage of 0.15 mg/kg/day until the total leucocyte count has fallen to 10,000 per μL. Treatment may be resumed 4 weeks after the end of the first course and continued at a dosage of 0.1 mg/kg/day.

In a proportion of patients, usually after about 2 years of treatment, the blood leucocyte count is reduced to the normal range, enlarged spleen and lymph nodes become impalpable and the proportion of lymphocytes in the bone marrow is reduced to less than 20 per cent. Patients with evidence of bone marrow failure should first be treated with prednisolone and evidence of marrow regeneration should be obtained before commencing treatment with Leukeran. Intermittent high dose therapy has been compared with daily Leukeran but no significant difference in therapeutic response or frequency of side effects was observed between the two treatment groups.

Waldenstrom's Macroglobulinaemia: Leukeran is the treatment of choice in this indication. Starting doses of 6-12 mg daily until leucopenia occurs are recommended followed by 2-8 mg daily indefinitely.

Children: Leukeran may be used in the management of Hodgkin's disease and non-Hodgkin's lymphomas in children. The dosage regimes are similar to those used in adults.

Use in the Elderly: No specific studies have been carried out in the elderly, however, it may be advisable to monitor renal or hepatic function and if there is serious impairment then caution should be exercised.

4.3 Contraindications

Hypersensitivity to chlorambucil or to any of the excipients.

4.4 Special warnings and special precautions for use

Leukeran is an active cytotoxic agent for use only under the direction of physicians experienced in the administration of such agents.

Safe Handling of Leukeran tablets:

See 6.6 Instructions for Use/Handling

Immunisation using a live organism vaccine has the potential to cause infection in immunocompromised hosts. Therefore, immunisations with live organism vaccines are not recommended.

Monitoring: Since Leukeran is capable of producing irreversible bone marrow suppression, blood counts should be closely monitored in patients under treatment.

At therapeutic dosage Leukeran depresses lymphocytes and has less effect on neutrophil and platelet counts and on haemoglobin levels. Discontinuation of Leukeran is not necessary at the first sign of a fall in neutrophils but it must be remembered that the fall may continue for 10 days or more after the last dose.

Leukeran should not be given to patients who have recently undergone radiotherapy or received other cytotoxic agents.

When lymphocytic infiltration of the bone marrow is present or the bone marrow is hypoplastic, the daily dose should not exceed 0.1 mg/kg body weight.

Children with nephrotic syndrome, patients prescribed high pulse dosing regimens and patients with a history of seizure disorder, should be closely monitored following administration of Leukeran, as they may have an increased risk of seizures.

Renal impairment:

Patients with evidence of impaired renal function should be carefully monitored as they are prone to additional myelosuppression associated with azotaemia.

Hepatic impairment:

The metabolism of Leukeran is still under investigation and consideration should be given to dose reduction in patients with gross hepatic dysfunction.

Mutagenicity and Carcinogenicity:

Leukeran has been shown to cause chromatid or chromosome damage in man.

Development of acute leukaemia after Leukeran therapy for chronic lymphocytic leukaemia has been reported. However, it was not clear whether the acute leukaemia was part of the natural history of the disease or if the chemotherapy was the cause.

A comparison of patients with ovarian cancer who received alkylating agents with those who did not, showed that the use of alkylating agents, including Leukeran, significantly increased the incidence of acute leukaemia.

Acute myelogenous leukaemia has been reported in a small proportion of patients receiving Leukeran as long term adjuvant therapy for breast cancer.

The leukaemogenic risk must be balanced against the potential therapeutic benefit when considering the use of Leukeran.

4.5 Interaction with other medicinal products and other forms of Interaction

Vaccinations with live organism vaccines are not recommended in immunocompromised individuals (see Section 4.4 Special Warnings and Precautions for use).

Patients receiving phenylbutazone may require a reduced dose of Leukeran.

4.6 Pregnancy and lactation

As with other cytotoxic agents Leukeran is potentially teratogenic. The use of Leukeran should be avoided whenever possible during pregnancy, particularly during the first trimester. In any individual case, the potential hazard to the foetus must be balanced against the expected benefit to the mother.

As with all cytotoxic chemotherapy, adequate contraceptive precautions should be advised when either partner is receiving Leukeran.

Mothers receiving Leukeran should not breast feed.

4.7 Effects on ability to drive and use machines

None known

4.8 Undesirable effects

For this product there is no modern clinical documentation which can be used as support for determining the frequency of undesirable effects. Undesirable effects may vary in their incidence depending on the dose received and also when given in combination with other therapeutic agents.

The following convention has been utilised for the classification of frequency: Very common ($\geqslant$1/10), common ($\geqslant$1/100 and $<$1/10), uncommon ($\geqslant$1/1000 and $<$1/100), rare ($\geqslant$1/10,000 and $<$1/1000) and very rare ($<$1/10,000).

Blood and lymphatic system disorders

Very common: Bone marrow suppression.

Very rare: Irreversible bone marrow failure.

Although bone marrow suppression frequently occurs, it is usually reversible if Leukeran is withdrawn early enough.

Immune system disorders

Uncommon: Rash.

Rare: Allergic reactions such as urticaria and angioneurotic oedema following initial or subsequent dosing. Stevens-Johnson syndrome and toxic epidermal necrolysis.

(See Skin and subcutaneous tissue disorders)

On rare occasions skin rash has been reported to progress to serious conditions including Stevens-Johnson Syndrome and toxic epidermal necrolysis.

Nervous system disorders

Common: Seizures in children with nephrotic syndrome.

Rare: Seizures#, focal and/or generalised in children and adults receiving therapeutic daily doses or high pulse dosing regimens of chlorambucil.

Very rare: Movement disorders including tremor, twitching and myoclonia in the absence of convulsions. Peripheral neuropathy.

#Patients with a history of seizure disorder may be particularly susceptible.

Respiratory, thoracic and mediastinal disorders

Very rare: Interstitial pulmonary fibrosis, interstitial pneumonia.

Severe interstitial pulmonary fibrosis has occasionally been reported in patients with chronic lymphocytic leukaemia on long-term Leukeran therapy. However, this may be reversible on withdrawal of Leukeran.

Gastrointestinal disorders

Common: Gastro-intestinal disturbances such as nausea and vomiting, diarrhoea and oral ulceration.

Hepatobiliary disorders

Rare: Hepatoxicity, jaundice.

Skin and subcutaneous tissue disorders

Uncommon: Rash.

Rare: Allergic reactions such as urticaria and angioneurotic oedema following initial or subsequent dosing. Stevens-Johnson syndrome and toxic epidermal necrolysis.

(See Immune system disorders)

On rare occasions skin rash has been reported to progress to serious conditions including Stevens-Johnson syndrome and toxic epidermal necrolysis.

Renal and urinary disorders

Very rare: Sterile cystitis.

General disorders and administration site conditions

Rare: Drug fever.

4.9 Overdose

Reversible pancytopenia was the main finding of inadvertent overdoses of Leukeran. Neurological toxicity ranging from agitated behaviour and ataxia to multiple grand mal seizures has also occurred. As there is no known antidote the blood picture should be closely monitored and general supportive measures should be instituted, together with appropriate blood transfusion if necessary.

5. PHARMACOLOGICAL PROPERTIES

5.1 Pharmacodynamic properties

Chlorambucil is an aromatic nitrogen mustard derivative which acts as a bifunctional alkylating agent. Alkylation takes place through the formation of a highly reactive ethylenimonium radical. A probable mode of action involves cross-linkage of the ethylenimonium derivative between 2 strands of helical DNA and subsequent interference with replication.

5.2 Pharmacokinetic properties

In a study of 12 patients administered chlorambucil 0.2 mg/kg body weight orally, the mean dose adjusted maximum plasma concentration (492 ± 160 ng/ml) occurred between 0.25 and 2 hours after administration. The mean (± SD) terminal plasma elimination half-life was 1.3 ± 0.5 hours.

After oral administration of [^{14}C]-chlorambucil, maximum plasma radioactivity occurs between 40 and 70 minutes later. Studies have shown that chlorambucil disappears from the plasma with a mean terminal phase life of 1.5 hours and that its urinary excretion is low. A high level of urinary radioactivity after oral or intravenous administration of [^{14}C]-chlorambucil indicates that the drug is well absorbed after oral dosage.

The metabolism of chlorambucil in man appears to be similar to that in laboratory animals and involves S-oxidation of the butyric acid side chain. Bis-2-chlorethyl-2(4-aminophenyl) acetic acid [phenylacetic acid mustard (PAAM)] is a major metabolite of chlorambucil. In a study of 12 patients administered chlorambucil 0.2 mg/kg body weight orally, the mean dose adjusted-peak plasma concentration of PAAM (306 ± 73 ng/ml) was reached within 1 - 3 hours. The mean terminal elimination plasma half-life was 1.8 ± 0.4 hours. The significant contribution of PAAM to the alkylating activity of the drug was evident as the mean area under the plasma concentration time curve (AUC) of PAAM was approximately 1.33 times greater than the AUC of chlorambucil.

5.3 Preclinical safety data

Mutagenicity and Carcinogenicity

As with other cytotoxic agents chlorambucil is mutagenic in *in vitro* and *in vivo* genotoxicity tests and carcinogenic in animals and humans.

Teratogenicity

See information under 'Pregnancy and Lactation' section.

Chlorambucil has been shown to induce skeletal abnormalities in the embryos of mice and rats following a single oral administration of 4-20 mg/kg. Chlorambucil has also been shown to induce renal abnormalities in the offspring of rats following a single intraperitoneal injection of 3-6 mg/kg.

Effects on fertility

Leukeran may cause suppression of ovarian function and amenorrhoea has been reported following Leukeran therapy.

Azoospermia has been observed as a result of therapy with Leukeran although it is estimated that a total dose of at least 400 mg is necessary.

Varying degrees of recovery of spermatogenesis have been reported in patients with lymphoma following treatment with Leukeran in total doses of 400-2600 mg.

In rats, chlorambucil has been shown to damage spermatogenesis and cause testicular atrophy.

6. PHARMACEUTICAL PARTICULARS

6.1 List of excipients

Tablet Core:

Microcrystalline cellulose

Anhydrous lactose

Colloidal anhydrous silica

Stearic acid

Tablet Film Coating:

Hypromellose

Titanium dioxide

Synthetic yellow iron oxide

Synthetic red iron oxide

Macrogol

6.2 Incompatibilities

None known.

6.3 Shelf life

3 years.

6.4 Special precautions for storage

Store at 2°C - 8°C.

6.5 Nature and contents of container

Leukeran are brown film-coated, round, biconvex tablets engraved "GX EG3" on one side and "L" on the other, supplied in amber glass bottles with a child resistant closure containing 25 tablets.

6.6 Instructions for use and handling

Leukeran is an active cytotoxic agent for use only under the direction of physicians experienced in the administration of such agents.

Safe handling of Leukeran Tablets: The handling of Leukeran Tablets should follow guidelines for the handling of cytotoxic drugs according to prevailing local recommendations and/or regulations (for example, Royal Pharmaceutical Society of Great Britain Working Party on the Handling of Cytotoxic Drugs).

Provided that the outer coating of the tablet is intact, there is no risk in handling Leukeran Tablets. Leukeran Tablets should not be divided.

Administrative Data

7. MARKETING AUTHORISATION HOLDER

The Wellcome Foundation Ltd

Glaxo Wellcome House

Berkeley Avenue

Greenford

Middlesex

trading as

GlaxoSmithKline UK

Stockley Park West

Uxbridge

Middlesex UB11 1BT

8. MARKETING AUTHORISATION NUMBER(S)

PL 00003/5264R

9. DATE OF FIRST AUTHORISATION/RENEWAL OF THE AUTHORISATION

6 July 1995

10. DATE OF REVISION OF THE TEXT

25th February 2005

11. Legal Status

POM

Leustat Injection.

(Janssen-Cilag Ltd)

1. NAME OF THE MEDICINAL PRODUCT

Leustat® Injection.

2. QUALITATIVE AND QUANTITATIVE COMPOSITION

LEUSTAT (cladribine) Injection is a synthetic antineoplastic agent for continuous intravenous infusion. It is a clear, colourless, sterile, preservative-free, isotonic solution. LEUSTAT Injection is available in single-use vials containing 10 mg (1 mg/ml) of cladribine, a chlorinated purine nucleoside analogue. Each millilitre of LEUSTAT Injection contains 1 mg of the active ingredient, cladribine, and 9 mg (0.15 mEq) of sodium chloride as an inactive ingredient. The solution has pH range of 5.5 to 8.0. Phosphoric acid and/or dibasic sodium phosphate may have been added to adjust the pH.

3. PHARMACEUTICAL FORM

A sterile, buffered solution in vials containing 10 mg (1 mg/ml) of cladribine for dilution and subsequent continuous intravenous infusion.

4. CLINICAL PARTICULARS

4.1 Therapeutic indications

LEUSTAT Injection is indicated for the primary or secondary treatment of patients with Hairy Cell Leukaemia (HCL).

LEUSTAT is also indicated for the treatment of patients with B-cell chronic lymphocytic leukaemia (CLL) who have not responded to, or whose disease has progressed during or after, treatment with at least one standard alkylating-agent-containing regimen.

4.2 Posology and method of administration

Usual dose:

Adults and elderly:

HCL: The recommended treatment for Hairy Cell Leukaemia is a single course of LEUSTAT given by continuous intravenous infusion for 7 consecutive days at a dose of 0.09 mg/kg/day (3.6 mg/m^2/day). Deviations from this dosage regimen are not advised. Physicians should consider delaying or discontinuing the drug if neurotoxicity or renal toxicity occurs.

CLL: In patients with CLL, the recommended treatment consists of a continuous intravenous infusion of LEUSTAT for 2 hours on days 1 to 5 of a 28 day cycle at a dose of 0.12 mg/kg/day (4.8 mg/m^2/day). The patient's response to therapy should be determined every two cycles of treatment. It is recommended that LEUSTAT Injection be administered in responding patients for 2 cycles after maximum response has occurred, up to a maximum of 6 cycles. Therapy should be discontinued after 2 cycles in non-responding patients. Response for this treatment decision is defined as a lymphocyte reduction of 50% or more, ie if lymphocyte count decreases by 50% or more, administer 2 more cycles and re-evaluate response for decision whether to continue with 2 more cycles up to a maximum of 6 cycles.

Children:

Safety and efficacy in children have not been established.

Specific risk factors predisposing to increased toxicity from LEUSTAT have not been defined. In view of the known toxicities of agents of this class, it would be prudent to proceed carefully in patients with known or suspected renal insufficiency or severe bone marrow impairment of any aetiology. Patients should be monitored closely for haematological and renal and hepatic toxicity.

Preparation and administration of intravenous solutions:

LEUSTAT Injection must be diluted with the designated diluent prior to administration. Since the product does not contain any anti-microbial preservative or bacteriostatic agent, aseptic technique and proper environmental precautions must be observed in preparation of a solution of LEUSTAT. For full details concerning preparation of an infusion solution, see 6.6 Instructions for Use/Handling.

4.3 Contraindications

LEUSTAT Injection is contraindicated in those patients who are hypersensitive to this drug or any of its components. LEUSTAT is contra-indicated in pregnant women and nursing mothers.

4.4 Special warnings and special precautions for use

LEUSTAT Injection is a potent antineoplastic agent with potentially significant toxic side effects. It should be administered under the supervision of a qualified physician experienced in the use of antineoplastic therapy.

CLL: The weight of evidence suggests that a patient whose disease has progressed while treated with fludarabine is unlikely to respond to treatment with LEUSTAT Injection and therefore use in such a patient is not recommended.

Patients should be monitored closely for infections. Patients with active infection should be treated for the underlying condition prior to receiving therapy with LEUSTAT Injection. Patients who are or who become Coombs' positive should be monitored carefully for occurrence of haemolysis.

Patients with high tumour burden or who are considered at risk for the development of hyperuricaemia as a result of tumour breakdown should receive appropriate prophylactic treatment.

4.4.1 Bone Marrow Suppression:

Suppression of bone marrow function should be anticipated. This is usually reversible and appears to be dose dependent. Severe bone marrow suppression, including neutropenia, anaemia and thrombocytopenia, has been commonly observed in patients treated with LEUSTAT, especially at high doses. At initiation of treatment, most patients in the clinical studies had haematological impairment as a manifestation of active Hairy Cell Leukaemia or Chronic Lymphocytic Leukaemia. Following treatment with LEUSTAT, further haematological impairment occurred before recovery of peripheral blood counts began. Proceed carefully in patients with severe bone marrow impairment of any aetiology since further suppression of bone marrow function should be anticipated.

HCL: During the first two weeks after treatment initiation, mean platelet count, absolute neutrophil count (ANC), and haemoglobin concentration declined and then subsequently increased with normalisation of mean counts by day 15, week 5 and week 8, respectively. The myelosuppressive effects of LEUSTAT were most notable during the first month following treatment. Forty three percent (43%) of patients received transfusions with RBCs and 13% received transfusions with platelets during month 1. Careful haematological monitoring, especially during the first 4 to 8 weeks after treatment with LEUSTAT is recommended. (See 4.8, Undesirable Effects).

CLL: During the first 2 cycles of therapy with LEUSTAT Injection, haemoglobin concentration, platelet count and absolute neutrophil count declined to a nadir usually observed in Cycle 2. There appeared to be no cumulative toxicity upon administration of further cycles of therapy. Careful haematological monitoring is recommended throughout administration of LEUSTAT Injection.

4.4.2 Neurotoxicity:

Serious neurological toxicity (including irreversible paraparesis and quadraparesis) has been reported in patients who received LEUSTAT Injection by continuous infusion at high doses (4 to 9 times the recommended dose for hairy cell leukaemia). Neurological toxicity appears to demonstrate a dose relationship; however, severe neurological toxicities have been reported rarely with the recommended dose. Physicians should consider delaying or discontinuing therapy if neurotoxicity occurs.

4.4.3 Fever/Infection:

HCL: Fever (temperature greater than or equal to 37.8°C) was associated with the use of LEUSTAT in approximately 72% (89/124) of patients. Most febrile episodes occurred during the first month. Although seventy percent (70%) of patients were treated empirically with parenteral antibiotics, less than a third of febrile events were associated with documented infection.

CLL: Pyrexia was reported in 22-24% of CLL patients during Cycle 1 of therapy with LEUSTAT Injection, and in less than 3% of patients during subsequent cycles. Forty of 123 patients (32.5%) reported at least one infection during Cycle 1. Infections that occurred in 5% or more were: respiratory infection/inflammation (8.9%), pneumonia (7.3%), bacterial infection (5.7%), and viral skin infections (5.7%). Approximately 70% of patients had at least one infection during the overall study period of 6 years, including treatment and follow-up.

Since the majority of fevers occurred in neutropenic patients, patients should be closely monitored during the first month of treatment and empirical antibiotics should be initiated as clinically indicated. Given the known myelosuppressive effects of LEUSTAT, practitioners should carefully evaluate the risks and benefits of administering this drug to patients with active infections. Since fever may be accompanied by increased fluid loss, patients should be kept well hydrated (See 4.8, Undesirable effects).

4.4.4

Rare cases of tumour lysis syndrome have been reported in patients with haematological malignancies having a high tumour burden.

4.4.5 Effect on Renal and Hepatic Function:

Acute renal insufficiency has developed in some patients receiving high doses of LEUSTAT. In addition, there are inadequate data on dosing of patients with renal or hepatic insufficiency. Until more information is available, caution is advised when administering the drug to patients with known or suspected renal or hepatic insufficiency. All patients should have their renal and hepatic function monitored regularly. (See 4.8.1.4, Effects of High Doses).

4.4.6

LEUSTAT Injection must be diluted in a designated intravenous solution prior to administration (See 6.6, Instructions for Use/Handling for full details concerning preparation of an infusion solution).

4.4.7 Laboratory Tests:

During and following treatment, the patient's haematological profile should be monitored regularly to determine the degree of haematopoietic suppression. In HCL patients, bone marrow aspiration and biopsy should be performed to confirm response to treatment with LEUSTAT after peripheral counts have normalised. Febrile events should be investigated with appropriate laboratory and radiological studies. As with other potent chemotherapeutic agents, monitoring of renal and hepatic function should be performed as clinically indicated, especially in patients with underlying kidney or liver dysfunction.

4.4.8 Carcinogenesis/Mutagenesis:

Please refer to section 5.3: Preclinical Safety Data

4.4.9 Impairment of Fertility:

When administered intravenously to Cynomolgus monkeys, LEUSTAT (cladribine) has been shown to cause suppression of rapidly generating cells, including testicular cells. The effect on human fertility is unknown.

4.4.10 Extravasation:

Should the drug accidentally be given extravenously, local tissue damage is unlikely. If extravasation occurs, the administration should be stopped immediately and restarted in another vein. Other recommended local measures include elevating the arm and applying an ice pack to reduce swelling.

4.5 Interaction with other medicinal products and other forms of Interaction

Caution should be exercised if LEUSTAT Injection is administered following or in conjunction with other drugs known to cause myelosuppression. Following administration of LEUSTAT Injection, caution should be exercised before administering other immunosuppressive or myelosuppressive therapy. (See 4.4.1 and 4.8.1.2 Bone Marrow Suppression).

4.6 Pregnancy and lactation

LEUSTAT Injection is teratogenic in mice and rabbits and consequently has the potential to cause foetal harm when administered to a pregnant woman. There are no human data, but LEUSTAT Injection is contra-indicated in pregnancy.

A significant increase in foetal variations was observed in mice receiving 1.5 mg/kg/day (4.5 mg/m^2) and increased resorptions, reduced litter size and increased foetal malformations were observed when mice received 3.0 mg/kg/day (9 mg/m^2). Foetal death and malformations were observed in rabbits that received 3.0 mg/kg/day (33.0 mg/m^2). No foetal effects were seen in mice at 0.5 mg/kg/day (1.5 mg/m^2) or in rabbits at 1.0 mg/kg/day (11.0 mg/m^2).

Although there is no evidence of teratogenicity in humans due to LEUSTAT, other drugs which inhibit DNA synthesis (eg methotrexate and aminopterin) have been reported to be teratogenic in humans. LEUSTAT has been shown to be embryotoxic in mice when given at doses equivalent to the recommended dose.

It is not known whether this drug is excreted in human milk. Because it may be excreted in human milk and because there is potential for serious adverse reactions in nursing infants, LEUSTAT should not be given to a nursing mother.

4.7 Effects on ability to drive and use machines

Given the patients underlying medical condition and the safety profile of LEUSTAT Injection, caution should be exercised when a patient is performing activities requiring substantial physical well-being (See 4.8, Undesirable Effects).

4.8 Undesirable effects

4.8.1 Clinical Trial Experience

4.8.1.1 Overview:

HCL: The following safety data are based on 124 patients with HCL enrolled in the pivotal studies. Severe neutropenia was noted in 70% of patients in month 1; fever in 72% at anytime; and infection was documented in 31% of patients in month 1. Other adverse experiences reported frequently during the first 14 days after initiating treatment included: fatigue (49%), nausea (29%), rash (31%), headache (23%) and decreased appetite (23%). Most non-haematological adverse experiences were mild to moderate in severity.

During the first 14 days, events reported by greater than 5% but less than 20% of patients included:

Body as a whole:	Chills (13%), asthenia (11%), diaphoresis (11%), malaise (8%), trunk pain (7%).
Gastro-intestinal:	Vomiting (14%), constipation (14%), diarrhoea (12%), abdominal pain (8%), flatulence (7%).
Haemic/Lymphatic:	Purpura (12%), petechia (9%).
Nervous System:	Dizziness (13%), insomnia (8%), anxiety (7%).
Cardiovascular System:	Oedema (8%), tachycardia (8%), heart murmur (7%).
Respiratory System:	Abnormal breath sounds (14%), cough (12%), abnormal chest sounds (12%), shortness of breath (7%).
Skin/Subcutaneous Tissue:	Injection site reaction (15%), pruritus (9%), pain (9%), erythema (8%).
Musculoskeletal System:	Myalgia (8%).

Injection site reactions (ie redness, swelling, pain), thrombosis and phlebitis appear usually to be related to the infusion procedure and/or indwelling catheter, rather than to the medication or the vehicle.

From day 15 to the last day of follow-up, the following effects were reported in greater than 5% of patients: fatigue (14%), rash (10%), headache (7%), oedema (7%), arthralgia (7%), malaise (6%), diaphoresis (6%).

CLL: The following safety data are based on 124 patients with CLL enrolled in an open-label safety study. Haematological parameters declined during Cycle 1 and Cycle 2, reaching nadir values in Cycle 2; the percentage of patients having a haemoglobin level below 8.5 g/dL in Cycle 2 was 46.1%. The percentage of patients with platelet counts below 20 × 10(9)/L was 22.5% during Cycle 2. Absolute neutrophil count was below 500 × 10(6)/L in 61.8% of patients in Cycle 2. Adverse experiences reported frequently during the first 14 days after initiating treatment included: skin reaction at the injection site (22.8%), pyrexia (17.9%), fatigue (16.3%), oedema (13.8%), headache (13.0%), cough (11.4%), purpura (10.6%), diaphoresis (8.9%), diarrhoea (7.3%), nausea (6.5%), coagulation defect (6.5%), abnormal breath sounds (5.7%), pneumonia (5.7%), and abnormal chest sounds (5.7%). Adverse experiences that occurred in 5% or more of patients during the remainder of follow-up for Cycle 1 were: pyrexia (6.7%), and preterminal events (6.7%). Drug-related adverse experiences reported during cycles of therapy subsequent to Cycle 1 were limited to the following: skin reaction at medication site (22.8%), phlebitis (5.0%), bacterial skin infection (2.0%), cellulitis (1.0%), nausea (1.0%), skin pain (1.0%), and bacterial infection (1.0%). Skin reactions at the injection site were felt to be more likely related to the indwelling IV catheter and not study drug related. LEUSTAT Injection was not associated with renal or hepatic toxicities.

4.8.1.2 Bone Marrow Suppression:

HCL: Myelosuppression was frequently observed during the first month after starting treatment with LEUSTAT Injection. Neutropenia (ANC less than 500 × 10^6/L) was noted in 69% of patients, compared with 25% in whom it was present initially. Severe anaemia (haemoglobin less than 8.5 g/dL) occurred in 41.1% of patients, compared with 12% initially and thrombocytopenia (platelets less than 20 × 10^9/L) occurred in 15% of patients, compared to 5% in whom it was noted initially.

Analysis of lymphocyte subsets indicates that treatment with cladribine is associated with prolonged depression of the CD4 counts. Prior to treatment, the mean CD4 count was 766/μl. The mean CD4 count nadir, which occurred 4 to 6 months following treatment, was 272/μl. Fifteen (15) months after treatment, mean CD4 counts remained below 500/μl. CD8 counts behaved similarly, though increasing counts were observed after 9 months. There were no serious opportunistic infections reported during this time. The clinical significance of the prolonged CD4 lymphopenia is unclear.

Prolonged bone marrow hypocellularity (< 35%) was observed. It is not known whether the hypocellularity is the result of disease related marrow fibrosis or LEUSTAT Injection toxicity.

CLL: Patients with CLL treated with LEUSTAT Injection were more severely myelosuppressed prior to therapy than HCL patients; increased myelo-suppression was observed during Cycle 1 and Cycle 2 of therapy, reaching a nadir during Cycle 2. The percentage of patients having a haemoglobin level below 8.5 g/dL was 16.9% at baseline, 37.9% in Cycle 1, and 46.1% in Cycle 2. The percentage of patients with platelet counts below 20 × 10(9)/L was 4.0% at baseline, 20.2% during Cycle 1, and 22.5% during Cycle 2. Absolute neutrophil count was below 500 × 10(6)/L in 19.0% of patients at baseline, 56.5% in Cycle 1, 61.8% in Cycle 2, 59.3% in Cycle 3 and 55.9% in Cycle 4. There appeared to be no cumulative toxicity upon administration of multiple cycles of therapy. Marked blood chemistry abnormalities noted during the study were preexisting, or were isolated abnormalities which resolved, or were associated with death due to the underlying disease.

4.8.1.3 Fever/Infection:

HCL: As with other agents having known immunosuppressive effects, opportunistic infections have occurred in the acute phase of treatment due to the immunosuppression mediated by cladribine. Fever was a frequently observed side effect during the first month of study.

During the first month, 12% of patients experienced severe fever (ie greater than or equal to 40°C). Documented infections were noted in fewer than one-third of all febrile episodes. Of the 124 patients treated, 11 were noted to have a documented infection in the month prior to treatment. In the month following treatment, 31% of patients had a documented infection: 13.7% of patients had bacterial infection, 6.5% had viral and 6.5% had fungal infections. Seventy percent (70%) of these patients were treated empirically with antibiotics.

During the first month, serious infections (eg septicaemia, pneumonia), were reported in 7% of all patients; the remainder were mild or moderate. During the second month, the overall rate of documented infection was 8%; these infections were mild to moderate and no severe systemic infections were seen. After the third month, the monthly incidence of infection was either less than or equal to that of the months immediately preceding LEUSTAT therapy.

CLL: During Cycle 1, 23.6% of patients experienced pyrexia, and 32.5% experienced at least one documented infection. Infections that occurred in 5% or more of the patients during Cycle 1 were: respiratory infection/inflammation (8.9%), pneumonia (7.3%), bacterial infection (5.6%), and viral skin infections (5.7%). In Cycles 2 through 9, 71.3% of the patients had at least one infection. Infections that occurred in 10% or more of patients were: pneumonia (28.7%), bacterial infection (21.8%), viral skin infection (20.8%), upper respiratory infection (12.9%), other intestinal infection/inflammation (12.9%), oral candidiasis (11.9%), urinary tract infection (11.9%), and other skin infections (11.9%). Overall, 72.4% of the patients had at least one infection during therapy with LEUSTAT Injection. Of these, 32.6% had been administered concomitant immunosuppressive therapy (prednisone).

4.8.1.4 Effects of High Doses:

In a Phase 1 study with 31 patients in which LEUSTAT Injection was administered at high doses (4 to 9 times that recommended for hairy cell leukaemia) for 7-14 days in conjunction with cyclophosphamide and total body irradiation as preparation for bone marrow transplantation, acute nephrotoxicity, delayed onset neurotoxicity, severe bone marrow suppression with neutropenia, anaemia, and thrombocytopenia and gastro-intestinal symptoms were reported.

Nephrotoxicity: Six patients (19%) developed manifestations of acute renal dysfunction/insufficiency (eg acidosis, anuria, elevated serum creatinine, etc) within 7 to 13 days after starting treatment with LEUSTAT, 5 of the affected patients required dialysis. Renal insufficiency was reversible in 2 of these patients. Evidence of tubular damage was noted at autopsy in 2 (of 4) patients whose renal function had not recovered at the time of death. Several of these patients had also been treated with other medications having known nephrotoxic potential.

Neurotoxicity: Eleven patients (35%) experienced delayed onset neurological toxicity. In the majority, this was characterised by progressive irreversible motor weakness, of the upper and/or lower extremities (paraparesis/quadraparesis), noted 35 to 84 days after starting high dose therapy.

Non-invasive neurological testing was consistent with demyelinating disease.

4.8.2 Post-marketing Experience:

The following additional adverse events have been reported since the drug became commercially available. These adverse events have been reported primarily in patients who received multiple courses of LEUSTAT Injection:

Haematological: bone marrow suppression with prolonged pancytopenia, including some reports of aplastic anaemia; haemolytic anaemia, which was reported in patients with lymphoid malignancies, occurring within the first few weeks following treatment; hypereosinophilia.

Hepatic: reversible, generally mild, increases in bilirubin and transaminases.

Nervous System: confusion, neuropathy, ataxia, insomnia and somnolence.

Respiratory System: pulmonary interstitial infiltrates, in most cases an infectious aetiology was identified.

Skin/Subcutaneous: urticaria.

Opportunistic infections have occurred in the acute phase of treatment due to the immunosuppression mediated by LEUSTAT Injection.

4.9 Overdose

High doses of LEUSTAT have been associated with serious neurological toxicity (including irreversible paraparesis/quadraparesis), acute nephrotoxicity, and severe bone marrow suppression resulting in neutropenia, anaemia and thrombocytopenia (See 4.4, Special Warnings and Special Precautions for Use). There is no known specific antidote to overdosage. It is not known whether the drug can be removed from the circulation by dialysis or haemofiltration. Treatment of overdosage consists of discontinuation of LEUSTAT Injection, careful observation and appropriate supportive measures.

5. PHARMACOLOGICAL PROPERTIES

5.1 Pharmacodynamic properties

LEUSTAT Injection (cladribine) is a synthetic antineoplastic agent.

Cellular Resistance and Sensitivity: The selective toxicity cladribine towards certain normal and malignant lymphocyte and monocyte populations is based on the relative activities of deoxycytidine kinase, deoxynucleotidase and adenosine deaminase. It is postulated that cells with high deoxycytidine kinase and low deoxynucleotidase activities will be selectively killed by cladribine as toxic deoxynucleotides accumulate intracellularly.

Cells containing high concentrations of deoxynucleotides are unable to properly repair single-strand DNA breaks. LEUSTAT Injection can be distinguished from other chemotherapeutic agents affecting purine metabolism in that it is cytotoxic to both actively dividing and quiescent lymphocytes and monocytes, inhibiting both DNA synthesis and repair.

5.2 Pharmacokinetic properties

When LEUSTAT Injection was given by continuous intravenous infusion over 7 days the mean steady-state serum concentration was estimated to be 5.7 ng/ml with an estimated systemic clearance of 663.5 ml/h/kg. Accumulation of LEUSTAT over the seven day treatment period was not noted.

Plasma concentrations are reported to decline multi-exponentially after intravenous infusions with terminal half-lives ranging from approximately 3-22 hours. In general, the apparent volume of distribution of cladribine is very large (mean approximately 9l/kg), indicating an extensive distribution of cladribine in body tissues. The mean half-life of cladribine in leukaemic cells has been reported to be 23 hours.

There is little information available on the metabolism or route of excretion of cladribine in man. An average of 18% of the administered dose has been reported to be excreted in urine of patients with solid tumours during a 5-day continuous intravenous infusion of 3.5-8.1 mg/m^2/day of LEUSTAT. The effect of renal and hepatic impairment on the elimination of cladribine has not been investigated in humans.

Cladribine penetrates into cerebrospinal fluid. One report indicates that concentrations are approximately 25% of those in plasma.

Cladribine is bound approximately 20% to plasma proteins.

5.3 Preclinical safety data

Carcinogenesis/Mutagenesis: No animal carcinogenicity studies have been conducted with cladribine. However, its carcinogenic potential cannot be excluded based on demonstrated genotoxicity of cladribine. Cladribine induced chromosomal effects when tested in both an *in vivo* bone marrow micronucleus assay in mice and an *in vitro* assay using CHO-WBL cells. Cladribine is mutagenic in mammalian cells in culture. Cladribine was not mutagenic to bacteria and did not induce unscheduled DNA synthesis in primary rat hepatocyte cultures.

Other preclinical safety data has been included in specific sections of SPC. However, a full tabulation is attached in Appendix 1.

6. PHARMACEUTICAL PARTICULARS

6.1 List of excipients

9.0 mg (0.15 mEq) of sodium chloride as an inactive ingredient. Phosphoric acid and/or dibasic sodium phosphate to adjust the pH to a range of 5.5 to 8.0.

6.2 Incompatibilities

Since limited compatibility data are available, adherence to the recommended diluents and infusion systems is advised.

Solutions containing LEUSTAT Injection should not be mixed with other intravenous drugs or additives or infused simultaneously via a common intravenous line, since compatibility testing has not been performed.

If the same intravenous line is used for sequential infusion of several different drugs, the line should be flushed with a compatible diluent before and after infusion of LEUSTAT (See 4.2 or 6.6).

The use of 5% dextrose as a diluent is not recommended because of increased degradation of cladribine.

6.3 Shelf life

The shelf life for LEUSTAT Injection is 3 years.

When stored in refrigerated conditions between 2° to 8°C (36° to 46°F) protected from light, unopened vials of LEUSTAT Injection are stable until the expiration date indicated on the package. Freezing does not adversely affect the solution.

If freezing occurs, thaw naturally to room temperature. DO NOT heat or microwave. Once thawed, the vial of LEUSTAT Injection is stable until expiry if refrigerated. DO NOT REFREEZE.

Once diluted, solutions containing LEUSTAT Injection should be administered promptly or stored in the refrigerator (2° to 8°C) for no more than 8 hours prior to start of administration.

6.4 Special precautions for storage

Store refrigerated at 2° to 8°C (36° to 46°F). Protect from light during storage.

6.5 Nature and contents of container

LEUSTAT Injection is supplied as a sterile, preservative-free, isotonic solution containing 10 mg (1 mg/ml) of cladribine (as 10 ml) in a single-use, flint glass 20 ml vial.

6.6 Instructions for use and handling

Preparation and administration of intravenous solutions: LEUSTAT Injection must be diluted with the designated diluent prior to administration. Since the drug product does not contain any anti-microbial preservative or bacteriostatic agent, aseptic technique and proper environmental precautions must be observed in preparation of a solution of LEUSTAT.

Parenteral drug products should be inspected visually for particulate matter and discoloration prior to administration, whenever solution and container permit. A precipitate may occur during the exposure of LEUSTAT to low temperatures; it may be resolubilised by allowing the solution to warm naturally to room temperature and by shaking vigorously. *DO NOT HEAT OR MICROWAVE.*

Table 1

	DOSE OF LEUSTAT	RECOMMENDED DILUENT	QUANTITY OF DILUENT
HCL: 24-hour infusion method	0.09 mg/kg/day	0.9% sodium chloride injection, PhEur	100 ml to 500 ml
CLL: 2-hour infusion method	0.12 mg/kg/day	0.9% sodium chloride injection, PhEur	100 ml to 500 ml

Table 2 INHIBITION OF THE GROWTH OF VARIOUS HUMAN CELLS TREATED WITH CLADRIBINE

Cell Line or Cells	Cell Type	IC50 or ID50 (nM)
CEM	T-lymphoblast	14
MOLT-3	T-lymphoblast	24
MOLT-4	T-lymphoblast	55
HL60	Myeloid	20
THP-1	Myeloid	24
U937	Myeloid	23
RAJI	B-lymphoblast	27
SB	B-lymphoblast	–
K562	Myeloid Progenitor	256
WI-38	Fibroblast	–
CCRF-CEM	T-lymphoblast	3
WI-L2	B-lymphoblast	35
WI-L2 (AKase deficient)	B-lymphoblast	35
WI-L2 (dCKase deficient)	B-lymphoblast	>2000
Monocycles*	Monocyte	27
Lymphocytes*	Lymphocyte	20
GM 01380	Fibroblast	–

Akase – adenosine kinase
dCKase – deoxycytidine kinase
– No concentration inhibited 50%
* Isolated Peripheral Blood Cells

Care must be taken to assure the sterility of prepared solutions. Once diluted, solutions of LEUSTAT Injection should be administered promptly or stored in the refrigerator (2° to 8°C) for no more than 8 hours prior to start of administration. Vials of LEUSTAT Injection are for single-use only. Any unused portion should be discarded in an appropriate manner.

The potential hazards associated with cytotoxic agents are well established and proper precautions should be taken when handling, preparing, and administering LEUSTAT Injection. The use of disposable gloves and protective garments is recommended. If LEUSTAT Injection contacts the skin or mucous membranes, wash the involved surface immediately with copious amounts of water.

Preparation of a Single Daily Dose:

HCL: Add the calculated dose for a 24 hour period (0.09 mg/kg or 0.09 ml/kg or 3.6 mg/m^2) of LEUSTAT Injection to an infusion bag containing 100 ml to 500 ml of 0.9% sodium chloride injection (PhEur). Infuse intravenously continuously over 24 hours. Repeat daily for a total of 7 consecutive days.

CLL: Add the calculated dose for a 2 hour period (0.12 mg/kg or 4.8 mg/m^2) of LEUSTAT Injection to an infusion bag containing 100 ml to 500 ml of 0.9% sodium chloride injection (PhEur). Infuse intravenously continuously over 2 hours. Repeat daily for a total of 5 consecutive days.

The use of 5% dextrose as a diluent is not recommended because of increased degradation of cladribine. Admixtures of LEUSTAT Injection are chemically and physically stable for at least 24 hours at room temperature under normal room fluorescent light in most commonly available PVC infusion containers.

(see Table 1 on previous page)

7. MARKETING AUTHORISATION HOLDER

Janssen-Cilag Ltd

Saunderton

High Wycombe

Buckinghamshire

HP14 4HJ

8. MARKETING AUTHORISATION NUMBER(S)

PL 0242/0232

9. DATE OF FIRST AUTHORISATION/RENEWAL OF THE AUTHORISATION

3 February 1995

10. DATE OF REVISION OF THE TEXT

February 2004

Legal category POM.

APPENDIX 1

Animal: *In Vivo Pharmacology*

In a pilot study, female Sprague-Dawley rats had cannulas implanted in both the femoral (administration) and jugular (sampling) veins. Cladribine (spiked with ^{3}H-2-CdA) was administered, at 1mg/kg, either by bolus (2 rats) or by a constant 1 hour infusion (2 rats). Immediately following bolus dosing, the total plasma radioactivity concentration was ~ 1.2μg-eq/ml. Since this sample was drawn immediately post dose, the radiolabelled concentration is likely to equate to the Cladribine concentration. In this case, Cladribine would distribute into an initial volume ~ 0.8 L/kg. At 1 hour circulating radioactivity concentrations were ~ 0.5 μg-eq/ml and remained essentially constant at that concentration for 96 hours. Following the end of the constant infusion, the plasma radioactivity concentration was ~0.6μg-eq/ml, and, as from bolus administration, showed minimal decline over 96 hours.

Since the above concentrations are based on radioactivity measurements, it can be assumed that this elimination profile does not reflect the actual decline of Cladribine from rat plasma. In man, following a 2-hour infusion, the terminal half-life of Cladribine has been estimated at ~5.4 hours.

In a pilot study rats treated with radiolabelled Cladribine, approximately 41% to 44% of the administered label was recovered in the urine in the first 6 hours from a 1mg/kg bolus or infusion. Only small amounts of radioactivity were recovered after 6 hours. Less than 1% of the administered radioactivity was excreted in the faeces following a bolus dose to rats. From preliminary profiling of the 0.6 hour urine in one rat, it would appear that three of the radioactivity peaks were associated with intact Cladribine, 2-CdAMP and 2-CA. Since it is recognised that 2-CA can be degradation product of Cladribine, it is possible that its detection in rat urine may be an artifact, as the samples were stored at –20°C for about 4-6 weeks prior to assay. Quantitatively, ~37 to 46 percent of the urinary radioactivity was associated with 2-CdA, which would infer that in the Sprague-Dawley rat Cladribine does undergo biotransformation to some extent.

In addition, in an earlier pilot study, <1 percent of the administered radioactivity was excreted in the faeces following bolus injection.

The metabolism of 2-chloro-2'-3'- dideoxyadenosine (2CddA) has been investigated in mice. The total urinary excretion of unchanged CdA for 24 hours, after exposure to 24 mg/kg, was 3.4 percent of the delivered dose. At least two possible CddA metabolites were detected in mouse urine, which did not co-elute with 2-chloro-'2-'3--dideoxyinosine, 2-CA or 2-chlorohypoxanthine.

Animal: *In Vitro Pharmacology*

The table on the next page summarises the data for the effects of Cladribine on human cell lines and peripheral blood cells. The IC50 or ID50 values (CEM cells) may vary with experimental protocols and duration of drug exposure.

INHIBITION OF THE GROWTH OF VARIOUS HUMAN CELLS TREATED WITH CLADRIBINE

(see Table 2 on previous page)

Freshly isolated human peripheral blood monocytes and lymphocytes, and normal human GM 01380 fibroblasts were cultured for 5 days with various concentrations of Cladribine. Viable monocytes and fibroblasts were measured by the MTT [3-(4,5-dimethylthiazol-2yl)-2,5diphenyl tetrazoliumbromide] reduction assay, and viable lymphocytes were enumerated by dye exclusion. The data indicate that lymphocytes and monocytes are sensitive to the cytotoxic effects of Cladribine, *in vitro*, at nanomolar concentrations, whereas the fibroblast line, GM 01380 is unaffected. This cytotoxicity of both peripheral blood cell populations is substantially prevented by deoxycytidine (Figure 4 and Reference 4). However, contrasting lymphocytes, monocyte lysis is not prevented by nicotinamide or 3-aminobenzamide, inhibitors of poly (ADP ribose) synthetase, suggesting that the cytotoxic mechanism differs in these two cell types.

Utilising a human tumour colony forming assay, the cytotoxic activity of Cladribine toward several human solid tumours was assessed. Overall, Cladribine, at concentrations of 1.0 and 10.0 μg/ml, reduced the tumour survival rate (defined as <50% survival of tumour colony forming units) by 8% and 23% respectively, when given in a 1 hour pulse; and by 11% and 31% respectively when given as a continuous exposure. The data indicate that Cladribine is much less active against solid tumours than against leukaemic lymphoblasts.

Whereas lymphoblasts are sensitive to nanomolar concentrations of Cladribine, the solid tumours required at least 100-fold greater concentrations. The data suggest that some solid tumours may respond to Cladribine therapy, *in vivo*, but the concentration of drug required to kill these tumour cells may be considerably higher than the concentrations required to kill lymphoid cells.

Cladribine has been examined *in vitro* for cytotoxic effects against normal bone marrow and a number of human leukaemia and lymphoma cells. In these studies the effects of the Cladribine on spontaneous thymidine uptake by 40 leukaemic or 20 normal human bone marrow suspensions were monitored. Twelve of 20 acute lymphoblastic leukaemia (ALL) cell suspensions bearing the common acute

Table 3 ACUTE TOXICITY STUDIES WITH CLADRIBINE

Strain/Species (# sex/group)	Age/ Weight	Administration Route	Dose Groups	Observations	Results
Crl:CD-1°(ICR)BR, VAF/Plus° Mice (5 M,F/group)	6wks/ M: 26 - 32 g F: 20 – 25 g	I.v	25mg/kg 2-CDA; [a]25 mg/kg 2-CdA+ 2-chloroadenine,[b] Vehicle: Saline	Clinical signs and symptoms. Mortality, body weight changes	No mortality. No treatment - induced signs of toxicity.
CDF1 Mice (3 or 4 F/group)	4 – 6 wks/ Wt NA	i.p.	30, 45, 60, 75, 90, 120, 150, 180, and 210 mg/kg[c] Vehicle: 0.9% NaCl	Mortality	MTD=120mg/kg LD_{50}=150 mg/kg $LD_{90}\leq$180mg/kg

a 1.0 mg/mL solution of 2-CdA in 0.9% NaCl at a dose volume of 25 mL/kg.

b 1.0 mg/mL 2-CdA + approximately 75 μg/ml 2-chloradenine (breakdown product observed in clinical formulation under some storage conditions) in 0.9% NaCl at a dose volume of 25 mL/kg.

* Administered as a 0.1% solution in 0.9% NaCl.

KEY:

wks = weeks; NA = not available; I.V. = intravenous; i.p = intraperitoneal;

MTD = maximum tolerated dose; wt = weight.

Table 4 REPEATED DOSE TOXICITY STUDIES WITH CLADRIBINE (subacute)

Strain/Species (~ sex/group)	Age/ Weight	Duration of Trt	Admin Route	Dose Groups	Observations	Results
CDF1/Mice (4 F/ group)	4-6wks/ Wt NA	5 Days	I.P.	50, 75, 100 and 125 mg/kg/ day[a]; Vehicle: 0.9% NaCl	Clinical signs, mortality.	MTD=120mg/kg LD_{50}=150 mg/kg $LD_{9}0\leq$180mg/kg
Cynomolgus Monkey/Macaca fascicularis (1 M/dose)	Age & Wt NA	7-10 Days	I.V cont. infusion	#1:1.0,2.0mg/ kg/ day[b] #2:1.0mg/kg/ day (10 days)	Mortality, clinical signs, serum chemistry necropsy and histopathology.	Moribund condition & mortality observed 2-3 days after end of treatment. Major signs of toxicity: anorexia, nausea & vomiting, seizures, ataxia, suppression of rapidly dividing tissues.
Cynomolgus Monkey/Macaca fascicularis (4 M,F/grp; 2M,F/0.1 mg/kg grp)	Age NA/ 1.8-4.9kg	14 Days followed by 6-week recovery period	I.V. cont. Infusion[c]	0.1, 0.3 & 0.6 mg/kg/day Vehicle: Saline	Mortality, clinical signs, body wt, food consumption, ECG, ophthalmoscopy, neurological exam, haematology & serum chemistry, FACS, necropsy and histopathology.	No mortality. Major signs of toxicity in 0.6 mg/kg/day group: body wt loss, reduced motor activity, diarrhoea in males: reduction in red & white cells (including lymphocyte & monocyte subsets). Marked suppression of proliferating tissues; cellular depletion of lymphoid tissues and bone marrow. Effects reversed following 6 weeks of recovery. 0.3 mg/kg/day group: leukopenia. 0.1 mg/kg/ day group: no toxicity.

a Administered as a 0.1% solution in 0.9% NaCl.

b 7 days for each, separated by a 7 day recovery period

c Infusion rate of 7.5mL/kg/day

Key: i.v.= intravenous; i.p.=intraperitoenal; wt=weight; #/group=number of animals per group; Admin=administration; Trt=Treatment; NA=not available; cont=continous; wks=weeks; M=male; F=female; ECG=electrocardiogram

lymphocytic leukaemia antigen (CALLA+), and 4 of 5 T and pre-T acute lymphoblastic leukaemia cell preparations, were more sensitive to the inhibitory effects of Cladribine (ID50$\leq$5nM) than any normal bone marrow. The pre-B cell acute lymphocytic leukaemias and the acute myelocytic leukaemias (AML) varied greatly in their sensitivity to Cladribine (2 nM to > 50 nM). These studies indicate that the CALLA-positive ALL specimens and the T and pre-T all specimens are significantly more sensitive to Cladribine than normal bone marrow. The data suggest that Cladribine inhibits the proliferation and survival of malignant T and non T, non-B lymphocytes at concentrations that spare normal bone marrow cells and other cell types.

Cladribine showed curative therapeutic activity (50% of mice were cured; i.e. survived >60 days) in mice bearing L1210 leukaemia, when administered at 15mg/kg every 3 hrs on days, 1, 5, and 9 after tumour inoculation. Increase in the life span of dying mice was dose dependent. Cladribine was most effective when administered via a multiple dosage schedule on days 1, 5, and 9 after tumour implantation. Neither single treatment nor a daily dose of 50 mg/kg over 6 days produced cures (survival beyond 60 days).

The degree of Cladribine binding to plasma proteins has been investigated in normal rat (male; Sprague-Dawley), dog (female; Beagle), monkey (male; cynomolgus) and human (male; fasted, no caffeine consumption for 24 hours prior to blood donation and not on any medication) plasma. For all species, heparin was used as the anticoagulant. In humans, the degree of Cladribine binding to serum proteins was also investigated. Cladribine solutions (spike with ^{3}H-2-CdA) were added to plasma/serum to achieve concentrations of 6.1 ng, 61.1 ng or 6.1 μg/ml and dialyzed to equilibrium at 37°C.

Cladribine was minimally bound to plasma proteins in all species (~10 to 20 percent) at each drug concentration tested. At the same Cladribine concentrations, human plasma and serum yielded similar results, indicating that the anti-coagulant (heparin) did not compete with Cladribine binding sites.

TOXICOLOGY

ACUTE TOXICITY STUDIES WITH CLADRIBINE

(see Table 3 on previous page)

REPEATED DOSE TOXICITY STUDIES WITH CLADRIBINE (subacute)

(see Table 4 on previous page)

REPRODUCTIVE TOXICITY STUDIES WITH CLADRIBINE

(see Table 5)

Mutagenesis

As expected for compounds in this class, the actions of Cladribine have been shown to yield DNA damage. The mutagencicity studies are summarised below.

MUTAGENICITY STUDIES WITH CLADRIBINE

(see Table 6)

Carcinogenesis

No animal carcinogenicity studies have been conducted with Cladribine.

Table 5 REPRODUCTIVE TOXICITY STUDIES WITH CLADRIBINE

Strain/Species (~ sex/group)	Route/Duration of Administration	Dose Groups	Observations	Results
Mouse/Crl: CD-1[a] (ICR) (BR) (30/group)	I.V. /Days 6-15 of gestation[b]	0.5, 1.5 & 3.0 mg/kg/day Vehicle: Saline	Maternal body weight and clinical signs. Number of corporea lutea/ implantations and early/late resorptions: foetal survival, foetal weight/sex; foetal alterations.	3 mg/kg/day: Mean maternal body weight sign. Reduced attributed to a sign, increase in number of resorptions and concomitant reduced number of live foetuses. Increases in incidence of foetal variations and malformations. 1.5 mg/kg/day: Increase in skeletal variations. 0.5 mg/kg/day: No effect on foetal development.
Rabbit/ New Zealand White (Hra: (NZW/SPF) (18/group	i.v/Days 7-19 of gestation[c]	0.3, 1.0 & 3.0 mg/kg/day Vehicle: Saline	Maternal body weight, food consumption & clinical signs. Number of corporea lutea/ implantations and early/late resorptions; foetal survival, foetal weight/sex; foetal alterations	3 mg/kg/day: Mean foetal weight. Sign. Reduced. Abnormalities of head, limbs and palate. 1.0 and 0.3 mg/kg/day: No effect on foetal development.

a All animals were female

b Dose volume of 10mL/kg at an infusion rate of 1 mL/min.

c Administered as a bolus injection in dose volume of 2.5 mL/kg.

KEY: i.v = intraveneous; sign. = significant(ly); #/group = number of animals per group

Table 6 MUTAGENICITY STUDIES WITH CLADRIBINE

Assay	Species/Cell Line	Dose Levels	Control Groups	Results
Ames Test	Salmonella typhimunum strains TA98, TA100, TA1535, TA1537, TA1538; Escherichia coli strain WP $_2$ uvrA	10, 50, 100, 250, 500, and 1000 μg/plate, +/- S-9 mix	Vehicle: Saline Positives [1]: MNNG, 9-aminoacridine-HCl, 2-anthramine, sodium azide	Cladribine negative for inducing mutations in bacteria
DNA Repair Assay	Primary rat hepatocyte cultures (*in vitro* assay)	1, 5, 10, 50, 100, 150, and 200 μg/ml	Vehicle: Saline Positive: 2-AAF	Cladribine negative for inducing unscheduled DNA synthesis
DNA Synthesis Inhibition	CCRF-CEM Cells (Human Lymphoblastic Cells)	0.3 μM	-[2]	Cladribine incorporated into DNA; 90% reduction in DNA synthesis (0.3 μM): Decreased levels of dNTPs
dNTP Imbalance: DNA Strand Breaks	Mouse mammary tumour FM3A cells (F28-7)	0.5, 1.0, 5.0, and 20.0 μM	-[2]	Intracellular dNTP imbalance: double strand DNA breaks: cell death
DNA Strand Breaks: NAD depletion	Human peripheral blood lymphocytes	0.1, 1, and 10 μM	-[2]	DNA strand breaks: inhibition of RNA synthesis; reduced intracellular NAD levels; reduced ATP pool; cell death [3]
DNA Repair Inhibition	Human peripheral blood lymphocytes	0.1, 1, 10, and 100 μM	Radiation	Blocked radiation induced unscheduled DNA synthesis (DNA repair)

1 Choice of positive control dependent on strain and/or presence or absence of S-9 mix.

2 No control groups identified.

3 Effects prevented by deoxycytidine, a competitive inhibitor of Cladribine phosphorylation; Nicotinamide (NAD precursor) and 3-aminobenzamide [both inhibitors of poly (ADP-ribose) synthetase] also protected the cells from Cladribine toxicity.

Key: S-9 mix = Aroclor® 1254-induced rat liver s-9 mix; MNNG = n-methyl-nitro-N-nitrosoguanidine; 2-AAF = 2-acetylaminofluorene, dNTP = deoxynucleotide triphosphate.

Levemir Cartridge 100 U/ml, Levemir Pre-filled Pen 100 U/ml

(Novo Nordisk Limited)

1. NAME OF THE MEDICINAL PRODUCT

Levemir▼ 100 U/ml solution for injection in a cartridge

Levemir▼ 100 U/ml solution for injection in a pre-filled pen

2. QUALITATIVE AND QUANTITATIVE COMPOSITION

1 ml contains 100 U of insulin detemir (produced by recombinant DNA technology in Saccharomyces cerevisiae).

1 cartridge contains 3 ml equivalent to 300 U.

1 pre-filled pen contains 3ml equivalent to 300 U.

One unit of insulin detemir contains 0.142 mg salt-free anhydrous insulin detemir. One unit (U) of insulin detemir corresponds to one IU of human insulin.

For excipients, see section 6.1.

3. PHARMACEUTICAL FORM

Solution for injection in a cartridge (Penfill)

Solution for injection in a pre-filled pen (FlexPen)

Levemir is a clear, colourless, neutral solution.

4. CLINICAL PARTICULARS

4.1 Therapeutic indications

Treatment of diabetes mellitus.

4.2 Posology and method of administration

Levemir is a long-acting insulin analogue used as basal insulin, in combination with meal-related short- or rapid acting insulin.

Dosage:

Dosage of Levemir should be adjusted individually.

Levemir should be administered once or twice daily depending on patients' needs.

For patients who require twice daily dosing to optimise blood glucose control, the evening dose can be administered in the evening or at bedtime.

Transfer from other insulins:

Transfer to Levemir from intermediate or long-acting insulins may require adjustment of dose and timing of administration (see section 4.4).

As with all insulins, close glucose monitoring is recommended during the transfer and in the initial weeks thereafter.

Concomitant antidiabetic treatment may need to be adjusted (dose and timing of concurrent short-acting insulins).

As with all insulins, in elderly patients and patients with renal or hepatic impairment, glucose monitoring should be intensified and insulin detemir dosage adjusted on an individual basis.

The efficacy and safety of Levemir were demonstrated in children and adolescents aged 6 to 17 years in studies up to 6 months.

The efficacy and safety of Levemir have not been studied in children below the age of 6 years.

Adjustment of dosage may also be necessary if patients undertake increased physical activity, change their usual diet or during concomitant illness.

Administration:

Subcutaneous use.

Levemir is administered subcutaneously by injection in the thigh, abdominal wall, or the upper arm. As with human insulins, the rate and extent of absorption of insulin detemir may be higher when administered s.c. in the abdomen or deltoid than in the thigh. Injection sites should therefore be alternated within the same region.

Levemir Penfill and Levemir FlexPen are accompanied by a package leaflet with detailed instruction for use to be followed.

Levemir Penfill is designed to be used with Novo Nordisk delivery systems and NovoFine needles. Detailed instruction accompanying the delivery system must be followed.

4.3 Contraindications

Hypersensitivity to insulin detemir or to any of the excipients.

4.4 Special warnings and special precautions for use

Inadequate dosing or discontinuation of treatment, especially in type 1 diabetes, may lead to hyperglycaemia and diabetic ketoacidosis. Usually the first symptoms of hyperglycaemia develop gradually over a period of hours or days. They include thirst, increased frequency of urination, nausea, vomiting, drowsiness, flushed dry skin, dry mouth, loss of appetite as well as acetone odour of breath. In type 1 diabetes, untreated hyperglycaemic events eventually lead to diabetic ketoacidosis, which is potentially lethal.

Hypoglycaemia may occur if the insulin dose is too high in relation to the insulin requirement (see section 4.8 and 4.9).

Omission of a meal or unplanned strenuous physical exercise may lead to hypoglycaemia.

Patients, whose blood glucose control is greatly improved, e.g. by intensified insulin therapy, may experience a change in their usual warning symptoms of hypoglycaemia, and should be advised accordingly. Usual warning symptoms may disappear in patients with longstanding diabetes.

Concomitant illness, especially infections and feverish conditions, usually increases the patient's insulin requirement.

Transferring a patient to another type or brand of insulin should be done under strict medical supervision. Changes in strength, brand (manufacturer), type, origin (animal, human, human insulin analogue) and/or method of manufacture (recombinant DNA versus animal source insulin) may result in the need for a change in dosage. Patients taking Levemir may require a change in dosage from that used with their usual insulin. If an adjustment is needed, it may occur with the first dose or during the first few weeks or months.

Levemir should not be administered intravenously as it may result in severe hypoglycaemia.

Intramuscular administration should be avoided.

If Levemir is mixed with other insulin preparations the profile of action of one or both individual components will change. Mixing Levemir with a rapid acting insulin analogue like insulin aspart, results in an action profile with a lower and delayed maximum effect compared to separate injections. Therefore, mixing of rapid acting insulin with Levemir should be avoided.

There are limited data in patients with severe hypoalbuminaemia. Careful monitoring is recommended in these patients.

Levemir is not to be used in insulin infusion pumps.

Levemir contains metacresol, which may cause allergic reactions.

4.5 Interaction with other medicinal products and other forms of Interaction

A number of medicinal products are known to interact with the glucose metabolism.

The following substances may reduce the insulin requirements:

Oral antidiabetic medicinal products, monoamine oxidase inhibitors (MAOI), non-selective beta-blocking agents, angiotensin converting enzyme (ACE) inhibitors, salicylates and alcohol.

The following substances may increase the insulin requirements:

Thiazides, glucocorticoids, thyroid hormones and beta-sympathomimetics, growth hormone and danazol.

Beta-blocking agents may mask the symptoms of hypoglycaemia and delay recovery from hypoglycaemia.

Octreotide/lanreotide may both increase and decrease insulin requirement.

Alcohol may intensify and prolong the hypoglycaemic effect of insulin.

4.6 Pregnancy and lactation

Pregnancy:

There is no clinical experience with insulin detemir during pregnancy.

Animal reproduction studies have not revealed any differences between insulin detemir and human insulin regarding embryotoxicity and teratogenicity. Caution should be exercised when prescribing to pregnant women.

In general, intensified blood glucose control and monitoring of pregnant women with diabetes are recommended throughout pregnancy and when contemplating pregnancy. Insulin requirements usually fall in the first trimester and increase subsequently during the second and third trimester. After delivery, insulin requirements normally return rapidly to pre-pregnancy values.

Lactation:

There is no clinical experience with insulin detemir during lactation. Caution should be exercised when prescribing to lactating women. Lactating women may require adjustments in insulin dose and diet.

4.7 Effects on ability to drive and use machines

The patient's ability to concentrate and react may be impaired as a result of hypoglycaemia. This may constitute a risk in situations where these abilities are of special importance (e.g. driving a car or operating machinery).

Patients should be advised to take precautions to avoid hypoglycaemia while driving. This is particularly important in those who have reduced or absent awareness of the warning signs of hypoglycaemia or have frequent episodes of hypoglycaemia. The advisability of driving should be considered in these circumstances.

4.8 Undesirable effects

Adverse drug reactions observed in patients using Levemir are mainly dose-dependent and due to the pharmacologic effect of insulin. Hypoglycaemia is a common undesirable effect. It may occur if the insulin dose is too high in relation to the insulin requirement. From clinical investigations it is known that major hypoglycaemia, defined as requirement for third party intervention, occurs in approximately 6% of the patients treated with Levemir. Severe hypoglycaemia may lead to unconsciousness and/or convulsions and may result in temporary or permanent impairment of brain function or even death.

Injection site reactions are commonly seen during treatment with Levemir, namely in 2% of patients. These reactions include redness, swelling and itching at the injection site and are usually of a transitory nature, i.e. they normally disappear during continued treatment.

The overall percentage of treated patients expected to experience adverse drug reactions is estimated to be 12%.

Frequencies of adverse drug reactions from clinical trials, which by an overall judgment are considered related to Levemir are listed below.

(see Table 1 below)

4.9 Overdose

A specific overdose for insulin cannot be defined, however, hypoglycaemia may develop over sequential stages if too high doses relative to the patient's requirement are administered:

- Mild hypoglycaemic episodes can be treated by oral administration of glucose or sugary products. It is therefore recommended that the diabetic patient always carries sugar containing products.
- Severe hypoglycaemic episodes, where the patient has become unconscious, can be treated by glucagon (0.5 to 1 mg) given intramuscularly or subcutaneously by a trained person, or by glucose given intravenously by a medical professional. Glucose must also be given intravenously, if the patient does not respond to glucagon within 10 to 15 minutes. Upon regaining consciousness, administration of oral carbohydrates is recommended for the patient in order to prevent a relapse.

5. PHARMACOLOGICAL PROPERTIES

5.1 Pharmacodynamic properties

Pharmacotherapeutic group: Drugs used in diabetes. Insulins and analogues, long-acting. ATC code: A10AE05.

Insulin detemir is a soluble, long-acting basal insulin analogue with a prolonged duration of effect.

The time action profile of insulin detemir is statistically significantly less variable and therefore more predictable than for NPH insulin as seen from the within-subject Coefficients of Variation (CV) for the total and maximum pharmacodynamic effect in Table 2.

Table 2. Within-Subject Variability of the time action profile of insulin detemir and NPH insulin

Pharmacodynamic Endpoint	Insulin detemir CV (%)	NPH insulin CV (%)
$AUC_{GIR,0\text{-}24h}$*	27	68
GIR_{max}**	23	46

*Area under the curve ** Glucose Infusion Rate p-value <0.001 for all comparisons with insulin detemir

The prolonged action of insulin detemir is mediated by the strong self-association of insulin detemir molecules at the injection site and albumin binding via the fatty acid side-chain. Insulin detemir is distributed more slowly to peripheral target tissues compared to NPH insulin. These

Table 1

Metabolism and nutrition disorders		
Common (>1/100, <1/10)		Hypoglycaemia:
		Symptoms of hypoglycaemia usually occur suddenly. They may include cold sweats, cool pale skin, fatigue, nervousness or tremor, anxiousness, unusual tiredness or weakness, confusion, difficulty in concentration, drowsiness, excessive hunger, vision changes, headache, nausea and palpitation. Severe hypoglycaemia may lead to unconsciousness and/or convulsions and may result in temporary or permanent impairment of brain function or even death.
General disorders and administration site conditions		
Common (>1/100, <1/10)		Injection site reactions:
		Injection site reactions (redness, swelling and itching at the injection site) may occur during treatment with insulin. These reactions are usually transitory and normally they disappear during continued treatment.
Uncommon (>1/1,000, <1/100)		Lipodystrophy:
		Lipodystrophy may occur at the injection site as a consequence of failure to rotate injection sites within an area.
		Oedema:
		Oedema may occur upon initiation of insulin therapy. These symptoms are usually of transitory nature.
Immune system disorders		
Uncommon (>1/1,000, <1/100)		Allergic reactions, urticaria, rash and eruptions:
		Such symptoms may be due to generalised hypersensitivity. Other signs of generalised hypersensitivity may be itching, sweating, gastrointestinal upset, angioneurotic oedema, difficulties in breathing, palpitation and reduction in blood pressure. Generalised hypersensitivity reactions are potentially life threatening.
Eye disorders		
Uncommon (>1/1,000, <1/100)		Refraction disorders:
		Refraction anomalies may occur upon initiation of insulin therapy. These symptoms are usually of transitory nature.
		Diabetic retinopathy:
		Long-term improved glycaemic control decreases the risk of progression of diabetic retinopathy. However, intensification of insulin therapy with abrupt improvement in glycaemic control may be associated with temporary worsening of diabetic retinopathy.
Nervous system disorders		
Rare (>1/10,000, <1/1,000)		Peripheral neuropathy:
		Fast improvement in blood glucose control may be associated with the condition "acute painful neuropathy", which is usually reversible.

Figure 1 Activity profiles of Levemir in patients with type 1 diabetes

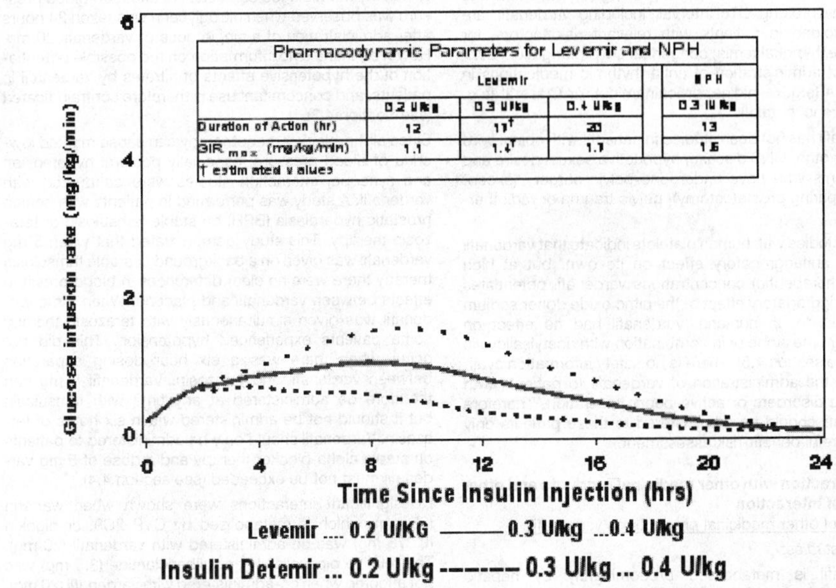

combined mechanisms of protraction provide a more reproducible absorption and action profile of insulin detemir compared to NPH insulin.

The blood glucose lowering effect of insulin detemir is due to the facilitated uptake of glucose following binding of insulin to receptors on muscle and fat cells and to the simultaneous inhibition of glucose output from the liver.

(see Figure 1 above)

The duration of action is up to 24 hours depending on dose providing an opportunity for once or twice daily administration. If administered twice daily, steady state will occur after 2-3 dose administrations. For doses in the interval of 0.2 – 0.4 U/kg, Levemir exerts more than 50% of its maximum effect from 3-4 hours and up to approximately 14 hours after dose administration.

Dose proportionality in pharmacodynamic response (maximum effect, duration of action, total effect) is observed after subcutaneous administration.

In long-term treatment trials, fasting plasma glucose in patients with type 1 diabetes was improved with Levemir compared with NPH insulin when given as basal/bolus therapy including in children and adolescents aged 6 to 17 years. Glycaemic control (HbA_{1c}) with Levemir is comparable to NPH insulin, with a lower risk of nocturnal hypoglycaemia and no associated weight gain.

Lower day-to-day variability in FPG was demonstrated during treatment with Levemir compared to NPH in long-term clinical trials.

The blood glucose lowering effect of Levemir has been demonstrated in clinical trials outside a basal bolus regimen. However, outside a basal bolus regimen non inferiority of HbA_{1c} compared to NPH has not been demonstrated.

In clinical trials, the overall rates of hypoglycaemia with Levemir and NPH insulin were similar. Analyses of nocturnal hypoglycaemia in type 1 diabetes showed a significantly lower risk of minor nocturnal hypoglycaemia (able to self-treat and confirmed by capillary blood glucose less than 2.8 mmol/L or 3.1 mmol/L if expressed as plasma glucose) than with NPH insulin, whereas no difference was seen in type 2 diabetes. Furthermore, the overall risk of nocturnal hypoglycaemia in children and adolescents aged 6 to 17 years with type 1 diabetes was significantly lower with Levemir compared to NPH insulin.

Unlike other insulins, intensive therapy with Levemir is not associated with undesirable weight gain.

5.2 Pharmacokinetic properties

Absorption:

Maximum serum concentration is reached between 6 and 8 hours after administration.

When administered twice daily, steady state serum concentrations are reached after 2-3 dose administrations.

Within-patient variation in absorption is lower for Levemir than for other basal insulin preparations.

There are no clinically relevant differences between genders in pharmacokinetic properties of insulin detemir.

The absolute bioavailability of insulin detemir when administered subcutaneous is approximately 60 %.

Distribution:

An apparent volume of distribution for insulin detemir (approximately 0.1 l/kg) indicates that a high fraction of insulin detemir is circulating in the blood.

Metabolism:

Degradation of insulin detemir is similar to that of human insulin; all metabolites formed are inactive.

The results of the *in vitro* and *in vivo* protein binding studies suggest that there is no clinically relevant interaction between insulin detemir and fatty acids or other protein bound medicinal products.

Elimination:

The terminal half-life after subcutaneous administration is determined by the rate of absorption from the subcutaneous tissue. The terminal half-life is between 5 and 7 hours depending on dose.

Linearity:

Dose proportionality in serum concentrations (maximum concentration, extent of absorption) is observed after subcutaneous administration in the therapeutic dose range.

Special Populations:

The pharmacokinetic properties of insulin detemir were investigated in children (6–12 years) and adolescents (13–17 years) and compared to adults with type 1 diabetes. There was no clinically relevant difference in pharmacokinetic properties.

There was no clinically relevant difference in pharmacokinetics of insulin detemir between elderly and young subjects or between subjects with renal or hepatic impairment and healthy subjects. No clinically relevant differences in the pharmacokinetics of insulin detemir are expected between healthy subjects and subjects with renal or hepatic impairment, based on the studies performed. As the pharmacokinetics of insulin detemir has not been studied extensively in these populations, it is advised to monitor plasma glucose closely in these populations.

5.3 Preclinical safety data

Preclinical data reveal no special hazard for humans based on conventional studies of safety pharmacology, repeated dose toxicity, genotoxicity and toxicity to reproduction. Receptor affinity data and *in-vitro* mitogenicity tests revealed no evidence of an increased mitogenic potential compared to human insulin.

6. PHARMACEUTICAL PARTICULARS

6.1 List of excipients

Mannitol

Phenol

Metacresol

Zinc acetate

Disodium phosphate dihydrate

Sodium chloride

Hydrochloric acid 2N (pH adjustment)

Sodium hydroxide 2N (pH adjustment)

Water for injections

6.2 Incompatibilities

Substances added to Levemir may cause degradation of insulin detemir, e.g. if the medicinal product contains thiols or sulphites. Levemir should not be added to infusion fluids.

6.3 Shelf life

2 years.

After first opening the product must be stored for a maximum of 6 weeks, not above 30°C.

6.4 Special precautions for storage

Store in a refrigerator (2°C - 8°C) not near a freezing compartment. Do not freeze.

Keep the container (cartridge) in the outer carton in order to protect from light.

Keep the pen cap on when Levemir FlexPen is not in use in order to protect from light.

During use: Do not refrigerate. Do not store above 30°C.

Levemir should be protected from excessive heat and sunlight.

6.5 Nature and contents of container

3 ml solution in a cartridge (Type I glass), with a plunger (bromobutyl) and a stopper (bromobutyl/polyisoprene) in a carton. Pack size of 1, 5 and 10 cartridges.

3ml solution in a cartridge (Type I glass) with a plunger (bromobutyl) and a stopper (bromobutyl/polyisoprene) contained in a pre-filled pen (multidose disposable pen) (polypropylene). Pack size of 1, 5 and 10 pre-filled pens.

Not all pack sizes may be marketed.

6.6 Instructions for use and handling

Levemir Penfill is designed to be used with Novo Nordisk delivery systems and NovoFine needles. Detailed instruction accompanying the delivery system must be followed.

Levemir is for use by one person only. The cartridge must not be refilled.

Levemir should not be used if it does not appear clear and colourless.

Levemir which has been frozen must not be used.

The patient should be advised to discard the needle after each injection.

Any unused product or waste material should be disposed of in accordance with local requirements.

7. MARKETING AUTHORISATION HOLDER

Novo Nordisk A/S

DK-2880 Bagsværd

Denmark

8. MARKETING AUTHORISATION NUMBER(S)

Levemir Penfill	EU/1/04/278/001-003
Levemir FlexPen	EU/1/04/278/004-006

9. DATE OF FIRST AUTHORISATION/RENEWAL OF THE AUTHORISATION

1 June 2004

10. DATE OF REVISION OF THE TEXT

4 July 2005

LEGAL CATEGORY

POM (Prescription Only Medicine)

Levitra

(Bayer plc)

1. NAME OF THE MEDICINAL PRODUCT

LEVITRA 5 mg film-coated tablets▼

LEVITRA 10 mg film-coated tablets▼

LEVITRA 20 mg film-coated tablets▼

2. QUALITATIVE AND QUANTITATIVE COMPOSITION

Each tablet contains 5 mg, 10 mg or 20 mg vardenafil (as hydrochloride trihydrate)

For excipients, see 6.1.

3. PHARMACEUTICAL FORM

Film-coated tablet

LEVITRA 5 mg film-coated tablets:

Orange round tablets marked with the BAYER-cross on one side and 5 on the other side.

LEVITRA 10 mg film-coated tablets:

Orange round tablets marked with the BAYER-cross on one side and 10 on the other side.

LEVITRA 20 mg film-coated tablets:

Orange round tablets marked with the BAYER-cross on one side and 20 on the other side.

4. CLINICAL PARTICULARS

4.1 Therapeutic indications

Treatment of erectile dysfunction, which is the inability to achieve or maintain a penile erection sufficient for satisfactory sexual performance.

In order for LEVITRA to be effective, sexual stimulation is required.

LEVITRA is not indicated for use by women.

4.2 Posology and method of administration

Oral use.

Adult men

The recommended dose is 10 mg taken as needed approximately 25 to 60 minutes before sexual activity. Based on efficacy and tolerability the dose may be increased to 20 mg or decreased to 5 mg. The maximum recommended dose is 20 mg. The maximum recommended dosing frequency is once per day. LEVITRA can be taken with or without food. The onset of activity may be delayed if taken with a high fat meal (see Section 5.2).

Elderly men

Since vardenafil clearance is reduced in elderly patients (see Section 5.2) a first dose of 5 mg should be used. Based on efficacy and tolerability the dose may be increased to 10 mg and 20 mg.

Children and adolescents

LEVITRA is not indicated for individuals below 18 years of age.

Use in patients with impaired hepatic function

A starting dose of 5 mg should be considered in patients with mild and moderate hepatic impairment (Child-Pugh A-B). Based on tolerability and efficacy, the dose may subsequently be increased. The maximum dose recommended in patients with moderate hepatic impairment (Child-Pugh B) is 10 mg. (see sections 4.3 and 5.2).

Use in patients with impaired renal function

No dosage adjustment is required in patients with mild to moderate renal impairment.

In patients with severe renal impairment (creatinine clearance < 30 ml/min), a starting dose of 5 mg should be considered. Based on tolerability and efficacy the dose may be increased to 10 mg and 20 mg.

Use in patients using other medicinal products

When used in combination with the CYP 3A4 inhibitor erythromycin, the dose of vardenafil should not exceed 5 mg (see Section 4.5).

4.3 Contraindications

The coadministration of vardenafil with nitrates or nitric oxide donors (such as amyl nitrite) in any form is contraindicated (see Section 4.5 and 5.1).

Agents for the treatment of erectile dysfunction should generally not be used in men for whom sexual activity is inadvisable (e.g. patients with severe cardiovascular disorders such as unstable angina or severe cardiac failure [New York Heart Association III or IV]).

The safety of vardenafil has not been studied in the following sub-groups of patients and its use is therefore contraindicated until further information is available: severe hepatic impairment (Child-Pugh C), endstage renal disease requiring dialysis, hypotension (blood pressure <90/50 mmHg), recent history of stroke or myocardial infarction (within the last 6 months), unstable angina and known hereditary retinal degenerative disorders such as retinitis pigmentosa.

Concomitant use of vardenafil with potent CYP 3A4 inhibitors ketoconazole and itraconazole (oral form) is contraindicated in men older than 75 years.

Concomitant use of vardenafil with HIV protease inhibitors such as ritonavir and indinavir is contraindicated, as they are very potent inhibitors of CYP 3A4 (see Section 4.5).

Hypersensitivity to vardenafil or to any of the excipients.

4.4 Special warnings and special precautions for use

A medical history and physical examination should be undertaken to diagnose erectile dysfunction and determine potential underlying causes, before pharmacological treatment is considered.

Prior to initiating any treatment for erectile dysfunction, physicians should consider the cardiovascular status of their patients, since there is a degree of cardiac risk associated with sexual activity (see Section 4.3). Vardenafil has vasodilator properties, resulting in mild and transient decreases in blood pressure (see Section 5.1). Patients with left ventricular outflow obstruction, e.g., aortic stenosis and idiopathic hypertrophic subaortic stenosis, can be sensitive to the action of vasodilators including Type 5 phosphodiesterase inhibitors.

Agents for the treatment of erectile dysfunction should be used with caution in patients with anatomical deformation of the penis (such as angulation, cavernosal fibrosis or Peyronie's disease), or in patients who have conditions which may predispose them to priapism (such as sickle cell anaemia, multiple myeloma or leukaemia).

The safety and efficacy of combinations of vardenafil with other treatments for erectile dysfunction have not been studied. Therefore the use of such combinations is not recommended.

The concomitant use of alpha-blockers and vardenafil may lead to symptomatic hypotension in some patients because both are vasodilators. Concomitant treatment with vardenafil should only be initiated if the patient has been stabilised on his alpha-blocker therapy. The maximum dose of vardenafil must not exceed 5 mg in such patients. In addition, vardenafil should not be taken within 6 hours of an alpha-blocker, with the exception of tamsulosin, for which this precaution should not be necessary (see section 4.5).

Concomitant use of vardenafil with potent CYP 3A4 inhibitors such as itraconazole and ketoconazole (oral form) should be avoided as very high plasma concentrations of vardenafil are reached if the drugs are combined (see Section 4.5 and 4.3).

Vardenafil dose adjustment might be necessary if the CYP 3A4 inhibitors, erythromycin, is given concomitantly (see Section 4.5 and Section 4.2).

Concomitant intake of grapefruit juice is expected to increase the plasma concentrations of vardenafil. The combination should be avoided (see Section 4.5).

Single oral doses of 10 mg and 80 mg of vardenafil have been shown to prolong the QTc interval by a mean of 8 msec and 10 msec, respectively (see Section 5.1). The clinical relevance of this finding is unknown and cannot be generalised to all patients under all circumstances, as it will depend on the individual risk factors and susceptibilities that may be present at any time in any given patient. Drugs that may prolong QTc interval, including vardenafil, are best avoided in patients with relevant risk factors, for example, hypokalaemia; congenital QT prolongation; concomitant administration of antiarrhythmic medications in Class 1A (e.g. quinidine, procainamide), or Class III (e.g. amiodarone, sotalol).

Vardenafil has not been studied in patients with spinal cord injury or other CNS disease, hypoactive sexual desire and in patients who have undergone pelvic surgery (except nerve-sparing prostatectomy), pelvic trauma or radiotherapy.

In vitro studies with human platelets indicate that vardenafil has no antiaggregatory effect on its own, but at high (super-therapeutic) concentrations vardenafil potentiates the antiaggregatory effect of the nitric oxide donor sodium nitroprusside. In humans, vardenafil had no effect on bleeding time alone or in combination with acetylsalicyclic acid (see section 4.5). There is no safety information available on the administration of vardenafil to patients with bleeding disorders or active peptic ulceration. Therefore vardenafil should be administered to these patients only after careful benefit-risk assessment.

4.5 Interaction with other medicinal products and other forms of Interaction

Effects of other medicinal products on vardenafil

In vitro studies:

Vardenafil is metabolised predominantly by hepatic enzymes via cytochrome P450 (CYP) isoform 3A4, with some contribution from CYP 3A5 and CYP 2C isoforms. Therefore, inhibitors of these isoenzymes may reduce vardenafil clearance.

In vivo studies:

Co-administration of the HIV protease inhibitor indinavir (800 mg t.i.d.), a potent CYP 3A4 inhibitor, with vardenafil (10 mg) resulted in a 16-fold increase in vardenafil AUC and a 7-fold increase in vardenafil C_{max}. At 24 hours, the plasma levels of vardenafil had fallen to approximately 4% of the maximum vardenafil plasma level (C_{max}).

Co-administration of vardenafil with ritonavir (600 mg b.i.d.) resulted in a 13-fold increase in vardenafil C_{max} and a 49-fold increase in vardenafil AUC_{0-24} when co-administered with vardenafil 5 mg The interaction is a consequence of blocking hepatic metabolism of LEVITRA by ritonavir, a highly potent CYP 3A4 inhibitor, which also inhibits CYP 2C9. Ritonavir significantly prolonged the half-life of LEVITRA to 25.7 hours (see Section 4.3).

Co-administration of ketoconazole (200 mg), a potent CYP 3A4 inhibitor, with vardenafil (5 mg) resulted in a 10-fold increase in vardenafil AUC and a 4-fold increase in vardenafil C_{max} (see Section 4.4).

Although specific interaction studies have not been conducted, the concomitant use of other potent CYP 3A4 inhibitors (such as itraconazole) can be expected to produce vardenafil plasma levels comparable to those produced by ketoconazole. Concomitant use of vardenafil with potent CYP 3A4 inhibitors such as itraconazole and ketoconazole (oral form) should be avoided (see Sections 4.3 and 4.4). In men older than 75 years the concomitant use of vardenafil with itraconazole or ketoconazole is contraindicated (see section 4.3).

Co-administration of erythromycin (500 mg t.i.d.), a CYP 3A4 inhibitor, with vardenafil (5 mg) resulted in a 4-fold increase in vardenafil AUC and a 3-fold increase in C_{max}. When used in combination with erythromycin, vardenafil dose adjustment might be necessary (see Section 4.2 and Section 4.4). Cimetidine (400 mg b.i.d.), a non-specific cytochrome P450 inhibitor, had no effect on vardenafil AUC and C_{max} when co-administered with vardenafil (20 mg) to healthy volunteers.

Grapefruit juice being a weak inhibitor of CYP 3A4 gut wall metabolism, may give rise to modest increases in plasma levels of vardenafil (see Section 4.4).

The pharmacokinetics of vardenafil (20 mg) was not affected by co-administration with the H2-antagonist ranitidine (150 mg b.i.d.), digoxin, warfarin, glibenclamide, alcohol (mean maximum blood alcohol level of 73 mg/dl) or single doses of antacid (magnesium hydroxide/aluminium hydroxide).

Although specific interaction studies were not conducted for all medicinal products, population pharmacokinetic analysis showed no effect on vardenafil pharmacokinetics of the following concomitant medicinal products: acetylsalicylic acid, ACE-inhibitors, beta-blockers, weak CYP 3A4 inhibitors, diuretics and medications for the treatment of diabetes (sulfonylureas and metformin).

Effects of vardenafil on other medicinal products

There are no data on the interaction of vardenafil and non-specific phosphodiesterase inhibitors such as theophylline or dipyridamole.

In vivo studies:

No potentiation of the blood pressure lowering effect of sublingual nitroglycerin (0.4 mg) was observed when vardenafil (10 mg) was given at varying time intervals (1 h to 24 h) prior to the dose of nitroglycerin in a study in 18 healthy male subjects. Vardenafil 20 mg potentiated the blood pressure lowering effect of sublingual nitroglycerin (0.4 mg) taken 1 and 4 hours after vardenafil administration to healthy middle aged subjects. No effect on blood pressure was observed when nitroglycerin was taken 24 hours after administration of a single dose of vardenafil 20 mg. However, there is no information on the possible potentiation of the hypotensive effects of nitrates by vardenafil in patients, and concomitant use is therefore contraindicated (see Section 4.3).

Since alpha-blocker monotherapy can cause marked lowering of blood pressure, especially postural hypotension and syncope, interaction studies were conducted with vardenafil. A study was performed in patients with benign prostatic hyperplasia (BPH) on stable tamsulosin or terazosin therapy. This study demonstrated that when 5 mg vardenafil was given on a background of stable tamsulosin therapy there were no clear differences in blood pressure effects between vardenafil and placebo. When 5 mg vardenafil was given simultaneously with terazosin therapy some patients experienced hypotension. This did not occur when there was a six hour dosing separation between vardenafil and terazosin. Vardenafil 5 mg can therefore be administered at any time with tamsulosin but it should not be administered within six hours of terazosin. Vardenafil should only be administered to patients on stable alpha-blocker therapy and a dose of 5 mg vardenafil must not be exceeded (see section 4.4).

No significant interactions were shown when warfarin (25 mg), which is metabolised by CYP 2C9, or digoxin (0.375 mg) was co-administered with vardenafil (20 mg). The relative bioavailability of glibenclamide (3.5 mg) was not affected when co-administered with vardenafil (20 mg). In a specific study, where vardenafil (20 mg) was co-administered with slow release nifedipine (30 mg or 60 mg) in hypertensive patients, there was an additional reduction on supine systolic blood pressure of 6 mmHg and supine diastolic blood pressure of 5 mmHg accompanied with an increase in heart rate of 4 bpm.

When vardenafil (20 mg) and alcohol (mean maximum blood alcohol level of 73 mg/dl) were taken together, vardenafil did not potentiate the effects of alcohol on blood pressure and heart rate and the pharmacokinetics of vardenafil were not altered.

Vardenafil (10 mg) did not potentiate the increase in bleeding time caused by acetylsalicylic acid (2 × 81 mg).

4.6 Pregnancy and lactation

LEVITRA is not indicated for use by women.

4.7 Effects on ability to drive and use machines

As dizziness and abnormal vision have been reported in clinical trials with vardenafil, patients should be aware of how they react to LEVITRA, before driving or operating machinery.

4.8 Undesirable effects

Over 9500 patients have received LEVITRA in clinical trials. The adverse reactions were generally transient and mild to moderate in nature. The most commonly reported adverse drug reactions occurring in ⩾ 10% of patients are headache and flushing.

The following adverse reactions have been reported in clinical trials:

(see Table 1 on next page)

Myocardial infarction have been reported in temporal association with the use of vardenafil and sexual activity, but it is not possible to determine whether myocardial infarction is related directly to vardenafil or to sexual activity, to the patient's underlying cardiovascular disease, or to a combination of these factors.

In a study evaluating visual function with twice the maximum recommended dose of vardenafil, some patients were found to have mild and transient impairment of colour discrimination in the blue/green range and in the purple range one hour after dosing. These changes had improved by six hours and no changes were present at 24 hours. The majority of these patients had no subjective visual symptoms.

Serious cardiovascular events, including cerebrovascular haemorrhage, sudden cardiac death, transient ischeamic attack and ventricular arrhythmia have been reported post marketing in temporal association with another medicinal product in this class.

4.9 Overdose

In single dose volunteer studies, doses up to and including 80 mg per day were tolerated without exhibiting serious adverse reactions.

When vardenafil was administered in higher doses and more frequently than the recommended dosing regimen (40 mg b.i.d.) cases of severe back pain have been reported. This was not associated with any muscle or neurological toxicity.

In cases of overdose, standard supportive measures should be adopted as required. Renal dialysis is not expected to accelerate clearance, as vardenafil is highly bound to plasma proteins and not significantly eliminated in the urine.

5. PHARMACOLOGICAL PROPERTIES

5.1 Pharmacodynamic properties

Pharmacotherapeutic group: Medicinal product used in erectile dysfunction, ATC code: G04B E09

Table 1

System Organ Class	Very Common (≥10%)	Common (≥1% < 10%)	Uncommon (≥0.1% < 1%)*	Rare (≥0.01% < 0.1%)*
Immune System Disorders				Hypersensitivity
Psychiatric Disorders				Anxiety
Nervous System Disorders	Headache	Dizziness	Somnolence	Syncope
Eye Disorders incl. Related Investigations			Lacrimation increased Visual Disturbance (incl. Visual brightness) Chromatopsia Conjunctivitis	Intraocular pressure increased
Cardiac Disorders incl. related Investigations			Tachycardia Palpitations	Angina Pectoris Myocardial ischemia
Vascular Disorders incl. related Investigations	Flushing		Hypertension Hypotension Orthostatic Hypotension	
Respiratory, Thoracic and Mediastinal Disorders		Nasal Congestion	Dyspnoea Epistaxis	Laryngeal oedema
Gastrointestinal Disorders incl. related Investigations		Dyspepsia Nausea	Abnormal liver function tests GGTP increased	
Skin and Subcutaneous Tissue Disorders			Photosensitivity reaction Face oedema Rash	
Musculoskeletal and Connective Tissue Disorders incl. Related Investigations			Blood creatine phosphokinase increased Myalgia Back Pain	Muscle Rigidity
Reproductive System and Breast Disorders				Priapism Erections increased (prolonged or painful erections)

*For adverse reactions reported in <1% of patients, only those which warrant special attention, because of their possible association with serious disease states or of otherwise clinical relevance are listed.

Vardenafil is an oral therapy for the improvement of erectile function in men with erectile dysfunction. In the natural setting, i.e. with sexual stimulation it restores impaired erectile function by increasing blood flow to the penis.

Penile erection is a haemodynamic process. During sexual stimulation, nitric oxide is released. It activates the enzyme guanylate cyclase, resulting in an increased level of cyclic guanosine monophosphate (cGMP) in the corpus cavernosum. This in turn results in smooth muscle relaxation, allowing increased inflow of blood into the penis. The level of cGMP is regulated by the rate of synthesis via guanylate cyclase and by the rate of degradation via cGMP hydrolysing phosphodiesterases (PDEs).

Vardenafil is a potent and selective inhibitor of the cGMP specific phosphodiesterase type 5 (PDE5), the most prominent PDE in the human corpus cavernosum. Vardenafil potently enhances the effect of endogenous nitric oxide in the corpus cavernosum by inhibiting PDE5. When nitric oxide is released in response to sexual stimulation, inhibition of PDE5 by vardenafil results in increased corpus cavernosum levels of cGMP. Sexual stimulation is therefore required for vardenafil to produce its beneficial therapeutic effects.

In vitro studies have shown that vardenafil is more potent on PDE5 than on other known phosphodiesterases (>15-fold relative to PDE6, >130-fold relative to PDE1, >300-fold relative to PDE11, and >1000-fold relative to PDE2, PDE3, PDE4, PDE7, PDE8, PDE9 and PDE10).

In a penile plesthysmography (RigiScan) study, vardenafil 20 mg produced erections considered sufficient for penetration (60% rigidity by RigiScan) in some men as early as 15 minutes after dosing. The overall response of these subjects to vardenafil became statistically significant, compared to placebo, 25 minutes after dosing.

Vardenafil causes mild and transient decreases in blood pressure which, in the majority of the cases, do not translate into clinical effects. The mean maximum decreases in supine systolic blood pressure following 20 mg and 40 mg vardenafil were – 6.9 mmHg under 20 mg and – 4.3 mmHg under 40 mg of vardenafil, when compared to placebo. These effects are consistent with the vasodilatory effects of PDE5-inhibitors and are probably due to increased cGMP levels in vascular smooth muscle cells. Single and multiple oral doses of vardenafil up to 40 mg produced no clinically relevant changes in the ECGs of normal male volunteers.

A single dose, double blind, crossover, randomised trial in 59 healthy males compared the effects on the QT interval of vardenafil (10 mg and 80 mg), sildenafil (50 mg and 400 mg) and placebo. Moxifloxacin (400 mg) was included as an active internal control. Effects on the QT interval were measured one hour post dose (average T_{max} for vardenafil). The primary objective of this study was to rule out a greater than 10 msec effect (i.e. to demonstrate lack of effect) of a single 80 mg oral dose of vardenafil on QTc interval compared to placebo, as measured by the change in Fridericia's correction formula (QTcF=QT/RR1/3) from baseline at the 1 hour post-dose time point. The vardenafil results showed an increase in QTc (Fridericia) of 8 msec (90% CI: 6-9) and 10 msec (90% CI: 8-11) at 10 and 80 mg doses compared to placebo and an increase in QTci of 4 msec (90% CI: 3-6) and 6 msec (90% CI: 4-7) at 10 and 80 mg doses compared to placebo, at one hour postdose. At T_{max}, only the mean change in QTcF for vardenafil 80 mg was out of the study established limit (mean 10 msec, 90% CI (8-11)). When using the individual correction formulae, none of the values were out of the limit. The actual clinical impact of these changes is unknown.

Further information on clinical trials

In clinical studies vardenafil was administered to over 3750 men with erectile dysfunction (ED) aged 18 - 89 years, many of whom had multiple co-morbid conditions. Over 1630 patients have been treated with LEVITRA for six months or longer. Of these, over 730 have been treated for one year or longer.

The following patient groups were represented: elderly (22%), patients with hypertension (35%), diabetes mellitus (29%), ischaemic heart disease and other cardiovascular diseases (7%), chronic pulmonary disease (5%), hyperlipidaemia (22%), depression (5%), radical prostatectomy (9%). The following groups were not well represented in clinical trials: elderly (>75 years, 2.4%), and patients with certain cardiovascular conditions (see Section 4.3). No clinical studies in spinal cord injury or other CNS diseases, patients with severe renal or hepatic impairment, pelvic surgery (except nerve-sparing prostatectomy) or trauma or radiotherapy and hypoactive sexual desire or penile anatomic deformities have been performed.

Across the pivotal trials, treatment with vardenafil resulted in an improvement of erectile function compared to placebo. In the small number of patients who attempted intercourse up to four to five hours after dosing the success rate for penetration and maintenance of erection was consistently greater than placebo.

In fixed dose studies in a broad population of men with erectile dysfunction, 68% (5 mg), 76% (10 mg) and 80% (20 mg) of patients experienced successful penetrations (SEP 2) compared to 49% on placebo over a three month study period. The ability to maintain the erection (SEP 3) in this broad ED population was given as 53% (5 mg), 63% (10 mg) and 65% (20 mg) compared to 29% on placebo.

In pooled data from the major efficacy trials, the proportion of patients experiencing successful penetration on vardenafil were as follows: psychogenic erectile dysfunction (77-87%), mixed erectile dysfunction (69-83%), organic erectile dysfunction (64-75%), elderly (52-75%), ischaemic heart disease (70-73%), hyperlipidemia (62-73%), chronic pulmonary disease (74-78%), depression (59-69%), and patients concomitantly treated with antihypertensives (62-73%).

In a clinical trial in patients with diabetes mellitus, vardenafil significantly improved the erectile function domain score, the ability to obtain and maintain an erection long enough for successful intercourse and penile rigidity compared to placebo at vardenafil doses of 10 mg and 20 mg. The response rates for the ability to obtain and maintain an erection was 61% and 49% on 10 mg and 64% and 54% on 20 mg vardenafil compared to 36% and 23% on placebo for patients who completed three months treatment.

In a clinical trial in patients post-prostatectomy patients, vardenafil significantly improved the erectile function domain score, the ability to obtain and maintain an erection long enough for successful intercourse and penile rigidity compared to placebo at vardenafil doses of 10 mg and 20 mg. The response rates for the ability to obtain and maintain an erection was 47% and 37% on 10 mg and 48% and 34% on 20 mg vardenafil compared to 22% and 10% on placebo for patients who completed three months treatment.

The safety and efficacy of vardenafil was maintained in long term studies.

5.2 Pharmacokinetic properties

Absorption

Vardenafil is rapidly absorbed with maximum observed plasma concentrations reached in some men as early as 15 minutes after oral administration. However, 90% of the time, maximum plasma concentrations are reached within 30 to 120 minutes (median 60 minutes) of oral dosing in the fasted state. The mean absolute oral bioavailability is 15 %. After oral dosing of vardenafil AUC and C_{max} increase almost dose proportionally over the recommended dose range (5 – 20 mg).

When vardenafil is taken with a high fat meal (containing 57% fat), the rate of absorption is reduced, with an increase in the median t_{max} of 1 hour and a mean reduction in C_{max} of 20%. Vardenafil AUC is not affected. After a meal containing 30% fat, the rate and extent of absorption of vardenafil (t_{max}, C_{max} and AUC) are unchanged compared to administration under fasting conditions.

Distribution

The mean steady state volume of distribution for vardenafil is 208 l, indicating distribution into the tissues. Vardenafil and its major circulating metabolite (M1) are highly bound to plasma proteins (approximately 95% for vardenafil or M1). For vardenafil as well as M1, protein binding is independent of total drug concentrations.

Based on measurements of vardenafil in semen of healthy subjects 90 minutes after dosing, not more than 0.00012% of the administered dose may appear in the semen of patients.

Metabolism

Vardenafil is metabolised predominantly by hepatic metabolism via cytochrome P450 (CYP) isoform 3A4 with some contribution from CYP 3A5 and CYP 2C isoforms.

In humans the one major circulating metabolite (M1) results from desethylation of vardenafil and is subject to further metabolism with a plasma elimination half life of approximately 4 hours. Parts of M1 are in the form of the glucuronide in systemic circulation. Metabolite M1 shows a phosphodiesterase selectivity profile similar to vardenafil and an *in vitro* potency for phosphodiesterase type 5 of approximately 28% compared to vardenafil, resulting in an efficacy contribution of about 7%.

Elimination

The total body clearance of vardenafil is 56 l/h with a resultant terminal half life of approximately 4-5 hours. After oral administration, vardenafil is excreted as metabolites predominantly in the faeces (approximately 91-95% of the administered dose) and to a lesser extent in the urine (approximately 2-6% of the administered dose).

Pharmacokinetics in special patient groups

Elderly

Hepatic clearance of vardenafil in healthy elderly volunteers (65 years and over) was reduced as compared to healthy younger volunteers (18 - 45 years). On average elderly males had a 52% higher AUC, and a 34% higher C_{max} than younger males (see Section 4.2).

Renal insufficiency

In volunteers with mild to moderate renal impairment (creatinine clearance 30 – 80 ml/min), the pharmacokinetics of vardenafil were similar to that of a normal renal function control group. In volunteers with severe renal impairment (creatinine clearance < 30 ml/min) the mean AUC was increased by 21% and the mean Cmax decreased by 23%, compared to volunteers with no renal impairment. No statistically significant correlation was observed between creatinine clearance and vardenafil exposure (AUC and C_{max}) (see Section 4.2). Vardenafil pharmacokinetics have not been studied in patients requiring dialysis (see section 4.3).

Hepatic insufficiency

In patients with mild to moderate hepatic impairment (Child-Pugh A and B), the clearance of vardenafil was reduced in proportion to the degree of hepatic impairment. In patients with mild hepatic impairment (Child-Pugh A), the mean AUC and C_{max} increased 17% and 22% respectively, compared to healthy control subjects. In patients with moderate impairment (Child-Pugh B), the mean AUC and C_{max} increased 160% and 133% respectively, compared to healthy control subjects (see Section 4.2). The pharmacokinetics of vardenafil in patients with severely impaired hepatic function (Child-Pugh C) have not been studied (see Section 4.3).

5.3 Preclinical safety data

Preclinical data reveal no special hazard for humans based on conventional studies of safety pharmacology, repeated dose toxicity, genotoxicity, carcinogenic potential, toxicity to reproduction.

6. PHARMACEUTICAL PARTICULARS

6.1 List of excipients

Tablet core:

Crospovidone,

Magnesium Stearate,

Microcrystalline cellulose,

Silica, colloidal anhydrous.

Film coat:

Macrogol 400,

Hypromellose,

Titanium dioxide (E171),

Ferric oxide yellow (E172),

Ferric oxide red (E172)

6.2 Incompatibilities

Not applicable.

6.3 Shelf life

3 years

6.4 Special precautions for storage

No special precautions for storage.

6.5 Nature and contents of container

PP/Aluminium foil blisters in cartons of 2, 4, 8 and 12 tablets.

Not all pack sizes may be marketed.

6.6 Instructions for use and handling

No special requirements.

7. MARKETING AUTHORISATION HOLDER

Bayer AG,

D-51368 Leverkusen,

Germany

8. MARKETING AUTHORISATION NUMBER(S)

EU/1/03/248/001 LEVITRA 5 mg film-coated tablet, pack size 2 tablets

EU/1/03/248/002 LEVITRA 5 mg film-coated tablet, pack size 4 tablets

EU/1/03/248/003 LEVITRA 5 mg film-coated tablet, pack size 8 tablets

EU/1/03/248/004 LEVITRA 5 mg film-coated tablet, pack size 12 tablets

EU/1/03/248/005 LEVITRA 10 mg film-coated tablet, pack size 2 tablets

EU/1/03/248/006 LEVITRA 10 mg film-coated tablet, pack size 4 tablets

EU/1/03/248/007 LEVITRA 10 mg film-coated tablet, pack size 8 tablets

EU/1/03/248/008 LEVITRA 10 mg film-coated tablet, pack size 12 tablets

EU/1/03/248/009 LEVITRA 20 mg film-coated tablet, pack size 2 tablets

EU/1/03/248/010 LEVITRA 20 mg film-coated tablet, pack size 4 tablets

EU/1/03/248/011 LEVITRA 20 mg film-coated tablet, pack size 8 tablets

EU/1/03/248/012 LEVITRA 20 mg film-coated tablet, pack size 12 tablets

9. DATE OF FIRST AUTHORISATION/RENEWAL OF THE AUTHORISATION

6 March 2003

10. DATE OF REVISION OF THE TEXT

29 March 2005

Levonelle One Step

(Schering Health Care Limited)

1. NAME OF THE MEDICINAL PRODUCT

Levonelle® One Step(TM) 1500 microgram tablet

2. QUALITATIVE AND QUANTITATIVE COMPOSITION

The tablet contains 1500 microgram of levonorgestrel. For excipients see 6.1

3. PHARMACEUTICAL FORM

Tablet

The tablet is round and white.

4. CLINICAL PARTICULARS

4.1 Therapeutic indications

Emergency contraception within 72 hours of unprotected sexual intercourse or failure of a contraceptive method.

Levonelle One Step is not recommended for use by young women under 16 years of age without medical supervision.

4.2 Posology and method of administration

For oral administration: One tablet should be taken as soon as possible, preferably within 12 hours and no later than 72 hours after unprotected intercourse (see section 5.1).

If vomiting occurs within three hours of taking the tablet another tablet should be taken immediately. The patient should contact her doctor, family planning clinic or pharmacist for advice and another tablet.

Levonelle One Step can be used at any time during the menstrual cycle unless menstrual bleeding is overdue.

After using emergency contraception it is recommended to use a barrier method (e.g. condom, diaphragm or cap) until the next menstrual period starts. The use of Levonelle One Step does not contraindicate the continuation of regular hormonal contraception.

Children: Levonelle One Step is not recommended for use by young women under 16 years of age without medical supervision.

4.3 Contraindications

Hypersensitivity to the active substance levonorgestrel or any of the excipients.

4.4 Special warnings and special precautions for use

Emergency contraception is an occasional method. It should in no instance replace a regular contraceptive method.

Emergency contraception does not prevent a pregnancy in every instance. If there is uncertainty about the timing of the unprotected intercourse or if the woman has had unprotected intercourse more than 72 hours earlier in the same menstrual cycle, conception may have occurred. Treatment with Levonelle One Step following the second act of intercourse may therefore be ineffective in preventing pregnancy. If menstrual periods are delayed by more than 5 days or abnormal bleeding occurs at the expected date of menstrual periods or pregnancy is suspected for any other reason, women should be referred to a doctor so that pregnancy may be excluded. If pregnancy occurs after treatment with Levonelle One Step, the possibility of an ectopic pregnancy should be considered. The absolute risk of ectopic pregnancy is likely to be low, as Levonelle One Step prevents ovulation and fertilisation. Ectopic pregnancy may continue, despite the occurrence of uterine bleeding.

Levonelle One Step is not recommended in patients with severe hepatic dysfunction.

Severe malabsorption syndromes, such as Crohn's disease, might impair the efficacy of Levonelle One Step. Women suffering from these conditions should be referred to a doctor for emergency contraception.

Levonelle One Step contains 142.5 mg lactose. This should be taken into account in women with rare hereditary problems of galactose intolerance, the Lapp lactase deficiency or glucose-galactose malabsorption.

After Levonelle One Step intake, menstrual periods are usually normal and occur at the expected date. They can sometimes occur earlier or later than expected by a few days. Women should be advised to make a medical appointment to initiate or adopt a method of regular contraception. If no withdrawal bleed occurs in the next pill-free period following the use of Levonelle One Step after regular hormonal contraception, pregnancy should be ruled out.

Repeated administration within a menstrual cycle is not advisable because of the possibility of disturbance of the cycle.

Levonelle One Step is not as effective as a conventional regular method of contraception and is suitable only as an emergency measure. Women who present for repeated courses of emergency contraception should be advised to consider long-term methods of contraception.

Use of emergency contraception does not replace the necessary precautions against sexually transmitted diseases.

4.5 Interaction with other medicinal products and other forms of Interaction

The metabolism of levonorgestrel is enhanced by concomitant use of liver enzyme inducers.

Drugs suspected of having the capacity to reduce the efficacy of levonorgestrel containing medication include barbiturates (including primidone), phenytoin, carbamazepine, herbal medicines containing Hypericum perforatum (St. John's Wort), rifampicin, ritonavir, rifabutin, griseofulvin. Women taking such drugs should be referred to their doctor for advice.

Medicines containing levonorgestrel may increase the risk of cyclosporin toxicity due to possible inhibition of cyclosporin metabolism. Women taking cyclosporin containing medication should be referred to their doctor for advice.

4.6 Pregnancy and lactation

Pregnancy

Levonelle One Step should not be given to pregnant women. It will not interrupt a pregnancy. In the case of continued pregnancy, limited epidemiological data indicate no adverse effects on the fetus but there are no clinical data on the potential consequences if doses greater than 1.5 mg of levonorgestrel are taken (see section 5.3.).

Lactation

Levonorgestrel is secreted into breast milk. Potential exposure of an infant to levonorgestrel can be reduced if the breast-feeding woman takes the tablet immediately after feeding and avoids nursing following Levonelle One Step administration.

4.7 Effects on ability to drive and use machines

No studies on the effect on the ability to drive and use machines have been reported.

4.8 Undesirable effects

The most commonly reported undesirable effect was nausea. The following undesirable effects were observed in two different studies[1, 2]

Body System	Frequency of adverse reactions	
	Very common >1/10)	**Common >1/100)**
Endocrine system	Bleeding not related to menses*	Delay of menses more than 7 days ** Irregular bleeding and spotting
Nervous system		Dizziness Headache
Gastrointestinal system	Nausea Low abdominal pain	Diarrhoea Vomiting
Reproductive system and breast		Breast tenderness
General	Fatigue	

[1] Task Force on post-ovulatory Methods of Fertility Regulation. Randomised controlled trial of levonorgestrel versus the Yuzpe regimen of combined oral contraceptives for emergency contraception. Lancet, 1998; 352:428-433

(n=977; data on 0.75 mg levonorgestrel tablet taken as two doses with a 12-hour interval)

[2] Hertzen et al. Low dose mifepristone and two regimens of levonorgestrel for emergency contraception: a WHO multicentre randomised trial. Lancet. 2002; 360:1803-1810

(n=1,359; data on Levonelle One Step taken as a single dose of 1.5 mg)

* n=1,011 out of 1,359

** n=1,334 out of 1,359

Bleeding patterns may be temporarily disturbed, but most women will have their next menstrual period within 7 days of the expected time.

If the next menstrual period is more than 5 days overdue, pregnancy should be excluded.

4.9 Overdose

Serious undesirable effects have not been reported following acute ingestion of large doses of oral contraceptives. Overdose may cause nausea, and withdrawal bleeding may occur. There are no specific antidotes and treatment should be symptomatic.

5. PHARMACOLOGICAL PROPERTIES

5.1 Pharmacodynamic properties

PROGESTOGENS

G03AC03

The precise mode of action of Levonelle One Step is not known.

At the recommended regimen, levonorgestrel is thought to work mainly by preventing ovulation and fertilisation if intercourse has taken place in the preovulatory phase, when the likelihood of fertilisation is the highest. It may also cause endometrial changes that discourage implantation. Levonelle One Step is not effective once the process of implantation has begun.

Efficacy: It was estimated from the results of an earlier clinical study (Lancet, 1998; 352: 428-433), that levonorgestrel, taken as two 750 microgram doses with a 12 hour interval, prevents 85% of expected pregnancies. Efficacy appears to decline with time of start of treatment after intercourse (95% within 24 hours, 85% 24-48 hours, 58% if started between 48 and 72 hours).

Results from a recent clinical study (Lancet 2002; 360: 1803-1810) showed that a 1500 microgram single dose of Levonelle One Step (taken within 72 hours of unprotected sex) prevented 84% of expected pregnancies (compared with 79% when the two 750 microgram tablets were taken 12 hours apart).

At the recommended regimen, levonorgestrel is not expected to induce significant modification of blood clotting factors, and lipid and carbohydrate metabolism.

5.2 Pharmacokinetic properties

Levonorgestrel: orally administered levonorgestrel is rapidly and almost completely absorbed.

The results of a pharmacokinetic study carried out with 15 healthy women showed that following ingestion of one tablet of Levonelle One Step maximum drug serum levels of levonorgestrel of 18.5 ng/ml were found at 2 hours. After reaching maximum serum levels, the concentration of levonorgestrel decreased with a mean elimination half-life of about 26 hours.

Levonorgestrel is not excreted in unchanged form but as metabolites. Levonorgestrel metabolites are excreted in about equal proportions with urine and faeces. The biotransformation follows the known pathways of steroid metabolism, the levonorgestrel is hydroxylated in the liver and the metabolites are excreted as glucuronide conjugates.

No pharmacologically active metabolites are known.

Levonorgestrel is bound to serum albumin and sex hormone binding globulin (SHBG). Only about 1.5% of the total serum levels are present as free steroid, but 65% are specifically bound to SHBG.

The absolute bioavailability of levonorgestrel was determined to be almost 100% of the dose administered.

About 0.1% of the maternal dose can be transferred via milk to the nursed infant.

5.3 Preclinical safety data

Animal experiments with levonorgestrel have shown virilisation of female fetuses at high doses.

6. PHARMACEUTICAL PARTICULARS

6.1 List of excipients

Potato starch, maize starch, colloidal silica anhydrous, magnesium stearate, talc, lactose monohydrate.

6.2 Incompatibilities

Not applicable.

6.3 Shelf life

2 years.

6.4 Special precautions for storage

Store in original container.

6.5 Nature and contents of container

The folded carton of Levonelle One Step contains one blister of one tablet. The blister is made of aluminium/PVC.

6.6 Instructions for use and handling

No special requirements.

7. MARKETING AUTHORISATION HOLDER

Medimpex UK Limited

127 Shirland Road

London W9 2EP

United Kingdom

8. MARKETING AUTHORISATION NUMBER(S)

PL05276/0020

9. DATE OF FIRST AUTHORISATION/RENEWAL OF THE AUTHORISATION

14th June 2004.

10. DATE OF REVISION OF THE TEXT

LEGAL CATEGORY

P

Levothyroxine Tablets BP 25, 50 and 100 micrograms

(Celltech Manufacturing Services Limited)

1. NAME OF THE MEDICINAL PRODUCT

Levothyroxine Tablets BP 100 micrograms

Levothyroxine Tablets BP 50 micrograms

Levothyroxine Tablets BP 25 micrograms

2. QUALITATIVE AND QUANTITATIVE COMPOSITION

Levothyroxine Sodium 111.2 micrograms per tablet.

Equivalent to Levothyroxine Sodium Anhydrous 100 micrograms per tablet.

Levothyroxine Sodium 55.6 micrograms per tablet.

Equivalent to Levothyroxine Sodium Anhydrous 50 micrograms per tablet.

Levothyroxine Sodium 27.8 micrograms per tablet.

Equivalent to Levothyroxine Sodium Anhydrous 25 micrograms per tablet.

3. PHARMACEUTICAL FORM

100 mcg

- Uncoated, white, biconvex tablet, engraved E 907 on one side, plain on the other.

50 mcg

- Uncoated, white, biconvex tablet, engraved E 905 on one side, plain on the other.

25 mcg

- Uncoated, white, biconvex tablet, engraved E 902 on one side, plain on the other.

4. CLINICAL PARTICULARS

4.1 Therapeutic indications

For the treatment of hypothyroidism (congenital or acquired), diffuse non toxic goitre or Hashimoto's thyroiditis and thyroid carcinoma.

4.2 Posology and method of administration

The treatment of any thyroid disorder should be determined on an individual basis, taking account of clinical response, biochemical tests and regular monitoring. A pre-therapy ECG is valuable as changes induced by hypothyroidism may be confused with evidence of ischaemia. If too rapid an increase of metabolism is produced (causing diarrhoea, nervousness, rapid pulse, insomnia, tremors and sometimes anginal pain where there is latent myocardial ischaemia), reduce the dose or withhold for 1-2 days and start again at a lower dose.

Levothyroxine is best taken as a single dose on an empty stomach, usually before breakfast.

Adults, children over 12 years

Initial dose:	50 - 100 micrograms daily before breakfast.
Usual maintenance dose:	100 - 200 micrograms daily.

The initial dose is adjusted by 25 to 50 microgram increments at 3 – 4 week intervals until clinical response and measurements of plasma thyroxine and thyroid stimulating hormone indicate that the thyroid deficiency is corrected and a maintenance dose established.

Elderly patients (over 50 years of age), or those with cardiac insufficiency or in those with severe hypothyroidism

Initial dose:	25 micrograms daily before breakfast.
Usual maintenance dose:	50 to 200 micrograms daily.

The initial dose is adjusted by 25 microgram increments at 4 week intervals until clinical response and measurements of plasma thyroxine and thyroid stimulating hormone indicate that the thyroid deficiency is corrected and a maintenance dose is established.

Children under 12 years

The initial dose for children up to 1 month is 5-10 micrograms/kg daily, and for children over 1 month is 5 micrograms/kg daily. This dose should be adjusted in steps of 25 micrograms every 2-4 weeks until mild toxic symptoms appear then the dose should be reduce slightly.

4.3 Contraindications

Thyrotoxicosis, hypersensitivity to any component. In patients with adrenal insufficiency without adequate corticosteroid cover.

4.4 Special warnings and special precautions for use

Thyroid treatments should be used with caution in patients with cardiovascular disorders, including myocardial insufficiency and hypertension.

Thyroid replacement therapy should be introduced gradually in elderly patients, and those with severe long standing hypothyroidism.

Special care is needed when there are symptoms of myocardial insufficiency or ECG evidence of myocardial infarction and for similar reasons the treatment of hypothyroidism in the elderly should be initiated cautiously. Patients with adrenal insufficiency may react unfavourably to levothyroxine treatment so it is advisable to initiate corticosteroid therapy before giving levothyroxine. Caution should also be exercised when administering levothyroxine to diabetics or digitalised patients.

Subclinical hyperthyroidism may be associated with bone loss. To minimise the risk of osteoporosis, dosage of levothyroxine sodium should be titrated to the lowest possible effective level.

Parents of children receiving a thyroid agent should be advised that partial loss of hair may occur during the first few months of therapy, but this effect is usually transient and subsequent regrowth usually occurs.

4.5 Interaction with other medicinal products and other forms of Interaction

The effects of warfarin, dicoumarol, nicoumalone, phenindione and probably other anticoagulants are increased by the concurrent use of thyroid compounds. The antidepressant response to imipramine, amitriptyline and possibly other tricyclic antidepressants can be accelerated by the concurrent use of levothyroxine.

The absorption of levothyroxine is reduced by sucralfate, sodium polystyrene sulphonate or colestyramine binding within the gut. Cimetidine, aluminium hydroxide, calcium carbonate and ferrous sulphate also reduce absorption of levothyroxine from the G.I. tract. Dosages should be separated by an interval of several hours.

The concurrent use of carbamazepine, phenytoin, phenobarbital, primadone or rifampicin with levothyroxine have been found to increase levothyroxine metabolism. A possible interaction occurs with hypoglycaemic agents, hence diabetic patients should be monitored for increased requirements of insulin or oral hypoglycaemic agents.

If levothyroxine therapy is initiated in digitalised patients, the dose of digoxin may require adjustment, hyperthyroid patients may need their digoxin dosage gradually increased as treatment proceeds, because initially patients are relatively sensitive to digoxin.

Isolated reports of marked hypertension and tachycardia has been reported with concurrent ketamine administration. Lovastatin has been reported to cause one case each of hypothyroidism and hyperthyroidism in two patients taking levothyroxine.

False low total plasma concentrations have been observed with concurrent anti-inflammatory treatment such as phenylbutazone or acetylsalicylic acid and levothyroxine therapy. Levothyroxine accelerates the metabolism of propranolol.

Oestrogen, oestrogen containing products and oral contraceptives may increase the requirement of thyroid therapy dosage. Conversely, androgens and corticosteroids may decrease serum concentrations of thyroxine-binding globulins.

Amiodarone may reduce the effects of thyroid hormones used in the treatment of hypothyroidism.

4.6 Pregnancy and lactation

Pregnancy

Women on a maintenance dose for hypothyroidism who become pregnant, must be monitored closely. Levothyroxine sodium does not readily cross the placenta in the second and third trimester, but may do so in the first. Levothyroxine sodium is not known to have either carcinogenic or tetragenic effects.

Lactation

Minimal concentrations of levothyroxine are excreted in breast milk and may mask hypothyroidism in a newborn baby. It is considered that there is insufficient thyroid hormone in breast milk to meet the needs of a suckling infant with a non-functioning thyroid gland.

4.7 Effects on ability to drive and use machines

None known.

4.8 Undesirable effects

The following side effects are usually due to excessive dosage, and correspond to symptoms of hyperthyroidism. They include arrhythmias, anginal pain, tachycardia, cramps in skeletal muscles, headache, restlessness, excitability, flushing, sweating, diarrhoea, excessive weight loss and muscular weakness, insomnia, tremor, fever, vomiting, palpitations and heat intolerance. These reactions usually disappear after dose reduction or withdrawal of treatment. Hypersensitivity reactions including rash, pruritus and oedema have also been reported.

Thyroid crisis have occasionally been reported following massive or chronic intoxication and cardiac arrhythmias, heart failure, coma and death have occurred.

4.9 Overdose

Symptoms of mild to moderate overdose: fever, angina, tachycardia, arrhythmias, muscle cramps, headache, restlessness, flushing, sweating, diarrhoea. Reduction of dose or withdrawal of therapy reverses mild overdose effects.

Symptoms of severe overdose: this may resemble thyroid crisis with collapse and coma.

Signs and symptoms of hyperthyroidism may be delayed for up to 5 days due to the gradual peripheral conversion of levothyroxine to triiodothyronine. Overdosage following recent ingestion of tablets can be treated using gastric lavage/emesis. Propranolol and other supportive measures are used to maintain the circulation. Antithyroid drugs such as propylthiouracil and lithium are unlikely to be of benefit to prevent thyrotoxic crisis due to delayed absorption/onset of action.

5. PHARMACOLOGICAL PROPERTIES

5.1 Pharmacodynamic properties

Thyroxine (T4) is a naturally occurring hormone containing iodine, produced by the thyroid gland. It is converted to its more active principle triiodothyronine (T3) in the peripheral tissues. Receptors for T3 are found on cell membranes, mitochondria and cell nuclei. Thyroid hormones are required for normal growth and development of the body, especially the nervous system. They increase the basal metabolic rate of the whole body and have stimulatory effects on the heart, skeletal muscle, liver and kidney.

5.2 Pharmacokinetic properties

Levothyroxine sodium is incompletely and variably absorbed from the gastro-intestinal tract. Levothyroxine is extensively metabolised in the thyroid, liver, kidney and anterior pituitary. Some enterohepatic re-circulation occurs. Part of the levothyroxine is metabolised to triiodothyronine. Levothyroxine is excreted in the urine and faeces, partly as free drug and partly as conjugates and deiodinated metabolites.

It has a half life of 7 days but this may be shortened or prolonged depending on the disease condition. Levothyroxine is almost completely bound to plasma protein, mainly thyroxine binding globulin, with approx. 0.03% of levothyroxine unbound. The unbound levothyroxine is converted to triiodothyronine.

There are four main pathways of metabolism:

1) Deiodination to triiodothyronine (active) - T3 or to reverse triiodothyronine (inactive). Further deiodination of T3 leads to the formation of thyroacetic acid.

2) Deamination to the tetrone.

3) Conjugation to the glucoronide or sulphate.

4) Ether bond cleavage to diiodotyrosines.

The most important metabolic pathway is deiodination. Between 30 - 55% of the levothyroxine dose is excreted in the urine and 20 - 40% in the faeces.

5.3 Preclinical safety data

Not applicable since Levothyroxine Tablets have been used in clinical practice for many years and its effects in man are well known.

6. PHARMACEUTICAL PARTICULARS

6.1 List of excipients

Lactose

Sucrose

Maize Starch

Magnesium Stearate

6.2 Incompatibilities

None known.

6.3 Shelf life

100 mcg

- 24 months in polypropylene containers, 18 months in blister packs.

50 mcg, 25 mcg -

24 months in polypropylene containers, 12 months in blister packs.

6.4 Special precautions for storage

Store below 25°C and protect from light.

6.5 Nature and contents of container

Opaque polypropylene containers having snap-on polythene lids, with integral tear-off security seals containing 7, 14, 21, 28, 30, 50, 56, 60, 84, 90, 100, 112, 120, 500 or 1000 tablets.

PVC/PVDC/aluminium blisters containing 14 tablets. Blisters are packaged into cartons to give packs of 28, 42, or 56 tablets.

Not all pack sizes may be marketed.

6.6 Instructions for use and handling

No special precautions are required.

7. MARKETING AUTHORISATION HOLDER

Celltech Manufacturing Services Limited

Vale of Bardsley

Ashton under Lyne

Lancashire

OL7 9RR

United Kingdom

8. MARKETING AUTHORISATION NUMBER(S)

100 mcg

- PL 18816/0017

50 mcg

- PL 18816/0016

25 mcg

- PL 18816/0015

9. DATE OF FIRST AUTHORISATION/RENEWAL OF THE AUTHORISATION

7 October 2001

10. DATE OF REVISION OF THE TEXT

June 2004

Lexpec Folic Acid Oral Solution 2.5mg/5ml

(Rosemont Pharmaceuticals Limited)

1. NAME OF THE MEDICINAL PRODUCT

Lexpec Folic Acid Oral Solution 2.5mg/5ml

2. QUALITATIVE AND QUANTITATIVE COMPOSITION

Folic Acid 2.5mg/5ml

3. PHARMACEUTICAL FORM

Oral Solution

4. CLINICAL PARTICULARS

4.1 Therapeutic indications

1. Folate deficient megaloblastic anaemia

2. Folate deficient megaloblastic anaemia in infants

3. Malabsorption syndromes

3.1 Tropical sprue

3.2 Coeliac disease

3.3 Non-tropical sprue

4. Megaloblastic anaemia in pregnancy

5. Megaloblastic anaemia associated with alcoholism

6. Megaloblastic anaemia associated with anti-convulsant therapy

7. Haemolytic anaemias e.g. Sickle Cell Anaemia

4.2 Posology and method of administration

For oral administration only.

Children:

May be given 5mg to 15mg daily, in divided doses, according to the severity of the deficiency state.

Adults:

Initial dose of 10mg to 20mg daily, in divided doses, for 14 days or until a haemopotoietic response has been obtained.

Maintenance dose is 2.5mg to 10mg daily.

Prophylactic dose in pregnancy 0.5mg (1ml) daily.

Elderly:

As for adults.

4.3 Contraindications

Known hypersensitivity to folic acid.

Known hypersensitivity to hydroxybenzoate esters.

4.4 Special warnings and special precautions for use

If folic acid is used indiscriminately, there is a danger that patients with pernicious anaemia, despite a haematological remission, may develop irreparable neurological lesions. Therefore a full clinical diagnosis should be made before initiating treatment.

Folic acid is removed by haemodialysis.

Excipients in the Formulation

This product contains hydroxybenzoate esters. These are known to cause urticaria, delayed type reactions such as contact dermatitis and rarely an immediate reaction with urticaria and bronchospasm.

4.5 Interaction with other medicinal products and other forms of Interaction

There are claims that folic acid partially reverses the anti-epileptic effects of phenytoin and primidone.

4.6 Pregnancy and lactation

There are no known hazards to the use of folic acid, indeed folic acid supplements are often necessary in pregnancy.

Folic acid is excreted in breast milk.

4.7 Effects on ability to drive and use machines

There are no known effects of this preparation on the ability to drive or use machines.

4.8 Undesirable effects

Allergenic reactions to folic acid have been reported.

Large doses may cause a yellow discolouration of the urine.

4.9 Overdose

Folic acid is non-toxic in man.

5. PHARMACOLOGICAL PROPERTIES

5.1 Pharmacodynamic properties

ATC Code: B03B B

After conversion into co-enzyme forms it is concerned in single carbon unit transfers in the synthesis of purines, pyrimidines and methionine.

5.2 Pharmacokinetic properties

About 70-80% of a 2mg oral solution of folic acid is absorbed. Larger doses are probably equally well absorbed. It is distributed into plasma and extracellular fluid. In plasma, folate is bound weakly to albumin (70%). There is a further high affinity binder for folate but this has a very low capacity and is barely detectable in normal sera. About 70% of small doses of folate (about 1mg) are retained and the rest excreted into the urine. With larger doses most is excreted into the urine. With a 5mg dose of folate, urinary excretion will be complete in about 5 hours. There is an enterohepatic circulation of folate. The retained folate is taken into cells and reduced by dihydrofolate to tetrahydrofolate. Folic acid is a relatively poor substrate for folate reduction, the normal substrate being dihydrofolate.

Folic acid itself does not occur in natural materials, it is entirely a pharmacological form of the compound. Once reduced, folate has additional glutamic acid residues added, a folate pentaglutamate being the dominant intracellular analogue. These polyglutamates are the active co-enzymes.

5.3 Preclinical safety data

Folic Acid is a drug on which extensive clinical experience has been obtained. Relevant information for the prescriber is provided elsewhere in the Summary of Product Characteristics.

6. PHARMACEUTICAL PARTICULARS

6.1 List of excipients

Mannitol (E421), glycerol (E422), methyl hydroxybenzoate (E218), ethyl hydroxybenzoate (E214), propyl hydroxybenzoate (E216), sodium dihydrogen phosphate, disodium hydrogen phosphate (E339), disodium ethylene diamine tetra acetic acid, strawberry flavour and purified water.

6.2 Incompatibilities

None stated.

6.3 Shelf life

2 years

6.4 Special precautions for storage

Do not store above 25°C

6.5 Nature and contents of container

Bottle: Amber (Type III) glass with 125ml or 150ml capacity.

Closure:

a) Aluminium, EPE wadded, roll-on pilfer-proof

b) HDPE, EPE wadded, tamper evident

c) HDPE, EPE wadded, tamper evident, child resistant.

6.6 Instructions for use and handling

Not applicable.

7. MARKETING AUTHORISATION HOLDER

Rosemont Pharmaceuticals Ltd, Rosemont House, Yorkdale Industrial Park, Braithwaite Street, Leeds, LS11 9XE, UK

8. MARKETING AUTHORISATION NUMBER(S)

PL 00427/0034

9. DATE OF FIRST AUTHORISATION/RENEWAL OF THE AUTHORISATION

30.10.74/17.4.02

10. DATE OF REVISION OF THE TEXT

October 2002

LIBRIUM CAPSULES 10MG

(Valeant Pharmaceuticals Ltd)

1. NAME OF THE MEDICINAL PRODUCT

Librium 10mg Capsules

2. QUALITATIVE AND QUANTITATIVE COMPOSITION

Each 10mg capsule contains 10mg of the active ingredient chlordiazepoxide

hydrochloride BP.

3. PHARMACEUTICAL FORM

Librium Capsules 10mg

4. CLINICAL PARTICULARS

4.1 Therapeutic indications

Short-term (2-4 weeks) symptomatic treatment of anxiety that is severe, disabling or subjecting the individual to unacceptable distress, occurring alone or in association with insomnia or short-term psychosomatic, organic or psychotic illness.

Muscle spasm of varied aetiology.

Symptomatic relief of acute alcohol withdrawal.

4.2 Posology and method of administration

Adults

Anxiety states	Usual dose	Up to 30mg daily in divided doses.
	Maximum dose	Up to 100mg daily in divided doses. Adjusted on an individual basis.
Insomnia associated with anxiety		10 to 30mg before retiring
Symptomatic relief of acute alcohol withdrawal		25 to 100mg repeated if necessary in 2 to 4 hours
Muscle spasm of varied aetiology		10 to 30mg daily in divided doses.

Elderly

Elderly or debilitated patients: doses should not exceed half those normally recommended.

Children

Librium is not for paediatric use.

The lowest dose which can control symptoms should be used. Treatment should not be continued at the full dose beyond four weeks.

Long-term chronic use is not recommended.

Treatment should always be tapered off gradually. Patients who have taken benzodiazepines for a prolonged time may require a longer period during which doses are reduced. Specialist help may be appropriate.

Librium capsules and tablets are for oral administration.

Treatment should be kept to a minimum and given only under close medical supervision. Little is known regarding the efficacy or safety of benzodiazepines in long-term use.

4.3 Contraindications

Patients with known sensitivity to benzodiazepines; acute pulmonary insufficiency; respiratory depression; phobic or obsessional states; chronic psychosis.

4.4 Special warnings and special precautions for use

In patients with chronic pulmonary insufficiency, and in patients with chronic renal or hepatic disease, dosage may need to be reduced.

Librium should not be used alone to treat depression or anxiety associated with depression, since suicide may be precipitated in such patients.

Amnesia may occur.

In cases of loss or bereavement, psychological adjustment may be inhibited by benzodiazepines.

The dependent potential of the benzodiazepines is low, particularly when limited to short-term use, but this increases when high doses are used, especially when given over long periods. This is particularly so in patients with a history of alcoholism or drug abuse or in patients with marked personality disorders. Regular monitoring in such patients is essential, routine repeat prescriptions should be avoided and treatment should be withdrawn gradually. Symptoms such as depression, nervousness, rebound insomnia, irritability, sweating, and diarrhoea have been reported following abrupt cessation of treatment in patients receiving even normal therapeutic doses for short periods of time.

In rare instances, withdrawal following excessive dosages may produce confusional states, psychotic manifestations and convulsions.

Abnormal psychological reactions to benzodiazepines have been reported. Rare behavioural effects include paradoxical aggressive outbursts, excitement, confusion, and the uncovering of depression with suicidal tendencies. Extreme caution should therefore be used in prescribing benzodiazepines to patients with personality disorders.

4.5 Interaction with other medicinal products and other forms of Interaction

If Librium is combined with centrally-acting drugs such as neuroleptics, tranquilisers, antidepressants, hypnotics, analgesics and anaesthetics, the sedative effects are likely to be intensified. The elderly require special supervision.

When Librium is used in conjunction with anti-epileptic drugs, side-effects and toxicity may be more evident, particularly with hydantoins or barbiturates or combinations including them. This requires extra care in adjusting dosage in the initial stages of treatment.

Known inhibitors of hepatic enzymes, eg cimetidine, have been shown to reduce the clearance of benzodiazepines and may potentiate their action and known inducers of hepatic enzymes, eg rifampicin, may increase the clearance of benzodiazepines.

Concomitant intake with alcohol should be avoided. The sedative effect may be enhanced when the product is used in combination with alcohol. This adversely affects the ability to drive or use machines.

4.6 Pregnancy and lactation

There is no evidence as to drug safety in human pregnancy, nor is there evidence from animal work that it is free from hazard. Do not use during pregnancy, especially during the first and last trimesters, unless there are compelling reasons.

If the product is prescribed to a woman of childbearing potential, she should be warned to contact her physician regarding discontinuance of the product if she intends to become or suspects that she is pregnant.

The administration of high doses or prolonged administration of low doses of benzodiazepines in the last trimester of pregnancy has been reported to produce irregularities in the foetal heart rate, and hypotonia, poor sucking and hypothermia in the neonate.

Moreover, infants born to mothers who took benzodiazepines chronically during the later stages of pregnancy may have developed physical dependence and may be at some risk for developing withdrawal symptoms in the postnatal period.

Chlordiazepoxide may appear in breast milk. If possible the use of Librium should be avoided during lactation.

4.7 Effects on ability to drive and use machines

Patients should be advised that, like all medicaments of this type, Librium may modify patients' performance at skilled tasks. Sedation, amnesia, impaired concentration and impaired muscle function may adversely affect the ability to drive or use machinery. If insufficient sleep duration occurs, the likelihood of impaired alertness may be increased. Patients should further be advised that alcohol may intensify any impairment, and should, therefore, be avoided during treatment.

4.8 Undesirable effects

Common adverse effects include drowsiness, sedation, unsteadiness and ataxia; these are dose-related and may persist into the following day even after a single dose. The elderly are particularly sensitive to the effects of centrally-depressant drugs and may experience confusion, especially if organic brain changes are present; the dosage of Librium should not exceed one-half that recommended for other adults.

Other adverse effects are rare and include headache, vertigo, hypotension, gastro-intestinal upsets, skin rashes, visual disturbances, changes in libido, and urinary retention. Isolated cases of blood dyscrasias and jaundice have also been reported.

4.9 Overdose

When taken alone in overdosage Librium presents few problems in management. Signs may include drowsiness, ataxia and dysarthria, with coma in severe cases. Treatment is symptomatic. Gastric lavage is useful only if performed soon after ingestion.

The value of dialysis has not been determined. Anexate is a specific IV antidote for use in emergency situation. Patients requiring such intervention should be monitored closely in hospital (see separate prescribing information).

If excitation occurs, barbiturates should not be used.

When taken with centrally-acting drugs, especially alcohol, the effects of overdosage are likely to be more severe and, in the absence of supportive measures, may prove fatal.

5. PHARMACOLOGICAL PROPERTIES

5.1 Pharmacodynamic properties

Librium has anxiolytic and central muscle relaxant properties. It has little autonomic activity.

5.2 Pharmacokinetic properties

Librium is well absorbed, with peak blood levels being achieved one or two hours after administration. The drug has a half-life of 6-30 hours. Steady-state levels are usually reached within three days.

Chlordiazepoxide is metabolised to desmethylchlordiazepoxide. Demoxepam and desmethyldiazepam are also found in the plasma of patients on continuous treatment. The active metabolite desmethylchloriazepoxide has an accumulation half-life of 10-18 hours; that of demoxepam has been recorded as 21-78 hours.

Steady-state levels of these active metabolites are reached after 10-15 days, with metabolite concentrations which are similar to those of the parent drug.

No clear correlation has been demonstrated between the blood levels of Librium and its clinical effects.

5.3 Preclinical safety data

None stated

6. PHARMACEUTICAL PARTICULARS

6.1 List of excipients

10mg capsules contain the following excipients: gelatine, starch maize white, talc purified, lactose, black iron oxide E172, titanium dioxide E171, yellow iron oxide E172 and indigo carmine E132.

6.2 Incompatibilities

None

6.3 Shelf life

PVDC blister pack 36 months

HDPE bottle 60 months

Plastic bottle 60 months

Amber glass bottle 60 months

6.4 Special precautions for storage

Librium capsules should not be stored above 30°C.

6.5 Nature and contents of container

PVDC Blister pack container 10 capsules

HDPE bottle with jay-cap (snap-fit) closure containing 100 capsules

Plastic bottle with screw cap containing 100 capsules

Amber glass bottle with screw cap containing 100 capsules

6.6 Instructions for use and handling

None

Administrative Data

7. MARKETING AUTHORISATION HOLDER

Valeant Pharmaceuticals Limited

Cedarwood

Chineham Business Park

Basingstoke

Hampshire

RG24 8WD

United Kingdom

8. MARKETING AUTHORISATION NUMBER(S)

PL 15142/0005

9. DATE OF FIRST AUTHORISATION/RENEWAL OF THE AUTHORISATION

1 March 1998

10. DATE OF REVISION OF THE TEXT

November 2004

LIBRIUM CAPSULES 5MG

(Valeant Pharmaceuticals Ltd)

1. NAME OF THE MEDICINAL PRODUCT

Librium 5mg Capsules

2. QUALITATIVE AND QUANTITATIVE COMPOSITION

Each 5mg capsule contains 5mg of the active ingredient chlordiazepoxide hydrochloride BP

3. PHARMACEUTICAL FORM

Librium Capsules 5mg

4. CLINICAL PARTICULARS

4.1 Therapeutic indications

Short-term (2-4 weeks) symptomatic treatment of anxiety that is severe, disabling or subjecting the individual to unacceptable distress, occurring alone or in association with insomnia or short-term psychosomatic, organic or psychotic illness.

Muscle spasm of varied aetiology.

Symptomatic relief of acute alcohol withdrawal.

4.2 Posology and method of administration

Adults

Anxiety states	Usual dose	Up to 30mg daily in divided doses.
	Maximum dose	Up to 100mg daily in divided doses. Adjusted on an individual basis.
Insomnia associated with anxiety		10 to 30mg before retiring
Symptomatic relief of acute alcohol withdrawal		25 to 100mg repeated if necessary in 2 to 4 hours
Muscle spasm of varied aetiology		10 to 30mg daily in divided doses.

Elderly

Elderly or debilitated patients: doses should not exceed half those normally recommended.

Children

Librium is not for paediatric use.

The lowest dose which can control symptoms should be used. Treatment should not be continued at the full dose beyond four weeks.

Long-term chronic use is not recommended.

Treatment should always be tapered off gradually. Patients who have taken benzodiazepines for a prolonged time may require a longer period during which doses are reduced. Specialist help may be appropriate.

Librium capsules and tablets are for oral administration.

Treatment should be kept to a minimum and given only under close medical supervision. Little is known regarding the efficacy or safety of benzodiazepines in long-term use.

4.3 Contraindications

Patients with known sensitivity to benzodiazepines; acute pulmonary insufficiency; respiratory depression; phobic or obsessional states; chronic psychosis.

4.4 Special warnings and special precautions for use

In patients with chronic pulmonary insufficiency, and in patients with chronic renal or hepatic disease, dosage may need to be reduced.

Librium should not be used alone to treat depression or anxiety associated with depression, since suicide may be precipitated in such patients.

Amnesia may occur.

In cases of loss or bereavement, psychological adjustment may be inhibited by benzodiazepines.

The dependent potential of the benzodiazepines is low, particularly when limited to short-term use, but this increases when high doses are used, especially when given over long periods. This is particularly so in patients with a history of alcoholism or drug abuse or in patients with marked personality disorders. Regular monitoring in such patients is essential, routine repeat prescriptions should be avoided and treatment should be withdrawn gradually. Symptoms such as depression, nervousness, rebound insomnia, irritability, sweating, and diarrhoea have been reported following abrupt cessation of treatment in patients receiving even normal therapeutic doses for short periods of time.

In rare instances, withdrawal following excessive dosages may produce confusional states, psychotic manifestations and convulsions.

Abnormal psychological reactions to benzodiazepines have been reported. Rare behavioural effects include paradoxical aggressive outbursts, excitement, confusion, and the uncovering of depression with suicidal tendencies. Extreme caution should therefore be used in prescribing benzodiazepines to patients with personality disorders.

4.5 Interaction with other medicinal products and other forms of Interaction

If Librium is combined with centrally-acting drugs such as neuroleptics, tranquilisers, antidepressants, hypnotics, analgesics and anaesthetics, the sedative effects are likely to be intensified. The elderly require special supervision.

When Librium is used in conjunction with anti-epileptic drugs, side-effects and toxicity may be more evident, particularly with hydantoins or barbiturates or combinations including them. This requires extra care in adjusting dosage in the initial stages of treatment.

Known inhibitors of hepatic enzymes, eg cimetidine, have been shown to reduce the clearance of benzodiazepines and may potentiate their action and known inducers of hepatic enzymes, eg rifampicin, may increase the clearance of benzodiazepines.

Concomitant intake with alcohol should be avoided. The sedative effect may be enhanced when the product is used in combination with alcohol. This adversely affects the ability to drive or use machines.

4.6 Pregnancy and lactation

There is no evidence as to drug safety in human pregnancy, nor is there evidence from animal work that it is free from hazard. Do not use during pregnancy, especially during the first and last trimesters, unless there are compelling reasons.

If the product is prescribed to a woman of childbearing potential, she should be warned to contact her physician regarding discontinuance of the product if she intends to become or suspects that she is pregnant.

The administration of high doses or prolonged administration of low doses of benzodiazepines in the last trimester of pregnancy has been reported to produce irregularities in the foetal heart rate, and hypotonia, poor sucking and hypothermia in the neonate.

Moreover, infants born to mothers who took benzodiazepines chronically during the later stages of pregnancy may have developed physical dependence and may be at some risk for developing withdrawal symptoms in the postnatal period.

Chlordiazepoxide may appear in breast milk. If possible the use of Librium should be avoided during lactation.

4.7 Effects on ability to drive and use machines

Patients should be advised that, like all medicaments of this type, Librium may modify patients' performance at skilled tasks. Sedation, amnesia, impaired concentration and impaired muscle function may adversely affect the ability to drive or use machinery. If insufficient sleep duration occurs, the likelihood of impaired alertness may be increased. Patients should further be advised that alcohol may intensify any impairment, and should, therefore, be avoided during treatment.

4.8 Undesirable effects

Common adverse effects include drowsiness, sedation, unsteadiness and ataxia; these are dose-related and may persist into the following day even after a single dose. The elderly are particularly sensitive to the effects of centrally-depressant drugs and may experience confusion, especially if organic brain changes are present; the dosage of Librium should not exceed one-half that recommended for other adults.

Other adverse effects are rare and include headache, vertigo, hypotension, gastro-intestinal upsets, skin rashes, visual disturbances, changes in libido, and urinary retention. Isolated cases of blood dyscrasias and jaundice have also been reported.

4.9 Overdose

When taken alone in overdosage Librium presents few problems in management. Signs may include drowsiness, ataxia and dysarthria, with coma in severe cases. Treatment is symptomatic. Gastric lavage is useful only if performed soon after ingestion.

The value of dialysis has not been determined. Anexate is a specific IV antidote for use in emergency situation. Patients requiring such intervention should be monitored closely in hospital (see separate prescribing information).

If excitation occurs, barbiturates should not be used.

When taken with centrally-acting drugs, especially alcohol, the effects of overdosage are likely to be more severe and, in the absence of supportive measures, may prove fatal.

5. PHARMACOLOGICAL PROPERTIES

5.1 Pharmacodynamic properties

Librium has anxiolytic and central muscle relaxant properties. It has little autonomic activity.

5.2 Pharmacokinetic properties

Librium is well absorbed, with peak blood levels being achieved one or two hours after administration. The drug has a half-life of 6-30 hours. Steady-state levels are usually reached within three days.

Chlordiazepoxide is metabolised to desmethylchlordiazepoxide. Demoxepam and desmethyldiazepam are also found in the plasma of patients on continuous treatment. The active metabolite desmethylchloriazepoxide has an accumulation half-life of 10-18 hours; that of demoxepam has been recorded as 21-78 hours.

Steady-state levels of these active metabolites are reached after 10-15 days, with metabolite concentrations which are similar to those of the parent drug.

No clear correlation has been demonstrated between the blood levels of Librium and its clinical effects.

5.3 Preclinical safety data

None stated

6. PHARMACEUTICAL PARTICULARS

6.1 List of excipients

5mg capsules contain the following excipients: gelatine, starch maize white, talc purified, lactose, yellow iron oxide E172, indigo carmine E132, titanium dioxide E171, quinoline yellow E104 and erythrosine E127.

6.2 Incompatibilities

None

6.3 Shelf life

PVDC blister pack 36 months

HDPE bottle 60 months

Plastic bottle 60 months

Amber glass bottle 60 months

6.4 Special precautions for storage

Librium capsules should not be stored above 30°C.

6.5 Nature and contents of container

PVDC Blister pack container 10 capsules

HDPE bottle with jay-cap (snap-fit) closure containing 100 capsules

Plastic bottle with screw cap containing 100 capsules

Amber glass bottle with screw cap containing 100 capsules

6.6 Instructions for use and handling

None

Administrative Data

7. MARKETING AUTHORISATION HOLDER

Valeant Pharmaceuticals Limited
Cedarwood
Chineham Business Park
Basingstoke
Hampshire
RG24 8WD
United Kingdom

8. MARKETING AUTHORISATION NUMBER(S)

PL 15142/0004

9. DATE OF FIRST AUTHORISATION/RENEWAL OF THE AUTHORISATION

1 March 1998

10. DATE OF REVISION OF THE TEXT

November 2004

Lidocaine Hydrochloride BP Laryngojet 4%

(International Medication Systems (UK) Ltd)

1. NAME OF THE MEDICINAL PRODUCT

Lidocaine Hydrochloride BP Laryngojet 4% w/v.

2. QUALITATIVE AND QUANTITATIVE COMPOSITION

Lidocaine Hydrochloride BP 160mg in 4ml.

3. PHARMACEUTICAL FORM

Sterile aqueous solution for topical application to the oral mucosa.

4. CLINICAL PARTICULARS

4.1 Therapeutic indications

For topical anaesthesia of the mucous membranes of the oropharynx, trachea, and respiratory tract, e.g. in bronchoscopy, bronchography, laryngoscopy, endotracheal intubation and biopsy in these areas.

4.2 Posology and method of administration

The lowest effective dose should be administered. The usual adult dose is 160mg (one pre-filled syringe). If less is required, the excess should be expelled before use to avoid inadvertent overdosage.

Adults: 1-5ml (40-200mg lidocaine).

Elderly: may need reduced dosage depending on physical state.

Children: up to 3mg/kg.

The solution may be sprayed, instilled (if a cavity) or applied with a swab. Anaesthesia usually occurs within 5 minutes.

4.3 Contraindications

Lidocaine is contraindicated in patients with known hypersensitivity to local anaesthetics of the amide type or in patients with porphyria.

4.4 Special warnings and special precautions for use

Topical application of lidocaine should be used with caution if the mucosa in the area of application has been traumatised or sepsis is present, as absorption will be high.

Use with caution in patients with epilepsy, liver disease, congestive heart failure, marked hypoxia, severe respiratory depression, hypovolaemia or shock and in patients with any form of heart block or sinus bradycardia, or myasthenia gravis.

It should be kept in mind that absorption of aqueous drugs from the respiratory tract may often be nearly as rapid and complete as that occurring with intravenous injection. If there are likely to be high blood levels, resuscitation equipment should be available.

Anaesthesia around the oral cavity may impair swallowing and thus increase the risk of aspiration.

4.5 Interaction with other medicinal products and other forms of Interaction

Propranolol and cimetidine may reduce the renal and hepatic clearance of lidocaine, thus increasing toxicity. The cardiac depressant effects of lidocaine are additive to those of other antiarrhythmic agents. Lidocaine prolongs the action of suxamethonium.

4.6 Pregnancy and lactation

The safe use of lidocaine has not been established with respect to possible adverse effects upon foetal development. Lidocaine is excreted into breast milk and so should therefore be used with caution in nursing women.

4.7 Effects on ability to drive and use machines

Not applicable.

4.8 Undesirable effects

Adverse effects are usually due to inadvertent intravenous administration or overdosage. Rarely, lidocaine may induce an allergic reaction including anaphylaxis.

The following systemic reactions have been reported in association with lidocaine:

Central nervous system: light-headedness, drowsiness, dizziness, apprehension, euphoria, tinnitus, blurred or double vision, nystagmus, vomiting, sensations of heat, cold or numbness, twitching, tremors, convulsions, unconsciousness, respiratory depression and arrest, nausea.

Cardiovascular system: hypotension, cardiovascular collapse and bradycardia which may lead to cardiac arrest.

4.9 Overdose

Symptoms: reactions due to overdose with lidocaine (high plasma levels) are systemic and involve the central nervous and cardiovascular systems. Effects include medullary depression, tonic and clonic convulsions and cardiovascular collapse.

Treatment: institute emergency resuscitative procedures and administer the drugs necessary to manage the severe reaction. For severe convulsions small increments of diazepam or an ultra-short acting barbiturate (thiopentone), or if not available, a short-acting barbiturate (pentobarbitone or quinalbarbitone), or if the patient is under anaesthesia, a short-acting muscle relaxant (suxamethonium) may be given intravenously. Patency of the airway and adequacy of ventilation must be assured.

Should circulatory depression occur vasopressors such as metaraminol may be used.

5. PHARMACOLOGICAL PROPERTIES

5.1 Pharmacodynamic properties

Lidocaine stabilises the neuronal membrane and prevents the initiation and transmission of nerve impulses, thereby effecting local anaesthetic action. The onset of action is rapid and the blockade may last from one to one and a half hours.

5.2 Pharmacokinetic properties

Lidocaine is rapidly distributed to all body tissues. About 65% is plasma bound. Lidocaine crosses the placenta and the blood brain barrier. The plasma half life is 1.6 hours. About 80% of the dose is metabolised in the liver; less than 10% is found unchanged in the urine.

5.3 Preclinical safety data

Not applicable since lidocaine has been used in clinical practice for many years and its effects in man are well known.

6. PHARMACEUTICAL PARTICULARS

6.1 List of excipients

Sodium Hydroxide NF

Water for Injection USP

6.2 Incompatibilities

None known.

6.3 Shelf life

36 months.

6.4 Special precautions for storage

Store below 25°C

6.5 Nature and contents of container

The solution is contained in a USP type I glass vial with an elastomeric closure which meets all the relevant USP specifications. The product is available as 4ml.

6.6 Instructions for use and handling

The container is specially designed for use with the IMS Laryngojet injector device.

7. MARKETING AUTHORISATION HOLDER

International Medication Systems (UK) Limited

208 Bath Road

Slough

Berkshire

SL1 3WE

UK

8. MARKETING AUTHORISATION NUMBER(S)

PL 03265/0040.

9. DATE OF FIRST AUTHORISATION/RENEWAL OF THE AUTHORISATION

Date first granted: 15 November 1977

Date renewed: 21 November 1997

10. DATE OF REVISION OF THE TEXT

June 2004

POM

Lidocaine Hydrochloride Injection BP Minijet 1%

(International Medication Systems (UK) Ltd)

1. NAME OF THE MEDICINAL PRODUCT

Lidocaine Hydrochloride Injection BP Minijet 1% w/v.

2. QUALITATIVE AND QUANTITATIVE COMPOSITION

Lidocaine Hydrochloride BP 10 mg per ml

3. PHARMACEUTICAL FORM

Sterile aqueous solution for infiltration injection or intravenous administration.

4. CLINICAL PARTICULARS

4.1 Therapeutic indications

For local anaesthesia by infiltration, intravenous regional anaesthesia and nerve blocks.

By intravenous injection for the emergency management of ventricular arrhythmias, particularly after myocardial infarction and cardiac surgery.

4.2 Posology and method of administration

For local anaesthesia:

The dosage varies depending upon the area to be anaesthetised, vascularity of the tissues, number of neuronal segments to be blocked, individual tolerance and the anaesthetic technique. The lowest dosage needed to provide anaesthesia should be administered.

Adults: the usual dose should not exceed 200 mg.

Children: the usual dose should not exceed 3 mg/kg.

For epidurals, a test dose should be administered at least 5 minutes before total dose to prevent inadvertent intravascular or subarachnoid injection.

For continuous epidural, caudal or paracervical anaesthesia, the maximal dose should not be repeated at intervals under 90 minutes.

For IV regional anaesthesia (Bier's block), the tourniquet should not be released until at least 20 minutes after administration.

For intravenous use in cardiac arrhythmias:

Adults: the usual dose is 50 to 100 mg administered intravenously under ECG monitoring. This dose may be injected at a rate of approximately 25 to 50 mg (2.5 to 5.0 ml 1% solution or 1.25 to 2.5 ml 2% solution) per minute. A sufficient period of time should be allowed to enable a slow circulation to carry the drug to the site of action. If the initial dose of 50 to 100 mg does not produce the desired response, a second dose may be given after 5 minutes. No more than 200 to 300 mg of lidocaine should be administered during a one hour period.

Following a single injection in those patients in whom arrhythmia tends to recur and who are incapable of receiving oral antiarrhythmic therapy, intravenous infusions of lidocaine may be administered at the rate of 1 to 4 mg/minute (20 to 50 mcg/kg/minute). IV infusions must be given under ECG monitoring to avoid potential overdosage and toxicity. The infusion should be terminated as soon as the patient's basic cardiac rhythm appears to be stable or at the earliest signs of toxicity. It should rarely be necessary to continue the infusion beyond 24 hours. As soon as possible, patients should be changed to an oral antiarrhythmic agent for maintenance therapy.

Children: experience with lidocaine is limited. A suggested paediatric dose is a loading dose of 0.8 to 1 mg/kg repeated if necessary up to 3-5 mg/kg, followed by continuous infusion of 10 to 50 mcg/kg/minute.

Elderly: doses may need to be reduced depending on age and physical state.

4.3 Contraindications

Lidocaine is contraindicated in patients with known hypersensitivity to local anaesthetics of the amide type and in patients with porphyria.

4.4 Special warnings and special precautions for use

Constant ECG monitoring is necessary during IV administration. Resuscitative equipment and drugs should be immediately available for the management of severe adverse cardiovascular, respiratory or central nervous system effects. If severe reactions occur, lidocaine should be discontinued.

Use with caution in patients with epilepsy, liver disease, congestive heart failure, severe renal disease, marked hypoxia, severe respiratory depression, hypovolaemia or shock and in patients with any form of heart block or sinus bradycardia. Hypokalaemia, hypoxia and disorders of acid-base balance should be corrected before treatment with lidocaine begins.

4.5 Interaction with other medicinal products and other forms of Interaction

Propranolol and cimetidine may reduce the renal and hepatic clearance of lidocaine, thus increasing toxicity. The cardiac depressant effects of lidocaine are additive to those of other antiarrhythmic agents. Lidocaine prolongs the action of suxamethonium.

4.6 Pregnancy and lactation

The safe use of lidocaine has not been established with respect to possible adverse effects upon foetal development. Lidocaine is excreted in breast milk and so should be used with caution in nursing women.

4.7 Effects on ability to drive and use machines

Not applicable; this preparation is intended for use only in emergencies.

4.8 Undesirable effects

Adverse effects are usually due to inadvertent intravenous administration or overdosage. Allergic reactions (including anaphylaxis) have been reported rarely.

The following systemic reactions have been reported in association with lidocaine:

Central nervous system: light-headedness, drowsiness, dizziness, apprehension, nervousness, euphoria, tinnitus, blurred or double vision, nystagmus, vomiting, sensations of heat, cold or numbness, twitching, tremors, paraesthesia, convulsions, unconsciousness, respiratory depression and arrest.

Cardiovascular system: hypotension, cardiovascular collapse and bradycardia which may lead to cardiac arrest.

4.9 Overdose

Symptoms: reactions due to overdose with lidocaine (high plasma levels) are systemic and involve the central nervous and cardiovascular systems. Effects include medullary depression, tonic and clonic convulsions and cardiovascular collapse.

Treatment: institute emergency resuscitative procedures and administer the drugs necessary to manage the severe reaction. For severe convulsions, small increments of diazepam or an ultra-short acting barbiturate (thiopentone), or if not available, a short-acting barbiturate (pentobarbitone or quinalbarbitone), or if the patient is under anaesthesia, a short-acting muscle relaxant (suxamethonium) may be given intravenously. Patency of the airway and adequacy of ventilation must be assured.

Should circulatory depression occur vasopressors such as metaraminol may be used.

5. PHARMACOLOGICAL PROPERTIES

5.1 Pharmacodynamic properties

Lidocaine stabilises the neuronal membrane and prevents the initiation and transmission of nerve impulses, thereby effecting local anaesthetic action. The onset of action is rapid and the blockade may last up to 2 hours.

In the heart, lidocaine reduces automaticity by decreasing the rate of diastolic (phase 4) depolarisation. Lidocaine is considered as a class 1b (membrane stabilising) antiarrhythmic agent. The duration of the action potential is decreased due to blockade of the sodium channel and the refractory period is shortened.

5.2 Pharmacokinetic properties

Lidocaine is rapidly distributed to all body tissues. About 65% is plasma bound. Lidocaine crosses the placenta and the blood brain barrier. The plasma half life is 1.6 hours. About 80% of the dose is metabolised in the liver; less than 10% is found unchanged in the urine.

5.3 Preclinical safety data

Not applicable since lidocaine has been used in clinical practice for many years and its effects in man are well known.

6. PHARMACEUTICAL PARTICULARS

6.1 List of excipients

Hydrochloric Acid BP

Sodium Chloride BP

Sodium Hydroxide BP

Water for Injection USP

6.2 Incompatibilities

None known.

6.3 Shelf life

3 years.

6.4 Special precautions for storage

Store below 25°C.

6.5 Nature and contents of container

The solution is contained in a USP type I glass vial with an elastomeric closure which meets all the relevant USP specifications. The product is available as a 1% solution in a 10ml vial.

6.6 Instructions for use and handling

The container is specially designed for use with the IMS Minijet injector.

7. MARKETING AUTHORISATION HOLDER

International Medication Systems (UK) Ltd

208 Bath Road

Slough

Berkshire

SL1 3WE

UK

8. MARKETING AUTHORISATION NUMBER(S)

PL 03265/0005R

9. DATE OF FIRST AUTHORISATION/RENEWAL OF THE AUTHORISATION

Date first granted: 28 February 1991

Date renewed: 29 November 1996

10. DATE OF REVISION OF THE TEXT

June 2004

POM

Lidocaine Hydrochloride Injection BP Minijet 2%

(International Medication Systems (UK) Ltd)

1. NAME OF THE MEDICINAL PRODUCT

Lidocaine Hydrochloride Injection BP Minijet 2% w/v.

2. QUALITATIVE AND QUANTITATIVE COMPOSITION

Lidocaine Hydrochloride BP 20 mg per ml

3. PHARMACEUTICAL FORM

Sterile aqueous solution for infiltration injection or intravenous administration.

4. CLINICAL PARTICULARS

4.1 Therapeutic indications

For local anaesthesia by infiltration, intravenous regional anaesthesia and nerve blocks.

By intravenous injection for the emergency management of ventricular arrhythmias, particularly after myocardial infarction and cardiac surgery.

4.2 Posology and method of administration

For local anaesthesia:

The dosage varies depending upon the area to be anaesthetised, vascularity of the tissues, number of neuronal segments to be blocked, individual tolerance and the anaesthetic technique. The lowest dosage needed to provide anaesthesia should be administered.

Adults: the usual dose should not exceed 200 mg.

Children: the usual dose should not exceed 3 mg/kg.

For epidurals, a test dose should be administered at least 5 minutes before total dose to prevent inadvertent intravascular or subarachnoid injection.

For continuous epidural, caudal or paracervical anaesthesia, the maximal dose should not be repeated at intervals under 90 minutes.

For IV regional anaesthesia (Bier's block), the tourniquet should not be released until at least 20 minutes after administration.

For intravenous use in cardiac arrhythmias:

Adults: the usual dose is 50 to 100 mg administered intravenously under ECG monitoring. This dose may be injected at a rate of approximately 25 to 50 mg (2.5 to 5.0 ml 1% solution or 1.25 to 2.5 ml 2% solution) per minute. A sufficient period of time should be allowed to enable a slow circulation to carry the drug to the site of action. If the initial dose of 50 to 100 mg does not produce the desired response, a second dose may be given after 5 minutes.

No more than 200 to 300 mg of lidocaine should be administered during a one hour period.

Following a single injection in those patients in whom arrhythmia tends to recur and who are incapable of receiving oral antiarrhythmic therapy, intravenous infusions of lidocaine may be administered at the rate of 1 to 4 mg/minute (20 to 50 mcg/kg/minute). IV infusions must be given under ECG monitoring to avoid potential overdosage and toxicity. The infusion should be terminated as soon as the patient's basic cardiac rhythm appears to be stable or at the earliest signs of toxicity. It should rarely be necessary to continue the infusion beyond 24 hours. As soon as possible, patients should be changed to an oral antiarrhythmic agent for maintenance therapy.

Children: experience with lidocaine is limited. A suggested paediatric dose is a loading dose of 0.8 to 1 mg/kg repeated if necessary up to 3-5 mg/kg, followed by continuous infusion of 10 to 50 mcg/kg/minute.

Elderly: doses may need to be reduced depending on age and physical state.

4.3 Contraindications

Lidocaine is contraindicated in patients with known hypersensitivity to local anaesthetics of the amide type and in patients with porphyria.

4.4 Special warnings and special precautions for use

Constant ECG monitoring is necessary during IV administration. Resuscitative equipment and drugs should be immediately available for the management of severe adverse cardiovascular, respiratory or central nervous system effects. If severe reactions occur, lidocaine should be discontinued.

Use with caution in patients with epilepsy, liver disease, congestive heart failure, severe renal disease, marked hypoxia, severe respiratory depression, hypovolaemia or shock and in patients with any form of heart block or sinus bradycardia. Hypokalaemia, hypoxia and disorders of acid-base balance should be corrected before treatment with lidocaine begins.

4.5 Interaction with other medicinal products and other forms of Interaction

Propranolol and cimetidine may reduce the renal and hepatic clearance of lidocaine, thus increasing toxicity. The cardiac depressant effects of lidocaine are additive to those of other antiarrhythmic agents. Lidocaine prolongs the action of suxamethonium.

4.6 Pregnancy and lactation

The safe use of lidocaine has not been established with respect to possible adverse effects upon foetal development. Lidocaine is excreted in breast milk and so should be used with caution in nursing women.

4.7 Effects on ability to drive and use machines

Not applicable; this preparation is intended for use only in emergencies.

4.8 Undesirable effects

Adverse effects are usually due to inadvertent intravenous administration or overdosage. Allergic reactions (including anaphylaxis) have been reported rarely.

The following systemic reactions have been reported in association with lidocaine:

Central nervous system: light-headedness, drowsiness, dizziness, apprehension, nervousness, euphoria, tinnitus, blurred or double vision, nystagmus, vomiting, sensations of heat, cold or numbness, twitching, tremors, paraesthesia, convulsions, unconsciousness, respiratory depression and arrest.

Cardiovascular system: hypotension, cardiovascular collapse and bradycardia which may lead to cardiac arrest.

4.9 Overdose

Symptoms: reactions due to overdose with lidocaine (high plasma levels) are systemic and involve the central nervous and cardiovascular systems. Effects include medullary depression, tonic and clonic convulsions and cardiovascular collapse.

Treatment: institute emergency resuscitative procedures and administer the drugs necessary to manage the severe reaction. For severe convulsions, small increments of diazepam or an ultra-short acting barbiturate (thiopentone), or if not available, a short-acting barbiturate (pentobarbitone or quinalbarbitone), or if the patient is under anaesthesia, a short-acting muscle relaxant (suxamethonium) may be given intravenously. Patency of the airway and adequacy of ventilation must be assured.

Should circulatory depression occur vasopressors such as metaraminol may be used.

5. PHARMACOLOGICAL PROPERTIES

5.1 Pharmacodynamic properties

Lidocaine stabilises the neuronal membrane and prevents the initiation and transmission of nerve impulses, thereby effecting local anaesthetic action. The onset of action is rapid and the blockade may last up to 2 hours.

In the heart, lidocaine reduces automaticity by decreasing the rate of diastolic (phase 4) depolarisation. Lidocaine is considered as a class 1b (membrane stabilising) antiarrhythmic agent. The duration of the action potential is decreased due to blockade of the sodium channel and the refractory period is shortened.

5.2 Pharmacokinetic properties

Lidocaine is rapidly distributed to all body tissues. About 65% is plasma bound. Lidocaine crosses the placenta and the blood brain barrier. The plasma half life is 1.6 hours. About 80% of the dose is metabolised in the liver; less than 10% is found unchanged in the urine.

5.3 Preclinical safety data

Not applicable since lidocaine has been used in clinical practice for many years and its effects in man are well known.

6. PHARMACEUTICAL PARTICULARS

6.1 List of excipients

Hydrochloric Acid BP

Sodium Chloride BP

Sodium Hydroxide BP

Water for Injection USP

6.2 Incompatibilities

None known.

6.3 Shelf life

3 years.

6.4 Special precautions for storage

Store below 25°C.

6.5 Nature and contents of container

The solution is contained in a USP type I glass vial with an elastomeric closure which meets all the relevant USP specifications. The product is available as a 2% solution in a 5ml vial.

6.6 Instructions for use and handling

The container is specially designed for use with the IMS Minijet injector.

7. MARKETING AUTHORISATION HOLDER

International Medication Systems (UK) Ltd

208 Bath Road

Slough

Berkshire

SL1 3WE

UK

8. MARKETING AUTHORISATION NUMBER(S)

PL 03265/0006R

9. DATE OF FIRST AUTHORISATION/RENEWAL OF THE AUTHORISATION

Date first granted: 28 February 1991

Date renewed: 29 November 1996

10. DATE OF REVISION OF THE TEXT

June 2004

11. Legal category

POM

Lioresal Intrathecal

(Novartis Pharmaceuticals UK Ltd)

1. NAME OF THE MEDICINAL PRODUCT

Lioresal ® Intrathecal Injection 50micrograms/1ml

Lioresal ® Intrathecal Infusion 10mg/20ml

Lioresal ® Intrathecal Infusion 10mg/5ml

2. QUALITATIVE AND QUANTITATIVE COMPOSITION

Active substance

b-(Aminomethyl)-p-chlorohydrocinnamic acid (= baclofen), a racemic mixture of the R, (-) and S, (+) isomers.

One ampoule of 1 ml contains 50 micrograms baclofen, (50 micrograms/ml).

One ampoule of 5 ml contains 10 mg baclofen, (2000 micrograms/ml).

One ampoule of 20 ml contains 10 mg baclofen, (500 micrograms/ml).

3. PHARMACEUTICAL FORM

Solutions for intrathecal injection and intrathecal infusion.

4. CLINICAL PARTICULARS

4.1 Therapeutic indications

Lioresal Intrathecal is indicated in patients with severe chronic spasticity of spinal or cerebral origin (associated with injury, multiple sclerosis, cerebral palsy) who are unresponsive to oral baclofen or other orally administered antispastic agents and/or those patients who experience unacceptable side-effects at effective oral doses.

Lioresal Intrathecal is not recommended for use in patients under 18 years of age with spasticity of spinal origin due to limited clinical experience in this age group.

In patients with spasticity due to head injury a delay of at least one year before treatment with Lioresal Intrathecal is recommended, to allow the symptoms of spasticity to stabilise.

Lioresal Intrathecal may be considered as an alternative to ablative neurosurgical procedures.

4.2 Posology and method of administration

Intrathecal administration of Lioresal through an implanted delivery system should only be undertaken by physicians with the necessary knowledge and experience. Specific instructions for implantation, programming and/or refilling of the implantable pump are given by the pump manufacturers, and must be strictly adhered to.

Adults, Children and the Elderly

Lioresal Intrathecal 50 micrograms/1ml is intended for administration in single bolus test injections via a lumbar puncture or intrathecal catheter. Lioresal Intrathecal 10mg/20ml and 10mg/5ml have been developed specifically for use with implantable pumps.

Individual titration of dosage is essential due to a high interindividual variability in response. Each patient must undergo an initial screening phase to determine the response to test bolus doses followed by a dose-titration phase to determine the optimum dose schedule for maintenance therapy with an appropriate implanted delivery system.

Respiratory function should be monitored and appropriate resuscitation facilities should be available during the introduction of treatment with Lioresal Intrathecal. Intrathecal administration using an implanted delivery system should only be undertaken by physicians with appropriate knowledge and experience. Specific instructions for using the implantable pump should be obtained from the pump manufacturers. Only pumps constructed of material known to be compatible with the product and incorporating an in-line bacterial retentive filter should be used.

Screening Phase

Prior to initiation of a chronic infusion, the patient's response to intrathecal bolus doses administered via a catheter or lumbar puncture must be assessed. Low concentration ampoules containing 50 micrograms baclofen in 1ml are available for the purpose. Patients should be infection-free prior to screening, as the presence of a systemic infection may prevent an accurate assessment of the response.

The usual initial test dose in adults is 25 or 50 micrograms, increasing step-wise by 25 microgram increments at intervals of not less than 24 hours until a response of approximately 4 to 8 hours duration is observed. The recommended initial test dose in children (patients under 18 years) is 25μg. Each dose should be given **slowly** (over at least one minute). In order to be considered a responder the patient must demonstrate a significant decrease in muscle tone and/or frequency and/or severity of muscle spasms.

The variability in sensitivity to intrathecal baclofen between patients is emphasised. Signs of severe overdose (coma) have been observed in an adult after a single test dose of 25 micrograms. It is recommended that the initial test dose is administered with resuscitative equipment on hand.

Patients who do not respond to a 100 micrograms test dose should not be given further dose increments or considered for continuous intrathecal infusion.

Monitoring of respiratory and cardiac function is essential during this phase, especially in patients with cardiopulmonary disease and respiratory muscle weakness or those being treated with benzodiazepine-type preparations or opiates, who are at higher risk of respiratory depression.

Dose-Titration Phase

Once the patient's responsiveness to Lioresal Intrathecal has been established, an intrathecal infusion may be introduced. Lioresal Intrathecal is most often administered using an infusion pump which is implanted in the chest wall or abdominal wall tissues. Implantation of pumps should only be performed in experienced centres to minimise risks during the perioperative phase.

Infection may increase the risk of surgical complications and complicate attempts to adjust the dose.

The initial total daily infused dose is determined by doubling the bolus dose which gave a significant response in the initial screening phase and administering it over a 24 hour period. However, if a prolonged effect (i.e. lasting more than 12 hours) is observed during screening the starting dose should be the unchanged screening dose delivered over 24 hours. No dose increases should be attempted during the first 24 hours.

After the initial 24 hour period dosage should be adjusted slowly to achieve the desired clinical effect. If a programmable pump is used the dose should be increased only once every 24 hours; for non-programmable multi-dose reservoir pumps intervals of 48 hours between dose adjustments are recommended. In either case increments should be limited as follows to avoid possible overdosage:

Patients with spasticity of spinal origin: 10-30% of the previous daily dose

Patients with spasticity of cerebral origin: 5-15% of the previous daily dose.

If the dose has been significantly increased without apparent clinical effect pump function and catheter patency should be investigated.

There is limited clinical experience using doses greater than 1000 micrograms/day.

It is important that patients are monitored closely in an appropriately equipped and staffed environment during screening and immediately following pump implantation. Resuscitative equipment should be available for immediate use in case of life-threatening adverse reactions.

Maintenance Therapy

The clinical goal is to maintain as normal a muscle tone as possible, and to minimise the frequency and severity of spasms without inducing intolerable side effects. The lowest dose producing an adequate response should be used. The retention of some spasticity is desirable to avoid a sensation of "paralysis" on the part of the patient. In addition, a degree of muscle tone and occasional spasms may help support circulatory function and possibly prevent the formation of deep vein thrombosis.

In patients with spasticity of spinal origin maintenance dosing for long-term continuous infusions of intrathecal baclofen has been found to range from 12 to 2003 micrograms/day, with most patients being adequately maintained on 300 to 800 micrograms/day.

In patients with spasticity of cerebral origin maintenance dosage has been found to range from 22 to 1400 micrograms/day, with a mean daily dosage of 276 micrograms per day at 12 months and 307 micrograms per day at 24 months. Paediatric patients under the age of 12 will generally require lower doses; maintenance dosage has been found to range from 24 to 1199 micrograms per day (mean daily dose of 274 micrograms per day).

Delivery specifications

Lioresal Intrathecal ampoules of 20ml containing 500 micrograms/ml and 5ml containing 2mg (2000micrograms)/ml are intended for use with infusion pumps. The concentration to be used depends on the dose requirements and size of pump reservoir. Use of the more concentrated solution obviates the need for frequent re-filling in patients with high dosage requirements.

Delivery regimen

Lioresal Intrathecal is most often administered in a continuous infusion mode immediately following implant. After the patient has stabilised with regard to daily dose and functional status, and provided the pump allows it, a more complex mode of delivery may be started to optimise control of spasticity at different times of the day. For example, patients who have increased spasm at night may require a 20 % increase in their hourly infusion rate. Changes in flow rate should be programmed to start two hours before the desired onset of clinical effect.

Most patients require gradual dose increases to maintain optimum response during chronic therapy due to decreased responsiveness or disease progression. In patients with spasticity of spinal origin the daily dose may be increased gradually by 10-30% to maintain adequate symptom control. Where the spasticity is of cerebral origin any increase in dose should be limited to 20% (range: 5-20%). In both cases the daily dose may also be reduced by 10-20% if patients suffer side effects.

A sudden requirement for substantial dose escalation is indicative of a catheter complication (i.e. a kink or dislodgement) or pump malfunction.

In order to prevent excessive weakness the dosage of Lioresal Intrathecal should be adjusted with caution whenever spasticity is required to maintain function.

During long-term treatment approximately 5% of patients become refractory to increasing doses. This can be due to tolerance or to drug delivery failure (see Section 4.4 – Special Warnings and Precautions for Use "Treatment Withdrawal" section). There is insufficient clinical experience on which to base firm recommendations for tolerance treatment, however This "tolerance" has been treated on occasion in hospital by a "drug holiday" consisting of the gradual reduction of Lioresal Intrathecal over 2 to 4 week period and switching to alternative methods of spasticity management eg. Intrathecal preservative-free morphine sulphate. Lioresal Intrathecal should be resumed at the initial continuous infusion dose followed by re-titration to avoid overdose. Caution should be exercised when switching from Lioresal Intrathecal to morphine and vice versa (see "Interactions").

Discontinuation

Except in overdose-dose related emergencies, the treatment with Lioresal Intrathecal should always be gradually discontinued by successively reducing the dosage. Lioresal Intrathecal should not be discontinued suddenly (see Section 4.4 – Special Warnings and Precautions for Use).

4.3 Contraindications

Known hypersensitivity to baclofen.

The drug should not be administered by any route other than intrathecal.

4.4 Special warnings and special precautions for use

Intrathecal baclofen therapy is valuable but hazardous. Careful pre-operative assessment is mandatory.

The patient must be given adequate information regarding the risks of this mode of treatment, and be physically and psychologically able to cope with the pump. It is essential that the responsible physicians and all those involved in the care of the patient receive adequate instruction on the signs and symptoms of overdose, procedures to be followed in the event of an overdose and the proper home care of the pump and insertion site.

Pump Implantation

Patients should be infection-free prior to pump implantation because the presence of infection may increase the risk of surgical complications. Moreover, a systemic infection may complicate attempts to adjust the dose. A local infection or catheter malplacement can also lead to drug delivery failure, which may result in sudden Lioresal Intrathecal withdrawal and its related symptoms (see Section 4.4 – Special Precautions for Use "Treatment Withdrawal" section).

Reservoir refilling

Reservoir refilling must be performed by trained and qualified personnel in accordance with the instructions provided by the pump manufacturer. Refills should be timed to avoid excessive depletion of the reservoir, as this would result in the return of spasticity or potentially life-threatening symptoms of Lioresal Intrathecal withdrawal (see Section 4.4 – Special Precautions for Use "Treatment Withdrawal" section.

When refilling the pump care should be taken to avoid discharging the contents of the catheter into the intrathecal space.

Strict asepsis is required to avoid microbial contamination and infection.

Extreme caution must be taken when filling a pump equipped with an injection port that allows direct access to the intrathecal catheter as a direct injection into the catheter through the access port could cause a life-threatening overdose.

Precautions in paediatric patients

Children should be of sufficient body mass to accommodate the implantable pump for chronic infusion. There is very limited clinical experience of the use of Lioresal Intrathecal in children under six. The safety of Lioresal Intrathecal in children under four has not yet been established.

Precautions in special patient populations

In patients with abnormal CSF flow the circulation of drug and hence antispastic activity may be inadequate.

Psychotic disorders, schizophrenia, confusional states or Parkinson's disease may be exacerbated by treatment with oral Lioresal. Patients suffering from these conditions should therefore be treated cautiously and kept under close surveillance.

Special attention should be given to patients known to suffer from epilepsy as seizures have occasionally been reported during overdose with, and withdrawal from, Lioresal Intrathecal as well as in patients maintained on therapeutic doses.

Lioresal Intrathecal should be used with caution in patients with a history of autonomic dysreflexia. The presence of nociceptive stimuli or abrupt withdrawal of Lioresal Intrathecal may precipitate an autonomic dysreflexic episode.

Lioresal should be used with caution in patients with cerebrovascular or respiratory insufficiency.

An effect of Lioresal Intrathecal on underlying, non-CNS related diseases is unlikely because its systemic availability is substantially lower than after oral administration. Observations after oral baclofen therapy suggest that caution should be exercised in patients with a history of peptic ulcers, pre-existing sphincter hypertonia and impaired renal function.

In rare instances elevated SGOT, alkaline phosphatase and glucose levels in the serum have been recorded when using oral Lioresal.

Several patients over the age of 65 years have been treated with intrathecal baclofen without specific problems, and as doses are individually titrated there are unlikely to be any specific problems in elderly patients.

Treatment withdrawal

Abrupt discontinuation of Lioresal Intrathecal, regardless of cause, manifested by increased spasticity, pruritus, paraethesia and hypotension, as resulted in sequelae including a hyperactive state with rapid uncontrolled spasms, hyperthermia and symptoms consistent with neuroleptic malignant syndrome, e.g. altered mental status and muscle rigidity. In rare cases this has advanced to seizures/status epilepticus, rhabdomyolysis, coagulopathy, multiple organ failure and death. All patients receiving intrathecal baclofen therapy are potentially at risk for withdrawal.

Patients and caregivers should be advised of the importance of keeping scheduled refill visits and should be educated on the signs and symptoms of baclofen withdrawal particularly those seen early in the withdrawal syndrome.

In most cases, symptoms of withdrawal appeared within hours to a few days following interruption of baclofen therapy. Common reasons for abrupt interruption intrathecal baclofen therapy included malfunction of the catheter (especially disconnection), low volume in the pump reservoir and end of pump battery life; human error may have played a causal or contributing role in some cases.

Prevention of abrupt discontinuation of intrathecal baclofen requires careful attention to programming and monitoring of the infusion system, refill scheduling and procedures, and pump alarms.

Instructions for implantation programming and/or refilling of the implantable pump given by the pump manufacturers must be strictly followed.

4.5 Interaction with other medicinal products and other forms of Interaction

The co-administration of other intrathecal agents with Lioresal Intrathecal is not recommended.

An attempt should be made to reduce or discontinue concomitant oral antispastic medications, preferably before initiating baclofen infusion. However, abrupt reduction or discontinuation during chronic intrathecal baclofen therapy should be avoided.

There is inadequate experience with Lioresal Intrathecal in combination with systemic medications to be able to predict specific drug-drug interactions, although it is suggested that the lower plasma baclofen levels produced by intrathecal administration should reduce the potential for interactions. Experience with oral baclofen would suggest that:

There may be increased sedation where Lioresal is taken concomitantly with other drugs acting on the CNS or with alcohol.

During concurrent treatment with tricyclic antidepressants, the effect of Lioresal may be potentiated, resulting in muscular hypotonia.

Since concomitant treatment with Lioresal and anti-hypertensives is likely to increase the fall in blood pressure, it may be necessary to reduce the dosage of antihypertensive medication.

In patients with Parkinson's disease receiving treatment with Lioresal and levodopa plus carbidopa mental confusion, hallucinations and agitation may occur.

The combined use of morphine and intrathecal baclofen has been responsible for hypotension in one patient; the potential for this combination to cause dyspnoea or other CNS symptoms cannot be excluded.

4.6 Pregnancy and lactation

There are no adequate and well-controlled studies in pregnant women. Oral baclofen increases the incidence of omphaloceles (ventral hernias) in the foetuses of rats at high doses. No teratogenic effects have been noted in mice or rabbits.

A dose related increase in the incidence of ovarian cysts, and a less marked increase in enlarged and/or haemorrhagic adrenals have been observed in female rats treated for 2 years. The clinical relevance of these findings is not known.

Lioresal Intrathecal should not be used during pregnancy unless the potential benefit is judged to outweigh the potential risk to the foetus. Baclofen crosses the placental barrier.

In mothers taking oral Lioresal in therapeutic doses the active substance passes into the breast milk, but in quantities so small that no undesirable effects on the infant are to be expected. It is not known whether detectable levels of drug are present in the breast milk of nursing mothers receiving Lioresal Intrathecal.

4.7 Effects on ability to drive and use machines

Drowsiness has been reported in some patients receiving intrathecal baclofen, and patients should be advised to exercise due caution. Operating equipment or machinery may be hazardous.

4.8 Undesirable effects

A causal link between the following observed events and the administration of baclofen cannot be reliably assessed in many cases, since many of the adverse events reported are known to occur in association with the underlying conditions being treated. Nonetheless, some of the more commonly reported reactions - drowsiness/somnolence, dizziness, headache, nausea, hypotension, hypotonia - appear to be drug-related.

Some of the adverse events listed below have been reported in patients with spasticity of spinal origin but could also occur in patients with spasticity of cerebral origin. Adverse events that are more frequent in either population are indicated below.

Adverse events are ranked under headings of frequency, the most frequent first, using the following convention: very common ≥ 10%, common ≥ 1% to < 10%, uncommon ≥ 0.1% to < 1%, rare ≥ 0.01% to < 0.1%, very rare < 0.01%.

(see Table 1 on next page)

Adverse events associated with the delivery system (eg. Catheter dislocation, pocket infection, meningitis, overdose due to wrong manipulation of the device) are not included here.

4.9 Overdose

Special attention should be given to recognising the signs and symptoms of overdosage at all times, but especially during the initial "screening" and "dose-titration" phases and also during reintroduction of Lioresal Intrathecal after an interruption of therapy.

Signs of overdose may appear suddenly or (more usually) insidiously.

Symptoms of overdose: excessive muscular hypotonia, drowsiness, lightheadedness, dizziness, somnolence,

Table 1

Central nervous system	
Very common:	drowsiness/somnolence
Common:	sedation, dizziness/ lightheadedness, seizures, headache, paraesthesia, accommodation disorders/blurred vision/double vision, slurred speech, lethargy, asthenia, respiratory depression, insomnia, confusion/ disorientation, anxiety/ agitation, depression
Uncommon:	hypothermia, nystagmus, dysphagia, ataxia, impaired memory, suicidal ideation and attempt, euphoria, dysphoria, hallucinations, paranoia.
(Seizures and headache occur more often in patients with spasticity of cerebral origin than in patients with spasticity of spinal origin).	
Cardiovascular system	
Common:	Hypotension.
Uncommon:	hypertension, bradycardia, deep vein thrombosis, skin flushing, paleness.
Musculoskeletal system	
Very common:	muscular hypotonia.
Common:	muscular hypertonia.
Gastroin intestinal tract	
Common:	nausea/vomiting, constipation, dry mouth, diarrhoea, decreased appetite, increased salivation.
Uncommon:	dehydration, ileus, decreased taste.
(Nausea and vomiting occur more often in patients with spasticity of cerebral origin than in patients with spasticity of spinal origin).	
Respiratory system	
Common:	dyspnoea, bradypnoea, pneumonia.
Renal and urinary	
Common:	urinary incontinence, urinary retention, sexual dysfunction.
(Intrathecal Lioresal may compromise erection and ejaculation. This effect is usually reversible on withdrawal of Lioresal Intrathecal. Urinary retention occurs more often in patients with spasticity of cerebral origin than in patients with spasticity of spinal origin).	
Skin	
Common:	urticaria/pruritus, facial or peripheral oedema.
Uncommon:	alopecia, diaphoresis.
Miscellaneous	
Common:	pain, fever/chills.
Rare:	Life threatening withdrawal symptoms due to drug delivery failure (see Section 4.4 – Special Warnings and Precautions for Use "Treatment Withdrawal").

seizures, loss of consciousness, excessive salivation, nausea and vomiting.

Respiratory depression, apnoea, and coma result from serious overdosage. Seizures may occur with increasing dosage or, more commonly, during recovery from an overdose. Serious overdose may occur through the inadvertent delivery of the catheter contents, errors in pump programming, excessively rapid dose increases or concomitant treatment with oral baclofen. Possible pump malfunction should also be investigated.

Treatment

There is no specific antidote for treating overdoses of intrathecal baclofen. Any instructions provided by the pump manufacturer should be followed, and the following steps should generally be undertaken:

Where a programmable continuous infusion pump is used further delivery of baclofen should be halted immediately by removal of residual drug solution from the reservoir.

If it is possible to do so without surgical intervention the intrathecal catheter should be disconnected from the pump as soon as possible, and infusion fluid allowed to drain back together with some CSF (up to 30-40ml is suggested).

Patients with respiratory depression should be intubated if necessary, and ventilated artificially if required. Cardiovascular functions should be supported and in the event of convulsions, iv diazepam cautiously administered.

Anecdotal reports suggest that intravenous physostigmine may assist in the reversal of central side effects (notably drowsiness and respiratory depression), but its use has been associated with the induction of seizures, bradycardia and cardiac conduction disturbances, and it should not be used in cases of severe overdose. In such cases intubation and ventilation are essential. In adults a total dose of 1-2mg physostigmine may be tried intravenously over 5-10 minutes. Patients should be monitored closely during this time. Repeated doses of 1mg may be administered at 30-60 minute intervals in an attempt to maintain adequate respiration in the absence of facilities for respiratory support.

In children a dose of 0.02mg/kg physostigmine may be administered iv at a rate not exceeding 0.5mg per minute. This dose may be repeated at 5 to 10 minute intervals until a therapeutic effect is obtained or a total dose of 2mg has been administered.

5. PHARMACOLOGICAL PROPERTIES

5.1 Pharmacodynamic properties

Antispastic with a spinal site of attack.

Baclofen depresses both monosynaptic and polysynaptic reflex transmission in the spinal cord by stimulating the $GABA_\beta$ receptors. Baclofen is a chemical analogue of the inhibitory neurotransmitter gamma-aminobutyric acid (GABA).

Neuromuscular transmission is not affected by baclofen. Baclofen exerts an antinociceptive effect. In neurological diseases associated with spasm of the skeletal muscles, the clinical effects of Lioresal take the form of a beneficial action on reflex muscle contractions and of marked relief from painful spasm, automatism, and clonus. Lioresal improves the patient's mobility, makes it easier for him/her to manage without aid, and facilitates physiotherapy.

Consequent important gains include improved ambulation, prevention and healing of decubitus ulcers, and better sleep patterns due to elimination of painful muscle spasms. In addition, patients experience improvement in bladder and sphincter function and catheterisation is made easier, all representing significant improvements in the patient's quality of life. Baclofen has been shown to have general CNS depressant properties, causing sedation, somnolence, and respiratory and cardiovascular depression.

Baclofen when introduced directly into the intrathecal space, permits effective treatment of spasticity wih doses at least 100 times smaller than those for oral administration.

Intrathecal bolus:

The onset of action is generally half an hour to one hour after administration of a single intrathecal dose. Peak spasmolytic effect is seen at approximately 4 hours after dosing, the effect lasting 4 to 8 hours. Onset, peak response, and duration of action may vary with individual patients depending on the dose and severity of symptoms and the method and speed of drug administration.

Continuous infusion:

Baclofen's antispastic action is first seen at 6 to 8 hours after initiation of continuous infusion. Maximum efficacy is observed within 24 to 48 hours.

5.2 Pharmacokinetic properties

The following kinetic parameters have to be interpreted in the light of intrathecal administration coupled with slow CSF circulation.

Absorption

Direct infusion into the spinal subarachnoid space bypasses absorption processes and allows exposure to the receptor sites in the dorsal horn of the spinal cord.

Distribution

After single intrathecal bolus injection/short-term infusion the volume of distribution, calculated from CSF levels, ranges from 22 to 157 ml.

With continuous intrathecal infusion daily doses of 50 to 1200 micrograms result in lumbar CSF concentrations of baclofen as high as 130 to 1240 ng/ml at steady state. According to the half-life measured in the CSF, CSF steady-state concentrations will be reached within 1-2 days. No paediatric data are available.

During intrathecal infusion the plasma concentrations do not exceed 5ng/ml (10ng/ml in paediatric patients), confirming that baclofen passes only slowly across the blood-brain barrier.

Elimination

The elimination half-life in the CSF after single intrathecal bolus injection/short-term infusion of 50 to 136 micrograms baclofen ranges from 1 to 5 hours. Elimination half-life of baclofen after having reached steady-state in the CSF has not been determined.

After both single bolus injection and chronic lumbar subarachnoid infusion using an implantable pump system, the mean CSF clearance was about 30 ml/h.

At steady-state conditions during continuous intrathecal infusion, a baclofen concentration gradient is built up in the range between 1.8: 1 and 8.7: 1 (mean:

4: 1) from lumbar to cisternal CSF. This is of clinical importance insofar as spasticity in the lower extremities can be effectively treated with little effect on the upper limbs and with fewer CNS adverse reactions due to effects on the brain centres.

5.3 Preclinical safety data

Subacute and subchronic studies with continuous intrathecal baclofen infusion in two species (rat, dog) revealed no signs of local irritation or inflammation on histological examination.

A 2-year rat study (oral administration) showed that baclofen is not carcinogenic. In the same study a dose-related increase in incidence of ovarian cysts and a less marked increase in enlarged and/or haemorrhagic adrenal glands was observed.

Ovarian cysts have been found by palpation in about 5% of the multiple sclerosis patients who were treated with oral Lioresal for up to one year. In most cases these cysts disappeared spontaneously while patients continued to receive the drug. Ovarian cysts are known to occur spontaneously in a proportion of the normal female population.

Mutagenicity assays in vitro and in vivo showed no evidence of mutagenic effects.

6. PHARMACEUTICAL PARTICULARS

6.1 List of excipients

Sodium chloride; water for injections

6.2 Incompatibilities

If alternative baclofen concentrations are required Lioresal Intrathecal may be diluted under aseptic conditions with sterile preservative-free sodium chloride for injections. The ampoules should not be mixed with other solutions for injection or infusion (dextrose has proved to be incompatible due to a chemical reaction with baclofen).

The compatibility of Lioresal Intrathecal with the components of the infusion pump (including the chemical stability of baclofen in the reservoir) and the presence of an in-line bacterial retentive filter should be confirmed with the pump manufacturer prior to use.

6.3 Shelf life

Lioresal ® Intrathecal Injection 50micrograms/1ml: 3 years

Lioresal ® Intrathecal Infusion 10mg/20ml: 3 years

Lioresal ® Intrathecal Infusion 10mg/5ml: 5 years

6.4 Special precautions for storage
Protect from heat (store below 30°C).

Medicines should be kept out of the reach of children.

6.5 Nature and contents of container
Colourless glass ampoules, glass type I, according to Ph. Eur.

6.6 Instructions for use and handling
Each ampoule is intended for single use only, and any unused solution should be discarded. Ampoules should not be either frozen or autoclaved.

7. MARKETING AUTHORISATION HOLDER
Novartis Pharmaceuticals UK Limited
Trading as Ciba Laboratories
Frimley Business Park
Frimley
Camberley
Surrey
GU16 7SR
England.

8. MARKETING AUTHORISATION NUMBER(S)
PL 00101/0500 – 2

9. DATE OF FIRST AUTHORISATION/RENEWAL OF THE AUTHORISATION
21 September 1997

10. DATE OF REVISION OF THE TEXT
13 June 2003

Legal Category
POM

Lioresal Liquid

(Cephalon UK Limited)

1. NAME OF THE MEDICINAL PRODUCT
Lioresal ® Liquid

2. QUALITATIVE AND QUANTITATIVE COMPOSITION
The active ingredient is: β-(Aminomethyl)-p-chlorohydrocinnamic acid (= baclofen), a racemic mixture of the R,(-) and S, (+) isomers.

The liquid contains 5mg/5ml baclofen Ph. Eur.

3. PHARMACEUTICAL FORM
Liquid

4. CLINICAL PARTICULARS
4.1 Therapeutic indications
Lioresal is indicated for the relief of spasticity of voluntary muscle resulting from such disorders as: multiple sclerosis, other spinal lesions, e.g. tumours of the spinal cord, syringomyelia, motor neurone disease, transverse myelitis, traumatic partial section of the cord.

Lioresal is also indicated in adults and children for the relief of spasticity of voluntary muscle arising from e.g. cerebrovascular accidents, cerebral palsy, meningitis, traumatic head injury.

Patient selection is important when initiating Lioresal therapy; it is likely to be of most benefit in patients whose spasticity constitutes a handicap to activities and/or physiotherapy. Treatment should not be commenced until the spastic state has become stabilised.

4.2 Posology and method of administration
Lioresal is given orally in either tablet or liquid form. These two formulations are bioequivalent. The liquid may be particularly suitable for children or those adults who are unable to take tablets. Dosage titration can be more precisely managed with the liquid.

Before starting treatment with Lioresal it is prudent to realistically assess the overall extent of clinical improvement that the patient may be expected to achieve. Careful titration of dosage is essential (particularly in the elderly) until the patient is stabilised. If too high a dose is initiated or if the dosage is increased too rapidly side effects may occur. This is particularly relevant if the patient is ambulant in order to minimise muscle weakness in the unaffected limbs or where spasticity is necessary for support.

Adults: The following gradually increasing dosage regimen is suggested, but should be adjusted to suit individual patient requirements.

5mg three times a day for three days

10mg three times a day for three days

15mg three times a day for three days

20mg three times a day for three days

Satisfactory control of symptoms is usually obtained with doses of up to 60mg daily, but a careful adjustment is often necessary to meet the requirements of each individual patient.

The dose may be increased slowly if required, but a maximum daily dose of more than 100mg is not advised unless the patient is in hospital under careful medical supervision. Small frequent dosage may prove better in some cases than larger spaced doses.

Also some patients benefit from the use of Lioresal only at night to counteract painful flexor spasm. Similarly a single dose given approximately 1 hour prior to performance of specific tasks such as washing, dressing, shaving, physiotherapy, will often improve mobility.

Once the maximum recommended dose has been reached, if the therapeutic effect is not apparent within 6 weeks a decision whether to continue with Lioresal should be taken.

Elderly: Elderly patients may be more susceptible to side effects, particularly in the early stages of introducing Lioresal. Small doses should therefore be used at the start of treatment, the dose being titrated gradually against the response, under careful supervision. There is no evidence that the eventual average maximum dose differs from that in younger patients.

Children: A dosage range of 0.75-2mg/kg body weight should be used. In children over 10 years of age, however a maximum daily dosage of 2.5mg/kg body weight may be given. Treatment is usually started with 2.5mg given 4 times daily. The dosage should be cautiously raised at about 3 day intervals, until it becomes sufficient for the child's individual requirements. The recommended daily dosages for maintenance therapy are as follows:

Children aged: 12 months - 2 years: 10-20mg

2 years - 6 years: 20-30mg

6 years - 10 years: 30-60mg

Patients with impaired renal function: In patients with impaired renal function or undergoing chronic haemodialysis, a particularly low dosage of Lioresal should be selected i.e. approx. 5mg daily. Signs of overdose have been observed in patients with renal impairment taking oral Lioresal at doses more than 5mg per day.

Patients with spastic states of cerebral origin: Unwanted effects are more likely to occur in these patients. It is therefore recommended that a very cautious dosage schedule be adopted and that patients be kept under appropriate surveillance.

4.3 Contraindications
Hypersensitivity to baclofen, peptic ulceration.

4.4 Special warnings and special precautions for use
Psychotic disorders, schizophrenia, depressive or manic disorders, confusional states or Parkinson's disease may be exacerbated by treatment with Lioresal. Patients suffering from these conditions should therefore be treated cautiously and kept under close surveillance.

Lioresal may also exacerbate epileptic manifestations but can be employed provided appropriate supervision and adequate anticonvulsive therapy are maintained. Lioresal should be used with extreme care in patients already receiving antihypertensive therapy, (see Interactions).

Lioresal should be used with caution in patients suffering from cerebrovascular accidents or from respiratory, hepatic or renal impairment.

Signs of overdose have been observed in patients with renal impairment taking oral Lioresal at doses of more than 5mg per day.

Under treatment with Lioresal neurogenic disturbances affecting emptying of the bladder may show an improvement. In patients with pre-existing sphincter hypertonia, acute retention of urine may occur; the drug should be used with caution in such cases.

Abrupt withdrawal:
Anxiety and confusional states, hallucinations, psychotic, manic or paranoid states, convulsions (status epilepticus), dyskinesia, tachycardia, hyperthermia and as rebound phenomenon temporary aggravation of spasticity have been reported with abrupt withdrawal of Lioresal, especially after long term medication. Treatment should always, (unless serious adverse effects occur), therefore be gradually discontinued by successively reducing the dosage over a period of about 1-2 weeks.

Since in rare instances elevated SGOT, alkaline phosphatase and glucose levels in serum have been recorded, appropriate laboratory tests should be performed in patients with liver diseases or diabetes mellitus in order to ensure that no drug induced changes in these underlying diseases have occurred.

4.5 Interaction with other medicinal products and other forms of Interaction
Where Lioresal is taken concomitantly with other drugs acting on the CNS with synthetic opiates or with alcohol, increased sedation may occur.

The risk of respiratory depression is also increased. Careful monitoring of respiratory and cardiovascular functions is essential especially in patients with cardiopulmonary disease and respiratory muscle weakness.

During concurrent treatment with tricyclic antidepressants, the effect of Lioresal may be potentiated, resulting in pronounced muscular hypotonia.

Since concomitant treatment with Lioresal and anti-hypertensives is likely to increase the fall in blood pressure, the dosage of antihypertensive medication should be adjusted accordingly. Hypotension has been reported in one patient receiving morphine and intrathecal baclofen.

Drugs which may produce renal insufficiency e.g. ibuprofen may reduce baclofen excretion leading to toxic effects.

In patients with Parkinson's disease receiving treatment with Lioresal and levodopa plus carbidopa, there have been reports of mental confusion, hallucinations, nausea and agitation.

4.6 Pregnancy and lactation
During pregnancy, especially in the first 3 months, Lioresal should only be employed if its use is of vital necessity. The benefits of the treatment for the mother must be carefully weighed against the possible risks for the child. Baclofen crosses the placental barrier.

In mothers taking Lioresal in therapeutic doses, the active substance passes into the breast milk, but in quantities so small that no undesirable effects on the infant are to be expected.

4.7 Effects on ability to drive and use machines
The patient's reactions may be adversely affected by Lioresal induced sedation or decreased alertness, patients should therefore exercise due caution. Operating equipment or machinery may be hazardous.

4.8 Undesirable effects
Side-effects: Unwanted effects occur mainly at the start of treatment, if the dosage is raised too rapidly, if large doses are employed, or in elderly patients. They are often transitory and can be attenuated or eliminated by reducing the dosage; they are seldom severe enough to necessitate withdrawal of the medication.

Should nausea persist following a reduction in dosage, it is recommended that Lioresal be ingested with food or a milk beverage.

In patients with a case history of psychiatric illness or with cerebrovascular disorders (e.g. stroke) as well as in elderly patients, adverse reactions may assume a more serious form.

Frequency estimates: frequent > 10%, occasional > 1%-10%, Rare > 0.001%-1%, isolated cases < 0.001%.

Central Nervous System:
Frequent: particularly at the start of treatment daytime sedation, drowsiness, and nausea may frequently occur.

Occasional: respiratory depression, light-headedness, lassitude, exhaustion, mental confusion, dizziness, headache, insomnia, euphoria, depression, muscular weakness, ataxia, tremor, hallucinations, nightmares, myalgia, nystagmus, dry mouth.

Rare: paraesthesia, dysarthria. Lowering of the convulsion threshold and convulsions may occur, particularly in epileptic patients.

Sense organs:
Occasional: accommodation disorders, visual disturbance.

Rare: dysgeusia.

Gastro-intestinal tract:
Frequent: nausea.

Occasional: mild gastro-intestinal disturbances, constipation, diarrhoea, retching and vomiting.

Rare: abdominal pain

Cardiovascular system:
Occasional: hypotension, diminished cardiovascular function.

Urogenital system:
Frequent: frequency of micturition, enuresis, dysuria.

Rare: urinary retention, impotence.

Liver:
Rare: disorders of hepatic function.

Skin:
Occasional: hyperhydrosis, skin rash.

Certain patients have shown increased spasticity as a paradoxical reaction to the medication.

An undesirable degree of muscular hypotonia - making it more difficult for patients to walk or fend for themselves - may occur and can usually be relieved by re-adjusting the dosage (i.e. by reducing the doses given during the day and possibly increasing the evening dose).

4.9 Overdose
Symptoms: Prominent features are signs of central nervous depression: drowsiness, impairment of consciousness, respiratory depression, coma. Also liable to occur are: confusion, hallucinations, agitation, accommodation disorders, absent pupillary reflex; generalised muscular hypotonia, myoclonia, hyporeflexia or areflexia; convulsions; peripheral vasodilatation, hypotension, bradycardia; hypothermia; nausea, vomiting, diarrhoea, hypersalivation; elevated LDH, SGOT and AP values.

Patients with renal impairment can develop signs of overdose even on low doses of oral Lioresal (see section 4.2 Posology and Method of administration and 4.4 Special warnings and special precautions for use.)

A deterioration in the condition may occur if various substances or drugs acting on the central nervous system (e.g. alcohol, diazepam, tricyclic antidepressants) have been taken at the same time.

Treatment: No specific antidote is known.

Elimination of the drug from the gastro-intestinal tract (induction of vomiting, gastric lavage; comatose patients should be intubated prior to gastric lavage), administration of activated charcoal; if necessary, saline aperient; in respiratory depression, administration of artificial respiration, also measures in support of cardiovascular functions. Since the drug is excreted chiefly via the kidneys, generous quantities of fluid should be given, possibly together with a diuretic. In the event of convulsions diazepam should be administered cautiously i.v.

5. PHARMACOLOGICAL PROPERTIES

5.1 Pharmacodynamic properties

Lioresal is an antispastic agent acting at the spinal level. A gamma-aminobutyric acid (GABA) derivative, Lioresal is chemically unrelated to other antispastic agents.

Lioresal depresses monosynaptic and polysynaptic reflex transmission, probably by stimulating the $GABA_B$ receptors, this stimulation in turn inhibiting the release of the excitatory amino acids glutamate and aspartate. Neuromuscular transmission is unaffected by Lioresal.

The major benefits of Lioresal stem from its ability to reduce painful flexor spasms and spontaneous clonus thereby facilitating the mobility of the patient, increasing his independence and helping rehabilitation.

Lioresal also exerts an antinociceptive effect. General well being is often improved and sedation is less often a problem than with centrally acting drugs.

Baclofen stimulates gastric acid secretion.

5.2 Pharmacokinetic properties

Absorption: Lioresal (baclofen) is rapidly and completely absorbed from the gastro-intestinal tract. No significant difference between the liquid and tablet formulations is observed in respect of t_{max}, c_{max} and bioavailability. Following oral administration of single doses (10-30mg) peak plasma concentrations are recorded after 0.5 to 1.5 hours and areas under the serum concentration curves are proportional to the dose.

Distribution: The volume of distribution of baclofen is 0.7 l/kg and the protein binding rate is approximately 30%. In cerebrospinal fluid active substance concentrations are approximately 8.5 times lower than in the plasma.

Biotransformation: Baclofen is metabolised to only a minor extent. Deamination yields the main metabolite, -(p-chlorophenyl)-4-hydroxybutyric acid, which is pharmacologically inactive.

Elimination/excretion: The plasma elimination half-life of baclofen averages 3 to 4 hours. The serum protein binding rate is approximately 30%.

Baclofen is eliminated largely in unchanged form. Within 72 hours, about 75% of the dose is excreted via the kidneys with about 5% of this amount as metabolites.

Elderly: The pharmacokinetics of baclofen in elderly patients are virtually the same as in young subjects. The peak plasma concentrations of baclofen in elderly patients are slightly lower and occur later than in healthy young subjects but the AUCs are similar in the two groups.

5.3 Preclinical safety data

Baclofen increases the incidence of omphaloceles (ventral hernias) in the foetuses of rats given approximately 13 times the maximum oral dose (on a mg/kg basis) recommended for human use. This was not seen in mice or rabbits.

An apparently dose related increase in the incidence of ovarian cysts, and a less marked increase in enlarged and/or haemorrhagic adrenals have been observed in female rats treated for 2 years. The clinical relevance of these findings is not known.

Experimental evidence to date suggests that baclofen does not possess either carcinogenic or mutagenic properties.

6. PHARMACEUTICAL PARTICULARS

6.1 List of excipients

Methylparahydroxybenzoate; propylparahydroxybenzoate; raspberry flavour; carmellose sodium, sorbitol; purified water.

Lioresal liquid contains no sucrose and is therefore suitable for diabetics and children.

6.2 Incompatibilities

None known.

6.3 Shelf life

3 years

6.4 Special precautions for storage

Protect from light. Store below 25C. Do not refrigerate.

Dilution: Lioresal liquid may be diluted with Purified Water BP and stored at room temperature for up to 14 days.

6.5 Nature and contents of container

Liquid 5mg/5ml: clear, very slightly yellow solution with a raspberry flavour.

Bottles of 300ml with child proof closures.

6.6 Instructions for use and handling

There is no specific instruction for use/handling.

7. MARKETING AUTHORISATION HOLDER

Novartis Pharmaceuticals UK Ltd,
Trading as:
Ciba Laboratories,
Frimley Business Park
Frimley
Camberley
Surrey
GU16 7SR

8. MARKETING AUTHORISATION NUMBER(S)

PL 00101 / 0503

9. DATE OF FIRST AUTHORISATION/RENEWAL OF THE AUTHORISATION

1 April 2001

10. DATE OF REVISION OF THE TEXT

22 February 2005

Legal Category

POM

Lioresal Tablets 10mg

(Cephalon UK Limited)

1. NAME OF THE MEDICINAL PRODUCT

Lioresal ® Tablets 10mg

2. QUALITATIVE AND QUANTITATIVE COMPOSITION

The active ingredient is: β-(Aminomethyl)-p-chlorohydrocinnamic acid (= baclofen), a racemic mixture of the R,(-) and S, (+) isomers.

One tablet contains 10mg baclofen Ph. Eur.

3. PHARMACEUTICAL FORM

Tablet scored

4. CLINICAL PARTICULARS

4.1 Therapeutic indications

Lioresal is indicated for the relief of spasticity of voluntary muscle resulting from such disorders as: multiple sclerosis, other spinal lesions, e.g. tumours of the spinal cord, syringomyelia, motor neurone disease, transverse myelitis, traumatic partial section of the cord.

Lioresal is also indicated in adults and children for the relief of spasticity of voluntary muscle arising from e.g. cerebrovascular accidents, cerebral palsy, meningitis, traumatic head injury.

Patient selection is important when initiating Lioresal therapy; it is likely to be of most benefit in patients whose spasticity constitutes a handicap to activities and/or physiotherapy. Treatment should not be commenced until the spastic state has become stabilised.

4.2 Posology and method of administration

Lioresal is given orally in either tablet or liquid form. These two formulations are bioequivalent. The liquid may be particularly suitable for children or those adults who are unable to take tablets. Dosage titration can be more precisely managed with the liquid.

Before starting treatment with Lioresal it is prudent to realistically assess the overall extent of clinical improvement that the patient may be expected to achieve. Careful titration of dosage is essential (particularly in the elderly) until the patient is stabilised. If too high a dose is initiated or if the dosage is increased too rapidly side effects may occur. This is particularly relevant if the patient is ambulant in order to minimise muscle weakness in the unaffected limbs or where spasticity is necessary for support.

Adults: The following gradually increasing dosage regimen is suggested, but should be adjusted to suit individual patient requirements.

5mg three times a day for three days

10mg three times a day for three days

15mg three times a day for three days

20mg three times a day for three days

Satisfactory control of symptoms is usually obtained with doses of up to 60mg daily, but a careful adjustment is often necessary to meet the requirements of each individual patient. The dose may be increased slowly if required, but a maximum daily dose of more than 100mg is not advised unless the patient is in hospital under careful medical supervision. Small frequent dosage may prove better in some cases than larger spaced doses. Also some patients benefit from the use of Lioresal only at night to counteract painful flexor spasm. Similarly a single dose given approximately 1 hour prior to performance of specific tasks such as washing, dressing, shaving, physiotherapy, will often improve mobility.

Once the maximum recommended dose has been reached, if the therapeutic effect is not apparent within 6 weeks a decision whether to continue with Lioresal should be taken.

Elderly: Elderly patients may be more susceptible to side effects, particularly in the early stages of introducing Lioresal. Small doses should therefore be used at the start of treatment, the dose being titrated gradually against the response, under careful supervision. There is no evidence that the eventual average maximum dose differs from that in younger patients.

Children: A dosage range of 0.75-2mg/kg body weight should be used. In children over 10 years of age, however a maximum daily dosage of 2.5mg/kg body weight may be given. Treatment is usually started with 2.5mg given 4 times daily. The dosage should be cautiously raised at about 3 day intervals, until it becomes sufficient for the child's individual requirements. The recommended daily dosages for maintenance therapy are as follows:

Children aged: 12 months - 2 years: 10-20mg

2 years - 6 years: 20-30mg

6 years - 10 years: 30-60mg

Patients with impaired renal function: In patients with impaired renal function or undergoing chronic haemodialysis, a particularly low dosage of Lioresal should be selected i.e. approx. 5mg daily. Signs of overdose have been observed in patients with renal impairment taking oral Lioresal at doses of more than 5mg per day.

Patients with spastic states of cerebral origin: Unwanted effects are more likely to occur in these patients. It is therefore recommended that a very cautious dosage schedule be adopted and that patients be kept under appropriate surveillance.

4.3 Contraindications

Hypersensitivity to baclofen, peptic ulceration.

4.4 Special warnings and special precautions for use

Psychotic disorders, schizophrenia, depressive or manic disorders, confusional states or Parkinson's disease may be exacerbated by treatment with Lioresal. Patients suffering from these conditions should therefore be treated cautiously and kept under close surveillance.

Lioresal may also exacerbate epileptic manifestations but can be employed provided appropriate supervision and adequate anticonvulsive therapy are maintained. Lioresal should be used with extreme care in patients already receiving antihypertensive therapy, (see Interactions).

Lioresal should be used with caution in patients suffering from cerebrovascular accidents or from respiratory, hepatic or renal impairment.

Signs of overdose have been observed in patients with renal impairment taking oral Lioresal at doses of more than 5mg per day.

Under treatment with Lioresal neurogenic disturbances affecting emptying of the bladder may show an improvement. In patients with pre-existing sphincter hypertonia, acute retention of urine may occur; the drug should be used with caution in such cases.

Abrupt withdrawal:

Anxiety and confusional states, hallucinations, psychotic, manic or paranoid states, convulsions (status epilepticus), dyskinesia, tachycardia, hyperthermia and as rebound phenomenon temporary aggravation of spasticity have been reported with abrupt withdrawal of Lioresal, especially after long term medication. Treatment should always, (unless serious adverse effects occur), therefore be gradually discontinued by successively reducing the dosage over a period of about 1-2 weeks.

Since in rare instances elevated SGOT, alkaline phosphatase and glucose levels in serum have been recorded, appropriate laboratory tests should be performed in patients with liver diseases or diabetes mellitus in order to ensure that no drug induced changes in these underlying diseases have occurred.

4.5 Interaction with other medicinal products and other forms of Interaction

Where Lioresal is taken concomitantly with other drugs acting on the CNS with synthetic opiates or with alcohol, increased sedation may occur.

The risk of respiratory depression is also increased. Careful monitoring of respiratory and cardiovascular functions is essential especially in patients with cardiopulmonary disease and respiratory muscle weakness.

During concurrent treatment with tricyclic antidepressants, the effect of Lioresal may be potentiated, resulting in pronounced muscular hypotonia.

Since concomitant treatment with Lioresal and anti-hypertensives is likely to increase the fall in blood pressure, the dosage of antihypertensive medication should be adjusted accordingly. Hypotension has been reported in one patient receiving morphine and intrathecal baclofen.

Drugs which may produce renal insufficiency e.g. ibuprofen may reduce baclofen excretion leading to toxic effects.

In patients with Parkinson's disease receiving treatment with Lioresal and levodopa plus carbidopa, there have been reports of mental confusion, hallucinations, nausea and agitation.

4.6 Pregnancy and lactation

During pregnancy, especially in the first 3 months, Lioresal should only be employed if its use is of vital necessity. The benefits of the treatment for the mother must be carefully weighed against the possible risks for the child. Baclofen crosses the placental barrier.

In mothers taking Lioresal in therapeutic doses, the active substance passes into the breast milk, but in quantities so small that no undesirable effects on the infant are to be expected.

4.7 Effects on ability to drive and use machines

The patient's reactions may be adversely affected by Lioresal induced sedation or decreased alertness, patients should therefore exercise due caution. Operating equipment or machinery may be hazardous.

4.8 Undesirable effects

Side-effects: Unwanted effects occur mainly at the start of treatment, if the dosage is raised too rapidly, if large doses are employed, or in elderly patients. They are often transitory and can be attenuated or eliminated by reducing the dosage; they are seldom severe enough to necessitate withdrawal of the medication.

Should nausea persist following a reduction in dosage, it is recommended that Lioresal be ingested with food or a milk beverage.

In patients with a case history of psychiatric illness or with cerebrovascular disorders (e.g. stroke) as well as in elderly patients, adverse reactions may assume a more serious form.

Frequency estimates: frequent > 10%, occasional > 1%-10%, Rare > 0.001%-1%, isolated cases < 0.001%.

Central Nervous System:

Frequent: particularly at the start of treatment daytime sedation, drowsiness, and nausea may frequently occur.

Occasional: respiratory depression, light-headedness, lassitude, exhaustion, mental confusion, dizziness,, headache, insomnia, euphoria, depression, muscular weakness, ataxia, tremor, hallucinations, nightmares, myalgia, nystagmus, dry mouth.

Rare: paraesthesia, dysarthria. Lowering of the convulsion threshold and convulsions may occur, particularly in epileptic patients.

Sense organs:

Occasional: accommodation disorders, visual disturbance.

Rare: dysgeusia.

Gastro-intestinal tract:

Frequent: nausea.

Occasional: mild gastro-intestinal disturbances constipation, diarrhoea, retching and vomiting.

Rare: abdominal pain

Cardiovascular system:

Occasional: hypotension, diminished cardiovascular function.

Urogenital system:

Frequent: frequency of micturition, enuresis, dysuria.

Rare: urinary retention, impotence.

Liver:

Rare: disorders of hepatic function.

Skin:

Occasional: hyperhydrosis, skin rash.

Certain patients have shown increased spasticity as a paradoxical reaction to the medication.

An undesirable degree of muscular hypotonia - making it more difficult for patients to walk or fend for themselves - may occur and can usually be relieved by re-adjusting the dosage (i.e. by reducing the doses given during the day and possibly increasing the evening dose).

4.9 Overdose

Symptoms: Prominent features are signs of central nervous depression: drowsiness, impairment of consciousness, respiratory depression, coma Also liable to occur are: confusion, hallucinations, agitation, accommodation disorders, absent pupillary reflex; generalised muscular hypotonia, myoclonia, hyporeflexia or areflexia; convulsions; peripheral vasodilatation, hypotension, bradycardia; hypothermia; nausea, vomiting, diarrhoea, hypersalivation; elevated LDH, SGOT and AP values. Patients with renal impairment can develop signs of overdose even on low doses of oral Lioresal (see section 4.2 Posology and Method of administration, 4.4 Special warnings and special precautions for use).

A deterioration in the condition may occur if various substances or drugs acting on the central nervous system (e.g. alcohol, diazepam, tricyclic antidepressants) have been taken at the same time.

Treatment: No specific antidote is known.

Elimination of the drug from the gastro-intestinal tract (induction of vomiting, gastric lavage; comatose patients should be intubated prior to gastric lavage), administration of activated charcoal; if necessary, saline aperient; in respiratory depression, administration of artificial respiration, also measures in support of cardiovascular functions. Since the drug is excreted chiefly via the kidneys, generous quantities of fluid should be given, possibly together with a diuretic. In the event of convulsions diazepam should be administered cautiously i.v.

5. PHARMACOLOGICAL PROPERTIES

5.1 Pharmacodynamic properties

Lioresal is an antispastic agent acting at the spinal level. A gamma-aminobutyric acid (GABA) derivative, Lioresal is chemically unrelated to other antispastic agents.

Lioresal depresses monosynaptic and polysynaptic reflex transmission, probably by stimulating the $GABA_B$-receptors, this stimulation in turn inhibiting the release of the excitatory amino acids glutamate and aspartate. Neuromuscular transmission is unaffected by Lioresal.

The major benefits of Lioresal stem from its ability to reduce painful flexor spasms and spontaneous clonus thereby facilitating the mobility of the patient, increasing his independence and helping rehabilitation.

Lioresal also exerts an antinociceptive effect. General well being is often improved and sedation is less often a problem than with centrally acting drugs.

Baclofen stimulates gastric acid secretion.

5.2 Pharmacokinetic properties

Absorption: Lioresal (baclofen) is rapidly and completely absorbed from the gastro-intestinal tract. No significant difference between the liquid and tablet formulations is observed in respect of t_{max}, c_{max} and bioavailability. Following oral administration of single doses (10-30mg) peak plasma concentrations are recorded after 0.5 to 1.5 hours and areas under the serum concentration curves are proportional to the dose.

Distribution: The volume of distribution of baclofen is 0.7 l/kg and the protein binding rate is approximately 30%. In cerebrospinal fluid active substance concentrations are approximately 8.5 times lower than in the plasma.

Biotransformation: Baclofen is metabolised to only a minor extent. Deamination yields the main metabolite, -(p-chlorophenyl)-4-hydroxybutyric acid, which is pharmacologically inactive.

Elimination/excretion: The plasma elimination half-life of baclofen averages 3 to 4 hours. The serum protein binding rate is approximately 30%.

Baclofen is eliminated largely in unchanged form. Within 72 hours, about 75% of the dose is excreted via the kidneys with about 5% of this amount as metabolites.

Elderly: The pharmacokinetics of baclofen in elderly patients are virtually the same as in young subjects. The peak plasma concentrations of baclofen in elderly patients are slightly lower and occur later than in healthy young subjects but the AUCs are similar in the two groups.

5.3 Preclinical safety data

Baclofen increases the incidence of omphaloceles (ventral hernias) in the foetuses of rats given approximately 13 times the maximum oral dose (on a mg/kg basis) recommended for human use. This was not seen in mice or rabbits.

An apparently dose related increase in the incidence of ovarian cysts, and a less marked increase in enlarged and/or haemorrhagic adrenals have been observed in female rats treated for 2 years. The clinical relevance of these findings is not known.

Experimental evidence to date suggests that baclofen does not possess either carcinogenic or mutagenic properties.

6. PHARMACEUTICAL PARTICULARS

6.1 List of excipients

Tablets: silica aerogel; microcryst.cellulose; magnesium stearate; povidone; wheat starch; deionised water.

6.2 Incompatibilities

None known.

6.3 Shelf life

4 years

6.4 Special precautions for storage

Lioresal tablets should be protected from heat (store below 25 °C) and moisture.

6.5 Nature and contents of container

Tablets 10mg: circular, flat, white to faint yellowish tablets, uncoated, with bevelled edges, having the monogram CG on one side and the letters KJ and a break line on the other.

In blister packs of 84 and 100 or securitainers of 84 and 200 or child-resistant/tamper evident loose fill packs of 84 and 200.

6.6 Instructions for use and handling

There is no specific instruction for use/handling.

7. MARKETING AUTHORISATION HOLDER

Novartis Pharmaceuticals UK Limited

Trading as:

Ciba Pharmaceuticals,

Frimley Business Park

Frimley

Camberley

Surrey

GU16 7SR

8. MARKETING AUTHORISATION NUMBER(S)

PL 00101/0504

9. DATE OF FIRST AUTHORISATION/RENEWAL OF THE AUTHORISATION

1 April 2001

10. DATE OF REVISION OF THE TEXT

22 February 2005

LEGAL CATEGORY

POM

Lipantil Micro 200

(Fournier Pharmaceuticals Limited)

1. NAME OF THE MEDICINAL PRODUCT

Lipantil® Micro 200 mg, capsules.

2. QUALITATIVE AND QUANTITATIVE COMPOSITION

Each capsule contains 200 mg fenofibrate.

For excipients, see 6.1

3. PHARMACEUTICAL FORM

Orange, hard gelatin capsule.

4. CLINICAL PARTICULARS

4.1 Therapeutic indications

Lipantil Micro 200 reduces elevated serum cholesterol and triglyceride and is of benefit in the treatment of severe dyslipidaemia in patients in whom dietary measures alone have failed to produce an adequate response. Lipantil Micro 200 is therefore indicated in appropriate cases of hyperlipidaemia (Fredrickson classification types IIa, IIb, III, IV and V).

Type	Major lipid elevated	Lipoproteins elevated
IIa	Cholesterol	LDL
IIb	Cholesterol, triglyceride	LDL, VLDL
III (rare)	Cholesterol, triglyceride	LDL and Chylomicron Remnants
IV	Triglyceride	VLDL
V (rare)	Triglyceride	Chylomicrons, VLDL

Lipantil Micro 200 should only be used in patients whose disease is unresponsive to dietary control and in whom a full investigation has been performed to define their abnormality, and where long-term risks associated with their condition warrant treatment. Other risk factors, such as hypertension and smoking, may also require management.

4.2 Posology and method of administration

Adults

The recommended initial dose is one capsule taken daily during a main meal. In elderly patients without renal impairment, the normal adult dose is recommended. Since it is less well absorbed from an empty stomach, Lipantil Micro 200 should always be taken with food. Dietary restrictions instituted before therapy should be continued.

Response to therapy should be monitored by determination of serum lipid values. Rapid reduction of serum lipid levels usually follows Lipantil Micro 200 treatment, but treatment should be discontinued if an adequate response has not been achieved within three months.

4.3 Contraindications

Lipantil Micro 200 is contra-indicated in children, in patients with severe liver dysfunction, gallbladder disease, biliary cirrhosis, severe renal disorders and in patients hypersensitive to fenofibrate or any component of this medication, known photoallergy or phototoxic reaction during treatment with fibrates or ketoprofen.

Use during pregnancy and lactation (see section 4.6).

4.4 Special warnings and special precautions for use

Renal Impairment

In renal dysfunction the dose of fenofibrate may need to be reduced, depending on the rate of creatinine clearance. In this case, Lipantil Micro 67 (micronised fenofibrate) should be used, e.g. 2 capsules of Lipantil Micro 67 daily for creatinine clearance levels of <60 ml/min and 1 capsule of Lipantil Micro 67 daily for creatinine clearance levels of <20 ml/min.

Use of Lipantil Micro 67 is also to be preferred in elderly patients with renal impairment where dosage reduction may be required.

Serum Transaminases

Moderately elevated levels of serum transaminases may be found in some patients but rarely interfere with treatment. However, it is recommended that serum transaminases should be monitored every three months during the first twelve months of treatment. Treatment should be interrupted in the event of ALAT (SGPT) or ASAT (SGOT) elevations to more than 3 times the upper limit of the normal range or more than one hundred international units.

Pancreatitis

Pancreatitis has been reported in patients taking fenofibrate. This occurrence may represent a failure of efficacy in patients with severe hypertriglyceridaemia, a direct drug effect, or a secondary phenomenon mediated through biliary tract stone or sludge formation, resulting in the obstruction of the common bile duct.

Myopathy

Patients with pre-disposing factors for rhabdomyolysis, including renal impairment, hypothyroidism and high alcohol intake, may be at an increased risk of developing rhabdomyolysis.

Muscle toxicity, including very rare cases of rhabdomyolysis, has been reported with administration of fibrates and other lipid-lowering agents. The incidence of this disorder increases in cases of hypoalbuminaemia and previous renal insufficiency. Muscle toxicity should be suspected in patients presenting diffuse myalgia, myositis, muscular cramps and weakness and/or marked increases in CPK (levels exceeding 5 times the normal range). In such cases treatment with fenofibrate should be stopped.

The risk of muscle toxicity may be increased if the drug is administered with another fibrate or an HMG-CoA reductase inhibitor, especially in cases of pre-existing muscular disease. Consequently, the co-prescription of fenofibrate with a statin should be reserved to patients with severe combined dyslipidaemia and high cardiovascular risk without any history of muscular disease. This combination therapy should be used with caution and patients should be monitored closely for signs of muscle toxicity.

For hyperlipidaemic patients taking oestrogens or contraceptives containing oestrogen it should be ascertained whether the hyperlipidaemia is of primary or secondary nature (possible elevation of lipid values caused by oral oestrogen).

For patients with rare hereditary problems of galactose intolerance, the Lapp lactase deficiency or glucose-galactose malabsorption: although the amount of lactose contained in Lipantil Micro 200 mg is low, caution should be exercised in these patients (as no study has been formally conducted in this special population).

4.5 Interaction with other medicinal products and other forms of Interaction

Oral Anti-coagulants

Fenofibrate enhances oral anti-coagulant effect and may increase risk of bleeding. In patients receiving oral anti-coagulant therapy, the dose of anti-coagulant should be reduced by about one-third at the commencement of treatment and then gradually adjusted if necessary according to INR (International Normalised Ratio) monitoring.

HMG-CoA reductase inhibitorsor Other Fibrates

The risk of serious muscle toxicity is increased if fenofibrate is used concomitantly with HMG-CoA reductase inhibitors or other fibrates. Such combination therapy should be used with caution and patients monitored closely for signs of muscle toxicity (see section 4.4.).

There is currently no evidence to suggest that fenofibrate affects the pharmacokinetics of simvastatin.

Cyclosporin

Some severe cases of reversible renal function impairment have been reported during concomitant administration of fenofibrate and cyclosporin. The renal function of these patients must therefore be closely monitored and the treatment with fenofibrate stopped in the case of severe alteration of laboratory parameters.

Other

No proven clinical interactions of fenofibrate with other drugs have been reported, although in vitro interaction studies suggest displacement of phenylbutazone from plasma protein binding sites. In common with other fibrates, fenofibrate induces microsomal mixed-function oxidases involved in fatty acid metabolism in rodents and may interact with drugs metabolised by these enzymes.

4.6 Pregnancy and lactation

There are no adequate data from the use of fenofibrate in pregnant women. Animal studies have not demonstrated any teratogenic effects. Embryotoxic effects have been shown at doses in the range of maternal toxicity (see section 5.3). The potential risk for humans is unknown.

There are no data on the excretion of fenofibrate and/or its metabolites into breast milk. It is therefore recommended that Lipantil Micro 200 should not be administered to women who are pregnant or are breast feeding.

4.7 Effects on ability to drive and use machines

No effect noted to date.

4.8 Undesirable effects

Adverse reactions observed during Lipantil Micro 200 treatment are not very frequent (2 - 4 % of cases): they are generally minor, transient and do not interfere with treatment.

The most commonly reported adverse reactions include:

Gastrointestinal: Digestive, gastric or intestinal disorders (abdominal pain, nausea, vomiting, diarrhoea, and flatulence) moderate in severity.

Skin: Reactions such as rashes, pruritus, urticaria or photosensitivity reactions; in individual cases (even after many months of uncomplicated use) cutaneous photosensitivity may occur with erythema, vesiculation or nodulation on parts of the skin exposed to sunlight or artificial UV light (e.g. sun lamp).

Neurological disorders: Headache.

General disorders: Fatigue.

Disorders of the ear: Vertigo.

Less frequently reported adverse reactions:

Liver: Moderately elevated levels of serum transaminases may be found in some patients but rarely interfere with treatment (see also section 4.4). Episodes of hepatitis have been reported very rarely. When symptoms (e.g. jaundice, pruritus) indicative of hepatitis occur, laboratory tests are to be conducted for verification and fenofibrate discontinued, if applicable (see Special Warnings). Development of gallstones has been reported.

Muscle: As with other lipid lowering agents, cases of muscle toxicity (diffuse myalgia, myositis, muscular cramps and weakness) and very rare cases of rhabdomyolysis have been reported. These effects are usually reversible when the drug is withdrawn (see Special Warnings).

In rare cases, the following effects are reported: Sexual asthenia and alopecia. Increases in serum creatinine and urea, which are generally slight, and also a slight decrease in haemoglobin and leukocytes may be observed.

Very rare cases of interstitial pneumopathies have been reported.

4.9 Overdose

No case of overdosage has been reported. No specific antidote is known. If overdose is suspected, treat symptomatically and institute appropriate supportive measures as required. Fenofibrate cannot be eliminated by haemodialysis.

5. PHARMACOLOGICAL PROPERTIES

5.1 Pharmacodynamic properties

Serum Lipid Reducing Agents/Cholesterol and Triglyceride Reducers/Fibrates. ATC code:C10 AB 05.

Lipantil Micro 200 is a formulation containing 200mg of micronised fenofibrate; the administration of this product results in effective plasma concentrations identical to those obtained with 3 capsules of Lipantil Micro 67 containing 67mg of micronised fenofibrate.

The lipid-lowering properties of fenofibrate seen in clinical practice have been explained in vivo in transgenic mice and in human hepatocyte cultures by activation of Peroxisome Proliferator Activated Receptor type α (PPARα). Through this mechanism, fenofibrate increases lipolysis and elimination of triglyceride rich particles from plasma by activating lipoprotein lipase and reducing production of Apoprotein C-III. Activation of PPARα also induces an increase in the synthesis of Apoproteins A-I, A-II and of HDL cholesterol.

Epidemiological studies have demonstrated a positive correlation between abnormally increased serum lipid levels and an increased risk of coronary heart disease. The control of such dyslipidaemia forms the rationale for treatment with Lipantil Micro 200. However the possible beneficial and adverse long term consequences of drugs used in the management of dyslipidaemia are still the subject of scientific discussion. Therefore the presumptive beneficial effect of Lipantil Micro 200 on cardiovascular morbidity and mortality is as yet unproven.

Studies with fenofibrate on lipoprotein fractions show decreases in levels of LDL and VLDL cholesterol. HDL cholesterol levels are frequently increased. LDL and VLDL triglycerides are reduced. The overall effect is a decrease in the ratio of low and very low density lipoproteins to high density lipoproteins, which epidemiological studies have correlated with a decrease in atherogenic risk. Apolipoprotein-A and apolipoprotein-B levels are altered in parallel with HDL and LDL and VLDL levels respectively.

Regression of xanthomata has been observed during fenofibrate therapy.

Plasma uric acid levels are increased in approximately 20% of hyperlipidaemic patients, particularly in those with type IV disease. Lipantil Micro 200 has a uricosuric effect and is therefore of additional benefit in such patients.

Patients with raised levels of fibrinogen and Lp(a) have shown significant reductions in these measurements during clinical trials with fenofibrate.

5.2 Pharmacokinetic properties

Absorption

The unchanged compound is not recovered in the plasma. Fenofibric acid is the major plasma metabolite. Peak plasma concentration occurs after a mean period of 5 hours following dosing.

Mean plasma concentration is 15μg/ml for a daily dose of 200mg of micronised fenofibrate, equivalent to 3 capsules of Lipantil Micro 67.

Steady state levels are observed throughout continuous treatments.

Fenofibric acid is highly bound to plasma albumin; it can displace antivitamin K compounds from protein binding sites and may potentiate their anti-coagulant effect.

The plasma half-life of elimination of fenofibric acid is approximately 20 hours.

Metabolism and excretion

The product is mainly excreted in the urine; 70% in 24 hours and 88% in 6 days, at which time the total excretion in urine and faeces reaches 93%. Fenofibrate is mainly excreted as fenofibric acid and its derived glucuroconjugate.

Kinetic studies after administration of repeated doses show the absence of accumulation of the product.

Fenofibric acid is not eliminated during haemodialysis.

5.3 Preclinical safety data

Chronic toxicity studies have yielded no relevant information about specific toxicity of fenofibrate.

Studies on mutagenicity of fenofibrate have been negative.

In rats and mice, liver tumours have been found at high dosages, which are attributable to peroxisome proliferation. These changes are specific to small rodents and have not been observed in other animal species. This is of no relevance to therapeutic use in man.

Studies in mice, rats and rabbits did not reveal any teratogenic effect. Embryotoxic effects were observed at doses in the range of maternal toxicity. Prolongation of the gestation period and difficulties during delivery were observed at high doses. No sign of any effect on fertility has been detected.

6. PHARMACEUTICAL PARTICULARS

6.1 List of excipients

Excipients: lactose monohydrate, pregelatinised starch, sodium laurilsulfate, crospovidone and magnesium stearate.

Composition of the capsule shell: gelatin, titanium dioxide (E171), ferrous oxide (E172) and erythrosine (E127).

6.2 Incompatibilities

No effect noted to date.

6.3 Shelf life

3 years.

6.4 Special precautions for storage

Store in the original package. Do not store above 30°C.

6.5 Nature and contents of container

Pack of 10,28,30 capsules in blisters (PVC/Aluminium).

*Not all pack sizes may be marketed.

6.6 Instructions for use and handling

-

7. MARKETING AUTHORISATION HOLDER

Fournier Pharmaceuticals Ltd

19-20 Progress Business Centre

Whittle Parkway

Slough SL1 6DQ, Berkshire, UK

8. MARKETING AUTHORISATION NUMBER(S)

PL 12509/0001

9. DATE OF FIRST AUTHORISATION/RENEWAL OF THE AUTHORISATION

November 1993/December 2003

10. DATE OF REVISION OF THE TEXT

December 2004

11. LEGAL CATEGORY

POM

Lipantil Micro 267

(Fournier Pharmaceuticals Limited)

1. NAME OF THE MEDICINAL PRODUCT

Lipantil® Micro 267 mg, capsules.

2. QUALITATIVE AND QUANTITATIVE COMPOSITION

Each capsule contains 267 mg fenofibrate.

For excipients, see 6.1

3. PHARMACEUTICAL FORM

Orange/ivory, hard gelatin capsule.

4. CLINICAL PARTICULARS

4.1 Therapeutic indications

Lipantil Micro 267 reduces elevated serum cholesterol and triglycerides and is of benefit in the treatment of severe dyslipidaemia in patients in whom dietary measures alone have failed to produce an adequate response. Lipantil Micro 267 is indicated in appropriate cases of dyslipidaemia (Fredrickson classification types IIa, IIb, III, IV and V).

Type	Major lipid elevated	Lipoproteins elevated
IIa	Cholesterol	LDL
IIb	Cholesterol, triglycerides	LDL, VLDL
III (rare)	Cholesterol, triglycerides	IDL and chylomicron remnants
IV	Triglyceride	VLDL
V (rare)	Triglyceride	Chylomicrons, VLDL

Lipantil Micro 267 should only be used in patients in whom a full investigation has been performed to define their abnormality. Other risk factors, such as hypertension and smoking, may also require management.

4.2 Posology and method of administration

Adults

The initial recommended dose is one capsule of Lipantil Micro 200 taken daily with food. However, in patients with severe dyslipidaemia, an increased dose of 267mg (Lipantil Micro 267), is recommended. Lipantil Micro 267 should always be taken with food, because it is less well absorbed from an empty stomach. Dietary measures instituted before therapy should be continued.

Children

This dosage is not recommended in children.

Elderly

In elderly patients without renal impairment, the normal adult dose is recommended.

Renal impairment

In renal dysfunction, the dosage may need to be reduced depending on the rate of creatinine clearance, for example:

Creatinine clearance (ml/min)	Dosage
< 60	One Lipantil Micro 140 mg capsule
< 20	One Lipantil Micro 67 mg capsule

4.3 Contraindications

Lipantil Micro 267 is contra-indicated in children, in patients with severe liver or renal dysfunction, gallbladder disease, biliary cirrhosis and in patients hypersensitive to fenofibrate or any component of this medication, known photoallergy or phototoxic reaction during treatment with fibrates or ketoprofen.

Use during pregnancy and lactation (see section 4.6).

4.4 Special warnings and special precautions for use

In renal impairment

In renal dysfunction the dose of fenofibrate may need to be reduced, depending on the rate of creatinine clearance, (see section 4.2). Dose reduction should be considered in elderly patients with impaired renal function.

Transaminases

Moderately elevated levels of serum transaminases may be found in some patients but rarely interfere with treatment. However, it is recommended that serum transaminases should be monitored every three months during the first twelve months of treatment. Treatment should be interrupted in the event of ALAT (SGPT) or ASAT (SGOT) elevations to more than 3 times the upper limit of the normal range or more than one hundred international units.

Pancreatitis

Pancreatitis has been reported in patients taking fenofibrate. This occurrence may represent a failure of efficacy in patients with severe hypertriglyceridaemia, a direct drug effect, or a secondary phenomenon mediated through biliary tract stone or sludge formation, resulting in the obstruction of the common bile duct.

Myopathy

Patients with pre-disposing factors for rhabdomyolysis, including renal impairment, hypothyroidism and high alcohol intake, may be at an increased risk of developing rhabdomyolysis.

Muscle toxicity, including very rare cases of rhabdomyolysis, has been reported with administration of fibrates and other lipid-lowering agents. The incidence of this disorder increases in cases of hypoalbuminaemia and previous renal insufficiency. Muscle toxicity should be suspected in patients presenting diffuse myalgia, myositis, muscular cramps and weakness and/or marked increases in CPK (levels exceeding 5 times the normal range). In such cases treatment with fenofibrate should be stopped.

The risk of muscle toxicity may be increased if the drug is administered with another fibrate or an HMG-CoA reductase inhibitor, especially in cases of pre-existing muscular disease. Consequently, the co-prescription of fenofibrate with a statin should be reserved to patients with severe combined dyslipidaemia and high cardiovascular risk without any history of muscular disease. This combination therapy should be used with caution and patients should be monitored closely for signs of muscle toxicity.

For hyperlipidaemic patients taking oestrogens or contraceptives containing oestrogen it should be ascertained whether the hyperlipidaemia is of primary or secondary nature (possible elevation of lipid values caused by oral oestrogen).

For patients with rare hereditary problems of galactose intolerance, the Lapp lactase deficiency or glucose-galactose malabsorption: although the amount of lactose contained in Lipantil Micro 267 mg is low, caution should be exercised in these patients (as no study has been formally conducted in this special population).

4.5 Interaction with other medicinal products and other forms of Interaction

Oral anti-coagulants

Fenofibrate enhances oral anti-coagulant effect and may increase risk of bleeding. In patients receiving oral anticoagulant therapy, the dose of anti-coagulant should be reduced by about one-third at the commencement of treatment and then gradually adjusted if necessaryaccording to INR (International Normalised Ratio) monitoring.

HMG-CoA reductase inhibitors or Other Fibrates

The risk of serious muscle toxicity is increased if fenofibrate is used concomitantly with HMG-CoA reductase inhibitors or other fibrates. Such combination therapy should be used with caution and patients monitored closely for signs of muscle toxicity (see section 4.4).

There is currently no evidence to suggest that fenofibrate affects the pharmacokinetics of simvastatin.

Cyclosporin

Some severe cases of reversible renal function impairment have been reported during concomitant administration of fenofibrate and cyclosporin. The renal function of these patients must therefore be closely monitored and the treatment with fenofibrate stopped in the case of severe alteration of laboratory parameters.

Other

No proven clinical interactions of fenofibrate with other drugs have been reported, although in vitro interaction studies suggest displacement of phenylbutazone from plasma protein binding sites. In common with other fibrates, fenofibrate induces microsomal mixed-function oxidases involved in fatty acid metabolism in rodents and may interact with drugs metabolised by these enzymes.

4.6 Pregnancy and lactation

There are no adequate data from the use of fenofibrate in pregnant women. Animal studies have not demonstrated any teratogenic effects. Embryotoxic effects have been shown at doses in the range of maternal toxicity (see section 5.3). The potential risk for humans is unknown.

There are no data on the excretion of fenofibrate and/or its metabolites into breast milk. It is therefore recommended that Lipantil Micro 267 should not be administered to women who are pregnant or are breast feeding.

4.7 Effects on ability to drive and use machines

No effect noted to date.

4.8 Undesirable effects

Fenofibrate is generally well tolerated. Adverse reactions observed during fenofibrate treatment are not very frequent; they are generally minor, transient and do not interfere with treatment.

The most commonly reported adverse reactions include:

Gastrointestinal: Digestive, gastric or intestinal disorders (abdominal pain, nausea, vomiting, diarrhoea, and flatulence) moderate in severity.

Skin: Reactions such as rashes, pruritus, urticaria or photosensitivity reactions; in individual cases (even after many months of uncomplicated use) cutaneous photosensitivity may occur with erythema, vesiculation or nodulation on parts of the skin exposed to sunlight or artificial UV light (e.g. sun lamp).

Neurological disorders: Headache

General disorders: Fatigue

Disorders of the ear: Vertigo

Less frequently reported adverse reactions:

Liver: Moderately elevated levels of serum transaminases may be found in some patients but rarely interfere with treatment (see also section 4.4). Episodes of hepatitis have been reported very rarely. When symptoms (e.g. jaundice, pruritus) indicative of hepatitis occur, laboratory tests are to be conducted for verification and fenofibrate discontinued, if applicable (see Special Warnings). Development of gallstones has been reported.

Muscle: As with other lipid lowering agents, cases of muscle toxicity (diffuse myalgia, myositis, muscular cramps and weakness) and very rare cases of rhabdomyolysis have been reported. These effects are usually reversible when the drug is withdrawn (see Special Warnings).

In rare cases, the following effects are reported: Sexual asthenia and alopecia. Increases in serum creatinine and urea, which are generally slight, and also a slight decrease in haemoglobin and leukocytes may be observed.

Very rare cases of interstitial pneumopathies have been reported.

4.9 Overdose

No case of overdosage has been reported. No specific antidote is known. If overdose is suspected, treat symptomatically and institute appropriate supportive measures as required. Fenofibrate cannot be eliminated by haemodialysis.

5. PHARMACOLOGICAL PROPERTIES

5.1 Pharmacodynamic properties

Serum Lipid Reducing Agents/Cholesterol and Triglyceride Reducers/Fibrates. ATC code:C10 AB 05

Lipantil Micro 267 is a formulation containing 267 mg of micronised fenofibrate.

The lipid lowering properties of fenofibrate seen in clinical practice have been explained in vivo in transgenic mice and in human hepatocyte cultures by activation of Peroxisome Proliferator Activated Receptor type α (PPARα). Through this mechanism, fenofibrate increases lipolysis and elimination of triglyceride-rich particles from plasma by activating lipoprotein lipase and reducing production of Apoprotein C-III. Activation of PPARα also induces an increase in the synthesis of Apoproteins A-I, A-II and of HDL cholesterol.

Epidemiological studies have demonstrated a positive correlation between increased serum lipid levels and an increased risk of coronary heart disease. The control of such dyslipidaemias forms the rationale for treatment with fenofibrate. However, the possible beneficial and adverse long-term consequences of drugs used in the management of dyslipidaemias are still the subject of scientific discussion. Therefore the presumptive beneficial effect of Lipantil Micro 267 on cardiovascular morbidity and mortality is as yet unproven.

Studies with fenofibrate consistently show decreases in levels of LDL-cholesterol. HDL-cholesterol levels are frequently increased. Triglyceride levels are also reduced. This results in a decrease in the ratio of low and very low density lipoproteins to high density lipoproteins, which has been correlated with a decrease in atherogenic risk in epidemiological studies. Apolipoprotein-A and apolipoprotein-B levels are altered in parallel with HDL and LDL and VLDL levels respectively.

Regression of xanthomata has been observed during fenofibrate therapy.

Plasma uric acid levels are increased in approximately 20% of hyperlipidaemic patients, particularly in those with type IV phenotype. Lipantil Micro 267 has a uricosuric effect and is therefore of additional benefit in such patients.

Patients with raised levels of fibrinogen and Lp(a) have shown significant reductions in these measurements during clinical trials with fenofibrate.

5.2 Pharmacokinetic properties

Absorption

The unchanged compound is not recovered in the plasma. Fenofibric acid is the major plasma metabolite. Peak plasma concentration occurs after a mean period of 5 hours following dosing.

Mean plasma concentration is 15 μg/ml for a daily dosage of 200 mg of micronised fenofibrate.

Steady state levels are observed throughout continuous treatments.

Fenofibric acid is highly bound to plasma albumin: it can displace antivitamin K compounds from the protein binding sites and potentiate their anti-coagulant effect.

Plasma half-life

The plasma half-life of elimination of fenofibric acid is approximately 20 hours.

Metabolism and excretion

The product is mainly excreted in the urine: 70% in 24 hours and 88% in 6 days, at which time total excretion in urine and faeces reaches 93%. Fenofibrate is mainly excreted as fenofibric acid and its derived glucuroconjugate.

Kinetic studies after administration of repeated doses show the absence of accumulation of the product.

Fenofibric acid is not eliminated during haemodialysis.

5.3 Preclinical safety data

Chronic toxicity studies have yielded no relevant information about specific toxicity of fenofibrate.

Studies on mutagenicity of fenofibrate have been negative.

In rats and mice, liver tumours have been found at high dosages, which are attributable to peroxisome proliferation. These changes are specific to small rodents and have not been observed in other animal species. This is of no relevance to therapeutic use in man.

Studies in mice, rats and rabbits did not reveal any teratogenic effect. Embryotoxic effects were observed at doses in the range of maternal toxicity. Prolongation of the gestation period and difficulties during delivery were observed at high doses. No sign of any effect on fertility has been detected.

6. PHARMACEUTICAL PARTICULARS

6.1 List of excipients

Excipients: lactose monohydrate, magnesium stearate, pregelatinised starch, sodium laurilsulfate, crospovidone.

Composition of the capsule shell: gelatin, titanium dioxide (E 171), yellow and red ferrous oxide (E 172).

6.2 Incompatibilities

No effect noted to date.

6.3 Shelf life

3 years.

6.4 Special precautions for storage

Store in the original package. Do not store above 30°C.

6.5 Nature and contents of container

Pack of 28,30 capsules in blisters (PVC/Aluminium).

*Not all pack sizes may be marketed.

6.6 Instructions for use and handling

Capsules should be swallowed whole with water.

7. MARKETING AUTHORISATION HOLDER

Fournier Pharmaceuticals Ltd

19-20 Progress Business Centre

Whittle Parkway

Slough SL1 6DQ, Berkshire, UK

8. MARKETING AUTHORISATION NUMBER(S)

PL 12509/0014

9. DATE OF FIRST AUTHORISATION/RENEWAL OF THE AUTHORISATION

3 February 1999/February 2004

10. DATE OF REVISION OF THE TEXT

December 2004

11. LEGAL CATEGORY

POM

Lipantil Micro 67

(Fournier Pharmaceuticals Limited)

1. NAME OF THE MEDICINAL PRODUCT

Lipantil® Micro 67 mg, capsules.

2. QUALITATIVE AND QUANTITATIVE COMPOSITION

Each capsule contains 67 mg fenofibrate.

For excipients, see 6.1

3. PHARMACEUTICAL FORM

Yellow, hard gelatin capsule.

4. CLINICAL PARTICULARS

4.1 Therapeutic indications

Lipantil Micro 67 reduces elevated serum cholesterol and triglycerides and is of benefit in the treatment of severe dyslipidaemia in patients in whom dietary measures alone have failed to produce an adequate response. Lipantil Micro 67 is indicated in appropriate cases of dyslipidaemia (Fredrickson classification types IIa, IIb, III, IV and V).

Type	Major lipid elevated	Lipoproteins elevated
IIa	Cholesterol	LDL
IIb	Cholesterol, triglycerides	LDL, VLDL
III (rare)	Cholesterol, triglycerides	LDL and chylomicron remnants
IV	Triglycerides	VLDL
V (rare)	Triglycerides	Chylomicrons, VLDL

Lipantil Micro 67 should only be used in patients in whom a full investigation has been performed to define their abnormality. Other risk factors, such as hypertension and smoking, may also require management.

4.2 Posology and method of administration

Adults

In adults, the recommended initial dose is 3 capsules taken daily in divided doses. Lipantil Micro 67 should always be taken with food, because it is less well absorbed from an empty stomach. Dietary measures instituted before therapy should be continued.

The response to therapy should be monitored by determination of serum lipid values and the dosage may be altered within the range 2-4 capsules of Lipantil Micro 67 daily.

Children

In children, the recommended dose is one capsule (67mg) micronised fenofibrate / day / 20kg body weight.

Elderly

In elderly patients without renal impairment, the normal adult dose is recommended.

Renal Impairment

In renal dysfunction, the dosage may need to be reduced depending on the rate of creatinine clearance, for example:

Creatinine clearance (ml/min)	Dosage
<60	Two 67mg capsules
<20	One 67mg capsule

4.3 Contraindications

Lipantil Micro 67 is contra-indicated in patients with severe liver or renal dysfunction, gallbladder disease, biliary cirrhosis and in patients hypersensitive to fenofibrate or any component of this medication, known photoallergy or phototoxic reaction during treatment with fibrates or ketoprofen.

Use during pregnancy and lactation (see section 4.6).

See also section 4.6 (Pregnancy and lactation)

4.4 Special warnings and special precautions for use

In renal impairment

In renal dysfunction the dose of fenofibrate may need to be reduced, depending on the rate of creatinine clearance, (see section 4.2). Dose reduction should be considered in elderly patients with impaired renal function.

Transaminases

Moderately elevated levels of serum transaminases may be found in some patients but rarely interfere with treatment. However, it is recommended that serum transaminases should be monitored every three months during the first twelve months of treatment. Treatment should be interrupted in the event of ALAT (SGPT) or ASAT (SGOT) elevations to more than 3 times the upper limit of the normal range or more than one hundred international units.

Pancreatitis

Pancreatitis has been reported in patients taking fenofibrate. This occurrence may represent a failure of efficacy in patients with severe hypertriglyceridaemia, a direct drug effect, or a secondary phenomenon mediated through biliary tract stone or sludge formation, resulting in the obstruction of the common bile duct.

Myopathy

Patients with pre-disposing factors for rhabdomyolysis, including renal impairment, hypothyroidism and high alcohol intake, may be at an increased risk of developing rhabdomyolysis.

Muscle toxicity, including very rare cases of rhabdomyolysis, has been reported with administration of fibrates and other lipid-lowering agents. The incidence of this disorder increases in cases of hypoalbuminaemia and previous renal insufficiency. Muscle toxicity should be suspected in patients presenting diffuse myalgia, myositis, muscular cramps and weakness and/or marked increases in CPK (levels exceeding 5 times the normal range). In such cases treatment with fenofibrate should be stopped.

The risk of muscle toxicity may be increased if the drug is administered with another fibrate or an HMG-CoA reductase inhibitor, especially in cases of pre-existing muscular disease. Consequently, the co-prescription of fenofibrate with a statin should be reserved to patients with severe combined dyslipidaemia and high cardiovascular risk without any history of muscular disease. This combination therapy should be used with caution and patients should be monitored closely for signs of muscle toxicity.

For hyperlipidaemic patients taking oestrogens or contraceptives containing oestrogen it should be ascertained whether the hyperlipidaemia is of primary or secondary nature (possible elevation of lipid values caused by oral oestrogen).

For patients with rare hereditary problems of galactose intolerance, the Lapp lactase deficiency or glucose-galactose malabsorption: although the amount of lactose contained in Lipantil Micro 67 mg is low, caution should be exercised in these patients (as no study has been formally conducted in this special population).

In children

Only an hereditary disease (familial hyperlipidaemia) justifies early treatment, and the precise nature of the hyperlipidaemia must be determined by genetic and laboratory investigations. It is recommended to begin treatment with controlled dietary restrictions for a period of at least 3 months. Proceeding to medicinal treatment should only be considered after specialist advice and only in severe forms with clinical signs of atherosclerosis and/or xanthomata and/or in cases where patients suffer from atherosclerotic cardiovascular disease before the age of 40.

4.5 Interaction with other medicinal products and other forms of Interaction

Oral anti-coagulants

Fenofibrate enhances oral anti-coagulant effect and may increase risk of bleeding. In patients receiving oralanti-coagulant therapy, the dose of anti-coagulant should be reduced by about one-third at the commencement of treatment and then gradually adjusted if necessary according to INR (International Normalised Ratio) monitoring.

HMG-CoA reductase inhibitors or Other Fibrates

The risk of serious muscle toxicity is increased if fenofibrate is used concomitantly with HMG-CoA reductase inhibitors or other fibrates. Such combination therapy should be used with caution and patients monitored closely for signs of muscle toxicity (see Section 4.4).

There is currently no evidence to suggest that fenofibrate affects the pharmacokinetics of simvastatin.

Cyclosporin

Some severe cases of reversible renal function impairment have been reported during concomitant administration of fenofibrate and cyclosporin. The renal function of these patients must therefore be closely monitored and the treatment with fenofibrate stopped in the case of severe alteration of laboratory parameters.

Other

No proven clinical interactions of fenofibrate with other drugs have been reported, although in vitro interaction studies suggest displacement of phenylbutazone from plasma protein binding sites. In common with other fibrates, fenofibrate induces microsomal mixed-function oxidases involved in fatty acid metabolism in rodents and may interact with drugs metabolised by these enzymes.

4.6 Pregnancy and lactation

There are no adequate data from the use of fenofibrate in pregnant women. Animal studies have not demonstrated any teratogenic effects. Embryotoxic effects have been shown at doses in the range of maternal toxicity (see section 5.3). The potential risk for humans is unknown.

There are no data on the excretion of fenofibrate and/or its metabolites into breast milk.

It is therefore recommended that Lipantil Micro 67 should not be administered to women who are pregnant or are breast feeding.

4.7 Effects on ability to drive and use machines

No effect noted to date.

4.8 Undesirable effects

Fenofibrate is generally well tolerated. Adverse reactions observed during fenofibrate treatment are not very frequent; they are generally minor, transient and do not interfere with treatment.

The most commonly reported adverse reactions include:

Gastrointestinal: Digestive, gastric or intestinal disorders (abdominal pain, nausea, vomiting, diarrhoea, and flatulence) moderate in severity.

Skin: Reactions such as rashes, pruritus, urticaria or photosensitivity reactions; in individual cases (even after many months of uncomplicated use) cutaneous photosensitivity may occur with erythema, vesiculation or nodulation on parts of the skin exposed to sunlight or artificial UV light (e.g. sun lamp).

Neurological disorders: Headache.

General disorders: Fatigue.

Disorders of the ear: Vertigo.

Less frequently reported adverse reactions:

Liver:Moderately elevated levels of serum transaminases may be found in some patients but rarely interfere with treatment (see also section 4.4). Episodes of hepatitis have been reported very rarely. When symptoms (e.g. jaundice, pruritus) indicative of hepatitis occur, laboratory tests are to be conducted for verification and fenofibrate discontinued, if applicable (see Special Warnings). Development of gallstones has been reported.

Muscle: As with other lipid lowering agents, cases of muscle toxicity (diffuse myalgia, myositis, muscular cramps and weakness) and very rare cases of rhabdomyolysis have been reported. These effects are usually reversible when the drug is withdrawn (see Special Warnings).

In rare cases, the following effects are reported: sexual asthenia and alopecia. Increases in serum creatinine and urea, which are generally slight, and also a slight decrease in haemoglobin and leukocytes may be observed.

Very rare cases of interstitial pneumopathies have been reported.

4.9 Overdose

No case of overdosage has been reported. No specific antidote is known. If overdose is suspected, treat symptomatically and institute appropriate supportive measures as required. Fenofibrate cannot be eliminated by haemodialysis.

5. PHARMACOLOGICAL PROPERTIES

5.1 Pharmacodynamic properties

Serum Lipid Reducing Agents/Cholesterol and Triglyceride Reducers/Fibrates. ATC code:C10 AB 05.

Lipantil Micro 67 is a formulation containing 67mg of micronised fenofibrate.

The lipid-lowering properties of fenofibrate seen in clinical practice have been explained in vivo in transgenic mice and in human hepatocyte cultures by activation of Peroxisome Proliferator Activated Receptor type α (PPARα). Through this mechanism, fenofibrate increases lipolysis and elimination of triglyceride rich particles from plasma by activating lipoprotein lipase and reducing production of Apoprotein C-III. Activation of PPARα also induces an increase in the synthesis of Apoproteins A-I, A-II and of HDL cholesterol.

Epidemiological studies have demonstrated a positive correlation between increased serum lipid levels and an increased risk of coronary heart disease. The control of such dyslipidaemias forms the rationale for treatment with fenofibrate. However, the possible beneficial and adverse long-term consequences of drugs used in the hyperlipidaemias are still the subject of scientific discussion. Therefore the presumptive beneficial effect of Lipantil Micro 67 on cardiovascular morbidity and mortality is as yet unproven.

Studies with fenofibrate consistently show decreases in levels of LDL-cholesterol. HDL-cholesterol levels are frequently increased. Triglyceride levels are also reduced. This results in a decrease in the ratio of low and very low density lipoproteins to high density lipoproteins, which has been correlated with a decrease in atherogenic risk in epidemiological studies. Apolipoprotein-A and apolipoprotein-B levels are altered in parallel with HDL and LDL and VLDL levels respectively.

Regression of xanthomata has been observed during fenofibrate therapy.

Plasma uric acid levels are increased in approximately 20% of hyperlipidaemic patients, particularly in those with type IV phenotype. Lipantil Micro 67 has a uricosuric effect and is therefore of additional benefit in such patients.

Patients with raised levels of fibrinogen and Lp(a) have shown significant reductions in these measurements during clinical trials with fenofibrate.

5.2 Pharmacokinetic properties

Absorption

The unchanged compound is not recovered in the plasma. Fenofibric acid is the major plasma metabolite. Peak plasma concentration occurs after a mean period of 5 hours following dosing.

Mean plasma concentration is 15μg/ml for a daily dosage of 200mg of micronised fenofibrate, equivalent to 3 capsules of Lipantil Micro 67.

Steady state levels are observed throughout continuous treatments.

Fenofibric acid is highly bound to plasma albumin: it can displace antivitamin K compounds from the protein binding sites and potentiate their anti-coagulant effect.

Plasma half-life

The plasma half-life of elimination of fenofibric acid is approximately 20 hours.

Metabolism and excretion

The product is mainly excreted in the urine: 70% in 24 hours and 88% in 6 days, at which time total excretion in urine and faeces reaches 93%. Fenofibrate is mainly excreted as fenofibric acid and its derived glucuroconjugate.

Kinetic studies after administration of repeated doses show the absence of accumulation of the product.

Fenofibric acid is not eliminated during haemodialysis.

5.3 Preclinical safety data

Chronic toxicity studies have yielded no relevant information about specific toxicity of fenofibrate. Studies on mutagenicity of fenofibrate have been negative. In rats and mice, liver tumours have been found at high dosages, which are attributable to peroxisome proliferation. These changes are specific to small rodents and have not been observed in other animal species. This is of no relevance to therapeutic use in man. Studies in mice, rats and rabbits did not reveal any teratogenic effect. Embryotoxic effects were observed at doses in the range of maternal toxicity. Prolongation of the gestation period and difficulties during delivery were observed at high doses. No sign of any effect on fertility has been detected.

6. PHARMACEUTICAL PARTICULARS

6.1 List of excipients

Excipients: lactose monohydrate, magnesium stearate, pregelatinised starch, sodium laurilsulfate, crospovidone.

Composition of the capsule shell: gelatin, titanium dioxide (E171), quinoline yellow (E104) and erythrosine (E127).

6.2 Incompatibilities

No effect noted to date.

6.3 Shelf life

3 years.

6.4 Special precautions for storage

Store in the original package. Do not store above 30°C.

6.5 Nature and contents of container

Pack of 28,56,84,90 capsules in blisters (PVC/Aluminium).

*Not all pack sizes may be marketed.

6.6 Instructions for use and handling

Capsules should be swallowed whole with water.

Administrative Data

7. MARKETING AUTHORISATION HOLDER

Fournier Pharmaceuticals Ltd
19-20 Progress Business Centre
Whittle Parkway
Slough SL1 6DQ, Berkshire, UK

8. MARKETING AUTHORISATION NUMBER(S)

PL 12509/0004

9. DATE OF FIRST AUTHORISATION/RENEWAL OF THE AUTHORISATION

11 September 1997/10th September 2002

10. DATE OF REVISION OF THE TEXT

December 2004

11. LEGAL CATEGORY

POM

Lipitor 10 mg, 20mg, 40mg, 80 mg Tablets.

(Pfizer Limited)

1. NAME OF THE MEDICINAL PRODUCT

Lipitor® 10 mg, 20mg, 40mg, 80 mg Tablets.

2. QUALITATIVE AND QUANTITATIVE COMPOSITION

Each tablet contains 10 mg, 20mg, 40mg, or 80mg atorvastatin as atorvastatin calcium trihydrate.

For excipients see section 6.1.

3. PHARMACEUTICAL FORM

Film-coated tablets.

White, elliptical, film-coated tablets debossed '10' on one side and 'PD 155' on the other side.

White, elliptical, film-coated tablets debossed '20' on one side and 'PD 156' on the other side.

White, elliptical, film-coated tablets debossed '40' on one side and 'PD 157' on the other side.

White, elliptical, film-coated tablets debossed '80' on one side and 'PD 158' on the other side.

4. CLINICAL PARTICULARS

4.1 Therapeutic indications

Lipitor is indicated as an adjunct to diet for reduction of elevated total cholesterol, LDL-cholesterol, apolipoprotein B, and triglycerides in adults and children aged 10 years and older with primary hypercholesterolaemia, heterozygous familial hypercholesterolaemia or combined (mixed) hyperlipidaemia when response to diet and other nonpharmacological measures is inadequate.

Lipitor also raises HDL-cholesterol and lowers the LDL/HDL and total cholesterol/HDL ratios.

Lipitor is also indicated as an adjunct to diet and other non-dietary measures in reducing elevated total cholesterol, LDL-cholesterol, and apolipoprotein B in patients with homozygous familial hypercholesterolaemia when response to these measures is inadequate.

4.2 Posology and method of administration

The patient should be placed on a standard cholesterol-lowering diet before receiving Lipitor and should continue on this diet during treatment with Lipitor. The usual starting dose is 10 mg once a day. Doses should be individualised according to baseline LDL-C levels, the goal of therapy, and patient response. Adjustment of dosage should be made at intervals of 4 weeks or more. The maximum dose is 80 mg once a day. Doses above 20mg/day have not been investigated in patients aged <18 years. Doses may be given at any time of day with or without food.

Primary Hypercholesterolaemia and Combined (Mixed) Hyperlipidaemia

Adults:

The majority of patients are controlled with 10 mg Lipitor once a day. A therapeutic response is evident within 2 weeks, and the maximum response is usually achieved within 4 weeks. The response is maintained during chronic therapy.

Current consensus guidelines should be consulted to establish treatment goals for individual patients.

Children aged 10-17 years:

Doses above 20mg/day have not been investigated.

Heterozygous Familial Hypercholesterolaemia

Adults:

Patients should be started with Lipitor 10 mg daily. Doses should be individualised and adjusted every 4 weeks to 40 mg daily. Thereafter, either the dose may be increased to a maximum of 80 mg daily or a bile acid sequestrant (eg, colestipol) may be combined with 40 mg Lipitor.

Children aged 10-17 years:

Doses above 20mg/day and combination therapies have not been investigated.

Homozygous Familial Hypercholesterolaemia

Adults: In a compassionate-use study of patients with homozygous familial hypercholesterolaemia, most patients responded to a dose of 80 mg of Lipitor (see Section 5.1 Pharmacodynamics).

Children: Treatment experience in a paediatric population with doses of Lipitor up to 80 mg/day is limited.

Dosage in Patients With Renal Insufficiency

Renal disease has no influence on the plasma concentrations nor lipid effects of Lipitor; thus, no adjustment of dose is required.

Dosage in Patients With Hepatic Dysfunction

In patients with moderate to severe hepatic dysfunction, the therapeutic response to Lipitor is unaffected but exposure to the drug is greatly increased. Cmax increases by approximately 16 fold and AUC (0-24) by approximately 11 fold. Therefore, caution should be exercised in patients who consume substantial quantities of alcohol and/or have a history of liver disease.

Geriatric Use

Adequate treatment experience in adults age 70 or older with doses of Lipitor up to 80 mg/day has been obtained. Efficacy and safety in older patients using recommended doses is similar to that seen in the general population.

4.3 Contraindications

Lipitor is contraindicated in patients with hypersensitivity to any component of this medication, active liver disease or unexplained persistent elevations of serum transaminases exceeding 3 times the upper limit of normal, during pregnancy, while breast-feeding, and in women of child-bearing potential not using appropriate contraceptive measures.

4.4 Special warnings and special precautions for use

Liver Effects

Liver function tests should be performed before the initiation of treatment and periodically thereafter. Patients who develop any signs or symptoms suggestive of liver injury should have liver function tests performed. Patients who develop increased transaminase levels should be monitored until the abnormality(ies) resolve. Should an increase in ALT or AST of greater than 3 times the upper limit of normal persist, reduction of dose or withdrawal of Lipitor is recommended.

Lipitor should be used with caution in patients who consume substantial quantities of alcohol and/or have a history of liver disease. Muscle effects

Treatment with HMG-CoA reductase inhibitors (statins) has been associated with the onset of myalgia, myopathy, and very rarely rhabdomyolysis. Myopathy must be considered in any patient under statin therapy presenting with unexplained muscle symptoms such as pain or tenderness, muscle weakness or muscle cramps. In such cases creatine kinase (CK) levels should be measured (see below).

Creatine phosphokinase measurement

Creatine phosphokinase (CPK) should not be measured following strenuous exercise or in the presence of any plausible alternative cause of CPK increase as this makes value interpretation difficult. If CPK levels are significantly elevated at baseline >5 times ULN), levels should be remeasured within 5 to 7 days later to confirm the results.

Before treatment

As with other statins atorvastatin should be prescribed with caution in patients with pre-disposing factors for rhabdomyolysis. A creatine phosphokinase (CPK) level should be measured before starting treatment in the following situations:

– Renal impairment

– Hypothyroidism

– Personal or familial history of hereditary muscular disorders

– Previous history of muscular toxicity with a statin or fibrate

– Previous history of liver disease and/or where substantial quantities of alcohol are consumed

– In elderly (age > 70 years), the necessity of such measurement should be considered, according to the presence of other predisposing factors for rhabdomyolysis

In such situations, the risk of treatment should be considered in relation to possible benefit and clinical monitoring is recommended. If CPK levels are significantly elevated >5 times ULN) at baseline, treatment should not be started.

Whilst on treatment

– If muscular pain, weakness or cramps occur whilst a patient is receiving treatment with a statin, their CPK levels should be measured. If these levels are found to be significantly elevated > 5 times ULN), treatment should be stopped.

– If muscular symptoms are severe and cause daily discomfort, even if CPK levels are elevated to ≤ 5 times ULN, treatment discontinuation should be considered.

– If symptoms resolve and CPK levels return to normal, then re-introduction of atorvastatin or introduction of an alternative statin may be considered at the lowest dose and with close monitoring.

These CPK elevations should be considered when evaluating the possibility of myocardial infarction in the differential diagnosis of chest pain.

The risk of myopathy during treatment with Lipitor may be increased with concurrent administration of certain other drugs, such as fibrates (e.g. gemfibrozil) and co-administration should only be undertaken with caution. (See Section 4.5 Interaction with other medicaments and other forms of interaction).

As with other drugs in this class, rhabdomyolysis with acute renal failure has been reported.

Children aged 10-17 years

In patients aged <18 years efficacy and safety have not been studied for treatment periods >52 weeks' duration and effects on long-term cardiovascular outcomes are unknown.

The effects of atorvastatin in children aged <10 years and premenarchal girls have not been investigated.

Long term effects on cognitive development, growth and pubertal maturation are unknown.

4.5 Interaction with other medicinal products and other forms of Interaction

The risk of myopathy during treatment with other drugs in this class is increased with concurrent administration of cyclosporin, fibric acid derivatives, erythromycin, azole antifungals, or niacin. This increase in risk may also occur when combining these drugs with Lipitor.

Phenazone (antipyrine) is a non-specific model for evaluation of drug metabolism by the hepatic microsomal enzyme system. Administration of multiple doses of Lipitor with phenazone showed little or no detectable effect on the pharmacokinetics of phenazone in healthy subjects (no change in the clearance of phenazone but the formation clearance of 4-hydroxyphenazone increased by 20% and that of norphenazone by 8%).

More specific in vitro studies using human hepatic microsomes and cells expressing human cytochrome P450 isozymes show that atorvastatin, like other HMG-CoA reductase inhibitors, is metabolised by cytochrome P450 3A4 indicating the possibility of an interaction with drugs also metabolised by this isozyme. When combining Lipitor with other drugs which are the substrate of this isozyme (eg, immunomodulators, many antiarrhythmic agents, some calcium channel antagonists and some benzodiazepines) the possibility of a change in the plasma drug levels of either drug should be considered. In clinical studies in which Lipitor was administered with antihypertensives (including ACE inhibitors, beta-blockers, calcium channel antagonists, and diuretics) or hypoglycaemic agents no clinically significant interactions were seen.

Based on experience with other HMG-CoA reductase inhibitors caution should also be exercised when Lipitor is administered with inhibitors of cytochrome P450 3A4 (eg, certain macrolide antibiotics and azole antifungals).

Increases and decreases in plasma phenytoin levels have been reported, but the relationship with Lipitor is unknown.

Inhibitors of P-glycoprotein: Atorvastatin and atorvastatin metabolites are substrates of P-glycoprotein. Inhibitors of the P-glycoprotein (e.g. cyclosporin) can increase the bioavailability of atorvastatin and thereby increase the risk of dose-related side-effects such as myopathy.

Gemfibrozil/fibric acid derivatives: The use of fibrates alone is occasionally associated with myopathy. An increased risk of muscle related adverse event has been described when fibrates are co-administered with HMG-CoA reductase inhibitors. The risk of atorvastatin induced myopathy may therefore be increased with concomitant use of fibric acid derivatives. Pre-clinical data suggest that gemfibrozil may also interact with atorvastatin by inhibiting its glucuronidation. Co-administration of atorvastatin with fibrates (especially gemfibrozil) should only be undertaken with caution.

Digoxin: When multiple doses of digoxin and 10 mg Lipitor were coadministered, steady state plasma digoxin concentrations were unaffected. However, digoxin concentrations increased approximately 20% following administration of digoxin with 80 mg Lipitor daily. Patients taking digoxin should be monitored appropriately.

Macrolide antibiotics:

Erythromycin, clarithromycin: Coadministration of Lipitor and erythromycin (500 mg QID), or clarithromycin (500 mg BID), known inhibitors of cytochrome P450 3A4, were associated with higher plasma concentrations of atorvastatin.

Azithromycin: Coadministration of Lipitor (10 mg OD) and azithromycin (500 mg OD) did not alter the plasma concentrations of atorvastatin.

Oral contraceptives: Administration of Lipitor with an oral contraceptive containing norethisterone and ethinyl oestradiol produced increases in plasma concentrations of norethisterone and ethinyl oestradiol. These increased concentrations should be considered when selecting oral contraceptive doses.

Amlodipine: Atorvastatin pharmacokinetics were not altered by the coadministration of Lipitor 80 mg and amlodipine 10 mg at steady state.

Colestipol: Plasma concentrations of atorvastatin were lower (approximately 25%) when colestipol was administered with Lipitor. However, lipid effects were greater when Lipitor and colestipol were administered together than when either drug was given alone.

Antacid: Administration of Lipitor with an oral antacid suspension containing magnesium and aluminium hydroxides decreased atorvastatin plasma concentrations approximately 35%; however, LDL-C reduction was not altered.

Warfarin: Administration of Lipitor with warfarin caused a minimal decrease in prothrombin time (mean ± SE of 1.7 ± 0.4 seconds) during the first 4 days of dosing with 80 mg Lipitor. Dosing continued for 15 days and prothrombin time returned to normal by the end of Lipitor treatment. Nevertheless, patients receiving warfarin should be closely monitored when Lipitor is added to their therapy.

Cimetidine: An interaction study with cimetidine and Lipitor was conducted, and no interaction was seen.

Grapefruit juice: Contains one or more components that inhibit CYP3A4 and can increase plasma concentrations of drugs metabolised by CYP3A4. Intake of one 240 ml glass of grapefruit juice resulted in an increase in atorvastatin AUC of 37 % and a decreased AUC of 20.4 % for the active orthohydroxy metabolite. However, large quantities of grapefruit juice (over 1.2L daily for 5 days) increased AUC of atorvastatin 2.5 fold and AUC of active (atorvastatin and metabolites) HMG-CoA reductase inhibitors 1.3 fold. Concomitant intake of large quantities of grapefruit juice and atorvastatin is therefore not recommended.

Protease inhibitors: Co-administration of atorvastatin and protease inhibitors, known inhibitors of cytochrome P450 3A4, was associated with an approximately two-fold increase in plasma concentrations of atorvastatin. Consideration should be given to starting atorvastatin at a lower dose (see section 4.2) when co-administered with a protease inhibitor.

4.6 Pregnancy and lactation

Lipitor is contraindicated in pregnancy and while breastfeeding. Women of child-bearing potential should use appropriate contraceptive measures.

An interval of 1 month should be allowed from stopping Lipitor treatment to conception in the event of planning a pregnancy.

In animal studies atorvastatin had no effect on fertility and was not teratogenic, however, at maternally toxic doses foetal toxicity was observed in rats and rabbits. The development of the rat offspring was delayed and post-natal survival reduced during exposure of the dams to atorvastatin equivalent to 6 and 21 times that expected in man, respectively.

In rats, plasma concentrations of atorvastatin are similar to those in milk. It is not known whether this drug or its metabolites is excreted in human milk.

4.7 Effects on ability to drive and use machines

There is no pattern of reported adverse events suggesting that patients taking Lipitor will have any impairment of ability to drive and use hazardous machinery.

4.8 Undesirable effects

Adverse reactions have usually been mild and transient. Less than 2% of patients were discontinued from clinical trials due to side effects attributed to Lipitor.

The most frequent (1% or more) adverse effects associated with Lipitor therapy, in patients participating in controlled clinical studies were:

Psychiatric Disorders: insomnia

Nervous System Disorders: headache

Gastrointestinal Disorders: abdominal pain, dyspepsia, nausea, flatulence, constipation, diarrhoea

Musculoskeletal and Connective Tissue Disorders: myalgia

General Disorders and Administration Site Conditions: asthenia

Elevated serum ALT levels have been reported in 1.3% of patients receiving Lipitor. Clinically important >3 times upper normal limit) elevations in serum ALT levels occurred in 19 of the 2483 (0.8%) patients on Lipitor. It was dose related and was reversible in all 19 patients. In 10 cases, the increase was first observed within 12 weeks of starting the treatment. Only 1 case occurred after 36 weeks and only 1 patient had symptoms suggestive of hepatitis. Treatment was discontinued in only 9 of these 19 cases.

Elevated serum CPK levels >3 times upper normal limit) occurred in 62 of the 2452 (2.5%) patients on Lipitor compared with 3.1% with other HMG-CoA reductase inhibitors in clinical trials. Levels above 10 times the normal upper range occurred in only 11 (0.4%) Lipitor-treated patients. Only 3 (0.1%) of these 11 patients had concurrent muscle pain, tenderness, or weakness.

Additional adverse events that have been reported in atorvastatin clinical trials are categorised below according to system organ class and frequency. Frequencies are defined as: very common (≥10%), common (≥1% and <10%), uncommon (≥0.1% and <1%), rare (≥0.01% and <0.1%) and very rare (<0.01%).

Metabolism and Nutrition Disorders	anorexia	uncommon
	hypoglycaemia	very rare
	hyperglycaemia	very rare
Nervous system Disorders	dizziness	common
	paresthesia	uncommon
	peripheral neuropathy	rare
Gastrointestinal Disorders	vomiting	uncommon
	pancreatitis	rare
Hepatobiliary Disorders	hepatitis	very rare
	cholestatic jaundice	very rare
Skin and Subcutaneous Tissue Disorders	alopecia	uncommon
	pruritis	uncommon
	rash	uncommon
Musculoskeletal and Connective Tissue Disorders	muscle cramps	uncommon
	myositis	rare
	myopathy	very rare
Reproductive System and Breast Disorders	impotence	uncommon
General Disorders and Administration Site Conditions	chest pain	common
	angina	common
	angioneurotic oedema	very rare

Post Marketing Experience

Adverse events that have been reported post-marketing that are not listed above are:

Blood and Lymphatic System Disorders	thrombocytopenia	uncommon
Immune System Disorders	allergic reactions (including anaphylaxis)	common
Metabolism and Nutrition Disorders	weight gain	uncommon
Nervous System Disorders	hypoesthesia	common
	amnesia	uncommon
Ear and Labyrinth Disorders	tinnitus	uncommon
Skin and Subcutaneous Tissue Disorders	urticaria	uncommon
	bullous rashes	rare
	erythema multiforme	very rare
	Stevens-Johnson syndrome	very rare
Musculoskeletal and Connective Tissue Disorders	arthralgia	common
	back pain	common
	rhabdomyolysis (see section 4.4).	very rare
General Disorders and Administration Site Conditions	malaise	uncommon
	peripheral oedema	rare

4.9 Overdose

Specific treatment is not available for Lipitor overdosage. Should an overdose occur, the patient should be treated symptomatically and supportive measures instituted, as required. Liver function tests and serum CPK levels should be monitored. Due to extensive drug binding to plasma proteins, haemodialysis is not expected to significantly enhance atorvastatin clearance.

5. PHARMACOLOGICAL PROPERTIES

5.1 Pharmacodynamic properties

Atorvastatin is a selective, competitive inhibitor of HMG-CoA reductase, the rate-limiting enzyme responsible for the conversion of 3-hydroxy-3-methyl-glutaryl-coenzyme A to mevalonate, a precursor of sterols, including cholesterol. Triglycerides and cholesterol in the liver are incorporated into VLDL and released into the plasma for delivery to peripheral tissues. Low-density lipoprotein (LDL) is formed from VLDL and is catabolised primarily through the high affinity LDL receptor.

Atorvastatin lowers plasma cholesterol and lipoprotein levels by inhibiting HMG-CoA reductase and cholesterol synthesis in the liver and increases the number of hepatic LDL receptors on the cell surface for enhanced uptake and catabolism of LDL.

Atorvastatin reduces LDL production and the number of LDL particles. Atorvastatin produces a profound and sustained increase in LDL receptor activity coupled with a beneficial change in the quality of circulating LDL particles.

Approximately 70% of circulating inhibitory activity for HMG-CoA reductase is attributed to active metabolites (see Section 5.2 Pharmacokinetic Properties).

Atorvastatin has been shown to reduce total-C, LDL-C, apolipoprotein B, and triglycerides while producing variable increases in HDL-C in a dose-response study as shown in Table 1 below.

(see Table 1 on next page)

Atorvastatin produced a variable but small increase in apolipoprotein A1. However, there was no clear dose response effect.

Review of the current clinical database of 24 complete studies shows that atorvastatin increases HDL-cholesterol and reduces the LDL/HDL and total cholesterol/HDL ratios.

These results are consistent in patients with heterozygous familial hypercholesterolaemia, nonfamilial forms of hypercholesterolaemia, and mixed hyperlipidaemia, including patients with noninsulin-dependent diabetes mellitus.

Lipitor is effective in reducing LDL-C in patients with homozygous familial hypercholesterolaemia, a population that has not usually responded to lipid-lowering medication. In a compassionate use study, 41 patients aged 6 to 51 years with homozygous familial hypercholesterolaemia or with severe hypercholesterolaemia, who had ≤15% reduction in LDL-C in response to previous maximum dose combination drug therapy, received daily doses of 40 to 80 mg of Lipitor. Twenty four patients with homozygous familial hypercholesterolaemia received 80 mg Lipitor. Nineteen of these 24 patients responded with a greater than 15% reduction of LDL-C (mean 26%, range 18% to 42%).

Atherosclerosis

In the Reversing Atherosclerosis with Aggressive Lipid-Lowering Study (REVERSAL), the effect of atorvastatin 80 mg and pravastatin 40 mg on coronary atherosclerosis was assessed by intravascular ultrasound (IVUS), during angiography, in patients with coronary heart disease. In this randomized, double-blind, multicenter, controlled clinical trial, IVUS was performed at baseline and at 18 months in 502 patients. In the atorvastatin group (n=253), there was no progression of atherosclerosis evaluated by the percentage change in atheroma volume in a pre-defined target vessel with a stenosis between 20% and 50%. The median percent change, from baseline, in total atheroma volume (the primary study criteria) was -0.4% (p=0.98) in the atorvastatin group and +2.7% (p=0.001) in the pravastatin group (n=249). When compared to pravastatin, the effects of atovastatin were statistically significant (p=0.02).

In the atorvastatin group, LDL-C was reduced to a mean of 2.04 mmol/L ± 0.8 (78.9 mg/dL ± 30) from baseline 3.89 mmol/L + 0.7 (150 mg/dL ± 28) and in the pravastatin group, LDL-C was reduced to a mean of 2.85 mmol/L + 0.7 (110 mg/dL ± 26) from baseline 3.89 mmol/L + 0.7 (150 mg/dL ± 26) (p<0.0001). Atorvastatin also significantly reduced mean TC by 34.1% (pravastatin: -18.4%, p<0.0001), mean TG levels by 20% (pravastatin: -6.8%, p<0.0009), and mean apolipoprotein B by 39.1% (pravastatin: -22.0%, p<0.0001). Atorvastatin increased mean HDL-C by 2.9% (pravastatin: +5.6%, p=*NS*). There was a 36.4% mean reduction in CRP in the atorvastatin group compared to a 5.2% reduction in the pravastatin group (p<0.0001).

Table 1 Dose Response in Patients with Primary Hypercholesterolaemia

Lipitor Dose (mg)	N	Total-C	LDL-C	Apo B	TG	HDL-C
Placebo	12	5	8	6	-1	-2
10	11	-30	-41	-34	-14	4
20	10	-35	-44	-36	-33	12
40	11	-38	-50	-41	-25	-3
80	11	-46	-61	-50	-27	3

Adjusted Mean % Change from Baseline

The safety and tolerability profiles of the two treatment groups were comparable.

The effect of intensive lipid lowering with atorvastatin on cardiovascular mortality and morbidity was not investigated in this 18-month study. Therefore, the clinical significance of these imaging results with regard to the primary and secondary prevention of cardiovascular events is unknown.

Heterozygous Familial Hypercholesterolaemia in Paediatric Patients

In a double-blind, placebo controlled study followed by an open-label phase, 187 boys and postmenarchal girls 10-17 years of age (mean age 14.1 years) with heterozygous familial hypercholesterolaemia (FH) or severe hypercholesterolaemia were randomised to atorvastatin (n=140) or placebo (n=47) for 26 weeks and then all received atorvastatin for 26 weeks. Inclusion in the study required 1) a baseline LDL-C level ≥4.91 mmol/l or 2) a baseline LDL-C ≥4.14 mmol/l and positive family history of FH or documented premature cardiovascular disease in a first- or second degree relative. The mean baseline LDL-C value was 5.65 mmol/l (range: 3.58-9.96 mmol/l) in the atorvastatin group compared to 5.95 mmol/l (range: 4.14-8.39 mmol/l) in placebo group. The dosage if atorvastatin (once daily) was 10mg for the first 4 weeks and up-titrated to 20mg if the LDL-C level was >3.36 mmol/l. The number of atorvastatin-treated patients who required up-titration to 20mg after Week 4 during the double-blind phase was 80 (57.1%).

Atorvastatin significantly decreased plasma levels of total-C, LDL-C, triglycerides, and apolipoprotein B during the 26 week double-blind phase (see Table 2).

(see Table 2 below)

The mean achieved LDL-C value was 3.38 mmol/l (range: 1.81-6.26 mmol/l) in the atorvastatin group compared to 5.91 mmol/l (range: 3.93-9.96 mmol/l) in the placebo group during the 26-week double-blind phase.

In this limited controlled study, there was no detectable effect on growth or sexual maturation in boys or on menstrual length in girls. Atorvastatin has not been studied in controlled clinical trials involving pre-pubertal patients or patients younger than 10 years of age. The safety and efficacy of doses above 20mg have not been studied in controlled trials in children. The long-term efficacy of atorvastatin therapy in childhood to reduce morbidity and mortality in adulthood has not been established.

5.2 Pharmacokinetic properties

Pharmacokinetics and Drug Metabolism

Absorption: Atorvastatin is rapidly absorbed after oral administration; maximum plasma concentrations occur within 1 to 2 hours. Extent of absorption increases in proportion to atorvastatin dose. Lipitor tablets are bioequivalent to atorvastatin solutions. The absolute bioavailability of atorvastatin is approximately 12% and the systemic availability of HMG-CoA reductase inhibitory activity is approximately 30%. The low systemic availability is attributed to presystemic clearance in gastrointestinal mucosa and/or hepatic first-pass metabolism.

Distribution: Mean volume of distribution of atorvastatin is approximately 381 L. Atorvastatin is ≥98% bound to plasma proteins.

Metabolism: Atorvastatin is metabolised by cytochrome P450 3A4 to ortho- and parahydroxylated derivatives and various beta-oxidation products. In vitro, inhibition of HMG-CoA reductase by ortho- and parahydroxylated metabolites is equivalent to that of atorvastatin. Approximately 70% of circulating inhibitory activity for HMG-CoA reductase is attributed to active metabolites.

Excretion: Atorvastatin and atorvastatin metabolites are substrates of P-glycoprotein (see section 4.5). Atorvastatin is eliminated primarily in bile following hepatic and/or extrahepatic metabolism. However, the drug does not appear to undergo significant enterohepatic recirculation. Mean plasma elimination half-life of atorvastatin in humans is approximately 14 hours. The half-life of inhibitory activity for HMG-CoA reductase is approximately 20 to 30 hours due to the contribution of active metabolites.

Special Populations

Geriatric: Plasma concentrations of atorvastatin are higher in healthy elderly subjects than in young adults while the lipid effects were comparable to those seen in younger patient populations.

Paediatric: Pharmacokinetic data in the paediatric population are not available.

Gender: Concentrations of atorvastatin in women differ (approximately 20% higher for Cmax and 10% lower for AUC) from those in men. These differences were of no clinical significance, resulting in no clinically significant differences in lipid effects among men and women.

Renal Insufficiency: Renal disease has no influence on the plasma concentrations or lipid effects of atorvastatin.

Hepatic Insufficiency: Plasma concentrations of atorvastatin are markedly increased (approximately 16-fold in Cmax and 11-fold in AUC) in patients with chronic alcoholic liver disease (Childs-Pugh B).

5.3 Preclinical safety data

Atorvastatin was not carcinogenic in rats. The maximum dose used was 63-fold higher than the highest human dose (80 mg/day) on a mg/kg body-weight basis and 8 to 16-fold higher based on AUC(0-24) values as determined by total inhibitory activity. In a 2-year study in mice, incidences of hepatocellular adenoma in males and hepatocellular carcinomas in females were increased at the maximum dose used, and the maximum dose used was 250-fold higher than the highest human dose on a mg/kg body-weight basis. Systemic exposure was 6- to 11-fold higher based on AUC(0-24). Atorvastatin did not demonstrate mutagenic or clastogenic potential in 4 in vitro tests with and without metabolic activation and in 1 in vivo assay.

6. PHARMACEUTICAL PARTICULARS

6.1 List of excipients

The 10-, 20-, and 40-mg dosage forms each contain the following excipients:

Calcium carbonate, E170

Microcrystalline cellulose, E460

Lactose monohydrate

Croscarmellose sodium

Polysorbate 80, E433

Hydroxypropyl cellulose, E463

Magnesium stearate, E572

Opadry White YS-1-7040 (containing hypromellose, E464, macrogol 8000, titanium dioxide, E171 and talc, E553b)

Simeticone Emulsion (containing simeticone, E900, macrogol stearate and sorbic acid, E200, water)

Candelilla wax

The 80-mg dosage form contains the following excipients:

Calcium carbonate, E170

Microcrystalline cellulose, E460

Lactose monohydrate

Croscarmellose sodium

Polysorbate 80, E433

Hydroxypropyl cellulose, E463

Magnesium stearate, E572

Opadry White YS-1-7040 (containing hypromellose, E464, macrogol 8000, titanium dioxide, E171 and talc, E553b)

Simeticone Emulsion (containing simeticone, E900, macrogol stearate and sorbic acid, E200, water)

6.2 Incompatibilities

Not applicable.

6.3 Shelf life

Three Years.

6.4 Special precautions for storage

No special precautions for storage.

6.5 Nature and contents of container

Foil/foil blisters consisting of a polyamide/aluminium foil/polyvinyl chloride unit-dose blister and a paper/polyester/aluminium foil/vinyl heat-seal coated backing or an aluminium foil/vinyl heat-seal coated backing.

Lipitor is supplied in packs of 28 tablets.

6.6 Instructions for use and handling

No special instructions needed.

7. MARKETING AUTHORISATION HOLDER

Pfizer Ireland Pharmaceuticals

Pottery Road

Dun Laoghaire

Co Dublin

Ireland

8. MARKETING AUTHORISATION NUMBER(S)

Lipitor 10mg PL 16051/0001

Lipitor 20mg PL 16051/0002

Lipitor 40mg PL 16051/0003

Lipitor 80mg PL 16051/0005

9. DATE OF FIRST AUTHORISATION/RENEWAL OF THE AUTHORISATION

Lipitor 10mg, 20mg, and 40mg Tablets: 8 September 1997

Lipitor 80mg Tablets: 15 August 2000

10. DATE OF REVISION OF THE TEXT

March 2005.

11. LEGAL CATEGORY

POM

REF: LRABCD_7_0.

Lipobase

(Astellas Pharma Limited)

1. NAME OF THE MEDICINAL PRODUCT

Lipobase.

2. QUALITATIVE AND QUANTITATIVE COMPOSITION

Lipobase contains no active ingredient.

3. PHARMACEUTICAL FORM

Cream.

4. CLINICAL PARTICULARS

4.1 Therapeutic indications

For use where it is desired by the physician to reduce gradually the topical dosage of Locoid Lipocream. It may also be used where a continuously alternating application of the active product and the base is required eg in prophylactic therapy. Application of the Lipobase is also recommended where it is felt by the physician that the use of a bland emollient base is preferable to the cessation of therapy with the active product. Lipobase may also be used as a diluent for the active product in those cases where dilution is regarded as necessary by the prescriber. Lipobase may also be used other than in conjunction with a topical corticosteroid for its emollient action, and for the treatment of mild skin lesions such as pruritus or dry, scaly skin, where topical corticosteroid is not warranted.

4.2 Posology and method of administration

For adults, children and the elderly: Lipobase may be used either by replacing an application of the active product or alternating the application of the active product and the base, gradually diminishing the application of the active product until therapy ceases, or by the application of the product for its emollient action.

4.3 Contraindications

None stated.

4.4 Special warnings and special precautions for use

None stated.

4.5 Interaction with other medicinal products and other forms of Interaction

None stated.

4.6 Pregnancy and lactation

None stated.

4.7 Effects on ability to drive and use machines

None stated.

4.8 Undesirable effects

None stated.

4.9 Overdose

None stated.

5. PHARMACOLOGICAL PROPERTIES

5.1 Pharmacodynamic properties

The product acts topically as an emollient cream.

5.2 Pharmacokinetic properties

Topical administration with no pharmacologically active constituents.

5.3 Preclinical safety data

No relevant preclinical safety data has been generated.

Table 2 Lipid Lowering effects of atorvastatin in adolescent boys and girls with heterozygous familial hypercholesterolaemia or severe hypocholesterolaemia (mean percent change from baseline at endpoint in intention- to-treat-population

DOSAGE	N	Total-C	LDL-C	HDL-C	TG	Apo B
Placebo	47	-1.5	-0.4	-1.9	1.0	0.7
Atorvastatin	140	-31.4	-39.6	2.8	-12.0	-34.0

6. PHARMACEUTICAL PARTICULARS

6.1 List of excipients

Cetostearyl alcohol

Macrogol cetostearyl ether

Light liquid paraffin

White soft paraffin

Methyl parahydroxybenzoate

Sodium citrate, anhydrous

Citric acid, anhydrous

Purified water

6.2 Incompatibilities

None stated.

6.3 Shelf life

30g, 50g, 100g and 200g packs, 5 years.

200g and 500g packs, 2 years

6.4 Special precautions for storage

Do not store above 25°C.

6.5 Nature and contents of container

Collapsible aluminium tube with plastic screw cap containing 30 g, 50 g, 100 g or 200 g; and pump dispenser containing 200 g or 500 g.

6.6 Instructions for use and handling

Not applicable.

7. MARKETING AUTHORISATION HOLDER

Yamanouchi Pharma Ltd

Yamanouchi House

Pyrford Road

West Byfleet

Surrey

KT14 6RA

8. MARKETING AUTHORISATION NUMBER(S)

Product licence 0166/0125

9. DATE OF FIRST AUTHORISATION/RENEWAL OF THE AUTHORISATION

First authorisation granted 19 February 1985

Renewal granted 23 January 2001.

10. DATE OF REVISION OF THE TEXT

Date of partial revision = 22nd February 2002

11. Legal category

P

Liposic

(Chauvin Pharmaceuticals Ltd)

1. NAME OF THE MEDICINAL PRODUCT

Liposic®, eye gel

2. QUALITATIVE AND QUANTITATIVE COMPOSITION

Each 1g of gel contains 2mg of carbomer

For excipients see 6.1

3. PHARMACEUTICAL FORM

Eye gel; white, turbid, highly viscous, dripable

4. CLINICAL PARTICULARS

4.1 Therapeutic indications

Symptomatic treatment of dry eye syndrome

4.2 Posology and method of administration

Therapy of dry eye conditions requires an individual dosage regimen.

According to the severity and intensity of the symptoms, instill one drop into the conjunctival sac 3-5 times daily; and approximately 30 minutes before going to bed (otherwise there is a risk of sticky eyelids).

Generally, an ophthalmologist should be consulted when treating keratoconjunctivitis sicca, which normally turns out to be long-term or permanent therapy.

An appropriate drop size is obtained when the tube is held in a vertical position above the eye during instillation.

4.3 Contraindications

Hypersensitivity to any component of this product

4.4 Special warnings and special precautions for use

Contact lenses should be removed prior to administration, and may be inserted again 30 minutes after Liposic has been instilled. Concomitant ocular medication should be administered 15 minutes prior to instillation of Liposic (see 4.5).

No specific studies with Liposic have been performed in children.

If the symptoms of the dry eye continue or worsen, treatment should be stopped and an ophthalmologist should be consulted.

4.5 Interaction with other medicinal products and other forms of Interaction

None known

Please note:

Liposic may prolong the contact-time of topically applied drugs in ophthalmology. Concomitant ocular medication should be administered 15 minutes prior to instillation of Liposic.

4.6 Pregnancy and lactation

Clinical data regarding the safety of Liposic in human pregnancy or lactation are not available. Preclinical data predict that the risk of Liposic use in human pregnancy or lactation is very low. But due to the lack of clinical data the use of Liposic during pregnancy or lactation can not be recommended.

4.7 Effects on ability to drive and use machines

Even when used as indicated, this medicinal product may impair visual acuity for about five minutes due to the formation of streaks after gel application, and patients should exercise caution when driving vehicles or operating machinery.

4.8 Undesirable effects

Ocular irritation may occur in rare cases due to the preservative contained. Intolerance reactions to one of the ingredients may be seen in isolated cases. Observed undesirable effects include burning, reddening of the eyes, sticky eyelids, palpebral giant papillary conjunctivitis, corneal stipples, episcleritis, blurred vision, itching, discomfort

4.9 Overdose

Any ocular overdosage or oral intake which might occur is of no clinical relevance. However, care should be taken to administer small drops to the eye to avoid sticky eyelids.

5. PHARMACOLOGICAL PROPERTIES

ATC code S01XA20

5.1 Pharmacodynamic properties

Liposic eye gel is based on a high molecular weight hydrophilic polymer. Its pH and osmolality are similar to those of the normal tear film. Due to its physical properties, the eye gel binds water and forms a translucent lubricating and wetting film on the surface of the eye. The gel structure is destroyed by the salts contained in the lacrimal fluid and releases moisture. A study in 54 patients with keratoconjunctivitis sicca found that Liposic therapy prolonged tear break-up time from a mean of 5.3 seconds to 11.2 seconds after 6 weeks. Schirmer I-test values were increased from a mean of 4.8 mm to 10.7 mm after 6 weeks.

5.2 Pharmacokinetic properties

No controlled animal nor human pharmacokinetic studies with this product are available. However, absorption or accumulation in eye tissues can presumably be excluded due to the high molecular weight of carbomer. Clinical studies performed with an essentially similar product have shown that ocular residence time can be assumed to be approximately up to 90 minutes.

5.3 Preclinical safety data

Preclinical data reveal no special hazard for humans based on studies of repeated dose toxicity, genotoxicity, carcinogenic potential, reproductive toxicity and pharmacological safety.

6. PHARMACEUTICAL PARTICULARS

6.1 List of excipients

Cetrimide, sorbitol, medium-chain triglycerides, sodium hydroxide (for pH adjustment), purified water

6.2 Incompatibilities

None known so far.

6.3 Shelf life

3 years

28 days after opening of the container

6.4 Special precautions for storage

Do not store above 25°C

6.5 Nature and contents of container

Tubes of 5 g eye gel. Packs with one or three tubes of 5 g eye gel.

Tubes of 10 g eye gel. Packs with one or three tubes of 10 g eye gel.

6.6 Instructions for use and handling

No special requirements

7. MARKETING AUTHORISATION HOLDER

Dr. Gerhard Mann

Chem.-Pharm. Fabrik GmbH

Brunsbuetteler Damm 165-173

13581 Berlin (Germany)

8. MARKETING AUTHORISATION NUMBER(S)

PL 13757/0001

9. DATE OF FIRST AUTHORISATION/RENEWAL OF THE AUTHORISATION

21 March 2000

10. DATE OF REVISION OF THE TEXT

26 October 2001

11. Legal Category

P

Lipostat 10 mg, 20 mg and 40 mg Tablets

(Bristol-Myers Squibb Pharmaceuticals Ltd)

1. NAME OF THE MEDICINAL PRODUCT

Lipostat 10mg tablets

Lipostat 20mg tablets

Lipostat 40mg tablets

2. QUALITATIVE AND QUANTITATIVE COMPOSITION

Lipostat 10mg tablets: Each tablet contains 10mg pravastatin sodium.

Lipostat 20mg tablets: Each tablet contains 20mg pravastatin sodium.

Lipostat 40mg tablets: Each tablet contains 40mg pravastatin sodium.

For excipients, see section 6.1.

3. PHARMACEUTICAL FORM

Tablet.

Lipostat 10mg tablets: Yellow, capsule shaped biconvex scored tablet with a "10" engraved on one side.

Lipostat 20mg tablets: Yellow, capsule shaped biconvex scored tablet with a "20" engraved on one side.

Lipostat 40mg tablets: Yellow, capsule shaped biconvex scored or unscored tablet with a "40" engraved on one side.

4. CLINICAL PARTICULARS

4.1 Therapeutic indications

Hypercholesterolaemia

Treatment of primary hypercholesterolaemia or mixed dyslipidaemia, as an adjunct to diet, when response to diet and other non-pharmacological treatments (e.g. exercise, weight reduction) is inadequate.

Primary prevention

Reduction of cardiovascular mortality and morbidity in patients with moderate or severe hypercholesterolaemia and at high risk of a first cardiovascular event, as an adjunct to diet (see section 5.1).

Secondary prevention

Reduction of cardiovascular mortality and morbidity in patients with a history of myocardial infarction or unstable angina pectoris and with either normal or increased cholesterol levels, as an adjunct to correction of other risk factors (see section 5.1).

Post transplantation

Reduction of post transplantation hyperlipidaemia in patients receiving immunosuppressive therapy following solid organ transplantation. (see sections 4.2, 4.5 and 5.1).

4.2 Posology and method of administration

Prior to initiating LIPOSTAT, secondary causes of hypercholesterolaemia should be excluded and patients should be placed on a standard lipid-lowering diet which should be continued during treatment.

LIPOSTAT is administered orally once daily preferably in the evening with or without food.

Hypercholesterolaemia: the recommended dose range is 10-40 mg once daily. The therapeutic response is seen within a week and the full effect of a given dose occurs within four weeks, therefore periodic lipid determinations should be performed and the dosage adjusted accordingly. The maximum daily dose is 40 mg.

Cardiovascular prevention: in all preventive morbidity and mortality trials, the only studied starting and maintenance dose was 40 mg daily.

Dosage after transplantation: following **organ transplantation** a starting dose of 20 mg per day is recommended in patients receiving immunosuppressive therapy (see section 4.5). Depending on the response of the lipid parameters, the dose may be adjusted up to 40 mg under close medical supervision (see section 4.5).

Children and adolescents (8-18 years of age) with heterozygous familial hypercholesterolaemia: the recommended dose range is 10-20 mg once daily between 8 and 13 years of age as doses greater than 20 mg have not been studied in this population and 10-40 mg daily between 14 and 18 years of age (for children and adolescent females of child-bearing potential, see section 4.6; for results of the study see section 5.1).

Elderly patients: there is no dose adjustment necessary in these patients unless there are predisposing risk factors (see section 4.4).

Renal or hepatic impairment: a starting dose of 10 mg a day is recommended in patients with moderate or severe renal impairment or significant hepatic impairment. The dosage should be adjusted according to the response of lipid parameters and under medical supervision.

Concomitant therapy: the lipid lowering effects of LIPOSTAT on total cholesterol and LDL-cholesterol are enhanced when combined with a bile acid-binding resin (e.g. colestyramine, colestipol). LIPOSTAT should be given either one hour before or at least four hours after the resin (see section 4.5).

For patients taking ciclosporin with or without other immunosuppressive medicinal products, treatment should begin with 20 mg of pravastatin once daily and titration to 40 mg should be performed with caution (see section 4.5).

4.3 Contraindications

- Hypersensitivity to the active substance or to any of the excipients.

- Active liver disease including unexplained persistent elevations of serum transaminase elevation exceeding 3 × the upper limit of normal (ULN) (see section 4.4).

- Pregnancy and lactation (see section 4.6).

4.4 Special warnings and special precautions for use

Pravastatin has not been evaluated in patients with homozygous familial hypercholesterolaemia. Therapy is not suitable when hypercholesterolaemia is due to elevated HDL-Cholesterol.

As for other HMG-CoA reductase inhibitors, combination of pravastatin with fibrates is not recommended.

In children before puberty, the benefit/risk of treatment should be carefully evaluated by physicians before treatment initiation.

Hepatic disorders: as with other lipid-lowering agents, moderate increases in liver transaminase levels have been observed. In the majority of cases, liver transaminase levels have returned to their baseline value without the need for treatment discontinuation. Special attention should be given to patients who develop increased transaminase levels and therapy should be discontinued if increases in alanine aminotransferase (ALT) and aspartate aminotransferase (AST) exceed three times the upper limit of normal and persist.

Caution should be exercised when pravastatin is administered to patients with a history of liver disease or heavy alcohol ingestion.

Muscle disorders: as with other HMG-CoA reductase inhibitors (statins), pravastatin has been associated with the onset of myalgia, myopathy and very rarely, rhabdomyolysis. Myopathy must be considered in any patient under statin therapy presenting with unexplained muscle symptoms such as pain or tenderness, muscle weakness, or muscle cramps. In such cases creatine kinase (CK) levels should be measured (see below). Statin therapy should be temporarily interrupted when CK levels are > 5 × ULN or when there are severe clinical symptoms. Very rarely (in about 1 case over 100,000 patient-years), rhabdomyolysis occurs, with or without secondary renal insufficiency. Rhabdomyolysis is an acute potentially fatal condition of skeletal muscle which may develop at any time during treatment and is characterised by massive muscle destruction associated with major increase in CK (usually > 30 or 40 × ULN) leading to myoglobinuria.

The risk of myopathy with statins appears to be exposure-dependent and therefore may vary with individual drugs (due to lipophilicity and pharmacokinetic differences), including their dosage and potential for drug interactions. Although there is no muscular contraindication to the prescription of a statin, certain predisposing factors may increase the risk of muscular toxicity and therefore justify a careful evaluation of the benefit/risk and special clinical monitoring. CK measurement is indicated before starting statin therapy in these patients (see below).

The risk and severity of muscular disorders during statin therapy is increased by the co-administration of interacting medicines. The use of fibrates alone is occasionally associated with myopathy. The combined use of a statin and fibrates should generally be avoided. The co-administration of statins and nicotinic acid should be used with caution. An increase in the incidence of myopathy has also been described in patients receiving other statins in combination with inhibitors of cytochrome P450 metabolism. This may result from pharmacokinetic interactions that have not been documented for pravastatin (see section 4.5). When associated with statin therapy, muscle symptoms usually resolve following discontinuation of statin therapy.

<u>Creatine kinase measurement and interpretation</u>:

Routine monitoring of creatine kinase (CK) or other muscle enzyme levels is not recommended in asymptomatic patients on statin therapy. However, measurement of CK is recommended before starting statin therapy in patients with special predisposing factors, and in patients developing muscular symptoms during statin therapy, as described below. If CK levels are significantly elevated at baseline > 5 × ULN), CK levels should be re measured about 5 to 7 days later to confirm the results. When measured, CK levels should be interpreted in the context of other potential factors that can cause transient muscle damage, such as strenuous exercise or muscle trauma.

<u>Before treatment initiation</u>: caution should be used in patients with predisposing factors such as renal impairment, hypothyroidism, previous history of muscular toxicity with a statin or fibrate, personal or familial history of hereditary muscular disorders, or alcohol abuse. In these cases, CK levels should be measured prior to initiation of therapy. CK measurement should also be considered before starting treatment in persons over 70 years of age especially in the presence of other predisposing factors in this population. If CK levels are significantly elevated > 5 × ULN) at baseline, treatment should not be started and the results should be re-measured after 5 - 7 days. The baseline CK levels may also be useful as a reference in the event of a later increase during statin therapy.

<u>During treatment</u>: patients should be advised to report promptly unexplained muscle pain, tenderness, weakness or cramps. In these cases, CK levels should be measured. If a markedly elevated > 5 × ULN) CK level is detected, statin therapy must be interrupted. Treatment discontinuation should also be considered if the muscular symptoms are severe and cause daily discomfort, even if the CK increase remains ⩽ 5 × ULN. If symptoms resolve and CK levels return to normal, then reintroduction of statin therapy may be considered at the lowest dose and with close monitoring. If a hereditary muscular disease is suspected in such patients, restarting statin therapy is not recommended.

Lactose: this product contains lactose. Patients with rare hereditary problems of galactose intolerance, the Lapp lactase deficiency or glucose-galactose malabsorption should not take this medicinal product.

4.5 Interaction with other medicinal products and other forms of Interaction

Fibrates: the use of fibrates alone is occasionally associated with myopathy. An increased risk of muscle related adverse events, including rhabdomyolysis, have been reported when fibrates are co-administered with other statins. These adverse events with pravastatin cannot be excluded; therefore the combined use of pravastatin and fibrates (e.g. gemfibrozil, fenofibrate) should generally be avoided (see section 4.4). If this combination is considered necessary, careful clinical and CK monitoring of patients on such regimen is required.

Colestyramine/Colestipol: concomitant administration resulted in approximately 40 to 50% decrease in the bioavailability of pravastatin. There was no clinically significant decrease in bioavailability or therapeutic effect when pravastatin was administered one hour before or four hours after colestyramine or one hour before colestipol (see section 4.2).

Ciclosporin: concomitant administration of pravastatin and ciclosporin leads to an approximately 4-fold increase in pravastatin systemic exposure. In some patients, however, the increase in pravastatin exposure may be larger. Clinical and biochemical monitoring of patients receiving this combination is recommended (see section 4.2).

Warfarin and other oral anticoagulants: bioavailability parameters at steady state for pravastatin were not altered following administration with warfarin. Chronic dosing of the two products did not produce any changes in the anticoagulant action of warfarin.

Products metabolised by cytochrome P450: pravastatin is not metabolised to a clinically significant extent by the cytochrome P450 system. This is why products that are metabolised by, or inhibitors of, the cytochrome P450 system can be added to a stable regimen of pravastatin without causing significant changes in the plasma levels of pravastatin, as have been seen with other statins. The absence of a significant pharmacokinetic interaction with pravastatin has been specifically demonstrated for several products, particularly those that are substrates/inhibitors of CYP3A4 e.g. diltiazem, verapamil, itraconazole, ketoconazole, protease inhibitors, grapefruit juice and CYP2C9 inhibitors (e.g. fluconazole).

In one of two interaction studies with pravastatin and erythromycin a statistically significant increase in pravastatin AUC (70%) and Cmax (121%) was observed. In a similar study with clarithromycin a statistically significant increase in AUC (110%) and Cmax (127%) was observed. Although these changes were minor, caution should be exercised when associating pravastatin with erythromycin or clarithromycin.

Other products: in interaction studies, no statistically significant differences in bioavailability were observed when pravastatin was administered with acetylsalicylic acid, antacids (when given one hour prior to pravastatin), nicotinic acid or probucol.

4.6 Pregnancy and lactation

Pregnancy: pravastatin is contraindicated during pregnancy and should be administered to women of childbearing potential only when such patients are unlikely to conceive and have been informed of the potential risk. Special caution is recommended in adolescent females of childbearing potential to ensure proper understanding of the potential risk associated with pravastatin therapy during pregnancy. If a patient plans to become pregnant or becomes pregnant, the doctor has to be informed immediately and pravastatin should be discontinued because of the potential risk to the foetus.

Lactation: a small amount of pravastatin is excreted in human breast milk, therefore pravastatin is contraindicated during breastfeeding (see section 4.3).

4.7 Effects on ability to drive and use machines

Pravastatin has no or negligible influence on the ability to drive and use machines. However, when driving vehicles or operating machines, it should be taken into account that dizziness may occur during treatment.

4.8 Undesirable effects

The frequencies of adverse events are ranked according to the following: very common (⩾ 1/10); common (⩾ 1/100, < 1/10); uncommon (⩾ 1/1,000, < 1/100); rare (⩾ 1/10,000, < 1/1,000); very rare (< 1/10,000).

Clinical trials: LIPOSTAT has been studied at 40 mg in seven randomised double-blind placebo-controlled trials involving over 21,000 patients treated with pravastatin (n = 10764) or placebo (n = 10719), representing over 47,000 patients years of exposure to pravastatin. Over 19,000 patients were followed for a median of 4.8 - 5.9 years.

The following adverse drug reactions were reported; none of them occurred at a rate in excess of 0.3% in the pravastatin group compared to the placebo group.

<u>Nervous system disorders</u>:

Uncommon: dizziness, headache, sleep disturbance, insomnia

<u>Eye disorders</u>:

Uncommon: vision disturbance (including blurred vision and diplopia)

<u>Gastrointestinal disorders</u>:

Uncommon: dyspepsia/heartburn, abdominal pain, nausea/vomiting, constipation, diarrhoea, flatulence

<u>Skin and subcutaneous tissue disorders</u>:

Uncommon: pruritus, rash, urticaria, scalp/hair abnormality (including alopecia)

<u>Renal and urinary disorders</u>:

Uncommon: abnormal urination (including dysuria, frequency, nocturia)

<u>Reproductive system and breast disorders</u>:

Uncommon: sexual dysfunction

<u>General disorders</u>:

Uncommon: fatigue

Events of special clinical interest

<u>Skeletal muscle</u>: effects on the skeletal muscle, e.g. musculoskeletal pain including arthralgia, muscle cramps, myalgia, muscle weakness and elevated CK levels have been reported in clinical trials. The rate of myalgia (1.4% pravastatin vs 1.4% placebo) and muscle weakness (0.1% pravastatin vs < 0.1% placebo) and the incidence of CK level > 3 × ULN and > 10 × ULN in CARE, WOSCOPS and LIPID was similar to placebo (1.6% pravastatin vs 1.6% placebo and 1.0% pravastatin vs 1.0% placebo, respectively) (see section 4.4).

<u>Liver effects</u>: elevations of serum transaminases have been reported. In the three long-term, placebo-controlled clinical trials CARE, WOSCOPS and LIPID, marked abnormalities of ALT and AST > 3 × ULN) occurred at similar frequency (⩽ 1.2%) in both treatment groups.

Post marketing

In addition to the above the following adverse events have been reported during post marketing experience of pravastatin:

<u>Nervous system disorders</u>:

Very rare: peripheral polyneuropathy, in particular if used for long period of time, paresthesia

<u>Immune system disorders</u>:

Very rare: hypersensitivity reactions: anaphylaxis, angioedema, lupus erythematous-like syndrome

<u>Gastrointestinal disorders</u>:

Very rare: pancreatitis

<u>Hepatobiliary disorders</u>:

Very rare: jaundice, hepatitis, fulminant hepatic necrosis

<u>Musculoskeletal and connective tissue disorders</u>:

Very rare: rhabdomyolysis, which can be associated with acute renal failure secondary to myoglobinuria, myopathy (see section 4.4)

Isolated cases of tendon disorders, sometimes complicated by rupture

4.9 Overdose

To date there has been limited experience with overdosage of pravastatin. There is no specific treatment in the event of overdose. In the event of overdose, the patient should be treated symptomatically and supportive measures instituted as required.

5. PHARMACOLOGICAL PROPERTIES

5.1 Pharmacodynamic properties

Pharmacotherapeutic group: serum lipid reducing agents/cholesterol and triglyceride reducers/HMG-CoA reductase inhibitors, ATC-Code: C10AA03

Mechanism of action:

Pravastatin is a competitive inhibitor of 3-hydroxy-3-methylglutaryl-coenzyme A (HMG-CoA) reductase, the enzyme catalysing the early rate-limiting step in cholesterol biosynthesis, and produces its lipid-lowering effect in two ways. Firstly, with the reversible and specific competitive inhibition of HMG-CoA reductase, it effects modest reduction in the synthesis of intracellular cholesterol. This results in an increase in the number of LDL-receptors on cell surfaces and enhanced receptor-mediated catabolism and clearance of circulating LDL-cholesterol.

Secondly, pravastatin inhibits LDL production by inhibiting the hepatic synthesis of VLDL-cholesterol, the LDL-cholesterol precursor.

In both healthy subjects and patients with hypercholesterolaemia, pravastatin sodium lowers the following lipid values: total cholesterol, LDL-cholesterol, apolipoprotein B, VLDL-cholesterol and triglycerides; while HDL-cholesterol and apolipoprotein A are elevated.

Clinical efficacy:

Primary prevention

The "West of Scotland Coronary Prevention Study (WOSCOPS)" was a randomised, double-blind, placebo-controlled trial among 6,595 male patients aged from 45 to 64 years with moderate to severe hypercholesterolaemia (LDL-C: 155-232 mg/dl [4.0-6.0 mmol/l]) and with no history of myocardial infarction, treated for an average duration of 4.8 years with either a 40 mg daily dose of pravastatin or placebo as an adjunct to diet. In pravastatin-treated patients, results showed:

- a decrease in the risk of mortality from coronary disease and of non-lethal myocardial infarction (relative risk reduction RRR was 31%; p = 0.0001 with an absolute risk of 7.9% in the placebo group, and 5.5% in pravastatin treated patients); the effects on these cumulative cardiovascular events rates being evident as early as 6 months of treatment;

- a decrease in the total number of deaths from a cardiovascular event (RRR 32%; p = 0.03);

- when risk factors were taken into account, a RRR of 24% (p = 0.039) in total mortality was also observed among patients treated with pravastatin;

- a decrease in the relative risk for undergoing myocardial revascularisation procedures (coronary artery bypass graft surgery or coronary angioplasty) by 37% (p = 0.009) and coronary angiography by 31% (p = 0.007).

The benefit of the treatment on the criteria indicated above is not known in patients over the age of 65 years, who could not be included in the study.

In the absence of data in patients with hypercholesterolaemia associated with a triglyceride level of more than 6 mmol/l (5.3 g/l) after a diet for 8 weeks, in this study, the benefit of pravastatin treatment has not been established in this type of patient.

Secondary prevention

The "Long-Term Intervention with Pravastatin in Ischemic Disease (LIPID)" study was a multi-center, randomised, double-blind, placebo-controlled study comparing the effects of pravastatin (40 mg OD) with placebo in 9014 patients aged 31 to 75 years for an average duration of 5.6 years with normal to elevated serum cholesterol levels (baseline total cholesterol = 155 to 271 mg/dl [4.0-7.0 mmol/l], mean total cholesterol = 219 mg/dl [5.66 mmol/l]) and with variable triglyceride levels of up to 443 mg/dl [5.0 mmol/l] and with a history of myocardial infarction or unstable angina pectoris in the preceding 3 to 36 months. Treatment with pravastatin significantly reduced the relative risk of CHD death by 24% (p = 0.0004, with an absolute risk of 6.4% in the placebo group, and 5.3% in pravastatin treated patients), the relative risk of coronary events (either CHD death or nonfatal MI) by 24% ($p < 0.0001$) and the relative risk of fatal or nonfatal myocardial infarction by 29% ($p < 0.0001$). In pravastatin-treated patients, results showed:

- a reduction in the relative risk of total mortality by 23% ($p < 0.0001$) and cardiovascular mortality by 25% ($p < 0.0001$);

- a reduction in the relative risk of undergoing myocardial revascularisation procedures (coronary artery bypass grafting or percutaneous transluminal coronary angioplasty) by 20% ($p < 0.0001$);

- a reduction in the relative risk of stroke by 19% (p = 0.048).

The "Cholesterol and Recurrent Events (CARE)" study was a randomised, double-blind, placebo-controlled study comparing the effects of pravastatin (40 mg OD) on coronary heart disease death and nonfatal myocardial infarction for an average of 4.9 years in 4,159 patients aged 21 to 75 years, with normal total cholesterol levels (baseline mean total cholesterol < 240 mg/dl), who had experienced a myocardial infarction in the preceding 3 to 20 months. Treatment with pravastatin significantly reduced:

- the rate of a recurrent coronary event (either coronary heart disease death or nonfatal MI) by 24% (p = 0.003, placebo 13.3%, pravastatin 10.4%);

- the relative risk of undergoing revascularisation procedures (coronary artery bypass grafting or percutaneous transluminal coronary angioplasty) by 27% ($p < 0.001$).

The relative risk of stroke was also reduced by 32% (p = 0.032), and stroke or transient ischaemic attack (TIA) combined by 27% (p = 0.02).

The benefit of the treatment on the above criteria is not known in patients over the age of 75 years, who could not be included in the CARE and LIPID studies.

In the absence of data in patients with hypercholesterolaemia associated with a triglyceride level of more than 4 mmol/l (3.5 g/l) or more than 5 mmol/l (4.45 g/l) after following a diet for 4 or 8 weeks, in the CARE and LIPID studies, respectively, the benefit of treatment with pravastatin has not been established in this type of patient.

In the CARE and LIPID studies, about 80% of patients had received ASA as part of their regimen.

Heart and kidney transplantation

The efficacy of pravastatin in patients receiving an immunosuppressant treatment following:

- Heart transplant was assessed in one prospective, randomised, controlled study (n = 97). Patients were treated concurrently with either pravastatin (20 - 40 mg) or not, and a standard immunosuppressive regimen of ciclosporin, prednisone and azathioprine. Treatment with pravastatin significantly reduced the rate of cardiac rejection with haemodynamic compromise at one year, improved one-year survival (p = 0.025), and lowered the risk of coronary vasculopathy in the transplant as determined by angiography and autopsy (p = 0.049).

- Renal transplant was assessed in one prospective not controlled, not randomised study (n = 48) of 4 months duration. Patients were treated concurrently with either pravastatin (20 mg) or not, and a standard immunosuppressive regimen of ciclosporin, and prednisone. In patients following kidney transplantation, pravastatin significantly reduced both the incidence of multiple rejection episodes and the incidence of biopsy-proved acute rejection episodes, and the use of pulse injections of both prednisolone and Muromonab-CD3.

Children and adolescents (8-18 years of age):

A double-blind placebo-controlled study in 214 paediatric patients with heterozygous familial hypercholesterolaemia was conducted over 2 years. Children (8-13 years) were randomised to placebo (n = 63) or 20 mg of pravastatin daily (n = 65) and the adolescents (aged 14-18 years) were randomised to placebo (n = 45) or 40 mg of pravastatin daily (n = 41).

Inclusion in this study required one parent with either a clinical or molecular diagnosis of familial hypercholesterolaemia. The mean baseline LDL-C value was 239 mg/dl (6.2 mmol/l) and 237 mg/dl (6.1 mmol/l) in the pravastatin (range 151-405 mg/dl [3.9-10.5 mmol/l]) and placebo (range 154-375 mg/dl [4.0-9.7 mmol/l]). There was a significant mean percent reduction in LDL-C of -22.9% and also in total cholesterol (-17.2%) from the pooled data analysis in both children and adolescents, similar to demonstrated efficacy in adults on 20 mg of pravastatin.

The effects of pravastatin treatment in the two age groups was similar. The mean achieved LDL-C was 186 mg/dl (4.8 mmol/l) (range: 67-363 mg/dl [1.7-9.4 mmol/l]) in the pravastatin group compared to 236 mg/dl (6.1 mmol/l) (range: 105-438 mg/dl [2.7-11.3 mmol/l]) in the placebo group. In subjects receiving pravastatin, there were no differences seen in any of the monitored endocrine parameters [ACTH, cortisol, DHEAS, FSH, LH, TSH, estradiol (girls) or testosterone (boys)] relative to placebo. There were no developmental differences, testicular volume changes or Tanner score differences observed relative to placebo. The power of this study to detect a difference between the two groups of treatment was low.

The long-term efficacy of pravastatin therapy in childhood to reduce morbidity and mortality in adulthood has not been established.

5.2 Pharmacokinetic properties

Absorption:

Pravastatin is administered orally in the active form. It is rapidly absorbed; peak serum levels are achieved 1 to 1.5 hours after ingestion. On average, 34% of the orally administered dose is absorbed, with an absolute bioavailability of 17%.

The presence of food in the gastrointestinal tract leads to a reduction in the bioavailability, but the cholesterol-lowering effect of pravastatin is identical whether taken with or without food.

After absorption, 66% of pravastatin undergoes a first-pass extraction through the liver, which is the primary site of its action and the primary site of cholesterol synthesis and clearance of LDL-cholesterol. *In vitro* studies demonstrated that pravastatin is transported into hepatocytes and with substantially less intake in other cells.

In view of this substantial first pass through the liver, plasma concentrations of pravastatin have only a limited value in predicting the lipid-lowering effect.

The plasma concentrations are proportional to the doses administered.

Distribution:

About 50% of circulating pravastatin is bound to plasma proteins.

The volume of distribution is about 0.5 l/kg.

A small quantity of pravastatin passes into the human breast milk.

Metabolism and elimination:

Pravastatin is not significantly metabolised by cytochrome P450 nor does it appear to be a substrate or an inhibitor of P-glycoprotein but rather a substrate of other transport proteins.

Following oral administration, 20% of the initial dose is eliminated in the urine and 70% in the faeces. Plasma elimination half-life of oral pravastatin is 1.5 to 2 hours.

After intravenous administration, 47% of the dose is eliminated by the renal excretion and 53% by biliary excretion and biotransformation. The major degradation product of pravastatin is the 3-α-hydroxy isomeric metabolite. This metabolite has one-tenth to one-fortieth the HMG-CoA reductase inhibitor activity of the parent compound.

The systemic clearance of pravastatin is 0.81 l/h/kg and the renal clearance is 0.38 l/h/kg indicating tubular secretion.

Populations at risk:

Paediatric subject: mean pravastatin Cmax and AUC values for paediatric subjects pooled across age and gender were similar to those values observed in adults after a 20 mg oral dose.

Hepatic failure: systemic exposure to pravastatin and metabolites in patients with alcoholic cirrhosis is enhanced by about 50% comparatively to patients with normal liver function.

Renal impairment: no significant modifications were observed in patients with mild renal impairment. However severe and moderate renal insufficiency may lead to a two-fold increase of the systemic exposure to pravastatin and metabolites.

5.3 Preclinical safety data

Based on conventional studies of safety pharmacology, repeated dose toxicity and toxicity on reproduction, there are no other risks for the patient than those expected due to the pharmacological mechanism of action.

Repeated dose studies indicate that pravastatin may induce varying degrees of hepatotoxicity and myopathy; in general, substantive effects on these tissues were only evident at doses 50 or more times the maximum human mg/kg dose.

In vitro and *in vivo* genetic toxicology studies have shown no evidence of mutagenic potential.

In mice, a 2-year carcinogenicity study with pravastatin demonstrates at doses of 250 and 500 mg/kg/day (≥ 310 times the maximum human mg/kg dose), statistically significant increases in the incidence of hepatocellular carcinomas in males and females, and lung adenomas in females only. In rats a 2-year carcinogenicity study demonstrates at a dose of 100 mg/kg/day (125 times the maximum human mg/kg/dose) a statistically significant increase in the incidence of hepatocellular carcinomas in males only.

6. PHARMACEUTICAL PARTICULARS

6.1 List of excipients

Croscarmellose sodium, lactose monohydrate, magnesium stearate, heavy magnesium oxide, microcrystalline cellulose, povidone, yellow ferric oxide E172.

6.2 Incompatibilities

Not applicable.

6.3 Shelf life

24 months

6.4 Special precautions for storage

Do not store above 30°C. Store in the original package.

6.5 Nature and contents of container

PVC/PE/PVDC/Aluminium blister packs of 10, 14, 20, 28, 30, 50, 60, 98, 100, 200, and 280 tablets.

Not all pack sizes may be marketed.

6.6 Instructions for use and handling

No special requirements.

7. MARKETING AUTHORISATION HOLDER

Bristol-Myers Squibb Pharmaceuticals Ltd.,
Uxbridge Business Park,
Sanderson Road,
Uxbridge,
Middlesex
UB8 1DH

8. MARKETING AUTHORISATION NUMBER(S)

PL 11184/0055
PL 11185/0056
PL 11184/0057

9. DATE OF FIRST AUTHORISATION/RENEWAL OF THE AUTHORISATION

10 January 1997 / 23 March 2003

10. DATE OF REVISION OF THE TEXT

September 2005

Liquifilm Tears

(Allergan Ltd)

1. NAME OF THE MEDICINAL PRODUCT

Liquifilm Tears

2. QUALITATIVE AND QUANTITATIVE COMPOSITION

Polyvinyl alcohol 1.4% w/v USP

3. PHARMACEUTICAL FORM

Eye Drops

4. CLINICAL PARTICULARS

4.1 Therapeutic indications

As an ocular lubricant for the relief of dry eye and dry eye symptoms.

4.2 Posology and method of administration

For all ages. One to two drops administered topically to the affected eye(s) as required.

4.3 Contraindications

Sensitivity to any of the ingredients. Not for use with soft contact lenses.

4.4 Special warnings and special precautions for use

None.

4.5 Interaction with other medicinal products and other forms of Interaction

None known.

4.6 Pregnancy and lactation

No untoward effect is anticipated, (product contains no pharmacologically active ingredient).

4.7 Effects on ability to drive and use machines

None.

4.8 Undesirable effects

None.

4.9 Overdose

None.

5. PHARMACOLOGICAL PROPERTIES

5.1 Pharmacodynamic properties

Not applicable. Liquifilm Tears contains no pharmacologically active ingredient.

5.2 Pharmacokinetic properties

Not applicable. Liquifilm Tears contains no pharmacologically active ingredient.

5.3 Preclinical safety data

The constituents of Liquifilm Tears have been used safely in pharmaceutical products for many years. Topical administration in animal studies showed no untoward effects.

6. PHARMACEUTICAL PARTICULARS

6.1 List of excipients

Sodium chloride EP

Sodium phosphate dibasic USP

Sodium phosphate monobasic USP

Benzalkonium chloride EP

Edetate disodium EP

Hydrochloric acid or sodium hydroxide (to adjust pH) EP

Purified water EP

6.2 Incompatibilities

None known

6.3 Shelf life

24 months unopened.

Discard 28 days after opening.

6.4 Special precautions for storage

None.

6.5 Nature and contents of container

Low density polyethylene (LDPE) bottle and tip and medium impact polystyrene (MIPS) screw cap. Safety seal to ensure integrity of the container.

Liquifilm Tears is available in 15ml bottles.

6.6 Instructions for use and handling

Not applicable.

Administrative Data

7. MARKETING AUTHORISATION HOLDER

Allergan Ltd.

Coronation Road

High Wycombe

Bucks HP12 3SH

8. MARKETING AUTHORISATION NUMBER(S)

PL 00426/0009R

9. DATE OF FIRST AUTHORISATION/RENEWAL OF THE AUTHORISATION

19th September 1974/22nd September 1998

10. DATE OF REVISION OF THE TEXT

23rd September 1998

Liquifilm Tears Preservative Free

(Allergan Ltd)

1. NAME OF THE MEDICINAL PRODUCT

Liquifilm® Tears Preservative Free or REFRESH OPHTHALMIC™.

2. QUALITATIVE AND QUANTITATIVE COMPOSITION

Polyvinyl alcohol 1.4% w/v.

3. PHARMACEUTICAL FORM

Eye drops, solution

4. CLINICAL PARTICULARS

4.1 Therapeutic indications

Symptomatic relief of dry eye and symptomatic relief of eye irritation associated with deficient tear production.

4.2 Posology and method of administration

Dosage schedule: Apply one or two drops in each eye as needed, or as directed. No special dosage for the elderly or for children.

Route of administration: Ocular instillation.

4.3 Contraindications

Hypersensitivity to any component of the formulation.

4.4 Special warnings and special precautions for use

If symptoms worsen or persist or other adverse effects occur, discontinue use and consult a doctor.

In order to avoid contamination, dropper should not be allowed to touch the eye or any other surface.

Use immediately after opening.

Do not store opened container.

4.5 Interaction with other medicinal products and other forms of Interaction

None known.

4.6 Pregnancy and lactation

The constituents of Liquifilm® Tears Preservative Free/ REFRESH OPHTHALMIC™ have been used as pharmaceutical agents for many years with no untoward effects. No special precautions are necessary for the use of Liquifilm® Tears Preservative Free/REFRESH OPHTHALMIC™ in pregnancy and lactation.

4.7 Effects on ability to drive and use machines

May cause transient blurring. Do not drive or use hazardous machinery unless vision is clear.

4.8 Undesirable effects

May cause transient stinging or irritation on instillation.

4.9 Overdose

Accidental overdose will not present any hazard.

5. PHARMACOLOGICAL PROPERTIES

5.1 Pharmacodynamic properties

Liquifilm® Tears Preservative Free/REFRESH OPHTHALMIC™ exerts a mechanical, not a pharmacological action. The viscosity enhancing agent is polyvinyl alcohol and the lubricating-enhancing agent is povidone.

5.2 Pharmacokinetic properties

Not applicable.

5.3 Preclinical safety data

The constituents of Liquifilm® Tears Preservative Free/ REFRESH OPHTHALMIC™ have been used safely in pharmaceutical products for many years. Topical administration in animals studies showed untoward effects.

6. PHARMACEUTICAL PARTICULARS

6.1 List of excipients

Povidone

Sodium chloride

Sodium hydroxide or hydrochloric acid (to adjust pH)

Purified water

6.2 Incompatibilities

None known.

6.3 Shelf life

24 months (unopened).

Do not store opened container.

6.4 Special precautions for storage

Store at 25°C or below.

6.5 Nature and contents of container

Low density polyethylene unit dose vials containing 0.4 ml of Liquifilm® Tears Preservative Free/REFRESH OPHTHALMIC™.

Cartons contain 2, 5, 10, 15, 30 or 50 units per pack.

6.6 Instructions for use and handling

Ensure container is intact. Twist off tab and apply eyedrops.

7. MARKETING AUTHORISATION HOLDER

Allergan Limited

Coronation Road

High Wycombe

Buckinghamshire

HP12 3SH

UK

8. MARKETING AUTHORISATION NUMBER(S)

PL 00426/0063

9. DATE OF FIRST AUTHORISATION/RENEWAL OF THE AUTHORISATION

14th August 2003

10. DATE OF REVISION OF THE TEXT

14th August 2003

Liquivisc

(Allergan Ltd)

1. NAME OF THE MEDICINAL PRODUCT

LIQUIVISC™ 2.5 mg/g, eye gel

2. QUALITATIVE AND QUANTITATIVE COMPOSITION

Carbomer 974P 2.5 mg/g

For excipients, see 6.1.

3. PHARMACEUTICAL FORM

Eye gel.

Slightly yellow and opalescent gel.

4. CLINICAL PARTICULARS

4.1 Therapeutic indications

Symptomatic treatment of dry eye syndrome.

4.2 Posology and method of administration

Ocular use.

Adults (including the elderly)

Instil one drop of the gel into the inferior conjunctival cul-de-sac 1 to 4 times daily according to the degree of ocular trouble.

Children: no specific studies with LIQUIVISC™ 2.5 mg/g, eye gel have been performed in children. It is recommended that LIQUIVISC™ 2.5 mg/g, eye gel should not be used in children until further data becomes available.

After instillation, the bottle should be stored vertically with the dropper downwards to facilitate the formation of drops when next used.

Do not touch the eye with the dropper tip. Replace the cap after use.

4.3 Contraindications

Hypersensitivity to any of the components of the product.

4.4 Special warnings and special precautions for use

Benzalkonium chloride is commonly used as a preservative in ophthalmic products and has been reported rarely to cause punctate keratopathy and/or ulcerative keratopathy.

Contact lenses:

Benzalkonium chloride may be absorbed by and discolour contact lenses and therefore the patients should be instructed to wait until 30 minutes after instillation of LIQUIVISC™ 2.5 mg/g, eye gel before inserting contact lenses.

If symptoms continue or worsen, the patient should be reviewed by a physician.

4.5 Interaction with other medicinal products and other forms of Interaction

In case of concomitant use with another eye drops, wait for 15 minutes between instillations.

LIQUIVISC 2.5 mg/g, eye gel should be the last medication instilled.

4.6 Pregnancy and lactation

LIQUIVISC 2.5 mg/g, eye gel was not studied in pregnant and breast-feeding women.

Caution should be exercised when prescribing to pregnant or breast-feeding women.

4.7 Effects on ability to drive and use machines

Vision may be blurred for a few minutes after the instillation.

If affected, the patient should be advised not to drive or operate hazardous machinery until normal vision is restored.

4.8 Undesirable effects

As for other eye drops, possibility of mild transient stinging or burning upon instillation.

Blurred vision may occur briefly after instillation until the gel is evenly distributed over the eye surface.

4.9 Overdose

Any ocular overdose or oral intake that could occur is of no clinical relevance.

5. PHARMACOLOGICAL PROPERTIES

5.1 Pharmacodynamic properties

TEAR SUBSTITUTE

- (S: Sensory organ (eye)

- Fluid eye gel based on a high molecular weight hydrophilic polymer (carbomer 974P).

- Due to its physical properties, this gel forms a transparent lubricating and wetting film on the surface of the eye, temporarily compensating for tear insufficiency.

- Its pH (7.3) and osmolality are similar to those of the normal tear film.

- Its viscosity (700 mPas) is greater than that of artificial tears, allowing less frequent administration.

5.2 Pharmacokinetic properties

Because of the relatively large size of the carbomer molecule, penetration through the cornea is unlikely.

The persistence time of the gel on the eye surface is about 30 minutes.

5.3 Preclinical safety data

Data from subacute toxicity and local tolerance studies do not show any relevant findings.

6. PHARMACEUTICAL PARTICULARS

6.1 List of excipients

Benzalkonium chloride, sorbitol, lysine monohydrate, sodium acetate, polyvinyl alcohol, water for injections

6.2 Incompatibilities

Not applicable

6.3 Shelf life
Shelf life prior to opening

30 months

In-use shelf life

4 weeks

6.4 Special precautions for storage
Do not store above 25°C. Store container in the outer carton, in order to protect from light.

6.5 Nature and contents of container
10 g in 10 ml bottle (PE) with dropper (PE).

6.6 Instructions for use and handling
No special requirements.

7. MARKETING AUTHORISATION HOLDER
Allergan Pharmaceuticals Ireland

Castlebar Road

Westport

County Mayo

Ireland

8. MARKETING AUTHORISATION NUMBER(S)
PL 05179/0005

9. DATE OF FIRST AUTHORISATION/RENEWAL OF THE AUTHORISATION
20th August 2003 / 13th October 2003

10. DATE OF REVISION OF THE TEXT
9th November 2004

Liskonum Tablets

(GlaxoSmithKline UK)

1. NAME OF THE MEDICINAL PRODUCT
Liskonum® Tablets

2. QUALITATIVE AND QUANTITATIVE COMPOSITION
Liskonum Tablets are available in one strength. Each tablet contains 450 mg lithium carbonate (12.2 mmol Li^+) in controlled-release form.

3. PHARMACEUTICAL FORM
White, oblong, film-coated tablets, with convex faces and a breakline on both sides.

4. CLINICAL PARTICULARS
4.1 Therapeutic indications
Liskonum is a controlled-release tablet, designed to reduce fluctuations in serum lithium levels and the likelihood of adverse reactions.

It is indicated for the treatment of acute episodes of mania or hypomania and for the prophylaxis of recurrent manic-depressive illness.

4.2 Posology and method of administration
Dosage:

Adults only: Liskonum should be given twice a day.

Treatment of acute mania or hypomania

Patients should be started on one or one-and-a-half tablets twice a day. Dosage should then be adjusted to achieve a serum lithium level of 0.8 to a maximum of 1.5 mmol/l. Serum concentration of lithium should be measured after four to seven days' treatment and then at least once a week until dosage has remained constant for four weeks. When the acute symptoms have been controlled, recommendations for prophylaxis should be followed.

Prophylaxis: The usual starting dosage is one tablet twice a day. Dosage should then be adjusted until a serum level of 0.5 to 1.0 mmol/l is maintained. Serum concentration of lithium should be measured after four to seven days' treatment and then every week until dosage has remained constant for four weeks. Frequency of monitoring may then be gradually decreased to a minimum of once every two months, but should be increased following any situation where changes in lithium levels are possible (see Section 4.4).

Blood samples for measurement of serum lithium concentration should be taken just before a dose is due and not less than 12 hours after the previous dose.

Levels of more than 2 mmol/l *must* be avoided.

Elderly: Use with caution. Start with half a tablet twice a day and adjust serum levels to the lower end of the above ranges (see also Section 4.4).

The full prophylactic effect of lithium may not be evident for six to 12 months, and treatment should be continued through any recurrence of the illness.

Children: Not recommended for use in children under 12 years of age

Administration:

Oral.

4.3 Contraindications
Do not use in patients with a history of hypersensitivity to lithium, impaired renal function, cardiac disease, or untreated hypothyroidism. Lithium should not be given to patients with low body sodium levels, including, for example, dehydrated patients, those on low sodium diets, or those with Addison's disease.

4.4 Special warnings and special precautions for use
Vomiting, diarrhoea, intercurrent infection, fluid deprivation and drugs likely to upset electrolyte balance, such as diuretics, may all reduce lithium excretion and thereby precipitate intoxication; reduction of dosage may be required. Use with care in elderly patients as lithium excretion may also be reduced.

The possibility of hypothyroidism and of renal dysfunction arising during prolonged treatment should be borne in mind and periodic assessments made.

Patients should be warned of the symptoms of impending intoxication (see Section 4.8), of the urgency of immediate action should these symptoms appear, and also of the need to maintain a constant and adequate salt and water intake. Treatment should be discontinued immediately on the first signs of toxicity (see Section 4.8). Acute renal failure has been reported rarely with lithium toxicity.

4.5 Interaction with other medicinal products and other forms of Interaction
Interactions which increase lithium concentrations:

- Metronidazole
- Non-steroidal anti-inflammatory drugs, including selective cyclo-oxygenase (COX) II inhibitors (monitor serum lithium concentrations more frequently if NSAID therapy is initiated or discontinued)
- ACE inhibitors
- Angiotensin II receptor antagonists.
- Diuretics (thiazides show a paradoxical antidiuretic effect resulting in possible water retention and lithium intoxication)

Interactions which decrease serum lithium concentrations:

- Urea
- Xanthines
- Sodium bicarbonate containing products
- Diuretics (carbonic anhydrase inhibitors)

Interactions causing neurotoxicity:

- Neuroleptics (particularly haloperidol at higher dosages)
- Methyldopa
- Selective Serotonin Re-uptake Inhibitors (e.g. fluvoxamine and fluoxetine) as this combination may precipitate a serotonergic syndrome.
- Calcium channel blockers

Lithium may prolong the effects of neuromuscular blocking agents. There have been reports of interaction between lithium and phenytoin.

4.6 Pregnancy and lactation
Lithium crosses the placental barrier. In animal studies, lithium has been reported to interfere with fertility, gestation and foetal development. There is epidemiological evidence that the drug may be harmful in human pregnancy. Lithium therapy should not be used during pregnancy, especially during the first trimester, unless considered essential. In certain cases where a severe risk to the patient could exist if treatment were to be stopped, lithium has been continued during pregnancy. If given, however, serum levels should be measured frequently because of the changes in renal function associated with pregnancy and parturition.

Since adequate human data on use during lactation and adequate animal reproduction studies are not available, bottle feeding is advisable.

4.7 Effects on ability to drive and use machines
As lithium may cause disturbances of the CNS, patients should be warned of the possible hazards when driving or operating machinery.

4.8 Undesirable effects
Initial therapy: Fine tremor of the hands, polyuria and thirst may occur

Body as a whole: Oedema, muscle weakness

Cardiovascular: Reported cardiovascular effects are cardiac arrhythmia, bradycardia, sinus node dysfunction, peripheral circulatory collapse, hypotension, oedema, Raynaud's phenomena and ECG changes.

CNS: ataxia, hyperactive deep tendon reflexes, extrapyramidal symptoms, seizures, slurred speech, dizziness, nystagmus, stupor, coma, pseudotumor cerebri, myasthenia gravis, vertigo, giddiness, dazed feeling.

Dermatological: alopecia, acne, folliculitis, pruritis, psoriasis exacerbation, rash, acneiform eruptions, papular skin disorder.

Endocrine: euthyroid goitre, hypothyroidism, hyperthyroidism, hyperparathyroidism.

Gastrointestinal: anorexia, nausea, vomiting, diarrhoea, gastritis, excessive salivation, dry mouth.

Haematological: leukocytosis.

Metabolic and Nutritional: hyperglycaemia, hypercalcaemia, weight gain.

Renal: polydipsia, symptoms of nephrogenic diabetes insipidus, histological renal changes with interstitial fibrosis after long term treatment.

Reproductive: sexual dysfunction.

Senses: scotomata, dysgeusia, blurred vision.

Intoxication (see 4.4): Vomiting, diarrhoea, drowsiness, lack of co-ordination and/or a coarse tremor of the extremities and lower jaw may occur, especially with serum levels above the therapeutic range. Ataxia, giddiness, blurred vision, dysarthria, tinnitus, muscle hyperirritability, choreoathetoid movements and toxic psychosis have also been described.

If any of the above symptoms appear, treatment should be stopped immediately and arrangements made for serum lithium measurement.

4.9 Overdose
Any overdose in a patient who has been taking chronic lithium therapy should be regarded as potentially serious. A single acute overdose usually carries low risk and patients tend to show mild symptoms only, irrespective of their serum lithium concentration. However more severe symptoms may occur after a delay if lithium elimination is reduced because of renal impairment, particularly if a slow-release preparation has been taken.

If an acute overdose has been taken by a patient on chronic lithium therapy, this can lead to serious toxicity occurring even after a modest overdose as the extravascular tissues are already saturated with lithium.

Symptoms

The onset of symptoms may be delayed, with peak effects not occurring for as long as 24 hours, especially in patients who are not receiving chronic lithium therapy, or following the use of a sustained release preparation.

Mild: Nausea, diarrhoea, vomiting, blurred vision, polyuria, light headedness, fine resting tremor, first degree heart block, muscular weakness and drowsiness.

Moderate: Increasing confusion, blackouts, fasciculation and increased deep tendon reflexes, myoclonic twitches and jerks, ataxia, choreoathetoid movements, urinary and faecal incontinence, increasing restlessness followed by stupor. Hypernatraemia.

Severe: Coma, convulsions, cerebellar signs, cardiac dysrhythmias including sino-atrial block, sinus and junctional bradycardia. Hypotension or rarely hypertension, circulatory collapse and renal failure.

Management

There is no known antidote.

Consider gastric lavage within 1 hour of an acute ingestion of non-sustained-release preparations by an adult or child. Slow-release tablets do not disintegrate in the stomach and most are too large to pass up a lavage tube. Gut decontamination is not useful for chronic accumulation. Whole bowel irrigation may be helpful in patients ingesting large quantities of slow-release preparation.

NOTE: activated charcoal does not adsorb lithium.

Haemodialysis is the treatment of choice for severe poisoning and should be considered in all patients with marked neurological features. It is the most efficient method of lowering lithium concentrations rapidly but substantial rebound increases can be expected when dialysis is stopped, and prolonged, or repeated treatments may be required. It should be considered also in acute, acute on chronic or chronic overdose in patients with severe symptoms regardless of serum lithium concentration; discuss with your local poisons service.

NOTE: Clinical improvement generally takes longer than reduction of serum lithium concentrations regardless of the method used.

5. PHARMACOLOGICAL PROPERTIES
5.1 Pharmacodynamic properties
Lithium carbonate is used as a source of lithium ions. The mechanism by which it exerts its effect in affective disorders is not known but may be related to inhibition of neurotransmitter receptor mediated processes involving beta-adrenoceptors. It is used in the treatment of acute episodes of mania or hypomania and for prophylaxis of recurrent manic depressive illness.

5.2 Pharmacokinetic properties
Lithium is readily absorbed from the gastrointestinal tract, and is distributed throughout the body over a period of several hours. Lithium is excreted almost exclusively in the kidneys but can also be detected in sweat and saliva. It is not bound to plasma proteins. It crosses the placenta, and is excreted in breast milk. The half-life of non-sustained lithium varies considerably, but generally is considered to be about 12 to 24 hours following a single dose. It is however increased for example in those with renal impairment and with age, and may increase significantly during long-term therapy.

5.3 Preclinical safety data
Not applicable

6. PHARMACEUTICAL PARTICULARS
6.1 List of excipients
Povidone Titanium Dioxide (E171)

Maize Starch Magnesium Stearate (E572)

Lactose Polyethylene Glycol 6000

Gelatin Eudragit E12.5

Calcium Carboxymethylcellulose

Talcum (E553Cb)

Calcium Arachinate

6.2 Incompatibilities
Not applicable.

6.3 Shelf life
Liskonum Tablets have a shelf-life of five years.

6.4 Special precautions for storage
Store below 25°C.

6.5 Nature and contents of container
Opaque Blister Packs (OP) of 60 (6 × 10) tablets.

6.6 Instructions for use and handling
Tablets may be halved but should not be chewed or broken up.

Administrative Data

7. MARKETING AUTHORISATION HOLDER
Smith Kline & French Laboratories Limited
Great West Road
Brentford
Middlesex TW8 9GS
Trading as:
GlaxoSmithKline UK,
Stockley Park West,
Uxbridge,
Middlesex, UB11 1BT

8. MARKETING AUTHORISATION NUMBER(S)
PL 0002/0083

9. DATE OF FIRST AUTHORISATION/RENEWAL OF THE AUTHORISATION
29.09.02

10. DATE OF REVISION OF THE TEXT
19 November 2004

Lisuride Tablets 200mcg

(Cambridge Laboratories)

1. NAME OF THE MEDICINAL PRODUCT
Lisuride Tablets 200 mcg

2. QUALITATIVE AND QUANTITATIVE COMPOSITION
Each tablet contains 200 micrograms Lisuride Maleate (equivalent to 149 micrograms Lisuride).

3. PHARMACEUTICAL FORM
Tablet

4. CLINICAL PARTICULARS
Lisuride is a selective dopamine agonist. Parkinson's disease, which is charaterised by a deficiency of dopamine in the nigro-striatal pathway, responds to Lisuride, which can be used either alone or in combination with levodopa, for the management of previously untreated patients and those exhibiting "on-off" phenomena. It is suitable for patients who cannot tolerate levodopa or whose response to levodopa is declining.

4.1 Therapeutic indications
For the treatment of Parkinson's disease.

4.2 Posology and method of administration
The following general rules apply: Lisuride should always be taken with food. The initial dose should preferably be taken at bedtime. Dosage should be low initially, increasing gradually to the appropriate final level, as determined by the efficacy and tolerance of the drug.

Adults and Elderly Patients:

Initially, one tablet at bedtime. After one week, the dosage may be increased to 200 micrograms at bedtime and 200 micrograms at midday. After a further week, an additional 200 micrograms may be added in the morning. The dosage should continue to be increased by 200 micrograms per week (beginning each sequence of three increases with the bedtime dose) until the optimum dosage is achieved.

The maximum daily dosage should not normally exceed 5 mg (25 tablets).

Children:

Lisuride is not recommended in children.

4.3 Contraindications
Severe disturbances of peripheral circulation, coronary insufficiency.

4.4 Special warnings and special precautions for use
Lisuride should be given with extreme caution to a patient who has, or has had treated, a pituitary tumour. Enlargement can occur, particularly during pregnancy, which may result in early visual field defects.

Psychiatric reactions have been seen with the use of Lisuride and this is more likely with high dosage and in patients who have a history of psychotic disturbance.

4.5 Interaction with other medicinal products and other forms of Interaction
The effects of some psychotropic drugs may possibly be impaired by the simultaneous use of Lisuride. Dopamine antagonists (e.g. haloperidol, sulpiride and metoclopramide) can weaken the effects and side-effects of Lisuride.

4.6 Pregnancy and lactation
Although many foetuses have been exposed to Lisuride, without evidence of teratogenicity in women of child bearing potential, the potential risks of use must be weighed against the benefits of treatment.

Lactation is unlikely to be inhibited if suckling or a breast pump is used.

4.7 Effects on ability to drive and use machines
The possibility of hypotensive reactions demands particular care in activities such as driving or operating machinery.

4.8 Undesirable effects
Nausea and vomiting are the most common side-effects experienced in patients with Parkinson's disease. In these patients domperidone can be freely used, since although it is an antidopaminergic drug it does not pass the blood brain barrier and therefore does not antagonise the anti-Parkinsonian effects of Lisuride. A sudden severe fall in blood pressure has been observed in isolated cases. Tolerance is rapidly acquired, and side-effects are most likely during the first few days of treatment. Dizziness, headache, lethargy, malaise and slight drowsiness are possible. There are occasional transient slightly itchy exanthemata. Abdominal pains and constipation occur rarely. Raynaud's phenomenon has been reported in one case so far. Psychiatric reactions, including hallucinations, have been reported occasionally.

4.9 Overdose
Expected symptoms of overdosage include severe nausea and vomiting, confusion, hallucinations and postural hypotension. Treatment should include the use of a specific dopamine antagonist as well as general supportive measures and maintenance of the blood pressure. Gastric lavage should be employed if overdosage is discovered soon enough.

5. PHARMACOLOGICAL PROPERTIES
5.1 Pharmacodynamic properties
Numerous pharmacological experiments have shown Lisuride to be a potent direct dopamine agonist. It has been shown to interact with peripheral 5-HT systems as an antagonist and with central 5-HT systems as an agonist. At higher doses, it also has alpha-adrenolytic and even beta-receptor-blocking activity.

Biochemical investigations have confirmed that it is one of the most potent dopamine- receptor agonists known, displaying very high affinity for both D_1 and D_2 receptors.

5.2 Pharmacokinetic properties
Absorption
In man, Lisuride is completely absorbed after oral administration with an absorption half-life of 1.2 ± 0.3 h. Lisuride maleate is a semi-synthetic ergot derivative with a high affinity for central dopamine receptors. Lisuride maleate is subject to a high first-pass metabolism.

Drug level/metabolic clearance
In man, following an intravenous bolus injection, the plasma concentration of Lisuride falls in three phases with half-lives of 3-5 minutes, 20 mins and 2-3. hours. Values found in younger and older healthy volunteers were almost identical. The basis pharmacokinetic data for Lisuride were unchanged in Parkinson patients. Metabolic clearance was 13 ml/kg/min in young healthy volunteers, 16 ml/kg/min in elderly volunteers and 11 ± 12.7 ml/kg/min in patients.

Bioavailability
Bioavailability is low in man and all animal species tested because of the high level of first-pass metabolism.

Elimination
In man, only 1.8% of the IV dose and 0.1% of the oral dose are recovered in the urine as unchanged metabolite. The metabolites of Lisuride are eliminated in almost equal portions via the kidney and liver.

5.3 Preclinical safety data
There are no pre-clinical data of relevance to the prescriber which are additional to that already included in other sections of the SPC.

6. PHARMACEUTICAL PARTICULARS
6.1 List of excipients
Tartaric acid, lactose, magnesium stearate, calcium disodium edetate, microcrystalline cellulose.

6.2 Incompatibilities
None known.

6.3 Shelf life
5 years.

6.4 Special precautions for storage
Recommended maximum storage temperature for Lisuride tablets is 25°C. Lisuride tablets should be stored in a dry place.

6.5 Nature and contents of container
Amber glass bottle with white polyethylene snap-in stopper, containing 100 tablets.

6.6 Instructions for use and handling
No special requirements.

7. MARKETING AUTHORISATION HOLDER
Cambridge Laboratories Limited
Deltic House
Kingfisher Way
Silverlink Business Park
Wallsend
Tyne & Wear
NE28 9NX

8. MARKETING AUTHORISATION NUMBER(S)
12070/0021

9. DATE OF FIRST AUTHORISATION/RENEWAL OF THE AUTHORISATION
16th June 1997

10. DATE OF REVISION OF THE TEXT
January 2001

Livial 2.5mg tablets

(Organon Laboratories Limited)

1. NAME OF THE MEDICINAL PRODUCT
Livial 2.5mg tablets

2. QUALITATIVE AND QUANTITATIVE COMPOSITION
Each Livial tablet contains as active substance 2.5mg of the steroid tibolone.

3. PHARMACEUTICAL FORM
Tablets for oral use.

4. CLINICAL PARTICULARS
4.1 Therapeutic indications
Treatment of oestrogen deficiency symptoms (including vasomotor symptoms, depressed mood, decreased libido) in postmenopausal women.

Second line therapy for prevention of osteoporosis in postmenopausal women at high risk of future fractures who are intolerant of, or contraindicated for, other medicinal products approved for the prevention of osteoporosis.

4.2 Posology and method of administration
Adults and the elderly
The dosage is one tablet per day without interruption. No dose adjustment is necessary for the elderly. The tablets should be swallowed without chewing with some water or other drink, preferably at the same time of day.

For treatment of postmenopausal symptoms, the lowest effective dose should be used.

HRT should only be continued as long as the benefit in alleviation of severe symptoms outweighs the risk.

Starting Livial

For the treatment of oestrogen deficiency symptoms and the prevention of osteoporosis -

- Women experiencing a natural menopause should commence treatment with Livial at least 12 months after their last natural bleed.
- Women experiencing a surgical menopause may commence treatment with Livial immediately.
- Women being treated with gonadotrophin releasing hormone (GnRH) analogues, for example, for endometriosis, may commence treatment with Livial immediately.

Switching from a Sequential or Continuous-combined HRT preparation

- If changing from a Sequential HRT preparation, the endometrium may already be stimulated, so induction of a withdrawal bleed with a progestogen is advisable. Treatment with Livial should start right after the withdrawal bleeding has ended.
- If changing from a Continuous-combined HRT preparation, treatment can start at any time.

Missed pills

A missed dose should be taken as soon as remembered, unless it is more than 12 hours overdue. In the latter case, the missed dose should be skipped and the next dose should be taken at the normal time.

Missing a dose may increase the likelihood of breakthrough bleeding and spotting.

Children

Not applicable.

4.3 Contraindications
- Pregnancy or lactation;
- Known, past or suspected breast cancer;
- Known or suspected oestrogen-dependent malignant tumours. (e.g. endometrial cancer);
- Undiagnosed vaginal bleeding;
- Untreated endometrial hyperplasia;
- Previous idiopathic or current venous thromboembolism (deep venous thrombosis, pulmonary embolism);
- Active or recent arterial thromboembolic disease (e.g. angina, myocardial infarction);

- Acute liver disease, or a history of liver disease as long as liver function tests have failed to return to normal;

- Known hypersensitivity to the active substance, or to any of the excipients;

- Porphyria.

4.4 Special warnings and special precautions for use

Women experiencing a natural menopause should commence treatment with Livial at least 12 months after their last natural bleed.

Medical examination and follow up

Before initiating or reinstituting Livial, a complete personal and family medical history should be taken. Physical (including pelvic and breast) examination should be guided by this and by the contraindications and warnings for use.

In women with an intact uterus, the benefits of the lower risk of endometrial hyperplasia and endometrial cancer due to adding a progestogen should be weighed against any increased risk of breast cancer. (*Livial has progestogenic actions in the endometrium. Therefore a separate progestogen is not needed with Livial treatment. see "Endometrial hyperplasia" below and section 4.8.)*

During treatment, periodic check-ups are recommended of a frequency and nature adapted to the individual woman. Women should be advised what changes in their breasts should be reported to their doctor or nurse (See "Breast cancer" below). Investigations, including mammography, should be carried out in accordance with currently accepted screening practices, modified to the clinical needs of the individual. A careful appraisal of the risks and benefits should be undertaken at least annually in women treated with Livial.

Conditions which need supervision

If any of the following conditions are present, have occurred previously and/or have been aggravated during pregnancy or previous hormone treatment, the patient should be closely supervised. It should be taken into account that these conditions may recur or be aggravated during treatment with Livial, in particular:

- Leiomyoma (uterine fibroids) or endometriosis;

- A history of, or risk factors for, thromboembolic disorders (see below);

- Risk factors for oestrogen dependent tumours, e.g. 1st degree heredity for breast cancer;

- Hypertension;

- Liver disorders (e.g. liver adenoma);

- Diabetes mellitus with or without vascular involvement;

- Cholelithiasis;

- Migraine or (severe) headache;

- Systemic lupus erythematosis;

- A history of endometrial hyperplasia (see below);

- Epilepsy;

- Asthma;

- Otosclerosis.

Reasons for immediate withdrawal of therapy:

Therapy should be discontinued when a contra-indication is discovered and in the following situations:

– Jaundice or deterioration in liver function;

– Significant increase in blood pressure;

– New onset of migraine-type headache;

Endometrial hyperplasia

– The risk of endometrial hyperplasia and carcinoma is increased when oestrogens are administered alone for prolonged periods. The addition of a progestogen for at least 12 days of the cycle in non-hysterectomised women reduces, but may not eliminate, this risk (see Section 4.8).

– Livial has progestogenic actions in the endometrium. Therefore a separate progestogen is not needed with Livial treatment.

– Observational study data on the endometrial safety of tibolone are inconclusive.

– Break-through bleeding and spotting may occur during the first months of treatment. If break-through bleeding or spotting is present after some time on therapy, or continued after treatment has been discontinued, the reason should be investigated, which may include endometrial biopsy to exclude endometrial malignancy.

Breast cancer

– Randomised controlled trials and epidemiological studies have reported an increased risk of breast cancer in women taking oestrogens or oestrogen-progestogen combinations for HRT for several years (see Section 4.8). A large observational study has shown that, compared to never-users, use of oestrogen-progestogen combined HRT is associated with a higher risk of breast cancer (RR = 2.00, 95%CI: 1.88-2.12) than use of estrogens alone (RR = 1.30, 95%CI: 1.21-1.40) or tibolone (RR = 1.45, 95%CI: 1.25-1.68).

For all HRT, an excess risk becomes apparent within 1-2 years of starting treatment and increases with duration of use of HRT but begins to decline when HRT is stopped and by 5 years reaches the same level as in women who have never taken HRT.

At present the effect of HRT on the diagnosis of breast tumours remains unclear – all women should be encouraged to report any changes in their breasts to their doctor or nurse.

Venous thromboembolism

– HRT is associated with a higher relative risk of developing venous thromboembolism (VTE), i.e. deep vein thrombosis or pulmonary embolism. One randomised controlled trial and epidemiological studies found a two- to threefold higher risk for users compared with non-users. For non-users, it is estimated that the number of cases of VTE that will occur over a 5 year period is about 3 per 1000 women aged 50-59 years and 8 per 1000 women aged between 60-69 years. It is estimated that in healthy women who use HRT for 5 years, the number of additional cases of VTE over a 5 year period will be between 2 and 6 (best estimate =4) per 1000 women aged 50-59 years and between 5 and 15 (best estimate = 9) per 1000 women aged 60-69 years. The occurrence of such an event is more likely in the first year of HRT than later.

– It is unknown whether Livial carries the same level of risk.

– Generally recognised risk factors for VTE include a personal history or family history, severe obesity (BMI> 30 kg/m2) and systemic lupus erythematosus (SLE). There is no consensus about the possible role of varicose veins in VTE.

– Patients with a history of VTE or known thrombophilic states have an increased risk of VTE. HRT may add to this risk. Personal or strong family history of thromboembolism or recurrent spontaneous abortion should be investigated in order to exclude a thrombophilic predisposition. Until a thorough evaluation of thrombophilic factors has been made or anticoagulant treatment initiated, use of HRT in such patients should be viewed as contraindicated. Those women already on anticoagulant treatment require careful consideration of the benefit-risk of use of HRT.

– The risk of VTE may be temporarily increased with prolonged immobilisation, major trauma or major surgery. As in all postoperative patients, scrupulous attention should be given to prophylactic measures to prevent VTE following surgery. Where prolonged immobilisation is liable to follow elective surgery, particularly abdominal or orthopaedic surgery to the lower limbs, consideration should be given to temporarily stopping HRT 4 to 6 weeks earlier, if possible. Treatment should not be restarted until the woman is completely mobilised.

– If VTE develops after initiating therapy, the drug should be discontinued. Patients should be told to contact their doctors immediately when they are aware of a potential thromboembolic symptom (eg, painful swelling of a leg, sudden pain in the chest, dyspnea).

Coronary artery disease (CAD)

– There is no evidence from randomised controlled trials of cardiovascular benefit with continuous combined conjugated oestrogens and MPA. Large clinical trials showed a possible increased risk of cardiovascular morbidity in the first year of use and no benefit thereafter. For other HRT products there are as yet no randomised controlled trials to date examining benefit in cardiovascular morbidity or mortality. Therefore it is uncertain whether these findings also extend to other HRT products, or tibolone.

-Stroke

- One large randomised clinical trial (WHI-trial) found, as a secondary outcome, an increased risk of stroke in healthy women during treatment with continuous combined conjugated oestrogens and MPA. For women who do not use HRT, it is estimated that the number of cases of stroke that will occur over a 5 year period is about 3 per 1000 women aged 50-59 years and 11 per 1000 women aged 60-69 years. It is estimated that for women who use conjugated oestrogens and MPA for 5 years, the number of additional cases will be between 0 and 3 (best estimate=1) per 1000 users aged 50-59 and between 1 and 9 (best estimate = 4) per 1000 users aged 60-69. It is unknown whether the increased risk also extends to other HRT products, or tibolone.

-Ovarian cancer

- Long-term (at least 5 to 10 years) use of oestrogen-only HRT products in hysterectomised women has been associated with an increased risk of ovarian cancer in some epidemiological studies. It is uncertain whether long-term use of combined HRT, or tibolone, confers a different risk than oestrogen-only products.

-Other conditions

- Oestrogens may cause fluid retention, and therefore patients with cardiac or renal dysfunction should be carefully observed.

- Women with pre-existing hypertriglyceridaemia should be followed closely during oestrogen replacement or hormone replacement therapy, since rare cases of large increases of plasma triglycerides leading to pancreatitis have been reported with oestrogen therapy in this condition.

- Treatment with Livial results in a very minor decrease of thyroid binding globulin (TBG) and total T4. Levels of total T3 are unaltered. Livial decreases the level of sex-hormone-binding globulin (SHBG), whereas the levels of corticoid binding globulin (CBG) and circulating cortisol are unaffected.

- Livial is not intended for contraceptive use.

- Patients with rare hereditary problems of galactose intolerance, the Lapp lactase deficiency or glucose-galactose malabsorption should not take this medicine.

4.5 Interaction with other medicinal products and other forms of Interaction

No examples of interactions between Livial and other medicines have been reported in clinical practice. However, the following potential interactions should be considered on a theoretical basis:

Enzyme inducing compounds such as barbiturates, carbamazepine, hydantoins and rifampicin may enhance the metabolism of tibolone and thus decrease its therapeutic effect.

Since Livial may increase blood fibrinolytic activity (lower fibrinogen levels, higher antithrombin III, plasminogen and fibrinolytic activity values) it may enhance the effect of anticoagulants, such as warfarin. Therefore the simultaneous use of Livial and warfarin should be monitored, especially when starting or stopping concurrent Livial treatment, and the warfarin dose should be appropriately adjusted.

4.6 Pregnancy and lactation

Livial is contraindicated during pregnancy and lactation (See section 4.3).

If pregnancy occurs during medication with Livial, treatment should be withdrawn immediately. For Livial no clinical data on exposed pregnancies are available.

Studies in animals have shown reproductive toxicity (see Section 5.3). The potential risk for humans is unknown.

The results of most epidemiological studies to date relevant to inadvertent foetal exposure to combinations of estrogens with progestogens indicate no teratogenic or foetotoxic effects

4.7 Effects on ability to drive and use machines

Livial is not known to have any effects on alertness and concentration.

4.8 Undesirable effects

Occasionally, vaginal bleeding or spotting may occur, mainly during the first months of treatment. Other adverse events that have been observed occasionally include:

dizziness, rash, pruritus, seborrhoeic dermatosis,, headache, migraine, visual disturbances (including blurred vision), gastrointestinal upset, depression, oedema, effects on the musculoskeletal system such as arthralgia or myalgia and changes in liver function parameters.

Clinical Trials Experience

This section describes undesirable effects, which were registered in 16 placebo-controlled studies, with 1463 women receiving therapeutic doses of tibolone, and 855 women receiving placebo. The duration of treatment in these studies ranged from 2 to 24 months. The following undesirable effects occurred statistically significantly more frequently during treatment with tibolone than with placebo.

Table 1 Undesirable effects of Livial

System organ class	**Common** >1%,<10%	**Uncommon** >0.1%,<1%
Gastro-intestinal disorders	Abdominal pain#	
Metabolic and nutritional disorders	Weight increase	
Reproductive disorders, female	Vaginal bleeding or spotting# Leukorrhoea Breast pain# Genital pruritus Genital moniliasis Vaginitis	
Skin and appendages disorders	Hypertrichosis	
Central and peripheral nervous system disorders		Amnesia

#Undesirable effects that occurred mainly during the first months of treatment and then subsided.

The risk of breast cancer increases with the number of years of HRT usage. According to data from a recent epidemiological study in about 829,000 postmenopausal women, the best estimate of the risk is that for women not using HRT, in total about 32 women in every 1000 women are expected to have breast cancer diagnosed between the ages of 50 and 65 years. Among those with current or recent use of oestrogen-only replacement therapy, it is estimated that the total number of additional cases during the corresponding period will be between 0 and 3 (best estimate = 1.5) per 1000 for 5 years use and between 3 and 7 (best estimate = 5) per 1000 for 10 years use (see table below).

Among those with current or recent use of oestrogen plus progestogen combined HRT, it is estimated that the total number of additional cases will be between 5 and 7 (best estimate = 6) per 1000 for 5 years use and between 18 and

20 (best estimate = 19) per 1000 for 10 years use (see section 4.4).

	No of additional cases of breast cancer diagnosed per 1000 users (95% confidence intervals)	
Type of HRT	**5 years of use**	**10 years of use**
Oestrogen-only	1.5 (0 - 3)	5 (3 - 7)
Combined	6 (5 – 7)	19 (18 – 20)

For tibolone, the increased risk in this study, compared with never-use (RR = 1.45; 95%CI 1.25-1.68) lies between that for oestrogen-only HRT (RR = 1.30; 95%CI 1.21-1.40) and combined oestrogen plus progestogen HRT (RR = 2.00; 95%CI 1.88-2.12).

The number of additional cases of breast cancer is broadly similar for women who start HRT irrespective of age at start of HRT use (between the ages of 45 - 65).

There have been reports of endometrial hyperplasia and endometrial cancer in patients treated with tibolone although a causal relationship has not been established.

Other adverse reactions reported in association with estrogen-progestogen treatment are:

- Estrogen-dependent neoplasms benign and malignant;
- Venous thromboembolism, i.e. deep leg or pelvic venous thrombosis and pulmonary embolism, is more frequent among hormone replacement therapy users than among non-users. For further information, see Section 4.3 Contraindications and 4.4 Special warnings and precautions for use;
- Myocardial infarction and stroke;
- Gall bladder disease;
- Skin and subcutaneous disorders: chloasma, erythema multiforme, erythema nodosum, vascular purpura.

4.9 Overdose

The acute toxicity of tibolone in animals is very low. Therefore toxic symptoms are not expected to occur even when several tablets are taken simultaneously. In cases of acute overdose, nausea, vomiting and withdrawal bleeding in females may develop. No specific antidote is known. Symptomatic treatment can be given if necessary.

5. PHARMACOLOGICAL PROPERTIES

5.1 Pharmacodynamic properties

ATC code: GO3D C05 urogenital system (including sex hormones)

After oral administration tibolone is rapidly metabolised into three compounds which all contribute to the pharmacological effects of Livial. Two of these metabolites (3α-OH-tibolone and 3β-OH-tibolone) have oestrogen-like activity, whereas the third metabolite (Δ4-isomer of tibolone) and the parent compound have predominantly progestogenic and androgenic activities.

In vitro studies suggest that tibolone is subject to tissue-selective local metabolism, with the Δ4-isomer mainly formed in endometrial tissue, and local effects on enzyme systems in breast tissue.

Tibolone substitutes for the loss of estrogen production in postmenopausal women, and alleviates menopausal symptoms. Livial prevents bone loss following menopause or ovariectomy.

Clinical trial information on Livial:

- Relief of estrogen-deficiency symptoms

- Improvement of symptoms generally occurs within a few weeks, but optimal results are obtained when therapy is continued for at least 3 months.

- Effects on the endometrium and bleeding patterns

- In the endometrium, tibolone and its estrogenic 3β-OH metabolite are converted to the progestogenic/androgenic Δ4-isomer. In addition, the Δ4-isomer cannot be reduced by the 5α-reductase enzyme to a less active progestogen. This considerably prolongs the presence of the Δ4-isomer and thus the progestogenic activity in the endometrium.

- The incidence of vaginal bleeding is no higher than that with placebo use. In women in whom some endogenous oestrogen is still produced, vaginal bleeding may occur during Livial therapy because of an apparently stimulated endometrium.

- Amenorrhea was seen in 88.4% of the women after 9 months of Livial treatment. Break through bleeding and/or spotting appeared in 32.6% of the women during the first three months of treatment and in 11.6% during the last 3 months of the 12 months observation period.

- Prevention of osteoporosis

- Estrogen deficiency at menopause is associated with an increasing bone turnover and decline in bone mass. Therefore, if possible, treatment for prevention of osteoporosis should start as soon as possible after the onset of menopause in women with increased risk for future osteoporotic fractures.

Protection appears to be effective for as long as treatment is continued.

- After 2 years of treatment with Livial, the increase in lumbar spine bone mineral density (BMD) was 2.6 ± 3.8%. The percentage of women who maintained or gained BMD in lumbar zone during treatment was 76%. A second study confirmed these results.

- Livial also had an effect on hip BMD. In one study, the increase after 2 years was 0.7 ± 3.9% at the femoral neck and 1.7 ± 3.0% at the total hip. The percentage of women who maintained or gained BMD in the hip region during treatment was 72.5%. A second study showed that the increase after 2 years was 1.3 ± 5.1% at the femoral neck and 2.9 ± 3.4% at the total hip. The percentage of women who maintained or gained BMD in the hip region during treatment was 84.7%.

- Effects on the breast

- *In vitro* data indicate that, in the breast, tibolone inhibits the sulfatase enzyme thereby reducing the levels of active estrogens in this tissue. In clinical studies mammographic density is not increased in women treated with Livial compared to placebo.

5.2 Pharmacokinetic properties

Following oral administration tibolone is rapidly and extensively absorbed.

The consumption of food has no significant effects on the extent of absorption.

Due to rapid metabolism the plasma levels of tibolone are very low.

The plasma levels of the Δ4-isomer of tibolone are also very low. Therefore some of the pharmacokinetic parameters could not be determined. Peak plasma levels of the 3α-OH and the 3β-OH metabolites are higher but accumulation does not occur.

Table 2 Pharmacokinetic parameters of Livial

(see Table 2 below)

Excretion of tibolone is mainly in the form of conjugated (mostly sulfated) metabolites. Part of the administered compound is excreted in the urine, but most is eliminated via the faeces.

The pharmacokinetic parameters for tibolone and its metabolites were found to be independent of renal function.

5.3 Preclinical safety data

Livial is not genotoxic. Although a carcinogenic effect was seen in certain strains of rat (hepatic tumours) and mouse (bladder tumours), the relevance of this evidence to man is uncertain.

In animal studies, tibolone had anti-fertility and embryotoxic activities by virtue of its hormonal properties. Tibolone was not teratogenic in mice and rats. It displayed teratogenic potential in the rabbit at near-abortive dosages. (See Section 4.6)

6. PHARMACEUTICAL PARTICULARS

6.1 List of excipients

Potato starch, magnesium stearate, ascorbyl palmitate and lactose.

6.2 Incompatibilities

None stated

6.3 Shelf life

When stored as indicated in 6.4 the tablets can be stored for up to two years.

6.4 Special precautions for storage

Livial tablets should be stored at room temperature (below 25°C), protected from moisture and light.

6.5 Nature and contents of container

Press-through strips of 28 or 30 tablets each containing 2.5mg of tibolone.

Cartons containing 1 strip or 3 strips.

6.6 Instructions for use and handling

Not applicable

7. MARKETING AUTHORISATION HOLDER

Organon Laboratories Limited, Science Park, Milton Road, Cambridge, CB4 OFL

8. MARKETING AUTHORISATION NUMBER(S)

0065/0086

9. DATE OF FIRST AUTHORISATION/RENEWAL OF THE AUTHORISATION

March 1991

10. DATE OF REVISION OF THE TEXT

December 2003

USLIV v10.5

Table 2 Pharmacokinetic parameters of Livial

	tibolone		3 α -OH metabolite		3 β -OH metabolite		Δ 4-isomer	
	SD	MD	SD	MD	SD	MD	SD	MD
C_{max} (ng/ml)	1.37	1.72	14.23	14.15	3.43	3.75	0.47	0.43
$C_{average}$	–	–	–	1.88	–	–	–	–
T_{max} (h)	1.08	1.19	1.21	1.15	1.37	1.35	1.64	1.65
$T_{1/2}$ (h)	–	–	5.78	7.71	5.87	–	–	–
C_{min} (ng/ml)	–	–	–	0.23	–	–	–	–
AUC_{0-24} (ng/ml.h)	–	–	53.23	44.73	16.23	9.20	–	–

SD = single dose; MD = multiple dose

Loceryl 0.25% Cream

(Galderma (U.K.) Ltd)

1. NAME OF THE MEDICINAL PRODUCT

Loceryl 0.25% cream

2. QUALITATIVE AND QUANTITATIVE COMPOSITION

Loceryl cream contains 0.25% w/w amorolfine in the form of hydrochloride. Amorolfine is chemically described as *cis*-4-[(RS)-3[4-(1,1-Dimethylpropyl)phenyl]-2-methylpropyl]-2,6-dimethylmorpholine.

Amorolfine hydrochloride HSE 0.279 w/w

(equivalent to 0.25% w/w base)

3. PHARMACEUTICAL FORM

Cream.

4. CLINICAL PARTICULARS

4.1 Therapeutic indications

Dermatomycoses caused by dermatophytes: tinea pedis (athlete's foot), tinea cruris, tinea inguinalis, tinea corporis, tinea manuum. Pityriasis versicolor.

4.2 Posology and method of administration

Dermatomycoses

Cream: To be applied to affected skin areas once daily following cleansing (in the evening).

The treatment should be continued without interruption until clinical cure, and for 3 - 5 days thereafter. The required duration of treatment depends on the species of fungi and on the localisation of the infection. In general, treatment should be continued for at least two to three weeks. With foot mycoses, up to six weeks of therapy may be necessary.

Elderly

There are no specific dosage recommendations for use in elderly patients.

Children

There are no specific dosage recommendations for children owing to the lack of clinical experience available to date.

4.3 Contraindications

Loceryl cream must not be reused by patients who have shown hypersensitivity to the treatment.

No experience exists of use during pregnancy and nursing, therefore, the use of Loceryl should be avoided during pregnancy and lactation.

4.4 Special warnings and special precautions for use

Avoid contact of Loceryl cream with eyes, ears and mucous membranes.

4.5 Interaction with other medicinal products and other forms of Interaction

There are no specific studies involving concomitant treatment with other topical medicines. Use of nail varnish or artificial nails should be avoided during treatment.

4.6 Pregnancy and lactation

Reproductive toxicology studies showed no evidence of teratogenicity in laboratory animals but embryotoxicity was observed at high oral doses. The systemic absorption of amorolfine during and after topical administration is very low and therefore the risk to the human foetus appears to be negligible. However, because there is no relevant experience Loceryl should be avoided during pregnancy and breast feeding.

4.7 Effects on ability to drive and use machines

None.

4.8 Undesirable effects

Rarely, skin irritation - presenting as erythema, pruritus or a burning sensation - has occurred during treatment with the cream. In exceptional cases, a slight, transient burning sensation in the area of the nails was observed after the application of nail lacquer.

4.9 Overdose

Accidental oral Ingestion

Loceryl is for topical use. In the event of accidental oral ingestion, an appropriate method of gastric emptying may be used.

5. PHARMACOLOGICAL PROPERTIES

5.1 Pharmacodynamic properties

Loceryl is a topical antimycotic. Amorolfine belongs to a new chemical class, and its fungicidal action is based on an alteration of the fungal cell membrane targeted primarily on sterol biosynthesis. The ergosterol content is reduced, and at the same time unusual sterically nonplanar sterols accumulate.

Amorolfine is a broad spectrum antimycotic. It is highly active (MIC < 2mcg/ml) *in vitro* against

yeasts:Candida, Cryptococcus, Malassezia

dermatophytes: Trichophyton, Microsporum, Epidermophyton

moulds: Hendersonula, Alternaria, Scopulariopsis

dematiacea: Cladosporium, Fonsecaea, Wangiella

dimorphic fungi: Coccidioides, Histoplasma, Sporothrix

With the exception of *Actinomyces*, bacteria are not sensitive to amorolfine. *Propionibacterium acnes* is only slightly sensitive.

5.2 Pharmacokinetic properties

Amorolfine from cream penetrates into the stratum corneum. Nevertheless, systemic absorption is extremely low during and after therapeutic use.

5.3 Preclinical safety data

None stated.

6. PHARMACEUTICAL PARTICULARS

6.1 List of excipients

Polyoxyl 40 stearate, stearyl alcohol, paraffin liquid, white soft paraffin, carbomer, sodium hydroxide, disodium edetate, 2 phenoxyethanol.

6.2 Incompatibilities

None.

6.3 Shelf life

3 years.

6.4 Special precautions for storage

Loceryl cream should be stored below 30°C.

6.5 Nature and contents of container

20g collapsible aluminium tube, sealed with an aluminium membrane and fitted with a plastic screw cap.

6.6 Instructions for use and handling

No special instructions.

7. MARKETING AUTHORISATION HOLDER

Galderma (UK) Limited

Galderma House

Church Lane

Kings Langley

Herts. WD4 8JP

8. MARKETING AUTHORISATION NUMBER(S)

PL 10590/0041

9. DATE OF FIRST AUTHORISATION/RENEWAL OF THE AUTHORISATION

April 1999

10. DATE OF REVISION OF THE TEXT

May 2001

Loceryl Nail Lacquer 5%

(Galderma (U.K.) Ltd)

1. NAME OF THE MEDICINAL PRODUCT

Loceryl Nail Lacquer 5%.

2. QUALITATIVE AND QUANTITATIVE COMPOSITION

Loceryl nail lacquer contains 5% w/v amorolfine in the form of hydrochloride. Amorolfine is chemically described as *cis*-4-[(RS)-3[4-(1,1-Dimethylpropyl)phenyl]-2-methylpropyl]-2,6-dimethylmorpholine.

Amorolfine hydrochloride HSE 6.40 w/w

3. PHARMACEUTICAL FORM

Lacquer.

4. CLINICAL PARTICULARS

4.1 Therapeutic indications

Onychomycoses caused by dermatophytes, yeasts and moulds.

4.2 Posology and method of administration

The nail lacquer should be applied to the affected finger or toe nails once weekly. Twice weekly application may prove beneficial in some cases.

The patient should apply the nail lacquer as follows:

1. Before the first application of Loceryl, it is essential that the affected areas of nail (particularly the nail surfaces) should be filed down as thoroughly as possible using the nail file supplied. The surface of the nail should then be cleansed and degreased using a cleaning pad (as supplied). Before repeat application of Loceryl, the affected nails should be filed down again as required, following cleansing with a cleaning pad to remove any remaining lacquer.

Caution: Nail files used for affected nails must not be used for healthy nails.

2. With one of the reusable applicators supplied, apply the nail lacquer to the entire surface of the affected nails and allow it to dry. After use, clean the applicator with the same cleaning pad used before for nail cleaning. Keep the bottle tightly closed.

For each nail to be treated, dip the applicator into the nail lacquer without wiping off any of the lacquer on the bottle neck.

Caution: When working with organic solvents (thinners, white spirit, etc.) wear impermeable gloves in order to protect the Loceryl lacquer on the nails.

Treatment should be continued without interruption until the nail is regenerated and the affected areas are finally cured. The required frequency and duration of treatment depends essentially on intensity and localisation of the infection. In general, it is six months (finger nails) and nine to twelve months (toe nails). A review of the treatment is recommended at intervals of approximately three months.

Co-existent tinea pedis should be treated with an appropriate antimycotic cream.

Elderly

There are no specific dosage recommendations for use in elderly patients.

Children

There are no specific dosage recommendations for children owing to the lack of clinical experience available to date.

4.3 Contraindications

Loceryl nail lacquer must not be reused by patients who have shown hypersensitivity to the treatment.

No experience exists of use during pregnancy and nursing, therefore, the use of Loceryl should be avoided during pregnancy and lactation.

4.4 Special warnings and special precautions for use

Avoid contact of the lacquer with eyes, ears and mucous membranes.

4.5 Interaction with other medicinal products and other forms of Interaction

There are no specific studies involving concomitant treatment with other topical medicines.

Use of nail varnish or artificial nails should be avoided during treatment.

4.6 Pregnancy and lactation

Reproductive toxicology studies showed no evidence of teratogenicity in laboratory animals but embryotoxicity was observed at high oral doses. The systemic absorption of amorolfine during and after topical administration is very low and therefore the risk to the human foetus appears to be negligible. However, because there is no relevant experience, Loceryl should be avoided during pregnancy and breast feeding.

4.7 Effects on ability to drive and use machines

None.

4.8 Undesirable effects

In exceptional cases, a slight, transient burning sensation in the area of the nails was observed after the application of nail lacquer.

Rare cases of nail disorders, i.e. nail discoloration, broken nails, brittle nails have been reported during treatment with Loceryl Nail Lacquer. However, these reactions can also be linked to the onychomycosis itself.

4.9 Overdose

Accidental oral ingestion

Loceryl is for topical use. In the event of accidental oral ingestion, an appropriate method of gastric emptying may be used.

5. PHARMACOLOGICAL PROPERTIES

5.1 Pharmacodynamic properties

Loceryl is a topical antimycotic. Amorolfine belongs to a new chemical class, and its fungicidal action is based on an alteration of the fungal cell membrane targeted primarily on sterol biosynthesis. The ergosterol content is reduced, and at the same time unusual sterically nonplanar sterols accumulate.

Amorolfine is a broad spectrum antimycotic. It is highly active (MIC < 2mcg/ml) *in vitro* against

yeasts:Candida, Cryptococcus, Malassezia

dermatophytes: Trichophyton, Microsporum, Epidermophyton

moulds: Hendersonula, Alternaria, Scopulariopsis

dematiacea: Cladosporium, Fonsecaea, Wangiella

dimorphic fungi: Coccidioides, Histoplasma, Sporothrix

With the exception of *Actinomyces*, bacteria are not sensitive to amorolfine. *Propionibacterium acnes* is only slightly sensitive.

5.2 Pharmacokinetic properties

Amorolfine from nail lacquer penetrates into and diffuses through the nail plate and is thus able to eradicate poorly accessible fungi in the nail bed. Systemic absorption of the active ingredient is very low with this type of application.

Following prolonged use of Loceryl Nail Lacquer, there is no indication of drug accumulation in the body.

5.3 Preclinical safety data

None stated.

6. PHARMACEUTICAL PARTICULARS

6.1 List of excipients

Ammonio methacrylate copolymer A, triacetin, butyl acetate, ethyl acetate, ethanol absolute.

6.2 Incompatibilities

None.

6.3 Shelf life

3 years.

6.4 Special precautions for storage

Loceryl nail lacquer should be stored below 30°C. Protect from heat. Keep bottle tightly closed after use.

6.5 Nature and contents of container

Amber glass container with screw thread and plastic screw closure.

Pack Sizes: 5.0 ml (1 × 5.0 ml)

All packs contain cleansing swabs, spatulas and nail files.

6.6 Instructions for use and handling

No special instructions.

Administrative Data

7. MARKETING AUTHORISATION HOLDER

Galderma (UK) Limited

Galderma House

Church Lane

Kings Langley

Herts. WD4 8JP

United Kingdom

8. MARKETING AUTHORISATION NUMBER(S)

PL 10590/0042

9. DATE OF FIRST AUTHORISATION/RENEWAL OF THE AUTHORISATION

April 1999

10. DATE OF REVISION OF THE TEXT

December 2004

Loceryl Nail Lacquer is a registered trade mark

Locoid C Cream

(Astellas Pharma Limited)

1. NAME OF THE MEDICINAL PRODUCT

LOCOID C CREAM

2. QUALITATIVE AND QUANTITATIVE COMPOSITION

Contains 0.1% w/w hydrocortisone butyrate and 3.0% w/w chlorquinaldol.

For excipients, see 6.1

3. PHARMACEUTICAL FORM

Cream

Buff to white aqueous-based cream.

4. CLINICAL PARTICULARS

4.1 Therapeutic indications

The product is recommended for clinical use in the treatment of conditions responsive to topical corticosteroids e.g. eczema, dermatitis and psoriasis where there is concurrent infection by a micro-organism susceptible to chlorquinaldol, or where such infection is to be prevented.

Topical corticosteroids are not generally indicated in psoriasis but may be acceptable in psoriasis excluding widespread plaque psoriasis provided warnings are given, see section 4.4 Special warnings and special precautions for use.

4.2 Posology and method of administration

For topical application.

Dosage: To be applied evenly and sparingly two or three times daily.

Application may be made under occlusion in the more resistant lesions such as thickened psoriatic plaques on elbows and knees.

Adults and the Elderly: The same dose is used for adults and the elderly, as clinical evidence would indicate that no special dosage regimen is necessary in the elderly.

Children: Long term treatment should be avoided where possible.

Infants: Therapy should be limited if possible to a maximum of seven days.

4.3 Contraindications

Hypersensitivity to hydrocortisone or to any of the ingredients of the cream.

This preparation is contraindicated in the presence of untreated viral or fungal infections, tubercular or syphilitic lesions, peri-oral dermatitis, acne vulgaris and rosacea and in bacterial infections (other than those responsive to topical chlorquinaldol at the site of application) unless used in connection with appropriate chemotherapy.

4.4 Special warnings and special precautions for use

Although generally regarded as safe, even for long-term administration in adults, there is a potential for adverse effects if over used in infancy. Extreme caution is required in dermatoses of infancy including napkin eruption. In such patients courses of treatment should not normally exceed 7 days.

Application under occlusion should be restricted to dermatoses involving limited areas.

As with all corticosteroids, application to the face, flexures and other areas of thin skin may cause skin atrophy and increased absorption and should be avoided.

Topical corticosteroids may be hazardous in psoriasis for a number of reasons including rebound relapses following development of tolerance, risk of generalised pustular psoriasis and local and systemic toxicity due to impaired barrier function of the skin. Steroids may have a place in psoriasis of the scalp and chronic plaque psoriasis of the hands and feet. Careful patient supervision is important.

Keep away from the eyes.

4.5 Interaction with other medicinal products and other forms of Interaction

None known.

4.6 Pregnancy and lactation

There is inadequate evidence of safety in human pregnancy. Topical administration of corticosteroids to pregnant animals can cause abnormalities of foetal development including cleft palate and intra-uterine growth retardation. There may therefore be a very small risk of such effects in the human foetus.

Theoretically, there is the possibility that if maternal systemic absorption occurred the infant's adrenal function could be affected.

The use of topical corticosteroids during lactation is unlikely to present a hazard to infants being breast-fed.

4.7 Effects on ability to drive and use machines

None known.

4.8 Undesirable effects

Local atrophic changes may occur in intertriginous areas or in nappy areas in young children where moist conditions favour hydrocortisone absorption. Systemic absorption from such sites may be sufficient to produce hypercorticism and suppression of the pituitary adrenal axis after prolonged treatment. This effect is more likely to occur in infants and children and if occlusive dressings are used or large areas of skin treated.

4.9 Overdose

Excessive use under occlusive dressings may produce adrenal suppression. No special procedures or antidote. Treat any adverse effects symptomatically.

5. PHARMACOLOGICAL PROPERTIES

5.1 Pharmacodynamic properties

The active substance is a well-established topical corticosteroid, with an activity classified as potent.

Chlorquinaldol is an established anti-infectious agent with an anti-bacterial and anti-fungal activity.

5.2 Pharmacokinetic properties

In-vivo studies have demonstrated the topical activity of the product, e.g. by the McKenzie-Stoughton test.

Chlorquinaldol acts topically at the site of application.

5.3 Preclinical safety data

No relevant pre-clinical safety data has been generated

6. PHARMACEUTICAL PARTICULARS

6.1 List of excipients

Macrogol cetostearyl ether

Cetostearyl alcohol

Light liquid paraffin

White soft paraffin

Sodium citrate (anhydrous)

Citric acid (anhydrous)

Purified water

6.2 Incompatibilities

None stated.

6.3 Shelf life

4 years

6.4 Special precautions for storage

Do not store above 25°C.

6.5 Nature and contents of container

Collapsible aluminium tube with plastic screw cap containing

30g or 50g.

6.6 Instructions for use and handling

No special requirements.

7. MARKETING AUTHORISATION HOLDER

Yamanouchi Pharma Ltd

Yamanouchi House

Pyrford Road

West Byfleet

Surrey

KT14 6RA

United Kingdom

8. MARKETING AUTHORISATION NUMBER(S)

Product Licence 0166/0056

9. DATE OF FIRST AUTHORISATION/RENEWAL OF THE AUTHORISATION

First authorisation granted 31 January 1980

Renewal granted 22 February 2001

10. DATE OF REVISION OF THE TEXT

December 2003

11. LEGAL CATEGORY

POM

Locoid C Ointment

(Astellas Pharma Limited)

1. NAME OF THE MEDICINAL PRODUCT

LOCOID C OINTMENT

2. QUALITATIVE AND QUANTITATIVE COMPOSITION

Contains 0.1% w/w hydrocortisone butyrate and 3.0% w/w chlorquinaldol.

For excipients, see 6.1

3. PHARMACEUTICAL FORM

Ointment

Buff coloured, translucent soft fatty ointment.

4. CLINICAL PARTICULARS

4.1 Therapeutic indications

The product is recommended for clinical use in the treatment of conditions responsive to topical corticosteroids e.g. eczema, dermatitis and psoriasis where there is concurrent infection by a micro-organism susceptible to chlorquinaldol, or where such infection is to be prevented.

Topical corticosteroids are not generally indicated in psoriasis but may be acceptable in psoriasis excluding widespread plaque psoriasis provided warnings are given, see section 4.4 Special warnings and special precautions for use.

4.2 Posology and method of administration

For topical application.

Dosage: To be applied evenly and sparingly two or three times daily.

Application may be made under occlusion in the more resistant lesions such as thickened psoriatic plaques on elbows and knees.

Adults and the Elderly: The same dose is used for adults and the elderly, as clinical advice would indicate that no special dosage regimen is necessary in the elderly.

Children: Long term treatment should be avoided where possible.

Infants: Therapy should be limited if possible to a maximum of seven days.

4.3 Contraindications

Hypersensitivity to hydrocortisone or to any of the ingredients of the ointment.

This preparation is contraindicated in the presence of untreated viral or fungal infections, tubercular or syphilitic lesions, peri-oral dermatitis, acne vulgaris and rosacea and in bacterial infections (other than those responsive to topical chlorquinaldol at the site of application) unless used in connection with appropriate chemotherapy.

4.4 Special warnings and special precautions for use

Although generally regarded as safe, even for long-term administration in adults, there is a potential for adverse effects if over used in infancy. Extreme caution is required in dermatoses of infancy including napkin eruption. In such patients courses of treatment should not normally exceed 7 days.

Application under occlusion should be restricted to dermatoses involving limited areas.

As with all corticosteroids, application to the face, flexures and other areas of thin skin may cause skin atrophy and increased absorption and should be avoided.

Topical corticosteroids may be hazardous in psoriasis for a number of reasons including rebound relapses following development of tolerance, risk of generalised pustular psoriasis and local and systemic toxicity due to impaired barrier function of the skin. Steroids may have a place in psoriasis of the scalp and chronic plaque psoriasis of the hands and feet. Careful patient supervision is important.

Keep away from the eyes.

4.5 Interaction with other medicinal products and other forms of Interaction

None known.

4.6 Pregnancy and lactation

There is inadequate evidence of safety in human pregnancy. Topical administration of corticosteroids to pregnant animals can cause abnormalities of foetal development including cleft palate and intra-uterine growth retardation. There may therefore be a very small risk of such effects in the human foetus.

Theoretically, there is the possibility that if maternal systemic absorption occurred the infant's adrenal function could be affected.

The use of topical corticosteroids during lactation is unlikely to present a hazard to infants being breast-fed.

4.7 Effects on ability to drive and use machines

None known.

4.8 Undesirable effects

Local atrophic changes may occur in intertriginous areas or in nappy areas in young children where moist conditions favour hydrocortisone absorption. Systemic absorption from such sites may be sufficient to produce hypercorticism and suppression of the pituitary adrenal axis after prolonged treatment. This effect is more likely to occur in infants and children and if occlusive dressings are used or large areas of skin treated.

4.9 Overdose

Excessive use under occlusive dressings may produce adrenal suppression. No special procedures or antidote. Treat any adverse effects symptomatically.

5. PHARMACOLOGICAL PROPERTIES

5.1 Pharmacodynamic properties

The active substance is a well-established topical corticosteroid, with an activity classified as potent.

Chlorquinaldol is an established anti-infectious agent with an anti-bacterial and anti-fungal activity.

5.2 Pharmacokinetic properties

In-vivo studies have demonstrated the topical activity of the product, e.g. by the McKenzie-Stoughton test.

Chlorquinaldol acts topically at the site of application.

5.3 Preclinical safety data

No relevant pre-clinical safety data has been generated.

The product acts topically as an emollient cream.

6. PHARMACEUTICAL PARTICULARS

6.1 List of excipients

Plastibase 50 W (containing liquid paraffin and polyethylene)

6.2 Incompatibilities

None stated.

6.3 Shelf life

Five years

6.4 Special precautions for storage

Do not store above 25°C.

6.5 Nature and contents of container

Collapsible aluminium tube with plastic screw cap containing

30g or 50g.

6.6 Instructions for use and handling

No special requirements.

7. MARKETING AUTHORISATION HOLDER

Yamanouchi Pharma Ltd

Yamanouchi House

Pyrford Road

West Byfleet

Surrey

KT14 6RA

8. MARKETING AUTHORISATION NUMBER(S)

Product Licence 0166/0057

9. DATE OF FIRST AUTHORISATION/RENEWAL OF THE AUTHORISATION

First authorisation granted 31 January 1980

Date of renewal approval 25 September 2002

10. DATE OF REVISION OF THE TEXT

Date of revision = December 2003

11. LEGAL CATEGORY

POM

Locoid Cream

(Astellas Pharma Limited)

1. NAME OF THE MEDICINAL PRODUCT

LOCOID CREAM

2. QUALITATIVE AND QUANTITATIVE COMPOSITION

Contains 0.1% w/w hydrocortisone butyrate.

For excipients, see 6.1

3. PHARMACEUTICAL FORM

Cream

White to practically white cream.

4. CLINICAL PARTICULARS

4.1 Therapeutic indications

The product is recommended for clinical use in the treatment of conditions responsive to topical corticosteroids e.g. eczema, dermatitis and psoriasis.

Topical corticosteroids are not generally indicated in psoriasis but may be acceptable in psoriasis excluding widespread plaque psoriasis provided warnings are given, see section 4.4 Special warnings and special precautions for use.

4.2 Posology and method of administration

For topical application.

Dosage: To be applied evenly and sparingly two or three times daily.

Application may be made under occlusion in the more resistant lesions such as thickened psoriatic plaques on elbows and knees.

Adults and the Elderly: The same dose is used for adults and the elderly, as clinical evidence would indicate that no special dosage regimen is necessary in the elderly.

Children: Long term treatment should be avoided where possible.

Infants: Therapy should be limited if possible to a maximum of seven days.

4.3 Contraindications

Hypersensitivity to hydrocortisone or to any of the ingredients of the cream.

This preparation is contraindicated in the presence of untreated viral or fungal infections, tubercular or syphilitic lesions, peri-oral dermatitis, acne vulgaris and rosacea and in bacterial infections unless used in connection with appropriate chemotherapy.

4.4 Special warnings and special precautions for use

Although generally regarded as safe, even for long-term administration in adults, there is a potential for adverse effects if over used in infancy. Extreme caution is required in dermatoses of infancy including napkin eruption. In such patients courses of treatment should not normally exceed 7 days.

Application under occlusion should be restricted to dermatoses involving limited areas.

As with all corticosteroids, application to the face, flexures and other areas of thin skin may cause skin atrophy and increased absorption and should be avoided.

Topical corticosteroids may be hazardous in psoriasis for a number of reasons including rebound relapses following development of tolerance, risk of generalised pustular psoriasis and local and systemic toxicity due to impaired barrier function of the skin. Steroids may have a place in psoriasis of the scalp and chronic plaque psoriasis of the hands and feet. Careful patient supervision is important.

Keep away from the eyes.

4.5 Interaction with other medicinal products and other forms of Interaction

None known.

4.6 Pregnancy and lactation

There is inadequate evidence of safety in human pregnancy. Topical administration of corticosteroids to pregnant animals can cause abnormalities of foetal development including cleft palate and intra-uterine growth retardation. There may therefore be a very small risk of such effects in the human foetus. Theoretically, there is the possibility that if maternal systemic absorption occurred the infant's adrenal function could be affected.

The use of topical corticosteroids during lactation is unlikely to present a hazard to infants being breast-fed.

4.7 Effects on ability to drive and use machines

None known.

4.8 Undesirable effects

Local atrophic changes may occur in intertriginous areas or in nappy areas in young children where moist conditions favour hydrocortisone absorption. Systemic absorption from such sites may be sufficient to produce hypercorticism and suppression of the pituitary adrenal axis after prolonged treatment. This effect is more likely to occur in infants and children and if occlusive dressings are used or large areas of skin treated.

4.9 Overdose

Excessive use under occlusive dressings may produce adrenal suppression. No special procedures or antidote. Treat any adverse effects symptomatically.

5. PHARMACOLOGICAL PROPERTIES

5.1 Pharmacodynamic properties

Hydrocortisone butyrate is a potent topical corticosteroid.

5.2 Pharmacokinetic properties

The topical activity has been demonstrated *in vivo* using the McKenzie-Stoughton test.

5.3 Preclinical safety data

No preclinical safety data have been generated.

6. PHARMACEUTICAL PARTICULARS

6.1 List of excipients

Cetostearyl alcohol, Macrogol Cetostearyl ether, Light Liquid Paraffin, White Soft Paraffin, Butyl parahydroxybenzoate, Propyl parahydroxybenzoate, Citric Acid (anhydrous), Sodium Citrate (anhydrous), Purified Water.

6.2 Incompatibilities

None stated.

6.3 Shelf life

3 years

6.4 Special precautions for storage

Do not store above 25°C. Do not refrigerate or freeze.

6.5 Nature and contents of container

Collapsible aluminium tubes containing either 30 G, 50 G, 100 G or 200G. Packed in a carton.

6.6 Instructions for use and handling

No special requirements.

7. MARKETING AUTHORISATION HOLDER

Yamanouchi Pharma Ltd

Yamanouchi House

Pyrford Road

West Byfleet

Surrey

KT14 6RA

England

8. MARKETING AUTHORISATION NUMBER(S)

PL 00166/0058R

9. DATE OF FIRST AUTHORISATION/RENEWAL OF THE AUTHORISATION

First authorised 28 September 1973, renewed 17th January 2001.

10. DATE OF REVISION OF THE TEXT

Date of revision = 9th February 2005.

11. LEGAL CATEGORY

POM

Locoid Crelo

(Astellas Pharma Limited)

1. NAME OF THE MEDICINAL PRODUCT

LOCOID CRELO

2. QUALITATIVE AND QUANTITATIVE COMPOSITION

Contains 0.1% w/w hydrocortisone butyrate.

For excipients, see 6.1

3. PHARMACEUTICAL FORM

Topical emulsion.

4. CLINICAL PARTICULARS

4.1 Therapeutic indications

The product is recommended for clinical use in the treatment of conditions responsive to topical corticosteroids, e.g. eczema, dermatitis and psoriasis. The product is intended for topical application especially to the scalp or hirsute skin.

Topical corticosteroids are not generally indicated in psoriasis but may be acceptable in psoriasis excluding widespread plaque psoriasis provided warnings are given, see section 4.4 Special warnings and special precautions for use.

4.2 Posology and method of administration

For topical application.

Dosage: To be applied evenly and sparingly two or three times daily.

Adults and the Elderly: The same dose is used for adults and the elderly, as clinical evidence would indicate that no special dosage regimen is necessary in the elderly.

Children: Long term treatment should be avoided where possible.

Infants: Therapy should be limited if possible to a maximum of seven days.

The formulation of the product makes it suitable for use in both scaly lesions and for moist, weeping lesions.

4.3 Contraindications

Hypersensitivity to hydrocortisone or to any of the ingredients of the lotion.

This preparation is contraindicated in the presence of untreated viral or fungal infections, tubercular or syphilitic lesions, peri-oral dermatitis, acne vulgaris and rosacea and in bacterial infections unless used in connection with appropriate chemotherapy.

4.4 Special warnings and special precautions for use

Although generally regarded as safe, even for long-term administration in adults, there is a potential for adverse effects if over used in infancy. Extreme caution is required in dermatoses of infancy including napkin eruption. In such patients, courses of treatment should not normally exceed 7 days.

As with all corticosteroids, application to the face, flexures and other areas of thin skin may cause skin atrophy and increased absorption and should be avoided.

Topical corticosteroids may be hazardous in psoriasis for a number of reasons including rebound relapses following development of tolerance, risk of generalised pustular psoriasis and local and systemic toxicity due to impaired barrier function of the skin. Steroids may have a place in psoriasis of the scalp and chronic plaque psoriasis of the hands and feet. Careful patient supervision is important.

Keep away from the eyes.

4.5 Interaction with other medicinal products and other forms of Interaction

None known.

4.6 Pregnancy and lactation

There is inadequate evidence of safety in human pregnancy. Topical administration of corticosteroids to pregnant animals can cause abnormalities of foetal development including cleft palate and intra-uterine growth retardation. There may therefore be a very small risk of such effects in the human foetus.

Theoretically, there is the possibility that if maternal systemic absorption occurred the infant's adrenal function could be affected.

The use of topical corticosteroids during lactation is unlikely to present a hazard to infants being breast-fed.

4.7 Effects on ability to drive and use machines

None known.

4.8 Undesirable effects

Local atrophic changes may occur in intertriginous areas or in nappy areas in young children where moist conditions favour hydrocortisone absorption. Systemic absorption from such sites may be sufficient to produce hypercorticism and suppression of the pituitary adrenal axis after prolonged treatment. This effect is more likely to occur in infants and children and if occlusive dressings are used or large areas of skin treated.

4.9 Overdose

Excessive use under occlusive dressings may produce adrenal suppression. No special procedures or antidote. Treat any adverse effects symptomatically.

5. PHARMACOLOGICAL PROPERTIES

5.1 Pharmacodynamic properties

The active constituent, hydrocortisone butyrate, is an established topical corticosteroid, equi-efficacious with those corticosteroids classified as potent.

5.2 Pharmacokinetic properties

In human in-vivo studies, the potency of this form of active ingredient has been shown to be of the same order as other topical corticosteroids classed as potent. The active ingredient metabolises to hydrocortisone and butyric acid.

5.3 Preclinical safety data

The well-established use of hydrocortisone 17-butyrate topical preparations over many years does not warrant further safety evaluation studies in animals.

6. PHARMACEUTICAL PARTICULARS

6.1 List of excipients

Macrogol cetostearyl ether

Cetostearyl Alcohol

White soft paraffin

Hard paraffin

Borage oil

Butylhydroxytoluene

Propyleneglycol

Sodium citrate

Anhydrous citric acid

Propyl parahydroxybenzoate

Butyl hydroxybenzoate

Purified water

6.2 Incompatibilities

None known.

6.3 Shelf life

2 years.

6.4 Special precautions for storage

Do not store above 25°C.

6.5 Nature and contents of container

White opaque low density polyethylene bottles of 15, 25, 30, 50 and 100 g capacity, equipped with a natural low density polyethylene dropper applicator, closed with a white polypropylene screw cap.

6.6 Instructions for use and handling

No special requirements.

7. MARKETING AUTHORISATION HOLDER

Yamanouchi Pharma Ltd

Yamanouchi House

Pyrford Road

West Byfleet

Surrey

KT14 6RA

8. MARKETING AUTHORISATION NUMBER(S)

Product licence 0166/0170.

9. DATE OF FIRST AUTHORISATION/RENEWAL OF THE AUTHORISATION

23 May 1995 / 15 January 2001

10. DATE OF REVISION OF THE TEXT
Date of revision = December 2003

11. LEGAL CATEGORY
POM

Locoid Lipocream

(Astellas Pharma Limited)

1. NAME OF THE MEDICINAL PRODUCT
LOCOID LIPOCREAM

2. QUALITATIVE AND QUANTITATIVE COMPOSITION
Contains 0.1% w/w hydrocortisone butyrate.

For excipients, see 6.1

3. PHARMACEUTICAL FORM
Cream

4. CLINICAL PARTICULARS

4.1 Therapeutic indications
The product is recommended for clinical use in the treatment of conditions responsive to topical corticosteroids e.g. eczema, dermatitis and psoriasis.

Topical corticosteroids are not generally indicated in psoriasis but may be acceptable in psoriasis excluding widespread plaque psoriasis provided warnings are given, see section 4.4 Special warnings and special precautions for use.

4.2 Posology and method of administration
For topical application.

Dosage: To be applied evenly and sparingly two or three times daily

Application may be made under occlusion in the more resistant lesions such as thickened psoriatic plaques on elbows and knees.

Adults and the Elderly: The same dose is used for adults and the elderly, as clinical evidence would indicate that no special dosage regimen is necessary in the elderly.

Children: Long term treatment should be avoided where possible.

Infants: Therapy should be limited if possible to a maximum of seven days.

Due to the formulation of the base the product may be used both for dry scaly lesions and for moist or weeping lesions.

4.3 Contraindications
Hypersensitivity to hydrocortisone or to any of the ingredients of the cream.

This preparation is contraindicated in the presence of untreated viral or fungal infections, tubercular or syphilitic lesions, peri-oral dermatitis, acne vulgaris and rosacea and in bacterial infections unless used in connection with appropriate chemotherapy.

4.4 Special warnings and special precautions for use
Although generally regarded as safe, even for long-term administration in adults, there is a potential for adverse effects if over used in infancy. Extreme caution is required in dermatoses of infancy including napkin eruption. In such patients courses of treatment should not normally exceed 7 days.

Application under occlusion should be restricted to dermatoses involving limited areas.

As with all corticosteroids, application to the face, flexures and other areas of thin skin may cause skin atrophy and increased absorption and should be avoided.

Topical corticosteroids may be hazardous in psoriasis for a number of reasons including rebound relapses following development of tolerance, risk of generalised pustular psoriasis and local and systemic toxicity due to impaired barrier function of the skin. Steroids may have a place in psoriasis of the scalp and chronic plaque psoriasis of the hands and feet. Careful patient supervision is important.

Keep away from the eyes.

4.5 Interaction with other medicinal products and other forms of Interaction
None known.

4.6 Pregnancy and lactation
There is inadequate evidence of safety in human pregnancy. Topical administration of corticosteroids to pregnant animals can cause abnormalities of foetal development including cleft palate and intra-uterine growth retardation. There may therefore be a very small risk of such effects in the human foetus. Theoretically, there is the possibility that if maternal systemic absorption occurred the infant's adrenal function could be affected.

The use of topical corticosteroids during lactation is unlikely to present a hazard to infants being breast-fed.

4.7 Effects on ability to drive and use machines
None known.

4.8 Undesirable effects
Local atrophic changes may occur in intertriginous areas or in nappy areas in young children where moist conditions favour hydrocortisone absorption. Systemic absorption from such sites may be sufficient to produce hypercorticism and suppression of the pituitary adrenal axis after prolonged treatment. This effect is more likely to occur in infants and children and if occlusive dressings are used or large areas of skin treated.

4.9 Overdose
Excessive use under occlusive dressings may produce adrenal suppression. No special procedures or antidote. Treat any adverse effects symptomatically

5. PHARMACOLOGICAL PROPERTIES

5.1 Pharmacodynamic properties
The active substance, hydrocortisone butyrate, is an established topical corticosteroid, equi-efficacious with those corticosteroids classified as potent.

5.2 Pharmacokinetic properties
In human in-vivo studies the potency of this formulation has been shown to be of the same order as other topical corticosteroids classified as potent. The active substance metabolises to hydrocortisone and butyric acid.

5.3 Preclinical safety data
No relevant pre-clinical safety data have been generated

6. PHARMACEUTICAL PARTICULARS

6.1 List of excipients
Macrogol cetostearyl ether

Cetostearyl alcohol

White soft paraffin

Light liquid paraffin

Sodium citrate anhydrous

Citric acid anhydrous

Methyl parahydroxybenzoate

Purified water

6.2 Incompatibilities
None stated.

6.3 Shelf life
Five years

6.4 Special precautions for storage
Do not store above 25°C.

6.5 Nature and contents of container
Collapsible aluminium tube with plastic screw cap containing

15g, 30g, 50g or 100 g.

6.6 Instructions for use and handling
No special requirements.

7. MARKETING AUTHORISATION HOLDER
Yamanouchi Pharma Ltd

Yamanouchi House

Pyrford Road

West Byfleet

Surrey

KT14 6RA

United Kingdom

8. MARKETING AUTHORISATION NUMBER(S)
PL 0166/0112

9. DATE OF FIRST AUTHORISATION/RENEWAL OF THE AUTHORISATION
3 May 1983; 18 September 1998.

10. DATE OF REVISION OF THE TEXT
December 2003

11. LEGAL CATEGORY
POM

Locoid Ointment

(Astellas Pharma Limited)

1. NAME OF THE MEDICINAL PRODUCT
LOCOID OINTMENT

2. QUALITATIVE AND QUANTITATIVE COMPOSITION
Contains 0.1% w/w hydrocortisone butyrate.

For excipients, see 6.1

3. PHARMACEUTICAL FORM
Ointment.

Translucent, light grey to whitish, soft fatty ointment.

4. CLINICAL PARTICULARS

4.1 Therapeutic indications
The product is recommended for clinical use in the treatment of conditions responsive to topical corticosteroids e.g. eczema, dermatitis and psoriasis.

Topical corticosteroids are not generally indicated in psoriasis but may be acceptable in psoriasis excluding widespread plaque psoriasis provided warnings are given, see section 4.4 Special warnings and special precautions for use.

4.2 Posology and method of administration
For topical application.

Dosage: To be applied evenly and sparingly two or three times daily.

Application may be made under occlusion in the more resistant lesions such as thickened psoriatic plaques on elbows and knees.

Adults and the Elderly: The same dose is used for adults and the elderly, as clinical evidence would indicate that no special dosage regimen is necessary in the elderly.

Children: Long term treatment should be avoided where possible.

Infants: Therapy should be limited if possible to a maximum of seven days.

4.3 Contraindications
Hypersensitivity to hydrocortisone or to any of the ingredients of the ointment.

This preparation is contraindicated in the presence of untreated viral or fungal infections, tubercular or syphilitic lesions, peri-oral dermatitis, acne vulgaris and rosacea and in bacterial infections unless used in connection with appropriate chemotherapy.

4.4 Special warnings and special precautions for use
Although generally regarded as safe, even for long-term administration in adults, there is a potential for adverse effects if over used in infancy. Extreme caution is required in dermatoses of infancy including napkin eruption. In such patients courses of treatment should not normally exceed 7 days.

Application under occlusion should be restricted to dermatoses involving limited areas.

As with all corticosteroids, application to the face, flexures and other areas of thin skin may cause skin atrophy and increased absorption and should be avoided.

Topical corticosteroids may be hazardous in psoriasis for a number of reasons including rebound relapses following development of tolerance, risk of generalised pustular psoriasis and local systemic toxicity due to impaired barrier function of the skin. Steroids may have a place in psoriasis of the scalp and chronic plaque psoriasis of the hands and feet. Careful patient supervision is important.

Keep away from the eyes.

4.5 Interaction with other medicinal products and other forms of Interaction
None known.

4.6 Pregnancy and lactation
There is inadequate evidence of safety in human pregnancy. Topical administration of corticosteroids to pregnant animals can cause abnormalities of foetal development including cleft palate and intra-uterine growth retardation. There may therefore be a very small risk of such effects in the human foetus.

Theoretically, there is the possibility that if maternal systemic absorption occurred the infant's adrenal function could be affected.

The use of topical corticosteroids during lactation is unlikely to present a hazard to infants being breast-fed.

4.7 Effects on ability to drive and use machines
None known.

4.8 Undesirable effects
Local atrophic changes may occur in intertriginous areas or in nappy areas in young children where moist conditions favour hydrocortisone absorption. Systemic absorption from such sites may be sufficient to produce hypercorticism and suppression of the pituitary adrenal axis after prolonged treatment. This effect is more likely to occur in infants and children and if occlusive dressings are used or large areas of skin treated.

4.9 Overdose
Excessive use under occlusive dressings may produce adrenal suppression. No special procedures or antidote. Treat any adverse effects symptomatically.

5. PHARMACOLOGICAL PROPERTIES

5.1 Pharmacodynamic properties
Hydrocortisone butyrate is a potent topical corticosteroid.

5.2 Pharmacokinetic properties
The topical activity has been demonstrated *in vivo* using the McKenzie-Stoughton test.

5.3 Preclinical safety data
No preclinical safety data have been generated.

6. PHARMACEUTICAL PARTICULARS

6.1 List of excipients
Polyethylene oleogel (liquid paraffin, polyethylene)

6.2 Incompatibilities
None stated.

6.3 Shelf life
5 years

6.4 Special precautions for storage
Do not store above 25°C.

6.5 Nature and contents of container
Collapsible aluminium tubes containing either 30 G, 50 G, 100 G or 200G. Packed in a carton.

6.6 Instructions for use and handling
No special requirements.

7. MARKETING AUTHORISATION HOLDER
Yamanouchi Pharma Ltd

Yamanouchi House

Pyrford Road

West Byfleet

Surrey

KT14 6RA. England

8. MARKETING AUTHORISATION NUMBER(S)
PL 00166/0059R

9. DATE OF FIRST AUTHORISATION/RENEWAL OF THE AUTHORISATION
First authorised 28 September 1973, renewed 17 January 2001.

10. DATE OF REVISION OF THE TEXT
Date of revision = December 2003

11. LEGAL CATEGORY
POM

Locoid Scalp Lotion

(Astellas Pharma Limited)

1. NAME OF THE MEDICINAL PRODUCT
LOCOID SCALP LOTION

2. QUALITATIVE AND QUANTITATIVE COMPOSITION
Contains 0.1% w/v hydrocortisone butyrate.

For excipients, see 6.1

3. PHARMACEUTICAL FORM
Cutaneous solution.

Clear, colourless solution.

4. CLINICAL PARTICULARS

4.1 Therapeutic indications
The product is recommended for clinical use in the treatment of scalp conditions responsive to topical corticosteroids e.g. eczema, dermatitis and psoriasis.

Topical corticosteroids are not generally indicated in psoriasis but may be acceptable in psoriasis excluding widespread plaque psoriasis provided warnings are given; see section 4.4 Special warnings and special precautions for use.

4.2 Posology and method of administration
For topical application to the scalp.

Dosage: To be applied evenly and sparingly two or three times daily

Adults and the Elderly: The same dose is used for adults and the elderly, as clinical evidence would indicate that no special dosage regimen is necessary in the elderly.

Children: Long term treatment should be avoided where possible.

Infants: Therapy should be limited if possible to a maximum of seven days.

4.3 Contraindications
Hypersensitivity to hydrocortisone or to any of the ingredients of the lotion.

This preparation is contraindicated in the presence of untreated viral or fungal infections, tubercular or syphilitic lesions, peri-oral dermatitis, acne vulgaris and rosacea and in bacterial infections unless used in connection with appropriate chemotherapy.

4.4 Special warnings and special precautions for use
Although generally regarded as safe, even for long-term administration in adults, there is a potential for adverse effects if over used in infancy. Extreme caution is required in dermatoses of infancy. In such patients courses of treatment should not normally exceed 7 days.

As with all corticosteroids, application to the face, flexures and other areas of thin skin may cause skin atrophy and increased absorption and should be avoided.

Topical corticosteroids may be hazardous in psoriasis for a number of reasons including rebound relapses following development of tolerance, risk of generalised pustular psoriasis and local and systemic toxicity due to impaired barrier function of the skin. Steroids may have a place in psoriasis of the scalp and chronic plaque psoriasis of the hands and feet. Careful patient supervision is important.

Keep away from eyes.

4.5 Interaction with other medicinal products and other forms of Interaction
None known.

4.6 Pregnancy and lactation
There is inadequate evidence of safety in human pregnancy. Topical administration of corticosteroids to pregnant animals can cause abnormalities of foetal development including cleft palate and intra-uterine growth retardation. There may therefore be a very small risk of such effects in the human foetus.

Theoretically, there is the possibility that if maternal systemic absorption occurred the infant's adrenal function could be affected.

The use of topical corticosteroids during lactation is unlikely to present a hazard to infants being breast-fed.

4.7 Effects on ability to drive and use machines
None known.

4.8 Undesirable effects
Local atrophic changes may occur in intertriginous areas or in nappy areas in young children where moist conditions favour hydrocortisone absorption. Systemic absorption from such sites may be sufficient to produce hypercorticism and suppression of the pituitary adrenal axis after prolonged treatment. This effect is more likely to occur in infants and children and if occlusive dressings are used or large areas of skin treated.

4.9 Overdose
Excessive use under occlusive dressings may produce adrenal suppression. No special procedures or antidote. Treat any adverse effects symptomatically.

5. PHARMACOLOGICAL PROPERTIES

5.1 Pharmacodynamic properties
Hydrocortisone butyrate is a potent topical corticosteroid.

5.2 Pharmacokinetic properties
The topical activity has been demonstrated *in vivo* using the McKenzie-Stoughton test.

5.3 Preclinical safety data
No preclinical safety data have been generated.

6. PHARMACEUTICAL PARTICULARS

6.1 List of excipients
Isopropyl alcohol, glycerol (85%), Povidone K90, anhydrous citric acid, anhydrous sodium citrate, purified water.

6.2 Incompatibilities
None stated.

6.3 Shelf life
2 years

6.4 Special precautions for storage
Do not store above 25°C.

6.5 Nature and contents of container
Plastic, dropper-necked screw cap vial.

Pack sizes: 30 ml and 100 ml.

6.6 Instructions for use and handling
No special requirements.

7. MARKETING AUTHORISATION HOLDER
Yamanouchi Pharma Ltd

Yamanouchi House

Pyrford Road

West Byfleet

Surrey

KT14 6RA

England

8. MARKETING AUTHORISATION NUMBER(S)
PL 00166/0060R

9. DATE OF FIRST AUTHORISATION/RENEWAL OF THE AUTHORISATION
First authorised 28 September 1973; renewed 17 January 2001.

10. DATE OF REVISION OF THE TEXT
Date of revision = 2 June 2004.

11. LEGAL CATEGORY
POM.

Locorten Vioform Ear Drops

(Amdipharm)

1. NAME OF THE MEDICINAL PRODUCT
Locorten Vioform Ear Drops

2. QUALITATIVE AND QUANTITATIVE COMPOSITION
Active ingredients: Flumetasone pivalate 0.02% w/v

Clioquinol BP 1.0% w/v

3. PHARMACEUTICAL FORM
Ear drops, solution.

4. CLINICAL PARTICULARS

4.1 Therapeutic indications
Inflammatory conditions of the external ear where a secondary infection is suspected. Otorrhoea.

4.2 Posology and method of administration
Instil 2 or 3 drops twice daily directly into the auditory canal of the affected ear. Treatment should be limited to 7-10 days.

If there is little improvement after 7 days treatment with Locorten Vioform, appropriate microbiological investigations should be carried out and local or systemic antibiotic treatment given.

Use in the elderly

There is no evidence to suggest that dosage should be different in the elderly.

Use in children

Locorten Vioform Ear Drops are contra-indicated in children below the age of two years.

Route of administration: Auricular use

4.3 Contraindications
Hypersensitivity to any component of the formulation or iodine. Primary bacterial, viral or fungal infections of the outer ear. Perforation of the tympanic membrane. Use in children below the age of two years.

4.4 Special warnings and special precautions for use
Long-term continuous topical therapy should be avoided since this can lead to adrenal suppression.

Topical application of clioquinol-containing preparations may lead to a marked increase in protein-bound iodine (PBI). The results of thyroid function tests, such as PBI, radioactive iodine and butanol extractable iodine, may be affected. However, other thyroid function tests, such as the T_3 resin sponge test or T_4 determination, are unaffected.

The ferric chloride test of phenylketonuria may yield a false-positive result when clioquinol is present in the urine. Locorten Vioform should not be allowed to come into contact with the conjunctiva.

4.5 Interaction with other medicinal products and other forms of Interaction
None known via this topical route.

4.6 Pregnancy and lactation
There is inadequate evidence of safety in human pregnancy. Topical administration of corticosteroids to pregnant animals can cause abnormalities of foetal development, including cleft palate and intra-uterine growth retardation. There may, therefore, be a very small risk of such effects in the human foetus.

It is not known whether the active substances of Locorten Vioform and/or their metabolite(s) pass into breast milk after topical administration. Use in lactating mothers should only be at the doctor's discretion.

4.7 Effects on ability to drive and use machines
None known.

4.8 Undesirable effects
Locorten Vioform is generally well tolerated, but occasionally at the site of application, there may be signs of irritation such as a burning sensation, itching or skin rash. Hypersensitivity reactions may also occasionally occur. Treatment should be discontinued if patients experience severe irritation or sensitisation.

Locorten Vioform may cause hair discoloration.

4.9 Overdose
Locorten Vioform is for topical (external) use only. If accidental ingestion of large quantities occurs, there is no specific antidote and general measures to eliminate the drug and reduce its absorption should be undertaken. Symptomatic treatment should be administered as appropriate.

5. PHARMACOLOGICAL PROPERTIES

5.1 Pharmacodynamic properties
Locorten Vioform Ear Drops combine the anti-fungal and anti-bacterial properties of clioquinol with the anti-inflammatory activity of flumetasone pivalate.

5.2 Pharmacokinetic properties
No pharmacokinetic data on Locorten Vioform Ear Drops are available.

5.3 Preclinical safety data
Not applicable.

6. PHARMACEUTICAL PARTICULARS

6.1 List of excipients
Polyethylene glycol.

6.2 Incompatibilities
None known.

6.3 Shelf life
36 months.

6.4 Special precautions for storage
Do not store above 25°C.

6.5 Nature and contents of container
Plastic dropper bottle containing 7.5 ml.

6.6 Instructions for use and handling
Medicines should be kept out of the reach of children.

7. MARKETING AUTHORISATION HOLDER
Amdipharm plc

Regency House

Miles Gray Road

Basildon

Essex

SS14 3AF

UK

8. MARKETING AUTHORISATION NUMBER(S)
PL 20072/0012

9. DATE OF FIRST AUTHORISATION/RENEWAL OF THE AUTHORISATION
11 October 2004

10. DATE OF REVISION OF THE TEXT
October 2004

Lodine SR

(Shire Pharmaceuticals Limited)

1. NAME OF THE MEDICINAL PRODUCT
Lodine™ SR Tablets 600mg.

2. QUALITATIVE AND QUANTITATIVE COMPOSITION
Etodolac 600mg.

3. PHARMACEUTICAL FORM
Lodine SR Tablets are for oral administration. Each tablet is capsular, oval shaped light grey film coated, impressed on one side with Lodine SR600 and contains etodolac 600mg in a sustained release formulation.

4. CLINICAL PARTICULARS
4.1 Therapeutic indications
Lodine (etodolac) is indicated for acute or long-term use in rheumatoid arthritis and osteoarthritis.

4.2 Posology and method of administration
Adults: Lodine SR Tablets 600mg

One tablet daily, swallowed whole with a tumblerful of water. If a lower dose is sufficient, conventional Lodine capsules or tablets may be used.

The safety of doses in excess of 600mg per day has not been established.

No occurrence of tolerance or tachyphylaxis has been reported.

Elderly: No change in initial dosage is generally required in the elderly (see precautions).

Children: Not recommended.

4.3 Contraindications
Lodine should not be used in patients who have previously shown hypersensitivity to it.

Lodine should not be used in patients with active peptic ulceration or a history of peptic ulcer disease (including gastrointestinal haemorrhage due to another non-steroidal anti-inflammatory drug).

Due to possible cross-reactivity, Lodine should not be administered to patients who experience asthma, rhinitis or urticaria during therapy with aspirin or other non-steroidal anti-inflammatory drugs.

4.4 Special warnings and special precautions for use
Caution is required if Lodine is administered to patients suffering from, or with a previous history of, bronchial asthma since NSAIDs have been reported to cause bronchospasm in such patients.

Although non-steroidal anti-inflammatory drugs do not have the same direct effects on platelets as does aspirin, all drugs which inhibit the biosynthesis of prostaglandins may interfere, to some extent, with platelet function. Patients receiving Lodine who may be adversely affected by such actions should be carefully observed.

In patients with renal, cardiac or hepatic impairment especially those taking diuretics, caution is required since the use of NSAIDs may result in deterioration of renal function. The dose should be kept as low as possible and renal function should be monitored. However, impairment of renal or hepatic functions due to other causes may alter drug metabolism; patients receiving concomitant long term therapy, especially the elderly, should be observed for potential side effects and their drug doses adjusted as needed, or the drug discontinued.

Serious gastrointestinal adverse effects such as bleeding, ulceration and perforation can occur at any time with or without warning symptoms in patients treated with NSAIDs. If any sign of gastrointestinal bleeding occurs, Lodine should be stopped immediately.

Patients on long-term treatment with Lodine should be regularly reviewed as a precautionary measure e.g. for changes in, renal function, haematological parameters, or hepatic function.

Lodine should be used with caution in patients with fluid retention, hypertension or heart failure.

4.5 Interaction with other medicinal products and other forms of Interaction
Since Lodine is extensively protein-bound, it may be necessary to modify the dosage of other highly protein-bound drugs.

The concomitant administration of warfarin and Lodine should not require a dosage adjustment of either drug, however it has rarely led to prolonged prothrombin times, therefore caution should be exercised when Lodine is administered with warfarin.

Bilirubin tests can give a false positive result due to the presence of phenolic metabolites of Lodine in the urine.

Concomitant use of cyclosporin, methotrexate, digoxin, or lithium with NSAIDs may cause an increase in serum levels of these compounds and associated toxicities.

Care should also be taken in patients treated with any of the following drugs as interactions have been reported in some patients:

Anti-hypertensives: reduced anti-hypertensive effect.

Mifepristone: NSAIDs should not be used for 8-12 days after mifepristone administration as NSAIDs can reduce the effect of mifepristone.

Other analgesics: avoid the concomitant use of two or more NSAIDs.

Corticosteroids: increased risk of gastrointestinal bleeding.

Quinolone antibiotics: animal data indicate that NSAIDs can increase the risk of convulsions associated with quinolone antibiotics. Patients taking NSAIDs and quinolones may have an increased risk of developing convulsions.

4.6 Pregnancy and lactation
Drugs which inhibit prostaglandin biosynthesis may cause dystocia and delayed parturition as evidenced by studies in pregnant animals. Some inhibitors of prostaglandin biosynthesis have been shown to interfere with the closure of the ductus arteriosus. Safety in human pregnancy has not been established and Lodine should not be used during pregnancy. Safety of Lodine use during lactation has not been established and as such its use in nursing mothers should be avoided.

4.7 Effects on ability to drive and use machines
Lodine can cause dizziness, drowsiness or abnormal vision. Patients need to be aware of how they react to this medicine before driving or operating machines.

4.8 Undesirable effects
Reported side effects include nausea, epigastric pain, diarrhoea, indigestion, heartburn, flatulence, abdominal pain, constipation, vomiting, ulcerative stomatitis, dyspepsia, gastritis, haematemesis, melaena, rectal bleeding, colitis, vasculitis, headaches, dizziness, abnormal vision, pyrexia, drowsiness, tinnitus, rash, pruritus, fatigue, depression, insomnia, confusion, paraesthesia, tremor, weakness/malaise, dyspnoea, oedema, palpitations, bilirubinuria, hepatic function abnormalities and jaundice, urinary frequency, dysuria, angioedema, anaphylactoid reaction, photosensitivity, urticaria and Stevens-Johnson syndrome.

More serious adverse reactions which may occasionally occur are gastrointestinal ulceration and peptic ulceration.

NSAIDs have been reported to cause nephrotoxicity in various forms and their use can lead to interstitial nephritis, nephrotic syndrome and renal failure. There have been reports of nephritis and renal failure with etodolac.

Occasionally blood disorders have been reported including: thrombocytopenia, neutropenia, agranulocytosis and anaemia.

4.9 Overdose
The standard practices of gastric lavage, activated charcoal administration and general supportive therapy should be undertaken.

5. PHARMACOLOGICAL PROPERTIES
5.1 Pharmacodynamic properties
Inhibition of prostaglandin synthesis and COX-2 selectivity: All non-steroidal anti-inflammatory drugs (NSAIDs) have been shown to inhibit the formation of prostaglandins. It is this action which is responsible both for their therapeutic effects and some of their side-effects. The inhibition of prostaglandin synthesis observed with etodolac differs from that of other NSAIDs. In an animal model at an established anti-inflammatory dose, cytoprotective PGE concentration in the gastric mucosa have been shown to be reduced to a lesser degree and for a shorter period than other NSAIDs. This finding is consistent with subsequent *in-vitro* studies which have found etodolac to be selective for induced cyclo-oxygenase 2 (COX-2, associated with inflammation) over COX-1 (cytoprotective).

Furthermore, studies in human cell models have confirmed that etodolac is selective for the inhibition of COX-2.

The clinical benefit of preferential COX-2 inhibition over COX-1 has yet to be proven.

Anti-inflammatory effects: Experiments have shown etodolac to have marked anti-inflammatory activity, being more potent than several clinically established NSAIDs.

5.2 Pharmacokinetic properties
In man, etodolac is well absorbed following oral administration.

Etodolac is highly bound to serum proteins.

The elimination half-life averages seven hours in man. The primary route of excretion is in the urine, mostly in the form of metabolites.

In subjects receiving daily doses of Lodine SR 400mg or 600mg to steady state levels over a three day period, the peak plasma concentrations were 7.5μg/ml at 7.9 hours and 11.9μg/ml at 7.8 hours.

5.3 Preclinical safety data
Nothing of note to the prescriber.

6. PHARMACEUTICAL PARTICULARS
6.1 List of excipients
Hydroxypropyl Methylcellulose USP

Dibasic Sodium Phosphate USP

Ethylcellulose USNF

Lactose Ph Eur

Magnesium Stearate Ph Eur

Hydroxypropyl cellulose

Macrogol 400

Macrogol 6000

Colourings - Titanium Dioxide (E171), Iron Oxide (E172)

6.2 Incompatibilities
None.

6.3 Shelf life
Lodine SR Tablets may be stored for up to 3 years.

6.4 Special precautions for storage
Store at room temperature, below 25°C.

6.5 Nature and contents of container
PVdC/PVC/Aluminium foil blister packs of 30 tablets.

6.6 Instructions for use and handling
None.

7. MARKETING AUTHORISATION HOLDER
Shire Pharmaceuticals Ltd

Hampshire International Business Park

Chineham

Basingstoke

Hampshire RG24 8EP

United Kingdom

8. MARKETING AUTHORISATION NUMBER(S)
PL 08557/0043

9. DATE OF FIRST AUTHORISATION/RENEWAL OF THE AUTHORISATION
1 September 2000

10. DATE OF REVISION OF THE TEXT
August 2002

LEGAL CATEGORY
POM

LOGYNON®

(Schering Health Care Limited)

Presentation The memo-pack holds six light brown tablets containing 30 micrograms ethinylestradiol and 50 micrograms levonorgestrel, five white tablets containing 40 micrograms ethinylestradiol and 75 micrograms levonorgestrel and ten ochre tablets containing 30 micrograms ethinylestradiol and 125 micrograms levonorgestrel.

All tablets have a lustrous, sugar coating.

Excipients: lactose, maize starch, povidone 25 000, talc, magnesium stearate, sucrose, povidone 700 000, polyethylene glycol 6000, calcium carbonate, montan glycol wax, titanium dioxide, glycerol, ferric oxide pigment (yellow and red).

Uses Oral contraception and the recognised gynaecological indications for such oestrogen-progestogen combinations. The mode of action includes the inhibition of ovulation by suppression of the mid-cycle surge of luteinising hormone, the inspissation of cervical mucus so as to constitute a barrier to sperm, and the rendering of the endometrium unreceptive to implantation.

Dosage and administration *First treatment cycle:* 1 tablet daily for 21 days, starting on the first day of the menstrual cycle. Contraceptive protection begins immediately.

Subsequent cycles: Tablet taking from the next pack of Logynon is continued after a 7-day interval, beginning on the same day of the week as the first pack.

Changing from 21-day combined oral contraceptives: The first tablet of Logynon should be taken on the first day immediately after the end of the previous oral contraceptive course. Additional contraceptive precautions are not required.

Changing from a combined Every Day pill (28 day tablets): Logynon should be started after taking the last active tablet from the Every Day Pill pack. The first Logynon tablet is taken the next day. Additional contraceptive precautions are not then required.

Changing from a progestogen-only pill (POP): The first tablet of Logynon should be taken on the first day of bleeding, even if a POP has already been taken on that day. Additional contraceptive precautions are not then required. The remaining progestogen-only pills should be discarded.

Post-partum and post-abortum use: After pregnancy, oral contraception can be started 21 days after a vaginal delivery, provided that the patient is fully ambulant and there are no puerperal complications. Additional contraceptive precautions will be required for the first 7 days of tablet taking. Since the first post-partum ovulation may precede the first bleeding, another method of contraception should be used in the interval between childbirth and the first course of tablets. After a first-trimester abortion, oral contraception may be started immediately in which case no additional contraceptive precautions are required.

Pregnancy and lactation: If pregnancy occurs during medication with oral contraceptives, the preparation should be withdrawn immediately.

The use of Logynon during lactation may lead to a reduction in the volume of milk produced and to a change in its composition. Minute amounts of the active substances are excreted with the milk. Mothers who are breast-feeding may be advised instead to use a progestogen-only pill.

Special circumstances requiring additional contraception

Incorrect administration: A single delayed tablet should be taken as soon as possible, and if this can be done within 12 hours of the correct time, contraceptive protection is maintained. With longer delays, additional contraception is needed. Only the most recently delayed tablet should be taken, earlier missed tablets being omitted, and additional non-hormonal methods of contraception (except the rhythm or temperature methods) should be used for the next 7 days, while the next 7 tablets are being taken. Additionally, therefore, if tablet(s) have been missed during the last 7 days of a pack, there should be no break before the next pack is started. In this situation, a withdrawal bleed should not be expected until the end of the second pack. Some breakthrough bleeding may occur on tablet taking days but this is not clinically significant. If the patient does not have a withdrawal bleed during the tablet-free interval following the end of the second pack, the possibility of pregnancy must be ruled out before starting the next pack.

Gastro-intestinal upset: Vomiting or diarrhoea may reduce the efficacy of oral contraceptives by preventing full absorption. Tablet-taking from the current pack should be continued. Additional non-hormonal methods of contraception (except the rhythm or temperature methods) should be used during the gastro-intestinal upset and for 7 days following the upset. If these 7 days overrun the end of a pack, the next pack should be started without a break. In this situation, a withdrawal bleed should not be expected until the end of the second pack. If the patient does not have a withdrawal bleed during the tablet-free interval following the end of the second pack, the possibility of pregnancy must be ruled out before starting the next pack. Other methods of contraception should be considered if the gastro-intestinal disorder is likely to be prolonged.

Interaction with other drugs: Hepatic enzyme inducers such as barbiturates, primidone, phenobarbitone, phenytoin, phenylbutazone, rifampicin, carbamazepine and griseofulvin can impair the efficacy of Logynon. For women receiving long-term therapy with hepatic enzyme inducers, another method of contraception should be used. The use of antibiotics may also reduce the efficacy of Logynon, possibly by altering the intestinal flora.

Women receiving short courses of enzyme inducers or broad spectrum antibiotics should take additional, non-hormonal (except the rhythm or temperature method) contraceptive precautions during the time of concurrent medication and for 7 days afterwards. If these 7 days overrun the end of a pack, the next pack should be started without a break. In this situation, a withdrawal bleed should not be expected until the end of the second pack. If the patient does not have a withdrawal bleed during the tablet-free interval following the end of the second pack, the possibility of pregnancy must be ruled out before resuming with the next pack. With rifampicin, additional contraceptive precautions should be continued for 4 weeks after treatment stops, even if only a short course was administered.

The requirement for oral antidiabetics or insulin can change as a result of the effect on glucose tolerance.

The herbal remedy St John's wort (Hypericum perforatum) should not be taken concomitantly with Logynon as this could potentially lead to a loss of contraceptive effect.

Contra-indications, warnings, etc

Contra-indications:

1. Pregnancy
2. Severe disturbances of liver function, jaundice or persistent itching during a previous pregnancy, Dubin-Johnson syndrome, Rotor syndrome, previous or existing liver tumours
3. Existing or a history of confirmed venous thromboembolism (VTE), family history of idiopathic VTE and other known risk factors for VTE.
4. Existing or previous arterial thrombotic or embolic processes.
5. Conditions which predispose to thromboembolism e.g. disorders of the clotting processes, valvular heart disease and atrial fibrillation
6. Sickle-cell anaemia
7. Mammary or endometrial carcinoma, or a history of these conditions
8. Severe diabetes mellitus with vascular changes
9. Disorders of lipid metabolism
10. History of herpes gestationis
11. Deterioration of otosclerosis during pregnancy
12. Undiagnosed abnormal vaginal bleeding

Figure 1

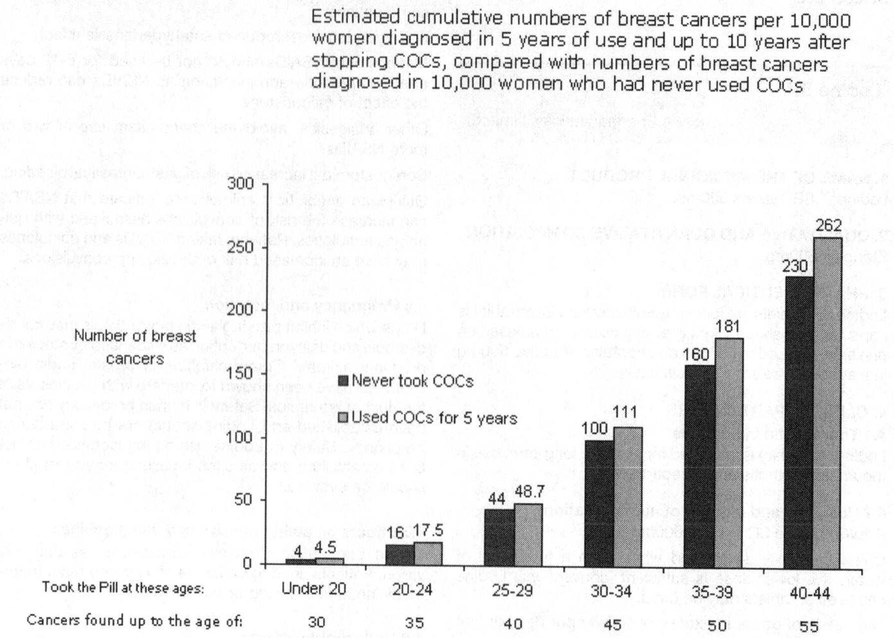

13. Hypersensitivity to any of the components of Logynon.

Warnings:

The use of any combined oral contraceptive carries an increased risk of venous thromboembolism (VTE) compared with no use. The excess risk of VTE is highest during the first year a woman ever uses a combined oral contraceptive. This increased risk is less than the risk of VTE associated with pregnancy which is estimated as 60 cases per 100 000 pregnancies. Some epidemiological studies have reported a greater risk of VTE for women using combined oral contraceptives containing desogestrel or gestodene (the so-called 'third generation' pills) than for women using pills containing levonorgestrel (the so-called 'second generation' pills).

The spontaneous incidence of VTE in healthy non-pregnant women (not taking any oral contraceptive) is about 5 cases per 100,000 per year. The incidence in users of second generation pills is about 15 per 100,000 women per year of use. The incidence in users of third generation pills is about 25 cases per 100,000 women per year of use; this excess incidence has not been satisfactorily explained by bias or confounding. This level of all these risks increases with age and is likely to be further increased in women with other known risk factors for VTE such as obesity.

The risk of venous and/or arterial thrombosis associated with combined oral contraceptives increases with:

- age;
- smoking (with heavier smoking and increasing age the risk further increases, especially in women over 35 years of age);
- a positive family history (i.e. venous or arterial thromboembolism ever in a sibling or parent at a relatively early age). If a hereditary predisposition is suspected, the woman should be referred to a specialist for advice before deciding about any COC use;
- obesity (body mass index over 30 kg/m^2);
- dyslipoproteinaemia;
- hypertension;
- valvular heart disease;
- atrial fibrillation;
- prolonged immobilisation, major surgery, any surgery to the legs, or major trauma. In these situations it is advisable to discontinue COC use (in the case of elective surgery at least six weeks in advance) and not to resume until two weeks after complete remobilisation.

- There is no consensus about the possible role of varicose veins and superficial thrombophlebitis in venous thromboembolism.
- The increased risk of thromboembolism in the puerperium must be considered (for information on "Pregnancy and Lactation" see Section 4.6).
- Other medical conditions which have been associated with adverse circulatory events include diabetes mellitus, systemic lupus erythematosus, haemolytic uraemic syndrome, chronic inflammatory bowel disease (Crohn's disease or ulcerative colitis), sickle cell disease and subarachnoid haemorrhage.
- An increase in frequency or severity of migraine during COC use (which may be prodromal of a cerebrovascular event) may be a reason for immediate discontinuation of the COC.
- Biochemical factors that may be indicative of hereditary or acquired predisposition for venous or arterial thrombosis include Activated Protein C (APC) resistance, hyperhomocysteinaemia, antithrombin-III deficiency, protein C deficiency, protein S deficiency, antiphospholipid antibodies (anticardiolipin antibodies, lupus anticoagulant).

When considering risk/benefit, the physician should take into account that adequate treatment of a condition may reduce the associated risk of thrombosis and that the risk associated with pregnancy is higher than that associated with COC use.

Numerous epidemiological studies have been reported on the risks of ovarian, endometrial, cervical and breast cancer in women using combined oral contraceptives. The evidence is clear that combined oral contraceptives offer substantial protection against both ovarian and endometrial cancer.

An increased risk of cervical cancer in long-term users of combined oral contraceptives has been reported in some studies, but there continues to be controversy about the extent to which this is attributable to the confounding effects of sexual behaviour and other factors.

A meta-analysis from 54 epidemiological studies reported that there is a slightly increased relative risk (RR = 1.24) of having breast cancer diagnosed in women who are currently using combined oral contraceptives (COCs). The observed pattern of increased risk may be due to an earlier diagnosis of breast cancer in COC users, the biological effects of COCs or a combination of both. The additional breast cancers diagnosed in current users of COCs or in women who have used COCs in the last ten years are more likely to be localised to the breast than those in women who never used COCs.

Breast cancer is rare among women under 40 years of age whether or not they take COCs. Whilst this background risk increases with age, the excess number of breast cancer diagnoses in current and recent COC users is small in relation to the overall risk of breast cancer (see bar chart).

The most important risk factor for breast cancer in COC users is the age women discontinue the COC; the older the age at stopping, the more breast cancers are diagnosed. Duration of use is less important and the excess risk gradually disappears during the course of the 10 years after stopping COC use such that by 10 years there appears to be no excess.

The possible increase in risk of breast cancer should be discussed with the user and weighed against the benefits of COCs taking into account the evidence that they offer substantial protection against the risk of developing certain other cancers (e.g. ovarian and endometrial cancer).

(see Figure 1 above)

The possibility cannot be ruled out that certain chronic diseases may occasionally deteriorate during the use of combined oral contraceptives (see *'Precautions'*).

In rare cases benign and, in even rarer cases, malignant liver tumours leading in isolated cases to life-threatening intra-abdominal haemorrhage have been observed after the use of hormonal substances such as those contained in Logynon. If severe upper abdominal complaints, liver enlargement or signs of intra-abdominal haemorrhage occur, the possibility of a liver tumour should be included in the differential diagnosis.

Reasons for stopping oral contraception immediately:

1. Occurrence for the first time, or exacerbation, of migrainous headaches or unusually frequent or unusually severe headaches

2. Sudden disturbances of vision or hearing or other perceptual disorders

3. First signs of thrombophlebitis or thromboembolic symptoms (e.g. unusual pains in or swelling of the leg(s), stabbing pains on breathing or coughing for no apparent reason). Feeling of pain and tightness in the chest

4. Six weeks before an elective major operation (e.g. abdominal, orthopaedic), any surgery to the legs, medical treatment for varicose veins or prolonged immobilisation, e.g. after accidents or surgery. Do not restart until 2 weeks after full ambulation. In case of emergency surgery, thrombotic prophylaxis is usually indicated e.g. subcutaneous heparin

5. Onset of jaundice, hepatitis, itching of the whole body

6. Increase in epileptic seizures

7. Significant rise in blood pressure

8. Onset of severe depression

9. Severe upper abdominal pain or liver enlargement

10. Clear exacerbation of conditions known to be capable of deteriorating during oral contraception or pregnancy

11. Pregnancy is a reason for stopping immediately because it has been suggested by some investigations that oral contraceptives taken in early pregnancy may slightly increase the risk of foetal malformations. Other investigations have failed to support these findings. The possibility therefore cannot be excluded, but it is certain that if a risk exists at all, it is very small.

Precautions:

Assessment of women prior to starting oral contraceptives (and at regular intervals thereafter) should include a personal and family medical history of each woman. Physical examination should be guided by this and by the contraindications, warnings etc for this product. The frequency and nature of these assessments should be based upon relevant guidelines and should be adapted to the individual woman, but should include measurement of blood pressure and, if judged appropriate by the clinician, breast, abdominal and pelvic examination including cervical cytology.

The following conditions require strict medical supervision during medication with oral contraceptives. Deterioration or first appearance of any of these conditions may indicate that use of the oral contraceptive should be discontinued: diabetes mellitus, or a tendency towards diabetes mellitus (e.g. unexplained glycosuria), hypertension, varicose veins, a history of phlebitis, otosclerosis, multiple sclerosis, epilepsy, porphyria, tetany, disturbed liver function, Sydenham's chorea, renal dysfunction, family history of clotting disorders, obesity, family history of breast cancer and patient history of benign breast disease, history of clinical depression, systemic lupus erythematosus, uterine fibroids and migraine, gall-stones, cardiovascular diseases, chloasma, asthma, an intolerance of contact lenses, or any disease that is prone to worsen during pregnancy

Some women may experience amenorrhoea or oligomenorrhoea after discontinuation of oral contraceptives, especially when these conditions existed prior to use. Women should be informed of this possibility.

Side-effects: In rare cases, headaches, gastric upsets, nausea, vomiting, breast tenderness, changes in body weight, changes in libido, depressive moods can occur.

In predisposed women, use of Logynon can sometimes cause chloasma which is exacerbated by exposure to sunlight. Such women should avoid prolonged exposure to sunlight.

Individual cases of poor tolerance of contact lenses have been reported with use of oral contraceptives. Contact lens wearers who develop changes in lens tolerance should be assessed by an ophthalmologist.

Menstrual changes:

1. Reduction of menstrual flow: This is not abnormal and it is to be expected in some patients. Indeed, it may be beneficial where heavy periods were previously experienced.

2. Missed menstruation: Occasionally, withdrawal bleeding may not occur at all. If the tablets have been taken correctly, pregnancy is very unlikely. If withdrawal bleeding fails to occur at the end of a second pack, the possibility of pregnancy must be ruled out before resuming with the next pack.

Intermenstrual bleeding: 'Spotting' or heavier 'breakthrough bleeding' sometimes occur during tablet taking, especially in the first few cycles, and normally cease spontaneously. Logynon should therefore, be continued even if irregular bleeding occurs. If irregular bleeding is persistent, appropriate diagnostic measures to exclude an organic cause are indicated and may include curettage. This also applies in the case of spotting which occurs at irregular intervals in several consecutive cycles or which occurs for the first time after long use of Logynon.

Effect on blood chemistry: The use of oral contraceptives may influence the results of certain laboratory tests including biochemical parameters of liver, thyroid, adrenal and renal function, plasma levels of carrier proteins and lipid/lipoprotein fractions, parameters of carbohydrate metabolism and parameters of coagulation and fibrinolysis. Laboratory staff should therefore be informed about oral contraceptive use when laboratory tests are requested.

Overdosage: Overdosage may cause nausea, vomiting and, in females, withdrawal bleeding. There are no specific antidotes and treatment should be symptomatic.

Pharmaceutical precautions Shelf-life - Five years

Legal category POM

Package quantities Individual packs containing three months' supply (OP)

Further information Nil

Product licence number 0053/0085

Date of last revision 16 July 2004

Logynon ED

(Schering Health Care Limited)

1. NAME OF THE MEDICINAL PRODUCT

Logynon® ED

2. QUALITATIVE AND QUANTITATIVE COMPOSITION

Calendar pack containing 6 light brown tablets, 5 white tablets and 10 ochre-coloured tablets containing the following active ingredients.

Light Brown Tablets

Levonorgestrel	50 micrograms
Ethinylestradiol	30 micrograms

White Tablets

Levonorgestrel	75 micrograms
Ethinylestradiol	40 micrograms

Ochre Tablets

Levonorgestrel	125 micrograms
Ethinylestradiol	30 micrograms

Loygnon ED also contains 7 large white placebo tablets.

3. PHARMACEUTICAL FORM

Sugar-coated tablets

4. CLINICAL PARTICULARS

4.1 Therapeutic indications

Oral contraception and the recognised gynaecological indications for such oestrogen-progestogen combinations.

4.2 Posology and method of administration

First treatment cycle: 1 tablet daily for 28 days, starting on the first day of the menstrual cycle. 21 (small) active tablets are taken followed by 7 (larger) placebo tablets. Contraceptive protection begins immediately.

Subsequent cycles: Tablet taking is continuous, which means that the next pack of Logynon ED follows immediately without a break. A withdrawal bleed usually occurs when the white placebo tablets are being taken.

Changing from 21-day combined oral contraceptives: The first tablet of Logynon ED should be taken on the first day immediately after the end of the previous oral contraceptive course. Additional contraceptive precautions are not required.

Changing from a combined Every Day pill (28 -day pill): Logynon ED should be started after taking the last active tablet from the previous Every Day pill pack. The first Logynon ED tablet is taken the next day. Additional contraceptive precautions are not then required.

Changing from a progestogen-only pill (POP):

The first tablet of Logynon ED should be taken on the first day of bleeding, even if a POP has already been taken on that day. Additional contraceptive precautions are not then required. The remaining progestogen-only pills should be discarded.

Post-partum and post-abortum use: After pregnancy, Logynon ED can be started 21 days after a vaginal delivery, provided that the patient is fully ambulant and there are no puerperal complications. Additional contraceptive precautions will be required for the first 7 days of tablet taking. Since the first post-partum ovulation may precede the first bleeding, another method of contraception should be used in the interval between childbirth and the first course of tablets. After a first-trimester abortion, oral contraception may be started immediately in which case no additional contraceptive precautions are required.

Special circumstances requiring additional contraception:

Incorrect administration: Errors in taking the 7 inactive white placebo tablets (i.e. the larger white tablets in the last row) can be ignored. A single delayed active (small) tablet should be taken as soon as possible, and if this can be done within 12 hours of the correct time, contraceptive protection is maintained.

With longer delays in taking active tablets, additional contraception is needed. Only the most recently delayed tablet should be taken, earlier missed tablets being omitted, and additional non-hormonal methods of contraception (except the rhythm or temperature methods) should be used for *the next 7 days, while the next 7 active (small) tablets are being taken.* Therefore, if the 7 days additional contraception will extend beyond the last active (small) tablet, the user should finish taking all the active tablets, discard the placebo tablets and start a new pack of Logynon ED the next day with an appropriate active (small) tablet. Thus, active tablet follows active tablet with no 7 day break. In this situation, a withdrawal bleed should not be expected until the end of the second pack. Some breakthrough bleeding may occur on pill taking days but this is not clinically significant. If the patient does not have a withdrawal bleed following the end of the second pack, the possibility of pregnancy must be ruled out before starting the next pack.

Gastro-intestinal upset: Vomiting or diarrhoea may reduce the efficacy of oral contraceptives by preventing full absorption. Tablet taking from the current pack should be continued. Additional non-hormonal methods of contraception (except the rhythm or temperature methods) should be used during the gastro-intestinal upset and for 7 days following the upset. If these 7 days extend beyond the last active (small) tablet the user should finish taking all the active tablets, discard the placebo tablets and start a new pack of Logynon ED the next day with an appropriate active (small) tablet. In this situation, a withdrawal bleed should not be expected until the end of the second pack. If the patient does not have a withdrawal bleed at the end of the second pack, the possibility of pregnancy must be ruled out before starting the next pack. Other methods of contraception should be considered if the gastro-intestinal disorder is likely to be prolonged.

4.3 Contraindications

1. Pregnancy

2. Severe disturbances of liver function, jaundice or persistent itching during a previous pregnancy, Dubin-Johnson syndrome, Rotor syndrome, previous or existing liver tumours

3. Existing or a history of confirmed venous thromboembolism (VTE), family history of idiopathic VTE and other known risk factors for VTE.

4. Existing or previous arterial thrombotic or embolic processes.

5. Conditions which predispose to them e.g. disorders of the clotting processes, valvular heart disease and atrial fibrillation

6. Sickle-cell anaemia

7. Mammary or endometrial carcinoma, or a history of these conditions

8. Severe diabetes mellitus with vascular changes

9. Disorders of lipid metabolism

10. History of herpes gestationis

11. Deterioration of otosclerosis during pregnancy

12. Undiagnosed abnormal vaginal bleeding

13. Hypersensitivity to any of the components of Logynon ED.

4.4 Special warnings and special precautions for use

Warnings:

The use of any combined oral contraceptive carries an increased risk of venous thromboembolism (VTE) compared with no use. The excess risk of VTE is highest during the first year a woman ever uses a combined oral contraceptive. This increased risk is less than the risk of VTE associated with pregnancy which is estimated as 60 cases per 100 000 pregnancies. Some epidemiological studies have reported a greater risk of VTE for women using combined oral contraceptives containing desogestrel or gestodene (the so-called 'third generation' pills) than for women using pills containing levonorgestrel (the so-called 'second generation' pills).

The spontaneous incidence of VTE in healthy non-pregnant women (not taking any oral contraceptive) is about 5 cases per 100,000 per year. The incidence in users of second generation pills is about 15 per 100,000 women per year of use. The incidence in users of third generation pills is about 25 cases per 100,000 women per year of use; this excess incidence has not been satisfactorily explained by bias or confounding. The level of all these risks increases with age and is likely to be further increased in women with other known risk factors for VTE such as obesity.

The risk of venous and/or arterial thrombosis associated with combined oral contraceptives increases with:

- age;
- smoking (with heavier smoking and increasing age the risk further increases, especially in women over 35 years of age);
- a positive family history (i.e. venous or arterial thromboembolism ever in a sibling or parent at a relatively early age). If a hereditary predisposition is suspected, the woman should be referred to a specialist for advice before deciding about any COC use;
- obesity (body mass index over 30 kg/m^2);
- dyslipoproteinaemia;

Figure 1

Estimated cumulative numbers of breast cancers per 10,000 women diagnosed in 5 years of use and up to 10 years after stopping COCs, compared with numbers of breast cancers diagnosed in 10,000 women who had never used COCs

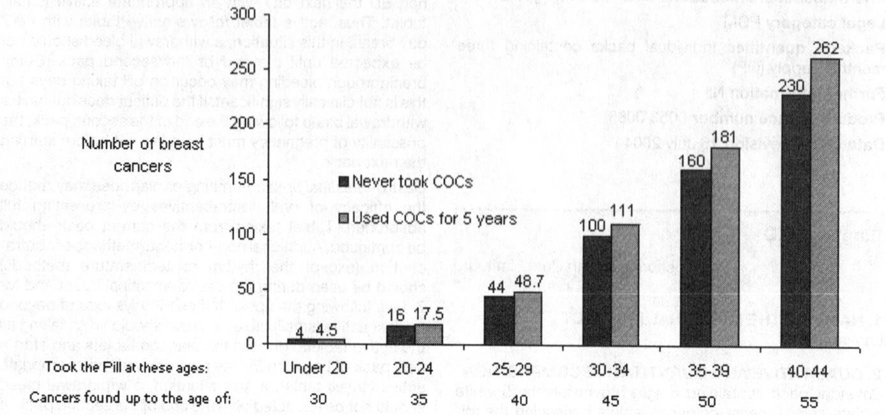

- hypertension;
- valvular heart disease;
- atrial fibrillation;
- prolonged immobilisation, major surgery, any surgery to the legs, or major trauma. In these situations it is advisable to discontinue COC use (in the case of elective surgery at least six weeks in advance) and not to resume until two weeks after complete remobilisation.
- There is no consensus about the possible role of varicose veins and superficial thrombophlebitis in venous thromboembolism.
- The increased risk of thromboembolism in the puerperium must be considered (for information on "Pregnancy and Lactation" see Section 4.6).
- Other medical conditions which have been associated with adverse circulatory events include diabetes mellitus, systemic lupus erythematosus, haemolytic uraemic syndrome, chronic inflammatory bowel disease (Crohn's disease or ulcerative colitis), sickle cell disease and subarachnoid haemorrhage.
- An increase in frequency or severity of migraine during COC use (which may be prodromal of a cerebrovascular event) may be a reason for immediate discontinuation of the COC.
- Biochemical factors that may be indicative of hereditary or acquired predisposition for venous or arterial thrombosis include Activated Protein C (APC) resistance, hyperhomocysteinaemia, antithrombin-III deficiency, protein C deficiency, protein S deficiency, antiphospholipid antibodies (anticardiolipin antibodies, lupus anticoagulant).

When considering risk/benefit, the physician should take into account that adequate treatment of a condition may reduce the associated risk of thrombosis and that the risk associated with pregnancy is higher than that associated with COC use.

Numerous epidemiological studies have been reported on the risks of ovarian, endometrial, cervical and breast cancer in women using combined oral contraceptives. The evidence is clear that combined oral contraceptives offer substantial protection against both ovarian and endometrial cancer.

An increased risk of cervical cancer in long-term users of combined oral contraceptives has been reported in some studies, but there continues to be controversy about the extent to which this is attributable to the confounding effects of sexual behaviour and other factors.

A meta-analysis from 54 epidemiological studies reported that there is a slightly increased relative risk (RR = 1.24) of having breast cancer diagnosed in women who are currently using combined oral contraceptives (COCs). The observed pattern of increased risk may be due to an earlier diagnosis of breast cancer in COC users, the biological effects of COCs or a combination of both. The additional breast cancers diagnosed in current users of COCs or in women who have used COCs in the last ten years are more likely to be localised to the breast than those in women who never used COCs.

Breast cancer is rare among women under 40 years of age whether or not they take COCs. Whilst this background risk increases with age, the excess number of breast cancer diagnoses in current and recent COC users is small in relation to the overall risk of breast cancer (see bar chart).

The most important risk factor for breast cancer in COC users is the age women discontinue the COC; the older the age at stopping, the more breast cancers are diagnosed. Duration of use is less important and the excess risk gradually disappears during the course of the 10 years after stopping COC use such that by 10 years there appears to be no excess.

The possible increase in risk of breast cancer should be discussed with the user and weighed against the benefits of COCs taking into account the evidence that they offer substantial protection against the risk of developing certain other cancers (e.g. ovarian and endometrial cancer).

(see Figure 1 above)

The possibility cannot be ruled out that certain chronic diseases may occasionally deteriorate during the use of combined oral contraceptives (see *'Precautions'*).

In rare cases benign and, in even rarer cases, malignant liver tumours leading in isolated cases to life-threatening intra-abdominal haemorrhage have been observed after the use of hormonal substances such as those contained in Logynon ED. If severe upper abdominal complaints, liver enlargement or signs of intra-abdominal haemorrhage occur, the possibility of a liver tumour should be included in the differential diagnosis.

Reasons for stopping oral contraception immediately:

1. Occurrence for the first time, or exacerbation, of migrainous headaches or unusually frequent or unusually severe headaches
2. Sudden disturbances of vision or hearing or other perceptual disorders
3. First signs of thrombophlebitis or thromboembolic symptoms (e.g. unusual pains in or swelling of the leg(s), stabbing pains on breathing or coughing for no apparent reason). Feeling of pain and tightness in the chest
4. Six weeks before an elective major operation (e.g. abdominal, orthopaedic), any surgery to the legs, medical treatment for varicose veins or prolonged immobilisation, e.g. after accidents or surgery. Do not restart until 2 weeks after full ambulation. In case of emergency surgery, thrombotic prophylaxis is usually indicated e.g. subcutaneous heparin
5. Onset of jaundice, hepatitis, itching of the whole body
6. Increase in epileptic seizures
7. Significant rise in blood pressure
8. Onset of severe depression
9. Severe upper abdominal pain or liver enlargement
10. Clear exacerbation of conditions known to be capable of deteriorating during oral contraception or pregnancy
11. Pregnancy is a reason for stopping immediately because it has been suggested by some investigations that oral contraceptives taken in early pregnancy may slightly increase the risk of foetal malformations. Other investigations have failed to support these findings. The possibility therefore cannot be excluded, but it is certain that if a risk exists at all, it is very small.

Precautions:

Assessment of women prior to starting oral contraceptives (and at regular intervals thereafter) should include a personal and family medical history of each woman. Physical examination should be guided by this and by the contraindications (section 4.3) and warnings (section 4.4) for this product. The frequency and nature of these assessments should be based upon relevant guidelines and should be adapted to the individual woman, but should include measurement of blood pressure and, if judged appropriate by the clinician, breast, abdominal and pelvic examination including cervical cytology.

<u>The following conditions require strict medical supervision</u> during medication with oral contraceptives. Deterioration or first appearance of some of these conditions may indicate that use of the oral contraceptive should be discontinued:

Diabetes mellitus, or a tendency towards diabetes mellitus (e.g. unexplained glycosuria), hypertension, varicose veins, a history of phlebitis, otosclerosis, multiple sclerosis, epilepsy, porphyria, tetany, disturbed liver function, Sydenham's chorea (chorea minor), renal dysfunction, family history of clotting disorders, obesity, family history of breast cancer and patient history of benign breast disease, history of clinical depression, systemic lupus erythematosus, uterine fibroids and migraine, gall-stones, cardiovascular diseases, chloasma, asthma, an intolerance of contact lenses, or any disease that is prone to worsen during pregnancy.

Some women may experience amenorrhoea or oligomenorrhoea after discontinuation of oral contraceptives, especially when these conditions existed prior to use. Women should be informed of this possibility.

4.5 Interaction with other medicinal products and other forms of Interaction

Hepatic enzyme inducers such as barbiturates, primidone, phenobarbitone, phenytoin, phenylbutazone, rifampicin, carbamazepine and griseofulvin can impair the efficacy of Logynon ED. For women receiving long-term therapy with hepatic enzyme inducers, another method of contraception should be used. The use of antibiotics may also reduce the efficacy of Logynon ED, possibly by altering the intestinal flora.

Women receiving short courses of enzyme inducers or broad spectrum antibiotics should take additional, non-hormonal (except the rhythm or temperature methods) contraceptive precautions during the time of concurrent medication and for 7 days afterwards. If these 7 days extend beyond the last active (small) tablet the user should finish taking all the active tablets, discard the placebo (large) tablets and start a new pack of Logynon ED the next day with an appropriate active (small) tablet. In this situation, a withdrawal bleed should not be expected until the end of the second pack. If the patient does not have a withdrawal bleed at the end of the second pack, the possibility of pregnancy must be ruled out before resuming with the next pack. With rifampicin, additional contraceptive precautions should be continued for 4 weeks after treatment stops, even if only a short course was administered.

The requirement for oral antidiabetics or insulin can change as a result of the effect on glucose tolerance.

The herbal remedy St John's wort (Hypericum perforatum) should not be taken concomitantly with Logynon ED as this could potentially lead to a loss of contraceptive effect.

4.6 Pregnancy and lactation

If pregnancy occurs during medication with oral contraceptives, the preparation should be withdrawn immediately (see 'Reasons for stopping oral contraception immediately').

The use of Logynon ED during lactation may lead to a reduction in the volume of milk produced and to a change in its composition. Minute amounts of the active substances are excreted with the milk. Mothers who are breast-feeding may be advised instead to use a progestogen-only pill.

4.7 Effects on ability to drive and use machines

None known.

4.8 Undesirable effects

In rare cases, headaches, gastric upsets, nausea, vomiting, breast tenderness, changes in body weight, changes in libido, depressive moods can occur.

In predisposed women, use of Logynon ED can sometimes cause chloasma which is exacerbated by exposure to sunlight. Such women should avoid prolonged exposure to sunlight.

Individual cases of poor tolerance of contact lenses have been reported with use of oral contraceptives. Contact lens wearers who develop changes in lens tolerance should be assessed by an ophthalmologist.

Menstrual changes:

1. Reduction of menstrual flow:

This is not abnormal and it is to be expected in some patients. Indeed, it may be beneficial where heavy periods were previously experienced.

2. Missed menstruation:

Occasionally, withdrawal bleeding may not occur at all. If the tablets have been taken correctly, pregnancy is very unlikely. If withdrawal bleeding fails to occur at the end of a second pack, the possibility of pregnancy must be ruled out before resuming with the next pack.

Intermenstrual bleeding: 'Spotting' or heavier 'breakthrough bleeding' sometimes occur during tablet taking, especially in the first few cycles, and normally cease spontaneously. Logynon ED should therefore be continued even if irregular bleeding occurs. If irregular bleeding is persistent, appropriate diagnostic measures to exclude an organic cause are indicated and may include curettage. This also applies in the case of spotting which occurs at irregular intervals in several consecutive cycles or which occurs for the first time after long use of Logynon ED.

Effect on blood chemistry: The use of oral contraceptives may influence the results of certain laboratory tests including biochemical parameters of liver, thyroid, adrenal and renal function, plasma levels of carrier proteins and lipid/lipoprotein fractions, parameters of carbohydrate metabolism and parameters of coagulation and fibrinolysis. Laboratory staff should therefore be informed about oral contraceptive use when laboratory tests are requested.

Refer to "Section 4.4 Special warnings and special precautions for use" for additional information.

4.9 Overdose

Overdosage may cause nausea, vomiting and, in females, withdrawal bleeding.

There are no specific antidotes and treatment should be symptomatic.

5. PHARMACOLOGICAL PROPERTIES

5.1 Pharmacodynamic properties

Logynon ED is an oestrogen-progestogen combination which acts by inhibiting ovulation by suppression of the mid-cycle surge of luteinizing hormone, the inspissation of cervical mucus so as to constitute a barrier to sperm, and the rendering of the endometrium unreceptive to implantation.

5.2 Pharmacokinetic properties

Levonorgestrel

Orally administered levonorgestrel is rapidly and completely absorbed. Following ingestion of 0.125mg levonorgestrel together with 0.03mg ethinylestradiol (which represents the combination with the highest levonorgestrel content of the tri-step formulation), maximum drug serum levels of about 4.3ng/ml are reached at 1.0 hour. Thereafter, levonorgestrel serum levels decrease in two phases, characterized by half-lives of 0.4 hours and about 22 hours. For levonorgestrel, a metabolic clearance rate from serum of about 1.5ml/min/kg was determined. Levonorgestrel is not excreted in unchanged form but as metabolites. Levonorgestrel metabolites are excreted in about equal proportions with urine and faeces. The biotransformation follows the known pathways of steroid metabolism. No pharmacologically active metabolites are known.

Levonorgestrel is bound to serum albumin and to SHBG. Only 1.4% of the total serum drug levels are present as free steroid, but 55% are specifically bound to SHBG. The relative distribution (free, albumin-bound, SHBG-bound) depends on the SHBG concentrations in the serum. Following induction of the binding protein, the SHBG-bound fraction increases while the unbound fractions decrease.

Following daily repeated administration of Logynon ED, levonorgestrel concentrations in the serum increase by a factor of about 4. Steady-state conditions are reached during the second half of a treatment cycle. The pharmacokinetics of levonorgestrel is influenced by SHBG serum levels. Under treatment with Logynon ED, an increase in the serum levels of SHBG by a factor of about 2 occurs during a treatment cycle. Due to the specific binding of levonorgestrel to SHBG, the increase in SHBG levels is accompanied by an almost parallel increase in levonorgestrel serum levels. The absolute bioavailability of levonorgestrel was determined to be almost 100% of the dose administered.

Ethinylestradiol

Orally administered ethinylestradiol is rapidly and completely absorbed. Following ingestion of 0.03mg ethinylestradiol together with 0.125mg levonorgestrel, maximum drug serum levels of about 116 pg/ml are reached at 1.3 hours. Thereafter, ethinylestradiol serum levels decrease in two phases characterized by half-lives of 1 - 2 hours and about 20 hours. For technical reasons, these parameters can only be calculated following the administration of higher doses. For ethinylestradiol an apparent volume of distribution of about 5 l/kg and a metabolic clearance rate from serum of about 5 ml/min/kg were determined. Ethinylestradiol is highly but non-specifically bound to serum albumin. About 2% of drug levels are present unbound. During absorption and first liver passage, ethinylestradiol is metabolized resulting in a reduced absolute and variable oral bioavailability. Unchanged drug is not excreted. Ethinylestradiol metabolites are excreted at a urinary to biliary ratio of 4:6 with a half-life of about 1 day.

Due to the half-life of the terminal disposition phase from serum and the daily ingestion, steady-state serum levels are reached after 3-4 days and are higher by 30 - 40% as compared to a single dose. The absolute bioavailability of ethinylestradiol is subject to a considerable interindividual variation. Following oral administration, the mean bioavailability was found to be about 40 - 60% of the administered dose.

During established lactation, 0.02% of the daily maternal dose could be transferred to the newborn via milk.

The systemic availability of ethinylestradiol might be influenced in both directions by other drugs. There is, however, no interaction with high doses of vitamin C. Ethinylestradiol induces the hepatic synthesis of SHBG and CBG during continuous use. The extent of SHBG induction, however, depends on the chemical structure and the dose of the co-administered progestogen. During treatment with Logynon ED, SHBG concentrations in the serum increased from about 76 nmol/l to 164 nmol/l and the serum concentrations of CBG increased from about 48 μg/ml to 111 μg/ml.

5.3 Preclinical safety data

There are no preclinical safety data which could be of relevance to the prescriber and which are not already included in other relevant sections of the SPC.

6. PHARMACEUTICAL PARTICULARS

6.1 List of excipients

Excipients included in both active and placebo tablets:

Active Tablets	*Placebo tablets*
lactose	lactose
maize starch	maize starch
povidone	povidone
magnesium stearate (E 572)	magnesium stearate (E 572)
sucrose	sucrose
polyethylene glycol 6000	polyethylene glycol 6000
calcium carbonate (E 170)	calcium carbonate (E 170)
talc	talc
montan glycol wax	montan glycol wax
glycerin (E 422)	
titanium dioxide (E171)	
ferric oxide pigment (red and yellow) (E172)	

6.2 Incompatibilities

None known

6.3 Shelf life

5 years

6.4 Special precautions for storage

Not applicable

6.5 Nature and contents of container

Deep drawn strips made of polyvinyl chloride film with counter-sealing foil made of aluminium with heat sealable coating.

Presentation:

Cartons containing 3 blister memo-packs. Each memo-pack contains 21 active tablets and 7 placebo tablets (total 28 tablets).

6.6 Instructions for use and handling

Keep out of the reach of children.

7. MARKETING AUTHORISATION HOLDER

Schering Health Care Limited

The Brow

Burgess Hill

West Sussex, RH15 9NE

8. MARKETING AUTHORISATION NUMBER(S)

0053/0115

9. DATE OF FIRST AUTHORISATION/RENEWAL OF THE AUTHORISATION

June 1980/16 November 1995

10. DATE OF REVISION OF THE TEXT

16 July 2004

LEGAL CATEGORY

POM

Lomont

(Rosemont Pharmaceuticals Limited)

1. NAME OF THE MEDICINAL PRODUCT

Lomont 70mg/5ml

2. QUALITATIVE AND QUANTITATIVE COMPOSITION

Active IngredientPer 5ml

Lofepramine Hydrochloride, 76.1mg

(equivalent to Lofepramine base) 70mg

3. PHARMACEUTICAL FORM

A white to pale yellow/orange suspension with odour of Cherry.

4. CLINICAL PARTICULARS

4.1 Therapeutic indications

For the treatment of symptoms of depressive illness.

4.2 Posology and method of administration

Adults: The usual dose 70mg twice daily (140mg) or three times daily (210mg) depending upon patient response.

Elderly: Elderly patients may respond to lower doses in some cases.

Children: Not recommended

4.3 Contraindications

Lofepramine should not be used in patients hypersensitive to dibenzazepines, in mania, severe liver impairment and/or severe renal impairment, heart block, cardiac arrhythmias, or during the recovery phase following a myocardial infarction.

4.4 Special warnings and special precautions for use

Lofepramine should be used with caution in patients with cardiovascular disease, impaired liver or renal function, narrow angle glaucoma, symptoms suggestive of prostatic hypertrophy, a history of epilepsy or recent convulsions, hyperthyroidism, blood dyscrasias or porphyria.

Hyponatraemia (usually in the elderly and possibly due to inappropriate secretion of antidiuretic hormone) has been associated with all types of antidepressants and should be considered in all patients who develop drowsiness, confusion or convulsions while taking lofepramine.

4.5 Interaction with other medicinal products and other forms of Interaction

Lofepramine should not be administered concurrently with or within 2 weeks of cessation of therapy of monamine oxidase inhibitors. It should then be introduced cautiously using a low initial dosage.

Lofepramine should not be given with sympathomimetic agents, central nervous depressants including alcohol or thyroid hormone therapy since its effects may be potentiated.

Lofepramine may decrease the antihypertensive effect of adrenergic neurone-blocking drugs; it is therefore advisable to review this form of antihypertensive therapy during treatment.

Anaesthetics given during tricyclic antidepressant therapy may increase the risk of arrhythmias and hypotension. If surgery is necessary, the anaesthetist should be informed that a patient is being so treated. Barbiturates may increase the rate of metabolism.

Possible interactions between lofepramine and warfarin, leading to an enhancement of anticoagulant effect, have been reported rarely.

4.6 Pregnancy and lactation

The safety of Lofepramine for use during pregnancy has not been established and there is evidence of harmful effects in pregnancy in animals when high doses are given. Lofepramine has been shown to be excreted in breast milk. The administration of Lofepramine in pregnancy and during breast feeding therefore, is not advised unless there are compelling medical reasons.

Adverse effects such as withdrawal symptoms, respiratory depression and agitation have been reported in neonates whose mothers have taken tricyclic antidepressants during the last trimester of pregnancy.

4.7 Effects on ability to drive and use machines

Ability to drive a car and operate machinery may be affected. Therefore caution should be exercised initially until the individual reaction to treatment is known.

4.8 Undesirable effects

Lofepramine has been shown to be well tolerated and side-effects, when they occur, tend to be mild. Comparative clinical trials have shown that Lofepramine is associated with a low incidence of anticholinergic side effects. The following side effects have been reported with Lofepramine:

Cardiovascular: Hypotension, tachycardia

CNS and neuromuscular: Dizziness, drowsiness, agitation, confusion, headache, malaise, paraesthesia, tinnitus and rarely hypomania and convulsions.(See section 4.4 Special Warnings and Precautions for Use)

Anticholinergic: Dryness of mouth, constipation, disturbances of accommodation, urinary hesitancy, urinary retention, sweating and tremor.

Allergic: Skin rash, allergic skin reactions, photosensitivity reactions

Gastro-intestinal: Nausea, vomiting

Endocrine: Rarely, inappropriate secretion of antidiuretic hormone, interference with sexual function.

Haematological/ biochemical: Rarely, bone marrow depression including isolated report of: agranulocytosis, eosinophilia, granuloctyopenia, leucopenia, pancytopenia, thrombocytopenia. Rises in liver enzymes have been observed in some patients usually occurring within the first three months of starting therapy. There have been a small number of reports of jaundice. These reactions are reversible on cessation of therapy. Hyponatraemia (usually in the elderly and possibly due to inappropriate antidiuretic hormone secretion see section 4.4 Special Warnings and Precautions for Use)

The following adverse effects have been encountered in patients under treatment with tricyclic antidepressants and should therefore be considered as theoretical hazards of Lofepramine even in the absence of substantiation: psychotic manifestations including mania and paranoid delusions may be exacerbated during treatment with tricyclic antidepressants; withdrawal symptoms may occur on abrupt cessation of therapy and include insomnia, irritability and excessive perspiration.

4.9 Overdose

Treatment of overdosage is symptomatic and supportive. It should include immediate gastric lavage and routine close monitoring of cardiac function. Reports of overdosage with Lofepramine, with quantities ranging from 0.7g up to 6.72g, have shown no serious sequelae directly attributable to the drug.

5. PHARMACOLOGICAL PROPERTIES

5.1 Pharmacodynamic properties

Lofepramine inhibits the re-uptake of monoamines in peripheral adrenergic nerves. Lofepramine produces a lesser increase in heart rate than that produced by Amitriptyline when administered to normal individuals.

5.2 Pharmacokinetic properties

Lofepramine is rapidly absorbed with peak plasma concentration being reached within 1 hour and having a plasma half-life of 5 hours. In common with Imipramine, Lofepramine appears to undergo significant presystemic metabolism.

Plasma protein binding is approximately 99%. After oral administration higher concentrations of Lofepramine and its metabolites can be found in blood, lungs, liver, kidney and brain.

Almost all of the drug is metabolized before excretion, which is mainly in the urine and in faeces. Lofepramine is metabolized by N-dealkylation, hydroxylation and glucuronidation. It is extensively metabolized to its principal metabolite, desmethylimipramine, on first pass through the liver. During chronic administration, the plasma level of desmethylimipramine is typically three times greater than that of lofepramine, except in the first few hours following administration of each dose, during which time the plasma level of the parent drug can exceed that of its metabolite. Desipramine, which is also an antidepressant is converted to 2-hydroxydesipramine in the liver. Both compounds are excreted mainly in the urine as glucuronides, but also by biliary excretion in the faeces. Less than 5% is excreted unchanged in the urine over 24 hours.

Neither renal disease or old age has any appreciable effect on the kinetics of desipramine. Elimination may be reduced and bioavailability increased in hepatic disease.

5.3 Preclinical safety data

Lofepramine Hydrochloride is a well established active substance.

Lofepramine, like other tricyclic antidepressants, has been shown to inhibit the neuronal uptake of noradrenaline and to potentiate serotonergic transmission.

The safety of Lofepramine for use during pregnancy has not been established and there is evidence of harmful effects in pregnancy in animals when high doses are given. Lofepramine has been shown to be excreted in breast milk. The administration of Lofepramine in pregnancy and breast feeding therefore, is not advised unless there are compelling medical reasons.

Adverse effects such as withdrawal symptoms, respiratory depression and agitation have been reported in neonates whose mothers have taken tricyclic antidepressants during the last trimester of pregnancy.

The toxological data available in the published literature on lofepramine have not revealed any hazards, which are likely to occur at the usual oral therapeutic dosage. The excipients in the formulation would not be anticipated to influence the pharmacology or toxicology of the drug.

6. PHARMACEUTICAL PARTICULARS

6.1 List of excipients

Purified water, sodium ascorbate, sorbitol solution 70% (non-crystallising), liquid maltitol, methyl hydroxybenzoate, propyl hydroxybenzoate, propylene glycol, ethanol (absolute), colloidal silicon dioxide (aerosil) and cherry flavour 28T7704.

6.2 Incompatibilities

None known

6.3 Shelf life

24 months

6.4 Special precautions for storage

Store between 4°C and 25°C. Protect from light.

6.5 Nature and contents of container

150ml, 200ml or 300ml amber (type III) glass bottles

Closures: - 1) Aluminium, EPE wadded, roll-on, pilfer-proof, or 2) HDPE, EPE wadded, tamper evident or 3) HDPE EPE wadded, tamper evident child resistant.

6.6 Instructions for use and handling

Keep out of the reach of children. Shake before use.

7. MARKETING AUTHORISATION HOLDER

Rosemont Pharmaceuticals Ltd

Rosemont House

Yorkdale Industrial Park

Braithwaite Street

Leeds

LS11 9XE

8. MARKETING AUTHORISATION NUMBER(S)

PL 0427/0094

9. DATE OF FIRST AUTHORISATION/RENEWAL OF THE AUTHORISATION

1 February 1996

10. DATE OF REVISION OF THE TEXT

January 2004

Lomustine "medac" 40 mg

(medac GmbH)

1. NAME OF THE MEDICINAL PRODUCT

Lomustine "medac" 40 mg

2. QUALITATIVE AND QUANTITATIVE COMPOSITION

Lomustine (CCNU) 40 mg per capsule

3. PHARMACEUTICAL FORM

Hard capsule

4. CLINICAL PARTICULARS

4.1 Therapeutic indications

As palliative or supplementary treatment, usually in combination with radiotherapy and/or surgery as part of multiple drug regimens in:

Brain tumours (primary or metastatic)

Lung tumours (especially oat-cell carcinoma)

Hodgkin's disease (resistant to conventional combination chemo-therapy)

Malignant melanoma (metastatic)

Lomustine "medac" may also be of value as second-line treatment in Non-Hodgkin's lymphoma, myelomatosis, gastrointestinal tumours, carcinoma of the kidney, the testis, the ovary, the cervix uteri and the breast.

4.2 Posology and method of administration

Dosage

Adults:

Lomustine "medac" is given by mouth. The recommended dose in patients with normally functioning bone marrow receiving Lomustine "medac" as their only chemotherapy is 120-130 mg/m^2 as a single dose every six to eight weeks (or as a divided dose over 3 days, e.g. 40 mg/m^2/day).

Dosage is reduced if:

(i) Lomustine "medac" is being given as part of a drug regimen which includes other marrow-depressant drugs, and

(ii) In the presence of leucopenia below 3,000/mm^3 or thrombocytopenia below 75,000/mm^3.

Marrow depression after Lomustine "medac" is sustained longer than after nitrogen mustards and recovery of white cell and platelet counts may not occur for six weeks or more. Blood elements depressed below the above levels should be allowed to recover to 4,000/mm^3 (WBC) and 100,000/mm^3 (platelets) before repeating Lomustine "medac" dosage.

Children:

Until further data is available, administration of Lomustine "medac" to children with malignancies other than brain tumours should be restricted to specialised centres and exceptional situations. Dosage in children, like that in adults, is based on body surface area (120 - 130 mg/m^2 every six to eight weeks, with the same qualifications as apply to adults).

Route of Adminstration:

Lomustine "medac" is given by mouth.

4.3 Contraindications

Lomustine can cause birth defects. Men and women are recommended to take contraceptive precautions during therapy with lomustine and for 6 months after treatment. Men should be informed about the risk for an irreversible infertility due to treatment with lomustine.

Lomustine "medac" should not be administered to patients who are pregnant or to mothers who are breast feeding.

Other contraindications are:

(i) Previous hypersensitivity to nitrosoureas;

(ii) Previous failure of the tumor to respond to other nitrosoureas;

(iii) Severe bone-marrow depression;

(iv) Severe renal impairment;

(v) Coeliac disease or wheat allergy.

4.4 Special warnings and special precautions for use

Patients receiving Lomustine "medac" chemotherapy should be under the care of doctors experienced in cancer treatment. Blood counts should be carried out before starting the drug and at frequent intervals (preferably weekly) during treatment. Treatment and dosage is governed principally by the haemoglobin, white cell count and platelet count. Liver and kidney function should also be assessed periodically.

4.5 Interaction with other medicinal products and other forms of Interaction

Lomustine "medac" use in combination with theophylline or with the H_2-receptor antagonist cimetidine may potentiate bone marrow toxicity. Cross resistance with other nitrosoureas is usual, but cross resistance with conventional alkylating agents is unusual.

Pre-treatment with phenobarbital can lead to a reduced antitumour effect of lomustine due to an accelerated elimination caused by induction of microsomal liver enzyms.

4.6 Pregnancy and lactation

Lomustine is contraindicated in women who are pregnant and mothers who are breast feeding.

4.7 Effects on ability to drive and use machines

Lomustine "medac" capsules can impair the ability to drive and use machines, e.g. because of nausea and vomiting.

4.8 Undesirable effects

Haematological

The principal adverse effect is marrow toxicity of a delayed or prolonged nature. Thrombocytopenia appears about four weeks after a dose of Lomustine "medac" and lasts one or two weeks at a level around 80-100,000/mm^3. Leucopenia appears after six weeks and persists for one or two weeks at about 4 - 5,000/mm^3.

The haematological toxicity may be cumulative, leading to successively lower white cell and platelet counts with successive doses of the drug.

Gastrointestinal

Nausea and vomiting usually occur four to six hours after a full single dose of Lomustine "medac" and last for 24-48 hours, followed by anorexia for two or three days. The effects are less troublesome if the 6 weekly dose is divided into three doses given on each of the first three days of the six week period. Gastrointestinal tolerance is usually good, however, if prophylactic antiemetics are given (e. g. metoclopramide or chlorpromazine). Disorders of liver function have been reported commonly. They are mild in most cases. In rare cases a cholestatic jaundice occurs. Transient elevation of liver enzymes (SGOT, SGPT, LDH or alkaline phosphatase) are occasionally observed.

More rarely patients are troubled by stomatitis and diarrhoea.

Neurologic system

Mild neurologic symptoms, like e.g. apathy, disorientation, confusion and stuttering can occur uncommonly in combination therapy with other antineoplastic drugs or radiation.

Pulmonary system

Interstitial pneunomia or lung fibrosis have been reported rarely.

Renal system

Renal failure has been reported in single cases after prolonged treatment with lomustine reaching a high cumulative total dose. Therefore it is recommended not to exceed a maximum cumulative total lomustine dose of 1000 mg/m^2.

Other Side Effects

Loss of scalp hair has been reported rarely.

In single cases an irreversible vision loss has been reported after a combined therapy of lomustine with radiation.

4.9 Overdose

Symptoms

Symptoms of overdosage with Lomustine "medac" will probably include bone-marrow toxicity, haematological toxicity, nausea and vomiting.

Emergency Procedures

Overdosage should be treated immediately by gastric lavage.

Antidote

There is no specific antidote to overdosage with Lomustine "medac". Treatment should be symptomatic and supportive. Appropriate blood product replacement should be given as clinically required.

5. PHARMACOLOGICAL PROPERTIES

5.1 Pharmacodynamic properties

The mode of action is believed to be partly as an alkylating agent and partly by inhibition of several steps in the synthesis of nucleic acid and inhibition of the repair of single strand breaks in DNA chains.

5.2 Pharmacokinetic properties

Lomustine "medac" is readily absorbed from the intestinal tract. A maximum plasma concentration of 0.5-2 ng/ml is reached after 3 hours following an oral dose of 30-100 mg/m^2.

The plasma-disappearance of the chloroethyl-group follows by a single phased course with a half-life of 72 hours. The cyclohexyl-group disappears according to a twofold plasma-disappearance with half-lives of 4 hours ($t_{1/2}\,\alpha$) and 50 hours ($t_{1/2}\,\beta$). After oral application of radioactive marked lomustine the blood-brain-barrier is passed. Approximately 15 to 30 % of the measured radioactivity in the plasma can be detected in the cerebrospinal fluid.

Lomustine "medac" is rapidly metabolised and metabolites are excreted mainly via the kidneys. Lomustine "medac" cannot be detected in its active form in the urine at any time.

5.3 Preclinical safety data

Not stated

6. PHARMACEUTICAL PARTICULARS

6.1 List of excipients

Capsule Contents:

Lactose

Wheat Starch

Talc

Magnesium Stearate

Capsule Shell:

Gelatin

Indigo carmine E132

Titanium Dioxide E171

6.2 Incompatibilities
None stated.

6.3 Shelf life
3 years as packaged for sale.

6.4 Special precautions for storage
Do not store above 25 °C.

Store in the original container protected from light and moisture.

6.5 Nature and contents of container
Securitainers containing 20 capsules.

6.6 Instructions for use and handling
None.

7. MARKETING AUTHORISATION HOLDER
medac - Gesellschaft fuer klinische Spezialpraeparate mbH

Fehlandtstrasse 3

20354 Hamburg, Germany

8. MARKETING AUTHORISATION NUMBER(S)
PL 11587/0003

9. DATE OF FIRST AUTHORISATION/RENEWAL OF THE AUTHORISATION
—

10. DATE OF REVISION OF THE TEXT
28 September 2001

Loniten Tablets 2.5 mg, 5 mg and 10mg

(Pharmacia Limited)

1. NAME OF THE MEDICINAL PRODUCT
Loniten Tablets 2.5 mg, 5 mg and 10mg

2. QUALITATIVE AND QUANTITATIVE COMPOSITION
Each Loniten Tablet contains 2.5 mg, 5 mg or 10 mg minoxidil USP.

3. PHARMACEUTICAL FORM
Tablet

4. CLINICAL PARTICULARS

4.1 Therapeutic indications
Loniten is indicated for the treatment of severe hypertension.

It should not be used as the sole agent to initiate therapy. It is a peripheral vasodilator and should be given in conjunction with a diuretic, to control salt and water retention, and a beta-adrenergic blocking agent, or appropriate substitute, to control reflex tachycardia.

4.2 Posology and method of administration
Oral Administration

Adults and Patients over 12 years of age: An initial daily dose of 5 mg, which may be given as a single or divided dosage, is recommended. This dose may first be increased to 10 mg daily and subsequent increases should be by increments of 10 mg in the daily dose. Dosage adjustments should be made at intervals of not less than three days, until optimum control of blood pressure is achieved. It is seldom necessary to exceed 50 mg per day although, in exceptional circumstances, doses up to 100 mg per day have been used. Twice-daily dosage is satisfactory. Where diastolic pressure reduction of less than 30 mm Hg is required, once daily dosing has been reported as effective.

Dosage requirements may be lower in dialysis patients. Minoxidil is removed from the blood by dialysis, but its pharmacological action, once established is not reversed. Therefore haemodialysis patients should take Loniten either after or at least two hours before dialysis.

Children: For patients of 12 years of age or under, the initial dose should be 200 micrograms per kilogram (0.2 mg/kg) given as a single or divided daily dosage. Incremental increases of 100 - 200 micrograms per kilogram (0.1-0.2 mg/kg) in the daily dose are recommended at intervals of not less than three days until optimum blood pressure control has been achieved, or the maximum daily dose of 1.0 mg/kg has been reached.

Rapid reduction of blood pressure: Under hospital monitoring conditions, rapid reduction of blood pressure can be achieved using continuous blood pressure monitoring and incremental doses of 5 mg every six hours.

Concomitant antihypertensive therapy: It is recommended that, where possible, antihypertensive therapy, other than a beta-adrenergic blocking agent and a diuretic be discontinued before Loniten treatment is started. It is recognised that some antihypertensive agents should not be abruptly discontinued. These drugs should be gradually discontinued during the first week of Loniten treatment.

Loniten causes sodium retention and if used alone can result in several hundred milli-equivalents of salt being retained together with a corresponding volume of water. Therefore, in all patients who are not on dialysis, Loniten must be given in conjunction with a diuretic in sufficient dosage to maintain salt and water balance. Examples of the daily dosages of diuretics commonly used when starting therapy with Loniten include:

1. Hydrochlorothiazide (100 mg) - or other thiazides at equi-effective dosage.

2. Chlorthalidone (100 mg).

3. Frusemide (80 mg).

If excessive water retention results in a weight gain of more than 3 pounds when a thiazide or chlorthalidone is being used, diuretic therapy should be changed to frusemide, the dose of which may be increased in accordance with the patient's requirements. Diuretic dosage in children should be proportionally less in relation to weight.

Patients will require a sympathetic nervous system suppressant to limit a Loniten-induced rise in heart rate. The preferred agent is a beta-blocker equivalent to an adult propranolol dosage of 80 - 160 mg/day. Higher doses may be required when pre-treated patients have an increase in heart rate exceeding 20 beats per minute or when simultaneous introduction causes an increase exceeding 10 beats per minute. When beta-blockers are contra-indicated, alternatives such as methyldopa may be used instead and should be started 24 hours prior to Loniten.

Elderly patients: At present there are no extensive clinical studies with minoxidil in patients over age 65. There is data indicating that elevated systolic and diastolic pressures are important risk factors for cardiovascular disease in individuals over age 65. However, elderly patients may be sensitive to the blood pressure lowering effect of minoxidil and thus caution is urged in initiating therapy as orthostatic hypotension may occur. It is suggested that 2.5 mg per day be used as the initial starting dose in patients over 65 years of age.

4.3 Contraindications
Loniten is contra-indicated in patients with a phaeochromocytoma.

4.4 Special warnings and special precautions for use
If used alone, Loniten can cause a significant retention of salt and water leading to positive physical signs such as oedema, and to clinical deterioration of some patients with heart failure. Diuretic treatment alone, or in combination with restricted salt intake is, therefore, necessary for all patients taking Loniten.

Patients who have had myocardial infarction should only be treated with Loniten after a stable post-infarction state has been established.

The physician should bear in mind that if not controlled by sympathetic suppressants, the rise in cardiac rate and output that follows the use of potent vasodilators may induce anginal symptoms in patients with undiagnosed coronary artery disease, or may aggravate pre-existing angina pectoris.

The effect of Loniten may be additive to concurrent antihypertensive agents. The interaction of Loniten with sympathetic-blocking agents such as guanethidine or bethanidine may produce excessive blood pressure reduction and/or orthostasis.

Hypertrichosis occurs in most patients treated with Loniten and all patients should be warned of this possibility before starting therapy. Spontaneous reversal to the pre-treatment state can be expected one to three months after cessation of therapy.

Soon after starting Loniten therapy approximately 60% of patients exhibit ECG alterations in the direction and magnitude of their T waves. Large changes may encroach on the ST segment, unaccompanied by evidence of ischaemia. These asymptomatic changes usually disappear with continuing Loniten treatment. The ECG reverts to the pre-treatment state if Loniten is discontinued.

Pericardial effusion has been detected in patients treated with a Loniten-containing regime. A cause and effect relationship has not been established. Most effusions have either been present before Loniten was given, or occurred among uraemic patients. However, it is suggested that Loniten-treated patients should be periodically monitored for signs or symptoms of pericardial effusion and appropriate therapy instituted if necessary.

Salt and water retention in excess of 2 to 3 pounds may diminish the effectiveness of Loniten. Patients should, therefore, be carefully instructed about compliance with diuretic therapy and a detailed record of body weight should be maintained.

4.5 Interaction with other medicinal products and other forms of Interaction
The effect of Loniten may be additive to concurrent antihypertensive agents. The interaction of Loniten with sympathetic-blocking agents such as guanethidine or bethanidine may produce excessive blood pressure reduction and/or orthostasis.

4.6 Pregnancy and lactation
The safety of Loniten in pregnancy remains to be established. Minoxidil has been shown to reduce the conception rate in rats and to show evidence of increased fetal absorption in rabbits. There was no evidence of teratogenic effects in rats and rabbits. Minoxidil has been reported to be secreted in breast milk. Therefore, breast-feeding should not be undertaken while a patient is on Loniten Tablets.

4.7 Effects on ability to drive and use machines
No adverse effects reported

4.8 Undesirable effects
Most patients receiving Loniten experience a diminution of pre-existing side-effects attributable to their disease or previous therapy. New events or side-effects likely to increase include peripheral oedema, associated with or independent of weight gain; increases in heart rate; hypertrichosis; and a temporary rise in creatinine and blood urea nitrogen. Gastro-intestinal intolerance, rash and breast tenderness are infrequently reported side-effects of Loniten therapy.

4.9 Overdose
If exaggerated hypotension is encountered, it is most likely to occur in association with residual sympathetic nervous system blockade (guanethidine-like effects or alpha-adrenergic blockade). Recommended treatment is intravenous administration of normal saline. Sympathomimetic drugs, such as noradrenaline or adrenaline, should be avoided because of their excessive cardiac-stimulating action. Phenylephrine, angiotensin II and vasopressin, which reverse the effect of Loniten, should be used only if inadequate perfusion of a vital organ is evident.

5. PHARMACOLOGICAL PROPERTIES

5.1 Pharmacodynamic properties
Minoxidil is an antihypertensive agent which acts predominantly by causing direct peripheral vasodilation of the arterioles.

5.2 Pharmacokinetic properties
About 90% of an oral dose of minoxidil has been reported to associated from the GI tract.

Following oral administration the maximum hypotensive effect usually occurs after 2-3 hours. The action may persist for up to 75 hours. The plasma half life is about 4.2 hours.

Minoxidil is not bound to plasma proteins. It is extensively metabolised in the liver primarily by conjugation with glucuronic acid and is excreted in the urine mainly in the form of metabolites.

6. PHARMACEUTICAL PARTICULARS

6.1 List of excipients
Lactose hydrous, microcrystalline cellulose, starch, colloidal silicon dioxide and magnesium stearate.

6.2 Incompatibilities
None

6.3 Shelf life
Shelf-life of the medicinal product as packaged for sale: 36 months.

6.4 Special precautions for storage
Store below 25°C.

6.5 Nature and contents of container
High density polyethylene (HDPE) bottles with LDPE caps. Each bottle contains 100 tablets.

20-25 micron aluminium foil/250 micron opaque pvc blister. Pack contains 60 tablets.

6.6 Instructions for use and handling
No special requirements.

7. MARKETING AUTHORISATION HOLDER
Pharmacia Limited, Davy Avenue, Milton Keynes, MK5 8PH, UK

8. MARKETING AUTHORISATION NUMBER(S)
PL 0032/0064 2.5mg

PL 0032/0065 5 mg

PL 0032/0066 10 mg

9. DATE OF FIRST AUTHORISATION/RENEWAL OF THE AUTHORISATION
24 May 1995.

10. DATE OF REVISION OF THE TEXT
April 2001

LEGAL CATEGORY
POM

Company Ref: LN 1_0

Lopid 300mg Capsules & 600mg Film-coated Tablets

(Pfizer Limited)

1. NAME OF THE MEDICINAL PRODUCT
Lopid® 300mg Capsules

Lopid™ 600mg Film-coated Tablets

2. QUALITATIVE AND QUANTITATIVE COMPOSITION
Each capsule contains 300 mg gemfibrozil.

Each film-coated tablet contains 600mg gemfibrozil.

For excipients, see 6.1.

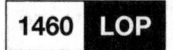

3. PHARMACEUTICAL FORM

Lopid 300mg capsules: A fine white powder contained in a hard gelatin capsule with a white opaque body and maroon cap, radially imprinted 'Lopid 300' on each capsule half.

Lopid 600mg film-coated tablets: A white, elliptical, film-coated tablet embossed with 'LOPID' on one side.

4. CLINICAL PARTICULARS

4.1 Therapeutic indications

Lopid is indicated as an adjunct to diet and other non-pharmacological treatment (e.g. exercise, weight reduction) for the following:

Treatment of dyslipidemia

Mixed dyslipidaemia characterised by hypertriglyceridaemia and/or low HDL-cholesterol. Primary hypercholesterolaemia, particularly when a statin is considered inappropriate or is not tolerated.

Primary prevention

Reduction of cardiovascular morbidity in males with increased non-HDL cholesterol and at high risk for a first cardiovascular event, particularly when a statin is considered inappropriate or is not tolerated (see section 5.1).

4.2 Posology and method of administration

Prior to initiating gemfibrozil, other medical problems such as hypothyroidism and diabetes mellitus must be controlled as best as possible and patients should be placed on a standard lipid-lowering diet, which should be continued during treatment. Lopid should be taken orally.

Adult

The dose range is 900 mg to 1200 mg daily.

The only dose with documented effect on morbidity is 1200 mg daily.

The 1200 mg dose is taken as 600 mg twice daily, half an hour before breakfast and half an hour before the evening meal.

The 900 mg dose is taken as a single dose half an hour before the evening meal.

Elderly (over 65 years old)

As for adults

Children and adolescents

Gemfibrozil therapy has not been investigated in children. Due to the lack of data the use of Lopid in children is not recommended.

Renal impairment

In patients with mild to moderate renal impairment (Glomerular filtration rate 50 - 80 and 30 - < 50 ml/min/1.73 m^2, respectively), start treatment at 900 mg daily and assess renal function before increasing dose. Lopid should not be used in patients with severely impaired renal function (see section 4.3).

Hepatic impairment

Gemfibrozil is contraindicated in hepatic impairment (see section 4.3).

4.3 Contraindications

Hypersensitivity to gemfibrozil or any of the excipients.

Hepatic impairment.

Severe renal impairment.

History of/or pre-existing gall bladder or biliary tract disease, including gallstones

Concomitant use of repaglinide (see section 4.5).

Patients with previous history of photoallergy or phototoxic reaction during treatment with fibrates.

4.4 Special warnings and special precautions for use

Muscle disorders (myopathy/rhabdomyolysis)

There have been reports of myositis, myopathy and markedly elevated creatine phosphokinase associated with gemfibrozil. Rhabdomyolysis has also been reported rarely.

Muscle damage must be considered in any patient presenting with diffuse myalgia, muscle tenderness and/or marked increase in muscle CPK levels >5x ULN); under these conditions treatment must be discontinued.

Concomitant HMG CoA reductase inhibitors

The risk of muscle damage may be increased in the event of combination with an HMG-CoA reductase inhibitor. Pharmacokinetic interactions may also be present (see also section 4.5) and dosage adjustments may be necessary.

The benefit of further alterations in lipid levels by the combined use of gemfibrozil and HMG-CoA reductase inhibitors should be carefully weighed against the potential risks of such combinations and clinical monitoring is recommended.

A creatine phosphokinase (CPK) level should be measured before starting such a combination in patients with predisposing factors for rhabdomyolysis as follows:

- renal impairment
- hypothyroidism
- alcohol abuse
- age > 70 years
- personal or family history of hereditary muscular disorders
- previous history of muscular toxicity with another fibrate or HMG-CoA reductase inhibitor

In most subjects who have had an unsatisfactory lipid response to either drug alone, the possible benefits of combined therapy with HMG-CoA reductase inhibitors and gemfibrozil does not outweigh the risks of severe myopathy, rhabdomylosis and acute renal failure.

Use in patients with gallstone formation

Gemfibrozil may increase cholesterol excretion into the bile raising the potential for gallstone formation. Cases of cholelithiasis have been reported with gemfibrozil therapy. If cholelithiasis is suspected, gallbladder studies are indicated. Gemfibrozil therapy should be discontinued if gallstones are found.

Monitoring serum lipids

Periodic determinations of serum lipids are necessary during treatment with gemfibrozil. Sometimes a paradoxical increase of (total and LDL) cholesterol can occur in patients with hypertriglyceridaemia. If the response is insufficient after 3 months of therapy at recommended doses treatment should be discontinued and alternative treatment methods considered.

Monitoring liver function

Elevated levels of ALAT, ASAT, alkaline phosphatase, LDH, CK and bilirubin have been reported. These are usually reversible when gemfibrozil is discontinued. Therefore liver function tests should be performed periodically. Gemfibrozil therapy should be terminated if abnormalities persist.

Monitoring blood counts

Periodic blood count determinations are recommended during the first 12 months of gemfibrozil administration. Anaemia, leucopenia, thrombocytopenia, eosinophilia and bone marrow hypoplasia have been reported rarely (see section 4.8).

Interactions with other medicinal products (see also sections 4.3 and 4.5).

Concomitant use with CYP2C8, CYP2C9, CYP2C19, CYP1A2, UGTA1 and UGTA3 substrates.

The interaction profile of gemfibrozil is complex resulting in increased exposure of many medicinal products if administered concomitantly with gemfibrozil.

Gemfibrozil potently inhibits CYP2C8, CYP2C9, CYP2C19, CYP1A2, UGTA1 and UGTA3 enzymes (see section 4.5)

Concomitant use with hypoglycaemic agents

There have been reports of hypoglycaemic reactions after concomitant use with gemfibrozil and hypoglycaemic agents (oral agents and insulin). Monitoring of glucose levels is recommended.

Concomitant oral anticoagulants

Gemfibrozil may potentiate the effects of oral anticoagulants, which necessitates careful monitoring of the anticoaglant dosing. Caution should be exercised when anticoagulants are given in conjunction with gemfibrozil. The dosage of the anticoagulant may need to be reduced to maintain desired prothrombin time levels (see Section 4.5.)

4.5 Interaction with other medicinal products and other forms of Interaction

The interaction profile of gemfibrozil is complex. In vivo studies indicate that gemfibrozil is a potent inhibitor of CYP2C8 (an enzyme important for the metabolism of e.g. repaglinide, rosiglitazone and paclitaxel). In vitro studies have shown that gemfibrozil is a strong inhibitor of CYP2C9 (an enzyme involved in the metabolism of e.g. warfarin and glimepiride), but also of CYP 2C19, CYP1A2 and UGTA1 and UGTA3 (see Section 4.4).

Repaglinide

The combination of gemfibrozil with repaglinide is contraindicated (see Section 4.3). Concomitant administration has resulted in 8-fold increase in repaglinide plasma concentration probably by inhibition of the CYP2C8 enzyme, resulting in hypoglycaemic reactions.

Rosiglitazone

The combination of gemfibrozil with rosiglitazone should be approached with caution. Co-administration with rosiglitazone has resulted in 2.3-fold increase in rosiglitazone systemic exposure, probably by inhibition of the CYP2C8 isozyme (see section 4.4).

HMG CoA reductase inhibitors

The combined use of gemfibrozil and a statin should generally be avoided (see section 4.4). The use of fibrates alone is occasionally associated with myopathy. An increased risk of muscle related adverse events, including rhabdomyolysis, has been reported when fibrates are co-administered with statins.

Gemfibrozil has also been reported to influence the pharmacokinetics of simvaststin, lovastatin, pravastatin and rosuvastatin. Gemfibrozil caused an almost 3-fold increased in AUC of simvastatin acid possibly due to inhibition of glucoronidation via UGTA1 and UGTA3, and a 3-fold increase in pravastatin AUC which may be due to interference with transport proteins. One study indicated that the co-administration of a single rosuvastatin dose of 80 mg to healthy volunteers on gemfibrozil (600 mg twice daily) resulted in a 2.2-fold increase in mean C_{max} and a 1.9-fold increase in mean AUC of rosuvastatin.

Oral anticoagulants

Gemfibrozil may potentiate the effects of oral anticoagulants, which necessitates careful monitoring of the anticoagulant dosing (see section 4.4).

Bexarotene

Concomitant administration of gemfibrozil with bexarotene is not recommended. A population analysis of plasma bexarotene concentrations in patients with cutaneous T-cell lymphoma (CTCL) indicated that concomitant administration of gemfibrozil resulted in substantial increases in plasma concentrations of bexarotene.

Bile Acid – Binding Resins

Reduced bioavailability of gemfibrozil may result when given simultaneously with resin-granule drugs such as colestipol. Administration of the products two hours or more apart is recommended.

Gemfibrozil is highly bound to plasma proteins and there is potential for displacement interactions with other drugs.

4.6 Pregnancy and lactation

Pregnancy

There are no adequate data on use of Lopid in pregnant women. Animal studies are insufficiently clear to allow conclusions to be drawn on pregnancy and foetal development (see section 5.3). The potential risk for humans is unknown. Lopid should not be used during pregnancy unless it is clearly necessary.

Lactation

There are no data on excretion of gemfibrozil in milk. Lopid should not be used when breast feeding.

4.7 Effects on ability to drive and use machines

No studies on the effects on the ability to drive and use machines have been performed. In isolated cases dizziness and visual disturbances can occur which may negatively influence driving.

4.8 Undesirable effects

Most commonly reported adverse reactions are of gastro-intestinal character and are seen in approximately 7% of the patients. These adverse reactions do not usually lead to discontinuation of the treatment.

Adverse reactions are ranked according to frequency using the following convention: Very common >1/10), Common >1/100, <1/10), Uncommon >1/1,000, <1/100), Rare >1/10,000, <1/1,000), Very rare (<1/10,000), including isolated reports:

Platelet, bleeding and clotting disorders

Rare: thrombocytopenia.

Red blood cell disorders

Rare: severe anaemia. Self-limiting, mild haemoglobin and haematocrit decrease have been observed on initiating gemfibrozil therapy.

White cell and reticuloendothelial system disorders

Rare: leucopoenia, eosinophilia, bone marrow hypoplasia. Self-limiting, white cell decrease has been observed on initiating gemfibrozil therapy.

Central and peripheral nervous system

Common: vertigo, headache.

Rare: dizziness, somnolence, paresthesia, peripheral neuritis, depression, decreased libido.

Vision disorders

Rare: blurred vision.

Heart rate and rhythm disorders

Uncommon: atrial fibrillation.

Gastro-intestinal system disorders

Very common: dyspepsia.

Common: abdominal pain, diarrhoea, flatulence, nausea, vomiting, constipation.

Rare: pancreatitis, acute appendicitis.

Liver and biliary system disorders

Rare: cholestatic jaundice, disturbed liver function, hepatitis, cholelithiasis, cholecystitis.

Skin and appendages disorders

Common: eczema, rash.

Rare: exfoliative dermatitis, dermatitis, pruritus, alopecia.

Musculoskeletal disorders

Rare: arthralgia, synovitis, myalgia, myopathy, myasthenia, painful extremities and myositis accompanied by increase in creatine kinase (CK), rhabdomyolysis.

Urinary system disorders

Rare: impotence.

Body as a whole-general disorders

Common: fatigue.

Rare: photosensitivity, angioedema, laryngeal edema, urticaria.

4.9 Overdose

Overdose has been reported. Symptoms reported with overdosage were abdominal cramps, abdominal LFT's, diarrhoea, increased CPK, joint muscle pain, nausea and vomiting. The patients fully recovered. Symptomatic supportive measures should be taken if overdose occurs.

5. PHARMACOLOGICAL PROPERTIES

5.1 Pharmacodynamic properties

Pharmacotherapeutic group: Serum-lipid lowering agent

Chemical subgroup: Fibrates

ATC code: C10A B04

Gemfibrozil is a non-halogenated phenoxypentanoic acid. Gemfibrozil is a lipid regulating agent which regulates lipid fractions.

Gemfibrozil's mechanism of action has not been definitively established. In man, gemfibrozil stimulates the peripheral lipolysis of triglyceride rich lipoproteins such as VLDL and cholymicrons (by stimulation of LPL). Gemfibrozil also inhibits synthesis of VLDL in the liver. Gemfibrozil increases the HDL_2 and HDL_3 subfractions as well as apolipoprotein A-I and A-II.

Animal studies suggest that the turnover and removal of cholesterol from the liver is increased by gemfibrozil.

In the Helsinki Heart Study, which was a large placebo-controlled study with 4081 male subjects, 40 to 55 years of age, with primary dyslipidaemia (predominantly raised non-HDL cholesterol +/- hypertriglyceridaemia), but no previous history of coronary heart disease, gemfibrozil 600 mg twice daily, produced a significant reduction in total plasma triglycerides, total and low density lipoprotein cholesterol and a significant increase in high density lipoprotein cholesterol. The cumulative rate of cardiac endpoints (cardiac death and non-fatal myocardial infarction) during a 5 year follow-up was 27.3/1000 in the gemfibrozil group (56 subjects) and 41.4/1000 in the placebo group (84 subjects) showing a relative risk reduction of 34.0% (95% confidence interval 8.2 to 52.6, $p<0.02$) and an absolute risk reduction of 1.4% in the gemfibrozil group compared to placebo. There was a 37% reduction in non-fatal myocardial infarction and a 26% reduction in cardiac deaths. The number of deaths from all causes was, however, not different (44 in the gemfibrozil group and 43 in the placebo group). Diabetes patients and patients with severe lipid fraction deviations showed a 68% and 71% reduction of CHD endpoints, respectively.

5.2 Pharmacokinetic properties

Absorption

Gemfibrozil is well absorbed from the gastro-intestinal tract after oral administration with a bioavailability close to 100%. As the presence of food alters the bioavailability slightly gemfibrozil should be taken 30 minutes before a meal. Peak plasma levels occur in one to two hours. After administration of 600 mg twice daily a C_{max} in the range 15 to 25 mg/ml is obtained.

Distribution

Volume of distribution at steady state is 9-13 l. The plasma protein binding of gemfibrozil and its main metabolite are at least 97%.

Biotransformation

Gemfibrozil undergoes oxidation of a ring methyl group to form successively a hydroxymethyl and a carboxyl metabolite (the main metabolite). This metabolite has a low activity compared to the mother compound gemfibrozil and an elimination half-life of approximately 20 hours.

The enzymes involved in the metabolism of gemfibrozil are not known. The interaction profile of gemfibrozil is complex (see sections 4.3, 4.4 and 4.5). In vitro and in vivo studies have shown that gemfibrozil inhibits CYP2C8, CYP2C9, CYP2C19, CYP1A2, UGTA1 and UGTA3.

Elimination

Gemfibrozil is eliminated mainly by metabolism. Approximately 70% of the administered human dose is excreted in the urine, mainly as conjugates of gemfibrozil and its metabolites. Less than 6% of the dose is excreteed unchanged in the urine. Six percent of the dose is found in faeces. The total clearance of gemfibrozil is in the range 100 to 160 ml/min, and the elimination half-life is in the range 1.3 to 1.5 hours. The pharmacokinetics is linear within the therapeutic dose range.

Special patient groups

No pharmacokinetic studies have been performed in patients with impaired hepatic function.

There are limited data on patients with mild, moderate and non-dialysed severe renal impairment. The limited data support the use of up to 1200 mg a day in patients with mild to moderate renal failure not receiving any other lipid lowering drug.

5.3 Preclinical safety data

In a 2-year study of gemfibrozil, subcapsular bilateral cataracts occurred in 10%, and unilateral in 6.3%, of male rats treated at 10 times the human dose.

In a mouse carcinogenicity study at dosages corresponding to 0.1 and 0.7 times the clinical exposure (based on AUC), there were no significant differences from controls in the incidence of tumors. In a rat carcinogenicity study at dosages corresponding to 0.2 and 1.3 times the clinical exposure (based on AUC), the incidence of benign liver nodules and liver carcinomas was significantly increased in high dose males, and the incidence of liver carcinomas increased also in the low dose males, but this increase was not statistically significant.

Liver tumours induced by gemfibrozil and other fibrates in small rodents are generally considered to be related to the extensive proliferation of peroxisomes in these species and, consequently, of minor clinical relevance.

In the male rat, gemfibrozil also induced benign Leydig cell tumors. The clinical relevance of this finding is minimal.

In reproductive toxicity studies, administration of gemfibrozil at approximately 2 times the human dose (based on body surface area) to male rats for 10 weeks resulted in decreased fertility. Fertility was restored after a drug-free period of 8 weeks. Gemfibrozil was not teratogenic in either rats or rabbits. Administration of 1 and 3 times the human dose (based on body surface area) of gemfibrozil to female rabbits during organogenesis caused a dose-related decrease in litter size. Administration of 0.6 and 2 times the human dose (based on body surface area) of gemfibrozil to female rats from gestation Day 15 through weaning caused dose-related decreases in birth weight and suppression of pup growth during lactation. Maternal toxicity was observed in both species and the clinical relevance of decreases in rabbit litter size and rat pup weight is uncertain.

6. PHARMACEUTICAL PARTICULARS

6.1 List of excipients

Polysorbate on silica, maize starch, titanium dioxide (E171), gelatin, erythrosine (E127), indigo carmine (E132), shellac, black iron oxide (E172), 2-ethoxyethanol, soya lecithin (E322) and dimethicone.

6.2 Incompatibilities

None Known.

6.3 Shelf life

3 years

6.4 Special precautions for storage

Lopid 300mg capsules: Do not store above 30°C.

Lopid 600 film-coated tablets: Do not store above 25 °C

6.5 Nature and contents of container

Not all pack sizes may be marketed

Securitainer with tamper evident polyethylene cap containing 100 capsules.

Tampertainer bottle with a white tamper evident cap containing 100 capsules.

Aluminium foil blister strips supplied in packs of 100 or 112 capsules.

6.6 Instructions for use and handling

No special instructions needed.

7. MARKETING AUTHORISATION HOLDER

Pfizer Limited

Ramsgate Road

Sandwich

Kent CT13 9NJ

United Kingdom

8. MARKETING AUTHORISATION NUMBER(S)

Lopid 300mg capsules: PL 00057/0534

Lopid 600mg film-coated tablets: PL 00057/0535

9. DATE OF FIRST AUTHORISATION/RENEWAL OF THE AUTHORISATION

3 April 2005

10. DATE OF REVISION OF THE TEXT

Partial revision of text 02 February 2005 and 17 March 2005, Sections 4.4, 4.5, 4.8, & 4.9

Ref: LP6_0 UK

Loprazolam 1mg tablets

(sanofi-aventis)

1. NAME OF THE MEDICINAL PRODUCT

Loprazolam 1mg Tablets

2. QUALITATIVE AND QUANTITATIVE COMPOSITION

Each tablet contains loprazolam mesylate equivalent to 1mg loprazolam.

3. PHARMACEUTICAL FORM

Pale yellow, biconvex tablets, 7mm in diameter, marked L1 on one face with breakline on reverse

4. CLINICAL PARTICULARS

4.1 Therapeutic indications

Loprazolam is indicated for the short-term treatment of insomnia including difficulty in falling asleep and/or frequent nocturnal awakenings. Benzodiazepines should be used to treat insomnia only when it is severe, disabling or subjecting the individual to extreme distress. An underlying cause of insomnia should be sought before deciding upon the use of benzodiazepines for symptomatic relief.

4.2 Posology and method of administration

Adults: The recommended dose is 1mg at bedtime. This may be increased to 1.5mg or 2mg if necessary.

Elderly:Dosage in the elderly should be limited to 1mg at bedtime.

Frail, debilitated or aged patients: A starting dose of a half tablet may be appropriate. Dosage should not exceed 1mg.

Treatment should if possible be intermittent.

The lowest dose to control symptoms should be used. Treatment should not normally be continued beyond 4 weeks.

Long term chronic use is not recommended.

Treatment should always be tapered off gradually.

Patients who have taken benzodiazepines for a long time may require a longer period during which doses are reduced.

Children: There is insufficient evidence to recommend the use of Loprazolam in children.

4.3 Contraindications

Sensitivity to benzodiazepines, acute pulmonary insufficiency, severe respiratory insufficiency, myasthenia gravis, phobic or obsessional states and sleep apnoea syndrome. Monotherapy in depression or anxiety associated with depression and chronic psychosis and alcohol intake.

4.4 Special warnings and special precautions for use

Disinhibiting effects may be manifested in various ways. Suicide may be precipitated in patients who are depressed and who exhibit aggressive behaviour towards self and others. Extreme caution should therefore be used in prescribing benzodiazepines in patients with personality disorders.

In general, the dependence potential of benzodiazepines is low but this increases when high doses are attained, especially when given over long periods and particularly in patients with a history of alcoholism or drug abuse. However, withdrawal symptoms occur even with normal therapeutic doses given for short periods of time. Withdrawal from benzodiazepines may be associated with physiological and psychological symptoms of withdrawal including depression, anxiety, tension, restlessness, confusion, irritability and headaches. Patients receiving benzodiazepines should be regularly monitored.

Rebound insomnia may also occur. It may be accompanied by other reactions such as changes in mood, anxiety, sleep disturbances and restlessness.

Loprazolam should be used with caution in chronic pulmonary insufficiency, cerebrovascular disease and chronic renal or hepatic impairment.

4.5 Interaction with other medicinal products and other forms of Interaction

Loprazolam may be potentiated by alcohol or other drugs acting on the CNS or with Cisapride. Additive synergy has been observed with neuromuscular depressants (curare-like drugs and muscle relaxants).

Combination with CNS depressants e.g. antipsychotics, hypnotics, anxiolytics/sedatives, antidepressant agents, narcotic analgesics, anti-epileptic drugs, anaesthetics and sedative antihistamines, causes enhancement of the central depressive effects of Loprazolam.

Concommitant intake with alcohol is not recommended. The sedative effects may be enhanced when the product is used in combination with alcohol. This affects the ability to drive or use machinery.

The risk of a withdrawal syndrome occurring is increased when loprazolam is combined with other benzodiazepines prescribed as anxiolytics or hypnotics.

4.6 Pregnancy and lactation

If the product is prescribed to a woman of childbearing potential, she should be warned to contact her physician regarding discontinuance of the product if she intends to become or suspects that she is pregnant.

If, for compelling medical reasons, the product is administered during the late phase of pregnancy, or during labour at high doses, effects on the neonate, such as hypothermia, hypotonia and moderate respiratory depression can be expected due to the pharmacological action of the compound.

Moreover, infants born to mothers who took benzodiazepines chronically during the latter stages of pregnancy may have developed physical dependency and may be at some risk for developing withdrawal symptoms in the postnatal period.

Since benzodiazepines are found in the breast milk, they should not be given to breast feeding mothers.

4.7 Effects on ability to drive and use machines

Attention should be drawn to the risk of drowsiness, sedation, amnesia, impaired concentration and muscular weakness, especially in drivers of vehicles and operators of machines, when taking the product (see also "Interactions").

4.8 Undesirable effects

In general, Loprazolam is very well tolerated. However, the common side effects of benzodiazepines, including headaches, nausea, drowsiness, hypotonia, blurring of vision, dizziness and ataxia may occur on the following day, particularly in unusually sensitive patients or when dosage has been excessive.

Rare behavioural adverse effects of benzodiazepines include paradoxical aggressive outbursts, excitement, confusion and the uncovering of depression with suicidal tendencies. If these reactions should occur, use of the drug should be discontinued. Even more rare side effects reported with some benzodiazepines have been hypotension, gastro-intestinal and visual disturbances, skin rashes, urinary retention, changes in libido, blood dyscrasias and jaundice.

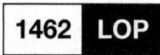

Benzodiazepines may induce anterograde amnesia. In cases of loss or bereavement, psychological adjustment may be inhibited by benzodiazepines.

4.9 Overdose

As with other benzodiazepines, overdosage does not usually present a threat to life. Treatment is symptomatic and gastric lavage may be of use if performed shortly after ingestion. Use of a specific antidote such as flumazenil in association with symptomatic treatment in hospital should be considered.

5. PHARMACOLOGICAL PROPERTIES

5.1 Pharmacodynamic properties

Benzodiazepines have a widespread action as a result of their enhancing the release of gamma-aminobutyric acid (GABA). They are effective as anti-convulsants, muscle relaxants, anti-anxiety agents, pre-medications and sedative hypnotics.

5.2 Pharmacokinetic properties

The pharmacokinetics of oral Loprazolam given in a single dose or in repeated doses on 7 consecutive nights were studied in a balanced cross-over trial in six healthy male subjects aged 22-37 years. The subjects were allocated randomly to the treatment phases which were separated by 2-week drug-free intervals. Loprazolam was administered as 1mg tablets.

On the night of administration of the single dose and the seventh repeated dose, venous blood samples were taken before and at intervals after treatment. Serum Loprazolam concentrations were measured using both a radioimmunoassay (RIA) and the more specific high pressure liquid chromatography and gas chromatography (HPLC/GC) technique. Maximum serum levels (Cmax) and the time taken to achieve them (Tmax) were measured, and the half-life (t1/2) was calculated. The area under the serum concentration-time curve (AUC) was determined using the trapezoidal rule. The ratios of AUC and Cmax after repeated doses to AUC and Cmax after single doses were used to assess possible accumulation of Loprazolam.

	MEAN (SD)	
SINGLE DOSES	**RIA data**	**HPLC/GC data**
Cmax (mcg/litre)	4.0 (1.2)	4.1 (2.2)
tmax (hours)	4.0 (2.1)	5.0 (3.6)
t1/2 (hours)	11.7 (4.7)	8.0 (3.4)*
AUC (mcg/litre hour)	60.0 (20.9)	35.5 (22.2)
REPEATED DOSES	**RIA data**	**HPLC/GC data**
Cmax (mcg/litre)	5.1 (1.2)	4.6 (2.1)
tmax (hours)	5.3 (3.7)	5.5 (2.7)
t1/2 (hours)	12.8 (4.9)	3.5 (0.2)**
AUC (mcg/litre hour)	75.6 (21.1)	50.0 (26.9)

n = 6 subjects, except for *n = 5, **n = 3.

5.3 Preclinical safety data

No additional data of relevance to the prescriber.

6. PHARMACEUTICAL PARTICULARS

6.1 List of excipients

Povidone, Lactose, Colloidal silicon dioxide, Maize starch, Microcrystalline cellulose and Magnesium stearate.

6.2 Incompatibilities

None.

6.3 Shelf life

60 months.

6.4 Special precautions for storage

Store below 25°C in a dry place. Protect from light.

6.5 Nature and contents of container

UPVC/PVdC/aluminium foil blisters, packaged in cartons of 28 tablets.

6.6 Instructions for use and handling

None stated.

7. MARKETING AUTHORISATION HOLDER

Aventis Pharma Ltd

50 Kings Hill Avenue

Kings Hill

West Malling

Kent

ME19 4AH

United Kingdom

8. MARKETING AUTHORISATION NUMBER(S)

PL 04425/0209

9. DATE OF FIRST AUTHORISATION/RENEWAL OF THE AUTHORISATION

14 May 2004

10. DATE OF REVISION OF THE TEXT

11 LEGAL CLASSIFICATION

POM

Lopresor SR

(Novartis Pharmaceuticals UK Ltd)

1. NAME OF THE MEDICINAL PRODUCT

Lopresor® SR.

2. QUALITATIVE AND QUANTITATIVE COMPOSITION

The active ingredient is Di-[(±)-1-(isopropylamino)-3-[p-2(methoxyethyl)phenoxy]-2-propanol] L(+)-tartrate (metoprolol tartrate). One coated slow release tablet contains 200mg metoprolol tartrate.

3. PHARMACEUTICAL FORM

Film coated tablets.

4. CLINICAL PARTICULARS

4.1 Therapeutic indications

For the treatment of hypertension, angina pectoris, prophylaxis of migraine.

4.2 Posology and method of administration

Lopresor SR Tablets should be administered orally and swallowed unchewed.

The dose must always be adjusted to the individual requirements of the patient but should not exceed 400mg/day.

The following are the guidelines:

Adults

Hypertension

One Lopresor SR Tablet should be given in the morning. Most patients may be expected to respond satisfactorily within 14 days. Further antihypertensive effect may be achieved by the addition of a diuretic or a vasodilator.

Lopresor SR may be administered with benefit to both previously untreated patients with hypertension and to those in whom the response to previous therapy is inadequate. In the latter type of patient therapy may be continued and Lopresor SR added into the regime with adjustment of previous therapy if necessary.

Angina pectoris

Initially, one Lopresor SR Tablet daily. The dose may be increased to two tablets once daily if required. In general a significant improvement in exercise tolerance and a reduction of anginal attacks may be expected with a dose of one Lopresor SR Tablet daily.

Prophylaxis of migraine

One tablet daily given in the morning.

Elderly

There is no evidence to suggest that dosage requirements are different in otherwise healthy elderly patients. However, caution is indicated in elderly patients as an excessive decrease in blood pressure or pulse rate may cause the blood supply to vital organs to fall to inadequate levels.

In patients with significant hepatic dysfunction the lower dosage recommendations will be more appropriate.

Children

Not recommended.

4.3 Contraindications

Known hypersensitivity to metoprolol and related derivatives or to any of the excipients, severe asthma or history of severe bronchospasm, atrioventricular block of second or third degree, uncontrolled heart failure, clinically relevant sinus bradycardia, sick-sinus syndrome, severe peripheral arterial disease, cardiogenic shock, hypotension, untreated phaeochromocytoma, metabolic acidosis.

Metoprolol is also contraindicated when myocardial infarction is complicated by significant bradycardia, first degree heart block, systolic hypotension (less than 100mmHg) and/or severe heart failure.

4.4 Special warnings and special precautions for use

A warning stating "Do not take this medicine if you have a history of wheezing or asthma" will appear on the label.

Although cardioselective beta-blockers may have less effect on lung function than non selective beta-blockers, as with all beta-blockers these should be avoided in patients with reversible obstructive airway disease unless there are compelling clinical reasons for their use. Therapy with a beta$_2$-stimulant may become necessary or current therapy require adjustment.

Metoprolol may aggravate bradycardia and symptoms of peripheral arterial circulatory disorders. If the patient develops increasing bradycardia (heart rate less than 50 to 55 beats/min), Lopresor SR should be given in lower doses or gradually withdrawn.

In addition, anaphylactic reactions precipitated by other agents may be particularly severe in patients taking β-blockers, and may be resistant to normal doses of adrenaline. Whenever possible, β-blockers should be avoided for patients who are at increased risk of anaphylaxis.

Abrupt cessation of therapy with a beta-blocker should be avoided, especially in patients with ischaemic heart disease. When possible, Lopresor SR should be withdrawn gradually over a period of 10 days, the doses diminishing to 25mg for the last 6 days. During its withdrawal the patient should be kept under close surveillance and replacement therapy should be initiated when required.

Beta-blockers should not be used in patients with untreated congestive heart failure (see Contraindications). This condition should first be stabilised. Additional therapy e.g. diuretics and/or digitalisation should also be considered for patients with a history of heart failure or patients who are known to have a poor cardiac reserve.

Because of their negative effect on atrioventricular conduction, β-blockers should be given only with caution to patients with first degree atrioventricular block (see Contraindications).

Beta-blockers mask some of the clinical signs of thyrotoxicosis. Therefore, Lopresor SR should be administered with caution to patients having, or suspected of developing, thyrotoxicosis, and both thyroid and cardiac function should be monitored closely

Lopresor SR should be used with caution in patients with diabetes mellitus, especially those who are receiving insulin or oral hypoglycaemic agents (see Interactions with other medicaments and other forms of interaction). In labile and insulin-dependent diabetes it may be necessary to adjust the hypoglycaemic therapy. Lopresor SR may mask some of the symptoms of hypoglycaemia by inhibition of sympathetic nerve functions and patients should be warned accordingly.

In patients with a treated phaeochromocytoma, an alpha-blocker should be given concomitantly.

In patients with significant hepatic dysfunction it may be necessary to adjust the dosage because metoprolol undergoes biotransformation in the liver.

The administration of adrenaline to patients undergoing beta-blockade can result in an increase in blood pressure and bradycardia although this is less likely to occur with beta$_1$-selective drugs.

Lopresor SR therapy should be brought to the attention of the anaesthetist prior to general anaesthesia. When it has been decided to interrupt a beta-blockade in preparation for surgery, therapy should be discontinued for at least 24 hours. Continuation of beta-blockade reduces the risk of arrhythmias during induction and intubation. However, the risk of hypertension may be increased. If treatment is continued, caution should be observed with the use of certain anaesthetic drugs. In a patient under beta-blockade, the anaesthetic selected should be one exhibiting as little negative inotropic activity as possible (halothane/nitrous oxide). The patient may be protected against vagal reactions by intravenous administration of atropine.

Beta-blockers may increase the number and duration of angina attacks in patients with Prinzmetal's angina (variant angina pectoris). However, relatively selective β_1-receptor blockers, such as Lopresor SR, can be used in such patients, but only with the utmost care.

The full oculomucocutaneous syndrome, as described elsewhere with practolol, has not been reported with Lopresor SR. However, part of this syndrome (dry eyes either alone or, occasionally, with skin rashes) has occurred. In most cases the symptoms cleared when Lopresor SR treatment was withdrawn. Patients should be observed carefully for potential ocular effects. If such effects occur, discontinuation of Lopresor SR should be considered (see advice about discontinuation above).

4.5 Interaction with other medicinal products and other forms of Interaction

The effects of metoprolol and other antihypertensive drugs on blood pressure are usually additive, and care should be taken to avoid hypotension. However, combinations of antihypertensive drugs may often be used with benefit to improve control of hypertension.

As beta-blockers may affect the peripheral circulation, care should be exercised when drugs with similar activity, e.g. ergotamine are given concurrently.

Care should also be exercised when beta-blockers are given in combination with sympathetic ganglion blocking agents, other beta blockers (also in the form of eye drops) or MAO inhibitors.

Prazosin

The acute postural hypotension that can follow the first dose of prazosin may be increased in patients already taking a beta-blocker.

Clonidine

If combination treatment with clonidine is to be discontinued metoprolol should be withdrawn several days before clonidine. This is because the hypertension that can follow withdrawal of clonidine may be increased in patients receiving concurrent beta-blocker treatment.

Calcium channel blockers

Calcium channel blockers such as verapamil and diltiazem may potentiate the depressant effects of β-blockers on blood pressure, heart rate, cardiac contractility and atrioventricular conduction. A calcium channel blocker of the verapamil (phenylalkylamine) type should not be given intravenously to patients receiving Lopresor SR because there is a risk of cardiac arrest in this situation. Patients taking an oral calcium channel blocker of the verapamil type in combination with Lopresor SR should be closely monitored.

Class I anti-arrhythmic drugs and amiodarone

Amiodarone, propafenone, and other class I anti-arrhythmic agents such as quinidine and disopyramide may potentiate the effects of beta-blockers on heart rate and atrioventricular conduction.

Nitroglycerin

Nitroglycerin may enhance the hypotensive effect of Lopresor SR.

Digitalis glycosides

Concurrent use of digitalis glycosides may result in excessive bradycardia and/or increase in atrioventricular conduction time

Sympathomimetics

Metoprolol will antagonise the beta$_1$ effects of sympathomimetic agents but should have little influence on the bronchodilator effects of beta$_2$-agonists at normal therapeutic doses.

Insulin and oral hypoglycaemic drugs

In diabetic patients who use insulin, beta-blocker treatment may be associated with increased or prolonged hypoglycaemia. Beta-blockers may also antagonise the hypoglycaemic effects of sulfonylureas. The risk of either effect is less with a beta$_1$-selective drug such as Lopresor SR than with a non-selective beta-blocker. However, diabetic patients receiving Lopresor SR should be monitored to ensure that diabetes control is maintained (see also Special warnings and special precautions for use)

Non-steroidal anti-inflammatory drugs

Concurrent treatment with non-steroidal anti-inflammatory drugs such as indomethacin may decrease the antihypertensive effect of metoprolol

Lignocaine

Metoprolol may impair the elimination of lignocaine.

General anaesthetics

Some inhalation anaesthetics may enhance the cardiodepressant effect of beta-blockers (see Special warnings and special precautions for use).

Hepatic enzyme inducers/inhibitors

Enzyme inducing agents (e.g. rifampicin) may reduce plasma concentrations of metoprolol, whereas enzyme inhibitors (e.g. cimetidine) may increase plasma concentrations.

Alcohol

During concomitant ingestion of alcohol and metoprolol the concentration of blood alcohol may reach higher levels and may decrease more slowly.

4.6 Pregnancy and lactation

Beta-blockers reduce placental perfusion which may result in intrauterine foetal death, immature and premature deliveries. Lopresor SR should not be used in pregnancy or lactation unless it is considered that the benefit outweighs the possible risk to the foetus/infant.

Metoprolol has, however, been used in pregnancy associated hypertension under close supervision after 20 weeks gestation. Although the drug crosses the placental barrier and is present in cord blood no evidence of foetal abnormalities have been reported. Animal experiments have shown neither teratogenic potential nor other adverse events on the embryo and/or foetus relevant to the safety assessment of the product.

The amount of metoprolol ingested via breast milk seems to be negligible with regard to its beta-blocking effects if the mother is treated in doses within the therapeutic range.

If Lopresor SR is used during pregnancy and lactation special attention should be paid to the foetus, neonate and breast-fed infant for undesirable effects of the drug's beta-blocking action (e.g. bradycardia, hypoglycaemia). The lowest possible dose should be used, and treatment should be discontinued at least 2 to 3 days before delivery to avoid increased uterine contractility and effects of β-blockade in the newborn baby.

4.7 Effects on ability to drive and use machines

As with all beta-blockers, metoprolol may affect patients ability to drive and operate machinery. Patients should be warned accordingly.

4.8 Undesirable effects

Frequency estimates:

very common $\geqslant$ 10%

common $\geqslant$ 1% and $<$ 10%

uncommon $\geqslant$ 0.1% and $<$ 1%

rare $\geqslant$ 0.01% and $<$ 0.1%

very rare $<$ 0.01%

Central and peripheral nervous system

Common: fatigue, dizziness, headache

Rare: paraesthesiae, muscle cramps, depression, decreased mental alertness, somnolence or insomnia, nightmares

Very rare: personality disorder, hallucinations

Cardiovascular system

Common: bradycardia, postural disorders (occasionally with syncope)

Rare: heart failure, cardiac arrhythmias, oedema, palpitation, Raynaud's phenomenon

Very rare: disturbances of cardiac conduction, precordial pain, gangrene in patients with pre-existing severe peripheral circulatory disorders

Gastrointestinal tract

Common: nausea and vomiting, abdominal pain

Rare: diarrhoea or constipation

Very rare: dryness of the mouth, liver function test abnormalities

Skin and appendages

Rare: skin rash (in the form of urticaria, psoriatiform and dystrophic skin lesions), occurrence of antinuclear antibodies (not associated with SLE).

Very rare: photosensitivity, increased sweating, loss of hair, worsening of psoriasis

Respiratory tract

Common: exertional dyspnoea

Rare: bronchospasm, also in patients without a history of obstructive lung disease

Very rare: rhinitis

Endocrine system and metabolism

Very rare: weight gain

Urogential system

Very rare: disturbances of libido and potency

Sense organs

Very rare: disturbances of vision, dry and/or irritated eyes, tinnitus, and, in doses exceeding those recommended, loss of hearing

Blood

Very rare: thrombocytopenia

Other organ systems

Very rare: arthritis

4.9 Overdose

Signs and symptoms

In more severe cases an overdosage of metoprolol may lead to severe hypotension, sinus bradycardia, atrioventricular block, heart failure, cardiogenic shock, cardiac arrest, bronchospasm, impairment of consciousness, coma, convulsions, nausea, vomiting, cyanosis, hypoglycaemia and occasionally hyperkalaemia.

The first manifestations of overdosage appear 20 minutes to 2 hours after ingestion of Lopresor SR. The effects of massive overdose may persist for several days, despite declining plasma concentrations.

Treatment

Patients should be admitted to hospital and, generally, should be managed in an intensive care setting, with continuous monitoring of cardiac function, blood gases, and blood biochemistry. Emergency supportive measures such as artificial ventilation or cardiac pacing should be instituted if appropriate. Even apparently well patients who have taken a small overdose should be closely observed for signs of poisoning for at least 4 hours.

In the event of a potentially life-threatening oral overdose, use induction of vomiting or gastric lavage (if within 4 hours after ingestion of Lopresor SR) and/or activated charcoal to remove the drug from the gastrointestinal tract. Metoprolol can not be effectively removed by haemodialysis.

Atropine may be given intravenously to control significant bradycardia. Intravenous β-agonists such as prenalterol or isoprenaline should be used to treat bradycardia and hypotension; very high doses may be needed to overcome the β-blockade. Dopamine, dobutamine or noradrenaline may be given to maintain blood pressure. Glucagon has positive inotropic and chronotropic effects on the heart that are independent of β-adrenergic receptors, and has proved effective in the treatment of resistant hypotension and heart failure associated with β-blocker overdose.

Diazepam is the drug of choice for controlling seizures. A β_2-agonist or aminophylline can be used to reverse bronchospasm; patients should be monitored for evidence of cardiac arrhythmias during and after administration of the bronchodilator.

5. PHARMACOLOGICAL PROPERTIES

5.1 Pharmacodynamic properties

Pharmacotherapeutic group

Lopresor SR is a cardioselective beta-adrenagergic receptor blocking agent.

Mechanism of action

It has a relatively greater blocking effect on beta$_1$-receptors (i.e. those mediating adrenergic stimulation of heart rate and contractility and release of free fatty acids from fat stores) than on beta$_2$-receptors, which are chiefly involved in broncho- and vasodilation.

It has no membrane-stabilising effect nor partial agonist (intrinsic sympathomimetic) activity.

The stimulant effect of catecholamines on the heart is reduced or inhibited by metoprolol. This leads to a decrease in heart rate, cardiac contractility and cardiac output.

5.2 Pharmacokinetic properties

Absorption

Lopresor SR is well absorbed after oral administration, peak plasma concentrations occurring 4-5 hours after dosing. The bioavailability of a single dose is approximately 50%, increasing to approximately 70% during repeated administration. The bioavailability also increases if metoprolol is given with food.

Distribution and Biotransformation

Approximately 10% of metoprolol in plasma is protein bound. Metoprolol crosses the placenta, and is found in breast milk (see "Pregnancy and lactation").

Metoprolol is extensively metabolised by enzymes of the cytochrome P450 system in the liver. The oxidative metabolism of metoprolol is under genetic control. None of the metabolites of metoprolol contribute significantly to its beta-blocking effect.

Elimination

Elimination is mainly by hepatic metabolism and the average elimination half-life is 3.5 hours (range 1 to 9 hours). Rates of metabolism vary between individuals, with poor metabolisers (approximately 10%) showing higher plasma concentrations and slower elimination than extensive metabolisers. Within individuals, however, plasma concentrations are stable and reproducible.

Characteristics in patients

Because of variation in rates of metabolism, the dose of metoprolol should always be adjusted to the individual requirements of the patient. At the therapeutic response, adverse effects and relative cardioselectivity are related to plasma concentration, poor metabolisers may require lower than normal doses. Dosage adjustment is not routinely required in the elderly or in patients with renal failure, but dosage may need to be reduced in patients with significant hepatic dysfunction when metoprolol elimination may be impaired.

5.3 Preclinical safety data

There are no further data of relevance to the prescriber which are additional to that already included in other sections of the Summary of Product Characteristics.

6. PHARMACEUTICAL PARTICULARS

6.1 List of excipients

The coated tablets contain silicon dioxide, microcrystalline cellulose, calcium phosphate, polyacrylic/methacrylic copolymer, magnesium stearate, stearic acid, hydroxypropyl methylcellulose, glyceryl palmitostearate, talc, titanium dioxide, polysorbate and yellow iron oxide.

6.2 Incompatibilities

None known.

6.3 Shelf life

Five years.

6.4 Special precautions for storage

No special recommendations.

Medicines should be kept out of reach of children.

6.5 Nature and contents of container

The tablets are pale yellow, capsule shaped, biconvex, film coated tablets, one face imprinted CG/CG, the other face with the letters CDC/CDC and packed in PVC/PVdC/foil bubble packs of 28 tablets.

6.6 Instructions for use and handling

None.

Administrative Data

7. MARKETING AUTHORISATION HOLDER

Novartis Pharmaceuticals UK Limited

Trading as Geigy Pharmaceuticals

Frimley Business Park

Frimley

Camberley

Surrey

GU16 7SR

8. MARKETING AUTHORISATION NUMBER(S)

PL 00101/0420.

9. DATE OF FIRST AUTHORISATION/RENEWAL OF THE AUTHORISATION

08 December 1980/ 09 April 2003

10. DATE OF REVISION OF THE TEXT

15 March 2001.

LEGAL CATEGORY

POM

Lopresor Tablets 100mg, 50mg

(Novartis Pharmaceuticals UK Ltd)

1. NAME OF THE MEDICINAL PRODUCT

Lopresor® Tablets 50mg & 100mg

2. QUALITATIVE AND QUANTITATIVE COMPOSITION
Each tablet contains 50mg or 100mg metoprolol tartrate BP

3. PHARMACEUTICAL FORM
Film coated tablet

4. CLINICAL PARTICULARS

4.1 Therapeutic indications
Hypertension and angina pectoris, cardiac arrhythmias, especially supraventricular tachyarrhythmias. Adjunct to treatment of thyrotoxicosis. Early intervention with Lopresor in myocardial infarction reduces infarct size and the incidence of ventricular fibrillation. Pain relief may also decrease the need for opiate analgesics. Lopresor has been shown to reduce mortality when administered to patients with acute myocardial infarction. Prophylaxis of migraine.

4.2 Posology and method of administration
Lopresor tablets should be administered orally and swallowed unchewed. The dose must always be adjusted to the individual requirements of the patient but should not exceed 400mg/day.

The following are the guidelines:

Adults

Hypertension

Initially a dose of 100mg per day should be prescribed either as single or divided doses. Depending upon the response the dosage may be increased by 100mg per day at weekly intervals to 200mg daily given in single or divided doses. Over the dosage range most patients may be expected to respond rapidly and satisfactorily. A further reduction in blood pressure may be achieved if Lopresor is used in conjunction with an antihypertensive diuretic or other hypotensive agent.

Lopresor may be administered with benefit both to previously untreated patients with hypertension and to those in whom the response to previous therapy is inadequate. In the latter type of patient the previous therapy may be continued and Lopresor added into the regime with adjustment of the previous therapy if necessary.

Angina Pectoris

50-100mg twice or three times daily

In general a significant improvement in exercise tolerance and reduction of anginal attacks may be expected with a dose of 50-100mg twice daily.

Cardiac Arrhythmias

A dosage of 50mg two or three times daily is usually sufficient. If necessary the dose can be increased up to 300mg per day administered in divided doses.

Hyperthyroidism

50mg four times daily. The dosage should be progressively reduced as euthyroid state is slowly achieved.

Myocardial Infarction

Early intervention: 50mg every 6 hours for 48 hours, preferably within 12 hours of the onset of chest pain.

Maintenance: the usual maintenance dose is 200mg daily given in divided doses. The treatment should be continued for at least 3 months.

Prophylaxis of Migraine

100-200mg daily, given in divided doses (morning and evening).

Elderly

There is no evidence to suggest that dosage requirements are different in otherwise healthy elderly patients. However, caution is indicated in elderly patients as an excessively pronounced decrease in blood pressure or pulse rate may cause the blood supply to vital organs to fall to inadequate levels.

In patients with significant hepatic dysfunction the lower dosage recommendations will be more appropriate.

Children

Not recommended

4.3 Contraindications
Known hypersensitivity to metoprolol and related derivatives or to any of the excipients, severe asthma or history of severe bronchospasm, atrioventricular block of second or third degree, uncontrolled heart failure, clinically relevant sinus bradycardia, sick-sinus syndrome, severe peripheral arterial disease, cardiogenic shock, hypotension, untreated phaeochromocytoma, metabolic acidosis.

Metoprolol is also contraindicated when myocardial infarction is complicated by significant bradycardia, first degree heart block, systolic hypotension (less than 100mmHg) and/or severe heart failure.

4.4 Special warnings and special precautions for use
A warning stating "Do not take this medicine if you have a history of wheezing or asthma" will appear on the label.

Although cardioselective beta-blockers may have less effect on lung function than non-selective beta-blockers, as with all beta-blockers these should be avoided in patients with reversible obstructive airway disease unless there are compelling clinical reasons for their use. Therapy with a beta$_2$- stimulant may become necessary or current therapy require adjustment.

Metoprolol may aggravate bradycardia and symptoms of peripheral arterial circulatory disorders. If the patient develops increasing bradycardia, (heart rate less than 50 to 55 beats/min) Lopresor should be given in lower doses or gradually withdrawn.

In addition, anaphylactic reactions precipitated by other agents may be particularly severe in patients taking beta-blockers, and may be resistant to normal doses of adrenaline. Whenever possible, beta-blockers should be avoided for patients who are at increased risk of anaphylaxis

Abrupt cessation of therapy with a beta-blocker should be avoided, especially in patients with ischaemic heart disease. When possible, Lopresor should be withdrawn gradually over a period of 10 days, the doses diminishing to 25mg for the last 6 days. During its withdrawal, the patient should be kept under close surveillance and replacement therapy should be initiated where required.

Beta-blockers should not be used in patients with untreated congestive heart failure (see "Contraindications"). This condition should first be stabilised. Additional therapy should also be considered for patients with a history of heart failure or patients who are known to have a poor cardiac reserve, e.g. diuretics and/or digitalisation.

Because of their negative effect on atrioventricular conduction, beta-blockers should be given only with caution to patients with first degree atrioventricular block (see "Contraindications")

Beta-blockers mask some of the clinical signs of thyrotoxicosis. Therefore, Lopresor should be administered with caution to patients having, or suspected of developing, thyrotoxicosis, and both thyroid and cardiac function should be monitored closely

Lopresor should be used with caution in patients with diabetes mellitus, especially those who are receiving insulin or oral hypoglycaemic agents (see "Interactions with other medicaments and other forms of interaction"). In labile and insulin-dependent diabetes it may be necessary to adjust the hypoglycaemic therapy. Lopresor may mask some of the symptoms of hypoglycaemia by inhibition of sympathetic nerve functions and patients should be warned accordingly.

In patients with a treated phaeochromocytoma, an alpha-blocker should be given concomitantly.

In patients with significant hepatic dysfunction it may be necessary to adjust the dosage because metoprolol undergoes biotransformation in the liver.

The administration of adrenaline to patients undergoing beta-blockade can result in an increase in blood pressure and bradycardia although this is less likely to occur with beta$_1$-selective drugs.

Lopresor therapy should be brought to the attention of the anaesthetist prior to general anaesthesia. When it has been decided to interrupt a beta-blockade in preparation for surgery, therapy should be discontinued for at least 24 hours. Continuation of beta-blockade reduces the risk of arrhythmias during induction and intubation. However, the risk of hypertension may be increased. If treatment is continued, caution should be observed with the use of certain anaesthetic drugs. In a patient under beta-blockade, the anaesthetic selected should be one exhibiting as little negative inotropic activity as possible (halothane/nitrous oxide). The patient may be protected against vagal reactions by intravenous administration of atropine.

Beta-blockers may increase the number and duration of angina attacks in patients with Prinzmetal's angina (variant angina pectoris). However, relatively selective β_1-receptor blockers, such as Lopresor, can be used in such patients, but only with the utmost care

Patients with anamnestically known psoriasis should take beta-blockers only after careful consideration.

The full oculomucocutaneous syndrome, as described elsewhere with practolol, has not been reported with Lopresor. However, part of this syndrome (dry eyes either alone or, occasionally, with skin rashes) has occurred. In most cases the symptoms cleared when Lopresor treatment was withdrawn. Patients should be observed carefully for potential ocular effects. If such effects occur, discontinuation of Lopresor should be considered. (see advice about discontinuation above).

4.5 Interaction with other medicinal products and other forms of Interaction
The effects of metoprolol and other antihypertensive drugs on blood pressure are usually additive, and care should be taken to avoid hypotension. However, combinations of antihypertensive drugs may often be used with benefit to improve control of hypertension.

As beta-blockers may affect the peripheral circulation, care should be exercised when drugs with similar activity, e.g. ergotamine are given concurrently.

Care should also be exercised when beta-blockers are given in combination with sympathetic ganglion blocking agents, other beta blockers (also in the form of eye drops) or MAO inhibitors.

Prazosin

The acute postural hypotension that can follow the first dose of prazosin may be increased in patients already taking a beta-blocker

Clonidine

If combination treatment with clonidine is to be discontinued metoprolol should be withdrawn several days before clonidine. This is because the hypertension that can follow withdrawal of clonidine may be increased in patients receiving concurrent beta-blocker treatment

Calcium channel blockers

Calcium channel blockers such as verapamil and diltiazem may potentiate the depressant effects of beta-blockers on blood pressure, heart rate, cardiac contractility and atrio-ventricular conduction. A calcium channel blocker of the verapamil (phenylalkylamine) type should not be given intravenously to patients receiving Lopresor because there is a risk of cardiac arrest in this situation. Patients taking an oral calcium channel blocker of the verapamil type in combination with Lopresor should be closely monitored

Class I anti-arrhythmic drugs and amiodarone

Amiodarone, propafenone, and other class I anti-arrhythmic agents such as quinidine and disopyramide may potentiate the effects of beta-blockers on heart rate and atrioventricular conduction

Nitroglycerin

Nitroglycerin may enhance the hypotensive effect of Lopresor.

Digitalis glycosides

Concurrent use of digitalis glycosides may result in excessive bradycardia and/or increase in atrioventricular conduction time

Sympathomimetics

Metoprolol will antagonise the beta$_1$ effects of sympathomimetic agents but should have little influence on the bronchodilator effects of beta$_2$-agonists at normal therapeutic doses.

Insulin and oral hypoglycaemic drugs

In diabetic patients who use insulin, beta-blocker treatment may be associated with increased or prolonged hypoglycaemia. Beta-blockers may also antagonise the hypoglycaemic effects of sulfonylureas. The risk of either effect is less with a beta$_1$-selective drug such as Lopresor than with a non-selective beta-blocker. However, diabetic patients receiving Lopresor should be monitored to ensure that diabetes control is maintained (see also "Special warnings and special precautions for use")

Non-steroidal anti-inflammatory drugs

Concurrent treatment with non-steroidal anti-inflammatory drugs such as indomethacin may decrease the antihypertensive effect of metoprolol

Lignocaine

Metoprolol may impair the elimination of lignocaine.

General anaesthetics

Some inhalation anaesthetics may enhance the cardiodepressant effect of beta-blockers (see "Special warnings and special precautions for use").

Hepatic enzyme inducers/inhibitors

Enzyme inducing agents (e.g. rifampicin) may reduce plasma concentrations of metoprolol, whereas enzyme inhibitors (e.g. cimetidine) may increase plasma concentrations.

Alcohol

During concomitant ingestion of alcohol and metoprolol the concentration of blood alcohol may reach higher levels and may decrease more slowly.

4.6 Pregnancy and lactation
Beta-blockers reduce placental perfusion which may result in intrauterine foetal death, immature and premature deliveries. Lopresor should not be used in pregnancy or lactation unless it is considered that the benefit outweighs the possible risk to the foetus/infant.

Metoprolol has, however, been used in pregnancy associated hypertension under close supervision after 20 weeks gestation. Although the drug crosses the placental barrier and is present in cord blood no evidence of foetal abnormalities have been reported. Animal experiments have shown neither teratogenic potential nor other adverse events on the embryo and/or foetus relevant to the safety assessment of the product.

The amount of metoprolol ingested via breast milk seems to be negligible with regard to its beta-blocking effects if the mother is treated in doses within the therapeutic range.

If Lopresor is used during pregnancy and lactation special attention should be paid to the foetus, neonate and breast-fed infant for undesirable effects of the drug's beta-blocking action (e.g. bradycardia, hypoglycaemia). The lowest possible dose should be used, and treatment should be discontinued at least 2 to 3 days before delivery to avoid increased uterine contractility and effects of beta-blockade in the newborn baby.

4.7 Effects on ability to drive and use machines
As with all beta-blockers, metoprolol may affect patients' ability to drive and operate machinery. Patients should be warned accordingly.

4.8 Undesirable effects
Frequency estimates:

very common ⩾ 10%

common $\geqslant$ 1% and < 10%
uncommon $\geqslant$ 0.1% and < 1%
rare $\geqslant$ 0.01% and < 0.1%
very rare < 0.01%.

Central and peripheral nervous system

Common: fatigue, dizziness, headache.

Rare: paraesthesiae, muscle cramps depression, decreased mental alertness, somnolence or insomnia, nightmares.

Very rare: personality disorder, hallucinations.

Cardiovascular system

Common: bradycardia, postural disorders (occasionally with syncope)

Rare: heart failure, cardiac arrhythmias, oedema palpitation, Raynaud's phenomenon

Very rare: disturbances of cardiac conduction, precordial pain, gangrene in patients with pre-existing severe peripheral circulatory disorders

Gastrointestinal tract

Common: nausea and vomiting, abdominal pain

Rare: diarrhoea or constipation

Very rare: dryness of the mouth, liver function test abnormalities

Skin and appendages

Rare: skin rash (in the form of urticaria, psoriasiform and dystrophic skin lesions), occurrence of antinuclear antibodies (not associated with SLE).

Very rare: photosensitivity, increased sweating, loss of hair, worsening of psoriasis

Respiratory tract

Common: exertional dyspnoea

Rare: bronchospasm, also in patients without a history of obstructive lung disease

Very rare: rhinitis

Endocrine system and metabolism

Very rare: weight gain

Urogential system

Very rare: disturbances of libido and potency

Sense organs

Very rare: disturbances of vision, dry and/or irritated eyes, tinnitus, and, in doses exceeding those recommended, loss of hearing

Blood

Very rare: thrombocytopenia

Other organ systems

Very rare: arthritis

4.9 Overdose

Signs and symptoms

In more severe cases an overdosage of metoprolol may lead to severe hypotension, sinus bradycardia, atrioventricular block, heart failure, cardiogenic shock, cardiac arrest, bronchospasm, impairment of consciousness, coma, convulsions, nausea, vomiting, cyanosis, hypoglycaemia and occasionally hyperkalaemia.

The first manifestations of overdosage appear 20 minutes to 2 hours after ingestion of Lopresor. The effects of massive overdose may persist for several days, despite declining plasma concentrations

Treatment

Patients should be admitted to hospital and, generally, should be managed in an intensive care setting, with continuous monitoring of cardiac function, blood gases, and blood biochemistry. Emergency supportive measures such as artificial ventilation or cardiac pacing should be instituted if appropriate. Even apparently well patients who have taken a small overdose should be closely observed for signs of poisoning for at least 4 hours.

In the event of a potentially life-threatening oral overdose, use induction of vomiting or gastric lavage (if within 4 hours after ingestion of Lopresor) and/or activated charcoal to remove the drug from the gastrointestinal tract. Metoprolol can not be effectively removed by haemodialysis.

Atropine may be given intravenously to control significant bradycardia. Intravenous beta-agonists such as prenalterol or isoprenaline should be used to treat bradycardia and hypotension; very high doses may be needed to overcome the beta-blockade. Dopamine, dobutamine or noradrenaline may be given to maintain blood pressure. Glucagon has positive inotropic and chronotropic effects on the heart that are independent of beta-adrenergic receptors, and has proved effective in the treatment of resistant hypotension and heart failure associated with beta-blocker overdose.

Diazepam is the drug of choice for controlling seizures. A β_2-agonist or aminophylline can be used to reverse bronchospasm; patients should be monitored for evidence of cardiac arrhythmias during and after administration of the bronchodilator.

5. PHARMACOLOGICAL PROPERTIES

5.1 Pharmacodynamic properties

Pharmacotherapeutic group

Lopresor is a cardioselective beta-adrenergic blocking agent.

Mechanism of Action

It has a relatively greater blocking effect on beta$_1$-receptors (i.e. those mediating adrenergic stimulation of heart rate and contractility and release of free fatty acids from fat stores) than on beta$_2$-receptors which are chiefly involved in broncho and vasodilation. It has no membrane-stabilising effect nor partial agonist (intrinsic sympathomimetic) activity.

The stimulant effect of catecholamines on the heart is reduced or inhibited by metoprolol. This leads to a decrease in heart rate, cardiac contractility and cardiac output.

5.2 Pharmacokinetic properties

Absorption

Metoprolol is well absorbed after oral administration, peak plasma concentrations occurring 1.5 - 2 hours after dosing. The bioavailability of a single dose is approximately 50%, increasing to approximately 70% during repeated administration. The bioavailability also increases if metoprolol is given with food.

Distribution and Biotransformation

Approximately 10% of metoprolol in plasma is protein bound. Metoprolol crosses the placenta, and is found in breast milk (see "Pregnancy and lactation").

Metoprolol is extensively metabolised by enzymes of the cytochrome P450 system in the liver. The oxidative metabolism of metoprolol is under genetic control None of the metabolites of metoprolol contribute significantly to its beta-blocking effect.

Elimination

Elimination is mainly by hepatic metabolism and the average elimination half-life is 3.5 hours (range 1 to 9 hours). Rates of metabolism vary between individuals, with poor metabolisers (approximately 10%) showing higher plasma concentrations and slower elimination than extensive metabolisers. Within individuals, however, plasma concentrations are stable and reproducible.

Characteristics in Patients

Because of variation in rates of metabolism, the dose of metoprolol should always be adjusted to the individual requirements of the patient. As the therapeutic response, adverse effects and relative cardioselectivity are related to plasma concentration, poor metabolisers may require lower than normal doses. Dosage adjustment is not routinely required in the elderly or in patients with renal failure, but dosage may need to be reduced in patients with significant hepatic dysfunction when metoprolol elimination may be impaired.

5.3 Preclinical safety data

There are no further data of relevance to the prescriber.

6. PHARMACEUTICAL PARTICULARS

6.1 List of excipients

Avicel PH101, povidone, Aerosil 200, sodium starch glycollate, magnesium stearate, hydroxypropylmethylcellulose, polysorbate 80, purified special talc, red iron oxide E172 (50mg tablets only), dispersed blue E132 (100mg tablets only), titanium dioxide (E171).

6.2 Incompatibilities

None known.

6.3 Shelf life

60 months.

6.4 Special precautions for storage

Protect from moisture.

6.5 Nature and contents of container

56 tablets in an Al/PVC(PVdC) blister pack.

6.6 Instructions for use and handling

Not applicable.

7. MARKETING AUTHORISATION HOLDER

Novartis Pharmaceuticals UK Limited
Trading as Geigy Pharmaceuticals
Frimley Business Park
Frimley
Camberley
Surrey
GU16 7SR

8. MARKETING AUTHORISATION NUMBER(S)

00101/0418 50mg tablets
00101/0419 100mg tablets

9. DATE OF FIRST AUTHORISATION/RENEWAL OF THE AUTHORISATION

06 June 1997 / 11 October 2000

10. DATE OF REVISION OF THE TEXT

17 July 2000

Legal Category

POM

Loron 520

(Roche Products Limited)

1. NAME OF THE MEDICINAL PRODUCT

Loron 520

2. QUALITATIVE AND QUANTITATIVE COMPOSITION

Each Loron 520 tablet contains 520mg disodium clodronate.

3. PHARMACEUTICAL FORM

Film-coated tablets for oral administration.

4. CLINICAL PARTICULARS

4.1 Therapeutic indications

Loron is indicated for the management of osteolytic lesions, hypercalcaemia and bone pain associated with skeletal metastases in patients with carcinoma of the breast or multiple myeloma. Loron 520 is also indicated for the maintenance of clinically acceptable serum calcium levels in patients with hypercalcaemia of malignancy initially treated with an intravenous infusion of disodium clodronate.

4.2 Posology and method of administration

Adults

The recommended dose is 2 tablets (1040mg disodium clodronate) daily. If necessary, the dosage may be increased but should not exceed a maximum of 4 tablets (2080mg disodium clodronate) daily.

The tablets may be taken as a single dose or in two equally divided doses if necessary to improve gastrointestinal tolerance. Loron tablets should be swallowed with a little fluid, but not milk, at least one hour before or one hour after food.

When changing therapy from Loron capsules (400mg) to Loron 520 tablets (520mg), it should be noted that two Loron capsules are equivalent to one Loron 520 tablet. This is due to greater bioavailability of the tablet formulation.

Elderly

No special dosage recommendations.

Children

Safety and efficacy in children has not been established.

Use in renal impairment

In patients with renal insufficiency with creatinine clearance between 10 and 30ml/min, the daily dose should be reduced to one half the recommended adult dose. Serum creatinine should be monitored during therapy. Disodium clodronate is contra-indicated in patients with creatinine clearance below 10ml/min.

The oral bioavailability of bisphosphonates is poor. Bioequivalence studies have shown appreciable differences in bioavailability between different oral formulations of disodium clodronate, as well as marked inter and intra patient variability. Dose adjustment may be required if the formulation is changed.

4.3 Contraindications

Hypersensitivity to disodium clodronate. Acute, severe inflammatory conditions of the gastrointestinal tract. Pregnancy and lactation. Renal failure with creatinine clearance below 10ml/min, except for short term use in the presence of purely functional renal insufficiency caused by elevated serum calcium levels. Concomitant use of other bisphosphonates.

4.4 Special warnings and special precautions for use

No information is available on the potential carcinogenicity of disodium clodronate, but patients have been treated in clinical trials for up to 2 years. The duration of the treatment is therefore at the discretion of the physician, according to the status of the underlying malignancy.

It is recommended that appropriate monitoring of renal function with serum creatinine be carried out during treatment. Serum calcium and phosphate should be monitored periodically. Monitoring of liver enzymes and white cells is advised (see side effects).

4.5 Interaction with other medicinal products and other forms of Interaction

No other bisphosphonate drugs should be given with Loron tablets.

The calcium-lowering action of clodronate can be potentiated by the administration of aminoglycosides either concomitantly or one to several weeks apart. Severe hypocalcaemia has been observed in some cases. Hypomagnesaemia may also occur simultaneously. Patients receiving NSAID's in addition to disodium clodronate have developed renal dysfunction. However, a synergistic action has not been established. There is no evidence from clinical experience that sodium clodronate interacts with other medication, such as steroids, diuretics, calcitonin, non NSAID analgesics, or chemotherapeutic agents. Calcium rich foods, mineral supplements and antacids may impair absorption.

4.6 Pregnancy and lactation

There are insufficient data either from animal studies or from experience in humans of the effects of disodium clodronate on the embryo and foetus. No studies have been conducted on excretion in breast milk. Consequently, disodium clodronate is contraindicated in pregnancy and lactation.

4.7 Effects on ability to drive and use machines

No known effects which would impair alertness.

4.8 Undesirable effects

Patients may experience a mild gastrointestinal upset, usually in the form of nausea or mild diarrhoea. The symptoms may respond to the use of a twice daily dosage regime rather than a single dose. It is not normally required to withdraw therapy or to provide medication to control these effects. Asymptomatic hypocalcaemia has been noted rarely. A reversible elevation of serum parathyroid hormone may occur. In a small proportion of patients, a mild, reversible increase in serum lactate dehydrogenase and a modest transient leucopenia have been reported although these may have been associated with concurrent chemotherapy. Renal dysfunction, including renal failure has been reported. Hypersensitivity reactions have been mainly confined to the skin: pruritus, urticaria and rarely exfoliative dermatitis. However, bronchospasm has been precipitated in patients with or without a previous history of asthma.

4.9 Overdose

Symptoms and signs:

There is no experience of acute overdosage in humans. The development of hypocalcaemia is possible for up to 2 or 3 days following the overdosage.

Treatment:

Serum calcium should be monitored and oral or parenteral calcium supplementation may be required. Acute overdosage may be associated with gastrointestinal symptoms such as nausea and vomiting. Treatment should be symptomatic.

5. PHARMACOLOGICAL PROPERTIES

5.1 Pharmacodynamic properties

Disodium clodronate is a bisphosphonate which has a high affinity to bone. It is mainly the portion of the dose adsorbed to bone which is pharmacologically active. The pharmacological effect of disodium clodronate is to suppress osteoclast mediated bone resorption as judged by bone histology and decreases in serum calcium, urine calcium and urinary excretion of hydroxyproline, without adversely affecting mineralisation.

5.2 Pharmacokinetic properties

Oral bioavailability is in the order of 2%.

Disodium clodronate is not metabolised. The volume of distribution is approximately 0.3L/kg. Elimination from serum is rapid, 75% of the dose is recovered unchanged in urine within 24 hours.

The elimination kinetics best fit a 3 compartment model. The first two compartments have relatively short half-lives. The third compartment is probably the skeleton. Elimination half life is approximately 12 - 13 hours.

5.3 Preclinical safety data

Disodium clodronate shows relatively little toxicity either on single oral administration or after daily oral administration for a period of up to 6 months. In rats, a dose of 200mg/kg/day in the chronic toxicity test is at the limit of tolerability. In dogs, 40mg/kg/day chronically is within the tolerated range.

On daily administration of 500mg/kg for 6 weeks to rats, signs of renal failure with a clear rise in BUN, and initial liver parenchymal reaction with rises of SGOT, SGPT and AP occurred. No significant haematological changes were found in the toxicological investigations.

Investigations for mutagenic properties did not show any indication of mutagenic potency.

Reproduction toxicology investigations did not provide any indication of peri and post natal disorders, teratogenic damage or disorders of fertility.

It is not known if disodium clodronate passes into the mother's milk or through the placenta.

6. PHARMACEUTICAL PARTICULARS

6.1 List of excipients

Loron 520 tablets also contain:

Core

Disodium clodronate, talc, maize starch, microcrystalline cellulose, magnesium stearate, sodium starch glycollate.

Coating

Methylhydroxypropylcellulose, poly(meth) acrylic acid esters (Eudragit NE 30D), polyoxyethylene alkyl ether (Macrogol 1000), lactose monohydrate, talc, titanium dioxide (E171), polysorbate 80, sodium citrate.

6.2 Incompatibilities

Not applicable.

6.3 Shelf life

PVC/aluminium blister packs:

5 years.

6.4 Special precautions for storage

None

6.5 Nature and contents of container

PVC/aluminium blister packs containing 10 or 60 tablets.

6.6 Instructions for use and handling

No special instructions.

7. MARKETING AUTHORISATION HOLDER

Roche Products Limited, 40 Broadwater Road, Welwyn Garden City, Hertfordshire, AL7 3AY.

8. MARKETING AUTHORISATION NUMBER(S)

PL 00031/0521

9. DATE OF FIRST AUTHORISATION/RENEWAL OF THE AUTHORISATION

1 July 1999

10. DATE OF REVISION OF THE TEXT

July 1999

11. LEGAL CATEGORY

POM

Loron is a registered trade mark

P469044/999

Losec Capsules 10mg, 20mg & 40mg

(AstraZeneca UK Limited)

1. NAME OF THE MEDICINAL PRODUCT

Losec Capsules 10mg.

Losec Capsules 20mg.

Losec Capsules 40mg.

2. QUALITATIVE AND QUANTITATIVE COMPOSITION

Each capsule contains: Omeprazole 10mg/20mg/40mg

For excipients, see 6.1

3. PHARMACEUTICAL FORM

Hard gelatin capsules.

Losec Capsules 10mg: hard gelatin capsules with an opaque pink body, marked 10 and an opaque pink cap marked A/OS in black ink. Each capsule contains omeprazole 10mg as enteric coated granules, with an aqueous based coating.

Losec Capsules 20mg: hard gelatin capsules with an opaque pink body, marked 20 and an opaque reddish-brown cap marked A/OM in black ink. Each capsule contains omeprazole 20mg as enteric coated granules, with an aqueous based coating.

Losec Capsules 40mg: hard gelatin capsules with an opaque reddish-brown body, marked 40 and an opaque reddish-brown cap marked A/OL in black ink. Each capsule contains omeprazole 40mg as enteric coated granules, with an aqueous based coating

4. CLINICAL PARTICULARS

4.1 Therapeutic indications

Treatment of oesophageal reflux disease. In reflux oesophagitis the majority of patients are healed after 4 weeks. Symptom relief is rapid.

Treatment of duodenal and benign gastric ulcers including those complicating NSAID therapy.

Helicobacter pylori eradication: Omeprazole should be used in combination with antibiotics for eradication of *Helicobacter pylori* (*Hp*) in peptic ulcer disease.

Relief of associated dyspeptic symptoms.

Prophylaxis of acid aspiration.

Zollinger-Ellison syndrome.

<u>For 10 and 20mg Capsules only</u>:

Relief of reflux-like symptoms (eg. heartburn) and/or ulcer-like symptoms (eg. epigastric pain) associated with acid-related dyspepsia.

Treatment and prophylaxis of NSAID-associated benign gastric ulcers, duodenal ulcers and gastroduodenal erosions in patients with a previous history of gastroduodenal lesions who require continued NSAID treatment.

4.2 Posology and method of administration

Adults:

<u>Oesophageal reflux disease includingreflux oesophagitis:</u> The usual dosage is 20 mg Losec once daily. The majority of patients are healed after 4 weeks. For those patients not fully healed after the initial course, healing usually occurs during a further 4-8 weeks treatment. Losec has also been used in a dose of 40 mg once daily in patients with reflux oesophagitis refractory to other therapy. Healing usually occurred within 8 weeks. Patients can be continued at a dosage of 20 mg once daily.

<u>Acid reflux disease:</u> For long-term management Losec 10 mg once daily is recommended, increasing to 20 mg if symptoms return.

<u>Duodenal and benign gastric ulcers:</u> The usual dose is 20 mg Losec once daily. The majority of patients with duodenal ulcer are healed after 4 weeks. The majority of patients with benign gastric ulcer are healed after 8 weeks. In severe or recurrent cases the dose may be increased to 40 mg Losec daily. Long-term therapy for patients with a history of recurrent duodenal ulcer is recommended at a dosage of 20 mg Losec once daily.

For prevention of relapse in patients with duodenal ulcer the recommended dose is Losec 10 mg, once daily, increasing to 20 mg, once daily if symptoms return.

The following groups are at risk from recurrent ulcer relapse; those with *Helicobacter pylori* infection, younger patients (<60 years), those whose symptoms persist for more than one year and smokers. These patients will require initial long-term therapy with Losec 20 mg once daily, reducing to 10mg once daily, if necessary.

<u>Helicobacter pylori (Hp) eradication regimens in peptic ulcer disease:</u> Losec is recommended at a dose of 40 mg once daily or 20 mg twice daily in association with antimicrobial agents as detailed below:

<u>Triple therapy regimens in duodenal ulcer disease:</u> Losec and the following antimicrobial combinations;

Amoxicillin 500 mg and metronidazole 400 mg both three times a day for one week.

or

Clarithromycin 250 mg and metronidazole 400 mg (or tinidazole 500 mg) both twice a day for one week.

or

Amoxicillin 1 g and clarithromycin 500 mg both twice a day for one week.

<u>Dual therapy regimens in duodenal ulcer disease:</u>

Losec and amoxicillin 750 mg to 1 g twice daily for two weeks. Alternatively Losec and clarithromycin 500 mg three times a day for two weeks.

<u>Dual therapy regimens in gastric ulcer disease:</u>

Losec and amoxicillin 750 mg to 1 g twice daily for two weeks

In each regimen if symptoms return and the patient is *Hp* positive, therapy may be repeated or one of the alternative regimens can be used; if the patient is *Hp* negative then see dosage instructions for acid reflux disease.

To ensure healing in patients with active peptic ulcer disease, see further dosage recommendations for duodenal and benign gastric ulcer.

<u>Prophylaxis of acid aspiration:</u> For patients considered to be at risk of aspiration of the gastric contents during general anaesthesia, the recommended dosage is Losec 40 mg on the evening before surgery followed by Losec 40 mg 2 - 6 hours prior to surgery.

<u>Zollinger-Ellison syndrome:</u> The recommended initial dosage is 60mg Losec once daily. The dosage should be adjusted individually and treatment continued as long as clinically indicated. More than 90% of patients with severe disease and inadequate response to other therapies have been effectively controlled on doses of 20-120mg daily. With doses above 80mg daily, the dose should be divided and given twice daily.

<u>For 10 & 20mg Capsules only:</u>

<u>Acid-related dyspepsia:</u> The usual dosage is Losec 10 mg or 20 mg once daily for 2-4 weeks depending on the severity and persistence of symptoms. Patients who do not respond after 4 weeks or who relapse shortly afterwards, should be investigated.

<u>For the treatment of NSAID-associated gastric ulcers, duodenal ulcers or gastroduodenal erosions:</u> The recommended dosage of Losec is 20 mg once daily. Symptom resolution is rapid and in most patients healing occurs within 4 weeks. For those patients who may not be fully healed after the initial course, healing usually occurs during a further 4 weeks treatment.

<u>For the prophylaxis of NSAID-associated gastric ulcers, duodenal ulcers, gastroduodenal erosions and dyspeptic symptoms in patients with a previous history of gastroduodenal lesions who require continued NSAID treatment:</u> The recommended dosage of Losec is 20 mg once daily.

Elderly:

Dose adjustment is not required in the elderly.

Children:

Experience of the use of Losec in children is limited. In children 1 year and above with severe ulcerating reflux oesophagitis, Losec is recommended for healing and symptom relief at the following doses:

<u>Weight</u>	<u>Dosage</u>
10-20 kg	Losec 10 mg once daily
>20 kg	Losec 20 mg once daily

If needed the dose may be increased to 20 mg and 40 mg respectively for 4-12 weeks.

Data suggest that approximately 65% of children will experience pain relief with this dose regimen. Treatment should be initiated by a paediatrician.

Impaired renal function:

Dose adjustment is not required in patients with impaired renal function.

Impaired hepatic function:

As bioavailability and half-life can increase in patients with impaired hepatic function, the dose requires adjustment with a maximum daily dose of 20mg.

<u>For patients (including children aged 1 year and above who can drink or swallow semi-solid food) who are unable to swallow Losec Capsules:</u>

The capsules may be opened and the contents swallowed directly with half a glass of water or suspended in 10 ml of non-carbonated water, any fruit juice with a pH less than 5 e.g. apple, orange, pineapple, or in applesauce or yoghurt and swallowed after gentle mixing. The dispersion should be taken immediately or within 30 minutes. Stir just before drinking and rinse it down with half a glass of water. Alternatively the actual capsules may be sucked and then swallowed with half a glass of water. There is no evidedence to support the use of sodium bicarbonate buffer as a delivery form. It is important that the contents of the capsules should not be crushed or chewed.

4.3 Contraindications

Known hypersensitivity to omeprazole or to any of the other constituents of the formulation.

When gastric ulcer is suspected, the possibility of malignancy should be excluded before treatment with Losec is instituted, as treatment may alleviate symptoms and delay diagnosis.

4.4 Special warnings and special precautions for use

Decreased gastric acidity due to any means, including proton-pump inhibitors, increases gastric counts of bacteria normally present in the gastrointestinal tract. Treatment with acid-reducing drugs may lead to a slightly increased risk of gastrointestinal infections, such as *Salmonella* and *Campylobacter*.

For severely ill children, who require long-term treatment with Losec, and may have borderline levels or body stores of B_{12}, it may be advisable to monitor serum B_{12} levels during long-term treatment (see section 4.8).

4.5 Interaction with other medicinal products and other forms of Interaction

Due to the decreased intragastric acidity the absorption of ketoconazole or itraconazole may be reduced during omeprazole treatment as it is during treatment with other acid secretion inhibitors.

As Losec is metabolised in the liver through cytochrome P450 it can prolong the elimination of diazepam, phenytoin and warfarin. Monitoring of patients receiving warfarin or phenytoin is recommended and a reduction of warfarin or phenytoin dose may be necessary. However concomitant treatment with Losec 20mg daily did not change the blood concentration of phenytoin in patients on continuous treatment with phenytoin. Similarly concomitant treatment with Losec 20mg daily did not change coagulation time in patients on continuous treatment with warfarin.

Plasma concentrations of omeprazole and clarithromycin are increased during concomitant administration. This is considered to be a useful interaction during *H. pylori* eradication. There is no interaction with metronidazole or amoxicillin. These antimicrobials are used together with omeprazole for eradication of Helicobacter *pylori*.

There is no evidence of an interaction with phenacetin, theophylline, caffeine, propranolol, metoprolol, ciclosporin, lidocaine, quinidine, estradiol or antacids. The absorption of Losec is not affected by alcohol or food.

There is no evidence of an interaction with piroxicam, diclofenac or naproxen. This is considered useful when patients are required to continue these treatments.

Simultaneous treatment with omeprazole and digoxin in healthy subjects lead to a 10% increase in the bioavailability of digoxin as a consequence of the increased intragastric pH.

4.6 Pregnancy and lactation

Pregnancy

The analysis of the results from three epidemiological studies has revealed no evidence of adverse events of omeprazole on pregnancy or on the health of the foetus / newborn child. Losec can be used during pregnancy.

Lactation

Omeprazole is excreted in breast milk but is not likely to influence the child when therapeutic doses are used.

4.7 Effects on ability to drive and use machines

No effects are foreseen.

4.8 Undesirable effects

Losec is well tolerated and adverse reactions have generally been mild and reversible. The following have been reported as adverse events in clinical trials or reported from routine use but in many cases a relationship to treatment with omeprazole has not been established.

The following definitions of frequencies are used:

Common	⩾ 1/100
Uncommon	⩾ 1/1000 and < 1/100
Rare	< 1/1000

Common	*Central and peripheral nervous system:*	Headache
	Gastrointestinal:	Diarrhoea, constipation, Abdominal pain, nausea/vomiting and flatulence
Uncommon	*Central and peripheral nervous system:*	Dizziness, paraesthesia, light headedness, feeling faint, somnolence, insomnia and vertigo.
	Hepatic:	Increased liver enzymes.
	Skin:	Rash and/or pruritus. Urticaria.
	Other:	Malaise.
Rare	*Central and peripheral nervous system:*	*Reversible mental confusion, agitation, aggression, depression and hallucinations, predominantly in severely ill patients.*
	Endocrine:	*Gynaecomastia.*
	Gastrointestinal:	*Dry mouth, stomatitis and gastrointestinal candidiasis.*
	Haematological:	*Leukopenia, thrombocytopenia, agranulocytosis and pancytopenia.*
	Hepatic	*Encephalopathy in patients with pre-existing severe liver disease; hepatitis with or without jaundice, hepatic failure.*
	Musculoskeletal	*Arthritic and myalgic symptoms and muscular weakness.*
	Reproductive system and breast disorders	*Impotence*
	Skin	*Photosensitivity, bullous eruption erythema multiforme, Stevens-Johnson syndrome, toxic epidermal necrolysis (TEN), alopecia.*
	Other	*Hypersensitivity reactions e.g. angioedema, fever, broncho-spasm, interstitial nephritis and anaphylactic shock [3]. Increased sweating, peripheral oedema, blurred vision, taste disturbance and hyponatraemia.*

The safety of omeprazole has been assessed in 310 children aged 0 to 16 years with acid related disease and 62 physiologically normal volunteers aged 2 years to 16 years. Omeprazole was generally well tolerated with an adverse event profile resembling that in adults.

In a study of 106 children aged 0-24 months with gastro-oesophageal reflux, treated with omeprazole, 11 patients had moderate elevations of serum liver enzymes (AST, ALT, GGT), but were clinically asymptomatic. In addition, 52 patients had mild to moderate reductions in neutrophil counts, although there was only one case of reduction in WBC.

There are limited long-term safety data from 46 children who received maintenance therapy of omeprazole during a clinical study for severe erosive oesophagitis for up to 749 days (see section 5.1). In this group, a retrospective review of patients showed that serum vitamin B12 levels decreased mildly in 18 children during 24 months of the study. In no patient did the level fall below normal limits. Iron- deficiency anaemia was reported in 12 patients. Elevations in serum gastrin levels were noted in 20 patients, and 4 children had argyophil (ECL) hyperplasia during this study.

4.9 Overdose

Rare reports have been received of overdosage with omeprazole. In the literature doses of up to 560 mg have been described and occasional reports have been received when single oral doses have reached up to 2400 mg omeprazole (120 times the usual recommended clinical dose). Nausea, vomiting, dizziness, abdominal pain, diarrhoea and headache have been reported from overdosage with omeprazole. Also apathy, depression and confusion have been described in single cases.

The symptoms described in connection to omeprazole overdosage have been transient, and no serious outcome due to omeprazole has been reported. The rate of elimination was unchanged (first order kinetics) with increased doses and no specific treatment has been needed.

5. PHARMACOLOGICAL PROPERTIES

5.1 Pharmacodynamic properties

Losec reduces gastric acid secretion through a unique mechanism of action. It is a specific inhibitor of the gastric proton pump in the parietal cell. It is rapidly acting and produces reversible control of gastric acid secretion with once daily dosing.

Oral dosing with 20mg Losec once daily provides for rapid and effective inhibition of gastric acid secretion with maximum effect being achieved within 4 days of treatment. In duodenal ulcer patients, a mean decrease of approximately 80% in 24-hour intragastric acidity is then maintained, with the mean decrease in peak acid output after pentagastrin stimulation being about 70%, twenty-four hours after dosing with Losec.

Clinical data for omeprazole in the prophylaxis of NSAID induced gastroduodenal lesions are derived from clinical studies of up to 6 months duration.

Helicobacter pylori(Hp) is associated with acid peptic disease including duodenal ulcer (DU) and gastric ulcer (GU) in which about 95% and 80% of patients respectively are infected with this bacterium. *Hp* is implicated as a major contributing factor in the development of gastritis and ulcers in such patients. Recent evidence also suggests a causative link between *Hp* and gastric carcinoma.

Omeprazole has been shown to have a bactericidal effect on *Hp* in vitro.

Eradication of *Hp* with omeprazole and antimicrobials is associated with rapid symptom relief, high rates of healing of any mucosal lesions, and long-term remission of peptic ulcer disease thus reducing complications such as gastro-intestinal bleeding as well as the need for prolonged anti-secretory treatment.

In recent clinical data in patients with acute peptic ulcer omeprazole *Hp* eradication therapy improved patients' quality of life.

During long-term treatment an increased frequency of gastric glandular cysts have been reported. These changes are a physiological consequence of pronounced inhibition of acid secretion. The cysts are benign and appear to be reversible. No other treatment related mucosal changes have been observed in patients treated continuously with omeprazole for periods up to 5 years.

Children

Treatment of non-erosive Gastroesophageal Reflux Disease

In a randomised study, with no comparator, the efficacy of 0.5 mg/kg, 1.0 mg/kg and 1.5 mg/kg of omeprazole was compared in 110 children aged 0-24 months with endoscopically and clinically diagnosed GORD. Due to the lack of placebo comparison no efficacy could be confirmed

Severe Erosive Oesophagitis

In an uncontrolled, open-label dose-titration study, healing of severe erosive oesophagitis in children aged 1- 16 years, approximately 65% of patients were healed with doses of 0.7-1.4 mg/kg.

Maintenance of Healing of Erosive Oesophagitis

In an uncontrolled, open-label study of omeprazole for the maintenance of healing of severe erosive oesophagitis in 46 children aged 1 to 16 yrs, 59% of patients relapsed on half their healing dose and they had to return to their healing dose.

Helicobacter pylori eradication

In a double-blind controlled parallel group study of 73 children aged 3 months to 15 years (mean age 10.5 years) with dyspeptic symptoms and *H. pylori* associated gastritis who were treated with triple therapy alone or in combination with omeprazole, the mean eradication rate was 74.2% in the omeprazole group compared with 9.4% in the placebo group. However, there was no evidence of clinical benefit demonstrated regarding dyspeptic symptoms.

Site and mechanism of action

Omeprazole is a weak base and is concentrated and converted to the active form in the acid environment of the intracellular canaliculi within the parietal cell, where it inhibits the enzyme H^+, K^+-ATPase - the proton pump. This effect on the final step of the gastric acid formation process is dose-dependent and provides for effective inhibition of both basal acid secretion and stimulated acid secretion irrespective of the stimulus.

All pharmacodynamic effects observed are explained by the effect of omeprazole on acid secretion.

5.2 Pharmacokinetic properties

Absorption and distribution

Omeprazole is acid labile and is administered orally as enteric-coated granules in capsules. Absorption takes place in the small intestine and is usually completed within 3-6 hours. The systemic bioavailability of omeprazole from a single oral dose of Losec is approximately 35%. After repeated once-daily administration, the bioavailability increases to about 60%. Concomitant intake of food has no influence on the bioavailability. The plasma protein binding of omeprazole is about 95%.

Elimination and metabolism

The average half-life of the terminal phase of the plasma concentration-time curve is approximately 40 minutes. There is no change in half-life during treatment. The inhibition of acid secretion is related to the area under the plasma concentration-time curve (AUC) but not to the actual plasma concentration at a given time.

Omeprazole is entirely metabolised mainly in the liver. Identified metabolites in plasma are the sulphone, the sulphide and hydroxy-omeprazole, these metabolites have no significant effect on acid secretion. About 80% of the metabolites are excreted in the urine and the rest in the faeces. The two main urinary metabolites are hydroxy-omeprazole and the corresponding carboxylic acid.

The systemic bioavailability of omeprazole is not significantly altered in patients with reduced renal function. The area under the plasma concentration-time curve is increased in patients with impaired liver function, but no tendency to accumulation of omeprazole has been found.

Children

Limited data from children aged 0-16 years suggest that the pharmacokinetics within the recommended doses are similar to those reported in adults.

5.3 Preclinical safety data

Animal Toxicology:

Gastric ECL-cell hyperplasia and carcinoids, have been observed in life-long studies in rats treated with omeprazole or subjected to partial fundectomy. These changes are the result of sustained hypergastrinaemia secondary to acid inhibition, and not from a direct effect of any individual drug.

6. PHARMACEUTICAL PARTICULARS

6.1 List of excipients

Mannitol, hyprolose, cellulose microcrystalline, lactose anhydrous, sodium laurilsulfate, disodium hydrogen phosphate dihydrate, hypromellose, methacrylic acid copolymer, macrogol, red iron oxide (E172), titanium dioxide (E171), gelatin and magnesium stearate.

6.2 Incompatibilities

None known.

6.3 Shelf life

3 years

Bottles: 3 month in use shelf-life

6.4 Special precautions for storage

Do not store above 30°C

Blisters: Store in the original container.

Bottles: Keep the container tightly closed.

6.5 Nature and contents of container

Losec Capsules are provided in high density polyethylene bottles with tamper-proof child resistant lids containing integral desiccant. Packs of 5, 7, 14, 28 Capsules.

OR

Losec Capsules are provided in Aluminium-PVC / Aluminium foil blister packs. Packs of 7, 14 and 28 capsules.

Not all pack sizes may be marketed.

6.6 Instructions for use and handling

The cap should be replaced firmly after use.

To be dispensed in original containers.

7. MARKETING AUTHORISATION HOLDER

AstraZeneca UK Ltd.,

600 Capability Green,

Luton, LU1 3LU, UK.

8. MARKETING AUTHORISATION NUMBER(S)

PL 17901/0132

PL 17901/0133

PL 17901/0134

9. DATE OF FIRST AUTHORISATION/RENEWAL OF THE AUTHORISATION

14th May 2002

10. DATE OF REVISION OF THE TEXT

22nd March 2005

Losec I.V. Injection 40mg

(AstraZeneca UK Limited)

1. NAME OF THE MEDICINAL PRODUCT

Losec® I.V. Injection 40mg▼

2. QUALITATIVE AND QUANTITATIVE COMPOSITION

a) Each vial of powder for solution for injection contains Omeprazole Sodium Ph. Eur., equivalent to Omeprazole 40mg.

b) Each ampoule contains 10ml of solvent for injection

3. PHARMACEUTICAL FORM

Powder and solvent for solution for injection.

4. CLINICAL PARTICULARS

4.1 Therapeutic indications

Prophylaxis of acid aspiration.

In patients who are unable to take oral therapy for the short term treatment (up to 5 days) of reflux oesophagitis, duodenal and benign gastric ulcers, including those complicating NSAID therapy e.g. peri-operative use.

4.2 Posology and method of administration

Dosage

Adults only

Prophylaxis of acid aspiration: Losec 40mg to be given slowly (over a period of 5 minutes) as an intravenous injection, one hour before surgery.

Treatment in patients where oral therapy is inappropriate e.g. in severely ill patients with either reflux oesophagitis, duodenal ulcer or gastric ulcer: Losec 40mg given as an intravenous injection once daily is recommended for up to 5 days.

Clinical experience in Zollinger-Ellison syndrome is limited (see section 5.1 Pharmacodynamic properties).

Administration

Losec powder and solvent for solution for injection is for intravenous administration ONLY and must NOT be given by any other route.

Losec powder and solvent for solution for injection should only be dissolved in the solvent provided. No other solvents for i.v. injection should be used.

After reconstitution outside validated aseptic conditions, use within 4 hours of preparation and any unused portion should be discarded.

The duration of administration should be over 5 minutes.

Use in the Elderly:

Dosage adjustment is not necessary.

Use in Children:

There is limited experience of use in children.

Impaired renal function:

Dose adjustment is not required in patients with impaired renal function.

Impaired hepatic function:

As half-life is increased in patients with impaired hepatic function, the dose requires adjustment and a daily dose of 10mg - 20mg may be sufficient.

4.3 Contraindications

Known hypersensitivity to any of the constituents of the formulation.

4.4 Special warnings and special precautions for use

When gastric ulcer is suspected the possibility of malignancy should be excluded before treatment with Losec is instituted, as treatment may alleviate symptoms and delay diagnosis.

Decreased gastric acidity due to any means including proton-pump inhibitors, increases gastric counts of bacteria normally present in the gastrointestinal tract. Treatment with acid-reducing drugs may lead to a slightly increased risk of gastrointestinal infections, such as *Salmonella* and *Campylobacter*.

4.5 Interaction with other medicinal products and other forms of Interaction

Due to the decreased intragastric acidity, the absorption of ketoconazole or itraconazole may be reduced during omeprazole therapy as it is during treatment with other acid secretion inhibitors.

As omeprazole is metabolised in the liver through cytochrome P450 it can prolong the elimination of diazepam, phenytoin and warfarin. Monitoring of patients receiving a phenytoin or warfarin is recommended and a reduction of phenytoin or warfarin dose may be necessary when Losec is added to treatment. However, concomitant treatment with Losec 20mg orally daily did not change the blood concentration of phenytoin in patients on continuous treatment with phenytoin. Similarly, concomitant treatment with Losec 20mg orally daily did not change coagulation time in patients on continuous treatment with warfarin.

Plasma concentrations of omeprazole and clarithromycin are increased during concomitant oral administration. There is no interaction with metronidazole or amoxicillin. These antimicrobials are used together with omeprazole for eradication of Helicobacter *pylori*.

There is no evidence of an interaction with phenacetin, theophylline, caffeine, propranolol, metoprolol, cyclosporin, lidocaine, quinidine, oestradiol, or antacids when Losec is given orally. The absorption of Losec given orally is not affected by alcohol or food.

There is no evidence of an interaction with piroxicam, diclofenac or naproxen, this is considered useful when patients are required to continue these treatments.

Simultaneous treatment with omeprazole and digoxin in healthy subjects led to a 10% increase in the bioavailability of digoxin as a consequence of the increased intragastric pH.

Interaction with other drugs also metabolised via the cytochrome P450 system cannot be excluded.

4.6 Pregnancy and lactation

Use in pregnancy

The analysis of the results from three epidemiological studies has revealed no evidence of adverse events of omeprazole on pregnancy or on the health of the fetus/newborn child. LOSEC® can be used during pregnancy.

Use in lactation

Omeprazole is excreted in breast milk but is not likely to influence the child when therapeutic doses are used.

4.7 Effects on ability to drive and use machines

No effects are foreseen.

4.8 Undesirable effects

Losec is well tolerated and adverse reactions have generally been mild and reversible. The following have been reported as adverse events in clinical trials or reported from routine use but in many cases a relationship to treatment with omeprazole has not been established.

The following definitions of frequencies are used:

Common $\geq$ 1/100

Uncommon $\geq$ 1/1000 and $<$ 1/100

Rare $<$ 1/1000

Common	Central and peripheral nervous system:	Headache
	Gastrointestinal:	Diarrhoea, constipation, abdominal pain, nausea/vomiting and flatulence
Uncommon	Central and peripheral nervous system:	Dizziness, paraesthesia, light headedness, feeling faint, somnolence, insomnia and vertigo.
	Hepatic:	Increased liver enzymes.
	Skin:	Rash and/or pruritus. Urticaria.
	Other:	Malaise.
Rare	Central and peripheral nervous system:	Reversible mental confusion, agitation, aggression, depression and hallucinations, predominantly in severely ill patients.
	Endocrine:	Gynaecomastia.
	Gastrointestinal:	Dry mouth, stomatitis and gastrointestinal candidiasis.
	Haematological:	Leukopenia, thrombocytopenia, agranulocytosis and pancytopenia.
	Hepatic	Encephalopathy in patients with pre-existing severe liver disease; hepatitis with or without jaundice, hepatic failure increased liver enzymes.
	Musculoskeletal	Arthritic and myalgic symptoms and muscular weakness.
	Reproductive system and breast disorders	Impotence
	Skin	Photosensitivity, bullous eruption, erythema multiforme, Stevens-Johnson syndrome, toxic epidermal necrolysis (TEN), alopecia.

Other	Hypersensitivity reactions e.g. angioedema, fever, broncho-spasm, interstitial nephritis and anaphylactic shock. Increased sweating, peripheral oedema, blurred vision, taste disturbance and hyponatraemia.

Isolated cases of irreversible visual impairment have been reported in critically ill patients who have received Losec Intravenous Injection, particularly at high doses, however no causal relationship has been established.

4.9 Overdose

Intravenous doses of up to 270mg on a single day and up to 650mg over a three-day period have been given in clinical trials without any dose related adverse effects.

5. PHARMACOLOGICAL PROPERTIES

5.1 Pharmacodynamic properties

Omeprazole reduces gastric acid secretion through a unique mechanism of action. It is a specific inhibitor of the gastric proton pump in the parietal cell. It is rapidly acting and produces reversible control of gastric acid secretion with once daily dosing.

Intravenous administration of omeprazole results in an immediate reduction of intragastric acidity and a mean decrease over 24 hours of approximately 90% in patients with duodenal ulcer disease. A single 40mg i.v. dose has similar effect on intragastric acidity over a 24 hour period as repeated oral dosing with 20mg once daily. A higher dose of 60mg i.v. twice daily has been used in a clinical study in patients with Zollinger - Ellison syndrome.

Site and mechanism of action

Omeprazole is a weak base and is concentrated and converted to the active form in the acid environment of the intracellular canaliculi within the parietal cell, where it inhibits the enzyme H^+, K^+,-ATPase - the proton pump. This effect on the final step of the gastric acid formation process is dose-dependent and provides for effective inhibition of both basal acid secretion and stimulated acid secretion irrespective of the stimulus.

All pharmacodynamic effects observed are explained by the effect of omeprazole on acid secretion. No tachyphylaxis has been observed during treatment with omeprazole.

5.2 Pharmacokinetic properties

Distribution

The apparent volume of distribution in healthy subjects is approximately 0.3 L/kg and a similar value is also seen in patients with renal insufficiency. In the elderly and in patients with hepatic insufficiency, the volume of distribution is slightly decreased. The plasma protein binding of omeprazole is about 95%.

Metabolism and excretion

The average half-life of the terminal phase of the plasma concentration-time curve following i.v. administration of omeprazole is approximately 40 minutes; the total plasma clearance is 0.3 to 0.6 L/min. There is no change in half-life during treatment.

Omeprazole is completely metabolised by the cytochrome P450 system, mainly in the liver. The major part of its metabolism is dependent on the polymorphically expressed, specific isoform CYP2C19 (S-mephenytoin hydroxylase), responsible for the formation of hydroxyomeprazole, the major metabolite in plasma.

No metabolite has been found to have any effect on gastric acid secretion. Almost 80% of an intravenously given dose is excreted as metabolites in the urine, and the remainder is found in the faeces, primarily originating from biliary secretion.

Elimination of omeprazole is unchanged in patients with reduced renal function. The elimination half-life is increased in patients with impaired liver function, but omeprazole has not shown any accumulation with once daily oral dosing.

5.3 Preclinical safety data

Animal Toxicology:

Gastric ECL-cell hyperplasia and carcinoids, have been observed in life-long studies in rats treated with omeprazole or subjected to partial fundectomy. These changes are the result of sustained hypergastrinaemia secondary to acid inhibition, and not from a direct effect of any individual drug.

6. PHARMACEUTICAL PARTICULARS

6.1 List of excipients

a) Vial: Sodium hydroxide.

b) Ampoule: Macrogol 400, Citric acid monohydrate and Water for injections.

6.2 Incompatibilities

No other drugs should be mixed with reconstituted Losec i.v. Injection solution.

6.3 Shelf life

Unopened packs: 2 years.

Reconstituted solution: 4 hours.

6.4 Special precautions for storage

Do not store above 25°C. Keep the containers in outer carton.

6.5 Nature and contents of container

Combination pack consisting of a clear, Type I, glass vial containing omeprazole sodium 42.6mg with grey bromobutyl rubber stopper, white polypropylene cap with aluminium frame and a clear, Type I, (OPC) glass ampoule containing solvent for intravenous administration, both packed together in a plastic tray in a hard cardboard box.

6.6 Instructions for use and handling

The entire contents of the vial should be completely dissolved with the 10ml of solvent provided in the ampoule. No other solvents for i.v. injection should be used.

Use on one patient during one treatment only.

DO NOT USE if any particles are present in the reconstituted solution.

Chemical and physical in use stability of the reconstituted product has been shown for 4 hours when stored at 25°C.

From a microbiological point of view, once opened and reconstituted the product may be stored for a maximum of 4 hours at 25°C. Other in-use storage times and conditions are the responsibility of the user.

Any unused portion should be discarded.

Preparation:

NOTE: Stages 1 to 5 should be done in immediate sequence.

With a syringe draw 10ml of solvent from the ampoule.

Add approximately 5ml of the solvent to the vial with freeze-dried omeprazole.

Withdraw as much air as possible from the vial back into the syringe in order to reduce positive pressure. This will make it easier to add the remaining solvent.

Add the remaining solvent into the vial, make sure that the syringe is empty.

Rotate and shake the vial to ensure all the freeze-dried omeprazole has dissolved.

7. MARKETING AUTHORISATION HOLDER

AstraZeneca UK Ltd.,

600 Capability Green,

Luton, LU1 3LU, UK.

8. MARKETING AUTHORISATION NUMBER(S)

PL 17901/0135

9. DATE OF FIRST AUTHORISATION/RENEWAL OF THE AUTHORISATION

18th June 2002

10. DATE OF REVISION OF THE TEXT

29th October 2004

Losec Infusion 40mg

(AstraZeneca UK Limited)

1. NAME OF THE MEDICINAL PRODUCT

Losec® Infusion 40mg▼

2. QUALITATIVE AND QUANTITATIVE COMPOSITION

Each vial of powder for solution for infusion contains Omeprazole Sodium Ph. Eur., equivalent to Omeprazole 40mg.

3. PHARMACEUTICAL FORM

Powder for solution for infusion.

4. CLINICAL PARTICULARS

4.1 Therapeutic indications

Prophylaxis of acid aspiration.

In patients who are unable to take oral therapy for the short term treatment (up to 5 days) of reflux oesophagitis, duodenal and benign gastric ulcers, including those complicating NSAID therapy e.g. peri-operative use.

4.2 Posology and method of administration

Dosage

Adults only

Prophylaxis of acid aspiration Losec 40mg given as an intravenous infusion to be completed one hour before surgery.

Treatment in patients where oral therapy is inappropriate e.g. in severely ill patients with either reflux oesophagitis, duodenal ulcer or gastric ulcer: Losec 40mg given as an intravenous infusion once daily is recommended for up to 5 days.

The i.v. infusion produces an immediate decrease in intragastric acidity and a mean decrease over 24 hours of approximately 90%.

Clinical experience in Zollinger Ellison syndrome is limited (see section 5.1 Pharmacodynamic properties).

Administration

Losec powder for solution for infusion is for intravenous administration ONLY and must NOT be given by any other route.

Losec powder for solution for infusion should only be dissolved in either 100ml normal saline for infusion or 100ml 5% dextrose for infusion. No other solutions for i.v. infusion should be used.

After reconstitution from a microbiological point of view, use immediately (i.e. within 3 hours) and any unused portion should be discarded.

The duration of administration should be 20-30 minutes.

Use in the Elderly:

Dosage adjustment is not necessary.

Use in Children:

There is limited experience of use in children.

Impaired renal function:

Dose adjustment is not required in patients with impaired renal function.

Impaired hepatic function:

As half-life is increased in patients with impaired hepatic function, the dose requires adjustment and a daily dose of 10mg - 20mg may be sufficient.

4.3 Contraindications

Known hypersensitivity to omeprazole or to any of the other constituents of the formulation.

4.4 Special warnings and special precautions for use

When gastric ulcer is suspected the possibility of malignancy should be excluded before treatment with Losec is instituted, as treatment may alleviate symptoms and delay diagnosis.

Decreased gastric acidity due to any means including proton-pump inhibitors, increases gastric counts of bacteria normally present in the gastrointestinal tract. Treatment with acid-reducing drugs may lead to a slightly increased risk of gastrointestinal infections, such as *Salmonella* and *Campylobacter*.

4.5 Interaction with other medicinal products and other forms of Interaction

Due to the decreased intragastric acidity, the absorption of ketoconazole or itraconazole may be reduced during omeprazole therapy as it is during treatment with other acid secretion inhibitors.

As omeprazole is metabolised in the liver through cytochrome P450 it can prolong the elimination of diazepam, phenytoin and warfarin. Monitoring of patients receiving phenytoin or warfarin is recommended and a reduction of phenytoin or warfarin dose may be necessary when Losec is added to treatment. However, concomitant treatment with Losec 20mg orally daily did not change the blood concentration of phenytoin in patients on continuous treatment with phenytoin. Similarly, concomitant treatment with Losec 20mg orally daily did not change coagulation time in patients on continuous treatment with warfarin.

Plasma concentrations of omeprazole and clarithromycin are increased during concomitant oral administration. There is no interaction with metronidazole or amoxicillin. These antimicrobials are used together with omeprazole for eradication of Helicobacter *pylori*.

There is no evidence of an interaction with phenacetin, theophylline, caffeine, propranolol, metoprolol, cyclosporin, lidocaine, quinidine, oestradiol, or antacids when Losec is given orally. The absorption of Losec given orally is not affected by alcohol or food.

There is no evidence of an interaction with piroxicam, diclofenac or naproxen, this is considered useful when patients are required to continue these treatments.

Simultaneous treatment with omeprazole and digoxin in healthy subjects led to a 10% increase in the bioavailability of digoxin as a consequence of the increased intragastric pH.

Interaction with other drugs also metabolised via the cytochrome P450 system cannot be excluded.

4.6 Pregnancy and lactation

Use in pregnancy

The analysis of the results from three epidemiological studies has revealed no evidence of adverse events of omeprazole on pregnancy or on the health of the fetus/newborn child. LOSEC® can be used during pregnancy.

Use in lactation

Omeprazole is excreted in breast milk but is not likely to influence the child when therapeutic doses are used.

4.7 Effects on ability to drive and use machines

No effects are foreseen.

4.8 Undesirable effects

Losec is well tolerated and adverse reactions have generally been mild and reversible. The following have been reported as adverse events in clinical trials or reported from routine use but in many cases a relationship to treatment with omeprazole has not been established.

The following definitions of frequencies are used:

Common $\geq$ 1/100

Uncommon $\geq$ 1/1000 and $<$ 1/100

Rare $<$ 1/1000

Common	Central and peripheral nervous system:	Headache
	Gastrointestinal:	Diarrhoea, constipation, abdominal pain, nausea/vomiting and flatulence
Uncommon	Central and peripheral nervous system:	Dizziness, paraesthesia, light headedness, feeling faint, somnolence, insomnia and vertigo.
	Hepatic:	Increased liver enzymes.
	Skin:	Rash and/or pruritus. Urticaria.
	Other:	Malaise.
Rare	Central and peripheral nervous system:	Reversible mental confusion, agitation, aggression, depression and hallucinations, predominantly in severely ill patients.
	Endocrine:	Gynaecomastia.
	Gastrointestinal:	Dry mouth, stomatitis and gastrointestinal candidiasis.
	Haematological:	Leukopenia, thrombocytopenia, agranulocytosis and pancytopenia.
	Hepatic:	Encephalopathy in patients with pre-existing severe liver disease; hepatitis with or without jaundice, hepatic failure increased liver enzymes.
	Musculoskeletal:	Arthritic and myalgic symptoms and muscular weakness.
	Reproductive system and breast disorders:	Impotence
	Skin:	Photosensitivity, erythema multiforme, Stevens-Johnson syndrome, toxic epidermal necrolysis (TEN), alopecia.
	Other:	Hypersensitivity reactions e.g. angioedema, fever, broncho-spasm, interstitial nephritis and anaphylactic shock. Increased sweating, peripheral oedema, blurred vision, taste disturbance and hyponatraemia.

Isolated cases of irreversible visual impairment have been reported in critically ill patients who have received Losec Intravenous Injection, particularly at high doses, however no causal relationship has been established.

4.9 Overdose

Intravenous doses of up to 270mg on a single day and up to 650mg over a three-day period have been given in clinical trials without any dose related adverse effects.

5. PHARMACOLOGICAL PROPERTIES

5.1 Pharmacodynamic properties

Omeprazole reduces gastric acid secretion through a unique mechanism of action. It is a specific inhibitor of the gastric proton pump in the parietal cell. It is rapidly acting and produces reversible control of gastric acid secretion with once daily dosing.

Intravenous administration of omeprazole results in an immediate reduction of intragastric acidity and a mean decrease over 24 hours of approximately 90% in patients with duodenal ulcer disease. A single 40mg i.v. dose has similar effect on intragastric acidity over a 24 hour period as repeated oral dosing with 20mg once daily. A higher dose of 60mg i.v. twice daily has been used in a clinical study in patients with Zollinger - Ellison syndrome.

Site and mechanism of action

Omeprazole is a weak base and is concentrated and converted to the active form in the acid environment of the intracellular canaliculi within the parietal cell, where it inhibits the enzyme H^+, K^+,-ATPase - the proton pump. This effect on the final step of the gastric acid formation process is dose-dependent and provides for effective inhibition of both basal acid secretion and stimulated acid secretion irrespective of the stimulus.

All pharmacodynamic effects observed are explained by the effect of omeprazole on acid secretion. No tachyphylaxis has been observed during treatment with omeprazole.

5.2 Pharmacokinetic properties

Distribution

The apparent volume of distribution in healthy subjects is approximately 0.3 L/kg and a similar value is also seen in patients with renal insufficiency. In the elderly and in patients with hepatic insufficiency, the volume of distribution is slightly decreased. The plasma protein binding of omeprazole is about 95%.

Metabolism and excretion

The average half-life of the terminal phase of the plasma concentration-time curve following i.v. administration of omeprazole is approximately 40 minutes; the total plasma clearance is 0.3 to 0.6 L/min. There is no change in half-life during treatment.

Omeprazole is completely metabolised by the cytochrome P450 system, mainly in the liver. The major part of its metabolism is dependent on the polymorphically expressed, specific isoform CYP2C19 (S-mephenytoin hydroxylase), responsible for the formation of hydroxyomeprazole, the major metabolite in plasma.

No metabolite has been found to have any effect on gastric acid secretion. Almost 80% of an intravenously given dose is excreted as metabolites in the urine, and the remainder is found in the faeces, primarily originating from biliary secretion.

Elimination of omeprazole is unchanged in patients with reduced renal function. The elimination half-life is increased in patients with impaired liver function, but omeprazole has not shown any accumulation with once daily oral dosing.

5.3 Preclinical safety data

Animal Toxicology:

Gastric ECL-cell hyperplasia and carcinoids, have been observed in life-long studies in rats treated with omeprazole or subjected to partial fundectomy. These changes are the result of sustained hypergastrinaemia secondary to acid inhibition, and not from a direct effect of any individual drug.

6. PHARMACEUTICAL PARTICULARS

6.1 List of excipients

Sodium hydroxide and disodium edetate.

6.2 Incompatibilities

No other drugs should be mixed with reconstituted Losec Infusion solution.

6.3 Shelf life

Unopened pack: 2 years.

Reconstituted solution: See section 6.6

6.4 Special precautions for storage

Do not store above 25°C. Keep container in outer carton.

6.5 Nature and contents of container

Pack of 5, clear, Type I, glass 10ml vials each containing omeprazole sodium 42.6mg with grey bromobutyl stopper, blue polypropylene cap and golden aluminium frame.

6.6 Instructions for use and handling

The entire contents of each vial should be dissolved in approximately 5ml and then immediately diluted to 100 ml. Normal saline for infusion or 5 % dextrose for infusion should be used. No other solutions for i.v. infusion should be used.

Use on one patient during one treatment only.

DO NOT USE if any particles are present in the reconstituted solution.

Chemical and physical in use stability of the product has been shown for 12 hours when dissolved in normal saline and 3 hours in 5% dextrose when stored at 25°C.

From a microbiological point of view, the product should be used immediately (i.e. within 3 hours).

Any unused portion should be discarded.

Preparation:

1. With a syringe draw approximately 5 ml of infusion solution from the infusion bottle or bag.
2. Add the infusion solution to the vial with the freeze dried omeprazole, mix thoroughly making sure all omeprazole is dissolved.
3. Draw the omeprazole solution back into the syringe.
4. Transfer the solution in the infusion bottle or bag.
5. Repeat 1-4 to make sure all omeprazole is transferred from the vial into the infusion bottle or bag.

Alternative preparation for infusions in flexible containers:

1. Use a double ended transfer needle and attach to the injection membrane of the infusion bag. Connect the other needle-end from the vial with freeze-dried omeprazole.
2. Dissolve the omeprazole substance by pumping the infusion solution back and forward between the infusion bag and the vial.
3. Make sure all omeprazole is dissolved.

(see Diagrams below)

7. MARKETING AUTHORISATION HOLDER

AstraZeneca UK Ltd.,
600 Capability Green,
Luton, LU1 3LU, UK.

8. MARKETING AUTHORISATION NUMBER(S)

PL 17901/0136

9. DATE OF FIRST AUTHORISATION/RENEWAL OF THE AUTHORISATION

14th May 2002

10. DATE OF REVISION OF THE TEXT

29th October 2004

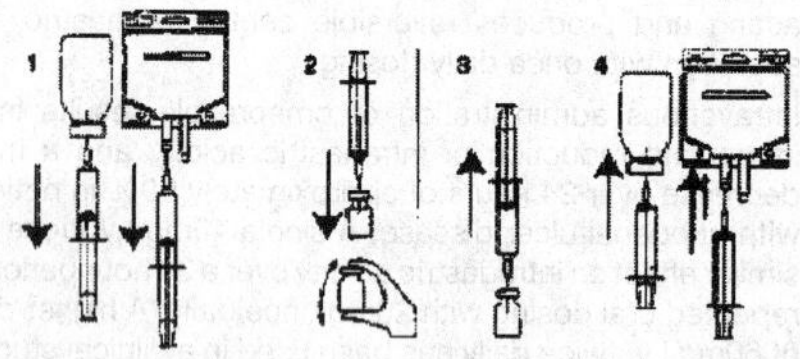

Losec IV Injection Solvent

(AstraZeneca UK Limited)

1. NAME OF THE MEDICINAL PRODUCT

Solvent for Losec® i.v. Injection 40 mg.

2. QUALITATIVE AND QUANTITATIVE COMPOSITION

Each ampoule contains 10ml of solvent for injection

3. PHARMACEUTICAL FORM

Solvent for solution for injection

4. CLINICAL PARTICULARS

4.1 Therapeutic indications

To be used as a Solvent for i.v. injection with 1 vial of powder for injection which contains Omeprazole sodium Ph. Eur., equivalent to Omeprazole 40mg

4.2 Posology and method of administration

Dosage and Administration

The intravenous solution is obtained by dissolving the lyophilised omeprazole in the solvent provided. No other solvent should be used and the solution must be given by intravenous injection and not added to any other solutions for injection. The injection should be given slowly over a period of 5 minutes. The solution should be used within 4 hours of preparation.

Use in the Elderly:

Dosage adjustment is not necessary.

Use in Children:

There is limited experience of use in children.

4.3 Contraindications

Known hypersensitivity macrogol (polyethylene glycol) and citric acid monohydrate.

4.4 Special warnings and special precautions for use

None stated

4.5 Interaction with other medicinal products and other forms of Interaction

None stated

4.6 Pregnancy and lactation

None stated

4.7 Effects on ability to drive and use machines

None stated

4.8 Undesirable effects

None stated

4.9 Overdose

None stated

5. PHARMACOLOGICAL PROPERTIES

5.1 Pharmacodynamic properties

None stated

5.2 Pharmacokinetic properties

Macrogols entering the systemic circulation are predominantly excreted unchanged in the urine, low molecular-weight macrogols may be partly metabolised.

5.3 Preclinical safety data

Citric acid and macrogols are commonly used in pharmaceutical preparations, no addition information is necessary.

6. PHARMACEUTICAL PARTICULARS

6.1 List of excipients

Macrogol 400, Citric acid monohydrate and water for injections.

6.2 Incompatibilities

None known.

6.3 Shelf life

Unopened pack: 2 years.

Reconstituted solution: 4 hours.

6.4 Special precautions for storage

Do not store above 25°C. Keep container in outer carton.

6.5 Nature and contents of container

A clear, Type I (OPC) glass ampoule containing solvent for intravenous administration, packed in a plastic tray with a glass vial in a hard cardboard box.

6.6 Instructions for use and handling

The solvent in the ampoule is used to reconstitute lyophilised powder to provide a solution for i.v. injection.

Use on one patient during one treatment only.

DO NOT USE if any particles are present in the reconstituted solution.

From a microbiological point of view, once opened and reconstituted the product may be stored for a maximum of 4 hours at 25°C. Other in-use storage times and conditions are the responsibility of the user.

Any unused portion should be discarded.

Preparation:

NOTE: Stages 1 to 5 should be done in immediate sequence.

1. With a syringe draw 10ml of solvent from the ampoule.
2. Add approximately 5ml of the solvent to the vial with the lyophilised powder.
3. Withdraw as much air as possible from the vial back into the syringe in order to reduce positive pressure. This will make it easier to add the remaining solvent.
4. Add the remaining solvent into the vial, make sure that the syringe is empty.
5. Rotate and shake the vial to ensure all the lyophilised powder has been dissolved.

Administrative Data

7. MARKETING AUTHORISATION HOLDER

AstraZeneca UK Ltd,

600 Capability Green,

Luton, LU1 3LU, UK.

8. MARKETING AUTHORISATION NUMBER(S)

PL 17901/0167

9. DATE OF FIRST AUTHORISATION/RENEWAL OF THE AUTHORISATION

18th June 2002

10. DATE OF REVISION OF THE TEXT

18th June 2002

(see Figure 1 below)

Figure 1

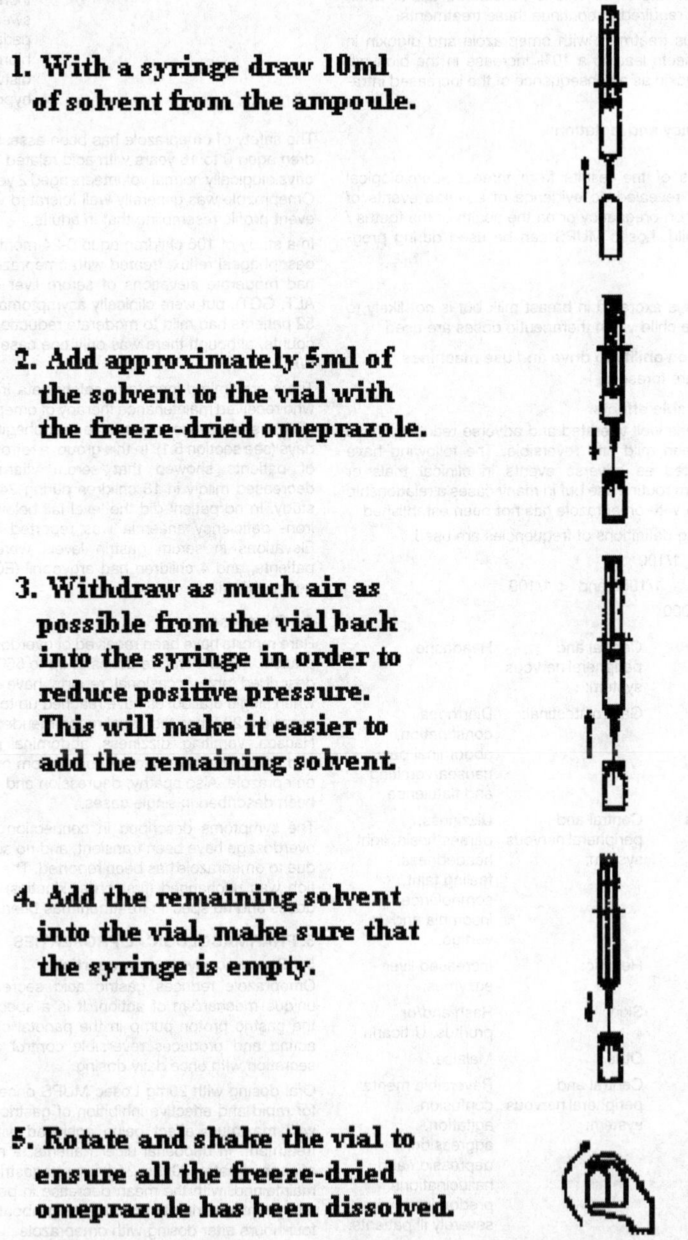
1. With a syringe draw 10ml of solvent from the ampoule.
2. Add approximately 5ml of the solvent to the vial with the freeze-dried omeprazole.
3. Withdraw as much air as possible from the vial back into the syringe in order to reduce positive pressure. This will make it easier to add the remaining solvent.
4. Add the remaining solvent into the vial, make sure that the syringe is empty.
5. Rotate and shake the vial to ensure all the freeze-dried omeprazole has been dissolved.

Losec MUPS Tablets 10mg, 20mg & 40mg

(AstraZeneca UK Limited)

1. NAME OF THE MEDICINAL PRODUCT

Losec MUPS® Tablets 10 mg.

Losec MUPS® Tablets 20 mg.

Losec MUPS® Tablets 40 mg.

2. QUALITATIVE AND QUANTITATIVE COMPOSITION

Each tablet contains either:

10.3mg omeprazole magnesium equivalent to 10mg omeprazole.

20.6mg omeprazole magnesium equivalent to 20mg omeprazole.

41.3mg omeprazole magnesium equivalent to 40mg omeprazole.

(The list of excipients is detailed in section 6.1).

3. PHARMACEUTICAL FORM

LOSEC MUPS® tablets 10mg: Light-pink, oblong, biconvex, film-coated tablets engraved with on one side and 10mg on the other side. Each tablet contains omeprazole magnesium 10.3mg as enteric coated pellets.

LOSEC MUPS® tablets 20mg: Pink, oblong, biconvex, film-coated tablets engraved with on one side and 20mg on the other side. Each tablet contains omeprazole magnesium 20.6mg as enteric coated pellets.

LOSEC MUPS® tablets 40mg: A red-brown, oblong, biconvex, film-coated tablet with a score and engraved with on one side and 40mg on the other side. Each tablet contains omeprazole magnesium 41.3mg as enteric coated pellets.

4. CLINICAL PARTICULARS

4.1 Therapeutic indications

Treatment of oesophageal reflux disease. In reflux oesophagitis the majority of patients are healed after 4 weeks. Symptom relief is rapid.

Treatment of duodenal and benign gastric ulcers including those complicating NSAID therapy.

Helicobacter pylori eradication: Omeprazole should be used in combination with antibiotics for eradication of *Helicobacter pylori (Hp)* in peptic ulcer disease.

Relief of associated dyspeptic symptoms.

Prophylaxis of acid aspiration.

Zollinger-Ellison syndrome.

10 mg and 20 mg tablets only:

Relief of reflux-like symptoms (e.g. heartburn) and/or ulcer-like symptoms (e.g. epigastric pain) associated with acid-related dyspepsia.

Treatment and prophylaxis of NSAID-associated benign gastric ulcers, duodenal ulcers and gastroduodenal erosions in patients with a previous history of gastroduodenal lesions who require continued NSAID treatment.

4.2 Posology and method of administration

Adults

Oesophageal reflux disease includingreflux oesophagitis: The usual dosage is 20mg Losec MUPS once daily. The majority of patients are healed after 4 weeks. For those patients not fully healed after the initial course, healing usually occurs during a further 4-8 weeks treatment. Losec MUPS can also been used at a dose of 40mg once daily in patients with reflux oesophagitis refractory to other therapy. Healing usually occurs within 8 weeks. Patients can be continued at a dosage of 20mg once daily.

Acid reflux disease: For long-term management, Losec MUPS 10mg once daily is recommended, increasing to 20mg if symptoms return.

Duodenal and benign gastric ulcers: The usual dose is 20mg Losec MUPS once daily. The majority of patients with duodenal ulcer are healed after 4 weeks. The majority of patients with benign gastric ulcer are healed after 8 weeks. In severe or recurrent cases the dose may be increased to 40mg Losec MUPS daily. Long-term therapy for patients with a history of recurrent duodenal ulcer is recommended at a dosage of 20mg Losec MUPS once daily.

For prevention of relapse in patients with duodenal ulcer the recommended dose is Losec MUPS 10mg, once daily, increasing to 20mg, once daily if symptoms return.

The following groups are at risk from recurrent ulcer relapse; those with Helicobacter pylori infection, younger patients (<60 years), those whose symptoms persist for more than one year and smokers. These patients will require initial long-term therapy with Losec MUPS 20mg once daily, reducing to 10mg once daily, if necessary.

Helicobacter pylori (Hp) eradication regimens in peptic ulcer disease: Losec MUPS is recommended at a dose of 40mg once daily or 20mg twice daily in association with antimicrobial agents as detailed below:

Triple therapy regimens in duodenal ulcer disease: Losec MUPS and the following antimicrobial combinations;

Amoxicillin 500mg and metronidazole 400mg both three times a day for one week.

or

Clarithromycin 250mg and metronidazole 400mg (or tinidazole 500mg) both twice a day for one week.

or

Amoxicillin 1g and clarithromycin 500mg both twice a day for one week.

Dual therapy regimens in duodenal ulcer disease:

Losec MUPS and amoxicillin 750mg to 1g twice daily for two weeks. Alternatively Losec MUPS and clarithromycin 500mg three times a day for two weeks.

Dual therapy regimens in gastric ulcer disease:

Losec MUPS and amoxicillin 750mg to 1g twice daily for two weeks

In each regimen if symptoms return and the patient is *Hp* positive, therapy may be repeated or one of the alternative regimens can be used; if the patient is *Hp* negative then see dosage instructions for acid reflux disease.

To ensure healing in patients with active peptic ulcer disease, see further dosage recommendations for duodenal and benign gastric ulcer.

Prophylaxis of acid aspiration: For patients considered to be at risk of aspiration of the gastric contents during general anaesthesia, the recommended dosage is Losec MUPS 40mg on the evening before surgery followed by Losec MUPS 40mg 2 - 6 hours prior to surgery.

Zollinger-Ellison syndrome: The recommended initial dosage is 60mg Losec MUPS once daily. The dosage should be adjusted individually and treatment continued as long as clinically indicated. More than 90% of patients with severe disease and inadequate response to other therapies have been effectively controlled on doses of 20-120mg daily. With doses above 80mg daily, the dose should be divided and given twice daily.

10 mg and 20 mg MUPS tablets only:

Acid-related dyspepsia: The usual dosage is Losec MUPS 10mg or 20mg once daily for 2-4 weeks depending on the severity and persistence of symptoms. Patients who do not respond after 4 weeks or who relapse shortly afterwards, should be investigated.

For the treatment of NSAID-associated gastric ulcers, duodenal ulcers or gastroduodenal erosions: The recommended dosage of Losec MUPS is 20mg once daily. Symptom resolution is rapid and in most patients healing occurs within 4 weeks. For those patients who may not be fully healed after the initial course, healing usually occurs during a further 4 weeks treatment.

For the prophylaxis of NSAID-associated gastric ulcers, duodenal ulcers, gastroduodenal erosions and dyspeptic symptoms in patients with a previous history of gastroduodenal lesions who require continued NSAID treatment: The recommended dosage of Losec MUPS is 20mg once daily.

Elderly: Dose adjustment is not required in the elderly.

Children: Experience of the use of Losec MUPS in children is limited. In children 1 year and above with severe ulcerating reflux oesophagitis, Losec MUPS is recommended for healing and symptom relief at the following doses:

Weight	Dosage
10-20kg	Losec MUPS 10mg once daily
>20kg	Losec MUPS 20mg once daily

If needed the dose may be increased to 20mg and 40mg respectively for 4 -12 weeks.

Data suggest that approximately 65% of children will experience pain relief with this dose regimen. Treatment should be initiated by a paediatrician.

Impaired renal function: Dose adjustment is not required in patients with impaired renal function.

Impaired hepatic function: As bioavailability and half-life can increase in patients with impaired hepatic function, the dose requires adjustment with a maximum daily dose of 20mg.

For patients (including children aged 1 year and above who can drink or swallow semi-solid food) who are unable to swallow Losec MUPS tablets:

The tablets may be dispersed in 10 ml of non-carbonated water and then suspended in a small amount of any fruit juice with a pH less than 5 e.g. apple, orange, pineapple or in applesauce or yoghurt after gentle mixing. Do not use milk or carbonated water. The dispersion should be taken immediately or within 30 minutes. Stir the dispersion just before drinking and rinse it down with half a glass of water. There is no evidendence to support the use of sodium bicarbonate buffer as a delivery form. It is important that the tablets should not be crushed or chewed.

4.3 Contraindications

Known hypersensitivity to omeprazole.

When gastric ulcer is suspected, the possibility of malignancy should be excluded before treatment with Losec MUPS is instituted, as treatment may alleviate symptoms and delay diagnosis.

4.4 Special warnings and special precautions for use

When treatment with Losec MUPS Tablets is instituted, patients on previous Losec capsules therapy should be monitored for any reports of 'flare up' of disease symptoms.

Decreased gastric acidity due to any means including proton-pump inhibitors, increases gastric counts of bacteria normally present in the gastrointestinal tract. Treatment with acid-reducing drugs may lead to slightly increased risk of gastrointestinal infections such as *Salmonella* or *Campylobacter*.

For severely ill children, who require long-term treatment with Losec, and may have borderline levels or body stores of B_{12}, it may be advisable to monitor serum B_{12} levels during long-term treatment (see section 4.8).

4.5 Interaction with other medicinal products and other forms of Interaction

Due to the decreased intragastric acidity, the absorption of ketoconazole or itraconazole may be reduced during omeprazole treatment as it is during treatment with other acid secretion inhibitors.

As omeprazole is metabolised in the liver through cytochrome P450 it can prolong the elimination of diazepam, phenytoin and warfarin. Monitoring of patients receiving warfarin or phenytoin is recommended and a reduction of warfarin or phenytoin dose may be necessary. However concomitant treatment with omeprazole 20mg daily did not change the blood concentration of phenytoin in patients on continuous treatment with phenytoin. Similarly concomitant treatment with omeprazole 20mg daily did not change coagulation time in patients on continuous treatment with warfarin.

Plasma concentrations of omeprazole and clarithromycin are increased during concomitant administration. This is considered to be a useful interaction during *H. pylori* eradication. There is no interaction with metronidazole or amoxicillin. These antimicrobials are used together with omeprazole for eradication of Helicobacter *pylori*.

There is no evidence of an interaction with phenacetin, theophylline, caffeine, propranolol, metoprolol, cyclosporin, lidocaine, quinidine, estradiol or antacids. The absorption of omeprazole is not affected by alcohol or food.

There is no evidence of an interaction with piroxicam, diclofenac or naproxen. This is considered useful when patients are required to continue these treatments.

Simultaneous treatment with omeprazole and digoxin in healthy subjects lead to a 10% increase in the bioavailability of digoxin as a consequence of the increased intragastric pH.

4.6 Pregnancy and lactation

Pregnancy

The analysis of the results from three epidemiological studies has revealed no evidence of adverse events of omeprazole on pregnancy or on the health of the foetus / newborn child. Losec MUPS can be used during pregnancy.

Lactation

Omeprazole is excreted in breast milk but is not likely to influence the child when therapeutic doses are used.

4.7 Effects on ability to drive and use machines

No effects are foreseen.

4.8 Undesirable effects

Omeprazole is well tolerated and adverse reactions have generally been mild and reversible. The following have been reported as adverse events in clinical trials or reported from routine use but in many cases a relationship to treatment with omeprazole has not been established.

The following definitions of frequencies are used:

Common ⩾ 1/100

Uncommon ⩾ 1/1000 and < 1/100

Rare < 1/1000

Common	Central and peripheral nervous system:	Headache
	Gastrointestinal:	Diarrhoea, constipation, abdominal pain, nausea/vomiting and flatulence
Uncommon	Central and peripheral nervous system:	Dizziness, paraesthesia, light headedness, feeling faint, somnolence, insomnia and vertigo.
	Hepatic:	Increased liver enzymes.
	Skin:	Rash and/or pruritus. Urticaria.
	Other:	Malaise.
Rare	Central and peripheral nervous system:	Reversible mental confusion, agitation, aggression, depression and hallucinations, predominantly in severely ill patients.
	Endocrine:	Gynaecomastia.
	Gastrointestinal:	Dry mouth, stomatitis and gastrointestinal candidiasis.
	Haematological:	Leukopenia, thrombocytopenia, agranulocytosis and pancytopenia.
	Hepatic	Encephalopathy in patients with pre-existing severe liver disease; hepatitis with or without jaundice, hepatic failure.
	Musculoskeletal	Arthritic and myalgic symptoms and muscular weakness.
	Reproductive system and breast disorders	Impotence
	Skin	Photosensitivity, bullous eruption erythema multiforme, Stevens-Johnson syndrome, toxic epidermal necrolysis (TEN), alopecia.
	Other	Hypersensitivity reactions e.g. angioedema, fever, broncho-spasm, interstitial nephritis and anaphylactic shock [3]. Increased sweating, peripheral oedema, blurred vision, taste disturbance and hyponatraemia.

The safety of omeprazole has been assessed in 310 children aged 0 to 16 years with acid related disease and 62 physiologically normal volunteers aged 2 years to 16 years. Omeprazole was generally well tolerated with an adverse event profile resembling that in adults.

In a study of 106 children aged 0-24 months with gastro-oesophageal reflux, treated with omeprazole, 11 patients had moderate elevations of serum liver enzymes (AST, ALT, GGT), but were clinically asymptomatic. In addition, 52 patients had mild to moderate reductions in neutrophil counts, although there was only one case of reduction in WBC.

There are limited long term safety data from 46 children who received maintenance therapy of omeprazole during a clinical study for severe erosive oesophagitis for up to 749 days (see section 5.1). In this group, a retrospective review of patients showed that serum vitamin B12 levels decreased mildly in 18 children during 24 months of the study. In no patient did the level fall below normal limits. Iron- deficiency anaemia was reported in 12 patients. Elevations in serum gastrin levels were noted in 20 patients, and 4 children had argyophil (ECL) hyperplasia during this study.

4.9 Overdose

Rare reports have been received of overdosage with omeprazole. In the literature doses of up to 560 mg have been described and occasional reports have been received when single oral doses have reached up to 2400 mg omeprazole (120 times the usual recommended clinical dose). Nausea, vomiting, dizziness, abdominal pain, diarrhoea and headache have been reported from overdosage with omeprazole. Also apathy, depression and confusion have been described in single cases.

The symptoms described in connection to omeprazole overdosage have been transient, and no serious outcome due to omeprazole has been reported. The rate of elimination was unchanged (first order kinetics) with increased doses and no specific treatment has been needed.

5. PHARMACOLOGICAL PROPERTIES

5.1 Pharmacodynamic properties

Omeprazole reduces gastric acid secretion through a unique mechanism of action. It is a specific inhibitor of the gastric proton pump in the parietal cell. It is rapidly acting and produces reversible control of gastric acid secretion with once daily dosing.

Oral dosing with 20mg Losec MUPS once daily provides for rapid and effective inhibition of gastric acid secretion with maximum effect being achieved within 4 days of treatment. In duodenal ulcer patients, a mean decrease of approximately 80% in 24-hour intragastric acidity is then maintained, with the mean decrease in peak acid output after pentagastrin stimulation being about 70%, twenty-four hours after dosing with omeprazole.

Clinical data for omeprazole in the prophylaxis of NSAID induced gastroduodenal lesions are derived from clinical studies of up to 6 months duration.

Helicobacter pylori(*Hp*) is associated with acid peptic disease including duodenal ulcer (DU) and gastric ulcer (GU) in which about 95% and 80% of patients respectively are infected with this bacterium. *Hp* is implicated as a major contributing factor in the development of gastritis and ulcers in such patients. Recent evidence also suggests a causative link between *Hp* and gastric carcinoma.

Omeprazole has been shown to have a bactericidal effect on *Hp* in vitro.

Eradication of *Hp* with omeprazole and antimicrobials is associated with rapid symptom relief, high rates of healing of any mucosal lesions, and long-term remission of peptic ulcer disease thus reducing complications such as gastrointestinal bleeding as well as the need for prolonged antisecretory treatment.

In clinical data in patients with acute peptic ulcer, omeprazole *Hp* eradication therapy improved patients' quality of life.

During long-term treatment an increased frequency of gastric glandular cysts have been reported. These changes are a physiological consequence of pronounced inhibition of acid secretion. The cysts are benign and appear to be reversible. No other treatment related mucosal changes have been observed in patients treated continuously with omeprazole for periods up to 5 years.

Children

Treatment of non-erosive Gastroesophageal Reflux Disease

In a randomised study, with no comparator, the efficacy of 0.5mg/kg, 1.0mg/kg and 1.5mg/kg of omeprazole was compared in 110 children aged 0-24 months with endoscopically and clinically diagnosed GORD. Due to the lack of placebo comparison no efficacy could be confirmed.

Severe Erosive Oesophagitis

In an uncontrolled, open-label dose-titration study, healing of severe erosive oesophagitis in children aged 1-16 years, approximately 65% of patients were healed with doses of 0.7-1.4mg/kg.

Maintenance of Healing of Erosive Oesophagitis

In an uncontrolled, open-label study of omeprazole for the maintenance of healing of severe erosive oesophagitis in 46 children aged 1 to 16 yrs, 59% of patients relapsed on half their healing dose and they had to return to their healing dose.

Helicobacter pylori eradication

In a double-blind controlled parallel group study of 73 children aged 3 months to 15 years (mean age 10.5 years) with dyspeptic symptoms and *H. pylori* associated gastritis who were treated with triple therapy alone or in combination with omeprazole, the mean eradication rate was 74.2% in the omeprazole group compared with 9.4% in the placebo group. However, there was no evidence of clinical benefit demonstrated regarding dyspeptic symptoms.

Site and mechanism of action

Omeprazole is a weak base and is concentrated and converted to the active form in the acid environment of the intracellular canaliculi within the parietal cell, where it inhibits the enzyme H^+, K^+-ATPase - the proton pump. This effect on the final step of the gastric acid formation process is dose-dependent and provides for effective inhibition of both basal acid secretion and stimulated acid secretion irrespective of the stimulus.

All pharmacodynamic effects observed are explained by the effect of omeprazole on acid secretion.

5.2 Pharmacokinetic properties

Absorption and distribution

Omeprazole and omeprazole magnesium are acid labile and are administered orally as enteric-coated granules in capsules or tablets. Bioequivalence between Losec® Capsules and Losec MUPS® Tablets based on omeprazole plasma concentration-time curve (AUC) has been demonstrated. Absorption of omeprazole takes place in the small intestine and is usually completed within 3-6 hours. The systemic bioavailability of omeprazole from a single oral dose of omeprazole is approximately 35%. After repeated once-daily administration, the bioavailability increases to about 60%. Concomitant intake of food has no influence on the bioavailability. The plasma protein binding of omeprazole is about 95%.

Metabolism and elimination

The average half-life of the terminal phase of the plasma concentration-time curve is approximately 40 minutes. There is no change in half-life during treatment. The inhibition of acid secretion is related to the area under the plasma concentration-time curve (AUC) but not to the actual plasma concentration at a given time.

Omeprazole is entirely metabolised, mainly in the liver. Identified metabolites in plasma are the sulphone, the sulphide and hydroxy-omeprazole, these metabolites have no significant effect on acid secretion. About 80% of the metabolites are excreted in the urine and the rest in the faeces. The two main urinary metabolites are hydroxy-omeprazole and the corresponding carboxylic acid.

The systemic bioavailability of omeprazole is not significantly altered in patients with reduced renal function. The area under the plasma concentration-time curve is increased in patients with impaired liver function, but no tendency to accumulation of omeprazole has been found.

Children

Limited data from children aged 0-16 years suggest that the pharmacokinetics within the recommended doses are similar to those reported in adults.

5.3 Preclinical safety data

Animal Toxicology:

Gastric ECL-cell hyperplasia and carcinoids, have been observed in life-long studies in rats treated with omeprazole or subjected to partial fundectomy.

These changes are the result of sustained hypergastrinaemia secondary to acid inhibition, and not from a direct effect of any individual drug.

6. PHARMACEUTICAL PARTICULARS

6.1 List of excipients

Microcrystalline cellulose, glyceryl monostearate, hydroxypropylcellulose, hydroxypropylmethylcellulose, magnesium stearate, methylacrylic acid co-polymer C, sugar spheres, paraffin, polyethylene glycol (Macrogol), polysorbate, polyvinylpyrrolidone crosslinked (Crospovidone), sodium stearyl fumarate, sodium hydroxide*, talc, triethyl citrate, iron oxide, titanium dioxide.

* May be added as a pH adjuster

6.2 Incompatibilities

None known.

6.3 Shelf life

3 years

6.4 Special precautions for storage

Do not store above 25°C.

Keep the container tightly closed (bottles)

or

Store in the original container (blisters)

6.5 Nature and contents of container

Losec MUPS Tablets are provided in high density polyethylene (HDPE) bottles with tamper-proof, child resistant, polypropylene (PP) lids containing integral desiccant. Packs of 7, 14, 28, 56, 230 and 560 tablets.

or

Losec MUPS Tablets are provided in press-through Aluminium-Polyamide-PVC/Aluminium foil calendarised blister packs. Packs of 7, 14, 28, 56 and 560 tablets.

Not all pack sizes may be marketed.

6.6 Instructions for use and handling

HDPE Bottles:

The cap should be replaced firmly after use.

To be dispensed in original containers.

7. MARKETING AUTHORISATION HOLDER

AstraZeneca UK Ltd.,

600 Capability Green,

Luton, LU1 3LU, UK

8. MARKETING AUTHORISATION NUMBER(S)

PL 17901/0137

PL 17901/0138

PL 17901/0139

9. DATE OF FIRST AUTHORISATION/RENEWAL OF THE AUTHORISATION

14th May 2002

10. DATE OF REVISION OF THE TEXT

22nd March 2005

Lotriderm Cream

(Pliva Pharma Ltd)

1. NAME OF THE MEDICINAL PRODUCT

LOTRIDERM Cream

2. QUALITATIVE AND QUANTITATIVE COMPOSITION

Betamethasone Dipropionate Ph.Eur 0.064% w/w

Clotrimazole Ph.Eur 1.0% w/w

3. PHARMACEUTICAL FORM

Cream

4. CLINICAL PARTICULARS

4.1 Therapeutic indications

Short-term topical treatment of tinea infections due to Trichophyton rubrum; T.mentagrophytes; Epidermophyton floccusum and Microsporum canis; candidiasis due to Candida albicans.

4.2 Posology and method of administration

Adults and children over the age of 12 years: Topical administration twice daily for two weeks (tinea cruris, tinea corporis and candidiasis) or for four weeks (tinea pedis).

Lotriderm cream is not recommended for children under the age of twelve years.

4.3 Contraindications

Lotriderm is contraindicated in those patients with a history of sensitivity to any of its components or to other corticosteroids or imidazoles.

If irritation or sensitisation develops with the use of Lotriderm cream, treatment should be discontinued and appropriate therapy instituted.

Lotriderm is contraindicated in facial rosacea, acne vulgaris, perioral dermatitis, napkin eruptions and bacterial or viral infections.

4.4 Special warnings and special precautions for use

Local and systemic toxicity is common especially following long continued use on large areas of damaged skin and in flexures. If used in children or on the face, courses should be limited to 5 days. Long term continuous therapy should be avoided in all children irrespective of age. Lotriderm cream should not be used with adhesive dressing.

The safety and effectiveness of Lotriderm cream has not been established in children below the age of 12.

LOTRIDERM CREAM SHOULD NOT BE USED WITH OCCLUSIVE DRESSING.

Topical corticosteroids may be hazardous in psoriasis for a number of reasons including rebound relapses following the development of tolerance, risk of generalised pustular psoriasis and local and systemic toxicity due to impaired barrier function of the skin.

Lotriderm Cream is not intended for ophthalmic use.

4.5 Interaction with other medicinal products and other forms of Interaction

There are no known interactions.

4.6 Pregnancy and lactation

There is inadequate evidence of safety in pregnancy. Clotrimazole has shown no teratogenic effect in animals but is foetotoxic at high oral doses.

Topical administration of corticosteroids to pregnant animals can cause abnormalities of foetal development including cleft palate and intra-uterine growth retardation. There may therefore be a very small risk of such effects in human foetus. Hence Lotriderm Cream should only be used in pregnancy if the benefit justifies the potential risk to the foetus and such use should not be extensive i.e. in large amounts or for long periods.

It is not known whether the components of Lotriderm are excreted in human milk and therefore caution should be exercised when treating nursing mothers.

4.7 Effects on ability to drive and use machines

None known.

4.8 Undesirable effects

Adverse reactions reported for Lotriderm include: burning and stinging, maculopapular rash, oedema and secondary infection.

Reported reactions to clotrimazole include erythema, stinging, blistering, peeling, oedema, pruritis, urticaria and general irritation of the skin.

Reactions to betamethasone dipropionate include: burning, itching, irritation, dryness, folliculitis, hypertrichosis, acneiform eruptions, hyperpigmentation, perioral dermatitis, allergic contact dermatitis, maceration of the skin, secondary infection, skin atrophy, striae and miliaria.

4.9 Overdose

Acute overdosage with topical application of Lotriderm cream is unlikely and would not be expected to lead to a life-threatening situation; however topically applied corticosteroids can be absorbed in sufficient amounts to produce systemic effects.

Toxic effects are unlikely to occur following accidental ingestion of Lotriderm cream. Signs of toxicology appearing after such accidental ingestion should be treated symptomatically.

5. PHARMACOLOGICAL PROPERTIES

5.1 Pharmacodynamic properties

Lotriderm Cream contains the dipropionate ester of betamethasone, a glucocorticoid exhibiting the general properties of corticosteroids, and clotrimazole which is an imidazole antifungal agent.

Topical corticosteroids are effective in the treatment of a range of dermatoses because of their anti-inflammatory anti-pruritic and vasoconstrictive actions.

Clotrimazole is a broad-spectrum antifungal agent with activity against Trichomones, Staphylococci and Bacteroides.

5.2 Pharmacokinetic properties

Lotriderm is intended for treatment of skin conditions and is applied topically. Thus there are minimal pharmacokinetic aspects related to bioavailability at the site of action.

Clotrimazole penetrates the epidermis after topical administration but there is little, if any, systemic absorption.

The extent of percutaneous absorption of topical corticosteroids is determined by many factors including vehicle, integrity of skin and use of occlusion.

Systemically absorbed topical corticosteroids are bound to plasma proteins metabolised in the liver and excreted by the kidneys. Some corticosteroids and their metabolites are also excreted in the bile.

5.3 Preclinical safety data
There are no pre-clinical data of relevance to the prescriber which are additional to that already included in other sections of this SmPC.

6. PHARMACEUTICAL PARTICULARS

6.1 List of excipients
Liquid paraffin, white soft paraffin, cetosteryl alcohol, Macrogol cetostearyl ether, benzyl alcohol, sodium dihydrogen phosphate dihydrate, phosphoric acid concentrated, sodium hydroxide, propylene glycol and purified water.

6.2 Incompatibilities
None known.

6.3 Shelf life
48 months.

6.4 Special precautions for storage
Do not store above 25° C.

6.5 Nature and contents of container
The product will be marketed in standard epoxy-lined aluminium tubes with low density polyethylene caps. Tubes will contain 2g or 5g (Professional Sample Packs), 15g, 30g or 50g,

6.6 Instructions for use and handling
There are no special instructions for use.

Administrative Data

7. MARKETING AUTHORISATION HOLDER
Schering-Plough Ltd
Shire Park
Welwyn Garden City
Hertfordshire AL7 1TW
UK

8. MARKETING AUTHORISATION NUMBER(S)
PL 0201/0081

9. DATE OF FIRST AUTHORISATION/RENEWAL OF THE AUTHORISATION
October 1992 / October 1997

10. DATE OF REVISION OF THE TEXT
June 2003

Distributed in the UK by PLIVA Pharma Ltd., Vision House, Bedford Road, Petersfield, Hampshire, GU32 3QB

Loxapac

(Wyeth Pharmaceuticals)

1. NAME OF THE MEDICINAL PRODUCT
Loxapac

LOXAPAC® CAPSULES 10mg LOXAPAC® CAPSULES 25mg LOXAPAC® CAPSULES 50mg

2. QUALITATIVE AND QUANTITATIVE COMPOSITION

10 mg Capsules:
Two piece, hard shell, opaque capsules with a yellow body and a green cap, printed with script "Lederle" over "L2" on one half and "10mg" on the other in grey ink, containing 10mg loxapine as loxapine succinate. The capsules have a locking feature.

25 mg Capsules:
Two piece, hard shell, opaque capsules with a light green body and a dark green cap, printed with script "Lederle" over "L3" on one half and "25mg" on the other in grey ink, containing 25mg loxapine as loxapine succinate. The capsules have a locking feature.

50 mg Capsules:
Two piece, hard shell, opaque capsules with a blue body and a dark green cap, printed with script "Lederle" over "L4" on one half and "50mg" on the other in grey ink, containing 50mg loxapine as loxapine succinate. The capsules have a locking feature.

3. PHARMACEUTICAL FORM
Capsules

4. CLINICAL PARTICULARS

4.1 Therapeutic indications
The treatment of acute and chronic psychotic states.

4.2 Posology and method of administration

Route of administration:
oral

Posology:

Adults:
Initially 20-50mg/day in two doses. Dosage is then increased over 7-10 days to the range 60-100mg/day in 2-4 doses, until there is effective control of psychotic symptoms.

Maximum daily dose:
250mg.

Maintenance doses should be adjusted to the needs of the patient, usually in the range of 20-100mg/day in divided doses.

Children:
Not recommended for use in children.

4.3 Contraindications
Use in comatose or semi-comatose patients or in severe drug-induced depressed states (alcohol, barbiturates, narcotics).

Use in individuals with known hypersensitivity to the drug.

4.4 Special warnings and special precautions for use

Precautions:
LOXAPAC may impair mental and/or physical abilities, especially during the first few days of therapy. Therefore, ambulatory patients should be warned about activities requiring alertness, (e.g. operating machinery or vehicles) and about concomitant use of alcohol and other CNS depressants.

LOXAPAC should be used with extreme caution in patients with a history of convulsive disorders, since it lowers the convulsive threshold. Seizures have been reported in epileptic patients receiving LOXAPAC at antipsychotic dose levels, and may occur even with maintenance of routine anticonvulsant drug therapy.

LOXAPAC has an antiemetic effect in animals. Since this effect may also occur in man, LOXAPAC may mask signs of overdosage of toxic drugs and may obscure conditions such as intestinal obstruction and brain tumour.

LOXAPAC should be used with caution in patients with cardiovascular disease. Increased pulse rates have been reported in the majority of patients receiving antipsychotic doses; transient hypotension has been reported. In the presence of severe hypotension requiring vasopressor therapy, the preferred drugs may be noradrenaline or angiotensin. Usual doses of adrenaline may be ineffective because of inhibition of its vasopressor effect by LOXAPAC.

The possibility of ocular toxicity from LOXAPAC cannot be excluded at this time. Therefore, careful observation should be made for pigmentary retinopathy and lenticular pigmentation, since these have been observed in some patients receiving certain other antipsychotic drugs for prolonged periods.

Because of possible anticholinergic action, the drug should be used cautiously in patients with glaucoma or a tendency to urinary retention, particularly with concomitant administration of anticholinergic type anti-Parkinson medication.

4.5 Interaction with other medicinal products and other forms of Interaction
LOXAPAC may increase the CNS depression produced by drugs such as alcohol, hypnotics, sedatives, antihistamines, strong analgesics or other anti-psychotics. There have been reports of respiratory depression with concurrent use of loxapine and lorazepam.

The anticholinergic effect of loxapine may be enhanced by other anticholinergic drugs. The possibility of occurrence of heat stroke, severe constipation, paralytic ileus and atropine-like psychoses should be noted. Neuroleptics may impair the anti-parkinsonian effect of l-dopa, while therapeutic efficacy of the neuroleptic may be reduced. Concurrent use of neuroleptics and tricyclic antidepressants may contribute to increased incidence of tardive dyskinesia.

Loxapine may reduce serum levels of phenytoin.

There have been rare reports of patients developing neurotoxicity when treated concurrently with lithium; lithium serum levels were within normal limits and the mechanism of action is unknown.

4.6 Pregnancy and lactation
LOXAPAC should not be used during pregnancy or lactation unless considered essential by the physician. Studies in animals do not indicate a teratogenic effect but there is no information on uses during human pregnancy. LOXAPAC crosses the placenta and is excreted in breast milk.

4.7 Effects on ability to drive and use machines
LOXAPAC may impair mental and/or physical abilities, especially during the first few days of therapy. Therefore, patients should be warned about the possible hazard of driving or operating machinery.

4.8 Undesirable effects

CNS effects:
Manifestations of adverse effects on the central nervous system (other than extrapyramidal effects; see below) have been seen infrequently. Drowsiness (usually mild) may occur at the beginning of therapy or when dosage is increased, and usually subsides with continued LOXAPAC therapy. Dizziness, faintness, staggering gait, muscle twitching, weakness, confusional states and seizures have been reported.

Extrapyramidal (neuromuscular) reactions during the administration of LOXAPAC have been reported frequently, often during the first few days of treatment. In most patients, these reactions involved Parkinson-like symptoms such as tremor, rigidity, excessive salivation, and a mask like face. Also, akathisia (motor restlessness) has been reported relatively frequently. These symptoms are usually not severe and can be controlled by reduction of dosage or by administration of anti-Parkinson drugs in usual dosage. Dystonias include spasms of muscles of the neck and face, tongue protrusion, and oculogyric choreoathetoid movements. Dyskinetic reaction has been described in the form of choreo-athetoid movements. These reactions sometimes require reduction or temporary withdrawal of LOXAPAC dosage in addition to appropriate counteractive drugs.

As with all antipsychotic agents, persistent tardive dyskinesia may appear in some patients on long term therapy or may appear after drug therapy has been discontinued. The risk appears to be greater in elderly patients on high-dose therapy, especially females. The symptoms are persistent and in some patients appear to be irreversible. The syndrome is characterised by rhythmical involuntary movement of the tongue, face, mouth or jaw (e.g. protrusion of tongue, puffing of cheeks, puckering of mouth, chewing movements). Sometimes these may be accompanied by involuntary movements of extremities.

There is no known effective treatment for tardive dyskinesia; anti-Parkinson agents usually do not alleviate the symptoms of this syndrome. It is suggested that all antipsychotic agents be discontinued if these symptoms appear.

Should it be necessary to reinstitute treatment, or increase the dose of the agent, or switch to a different antipsychotic agent, the syndrome may be masked. It has been suggested that fine vermicular movements of the tongue may be an early sign of the syndrome, and, if the medication is stopped at that time, the syndrome may not develop.

Cardiovascular effects:
Tachycardia, hypotension, hypertension, lightheadedness and syncope have been reported. A few cases of ECG changes similar to those seen with phenothiazines have been reported. It is not known whether these were related to administration.

Skin:
Dermatitis, oedema (puffiness of face), pruritis, and seborrhoea have been reported with LOXAPAC. The possibility of photosensitivity and/or phototoxicity occurring has not been excluded; skin rashes of uncertain aetiology have been observed in a few patients during hot summer months.

Endocrine effects:
Hormonal effects of anti-psychotic neuroleptic drugs include hyperprolactinaemia. Galactorrhoea, hyperprolactinaemia and amenorrhoea have been reported rarely.

Anticholinergic effects:
Dry mouth, nasal congestion, constipation, and blurred vision have occurred; these are more likely to occur with concomitant use of anti-Parkinson agents.

Other adverse reactions:
Nausea, vomiting, weight gain, weight loss, dyspnoea, ptosis, hyperpyrexia, flushed facies, headache, paraesthesia, and polydipsia have been reported in some patients. Transient abnormalities of liver function tests have been reported rarely. Jaundice has been reported in patients taking neuroleptic medication.

Neuroleptic Malignant Syndrome has been reported rarely following the use of LOXAPAC. This syndrome is potentially fatal and presents with symptoms of hyperpyrexia, muscle rigidity, altered mental status and evidence of autonomic instability. If a patient is diagnosed as suffering from Neuroleptic Malignant Syndrome, the management should include: (1) immediate discontinuation of antipsychotic drugs and other drugs not essential to concurrent therapy (2) symptomatic treatment and monitoring of vital signs and (3) treatment of any concomitant serious medical problems.

4.9 Overdose
Signs and symptoms of overdosage might be expected to include convulsive seizures and range from mild depression of the CNS and cardiovascular systems to profound hypotension, respiratory depression and unconsciousness. Renal failure has been reported following LOXAPAC administration. Severe extrapyramidal reactions should be treated with anticholinergic anti-Parkinson agents or diphenhydramine hydrochloride, and anticonvulsant therapy should be initiated as indicated.

The treatment of overdosage would be essentially symptomatic and supportive. Early gastric lavage and extended dialysis might be expected to be beneficial. Centrally acting emetics may have little effect because of the antiemetic action of loxapine. Avoid analeptics, such as picrotoxin and pentylenetetrazole, which may cause convulsions. Severe hypotension might be expected to respond to the administration of levarterenol or phenylephrine. ADRENALINE SHOULD NOT BE USED SINCE ITS USE IN A PATIENT WITH PARTIAL ADRENERGIC BLOCKADE MAY FURTHER LOWER THE BLOOD PRESSURE. Additional measures include oxygen and intravenous fluids.

5. PHARMACOLOGICAL PROPERTIES

5.1 Pharmacodynamic properties
Loxapine is a dibenzoxazepine with anti-psychotic actions similar to those of chlorpromazine. It is given by mouth as the succinate but the dose is expressed in terms of the base.

5.2 Pharmacokinetic properties
Loxapine is readily absorbed in the gastrointestinal tract. It is rapidly and extensively metabolised, with the possibility that one or more of its metabolites may be pharmacologically active: excretion occurs mainly in the first 24 hours. It is mainly excreted in the urine as conjugated metabolites with smaller amounts excreted in the faeces as unconjugated metabolites. Loxapine is widely distributed and

animal studies have indicated that it crosses the blood-brain barrier.

5.3 Preclinical safety data
Nothing of relevance to the prescriber.

6. PHARMACEUTICAL PARTICULARS

6.1 List of excipients
Lactose monohydrate, magnesium stearate, gelatin and colourings: quinoline yellow (E104), erythrosine (E127; 10mg and 50mg capsules only), Patent Blue V (E131), indicotine (E132; 25mg capsules only), titanium dioxide (E171).

6.2 Incompatibilities
None

6.3 Shelf life
60 months

6.4 Special precautions for storage
Store at room temperature.

6.5 Nature and contents of container
Polypropylene bottles of 28 (50mg strength only) or 56 (10mg and 25mg strengths) capsules.

6.6 Instructions for use and handling
None

7. MARKETING AUTHORISATION HOLDER
Cyanamid of Great Britain Limited Fareham Road

Gosport

Hampshire PO13 0AS

8. MARKETING AUTHORISATION NUMBER(S)

Loxapac Capsules 10mg:	PL 000095/0036
Loxapac Capsules 25mg:	PL 000095/0037
Loxapac Capsules 50mg:	PL 000095/0038

9. DATE OF FIRST AUTHORISATION/RENEWAL OF THE AUTHORISATION

First Authorisation	:	23 November 1977
Last Renewal	:	15 February 1999

10. DATE OF REVISION OF THE TEXT
15 February 1999

Lumigan

(Allergan Ltd)

1. NAME OF THE MEDICINAL PRODUCT
Lumigan▼ 0.3 mg/ml eye drops, solution

2. QUALITATIVE AND QUANTITATIVE COMPOSITION
One ml contains 0.3 mg bimatoprost.

For excipients, see 6.1.

3. PHARMACEUTICAL FORM
Eye drops, solution.

4. CLINICAL PARTICULARS

4.1 Therapeutic indications
Reduction of elevated intraocular pressure in chronic open-angle glaucoma and ocular hypertension (as monotherapy or as adjunctive therapy to beta-blockers).

4.2 Posology and method of administration
The recommended dose is one drop in the affected eye(s) once daily, administered in the evening. The dose should not exceed once daily as more frequent administration may lessen the intraocular pressure lowering effect.

If more than one topical ophthalmic medicinal product is being used, each one should be administered at least 5 minutes apart.

Use in children and adolescents (under the age of 18):

Lumigan has only been studied in adults and therefore its use is not recommended in children or adolescents.

Use in hepatic and renal impairment:

Lumigan has not been studied in patients with renal or moderate to severe hepatic impairment and should therefore be used with caution in such patients. In patients with a history of mild liver disease or abnormal ALT, AST and/or bilirubin at baseline, Lumigan had no adverse effect on liver function over 24 months.

4.3 Contraindications
Hypersensitivity to bimatoprost or to any of the excipients.

4.4 Special warnings and special precautions for use
Before treatment is initiated, patients should be informed of the possibility of eyelash growth, darkening of the eyelid skin and increased iris pigmentation since these have been observed during treatment with Lumigan. Some of these changes may be permanent, and may lead to differences in appearance between the eyes when only one eye is treated. The change in iris pigmentation occurs slowly and may not be noticeable for several months. At 12 months, the incidence was 1.5% and did not increase following 3 years treatment.

Lumigan contains the preservative benzalkonium chloride, which may be absorbed by soft contact lenses. Contact lenses should be removed prior to instillation and may be reinserted 15 minutes following administration.

Benzalkonium chloride, which is commonly used as a preservative in ophthalmic products, has been reported to cause punctate keratopathy and/or toxic ulcerative keratopathy. Since Lumigan contains benzalkonium chloride, monitoring is required with frequent or prolonged use in dry eye patients or where the cornea is compromised.

Lumigan has not been studied in patients with compromised respiratory function and should therefore be used with caution in such patients. In clinical studies, in those patients with a history of a compromised respiratory function, no significant untoward respiratory effects have been seen.

Lumigan has not been studied in patients with heart block more severe than first degree or uncontrolled congestive heart failure.

Lumigan has not been studied in patients with inflammatory ocular conditions, neovascular, inflammatory, angle-closure glaucoma, congenital glaucoma or narrow-angle glaucoma.

Cystoid macular oedema has been uncommonly reported (>0.1% to <1%) following treatment with Lumigan and should therefore be used with caution in patients with known risk factors for macular oedema (e.g. aphakic patients, pseudophakic patients with a torn posterior lens capsule).

4.5 Interaction with other medicinal products and other forms of Interaction
No interactions are anticipated in humans, since systemic concentrations of bimatoprost are extremely low (less than 0.2 ng/ml) following ocular dosing. Bimatoprost is biotransformed by any of multiple enzymes and pathways, and no effects on hepatic drug metabolising enzymes were observed in preclinical studies. Therefore, specific interaction studies with other medicinal products have not been performed with Lumigan.

In clinical studies, Lumigan was used concomitantly with a number of different ophthalmic beta-blocking agents without evidence of interactions.

Concomitant use of Lumigan and antiglaucomatous agents other than topical beta-blockers has not been evaluated during adjunctive glaucoma therapy.

4.6 Pregnancy and lactation

Pregnancy

The safety of Lumigan has not been studied in pregnant women. Studies in rodents produced species-specific abortion at systemic exposure levels 33- to 97-times that achieved in humans after ocular administration. No drug related developmental effects were observed (see section 5.3). Lumigan should not be used during pregnancy unless clearly necessary.

Lactation

It is not known if bimatoprost is excreted in human milk, however, this substance is excreted in rat milk after intravenous administration. It is recommended that Lumigan is not used in nursing mothers.

4.7 Effects on ability to drive and use machines
Bimatoprost is not expected to affect the ability to drive and use machines. As with any ocular treatment, if transient blurred vision occurs at instillation, the patient should wait until the vision clears before driving or using machinery.

4.8 Undesirable effects
In clinical studies, over 1800 patients have been treated with Lumigan. On combining the data from phase III monotherapy and adjunctive Lumigan usage, the most frequently reported treatment-related adverse events were: growth of eyelashes in up to 45% in the first year with the incidence of new reports decreasing to 7% at 2 years and 2% at 3 years, conjunctival hyperaemia (mostly trace to mild and thought to be of a non-inflammatory nature) in up to 44% in the first year with the incidence of new reports decreasing to 13% at 2 years and 12% at 3 years and ocular pruritus in up to 14% of patients in the first year with the incidence of new reports decreasing to 3% at 2 years and 0% at 3 years. Less than 9% of patients discontinued due to any adverse event in the first year with the incidence of additional patient discontinuations being 3% at both 2 and 3 years.

The following undesirable effects definitely, probably or possibly related to treatment were reported during clinical trials with Lumigan. Most were ocular, mild to moderate, and none was serious:

Ocular effects

Very common (>10%): conjunctival hyperaemia, growth of eyelashes, ocular pruritus

Common (>1% to <10%): allergic conjunctivitis, asthenopia, blepharitis, cataract, conjunctival oedema, corneal erosion, eye discharge, eyelash darkening, eyelid erythema, eyelid pruritus, eye pain, foreign body sensation, increased iris pigmentation, ocular burning, ocular dryness, ocular irritation, photophobia, pigmentation of periocular skin, superficial punctate keratitis, tearing, visual disturbance and worsening of visual acuity

Uncommon (>0.1% to <1%): blepharospasm, cystoid macular oedema, eyelid oedema, eyelid retraction, iritis, retinal haemorrhage, uveitis.

Systemic effects

Body as a whole

Common (>1% to <10%): headache

Uncommon (>0.1% to <1%): asthenia, infection (primarily colds and upper respiratory tract infections)

Gastrointestinal effects

Common (>1% to <10%): elevated liver function

Nervous system effects

Uncommon (>0.1% to <1%): dizziness

Cardiovascular

Common (>1% to <10%): hypertension

Metabolic

Uncommon (>0.1% to <1%): peripheral oedema

Skin

Uncommon (>0.1% to <1%): hirsutism.

4.9 Overdose
No case of overdose has been reported, and is unlikely to occur after ocular administration.

If overdosage occurs, treatment should be symptomatic and supportive. If Lumigan is accidentally ingested, the following information may be useful: in two-week oral rat and mouse studies, doses up to 100 mg/kg/day did not produce any toxicity. This dose expressed as mg/m^2 is at least 70-times higher than the accidental dose of one bottle of Lumigan in a 10 kg child.

5. PHARMACOLOGICAL PROPERTIES

5.1 Pharmacodynamic properties
Pharmacotherapeutic group: other antiglaucoma preparations;

ATC code: S01EE03

The mechanism of action by which bimatoprost reduces intraocular pressure in man is by increasing aqueous humour outflow through the trabecular meshwork and enhancing uveoscleral outflow. Reduction of the intraocular pressure starts approximately 4 hours after the first administration and maximum effect is reached within approximately 8 to 12 hours. The duration of effect is maintained for at least 24 hours.

Bimatoprost is a potent ocular hypotensive agent. It is a synthetic prostamide, structurally related to prostaglandin $F_{2\alpha}$ ($PGF_{2\alpha}$), that does not act through any known prostaglandin receptors. Bimatoprost selectively mimics the effects of newly discovered biosynthesised substances called prostamides. The prostamide receptor, however, has not yet been structurally identified.

During 12 months' monotherapy treatment, versus timolol, mean change from baseline in morning (08:00) intraocular pressure ranged from -7.9 to -8.8 mm Hg. At any visit, the mean diurnal IOP values measured over the 12-month study period differed by no more than 1.3 mmHg throughout the day and were never greater than 18.0 mmHg.

In a 6-month clinical study, versus latanoprost, a statistically superior reduction in morning mean IOP (ranging from -7.6 to -8.2 mmHg for bimatoprost versus -6.0 to -7.2 mmHg for latanoprost) was observed at all visits throughout the study. Conjunctival hyperaemia, growth of eyelashes, and eye pruritus were statistically significantly higher with bimatoprost than with latanoprost, however, the discontinuation rates due to adverse events were low with no statistically significant difference.

Compared to treatment with beta-blocker alone, adjunctive therapy with beta-blocker and bimatoprost lowered mean morning (08:00) intraocular pressure by -6.5 to -8.1 mmHg.

Limited experience is available with the use in patients with open-angle glaucoma with pseudoexfoliative and pigmentary glaucoma, and chronic angle-closure glaucoma with patent iridotomy.

No clinically relevant effects on heart rate and blood pressure have been observed in clinical trials.

5.2 Pharmacokinetic properties
Bimatoprost penetrates the human cornea and sclera well *in vitro*. After ocular administration, the systemic exposure of bimatoprost is very low with no accumulation over time. After once daily ocular administration of one drop of 0.03% bimatoprost to both eyes for two weeks, blood concentrations peaked within 10 minutes after dosing and declined to below the lower limit of detection (0.025 ng/ml) within 1.5 hours after dosing. Mean C_{max} and $AUC_{0\text{-}24hrs}$ values were similar on days 7 and 14 at approximately 0.08 ng/ml and 0.09 ng•hr/ml respectively, indicating that a steady drug concentration was reached during the first week of ocular dosing.

Bimatoprost is moderately distributed into body tissues and the systemic volume of distribution in humans at steady-state was 0.67 l/kg. In human blood, bimatoprost resides mainly in the plasma. The plasma protein binding of bimatoprost is approximately 88%.

Bimatoprost is the major circulating species in the blood once it reaches the systemic circulation following ocular dosing. Bimatoprost then undergoes oxidation,

N-deethylation and glucuronidation to form a diverse variety of metabolites.

Bimatoprost is eliminated primarily by renal excretion, up to 67% of an intravenous dose administered to healthy volunteers was excreted in the urine, 25% of the dose was excreted via the faeces. The elimination half-life, determined after intravenous administration, was approximately 45 minutes; the total blood clearance was 1.5 l/hr/kg.

Characteristics in elderly patients:

After twice daily dosing, the mean AUC_{0-24hr} value of 0.0634 ng•hr/ml bimatoprost in the elderly (subjects 65 years or older) were significantly higher than 0.0218 ng•hr/ml in young healthy adults. However, this finding is not clinically relevant as systemic exposure for both elderly and young subjects remained very low from ocular dosing. There was no accumulation of bimatoprost in the blood over time and the safety profile was similar in elderly and young patients.

5.3 Preclinical safety data

Monkeys administered ocular bimatoprost concentrations of ⩾0.03% daily for 1 year had an increase in iris pigmentation and reversible dose-related periocular effects characterised by a prominent upper and/or lower sulcus and widening of the palpebral fissure. The increased iris pigmentation appears to be caused by increased stimulation of melanin production in melanocytes and not by an increase in melanocyte number. No functional or microscopic changes related to the periocular effects have been observed, and the mechanism of action for the periocular changes is unknown.

Bimatoprost was not mutagenic or carcinogenic in a series of *in vitro* and *in vivo* studies.

Bimatoprost did not impair fertility in rats up to doses of 0.6 mg/kg/day (approximately 103-times the intended human exposure). In embryo/foetal developmental studies abortion, but no developmental effects were seen in mice and rats at doses that were at least 860-times or 1700-times higher than the dose in humans, respectively. These doses resulted in systemic exposures of at least 33- or 97-times higher, respectively, than the intended human exposure. In rat peri/postnatal studies, maternal toxicity caused reduced gestation time, foetal death, and decreased pup body weights at ⩾0.3 mg/kg/day (at least 41-times the intended human exposure). Neurobehavioural functions of offspring were not affected.

6. PHARMACEUTICAL PARTICULARS

6.1 List of excipients

Benzalkonium chloride

Sodium chloride

Sodium phosphate dibasic heptahydrate

Citric acid monohydrate

Hydrochloric acid or sodium hydroxide (to adjust pH)

Purified water

6.2 Incompatibilities

None known.

6.3 Shelf life

2 years.

4 weeks after first opening.

6.4 Special precautions for storage

No special precautions for storage.

Chemical and physical in-use stability has been demonstrated for 28 days at 25°C. From a microbiological point of view, the in-use storage times and conditions are the responsibility of the user and would normally not be longer than 28 days at 25°C.

6.5 Nature and contents of container

White opaque low density polyethylene bottles with polystyrene screw cap. Each bottle has a fill volume of 3 ml.

The following pack sizes are available: cartons containing 1 or 3 bottles of 3 ml. Not all pack sizes may be marketed.

6.6 Instructions for use and handling

None.

7. MARKETING AUTHORISATION HOLDER

Allergan Pharmaceuticals Ireland

Castlebar Road

Westport

Co. Mayo

Ireland

8. MARKETING AUTHORISATION NUMBER(S)

EU/1/02/205/001-002

9. DATE OF FIRST AUTHORISATION/RENEWAL OF THE AUTHORISATION

8 March 2002

10. DATE OF REVISION OF THE TEXT

20 January 2004

Lustral

(Pfizer Limited)

1. NAME OF THE MEDICINAL PRODUCT

LUSTRAL®

2. QUALITATIVE AND QUANTITATIVE COMPOSITION

Each tablet contains Sertraline hydrochloride equivalent to 50 mg or 100 mg sertraline.

3. PHARMACEUTICAL FORM

Film-coated tablet

50mg white, capsular shaped, film-coated scored tablets coded 'LTL-50' on one side and 'PFIZER' on the other.

100mg white, capsular shaped, film-coated tablets coded 'LTL-100' on one side and 'PFIZER' on the other.

4. CLINICAL PARTICULARS

4.1 Therapeutic indications

Lustral is indicated for the treatment of symptoms of depressive illness, including accompanying symptoms of anxiety. Following satisfactory response, continuation with Lustral therapy is effective in preventing relapse of the initial episode of depression or recurrence of further depressive episodes, including accompanying symptoms of anxiety.

Lustral is also indicated for the treatment of obsessive compulsive disorder (OCD). Following initial response, Lustral has been associated with sustained efficacy, safety and tolerability in up to two years treatment of OCD.

Lustral is also indicated for the treatment of paediatric patients with OCD.

Clinical trials in PTSD demonstrated efficacy in female patients but no evidence of efficacy was seen in males. Treatment with Lustral cannot normally therefore be recommended for male patients with PTSD. A therapeutic trial in males might on occasion be justified, but treatment should subsequently be withdrawn unless there is clear evidence of therapeutic benefit.

Lustral is not indicated for use in children and adolescents under the age of 18 years with Major Depressive Disorder.

In particular, controlled clinical studies failed to demonstrate efficacy and do not support the use of Lustral in the treatment of children and adolescents with Major Depressive Disorder (See sections 4.3, Contra-Indications and 4.8, Undesirable effects).

4.2 Posology and method of administration

Lustral should be given as a single daily dose. Lustral tablets can be administered with or without food.

Adults

Depression (including accompanying symptoms of anxiety): The starting dose is 50mg daily and the usual antidepressant dose is 50mg daily. In some patients, doses higher than 50mg may be required.

Obsessive Compulsive Disorder: The starting dose is 50mg daily, and the therapeutic dose range is 50-200mg daily.

Post-Traumatic Stress Disorder: Treatment for PTSD should be initiated at 25mg/day. After one week, the dose should be increased to 50mg once daily. PTSD is a heterogeneous illness and some patient groups fulfilling the criteria for PTSD do not appear to be responsive to treatment with Lustral. Dosing should be reviewed periodically by the prescribing physician to determine response to therapy and treatment should be withdrawn if there is no clear evidence of efficacy.

Depression (including accompanying symptoms of anxiety), OCD and PTSD: In some patients doses higher than 50mg daily may be required. In patients with incomplete response but good toleration at lower doses, dosage adjustments should be made in 50mg increments over a period of weeks to a maximum of 200mg daily.

Once optimal therapeutic response is achieved the dose should be reduced, depending on therapeutic response, to the lowest effective level. Dosage during prolonged maintenance therapy should be kept at the lowest effective level, with subsequent adjustments depending on therapeutic response. The onset of therapeutic effect may be seen within 7 days, although 2-4 weeks (and even longer in OCD) are usually necessary for full activity. A longer treatment period, even beyond 12 weeks in some cases, may be required in the case of a therapeutic trial in PTSD.

Use in children aged 6-17 years Treatment should only be *initiated* by specialists. The safety and efficacy of Lustral has been established in paediatric OCD patients (aged 6-17). The administration of Lustral to paediatric OCD patients (aged 13-17) should commence at 50 mg/day. Therapy for paediatric OCD patients (aged 6-12) should commence at 25mg/day increasing to 50mg/day after 1 week. Subsequent doses may be increased in case of lack of response in 50mg/day increments up to 200mg/day as needed. However, the generally lower body weights of children compared to adults should be taken into consideration in advancing the dose from 50mg, in order to avoid excessive dosing. Given the 24 hour elimination half-life of sertraline, dose changes should not occur at intervals of less than 1 week.

The efficacy and safety of Lustral in children and adolescents under the age of 18 years with Major Depressive Disorder have not been established. Controlled clinical studies failed to demonstrate efficacy and do not support the use of Lustral in the treatment of children and adolescents with Major Depressive Disorder (See sections 4.3, Contra-Indications and 4.8, Undesirable effects).

Children aged less than six years Lustral is not recommended in children under six years of age since safety and efficacy have not been established. See also 'Pharmacological Properties'.

Use in the elderly No special precautions are required. The usual adult dose is recommended. Several hundred elderly patients have participated in clinical studies with Lustral. The pattern and incidence of adverse reactions in the elderly is similar to that in younger patients.

Lustral tablets are for oral administration only.

4.3 Contraindications

Lustral is contra-indicated in patients with a known hypersensitivity to sertraline.

Monoamine oxidase inhibitors: Cases of serious and sometimes fatal reactions have been reported in patients receiving an SSRI in combination with a monoamine oxidase inhibitor (MAOI), including the selective MAOI selegiline and the reversible MAOI (RIMA) moclobemide and in patients who have recently discontinued an SSRI and have been started on a MAOI.

Some cases presented with features resembling serotonin syndrome. Symptoms of a drug interaction with a MAOI include: hyperthermia, rigidity, myoclonus, autonomic instability with possible rapid fluctuations of vital signs, mental status changes that include confusion, irritability and extreme agitation progressing to delirium and coma.

Lustral should not be used in combination with a MAOI. Lustral may be started 14 days after discontinuing treatment with an irreversible MAOI and at least one day after discontinuing treatment with the reversible MAOI (RIMA), moclobemide. At least 14 days should elapse after discontinuing Lustral treatment before starting a MAOI or RIMA.

Use in hepatic impairment: There is insufficient clinical experience in patients with significant hepatic dysfunction and accordingly Lustral should not be used in such patients.

Concomitant use in patients taking pimozide is contra-indicated (see section 4.5 - Interaction with Other Medicaments and Other Forms of Interaction.

Lustral should not be used in children and adolescents under the age of 18 years with Major Depressive Disorder. (See section 4.8, Undesirable effects).

4.4 Special warnings and special precautions for use

Monoamine oxidase inhibitors See 'Contra-indications'.

Use in patients with renal or hepatic impairment As with many other medications, sertraline should be used with caution in patients with renal and hepatic impairment (see 'Contra-indications').

Since sertraline is extensively metabolised, excretion of unchanged drug in urine is a minor route of elimination. In patients with mild to moderate renal impairment (creatinine clearance 20-50ml/min) or severe renal impairment (creatinine clearance <20ml/min), single dose pharmacokinetic parameters were not significantly different compared with controls. However, steady state pharmacokinetics of sertraline have not been adequately studied in this patient population and caution is advised when treating patients with renal impairment.

Sertraline is extensively metabolised by the liver. A multiple dose pharmacokinetic study in subjects with mild, stable cirrhosis demonstrated a prolonged elimination half-life and approximately three-fold greater AUC and C_{max} in comparison with normal subjects. There were no significant differences in plasma protein binding observed between the two groups. The use of sertraline in patients with hepatic disease should be approached with caution. A lower or less frequent dose should be used in patients with hepatic impairment.

DiabetesIn patients with diabetes, treatment with an SSRI may alter glycaemic control, possibly due to improvement of depressive symptoms. Insulin and/or oral hypoglycaemic dosage may be needed to be adjusted.

Seizures Seizures are a potential risk with antidepressant or antiobsessional drugs. The drug should be discontinued in any patient who develops seizures. Lustral should be avoided in patients with unstable epilepsy and patients with controlled epilepsy should be carefully monitored. Lustral should be discontinued if there is an increase in seizure frequency.

Electroconvulsive therapy (ECT) Since there is little clinical experience of concurrent administration of Lustral and ECT, caution is advisable.

ManiaLustral should be used with caution in patients with a history of mania/hypomania. Lustral should be discontinued in any patient entering a manic phase.

SuicideAs improvement may not occur during the first few weeks or more of treatment, patients should be closely monitored during this period. The possibility of a suicide attempt is inherent in depression and may persist until significant therapeutic effect is achieved and it is general clinical experience with all antidepressant therapies that the risk of suicide may increase in the early stages of recovery.

Haemorrhage There have been reports of cutaneous bleeding abnormalities such as ecchymoses and purpura with SSRIs.

Caution is advised in patients taking SSRIs, particularly in concomitant use with drugs known to affect platelet function (*e.g.* atypical antipsychotics and phenothiazines, most tricyclic antidepressants, aspirin and non-steroidal anti-inflammatory drugs (NSAIDs)) as well as in patients with a history of bleeding disorders.

Use in the elderly Several hundred elderly patients have participated in clinical studies with Lustral. The pattern and incidence of adverse reactions in the elderly is similar to that in younger patients.

Use in Children more than 250 paediatric OCD patients have been exposed to Lustral in completed and ongoing studies. The safety profile of Lustral in these paediatric studies is comparable to that observed in the adult OCD studies. The efficacy of Lustral in paediatric patients with depression or panic disorder has not been demonstrated in controlled trials. Safety and effectiveness in paediatric patients below the age of 6 have not been established.

There is limited knowledge with respect to an effect on sexual development in children.

4.5 Interaction with other medicinal products and other forms of Interaction

Monoamine oxidase inhibitors See 'Contra-indications'.

Centrally active medication Caution is advised if Lustral is administered with other centrally active medication. In particular, SSRIs have the potential to interact with tricyclic antidepressants leading to an increase in plasma levels of the tricyclic antidepressant. A possible mechanism for this interaction is the inhibitory effect of SSRIs on the CYP2D6 isoenzyme. There is variability among the SSRIs in the extent to which they inhibit the activity of CYP2D6. The clinical significance of this depends on the extent of inhibition and the therapeutic index of the co-administered drug. In formal interaction studies, chronic dosing with sertraline 50mg daily showed minimal elevation (mean 23-37%) of steady state plasma desipramine levels (a marker of CYP2D6 isoenzyme activity).

Pimozide – Increased pimozide levels have been demonstrated in a study of a single low dose pimozide (2mg) with sertraline coadministration. These increased levels were not associated with any changes in ECG. While the mechanism of this interaction is unknown, due to the narrow therapeutic index of pimozide, concomitant of pimozide and sertraline is contra-indicated.

Alcohol In 11 healthy subjects administered Lustral (200mg daily) for 9 days, there was no adverse effect on cognitive or psychomotor performance relative to placebo, following a single dose of 500mg/kg alcohol. However, the concomitant use of Lustral and alcohol in depressed patients is not recommended.

Lithium and Tryptophan In placebo-controlled trials in normal volunteers, the co-administration of Lustral and lithium did not significantly alter lithium pharmacokinetics.

Co-administration of Lustral with lithium did result in an increase in tremor relative to placebo, indicating a possible pharmacodynamic interaction. There have been other reports of enhanced effects when SSRIs have been given with lithium or tryptophan and therefore the concomitant use of SSRIs with these drugs should be undertaken with caution.

Serotonergic drugs There is limited controlled experience regarding the optimal timing of switching from other antidepressant or antiobsessional drugs to Lustral. Care and prudent medical judgement should be exercised when switching, particularly from long-acting agents. The duration of washout period which should intervene before switching from one selective serotonin reuptake inhibitor (SSRI) to another has not been established.

Until further data are available, serotonergic drugs, such as tramadol, sumatriptan or fenfluramine, should not be used concomitantly with Lustral, due to a possible enhancement of 5-HT associated effects.

St John's Wort Concomitant use of the herbal remedy St John's wort (Hypericum perforatum) in patients receiving SSRIs should be avoided since there is a possibility of serotonergic potentiation.

Drugs that affect platelet function, such as NSAIDs See 'Special warnings and special precautions for use (*Haemorrhage*)'.

Other drug interactions Since Lustral is bound to plasma proteins, the potential of Lustral to interact with other plasma protein bound drugs should be borne in mind.

Formal drug interaction studies have been performed with Lustral. Co-administration of Lustral (200mg daily) with diazepam or tolbutamide resulted in small, statistically significant changes in some pharmacokinetic parameters. Co-administration with cimetidine caused a substantial decrease in sertraline clearance. The clinical significance of these changes is unknown. Lustral had no effect on the beta-adrenergic blocking ability of atenolol. No interaction with Lustral (200mg daily) was observed with glibenclamide or digoxin.

Co-administration of Lustral (200mg daily) with warfarin resulted in a small but statistically significant increase in prothrombin time, the clinical significance of which is unknown. Accordingly, prothrombin time should be carefully monitored when Lustral therapy is initiated or stopped.

Lustral (200mg daily), did not potentiate the effects of carbamazepine, haloperidol or phenytoin on cognitive and psychomotor performance in healthy subjects.

4.6 Pregnancy and lactation

Pregnancy Although animal studies did not provide any evidence of teratogenicity, the safety of Lustral during human pregnancy has not been established. As with all drugs Lustral should only be used in pregnancy if the potential benefits of treatment to the mother outweigh the possible risks to the developing foetus.

Lactation Lustral is known to be excreted in breast milk. Its effects on the nursing infant have not yet been established. If treatment with Lustral is considered necessary, discontinuation of breast feeding should be considered.

4.7 Effects on ability to drive and use machines

Clinical pharmacology studies have shown that Lustral has no effect on psychomotor performance. However, since antidepressant or antiobsessional drugs may impair the abilities required to perform potentially hazardous tasks such as driving a car or operating machinery, the patient should be cautioned accordingly. Lustral should not be administered with benzodiazepines or other tranquillizers in patients who drive or operate machinery.

4.8 Undesirable effects

Side-effects which occurred significantly more frequently with sertraline than placebo in multiple dose studies were: nausea, diarrhoea/loose stools, anorexia, dyspepsia, tremor, dizziness, insomnia, somnolence, increased sweating, dry mouth and sexual dysfunction (principally ejaculatory delay in males).

The side-effect profile commonly observed in double-blind, placebo-controlled studies in patients with OCD and PTSD was similar to that observed in patients with depression.

In paediatric OCD patients, side-effects which occurred significantly more frequently with sertraline than placebo were: headache, insomnia, agitation, anorexia, tremor. Most were of mild to moderate severity.

Post-marketing spontaneous reports include the following:

Cardiovascular Blood pressure disturbances including postural hypotension, tachycardia.

Eye disorders Abnormal vision.

Gastro-intestinal Vomiting, abdominal pain.

Nervous system Amnesia, headache, drowsiness, movement disorders, paraesthesia, hypoaesthesia, depressive symptoms, hallucinations, aggressive reaction, agitation, anxiety, psychosis, depersonalisation, nervousness, panic reaction and signs and symptoms associated with serotonin syndrome which include fever, rigidity, confusion, agitation, diaphoresis, tachycardia, hypertension and diarrhoea.

There have also been reports of manic reaction, although this phenomenon may be part of the underlying disease.

Convulsions (Seizures) Lustral should be discontinued in any patient who develops seizures (See 'Special warnings and special precautions for use').

MusculoskeletalArthralgia, myalgia.

Hepatic/pancreatic Rarely, pancreatitis and serious liver events (including hepatitis, jaundice and liver failure). Asymptomatic elevations in serum transaminases (SGOT and SGPT) have been reported in association with sertraline administration (0.8 – 1.3%), with an increased risk associated with the 200mg daily dose. The abnormalities usually occurred within the first 1 to 9 weeks of drug treatment and promptly diminished upon drug discontinuation.

Renal & urinary disorders Urinary retention.

ReproductiveHyperprolactinemia, galactorrhoea, menstrual irregularities, anorgasmy.

Skin and allergic reactions Rash (including rare reports of erythema multiforme, photosensitivity), angioedema, ecchymoses, pruritus and anaphylactoid reactions.

MetabolicRare cases of hyponatremia have been reported and appeared to be reversible when sertraline was discontinued. Some cases were possibly due to the syndrome of inappropriate antidiuretic hormone secretion. The majority of reports were associated with older patients, and patients taking diuretics or other medications.

HaematologicThere have been rare reports of altered platelet function and/or abnormal clinical laboratory results in patients taking sertraline. While there have been reports of thrombocytopenia, abnormal bleeding or purpura in several patients taking sertraline, it is unclear whether sertraline had a causative role. See also 'Special warnings and special precautions for use'.

GeneralMalaise.

OtherWithdrawal reactions have been reported with Lustral. Common symptoms include dizziness, paraesthesia, headache, anxiety and nausea. Abrupt discontinuation of treatment with Lustral should be avoided. The majority of symptoms experienced on withdrawal of Lustral are non-serious and self-limiting.

Adverse events from paediatric clinical trials

In paediatric clinical trials in depression the following adverse events were reported at a frequency of at least 2% of patients and occurred at a rate of at least twice that of placebo: dry mouth (2.1% vs 0.5%), hyperkinesia (2.6% vs 0.5%), tremor (2.1% vs 0%), diarrhoea (9.5% vs 1.6%), vomiting (4.2% vs 1.1%), agitation (6.3% vs 1.1%), anorexia (5.3% vs 1.1%) and urinary incontinence (2.1% vs 0%).

Suicidal thoughts and suicide attempts were mainly observed in clinical trials with Major Depressive Disorder.

4.9 Overdose

On the evidence available, Lustral has a wide margin of safety in overdose. Overdoses of Lustral alone of up to 8g have been reported. Deaths involving overdoses of Lustral in combination with other drugs and/or alcohol have been reported. Therefore, any overdosage should be treated aggressively.

Symptoms of overdose include serotonin-mediated side-effects such as somnolence, gastrointestinal disturbances (such as nausea and vomiting), tachycardia, tremor, agitation and dizziness. Less frequently reported was coma.

No specific therapy is recommended and there are no specific antidotes to Lustral. Establish and maintain an airway, ensure adequate oxygenation and ventilation. Activated charcoal, which may be used with sorbitol, may be as or more effective than emesis or lavage, and should be considered in treating overdose. Cardiac and vital signs monitoring is recommended along with general symptomatic and supportive measures. Due to the large volume of distribution of sertraline, forced diuresis, dialysis, haemoperfusion and exchange transfusion are unlikely to be of benefit.

5. PHARMACOLOGICAL PROPERTIES

5.1 Pharmacodynamic properties

Sertraline is a potent and specific inhibitor of neuronal serotonin (5-HT) uptake *in vitro* and *in vivo*, but is without affinity for muscarinic, serotonergic, dopaminergic, adrenergic, histaminergic, GABA or benzodiazepine receptors.

Sertraline is devoid of stimulant, sedative or anticholinergic activity or cardiotoxicity in animals.

Unlike tricyclic antidepressants, no weight gain is observed with treatment for depression.

Lustral has not been observed to produce physical or psychological dependence.

Lustral has been evaluated in paediatric OCD patients aged 6 to 17 in a 12 week placebo-controlled study. Therapy for paediatric OCD patients (aged 6-12) commenced at 25mg/day increasing to 50mg/day after 1 week. Side-effects which occurred significantly more frequently with sertraline than placebo were: headache, insomnia, agitation [6-12 years]; insomnia, anorexia, tremor [13-17 years]. There is limited evidence of efficacy and safety beyond 12 weeks of treatment.

5.2 Pharmacokinetic properties

Sertraline exhibits dose proportional pharmacokinetics over a range of 50-200mg. After oral administration of sertraline in man, peak blood levels occur at about 4.5 - 8.4 hours. Daily doses of sertraline achieve steady-state after one week. Sertraline has a plasma half-life of approximately 26 hours with a mean half-life for young and elderly adults ranging from 22-36 hours. Sertraline is approximately 98% bound to plasma proteins. The principal metabolite, N-desmethylsertraline, is inactive in *in vivo* models of depression and has a half-life of approximately 62-104 hours. Sertraline and N-desmethylsertraline are both extensively metabolised in man and the resultant metabolites excreted in faeces and urine in equal amounts. Only a small amount (<0.2%) of unchanged sertraline is excreted in the urine.

The pharmacokinetics of sertraline in paediatric OCD patients have been shown to be comparable with adults (although paediatric patients metabolise sertraline with slightly greater efficiency). However, lower doses may be advisable for paediatric patients given their lower body weights (especially 6-12 years), in order to avoid excessive plasma levels.

A clear relationship between sertraline concentration and the magnitude of therapeutic response has not been established.

The pharmacokinetics of sertraline in elderly patients are similar to younger adults.

Food does not significantly change the bioavailability of Lustral tablets.

5.3 Preclinical safety data

Extensive chronic safety evaluation studies in animals show that sertraline is generally well tolerated at doses that are appreciable multiples of those that are clinically effective.

6. PHARMACEUTICAL PARTICULARS

6.1 List of excipients

Sertraline tablets include the following inert ingredients:

Tablet cores:

calcium hydrogen phosphate

microcrystalline cellulose

hydroxypropylcellulose

sodium starch glycollate

magnesium stearate

Film coating:
-Opadry® White
- titanium dioxide (E171)
- hypromellose
- macrogol 400
- polysorbate-80
- Opadry® Clear
- hypromellose
- macrogol 400
- macrogol 6000

6.2 Incompatibilities
None.

6.3 Shelf life
5 years.

6.4 Special precautions for storage
None

6.5 Nature and contents of container
Lustral is available as:

Calendar packs of 28 tablets. Aluminium/PVC blister strips, 14 tablets/strip, 2 strips in a carton box.

6.6 Instructions for use and handling
No special requirements.

7. MARKETING AUTHORISATION HOLDER
Pfizer Limited
Ramsgate Road
Sandwich
Kent CT13 9NJ
United Kingdom

8. MARKETING AUTHORISATION NUMBER(S)
Lustral Tablets 50mg PL 0057/0308
Lustral Tablets 100mg PL 0057/0309

9. DATE OF FIRST AUTHORISATION/RENEWAL OF THE AUTHORISATION
30 September 1997

10. DATE OF REVISION OF THE TEXT
10 December 2003

LEGAL CATEGORY
POM

Luveris 75 IU

(Serono Ltd)

1. NAME OF THE MEDICINAL PRODUCT
Luveris 75 IU, powder and solvent for solution for injection.

2. QUALITATIVE AND QUANTITATIVE COMPOSITION
One vial contains 75 IU of lutropin alfa (recombinant human luteinising hormone {LH}). Lutropin alfa is produced in genetically engineered Chinese hamster ovary (CHO) cells.

For excipients, see 6.1.

3. PHARMACEUTICAL FORM
Powder and solvent for solution for injection.

Appearance of the powder: white lyophilised pellet

Appearance of the solvent: clear colourless solution

4. CLINICAL PARTICULARS

4.1 Therapeutic indications
Luveris in association with a follicle stimulating hormone (FSH) preparation is recommended for the stimulation of follicular development in women with severe LH and FSH deficiency. In clinical trials these patients were defined by an endogenous serum LH level <1.2 IU/l.

4.2 Posology and method of administration
Treatment with Luveris should be initiated under the supervision of a physician experienced in the treatment of fertility problems. Self-administration of Luveris should only be performed by patients who are well-motivated, adequately trained and with access to expert advice.

In LH and FSH deficient women, the objective of Luveris therapy in association with FSH is to develop a single mature Graafian follicle from which the oocyte will be liberated after the administration of human chorionic gonadotrophin (hCG). Luveris should be given as a course of daily injections simultaneously with FSH. Since these patients are amenorrhoeic and have low endogenous oestrogen secretion, treatment can commence at any time.

All clinical experience to date with Luveris in this indication has been gained with concomitant administration of follitropin alfa.

Luveris is intended for subcutaneous administration. The powder should be reconstituted, immediately prior to use, with the solvent provided.

Treatment should be tailored to the individual patient's response as assessed by measuring (i) follicle size by ultrasound and (ii) oestrogen response. A recommended regimen commences at 75 IU of lutropin alfa (ie. one vial of Luveris) daily with 75-150 IU FSH.

If an FSH dose increase is deemed appropriate, dose adaptation should preferably be after 7-14 day intervals and preferably by 37.5 IU-75 IU increments. It may be acceptable to extend the duration of stimulation in any one cycle to up to 5 weeks.

When an optimal response is obtained, a single injection of 5,000 IU to 10,000 IU hCG should be administered 24-48 hours after the last Luveris and FSH injections. The patient is recommended to have coitus on the day of, and on the day following, hCG administration.

Alternatively, intrauterine insemination (IUI) may be performed.

Luteal phase support may be considered since lack of substances with luteotrophic activity (LH/hCG) after ovulation may lead to premature failure of the corpus luteum.

If an excessive response is obtained, treatment should be stopped and hCG withheld. Treatment should recommence in the next cycle at a dose of FSH lower than that of the previous cycle.

4.3 Contraindications
Luveris is contraindicated in patients with:

- hypersensitivity to gonadotrophins or to any of the excipients.
- ovarian, uterine, or mammary carcinoma;
- active, untreated tumours of the hypothalamus and pituitary gland;
- ovarian enlargement or cyst not due to polycystic ovarian disease;
- gynaecological haemorrhages of unknown origin

4.4 Special warnings and special precautions for use
Before starting treatment, the couple's infertility should be assessed as appropriate and putative contraindications for pregnancy evaluated. This medicinal product should not be used when an effective response cannot be obtained, such as ovarian failure, malformation of the sexual organs incompatible with pregnancy or fibroid tumours of the uterus incompatible with pregnancy. In addition, patients should be evaluated for hypothyroidism, adrenocortical deficiency, hyperprolactinemia and pituitary or hypothalamic tumours, and appropriate specific treatment given.

Patients undergoing stimulation of follicular growth are at an increased risk of developing hyperstimulation in view of possible excessive oestrogen response and multiple follicular development.

Ovarian hyperstimulation syndrome (OHSS) can become a serious medical event characterised by large ovarian cysts which are prone to rupture. Excessive ovarian response seldom gives rise to significant hyperstimulation unless hCG is administered to induce ovulation. It is therefore prudent to withhold hCG in such cases and advise the patient to refrain from coitus or use barrier methods for at least 4 days.

Careful monitoring of ovarian response, based on ultrasound is recommended prior to and during stimulation therapy, especially in patients with polycystic ovaries.

In patients undergoing induction of ovulation, the incidence of multiple pregnancies and births is increased compared with natural conception.

To minimise the risk of OHSS or of multiple pregnancy, ultrasound scans as well as oestradiol measurements are recommended. In anovulation the risk of OHSS is increased by a serum oestradiol level > 900 pg/ml (3300 pmol/l) and by the presence of more than 3 follicles of 14 mm or more in diameter.

Adherence to recommended Luveris and FSH dosage and regimen of administration and careful monitoring of therapy will minimise the incidence of ovarian hyperstimulation and multiple pregnancy.

In clinical trials, the medicinal product has been shown to increase the ovarian sensitivity to follitropin alfa. If an FSH dose increase is deemed appropriate, dose adaptation should preferably be at 7-14 day intervals and preferably with 37.5-75 IU increments.

In clinical trials, there have been no reports of hypersensitivity to lutropin alfa.

No direct comparison of Luveris/FSH versus human menopausal gonadotrophin (hMG) has been performed. Comparison with historical data suggests that the ovulation rate obtained with Luveris/FSH is similar to what can be obtained with hMG.

4.5 Interaction with other medicinal products and other forms of Interaction
Luveris should not be administered as a mixture with other medicinal products, in the same injection, except follitropin alfa for which studies have shown that co-administration does not significantly alter the activity, stability, pharmacokinetic nor pharmacodynamic properties of the active substances.

4.6 Pregnancy and lactation
Luveris should not be administered during pregnancy or lactation.

4.7 Effects on ability to drive and use machines
Luveris does not interfere with the patient's ability to drive or use machines.

4.8 Undesirable effects
a) General description

Lutropin alfa is used for the stimulation of follicular development in association with follitropin - alfa. In this context, it is difficult to attribute undesirable effects to any one of the substances used.

There is considerable post-marketing safety experience with human luteinising hormone (hLH)-containing medicinal products of urinary origin. The safety profile of Luveris is expected to be very similar to that of urine derived hLH, with the exception of hypersensitivity reactions and application site disorders.

In a clinical trial, mild and moderate injection site reactions (bruising, pain, redness, itching or swelling) were reported in 7.4% and 0.9% of the injections, respectively. No severe injection site reactions were reported. To date no systemic allergic reactions have been reported following Luveris administration.

Ovarian hyperstimulation syndrome was observed in less than 6% of patients treated with Luveris. No severe ovarian hyperstimulation syndrome was reported (section 4.4 Special warnings and special precautions for use).

In rare instances, thromboembolisms, adnexal torsion (a complication of ovarian enlargement), and haemoperitoneum have been associated with human menopausal gonadotrophin therapy. Although these adverse events were not observed, there is the possibility that they may also occur with Luveris.

Ectopic pregnancy may also occur, especially in women with a history of prior tubal disease.

b) Undesirable effects

The following convention was used for the frequency (events/ no. of patients): very rare: <1/10000, rare: >1/10000, <1/1000, uncommon: >1/1000, <1/100, common: >1/100, <1/10, very common: >1/10

After best evidence assessment, the following undesirable effects may be observed after administration of Luveris.

Common

Application site disorders: injection site reaction

General disorders: headache, somnolence

Gastro-intestinal system disorders: nausea, abdominal pain, pelvic pain

Reproductive disorders: ovarian hyperstimulation syndrome, ovarian cyst, breast pain

The reported undesirable effects are in agreement with those reported for other hLH-containing medicinal products, except for injection site reactions where the incidence was significantly lower with Luveris treatment.

4.9 Overdose
The effects of an overdose of lutropin alfa are unknown, nevertheless there is a possibility that ovarian hyperstimulation syndrome may occur, which is further described in 'Special warnings and special precautions for use'.

Single doses of up to 40,000 IU of lutropin alfa have been administered to healthy female volunteers without serious adverse events and were well tolerated.

5. PHARMACOLOGICAL PROPERTIES

5.1 Pharmacodynamic properties
Pharmacotherapeutic group: gonadotrophins. ATC code: G03G

Lutropin alfa is a recombinant human luteinising hormone, a glycoprotein composed of non-covalently bound α- and β-subunits. Luteinising hormone binds on the ovarian theca (and granulosa) cells and testicular Leydig cells, to a receptor shared with human chorionic gonadotrophin hormone (hCG). This LH/CG transmembrane receptor is a member of the super-family of G protein-coupled receptors; specifically, it has a large extra-cellular domain. *In vitro* the affinity binding of recombinant hLH to the LH/CG receptor on Leydig tumour cells (MA-10) is between that for hCG and that of pituitary hLH, but within the same order of magnitude.

In the ovaries, during the follicular phase, LH stimulates theca cells to secrete androgens, which will be used as the substrate by granulosa cell aromatase enzyme to produce oestradiol, supporting FSH-induced follicular development. At mid-cycle, high levels of LH trigger corpus luteum formation and ovulation. After ovulation, LH stimulates progesterone production in the corpus luteum by increasing the conversion of cholesterol to pregnenolone.

In the stimulation of follicular development in anovulatory women deficient in LH and FSH, the primary effect resulting from administration of lutropin alfa is an increase in oestradiol secretion by the follicles, the growth of which is stimulated by FSH.

In clinical trials, patients were defined by an endogenous serum LH level <1.2 IU/l as measured in a central laboratory. However, it should be taken into account that there are variations between LH measurements performed in different laboratories.

In these trials the ovulation rate per cycle was 70-75%. The combination of r-hLH and r-hFSH has not been directly compared with treatment with hMG.

5.2 Pharmacokinetic properties
The pharmacokinetics of lutropin alfa have been studied in pituitary desensitised female volunteers from 75 IU up to 40,000 IU.

The pharmacokinetic profile of lutropin alfa is similar to that of urinary-derived hLH. Following intravenous administration, lutropin alfa is rapidly distributed with an initial half-life of approximately one hour and eliminated from the body with a terminal half-life of about 10-12 hours. The steady state volume of distribution is around 10-14 l. Lutropin alfa shows linear pharmacokinetics, as assessed by AUC which is directly proportional to the dose administered. Total clearance is around 2 l/h, and less than 5% of the dose is excreted in the urine. The mean residence time is approximately 5 hours.

Following subcutaneous administration, the absolute bioavailability is approximately 60%; the terminal half-life is slightly prolonged. The lutropin alfa pharmacokinetics following single and repeated administration of Luveris are comparable and the accumulation ratio of lutropin alfa is minimal. There is no pharmacokinetic interaction with follitropin alfa when administered simultaneously.

5.3 Preclinical safety data
Extensive toxicology studies have been carried out with lutropin alfa in a range of animal models. These include the daily treatment of rats and monkeys with lutropin alfa for a duration of three months which resulted in well known pharmacological and morphological effects related to LH. No toxicity was observed in either species. As expected from the heterologous protein nature of the hormone, lutropin alfa raised an antibody response in experimental animals after a period that reduced the measurable serum LH levels but did not fully prevent its biological action. No signs of toxicity due to the development of antibodies to lutropin alfa were observed.

At doses of 10 IU/kg/day and greater, repeated administration of lutropin alfa to pregnant rats and rabbits caused impairment of reproductive function including resorption of foetuses and reduced body weight gain of the dams. However, drug-related teratogenesis was not observed in either animal model.

Other studies have shown that lutropin alfa is not mutagenic.

After intravenous administration of radiolabelled lutropin alfa to rats, tissue uptake paralleled the plasma profile of radioactivity with only a strong affinity to the ovaries in pregnant animals. Foetal penetration of radioactivity was low. In lactating rats, radioactivity in milk was greater than or equal to that in plasma. Due to its heterologous protein nature, lutropin alfa produced moderate allergenic reactions in guinea pigs after intravenous challenge. For the same reason, a mild sensitisation was observed in guinea pigs after intradermal challenge.

6. PHARMACEUTICAL PARTICULARS

6.1 List of excipients
Sucrose
Disodium phosphate dihydrate
Sodium dihydrogen phosphate monohydrate
Polysorbate 20
Phosphoric acid, concentrated
Sodium hydroxide
Methionine
Nitrogen
Solvent: Water for injections

6.2 Incompatibilities
This medicinal product must not be mixed with other medicinal products except those mentioned in 6.6.

6.3 Shelf life
36 months.

6.4 Special precautions for storage
Do not store above 25°C. Store in the original package.

6.5 Nature and contents of container
The powder is packaged in 3 ml neutral colourless glass (type I) vials. The vials are sealed with bromobutyl stoppers protected by aluminium seal rings and flip-off caps. The solvent is packaged either in 2 ml neutral colourless glass (type I) vials with a Teflon-coated rubber stopper or in 2 ml neutral colourless glass (type I) ampoules.

The product is supplied in packs of 1, 3 or 10 vials with the corresponding number of solvent vials or ampoules. Not all pack sizes may be marketed.

6.6 Instructions for use and handling
For immediate and single use following first opening and reconstitution.

The powder must be reconstituted with the solvent before use by gentle swirling.

The reconstituted solution should not be administered if it contains particles or is not clear.

Luveris may be mixed with follitropin alfa and co-administered as a single injection.

In this case Luveris should be reconstituted first and then used to reconstitute the follitropin alfa powder.

In order to avoid the injection of large volumes, one vial of Luveris can be reconstituted together with one or two ampoule(s)/vial(s) of follitropin alfa, 37.5 IU, 75 IU or 150 IU, in 1 ml of solvent.

Any unused product or waste material should be disposed of in accordance with local requirements.

7. MARKETING AUTHORISATION HOLDER
Serono Europe Limited
56, Marsh Wall
London E14 9TP
United Kingdom

8. MARKETING AUTHORISATION NUMBER(S)

Authorisation number	Presentations
EU/1/00/155/001	Luveris – 75 IU - Powder and solvent for solution for injection – Subcutaneous use – Powder: vial (glass), Solvent: ampoule (glass) (1 ml) – 1 vial + 1 ampoule
EU/1/00/155/002	Luveris – 75 IU - Powder and solvent for solution for injection – Subcutaneous use – Powder: vials (glass), Solvent: ampoules (glass) (1 ml) – 3 vials + 3 ampoules
EU/1/00/155/003	Luveris – 75 IU - Powder and solvent for solution for injection – Subcutaneous use – Powder: vials (glass), Solvent: ampoules (glass) (1 ml) – 10 vials + 10 ampoules
EU/1/00/155/004	Luveris – 75 IU - Powder and solvent for solution for injection – Subcutaneous use – Powder: vial (glass), Solvent: vial (glass) (1 ml) – 1 vial + 1 vial
EU/1/00/155/005	Luveris – 75 IU - Powder and solvent for solution for injection – Subcutaneous use – Powder: vials (glass), Solvent: vials (glass) (1 ml) – 3 vials + 3 vials
EU/1/00/155/006	Luveris – 75 IU - Powder and solvent for solution for injection – Subcutaneous use – Powder: vials (glass), Solvent: vials (glass) (1 ml) – 10 vials + 10 vials

9. DATE OF FIRST AUTHORISATION/RENEWAL OF THE AUTHORISATION
29th November 2000

10. DATE OF REVISION OF THE TEXT
26th May 2004

LEGAL STATUS POM

NAME AND ADDRESS OF DISTRIBUTOR IN UK
Serono Ltd
Bedfont Cross
Stanwell Road
Feltham
Middlesex
TW14 8NX
Tel 020 8818 7200

NAME AND ADDRESS OF DISTRIBUTOR IN IRELAND
Allphar Services Limited
Pharmaceutical Agents and Distributors
Belgard Road
Tallaght
Dublin 24

Lyflex 5mg/5ml Oral Solution

(Chemidex Pharma Ltd.)

1. NAME OF THE MEDICINAL PRODUCT
Lyflex 5mg/5ml Oral Solution

2. QUALITATIVE AND QUANTITATIVE COMPOSITION
Each 5ml of oral solution contains 5mg Baclofen.

For excipients see Section 6.1

3. PHARMACEUTICAL FORM
Oral Solution

Clear yellowish liquid with an odour and flavour of raspberry

4. CLINICAL PARTICULARS

4.1 Therapeutic indications
Baclofen is indicated for the relief of voluntary muscle spasticity resulting from disorders such as: multiple sclerosis, other spinal lesions, e.g. tumours of the spinal cord, syringomyelia, motor neurone disease, transverse myelitis, traumatic partial section of the cord.

Baclofen Oral Solution is also indicated in adults and children for the relief of spasticity of voluntary muscle arising from e.g. cerebrovascular accidents, cerebral palsy, meningitis, traumatic head injury.

Patient selection is important when initiating treatment with Baclofen Oral Solution; it is likely to be of most benefit in patients whose spasticity constitutes a handicap to activities and/or physiotherapy. Treatment should not be commenced until the spastic state has become stabilised.

4.2 Posology and method of administration
Baclofen Oral Solution is particularly suitable for children or those adults who are unable to take tablets. Dosage titration can be achieved more precisely with the oral solution.

Before initiating treatment with Baclofen Oral Solution it is advisable to assess realistically the overall extent of clinical improvement that the patient may be expected to achieve with treatment. Careful titration of dosage is essential (particularly in the elderly) until the patient is stabilised. If too high a dose is used initially or if increases in dosage are too rapid side effects may occur. This is particularly relevant if the patient is ambulant in order to minimise muscle weakness in the unaffected limbs or where spasticity is necessary for support.

Adults:

It is recommended that treatment is started with a gradually increasing dosage regimen as follows. However this may be adjusted to meet individual patient requirements:

5mg three times a day for three days
10mg three times a day for three days
15mg three times a day for three days
20mg three times a day for three days

Satisfactory control of symptoms is usually obtained with doses of up to 60mg daily, but a careful adjustment is often necessary to meet the requirements of each individual patient. The dose may be increased slowly if required, but a maximum daily dose of more than 100mg is not advised unless the patient is in hospital under careful medical supervision. Small frequent doses may prove better in some cases than larger spaced doses. Also some patients benefit from the use of Baclofen Oral Solution only at night to counteract painful flexor spasm. Similarly a single dose given approximately 1 hour prior to performance of specific tasks such as washing, dressing, shaving, physiotherapy, will often improve mobility.

Once the maximum recommended dose has been reached, if the therapeutic effect is not apparent within 6 weeks consideration should be made by the physician as to whether to continue treatment with Baclofen Oral Solution.

Elderly:

Elderly patients may be more susceptible to side effects, particularly in the early stages of starting treatment with Baclofen Oral Solution. Small doses should therefore be used at the start of treatment, the dose being titrated gradually against the response, under careful supervision. There is no evidence that the eventual average maximum dose differs from that in younger patients.

Children:

A dosage range of 0.75-2mg/kg body weight should be used. In children over 10 years of age, however a maximum daily dosage of 2.5mg/kg body weight may be given. Treatment is usually started with 2.5mg given 4 times daily. The dosage should be increased cautiously at about 3 day intervals, until it becomes sufficient for the child's individual requirements. The recommended daily dosages for maintenance therapy are as follows:

Children aged, 12 months – 2 years: 10-20mg;
2 years – 6 years: 20-30mg;
6 years – 10 years: 30-60mg

Patients with impaired renal function:

In patients with impaired renal function or undergoing chronic haemodialysis, a particularly low dosage of Baclofen should be selected i.e. approx. 5mg daily.

Patients with spastic states of cerebral origin:

Unwanted effects are more likely to occur in these patients. It is therefore recommended that a very cautious dosage schedule be adopted and that patients be kept under appropriate surveillance.

4.3 Contraindications
Hypersensitivity to baclofen or any of the ingredients of the oral solution, peptic ulceration.

4.4 Special warnings and special precautions for use
Psychotic disorders, schizophrenia, depressive or manic disorders, confusional states or Parkinson's disease may be exacerbated by treatment with baclofen. Patients suffering from these conditions should therefore be treated cautiously and kept under close surveillance.

Baclofen may also exacerbate epileptic manifestations but can be used provided appropriate supervision and adequate anticonvulsive therapy are maintained. Baclofen should be used with extreme care in patients already receiving antihypertensive therapy, (see Interactions).

Baclofen should be used with caution in patients suffering from cerebrovascular accidents or from respiratory, hepatic or renal impairment.

During treatment with baclofen, neurogenic disturbances affecting emptying of the bladder may show an improvement. In patients with pre-existing sphincter hypertonia, acute retention of urine may occur; the drug should be used with caution in such cases.

This medicine contains sorbitol. Patients with rare hereditary problems should not take this medicine. Calorific value 2.6kcal/g sorbitol".

Abrupt withdrawal:

Anxiety and confusional states, hallucinations, psychotic, manic or paranoid states, convulsions (status epilepticus), dyskinesia, tachycardia, hyperthermia and as rebound phenomenon temporary aggravation of spasticity have been reported with abrupt withdrawal of baclofen, especially after long term medication. Treatment should always, (unless serious adverse effects occur), be gradually discontinued by successively reducing the dosage over a period of about 1-2 weeks.

Since in rare instances elevated SGOT, alkaline phosphatase and glucose levels in serum have been recorded, appropriate laboratory tests should be performed in patients with liver diseases or diabetes mellitus in order to ensure that no drug induced changes in these underlying diseases have occurred.

4.5 Interaction with other medicinal products and other forms of Interaction

Where baclofen is taken concomitantly with other drugs acting on the CNS with synthetic opiates or with alcohol, increased sedation may occur.

The risk of respiratory depression is also increased. Careful monitoring of respiratory and cardiovascular functions is essential especially in patients with cardiopulmonary disease and respiratory muscle weakness.

During concurrent treatment with tricyclic antidepressants, the effect of baclofen may be potentiated, resulting in pronounced muscular hypotonia.

Since concomitant treatment with baclofen and antihypertensives is likely to increase the fall in blood pressure, the dosage of antihypertensive medication should be adjusted accordingly. Hypotension has been reported in one patient receiving morphine and intrathecal baclofen.

Drugs which may produce renal insufficiency e.g. ibuprofen may reduce baclofen excretion leading to toxic effects. In patients with Parkinson's disease receiving treatment with baclofen and levodopa plus carbidopa, there have been reports of mental confusion, hallucinations, nausea and agitation.

4.6 Pregnancy and lactation

During pregnancy, especially in the first 3 months, baclofen should only be used if its use is of vital necessity. The benefits of the treatment for the mother must be carefully weighed against the possible risks for the child. Baclofen crosses the placental barrier.

In mothers taking baclofen in therapeutic doses, the active substance passes into the breast milk, but in quantities so small that no undesirable effects on the infant would be expected.

4.7 Effects on ability to drive and use machines

The patient's reactions may be adversely affected by baclofen induced sedation or decreased alertness. Patients should therefore exercise due caution. Operating equipment or machinery may be hazardous.

4.8 Undesirable effects

Unwanted effects occur mainly at the start of treatment, if the dosage is raised too rapidly, if large doses are employed, or in elderly patients. They are often transitory and can be attenuated or eliminated by reducing the dosage; they are seldom severe enough to necessitate withdrawal of the medication.

Should nausea persist following a reduction in dosage, it is recommended that baclofen be ingested with food or a milk beverage.

In patients with a case history of psychiatric illness or with cerebrovascular disorders (e.g. stroke) as well as in elderly patients, adverse reactions may assume a more serious form.

Central Nervous System:

Frequent (>10%): particularly at the start of treatment daytime sedation, drowsiness, and nausea.

Occasional (> 1%, <10%): respiratory depression, lightheadedness, lassitude, exhaustion, mental confusion, dizziness, headache, insomnia, euphoria, depression, muscular weakness, ataxia, tremor, hallucinations, nightmares, myalgia, nystagmus, dry mouth.

Rare (> 0.001%, <1%): paraesthesia, dysarthria. Lowering of the convulsion threshold and convulsions may occur, particularly in epileptic patients.

Sense organs:

Occasional (> 1%, <10%): accommodation disorders, visual disturbance.

Rare (> 0.001%, <1%): dysgeusia.

Gastro-intestinal tract:

Frequent (>10%): nausea.

Occasional (> 1%, <10%): mild gastro-intestinal disturbances constipation, diarrhoea, retching and vomiting.

Rare (> 0.001%, <1%): abdominal pain

Cardiovascular system:

Occasional (> 1%, <10%): hypotension, diminished cardiovascular function.

Urogenital system:

Frequent (>10%): frequency of micturition, enuresis, dysuria.

Rare (> 0.001%, <1%): urinary retention, impotence.

Liver:

Rare (> 0.001%, <1%): disorders of hepatic function.

Skin:

Occasional (> 1%, <10%): hyperhydrosis, skin rash.

Certain patients have shown increased spasticity as a paradoxical reaction to the medication.

An undesirable degree of muscular hypotonia – making it more difficult for patients to walk or fend for themselves – may occur and can usually be relieved by re-adjusting the dosage (i.e. by reducing the doses given during the day and possibly increasing the evening dose).

The excipient sorbitol may have a mild laxative effect when taken in large amounts and hydroxybenzoates may cause allergic reactions which may be possibly delayed.

4.9 Overdose

Symptoms:

Prominent features of overdosage are signs of central nervous depression: drowsiness, impairment of consciousness, respiratory depression, coma. Also liable to occur are: confusion, hallucinations, agitation, accommodation disorders, absent pupillary reflex; generalised muscular hypotonia, myoclonia, hyporeflexia or areflexia; convulsions; peripheral vasodilatation, hypotension, bradycardia; hypothermia; nausea, vomiting, diarrhoea, hypersalivation; elevated LDH, SGOT and AP values.

A deterioration in the condition may occur if various substances or drugs acting on the central nervous system (e.g. alcohol, diazepam, tricyclic antidepressants) have been taken at the same time.

Treatment:

No specific antidote is known.

Elimination of the drug from the gastro-intestinal tract (induction of vomiting, gastric lavage; comatose patients should be intubated prior to gastric lavage), administration of activated charcoal; if necessary, saline aperient; in respiratory depression, administration of artificial respiration, also measures in support of cardiovascular functions. Since the drug is excreted chiefly via the kidneys, generous quantities of fluid should be given, possibly together with a diuretic. In the event of convulsions diazepam should be administered cautiously i.v.

5. PHARMACOLOGICAL PROPERTIES

5.1 Pharmacodynamic properties

Baclofen is an antispastic agent acting at the spinal level. It is a gamma-aminobutyric acid (GABA) derivative, with a similar chemical structure, but differing in action.

Baclofen depresses monosynaptic and polysynaptic reflex transmission, probably by stimulating the GABA beta receptors, this stimulation in turn inhibiting the release of the excitatory amino acids glutamate and aspartate. Neuromuscular transmission is unaffected by baclofen.

The major benefits of baclofen stem from its ability to reduce painful flexor spasms and spontaneous clonus thereby facilitating the mobility of the patient, increasing their independence and helping rehabilitation.

Baclofen also exerts an antinociceptive effect. General well being is often improved and sedation is less often a problem than with centrally acting drugs.

Baclofen stimulates gastric acid secretion.

5.2 Pharmacokinetic properties

Absorption:

Baclofen is rapidly and completely absorbed from the gastro-intestinal tract. No significant difference between the liquid and tablet formulations is observed in respect of t_{max}, C_{max} and bioavailability.

Following oral administration of single doses (10-30mg) peak plasma concentrations are reached after 0.5 to 3.0 hours and the areas under the serum concentration curves are proportional to the dose.

Distribution:

The volume of distribution of baclofen is 0.7 l/kg and the protein binding rate is approximately 30%. In cerebrospinal fluid active substance concentrations are approximately 8.5 times lower than in the plasma.

Biotransformation:

Baclofen is metabolised to only a minor extent. Deamination yields the main metabolite, β-(p-chlorophenyl)-4-hydroxybutyric acid, which is pharmacologically inactive.

Elimination / excretion:

The plasma elimination half-life of baclofen averages 3 to 4 hours. The serum protein binding rate is approximately 30%.

Baclofen is eliminated largely in unchanged form. Within 72 hours, about 75% of the dose is excreted via the kidneys with about 5% of this amount as metabolites.

Elderly:

The pharmacokinetics of baclofen in elderly patients are virtually the same as in young subjects. The peak plasma concentrations of baclofen in elderly patients are slightly lower and occur later than in healthy young subjects but the AUCs are similar in the two groups.

5.3 Preclinical safety data

Baclofen increases the incidence of omphaloceles (ventral hernias) in the foetuses of rats given approximately 13 times the maximum oral dose (on a mg/kg basis) recommended for human use. This was not seen in mice or rabbits.

A dose related increase in the incidence of ovarian cysts, and a less marked increase in enlarged and/or haemorrhagic adrenals have been observed in female rats treated for 2 years. The clinical relevance of these findings is not known.

Experimental evidence to date suggests that baclofen does not possess either carcinogenic or mutagenic properties.

6. PHARMACEUTICAL PARTICULARS

6.1 List of excipients

70% Sorbitol Solution

Methyl hydroxybenzoate,

Propyl hydroxybenzoate,

Raspberry flavour (contains propylene glycol),

Carmellose Sodium,

Purified water.

Baclofen Oral Solution is sugar free.

6.2 Incompatibilities

None known.

6.3 Shelf life

24 months

Once opened use within 56 days of first opening

Baclofen Oral Solution may be diluted with purified water. The shelf life of the diluted solution is 14 days when stored not above 25°C.

6.4 Special precautions for storage

Do not store above 25°C

Store in the original container

Do not refrigerate or freeze

6.5 Nature and contents of container

Pharmaceutical grade type III amber glass bottle with child resistant and tamper evident polypropylene faced cap with an EPE liner

6.6 Instructions for use and handling

There is no specific instruction for use/handling.

7. MARKETING AUTHORISATION HOLDER

Chemidex Pharma Limited,

Egham Business Village,

Crabtree Road,

Egham,

Surrey,

TW20 8RB

8. MARKETING AUTHORISATION NUMBER(S)

PL 17736 / 0061

9. DATE OF FIRST AUTHORISATION/RENEWAL OF THE AUTHORISATION

24 May 2004

10. DATE OF REVISION OF THE TEXT

10 June 2004

Lyrica Capsules

(Pfizer Limited)

1. NAME OF THE MEDICINAL PRODUCT

LYRICA▼ 25 mg hard capsules

LYRICA▼ 50 mg hard capsules

LYRICA▼ 75 mg hard capsules

LYRICA▼ 100 mg hard capsules

LYRICA▼ 150 mg hard capsules

LYRICA▼ 200 mg hard capsules

LYRICA▼ 300 mg hard capsules

2. QUALITATIVE AND QUANTITATIVE COMPOSITION

Each hard capsule contains 25 mg, 50 mg, 75 mg, 100 mg, 150 mg, 200 mg, or 300 mg of pregabalin.

For excipients, see section 6.1.

3. PHARMACEUTICAL FORM

Hard capsule

25 mg capsule: White hard gelatine capsule, marked "Pfizer" on the cap and "PGN 25" on the body with black ink.

50 mg capsule: White hard gelatine capsule, marked "Pfizer" on the cap and "PGN 50" on the body with black ink. The body is also marked with a black band.

75 mg capsule: White and orange hard gelatine capsule, marked "Pfizer" on the cap and "PGN 75" on the body with black ink.

100 mg capsule: Orange hard gelatine capsules, marked "Pfizer" on the cap and "PGN 100" on the body with black ink.

150 mg capsule: White hard gelatine capsule, marked "Pfizer" on the cap and "PGN 150" on the body with black ink.

Table 1 Pregabalin dosage adjustment based on renal function

Creatinine Clearance (CL_{cr}) (ml/min)	Total Pregabalin Daily dose *		Dose Regimen
	Starting dose (mg/day)	Maximum dose (mg/day)	
⩾ 60	150	600	BID or TID
⩾30 - <60	75	300	BID or TID
⩾15 - <30	25 – 50	150	Once Daily or BID
< 15	25	75	Once Daily
Supplementary dosage following haemodialysis (mg)			
	25	100	Single dose⁺

TID = Three divided doses

BID = Two divided doses

* Total daily dose (mg/day) should be divided as indicated by dose regimen to provide mg/dose

⁺ Supplementary dose is a single additional dose

200 mg capsule: Light orange hard gelatine capsules, marked "Pfizer" on the cap and "PGN 200" on the body with black ink.

300 mg capsule: White and orange hard gelatine capsule, marked "Pfizer" on the cap and "PGN 300" on the body with black ink.

4. CLINICAL PARTICULARS

4.1 Therapeutic indications

Neuropathic pain

Lyrica is indicated for the treatment of peripheral neuropathic pain in adults.

Epilepsy

Lyrica is indicated as adjunctive therapy in adults with partial seizures with or without secondary generalisation.

4.2 Posology and method of administration

The dose range is 150 to 600 mg per day given in either two or three divided doses.

Lyrica may be taken with or without food.

Neuropathic pain

Pregabalin treatment can be started at a dose of 150 mg per day. Based on individual patient response and tolerability, the dosage may be increased to 300 mg per day after an interval of 3 to 7 days, and if needed, to a maximum dose of 600 mg per day after an additional 7-day interval.

Epilepsy

Pregabalin treatment can be started with a dose of 150 mg per day. Based on individual patient response and tolerability, the dosage may be increased to 300 mg per day after 1 week. The maximum dosage of 600 mg per day may be achieved after an additional week.

Discontinuation of pregabalin

In accordance with current clinical practice, if pregabalin has to be discontinued either in neuropathic pain or epilepsy, it is recommended this should be done gradually over a minimum of 1 week

Patients with renal impairment

Pregabalin is eliminated from the systemic circulation primarily by renal excretion as unchanged drug. As pregabalin clearance is directly proportional to creatinine clearance (see section 5.2), dosage reduction in patients with compromised renal function must be individualised according to creatinine clearance (CLcr), as indicated in Table 1 determined using the following formula:

$$CL_{cr}(ml/min) = \frac{[140 - age(years)] \times weight(kg)}{72 \times serum\ creatinine\ (mg/dl)} (\times 0.85 \text{ for female patients})$$

Pregabalin is removed effectively from plasma by haemodialysis (50% of drug in 4 hours). For patients receiving haemodialysis, the pregabalin daily dose should be adjusted based on renal function. In addition to the daily dose, a supplementary dose should be given immediately following every 4-hour haemodialysis treatment (see Table 1).

Table 1. Pregabalin dosage adjustment based on renal function

(see Table 1 above)

Use in patients with hepaticimpairment

No dosage adjustment is required for patients with hepatic impairment (see section 5.2).

Use in children and adolescents (12 to 17 years of age)

The safety and effectiveness of pregabalin in paediatric patients below the age of 12 years and adolescents has not been established.

The use in children is not recommended (see section 5.3)

Use in the elderly (over 65 years of age)

Elderly patients may require a dose reduction of pregabalin due to a decreased renal function (see patients with renal impairment).

4.3 Contraindications

Hypersensitivity to the active substance or to any of the excipients.

4.4 Special warnings and special precautions for use

Patients with rare hereditary problems of galactose intolerance, the Lapp lactase deficiency or glucose-galactose malabsorption should not take this medicine.

In accordance with current clinical practice, some diabetic patients who gain weight on pregabalin treatment may need to adjust hypoglycaemic medications.

Pregabalin treatment has been associated with dizziness and somnolence, which could increase the occurrence of accidental injury (fall) in the elderly population. Therefore, patients should be advised to exercise caution until they are familiar with the potential effects of the medication.

There are insufficient data for the withdrawal of concomitant antiepileptic medicinal products, once seizure control with pregabalin in the add-on situation has been reached, in order to reach monotherapy on pregabalin.

4.5 Interaction with other medicinal products and other forms of Interaction

Since pregabalin is predominantly excreted unchanged in the urine, undergoes negligible metabolism in humans (<2% of a dose recovered in urine as metabolites), does not inhibit drug metabolism *in vitro*, and is not bound to plasma proteins, it is unlikely to produce, or be subject to, pharmacokinetic interactions.

Accordingly, in *in vivo* studies no clinically relevant pharmacokinetic interactions were observed between pregabalin and phenytoin, carbamazepine, valproic acid, lamotrigine, gabapentin, lorazepam, oxycodone or ethanol. Population pharmacokinetic analysis indicated that oral antidiabetics, diuretics, insulin, phenobarbital, tiagabine and topiramate had no clinically significant effect on pregabalin clearance.

Co-administration of pregabalin with the oral contraceptives norethisterone and/or ethinyl oestradiol does not influence the steady-state pharmacokinetics of either substance.

Multiple oral doses of pregabalin co-administered with oxycodone, lorazepam, or ethanol did not result in clinically important effects on respiration. Pregabalin appears to be additive in the impairment of cognitive and gross motor function caused by oxycodone. Pregabalin may potentiate the effects of ethanol and lorazepam.

No specific pharmacodynamic interaction studies were conducted in elderly volunteers.

4.6 Pregnancy and lactation

There are no adequate data on the use of pregabalin in pregnant women.

Studies in animals have shown reproductive toxicity (see section 5.3). The potential risk to humans is unknown. Therefore, Lyrica should not be used during pregnancy unless the benefit to the mother clearly outweighs the potential risk to the foetus. Effective contraception must be used in women of child bearing potential.

It is not known if pregabalin is excreted in the breast milk of humans; however, it is present in the milk of rats. Therefore, breast-feeding is not recommended during treatment with pregabalin.

4.7 Effects on ability to drive and use machines

Lyrica may cause dizziness and somnolence and therefore may influence the ability to drive or use machines. Patients are advised not to drive, operate complex machinery or engage in other potentially hazardous activities until it is known whether this medication affects their ability to perform these activities.

4.8 Undesirable effects

The pregabalin clinical programme involved over 9000 patients who were exposed to pregabalin, of whom over 5000 were in double-blind placebo controlled trials. The most commonly reported adverse reactions were dizziness and somnolence. Adverse reactions were usually mild to moderate in intensity. In all controlled studies, the discontinuation rate due to adverse reactions was 13% for patients receiving pregabalin and 7% for patients receiving placebo. The most common adverse reactions resulting in discontinuation from pregabalin treatment groups were dizziness and somnolence.

In the table below all adverse reactions, which occurred at an incidence greater than placebo and in more than one patient, are listed by class and frequency (very common > 1/10), common > 1/100, < 1/10), uncommon >1/1000, <1/100) and rare (<1/1000)).

The adverse reactions listed may also be associated with the underlying disease and / or concomitant medications.

Body System	Adverse drug reactions
Blood and lymphatic system disorders	
Rare	Neutropenia
Metabolism and nutrition disorders	
Common	Appetite increased
Uncommon	Anorexia
Rare	Hypoglycaemia
Psychiatric disorders	
Common	Euphoric mood, confusion, libido decreased, irritability
Uncommon	Depersonalisation, anorgasmia, restlessness, depression, agitation, mood swings, insomnia exacerbated, depressed mood, word finding difficulty, hallucination, abnormal dreams, libido increased, panic attack, apathy
Rare	Disinhibition, elevated mood
Nervous system disorders	
Very Common	Dizziness, somnolence
Common	Ataxia, disturbance in attention, coordination abnormal, memory impairment, tremor, dysarthria, paraesthesia
Uncommon	Cognitive disorder, hypoaesthesia, visual field defect, nystagmus, speech disorder, myoclonus, hyporeflexia, dyskinesia, psychomotor hyperactivity, dizziness postural, hyperaesthesia, ageusia, burning sensation, intention tremor, stupor, syncope
Rare	Hypokinesia, parosmia, dysgraphia
Eye disorders	
Common	Vision blurred, diplopia
Uncommon	Visual disturbance, dry eye, eye swelling, visual acuity reduced, eye pain, asthenopia, lacrimation increased
Rare	Photopsia, eye irritation, mydriasis, oscillopsia, altered visual depth perception, peripheral vision loss, strabismus, visual brightness
Ear and labyrinth disorders	
Common	Vertigo
Rare	Hyperacusis
Cardiac disorders	
Uncommon	Tachycardia
Rare	Atrioventricular block first degree, sinus tachycardia, sinus arrhythmia, sinus bradycardia
Vascular disorders	
Uncommon	Flushing, hot flushes
Rare	Hypotension, peripheral coldness, hypertension

Respiratory, thoracic and mediastinal disorders	
Uncommon	Dyspnoea, nasal dryness
Rare	Nasopharyngitis, cough, nasal congestion, epistaxis, rhinitis, snoring, throat tightness
Gastrointestinal disorders	
Common	Dry mouth, constipation, vomiting, flatulence
Uncommon	Abdominal distension, salivary hypersecretion, gastroesophageal reflux disease, hypoaesthesia oral
Rare	Ascites, dysphagia, pancreatitis
Skin and subcutaneous tissue disorders	
Uncommon	Sweating, rash papular
Rare	Cold sweat, urticaria
Musculoskeletal and connective tissue disorders	
Uncommon	Muscle twitching, joint swelling, muscle cramp, myalgia, arthralgia, back pain, pain in limb, muscle stiffness
Rare	Cervical spasm, neck pain, rhabdomyolysis
Renal and urinary disorders	
Uncommon	Dysuria, urinary incontinence
Rare	Oliguria, renal failure
Reproductive system and breast disorders	
Common	Erectile dysfunction
Uncommon	Ejaculation delayed, sexual dysfunction
Rare	Amenorrhoea, breast pain, breast discharge, dysmenorrhoea, hypertrophy breast
General disorders and administration site conditions	
Common	Fatigue, oedema peripheral, feeling drunk, oedema, gait abnormal
Uncommon	Asthenia, fall, thirst, chest tightness
Rare	Pain exacerbated anasarca, pyrexia, rigors
Investigations	
Common	Weight increased
Uncommon	Alanine aminotransferase increased, blood creatine phosphokinase increased, aspartate aminotransferase increased, platelet count decreased
Rare	Blood glucose increased, blood creatinine increased, blood potassium decreased, weight decreased, white blood cell count decreased

4.9 Overdose

In overdoses up to 15 g, no unexpected adverse reactions were reported. Treatment of pregabalin overdose should include general supportive measures and may include haemodialysis if necessary (see section 4.2 Table 1).

5. PHARMACOLOGICAL PROPERTIES

5.1 Pharmacodynamic properties

Pharmacotherapeutic group: Antiepileptics, ATC code: N03AX16

The active substance, pregabalin, is a gamma-aminobutyric acid analogue ((S)-3-(aminomethyl)-5-methylhexanoic acid).

Mechanism of action

Pregabalin binds to an auxiliary subunit (α_2-δ protein) of voltage-gated calcium channels in the central nervous system, potently displacing [^{3}H]-gabapentin.

Clinical experience

Neuropathic pain

Efficacy has been shown in studies in diabetic neuropathy and post herpetic neuralgia. Efficacy has not been studied in other models of neuropathic pain.

Pregabalin has been studied in 9 controlled clinical studies of up to 13 weeks with twice a day dosing (BID) and up to 8 weeks with three times a day (TID) dosing. Overall, the safety and efficacy profiles for BID and TID dosing regimens were similar.

In clinical trials up to 13 weeks, a reduction in pain was seen by week 1 and was maintained throughout the treatment period.

In controlled clinical trials 35% of the pregabalin treated patients and 18% of the patients on placebo had a 50% improvement in pain score. For patients not experiencing somnolence, such an improvement was observed in 33% of patients treated with pregabalin and 18% of patients on placebo. For patients who experienced somnolence the responder rates were 48% on pregabalin and 16% on placebo.

Epilepsy

Pregabalin has been studied in 3 controlled clinical studies of 12 week duration with either twice a day dosing (BID) or three times a day (TID) dosing. Overall, the safety and efficacy profiles for BID and TID dosing regimens were similar.

A reduction in seizure frequency was observed by Week 1.

5.2 Pharmacokinetic properties

Pregabalin steady-state pharmacokinetics are similar in healthy volunteers, patients with epilepsy receiving anti-epileptic drugs and patients with chronic pain.

Absorption:

Pregabalin is rapidly absorbed when administered in the fasted state, with peak plasma concentrations occurring within 1 hourfollowing both single and multiple dose administration. Pregabalin oral bioavailability is estimated to be ≥90% and is independent of dose. Following repeated administration, steady state is achieved within 24 to 48 hours. The rate of pregabalin absorption is decreased when given with food resulting in a decrease in C_{max} by approximately 25-30% and a delay in t_{max} to approximately 2.5 hours. However, administration of pregabalin with food has no clinically significant effect on the extent of pregabalin absorption.

Distribution:

In preclinical studies, pregabalin has been shown to cross the blood brain barrier in mice, rats, and monkeys. Pregabalin has been shown to cross the placenta in rats and is present in the milk of lactating rats. In humans, the apparent volume of distribution of pregabalin following oral administration is approximately 0.56 l/kg. Pregabalin is not bound to plasma proteins.

Metabolism:

Pregabalin undergoes negligible metabolism in humans. Following a dose of radiolabelled pregabalin, approximately 98% of the radioactivity recovered in the urine was unchanged pregabalin. The N-methylated derivative of pregabalin, the major metabolite of pregabalin found in urine, accounted for 0.9% of the dose. In preclinical studies, there was no indication of racemisation of pregabalin S-enantiomer to the R-enantiomer.

Elimination:

Pregabalin is eliminated from the systemic circulation primarily by renal excretion as unchanged drug.

Pregabalin mean elimination half-life is 6.3 hours. Pregabalin plasma clearance and renal clearance are directly proportional to creatinine clearance (see section 5.2 Renal impairment).

Dosage adjustment in patients with reduced renal function or undergoing haemodialysis is necessary (see Section 4.2 Table 1).

Linearity / non-linearity:

Pregabalin pharmacokinetics are linear over the recommended daily dose range. Inter-subject pharmacokinetic variability for pregabalin is low (<20%). Multiple dose pharmacokinetics are predictable from single-dose data. Therefore, there is no need for routine monitoring of plasma concentrations of pregabalin.

Pharmacokinetics in special patient groups

Gender

Clinical trials indicate that gender does not have a clinically significant influence on the plasma concentrations of pregabalin.

Renal impairment

Pregabalin clearance is directly proportional to creatinine clearance. In addition, pregabalin is effectively removed from plasma by haemodialysis (following a 4 hour haemodialysis treatment plasma pregabalin concentrations are reduced by approximately 50%). Because renal elimination is the major elimination pathway, dosage reduction in patients with renal impairment and dosage supplementation following haemodialysis is necessary (see section 4.2 Table 1).

Hepatic impairment

No specific pharmacokinetic studies were carried out in patients with impaired liver function. Since pregabalin does not undergo significant metabolism and is excreted predominantly as unchanged drug in the urine, impaired liver function would not be expected to significantly alter pregabalin plasma concentrations.

Elderly (over 65 years of age)

Pregabalin clearance tends to decrease with increasing age. This decrease in pregabalin oral clearance is consistent with decreases in creatinine clearance associated with increasing age. Reduction of pregabalin dose may be required in patients who have age related compromised renal function (see section 4.2 Table 1).

5.3 Preclinical safety data

In conventional safety pharmacology studies in animals, pregabalin was well-tolerated at clinically relevant doses. In repeated dose toxicity studies in rats and monkeys CNS effects were observed, including hypoactivity, hyperactivity and ataxia. An increased incidence of retinal atrophy commonly observed in aged albino rats was seen after long term exposure to pregabalin at exposures≥ 5 times the mean human exposure at the maximum recommended clinical dose.

Pregabalin was not teratogenic in mice, rats or rabbits. Foetal toxicity in rats and rabbits occurred only at exposures sufficiently above human exposure. In prenatal/postnatal toxicity studies, pregabalin induced offspring developmental toxicity in rats at exposures >2 times the maximum recommended human exposure.

Pregabalin is not genotoxic based on results of a battery of *in vitro* and *in vivo* tests.

Two-year carcinogenicity studies with pregabalin were conducted in rats and mice. No tumours were observed in rats at exposures up to 24 times the mean human exposure at the maximum recommended clinical dose of 600 mg/day. In mice, no increased incidence of tumours was found at exposures similar to the mean human exposure, but an increased incidence of haemangiosarcoma was observed at higher exposures. The non-genotoxic mechanism of pregabalin-induced tumour formation in mice involves platelet changes and associated endothelial cell proliferation. These platelet changes were not present in rats or in humans based on short term and limited long term clinical data. There is no evidence to suggest an associated risk to humans.

In juvenile rats the types of toxicity do not differ qualitatively from those observed in adult rats. However, juvenile rats are more sensitive. At therapeutic exposures, there was evidence of CNS clinical signs of hyperactivity and bruxism and some changes in growth (transient body weight gain suppression). Effects on the oestrus cycle were observed at 5-fold the human therapeutic exposure. Neurobehavioural/cognitive effects were observed in juvenile rats 1-2 weeks after exposure >2 times (acoustic startle response) or >5 times (learning/memory) the human therapeutic exposure.

6. PHARMACEUTICAL PARTICULARS

6.1 List of excipients

Capsule content:

Lactose monohydrate

Maize starch

Talc

Capsule shell:

Gelatin

Titanium Dioxide (E171)

Sodium Laurilsulfate

Silica, colloidal anhydrous

Purified water

75 mg, 100 mg, 200 mg and 300 mg shells only:

Red Iron Oxide (E172)

Printing Ink:

Shellac

Black Iron Oxide (E172)

Propylene Glycol

Potassium Hydroxide

6.2 Incompatibilities

Not applicable.

6.3 Shelf life

3 years.

6.4 Special precautions for storage

This medicinal product does not require any special storage conditions

6.5 Nature and contents of container

PVC/Aluminium blisters containing 14, 21, 56, 84 or 112 (2 × 56) hard capsules.

PVC/Aluminium perforated unit dose blisters containing 100 × 1 hard capsules.

HDPE bottle containing 200 hard capsules.

Not all pack sizes may be marketed

6.6 Instructions for use and handling

No special requirements.

7. MARKETING AUTHORISATION HOLDER
Pfizer Limited,
Ramsgate Road,
Sandwich,
Kent
CT13 9NJ
UK

8. MARKETING AUTHORISATION NUMBER(S)
EU/1/04/279/001 - 032

9. DATE OF FIRST AUTHORISATION/RENEWAL OF THE AUTHORISATION
July 2004

10. DATE OF REVISION OF THE TEXT
July 2005

11. LEGAL CATEGORY
POM

Lyrinel XL prolonged release tablet

(Janssen-Cilag Ltd)

1. NAME OF THE MEDICINAL PRODUCT
Lyrinel XL® 5 mg prolonged release tablet
Lyrinel XL® 10 mg prolonged release tablet

2. QUALITATIVE AND QUANTITATIVE COMPOSITION
Each tablet contains oxybutynin hydrochloride 5 mg
Each tablet contains oxybutynin hydrochloride 10 mg
For excipients, see Section 6.1.

3. PHARMACEUTICAL FORM
Prolonged release tablet.

Lyrinel XL 5 mg: Round yellow coloured tablet printed "5 XL" with black ink.

Lyrinel XL 10 mg: Round pink coloured tablet printed "10 XL" with black ink.

4. CLINICAL PARTICULARS

4.1 Therapeutic indications
For the symptomatic treatment of urge incontinence and/or increased urinary frequency associated with urgency as may occur in patients with unstable bladder.

4.2 Posology and method of administration
Dosage (adults and elderly)
Starting dose: the recommended starting dose is one 5 mg tablet once daily.

Maintenance dose/dose adjustment: In order to achieve a maintenance dose giving an optimal balance of efficacy and tolerability, after at least one week on 5 mg daily, the dose may be increased to 10 mg once daily, with subsequent incremental increases or decreases of 5 mg/day. There should be an interval of at least one week between dose changes.

Maximum dose: in patients requiring a higher dose, the total daily dose should not exceed 20 mg.

For patients currently taking oxybutynin immediate release, clinical judgement should be exercised in selecting the appropriate dose of Lyrinel XL. The dosage should be adjusted to the minimum dose that achieves an optimal balance of efficacy and tolerability, taking into account the current immediate-release dose.

The safety and efficacy of Lyrinel XL have not been established in patients under 18 years. The use of Lyrinel XL in children is not recommended.

Method of administration
Lyrinel XL must be swallowed whole with the aid of liquid, and must not be chewed, divided, or crushed.

Patients should be advised that the tablet membrane may pass through the gastrointestinal tract unchanged. This has no bearing on the efficacy of the product.

Lyrinel XL may be administered with or without food (cf. 5.2 Pharmacokinetics).

4.3 Contraindications
- Hypersensitivity to oxybutynin or any of the excipients
- Narrow-angle glaucoma or shallow anterior chamber
- Myasthenia gravis
- Patients with urinary retention
- Gastrointestinal obstructive disorder, paralytic ileus or intestinal atony
- Severe ulcerative colitis
- Toxic megacolon
- Urinary frequency and nocturia due to heart or renal failure

4.4 Special warnings and special precautions for use
Oxybutynin should be used with caution in the frail elderly who may be more sensitive to the effects of oxybutynin, in patients with gastro-intestinal motility disorders, particularly gastroesophageal reflux, and in patients with hepatic or renal impairment.

Oxybutynin should be used with caution in patients with clinically significant bladder outflow obstruction since anticholinergic drugs may aggravate bladder outflow and cause retention.

If urinary tract infection is present, an appropriate antibacterial therapy should be started.

Oxybutynin may aggravate the symptoms of hyperthyroidism, congestive heart failure, cardiac arrhythmia, tachycardia, hypertension and prostatic hypertrophy.

When oxybutynin is used in patients with fever or in high environmental temperatures, this can cause heat prostration due to decreased sweating.

Patients with rare hereditary problems of galactose intolerance, the Lapp lactase deficiency or glucose-galactose malabsorption should not take this medicine.

Oxybutynin may lead to decreased salivary secretions which could result in tooth caries, periodontitis, or oral candidiasis.

4.5 Interaction with other medicinal products and other forms of Interaction
The concomitant use of oxybutynin with other anticholinergic medicinal products or drugs with anticholinergic activity, such as amantadine and other anticholinergic antiparkinsonian drugs (e.g. biperiden, levodopa), antihistamines, antipsychotics (e.g. phenothiazines, butyrophenones, clozapine), quinidine, tricyclic antidepressants, atropine and related compounds like atropine antispasmodics, dipyridamole, may increase the frequency or severity of dry mouth, constipation and drowsiness.

Anticholinergic agents may potentially alter the absorption of some concomitantly administered drugs due to anticholinergic effects on gastrointestinal motility.

Oxybutynin is metabolised by cytochrome P450 isoenzyme CYP3A4. Mean oxybutynin chloride concentrations were approximately 2 fold higher when Lyrinel XL was administered with ketoconazole, a potent CYP3A4 inhibitor. Other inhibitors of cytochrome P450 3A4 enzyme system, such as antimycotic agents (e.g. itraconazole and fluconazole) or macrolide antibiotics (e.g. erythromycin), may alter oxybutynin pharmacokinetics. The clinical relevance of such potential interaction is not known. Caution should be used when such drugs are co-administered.

The effect of prokinetics may be decreased by anticholinergic agents. However, the interaction between prokinetics and oxybutynin has not been studied.

4.6 Pregnancy and lactation
Pregnancy
There are no adequate data on the use of oxybutynin in pregnant women. Studies in animals have shown minor reproductive toxicity (see Section 5.3). Lyrinel XL should only be used during pregnancy if the expected benefit outweighs the risk.

Lactation
When oxybutynin is used during lactation, a small amount is excreted in the mother's milk. Breast feeding while using oxybutynin is therefore not recommended.

4.7 Effects on ability to drive and use machines
As oxybutynin may produce drowsiness or blurred vision, the patient should be cautioned regarding activities requiring mental alertness such as driving, operating machinery or performing hazardous work while taking this drug.

4.8 Undesirable effects
In clinical trials with Lyrinel XL (n=1006), adverse reactions were caused mainly by the anticholinergic actions of oxybutynin. As with other oxybutynin formulations, dry mouth was the most frequently reported adverse reaction.

Frequency estimate: Very Common $>$ 10%; Common $>$ 1% to $<$ 10%; Uncommon $>$ 0.1% to $<$ 1%; Rare $>$ 0.01% to $<$ 0.1%; Very Rare $<$ 0.01%.

Blood and Lymphatic system disorders: Rare: Leukopenia, thrombocytopenia.

Cardiac Disorders: Common: Palpitation. Uncommon: Tachycardia. Rare: Arrhythmia, atrial arrhythmia, bradycardia, bundle branch block, nodal arrhythmia, supraventricular extrasystoles.

Eye disorders: Common: Vision blurred, dry eye. Uncommon: Conjunctivitis. Rare: Diplopia, glaucoma, photophobia.

Gastrointestinal Disorders: Very common: Dry mouth. Common: constipation, diarrhoea, nausea, dyspepsia, abdominal pain, dysgeusia, flatulence, gastrooesophageal reflux. Uncommon: dysphagia, vomiting, mouth ulceration, abdominal distension, glossitis, stomatitis. Rare: Faecal abnormality, oesophageal stenosis acquired, gastritis, gastroenteritis viral, hernia, rectal disorder, gastric atony, tongue disorder, tongue oedema.

General Disorders: Common: Asthenia, mucosal dryness. Uncommon: Chest pain, thirst. Rare: Rigor, pyrexia, influenza like illness, malaise, pelvic pain.

Immune System Disorder: Rare: Hypersensitivity

Investigations: Uncommon: Electrocardiogram abnormal, blood urea increased, blood creatinine increased. Rare: Blood alkaline phosphatase increased, blood lactase dehydrogenase increased, blood aspartate aminotransferase increased, blood alanine aminotransferase increased.

Metabolic and nutrition disorders: Common: Oedema peripheral. Uncommon: Anorexia, oedema, dehydration, hyperglycaemia. Rare: appetite increased.

Musculoskeletal and connective tissue disorders: Uncommon: Muscle cramps, back pain, myalgia. Rare: Arthralgia, arthritis.

Nervous system disorders: Common: Somnolence, headache, dizziness, insomnia, nervousness, confusional state. Uncommon: Abnormal dreams, paraesthesia, vertigo. Rare: Hypertonia, tremor, tinnitus.

Psychiatric disorders: Uncommon: Anxiety, depression.

Renal and Urinary disorders: Common: Micturition disorder, residual urine volume, urinary retention, urinary tract infection, dysuria. Uncommon: Urinary frequency, cystitis, urinary tract disorder, haematuria, nocturia, pyuria, micturition urgency. Rare: Urinary incontinence, urine abnormal, urogenital disorder.

Reproductive system and breast disorders: Uncommon: Breast pain, vaginitis. Rare: Vulvovaginal disorder, uterine cervical disorder, genital discharge.

Respiratory, thoracic and mediastinal disorders: Common: pharyngitis. Uncommon: Cough, rhinitis, hoarseness, epistaxis, upper respiratory tract infection, dyspnoea, sinusitis. Rare: Bronchitis, laryngitis, laryngeal oedema, respiratory disorder, sputum increased.

Skin and subcutaneous tissue disorders: Common: Dry skin. Uncommon: Pruritus, rash, acne, urticaria, face oedema, alopecia, eczema, nail disorder, skin discolouration, anhidrosis. Rare: Hair disorder, rash maculo-papular, granuloma, sweating increased, photosensitivity reaction.

Vascular disorders: Uncommon: Hypertension, vasodilatation, migraine. Rare: Hypotension, phlebitis, ecchymosis.

In clinical studies, dry mouth has been less frequently reported with Lyrinel XL than with oxybutynin immediate release formulations.

Adverse events were generally dose related. For patients who required final doses of 5 or 10 mg of Lyrinel XL, the relative incidence of dry mouth that occurred at any dose level was 1.8 times lower compared with patients who required final doses $>$ 10 mg.

Post-marketing experience with Lyrinel XL:

Additional rare adverse events reported from worldwide post-marketing experience with oxybutynin chloride include hallucinations, convulsions and erectile dysfunction.

4.9 Overdose
The symptoms of overdosage with oxybutynin progress from an intensification of the usual CNS disturbances (from restlessness and excitement to psychotic behaviour), circulatory changes (flushing, fall in blood pressure, circulatory failure etc.), respiratory failure, paralysis and coma.

Measures to be taken are:

1) administration of activated charcoal

2) physostigmine by slow intravenous injection:

Adults: 0.5 to 2.0 mg i.v. slowly, repeated after 5 minutes if necessary, up to a maximum of 5 mg.

Fever should be treated symptomatically with tepid sponging or ice packs.

In pronounced restlessness or excitation, diazepam 10 mg may be given by intravenous injection. Tachycardia may be treated with intravenous propranolol and urinary retention managed by bladder catheterisation.

In the event of progression of curare-like effects to paralysis of the respiratory muscles, mechanical ventilation will be required.

The continuous release of oxybutynin from Lyrinel XL should be considered in the treatment of overdosage. Patients should be monitored for at least 24 hours.

5. PHARMACOLOGICAL PROPERTIES

5.1 Pharmacodynamic properties
Pharmacotherapeutic group: urinary antispasmodic, ATC code: G04B D04.

Mechanism of action: oxybutynin acts as a competitive antagonist of acetylcholine at post-ganglionic muscarinic receptors, resulting in relaxation of bladder smooth muscle.

Pharmacodynamic effects: in patients with overactive bladder, characterized by detrusor muscle instability or hyperreflexia, cystometric studies have demonstrated that oxybutynin increases maximum urinary bladder capacity and increases the volume to first detrusor contraction. Oxybutynin thus decreases urinary urgency and frequency of both incontinence episodes and voluntary urination.

Oxybutynin is a racemic (50:50) mixture of R- and S-isomers. Antimuscarinic activity resides predominantly in the R-isomer. The R-isomer of oxybutynin shows greater selectivity for the M_1 and M_3 muscarinic subtypes (predominant in bladder detrusor muscle and parotid gland) compared to the M_2 subtype (predominant in cardiac tissue). The active metabolite, N-desethyloxybutynin, has pharmacological activity on the human detrusor muscle that is similar to that of oxybutynin *in vitro* studies, but has a greater binding affinity for parotid tissue than oxybutynin. The free base form of oxybutynin is pharmacologically equivalent to oxybutynin hydrochloride.

5.2 Pharmacokinetic properties
Following the first dose of Lyrinel XL, oxybutynin plasma concentrations rise for 4 to 6 hours; thereafter, concentrations are maintained for up to 24 hours, thus reducing the

fluctuations between peak and trough concentrations associated with oxybutynin immediate release formulations.

The relative bioavailabilities of R-oxybutynin and S-oxybutynin from Lyrinel XL are 156% and 187% respectively, compared with oxybutynin immediate release. After a 10 mg single dose of Lyrinel XL, the peak plasma concentrations of R-oxybutynin and S-oxybutynin, achieved after 12.7±5.4 and 11.8±5.3 hours respectively, are 1.0±0.6 and 1.8±1.0 ng/ml, and the plasma concentration time profiles of both enantiomers are similar in shape. The elimination half-life is 13.2±10.3 hours for R-oxybutynin and 12.4±6.1 hours for S-oxybutynin.

Steady state oxybutynin plasma concentrations are achieved by Day 3 of repeated Lyrinel XL dosing, with no observed change in oxybutynin and desethyloxybutynin pharmacokinetic parameters over time.

Pharmacokinetic parameters of oxybutynin and desethyloxybutynin (C_{max} and AUC) are dose proportional following administration of 5-20 mg of Lyrinel XL.

The pharmacokinetics of Lyrinel XL were similar in all patients studied, irrespective of gender or age and are unaffected by food intake.

The pharmacokinetics of Lyrinel XL tablets have not been investigated in children, nor in patients with renal or hepatic insufficiency.

Oxybutynin is extensively metabolised by the liver, primarily by the cytochrome P450 enzyme system, particularly CYP3A4 found mostly in the liver and gut wall. Absolute bioavailability of immediate release oxybutynin has been estimated to be 2-11%. Following intravenous administration of 5 mg oxybutynin, clearance and volume of distribution were estimated to be 26 L/h and 193 L, respectively. Less than 0.1% of the administered dose is excreted unchanged in the urine. Its metabolic products include phenylcyclohexylglycolic acid, which is pharmacologically inactive, and desethyloxybutynin, which is pharmacologically active. Following Lyrinel XL administration, area under the plasma concentrations profiles of R- and S-desethyloxybutynin are 73% and 92% respectively of those observed with oxybutynin immediate release formulations.

The binding of oxybutynin to plasma proteins is unknown.

5.3 Preclinical safety data

Preclinical data reveal no special hazard for humans based on studies of acute toxicity, repeat dose toxicity, genotoxicity, carcinogenic potential and local toxicity. In a fertility study of subcutaneous oxybutynin injections in rats, female fertility was impaired while no effect was noted in male animals. In a rabbit embryotoxicity study, organ anomalies were observed in the presence of maternal toxicity at a dose of 0.4 mg/kg/day s.c. The relevance to human safety is unknown.

6. PHARMACEUTICAL PARTICULARS

6.1 List of excipients

5 mg

Butylhydroxytoluene (E321), cellulose acetate, hypromellose, macrogol 3350, magnesium stearate, polyethylene oxides, sodium chloride, black iron oxide (E172), ferric oxide yellow (E172) and lactose anhydrous.

Film coat: ferric oxide yellow (E172), hypromellose, macrogol 400, polysorbate 80 and titanium dioxide (E171)

Printing Ink: black iron oxide (E172), hypromellose, and propylene glycol.

10 mg

Butylhydroxytoluene (E321), cellulose acetate, hypromellose, macrogol 3350, magnesium stearate, polyethylene oxide, sodium chloride, black iron oxide (E172), ferric oxide red (E172) and lactose anhydrous.

Film coat: ferric oxide red (E172), hypromellose, macrogol 400, polysorbate 80 and titanium dioxide (E171)

Printing Ink: black iron oxide (E172), hypromellose and propylene glycol.

6.2 Incompatibilities

Not applicable.

6.3 Shelf life

Lyrinel XL5: 2 years

Lyrinel XL10: 18 months

6.4 Special precautions for storage

Keep the container tightly closed in order to protect from moisture. Do not store above 25°C.

6.5 Nature and contents of container

High density polyethylene bottles with child resistant closure (polypropylene) and desiccant.

Pack sizes 3, 7, 10, 14, 30, 50, 60, 90 or 100 tablets.

Not all pack sizes may be marketed.

6.6 Instructions for use and handling

No special requirements.

7. MARKETING AUTHORISATION HOLDER

Janssen-Cilag Limited
Saunderton
High Wycombe
Buckinghamshire
HP14 4HJ
UK

8. MARKETING AUTHORISATION NUMBER(S)

PL 0242/0385

PL 0242/0386

9. DATE OF FIRST AUTHORISATION/RENEWAL OF THE AUTHORISATION

1st August 2002

10. DATE OF REVISION OF THE TEXT

17th December 2004

Lysodren 500 mg tablets

(Laboratoire HRA Pharma)

1. NAME OF THE MEDICINAL PRODUCT

Lysodren 500 mg tablets

2. QUALITATIVE AND QUANTITATIVE COMPOSITION

Each tablet contains 500 mg of mitotane

For excipients, see section 6.1.

3. PHARMACEUTICAL FORM

Tablet.

White, biconvex, round, scored tablets.

4. CLINICAL PARTICULARS

4.1 Therapeutic indications

Symptomatic treatment of advanced (unresectable, metastatic or relapsed) adrenal cortical carcinoma. The effect of Lysodren on non-functional adrenal cortical carcinoma is not established.

4.2 Posology and method of administration

Treatment should be initiated by a suitably experienced specialist until a stable dosage regimen is achieved.

Adult patients

Treatment should be started with 2-3 g of Lysodren per day. The total daily dose may be divided in two or three doses according to patient's convenience. Lysodren should be preferably taken during meals (see section 4.5).

Doses may be reduced to 1-2 g per day after two months of treatment (cumulative dose of 200 g) or in case of toxicity.

If serious adverse reactions occur, such as neurotoxicity, treatment with mitotane may need to be transiently interrupted. In case of mild toxicity, dosage should be reduced until the maximum tolerated dosage is attained.

Monitoring of plasma level, if available, may be considered. Neurologic toxicity has been associated with levels above 18-20 mg/l and, therefore, this threshold should not be reached. Weaker evidence has suggested that drug plasma levels above 14 mg/l may result in enhanced efficacy. In dose readjustments, it should be taken into account that they do not produce immediate changes in plasma levels of mitotane. In case that plasma monitoring is available, the starting dose of Lysodren could be as high as 4-6 g daily in divided doses until a cumulative dose of 75 g is reached (approximately in 15 days). Thereafter, a monitoring schedule of once a month until a stable dosage is achieved is reasonable (see section 4.4).

Treatment with Lysodren should be continued as long as clinical benefits are observed. If no clinical benefits are observed after 3 months at optimal dose (based on empirical and/or drug monitoring criteria) and if no toxicity is observed, dose escalation up to 6 g per day may be considered.

Paediatric patients

The safety and efficacy of mitotane in patients under the age of 18 years have not been established and, at present only very limited data are available in this age group.

The paediatric dosage of mitotane has not been well characterised but appears equivalent to that of adults: treatment should be initiated at 1.5 to 3.5 g/m^2/day in children and adolescents and may be reduced after 2 or 3 months according to the plasma mitotane levels. Doses should be reduced in case of serious toxicity as in adults (see above).

The total daily dose may be divided in two or three doses according to patient's convenience. Lysodren should be preferably taken during meals.

Liver impairment

Since mitotane is mainly metabolised through the liver, mitotane plasma levels are expected to increase if liver function is impaired. There is no experience in the use of mitotane in patients with hepatic impairment, so data are insufficient to give a dose recommendation in this group. Until further data are available, the use of mitotane in patients with severe hepatic impairment is not recommended and, in cases of mild to moderate hepatic impairment, caution should be exercised. Monitoring of plasma mitotane levels is specially recommended in these patients (see section 4.4).

Renal impairment

There is no experience in the use of mitotane in patients with renal impairment, so data are insufficient to give a dose recommendation in this group. Until further data are available, the use of mitotane in patients with severe renal impairment is not recommended and, in cases of mild to moderate renal impairment, caution should be exercised. Monitoring of plasma mitotane levels is specially recommended in these patients (see section 4.4).

Elderly patients

There is no experience on the use of mitotane in elderly patients, so data are insufficient to give a dose recommendation in this group. Until further data are available caution should be exercised and frequent monitoring of plasma mitotane levels is highly recommended.

4.3 Contraindications

Hypersensitivity to the active substance or to any of the excipients.

Breast-feeding is contra-indicated while taking mitotane. The prolonged elimination of mitotane from the body after discontinuation of Lysodren should be considered (see section 4.6).

Lysodren and spironolactone must not be used concomitantly (see section 4.5).

4.4 Special warnings and special precautions for use

Before the initiation of the treatment: All possible tumour tissues should be surgically removed from large metastatic masses before mitotane administration is instituted. This is necessary to minimise the possibility of infarction and haemorrhage in the tumour due to a rapid cytotoxic effect of mitotane.

Shock, severe trauma or infection: Mitotane should be temporarily discontinued immediately following shock, severe trauma or infection, since adrenal suppression is its prime action. Exogenous steroids should be administered in such circumstances, since the depressed adrenal gland may not immediately start to secrete steroids. Because of an increased risk of acute adrenocortical insufficiency, patients should be instructed to contact their physician immediately if injury, infection, or other illness occurs. Patients should carry with them the card provided with the package leaflet indicating that they are prone to adrenal insufficiency and that in case of emergency care, adequate precautionary measures should be taken.

Monitoring of plasma levels: Monitoring of the plasma levels of mitotane may be used to guide Lysodren dosing. It may be especially useful in cases where administration of higher starting doses is considered necessary in order to reach earlier the desired therapeutic levels (e.g. highly symptomatic patients). The therapeutic window of mitotane lies between 14 mg/l and 20 mg/l. A dose adjustment may be necessary to achieve the correct therapeutic level and avoid specific adverse reactions. Plasma levels higher than 20 mg/l may be associated with severe undesirable effects and offer no further benefit in terms of efficacy.

Monitoring of plasma levels is particularly recommended in patients with liver impairment and/or renal insufficiency (see section 4.2) for whom treatment with Lysodren is considered necessary.

In patients with severe liver disease or severe renal impairment, there are insufficient data to support the use of mitotane (see section 4.2). In patients with mild or moderate hepatic impairment and in patients with mild or moderate renal impairment, caution should be exercised.

Since mitotane is mainly stored in fat tissues, caution should be taken when treating overweight patients as prolonged release of mitotane can occur.

Central nervous system disorders: Long-term continuous administration of high doses of mitotane may lead to reversible brain damage and impairment of function. Behavioural and neurological assessments should be made at regular intervals especially when plasma mitotane levels exceed 20 mg/l (see section 4.8).

Risk of adrenal insufficiency: A substantial percentage of patients treated show signs of adrenal insufficiency. Therefore steroid replacement may be necessary in these patients. Since mitotane increases plasma levels of steroid binding proteins, free cortisol and corticotropin (ACTH) determinations are necessary for optimal dosing of steroid substitution (see section 4.8).

Women of childbearing potential: Women of childbearing potential should be advised to use effective contraception during treatment with mitotane (see section 4.6).

Bleeding time: Prolonged bleeding time has been reported in patients treated with mitotane and this should be taken into account when surgery is considered (see section 4.8).

Warfarin and coumarin-like anticoagulants: physicians should closely monitor patients for a change in anticoagulant dosage requirements when administering mitotane to patients on coumarin-like anticoagulants (see section 4.5).

Mitotane is a hepatic enzyme inducer and it should be used with caution in case of concomitant use of medicinal products influenced by hepatic enzyme induction (see section 4.5).

Paediatric population:

In children, neuro-psychological retardation can be observed during mitotane treatment. In such cases, thyroid function should be investigated in order to identify a possible thyroid impairment linked to mitotane treatment.

4.5 Interaction with other medicinal products and other forms of Interaction

Spironolactone: Mitotane should not be given in combination with spironolactone since this drug may block the action of mitotane (see section 4.3).

Warfarin and coumarin-like anticoagulants: Mitotane has been reported to accelerate the metabolism of warfarin by the mechanism of hepatic microsomal enzyme induction, leading to an increase in dosage requirements for warfarin. Therefore, physicians should closely monitor patients for a change in anticoagulant dosage requirements when administering mitotane to patients on coumarin-like anticoagulants.

Substances metabolised through cytochrome P450: Mitotane has been shown to have an inductive effect on cytochrome P450 enzymes. Therefore the plasma concentrations of the products metabolised via cytochrome P450 may be modified. In the absence of information on the specific P450 isoenzymes involved, caution should be taken when coprescribing active substances metabolised by this route such as, among others, anticonvulsants, rifabutin, rifampicin, griseofulvin and St. John's Wort (*Hypericum perforatum*).

Mitotane can give rise to central nervous system undesirable effects at high concentrations (see section 4.8). Although no specific information on pharmacodynamic interactions in the central nervous system is available, this should be borne in mind when coprescribing medicinal products with central nervous system depressant action.

Data with various mitotane formulations suggest that administration with food and/or oil enhance absorption (see section 5.2).

Mitotane has been shown to increase plasma hormone binding protein: this should be taken into account when interpreting the results of hormonal assays.

4.6 Pregnancy and lactation

Pregnancy

Data on a limited number of exposed pregnancies indicate adverse reactions of mitotane on the health of the foetus. Animal reproduction studies have not been conducted with mitotane. Animal studies with similar substances have shown reproductive toxicity (see section 5.3). Lysodren should be given to a pregnant woman only if clearly needed and if the clinical benefit clearly outweighs any potential risk to the foetus.

Women of childbearing potential should be advised to use effective contraception during treatment. The prolonged elimination of mitotane from the body after discontinuation of Lysodren should be considered.

Lactation

Due to the lipophilic nature of mitotane, it is likely to be excreted in breast milk. Breastfeeding is contra-indicated while taking mitotane (see section 4.3). A decision should be made whether to discontinue breast-feeding or to discontinue Lysodren taking into account, on an individual basis, the importance of the treatment to the mother.

The prolonged elimination of mitotane from the body after discontinuation of Lysodren should be considered.

4.7 Effects on ability to drive and use machines

Lysodren has a major influence on the ability to drive and use machines. Since sedation, lethargy, vertigo, and other central nervous system undesirable effects can occur, ambulatory patients should be cautioned about driving, operating machines, and other hazardous pursuits requiring mental and physical alertness.

4.8 Undesirable effects

More than 80 % of patients treated with mitotane have shown at least one type of undesirable effect. The main types of adverse reactions consist of the following:

(see Table 1)

Table 1

System Organ Class	Undesirable effect (frequency) *Very common (> 1 / 10)*	*Common (> 1/100, < 1 / 10)*	*Rare (> 1/10,000, < 1/1,000) or very rare (< 1/10,000), including isolated reports*
Infections and infestations			Opportunistic mycoses
Blood and lymphatic system disorders	Bleeding time prolonged Leucopoenia	Thrombocytopenia Anaemia	
Metabolism and nutrition disorders	Hypercholesterolemia Hypertriglyceridaemia		Hypouricaemia
Nervous system and psychiatric disorders	Anorexia Asthenia Myasthenia Paresthesia Confusion Vertigo Sleepiness Ataxia	Dizziness Mental impairment Headache Polyneuropathy Movement disorder	
Eye disorders			Visual impairment Maculopathy Vision blurred Diplopia Lens opacity Retinal toxicity
Cardiac and vascular disorders			Hypertension Orthostatic hypotension Flushing
Gastrointestinal disorders	Nausea Epigastric discomfort Diarrhoea Vomiting Mucositis		Salivary hypersecretion
Hepato-biliary disorders		Autoimmune hepatitis	
Skin and subcutaneous tissue disorders	Skin rash		
Renal and urinary disorders			Haematuria Haemorrhagic cystitis Proteinuria
Reproductive system and breast disorders	Gynaecomastia		
General disorders and administration site conditions			Hyperpyrexia
Investigations	Plasma cholesterol increased Plasma triglycerides increased Elevated liver enzymes		Blood uric acid decreased

•Gastrointestinal disorders are the most frequently reported (10 to 100 % of patients) and are reversible when the dose is reduced. Some of these effects (anorexia) may constitute the hallmark of initial central nervous system impairment.

•Nervous system undesirable effects occur in approximately 40 % of the patients. Other undesirable central nervous effects have been reported in literature such as memory defects, aggressiveness, central vestibular syndrome, dysarthria, or Parkinson syndrome. Serious undesirable effects appear linked to the cumulative exposure to mitotane and are most likely to occur when plasma mitotane levels are at 20 mg/l or above. At high doses and after prolonged utilization, brain function impairment can occur. Nervous system undesirable effects appear reversible after cessation of mitotane treatment and decrease in plasma levels (see section 4.4).

•Metabolic disorders such as increases in plasma cholesterol or triglycerides are very common.

•Skin rashes which have been reported in 5 to 25 % of the cases do not seem to be dose related.

•Leucopenia has been reported in 8 to 12 % of patients. Prolonged bleeding time appears a frequent finding (90 percent of the cases): although the exact mechanism of such an effect is unknown and its relation with mitotane or with the underlying disease is uncertain, it should be taken into account when surgery is considered.

•The activity of liver enzymes (gamma-GT, aminotransferase, alkaline phosphatase) is commonly increased. Autoimmune hepatitis has been reported in 7 % of patients with no other information on mechanism. Liver enzymes normalize when the mitotane dose is decreased.

•Other isolated undesirable effects have been reported involving: the eye (visual impairment, maculopathy, vision blurred, diplopia, lens opacity, retinal toxicity); the renal and urinary system (haematuria, haemorrhagic cystitis, proteinuria); cardiovascular system (hypertension, or orthostatic hypotension, and flushing); and some miscellaneous effects including generalized aching; hyperpyrexia; decreased plasma uric acid.

•Because of its adrenolytic activity and its action on cortisol metabolism, mitotane treatment induces a state of functional adrenal insufficiency, which necessitates hormone supplementation. Since mitotane increases plasma level of steroid binding proteins, free cortisol and ACTH determinations are necessary for optimal dosing of steroid substitution (see section 4.4).

In paediatric patients:

Nervous system disorders: neuro-psychological retardation may be observed during mitotane treatment. In such cases, thyroid function should be investigated in order to identify a possible thyroid impairment linked to mitotane treatment.

Hypothyroidism and growth retardation may be also observed during mitotane treatment.

4.9 Overdose

Mitotane overdose may lead to central nervous system impairment especially if plasma mitotane levels are above 20 mg/l. No proven antidotes have been established for mitotane overdose. The patient should be followed closely, taking into account that impairment is reversible but given the long half-life and the lipophilic nature of mitotane it may take weeks to return to normal. Other effects should be treated symptomatically. Because of its lipophilic nature, mitotane is not likely to be dialysable.

5. PHARMACOLOGICAL PROPERTIES

5.1 Pharmacodynamic properties

Pharmacotherapeutic group: Other antineoplastic agents. ATC code: L01XX23

Mitotane is an adrenal cytotoxic active substance, although it can cause adrenal inhibition, apparently without cellular destruction. Its biochemical mechanism of action is unknown. Data are available to suggest that mitotane modifies the peripheral metabolism of steroids as well as directly suppressing the adrenal cortex. The administration of mitotane alters the extra-adrenal metabolism of cortisol in man, leading to a reduction in measurable 17-hydroxy corticosteroids, even though plasma levels of corticosteroids do not fall. Mitotane apparently causes increased formation of 6-beta-hydroxyl cholesterol.

Mitotane has not been studied in a clinical therapeutic program. Available clinical information comes mainly from published data in patients with inoperable or metastatic adrenal carcinoma. In terms of overall survival, four studies conclude that mitotane treatment does not increase the survival rate whereas five find an increase in the survival rate. Among the latter, three studies find such an increase only in patients in whom plasma mitotane is above 14 mg/l. In terms of total or partial tumour and/or metastasis regression, eleven studies have shown some degree of improvement and sometimes occasional prolonged remissions. However, in several studies, the objective criteria for evaluating tumour response are missing or not reported. There are nevertheless some studies which provide accurate information on tumour regression or disappearance and demonstrate that the threshold of 14 mg/l appears necessary to induce an objective tumour regression. In addition, mitotane induces a state of adrenal insufficiency which leads to the disappearance of Cushing syndrome in patients with secreting adrenal carcinoma and necessitates substitution hormonotherapy.

Paediatric population: clinical information comes mainly from a large retrospective trial in children (median age, 4 years) who had an unresectable primary tumour or who presented a tumour recurrence or a metastasic disease; most of the children (75%) presented with endocrine symptoms.

Mitotane was given alone or combined with chemotherapy with various agents. Overall, the disease-free interval was 7 months (2 to 16 months). There were recurrences in 40% of children; the survival rate at 5 years was 49%.

The observed undesirable effects were almost comparable to those in adults; however, neuro-psychological retardation, hypothyroidism and growth retardation can also be observed.

5.2 Pharmacokinetic properties

In a study performed in patients with adrenal carcinoma treated with 2 to 3 g daily of mitotane, a highly significant correlation was found between plasma mitotane concentration and the total mitotane dose. The target plasma mitotane concentration (14 mg/l) was reached in all patients within 3 to 5 months and the total Lysodren dose ranged between 283 and 387 g × days of treatment (median value: 363 g × days of treatment). The threshold of 20 mg/l was reached for cumulative amounts of mitotane of approximately 500 g. In another study, 3 patients with adrenal carcinoma received Lysodren according to a precise protocol allowing fast introduction of a high dose if the product was well tolerated: 3 g (as 3 intakes) on day 1, 4.5 g on day 2, 6 g on day 3, 7.5 g on day 4 and 9 g on day 5. This dose of Lysodren was continued or decreased in function of side effects and plasma mitotane levels. There was a positive linear correlation between the cumulative dose of Lysodren and the plasma levels of mitotane. In two of the 3 patients, plasma levels of more than 14 mg/l were achieved within 15 days and in one of them levels above 20 mg/l were achieved within approximately 30 days. In addition, in both studies, in some patients, the plasma mitotane levels continued to rise despite maintenance or a decrease of the daily dose of mitotane.

Administration of Lysodren tablets with food increased absorption (see section 4.2), although no quantitative measure of relative bioavailability was made.

Autopsy data from patients show that mitotane is found in most tissues of the body, with fat as the primary site of storage.

Metabolism studies in man have identified the corresponding acid, *o,p'*-DDA, as the major circulating metabolite, together with smaller quantities of the *o,p'*-DDE analogue of mitotane. No unchanged mitotane has been found in bile or in urine, where *o,p'*-DDA predominates, together with several of its hydroxylated derivatives.

After intravenous administration, 25% of the dose was excreted as metabolite within 24 hours. Following discontinuation of mitotane treatment, it is slowly released from storage sites in fat, leading to reported terminal plasma half-lives ranging from 18 to 159 days.

For induction with cytochrome P450, see section 4.5.

5.3 Preclinical safety data

Preclinical data on the general toxicity of mitotane is limited. Reproductive toxicity studies have not been performed with mitotane. However, DDT and other polychlorinated biphenyl analogues are recognised to have deleterious effects on fertility, pregnancy and development, and mitotane could be expected to share these properties. The genotoxic and carcinogenic potential of mitotane have not been investigated.

6. PHARMACEUTICAL PARTICULARS

6.1 List of excipients

Maize starch

Microcrystalline cellulose (E 460)

Macrogol 3350

Anhydrous colloidal silica.

6.2 Incompatibilities

Not applicable.

6.3 Shelf life

3 years.

After opening: 1 year.

6.4 Special precautions for storage

Store in the original container.

6.5 Nature and contents of container

Square opaque white HDPE bottle containing 100 tablets. Packs of 1 bottle.

6.6 Instructions for use and handling

This medicinal product should not be handled by persons other than the patient and his/her caregivers and especially not by pregnant women. Caregivers should wear disposable gloves when handling the tablets.

Do not use any tablet which shows signs of deterioration; these should be disposed of in accordance with local requirements.

Unused containers or partially empty bottles should be disposed of in accordance with local requirements.

7. MARKETING AUTHORISATION HOLDER

Laboratoire HRA Pharma

15 rue Béranger

75003 Paris

France

8. MARKETING AUTHORISATION NUMBER(S)

EU/1/04/273/001

9. DATE OF FIRST AUTHORISATION/RENEWAL OF THE AUTHORISATION

28/04/2004

10. DATE OF REVISION OF THE TEXT

Lysovir 100mg Capsules

(Alliance Pharmaceuticals)

1. NAME OF THE MEDICINAL PRODUCT

Lysovir 100mg Capsules

2. QUALITATIVE AND QUANTITATIVE COMPOSITION

Amantadine hydrochloride PhEur 100 mg.

3. PHARMACEUTICAL FORM

Capsule.

Reddish-brown hard gelatin capsules, printed SYMM in white on both the cap and body.

4. CLINICAL PARTICULARS

4.1 Therapeutic indications

Prophylaxis and treatment of signs and symptoms of infection caused by influenza A virus. It is suggested that Lysovir be given to patients suffering from clinical influenza in which complications might be expected to occur. In addition, Lysovir is recommended prophylactically in cases particularly at risk. This can include those with chronic respiratory disease or debilitating conditions, the elderly and those living in crowded conditions. It can also be used for individuals in families where influenza has already been diagnosed, for control of institutional outbreaks or for those in essential services who are unvaccinated or when vaccination is unavailable or contraindicated.

Lysovir does not completely prevent the host immune response to influenza A infection, so individuals who take this drug still develop immune responses to the natural disease or vaccination and may be protected when later exposed to antigenically related viruses. Lysovir may also be used in post-exposure prophylaxis in conjunction with inactivated vaccine during an outbreak until protective antibodies develop, or in patients who are not expected to have a substantial antibody response (immunosuppression).

4.2 Posology and method of administration

Treatment: It is advisable to start treating influenza as early as possible and to continue for 4 to 5 days. When amantadine is started within 48 hours of symptoms appearing, the duration of fever and other effects is reduced by one or two days and the inflammatory reaction of the bronchial tree that usually accompanies influenza resolves more quickly. ***Prophylaxis:*** Treat daily for as long as protection from infection is required. In most instances this is expected to be for 6 weeks. When used with inactivated influenza A vaccine, amantadine is continued for 2 to 3 weeks following inoculation.

Adults: 100mg daily for the recommended period.

Children aged 10-15 years: 100mg daily for the recommended period.

Children under 10 years of age: Dosage not established.

Adults over 65 years of age: Plasma amantadine concentrations are influenced by renal function. In elderly patients, the elimination half-life is longer and renal clearance of the compound is diminished in comparison to young people. A daily dose of less than 100mg, or 100mg given at intervals of greater than one day, may be appropriate.

In patients with ***renal impairment*** the dose of amantadine should be reduced. This can be achieved by either reducing the total daily dose, or by increasing the dosage interval in accordance with the creatinine clearance. For example,

Creatinine clearance (ml/min)	Dose
< 15	Lysovir contra-indicated.
15 – 35	100mg every 2 to 3 days.
> 35	100mg every day

The above recommendations are for guidance only and physicians should continue to monitor their patients for signs of unwanted effects.

4.3 Contraindications

Known hypersensitivity to amantadine or any of the excipients. Individuals subject to convulsions. A history of gastric ulceration. Severe renal disease. Pregnancy.

4.4 Special warnings and special precautions for use

Lysovir should be used with caution in patients with confusional or hallucinatory states or underlying psychiatric disorders, in patients with liver or kidney disorders, and those suffering from, or who have a history of, cardiovascular disorders. Caution should be applied when prescribing Lysovir with other medications having an effect on the CNS (See Section 4.5, Interactions with other medicaments and other forms of interaction).

Lysovir should not be stopped abruptly in patients who are treated concurrently with neuroleptics. There have been isolated reports of precipitation or aggravation of neuroleptic malignant syndrome or neuroleptic-induced catatonia following the withdrawal of amantadine in patients taking neuroleptic agents.

Resistance to amantadine occurs during serial passage of influenza virus strains *in vitro* or *in vivo* in the presence of the drug. Apparent transmission of drug-resistant viruses may have been the cause of failure of prophylaxis and treatment in household contacts and in nursing-home patients. However, there is no evidence to date that the resistant virus produces a disease that is in any way different from that produced by sensitive viruses.

As some individuals have attempted suicide with amantadine, prescriptions should be written for the smallest quantity consistent with good patient management.

Peripheral oedema (thought to be due to an alteration in the responsiveness of peripheral vessels) may occur in some patients during chronic treatment (not usually before 4 weeks) with amantadine. This should be taken into account in patients with congestive heart failure.

4.5 Interaction with other medicinal products and other forms of Interaction

Concurrent administration of amantadine and anticholinergic agents or levodopa may increase confusion, hallucinations, nightmares, gastro-intestinal disturbances, or other atropine-like side effects (see Section 4.9 "Overdose"). Psychotic reactions have been observed in patients receiving amantadine and levodopa.

In isolated cases, worsening of psychotic symptoms has been reported in patients receiving amantadine and concomitant neuroleptic medication.

Concurrent administration of amantadine and drugs or substances (e.g. alcohol) acting on the CNS may result in additive CNS toxicity. Close observation is recommended (see Section 4.9 "Overdose").

There have been isolated reports of a suspected interaction between amantadine and combination diuretics (hydrochlorothiazide + potassium sparing diuretics). One or both of the components apparently reduce the clearance of amantadine, leading to higher plasma concentrations and toxic effects (confusion, hallucinations, ataxia, myoclonus).

4.6 Pregnancy and lactation

Amantadine-related complications during pregnancy have been reported. Lysovir is contra-indicated during pregnancy and in women wishing to become pregnant. Amantadine passes into breast milk. Undesirable effects have been reported in breast-fed infants. Nursing mothers should not take Lysovir.

4.7 Effects on ability to drive and use machines

Patients should be warned of the potential hazards of driving or operating machinery if they experience side effects such as dizziness or blurred vision. If taken concomitantly with other products affecting the CNS, additive adverse effects could be seen.

4.8 Undesirable effects

Amantadine's undesirable effects are often mild and transient, usually appearing within the first 2 to 4 days of treatment and promptly disappearing 24 to 48 hours after discontinuation. A direct relationship between dose and incidence of side effects has not been demonstrated, although there seems to be a tendency towards more frequent undesirable effects (particularly affecting the CNS) with increasing doses.

The side effects reported after the pivotal clinical studies in influenza in over 1200 patients receiving amantadine at 100mg daily were mostly mild, transient, and equivalent to placebo. Only 7% of subjects reported adverse events, many being similar to the effects of influenza itself. The most commonly reported effects were gastro-intestinal disturbances (anorexia, nausea), CNS effects (loss of concentration, dizziness, agitation, nervousness, depression, insomnia, fatigue, weakness), or myalgia.

Side effects reported after higher doses or chronic use, in addition to those already stated, include:

Frequency estimates: frequent > 10%, occasional 1%-10%, rare 0.001%-1%, isolated cases < 0.001%.

Central nervous system: Occasional: anxiety, elevation of mood, lightheadedness, headache, lethargy, hallucinations, nightmares, ataxia, slurred speech, blurred vision. Hallucinations, confusion and nightmares are more common when amantadine is administered concurrently with anticholinergic agents or when the patient has an underlying psychiatric disorder. Rare: confusion, disorientation, psychosis, tremor, dyskinesia, convulsions. Delirium, hypomanic state and mania have been reported but their incidence cannot be readily deduced from the literature.

Cardiovascular system: Frequent: oedema of ankles, livedo reticularis (usually after very high doses or use over many months). Occasional: palpitations, orthostatic hypotension. Isolated cases: heart insufficiency/failure. *Blood*: Isolated cases: leucopenia, reversible elevation of liver enzymes. *Gastrointestinal tract:* Occasional: dry mouth, anorexia, nausea, vomiting, constipation. Rare: diarrhoea. *Skin and appendages:* Occasional: diaphoresis. Rare: exanthema. Isolated cases: photosensitisation. *Sense organs*: Rare: corneal lesions, e.g. punctate subepithelial opacities which might be associated with superficial punctate keratitis, corneal epithelial oedema, and markedly reduced visual acuity. *Urogenital tract:* Rare: urinary retention, urinary incontinence.

4.9 Overdose

Signs and symptoms: *Neuromuscular* disturbances and symptoms of acute psychosis are prominent. *Central nervous system:* Hyperreflexia, motor restlessness, convulsions, extrapyramidal signs, torsion spasms, dystonic posturing, dilated pupils, confusion, disorientation, delirium, visual hallucinations. *Respiratory system*: hyperventilation, pulmonary oedema, respiratory distress, including adult respiratory distress syndrome. *Cardiovascular system*: sinus tachycardia, arrhythmia. *Gastrointestinal system*: nausea, vomiting, dry mouth. *Renal function*: urine retention, renal dysfunction, including increase in BUN and decreased creatinine clearance.

Overdose from combined drug treatment: the effects of anticholinergic drugs are increased by amantadine. Acute psychotic reactions (which may be identical to those of atropine poisoning) may occur when large doses of anticholinergic agents are used. Where alcohol or central nervous stimulants have been taken at the same time, the signs and symptoms of acute poisoning with amantadine may be aggravated and/or modified.

Management: There is no specific antidote. Induction of vomiting and/or gastric aspiration (and lavage if patient is conscious), activated charcoal or saline cathartic may be used if judged appropriate. Since amantadine is excreted mainly unchanged in the urine, maintenance of renal function and copious diuresis (forced diuresis if necessary) are effective ways to remove it from the blood stream. Acidification of the urine favours its excretion. Haemodialysis does not remove significant amounts of amantadine.

Monitor the blood pressure, heart rate, ECG, respiration and body temperature, and treat for possible hypotension and cardiac arhythmias, as necessary. *Convulsions and excessive motor restlessness*: administer anticonvulsants such as diazepam iv, paraldehyde im or per rectum, or phenobarbital im. *Acute psychotic symptoms, delirium, dystonic posturing, myoclonic manifestations*: physostigmine by slow iv infusion (1mg doses in adults, 0.5mg in children) repeated administration according to the initial response and the subsequent need, has been reported. *Retention of urine*: bladder should be catheterised; an indwelling catheter can be left in place for the time required.

5. PHARMACOLOGICAL PROPERTIES

5.1 Pharmacodynamic properties

Amantadine specifically inhibits the replication of influenza A viruses at low concentrations. If using a sensitive plaque-reduction assay, human influenza viruses, including H_1N_1, H_2N_2 and H_3N_2 subtypes, are inhibited by $\leqslant 0.4\mu g/ml$ of amantadine. Amantadine inhibits an early stage in viral replication by blocking the proton pump of the M_2 protein in the virus. This has two actions; it stops the virus uncoating and inactivates newly synthesised viral haemagglutinin. Effects on late replicative steps have been found for representative avian influenza viruses.

Data from tests with representative strains of influenza A virus indicate that Lysovir is likely to be active against previously unknown strains, and could be used in the early stages of an epidemic, before a vaccine against the causative strain is generally available.

5.2 Pharmacokinetic properties

Absorption: Amantadine is absorbed slowly but almost completely. Peak plasma concentrations of approximately 250ng/ml and 500ng/ml are attained within 3 to 4 hours after single oral administration of 100mg and 200mg amantadine, respectively. Following repeated administration of 200mg daily, the steady-state plasma concentration settles at 300ng/ml within 3 days.

Distribution: Amantadine accumulates after several hours in nasal secretions and crosses the blood-brain barrier (this has not been quantified). *In vitro*, 67% is bound to plasma proteins, with a substantial amount bound to red blood cells. The concentration in erythrocytes in normal healthy volunteers is 2.66 times the plasma concentration. The apparent volume of distribution is 5 to 10L/kg, suggesting extensive tissue binding. This declines with increasing doses. The concentrations in the lung, heart, kidney, liver and spleen are higher than in the blood.

Biotransformation: Amantadine is metabolised to a minor extent, principally by N-acetylation.

Elimination: The drug is eliminated in healthy young adults with a mean plasma elimination half-life of 15 hours (10 to 31 hours). The total plasma clearance is about the same as renal clearance (250ml/min). The renal amantadine clearance is much higher than the creatinine clearance, suggesting renal tubular secretion. After 4 to 5 days, 90% of the dose appears unchanged in urine. The rate is considerably influenced by urinary pH: a rise in pH brings about a fall in excretion.

Characteristics in special patient populations:

Elderly patients: compared with healthy young adults, the half-life may be doubled and renal clearance diminished. Tubular secretion diminishes more than glomerular filtration in the elderly. In elderly patients with renal impairment, repeated administration of 100mg daily for 14 days raised the plasma concentration into the toxic range.

Renal impairment: amantadine may accumulate in renal failure, causing severe side effects. The rate of elimination from plasma correlates to creatinine clearance divided by body surface area, although total renal elimination exceeds this value (possibly due to tubular secretion). The effects of reduced kidney function are dramatic: a reduction of creatinine clearance to 40ml/min may result in a five-fold increase in elimination half-life. The urine is the almost exclusive route of excretion, even with renal failure, and amantadine may persist in the plasma for several days. Haemodialysis does not remove significant amounts of amantadine, possibly due to extensive tissue binding.

5.3 Preclinical safety data

Reproductive toxicity studies were performed in rats and rabbits. In rat oral doses of 50 and 100 mg/kg proved to be teratogenic. This is 33-fold the recommended dose of 100mg for influenza. The maximum recommended dose, of 400mg in Parkinson's disease, is less than 6mg/kg.

There are no other pre-clinical data of relevance to the prescriber, which are additional to those already included in other sections of the Summary of Product Characteristics.

6. PHARMACEUTICAL PARTICULARS

6.1 List of excipients

Lactose, povidone, magnesium stearate. Capsule shell: gelatin, titanium dioxide (E171), red iron oxide (E172). White printing ink: Opacode S-1-7020 containing, Shellac, I.M.S. 74 OP, purified water, soya lecithin (E322), 2-ethoxyethanol, antifoam DC 1510, titanium dioxide (E171).

6.2 Incompatibilities

None known.

6.3 Shelf life

Five years.

6.4 Special precautions for storage

Store in the original package.

6.5 Nature and contents of container

PVC/PVdC blister packs of 5 or 14 capsules.

6.6 Instructions for use and handling

None.

7. MARKETING AUTHORISATION HOLDER

Alliance Pharmaceuticals Ltd

Avonbridge House, Bath Road

Chippenham, Wiltshire SN15 2BB

8. MARKETING AUTHORISATION NUMBER(S)

PL16853/0035

9. DATE OF FIRST AUTHORISATION/RENEWAL OF THE AUTHORISATION

January 2000

10. DATE OF REVISION OF THE TEXT

July 2005

Legal Status

POM

MabCampath 30mg/ml concentrate for solution for infusion

(Schering Health Care Limited)

1. NAME OF THE MEDICINAL PRODUCT
▼MabCampath 30 mg/ml concentrate for solution for infusion.

2. QUALITATIVE AND QUANTITATIVE COMPOSITION
Each vial contains 30 mg alemtuzumab.

Alemtuzumab is a genetically engineered humanised IgG1 kappa monoclonal antibody specific for a 21-28 kD lymphocyte cell surface glycoprotein (CD52). The antibody is produced in mammalian cell (Chinese Hamster ovary) suspension culture in a nutrient medium.

For excipients, see Section 6.1.

3. PHARMACEUTICAL FORM
Concentrate for solution for infusion.

4. CLINICAL PARTICULARS
4.1 Therapeutic indications
MabCampath is indicated for the treatment of patients with chronic lymphocytic leukaemia (CLL) who have been treated with alkylating agents and who have failed to achieve a complete or partial response or achieved only a short remission (less than 6 months) following fludarabine phosphate therapy.

4.2 Posology and method of administration
MabCampath should be administered under the supervision of a physician experienced in the use of cancer therapy.

The MabCampath solution must be prepared according to the instructions provided in Section 6.6. All doses should be administered by intravenous infusion over approximately 2 hours.

Patients should be premedicated with an appropriate antihistamine and analgesic prior to the first dose at each escalation and prior to subsequent infusions, as clinically indicated (see Section 4.4).

Antibiotics and antivirals should be administered routinely to all patients throughout and following treatment (see Section 4.4).

During the first week of treatment, MabCampath should be administered in escalating doses: 3 mg on day 1, 10 mg on day 2 and 30 mg on day 3 assuming that each dose is well tolerated. Thereafter, the recommended dose is 30 mg daily administered 3 times weekly on alternate days up to a maximum of 12 weeks.

In most patients, dose escalation to 30 mg can be accomplished in 3-7 days. However, if acute moderate to severe adverse reactions due to cytokine release (hypotension, rigors, fever, shortness of breath, chills, rashes and bronchospasm) occur at either the 3 mg or 10 mg dose levels, then those doses should be repeated daily until they are well tolerated or before further dose escalation is attempted (see Section 4.4).

The majority of major responses to MabCampath have been achieved with treatment durations of 4 - 12 weeks. Once a patient meets all laboratory and clinical criteria for a complete response, MabCampath should be discontinued and the patient monitored. If a patient improves (i.e. achieves a partial response or stable disease) and then reaches a plateau without further improvement for 4 weeks or more, then MabCampath should be discontinued and the patient monitored. Therapy should be discontinued if there is evidence of disease progression.

In the event of serious infection or severe haematological toxicity MabCampath should be discontinued until the event resolves. It is recommended that MabCampath should be discontinued in patients whose platelet count falls to $< 25{,}000/\mu l$ or whose absolute neutrophil count (ANC) drops to $< 250/\mu l$. MabCampath may be reinstituted after the infection or toxicity has resolved. The following table outlines the recommended procedure for dose modification following the occurrence of haematological toxicity while on therapy:

Haematological Toxicity (platelets $< 25{,}000/\mu l$ and/or ANC $< 250/\mu l$)	**Reinstitution of MabCampath**
First occurrence	After resolution, reinstitute at 30 mg*
Second occurrence	After resolution, reinstitute at 10 mg*
Third occurrence	Permanent discontinuation

*If therapy has been withheld for more than 7 days, MabCampath must be reinstituted by gradual dose escalation

Children and adolescents (below 17 years of age):
No studies have been conducted (see Section 4.4).

Elderly (over 65 years of age):
Recommendations are as stated above for adults. Patients should be monitored carefully (see Section 4.4).

Patients with renal or hepatic impairment:
No studies have been conducted (see Section 4.4).

4.3 Contraindications
- hypersensitivity or anaphylactic reactions to alemtuzumab, to murine proteins or to any of the excipients;
- in patients with active systemic infections;
- in patients infected with HIV;
- in patients with active secondary malignancies;
- pregnancy and breast-feeding.

4.4 Special warnings and special precautions for use
Acute adverse reactions, which may occur during initial dose escalation due to the release of cytokines, include hypotension, rigors, fever, shortness of breath, chills and rashes. If these events are moderate to severe, then dosing should continue at the same level prior to each dose escalation, with appropriate premedication, until each dose is well tolerated. If therapy is withheld for more than 7 days, MabCampath should be reinstituted with gradual dose escalation.

Transient hypotension has occurred in patients receiving MabCampath. Caution should be used in treating patients with ischaemic heart disease, angina and/or in patients receiving antihypertensive medication. Myocardial infarction and cardiac arrest have been observed in association with MabCampath infusion in this patient population.

It is recommended that patients be premedicated with oral or intravenous steroids 30-60 minutes prior to each MabCampath infusion during dose escalation and as clinically indicated. The recommended premedication is hydrocortisone 100-200 mg, or equivalent, which may be reduced once dose escalation has been achieved. In addition, an oral antihistamine, e.g. diphenhydramine 50 mg, and an analgesic, e.g. paracetamol 500 mg, may be given. In the event that acute infusion reactions persist, the infusion time may be extended up to 8 hours from the time of reconstitution of MabCampath in solution for infusion.

Profound lymphocyte depletion, an expected pharmacological effect of MabCampath, inevitably occurs and may be prolonged. CD4 and CD8 T-cell counts begin to rise from weeks 8-12 during treatment and continue to recover for several months following the discontinuation of treatment. The median time to reach a level of 200 cells/μl is 2 months following last infusion with MabCampath but may take 6 months or longer to approximate pretreatment levels. This may predispose patients to opportunistic infections. It is highly recommended that anti-infective prophylaxis (e.g. trimethoprim/sulfamethoxazole 1 tablet twice daily, 3 times weekly, or other prophylaxis against *Pneumocystis carinii* pneumonia (PCP) and an effective oral antiherpes agent, such as famciclovir, 250 mg twice daily) should be initiated while on therapy and continued following the completion of treatment with MabCampath until the CD4+ count has recovered to 200 cells/μl or greater. If CD4 counts are not obtainable, then patients should remain on anti-infective prophylaxis for 4 months. It is not necessary to discontinue MabCampath in the event that an opportunistic infection occurs during treatment, since the T-cell population will already be depleted.

Because of the potential for GVHD in severely lymphopenic patients, blood products should be irradiated prior to use until lymphopenia has resolved, and particularly until the T-cells are adequately repopulated to at least 200 cells/μl or greater.

Transient grade 3 or 4 neutropenia occurs very commonly by weeks 5-8 following initiation of treatment. Transient grade 3 or 4 thrombocytopenia occurs very commonly during the first 2 weeks of therapy and then begins to improve in most patients. Therefore, haematological monitoring of patients is indicated. If a severe haematological toxicity develops, MabCampath treatment should be discontinued until the event resolves. MabCampath treatment may be reinstituted following resolution of the haematological toxicity (see Section 4.2).

Complete blood counts and platelet counts should be obtained at regular intervals during MabCampath therapy and more frequently in patients who develop cytopenias.

It is not proposed that regular and systematic monitoring of CD52 expression should be carried out as routine clinical practice. However, if retreatment is considered, it may be prudent to confirm the presence of CD52 expression.

Patients may have allergic or hypersensitivity reactions to MabCampath and to murine or chimeric monoclonal antibodies.

Males and females of childbearing potential should use effective contraceptive measures during treatment and for 6 months following MabCampath therapy (see Sections 4.6 and 5.3).

No studies have been conducted which specifically address the effect of age on MabCampath disposition and toxicity. In general, older patients (over 65 years of age) tolerate cytotoxic therapy less well than younger individuals. Since CLL occurs commonly in this older age group, these patients should be monitored carefully (see Section 4.2).

No studies have been conducted to investigate the safety and efficacy of MabCampath in children and in patients with renal and hepatic impairment (see Section 4.2).

4.5 Interaction with other medicinal products and other forms of Interaction
No formal drug interaction studies have been performed with MabCampath. There are no known clinically significant interactions of MabCampath with other medicinal products. However, it is recommended that MabCampath should not be given within 3 weeks of other chemotherapeutic agents.

Although it has not been studied, it is recommended that patients should not receive live viral vaccines in, at least, the 12 months following MabCampath therapy. The ability to generate a primary or anamnestic humoral response to any vaccine has not been studied.

4.6 Pregnancy and lactation
Males and females of childbearing capacity should use effective contraceptive measures during treatment and for 6 months following MabCampath therapy.

Pregnancy:
MabCampath is contraindicated during pregnancy. Human IgG is known to cross the placental barrier; MabCampath may cross the placental barrier as well and thus potentially cause foetal B and T cell lymphocyte depletion. Animal reproduction studies have not been conducted with MabCampath. It is not known whether MabCampath can cause foetal harm when administered to a pregnant woman or whether it can affect reproductive capacity.

Lactation:
MabCampath is contraindicated during breast-feeding. It is not known whether MabCampath is excreted in human milk. Breast-feeding should be discontinued during treatment and for at least 4 weeks following MabCampath therapy.

4.7 Effects on ability to drive and use machines
No studies on the effects on the ability to drive and use machines have been performed. However, caution should be exercised as confusion and somnolence have been reported.

4.8 Undesirable effects
More than 80% patients may be expected to experience adverse reactions; the most commonly reported reactions usually occur during the first week of therapy.

The frequencies of the adverse reactions reported below (very common $>10\%$, common $>1\text{-}10\%$, uncommon $> 0.1\text{-}1\%$, rare $> 0.01\text{-}0.1\%$, very rare $< 0.01\%$) are based on clinical trial data in CLL patients (refer to the table) and post-marketing data.

Infusion-related reactions: very commonly reported reactions (due to release of cytokines) have been acute infusion-related reactions including fever, rigors, nausea, vomiting, hypotension, fatigue, rash, urticaria, dyspnoea, headache, pruritus and diarrhoea. The majority of these reactions are mild to moderate in severity. Serious reactions, including bronchospasm, syncope, pulmonary infiltrates, acute respiratory distress syndrome, respiratory arrest, myocardial infarction and cardiac arrest, have occurred in association with cytokine release, with fatal outcome in rare cases. Acute infusion-related reactions usually occur during the first week of therapy and substantially decline thereafter. Grade 3 or 4 infusion-related reactions are uncommon after the first week of therapy. These symptoms can be ameliorated or avoided if premedication and dose escalation are utilised (see Section 4.4).

Infections: grade 3 or 4 infections have been reported very commonly including herpes simplex and pneumonia of grade 3 or 4 severity. Opportunistic infections, including *Pneumocystis carinii* pneumonia (PCP), cytomegalovirus (CMV), *Aspergillus* pneumonia and herpes zoster occur commonly. Rhinocerebral mucormycosis has been reported but is uncommon. Other serious and sometimes fatal viral (e.g. adenovirus, parainfluenza, hepatitis B), bacterial (including tuberculosis and atypical mycobacterioses, nocardiosis), and fungal infections have occurred during post-marketing surveillance. The recommended anti-infective prophylaxis treatment appears to be effective in reducing the risk of PCP and herpes zoster infections (see Section 4.4).

Haematological reactions: severe bleeding reactions have been reported commonly. Pancytopenia has been reported commonly and may be grade 3 or 4 in severity or serious in nature. Autoimmune haemolytic anaemia and autoimmune thrombocytopenia have occurred with fatal outcome in rare cases.

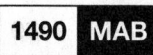

The table below details reports adverse reactions reported in the CLL clinical trials by body system and in descending order of severity:

(see Table 1)

Additional post-marketing data

Metabolism and nutritional disorders: tumour lysis syndrome has occurred in rare cases.

Central and peripheral nervous system disorders: intracranial haemorrhage has occurred in rare cases.

4.9 Overdose

Patients have received repeated unit doses of up to 240 mg of MabCampath. The frequency of grade 3 or 4 adverse events, such as fever, hypotension and anaemia, may be higher in these patients. There is no known specific antidote for MabCampath overdosage. Treatment consists of discontinuation of MabCampath and supportive therapy.

5. PHARMACOLOGICAL PROPERTIES

5.1 Pharmacodynamic properties

Pharmacotherapeutic group: monoclonal antibody, ATC code: L01X C.

Alemtuzumab is a genetically engineered humanised IgG1 kappa monoclonal antibody specific for a 21-28 kD lymphocyte cell surface glycoprotein (CD52) expressed primarily on the surface of normal and malignant peripheral blood B and T cell lymphocytes. Alemtuzumab was generated by the insertion of six complementarity-determining regions from an IgG2a rat monoclonal antibody into a human IgG1 immunoglobulin molecule.

Alemtuzumab causes the lysis of lymphocytes by binding to CD52, a highly expressed, non-modulating antigen which is present on the surface of essentially all B and T cell lymphocytes as well as monocytes, thymocytes and macrophages. The antibody mediates the lysis of lymphocytes via complement fixation and antibody-dependent cell mediated cytotoxicity. The antigen has been found on a small percentage (< 5%) of granulocytes, but not on erythrocytes or platelets. Alemtuzumab does not appear to damage haematopoietic stem cells or progenitor cells.

Determination of the efficacy of MabCampath is based on overall response and survival rates. Data available from three uncontrolled B-CLL studies are summarised in the following table:

(see Table 2 on next page)

5.2 Pharmacokinetic properties

Pharmacokinetics were characterised in MabCampath-naive patients with B-cell chronic lymphocytic leukaemia (B-CLL) who had failed previous therapy with purine analogues. MabCampath was administered as a 2 hour intravenous infusion, at the recommended dosing schedule, starting at 3 mg and increasing to 30 mg, 3 times weekly, for up to 12 weeks. MabCampath pharmacokinetics followed a 2-compartment model and displayed non-linear elimination kinetics. After the last 30 mg dose, the median volume of distribution at steady-state was 0.15 l/kg (range: 0.1-0.4 l/kg), indicating that distribution was primarily to the extracellular fluid and plasma compartments. Systemic clearance decreased with repeated administration due to decreased receptor-mediated clearance (i.e. loss of CD52 receptors in the periphery). With repeated administration and consequent plasma concentration accumulation, the rate of elimination approached zero-order kinetics. As such, half-life was 8 hours (range: 2-32 hours) after the first 30 mg dose and was 6 days (range: 1-14 days) after the last 30 mg dose. Steady-state concentrations were reached after about 6 weeks of dosing. No apparent difference in pharmacokinetics between males and females was observed nor was any apparent age effect observed.

5.3 Preclinical safety data

Preclinical evaluation of alemtuzumab in animals has been limited to the cynomolgus monkey because of the lack of expression of the CD52 antigen on non-primate species.

Lymphocytopenia was the most common treatment-related effect in this species. A slight cumulative effect on the degree of lymphocyte depletion was seen in repeated dose studies compared to single dose studies. Lymphocyte depletion was rapidly reversible after cessation of dosing. Reversible neutropenia was seen following daily intravenous or subcutaneous dosing for 30 days, but not following single doses or daily dosing for 14 days. Histopathology results from bone marrow samples revealed no remarkable changes attributable to treatment. Single intravenous doses of 10 and 30 mg/kg produced moderate to severe dose related hypotension accompanied by a slight tachycardia.

MabCampath Fab binding was observed in lymphoid tissues and the mononuclear phagocyte system. Significant Fab binding was also observed in the male reproductive tract (epididymis, sperm, seminal vesicle) and the skin.

No other findings, in the above toxicity studies, provide information of significant relevance to clinical use.

No short or long term animal studies have been conducted with MabCampath to assess carcinogenic and mutagenic potential.

Table 1

Body System	Adverse Reactions and Infections		
	Very Common	**Common**	**Uncommon**
Application site		Injection site reaction	Injection site bruising Injection site dermatitis Injection site pain
Body as a whole - general	Rigors Fever Fatigue Anorexia	Back pain Neutropenic fever Chest Pain Pain Oedema mouth Asthenia Malaise Influenza-like symptoms Oedema Temperature change sensation	Syncope Oedema peripheral Leg pain Allergic reaction
Cardiovascular	Hypotension	Hypertension Tachycardia Vasospasm Flushing Palpitation	Cardiac arrest Myocardial infarction Fibrillation atrial Tachycardia supraventricular ECG abnormal Arrhythmia Bradycardia Peripheral ischaemia
Central & peripheral nervous including vision, hearing & special senses	Headache	Taste loss Tremor Hypoaesthesia Dizziness Hyperkinesia Conjunctivitis Paraesthesia Vertigo	Gait abnormal Endophthalmitis Dystonia Hyperaesthesia Hypertonia Deafness Tinnitus Taste perversion Neuropathy
Gastro-intestinal, liver & biliary	Vomiting Nausea Diarrhoea	Abdominal pain Gastro-intestinal haemorrhage Stomatitis Mucositis Hepatic function abnormal Constipation Dyspepsia Stomatitis ulcerative Flatulence	Gastroenteritis Gingivitis Eructation Hiccup Mouth dry Mucosal ulceration Tongue ulceration
Haematological	Granulocytopenia Thrombocytopenia Anaemia	Pancytopenia Leukopenia Lymphopenia Purpura	Aplasia bone marrow Haptoglobin decreased Dissem. intravascular coagulation Anaemia haemolytic Marrow depression Epistaxis Gingival bleeding Haematology value abnormal
Metabolic & nutritional		Hyponatraemia Dehydration Weight decrease Hypocalcaemia Thirst	Diabetes mellitus aggravated Oedema periorbital Hypokalaemia
Musculo-skeletal		Skeletal pain Arthralgia Myalgia	
Neoplasm			Lymphoma-like disorder
Psychiatric		Confusion Anxiety Somnolence Depression Insomnia	Nervousness Thinking abnormal Depersonalisation Impotence Personality disorder
Resistance mechanism	Sepsis Herpes simplex	Cytomegalovirus infection *Pneumocystis carinii* infection Moniliasis Herpes zoster Infection Infection fungal Abscess	Infection viral Infection bacterial
Respiratory	Pneumonia Dyspnoea	Pneumonitis Bronchospasm Sinusitis Coughing Hypoxia Upper tract infection Bronchitis Pharyngitis Haemoptysis	Pulmonary oedema Stridor Pulmonary infiltration Respiratory disorder Breath sounds decreased Laryngitis Rhinitis Throat tightness Pleural effusion
Skin & appendages	Urticaria Rash Pruritus Sweating increased	Rash erythematous Bullous eruption	Dermatitis fungal Onychomycosis Rash maculo-papular Skin disorder
Urinary		Urinary tract infection	Renal function abnormal Polyuria Haematuria Urinary incontinence Urine flow decreased

Table 2

Efficacy Parameters	Study 1	Study 2	Study 3
Number of Patients	93	32	24
Diagnostic Group	B-CLL pts who had received an alkylating agent and had failed fludarabine	B-CLL pts who had failed to respond or relapsed following treatment with conventional chemotherapy	B-CLL (plus a PLL) pts who had failed to respond or relapsed following treatment with fludarabine
Median Age (years)	66	57	62
Disease Characteristics (%) Rai Stage III/IV B Symptoms	 76 42	 72 31	 71 21
Prior Therapies (%): Alkylating Agents Fludarabine	 100 100	 100 34	 92 100
Number of Prior Regimens (range)	3 (2-7)	3 (1-10)	3 (1-8)
Initial Dosing Regimen	Gradual escalation from 3 to 10 to 30 mg	Gradual escalation from 10 to 30 mg	Gradual escalation from 10 to 30 mg
Final Dosing Regimen	30 mg iv 3 × weekly	30 mg iv 3 × weekly	30 mg iv 3 × weekly
Overall Response Rate (%) (95% Confidence Interval) Complete Response Partial Response	33 (23-43) 2 31	21 (8-33) 0 21	29 (11-47) 0 29
Median Duration of Response (months) (95% Confidence Interval)	7 (5-8)	7 (5-23)	11 (6-19)
Median time to Response (months) (95% Confidence Interval)	2 (1-2)	4 (1-5)	4 (2-4)
Progression-Free Survival (months) (95% Confidence Interval)	4 (3-5)	5 (3-7)	7 (3-9)
Survival (months): (95% Confidence Interval) All patients Responders	 16 (12-22) 33 (26-NR)	 26 (12-44) 44 (28-NR)	 28 (7-33) 36 (19-NR)

NR = not reached

6. PHARMACEUTICAL PARTICULARS

6.1 List of excipients

Disodium edetate

Polysorbate 80

Phosphate buffered saline consisting of:

Potassium chloride

Potassium dihydrogen phosphate

Sodium chloride

Dibasic sodium phosphate

Water for injections

6.2 Incompatibilities

This medicinal product should not be reconstituted with solvents other than those mentioned in Section 6.6.

There are no known incompatibilities with other medicinal products.

6.3 Shelf life

3 years.

Reconstituted solution: MabCampath contains no antimicrobial preservative. MabCampath should be used within 8 hours after dilution. Solutions may be stored at 15°C-30°C or refrigerated. This can only be accepted if preparation of the solution takes place under strictly aseptic conditions and the solution is protected from light.

6.4 Special precautions for storage

Store in a refrigerator (2°C-8°C).

Do not freeze.

Protect from light.

6.5 Nature and contents of container

Vials of 2 ml, clear, glass type I, containing 1 ml colourless concentrate.

Pack size: carton of 3 vials.

6.6 Instructions for use and handling

The vial contents should be inspected for particulate matter and discolouration prior to administration. If particulate matter is present or the concentrate is coloured, then the vial should not be used.

MabCampath contains no antimicrobial preservatives, therefore, it is recommended that itshould be prepared using aseptic techniques and that the diluted solution for infusion should be administered within 8 hours after preparation. The required amount of the vial contents should be added to 100 ml of 0.9% sodium chloride solution or 5% glucose solution. The bag should be inverted gently to mix the solution.

Other medicinal products should not be added to the MabCampath infusion solution or simultaneously infused through the same intravenous line.

Women who are pregnant or trying to become pregnant should not handle MabCampath.

Procedures for proper handling and disposal should be observed. Any spillage or waste material should be disposed of by incineration.

Caution should be exercised in the handling and preparation of the MabCampath solution. The use of latex gloves and safety glasses is recommended to avoid exposure in case of breakage of the vial or other accidental spillage.

7. MARKETING AUTHORISATION HOLDER

Genzyme Europe BV

Gooimeer 10

1411 DD Naarden

Netherlands

8. MARKETING AUTHORISATION NUMBER(S)

EU/1/01/193/002

9. DATE OF FIRST AUTHORISATION/RENEWAL OF THE AUTHORISATION

29/10/2004

10. DATE OF REVISION OF THE TEXT

September 2005

LEGAL CATEGORY

POM

Mabthera 100mg

(Roche Products Limited)

1. NAME OF THE MEDICINAL PRODUCT

MabThera 100 mg

Concentrate for solution for infusion

2. QUALITATIVE AND QUANTITATIVE COMPOSITION

1 single-use vial contains 100 mg of rituximab in 10 ml (10 mg/ml).

Rituximab is a genetically engineered chimeric mouse/human monoclonal antibody representing a glycosylated immunoglobulin with human IgG1 constant regions and murine light-chain and heavy-chain variable region sequences. The antibody is produced by mammalian (Chinese hamster ovary) cell suspension culture and purified by affinity chromatography and ion exchange, including specific viral inactivation and removal procedures.

For excipients, see section 6.1.

3. PHARMACEUTICAL FORM

Concentrate for solution for infusion.

MabThera is a clear, colourless liquid.

4. CLINICAL PARTICULARS

4.1 Therapeutic indications

MabThera is indicated for treatment of patients with stage III-IV follicular lymphoma who are chemoresistant or are in their second or subsequent relapse after chemotherapy.

MabThera is indicated for the treatment of previously untreated patients with stage III-IV follicular lymphoma in combination with CVP chemotherapy.

MabThera is indicated for the treatment of patients with CD20 positive diffuse large B cell non-Hodgkin's lymphoma in combination with CHOP chemotherapy.

See section 5.1 (Pharmacodynamic properties) for further information.

4.2 Posology and method of administration

Standard dosage

The prepared MabThera solution should be administered as an IV infusion through a dedicated line.

MabThera infusions should be administered in a hospital environment where full resuscitation facilities are immediately available, and under the close supervision of an experienced oncologist/haematologist.

Premedication consisting of a pain-reliever and an antihistaminic, e.g. paracetamol and diphenhydramine, should always be administered before each infusion of MabThera. Premedication with corticosteroids should also be considered if MabThera is not given in combination with CHOP chemotherapy.

Patients should be closely monitored for the onset of cytokine release syndrome (see section 4.4). Patients who develop evidence of severe reactions, especially severe dyspnoea, bronchospasm or hypoxia should have the infusion interrupted immediately. The patient should then be evaluated for evidence of tumour lysis syndrome including appropriate laboratory tests and, for pulmonary infiltration, with a chest x-ray. The infusion should not be restarted until complete resolution of all symptoms, and normalisation of laboratory values and chest x-ray findings. At this time, the infusion can be initially resumed at not more than one-half the previous rate. If the same severe adverse reactions occur for a second time, the decision to stop the treatment should be seriously considered on a case by case basis.

Mild or moderate infusion-related reactions (section 4.8) usually respond to a reduction in the rate of infusion. The infusion rate may be increased upon improvement of symptoms.

Follicular non-Hodgkin's lymphoma

The recommended dosage of MabThera used as a single agent for adult patients is 375 mg/m² body surface, administered as an IV infusion once weekly for four weeks.

The recommended dosage of MabThera in combination with CVP chemotherapy is 375 mg/m² body surface area for 8 cycles (21 days/cycle), administered on day 1 of each chemotherapy cycle after IV administration of the corticosteroid component of CVP.

Retreatment following relapse in non-Hodgkin's lymphoma: Patients who have responded to MabThera initially have been treated again with MabThera at a dose of 375 mg/m² body surface area, administered as an IV infusion once weekly for four weeks (see section 5.1).

Diffuse large B cell non-Hodgkin's lymphoma

MabThera should be used in combination with CHOP chemotherapy. The recommended dosage is 375 mg/m² body surface area, administered on day 1 of each chemotherapy cycle for 8 cycles after IV administration of the corticosteroid component of CHOP. Safety and efficacy of MabThera have not been established in combination with other chemotherapies.

First infusion: The recommended initial rate for infusion is 50 mg/hr; after the first 30 minutes, it can be escalated in 50 mg/hr increments every 30 minutes, to a maximum of 400 mg/hr.

Subsequent infusions: Subsequent doses of MabThera can be infused at an initial rate of 100 mg/hr, and increased by 100 mg/hr increments at 30 minutes intervals, to a maximum of 400 mg/hr.

Dosage adjustments during treatment

No dose reductions of MabThera are recommended. When MabThera is given in combination with CHOP or CVP chemotherapy, standard dose reductions for the chemotherapeutic medicinal products should be applied.

4.3 Contraindications

MabThera is contraindicated in patients with known hypersensitivity to any component of this product or to murine proteins.

4.4 Special warnings and special precautions for use
Patients with a high tumour burden or with a high number (≥ 25 × 10^9/l) of circulating malignant cells, who may be at higher risk of especially severe cytokine release syndrome, should only be treated with extreme caution and when other therapeutic alternatives have been exhausted. These patients should be very closely monitored throughout the first infusion. Consideration should be given to the use of a reduced infusion rate for the first infusion in these patients.

Severe cytokine release syndrome is characterised by severe dyspnoea, often accompanied by bronchospasm and hypoxia, in addition to fever, chills, rigors, urticaria, and angioedema. This syndrome may be associated with some features of ***tumour lysis syndrome*** such as hyperuricaemia, hyperkalaemia, hypocalcaemia, acute renal failure, elevated LDH and may be associated with acute respiratory failure and death. The acute respiratory failure may be accompanied by events such as pulmonary interstitial infiltration or oedema, visible on a chest x-ray. The syndrome frequently manifests itself within one or two hours of initiating the first infusion. Patients with a history of pulmonary insufficiency or those with pulmonary tumour infiltration may be at greater risk of poor outcome and should be treated with increased caution. Patients who develop severe cytokine release syndrome should have their infusion interrupted immediately (see section 4.2) and should receive aggressive symptomatic treatment. Since initial improvement of clinical symptoms may be followed by deterioration, these patients should be closely monitored until tumour lysis syndrome and pulmonary infiltration have been resolved or ruled out. Further treatment of patients after complete resolution of signs and symptoms has rarely resulted in repeated severe cytokine release syndrome.

Infusion related adverse reactions including cytokine release syndrome (see section 4.8) accompanied by hypotension and bronchospasm have been observed in 10 % of patients treated with MabThera. These symptoms are usually reversible with interruption of MabThera infusion and administration of a pain-reliever, an antihistaminic, and, occasionally, oxygen, IV saline or bronchodilators, and corticosteroids if required. Please see cytokine release syndrome above for severe reactions.

Anaphylactic and other hypersensitivity reactions have been reported following the IV administration of proteins to patients. In contrast to cytokine release syndrome, true hypersensitivity reactions typically occur within minutes after starting infusion. Medicinal products for the treatment of hypersensitivity reactions, e.g., epinephrine, antihistamines and corticosteroids, should be available for immediate use in the event of an allergic reaction during administration of MabThera. Clinical manifestations of anaphylaxis may appear similar to clinical manifestations of the cytokine release syndrome (described above). Reactions attributed to hypersensitivity have been reported less frequently than those attributed to cytokine release.

Since hypotension may occur during MabThera infusion, consideration should be given to withholding anti-hypertensive medications 12 hours prior to the MabThera infusion.

Angina pectoris, or cardiac arrhythmias such as atrial flutter and fibrillation heart failure or myocardial infarction have occurred in patients treated with MabThera. Therefore patients with a history of cardiac disease and/or cardiotoxic chemotherapy should be monitored closely.

Although MabThera is not myelosuppressive in monotherapy, caution should be exercised when considering treatment of patients with neutrophils < 1.5 × 10^9/l and/or platelet counts < 75 × 10^9/l, as clinical experience in this population is limited. MabThera has been used in 21 patients who underwent autologous bone transplantation and other risk groups with a presumable reduced bone marrow function without inducing myelotoxicity.

Consideration should be given to the need for regular full blood counts, including platelet counts, during monotherapy with MabThera. When MabThera is given in combination with CHOP or CVP chemotherapy, regular full blood counts should be performed according to usual medical practice.

Very rare cases of hepatitis B reactivation, including reports of fulminant hepatitis, have been reported in subjects receiving rituximab, although these subjects were also exposed to cytotoxic chemotherapy. The reports are confounded by both the underlying disease state and the cytotoxic chemotherapy. Patients with a history of hepatitis B infection should be carefully monitored for signs of active hepatitis B infection when rituximab is used in association with cytotoxic chemotherapy.

Do not administer the prepared infusion solutions as an IV push or bolus.

Paediatric Use

The safety and efficacy of MabThera in children have not been established.

4.5 Interaction with other medicinal products and other forms of Interaction
Currently, no data are available on possible drug interactions with MabThera. Patients with human anti-mouse antibody or human anti-chimeric antibody (HAMA/HACA) titres may have allergic or hypersensitivity reactions when treated with other diagnostic or therapeutic monoclonal antibodies.

The tolerability of simultaneous or sequential combination of MabThera with chemotherapy other than CHOP or CVP, or agents which are liable to cause depletion of normal B cells is not well defined.

4.6 Pregnancy and lactation
Pregnancy
Animal reproduction studies have not been conducted with rituximab. It is also not known whether MabThera can cause foetal harm when administered to a pregnant woman or whether it can affect reproductive capacity. However, since IgG is known to pass the placental barrier, rituximab may cause B cell depletion in the foetus. For these reasons MabThera should not be given to a pregnant woman unless the potential benefit outweighs the potential risk.

Due to the long retention time of rituximab in B cell depleted patients, women of childbearing potential should use effective contraceptive methods during treatment and up to 12 months following MabThera therapy.

Lactation

Whether rituximab is excreted in human milk is not known. However, because maternal IgG is excreted in human milk, MabThera should not be given to women who are breast-feeding.

4.7 Effects on ability to drive and use machines
No studies on the effects on the ability to drive and use machines have been performed, although the pharmacological activity and adverse events reported to date do not indicate that such an effect is likely.

4.8 Undesirable effects
Monotherapy
The following data are based on 356 patients treated in single-arm studies of MabThera administered as single agent (see section 5.1). Most patients received MabThera 375 mg/m^2 weekly for 4 doses. These include 39 patients with bulky disease (lesions ≥ 10 cm) and 58 patients who received more than one course of MabThera (60 re-treatments). Thirty-seven patients received 375 mg/m^2 for eight doses and 25 patients received doses other than 375 mg/m^2 for four doses and up to 500 mg/m^2 single dose in the Phase I setting.

The following table shows adverse events that were considered to be at least possibly related to MabThera during or up to 12 months after treatment. Adverse events were graded according to the four-scale National Cancer Institute (NCI) Common Toxicity Criteria.

Table 1. Summary of adverse events reported in ≥ 1 % of 356 patients receiving MabThera monotherapy in clinical trials

	All grades	Grade 3 and 4
Body system Adverse event	%	%
Any adverse event	91.0	17.7
Body as a whole		
Fever	48.3	0.6
Chills	31.7	2.2
Asthenia	18.0	0.3
Headache	12.6	0.6
Throat irritation	7.6	-
Abdominal pain	7.0	0.6
Back pain	4.5	0.3
Pain	4.2	-
Flushing	4.2	-
Chest pain	2.2	-
Malaise	2.0	-
Tumour pain	1.7	-
Cold syndrome	1.4	-
Neck pain	1.1	-
Cardiovascular system		
Hypotension	9.8	0.8
Hypertension	4.5	0.3
Tachycardia	1.4	-
Arrhythmia	1.4	0.6
Orthostatic hypotension	1.1	-
Digestive system		
Nausea	17.1	0.3
Vomiting	6.7	0.3
Diarrhoea	4.2	-
Dyspepsia	2.8	-
Anorexia	2.8	-
Dysphagia	1.4	0.3
Stomatitis	1.4	-
Constipation	1.1	-
Blood and lymphatic system		
Leucopenia	12.4	2.8
Neutropenia	11.2	4.2
Thrombocytopenia	9.6	1.7
Anaemia	3.7	1.1
Metabolic and nutritional disorders		
Angioedema	10.7	0.3
Hyperglycaemia	5.3	0.3
Peripheral oedema	4.8	-
LDH increase	2.2	-
Hypocalcaemia	2.2	-
Facial oedema	1.1	-
Weight decrease	1.1	-
Musculoskeletal system		
Myalgia	8.1	0.3
Arthralgia	5.9	0.6
Hypertonia	1.4	-
Pain	1.1	0.3
Nervous system		
Dizziness	7.3	-
Paraesthesia	2.5	-
Anxiety	2.2	-
Insomnia	2.2	-
Vasodilatation	1.7	-
Hypoaesthesia	1.4	-
Agitation	1.4	-
Respiratory system		
Bronchospasm	7.9	1.4
Rhinitis	7.3	0.3
Increased cough	5.1	0.3
Dyspnoea	2.2	0.8
Chest pain	1.1	-
Respiratory disease	1.1	-
Skin and appendages		
Pruritus	12.4	0.3

Rash	11.2	0.3
Urticaria	7.3	0.8
Night sweats	2.8	-
Sweating	2.8	-
Special senses		
Lacrimation disorder	3.1	-
Conjunctivitis	1.4	-
Ear pain	1.1	-
Tinnitus	1.1	-

The following adverse events were also reported (< 1 %): coagulation disorders, asthma, lung disorder, bronchiolitis obliterans, hypoxia, abdominal enlargement, pain at the infusion site, bradycardia, lymphadenopathy, nervousness, depression, dysgeusia.

Infusion-related reactions: Infusion-related reactions occurred in more than 50 % of patients, and were predominantly seen during the first infusion, usually during the first one to two hours. These events mainly comprised fever, chills, and rigors. Other symptoms included flushing, angioedema, nausea, urticaria/rash, fatigue, headache, throat irritation, rhinitis, vomiting, and tumour pain. These symptoms were accompanied by hypotension and bronchospasm in about 10 % of the cases. Less frequently, patients experienced an exacerbation of pre-existing cardiac conditions such as angina pectoris or congestive heart failure. The incidence of infusion-related symptoms decreases substantially with subsequent infusions (see section 4.4).

Infections: MabThera induced B cell depletion in 70 % to 80 % of patients but was associated with decreased serum immunoglobulins only in a minority of patients. Infectious events, irrespective of causal assessment, occurred in 30.3 % of 356 patients: 18.8 % of patients had bacterial infections, 10.4 % had viral infections, 1.4 % had fungal infections, and 5.9 % had infections of unknown aetiology. Severe infectious events (grade 3 or 4), including sepsis occurred in 3.9 % of patients; in 1.4 % during the treatment period and in 2.5 % during the follow up period. As these were single-arm trials, the contributory role of MabThera or of the underlying NHL and its previous treatment to the development of these infectious events cannot be determined.

Haematologic Adverse Reactions: Haematological abnormalities occurred in a minority of patients and are usually mild and reversible. Severe (grade 3 and 4) thrombocytopenia and neutropenia were reported in 1.7 % and 4.2 % of patients respectively, and severe anaemia was reported in 1.1 % of patients. A single occurrence of transient aplastic anaemia (pure red cell aplasia) and infrequent occurrences of haemolytic anaemia following MabThera treatment were reported.

Cardiovascular events: Cardiovascular events were reported in 18.8 % of patients during the treatment period. The most frequently reported events were hypotension and hypertension. Two patients (0.6 %) experienced grade 3 or 4 arrhythmia (including ventricular and supraventricular tachycardia) during a MabThera infusion and one patient with a history of myocardial infarction experienced angina pectoris, evolving into myocardial infarction 4 days later.

Subpopulations:

Elderly patients: (≥ 65 years): The incidence of any adverse event and of grade 3 and 4 adverse events was similar in elderly (N=94) and younger (N=237) patients (88.3 % versus 92.0 % for any adverse event and 16.0 % versus 18.1 % for grade 3 and 4 adverse events).

Bulky disease: Patients with bulky disease (N=39) had a higher incidence of grade 3 and 4 adverse events than patients without bulky disease (N=195) (25.6 % versus 15.4 %). The incidence of any adverse event was similar in these two groups (92.3 % in bulky disease versus 89.2 % in non-bulky disease).

Re-treatment: The percentage of patients reporting any adverse event and grade 3 and 4 adverse events upon re-treatment (N=60) with further courses of MabThera was similar to the percentage of patients reporting any adverse event and grade 3 and 4 adverse events upon initial exposure (N=203) (95.0 % versus 89.7 % for any adverse event and 13.3 % versus 14.8 % for grade 3 and 4 adverse events).

Adverse reactions reported in other monotherapy clinical trials: One case of serum sickness has been reported in a clinical trial using MabThera monotherapy for treatment of diffuse large B cell lymphoma.

In combination with CVP chemotherapy

The following data are based on 321 patients from a randomised phase III clinical trial comparing MabThera plus CVP (R-CVP) to CVP alone (162 R-CVP, 159 CVP).

Differences between the treatment groups with respect to the type and incidence of adverse event were mainly accounted for by typical adverse events associated with MabThera monotherapy.

The following grade 3 to 4 clinical adverse events were reported in ≥ 2 % higher incidence in patients receiving R-CVP compared to CVP treatment group and therefore may be attributable to R-CVP. Adverse events were graded according to the four-scale National Cancer Institute (NCI) Common Toxicity Criteria:

- Fatigue: 3.7 % (R-CVP), 1.3 % (CVP)
- Neutropenia: 3.1 % (R-CVP), 0.6 % (CVP)

Infusion-related reactions: The signs and symptoms of severe or life-threatening (NCI CTC grades 3 and 4) infusion-related reactions (defined as starting during or within one day of an infusion with MabThera) occurred in 9 % of all patients who received R-CVP. These results are consistent with those observed during monotherapy (see section 4.4 and 4.8, Undesirable effects, monotherapy), and included rigors, fatigue, dyspnoea, dyspepsia, nausea, rash NOS, flushing.

Infections: The overall proportion of patients with infections or infestations during treatment and for 28 days after trial treatment end was comparable between the treatment groups (33 % R-CVP, 32 % CVP). The most common infections were upper respiratory tract infections which were reported for 12.3 % patients on R-CVP and 16.4 % patients receiving CVP; most of these infections were nasopharyngitis.

Serious infections were reported in 4.3 % of the patients receiving R-CVP and 4.4 % of the patients receiving CVP. No life threatening infections were reported during this study.

Haematologic laboratory abnormalities: 24 % of patients on R-CVP and 14 % of patients on CVP experienced grade 3 or 4 neutropenia during treatment. The proportion of patients with grade 4 neutropenia was comparable between the treatment groups. These laboratory findings were reported as adverse events and resulted in medical intervention in 3.1 % of patients on R-CVP and 0.6 % of patients on CVP. All other laboratory abnormalities were not treated and resolved without any intervention. In addition, the higher incidence of neutropenia in the R-CVP group was not associated with a higher incidence of infections and infestations.

No relevant difference between the two treatment arms was observed with respect to grade 3 and 4 anaemia (0.6 % R-CVP and 1.9 % CVP) and thrombocytopenia (1.2 % in the R-CVP group and no events reported in the CVP group).

Cardiac events: The overall incidence of cardiac disorders in the safety population was low (4 % R-CVP, 5 % CVP), with no relevant differences between the treatment groups.

In combination with CHOP chemotherapy

The following table shows grade 3 to 4 clinical adverse events, including grade 2 infections, from a randomised phase III clinical trial comparing MabThera plus CHOP (R-CHOP) to CHOP alone in a safety population of 398 patients. Events shown were reported at a greater than 2 % higher incidence with R-CHOP when compared to CHOP alone and therefore may be attributable to R-CHOP (absolute incidence cut off at 2 %). Adverse events were graded according to the four-scale National Cancer Institute of Canada (NCIC) Common Toxicity Criteria.

Table 2: Excess incidence (> = 2 %) of grade 3 and 4 adverse events (including grade 2 infections) with R-CHOP compared with CHOP (overall cut off of 2 %)

	R-CHOP	CHOP
	N=202	N=196
	%	%
Infections and infestations		
Bronchitis	11.9	8.2
Herpes zoster	4.0	1.5
Acute bronchitis	2.5	0.5
Sinusitis	2.5	-
Respiratory disorders		
Dyspnoea	8.9	3.6
General disorders and administration site disorders		
Shivering	3.5	1.0
Vascular disorders		
Hypertension	2.5	0.5
Cardiac disorder		
Atrial fibrillation	2.5	0.5

Infusion-related reactions: Grade 3 and 4 infusion-related reactions (defined as starting during or within one day of an infusion with MabThera) occurred in approximately 9 % of patients at the time of the first cycle of R-CHOP. The incidence of grade 3 and 4 infusion-related reactions decreased to less than 1 % by the eighth cycle of R-CHOP. The signs and symptoms were consistent with those observed during monotherapy (see section 4.4 and 4.8, Undesirable effects, monotherapy), and included fever, chills, hypotension, hypertension, tachycardia, dyspnoea, bronchospasm, nausea, vomiting, pain and features of tumour lysis syndrome. Additional reactions reported in isolated cases at the time of R-CHOP therapy were myocardial infarction, atrial fibrillation and pulmonary oedema.

Infections: The proportion of patients with grade 2 to 4 infections and/or febrile neutropenia was 55.4 % in the R-CHOP group and 51.5 % in the CHOP group. Febrile neutropenia (i.e. no report of concomitant documented infection) was reported only during the treatment period, in 20.8 % in the R-CHOP group and 15.3 % in the CHOP group. The overall incidence of grade 2 to 4 infections was 45.5 % in the R-CHOP group and 42.3 % in the CHOP group with no difference in the incidence of systemic bacterial and fungal infections. Grade 2 to 4 fungal infections were more frequent in the R-CHOP group (4.5 % vs 2.6 % in the CHOP group); this difference was due to a higher incidence of localised Candida infections during the treatment period. The incidence of grade 2 to 4 herpes zoster, including ophthalmic herpes zoster, was higher in the R-CHOP group (4.5 %) than in the CHOP group (1.5 %), with 7 of a total of 9 cases in the R-CHOP group occurring during the treatment phase.

Haematologic events: After each treatment cycle, grade 3 and 4 leucopenia (88 % vs 79 %) and neutropenia (97 % vs 88 %) occurred more frequently in the R-CHOP group than in the CHOP group. There was no evidence that neutropenia was more prolonged in the R-CHOP group. No difference between the two treatment arms was observed with respect to grade 3 and 4 anaemia (19 % in the CHOP group vs 14 % in the R-CHOP group) and thrombocytopenia (16 % in the CHOP group vs 15 % in the R-CHOP group). The time to recovery from all haematological abnormalities was comparable in the two treatment groups.

Cardiac events: The incidence of grade 3 and 4 cardiac arrhythmias, predominantly supraventricular arrhythmias such as tachycardia and atrial flutter/fibrillation, was higher in the R-CHOP group (14 patients, 6.9 %) as compared to the CHOP group (3 patients, 1.5 %). All of these arrhythmias either occurred in the context of a MabThera infusion or were associated with predisposing conditions such as fever, infection, acute myocardial infarction or pre-existing respiratory and cardiovascular disease. No difference between the R-CHOP and CHOP group was observed in the incidence of other grade 3 and 4 cardiac events including heart failure, myocardial disease and manifestations of coronary artery disease.

Neurologic events: During the treatment period, four patients (2 %) in the R-CHOP group, all with cardiovascular risk factors, experienced thromboembolic cerebrovascular accidents during the first treatment cycle. There was no difference between the treatment groups in the incidence of other thromboembolic events. In contrast, three patients (1.5 %) had cerebrovascular events in the CHOP group, all of which occurred during the follow-up period.

Post-marketing experience

As part of the continuing post-marketing surveillance of MabThera safety, the following serious adverse reactions have been observed:

Blood and lymphatic system disorders	
Rare (≥ 1/10,000, < 1/1000):	Late neutropenia[1]
Very rare (< 1/10,000):	Pancytopenia Aplastic anaemia Transient increase in serum IgM levels[2]
Cardiovascular system	
Rare (≥ 1/10,000, < 1/1000):	*Severe cardiac events[3]
Very rare (< 1/10,000):	*Heart failure[3] *Myocardial infarction[3]
Ear and labyrinth disorders	
Very rare (< 1/10,000):	†Hearing loss
Eye disorders	
Very rare (< 1/10,000):	†Severe vision loss
General disorders and administration site conditions	
Very rare (< 1/10,000):	*Multi-organ failure

Immune system disorders	
Uncommon (⩾ 1/1000, < 1/100):	Infusion related reactions
Rare (⩾ 1/10,000, < 1/1000):	Anaphylaxis
Very rare (< 1/10,000):	*Tumour lysis syndrome *Cytokine release syndrome Serum sickness Hepatitis B reactivation[4]
Nervous system disorders	
Very rare (< 1/10,000):	Cranial neuropathy Peripheral neuropathy †Facial nerve palsy †Loss of other senses
Renal and urinary disorders	
Very rare (< 1/10,000):	*Renal failure
Respiratory, thoracic and mediastinal disorders	
Rare (⩾ 1/10,000, < 1/1000):	*Bronchospasm
Very rare (< 1/10,000):	*Respiratory failure Pulmonary infiltrates Interstitial pneumonitis
Skin and subcutaneous tissue disorders	
Very rare (< 1/10,000):	Severe bullous skin reactions Toxic epidermal necrolysis[5]
Vascular disorders	
Very rare (< 1/10,000):	Vasculitis (predominately cutaneous) Leucocytoclastic vasculitis

*Associated with infusion-related reactions. Rarely fatal cases reported

† Signs and symptoms of cranial neuropathy. Occurred at various times up to several months after completion of MabThera therapy

[1] Neutropenia that has occurred more than four weeks after the last infusion of MabThera.

[2] In post-marketing studies of rituximab in patients with Waldenstrom's macroglobulinaemia, transient increases in serum IgM levels have been observed following treatment initiation, which may be associated with hyperviscosity and related symptoms. The transient IgM increase usually returned to at least baseline level within 4 months.

[3] Observed mainly in patients with prior cardiac condition and/or cardiotoxic chemotherapy and were mostly associated with infusion-related reactions

[4] Very rare cases of hepatitis B reactivation, have been reported in subjects receiving rituximab in combination with cytotoxic chemotherapy.

[5] Including fatal cases

4.9 Overdose

There has been no experience of overdose in human clinical trials. However, single doses higher than 500 mg/m^2 body surface have not been tested in controlled clinical trials.

5. PHARMACOLOGICAL PROPERTIES

5.1 Pharmacodynamic properties

Pharmacotherapeutic group: Antineoplastic Agents, ATC code: L01X C02

Rituximab binds specifically to the transmembrane antigen, CD20, a non-glycosylated phosphoprotein, located on pre-B and mature B lymphocytes. The antigen is expressed on >95 % of all B cell non-Hodgkin's lymphomas (NHLs).

CD20 is found on both normal and malignant B cells, but not on haematopoietic stem cells, pro-B cells, normal plasma cells or other normal tissue. This antigen does not internalise upon antibody binding and is not shed from the cell surface. CD20 does not circulate in the plasma as a free antigen and, thus, does not compete for antibody binding.

The Fab domain of rituximab binds to the CD20 antigen on B lymphocytes and the Fc domain can recruit immune effector functions to mediate B cell lysis. Possible mechanisms of effector-mediated cell lysis include complement-dependent cytotoxicity (CDC) resulting from C1q binding, and antibody-dependent cellular cytotoxicity (ADCC) mediated by one or more of the Fcγ receptors on the surface of granulocytes, macrophages and NK cells. Rituximab binding to CD 20 antigen on B lymphocytes has also been demonstrated to induce cell death via apoptosis.

Median peripheral B cell counts declined below normal following completion of the first dose, with recovery beginning after 6 months. B cell levels returned to normal between 9 and 12 months following completion of therapy.

Follicular non-Hodgkin's lymphoma:

Monotherapy:*Initial treatment, weekly for 4 doses:* In the pivotal study, 166 patients with relapsed or chemoresistant low-grade or follicular B cell NHL received 375 mg/m^2 of MabThera as an IV infusion once weekly for four weeks. The overall response rate (ORR) in the intent-to-treat (ITT) population was 48 % ($CI_{95\ \%}$ 41 % - 56 %) with a 6 % complete response (CR) and a 42 % partial response (PR) rate. The projected median time to progression (TTP) for responding patients was 13.0 months. In a subgroup analysis, the ORR was higher in patients with IWF B, C, and D histological subtypes as compared to IWF A subtype (58 % vs. 12 %), higher in patients whose largest lesion was < 5 cm vs. > 7 cm in greatest diameter (53 % vs. 38 %), and higher in patients with chemosensitive relapse as compared to chemoresistant (defined as duration of response < 3 months) relapse (50 % vs. 22 %). ORR in patients previously treated with autologous bone marrow transplant (ABMT) was 78 % versus 43 % in patients with no ABMT. Neither age, sex, lymphoma grade, initial diagnosis, presence or absence of bulky disease, normal or high LDH nor presence of extranodal disease had a statistically significant effect (Fisher's exact test) on response to MabThera. A statistically significant correlation was noted between response rates and bone marrow involvement. 40 % of patients with bone marrow involvement responded compared to 59 % of patients with no bone marrow involvement (p=0.0186). This finding was not supported by a stepwise logistic regression analysis in which the following factors were identified as prognostic factors: histological type, bcl-2 positivity at baseline, resistance to last chemotherapy and bulky disease.

Initial treatment, weekly for 8 doses: In a multi-centre, single-arm study, 37 patients with relapsed or chemoresistant, low grade or follicular B cell NHL received 375 mg/m^2 of MabThera as IV infusion weekly for eight doses. The ORR was 57 % ($CI_{95\ \%}$ 41 % – 73 %; CR 14 %, PR 43 %) with a projected median TTP for responding patients of 19.4 months (range 5.3 to 38.9 months).

Initial treatment, bulky disease, weekly for 4 doses: In pooled data from three studies, 39 patients with relapsed or chemoresistant, bulky disease (single lesion ⩾ 10 cm in diameter), low grade or follicular B cell NHL received 375 mg/m^2 of MabThera as IV infusion weekly for four doses. The ORR was 36 % ($CI_{95\ \%}$ 21 % – 51 %; CR 3 %, PR 33 %) with a median TTP for responding patients of 9.6 months (range 4.5 to 26.8 months).

Re-treatment, weekly for 4 doses: In a multi-centre, single-arm study, 58 patients with relapsed or chemoresistant low grade or follicular B cell NHL, who had achieved an objective clinical response to a prior course of MabThera, were re-treated with 375 mg/m^2 of MabThera as IV infusion weekly for four doses. Three of the patients had received two courses of MabThera before enrollment and thus were given a third course in the study. Two patients were re-treated twice in the study. For the 60 re-treatments on study, the ORR was 38 % ($CI_{95\ \%}$ 26 % – 51 %; 10 % CR, 28 % PR) with a projected median TTP for responding patients of 17.8 months (range 5.4 – 26.6). This compares favourably with the TTP achieved after the prior course of MabThera (12.4 months).

Initial treatment, in combination with CVP: In an open-label randomised trial, a total of 322 previously untreated low-grade or follicular B cell NHL patients were randomised to receive either CVP chemotherapy (cyclophosphamide 750 mg/m^2, vincristine 1.4 mg/m^2 up to a maximum of 2 mg on day 1, and prednisolone 40 mg/m^2/day on days 1 – 5) every 3 weeks for 8 cycles or MabThera 375 mg/m^2 in combination with CVP (R-CVP). MabThera was administered on the first day of each treatment cycle. A total of 321 patients (162 R-CVP, 159 CVP) received therapy and were analysed for efficacy. At the time of the analysis, the median observation time was 18 months. R-CVP led to a significant benefit over CVP for the primary endpoint, time to treatment failure (25.9 months vs. 6.7 months, p < 0.0001, log-rank test). The risk of experiencing a treatment failure event was reduced by 67 % (95 % CI: 56 % - 76 %) with R-CVP compared with CVP alone, using a Cox regression analysis. The Kaplan-Meier estimated event free rate at 12 months was 69 % in the R-CVP group compared with 32 % in the CVP group. The proportion of patients with a tumour response (CR, CRu, PR) was significantly higher (p< 0.0001 Chi-Square test) in the R-CVP group (80.9 %) than the CVP group (57.2 %). At 18 months, the median duration of response had not been reached in the R-CVP group and was 9.8 months in the CVP group (p < 0.0001, log-rank test). Amongst responding patients, Cox regression analysis showed that the risk of relapse was reduced by 70 % (95 % CI: 55 % - 81 %) in the R-CVP group compared to the CVP group.

The time to institution of new lymphoma treatment or death was significantly longer in the R-CVP group (not estimable), compared to the CVP group (12.3 months) (p < 0.0001, log-rank test). Treatment with R-CVP significantly prolonged the time to disease progression compared to CVP, 27 months and 14.5 months, respectively. At 12 months, 81 % in the R-CVP group had not relapsed compared to 58 % of patients receiving CVP.

The benefit of adding rituximab to CVP was seen consistently throughout the population recruited in study M39021 (randomised according to BNLI criteria (no versus yes), age (⩽ 60 years, > 60 years), number of extra-nodal sites (0-1 versus > 1), bone marrow involvement (no versus yes), LDH (elevated, not elevated), β_2-microglobulin (elevated, not elevated), B symptoms (absent, present), bulky disease (absent, present), number of nodal sites (< 5 versus ⩾ 5), haemoglobin (⩽ 12 g/dL versus > 12 g/dL), IPI (⩽ 1 versus > 1), and FLIPI index (0-2 versus 3-5)).

Due to the number of events at the time of analysis and the relatively short observation time of 18 months, conclusion regarding differences for overall survival cannot be drawn.

Diffuse large B cell non-Hodgkin's lymphoma: In a randomised, open-label trial, a total of 399 previously untreated elderly patients (age 60 to 80 years) with diffuse large B cell lymphoma received standard CHOP chemotherapy (cyclophosphamide 750 mg/m^2, doxorubicin 50 mg/m^2, vincristine 1.4 mg/m^2 up to a maximum of 2 mg on day 1, and prednisone 40 mg/m^2/day on days 1-5) every 3 weeks for eight cycles, or MabThera 375 mg/m^2 plus CHOP (R-CHOP). MabThera was administered on the first day of the treatment cycle.

The final efficacy analysis included all randomised patients (197 CHOP, 202 R-CHOP), and had a median follow-up duration of approximately 31 months. The two treatment groups were well balanced in baseline disease characteristics and disease status. The final analysis confirmed that R-CHOP treatment was associated with a clinically relevant and statistically significant improvement in the duration of event-free survival (the primary efficacy parameter; where events were death, relapse or progression of lymphoma, or institution of a new anti-lymphoma treatment) (p = 0.0001). Kaplan Meier estimates of the median duration of event-free survival were 35 months in the R-CHOP arm compared to 13 months in the CHOP arm, representing a risk reduction of 41 %. At 24 months, estimates for overall survival were 68.2 % in the R-CHOP arm compared to 57.4 % in the CHOP arm. A subsequent analysis of the duration of overall survival, carried out with a median follow-up duration of 38 months, confirmed the benefit of R-CHOP over CHOP treatment (p=0.0094), representing a risk reduction of 33 %.

The analysis of all secondary parameters (response rates, progression-free survival, disease-free survival, duration of response) verified the treatment effect of R-CHOP compared to CHOP. The complete response rate after cycle 8 was 76.2 % in the R-CHOP group and 62.4 % in the CHOP group (p=0.0028). The risk of disease progression was reduced by 46 % and the risk of relapse by 51 %.

In all patients subgroups (gender, age, age adjusted IPI, Ann Arbor stage, ECOG, β2 microglobulin, LDH, albumin, B symptoms, bulky disease, extranodal sites, bone marrow involvement), the risk ratios for event-free survival and overall survival (R-CHOP compared with CHOP) were less than 0.83 and 0.95 respectively. R-CHOP was associated with improvements in outcome for both high- and low-risk patients according to age adjusted IPI.

Clinical Laboratory Findings

Of 67 patients evaluated for human anti-mouse antibody (HAMA), no responses were noted. Of 356 patients evaluated for HACA, 1.1 % (4 patients) were positive.

5.2 Pharmacokinetic properties

Pharmacokinetic studies performed in a phase I study in which patients (n=15) with relapsed B cell lymphoma were given single doses of rituximab at 10, 50, 100 or 500 mg/m^2 indicated that serum levels and half-life of rituximab were proportional to dose. In a cohort of 14 patients among the 166 patients with relapsed or chemoresistant low-grade or follicular non-Hodgkin's lymphoma enrolled in the phase III pivotal trial and given rituximab 375 mg/m^2 as an IV infusion for 4 weekly doses, the mean serum half-life was 76.3 hours (range, 31.5 to 152.6 hours) after the first infusion and 205.8 hours (range, 83.9 to 407.0 hours) after the fourth infusion. The mean C_{max} after the first and fourth infusion were 205.6 ± 59.9 μg/ml and 464.7 ± 119.0 μg/ml, respectively. The mean plasma clearance after the first and fourth infusion was 0.0382 ± 0.0182 L/h and 0.0092 ± 0.0033 L/h, respectively. However, variability in serum levels was large.

Rituximab serum concentrations were statistically significantly higher in responding patients compared to non-responding patients just prior to and after the fourth infusion and post treatment. Serum concentrations were negatively correlated with tumour burden and the number of circulating B cells at baseline. Typically, rituximab was detectable for 3 to 6 months.

Elimination and distribution have not been extensively studied in patients with diffuse large B cell non-Hodgkin's lymphoma, but available data indicate that serum levels of rituximab in these patients are comparable to those in patients with follicular non-Hodgkin's lymphoma following treatment with similar doses.

5.3 Preclinical safety data

Rituximab has shown to be highly specific to the CD20 antigen on B cells. Toxicity studies in cynomolgus monkeys have shown no other effect than the expected pharmacological depletion of B cells in peripheral blood and in lymphoid tissue. The recovery of the peripheral B-cells was marked by large intraindividual variability. However, peripheral B cell recovery usually started two weeks after treatment, and median B cells counts reached 40 % of baseline levels after a 3 month period. No adverse reactions unrelated to the targeted effect were seen, whether in single or in multiple dose studies in the cynomolgus monkey.

No long-term animal studies have been performed to establish the carcinogenic potential of rituximab, or to determine its effects on fertility in males or females. Standard tests to investigate mutagenicity have not been carried out, since such tests are not relevant for this molecule. However, due to its character it is unlikely that rituximab has any mutagenic potential.

6. PHARMACEUTICAL PARTICULARS

6.1 List of excipients
Sodium citrate

Polysorbate 80

Sodium chloride

Sodium hydroxide

Hydrochloric acid

Water for injections

6.2 Incompatibilities
No incompatibilities between MabThera and polyvinyl chloride or polyethylene bags or infusion sets have been observed.

6.3 Shelf life
30 months

The prepared infusion solution of MabThera is physically and chemically stable for 24 hours at 2 °C – 8 °C and subsequently 12 hours at room temperature.

6.4 Special precautions for storage
Store vials at 2 °C - 8 °C (in a refrigerator). Keep the container in the outer carton in order to protect from light.

The prepared infusion solution of MabThera is physically and chemically stable for 24 hours at 2 °C – 8 °C and subsequently 12 hours at room temperature.

From a microbiological point of view, the prepared infusion solution should be used immediately. If not used immediately, in-use storage times and conditions prior to use are the responsibility of the user and would normally not be longer than 24 hours at 2 °C – 8 °C, unless dilution has taken place in controlled and validated aseptic conditions.

6.5 Nature and contents of container
Single-use, preservative-free, clear Type I glass vials with butyl rubber stopper containing 100 mg of rituximab in 10 ml (10 mg/ml).

Packs of 2 vials.

6.6 Instructions for use and handling
MabThera is provided in sterile, preservative-free, non-pyrogenic, single use vials.

Aseptically withdraw the necessary amount of MabThera, and dilute to a calculated concentration of 1 to 4 mg/ml rituximab into an infusion bag containing sterile, pyrogen-free 0.9 % Sodium Chloride or 5 % Dextrose in water. For mixing the solution, gently invert the bag in order to avoid foaming. Care must be taken to ensure the sterility of prepared solutions. Since the drug product does not contain any anti-microbial preservative or bacteriostatic agents, aseptic technique must be observed. Parenteral drug products should be inspected visually for particulate matter and discoloration prior to administration.

Any unused product or waste material should be disposed of in accordance with local requirements.

7. MARKETING AUTHORISATION HOLDER
Roche Registration Limited

40 Broadwater Road

Welwyn Garden City

Hertfordshire, AL7 3AY

United Kingdom

8. MARKETING AUTHORISATION NUMBER(S)
EU/1/98/067/001

9. DATE OF FIRST AUTHORISATION/RENEWAL OF THE AUTHORISATION
2 June 1998 / 28 July 2003

10. DATE OF REVISION OF THE TEXT
March 2005

Mabthera 500mg

(Roche Products Limited)

1. NAME OF THE MEDICINAL PRODUCT
MabThera 500 mg

Concentrate for solution for infusion.

2. QUALITATIVE AND QUANTITATIVE COMPOSITION
1 single-use vial contains 500 mg of rituximab in 50 ml (10 mg/ml).

Rituximab is a genetically engineered chimeric mouse/human monoclonal antibody representing a glycosylated immunoglobulin with human IgG1 constant regions and murine light-chain and heavy-chain variable region sequences. The antibody is produced by mammalian (Chinese hamster ovary) cell suspension culture and purified by affinity chromatography and ion exchange, including specific viral inactivation and removal procedures.

For excipients, see section 6.1.

3. PHARMACEUTICAL FORM
Concentrate for solution for infusion.

MabThera is a clear, colourless liquid.

4. CLINICAL PARTICULARS

4.1 Therapeutic indications
MabThera is indicated for treatment of patients with stage III-IV follicular lymphoma who are chemoresistant or are in their second or subsequent relapse after chemotherapy.

MabThera is indicated for the treatment of previously untreated patients with stage III-IV follicular lymphoma in combination with CVP chemotherapy.

MabThera is indicated for the treatment of patients with CD20 positive diffuse large B cell non-Hodgkin's lymphoma in combination with CHOP chemotherapy.

See section 5.1 (Pharmacodynamic properties) for further information.

4.2 Posology and method of administration
Standard dosage

The prepared MabThera solution should be administered as an IV infusion through a dedicated line.

MabThera infusions should be administered in a hospital environment where full resuscitation facilities are immediately available, and under the close supervision of an experienced oncologist/haematologist.

Premedication consisting of a pain-reliever and an antihistaminic, e.g. paracetamol and diphenhydramine, should always be administered before each infusion of MabThera. Premedication with corticosteroids should also be considered if MabThera is not given in combination with CHOP chemotherapy.

Patients should be closely monitored for the onset of cytokine release syndrome (see section 4.4). Patients who develop evidence of severe reactions, especially severe dyspnoea, bronchospasm or hypoxia should have the infusion interrupted immediately. The patient should then be evaluated for evidence of tumour lysis syndrome including appropriate laboratory tests and, for pulmonary infiltration, with a chest x-ray. The infusion should not be restarted until complete resolution of all symptoms, and normalisation of laboratory values and chest x-ray findings. At this time, the infusion can be initially resumed at not more than one-half the previous rate. If the same severe adverse reactions occur for a second time, the decision to stop the treatment should be seriously considered on a case by case basis.

Mild or moderate infusion-related reactions (section 4.8) usually respond to a reduction in the rate of infusion. The infusion rate may be increased upon improvement of symptoms.

Follicular non-Hodgkin's lymphoma

The recommended dosage of MabThera used as a single agent for adult patients is 375 mg/m^2 body surface, administered as an IV infusion once weekly for four weeks.

The recommended dosage of MabThera in combination with CVP chemotherapy is 375 mg/m^2 body surface area for 8 cycles (21 days/cycle), administered on day 1 of each chemotherapy cycle after IV administration of the corticosteroid component of CVP.

Retreatment following relapse in non-Hodgkin's lymphoma: Patients who have responded to MabThera initially have been treated again with MabThera at a dose of 375 mg/m^2 body surface area, administered as an IV infusion once weekly for four weeks (see section 5.1).

Diffuse large B cell non-Hodgkin's lymphoma

MabThera should be used in combination with CHOP chemotherapy. The recommended dosage is 375 mg/m^2 body surface area, administered on day 1 of each chemotherapy cycle for 8 cycles after IV administration of the corticosteroid component of CHOP. Safety and efficacy of MabThera have not been established in combination with other chemotherapies.

First infusion: The recommended initial rate for infusion is 50 mg/hr; after the first 30 minutes, it can be escalated in 50 mg/hr increments every 30 minutes, to a maximum of 400 mg/hr.

Subsequent infusions: Subsequent doses of MabThera can be infused at an initial rate of 100 mg/hr, and increased by 100 mg/hr increments at 30 minutes intervals, to a maximum of 400 mg/hr.

Dosage adjustments during treatment

No dose reductions of MabThera are recommended. When MabThera is given in combination with CHOP or CVP chemotherapy, standard dose reductions for the chemotherapeutic medicinal products should be applied.

4.3 Contraindications
MabThera is contraindicated in patients with known hypersensitivity to any component of this product or to murine proteins.

4.4 Special warnings and special precautions for use
Patients with a high tumour burden or with a high number ($\geqslant 25 \times 10^9$/l) of circulating malignant cells, who may be at higher risk of especially severe cytokine release syndrome, should only be treated with extreme caution and when other therapeutic alternatives have been exhausted. These patients should be very closely monitored throughout the first infusion. Consideration should be given to the use of a reduced infusion rate for the first infusion in these patients.

Severe cytokine release syndrome is characterised by severe dyspnoea, often accompanied by bronchospasm and hypoxia, in addition to fever, chills, rigors, urticaria, and angioedema. This syndrome may be associated with some features of ***tumour lysis syndrome*** such as hyperuricaemia, hyperkalaemia, hypocalcaemia, acute renal failure, elevated LDH and may be associated with acute respiratory failure and death. The acute respiratory failure may be accompanied by events such as pulmonary interstitial infiltration or oedema, visible on a chest x-ray. The syndrome frequently manifests itself within one or two hours of initiating the first infusion. Patients with a history of pulmonary insufficiency or those with pulmonary tumour infiltration may be at greater risk of poor outcome and should be treated with increased caution. Patients who develop severe cytokine release syndrome should have their infusion interrupted immediately (see section 4.2) and should receive aggressive symptomatic treatment. Since initial improvement of clinical symptoms may be followed by deterioration, these patients should be closely monitored until tumour lysis syndrome and pulmonary infiltration have been resolved or ruled out. Further treatment of patients after complete resolution of signs and symptoms has rarely resulted in repeated severe cytokine release syndrome.

Infusion related adverse reactions including cytokine release syndrome (see section 4.8) accompanied by hypotension and bronchospasm have been observed in 10 % of patients treated with MabThera. These symptoms are usually reversible with interruption of MabThera infusion and administration of a pain-reliever, an antihistaminic, and, occasionally, oxygen, IV saline or bronchodilators, and corticosteroids if required. Please see cytokine release syndrome above for severe reactions.

Anaphylactic and other hypersensitivity reactions have been reported following the IV administration of proteins to patients. In contrast to cytokine release syndrome, true hypersensitivity reactions typically occur within minutes after starting infusion. Medicinal products for the treatment of hypersensitivity reactions, e.g., epinephrine, antihistamines and corticosteroids, should be available for immediate use in the event of an allergic reaction during administration of MabThera. Clinical manifestations of anaphylaxis may appear similar to clinical manifestations of the cytokine release syndrome (described above). Reactions attributed to hypersensitivity have been reported less frequently than those attributed to cytokine release.

Since hypotension may occur during MabThera infusion, consideration should be given to withholding anti-hypertensive medications 12 hours prior to the MabThera infusion.

Angina pectoris, or cardiac arrhythmias such as atrial flutter and fibrillation, heart failure or myocardial infarction have occurred in patients treated with MabThera. Therefore patients with a history of cardiac disease and/or cardiotoxic chemotherapy should be monitored closely.

Although MabThera is not myelosuppressive in monotherapy, caution should be exercised when considering treatment of patients with neutrophils $< 1.5 \times 10^9$/l and/or platelet counts $< 75 \times 10^9$/l, as clinical experience in this population is limited. MabThera has been used in 21 patients who underwent autologous bone transplantation and other risk groups with a presumable reduced bone marrow function without inducing myelotoxicity.

Consideration should be given to the need for regular full blood counts, including platelet counts, during monotherapy with MabThera. When MabThera is given in combination with CHOP or CVP chemotherapy, regular full blood counts should be performed according to usual medical practice

Very rare cases of hepatitis B reactivation, including reports of fulminant hepatitis, have been reported in subjects receiving rituximab, although these subjects were also exposed to cytotoxic chemotherapy. The reports are confounded by both the underlying disease state and the cytotoxic chemotherapy. Patients with a history of hepatitis B infection should be carefully monitored for signs of active hepatitis B infection when rituximab is used in association with cytotoxic chemotherapy.

Do not administer the prepared infusion solutions as an IV push or bolus.

Paediatric Use

The safety and efficacy of MabThera in children have not been established.

4.5 Interaction with other medicinal products and other forms of Interaction
Currently, no data are available on possible drug interactions with MabThera. Patients with human anti-mouse antibody or human anti-chimeric antibody (HAMA/HACA) titres may have allergic or hypersensitivity reactions when treated with other diagnostic or therapeutic monoclonal antibodies.

The tolerability of simultaneous or sequential combination of MabThera with chemotherapy other than CHOP or

CVP, or agents which are liable to cause depletion of normal B cells is not well defined.

4.6 Pregnancy and lactation

Pregnancy

Animal reproduction studies have not been conducted with rituximab. It is also not known whether MabThera can cause foetal harm when administered to a pregnant woman or whether it can affect reproductive capacity. However, since IgG is known to pass the placental barrier, rituximab may cause B cell depletion in the foetus. For these reasons MabThera should not be given to a pregnant woman unless the potential benefit outweighs the potential risk.

Due to the long retention time of rituximab in B cell depleted patients, women of childbearing potential should use effective contraceptive methods during treatment and up to 12 months following MabThera therapy.

Lactation

Whether rituximab is excreted in human milk is not known. However, because maternal IgG is excreted in human milk, MabThera should not be given to women who are breast-feeding.

4.7 Effects on ability to drive and use machines

No studies on the effects on the ability to drive and use machines have been performed, although the pharmacological activity and adverse events reported to date do not indicate that such an effect is likely.

4.8 Undesirable effects

Monotherapy

The following data are based on 356 patients treated in single-arm studies of MabThera administered as single agent (see section 5.1). Most patients received MabThera 375 mg/m^2 weekly for 4 doses. These include 39 patients with bulky disease (lesions ⩾ 10 cm) and 58 patients who received more than one course of MabThera (60 re-treatments). Thirty-seven patients received 375 mg/m^2 for eight doses and 25 patients received doses other than 375 mg/m^2 for four doses and up to 500 mg/m^2 single dose in the Phase I setting.

The following table shows adverse events that were considered to be at least possibly related to MabThera during or up to 12 months after treatment. Adverse events were graded according to the four-scale National Cancer Institute (NCI) Common Toxicity Criteria.

Table 1. Summary of adverse events reported in ⩾ 1 % of 356 patients receiving MabThera monotherapy in clinical trials

	All grades	Grade 3 and 4
Body system Adverse event	%	%
Any adverse event	91.0	17.7
Body as a whole		
Fever	48.3	0.6
Chills	31.7	2.2
Asthenia	18.0	0.3
Headache	12.6	0.6
Throat irritation	7.6	-
Abdominal pain	7.0	0.6
Back pain	4.5	0.3
Pain	4.2	-
Flushing	4.2	-
Chest pain	2.2	-
Malaise	2.0	-
Tumour pain	1.7	-
Cold syndrome	1.4	-
Neck pain	1.1	-
Cardiovascular system		
Hypotension	9.8	0.8
Hypertension	4.5	0.3
Tachycardia	1.4	-
Arrhythmia	1.4	0.6
Orthostatic hypotension	1.1	-
Digestive system		
Nausea	17.1	0.3
Vomiting	6.7	0.3
Diarrhoea	4.2	-
Dyspepsia	2.8	-
Anorexia	2.8	-
Dysphagia	1.4	0.3
Stomatitis	1.4	-
Constipation	1.1	-
Blood and lymphatic system		
Leucopenia	12.4	2.8
Neutropenia	11.2	4.2
Thrombocytopenia	9.6	1.7
Anaemia	3.7	1.1
Metabolic and nutritional disorders		
Angioedema	10.7	0.3
Hyperglycaemia	5.3	0.3
Peripheral oedema	4.8	-
LDH increase	2.2	-
Hypocalcaemia	2.2	-
Facial oedema	1.1	-
Weight decrease	1.1	-
Musculoskeletal system		
Myalgia	8.1	0.3
Arthralgia	5.9	0.6
Hypertonia	1.4	-
Pain	1.1	0.3
Nervous system		
Dizziness	7.3	-
Paraesthesia	2.5	-
Anxiety	2.2	-
Insomnia	2.2	-
Vasodilatation	1.7	-
Hypoaesthesia	1.4	-
Agitation	1.4	-
Respiratory system		
Bronchospasm	7.9	1.4
Rhinitis	7.3	0.3
Increased cough	5.1	0.3
Dyspnoea	2.2	0.8
Chest pain	1.1	-
Respiratory disease	1.1	-
Skin and appendages		
Pruritus	12.4	0.3
Rash	11.2	0.3
Urticaria	7.3	0.8
Night sweats	2.8	-
Sweating	2.8	-
Special senses		
Lacrimation disorder	3.1	-
Conjunctivitis	1.4	-
Ear pain	1.1	-
Tinnitus	1.1	-

The following adverse events were also reported (< 1 %): coagulation disorders, asthma, lung disorder, bronchiolitis obliterans, hypoxia, abdominal enlargement, pain at the infusion site, bradycardia, lymphadenopathy, nervousness, depression, dysgeusia.

Infusion-related reactions: Infusion-related reactions occurred in more than 50 % of patients, and were predominantly seen during the first infusion, usually during the first one to two hours. These events mainly comprised fever, chills, and rigors. Other symptoms included flushing, angioedema, nausea, urticaria/rash, fatigue, headache, throat irritation, rhinitis, vomiting, and tumour pain. These symptoms were accompanied by hypotension and bronchospasm in about 10 % of the cases. Less frequently, patients experienced an exacerbation of pre-existing cardiac conditions such as angina pectoris or congestive heart failure. The incidence of infusion-related symptoms decreases substantially with subsequent infusions (see section 4.4).

Infections: MabThera induced B cell depletion in 70 % to 80 % of patients but was associated with decreased serum immunoglobulins only in a minority of patients. Infectious events, irrespective of causal assessment, occurred in 30.3 % of 356 patients: 18.8 % of patients had bacterial infections, 10.4 % had viral infections, 1.4 % had fungal infections, and 5.9 % had infections of unknown aetiology. Severe infectious events (grade 3 or 4), including sepsis occurred in 3.9 % of patients; in 1.4 % during the treatment period and in 2.5 % during the follow up period. As these were single-arm trials, the contributory role of MabThera or of the underlying NHL and its previous treatment to the development of these infectious events cannot be determined.

Haematologic Adverse Reactions: Haematological abnormalities occurred in a minority of patients and are usually mild and reversible. Severe (grade 3 and 4) thrombocytopenia and neutropenia were reported in 1.7 % and 4.2 % of patients respectively, and severe anaemia was reported in 1.1 % of patients. A single occurrence of transient aplastic anaemia (pure red cell aplasia) and infrequent occurrences of haemolytic anaemia following MabThera treatment were reported.

Cardiovascular events: Cardiovascular events were reported in 18.8 % of patients during the treatment period. The most frequently reported events were hypotension and hypertension. Two patients (0.6 %) experienced grade 3 or 4 arrhythmia (including ventricular and supraventricular tachycardia) during a MabThera infusion and one patient with a history of myocardial infarction experienced angina pectoris, evolving into myocardial infarction 4 days later.

Subpopulations:

Elderly patients: (⩾ 65 years): The incidence of any adverse event and of grade 3 and 4 adverse events was similar in elderly (N=94) and younger (N=237) patients (88.3 % versus 92.0 % for any adverse event and 16.0 % versus 18.1 % for grade 3 and 4 adverse events).

Bulky disease: Patients with bulky disease (N=39) had a higher incidence of grade 3 and 4 adverse events than patients without bulky disease (N=195) (25.6 % versus 15.4 %). The incidence of any adverse event was similar in these two groups (92.3 % in bulky disease versus 89.2 % in non-bulky disease).

Re-treatment: The percentage of patients reporting any adverse event and grade 3 and 4 adverse events upon re-treatment (N=60) with further courses of MabThera was similar to the percentage of patients reporting any adverse event and grade 3 and 4 adverse events upon initial exposure (N=203) (95.0 % versus 89.7 % for any adverse event and 13.3 % versus 14.8 % for grade 3 and 4 adverse events).

Adverse reactions reported in other monotherapy clinical trials: One case of serum sickness has been reported in a clinical trial using MabThera monotherapy for treatment of diffuse large B cell lymphoma.

In combination with CVP chemotherapy

The following data are based on 321 patients from a randomised phase III clinical trial comparing MabThera plus CVP (R-CVP) to CVP alone (162 R-CVP, 159 CVP).

Differences between the treatment groups with respect to the type and incidence of adverse event were mainly accounted for by typical adverse events associated with MabThera monotherapy.

The following grade 3 to 4 clinical adverse events were reported in ⩾ 2 % higher incidence in patients receiving R-CVP compared to CVP treatment group and therefore may be attributable to R-CVP. Adverse events were graded according to the four-scale National Cancer Institute (NCI) Common Toxicity Criteria:

- Fatigue: 3.7 % (R-CVP), 1.3 % (CVP)
- Neutropenia: 3.1 % (R-CVP), 0.6 % (CVP)

Infusion-related reactions: The signs and symptoms of severe or life-threatening (NCI CTC grades 3 and 4) infusion-related reactions (defined as starting during or within one day of an infusion with MabThera) occurred in 9 % of all patients who received R-CVP. These results are consistent with those observed during monotherapy (see section 4.4 and 4.8, Undesirable effects, monotherapy), and included rigors, fatigue, dyspnoea, dyspepsia, nausea, rash NOS, flushing.

Infections: The overall proportion of patients with infections or infestations during treatment and for 28 days after trial treatment end was comparable between the treatment groups (33 % R-CVP, 32 % CVP). The most common infections were upper respiratory tract infections which were reported for 12.3 % patients on R-CVP and 16.4 % patients receiving CVP; most of these infections were nasopharyngitis.

Serious infections were reported in 4.3 % of the patients receiving R-CVP and 4.4 % of the patients receiving CVP. No life threatening infections were reported during this study.

Haematologic laboratory abnormalities: 24 % of patients on R-CVP and 14 % of patients on CVP experienced grade 3 or 4 neutropenia during treatment. The proportion of patients with grade 4 neutropenia was comparable between the treatment groups. These laboratory findings were reported as adverse events and resulted in medical intervention in 3.1 % of patients on R-CVP and 0.6 % of patients on CVP. All other laboratory abnormalities were not treated and resolved without any intervention. In addition, the higher incidence of neutropenia in the R-CVP group was not associated with a higher incidence of infections and infestations.

No relevant difference between the two treatment arms was observed with respect to grade 3 and 4 anaemia (0.6 % R-CVP and 1.9 % CVP) and thrombocytopenia (1.2 % in the R-CVP group and no events reported in the CVP group).

Cardiac events: The overall incidence of cardiac disorders in the safety population was low (4 % R-CVP, 5 % CVP), with no relevant differences between the treatment groups.

<u>In combination with CHOP chemotherapy</u>

The following table shows grade 3 to 4 clinical adverse events, including grade 2 infections, from a randomised phase III clinical trial comparing MabThera plus CHOP (R-CHOP) to CHOP alone in a safety population of 398 patients. Events shown were reported at a greater than 2 % higher incidence with R-CHOP when compared to CHOP alone and therefore may be attributable to R-CHOP (absolute incidence cut off at 2 %). Adverse events were graded according to the four-scale National Cancer Institute of Canada (NCIC) Common Toxicity Criteria.

Table 2: Excess incidence (>= 2 %) of grade 3 and 4 adverse events (including grade 2 infections) with R-CHOP compared with CHOP (overall cut off of 2 %)

	R-CHOP	CHOP
	N=202	N=196
	%	%
Infections and infestations		
Bronchitis	11.9	8.2
Herpes zoster	4.0	1.5
Acute bronchitis	2.5	0.5
Sinusitis	2.5	-
Respiratory disorders		
Dyspnoea	8.9	3.6
General disorders and administration site disorders		
Shivering	3.5	1.0
Vascular disorders		
Hypertension	2.5	0.5
Cardiac disorder		
Atrial fibrillation	2.5	0.5

Infusion-related reactions: Grade 3 and 4 infusion-related reactions (defined as starting during or within one day of an infusion with MabThera) occurred in approximately 9 % of patients at the time of the first cycle of R-CHOP. The incidence of grade 3 and 4 infusion-related reactions decreased to less than 1 % by the eighth cycle of R-CHOP. The signs and symptoms were consistent with those observed during monotherapy (see section 4.4 and 4.8, Undesirable effects, monotherapy), and included fever, chills, hypotension, hypertension, tachycardia, dyspnoea, bronchospasm, nausea, vomiting, pain and features of tumour lysis syndrome. Additional reactions reported in isolated cases at the time of R-CHOP therapy were myocardial infarction, atrial fibrillation and pulmonary oedema.

Infections: The proportion of patients with grade 2 to 4 infections and/or febrile neutropenia was 55.4 % in the R-CHOP group and 51.5 % in the CHOP group. Febrile neutropenia (i.e. no report of concomitant documented infection) was reported only during the treatment period, in 20.8 % in the R-CHOP group and 15.3 % in the CHOP group. The overall incidence of grade 2 to 4 infections was 45.5 % in the R-CHOP group and 42.3 % in the CHOP group with no difference in the incidence of systemic bacterial and fungal infections. Grade 2 to 4 fungal infections were more frequent in the R-CHOP group (4.5 % vs 2.6 % in the CHOP group); this difference was due to a higher incidence of localised Candida infections during the treatment period. The incidence of grade 2 to 4 herpes zoster, including ophthalmic herpes zoster, was higher in the R-CHOP group (4.5 %) than in the CHOP group (1.5 %), with 7 of a total of 9 cases in the R-CHOP group occurring during the treatment phase.

Haematologic events: After each treatment cycle, grade 3 and 4 leucopenia (88 % vs 79 %) and neutropenia (97 % vs 88 %) occurred more frequently in the R-CHOP group than in the CHOP group. There was no evidence that neutropenia was more prolonged in the R-CHOP group. No difference between the two treatment arms was observed with respect to grade 3 and 4 anaemia (19 % in the CHOP group vs 14 % in the R-CHOP group) and thrombocytopenia (16 % in the CHOP group vs 15 % in the R-CHOP group). The time to recovery from all haematological abnormalities was comparable in the two treatment groups.

Cardiac events: The incidence of grade 3 and 4 cardiac arrhythmias, predominantly supraventricular arrhythmias such as tachycardia and atrial flutter/fibrillation, was higher in the R-CHOP group (14 patients, 6.9 %) as compared to the CHOP group (3 patients, 1.5 %). All of these arrhythmias either occurred in the context of a MabThera infusion or were associated with predisposing conditions such as fever, infection, acute myocardial infarction or pre-existing respiratory and cardiovascular disease. No difference between the R-CHOP and CHOP group was observed in the incidence of other grade 3 and 4 cardiac events including heart failure, myocardial disease and manifestations of coronary artery disease.

Neurologic events: During the treatment period, four patients (2 %) in the R-CHOP group, all with cardiovascular risk factors, experienced thromboembolic cerebrovascular accidents during the first treatment cycle. There was no difference between the treatment groups in the incidence of other thromboembolic events. In contrast, three patients (1.5 %) had cerebrovascular events in the CHOP group, all of which occurred during the follow-up period.

<u>**Post-marketing experience**</u>

As part of the continuing post-marketing surveillance of MabThera safety, the following serious adverse reactions have been observed:

Blood and lymphatic system disorders	
Rare (≥ 1/10,000, < 1/1000):	Late neutropenia[1]
Very rare (< 1/10,000):	Pancytopenia Aplastic anaemia Transient increase in serum IgM levels[2]
Cardiovascular system	
Rare (≥ 1/10,000, < 1/1000):	*Severe cardiac events[3]
Very rare (< 1/10,000):	*Heart failure[3] *Myocardial infarction[3]
Ear and labyrinth disorders	
Very rare (< 1/10,000):	†Hearing loss
Eye disorders	
Very rare (< 1/10,000):	†Severe vision loss
General disorders and administration site conditions	
Very rare (< 1/10,000):	*Multi-organ failure
Immune system disorders	
Uncommon (≥ 1/1000, < 1/100):	Infusion related reactions
Rare (≥ 1/10,000, < 1/1000):	Anaphylaxis
Very rare (< 1/10,000):	*Tumour lysis syndrome *Cytokine release syndrome Serum sickness Hepatitis B reactivation[4]
Nervous system disorders	
Very rare (< 1/10,000):	Cranial neuropathy Peripheral neuropathy †Facial nerve palsy †Loss of other senses
Renal and urinary disorders	
Very rare (< 1/10,000):	*Renal failure
Respiratory, thoracic and mediastinal disorders	
Rare (≥ 1/10,000, < 1/1000):	*Bronchospasm
Very rare (< 1/10,000):	*Respiratory failure Pulmonary infiltrates Interstitial pneumonitis
Skin and subcutaneous tissue disorders	
Very rare (< 1/10,000):	Severe bullous skin reactions Toxic epidermal necrolysis[5]
Vascular disorders	
Very rare (< 1/10,000):	Vasculitis (predominately cutaneous) Leucocytoclastic vasculitis

*Associated with infusion-related reactions. Rarely fatal cases reported

† Signs and symptoms of cranial neuropathy. Occurred at various times up to several months after completion of MabThera therapy

[1] Neutropenia that has occurred more than four weeks after the last infusion of MabThera.

[2] In post-marketing studies of rituximab in patients with Waldenstrom's macroglobulinaemia, transient increases in serum IgM levels have been observed following treatment initiation, which may be associated with hyperviscosity and related symptoms. The transient IgM increase usually returned to at least baseline level within 4 months.

[3] Observed mainly in patients with prior cardiac condition and/or cardiotoxic chemotherapy and were mostly associated with infusion-related reactions

[4] Very rare cases of hepatitis B reactivation, have been reported in subjects receiving rituximab in combination with cytotoxic chemotherapy.

[5] Including fatal cases

4.9 Overdose

There has been no experience of overdose in human clinical trials. However, single doses higher than 500 mg/m^2 body surface have not been tested in controlled clinical trials.

5. PHARMACOLOGICAL PROPERTIES

5.1 Pharmacodynamic properties

Pharmacotherapeutic group: Antineoplastic Agents, ATC code: L01X C02

Rituximab binds specifically to the transmembrane antigen, CD20, a non-glycosylated phosphoprotein, located on pre-B and mature B lymphocytes. The antigen is expressed on >95 % of all B cell non-Hodgkin's lymphomas (NHLs).

CD20 is found on both normal and malignant B cells, but not on haematopoietic stem cells, pro-B-cells, normal plasma cells or other normal tissue. This antigen does not internalise upon antibody binding and is not shed from the cell surface. CD20 does not circulate in the plasma as a free antigen and, thus, does not compete for antibody binding.

The Fab domain of rituximab binds to the CD20 antigen on B lymphocytes and the Fc domain can recruit immune effector functions to mediate B cell lysis. Possible mechanisms of effector-mediated cell lysis include complement-dependent cytotoxicity (CDC) resulting from C1q binding, and antibody-dependent cellular cytotoxicity (ADCC) mediated by one or more of the Fcγ receptors on the surface of granulocytes, macrophages and NK cells. Rituximab binding to CD 20 antigen on B lymphocytes has also been demonstrated to induce cell death via apoptosis.

Median peripheral B cell counts declined below normal following completion of the first dose, with recovery beginning after 6 months. B cell levels returned to normal between 9 and 12 months following completion of therapy.

Follicular non-Hodgkin's lymphoma:

Monotherapy: *Initial treatment, weekly for 4 doses:* In the pivotal study, 166 patients with relapsed or chemoresistant low-grade or follicular B cell NHL received 375 mg/m^2 of MabThera as an IV infusion once weekly for four weeks. The overall response rate (ORR) in the intent-to-treat (ITT) population was 48 % ($CI_{95\ \%}$ 41 % - 56 %) with a 6 % complete response (CR) and a 42 % partial response (PR) rate. The projected median time to progression (TTP) for responding patients was 13.0 months. In a subgroup analysis, the ORR was higher in patients with IWF B, C, and D histological subtypes as compared to IWF A subtype (58 % vs. 12 %), higher in patients whose largest lesion was < 5 cm vs. > 7 cm in greatest diameter (53 % vs. 38 %), and higher in patients with chemosensitive relapse as compared to chemoresistant (defined as duration of response < 3 months) relapse (50 % vs. 22 %). ORR in patients previously treated with autologous bone marrow transplant (ABMT) was 78 % versus 43 % in patients with no ABMT. Neither age, sex, lymphoma grade, initial diagnosis, presence or absence of bulky disease, normal or high LDH nor presence of extranodal disease had a statistically significant effect (Fisher's exact test) on response to MabThera. A statistically significant correlation was noted between response rates and bone marrow involvement. 40 % of patients with bone marrow involvement responded compared to 59 % of patients with no bone marrow involvement (p=0.0186). This finding was not supported by a stepwise logistic regression analysis in which the following factors were identified as prognostic factors: histological type, bcl-2 positivity at baseline, resistance to last chemotherapy and bulky disease.

Initial treatment, weekly for 8 doses: In a multi-centre, single-arm study, 37 patients with relapsed or chemoresistant, low grade or follicular B cell NHL received 375 mg/m^2 of MabThera as IV infusion weekly for eight doses. The ORR was 57 % ($CI_{95\ \%}$ 41 % – 73 %; CR 14 %, PR 43 %) with a projected median TTP for responding patients of 19.4 months (range 5.3 to 38.9 months).

Initial treatment, bulky disease, weekly for 4 doses: In pooled data from three studies, 39 patients with relapsed or chemoresistant, bulky disease (single lesion ⩾ 10 cm in diameter), low grade or follicular B cell NHL received 375 mg/m^2 of MabThera as IV infusion weekly for four doses. The ORR was 36 % ($CI_{95\ \%}$ 21 % – 51 %; CR 3 %, PR 33 %) with a median TTP for responding patients of 9.6 months (range 4.5 to 26.8 months).

Re-treatment, weekly for 4 doses: In a multi-centre, single-arm study, 58 patients with relapsed or chemoresistant low grade or follicular B cell NHL, who had achieved an objective clinical response to a prior course of MabThera, were re-treated with 375 mg/m^2 of MabThera as IV infusion weekly for four doses. Three of the patients had received two courses of MabThera before enrollment and thus were given a third course in the study. Two patients were re-treated twice in the study. For the 60 re-treatments on study, the ORR was 38 % ($CI_{95\ \%}$ 26 % – 51 %; 10 % CR, 28 % PR) with a projected median TTP for responding patients of 17.8 months (range 5.4 – 26.6). This compares favourably with the TTP achieved after the prior course of MabThera (12.4 months).

Initial treatment, in combination with CVP: In an open-label randomised trial, a total of 322 previously untreated low-grade or follicular B cell NHL patients were randomised to receive either CVP chemotherapy (cyclophosphamide 750 mg/m^2, vincristine 1.4 mg/m^2 up to a maximum of 2 mg on day 1, and prednisolone 40 mg/m^2/day on days 1 – 5) every 3 weeks for 8 cycles or MabThera 375 mg/m^2 in combination with CVP (R-CVP). MabThera was administered on the first day of each treatment cycle. A total of 321 patients (162 R-CVP, 159 CVP) received therapy and were analysed for efficacy. At the time of the analysis, the median observation time was 18 months. R-CVP led to a significant benefit over CVP for the primary endpoint, time to treatment failure (25.9 months vs. 6.7 months, p < 0.0001, log-rank test). The risk of experiencing a treatment failure event was reduced by 67 % (95 % CI: 56 % - 76 %) with R-CVP compared with CVP alone, using a Cox regression analysis. The Kaplan-Meier estimated event free rate at 12 months was 69 % in the R-CVP group compared with 32 % in the CVP group. The proportion of patients with a tumour response (CR, CRu, PR) was significantly higher (p< 0.0001 Chi-Square test) in the R-CVP group (80.9 %) than the CVP group (57.2 %). At 18 months, the median duration of response had not been reached in the R-CVP group and was 9.8 months in the CVP group (p < 0.0001, log-rank test). Amongst responding patients, Cox regression analysis showed that the risk of relapse was reduced by 70 % (95 % CI: 55 % - 81 %) in the R-CVP group compared to the CVP group.

The time to institution of new lymphoma treatment or death was significantly longer in the R-CVP group (not estimable), compared to the CVP group (12.3 months) (p < 0.0001, log-rank test). Treatment with R-CVP significantly prolonged the time to disease progression compared to CVP, 27 months and 14.5 months, respectively. At 12 months, 81 % in the R-CVP group had not relapsed compared to 58 % of patients receiving CVP.

The benefit of adding rituximab to CVP was seen consistently throughout the population recruited in study M39021 (randomised according to BNLI criteria (no versus yes), age (⩽ 60 years, > 60 years), number of extra-nodal sites (0-1 versus > 1), bone marrow involvement (no versus yes), LDH (elevated, not elevated), β_2-microglobulin (elevated, not elevated), B symptoms (absent, present), bulky disease (absent, present), number of nodal sites (< 5 versus ⩾ 5), haemoglobin (⩽ 12 g/dL versus > 12 g/dL), IPI (⩽ 1 versus > 1), and FLIPI index (0-2 versus 3-5)).

Due to the number of events at the time of analysis and the relatively short observation time of 18 months, conclusion regarding differences for overall survival cannot be drawn.

Diffuse large B cell non-Hodgkin's lymphoma: In a randomised, open-label trial, a total of 399 previously untreated elderly patients (age 60 to 80 years) with diffuse large B cell lymphoma received standard CHOP chemotherapy (cyclophosphamide 750 mg/m^2, doxorubicin 50 mg/m^2, vincristine 1.4 mg/m^2 up to a maximum of 2 mg on day 1, and prednisone 40 mg/m^2/day on days 1-5) every 3 weeks for eight cycles, or MabThera 375 mg/m^2 plus CHOP (R-CHOP). MabThera was administered on the first day of the treatment cycle.

The final efficacy analysis included all randomised patients (197 CHOP, 202 R-CHOP), and had a median follow-up duration of approximately 31 months. The two treatment groups were well balanced in baseline disease characteristics and disease status. The final analysis confirmed that R-CHOP treatment was associated with a clinically relevant and statistically significant improvement in the duration of event-free survival (the primary efficacy parameter; where events were death, relapse or progression of lymphoma, or institution of a new anti-lymphoma treatment) (p = 0.0001). Kaplan Meier estimates of the median duration of event-free survival were 35 months in the R-CHOP arm compared to 13 months in the CHOP arm, representing a risk reduction of 41 %. At 24 months, estimates for overall survival were 68.2 % in the R-CHOP arm compared to 57.4 % in the CHOP arm. A subsequent analysis of the duration of overall survival, carried out with a median follow-up duration of 38 months, confirmed the benefit of R-CHOP over CHOP treatment (p=0.0094), representing a risk reduction of 33 %.

The analysis of all secondary parameters (response rates, progression-free survival, disease-free survival, duration of response) verified the treatment effect of R-CHOP compared to CHOP. The complete response rate after cycle 8 was 76.2 % in the R-CHOP group and 62.4 % in the CHOP group (p=0.0028). The risk of disease progression was reduced by 46 % and the risk of relapse by 51 %.

In all patients subgroups (gender, age, age adjusted IPI, Ann Arbor stage, ECOG, β2 microglobulin, LDH, albumin, B symptoms, bulky disease, extranodal sites, bone marrow involvement), the risk ratios for event-free survival and overall survival (R-CHOP compared with CHOP) were less than 0.83 and 0.95 respectively. R-CHOP was associated with improvements in outcome for both high- and low-risk patients according to age adjusted IPI.

Clinical Laboratory Findings

Of 67 patients evaluated for human anti-mouse antibody (HAMA), no responses were noted. Of 356 patients evaluated for HACA, 1.1 % (4 patients) were positive.

5.2 Pharmacokinetic properties

Pharmacokinetic studies performed in a phase I study in which patients (n=15) with relapsed B cell lymphoma were given single doses of rituximab at 10, 50, 100 or 500 mg/m^2 indicated that serum levels and half-life of rituximab were proportional to dose. In a cohort of 14 patients among the 166 patients with relapsed or chemoresistant low-grade or follicular non-Hodgkin's lymphoma enrolled in the phase III pivotal trial and given rituximab 375 mg/m^2 as an IV infusion for 4 weekly doses, the mean serum half-life was 76.3 hours (range, 31.5 to 152.6 hours) after the first infusion and 205.8 hours (range, 83.9 to 407.0 hours) after the fourth infusion. The mean C_{max} after the first and fourth infusion were 205.6 ± 59.9 μg/ml and 464.7 ± 119.0 μg/ml, respectively. The mean plasma clearance after the first and fourth infusion was 0.0382 ± 0.0182 L/h and 0.0092 ± 0.0033 L/h, respectively. However, variability in serum levels was large.

Rituximab serum concentrations were statistically significantly higher in responding patients compared to non-responding patients just prior to and after the fourth infusion and post treatment. Serum concentrations were negatively correlated with tumour burden and the number of circulating B cells at baseline. Typically, rituximab was detectable for 3 to 6 months.

Elimination and distribution have not been extensively studied in patients with diffuse large B cell non-Hodgkin's lymphoma, but available data indicate that serum levels of rituximab in these patients are comparable to those in patients with follicular non-Hodgkin's lymphoma following treatment with similar doses.

5.3 Preclinical safety data

Rituximab has shown to be highly specific to the CD20 antigen on B cells. Toxicity studies in cynomolgus monkeys have shown no other effect than the expected pharmacological depletion of B cells in peripheral blood and in lymphoid tissue. The recovery of the peripheral B cells was marked by large intraindividual variability. However, peripheral B cell recovery usually started two weeks after treatment, and median B cells counts reached 40 % of baseline levels after a 3 month period. No adverse reactions unrelated to the targeted effect were seen, whether in single or in multiple dose studies in the cynomolgus monkey.

No long-term animal studies have been performed to establish the carcinogenic potential of rituximab, or to determine its effects on fertility in males or females. Standard tests to investigate mutagenicity have not been carried out, since such tests are not relevant for this molecule. However, due to its character it is unlikely that rituximab has any mutagenic potential.

6. PHARMACEUTICAL PARTICULARS

6.1 List of excipients

Sodium citrate

Polysorbate 80

Sodium chloride

Sodium hydroxide

Hydrochloric acid

Water for injections

6.2 Incompatibilities

No incompatibilities between MabThera and polyvinyl chloride or polyethylene bags or infusion sets have been observed.

6.3 Shelf life

30 months

The prepared infusion solution of MabThera is physically and chemically stable for 24 hours at 2 °C - 8 °C and subsequently 12 hours at room temperature.

6.4 Special precautions for storage

Store vials at 2 °C- 8 °C (in a refrigerator). Keep the container in the outer carton in order to protect from light.

The prepared infusion solution of MabThera is physically and chemically stable for 24 hours at 2 °C - 8 °C and subsequently 12 hours at room temperature.

From a microbiological point of view, the prepared infusion solution should be used immediately. If not used immediately, in-use storage times and conditions prior to use are the responsibility of the user and would normally not be longer than 24 hours at 2 °C - 8 °C, unless dilution has taken place in controlled and validated aseptic conditions.

6.5 Nature and contents of container

Single-use, preservative-free, clear Type I glass vials with butyl rubber stopper containing 500 mg of rituximab in 50 ml (10 mg/ml).

Packs of 1 vial.

6.6 Instructions for use and handling

MabThera is provided in sterile, preservative-free, non-pyrogenic, single use vials.

Aseptically withdraw the necessary amount of MabThera, and dilute to a calculated concentration of 1 to 4 mg/ml rituximab into an infusion bag containing sterile, pyrogen-free 0.9 % Sodium Chloride or 5 % Dextrose in water. For mixing the solution, gently invert the bag in order to avoid foaming. Care must be taken to ensure the sterility of prepared solutions. Since the drug product does not contain any anti-microbial preservative or bacteriostatic agents, aseptic technique must be observed. Parenteral drug products should be inspected visually for particulate matter and discoloration prior to administration.

Any unused product or waste material should be disposed of in accordance with local requirements.

7. MARKETING AUTHORISATION HOLDER

Roche Registration Limited

40 Broadwater Road

Welwyn Garden City

Hertfordshire, AL7 3AY

United Kingdom

8. MARKETING AUTHORISATION NUMBER(S)

EU/1/98/067/002

9. DATE OF FIRST AUTHORISATION/RENEWAL OF THE AUTHORISATION

2 June 1998 / 28 July 2003

10. DATE OF REVISION OF THE TEXT

March 2005

Mackenzies Smelling Salts

(Alpharma Limited)

1. NAME OF THE MEDICINAL PRODUCT

MACKENZIES SMELLING SALTS

2. QUALITATIVE AND QUANTITATIVE COMPOSITION

Contains not less than 8.698g Ammonia Liquor 880/890 and 0.5g Eucalyptus Oil BP

3. PHARMACEUTICAL FORM

White granules.

4. CLINICAL PARTICULARS

4.1 Therapeutic indications

Traditionally used for the symptomatic relief of catarrh and head colds.

4.2 Posology and method of administration

Posology

Inhale vapour through nostrils as required.

Do not use for children under 3 months of age.

Method of Administration

Inhalant.

4.3 Contraindications
Do not use for children under 3 months of age.

4.4 Special warnings and special precautions for use
None known.

The product labelling includes the following statements:

Not to be taken.

If symptoms persist consult your doctor.

Keep out of the reach and sight of children.

4.5 Interaction with other medicinal products and other forms of Interaction
None known.

4.6 Pregnancy and lactation
No special precautions are considered necessary.

4.7 Effects on ability to drive and use machines
None known.

4.8 Undesirable effects
None known.

4.9 Overdose
No special requirements are anticipated.

5. PHARMACOLOGICAL PROPERTIES
5.1 Pharmacodynamic properties
ATC code: R01A X

Ammonia is employed in the product as a reflex stimulant.

Eucalyptus oil is an essential oil.

5.2 Pharmacokinetic properties
Not applicable.

5.3 Preclinical safety data
There are no pre-clinical data of relevance to the prescriber which are additional to that already included in other sections of the SPC.

6. PHARMACEUTICAL PARTICULARS
6.1 List of excipients
Also contains glycerol, soft soap, tapioca, water.

6.2 Incompatibilities
None known.

6.3 Shelf life
Shelf-life

Three years from the date of manufacture.

Shelf-life after dilution/reconstitution

Not applicable.

Shelf-life after first opening

Not applicable.

6.4 Special precautions for storage
Store in a cool place.

6.5 Nature and contents of container
The product container is a uniquely-shaped amber glass bottle with black polypropylene cap with foil wad or black urea formaldehyde cap with polycone.

Pack size: 17ml

6.6 Instructions for use and handling
Not applicable.

Administrative Data
7. MARKETING AUTHORISATION HOLDER
Name or style and permanent address of registered place of business of the holder of the Marketing Authorisation:

Alpharma Limited

(Trading styles: Alpharma, Cox Pharmaceuticals)

Whiddon Valley

BARNSTAPLE

N Devon EX32 8NS

8. MARKETING AUTHORISATION NUMBER(S)
PL 0142/5010 R

9. DATE OF FIRST AUTHORISATION/RENEWAL OF THE AUTHORISATION
16.10.86 (Product Licence of Right issued: 27.7.73)

Renewed: 14.5.92; 11.7.97

10. DATE OF REVISION OF THE TEXT
February 2002

Madopar Capsules

(Roche Products Limited)

1. NAME OF THE MEDICINAL PRODUCT
Madopar® 62.5 Capsules
Madopar® 125 Capsules
Madopar® 250 Capsules

2. QUALITATIVE AND QUANTITATIVE COMPOSITION
Each 62.5 capsule contains 50.0mg levodopa Ph. Eur. and 14.25mg benserazide hydrochloride Ph. Eur. (equivalent to 12.5mg of the base).

Each 125 capsule contains 100.0mg levodopa Ph. Eur. and 28.5mg benserazide hydrochloride Ph. Eur. (equivalent to 25mg of the base).

Each 250 capsule contains 200.0mg levodopa Ph. Eur. and 57.0mg benserazide hydrochloride Ph. Eur (equivalent to 50mg of the base).

3. PHARMACEUTICAL FORM
Hard capsules.

4. CLINICAL PARTICULARS
4.1 Therapeutic indications
Parkinsonism - idiopathic post-encephalitic.

Previous neurosurgery is not a contra-indication to Madopar.

4.2 Posology and method of administration
Dosage and administration are variable and no more than a guide can be given.

Adults

Patients not previously treated with levodopa

The recommended initial dose is one capsule or dispersible tablet of Madopar 62.5 three or four times daily. If the disease is at an advanced stage, the starting dose should be one capsule or dispersible tablet of Madopar 125 three times daily.

The daily dosage should then be increased by one capsule or dispersible tablet of Madopar 125, or their equivalent, once or twice weekly until a full therapeutic effect is obtained, or side-effects supervene.

In some elderly patients, it may suffice to initiate treatment with one capsule or dispersible tablet of Madopar 62.5 once or twice daily, increasing by one capsule or dispersible tablet every third or fourth day.

The effective dose usually lies within the range of four to eight capsules or dispersible tablets of Madopar 125 (two to four capsules of Madopar 250) daily in divided doses, most patients requiring no more than six capsules or dispersible tablets of Madopar 125 daily.

Optimal improvement is usually seen in one to three weeks but the full therapeutic effect of Madopar may not be apparent for some time. It is advisable, therefore, to allow several weeks to elapse before contemplating dosage increments above the average dose range. If satisfactory improvement is still not achieved, the dose of Madopar may be increased but with caution. It is rarely necessary to give more than ten capsules or dispersible tablets of Madopar 125 (five capsules of Madopar 250) per day.

Treatment should be continued for at least six months before failure is concluded from the absence of a clinical response.

Madopar 62.5 capsules or dispersible tablets may be used to facilitate adjustment of dosage to the needs of the individual patient. Patients who experience fluctuations in response may be helped by dividing the dosage into smaller, more frequent doses with the aid of Madopar 62.5 capsules or dispersible tablets without, however, altering the total daily dose.

Madopar 250 capsules are only for maintenance therapy once the optimal dosage has been determined using Madopar 125 capsules or dispersible tablets.

Patients previously treated with levodopa

The following procedure is recommended: levodopa alone should be discontinued and Madopar started on the following day. The patient should be initiated on a total of one less Madopar 125 capsule or dispersible tablet daily than the total number of 500mg levodopa tablets or capsules previously taken (for example, if the patient had previously taken 2g levodopa daily, then he should start on three capsules or dispersible tablets Madopar 125 daily on the following day). Observe the patient for one week and then, if necessary, increase the dosage in the manner described for new patients.

Patients previously treated with other levodopa/decarboxylase inhibitor combinations

Previous therapy should be withdrawn for 12 hours. In order to minimise the potential for any effects of levodopa withdrawal, it may be beneficial to discontinue previous therapy at night and institute Madopar therapy the following morning. The initial Madopar dose should be one capsule or dispersible tablet of Madopar 62.5 three or four times daily. This dose may then be increased in the manner described for patients not previously treated with levodopa.

Other anti-Parkinsonian drugs may be given with Madopar. Existing treatment with other anti-Parkinsonian drugs, e.g. anticholinergics or amantadine, should be continued during initiation of Madopar therapy. However, as treatment with Madopar proceeds and the therapeutic effect becomes apparent, the dosage of the other drugs may need to be reduced or the drugs gradually withdrawn.

Elderly

Although there may be an age-related decrease in tolerance to levodopa in the elderly, Madopar appears to be well-tolerated and side-effects are generally not troublesome.

Children

Not to be given to patients under 25 years of age: therefore, no dosage recommendations are made for the administration of Madopar to children.

Madopar capsules are for oral administration. They should be taken with, or immediately after, meals.

4.3 Contraindications
Madopar must not be given to patients with known hypersensitivity to levodopa or benserazide.

Madopar is contra-indicated in narrow-angle glaucoma (it may be used in wide-angle glaucoma provided that the intra-ocular pressure remains under control); severe psychoneuroses or psychoses; severe endocrine, renal, hepatic or cardiac disorders.

It should not be given in conjunction with, or within 2 weeks of withdrawal of, monoamine oxidase (MAO) inhibitors, except selective MAO-B inhibitors (e.g. selegiline) or selective MAO-A inhibitors (e.g. moclobemide).

It should not be given to patients under 25 years of age.

It should not be given to pregnant women or to women of childbearing potential in the absence of adequate contraception. If pregnancy occurs in a woman taking Madopar, the drug must be discontinued.

Suspicion has arisen that levodopa may activate a malignant melanoma. Therefore, Madopar should not be used in persons who have a history of, or who may be suffering from, a malignant melanoma.

4.4 Special warnings and special precautions for use
When other drugs must be given in conjunction with Madopar, the patient should be carefully observed for unusual side-effects or potentiating effects.

In the event of general anaesthesia being required, Madopar therapy may be continued as long as the patient is able to take fluids and medication by mouth. If therapy is temporarily interrupted, the usual daily dosage may be administered as soon as the patient is able to take oral medication. Whenever therapy has been interrupted for longer periods, dosage should again be adjusted gradually; however, in many cases the patient can rapidly be returned to his previous therapeutic dosage.

If a patient has to undergo surgery, when Madopar has not been withdrawn, anaesthesia with halothane should be avoided.

There have been occasional reports of a neuroleptic malignant-like syndrome, involving hyperthermia, on abrupt withdrawal of levodopa preparations. Sudden discontinuation of Madopar, without close supervision, or "drug holidays" should therefore be avoided.

Pyridoxine (vitamin B_6) may be given with Madopar since the presence of a decarboxylase inhibitor protects against the peripheral levodopa transformation facilitated by pyridoxine.

Levodopa has been associated with somnolence and episodes of sleep onset. Sudden onset of sleep during daily activities, in some cases without awareness or warning signs, has been reported very rarely. Patients must be informed of this and advised to exercise caution while driving or operating machines during treatment with levodopa. Patients who have experienced somnolence and/or an episode of sudden sleep onset must refrain from driving or operating machines. Furthermore a reduction of dosage or termination of therapy may be considered.

Care should be taken when using Madopar in the following circumstances: in endocrine, renal, pulmonary or cardiovascular disease, particularly where there is a history of myocardial infarction or arrhythmia; psychiatric disturbances (e.g. depression); hepatic disorder; peptic ulcer; osteomalacia; where sympathomimetic drugs may be required (e.g. bronchial asthma), due to possible potentiation of the cardiovascular effects of levodopa; where antihypertensive drugs are being used, due to possible increased hypotensive action.

Periodic evaluation of hepatic, haemopoietic, renal and cardiovascular functions is advised.

Patients with diabetes should undergo frequent blood sugar tests and the dosage of anti-diabetic agents should be adjusted to blood sugar levels.

Patients who improve on Madopar therapy should be advised to resume normal activities gradually as rapid mobilisation may increase the risk of injury.

4.5 Interaction with other medicinal products and other forms of Interaction
Ferrous sulphate decreases the maximum plasma concentration and the AUC of levodopa by 30 - 50%. The pharmacokinetic changes observed during co-treatment with ferrous sulphate appeared to be clinically significant in some but not all patients.

Opioids and drugs which interfere with central amine mechanisms, such as rauwolfia alkaloids (reserpine), tetrabenazine (Nitoman), metoclopramide, phenothiazines, thioxanthenes, butyrophenones, amphetamines and papaverine, should be avoided where possible. If, however, their administration is considered essential, extreme care should be exercised and a close watch kept for any signs of potentiation, antagonism or other interactions and for unusual side-effects. Metoclopramide has been shown to increase the rate of levodopa absorption.

Co-administration of the anticholinergic drug trihexyphenidyl with Madopar reduces the rate, but not the extent, of levodopa absorption.

Combination with other anti-Parkinsonian agents (anticholinergics, amantadine, dopamine agonists) is permissible, though both the desired and undesired effects of treatment may be intensified. It may be necessary to reduce the dosage of Madopar or the other substance. When initiating an adjuvant treatment with a COMT inhibitor, a reduction of the dosage of Madopar may be necessary. Anticholinergics should not be withdrawn abruptly when Madopar therapy is instituted, as levodopa does not begin to take effect for some time.

There have been rare reports of possible antagonism of levodopa by diazepam. Isolated cases of hypertensive crisis have been reported with concomitant use of tricyclic antidepressants. Madopar must not be given in conjunction with MAO inhibitors (see section *4.3 Contra-indications*)

Use with antihypertensive agents may increase the hypotensive response, while sympathomimetics may increase the cardiovascular side-effects of levodopa.

Levodopa may interfere chemically with several diagnostic laboratory tests including those for glucose, ketone bodies or catecholamines in urine and for glucose or uric acid in blood. Levodopa therapy has been reported to inhibit the response to protirelin in tests of thyroid function. Coombs' tests may give a false-positive result in patients taking Madopar.

4.6 Pregnancy and lactation
Madopar is contra-indicated in pregnancy and in women of childbearing potential in the absence of adequate contraception, since there is evidence of harmful effects in studies in pregnant rabbits and the benserazide component has been found to be associated with skeletal malformations in the rat. If pregnancy occurs in a woman taking Madopar, the drug must be discontinued. Patients taking Madopar should not breast-feed their infants.

4.7 Effects on ability to drive and use machines
Patients being treated with levodopa and presenting with somnolence and/or sudden sleep episodes must be informed to refrain from driving or engaging in activities where impaired alertness may put themselves or others at risk of serious injury or death (e.g. operating machines) until such recurrent episodes and somnolence have resolved (see Section *4.4*).

4.8 Undesirable effects
- Gastrointestinal:

- Anorexia, nausea, vomiting, diarrhoea (less commonly than with levodopa) mainly occurring in the early stages of treatment. May be controlled by taking Madopar with some food or liquid or increasing the dose slowly.

- Gastro-intestinal bleeding has been reported with levodopa therapy.

- Isolated cases of loss or alterations of taste.

- Skin:

- rarely allergic reactions such as pruritus and rash.

- Cardiovascular:

- Occasional reports of cardiac arrhythmias and orthostatic hypotension (less frequently than with levodopa alone). Orthostatic disorders usually improve following dosage reduction.

- Haematological:

- Rare cases of haemolytic anaemia, transient leucopenia and thrombocytopenia.

- Neuropsychiatric:

- Psychiatric disturbances are common in Parkinsonian patients, including those treated with levodopa, including mild elation, anxiety, agitation, insomnia, drowsiness, depression, aggression, delusions, hallucinations, temporal disorientation and "unmasking" of psychoses.

- Levodopa is associated with somnolence and has been associated very rarely with excessive daytime somnolence and sudden sleep onset episodes.

- Involuntary movements (e.g. choreiform or athetotic, oral dyskinesias, "paddling" foot) are common, particularly on long-term administration. These are usually dose-dependant and may disappear or become tolerable after dose adjustment.

- Laboratory abnormalities:

- Transient rises in SGOT, SGPT and alkaline phosphatase values have been noted.

- Serum uric acid and blood urea nitrogen levels are occasionally increased.

- Others:

- Flushing and sweating have been reported with levodopa.

- Urine passed during treatment may be altered in colour; usually red-tinged, this will turn dark on standing. These changes are due to metabolites and are no cause for concern.

Tolerance to Madopar varies widely between patients and is often related to the rate of dosage increases. With long-term administration, fluctuations in the therapeutic response may be encountered. They include "freezing" episodes, end-of-dose deterioration and the so-called "on-off" effect. Patients may be helped by dosage reduction or by giving smaller and more frequent doses.

4.9 Overdose
Symptoms of overdosage are qualitatively similar to the side-effects but may be of greater magnitude.

Treatment should include gastric lavage, general supportive measures, intravenous fluids and the maintenance of an adequate airway.

Electrocardiographic monitoring should be instituted and the patient carefully observed for the possible development of arrhythmias. If necessary, anti-arrhythmic therapy should be given and other symptoms treated as they arise.

5. PHARMACOLOGICAL PROPERTIES

5.1 Pharmacodynamic properties
Madopar is an anti-Parkinsonian agent. Levodopa is the metabolic precursor of dopamine. The latter is severely depleted in the striatum, pallidum and substantia nigra of Parkinsonian patients and it is considered that administration of levodopa raises the level of available dopamine in these centres. However, conversion of levodopa into dopamine by the enzyme dopa decarboxylase also takes place in extracerebral tissues. As a consequence the full therapeutic effect may not be obtained and side-effects occur.

Administration of a peripheral decarboxylase inhibitor, which blocks the extracerebral decarboxylation of levodopa, in conjunction with levodopa has significant advantages; these include reduced gastro-intestinal side-effects, a more rapid response at the initiation of therapy and a simpler dosage regimen. Madopar is a combination of levodopa and benserazide in the ratio 4:1 which in clinical trials has been shown to be the most satisfactory.

Like every replacement therapy, chronic treatment with Madopar will be necessary.

5.2 Pharmacokinetic properties
Absorption

Low levels of endogenous levodopa are detectable in pre-dose blood samples. After oral administration of Madopar, levodopa and benserazide are rapidly absorbed, mainly in the upper regions of the small intestine and absorption there is independent of the site. Interaction studies indicate that a higher proportion of levodopa is absorbed when administered in combination with benserazide, compared with levodopa administered alone. Maximum plasma concentrations of levodopa are reached approximately one hour after ingestion of Madopar. The absolute bioavailability of levodopa from standard Madopar is approximately 98%.

The maximum plasma concentration of levodopa and the extent of absorption (AUC) increase proportionally with dose (50 – 200mg levodopa). The peak levodopa plasma concentration is 30% lower and occurs later when Madopar is administered after a standard meal. Food intake generally reduces the extent of levodopa absorption by 15% but this can be variable.

Distribution

Levodopa crosses the blood-brain barrier by a saturable transport system. It is not bound to plasma proteins. Benserazide does not cross the blood-brain barrier at therapeutic doses. Benserazide is concentrated mainly in the kidneys, lungs, small intestine and liver.

Metabolism

The 2 major routes of metabolism of levodopa are decarboxylation to form dopamine, which in turn is converted to a minor degree to norepinephrine and to a greater extent, to inactive metabolites, and O-methylation, forming 3-O-methyldopa, which has an elimination half-life of approximately 15 hours and accumulates in patients receiving therapeutic doses of Madopar. Decreased peripheral decarboxylation of levodopa when it is administered with benserazide is reflected in higher plasma levels of levodopa and 3-O-methyldopa.

Benserazide is hydroxylated to trihydroxybenzylhydrazine in the intestinal mucosa and the liver. This metabolite is a potent inhibitor of the aromatic amino acid decarboxylase.

Elimination

In the presence of the peripheral decarboxylase inhibitor, benserazide, the elimination half-life of levodopa is approximately 1.5 hours. In elderly patients the elimination half-life is slightly (25%) longer. Clearance of levodopa is 430ml/min.

Benserazide is almost entirely eliminated by metabolism. The metabolites are mainly excreted in the urine (64%) and to a small extent in faeces (24%).

5.3 Preclinical safety data
See section *4.6 Pregnancy and lactation*.

6. PHARMACEUTICAL PARTICULARS

6.1 List of excipients
Each capsule contains:

Microcrystalline cellulose

Povidone

Purified talc

Magnesium stearate

Mannitol

Gelatin

and the colouring agents E132, E171 and E172.

6.2 Incompatibilities
None known.

6.3 Shelf life
3 years.

6.4 Special precautions for storage
Do not store above 25°C. Keep container tightly closed.

6.5 Nature and contents of container
Madopar 62.5 and 125 Capsules:

Amber glass bottles with HDPE cap and integral desiccant containing 100 capsules.

Madopar 250 Capsules:

Amber glass bottles with polypropylene cap with loose desiccant containing 100 capsules.

6.6 Instructions for use and handling
No special requirements.

7. MARKETING AUTHORISATION HOLDER
Roche Products Limited, 40 Broadwater Road, Welwyn Garden City, Hertfordshire, AL7 3AY.

8. MARKETING AUTHORISATION NUMBER(S)
Madopar 62.5 Capsules: PL 0031/0125

Madopar 125 Capsules: PL 0031/0073

Madopar 250 Capsules: PL 0031/0074

9. DATE OF FIRST AUTHORISATION/RENEWAL OF THE AUTHORISATION
March 1995

10. DATE OF REVISION OF THE TEXT
December 2002

Madopar is a registered trade mark

P522578/103

Madopar CR Capsules 125

(Roche Products Limited)

1. NAME OF THE MEDICINAL PRODUCT
Madopar® CR Capsules "125".

2. QUALITATIVE AND QUANTITATIVE COMPOSITION
Each capsule contains 100.0mg levodopa Ph. Eur. and 28.5mg benserazide hydrochloride Ph. Eur. (equivalent to 25mg of the base) in a controlled release formulation.

3. PHARMACEUTICAL FORM
Prolonged-release hard capsules.

4. CLINICAL PARTICULARS

4.1 Therapeutic indications
Treatment of all stages of Parkinson's disease. Patients with fluctuations related to levodopa plasma concentrations or timing of dose, e.g. end of dose deterioration or wearing-off effects, are more likely to benefit from switching to Madopar CR.

4.2 Posology and method of administration
Adults, including the elderly

Dosage and administration are very variable and must be titrated to the needs of the individual patient.

Madopar CR capsules must always be swallowed whole, preferably with a little water. They may be taken with or without food but antacid preparations should be avoided.

In patients with nocturnal immobility, positive effects have been reported after gradually increasing the last evening dose to 250mg Madopar CR on retiring.

Patients not currently treated with levodopa

In patients with mild to moderate disease, the initial recommended dose is one capsule of Madopar CR three times daily with meals. Higher doses, in general, of Madopar CR will be required than with conventional levodopa-decarboxylase inhibitor combinations as a result of the reduced bioavailability. The initial dosages should not exceed 600mg per day of levodopa.

Some patients may require a supplementary dose of conventional Madopar, or Madopar Dispersible, together with the first morning dose of Madopar CR to compensate for the more gradual onset of the CR formulation.

In cases of poor response to Madopar CR at total daily doses of Madopar CR plus any supplementary conventional Madopar corresponding to 1200mg levodopa, administration of Madopar CR should be discontinued and alternative therapy considered.

Patients currently treated with levodopa

Madopar CR should be substituted for the standard levodopa-decarboxylase inhibitor preparation by one capsule Madopar CR 125 per 100mg levodopa. For example, where a patient previously received daily doses of 200mg levodopa with a decarboxylase inhibitor, then therapy should be initiated with two capsules Madopar CR 125. Therapy should continue with the same frequency of doses as previously.

With Madopar CR, *on average*, a 50% increase in daily levodopa dosage compared with previous therapy has been found to be appropriate. The dosage should be titrated every 2 to 3 days using dosage increments of Madopar CR 125 capsules and a period of up to 4 weeks should be allowed for optimisation of dosage.

Patients already on levodopa therapy should be informed that their condition may deteriorate initially until the optimal dosage regimen has been found. Close medical supervision of the patient is advisable during the initial period whilst adjusting the dosage.

Children

Not to be given to patients under 25 years of age: therefore, no dosage recommendations are made for the administration of Madopar CR to children.

4.3 Contraindications

Madopar must not be given to patients with known hypersensitivity to levodopa or benserazide.

Madopar is contra-indicated in narrow-angle glaucoma (it may be used in wide-angle glaucoma provided that the intra-ocular pressure remains under control); severe psychoneuroses or psychoses; severe endocrine, renal, hepatic or cardiac disorders.

It should not be given in conjunction with, or within 2 weeks of withdrawal of, monoamine oxidase (MAO) inhibitors, except selective MAO-B inhibitors (e.g. selegiline) or selective MAO-A inhibitors (e.g. moclobemide).

It should not be given to patients under 25 years of age.

It should not be given to pregnant women or to women of childbearing potential in the absence of adequate contraception. If pregnancy occurs in a woman taking Madopar, the drug must be discontinued.

Suspicion has arisen that levodopa may activate a malignant melanoma. Therefore, Madopar should not be used in persons who have a history of, or who may be suffering from, a malignant melanoma.

4.4 Special warnings and special precautions for use

When other drugs must be given in conjunction with Madopar, the patient should be carefully observed for unusual side-effects or potentiating effects.

In the event of general anaesthesia being required, Madopar therapy may be continued as long as the patient is able to take fluids and medication by mouth. If therapy is temporarily interrupted, the usual daily dosage may be administered as soon as the patient is able to take oral medication. Whenever therapy has been interrupted for longer periods, dosage should again be adjusted gradually; however, in many cases the patient can rapidly be returned to his previous therapeutic dosage.

If a patient has to undergo surgery, when Madopar has not been withdrawn, anaesthesia with halothane should be avoided.

There have been occasional reports of a neuroleptic malignant-like syndrome, involving hyperthermia, on abrupt withdrawal of levodopa preparations. Sudden discontinuation of Madopar, without close supervision, or "drug holidays" should therefore be avoided.

Pyridoxine (vitamin B_6) may be given with Madopar since the presence of a decarboxylase inhibitor protects against the peripheral levodopa transformation facilitated by pyridoxine.

Levodopa has been associated with somnolence and episodes of sudden sleep onset. Sudden onset of sleep during daily activities, in some cases without awareness or warning signs, has been reported very rarely. Patients must be informed of this and advised to exercise caution while driving or operating machines during treatment with levodopa. Patients who have experienced somnolence and/or an episode of sudden sleep onset must refrain from driving or operating machines. Furthermore a reduction of dosage or termination of therapy may be considered.

Care should be taken when using Madopar in the following circumstances: in endocrine, renal, pulmonary or cardiovascular disease, particularly where there is a history of myocardial infarction or arrhythmia; psychiatric disturbances (e.g. depression); hepatic disorder; peptic ulcer; osteomalacia; where sympathomimetic drugs may be required (e.g. bronchial asthma), due to possible potentiation of the cardiovascular effects of levodopa; where antihypertensive drugs are being used, due to possible increased hypotensive action.

Periodic evaluation of hepatic, haemopoietic, renal and cardiovascular functions is advised.

Patients who improve on Madopar therapy should be advised to resume normal activities gradually as rapid mobilisation may increase the risk of injury.

Patients with diabetes should undergo frequent blood sugar tests and the dosage of antidiabetic agents should be adjusted to blood sugar levels.

4.5 Interaction with other medicinal products and other forms of Interaction

Ferrous sulphate decreases the maximum plasma concentration and the AUC of levodopa by 30 – 50%. The pharmacokinetic changes observed during co-treatment with ferrous sulphate appeared to be clinically significant in some but not all patients.

Opioids and drugs which interfere with central amine mechanisms, such as rauwolfia alkaloids (reserpine), tetrabenazine (Nitoman), metoclopramide, phenothiazines, thioxanthenes, butyrophenones, amphetamines and papaverine, should be avoided where possible. If, however, their administration is considered essential, extreme care should be exercised and a close watch kept for any signs of potentiation, antagonism or other interactions and for unusual side-effects. Metoclopramide has been shown to increase the rate of levodopa absorption.

Combination with other anti-Parkinsonian agents (anticholinergics, amantadine, dopamine agonists) is permissible, though both the desired and undesired effects of treatment may be intensified. It may be necessary to reduce the dosage of Madopar or the other substance. When initiating an adjuvant treatment with a COMT inhibitor, a reduction of the dosage of Madopar may be necessary. Anticholinergics should not be withdrawn abruptly when Madopar therapy is instituted, as levodopa does not begin to take effect for some time.

There have been rare reports of possible antagonism of levodopa by diazepam. Isolated cases of hypertensive crisis have been reported with concomitant use of tricyclic antidepressants. Madopar must not be given in conjunction with MAO inhibitors (see section *4.3 Contra-indications*)

Use with antihypertensive agents may increase the hypotensive response, while sympathomimetics may increase the cardiovascular side-effects of levodopa.

Levodopa may interfere chemically with several diagnostic laboratory tests including those for glucose, ketone bodies, or catecholamines in urine and for glucose or uric acid in blood. Levodopa therapy has been reported to inhibit the response to protirelin in tests of thyroid function. Coombs' tests may give a false-positive result in patients taking Madopar.

When Madopar CR is given with antacid preparations the bioavailability of levodopa is reduced, in comparison with conventional Madopar.

4.6 Pregnancy and lactation

Madopar is contra-indicated in pregnancy and in women of childbearing potential in the absence of adequate contraception.

Since there is evidence of harmful effects in studies in pregnant rabbits and the benserazide component has been found to be associated with skeletal malformations in the rat. If pregnancy occurs in a woman taking Madopar, the drug must be discontinued. Patients taking Madopar should not breast-feed their infants.

4.7 Effects on ability to drive and use machines

Patients being treated with levodopa and presenting with somnolence and /or sudden sleep episodes must be informed to refrain from driving or engaging in activities where impaired alertness may put themselves or others at risk of serious injury or death (e.g. operating machines) until such recurrent episodes and somnolence have resolved (see Section 4.4).

4.8 Undesirable effects

Gastro-intestinal:

– Anorexia, nausea, vomiting, diarrhoea (less commonly than with levodopa) mainly occurring in the early stages of treatment may be controlled by taking Madopar with some food or liquid or increasing the dose slowly.

– Gastro-intestinal bleeding has been reported with levodopa therapy.

– Isolated cases of loss or alterations of taste.

Skin:

– Rarely allergic reactions such as pruritus and rash.

Cardiovascular:

– Occasional reports of cardiac arrhythmias and orthostatic hypotension (less frequently than with levodopa alone). Orthostatic disorders usually improve following dosage reduction.

Haematological:

– Rare cases of haemolytic anaemia, transient leucopenia and thrombocytopenia.

Neuropsychiatric:

– Psychiatric disturbances are common in Parkinsonian patients, including those treated with levodopa, including mild elation, anxiety, agitation, insomnia, drowsiness, depression, aggression, delusions, hallucinations, temporal disorientation and "unmasking" of psychoses.

– Levodopa is associated with somnolence and has been associated very rarely with excessive daytime somnolence and sudden sleep onset episodes.

– Involuntary movements (e.g. choreiform or athetotic, oral dyskinesias, "paddling" foot) are common, particularly on long-term administration. These are usually dose-dependent and may disappear or become tolerable after dose adjustment.

Laboratory abnormalities:

– Transient rises in SGOT, SGPT and alkaline phosphatase values have been noted.

– Serum uric acid and blood urea nitrogen levels are occasionally increased.

Others:

– Flushing and sweating have been reported with levodopa.

– Urine passed during treatment may be altered in colour; usually red-tinged, this will turn dark on standing. These changes are due to metabolites and are no cause for concern.

Tolerance to Madopar varies widely between patients and is often related to the rate of dosage increases.

4.9 Overdose

Symptoms of overdosage are qualitatively similar to the side-effects but may be of greater magnitude.

Treatment should include gastric lavage, general supportive measures, intravenous fluids and the maintenance of an adequate airway.

Electrocardiographic monitoring should be instituted and the patient carefully observed for the possible development of arrhythmias. If necessary, anti-arrhythmic therapy should be given and other symptoms treated as they arise.

5. PHARMACOLOGICAL PROPERTIES

5.1 Pharmacodynamic properties

Madopar is an anti-Parkinsonian agent. Levodopa is the metabolic precursor of dopamine. The latter is severely depleted in the striatum, pallidum and substantia nigra of Parkinsonian patients and it is considered that administration of levodopa raises the level of available dopamine in these centres. However, conversion of levodopa into dopamine by the enzyme dopa decarboxylase also takes place in extracerebral tissues. As a consequence the full therapeutic effect may not be obtained and side-effects occur.

Administration of a peripheral decarboxylase inhibitor, which blocks the extracerebral decarboxylation of levodopa, in conjunction with levodopa has significant advantages; these include reduced gastro-intestinal side-effects, a more rapid response at the initiation of therapy and a simpler dosage regimen. Madopar consists of levodopa and the peripheral decarboxylase inhibitor benserazide in the ratio 4:1 which in clinical trials has been shown to be the most satisfactory combination.

Like every replacement therapy, chronic treatment with Madopar will be necessary.

5.2 Pharmacokinetic properties

Madopar CR is a controlled-release form which provides more prolonged, but lower, peak plasma concentrations of levodopa than standard Madopar or other conventional formulations of levodopa.

Absorption

The active ingredients of Madopar CR are released slowly in the stomach and the maximum levodopa plasma concentration is reached approximately 3 hours after ingestion. The plasma concentration-time curve for levodopa shows a longer "half-duration" (= time-span when plasma concentrations are equal to or higher than half the maximum concentration) than that of standard Madopar, which indicates pronounced controlled-release properties. Madopar CR bioavailability is approximately 60% that of standard Madopar and is not affected by food. Maximum plasma concentrations of levodopa are not affected by food but occur later (five hours) after postprandial administration. Co-administration of an antacid with Madopar CR reduces the extent of levodopa absorption by 32%.

Distribution

Levodopa crosses the blood-brain barrier by a saturable transport system. It is not bound to plasma proteins. Benserazide does not cross the blood-brain barrier at therapeutic doses. Benserazide is concentrated mainly in the kidneys, lungs, small intestine and liver.

Metabolism

The 2 major routes of metabolism of levodopa are decarboxylation to form dopamine, which in turn is converted to a minor degree to norepinephrine and to a greater extent, to inactive metabolites, and O-methylation, forming 3-O-methyldopa, which has an elimination half-life of approximately 15 hours and accumulates in patients receiving therapeutic doses of Madopar. Decreased peripheral decarboxylation of levodopa when it is administered with benserazide is reflected in higher plasma levels of levodopa and 3-O-methyldopa.

Benserazide is hydroxylated to trihydroxybenzylhydrazine in the intestinal mucosa and the liver. This metabolite is a potent inhibitor of the aromatic amino acid decarboxylase.

Elimination

In the presence of the peripheral decarboxylase inhibitor, benserazide, the elimination half-life of levodopa is approximately 1.5 hours. In elderly patients the elimination half-life is slightly (25%) longer. Clearance of levodopa is 430 ml/min.

Benserazide is almost entirely eliminated by metabolism. The metabolites are mainly excreted in the urine (64%) and to a small extent in faeces (24%).

6. PHARMACEUTICAL PARTICULARS

6.1 List of excipients

Each capsule contains:

Hydroxypropyl methylcellulose

Hydrogenated vegetable oil

Calcium phosphate, dibasic anhydrous

Mannitol

Talc

Povidone

Magnesium stearate

Gelatin

and the colouring agents E132, E171 and E172

6.2 Incompatibilities

None known.

6.3 Shelf life
3 years.

6.4 Special precautions for storage
Do not store above 25°C. Keep container tightly closed.

6.5 Nature and contents of container
Amber glass bottles with polyethylene closure and integrated desiccant containing 100 capsules.

6.6 Instructions for use and handling
No special requirements.

7. MARKETING AUTHORISATION HOLDER
Roche Products Limited, 40 Broadwater Road, Welwyn Garden City, Hertfordshire, AL7 3AY.

8. MARKETING AUTHORISATION NUMBER(S)
PL 0031/0227

9. DATE OF FIRST AUTHORISATION/RENEWAL OF THE AUTHORISATION
Last renewal approved 09 March 1999

10. DATE OF REVISION OF THE TEXT
December 2002

Madopar is a registered trade mark

P522579/103

Madopar Dispersible

(Roche Products Limited)

1. NAME OF THE MEDICINAL PRODUCT
Madopar® 62.5 Dispersible Tablets

Madopar® 125 Dispersible Tablets

2. QUALITATIVE AND QUANTITATIVE COMPOSITION
Madopar 62.5 dispersible tablets: Round, white tablets with ROCHE 62.5 imprinted on one face and a single break bar on the other, containing 50mg levodopa Ph. Eur. and 14.25mg benserazide hydrochloride Ph. Eur. (equivalent to 12.5mg of the base).

Madopar 125 Dispersible Tablets: Round, white tablets with ROCHE 125 imprinted on one face and a single break bar on the other, containing 100mg levodopa Ph. Eur and 28.5mg benserazide hydrochloride Ph. Eur (equivalent to 25mg of the base).

3. PHARMACEUTICAL FORM
Madopar 62.5 Dispersible tablets.

Madopar 125 Dispersible tablets.

4. CLINICAL PARTICULARS

4.1 Therapeutic indications
Parkinsonism - idiopathic, post-encephalitic. Previous neurosurgery is not a contra-indication to Madopar. Patients requiring a more rapid onset of action, e.g. patients suffering from early morning or afternoon akinesia, or who exhibit "delayed on" or "wearing off" phenomena, are more likely to benefit from Madopar Dispersible.

4.2 Posology and method of administration
Dosage and administration are variable and no more than a guide can be given.

Adults

Patients not previously treated with levodopa

The recommended initial dose is one capsule or dispersible tablet of Madopar 62.5 three or four times daily. If the disease is at an advanced stage, the starting dose should be one capsule or dispersible tablet of Madopar 125 three times daily.

The daily dosage should then be increased by one capsule or dispersible tablet of Madopar 125, or their equivalent, once or twice weekly until a full therapeutic effect is obtained, or side-effects supervene.

In some elderly patients, it may suffice to initiate treatment with one capsule or dispersible tablet of Madopar 62.5 once or twice daily, increasing by one capsule or dispersible tablet every third or fourth day.

The effective dose usually lies within the range of four to eight capsules or dispersible tablets of Madopar 125 (two to four capsules of Madopar 250) daily in divided doses, most patients requiring no more than six capsules or dispersible tablets of Madopar 125 daily.

Optimal improvement is usually seen in one to three weeks but the full therapeutic effect of Madopar may not be apparent for some time. It is advisable, therefore, to allow several weeks to elapse before contemplating dosage increments above the average dose range. If satisfactory improvement is still not achieved, the dose of Madopar may be increased but with caution. It is rarely necessary to give more than ten capsules or dispersible tablets of Madopar 125 (five capsules of Madopar 250) per day.

Treatment should be continued for at least six months before failure is concluded from the absence of a clinical response.

Madopar 62.5 capsules or dispersible tablets may be used to facilitate adjustment of dosage to the needs of the individual patient. Patients who experience fluctuations in response may be helped by dividing the dosage into smaller, more frequent doses with the aid of Madopar 62.5 capsules or dispersible tablets without, however, altering the total daily dose.

Madopar 250 capsules are only for maintenance therapy once the optimal dosage has been determined using Madopar 125 capsules or dispersible tablets.

Patients previously treated with levodopa

The following procedure is recommended: Levodopa alone should be discontinued and Madopar started on the following day. The patient should be initiated on a total of one less Madopar 125 capsule or dispersible tablet daily than the total number of 500mg levodopa tablets or capsules previously taken (for example, if the patient had previously taken 2g levodopa daily, then he should start on three capsules or dispersible tablets Madopar 125 daily on the following day). Observe the patient for one week and then, if necessary, increase the dosage in the manner described for new patients.

Patients previously treated with other levodopa/decarboxylase inhibitor combinations

Previous therapy should be withdrawn for 12 hours. In order to minimise the potential for any effects of levodopa withdrawal, it may be beneficial to discontinue previous therapy at night and institute Madopar therapy the following morning. The initial Madopar dose should be one capsule or dispersible tablet of Madopar 62.5 three or four times daily. This dose may then be increased in the manner described for patients not previously treated with levodopa.

Other anti-Parkinsonian drugs may be given with Madopar. Existing treatment with other anti-Parkinsonian drugs, e.g. anticholinergics or amantadine, should be continued during initiation of Madopar therapy. However, as treatment with Madopar proceeds and the therapeutic effect becomes apparent, the dosage of the other drugs may need to be reduced or the drugs gradually withdrawn.

Elderly

Although there may be an age-related decrease in tolerance to levodopa in the elderly, Madopar appears to be well-tolerated and side effects are generally not troublesome.

Children

Not to be given to patients under 25 years of age, therefore, no dosage recommendations are made for the administration of Madopar to children.

Madopar capsules and dispersible tablets are for oral administration. They should be taken with, or immediately after, meals.

Madopar dispersible tablets may be swallowed whole or dispersed in at least 25ml water per tablet. They may be taken in dilute orange squash (at least 25ml per tablet) if preferred. However, orange juice should not be used. Madopar dispersible tablets are particularly suitable for patients who dislike taking capsules or have difficulty in swallowing solid dosage forms.

4.3 Contraindications
Madopar must not be given to patients with known hypersensitivity to levodopa or benserazide.

Madopar is contra-indicated in narrow-angle glaucoma (it may be used in wide-angle glaucoma provided that the intra-ocular pressure remains under control); severe psychoneuroses or psychoses; severe endocrine, renal, hepatic or cardiac disorders.

It should not be given in conjunction with, or within 2 weeks of withdrawal of, monoamine oxidase (MAO) inhibitors, except selective MAO-B inhibitors (e.g. selegiline) or selective MAO-A inhibitors (e.g. moclobemide).

It should not be given to patients under 25 years of age.

It should not be given to pregnant women or to women of childbearing potential in the absence of adequate contraception. If pregnancy occurs in a woman taking Madopar, the drug must be discontinued.

Suspicion has arisen that levodopa may activate a malignant melanoma. Therefore, Madopar should not be used in persons who have a history of, or who may be suffering from, a malignant melanoma.

4.4 Special warnings and special precautions for use
When other drugs must be given in conjunction with Madopar, the patient should be carefully observed for unusual side-effects or potentiating effects.

In the event of general anaesthesia being required, Madopar therapy may be continued as long as the patient is able to take fluids and medication by mouth. If therapy is temporarily interrupted, the usual daily dosage may be administered as soon as the patient is able to take oral medication. Whenever therapy has been interrupted for longer periods, dosage should again be adjusted gradually; however, in many cases the patient can rapidly be returned to his previous therapeutic dosage.

If a patient has to undergo surgery, when Madopar has not been withdrawn, anaesthesia with halothane should be avoided.

There have been occasional reports of a neuroleptic malignant-like syndrome, involving hyperthermia, on abrupt withdrawal of levodopa preparations. Sudden discontinuation of Madopar, without close supervision, or "drug holidays" should therefore be avoided.

Pyridoxine (vitamin B_6) may be given with Madopar since the presence of a decarboxylase inhibitor protects against the peripheral levodopa transformation facilitated by pyridoxine.

Levodopa has been associated with somnolence and episodes of sleep onset. Sudden onset of sleep during daily activities, in some cases without awareness or warning signs, has been reported very rarely. Patients must be informed of this and advised to exercise caution while driving or operating machines during treatment with levodopa. Patients who have experienced somnolence and/or an episode of sudden sleep onset must refrain from driving or operating machines. Furthermore a reduction of dosage or termination of therapy may be considered.

Care should be taken when using Madopar in the following circumstances: In endocrine, renal, pulmonary or cardiovascular disease, particularly where there is a history of myocardial infarction or arrhythmia; psychiatric disturbances (e.g. depression); hepatic disorder; peptic ulcer; osteomalacia; where sympathomimetic drugs may be required (e.g. bronchial asthma), due to possible potentiation of the cardiovascular effects of levodopa; where antihypertensive drugs are being used, due to possible increased hypotensive action.

Periodic evaluation of hepatic, haemopoietic, renal and cardiovascular functions is advised.

Patients with diabetes should undergo frequent blood sugar tests and the dosage of anti-diabetic agents should be adjusted to blood sugar levels.

Patients who improve on Madopar therapy should be advised to resume normal activities gradually as rapid mobilisation may increase the risk of injury.

4.5 Interaction with other medicinal products and other forms of Interaction
Ferrous sulphate decreases the maximum plasma concentration and the AUC of levodopa by 30 - 50%. The pharmacokinetic changes observed during co-treatment with ferrous sulphate appeared to be clinically significant in some but not all patients.

Opioids and drugs which interfere with central amine mechanisms, such as rauwolfia alkaloids (reserpine), tetrabenazine (Nitoman), metoclopramide, phenothiazines, thioxanthenes, butyrophenones, amphetamines and papaverine, should be avoided where possible. If, however, their administration is considered essential, extreme care should be exercised and a close watch kept for any signs of potentiation, antagonism or other interactions and for unusual side-effects. Metoclopramide has been shown to increase the rate of levodopa absorption.

Co-administration of the anticholinergic drug trihexyphenidyl with Madopar reduces the rate, but not the extent, of levodopa absorption.

Combination with other anti-Parkinsonian agents (anticholinergics, amantadine, dopamine agonists) is permissible, though both the desired and undesired effects of treatment may be intensified. It may be necessary to reduce the dosage of Madopar or the other substance. When initiating an adjuvant treatment with a COMT inhibitor, a reduction of the dosage of Madopar may be necessary. Anticholinergics should not be withdrawn abruptly when Madopar therapy is instituted, as levodopa does not begin to take effect for some time.

There have been rare reports of possible antagonism of levodopa by diazepam. Isolated cases of hypertensive crisis have been reported with concomitant use of tricyclic antidepressants. Madopar must not be given in conjunction with MAO inhibitors (see section *4.3 Contra-indications*)

Use with antihypertensive agents may increase the hypotensive response, while sympathomimetics may increase the cardiovascular side-effects of levodopa.

Levodopa may interfere chemically with several diagnostic laboratory tests including those for glucose, ketone bodies or catecholamines in urine and for glucose or uric acid in blood. Levodopa therapy has been reported to inhibit the response to protirelin in tests of thyroid function. Coombs' tests may give a false-positive result in patients taking Madopar.

4.6 Pregnancy and lactation
Madopar is contra-indicated in pregnancy and in women of childbearing potential in the absence of adequate contraception, since there is evidence of harmful effects in studies in pregnant rabbits and the benserazide component has been found to be associated with skeletal malformations in the rat. If pregnancy occurs in a woman taking Madopar, the drug must be discontinued. Patients taking Madopar should not breast-feed their infants.

4.7 Effects on ability to drive and use machines
Patients being treated with levodopa and presenting with somnolence and/or sudden sleep episodes must be informed to refrain from driving or engaging in activities where impaired alertness may put themselves or others at risk of serious injury or death (e.g. operating machines) until such recurrent episodes and somnolence have resolved (see Section *4.4*).

4.8 Undesirable effects
-Gastrointestinal:

- Anorexia, nausea, vomiting, diarrhoea (less commonly than with levodopa) mainly occurring in the early stages of treatment. May be controlled by taking Madopar with some food or liquid or increasing the dose slowly.

- Gastro-intestinal bleeding has been reported with levodopa therapy.

- Isolated cases of loss or alterations of taste.

-Skin:
- rarely allergic reactions such as pruritus and rash.

-Cardiovascular:

- Occasional reports of cardiac arrhythmias and orthostatic hypotension (less frequently than with levodopa alone). Orthostatic disorders usually improve following dosage reduction.

-Haematological:

- Rare cases of haemolytic anaemia, transient leucopenia and thrombocytopenia.

-Neuropsychiatric:

- Psychiatric disturbances are common in Parkinsonian patients, including those treated with levodopa, including mild elation, anxiety, agitation, insomnia, drowsiness, depression, aggression, delusions, hallucinations, temporal disorientation and "unmasking" of psychoses.

- Levodopa is associated with somnolence and has been associated very rarely with excessive daytime somnolence and sudden sleep onset episodes.

- Involuntary movements (e.g. choreiform or athetotic, oral dyskinesias, "paddling" foot) are common, particularly on long-term administration. These are usually dose-dependant and may disappear or become tolerable after dose adjustment.

-Laboratory abnormalities:

- Transient rises in SGOT, SGPT and alkaline phosphatase values have been noted.

- Serum uric acid and blood urea nitrogen levels are occasionally increased.

-Others:

- Flushing and sweating have been reported with levodopa.

- Urine passed during treatment may be altered in colour; usually red-tinged, this will turn dark on standing. These changes are due to metabolites and are no cause for concern.

Tolerance to Madopar varies widely between patients and is often related to the rate of dosage increases. With long-term administration, fluctuations in the therapeutic response may be encountered. They include "freezing" episodes, end-of-dose deterioration and the so-called "on-off" effect. Patients may be helped by dosage reduction or by giving smaller and more frequent doses.

4.9 Overdose
Symptoms of overdosage are qualitatively similar to the side-effects but may be of greater magnitude.

Treatment should include gastric lavage, general supportive measures, intravenous fluids and the maintenance of an adequate airway. Electrocardiographic monitoring should be instituted and the patient carefully observed for the possible development of arrhythmias. If necessary, anti-arrhythmic therapy, should be given and other symptoms treated as they arise.

5. PHARMACOLOGICAL PROPERTIES
5.1 Pharmacodynamic properties
Madopar is an anti-Parkinsonian agent. Levodopa is the metabolic precursor of dopamine. The latter is severely depleted in the striatum, pallidum and substantia nigra of Parkinsonian patients and it is considered that administration of levodopa raises the level of available dopamine in these centres. However, conversion of levodopa into dopamine by the enzyme dopa decarboxylase also takes place in extracerebral tissues. As a consequence the full therapeutic effect may not be obtained and side-effects occur.

Administration of a peripheral decarboxylase inhibitor, which blocks the extracerebral decarboxylation of levodopa, in conjunction with levodopa has significant advantages; these include reduced gastro-intestinal side-effects, a more rapid response at the initiation of therapy and a simpler dosage regimen. Madopar is a combination of levodopa and benserazide in the ratio 4:1 which in clinical trials has been shown to be the most satisfactory.

Like every replacement therapy, chronic treatment with Madopar will be necessary.

5.2 Pharmacokinetic properties
Absorption

Low levels of endogenous levodopa are detectable in pre-dose blood samples. After oral administration of Madopar, levodopa and benserazide are rapidly absorbed, mainly in the upper regions of the small intestine and absorption there is independent of the site. Interaction studies indicate that a higher proportion of levodopa is absorbed when administered in combination with benserazide, compared with levodopa administered alone. Maximum plasma concentrations of levodopa are reached approximately one hour after ingestion of Madopar. The absolute bioavailability of levodopa from standard Madopar is approximately 98%.

The maximum plasma concentration of levodopa and the extent of absorption (AUC) increase proportionally with dose (50 – 200mg levodopa). The peak levodopa plasma concentration is 30% lower and occurs later when Madopar is administered after a standard meal. Food intake generally reduces the extent of levodopa absorption by 15% but this can be variable.

Distribution

Levodopa crosses the blood-brain barrier by a saturable transport system. It is not bound to plasma proteins. Benserazide does not cross the blood-brain barrier at therapeutic doses. Benserazide is concentrated mainly in the kidneys, lungs, small intestine and liver.

Metabolism

The 2 major routes of metabolism of levodopa are decarboxylation to form dopamine, which in turn is converted to a minor degree to norepinephrine and to a greater extent, to inactive metabolites, and O-methylation, forming 3-O-methyldopa, which has an elimination half-life of approximately 15 hours and accumulates in patients receiving therapeutic doses of Madopar. Decreased peripheral decarboxylation of levodopa when it is administered with benserazide is reflected in higher plasma levels of levodopa and 3-O-methyldopa.

Benserazide is hydroxylated to trihydroxybenzylhydrazine in the intestinal mucosa and the liver. This metabolite is a potent inhibitor of the aromatic amino acid decarboxylase.

Elimination

In the presence of the peripheral decarboxylase inhibitor, benserazide, the elimination half-life of levodopa is approximately 1.5 hours. In elderly patients the elimination half-life is slightly (25%) longer. Clearance of levodopa is 430ml/min.

Benserazide is almost entirely eliminated by metabolism. The metabolites are mainly excreted in the urine (64%) and to a small extent in faeces (24%).

5.3 Preclinical safety data
None stated.

6. PHARMACEUTICAL PARTICULARS
6.1 List of excipients
Each dispersible tablet also contains: Anhydrous granular citric acid, starch maize modified, microcrystalline cellulose and magnesium stearate.

6.2 Incompatibilities
None known.

6.3 Shelf life
3 years.

6.4 Special precautions for storage
Do not store above 25°C. Keep container tightly closed.

6.5 Nature and contents of container
Amber glass bottles with HDPE cap with integral desiccant, containing 100 dispersible tablets.

6.6 Instructions for use and handling
No special requirements.

7. MARKETING AUTHORISATION HOLDER
Roche Products Limited, 40 Broadwater Road, Welwyn Garden City, Hertfordshire, AL7 3AY.

8. MARKETING AUTHORISATION NUMBER(S)
Madopar 62.5 Dispersible Tablets: PL 0031/0220

Madopar 125 Dispersible Tablets: PL 0031/0221

9. DATE OF FIRST AUTHORISATION/RENEWAL OF THE AUTHORISATION
April 1987

10. DATE OF REVISION OF THE TEXT
December 2002

Madopar is a registered trade mark

P522586/103

Magnapen Capsules

(Wockhardt UK Ltd)

1. NAME OF THE MEDICINAL PRODUCT
Magnapen Capsules or Co-fluampicil Capsules

2. QUALITATIVE AND QUANTITATIVE COMPOSITION
Co-fluampicil Capsules contain 250mg ampicillin as ampicillin trihydrate with 250mg flucloxacillin as flucloxacillin sodium (co-fluampicil 250/250).

3. PHARMACEUTICAL FORM
Capsules

Black and turquoise capsules overprinted Magnapen/ Magnapen or CF500/CP

4. CLINICAL PARTICULARS
4.1 Therapeutic indications
Co-fluampicil is indicated for the treatment of severe infections where the causative organism is unknown, and for mixed infections involving β-lactamase-producing staphylococci. Typical indications include:

In general practice: Chest infections, ENT infections, skin and soft tissue infections, and infections in patients whose underlying pathology places them at special risk.

In hospital (prior to laboratory results being available): severe respiratory tract infections, post-operative chest and wound infections, septic abortion, puerperal fever; septicaemia, prophylaxis in major surgery, infections in patients receiving immuno-suppressive therapy.

The spectrum of activity of co-fluampicil also makes it suitable for the treatment of many mixed infections, particularly those where β-lactamase-producing staphylococci are suspected or confirmed.

Parenteral usage is indicated where oral dosage is inappropriate.

4.2 Posology and method of administration
Usual adult dosage (including elderly patients and children over 10 years):

Oral: 1 capsule four times a day.

Usual children's dosage:

Oral: Under 10 years: half adult dose, using Co-fluampicil Syrup.

The above dosages for adults and children may be doubled where necessary.

Oral doses should be administered half to one hour before meals.

4.3 Contraindications
Co-fluampicil contains ampicillin and flucloxacillin which are penicillins, and should not be given to patients with a history of hypersensitivity to β-lactam antibiotics (e.g. penicillins, cephalosporins).

Co-fluampicil is contraindicated in patients with a history of flucloxacillin-associated jaundice/hepatic dysfunction.

4.4 Special warnings and special precautions for use
Before initiating therapy with co-fluampicil careful enquiries should be made concerning previous hypersensitivity reactions to β-lactam antibiotics.

Serious and occasionally fatal hypersensitivity reactions (anaphylaxis) have been reported in patients receiving β-lactam antibiotics. Although anaphylaxis is more frequent following parenteral therapy, it has occurred in patients on oral therapy. These reactions are more likely to occur in individuals with a hypersensitivity to β-lactam antibiotics.

Co-fluampicil contains ampicillin and should be avoided if infectious mononucleosis and/or acute or chronic leukaemia of lymphoid origin are suspected. The occurrence of a skin rash has been associated with these conditions following the administration of ampicillin.

Co-fluampicil should be used with caution in patients with evidence of hepatic dysfunction (see Section 4.8).

During prolonged treatments (e.g. osteomyelitis, endocarditis), regular monitoring of hepatic and renal functions is recommended.

Prolonged use may occasionally result in the selection of resistant strains of organisms.

Sodium Content: Co-fluampicil Capsules contain 13.0mg sodium per capsule. This should be included in the daily allowance of patients on sodium restricted diets.

4.5 Interaction with other medicinal products and other forms of Interaction
Bacteriostatic drugs may interfere with the bactericidal action of ampicillin and flucloxacillin.

In common with other oral broad-spectrum antibiotics, co-fluampicil may reduce the efficacy of oral contraceptives and patients should be warned accordingly.

Probenecid decreases the renal tubular secretion of co-fluampicil. Concurrent use with co-fluampicil may result in increased and prolonged blood levels of both ampicillin and flucloxacillin.

Concurrent administration of allopurinol during treatment with ampicillin can increase the likelihood of allergic skin reactions.

Co-fluampicil contains ampicillin. It is recommend that when testing for the presence of glucose in urine during ampicillin treatment, enzymatic glucose oxidase methods should be used because false positive readings are common with chemical methods due to the high urinary concentrations of ampicillin.

4.6 Pregnancy and lactation
Pregnancy: Animal studies with co-fluampicil have shown no teratogenic effects. The product has been in clinical use since 1971 and the limited number of reported cases of use in human pregnancy have shown no evidence of untoward effects. The decision to administer any drug during pregnancy should be taken with the utmost care. Therefore co-fluampicil should only be used in pregnancy when the potential benefits outweigh the potential risks associated with treatment.

Lactation: Trace quantities of ampicillin and flucloxacillin can be detected in breast milk. The possibility of hypersensitivity reactions must be considered in breast-fed infants. Therefore co-fluampicil should only be administered to a breast-feeding mother when the potential benefit outweigh the potential risks associated with treatment.

4.7 Effects on ability to drive and use machines
Adverse effects on the ability to drive or operate machinery have not been observed.

4.8 Undesirable effects
Hypersensitivity reactions:

If any hypersensitivity reaction occurs, the treatment should be discontinued.

Skin rash, puritis and urticaria have been reported occasionally. The incidence of rash is higher in patients suffering from infectious mononucleosis and acute or chronic leukaemia of lymphoid origin. Purpura, fever, eosinophilia and sometimes angioneurotic oedema have also been reported. Rarely, skin reactions such as erythema multiforme, Stevens-Johnson syndrome, and toxic epidermal necrolysis have been reported. Reactions such as fever, arthralgia, and myalgia can develop more than 48 hours after the start of the treatment.

Anaphylaxis (see Item 4.4-Warnings) has been reported rarely.

Gastrointestinal reactions:

Minor gastrointestinal disturbances, including occasionally nausea, vomiting and diarrhoea may occur during treatment. Pseudomembranous colitis has been reported rarely.

Hepatic effects:

Hepatitis and cholestatic jaundice have been reported rarely. These may be delayed for up to two months after withdrawal of treatment. In some cases the course of these conditions has been protracted and lasted for several months. Very rarely deaths have been reported from hepatic effects but are mostly limited to patients with serious underlying disease.

As with most other antibiotics, a moderate transient increase in transaminases has been reported.

Renal effects:

Interstitial nephritis may occur.

Haematological effects:

As with other β-lactam antibiotic, haematological effects including reversible leucopenia, reversible thrombocytopenia and haemolytic anaemia have been reported rarely.

4.9 Overdose
Gastrointestinal effects such as nausea, vomiting and diarrhoea may be evident and should be treated symptomatically.

Co-fluampicil contains flucloxacillin. Haemodialysis does not lower the serum levels of flucloxacillin.

Co-fluampicil contains ampicillin, which may be removed from the circulation by haemodialysis.

5. PHARMACOLOGICAL PROPERTIES
5.1 Pharmacodynamic properties
Infections encountered in medical practice can involve mixed strains of bacteria and may include β-lactamase-producing strains. Co-fluampicil provides broad spectrum activity.

5.2 Pharmacokinetic properties
Co-fluampicil is excreted via the kidneys with a plasma half-life of approximately one hour.

5.3 Preclinical safety data
Not relevant

6. PHARMACEUTICAL PARTICULARS
6.1 List of excipients
Capsules: Magnesium Stearate:

Capsule Shells: Gelatin, Black Iron Oxide (E172), Titanium Dioxide (E171), Patent Blue V (E131), Quinoline Yellow (E104).

6.2 Incompatibilities
None known

6.3 Shelf life
Two years

6.4 Special precautions for storage
Do not store above 25°C

Store in the original package

6.5 Nature and contents of container
Capsules: Standard polypropylene tube with a polythene closure or standard aluminium canisters or glass bottles fitted with a screw cap with a waxed pulpboard wad. Pack sizes of 20, 50, 100 or 500.

Aluminium foil pack. Pack size 12 capsules.

Aluminium/PVDC blister pack with aluminium overseal. Pack size 20, 28 and 100 capsules.

6.6 Instructions for use and handling
None

Administrative Data
7. MARKETING AUTHORISATION HOLDER
CP Pharmaceuticals Ltd

Ash Road North

Wrexham

LL13 9UF

United Kingdom.

8. MARKETING AUTHORISATION NUMBER(S)
PL 04543/0430

9. DATE OF FIRST AUTHORISATION/RENEWAL OF THE AUTHORISATION
8 May 2000

10. DATE OF REVISION OF THE TEXT
March 2002

Legal Category
POM

Magnapen Syrup

(Wockhardt UK Ltd)

1. NAME OF THE MEDICINAL PRODUCT
Magnapen Syrup or Co-fluampicil Syrup

2. QUALITATIVE AND QUANTITATIVE COMPOSITION
When reconstituted each 5ml contains 125mg ampicillin as Ampicillin Trihydrate BP with 125mg flucloxacillin as Flucloxacillin Magnesium BP (co-fluampicil 125/125).

3. PHARMACEUTICAL FORM
Bottle containing powder for the preparation of 100ml suspension.

4. CLINICAL PARTICULARS
4.1 Therapeutic indications
Co-fluampicil is indicated for the treatment of severe infections where the causative organism is unknown, and for mixed infections involving β-lactamase-producing staphylococci. Typical indications include:

In general practice: Chest infections, ENT infections, skin and soft tissue infections, and infections in patients whose underlying pathology places them at special risk.

In hospital (prior to laboratory results being available): severe respiratory tract infections, post-operative chest and wound infections, septic abortion, puerperal fever; septicaemia, prophylaxis in major surgery, infections in patients receiving immuno-suppressive therapy.

The spectrum of activity of co-fluampicil also makes it suitable for the treatment of many mixed infections, particularly those where β-lactamase-producing staphylococci are suspected or confirmed.

4.2 Posology and method of administration
Usual adult dosage (including elderly patients and children over 10 years):

Oral: 10ml syrup four times a day.

Usual children's dosage:

Oral: Under 10 years: 5ml syrup four times a day.

The above dosages for adults and children may be doubled where necessary.

Oral doses should be administered half to one hour before meals.

4.3 Contraindications
Co-fluampicil contains ampicillin and flucloxacillin which are penicillins, and should not be given to patients with a history of hypersensitivity to β-lactam antibiotics (e.g. penicillins, cephalosporins).

Co-fluampicil is contraindicated in patients with a history of flucloxacillin-associated jaundice/hepatic dysfunction.

4.4 Special warnings and special precautions for use
Before initiating therapy with co-fluampicil careful enquiries should be made concerning previous hypersensitivity reactions to β-lactam antibiotics.

Serious and occasionally fatal hypersensitivity reactions (anaphylaxis) have been reported in patients receiving β-lactam antibiotics. Although anaphylaxis is more frequent following parenteral therapy, it has occurred in patients on oral therapy. These reactions are more likely to occur in individuals with a history of hypersensitivity to β-lactam antibiotics.

Co-fluampicil contains ampicillin and should be avoided if infectious mononucleosis and/or acute or chronic leukaemia of lymphoid origin are suspected. The occurrence of a skin rash has been associated with these conditions following the administration of ampicillin.

Co-fluampicil should be used with caution in patients with evidence of hepatic dysfunction (see Section 4.8).

Special caution is essential in the newborn because of the risk of hyperbilirubinemia. Studies have shown that, at high dose following parenteral administration, flucloxacillin can displace bilirubin from plasma protein binding sites, and may therefore predispose to kernicterus in a jaundiced baby. In addition, special caution is essential in the newborn because of the potential for high serum levels of flucloxacillin due to a reduced rate of renal excretion.

During prolonged treatments (e.g osteomyelitis, endocarditis), regular monitoring of hepatic and renal functions is recommended.

Prolonged use may occasionally result in the selection of resistant strains of organisms.

Magnesium Content: Co-fluampicil Syrup contains 6.9mg magnesium per 5ml. This should be considered for patients with impaired renal function (creatinine clearance of less than 30ml/min).

4.5 Interaction with other medicinal products and other forms of Interaction
Bacteriostatic drugs may interfere with the bactericidal action of ampicillin and flucloxacillin.

In common with other oral broad-spectrum antibiotics, co-fluampicil may reduce the efficacy of oral contraceptives and patients should be warned accordingly.

Probenecid decreases the renal tubular secretion of co-fluampicil. Concurrent use with co-fluampicil may result in increased and prolonged blood levels of both ampicillin and flucloxacillin.

Concurrent administration of all allopurinol during treatment with ampicillin can increase the likelihood of allergic skin reactions.

Co-fluampicil contains ampicillin. It is recommended that when testing for the presence of glucose in urine during ampicillin treatment, enzymatic glucose oxidase methods should be used because false positive readings are common with chemical methods due to the high urinary concentrations of ampicillin.

4.6 Pregnancy and lactation
Pregnancy: Animal studies with co-fluampicil have shown no teratogenic effects. The product has been in clinical use since 1971 and the limited number of reported cases of use in human pregnancy have shown no evidence of untoward effects. The decision to administer any drug during pregnancy should be taken with the utmost care. Therefore co-fluampicil should only be used in pregnancy when the potential benefits outweigh the potential risks associated with treatment.

Lactation: Trace quantities of ampicillin and flucloxacillin can be detected in breast milk. The possibility of hypersensitivity reactions must be considered in breast-fed infants. Therefore co-fluampicil should only be administered to a breast-feeding mother when the potential benefit outweigh the potential risks associated with treatment.

4.7 Effects on ability to drive and use machines
Adverse effects on the ability to drive or operate machinery have not been observed.

4.8 Undesirable effects
Hypersensitivity reactions:

If any hypersensitivity reaction occurs, the treatment should be discontinued.

Skin rash, puritis and urticaria have been reported occasionally. The incidence of rash is higher in patients suffering from infectious mononucleosis and acute or chronic leukaemia of lymphoid origin. Purpura, fever, eosinophilia and sometimes angioneurotic oedema have also been reported. Rarely, skin reactions such as erythema multiforme, Stevens-Johnson syndrome, and toxic epidermal necrolysis have been reported. Reactions such as fever, arthralgia and myalgia can develop more than 48 hours after the start of the treatment.

Anaphylaxis (see Item 4.4 -Warnings) has been reported rarely.

Gastrointestinal reactions:

Minor gastrointestinal disturbances, including occasionally nausea, vomiting and diarrhoea may occur during treatment. Pseudomembranous colitis has been reported rarely.

Hepatic effects:

Hepatitis and cholestatic jaundice have been reported rarely. These may be delayed for up to two months after withdrawal of treatment. In some cases the course of these conditions has been protracted and lasted for several months. Very rarely deaths have been reported from hepatic effects but are mostly limited to patients with serious underlying disease.

A moderate transient increase in transaminases has been reported.

Renal effects:

Interstitial nephritis may occur but it is reversible when treatment is discontinued.

Haematological effects:

As with other β-lactam antibiotics, haematological effects including reversible leucopenia, reversible thrombocytopenia and haemolytic anaemia have been reported rarely

4.9 Overdose
Gastrointestinal effects such as nausea, vomiting and diarrhoea may be evident and should be treated symptomatically.

Co-fluampicil contains flucloxacillin. Haemodialysis does not lower the serum levels of flucloxacillin.

Co-fluampicil contains ampicillin, which may be removed from the circulation by haemodialysis.

5. PHARMACOLOGICAL PROPERTIES
5.1 Pharmacodynamic properties
Infections encountered in medical practice can involve mixed strains of bacteria and may includeβ-lactamase-producing strains. Co-fluampicil provides broad spectrum activity.

5.2 Pharmacokinetic properties

Both ampicillin and flucloxacillin have been shown to attain therapeutic serum levels following oral administration of co-fluampicil and the serum levels achieved are comparable with those which could be expected as a result of administering each antibiotic separately.

5.3 Preclinical safety data

Not relevant

6. PHARMACEUTICAL PARTICULARS

6.1 List of excipients

Disodium Edetate

Blood Orange Dry Flavour

Menthol Dry Flavour

Monoammonium Glycyrrhizinate

Sodium Benzoate (E211)

Carmellose Sodium Dried

Sodium Citrate, Anhydrous

Saccharin Sodium, Dried

Sucrose.

6.2 Incompatibilities

None known

6.3 Shelf life

Powder: Three years

Once dispensed, Co-fluampicil Syrup remains stable for 14 days.

6.4 Special precautions for storage

Co-fluampicil Syrup powder should be stored in a dry place at, or below 25°C.

Once dispensed Co-fluampicil Syrup should be stored at 2-8°C.

6.5 Nature and contents of container

Clear glass Winchester bottles fitted with 28mm Flavor-Lok caps. Original pack of 100ml with Patient Information Leaflet.

6.6 Instructions for use and handling

If dilution of the reconstituted suspension is required, Syrup BP should be used.

Administrative Data

7. MARKETING AUTHORISATION HOLDER

CP Pharmaceuticals Ltd

Ash Road North

Wrexham

LL13 9UF

United Kingdom

8. MARKETING AUTHORISATION NUMBER(S)

PL 04543/0431

9. DATE OF FIRST AUTHORISATION/RENEWAL OF THE AUTHORISATION

8th May 2000

10. DATE OF REVISION OF THE TEXT

April 2001

Legal Category

POM

Magnapen Vials for Injection

(Wockhardt UK Ltd)

1. NAME OF THE MEDICINAL PRODUCT

Magnapen Vials for Injection or Co-fluampicil Vials for Injection

2. QUALITATIVE AND QUANTITATIVE COMPOSITION

Co-fluampilcil 500mg Vials contain 250mg ampicillin as Ampicillin Sodium BP with 250mg flucloxacillin as Flucloxacillin Sodium BP (co-fluampicil 250/250).

3. PHARMACEUTICAL FORM

Vials containing powder for reconstitution for parenteral administration.

4. CLINICAL PARTICULARS

4.1 Therapeutic indications

Co-fluampicil is indicated for the treatment of severe infections where the causative organism is unknown, and for mixed infections involving β-lactamase-producing staphylococci. Typical indications include:

In general practice: Chest infections, ENT infections, skin and soft tissue infections, and infections in patients whose underlying pathology places them at special risk.

In hospital (prior to laboratory results being available): severe respiratory tract infections, post-operative chest and wound infections, septic abortion, puerperal fever; septicaemia, prophylaxis in major surgery, infections in patients receiving immuno-suppressive therapy.

The spectrum of activity of co-fluampicil also makes it suitable for the treatment of many mixed infections, particularly those where β-lactamase-producing staphylococci are suspected or confirmed.

Parenteral usage is indicated where oral dosage is inappropriate.

4.2 Posology and method of administration

Usual adult dosage (including elderly patients and children over ten years):

Intramuscular/Intravenous: 500mg four times a day.

Usual children's dosage:

Intramuscular/Intravenous: Under 2 years: quarter adult dose, four times a day.

2-10 years: half adult dose, four times a day.

The above dosages for adults and children may be doubled where necessary.

Therapy may be continued for as long as it is indicated by the nature of infection.

Administration:

Intramuscular: Add 1.5ml Water for Injections BP to vial contents.

Intravenous: Dissolve 500mg in 10ml Water for Injections BP.

Administer by slow intravenous injection.

Co-fluampicil Injection may be added to infusion fluids or injected, suitably diluted into the drip tube over a period of 3-4 minutes.

4.3 Contraindications

Co-fluampicil contains ampicillin and flucloxacillin which are penicillins, and should not be given to patients with a history of hypersensitivity to β-lactam antibiotics (e.g. penicillins, cephalosporins).

Co-fluampicil is contraindicated in patients with a history of flucloxacillin-associated jaundice/hepatic dysfunction.

Ocular administration.

4.4 Special warnings and special precautions for use

Before initiating therapy with co-fluampicil careful enquiries should be made concerning previous hypersensitivity reactions to β-lactam antibiotics.

Serious and occasionally fatal hypersensitivity reactions (anaphylaxis) have been reported in patients receiving β-lactam antibiotics. Although anaphylaxis is more frequent following parenteral therapy, it has occurred in patients on oral therapy. These reactions are more likely to occur in individuals with hypersensitivity to β-lactam antibiotics.

Co-fluampicil contains ampicillin and should be avoided if infectious mononucleosis and/or acute or chronic leukaemia of lymphoid origin are suspected. The occurrence of a skin rash has been associated with these conditions following the administration of ampicillin.

Co-fluampicil should be used with caution in patients with evidence of hepatic dysfunction (see Section 4.8).

Special caution is essential in the newborn because of the risk of hyperbilirubinemia. Studies have shown that, at high dose following parenteral administration, flucloxacillin can displace bilirubin from plasma protein binding sites, and may therefore predispose to kernicterus in a jaundiced baby. In addition, special caution is essential in the newborn because of the potential for high serum levels of flucloxacillin due to a reduced rate of renal excretion.

During prolonged treatments (e.g osteomyelitis, endocarditis), regular monitoring of hepatic and renal functions is recommended.

Prolonged use may occasionally result in the selection of resistant strains of organisms.

Sodium Content: Co-fluampicil 500mg vials contains 29.9mg sodium per vial. This should be included in the daily allowance of patients on sodium restricted diets.

4.5 Interaction with other medicinal products and other forms of Interaction

Bacteriostatic drugs may interfere with the bactericidal action of ampicillin and flucloxacillin.

In common with other oral broad-spectrum antibiotics, co-fluampicil may reduce the efficacy of oral contraceptives and patients should be warned accordingly.

Probenecid decreases the renal tubular secretion of co-fluampicil. Concurrent use with co-fluampicil may result in increased and prolonged blood levels of both ampicillin and flucloxacillin.

Concurrent administration of allopurinol during treatment with ampicillin can increase the likelihood of allergic skin reactions.

Co-fluampicil contains ampicillin. It is recommended that when testing for the presence of glucose in urine during ampicillin treatment, enzymatic glucose oxidase methods should be used, because false positive readings are common with chemical methods due to the high urinary concentrations of ampicillin.

4.6 Pregnancy and lactation

Pregnancy: Animal studies with co-fluampicil have shown no teratogenic effects. The product has been in clinical use since 1971 and the limited number of reported cases of use in human pregnancy have shown no evidence of untoward effects. The decision to administer any drug during pregnancy should be taken with the utmost care. Therefore co-fluampicil should only be used in pregnancy when the potential benefits outweigh the potential risks associated with treatment.

Lactation: Trace quantities of ampicillin and flucloxacillin can be detected in breast milk. The possibility of hypersensitivity reactions must be considered in breast-fed infants. Therefore co-fluampicil should only be administered to a breast-feeding mother when the potential benefit outweigh the potential risks associated with treatment.

4.7 Effects on ability to drive and use machines

Adverse effects on the ability to drive or operate machinery have not been observed.

4.8 Undesirable effects

Hypersensitivity reactions:

If any hypersensitivity reaction occurs, the treatment should be discontinued.

Skin rash, puritis and urticaria have been reported occasionally. The incidence of rash is higher in patients suffering from infectious mononucleosis and acute or chronic leukaemia of lymphoid origin. Purpura, fever, eosinophilia and sometimes angioneurotic oedema have also been reported. Rarely, skin reactions such as erythema multiforme, Stevens-Johnson syndrome, and toxic epidermal necrolysis have been reported. Reactions such as fever, arthralgia, and myalgia can develop more than 48 hours after the start of the treatment.

Anaphylaxis (see Item 4.4-Warnings) has been reported rarely.

Gastrointestinal reactions:

Minor gastrointestinal disturbances, including occasionally nausea, vomiting and diarrhoea may occur during treatment. Pseudomembranous colitis has been reported rarely.

Hepatic effects:

Hepatitis and cholestatic jaundice have been reported rarely. These may be delayed for up to two months after withdrawal of treatment. In some cases the course of these conditions has been protracted and lasted for several months. Very rarely deaths have been reported from hepatic effects but are mostly limited to patients with serious underlying disease.

As with most other antibiotics, a moderate transient increase in transaminases has been reported.

Renal effects:

Interstitial nephritis may occur.

Neurological effects:

Convulsions may be associated with IV administration of high doses to patients with underlying renal failure.

Haematological effects:

As with other β-lactam antibiotics haematological effects including reversible leucopenia, reversible thrombocytopenia and haemolytic anaemia have been reported rarely.

4.9 Overdose

Gastrointestinal effects such as nausea, vomiting and diarrhoea may be evident and should be treated symptomatically.

Co-fluampicil contains flucloxacillin. Haemodialysis does not lower the serum levels of flucloxacillin.

Co-fluampicil contains ampicillin, which may be removed from the circulation by haemodialysis.

5. PHARMACOLOGICAL PROPERTIES

5.1 Pharmacodynamic properties

Co-fluampicil is indicated for the treatment of severe infections where the causative organism is unknown, and for mixed infections involving β-lactamase-producing staphylococci.

5.2 Pharmacokinetic properties

Co-fluampicil is excreted via the kidneys with a plasma half life of approximately one hour.

5.3 Preclinical safety data

Not relevant

6. PHARMACEUTICAL PARTICULARS

6.1 List of excipients

None

6.2 Incompatibilities

Co-fluampicil should not be mixed with blood products or other proteinaceous fluids (e.g. protein hydrolysates) or with intravenous lipid emulsions.

If co-fluampicil is prescribed concurrently with an aminoglycoside, the antibiotics should not be mixed in the syringe, intravenous fluid container or giving set because of loss of activity of the aminoglycoside can occur under these conditions.

6.3 Shelf life

Three years.

See also Section 6.6.

6.4 Special precautions for storage

Co-fluampicil Vials for Injection should be stored in a dry place at, or below 25°C.

6.5 Nature and contents of container

5 or 10 ml glass vials fitted with butyl rubber disc and an aluminium seal. Boxes of 10 vials with instructions for use.

6.6 Instructions for use and handling

Co-fluampicil solutions for injection should be used immediately. Co-fluampicil may be added to most intravenous fluids (e.g. Water for Injections, sodium chloride 0.9%, glucose 5%, sodium chloride 0.18% with glucose 4%). In intravenous solutions containing glucose or other carbohydrates, co-fluampicil should be infused within two hours of preparation. Intravenous solutions of co-fluampicil in Water for Injections or sodium chloride 0.9% should be infused within 24 hours of preparation. Full particulars are given in the package enclosure leaflet. Preparation of co-fluampicil infusion solutions must be carried out under appropriate aseptic conditions if these extended storage periods are required.

Administrative Data

7. MARKETING AUTHORISATION HOLDER
CP Pharmaceuticals Ltd

Ash Road North

Wrexham

LL13 9UF

United Kingdom

8. MARKETING AUTHORISATION NUMBER(S)
PL 04543/0432

9. DATE OF FIRST AUTHORISATION/RENEWAL OF THE AUTHORISATION
8 May 2000

10. DATE OF REVISION OF THE TEXT
April 2001

Magnesium Sulphate Injection 50%

(UCB Pharma Limited)

1. NAME OF THE MEDICINAL PRODUCT
Magnesium Sulphate Injection 50%

2. QUALITATIVE AND QUANTITATIVE COMPOSITION
Magnesium Sulphate BP 50% w/v

3. PHARMACEUTICAL FORM
Sterile solution for parenteral use.

4. CLINICAL PARTICULARS

4.1 Therapeutic indications
Treatment of magnesium deficiency where the oral route of administration may be inappropriate, which may be due to malabsorption syndromes, chronic alcoholism, malnutrition, severe diarrhoea or patients on total parenteral nutrition.

4.2 Posology and method of administration
Magnesium sulphate injection may be administered by intramuscular or intravenous routes. For intravenous administration, a concentration of 20% or less should be used; the rate of injection not exceeding 1.5ml/minute of a 10% solution or its equivalent.

Adults

The dosage should be individualised according to patient's needs and responses.

Mild magnesium deficiency

1g intramuscularly every 6 hours for 4 doses.

Severe magnesium deficiency

Up to 250mg/kg intramuscularly given over 4 hours or 5g/litre of infusion solution intravenously over 3 hours.

Children

It is recommended that the solution be diluted to 20% w/v prior to intramuscular injection.

Elderly

No special recommendations.

4.3 Contraindications
Magnesium sulphate is contraindicated in patients with heart block, myocardial damage or impaired renal function.

4.4 Special warnings and special precautions for use
Magnesium sulphate must be used with caution in patients suspected of or known to have renal impairment.

4.5 Interaction with other medicinal products and other forms of Interaction
Administer with caution to patients receiving digitalis glycosides. Effects of neuromuscular blocking agents may be enhanced. Magnesium sulphate should not be administered concomitantly with high doses of barbiturates, opioids or hypnotics due to the risk of respiratory depression.

Concomitant use of nifedipine may very rarely lead to a calcium ion imbalance and could result in abnormal muscle function.

4.6 Pregnancy and lactation
Safety in human pregnancy and during breastfeeding has not been established, therefore, as with all drugs it is not advisable to administer magnesium sulphate during pregnancy or breastfeeding unless considered essential, and it must be administered under medical supervision.

4.7 Effects on ability to drive and use machines
None known.

4.8 Undesirable effects
Hypermagnesaemia characterised by flushing, thirst, hypotension, drowsiness, nausea, vomiting, confusion, loss of tendon reflexes due to neuromuscular blockade, muscle weakness, respiratory depression, cardiac arrhythmias, coma and cardiac arrest.

There is a risk of respiratory depression if magnesium sulphate is administered concomitantly with high doses of barbiturates, opioids or hypnotics (see 'Interactions').

4.9 Overdose
Symptoms: Hypermagnesaemia characterised by flushing, thirst, hypotension, drowsiness, nausea, vomiting, confusion, loss of tendon reflexes due to neuromuscular blockade, muscle weakness, respiratory depression, cardiac arrhythmias, coma and cardiac arrest.

Treatment: Maintain respiration with 10% calcium gluconate administered intravenously in a dose of 10-20ml. If renal function is normal adequate fluids should be given to assist removal of magnesium from the body. Dialysis may be necessary in patients with renal impairment or severe hypermagnesaemia.

5. PHARMACOLOGICAL PROPERTIES

5.1 Pharmacodynamic properties
Magnesium is the second most abundant cation in intracellular fluid and is an essential body electrolyte. Magnesium is a factor in a number of enzyme systems, and is involved in neurochemical transmission and muscular excitability.

Parenterally administered magnesium sulphate exerts a depressant effect on the central nervous system and acts peripherally to produce vasodilation.

5.2 Pharmacokinetic properties
Following intravenous administration, the onset of action is immediate and the duration approximately 30 minutes. Following intramuscular administration the onset of action occurs after approximately one hour and the duration of action is 3-4 hours.

Magnesium sulphate is excreted by the kidneys with small amounts being excreted in breast milk and saliva.

5.3 Preclinical safety data
None stated.

6. PHARMACEUTICAL PARTICULARS

6.1 List of excipients
Sodium hydroxide BP

Sulphuric acid BP

Water for injections HSE

6.2 Incompatibilities
Magnesium sulphate is incompatible with alkali hydroxides (forming insoluble magnesium hydroxide), alkali carbonates (forming insoluble magnesium carbonate) and salicylates. Streptomycin sulphate and tetramycin sulphate activity is inhibited by magnesium ions.

6.3 Shelf life
36 months.

6.4 Special precautions for storage
Store below 25°C.

6.5 Nature and contents of container
Neutral Type I glass ampoules containing 2ml, 4ml or 40ml, supplied in packs of 1, 5 or 10 units.

Not all pack sizes may be marketed.

6.6 Instructions for use and handling
None stated.

7. MARKETING AUTHORISATION HOLDER
UCB Pharma Limited

208 Bath Road

Slough

Berkshire

SL1 3 WE

UK

8. MARKETING AUTHORISATION NUMBER(S)
PL 00039/5903R

9. DATE OF FIRST AUTHORISATION/RENEWAL OF THE AUTHORISATION
2 June 1987 / 3 September 1997

10. DATE OF REVISION OF THE TEXT
June 2005

POM

Malarone

(GlaxoSmithKline UK)

1. NAME OF THE MEDICINAL PRODUCT
Malarone ® Tablets.

2. QUALITATIVE AND QUANTITATIVE COMPOSITION
Each Malarone tablet contains:

Atovaquone 250mg

Proguanil hydrochloride 100mg

For excipients, see Section 6.1

3. PHARMACEUTICAL FORM
Film coated tablets.

Round, biconvex, pink tablets.

4. CLINICAL PARTICULARS

4.1 Therapeutic indications
Malarone is a fixed dose combination of atovaquone and proguanil hydrochloride which acts as a blood schizonticide and also has activity against hepatic schizonts of Plasmodium falciparum. It is indicated for:

Prophylaxis of *Plasmodium falciparum* malaria.

Treatment of acute, uncomplicated *Plasmodium falciparum* malaria.

Because Malarone is effective against drug sensitive and drug resistant *P. falciparum* it is especially recommended for prophylaxis and treatment of *P. falciparum* malaria where the pathogen may be resistant to other antimalarials.

Official guidelines and local information on the prevalence of resistance to antimalarial drugs should be taken into consideration. Official guidelines will normally include WHO and public health authorities guidelines.

4.2 Posology and method of administration
The daily dose should be taken with food or a milky drink (to ensure maximum absorption) at the same time each day.

If patients are unable to tolerate food, Malarone should be administered, but systemic exposure of atovaquone will be reduced. In the event of vomiting within 1 hour of dosing a repeat dose should be taken.

PROPHYLAXIS:

Prophylaxis should

- commence 24 or 48 hours prior to entering a malaria-endemic area,
- continue during the period of the stay, **which should not exceed 28 days,**
- continue for 7 days after leaving the area.

In residents (semi-immune subjects) of endemic areas, the safety and effectiveness of Malarone has been established in studies of up to 12 weeks.

Dosage in Adults

One Malarone tablet daily.

Malarone tablets are not recommended for malaria prophylaxis in persons under 40kg bodyweight.

TREATMENT

Dosage in Adults

Four Malarone tablets as a single dose for three consecutive days.

Dosage in Children

11-20kg bodyweight. One tablet daily for three consecutive days.

21-30kg bodyweight. Two tablets as a single dose for three consecutive days.

31-40kg bodyweight. Three tablets as a single dose for three consecutive days.

> 40kg bodyweight. Dose as for adults.

Dosage in the Elderly

A pharmacokinetic study indicates that no dosage adjustments are needed in the elderly (See Section 5.2).

Dosage in Hepatic Impairment

A pharmacokinetic study indicates that no dosage adjustments are needed in patients with mild to moderate hepatic impairment. Although no studies have been conducted in patients with severe hepatic impairment, no special precautions or dosage adjustment are anticipated (See Section 5.2).

Dosage in Renal Impairment

Pharmacokinetic studies indicate that no dosage adjustments are needed in patients with mild to moderate renal impairment. In patients with severe renal impairment (creatinine clearance < 30mL/min) alternatives to Malarone for treatment of acute *P. falciparum* malaria should be recommended whenever possible (See Sections 4.4 and 5.2). For prophylaxis of *P. falciparum* malaria in patients with severe renal impairment see Section 4.3.

4.3 Contraindications
Malarone is contra-indicated in individuals with known hypersensitivity to atovaquone or proguanil hydrochloride or any component of the formulation.

Malarone is contra-indicated for prophylaxis of *P. falciparum* malaria in patients with severe renal impairment (creatinine clearance < 30mL/min).

4.4 Special warnings and special precautions for use
Safety and effectiveness of Malarone for prophylaxis of malaria in patients who weigh less than 40kg has not been established.

Persons taking Malarone for prophylaxis or treatment of malaria should take a repeat dose if they vomit within 1 hour of dosing. In the event of diarrhoea, normal dosing should be continued. Absorption of atovaquone may be reduced in patients with diarrhoea or vomiting, but diarrhoea or vomiting was not associated with reduced efficacy in clinical trials of Malarone for malaria prophylaxis. However, as with other antimalarial agents, subjects with diarrhoea or vomiting should be advised to continue to comply with personal protection measures (repellants, bednets).

In patients with acute malaria who present with diarrhoea or vomiting, alternative therapy should be considered. If Malarone is used to treat malaria in these patients, parasitaemia should be closely monitored.

Safety and effectiveness of Malarone for treatment of malaria in paediatric patients who weigh less than 11kg has not been established.

Malarone has not been evaluated for the treatment of cerebral malaria or other severe manifestations of complicated malaria including hyperparasitaemia, pulmonary oedema or renal failure.

Parasite relapse occurred commonly when *P. vivax* malaria was treated with Malarone alone. Travellers with intense exposure to *P. vivax* or *P. ovale*, and those who develop malaria caused by either of these parasites, will require additional treatment with a drug that is active against hypnozoites.

In the event of recrudescent infections due to *P. falciparum* after treatment with Malarone, or failure of chemoprophylaxis, patients should be treated with a different blood schizonticide.

Parasitaemia should be closely monitored in patients receiving concurrent metoclopramide or tetracycline (See Section 4.5).

The concomitant administration of Malarone and rifampicin or rifabutin is not recommended (See Section 4.5).

In patients with severe renal impairment (creatinine clearance < 30mL/min) alternatives to Malarone for treatment of acute *P. falciparum* malaria should be recommended whenever possible (See Sections 4.2, 4.3 and 5.2).

4.5 Interaction with other medicinal products and other forms of Interaction

Concomitant treatment with metoclopramide and tetracycline have been associated with significant decreases in plasma concentrations of atovaquone (See Section 4.4).

Concomitant administration of atovaquone and indinavir results in a decrease in the C_{min} of indinavir (23% decrease; 90% CI 8-35%). Caution should be exercised when prescribing atovaquone with indinavir due to the decrease in the trough levels of indinavir.

Concomitant administration of rifampicin or rifabutin is known to reduce atovaquone levels by approximately 50% and 34%, respectively.

(See Section 4.4).

Atovaquone is highly protein bound (> 99%) but does not displace other highly protein bound drugs *in vitro*, indicating significant drug interactions arising from displacement are unlikely.

4.6 Pregnancy and lactation

The safety of atovaquone and proguanil hydrochloride when administered concurrently for use in human pregnancy has not been established and the potential risk is unknown.

Animal studies showed no evidence for teratogenicity of the combination. The individual components have shown no effects on parturition or pre- and post-natal development. Maternal toxicity was seen in pregnant rabbits during a teratogenicity study (See Section 5.3). The use of Malarone in pregnancy should only be considered if the expected benefit to the mother outweighs any potential risk to the foetus.

The proguanil component of Malarone acts by inhibiting parasitic dihydrofolate reductase. There are no clinical data indicating that folate supplementation diminishes drug efficacy. For women of childbearing age receiving folate supplements to prevent neural tube birth defects, such supplements should be continued while taking Malarone.

Lactation

The atovaquone concentrations in milk, in a rat study, were 30% of the concurrent atovaquone concentrations in maternal plasma. It is not known whether atovaquone is excreted in human milk.

Proguanil is excreted in human milk in small quantities.

Malarone should not be taken by breast-feeding women.

4.7 Effects on ability to drive and use machines

Dizziness has been reported. Patients should be warned that if affected they should not drive, operate machinery or take part in activities where this may put themselves or others at risk.

4.8 Undesirable effects

As Malarone contains atovaquone and proguanil hydrochloride adverse events associated with each of these compounds may be expected with Malarone. At the doses employed for both treatment and prophylaxis of malaria, adverse events are generally mild and of limited duration. There is no evidence of added toxicity following concurrent administration of atovaquone and proguanil.

A summary of adverse events associated with the use of Malarone, atovaquone or proguanil hydrochloride is provided below:

Blood & Lymphatic: Anaemia, neutropenia, Pancytopenia in patients with severe renal impairment

Endocrine & Metabolic: Anorexia, hyponatraemia

Gastrointestinal: Abdominal pain, nausea, vomiting, diarrhoea, gastric intolerance, oral ulceration, stomatitis

Hepatobiliary Tract & Pancreas: Elevated liver enzyme levels, elevated amylase levels. Clinical trial data for Malarone indicated that abnormalities in liver function tests were reversible and not associated with untoward clinical events

Lower Respiratory: Cough

Neurology: Headache, insomnia, dizziness

Non-Site Specific: Fever

Skin/hypersensitivity: Allergic reactions: including rash, urticaria, angioedema and isolated reports of anaphylaxis. Hair loss.

In clinical trials for prophylaxis of malaria, the most commonly reported adverse events, independent of attributability, were headache, abdominal pain and diarrhoea, and were reported in a similar proportion of subjects receiving Malarone or placebo.

In clinical trials for treatment of malaria, the most commonly reported adverse events, independent of attributability, were abdominal pain, headache, anorexia, nausea, vomiting, diarrhoea and coughing, and were generally reported in a similar proportion of patients receiving Malarone or a comparator antimalarial drug.

4.9 Overdose

There have been no reports of overdosage with Malarone. In cases of suspected overdosage symptomatic and supportive therapy should be given as appropriate.

5. PHARMACOLOGICAL PROPERTIES

5.1 Pharmacodynamic properties

Pharmacotherapeutic Group: Antimalarials

ATC Code: P01B B51

Mode of Action

The constituents of Malarone, atovaquone and proguanil hydrochloride, interfere with two different pathways involved in the biosynthesis of pyrimidines required for nucleic acid replication. The mechanism of action of atovaquone against *P. falciparum* is via inhibition of mitochondrial electron transport, at the level of the cytochrome bc_1 complex, and collapse of mitochondrial membrane potential. One mechanism of action of proguanil, via its metabolite cycloguanil, is inhibition of dihydrofolate reductase, which disrupts deoxythymidylate synthesis. Proguanil also has antimalarial activity independent of its metabolism to cycloguanil, and proguanil, but not cycloguanil, is able to potentiate the ability of atovaquone to collapse mitochondrial membrane potential in malaria parasites. This latter mechanism may explain the synergy seen when atovaquone and proguanil are used in combination.

Microbiology

Atovaquone has potent activity against *Plasmodium spp* (*in vitro* IC_{50} against *P. falciparum* 0.23-1.43ng/mL).

Atovaquone is not cross-resistant with any other antimalarial drugs in current use. Among more than 30 *P. falciparum* isolates, *in vitro* resistance was detected against chloroquine (41% of isolates), quinine (32% of isolates), mefloquine (29% of isolates), and halofantrine (48% of isolates) but not atovaquone (0% of isolates).

The antimalarial activity of proguanil is exerted via the primary metabolite cycloguanil (*in vitro* IC_{50} against various *P. falciparum* strains of 4-20ng/mL; some activity of proguanil and another metabolite, 4-chlorophenylbiguanide, is seen *in vitro* at 600-3000ng/mL).

In *in vitro* studies of *P. falciparum* the combination of atovaquone and proguanil was shown to be synergistic. This enhanced efficacy was also demonstrated in clinical studies in both immune and non-immune patients.

5.2 Pharmacokinetic properties

There are no pharmacokinetic interactions between atovaquone and proguanil at the recommended dose. In clinical trials, where children have received Malarone dosed by body weight, trough levels of atovaquone, proguanil and cycloguanil in children are generally within the range observed in adults.

Absorption

Atovaquone is a highly lipophilic compound with low aqueous solubility. In HIV-infected patients, the absolute bioavailability of a 750 mg single dose of atovaquone tablets taken with food is 23% with an inter-subject variability of about 45%.

Dietary fat taken with atovaquone increases the rate and extent of absorption, increasing AUC 2-3 times and C_{max} 5 times over fasting. Patients are recommended to take Malarone tablets with food or a milky drink (See Section 4.2).

Proguanil hydrochloride is rapidly and extensively absorbed regardless of food intake.

Distribution

Apparent volume of distribution of atovaquone and proguanil is a function of bodyweight.

Atovaquone is highly protein bound (> 99%) but does not displace other highly protein bound drugs *in vitro*, indicating significant drug interactions arising from displacement are unlikely.

Following oral administration, the volume of distribution of atovaquone in adults and children is approximately 8.8 L/Kg.

Proguanil is 75% protein bound. Following oral administration, the volume of distribution of proguanil in adults and children ranged from 20 to 42 L/kg.

In human plasma the binding of atovaquone and proguanil were unaffected by the presence of the other.

Metabolism

There is no evidence that atovaquone is metabolised and there is negligible excretion of atovaquone in urine with the parent drug being predominantly (> 90%) eliminated unchanged in faeces.

Proguanil hydrochloride is partially metabolised, primarily by the polymorphic cytochrome P450 isoenzyme 2C19, with less than 40% being excreted unchanged in the urine. Its metabolites cycloguanil and 4-chlorophenylbiguanide are also excreted in the urine.

During administration of Malarone at recommended doses proguanil metabolism status appears to have no implications for treatment or prophylaxis of malaria.

Elimination

The elimination half life of atovaquone is about 2-3 days in adults and 1-2 days in children.

The elimination half lives of proguanil and cycloguanil are about 12-15 hours in both adults and children.

Oral clearance for atovaquone and proguanil increases with increased body weight and is about 70% higher in an 80 kg subject relative to a 40 kg subject. The mean oral clearance in paediatric and adult patients weighing 10 to 80 kg ranged from 0.8 to 10.8 L/h for atovaquone and from 15 to 106 L/h for proguanil.

Pharmacokinetics in the elderly

There is no clinically significant change in the average rate or extent of absorption of atovaquone or proguanil between elderly and young patients. Systemic availability of cycloguanil is higher in the elderly compared to the young patients (AUC is increased by 140% and Cmax is increased by 80%), but there is no clinically significant change in its elimination half-life (see Section 4.2).

Pharmacokinetics in renal impairment

In patients with mild to moderate renal impairment, oral clearance and/or AUC data for atovaquone, proguanil and cycloguanil are within the range of values observed in patients with normal renal function.

Atovaquone Cmax and AUC are reduced by 64% and 54%, respectively, in patients with severe renal impairment.

In patients with severe renal impairment, the elimination half lives for proguanil ($t_{1/2}$ 39h) and cycloguanil ($t_{1/2}$ 37h) are prolonged, resulting in the potential for drug accumulation with repeated dosing (see Section 4.2 and 4.4).

Pharmacokinetics in hepatic impairment

In patients with mild to moderate hepatic impairment there is no clinically significant change in exposure to atovaquone when compared to healthy patients.

In patients with mild to moderate hepatic impairment there is an 85% increase in proguanil AUC with no change in elimination half life and there is a 65-68% decrease in Cmax and AUC for cycloguanil.

No data are available in patients with severe hepatic impairment (see Section 4.2).

5.3 Preclinical safety data

Repeat dose toxicity:

Findings in repeat dose toxicity studies with atovaquone:-proguanil hydrochloride combination were entirely proguanil related and were observed at doses providing no significant margin of exposure in comparison with the expected clinical exposure. As proguanil has been used extensively and safely in the treatment and prophylaxis of malaria at doses similar to those used in the combination, these findings are considered of little relevance to the clinical situation.

Reproductive toxicity studies:

In rats and rabbits there was no evidence of teratogenicity for the combination. No data are available regarding the effects of the combination on fertility or pre- and post-natal development, but studies on the individual components of Malarone have shown no effects on these parameters. In a rabbit teratogenicity study using the combination, unexplained maternal toxicity was found at a systemic exposure similar to that observed in humans following clinical use.

Mutagenicity:

A wide range of mutagenicity tests have shown no evidence that atovaquone or proguanil have mutagenic activity as single agents.

Mutagenicity studies have not been performed with atovaquone in combination with proguanil.

Cycloguanil, the active metabolite of proguanil, was also negative in the Ames test, but was positive in the Mouse Lymphoma assay and the Mouse Micronucleus assay. These positive effects with cycloguanil (a dihydrofolate antagonist) were significantly reduced or abolished with folinic acid supplementation.

Carcinogenicity:

Oncogenicity studies of atovaquone alone in mice showed an increased incidence of hepatocellular adenomas and carcinomas. No such findings were observed in rats and mutagenicity tests were negative. These findings appear to be due to the inherent susceptibility of mice to atovaquone and are considered of no relevance in the clinical situation.

Oncogenicity studies on proguanil alone showed no evidence of carcinogenicity in rats and mice.

Oncogenicity studies on proguanil in combination with atovaquone have not been performed.

6. PHARMACEUTICAL PARTICULARS

6.1 List of excipients

Core

Poloxamer 188 BP

Microcrystalline Cellulose Ph.Eur

Low-substituted Hydroxypropyl Cellulose USNF

Povidone K30 Ph.Eur

Sodium Starch Glycollate Ph.Eur

Magnesium Stearate Ph.Eur

Coating

Methylhydroxypropyl cellulose Ph.Eur

Titanium Dioxide Ph.Eur

Iron Oxide Red E172

Macrogol 400 Ph.Eur

Polyethylene Glycol 8000 USNF

6.2 Incompatibilities

Not applicable.

6.3 Shelf life

5 years.

6.4 Special precautions for storage

No special precautions for storage.

6.5 Nature and contents of container

PVC aluminium foil blister pack/s containing 12 tablets.

6.6 Instructions for use and handling

No special requirements.

Administrative Data

7. MARKETING AUTHORISATION HOLDER

Glaxo Wellcome UK Ltd, trading as GlaxoSmithKline UK.

Stockley Park West

Uxbridge

Middlesex

UB11 1BT

8. MARKETING AUTHORISATION NUMBER(S)

PL 10949/0258

9. DATE OF FIRST AUTHORISATION/RENEWAL OF THE AUTHORISATION

21 October 1996

10. DATE OF REVISION OF THE TEXT

21 March 2005

11. Legal Status

POM

Malarone Paediatric Tablets

(GlaxoSmithKline UK)

1. NAME OF THE MEDICINAL PRODUCT

MALARONE ▼Paediatric Tablets.

2. QUALITATIVE AND QUANTITATIVE COMPOSITION

Each Tablet contains:

Atovaquone 62.5mg

Proguanil hydrochloride 25mg

For excipients, see 6.1

3. PHARMACEUTICAL FORM

Film coated tablets.

Round, biconvex, pink tablets engraved 'GX CG7' on one side.

4. CLINICAL PARTICULARS

4.1 Therapeutic indications

MALARONE Paediatric Tablets contain a fixed dose combination of atovaquone and proguanil hydrochloride, which acts as a blood schizontocide and also has activity against hepatic schizonts of *Plasmodium falciparum*. They are indicated for:

Prophylaxis of *P. falciparum* malaria in individuals weighing 11-40kg.

(For treatment of acute, uncomplicated *P. falciparum* malaria in individuals weighing 11-40kg please refer to the Summary of Product Characteristics for MALARONE tablets).

MALARONE may be active against *P. falciparum* that are resistant to one or more other antimalarial agents. Therefore, MALARONE may be particularly suitable for prophylaxis against *P. falciparum* infections in areas where this species is known to be commonly resistant to one or more other antimalarial agents

Official guidelines and local information on the prevalence of resistance to antimalarial drugs should be taken into consideration. Official guidelines will normally include WHO and public health authorities' guidelines.

4.2 Posology and method of administration

Posology

Dosage in individuals weighing 11-40kg (see Table 1 below)

The safety and effectiveness of MALARONE Paediatric Tablets for prophylaxis of malaria in children who weigh less than 11 kg has not been established.

Prophylaxis should

- commence 24 or 48 hours prior to entering a malaria-endemic area,
- continue during the period of the stay, which should not exceed 28 days,
- continue for 7 days after leaving the area.

The safety and effectiveness of MALARONE Paediatric Tablets have been established in studies of up to 12 weeks in residents (semi-immune) of endemic areas. (see section 5.1 Pharmacodynamic Properties)

Dosage in Hepatic Impairment

There are no studies in children with hepatic impairment. However, a pharmacokinetic study in adults indicates that no dosage adjustments are needed in patients with mild to moderate hepatic impairment. Although no studies have been conducted in patients with severe hepatic impairment, no special precautions or dosage adjustment are anticipated (See Section 5.2 Pharmacokinetics).

Dosage in Renal Impairment

There are no studies in children with renal impairment. However, pharmacokinetic studies in adults indicate that no dosage adjustments are needed in those with mild to moderate renal impairment. Due to the lack of information regarding appropriate dosing, MALARONE is contraindicated for the prophylaxis of malaria in adults and children with severe renal impairment (creatinine clearance < 30mL/min; see Section 4.3 Contra-indications and Section 5.2 Pharmacokinetics).

Method of Administration

The daily dose should be taken once daily with food or a milky drink (to ensure maximum absorption) at the same time each day.

If patients are unable to tolerate food, MALARONE Paediatric Tablets should be administered, but systemic exposure of atovaquone will be reduced. In the event of vomiting within 1 hour of dosing a repeat dose should be taken.

MALARONE Paediatric Tablets should preferably be swallowed whole. If difficulties are encountered when dosing young children, the tablets may be crushed and administered with food.

4.3 Contraindications

Hypersensitivity to atovaquone or proguanil hydrochloride or any of the excipients.

MALARONE Paediatric Tablets are contra-indicated for prophylaxis of *P. falciparum* malaria in patients with severe renal impairment (creatinine clearance < 30mL/min).

4.4 Special warnings and special precautions for use

Individuals taking MALARONE Paediatric Tablets for prophylaxis of malaria should take a repeat dose if they vomit within 1 hour of dosing. In the event of diarrhoea, normal dosing should be continued. Absorption of atovaquone may be reduced in individuals with diarrhoea or vomiting, but diarrhoea or vomiting was not associated with reduced efficacy in clinical trials of MALARONE for malaria prophylaxis in adults. However, as with other antimalarial agents, individuals with diarrhoea or vomiting should be advised to continue to comply with personal protection measures (repellants, bednets).

Safety and effectiveness of MALARONE Paediatric Tablets for prophylaxis of malaria in children who weigh less than 11kg has not been established.

MALARONE Paediatric Tablets are not suitable for the treatment of acute uncomplicated *P. falciparum* malaria in individuals weighing 11-40 kg. MALARONE Tablets (250/100mg) should be used in these individuals

Parasite relapse occurred commonly when *P. vivax* malaria was treated with MALARONE alone. Travellers with intense exposure to *P. vivax* or *P. ovale*, and those who develop malaria caused by either of these parasites, will require additional treatment with a drug that is active against hypnozoites.

In the event of failure of chemoprophylaxis with MALARONE Paediatric Tablets, individuals should be treated with a different blood schizonticide.

4.5 Interaction with other medicinal products and other forms of Interaction

Metoclopramide and tetracycline have been associated with significant decreases in plasma concentrations of atovaquone when administered concomitantly. Although some children have received concomitant MALARONE and metoclopramide in clinical trials without any evidence of decreased protection against malaria, the possibility of a clinically significant drug interaction cannot be ruled out.

Concomitant administration of atovaquone and indinavir results in a decrease in the C_{min} of indinavir (23% decrease; 90% CI 8-35%). Caution should be exercised when prescribing atovaquone with indinavir due to the decrease in the trough levels of indinavir.

Concomitant administration of MALARONE with rifampicin or rifabutin should be avoided due to the reduction in plasma levels of atovaquone by approximately 50% and 34%, respectively.

Atovaquone is highly protein bound > 99%) but does not displace other highly protein bound drugs *in vitro*, indicating significant drug interactions arising from displacement are unlikely.

4.6 Pregnancy and lactation

The safety of atovaquone and proguanil hydrochloride when administered concurrently for use in human pregnancy has not been established and the potential risk is unknown.

Animal studies showed no evidence for teratogenicity of the combination. The individual components have shown no effects on parturition or pre- and post-natal development. Maternal toxicity was seen in pregnant rabbits during a teratogenicity study (See Section 5.3 Preclinical Safety Data). The use of MALARONE Paediatric Tablets in pregnancy should only be considered if the expected benefit to the mother outweighs any potential risk to the foetus.

Proguanil acts by inhibiting parasitic dihydrofolate reductase. There are no clinical data indicating that folate supplementation diminishes drug efficacy. For women of childbearing age receiving folate supplements to prevent neural tube birth defects, such supplements should be continued while taking MALARONE Paediatric Tablets.

Lactation

The atovaquone concentrations in milk, in a rat study, were 30% of the concurrent atovaquone concentrations in maternal plasma. It is not known whether atovaquone is excreted in human milk.

Proguanil is excreted in human milk in small quantities.

MALARONE Paediatric Tablets should not be taken by breast-feeding women.

4.7 Effects on ability to drive and use machines

There have been no studies to investigate the effect of MALARONE Paediatric Tablets on driving performance or the ability to operate machinery but a detrimental effect on such activities is not predicted from the pharmacology of the component drugs.

4.8 Undesirable effects

In clinical trials of MALARONE Paediatric Tablets for prophylaxis of malaria, 357 children or adolescents ⩽ 40 kg body weight received MALARONE Paediatric Tablets. Most of these were residents of endemic areas and took MALARONE Paediatric tablets for about 12 weeks. The rest were travelling to endemic areas, and most took MALARONE Paediatric Tablets for 2-4 weeks.

In clinical trials, commonly reported (greater than 1/100) adverse events included abdominal pain, diarrhoea, fever, nausea, vomiting and headache. However, in placebo controlled trials all these events occurred at similar rates in the MALARONE and placebo groups.

A summary of other adverse events associated with the use of MALARONE or MALARONE Paediatric Tablets, atovaquone or proguanil hydrochloride is provided below:

Non-Site Specific: Fever

Blood & Lymphatic: Anaemia, neutropenia,

Pancytopenia in patients with severe renal impairment

Table 1 Dosage in individuals weighing 11-40kg

Body Weight Range (kg)	Dosage/day Atovaquone (mg)	Proguanil (mg)	No of Tablets
11-20	62.5	25	One MALARONE Paediatric Tablet
21-30	125	50	Two MALARONE Paediatric Tablets
31-40	187.5	75	Three MALARONE Paediatric Tablet
>40	250	100	Subjects of > 40 kg should receive ONE MALARONE 250/100mg Tablet daily

Endocrine & Metabolic: Anorexia, hyponatraemia

Gastrointestinal: Abdominal pain, nausea, vomiting, diarrhoea, gastric intolerance, oral ulceration, stomatitis

Hepatobiliary Tract

& Pancreas: Elevated liver enzyme levels, elevated amylase levels.

Clinical trial data for MALARONE Tablets indicated that abnormalities in liver function tests were reversible and not associated with untoward clinical events

Lower Respiratory: Cough

Neurology: Headache, insomnia, dizziness

Skin/hypersensitivity: Allergic reactions: including rash, urticaria, pruritus, angioedema and isolated reports of anaphylaxis, Hair loss.

4.9 Overdose

There have been no reports of overdosage with MALARONE or MALARONE Paediatric Tablets. In cases of suspected overdosage, symptomatic and supportive therapy should be given as appropriate.

5. PHARMACOLOGICAL PROPERTIES

5.1 Pharmacodynamic properties

Pharmacotherapeutic Group: Antimalarials

ATC Code: P01B B51

Mode of Action

The constituents of MALARONE Paediatric Tablets, atovaquone and proguanil hydrochloride, interfere with two different pathways involved in the biosynthesis of pyrimidines required for nucleic acid replication. The mechanism of action of atovaquone against *P. falciparum* is via inhibition of mitochondrial electron transport, at the level of the cytochrome bc_1 complex, and collapse of mitochondrial membrane potential. One mechanism of action of proguanil, via its metabolite cycloguanil, is inhibition of dihydrofolate reductase, which disrupts deoxythymidylate synthesis. Proguanil also has antimalarial activity independent of its metabolism to cycloguanil. Proguanil, but not cycloguanil, is able to potentiate the ability of atovaquone to collapse mitochondrial membrane potential in malaria parasites. This latter mechanism may contribute to the antimalarial synergy seen when atovaquone and proguanil are used in combination.

Microbiology

Atovaquone has activity against *Plasmodium spp* (*in vitro* IC_{50} against *P. falciparum* 0.23-1.43ng/mL).

Cross-resistance between atovaquone and antimalarial agents of other drug classes was not detected among more than 30 *P. falciparum* isolates that demonstrated resistance *in vitro* to one or more of chloroquine (41% of isolates), quinine (32% of isolates), mefloquine (29% of isolates), and halofantrine (48% of isolates).

The IC_{50} of the primarily metabolite of proguanil-cycloguanil - against various *P. falciparum* strains was 4-20ng/mL; some activity of proguanil and another metabolite, 4-chlorophenylbiguanide, is seen *in vitro* at 600-3000ng/mL).

The combination of atovaquone and proguanil was shown to be synergistic against *P. falciparum in vitro.* The combination was more effective than either drug alone in clinical studies of the treatment of malaria in both immune and non-immune patients.

The efficacy in non-immune paediatric travellers has not been directly established, but may be assumed through extrapolation by the results on safety and efficacy in studies of up to 12 weeks in paediatric residents (semi-immune) of endemic areas, and from results of safety and efficacy in both semi immune and non immune adults.

Data in the paediatric population are available from two trials that primarily evaluated the safety of Malarone Paediatric tablets in (non-immune) travellers to endemic areas. In these trials, a total of 93 travellers weighing < 40 kg were given Malarone and 93 received another prophylactic antimalarial regimen (81 chloroquine/proguanil and 12 mefloquine). The majority of travellers went to Africa and the mean duration of stay was between 2-3 weeks. There were no cases of malaria recorded in any subjects who took part in these studies.

5.2 Pharmacokinetic properties

There are no pharmacokinetic interactions between atovaquone and proguanil at the recommended doses.

In clinical trialswhere children have received Malarone dosed by body weight, trough levels of atovaquone, proguanil and cycloguanil in children are generally within the range observed in adults (see following table).

Trough Plasma Concentrations [Mean ± SD, (range)] of Atovaquone, Proguanil and Cycloguanil during Prophylaxis with MALARONE in Children* and Adults

(see Table 2 below)

• Pooled data from two studies

Absorption

Atovaquone is a highly lipophilic compound with low aqueous solubility. Although there are no atovaquone bioavailability data in healthy subjects, in HIV-infected patients the absolute bioavailability of a 750 mg single dose of atovaquone tablets taken with food is 21% (90% CI: 17% - 27%).

Dietary fat taken with atovaquone increases the rate and extent of absorption, increasing AUC 2-3 times and C_{max} 5 times over fasting. Patients are recommended to take MALARONE tablets with food or a milky drink (See Section 4.2 Posology and Method of Administration).

Proguanil hydrochloride is rapidly and extensively absorbed regardless of food intake.

Distribution

Apparent volume of distribution of atovaquone and proguanil is a function of body weight.

Atovaquone is highly protein bound > 99%) but does not displace other highly protein bound drugs *in vitro*, indicating significant drug interactions arising from displacement are unlikely.

Following oral administration, the volume of distribution of atovaquone in adults and children is approximately 8.8 L/kg.

Proguanil is 75% protein bound. Following oral administration, the volume of distribution of proguanil in adults and children ranged from 20 to 42 L/kg.

In human plasma the binding of atovaquone and proguanil were unaffected by the presence of the other.

Metabolism

There is no evidence that atovaquone is metabolised, and there is negligible excretion of atovaquone in urine with the parent drug being predominantly > 90%) eliminated unchanged in faeces.

Proguanil hydrochloride is partially metabolised, primarily by the polymorphic cytochrome P450 isoenzyme 2C19, with less than 40% being excreted unchanged in the urine. Its metabolites, cycloguanil and 4-chlorophenylbiguanide, are also excreted in the urine.

During administration of MALARONE at recommended doses proguanil metabolism status appears to have no implications for treatment or prophylaxis of malaria.

Elimination

The elimination half life of atovaquone is 1-2 days in children.

The elimination half lives of proguanil and cycloguanil are each about 12-15 hours in children.

Oral clearance for atovaquone and proguanil increases with increased body weight and is about 70% higher in a 40 kg subject relative to a 20 kg subject. The mean oral clearance in paediatric and adult patients weighing 10 to 40 kg ranged from 0.8 to 6.3.8 L/h for atovaquone and from 15 to 64 L/h for proguanil.

Pharmacokinetics in renal impairment

There are no studies in children with renal impairment.

In adult patients with mild to moderate renal impairment, oral clearance and/or AUC data for atovaquone, proguanil and cycloguanil are within the range of values observed in patients with normal renal function.

Atovaquone Cmax and AUC are reduced by 64% and 54%, respectively, in adult patients with severe renal impairment (< 30 mL/min/1.73 m^2).

Table 2 Trough Plasma Concentrations [Mean ± SD, (range)] of Atovaquone, Proguanil and Cycloguanil during Prophylaxis with MALARONE in Children* and Adults

Atovaquone:Proguanil HCl Daily Dose	62.5 mg:25 mg	125 mg:50 mg	187.5 mg:75 mg	250mg:100 mg
[Weight Category]	[11-20 kg]	[21-30 kg]	[31-40 kg]	Adult >40 kg)
Atovaquone (μ g/mL)	2.2 ± 1.1 (0.2-5.8)	3.2 ± 1.8 (0.2-10.9)	4.1 ± 1.8 (0.7-8.8)	2.1 + 1.2 (0.1-5.7)
No. Subjects	*n=87*	*n=88*	*n=76*	*n=100*
Proguanil (ng/mL)	12.3 ± 14.4 (<5.0-14.3)	18.8 ± 11.2 (<5.0-87.0)	26.8 ± 17.1 (5.1-55.9)	26.8 + 14.0 (5.2-73.2)
No. Subjects	*n=72*	*n=83*	*n=75*	*n=95*
Cycloguanil (ng/mL)	7.7 ± 7.2 (<5.0-43.5)	8.1 ± 6.3 (<5.0-44.1)	8.7 ± 7.3 (6.4-17.0)	10.9 + 5.6 (5.0-37.8)
No. Subjects	*n=58*	*n=69*	*n=66*	*n=95*

In adult patients with severe renal impairment, the elimination half lives for proguanil ($t_{½}$ 39h) and cycloguanil ($t_{½}$ 37h) are prolonged, resulting in the potential for drug accumulation with repeated dosing (see Section 4.2 Posology and Method of Administration and 4.4 Special Warnings and Special Precautions for Use).

Pharmacokinetics in hepatic impairment

There are no studies in children with hepatic impairment.

In adult patients with mild to moderate hepatic impairment, there is no clinically significant change in exposure to atovaquone when compared to healthy patients.

In adult patients with mild to moderate hepatic impairment there is an 85% increase in proguanil AUC, with no change in elimination half life, and there is a 65-68% decrease in Cmax and AUC for cycloguanil.

No data are available in adult patients with severe hepatic impairment (see Section 4.2 Posology and Method of Administration).

5.3 Preclinical safety data

Repeat dose toxicity:

Findings in repeat dose toxicity studies with atovaquone/proguanil hydrochloride combination were entirely proguanil-related and were observed at doses providing no significant margin of exposure in comparison with the expected clinical exposure. However, as proguanil has been used extensively and safely in the treatment and prophylaxis of malaria at doses similar to those used in the combination, these findings are considered of little relevance to the clinical situation.

Reproductive toxicity studies:

In rats and rabbits there was no evidence of teratogenicity for the combination. No data are available regarding the effects of the combination on fertility or pre- and post-natal development, but studies on the individual components of MALARONE Paediatric Tablets have shown no effects on these parameters. In a rabbit teratogenicity study using the combination, unexplained maternal toxicity was found at a systemic exposure similar to that observed in humans following clinical use.

Mutagenicity:

A wide range of mutagenicity tests have shown no evidence that atovaquone or proguanil have mutagenic activity as single agents.

Mutagenicity studies have not been performed with atovaquone in combination with proguanil.

Cycloguanil, the active metabolite of proguanil, was also negative in the Ames test, but was positive in the Mouse Lymphoma assay and the Mouse Micronucleus assay. These positive effects with cycloguanil (a dihydrofolate antagonist) were significantly reduced or abolished with folinic acid supplementation.

Carcinogenicity:

Oncogenicity studies of atovaquone alone in mice showed an increased incidence of hepatocellular adenomas and carcinomas. No such findings were observed in rats and mutagenicity tests were negative. These findings appear to be due to the inherent susceptibility of mice to atovaquone and are considered of no relevance in the clinical situation.

Oncogenicity studies on proguanil alone showed no evidence of carcinogenicity in rats and mice.

Oncogenicity studies on proguanil in combination with atovaquone have not been performed.

6. PHARMACEUTICAL PARTICULARS

6.1 List of excipients

Core

Poloxamer 188

Microcrystalline Cellulose

Low-substituted Hydroxypropyl Cellulose

Povidone K30

Sodium Starch Glycollate (Type A)

Magnesium Stearate

Coating

Hypromellose

Titanium Dioxide E171

Iron Oxide Red E172

Macrogol 400

Polyethylene Glycol 8000

6.2 Incompatibilities

Not applicable.

6.3 Shelf life

5 years.

6.4 Special precautions for storage

No special precautions for storage.

6.5 Nature and contents of container

PVC aluminium foil blister pack containing 12 tablets.

6.6 Instructions for use and handling

No special requirements.

Administrative Data

7. MARKETING AUTHORISATION HOLDER

Glaxo Wellcome UK Ltd.

Trading as

GlaxoSmithKline UK, Stockley Park West

Stockley Park West

Uxbridge

Middlesex

UB11 1BT

8. MARKETING AUTHORISATION NUMBER(S)

PL 10949/0363

9. DATE OF FIRST AUTHORISATION/RENEWAL OF THE AUTHORISATION

15 July 2002

10. DATE OF REVISION OF THE TEXT

21 March 2005

11. Legal Entity

POM

Manerix

(Roche Products Limited)

1. NAME OF THE MEDICINAL PRODUCT

Manerix

2. QUALITATIVE AND QUANTITATIVE COMPOSITION

1 film-coated 150mg tablet contains 150mg moclobemide.

1 film-coated 300mg tablet contains 300mg moclobemide.

3. PHARMACEUTICAL FORM

Film-coated tablets containing 150mg or 300mg of moclobemide.

4. CLINICAL PARTICULARS

4.1 Therapeutic indications

Major depression.

Treatment of social phobia.

4.2 Posology and method of administration

Manerix tablets are for oral administration.

The tablets should be taken at the end of a meal.

Adults

Major depression

The recommended initial dose is 300mg daily, usually administered in divided doses. The dose may be increased up to 600mg/day depending on the severity of the depression.

The individual response may allow a reduction of the daily dose to 150mg.

Treatment of social phobia

The recommended dose of moclobemide is 600mg/day, given in 2 divided doses. The moclobemide dose should be started at 300mg/day and should be increased to 600mg/day on day 4. Continuing the 300mg/day dose for longer than 3 days is not recommended, as the efficacious dose is 600mg/day. Treatment with 600mg/day should continue for 8 - 12 weeks in order to assess the efficacy of the drug. Social phobia may be a chronic condition and it is reasonable to consider continuation of treatment for a responding patient. Patients should be periodically re-evaluated to determine need for further treatment.

Elderly

Elderly patients do not require a special dose adjustment of Manerix.

Children

In view of the lack of clinical data available, Manerix is not recommended for use in children.

Renal/hepatic impairment

Patients with reduced renal function do not require a special dose adjustment of Manerix. When hepatic metabolism is severely impaired by hepatic disease or a drug that inhibits microsomal mono-oxygenase activity (e.g. cimetidine), normal plasma levels are achieved by reducing the daily dose of Manerix to half or one third (see section *5.2 Pharmacokinetics in special populations*).

4.3 Contraindications

Manerix is contra-indicated in patients with known hypersensitivity to the drug or to any component of the product, in acute confusional states and in patients with phaeochromocytoma.

Manerix should not be co-administered with pethidine or selegiline.

Manerix should not be co-administered with 5-HT re-uptake inhibitors (including those which are tricyclic antidepressants) in order to prevent precipitation of serotonergic overactivity (see section *4.4 Special warnings and special precautions for use* and section *4.5 Interaction with other medicaments and other forms of interaction*). After stopping treatment with 5-HT re-uptake inhibitors a time period equal to 4 - 5 half lives of the drug or any active metabolite should elapse between stopping therapy and starting therapy with Manerix.

Manerix should not be co-administered with dextromethorphan, contained in many proprietary cough medicines, as isolated cases of severe central nervous system adverse reactions have been reported after co-administration.

Manerix should not be administered to children for the time being as clinical experience in this category is lacking.

4.4 Special warnings and special precautions for use

Manerix is a reversible inhibitor of monoamine oxidase type A (RIMA). It causes less potentiation of tyramine than traditional irreversible MAOIs, and therefore Manerix does not generally necessitate the special dietary restrictions required for these irreversible MAOIs. However, as a few patients may be especially sensitive to tyramine, all patients should be advised to avoid the consumption of large amounts of tyramine rich food (mature cheese, yeast extracts and fermented soya bean products).

Patients should be advised to avoid sympathomimetic agents such as ephedrine, pseudoephedrine and phenylpropanolamine (contained in many proprietary cough and cold medications) (see section *4.5 Interaction with other medicaments and other forms of interaction*).

Depressive patients with excitation or agitation as the predominant clinical feature should either not be treated with Manerix or only in combination with a sedative (e.g. a benzodiazepine). The sedative should only be used for a maximum of 2 to 3 weeks.

Patients with suicidal tendencies should be closely monitored at the start of treatment.

If a depressive episode is treated in bipolar disorders, manic episodes can be provoked.

Due to the lack of clinical data, patients with concomitant schizophrenia or schizo-affective organic disorders should not be treated with Manerix.

Theoretical pharmacological considerations indicate that MAO inhibitors may precipitate a hypertensive reaction in patients with thyrotoxicosis. As experience with Manerix in this population group is lacking, caution should be exercised before prescribing Manerix.

In patients receiving Manerix, caution should be exercised when co-administering drugs that enhance serotonin in order to prevent precipitation of serotoninergic syndrome (see section *4.3 Contra-indications* and section *4.5 Interaction with other medicaments and other forms of interaction*).

Hypersensitivity may occur in susceptible individuals. Symptoms may include rash and oedema.

Hyponatraemia, (usually in the elderly and possibly due to inappropriate secretion of antidiuretic hormone) has been associated with all types of antidepressants, although very rarely with Manerix (see *4.8 Undesirable effects*), and should be considered in all patients who develop drowsiness, confusion or convulsions while taking an antidepressant.

4.5 Interaction with other medicinal products and other forms of Interaction

In animals, Manerix potentiates the effects of opiates. Opiate analgesics, such as, Morphine and fentanyl should be used with caution. A dosage adjustment may be necessary for these drugs.

Cimetidine prolongs the metabolism of Manerix. The normal dose of Manerix should therefore be reduced to half the dose in patients taking cimetidine.

In patients receiving Manerix, additional drugs that enhance serotonin, such as many other antidepressants, particularly in multiple-drug combinations, should be given with caution. In isolated cases there have been combinations of serious symptoms and signs, including hyperthermia, confusion, hyperreflexia and myoclonus, which are indicative of serotonergic overactivity (see section *4.3 Contra-indications* and section *4.4 Special warnings and special precautions for use*). Should such combined symptoms occur, the patient should be closely observed by a physician (and if necessary hospitalised) and appropriate treatment given.

The pharmacologic action of systemic regimens of sympathomimetic agents may possibly be intensified and prolonged by concurrent treatment with moclobemide.

4.6 Pregnancy and lactation

Reproduction studies in animals have not revealed any risk to the foetus, but the safety of Manerix in human pregnancy has not been established. Therefore the benefits of drug therapy during pregnancy should be weighed against possible risk to the foetus.

Since only a small amount of Manerix passes into breast milk (approximately $^1/_{30}$ of the maternal dose), the benefits of continuing drug therapy during nursing should be weighed against possible risks to the child.

4.7 Effects on ability to drive and use machines

Impairment of performance in activities requiring complete mental alertness (e.g. driving a motor vehicle) is generally not to be expected with Manerix. The individual reaction should however be monitored during early treatment.

4.8 Undesirable effects

The following undesirable effects have been observed: sleep disturbances, agitation, feelings of anxiety, restlessness, irritability, dizziness, headache, paraesthesia, dry mouth, visual disturbances, nausea, diarrhoea, constipation, vomiting, oedema and skin reactions such as rash, pruritus, urticaria and flushing. Confusional states have been observed, but these have disappeared rapidly on discontinuation of therapy.

In clinical trials, there was a low incidence of raised liver enzymes without associated clinical sequelae.

Hyponatraemia has very rarely been reported (see *4.4 Special warnings and precautions for use*).

4.9 Overdose

Overdoses of moclobemide alone induce generally mild and reversible signs of CNS and gastro-intestinal irritation.

Treatment of overdose should be aimed primarily at maintenance of the vital functions.

As with other antidepressants, mixed overdoses of moclobemide with other drugs (e.g. other CNS-acting drugs) could be life-threatening. Therefore, patients should be hospitalised and closely monitored so that appropriate treatment may be given.

5. PHARMACOLOGICAL PROPERTIES

5.1 Pharmacodynamic properties

Manerix is an antidepressant which affects the monoaminergic cerebral neurotransmitter system by means of a reversible inhibition of monoamine oxidase preferentially of type A (RIMA). The metabolism of noradrenaline, dopamine and serotonin (5-HT) is decreased by this effect, and this leads to increased extracellular concentrations of these neuronal transmitters.

5.2 Pharmacokinetic properties

Absorption

After oral administration, moclobemide is completely absorbed from the gastrointestinal tract into the portal blood. Peak plasma concentrations of the drug are usually reached within one hour of dosage. A hepatic first-pass effect reduces the systemically available dose fraction (bioavailability F). This reduction is more pronounced after single (F: 60%) than after multiple (F: 80%) doses. After multiple dosing, plasma concentrations of moclobemide increase over the first week of therapy and remain stable thereafter. When the daily dose is increased, there is a more than proportional increase in steady-state concentrations.

Distribution

Due to its lipophilic nature, moclobemide is extensively distributed in the body. The volume of distribution (V_{ss}) is about 1.0 l/kg. Binding of the drug to plasma proteins, mainly albumin, is low (50%).

Metabolism

The drug is almost entirely metabolised before its elimination from the body. Metabolism occurs largely via oxidative reactions on the morpholine moiety of the molecule. Degradation products with pharmacological activity are present in the systemic circulation in man at very low concentrations only. The major metabolites present in plasma are a lactam derivative and an N-oxide derivative. Moclobemide has been shown to be metabolised in part by the polymorphic isoenzymes CYP2C19 and CYP2D6. Thus, in genetically or drug-induced (via metabolic inhibitors) poor metabolisers, metabolism of the drug may be affected. Two studies conducted to investigate the magnitude of these effects suggested that, due to the presence of multiple alternative metabolic pathways, they are of no clinical significance and should not necessitate dosage modification.

Elimination

Moclobemide is rapidly eliminated by metabolic processes. Total clearance is approximately 20 - 50 l/hour. The mean elimination half-life during multiple dosing (300mg b.i.d) is approximately 3 hours and generally ranges from 2 – 4 hours in most patients. Less than 1% of a dose is excreted renally in unchanged form. The metabolites formed are eliminated renally. Insignificant amounts are excreted in human breast milk.

Pharmacokinetics in special populations

Elderly

Absorption and disposition parameters are unchanged in the elderly.

Patients with renal impairment

Renal disease does not alter the elimination characteristics of moclobemide.

Patients with hepatic impairment

In advanced liver insufficiency, the metabolism of moclobemide is reduced (see section *4.2 Posology and method of administration*).

5.3 Preclinical safety data

Not applicable.

6. PHARMACEUTICAL PARTICULARS

6.1 List of excipients

Lactose, maize starch, povidone K30, sodium starch glycollate, magnesium stearate, hydroxypropyl methylcellulose, ethylcellulose, polyethylene glycol 6000, talc and titanium dioxide (E171). The 150mg tablets also contain yellow iron oxide (E172).

6.2 Incompatibilities

Not applicable.

6.3 Shelf life
5 years.

6.4 Special precautions for storage
No special precautions for storage.

6.5 Nature and contents of container
Blister packing.
Pack sizes: 28, 30, 84 and 100 tablets (150mg tablets)
30 and 60 tablets (300mg tablets)

6.6 Instructions for use and handling
Not applicable.

7. MARKETING AUTHORISATION HOLDER
Roche Products Limited, 40 Broadwater Road, Welwyn Garden City, Hertfordshire, AL7 3AY.

8. MARKETING AUTHORISATION NUMBER(S)
PL 0031/0275 (150mg tablets)
PL 0031/0347 (300mg tablets)

9. DATE OF FIRST AUTHORISATION/RENEWAL OF THE AUTHORISATION
150 mg tablets:
First approved 19 June 1991
300 mg tablets:
First approved 5 July 1994

10. DATE OF REVISION OF THE TEXT
May 2004
Manerix is a registered trade mark
P999788/804

Manusept
(Medlock Medical Ltd)

1. NAME OF THE MEDICINAL PRODUCT
Manusept Antibacterial Hand Rub.

2. QUALITATIVE AND QUANTITATIVE COMPOSITION
Isopropyl Alcohol 70% v/v; Triclosan 0.5% w/v.

3. PHARMACEUTICAL FORM
Topical solution.

4. CLINICAL PARTICULARS

4.1 Therapeutic indications
For the disinfection of physically clean hands. For the pre-operative disinfection of physically clean hands. For the disinfection of skin prior to surgery, injection or venepuncture.

4.2 Posology and method of administration
Route of Administration: Cutaneous use. *For the disinfection of physically clean hands:* Dispense 3ml of Manusept into the cupped palm of one hand. Spread thoroughly over both hands and wrists, rub vigorously until dry. *For the pre-operative disinfection of physically clean hands:*
Apply as above but using 5ml of Manusept and include the forearms. Repeat the procedure once more. *For the disinfection of skin prior to surgery, injection or venepuncture:* Apply a quantity of Manusept with cotton wool swabs, rub vigorously until dry.

4.3 Contraindications
Avoid contact with the eyes. If swallowed, gastric aspiration and lavage avoiding pulmonary aspiration. Apomorphine should not be used.

4.4 Special warnings and special precautions for use
Keep away from the eyes. Do not use in the vicinity of naked flames. For external use only.

4.5 Interaction with other medicinal products and other forms of Interaction
None stated.

4.6 Pregnancy and lactation
None stated.

4.7 Effects on ability to drive and use machines
None stated.

4.8 Undesirable effects
None stated.

4.9 Overdose
Not applicable.

5. PHARMACOLOGICAL PROPERTIES

5.1 Pharmacodynamic properties
Triclosan is a bactericide. Isopropyl alcohol is a bactericide.

5.2 Pharmacokinetic properties
None stated.

5.3 Preclinical safety data
There are no pre-clinical data of relevance to the prescriber which are additional to that already included in other sections of the summary.

6. PHARMACEUTICAL PARTICULARS

6.1 List of excipients
Isopropyl myristate; purified water.

6.2 Incompatibilities
None stated.

6.3 Shelf life
36 months unopened.

6.4 Special precautions for storage
Do not store above 25°C.

6.5 Nature and contents of container
HDPE bottles with compression moulded polypropylene screw caps with steran faced pulp board wads containing 100, 250 or 500ml of product.

6.6 Instructions for use and handling
Not applicable.

7. MARKETING AUTHORISATION HOLDER
Medlock Medical Limited, Tubiton House, Medlock Street, Oldham, OL1 3HS.

8. MARKETING AUTHORISATION NUMBER(S)
PL 21248/0019.

9. DATE OF FIRST AUTHORISATION/RENEWAL OF THE AUTHORISATION
3rd July 2005.

10. DATE OF REVISION OF THE TEXT
July 2005.

Marcain Heavy, 0.5% solution for injection.
(AstraZeneca UK Limited)

1. NAME OF THE MEDICINAL PRODUCT
Marcain Heavy, 0.5% solution for injection.

2. QUALITATIVE AND QUANTITATIVE COMPOSITION
Bupivacaine Hydrochloride BP 5.28mg/ml equivalent to 5.0mg/ml bupivacaine hydrochloride anhydrous.
For excipients, see 6.1

3. PHARMACEUTICAL FORM
Solution for injection.
Clear, colourless solution.

4. CLINICAL PARTICULARS

4.1 Therapeutic indications
Intrathecal (subarachnoid) spinal anaesthesia for surgery (urological and lower limb surgery lasting 2-3 hours, abdominal surgery lasting 45-60 minutes).

Bupivacaine is a long acting anaesthetic agent of the amide type. Marcain Heavy has a rapid onset of action and long duration. The duration of analgesia in the T_{10}-T_{12} segments is 2-3 hours.

Marcain Heavy produces a moderate muscular relaxation of the lower extremities lasting 2-2.5 hours. The motor blockade of the abdominal muscles makes the solution suitable for performance of abdominal surgery lasting 45-60 minutes. The duration of the motor blockade does not exceed the duration of analgesia. The cardiovascular effects of Marcain Heavy are similar or less than those seen with other spinal agents. Bupivacaine 5mg/ml with glucose 80mg/ml is exceptionally well tolerated by all tissues with which it comes in contact.

4.2 Posology and method of administration
Route of administration: For intrathecal injection.

The doses recommended below should be regarded as a guide for use in the average adult.

Intrathecal anaesthesia for surgery:

2-4ml (10-20mg bupivacaine hydrochloride).

The dose should be reduced in the elderly and in patients in the late stages of pregnancy, see Section 4.4.

The spread of anaesthesia obtained with Marcain Heavy depends on several factors including the volume of solution and the position of the patient during and following the injection.

When injected at the L_3-L_4 intervertebral space, with the patient in the sitting position, 3ml of Marcain Heavy spreads to the T_7-T_{10} spinal segments. With the patient receiving the injection in the horizontal position and then turned supine, the blockade spreads to T_4-T_7 spinal segments. It should be understood that the level of spinal anaesthesia achieved with any local anaesthetic can be unpredictable in a given patient.

The recommended site of injection is below L3.

The effects of injections of Marcain Heavy exceeding 4ml have not yet been studied and such volumes can therefore not be recommended.

4.3 Contraindications
Hypersensitivity to local anaesthetics of the amide type or to any of the excipients.

Intrathecal anaesthesia, regardless of the local anaesthetic used, has its own contra-indications which include:

Active disease of the central nervous system such as meningitis, poliomyelitis, intracranial haemorrhage, sub-acute combined degeneration of the cord due to pernicious anaemia and cerebral and spinal tumours.

Spinal stenosis and active disease (e.g. spondylitis, tuberculosis, tumour) or recent trauma (e.g. fracture) in the vertebral column.

Septicaemia.

Pyogenic infection of the skin at or adjacent to the site of lumbar puncture.

Cardiogenic or hypovolaemic shock.

Coagulation disorders or ongoing anticoagulation treatment.

4.4 Special warnings and special precautions for use
Intrathecal anaesthesia should only be undertaken by clinicians with the necessary knowledge and experience.

Regional anaesthetic procedures should always be performed in a properly equipped and staffed area. Resuscitative equipment and drugs should be immediately available and the anaesthetist should remain in constant attendance.

Intravenous access, e.g. an i.v. infusion, should be in place before starting the intrathecal anaesthesia. The clinician responsible should take the necessary precautions to avoid intravascular injection and be appropriately trained and familiar with the diagnosis and treatment of side effects, systemic toxicity and other complications. If signs of acute systemic toxicity or total spinal block appear, injection of the local anaesthetic should be stopped immediately, see Section 4.9.

Like all local anaesthetic drugs, bupivacaine may cause acute toxicity effects on the central nervous and cardiovascular systems, if utilised for local anaesthetic procedures resulting in high blood concentrations of the drug. This is especially the case after unintentional intravascular administration or injection into highly vascular areas.

Ventricular arrhythmia, ventricular fibrillation, sudden cardiovascular collapse and death have been reported in connection with high systemic concentrations of bupivacaine. Should cardiac arrest occur, a successful outcome may require prolonged resuscitative efforts. High systemic concentrations are not expected with doses normally used for intrathecal anaesthesia.

There is an increased risk of high or total spinal blockade, resulting in cardiovascular and respiratory depression, in the elderly and in patients in the late stages of pregnancy. The dose should therefore be reduced in these patients.

Intrathecal anaesthesia with any local anaesthetic can cause hypotension and bradycardia which should be anticipated and appropriate precautions taken. These may include preloading the circulation with crystalloid or colloid solution. If hypotension develops it should be treated with a vasopressor such as ephedrine 10-15mg intravenously. Severe hypotension may result from hypovolaemia due to haemorrhage or dehydration, or aorto-caval occlusion in patients with massive ascites, large abdominal tumours or late pregnancy. Marked hypotension should be avoided in patients with cardiac decompensation.

Patients with hypovolaemia due to any cause can develop sudden and severe hypotension during intrathecal anaesthesia.

Intrathecal anaesthesia can cause intercostal paralysis and patients with pleural effusions may suffer respiratory embarrassment. Septicaemia can increase the risk of intraspinal abscess formation in the postoperative period.

Before treatment is instituted, consideration should be taken if the benefits outweigh the possible risks for the patient.

Patients in poor general condition due to ageing or other compromising factors such as partial or complete heart conduction block, advanced liver or renal dysfunction require special attention, although regional anaesthesia may be the optimal choice for surgery in these patients.

4.5 Interaction with other medicinal products and other forms of Interaction
Bupivacaine should be used with caution in patients receiving other local anaesthetics or agents structurally related to amide-type local anaesthetics, e.g. certain anti-arrhythmics, since the systemic toxic effects are additive.

4.6 Pregnancy and lactation
There is no evidence of untoward effects in human pregnancy. In large doses there is evidence of decreased pup survival in rats and an embryological effect in rabbits if Marcain is administered in pregnancy. Marcain should not therefore be given in early pregnancy unless the benefits are considered to outweigh the risks.

It should be noted that the dose should be reduced in patients in the late stages of pregnancy, see Section 4.4.

Bupivacaine enters the mother's milk, but in such small quantities that there is generally no risk of affecting the child at therapeutic dose levels.

4.7 Effects on ability to drive and use machines
Besides the direct anaesthetic effect, local anaesthetics may have a very mild effect on mental function and coordination even in the absence of overt CNS toxicity and may temporarily impair locomotion and alertness.

4.8 Undesirable effects

General

The adverse reaction profile for Marcain Heavy is similar to those for other long acting local anaesthetics used for intrathecal anaesthesia

Table of Adverse Drug Reactions

Very Common (>1/10)

Cardiac disorders: Hypotension, bradycardia

Gastrointestinal disorders: Nausea

Common (>1/100 <1/10)

Nervous system disorders: Postdural puncture headache

Gastrointestinal disorders: Vomiting

Renal and urinary disorders: Urinary retention, urinary incontinence

Uncommon (>1/1000 <1/100)

Nervous system disorders: Paraesthesia, paresis, dysaesthesia

Musculoskeletal, connective tissue and bone disorders: Muscle weakness, back pain

Rare (<1/1000)

Cardiac disorders: Cardiac arrest

Immune system disorders: Allergic reactions, anaphylactic shock

Nervous system disorders: Total spinal block unintentional, paraplegia, paralysis, neuropathy, arachnoiditis

Respiratory disorders: Respiratory depression

Adverse reactions caused by the drug *per se* are difficult to distinguish from the physiological effects of the nerve block (e.g. decrease in blood pressure, bradycardia, temporary urinary retention), events caused directly (e.g. spinal haematoma) or indirectly (e.g. meningitis, epidural abcess) by needle puncture or events associated to cerebrospinal leakage (e.g. postdural puncture headache).

Treatment of side-effects: High or total spinal blockade causing respiratory paralysis should be treated by ensuring and maintaining a patent airway and giving oxygen by assisted or controlled ventilation.

Hypotension should be treated by the use of vasopressors, e.g. ephedrine 10-15mg intravenously and repeated until the desired level of arterial pressure is reached. Intravenous fluids, both electrolytes and colloids, given rapidly can also reverse hypotension. See Section 4.9, Overdosage.

4.9 Overdose

Marcain Heavy, used as recommended, is not likely to cause blood levels high enough to cause systemic toxicity. However, if other local anaesthetics are concomitantly administered, toxic effects are additive and may cause systemic toxic reactions.

Systemic toxicity is rarely associated with spinal anaesthesia but might occur after accidental intravascular injection. Systemic adverse reactions are characterised by numbness of the tongue, light-headedness, dizziness and tremors, followed by convulsions and cardiovascular disorders.

Treatment of systemic toxicity: No treatment is required for milder symptoms of systemic toxicity but if convulsions occur then it is important to ensure adequate oxygenation and to arrest the convulsions if they last more than 15-30 seconds. Oxygen should be given by face mask and the respiration assisted or controlled if necessary. Convulsions can be arrested by injection of thiopentone 100-150mg intravenously or with diazepam 5-10mg intravenously. Alternatively, succinylcholine 50-100mg intravenously may be given but only if the clinician has the ability to perform endotracheal intubation and to manage a totally paralysed patient.

5. PHARMACOLOGICAL PROPERTIES

5.1 Pharmacodynamic properties

Bupivacaine is a long acting local anaesthetic agent of the amide type.

Moderate muscular relaxation of lower extremities.

Motor blockade of the abdominal muscles.

5.2 Pharmacokinetic properties

Rapid onset of action and long duration i.e. T_{10}-T_{12} segments - duration 2-3 hours.

Muscular relaxation of lower extremities lasts 2-2.5 hours.

Blockade of the abdominal muscles lasts 45-60 minutes. The duration of motor blockade does not exceed duration of analgesia.

5.3 Preclinical safety data

Bupivacaine hydrochloride is a well established active ingredient.

6. PHARMACEUTICAL PARTICULARS

6.1 List of excipients

Glucose Anhydrous, Sodium hydroxide and Water for Injections

6.2 Incompatibilities

None known.

6.3 Shelf life

3 years.

6.4 Special precautions for storage

Do not store above 25°C.

6.5 Nature and contents of container

4ml sterile wrapped glass ampoules or One Point Cut ampoules.

6.6 Instructions for use and handling

The solution should be used immediately after opening of the ampoule. Any remaining solution should be discarded.

7. MARKETING AUTHORISATION HOLDER

AstraZeneca UK Ltd.,

600 Capability Green,

Luton, LU1 3LU, UK.

8. MARKETING AUTHORISATION NUMBER(S)

PL 17901/0142

9. DATE OF FIRST AUTHORISATION/RENEWAL OF THE AUTHORISATION

20th September 2004

10. DATE OF REVISION OF THE TEXT

13th April 2005

Marcain Polyamp Steripack 0.25% & 0.5%

(AstraZeneca UK Limited)

1. NAME OF THE MEDICINAL PRODUCT

Marcain Polyamp Steripack 0.25%.

Marcain Polyamp Steripack 0.5%.

2. QUALITATIVE AND QUANTITATIVE COMPOSITION

Marcain Polyamp Steripack 0.25% contains Bupivacaine Hydrochloride BP 2.64mg/ml equivalent to bupivacaine hydrochloride anhydrous 2.5mg/ml.

Marcain Polyamp Steripack 0.5% contains Bupivacaine Hydrochloride BP 5.28mg/ml equivalent to bupivacaine hydrochloride anhydrous 5.0mg/ml.

3. PHARMACEUTICAL FORM

Injection.

4. CLINICAL PARTICULARS

4.1 Therapeutic indications

Marcain 0.25% and 0.5% solutions are used for the production of local anaesthesia by percutaneous infiltration, peripheral nerve block(s) and central neural block (caudal or epidural), that is, for specialist use in situations where prolonged anaesthesia is required. Because sensory nerve block is more marked than motor block, Marcain is especially useful in the relief of pain, e.g. during labour.

A list of indications and the suggested dose and strength of solution appropriate for each are shown in the table below.

4.2 Posology and method of administration

The utmost care should be taken to prevent an accidental intravascular injection, always including careful aspiration. For epidural anaesthesia, a test dose of 3-5ml of bupivacaine containing adrenaline should be administered, since an intravascular injection of adrenaline will be quickly recognised by an increase in heart rate. Verbal contact and repeated measurement of heart rate should be maintained throughout a period of 5 minutes following the test dose. Aspiration should be repeated prior to administration of the total dose. The main dose should be injected slowly, 25-50mg/min, in incremental doses under constant contact with the patient. If mild toxic symptoms occur, the injection should be stopped immediately.

When prolonged blocks are used, either by continuous infusion or by repeated bolus administration, the risks of reaching a toxic plasma concentration or inducing a local neural injury must be considered.

The dosage varies and depends upon the area to be anaesthetised, the vascularity of the tissues, the number of neuronal segments to be blocked, individual tolerance and the technique of anaesthesia used. The lowest dosage needed to provide effective anaesthesia should be administered. For most indications, the duration of anaesthesia with Marcain solutions is such that a single dose is sufficient.

The maximum dosage must be determined by evaluating the size and physical status of the patient and considering the usual rate of systemic absorption from a particular injection site. Experience to date indicates a single dose of up to 150mg bupivacaine hydrochloride. Doses of up to 50mg 2-hourly may subsequently be used. A total dose of up to 500 mg bupivacaine over 24 hours, which does not include the initial bolus dose, has been used routinely for many years without reports of toxicity. The dosages in the following table are recommended as a guide for use in the average adult. For young, elderly or debilitated patients, these doses should be reduced.

(see Table 1 below)

4.3 Contraindications

Bupivacaine hydrochloride solutions are contra-indicated in patients with hypersensitivity to local anaesthetic agents of the amide type or to any of the excipients.

Solutions of bupivacaine hydrochloride are contra-indicated for intravenous regional anaesthesia (Bier's-block).

Epidural anaesthesia, regardless of the local anaesthetic used, has its own contra-indications which include:

Active disease of the central nervous system such as meningitis, poliomyelitis, intracranial haemorrhage, subacute combined degeneration of the cord due to pernicious anaemia and cerebral and spinal tumours; tuberculosis of the spine; pyogenic infection of the skin at or adjacent to the site of lumbar puncture; cardiogenic or hypovolaemic shock; coagulation disorders or ongoing anticoagulation treatment.

4.4 Special warnings and special precautions for use

There have been reports of cardiac arrest during the use of bupivacaine for epidural anaesthesia or peripheral nerve blockade where resuscitative efforts have been difficult, and were required to be prolonged before the patient responded. However, in some instances resuscitation has proven impossible despite apparently adequate preparation and appropriate management.

Like all local anaesthetic drugs, bupivacaine may cause acute toxicity effects on the central nervous and cardiovascular systems if utilised for local anaesthetic procedures resulting in high blood concentrations of the drug. This is especially the case after unintentional intravascular administration. Ventricular arrhythmia, ventricular fibrillation, sudden cardiovascular collapse and death have been reported in connection with high systemic concentrations of bupivacaine.

Major peripheral nerve blocks may require the administration of a large volume of local anaesthetic in areas of high vascularity, often close to large vessels where there is an increased risk of intravascular injection and/or systemic absorption. This may lead to high plasma concentrations.

Before any nerve block is attempted, intravenous access for resuscitation purposes should be established.

Table 1

TYPE OF BLOCK	% CONC.	EACH DOSE ML	MG	MOTOR BLOCK*
LOCAL INFILTRATION	0.25	UP TO 60	UP TO 150	-
LUMBAR EPIDURAL				
SURGICAL OPERATIONS	0.5	10 TO 20	50 TO 100	MODERATE TO COMPLETE
ANALGESIA IN LABOUR	0.5	6 to 12	30 TO 60	MODERATE TO COMPLETE
	0.25	6 to 12	15 TO 30	MINIMAL
CAUDAL EPIDURAL				
SURGICAL operations	0.5	15 TO 30	75 TO 150	MODERATE TO COMPLETE
CHILDREN (AGED UP TO 10 YEARS):				
UP TO LOWER THORACIC (T10)	0.25	0.3 - 0.4 ml/kg	0.75 - 1.0 mg/kg	
UP TO MID-THORACIC (T6)	0.25	0.4 - 0.6 ML/KG	1.0 - 1.5 MG/KG	
IF TOTAL AMOUNT GREATER THAN 20ML REDUCE CONCENTRATION TO 0.2%.				
ANALGESIA IN LABOUR	0.5	10 TO 20	50 TO 100	MODERATE TO COMPLETE
	0.25	10 TO 20	25 TO 50	MODERATE
PERIPHERAL NERVES	0.5	UP TO 30	UP TO 150	MODERATE TO COMPLETE
	0.25	UP TO 60	UP TO 150	SLIGHT TO MODERATE
SYMPATHETIC BLOCKS	0.25	20 TO 50	50 TO 125	-

* With continuous (intermittent) techniques, repeat doses increase the degree of motor block. The first repeat dose of 0.5% may produce complete motor block for intra-abdominal surgery.

Clinicians should have received adequate and appropriate training in the procedure to be performed and should be familiar with the diagnosis and treatment of side effects, systemic toxicity or other complications (see 4.9).

Adequate resuscitation equipment should be available whenever local or general anaesthesia is administered. The clinician responsible should take the necessary precautions to avoid intravascular injection (see 4.2).

Overdosage or accidental intravenous injection may give rise to toxic reactions.

Injection of repeated doses of bupivacaine hydrochloride may cause significant increases in blood levels with each repeated dose due to slow accumulation of the drug. Tolerance varies with the status of the patient.

Debilitated, elderly or acutely ill patients should be given reduced doses commensurate with their physical status.

Patients treated with anti-arrhythmic drugs class III (e.g. amiodarone) should be under close surveillance and ECG monitoring, since cardiac effects may be additive.

Only in rare cases have amide local anaesthetics been associated with allergic reactions (in most severe instances anaphylactic shock).

Patients allergic to ester-type local anaesthetic drugs (procaine, tetracaine, benzocaine, etc.) have not shown cross-sensitivity to agents of the amide type such as bupivacaine.

Local anaesthetics should be used with caution for epidural anaesthesia in patients with impaired cardiovascular function since they may be less able to compensate for functional changes associated with the prolongation of A-V conduction produced by these drugs.

Since bupivacaine is metabolised in the liver, it should be used cautiously in patients with liver disease or with reduced liver blood flow.

The physiological effects generated by a central neural blockade are more pronounced in the presence of hypotension. Patients with hypovolaemia due to any cause can develop sudden and severe hypotension during epidural anaesthesia. Epidural anaesthesia should therefore be avoided or used with caution in patients with untreated hypovolaemia or significantly impaired venous return.

Epidural anaesthesia with any local anaesthetic can cause hypotension and bradycardia which should be anticipated and appropriate precautions taken. These may include pre-loading the circulation with crystalloid or colloid solution. If hypotension develops it should be treated with a vasopressor such as ephedrine 10-15mg intravenously. Severe hypotension may result from hypovolaemia due to haemorrhage or dehydration, or aorto-caval occlusion in patients with massive ascites, large abdominal tumours or late pregnancy. Marked hypotension should be avoided in patients with cardiac decompensation.

Patients with hypovolaemia due to any cause can develop sudden and severe hypotension during epidural anaesthesia.

Epidural anaesthesia can cause intercostal paralysis and patients with pleural effusions may suffer respiratory embarrassment. Septicaemia can increase the risk of intraspinal abscess formation in the postoperative period.

Paracervical block may have a greater adverse effect on the foetus than other nerve blocks used in obstetrics. Due to the systemic toxicity of bupivacaine special care should be taken when using bupivacaine for paracervical block.

Small doses of local anaesthetics injected into the head and neck, including retrobulbar, dental and stellate ganglion blocks, may produce systemic toxicity due to inadvertent intra-arterial injection.

Retrobulbar injections may very rarely reach the cranial subarachnoid space causing serious/severe reactions, including temporary blindness, cardiovascular collapse, apnoea, convulsions.

Retro- and peribulbar injections of local anaesthetics carry a low risk of persistent ocular muscle dysfunction. The primary causes include trauma and/or local toxic effects on muscles and/or nerves. The severity of such tissue reactions is related to the degree of trauma, the concentration of the local anaesthetic and the duration of exposure of the tissue to the local anaesthetic. For this reason, as with all local anaesthetics, the lowest effective concentration and dose of local anaesthetic should be used.

4.5 Interaction with other medicinal products and other forms of Interaction

Bupivacaine should be used with caution in patients receiving other local anaesthetics or agents structurally related to amide-type local anaesthetics, e.g. certain anti-arrhythmics, such as lidocane, since the systemic toxic effects are additive.

Specific interaction studies with bupivacaine and anti-arrhythmic drugs class III (e.g. amiodarone) have not been performed, but caution should be advised. (see also 4.4)

4.6 Pregnancy and lactation

There is no evidence of untoward effects in human pregnancy. In large doses there is evidence of decreased pup survival in rats and an embryological effect in rabbits if Marcain is administered in pregnancy. Marcain should not therefore be given in early pregnancy unless the benefits are considered to outweigh the risks.

Foetal adverse effects due to local anaesthetics, such as foetal bradycardia, seem to be most apparent in paracervical block anaesthesia. Such effects may be due to high concentrations of anaesthetic reaching the foetus. (see also Section 4.4)

Bupivacaine enters the mother's milk, but in such small quantities that there is no risk of affecting the child at therapeutic dose levels.

4.7 Effects on ability to drive and use machines

Besides the direct anaesthetic effect, local anaesthetics may have a very mild effect on mental function and co-ordination even in the absence of overt CNS toxicity, and may temporarily impair locomotion and alertness.

4.8 Undesirable effects

Serious systemic adverse reactions are rare, but may occur in connection with overdosage (see also Section 4.9) or unintentional intravascular injection.

Bupivacaine causes systemic toxicity similar to that observed with other local anaesthetic agents. It is caused by high plasma concentrations as a result of excessive dosage, rapid absorption or, most commonly, inadvertent intravascular injection. Pronounced acidosis or hypoxia may increase the risk and severity of toxic reactions. Such reactions involve the central nervous system and the cardiovascular system. CNS reactions are characterised by numbness of the tongue, light-headedness, dizziness, blurred vision and muscle twitch, followed by drowsiness, convulsions, unconsciousness and possibly respiratory arrest.

Cardiovascular reactions are related to depression of the conduction system of the heart and myocardium leading to decreased cardiac output, heart block, hypotension, bradycardia and sometimes ventricular arrhythmias, including ventricular tachycardia, ventricular fibrillation and cardiac arrest. Usually these will be preceded or accompanied by major CNS toxicity, i.e. convulsions, but in rare cases cardiac arrest has occurred without prodromal CNS effects.

Epidural anaesthesia itself can cause adverse reactions regardless of the local anaesthetic agent used. These include hypotension and bradycardia due to sympathetic blockade and/or vasovagal fainting.

In severe cases cardiac arrest may occur.

Accidental sub-arachnoid injection can lead to very high spinal anaesthesia possibly with apnoea and severe hypotension.

Neurological damage is a rare but well recognised consequence of regional and particularly epidural and spinal anaesthesia. It may be due to several causes, e.g. direct injury to the spinal cord or spinal nerves, anterior spinal artery syndrome, injection of an irritant substance, or an injection of a non-sterile solution. These may result in localised areas of paraesthesia or anaesthesia, motor weakness, loss of sphincter control and paraplegia. Occasionally these are permanent.

Hepatic dysfunction, with reversible increases of SGOT, SGPT, alkaline phosphates and bilirubin, has been observed following repeated injections or long-term infusions of bupivacaine. If signs of hepatic dysfunction are observed during treatment with bupivacaine, the drug should be discontinued.

4.9 Overdose

4.9.1 Acute Systemic Toxicity

Central nervous system toxicity is a graded response with symptoms and signs of escalating severity. The first symptoms are usually light-headedness, circumoral paraesthesia, numbness of the tongue, hyperacusis, tinnitus and visual disturbances.

Dysarthria, muscular twitching or tremors are more serious and precede the onset of generalised convulsions. These signs must not be mistaken for a neurotic behaviour. Unconsciousness and grand mal convulsions may follow which may last from a few seconds to several minutes. Hypoxia and hypercarbia occur rapidly following convulsions due to the increased muscular activity, together with the interference with respiration. In severe cases apnoea may occur. Acidosis, hyperkalaemia and hypoxia increase and extend the toxic effects of local anaesthetics.

Recovery is due to redistribution of the local anaesthetic drug from the central nervous system and subsequent metabolism and excretion. Recovery may be rapid unless large amounts of the drug have been injected.

Cardiovascular system toxicity may be seen in severe cases and is generally preceded by signs of toxicity in the central nervous system. In patients under heavy sedation or receiving a general anaesthetic, prodromal CNS symptoms may be absent.

Hypotension, bradycardia, arrhythmia and even cardiac arrest may occur as a result of high systemic concentrations of local anaesthetics, but in rare cases cardiac arrest has occurred without prodromal CNS effects.

4.9.2 Treatment of Acute Toxicity

If signs of acute systemic toxicity appear, injection of the local anaesthetic should be immediately stopped.

Treatment of a patient with systemic toxicity consists of arresting convulsions and ensuring adequate ventilation with oxygen, if necessary by assisted or controlled ventilation (respiration). If convulsions occur they must be treated promptly by intravenous injection of thiopentone 100 to 200mg or diazepam 5 to 10mg. Alternatively succinylcholine 50mg - 100mg i.v. may be used providing the clinician is capable of performing endotracheal intubation and managing a fully paralysed patient.

Once convulsions have been controlled and adequate ventilation of the lungs ensured, no other treatment is generally required

Cardiac arrest due to bupivacaine can be resistant to electrical defibrillation and resuscitation must be continued energetically for a prolonged period.

High or total spinal blockade causing respiratory paralysis and hypotension during epidural anaesthesia should be treated by ensuring and maintaining a patent airway and giving oxygen by assisted or controlled ventilation.

Hypotension should be treated by the use of vasopressors, e.g. ephedrine 10-15mg intravenously and repeated until the desired level of arterial pressure is reached. Intravenous fluids, both electrolytes and colloids, given rapidly can also reverse hypotension.

5. PHARMACOLOGICAL PROPERTIES

5.1 Pharmacodynamic properties

Bupivacaine is a potent amide local anaesthetic with a prolonged duration of action. It affects sensory nerves more than motor nerves and is ideal for producing analgesia without motor blockade.

5.2 Pharmacokinetic properties

In adults, the terminal half-life of bupivacaine is 3.5 hours. The maximum blood concentration varies with the site of injection and is highest after intercostal nerve blockade.

Total dose, rather than concentration, is an important determinant of peak blood levels.

Bupivacaine is biodegraded in the liver and only 6% is excreted unchanged in the urine.

5.3 Preclinical safety data

Bupivacaine hydrochloride is a well established active ingredient.

6. PHARMACEUTICAL PARTICULARS

6.1 List of excipients

Sodium chloride, sodium hydroxide and water for injections.

6.2 Incompatibilities

None stated.

6.3 Shelf life

24 months.

6.4 Special precautions for storage

Store below 30°C.

6.5 Nature and contents of container

10ml and 20ml polypropylene ampoules (Steripack). Cartons contain 5 or 10 ampoules.

6.6 Instructions for use and handling

For single use only. Discard any unused solution.

7. MARKETING AUTHORISATION HOLDER

AstraZeneca UK Ltd.,

600 Capability Green,

Luton, LU1 3LU, UK.

8. MARKETING AUTHORISATION NUMBER(S)

Marcain Polyamp Steripack 0.25% - PL 17901/0144

Marcain Polyamp Steripack 0.5% - PL 17901/0145

9. DATE OF FIRST AUTHORISATION/RENEWAL OF THE AUTHORISATION

4th June 2002

10. DATE OF REVISION OF THE TEXT

4th March 2005

MASTAFLU

(MASTA Ltd)

1. NAME OF THE MEDICINAL PRODUCT

MASTAFLU®, suspension for injection (influenza vaccine, surface antigen, inactivated)

2. QUALITATIVE AND QUANTITATIVE COMPOSITION

Influenza virus surface antigens (haemagglutinin and neuraminidase)* of strains:

- A/California/7/2004 (H_3N_2)-like strain

(A/New York/55/2004 NYMC X-157 reass.) 15 micrograms**

- A/New Caledonia/20/99 (H_1N_1)-like strain

(A/New Caledonia/20/99 IVR-116 reass.) 15 micrograms

- B/Shanghai/361/2002-like strain

(B/Jiangsu/10/2003) 15 micrograms

per 0.5 ml dose.

* propagated in hens' eggs

** haemagglutinin

This vaccine complies with the WHO recommendation (northern hemisphere), and the decision of the EU for the 2005/2006 season.

For excipients, see 6.1.

3. PHARMACEUTICAL FORM
Suspension for injection in pre-filled syringes.

4. CLINICAL PARTICULARS

4.1 Therapeutic indications
Prophylaxis of influenza, especially in those who run an increased risk of associated complications.

4.2 Posology and method of administration
Adults and children from 36 months: 0.5 ml.

Children from 6 months to 35 months: Clinical data are limited; doses of 0.25 ml or 0.5 ml have been used.

For children who have not previously been vaccinated, a second dose should be given after an interval of at least 4 weeks.

Immunisation should be carried out by intramuscular or deep subcutaneous injection.

4.3 Contraindications
Hypersensitivity to the active substances, to any of the excipients and to eggs, chicken protein, formaldehyde, cetyltrimethylammonium bromide, polysorbate 80, or gentamicin.

Immunisation shall be postponed in patients with febrile illness or acute infection.

4.4 Special warnings and special precautions for use
As with all injectable vaccines, appropriate medical treatment and supervision should always be readily available in case of a rare anaphylactic event following the administration of the vaccine.

MASTAFLU should under no circumstances be administered intravascularly.

Antibody response in patients with endogenous or iatrogenic immunosuppression may be insufficient.

4.5 Interaction with other medicinal products and other forms of Interaction
MASTAFLU may be given at the same time as other vaccines. Immunisation should be carried out on separate limbs. It should be noted that the adverse reactions may be intensified.

The immunological response may be diminished if the patient is undergoing immunosuppressant treatment.

Following influenza vaccination, false positive results in serology tests using the ELISA method to detect antibodies against HIV1, Hepatitis C and especially HTLV1 have been observed. The Western Blot technique disproves the results. The transient false positive reactions could be due to the IgM response by the vaccine.

4.6 Pregnancy and lactation
Limited data from vaccinations in pregnant women do not indicate that adverse fetal and maternal outcomes were attributable to the vaccine. The use of this vaccine may be considered from the second trimester of pregnancy. For pregnant women with medical conditions that increase their risk of complications from influenza, administration of the vaccine is recommended, irrespective of their stage of pregnancy.

MASTAFLU may be used during lactation.

4.7 Effects on ability to drive and use machines
MASTAFLU is unlikely to produce an effect on the ability to drive and use machines.

4.8 Undesirable effects
Adverse events from clinical trials:

The safety of trivalent inactivated influenza vaccines is assessed in open label, uncontrolled clinical trials performed as annual update requirement, including at least 50 adults aged 18-60 and at least 50 elderly subjects aged 60 or older. Safety evaluation is performed during the first 3 days following vaccination.

Undesirable effects reported are listed according to the following frequency:

Adverse events from clinical trials:

Common >1/100, <1/10)

Local reactions: redness, swelling, pain, ecchymosis, induration.

Systemic reactions: fever, malaise, shivering, fatigue, headache, sweating, myalgia, arthralgia. These reactions usually disappear within 1-2 days without treatment.

From post-marketing surveillance additionally, the following adverse events have been reported:

Uncommon >1/1,000, <1/100)

Generalised skin reactions including pruritus, urticaria or non-specific rash.

Rare >1/10,000, <1/1,000)

Neuralgia, paraesthesia, convulsions, transient thrombocytopenia.

Allergic reactions, in rare cases leading to shock, have been reported.

Very rare (<1/10,000)

Vasculitis with transient renal involvement. Neurological disorders, such as encephalomyelitis, neuritis and Guillain Barré syndrome.

4.9 Overdose
Overdosage is unlikely to have any untoward effect.

5. PHARMACOLOGICAL PROPERTIES

5.1 Pharmacodynamic properties
Seroprotection is generally obtained within 2 to 3 weeks. The duration of postvaccinal immunity to homologous strains or to strains closely related to the vaccine strains varies but is usually 6-12 months.

5.2 Pharmacokinetic properties
Not applicable.

5.3 Preclinical safety data
Not applicable.

6. PHARMACEUTICAL PARTICULARS

6.1 List of excipients
Potassium chloride, potassium dihydrogen phosphate, disodium phosphate dihydrate, sodium chloride, calcium chloride, magnesium chloride hexahydrate and water for injections.

6.2 Incompatibilities
In the absence of compatibility studies, this medicinal product must not be mixed with other medicinal products.

6.3 Shelf life
1 year.

6.4 Special precautions for storage
MASTAFLU should be stored at +2°C to +8°C (in a refrigerator). Do not freeze. Protect from light.

6.5 Nature and contents of container
0.5 ml suspension for injection in pre-filled syringe (glass, type 1), pack of 1 or 10.

Not all pack sizes may be marketed.

6.6 Instructions for use and handling
MASTAFLU should be allowed to reach room temperature before use. Shake before use.

For administration of a 0.25 ml dose from a syringe, push the front side of the plunger exactly to the edge of the hub (the knurled polypropylene ring); a reproducible volume of vaccine remains in the syringe, suitable for administration.

7. MARKETING AUTHORISATION HOLDER
Solvay Healthcare Limited
Mansbridge Road
West End
Southampton
SO18 3JD

8. MARKETING AUTHORISATION NUMBER(S)
PL 00512/0170

9. DATE OF FIRST AUTHORISATION/RENEWAL OF THE AUTHORISATION
14 June 2000

10. DATE OF REVISION OF THE TEXT
22 August 2005

Legal category
POM

Maxalt 5mg, 10mg Tablets, Maxalt Melt 10mg Oral Lyophilisates

(Merck Sharp & Dohme Limited)

1. NAME OF THE MEDICINAL PRODUCT
MAXALT® 5 mg Tablets
MAXALT® 10 mg Tablets
MAXALT® Melt 10 mg oral lyophilisates

2. QUALITATIVE AND QUANTITATIVE COMPOSITION
Each tablet contains 7.265 mg of rizatriptan benzoate (corresponding to 5 mg of the rizatriptan).

Each tablet contains 14.53 mg of rizatriptan benzoate (corresponding to 10 mg of the rizatriptan).

Each oral lyophilisate contains 14.53 mg of rizatriptan benzoate (corresponding to 10 mg of the rizatriptan).

For excipients see 6.1.

3. PHARMACEUTICAL FORM
Tablets.

5 mg tablets are pale pink, capsule-shaped, coded MSD on one side and 266 on the other.

10 mg tablets are pale pink, capsule-shaped, coded MAXALT on one side and MSD 267 on the other.

Oral lyophilisates.

10 mg oral lyophilisates are white to off-white, round with a modified square on one side, with a peppermint flavour.

4. CLINICAL PARTICULARS

4.1 Therapeutic indications
Acute treatment of the headache phase of migraine attacks, with or without aura.

4.2 Posology and method of administration
General

'Maxalt' should not be used prophylactically.

The oral tablets should be swallowed whole with liquid.

Effects of food: The absorption of rizatriptan is delayed by approximately 1 hour when administered together with food. Therefore, onset of effect may be delayed when rizatriptan is administered in the fed state. (See also 5.2 'Pharmacokinetic properties', *Absorption*).

'Maxalt' Melt oral lyophilisates need not be taken with liquid.

The oral lyophilisate is packaged in a blister within an outer aluminium sachet. Patients should be instructed not to remove the blister from the outer sachet until just prior to dosing. The blister pack should then be peeled open with dry hands and the oral lyophilisate placed on the tongue, where it will dissolve and be swallowed with the saliva.

The oral lyophilisate can be used in situations in which liquids are not available, or to avoid the nausea and vomiting that may accompany the ingestion of tablets with liquids.

Adults 18 years of age and older

The recommended dose is 10 mg.

Redosing: doses should be separated by at least two hours; no more than two doses should be taken in any 24-hour period.

– *for headache recurrence within 24 hours*: if headache returns after relief of the initial attack, one further dose may be taken. The above dosing limits should be observed.

– *after non-response*: the effectiveness of a second dose for treatment of the same attack, when an initial dose is ineffective, has not been examined in controlled trials. Therefore, if a patient does not respond to the first dose, a second dose should not be taken for the same attack.

Clinical studies have shown that patients who do not respond to treatment of an attack are still likely to respond to treatment for subsequent attacks.

Some patients should receive the lower (5 mg) dose of 'Maxalt', in particular the following patient groups:

– patients on propranolol. Administration of rizatriptan should be separated by at least two hours from administration of propranolol. (See also 4.5 'Interaction with other medicinal products and other forms of interaction'.)

– patients with mild or moderate renal insufficiency,

– patients with mild to moderate hepatic insufficiency.

Doses should be separated by at least two hours; no more than two doses should be taken in any 24-hour period.

Paediatric patients

Children (under 12 years of age)

The use of 'Maxalt' in patients under 12 years of age is not recommended. There are no data available on the use of rizatriptan in children under 12 years of age.

Tablets: adolescents (12-17 years of age)

The use of 'Maxalt' Tablets in patients under 18 years of age is not recommended. In a placebo controlled study, the efficacy of 'Maxalt' Tablets (5 mg) was not superior to placebo. The efficacy of 'Maxalt' in patients under 18 years of age has not been established.

Oral lyophilisates: adolescents (12-17 years of age)

The use of 'Maxalt' Melt oral lyophilisates in patients under 18 years of age is not recommended. Safety and effectiveness of 'Maxalt' Melt oral lyophilisates in paediatric patients have not been evaluated.

Patients older than 65 years

The safety and effectiveness of rizatriptan in patients older than 65 years have not been systematically evaluated.

4.3 Contraindications
Hypersensitivity to rizatriptan or any of the ingredients.

Concurrent administration of monoamine oxidase (MAO) inhibitors or use within two weeks of discontinuation of MAO inhibitor therapy. (See 4.5 'Interaction with other medicinal products and other forms of interaction'.)

'Maxalt' is contraindicated in patients with severe hepatic or severe renal insufficiency.

'Maxalt' is contraindicated in patients with a previous cerebrovascular accident (CVA) or transient ischaemic attack (TIA).

Moderately severe or severe hypertension, or untreated mild hypertension.

Established coronary artery disease, including ischaemic heart disease (angina pectoris, history of myocardial infarction, or documented silent ischaemia), signs and symptoms of ischaemic heart disease, or Prinzmetal's angina.

Peripheral vascular disease.

Concomitant use of rizatriptan and ergotamine, ergot derivatives (including methysergide), or other $5\text{-HT}_{1B/1D}$ receptor agonists. (See also 4.5 'Interaction with other medicinal products and other forms of interaction').

4.4 Special warnings and special precautions for use
'Maxalt' should only be administered to patients in whom a clear diagnosis of migraine has been established. 'Maxalt' should not be administered to patients with basilar or hemiplegic migraine.

'Maxalt' should not be used to treat 'atypical' headaches, i.e. those that might be associated with potentially serious medical conditions, (e.g. CVA, ruptured aneurysm) in which cerebrovascular vasoconstriction could be harmful.

Rizatriptan can be associated with transient symptoms including chest pain and tightness which may be intense and involve the throat (see 4.8 'Undesirable effects'). Where such symptoms are thought to indicate ischaemic heart disease, no further dose should be taken and appropriate evaluation should be carried out.

As with other 5-$HT_{1B/1D}$ receptor agonists, rizatriptan should not be given, without prior evaluation, to patients in whom unrecognised cardiac disease is likely or to patients at risk for coronary artery disease (CAD) [e.g. patients with hypertension, diabetics, smokers or users of nicotine substitution therapy, men over 40 years of age, post-menopausal women, patients with bundle branch block, and those with strong family history for CAD]. Cardiac evaluations may not identify every patient who has cardiac disease and, in very rare cases, serious cardiac events have occurred in patients without underlying cardiovascular disease when 5-HT_1 agonists have been administered. Those in whom CAD is established should not be given 'Maxalt'. (See 4.3 'Contraindications'.)

5-$HT_{1B/1D}$ receptor agonists have been associated with coronary vasospasm. In rare cases, myocardial ischaemia or infarction have been reported with 5-$HT_{1B/1D}$ receptor agonists including 'Maxalt' (see 4.8 'Undesirable effects'.)

Other 5-$HT_{1B/1D}$ agonists, (e.g. sumatriptan) should not be used concomitantly with 'Maxalt'. (See also 4.5 'Interaction with other medicinal products and other forms of interaction').

It is advised to wait at least six hours following use of rizatriptan before administering ergotamine-type medications, (e.g. ergotamine, dihydro-ergotamine or methysergide). At least 24 hours should elapse after the administration of an ergotamine-containing preparation before rizatriptan is given. Although additive vasospastic effects were not observed in a clinical pharmacology study in which 16 healthy males received oral rizatriptan and parenteral ergotamine, such additive effects are theoretically possible, (see 4.3 'Contraindications'.)

Undesirable effects may be more common during concomitant use of triptans (5-$HT_{1B/1D}$ agonists) and herbal preparations containing St John's wort (Hypericum perforatum).

Angioedema (e.g. facial oedema, tongue swelling and pharyngeal oedema) may occur in patients treated with triptans, among which rizatriptan. If angioedema of the tongue or pharynx occurs, the patient should be placed under medical supervision until symptoms have resolved. Treatment should promptly be discontinued and replaced by an agent belonging to another class of drugs.

The quantity of lactose in each tablet (30.25 mg in the 5 mg tablet and 60.50 mg in the 10 mg tablet) is probably not sufficient to induce specific symptoms of lactose intolerance.

Phenylketonurics: Phenylketonuric patients should be informed that 'Maxalt' Melt oral lyophilisates contain phenylalanine (a component of aspartame). Each 10 mg oral lyophilisate contains 2.10 mg phenylalanine.

The potential for interaction should be considered when rizatriptan is administered to patients taking CYP 2D6 substrates (see 4.5 'Interaction with other medicinal products and other forms of interaction'.)

As with other acute migraine treatments, chronic daily headache/exacerbation of headache has been reported with overuse of rizatriptan, which may necessitate a drug withdrawal.

4.5 Interaction with other medicinal products and other forms of Interaction

Ergotamine, ergot derivatives (including methylsergide), other 5 HT $_{1B/1D}$ receptor agonists: Due to an additive effect, the concomitant use of rizatriptan and ergotamine, ergot derivatives (including methylsergide), or other 5 HT $_{1B/1D}$ receptor agonists (e.g. sumatriptan, zolmitriptan, naratriptan) increase the risk of coronary artery vasoconstriction and hypertensive effects. This combination is contraindicated (See also 4.2 'Contraindications').

Monoamine oxidase inhibitors: Rizatriptan is principally metabolised via monoamine oxidase, 'A' subtype (MAO-A). Plasma concentrations of rizatriptan and its active N-monodesmethyl metabolite were increased by concomitant administration of a selective, reversible MAO-A inhibitor. Similar or greater effects are expected with non-selective, reversible (e.g. linezolid) and irreversible MAO inhibitors. Due to a risk of coronary artery vasoconstriction and hypertensive episodes, administration of 'Maxalt' to patients taking inhibitors of MAO is contraindicated. (See 4.3 'Contraindications'.)

Beta-blockers: Plasma concentrations of rizatriptan may be increased by concomitant administration of propranolol. This increase is most probably due to first-pass metabolic interaction between the two drugs, since MAO-A plays a role in the metabolism of both rizatriptan and propranolol. This interaction leads to a mean increase in AUC and C_{max} of 70-80%. In patients receiving propranolol, the 5 mg dose of 'Maxalt' should be used. (See 4.2 also 'Posology and method of administration'.)

In a drug-interaction study, nadolol and metoprolol did not alter plasma concentrations of rizatriptan.

Selective serotonin-reuptake inhibitors (SSRIs): No pharmacodynamic or pharmacokinetic interactions were observed when rizatriptan was administered with paroxetine. However the theoretical possibility regarding the occurrence of a serotonin syndrome (weakness, hyperreflexia, co-ordination disturbances) in case of concomitant treatment with SSRIs cannot be ruled out.

In vitro studies indicate that rizatriptan inhibits cytochrome P450 2D6 (CYP 2D6). Clinical interaction data are not available. The potential for interaction should be considered when rizatriptan is administered to patients taking CYP 2D6 substrates.

4.6 Pregnancy and lactation

Use during pregnancy

The safety of rizatriptan for the use in human pregnancy has not been established. Animal studies do not indicate harmful effects at dose levels that exceed therapeutic dose levels with respect to the development of the embryo or foetus, or the course of gestation, parturition and postnatal development.

Because animal reproductive and developmental studies are not always predictive of human response, 'Maxalt' should be used during pregnancy only if clearly needed.

Use during lactation

Studies in rats indicated that very high milk transfer of rizatriptan occurred. Transient, very slight decreases in pre-weaning pup body weights were observed only when the mother's systemic exposure was well in excess of the maximum exposure level for humans. No data exist in humans.

Therefore, caution should be exercised when administering rizatriptan to women who are breast-feeding. Infant exposure should be minimised by avoiding breast-feeding for 24 hours after treatment.

4.7 Effects on ability to drive and use machines

Migraine or treatment with 'Maxalt' may cause somnolence in some patients. Dizziness has also been reported in some patients receiving 'Maxalt'. Patients should, therefore, evaluate their ability to perform complex tasks during migraine attacks and after administration of 'Maxalt'.

4.8 Undesirable effects

'Maxalt' (as the tablet and oral lyophilisate formulation) was evaluated in over 3,600 patients for up to one year in controlled clinical studies. The most common side effects evaluated in clinical studies were dizziness, somnolence, and asthenia/fatigue.

Additional side effects evaluated in clinical studies and reported in post-marketing experience include:

(*Common*: >1/100, <1/10], *Uncommon*: >1/1000, <1/100] and Rare: >1/10,000 <1/1,000]).

Nervous system and psychiatric disorders:

Common: paresthesia, headache, hypesthesia, decreased mental acuity, tremor.

Uncommon: ataxia, disorientation, insomnia, nervousness, vertigo.

Rare: syncope, dysgeusia/bad taste.

Eye disorders:

Uncommon: blurred vision.

Cardiac disorders:

Common: palpitation, tachycardia

Rare: Myocardial ischaemia or infarction, cerebrovascular accident. Most of these adverse reactions have been reported in patients with risk factors predictive of coronary artery disease.

Vascular disorders:

Common: hot flushes/flashes

Uncommon: hypertension.

Respiratory, thoracic and mediastinal disorders:

Common: pharyngeal discomfort, dyspnea

Rare: wheezing.

Gastrointestinal disorders:

Common: nausea, dry mouth, vomiting, diarrhoea

Uncommon: thirst, dyspepsia.

Skin and subcutaneous tissue disorders:

Common: flushing, sweating

Uncommon: pruritus, urticaria

Rare: angioedema (e.g. facial oedema, tongue swelling, pharyngeal oedema), rash, toxic epidermal necrolysis (for angioedema see also section 4.4 'Special warnings and precautions for use').

Musculoskeletal, connective tissue and bone disorders:

Common: regional heaviness

Uncommon: neck pain, regional tightness, stiffness, muscle weakness.

Rare: facial pain.

General disorders and administration site conditions:

Common: pain in abdomen or chest.

4.9 Overdose

Rizatriptan 40 mg (administered as either a single tablet dose or as two doses with a two-hour interdose interval) was generally well tolerated in over 300 patients; dizziness and somnolence were the most common drug-related adverse effects.

In a clinical pharmacology study in which 12 subjects received rizatriptan, at total cumulative doses of 80 mg (given within four hours), two subjects experienced syncope and/or bradycardia. One subject, a female aged 29 years, developed vomiting, bradycardia, and dizziness beginning three hours after receiving a total of 80 mg rizatriptan (administered over two hours). A third-degree AV block, responsive to atropine, was observed an hour after the onset of the other symptoms. The second subject, a 25 year-old male, experienced transient dizziness, syncope, incontinence, and a five-second systolic pause (on ECG monitor) immediately after a painful venipuncture. The venipuncture occurred two hours after the subject had received a total of 80 mg rizatriptan (administered over four hours).

In addition, based on the pharmacology of rizatriptan, hypertension or other more serious cardiovascular symptoms could occur after overdosage. Gastro-intestinal decontamination, (e.g. gastric lavage followed by activated charcoal) should be considered in patients suspected of an overdose with 'Maxalt'. Clinical and electrocardiographic monitoring should be continued for at least 12 hours, even if clinical symptoms are not observed.

The effects of haemo- or peritoneal dialysis on serum concentrations of rizatriptan are unknown.

5. PHARMACOLOGICAL PROPERTIES

5.1 Pharmacodynamic properties

Mechanism of action

ATC-code: N02C C04

Rizatriptan binds selectively with high affinity to human 5-HT_{1B} and 5-HT_{1D} receptors and has little or no effect or pharmacological activity at 5-HT_2, 5-HT_3; adrenergic $alpha_1$, $alpha_2$ or beta; D_1, D_2, dopaminergic, histaminic H_1; muscarinic; or benzodiazepine receptors.

The therapeutic activity of rizatriptan in treating migraine headache may be attributed to its agonist effects at 5-HT_{1B} and 5-HT_{1D} receptors on the extracerebral intracranial blood vessels that are thought to become dilated during an attack and on the trigeminal sensory nerves that innervate them. Activation of these 5-HT_{1B} and 5-HT_{1D} receptors may result in constriction of pain-producing intracranial blood vessels and inhibition of neuropeptide release that leads to decreased inflammation in sensitive tissues and reduced central trigeminal pain signal transmission.

Pharmacodynamic effects

Tablets

The efficacy of 'Maxalt' Tablets in the acute treatment of migraine attacks was established in four multicentre, placebo-controlled trials that included over 2,000 patients who received 'Maxalt' 5 or 10 mg for up to one year. Headache relief occurred as early as 30 minutes following dosing, and response rates, (i.e. reduction of moderate or severe headache pain to no or mild pain) two hours after treatment were 67-77% with the 10 mg tablet, 60-63% with the 5 mg tablet, and 23-40% with placebo. Although patients who did not respond to initial treatment with 'Maxalt' were not redosed for the same attack, they were still likely to respond to treatment for a subsequent attack. 'Maxalt' reduced the functional disability and relieved the nausea, photophobia, and phonophobia associated with migraine attacks.

'Maxalt' remains effective in treating menstrual migraine, i.e. migraine that occurs within 3 days before or after the onset of menses.

Oral lyophilisates

The efficacy of 'Maxalt' Melt oral lyophilisates in the acute treatment of migraine attacks was established in two multicentre, randomised, placebo-controlled trials that were similar in design to the trials of 'Maxalt' Tablets. In one study (n=311), by two hours post-dosing, relief rates in patients treated with 'Maxalt' Melt oral lyophilisates were approximately 66% for rizatriptan 5 mg and 10 mg, compared to 47% in the placebo group. In a larger study (n=547), by two hours post-dosing, relief rates were 59% in patients treated with 'Maxalt' Melt oral lyophilisates 5 mg, and 74% after 10 mg, compared to 28% in the placebo group. 'Maxalt' Melt oral lyophilisates also relieved the disability, nausea, photophobia, and phonophobia which accompanied the migraine episodes. A significant effect on pain relief was observed as early as 30 minutes post-dosing in one of the two clinical trials for the 10 mg dose (see also 5.2 'Pharmacokinetic properties', *Absorption*).

Based on studies with the oral tablet, rizatriptan remains effective in treating menstrual migraine, i.e. migraine that occurs within 3 days before or after the onset of menses.

'Maxalt' Melt oral lyophilisates enables migraine patients to treat their migraine attacks without having to swallow liquids. This may allow patients to administer their medication earlier, for example, when liquids are not available, and to avoid possible worsening of GI symptoms by swallowing liquids.

5.2 Pharmacokinetic properties

Absorption

Rizatriptan is rapidly and completely absorbed following oral administration.

Tablets: The mean oral bioavailability of the tablet is approximately 40-45%, and mean peak plasma concentrations (C_{max}) are reached in approximately 1-1.5 hours (T_{max}). Administration of an oral tablet dose with a high-fat breakfast had no effect on the extent of rizatriptan absorption, but absorption was delayed for approximately one hour.

Oral lyophilisates: The mean oral bioavailability of the oral lyophilisate is approximately 40-45%, and mean peak plasma concentrations (C_{max}) are reached in approximately 1.6-2.5 hours (T_{max}). The time to maximum plasma concentration following administration of rizatriptan as the oral lyophilisate formulation is delayed by 30-60 minutes relative to the tablet.

Effect of food: The effect of food on the absorption of rizatriptan from the oral lyophilisate has not been studied. For the rizatriptan tablets, T_{max} is delayed by approximately 1 hour when the tablets are administered in the fed state. A further delay in the absorption of rizatriptan may occur when the oral lyophilisate is administered after meals. (See also 4.2 'Posology and method of administration').

Distribution

Rizatriptan is minimally bound (14%) to plasma proteins. The volume of distribution is approximately 140 litres in male subjects, and 110 litres in female subjects.

Biotransformation

The primary route of rizatriptan metabolism is via oxidative deamination by monoamine oxidase-A (MAO-A) to the indole acetic acid metabolite, which is not pharmacologically active. N-monodesmethyl-rizatriptan, a metabolite with activity similar to that of parent compound at the 5-$HT_{1B/1D}$ receptor, is formed to a minor degree, but does not contribute significantly to the pharmacodynamic activity of rizatriptan. Plasma concentrations of N-monodesmethyl-rizatriptan are approximately 14% of those of parent compound, and it is eliminated at a similar rate. Other minor metabolites include the N-oxide, the 6-hydroxy compound, and the sulphate conjugate of the 6-hydroxy metabolite. None of these minor metabolites is pharmacologically active. Following oral administration of ^{14}C-labelled rizatriptan, rizatriptan accounts for about 17% of circulating plasma radioactivity.

Elimination

Following intravenous administration, AUC in men increases proportionally and in women near-proportionally with the dose over a dose range of 10-60 mcg/kg. Following oral administration, AUC increases near-proportionally with the dose over a dose range of 2.5-10 mg. The plasma half-life of rizatriptan in males and females averages 2-3 hours. The plasma clearance of rizatriptan averages about 1,000-1,500 ml/min in males and about 900-1,100 ml/min in females; about 20-30% of this is renal clearance. Following an oral dose of ^{14}C-labelled rizatriptan, about 80% of the radioactivity is excreted in urine, and about 10% of the dose is excreted in faeces. This shows that the metabolites are excreted primarily via the kidneys.

Consistent with its first pass metabolism, approximately 14% of an oral dose is excreted in urine as unchanged rizatriptan while 51% is excreted as indole acetic acid metabolite. No more than 1% is excreted in urine as the active N-monodesmethyl metabolite.

If rizatriptan is administered according to the maximum dosage regimen, no drug accumulation in the plasma occurs from day to day.

Characteristics in patients

The following data are based on studies with the oral tablet formulation.

Patients with a migraine attack: A migraine attack does not affect the pharmacokinetics of rizatriptan.

Gender: The AUC of rizatriptan (10 mg orally) was about 25% lower in males as compared to females, C_{max} was 11% lower, and T_{max} occurred at approximately the same time. This apparent pharmacokinetic difference was of no clinical significance.

Elderly: The plasma concentrations of rizatriptan observed in elderly subjects (age range 65 to 77 years) after tablet administration were similar to those observed in young adults.

Hepatic impairment (Child-Pugh's score 5-6): Following oral tablet administration in patients with hepatic impairment caused by mild alcoholic cirrhosis of the liver, plasma concentrations of rizatriptan were similar to those seen in young male and female subjects. A significant increase in AUC (50%) and C_{max} (25%) was observed in patients with moderate hepatic impairment (Child-Pugh's score 7). Pharmacokinetics were not studied in patients with Child-Pugh's score >7 (severe hepatic impairment).

Renal impairment: In patients with renal impairment (creatinine clearance 10-60 ml/min/1.73 m^2), the AUC of rizatriptan after tablet administration was not significantly different from that in healthy subjects. In haemodialysis patients (creatinine clearance <10 ml/min/1.73 m^2), the AUC for rizatriptan was approximately 44% greater than that in patients with normal renal function. The maximal plasma concentration of rizatriptan in patients with all degrees of renal impairment was similar to that in healthy subjects.

5.3 Preclinical safety data

Preclinical data indicate no risk for humans based on conventional studies of repeat dose toxicity, genotoxicity, carcinogenic potential, reproductive and developmental toxicity, safety pharmacology, and pharmacokinetics and metabolism.

6. PHARMACEUTICAL PARTICULARS

6.1 List of excipients

Tablets: Lactose monohydrate, microcrystalline cellulose, pregelatinised corn starch, ferric oxide red (E 172), and magnesium stearate.

Oral lyophilisates: Gelatin, mannitol, glycine, aspartame, and peppermint flavour (peppermint oil and maltodextrin).

6.2 Incompatibilities

Not applicable.

6.3 Shelf life

3 years.

6.4 Special precautions for storage

Do not store above 30°C.

6.5 Nature and contents of container

5 mg tablets:

All aluminium blister push through, packs with 6 tablets.

10 mg tablets:

All aluminium blister push through, packs with 3 or 6 tablets.

10 mg oral lyophilisates:

PVC/PVDC blister with one oral lyophilisate within an aluminium sachet. Packs with 3 or 6 oral lyophilisates.

6.6 Instructions for use and handling

No special requirements.

7. MARKETING AUTHORISATION HOLDER

Merck Sharp & Dohme Limited

Hertford Road, Hoddesdon, Hertfordshire EN11 9BU, UK

8. MARKETING AUTHORISATION NUMBER(S)

Tablet 5 mg PL 0025/0369

Tablet 10 mg PL 0025/0370

Oral lyophilisate 10 mg PL 0025/0372

9. DATE OF FIRST AUTHORISATION/RENEWAL OF THE AUTHORISATION

Date first authorised: June 1998.

Date last renewed: 11 February 2003.

10. DATE OF REVISION OF THE TEXT

April 2003

LEGAL CATEGORY

POM

® denotes registered trademark of Merck & Co., Inc., Whitehouse Station, NJ, USA.

SPC.MXT/M.03.UK.0876(N01) FT 190104

Maxolon High Dose

(Shire Pharmaceuticals Limited)

1. NAME OF THE MEDICINAL PRODUCT

Maxolon® High Dose

2. QUALITATIVE AND QUANTITATIVE COMPOSITION

Each 20ml ampoule contains Metoclopramide Hydrochloride BP equivalent to 100mg of the anhydrous substance.

3. PHARMACEUTICAL FORM

Clear colourless solution for intravenous infusion.

4. CLINICAL PARTICULARS

4.1 Therapeutic indications

Maxolon High Dose is indicated for the treatment of nausea and vomiting associated with intolerance to cytotoxic drugs.

4.2 Posology and method of administration

Maxolon High Dose is administered by IV infusion, suitably diluted. The recommended method of administration is by continuous infusion which allows steady serum levels of metoclopramide to be maintained.

Continuous infusion (recommended method):

Maxolon High Dose is given by IV infusion as a loading dose followed by a continuous infusion to maintain a metoclopramide serum concentration of 0.85μg - 1.0μg/ml. The loading dose should be given before starting cytotoxic chemotherapy.

(see Table 1 below)

Total dosage in any 24 hour period should not normally exceed 10 mg/kg body weight.

Where cisplatin is to be used the loading dose of Maxolon High Dose should be at least 3 mg/kg body weight and the maintenance dose at least 4 mg/kg body weight.

Intermittent Infusion (alternative regimen):

Maxolon High Dose can be given by intermittent IV infusion suitably diluted.

The initial dose should be given before starting cytotoxic chemotherapy.

(see Table 2 below)

Total dosage in any 24 hour period should not normally exceed 10 mg/kg body weight.

Abnormal renal or hepatic function:

In patients with clinically significant degrees of renal or hepatic impairment, therapy should be at reduced dosage. Metoclopramide is metabolised in the liver and the predominant route of elimination of metoclopramide and its metabolites is via the kidney.

Compatibility with cytotoxic agents:

Maxolon High Dose is compatible with a number of cytotoxic drugs; however it should not be mixed in solution with therapeutic agents other than those stated. Maxolon High Dose is compatible with cisplatin, cyclophosphamide and doxorubicin hydrochloride and is stable over the concentration ranges listed below for 24 hours at room temperature when protected from light.

40-200 ml cisplatin (1 mg/ml) per 100 mg/20 ml of Maxolon High Dose in 1 litre of sodium chloride 0.9%.

Up to 40 mg doxorubicin hydrochloride (powder) per 100 mg/20 ml of Maxolon High Dose.

Up to 4 g cyclophosphamide (1 g/50 ml) per 100 mg/20 ml of Maxolon High Dose.

Compatibility with morphine/diamorphine:

Maxolon High Dose is compatible with morphine hydrochloride and diamorphine hydrochloride and is stable over the concentration ranges listed below for 48 hours at room temperature under normal fluorescent lighting.

Up to 100 mg of morphine hydrochloride per 100 mg/20 ml of Maxolon High Dose.

Up to 50 mg of diamorphine hydrochloride per 100 mg/20 ml of Maxolon High Dose.

Maxolon High Dose 100 mg/20 ml also remains stable for 48 hours at room temperature with 100 mg of morphine hydrochloride, or 50 mg diamorphine hydrochloride, when diluted 1 in 10 with sodium chloride 0.9%.

Stability in intravenous fluids:

Ideally intravenous solutions should be prepared at the time of infusion. However, Maxolon High Dose has been shown to be stable for at least 48 hours at room temperature in the following solutions when administered in a PVC infusion bag (e.g. Viaflex[R] Travenol).

Sodium chloride intravenous infusion BP (0.9% w/v)

Glucose intravenous infusion BP (5% w/v)

Sodium chloride and glucose intravenous infusion BP (sodium chloride 0.18% w/v; glucose 4% w/v)

Compound sodium lactate intravenous infusion BP (ringer-lactate solution; Hartmann's solution)

Note: preparation must be under appropriate aseptic conditions if the above extended storage periods are required. The high dose ampoule presentation is not suitable for multidose use.

Elderly patients:

As for adults. To avoid adverse reactions adhere strictly to dosage recommendations.

Young adults and children:

Maxolon should only be used after careful examination to avoid masking an underlying disorder, e.g. cerebral irritation. In the dosage of this patient group attention should be given primarily to body weight.

4.3 Contraindications

Maxolon should not be used in patients with phaeochromocytoma as it may induce an acute hypertensive response.

Maxolon should not be used during the first three to four days following operations such as pyloroplasty or gut anastomosis as vigorous muscular contractions may not help healing.

Maxolon should not be administered to patients with gastrointestinal obstruction, perforation or haemorrhage.

Table 1

	Maxolon High Dose	Volume of Diluent	IV Infusion Time
Loading dose	2-4 mg/kg body weight	50-100 ml	15-20 minutes
Maintenance dose	3-5 mg/kg body weight	500 ml	8-12 hours

Table 2

	Maxolon High Dose	Volume of Diluent	IV Infusion Time
Initial dose	Up to 2 mg/kg body weight	at least 50 ml	at least 15 minutes
Repeat doses at 2 hourly intervals	Up to 2 mg/kg body weight	at least 50 ml	at least 15 minutes

Maxolon is contra-indicated in patients who have previously shown hypersensitivity to metoclopramide or any of its components.

4.4 Special warnings and special precautions for use

Precautions

Care should be exercised in epileptic patients and patients being treated with other centrally acting drugs.

Since extrapyramidal symptoms may occur with both metoclopramide and neuroleptics such as the phenothiazines, particular care should be exercised in the event of these drugs being prescribed concurrently.

The neuroleptic malignant syndrome has been reported with metoclopramide in combination with neuroleptics as well as with metoclopramide monotherapy (see section 4.8 Undesirable effects).

Special care should be taken in cases of severe renal and hepatic insufficiency (see also section 4.2 Posology and method of administration).

Care should be exercised when using Maxolon in patients with porphyria.

4.5 Interaction with other medicinal products and other forms of Interaction

The action of Maxolon on the gastro-intestinal tract is antagonised by Anticholinergics and Opioid Analgesics.

The absorption of any concurrently administered oral medication may be modified by the effect of Maxolon on gastric motility. Drugs known to be affected in this way include aspirin and paracetamol.

Since extrapyramidal reactions may occur with Maxolon, Phenothiazines and Tetrabenazine, care should be exercised in the event of co-administration of these drugs.

Maxolon should be used with care in association with other drugs acting at central dopamine receptors, such as levodopa, bromocriptine and pergolide.

Maxolon may reduce plasma concentrations of atovaquone.

4.6 Pregnancy and lactation

Animal tests in several mammalian species and clinical experience have not indicated a teratogenic effect. Nevertheless Maxolon should only be used when there are compelling reasons and is not advised during the first trimester.

During lactation metoclopramide is found in breast milk, therefore it should not be used during lactation.

4.7 Effects on ability to drive and use machines

None but see 4.8.

4.8 Undesirable effects

When given at high dose in association with cancer chemotherapy, Maxolon has been found to be well tolerated with few adverse events. Various extrapyramidal reactions to Maxolon, usually of the dystonic type, have been reported. Studies of Maxolon given in doses up to 10mg/kg body weight/day by IV infusion report an incidence of extrapyramidal reactions of less than 10%. The incidence of such reactions may be increased in the younger patient. Reactions to Maxolon have included spasm of the facial muscles, trismus, rhythmic protrusion of the tongue, a bulbar type of speech, spasm of extra-ocular muscles including oculogyric crises, unnatural positioning of the head and shoulders and opisthotonos. There may be a generalised increase in muscle tone. The majority of reactions occur within 36 hours of starting treatment and the effects usually disappear within 24 hours of withdrawal of the drug. Should treatment of a dystonic reaction be required an anticholinergic anti-Parkinsonian drug, or a benzodiazepine may be used.

Very rare occurrences of the neuroleptic malignant syndrome have been reported. This syndrome is potentially fatal and comprises hyperpyrexia, altered consciousness, muscle rigidity, autonomic instability and elevated levels of creatine phosphokinase (CPK) and must be treated urgently (recognised treatments include dantrolene and bromocriptine). Metoclopramide should be stopped immediately if this syndrome occurs.

There have been very rare reports of abnormalities of cardiac conduction (such as bradycardia and heart block) in association with intravenous metoclopramide.

Mild drowsiness, confusion and diarrhoea have been noted. Depression has been reported extremely rarely.

Raised serum prolactin levels have been observed during metoclopramide therapy: this may result in galactorrhoea, irregular periods and gynaecomastia.

Extremely rarely cases of red cell disorders such as methaemoglobinaemia and sulphaemoglobinaemia have been reported, particularly at high doses of metoclopramide. If this occurs the drug should be withdrawn. Methaemoglobinaemia may be treated using methylene blue.

A small number of skin reactions such as rashes, urticaria, pruritus and oedema have also been reported.

4.9 Overdose

In cases of overdosage, acute dystonic reactions have occurred. Very rarely AV block has been observed. Should treatment of a dystonic reaction be required, an anticholinergic anti-Parkinsonian drug or a benzodiazepine may be used.

5. PHARMACOLOGICAL PROPERTIES

5.1 Pharmacodynamic properties

Maxolon High Dose is indicated for the treatment of nausea and vomiting associated with intolerance to cytotoxic drugs. It is specially formulated to ensure compatibility in solution with cisplatin.

Maxolon exerts a three-fold anti-emetic action: by inhibiting central dopamine receptors Maxolon raises the threshold of the chemoreceptor trigger zone, and reduces the reaction of the adjacent vomiting centre to centrally-acting emetics. Maxolon decreases the sensitivity of the visceral afferent nerves to the vomiting centre, reducing the effect of locally-acting emetics and irritant substances. In the upper gastro-intestinal tract Maxolon promotes normal gastric emptying and it may thus abolish gastric stasis which is part of the vomiting reflex.

Maxolon High Dose is not intended for use in the wider range of indications for which Maxolon at standard dose is indicated.

5.2 Pharmacokinetic properties

Based on current literature, a metoclopramide concentration range of about 0.85 μg/ml would appear desirable for the control of cytotoxic drug induced emesis. Such plasma concentrations may be achieved by the administration of a loading dose of 2-4 mg/kg infused over 15-30 minutes prior to cytotoxic drug therapy followed by a maintenance continuous infusion of 3-5 mg/kg over 8-12 hours.

Metoclopramide is metabolised in the liver and the predominant route of elimination of metoclopramide and its metabolites is via the kidney. In patients with clinically significant degrees of renal or hepatic impairment, therapy should be at reduced dosage.

5.3 Preclinical safety data

No additional data available.

6. PHARMACEUTICAL PARTICULARS

6.1 List of excipients

Sodium chloride

Water for injections.

6.2 Incompatibilities

Not applicable.

6.3 Shelf life

Thirty six months.

6.4 Special precautions for storage

If ampoules are removed from their carton, they should be stored away from light. If inadvertent exposure occurs, ampoules showing discolouration must be discarded.

6.5 Nature and contents of container

Clear glass 20 ml ampoules (Ph. Eur. Type I neutral glass) packed in boxes of 10.

6.6 Instructions for use and handling

Protect from light.

7. MARKETING AUTHORISATION HOLDER

Monmouth Pharmaceuticals Limited

Hampshire International Business Park

Chineham

Basingstoke

Hampshire RG24 8EP

United Kingdom

8. MARKETING AUTHORISATION NUMBER(S)

PL 10536/0035

9. DATE OF FIRST AUTHORISATION/RENEWAL OF THE AUTHORISATION

16 June 1995

10. DATE OF REVISION OF THE TEXT

March 2001

LEGAL CATEGORY

POM

Maxolon Injection

(Shire Pharmaceuticals Limited)

1. NAME OF THE MEDICINAL PRODUCT

Maxolon™ Injection

2. QUALITATIVE AND QUANTITATIVE COMPOSITION

Each 2ml ampoule contains Metoclopramide Hydrochloride BP equivalent to 10mg of the anhydrous substance.

3. PHARMACEUTICAL FORM

Clear colourless solution for intramuscular or intravenous administration.

4. CLINICAL PARTICULARS

4.1 Therapeutic indications

Adults (20 years and over)

Digestive disorders:

Maxolon restores normal co-ordination and tone to the upper digestive tract.

Maxolon relieves the symptoms of gastro-duodenal dysfunction including:

Dyspepsia	Heartburn
Flatulence	Sickness
Regurgitation of bile	Pain

These symptoms may be associated with such conditions as:

Peptic ulcer	Duodenitis
Reflux oesophagitis	Hiatus hernia
Gastritis	Cholelithiasis and Post-cholecystectomy dyspepsia

Nausea and vomiting:

Maxolon is indicated for the treatment of the nausea and vomiting associated with:

Gastro-intestinal disorders

Cyclical vomiting

Intolerance to cytotoxic drugs

Congestive heart failure

Deep x-ray or cobalt therapy

Post-anaesthetic vomiting

Migraine:

Maxolon relieves symptoms of nausea and vomiting, and overcomes gastric stasis associated with attacks of migraine. This improvement in gastric emptying assists the absorption of concurrently administered oral anti-migraine therapy (e.g. paracetamol) which may otherwise be impaired in such patients.

Post-operative conditions:

Post-operative gastric hypotonia

Post-vagotomy syndrome

Maxolon promotes normal gastric emptying and restores motility in vagotomised patients, and where post-operative symptoms suggest gastro-duodenal dysfunction.

Diagnostic procedures:

Radiology

Duodenal intubation

Maxolon speeds up the passage of a barium meal by decreasing gastric emptying time, co-ordinating peristalsis and dilating the duodenal bulb. Maxolon also facilitates duodenal intubation procedures.

Young adults and children

The use of Maxolon in patients under 20 years should be restricted to the following:

Severe intractable vomiting of known cause, vomiting associated with radiotherapy and intolerance to cytotoxic drugs, as an aid to gastro-intestinal intubation, and as part of the premedication before surgical procedures.

4.2 Posology and method of administration

Route of administration:

Maxolon injection may be administered either intramuscularly or by slow intravenous injection (1-2 minutes).

The dosage recommendations given below should be strictly adhered to if side effects of the dystonic type are to be avoided. It should be noted that total daily dosage of Maxolon, especially for children and young adults, should not normally exceed 0.5 mg/kg body weight.

In patients with clinically significant degrees of renal or hepatic impairment, therapy should be at reduced dosage. Metoclopramide is metabolised in the liver and the predominant route of elimination of metoclopramide and its metabolites is via the kidney.

Medical indications:

Adults 20 years and over: 10mg three times daily.

For patients of less than 60 kg see below.

Elderly patients:

As for adults. To avoid adverse reactions adhere strictly to dosage recommendations and where prolonged therapy is considered necessary, patients should be regularly reviewed.

Young adults and children:

Maxolon should only be used after careful examination to avoid masking an underlying disorder, e.g. cerebral irritation. In the treatment of this group attention should be given primarily to body weight and treatment should commence at the lower dosage where stated.

Young adults:	15-19 years, 60 kg and over	10mg three times daily
	30-59kg	5mg three times daily
Children:	9-14 years, 30 kg and over	5mg three times daily
	5-9 years, 20-29 kg	2½mg three times daily
	3-5 years, 15-19 kg	2mg two to three times daily
	1-3 years, 10-14 kg	1mg two to three times daily
	Under 1 year up to 10kg	1mg twice daily

Diagnostic indications:
A single dose of Maxolon may be given 5-10 minutes before the examination. Subject to body weight consideration, (see above), the following dosages are recommended.

Adults:	20 years and over	10-20mg
Young adults:	15-19 years	10mg
Children:	9-14 years	5mg
	5-9 years	2½mg
	3-5 years	2mg
	Under 3 years	1mg

4.3 Contraindications
Maxolon should not be used in patients with phaeochromocytoma as it may induce an acute hypertensive response.

Maxolon should not be used during the first three to four days following operations such as pyloroplasty or gut anastomosis as vigorous muscular contractions may not help healing.

Maxolon should not be administered to patients with gastrointestinal obstruction, perforation or haemorrhage.

Maxolon is contra-indicated in patients who have previously shown hypersensitivity to metoclopramide or any of its components.

4.4 Special warnings and special precautions for use
Precautions:

If vomiting persists the patient should be reassessed to exclude the possibility of an underlying disorder e.g. cerebral irritation.

Care should be exercised in epileptic patients and patients being treated with other centrally acting drugs.

Since extrapyramidal symptoms may occur with both metoclopramide and neuroleptics such as the phenothiazines, particular care should be exercised in the event of these drugs being prescribed concurrently.

The neuroleptic malignant syndrome has been reported with metoclopramide in combination with neuroleptics as well as with metoclopramide monotherapy (see section 4.8 Undesirable effects).

Special care should be taken in cases of severe renal and hepatic insufficiency (see also section 4.2 Posology and method of administration).

Care should be exercised when using Maxolon in patients with porphyria.

4.5 Interaction with other medicinal products and other forms of Interaction
The action of Maxolon on the gastro-intestinal tract is antagonised by anticholinergics and opioid analgesics. The absorption of any concurrently administered oral medication may be modified by the effect of Maxolon on gastric motility. Drugs known to be affected in this way include aspirin and paracetamol.

Since extrapyramidal reactions may occur with Maxolon, Phenothiazines and Tetrabenazine, care should be exercised in the event of co-administration of these drugs.

Maxolon should be used with care in association with other drugs acting at central dopamine receptors, such as levodopa, bromocriptine and pergolide.

Maxolon may reduce plasma concentrations of atovaquone.

4.6 Pregnancy and lactation
Animal tests in several mammalian species and clinical experience have not indicated a teratogenic effect. Nevertheless Maxolon should only be used when there are compelling reasons and is not advised during the first trimester.

During lactation metoclopramide is found in breast milk, therefore it should not be used during lactation.

4.7 Effects on ability to drive and use machines
None but see 4.8.

4.8 Undesirable effects
Various extrapyramidal reactions to Maxolon, usually of the dystonic type, have been reported. The incidence of dystonic reactions, particularly in children and young adults, is increased if daily dosages higher than 0.5mg per kg body weight are administered. Dystonic reactions include: spasm of the facial muscles, trismus, rhythmic protrusion of the tongue, a bulbar type of speech, spasm of extra-ocular muscles including oculogyric crises, unnatural positioning of the head and shoulders and opisthotonos. There may be a generalised increase in muscle tone. The majority of reactions occur within 36 hours of starting treatment and the effects usually disappear within 24 hours of withdrawal of the drug. Should treatment of a dystonic reaction be required an anticholinergic anti-Parkinsonian drug, or a benzodiazepine may be used.

Very rare occurrences of the neuroleptic malignant syndrome have been reported. This syndrome is potentially fatal and comprises hyperpyrexia, altered consciousness, muscle rigidity, autonomic instability and elevated levels of creatine phosphokinase (CPK) and must be treated urgently (recognised treatments include dantrolene and bromocriptine). Metoclopramide should be stopped immediately if this syndrome occurs.

There have been very rare reports of abnormalities of cardiac conduction (such as bradycardia and heart block) in association with intravenous metoclopramide.

Tardive dyskinesia has been reported during prolonged treatment in a small number of mainly elderly patients. Patients on prolonged treatment should be regularly reviewed.

Rarely, drowsiness, restlessness, confusion and diarrhoea have been reported in patients receiving metoclopramide therapy. Depression has been reported extremely rarely.

Raised serum prolactin levels have been observed during metoclopramide therapy: this may result in galactorrhoea, irregular periods and gynaecomastia.

Extremely rarely cases of red cell disorders such as methaemoglobinaemia and sulphaemoglobinaemia have been reported, particularly at high doses of metoclopramide. If this occurs the drug should be withdrawn. Methaemoglobinaemia may be treated using methylene blue.

A small number of skin reactions such as rashes, urticaria, pruritus and oedema have also been reported.

4.9 Overdose
In cases of overdosage, acute dystonic reactions have occurred. Very rarely AV block has been observed. Should treatment of a dystonic reaction be required, an anticholinergic anti-Parkinsonian drug or a benzodiazepine may be used.

5. PHARMACOLOGICAL PROPERTIES

5.1 Pharmacodynamic properties
The action of metoclopramide is closely associated with parasympathetic nervous control of the upper gastro-intestinal tract, where it has the effect of encouraging normal peristaltic action. This provides for a fundamental approach to the control of those conditions where disturbed gastro-intestinal motility is a common underlying factor.

5.2 Pharmacokinetic properties
Metoclopramide is metabolised in the liver and the predominant route of elimination of metoclopramide and its metabolites is via the kidney.

5.3 Preclinical safety data
No additional data available.

6. PHARMACEUTICAL PARTICULARS

6.1 List of excipients
Sodium chloride, Sodium metabisulphite, Water for injection.

6.2 Incompatibilities
Not applicable.

6.3 Shelf life
Sixty months.

6.4 Special precautions for storage
Do not store above 25°C. If ampoules are removed from their carton, they should be stored away from light. If inadvertent exposure occurs, ampoules showing discolouration must be discarded.

6.5 Nature and contents of container
Clear glass 2ml ampoules (Ph. Eur. Type I neutral glass) in packs of 12 ampoules.

6.6 Instructions for use and handling
Protect from light.

7. MARKETING AUTHORISATION HOLDER
Monmouth Pharmaceuticals Limited
Hampshire International Business Park
Chineham
Basingstoke
Hampshire RG24 8EP
United Kingdom

8. MARKETING AUTHORISATION NUMBER(S)
PL 10536/0034

9. DATE OF FIRST AUTHORISATION/RENEWAL OF THE AUTHORISATION
16 June 1995

10. DATE OF REVISION OF THE TEXT
March 2001

LEGAL CATEGORY
POM

Maxolon Paediatric Liquid

(Shire Pharmaceuticals Limited)

1. NAME OF THE MEDICINAL PRODUCT
Maxolon™ Paediatric Liquid

2. QUALITATIVE AND QUANTITATIVE COMPOSITION
The liquid contains Metoclopramide Hydrocloride BP equivalent to 1mg/ml of the anhydrous substance.

3. PHARMACEUTICAL FORM
Clear colourless lemon-lime flavoured solution.

4. CLINICAL PARTICULARS

4.1 Therapeutic indications
Young adults and children
The use of Maxolon in patients under 20 years should be restricted to the following:

Severe intractable vomiting of known cause, vomiting associated with radiotherapy and intolerance to cytotoxic drugs, as an aid to gastro-intestinal intubation, and as part of the premedication before surgical procedures.

4.2 Posology and method of administration
Route of administration:
Oral

The dosage recommendations given below should be strictly adhered to if side effects of the dystonic type are to be avoided. It should be noted that total daily dosage of Maxolon, especially for children and young adults, should not normally exceed 0.5 mg/kg body weight.

In patients with clinically significant degrees of renal or hepatic impairment, therapy should be at reduced dosage. Metoclopramide is metabolised in the liver and the predominant route of elimination of metoclopramide and its metabolites is via the kidney.

Medical indications:
Young adults and children:

Maxolon should only be used after careful examination to avoid masking an underlying disorder, e.g. cerebral irritation. In the treatment of this group attention should be given primarily to body weight and treatment should commence at the lower dosage where stated.

Young adults:	15-19 years, 60 kg and over	10mg three times daily
	30-59 kg	5mg three times daily
Children:	9-14 years, 30 kg and over	5mg three times daily
	5-9 years, 20-29 kg	2½mg three times daily
	3-5 years, 15-19 kg	2mg two to three times daily
	1-3 years, 10-14 kg	1mg two to three times daily
	Under 1 year up to 10 kg	1mg twice daily

Tablets should not be used in children under the age of 15. A liquid presentation should be used in the younger age groups; more accurate dosage is facilitated by the use of the Paediatric Liquid.

Diagnostic indications:
A single dose of Maxolon may be given 5-10 minutes before the examination subject to body weight consideration (see above), the following dosages are recommended.

Young adults:	15-19 years	10mg
Children:	9-14 years	5mg
	5-9 years	2½mg
	3-5 years	2mg
	Under 3 years	1mg

A liquid presentation should be used in the younger age groups; more accurate dosage is facilitated by the use of the Paediatric liquid.

4.3 Contraindications
Maxolon should not be used in patients with phaeochromocytoma as it may induce an acute hypertensive response.

Maxolon should not be used during the first three to four days following operations such as pyloroplasty or gut anastomosis as vigorous muscular contractions may not help healing.

Maxolon should not be administered to patients with gastrointestinal obstruction, perforation or haemorrhage.

Maxolon is contra-indicated in patients who have previously shown hypersensitivity to metoclopramide or any of its components.

4.4 Special warnings and special precautions for use
Precautions:

If vomiting persists the patient should be reassessed to exclude the possibility of an underlying disorder e.g. cerebral irritation.

Care should be exercised in epileptic patients and patients being treated with other centrally acting drugs.

Since extrapyramidal symptoms may occur with both metoclopramide and neuroleptics such as the phenothiazines, particular care should be exercised in the event of these drugs being prescribed concurrently.

The neuroleptic malignant syndrome has been reported with metoclopramide in combination with neuroleptics as well as with metoclopramide monotherapy (see section 4.8 Undesirable effects).

Special care should be taken in cases of severe renal or hepatic insufficiency (see also section 4.2 Posology and method of administration).

Care should be exercised when using Maxolon in patients with porphyria.

4.5 Interaction with other medicinal products and other forms of Interaction
The action of Maxolon on the gastro-intestinal tract is antagonised by anticholinergics and opioid analgesics. The absorption of any concurrently administered oral medication may be modified by the effect of Maxolon on gastric motility. Drugs known to be affected in this way include aspirin and paracetamol.

Since extrapyramidal reactions may occur with Maxolon, Phenothiazines and Tetrabenazine, care should be exercised in the event of co-administration of these drugs.

Maxolon should be used with care in association with other drugs acting at central dopamine receptors, such as levodopa, bromocriptine and pergolide.

Maxolon may reduce plasma concentrations of atovaquone.

4.6 Pregnancy and lactation
Animal tests in several mammalian species and clinical experience have not indicated a teratogenic effect. Nevertheless Maxolon should only be used when there are compelling reasons and is not advised during the first trimester.

During lactation metoclopramide is found in breast milk, therefore it should not be used during lactation.

4.7 Effects on ability to drive and use machines
None but see 4.8.

4.8 Undesirable effects
Various extrapyramidal reactions to Maxolon, usually of the dystonic type, have been reported. The incidence of dystonic reactions, particularly in children and young adults, is increased if daily dosages higher than 0.5mg per kg body weight are administered. Dystonic reactions include: spasm of the facial muscles, trismus, rhythmic protrusion of the tongue, a bulbar type of speech, spasm of extra-ocular muscles including oculogyric crises, unnatural positioning of the head and shoulders and opisthotonos. There may be a generalised increase in muscle tone.

The majority of reactions occur within 36 hours of starting treatment and the effects usually disappear within 24 hours of withdrawal of the drug. Should treatment of a dystonic reaction be required an anticholinergic anti-Parkinsonian drug, or a benzodiazepine may be used.

Very rare occurrences of the neuroleptic malignant syndrome have been reported. This syndrome is potentially fatal and comprises hyperpyrexia, altered consciousness, muscle rigidity, autonomic instability and elevated levels of creatine phosphokinase (CPK) and must be treated urgently (recognised treatments include dantrolene and bromocriptine). Metoclopramide should be stopped immediately if this syndrome occurs.

Tardive dyskinesia has been reported during prolonged treatment in a small number of mainly elderly patients. Patients on prolonged treatment should be regularly reviewed.

Rarely, drowsiness, restlessness, confusion and diarrhoea have been reported in patients receiving metoclopramide therapy. Depression has been reported extremely rarely.

Raised serum prolactin levels have been observed during metoclopramide therapy: this may result in galactorrhoea, irregular periods and gynaecomastia.

Extremely rarely cases of red cell disorders such as methaemoglobinaemia and sulphaemoglobinaemia have been reported, particularly at high doses of metoclopramide. If this occurs the drug should be withdrawn. Methaemoglobinaemia may be treated using methylene blue.

A small number of skin reactions such as rashes, urticaria, pruritus and oedema have also been reported.

4.9 Overdose
In cases of overdosage, acute dystonic reactions have occurred. Overdosage should be treated by gastric lavage with appropriate supportive measures. Should treatment of a dystonic reaction be required, an anticholinergic anti-Parkinsonian drug or a benzodiazepine may be used.

5. PHARMACOLOGICAL PROPERTIES

5.1 Pharmacodynamic properties
The action of metoclopramide is closely associated with parasympathetic nervous control of the upper gastro-intestinal tract, where it has the effect of encouraging normal peristaltic action. This provides for a fundamental approach to the control of those conditions where disturbed gastro-intestinal motility is a common underlying factor.

5.2 Pharmacokinetic properties
Metoclopramide is metabolised in the liver and the predominant route of elimination of metoclopramide and its metabolites is via the kidney.

5.3 Preclinical safety data
No additional data available.

6. PHARMACEUTICAL PARTICULARS

6.1 List of excipients
Hydroxyethylcellulose, Methyl parahydroxybenzoate, Propyl parahydroxybenzoate, Saccharin sodium, Citric acid monohydrate, Soluble lemon oil, No.1 lime flavour, Purified water.

6.2 Incompatibilities
Not applicable.

6.3 Shelf life
Thirty six months. The liquid should be used within 14 days of opening.

6.4 Special precautions for storage
Protect from light.

6.5 Nature and contents of container
Amber glass bottles with pipette administration device of 15ml liquid.

6.6 Instructions for use and handling
None.

7. MARKETING AUTHORISATION HOLDER
Monmouth Pharmaceuticals Limited
Hampshire International Business Park
Chineham
Basingstoke
Hampshire RG24 8EP
United Kingdom

8. MARKETING AUTHORISATION NUMBER(S)
PL 10536/0033

9. DATE OF FIRST AUTHORISATION/RENEWAL OF THE AUTHORISATION
16 June 1995

10. DATE OF REVISION OF THE TEXT
March 2001

LEGAL CATEGORY
POM

Maxolon SR

(Shire Pharmaceuticals Limited)

1. NAME OF THE MEDICINAL PRODUCT
Maxolon™ SR

2. QUALITATIVE AND QUANTITATIVE COMPOSITION
Each capsule contains Metoclopramide Hydrochloride BP equivalent to 15 mg of the anhydrous substance.

3. PHARMACEUTICAL FORM
Colourless, transparent capsules, overprinted 'Maxolon SR 15', containing white sustained release microgranules.

Maxolon SR does not contain tartrazine or any other azo dyes.

4. CLINICAL PARTICULARS

4.1 Therapeutic indications
Digestive disorders:

Maxolon SR restores normal co-ordination and tone to the upper digestive tract. Maxolon SR relieves symptoms of gastro-duodenal dysfunction, including: dyspepsia, heartburn, flatulence, sickness, pain, regurgitation of bile. These symptoms may be associated with such conditions as: reflux, oesophagitis, hiatus hernia, gastritis, duodenitis, peptic ulcer, cholelithiasis and post-cholecystectomy dyspepsia.

Nausea and vomiting:

Maxolon SR is indicated for the treatment of the nausea and vomiting associated with gastro-intestinal disorders and intolerance to cytotoxic drugs.

4.2 Posology and method of administration
Adults
In adults 20 years and over: 1 capsule (15 mg) twice daily, swallowed whole. Total daily dosage of Maxolon SR should not normally exceed 0.5 mg/kg body weight.

Elderly:
As for adults. To avoid adverse reactions adhere strictly to dosage recommendations and where prolonged therapy is considered necessary, patients should be regularly reviewed.

The interval between doses may need to be extended in patients with clinically significant degrees of renal or hepatic impairment. The predominant route of elimination is via the kidney.

Children and young adults:
A presentation of Maxolon SR suitable for patients under 20 years of age is not available.

4.3 Contraindications
Maxolon SR is contra-indicated in patients under 20 years since the dose level cannot be reduced.

Maxolon should not be used in patients with phaeochromocytoma as it may induce an acute hypertensive response.

Maxolon should not be used during the first three to four days following operations such as pyloroplasty or gut anastomosis as vigorous muscular contractions may not help healing.

Maxolon should not be administered to patients with gastrointestinal obstruction, perforation or haemorrhage.

Maxolon is contra-indicated in patients who have previously shown hypersensitivity to metoclopramide or any of its components.

4.4 Special warnings and special precautions for use
Precautions

If vomiting persists the patient should be reassessed to exclude the possibility of an underlying disorder e.g. cerebral irritation.

Care should be exercised in epileptic patients and patients being treated with other centrally-acting drugs.

Since extrapyramidal symptoms may occur with both metoclopramide and neuroleptics such as the phenothiazines, particular care should be exercised in the event of these drugs being prescribed concurrently.

The neuroleptic malignant syndrome has been reported with metoclopramide in combination with neuroleptics as well as with metoclopramide monotherapy (see section 4.8 Undesirable effects).

Special care should be taken in cases of severe renal or hepatic insufficiency (see also section 4.2 Posology and method of administration).

Care should be exercised when using Maxolon in patients with porphyria.

4.5 Interaction with other medicinal products and other forms of Interaction
The action of metoclopramide on gastro-intestinal tract is antagonised by anticholinergics and opioid analgesics. The absorption of any concurrently administered oral medication may be modified by the effect of metoclopramide on motility. Drugs known to be affected in this way include aspirin and paracetamol. See also under 4.4.

Since extrapyramidal reactions may occur with Maxolon, Phenothiazines and Tetrabenazine, care should be exercised in the event of co-administration of these drugs.

Maxolon should be used with care in association with other drugs acting at central dopamine receptors, such as levodopa, bromocriptine and pergolide.

Maxolon may reduce plasma concentrations of atovaquone.

4.6 Pregnancy and lactation
Animal tests in several mammalian species and clinical experience have not indicated a teratogenic effect. Nevertheless Maxolon SR should only be used when there are compelling reasons and is not advised during the first trimester.

During lactation metoclopramide is found in breast milk, therefore it should not be used during lactation.

4.7 Effects on ability to drive and use machines
None but see 4.8.

4.8 Undesirable effects
Various extrapyramidal reactions to metoclopramide, usually of the dystonic type, have been reported. The incidence of these reactions may be increased if daily dosages higher than 0.5 mg per kg body weight are administered. Dystonic reactions include: spasm of the facial muscles, trismus, rhythmic protrusion of the tongue, a bulbar type of speech, spasm of extra-ocular muscles including oculogyric crises, unnatural positioning of the head and shoulders and opisthotonos. There may be a generalised increase in muscle tone. The majority of reactions occur within 36 hours of starting treatment and the effects usually disappear within 24 hours of withdrawal of the drug. Should treatment of a dystonic reaction be required an anticholinergic anti-Parkinsonian drug, or a benzodiazepine may be used.

Very rare occurrences of the neuroleptic malignant syndrome have been reported. This syndrome is potentially fatal and comprises hyperpyrexia, altered consciousness, muscle rigidity, autonomic instability and elevated levels of creatine phosphokinase (CPK) and must be treated urgently (recognised treatments include dantrolene and bromocriptine). Metoclopramide should be stopped immediately if this syndrome occurs.

Tardive dyskinesia has been reported during prolonged treatment in a small number of mainly elderly patients. Patients on prolonged treatment should be regularly reviewed.

Rarely, drowsiness, restlessness, confusion and diarrhoea have been reported in patients receiving metoclopramide therapy. Depression has been reported extremely rarely.

Raised serum prolactin levels have been observed during metoclopramide therapy: this may result in galactorrhoea, irregular periods and gynaecomastia.

Extremely rarely cases of red cell disorders such as methaemoglobinaemia and sulphaemoglobinaemia have been reported, particularly at high doses of metoclopramide. If this occurs the drug should be withdrawn. Methaemoglobinaemia may be treated using methylene blue.

A small number of skin reactions such as rashes, urticaria, pruritus and oedema have also been reported.

4.9 Overdose
In cases of overdosage, acute dystonic reactions have occurred. Overdosage should be treated by gastric lavage with appropriate supportive measures. Should treatment of a dystonic reaction be required, an anticholinergic anti-Parkinsonian drug or a benzodiazepine may be used.

5. PHARMACOLOGICAL PROPERTIES

5.1 Pharmacodynamic properties

The action of metoclopramide is closely associated with parasympathetic nervous control of the upper gastro-intestinal tract, where it has the effect of encouraging normal peristaltic action. This provides for a fundamental approach to the control of those conditions where disturbed gastro-intestinal motility is a common underlying factor.

5.2 Pharmacokinetic properties

The following pharmacokinetic parameters for Maxolon SR after a single administration have been established.

C_{max} 102.5 nmol/l

T_{max} 4.5 hours

AUC 1514.25 nmol.hr/l

$t_{½}$ (elim) 7.04 hours

$C_{12\ hrs}$ 54.75 nmol/l

On repeated administration the following parameters have been established.

C_{max} 188 nmol/l

C_{min} 109 nmol/l

5.3 Preclinical safety data

No relevant information available.

6. PHARMACEUTICAL PARTICULARS

6.1 List of excipients

Sucrose

Maize starch

Dibutyl phthalate

Talc

Polymethacrylates

Gelatin

Black iron oxide

6.2 Incompatibilities

Not applicable.

6.3 Shelf life

See under 6.5.

6.4 Special precautions for storage

Protect from direct light.

6.5 Nature and contents of container

56 capsules are available in polypropylene containers with polyethylene caps. Shelf life 36 months.

6.6 Instructions for use and handling

None.

7. MARKETING AUTHORISATION HOLDER

Monmouth Pharmaceuticals Limited

Hampshire International Business Park

Chineham

Basingstoke

Hampshire RG24 8EP

United Kingdom

8. MARKETING AUTHORISATION NUMBER(S)

PL 10536/0030

9. DATE OF FIRST AUTHORISATION/RENEWAL OF THE AUTHORISATION

16 June 1995

10. DATE OF REVISION OF THE TEXT

March 2001

LEGAL CATEGORY

POM

Maxolon Syrup

(Shire Pharmaceuticals Limited)

1. NAME OF THE MEDICINAL PRODUCT

Maxolon™ Syrup

2. QUALITATIVE AND QUANTITATIVE COMPOSITION

The syrup contains Metoclopramide Hydrochloride BP equivalent to 1mg/ml of the anhydrous substance.

3. PHARMACEUTICAL FORM

Clear colourless lemon-lime solution for oral administration.

4. CLINICAL PARTICULARS

4.1 Therapeutic indications

Adults (20 years and over)

Digestive disorders:

Maxolon restores normal co-ordination and tone to the upper digestive tract.

Maxolon relieves the symptoms of gastro-duodenal dysfunction including:

Dyspepsia	Heartburn
Flatulence	Sickness
Regurgitation of bile	Pain

These symptoms may be associated with such conditions as:

Peptic ulcer	Duodenitis
Reflux oesophagitis	Hiatus hernia
Gastritis	Cholelithiasis and Post-cholecystectomy dyspepsia

Nausea and vomiting:

Maxolon is indicated for the treatment of the nausea and vomiting associated with:

Gastro-intestinal disorders

Cyclical vomiting

Intolerance to cytotoxic drugs

Congestive heart failure

Deep x-ray or cobalt therapy

Post-anaesthetic vomiting

Migraine:

Maxolon relieves symptoms of nausea and vomiting, and overcomes gastric stasis associated with attacks of migraine. This improvement in gastric emptying assists the absorption of concurrently administered oral anti-migraine therapy (e.g. paracetamol) which may otherwise be impaired in such patients.

Post-operative conditions:

Post-operative gastric hypotonia

Post-vagotomy syndrome

Maxolon promotes normal gastric emptying and restores motility in vagotomised patients, and where post-operative symptoms suggest gastro-duodenal dysfunction.

Diagnostic procedures:

Radiology

Duodenal intubation

Maxolon speeds up the passage of a barium meal by decreasing gastric emptying time, co-ordinating peristalsis and dilating the duodenal bulb. Maxolon also facilitates duodenal intubation procedures.

Young adults and children

The use of Maxolon in patients under 20 years should be restricted to the following:

Severe intractable vomiting of known cause, vomiting associated with radiotherapy and intolerance to cytotoxic drugs, as an aid to gastro-intestinal intubation, and as part of the premedication before surgical procedures.

4.2 Posology and method of administration

Route of administration:

Oral

The dosage recommendations given below should be strictly adhered to if side effects of the dystonic type are to be avoided. It should be noted that total daily dosage of Maxolon, especially for children and young adults, should not normally exceed 0.5 mg/kg body weight.

In patients with clinically significant degrees of renal or hepatic impairment, therapy should be at reduced dosage. Metoclopramide is metabolised in the liver and the predominant route of elimination of metoclopramide and its metabolites is via the kidney.

Medical indications:

Adults 20 years and over: 10mg three times daily.

For patients of less than 60 kg see below.

Elderly patients:

As for adults. To avoid adverse reactions adhere strictly to dosage recommendations and where prolonged therapy is considered necessary, patients should be regularly reviewed.

Young adults and children:

Maxolon should only be used after careful examination to avoid masking an underlying disorder, e.g. cerebral irritation. In the treatment of this group attention should be given primarily to body weight and treatment should commence at the lower dosage where stated.

Young adults:	15-19 years, 60 kg and over	10mg three times daily
	30-59kg	5mg three times daily
Children:	9-14 years, 30 kg and over	5mg three times daily
	5-9 years, 20-29 kg	2½mg three times daily
	3-5 years, 15-19 kg	2mg two to three times daily
	1-3 years, 10-14 kg	1mg two to three times daily
	Under 1 year up to 10kg	1mg twice daily

Tablets should not be used in children under the age of 15. A liquid presentation should be used in the younger age groups; more accurate dosage is facilitated by the use of the Paediatric Liquid.

Diagnostic indications:

A single dose of Maxolon may be given 5-10 minutes before the examination subject to body weight consideration (see above), the following dosages are recommended.

Adults:	20 years and over	10-20mg
Young adults:	15-19 years	10mg
Children:	9-14 years	5mg
	5-9 years	2½mg
	3-5 years	2mg*
	Under 3 years	1mg*

* more accurate dosage is facilitated by the use of the Paediatric liquid.

4.3 Contraindications

Maxolon should not be used in patients with phaeochromocytoma as it may induce an acute hypertensive response.

Maxolon should not be used during the first three to four days following operations such as pyloroplasty or gut anastomosis as vigorous muscular contractions may not help healing.

Maxolon should not be administered to patients with gastrointestinal obstruction, perforation or haemorrhage.

Maxolon is contra-indicated in patients who have previously shown hypersensitivity to metoclopramide or any of its components.

4.4 Special warnings and special precautions for use

Precautions:

If vomiting persists the patient should be reassessed to exclude the possibility of an underlying disorder e.g. cerebral irritation.

Care should be exercised in epileptic patients and patients being treated with other centrally acting drugs.

Since extrapyramidal symptoms may occur with both metoclopramide and neuroleptics such as the phenothiazines, particular care should be exercised in the event of these drugs being prescribed concurrently.

The neuroleptic malignant syndrome has been reported with metoclopramide in combination with neuroleptics as well as with metoclopramide monotherapy (see section 4.8 Undesirable effects).

Special care should be taken in cases of severe renal or hepatic insufficiency (see also section 4.2 Posology and method of administration).

Care should be exercised when using Maxolon in patients with porphyria.

4.5 Interaction with other medicinal products and other forms of Interaction

The action of Maxolon on the gastro-intestinal tract is antagonised by Anticholinergics and Opioid Analgesics. The absorption of any concurrently administered oral medication may be modified by the effect of Maxolon on gastric motility. Drugs known to be affected in this way include aspirin and paracetamol.

Since extrapyramidal reactions may occur with Maxolon, Phenothiazines and Tetrabenazine, care should be exercised in the event of co-administration of these drugs.

Maxolon should be used with care in association with other drugs acting at central dopamine receptors, such as levodopa, bromocriptine and pergolide.

Maxolon may reduce plasma concentrations of atovaquone.

4.6 Pregnancy and lactation

Animal tests in several mammalian species and clinical experience have not indicated a teratogenic effect. Nevertheless Maxolon should only be used when there are compelling reasons and is not advised during the first trimester.

During lactation metoclopramide is found in breast milk, therefore it should not be used during lactation.

4.7 Effects on ability to drive and use machines

None but see 4.8.

4.8 Undesirable effects

Various extrapyramidal reactions to Maxolon, usually of the dystonic type, have been reported. The incidence of dystonic reactions, particularly in children and young adults, is increased if daily dosages higher than 0.5mg per kg body weight are administered. Dystonic reactions include: spasm of the facial muscles, trismus, rhythmic protrusion of the tongue, a bulbar type of speech, spasm of extra-ocular muscles including oculogyric crises, unnatural positioning of the head and shoulders and opisthotonos. There may be a generalised increase in muscle tone. The majority of reactions occur within 36 hours of starting treatment and the effects usually disappear within 24 hours of withdrawal of the drug. Should treatment of a dystonic reaction be required an anticholinergic anti-Parkinsonian drug, or a benzodiazepine may be used.

Very rare occurrences of the neuroleptic malignant syndrome have been reported. This syndrome is potentially fatal and comprises hyperpyrexia, altered consciousness, muscle rigidity, autonomic instability and elevated levels of creatine phosphokinase (CPK) and must be treated urgently (recognised treatments include dantrolene and bromocriptine). Metoclopramide should be stopped immediately if this syndrome occurs.

Tardive dyskinesia has been reported during prolonged treatment in a small number of mainly elderly patients. Patients on prolonged treatment should be regularly reviewed.

Rarely, drowsiness, restlessness, confusion and diarrhoea have been reported in patients receiving metoclopramide therapy. Depression has been reported extremely rarely.

Raised serum prolactin levels have been observed during metoclopramide therapy: this may result in galactorrhoea, irregular periods and gynaecomastia.

Extremely rarely cases of red cell disorders such as methaemoglobinaemia and sulphaemoglobinaemia have been reported, particularly at high doses of metoclopramide. If this occurs the drug should be withdrawn. Methaemoglobinaemia may be treated using methylene blue.

A small number of skin reactions such as rashes, urticaria, pruritus and oedema have also been reported.

4.9 Overdose

In cases of overdosage, acute dystonic reactions have occurred. Overdosage should be treated by gastric lavage with appropriate supportive measures. Should treatment of a dystonic reaction be required, an anticholinergic anti-Parkinsonian drug or a benzodiazepine may be used.

5. PHARMACOLOGICAL PROPERTIES

5.1 Pharmacodynamic properties

The action of metoclopramide is closely associated with parasympathetic nervous control of the upper gastro-intestinal tract, where it has the effect of encouraging normal peristaltic action. This provides for a fundamental approach to the control of those conditions where disturbed gastro-intestinal motility is a common underlying factor.

5.2 Pharmacokinetic properties

Metoclopramide is metabolised in the liver and the predominant route of elimination of metoclopramide and its metabolites is via the kidney.

5.3 Preclinical safety data

No additional data available.

6. PHARMACEUTICAL PARTICULARS

6.1 List of excipients

Hydroxyethylcellulose, Methyl parahydroxybenzoate, Propyl parahydroxybenzoate, Saccharin sodium, Citric acid monohydrate, Soluble lemon oil, No.1 lime flavour, Purified water.

6.2 Incompatibilities

Not applicable.

6.3 Shelf life

Thirty six months.

Maxolon Syrup may be diluted with purified water BP to half strength but should not be stored diluted for more than 1 month.

6.4 Special precautions for storage

Do not store above 30°C. Protect from light.

6.5 Nature and contents of container

Amber glass bottles of 200ml.

6.6 Instructions for use and handling

None.

7. MARKETING AUTHORISATION HOLDER

Monmouth Pharmaceuticals Limited
Hampshire International Business Park
Chineham
Basingstoke
Hampshire RG24 8EP
United Kingdom

8. MARKETING AUTHORISATION NUMBER(S)

PL 10536/0032

9. DATE OF FIRST AUTHORISATION/RENEWAL OF THE AUTHORISATION

16 June 1995

10. DATE OF REVISION OF THE TEXT

March 2001

LEGAL CATEGORY

POM

Maxolon Tablets

(Shire Pharmaceuticals Limited)

1. NAME OF THE MEDICINAL PRODUCT

Maxolon® Tablets 10mg

2. QUALITATIVE AND QUANTITATIVE COMPOSITION

Each tablet contains Metoclopramide Hydrochloride BP equivalent to 10mg of the anhydrous substance.

3. PHARMACEUTICAL FORM

White uncoated tablets scored and engraved 'Maxolon'.

4. CLINICAL PARTICULARS

4.1 Therapeutic indications

Adults (20 years and over)

Digestive disorders:

Maxolon restores normal co-ordination and tone to the upper digestive tract.

Maxolon relieves the symptoms of gastro-duodenal dysfunction including:

Dyspepsia,	Heartburn,
Flatulence,	Sickness,
Regurgitation of bile,	Pain

These symptoms may be associated with such conditions as:

Peptic ulcer,	Duodenitis,
Reflux oesophagitis,	Hiatus hernia,
Gastritis,	Cholelithiasis and
	Post-cholecystectomy dyspepsia

Nausea and vomiting:

Maxolon is indicated for the treatment of the nausea and vomiting associated with:

Gastro-intestinal disorders
Cyclical vomiting
Intolerance to cytotoxic drugs
Congestive heart failure
Deep x-ray or cobalt therapy
Post-anaesthetic vomiting

Migraine:

Maxolon relieves symptoms of nausea and vomiting, and overcomes gastric stasis associated with attacks of migraine. This improvement in gastric emptying assists the absorption of concurrently administered oral anti-migraine therapy (e.g. paracetamol) which may otherwise be impaired in such patients.

Post-operative conditions:

Post operative gastric hypotonia
Post vagotomy syndrome

Maxolon promotes normal gastric emptying and restores motility in vagotomised patients, and where post-operative symptoms suggest gastro-duodenal dysfunction.

Diagnostic procedures:

Radiology
Duodenal intubation

Maxolon speeds up the passage of a barium meal by decreasing gastric emptying time, co-ordinating peristalsis and dilating the duodenal bulb.

Maxolon also facilitates duodenal intubation procedures.

Young adults and children

The use of Maxolon in patients under 20 years should be restricted to the following:

Severe intractable vomiting of known cause, vomiting associated with radiotherapy and intolerance to cytotoxic drugs, as an aid to gastro-intestinal intubation, and as part of the premedication before surgical procedures.

4.2 Posology and method of administration

Route of administration:

Oral

The dosage recommendations given below should be strictly adhered to if side effects of the dystonic type are to be avoided. It should be noted that total daily dosage of Maxolon, especially for children and young adults, should not normally exceed 0.5mg/kg body weight.

In patients with clinically significant degrees of renal or hepatic impairment, therapy should be at reduced dosage. Metoclopramide is metabolised in the liver and the predominant route of elimination of metoclopramide and its metabolites is via the kidney.

Medical indications:

Adults 20 years and over: 10mg three times daily.

For patients of less than 60 kg see below.

Elderly patients:

As for adults. To avoid adverse reactions adhere strictly to dosage recommendations and where prolonged therapy is considered necessary, patients should be regularly reviewed.

Young adults and children:

Maxolon should only be used after careful examination to avoid masking an underlying disorder, e.g. cerebral irritation. In the treatment of this group attention should be given primarily to body weight and treatment should commence at the lower dosage where stated.

Young adults:	15-19 years,	60 kg and over	10mg three times daily
		30-59kg	5mg three times daily

Tablets should not be used in children under the age of 15. A liquid presentation should be used in the younger age groups; more accurate dosage is facilitated by the use of the Paediatric Liquid.

Diagnostic indications:

A single dose of Maxolon may be given 5-10 minutes before the examination subject to body weight consideration, (see above), the following dosages are recommended.

Adults:	20 years and over	10-20mg
Young adults:	15-19 years	10mg

A liquid presentation should be used in the younger age groups; more accurate dosage is facilitated by the use of the Paediatric Liquid.

4.3 Contraindications

Maxolon should not be used in patients with phaeochromocytoma as it may induce an acute hypertensive response.

Maxolon should not be used during the first three to four days following operations such as pyloroplasty or gut anastomosis as vigorous muscular contractions may not help healing.

Maxolon should not be administered to patients with gastrointestinal obstruction, perforation or haemorrhage.

Maxolon is contraindicated in patients who have previously shown hypersensitivity to metoclopramide or any of its components.

4.4 Special warnings and special precautions for use

Precautions:

If vomiting persists the patient should be reassessed to exclude the possibility of an underlying disorder e.g. cerebral irritation.

Care should be exercised in epileptic patients and patients being treated with other centrally acting drugs.

Since extrapyramidal symptoms may occur with both metoclopramide and neuroleptics such as the phenothiazines, particular care should be exercised in the event of these drugs being prescribed concurrently.

The neuroleptic malignant syndrome has been reported with metoclopramide in combination with neuroleptics as well as with metoclopramide monotherapy (see section 4.8 Undesirable effects).

Special care should be taken in cases of severe renal and hepatic insufficiency (see also section 4.2 Posology and method of administration).

Care should be exercised when using Maxolon in patients with porphyria.

4.5 Interaction with other medicinal products and other forms of Interaction

The action of Maxolon on the gastro-intestinal tract is antagonised by anticholinergics and opioid analgesics. The absorption of any concurrently administered oral medication may be modified by the effect of Maxolon on gastric motility. Drugs known to be affected in this way include aspirin and paracetamol.

Since extrapyramidal reactions may occur with Maxolon, phenothiazines and tetrabenazine, care should be exercised in the event of co-administration of these drugs.

Maxolon should be used with care in association with other drugs acting at central dopamine receptors, such as levodopa, bromocriptine and pergolide.

Maxolon may reduce plasma concentrations of atovaquone.

4.6 Pregnancy and lactation

Animal tests in several mammalian species and clinical experience have not indicated a teratogenic effect. Nevertheless Maxolon should only be used when there are compelling reasons and is not advised during the first trimester.

During lactation metoclopramide is found in breast milk, therefore it should not be used during lactation.

4.7 Effects on ability to drive and use machines

None but see 4.8.

4.8 Undesirable effects

Various extrapyramidal reactions to Maxolon, usually of the dystonic type, have been reported. The incidence of dystonic reactions, particularly in children and young adults, is increased if daily dosages higher than 0.5mg per kg body weight are administered. Dystonic reactions include: spasm of the facial muscles, trismus, rhythmic protrusion of the tongue, a bulbar type of speech, spasm of extra-ocular muscles including oculogyric crises, unnatural positioning of the head and shoulders and opisthotonos. There may be a generalised increase in muscle tone. The majority of reactions occur within 36 hours of starting treatment and the effects usually disappear within 24 hours of withdrawal of the drug. Should treatment of a dystonic reaction be required an anticholinergic anti-Parkinsonian drug, or a benzodiazepine may be used.

Very rare occurrences of the neuroleptic malignant syndrome have been reported. This syndrome is potentially fatal and comprises hyperpyrexia, altered consciousness, muscle rigidity, autonomic instability and elevated levels of creatine phosphokinase (CPK) and must be treated urgently (recognised treatments include dantrolene and bromocriptine). Metoclopramide should be stopped immediately if this syndrome occurs.

Tardive dyskinesia has been reported during prolonged treatment in a small number of mainly elderly patients. Patients on prolonged treatment should be regularly reviewed.

Rarely, drowsiness, restlessness, confusion and diarrhoea have been reported in patients receiving metoclopramide therapy. Depression has been reported extremely rarely.

Raised serum prolactin levels have been observed during metoclopramide therapy: this may result in galactorrhoea, irregular periods and gynaecomastia.

Extremely rarely cases of red cell disorders such as methaemoglobinaemia and sulphaemoglobinaemia have been reported, particularly at high doses of metoclopramide. If this occurs the drug should be withdrawn. Methaemoglobinaemia may be treated using methylene blue.

A small number of skin reactions such as rashes, urticaria, pruritus and oedema have also been reported.

4.9 Overdose

In cases of overdosage, acute dystonic reactions have occurred. Overdosage should be treated by gastric lavage with appropriate supportive measures. Should treatment of a dystonic reaction be required, an anticholinergic anti-Parkinsonian drug or a benzodiazepine may be used.

5. PHARMACOLOGICAL PROPERTIES

5.1 Pharmacodynamic properties

The action of metoclopramide is closely associated with parasympathetic nervous control of the upper gastro-intestinal tract, where it has the effect of encouraging normal peristaltic action. This provides for a fundamental approach to the control of those conditions where disturbed gastro-intestinal motility is a common underlying factor.

5.2 Pharmacokinetic properties

Metoclopramide is metabolised in the liver and the predominant route of elimination of metoclopramide and its metabolites is via the kidney.

5.3 Preclinical safety data

No additional data available.

6. PHARMACEUTICAL PARTICULARS

6.1 List of excipients

Maize starch (dried)

Colloidal silicon dioxide

Magnesium stearate

Pregelatinised maize starch

Lactose

6.2 Incompatibilities

Not applicable.

6.3 Shelf life

Sixty months.

6.4 Special precautions for storage

Do not store above 30°C.

6.5 Nature and contents of container

Plastic recloseable containers packed into cartons of 500 tablets.

PVC blister (300 microns) of 84 tablets backed with aluminium foil (20 microns). The underside of the foil is coated with vinyl based lacquer.

6.6 Instructions for use and handling

None.

7. MARKETING AUTHORISATION HOLDER

Monmouth Pharmaceuticals Limited

Hampshire International Business Park

Chineham

Basingstoke

Hampshire

RG24 8EP

United Kingdom

8. MARKETING AUTHORISATION NUMBER(S)

PL 10536/0031

9. DATE OF FIRST AUTHORISATION/RENEWAL OF THE AUTHORISATION

16 June 1995/8 September 2000

10. DATE OF REVISION OF THE TEXT

March 2001

LEGAL CATEGORY

POM

Maxtrex Tablets 10 mg

(Pharmacia Limited)

1. NAME OF THE MEDICINAL PRODUCT

Maxtrex Tablets 10.0 mg

2. QUALITATIVE AND QUANTITATIVE COMPOSITION

Each tablet contains methotrexate Ph. Eur. 10.0 mg.

For excipients, see 6.1.

3. PHARMACEUTICAL FORM

Tablet.

'Capsule-shaped', uncoated, convex deep yellow tablets marked with 'M10' on one side and scored on the other.

4. CLINICAL PARTICULARS

4.1 Therapeutic indications

Methotrexate is a folic acid antagonist and is classified as an antimetabolite cytotoxic agent.

Methotrexate has been used to produce regression in a wide range of neoplastic conditions including acute leukaemias, non-Hodgkin's lymphoma, soft-tissue and osteogenic sarcomas, and solid tumours particularly breast, lung, head and neck, bladder, cervical, ovarian, and testicular carcinoma.

Methotrexate has also been used in the treatment of severe, uncontrolled psoriasis which is not responsive to other therapy.

4.2 Posology and method of administration

Method of Administration: Oral.

Dosage for cancer treatment:

A test dose of 5 - 10 mg parenterally is recommended, one week prior to therapy to detect idiosyncratic adverse events. Single doses, not exceeding 30 mg/m^2, on not more than 5 consecutive days. A rest period of at least two weeks is recommended between treatments, in order to allow the bone marrow to return to normal.

Doses in excess of 100 mg are usually given parenterally, when the injectable preparation should be used. Doses in excess of 70 mg/m^2 should not be administered without leucovorin rescue (folinic acid rescue) or assay of serum methotrexate levels 24 - 48 hours after dosing.

If methotrexate is administered in combination chemotherapy regimens, the dosage should be reduced, taking into consideration any overlapping toxicity of the other drug components.

Dosage for psoriasis:

For the treatment of severe psoriasis 10 - 25 mg orally, once weekly, is recommended. Dosage should be adjusted according to the patient's response and the haematological toxicity.

4.3 Contraindications

Methotrexate is contra-indicated in the presence of severe/significant renal or significanthepatic impairment, liver disease including fibrosis, cirrhosis, recent or active hepatitis; active infectious disease; and overt or laboratory evidence of immunodeficiency syndrome(s) and serious anaemia, leucopenia or thrombocytopenia. Maxtrex should not be used concomitantly with drugs with antifolate properties (see section 4.5, Interactions with other Medicinal Products and other forms of Interaction). Methotrexate is teratogenic and should not be given during pregnancy or to mothers who are breast feeding (see Section 4.6., Pregnancy and Lactation).

Following administration to a man or woman conception should be avoided by using an effective contraceptive method for at least 3 months after using Maxtrex Tablets 10mg (see section 4.4, Special Warnings and Special Precautions for Use).

Patients with a known allergic hypersensitivity to methotrexate or any of the excipients should not receive methotrexate.

4.4 Special warnings and special precautions for use

Methotrexate should be used with extreme caution in patients with haematological depression, renal impairment, diarrhoea, ulcerative disorders of the GI tract and psychiatric disorders. Hepatic toxicity has been observed, usually associated with chronic hepatic disease. Renal lesions may develop if the urinary flow is impeded and urinary pH is low, especially if large doses have been administered.

The administration of low doses of methotrexate for prolonged periods may give rise, in particular, to hepatic toxicity.

Particular care and possible cessation of treatment are indicated if stomatitis or GI toxicity occurs as haemorrhagic enteritis and intestinal perforation may result.

Liver function shouldbeclosely monitored. If hepatic function abnormalities develop, methotrexate dosing should be suspended for at least two weeks. It is only appropriate to restart methotrexate provided the abnormalities return to normal and the re-exposure is deemed appropriate. Renal function should be closely monitored before, during and after treatment. Reduce dose of methotrexate in patients with renal impairment. High doses may cause the precipitation of methotrexate or its metabolites in the renal tubules. A high fluid throughput and alkalinisation of the urine to pH 6.5 – 7 by oral or intravenous administration of sodium bicarbonate (5x625mg tablets every three hours) is recommended as a preventative measure.

Haematopoietic suppression caused by methotrexate may occur abruptly and with apparently safe dosages. Full blood counts should be closely monitored before, during and after treatment. If a clinically significant drop in white cell or platelet count develops, methotrexate therapy should be withdrawn immediately and appropriate supportive therapy given (see section 4.8, Undesirable Effects). Patients should be advised to report all symptoms or signs suggestive of infection.

Malignant lymphomas may occur in patients receiving low dose methotrexate, in which case therapy must be discontinued. Failure of the lymphoma to show signs of spontaneous regression requires the initiation of cytotoxic therapy.

Methotrexate has been shown to be teratogenic; it has been reported to cause foetal death and/or congenital abnormalities. Therefore, it is not recommended in women of childbearing potential unless the benefits can be expected to outweigh the considered risks. If this drug is used during pregnancy for antineoplastic indications, or if the patient becomes pregnant while taking this drug, the patient should be appraised of the potential hazard to the foetus.

Following administration to a man or woman conception should be avoided by using an effective contraceptive method for at least 3 months after using Maxtrex Tablets 10mg (see section 4.3, Contraindications).

Methotrexate has some immunosuppressive activity and therefore the immunological response to concurrent vaccination may be decreased. In addition, concomitant use of a live vaccine could cause severe antigenic reaction.

Methotrexate should only be used by clinicians that are familiar with the various characteristics of the drug and its mode of action. Before beginning methotrexate therapy or reinstituting methotrexate after a rest period, a chest x-ray, assessment of renal function, liver function and blood elements should be made by history, physical examination and laboratory tests. This will include a routine examination of lymph nodes and patients should report any unusual swelling to the doctor.

Patients receiving low-dose methotrexate should:

- Have a full blood count and renal and liver function tests before starting treatment. These should be repeated weekly until therapy is stabilised, thereafter patients should be monitored every 2-3 months throughout treatment.
- Patients should report all symptoms and signs suggestive of infection, especially sore throat.

If acute methotrexate toxicity occurs, patients may require treatment with folinic acid.

The disappearance of methotrexate from plasma should be monitored, if possible. This is recommended in particular when high, or very high doses are administered in order to permit calculation of an adequate dose of leucovorin (folinic acid) rescue.

Patients with pleural effusions and ascites should be drained prior to initiation of methotrexate therapy. A chest x-ray is recommended prior to initiation of methotrexate therapy or treatment should be withdrawn.

Methotrexate given concomitantly with radiotherapy may increase the risk of soft tissue necrosis and osteonecrosis.

Interstitial pulmonary fibrosis may occur, particularly after long-term treatment.

Acute or chronic pneumonitis, often associated with blood eosinophilia, may occur and deaths have been reported. Symptoms typically include dyspnoea, cough (especially a dry productive cough) and fever for which patients should be monitored at each follow-up visit. Patients should be informed of the risk of pneumonitis and advised to contact their doctor immediately should they develop persistent cough or dyspnoea.

Methotrexate should be withdrawn from patients with pulmonary symptoms, and a thorough investigation should be made to exclude infection. If methotrexate induced lung disease is suspected, treatment with corticosteroids should be initiated and treatment with methotrexate should not be restarted.

Lung manifestations of RA and other connective tissue disorders are recognised to occur. In patients with RA, the physician should be specifically alerted to the potential for methotrexate induced adverse effects on the pulmonary system.

4.5 Interaction with other medicinal products and other forms of Interaction

Methotrexate is immunosuppressive and may therefore reduce immunological response to concurrent vaccination. Severe antigenic reactions may occur if a live vaccine is given concurrently.

Methotrexate is extensively protein bound and may displace, or be displaced by, other acidic drugs. The concurrent administration of agents such as p-aminobenzoic acid, chloramphenicol, diphenylhydantoins, acidic anti-inflammatory agents, salicylates, sulphonamides, tetracyclines, thiazide diuretics, probenicid, sulphinpyrazone or oral hypoglycaemicswill decrease the methotrexate transport function of renal tubules, thereby reducing excretion and almost certainly increasing methotrexate toxicity. Methotrexate dosage should be monitored if concomitant treatment with NSAIDs is commenced, as concomitant use of NSAID's has been associated with fatal methotrexate toxicity. Concomitant administration of folate antagonists such as trimethoprim, co-trimoxazole and nitrous oxide should be avoided. Hepatic and nephrotoxic drugs should be avoided.

Acitretin (a treatment for psoriasis) is metabolised to eretinate. Methotrexate levels may be increased by eretinate and severe hepatitis has been reported following concomitant use.

Vitamin preparations containing folic acid or its derivatives may alter response to methotrexate.

4.6 Pregnancy and lactation

Methotrexate is contra-indicated in pregnancy. Methotrexate affects spermatogenesis and oogenesis and may therefore decrease fertility. This effect appears to be reversible after discontinuation of therapy. Patients and their partners should be advised to avoid pregnancy until 3 months after cessation of methotrexate therapy.

Patients should not breast feed whilst taking methotrexate.

Methotrexate causes embryotoxicity, abortion and foetal defects in humans. Therefore, the possible risks of effects on reproduction should be discussed with patients of child bearing potential (see section 4.4, Special Warnings and Special Precautions for Use and section 4.3, Contraindications).

4.7 Effects on ability to drive and use machines

None known.

4.8 Undesirable effects

In general, the incidence and severity of side effects are considered to be dose-related. Adverse reactions for the various systems are as follows:

Skin:

Stevens-Johnson Syndrome, epidermal necrolysis, erythematous rashes, pruritus, urticaria, photosensitivity, pigmentary changes, alopecia, ecchymosis, telangiectasia, acne, furunculosis. Lesions of psoriasis may be aggravated by concomitant exposure to ultraviolet radiation. Skin ulceration in psoriatic patients and rarely painful erosion of psoriatic plaques has been reported. The recall phenomenon has been reported in both radiation and solar damaged skin.

Haematopoietic:

Bone marrow depression is most frequently manifested by leucopenia, thrombocytopenia (which are usually reversible) and anaemia, or any combination may occur. Infection or hypogammaglobulinaemia has been reported.

Alimentary System:

Mucositis (most frequently stomatitis although gingivitis, pharyngitis and even enteritis, intestinal ulceration and bleeding) may occur. In rare cases the effect of Methotrexate on the intestinal mucosa has led to malabsorption or toxic megacolon. Nausea, anorexia and vomiting and/or diarrhoea may also occur.

Hepatic:

Hepatic toxicity resulting in significant elevations of liver enzymes, acute liver atrophy, necrosis, fatty metamorphosis, periportal fibrosis or cirrhosis or death may occur, usually following chronic administration.

Urogenital System:

Renal failure and uraemia may follow methotrexate administration, particularly after high doses or prolonged administration. Vaginitis, vaginal ulcers, cystitis, haematuria and nephropathy have also been reported. Methotrexate can decrease fertility. This effect appears to be reversible after discontinuation of therapy (see section 4.6, Pregnancy and Lactation).

Pulmonary System:

Acute or chronic interstitial pneumonitis, often associated with blood eosinophilia, may occur and deaths have been reported (see Section 4.4, Special Warnings and Special Precautions for Use).

Acute pulmonary oedema has also been reported after oral and intrathecal use. Pulmonary fibrosis is rare. A syndrome consisting of pleuritic pain and pleural thickening has been reported following high doses.

In the treatment of rheumatoid arthritis, methotrexate induced lung disease is a potentially serious adverse drug reaction which may occur acutely at any time during therapy. It is not always fully reversible. Pulmonary symptoms (especially a dry, non productive cough) may require interruption of treatment and careful investigation.

Central Nervous System:

Headaches, drowsiness, ataxia and blurred vision have occurred following low doses of methotrexate, transient subtle cognitive dysfunction, mood alteration, or unusual cranial sensations have been reported occasionally. Aphasia, paresis, hemiparesis, and convulsions have also occurred following administration of higher doses.

There have been reports of leucoencephalopathy following intravenous methotrexate in high doses, or low doses following cranial-spinal radiation.

Other reports include eye irritation, malaise, undue fatigue, vasculitis, sepsis, arthralgia/myalgia, chills and fever, dizziness, loss of libido/impotence and decreased resistance to infection. Also opportunistic infections such as herpes zoster. Osteoporosis, abnormal (usually "megaloblastic") red cell morphology, precipitation of diabetes, other metabolic changes, and sudden death in relation to or attributed to the use of methotrexate.

4.9 Overdose

Leucovorin is a specific antidote for methotrexate and, following accidental overdosage, should be administered within one hour at a dosage equal to, or greater than, the methotrexate dose. It may be administered by i.v. bolus or infusion. Further doses may be required. The patient should be observed carefully and blood transfusions, renal dialysis and reverse barrier nursing may be necessary.

In cases of massive overdose, hydration and urinary alkalisation may be necessary to prevent precipitation of methotrexate and/or its metabolites in the renal tubules. Neither haemodialysis nor peritoneal dialysis has been shown to improve methotrexate elimination. Effective clearance of methotrexate has been reported with acute, intermittent haemodialysis using a high flux dialyser.

5. PHARMACOLOGICAL PROPERTIES

5.1 Pharmacodynamic properties

Methotrexate is a folic acid antagonist and its major site of action is the enzyme dihydrofolate reductase. Its main effect is inhibition of DNA synthesis but it also acts directly both on RNA and protein synthesis. Methotrexate is a phase specific substance, the main effect being directed during the S-phase of cell division.

The inhibition of dihydrofolate reductase can be circumvented by the use of leucovorin (folinic acid; citrovorum factor) and protection of normal tissues can be carried out by properly timed administration of leucovorin calcium.

5.2 Pharmacokinetic properties

When given in low doses, methotrexate is rapidly absorbed from the GI tract giving plasma concentrations equivalent to those achieved after i.v. administration. Higher doses are less well absorbed. About 50% has been shown to be protein bound. Biphasic and triphasic plasma clearance has been shown. The majority of the dose is excreted within 24 hours in the urine mainly as unchanged drug.

5.3 Preclinical safety data

No further preclinical safety data are available.

6. PHARMACEUTICAL PARTICULARS

6.1 List of excipients

Maize starch

Lactose

Pregelatinised starch

Polysorbate 80

Microcrystalline cellulose

Magnesium stearate

Purified water

6.2 Incompatibilities

None stated.

6.3 Shelf life

60 months.

6.4 Special precautions for storage

None stated.

6.5 Nature and contents of container

White high density polyethylene container with high density polyethylene screw closure containing 100 tablets.

6.6 Instructions for use and handling

None.

7. MARKETING AUTHORISATION HOLDER

Pharmacia Limited

Davy Avenue

Milton Keynes

MK5 8PH

United Kingdom

8. MARKETING AUTHORISATION NUMBER(S)

PL 0032/0342

9. DATE OF FIRST AUTHORISATION/RENEWAL OF THE AUTHORISATION

17 July 2002

10. DATE OF REVISION OF THE TEXT

September 2004

Maxtrex Tablets 2.5 mg

(Pharmacia Limited)

1. NAME OF THE MEDICINAL PRODUCT

Maxtrex Tablets 2.5 mg.

2. QUALITATIVE AND QUANTITATIVE COMPOSITION

Each tablet contains methotrexate Ph. Eur. 2.5 mg.

For excipients, see 6.1

3. PHARMACEUTICAL FORM

Round, uncoated, convex deep yellow tablets marked with 'M2.5' on one side.

4. CLINICAL PARTICULARS

4.1 Therapeutic indications

Methotrexate is a folic acid antagonist and is classified as an antimetabolite cytotoxic agent.

Methotrexate is used in the treatment of adults with severe, active, classical or definite rheumatoid arthritis who are unresponsive or intolerant to conventional therapy.

Methotrexate has also been used in the treatment of severe, uncontrolled psoriasis, which is not responsive to other therapy.

Methotrexate has been used to produce regression in a wide range of neoplastic conditions including acute leukaemias, non-Hodgkin's lymphoma, soft-tissue and osteogenic sarcomas, and solid tumours particularly breast, lung, head and neck, bladder, cervical, ovarian, and testicular carcinoma.

4.2 Posology and method of administration

Method of Administration: Oral

Dosage and Administration with reference to Rheumatoid arthritis and Psoriasis

Dosage for Rheumatoid arthritis

Adults:

In adults with severe, active, classical or definite rheumatoid arthritis who are unresponsive or intolerant to conventional therapy 7.5 mg orally once weekly or divided oral doses of 2.5 mg at 12 hour intervals for 3 doses (7.5 mg) as a course once weekly. The schedule may be adjusted gradually to achieve an optimal response but should not exceed a total weekly dose of 20 mg. Once response has been achieved, the schedule should be reduced to the lowest possible effective dose.

Elderly:

Methotrexate should be used with extreme caution in elderly patients, a reduction in dosage should be considered.

Children:

Safety and effectiveness in children have not been established, other than in cancer chemotherapy.

Dosage for psoriasis:

For the treatment of severe psoriasis 10 - 25 mg orally, once weekly, is recommended. Dosage should be adjusted according to the patient's response and the haematological toxicity.

Dosage for cancer treatment:

A test dose of 5 - 10 mg parenterally is recommended, one week prior to therapy to detect idiosyncratic adverse events. Single doses, not exceeding 30 mg/m^2, on not more than 5 consecutive days. A rest period of at least two weeks is recommended between treatments, in order to allow the bone marrow to return to normal.

Doses in excess of 100 mg are usually given parenterally, when the injectable preparation should be used. Doses in excess of 70 mg/m^2 should not be administered without leucovorin rescue (folinic acid rescue) or assay of serum methotrexate levels 24 - 48 hours after dosing.

If methotrexate is administered in combination chemotherapy regimens, the dosage should be reduced, taking into consideration any overlapping toxicity of the other drug components.

4.3 Contraindications

Methotrexate is contra-indicated in the presence of severe/significant renal or significant hepatic impairment. Liver disease including fibrosis, cirrhosis, recent or active hepatitis; active infectious disease; and overt or laboratory evidence of immunodeficiency syndrome(s). Serious cases of anaemia, leucopenia or thrombocytopenia. Maxtrex should not be used concomitantly with drugs with antifolate properties (eg co-trimoxazole). Methotrexate is teratogenic and should not be given during pregnancy or to mothers who are breast feeding.

Following administration to a man or woman conception should be avoided by using an effective contraceptive method for at least 3 months after using Maxtrex Tablets 2.5mg (see section 4.4, Special Warnings).

Patients with a known allergic hypersensitivity to methotrexate should not receive methotrexate.

4.4 Special warnings and special precautions for use

Methotrexate should be used with extreme caution in patients with haematological depression, renal impairment, diarrhoea, and ulcerative disorders of the GI tract and psychiatric disorders. Hepatic toxicity has been observed, usually associated with chronic hepatic disease. The administration of low doses of methotrexate for prolonged periods may give rise, in particular, to hepatic toxicity. Liver function should be closely monitored. If hepatic function abnormalities develop, methotrexate dosing should be suspended for at least two weeks. It is only appropriate to restart methotrexate provided the abnormalities return to normal and the re-exposure is deemed appropriate

Particular care and possible cessation of treatment are indicated if stomatitis or GI toxicity occurs as haemorrhagic enteritis and intestinal perforation may result.

Reversible eosinophilic pulmonary reactions and treatment-resistant, interstitial fibrosis may occur, particularly after long-term treatment.

Renal lesions may develop if the urinary flow is impeded and urinary pH is low, especially if large doses have been administered. Renal function should be closely monitored before, during and after treatment. Reduce dose of methotrexate in patients with renal impairment. High doses may cause the precipitation of methotrexate or its metabolites in the renal tubules. A high fluid throughput and alkalinisation of the urine to pH 6.5 – 7 by oral or intravenous administration of sodium bicarbonate (5x625mg tablets every three hours) is recommended as a preventative measure.

Haematopoietic suppression caused by Methotrexate may occur abruptly and with apparently safe dosages. Full blood counts should be closely monitored before, during and after treatment. If a clinically significant drop in white cell or platelet count develops, methotrexate therapy should be withdrawn immediately and appropriate supportive therapy given (see Undesirable Effects section). Patients should be advised to report all symptoms or signs suggestive of infection.

Malignant lymphomas may occur in patients receiving low dose methotrexate, in which case therapy must be discontinued. Failure of the lymphoma to show signs of spontaneous regression requires the initiation of cytotoxic therapy.

Methotrexate has been shown to be teratogenic; it has been reported to cause foetal death and/or congenital abnormalities. Therefore, it is not recommended in women of childbearing potential unless the benefits can be expected to outweigh the considered risks. If this drug is used during pregnancy for antineoplastic indications, or if the patient becomes pregnant while taking this drug, the patient should be appraised of the potential hazard to the foetus.

Following administration to a man or woman conception should be avoided by using an effective contraceptive method for at least 3 months after using Maxtrex Tablets 2.5mg (see section 4.3, Contraindications).

Methotrexate has some immunosuppressive activity and therefore the immunological response to concurrent vaccination may be decreased. In addition, concomitant use of a live vaccine could cause severe antigenic reaction.

Methotrexate should only be used by clinicians that are familiar with the various characteristics of the drug and its mode of action. Before beginning Methotrexate therapy or reinstituting Methotrexate after a rest period, a chest x-ray, assessment of renal function, liver function and blood elements should be made by history, physical examination and laboratory tests. This will include a routine examination of lymph nodes and patients should report any unusual swelling to the doctor.

Patients receiving low-dose methotrexate should:

- Have a full blood count and renal and liver function tests before starting treatment. These should be repeated weekly until therapy is stabilised, thereafter patients should be monitored every 2-3 months throughout treatment.
- Patients should report all symptoms and signs suggestive of infection, especially sore throat.

If acute methotrexate toxicity occurs, patients may require treatment with folinic acid.

The disappearance of methotrexate from plasma should be monitored, if possible. This is recommended in particular when high, or very high doses are administered in order to permit calculation of an adequate dose of leucovorin (folinic acid) rescue.

Patients with pleural effusions and ascites should be drained prior to initiation of methotrexate therapy or treatment should be withdrawn.

When to perform a liver biopsy in rheumatoid arthritis patients has not been established either in terms of a cumulative Methotrexate dose or duration of therapy.

Pleuropulmonary manifestation of rheumatoid arthritis has been reported in the literature. In patients with rheumatoid arthritis, the physician should be specifically alerted to the potential for Methotrexate induced adverse effects in the pulmonary system. Patients should be advised to contact their physicians immediately should they develop a cough or dyspnoea (see Undesirable Effects section).

Methotrexate given concomitantly with radiotherapy may increase the risk of soft tissue necrosis and osteonecrosis.

Acute or chronic interstitial pneumonitis, often associated with blood eosinophilia, may occur and deaths have been reported. Symptoms typically include dyspnoea, cough (especially a dry non-productive cough) and fever for which patients should be monitored at each follow-up visit. Patients should be informed of the risk of pneumonitis and advised to contact their doctor immediately should they develop persistent cough or dyspnoea.

Methotrexate should be withdrawn from patients pulmonary symptoms, and a thorough investigation should be made to exclude infection. If methotrexate induced lung disease is suspected, treatment with corticosteroids should be initiated and treatment with methotrexate should not be restarted.

Lung manifestations of RA and other connective tissue disorders are recognised to occur. In patients with RA, the physician should be specifically alerted to the potential for methotrexate induced adverse effects on the pulmonary system.

4.5 Interaction with other medicinal products and other forms of Interaction

Methotrexate is immunosuppressive and may therefore reduce immunological response to concurrent vaccination. Severe antigenic reactions may occur if a live vaccine is given concurrently.

Methotrexate is extensively protein bound and may displace, or be displaced by, other acidic drugs. The concurrent administration of agents such as p-aminobenzoic acid, chloramphenicol, diphenylhydantoins, acidic anti-inflammatory agents, salicylates, sulphonamides, tetracyclines, thiazide diuretics, probenicid or sulphinpyrazone or oral hypoglycaemics will decrease the methotrexate transport function of renal tubules, thereby reducing excretion and almost certainly increasing methotrexate toxicity. Methotrexate dosage should be monitored if concomitant treatment with NSAID's is commenced, as concomitant use of NSAID's has been associated with fatal methotrexate toxicity. Concomitant administration of folate antagonists such as trimethoprim, cotrimoxazole and nitrous oxide should be avoided. Hepatic and nephrotoxic drugs should be avoided.

Acitretin (a treatment for psoriasis) is metabolised to eretinate. Methotrexate levels may be increased by eretinate and severe hepatitis has been reported following concomitant use.

Vitamin preparations containing folic acid or its derivatives may alter response to Methotrexate.

4.6 Pregnancy and lactation

Methotrexate is contra-indicated in pregnancy. Methotrexate affects spermatogenesis and oogenesis and may therefore decrease fertility. This effect appears to be reversible after discontinuation of therapy. Patients and their partners should be advised to avoid pregnancy until 3 months after cessation of methotrexate therapy.

Patients should not breast feed whilst taking methotrexate. Methotrexate causes embryotoxicity, abortion and foetal defects in humans. Therefore, the possible risks of effects on reproduction should be discussed with patients of child bearing potential (see Special Warnings sections).

4.7 Effects on ability to drive and use machines

None known.

4.8 Undesirable effects

In general, the incidence and severity of side effects are considered to be dose-related. Adverse reactions for the various systems are as follows:

Skin:

Stevens-Johnson Syndrome, epidermal necrolysis, erythematous rashes, pruritus, urticaria, photosensitivity, pigmentary changes, alopecia, ecchymosis, telangiectasia, acne, furunculosis. Lesions of psoriasis may be aggravated by concomitant exposure to ultraviolet radiation. Skin ulceration in psoriatic patients and rarely painful erosion of psoriatic plaques has been reported. The recall phenomenon has been reported in both radiation and solar damaged skin.

Haematopoietic:

Bone marrow depression is most frequently manifested by leucopenia, thrombocytopenia (which are usually reversible) and anaemia, or any combination may occur. Infection or Hypogammaglobulinaemia has been reported.

Alimentary System:

Mucositis (most frequently stomatitis although gingivitis, pharyngitis and even enteritis, intestinal ulceration and bleeding) may occur. In rare cases the effect of Methotrexate on the intestinal mucosa has led to malabsorption or toxic megacolon. Nausea, anorexia and vomiting and/or diarrhoea may also occur.

Hepatic:

Hepatic toxicity resulting in significant elevations of liver enzymes, acute liver atrophy, necrosis, fatty metamorphosis, periportal fibrosis or cirrhosis or death may occur, usually following chronic administration.

Urogenital System:

Renal failure and uraemia may follow Methotrexate administration, particularly after high doses or prolonged administration. Vaginitis, vaginal ulcers, cystitis, haematuria and nephropathy have also been reported. Methotrexate can decrease fertility. This effect appears to be reversible after discontinuation of therapy (see Pregnancy and Lactation section).

Pulmonary System:

Infrequently an acute or chronic interstitial pneumonitis, often associated with blood eosinophilia, may occur and deaths have been reported. Acute pulmonary oedema has also been reported after oral and intrathecal use. Pulmonary fibrosis is rare. A syndrome consisting of pleuritic pain and pleural thickening has been reported following high doses.

In the treatment of rheumatoid arthritis, Methotrexate induced lung disease is a potentially serious adverse drug reaction which may occur acutely at any time during therapy. It is not always fully reversible. Pulmonary symptoms (especially a dry, non productive cough) may require interruption of treatment and careful investigation.

Acute or chronic interstitial pneumonitis, often associated with blood eosinophilia, may occur and deaths have been reported (see Section 4.4 Warnings and Precautions for Use).

Central Nervous System:

Headaches, drowsiness, ataxia and blurred vision have occurred following low doses of Methotrexate, transient subtle cognitive dysfunction, mood alteration, or unusual cranial sensations have been reported occasionally. Aphasia, paresis, hemiparesis, and convulsions have also occurred following administration of higher doses.

There have been reports of leucoencephalopathy following intravenous Methotrexate in high doses, or low doses following cranial-spinal radiation.

Other reports include eye irritation, malaise, undue fatigue, vasculitis, sepsis, arthralgia/myalgia, chills and fever, dizziness, loss of libido/impotence and decreased resistance to infection. Also opportunistic infections such as herpes zoster. Osteoporosis, abnormal (usually "megaloblastic") red cell morphology, precipitation of diabetes, other metabolic changes, and sudden death in relation to or attributed to the use of Methotrexate.

4.9 Overdose

Leucovorin is a specific antidote for methotrexate and, following accidental overdosage, should be administered within one hour at a dosage equal to, or greater than, the methotrexate dose. It may be administered by i.v. bolus or infusion. Further doses may be required. The patient should be observed carefully and blood transfusions, renal dialysis and reverse barrier nursing may be necessary.

In cases of massive overdose, hydration and urinary alkalisation may be necessary to prevent precipitation of methotrexate and/or its metabolites in the renal tubules. Neither haemodialysis nor peritoneal dialysis has been shown to improve methotrexate elimination. Effective clearance of methotrexate has been reported with acute, intermittent haemodialysis using a high flux dialyser.

5. PHARMACOLOGICAL PROPERTIES

5.1 Pharmacodynamic properties

Methotrexate is a folic acid antagonist and its major site of action is the enzyme dihydrofolate reductase. Its main effect is inhibition of DNA synthesis but it also acts directly both on RNA and protein synthesis. Methotrexate is a phase specific substance, the main effect being directed during the S-phase of cell division.

The inhibition of dihydrofolate reductase can be circumvented by the use of leucovorin (folinic acid; citrovorum factor) and protection of normal tissues can be carried out by properly timed administration of leucovorin calcium.

5.2 Pharmacokinetic properties

When given in low doses, methotrexate is rapidly absorbed from the GI tract giving plasma concentrations equivalent to those achieved after i.v. administration. Higher doses are less well absorbed. About 50% has been shown to be protein bound. Biphasic and triphasic plasma clearance has been shown. The majority of the dose is excreted within 24 hours in the urine mainly as unchanged drug.

5.3 Preclinical safety data

No further preclinical safety data are available.

6. PHARMACEUTICAL PARTICULARS

6.1 List of excipients

Maize starch

Lactose

Pregelatinised starch

Polysorbate 80

Microcrystalline cellulose

Magnesium stearate

Purified water

6.2 Incompatibilities

None stated.

6.3 Shelf life

60 months.

6.4 Special precautions for storage

None.

6.5 Nature and contents of container

White high density polyethylene container with high density polyethylene screw closure.

Pack size: 100 tablets

6.6 Instructions for use and handling

None stated.

Administrative Data

7. MARKETING AUTHORISATION HOLDER

Pharmacia Limited

Davy Avenue

Milton Keynes

MK5 8PH

UK

8. MARKETING AUTHORISATION NUMBER(S)

PL 00032/0343

9. DATE OF FIRST AUTHORISATION/RENEWAL OF THE AUTHORISATION

13/08/2002

10. DATE OF REVISION OF THE TEXT
March 2004

Legal Category: **POM**

Version Number: **MX 1_0**

MCR-50

(Pharmacia Limited)

1. NAME OF THE MEDICINAL PRODUCT
MCR-50

2. QUALITATIVE AND QUANTITATIVE COMPOSITION
Isosorbide 5-mononitrate 50.0 mg

3. PHARMACEUTICAL FORM
A modified release capsule intended for oral administration.

4. CLINICAL PARTICULARS

4.1 Therapeutic indications
MCR-50 is intended for prophylactic treatment and maintenance of angina pectoris.

4.2 Posology and method of administration

Children:

The safety and efficacy of MCR-50 has yet to be established in children.

Adults:

One capsule to be taken in the morning swallowed whole.

Elderly:

As for adult dose.

4.3 Contraindications
MCR-50 should not be used in cases of acute myocardial infarction with low filling pressures, acute circulatory failure (shock, vascular collapse) or very low blood pressure. This product should not be given to patients with a known sensitivity to nitrates, marked anaemia, head trauma, cerebral haemorrhage, severe hypotension or hypovolaemia. Sildenafil has been shownto potentiate the hypotensive effects of nitrates, and it is co-administration with nitrates, or notric oxide donors is therefore contra-indicated.

4.4 Special warnings and special precautions for use
MCR-50 should be used with caution in patients who are predisposed to closed angle glaucoma or are suffering from hypothyroidism, malnutrition, severe liver disease or severe renal disease. Symptoms of circulatory collapse may arise after first dose, particularly in patients with labile circulation.

4.5 Interaction with other medicinal products and other forms of Interaction
Some of the effects of alcohol and the action of hypotensive agents may be potentiated by this product. The hypotensive effects of nitrates are potemtiated by concurrent administration of sildneafil.

4.6 Pregnancy and lactation
There is inadequate evidence of safety of the drug in human pregnancy but nitrates have been used widely in the treatment of angina for many years without apparent ill consequence, animal studies having shown no hazard, nevertheless, it is not advisable to use this drug during pregnancy and lactation.

4.7 Effects on ability to drive and use machines
None stated.

4.8 Undesirable effects
A headache may occurat the start of treatment, but this usually disappears after a few days.

4.9 Overdose
Overdosage may lead to vascular collapse and gastric lavage is indicated in severe cases. Further measures to support the circulation are recommended e.g. elevating the legs and/or treatment with hypertensive agents.

5. PHARMACOLOGICAL PROPERTIES

5.1 Pharmacodynamic properties
Isosorbide mononitrate is a vasodilator.

5.2 Pharmacokinetic properties

(i) Parameter	Value (± 0)	Units
T_{max}	5.0 (± 3)	Hrs
C_{max}	488.1 (± 128.6)	ng.ml
$T_{½}$	5.02 (± 0.68)	Hrs
Apparent VD	73.21 (± 16.28)	L
Apparent clearance	10.46 (± 2.26)	$l.h^{-1}$

(ii) Kinetics are aooroximately linear around the proposed dose range.

(iii) The extraction rate is zero (F = 1)

(iv) In patients with cirrhotic disease or cardiac failure or renal failure, pharmacokinetic parameters were similar to those obtained in healthy volunteers.

5.3 Preclinical safety data
None given.

6. PHARMACEUTICAL PARTICULARS

6.1 List of excipients

Lactose	Ph. Eur
Hydroxy propyl cellulose	USP
Poly ()-ethyl) cellulose	USP
Polyethylene glycol 20000	
Talc	Ph. Eur
Sugar spheres (non-pareil seeds 0.60-0.71mm)	
Sucrose 70% (M/M)	
Corn starch 23% (M/M)	
Glucose Syrup 7% (M/M)	
Acetone	USP
Water	
Hard gelatin capsule cap:	
Gelatin	Ph Eur
Titanium dioxide	Ph Eur
Iron oxide red E171	
Iron oxide black E172	
Hard gelatin capsule body:	
Titanium dioxide E171	Ph Eur
Iron oxide red E172	
Gelatin	Ph Eur

6.2 Incompatibilities
None known.

6.3 Shelf life
48 months.

6.4 Special precautions for storage
None stated.

6.5 Nature and contents of container
Blisters of PVC/Aluminium foil strips. 28 capsules per cardboard carton.

6.6 Instructions for use and handling
There are no special instructions for handling.

7. MARKETING AUTHORISATION HOLDER
J B Tillott Ltd (Trading as Tillotts Laboratories)
Davy Avenue
Milton Keynes
MK5 8PH

8. MARKETING AUTHORISATION NUMBER(S)
PL 0424/0081

9. DATE OF FIRST AUTHORISATION/RENEWAL OF THE AUTHORISATION
5 August 1988 / 18 September 1998.

10. DATE OF REVISION OF THE TEXT
October 1999

LEGAL CATEGORY
POM

Company Ref: MC1_0

Medac Disodium Pamidronate 3 mg/ml, sterile concentrate

(medac GmbH)

1. NAME OF THE MEDICINAL PRODUCT
Medac Disodium Pamidronate 3 mg/ml, sterile concentrate

2. QUALITATIVE AND QUANTITATIVE COMPOSITION
Each ml sterile concentrate contains 3 mg pamidronate disodium as pamidronic acid 2,527 mg.

1 vial with 5 ml sterile concentrate contains 15 mg pamidronate disodium.

1 vial with 10 ml sterile concentrate contains 30 mg pamidronate disodium.

1 vial with 20 ml sterile concentrate contains 60 mg pamidronate disodium.

1 vial with 30 ml sterile concentrate contains 90 mg pamidronate disodium.

For excipients, see section 6.1.

3. PHARMACEUTICAL FORM
Sterile concentrate.

Clear and colourless solution, free from visible particles.

4. CLINICAL PARTICULARS

4.1 Therapeutic indications
Treatment of conditions associated with increased osteoclast activity:

- Tumour-induced hypercalcaemia
- Osteolytic lesions in patients with bone metastases associated with breast cancer
- Multiple myeloma stage III

4.2 Posology and method of administration
Medac Disodium Pamidronate 3 mg/ml is a sterile concentrate and must therefore always be diluted in a calcium-free infusion solution (0.9 % sodium chloride or 5 % glucose) before use. The resulting solution must be infused slowly (see also section 4.4).

For information concerning compatibility with infusion solutions, see section 6.6.

The infusion rate should never exceed 60 mg/hour (1 mg/min), and the concentration of pamidronate disodium in the infusion solution should not exceed 90 mg/250 ml. A dose of 90 mg must usually be administered as a 2 hour infusion in a 250 ml solution for infusion.

In patients with multiple myeloma and patients with tumour induced hypercalcaemia, it is recommended that the infusion rate does not exceed 90 mg in 500 ml over 4 hours. In order to minimise local reactions at the infusion site, the cannula should be inserted carefully into a relatively large vein.

Pamidronate disodium should be given under the supervision of a physician with the facilities to monitor the clinical and biochemical effects.

Use only freshly prepared and clear dilutions!

Children and adolescents (< 18 years):

There is not enough clinical experience available for the use of pamidronate disodium in children and adolescents (< 18 years) (see section 4.4).

Tumour-induced hypercalcaemia:

It is recommended that patients be rehydrated with 0.9% w/v sodium chloride solution before or and during treatment(see section 4.4).

The total dose of pamidronate disodium to be used for a treatment course depends on the patient's initial serum calcium levels. The following guidelines are derived from clinical data on uncorrected calcium values. However, doses within the ranges given are also applicable for calcium values corrected for serum protein or albumin in rehydrated patients.

(see Table 1 on next page)

The total dose of pamidronate disodium may be administered either in a single infusion or in multiple infusions over 2-4 consecutive days. The maximum dose per treatment course is 90 mg for both initial and repeat courses. Higher doses did not improve clinical response.

A significant decrease in serum calcium is generally observed 24-48 hours after administration of pamidronate disodium, and normalisation is usually achieved within 3 to 7 days. If normocalcaemia is not achieved within this time, a further dose may be given. The duration of the response may vary from patient to patient, and treatment can be repeated whenever hypercalcaemia recurs. Clinical experience to date suggests that pamidronate disodium may become less effective as the number of treatments increases.

Osteolytic lesions in multiple myeloma:

The recommended dose is 90 mg every 4 weeks.

Osteolytic lesions in bone metastases associated with breast cancer:

The recommended dose is 90 mg every 4 weeks. This dose may also be administered at 3 weekly intervals to coincide with chemotherapy if desired.

Treatment should be continued until there is evidence of a substantial decrease in a patient's general performance status.

(see Table 2 on next page)

Renal Impairment:

Medac Disodium Pamidronate 3 mg/ml should not be administered to patients with severe renal impairment (creatinine clearance < 30 mL/min) unless in case of life-threatening tumour induced hypercalcaemia where the benefit outweighs the potential risk (see also section 4.4 and 5.2).

Dose adjustment is not necessary in mild (creatinine clearance 61-90 mL/min) to moderate renal impairment (creatinine clearance 30-60 mL/min). In such patients, the infusion rate should not exceed 90 mg/4h (approximately 20-22 mg/h).

As with other intravenous bisphosphonates, monitoring of renal function is recommended, for instance, measurements of serum creatinine prior to each dose of pamidronate disodium. In patients receiving pamidronate disodium for bone metastases who show evidence of deterioration in renal function, treatment with pamidronate disodium should be withheld until renal function returns to within 10 % of the baseline value.

Liver impairment:

There are no published data for the use of pamidronate disodium in patients with hepatic impairment available. Therefore no specific recommendations can be given for Pamidronate disodium in such patients (see section 5.2).

4.3 Contraindications
Known or suspected hypersensitivity to pamidronate disodium or other bisphosphonates or to any of the excipients.

Breast feeding is contraindicated (see also section 4.6).

Table 1

Initial plasma calcium level		Recommended total dose of pamidronate disodium	Concentration of solution for infusion	Maximum infusion rate
(mmol/l)	(mg %) (mg/100ml)	(mg)	mg/ml	mg/h
< 3.0	< 12.0	15-30	30/125	22.5
3.0-3.5	12.0-14.0	30-60	30/125 60/250	22.5
3.5-4.0	14.0-16.0	60-90	60/250 90/500	22.5
> 4.0	>16.0	90	90/500	22.5

Table 2

Indication	Treatment scheme	Solution for infusion (mg/ml)	Infusion rate (mg/h)
Bone metastases	90 mg/2h every 4 weeks	90/ 250	45
Multiple Myeloma	90 mg/4h every 4 weeks	90/ 500	22,5

4.4 Special warnings and special precautions for use

Warnings

Medac Disodium Pamidronate 3 mg/ml is a sterile concentrate and must therefore always be diluted and then given as a slow intravenous infusion (see section 4.2). Medac Disodium Pamidronate 3 mg/ml should be given only as an intravenous infusion.

The medicinal product contains 0.65 mmol sodium per maximum dose (90 mg). To be taken into consideration by patients on a controlled sodium diet.

Do not co-administer Medac Disodium Pamidronate 3 mg/ml with other bisphosphonates. If other calcium lowering agents are used in conjunction with pamidronate disodium, significant hypocalcaemia may result.

Convulsions have been occurred in some patients with tumour-induced hypercalcaemia due to electrolyte changes associated with this condition and its effective treatment.

Precautions

Serum electrolytes, calcium and phosphate should be monitored following initiation of therapy with Medac Disodium Pamidronate 3 mg/ml. Patients with anaemia, leukopenia or thrombocytopenia should have regular haematology assessments.

Patients who have undergone thyroid surgery may be particularly susceptible to develop hypocalcaemia due to relative hypoparathyroidism.

Although pamidronate is excreted unchanged by the kidneys, the medicinal product has been used without apparent increase in adverse effects in patients with significantly elevated plasma creatinine levels (including patients undergoing renal replacement therapy with both haemodialysis and peritoneal dialysis). However, experience with pamidronate disodium in patients with severe renal impairment (serum creatinine >440 micromol/l, or 5 mg/dl in TIH [Tumour-induced hypercalcaemia] patients; 180 micromol/l, or 2 mg/dl in multiple myeloma patients) is limited. If clinical judgement determines that the potential benefits outweigh the risk in such cases, Medac Disodium Pamidronate 3 mg/ml should be used cautiously and renal function carefully monitored.

Fluid balance (urine output, daily weights) should also be followed carefully. There is very little experience of the use of pamidronate disodium in patients receiving haemodialysis.

No specific recommendation on patients with severe liver impairment can be given as there are no clinical data available.

Patients should have standard laboratory (serum creatinine and BUN [blood urea nitrogen]) and clinical renal function parameters periodically evaluated, especially those receiving frequent pamidronate disodium infusions over a prolonged period of time, and those with pre-existing renal disease or a predisposition to renal impairment (e.g. patients with multiple myeloma and/or tumour-induced hypercalcaemia). If there is deterioration of renal function during pamidronate therapy, the infusion must be stopped. Deterioration of renal function (including renal failure) has been reported following long-term treatment with pamidronate disodium in patients with multiple myeloma. However, underlying disease progression and/or concomitant complications were also present and therefore a causal relationship with pamidronate disodium is unproven.

It is essential in the initial treatment of tumour induced hypercalcaemia that intravenous rehydration be instituted to restore urine output. Patients should be hydrated adequately throughout treatment but overhydration must be avoided. In patients with cardiac disease, especially in the elderly, additional saline overload may precipitate cardiac failure (left ventricular failure or congestive heart failure). Fever (influenza-like symptoms) may also contribute to this deterioration.

The safety and efficacy of pamidronate disodium in children and adolescents (< 18 years) has not been established.

Osteonecrosis of the jaw

Osteonecrosis of the jaw has been reported in patients with cancer receiving treatment regimens including Pamidronate. Osteonecrosis of the jaw has multiple well documented risk factors including cancer, concomitant therapies (e.g., chemotherapy, radiotherapy, corticosteroids) and co-morbid conditions (e.g., anemia, coagulopathies, infection, pre-existing oral disease).

The majority of reported cases have been associated with dental procedures such as tooth extraction. Many of these patients were also receiving chemotherapy or corticosteroids and had signs of local infection including osteomyelitis.

A dental examination with appropriate advice should be considered prior to treatment with Pamidronate.

While on treatment, these patients should avoid invasive dental procedures if possible. For patients who develop osteonecrosis of the jaw while on Pamidronate therapy, dental surgery may exacerbate the condition. For patients requiring dental procedures, there are no data available to suggest whether discontinuation of Pamidronate treatment reduces the risk of osteonecrosis of the jaw. Clinical judgement of the treating physician should guide the management plan of each patient based on individual benefit/risk assessment.

4.5 Interaction with other medicinal products and other forms of Interaction

Pamidronate disodium has been administered concomitantly with commonly used anti-tumour medicinal products without significant interactions.

Medac Disodium Pamidronate 3 mg/ml should not be used concomitantly with other bisphosphonates (see also section 4.4.).

Concomitant use of other bisphosphonates, other antihypercalcaemic agents and calcitonin may lead to hypocalcaemia with associated clinical symptoms (paraesthesia, tetany, hypotension).

In patients with severe hypercalcaemia, pamidronate disodium has been successfully combined with both calcitonin and mithramycin to accelerate and potentiate the calcium lowering effect.

Caution is warranted when pamidronate disodium is used with other potentially nephrotoxic medicinal products.

4.6 Pregnancy and lactation

Use in pregnancy:

There are no adequate data from the use of pamidronate disodium in pregnant women. There is no unequivocal evidence for teratogenicity in animal studies. Pamidronate may pose a risk to the foetus/newborn child through its pharmacological action on calcium homeostasis. When administered during the wholeperiod of gestation in animals, pamidronate can cause bone mineralization disorder especially of long bones resulting in angular distortion.

The potential risk for humans is unknown. Therefore, pamidronate disodium should not be used during pregnancy except in cases of life-threatening hypercalcaemia.

Use in lactation:

It is unknown whether Medac Disodium Pamidronate 3 mg/ml is excreted in human breast milk. Animal studies have shown excretion of pamidronate disodium in breast milk and a risk to the breast-fed child cannot be excluded. Therefore, breast-feeding is contraindicated in women treated with pamidronate disodium (see also section 4.3).

4.7 Effects on ability to drive and use machines

Pamidronate disodium has minor or moderate influence on the ability to drive and use machines.

Patients should be warned that in rare cases somnolence and/or dizziness may occur following pamidronate disodium infusion, in which case they should not drive, operate potentially dangerous machinery, or engage in other activities that may be hazardous because of decreased alertness.

4.8 Undesirable effects

Adverse reactions to pamidronate disodium are usually mild and transient. The most common >1/10) symptomatic adverse reactions are influenza-like symptoms and mild fever. This mild fever (an increase in body temperature of 1-2° C) usually occurs within the first 48 hours as a first-dose, dose-related, self-limiting reaction, often without further concomitant symptoms, and usually lasts no longer than 24 hours.

Acute "influenza-like" reactions usually occur only with the first pamidronate infusion. Local soft tissue inflammation at the infusion site occurs commonly >1/100, <1/10), especially at the highest dose.

Osteonecrosis primarily involving the jaws has been reported rarely (see 4.4. Precautions).

Symptomatic hypocalcaemia is very rare (<1/10,000).

Frequency estimate:

Very common >1/10)

Common >1/100, <1/10)

Uncommon >1/1,000, <1/100)

Rare >1/10,000, <1/1,000)

Very rare (<1/10,000), including isolated reports

(see Table 3 on next page)

Many of the above listed undesirable effects may have been related to the underlying disease.

4.9 Overdose

Patients who have received doses higher than those recommended should be carefully monitored. In the event of clinically significant hypocalcaemia with paraesthesia, tetany and hypotension, reversal may be achieved with an infusion of calcium gluconate. Acute hypocalcaemia is not expected to occur with pamidronate since plasma calcium levels fall progressively for several days after treatment.

There is no available information for overdose of pamidronate disodium.

5. PHARMACOLOGICAL PROPERTIES

5.1 Pharmacodynamic properties

Pharmacotherapeutic group: Medicinal products affecting bone structure and mineralisation, Bisphosphonates

ATC: M05 BA 03

Pamidronate disodium, active substance of Medac Disodium Pamidronate 3 mg/ml, is a potent inhibitor of osteoclastic bone resorption. It binds strongly to hydroxyapatite crystals and inhibits the formation and dissolution of these crystals *in vitro*. Inhibition of osteoclastic bone resorption *in vivo* may be at least partly due to binding of the medicinal product to the bone mineral.

Pamidronate suppresses the accession of osteoclast precursors onto the bone and the so induced transformation to mature absorbing osteoclasts. However, the local and direct antiresorptive effect of bone-bound biphosphonate appears to be the predominant mode of action *in vitro* and *in vivo*.

Experimental studies have demonstrated that pamidronate inhibits tumour-induced osteolysis when given prior to or at the time of inoculation or transplantation with tumour cells. Biochemical changes reflecting the inhibitory effect of pamidronate disodium on tumour-induced hypercalcaemia, are characterised by a decrease in serum calcium and phosphate and secondarily by decreases in urinary excretion of calcium, phosphate and hydroxyproline. A dose of 90mg achieves normocalcaemia in more than 90% of patients.

The normalisation of the plasma-calcium-level can also normalise the plasma-parathyroid-hormone-level in adequately rehydrated patients.

Serum levels of parathyroid hormone-related protein (PTHrP) inversely correlate with response to pamidronate. Medicinal products that inhibit tubular reabsorption of calcium or PTHrP secretion may help in patients who do not respond to pamidronate.

Hypercalcaemia can lead to a depletion in the volume of extracellular fluid and a reduction in the glomerular filtration rate (GFR). By controlling hypercalcaemia, pamidronate disodium improves GFR and lowers elevated serum creatinine levels in most patients.

When used in addition to systemic antineoplastic therapy pamidronate reduces skeletal complications of non-vertebral fracture, radiotherapy / surgery for bone complications and increases the time to first skeletal event.

Pamidronate may also reduce bone pain in about 50% women with advanced breast cancer and clinically evident bone metastases. In women with abnormal bone scans but

Table 3

Blood and lymphatic system disorders	Common >1/100, <1/10) Lymphopenia Uncommon >1/1,000, <1/100) Anaemia, leukopenia Very rare (<1/10,000), including isolated reports Thrombocytopenia
Immune system disorders	Uncommon >1/1,000, <1/100) Hypersensitivity including anaphylactic reactions, bronchospasm, dyspnoea, angioneurotic oedema Very rare (<1/10,000), including isolated reports Anaphylactic shock, reactivation of herpes simplex and herpes zoster
Metabolism and nutrition disorders	Very common >1/10) Hypocalcaemia, hypophosphataemia Common >1/100, <1/10) Hypomagnesaemia Uncommon >1/1,000, <1/100) Hyperkalaemia, hypokalaemia, hypernatraemia Very rare (<1/10,000), including isolated reports Hypernatraemia with confusional state
Nervous system disorders	Common >1/100, <1/10) Headache Uncommon >1/1,000, <1/100) Agitation, confusional state, dizziness, insomnia,somnolence, lethargy Very rare (<1/10,000), including isolated reports Seizures, visual hallucinations, symptomatic hypocalcaemia (paraesthesia, tetany, muscle cramps)
Eye disorders	Uncommon >1/1,000, <1/100) Uveitis (iritis, iridocyclitis), scleritis, episcleritis, conjunctivitis Very rare (<1/10,000), including isolated reports Xanthopsia, orbital inflammation
Cardiac disorders / Vascular disorders	Uncommon >1/1,000, <1/100) Hypertension Very rare (<1/10,000), including isolated reports Hypotension, heart disease aggravated (left ventricular failure / congestive cardial failure) with dyspnoea, pulmonary oedema due to fluid overload
Gastrointestinal disorders	Common >1/100, <1/10) Nausea, vomiting Uncommon >1/1,000, <1/100) Abdominal pain, anorexia, diarrhoea, constipation, dyspepsia Very rare (<1/10,000), including isolated reports Gastritis
Skin and subcutaneous tissue disorders	Uncommon >1/1,000, <1/100) Rash, pruritus
Musculoskeletal and connective tissue disorders	Common >1/100, <1/10) Transient bone pain, arthralgia, myalgia Uncommon >1/1,000, <1/100) Muscle cramp Rare >1/10,000, <1/1,000) Osteonecrosis primarily involving the jaws
Renal and urinary disorders	Rare >1/10,000, <1/1,000) Focal segmental glomerulosclerosis including the collapsing variant, nephrotic syndrome, renal tubular disorder, glomerulonephropathy, tubulointerstitial nephritis Very rare (<1/10,000), including isolated reports Renal function aggravated in patients with multiple myeloma, haematuria, renal failure acute, renal function aggravated in patients with pre-existing renal disease.
General disorders and administration site conditions	Very common >1/10) Fever and influenza like symptoms sometimes accompanied by malaise, rigors, fatigue and flushing Common >1/100, <1/10) Infusion site reactions like infusion site pain, infusion site rash, infusion site swelling, infusion site induration, infusion site phlebitis, thrombophlebitis, general body pain
Investigations	Very rare (<1/10,000), including isolated reports Liver function test abnormal, blood creatinine increased, blood urea increased

normal plain radiographs pain should be the primary guide to treatment.

Pamidronate has been shown to reduce pain, decrease the number of pathological fractures and the need for radiotherapy, correct hypercalcaemia and improve Quality of Life in patients with advanced multiple myeloma.

A meta-analysis of bisphosphonates in >1100 patients with multiple myeloma showed the NNT (number of patients needed to treat)to prevent one vertebral fracture was 10 and NNT to prevent one patient experiencing pain was 11 with best effects seen with pamidronate and clodronate.

5.2 Pharmacokinetic properties

General characteristics:

Pamidronate has a strong affinity for calcified tissues, and total elimination of pamidronate from the body is not observed within the time-frame of experimental studies. Calcified tissues are therefore regarded as site of "apparent elimination".

Absorption:

Pamidronate disodium is given by intravenous infusion. By definition, absorption is complete at the end of the infusion.

Distribution:

Plasma concentrations of pamidronate rise rapidly after the start of an infusion and fall rapidly when the infusion is stopped. The apparent distribution half-life in plasma is about 0.8 hours. Apparent steady-state concentrations are therefore achieved with infusions of more than about 2-3 hours duration. Peak plasma pamidronate concentrations of about 10 nmol/ml are achieved after an intravenous infusion of 60 mg given over 1 hour.

A similar percentage (approximately 50%) of the dose is retained in the body after admini-stra-tion of different doses (30-90 mg) of pamidronate disodium independent of infusion time (4 or 24 hours) Thus the accumulation of pamidronate in bone is not capacity-limited, and is dependent solely on the total cumulative dose administered. The percentage of circulating pamidronate bound to plasma proteins is relatively low (less than 50 %) and increases when calcium concentrations are pathologically elevated.

Elimination:

Pamidronate does not appear to be eliminated by biotransformation. After an intravenous infusion, about 20-55 % of the dose is recovered in the urine within 72 hours as unchanged pamidronate. Within the time-frame of experimental studies the remaining fraction of the dose is retained in the body. From the urinary elimination of pamidronate, two decay phases with apparent half-lives of about 1.6 and 27 hours, can be observed. The total plasma and renal clearance has been reported to be 88-254 ml/min and 38-60 ml/min, respectively. The apparent plasma clearance is about 180 ml/min. The apparent renal clearance is about 54 ml/min, and there is a tendency for the renal clearance to correlate with creatinine clearance.

Characteristics in patients:

Hepatic and metabolic clearance of pamidronate are insignificant. Impairment of liver function is therefore not expected to influence the pharmacokinetics of pamidronate disodium, although as there are no clinical data available in patients with severe liver impairment, no specific recommendations can be given for this patient population. Medac Disodium Pamidronate 3 mg/ml displays little potential for drug-drug interactions both at the metabolic level and at the level of protein binding (see section 5.2 above).

A pharmacokinetic study conducted in patients with cancer showed no differences in plasma AUC of pamidronate between patients with normal renal function and patients with mild to moderate renal impairment. In patients with severe renal impairment (creatinine clearance < 30 mL/min), the AUC of pamidronate was approximately 3 times higher than in patients with normal renal function (creatinine clearance > 90 mL/min).

5.3 Preclinical safety data

In pregnant rats, pamidronate has been shown to cross the placenta and accumulate in foetal bone in a manner similar to that observed in adult animals. Pamidronate disodium has been shown to increase the length of gestation and parturition in rats resulting in an increasing pup mortality when given orally at daily doses of 60 mg/kg (approximately equivalent to 1.2 mg/kg intravenously) and above (0.7 times the highest recommended human dose for a single intravenous infusion).

There was no unequivocal evidence for teratogenicity in studies with intravenous administration of pamidronate disodium to pregnant rats, although high doses (12 and 15 mg/kg/day) were associated with maternal toxicity and foetal developmental abnormalities (foetal oedema and shortened bones) and doses of 6 mg/kg and above with reduced ossification. Lower intravenous pamidronate disodium doses (1-6 mg/kg/day) interfered (pre-partum distress and fetotoxicity) with normal parturition in the rat. These effects: foetal developmental abnormalities, prolonged parturition and reduced survival rate of pups were probably caused by a decrease in maternal serum calcium levels.

Only low intravenous doses have been investigated in pregnant rabbits, because of maternal toxicity, but the highest dose used (1.5 mg/kg/day) was associated with an increased resorption rate and reduced ossification. However there was no evidence for teratogenicity.

The toxicity of pamidronate is characterised by direct (cytotoxic) effects on organs with a copious blood supply such as the stomach, lungs and kidneys. In animal studies with intravenous administration, renal tubular lesions were the prominent and consistent untoward effects of treatment.

Carcinogenesis and Mutagenesis:

Pamidronate disodium by daily oral administration was not carcinogenic in an 80 week or a 104 week study in mice.

Pamidronate disodium showed no genotoxic activity in a standard battery of assays for gene mutations and chromosomal damage.

6. PHARMACEUTICAL PARTICULARS

6.1 List of excipients

Sodium hydroxide (for pH adjustment)

Hydrochloric acid (for pH adjustment)

Water for Injections

6.2 Incompatibilities

Pamidronate will form complexes with divalent cations and should not be added to calcium-containing intravenous solutions.

The medicinal product should not be mixed with other products except those mentioned in section 6.6.

Solutions of pamidronate disodium are not soluble in lipophilic nutrition solutions, e. g. soya-bean oil.

6.3 Shelf life

Unopened vial: 36 months

Shelf life after dilution in 5 % glucose solution or in 0,9 % sodium chloride solution:

chemical and physical in-use stability has been demonstrated for 96 hours at 25°C.

From a microbiological point of view, the product should be used immediately. If not used immediately, in use storage times and conditions prior to use are the responsibility of the user and would normally not be longer than 24 hours at 2 to 8°C, unless dilution has taken place in controlled and validated aseptic conditions.

6.4 Special precautions for storage

No special precautions for storage.

6.5 Nature and contents of container
Colourless 5 ml/10 ml/20 ml/30 ml glass vials (Ph. Eur., Type 1) and bromobutylrubber stoppers (Ph. Eur., Type 1).

Pack sizes:

1, 4 or 10 vials containing 5 ml sterile concentrate

1, 4 or 10 vials containing 10 ml sterile concentrate

1, 4 or 10 vials containing 20 ml sterile concentrate

1, 4 or 10 vials containing 30 ml sterile concentrate

Not all pack sizes may be marketed.

6.6 Instructions for use and handling
Must be diluted with 5% glucose solution or 0.9% sodium chloride solution prior to administration.

The concentration of pamidronate disodium in the infusion solution should not exceed 90 mg/250 ml.

Do not use solution if particles are present.

Any portion of the contents remaining after use should be discarded.

Medac Disodium Pamidronate 3 mg/ml, sterile concentrate is for single use only.

The diluted solution for infusion should be visually inspected and only clear solutions practically free from particles should be used.

7. MARKETING AUTHORISATION HOLDER
medac

Gesellschaft für klinische Spezialpraeparate mbH

Fehlandtstraße 3

D-20354 Hamburg

Germany

8. MARKETING AUTHORISATION NUMBER(S)
PL 11587/0027

9. DATE OF FIRST AUTHORISATION/RENEWAL OF THE AUTHORISATION
7 September 2004

10. DATE OF REVISION OF THE TEXT
17 June 2005

Medinol Over 6 Paracetamol Oral Suspension BP 250mg/5ml.

(SSL International plc)

1. NAME OF THE MEDICINAL PRODUCT
Medinol Over 6 Paracetamol Oral Suspension.

2. QUALITATIVE AND QUANTITATIVE COMPOSITION
Paracetamol BP 250mg/5ml.

3. PHARMACEUTICAL FORM
Oral suspension.

4. CLINICAL PARTICULARS

4.1 Therapeutic indications
For the relief of mild to moderate pain including headache, migraine, neuralgia, toothache and sore throat. Symptomatic relief of rheumatic aches and pains. Symptomatic relief of influenza, feverishness and colds.

4.2 Posology and method of administration
Oral. To be taken four times daily. Do not repeat doses more frequently than every four hours.

Adults, the elderly and children over 12 years of age: two to four 5ml spoonfuls. Children 6 to 12 years: one to two 5ml spoonfuls. Not to be given to children under 6 years of age. Do not take more than 4 doses in 24 hours

4.3 Contraindications
Should be used with caution in patients with impaired kidney or liver function. Hypersensitivity to paracetamol and/or other constituents.

4.4 Special warnings and special precautions for use
Care is advised in the administration of paracetamol to patients with severe renal or severe hepatic impairment and in those with non-cirrhotic alcoholic liver disease. The hazards of overdose are greater in those with alcoholic liver disease. If pain or fever persists for more than 3 days, consult your doctor. Prolonged use without medical supervision may be harmful. Do not exceed the stated dose. Keep out of the reach of children.

The labels state: Do not give with any other paracetamol-containing products. Immediate medical advice should be sought in the event of an overdose, even if the child seems well.

The leaflet states: Immediate medical advice should be sought in the event of an overdose, even if the child seems well, because of the risk of delayed serious liver damage.

4.5 Interaction with other medicinal products and other forms of Interaction
Alcohol, barbiturates, anticonvulsants and tricyclic antidepressants may increase hepatotoxicity of paracetamol, particularly after an overdose. Paracetamol may increase the half life of chloramphenicol. The speed of absorption of paracetamol may be increased by metoclopramide or domperidone and absorption reduced by cholestyramine. The anticoagulant effect of warfarin and other coumarins may be enhanced by prolonged regular use of paracetamol with increased risk of bleeding.

4.6 Pregnancy and lactation
Epidemiological studies in human pregnancy have shown no effects due to paracetamol used in the recommended dosage. However, paracetamol should be avoided in pregnancy unless considered essential by the physician.

Paracetamol is excreted in breast milk but not in a clinically significant amount. Available published data do not contraindicate breast feeding.

4.7 Effects on ability to drive and use machines
None known.

4.8 Undesirable effects
Adverse effects of paracetamol are rare but hypersensitivity including skin rash may occur. There have been reports of blood dyscrasias including thrombocytopaenia and agranulocytosis, and of acute pancreatitis.

4.9 Overdose
Symptoms of overdosage in the first 24 hours are pallor, nausea, vomiting, anorexia, and abdominal pain. Liver damage may become apparent 12 to 48 hours after ingestion. Abnormalities of glucose metabolism and metabolic acidosis may occur. In severe poisoning, hepatic failure may progress to encephalopathy, coma and death. Acute renal failure with acute tubular necrosis may develop even in the absence of severe liver damage. Cardiac arrhythmias have been reported. Liver damage is likely in adults who have taken 10g or more of paracetamol. It is considered that excess quantities of a toxic metabolite (usually adequately detoxified by gluthathione when normal doses of paracetamol are ingested), become irreversibly bound to liver tissue.

Treatment: Immediate treatment is essential in the management of a paracetamol overdose. Despite a lack of significant early symptoms, patients should be referred to hospital urgently for immediate medical attention and any patient who has ingested around 7.5g or more of paracetamol in the preceding 4 hours should undergo gastric lavage. Administration of oral methionine or intravenous N-acetylcysteine, which may have a beneficial effect up to at least 48 hours after the overdose, may be required. General supportive measures must be available.

5. PHARMACOLOGICAL PROPERTIES

5.1 Pharmacodynamic properties
Paracetamol has analgesic and antipyretic properties.

5.2 Pharmacokinetic properties
Paracetamol is readily absorbed from the gastrointestinal tract with peak plasma concentrations occurring 30 minutes to 2 hours after ingestion. It is metabolised in the liver and excreted in the urine mainly as the glucuronide and sulphate conjugates. The elimination half-life varies from 1 to 4 hours.

5.3 Preclinical safety data
There are no pre-clinical data of relevance to the prescriber that are additional to that already included in other sections of the Summary of Product Characteristics.

6. PHARMACEUTICAL PARTICULARS

6.1 List of excipients
Sodium Methylhydroxybenzoate BP; Sodium Propylhydroxybenzoate BP; Sodium Saccharin BP; Sodium Cyclamate 1968 BP; Tragacanth BP; Lycasin 80/55; Strawberry Flavour PFW 500253E; Purified Water.

6.2 Incompatibilities
None known.

6.3 Shelf life
36 months.

6.4 Special precautions for storage
Store below 25°C.

6.5 Nature and contents of container
Amber glass sirop bottle with tamper evident cap fitted with polycone liner, containing 100 or 200ml of product.

6.6 Instructions for use and handling
Not applicable.

7. MARKETING AUTHORISATION HOLDER
Cupal Limited, Tubiton House, Oldham, OL1 3HS.

8. MARKETING AUTHORISATION NUMBER(S)
PL 0338/0069.

9. DATE OF FIRST AUTHORISATION/RENEWAL OF THE AUTHORISATION
10th November 1989 / 20th September 2004

10. DATE OF REVISION OF THE TEXT
September 2004

Medinol Paediatric Paracetamol Oral Suspension BP 120mg/5ml

(SSL International plc)

1. NAME OF THE MEDICINAL PRODUCT
Medinol Paediatric Paracetamol Oral Suspension BP 120mg/5ml.

2. QUALITATIVE AND QUANTITATIVE COMPOSITION
Paracetamol BP 120mg/5ml.

3. PHARMACEUTICAL FORM
Oral suspension.

4. CLINICAL PARTICULARS

4.1 Therapeutic indications
For the relief of pain and to relieve or reduce fever.

4.2 Posology and method of administration
Route of administration: oral. To be taken four times daily. Do not repeat dose more frequently than every four hours. Infants under 3 months: on doctors advice only (10mg/kg). A 2.5ml dose is suitable for babies who develop a fever following vaccination at 2 months. In all other cases use only under medical supervision. Infants 3 months to 1 year: half to one 5ml spoonful (60-120mg). Children 1-6 years: one or two 5ml spoonfuls (120-240mg). Children over 6 years: two or four 5ml spoonfuls (240-480mg). Do not give more than four doses in 24 hours. Not to be given to infants under 3 months except on medical advice.

4.3 Contraindications
Hypersensitivity to paracetamol and/or other constituents. Impaired kidney and liver function.

4.4 Special warnings and special precautions for use
If pain or fever persists for more than 3 days consult a doctor. Prolonged use without medical supervision may be harmful. Do not give with other product containing paracetamol concurrently.

If your baby was born prematurely and is less than 3 months old consult your doctor before use.

In cases of accidental overdose seek medical attention immediately. Care is advised in the administration of paracetamol to patients with severe renal or severe hepatic impairment. The hazards of overdose are greater in those with (non-cirrhotic) alcoholic liver disease.

Keep out of the reach of children. Do not exceed the stated dose.

4.5 Interaction with other medicinal products and other forms of Interaction
Cholestyramine may reduce absorption of paracetamol. Metoclopramide and domperidone may accelerate absorption of paracetamol. Alcohol, barbiturates, anticonvulsants and tricyclic antidepressants may increase the hepatoxicity of paracetamol particularly after an overdose. The anticoagulant effect of warfarin and other coumarins may be enhanced by prolonged regular use of paracetamol with increased risk of bleeding; occasional doses have no significant effect.

4.6 Pregnancy and lactation
Epidemiological studies in human pregnancy have shown no ill effects due to paracetamol used in the recommended dosage, but patients should follow the advice of their doctor regarding its use. Paracetamol is excreted in breast milk but not in a clinically significant amount. Available published data do not contraindicate breast-feeding. This product may, therefore, be taken during pregnancy and lactation.

4.7 Effects on ability to drive and use machines
None stated.

4.8 Undesirable effects
Adverse effects of paracetamol are rare but hypersensitivity including skin rash may occur. There have been reports of blood dyscrasias including thrombocytopaenia and agranulocytosis, but these were not necessarily causally related to paracetamol. If given in therapeutic doses side effects are rare. Haematological reactions have been reported. Most reports of adverse reactions to paracetamol relate to overdosage with the drug.

4.9 Overdose
Symptoms of paracetamol overdosage in the first 24 hours are pallor, nausea, vomiting, anorexia and abdominal pain. Liver damage may become apparent 12 to 48 hours after ingestion. Abnormalities of glucose metabolism and metabolic acidosis may occur. In severe poisoning, hepatic failure may progress to encephalopathy, coma and death. Acute renal failure with acute tubular necrosis may develop even in the absence of severe liver damage. Cardiac arrhythmias and pancreatitis have been reported. Liver damage is possible in adults who have taken 10g or more of paracetamol.

Treatment: Immediate treatment is essential in the management of paracetamol overdose. Despite a lack of significant early symptoms, patients should be referred to hospital urgently for immediate medical attention and any patient who has ingested around 7.5g or more of paracetamol in the preceding 4 hours should undergo gastric lavage. General supportive measures must be available. After gastric lavage a suitable antidote such as acetylcysteine or methionine should be given. Acetylcysteine is given by intravenous infusion in an initial dose of 150mg/kg body weight over 15 minutes, followed by 50mg/kg over 4 hours and then by 100mg/kg over the next 16 hours. Alternatively, methionine 2.5g may be given by mouth every four hours to a total of 4 doses. The blood paracetamol levels should be monitored to determine whether further therapy is necessary. In severe poisoning, hepatic failure may progress to encephalopathy, coma and death.

5. PHARMACOLOGICAL PROPERTIES

5.1 Pharmacodynamic properties

Analgesic/antipyretic.

5.2 Pharmacokinetic properties

Not applicable.

5.3 Preclinical safety data

None stated.

6. PHARMACEUTICAL PARTICULARS

6.1 List of excipients

Methylhydroxybenzoate BP; Propylhydroxybenzoate BP; Sodium Saccharin BP; Sodium Cyclamate 1968 BP; Tragacanth BP; Lycasin 80/55; Strawberry Flavour PFW 500253E; Water.

6.2 Incompatibilities

None stated.

6.3 Shelf life

36 months unopened.

6.4 Special precautions for storage

Avoid extremes of temperatures.

6.5 Nature and contents of container

Amber glass sirop bottle with tamper evident cap with fitted polycone liner containing containing 70 or 140ml of product. Supplied in a carton with a 5ml CE marked polystyrene measuring spoon.

6.6 Instructions for use and handling

Not applicable.

7. MARKETING AUTHORISATION HOLDER

Cupal Limited, Tubiton House, Oldham, OL1 3HS.

8. MARKETING AUTHORISATION NUMBER(S)

PL 0338/0033.

9. DATE OF FIRST AUTHORISATION/RENEWAL OF THE AUTHORISATION

10th February 1987 / 12th February 1992.

10. DATE OF REVISION OF THE TEXT

May 2004

Medinol Under 6 Paracetamol Oral Suspension BP 120mg/5ml

(SSL International plc)

1. NAME OF THE MEDICINAL PRODUCT

Medinol Under 6 Paracetamol Oral Suspension BP 120mg/5ml.

2. QUALITATIVE AND QUANTITATIVE COMPOSITION

Paracetamol BP 120mg/5ml.

3. PHARMACEUTICAL FORM

Oral suspension.

4. CLINICAL PARTICULARS

4.1 Therapeutic indications

For the relief of pain and to relieve or reduce fever.

4.2 Posology and method of administration

Route of administration: oral. To be taken four times daily. Do not repeat dose more frequently than every four hours. Infants under 3 months: on doctors advice only (10mg/kg). A 2.5ml dose is suitable for babies who develop a fever following vaccination at 2 months. In all other cases use only under medical supervision. Infants 3 months to 1 year: half to one 5ml spoonful (60-120mg). Children 1-6 years: one or two 5ml spoonfuls (120-240mg). Children over 6 years: two or four 5ml spoonfuls (240-480mg). Do not give more than four doses in 24 hours. Not to be given to infants under 3 months except on medical advice.

4.3 Contraindications

Hypersensitivity to paracetamol and/or other constituents. Impaired kidney and liver function.

4.4 Special warnings and special precautions for use

If pain or fever persists for more than 3 days consult a doctor. Prolonged use without medical supervision may be harmful. Do not give with other product containing paracetamol concurrently.

If your baby was born prematurely and is less than 3 months old consult your doctor before use.

In cases of accidental overdose seek medical attention immediately. Care is advised in the administration of paracetamol to patients with severe renal or severe hepatic impairment. The hazards of overdose are greater in those with (non-cirrhotic) alcoholic liver disease. Keep out of the reach of children. Do not exceed the stated dose.

4.5 Interaction with other medicinal products and other forms of Interaction

Cholestyramine may reduce absorption of paracetamol. Metoclopramide and domperidone may accelerate absorption of paracetamol. Alcohol, barbiturates, anticonvulsants and tricyclic antidepressants may increase the hepatoxicity of paracetamol particularly after an overdose. The anticoagulant effect of warfarin and other coumarins may be enhanced by prolonged regular use of paracetamol with increased risk of bleeding; occasional doses have no significant effect.

4.6 Pregnancy and lactation

Epidemiological studies in human pregnancy have shown no ill effects due to paracetamol used in the recommended dosage, but patients should follow the advice of their doctor regarding its use. Paracetamol is excreted in breast milk but not in a clinically significant amount. Available published data do not contraindicate breast-feeding. This product may, therefore, be taken during pregnancy and lactation.

4.7 Effects on ability to drive and use machines

None stated.

4.8 Undesirable effects

Adverse effects of paracetamol are rare but hypersensitivity including skin rash may occur. There have been reports of blood dyscrasias including thrombocytopaenia and agranulocytosis, but these were not necessarily causally related to paracetamol. If given in therapeutic doses side effects are rare. Haematological reactions have been reported. Most reports of adverse reactions to paracetamol relate to overdosage with the drug.

4.9 Overdose

Symptoms of paracetamol overdosage in the first 24 hours are pallor, nausea, vomiting, anorexia and abdominal pain. Liver damage may become apparent 12 to 48 hours after ingestion. Abnormalities of glucose metabolism and metabolic acidosis may occur. In severe poisoning, hepatic failure may progress to encephalopathy, coma and death. Acute renal failure with acute tubular necrosis may develop even in the absence of severe liver damage. Cardiac arrhythmias and pancreatitis have been reported. Liver damage is possible in adults who have taken 10g or more of paracetamol.

Treatment: Immediate treatment is essential in the management of paracetamol overdose. Despite a lack of significant early symptoms, patients should be referred to hospital urgently for immediate medical attention and any patient who has ingested around 7.5g or more of paracetamol in the preceding 4 hours should undergo gastric lavage. General supportive measures must be available. After gastric lavage a suitable antidote such as acetylcysteine or methionine should be given. Acetylcysteine is given by intravenous infusion in an initial dose of 150mg/kg body weight over 15 minutes, followed by 50mg/kg over 4 hours and then by 100mg/kg over the next 16 hours. Alternatively, methionine 2.5g may be given by mouth every four hours to a total of 4 doses. The blood paracetamol levels should be monitored to determine whether further therapy is necessary. In severe poisoning, hepatic failure may progress to encephalopathy, coma and death.

5. PHARMACOLOGICAL PROPERTIES

5.1 Pharmacodynamic properties

Analgesic/antipyretic

5.2 Pharmacokinetic properties

Not applicable.

5.3 Preclinical safety data

None stated.

6. PHARMACEUTICAL PARTICULARS

6.1 List of excipients

Methylhydroxybenzoate BP; Propylhydroxybenzoate BP; Sodium Saccharin BP; Sodium Cyclamate 1968 BP; Tragacanth BP; Lycasin 80/55; Strawberry Flavour PFW 500253E; Water.

6.2 Incompatibilities

None stated.

6.3 Shelf life

36 months unopened.

6.4 Special precautions for storage

Avoid extremes of temperatures.

6.5 Nature and contents of container

Amber glass sirop bottle with tamper evident cap with fitted polycone liner containing containing 70 or 140ml of product. Supplied in a carton with a 5ml CE marked polystyrene measuring spoon.

6.6 Instructions for use and handling

Not applicable.

7. MARKETING AUTHORISATION HOLDER

Cupal Limited, Tubiton House, Oldham, OL1 3HS.

8. MARKETING AUTHORISATION NUMBER(S)

PL 0338/0033.

9. DATE OF FIRST AUTHORISATION/RENEWAL OF THE AUTHORISATION

10th February 1987 / 12th February 1992.

10. DATE OF REVISION OF THE TEXT

May 2004

Medised for Children

(SSL International plc)

1. NAME OF THE MEDICINAL PRODUCT

Medised For Children

2. QUALITATIVE AND QUANTITATIVE COMPOSITION

Paracetamol BP 120mg/5ml; Diphenhydramine Hydrochloride 12.5mg/5ml.

3. PHARMACEUTICAL FORM

Oral solution. Clear to pale pink liquid.

4. CLINICAL PARTICULARS

4.1 Therapeutic indications

For the treatment of mild to moderate pain including teething pain, headache, sore throat, aches and pains. For the symptomatic relief of influenza, feverishness, and feverish colds. Controls excessive mucous secretion and eases nasal irritation. Also helps restful sleep.

4.2 Posology and method of administration

Route of Administration: Oral. Recommended Dosage and Dosage Schedules: 3 months to under 1 year: 2.5ml-5ml (0.5 to 1 teaspoonful) 3-4 times daily; 1 year to under 6 years: 5ml-10ml (1-2 teaspoonful) 3-4 times daily; 6 years to under 12 years: 10ml-20ml (2-4 teaspoonful) 3 times daily.

4.3 Contraindications

Hypersensitivity to paracetamol, and/or any other constituents. Large doses of antihistamines may precipitate fits in epileptics.

4.4 Special warnings and special precautions for use

Do not exceed the stated dose. Immediate medical advice should be sought in the event of an overdose, even if the patient feels well because of the risk of delayed serious liver damage. Do not take with any other paracetamol containing products. This product should not be given to children under the age of three months except on the advice of a doctor. Dose should not be repeated more frequently than four hour intervals. Not more than 4 doses should be taken in 24 hours. Dosage should not be continued for more than three days without consulting a doctor.

This product should be administered with caution to patients with known renal or hepatic impairment. The hazards of overdose are greater in those with alcoholic liver disease. Keep out of the reach of children.

4.5 Interaction with other medicinal products and other forms of Interaction

The speed of absorption of paracetamol may be increased by metoclopramide or domperidone and absorption reduced by cholestyramine. The anticoagulant effect of warfarin and other coumarins may be enhanced by prolonged regular daily use of paracetamol with increased risk of bleeding. Effects of alcohol and sedatives may be potentiated.

4.6 Pregnancy and lactation

Safety in pregnancy has not been established. Epidemiological studies in human pregnancy have shown no effects due to paracetamol used in the recommended dosage, but patients should follow the advice of their doctor regarding its use. Paracetamol is excreted in breast milk, but not a clinically significant amount. Available published data does not contraindicate breast feeding.

4.7 Effects on ability to drive and use machines

May cause drowsiness. If affected do not drive or operate machinery.

4.8 Undesirable effects

Adverse effects of paracetamol are rare but hypersensitivity, including skin rash, may occur. There have been a few reports of blood dyscrasias including thrombocytopenia and agranulocytosis but these were not necessarily causally related to paracetamol.

4.9 Overdose

The features of overdose are: sedation, pallor, nausea, vomiting, diarrhoea, anorexia, and abdominal pain; liver damage may become apparent in 12 to 48 hours. In some children overdose may cause cerebral stimulation resulting in convulsions and hyperpyrexia.

Abnormalities of glucose metabolism and metabolic acidosis may occur. In severe poisoning, hepatic failure may progress to encephalopathy, coma and death. Acute renal failure with acute tubular necrosis may develop even in the absence of severe liver damage. Cardiac arrhythmias and pancreatitis have been reported. Liver damage is likely in adults who have taken 10g or more of paracetamol. It is considered that excess quantities of a toxic metabolite (usually adequately detoxified by glutathione when normal doses of paracetamol are ingested), become irreversibly bound to liver tissue. Immediate treatment is essential in the management of paracetamol overdose. Despite a lack of significant early symptoms, patients should be referred to hospital urgently for immediate medical attention and any patient who has ingested around 7.5g or more of paracetamol in the preceeding four hours should undergo gastric lavage. Administration of oral methionine or intravenous N-acetylcysteine which may have a beneficial effect up to at least 48 hours after the overdose, may be required. General supportive measures must be available.

5. PHARMACOLOGICAL PROPERTIES

5.1 Pharmacodynamic properties

Paracetamol is an antipyretic and analgesic. Diphenhydramine hydrochloride is an antihistamine with anti-cholinergic, anti-emetic, anti-allergic and sedative effects.

5.2 Pharmacokinetic properties

Paracetamol and diphenhydramine hydrochloride are both readily absorbed from the gastrointestinal tract. Both are widely distributed throughout the body. Both are metabolised in the liver and excreted in the urine. As Medised Infant is a solution, absorption of actives is rapid following oral ingestion.

5.3 Preclinical safety data

Paracetamol and diphenhydramine hydrochloride are well established drug substances whose pre-clinical profiles have been investigated and are thoroughly established.

6. PHARMACEUTICAL PARTICULARS

6.1 List of excipients

Macrogol 4000; Glycerol; Propylene Glycol; Sorbitol Solution (non crystallising) 70%; Lycasin 80/55 (Maltitol Solution); Sodium Cyclamate; Sodium Saccharin; Nipasept (Methylhydroxybenzoate, Ethylhydroxybenzoate and Parahydroxybenzoate); Strawberry Flavour 513805E; Sugar Module 555049E; Water, Purified.

6.2 Incompatibilities

Not applicable.

6.3 Shelf life

36 months.

6.4 Special precautions for storage

Do not store above 25°C. Do not refrigerate. Keep container in outer carton.

6.5 Nature and contents of container

Amber type III glass and plastic clic loc cap with expanded polyethylene wadding. 100ml and 200ml. Supplied with a 5ml CE marked polystyrene measuring spoon.

6.6 Instructions for use and handling

None.

7. MARKETING AUTHORISATION HOLDER

Seton Products Limited, Tubiton House, Oldham, OL1 3HS.

8. MARKETING AUTHORISATION NUMBER(S)

PL 11314/0135.

9. DATE OF FIRST AUTHORISATION/RENEWAL OF THE AUTHORISATION

13th September 1999.

10. DATE OF REVISION OF THE TEXT

July 2004

Medrone Tablets 100mg

(Pharmacia Limited)

1. NAME OF THE MEDICINAL PRODUCT

Medrone® Tablets 100 mg.

2. QUALITATIVE AND QUANTITATIVE COMPOSITION

Each Medrone Tablet contains 100 mg methylprednisolone Ph. Eur.

3. PHARMACEUTICAL FORM

Tablet

4. CLINICAL PARTICULARS

4.1 Therapeutic indications

Medrone is a potent corticosteroid with an anti-inflammatory activity at least five times that of hydrocortisone. An enhanced separation of glucocorticoid and mineralocorticoid effect results in a reduced incidence of sodium and water retention.

Medrone is indicated for conditions requiring glucocorticoid activity such as:-

1. Collagen diseases/arteritis

Systemic lupus erythematosus

Systemic dermatomyositis (polymyositis)

Rheumatic fever with severe carditis

Giant cell arteritis/polymyalgia rheumatica

2. Dermatological diseases

Pemphigus vulgaris

3. Allergic states

Bronchial asthma

4. Respiratory diseases

Pulmonary sarcoid

5. Haematological disorders

Idiopathic thrombocytopenic purpura

Haemolytic anaemia (autoimmune)

6. Neoplastic diseases

Leukaemia (acute and lymphatic)

Malignant lymphoma

7. Gastro-intestinal diseases

Crohn's disease

8. Miscellaneous

Tuberculous meningitis (with appropriate antituberculous chemotherapy)

Transplantation

4.2 Posology and method of administration

The dosage recommendations shown in the table below are suggested initial daily doses and are intended as guides. The average total daily dose recommended may be given either as a single dose or in divided doses (excepting in alternate day therapy when the minimum effective daily dose is doubled and given every other day at 8.00 a.m.). It is envisaged that the 100 mg tablet will be used for high initial daily or alternate day doses in acute situations, with tapering of dosage achieved by using the 16 mg tablet.

Undesirable effects may be minimised by using the lowest effective dose for the minimum period (see Special warnings and special precautions for use).

The initial suppressive dose level may vary depending on the condition being treated. As soon as a satisfactory clinical response is obtained, the daily dose should be reduced gradually, either to termination of treatment in the case of acute conditions or to the minimal effective maintenance dose level in the case of chronic conditions. In chronic conditions it is important that the reduction in dosage from initial to maintenance dose levels be accomplished as clinically appropriate.

In alternate-day therapy, the minimum daily corticoid requirement is doubled and administered as a single dose every other day at 8.00 a.m. Dosage requirements depend on the condition being treated and response of the patient.

Elderly patients: Treatment of elderly patients, particularly if long-term, should be planned bearing in mind the more serious consequences of the common side-effects of corticosteroids in old age and close clinical supervision is required (see Special warnings and special precautions for use).

Children: In general, dosage for children should be based upon clinical response and is at the discretion of the clinician. Treatment should be limited to the minimum dosage for the shortest period of time. If possible, treatment should be administered as a single dose on alternate days (see Special warnings and special precautions for use).

Dosage Recommendations:

Indications	Recommended initial daily dosage
Systemic lupus erythematosus	20-100 mg
Systemic dermatomyositis	48 mg
Acute rheumatic fever	48 mg until ESR normal for one week.
Giant cell arteritis/polymyalgia rheumatica	64 mg
Pemphigus vulgaris	80-360 mg
Bronchial asthma	up to 64 mg single dose/alternate day up to 100 mg maximum.
Pulmonary sarcoid	32-48 mg on alternate days.
Haematological disorders and leukaemias	16-100 mg
Malignant lymphoma	16-100 mg
Crohn's disease	up to 48 mg per day in acute episodes.
Organ transplantation	up to 3.6 mg/kg/day

4.3 Contraindications

Medrone is contra-indicated where there is known hypersensitivity to components and in systemic fungal infection unless specific anti-infective therapy is employed.

4.4 Special warnings and special precautions for use

Warnings and Precautions:

1. A Patient Information Leaflet is provided in the pack by the manufacturer.

2. Undesirable effects may be minimised by using the lowest effective dose for the minimum period, and by administering the daily requirement as a single morning dose or whenever possible as a single morning dose on alternative days. Frequent patient review is required to appropriately titrate the dose against disease activity (see Posology and method of administration).

3. Adrenal cortical atrophy develops during prolonged therapy and may persist for months after stopping treatment. In patients who have received more than physiological doses of systemic corticosteroids (approximately 6 mg methylprednisolone) for greater than 3 weeks, withdrawal should not be abrupt. How dose reduction should be carried out depends largely on whether the disease is likely to relapse as the dose of systemic corticosteroids is reduced. Clinical assessment of disease activity may be needed during withdrawal. If the disease is unlikely to relapse on withdrawal of systemic corticosteroids, but there is uncertainty about HPA suppression, the dose of systemic corticosteroid may be reduced rapidly to physiological doses. Once a daily dose of 6 mg methylprednisolone is reached, dose reduction should be slower to allow the HPA-axis to recover.

Abrupt withdrawal of systemic corticosteroid treatment, which has continued up to 3 weeks is appropriate if it considered that the disease is unlikely to relapse. Abrupt withdrawal of doses up to 32 mg daily of methylprednisolone for 3 weeks is unlikely to lead to clinically relevant HPA-axis suppression, in the majority of patients. In the following patient groups, gradual withdrawal of systemic corticosteroid therapy should be *considered* even after courses lasting 3 weeks or less:

• Patients who have had repeated courses of systemic corticosteroids, particularly if taken for greater than 3 weeks.

• When a short course has been prescribed within one year of cessation of long-term therapy (months or years).

• Patients who may have reasons for adrenocortical insufficiency other than exogenous corticosteroid therapy.

• Patients receiving doses of systemic corticosteroid greater than 32 mg daily of methylprednisolone.

• Patients repeatedly taking doses in the evening.

4. Since mineralocorticoid secretion may be impaired, salt and/or a mineralocorticoid should be administered concurrently.

5. Patients should carry 'Steroid Treatment' cards which give clear guidance on the precautions to be taken to minimise risk and which provide details of prescriber, drug, dosage and the duration of treatment.

6. Corticosteroids may mask some signs of infection, and new infections may appear during their use. Suppression of the inflammatory response and immune function increases the susceptibility to fungal, viral and bacterial infections and their severity. The clinical presentation may often be atypical and may reach an advanced stage before being recognised.

7. Chickenpox is of serious concern since this normally minor illness may be fatal in immunosuppressed patients. Patients (or parents of children) without a definite history of chickenpox should be advised to avoid close personal contact with chickenpox or herpes zoster and if exposed they should seek urgent medical attention. Passive immunization with varicella/zoster immunoglobin (VZIG) is needed by exposed non-immune patients who are receiving systemic corticosteroids or who have used them within the previous 3 months; this should be given within 10 days of exposure to chickenpox. If a diagnosis of chickenpox is confirmed, the illness warrants specialist care and urgent treatment. Corticosteroids should not be stopped and the dose may need to be increased.

8. Exposure to measles should be avoided. Medical advice must be sought immediately if exposure occurs. Prophylaxis with normal intramuscular immunoglobulin may be needed.

9. Live vaccines should not be given to individuals with impaired immune responsiveness. The antibody response to other vaccines may be diminished.

10. The use of Medrone in active tuberculosis should be restricted to those cases of fulminating or disseminated tuberculosis in which the corticosteroid is used for the management of the disease in conjunction with an appropriate antituberculous regimen. If corticosteroids are indicated in patients with latent tuberculosis or tuberculin reactivity, close observation is necessary as reactivation of the disease may occur. During prolonged corticosteroid therapy, these patients should receive chemoprophylaxis.

11. Care should be taken for patients receiving cardioactive drugs such as digoxin because of steroid induced electrolyte disturbance/potassium loss (see Undesirable effects).

Special precautions:

Particular care is required when considering the use of systemic corticosteroids in patients with the following conditions and frequent patient monitoring is necessary.

1. Osteoporosis (post-menopausal females are particularly at risk).
2. Hypertension or congestive heart failure.
3. Existing or previous history of severe affective disorders (especially previous steroid psychosis).
4. Diabetes mellitus (or a family history of diabetes).
5. History of tuberculosis.
6. Glaucoma (or a family history of glaucoma).
7. Previous corticosteroid-induced myopathy.
8. Liver failure or cirrhosis.
9. Renal insufficiency.
10. Epilepsy.
11. Peptic ulceration.
12. Fresh intestinal anastomoses.
13. Predisposition to thrombophlebitis.
14. Abscess or other pyogenic infections.
15. Ulcerative colitis.
16. Diverticulitis.
17. Myasthenia gravis.
18. Ocular herpes simplex, for fear of corneal perforation.
19. Hypothyroidism.
20. Recent myocardial infarction (myocardial rupture has been reported).
21. Kaposi's sarcoma has been reported to occur in patients receiving corticosteroid therapy. Discontinuation of corticosteroids may result in clinical remission.

Use in children: Corticosteroids cause growth retardation in infancy, childhood and adolescence. Treatment should be limited to the minimum dosage for the shortest possible time. In order to minimise suppression of the hypothalamo-pituitary-adrenal axis and growth retardation, treatment should be administered where possible as a single dose on alternate days.

Use in the elderly: The common adverse effects of systemic corticosteroids may be associated with more serious consequences in old age, especially osteoporosis, hypertension, hypokalaemia, diabetes, susceptibility to infection and thinning of the skin. Close clinical supervision is required to avoid life-threatening reactions.

4.5 Interaction with other medicinal products and other forms of Interaction

1. Convulsions have been reported with concurrent use of methylprednisolone and cyclosporin. Since concurrent administration of these agents results in a mutual inhibition of metabolism, it is possible that convulsions and other adverse effects associated with the individual use of either drug may be more apt to occur.

2. Drugs that induce hepatic enzymes, such as rifampicin, rifabutin, carbamazepine, phenobarbitone, phenytoin, primidone, and aminoglutethimide enhance the metabolism of corticosteroids and its therapeutic effects may be reduced.

3. Drugs which inhibit the CYP3A4 enzyme, such as cimetidine, erythromycin, ketoconazole, itraconazole, diltiazem and mibefradil, may decrease the rate of metabolism of corticosteroids and hence increase the serum concentration.

4. Steroids may reduce the effects of anticholinesterases in myasthenia gravis. The desired effects of hypoglycaemic agents (including insulin), anti-hypertensives and diuretics are antagonised by corticosteroids, and the hypokalaemic effects of acetazolamide, loop diuretics, thiazide diuretics and carbenoxolone are enhanced.

5. The efficacy of coumarin anticoagulants may be enhanced by concurrent corticosteroid therapy and close monitoring of the INR or prothrombin time is required to avoid spontaneous bleeding.

6. The renal clearance of salicylates is increased by corticosteroids and steroid withdrawal may result in salicylate intoxication. Salicylates and non-steroidal anti-inflammatory agents should be used cautiously in conjunction with corticosteroids in hypothrombinaemia.

7. Steroids have been reported to interact with neuromuscular blocking agents such as pancuronium with partial reversal of the neuromuscular block.

4.6 Pregnancy and lactation

Pregnancy

The ability of corticosteroids to cross the placenta varies between individual drugs, however, methylprednisolone does cross the placenta.

Administration of corticosteroids to pregnant animals can cause abnormalities of foetal development including cleft palate, intra-uterine growth retardation and affects on brain growth and development. There is no evidence that corticosteroids result in an increased incidence of congenital abnormalities, such as cleft palate in man, however, when administered for long periods or repeatedly during pregnancy, corticosteroids may increase the risk of intra-uterine growth retardation. Hypoadrenalism may, in theory, occur in the neonate following prenatal exposure to corticosteroids but usually resolves spontaneously following birth and is rarely clinically important. As with all drugs, corticosteroids should only be prescribed when the benefits to the mother and child outweigh the risks. When corticosteroids are essential, however, patients with normal pregnancies may be treated as though they were in the non-gravid state.

Lactation

Corticosteroids are excreted in small amounts in breast milk, however, doses of up to 40 mg daily of methylprednisolone are unlikely to cause systemic effects in the infant. Infants of mothers taking higher doses than this may have a degree of adrenal suppression, but the benefits of breast-feeding are likely to outweigh any theoretical risk.

4.7 Effects on ability to drive and use machines

None stated.

4.8 Undesirable effects

The incidence of predictable undesirable side-effects associated with the use of corticosteroids, including hypothalamic-pituitary-adrenal suppression correlates with the relative potency of the drug, dosage, timing of administration and duration of treatment (see Special warnings and special precautions for use).

GASTRO-INTESTINAL - Dyspepsia, peptic ulceration with perforation and haemorrhage, abdominal distension, oesophageal ulceration, oesophageal candidiasis, acute pancreatitis, perforation of bowel, gastric haemorrhage.

Increases in alanine transaminase (ALT, SGPT) aspartate transaminase (AST, SGOT) and alkaline phosphatase have been observed following corticosteroid treatment. These changes are usually small, not associated with any clinical syndrome and are reversible upon discontinuation.

ANTI-INFLAMMATORY AND IMMUNOSUPPRESSIVE EFFECTS - Increased susceptibility and severity of infections with suppression of clinical symptoms and signs, opportunistic infections, may suppress reactions to skin tests, recurrence of dormant tuberculosis (see Special warnings and special precautions for use).

MUSCULOSKELETAL - Proximal myopathy, osteoporosis, vertebral and long bone fractures, avascular osteonecrosis, tendon rupture, muscle weakness.

FLUID AND ELECTROLYTE DISTURBANCE - Sodium and water retention, hypertension, hypokalaemic alkalosis, potassium loss, congestive heart failure in susceptible patients.

DERMATOLOGICAL - Impaired healing, skin atrophy, bruising, striae, telangiectasia, acne, petechiae and ecchymosis. Kaposi's sarcoma has been reported in patients receiving corticosteroid therapy.

ENDOCRINE/METABOLIC - Suppression of the hypothalamo-pituitary-adrenal axis, growth suppression in infancy, childhood and adolescence, menstrual irregularity and amenorrhoea. Cushingoid facies, hirsutism, weight gain, impaired carbohydrate tolerance with increased requirement for antidiabetic therapy, negative nitrogen and calcium balance. Increased appetite.

NEUROPSYCHIATRIC - Euphoria, psychological dependence, mood swings, depression, personality changes, insomnia. Increased intra-cranial pressure with papilloedema in children (pseudotumour cerebri), usually after treatment withdrawal. Psychosis, aggravation of schizophrenia, seizures.

OPHTHALMIC - Increased intra-ocular pressure, glaucoma, papilloedema with possible damage to the optic nerve, cataracts, corneal or scleral thinning, exacerbation of ophthalmic viral or fungal disease, exophthalmos.

CARDIOVASCULAR – Myocardial rupture following a myocardial infarction.

GENERAL - Leucocytosis, hypersensitivity reactions including anaphylaxis, thrombo-embolism, nausea, malaise, persistent hiccups with high dose corticosteroids.

WITHDRAWAL SYMPTOMS - Too rapid a reduction of corticosteroid dosage following prolonged treatment can lead to acute adrenal insufficiency, hypotension and death (see Special warnings and special precautions for use).

A 'withdrawal syndrome' may also occur including, fever, myalgia, arthralgia, rhinitis, conjunctivitis, painful itchy skin nodules and loss of weight.

4.9 Overdose

Administration of Medrone should not be discontinued abruptly but tailed off over a period of time. Appropriate action should be taken to alleviate the symptoms produced by any side-effect that may become apparent. It may be necessary to support the patient with corticosteroids during any further period of trauma occurring within two years of overdosage.

There is no clinical syndrome of acute overdose with Medrone. Methylprednisolone is dialysable.

5. PHARMACOLOGICAL PROPERTIES

5.1 Pharmacodynamic properties

Methylprednisolone is a potent anti-inflammatory steroid. It has greater anti-inflammatory potency than prednisolone and less tendency than prednisolone to induce sodium and water retention. The relative potency of methylprednisolone to hydrocortisone is at least four to one.

5.2 Pharmacokinetic properties

The mean elimination half-life ranges from 2.4 to 3.5 hours in normal, healthy adults and appears to be independent of the route of administration.

Methylprednisolone is metabolised in the liver to inactive metabolites, the major ones being 20 b-hydroxymethylprednisolone and 20 b-hydroxy-a-methylprednisolone.

Methylprednisolone clearance is altered by concurrent administration of troleandomycin, erythromycin, rifampicin, anticonvulsants and theophylline. No dosing adjustments are necessary in renal failure. Methylprednisolone is haemodialyzable.

5.3 Preclinical safety data

None.

6. PHARMACEUTICAL PARTICULARS

6.1 List of excipients

Methylcellulose, sodium starch glycolate, microcrystalline cellulose, magnesium stearate and E132.

6.2 Incompatibilities

None stated.

6.3 Shelf life

48 months.

6.4 Special precautions for storage

Store below 25°C.

6.5 Nature and contents of container

Amber glass bottle with LDPE cap and bulb or HDPE screw cap - each bottle contains 20 25, 30 or 100 tablets.

Flint glass bottle with LDPE cap and bulb or HDPE screw cap (child-resistant) - each bottle contains 25, 30 or 100 tablets.

Polypropylene bottle with LDPE closure or HDPE screw cap (child resistant) - each bottle contains 25, 30 or 100 tablets.

PVC blister/aluminium foil (10 tablet strip) - each pack contains 20, 30 or 100 tablets.

6.6 Instructions for use and handling

No special requirements.

7. MARKETING AUTHORISATION HOLDER

Pharmacia Limited
Davy Avenue
Milton Keynes
MK5 8PH
UK

8. MARKETING AUTHORISATION NUMBER(S)

PL 0032/0145

9. DATE OF FIRST AUTHORISATION/RENEWAL OF THE AUTHORISATION

Date of first authorisation: 3 May 1991

Last renewal dates: 25 March 1997

10. DATE OF REVISION OF THE TEXT

January 2003

LEGAL CATEGORY: POM

Medrone Tablets 16mg

(Pharmacia Limited)

1. NAME OF THE MEDICINAL PRODUCT

Medrone Tablets 16 mg.

2. QUALITATIVE AND QUANTITATIVE COMPOSITION

Each Medrone Tablet contains 16 mg methylprednisolone Ph. Eur.

3. PHARMACEUTICAL FORM

Tablet

4. CLINICAL PARTICULARS

4.1 Therapeutic indications

Medrone is indicated for conditions requiring glucocorticoid activity such as:-

1. Endocrine disorders

Primary and secondary adrenal insufficiency

Congenital adrenal hyperplasia

2. Rheumatic disorders

Rheumatoid arthritis

Juvenile chronic arthritis

Ankylosing spondylitis

3. Collagen diseases/arteritis

Systemic lupus erythematosus

Systemic dermatomyositis (polymyositis)

Rheumatic fever with severe carditis

Giant cell arteritis/polymyalgia rheumatica

4. Dermatological diseases

Pemphigus vulgaris

5. Allergic states

Severe seasonal and perennial allergic rhinitis

Drug hypersensitivity reactions

Serum sickness

Allergic contact dermatitis

Bronchial asthma

6. Ophthalmic diseases

Anterior uveitis (iritis, iridocyclitis)

Posterior uveitis

Optic neuritis

7. Respiratory diseases

Pulmonary sarcoid

Fulminating or disseminated tuberculosis (with appropriate anti-tuberculous chemotherapy)

Aspiration of gastric contents

8. Haematological disorders

Idiopathic thrombocytopenic purpura

Haemolytic anaemia (autoimmune)

9. Neoplastic diseases

Leukaemia (acute and lymphatic)

Malignant lymphoma

10. Gastro-intestinal diseases

Ulcerative colitis

Crohn's disease

11. Miscellaneous

Tuberculous meningitis (with appropriate anti-tuberculous chemotherapy)

Transplantation

4.2 Posology and method of administration

The dosage recommendations shown in the table below are suggested initial daily doses and are intended as guides. The average total daily dose recommended may be given either as a single dose or in divided doses (excepting in alternate day therapy when the minimum effective daily dose is doubled and given every other day at 8.00 am).

Undesirable effects may be minimised by using the lowest effective dose for the minimum period (see Special warnings and special precautions for use).

The initial suppressive dose level may vary depending on the condition being treated. This is continued until a satisfactory clinical response is obtained, a period usually of three to seven days in the case of rheumatic diseases (except for acute rheumatic carditis), allergic conditions affecting the skin or respiratory tract and ophthalmic diseases. If a satisfactory response is not obtained in seven days, re-evaluation of the case to confirm the original diagnosis should be made. As soon as a satisfactory clinical response is obtained, the daily dose should be reduced gradually, either to termination of treatment in the case of acute conditions (e.g. seasonal asthma, exfoliative dermatitis, acute ocular inflammations) or to the minimal effective maintenance dose level in the case of chronic conditions (e.g. rheumatoid arthritis, systemic lupus erythematosus, bronchial asthma, atopic dermatitis). In chronic conditions, and in rheumatoid arthritis especially, it is important that the reduction in dosage from initial to maintenance dose levels be accomplished as clinically appropriate. Decrements of not more than 2 mg at intervals of 7 - 10 days are suggested. In rheumatoid arthritis, maintenance steroid therapy should be at the lowest possible level.

In alternate-day therapy, the minimum daily corticoid requirement is doubled and administered as a single dose every other day at 8.00 am. Dosage requirements depend on the condition being treated and response of the patient.

Elderly patients: Treatment of elderly patients, particularly if long-term, should be planned bearing in mind the more serious consequences of the common side-effects of corticosteroids in old age, particularly osteoporosis, diabetes, hypertension, susceptibility to infection and thinning of skin (see Special warnings and special precautions for use).

Children: In general, dosage for children should be based upon clinical response and is at the discretion of the physician. Treatment should be limited to the minimum dosage for the shortest period of time. If possible, treatment should be administered as a single dose on alternate days (see Special warnings and special precautions for use).

Dosage Recommendations:

<u>IndicationsRecommended initial daily dosage</u>

Rheumatoid arthritis

severe 12 - 16 mg

moderately severe 8 - 12 mg

moderate 4 - 8 mg

children 4 - 8 mg

Systemic dermatomyositis 48 mg

Systemic lupus erythematosus 20 - 100 mg

Acute rheumatic fever 48 mg until ESR normal for one week.

Allergic diseases 12 - 40 mg

Bronchial asthma up to 64 mg single dose/alternate day up to 100 mg maximum.

Ophthalmic diseases 12 - 40 mg

Haematological disorders and leukaemias 16 - 100 mg

Malignant lymphoma 16 - 100 mg

Ulcerative colitis 16 - 60 mg

Crohn's disease up to 48 mg per day in acute episodes.

Organ transplantation up to 3.6 mg/kg/day

Pulmonary sarcoid 32 - 48 mg on alternate days.

Giant cell arteritis/polymyalgia rheumatica 64 mg

Pemphigus vulgaris 80 - 360 mg

4.3 Contraindications

Medrone is contra-indicated where there is known hypersensitivity to components and in systemic infection unless specific anti-infective therapy is employed.

4.4 Special warnings and special precautions for use

Warnings and precautions:

1. A Patient Information Leaflet is provided in the pack by the manufacturer.

2. Undesirable effects may be minimised by using the lowest effective dose for the minimum period, and by administering the daily requirement as a single morning dose or whenever possible as a single morning dose on alternative days. Frequent patient review is required to appropriately titrate the dose against disease activity (see Posology and method of administration).

3. Adrenal cortical atrophy develops during prolonged therapy and may persist for months after stopping treatment. In patients who have received more than physiological doses of systemic corticosteroids (approximately 6 mg methylprednisolone) for greater than 3 weeks, withdrawal should not be abrupt. How dose reduction should be carried out depends largely on whether the disease is likely to relapse as the dose of systemic corticosteroids is reduced. Clinical assessment of disease activity may be needed during withdrawal. If the disease is unlikely to relapse on withdrawal of systemic corticosteroids, but there is uncertainty about HPA suppression, the dose of systemic corticosteroid <u>may</u> be reduced rapidly to physiological doses. Once a daily dose of 6 mg methylprednisolone is reached, dose reduction should be slower to allow the HPA-axis to recover.

Abrupt withdrawal of systemic corticosteroid treatment, which has continued up to 3 weeks is appropriate if it considered that the disease is unlikely to relapse. Abrupt withdrawal of doses up to 32 mg daily of methylprednisolone for 3 weeks is unlikely to lead to clinically relevant HPA-axis suppression, in the majority of patients. In the following patient groups, gradual withdrawal of systemic corticosteroid therapy should be ***considered*** even after courses lasting 3 weeks or less:

- Patients who have had repeated courses of systemic corticosteroids, particularly if taken for greater than 3 weeks.
- When a short course has been prescribed within one year of cessation of long-term therapy (months or years).
- Patients who may have reasons for adrenocortical insufficiency other than exogenous corticosteroid therapy.
- Patients receiving doses of systemic corticosteroid greater than 32 mg daily of methylprednisolone.
- Patients repeatedly taking doses in the evening.

4. Since mineralocorticoid secretion may be impaired, salt and/or a mineralocorticoid should be administered concurrently.

5. Patients should carry 'Steroid Treatment' cards which give clear guidance on the precautions to be taken to minimise risk and which provide details of prescriber, drug, dosage and the duration of treatment.

6. Corticosteroids may mask some signs of infection, and new infections may appear during their use. Suppression of the inflammatory response and immune function increases the susceptibility to fungal, viral and bacterial infections and their severity. The clinical presentation may often be atypical and may reach an advanced stage before being recognised.

7. Chickenpox is of serious concern since this normally minor illness may be fatal in immunosuppressed patients. Patients (or parents of children) without a definite history of chickenpox should be advised to avoid close personal contact with chickenpox or herpes zoster and if exposed they should seek urgent medical attention. Passive immunization with varicella/zoster immunoglobulin (VZIG) is needed by exposed non-immune patients who are receiving systemic corticosteroids or who have used them within the previous 3 months; this should be given within 10 days of exposure to chickenpox. If a diagnosis of chickenpox is confirmed, the illness warrants specialist care and urgent treatment. Corticosteroids should not be stopped and the dose may need to be increased.

8. Exposure to measles should be avoided. Medical advice must be sought immediately if exposure occurs. Prophylaxis with normal intramuscular immunoglobulin may be needed.

9. Live vaccines should not be given to individuals with impaired immune responsiveness. The antibody response to other vaccines may be diminished.

10. The use of Medrone in active tuberculosis should be restricted to those cases of fulminating or disseminated tuberculosis in which the corticosteroid is used for the management of the disease in conjunction with an appropriate antituberculous regimen. If corticosteroids are indicated in patients with latent tuberculosis or tuberculin reactivity, close observation is necessary as reactivation of the disease may occur. During prolonged corticosteroid therapy, these patients should receive chemoprophylaxis.

11. Care should be taken for patients receiving cardioactive drugs such as digoxin because of steroid induced electrolyte disturbance/potassium loss (see Undesirable effects).

Special precautions:

Particular care is required when considering the use of systemic corticosteroids in patients with the following conditions and frequent patient monitoring is necessary.

1. Osteoporosis (post-menopausal females are particularly at risk).
2. Hypertension or congestive heart failure.
3. Existing or previous history of severe affective disorders (especially previous steroid psychosis).
4. Diabetes mellitus (or a family history of diabetes).
5. History of tuberculosis.
6. Glaucoma (or a family history of glaucoma).
7. Previous corticosteroid-induced myopathy.
8. Liver failure or cirrhosis.
9. Renal insufficiency.
10. Epilepsy.
11. Peptic ulceration.
12. Fresh intestinal anastomoses.
13. Predisposition to thrombophlebitis.
14. Abscess or other pyogenic infections.
15. Ulcerative colitis.
16. Diverticulitis.
17. Myasthenia gravis.
18. Ocular herpes simplex, for fear of corneal perforation.
19. Hypothyroidism.
20. Recent myocardial infarction (myocardial rupture has been reported).
21. Kaposi's sarcoma has been reported to occur in patients receiving corticosteroid therapy. Discontinuation of corticosteroids may result in clinical remission.

Use in children: Corticosteroids cause growth retardation in infancy, childhood and adolescence. Treatment should be limited to the minimum dosage for the shortest possible time. In order to minimise suppression of the hypothalamo-pituitary-adrenal axis and growth retardation, treatment should be administered where possible as a single dose on alternate days.

Use in the elderly: The common adverse effects of systemic corticosteroids may be associated with more serious consequences in old age, especially osteoporosis, hypertension, hypokalaemia, diabetes, susceptibility to infection and thinning of the skin. Close clinical supervision is required to avoid life-threatening reactions.

4.5 Interaction with other medicinal products and other forms of Interaction

1. Convulsions have been reported with concurrent use of methylprednisolone and ciclosporin. Since concurrent administration of these agents results in a mutual inhibition of metabolism, it is possible that convulsions and other adverse effects associated with the individual use of either drug may be more apt to occur.

2. Drugs that induce hepatic enzymes, such as rifampicin, rifabutin, carbamazepine, phenobarbitone, phenytoin, primidone, and aminoglutethimide enhance the metabolism of corticosteroids and its therapeutic effects may be reduced.

3. Drugs which inhibit the CYP3A4 enzyme, such as cimetidine, erythromycin, ketoconazole, itraconazole, diltiazem and mibefradil, may decrease the rate of metabolism of corticosteroids and hence increase the serum concentration.

4. Steroids may reduce the effects of anticholinesterases in myasthenia gravis. The desired effects of hypoglycaemic agents (including insulin), anti-hypertensives and diuretics are antagonised by corticosteroids, and the hypokalaemic effects of acetazolamide, loop diuretics, thiazide diuretics and carbenoxolone are enhanced.

5. The efficacy of coumarin anticoagulants may be enhanced by concurrent corticosteroid therapy and close monitoring of the INR or prothrombin time is required to avoid spontaneous bleeding.

6. The renal clearance of salicylates is increased by corticosteroids and steroid withdrawal may result in salicylate intoxication. Salicylates and non-steroidal anti-inflammatory agents should be used cautiously in conjunction with corticosteroids in hypothrombinaemia.

7. Steroids have been reported to interact with neuromuscular blocking agents such as pancuronium with partial reversal of the neuromuscular block.

4.6 Pregnancy and lactation

Pregnancy

The ability of corticosteroids to cross the placenta varies between individual drugs, however, methylprednisolone does cross the placenta.

Administration of corticosteroids to pregnant animals can cause abnormalities of foetal development including cleft palate, intra-uterine growth retardation and effects on brain growth and development. There is no evidence that corticosteroids result in an increased incidence of congenital abnormalities, such as cleft palate in man, however, when administered for long periods or repeatedly during pregnancy, corticosteroids may increase the risk of intra-uterine growth retardation. Hypoadrenalism may, in theory, occur in the neonate following prenatal exposure to corticosteroids but usually resolves spontaneously following birth and is rarely clinically important. As with all drugs, corticosteroids should only be prescribed when the benefits to the mother and child outweigh the risks. When corticosteroids are essential, however, patients with normal pregnancies may be treated as though they were in the non-gravid state.

Lactation

Corticosteroids are excreted in small amounts in breast milk, however, doses of up to 40 mg daily of methylprednisolone are unlikely to cause systemic effects in the infant. Infants of mothers taking higher doses than this may have a degree of adrenal suppression, but the benefits of breastfeeding are likely to outweigh any theoretical risk.

4.7 Effects on ability to drive and use machines

None stated.

4.8 Undesirable effects

The incidence of predictable undesirable side-effects associated with the use of corticosteroids, including hypothalamic-pituitary-adrenal suppression correlates with the relative potency of the drug, dosage, timing of administration and duration of treatment (see Special warnings and special precautions for use).

GASTRO-INTESTINAL - Dyspepsia, peptic ulceration with perforation and haemorrhage, abdominal distension, oesophageal ulceration, oesophageal candidiasis, acute pancreatitis, perforation of bowel, gastric haemorrhage.

Increases in alanine transaminase (ALT, SGPT) aspartate transaminase (AST, SGOT) and alkaline phosphatase have been observed following corticosteroid treatment. These changes are usually small, not associated with any clinical syndrome and are reversible upon discontinuation.

ANTI-INFLAMMATORY AND IMMUNOSUPPRESSIVE EFFECTS - Increased susceptibility and severity of infections with suppression of clinical symptoms and signs, opportunistic infections, may suppress reactions to skin tests, recurrence of dormant tuberculosis (see Special warnings and special precautions for use).

MUSCULOSKELETAL - Proximal myopathy, osteoporosis, vertebral and long bone fractures, avascular osteonecrosis, tendon rupture, muscle weakness.

FLUID AND ELECTROLYTE DISTURBANCE - Sodium and water retention, hypertension, hypokalaemic alkalosis, potassium loss, congestive heart failure in susceptible patients.

DERMATOLOGICAL - Impaired healing, skin atrophy, bruising, striae, telangiectasia, acne, petechiae and ecchymosis. Kaposi's sarcoma has been reported in patients receiving corticosteroid therapy.

ENDOCRINE/METABOLIC - Suppression of the hypothalamo-pituitary-adrenal axis, growth suppression in infancy, childhood and adolescence; menstrual irregularity and amenorrhoea. Cushingoid facies, hirsutism, weight gain, impaired carbohydrate tolerance with increased requirement for antidiabetic therapy, negative nitrogen and calcium balance. Increased appetite.

NEUROPSYCHIATRIC - Euphoria, psychological dependence, mood swings, depression, personality changes, insomnia. Increased intra-cranial pressure with papilloedema in children (pseudotumour cerebri), usually after treatment withdrawal. Psychosis, aggravation of schizophrenia, seizures.

OPHTHALMIC - Increased intra-ocular pressure, glaucoma, papilloedema with possible damage to the optic nerve, cataracts, corneal or scleral thinning, exacerbation of ophthalmic viral or fungal disease, exophthalmos.

CARDIOVASCULAR – Myocardial rupture following myocardial infarction.

GENERAL - Leucocytosis, hypersensitivity reactions including anaphylaxis, thrombo-embolism, nausea, malaise, persistent hiccups with high doses of corticosteroids.

WITHDRAWAL SYMPTOMS - Too rapid a reduction of corticosteroid dosage following prolonged treatment can lead to acute adrenal insufficiency, hypotension and death (see Special warnings and special precautions for use).

A 'withdrawal syndrome' may also occur including, fever, myalgia, arthralgia, rhinitis, conjunctivitis, painful itchy skin nodules and loss of weight.

4.9 Overdose

Administration of Medrone should not be discontinued abruptly but tailed off over a period of time. Appropriate action should be taken to alleviate the symptoms produced by any side-effect that may become apparent. It may be necessary to support the patient with corticosteroids during any further period of trauma occurring within two years of overdosage.

There is no clinical syndrome of acute overdose with Medrone. Methylprednisolone is dialysable.

5. PHARMACOLOGICAL PROPERTIES

5.1 Pharmacodynamic properties

Medrone is a potent corticosteroid with an anti-inflammatory activity at least five times that of hydrocortisone. An enhanced separation of glucocorticoid and mineralocorticoid effect results in a reduced incidence of sodium and water retention.

5.2 Pharmacokinetic properties

Corticosteroids are absorbed from the gastro-intestinal tract. In the circulation they are extensively bound to plasma proteins and are metabolised mainly in the liver but also in the kidney and are excreted in the urine.

The half-life of methylprednisolone has been reported to be slightly longer than that of prednisolone.

5.3 Preclinical safety data

None.

6. PHARMACEUTICAL PARTICULARS

6.1 List of excipients

Lactose, sucrose, maize starch, mineral oil and calcium stearate.

6.2 Incompatibilities

None stated.

6.3 Shelf life

Bottles - 60 months

Blister packs - 36 months.

6.4 Special precautions for storage

Store below 25°C.

6.5 Nature and contents of container

20-25 micron hard tempered aluminium foil/lacquer, 250 micron opaque polyvinyl chloride film blister. Pack contains 60 tablets.

6.6 Instructions for use and handling

No special requirements.

7. MARKETING AUTHORISATION HOLDER

Pharmacia Ltd

Davy Avenue

Milton Keynes

MK5 8PH

UK

8. MARKETING AUTHORISATION NUMBER(S)

PL 0032/0024R

9. DATE OF FIRST AUTHORISATION/RENEWAL OF THE AUTHORISATION

19 April 1989

10. DATE OF REVISION OF THE TEXT

June 2004

Legal category: POM

Medrone Tablets 2mg, 4mg

(Pharmacia Limited)

1. NAME OF THE MEDICINAL PRODUCT

Medrone Tablets 2 mg.

Medrone Tablets 4mg

2. QUALITATIVE AND QUANTITATIVE COMPOSITION

Medrone Tablets 2mg: each tablet contains 2 mg methylprednisolone Ph. Eur.

Medrone Tablets 4mg: each tablet contains 4 mg methylprednisolone Ph. Eur.

3. PHARMACEUTICAL FORM

Tablet

4. CLINICAL PARTICULARS

4.1 Therapeutic indications

Medrone is indicated for conditions requiring glucocorticoid activity such as:-

1. Endocrine disorders

Primary and secondary adrenal insufficiency

Congenital adrenal hyperplasia

2. Rheumatic disorders

Rheumatoid arthritis

Juvenile chronic arthritis

Ankylosing spondylitis

3. Collagen diseases/arteritis

Systemic lupus erythematosus

Systemic dermatomyositis (polymyositis)

Rheumatic fever with severe carditis

Giant cell arteritis/polymyalgia rheumatica

4. Dermatological diseases

Pemphigus vulgaris

5. Allergic states

Severe seasonal and perennial allergic rhinitis

Drug hypersensitivity reactions

Serum sickness

Allergic contact dermatitis

Bronchial asthma

6. Ophthalmic diseases

Anterior uveitis (iritis, iridocyclitis)

Posterior uveitis

Optic neuritis

7. Respiratory diseases

Pulmonary sarcoid

Fulminating or disseminated tuberculosis (with appropriate anti-tuberculous chemotherapy)

Aspiration of gastric contents

8. Haematological disorders

Idiopathic thrombocytopenic purpura

Haemolytic anaemia (autoimmune)

9. Neoplastic diseases

Leukaemia (acute and lymphatic)

Malignant lymphoma

10. Gastro-intestinal diseases

Ulcerative colitis

Crohn's disease

11. Miscellaneous

Tuberculous meningitis (with appropriate anti-tuberculous chemotherapy)

Transplantation

4.2 Posology and method of administration

The dosage recommendations shown in the table below are suggested initial daily doses and are intended as guides. The average total daily dose recommended may be given either as a single dose or in divided doses (excepting in alternate day therapy when the minimum effective daily dose is doubled and given every other day at 8.00 am).

Undesirable effects may be minimised by using the lowest effective dose for the minimum period (see Special warnings and special precautions for use).

The initial suppressive dose level may vary depending on the condition being treated. This is continued until a satisfactory clinical response is obtained, a period usually of three to seven days in the case of rheumatic diseases (except for acute rheumatic carditis), allergic conditions affecting the skin or respiratory tract and ophthalmic diseases. If a satisfactory response is not obtained in seven days, re-evaluation of the case to confirm the original diagnosis should be made. As soon as a satisfactory clinical response is obtained, the daily dose should be reduced gradually, either to termination of treatment in the case of acute conditions (e.g. seasonal asthma, exfoliative dermatitis, acute ocular inflammations) or to the minimal effective maintenance dose level in the case of chronic conditions (e.g. rheumatoid arthritis, systemic lupus erythematosus, bronchial asthma, atopic dermatitis). In chronic conditions, and in rheumatoid arthritis especially, it is important that the reduction in dosage from initial to maintenance dose levels be accomplished as clinically appropriate. Decrements of not more than 2 mg at intervals of 7 - 10 days are suggested. In rheumatoid arthritis, maintenance steroid therapy should be at the lowest possible level.

In alternate-day therapy, the minimum daily corticoid requirement is doubled and administered as a single dose every other day at 8.00 am. Dosage requirements depend on the condition being treated and response of the patient.

Elderly patients: Treatment of elderly patients, particularly if long-term, should be planned bearing in mind the more serious consequences of the common side-effects of corticosteroids in old age, particularly osteoporosis, diabetes, hypertension, susceptibility to infection and thinning of skin (see Special warnings and special precautions for use).

Children: In general, dosage for children should be based upon clinical response and is at the discretion of the physician. Treatment should be limited to the minimum dosage for the shortest period of time. If possible, treatment should be administered as a single dose on alternate days (see Special warnings and special precautions for use).

Dosage Recommendations:

IndicationsRecommended initial daily dosage

Rheumatoid arthritis

severe 12 - 16 mg

moderately severe 8 - 12 mg

moderate 4 - 8 mg

children 4 - 8 mg

Systemic dermatomyositis 48 mg

Systemic lupus erythematosus 20 - 100 mg

Acute rheumatic fever 48 mg until ESR normal for one week.

Allergic diseases 12 - 40 mg

Bronchial asthma up to 64 mg single dose/alternate day up to 100 mg maximum.

Ophthalmic diseases 12 - 40 mg

Haematological disorders and leukaemias 16 - 100 mg

Malignant lymphoma 16 - 100 mg

Ulcerative colitis 16 - 60 mg

Crohn's disease up to 48 mg per day in acute episodes.

Organ transplantation up to 3.6 mg/kg/day

Pulmonary sarcoid 32 - 48 mg on alternate days.

Giant cell arteritis/polymyalgia rheumatica 64 mg

Pemphigus vulgaris 80 - 360 mg

4.3 Contraindications

Medrone is contra-indicated where there is known hypersensitivity to components and in systemic infection unless specific anti-infective therapy is employed.

4.4 Special warnings and special precautions for use

Warnings and precautions:

1. A Patient Information Leaflet is provided in the pack by the manufacturer.

2. Undesirable effects may be minimised by using the lowest effective dose for the minimum period, and by administering the daily requirement as a single morning dose or whenever possible as a single morning dose on alternative days. Frequent patient review is required to appropriately titrate the dose against disease activity (see Posology and method of administration).

3. Adrenal cortical atrophy develops during prolonged therapy and may persist for months after stopping treatment. In patients who have received more than physiological doses of systemic corticosteroids (approximately 6 mg methylprednisolone) for greater than 3 weeks, withdrawal should not be abrupt. How dose reduction should be carried out depends largely on whether the disease is likely to relapse as the dose of systemic corticosteroids is reduced. Clinical assessment of disease activity may be needed during withdrawal. If the disease is unlikely to relapse on withdrawal of systemic corticosteroids, but there is uncertainty about HPA suppression, the dose of systemic corticosteroid may be reduced rapidly to physiological doses. Once a daily dose of 6 mg

methylprednisolone is reached, dose reduction should be slower to allow the HPA-axis to recover.

Abrupt withdrawal of systemic corticosteroid treatment, which has continued up to 3 weeks is appropriate if it considered that the disease is unlikely to relapse. Abrupt withdrawal of doses up to 32 mg daily of methylprednisolone for 3 weeks is unlikely to lead to clinically relevant HPA-axis suppression, in the majority of patients. In the following patient groups, gradual withdrawal of systemic corticosteroid therapy should be ***considered*** even after courses lasting 3 weeks or less:

- Patients who have had repeated courses of systemic corticosteroids, particularly if taken for greater than 3 weeks.
- When a short course has been prescribed within one year of cessation of long-term therapy (months or years).
- Patients who may have reasons for adrenocortical insufficiency other than exogenous corticosteroid therapy.
- Patients receiving doses of systemic corticosteroid greater than 32 mg daily of methylprednisolone.
- Patients repeatedly taking doses in the evening.

4. Since mineralocorticoid secretion may be impaired, salt and/or a mineralocorticoid should be administered concurrently.

5. Patients should carry 'Steroid Treatment' cards which give clear guidance on the precautions to be taken to minimise risk and which provide details of prescriber, drug, dosage and the duration of treatment.

6. Corticosteroids may mask some signs of infection, and new infections may appear during their use. Suppression of the inflammatory response and immune function increases the susceptibility to fungal, viral and bacterial infections and their severity. The clinical presentation may often be atypical and may reach an advanced stage before being recognised.

7. Chickenpox is of serious concern since this normally minor illness may be fatal in immunosuppressed patients. Patients (or parents of children) without a definite history of chickenpox should be advised to avoid close personal contact with chickenpox or herpes zoster and if exposed they should seek urgent medical attention. Passive immunization with varicella/zoster immunoglobulin (VZIG) is needed by exposed non-immune patients who are receiving systemic corticosteroids or who have used them within the previous 3 months; this should be given within 10 days of exposure to chickenpox. If a diagnosis of chickenpox is confirmed, the illness warrants specialist care and urgent treatment. Corticosteroids should not be stopped and the dose may need to be increased.

8. Exposure to measles should be avoided. Medical advice must be sought immediately if exposure occurs. Prophylaxis with normal intramuscular immunoglobulin may be needed.

9. Live vaccines should not be given to individuals with impaired immune responsiveness. The antibody response to other vaccines may be diminished.

10. The use of Medrone in active tuberculosis should be restricted to those cases of fulminating or disseminated tuberculosis in which the corticosteroid is used for the management of the disease in conjunction with an appropriate antituberculous regimen. If corticosteroids are indicated in patients with latent tuberculosis or tuberculin reactivity, close observation is necessary as reactivation of the disease may occur. During prolonged corticosteroid therapy, these patients should receive chemoprophylaxis.

11. Care should be taken for patients receiving cardioactive drugs such as digoxin because of steroid induced electrolyte disturbance/potassium loss (see Undesirable effects).

Special precautions:

Particular care is required when considering the use of systemic corticosteroids in patients with the following conditions and frequent patient monitoring is necessary.

1. Osteoporosis (post-menopausal females are particularly at risk).
2. Hypertension or congestive heart failure.
3. Existing or previous history of severe affective disorders (especially previous steroid psychosis).
4. Diabetes mellitus (or a family history of diabetes).
5. History of tuberculosis.
6. Glaucoma (or a family history of glaucoma).
7. Previous corticosteroid-induced myopathy.
8. Liver failure or cirrhosis.
9. Renal insufficiency.
10. Epilepsy.
11. Peptic ulceration.
12. Fresh intestinal anastomoses.
13. Predisposition to thrombophlebitis.
14. Abscess or other pyogenic infections.
15. Ulcerative colitis.
16. Diverticulitis.
17. Myasthenia gravis.
18. Ocular herpes simplex, for fear of corneal perforation.
19. Hypothyroidism.
20. Recent myocardial infarction (myocardial rupture has been reported).
21. Kaposi's sarcoma has been reported to occur in patients receiving corticosteroid therapy. Discontinuation of corticosteroids may result in clinical remission.

Use in children: Corticosteroids cause growth retardation in infancy, childhood and adolescence. Treatment should be limited to the minimum dosage for the shortest possible time. In order to minimise suppression of the hypothalamo-pituitary-adrenal axis and growth retardation, treatment should be administered where possible as a single dose on alternate days.

Use in the elderly: The common adverse effects of systemic corticosteroids may be associated with more serious consequences in old age, especially osteoporosis, hypertension, hypokalaemia, diabetes, susceptibility to infection and thinning of the skin. Close clinical supervision is required to avoid life-threatening reactions.

4.5 Interaction with other medicinal products and other forms of Interaction

1. Convulsions have been reported with concurrent use of methylprednisolone and ciclosporin. Since concurrent administration of these agents results in a mutual inhibition of metabolism, it is possible that convulsions and other adverse effects associated with the individual use of either drug may be more apt to occur.

2. Drugs that induce hepatic enzymes, such as rifampicin, rifabutin, carbamazepine, phenobarbitone, phenytoin, primidone, and aminoglutethimide enhance the metabolism of corticosteroids and its therapeutic effects may be reduced.

3. Drugs which inhibit the CYP3A4 enzyme, such as cimetidine, erythromycin, ketoconazole, itraconazole, diltiazem and mibefradil, may decrease the rate of metabolism of corticosteroids and hence increase the serum concentration.

4. Steroids may reduce the effects of anticholinesterases in myasthenia gravis. The desired effects of hypoglycaemic agents (including insulin), anti-hypertensives and diuretics are antagonised by corticosteroids, and the hypokalaemic effects of acetazolamide, loop diuretics, thiazide diuretics and carbenoxolone are enhanced.

5. The efficacy of coumarin anticoagulants may be enhanced by concurrent corticosteroid therapy and close monitoring of the INR or prothrombin time is required to avoid spontaneous bleeding.

6. The renal clearance of salicylates is increased by corticosteroids and steroid withdrawal may result in salicylate intoxication. Salicylates and non-steroidal anti-inflammatory agents should be used cautiously in conjunction with corticosteroids in hypothrombinaemia.

7. Steroids have been reported to interact with neuromuscular blocking agents such as pancuronium with partial reversal of the neuromuscular block.

4.6 Pregnancy and lactation

Pregnancy

The ability of corticosteroids to cross the placenta varies between individual drugs, however, methylprednisolone does cross the placenta.

Administration of corticosteroids to pregnant animals can cause abnormalities of foetal development including cleft palate, intra-uterine growth retardation and effects on brain growth and development. There is no evidence that corticosteroids result in an increased incidence of congenital abnormalities, such as cleft palate in man, however, when administered for long periods or repeatedly during pregnancy, corticosteroids may increase the risk of intra-uterine growth retardation. Hypoadrenalism may, in theory, occur in the neonate following prenatal exposure to corticosteroids but usually resolves spontaneously following birth and is rarely clinically important. As with all drugs, corticosteroids should only be prescribed when the benefits to the mother and child outweigh the risks. When corticosteroids are essential, however, patients with normal pregnancies may be treated as though they were in the non-gravid state.

Lactation

Corticosteroids are excreted in small amounts in breast milk, however, doses of up to 40 mg daily of methylprednisolone are unlikely to cause systemic effects in the infant. Infants of mothers taking higher doses than this may have a degree of adrenal suppression, but the benefits of breastfeeding are likely to outweigh any theoretical risk.

4.7 Effects on ability to drive and use machines

None stated.

4.8 Undesirable effects

The incidence of predictable undesirable side-effects associated with the use of corticosteroids, including hypothalamic-pituitary-adrenal suppression correlates with the relative potency of the drug, dosage, timing of administration and duration of treatment (see Special warnings and special precautions for use).

GASTRO-INTESTINAL - Dyspepsia, peptic ulceration with perforation and haemorrhage, abdominal distension, oesophageal ulceration, oesophageal candidiasis, acute pancreatitis, perforation of bowel, gastric haemorrhage.

Increases in alanine transaminase (ALT, SGPT) aspartate transaminase (AST, SGOT) and alkaline phosphatase have been observed following corticosteroid treatment. These changes are usually small, not associated with any clinical syndrome and are reversible upon discontinuation.

ANTI-INFLAMMATORY AND IMMUNOSUPPRESSIVE EFFECTS - Increased susceptibility and severity of infections with suppression of clinical symptoms and signs, opportunistic infections, may suppress reactions to skin tests, recurrence of dormant tuberculosis (see Special warnings and special precautions for use).

MUSCULOSKELETAL - Proximal myopathy, osteoporosis, vertebral and long bone fractures, avascular osteonecrosis, tendon rupture, muscle weakness.

FLUID AND ELECTROLYTE DISTURBANCE - Sodium and water retention, hypertension, hypokalaemic alkalosis, potassium loss, congestive heart failure in susceptible patients.

DERMATOLOGICAL - Impaired healing, skin atrophy, bruising, striae, telangiectasia, acne, petechiae and ecchymosis. Kaposi's sarcoma has been reported in patients receiving corticosteroid therapy.

ENDOCRINE/METABOLIC - Suppression of the hypothalamo-pituitary-adrenal axis, growth suppression in infancy, childhood and adolescence; menstrual irregularity and amenorrhoea. Cushingoid facies, hirsutism, weight gain, impaired carbohydrate tolerance with increased requirement for antidiabetic therapy, negative nitrogen and calcium balance. Increased appetite.

NEUROPSYCHIATRIC - Euphoria, psychological dependence, mood swings, depression, personality changes, insomnia. Increased intra-cranial pressure with papilloedema in children (pseudotumour cerebri), usually after treatment withdrawal. Psychosis, aggravation of schizophrenia, seizures.

OPHTHALMIC - Increased intra-ocular pressure, glaucoma, papilloedema with possible damage to the optic nerve, cataracts, corneal or scleral thinning, exacerbation of ophthalmic viral or fungal disease, exophthalmos.

CARDIOVASCULAR – Myocardial rupture following myocardial infarction.

GENERAL - Leucocytosis, hypersensitivity reactions including anaphylaxis, thrombo-embolism, nausea, malaise, persistent hiccups with high doses of corticosteroids.

WITHDRAWAL SYMPTOMS - Too rapid a reduction of corticosteroid dosage following prolonged treatment can lead to acute adrenal insufficiency, hypotension and death (see Special warnings and special precautions for use).

A 'withdrawal syndrome' may also occur including, fever, myalgia, arthralgia, rhinitis, conjunctivitis, painful itchy skin nodules and loss of weight.

4.9 Overdose

Administration of Medrone should not be discontinued abruptly but tailed off over a period of time. Appropriate action should be taken to alleviate the symptoms produced by any side-effect that may become apparent. It may be necessary to support the patient with corticosteroids during any further period of trauma occurring within two years of overdosage.

There is no clinical syndrome of acute overdose with Medrone. Methylprednisolone is dialysable.

5. PHARMACOLOGICAL PROPERTIES

5.1 Pharmacodynamic properties

Medrone is a potent corticosteroid with an anti-inflammatory activity at least five times that of hydrocortisone. An enhanced separation of glucocorticoid and mineralocorticoid effect results in a reduced incidence of sodium and water retention.

5.2 Pharmacokinetic properties

Corticosteroids are absorbed from the gastro-intestinal tract. In the circulation they are extensively bound to plasma proteins and are metabolised mainly in the liver but also in the kidney and are excreted in the urine.

The half-life of methylprednisolone has been reported to be slightly longer than that of prednisolone.

5.3 Preclinical safety data

None.

6. PHARMACEUTICAL PARTICULARS

6.1 List of excipients

Medrone Tablets 2mg: Lactose, rose colour, sucrose, maize starch and calcium stearate.

Medrone Tablets 4mg: Lactose, sucrose, maize starch and calcium stearate.

6.2 Incompatibilities

None stated.

6.3 Shelf life

Bottles - 60 months

Blister packs - 36 months.

6.4 Special precautions for storage

Store below 25°C.

6.5 Nature and contents of container

20-25 micron hard tempered aluminium foil/lacquer, 250 micron opaque polyvinyl chloride film blister. Pack contains 30 tablets.

6.6 Instructions for use and handling
No special requirements.

7. MARKETING AUTHORISATION HOLDER
Pharmacia Ltd
Davy Avenue
Milton Keynes
MK5 8PH
UK

8. MARKETING AUTHORISATION NUMBER(S)
Medrone Tablets 2mg: PL 0032/5017R
Medrone Tablets 4mg: PL 0032/5018R

9. DATE OF FIRST AUTHORISATION/RENEWAL OF THE AUTHORISATION
Date of first authorisation Medrone Tablets 2mg: 24 April 1996.

Date of first authorisation Medrone Tablets 4mg: 1 December 1989.

10. DATE OF REVISION OF THE TEXT
June 2004

Legal category: POM

Megace 40 mg and 160 mg Tablets

(Bristol-Myers Pharmaceuticals)

1. NAME OF THE MEDICINAL PRODUCT
Megace 40mg & 160mg Tablets

2. QUALITATIVE AND QUANTITATIVE COMPOSITION
Each tablet contains Megestrol Acetate BP 40 or 160 mg.

3. PHARMACEUTICAL FORM
Oral Tablets

4. CLINICAL PARTICULARS

4.1 Therapeutic indications
Megace is a progestational agent, indicated for the treatment of certain hormone dependent neoplasms, such as a endometrial or breast cancer.

4.2 Posology and method of administration
Breast cancer:

160 mg/day (40 mg qid or 160 mg taken once daily).

Endometrial cancer:

40-320 mg/day in divided doses (40-80 mg one to four times daily or one to two 160 mg tablets daily).

At least two months of continuous treatment is considered an adequate period for determining the efficacy of Megace.

Children:

Megace is not recommended for use in children.

Elderly:

No dosage adjustments is necessary.

4.3 Contraindications
Megace is contra-indicated in patients who have demonstrated hypersensitivity to the drug.

4.4 Special warnings and special precautions for use
Precautions:

Megace should be used with caution in patients with a history of thrombophlebitis and in patients with severe impaired liver function.

4.5 Interaction with other medicinal products and other forms of Interaction
None stated.

4.6 Pregnancy and lactation
Megace should not normally be administered to women who are pregnant or to mothers who are breast feeding.

Fertility and reproduction studies with high doses of megestrol acetate have shown a reversible feminising effect on some male rat foetuses.

Several reports suggest an association between intrauterine exposure to progestational drugs in the first trimester of pregnancy and genital abnormalities in male and female foetuses. The risk of hypospadias in male foetuses may be approximately doubled with the exposure to progestational drugs. There are insufficient data to quantify the risk to exposed female foetuses, however some of these drugs induce mild virilisation of the external genitalia of the female foetuses.

If a patient is exposed to Megace during the first four months of pregnancy or if she becomes pregnant whilst taking Megace, she should be apprised of the potential risks to the foetus.

Women of child bearing potential should be advised to avoid becoming pregnant.

Because of the potential for adverse effects, nursing should be discontinued during treatment with Megace.

4.7 Effects on ability to drive and use machines
None stated.

4.8 Undesirable effects
The major side-effect experienced by patients while taking megestrol acetate, particularly at high doses, is weight gain, which is usually not associated with water retention, but which is secondary to an increased appetite and food intake. Other occasionally noted side effects are nausea, vomiting oedema and breakthrough uterine bleeding. Reports have been received of patients developing dyspnoea, heart failure, hypertension, hot flushes, mood changes, Cushingoid facies, tumour flare (with or without hypercalcaemia), hyperglycaemia, alopecia and carpal tunnel syndrome while taking megestrol acetate. Thromboembolic phenomena including thrombophlebitis and pulmonary embolism (in some cases fatal) have been reported. A rarely encountered side effect of prolonged administration of megestrol acetate is urticaria, presumably an idiosyncratic reaction to the drug. The drug is devoid of the myelosuppressive activity characteristic of many cytotoxic drugs and it causes no significant changes in haematology, blood chemistry or urinalysis.

Pituitary adrenal axis abnormalities including glucose intolerance, and Cushing's syndrome have been reported with the use of megestrol acetate. Clinically apparent adrenal insufficiency has been rarely reported in patients shortly after discontinuing megestrol acetate. The possibility of adrenal suppression should be considered in all patients taking or withdrawing from chronic megestrol acerate therapy. Replacement stress doses of glucocorticoids may be indicated.

4.9 Overdose
No serious side effects have resulted from studies involving Megace (megestrol acetate) administered in dosages as high as 1600 mg/day.

There is no specific antidote to overdosage and treatment should therefore be symptomatic.

5. PHARMACOLOGICAL PROPERTIES

5.1 Pharmacodynamic properties
Megace (megestrol acetate) possesses pharmacologic properties similar to those of natural progesterone. Its progestational activity is slightly greater than that of medroxyprogesterone acetate, norethindrone, norethindrone acetate and norethynodrel; slightly less than that of chlormadinone acetate; and substantially less than that of norgestrel.

Megestrol acetate is a potent progestogen that exerts significant anti-oestrogenic effects. It has no androgenic or oestrogenic properties. It has anti-gonadotropic, anti-uterotropic and anti-androgenic/anti-myotropic actions. It has a slight but significant glucocorticoid effect and a very slight mineralocorticoid effect.

The progestational activity of megestrol acetate has been assessed in a number of standard tests, including Clauberg - McPhail, McGinty, uterotropic and carbonic anhydrase tests in rabbits; pregnancy maintenance and delay-of-implantation tests in rats; endometrial response in rhesus monkeys; conversion of an oestrogen-primed endometrium to a secretory one in normal women and in those with secondary amenorrhea with resultant withdrawal bleeding; induction of pseudopregnancy for treatment of endometriosis; and the delay-of-menses and thermogenic tests. In all these tests, progestational activity was high.

It has been demonstrated that megestrol acetate blocks oestrogen effects in the uteri of rats and mice in human cervical mucus and vaginal mucosa. Anti-gondotropic activity has been demonstrated in rats of both sexes.

5.2 Pharmacokinetic properties
Animal:

Peak plasma levels occur four to six hours after oral administration of radioactively labelled megestrol acetate to female rats. High concentrations are found in the liver, fat, adrenal glands, ovaries and kidneys. Radioactivity is almost wholly cleared within a week, chiefly by biliary excretion to the faeces.

In dogs, megestrol acetate metabolites are excreted primarily in the faeces. In rabbits, the principal route of metabolic excretion is urinary and the major metabolites are the 2-alpha-hydroxy-6-hydroxymethyl and 6-hydroxymethyl derivatives.

Human:

Peak plasma levels of tritiated megestrol acetate and metabolites occur one to three hours after oral administration. When 4 to 91mg of c-labelled megestrol acetate were administered orally to women, the major route of drug elimination was in the urine. The urinary and fecal recovery of total radioactivity within 10 days ranged from 56.6% to 78.4% (mean 66.4%) and 7.7% to 30.3% (mean 19.8%), respectively. The total recovered radioactivity varied between 83.1% and 94.7% (mean 86.2%). Megestrol acetate metabolites, which were identified in the urine as glucuronide conjugates, were 17-alpha-acetoxy-2-alpha hydroxy-6-methylpregna-4, 6-diene-3, 20-dione; 17-alpha-acetoxy-6-hydroxymethylpregna-4, 6-diene-3, 20-dione; and 17-alpha-acetoxy-2 alpha-hydroxy-6-hydromethylpregna-4, 6-diene-3, 20-dione; these identified metabolites accounted for only 5-8% of the administered dose.

Serum concentrations were measured after the administration of single and multiple oral doses of megestrol acetate. Adult male and post-menopausal female volunteers, no more than 65 years of age participated in the study.

Megestrol acetate is readily absorbed following oral administration of 20, 40, 80 and 200 mg doses. Megestrol serum concentrations increase with increasing doses, the relationship between increasing dosage and increasing serum levels not being arithmetically proportional. Average peak serum concentrations for the four doses tested were 89, 190, 209 and 465 ng/ml.

Mean peak serum concentrations are found three hours after single-dose administration for all dosage levels studied. The serum concentration curve appears biphasic, and the beta-phase half-life is 15 to 20 hours long.

After multiple doses over a three-day period, serum levels increase each day and are estimated to reach 80% to 90% predicted steady-state levels on the third day.

5.3 Preclinical safety data
No further relevant data.

6. PHARMACEUTICAL PARTICULARS

6.1 List of excipients

40mg Tablet:	Acacia, calcium hydrogen phosphate, lactose, magnesium stearate, maize starch, silicon dioxide.
160mg Tablet:	Colloidal silicon dioxide, lactose monohydrate, magnesium stearate, microcrystalline cellulose, povidone, sodium starch glycollate

6.2 Incompatibilities
None stated.

6.3 Shelf life
36 months - Blister packs

6.4 Special precautions for storage
Do not store Megace tablets above 25°C.

6.5 Nature and contents of container

40 mg Tablet:	blister packs of 120 tablets
160 mg Tablet:	blister packs of 30 tablets.

6.6 Instructions for use and handling
None

7. MARKETING AUTHORISATION HOLDER
Bristol-Myers Squibb Holdings Limited
t/a Bristol-Myers Pharmaceuticals
Uxbridge Business Park,
Sanderson Road,
Uxbridge,
Middlesex
UB8 1DH

8. MARKETING AUTHORISATION NUMBER(S)

40 mg Tablet:	PL 0125/0144
160 mg Tablet:	PL 0125/0173

9. DATE OF FIRST AUTHORISATION/RENEWAL OF THE AUTHORISATION

40 mg Tablet:	4 November 1982 / 2 November 1992
160 mg Tablet:	20 November 1985 / 25 April 2002

10. DATE OF REVISION OF THE TEXT
22 July 2005

Meltus Decongestant

(SSL International plc)

1. NAME OF THE MEDICINAL PRODUCT
Meltus Decongestant.

2. QUALITATIVE AND QUANTITATIVE COMPOSITION
Pseudoephedrine Hydrochloride BP 30.00mg/5ml.

3. PHARMACEUTICAL FORM
Oral Solution.

4. CLINICAL PARTICULARS

4.1 Therapeutic indications
Meltus Decongestant is a decongestant of the mucous membranes of the upper respiratory tract, especially the nasal mucosa and sinuses. It is indicated for the symptomatic relief of conditions such as the common cold, influenza, hay fever, allergic and vasomotor rhinitis. It is intended for the relief of such symptoms as blocked sinuses, stuffed up noses and catarrh.

4.2 Posology and method of administration
Route of administration: Oral. To be taken three times a day. Adults and children over 12 years: Two 5ml spoonfuls. Children 6 - 12 years: One 5ml spoonful. Children 2 - 5 years: One 2.5ml spoonful.

4.3 Contraindications
Contraindicated in patients who have previously shown intolerance to pseudoephedrine. It is contraindicated in persons under treatment with MAOIs, and within two weeks of stopping such treatment. It is also contraindicated in patients with severe hypertension or severe coronary artery disease.

4.4 Special warnings and special precautions for use

Although pseudoephedrine has virtually no pressor effects in patients with normal blood pressure, Meltus Decongestant should be used with caution in patients taking antihypertensive agents, tricyclic antidepressants, other sympathomimetic agents, such as decongestants, appetite suppressants, and amphetamine-like psycho-stimulants. The effects of a single dose on the blood pressure of these patients should be observed before recommending repeated or unsupervised treatment. As with other sympathomimetic agents, caution should be exercised in patients with uncontrolled diabetes, hyperthyroidism, elevated intraocular pressure and prostatic enlargement.

4.5 Interaction with other medicinal products and other forms of Interaction

The effect of antihypertensive agents which modify sympathetic activity may be partially reversed by Meltus Decongestant. Concomitant use with other sympathomimetic agents such as decongestants, tricyclic antidepressants, appetite suppressants and amphetamine like psycho-stimulants or with MAIOs which interfere with the catabolism of sympathomimetic amines, may occasionally cause a rise in high blood pressure.

The antibacterial agent furazolidine is known to cause a dose related inhibition of monoamine oxidase inhibitors and although there are no reports of hypertensive crises having occurred, it should not be administrated at the same time as Meltus Decongestant.

4.6 Pregnancy and lactation

Pseudoephedrine has been in widespread use for many years without apparent ill consequences. Caution should, therefore, be exercised by balancing the potential benefit of treatment against any possible hazards. Systemic administration of pseudoephedrine up to 50 times the human dose in rats and up to 35 times the human dose in rabbits did not produce teratogenic effects. It has been estimated that approximately 0.5-0.7% of a single dose of pseudoephedrine ingested by a mother will be excreted in the breast milk over 24 hours.

4.7 Effects on ability to drive and use machines

None reported.

4.8 Undesirable effects

Side effects are uncommon. In some patients pseudoephedrine may occasionally cause insomnia. Rarely, sleep disturbances and hallucinations have been reported. A fixed drug eruption to pseudoephedrine, taking the form of erythmatous nummular patches has been reported, but is rare occurrence. Urinary retention has been reported in male patients in whom prostatic enlargement could have been an important predisposing factor.

4.9 Overdose

Irritability, restlessness, tremor, convulsions, palpitations, hypertension and difficulty in micturation.

Treatment: Gastric lavage and supportive measures for respiration and circulation should be performed if indicated. Convulsions should be controlled with an anti-convulsant. Catheterisation of the bladder may be necessary. If desired the elimination of pseudoephedrine can be accelerated by acid diuresis or by dialysis.

5. PHARMACOLOGICAL PROPERTIES

5.1 Pharmacodynamic properties

Pseudoephedrine has direct and indirect sympathomimetic activity and is an orally effective upper respiratory tract decongestant.

5.2 Pharmacokinetic properties

Pseudoephedrine is readily and completely absorbed from the gastrointestinal tract following oral administration, with no pre-systemic metabolism. It achieves peak plasma concentration between one and three hours after oral dosing. It is eliminated, largely unchanged, in the urine (55-90%) in 24 hours, although there is some metabolism in the liver (<1%) by N-demethylation. It has a plasma half life of 5-8 hours following oral dosing, but its urinary elimination and hence its half life, is pH dependant such that elimination will be increased in subjects with acidic urine and decreased in patients with alkaline urine.

Pseudoephedrine is rapidly distributed throughout the body. Its volume of distribution is 2-3 L/Kg body weight but there are no reports of the extent of plasma binding and similarly, although CNS effects are observed, there is no specific information concerning its penetration into the CNS.

It is excreted in the breast milk at concentrations consistently higher than those in maternal plasma. The fraction of dose excreted in the milk has been estimated at approximately 0.5% of a single oral dose over 24 hours. Pseudoephedrine is likely to cross the placenta. The elimination of pseudoephedrine is reduced in renal impairment and with deteriorating renal function in the elderly.

Oral absorption: >95%

Presystemic metabolism: negligible

Plasma half-life: 5.4 - 8 hours

Volume of distribution: 2 - 3 L/Kg

Plasma protein binding: -

5.3 Preclinical safety data

There are no preclinical data of relevance to the prescriber which are additional to that already included in other sections of the SPC.

6. PHARMACEUTICAL PARTICULARS

6.1 List of excipients

Sorbitol Solution Non Crystallising BP; Menthol BP; Loganberry Flavour 500195E; Methylhydroxybenzoate BP; Propylhydroxybenzoate BP; Alcohol 96% BP; Glycerin BP; Sodium Saccharin BP; Sodium Cyclamate 1968 BP; Carmellose Sodium BP; Water.

6.2 Incompatibilities

Not applicable.

6.3 Shelf life

36 months unopened.

6.4 Special precautions for storage

Store at or below 25°C. Protect from light.

6.5 Nature and contents of container

Amber glass sirop bottle with tamper evident cap with fitted polycone liner packed into an outer carton containing a 5ml CE marked polystyrene measuring spoon with a 2.5ml graduation – bottle contains 100ml of product.

6.6 Instructions for use and handling

Not applicable.

7. MARKETING AUTHORISATION HOLDER

Cupal Limited, Tubiton House, Oldham, OL1 3HS.

8. MARKETING AUTHORISATION NUMBER(S)

PL 0338/0082.

9. DATE OF FIRST AUTHORISATION/RENEWAL OF THE AUTHORISATION

3rd September 1992 /29th January 2004.

10. DATE OF REVISION OF THE TEXT

January 2004

Menadiol Diphosphate Tablets 10mg

(Cambridge Laboratories)

1. NAME OF THE MEDICINAL PRODUCT

Menadiol Diphosphate Tablets 10mg

2. QUALITATIVE AND QUANTITATIVE COMPOSITION

Each tablet contains 10mg of Menadiol Diphosphate (as Menadiol Sodium Diphosphate USP).

3. PHARMACEUTICAL FORM

Tablets.

The tablets are round, white to pale pink with CL 1L3 imprinted on one face and a single break bar on the other.

4. CLINICAL PARTICULARS

4.1 Therapeutic indications

For the treatment of haemorrhage or threatened haemorrhage associated with a low blood level of prothrombin or factor vii. The main indication is obstructive jaundice (before and after surgery).

4.2 Posology and method of administration

Menadiol Diphosphate Tablets 10mg are for oral administration.

Adults

Usual therapeutic dose: 10-40mg daily

Children

If, on the recommendation of a physician, a children's dosage is required, it is suggested that 5-20mg daily be given.

The elderly

Recommendations for use in the elderly do not differ from those for other adults.

4.3 Contraindications

Administration to neonates, infants or to mothers in the pre- and post-natal periods.

4.4 Special warnings and special precautions for use

None.

4.5 Interaction with other medicinal products and other forms of Interaction

Large doses of menadiol sodium diphosphate may decrease patient sensitivity to anticoagulants.

4.6 Pregnancy and lactation

There is evidence of hazard if menadiol sodium diphosphate is used in human pregnancy. It is known to be associated with a small risk of haemolytic anaemia, hyperbilirubinaemia and kernicterus in the infant if administered to the mother in late pregnancy or during labour. Menadiol sodium diphosphate is therefore contra-indicated during late pregnancy.

4.7 Effects on ability to drive and use machines

None known.

4.8 Undesirable effects

Menadiol sodium diphosphate may induce haemolysis (especially in the newborn infant) in the presence of erythrocyte glucose-6-phosphate dehydrogenase deficiency or low concentrations of alpha-tocopherol in the blood.

4.9 Overdose

No information is available.

5. PHARMACOLOGICAL PROPERTIES

5.1 Pharmacodynamic properties

Menadiol sodium diphosphate is a water-soluble vitamin K analogue. The presence of vitamin K is essential for the formation within the body of prothrombin, factor VII, factor IX and factor X. Lack of vitamin K leads to increased tendency to haemorrhage.

5.2 Pharmacokinetic properties

Menadione is absorbed from the gastro-intestinal tract without being dependent upon the presence of bile salts. Vitamin K is rapidly metabolised and excreted by the body.

5.3 Preclinical safety data

There are no pre-clinical data of relevance to the prescriber which are additional to that already included in other sections of the SPC.

6. PHARMACEUTICAL PARTICULARS

6.1 List of excipients

Lactose

Maize starch

Talc

Magnesium stearate

6.2 Incompatibilities

No information is available.

6.3 Shelf life

Three years.

6.4 Special precautions for storage

Recommended maximum storage temperature 30°C.

Protect from light.

6.5 Nature and contents of container

White HDPE bottles containing 100 tablets.

6.6 Instructions for use and handling

None.

7. MARKETING AUTHORISATION HOLDER

Cambridge Laboratories Limited

Deltic House

Kingfisher Way

Silverlink Business Park

Wallsend

Tyne & Wear

NE28 9NX

8. MARKETING AUTHORISATION NUMBER(S)

PL 12070/0007

9. DATE OF FIRST AUTHORISATION/RENEWAL OF THE AUTHORISATION

30 April 1992

10. DATE OF REVISION OF THE TEXT

March 2000

Mengivac A+C

(Sanofi Pasteur MSD)

1. NAME OF THE MEDICINAL PRODUCT

Mengivac A+C®

Meningococcal Polysaccharide Vaccine BP

2. QUALITATIVE AND QUANTITATIVE COMPOSITION

Each 0.5 millilitre dose of vaccine contains:

Active Ingredients:

Neisseria meningitidis serogroup A polysaccharide...... 50 micrograms

Neisseria meningitidis serogroup C polysaccharide...... 50 micrograms

3. PHARMACEUTICAL FORM

Lyophilised powder for injection following reconstitution with isotonic buffered diluent.

4. CLINICAL PARTICULARS

4.1 Therapeutic indications

Active immunisation against meningococcal meningitis caused by *N.meningitidis* serogroups A and C.

a. *Travel:* Vaccination should be offered to travellers visiting parts of the world where the risk of contracting meningococcal meningitis is high. These regions include countries within the African meningitis belt (countries whose borders are between The Equator and latitude 15° North), parts of the Middle East and parts of the Indian Sub-Continent.

b. *Contacts of cases:* Family members and close contacts of disease cases of group A and group C meningococcal meningitis should be immunised. The vaccine does not protect against group B disease.

c. *Local outbreaks:* To help control local outbreaks of meningococcal group A and group C disease, vaccination may be recommended by appropriate Public Health Authorities.

Post vaccination immunity lasts at least 3 years.

4.2 Posology and method of administration
Administer by deep subcutaneous or intramuscular injection.

Adults, elderly and children over 18 months of age: a single dose of 0.5 millilitre of reconstituted vaccine.

Children under 18 months of age: Mengivac A+C® should not generally be given to children under 18 months except during epidemics (see Section 4.4).

4.3 Contraindications
Hypersensitivity to the vaccine or any component of the vaccine.

Vaccination should be delayed in the presence of acute infectious illness.

4.4 Special warnings and special precautions for use
As with any vaccine, appropriate medical treatment, including epinephrine (adrenaline) should be readily available for immediate use in case of anaphylactic reaction following injection.

Mengivac A+C® confers protection against meningitis caused by meningococci of serogroups A and C. Immunisation does not protect against meningococci of other serogroups or against meningitis caused by other organisms.

Mengivac A+C® should not generally be given to children under 18 months except during epidemics. Clinical data has confirmed the efficacy of the A component over 3 months of age. The response to the C component is only transitory but can be of limited value during a severe epidemic.

4.5 Interaction with other medicinal products and other forms of Interaction
None known.

4.6 Pregnancy and lactation
No studies have been performed in pregnant animals. There is insufficient data in humans to recommend the use of the vaccine in pregnancy and lactation unless the benefit outweighs the risk, e.g. in the event of an epidemic.

4.7 Effects on ability to drive and use machines
None known.

4.8 Undesirable effects
The adverse reactions reported during clinical trials and post-marketing surveillance studies were generally mild and transient.

Local reactions at the injection site: Transient local pain sometimes associated with oedema or erythema are reported. More severe local reactions are uncommon.

Systemic adverse events: Allergic-type reactions (urticaria, erythematous rash), fever, headache, myalgia or arthralgia and gastro-intestinal disorders are very rarely observed. Exceptionally, more severe hypersensitivity reactions such as anaphylaxis were reported. Very rare cases of neurological reactions (paraesthesia, meningism, convulsions or blurred vision) were observed. No causal relationship with the vaccine could be established.

4.9 Overdose
Not applicable.

5. PHARMACOLOGICAL PROPERTIES

5.1 Pharmacodynamic properties
Mengivac A+C® contains purified polysaccharides from *Neisseria meningitidis* serogroups A and C, and confers protection against meningococcal meningitis caused by *N. meningitidis* serogroup A and serogroup C.

5.2 Pharmacokinetic properties
Not applicable.

5.3 Preclinical safety data
No further information.

6. PHARMACEUTICAL PARTICULARS

6.1 List of excipients
Lactose.

6.2 Incompatibilities
None known.

6.3 Shelf life
36 months when stored between +2°C and +8°C.

6.4 Special precautions for storage
Store between +2°C and +8°C. Do not freeze diluent.

6.5 Nature and contents of container

Lyophilised vaccine	single or multidose (ten dose) type 1 glass vial with a siliconised rubber stopper and aluminium overcap.
Diluent	single dose prefilled syringe (type 1 glass) or multidose type 1 glass vial.

6.6 Instructions for use and handling
After reconstitution, use within one hour. Shake well immediately before use.

7. MARKETING AUTHORISATION HOLDER
Aventis Pasteur MSD Limited
Mallards Reach
Bridge Avenue
Maidenhead
Berkshire
SL6 1QP

8. MARKETING AUTHORISATION NUMBER(S)
PL 6745/0048 - Lyophilised vaccine

PL 6745/0029 - Diluent

9. DATE OF FIRST AUTHORISATION/RENEWAL OF THE AUTHORISATION
7 February 1994

10. DATE OF REVISION OF THE TEXT
March 2000

11. LEGAL CATEGORY
POM

® Registered trademark

4006241/MGV/RA271/0300/A

Meningitec

(Wyeth Pharmaceuticals)

1. NAME OF THE MEDICINAL PRODUCT
Meningitec suspension for injection

Meningococcal group C oligosaccharide conjugate vaccine (adsorbed).

2. QUALITATIVE AND QUANTITATIVE COMPOSITION
One dose (0.5ml) contains:

Neisseria meningitidis (strain C11)

Group C oligosaccharide......................... 10 micrograms

Conjugated to *Corynebacterium diphtheriae*

CRM_{197} protein................ approximately 15 micrograms

Adsorbed on aluminium phosphate .... 0.125 mg Al^{3+}

For excipients, see section 6.1.

3. PHARMACEUTICAL FORM
Suspension for injection. After shaking, the vaccine is a homogeneous, white suspension.

4. CLINICAL PARTICULARS

4.1 Therapeutic indications
Active immunisation of children from 2 months of age, adolescents and adults for the prevention of invasive disease caused by *Neisseria meningitidis* serogroup C.

The use of Meningitec should be determined on the basis of official recommendations.

4.2 Posology and method of administration

Posology

There are no data on the use of different meningococcal group C conjugate vaccines within the primary series or for boosting. Whenever possible, the same vaccine should be used throughout.

<u>Primary immunisation</u>

Infants up to the age of 12 months: two doses, each of 0.5 ml, the first dose given not earlier than 2 months of age and with an interval of at least 2 months between doses.

Children over the age of 12 months, adolescents and adults: a single dose of 0.5 ml.

<u>Booster doses</u>

It is recommended that a booster dose should be given after completion of the primary immunisation series in infants. The timing of this dose should be in accordance with available official recommendations. Information on responses to booster doses and on co-administration with other childhood vaccines is given in sections 5.1 and 4.5, respectively.

The need for booster doses in subjects primed with a single dose (i.e. aged 12 months or more when first immunised) has not yet been established.

Method of administration

Meningitec is for intramuscular injection, preferably in the anterolateral thigh in infants and in the deltoid region in older children, adolescents and adults. Meningitec should not be injected in the gluteal area.

Avoid injection into or near nerves and blood vessels.

The vaccine must not be administered intradermally, subcutaneously or intravenously (see section 4.4).

Separate injection sites should be used if more than one vaccine is being administered (see section 4.5). This vaccine must not be mixed with other vaccines in the same syringe.

4.3 Contraindications

- Persons who are hypersensitive to any component of the vaccine.
- Persons who have shown signs of hypersensitivity to any vaccine containing diphtheria toxoid or non-toxic diphtheria toxin protein.
- Persons who have shown signs of hypersensitivity after previous administration of Meningitec.
- Persons suffering from an acute severe febrile illness. As with other vaccines, the administration of Meningitec should be postponed in these persons.

4.4 Special warnings and special precautions for use
As with all injectable vaccines, appropriate medical treatment and supervision should always be readily available in case of a rare anaphylactoid/anaphylactic event following the administration of the vaccine (see section 4.8 Undesirable effects).

As with any intramuscular injection, the vaccine should be given with caution to individuals with thrombocytopenia or any coagulation disorder or to those receiving anticoagulation therapy.

The vial stopper contains dry natural rubber. This may elicit hypersensitivity reactions if handled during vaccine administration by healthcare personnel who have a history of allergy to latex. In addition, hypersensitivity reactions may occur in vaccinees with a history of allergy to latex.

Meningitec will only confer protection against group C of *Neisseria meningitidis* and may not completely prevent meningococcal group C disease. It will not protect against other groups of *Neisseria meningitidis* or other organisms that cause meningitis or septicaemia. In the event of petechiae and/or purpura following vaccination (see section 4.8), the aetiology should be thoroughly investigated. Both infective and non-infective causes should be considered.

Although symptoms of meningism such as neckpain/stiffness or photophobia have been reported there is no evidence that the vaccine causes meningococcal C meningitis. Clinical alertness to the possibility of co-incidental meningitis should therefore be maintained.

Consideration should be given to the risk of *Neisseria meningitidis* serogroup C disease in a given population and the perceived benefits of immunisation before the institution of a widespread immunisation programme.

No data on the applicability of the vaccine to outbreak control are available.

The safety and immunogenicity have not been established in infants below the age of two months (see section 5.1 Pharmacodynamic properties).

There are limited data on safety and immunogenicity of the vaccine in the adult population and there are no data in adults aged 65 years and older (see section 5.1).

Limited data are available on the use of Meningitec in immunodeficient subjects. In individuals with impaired immune responsiveness (whether due to the use of immunosuppressive therapy, a genetic defect, human immunodeficiency virus (HIV) infection, or other causes) the expected immune response to meningococcal serogroup C conjugate vaccines may not be obtained. The implications for the actual degree of protection against infection are unknown, since this will depend also on whether the vaccine has elicited an immunological memory response. Individuals with complement deficiencies and individuals with functional or anatomical asplenia may mount an immune response to meningococcal C conjugate vaccines; however, the degree of protection that would be afforded is unknown.

Immunisation with this vaccine does not substitute for routine diphtheria vaccination.

Meningitec SHOULD UNDER NO CIRCUMSTANCES BE ADMINISTERED INTRAVENOUSLY.

4.5 Interaction with other medicinal products and other forms of Interaction
Meningitec must not be mixed with other vaccines in the same syringe. Separate injection sites should be used if more than one vaccine is being administered.

Administration of Meningitec at the same time as (but, for injected vaccines, at a different injection site) the following vaccines did not reduce the immunological response to any of these other antigens in clinical trials:

Oral polio vaccine (OPV); inactivated polio vaccine (IPV); hepatitis B vaccine (HBV);diphtheria and tetanus alone (D or T), in combination (DT or dT), or in combination with whole cell or acellular pertussis (DTwP or DTaP); *Haemophilus influenzae* type b (hib alone or in combination with other antigens) or combined measles, mumps, and rubella (MMR). Minor variations in geometric mean antibody concentrations (GMCs) or titres (GMTs) were observed between studies; however, the clinical significance, if any, of these observations is not established.

Data that support concomitant administration of Meningitec and an acellular pertussis vaccine (i.e. DTaP) or an inactivated polio vaccine (IPV) are derived from studies in which subjects received either Meningitec or the same meningococcal serogroup C conjugate as in Meningitec combined with an investigational pneumococcal conjugate vaccine and from a study of concomitant administration with a pediatric combination vaccine (DTaP-HBV-IPV/Hib).

In various studies with different vaccines, concomitant administration of meningococcal serogroup C conjugates with combinations containing acellular pertussis components (with or without inactivated polio viruses, hepatitis B surface antigen or hib conjugates) has been shown to result in lower SBA GMTs compared to separate administrations or to co-administration with whole cell pertussis vaccines. The proportions reaching SBA titres of at least 1:8 or 1:128 are not affected. At present, the potential implications of these observations for the duration of protection are not known.

4.6 Pregnancy and lactation

Pregnancy

There are no clinical data on the use of this vaccine in pregnant women. Animal studies are insufficient with respect to effects on pregnancy and embryonal/foetal development, parturition and postnatal development (see 5.3. Preclinical safety data). The potential risk for humans is unknown.

Nevertheless, considering the severity of meningococcal C disease, pregnancy should not preclude vaccination when the risk of exposure is clearly defined.

Lactation

The risk-benefit relationship should also be examined before making the decision as to whether to immunise during lactation.

4.7 Effects on ability to drive and use machines

Some of the effects mentioned under section 4.8 (Undesirable effects) such as dizziness and somnolence may affect the ability to drive or operate machinery.

4.8 Undesirable effects

Note: the following descriptions of frequency have been defined as: Very common (≥10%); Common (≥1% and <10%); Uncommon (≥0.1% and <1%); Rare (≥0.01% and <0.1%); Very rare (<0.01%).

Adverse Reactions from Clinical Trials

Adverse reactions reported across all age groups are provided below. Adverse reactions were collected on the day of vaccination and the following three days. The majority of reactions were self-limiting and resolved within the follow-up period.

In all age groups injection site reactions (including redness, swelling and tenderness/pain) were very common. However, these were not usually clinically significant. Redness or swelling of at least 3 cm and tenderness interfering with movement for more than 48 hours was infrequent where studied. Transient injection site tenderness was reported in 70% of adults during clinical trials.

Fever of at least 38.0°C was common in infants and toddlers and very common in pre-school children, but did not usually exceed 39.1°C, particularly in older age groups.

In infants and toddlers crying was common after vaccination while drowsiness, impaired sleeping, anorexia, diarrhoea and vomiting were very common. Irritability was very common in infants and in toddlers and common in children aged between 3.5 and 6 years. There was no evidence that these were related to Meningitec rather than concomitant vaccines, particularly DTP.

In trials that evaluated three-dose schedules (2, 3 and 4 months or 2, 4 and 6 months) in infants, rates of adverse events did not increase with successive doses with the exception of fever ≥38°C. However, it should be noted that infants received other scheduled vaccines concomitantly with Meningitec in these studies.

Myalgia was common in adults. Somnolence was commonly reported in children between 3.5 and 6 years of age and in adults. Headache was common in children between 3.5 and 6 years of age and was very common in adults.

Adverse reactions reported across all age groups are provided below.

General Disorders and Administration Site Conditions:

Very common: Injection site reactions (e.g. redness, swelling, pain/tenderness)

Common: Fever ≥ 38 °C

Additional reactions reported in infants (first year of life) and toddlers (second year of life) are provided below.

Metabolism and Nutrition disorders:

Very common: Anorexia

Psychiatric Disorders:

Very common: Irritability

Common: Crying

Nervous System Disorders:

Very common: Drowsiness, impaired sleeping

Gastrointestinal Disorders:

Very common: Vomiting, diarrhoea

Additional reactions reported in older age groups including adults (4 to 60 years) included:

Psychiatric Disorders:

Common: Irritability (children between 3.5 and 6 years of age)

Nervous System Disorders:

Very common: Headache (adults)

Common: Somnolence, headache (children between 3.5 and 6 years of age)

Musculoskeletal Connective Tissue and Bone Disorders:

Common: Myalgia (adults)

Adverse Reactions from Post-Marketing Surveillance (for all age groups)

These frequencies are based on spontaneous reporting rates and have been calculated using number of reports and number of doses distributed.

Blood and Lymphatic System Disorders:

Very rare: Lymphadenopathy

Immune System Disorders:

Very rare: Anaphylactoid/anaphylactic reactions including shock, hypersensitivity reactions including bronchospasm, facial oedema and angioedema

Nervous System Disorders:

Very rare: Dizziness, faints, seizures (convulsions) including febrile seizures and seizures in patients with pre-existing seizure disorders, hypoaesthesia, paraesthesia and hypotonia

There have been very rare reports of seizures following Meningitec vaccination; individuals have usually rapidly recovered. Some of the reported seizures may have been faints. The reporting rate of seizures was below the background rate of epilepsy in children. In infants seizures were usually associated with fever and were likely to be febrile convulsions.

Gastrointestinal Disorders:

Very rare: Vomiting, nausea, abdominal pain

Skin and Subcutaneous Tissue Disorders:

Very rare: Rash, urticaria, pruritus, erythema multiforme, Stevens-Johnson syndrome

Musculoskeletal Connective Tissue and Bone Disorders:

Very rare: Arthralgia

Renal and Urinary Disorders:

Relapse of nephrotic syndrome has been reported in association with meningococcal group C conjugate vaccines.

Very rarely, petechiae and/or purpura have been reported following immunisation (see also section 4.4).

4.9 Overdose

There have been reports of overdose with Meningitec, including cases of administration of a higher than recommended dose at one visit, cases of subsequent doses administered closer than recommended to the previous dose, and cases in which the recommended total number of doses has been exceeded. Most individuals were asymptomatic. In general, adverse events reported with overdosage have also been reported with recommended single doses of Meningitec.

5. PHARMACOLOGICAL PROPERTIES

5.1 Pharmacodynamic properties

Pharmacotherapeutic Group: *Meningococcal vaccines*, ATC code: *J07AH*

Immunogenicity

No prospective efficacy trials have been performed.

Serological correlates for protection have not been definitively established for conjugated meningococcal C vaccines; these are under study.

The serum bactericidal antibody (SBA) assay referenced in the text below, used rabbit serum as a source of complement.

Primary Series in Infants

Two doses in infants provided SBA antibody titres (using baby rabbit complement) ≥1:8 in 98-99.5% of infants, as shown in the table below. A two-dose infant schedule primed for a memory response to a booster dose given at 12 months of age.

% of subjects achieving ≥1:8 SBA titres (GMT)

Study with Meningitec given at age	After 2nd dose	After 12-month booster
2, 3, 4 months with concomitant DTwP-Hib and OPV	98% (766) n=55	(Not studied)
3, 5, 7 months given alone	99.5% (1591)# n=214	(Not studied)
2, 4, 6 months with concomitant DTaP-HBV-IPV/Hib*	99.5% (1034)# n=218	(Not studied)
3, 5 months administered as 9vPnC-MnCC with concomitant DTaP-IPV/Hib	98.2% (572) n=56	100% (1928) n=23 (9vPnC-MnCC booster)
		100% (2623) n=28 (Meningite-c+23vPnPS booster)

* See section 4.5

measured at two months after the second dose

MnCC = meningococcal serogroup C conjugate vaccine (which is the active component in Meningitec)

DTwP = whole cell pertussis vaccine with diphtheria and tetanus toxoids

OPV = oral polio virus vaccine

DTaP-IPV/Hib = acellular pertussis components, diphtheria and tetanus toxoids, inactivated polioviruses and a hib conjugate (tetanus toxoid carrier protein)

DTaP-HBV-IPV/Hib = as above plus recombinant hepatitis B surface antigen in a hexavalent formulation

9v-PnC-MnCC = investigational 9-valent pneumococcal conjugate vaccine (not licensed) formulated with meningococcal serogroup C conjugate vaccine (which is the active component in Meningitec)

23vPnPS = 23-valent pneumococcal polysaccharide vaccine

Immunogenicity of a single primary dose in toddlers

91% of 75 toddlers of 13 months of age developed SBA titres ≥ 1/8 and 89% of these 75 subjects showed a four-fold increase over their pre-vaccination antibody titre after receiving a single dose of Meningitec.

Immunogenicity of a single primary dose in adults

All the 15 adults of 18-60 years who received a single dose of Meningitec achieved SBA titres ≥ 1/8 and a four-fold rise in antibody titre.

There are no data in adults aged 65 years and older.

Post-marketing surveillance following an immunisation campaign in the UK

Estimates of vaccine effectiveness from the UK's routine immunisation programme (using various quantities of three meningococcal serogroup C conjugate vaccines) covering the period from introduction at the end of 1999 to March 2004 have demonstrated the need for a booster dose after completion of the primary series (three doses administered at 2, 3 and 4 months). Within one year of completion of the primary series, vaccine effectiveness in the infant cohort was estimated at 93% (95% CI: 67, 99). However, more than one year after completion of the primary series, there was clear evidence of waning protection. Estimates of effectiveness based on a small number of cases to date indicate that there may also be waning protection in children who received a single priming dose as toddlers. Effectiveness in all other age groups (up to 18 years) primed with a single dose has so far remained around 90% or more within and more than one year after vaccination.

5.2 Pharmacokinetic properties

Evaluation of pharmacokinetic properties is not required for vaccines.

5.3 Preclinical safety data

Female mice were immunised intramuscularly with twice the clinical dose of meningococcal group C conjugate vaccine, either prior to mating or during the gestation period. Gross necropsy of viscera was performed on each mouse. All mice survived to either delivery or caesarean section. No adverse clinical signs were present in any mouse and no parameters that were evaluated were affected by administration of the vaccine, in either the adult or foetal mice.

6. PHARMACEUTICAL PARTICULARS

6.1 List of excipients

Sodium chloride.

Water for injections.

6.2 Incompatibilities

In the absence of compatibility studies, this medicinal product must not be mixed with other medicinal products.

6.3 Shelf life

3 years

6.4 Special precautions for storage

Store at 2°C to 8°C (in a refrigerator). Do not freeze. Discard if the vaccine has been frozen.

Store in the original package.

6.5 Nature and contents of container

0.5 ml of suspension in a vial (type I glass) with a stopper (butyl rubber). Pack sizes of 1 and 10 vials without syringe/needles. Pack size of 1 vial with a syringe and 2 needles (1 for withdrawal, 1 for injection).

Not all pack sizes may be marketed.

6.6 Instructions for use and handling

Upon storage, a white deposit and clear supernatant can be observed.

The vaccine should be well shaken in order to obtain a homogeneous white suspension and visually inspected for any foreign particulate matter and/or variation of physical aspect prior to administration. If this is observed, discard the vaccine. The vaccine must be administered immediately after being drawn up into a syringe. Any unused product or waste material should be disposed of in accordance with local requirements.

7. MARKETING AUTHORISATION HOLDER

John Wyeth & Brother Ltd

Huntercombe Lane South

Taplow, Maidenhead

Berkshire SL6 0PH

UK

8. MARKETING AUTHORISATION NUMBER(S)

UK: PL 00011/0245

Ireland: PA 22/78/1

MRP: UK/H/356/1

9. DATE OF FIRST AUTHORISATION/RENEWAL OF THE AUTHORISATION

UK: 15th October 1999

Ireland: 21st July 2000

10. DATE OF REVISION OF THE TEXT

08 June 2005

MENJUGATE

(Sanofi Pasteur MSD)

1. NAME OF THE MEDICINAL PRODUCT

MENJUGATE® powder and solvent for suspension for injection. Meningococcal group C oligosaccharide conjugate vaccine (adsorbed).

2. QUALITATIVE AND QUANTITATIVE COMPOSITION

One dose (0.5 ml of the reconstituted vaccine) contains:

Neisseria meningitidis group C (strain C11) oligosaccharide..........10 micrograms

Conjugated to

Corynebacterium diphtheriae CRM-197 protein.....12.5 to 25.0 micrograms

adsorbed on aluminium hydroxide.......... 3 to 0.4 mg Al^{3+}

For excipients, see 6.1.

3. PHARMACEUTICAL FORM

Powder and solvent for suspension for injection.

The product consists of two vials, one containing a white to off-white lyophilised powder and the other a white, aqueous aluminium hydroxide suspension.

4. CLINICAL PARTICULARS

4.1 Therapeutic indications

Active immunisation of children from 2 months of age, adolescents and adults, for the prevention of invasive disease caused by *Neisseria meningitidis* serogroup C.

4.2 Posology and method of administration

Posology

Infants up to the age of 12 months: three doses, each of 0.5 ml, the first dose given not earlier than 2 months and with an interval of at least 1 month between doses.

Children over the age of 12 months, adolescents and adults: a single dose of 0.5 ml.

Due to the limited data the necessity for a booster dose has not been established (see 5.1)

Method of Administration

Intramuscular injection. The vaccine (0.5 ml) is intended for deep intramuscular injection, preferably in the anterolateral thigh in infants and in the deltoid region in older children, adolescents and adults.

The vaccine must not be injected intravenously, subcutaneously or intradermally.

Menjugate® should not be mixed with other vaccines in the same syringe. Separate injection sites should be used if more than one vaccine is being administered.

4.3 Contraindications

Hypersensitivity to any component of the vaccine, including diphtheria toxoid.

Persons who have shown signs of hypersensitivity after previous administration of Menjugate®.

As with other vaccines, administration of Menjugate® should be postponed in subjects with an acute severe febrile illness.

4.4 Special warnings and special precautions for use

Before the injection of any vaccine, the person responsible for administration should take all precautions known for the prevention of allergic or any other reactions. As with all injectable vaccines, appropriate medical treatment and supervision should always be readily available in case of a rare anaphylactic event following administration of the vaccine.

Prior to administration of any dose of Menjugate®, the parent or guardian should be asked about the personal history, family history, and recent health status of the vaccine recipient, including immunisation history, current health status and any adverse event after previous immunisations.

The benefits of vaccination with meningococcal serogroup C conjugate vaccine should be reviewed in light of the incidence of N. meningitidis serogroup C infection in a given population before the institution of a widespread immunisation campaign.

Menjugate® will not protect against meningococcal diseases caused by any of the other types of meningococcal bacteria (A, B, 29-E, H, I, K, L, W-135, X, Y, or Z, including non-typed). Complete protection against meningococcal serogroup C infection cannot be guaranteed.

No data on the applicability of the vaccine for post-exposure outbreak control are as yet available.

There are no data in adults aged 65 years and older (see section 5.1)

In individuals deficient in producing antibodies, vaccination may not result in an appropriate protective antibody response. While HIV infection is not a contraindication, Menjugate® has not been specifically evaluated in the immunocompromised. Individuals with complement deficiencies and individuals with functional or anatomical asplenia may mount an immune response to meningococcal C conjugate vaccines; however, the degree of protection that would be afforded is unknown.

Although symptoms of meningism such as neck pain/stiffness or photophobia have been reported there is no evidence that the vaccine causes meningococcal C meningitis. Clinical alertness to the possibility of co-incidental meningitis should therefore be maintained.

Conjugate vaccines containing Cross Reacting Material 197 (CRM197) should not be considered as immunising agents against diphtheria. No changes in the schedule for administering vaccines containing Diphtheria Toxoid are recommended.

Any acute infection or febrile illness is reason for delaying the use of Menjugate® except when, in the opinion of the physician, withholding the vaccine entails a greater risk. A minor afebrile illness, such as a mild upper respiratory infection, is not usually reason to defer immunisation.

The vaccine must not be injected intravenously, subcutaneously or intradermally.

Menjugate® has not been evaluated in persons with thrombocytopenia or bleeding disorders. The risk versus benefit for persons at risk of haemorrhage following intramuscular injection must be evaluated.

Parents should be informed of the immunisation schedule for this vaccine. Precautions such as useful antipyretic measures for this vaccine should be relayed to the parent or guardian and the need to report any adverse event should be stressed.

4.5 Interaction with other medicinal products and other forms of Interaction

Menjugate® must not be mixed with other vaccines in the same syringe. Separate injection sites should be used if more than one vaccine is being administered.

Administration of Menjugate® at the same time as (but, for injected vaccines, at a different injection site) the following vaccines does not reduce the immunological response to any of these other antigens:

Polio (inactivated polio vaccine and oral polio vaccine); Diphtheria and Tetanus alone or in combination with whole cell or acellular Pertussis; Haemophilus Influenzae type B (Hib) or combined Measles, Mumps, and Rubella.

Minor variations in GMT antibody titers were observed between studies; however, the clinical significance, if any, of these observations is not established.

There is no information on co-administration of Menjugate® with Hepatitis B vaccine, or with pneumococcal conjugate vaccine. Concomitant use of Menjugate® with hepatitis B or pneumococcal conjugate vaccines should only be considered if medically important and not on a routine basis.

4.6 Pregnancy and lactation

Pregnancy

There are no data on the use of this vaccine in pregnant women. Animal studies in rabbit at different stages of gestation have not demonstrated a risk to the fetus following administration of Menjugate®. Nevertheless, considering the severity of meningococcal C disease pregnancy should not preclude vaccination when the risk of exposure is clearly defined.

Lactation

Information on the safety of the vaccine during lactation is not available. The risk-benefit ratio should be examined before making the decision as to whether to immunise during lactation.

4.7 Effects on ability to drive and use machines

Dizziness has been very rarely reported following vaccination. This may temporarily affect the ability to drive or use machines.

4.8 Undesirable effects

Adverse Reactions from Clinical Trials

Adverse reactions reported across all age groups are provided below. Note the following descriptions of frequency have been defined as: Very common (≥10%); common (≥1% and <10%); uncommon (≥0.1% and <1%); rare (≥0.01% and <0.1%); very rare (<0.01%). Adverse reactions were collected on the day of vaccination and each day following for at least 3 and up to 6 days. The majority of reactions were self-limiting and resolved within the follow-up period.

In all age groups injection site reactions (including redness, swelling and tenderness/pain) were very common (ranging from 1 in 3 older children to 1 in 10 pre-school children). However, these were not usually clinically significant. Redness or swelling of at least 3cm and tenderness interfering with movement for more than 48 hours was infrequent where studied.

Fever of at least 38.0°C is common (ranging from 1 in 20 in infants and toddlers to 1 in 10 in pre-school children), but does not usually exceed 39.1°C, particularly in older age groups.

In infants and toddlers symptoms including crying and vomiting (toddlers) were common after vaccination. Irritability, drowsiness, impaired sleeping, anorexia, diarrhoea and vomiting (infants) were very common after vaccination. There was no evidence that these were related to Menjugate® rather than concomitant vaccines, particularly DTP.

Very commonly reported adverse events include myalgia and arthralgia in adults. Drowsiness was commonly reported in younger children. Headache was very common in secondary school children and common in primary school children.

Adverse reactions reported across all age groups are provided below.

General disorders	
Common (≥1% and <10%)	Fever ≥ 38.0°C
Injection site reactions	
Very common (≥10%)	Redness, swelling and tenderness/pain

Additional reactions reported in infants (first year of life) and toddlers (second year of life)

General disorders	
Very common (≥10%)	Irritability, drowsiness and impaired sleeping
Common (≥1% and <10%)	Crying
Gastrointestinal disorders	
Very common (≥10%)	Diarrhoea and anorexia Vomiting (infants)
Common (≥1% and <10%)	Vomiting (toddlers)

Additional reactions reported in older children and adults

General disorders	
Very common (≥10%)	Malaise Headache (secondary school children)
Common (≥1% and <10%)	Headache (primary school children)

Muscoskeletal, connective and bone disorders	
Very common (≥10%)	Myalgia and arthralgia

Gastrointestinal disorders	
Very common (≥10%)	Nausea (adults)

Adverse Reactions from Post Marketing Surveillance (for all age groups)

The most commonly reported suspected reactions in post marketing surveillance include dizziness, pyrexia, headache, nausea, vomiting and faints.

The frequencies given below are based on spontaneous reporting rates, for this and other Meningococcal C Conjugate vaccines and have been calculated using the

Table 1 Comparison of the Percentage of Subjects with Antimeningococcal C Serum Bactericidal Titres ⩾1:8 (Human Complement) at One Month Following One Immunization of Menjugate® or a Licensed Unconjugated Meningococcal Polysaccharide Vaccine, by Age Group at Enrolment

	Age 1-2 years		Age 3-5 years		Age 11-17 years		Age 18-64 years	
	Menjugate n=237	MenPS (1) n=153	Menjugate n=80	MenPS (1) n=80	Menjugate n=90	MenPS (2) n=90	Menjugate n=136	MenPS (2) n=130
BCA % ⩾1:8 (95% CI) Human Complement	78% (72-83)	19% (13-26)	79% (68-87)	28% (18-39)	84% (75-91)	68% (57-77)	90% (84-95)	88% (82-93)

MenPS = licensed unconjugated Meningococcal polysaccharide vaccine.

(1) = serogroups A, C W-135 and Y, containing 50μg of serogroup C per dose.

(2) = serogroups A and C, containing 50μg of serogroup C per dose.

number of reports received as the numerator and the total number of doses distributed as the denominator.

Immune System Disorders:

Very rare (<0.01%): lymphadenopathy, anaphylaxis, hypersensitivity reactions including bronchospasm, facial oedema and angioedema.

Nervous System Disorders:

Very rare (<0.01%): dizziness, convulsions including febrile convulsions, faints, hypoaesthesia and paraesthesia, hypotonia.

There have been very rare reports of seizures following Menjugate® vaccination; individuals have usually rapidly recovered. Some of the reported seizures may have been faints. The reporting rate of seizures was below the background rate of epilepsy in children. In infants seizures were usually associated with fever and were likely to be febrile convulsions.

Gastrointestinal Disorders:

Very rare (<0.01%): vomiting and nausea.

Skin and Subcutaneous Tissue Disorders:

Very rare (<0.01%): rash, urticaria, pruritis, purpura, erythema multiforme, and Stevens-Johnson Syndrome

Muscoskeletal, connective tissue and bone disorders:

Very rare (<0.01%): myalgia and arthralgia

4.9 Overdose
There is no experience of overdosage with Menjugate®.

5. PHARMACODYNAMIC PROPERTIES
5.1 Pharmacodynamic properties
Pharmacotherapeutic group: Meningococcal vaccines, ATC code: J07A H.

Immunogenicity

No prospective efficacy trials have been performed.

Standardised serological correlates for protection have not been definitively established for conjugated meningococcal C vaccines; these are under study. The serum bactericidal assay (BCA) referenced in the text below used human serum as a source of complement. Serum bactericidal assay (BCA) results achieved with human serum as a source of complement are not directly comparable with those achieved with rabbit serum as a source of complement.

Data from trials in 540 infants using a 2, 3, 4 month schedule and 175 infants using a 2, 4, 6 month schedule demonstrate that >98% of infants developed serum bactericidal antibody titres of at least 1:8 (human complement) one month after the second and third dose. A booster dose in the second year of life induces an anamnestic response. Currently the necessity for a booster dose has not been established but is under evaluation.

A second dose may be considered for toddlers (second year of life) who are at an increased risk of meningococcal infection.

Compared to licensed unconjugated meningococcal polysaccharide vaccines in clinical studies, the immune response induced by Menjugate® was shown to be superior in toddlers, children and adolescents, and was comparable in adults (see table). Additionally, unlike unconjugated polysaccharide vaccines, Menjugate® induces immunologic memory after vaccination, although the duration of protection is not yet established.

There are no data in adults aged 65 years or older.

(see Table 1 above)

No pharmacodynamic studies have been conducted with Menjugate®, in accordance with its status as a vaccine.

5.2 Pharmacokinetic properties
No pharmacokinetic studies have been conducted with Menjugate®, in accordance with its status as a vaccine.

5.3 Preclinical safety data
Acute and subacute toxicity studies in mice, guinea pigs and rabbits demonstrated only local histologic changes secondary to vaccine injections. Embryofetal studies did not reveal evidence of toxicity.

6. PHARMACEUTICAL PARTICULARS
6.1 List of excipients
Vial containing MenC-CRM197 Conjugate

Mannitol, sodium dihydrogen phosphate monohydrate, disodium phosphate - heptahydrate.

Vial containing aluminium hydroxide

sodium chloride, water for injections.

6.2 Incompatibilities
This medicinal product must not be mixed with other medicinal products in the same syringe.

6.3 Shelf life
36 months

Following reconstitution, the product should be used immediately.

The two components of the product may have different expiry dates. The outer carton bears the earlier of the two dates and this date must be respected. The carton and ALL its contents should be discarded on reaching this outer carton expiry date.

6.4 Special precautions for storage
Store at +2°C to +8°C (in a refrigerator). Do not freeze. Protect from light.

6.5 Nature and contents of container
Menjugate® is presented as two Type I glass vials, with bromobutyl rubber stoppers. Menjugate® is supplied in packs containing one dose, five doses or ten doses.

6.6 Instructions for use and handling
The lyophilised vaccine will require preparation by reconstitution with liquid aluminium hydroxide diluent.

Gently agitate the aluminium hydroxide diluent vial. Withdraw 0.6 ml of the suspension and use to reconstitute the Meningococcal C-CRM197 Conjugate vial. Gently shake the reconstituted vial until vaccine is dissolved (this will ensure the antigen is bound to the adjuvant). Using a new suitable gauge needle, withdraw 0.5 ml of reconstituted product, ensuring no air bubbles are present. Following reconstitution the vaccine is a slightly opaque colourless to light yellow suspension, free from visible foreign particles. In the event of any foreign particulate matter and/or variation of physical aspect being observed, discard the vaccine

Any unused product or waste material should be disposed in accordance with local requirements.

7. MARKETING AUTHORISATION HOLDER
Chiron S.r.l., Via Fiorentina 1, 53100 Siena, Italy.

8. MARKETING AUTHORISATION NUMBER(S)
Menjugate® PL/13767/0013

Aluminium hydroxide Solvent (Single-dose) PL/13767/0014

9. DATE OF FIRST AUTHORISATION/RENEWAL OF THE AUTHORISATION
March 2002

10. DATE OF REVISION OF THE TEXT
March 2003

Menogon

(Ferring Pharmaceuticals Ltd)

1. NAME OF THE MEDICINAL PRODUCT
Menogon

2. QUALITATIVE AND QUANTITATIVE COMPOSITION
Active ingredient

Each ampoule with dry substance contains menotrophin (human menopausal gonadotrophin, HMG) corresponding to 75 IU human follicle stimulating hormone (FSH) and 75 IU human luteinising hormone (LH).

3. PHARMACEUTICAL FORM
Powder for injection; and solvent for parenteral use.

4. CLINICAL PARTICULARS
4.1 Therapeutic indications
Treatment of female and male infertility in the following groups of patients:

- Anovulatory women: Menogon can be used to stimulate follicle development in amenorrhoeic patients. Clomiphene (or a similar ovulation inducing agent which influences steroid feed-back mechanisms) is the preferred treatment for women with a variety of menstrual cycle disturbances, including luteal phase insufficiency with anovulatory cycles and with normal prolactin, and also amenorrhoeic patients with evidence of endogenous oestrogen production but normal prolactin and normal gonadotrophin levels. Non-responders may then be selected for menotrophin therapy.

- Women undergoing superovulation within a medically assisted fertilisation programme: Menogon can be used to induce multiple follicular development in patients undergoing an assisted conception technique such as in-vitro fertilisation (IVF).

- Hypogonadotrophic hypogonadism in men: Menogon may be given in combination with human chorionic gonadotrophin (e.g. Choragon) for the stimulation of spermatogenesis. Patients with primary testicular failure are usually unresponsive.

4.2 Posology and method of administration
Anovulatory infertility:

Menotrophin is administered to induce follicular maturation and is followed by treatment with chorionic gonadotrophin to stimulate ovulation and corpus luteum formation.

The dosage and schedule of treatment must be determined according to the needs of each patient. Response is monitored by studying the patient's urinary oestrogen excretion or by ultrasound visualisation of follicles. Menotrophin may be given daily by intramuscular injection to provide a dose of 75 to 150 units of FSH and 75 to 150 units of LH, and gradually adjusted if necessary until an adequate response is achieved, followed after 1 or 2 days by chorionic gonadotrophin. In menstruating patients treatment should be started within the first 7 days of the menstrual cycle. The treatment course should be abandoned if no response is seen in 3 weeks. This treatment cycle may be repeated at least twice more if necessary. Alternatively, three equal doses of menotrophin, each providing 225 to 375 units of FSH with 225 to 375 units of LH, may be given on alternate days followed by chorionic gonadotrophin one week after the first dose.

In the daily therapy schedule, the dose is gradually increased until oestrogen levels start to rise. The effective dose is then maintained until adequate pre-ovulatory oestrogen levels are reached. If oestrogen levels rise too rapidly, the dose should be decreased.

As a measure of follicle maturity the following values can be taken:

- total urinary oestrogen: 75-150 microgram (270 – 540 nmol)/24 hours:

- plasma 17 beta-oestradiol: 400-800 picogram/ml (1500 – 3000 pmol/L).

When adequate pre-ovulatory oestrogen levels have been reached, administration of Menogon is stopped, and ovulation may then be induced by administering human chorionic gonadotrophin at a dose of 5000 – 10000 IU.

Women undergoing superovulation in IVF or other assisted conception techniques:

In in-vitro fertilisation procedures or other assisted conception techniques menotrophin is used in conjunction with chorionic gonadotrophin and sometimes also clomiphene citrate or a gonadorelin agonist. Stimulation of follicular growth is produced by menotrophin in a dose providing 75 to 300 units of FSH with 75 to 300 units of LH daily. Treatment with menotrophin, either alone or in conjunction with clomiphene or a gonadorelin agonist, is continued until an adequate response is obtained and the final injection of menotrophin is followed 1 or 2 days later with up to 10000 units of chorionic gonadotrophin.

Maturation of follicles is monitored by measurement of oestrogen levels, ultrasound and/or clinical evaluation of oestrogen activity. It is recommended there should be at least 3 follicles greater than 17 mm in diameter with 17-beta oestradiol levels of at least 3500 pmol/L (920 picogram/ml). Egg maturation occurs by administration of human chorionic gonadotrophin in a dose of 5000-10000 IU, 30 – 40 hours after the last Menogon injection. Human chorionic gonadotrophin should not be administered if these criteria have not been met. Egg retrieval is carried out 32-36 hours after the human chorionic gonadotrophin injection.

Male infertility:

Spermatogenesis is stimulated with chorionic gonadotrophin (1000 – 2000 IU two to three times a week) and then menotrophin is given in a dose of 75 or 150 units of FSH with 75 or 150 units of LH two or three times weekly. Treatment should be continued for at least 3 or 4 months.

Children:

Not recommended for use in children.

Elderly

Not recommended for use in the elderly.

Method of Administration:

By intramuscular use.

The dry substance must be reconstituted with the diluent prior to use.

4.3 Contraindications
- Pregnancy.
- Enlargement of the ovaries or cysts not caused by polycystic ovarian syndrome.
- Gynaecological bleeding of unknown cause.
- Tumours in the uterus, ovaries, breasts, or testes.
- Carcinoma of the prostate.
- Structural abnormalities in which a satisfactory outcome cannot be expected, for example, tubal occlusion (unless superovulation is to be induced for IVF), ovarian dysgenesis, absent uterus or premature menopause.

4.4 Special warnings and special precautions for use
The following conditions should be properly treated and excluded as the cause of infertility before menotrophin therapy is initiated:-
- dysfunction of the thyroid gland and cortex of the suprarenal gland.
- hyperprolactinaemia.
- tumours in the pituitary or hypothalmic glands.

In the treatment of female infertility, ovarian activity should be checked (by ultrasound and plasma 17 beta-oestradiol measurement) prior to Menogon administration. During treatment, these tests and urinary oestrogen measurement should be carried out at regular intervals, until stimulation occurs. Close supervision is imperative during treatment. See "posology and administration" for optimum response levels of urinary oestrogens and plasma 17 beta-oestradiol. Values below these ranges may indicate inadequate follicular development. If urinary oestrogen levels exceed 540 nmol (150 micrograms)/24 hours, or if plasma 17 beta-oestradiol levels exceed 3000 pmol/L (800 picograms/ml), or if there is any steep rise in values, there is an increased risk of hyperstimulation and Menogon treatment should be immediately discontinued and human chorionic gonadotrophin withheld. Ultrasound will reveal any excessive follicular development and unintentional hyperstimulation. In the event of hyperstimulation, the patient should refrain from sexual intercourse until they are no longer at risk.

If during ultrasound, several mature follicles are visualised, human chorionic gonadotrophin should not be given as there is a risk of multiple ovulation and the occurrence of hyperstimulation syndrome.

Patients undergoing superovulation may be at an increased risk of developing hyperstimulation in view of the excessive oestrogen response and multiple follicular development. Aspiration of all follicles, prior to ovulation, may reduce the incidence of hyperstimulation syndrome.

The severe form of hyperstimulation syndrome may be life-threatening and is characterised by large ovarian cysts (prone to rupture), acute abdominal pain, ascites, very often hydrothorax and occasionally thromboembolic phenomena.

Prior to treatment with Menogon, primary ovarian failure should be excluded by the determination of gonadotrophin levels.

There have been reports of ectopic pregnancy in women receiving Menotrophin who have undergone assisted conception. One predisposing factor for ectopic pregnancy is tubal disease/occlusion, which women undergoing assisted conception may have. No causal relationship between ectopic pregnancy and the use of menotrophin has been established.

4.5 Interaction with other medicinal products and other forms of Interaction
None known.

4.6 Pregnancy and lactation
Menogon should not be given during pregnancy or to lactating mothers.

4.7 Effects on ability to drive and use machines
None known.

4.8 Undesirable effects
Treatment with menotrophin can often lead to ovarian hyperstimulation. This, however, mostly becomes clinically relevant only after human chorionic gonadotrophin has been administered to induce ovulation. This can lead to the formation of large ovarian cysts that tend to rupture and can cause intra-abdominal bleeding. In addition, ascites, hydrothorax, oliguria, hypotension, and thromboembolic phenomena can occur. Treatment should be immediately discontinued when the first signs of hyperstimulation can be detected by ultrasound or physically (abdominal pain and distension). With pregnancy, these side effects can intensify, continue over a long period of time, and be life threatening.

Local reactions including pain, itching, redness and swelling may occur at the site of injection.

Occasional adverse effects of menotrophin treatment, are nausea and vomiting.

There is an increased risk of miscarriage and also multiple pregnancies with menotrophin therapy.

Rarely reported side effects are fever and joint pain and hypersensitivity reactions (skin rash).

In very rare cases, long term use of menotrophin can lead to the formation of antibodies making treatment ineffectual.

4.9 Overdose
The acute toxicity of menotrophin has been shown to be very low. However, too high a dosage for more than one day may lead to hyperstimulation, which is categorised as mild, moderate or severe. Symptoms of overdosage usually appear 3-6 days after treatment with human chorionic gonadotrophin.

Mild hyperstimulation - Symptoms include some abdominal swelling and pain; ovaries enlarged to about 5 cm diameter. Therapy - rest; careful observation and symptomatic relief. Ovarian enlargement declines rapidly.

Moderate hyperstimulation - Symptoms include more pronounced abdominal distension and pain; nausea; vomiting; occasional diarrhoea; ovaries enlarged up to 12 cm diameter. Therapy - bed rest; close observation especially in the case of conception occurring, to detect any progression to severe hyperstimulation.

Pelvic examination of enlarged ovaries should be gentle in order to avoid rupture of the cysts. Symptoms subside spontaneously over 2-3 weeks.

Severe hyperstimulation - This is a rare but serious complication - symptoms include pronounced abdominal distension and pain; ascites; pleural effusion; decreased blood volume; reduced urine output; electrolyte imbalance and sometimes shock; ovaries enlarge to in excess of 12 cm diameter. Therapy - hospitalisation; treatment should be conservative and concentrate on restoring blood volume and preventing shock. Acute symptoms subside over several days and ovaries return to normal over 20-40 days if conception does not occur - symptoms may be prolonged if conception occurs.

5. PHARMACOLOGICAL PROPERTIES

5.1 Pharmacodynamic properties
Menotrophin is a gonadotrophin extracted from the urine of postmenopausal women and having both luteinising hormone and follicle stimulating hormone activity. It is given by intramuscular injection in the treatment of male and female infertility.

Menotrophin (HMG) directly affects the ovaries and the testes. HMG has a gametropic and steroidogenic effect.

In the ovaries, the FSH-component in HMG induces an increase in the number of growing follicles and stimulates their development. FSH increases the production of oestradiol in the granulosa cells by aromatising androgens that originate in the Theca cells under the influence of the LH-component.

In the testes, FSH induces the transformation of premature to mature Sertoli cells. It mainly causes the maturation of the seminal canals and the development of the spermatozoa. However, a high concentration of androgens within the testes is necessary and can be attained by a prior treatment using hCG.

5.2 Pharmacokinetic properties
HMG is not effective when taken orally and is injected i.m. The biological effectiveness of HMG is mainly due to its FSH content. The pharmacokinetics of HMG following i.m. administration show great individual variation. The maximum serum level of FSH is reached 6 - 24 hours after injection. After that, the serum level decreases by a half-life of 4 - 12 hours.

Excretion of HMG, following administration, is predominantly renal.

5.3 Preclinical safety data
Toxic effects caused by HMG are unknown in humans.

There is no evidence of teratogenic, mutagenic or carcinogenic activity of HMG. Antibodies against HMG can be built up in single cases following repeated cyclical administration of HMG, causing the treatment to be ineffectual.

6. PHARMACEUTICAL PARTICULARS

6.1 List of excipients
Dry substance: lactose, sodium hydroxide for pH-adjustment.

6.2 Incompatibilities
None known.

6.3 Shelf life
Two years as packaged for sale.

The reconstituted product should be used immediately and any remaining solution should be discarded.

6.4 Special precautions for storage
Protect from light. Store at a temperature not exceeding 25°C.

6.5 Nature and contents of container
Dry substance: 2ml glass ampoule

6.6 Instructions for use and handling
The dry substance must be reconstituted with the diluent prior to use.

Use immediately after reconstitution.

7. MARKETING AUTHORISATION HOLDER
Ferring Pharmaceuticals Limited,

The Courtyard,

Waterside Drive,

Langley,

Berkshire SL3 6EZ

8. MARKETING AUTHORISATION NUMBER(S)
PL 03194/0059

9. DATE OF FIRST AUTHORISATION/RENEWAL OF THE AUTHORISATION
26 August 1997

10. DATE OF REVISION OF THE TEXT
April 2002

Menopur
(Ferring Pharmaceuticals Ltd)

1. NAME OF THE MEDICINAL PRODUCT
Menopur

2. QUALITATIVE AND QUANTITATIVE COMPOSITION
Active ingredient

Each vial with dry substance contains highly purified menotrophin (human menopausal gonadotrophin, HMG) corresponding to 75IU human follicle stimulating hormone (FSH) and 75IU human luteinising hormone (LH).

3. PHARMACEUTICAL FORM
Powder for injection; and solvent for parenteral use.

4. CLINICAL PARTICULARS

4.1 Therapeutic indications
Treatment of female and male infertility in the following groups of patients:

- Anovulatory women: Menopur can be used to stimulate follicle development in amenorrhoeic patients. Clomiphene (or a similar ovulation inducing agent which influences steroid feed-back mechanisms) is the preferred treatment for women with a variety of menstrual cycle disturbances, including luteal phase insufficiency with anovulatory cycles and with normal prolactin, and also amenorrhoeic patients with evidence of endogenous oestrogen production but normal prolactin and normal gonadotrophin levels. Non-responders may then be selected for menotrophin therapy.
- Women undergoing superovulation within a medically assisted fertilisation programme: Menopur can be used to induce multiple follicular development in patients undergoing an assisted conception technique such as in-vitro fertilisation (IVF).
- Hypogonadotrophic hypogonadism in men: Menopur may be given in combination with human chorionic gonadotrophin (e.g. Choragon) for the stimulation of spermatogenesis. Patients with primary testicular failure are usually unresponsive.

4.2 Posology and method of administration
Anovulatory infertility:

Menotrophin is administered to induce follicular maturation and is followed by treatment with chorionic gonadotrophin to stimulate ovulation and corpus luteum formation.

The dosage and schedule of treatment must be determined according to the needs of each patient. Response is monitored by studying the patient's urinary oestrogen excretion or by ultrasound visualisation of follicles. Menotrophin may be given daily by either intramuscular or subcutaneous injection to provide a dose of 75 to 150 units of FSH and 75 to 150 units of LH, and gradually adjusted if necessary until an adequate response is achieved, followed after 1 or 2 days by chorionic gonadotrophin. In menstruating patients treatment should be started within the first 7 days of the menstrual cycle. The treatment course should be abandoned if no response is seen in 3 weeks. This treatment cycle may be repeated at least twice more if necessary. Alternatively, three equal doses of menotrophin, each providing 225 to 375 units of FSH with 225 to 375 units of LH, may be given on alternate days followed by chorionic gonadotrophin one week after the first dose.

In the daily therapy schedule, the dose is gradually increased until oestrogen levels start to rise. The effective dose is then maintained until adequate pre-ovulatory oestrogen levels are reached. If oestrogen levels rise too rapidly, the dose should be decreased.

As a measure of follicle maturity the following values can be taken:

- total urinary oestrogen: 75 - 150 microgram (270 - 540 nmol)/24 hours:
- plasma 17 beta-oestradiol: 400 - 800 picogram/ml (1500 - 3000 pmol/L).

When adequate pre-ovulatory oestrogen levels have been reached, administration of Menopur is stopped, and ovulation may then be induced by administering human chorionic gonadotrophin at a dose of 5000 - 10000 IU.

Women undergoing superovulation in IVF or other assisted conception techniques:

In in-vitro fertilisation procedures or other assisted conception techniques menotrophin is used in conjunction with chorionic gonadotrophin and sometimes also clomiphene citrate or a gonadorelin agonist. Stimulation of follicular growth is produced by menotrophin in a dose providing 75 to 300 units of FSH with 75 to 300 units of LH daily. Treatment with menotrophin, either alone or in conjunction with clomiphene or a gonadorelin agonist, is continued until an adequate response is obtained and the final injection of menotrophin is followed 1 or 2 days later with up to 10000 units of chorionic gonadotrophin.

Maturation of follicles is monitored by measurement of oestrogen levels, ultrasound and/or clinical evaluation of oestrogen activity. It is recommended there should be at least 3 follicles greater than 17 mm in diameter with 17-beta oestradiol levels of at least 3500 pmol/L (920 picogram/ml). Egg maturation occurs by administration of human chorionic gonadotrophin in a dose of 5000-10000IU, 30 - 40 hours after the last Menopur injection. Human chorionic gonadotrophin should not be administered if these criteria have not been met. Egg retrieval is carried out 32 - 36 hours after the human chorionic gonadotrophin injection.

Male infertility:

Spermatogenesis is stimulated with chorionic gonadotrophin (1000 - 2000IU two to three times a week) and then menotrophin is given in a dose of 75 or 150 units of FSH with 75 or 150 units of LH two or three times weekly. Treatment should be continued for at least 3 or 4 months.

Children:

Not recommended for use in children.

Elderly:

Not recommended for use in the elderly.

Method of Administration:

By intramuscular or subcutaneous use.

The dry substance must be reconstituted with the diluent prior to use.

4.3 Contraindications

- Pregnancy.
- Enlargement of the ovaries or cysts not caused by polycystic ovarian syndrome.
- Gynaecological bleeding of unknown cause.
- Tumours in the uterus, ovaries, breasts, or testes.
- Carcinoma of the prostate.
- Structural abnormalities in which a satisfactory outcome cannot be expected, for example, tubal occlusion (unless superovulation is to be induced for IVF), ovarian dysgenesis, absent uterus or premature menopause.

4.4 Special warnings and special precautions for use

The following conditions should be properly treated and excluded as the cause of infertility before menotrophin therapy is initiated:-

- dysfunction of the thyroid gland and cortex of the suprarenal gland.
- hyperprolactinaemia.
- tumours in the pituitary or hypothalamic glands.

In the treatment of female infertility, ovarian activity should be checked (by ultrasound and plasma 17 beta-oestradiol measurement) prior to Menopur administration. During treatment, these tests and urinary oestrogen measurement should be carried out at regular intervals, until stimulation occurs. Close supervision is imperative during treatment. See "posology and administration" for optimum response levels of urinary oestrogens and plasma 17 beta-oestradiol. Values below these ranges may indicate inadequate follicular development. If urinary oestrogen levels exceed 540 nmol (150 micrograms)/24 hours, or if plasma 17 beta-oestradiol levels exceed 3000 pmol/L (800 picograms/ml), or if there is any steep rise in values, there is an increased risk of hyperstimulation and Menopur treatment should be immediately discontinued and human chorionic gonadotrophin withheld. Ultrasound will reveal any excessive follicular development and unintentional hyperstimulation. In the event of hyperstimulation, the patient should refrain from sexual intercourse until they are no longer at risk.

If during ultrasound, several mature follicles are visualised, human chorionic gonadotrophin should not be given as there is a risk of multiple ovulation and the occurrence of hyperstimulation syndrome.

Patients undergoing superovulation may be at an increased risk of developing hyperstimulation in view of the excessive oestrogen response and multiple follicular development. Aspiration of all follicles, prior to ovulation, may reduce the incidence of hyperstimulation syndrome.

The severe form of hyperstimulation syndrome may be life-threatening and is characterised by large ovarian cysts (prone to rupture), acute abdominal pain, ascites, very often hydrothorax and occasionally thromboembolic phenomena.

Prior to treatment with Menotrophin, primary ovarian failure should be excluded by the determination of gonadotrophin levels.

There have been reports of ectopic pregnancy in women receiving Menotrophin who have undergone assisted conception. One predisposing factor for ectopic pregnancy is tubal disease/occlusion, which women undergoing assisted conception may have. No causal relationship between ectopic pregnancy and the use of menotrophin has been established.

4.5 Interaction with other medicinal products and other forms of Interaction

None known.

4.6 Pregnancy and lactation

Menopur should not be given during pregnancy or to lactating mothers.

4.7 Effects on ability to drive and use machines

None known.

4.8 Undesirable effects

Treatment with menotrophin can often lead to ovarian hyperstimulation. This, however, mostly becomes clinically relevant only after human chorionic gonadotrophin has been administered to induce ovulation. This can lead to the formation of large ovarian cysts that tend to rupture and can cause intra-abdominal bleeding. In addition, ascites, hydrothorax, oliguria, hypotension, and thromboembolic phenomena can occur. Treatment should be immediately discontinued when the first signs of hyperstimulation can be detected by ultrasound or physically (abdominal pain and distension). With pregnancy, these side effects can intensify, continue over a long period of time, and be life threatening.

Occasional adverse effects of menotrophin treatment, are nausea and vomiting.

There is an increased risk of miscarriage and also multiple pregnancies with menotrophin therapy.

Rarely reported side effects are fever and joint pain, hypersensitivity reactions (skin rash) and local reactions such as pain, itching, redness and swelling at the site of injection.

In very rare cases, long term use of menotrophin can lead to the formation of antibodies making treatment ineffectual.

4.9 Overdose

The acute toxicity of menotrophin has been shown to be very low. However, too high a dosage for more than one day may lead to hyperstimulation, which is categorised as mild, moderate or severe. Symptoms of overdosage usually appear 3 - 6 days after treatment with human chorionic gonadotrophin.

Mild hyperstimulation - Symptoms include some abdominal swelling and pain, ovaries enlarged to about 5 cm diameter. Therapy - rest; careful observation and symptomatic relief. Ovarian enlargement declines rapidly.

Moderate hyperstimulation - Symptoms include more pronounced abdominal distension and pain, nausea, vomiting, occasional diarrhoea, ovaries enlarged up to 12 cm diameter. Therapy - bed rest; close observation especially in the case of conception occurring, to detect any progression to severe hyperstimulation.

Pelvic examination of enlarged ovaries should be gentle in order to avoid rupture of the cysts. Symptoms subside spontaneously over 2 - 3 weeks.

Severe hyperstimulation - This is a rare but serious complication - symptoms include pronounced abdominal distension and pain, ascites, pleural effusion, decreased blood volume, reduced urine output, electrolyte imbalance and sometimes shock, ovaries enlarge to in excess of 12 cm diameter. Therapy - hospitalisation; treatment should be conservative and concentrate on restoring blood volume and preventing shock. Acute symptoms subside over several days and ovaries return to normal over 20 - 40 days if conception does not occur - symptoms may be prolonged if conception occurs.

5. PHARMACOLOGICAL PROPERTIES

5.1 Pharmacodynamic properties

Menotrophin is a gonadotrophin extracted from the urine of postmenopausal women and having both luteinising hormone and follicle stimulating hormone activity. It is given by intramuscular or subcutaneous injection in the treatment of male and female infertility.

Menotrophin (HMG) directly affects the ovaries and the testes. HMG has a gametropic and steroidogenic effect.

In the ovaries, the FSH-component in HMG induces an increase in the number of growing follicles and stimulates their development. FSH increases the production of oestradiol in the granulosa cells by aromatising androgens that originate in the Theca cells under the influence of the LH-component.

In the testes, FSH induces the transformation of premature to mature Sertoli cells. It mainly causes the maturation of the seminal canals and the development of the spermatozoa. However, a high concentration of androgens within the testes is necessary and can be attained by a prior treatment using hCG.

5.2 Pharmacokinetic properties

HMG is not effective when taken orally and is injected either intramuscularly or subcutaneously. The biological effectiveness of HMG is mainly due to its FSH content. The pharmacokinetics of HMG following intramuscular or subcutaneous administration show great individual variation. The maximum serum level of FSH is reached approximately 18 hours after intramuscular injection and 12 hours after subcutaneous injection. After that, the serum level decreases by a half-life of approximately 55 hours following intramuscular administration and 50 hours following subcutaneous administration.

Excretion of HMG, following administration, is predominantly renal.

5.3 Preclinical safety data

Toxic effects caused by HMG are unknown in humans.

There is no evidence of teratogenic, mutagenic or carcinogenic activity of HMG. Antibodies against HMG can be built up in single cases following repeated cyclical administration of HMG, causing the treatment to be ineffectual.

6. PHARMACEUTICAL PARTICULARS

6.1 List of excipients

Dry substance: lactose, polysorbate 20, sodium hydroxide and hydrochloric acid for pH-adjustment.

Solvent: isotonic sodium chloride solution, dilute hydrochloric acid for pH adjustment.

6.2 Incompatibilities

None known.

6.3 Shelf life

Two years as packaged for sale.

The reconstituted product should be used immediately and any remaining solution should be discarded.

6.4 Special precautions for storage

Protect from light. Store at a temperature not exceeding 25°C.

6.5 Nature and contents of container

Dry substance: 2ml glass vial

6.6 Instructions for use and handling

The dry substance must be reconstituted with the diluent prior to use.

Use immediately after reconstitution.

7. MARKETING AUTHORISATION HOLDER

Ferring Pharmaceuticals Limited

The Courtyard

Waterside Drive

Langley

Berkshire SL3 6EZ

United Kingdom

8. MARKETING AUTHORISATION NUMBER(S)

PL 03194/0074

9. DATE OF FIRST AUTHORISATION/RENEWAL OF THE AUTHORISATION

19 November 1999

10. DATE OF REVISION OF THE TEXT

April 2002

Meptid Injection 100mg/ml

(Shire Pharmaceuticals Limited)

1. NAME OF THE MEDICINAL PRODUCT

Meptid ™ Injection 100 mg/ml

2. QUALITATIVE AND QUANTITATIVE COMPOSITION

Each ampoule contains 100 mg of meptazinol base as meptazinol hydrochloride.

3. PHARMACEUTICAL FORM

Solution for injection.

4. CLINICAL PARTICULARS

4.1 Therapeutic indications

For the treatment of moderate to severe pain, including post-operative pain, obstetric pain and the pain of renal colic.

4.2 Posology and method of administration

Adults

Intramuscular dosage: 75-100 mg Meptid. The injection may be repeated 2-4 hourly as required. For obstetric pain a dose of 100-150 mg should be used according to weight. This dose should approximate 2 mg/kg.

Intravenous dosage: 50-100 mg Meptid by slow intravenous injection. The injection may be repeated 2-4 hourly as required. If vomiting occurs, a suitable antiemetic should be given.

Epidural/intrathecal use: This formulation is not suitable for these routes.

Elderly

The adult dosage schedule can be used in the elderly.

Children

Meptid Injection has not been evaluated for use in children.

4.3 Contraindications

None known, except for individuals with known sensitivity to the product.

4.4 Special warnings and special precautions for use

Caution should be observed in treating patients with hepatic or renal insufficiency.

Clinical studies have indicated absence of clinically significant respiratory depression but caution should be exercised in patients already severely compromised.

Safety for use in myocardial infarction has not been established.

Meptid Injection is a useful analgesic in labour, but in accordance with general medical principles, it should not be given in other stages of pregnancy unless considered essential by the physician. There is no evidence from animal reproductive studies to anticipate a teratogenic risk.

Meptid should be used cautiously in patients with head injuries as other drugs of this class have the potential to elevate cerebrospinal fluid pressure and to obscure the clinical course of such patients.

4.5 Interaction with other medicinal products and other forms of Interaction
None known.

4.6 Pregnancy and lactation
Meptid Injection is a useful analgesic in labour, but in accordance with general medical principles, it should not be given in other stages of pregnancy unless considered essential by the physician. There is no evidence from animal reproductive studies to anticipate a teratogenic risk. Meptid should not be given to lactating women unless considered essential by the physician.

4.7 Effects on ability to drive and use machines
Since dizziness and occasionally drowsiness have been reported, patients should be cautioned against driving or operating machinery until it is established that they do not become dizzy or drowsy whilst taking meptazinol.

4.8 Undesirable effects
The most commonly reported adverse reactions after treatment with meptazinol are nausea, vomiting, dizziness, diarrhoea and increased sweating, abdominal pain, rash, vertigo, headache, somnolence and dyspepsia.

Occasional reports of psychiatric disorders (hallucination, confusion, depression) have been received, but any causal relationship with the use of meptazinol has not been established.

4.9 Overdose
Overdose with Meptid Injection has not been reported. Large doses, including seven times the recommended therapeutic dose, have been given in balanced and total intravenous anaesthesia without significant respiratory depressant effects. In the event of cardiovascular and respiratory collapse, normal resuscitative procedures should be employed. Respiratory depression caused by overdosage with meptazinol may be reversed in part with therapeutic doses of naloxone.

5. PHARMACOLOGICAL PROPERTIES

5.1 Pharmacodynamic properties
Meptid (meptazinol) is a centrally acting analgesic belonging to the hexahydroazepine series, which has demonstrated mixed agonist and antagonist activity at opioid receptors.

Receptor binding studies have shown that although meptazinol displays only a low affinity for d (delta) and k (kapa) opioid receptor sites, it has a somewhat higher affinity for the subpopulation of μ sites. These binding sites also display a high affinity for the endogenous opioid peptides, and are thought to be responsible for, among other things, analgesia, but not for the mediation of respiratory depression. A component of its analgesic action is also attributable, in mice at least, to an effect on central cholinergic transmission. In this respect it differs from all conventional analgesic drugs which have been examined.

5.2 Pharmacokinetic properties
After intramuscular administration, meptazinol is rapidly absorbed and peak plasma levels are reached within 30 minutes. The plasma half-life is approximately 2 hours. The peak analgesic effect is seen within 30-60 minutes and lasts about 3-4 hours. After intravenous administration, the onset of action is immediate, occurring within minutes, and lasts a minimum of one hour.

The major route of metabolism is via the glucuronidation pathway and excretion occurs mainly in the urine.

5.3 Preclinical safety data
None given.

6. PHARMACEUTICAL PARTICULARS

6.1 List of excipients
Glucose

Water for injections.

6.2 Incompatibilities
Meptid Injection should not be mixed with other drugs in the same infusion solution or in the same syringe. Meptid Injection is an acidic solution of the hydrochloride salt of meptazinol and is therefore pharmaceutically incompatible with injection solutions known to be strongly basic (for example thiopentone) as precipitation of the meptazinol base may occur.

6.3 Shelf life
36 months.

6.4 Special precautions for storage
Store below 25°C.

6.5 Nature and contents of container
1ml clear glass ampoules. The glass complies with the requirements of the European Pharmacopoeia Type I. The ampoules are packed in cartons of 10.

6.6 Instructions for use and handling
None given.

7. MARKETING AUTHORISATION HOLDER
Monmouth Pharmaceuticals Limited

Hampshire International Business Park

Chineham

Basingstoke

Hampshire RG24 8EP

United Kingdom

8. MARKETING AUTHORISATION NUMBER(S)
PL 10536/0008

9. DATE OF FIRST AUTHORISATION/RENEWAL OF THE AUTHORISATION
16 December 1992

10. DATE OF REVISION OF THE TEXT
March 2001

LEGAL CATEGORY
POM

Meptid Tablets 200mg

(Shire Pharmaceuticals Limited)

1. NAME OF THE MEDICINAL PRODUCT
Meptid™ Tablets 200mg

2. QUALITATIVE AND QUANTITATIVE COMPOSITION
Each tablet contains 200mg of meptazinol base as meptazinol hydrochloride.

3. PHARMACEUTICAL FORM
Orange film coated tablets. The tablets are engraved "MPL023" on one side.

4. CLINICAL PARTICULARS

4.1 Therapeutic indications
For the short term treatment of moderate pain.

4.2 Posology and method of administration
Adults

200mg 3-6 hourly as required. Usually one tablet 4 hourly.

Elderly

The adult dosage schedule can be used in the elderly.

Children

Meptid Tablets have not been evaluated for use in children.

4.3 Contraindications
None known, except for individuals with known sensitivity to the product.

4.4 Special warnings and special precautions for use
Caution should be observed in treating patients with hepatic or renal insufficiency. Clinical studies have indicated absence of clinically significant respiratory depression but caution should be exercised in patients already severely compromised.

Safety for use in myocardial infarction has not yet been established. Meptid should be used cautiously in patients with head injuries as other drugs of this class have the potential to elevate cerebrospinal fluid pressure and to obscure the clinical course of some patients.

4.5 Interaction with other medicinal products and other forms of Interaction
None known.

4.6 Pregnancy and lactation
In accordance with general medical principles, Meptid Tablets should not be given to pregnant or lactating women unless considered essential by the physician. There is no evidence from animal reproductive studies to anticipate a teratogenic risk.

4.7 Effects on ability to drive and use machines
Since dizziness and occasionally drowsiness have been reported, patients should be cautioned against driving or operating machinery until it is established that they do not become dizzy or drowsy whilst taking meptazinol.

4.8 Undesirable effects
The most commonly reported adverse reactions after treatment with meptazinol are nausea, vomiting, dizziness, diarrhoea and increased sweating, abdominal pain, rash, vertigo, headache, somnolence and dyspepsia.

Occasional reports of psychiatric disorders (hallucination, confusion, depression) have been received, but any causal relationship with the use of meptazinol has not been established.

4.9 Overdose
Meptid Tablets are subject to hepatic first pass metabolism which prevents systemic concentrations of the drug reaching levels achieved by parenteral administration. In the unlikely event of overdose producing respiratory depression, naloxone is the treatment of choice. Recommended treatment includes gastric lavage, supportive therapy and naloxone if required.

5. PHARMACOLOGICAL PROPERTIES

5.1 Pharmacodynamic properties
Meptid (meptazinol) is a centrally acting analgesic belonging to the hexahydroazepine series, which has demonstrated mixed agonist and antagonist activity at opioid receptors.

Receptor binding studies have shown that although meptazinol displays only a low affinity for δ and κ opioid receptor sites, it has a somewhat higher affinity for the subpopulation of μ sites. These binding sites also display a high affinity for the endogenous opioid peptides, and are thought to be responsible for, among other things, analgesia, but not for the mediation of respiratory depression. A component of its analgesic action is also attributable, in mice at least, to an effect on central cholinergic transmission. In this respect it differs from all conventional analgesic drugs which have been examined.

5.2 Pharmacokinetic properties
After oral administration, meptazinol is rapidly absorbed and peak plasma levels are reached within 90 minutes. The plasma elimination half-life is variable (1.4-4 hours). The peak analgesic effect is seen within 30-60 minutes and lasts about 3-4 hours.

The drug is rapidly metabolised to the glucuronide, and mostly excreted in the urine.

5.3 Preclinical safety data
None given.

6. PHARMACEUTICAL PARTICULARS

6.1 List of excipients
Meptid Tablets 200mg contain Avicel PH101, Amberlite IRP88, and Magnesium Stearate. The coating contains hydroxypropylmethyl cellulose 2190, polyethylene glycol 400 and opaspray pigment M-1-3476 B.

6.2 Incompatibilities
Not applicable.

6.3 Shelf life
36 months.

6.4 Special precautions for storage
Do not store above 25°C.

6.5 Nature and contents of container
Cartons containing PVC blister packs of 112 tablets.

6.6 Instructions for use and handling
None given.

7. MARKETING AUTHORISATION HOLDER
Monmouth Pharmaceuticals Limited

Hampshire International Business Park

Chineham

Basingstoke

Hampshire RG24 8EP

United Kingdom

8. MARKETING AUTHORISATION NUMBER(S)
PL 10536/0007

9. DATE OF FIRST AUTHORISATION/RENEWAL OF THE AUTHORISATION
17 December 1992

10. DATE OF REVISION OF THE TEXT
March 2001

LEGAL CATEGORY
POM

Merbentyl Syrup

(sanofi-aventis)

1. NAME OF THE MEDICINAL PRODUCT
Merbentyl Syrup

2. QUALITATIVE AND QUANTITATIVE COMPOSITION
Dicycloverine Hydrochloride 10mg

3. PHARMACEUTICAL FORM
Syrup

4. CLINICAL PARTICULARS

4.1 Therapeutic indications
Merbentyl is a smooth muscle antispasmodic primarily indicated for treatment of functional conditions involving smooth muscle spasm of the gastrointestinal tract. The commonest of these are irritable colon (mucous colitis, spastic colon).

4.2 Posology and method of administration
Adults

One to two 5ml spoonfuls (10 - 20mg) three times daily before or after meals.

Children (2-12 years):

One 5ml spoonful (10mg) three times daily.

Children (6 months - 2 years)

5 - 10mg three or four times daily, 15 minutes before feeds. Do not exceed a daily dose of 40mg. If it is necessary to dilute Merbentyl Syrup this may be done using Syrup or if diluted immediately prior to use with water.

4.3 Contraindications
Known idiosyncrasy to dicycloverine hydrochloride. Infants under 6 months of age.

4.4 Special warnings and special precautions for use
Products containing dicycloverine hydrochloride should be used with caution in any patient with or suspected of having glaucoma or prostatic hypertrophy. Use with care in patients with hiatus hernia associated with reflux oesophagitis because anticholinergic drugs may aggravate the condition. There are reports of infants, 3 months of age and under, administered dicycloverine hydrochloride syrup who have evidenced respiratory symptoms (breathing difficulty, shortness of breath, breathlessness, respiratory collapse, apnoea) as well as seizures, syncope, asphyxia, pulse rate fluctuations, muscular hypotonia and coma. The above symptoms have occurred within minutes of ingestion and lasted 20-30 minutes. The symptoms were reported in association with dicycloverine hydrochloride syrup therapy but the cause and effect relationship has neither been disproved or proved. The timing and nature of the reactions suggest that they were a consequence of local irritation and/or aspiration, rather than to a direct pharmacological effect. Although no causal relationship between these effects, observed in infants and dicycloverine administration has been established, dicycloverine hydrochloride is contra-indicated in infants under 6 months of age.

4.5 Interaction with other medicinal products and other forms of Interaction
None stated.

4.6 Pregnancy and lactation
Epidemiological studies in pregnant women with products containing dicycloverine hydrochloride (at doses up to 40mg/day) have not shown that dicycloverine hydrochloride increases the risk of foetal abnormalities if administered during the first trimester of pregnancy. Reproduction studies have been performed in rats and rabbits at doses of up to 100 times the maximum recommended dose (based on 60mg per day for an adult person) and have revealed no evidence of impaired fertility or harm to the foetus due to dicycloverine. Since the risk of teratogenicity cannot be excluded with absolute certainty for any product, the drug should be used during pregnancy only if clearly needed.

It is not known whether dicycloverine is secreted in human milk. Because many drugs are excreted in human milk, caution should be exercised when dicycloverine is administered to a nursing mother.

4.7 Effects on ability to drive and use machines
None stated.

4.8 Undesirable effects
Side-effects seldom occur with Merbentyl. However, in susceptible individuals, dry mouth, thirst and dizziness may occur. On rare occasions, fatigue, sedation, blurred vision, rash, constipation, anorexia, nausea and vomiting, headache and dysuria have also been reported.

4.9 Overdose
Symptoms of Merbentyl overdosage are headache, dizziness, nausea, dry mouth, difficulty in swallowing, dilated pupils and hot dry skin. Treatment may include emetics, gastric lavage and symptomatic therapy if indicated.

5. PHARMACOLOGICAL PROPERTIES

5.1 Pharmacodynamic properties
Dicycloverine hydrochloride relieves smooth muscle spasm of the gastrointestinal tract.

Animal studies indicate that this action is achieved via a dual mechanism;

(1) a specific anticholinergic effect (antimuscarinic at the ACh-receptor sites) and

(2) a direct effect upon smooth muscle (musculotropic).

5.2 Pharmacokinetic properties
After a single oral 20mg dose of dicycloverine hydrochloride in volunteers, peak plasma concentration reached a mean value of 58ng/ml in 1 to 1.5 hours. ^{14}C labelled studies demonstrated comparable bioavailability from oral and intravenous administration. The principal route of elimination is via the urine.

5.3 Preclinical safety data
None stated.

6. PHARMACEUTICAL PARTICULARS

6.1 List of excipients
Invert Syrup Medium

Citric Acid Monohydrate

Sodium Benzoate

Raspberry Flavour

Wild Cherry Bark Flavour

Blackcurrant Essence

Vanilla Essence

Purified water

6.2 Incompatibilities
None stated.

6.3 Shelf life
3 years.

6.4 Special precautions for storage
Do not store above 25°C. Should be stored and dispensed in amber glass bottles.

6.5 Nature and contents of container
Type III, EP amber glass bottles sealed with a polyethylene screw cap equiped with a polyethylene seal and pilferproof closure.

Pack size: 1 bottle containing 120ml syrup.

6.6 Instructions for use and handling
None stated.

7. MARKETING AUTHORISATION HOLDER
Aventis Pharma Ltd

Aventis House

50, Kings Hill Avenue

Kings Hill

West Malling

Kent, ME19 4AH.

8. MARKETING AUTHORISATION NUMBER(S)
PL 04425/0047

9. DATE OF FIRST AUTHORISATION/RENEWAL OF THE AUTHORISATION
Date of first authorisation: 13th July 1983

Date of renewal: 31 July 2001

10. DATE OF REVISION OF THE TEXT
November 2004

Legal category: POM

Merbentyl Tablets

(sanofi-aventis)

1. NAME OF THE MEDICINAL PRODUCT
Merbentyl 10mg Tablets

Merbentyl 20mg Tablets

2. QUALITATIVE AND QUANTITATIVE COMPOSITION
Dicycloverine hydrochloride 10mg or 20mg

3. PHARMACEUTICAL FORM
Tablets

4. CLINICAL PARTICULARS

4.1 Therapeutic indications
Smooth muscle antispasmodic primarily indicated for treatment of functional conditions involving smooth muscle spasm of the gastrointestinal tract.

4.2 Posology and method of administration
Route of administration: Oral

Adults: 10-20mg three times daily before or after meals.

Children (2-12 years): 10mg three times daily.

4.3 Contraindications
Known idiosyncrasy to dicycloverine hydrochloride.

4.4 Special warnings and special precautions for use
Products containing dicycloverine hydrochloride should be used with caution in any patient with or suspected of having glaucoma or prostatic hypertrophy. Use with care in patients with hiatus hernia associated with reflux oesophagitis because anticholinergic drugs may aggravate the condition.

4.5 Interaction with other medicinal products and other forms of Interaction
None stated.

4.6 Pregnancy and lactation
Epidemiological studies in pregnant women with products containing dicycloverine hydrochloride (at doses up to 40mg/day) have not shown that dicycloverine hydrochloride increases the risk of foetal abnormalities if administered during the first trimester of pregnancy. Reproduction studies have been performed in rats and rabbits at doses of up to 100 times the maximum recommended dose (based on 60mg per day for an adult person) and have revealed no evidence of impaired fertility or harm to the foetus due to dicycloverine. Since the risk of teratogenicity cannot be excluded with absolute certainty for any product, the drug should be used during pregnancy only if clearly needed.

It is not known whether dicycloverine is secreted in human milk. Because many drugs are excreted in human milk, caution should be exercised when dicycloverine is administered to a nursing mother.

4.7 Effects on ability to drive and use machines
None stated.

4.8 Undesirable effects
Side-effects seldom occur with Merbentyl tablets. However, in susceptible individuals, dry mouth, thirst and dizziness may occur. On rare occasions, fatigue, sedation, blurred vision, rash, constipation, anorexia, nausea and vomiting, headache and dysuria have also been reported.

4.9 Overdose
Symptoms of Merbentyl overdosage are headache, dizziness, nausea, dry mouth, difficulty in swallowing, dilated pupils and hot dry skin. Treatment may include emetics, gastric lavage and symptomatic therapy if indicated.

5. PHARMACOLOGICAL PROPERTIES

5.1 Pharmacodynamic properties
Dicycloverine hydrochloride relieves smooth muscle spasm of the gastrointestinal tract.

Animal studies indicate that this action is achieved via a dual mechanism;

(1) a specific anticholinergic effect (antimuscarinic at the ACh-receptor sites) and

(2) a direct effect upon smooth muscle (musculotropic).

5.2 Pharmacokinetic properties
After a single oral 20mg dose of dicycloverine hydrochloride in volunteers, peak plasma concentration reached a mean value of 58ng/ml in 1 to 1.5 hours. ^{14}C labelled studies demonstrated comparable bioavailability from oral and intravenous administration. The principal route of elimination is via the urine.

5.3 Preclinical safety data
None stated.

6. PHARMACEUTICAL PARTICULARS

6.1 List of excipients
Lactose

Calcium Hydrogen Phosphate

Icing Sugar*

Maize Starch

Glucose Liquid**

Magnesium Stearate

Purified Water

* mixture of Sucrose 97%

Starch 3%

** equivalent to 4.8mg Glucose Solids

6.2 Incompatibilities
None stated.

6.3 Shelf life
5 years.

6.4 Special precautions for storage
Do not store above 25°C.

6.5 Nature and contents of container
Container: opaque blue 250 micron PVC blisters with aluminium foil 20 micron.

Pack sizes: 10mg - 100 tablets.

20mg – 84 tablets.

6.6 Instructions for use and handling
None stated.

7. MARKETING AUTHORISATION HOLDER
Aventis Pharma Ltd

Aventis House

50, Kings Hill Avenue

Kings Hill

West Malling

Kent, ME19 4AH

8. MARKETING AUTHORISATION NUMBER(S)
Merbentyl 10mg: PL 04425/0035

Merbentyl 20mg: PL04425/0081

9. DATE OF FIRST AUTHORISATION/RENEWAL OF THE AUTHORISATION
Date of first authorisation: 10mg - 27th September 1982

20mg – 13 February 1986

Date of renewal: 10mg - 14th April 1994

20mg – 13 February 1991

10. DATE OF REVISION OF THE TEXT
August 2004

Legal category: POM

Merocaine

(SSL International plc)

1. NAME OF THE MEDICINAL PRODUCT
Merocaine.

2. QUALITATIVE AND QUANTITATIVE COMPOSITION
Cetylpyridinium Chloride BP 1.40mg; Benzocaine Ph Eur 10.00mg.

3. PHARMACEUTICAL FORM
Lozenge.

4. CLINICAL PARTICULARS

4.1 Therapeutic indications
Merocaine provides rapid and profound local anaesthetic action and topical antibacterial effects for the temporary relief of pain and discomfort in sore throat and superficial mouth infections. Indicated for the relief of minor throat irritations and adjunctively, for symptomatic relief of pain

and discomfort in more serious throat infections, such as tonsillitis and pharyngitis.

4.2 Posology and method of administration

Route of administration: Oral. Adults and children over 12 years: Allow to dissolve slowly in the mouth. One lozenge every 2 hours as needed but not more than 8 lozenges in 24 hours.

4.3 Contraindications

Idiosyncrasy to any of the ingredients.

4.4 Special warnings and special precautions for use

None known.

4.5 Interaction with other medicinal products and other forms of Interaction

None known.

4.6 Pregnancy and lactation

There is no or inadequate evidence of safety of cetylpyridinium chloride or benzocaine in human pregnancy, but they have been widely used for many years without apparent ill-consequence. No data are available on the use of Merocaine lozenges during pregnancy and lactation.

4.7 Effects on ability to drive and use machines

Not applicable.

4.8 Undesirable effects

Allergic reactions and methaemoglobinaemia have been reported with benzocaine. If symptoms persist, or are severe, or are accompanied by fever, headache, nausea and vomiting, consult a doctor.

4.9 Overdose

No experience of overdosage. Treatment: No experience of overdosage but normal procedures of gastric lavage and maintenance of respiration and circulation (using vasopressor drugs if necessary) should apply.

5. PHARMACOLOGICAL PROPERTIES

5.1 Pharmacodynamic properties

Cetylpyridinium Chloride: topical antibacterial agent. Benzocaine: local anaesthetic.

5.2 Pharmacokinetic properties

Not applicable.

5.3 Preclinical safety data

Not applicable.

6. PHARMACEUTICAL PARTICULARS

6.1 List of excipients

Lime Oil; Lemon Oil; Sucrose, Granular; Glucose Liquid; Quinoline Yellow E104; FD & C Blue No 2; Isopropyl Alcohol; Ethyl Alcohol; Purified Water.

6.2 Incompatibilities

None known.

6.3 Shelf life

36 months unopened.

6.4 Special precautions for storage

Do not store above 25°C.

6.5 Nature and contents of container

Packs of 24 lozenges. PVC/PVdC/aluminium foli laminate blister in cardboard cartons.

6.6 Instructions for use and handling

None stated.

7. MARKETING AUTHORISATION HOLDER

Seton Products Limited, Tubiton House, Oldham, OL1 3HS.

8. MARKETING AUTHORISATION NUMBER(S)

PL 11314/0105.

9. DATE OF FIRST AUTHORISATION/RENEWAL OF THE AUTHORISATION

30th June 1997 / 29th August 2003.

10. DATE OF REVISION OF THE TEXT

August 2003.

Meronem IV 500mg & 1g

(AstraZeneca UK Limited)

1. NAME OF THE MEDICINAL PRODUCT

Meronem IV (Meropenem).

2. QUALITATIVE AND QUANTITATIVE COMPOSITION

Vial for IV injection or infusion	Meronem	Meronem
	500 mg	1000 mg
Active ingredient:		
Meropenem trihydrate	570 mg	1140 mg
equivalent to anhydrous meropenem	500 mg	1000 mg
Excipient:		
Anhydrous sodium carbonate	104 mg	208 mg

For each gram of meropenem (anhydrous potency) the vial contains 90 mg (3.9 mmol) of sodium.

3. PHARMACEUTICAL FORM

Powder for constitution for intravenous administration.

4. CLINICAL PARTICULARS

4.1 Therapeutic indications

Meronem IV is indicated for treatment, in adults and children, of the following infections caused by single or multiple bacteria sensitive to meropenem.

- Pneumonias and Nosocomial Pneumonias
- Urinary Tract Infections
- Intra-abdominal Infections
- Gynaecological Infections, such as endometritis.
- Skin and Skin Structure Infections
- Meningitis
- Septicaemia
- Empiric treatment, for presumed infections in adult patients with febrile neutropenia, used as monotherapy or in combination with anti-viral or anti-fungal agents.

Meronem has proved efficacious alone or in combination with other antimicrobial agents in the treatment of polymicrobial infections.

Intravenous meropenem has been used effectively in patients with cystic fibrosis and chronic lower respiratory tract infections, either as monotherapy or in combination with other antibacterial agents. Eradication of the organism was not always established.

There is no experience in paediatric patients with neutropenia or primary or secondary immunodeficiency.

4.2 Posology and method of administration

Adults

The dosage and duration of therapy shall be established depending on type and severity of infection and the condition of the patient.

The recommended daily dosage is as follows:-

500 mg IV every 8 hours in the treatment of pneumonia, UTI, gynaecological infections such as endometritis, skin and skin structure infections.

1 g IV every 8 hours in the treatment of nosocomial pneumonias, peritonitis, presumed infections in neutropenic patients, septicaemia.

In cystic fibrosis, doses up to 2 g every 8 hours have been used; most patients have been treated with 2 g every 8 hours.

In meningitis the recommended dosage is 2 g every 8 hours.

As with other antibiotics, particular caution is recommended in using meropenem as monotherapy in critically ill patients with known or suspected *Pseudomonas aeruginosa* lower respiratory tract infection.

Regular sensitivity testing is recommended when treating *Pseudomonas aeruginosa* infection.

Dosage Schedule for Adults with Impaired Renal Function

Dosage should be reduced in patients with creatinine clearance less than 51 ml/min, as scheduled below.

Table 1

Creatinine Clearance (ml/min)	Dose (based on unit doses of 500 mg, 1 g, 2 g)	Frequency
26-50	one unit dose	every 12 hours
10-25	one-half unit dose	every 12 hours
<10	one-half unit dose	every 24 hours

Meropenem is cleared by haemodialysis; if continued treatment with Meronem is necessary, it is recommended that the unit dose (based on the type and severity of infection) is administered at the completion of the haemodialysis procedure to restore therapeutically effective plasma concentrations.

There is no experience with the use of Meronem in patients under peritoneal dialysis.

Dosage in Adults with Hepatic Insufficiency

No dosage adjustment is necessary in patients with hepatic insufficiency (See Section 4.4).

Elderly Patients

No dosage adjustment is required for the elderly with normal renal function or creatinine clearance values above 50 ml/min.

Children

For children over 3 months and up to 12 years of age the recommended dose is 10 to 20 mg/kg every 8 hours depending on type and severity of infection, susceptibility of the pathogen and the condition of the patient. In children over 50 kg weight, adult dosage should be used.

For children aged 4 to 18 years with cystic fibrosis, doses ranging from 25 to 40 mg/kg every 8 hours have been used to treat acute exacerbations of chronic lower respiratory tract Infections.

In meningitis the recommended dose is 40 mg/kg every 8 hours.

There is no experience in children with renal impairment.

Method of Administration

Meronem IV can be given as an intravenous bolus injection over approximately 5 minutes or by intravenous infusion over approximately 15 to 30 minutes using the specific available presentations.

Meronem IV to be used for bolus intravenous injection should be constituted with sterile Water for Injections (5 ml per 250 mg meropenem). This provides an approximate concentration of 50 mg/ml. Constituted solutions are clear, and colourless or pale yellow.

Meronem IV for intravenous infusion may be constituted with compatible infusion fluids (50 to 200 ml) (see Sections 6.2 and 6.4).

4.3 Contraindications

Meronem is contraindicated in patients who have demonstrated hypersensitivity to this product.

4.4 Special warnings and special precautions for use

There is some clinical and laboratory evidence of partial cross-allergenicity between other carbapenems and beta-lactam antibiotics, penicillins and cephalosporins. As with all beta-lactam antibiotics, rare hypersensitivity reactions have been reported (see Section 4.8). Before initiating therapy with meropenem, careful inquiry should be made concerning previous hypersensitivity reactions to beta-lactam antibiotics. Meronem should be used with caution in patients with such a history. If an allergic reaction to meropenem occurs, the drug should be discontinued and appropriate measures taken.

Use of Meronem in patients with hepatic disease should be made with careful monitoring of transaminase and bilirubin levels.

As with other antibiotics, overgrowth of non-susceptible organisms may occur and, therefore, continuous monitoring of each patient is necessary.

Use in infections caused by methicillin resistant staphylococci is not recommended.

Rarely, pseudomembranous colitis has been reported on Meronem as with practically all antibiotics and may vary in severity from slight to life-threatening. Therefore, antibiotics should be prescribed with care for individuals with a history of gastro-intestinal complaints, particularly colitis.

It is important to consider the diagnosis of pseudomembranous colitis in the case of patients who develop diarrhoea in association with the use of Meronem. Although studies indicate that a toxin produced by *Clostridium difficile* is one of the main causes of antibiotic-associated colitis, other causes should be considered.

The co-administration of Meronem with potentially nephrotoxic drugs should be considered with caution. For dosage see Section 4.2.

Paediatric use

Efficacy and tolerability in infants under 3 months old have not been established; therefore, Meronem is not recommended for use below this age. There is no experience in children with altered hepatic or renal function.

Keep all medicines away from children.

4.5 Interaction with other medicinal products and other forms of Interaction

Probenecid competes with meropenem for active tubular secretion and thus inhibits the renal excretion, with the effect of increasing the elimination half-life and plasma concentration of meropenem. As the potency and duration of action of Meronem dosed without probenecid are adequate, the co-administration of probenecid with Meronem is not recommended.

The potential effect of Meronem on the protein binding of other drugs or metabolism has not been studied. The protein binding of Meronem is low (approximately 2%) and therefore no interactions with other compounds based on displacement from plasma proteins would be expected.

Meronem may reduce serum valproic acid levels. Subtherapeutic levels may be reached in some patients.

Meronem has been administered concomitantly with other medications without adverse pharmacological interactions. However, no other specific data regarding potential drug interactions is available (apart from probenecid as mentioned above).

4.6 Pregnancy and lactation

Pregnancy

The safety of Meronem in human pregnancy has not been evaluated. Animal studies have not shown any adverse effect on the developing foetus. The only adverse effect observed in animal reproductive studies was an increased incidence of abortions in monkeys at 13 times the expected exposure in man. Meronem should not be used in pregnancy unless the potential benefit justifies the potential risk to the foetus. In every case, it should be used under the direct supervision of the physician.

Lactation

Meropenem is detectable at very low concentrations in animal breast milk. Meronem should not be used in breast-feeding women unless the potential benefit justifies the potential risk to the baby.

4.7 Effects on ability to drive and use machines

No data are available, but it is not anticipated that Meronem will affect the ability to drive and use machines.

4.8 Undesirable effects

Serious adverse events are rare. During the clinical trials the following adverse events have been reported:

• Local intravenous injection site reactions: inflammation, thrombophlebitis, pain at the site of injection;

• Systemic allergic reactions: rarely, systemic allergic reactions (hypersensitivity) may occur following administration of meropenem. These reactions may include angioedema and manifestations of anaphylaxis;

• Skin reactions: rash, pruritus, urticaria. Rarely, severe skin reactions such as erythema multiforme, Stevens-Johnson Syndrome and toxic epidermal necrolysis have been observed;

• Gastro-intestinal: abdominal pain, nausea, vomiting, diarrhoea. Pseudomembranous colitis has been reported;

• Blood: Reversible thrombocythaemia, eosinophilia, thrombocytopenia, leucopenia and neutropenia (including very rare cases of agranulocytosis). A positive direct or indirect Coombs test may develop in some subjects; there have been reports of reduction in partial thromboplastin time;

• Liver function: Increases in serum concentrations of bilirubin, transaminases, alkaline phosphatase and lactic dehydrogenase alone or in combination have been reported;

• Central nervous system: headache, paraesthesiae. Convulsions have been reported but a causal link with Meronem has not been established;

• Other: Oral and vaginal candidosis.

4.9 Overdose

Accidental overdosage could occur during therapy, particularly in patients with renal impairment. Treatment of overdosage should be symptomatic. In normal individuals, rapid renal elimination will occur; in subjects with renal impairment, haemodialysis will remove meropenem and its metabolite.

5. PHARMACOLOGICAL PROPERTIES

5.1 Pharmacodynamic properties

Meropenem is a carbapenem antibiotic for parenteral use, that is relatively stable to human dehydropeptidase-1 (DHP-1) and therefore does not require the addition of an inhibitor of DHP-1.

Meropenem exerts its bactericidal action by interfering with vital bacterial cell wall synthesis. The ease with which it penetrates bacterial cell walls, its high level of stability to all serine beta-lactamases and its marked affinity for the Penicillin Binding Proteins (PBPs) explain the potent bactericidal action of meropenem against a broad spectrum of aerobic and anaerobic bacteria. Minimum bactericidal concentrations (MBC) are commonly the same as the minimum inhibitory concentrations (MIC). For 76% of the bacteria tested, the MBC:MIC ratios were 2 or less.

Meropenem is stable in susceptibility tests and these tests can be performed using normal routine methods. In vitro tests show that meropenem acts synergistically with various antibiotics. It has been demonstrated both in vitro and in vivo that meropenem has a post-antibiotic effect.

A single set of meropenem susceptibility criteria are recommended based on pharmacokinetics and correlation of clinical and microbiological outcomes with zone diameter and minimum inhibitory concentrations (MIC) of the infecting organisms.

Table 2

CATEGORISATION	METHOD OF ASSESSMENT	
	Zone Diameter (mm)	MIC breakpoints (mg/L)
Susceptible	⩾ 14	⩽ 4
Intermediate	12 to 13	8
Resistant	⩽ 11	⩾ 16

The in vitro antibacterial spectrum of meropenem includes the majority of clinically significant Gram-positive and Gram-negative, aerobic and anaerobic strains of bacteria, as shown below:

Gram-positive aerobes:

Bacillus spp., Corynebacterium diphtheriae, Enterococcus faecalis, Enterococcus liquifaciens, Enterococcus avium, Listeria monocytogenes, Lactobacillus spp., Nocardia asteroides, Staphylococcus aureus (penicillinase negative and positive), *Staphylococci-coagulase-negative;* including, *Staphylococcus epidermidis, Staphylococcus saprophyticus, Staphylococcus capitis, Staphylococcus cohnii, Staphylococcus xylosus, Staphylococcus warneri, Staphylococcus hominis, Staphylococcus simulans, Staphylococcus intermedius, Staphylococcus sciuri, Staphylococcus lugdunensis, Streptococcus pneumoniae* (penicillin susceptible and resistant), *Streptococcus agalactiae, Streptococcus pyogenes, Streptococcus equi, Streptococcus bovis, Streptococcus mitis, Streptococcus mitior, Streptococcus milleri, Streptococcus sanguis, Streptococcus viridans, Streptococcus salivarius, Streptococcus morbillorum, Streptococcus Group G, Streptococcus Group F, Rhodococcus equi.*

Gram-negative aerobes:

Achromobacter xylosoxidans, Acinetobacter anitratus, Acinetobacter lwoffii, Acinetobacter baumannii, Aeromonas hydrophila, Aeromonas sorbria, Aeromonas caviae, Alcaligenes faecalis, Bordetella bronchiseptica, Brucella melitensis, Campylobacter coli, Campylobacter jejuni, Citrobacter freundii, Citrobacter diversus, Citrobacter koseri, Citrobacter amalonaticus, Enterobacter aerogenes, Enterobacter (Pantoea) agglomerans, Enterobacter cloacae, Enterobacter sakazakii, Escherichia coli, Escherichia hermannii, Gardnerella vaginalis, Haemophilus influenzae (including beta-lactamase positive and ampicillin resistant strains), *Haemophilus parainfluenzae, Haemophilus ducreyi, Helicobacter pylori, Neisseria meningitidis, Neisseria gonorrhoeae* (including beta-lactamase positive, penicillin resistant and spectinomycin resistant strains), *Hafnia alvei, Klebsiella pneumoniae, Klebsiella aerogenes, Klebsiella ozaenae, Klebsiella oxytoca, Moraxella (Branhamella) catarrhalis, Morganella morganii, Proteus mirabilis, Proteus vulgaris, Proteus penneri, Providencia rettgeri, Providencia stuartii, Providencia alcalifaciens, Pasteurella multocida, Plesiomonas shigelloides, Pseudomonas aeruginosa, Pseudomonas putida, Pseudomonas alcaligenes, Burkholderia (Pseudomonas) cepacia, Pseudomonas fluorescens, Pseudomonas stutzeri, Pseudomonas pseudomallei, Pseudomonas acidovorans, Salmonella spp.* including *Salmonella enteritidis/typhi, Serratia marcescens, Serratia liquefaciens, Serratia rubidaea, Shigella sonnei, Shigella flexneri, Shigella boydii, Shigella dysenteriae, Vibrio cholerae, Vibrio parahaemolyticus, Vibrio vulnificus, Yersinia enterocolitica.*

Anaerobic bacteria:

Actinomyces odontolyticus, Actinomyces meyeri, Bacteroides-Prevotella-Porphyromonas spp., Bacteroides fragilis, Bacteroides vulgatus, Bacteroides variabilis, Bacteroides pneumosintes, Bacteroides coagulans, Bacteroides uniformis, Bacteroides distasonis, Bacteroides ovatus, Bacteroides thetaiotaomicron, Bacteroides eggerthii, Bacteroides capsillosis, Prevotella buccalis, Prevotella corporis, Bacteroides gracilis, Prevotella melaninogenica, Prevotella intermedia, Prevotella bivia, Prevotella splanchnicus, Prevotella oralis, Prevotella disiens, Prevotella rumenicola, Bacteroides ureolyticus, Prevotella oris, Prevotella buccae, Prevotella denticola, Bacteroides levii, Porphyromonas asaccharolytica, Bifidobacterium spp., Bilophila wadsworthia, Clostridium perfringens, Clostridium bifermentans, Clostridium ramosum, Clostridium sporogenes, Clostridium cadaveris, Clostridium sordellii, Clostridium butyricum, Clostridium clostridiiformis, Clostridium innocuum, Clostridium subterminale, Clostridium tertium, Eubacterium lentum, Eubacterium aerofaciens, Fusobacterium mortiferum, Fusobacterium necrophorum, Fusobacterium nucleatum, Fusobacterium varium, Mobiluncus curtisii, Mobiluncus mulieris, Peptostreptococcus anaerobius, Peptostreptococcus micros, Peptostreptococcus saccharolyticus, Peptococcus saccharolyticus, Peptostreptococcus asaccharolyticus, Peptostreptococcus magnus, Peptostreptococcus prevotii, Propionibacterium acnes, Propionibacterium avidum, Propionibacterium granulosum.

Stenotrophomonas maltophilia, Enterococcus faecium and methicillin-resistant staphylococci have been found to be resistant to meropenem.

5.2 Pharmacokinetic properties

A 30 minute intravenous infusion of a single dose of Meronem in healthy volunteers results in peak plasma levels of approximately 11 microgram/ml for the 250 mg dose, 23 microgram/ml for the 500 mg dose and 49 microgram/ml for the 1g dose.

However, there is no absolute pharmacokinetic proportionality with the administered dose both as regards Cmax and AUC. Furthermore, a reduction in plasma clearance from 287 to 205 ml/min for the range of dosage 250 mg to 2 g has been observed.

A 5 minute intravenous bolus injection of Meronem in healthy volunteers results in peak plasma levels of approximately 52 microgram/ml for the 500 mg dose and 112 microgram/ml for the 1g dose.

Intravenous infusions of 1 g over 2 minutes, 3 minutes and 5 minutes were compared in a three-way crossover trial. These durations of infusion resulted in peak plasma levels of 110, 91 and 94 microgram/ml, respectively.

After an IV dose of 500 mg, plasma levels of meropenem decline to values of 1 microgram/ml or less, 6 hours after administration.

When multiple doses are administered at 8 hourly intervals to subjects with normal renal function, accumulation of meropenem does not occur.

In subjects with normal renal function, meropenem's elimination half-life is approximately 1 hour.

Plasma protein binding of meropenem is approximately 2%.

Approximately 70% of the administered dose is recovered as unchanged meropenem in the urine over 12 hours, after which little further urinary excretion is detectable. Urinary concentrations of meropenem in excess of 10 microgram/ml are maintained for up to 5 hours after the administration of a 500 mg dose. No accumulation of meropenem in plasma or urine was observed with regimens using 500 mg administered every 8 hours or 1 g administered every 6 hours in volunteers with normal renal function.

The only metabolite of meropenem is microbiologically inactive.

Meropenem penetrates well into most body fluids and tissues including cerebrospinal fluid of patients with bacterial meningitis, achieving concentrations in excess of those required to inhibit most bacteria.

Studies in children have shown that the pharmacokinetics of Meronem in children are similar to those in adults. The elimination half-life for meropenem was approximately 1.5 to 2.3 hours in children under the age of 2 years and the pharmacokinetics are linear over the dose range of 10 to 40 mg/kg.

Pharmacokinetic studies in patients with renal insufficiency have shown the plasma clearance of meropenem correlates with creatinine clearance. Dosage adjustments are necessary in subjects with renal impairment.

Pharmacokinetic studies in the elderly have shown a reduction in plasma clearance of meropenem which correlated with age-associated reduction in creatinine clearance.

Pharmacokinetic studies in patients with liver disease have shown no effects of liver disease on the pharmacokinetics of meropenem.

5.3 Preclinical safety data

Animal studies indicate that meropenem is well tolerated by the kidney. In animal studies meropenem has shown nephrotoxic effects, only at high dose levels (500 mg/kg).

Effects on the CNS; convulsions in rats and vomiting in dogs, were seen only at high doses >2000 mg/kg).

For an IV dose the LD_{50} in rodents is greater than 2000 mg/kg. In repeat dose studies (up to 6 months) only minor effects were seen including a small decrease in red cell parameters and an increase in liver weight in dogs treated with doses of 500 mg/kg.

There was no evidence of mutagenic potential in the 5 tests conducted and no evidence of reproductive and teratogenic toxicity in studies at the highest possible doses in rats and monkeys; the no effect dose level of a (small) reduction in F_1 body weight in rat was 120 mg/kg. There was an increased incidence of abortions at 500 mg/kg in a preliminary study in monkeys.

There was no evidence of increased sensitivity to meropenem in juveniles compared to adult animals. The intravenous formulation was well tolerated in animal studies.

The sole metabolite of meropenem had a similar profile of toxicity in animal studies.

6. PHARMACEUTICAL PARTICULARS

6.1 List of excipients

Meronem for IV injection and infusion includes the excipient anhydrous sodium carbonate.

6.2 Incompatibilities

Meronem should not be mixed with or added to other drugs.

Meronem is compatible with the following infusion fluids:

0.9% Sodium Chloride solution

5% or 10% Glucose solution

5% Glucose solution with 0.02% Sodium Bicarbonate

0.9% Sodium Chloride and 5% Glucose solution

5% Glucose with 0.225% Sodium Chloride solution

5% Glucose with 0.15% Potassium Chloride solution

Mannitol 2.5% or 10% solution.

6.3 Shelf life

Meronem has a shelf life of 4 years.

6.4 Special precautions for storage

Do not store above 30°C.

Do not freeze.

It is recommended to use freshly prepared solutions of Meronem for IV injection and infusion. Reconstituted product should be used immediately and must be stored for no longer than 24 hours under refrigeration, only if necessary.

Diluent	Hours stable up to 25°C	4°C
Solutions (1 to 20 mg/ml) prepared with:		
* 0.9% sodium chloride	8	48
* 5% glucose	3	14
* 5% glucose and 0.225% sodium chloride	3	14
* 5% glucose and 0.9% sodium chloride	3	14

* 5% glucose and 0.15% potassium chloride	3	14
* 2.5% or 10% mannitol intravenous infusion	3	14
* 10% glucose	2	8
* 5% glucose and 0.02% sodium bicarbonate		
Intravenous Infusion	2	8

6.5 Nature and contents of container

Type 1 glass vials closed with halobutilic rubber stopper and sealed with an aluminium cap.

Packs for intravenous administration

Pack of 10 vials containing 500 mg or 1 g meropenem.

6.6 Instructions for use and handling

Refer to Section 4.2 "Dosage and Administration" above. Standard aseptic technique should be employed during constitution. Shake constituted solution before use.

All vials are for single use only.

7. MARKETING AUTHORISATION HOLDER

AstraZeneca UK Limited

600 Capability Green,

Luton, LU1 3LU, UK.

8. MARKETING AUTHORISATION NUMBER(S)

Meronem IV 500 mg – PL17901/0029

Meronem IV 1 g – PL17901/0030

9. DATE OF FIRST AUTHORISATION/RENEWAL OF THE AUTHORISATION

11 May 2001

10. DATE OF REVISION OF THE TEXT

21 January 2004

Mestinon 60 mg Tablets

(Valeant Pharmaceuticals Ltd)

1. NAME OF THE MEDICINAL PRODUCT

Mestinon 60 mg Tablets

2. QUALITATIVE AND QUANTITATIVE COMPOSITION

Each tablet contains 62.5mg pyridostigmine bromide (equivalent to 60.0mg of the base).

3. PHARMACEUTICAL FORM

Tablets for oral administration.

4. CLINICAL PARTICULARS

4.1 Therapeutic indications

Myasthenia gravis, paralytic ileus and post-operative urinary retention.

4.2 Posology and method of administration

Myasthenia gravis Adults

Doses of 30 to 120mg are given at intervals throughout the day when maximum strength is needed (for example, on rising and before mealtimes). The usual duration of action of a dose is 3 to 4 hours in the daytime but a longer effect (6 hours) is often obtained with a dose taken on retiring for bed.

The total daily dose is usually in the range of 5 – 20 tablets but doses higher than these may be needed by some patients.

Children

Children under 6 years old should receive an initial dose of half a tablet (30mg) of Mestinon; children 6 – 12 years old should receive one tablet (60mg). Dosage should be increased gradually, in increments of 15 – 30mg daily, until maximum improvement is obtained. Total daily requirements are usually in the range to 30 – 360mg.

The requirement for Mestinon is usually markedly decreased after thymectomy or when additional therapy (steroids, immunosuppressant drugs) is given.

When relatively large doses of Mestinon are taken by myasthenic patients it may be necessary to give atropine or other anticholinergic drugs to counteract the muscarinic effects. It should be noted that the slower gastro-intestinal motility caused by these drugs may affect the absorption of Mestinon.

In all patients the possibility of "cholinergic crisis", due to overdosage of Mestinon, and its differentiation from "myasthenic crisis", due to increased severity of the disease, must be borne in mind. Both types of crisis are manifested by increased muscle weakness, but whereas myasthenic crisis may require more intensive anticholinesterase treatment, cholinergic crisis calls for immediate discontinuation of this treatment and institution of appropriate supportive measures, including respiratory assistance.

Other Indications Adults

The usual dose is 1 to 4 tablets (60 – 240mg).

Children

15 – 60mg.

The frequency of these doses may be varied according to the needs of the patient.

Elderly

There are no specific dosage recommendation for Mestinon in elderly patients.

4.3 Contraindications

Mestinon should not be given to patients with mechanical gastro-intestinal or urinary obstruction. Mestinon is contraindicated in patients with known hypersensitivity to the drug and to bromides.

4.4 Special warnings and special precautions for use

Extreme caution is required when administering Mestinon to patients with bronchial asthma.

Care should also be taken in patients with bradycardia, recent coronary occlusion, hypotension, vagotonia, peptic ulcer, epilepsy or Parkinsonism.

There is no evidence to suggest that Mestinon has any special effects on the elderly. However, elderly patients may be more susceptible to dysrhythmias than the young adult.

Mestinon is mainly excreted unchanged by the kidney, therefore lower doses may be required in patients with renal disease and treatment should be based on titration of drug dosage to effect.

4.5 Interaction with other medicinal products and other forms of Interaction

Antimuscarinics:

Atropine and Hyoscine antagonise the muscarinic effects of pyridostigmine bromide.

Muscle Relaxants:

Pyridostigmine antagonises the effect of non-depolarising muscle relaxants (e.g. pancuronium and vecuronium). Pyridostigmine may prolong the effect of depolarising muscle relaxants (e.g. suxamethonium)

4.6 Pregnancy and lactation

The safety of Mestinon during pregnancy or lactation has not been established. Although the possible hazards to mother and child must be weighed against the potential benefits in every case, experience with Mestinon in pregnant patients with myasthenia gravis has revealed no untoward effect of the drug on the course of pregnancy.

As the severity of myasthenia gravis often fluctuates considerably, particular care is required to avoid cholinergic crisis, due to overdosage of the drug, but otherwise management is no different form that in non-pregnant patients.

Observations indicate that only negligible amounts of Mestinon are excreted in breast milk; nevertheless, due regard should be paid to possible effects on the breast-feeding infant.

4.7 Effects on ability to drive and use machines

None known.

4.8 Undesirable effects

These may include nausea and vomiting, increased salivation, diarrhoea and abdominal cramps.

4.9 Overdose

Signs of overdosage due to muscarinic effects may include abdominal cramps, increased peristalsis, diarrhoea, nausea and vomiting, increased bronchial secretions, salivation, diaphoresis and miosis. Nicotinic effects consist of muscular cramps, fasciculations and general weakness. Bradycardia and hypotension may also occur.

Artificial ventilation should be instituted if respiration is severely depressed. Atropine sulphate 1 to 2mg intravenously is an antidote to the muscarinic effects.

5. PHARMACOLOGICAL PROPERTIES

5.1 Pharmacodynamic properties

Mestinon is an antagonist to cholinesterase, the enzyme which normally destroys acetylcholine. The action of Mestinon can briefly be described, therefore, as the potentiation of naturally occurring acetylcholine. Mestinon has a more prolonged action than Prostigmin (neostigmine) although it is somewhat slower to take effect (generally taking 30 – 60 minutes). Because it has a weaker "muscarinic" action than Prostigmin, it is usually much better tolerated by myasthenic patients in whom the longer action is also an advantage.

5.2 Pharmacokinetic properties

Oral pyridostigmine is poorly absorbed. Maximum plasma concentrations occur at 1 to 2 hours and it is eliminated by the kidney largely unchanged with a half-life of 3 to 4 hours.

5.3 Preclinical safety data

Not applicable.

6. PHARMACEUTICAL PARTICULARS

6.1 List of excipients

Each tablet contains:

Lactose BP

Starch BP

Precipitated Silica

Talc BP

Magnesium Stearate BP

Purified Water BP

6.2 Incompatibilities

None known.

6.3 Shelf life

3 years.

6.4 Special precautions for storage

Recommend maximum storage temperature 25°C. Protect from light and moisture.

6.5 Nature and contents of container

Amber glass bottles with aluminium screw caps and desiccant containing 200 tablets.

6.6 Instructions for use and handling

No special requirements.

7. MARKETING AUTHORISATION HOLDER

Valeant Pharmaceuticals Limited

Cedarwood

Chineham Business Park

Crockford Lane

Basingstoke

Hampshire RG24 8WD

United Kingdom

8. MARKETING AUTHORISATION NUMBER(S)

PL 15142/0006

PA 1096/6/1

9. DATE OF FIRST AUTHORISATION/RENEWAL OF THE AUTHORISATION

1 March 1998

10. DATE OF REVISION OF THE TEXT

May 2004

Metalyse

(Boehringer Ingelheim Limited)

1. NAME OF THE MEDICINAL PRODUCT

Metalyse 8,000 units:

Powder and solvent for solution for injection

Metalyse 10,000 units:

Powder and solvent for solution for injection

2. QUALITATIVE AND QUANTITATIVE COMPOSITION

Metalyse 8,000 units:

1 vial contains 8,000 units (40 mg) tenecteplase.

1 prefilled syringe contains 8 ml water for injections.

Metalyse 10,000 units:

1 vial contains 10,000 units (50 mg) tenecteplase.

1 prefilled syringe contains 10 ml water for injections.

The reconstituted solution contains 1,000 units (5 mg) tenecteplase per ml.

Potency of tenecteplase is expressed in units (U) by using a reference standard which is specific for tenecteplase and is not comparable with units used for other thrombolytic agents.

Tenecteplase is a recombinant fibrin-specific plasminogen activator.

For excipients, see 6.1.

3. PHARMACEUTICAL FORM

Powder and solvent for solution for injection.

The powder is white to off-white.

The reconstituted preparation results in a colourless to pale yellow, clear solution.

4. CLINICAL PARTICULARS

4.1 Therapeutic indications

Metalyse is indicated for the thrombolytic treatment of suspected myocardial infarction with persistent ST elevation or recent left Bundle Branch Block within 6 hours after the onset of acute myocardial infarction (AMI) symptoms.

4.2 Posology and method of administration

Metalyse should be prescribed by physicians experienced in the use of thrombolytic treatment and with the facilities to monitor that use.

Treatment with Metalyse should be initiated as soon as possible after onset of symptoms.

Metalyse should be administered on the basis of body weight, with a maximum dose of 10,000 units (50 mg tenecteplase). The volume required to administer the correct dose can be calculated from the following scheme:

(see Table 1 on next page)

The required dose should be administered as a single intravenous bolus over approximately 10 seconds.

A pre-existing intravenous line may be used for administration of Metalyse in 0.9% sodium chloride solution only. Metalyse is incompatible with dextrose solution.

No other medicinal product should be added to the injection solution.

Adjunctive therapy

Acetylsalicylic acid (ASA) and heparin should be administered as soon as possible after diagnosis to inhibit the thrombogenic process.

Table 1

Patients' body weight category (kg)	Tenecteplase (U)	Tenecteplase (mg)	Corresponding volume of reconstituted solution (ml)
< 60	6,000	30	6
⩾ 60 to < 70	7,000	35	7
⩾ 70 to < 80	8,000	40	8
⩾ 80 to < 90	9,000	45	9
⩾ 90	10,000	50	10

see section 6.6.: Instructions for use and handling

ASA should be administered as soon as possible after AMI symptom onset and continued as long-term treatment. The recommended initial oral dose is between 150 and 325 mg per day. If the patient is unable to ingest tablets, an initial dose of 100-250 mg may be given intravenously if available. The ASA dosage during the following days will be at the discretion of the treating physician.

Heparin should be administered as soon as possible after the diagnosis of AMI has been confirmed, and continued for at least 48 hours on a body weight adjusted basis. For patients weighing 67 kg or less, an initial intravenous heparin bolus not exceeding 4,000 IU is recommended followed initially by not more than an 800 IU/hour infusion. For patients weighing more than 67 kg, an initial intravenous heparin bolus not exceeding 5,000 IU is recommended followed initially by not more than 1,000 IU/hour infusion. For patients already receiving heparin treatment, the initial bolus should not be given. The infusion rate should be adjusted to maintain an aPTT of 50-75 seconds (1.5 to 2.5 times control or a heparin plasma level of 0.2 to 0.5 IU/ml).

4.3 Contraindications

Metalyse is contraindicated in the following situations because thrombolytic therapy is associated with a higher risk of bleeding:

- Significant bleeding disorder either at present or within the past 6 months
- Patients with current concomitant oral anticoagulant therapy (INR> 1.3)
- Any history of central nervous system damage (i.e. neoplasm, aneurysm, intracranial or spinal surgery)
- Known haemorrhagic diathesis
- Severe uncontrolled hypertension
- Major surgery, biopsy of a parenchymal organ, or significant trauma within the past 2 months (this includes any trauma associated with the current AMI)
- Recent trauma to the head or cranium
- Prolonged cardiopulmonary resuscitation (> 2 minutes) within the past 2 weeks
- Acute pericarditis and/or subacute bacterial endocarditis
- Acute pancreatitis
- Severe hepatic dysfunction, including hepatic failure, cirrhosis, portal hypertension (oesophageal varices) and active hepatitis
- Active peptic ulceration
- Arterial aneurysm and known arterial/venous malformation
- Neoplasm with increased bleeding risk
- Any known history of stroke or transient ischaemic attack or dementia
- Hypersensitivity to the active substance tenecteplase and to any of the excipients

4.4 Special warnings and special precautions for use

Bleeding

The most common complication encountered during Metalyse therapy is bleeding. The concomitant use of heparin anticoagulation may contribute to bleeding. As fibrin is lysed during Metalyse therapy, bleeding from recent puncture site may occur. Therefore, thrombolytic therapy requires careful attention to all possible bleeding sites (including catheter insertion sites, arterial and venous puncture sites, cutdown sites and needle puncture sites). The use of rigid catheters as well as intramuscular injections and non-essential handling of the patient should be avoided during treatment with Metalyse.

Most frequently haemorrhage at the injection site, and occasionally genitourinary and gingival bleeding were observed.

Should serious bleeding occur, in particular cerebral haemorrhage, concomitant heparin administration should be terminated immediately. Administration of protamine should be considered if heparin has been administered within 4 hours before the onset of bleeding. In the few patients who fail to respond to these conservative measures, judicious use of transfusion products may be indicated. Transfusion of cryoprecipitate, fresh frozen plasma, and platelets should be considered with clinical and laboratory reassessment after each administration. A target fibrinogen level of 1 g/l is desirable with cryoprecipitate infusion. Antifibrinolytic agents are available as a last alternative. In the following conditions, the risk of Metalyse therapy may be increased and should be weighed against the anticipated benefits:

- Systolic blood pressure > 160 mm Hg
- Cerebrovascular disease
- Recent gastrointestinal or genitourinary bleeding (within the past 10 days)
- High likelihood of left heart thrombus, e.g., mitral stenosis with atrial fibrillation
- Any known recent (within the past 2 days) intramuscular injection
- Advanced age, i.e. over 75 years
- Low body weight < 60 kg

Arrhythmias

Coronary thrombolysis may result in arrhythmias associated with reperfusion. It is recommended that antiarrhythmic therapy for bradycardia and/or ventricular tachyarrhythmias (pacemaker, defibrillator) be available when Metalyse is administered.

GPIIb/IIIa antagonists

There is no experience with the use of GPIIb/IIIa antagonists within the first 24 hours after start of treatment.

Re-administration

Since at present there is no experience with re-administration of Metalyse, the re-administration is not recommended. However, no antibody formation to the tenecteplase molecule has been observed. If an anaphylactoid reaction occurs, the injection should be discontinued immediately and appropriate therapy should be initiated. In any case, tenecteplase should not be re-administered before assessment of haemostatic factors like fibrinogen, plasminogen and alpha2-antiplasmin.

4.5 Interaction with other medicinal products and other forms of Interaction

No formal interaction studies with Metalyse and medicinal products commonly administered in patients with AMI have been performed. However, the analysis of data from more than 12,000 patients treated during phase I, II and III did not reveal any clinically relevant interactions with medicinal products commonly used in patients with AMI and concomitantly used with Metalyse.

Medicinal products that affect coagulation or those that alter platelet function (e.g. ticlopidine, clopidogrel, LMWH) may increase the risk of bleeding prior to, during or after Metalyse therapy.

4.6 Pregnancy and lactation

No experience in pregnant women is available for tenecteplase. Because animal studies (see also section 5.3.) have shown a high risk of vaginal bleeding presumably from the placenta and of pregnancy loss, the benefit of treatment has to be evaluated against the potential risks which may aggravate an acute life-threatening situation.

It is not known if tenecteplase is excreted into breast milk. Breast milk should be discarded within the first 24 hours after thrombolytic therapy.

4.7 Effects on ability to drive and use machines

Not applicable.

4.8 Undesirable effects

Haemorrhage is a very common undesirable effect associated with the use of tenecteplase. The type of haemorrhage is predominantly superficial at the injection site. Ecchymoses are observed commonly but usually do not require any specific action. Death and permanent disability are reported in patients who have experienced stroke (including intracranial bleeding) and other serious bleeding episodes.

Immune system disorders

Uncommon: Anaphylactoid reactions (including rash, urticaria, bronchospasm, laryngeal oedema)

Nervous system disorders

Uncommon: Intracranial haemorrhage (including associated symptoms as somnolence, aphasia, convulsion)

Cardiac disorders

Very common: Reperfusion arrhythmias

Rare: Haemopericardium

Vascular disorders

Very common: Bleeding, Hypotension

Common: Ecchymosis

Uncommon: Thrombotic embolisation

Very rare: Eye haemorrhage, Cholesterol crystal embolism

Respiratory, thoracic and mediastinal disorders

Common: Epistaxis

Uncommon: Pulmonary haemorrhage

Gastrointestinal disorders

Common: Bleeding into gastrointestinal tract, nausea, vomiting

Uncommon: Bleeding into retroperitoneum

Renal and urinary disorders

Common: Bleeding into urogenital tract

General disorders and administration site conditions

Very common: Superficial bleeding, normally from punctures or damaged blood vessels

Common: Increased temperature

As with other thrombolytic agents, the following events have been reported as sequelae of myocardial infarction and/or thrombolytic administration:

- very common (>10%): hypotension, heart rate and rhythm disorders, angina pectoris
- common (>1%, <10%): recurrent ischaemia, heart failure, reinfarction, cardiogenic shock, pericarditis, pulmonary oedema
- uncommon (>0.1%, <1%): cardiac arrest, mitral insufficiency, pericardial effusion, venous thrombosis, cardiac tamponade, myocardial rupture
- rare (>0.01%, <0.1%): pulmonary embolism

These cardiovascular events can be life-threatening and may lead to death.

4.9 Overdose

In the event of overdose there may be an increased risk of bleeding. In case of severe prolonged bleeding substitution therapy may be considered (plasma, platelets), see also section 4.4.

5. PHARMACOLOGICAL PROPERTIES

5.1 Pharmacodynamic properties

Pharmacotherapeutic group: antithrombotic agents, ATC code: B01A D

Mechanism of action

Tenecteplase is a recombinant fibrin-specific plasminogen activator that is derived from native t-PA by modifications at three sites of the protein structure. It binds to the fibrin component of the thrombus (blood clot) and selectively converts thrombus-bound plasminogen to plasmin, which degrades the fibrin matrix of the thrombus. Tenecteplase has a higher fibrin specificity and greater resistance to inactivation by its endogenous inhibitor (PAI-1) compared to native t-PA.

Pharmacodynamic effects

After administration of tenecteplase dose dependent consumption of α2-antiplasmin (the fluid-phase inhibitor of plasmin) with consequent increase in the level of systemic plasmin generation have been observed. This observation is consistent with the intended effect of plasminogen activation. In comparative studies a less than 15% reduction in fibrinogen and a less than 25% reduction in plasminogen were observed in subjects treated with the maximum dose of tenecteplase (10,000 U, corresponding to 50 mg), whereas alteplase caused an approximately 50% decrease in fibrinogen and plasminogen levels. No clinically relevant antibody formation was detected at 30 days.

Clinical effects

Patency data from the phase I and II angiographic studies suggest that tenecteplase, administered as a single intravenous bolus, is effective in dissolving blood clots in the infarct-related artery of subjects experiencing an AMI on a dose related basis.

A large scale mortality trial (ASSENT II) in approx. 17,000 patients showed that tenecteplase is therapeutically equivalent to alteplase in reducing mortality (6.2% for both treatments, at 30 days, upper limit of the 95% CI for the relative risk ratio 1.124) and that the use of tenecteplase is associated with a significantly lower incidence of non-intracranial bleedings (26.4% vs. 28.9%, p=0.0003). This translates into a significantly lower need of transfusions (4.3% vs. 5.5%, p=0.0002). Intracranial haemorrhage occurred at a rate of 0.93% vs. 0.94% for tenecteplase and alteplase, respectively.

Coronary patency and limited clinical outcome data showed that AMI patients have been successfully treated later than 6 hours after symptom onset.

5.2 Pharmacokinetic properties

Tenecteplase is an intravenously administered, recombinant protein that activates plasminogen. Tenecteplase is cleared from circulation by binding to specific receptors in the liver followed by catabolism to small peptides. Binding to hepatic receptors is, however, reduced compared to native t-PA, resulting in a prolonged half-life. Data on tissue distribution and elimination were obtained in studies with radioactively labeled tenecteplase in rats. The main organ to which tenecteplase distributed was the liver. It is not

Table 2

Patients' body weight category (kg)	Volume of reconstituted solution (ml)	Tenecteplase (U)	Tenecteplase (mg)
< 60	6	6,000	30
≥ 60 to < 70	7	7,000	35
≥ 70 to < 80	8	8,000	40
≥ 80 to < 90	9	9,000	45
≥ 90	10	10,000	50

known whether and to what extent tenecteplase binds to plasma proteins in humans.

After single intravenous bolus injection of tenecteplase in patients with acute myocardial infarction, tenecteplase antigen exhibits biphasic elimination from plasma. There is no dose dependence of tenecteplase clearance in the therapeutic dose range. The initial, dominant half life is 24 ± 5.5 (mean +/-SD) min, which is 5 times longer than native t-PA. The terminal half-life is 129 ± 87 min, and plasma clearance is 119 ± 49 ml/min.

Increasing body weight resulted in a moderate increase of tenecteplase clearance, and increasing age resulted in a slight decrease of clearance. Women exhibit in general lower clearance than men, but this can be explained by the generally lower body weight of women.

The effect of renal and hepatic dysfunction on pharmacokinetics of tenecteplase in humans is not known. There is no specific experience to guide the adjustment to tenecteplase dose in patients with hepatic and severe renal insufficiency. However, based on animal data it is not expected that renal dysfunction will affect the pharmacokinetics.

5.3 Preclinical safety data

Intravenous single dose administration in rats, rabbits and dogs resulted only in dose-dependent and reversible alterations of the coagulation parameters with local haemorrhage at the injection site, which was regarded as a consequence of the pharmacodynamic effect of tenecteplase. Multiple-dose toxicity studies in rats and dogs confirmed these above-mentioned observations, but the study duration was limited to two weeks by antibody formation to the human protein tenecteplase, which resulted in anaphylaxis.

Safety pharmacology data in cynomolgus monkeys revealed reduction of blood pressure followed by changes of ECG, but these occurred at exposures that were considerably higher than the clinical exposure.

With regard to the indication and the single dose administration in humans, reproductive toxicity testing was limited to an embryotoxicity study in rabbits as a sensitive species. Tenecteplase induced total litter deaths during the mid-embryonal period. When tenecteplase was given during the mid- or late-embryonal period maternal animals showed vaginal bleeding on the day after the first dose. Secondary mortality was observed 1-2 days later. Data on the foetal period are not available.

Mutagenicity and carcinogenicity are not expected for this class of recombinant proteins and genotoxicity and carcinogenicity testing were not necessary.

No local irritation of the blood vessel was observed after intravenous, intra-arterial or paravenous administration of the final formulation of tenecteplase.

6. PHARMACEUTICAL PARTICULARS

6.1 List of excipients

Powder: L-arginine, phosphoric acid, polysorbate 20.

Solvent: water for injections

6.2 Incompatibilities

Metalyse is incompatible with dextrose infusion solutions.

6.3 Shelf life

Shelf life as packaged for sale

2 years

Reconstituted solution

Chemical and physical in-use stability has been demonstrated for up to 24 hours at 2 - 8° C and 8 hours at 30° C. From a microbiological point of view, the product should be used immediately after reconstitution. If not used immediately, in-use storage times and conditions prior to use are the responsibility of the user and would normally not be longer than 24 hours at 2-8° C.

6.4 Special precautions for storage

Do not store above 30° C. Keep the container in the outer carton.

6.5 Nature and contents of container

20 ml glass vial type I, with a coated (B2-42) grey rubber stopper and a flip off cap filled with powder for solution for injection.

10 ml plastic syringe pre-filled with 8 ml or 10 ml of water for injections for reconstitution.

Sterile vial adapter.

Sterile needle for single use.

6.6 Instructions for use and handling

Metalyse should be reconstituted by adding the complete volume of water for injections from the pre-filled syringe to the vial containing the powder for injection.

1. Ensure that the appropriate vial size is chosen according to the body weight of the patient.

(see Table 2 above)

2. Check that the cap of the vial is still intact.

3. Remove the flip-off cap from the vial.

4. Remove the tip-cap from the syringe. Then immediately screw the pre-filled syringe on the vial adapter and penetrate the vial stopper in the middle with the spike of the vial adapter.

5. Add the water for injections into the vial by pushing the syringe plunger down slowly to avoid foaming.

6. Reconstitute by swirling gently.

7. The reconstituted preparation results in a colourless to pale yellow, clear solution. Only clear solution without particles should be used.

8. Directly before the solution will be administered, invert the vial with the syringe still attached, so that the syringe is below the vial.

9. Transfer the appropriate volume of reconstituted solution of Metalyse into the syringe, based on the patient's weight.

10. Disconnect the syringe from the vial adapter.

11. Metalyse is to be administered to the patient, intravenously in about 10 seconds. It should not be administered in a line containing dextrose.

12. Any unused solution should be discarded.

Alternatively the reconstitution can be performed with the included needle.

7. MARKETING AUTHORISATION HOLDER

Boehringer Ingelheim International GmbH

Binger Strasse 173

D-55216 Ingelheim am Rhein

Germany

8. MARKETING AUTHORISATION NUMBER(S)

EU/1/00/169/002 EU/1/00/169/005

EU/1/00/169/003 EU/1/00/169/006

9. DATE OF FIRST AUTHORISATION/RENEWAL OF THE AUTHORISATION

23 February 2001

10. DATE OF REVISION OF THE TEXT

January 2004

M10/B/SPC/5

Meted Shampoo

(Alliance Pharmaceuticals)

1. NAME OF THE MEDICINAL PRODUCT

Meted Shampoo

2. QUALITATIVE AND QUANTITATIVE COMPOSITION

Salicylic acid	USP 3.0%
Colloidal sulphur	HSE 6.25%
(equivalent to sulphur 5.0%)	

3. PHARMACEUTICAL FORM

Shampoo

4. CLINICAL PARTICULARS

4.1 Therapeutic indications

For the relief of itching, irritation, redness, flaking and/or scaling due to dandruff, seborrhoeic dermatitis, or psoriasis of the scalp.

4.2 Posology and method of administration

For topical administration.

Adults:

The hair should be thoroughly wetted and sufficient Meted Shampoo applied to produce an abundant lather. The hair should be rinsed and the procedure repeated.

Use at least twice weekly or as directed by a physician.

Children:

As for adults.

Elderly:

As for adults.

4.3 Contraindications

Meted Shampoo is contra-indicated in persons with a sensitivity to any of the ingredients.

4.4 Special warnings and special precautions for use

Avoid contact with the eyes. If shampoo gets into the eyes rinse thoroughly with water.

If the condition worsens or does not improve after regular use of the product as directed, consult a physician.

Excessive prolonged use may result in symptoms of salicylism.

4.5 Interaction with other medicinal products and other forms of Interaction

None known.

4.6 Pregnancy and lactation

No limitations to the use of Meted Shampoo during pregnancy or lactation are known.

Safety has not been established in either humans or animals during pregnancy and lactation. However, with the small amounts of salicylic acid absorbed transdermally from Meted it is unlikely that use will cause any adverse effects.

4.7 Effects on ability to drive and use machines

None known.

4.8 Undesirable effects

There have been no reports of adverse effects following the use of Meted Shampoo. However, salicylic acid is a mild irritant and may cause dermatitis.

As with other topical preparations containing salicylic acid prolonged use may result in symptoms of salicylism.

4.9 Overdose

There is no evidence of systemic absorption following the use of this shampoo. There are no reports available of its ingestion.

Early symptoms are ringing in the ear tinnitus with deafness, epistaxis, nausea, vomiting, sensitivity and dryness of the mucous membranes. If this occurs treatment must be stopped immediately.

5. PHARMACOLOGICAL PROPERTIES

5.1 Pharmacodynamic properties

Sulphur is a keratolytic and mild antiseptic.

Salicylic acid has keratolytic and fungicidal properties.

5.2 Pharmacokinetic properties

There is no evidence of systemic absorption of sulphur or salicylic acid following use of Meted Shampoo.

5.3 Preclinical safety data

None presented.

6. PHARMACEUTICAL PARTICULARS

6.1 List of excipients

Magnesium aluminium silicate

Hydroxypropyl methyl cellulose

Panthenol

Sodium laureth sulphate

Sodium cocoyl sarcosinate

Cocamido propyl betaine

Fragrance - Firmenich 430 015

Purified water

6.2 Incompatibilities

None known.

6.3 Shelf life

36 months.

6.4 Special precautions for storage

Store below 30 deg C.

6.5 Nature and contents of container

Meted Shampoo is supplied in a white HDPE bottle with a white polypropylene screw cap. Each bottle contains either 30ml or 120ml of Meted Shampoo.

6.6 Instructions for use and handling

For external use only.

Keep out of reach of children.

7. MARKETING AUTHORISATION HOLDER

Alliance Pharmaceuticals Ltd

Avonbridge House

Bath Road

Chippenham

Wiltshire

SN15 2BB

8. MARKETING AUTHORISATION NUMBER(S)

PL 16853/0072

9. DATE OF FIRST AUTHORISATION/RENEWAL OF THE AUTHORISATION

1st July 1999

10. DATE OF REVISION OF THE TEXT
May 2005

Metenix 5 Tablets

(sanofi-aventis)

1. NAME OF THE MEDICINAL PRODUCT
Metenix 5 Tablets

2. QUALITATIVE AND QUANTITATIVE COMPOSITION
Metolazone 5 mg

3. PHARMACEUTICAL FORM
Tablet

4. CLINICAL PARTICULARS

4.1 Therapeutic indications
Metenix 5 is a diuretic for use in the treatment of mild and moderate hypertension. Metenix 5 may be used in conjunction with non-diuretic antihypertensive agents and, in these circumstances, it is usually possible to achieve satisfactory control of blood pressure with a reduced dose of the non-diuretic agent. Patients who have become resistant to therapy with these agents may respond to the addition of Metenix 5 to their antihypertensive regimen.

Metenix 5 may also be used for the treatment of cardiac, renal and hepatic oedema, ascites or toxaemia of pregnancy.

4.2 Posology and method of administration
Route of administration: Oral

Hypertension: The recommended initial dose in mild and moderate hypertension is 5 mg daily. After three to four weeks, the dose may be reduced if necessary to 5 mg on alternate days as maintenance therapy.

Oedema: In oedematous conditions, the normal recommended dose is 5–10 mg daily, given as a single dose. In resistant conditions, this may be increased to 20 mg daily or above. However, no more than 80 mg should be given in any 24–hour period.

Children: There is insufficient knowledge of the effects of Metenix 5 in children for any dosage recommendations to be made.

Elderly: Metolazone may be excreted more slowly in the elderly.

4.3 Contraindications
Metenix 5 is contra-indicated in electrolyte deficiency states, anuria, coma or pre-comatose states associated with liver cirrhosis; also in patients with known allergy or hypersensitivity to metolazone.

4.4 Special warnings and special precautions for use
Because of the antihypertensive effects of metolazone the dosage of concurrently administered non-diuretic antihypertensive agents may need to be reduced.

Caution should be exercised during Metenix 5 therapy in patients liable to electrolyte deficiency.

Chloride deficit, hyponatraemia and a low salt syndrome may also occur, particularly when the patient is also on a diet with restricted salt intake. Hypomagnesaemia has been reported as a consequence of prolonged diuretic therapy.

Prolonged therapy with Metenix 5 may result in hypokalaemia. Serum potassium levels should be determined at regular intervals and, if necessary, potassium supplementation should be instituted.

Fluid and electrolyte balance should be carefully monitored during therapy especially if Metenix 5 is used concurrently with other diuretics. In particular, Metenix 5 may potentiate the diuresis produced by frusemide and, if the two agents are used concurrently, patients should be carefully monitored.

4.5 Interaction with other medicinal products and other forms of Interaction
The dosage of concurrently administered cardiac glycosides may require adjustment. Metenix 5 may aggravate the increased potassium excretion associated with steroid therapy or diseases such as cirrhosis or severe ischaemic heart disease. Latent diabetes may become manifest or the insulin requirements of diabetic patients may increase.

Non steroidal anti-inflammatory drugs (e.g. Indomethacin, Sulindac) may attenuate the action of Metolazone.

Prolongation of bleeding time has been reported during concomitant administration of Metenix and warfarin.

4.6 Pregnancy and lactation
There is little evidence of safety of the drug in human pregnancy, but it has been in wide, general use for many years without apparent ill consequence, animal studies having shown no hazard.

If Metenix 5 is given to nursing mothers, metolazone may be present in the breast milk.

4.7 Effects on ability to drive and use machines
None known.

4.8 Undesirable effects
Metenix 5 is generally well tolerated. There have been occasional reports of headache, anorexia, vomiting, abdominal discomfort, muscle cramps and dizziness. There have been isolated reports of urticaria, leucopenia, tachycardia, chills and chest pain.

Hyperuricaemia or azotaemia may occur during treatment with Metenix 5, particularly in patients with impaired renal function. On rare occasions, clinical gout has been reported.

4.9 Overdose
In cases of overdose there is a danger of dehydration and electrolyte depletion. Treatment should therefore be aimed at fluid replacement and correction of the electrolyte imbalance.

5. PHARMACOLOGICAL PROPERTIES

5.1 Pharmacodynamic properties
Metolazone is a substituted quinazolinone diuretic.

5.2 Pharmacokinetic properties
Diuresis and saluresis begin within one hour of administration of Metenix 5 tablets, reaching a maximum in two hours and continuing for 12–24 hours according to dosage.

5.3 Preclinical safety data
None applicable.

6. PHARMACEUTICAL PARTICULARS

6.1 List of excipients
Microcrystalline cellulose, magnesium stearate, F D and C blue no 2 lake (E132)

6.2 Incompatibilities
None.

6.3 Shelf life
5 years.

6.4 Special precautions for storage
Metenix 5 tablets should be stored protected from light, in the original container or in containers similar to those of the manufacturer.

6.5 Nature and contents of container
Blister pack of 30 or 100 tablets.

6.6 Instructions for use and handling
None.

Administrative Data

7. MARKETING AUTHORISATION HOLDER
Aventis Pharma Limited
50 Kings Hill Avenue
Kings Hill
West Malling
Kent ME19 4AH

8. MARKETING AUTHORISATION NUMBER(S)
PL 04425/0212

9. DATE OF FIRST AUTHORISATION/RENEWAL OF THE AUTHORISATION
5 November 2001

10. DATE OF REVISION OF THE TEXT
November 2001

11. Legal Category
POM

Methadone Injection BP 1%

(Wockhardt UK Ltd)

1. NAME OF THE MEDICINAL PRODUCT
Methadone Injection BP 1%

2. QUALITATIVE AND QUANTITATIVE COMPOSITION
Methadone Hydrochloride 10mg in 1ml

3. PHARMACEUTICAL FORM
Solution for injection

A clear and colourless solution

4. CLINICAL PARTICULARS

4.1 Therapeutic indications
Methadone injection may be used in the management of opioid dependence; as an analgesic for moderate to severe pain as an alternative to morphine.

4.2 Posology and method of administration
Adults:

Opioid drug dependence: by intramuscular or subcutaneous injection.

The dose is adjusted according to the degree of dependence.

Initially 10-20 mg daily increased by 10-20 mg daily until no signs of withdrawal or intoxication. The usual dose is 40-60 mg daily. After stabilisation, the dose is gradually decreased until total withdrawal is achieved.

Elderly: Repeated doses should only be given with extreme caution in the case of elderly or debilitated patients.

Children: Not suitable for use.

As an analgesic: by intramuscular or subcutaneous injection.

Initially a single dose of 5-10 mg at six to eight hourly intervals, adjusted according to response.

Elderly: Repeated doses should only be given with extreme caution in the case of elderly or debilitated patients.

Children: Not suitable for use.

4.3 Contraindications
Respiratory depression or respiratory failure; airways obstruction. Use during an acute asthma attack is not advisable.

Methadone should not be administered to patients with head injuries or raised intracranial pressure as there is a risk of respiratory depression which may lead to a further elevation of CSF pressure. The sedation and pupillary changes produced may interfere with accurate monitoring of the patient.

Monoamine oxidase inhibitor drugs given concurrently or within two weeks of discontinuation.

Obstetric use is not recommended because of the increased risk of neonatal depression due to the long duration of action.

4.4 Special warnings and special precautions for use
Methadone has a long half life and accumulation may occur with repeated doses, especially in elderly or debilitated patients.

Care should be taken in assessing tolerance in dependent patients during induction.

Repeated administration of methadone may lead to dependence and tolerance developing. Abrupt withdrawal in patients who have developed dependence may precipitate a withdrawal syndrome.

Even at low doses methadone is a **special hazard** to children if ingested accidentally.

4.5 Interaction with other medicinal products and other forms of Interaction
Alcohol may induce serious respiratory depression and hypotension.

Monoamine oxidase inhibitors (MAOIs) may prolong and enhance the respiratory depressant effects of methadone and lead to CNS excitation or depression. Other agents with central nervous system depressant activity such as sedatives, hypnotics, antipsychotics, anxiolytics and barbiturates may result in increased CNS depression, respiratory depression and hypotension. Hyperpyrexia and CNS toxicity has been reported when selegiline was coadministered with opioid analgesics.

Methadone is metabolised in the liver and interactions are likely with enzyme inhibitors or inducers; for example, cimetidine may enhance the effects of methadone, while phenytoin may increase its metabolism; Similarly, an increase in its urinary excretion has been reported with rifampicin.

Based on the known metabolism of methadone, nevirapine may decrease plasma concentrations of methadone by increasing its hepatic metabolism. Narcotic withdrawal syndrome has been reported in patients treated with nevirapine and methadone concomitantly. Methadone maintained patients beginning nevirapine therapy should be monitored for evidence of withdrawal and methadone dose should be adjusted accordingly.

Administration of naltrexone to a patient addicted to methadone will rapidly precipitate long term withdrawal symptoms.

Administration of buprenorphine and pentazocine may precipitate withdrawal symptoms in the addicted patient.

Drugs that acidify or alkalinise the urine may affect methadone clearance which is increased at acidic pH.

4.6 Pregnancy and lactation
There is inadequate evidence of safety in human pregnancy.

Methadone should not be used during labour (see contra-indications). Methadone is excreted in breast milk.

4.7 Effects on ability to drive and use machines
Methadone may severely impair the ability to drive and use machinery. The physician must decide the time after which activities may be safely resumed.

4.8 Undesirable effects
The most common side effects are nausea, vomiting, drowsiness, constipation, confusion and euphoria.

Other side effects which occur more commonly in ambulant patients, include pruritus, urticaria, dry mouth, urinary retention, vertigo, bradycardia, orthostatic hypotension, palpitations, sweating, facial flushing, hypothermia, restlessness, changes of mood, hallucinations and miosis. Raised intracranial pressure and muscle rigidity have been reported.

Methadone causes pain at injection sites. Local irritation has been observed at the injection site and induration may occur with repeated subcutaneous injection.

4.9 Overdose
a) Symptoms
Serious overdosage is characterised by respiratory depression and drowsiness which progress to coma or stupor, constricted pupils, cold clammy skin and occasionally bradycardia and hypotension.

b) Treatment
Treatment consists of the establishment of a patent airway and other supportive measures. Oxygen and assisted

ventilation should be administered as necessary. Naloxone should be given if coma or bradycardia are present.

Administration of a narcotic antagonist will precipitate an acute withdrawal syndrome in a patient physically dependent upon narcotics. Use of the antagonist in such a person should be avoided if possible and should only be administered with great care.

5. PHARMACOLOGICAL PROPERTIES

5.1 Pharmacodynamic properties

Methadone is an opioid agonist with the general properties of morphine. It has analgesic properties and an extended duration of activity in suppressing withdrawal symptoms in physically dependant individuals. It is predominantly a central nervous depressant but it has stimulant actions resulting in nausea, vomiting and miosis.

5.2 Pharmacokinetic properties

Methadone is one of the more lipid soluble opioids and is well absorbed from the gastrointestinal tract but undergoes fairly extensive first pass metabolism. There is extensive binding to plasma and tissue proteins and fairly slow transfer between some parts of the tissue reservoir and the plasma. Methadone is distributed in skeletal muscle, kidney, lung, liver and spleen. Peak plasma concentration levels are reached in one hour with a half life of 6-8 hours for a single intramuscular dose, this figure reflecting distribution into tissue stores as well as renal and hepatic clearance. With regular doses the tissue reservoir is partially filled and the half life is extended to 13-47 hours reflecting only clearance. Approx 15-60% is recovered from the urine and as the dose is increased so a higher proportion of non-metabolised methadone is found there. Acidification of the urine can increase renal clearance by a factor of at least three and thus appreciably reduce the half life of elimination.

5.3 Preclinical safety data

The LD_{50} in rats is 95mg kg^{-1} and the intravenous LD_{50} in mice is 20mg kg^{-1}. Little detailed information on toxicology has been published.

6. PHARMACEUTICAL PARTICULARS

6.1 List of excipients

Hydrochloric Acid 0.1M

Sodium Hydroxide Solution 0.01M

Water for Injections

6.2 Incompatibilities

Physical incompatibility as judged by loss of clarity was reported when an intravenous solution of methadone hydrochloride was mixed with those of aminophylline, ammonium chloride, amylobarbitone sodium, chlorothiazide sodium, heparin sodium, methicillin sodium, nitrofurantoin sodium, novobiocin sodium, pentobarbitone sodium, phenobarbitone sodium, phenytoin sodium, quinalbarbitone sodium, sodium bicarbonate, sodium iodide, sulphadiazine sodium, sulphafurazole diethanolamine or thiopentone sodium.

6.3 Shelf life

36 months (unopened)

6.4 Special precautions for storage

Protect from light

Do not store above 25°C

6.5 Nature and contents of container

Pack of 10 neutral glass ampoules. Each ampoule contains 1, 2, 3.5, 5, 7.5 or 10ml of solution.

6.6 Instructions for use and handling

Methadone is controlled under the Misuse of Drugs Act 1971.

Administrative Data

7. MARKETING AUTHORISATION HOLDER

CP Pharmaceuticals Ltd

Ash Road North

Wrexham

LL13 9UF

8. MARKETING AUTHORISATION NUMBER(S)

PL 4543/0361

9. DATE OF FIRST AUTHORISATION/RENEWAL OF THE AUTHORISATION

10th June 1996

10. DATE OF REVISION OF THE TEXT

April 2000

Methionine Tablets 250mg

(UCB Pharma Limited)

1. NAME OF THE MEDICINAL PRODUCT

Methionine Tablets 250mg

2. QUALITATIVE AND QUANTITATIVE COMPOSITION

Methionine (DL) 250 mg

3. PHARMACEUTICAL FORM

Tablet

4. CLINICAL PARTICULARS

4.1 Therapeutic indications

Methionine is given, by mouth, for the treatment of paracetamol overdose if n-acetyl cysteine is not available or if the patient cannot tolerate n-acetyl cysteine.

4.2 Posology and method of administration

Paracetamol Overdose

Give within 10 hours of paracetamol ingestion, subsequent to any emesis being induced.

Adults and the elderly: 2.5g (10 tablets) every 4 hours to a maximum of 10g

Children (up to 6 years) 1g (4 tablets) every 4 hours to a maximum of 4g

Children (6 years and over) As adult dose

4.3 Contraindications

Methionine should not be used for the treatment of paracetamol overdosage if more than 10 hours have elapsed since the time of the overdose.

Do not use in patients with metabolic acidosis.

4.4 Special warnings and special precautions for use

Use methionine with care in patients with established liver disease as hepatic encephalopathy may be precipitated.

Use with caution in patients with schizophrenia as daily methionine doses of 10 to 20g have been reported to precipitate acute exacerbation of symptoms in such patients.

4.5 Interaction with other medicinal products and other forms of Interaction

The anti-parkinsonism effects of levodopa may be reduced by methionine, especially if large doses of methionine are given.

4.6 Pregnancy and lactation

The safety, in human pregnancy or during lactation, of the ingestion of higher levels of methionine than would normally be encountered in the diet, has not been established. Methionine should only be used during pregnancy or lactation if the benefit of its use has been weighed against any potential risks.

4.7 Effects on ability to drive and use machines

Patients should be advised that methionine may cause drowsiness and their ability to drive or operate machinery may be affected.

4.8 Undesirable effects

Oral doses of methionine may cause nausea, vomiting, drowsiness and irritability. Daily doses of 6 to 20g can cause neurological changes and precipitate Encephalopathy in patients with heptic cirrhosis especially if portal hypertension is present.

4.9 Overdose

Overdosage with methionine may be associated with the appearance of the above mentioned side-effects (nausea, vomiting, drowsiness, irritability). As methionine forms part of the normal diet, no specific recommendations for treatment of overdose are available. General support measures may be appropriate.

5. PHARMACOLOGICAL PROPERTIES

5.1 Pharmacodynamic properties

Methionine is an essential amino acid that plays a vital role in intermediary metabolism. It is the primary donor of methyl groups for biosynthetic reactions but must first be converted to s-adenosylmethionine, its active moiety. It is then involved in the transmethylation of nucleic acids, proteins, lipids and other metabolites and in the synthesis of choline. Methionine is converted to cysteine, a precursor of glutathione, in the liver. Methionine is thought to prevent liver damage in paracetamol overdose by facilitating glutathione synthesis. Methionine has a lipotropic action which prevents the development of fatty liver and it also stimulates pancreatic insulin release.

5.2 Pharmacokinetic properties

Adsorption

Methionine is absorbed from the gastro-intestinal tract. Absorption is unpredictable in patients who are vomiting.

Half-Life

Not known

Distribution

Not known

Metabolism

Methionine is metabolised via s-adenosylmethionine to homocysteine. About 80% is further converted to cysthathionine, cysteine, taurine and inorganic sulphate.

Excretion

Methionine is excreted in the urine as an inorganic sulphate.

5.3 Preclinical safety data

None stated

6. PHARMACEUTICAL PARTICULARS

6.1 List of excipients

Alginic acid

Starch maize

Tragacanth powdered

Magnesium stearate

Talc

Coating:

Acacia syrup solution

Talc

Light calcium carbonate

Acacia mucilage

Titanium dioxide 1700 ansteads

Opaglos AG 7350 containing:

Beeswax white

Carnauba wax yellow

Polysorbate 20

Sorbic acid (E200)

Purified water

Opacode S-1-8100HV Black containing:

Industrial Methylated Spirits

Shellac (E904)

Iron Oxide Black (E172)

Purified Water

2-Ethoxyethanol

Soya Lecithin MC Thin (E322)

Antifoam DC 1510

6.2 Incompatibilities

None known

6.3 Shelf life

36 months

6.4 Special precautions for storage

Store at room temperature

6.5 Nature and contents of container

Pigmented polypropylene container with tamper-evident closure of low density polyethylene. Containers hold either 50, 200 or 250 tablets

6.6 Instructions for use and handling

None stated

7. MARKETING AUTHORISATION HOLDER

UCB Pharma Ltd

208 Bath Road

Slough

Berkshire

SL1 3WE

8. MARKETING AUTHORISATION NUMBER(S)

PL 00039/0553

9. DATE OF FIRST AUTHORISATION/RENEWAL OF THE AUTHORISATION

4 July 2005

10. DATE OF REVISION OF THE TEXT

July 2005

Methotrexate 100 mg/ml Injection

(Wockhardt UK Ltd)

1. NAME OF THE MEDICINAL PRODUCT

Methotrexate 100 mg/ml Injection BP

2. QUALITATIVE AND QUANTITATIVE COMPOSITION

1ml contains 100mg methotrexate

1 vial of 10ml contains 1000mg of methotrexate.

1 vial of 50ml contains 5000mg of methotrexate

For excipients, see 6.1

3. PHARMACEUTICAL FORM

Solution for injection

The solution is a clear yellow solution free from particles.

4. CLINICAL PARTICULARS

4.1 Therapeutic indications

Methotrexate is indicated in the treatment of neoplastic disease, such as trophoblastic neoplasms and leukaemia, and the symptomatic treatment of severe recalcitrant disabling psoriasis which is not adequately responsive to other forms of therapy.

4.2 Posology and method of administration

Methotrexate injection may be given by the intramuscular, intravenous or intra-arterial routes.

Note: Methotrexate injection 1000mg /10ml presentation and 5000mg/50ml are hypertonic and therefore not suitable for intrathecal use.

Adults, elderly and children

Antineoplastic Chemotherapy

Methotrexate is active parenterally. Methotrexate injection may be given by the intramuscular, intravenous or intra-arterial routes. Dosage is related to the patient's body weight or surface area. Methotrexate has been used with beneficial effect in a wide variety of neoplastic diseases, alone and in combination with other cytotoxic agents.

Note: Methotrexate injection 1000mg /10ml presentation and 5000mg/50ml are hypertonic and therefore not suitable for intrathecal use.

Choriocarcinoma and Similar Trophoblastic Diseases

Methotrexate is administered intramuscularly in doses of 15-30mg daily for a five day course. Such courses may be repeated 3-5 times as required, with rest periods of one or more weeks interposed between courses until any manifesting toxic symptoms subside.

The effectiveness of therapy can be evaluated by 24 hours quantitative analysis of urinary chorionic gonadotrophin hormone (HCG). Combination therapy with other cytotoxic drugs has also been reported as useful.

Hydatidiform mole may precede or be followed by choriocarcinoma, and methotrexate has been used in similar doses for the treatment of hydatidiform mole and chorioadenoma destruens.

Breast Carcinoma

Prolonged cyclic combination with cyclophosphamide, methotrexate and fluorouracil has given good results when used as adjuvant treatment to radical mastectomy in primary breast cancer with positive axillary lymph nodes. Methotrexate dosage was 40mg/m^2 intravenously on the first and eighth days.

Leukaemia

Acute granulocytic leukaemia is rare in children but common in adults and it is not particularly sensitive to methotrexate but responds to other combination chemotherapy agents.

Methotrexate is not generally a drug of choice for induction of remission of lymphoblastic leukaemia. After a remission is attained, methotrexate in a maintenance dosage of 20-30mg/m^2 by I.M. injection has been administered twice weekly. Twice weekly doses appear to be more effective than daily drug administration. Alternatively, 2.5mg/kg has been administered I.V. every 14 days.

Meningeal Leukaemia

Some patients with leukaemia are subject to leukaemic invasions of the central nervous system and the CSF should be examined in all cases of acute lymphoblastic leukaemia and some cases of acute myeloblastic leukaemia.

Methotrexate may be given in a prophylactic regimen in all cases of acute lymphoblastic leukaemia. Methotrexate is administered by intrathecal injection in doses of 200-500 microgram/kg body weight. The administration is at intervals of two to five days and is usually until clearance of blasts in the CSF. At this point one additional dose is advised. Alternatively, methotrexate 12mg/m^2 can be given once weekly for two weeks and then once monthly. Large doses may cause convulsions and untoward side effects, commonly neurological in character, occur as with any intrathecal injection.

Note: Methotrexate injection 1000mg /10ml presentation and 5000mg/50ml are hypertonic and therefore not suitable for intrathecal use..

Lymphomas

In stage 3, methotrexate is commonly given concomitantly with other antitumour agents. Treatment in all stages usually consists of several courses of the drug interposed with seven to ten day rest periods, and in stage 3 combined drug therapy is given with methotrexate in doses of 0.625mg to 2.5mg/kg daily. Hodgkin's Disease does not usually respond to methotrexate but can have a substantial response to the use of other combination chemotherapy agents.

Mycosis Fungoides

Therapy with methotrexate appears to produce clinical remissions in one half of the cases treated adjusted according to the patient's response and haematological monitoring. Methotrexate has been given intramuscularly in doses of 50mg once weekly or 25mg twice weekly.

Psoriasis Chemotherapy

Cases of severe uncontrolled psoriasis, unresponsive to conventional therapy, have responded to weekly single, I.M. or I.V. doses of 10-25mg per week, adjusted according to the patient's response. An initial test dose one week prior to initiation of therapy is recommended to detect any idiosyncrasy. A suggested dose range is 5-10mg.

The patient should be fully informed of the risks involved and the clinician should pay particular attention to the appearance of liver toxicity by carrying out liver function tests before starting methotrexate treatment, and repeating these at two to four month intervals during therapy. The aim of therapy should be to reduce the dose to the lowest possible level with the longest possible rest period. The use of methotrexate may permit the return to conventional topical therapy which should be encouraged.

Renal Impairment (see 4.4. Special Warnings and Special Precautions for use).

Reduce dose in patients with renal impairment.

4.3 Contraindications

Significantly impaired renal function.

Significantly impaired hepatic function

Pre-existing blood dyscrasias, such as significant marrow hypoplasia, leukopenia, thrombocytopenia or anaemia.

Methotrexate is contraindicated in pregnancy.

Because of the potential for serious adverse reactions from methotrexate in breast fed infants, breast feeding is contraindicated in women taking methotrexate.

Patients with a known allergic hypersensitivity to methotrexate or any of the other ingredients should not receive methotrexate.

4.4 Special warnings and special precautions for use

WARNINGS

Methotrexate must be used only by physicians experienced in antimetabolite chemotherapy.

Because of the possibility of fatal or severe toxic reactions, the patient should be fully informed by the physician of the risks involved and be under his constant supervision.

Deaths have been reported with the use of methotrexate in the treatment of psoriasis.

In the treatment of psoriasis, methotrexate should be restricted to severe recalcitrant, disabling psoriasis which is not adequately responsive to other forms of therapy, and only when the diagnosis has been established by biopsy and/or after dermatological consultation.

1. Full blood counts should be closely monitored before, during and after treatment. If a clinically significant drop in white-cell or platelet count develops, methotrexate should be withdrawn immediately. Patients should be advised to report all symptoms or signs suggestive of infection.

2. Methotrexate may be hepatotoxic, particularly at high dosage or with prolonged therapy. Liver atrophy, necrosis, cirrhosis, fatty changes, and periportal fibrosis have been reported. Since changes may occur without previous signs of gastrointestinal or haematological toxicity, it is imperative that hepatic function be determined prior to initiation of treatment and monitored regularly throughout therapy. If substantial hepatic function abnormalities develop, methotrexate dosing should be suspended for at least two weeks. Special caution is indicated in the presence of pre-existing liver damage or impaired hepatic function. Concomitant use of other drugs with hepatotoxic potential (including alcohol) should be avoided.

3. Methotrexate has been shown to be teratogenic; it has caused foetal death and/or congenital anomalies. Therefore it is not recommended in women of childbearing potential unless there is appropriate medical evidence that the benefits can be expected to outweigh the considered risks. Pregnant psoriatic patients should not receive methotrexate.

4. Renal function should be closely monitored before, during and after treatment. Caution should be exercised if significant renal impairment is disclosed. Reduce dose of methotrexate in patients with renal impairment. High doses may cause the precipitation of methotrexate or its metabolites in the renal tubules. A high fluid throughput and alkalinisation of the urine to pH 6.5 – 7.0, by oral or intravenous administration of sodium bicarbonate (5 × 625mg tablets every three hours) or acetazolamide (500mg orally four times a day) is recommended as a preventative measure. Methotrexate is excreted primarily by the kidneys. Its use in the presence of impaired renal function may result in accumulation of toxic amounts or even additional renal damage.

5. Diarrhoea and ulcerative stomatitis are frequent toxic effects and require interruption of therapy, otherwise haemorrhagic enteritis and death from intestinal perforation may occur.

6. Methotrexate affects gametogenesis during the period of its administration and may result in decreased fertility which is thought to be reversible on discontinuation of therapy. Conception should be avoided during the period of methotrexate administration and for at least six months thereafter. Patients and their partners should be advised to this effect.

7. Methotrexate has some immunosuppressive activity and immunological responses to concurrent vaccination may be decreased. The immunosuppressive effect of methotrexate should be taken into account when immune responses of patients are important or essential.

8. Pleural effusions and ascites should be drained prior to initiation of methotrexate therapy.

9. Deaths have been reported with the use of methotrexate. Serious adverse reactions including deaths have been reported with concomitant administration of methotrexate (usually in high doses) along with some non-steroidal anti-inflammatory drugs (NSAIDs), (see 4.5 Interactions with other Medicaments and other forms of Interaction).

10. Concomitant administration of folate antagonists such as trimethoprim/sulphamethoxazole has been reported to cause an acute megaloblastic pancytopenia in rare instances.

11. Systemic toxicity may occur following intrathecal administration. Blood counts should be monitored closely.

12. A chest X-ray is recommended prior to initiation of methotrexate therapy.

13. If acute methotrexate toxicity occurs, patients may require folinic acid.

PRECAUTIONS

Methotrexate has a high potential toxicity, usually dose related, and should be used only by physicians experienced in antimetabolite chemotherapy, in patients under their constant supervision. The physician should be familiar with the various characteristics of the drug and its established clinical usage.

Before beginning methotrexate therapy or reinstituting methotrexate after a rest period, assessment of renal function, liver function and blood elements should be made by history, physical examination and laboratory tests.

It should be noted that intrathecal doses are transported into the cardiovascular system and may give rise to systemic toxicity. Systemic toxicity of methotrexate may also be enhanced in patients with renal dysfunction, ascites, or other effusions, due to prolongation of serum half-life.

Carcinogenesis, mutagenesis, and impairment of fertility: animal carcinogenicity studies have demonstrated methotrexate to be free of carcinogenic potential. Although methotrexate has been reported to cause chromosomal damage to animal somatic cells and bone marrow cells in humans, these effects are transient and reversible. In patients treated with methotrexate, evidence is insufficient to permit conclusive evaluation of any increased risk of neoplasia.

Methotrexate has been reported to cause impairment of fertility, oligospermia, menstrual dysfunction and amenorrhoea in humans, during and for a short period after cessation of therapy. In addition, methotrexate causes embryotoxicity, abortion and foetal defects in humans. Therefore the possible risk of effects on reproduction should be discussed with patients of childbearing potential (see 'Warnings').

Patients undergoing therapy should be subject to appropriate supervision so that signs or symptoms of possible toxic effects or adverse reactions may be detected and evaluated with minimal delay. Pretreatment and periodic haematological studies are essential to the use of methotrexate in chemotherapy because of its common adverse effect of haematopoietic suppression. This may occur abruptly and on apparent safe dosage, and any profound drop in blood cell count indicates immediate stopping of the drug and appropriate therapy. In patients with malignant disease who have pre-existing bone marrow aplasia, leukopenia, thrombocytopenia or anaemia, methotrexate should be used with caution, if at all.

In general, the following laboratory tests are recommended as part of essential clinical evaluation and appropriate monitoring of patients chosen for or receiving methotrexate therapy: complete haemogram; haematocrit; urinalysis; renal function tests; liver function tests and chest X-ray.

The purpose is to determine any existing organ dysfunction or system impairment. The tests should be performed prior to therapy, at appropriate periods during therapy and after termination of therapy.

Liver biopsy may be considered after cumulative doses >1.5g have been given, if hepatic impairment is suspected.

After absorption, methotrexate is bound in part to serum albumin and toxicity may be increased because of displacement by certain drugs such as salicylates, sulphonamides, phenytoin, and some antibacterials such as tetracycline, chloramphenicol and para-aminobenzoic acid (see 4.5 Interactions with other Medicaments and other forms of Interaction). These drugs, especially salicylates and sulphonamides, whether antibacterial, hypoglycaemic or diuretic, should not be given concurrently until the significance of these findings is established.

Vitamin preparations containing folic acid or its derivatives may alter response to methotrexate.

Methotrexate should be used with extreme caution in the presence of infection, peptic ulcer, ulcerative colitis, debility, and in extreme youth and old age. If profound leukopenia occurs during therapy, bacterial infection may occur or become a threat. Cessation of the drug and appropriate antibiotic therapy is usually indicated. In severe bone marrow depression, blood or platelet transfusions may be necessary.

Since it is reported that methotrexate may have an immunosuppressive action, this factor must be taken into consideration in evaluating the use of the drug where immune responses in a patient may be important or essential.

In all instances where the use of methotrexate is considered for chemotherapy, the physician must evaluate the need and usefulness of the drug against the risks of toxic effects or adverse reactions. Most such adverse reactions are reversible if detected early. When such effects or reactions do occur, the drug should be reduced in dosage or discontinued and appropriate corrective measures should be taken according to the clinical judgement of the physician. Reinstitution of methotrexate therapy should be carried out with caution, with adequate consideration of further need for the drug and alertness as to the possible recurrence of toxicity.

Methotrexate given concomitantly with radiotherapy may increase the risk of soft tissue necrosis and osteonecrosis.

Acute or chronic interstitial pneumonitis, often associated with blood eosinophilia, may occur and deaths have been reported. Symptoms typically include dyspnoea, cough (especially a dry non-productive cough) and fever for which patients should be monitored at each follow-up visit.

Patientsshould beinformed of the risk of pneumonitis and advised to contact their doctor immediately should they develop persistent cough or dyspnoea.

Methotrexate should be withdrawn from patients with pulmonary symptoms and a thorough investigation should be made to exclude infection. If methotrexate induced lung disease is suspected treatment with corticosteroids should be initiated and treatment with methotrexate should be restarted.

4.5 Interaction with other medicinal products and other forms of Interaction

Methotrexate is extensively protein bound and may be displaced by certain drugs such as salicylates, hypoglycaemics, diuretics, sulphonamides, diphenylhydantoins, tetracyclines, chloramphenicol and p-aminobenzoic acid, and the acidic anti-inflammatory agents, so causing a potential for increased toxicity when used concurrently (see 4.4. Special Warnings and Precautions for Use).

Concomitant use of other drugs with nephrotoxic or hepatotoxic potential (including alcohol) should be avoided.

Vitamin preparations containing folic acid or its derivatives may decrease the effectiveness of methotrexate.

Caution should be used when NSAIDs and salicylates are administered concomitantly with methotrexate (see 4.4. Special Warnings and Precautions for Use). These drugs have been reported to reduce the tubular secretion of methotrexate and thereby may enhance its toxicity. Concomitant use of NSAIDs and salicylates has been associated with fatal methotrexate toxicity.

However, patients using constant dosage regimens of NSAIDs have received concurrent doses of methotrexate without an problems being observed.

Renal tubular transport is also diminished by probenecid and penicillins; use of these with methotrexate should be carefully monitored.

Severe bone marrow depression has been reported following the concurrent use of methotrexate and co-trimoxazole or trimethoprim. Concurrent use should probably be avoided.

Methotrexate-induced stomatitis and other toxic effects may be increased by the use of nitrous oxide.

An increased risk of hepatitis has been reported following the use of methotrexate and the acitretin metabolite, etretinate. Consequently, the concomitant use of methotrexate and acitretin should be avoided.

4.6 Pregnancy and lactation

Abortion, foetal death, and/or congenital anomalies have occurred in pregnant women receiving methotrexate, especially during the first trimester of pregnancy. Methotrexate is contraindicated in the management of psoriasis or rheumatoid arthritis in pregnant women. Women of childbearing potential should not receive methotrexate until pregnancy is excluded. For the management of psoriasis or rheumatoid arthritis, methotrexate therapy in women should be started immediately following a menstrual period and appropriate measures should be taken in men or women to avoid conception during and for at least six months following cessation of methotrexate therapy.

Both men and women receiving methotrexate should be informed of the potential risk of adverse effects on reproduction. Women of childbearing potential should be fully informed of the potential hazard to the foetus should they become pregnant during methotrexate therapy. In cancer chemotherapy, methotrexate should not be used in pregnant women or women of childbearing potential who might become pregnant unless the potential benefits to the mother outweigh the possible risks to the foetus.

Defective oogenesis or spermatogenesis, transient oligospermia, menstrual dysfunction, and infertility have been reported in patients receiving methotrexate.

Methotrexate is distributed into breast milk. Because of the potential for serious adverse reactions to methotrexate in nursing infants, a decision should be made whether to discontinue nursing or the drug, taking into account the importance of the drug to the woman.

4.7 Effects on ability to drive and use machines

Methotrexate is not known to affect ability to drive or use machines.

4.8 Undesirable effects

The most common adverse reactions include ulcerative stomatitis, leukopenia, nausea and abdominal distress. Although very rare, anaphylactic reactions to methotrexate have occurred. Others reported are malaise, undue fatigue, chills and fever, dizziness and decreased resistance to infection. In general, the incidence and severity of side effects are considered to be dose-related. Adverse reactions as reported for the various systems are as follows:

Skin: Stevens-Johnson syndrome, epidermal necrolysis, erythematous rashes, pruritus, urticaria, photosensitivity, pigmentary changes, alopecia, ecchymosis, telangiectasia, acne, furunculosis. Lesions of psoriasis may be aggravated by concomitant exposure to ultraviolet radiation. Skin ulceration in psoriatic patients and rarely painful erosion of psoriatic plaques have been reported. The recall phenomenon has been reported in both radiation and solar damaged skin.

Blood: Bone marrow depression, leukopenia, thrombocytopenia, anaemia, hypogammaglobulinaemia, haemorrhage from various sites, septicaemia.

Alimentary System: Gingivitis, pharyngitis, stomatitis, anorexia, vomiting, diarrhoea, haematemesis, melaena, gastrointestinal ulceration and bleeding, enteritis, hepatic toxicity resulting in active liver atrophy, necrosis, fatty metamorphosis, periportal fibrosis, or hepatic cirrhosis. In rare cases the effect of methotrexate on the intestinal mucosa has led to malabsorption or toxic megacolon.

Hepatic: Hepatic toxicity resulting in significant elevations of liver enzymes, acute liver atrophy, necrosis, fatty metamorphosis, periportal fibrosis or cirrhosis or death may occur, usually following chronic administration.

Urogenital System: Renal failure, azotaemia, cystitis, haematuria, defective oogenesis or spermatogenesis, transient oligospermia, menstrual dysfunction, infertility, abortion, foetal defects, severe nephropathy. Vaginitis, vaginal ulcers, and nephropathy have also been reported.

Pulmonary System: Infrequently an acute or chronic interstitial pneumonitis, often associated with blood eosinophilia, may occur and deaths have been reported. Acute pulmonary oedema has also been reported after intrathecal use. Pulmonary fibrosis is rare. A syndrome consisting of pleuritic pain and pleural thickening has been reported following high doses.

Central Nervous System: Headaches, drowsiness, blurred vision, aphasia, hemiparesis and convulsions have occurred possibly related to haemorrhage or to complications from intra-arterial catheterization. Convulsion, paresis, Guillain-Barré syndrome and increased cerebrospinal fluid pressure have followed intrathecal administration.

Other reactions related to, or attributed to the use of methotrexate such as pneumonitis, metabolic changes, precipitation of diabetes, osteoporotic effects, abnormal changes in tissue cells, abnormal (usually 'megaloblastic') red cell morphology and even sudden death have been reported.

There have been reports of leukoencephalopathy following intravenous methotrexate in high doses, or low doses following cranial-spinal radiation.

Adverse reactions following intrathecal methotrexate are generally classified into three groups, acute, subacute, and chronic. The acute form is a chemical arachnoiditis manifested by headache, back or shoulder pain, nuchal rigidity, and fever. The subacute form may include paresis, usually transient, paraplegia, nerve palsies, and cerebellar dysfunction. The chronic form is a leukoencephalopathy manifested by irritability, confusion, ataxia, spasticity, occasionally convulsions, dementia, somnolence, coma, and rarely, death. There is evidence that the combined use of cranial radiation and intrathecal methotrexate increases the incidence of leukoencephalopathy.

Acute or chronic interstitial pneumonitis, often associated with blood eosinophilia, may occur and deaths have been reported. (see Section 4.4 Warnings And Precautions for Use)

4.9 Overdose

Calcium Folinate (Calcium Leucovorin) is a potent agent for neutralizing the immediate toxic effects of methotrexate on the haematopoietic system. Where large doses or overdoses are given, calcium folinate may be administered by intravenous infusion in doses up to 75mg within 12 hours, followed by 12mg intramuscularly every six hours for four doses. Where average doses of methotrexate appear to have an adverse effect, 6-12mg of calcium folinate may be given intramuscularly every six hours for four doses. In general, where overdosage is suspected, the dose of calcium folinate should be equal to, or higher than, the offending dose of methotrexate and should be administered as soon as possible; preferably within the first hour and certainly within four hours, after which it may not be effective.

Other supporting therapy such as blood transfusion and renal dialysis may be required. Effective clearance of methotrexate has been reported with acute, intermittent haemodialysis using a high flux dialyser.

5. PHARMACOLOGICAL PROPERTIES

5.1 Pharmacodynamic properties

Methotrexate is an antimetabolite, which acts principally by competitively inhibiting the enzyme, dihydrofolate reductase. In the process of DNA synthesis and cellular replication, folic acid must be reduced to tetrahydrofolic acid by this enzyme, and inhibition by methotrexate interferes with tissue cell reproduction. Actively proliferating tissues such as malignant cells are generally more sensitive to this effect of methotrexate. It also inhibits antibody synthesis.

Methotrexate also has immunosuppressive activity, in part possibly as a result of inhibition of lymphocyte multiplication. The mechanism(s) of action of the drug in the management of rheumatoid arthritis is not known, although suggested mechanisms have included immunosuppressive and/or anti-inflammatory effect.

5.2 Pharmacokinetic properties

Peak serum concentrations are achieved within 0.5 - 2 hours following I.V. / I.M. or intra-arterial administration.

Methotrexate is actively transported across cell membranes. The drug is widely distributed into body tissues with highest concentrations in the kidneys, gall bladder, spleen, liver and skin. Methotrexate is retained for several weeks in the kidneys and for months in the liver. Sustained serum concentrations and tissue accumulation may result from repeated daily doses. Methotrexate crosses the placental barrier and is distributed into breast milk. Approximately 50% of the drug in the blood is bound to serum proteins.

In one study, methotrexate had a serum half-life of 2-4 hours following I.M. administration.

Methotrexate does not appear to be appreciably metabolised. The drug is excreted primarily by the kidneys via glomerular filtration and active transport. Small amounts are excreted in the faeces, probably via the bile. Methotrexate has a biphasic excretion pattern. If methotrexate excretion is impaired accumulation will occur more rapidly in patients with impaired renal function. In addition, simultaneous administration of other weak organic acids such as salicylates may suppress methotrexate clearance.

5.3 Preclinical safety data

There are no pre-clinical data of relevance to the prescriber which are additional to those included in other sections.

6. PHARMACEUTICAL PARTICULARS

6.1 List of excipients

Sodium hydroxide

Water for injections

6.2 Incompatibilities

Immediate precipitation or turbidity results when combined with certain concentrations of droperidol, heparin sodium, metoclopramide hydrochloride or ranitidine hydrochloride in the syringe.

As with all parenteral solutions, incompatibility of the additive medications with the solution must be addressed before addition. In the absence of compatibility studies, this solution must not be mixed with other medicinal products, except sodium chloride solution 0.9% and glucose solution 5% (see Section 6.4, Special precautions for storage).

6.3 Shelf life

Two years

After dilution (see section 6.4. and 6.6.): 24 hours.

Any unused solution should be discarded immediately after use.

6.4 Special precautions for storage

Do not store above 25 °C. Store in the original container.

After dilution (see section 6.6.):

Chemical and physical in-use stability has been demonstrated for 24 hours at 25 °C for solutions with a final concentration of methotrexate 5mg/ml or 20mg/ml after dilution of the methotrexate 100mg/ml with one of the following solutions:

- sodium chloride solution 0.9%;
- glucose solution 5%

From a microbiological point of view, the product should be used immediately. If not used immediately, in-use storage times and conditions prior to use are the responsibility of the user and would normally not be longer than 24 hours at 2 to 8 C, unless dilution has taken place in controlled and validated aseptic conditions.

6.5 Nature and contents of container

Colourless vials of hydrolytic type I glass, packed in a carton.

Vials are closed with a rubber stopper with an aluminium crimp cap with flip-off.

Packs of 1 vial containing 1000mg/10ml of methotrexate.

Packs of 1 vial containing 5000mg/50ml of methotrexate

6.6 Instructions for use and handling

Cytotoxic drugs should only be handled by trained personnel in a designated area. The work surface should be covered with disposable plastic-backed absorbent paper. Protective gloves and goggles should be worn to avoid the drug accidentally coming into contact with the skin or eyes. Methotrexate is not a vesicant and should not cause harm if it comes into contact with the skin. It should of course be washed off with water immediately. Any transient stinging may be treated with bland cream. If there is any danger of systemic absorption of significant quantities of methotrexate, by any route, calcium folinate cover should be given.

Cytotoxic preparations should not be handled by pregnant staff.

Adequate care should be taken in the disposal of any unwanted product, syringes and containers. Any spillage or waste material may be disposed of by incineration. We do not make any specific recommendations with regard to the temperature of the incinerator.

Administrative Data

7. MARKETING AUTHORISATION HOLDER

CP Pharmaceuticals Ltd

Ash Road North

Wrexham LL13 9UF

United Kingdom

8. MARKETING AUTHORISATION NUMBER(S)
PL 04543/0457 (1,000mg in10ml)

PL 04543/0458 (5,000mg in 5ml)

9. DATE OF FIRST AUTHORISATION/RENEWAL OF THE AUTHORISATION
28 April 2004

10. DATE OF REVISION OF THE TEXT
March 2004

Methotrexate 10mg Tablets

(Wockhardt UK Ltd)

1. NAME OF THE MEDICINAL PRODUCT
Methotrexate 10mg Tablets BP

2. QUALITATIVE AND QUANTITATIVE COMPOSITION
Methotrexate 10mg

For excipients see 6.1

3. PHARMACEUTICAL FORM
Tablet

Methotrexate 10mg Tablets are light yellow, capsule shaped tablets with a score on one side, with a major axis of 15mm and a minor axis of 7mm; may contain yellow to red sprinkles.

4. CLINICAL PARTICULARS

4.1 Therapeutic indications
The treatment of acute lymphoblastic leukaemia and Burkitt's lymphoma. The treatment of severe cases of uncontrolled psoriasis, unresponsive to conventional therapy.

4.2 Posology and method of administration
For oral administration. Dosages are based on the patient's body weight or surface area. Doses should be reduced in cases of haematological deficiency and hepatic or renal impairment.

Acute Lymphocytic Leukaemia:

Children

In acute lymphocytic leukaemia remissions are usually best induced with a combination of corticosteroids and other cytotoxic agents.

Methotrexate 15mg/m^2, given orally once weekly, in combination with other drugs, appears to be the treatment of choice for maintenance of drug-induced remissions.

Burkitt's Lymphoma:

Children

Some cases of Burkitt's lymphoma, when treated in the early stages with courses of 15mg/m^2 daily orally for five days, have shown prolonged remissions. Combination chemotherapy is also commonly used in all stages of the disease.

Psoriasis:

Adults

It is recommended that a test dose of 5-10mg should be administered, one week prior to therapy to detect idiosyncratic adverse reactions.

In most cases of severe uncontrolled psoriasis, unresponsive to conventional therapy, 10-25mg orally once a week and adjusted by the patient's response is recommended.

The use of methotrexate in psoriasis may permit the return to conventional topical therapy which should be encouraged.

Elderly

Methotrexate should be used with extreme caution in elderly patients: a reduction in dosage be considered (see 4.4 Special Warnings and Special Precautions for Use).

Children

Safety and effectiveness in children have not been established, other than in cancer chemotherapy.

4.3 Contraindications
Profound impairment of renal or hepatic function or haematological impairment. Liver disease including fibrosis, cirrhosis, recent or active hepatitis; active infectious disease; and overt or laboratory evidence of immunodeficiency syndrome(s). Serious cases of anaemia, leucopenia, or thrombocytopenia. Methotrexate is contra-indicated in pregnant patients. Because of the potential for serious adverse reactions from methotrexate in breast fed infants, breast feeding is contra-indicated in women taking methotrexate. Patients with a known allergic hypersensitivity to methotrexate should not receive methotrexate.

4.4 Special warnings and special precautions for use
Warnings:

Methotrexate should be used with extreme caution in patients with haematological depression, renal impairment, peptic ulcer, ulcerative colitis, ulcerative stomatitis, diarrhoea, debility and in young children and the elderly. (See 4.2 Posology and Method of Administration).

Patients with pleural effusions or ascites should have these drained if appropriate before treatment or treatment should be withdrawn.

Symptoms of gastro-intestinal toxicity, usually first manifested by stomatitis, indicate that therapy should be interrupted otherwise haemorrhagic enteritis and death from intestinal perforation may occur.

Methotrexate has some immunosuppressive activity and therefore the immunological response to concurrent vaccination may be decreased. In addition, concomitant use of a live vaccine could cause a severe antigenic reaction.

Acute or chronic interstitial pneumonitis, often associated with blood eosinophilia, may occur and deaths have been reported. Symptoms typically include dyspnoea, cough (especially a dry non-productive cough) and fever for which patients should be monitored at each follow-up visit. Patients should be informed of the risk of pneumonitis and advised to contract their doctor immediately should they develop persistent cough or dyspnoea.

Methotrexate should be withdrawn from patients with pulmonary symptoms and a through investigation should be made to exclude infection. If Methotrexate induced lung disease is suspected treatment with corticosteroids should be initiated and treatment with Methotrexate should not be restarted.

Precautions:

Methotrexate should only be used by clinicians who are familiar with the various characteristics of the drug and its mode of action. Before beginning methotrexate therapy or reinstituting methotrexate after a rest period, a chest x-ray, assessment of renal function, liver function and blood elements should be made by history, physical examination and laboratory tests. Patients undergoing therapy should be subject to appropriate supervision every 2-3 months so that signs of possible toxic effects or adverse reactions may be detected and evaluated with minimal delay. Renal function and full blood counts should be closely monitored before, during and after treatment.

It is essential that the following laboratory tests are included regularly (every 2-3 months) in the clinical evaluation and monitoring of patients receiving methotrexate: complete haematological analysis, urinalysis, renal function tests, liver function tests and, when high doses are administered, determination of plasma levels of methotrexate.

Particular attention should be given to the appearance of liver toxicity which may occur without correlative changes in liver function tests. Treatment should not be instituted, or should be discontinued, if any abnormality in liver function tests or liver biopsy is present or develops during therapy. Such abnormalities should return to normal within two weeks, after which treatment may be recommenced at the discretion of the physician.

When to perform a liver biopsy in rheumatoid arthritis patients has not been established either in terms of a cumulative methotrexate dose or duration of therapy.

Pleuropulmonary manifestations of rheumatoid arthritis have been reported in the literature. In patients with rheumatoid arthritis, the physician should be specifically alerted to the potential for methotrexate induced adverse effects in the pulmonary system. Patients should be advised to contact their physicians immediately should they develop a cough or dyspnoea (see 4.8 Undesirable Effects).

Haematopoietic suppression caused by methotrexate may occur abruptly and with apparently safe dosages. Any profound drop in white-cell or platelet counts indicates immediate withdrawal of the drug and appropriate supportive therapy (see 4.8 Undesirable Effects). Patients should be advised to report all signs and symptoms suggestive of infection.

Systemic toxicity of methotrexate may also be enhanced in patients with renal dysfunction, ascites or other effusions due to prolongation of serum half-life.

High doses may cause the precipitation of methotrexate or its metabolites in the renal tubules. A high fluid throughput and alkalinisation of the urine to pH 6.5-7.0 by oral or intravenous administration of sodium bicarbonate (5x 625mg tablets every three hours) or acetazolamide (500mg orally four times a day) is recommended as a preventive measure.

Malignant lymphomas may occur in patients receiving low dose methotrexate, in which case therapy must be discontinued. Failure of the lymphoma to show signs of spontaneous regression requires the initiation of cytotoxic therapy.

Methotrexate given concomitantly with radiotherapy may increase the risk of soft tissue necrosis and osteonecrosis.

Patients with rare hereditary problems of galactose intolerance, the Lapp lactose deficiency or glucose-galactose malabsorption should not take this medicine.

4.5 Interaction with other medicinal products and other forms of Interaction
Methotrexate is extensively protein bound and may be displaced by certain drugs such as salicylates, sulphonamides, diuretics, hypoglycaemics, diphenylhydantoins, tetracyclines, chloramphenicol, p-aminobenzoic acid, and the acidic anti-inflammatory drugs, so causing a potential for increased toxicity when used concurrently. Concomitant use of other drugs with nephrotoxic or hepatotoxic potential (including alcohol) should generally be avoided, unless considered clinically justified, in which case the patient should be closely monitored.

Renal tubular transport is also diminished by probenecid and penicillins; use of methotrexate with these drugs should be carefully monitored.

NSAIDs should not be administered prior to, or concomitantly with, high dose methotrexate as fatal methotrexate toxicity has been reported. Caution is also advised when NSAIDs and salicylates are administered concomitantly with lower doses of methotrexate. These drugs have been reported to reduce the tubular secretion of methotrexate in an animal model and thereby may enhance its toxicity. It is recommended that methotrexate dosage be carefully controlled during treatment with NSAIDs.

Concomitant administration of folate antagonists, such as co-trimoxazole, have been reported to cause acute megaloblastic pancytopenia in rare instances. Methotrexate should be used with caution in patients taking drugs with an anti-folate potential, including nitrous oxide.

Vitamin preparations containing folic acid or its derivatives may alter response to methotrexate.

Existing data suggest that etretinate is formed from acitretin after ingestion of alcoholic beverages. However the formation of etretinate without concurrent alcohol intake cannot be excluded. Serum levels of methotrexate may be increased by etretinate and severe hepatitis has been reported following concurrent use.

4.6 Pregnancy and lactation
Methotrexate affects spermatogenesis and oogenesis during the period of its administration which may result in decreased fertility. To date, this effect appears to be reversible on discontinuing therapy. Conception should be avoided for at least three months after treatment with methotrexate has ceased. Patients receiving methotrexate and their partners should be advised appropriately.

Methotrexate has been shown to be teratogenic; it has been reported to cause foetal death and/or congenital abnormalities. Therefore, it is not recommended in women of childbearing potential unless the benefits can be expected to outweigh the considered risks. If this drug is used during pregnancy for antineoplastic indications, or if the patient becomes pregnant while taking this drug, the patient should be appraised of the potential hazard to the foetus.

Because of the potential for serious adverse reactions from methotrexate in breast fed infants, breast feeding is contra-indicated in women taking methotrexate.

4.7 Effects on ability to drive and use machines
Methotrexate is not known to affect ability to drive or use machines.

4.8 Undesirable effects
The most common adverse reactions include ulcerative stomatitis, leucopenia, nausea and abdominal distress. Although very rare, anaphylactic reactions to methotrexate have occurred. Others reported are eye irritation, malaise, undue fatigue, vasculitis, sepsis, arthralgia/myalgia, chills and fever, dizziness, loss of libido/impotence and decreased resistance to infection. Opportunistic infections such as herpes zoster have been reported in relation to or attributed to the use of methotrexate. In general, the incidence and severity of side effects are considered to be dose-related. Adverse reactions for the various systems are as follows:

Integument:

Stevens-Johnson Syndrome, epidermal necrolysis, erythematous rashes, pruritus, urticaria, photosensitivity, pigmentary changes, alopecia, ecchymosis, telangiectasia, acne, furunculosis. Lesions of psoriasis may be aggravated by concomitant exposure to ultraviolet radiation. Skin ulceration in psoriatic patients and rarely painful erosion of psoriatic plaques have been reported. The recall phenomenon has been reported in both radiation and solar damaged skin.

Haematopoietic:

Bone marrow depression is most frequently manifested by leucopenia, but thrombocytopenia, anaemia, or any combination may occur. Infection or septicemia and haemorrhage from various sites may result. Hypogammaglobulinaemia has been reported.

Alimentary System:

Mucositis (most frequently stomatitis although gingivitis, pharyngitis and even enteritis, intestinal ulceration and bleeding) may occur. In rare cases the effect of methotrexate on the intestinal mucosa has led to malabsorption or toxic megacolon. Nausea, anorexia and vomiting and/or diarrhoea may also occur.

Hepatic:

Hepatic toxicity resulting in significant elevations of liver enzymes, acute liver atrophy, necrosis, fatty metamorphosis, periportal fibrosis or cirrhosis or death may occur, usually following chronic administration.

Urogenital System:

Renal failure and uraemia may follow methotrexate administration, usually in high doses. Vaginitis, vaginal ulcers, cystitis, haematuria and nephropathy have also been reported.

Methotrexate has been reported to cause impairment of fertility, oligospermia, menstrual dysfunction and amenorrhoea in humans, during and for a short period after cessation of therapy. In addition, methotrexate causes embryotoxicity, abortion and foetal defects in humans. Therefore, the possible risks of effects on reproduction should be discussed with patients of child-bearing potential (See 4.6 Pregnancy and Lactation).

Pulmonary System:

Infrequently an acute or chronic interstitial pneumonitis, often associated with blood eosinophilia, may occur and deaths have been reported. Acute pulmonary oedema has also been reported after oral use. Pulmonary fibrosis is rare. A syndrome consisting of pleuritic pain and pleural thickening has been reported following high doses.

In the treatment of rheumatoid arthritis, methotrexate induced lung disease is a potentially serious adverse drug reaction which may occur acutely at any time during therapy. It is not always fully reversible. Pulmonary symptoms (especially a dry, non productive cough) may require interruption of treatment and careful investigation.

Central Nervous System:

Headaches, drowsiness and blurred vision have occurred. Following low doses of methotrexate, transient subtle cognitive dysfunction, mood alteration, or unusual cranial sensations have been reported occasionally. Aphasia, paresis, hemiparesis, and convulsions have also occurred following administration of higher doses.

Additional reactions related to or attributed to the use of methotrexate such as osteoporosis, abnormal (usually "megaloblastic") red cell morphology, precipitation of diabetes, other metabolic changes, and sudden death have been reported.

Carcinogenesis and mutagenesis:

Animal carcinogenicity studies have demonstrated methotrexate to be free of carcinogenic potential. Although methotrexate has been reported to cause chromosomal damage to animal somatic cells and bone marrow cells in humans, these effects are transient and reversible. In patients treated with methotrexate, evidence is insufficient to permit conclusive evaluation of any increased risk of neoplasia.

4.9 Overdose

Calcium folinate is the antidote for neutralising the immediate toxic effects of methotrexate on the haematopoietic system. It may be administered orally, intramuscularly, or by an intravenous bolus injection or infusion. In cases of accidental overdosage, a dose of calcium folinate equal to or higher than the offending dose of methotrexate should be administered within one hour and dosing continued until the serum levels of methotrexate are below 10^{-7}M. Other supporting therapy such as a blood transfusion and renal dialysis may be required.

In cases of massive overdose, hydration and urinary alkalisation may be necessary to prevent precipitation of methotrexate and/or its metabolites in the renal tubules. Neither haemodialysis nor peritoneal dialysis has been shown to improve methotrexate elimination. Effective clearance of methotrexate has been reported with acute, intermittent haemodialysis using a high flux dialyser.

5. PHARMACOLOGICAL PROPERTIES

5.1 Pharmacodynamic properties

Methotrexate, a derivative of folic acid, belongs to the class of cytotoxic agents known as antimetabolites. It acts principally during the 'S' phase of cell division, by the competitive inhibition of the enzyme dihydrofolate reductase, thus preventing the reduction of dihydrofolate to tetrahydrofolate, a necessary step in the process of DNA synthesis and cellular replication. Actively proliferating tissues such as malignant cells, bone marrow, foetal cells, buccal and intestinal mucosa, and cells of the urinary bladder are generally more sensitive to the effects of methotrexate. When cellular proliferation in malignant tissues is greater than in most normal tissues, methotrexate may impair malignant growth without irreversible damage to normal tissues.

The mechanism of action in rheumatoid arthritis is unknown; it may affect immune function. Clarification of the effect of methotrexate on immune activity and its relation to rheumatoid immunopathogenesis await further investigation.

In psoriasis, the rate of production of epithelial cells in the skin is greatly increased over normal skin. This differential in proliferation rates is the basis for the use of methotrexate to control the psoriatic process.

5.2 Pharmacokinetic properties

In doses of 0.1mg (of methotrexate) per kg, methotrexate is completely absorbed from the G.I. tract; larger oral doses may be incompletely absorbed. Serum concentrations following oral administration of methotrexate may be slightly lower than those following I.V. injection.

Methotrexate is actively transported across cell membranes. The drug is widely distributed into body tissues with highest concentrations in the kidneys, gall bladder, spleen, liver and skin. Methotrexate is retained for several weeks in the kidneys and for months in the liver. Sustained serum concentrations and tissue accumulation may result from repeated daily doses. Methotrexate crosses the placental barrier and is distributed into breast milk. Approximately 50% of the drug in the blood is bound to serum proteins.

Following oral doses of 0.06mg/kg or more, the drug had a serum half-life of 2-4 hours, but the serum half-life was reported to be increased to 8-10 hours when oral doses of 0.037mg/kg were given.

Methotrexate does not appear to be appreciably metabolised. The drug is excreted primarily by the kidneys via glomerular filtration and active transport. Small amounts are excreted in the faeces, probably via the bile. Methotrexate has a biphasic excretion pattern. If methotrexate excretion is impaired, accumulation will occur more rapidly, e.g. in patients with impaired renal function. In addition, simultaneous administration of other weak organic acids such as salicylates may suppress methotrexate clearance.

5.3 Preclinical safety data

There are no pre-clinical data of any relevance to the prescriber that are additional to those already included in other sections.

6. PHARMACEUTICAL PARTICULARS

6.1 List of excipients

Maize starch

Colloidal anhydrous silica

Magnesium stearate

Lactose monohydrate

Microcrystalline cellulose Potato starch

6.2 Incompatibilities

Not applicable

6.3 Shelf life

Three years

6.4 Special precautions for storage

This medicinal product does not require any special storage conditions.

Keep out the reach and sight of children.

6.5 Nature and contents of container

4, 8, 10, 12, 16, 20, 24, 28, 50 or 100 tablets in white polypropylene tablet containers sealed with a white polyethylene tamper evident lid in cartons.

6.6 Instructions for use and handling

Cytotoxic drugs should only be handled by trained personnel in a designated area. The work surface should be covered with disposable plastic-backed absorbent paper. Protective gloves and goggles should be worn to avoid the drug accidentally coming into contact with the skin or eyes. Methotrexate is not a vesicant and should not cause harm if it comes into contact with the skin. It should of course be washed off with water immediately. Any transient stinging may be treated with bland cream. If there is any danger of systemic absorption of significant quantities of methotrexate, by any route, calcium folinate cover should be given.

Cytotoxic preparations should not be handled by pregnant staff.

Adequate care should be taken in the disposal of any unwanted product and containers. Any waste material may be disposed of by incineration. We do not make any specific recommendations with regard to the temperature of the incinerator.

Administrative Data

7. MARKETING AUTHORISATION HOLDER

CP Pharmaceuticals Ltd

Ash Road North

Wrexham LL13 9UF

United Kingdom

8. MARKETING AUTHORISATION NUMBER(S)

PL 04543/0451

9. DATE OF FIRST AUTHORISATION/RENEWAL OF THE AUTHORISATION

6 May 2005

10. DATE OF REVISION OF THE TEXT

1st June 2005

Methotrexate 2.5mg Tablets

(Wockhardt UK Ltd)

1. NAME OF THE MEDICINAL PRODUCT

Methotrexate 2.5mg Tablets BP

2. QUALITATIVE AND QUANTITATIVE COMPOSITION

Methotrexate 2.5mg

For excipients see 6.1

3. PHARMACEUTICAL FORM

Tablet

Methotrexate 2.5mg Tablets are light yellow round shaped tablets with a diameter of 7mm; may contain yellow to red sprinkles

4. CLINICAL PARTICULARS

4.1 Therapeutic indications

The treatment of acute lymphoblastic leukaemia and Burkitt's lymphoma. The treatment of severe cases of uncontrolled psoriasis, unresponsive to conventional therapy.

The treatment of adults with severe, active, classical or definite rheumatoid arthritis who are unresponsive or intolerant to conventional therapy.

4.2 Posology and method of administration

For oral administration. Dosages are based on the patient's body weight or surface area. Doses should be reduced in cases of haematological deficiency and hepatic or renal impairment.

Acute Lymphocytic Leukaemia:

Children

In acute lymphocytic leukaemia remissions are usually best induced with a combination of corticosteroids and other cytotoxic agents.

Methotrexate 15mg/m^2, given orally once weekly, in combination with other drugs, appears to be the treatment of choice for maintenance of drug-induced remissions.

Burkitt's Lymphoma:

Children

Some cases of Burkitt's lymphoma, when treated in the early stages with courses of 15mg/m^2 daily orally for five days, have shown prolonged remissions. Combination chemotherapy is also commonly used in all stages of the disease.

Psoriasis:

Adults

It is recommended that a test dose of 5-10mg should be administered, one week prior to therapy to detect idiosyncratic adverse reactions.

In most cases of severe uncontrolled psoriasis, unresponsive to conventional therapy, 10-25mg orally once a week and adjusted by the patient's response is recommended.

The use of methotrexate in psoriasis may permit the return to conventional topical therapy which should be encouraged.

Rheumatoid arthritis:

Adults

It is recommended that a test dose of 5-10mg should be administered, one week prior to therapy to detect idiosyncratic adverse reactions.

In adults with severe, acute, classical or definite rheumatoid arthritis who are unresponsive or intolerant to conventional therapy, 7.5mg orally once weekly or divided oral doses of 2.5mg at 12 hour intervals for three doses (7.5mg) as a course once weekly. The schedule may be adjusted gradually to achieve an optimal response but should not exceed a total weekly dose of 20mg. Once response has been achieved, the schedule should be reduced to the lowest possible effective dose.

Elderly

Methotrexate should be used with extreme caution in elderly patients; a reduction in dosage should be considered (see 4.4 Special Warnings and Special Precautions for Use).

Children

Safety and effectiveness in children have not been established, other than in cancer chemotherapy.

4.3 Contraindications

Profound impairment of renal or hepatic function or haematological impairment. Liver disease including fibrosis, cirrhosis, recent or active hepatitis; active infectious disease; and overt or laboratory evidence of immunodeficiency syndrome(s). Serious cases of anaemia, leucopenia, or thrombocytopenia. Methotrexate is contra-indicated in pregnant patients. Because of the potential for serious adverse reactions from methotrexate in breast fed infants, breast feeding is contra-indicated in women taking methotrexate. Patients with a known allergic hypersensitivity to methotrexate should not receive methotrexate.

4.4 Special warnings and special precautions for use

Warnings:

Methotrexate should be used with extreme caution in patients with haematological depression, renal impairment, peptic ulcer, ulcerative colitis, ulcerative stomatitis, diarrhoea, debility and in young children and the elderly. (See 4.2 Posology and Method of Administration).

Patients with pleural effusions or ascites should have these drained if appropriate before treatment or treatment should be withdrawn.

Symptoms of gastro-intestinal toxicity, usually first manifested by stomatitis, indicate that therapy should be interrupted otherwise haemorrhagic enteritis and death from intestinal perforation may occur.

Methotrexate has some immunosuppressive activity and therefore the immunological response to concurrent vaccination may be decreased. In addition, concomitant use of a live vaccine could cause a severe antigenic reaction.

Acute or chronic interstitial pneumonitis, often associated with blood eosinophilia, may occur and deaths have been reported. Symptoms typically include dyspnoea, cough (especially a dry non-productive cough) and fever for which patients should be monitored at each follow-up visit. Patients should be informed of the risk of pneumonitis and advised to contract their doctor immediately should they develop persistent cough or dyspnoea.

Methorexate should be withdrawn from patients with pulmonary symptoms and a through investigation should be made to exclude infection. If Methotrexate induced lung disease is suspected treatment with corticosteroids should be initiated and treatment with Methotrexate should not be restarted.

Precautions:

Methotrexate should only be used by clinicians who are familiar with the various characteristics of the drug and its mode of action. Before beginning methotrexate therapy or reinstituting methotrexate after a rest period, a chest x-ray, assessment of renal function, liver function and blood elements should be made by history, physical examination and laboratory tests. Patients undergoing therapy should be subject to appropriate supervision every 2-3 months so that signs of possible toxic effects or adverse reactions may be detected and evaluated with minimal delay. Renal function and full blood counts should be closely monitored before, during and after treatment.

It is essential that the following laboratory tests are included regularly (every 2-3 months) in the clinical evaluation and monitoring of patients receiving methotrexate: complete haematological analysis, urinalysis, renal function tests, liver function tests and, when high doses are administered, determination of plasma levels of methotrexate.

Particular attention should be given to the appearance of liver toxicity which may occur without correlative changes in liver function tests. Treatment should not be instituted, or should be discontinued, if any abnormality in liver function tests or liver biopsy is present or develops during therapy. Such abnormalities should return to normal within two weeks, after which treatment may be recommenced at the discretion of the physician.

When to perform a liver biopsy in rheumatoid arthritis patients has not been established either in terms of a cumulative methotrexate dose or duration of therapy.

Pleuropulmonary manifestations of rheumatoid arthritis have been reported in the literature. In patients with rheumatoid arthritis, the physician should be specifically alerted to the potential for methotrexate induced adverse effects in the pulmonary system. Patients should be advised to contact their physicians immediately should they develop a cough or dyspnoea (see 4.8 Undesirable Effects).

Haematopoietic suppression caused by methotrexate may occur abruptly and with apparently safe dosages. Any profound drop in white-cell or platelet counts indicates immediate withdrawal of the drug and appropriate supportive therapy (see 4.8 Undesirable Effects). Patients should be advised to report all signs and symptoms suggestive of infection.

Systemic toxicity of methotrexate may also be enhanced in patients with renal dysfunction, ascites or other effusions due to prolongation of serum half-life.

High doses may cause the precipitation of methotrexate or its metabolites in the renal tubules. A high fluid throughput and alkalinisation of the urine to pH 6.5-7.0 by oral or intravenous administration of sodium bicarbonate (5x 625mg tablets every three hours) or acetazolamide (500mg orally four times a day) is recommended as a preventive measure.

Malignant lymphomas may occur in patients receiving low dose methotrexate, in which case therapy must be discontinued. Failure of the lymphoma to show signs of spontaneous regression requires the initiation of cytotoxic therapy.

Methotrexate given concomitantly with radiotherapy may increase the risk of soft tissue necrosis and osteonecrosis.

Patients with rare hereditary problems of galactose intolerance, the Lapp lactose deficiency or glucose-galactose malabsorption should not take this medicine.

4.5 Interaction with other medicinal products and other forms of Interaction

Methotrexate is extensively protein bound and may be displaced by certain drugs such as salicylates, sulphonamides, diuretics, hypoglycaemics, diphenylhydantoins, tetracyclines, chloramphenicol, p-aminobenzoic acid, and the acidic anti-inflammatory drugs, so causing a potential for increased toxicity when used concurrently. Concomitant use of other drugs with nephrotoxic or hepatotoxic potential (including alcohol) should generally be avoided, unless considered clinically justified, in which case the patient should be closely monitored.

Renal tubular transport is also diminished by probenecid and penicillins; use of methotrexate with these drugs should be carefully monitored.

NSAIDs should not be administered prior to, or concomitantly with, high dose methotrexate as fatal methotrexate toxicity has been reported. Caution is also advised when NSAIDs and salicylates are administered concomitantly with lower doses of methotrexate. These drugs have been reported to reduce the tubular secretion of methotrexate in an animal model and thereby may enhance its toxicity. It is recommended that methotrexate dosage be carefully controlled during treatment with NSAIDs.

Concomitant administration of folate antagonists, such as co-trimoxazole, have been reported to cause acute megaloblastic pancytopenia in rare instances. Methotrexate should be used with caution in patients taking drugs with an anti-folate potential, including nitrous oxide.

Vitamin preparations containing folic acid or its derivatives may alter response to methotrexate.

Existing data suggest that etretinate is formed from acitretin after ingestion of alcoholic beverages. However the formation of etretinate without concurrent alcohol intake cannot be excluded. Serum levels of methotrexate may be increased by etretinate and severe hepatitis has been reported following concurrent use.

4.6 Pregnancy and lactation

Methotrexate affects spermatogenesis and oogenesis during the period of its administration which may result in decreased fertility. To date, this effect appears to be reversible on discontinuing therapy. Conception should be avoided for at least three months after treatment with methotrexate has ceased. Patients receiving methotrexate and their partners should be advised appropriately.

Methotrexate has been shown to be teratogenic; it has been reported to cause foetal death and/or congenital abnormalities. Therefore, it is not recommended in women of childbearing potential unless the benefits can be expected to outweigh the considered risks. If this drug is used during pregnancy for antineoplastic indications, or if the patient becomes pregnant while taking this drug, the patient should be appraised of the potential hazard to the foetus.

Because of the potential for serious adverse reactions from methotrexate in breast fed infants, breast feeding is contraindicated in women taking methotrexate.

4.7 Effects on ability to drive and use machines

Methotrexate is not known to affect ability to drive or use machines.

4.8 Undesirable effects

The most common adverse reactions include ulcerative stomatitis, leucopenia, nausea and abdominal distress. Although very rare, anaphylactic reactions to methotrexate have occurred. Others reported are eye irritation, malaise, undue fatigue, vasculitis, sepsis, arthralgia/myalgia, chills and fever, dizziness, loss of libido/impotence and decreased resistance to infection. Opportunistic infections such as herpes zoster have been reported in relation to or attributed to the use of methotrexate. In general, the incidence and severity of side effects are considered to be dose-related. Adverse reactions for the various systems are as follows:

Integument:

Stevens-Johnson Syndrome, epidermal necrolysis, erythematous rashes, pruritus, urticaria, photosensitivity, pigmentary changes, alopecia, ecchymosis, telangiectasia, acne, furunculosis. Lesions of psoriasis may be aggravated by concomitant exposure to ultraviolet radiation. Skin ulceration in psoriatic patients and rarely painful erosion of psoriatic plaques have been reported. The recall phenomenon has been reported in both radiation and solar damaged skin.

Haematopoietic:

Bone marrow depression is most frequently manifested by leucopenia, but thrombocytopenia, anaemia, or any combination may occur. Infection or septicemia and haemorrhage from various sites may result. Hypogammaglobulinaemia has been reported.

Alimentary System:

Mucositis (most frequently stomatitis although gingivitis, pharyngitis and even enteritis, intestinal ulceration and bleeding) may occur. In rare cases the effect of methotrexate on the intestinal mucosa has led to malabsorption or toxic megacolon. Nausea, anorexia and vomiting and/or diarrhoea may also occur.

Hepatic:

Hepatic toxicity resulting in significant elevations of liver enzymes, acute liver atrophy, necrosis, fatty metamorphosis, periportal fibrosis or cirrhosis or death may occur, usually following chronic administration.

Urogenital System:

Renal failure and uraemia may follow methotrexate administration, usually in high doses. Vaginitis, vaginal ulcers, cystitis, haematuria and nephropathy have also been reported.

Methotrexate has been reported to cause impairment of fertility, oligospermia, menstrual dysfunction and amenorrhoea in humans, during and for a short period after cessation of therapy. In addition, methotrexate causes embryotoxicity, abortion and foetal defects in humans. Therefore, the possible risks of effects on reproduction should be discussed with patients of child-bearing potential (See 4.6 Pregnancy and Lactation).

Pulmonary System:

Infrequently an acute or chronic interstitial pneumonitis, often associated with blood eosinophilia, may occur and deaths have been reported. Acute pulmonary oedema has also been reported after oral use. Pulmonary fibrosis is rare. A syndrome consisting of pleuritic pain and pleural thickening has been reported following high doses.

In the treatment of rheumatoid arthritis, methotrexate induced lung disease is a potentially serious adverse drug reaction which may occur acutely at any time during therapy. It is not always fully reversible. Pulmonary symptoms (especially a dry, non productive cough) may require interruption of treatment and careful investigation.

Central Nervous System:

Headaches, drowsiness and blurred vision have occurred. Following low doses of methotrexate, transient subtle cognitive dysfunction, mood alteration, or unusual cranial sensations have been reported occasionally. Aphasia, paresis, hemiparesis, and convulsions have also occurred following administration of higher doses.

Additional reactions related to or attributed to the use of methotrexate such as osteoporosis, abnormal (usually "megaloblastic") red cell morphology, precipitation of diabetes, other metabolic changes, and sudden death have been reported.

Carcinogenesis and mutagenesis:

Animal carcinogenicity studies have demonstrated methotrexate to be free of carcinogenic potential. Although methotrexate has been reported to cause chromosomal damage to animal somatic cells and bone marrow cells in humans, these effects are transient and reversible. In patients treated with methotrexate, evidence is insufficient to permit conclusive evaluation of any increased risk of neoplasia.

4.9 Overdose

Calcium folinate is the antidote for neutralising the immediate toxic effects of methotrexate on the haematopoietic system. It may be administered orally, intramuscularly, or by an intravenous bolus injection or infusion. In cases of accidental overdosage, a dose of calcium folinate equal to or higher than the offending dose of methotrexate should be administered within one hour and dosing continued until the serum levels of methotrexate are below 10^{-7}M. Other supporting therapy such as a blood transfusion and renal dialysis may be required.

In cases of massive overdose, hydration and urinary alkalisation may be necessary to prevent precipitation of methotrexate and/or its metabolites in the renal tubules. Neither haemodialysis nor peritoneal dialysis has been shown to improve methotrexate elimination. Effective clearance of methotrexate has been reported with acute, intermittent haemodialysis using a high flux dialyser.

5. PHARMACOLOGICAL PROPERTIES

5.1 Pharmacodynamic properties

Methotrexate, a derivative of folic acid, belongs to the class of cytotoxic agents known as antimetabolites. It acts principally during the 'S' phase of cell division, by the competitive inhibition of the enzyme dihydrofolate reductase, thus preventing the reduction of dihydrofolate to tetrahydrofolate, a necessary step in the process of DNA synthesis and cellular replication. Actively proliferating tissues such as malignant cells, bone marrow, foetal cells, buccal and intestinal mucosa, and cells of the urinary bladder are generally more sensitive to the effects of methotrexate. When cellular proliferation in malignant tissues is greater than in most normal tissues, methotrexate may impair malignant growth without irreversible damage to normal tissues.

The mechanism of action in rheumatoid arthritis is unknown; it may affect immune function. Clarification of the effect of methotrexate on immune activity and its relation to rheumatoid immunopathogenesis await further investigation.

In psoriasis, the rate of production of epithelial cells in the skin is greatly increased over normal skin. This differential in proliferation rates is the basis for the use of methotrexate to control the psoriatic process.

5.2 Pharmacokinetic properties

In doses of 0.1mg (of methotrexate) per kg, methotrexate is completely absorbed from the G.I. tract; larger oral doses may be incompletely absorbed. Serum concentrations following oral administration of methotrexate may be slightly lower than those following I.V. injection.

Methotrexate is actively transported across cell membranes. The drug is widely distributed into body tissues with highest concentrations in the kidneys, gall bladder, spleen, liver and skin. Methotrexate is retained for several weeks in the kidneys and for months in the liver. Sustained serum concentrations and tissue accumulation may result from repeated daily doses. Methotrexate crosses the placental barrier and is distributed into breast milk. Approximately 50% of the drug in the blood is bound to serum proteins.

Following oral doses of 0.06mg/kg or more, the drug had a serum half-life of 2-4 hours, but the serum half-life was reported to be increased to 8-10 hours when oral doses of 0.037mg/kg were given.

Methotrexate does not appear to be appreciably metabolised. The drug is excreted primarily by the kidneys via glomerular filtration and active transport. Small amounts are excreted in the faeces, probably via the bile. Methotrexate has a biphasic excretion pattern. If methotrexate excretion is impaired, accumulation will occur more rapidly, e.g. in patients with impaired renal function. In addition, simultaneous administration of other weak organic acids such as salicylates may suppress methotrexate clearance.

5.3 Preclinical safety data
There are no pre-clinical data of any relevance to the prescriber that are additional to those already included in other sections.

6. PHARMACEUTICAL PARTICULARS

6.1 List of excipients
Maize starch

Colloidal anhydrous silica

Magnesium stearate

Lactose monohydrate

Microcrystalline cellulose

Potato starch

6.2 Incompatibilities
Not applicable

6.3 Shelf life
Three years

6.4 Special precautions for storage
This medicinal product does not require any special storage conditions

Keep out the reach and sight of children.

6.5 Nature and contents of container
4, 8, 10, 12, 16, 20, 24, 28, 50 or 100 tablets in white polypropylene tablet containers sealed with a white polyethylene tamper evident lid in cartons.

6.6 Instructions for use and handling
Cytotoxic drugs should only be handled by trained personnel in a designated area. The work surface should be covered with disposable plastic-backed absorbent paper. Protective gloves and goggles should be worn to avoid the drug accidentally coming into contact with the skin or eyes. Methotrexate is not a vesicant and should not cause harm if it comes into contact with the skin. It should of course be washed off with water immediately. Any transient stinging may be treated with bland cream. If there is any danger of systemic absorption of significant quantities of methotrexate, by any route, calcium folinate cover should be given.

Cytotoxic preparations should not be handled by pregnant staff.

Adequate care should be taken in the disposal of any unwanted product and containers. Any waste material may be disposed of by incineration. We do not make any specific recommendations with regard to the temperature of the incinerator.

Administrative Data

7. MARKETING AUTHORISATION HOLDER
CP Pharmaceuticals Ltd

Ash Road North

Wrexham LL13 9UF

United Kingdom

8. MARKETING AUTHORISATION NUMBER(S)
PL 04543/0444

9. DATE OF FIRST AUTHORISATION/RENEWAL OF THE AUTHORISATION
6 May 2005

10. DATE OF REVISION OF THE TEXT
1st June 2005

Methotrexate Injection

(Wyeth Pharmaceuticals)

1. NAME OF THE MEDICINAL PRODUCT
Methotrexate Injection 25mg/ml

2. QUALITATIVE AND QUANTITATIVE COMPOSITION
Each 1ml of Methotrexate Injection contains:

methotrexate sodium (BP) equivalent to 25mg methotrexate per ml.

For excipients see 6.1.

3. PHARMACEUTICAL FORM
A clear, yellowish solution for injection or infusion.

4. CLINICAL PARTICULARS

4.1 Therapeutic indications
Methotrexate is indicated in the treatment of neoplastic disease.

4.2 Posology and method of administration
Routes of administration: Methotrexate Injection may be given by intramuscular, intravenous (bolus injection or infusion), intrathecal, and intra-arterial routes of administration.

Dosage:

Adults and Children: Dosages are based on the patient's bodyweight or surface area except in the case of intrathecal administration when a maximum dose of 15mg is recommended. Doses should be reduced in cases of haematological deficiency and hepatic or renal impairment. Larger doses (greater than 100mg) are usually given by intravenous infusion over periods not exceeding 24 hours. Part of the dose may be given as an initial rapid intravenous infusion.

Methotrexate has been used with beneficial effects in a wide variety of neoplastic diseases, alone and in combination with other cytotoxic agents, hormones, radiotherapy or surgery. Dosage schedules therefore vary considerably, depending on the clinical use, particularly when intermittent high-dose regimes are followed by the administration of calcium leucovorin (calcium folinate) to rescue normal cells from toxic effects.

Examples of doses of methotrexate that have been used for particular indications are given below.

Choriocarcinoma and other trophoblastic tumours: Non-metastatic gestational trophoblastic neoplasms have been treated successfully with 0.25-1mg/kg up to a maximum of 60mg intramuscularly every 48 hours for four doses, followed by calcium leucovorin rescue. This course of treatment is repeated at seven day intervals until levels of urinary chorionic gonadotrophin hormone return to normal. Not less than four courses of treatment are usually necessary. Patients with complications, such as extensive metastases, may be treated with methotrexate in combination with other cytotoxic drugs.

Methotrexate has also been used in similar doses for the treatment of hydatidiform mole and chorioadenoma destruens.

Leukaemia in children: In acute lymphocytic leukaemia remissions are usually best induced with a combination of corticosteroids and other cytotoxic agents.

Methotrexate 15mg/m^2, given parenterally or orally once weekly, in combination with other drugs appears to be the treatment of choice for maintenance of drug-induced remissions.

Meningeal leukaemia in children: Doses up to 15mg, intrathecally, at weekly intervals, until the CSF appears normal (usually two to three weeks), have been found useful for the treatment of meningeal leukaemia.

Although intravenous doses of the order of 50mg/m^2 of methotrexate do not appreciably penetrate the CSF, larger doses of the order of 500mg/m^2 or greater do produce cytotoxic levels of methotrexate in the CSF. This type of therapy has been used in short courses, followed by administration of calcium leucovorin, as initial maintenance therapy to prevent leukaemic invasion of the central nervous system in children with poor prognosis lymphocytic leukaemia.

Lymphoma: Non-Hodgkin's lymphoma, e.g. childhood lymphosarcoma has recently been treated with 3-30mg/kg (approximately 90-900mg/m^2) of methotrexate given by intravenous injection and infusion followed by administration of calcium leucovorin with the higher doses. Some cases of Burkitt's lymphoma, when treated in the early stages with courses of 15mg/m^2 daily orally for five days, have shown prolonged remissions. Combination chemotherapy is also commonly used in all stages of the disease.

Breast cancer: Methotrexate, in intravenous doses of 10-60mg/m^2, is commonly included in cyclical combination regimes with other cytotoxic drugs in the treatment of advanced breast cancer. Similar regimes have also been used as adjuvant therapy in early cases following mastectomy and/or radiotherapy.

Osteogenic sarcoma: The use of methotrexate alone and in cyclical combination regimes has recently been introduced as an adjuvant therapy to the primary treatment of osteogenic sarcoma by amputation with or without prosthetic bone replacement. This has involved the use of intravenous infusions of 20-300mg/kg (approximately 600-9,000mg/m^2) of methotrexate followed by calcium leucovorin rescue. Methotrexate has also been used as the sole treatment in metastatic cases of osteogenic sarcoma.

Bronchogenic carcinoma: Intravenous infusions of 20-100mg/m^2 of methotrexate have been included in cyclical combination regimes for the treatment of advanced tumours. High doses with calcium leucovorin rescue have also been employed as the sole treatment.

Head and neck cancer: Intravenous infusions of 240-1,080mg/m^2 with calcium leucovorin rescue have been used both as pre-operative adjuvant therapy and in the treatment of advanced tumours. Intra-arterial infusions of methotrexate have been used in the treatment of head and neck cancers.

Bladder carcinoma: Intravenous injections or infusions of methotrexate in doses up to 100mg every one or two weeks have been used in the treatment of bladder carcinoma with promising results, varying from only symptomatic relief to complete though unsustained regressions. The use of high doses of methotrexate with calcium leucovorin rescue is currently being evaluated.

Elderly: Due to diminished hepatic and renal function and decreased folate stores, Methotrexate should be used with extreme caution in elderly patients, a reduction in dosage should be considered and these patients should be closely monitored for early signs of toxicity.

4.3 Contraindications
Profound impairment of renal or hepatic function or haematological impairment.

Alcoholism. Liver disease including alcoholic liver disease, fibrosis, cirrhosis, recent or active hepatitis; active infectious disease; and overt or laboratory evidence of immunodeficiency syndrome(s).

Pre-existing blood dyscrasias, such as bone marrow hypoplasia, anaemia, leucopenia or thrombocytopenia. Methotrexate is contra-indicated in pregnant patients. Because of the potential for serious adverse reactions from methotrexate in breast fed infants, breast feeding is contra-indicated in women taking methotrexate.

Patients with a known allergic hypersensitivity to methotrexate or any of the excipients in the formulation should not receive methotrexate.

Diluents containing preservatives must not be used for intrathecal or high dose methotrexate therapy.

4.4 Special warnings and special precautions for use
Deaths have been reported with the use of methotrexate in the treatment of malignancy, therefore it should only be used in life threatening neoplastic diseases.

Methotrexate should be used with extreme caution in patients with haematological depression, renal impairment, peptic ulcer, ulcerative colitis, ulcerative stomatitis, diarrhoea, debility and in young children and the elderly.

Haematologic and gastrointestinal toxicity have been observed in combination with high and low dose methotrexate.

Initiation
Methotrexate should only be used by clinicians who are familiar with the various characteristics of the drug and its mode of action. Before beginning methotrexate therapy or reinstituting methotrexate after a rest period, a chest x-ray, assessment of renal function, liver function and blood elements should be made by history, physical examination and laboratory tests. Patients undergoing therapy should be subject to appropriate supervision every 2-3 months so that signs of possible toxic effects or adverse reactions may be detected and evaluated with minimal delay. Renal function and full blood counts should be closely monitored before, during and after treatment.

Patients with pleural effusions or ascites should have these drained if appropriate before treatment and their plasma methotrexate levels monitored, or treatment should be withdrawn. The reason being that Methotrexate exits slowly from third party compartments (e.g. pleural effusions, ascites). This results in a prolonged terminal half-life and unexpected toxicity.

It should be noted that intrathecal doses are transported into the cardiovascular system and may give rise to systemic toxicity. Systemic toxicity of methotrexate may also be enhanced in patients with renal dysfunction, ascites or other effusions due to prolongation of serum half-life.

Monitoring
It is essential that the following laboratory tests are included regularly (every 2-3 months) in the clinical evaluation and monitoring of patients receiving methotrexate: complete haematological analysis, urinalysis, renal function tests, liver function tests and, when high doses are administered, determination of plasma levels of methotrexate.

It is necessary to monitor patients on methotrexate closely. Methotrexate has the potential for serious toxicity. Toxic effects may be related in frequency and severity to dose or frequency of administration, but has been seen at all doses and can occur at any time during therapy. Most adverse reactions are reversible if detected early. When such reactions do occur, the dosage should be reduced or discontinued and appropriate corrective measures should be taken. If methotrexate therapy is reinstituted, it should be carried out with caution, with adequate consideration of further need for the drug, and with increased alertness as to possible recurrence of toxicity.

Hepatic System
Methotrexate causes hepatotoxicity, liver fibrosis, and cirrhosis, but generally only after prolonged use. Particular attention should be given to the appearance of liver toxicity by carrying out liver function tests before starting methotrexate treatment and repeating these at two to three month intervals during therapy. Treatment should not be instituted or should be discontinued if any abnormality of liver function tests, or liver biopsy, is present or develops during therapy. Such abnormalities should return to normal within two weeks after which treatment may be recommenced at the discretion of the physician.

Acutely, liver enzyme elevations are frequently seen. These are usually transient and asymptomatic, and do not appear predictive of subsequent hepatic disease. Persistent liver abnormalities and/or decrease of serum albumin may be indicators of serious liver toxicity. Liver biopsy after sustained use often shows histological changes, and fibrosis and cirrhosis have been reported.

Renal System
Methotrexate therapy in patients with impaired renal function should be undertaken with extreme caution, and at reduced dosages because impairment of renal function will decrease methotrexate elimination.

High doses may cause the precipitation of methotrexate or its metabolites in the renal tubules. A high fluid throughput and alkalinisation of the urine to pH 6.5-7.0 by oral or intravenous administration of sodium bicarbonate (5 × 625mg tablets every three hours) or Diamox* (500mg orally four times a day) is recommended as a preventive measure.

Methotrexate may cause renal damage that may lead to acute renal failure. Close attention to renal function including adequate hydration, urine alkalinisation, and measurement of serum methotrexate and renal function are recommended.

Respiratory System

Acute or chronic interstitial pneumonitis, often associated with blood eosinophilia may occur and deaths have been reported. Symptoms typically include dyspnoea, cough (especially a dry, non-productive cough), fever, chest pain, and hypoxemia for which patients should be monitored at each follow-up visit. Patients should be informed of the risk of pneumonitis and advised to contact their doctor immediately should they develop persistent cough or dyspnoea.

Pulmonary lesions can occur at any time during therapy and have been reported at all dosages, even doses as low as 7.5mg/week. Methotrexate should be withdrawn from patients with pulmonary symptoms and a thorough investigation should be made to exclude infection. If methotrexate induced lung disease is suspected treatment with corticosteroids should be initiated and treatment with methotrexate should not be restarted.

Potentially fatal opportunistic infections, including Pneumocystis carinii pneumonia, may occur with methotrexate therapy. When a patient presents with pulmonary symptoms the possibility of Pneumocystis carinii pneumonia should be considered.

Gastrointestinal System

Symptoms of gastro-intestinal toxicity, usually first manifested by diarrhoea and ulcerative stomatitis, indicate interruption of therapy otherwise haemorrhagic enteritis and death from intestinal perforation may occur.

If vomiting resulting in dehydration happens, methotrexate should be discontinued until recovery occurs.

Metabolism and Nutrition

Folate deficiency states may increase methotrexate toxicity.

Immune System

Methotrexate has some immunosuppressive activity and therefore the immunological response to concurrent vaccination may be decreased. In addition, concomitant use of a live vaccine could cause a severe antigenic reaction and is therefore not generally recommended. There have been reports of disseminated vaccinia infections after smallpox immunisation in patients receiving methotrexate therapy.

Blood and Lymphatic System

Methotrexate can suppress haematopoiesis and cause anaemia, aplastic anaemia, pancytopenia, leucopenia, neutropenia and/or thrombocytopenia. Haematopoietic suppression caused by Methotrexate may occur abruptly and with apparently safe dosages. In the treatment of neoplastic diseases, methotrexate should be continued only if the potential benefit outweighs the risk of severe myelosuppression. Any profound drop in white-cell or platelet counts should result in immediate withdrawal of the drug and appropriate supportive therapy (see Undesirable Effects). Patients should be advised to report all signs and symptoms suggestive of infection.

Neoplasms Benign and Malignant

Like other cytotoxic drugs, methotrexate may induce 'tumour lysis syndrome' in patients with rapidly growing tumours. Appropriate supportive and pharmacologic measures may prevent or alleviate this condition.

Malignant lymphomas may occur in patients receiving low-dose methotrexate, in which case therapy must be discontinued. Failure of the lymphoma to show signs of spontaneous regression requires the initiation of cytotoxic therapy.

Methotrexate given concomitantly with radiotherapy may increase the risk of soft tissue necrosis and osteonecrosis.

The use of methotrexate high-dose regimens recommended for osteosarcoma requires meticulous care due to the potential for additive or synergistic renal toxcitiy. High dosage regimens for other neoplastic diseases are investigational and a therapeutic advantage has not been established.

Skin and Subcutaneous tissue

Severe, occasionally fatal, skin reactions such as Stevens-Johnson Syndrome, toxic epidermal necrolysis (Lyell's syndrome) and erythema multiforme have been reported within days of administering single or multiple doses of methotrexate.

4.5 Interaction with other medicinal products and other forms of Interaction

Methotrexate is extensively protein bound and may be displaced by certain drugs such as salicylates, sulphonamides, phenylbutazone, diuretics, hypoglycaemics, diphenylhydantoins, tetracyclines, chloramphenicol, p-aminobenzoic acid, and the acidic anti-inflammatory drugs, so causing a potential for increased toxicity when used concurrently. Concomitant use of other drugs with nephrotoxic potential should generally be avoided, unless considered clinically justified, in which case the patient should be closely monitored.

The potential for increased hepatototoxicity when methotrexate is administered with other hepatotoxic agents has not been evaluated. However, hepatotoxicity has been reported in such cases. Therefore, combination use of methotrexate and other potential hepatotoxic agents (e.g. alcohol, leflunomide, azathioprine, sulfasalazine, retinoids) should generally be avoided, unless clinically justified, in which case the patient should be closely monitored for possible increased risk of hepatotoxicity.

Enhancement of nephrotoxicity may be seen when high-dose methotrexate is administered in combination with a potentially nephrotoxic chemotherapeutic agent (e.g. cisplatin).

Renal tubular transport is also diminished by probenecid, penicillins, and omeprazole, which may result in potentially toxic methotrexate levels. The use of methotrexate with these drugs should be carefully monitored.

NSAIDs should not be administered prior to, or concomitantly with, high dose methotrexate as fatal methotrexate toxicity has been reported. Caution is also advised when NSAIDs and salicylates are administered concomitantly with lower doses of methotrexate. These drugs have been reported to reduce the tubular secretion of methotrexate in an animal model and thereby may enhance its toxicity. It is recommended that methotrexate dosage be carefully controlled during treatment with NSAIDs.

Methotrexate increases the plasma levels of mercaptopurine. Combinations of methotrexate and mercaptopurine may therefore require dose adjustment.

Concomitant administration of folate antagonists, such as co-trimoxazole, have been reported to cause acute megaloblastic pancytopenia in rare instances. Methotrexate should be used with caution in patients taking drugs with an anti-folate potential including nitrous oxide and trimethoprim.

Vitamin preparations containing folic acid or its derivatives may alter response to methotrexate. Folate deficiency states may increase methotrexate toxicity. High doses of leucovorin may reduce the efficacy of intrathecally administered methotrexate.

Existing data suggests that etretinate is formed from acitretin after ingestion of alcoholic beverages. However, the formation of etretinate without concurrent alcohol intake cannot be excluded. Serum levels of methotrexate may be increased by etretinate; severe hepatitis has been reported following concurrent use.

Oral antibiotics, such as tetracycline, chloramphenicol, and non-absorbable broad spectrum antibiotics, may decrease intestinal absorption of methotrexate or interfere with the enterohepatic circulation by inhibiting bowel flora and suppressing metabolism of methotrexate by bacteria.

Methotrexate may decrease the clearance of theophylline; theophylline levels should be monitored when used concurrently with methotrexate.

4.6 Pregnancy and lactation

Methotrexate has been shown to be teratogenic; it has been reported to cause foetal death and/or congenital abnormalities. Therefore it is not recommended in women of childbearing potential unless the benefits can be expected to outweigh the considered risks. Women of childbearing potential should not be started on methotrexate until pregnancy is excluded. If this drug is used during pregnancy for antineoplastic indications, or if the patient becomes pregnant while taking this drug, the patient should be appraised of the potential hazard to the foetus.

Methotrexate affects spermatogenesis and oogenesis during the period of its administration which may result in decreased fertility. To date, this effect appears to be reversible on discontinuing therapy. Conception should be avoided for at least three months after treatment with methotrexate has ceased. Patients receiving methotrexate and their partners should be advised appropriately.

Methotrexate has been detected in human breast milk and is contra-indicated during breastfeeding.

4.7 Effects on ability to drive and use machines

Methotrexate can cause dizziness, fatigue, blurred vision and eye-irritation which may affect the ability to drive or operate machinery.

4.8 Undesirable effects

The most common adverse reactions include ulcerative stomatitis, leucopenia, nausea and abdominal distress. Although very rare, anaphylactic reactions to methotrexate have occurred. Others reported are eye-irritation, malaise, undue fatigue, vasculitis, sepsis, arthralgia/myalgia, chills and fever, dizziness, loss of libido/impotence and decreased resistance to infection. In general, the incidence and severity of side-effects are considered to be dose-related.

Opportunistic infections (sometimes fatal e.g. fatal sepsis) have been reported in patients receiving methotrexate therapy for neoplastic and non-neoplastic diseases, Pneumocystis carinii pneumonia being the most common. Other reported infections include pneumonia, nocardiosis, histoplasmosis, cryptococcosis, Herpes zoster, H. simplex hepatitis and disseminated H. simplex and cytomegalovirus infection, including cytomegaloviral pneumonia.

Conjunctivitis and serious visual changes of unknown etiology have been reported.

Additional reactions related to or attributed to the use of methotrexate such as osteoporosis, stress fractures, nodulosis, lymphoma including reversible lymphomas, tumour lysis syndrome, abnormal (usually 'megaloblastic') red cell morphology, precipitation of diabetes, other metabolic changes, anaphylactoid reactions and sudden death have been reported.

Adverse reactions for the various systems are as follows:-

Integument: Stevens-Johnson Syndrome, toxic epidermal necrolysis (Lyell's Syndrome), erythematous rashes, pruritus, urticaria, photosensitivity, pigmentary changes, alopecia, ecchymosis, telangiectasia, acne, furunculosis, erythema multiforme. Lesions of psoriasis may be aggravated by concomitant exposure to ultraviolet radiation. Skin ulceration in psoriatic patients and rarely painful erosion of psoriatic plaques have been reported. The recall phenomenon has been reported in both radiation and solar damaged skin.

Haematopoietic: Bone marrow depression is most frequently manifested by leucopenia, but thrombocytopenia, anaemia, or any combination may occur. Infection (e.g. pneumonia) or septicaemia and haemorrhage from various sites may result. Aplastic anaemia, pancytopenia and neutropenia, agranulocytosis, eosinophilia, lymphadenopathy, lymphoproliferative disorders (including reversible) have been reported, as has hypogammaglobulinaemia.

Alimentary System: Mucositis (most frequently stomatitis although gingivitis, pharyngitis and even enteritis, intestinal ulceration and bleeding) may occur. In rare cases the effect of methotrexate on the intestinal mucosa has led to malabsorption or toxic megacolon. Melena, heamatemesis, nausea, anorexia and vomiting and/or diarrhoea may also occur.

Hepatic: Hepatic toxicity resulting in significant elevations of liver enzymes, decrease in serum albumin, acute liver atrophy, necrosis, acute hepatitis, fatty metamorphosis, periportal fibrosis or cirrhosis, hepatic failure or death may occur, usually following chronic administration.

Urogenital System: Renal failure and uraemia may follow methotrexate administration, usually in high doses. Vaginitis, vaginal discharge, vaginal ulcers, cystitis, azotemia, dysuria, haematuria, proteinuria and severe nephropathy have also been reported.

Pulmonary System: Acute or chronic interstitial pneumonitis, often associated with blood eosinophilia, may occur and deaths have been reported (see Section 4.4 Warnings and Precautions for Use). Acute pulmonary oedema has also been reported after oral and intrathecal use. Pulmonary fibrosis, respiratory failure and chronic interstitial pulmonary disease has been reported. A syndrome consisting of pleuritic pain and pleural thickening has been reported following high doses.

Central Nervous System: Headaches, drowsiness and blurred vision have occurred. Following low doses of methotrexate, transient subtle cognitive dysfunction, mood alteration, or unusual cranial sensations have been reported occasionally. Dysarthria and aphasia, paresis, hemiparesis, and convulsions have also occurred following administration of higher doses.

There have been reports of leucoencephalopathy following intravenous methotrexate in high doses, or low doses following cranial-spinal radiation.

Serious neurotoxicity, frequently manifested as generalised or focal seizures has been reported with unexpectedly increased frequency among paediatric patients with acute lymphoblastic leukaemia who were treated with intermediate-dose intravenous methotrexate (1 gm/m^2).

Symptomatic patients were commonly noted to have leucoencephalopathy and/or microangiopathic calcifications on diagnostic imaging studies. Chronic leucoencephalopathy has also been reported in patients who received repeated doses of high-dose methotrexate with leucovorin rescue even without cranial irradiation. Discontinuation of methotrexate does not always result in complete recovery.

A transient acute neurologic syndrome has been observed in patients treated with high dosage regimens. Manifestations of this neurologic syndrome may include behavioural abnormalities, focal sensorimotor signs, including transient blindness or vision loss, and abnormal reflexes. The exact cause is unknown.

Cardiac: Pericarditis, pericardial effusion, hypotension, and thromboembolic events including arterial thrombosis, cerebral thrombosis, thrombophlebitis, deep vein thrombosis, retinal vein thrombosis and pulmonary embolus.

Adverse reactions following intrathecal methotrexate are generally classified into three groups; acute, subacute and chronic. The acute form is a chemical arachnoiditis manifested by headache, back or shoulder pain, nuchal rigidity, and fever. The subacute form may include paresis, usually transient, paraparesis/paraplegia associated with involvement with one or more spinal nerve roots, nerve palsies, and cerebellar dysfunction. The chronic form is a leucoencephalopathy manifested by irritability, confusion, ataxia, spasticity, occasionally convulsions, dementia, somnolence, coma, and rarely, death. This central nervous system toxicity can be progressive. There is evidence that the combined use of cranial radiation and intrathecal methotrexate increases the incidence of leucoencephalopathy. Signs of neurotoxicity (meningeal irritation, transient or permanent paresis, encephalopathy) should be monitored following intrathecal administration of methotrexate.

Carcinogenesis, mutagenesis, and impairment of fertility: Animal carcinogenicity studies have demonstrated methotrexate to be free of carcinogenic potential. Although methotrexate has been reported to cause chromosomal damage to animal somatic cells and bone marrow cells in humans, these effects are transient and reversible. In patients treated with methotrexate, evidence is insufficient to permit conclusive evaluation of any increased risk of neoplasia. Methotrexate has been reported to cause impairment of fertility, oligospermia, menstrual dysfunction and amenorrhoea in humans, during and for a short period after cessation.

In addition, methotrexate causes embryotoxicity, abortion and foetal defects in humans and may cause foetal death. Therefore, the possible risks of effects on reproduction should be discussed with patients of child-bearing potential.

4.9 Overdose

In postmarketing experience, overdose with methotrexate has generally occurred with oral and intrathecal administration, although intravenous and intramuscular overdosage has also been reported.

Symptoms of intrathecal overdose are generally CNS symptoms, including headache, nausea and vomiting, seizure or convulsion, and acute toxic encephalopathy. In some cases, no symptoms were reported. There have been reports of death following intrathecal overdose. In these cases, cerebellar herniation associated with increased intracranial pressure, and acute toxic encephalopathy have also been reported.

Calcium leucovorin is the antidote for neutralising the immediate toxic effects of methotrexate on the haematopoietic system. It may be administered orally, intramuscularly, or by an intravenous bolus injection or infusion. In cases of accidental overdosage, a dose of calcium leucovorin equal to or higher than the offending dose of methotrexate should be administered within one hour and dosing continued until the serum levels of methotrexate are below 10^{-7}M. Other supporting therapy such as a blood transfusion and renal dialysis may be required. Calcium Leucovorin administration should begin as promptly as possible. As the time interval between methotrexate administration and leucovorin initiation increases the effectiveness of leucovorin in counteracting toxicity decreases. Monitoring of the serum methotrexate concentration is essential in determining the optimal dose and duration of treatment with leucovorin.

In cases of massive overdose, hydration and urinary alkalization may be necessary to prevent precipitation of methotrexate and/or its metabolites in the renal tubules. Neither haemodialysis nor peritoneal dialysis has been shown to improve methotrexate elimination. Effective clearance of methotrexate has been reported with acute, intermittent haemodialysis using a high flux dialyser.

Following intrathecal overdose, CSF drainage may remove up to 95% of the dose if commenced within 15 minutes of administration, although this falls to 20% after 2 hours. For intrathecal doses over 100mg ventriculolumbar perfusion should accompany CSF drainage. In addition, high dose systemic leucovorin or alkaline diuresis may be required.

There are published case reports of intravenous and intrathecal carboxypeptidase G2 treatment to hasten clearance of methotrexate in cases of overdose.

5. PHARMACOLOGICAL PROPERTIES

5.1 Pharmacodynamic properties

Methotrexate, a derivative of folic acid, belongs to the class of cytotoxic agents known as antimetabolites. It acts principally during the 'S' phase of cell division, by the competitive inhibition of the enzyme dihydrofolate reductase, thus preventing the reduction of dihydrofolate to tetrahydrofolate, a necessary step in the process of DNA synthesis and cellular replication.

5.2 Pharmacokinetic properties

Methotrexate distributes rapidly following a bolus intravenous injection; its disappearance from the plasma compartment is a triphasic: t½ (alpha) = 0.25-0.7 hour; t½ (beta) = 2.0-3.5 hours; t½ (gamma) = 10-15 hours. The initial plasma half-life value is often obscured because methotrexate is infused over 2 to 12 hour periods.

Methotrexate metabolites account for less than 10% of the total dose if the drug is given intravenously at 30mg/m². The two major metabolites are 2,4-diamino-N^{10}-methylpteroic acid (DAMPA) and 7-hydroxy-methotrexate (7-OH MTX). Both metabolites are biologically inactive. The 7-OH MTH in the kidney tubules may contribute to nephrotoxicity especially with high-dose therapy.

Under conditions of normal renal function, drug clearance from plasma is 103ml/min/m². Young children are able to tolerate considerably more systemic methotrexate, presumably because of improved renal clearance.

Methotrexate is concentrated in the liver and bile, and can reach bile:plasma ratios as high as 200:1. However, the actual amount of methotrexate excreted by this route has been reported to be only 6.3% because most biliary methotrexate is reabsorbed from the GI tract.

With intrathecal administration, the slow rate of release of methotrexate from the CSF is rate controlling, therefore the elimination from the body is delayed. T½ (beta) for methotrexate following intrathecal administration is 5.2-7.8 hours. The terminal elimination phase is greatly prolonged (t½ (gamma) = 52-78 hours).

Methotrexate is distributed mainly in the extracellular spaces but a proportion penetrates cell membranes and is strongly bound to dihydrofolate reductase. About 50% is bound to plasma proteins. Bound methotrexate may be retained in the body for many months.

5.3 Preclinical safety data

There are no other preclinical safety data of relevance to the prescriber apart from those already detailed in the SPC.

6. PHARMACEUTICAL PARTICULARS

6.1 List of excipients

Sodium hydroxide

Sodium chloride

Hydrochloric acid

Water for injection

6.2 Incompatibilities

It is inadvisable to mix fluorouracil and methotrexate. Other drugs should not be mixed with methotrexate in the same infusion container.

6.3 Shelf life

24 months.

Parenteral methotrexate preparations do not contain an antimicrobial preservative. Any unused injection should be discarded.

6.4 Special precautions for storage

Methotrexate preparations should be stored below 25°C and stored in the original package.

6.5 Nature and contents of container

Type I clear glass vial with grey butyl rubber stopper, aluminium ring seal and plastic 'flip-off' cover. Supplied in boxes of 1 vial containing 1, 2, 4, 8, 20, 40 or 200ml.

6.6 Instructions for use and handling

Handling of Cytotoxic drugs

Cytotoxic drugs should only be handled by trained personnel in a designated area. The work surface should be covered with disposable plastic-backed absorbent paper. Protective gloves and goggles should be worn to avoid the drug accidentally coming into contact with the skin or eyes. Methotrexate is not a vesicant and should not cause harm if it comes into contact with the skin. It should of course be washed off with water immediately. Any transient stinging may be treated with bland cream. If there is any danger of systemic absorption of significant quantities of methotrexate, by any route, calcium leucovorin cover should be given.

Cytotoxic preparations should not be handled by pregnant staff.

Any spillage or waste material may be disposed of by incineration. We do not make any specific recommendations with regard to the temperature of the incinerator.

7. MARKETING AUTHORISATION HOLDER

Cyanamid of Great Britain

Fareham Rd

Gosport

Hants PO13 0AS

UK

8. MARKETING AUTHORISATION NUMBER(S)

PL 0095/0016R

9. DATE OF FIRST AUTHORISATION/RENEWAL OF THE AUTHORISATION

18th July 1995

10. DATE OF REVISION OF THE TEXT

19 January 2005

Methotrexate sodium tablets 2.5 mg

(Wyeth Pharmaceuticals)

1. NAME OF THE MEDICINAL PRODUCT

Methotrexate sodium tablets 2.5mg.

2. QUALITATIVE AND QUANTITATIVE COMPOSITION

Methotrexate sodium equivalent to 2.5mg of methotrexate per tablet.

For excipients see 6.1.

3. PHARMACEUTICAL FORM

Tablet.

Round convex, scored, uncoated, yellow tablets embossed '2.5' and 'MI'.

4. CLINICAL PARTICULARS

4.1 Therapeutic indications

The treatment of neoplastic disease. The treatment of severe cases of uncontrolled psoriasis, unresponsive to conventional therapy.

The treatment of adults with severe, active, classical or definite rheumatoid arthritis who are unresponsive or intolerant to conventional therapy.

4.2 Posology and method of administration

Adults and Children

Methotrexate may be given by oral, intramuscular, intravenous (bolus injection or infusion), intrathecal andintra-arterial routes of administration. Dosages are based on the patient's body weight or surface area except in the case of intrathecal administration when a maximum dose of 15mg is recommended. Doses should be reduced in cases of haematological deficiency and hepatic or renal impairment. Larger doses (greater than 100mg) are usually given by intravenous infusion over periods not exceeding 24 hours. Part of the dose may be given in an initial rapid intravenous injection.

Methotrexate has been used with beneficial effects in a wide variety of neoplastic diseases, alone and in combination with other cytotoxic agents, hormones, radiotherapy or surgery. Dosage schedules therefore vary considerably, depending on the clinical use, particularly when intermittent high-dose regimes are followed by the administration of Calcium Leucovorin (calcium folinate) to rescue normal cells from toxic effects.

Examples of doses of Methotrexate that have been used for particular indications are given below.

Choriocarcinoma and other trophoblastic tumours: Non-metastatic gestational trophoblastic neoplasms have been treated successfully with 0.25-1mg/kg up to a maximum of 60mg intramuscularly every 48 hours for four doses, followed by Calcium Leucovorin rescue. This course of treatment is repeated at seven day intervals until levels of urinary chorionic gonadotrophin hormone return to normal. Not less than four courses of treatment are usually necessary. Patients with complications, such as extensive metastases, may be treated with methotrexate in combination with other cytotoxic drugs.

Methotrexate has also been used in similar doses for the treatment of hydatidiform mole and chorio-adenoma destruens.

Leukaemia in children: In acute lymphocytic leukaemia remissions are usually best induced with a combination of corticosteroids and other cytotoxic agents.

Methotrexate 15mg/m², given parenterally or orally once weekly, in combination with other drugs appears to be the treatment of choice for maintenance of drug-induced remissions.

Meningeal leukaemia in children: Doses up to 15mg, intrathecally, at weekly intervals, until the CSF appears normal (usually two to three weeks), have been found useful for the treatment of meningeal leukaemia.

Although intravenous doses of the order of 50mg/m² of methotrexate do not appreciably penetrate the CSF, larger doses of the order of 500mg/m² or greater do produce cytotoxic levels of methotrexate in the CSF. This type of therapy has been used in short courses, followed by administration of Calcium Leucovorin, as initial maintenance therapy to prevent leukaemic invasion of the central nervous system in children with poor prognosis lymphocytic leukaemia.

Lymphoma: Non-Hodgkin's lymphoma, e.g. childhood lymphosarcoma has recently been treated with 3-30mg/kg (approximately 90-900mg/m²) of methotrexate given by intravenous injection and infusion followed by administration of Calcium Leucovorin with the higher doses. Some cases of Burkitt's lymphoma, when treated in the early stages with courses of 15mg/m² daily orally for five days, have shown prolonged remissions. Combination chemotherapy is also commonly used in all stages of the disease.

Breast cancer: Methotrexate, in intravenous doses of 10-60mg/m², is commonly included in cyclical combination regimes with other cytotoxic drugs in the treatment of advanced breast cancer. Similar regimes have also been used as adjuvant therapy in early cases following mastectomy and/or radiotherapy.

Osteogenic sarcoma: The use of methotrexate alone and in cyclical combination regimes has recently been introduced as an adjuvant therapy to the primary treatment of osteogenic sarcoma by amputation with or without prosthetic bone replacement. This has involved the use of intravenous infusions of 20-300mg/kg (approximately 600-9,000mg/m²) of methotrexate followed by Calcium Leucovorin rescue. Methotrexate has also been used as the sole treatment in metastatic cases of osteogenic sarcoma.

Bronchogenic carcinoma: Intravenous infusions of 20-100mg/m² of methotrexate have been included in cyclical combination regimes for the treatment of advanced tumours. High doses with Calcium Leucovorin Rescue have also been employed as the sole treatment.

Head and neck cancer: Intravenous infusions of 240-1,080mg/m² with Calcium Leucovorin rescue have been used both as pre-operative adjuvant therapy and in the treatment of advanced tumours. Intra-arterial infusions of methotrexate have been used in the treatment of head and neck cancers.

Bladder carcinoma: Intravenous injections or infusions of methotrexate in doses up to 100mg every one or two weeks have been used in the treatment of bladder carcinoma with promising results, varying from only symptomatic relief to complete though unsustained regressions. The use of high doses of methotrexate with Calcium Leucovorin Rescue is currently being evaluated.

Psoriasis: It is recommended that a test dose of 5-10mg should be administered, one week prior to therapy to detect idiosyncratic adverse reactions.

In most cases of severe uncontrolled psoriasis, unresponsive to conventional therapy, 10-25mg orally once a week and adjusted by the patient's response is recommended.

The use of methotrexate in psoriasis may permit the return to conventional topical therapy which should be encouraged.

Rheumatoid arthritis: It is recommended that a test dose of 5-10mg should be administered, one week prior to therapy to detect idiosyncratic adverse reactions.

In adults with severe, acute, classical or definite rheumatoid arthritis who are unresponsive or intolerant to conventional therapy, 7.5mg orally once weekly or divided oral doses of 2.5mg at 12 hour intervals for 3 doses (7.5mg) as a course once weekly. The schedule may be adjusted gradually to achieve an optimal response but should not exceed a total weekly dose of 20mg. Once response has been achieved, the schedule should be reduced to the lowest possible effective dose.

Elderly:

Due to diminished hepatic and renal function and decreased folate stores, methotrexate should be used with extreme caution in elderly patients, a reduction in dosage should be considered and these patients should be closely monitored for early signs of toxicity.

Children:

Safety and effectiveness in children have not been established, other than in cancer chemotherapy.

4.3 Contraindications

Profound impairment of renal or hepatic function or haematological impairment.

Alcoholism, liver disease including alcoholic liver disease, fibrosis, cirrhosis, recent or active hepatitis; active infectious disease; and overt or laboratory evidence of immunodeficiency syndrome(s). Pre-existing blood dyscrasias, such as bone marrowhypoplasia, anaemia, leucopenia, or thrombocytopenia. Methotrexate is contra-indicated in pregnant patients. Because of the potential for serious adverse reactions from methotrexate in breast fed infants, breast feeding is contra-indicated in women taking methotrexate.

Patients with a known allergic hypersensitivity to methotrexate or any of theexcipientsin the formulationshould not receive methotrexate.

4.4 Special warnings and special precautions for use

Deaths have been reported with the use of methotrexate in the treatment of malignancy, psoriasis and rheumatoid arthritis. Therefore it should only be used in life threatening neoplastic diseases; or in patients with psoriasis or rheumatoid arthritis with severe, recalcitrant, disabling disease that is not adequately responsive to other forms of therapy.

Methotrexate should be used with extreme caution in patients with haematological depression, renal impairment, peptic ulcer, ulcerative stomatitis, diarrhoea, debility and in young children and the elderly.

Haematologic and gastrointestinal toxicity have been observed in combination with high and low dose methotrexate.

Initiation:

Methotrexate should only be used by clinicians who are familiar with the various characteristics of the drug and its mode of action. Before beginning methotrexate therapy or reinstituting methotrexate after a rest period, a chest x-ray, assessment of renal function, liver function and blood elements should be made by history, physical examination and laboratory tests. Patients undergoing therapy should be subject to appropriate supervision so that signs of possible toxic effects or adverse reactions may be detected and evaluated with minimal delay. Renal function and full blood counts should be closely monitored before, during and after treatment.

Patients with pleural effusions or ascites should have these drained if appropriate before treatment and their plasma methotrexate levels monitored, or treatment should be withdrawn. The reason being that methotrexate exits slowly from third party compartments (e.g. pleural effusions, ascites). This results in a prolonged terminal half-life and unexpected toxicity.

It should be noted that intrathecal doses are transported into the cardiovascular system and may give rise to systemic toxicity. Systemic toxicity of methotrexate may also be enhanced in patients with renal dysfunction, ascites or other effusions due to prolongation of serum half-life.

Monitoring:

It is essential that the following laboratory tests are included regularly (every 2-3 months) in the clinical evaluation and monitoring of patients receiving methotrexate: complete haematological analysis, urinalysis, renal function tests, liver function tests and, when high doses are administered, determination of plasma levels of methotrexate.

It is necessary to monitor patients on methotrexate closely. Methotrexate has the potential for serious toxicity. Toxic effects may be related in frequency and severity to dose or frequency of administration, but has been seen at all doses and can occur at any time during therapy. Most adverse reactions are reversible if detected early. When such reactions do occur, the dosage should be reduced or discontinued and appropriate corrective measures should be taken. If methotrexate therapy is reinstituted, it should be carried out with caution, with adequate consideration of further need for the drug and with increased alertness as to possible recurrence of toxicity.

Hepatic system:

Methotrexate causes hepatotoxicity, liver fibrosis, and cirrhosis, but generally only after prolonged use. Particular attention should be given to the appearance of liver toxicity which may occur without correlative changes in liver function tests. Treatment should not be instituted, or should be discontinued, if any abnormality in liver function tests or liver biopsy is present or develops during therapy. Suchabnormalities should return to normal within two weeks, after which treatment may be recommenced at the discretion of the physician.

Acutely, liver enzyme elevations are frequently seen. These are usually transient and asymptomatic, and do not appear predictive of subsequent hepatic disease. Persistent liver abnormalities and/or decrease of serum albumin may be indicators of serious liver toxicity. Liver biopsy after sustained use often shows histological changes, and fibrosis and cirrhosis have been reported.

In Rheumatoid arthritis:

When to perform a liver biopsy in rheumatoid arthritis patients has not been established either in terms of a cumulative methotrexate dose or duration of therapy.

Renal system:

Methotrexate therapy in patients with impaired renal function should be undertaken with extreme caution, and at reduced dosages because impairment of renal function will decrease methotrexate elimination.

High doses may cause the precipitation of methotrexate or its metabolites in the renal tubules. A high fluid throughput and alkalinisation of the urine to pH 6.5-7.0 by oral or intravenous administration of sodium bicarbonate (5 × 625mg tablets every three hours) or Diamox* (500mg orally four times a day) is recommended as a preventive measure.

Methotrexate may cause renal damage that may lead to acute renal failure. Close attention to renal function including adequate hydration, urine alkalinisation, and measurement of serum methotrexate and renal function are recommended.

Respiratory system:

Acute or chronic interstitial pneumonitis, often associated with blood eosinophilia may occur and deaths have been reported. Symptoms typically include dyspnoea, cough (especially a dry, non-productive cough), fever, chest pain, and hypoxemia for which patients should be monitored at each follow-up visit. Patients should be informed of the risk of pneumonitis and advised to contact their doctor immediately should they develop persistent cough or dyspnoea.

Pulmonary lesions can occur at any time during therapy and have been reported at all dosages, even doses as low as 7.5mg/week. Methotrexate should be withdrawn from patients with pulmonary symptoms and a thorough investigation should be made to exclude infection. If methotrexate induced lung disease is suspected treatment with corticosteroids should be initiated and treatment with methotrexate should not be restarted.

Potentially fatal opportunistic infections, including Pneumocystis carinii pneumonia, may occur with methotrexate therapy. When a patient presents with pulmonary symptoms the possibility of Pneumocystis carinii pneumonia should be considered.

In Rheumatoid arthritis:

Pleuropulmonary manifestation of rheumatoid arthritis and other connective tissue disorders have been reported in the literature. In patients with rheumatoid arthritis, the physician should be specifically alerted to the potential for methotrexate induced adverse effects in the pulmonary system. Patients should be advised to contact their physicians immediately should they develop a cough or dyspnoea.

Gastrointestinal system:

Symptoms of gastro-intestinal toxicity, usually first manifested by diarrhoea and ulcerative stomatitis, indicate interruption of therapy otherwise haemorrhagic enteritis and death from intestinal perforation may occur.

If vomiting resulting in dehydration happens, methotrexate should be discontinued until recovery occurs.

Metabolism and Nutrition:

Folate deficiency states may increase methotrexate toxicity.

Immune system:

Methotrexate has some immunosuppressive activity and therefore the immunological response to concurrent vaccination may be decreased. In addition, concomitant use of a live vaccine could create a severe antigenic reactionand is therefore not generally recommended. There have been reports of disseminated vaccinia infections after smallpox immunisation in patients receiving therapy.

Blood and Lymphatic system:

Methotrexate can suppress haematopoiesis and cause anaemia, aplastic anaemia, pancytopenia, leucopenia, neutropenia and/or thrombocytopenia. Haematopoietic suppression caused by methotrexate may occur abruptly and with apparently safe dosages. In the treatment of neoplastic diseases, methotrexate should be continued only if the potential benefit outweighs the risk of severe myelosuppression. Any profound drop in white-cell or platelet counts should result inimmediate withdrawal of the drug and appropriate supportive therapy. Patients should be advised to report all signs and symptoms suggestive of infection.

Neoplasms Benign and Malignant:

Like other cytotoxic drugs, methotrexate may induce 'tumour lysis syndrome' in patients with rapidly growing tumours. Appropriate supportive and pharmacologic measures may prevent or alleviate this condition.

Malignant lymphomas may occur in patients receiving low dose methotrexate, in which case therapy must be discontinued. Failure of the lymphoma to show signs of spontaneous regression requires the initiation of cytotoxic therapy.

Methotrexate given concomitantly with radiotherapy may increase the risk of soft tissue necrosis and osteonecrosis.

The use of methotrexate high-dose regimens recommended for osteosarcoma requires meticulous care due to the potential for additive or synergistic renal toxicity. High dosage regimens for other neoplastic diseases are investigational and a therapeutic advantage has not been established.

Skin and Subcutaneous tissue:

Severe, occasionally fatal, skin reactions such as Stevens-Johnson Syndrome, toxic epidermal necrolysis (Lyell's syndrome) and erythema multiforme have been reported within days of administering single or multiple doses of methotrexate.

The label will state: " Check dose and frequency – methotrexate is usually given once a week."

4.5 Interaction with other medicinal products and other forms of Interaction

Methotrexate is extensively protein bound and may be displaced by certain drugs such as salicylates, sulphonamides, phenylbutazone, diuretics, hypoglycaemics, diphenylhydantoins, tetracyclines, chloramphenicol, p-aminobenzoic acid, and the acidic anti-inflammatory drugs, so causing a potential for increased toxicity when used concurrently. Concomitant use of other drugs with nephrotoxic potential should generally be avoided unless considered clinically justified, in which case the patient should be closely monitored.

The potential for increased hepatotoxicity when methotrexate is administered with hepatotoxic agents has not been evaluated. However, hepatotoxicity has been reported in such cases. Therefore, combination use of methotrexate and other potential hepatotoxic agents (e.g. alcohol, leflunomide, azathioprine, sulphasalazine, retinoids) should generally be avoided, unless clinically justified, in which case the patient should be closely monitored for possible increased risk of hepatotoxicity.

Enhancement of nephrotoxicity may be seen with high-dose methotrexate is administered in combination with a potentially nephrotoxic chemotherapeutic agent (e.g. cisplatin).

Renal tubular transport is also diminished by probenecid, penicillins and omeprazole, which may result in potentially toxic methotrexate levels. The use of methotrexate with these drugs should be carefully monitored.

NSAIDs should not be administered prior to, or concomitantly with, high dose methotrexate as fatal methotrexate toxicity has been reported. Caution is also advised when NSAIDs and salicylates are administered concomitantly with lower doses of methotrexate. These drugs have been reported to reduce the tubular secretion of methotrexate in an animal model and thereby may enhance its toxicity. It is recommended that methotrexate dosage be carefully controlled during treatment with NSAIDs.

Methotrexate increases the plasma levels of mercaptopurine. Combinations of methotrexate and mercaptopurine may therefore require dose adjustment.

Concomitant administration of folate antagonists, such as co-trimoxazole, have been reported to cause acute megaloblastic pancytopenia in rare instances. Methotrexate should be used with caution in patients taking drugs known to have antifolate potential including nitrous oxide and trimethoprim.

Vitamin preparations containing folic acid or its derivatives may alter response to methotrexate. Folate deficiency states may increase methotrexate toxicity. High doses of leucovorin may reduce the efficacy of intrathecally administered methotrexate.

Existing data suggests that etretinate is formed from acitretin after ingestion of alcoholic beverages. However, the formation of etretinate without concurrent alcohol intake cannot be excluded. Serum levels of methotrexate may be increased by etretinate and severe hepatitis has been reported following concurrent use.

Oral antibiotics, such as tetracycline, chloramphenicol, and non-absorbable broad spectrum antibiotics, may decrease intestinal absorption of methotrexate or interfere with the enterohepatic circulation by inhibiting bowel flora and suppressing metabolism of methotrexate by bacteria.

Methotrexate may decrease the clearance of theophylline; theophylline levels should be monitored when used concurrently with methotrexate.

4.6 Pregnancy and lactation
Methotrexate has been shown to be teratogenic; it has been reported to cause foetal death and/or congenital abnormalities. Therefore, it is not recommended in women of childbearing potential unless the benefits can be expected to outweigh the considered risks. Women of childbearing potential should not be started on methotrexate until pregnancy is excluded. If this drug is used during pregnancy for antineoplastic indications, or if the patient becomes pregnant while taking this drug, the patient should be appraised of the potential hazard to the foetus.

Methotrexate affects spermatogenesis and oogenesis during the period of its administration which may result in decreased fertility. To date, this effect appears to be reversible on discontinuing therapy. Conception should be avoided for at least three months after treatment with methotrexate has ceased. Patients receiving methotrexate and their partners should be advised appropriately.

Pregnancy should be avoided if either the male or female partner is currently receiving, or has at any time in the last three months received methotrexate (see Section 4.4 Special Warnings and Precautions for Use).

Methotrexate has been detected in human breast milk and is contra-indicated during breastfeeding.

4.7 Effects on ability to drive and use machines
Methotrexate can cause dizziness, fatigue, blurred vision and eye-irritation, which may affect the ability to drive or operate machinery.

4.8 Undesirable effects
The most common adverse reactions include ulcerative stomatitis, leucopenia, nausea and abdominal distress. Although very rare, anaphylactic reactions to methotrexate have occurred. Others reported are eye irritation, malaise, undue fatigue, vasculitis, sepsis (including fatal infections), arthralgia/myalgia, chills and fever, dizziness, loss of libido/impotence and decreased resistance to infection. In general, the incidence and severity of side effects are considered to be dose-related.

Opportunistic infections (sometimes fatal e.g. fatal sepsis) have been reported in patients receiving methotrexate therapy for neoplastic and non-neoplastic diseases, Pneumocystic carinii pneumonia being the most common. Other reported infections include pneumonia, nocardiosis, histoplasmosis, cryptococcosis, Herpes zoster, H. simplex hepatitis and disseminated H. simplex and cytmomegalvirus infection, including cytomegaloviral pneumonia.

Conjunctivitis and serious visual changes of unknown etiology have been reported.

Additional reactions related to or attributed to the use of methotrexate such as osteoporosis, stress fractures, nodulosis, lymphoma including reversible lymphomas, tumour lysissyndrome, abnormal (usually "megaloblastic") red cell morphology, precipitation of diabetes, other metabolic changes, anaphylactoid reactionsand sudden death have been reported.

Adverse reactions for the various systems are as follows:

Integument: Stevens-Johnson Syndrome, toxicepidermal necrolysis (Lyell'sSyndrome), erythematous rashes, pruritus, urticaria, photosensitivity, pigmentary changes, alopecia, ecchymosis, telangiectasia, acne, furunculosis, erythemamultiforme. Lesions of psoriasis may be aggravated by concomitant exposure to ultraviolet radiation. Skin ulceration in psoriatic patients and rarely painful erosion of psoriatic plaques have been reported. The recall phenomenon has been reported in both radiation and solar damaged skin.

Haematopoietic: Bone marrow depression is most frequently manifested by leucopenia, but agranulocytosis, thrombocytopenia, anaemia, or any combination may occur. Infection (e.g pneumonia) or septicemia and haemorrhage from various sites may result. Aplastic anaemia, pancytopenia, neutropenia, agranulocytosis, eosinophilia, lymphadenopathy andlymphoproliferative disorders (including reversible) have been reported, as has hypogammaglobulinaemia.

Alimentary System: Mucositis (most frequently stomatitis although gingivitis, pharyngitis and even enteritis, intestinal ulceration and bleeding) may occur. In rare cases the effect of methotrexate on the intestinal mucosa has led to malabsorption or toxic megacolon. Melena, haematemesis, nausea, anorexia and vomiting and/or diarrhoea may also occur.

Hepatic: Hepatic toxicity resulting in significant elevations of liver enzymes, decrease in serum albumin, acute liver atrophy, necrosis, acute hepatitis, fatty metamorphosis, periportal fibrosis or cirrhosis, hepatic failure or death may occur, usually following chronic administration.

Urogenital System: Renal failure and uraemia may follow methotrexate administration, usually in high doses. Vaginitis, vaginal discharge, vaginal ulcers, cystitis, azotemia, dysuria, haematuria, proteinuria and severe nephropathy have also been reported.

Pulmonary System: Acute or chronic interstitial pneumonitis, often associated with blood eosinophilia, may occur and deaths have been reported (see Section 4.4 Warning and Precautions for Use). Acute pulmonary oedema has also been reported after oral and intrathecal use. Pulmonary fibrosis, alveolitis, respiratory failure and chronic interstitialpulmonary disease has been reported. A syndrome consisting of pleuritic pain and pleural thickening has been reported following high doses.

In the treatment of rheumatoid arthritis, methotrexate induced lung disease is a potentially serious adverse drug reaction which may occur acutely at any time during therapy. It is not always fully reversible. Pulmonary symptoms (especially a dry, non productive cough) may require interruption of treatment and careful investigation.

Central Nervous System: Headaches, drowsiness and blurred vision have occurred. Following low doses of methotrexate, transient subtle cognitive dysfunction, mood alteration, or unusual cranial sensations have been reported occasionally. Dysarthria and aphasia, paresis, hemiparesis, and convulsions have also occurred following administration of higher doses.

There have been reports of leucoencephalopathy following intravenous methotrexate in high doses, or low doses following cranial-spinal radiation.

Serious neurotoxicity, frequently manifested as generalised or focal seizures has been reported with unexpectedly increased frequency among paediatric patients with acute lymphoblastic leukaemia who were treated with intermediate-dose intravenous methotrexate (1 gm/m^2).

Symptomatic patients were commonly noted to have leucoencephalopathy and/or microangiopathic calcifications on diagnostic imaging studies. Chronic leucoencephalopathy has also been reported in patients who received repeated doses of high-dose methotrexate with leucovorin rescue even without cranial irradiation. Discontinuation of methotrexate does not always results in complete recovery.

A transient acute neurologic syndrome has been observed in patients treated with high dosage regimens. Manifestations of this neurologic syndrome may include behavioural abnormalities, focal sensorimotor signs, including transient blindness or vision loss, and abnormal reflexes. The exact cause is unknown.

Cardiac: Pericarditis, pericardial effusion, hypotension, and thromboembolic events including arterial thrombosis, cerebral thrombosis, thrombophlebitis, deep vein thrombosis, retinal vein thrombosis and pulmonary embolus.

Adverse reactions following intrathecal methotrexate: These are generally classified into three groups, acute, subacute, and chronic. The acute form is a chemical arachnoiditis manifested by headache, back or shoulder pain, nuchal rigidity, and fever. The subacute form may include paresis, usually transient, paraparesis/paraplegia associated with involvement with one or more spinal nerve roots, nerve palsies, and cerebellar dysfunction. The chronic form is a leucoencephalopathy manifested by irritability, confusion, ataxia, spasticity, occasionally convulsions, dementia, somnolence, coma, and rarely, death. This central nervous system toxicity can be progressive. There is evidence that the combined use of cranial radiation and intrathecal methotrexate increases the incidence of leucoencephalopathy. Signs of neurotoxicity (meningeal irritation, transient or permanent paresis, encephalopathy) should be monitored following intrathecal administration of Methotrexate.

Carcinogenesis, mutagenesis, and impairment of fertility: Animal carcinogenicity studies have demonstrated methotrexate to be free of carcinogenic potential. Although methotrexate has been reported to cause chromosomal damage to animal somatic cells and bone marrow cells in humans, these effects are transient and reversible. In patients treated with methotrexate, evidence is insufficient to permit conclusive evaluation of any increased risk of neoplasia. Methotrexate has been reported to cause impairment of fertility, oligospermia, menstrual dysfunction and amenorrhoea in humans, during and for a short period after cessation.

In addition, methotrexate causes embryotoxicity, abortion and foetal defects in humans and may cause foetal death. Therefore, the possible risks of effects on reproduction should be discussed with patients of child-bearing potential.

4.9 Overdose
In postmarketing experience, overdose with methotrexate has generally occurred with oral and intrathecal administration, although intravenous and intramuscular overdosage has also been reported.

Symptoms of intrathecal overdose are generally CNS symptoms, including headache, nausea and vomiting, seizure or convulsion, and acute toxic encephalopathy. In some cases, no symptoms were reported. There have been reports of death following intrathecal overdose. In these cases, cerebella herniation associated with increased intracranial pressure, and acute toxic encephalopathy have also been reported.

Calcium Leucovorin is the antidote for neutralising the immediate toxic effects of methotrexate on the haematopoietic system. It may be administered orally, intramuscularly, or by an intravenous bolus injection or infusion. In cases of accidental overdosage, a dose of Calcium Leucovorin equal to or higher than the offending dose of methotrexate should be administered within one hour and dosing continued until the serum levels of methotrexate are below 10^{-7}M. Other supporting therapy such as a blood transfusion and renal dialysis may be required. Calcium Leucovorin administration should begin as promptly as possible. As the time interval between methotrexate administration and leucovorin initiation increases the effectiveness of leucovorin in counteracting toxicity decreases. Monitoring of the serum methotrexate concentration is essential in determining the optimal dose and duration of treatment with leucovorin.

In cases of massive overdose, hydration and urinary alkalisation may be necessary to prevent precipitation of methotrexate and/or its metabolites in the renal tubules. Neither haemodialysis nor peritoneal dialysis has been shown to improve methotrexate elimination. Effective clearance of methotrexate has been reported with acute, intermittent haemodialysis using a high flux dialyser.

Following intrathecal overdose, CSF drainage may remove up to 95% of the dose if commenced within 15 minutes of administration, although this falls to 20% after 2 hours. For intrathecal doses over 100mg ventriculolumbar perfusion should accompany CSF drainage. In addition, high dose systemic leucovorin or alkaline diuresis may be required.

There are published case reports of intravenous and intrathecal carboxypeptidase G2 treatment to hasten clearance of methotrexate in cases of overdose.

5. PHARMACOLOGICAL PROPERTIES

5.1 Pharmacodynamic properties
Methotrexate is an antineoplastic agent which acts as an antimetabolite of folic acid. It also has immunosuppressant properties. Within the cell, folic acid is reduced to dihydrofolic and then tetrahydrofolic acid. Methotrexate competitively inhibits the enzyme dihydrofolate reductase and prevents the formation of tetrahydrofolate which is necessary for purine and pyrimidine synthesis and consequently the formation of DNA and RNA.

5.2 Pharmacokinetic properties
Gastro-intestinal absorption is dose-dependent, peak serum concentrations occur 1 to 2 hours after doses below 30mg/m^2 body surface. Higher doses are less well absorbed.

Methotrexate is distributed mainly in the extracellular spaces but a proportion penetrates cell membranes and is strongly bound to dihydrofolate reductase. Only small amounts of methotrexate diffuse into the cerebrospinal fluid but higher concentrations are achieved with higher doses. About 50% is bound to plasma proteins. Biphasic and triphasic clearance form plasma has been reported. The majority of a dose is excreted unchanged in the urine within 24 hours and up to 15% may appear in the bile although because of reabsorption less may be excreted in the faeces. Bound methotrexate may be retained in the body for many months.

5.3 Preclinical safety data
Nothing of note to the prescriber.

6. PHARMACEUTICAL PARTICULARS

6.1 List of excipients
Lactose Monohydrate, Magnesium Stearate and Pregelatinised Starch.

6.2 Incompatibilities
It is inadvisable to mix flurouracil and methotrexate. Other drugs should not be mixed with methotrexate in the same infusion container.

6.3 Shelf life
5 years.

6.4 Special precautions for storage
Do not store above 25°C.

6.5 Nature and contents of container
Polypropylene bottles - 28 or 100 tablets

HDPE bottles - 28 or 100 tablets

PVC/Aluminium blisters - 28 or 30 tablets

6.6 Instructions for use and handling
Cytotoxic drugs should only be handled by trained personnel in a designated area. The work surface should be covered with disposable plastic-backed absorbent paper.

Protective gloves and goggles should be worn to avoid the drug accidentally coming into contact with the skin or eyes.

Methotrexate is not vesicant and should not cause harm if it comes in contact with the skin. It should, of course, be washed off with water immediately. Any transient stinging may be treated with bland cream. If there is any danger of systemic absorption of significant quantities of methotrexate, by any route, Calcium Leucovorin cover should be given.

Cytotoxic preparations should not be handled by pregnant staff.

Any spillage or waste material may be disposed of by incineration. We do not make any specific recommendations with regards to the temperature of the incinerator.

7. MARKETING AUTHORISATION HOLDER
Cyanamid of Great Britain Ltd

154 Fareham Road

Gosport

Hampshire

United Kingdom

PO13 0AS

8. MARKETING AUTHORISATION NUMBER(S)
PL 00095/5079R

9. DATE OF FIRST AUTHORISATION/RENEWAL OF THE AUTHORISATION
27th September 1989

10. DATE OF REVISION OF THE TEXT
27 August 2004

Metopirone Capsules 250 mg

(Alliance Pharmaceuticals)

1. NAME OF THE MEDICINAL PRODUCT
Metopirone® Capsules 250mg

2. QUALITATIVE AND QUANTITATIVE COMPOSITION
Metyrapone BP 250mg.

3. PHARMACEUTICAL FORM
Yellowish-white, oblong, opaque, soft gelatin capsules printed 'CIBA' on one side and 'LN' on the other in brown ink.

4. CLINICAL PARTICULARS

4.1 Therapeutic indications
A diagnostic aid in the differential diagnosis of ACTH-dependent Cushing's syndrome. The management of patients with Cushing's syndrome.

In conjunction with glucocorticosteroids in the treatment of resistant oedema due to increased aldosterone secretion in patients suffering from cirrhosis, nephrosis and congestive heart failure.

4.2 Posology and method of administration
Adults:

The capsules should be taken with milk or after a meal, to minimise nausea and vomiting, which can lead to impaired absorption.

For use as a diagnostic aid: the patient must be hospitalised. Urinary 17-oxygenic steroid excretion is measured over 24 hours on each of 4 consecutive days. The first 2 days serve as a control period. On the third day, 750mg Metopirone (3 capsules) must be given at four-hourly intervals to give a total of 6 doses (ie 4.5g). Maximum urine steroid excretion may occur on the fourth day. If urinary steroid excretion increases in response to Metopirone, this suggests the high levels of circulatory cortisol are due to adrenocortical hyperplasia following excessive ACTH production rather than a cortisol-producing adrenal tumour.

For therapeutic use: for the management of Cushing's syndrome, the dosage must be adjusted to meet the patient's requirements; a daily dosage from 250mg to 6g may be required to restore normal cortisol levels.

For the treatment of resistant oedema: The usual daily dose of 3g (12 capsules) should be given in divided doses in conjunction with a glucocorticoid.

Children: Children should be given a smaller amount based upon 6 four-hourly doses of 15mg/kg, with a minimum dose of 250mg every four hours.

Elderly: Clinical evidence would indicate that no special dosage regimen is necessary.

4.3 Contraindications
Primary adrenocorticol insufficiency. Hypersensitivity to Metopirone or to any of the excipients. Pregnancy.

4.4 Special warnings and special precautions for use
In relation to use as a diagnostic aid: anticonvulsants (eg phenytoin, barbiturates), anti-depressants and neuroleptics (eg amitriptyline, chlorpromazine), hormones that affect the hypothalamo-pituitary axis and anti-thyroid agents may influence the results of the Metopirone test. If these drugs cannot be withdrawn, the necessity of carrying out the Metopirone test should be reviewed.

If adrenocortical or anterior pituitary function is more severely compromised than indicated by the results of the test, Metopirone may trigger transient adrenocortical insufficiency. This can be rapidly corrected by giving appropriate doses of corticosteroids.

Long-term treatment with Metopirone can cause hypertension as the result of excessive secretion of desoxycorticosterone.

The ability of the adrenal cortex to respond to exogenous ACTH should be demonstrated before Metopirone is employed as a test, as Metopirone may induce acute adrenal insufficiency in patients with reduced adrenal secretory capacity, as well as in patients with gross hypopituitarism.

Patients with liver cirrhosis often show a delayed response to Metopirone, due to liver damage delaying the metabolism of cortisol.

In cases of thyroid hypofunction, urinary steroid levels may rise very slowly, or not at all, in response to Metopirone.

4.5 Interaction with other medicinal products and other forms of Interaction
In some cases concomitant medication may affect the results of the Metopirone test (see Section 4.4, Special warnings and precautions for use).

4.6 Pregnancy and lactation
No data are available from animal reproduction studies. Metopirone should not be administered during pregnancy since the drug can impair the biosynthesis of foetal-placental steroids. It is not known whether metyrapone passes into the breast milk, therefore nursing mothers should refrain from breast-feeding their infants during treatment with Metopirone.

4.7 Effects on ability to drive and use machines
Patients should be warned of the potential hazards of driving or operating machinery if they experience side effects such as dizziness and sedation.

4.8 Undesirable effects
Gastrointestinal tract: Occasional: nausea, vomiting. Rare: abdominal pain.

Central nervous system: Occasional: dizziness, sedation, headache.

Cardiovascular system: Occasional: hypotension.

Skin: Rare: allergic skin reactions.

Endocrine system: Rare: hypoadrenalism, hirsutism.

4.9 Overdose
Signs and symptoms: The clinical picture of acute Metopirone poisoning is characterised by gastrointestinal symptoms and acute adrenocortical insufficiency. Laboratory findings: hyponatraemia, hypochloraemia, hyperkalaemia. In patients under treatment with insulin or oral antidiabetics, the signs and symptoms of acute poisoning with Metopirone may be aggravated or modified.

Treatment: There is no specific antidote. Gastric lavage and forced emesis should be employed to reduce the absorption of the drug. In addition to general measures, a large dose of hydrocortisone should be administered at once, together with iv saline and glucose. This should be repeated as necessary in accordance with the patient's clinical condition. For a few days, blood pressure and fluid and electrolyte balance should be monitored.

5. PHARMACOLOGICAL PROPERTIES

5.1 Pharmacodynamic properties
Metopirone inhibits the enzyme responsible for the 11β-hydroxylation stage in the biosynthesis of cortisol and to a lesser extent, aldosterone. The fall in plasma concentration of circulating glucocorticoids stimulates ACTH secretion, via the feedback mechanism which accelerates steroid biosynthesis. As a result, 11-desoxycortisol, the precursor of cortisol, is released into the circulation, metabolised by the liver and excreted in the urine. Unlike cortisol, 11-desoxycortisol does not suppress ACTH secretion and its urinary metabolites may be measured.

These metabolites can easily be determined by measuring urinary 17-hydroxycorticosteroids (17-OHCS) or 17-ketogenic steroids (17-KGS). Metopirone is used as a diagnostic test on the basis of these properties, with plasma 11-desoxycortisol and urinary 17-OHCS measured as an index of pituitary ACTH responsiveness. Metopirone may also suppress biosynthesis of aldosterone, resulting in mild natriuresis.

5.2 Pharmacokinetic properties
Metyrapone is rapidly absorbed and eliminated from the plasma. Peak plasma levels usually occur one hour after ingestion of Metopirone; after a dose of 750mg Metopirone, plasma drug levels average 3.7μg/ml. Plasma drug levels decrease to a mean value of 0.5μg/ml 4 hours after dosing. The half-life of elimination of Metopirone from the plasma is 20 to 26 minutes.

Metyrapol, the reduced form of metyrapone, is the main active metabolite. Eight hours after a single oral dose, the ratio of metyrapone to metyrapol in the plasma is 1:1.5. Metyrapol takes about twice as long as metyrapone to be eliminated in the plasma.

Seventy-two hours after a first daily dose of 4.5g Metopirone (750mg every 4 hours), 5.3% of the total dose was excreted in the urine as metyrapone (9.2% in free form and 90.8% conjugated with glucuronic acid), and 38.5% in the form of metyrapol (8.1% in free form and 91.9% conjugated with glucuronic acid).

5.3 Preclinical safety data
There are no pre-clinical data of relevance to the prescriber which are additional to those already included in other sections of the Summary of Product Characteristics.

6. PHARMACEUTICAL PARTICULARS

6.1 List of excipients
Capsule contents: Glycerin, polyethylene glycol 400, polyethylene glycol 4000 and water. Capsule shell: Sodium ethylparaben, ethyl vanillin, gelatin, glycerin 85%, p-methoxy acetophenone, sodium propylparaben and titanium oxide (E171).

6.2 Incompatibilities
None stated.

6.3 Shelf life
5 years

6.4 Special precautions for storage
Protect from moisture and heat. Store below 30°C.

6.5 Nature and contents of container
High density polyethylene bottles of 100 capsules.

6.6 Instructions for use and handling
None stated.

Administrative Details

7. MARKETING AUTHORISATION HOLDER
Alliance Pharmaceuticals Ltd
Avonbridge House
Bath Road
Chippenham
Wiltshire
SN15 2BB

8. MARKETING AUTHORISATION NUMBER(S)
PL16853/0010

9. DATE OF FIRST AUTHORISATION/RENEWAL OF THE AUTHORISATION
June 1998

10. DATE OF REVISION OF THE TEXT
February 2005

11. Legal status
POM

Alliance, Alliance Pharmaceuticals and associated devices are registered Trademarks of Alliance Pharmaceuticals Ltd.

Metrogel

(Galderma (U.K.) Ltd)

1. NAME OF THE MEDICINAL PRODUCT
Metrogel

2. QUALITATIVE AND QUANTITATIVE COMPOSITION
Metronidazole BP 0.75%.

3. PHARMACEUTICAL FORM
Aqueous gel for cutaneous use.

4. CLINICAL PARTICULARS

4.1 Therapeutic indications
For the treatment of acute inflammatory exacerbation of rosacea.

For the deodorisation of the smell associated with malodorous fungating tumours.

4.2 Posology and method of administration
For the treatment of rosacea:

Adults and elderly:

Apply to the affected skin of the face in a thin film twice daily for a period of eight to nine weeks. Thereafter, further applications may be necessary depending upon the severity of the condition.

Children:

Not recommended.

For the deodorisation of malodorous fungating tumours:

Adults and elderly:

Clean the wound thoroughly. Apply the gel over the complete area and cover with a non-adherent dressing. Use once or twice daily as necessary.

Children:

Not recommended.

4.3 Contraindications
Contraindicated in individuals with a history of hypersensitivity to Metronidazole, or other ingredients of the formulation.

4.4 Special warnings and special precautions for use
Metrogel has been reported to cause lacrimation of the eyes, therefore, contact with the eyes should be avoided. If a reaction suggesting local irritation occurs patients should be directed to use the medication less frequently, discontinue use temporarily or discontinue use until further instructions. Metronidazole is a nitroimidazole and should be used with care in patients with evidence of, or history of, blood dyscrasia. Exposure of treated sites to ultraviolet or strong sunlight should be avoided during use of metronidazole.

Unnecessary and prolonged use of this medication should be avoided.

4.5 Interaction with other medicinal products and other forms of Interaction
Interaction with systemic medication is unlikely because absorption of metronidazole following cutaneous application of Metrogel is low. Oral metronidazole has been reported to potentiate the effect of warfarin and other coumarin anticoagulants, resulting in a prolongation of prothrombin time. The effect of topical metronidazole on prothrombin is not known. However, very rare cases of modification of the INR values have been reported with concomitant use of Metrogel and coumarin anticoagulants.

4.6 Pregnancy and lactation
The safety of metronidazole in pregnancy and lactation had not been adequately established. The gel should therefore not be used in these circumstances unless the physician

considers it essential. Medication should be stopped if pregnancy occurs.

4.7 Effects on ability to drive and use machines
None.

4.8 Undesirable effects
Because of the minimal absorption of metronidazole and consequently its insignificant plasma concentration after topical administration, the adverse experiences reported with the oral form of the drug have not been reported with Metrogel. Adverse reactions reported with Metrogel have been only local and mild, and include skin discomfort (burning and stinging), erythema, pruritis, skin irritation, worsening of rosacea, nausea, metallic taste and tingling or numbness of the extremities, and watery eyes if applied too closely to this area.

4.9 Overdose
No data exists about overdosage in humans. Acute oral toxicity studies with a topical gel formulation containing 0.75% w/w metronidazole in rats have shown no toxic action with doses of up to 5 g of finished product per kilogram body weight, the highest dose used. This dose is equivalent to the oral intake of 12 tubes of 30g packaging Metrogel for an adult weighing 72 kg, and 2 tubes of Metrogel for a child weighing 12 kg.

5. PHARMACOLOGICAL PROPERTIES

5.1 Pharmacodynamic properties
The etiology of rosacea is unknown although a variety of hypotheses have been reported.

5.2 Pharmacokinetic properties
The systemic concentration of Metronidazole following the topical administration of 1 g of a 0.75% Metronidazole gel to 10 patients with rosacea ranged from 25 ng/ml (limit of detection), to 66 mg/ml with a mean Cmax of 40.6 ng/ml.

The corresponding mean Cmax following the oral administration of a solution containing 30 mg of metronidazole was 850 ng/ml (equivalent to 212 ng/ml if dose corrected. The mean Tmax for the topical formulation was 6.0 hours compared to 0.97 hours for the oral solution.

5.3 Preclinical safety data
Metronidazole is a well established pharmaceutical active ingredient and to the subject of pharmacopoeial monograph in both the BP and Ph.Eur.

6. PHARMACEUTICAL PARTICULARS

6.1 List of excipients
Bronopol BP,

Hydroxybenzoic acid esters HSE,

Hydroxyethylcellulose HSE,

Propylene glycol Ph.Eur,

Phosphoric acid Ph.Eur,

Purified water Ph.Eur.

6.2 Incompatibilities
None known

6.3 Shelf life
2 years.

6.4 Special precautions for storage
Store between 15°C and 25°C in a dry place.

6.5 Nature and contents of container
Tube: Internally lacquered, membrane sealed aluminium.

Cap: low density polyethylene

Pack sizes available: 25 g and 40 g.

6.6 Instructions for use and handling
There are no special instructions for use/handling.

7. MARKETING AUTHORISATION HOLDER
Galderma (UK) Limited

Galderma House

Church Lane

Kings Langley

Herts WD4 8JP

England

Distributed by Novartis Pharmaceuticals UK Limited (T/A Sandoz Pharmaceuticals)

Frimley Business Park

Frimley

Camberley

Surrey GU16 5SG

8. MARKETING AUTHORISATION NUMBER(S)
PL 10590/0035

9. DATE OF FIRST AUTHORISATION/RENEWAL OF THE AUTHORISATION
27 February 1998

10. DATE OF REVISION OF THE TEXT
May 2004

11. Legal category
POM

Metrotop

(Medlock Medical Ltd)

1. NAME OF THE MEDICINAL PRODUCT
Metrotop.

2. QUALITATIVE AND QUANTITATIVE COMPOSITION
Metronidazole BP 0.8% w/v.

3. PHARMACEUTICAL FORM
A colourless aqueous gel.

4. CLINICAL PARTICULARS

4.1 Therapeutic indications
For the treatment of malodorous fungating tumours, gravitational ulcers and decubitus ulcers (pressure sores).

4.2 Posology and method of administration
For external use only. Adults: All wounds should be cleaned thoroughly. Flat wounds require a liberal application of the gel over the complete area. Cavities should be loosely packed with paraffin gauze which has been smeared in the gel. All wounds should be covered with a non-adherent dressing and a pad of lint or gauze. Sticking may occur if the appropriate dressing is not used. Use once or twice daily as necessary. Elderly: No specific instructions. Children: Where necessary, instructions apply as for adults.

4.3 Contraindications
Known hypersensitivity to metronidazole.

4.4 Special warnings and special precautions for use
The following statements take into account the possibility that metronidazole may be absorbed after topical application. However, there is no evidence of any significant systemic concentrations of metronidazole following topical applications. Peripheral neuropathy has been reported in association with prolonged use of metronidazole. The elimination half-life of metronidazole remains unchanged in the presence of renal failure. Such patients, however, retain the metabolite of metronidazole. The clinical significance of this is not known at present. However, in patients undergoing dialysis, metronidazole and metabolites are efficiently removed.

4.5 Interaction with other medicinal products and other forms of Interaction
Some potentiation of anticoagulant therapy has been reported when metronidazole has been used with the warfarin type oral anticoagulants. Patients receiving phenobarbitone metabolise metronidazole at a much faster rate than normal, reducing the half-life to approximately 3 hours. Patients are advised not to take alcohol during systemic metronidazole therapy because of the possibility of a disulfiram-like reaction.

4.6 Pregnancy and lactation
There is inadequate evidence of the use of metronidazole in pregnancy. Metronidazole gel cannot therefore be recommended during pregnancy or lactation where significant systemic absorption may occur unless the physician considers it essential.

4.7 Effects on ability to drive and use machines
None known.

4.8 Undesirable effects
No adverse effects have been reported. Systemic metronidazole therapy may occasionally cause an unpleasant taste in the mouth, furred tongue, nausea, vomiting, gastrointestinal disturbance, urticaria, angioedema and anaphylaxis. Drowsiness, dizziness, headache, ataxia, skin rash, pruritus, and darkening of the urine have been reported, but rarely.

4.9 Overdose
There is no specific treatment for gross overdosage of metronidazole. Gastric lavage is recommended in cases of accidental ingestion. Uneventful recovery has followed overdosage of up to 12g taken orally. Metronidazole is readily removed from the plasma by dialysis.

5. PHARMACOLOGICAL PROPERTIES

5.1 Pharmacodynamic properties
Metronidazole is a potent agent against the anaerobic bacteria which are believed to produce odorous metabolites as a result of localised tissue colonisation. The aim of the product is to provide a high concentration of metronidazole at and around the site of colonisation in a water-miscible base. This form allows surface spread and penetration within the wound accompanied by ease of aseptic application and up to 24 hours duration of action.

5.2 Pharmacokinetic properties
There is presently no evidence of any systemic concentrations of metronidazole following topical application.

5.3 Preclinical safety data
No further data given.

6. PHARMACEUTICAL PARTICULARS

6.1 List of excipients
Hypromellose (4500); benzalkonium chloride solution; purified water.

6.2 Incompatibilities
None known.

6.3 Shelf life
The shelf life shall not exceed 24 months from the date of manufacture.

6.4 Special precautions for storage
Do not store above 25°C. Once opened the contents should be used within 28 days of opening.

6.5 Nature and contents of container
Polypropylene tubes each fitted with a plastic screw cap and tamper-evident seal and enclosed within a printed cardboard carton. Single tubes may sometimes be supplied without a carton. Pack sizes: The 15g, 30g and 60g tubes are available singly or in boxes of 12.

6.6 Instructions for use and handling
None given.

7. MARKETING AUTHORISATION HOLDER
Medlock Medical Limited, Tubiton House, Medlock Street, Oldham, OL1 3HS.

8. MARKETING AUTHORISATION NUMBER(S)
PL 21248/0040.

9. DATE OF FIRST AUTHORISATION/RENEWAL OF THE AUTHORISATION
16th September 2005.

10. DATE OF REVISION OF THE TEXT
September 2005.

Metvix 160 mg/g cream

(Galderma (U.K.) Ltd)

1. NAME OF THE MEDICINAL PRODUCT
Metvix 160 mg/g cream ▼

2. QUALITATIVE AND QUANTITATIVE COMPOSITION
Metvix cream contains 160 mg/g of methyl aminolevulinate (as hydrochloride) equivalent to 16.0% of methyl aminolevulinate (as hydrochloride).

For excipients, see 6.1.

3. PHARMACEUTICAL FORM
Cream.

The colour is cream to pale yellow.

4. CLINICAL PARTICULARS

4.1 Therapeutic indications
Treatment of thin or non-hyperkeratotic and non-pigmented actinic keratoses on the face and scalp when other therapies are considered less appropriate.

Only for treatment of superficial and/or nodular basal cell carcinoma unsuitable for other available therapies due to possible treatment related morbidity and poor cosmetic outcome; such as lesions on the mid-face or ears, lesions on severely sun damaged skin, large lesions, or recurrent lesions.

4.2 Posology and method of administration
Adults (including the elderly)

For treatment of actinic keratoses (AK) one session of photodynamic therapy should be administered. Treated lesions should be evaluated after three months and if needed be repeated with a second therapy session. For treatment of basal cell carcinoma (BCC) two sessions should be administered with an interval of one week between sessions. Before applying Metvix cream, the surface of AK and superficial BCC lesions should be prepared to remove scales and crusts and roughen the surface of the lesions. Nodular BCC lesions are often covered by an intact epidermal keratin layer which should be removed. Exposed tumour material should be removed gently without any attempt to excise beyond the tumour margins.

Apply a layer of Metvix cream (about 1 mm thick) by using a spatula to the lesion and the surrounding 5-10 mm of normal skin. Cover the treated area with an occlusive dressing for 3 hours.

Remove the dressing, and clean the area with saline and immediately expose the lesion to red light with a continuous spectrum of 570-670 nm and a total light dose of 75 J/cm^2 at the lesion surface. Red light with a narrower spectrum giving the same activation of accumulated porphyrins may be used. The light intensity at the lesion surface should not exceed 200 mW/cm^2.

Only CE marked lamps should be used, equipped with necessary filters and/or reflecting mirrors to minimize exposure to heat, blue light and UV radiation. It is important to ensure that the correct light dose is administered. The light dose is determined by factors such as the size of the light field, the distance between lamp and skin surface and illumination time. These factors vary with lamp type, and the lamp should be used according to the user manual. The light dose delivered should be monitored if a suitable detector is available.

Patient and operator should adhere to safety instructions provided with the light source. During illumination patient and operator should wear protective goggles which correspond to the lamp light spectrum.

Healthy untreated skin surrounding the lesion does not need to be protected during illumination.

Multiple lesions may be treated during the same treatment session. Lesion response should be assessed after three months, and it is recommended to confirm the response of BCC lesions by histological biopsy. At this response evaluation, AK and BCC lesion sites that show non-complete response may be retreated if desired.

Children and adolescents:

There is no experience of treating patients below the age of 18 years.

4.3 Contraindications
Hypersensitivity to the active substance or to any of the excipients which includes arachis oil.

Morpheaform basal cell carcinoma.

Porphyria.

4.4 Special warnings and special precautions for use
Metvix should only be administered in the presence of a physician, a nurse or other health care professionals trained in the use of photodynamic therapy with Metvix.

Metvix is not recommended during pregnancy (see 4.6).

There is no experience of treating pigmented or highly infiltrating lesions with Metvix cream. Thick (hyperkeratotic) actinic keratoses should not be treated with Metvix.

Methyl aminolevulinate may cause sensitization by skin contact. The excipient cetostearyl alcohol may cause local skin reactions (e.g. contact dermatitis), methyl- and propylparahydroxybenzoate (E218, E216) may cause allergic reactions (possibly delayed).

Any UV-therapy should be discontinued before treatment. As a general precaution, sun exposure on the treated lesion sites and surrounding skin has to be avoided for a couple of days following treatment.

Direct eye contact with Metvix cream should be avoided.

4.5 Interaction with other medicinal products and other forms of Interaction
No specific interaction studies have been performed with methyl aminolevulinate.

4.6 Pregnancy and lactation
Pregnancy

For methyl aminolevulinate, no clinical data on exposed pregnancies are available. Reproductive toxicity studies in animals have not been performed. Metvix is not recommended during pregnancy (see 4.4).

Lactation

The amount of methyl aminolevulinate excreted into human breast milk following topical administration of Metvix cream is not known. In the absence of clinical experience, breast-feeding should be discontinued for 48 hours after application of Metvix cream.

4.7 Effects on ability to drive and use machines
Not applicable.

4.8 Undesirable effects
Between 60 % and 80% of patients in clinical trials experienced reactions localised to the treatment site that are attributable to toxic effects of the photodynamic therapy (phototoxicity) or to preparation of the lesion. The most frequent symptoms are painful skin sensations. The severity is usually mild or moderate, but rarely, it may require early termination of illumination. Typically it begins at the time of illumination or soon after and lasts for a few hours, generally resolving on the day of treatment. Other frequent signs of phototoxicity are erythema and oedema which may persist for 1 to 2 weeks or occasionally for longer. In two cases they persisted for more than one year. The incidence of local adverse reactions is shown in the table below.

Skin and appendages disorders	Very common (>1/10)	Pain and discomfort described as pain, burning, warm, stinging, pricking and tingling skin, erythema, itching, oedema
	Common (>1/100, <1/10)	Crusting, ulceration, blisters, suppuration, infection peeling, application site reactions, bleeding skin, hypo/hyperpigmentation
	Uncommon (>1/1000 <1/100)	Rash, urticaria, eczema

Uncommon (<1%) non-local adverse events are headache, nausea, eye pain, eye irritation, fatigue and dizziness. There were isolated reports of scar where a relationship to treatment was uncertain.

Repeated use did not increase the frequency or intensity of the local phototoxic reactions.

4.9 Overdose
The severity of local phototoxic reactions such as erythema, pain and burning sensation may increase in case of prolonged application time or very high light intensity.

5. PHARMACOLOGICAL PROPERTIES

5.1 Pharmacodynamic properties
Pharmacotherapeutic group:

Antineoplastic agent, ATC Code: L01X D03

Mechanism of Action:

After topical application of methyl aminolevulinate, porphyrins will accumulate intracellularly in the treated skin lesions. The intracellular porphyrins (including PpIX) are phtoactive, fluorescing compounds and, upon light activation in the presence of oxygen, singlet oxygen is formed which causes damage to cellular compartments, in particular the mitochonidria. Light activation of accumulated porphyrins leads to a photochemical reaction and thereby phototoxicity to the light-exposed target cells.

Efficacy and safety has been investigated in studies for up to 3-6 months for actinic keratosis and up to 12 months for basal cell carcinoma. Experience of long term efficacy is limited.

5.2 Pharmacokinetic properties
In vitro dermal absorption of radiolabelled methyl aminolevulinate applied to human skin has been studied. After 24 hours the mean cumulative absorption through human skin was 0.26 % of the administered dose. A skin depot containing 4.9 % of the dose was formed. No corresponding studies in human skin with damage similar to actinic keratosis lesions and additionally roughened surface or without stratum corneum were performed.

In humans, a higher degree of accumulation of porphyrins in lesions compared to normal skin has been demonstrated with Metvix cream. After application of the cream for 3 hours and subsequent illumination with non-coherent light of 570-670 nm wavelength and a total light dose of 75 J/cm^2, complete photobleaching occurs with levels of porphyrins returning to pre-treatment values.

5.3 Preclinical safety data
Preclinical studies on general toxicity and genotoxicity studies in the presence or absence of photoactivation, do not indicate potential risks for man. Carcinogenicity studies or studies on the reproductive function have not been performed with methyl aminolevulinate.

6. PHARMACEUTICAL PARTICULARS

6.1 List of excipients
Self-emulsifying glyceryl monostearate

cetostearyl alcohol

poloxyl 40 stearate

methyl parahydroxybenzoate

propyl parahydroxybenzoate

disodium edetate

glycerol

white soft paraffin

cholesterol

isopropyl myristate

arachis oil

refined almond oil

oleyl alcohol

purified water.

6.2 Incompatibilities
Not applicable.

6.3 Shelf life
1 year.

1 week after first opening of the container.

6.4 Special precautions for storage
Store at 2 °C - 8 °C (in a refrigerator).

6.5 Nature and contents of container
Aluminium tube with internal protective lacquer and a latex seal. Screw cap of HDPE.

Metvix cream is supplied in a tube containing 2 g cream.

6.6 Instructions for use and handling
No special requirements.

7. MARKETING AUTHORISATION HOLDER
Galderma (UK) Ltd.

Galderma House

Church Lane

Kings Langley

Hertfordshire WD4 8JP

United Kingdom

8. MARKETING AUTHORISATION NUMBER(S)
PL 10590/0048 & PA 590/20/1

9. DATE OF FIRST AUTHORISATION/RENEWAL OF THE AUTHORISATION
17th May 2002

10. DATE OF REVISION OF THE TEXT

Mexitil Ampoules

(Boehringer Ingelheim Limited)

1. NAME OF THE MEDICINAL PRODUCT
Mexitil Ampoules.

2. QUALITATIVE AND QUANTITATIVE COMPOSITION
Colourless, glass, ampoules containing 250 mg mexiletine hydrochloride (equivalent to 207.7 mg of mexiletine) in 10 ml of solution.

3. PHARMACEUTICAL FORM
Ampoules for intravenous injection.

4. CLINICAL PARTICULARS

4.1 Therapeutic indications
For the treatment of ventricular arrhythmias which are considered as life-threatening by the physician.

Note: In deciding about the use of Mexitil it should be borne in mind that no anti-arrhythmic agents of Vaughan Williams classification 1 used in the long-term treatment of arrhythmias has been shown to prolong life.

4.2 Posology and method of administration
Plasma elimination half-life may be prolonged in moderate to severe hepatic disease, and in patients with creatinine clearance of less than 10 ml/min: individual dose titration is advised in these conditions.

1 Intravenous Mexitil

Mexitil should never be injected in bolus form.

(a) Loading Dose

IV injection of 4 - 10 ml (100 - 250 mg) Mexitil given at a suggested rate of 1 ml per minute (25 mg per minute). THEN

Add 500 mg (2 ampoules) Mexitil to 500 ml of a suitable infusion solution. Administer the first 250 ml by IV infusion over 1 hour (4 ml per minute). THEN

Administer the second 250 ml by IV infusion over 2 hours (2 ml per minute).

(b) Maintenance Dose

Add 250 mg (1 ampoule) Mexitil to 500 ml of suitable infusion solution. Administer at a suggested rate of 1 ml per minute (0.5 mg per minute), according to patient response. Continue for as long as required or until oral maintenance therapy is commenced.

2 Alternative Loading Dose Regimes

(a) Combination IV Mexitil and Oral Mexitil Loading Dose

IV injection of 8 ml (200 mg) Mexitil given at a suggested rate of 1 ml per minute. On completion of injection or infusion give 400 mg Mexitil orally.

(b) Maintenance Dose

As in 1(b) above.

3 Change over from IV to Oral Mexitil Maintenance

(a) From IV to Capsules

On discontinuing the IV infusion, commence the maintenance dose. The first capsule should be taken at, or shortly before, the end of the infusion. (An oral loading dose should not be given).

(b) From IV to Perlongets

One to two hours before the end of the infusion commence the oral maintenance therapy. (An oral loading dose should not be given).

Notes:

1 The loading dose regime is designed to compensate for the rapid phase of tissue distribution, which occurs especially with IV loading.

2 Side-effects are more likely to be encountered during the initial tissue loading phase, in which case the rate of infusion should be reduced.

3 If the optimum therapeutic affect is not achieved, the rate of infusion or oral dosage may be increased, side-effects permitting.

4 When mexiletine therapy is commenced, patients should be monitored closely (e.g. ECG, blood pressure and routine laboratory tests) over a period of at least 24 hours, and dosage adjustment made on the basis of this. Monitoring is particularly recommended in the following situations: sinus node dysfunction, conduction defects, bradycardia, hypotension or cardiac, renal or hepatic failure. There may be potentiation of tremor in patients with parkinsonism.

Regular monitoring of cardiac function throughout treatment is advisable.

The duration of treatment required in any patient is of necessity variable, and although no precise guide can be given, withdrawal may be attempted after a suitable period free of arrhythmia. Gradual withdrawal i.e. over 1 - 2 weeks, is preferable as arrhythmias which have been satisfactorily controlled may recur.

No specific information on the use of this product in the elderly or children is available. Clinical trials have included patients over 65 years and no adverse reactions specific to this age group have been reported.

Mexitil solution for injection is known to be compatible with the following infusion solutions: sodium chloride 0.9 %, sodium chloride 0.9 % with potassium chloride 0.3 % or

0.6 %, dextrose 5 %, sodium bicarbonate, sodium lactate (M/6).

Diluted Mexitil should not be stored for longer than 8 hours.

4.3 Contraindications

Mexitil should not be used in the first three months following myocardial infarction or where cardiac output is limited (left ventricular ejection fraction of less than 35 %), except in patients with life-threatening ventricular arrhythmias.

Mexitil is contraindicated in the presence of cardiogenic shock or pre-existing second- or third- degree AV block if no pacemaker is present.

Hypersensitivity to mexiletine or local anaesthetics e.g. lidocaine (lignocaine).

4.4 Special warnings and special precautions for use

(i) If the drug is used in the following situations, the patient should be carefully monitored and the dosage may need to be reduced: sinus node dysfunction, conduction defect, bradycardia, hypotension or cardiac failure.

(ii) Plasma elimination half-life may be prolonged in moderate to severe hepatic disease, and in patients with creatinine clearance of less than 10 ml/min: individual dose titration is advised in these conditions.

(iii) Patients in whom pathologically high liver values have been established or who have signs or symptoms of impaired liver function, should be monitored carefully.

4.5 Interaction with other medicinal products and other forms of Interaction

(i) Where there is concurrent administration of Mexitil and some other anti-arrhythmic drugs, an increased effect on conduction and pumping of the heart is to be expected. Mexitil may be used concurrently with the cardiovascular drugs digoxin, amiodarone, quinidine and beta-adrenergic blocking agents.

(ii) Since Mexitil is metabolised mainly in the liver, substances that influence liver enzyme function may alter the concentration of Mexitil in the blood. In particular, interactions with the two cytochrome P450 isozymes CYP1A2 and CYP2D6 have to be considered. It may be necessary to reduce the dose of Mexitil in cases of concomitant administration of substances that lead to enzyme inhibition in the liver.

In cases of concurrent therapy with substances that lead to enzyme induction, it may be necessary to increase the dose of Mexitil since it is metabolised at a faster rate.

(iii) Concurrent administration of mexiletine may increase plasma levels of theophylline and caffeine.

(iv) Drugs which markedly acidify or alkalise urine, should be avoided because they may enhance or reduce (respectively) the rate of drug excretion, and correspondingly affect the plasma concentration of mexiletine.

(v) Concomitant administration of Mexitil with warfarin may increase the risk of bleeding.

(vi) Local anaesthetic toxicity may occur in patients who receive Mexitil and local anaesthetic agents concurrently.

4.6 Pregnancy and lactation

Mexiletine freely crosses the placenta. Therefore, Mexitil should only be used in pregnancy if the potential benefit justifies the potential risk.

Mexiletine appears in breast milk in concentrations which may have an effect on the infant. Therefore, if the use of Mexitil is deemed essential for the mother, an alternative method of infant feeding should be considered.

4.7 Effects on ability to drive and use machines

Mexitil may impair the ability to drive or operate machinery, especially when taken in combination with alcohol.

4.8 Undesirable effects

Side-effects are mainly related to blood concentration and may, therefore be seen during the initial phases of both IV and oral treatment when fluctuation may occur before the blood and tissue concentrations reach equilibrium. Reducing the rate of injection of infusion or delaying the next oral dose allows the blood concentration to fall and usually reduces side-effects. Generally side-effects are of five types:

Gastrointestinal Nausea, vomiting, indigestion, constipation, diarrhoea, dry mouth, unpleasant taste, hiccoughs. Oesophageal ulceration may occur if oral Mexitil is swallowed without adequate liquid and is lodged in the oesophagus.

Central nervous system Drowsiness, dizziness, diplopia, blurred vision, nystagmus, dysarthria, ataxia, tremor, paraesthesiae, convulsion, psychiatric disorders, confusional state, insomnia.

Cardiovascular Hypotension, sinus bradycardia, atrial fibrillation, palpitation and conduction defects. Exacerbation of arrhythmias, pre-existing heart failure and torsade de pointes.

When hypotension has occurred this has tended to be in patients with severe illness who have already been given a variety of anti-arrhythmic or other preparations and, if associated with bradycardia, may be reduced by the use of atropine.

Pulmonary infiltrates, interstitial lung disease and pulmonary fibrosis have been observed in isolated cases.

Haematological Rash, arthralgia, fever, thrombocytopenia and appearance of positive but symptomless antinuclear factor titres. Leucopenia has been observed rarely. Rare cases of Stevens-Johnson Syndrome, some with liver involvement, have been reported in Japan. Isolated cases of erythroderma have also been reported.

Hepatic Liver damage has been observed following Mexitil administration; jaundice has been reported.

4.9 Overdose

The minimum fatal dose is unknown but 4.40g proved fatal in a healthy young adult.

The clinical features include nausea, vomiting, drowsiness, confusion, ataxia and convulsions. Blurred vision and paraesthesiae have also been reported. Hypotension, sinus bradycardia, atrial fibrillation and cardiac arrest are more specific effects.

Therapy:

General symptomatic treatment is advisable.

Arrhythmias should be treated as appropriate and intravenous diazepam may be useful to control convulsions. In the event of serious bradycardia and hypotension, it is advisable to first administer an IV dose of 0.5 - 1.0 mg atropine.

Acidification of the urine enhances the rate of drug elimination and so may be useful.

5. PHARMACOLOGICAL PROPERTIES

5.1 Pharmacodynamic properties

Mexitil (mexiletine hydrochloride) is a Class 1b anti-arrhythmic agent based on the Vaughan Williams classification with local anaesthetic properties, similar in structure and activity to lidocaine (lignocaine). Mexiletine depresses the maximum rate of depolarisation with little or no modification of resting potentials or the duration of action potentials.

5.2 Pharmacokinetic properties

Mexiletine is metabolised in the liver to a number of metabolites. It is excreted in the urine, mainly in the form of its metabolites with a small proportion of unchanged mexiletine; the clearance of mexiletine is increased in acid urine. Mexiletine is widely distributed throughout the body and is about 50-70 % bound to plasma proteins. It has a plasma half life of 5-17 hours in healthy subjects but this may be prolonged in patients with heart disease.

5.3 Preclinical safety data

There are no additional preclinical data of help to the prescriber.

6. PHARMACEUTICAL PARTICULARS

6.1 List of excipients

Sodium chloride

Water for Injection

6.2 Incompatibilities

None stated

6.3 Shelf life

The ampoules have a shelf life expiry date of 5 years from the date of manufacture. Diluted Mexitil should be discarded after 8 hours.

6.4 Special precautions for storage

Store below 25 °C. Protect from light.

6.5 Nature and contents of container

Cartons containing 5 × 10 ml colourless glass ampoules.

6.6 Instructions for use and handling

None stated.

7. MARKETING AUTHORISATION HOLDER

Boehringer Ingelheim Limited, Ellesfield Avenue, Bracknell, Berkshire, RG12 8YS, United Kingdom.

8. MARKETING AUTHORISATION NUMBER(S)

PL 00015/0065R

9. DATE OF FIRST AUTHORISATION/RENEWAL OF THE AUTHORISATION

05.06.85 / 24.04.97

10. DATE OF REVISION OF THE TEXT

October 1999.

11. Legal category

POM

Ref: M4a/UK/SPC/2

Mexitil Capsules 200mg

(Boehringer Ingelheim Limited)

1. NAME OF THE MEDICINAL PRODUCT

Mexitil Capsules 200 mg

2. QUALITATIVE AND QUANTITATIVE COMPOSITION

Red hard gelatin capsules containing mexiletine hydrochloride 200 mg (equivalent to mexiletine base 166.2 mg).

3. PHARMACEUTICAL FORM

Capsules for oral administration.

4. CLINICAL PARTICULARS

4.1 Therapeutic indications

For the treatment of ventricular arrhythmias which are considered as life-threatening by the physician.

Note:

In deciding about the use of Mexitil it should be borne in mind that no anti-arrhythmic agents of Vaughan Williams classification 1 used in the long-term treatment of arrhythmias has been shown to prolong life.

4.2 Posology and method of administration

Plasma elimination half-life may be prolonged in moderate to severe hepatic disease, and in patients with a creatinine clearance of less than 10 ml/min; individual dose titration is advised in these conditions.

The dosage of Mexitil must be individualised on the basis of response and tolerance, both of which are dose related.

(a) Capsules should be swallowed whole with ample liquid, preferably with the patient in an upright position. It is advisable to take Mexitil after food.

(i) *Loading dose:* Initially, if more rapidly effective blood levels are required, a loading dose, usually 400 mg may be desirable.

(ii) *Maintenance dose:* Give 200-250 mg Mexitil three to four times daily. Commencing 2 hours after the loading dose. The usual daily dose is between 600-800 mg in divided doses; optimal doses range from 300-1200 mg daily in divided doses.

NOTE: Mexitil is absorbed in the upper part of the small intestine. In acute myocardial infarction and particularly when opiates have been given, rate of absorption but not bioavailability may be delayed and therefore, a larger loading dose e.g. 600 mg may be preferable.

(b) **Alternative loading dose regimes**

(i) Combination IV Mexitil and oral Mexitil loading dose: IV injection of 8 ml (200 mg) Mexitil given at a suggested rate of 1 ml per minute. On completion of injection or infusion give 400 mg Mexitil orally.

Maintenance dose: As in (aii).

(ii) Combination IV lidocaine (lignocaine) and oral Mexitil loading dose: Give IV lidocaine (lignocaine) according to manufacturer's instructions. On completion of injection give 400 mg Mexitil orally.

Maintenance dose: As in (aii).

(c) **Change over from IV to oral maintenance:**

On discontinuing the IV infusion commence the maintenance dose. The first capsule should be taken at, or shortly before, the end of the infusion (an oral loading dose should not be given). Give 200 – 250 mg Mexitil orally three or four times a day.

(d) **Change over from Capsules to Perlongets:**

Give the first Perlonget in the evening, in place of the capsule. Alternatively, the first Perlonget may be given together with the last capsule in the morning.

NOTES:

1 The loading dose regime is designed to compensate for the rapid phase of tissue distribution which occurs especially with IV loading.

2 If the optimum therapeutic effect is not achieved, the rate of infusion or oral dosage may be increased, side effects permitting.

3 Gastric emptying time may be delayed in patients with myocardial infarction and/or to whom opiates have been given and thus, it may be necessary to titrate the dose against therapeutic effects and side effects.

4 The 50 mg capsule is available in order that a more precise dose titration may be undertaken should this be required. Small increments will also reduce the incidence of side effects.

5 When mexiletine therapy is commenced, patients should be monitored closely (ECG, blood pressure and routine laboratory tests) over a period of at least 24 hours, and dosage adjustment made on the basis of this. Monitoring is particularly recommended in the following situations: sinus node dysfunction, conduction defects, bradycardia, hypotension or cardiac, renal or hepatic failure. There may be a potentiation of tremor in patients with Parkinsonism.

Regular monitoring of cardiac function throughout treatment is advisable.

The duration of treatment required in any patient is of necessity variable, and although no precise guide can be given, withdrawal of treatment may be attempted after a suitable period free of arrhythmia. Gradual withdrawal i.e. over 1-2 weeks, is preferable as arrhythmias which have been satisfactorily controlled may recur.

No specific information on the use of this product in the elderly or children is available. Clinical trials have included patients over 65 years and no adverse reactions specific to this age group have been reported.

4.3 Contraindications

Mexitil should not be used in the first three months following myocardial infarction or where cardiac output is limited (left ventricular ejection fraction of less than 35 %), except in patients with life-threatening ventricular arrhythmias

Mexitil is contraindicated in the presence of cardiogenic shock or pre-existing second- or third- degree AV block if no pacemaker is present.

Mexitil should not be used in known cases of hypersensitivity to mexiletine or one of the excipients of the product, or local anaesthetics e.g. lidocaine (lignocaine).

4.4 Special warnings and special precautions for use

(i) If the drug is used in the following situations, the patient should be carefully monitored and the dosage may need to be reduced: sinus node dysfunction, conduction defect, bradycardia, hypotension or cardiac failure.

(ii) Myocardial infarction results in prolonged absorption half-life of oral mexiletine

(iii) Plasma elimination half-life may be prolonged in moderate to severe hepatic disease, and in patients with creatinine clearance of less than 10 ml/min: individual dose titration is advised in these conditions.

(iv) Patients in whom pathologically high liver values have been established or who have signs or symptoms of impaired liver function, should be monitored carefully.

4.5 Interaction with other medicinal products and other forms of Interaction

(i) Where there is concurrent administration of Mexitil and some other anti-arrhythmic drugs, an increased effect on conduction and pumping of the heart is to be expected. Mexitil may be used concurrently with the cardiovascular drugs digoxin, amiodarone, quinidine and beta-adrenergic blocking agents.

(ii) All medicines that affect gastrointestinal movement may affect the absorption of oral Mexitil.

Drugs that delay gastric emptying (e.g. opiates, antacids and atropine) may delay the absorption of Mexitil. Similarly, drugs that accelerate gastric emptying (e.g. metoclopramide) will reduce the time to peak mexiletine concentrations and increase peak concentrations.

(iii) Since Mexitil is metabolised mainly in the liver, substances that influence liver enzyme function may alter the concentration of Mexitil in the blood. In particular, interactions with the two cytochrome P450 isozymes CYP1A2 and CYP2D6 have to be considered. It may be necessary to reduce the dose of Mexitil in cases of concomitant administration of substances that lead to enzyme inhibition in the liver.

In cases of concurrent therapy with substances that lead to enzyme induction it may be necessary to increase the dose of Mexitil since it is metabolised at a faster rate.

(iv) Concurrent administration of mexiletine may increase plasma levels of theophylline and caffeine.

(v) Drugs which markedly acidify, or alkalise urine should be avoided because they may enhance or reduce (respectively) the rate of drug excretion and correspondingly affect the plasma concentration of mexiletine.

(vi) Concomitant administration of Mexitil with warfarin may increase the risk of bleeding.

(vii) Local anaesthetic toxicity may occur in patients who receive Mexitil and local anaesthetic agents concurrently.

4.6 Pregnancy and lactation

Mexiletine freely crosses the placenta. Therefore, Mexitil should only be used in pregnancy if the potential benefit justifies the potential risk.

Mexitil appears in breast milk in concentrations, which may have an effect on the infant. Therefore, if the use of Mexitil is deemed essential for the mother, an alternative method of infant feeding should be considered.

4.7 Effects on ability to drive and use machines

Mexitil may impair the ability to drive or operate machinery, especially when taken in combination with alcohol.

4.8 Undesirable effects

Side-effects are mainly related to blood concentration and may therefore be seen during the initial phases of both IV and oral treatment when fluctuation may occur before the blood and tissue concentrations reach equilibrium. Reducing the rate of injection of infusion or delaying the next oral dose allows the blood concentration to fall and usually reduces side-effects. Generally side-effects are of five types:

Gastro-Intestinal: Nausea, vomiting, indigestion, constipation, diarrhoea, dry mouth, unpleasant taste, hiccoughs. Oesophageal ulceration may occur if oral Mexitil is swallowed without adequate liquid and is lodged in the oesophagus.

Central Nervous System: Drowsiness, dizziness, diplopia, blurred vision, nystagmus, dysarthria, ataxia, tremor, paraesthesiae, convulsion, psychiatric disorders, confusional state, insomnia.

Cardiovascular: Hypotension, sinus bradycardia, atrial fibrillation, palpitation and conduction defects. Exacerbation of arrhythmias, pre-existing heart failure and torsade de pointes.

When hypotension has occurred this has tended to be in patients with severe illness who have already been given a variety of anti-arrhythmic or other preparations and, if associated with bradycardia, may be reduced by the use of atropine.

Pulmonary infiltrates, interstitial lung disease and pulmonary fibrosis have been observed in isolated cases.

Haematologica: Rash, arthralgia, fever, thrombocytopenia and appearance of positive but symptomless antinuclear factor titres. Leucopenia has been observed rarely. Rare cases of Stevens-Johnson syndrome, some with liver involvement, have been reported in Japan. Isolated cases of erythroderma have also been reported.

Hepatic: Liver damage has been observed following Mexitil administration; jaundice has been reported.

4.9 Overdose

The minimum fatal dose is unknown but 4.40 g proved fatal in a healthy young adult.

The clinical features include: nausea, vomiting, drowsiness, confusion, ataxia and convulsions. Blurred vision and paraesthesiae have also been reported. Hypotension, sinus bradycardia, atrial fibrillation and cardiac arrest are more specific effects.

Therapy

General symptomatic treatment is advisable. Gastric lavage should be performed where appropriate and the patient should be transferred to an intensive / coronary care unit for possible cardio-pulmonary support.

Arrhythmias should be treated as appropriate and intravenous diazepam may be useful to control convulsions. In the event of serious bradycardia and hypotension it is advisable to first administer an IV dose of 0.5 - 1.0 mg atropine.

Acidification of the urine enhances the rate of drug elimination and so may be useful.

5. PHARMACOLOGICAL PROPERTIES

5.1 Pharmacodynamic properties

Mexitil (mexiletine hydrochloride) is a Class 1b anti-arrhythmic agent based on the Vaughan Williams classification with local anaesthetic properties, similar in structure and activity to lidocaine (lignocaine). Mexiletine depresses the maximum rate of depolarisation with little or no modification of resting potentials or the duration of action potentials.

5.2 Pharmacokinetic properties

Mexiletine is primarily absorbed in the upper portion of the small intestine. Peak plasma levels are reached 2 - 3hours after administration to normal subjects; absorption is slower after myocardial infarction. Mexiletine shows a fast distribution phase, a slow distribution phase and a slow elimination phase. Tissue up-take is substantial. Bioavailability is about 80 ± 8 %. Renal clearance varies with urine pH but this is unlikely to have clinical significance. In patients the elimination half-life is 5 - 17 hours.

5.3 Preclinical safety data

There are no additional preclinical data of help to the prescriber.

6. PHARMACEUTICAL PARTICULARS

6.1 List of excipients

Dried Maize starch EP

Colloidal silica EP

Magnesium stearate BP

Ethanol

Gelatin

Erythrosine (E127)

Indigo carmine (E132)

Titanium dioxide (E171)

6.2 Incompatibilities

None stated

6.3 Shelf life

The capsules have a shelf-life expiry of 5 years from date of manufacture.

6.4 Special precautions for storage

Store below 25 °C

6.5 Nature and contents of container

White polypropylene securitainer of 100 and PVC blisters (backed with PVC-lacquered aluminium) of 100.

6.6 Instructions for use and handling

None stated.

7. MARKETING AUTHORISATION HOLDER

Boehringer Ingelheim Limited, Ellesfield Avenue, Bracknell, Berkshire, RG12 8YS, United Kingdom

8. MARKETING AUTHORISATION NUMBER(S)

PL 0015/0064R

9. DATE OF FIRST AUTHORISATION/RENEWAL OF THE AUTHORISATION

6 October 1975 / 21 April 1997

10. DATE OF REVISION OF THE TEXT

October 1999

11. Legal category

POM

Ref: M4b;200/UK/SPC/1

Miacalcic Ampoules, Multidose Vials

(Novartis Pharmaceuticals UK Ltd)

1. NAME OF THE MEDICINAL PRODUCT

MIACALCIC® 50 IU/ml Ampoules

MIACALCIC® 100 IU/ml Ampoules

MIACALCIC® 400 IU/2ml Multidose vials

2. QUALITATIVE AND QUANTITATIVE COMPOSITION

MIACALCIC® 50 IU/ml: Ampoules containing salcatonin BP 50IU/ml

MIACALCIC® 100 IU/ml: Ampoules containing salcatonin BP 100IU/ml

MIACALCIC® 400 IU/2ml: Multidose vials containing salcatonin BP 200IU/ml

For excipients, see 6.1.

3. PHARMACEUTICAL FORM

Solution for injection

4. CLINICAL PARTICULARS

4.1 Therapeutic indications

Calcitonin is indicated for:

- Prevention of acute bone loss due to sudden immobilisation such as in patients with recent osteoporotic fractures
- Paget's disease
- Hypercalcemia of malignancy

4.2 Posology and method of administration

For subcutaneous, intramuscular or intravenous use in individuals aged 18 years or more.

Salmon calcitonin may be administered at bedtime to reduce the incidence of nausea or vomiting which may occur, especially at the initiation of therapy.

Prevention of acute bone loss:

The recommended dosage is 100 I.U. daily or 50 I.U. twice daily for 2 to 4 weeks, administered subcutaneously or intramuscularly. The dose may be reduced to 50 I.U. daily at the start of remobilisation. The treatment should be maintained until patients are fully mobilised.

Paget's Disease:

The recommended dosage is 100 I.U. per day administered subcutaneously or intramuscularly, however a minimum dosage regimen of 50 I.U. three times a week has achieved clinical and biochemical improvement. Dosage is to be adjusted to the individual patient's needs. The duration of treatment depends on the indication for treatment and the patient's response. The effect of calcitonin may be monitored by measurement of suitable markers of bone remodelling, such as serum alkaline phosphatase or urinary hydroxyproline or deoxypyridinoline. The dose may be reduced after the condition of the patient has improved.

Hypercalcemia of malignancy:

The recommended starting dose is 100 I.U. every 6 to 8 hours by subcutaneous or intramuscular injection. In addition, salmon calcitonin could be administered by intravenous injection after previous rehydration.

If the response is not satisfactory after one or two days, the dose may be increased to a maximum of 400 I.U. every 6 to 8 hours. In severe or emergency cases, intravenous infusion with up to 10 I.U./kg body weight in 500 ml 0.9% w/v sodium chloride solution may be administered over a period of at least 6 hours.

Use in elderly, hepatic and renal impairment patients

Experience with the use of calcitonin in the elderly has shown no evidence of reduced tolerability or altered dosage requirements. The same applies to patients with altered hepatic function. The metabolic clearance is much lower in patients with end-stage renal failure than in healthy subjects. However, the clinical relevance of this finding is not known. (see section 5.2).

4.3 Contraindications

Hypersensitivity to the active substance or to any of the excipients.

Calcitonin is also contraindicated in patients with hypocalcaemia.

4.4 Special warnings and special precautions for use

Because calcitonin is a peptide, the possibility of systemic allergic reactions exists and allergic-type reactions including isolated cases of anaphylactic shock have been reported in patients receiving calcitonin. Such reactions should be differentiated from generalised or local flushing, which are common non-allergic effects of calcitonin (see 4.8). Skin testing should be conducted in patients with suspected sensitivity to calcitonin prior to their treatment with calcitonin.

4.5 Interaction with other medicinal products and other forms of Interaction

Serum calcium levels may be transiently decreased to below normal levels following administration of calcitonin, notably upon initiation of therapy in patients with abnormally high rates of bone turnover. This effect is diminished as osteoclastic activity is reduced. However, care should be exercised in patients receiving concurrent treatment with cardiac glycosides or calcium channel blocking agents. Dosages of these drugs may require adjustment in view of the fact that their effects may be modified by changes in cellular electrolyte concentrations.

The use of calcitonin in combination with bisphosphonates may result in an additive calcium-lowering effect.

4.6 Pregnancy and lactation

Calcitonin has not been studied in pregnant women. Calcitonin should be used during pregnancy only if treatment is considered absolutely essential by the physician.

It is not known if the substance is excreted in human milk. In animals, salmon calcitonin has been shown to decrease lactation and to be excreted in milk (see 5.3). Therefore, breast-feeding is not recommended during treatment.

4.7 Effects on ability to drive and use machines
No data exist on the effects of Miacalcic on the ability to drive and use machines. Miacalcic may cause dizziness (see 4.8 Undesirable effects) which may impair the reaction of the patient. Patients must therefore be warned that dizziness may occur, in which case they should not drive or use machines.

4.8 Undesirable effects
Frequency categories:

Very common (> 1/10); common (> 1/100, < 1/10); uncommon (> 1/1000, < 1/100); rare (> 1/10,000, < 1/ 1,000); very rare (< 1/10,000), including isolated reports.

Gastrointestinal disorder:

Very common: Nausea with or without vomiting is noted in approximately 10% of patients treated with calcitonin. The effect is more evident on initiation of therapy and tends to decrease or disappear with continued administration or a reduction in dose. An antiemetic may be administered, if required. Nausea/vomiting are less frequent when the injection is done in the evening and after meals.

Uncommon: diarrhoea

Vascular disorders:

Very common: skin flushes (facial or upper body). These are not allergic reactions but are due to a pharmacological effect, and are usually observed 10 to 20 minutes after administration.

General disorders and administration site conditions:

Uncommon: local inflammatory reactions at the site of subcutaneous or intramuscular injection.

Skin and subcutaneous tissue disorders:

Uncommon: skin rash

Nervous system disorders:

Uncommon: metallic taste in the mouth; dizziness

Renal and urinary disorders:

Uncommon: diuresis

Metabolic and nutrition disorders:

Rare: In case of patients with high bone remodelling (Paget's disease and young patients) a transient decrease of calcemia may occur between the 4th and the 6th hour after administration, usually asymptomatic.

Investigations:

Rare: Neutralising antibodies to calcitonin rarely develop. The development of these antibodies is not usually related to loss of clinical efficacy, although their presence in a small percentage of patients following long-term therapy with calcitonin may result in a reduced response to the product. The presence of antibodies appears to bear no relationship to allergic reactions, which are rare. Calcitonin receptor down-regulation may also result in a reduced clinical response in a small percentage of patients following long term therapy.

Immune system disorders:

Very rare: serious allergic-type reactions such as bronchospasm, swelling of the tongue and throat, and in isolated cases, anaphylaxis.

4.9 Overdose
Nausea, vomiting, flushing and dizziness are known to be dose dependent when calcitonin is administered parenterally. Single doses (up to 10,000 I.U.) of injectable salmon calcitonin have been administered without adverse reactions, other than nausea and vomiting, and exacerbation of pharmacological effects.

Should symptoms of overdose appear, treatment should be symptomatic.

5. PHARMACOLOGICAL PROPERTIES
Pharmacotherapeutic group: antiparathyroid hormone, ATC code: H05BA01 (calcitonin, salmon).

The pharmacological properties of the synthetic and recombinant peptides have been demonstrated to be qualitatively and quantitatively equivalent.

5.1 Pharmacodynamic properties
Calcitonin is a calciotropic hormone, which inhibits bone resorption by a direct action on osteoclasts. By inhibiting osteoclast activity via its specific receptors, salmon calcitonin decreases bone resorption. In pharmacological studies, calcitonin has been shown to have analgesic activity in animal models.

Calcitonin markedly reduces bone turnover in conditions with an increased rate of bone resorption such as Paget's disease and acute bone loss due to sudden immobilisation. The absence of mineralisation defect with calcitonin has been demonstrated by bone histomorphometric studies both in man and in animals.

Decreases in bone resorption as judged by a reduction in urinary hydroxylproline and deoxypyridinoline are observed following calcitonin treatment in both normal volunteers and patients with bone-related disorders, including Paget's disease and osteoporosis.

The calcium-lowering effect of calcitonin is caused both by a decrease in the efflux of calcium from the bone to the ECF and inhibition of renal tubular reabsorption of calcium.

5.2 Pharmacokinetic properties
General characteristics of the active substance

Salmon calcitonin is rapidly absorbed and eliminated. Peak plasma concentrations are attained within the first hour of administration.

Animal studies have shown that calcitonin is primarily metabolised via proteolysis in the kidney following parenteral administration. The metabolites lack the specific biological activity of calcitonin. Bioavailability following subcutaneous and intramuscular injection in humans is high and similar for the two routes of administration (71% and 66%, respectively).

Calcitonin has short absorption and elimination half-lives of 10-15 minutes and 50-80 minutes, respectively. Salmon calcitonin is primarily and almost exclusively degraded in the kidneys, forming pharmacologically inactive fragments of the molecule. Therefore, the metabolic clearance is much lower in patients with end-stage renal failure than in healthy subjects. However, the clinical relevance of this finding is not known.

Plasma protein binding is 30 to 40%.

Characteristics in patients

There is a relationship between the subcutaneous dose of calcitonin and peak plasma concentrations. Following parenteral administration of 100 I.U. calcitonin, peak plasma concentration lies between about 200 and 400 pg/ml. Higher blood levels may be associated with increased incidence of nausea and vomiting.

5.3 Preclinical safety data
Conventional long term toxicity, reproduction, mutagenicity and carcinogenicity studies have been performed in laboratory animals. Salmon calcitonin is devoid of embryotoxic, teratogenic and mutagenic potential.

An increased incidence of pituitary adenomas has been reported in rats given synthetic salmon calcitonin for 1 year. This is considered a species-specific effect and of no clinical relevance. Salmon calcitonin does not cross the placental barrier.

In lactating animals given calcitonin, suppression of milk production has been observed. Calcitonin is secreted into the milk.

6. PHARMACEUTICAL PARTICULARS

6.1 List of excipients
Ampoules: glacial acetic acid, sodium acetate trihydrate, sodium chloride, water for injection.

Multidose vials: glacial acetic acid, sodium acetate trihydrate, sodium chloride, water for injection, phenol.

6.2 Incompatibilities
None

6.3 Shelf life
Ampoules - 60 months

Multidose vials - 48 months (1 month after initial use).

6.4 Special precautions for storage
Store in a refrigerator (2-8 ° C). Do not freeze.

Allow to reach room temperature before subcutaneous or intramuscular use.

Multidose vials - Discard unused portion of contents one month after initial use. Once started, the MDV can be stored at room temperature.

6.5 Nature and contents of container
MIACALCIC® 50 IU/ml and 100 IU/ml: Glass ampoule – uncoloured

MIACALCIC® 400 IU/2ml Multidose vials: Uncoloured type I glass vial, with latex free rubber stopper.

6.6 Instructions for use and handling
Allow to reach room temperature before intramuscular or subcutaneous use. Solutions for infusions should be prepared immediately before use and glass or hard plastic containers should not be used.

7. MARKETING AUTHORISATION HOLDER
Novartis Pharmaceuticals UK Limited

Trading as: Sandoz Pharmaceuticals

Frimley Business Park

Frimley

Camberley

Surrey

GU16 7SR

8. MARKETING AUTHORISATION NUMBER(S)
50IU/ml Ampoule - PL 0101/0202

100IU/ml Ampoule - PL 0101/0095R

400IU/2ml MDV - PL 0101/0203

9. DATE OF FIRST AUTHORISATION/RENEWAL OF THE AUTHORISATION
50IU/ml Ampoule - 16 July 1990 / 30 October 1996

100IU/ml Ampoule - 8 December 1975 / 30 October 1996

400IU/2ml MDV - 23 July 1990 / 30 October 1996

10. DATE OF REVISION OF THE TEXT
6 October 2004

LEGAL CATEGORY:
POM

MIACALCIC Nasal Spray

(Novartis Pharmaceuticals UK Ltd)

1. NAME OF THE MEDICINAL PRODUCT
Miacalcic® 200 I.U. Nasal Spray. ▼

2. QUALITATIVE AND QUANTITATIVE COMPOSITION
One metered dose delivers 33.3 micrograms of calcitonin (salmon, synthetic), as free peptide, which corresponds to 200 I.U. of the drug substance.

For excipients, see 6.1.

3. PHARMACEUTICAL FORM
Nasal Spray, solution.

4. CLINICAL PARTICULARS

4.1 Therapeutic indications
Treatment of established post-menopausal osteoporosis, in order to reduce the risk of vertebral fractures. A reduction in hip fractures has not been demonstrated.

4.2 Posology and method of administration
The recommended dosage of Miacalcic Nasal Spray for the treatment of established post-menopausal osteoporosis is 200 I.U. once a day. Use of Miacalcic Nasal Spray is recommended in conjunction with an adequate calcium and vitamin D intake.

Treatment is to be administered on a long-term basis (see point 5.1., Pharmacodynamic properties).

Use in elderly patients, in hepatic impairment and in renal insufficiency

Extensive experience with the use of Miacalcic Nasal Spray in the elderly has shown no evidence of reduced tolerability or altered dosage requirements. The same applies to patients with altered renal or hepatic function.

Use in children

As intranasal calcitonin is indicated for postmenopausal women, its use in children is not appropriate.

Note

Full instructions for use by the patient are given in the patient leaflet.

4.3 Contraindications
Hypersensitivity to calcitonin (see section 4.8. Undesirable effects) or to any of the excipients of the formulation (see 6.1. List of excipients).

Calcitonin is also contra-indicated in patients with hypocalcaemia.

4.4 Special warnings and special precautions for use
Nasal examinations should be performed before treatment begins and in the case of nasal complaints medication should not be started. If severe ulceration of the nasal mucosa occurs (e.g. penetration below the mucosa or association with heavy bleeding), Miacalcic Nasal Spray is to be discontinued. In case of mild ulceration, medication is to be interrupted temporarily until healing occurs.

Because calcitonin is a peptide, the possibility of systemic allergic reactions exists and allergic-type reactions including isolated cases of anaphylactic shock have been reported in patients receiving Miacalcic Nasal Spray. In patients with suspected sensitivity to calcitonin, skin testing should be considered prior to treatment.

The excipient benzalkonium chloride is an irritant and may cause irritation of the nasal mucosa.

4.5 Interaction with other medicinal products and other forms of Interaction
No drug interactions with intranasal salmon calcitonin have been reported.

4.6 Pregnancy and lactation
As Miacalcic Nasal Spray is indicated for postmenopausal women, no studies have been carried out in pregnant women or nursing mothers. Therefore, Miacalcic Nasal Spray is not to be administered to such patients. However, animal studies have shown no embryotoxic and teratogenic potential. It appears that salmon calcitonin does not cross the placental barrier in animals.

It is not known whether salmon calcitonin is excreted into human breast milk. In animals, salmon calcitonin has been shown to decrease lactation and to be excreted in milk.

4.7 Effects on ability to drive and use machines
No data exist on the effects of Miacalcic Nasal Spray on the ability to drive and use machines. Miacalcic Nasal Spray may cause transient dizziness (see section 4.8. Undesirable effects) which may impair the reaction of the patient. Patients must therefore be warned that transient dizziness may occur, in which case they are not to drive or use machines.

4.8 Undesirable effects
Frequency estimates:

Very common (> 1/10); common (> 1/100, < 1/10); uncommon (> 1/1000, < 1/100); rare (> 1/10,000, < 1/ 1,000); very rare (< 1/10,000), including isolated reports.

Gastrointestinal disorders:

Common: nausea, diarrhoea, abdominal pain

Uncommon: vomiting

Vascular disorders:

Common: flushing

Uncommon: hypertension

Respiratory disorders:

Very common: rhinitis (including dry nose, nasal oedema, nasal congestion, sneezing, allergic rhinitis), unspecified symptoms of the nose (e.g., nasal passage irritation, rash papular, parosmia, erythema, abrasion).

Common: rhinitis ulcerative, sinusitis, epistaxis, pharyngitis.

Uncommon: cough

These events are generally mild (in about 80% of reports) and require discontinuation of the treatment in less than 5% of cases.

Nervous system disorders:

Common: dizziness, headache, dysgeusia.

Sense Organ disorders:

Uncommon: vision disturbance

Skin and subcutaneous tissue disorders:

Uncommon: oedema (face oedema, oedema peripheral and ansarca)

Musculoskeletal disorders:

Common: musculoskeletal pain

Uncommon: arthralgia

Immune system disorders:

Uncommon: hypersensitivity reactions such as generalised skin reactions, flushing, oedema (face oedema, oedema peripheral and ansarca), hypertension, arthralgia and pruritus.

Very rare: allergic and anaphylactoid-like reactions such as tachycardia, hypotension, circulatory collapse and anaphylactic shock.

Investigations:

Rare: development of neutralising antibodies to calcitonin. The development of these antibodies is not usually related to loss of clinical efficacy, although their presence in a small percentage of patients following long-term therapy with high doses of calcitonin may result in a reduced response to the product. The presence of antibodies appears to bear no relationship to allergic reactions, which are rare. Calcitonin receptor down-regulation may also result in a reduced clinical response in a small percentage of patients following long term therapy with high doses.

General disorders:

Common: fatigue

Uncommon: influenza-like illness

4.9 Overdose

Nausea, vomiting, flushing and dizziness are known to be dose dependent when calcitonin is administered parenterally. Single doses (up to 10,000 I.U) of salmon calcitonin have been administered parenterally without adverse effects other than nausea and vomiting and exacerbation of pharmacological effects. Such events might therefore also be expected to occur in association with an overdose of Miacalcic Nasal Spray. However, Miacalcic Nasal Spray has been administered at up to 1600 I.U. as a single dose and up to 800 I.U. per day for three days without causing any serious adverse event. If symptoms of overdose appear, treatment is to be symptomatic.

5. PHARMACOLOGICAL PROPERTIES

Pharmacotherapeutic group: antiparathyroid hormone, ATC code: H05B A01 (calcitonin, salmon).

5.1 Pharmacodynamic properties

Calcitonin is a calciotropic hormone, which inhibits bone resorption by a direct action on osteoclasts. By inhibiting osteoclast activity via its specific receptors, salmon calcitonin decreases bone resorption. Calcitonin markedly reduces bone turnover in conditions with an increased rate of bone resorption such as osteoporosis.

The absence of mineralisation defect with calcitonin has been demonstrated by bone histomorphometric studies both in man and in animals.

In pharmacological studies, calcitonin has been shown to have analgesic activity in animal models. Intranasal calcitonin produces a clinically relevant biological response in humans, as shown by an increase in the urinary excretion of calcium, phosphorus, and sodium (by reducing their tubular re-uptake) and a decrease in the urinary excretion of hydroxyproline. Long-term administration of intranasal calcitonin significantly suppresses biochemical markers of bone turnover such as serum C-telopeptides (sCTX) an skeletal isoenzymes of alkaline phosphatase.

Miacalcic Nasal Spray results in a statistically significant 1-2% increase in lumbar spine Bone Mineral Density (BMD) which is evident from year 1 and is sustained for up to 5 years. Hip BMD is preserved.

In a 5 year trial in postmenopausal women (PROOF study), administration of 200 I.U. Miacalcic Nasal Spray resulted in a reduction of 33% in the relative risk of developing vertebral fractures. The relative risk of developing vertebral fractures, compared to placebo (treatment with vitamin D and calcium alone) in all patients treated with daily doses of 200 I.U. was 0.67 (95% CI: 0.47-0.97). The absolute risk of developing vertebral fractures over 5 years was reduced from 25.9% in the placebo group to 17.8% in the 200 I.U group. A reduction in hip fractures has not been demonstrated. The recommended dosage of intranasal salmon calcitonin for the treatment of established postmenopausal osteoporosis is 200 I.U. once a day. Higher dosages were not more effective.

5.2 Pharmacokinetic properties

Pharmacokinetic parameters of intranasally administered salmon calcitonin are difficult to quantitate due to the inadequate sensitivity and uncertain specificity of the available immunoassay methods used in the studies performed to date. The bioavailability of a 200 I.U. dose relative to parenteral administration is between 2 and 15%. Miacalcic is absorbed rapidly through the nasal mucosa and peak plasma concentrations are attained within the first hour of administration. The half-life of elimination has been calculated to be approximately 16 to 43 minutes and no evidence of accumulation was observed with multiple dosing. Doses higher than the recommended dose result in higher blood levels (as shown by an increase in AUC) but relative bioavailability does not increase. As is the case with other polypeptide hormones, there is very little value in monitoring plasma levels of salmon calcitonin since these are not directly predictive of the therapeutic response. Hence, calcitonin activity is to be evaluated by using clinical parameters of efficacy.

Plasma protein binding is 30 to 40%.

5.3 Preclinical safety data

Conventional long-term toxicity, reproduction, mutagenicity and carcinogenicity studies have been performed in laboratory animals. In addition, nasal tolerance was investigated in dogs and monkeys.

Salmon calcitonin is devoid of embryotoxic, teratogenic and mutagenic potential. Daily intranasal administration of high doses of a calcitonin formulation containing 0.01% benzalkonium chloride for 26 weeks was well tolerated by monkeys.

An increased incidence of pituitary adenomas has been reported in rats given synthetic salmon calcitonin for 1 year. This is considered a species-specific effect and of no clinical relevance.

Salmon calcitonin does not cross the placental barrier.

In lactating animals given calcitonin, suppression of milk production has been observed. Calcitonins are secreted into the milk.

6. PHARMACEUTICAL PARTICULARS

6.1 List of excipients

Benzalkonium chloride, sodium chloride, hydrochloric acid, purified water.

6.2 Incompatibilities

Not applicable.

6.3 Shelf life

Unopened, 3 years.

After opening: it should be used within 4 weeks.

6.4 Special precautions for storage

Store at 2-8°C (in a refrigerator) before opening. Do not freeze.

Once opened, store at room temperature. Do not store above 25°C.

Keep the bottle upright at all times to reduce the risk of air bubbles getting into the dip tube.

6.5 Nature and contents of container

The device is composed of a clear, uncoloured glass bottle (glass type I) and a spray mechanism containing an integrated, automatic dose-counting mechanism and a built-in mechanical stop. The pack contains 1 bottle with 2 ml of spray solution, delivering at least 14 metered doses of 200 I.U.

6.6 Instructions for use and handling

No special requirements.

7. MARKETING AUTHORISATION HOLDER

Novartis Pharmaceuticals UK Limited

Frimley Business Park

Frimley

Camberley

Surrey, UK

GU 16 7SR

8. MARKETING AUTHORISATION NUMBER(S)

PL 00101/0586

9. DATE OF FIRST AUTHORISATION/RENEWAL OF THE AUTHORISATION

18 September 2000

10. DATE OF REVISION OF THE TEXT

6 October 2004

LEGAL CATEGORY

POM

Micardis 20mg, 40mg and 80mg tablets

(Boehringer Ingelheim Limited)

1. NAME OF THE MEDICINAL PRODUCT

Micardis 20 mg tablets

Micardis 40 mg tablets

Micardis 80 mg tablets

2. QUALITATIVE AND QUANTITATIVE COMPOSITION

Each tablet contains 20 mg or 40 mg or 80 mg of telmisartan

For excipients, see section 6.1.

3. PHARMACEUTICAL FORM

Tablet

20 mg: White round tablets engraved with the code number 50H on one side and the company symbol on the other side.

40 mg: White oblong tablets engraved with the code number 51H on one side and the company symbol on the other side.

80 mg: White oblong tablets engraved with the code number 52H on one side and the company symbol on the other side.

4. CLINICAL PARTICULARS

4.1 Therapeutic indications

Treatment of essential hypertension.

4.2 Posology and method of administration

Adults

The usually effective dose is 40 mg once daily. Some patients may already benefit at a daily dose of 20 mg. In cases where the target blood pressure is not achieved, telmisartan dose can be increased to a maximum of 80 mg once daily. Alternatively, telmisartan may be used in combination with thiazide-type diuretics such as hydrochlorothiazide which has been shown to have an additive blood pressure lowering effect with telmisartan. When considering raising the dose, it must be borne in mind that the maximum antihypertensive effect is generally attained four-eight weeks after the start of treatment (see section 5.1).

Renal impairment: no posology adjustment is required for patients with mild to moderate renal impairment. Limited experience is available in patients with severe renal impairment or haemodialysis. A lower starting dose of 20 mg is recommended in these patients (see section 4.4).

Hepatic impairment: in patients with mild to moderate hepatic impairment the posology should not exceed 40 mg once daily (see section 4.4).

Elderly

No dosing adjustment is necessary.

Children and adolescents

Safety and efficacy of Micardis have not been established in children and adolescents up to 18 years.

4.3 Contraindications

- Hypersensitivity to the active substance or to any of the excipients (see section 6.1).
- Second and third trimesters of pregnancy and lactation (see section 4.6).
- Biliary obstructive disorders.
- Severe hepatic impairment.

4.4 Special warnings and special precautions for use

Hepatic impairment:

Micardis should not be given to patients with cholestasis, biliary obstructive disorders or severe hepatic insufficiency (see section 4.3) since telmisartan is mostly eliminated with the bile. These patients can be expected to have reduced hepatic clearance for telmisartan. Micardis should be used only with caution in patients with mild to moderate hepatic impairment.

Renovascular hypertension:

There is an increased risk of severe hypotension and renal insufficiency when patients with bilateral renal artery stenosis or stenosis of the artery to a single functioning kidney are treated with medicinal products that affect the renin-angiotensin-aldosterone system.

Renal impairment and kidney transplant:

When Micardis is used in patients with impaired renal function, a periodic monitoring of potassium and creatinine serum levels is recommended. There is no experience regarding the administration of Micardis in patients with a recent kidney transplant.

Intravascular volume depletion:

Symptomatic hypotension, especially after the first dose, may occur in patients who are volume and/or sodium depleted by vigorous diuretic therapy, dietary salt restriction, diarrhoea or vomiting. Such conditions should be corrected before the administration of Micardis. Volume and/or sodium depletion should be corrected prior to administration of Micardis.

Other conditions with stimulation of the renin-angiotensin-aldosterone system:

In patients whose vascular tone and renal function depend predominantly on the activity of the renin-angiotensin-aldosterone system (e.g. patients with severe congestive heart failure or underlying renal disease, including renal artery stenosis), treatment with other medicinal products that affect this system has been associated with acute hypotension, hyperazotaemia, oliguria, or rarely acute renal failure.

Primary aldosteronism:

Patients with primary aldosteronism generally will not respond to antihypertensive medicinal products acting through inhibition of the renin-angiotensin system. Therefore, the use of telmisartan is not recommended.

Aortic and mitral valve stenosis, obstructive hypertrophic cardiomyopathy:

As with other vasodilators, special caution is indicated in patients suffering from aortic or mitral stenosis, or obstructive hypertrophic cardiomyopathy.

Electrolyte imbalance: Hyperkalaemia:

During treatment with other medicinal products that affect the renin-angiotensin-aldosterone system hyperkalaemia may occur, especially in the presence of renal impairment and/or heart failure and diabetes mellitus. Adequate monitoring of serum potassium in patients at risk is recommended.

Based on experience with the use of other medicinal products that affect the renin-angiotensin system, concomitant use with potassium-sparing diuretics, potassium supplements, salt substitutes containing potassium or other medicinal products that may increase the potassium level (heparin, etc.) may lead to an increase in serum potassium and should therefore be co-administered cautiously with Micardis (see section 4.5).

Sorbitol:

A recommended daily dose of Micardis 20 mg tablets contains 84.5 mg sorbitol. A recommended daily dose of Micardis 40 mg tablets contains 169 mg sorbitol. A recommended daily dose of Micardis 80 mg tablets contains 338 mg sorbitol. Patients with hereditary problems of fructose intolerance should not take Micardis.

Other:

As observed for angiotensin converting enzyme inhibitors, telmisartan and the other angiotensin antagonists are apparently less effective in lowering blood pressure in black people than in non-blacks, possibly because of higher prevalence of low-renin states in the black hypertensive population.

As with any antihypertensive agent, excessive reduction of blood pressure in patients with ischaemic cardiopathy or ischaemic cardiovascular disease could result in a myocardial infarction or stroke.

4.5 Interaction with other medicinal products and other forms of Interaction

Lithium:

Reversible increases in serum lithium concentrations and toxicity have been reported during concomitant administration of lithium with angiotensin converting enzyme inhibitors. Very rare cases have also been reported with angiotensin II receptor antagonists. Co-administration of lithium and Micardis should be done with caution. If this combination proves essential, serum lithium level monitoring is recommended during concomitant use.

Medicinal products that may increase potassium levels or induce hyperkalaemia (e.g. ACE inhibitors, potassium-sparing diuretics, potassium supplements, salt substitutes containing potassium, cyclosporin or other medicinal products such as heparin sodium): If these medicinal products are to be prescribed with telmisartan, monitoring of potassium plasma levels is advised. Based on the experience with the use of other medicinal products that blunt the renin-angiotensin system, concomitant use of the above medicinal products may lead to increases in serum potassium (see section 4.4).

Compounds, which have been studied in pharmacokinetic trials include digoxin, warfarin, hydrochlorothiazide, glibenclamide, ibuprofen, paracetamol and amlodipine. For digoxin a 20% increase in median plasma digoxin trough concentration has been observed (39% in a single case), monitoring of plasma digoxin levels should be considered.

Telmisartan may increase the hypotensive effect of other antihypertensive agents. Other interactions of clinical significance have not been identified.

Based on their pharmacological properties it can be expected that the following drugs may potentiate the hypotensive effects of all antihypertensives including telmisartan: Baclofen, amifostine. Futhermore, orthostatic hypotension may be potentiated by alcohol, barbiturates, narcotics or antidepressants.

The metabolite of simvastatin (simvastatin acid) has been shown to have a small increase in C_{max} (by a factor of 1.34) and more rapid elimination when co-administered with telmisartan.

4.6 Pregnancy and lactation

Use in pregnancy (See section 4.3)

There are no adequate data on the use of telmisartan in pregnant women. Animal studies do not indicate teratogenic effect, but have shown foetotoxicity. Therefore as a precautionary measure, telmisartan should preferably not be used during the first trimester of pregnancy. A switch to a suitable alternative treatment should be carried out in advance of a planned pregnancy.

In the second and third trimesters, substances that act directly on the renin-angiotensin-system can cause injury and even death in the developing foetus (See also section 5.3), therefore, telmisartan is contraindicated in the second and third trimesters of pregnancy. If pregnancy is diagnosed telmisartan should be discontinued as soon as possible.

Use in lactation (See section 4.3)

Telmisartan is contraindicated during lactation since it is not known whether it is excreted in human milk.

4.7 Effects on ability to drive and use machines

No studies on the effects on the ability to drive and use machines have been performed. However, when driving vehicles or operating machinery it must be borne in mind that dizziness or drowsiness may occasionally occur when taking antihypertensive therapy.

4.8 Undesirable effects

The overall incidence of adverse events reported with telmisartan (41.4%) was usually comparable to placebo (43.9%) in placebo controlled trials. The incidence of adverse events was not dose related and showed no correlation with gender, age or race of the patients.

The adverse drug reactions listed below have been accumulated from all clinical trials including 5788 hypertensive patients treated with telmisartan.

Adverse reactions have been ranked under headings of frequency using the following convention:

very common ($\geqslant$1/10); common ($\geqslant$1/100, $<$1/10); uncommon ($\geqslant$1/1000, $<$1/100);

rare ($\geqslant$1/10000, $<$1/1000); very rare ($<$ 1/10000)

Infections and infestations:

Common: symptoms of infection (e.g. urinary tract infections including cystitis), upper respiratory tract infections including pharyngitis and sinusitis

Psychiatric disorders:

Uncommon: Anxiety

Eye disorders:

Uncommon: Abnormal vision

Ear and labyrinth disorders:

Uncommon: Vertigo

Gastrointestinal disorders:

Common: Abdominal pain, diarrhoea, dyspepsia, gastrointestinal disorders

Uncommon: Dry mouth, flatulence

Skin and subcutaneous tissue disorders:

Common: Skin disorders like eczema

Uncommon: Sweating increased

Musculoskeletal, connective tissue and bone disorders:

Common: Arthralgia, back pain (e.g. sciatica), cramps in legs or leg pain, myalgia

Uncommon: Tendinitus like symptoms

General disorders and administration site conditions:

Common: Chest pain, influenza-like symptoms

In addition, since the introduction of telmisartan in the market, cases of erythema, pruritus, faintness, insomnia, depression, stomach upset, vomiting, hypotension, bradycardia, tachycardia, dyspnoea, eosinophilia, thrombocytopenia, weakness and lack of efficacy have been reported rarely.

As with other angiotensin II antagonists isolated cases of angioedema, urticaria and other related events have been reported.

Laboratory findings

Infrequently, a decrease in haemoglobin or an increase in uric acid have been observed which occur more often during treatment with telmisartan than with placebo. Increases in creatinine or liver enzymes have been observed during treatment with telmisartan but these changes in laboratory findings occurred with a frequency similar to or lower than placebo.

4.9 Overdose

No case of overdose has been reported. The most likely manifestations of telmisartan overdosage are expected to be hypotension and tachycardia; bradycardia might also occur. Telmisartan is not removed by haemodialysis. The patient should be closely monitored, and the treatment should be symptomatic and supportive. Management depends on the time since ingestion and the severity of the symptoms. Suggested measures include induction of emesis and / or gastric lavage. Activated charcoal may be useful in the treatment of overdosage. Serum electrolytes and creatinine should be monitored frequently. If hypotension occurs, the patient should be placed in a supine position, with salt and volume replacement given quickly.

5. PHARMACOLOGICAL PROPERTIES

5.1 Pharmacodynamic properties

Pharmacotherapeutic group: Angiotensin II Antagonists, ATC Code: C09CA07.

Telmisartan is an orally effective and specific angiotensin II receptor (type AT_1) antagonist. Telmisartan displaces angiotensin II with very high affinity from its binding site at the AT_1 receptor subtype, which is responsible for the known actions of angiotensin II. Telmisartan does not exhibit any partial agonist activity at the AT_1 receptor. Telmisartan selectively binds the AT_1 receptor. The binding is long-lasting. Telmisartan does not show affinity for other receptors, including AT_2 and other less characterised AT receptors. The functional role of these receptors is not known, nor is the effect of their possible overstimulation by angiotensin II, whose levels are increased by telmisartan. Plasma aldosterone levels are decreased by telmisartan. Telmisartan does not inhibit human plasma renin or block ion channels. Telmisartan does not inhibit angiotensin converting enzyme (kininase II), the enzyme which also degrades bradykinin. Therefore it is not expected to potentiate bradykinin-mediated adverse effects.

In man, an 80 mg dose of telmisartan almost completely inhibits the angiotensin II evoked blood pressure increase. The inhibitory effect is maintained over 24 hours and still measurable up to 48 hours.

After the first dose of telmisartan, the antihypertensive activity gradually becomes evident within 3 hours. The maximum reduction in blood pressure is generally attained 4-8 weeks after the start of treatment and is sustained during long-term therapy.

The antihypertensive effect persists constantly over 24 hours after dosing and includes the last 4 hours before the next dose as shown by ambulatory blood pressure measurements. This is confirmed by trough to peak ratios consistently above 80% seen after doses of 40 and 80 mg of telmisartan in placebo controlled clinical studies.

There is an apparent trend to a dose relationship to a time to recovery of baseline SBP. In this respect data concerning DBP are inconsistent.

In patients with hypertension telmisartan reduces both systolic and diastolic blood pressure without affecting pulse rate. The contribution of the drug's diuretic and natriuretic effect to its hypotensive activity has still to be defined. The antihypertensive efficacy of telmisartan is comparable to that of agents representative of other classes of antihypertensive drugs (demonstrated in clinical trials comparing telmisartan to amlodipine, atenolol, enalapril, hydrochlorothiazide, and lisinopril).

Upon abrupt cessation of treatment with telmisartan, blood pressure gradually returns to pre-treatment values over a period of several days without evidence of rebound hypertension.

The incidence of dry cough was significantly lower in patients treated with telmisartan than in those given angiotensin converting enzyme inhibitors in clinical trials directly comparing the two antihypertensive treatments.

Beneficial effects of telmisartan on mortality and cardiovascular morbidity are currently unknown.

5.2 Pharmacokinetic properties

Absorption:

Absorption of telmisartan is rapid although the amount absorbed varies. The mean absolute bioavailability for telmisartan is about 50%. When telmisartan is taken with food, the reduction in the area under the plasma concentration-time curve ($AUC_{0-\infty}$) of telmisartan varies from approximately 6% (40 mg dose) to approximately 19% (160 mg dose). By 3 hours after administration plasma concentrations are similar whether telmisartan is taken fasting or with food.

The small reduction in AUC is not expected to cause a reduction in the therapeutic efficacy.

There is no linear relationship between doses and plasma levels. C_{max} and to a lesser extent AUC increase disproportionately at doses above 40 mg.

Gender differences in plasma concentrations were observed, C_{max} and AUC being approximately 3-and 2-fold higher, respectively, in females compared to males.

Distribution:

Telmisartan is largely bound to plasma protein > 99.5%), mainly albumin and alpha-1 acid glycoprotein. The mean steady state apparent volume of distribution (V_{dss}) is approximately 500 l.

Metabolism:

Telmisartan is metabolised by conjugation to the glucuronide. No pharmacological activity has been shown for the conjugate.

Elimination:

Telmisartan is characterised by biexponential decay pharmacokinetics with a terminal elimination half-life of >20 hours. The maximum plasma concentration (C_{max}) and, to a smaller extent, area under the plasma concentration-time curve (AUC) increase disproportionately with dose. There is no evidence of clinically relevant accumulation of telmisartan taken at the recommended dose. Plasma concentrations were higher in females than in males, without relevant influence on efficacy.

After oral (and intravenous) administration telmisartan is nearly exclusively excreted with the faeces, mainly as unchanged compound. Cumulative urinary excretion is < 1% of dose. Total plasma clearance (Cl_{tot}) is high (approximately 1000 ml/min) compared with hepatic blood flow (about 1500 ml/min).

Special Populations

Elderly patients:

The pharmacokinetics of telmisartan do not differ in young and elderly patients.

Patients with renal impairment:

In mild to moderate and severe renal impairment patients doubling of plasma concentrations was observed. However, lower plasma concentrations were observed in patients with renal insufficiency undergoing dialysis. Telmisartan is highly bound to plasma protein in renal-insufficient subjects and cannot be removed by dialysis. The elimination half-life is not changed in patients with renal impairment.

Patients with hepatic impairment:

Pharmacokinetic studies in patients with hepatic impairment showed an increase in absolute bioavailability up to nearly 100%. The elimination half-life is not changed in patients with hepatic impairment.

5.3 Preclinical safety data

In preclinical safety studies doses producing exposure comparable to that in the clinical therapeutic range caused reduced red cell parameters (erythrocytes, haemoglobin, haematocrit) and changes in renal haemodynamics (increased blood urea nitrogen and creatinine), as well as increased serum potassium in normotensive animals. In dogs renal tubular dilation and atrophy were observed. Gastric mucosal injury (erosion, ulcers or inflammation) also was noted in rats and dogs. These pharmacologically-mediated undesirable effects, known from preclinical studies with both angiotensin converting enzyme inhibitors and angiotensin II antagonists, were prevented by oral saline supplementation.

In both species, increased plasma renin activity and hypertrophy/hyperplasia of the renal juxtaglomerular cells were observed. These changes, also a class effect of angiotensin converting enzyme inhibitors and other angiotensin II antagonists, do not appear to have clinical significance.

There is no evidence of teratogenic effect but animal studies indicated some hazardous potential of telmisartan to the postnatal development of the offspring: lower body weight, delayed eye opening, higher mortality.

There was no evidence of mutagenicity and relevant clastogenic activity in in vitro studies and no evidence of carcinogenicity in rats and mice.

6. PHARMACEUTICAL PARTICULARS

6.1 List of excipients

Povidone, meglumine, sodium hydroxide, sorbitol, magnesium stearate.

6.2 Incompatibilities

Not applicable.

6.3 Shelf life

20 mg tablets: 3 years

40 mg and 80 mg tablets: 4 years

6.4 Special precautions for storage

Store in the original package in order to protect from moisture.

6.5 Nature and contents of container

20 mg, 40 mg and 80 mg tablets:

14 tablets

28 tablets

56 tablets

98 tablets

Polyamide/aluminium/PVC blisters

40 mg and 80 mg tablets:

28 × 1 tablets

Polyamide/aluminium/PVC perforated unit dose blisters

Not all pack sizes may be marketed.

6.6 Instructions for use and handling

No special requirements

7. MARKETING AUTHORISATION HOLDER

Boehringer Ingelheim International GmbH

Binger Str. 173

D-55216 Ingelheim am Rhein

Germany

8. MARKETING AUTHORISATION NUMBER(S)

Micardis 20 mg tablets:

EU/1/98/090/009 (14 tablets)

EU/1/98/090/010 (28 tablets)

EU/1/98/090/011 (56 tablets)

EU/1/98/090/012 (98 tablets)

Micardis 40 mg tablets:

EU/1/98/090/001 (14 tablets)

EU/1/98/090/002 (28 tablets)

EU/1/98/090/003 (56 tablets)

EU/1/98/090/004 (98 tablets)

EU/1/98/090/013 (28 × 1 tablets)

Micardis 80 mg tablets:

EU/1/98/090/005 (14 tablets)

EU/1/98/090/006 (28 tablets)

EU/1/98/090/007 (56 tablets)

EU/1/98/090/008 (98 tablets)

EU/1/98/090/014 (28 × 1 tablets)

9. DATE OF FIRST AUTHORISATION/RENEWAL OF THE AUTHORISATION

Micardis 20 mg tablets

Date of first authorisation: 7 September 1999

Date of last renewal: 21 December 2003

Micardis 40 mg tablets

Date of first authorisation: 16 December 1998

Date of last renewal: 21 December 2003

Micardis 80 mg tablets

Date of first authorisation: 16 December 1998

Date of last renewal: 21 December 2003

10. DATE OF REVISION OF THE TEXT

December 2004

11. Legal Category

POM

M3a/UK/SPC/9

MicardisPlus

(Boehringer Ingelheim Limited)

1. NAME OF THE MEDICINAL PRODUCT

MicardisPlus▼ 40/12.5 mg tablets

MicardisPlus▼ 80/12.5 mg tablets

2. QUALITATIVE AND QUANTITATIVE COMPOSITION

Each tablet contains 40 mg telmisartan and 12.5 mg hydrochlorothiazide or 80 mg telmisartan and 12.5 mg hydrochlorothiazide.

For excipients, see 6.1

3. PHARMACEUTICAL FORM

Tablet.

Red and white oval shaped two layer tablet engraved with the company logo and the code H4 or H8.

4. CLINICAL PARTICULARS

4.1 Therapeutic indications

Treatment of essential hypertension.

MicardisPlus fixed dose combination (40 mg telmisartan/12.5 mg hydrochlorothiazide or 80 mg telmisartan/12.5 mg hydrochlorothiazide) is indicated in patients whose blood pressure is not adequately controlled on telmisartan alone.

4.2 Posology and method of administration

Adults

MicardisPlus should be taken once daily with liquid, with or without food in patients whose blood pressure is not adequately controlled by telmisartan alone. Individual dose titration with each of the two components is recommended before changing to the fixed dose combination.

When clinically appropriate, direct change from monotherapy to the fixed combination may be considered

- MicardisPlus 40/12.5 mg may be administered in patients whose blood pressure is not adequately controlled by Micardis 40 mg.

- MicardisPlus 80/12.5 mg may be administered in patients whose blood pressure is not adequately controlled by Micardis 80 mg.

Renal Impairment:

Periodic monitoring of renal function is advised (see 4.4 Special Warnings and Special Precautions for Use).

Hepatic Impairment:

In patients with mild to moderate hepatic impairment the posology should not exceed MicardisPlus 40/12.5 mg once daily. MicardisPlus is not indicated in patients with severe hepatic impairment. Thiazides should be used with caution in patients with impaired hepatic function (see 4.4 Special Warnings and Precautions for Use).

Elderly

No dosage adjustment is necessary.

Children and Adolescents

Safety and efficacy of MicardisPlus have not been established in children and adolescents up to 18 years.

4.3 Contraindications

- Hypersensitivity to any of the active substances or to any of the excipients (see 6.1 List of Excipients).

- Hypersensitivity to other sulphonamide-derived substances (since hydrochlorothiazide is a sulphonamide-derived medicinal product).

- Second and third trimesters of pregnancy and lactation (see 4.6 Pregnancy and Lactation).

- Cholestasis and biliary obstructive disorders.

- Severe hepatic impairment.

- Severe renal impairment (creatinine clearance < 30 ml/min).

- Refractory hypokalaemia, hypercalcaemia.

4.4 Special warnings and special precautions for use

Hepatic Impairment

MicardisPlus should not be given to patients with cholestasis, biliary obstructive disorders or severe hepatic insufficiency (see 4.3 Contraindications) since telmisartan is mostly eliminated with the bile. These patients can be expected to have reduced hepatic clearance for telmisartan.

In addition, MicardisPlus should be used with caution in patients with impaired hepatic function or progressive liver disease, since minor alterations of fluid and electrolyte balance may precipitate hepatic coma. There is no clinical experience with MicardisPlus in patients with hepatic impairment.

Renovascular Hypertension

There is an increased risk of severe hypotension and renal insufficiency when patients with bilateral renal artery stenosis or stenosis of the artery to a single functioning kidney are treated with medicinal products that affect the renin-angiotensin-aldosterone system.

Renal Impairment and Kidney Transplantation

MicardisPlus should not be used in patients with severe renal impairment (creatinine clearance < 30 ml/min) (see 4.3 Contraindications). There is no experience regarding the administration of MicardisPlus in patients with a recent kidney transplant. Experience with MicardisPlus is modest in the patients with mild to moderate renal impairment, therefore periodic monitoring of potassium, creatinine and uric acid serum levels is recommended. Thiazide diuretic-associated azotaemia may occur in patients with impaired renal function.

Intravascular Volume Depletion

Symptomatic hypotension, especially after the first dose, may occur in patients who are volume and/or sodium depleted by vigorous diuretic therapy, dietary salt restriction, diarrhoea or vomiting. Such conditions should be corrected before the administration of MicardisPlus.

Other Conditions with Stimulation of the Renin-Angiotensin-Aldosterone System

In patients whose vascular tone and renal function depend predominantly on the activity of the renin-angiotensin-aldosterone system (e.g. patients with severe congestive heart failure or underlying renal disease, including renal artery stenosis), treatment with other medicinal products that affect this system has been associated with acute hypotension, hyperazotaemia, oliguria, or rarely acute renal failure.

Primary Aldosteronism

Patients with primary aldosteronism generally will not respond to antihypertensive medicinal products acting through inhibition of the renin-angiotensin system. Therefore, the use of MicardisPlus is not recommended.

Aortic and Mitral Valve Stenosis, Obstructive Hypertrophic Cardiomyopathy

As with other vasodilators, special caution is indicated in patients suffering from aortic or mitral stenosis, or obstructive hypertrophic cardiomyopathy.

Metabolic and Endocrine Effects

Thiazide therapy may impair glucose tolerance. In diabetic patients dosage adjustments of insulin or oral hypoglycaemic agents may be required. Latent diabetes mellitus may become manifest during thiazide therapy.

Increase in cholesterol and triglyceride levels have been associated with thiazide diuretic therapy; however, at the 12.5 mg dose contained in MicardisPlus, minimal or no effects were reported. Hyperuricaemia may occur or frank gout may be precipitated in some patients receiving thiazide therapy.

Electrolyte Imbalance

As for any patient receiving diuretic therapy, periodic determination of serum electrolytes should be performed at appropriate intervals. Thiazides, including hydrochlorothiazide, can cause fluid or electrolyte imbalance (including hypokalaemia, hyponatraemia and hypochloraemic alkalosis). Warning signs of fluid or electrolyte imbalance are dryness of mouth, thirst, weakness, lethargy, drowsiness, restlessness, muscle pain or cramps, muscular fatigue, hypotension, oliguria, tachycardia, and gastrointestinal disturbances such as nausea or vomiting (see section 4.8 Undesirable Effects).

- Hypokalaemia

Although hypokalaemia may develop with the use of thiazide diuretics, concurrent therapy with telmisartan may reduce diuretic-induced hypokalaemia. The risk of hypokalaemia is greater in patients with cirrhosis of liver, in patients experiencing brisk diuresis, in patients who are receiving inadequate oral intake of electrolytes and in patients receiving concomitant therapy with corticosteroids or ACTH (see also section 4.5 Interactions with other Medicaments and other forms of Interaction).

- Hyperkalaemia

Conversely, due to the antagonism of the angiotensin II (AT1) receptors by the telmisartan component of MicardisPlus, hyperkalaemia might occur. Although clinically significant hyperkalaemia has not been documented with MicardisPlus, risk factors for the development of hyperkalaemia include renal insufficiency and/or heart failure, and diabetes mellitus. Potassium-sparing diuretics, potassium supplements or potassium-containing salt substitutes should be co-administered cautiously with MicardisPlus (see 4.5 Interactions with other Medicaments and other forms of Interaction).

- Hyponatraemia and Hypochloraemic Alkalosis

There is no evidence that MicardisPlus would reduce or prevent diuretic-induced hyponatraemia. Chloride deficit is generally mild and usually does not require treatment.

- Hypercalcaemia

Thiazides may decrease urinary calcium excretion and cause an intermittent and slight elevation of serum calcium in the absence of known disorders of calcium metabolism. Marked hypercalcaemia may be evidence of hidden hyperparathyroidism. Thiazides should be discontinued before carrying out tests for parathyroid function.

- Hypomagnesaemia

Thiazides have been shown to increase the urinary excretion of magnesium, which may result in hypomagnesaemia (see also section 4.5 Interactions with other Medicaments and other forms of Interaction).

Sorbitol

A recommended daily dose of MicardisPlus 40/12.5 mg tablets contains 169 mg sorbitol. A recommended daily dose of MicardisPlus 80/12.5 mg tablets contains 338 mg sorbitol. MicardisPlus is therefore unsuitable for patients with hereditary fructose intolerance.

Ethnic Differences

As with all other angiotensin antagonists telmisartan is apparently less effective in lowering blood pressure in black patients than in non blacks, possibly because of higher prevalence of low renin states in the black hypertensive population.

Other

As with any antihypertensive agent, excessive reduction of blood pressure in patients with ischaemic cardiopathy or ischaemic cardiovascular disease could result in a myocardial infarction or stroke.

General

Hypersensitivity reactions to hydrochlorothiazide may occur in patients with or without a history of allergy or bronchial asthma, but are more likely in patients with such a history.

Exacerbation or activation of systemic lupus erythematosus has been reported with the use of thiazide diuretics.

4.5 Interaction with other medicinal products and other forms of Interaction

Lithium

Reversible increases in serum lithium concentrations and toxicity have been reported during concomitant administration of lithium with angiotensin converting enzyme inhibitors. Very rare cases have also been reported with angiotensin II receptor antagonists. In addition, renal clearance of lithium is reduced by thiazides as a consequence the risk of lithium toxicity may be increased with MicardisPlus. Co-administration of lithium and MicardisPlus should only be allowed under strict medical supervision and should not be recommended. If this combination proves essential, serum lithium level monitoring is recommended during concomitant use.

Medicinal Products associated with Potassium Loss and Hypokalaemia (e.g. other kaliuretic diuretics, laxatives, corticosteroids, ACTH, amphotericin, carbenoxolone, penicillin G sodium, salicylic acid and derivatives)

If these drugs are to be prescribed with the hydrochlorothiazide-telmisartan combination, monitoring of potassium plasma levels is advised. These medicinal products may potentiate the effect of hydrochlorothiazide on serum potassium (see section 4.4 Special Warnings and Precautions for Use).

Medicinal Products that may increase Potassium Levels or Induce Hyperkalaemia (e.g. ACE inhibitors, potassium-sparing diuretics, potassium supplements, salt substitutes containing potassium, cyclosporin or other medicinal products such as heparin sodium)

If these medicinal products are to be prescribed with the hydrochlorothiazide-telmisartan combination, monitoring of potassium plasma levels is advised. Based on the experience with the use of other medicinal products that blunt the renin-angiotensin system, concomitant use of the above medicinal products may lead to increases in serum potassium (see section 4.4 Special Warnings and Precautions for Use).

Medicinal Products affected by Serum Potassium Disturbances:

Periodic monitoring of serum potassium and ECG is recommended when MicardisPlus is administered with drugs affected by serum potassium disturbances (e.g. digitalis glycosides, antiarrhythmics) and the following torsades de pointes inducing drugs (which include some antiarrhythmics), hypokalaemia being a predisposing factor to torsades de pointes.

- Class Ia antiarrythmics (e.g. quinidine, hydroquinidine, disopyramide).

- Class III antiarrythmics (e.g. amiodarone, sotalol, dofetilide, ibutilide).

– Some antipsychotics (e.g. thioridazine, chlorpromazine, levomepromazine, trifluoperazine, cyamemazine, sulpiride, sultopride, amisulpride, tiapride, pimozide, haloperidol, droperidol).

- Others (e.g. bepridil, cisapride, diphemanil, erythromycin IV, halofantrin, mizolastin, pentamidine, sparfloxacine, terfenadine, vincamine IV.)

Digitalis Glycosides

Thiazide-induced hypokalaemia or hypomagnesaemia favours the onset of digitalis-induced cardiac arrhythmias (see 4.4 Special Warnings and Precautions for Use).

Other Antihypertensive Agents

Telmisartan may increase the hypotensive effect of other antihypertensive agents.

Alcohol, Barbiturates, Narcotics or Antidepressants

Potentiation of orthostatic hypotension may occur.

Baclofen, Amifostine

Potentiation of antihypertensive effect may occur.

Antidiabetic Drugs (oral agents and insulin)

Dosage adjustment of the antidiabetic drug may be required (see 4.4 Special Warnings and Precautions for Use).

Metformin

Metformin should be used with precaution: risk of lactic acidosis induced by a possible functional renal failure linked to hydrochlorothiazide.

Cholestyramine and Colestipol Resins

Absorption of hydrochlorothiazide is impaired in the presence of anionic exchange resins.

Non-Steroidal Anti-Inflammatory Drugs

The administration of a non-steroidal anti-inflammatory drug may reduce the diuretic, natriuretic and antihypertensive effects of thiazide diuretics in some patients. In elderly patients and patients which may be dehydrated there is a risk of acute renal failure, therefore monitoring of renal function at the initiation of treatment is recommended.

Pressor Amines (e.g. noradrenaline)

The effect of pressor amines may be decreased.

Non-Depolarizing Skeletal Muscle Relaxants (e.g. tubocurarine)

The effect of nondepolarizing skeletal muscle relaxants may be potentiated by hydrochlorothiazide.

Medicinal Products used in the Treatment for Gout (probenecid, sulfinpyrazone and allopurinol)

Dosage adjustment of uricosuric medications may be necessary as hydrochlorothiazide may raise the level of serum uric acid. Increase in dosage of probenecid or sulfinpyrazone may be necessary. Co-administration of thiazide may increase the incidence of hypersensitivity reactions of allopurinol.

Calcium Salts

Thiazide diuretics may increase serum calcium levels due to the decreased excretion. If calcium supplements must be prescribed, serum calcium levels should be monitored and calcium dosage adjusted accordingly.

Beta-Blockers and Diazoxide:

The hyperglycaemic effect of beta-blockers and diazoxide may be enhanced by thiazides.

Anticholinergic Agents (e.g. atropine, biperiden)

May increase the bioavailability of thiazide-type diuretics by decreasing gastrointestinal motility and stomach emptying rate.

Amantadine

Thiazides may increase the risk of adverse effects caused by amantadine.

Cytotoxic Agents (e.g. cyclophosphamide, methotrexate)

Thiazides may reduce the renal excretion of cytotoxic drugs and potentiate their myelosuppressive effects.

4.6 Pregnancy and lactation

Pregnancy (See 4.3 Contraindications)

There are no adequate data on the use of MicardisPlus in pregnant women. Animal studies do not indicate a teratogenic effect, but have shown foetotoxicity. Therefore, as a precautionary measure MicardisPlus should preferably not be used during the first trimester of pregnancy. A switch to a suitable alternative treatment should be carried out in advance of a planned pregnancy.

In the second and third trimesters, substances that act directly on the renin-angiotensin-system can cause injury and even death in the developing foetus, therefore, MicardisPlus is contraindicated in the second and third trimesters of pregnancy. If pregnancy is diagnosed MicardisPlus should be discontinued as soon as possible.

Thiazides cross the placental barrier and appear in cord blood. They may cause foetal electrolyte disturbances and possibly other reactions that have occurred in the adults. Cases of neonatal thrombocytopenia, of foetal or neonatal jaundice have been reported with maternal thiazide therapy.

Lactation (see 4.3 Contraindications)

MicardisPlus is contraindicated during lactation since it is not known whether telmisartan is excreted in human milk. Thiazides appear in human milk and may inhibit lactation.

4.7 Effects on ability to drive and use machines

No studies on the effect on the ability to drive and use machines have been performed. However, when driving vehicles or operating machinery it must be borne in mind that dizziness or drowsiness may occasionally occur when taking antihypertensive therapy.

4.8 Undesirable effects

Fixed Dose Combination

The overall incidence of adverse events reported with MicardisPlus was comparable to those reported with telmisartan alone in randomised controlled trials involving 1471 patients randomised to receive telmisartan plus hydrochlorothiazide (835) or telmisartan alone (636). Dose-relationship of undesirable effects was not established and they showed no correlation with gender, age or race of the patients.

Adverse reactions reported in all clinical trials and occurring more frequently ($p \leqslant 0.05$) with telmisartan plus hydrochlorothiazide than with placebo are shown below according to system organ class. Adverse reactions known to occur with each component given singly but which have not been seen in clinical trials may occur during treatment with MicardisPlus.

Adverse reactions have been ranked under headings of frequency using the following convention:

very common ($\geqslant$ 1/10); common ($\geqslant$ 1/100, $<$1/10); uncommon ($\geqslant$ 1/1000, $<$1/100); rare ($\geqslant$ 1/10000, $<$ 1/1000); very rare ($<$ 1/10000)

Autonomic Nervous System Common:	Impotence
Body as a Whole, General Common: Uncommon:	Back pain, influenza-like symptoms, pain Allergy, leg pain
Central and Peripheral Nervous System Common:	Dizziness, vertigo
Gastro-intestinal System Common: Uncommon:	Abdominal pain, diarrhoea, dyspepsia, gastritis Gastro-intestinal disorder
Metabolic and Nutritional System Common: Uncommon:	Hypercholesterolaemia, hypokalaemia Loss of diabetic control, hyperuricaemia
Musculo-Skeletal System Common:	Arthralgia, arthrosis, myalgia
Psychiatric System Common:	Anxiety
Respiratory System Common:	Bronchitis, pharyngitis, sinusitis, upper respiratory tract infection
Skin and Appendages System Common: Uncommon:	Eczema Skin disorder
Urinary System Common:	Urinary tract infection

As with other angiotensin II antagonists isolated cases of angioedema, urticaria and other related reactions have been reported.

Laboratory Findings

Changes in laboratory findings that were seen in clinical trials of telmisartan plus hydrochlorothiazide are included above. (see also section 4.4 Special Warnings and Precautions for Use).

Additional Information on Individual Components

Undesirable effects previously reported with one of the individual components may be potential undesirable effects with MicardisPlus, even if not observed in clinical trials with this product.

Telmisartan

Undesirable effects occurred with similar frequency in placebo and telmisartan treated patients.

The overall incidence of adverse events reported with telmisartan (41.4%) was usually comparable to placebo (43.9%) in placebo controlled trials. The following adverse drug reactions listed below have been accumulated from all clinical trials including 5788 hypertensive patients treated with telmisartan:

Body as a Whole, General Common: Uncommon:	Back pain (e.g.sciatica), chest pain, influenza- like symptoms, symptoms of infection (e.g. urinary tract infections including cystitis) Abnormal vision, sweating increased

Central and Peripheral Nervous System Uncommon:	Vertigo
Gastro-intestinal System Common: Uncommon:	Abdominal pain, diarrhoea, dyspepsia, gastro- intestinal disorders Dry mouth, flatulence
Musculo-Skeletal System Common: Uncommon:	Arthralgia, cramps in legs or leg pain, myalgia Tendinitis like symptoms
Psychiatric System Uncommon:	Anxiety
Respiratory System Common:	Upper respiratory tract infections including pharyngitis and sinusitis
Skin and Appendages System Common:	Skin disorders like eczema

In addition, since the introduction of telmisartan in the market, cases of erythema, pruritus, faintness, insomnia, depression, stomach upset, vomiting, hypotension, bradycardia, tachycardia, dyspnoea, eosinophilia, thrombocytopenia, weakness, and lack of efficacy have been reported rarely.

Laboratory Findings

Infrequently, a decrease in haemoglobin or an increase in uric acid have been observed which occur more often during treatment with telmisartan than with placebo. Increases in creatinine or liver enzymes have been observed during treatment with telmisartan but these changes in laboratory findings occurred with a frequency similar to or lower than placebo (see also section 4.4 Special Warnings and Precautions for Use).

Hydrochlorothiazide

Hydrochlorothiazide may cause or exacerbate volume depletion which could lead to electrolyte imbalance (see also section 4.4 Special Warnings and Precautions for Use).

Adverse events reported with the use of hydrochlorothiazide alone include:

Gastrointestinal system	Anorexia, loss of appetite, gastric irritation, diarrhoea, constipation, sialadenitis, pancreatitis
Hepatobiliary disorders	Jaundice (intrahepatic cholestatic jaundice)
Eye disorders	Xanthopsia, transient blurred vision
Blood and lymphatic system	Leukopenia, neutropenia/ agranulocytosis, thrombocytopenia, aplastic anaemia, haemolytic anaemia, bone marrow depression
Skin and subcutaneous tissue disorders	Photosensitivity reactions, rash, cutaneous lupus erythematosus-like reactions, reactivation of cutaneous lupus, erythematosus, urticaria, necrotizing angiitis (vasculitis, cutaneous vasculitis), anaphylactic reactions, toxic epidermal necrolysis
General disorders	Fever
Respiratory disorders	Respiratory distress (including pneumonitis and pulmonary oedema)
Renal and urinary disorders	Renal dysfunction, interstitial nephritis
Musculoskeletal disorders	Muscle spasm, weakness
Nervous system disorders	Restlessness, light-headedness, vertigo, paraesthesia
Vascular disorders	Postural hypotension
Cardiac disorders	Cardiac arrhythmias
Psychiatric disorders	Sleep disturbances, depression

Laboratory Findings

Hyperglycaemia, glycosuria, hyperuricaemia, electrolyte imbalance (including hyponatraemia and hypokalaemia), increases in cholesterol and triglycerides.

4.9 Overdose

The patient should be closely monitored, and the treatment should be symptomatic and supportive. Management depends on the time since ingestion and the severity of the symptoms. Suggested measures include induction of emesis and/or gastric lavage. Activated charcoal may be useful in the treatment of overdosage. Serum electrolytes and creatinine should be monitored frequently. If hypotension occurs, the patient should be placed in a supine position, with salt and volume replacements given quickly.

The most likely manifestations of telmisartan overdosage are expected to be hypotension and tachycardia; bradycardia might also occur. Overdosage with hydrochlorothiazide is associated with electrolyte depletion (hypokalaemia, hypochloraemia) and dehydration resulting from excessive diuresis. The most common signs and symptoms of overdosage are nausea and somnolence. Hypokalaemia may result in muscle spasm and/or accentuate cardiac arrhythmias associated with the concomitant use of digitalis glycosides or certain anti-arrhythmic drugs. No data are available for telmisartan with regard to overdose in humans. Telmisartan is not removed by haemodialysis. The degree to which hydrochlorothiazide is removed by haemodialysis has not been established.

5. PHARMACOLOGICAL PROPERTIES

5.1 Pharmacodynamic properties

Pharmacotherapeutic Group: Angiotensin II antagonists and diuretics, ATC code: C09D A

MicardisPlus is a combination of an angiotensin II receptor antagonist, telmisartan, and a thiazide diuretic, hydrochlorothiazide. The combination of these ingredients has an additive antihypertensive effect, reducing blood pressure to a greater degree than either component alone. MicardisPlus once daily produces effective and smooth reductions in blood pressure across the therapeutic dose range.

Telmisartan is an orally effective and specific angiotensin II receptor subtype 1 (AT_1) antagonist.

Telmisartan displaces angiotensin II with very high affinity from its binding site at the AT_1 receptor subtype, which is responsible for the known actions of angiotensin II. Telmisartan does not exhibit any partial agonist activity at the AT_1 receptor. Telmisartan selectively binds the AT_1 receptor. The binding is long-lasting. Telmisartan does not show affinity for other receptors, including AT_2 and other less characterised AT receptors. The functional role of these receptors is not known, nor is the effect of their possible overstimulation by angiotensin II, whose levels are increased by telmisartan. Plasma aldosterone levels are decreased by telmisartan. Telmisartan does not inhibit human plasma renin or block ion channels. Telmisartan does not inhibit angiotensin converting enzyme (kininase II), the enzyme which also degrades bradykinin. Therefore, it is not expected to potentiate bradykinin-mediated adverse effects.

An 80 mg dose of telmisartan administered to healthy volunteers almost completely inhibits the angiotensin II evoked blood pressure increase. The inhibitory effect is maintained over 24 hours and still measurable up to 48 hours.

After the first dose of telmisartan, the antihypertensive activity gradually becomes evident within 3 hours. The maximum reduction in blood pressure is generally attained 4-8 weeks after the start of treatment and is sustained during long-term therapy. The antihypertensive effect persists constantly over 24 hours after dosing and includes the last 4 hours before the next dose as shown by ambulatory blood pressure measurements. This is confirmed by measurements made at the point of maximum effect and immediately prior to the next dose (trough to peak ratios consistently above 80 % after doses of 40 and 80 mg of telmisartan in placebo controlled clinical studies).

In patients with hypertension telmisartan reduces both systolic and diastolic blood pressure without affecting pulse rate. The antihypertensive efficacy of telmisartan is comparable to that of agents representative of other classes of antihypertensive drugs (demonstrated in clinical trials comparing telmisartan to amlodipine, atenolol, enalapril, hydrochlorothiazide, and lisinopril).

Upon abrupt cessation of treatment with telmisartan, blood pressure gradually returns to pre-treatment values over a period of several days without evidence of rebound hypertension.

The incidence of dry cough was significantly lower in patients treated with telmisartan than in those given angiotensin converting enzyme inhibitors in clinical trials directly comparing the two antihypertensive treatments.

The effects of telmisartan on mortality and cardiovascular morbidity are currently unknown.

Hydrochlorothiazide is a thiazide diuretic. The mechanism of the antihypertensive effect of thiazide diuretics is not fully known. Thiazides effect the renal tubular mechanisms of electrolyte reabsorption, directly increasing excretion of sodium and chloride in approximately equivalent amounts. The diuretic action of hydrochlorothiazide reduces plasma volume, increases plasma renin activity, increases aldosterone secretion, with consequent increases in urinary potassium and bicarbonate loss, and decreases in serum potassium. Presumably through blockade of the renin-angiotensin-aldosterone system, co-administration of telmisartan tends to reverse the potassium loss associated with these diuretics. With hydrochlorothiazide, onset of diuresis occurs in 2 hours, and peak effect occurs at about 4 hours, while the action persists for approximately 6-12 hours.

Epidemiological studies have shown that long-term treatment with hydrochlorothiazide reduces the risk of cardiovascular mortality and morbidity.

The effects of Fixed Dose Combination of telmisartan/ hydrochlorothiazide on mortality and cardiovascular morbidity are currently unknown.

5.2 Pharmacokinetic properties

Concomitant administration of hydrochlorothiazide and telmisartan does not appear to affect the pharmacokinetics of either drug in healthy subjects.

Absorption

Telmisartan: Following oral administration peak concentrations of telmisartan are reached in 0.5 – 1.5 h after dosing. The absolute bioavailability of telmisartan at 40 mg and 160 mg was 42 % and 58 %, respectively. Food slightly reduces the bioavailability of telmisartan with a reduction in the area under the plasma concentration time curve (AUC) of about 6 % with the 40 mg tablet and about 19 % after a 160 mg dose. By 3 hours after administration plasma concentrations are similar whether telmisartan is taken fasting or with food. The small reduction in AUC is not expected to cause a reduction in the therapeutic efficacy. The pharmacokinetics of orally administered telmisartan are non-linear over doses from 20 – 160 mg with greater than proportional increases of plasma concentrations (C_{max} and AUC) with increasing doses. Telmisartan does not accumulate significantly in plasma on repeated administration.

Hydrochlorothiazide: Following oral administration of MicardisPlus peak concentrations of hydrochlorothiazide are reached in approximately 1.0 – 3.0 hours after dosing. Based on cumulative renal excretion of hydrochlorothiazide the absolute bioavailability was about 60%.

Distribution

Telmisartan is highly bound to plasma proteins (>99.5 %) mainly albumin and alpha I-acid glycoprotein. The apparent volume of distribution for telmisartan is approximately 500 litres indicating additional tissue binding.

Hydrochlorothiazide is 68 % protein bound in the plasma and its apparent volume of distribution is 0.83 – 1.14 l/kg.

Biotransformation and Elimination

Telmisartan: Following either intravenous or oral administration of $_{14}$C-labelled telmisartan most of the administered dose (> 97 %) was eliminated in faeces via biliary excretion. Only minute amounts were found in urine. Telmisartan is metabolised by conjugation to form a pharmacologically inactive acylglucuronide. The glucuronide of the parent compound is the only metabolite that has been identified in humans. After a single dose of $_{14}$C-labelled telmisartan the glucuronide represents approximately 11% of the measured radioactivity in plasma. The cytochrome P450 isoenzymes are not involved in the metabolism of telmisartan. Total plasma clearance of telmisartan after oral administration is > 1500 ml/min. Terminal elimination half-life was > 20 hours.

Hydrochlorothiazide: Hydrochlorothiazide is not metabolised in man and is excreted almost entirely as unchanged drug in urine. About 60 % of the oral dose are eliminated as unchanged drug within 48 hours. Renal clearance is about 250 – 300 ml/min. The terminal elimination half-life of hydrochlorothiazide is 10 – 15 hours.

Special Populations

Elderly patients: Pharmacokinetics of telmisartan do not differ between the elderly and those younger than 65 years.

Gender: Plasma concentrations of telmisartan are generally 2 – 3 times higher in females than in males. In clinical trials however, no significant increases in blood pressure response or in the incidence of orthostatic hypotension were found in women. No dosage adjustment is necessary. There was a trend towards higher plasma concentrations of hydrochlorothiazide in female than in male subjects. This is not considered to be of clinical relevance.

Patients with renal impairment: Renal excretion does not contribute to the clearance of telmisartan. Based on modest experience in patients with mild to moderate renal impairment (creatinine clearance of 30 – 60 ml/min, mean about 50 ml/min) no dosage adjustment is necessary in patients with decreased renal function. Telmisartan is not removed from blood by haemodialysis. In patients with impaired renal function the rate of hydrochlorothiazide elimination is reduced. In a typical study in patients with a mean creatinine clearance of 90 ml/min the elimination half-life of hydrochlorothiazide was increased. In functionally anephric patients the elimination half-life is about 34 hours.

Patients with hepatic impairment: Pharmacokinetic studies in patients with hepatic impairment showed an increase in absolute bioavailability up to nearly 100 %. The elimination half-life is not changed in patients with hepatic impairment.

5.3 Preclinical safety data

In preclinical safety studies performed with co-administration of telmisartan and hydrochlorothiazide in normotensive rats and dogs, doses producing exposure comparable to that in the clinical therapeutic range caused no additional findings not already observed with administration of either substance alone. The toxicological findings observed appear to have no relevance to human therapeutic use.

Toxicological findings also well known from preclinical studies with angiotensin converting enzyme inhibitors and angiotensin II receptor antagonists were: a reduction of red cell parameters (erythrocytes, haemoglobin, haematocrit), changes of renal haemodynamics (increased blood urea nitrogen and creatinine), increased plasma renin activity, hypertrophy/hyperplasia of the juxtaglomerular cells and gastric mucosal injury. Gastric lesions could be prevented/ameliorated by oral saline supplementation and group housing of animals. In dogs renal tubular dilation and atrophy were observed. These findings are considered to be due to the pharmacological activity of telmisartan.

Telmisartan showed no evidence of mutagenicity and relevant clastogenic activity in in vitro studies and no evidence of carcinogenicity in rats and mice. Studies with hydrochlorothiazide have shown equivocal evidence for a genotoxic or carcinogenic effect in some experimental models. However, the extensive human experience with hydrochlorothiazide has failed to show an association between its use and an increase in neoplasms.

For the foetotoxic potential of the telmisartan/hydrochlorothiazide combination see 4.6 Pregnancy and Lactation.

6. PHARMACEUTICAL PARTICULARS

6.1 List of excipients

Lactose monohydrate,

magnesium stearate,

maize starch,

meglumine,

microcrystalline cellulose,

povidone (K25),

red ferric oxide (E172),

sodium hydroxide,

sodium starch glycollate (type A),

sorbitol (E420).

6.2 Incompatibilities

Not applicable.

6.3 Shelf life

2 years

6.4 Special precautions for storage

Store in the original package in order to protect from moisture

6.5 Nature and contents of container

14 tablets

28 tablets

56 tablets

98 tablets

Polyamide/aluminium/PVC blisters

28 × 1 tablets

Polyamide/aluminium/PVC perforated unit dose blisters

Not all package sizes may be marketed

6.6 Instructions for use and handling

Occasionally, the outer layer of the blister pack has been observed to separate from the inner layer between the blister pockets. No action need be taken if this is observed.

7. MARKETING AUTHORISATION HOLDER

Boehringer Ingelheim International GmbH

Binger Str. 173

D-55216 Ingelheim am Rhein

Germany

8. MARKETING AUTHORISATION NUMBER(S)

MicardisPlus 40/12.5 mg tablets:

EU/1/02/213/001 (14 tablets)

EU/1/02/213/002 (28 tablets)

EU/1/02/213/003 (28 × 1 tablets)

EU/1/02/213/004 (56 tablets)

EU/1/02/213/005 (98 tablets)

MicardisPlus 80/12.5 mg tablets:

EU/1/02/213/006 (14 tablets)

EU/1/02/213/007 (28 tablets)

EU/1/02/213/008 (28 × 1 tablets)

EU/1/02/213/009 (56 tablets)

EU/1/02/213/010 (98 tablets)

9. DATE OF FIRST AUTHORISATION/RENEWAL OF THE AUTHORISATION

19th April 2002

10. DATE OF REVISION OF THE TEXT

11. Legal Category

POM

Micralax Micro-Enema

(UCB Pharma Limited)

1. NAME OF THE MEDICINAL PRODUCT

Micralax Micro-enema

2. QUALITATIVE AND QUANTITATIVE COMPOSITION

Sodium alkylsulphoacetate 0.90% w/v; sodium citrate BP 9.0% w/v

3. PHARMACEUTICAL FORM

A colourless viscous liquid

4. CLINICAL PARTICULARS

4.1 Therapeutic indications

Micralax is indicated whenever an enema is necessary to relieve constipation: in dyschezia, especially in bedridden patients; in geriatrics, paediatrics and obstetrics; and in preparation for X-ray examination, proctoscopy and sigmoidoscopy.

4.2 Posology and method of administration

Adults and children aged 3 years and over: Administer the contents of one micro-enema rectally, inserting the full length of the nozzle. No lubricant is needed as a drop of the mixture is sufficient.

4.3 Contraindications

Do not use in patients with inflammatory bowel disease.

4.4 Special warnings and special precautions for use

None.

4.5 Interaction with other medicinal products and other forms of interaction

None.

4.6 Pregnancy and lactation

No special recommendations.

4.7 Effects on ability to drive and use machines

None.

4.8 Undesirable effects

No side effects have been reported. Excessive use may cause diarrhoea and fluid loss, which should be treated symptomatically.

4.9 Overdose

Not applicable.

5. PHARMACOLOGICAL PROPERTIES

5.1 Pharmacodynamic properties

Micralax combines the action of sodium citrate, a peptidising agent which can displace bound water present in the faeces; sorbitol, which enhances this action, and sodium alkylsulphoacetate, a wetting agent.

5.2 Pharmacokinetic properties

Not applicable.

5.3 Preclinical safety data

Not applicable.

6. PHARMACEUTICAL PARTICULARS

6.1 List of excipients

Sorbitol Solution 70% w/v BP, Glycerin PhEur, Sorbic Acid BP and Purified Water PhEur.

6.2 Incompatibilities

None.

6.3 Shelf life

60 months.

6.4 Special precautions for storage

Store at a temperature not exceeding 25°C.

6.5 Nature and contents of container

Polythene micro-enema tubes, capped, and with elongated nozzles.

6.6 Instructions for use and handling

Micralax usually works within 5 to 15 minutes, so make sure you are near a toilet before using it.

Always use a fresh tube of Micralax every time.

1. Lie down on your side with your knees drawn up towards your tummy or, if you prefer, sit on the toilet.

2. Pull or twist the black cap off the tube.

3. If you want to lubricate the nozzle before inserting it, squeeze a drop of liquid out onto the nozzle.

4. Insert the full length of the nozzle into your back passage.

5. Gently squeeze the tube until it is empty.

6. **Keep squeezing**
the tube as you pull the nozzle out of your back passage. This is to stop the medicine being drawn back into the tube.

7. Wait for the laxative to work (5-15 minutes)

7. MARKETING AUTHORISATION HOLDER

UCB Pharma Limited

208 Bath Road

Slough

Berkshire

SL1 3WE

UK

8. MARKETING AUTHORISATION NUMBER(S)

PL 00039/0368

9. DATE OF FIRST AUTHORISATION/RENEWAL OF THE AUTHORISATION

28 June 1991/28 May 1997

10. DATE OF REVISION OF THE TEXT

June 2005

P

MICROGYNON*30

(Schering Health Care Limited)

Presentation Each beige sugar-coated tablet contains 150 micrograms levonorgestrel and 30 micrograms ethinylestradiol.

Excipients:

lactose, maize starch, povidone 25 000, talc, magnesium stearate, sucrose, povidone 700 000, macrogol 6000, calcium carbonate, talc, titanium dioxide, glycerin, montan glycol wax, ferric oxide pigment yellow.

Uses Oral contraception and the recognised gynaecological indications for such oestrogen-progestogen combinations. The mode of action includes the inhibition of ovulation by suppression of the mid-cycle surge of luteinising hormone, the inspissation of cervical mucus so as to constitute a barrier to sperm, and the rendering of the endometrium unreceptive to implantation.

Dosage and administration

First treatment cycle: 1 tablet daily for 21 days, starting on the first day of the menstrual cycle. Contraceptive protection begins immediately.

Subsequent cycles: Tablet taking from the next pack of Microgynon 30 is continued after a 7-day interval, beginning on the same day of the week as the first pack.

Changing from 21-day combined oral contraceptives: The first tablet of Microgynon 30 should be taken on the first day immediately after the end of the previous oral contraceptive course. Additional contraceptive precautions are not required.

Changing from a combined Every Day pill (28 day tablets): Microgynon 30 should be started after taking the last active tablet from the Every Day Pill pack. The first Microgynon 30 tablet is taken the next day. Additional contraceptive precautions are not then required.

Changing from a progestogen-only pill (POP): The first tablet of Microgynon 30 should be taken on the first day of bleeding, even if a POP has already been taken on that day. Additional contraceptive precautions are not then required. The remaining progestogen-only pills should be discarded.

Post-partum and post-abortum use: After pregnancy, oral contraception can be started 21 days after a vaginal delivery, provided that the patient is fully ambulant and there are no puerperal complications. Additional contraceptive precautions will be required for the first 7 days of tablet taking. Since the first post-partum ovulation may precede the first bleeding, another method of contraception should be used in the interval between childbirth and the first course of tablets. After a first-trimester abortion, oral contraception may be started immediately, in which case no additional contraceptive precautions are required.

Pregnancy and lactation: If pregnancy occurs during medication with oral contraceptives, the preparation should be withdrawn immediately (see 'Reasons for stopping oral contraception immediately').

The use of Microgynon 30 during lactation may lead to a reduction in the volume of milk produced and to a change in its composition. Minute amounts of the active substances are excreted with the milk. Mothers who are breast-feeding may be advised instead to use a progestogen-only pill.

Special circumstances requiring additional contraception:

Incorrect administration: A single delayed tablet should be taken as soon as possible, and if this can be done within 12 hours of the correct time, contraceptive protection is maintained.

With longer delays, additional contraception is needed. Only the most recently delayed tablet should be taken, earlier missed tablets being omitted, and additional non-hormonal methods of contraception (except the rhythm or temperature methods) should be used for the next 7 days, while the next 7 tablets are being taken. Additionally, therefore, if tablet(s) have been missed during the last 7 days of a pack, there should be no break before the next pack is started. In this situation, a withdrawal bleed should not be expected until the end of the second pack. Some breakthrough bleeding may occur on tablet taking days but this is not clinically significant. If the patient does not have a withdrawal bleed during the tablet-free interval following the end of the second pack, the possibility of pregnancy must be ruled out before starting the next pack.

Gastro-intestinal upset: Vomiting or diarrhoea may reduce the efficacy of oral contraceptives by preventing full absorption. Tablet-taking from the current pack should be continued. Additional non-hormonal methods of contraception (except the rhythm or temperature methods) should be used during the gastro-intestinal upset and for 7 days following the upset. If these 7 days overrun the end of a pack, the next pack should be started without a break. In this situation, a withdrawal bleed should not be expected until the end of the second pack. If the patient does not have a withdrawal bleed during the tablet-free interval following the end of the second pack, the possibility of pregnancy must be ruled out before starting the next pack. Other methods of contraception should be considered if the gastro-intestinal disorder is likely to be prolonged.

Interaction with other drugs: Hepatic enzyme inducers such as barbiturates, primidone, phenobarbitone, phenytoin, phenylbutazone, rifampicin, carbamazepine and griseofulvin can impair the efficacy of Microgynon 30. For women receiving long-term therapy with hepatic enzyme inducers, another method of contraception should be used. The use of ampicillin and other antibiotics may also reduce the efficacy of Microgynon 30, possibly by altering the intestinal flora. Women receiving short courses of enzyme inducers or broad spectrum antibiotics should take additional, non-hormonal (except rhythm or temperature method) contraceptive precautions during the time of concurrent medication and for 7 days afterwards. If these 7 days overrun the end of a pack, the next pack should be started without a break. In this situation, a withdrawal bleed should not be expected until the end of the second pack. If the patient does not have a withdrawal bleed during the tablet-free interval following the end of the second pack, the possibility of pregnancy must be ruled out before resuming with the next pack. With rifampicin, additional contraceptive precautions should be continued for 4 weeks after treatment stops, even if only a short course was administered.

The requirement for oral antidiabetics or insulin can change as a result of the effect on glucose tolerance. The herbal remedy St John's wort (Hypericum perforatum) should not be taken concomitantly with Microgynon 30 as this could potentially lead to a loss of contraceptive effect.

Contra-indications, warnings etc

Contra-indications:

1. Pregnancy
2. Severe disturbances of liver function, jaundice or persistent itching during a previous pregnancy, Dubin-Johnson syndrome, Rotor syndrome, previous or existing liver tumours.
3. Existing or a history of confirmed venous thromboembolism (VTE), family history of idiopathic VTE, other known risk factors for VTE.
4. Existing or previous arterial thrombotic or embolic processes.
5. Conditions which predispose to thromboembolism e.g. disorders of the clotting processes, valvular heart disease and atrial fibrillation.
6. Sickle-cell anaemia.
7. Mammary or endometrial carcinoma, or a history of these conditions.
8. Severe diabetes mellitus with vascular changes.
9. Disorders of lipid metabolism.
10. History of herpes gestationis.
11. Deterioration of otosclerosis during pregnancy.
12. Undiagnosed abnormal vaginal bleeding.
13. Hypersensitivity to any of the components of Microgynon 30.

Warnings:

The use of any combined oral contraceptive carries an increased risk of venous thromboembolism (VTE) compared with no use. The excess risk of VTE is highest during the first year a woman ever uses a combined oral contraceptive. This increased risk is less than the risk of VTE associated with pregnancy which is estimated as 60 cases per 100 000 pregnancies. Some epidemiological studies have reported a greater risk of VTE for women using combined oral contraceptives containing desogestrel or gestodene (the so-called 'third generation' pills) than for women using pills containing levonorgestrel (the so-called 'second generation' pills).

The spontaneous incidence of VTE in healthy non-pregnant women (not taking any oral contraceptive) is about 5 cases per 100,000 per year. The incidence in users of second generation pills is about 15 per 100,000 women per year of use. The incidence in users of third generation pills is about 25 cases per 100,000 women per year of use; this excess incidence has not been satisfactorily explained by bias or confounding. This level of all these risks increases with age and is likely to be further increased in women with other known risk factors for VTE such as obesity.

The risk of venous and/or arterial thrombosis associated with combined oral contraceptives increases with:

- age;

Figure 1

Estimated cumulative numbers of breast cancers per 10,000 women diagnosed in 5 years of use and up to 10 years after stopping COCs, compared with numbers of breast cancers diagnosed in 10,000 women who had never used COCs

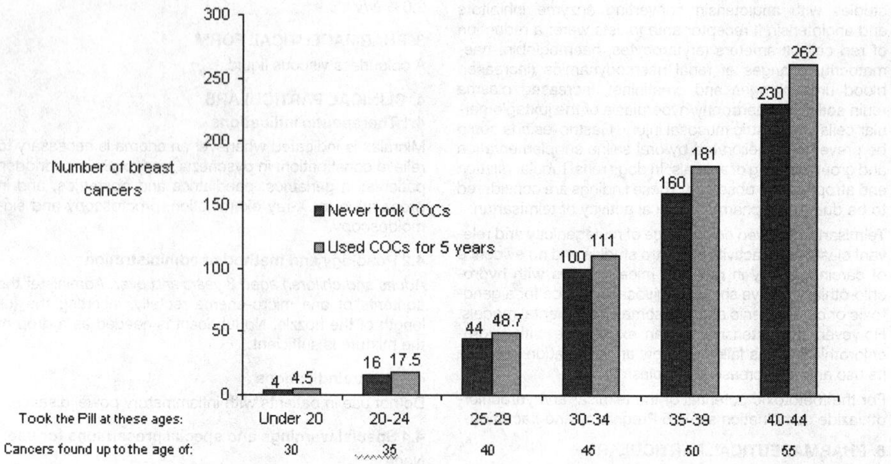

- smoking (with heavier smoking and increasing age the risk further increases, especially in women over 35 years of age);
- a positive family history (i.e. venous or arterial thromboembolism ever in a sibling or parent at a relatively early age). If a hereditary predisposition is suspected, the woman should be referred to a specialist for advice before deciding about any COC use;
- obesity (body mass index over 30 kg/m2);
- dyslipoproteinaemia;
- hypertension;
- valvular heart disease;
- atrial fibrillation;
- prolonged immobilisation, major surgery, any surgery to the legs, or major trauma. In these situations it is advisable to discontinue COC use (in the case of elective surgery at least six weeks in advance) and not to resume until two weeks after complete remobilisation.
- There is no consensus about the possible role of varicose veins and superficial thrombophlebitis in venous thromboembolism.
- The increased risk of thromboembolism in the puerperium must be considered (for information on "Pregnancy and Lactation" see Section 4.6).
- Other medical conditions which have been associated with adverse circulatory events include diabetes mellitus, systemic lupus erythematosus, haemolytic uraemic syndrome, chronic inflammatory bowel disease (Crohn's disease or ulcerative colitis), sickle cell disease and subarachnoid haemorrhage.
- An increase in frequency or severity of migraine during COC use (which may be prodromal of a cerebrovascular event) may be a reason for immediate discontinuation of the COC.
- Biochemical factors that may be indicative of hereditary or acquired predisposition for venous or arterial thrombosis include Activated Protein C (APC) resistance, hyperhomocysteinaemia, antithrombin-III deficiency, protein C deficiency, protein S deficiency, antiphospholipid antibodies (anticardiolipin antibodies, lupus anticoagulant).

When considering risk/benefit, the physician should take into account that adequate treatment of a condition may reduce the associated risk of thrombosis and that the risk associated with pregnancy is higher than that associated with COC use.

Numerous epidemiological studies have been reported on the risks of ovarian, endometrial, cervical and breast cancer in women using combined oral contraceptives. The evidence is clear that combined oral contraceptives offer substantial protection against both ovarian and endometrial cancer. An increased risk of cervical cancer in long-term users of combined oral contraceptives has been reported in some studies, but there continues to be controversy about the extent to which this is attributable to the confounding effects of sexual behaviour and other factors. A meta-analysis from 54 epidemiological studies reported that there is a slightly increased relative risk (RR = 1.24) of having breast cancer diagnosed in women who are currently using combined oral contraceptives (COCs). The observed pattern of increased risk may be due to an earlier diagnosis of breast cancer in COC users, the biological effects of COCs or a combination of both. The additional breast cancers diagnosed in current users of COCs or in women who have used COCs in the last ten years are more likely to be localised to the breast than those in women who never used COCs. Breast cancer is rare among women under 40 years of age whether or not they take COCs. Whilst this background risk increases with age, the excess number of breast cancer diagnoses in current and recent COC users is small in relation to the overall risk of breast cancer (see bar chart). The most important risk factor for breast cancer in COC users is the age women discontinue the COC; the older the age at stopping, the more breast cancers are diagnosed. Duration of use is less important and the excess risk gradually disappears during the course of the 10 years after stopping COC use such that by 10 years there appears to be no excess.

The possible increase in risk of breast cancer should be discussed with the user and weighed against the benefits of COCs taking into account the evidence that they offer substantial protection against the risk of developing certain other cancers (e.g. ovarian and endometrial cancer).

(see Figure 1 above)

The possibility cannot be ruled out that certain chronic diseases may occasionally deteriorate during the use of combined oral contraceptives (see '*Precautions*').

In rare cases benign and, in even rarer cases, malignant liver tumours leading in isolated cases to life-threatening intra-abdominal haemorrhage have been observed after the use of hormonal substances such as those contained in Microgynon 30. If severe upper abdominal complaints, liver enlargement or signs of intra-abdominal haemorrhage occur, the possibility of a liver tumour should be included in the differential diagnosis.

Reasons for stopping oral contraception immediately:

1. Occurrence for the first time, or exacerbation, of migrainous headaches or unusually frequent or unusually severe headaches.
2. Sudden disturbances of vision or hearing or other perceptual disorders.
3. First signs of thrombophlebitis or thromboembolic symptoms (e.g. unusual pains in or swelling of the leg(s), stabbing pains on breathing or coughing for no apparent reason). Feeling of pain and tightness in the chest.
4. Six weeks before an elective major operation (e.g. abdominal, orthopaedic), any surgery to the legs, medical treatment for varicose veins or prolonged immobilisation, e.g. after accidents or surgery. Do not restart until 2 weeks after full ambulation. In case of emergency surgery, thrombotic prophylaxis is usually indicated e.g. subcutaneous heparin.
5. Onset of jaundice, hepatitis, itching of the whole body.
6. Increase in epileptic seizures.
7. Significant rise in blood pressure.
8. Onset of severe depression.
9. Severe upper abdominal pain or liver enlargement.
10. Clear exacerbation of conditions known to be capable of deteriorating during oral contraception or pregnancy.
11. Pregnancy is a reason for stopping immediately because it has been suggested by some investigations that oral contraceptives taken in early pregnancy may slightly increase the risk of foetal malformations. Other investigations have failed to support these findings. The possibility therefore cannot be excluded, but it is certain that if a risk exists at all, it is very small.

Precautions:

Assessment of women prior to starting oral contraceptives (and at regular intervals thereafter) should include a personal and family medical history of each woman. Physical examination should be guided by this and by the contraindications, warnings etc for this product. The frequency and nature of these assessments should be based upon relevant guidelines and should be adapted to the individual woman, but should include measurement of blood pressure and, if judged appropriate by the clinician, breast, abdominal and pelvic examination including cervical cytology.

The following conditions require strict medical supervision during medication with oral contraceptives. Deterioration or first appearance of any of these conditions may indicate that use of the oral contraceptive should be discontinued: diabetes mellitus, or a tendency towards diabetes mellitus (e.g. unexplained glycosuria), hypertension, varicose veins, a history of phlebitis, otosclerosis, multiple sclerosis, epilepsy, porphyria, tetany, disturbed liver function, Sydenham's chorea, renal dysfunction, family history of clotting disorders, obesity, family history of breast cancer and patient history of benign breast disease, history of clinical depression, systemic lupus erythematosus, uterine fibroids and migraine, gall-stones, cardiovascular diseases, chloasma, asthma, an intolerance of contact lenses, or any disease that is prone to worsen during pregnancy. Some women may experience amenorrhoea or oligomenorrhoea after discontinuation of oral contraceptives, especially when these conditions existed prior to use. Women should be informed of this possibility.

Side-effects: In rare cases, headaches, gastric upsets, nausea, vomiting, breast tenderness, changes in body weight, changes in libido, depressive moods can occur. In predisposed women, use of Microgynon 30 can sometimes cause chloasma which is exacerbated by exposure to sunlight. Such women should avoid prolonged exposure to sunlight. Individual cases of poor tolerance of contact lenses have been reported with use of oral contraceptives. Contact lens wearers who develop changes in lens tolerance should be assessed by an ophthalmologist.

Menstrual changes:

1. Reduction of menstrual flow: This is not abnormal and it is to be expected in some patients. Indeed, it may be beneficial where heavy periods were previously experienced.

2. *Missed menstruation:* Occasionally, withdrawal bleeding may not occur at all. If the tablets have been taken correctly, pregnancy is very unlikely. If withdrawal bleeding fails to occur at the end of a second pack, the possibility of pregnancy must be ruled out before resuming with the next pack.

Intermenstrual bleeding: 'Spotting' or heavier 'breakthrough bleeding' sometimes occur during tablet taking, especially in the first few cycles, and normally cease spontaneously. Microgynon 30 should therefore be continued even if irregular bleeding occurs. If irregular bleeding is persistent, appropriate diagnostic measures to exclude an organic cause are indicated and may include curettage. This also applies in the case of spotting which occurs at irregular intervals in several consecutive cycles or which occurs for the first time after long use of Microgynon 30.

Effect on blood chemistry: The use of oral contraceptives may influence the results of certain laboratory tests including biochemical parameters of liver, thyroid, adrenal and renal function, plasma levels of carrier proteins and lipid/lipoprotein fractions, parameters of carbohydrate metabolism and parameters of coagulation and fibrinolysis. Laboratory staff should therefore be informed about oral contraceptive use when laboratory tests are requested.

Overdosage: Overdosage may cause nausea, vomiting and, in females, withdrawal bleeding. There are no specific antidotes and treatment should be symptomatic.

Pharmaceutical precautions *Shelf-life:* Five years.

Legal category POM

Package quantities Available in packs containing three months' supply

Further information Nil

Product licence number 0053/0064

Revision date: 12th October 2001

Microgynon 30 ED

(Schering Health Care Limited)

1. NAME OF THE MEDICINAL PRODUCT

Microgynon® 30 ED

2. QUALITATIVE AND QUANTITATIVE COMPOSITION

Each memo-pack contains 21 beige active tablets and 7 white placebo tablets which are larger.

Each active tablet contains 150 micrograms levonorgestrel and 30 micrograms ethinylestradiol.

3. PHARMACEUTICAL FORM

Sugar-coated tablets

4. CLINICAL PARTICULARS

4.1 Therapeutic indications

Oral contraception and the recognised gynaecological indications for such oestrogen-progestogen combinations.

4.2 Posology and method of administration

First treatment cycle: 1 tablet daily for 28 days, starting on the first day of the menstrual cycle. 21 (small) active tablets are taken followed by 7 (larger) placebo tablets. Contraceptive protection begins immediately.

Subsequent cycles: Tablet-taking is continuous, which means that the next pack of Microgynon 30 ED follows immediately without a break. A withdrawal bleed usually occurs when the placebo tablets are being taken.

Changing from 21-day combined oral contraceptives: The first tablet of Microgynon 30 ED should be taken on the first day immediately after the end of the previous oral contraceptive course. Additional contraceptive precautions are not required.

Changing from a combined Every Day pill (28 -day pill): Microgynon 30 ED should be started after taking the last active tablet from the previous Every Day pill pack. The first Microgynon 30 ED tablet is taken the next day. Additional contraceptive precautions are not then required.

Changing from a progestogen-only pill (POP):

The first tablet of Microgynon 30 ED should be taken on the first day of bleeding, even if a POP has already been taken on that day. Additional contraceptive precautions are not then required. The remaining progestogen-only pills should be discarded.

Post-partum and post-abortum use: After pregnancy, oral contraception can be started 21 days after a vaginal delivery, provided that the patient is fully ambulant and there are no puerperal complications. Additional contraceptive precautions will be required for the first 7 days of tablet taking to ensure adequate contraceptive cover if early ovulation has occurred. Since the first post-partum ovulation may precede the first bleeding, another method of contraception should be used in the interval between childbirth and the first course of tablets. After a first-trimester abortion, oral contraception may be started immediately in which case no additional contraceptive precautions are required.

Special circumstances requiring additional contraception

Incorrect administration: Errors in taking the 7 placebo tablets (i.e. the larger white tablets in the last row) can be ignored.

A single delayed active (small) tablet should be taken as soon as possible, and if this can be done within 12 hours of the correct time, contraceptive protection is maintained.

With longer delays in taking active tablets, additional contraception is needed. Only the most recently delayed tablet should be taken, earlier missed tablets being omitted, and additional non-hormonal methods of contraception (except the rhythm or temperature methods) should be used for *the next 7 days, while the next 7 active (small) tablets are being taken.* Therefore, if the 7 days additional contraception extend beyond the last active (small) tablet, the user should finish taking all the active tablets, discard the placebo tablets and start a new pack of Microgynon 30 ED the next day with an appropriate active (small) tablet. Thus, active tablet follows active tablet with no 7 day break. In this situation, a withdrawal bleed should not be expected until the end of the second pack. Some breakthrough bleeding may occur on tablet taking days but this is not clinically significant. If the patient does not have a withdrawal bleed following the end of the second pack, the possibility of pregnancy must be ruled out before starting the next pack.

Gastro-intestinal upset: Vomiting or diarrhoea may reduce the efficacy of oral contraceptives by preventing full absorption. Tablet-taking from the current pack should be continued. Additional non-hormonal methods of contraception (except the rhythm or temperature methods) should be used during the gastro-intestinal upset and for 7 days following the upset. If these 7 days extend beyond the last active (small) tablet the user should finish taking all the active tablets, discard the placebo tablets and start a new pack of Microgynon 30 ED the next day with an appropriate active (small) tablet. In this situation, a withdrawal bleed should not be expected until the end of the second pack. If the patient does not have a withdrawal bleed at the end of the second pack, the possibility of pregnancy must be ruled out before starting the next pack. Other methods of contraception should be considered if the gastro-intestinal disorder is likely to be prolonged.

Children and the elderly: Microgynon 30 ED is an oral contraceptive and is not applicable in children or the elderly.

4.3 Contraindications

1. Pregnancy

2. Severe disturbances of liver function, jaundice or persistent itching during a previous pregnancy, Dubin-Johnson syndrome, Rotor syndrome, previous or existing liver tumours

Existing or a history of confirmed venous thromboembolism (VTE), family history of idiopathic VTE and other known risk factors for VTE.

Existing or previous arterial thrombotic or embolic processes, conditions which predispose to them e.g. disorders of the clotting processes, valvular heart disease and atrial fibrillation

5. Sickle-cell anaemia

6. Mammary or endometrial carcinoma, or a history of these conditions

7. Severe diabetes mellitus with vascular changes

8. Disorders of lipid metabolism

9. History of herpes gestationis

10. Deterioration of otosclerosis during pregnancy

11. Undiagnosed abnormal vaginal bleeding

12. Hypersensitivity to any of the components of Microgynon 30 ED.

4.4 Special warnings and special precautions for use

Warnings:

The use of any combined oral contraceptive carries an increased risk of venous thromboembolism (VTE) compared with no use. The excess risk of VTE is highest during the first year a woman ever uses a combined oral contraceptive. This increased risk is less than the risk of VTE associated with pregnancy which is estimated as 60 cases per 100 000 pregnancies. Some epidemiological studies have reported a greater risk of VTE for women using combined oral contraceptives containing desogestrel or gestodene (the so-called 'third generation' pills) than for women using pills containing levonorgestrel (the so-called 'second generation' pills).

The spontaneous incidence of VTE in healthy non-pregnant women (not taking any oral contraceptive) is about 5 cases per 100,000 per year. The incidence in users of second generation pills is about 15 per 100,000 women per year of use. The incidence in users of third generation pills is about 25 cases per 100,000 women per year of use; this excess incidence has not been satisfactorily explained by bias or confounding. The level of all these risks of VTE increases with age and is likely to be further increased in women with other known risk factors for VTE such as obesity.

The risk of venous and/or arterial thrombosis associated with combined oral contraceptives increases with:

- age;
- smoking (with heavier smoking and increasing age the risk further increases, especially in women over 35 years of age);
- a positive family history (i.e. venous or arterial thromboembolism ever in a sibling or parent at a relatively early age). If a hereditary predisposition is suspected, the woman should be referred to a specialist for advice before deciding about any COC use;
- obesity (body mass index over 30 kg/m2);
- dyslipoproteinaemia;
- hypertension;
- valvular heart disease;
- atrial fibrillation;
- prolonged immobilisation, major surgery, any surgery to the legs, or major trauma. In these situations it is advisable to discontinue COC use (in the case of elective surgery at least six weeks in advance) and not to resume until two weeks after complete remobilisation.
- There is no consensus about the possible role of varicose veins and superficial thrombophlebitis in venous thromboembolism.
- The increased risk of thromboembolism in the puerperium must be considered (for information on Pregnancy and Lactation see Section 4.6).
- Other medical conditions which have been associated with adverse circulatory events include diabetes mellitus, systemic lupus erythematosus, haemolytic uraemic syndrome, chronic inflammatory bowel disease (Crohn's disease or ulcerative colitis), sickle cell disease and subarachnoid haemorrhage.
- An increase in frequency or severity of migraine during COC use (which may be prodromal of a cerebrovascular event) may be a reason for immediate discontinuation of the COC.
- Biochemical factors that may be indicative of hereditary or acquired predisposition for venous or arterial thrombosis include Activated Protein C (APC) resistance, hyperhomocysteinaemia, antithrombin-III deficiency, protein C deficiency, protein S deficiency, antiphospholipid antibodies (anticardiolipin antibodies, lupus anticoagulant).

When considering risk/benefit, the physician should take into account that adequate treatment of a condition may reduce the associated risk of thrombosis and that the risk associated with pregnancy is higher than that associated with COC use.

Numerous epidemiological studies have been reported on the risks of ovarian, endometrial, cervical and breast cancer in women using combined oral contraceptives. The evidence is clear that combined oral contraceptives offer substantial protection against both ovarian and endometrial cancer.

An increased risk of cervical cancer in long-term users of combined oral contraceptives has been reported in some studies, but there continues to be controversy about the

Figure 1 Estimated cumulative numbers of breast cancers per 10,000 women diagnosed in 5 years of use and up to 10 years after stopping COCs, compared with numbers of breast cancers diagnosed in 10,000 women who had never used COCs

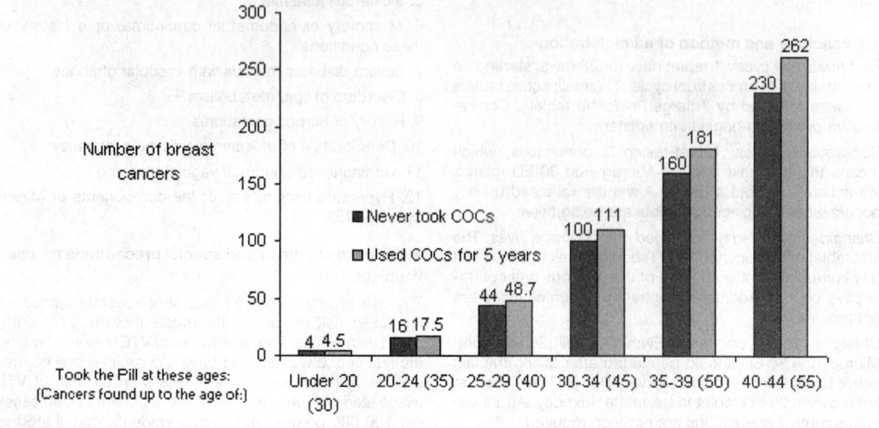

extent to which this is attributable to the confounding effects of sexual behaviour and other factors.

A meta-analysis from 54 epidemiological studies reported that there is a slightly increased relative risk (RR = 1.24) of having breast cancer diagnosed in women who are currently using combined oral contraceptives (COCs). The observed pattern of increased risk may be due to an earlier diagnosis of breast cancer in COC users, the biological effects of COCs or a combination of both. The additional breast cancers diagnosed in current users of COCs or in women who have used COCs in the last ten years are more likely to be localised to the breast than those in women who never used COCs.

Breast cancer is rare among women under 40 years of age whether or not they take COCs. Whilst this background risk increases with age, the excess number of breast cancer diagnoses in current and recent COC users is small in relation to the overall risk of breast cancer (see bar chart).

The most important risk factor for breast cancer in COC users is the age women discontinue the COC; the older the age at stopping, the more breast cancers are diagnosed. Duration of use is less important and the excess risk gradually disappears during the course of the 10 years after stopping COC use such that by 10 years there appears to be no excess.

The possible increase in risk of breast cancer should be discussed with the user and weighed against the benefits of COCs taking into account the evidence that they offer substantial protection against the risk of developing certain other cancers (e.g. ovarian and endometrial cancer).

Estimated cumulative numbers of breast cancers per 10,000 women diagnosed in 5 years of use and up to 10 years after stopping COCs, compared with numbers of breast cancers diagnosed in 10,000 women who had never used COCs

(see Figure 1 above)

The possibility cannot be ruled out that certain chronic diseases may occasionally deteriorate during the use of combined oral contraceptives (see '*Precautions*').

In rare cases benign and, in even rarer cases, malignant liver tumours leading in isolated cases to life-threatening intra-abdominal haemorrhage have been observed after the use of hormonal substances such as those contained in Microgynon 30 ED. If severe upper abdominal complaints, liver enlargement or signs of intra-abdominal haemorrhage occur, the possibility of a liver tumour should be included in the differential diagnosis.

Reasons for stopping oral contraception immediately:

1. Occurrence for the first time, or exacerbation, of migrainous headaches or unusually frequent or unusually severe headaches

2. Sudden disturbances of vision or hearing or other perceptual disorders

3. First signs of thrombophlebitis or thromboembolic symptoms (e.g. unusual pains in or swelling of the leg(s), stabbing pains on breathing or coughing for no apparent reason). Feeling of pain and tightness in the chest

4. Six weeks before an elective major operation (e.g. abdominal, orthopaedic), any surgery to the legs, medical treatment for varicose veins or prolonged immobilisation, e.g. after accidents or surgery. Do not restart until 2 weeks after full ambulation. In case of emergency surgery, thrombotic prophylaxis is usually indicated e.g. subcutaneous heparin

5. Onset of jaundice, hepatitis, itching of the whole body

6. Increase in epileptic seizures

7. Significant rise in blood pressure

8. Onset of severe depression

9. Severe upper abdominal pain or liver enlargement

10. Clear exacerbation of conditions known to be capable of deteriorating during oral contraception or pregnancy

11. Pregnancy is a reason for stopping immediately because it has been suggested by some investigations that oral contraceptives taken in early pregnancy may slightly increase the risk of foetal malformations. Other investigations have failed to support these findings. The possibility therefore cannot be excluded, but it is certain that if a risk exists at all, it is very small.

Precautions:

Assessment of women prior to starting oral contraceptives (and at regular intervals thereafter) should include a personal and family medical history of each woman. Physical examination should be guided by this and by the contraindications (section 4.3) and warnings (section 4.4) for this product. The frequency and nature of these assessments should be based upon relevant guidelines and should be adapted to the individual woman, but should include measurement of blood pressure and, if judged appropriate by the clinician, breast, abdominal and pelvic examination including cervical cytology.

<u>The following conditions require strict medical supervision during medication with oral contraceptives.</u> Deterioration or first appearance of any of these conditions may indicate that use of the oral contraceptive should be discontinued:

Diabetes mellitus, or a tendency towards diabetes mellitus (e.g. unexplained glycosuria), hypertension, varicose veins, a history of phlebitis, otosclerosis, multiple sclerosis, epilepsy, porphyria, tetany, disturbed liver function, Sydenham's chorea, renal dysfunction, family history of clotting disorders, obesity, family history of breast cancer and patient history of benign breast disease, history of clinical depression, systemic lupus erythematosus, uterine fibroids and migraine, gall-stones, cardiovascular diseases, chloasma, asthma, an intolerance of contact lenses, or any disease that is prone to worsen during pregnancy.

Some women may experience amenorrhoea or oligomenorrhoea after discontinuation of oral contraceptives, especially when these conditions existed prior to use. Women should be informed of this possibility.

4.5 Interaction with other medicinal products and other forms of Interaction

Hepatic enzyme inducers such as barbiturates, primidone, phenobarbitone, phenytoin, phenylbutazone, rifampicin, carbamazepine and griseofulvin can impair the efficacy of Microgynon 30 ED. For women receiving long-term therapy with hepatic enzyme inducers, another method of contraception should be used. The use of ampicillin and other antibiotics may also reduce the efficacy of Microgynon 30 ED, possibly by altering the intestinal flora.

Women receiving short courses of enzyme inducers or broad spectrum antibiotics should take additional, non-hormonal (except rhythm or temperature method) contraceptive precautions during the time of concurrent medication and for 7 days afterwards. If these 7 days extend beyond the last active (small) tablet the user should finish taking all the active tablets, discard the placebo (large) tablets and start a new pack of Microgynon 30 ED the next day with an appropriate active (small) tablet. In this situation, a withdrawal bleed should not be expected until the end of the second pack. If the patient does not have a withdrawal bleed at the end of the second pack, the possibility of pregnancy must be ruled out before resuming with the next pack. With rifampicin, additional contraceptive precautions should be continued for 4 weeks after treatment stops, even if only a short course was administered.

The requirement for oral antidiabetics or insulin can change as a result of the effect on glucose tolerance.

The herbal remedy St John's wort (Hypericum perforatum) should not be taken concomitantly with Microgynon 30 ED as this could potentially lead to a loss of contraceptive effect.

4.6 Pregnancy and lactation

If pregnancy occurs during medication with oral contraceptives, the preparation should be withdrawn immediately (see Section 4.4. 'Reasons for stopping oral contraception immediately').

The use of Microgynon 30 ED during lactation may lead to a reduction in the volume of milk produced and to a change in its composition. Minute amounts of the active substances are excreted with the milk. Mothers who are breast-feeding may be advised instead to use a progestogen-only pill.

4.7 Effects on ability to drive and use machines

None known.

4.8 Undesirable effects

In rare cases, headaches, gastric upsets, nausea, vomiting, breast tenderness, changes in body weight, changes in libido, depressive moods can occur.

In predisposed women, use of Microgynon 30 ED can sometimes cause chloasma which is exacerbated by exposure to sunlight. Such women should avoid prolonged exposure to sunlight.

Individual cases of poor tolerance of contact lenses have been reported with use of oral contraceptives. Contact lens wearers who develop changes in lens tolerance should be assessed by an ophthalmologist.

Menstrual changes:

1. Reduction of menstrual flow:

This is not abnormal and it is to be expected in some patients. Indeed, it may be beneficial where heavy periods were previously experienced.

2. Missed menstruation:

Occasionally, withdrawal bleeding may not occur at all. If the tablets have been taken correctly, pregnancy is very unlikely. If withdrawal bleeding fails to occur at the end of a second pack, the possibility of pregnancy must be ruled out before resuming with the next pack.

Intermenstrual bleeding: 'Spotting' or heavier 'breakthrough bleeding' sometimes occur during tablet taking, especially in the first few cycles, and normally cease spontaneously. Microgynon 30 ED should therefore, be continued even if irregular bleeding occurs. If irregular bleeding is persistent, appropriate diagnostic measures to exclude an organic cause are indicated and may include curettage. This also applies in the case of spotting which occurs at irregular intervals in several consecutive cycles or which occurs for the first time after long use of Microgynon 30 ED.

Effect on blood chemistry: The use of oral contraceptives may influence the results of certain laboratory tests including biochemical parameters of liver, thyroid, adrenal and renal function, plasma levels of carrier proteins and lipid/lipoprotein fractions, parameters of carbohydrate metabolism and parameters of coagulation and fibrinolysis. Laboratory staff should therefore be informed about oral contraceptive use when laboratory tests are requested.

Refer to Section 4.4. 'Special warnings and special precautions for use' for additional information.

4.9 Overdose

Overdosage may cause nausea, vomiting and, in females, withdrawal bleeding.

There are no specific antidotes and treatment should be symptomatic.

5. PHARMACOLOGICAL PROPERTIES

5.1 Pharmacodynamic properties

Microgynon 30 ED is an oestrogen-progestogen combination which acts by inhibiting ovulation by suppression of the mid-cycle surge of luteinizing hormone, the inspissation of cervical mucus so as to constitute a barrier to sperm, and the rendering of the endometrium unreceptive to implantation.

5.2 Pharmacokinetic properties

Levonorgestrel

Levonorgestrel is absorbed quickly and completely. Maximum active substance levels of approx. 3 ng/ml were reached in serum just one hour after ingestion of Microgynon 30 ED. The serum concentrations subsequently fell in 2 phases with half-lives of around 0.5 hours and 20 hours. The metabolic clearance rate from plasma is approx. 1.5 ml/min/kg.

Levonorgestrel is eliminated not in unchanged form, but in the form of metabolites with a half-life of around one day and in almost equal proportions via the kidney and bile. Biotransformation takes place via the familiar pathways of steroid metabolism. There are no known pharmacologically active products of metabolism.

Levonorgestrel is bound to serum albumin and SHBG. Only around 1.5% of the respective total concentration is present in unbound form, while approx. 65% is bound to SHBG. The relative proportions (free, albumin-bound, SHBG-bound) depend on the concentration of SHBG. After induction of the binding protein, the portion bound to SHBG increases, while the free portion and that bound to albumin decreases.

After daily repeated ingestion, levonorgestrel accumulates by about the factor 2. A steady state is reached during the second half of the treatment cycle. The pharmacokinetics of levonorgestrel are dependent on the concentration of SHBG in plasma. Under treatment with Microgynon 30 ED, an increase in the serum levels of SHBG effect a concomitant increase in the specific binding capacity and therefore also an increase in levonorgestrel serum levels.

The levonorgestrel serum levels do not change any further after 1 - 3 cycles of use owing to the fact that SHBG induction is concluded. Compared to a single administration, 3 - 4 fold higher levonorgestrel serum levels are reached in the steady state.

The absolute bioavailability of levonorgestrel amounts to almost 100%.

Approx. 0.1% of the maternal dose can be passed on to a baby with the breast milk.

Ethinylestradiol

Orally administered ethinylestradiol is absorbed quickly and completely. Ingestion of Microgynon 30 ED leads to maximum plasma levels of approx. 100 pg/ml after 1 - 2 hours. The substance concentration then falls in 2 phases for which half-lives of around 1 - 2 hours and about 20 hours have been determined. For technical reasons, these data can only be calculated at higher dosages.

An imaginary distribution volume of around 5 l/kg and a metabolic clearance rate from plasma of approx. 5 ml/min/kg have been determined for ethinylestradiol. Ethinylestradiol is bound non-specifically to serum albumin to the extent of 98%.

Ethinylestradiol is metabolised even during its absorption phase and during its first liver transit, leading to reduced and individually varying oral bioavailability. Ethinylestradiol is eliminated not in unchanged form, but in the form of metabolites with a half-life of around one day. The excretion ratio is 40 (urine): 60 (bile).

Because of the half-life of the terminal elimination phase from plasma, a steady state characterised by a 30 - 40% higher plasma substance level becomes established after approx. 5 - 6 daily administrations.

The absolute bioavailability of ethinylestradiol is subject to considerable interindividual variations. After oral ingestion, it amounts to around 40 - 60% of the dose.

In women with fully established lactation, around 0.02% of the maternal dose can be passed on to the baby with the breast milk.

Other drugs can have a negative or positive effect on the systemic availability of ethinylestradiol. No interaction with vitamin C takes place. On continuous use, ethinylestradiol induces the hepatic synthesis of CBG and SHBG, the extent of SHBG induction being dependent on the type and dose of the simultaneously administered progestogen.

5.3 Preclinical safety data

There are no preclinical safety data which could be of relevance to the prescriber and which are not already included in other relevant sections of the SPC.

6. PHARMACEUTICAL PARTICULARS

6.1 List of excipients

Active tablets	*Placebo tablets*
lactose	lactose
maize starch	maize starch
povidone	povidone
magnesium stearate (E 572)	magnesium stearate (E 572)
sucrose	sucrose
polyethylene glycol 6000	polyethylene glycol 6000
calcium carbonate (E 170)	calcium carbonate (E 170)
talc	talc
montan glycol wax	montan glycol wax
titanium dioxide (E 171)	
ferric oxide pigment yellow (E 172)	
glycerin (E 422)	

6.2 Incompatibilities

None known.

6.3 Shelf life

5 years.

6.4 Special precautions for storage

Not applicable.

6.5 Nature and contents of container

Deep drawn strips made of polyvinyl chloride film with counter-sealing foil made of aluminium with heat sealable coating.

Presentation:

Each carton contains either 1 or 3 blister memo-packs. Each blister memo-pack contains 21 active tablets and 7 placebo tablets.

6.6 Instructions for use and handling

Keep out of the reach of children.

7. MARKETING AUTHORISATION HOLDER

Schering Health Care Limited

The Brow

Burgess Hill

West Sussex RH15 9NE

8. MARKETING AUTHORISATION NUMBER(S)

0053/0260

9. DATE OF FIRST AUTHORISATION/RENEWAL OF THE AUTHORISATION

12th June 1996

10. DATE OF REVISION OF THE TEXT

12th October 2001

LEGAL CATEGORY

POM

Micronor HRT

(Janssen-Cilag Ltd)

1. NAME OF THE MEDICINAL PRODUCT

Micronor HRT

2. QUALITATIVE AND QUANTITATIVE COMPOSITION

Norethisterone 1.0 mg.

3. PHARMACEUTICAL FORM

Tablet.

4. CLINICAL PARTICULARS

4.1 Therapeutic indications

The progestogenic opposition of menopausal oestrogen replacement therapy in women with an intact uterus.

4.2 Posology and method of administration

Adult females: One tablet should be taken by mouth each day on days 15-26 of each 28 day cycle of oestrogen replacement therapy.

Children: Micronor HRT tablets are not indicated for use in children.

4.3 Contraindications

Micronor HRT tablets should not be used for contraception. Use is not recommended during pregnancy or lactation, severe disturbance of liver function, Dubin-Johnson and Rotor syndromes, history during pregnancy of idiopathic jaundice, severe pruritus, pemphigoid gestationis, or known or suspected cancer of the breast.

4.4 Special warnings and special precautions for use

Assessment of each woman prior to using hormone replacement therapy (and at regular intervals thereafter) should include a personal and family medical history. Physical examination should be guided by this and by the Contra-indications (Section 4.3) and Warnings (Section 4.4) for this product. During assessment of each individual woman clinical examination of the breasts and pelvic examination should be performed where clinically indicated rather than as a routine procedure. Women should be encouraged to participate in the national breast cancer screening programme (mammography) and the national cervical cancer screening programme (cervical cytology) as appropriate for their age. Breast awareness should also be encouraged and women advised to report any changes in their breasts to their doctor or nurse.

Close monitoring is recommended in patients with epilepsy, diabetes or hypertension, disturbances or impairment of liver function, mastopathy, or a strong family history of mammary cancer, uterine fibroids, cholelithiasis, multiple sclerosis, systemic lupus erythematosus, porphyria, melanoma and asthma. Repeated breakthrough bleeding should be investigated including endometrial biopsy.

A re-analysis of original data from 51 epidemiological studies reported a small or moderate increase in the probability of having breast cancer *diagnosed* in women currently or recently using HRT. The findings may be due to biological effects of HRT, earlier diagnosis, or a combination of both. The relative risk increased with duration of treatment (by 2.3% per year of use) and returned to normal in the course of five years after cessation of HRT use. This is comparable to the increase in relative risk when natural menopause is delayed in the absence of HRT. Breast cancers diagnosed in current or recent users of HRT are more likely to be localised to the breast than those found in non-users. HRT use may not be associated with increased mortality from breast cancer.

Between the ages of 50 and 70, about 45 women in every 1,000 not using HRT will have breast cancer diagnosed. It is estimated that among those who use HRT for 5 years starting at age 50, 2 extra cases of breast cancer will be detected by age 70 in every 1,000 women. For those who use HRT for 10 years, there will be 6 extra cases of breast cancer, and for 15 years use, 12 extra cases of breast cancer in every 1,000 women during the 20 year period until age 70.

It is important that the increased risk of being diagnosed with breast cancer is discussed with the patient and weighed against the known benefits of HRT.

Administration of unopposed oestrogen therapy in patients with an intact uterus has been reported to increase the risk of endometrial hyperplasia.

There is no indication from published studies that the risk of thrombo-embolic disease, including myocardial infarction, stroke and thrombophlebitis, is increased with hormone replacement therapy at the current recommended low dosage in apparently normal women. However, treatment should be discontinued immediately following the occurrence of an acute vascular thrombo-embolic event during therapy. There is no evidence that a past history of deep vein thrombosis, pulmonary embolism, stroke, or myocardial infarction should be a contra-indication to hormone replacement therapy when associated with recognised risk factors such as immobilisation (eg post-partum or post trauma) or post-operative (eg in particular after pelvic surgery) but in the absence of specific data, hormone replacement therapy should be used with caution.

4.5 Interaction with other medicinal products and other forms of Interaction

Barbiturates, hydantoins, carbamazepine, meprobamate, phenylbutazone, antibiotics (including rifampicin) and activated charcoal, may impair the activity of oestrogen and progestogens (irregular bleeding and recurrence of symptoms may occur).

4.6 Pregnancy and lactation

Micronor HRT tablets are contra-indicated in pregnancy and lactation.

4.7 Effects on ability to drive and use machines

In normal use, Micronor HRT tablets are not expected to have any effect on the ability to drive or use machinery.

4.8 Undesirable effects

Minor effects of oestrogen and combined oestrogen/progestogen hormone replacement therapy which do not usually preclude continuation of therapy include headaches, nausea and breast tenderness. The following side effects have been reported with oestrogen/progestogen therapy:-

Genito-urinary system - pre-menstrual-like syndrome, increase in size of uterine fibromyomata, vaginal candidiasis, change in cervical erosion and degree of cervical secretion, cystitis-like syndrome.

Breasts - tenderness, enlargement, secretion.

Gastro-intestinal - nausea, vomiting, abdominal cramps, bloating, cholestatic jaundice.

Skin - chloasma which may persist when drug is discontinued, erythema multiforme, erythema nodosum, haemorrhagic eruption, loss of scalp hair, hirsutism.

Eyes - steepening of corneal curvature, intolerance to contact lenses.

CNS - headaches, migraine, dizziness, mental depression, chorea.

Miscellaneous - increase or decrease in weight, reduced carbohydrate tolerance, aggravation of porphyria, oedema, changes in libido, leg cramps.

4.9 Overdose

There have been no reports of serious ill-effects from overdosage with norethisterone and treatment is usually unnecessary. Nausea and vomiting may occur.

There is no special antidote and treatment should be symptomatic.

5. PHARMACOLOGICAL PROPERTIES

5.1 Pharmacodynamic properties

Norethisterone is a progesterone and causes progestational effects by converting the oestrogen primed proliferative endometrium into secretory endometrium which, on withdrawal of norethisterone at the end of each cycle, causes a withdrawal bleed in most patients.

5.2 Pharmacokinetic properties

Norethisterone is rapidly and completely absorbed from the gastro-intestinal tract following oral administration and follows a two compartment model. Mean peak plasma levels are observed at 1-2 hours post dose and the elimination half-life is 7-9 hours with detectable levels in the urine at 5 days.

Norethisterone is rapidly and widely distributed throughout the body tissues, with the highest levels accumulating and being metabolised in the liver and kidneys.

Due to non-linear pharmacokinetic properties, the bioavailability of norethisterone decreases proportionally with increasing dose within the therapeutic dose range.

Norethisterone is subject to extensive first pass metabolism and 95% of norethisterone exists bound to protein, with only 5% free. About 60% of the dose of norethisterone is excreted as metabolites in urine and faeces.

5.3 Preclinical safety data

In both rats and mice, the acute LD_{50} is in excess of 4 g/kg. Single doses of norethisterone have produced minimal toxicity, limited to typical and expected progestational responses. Dosages as high as 225 mg/kg/day (equivalent to more than 12000 mg/day in an average 55 kg woman) have rarely resulted in animal deaths.

Chronic studies of up to 3 years duration have been conducted in male and female rats, dogs and monkeys. The major toxic effects seen are related to those that might be expected for progestogens, for example, the pituitary observable dose related effects consisted of a slight reduction in food intake and a slight decrease in weight.

Female beagles given extremely high doses (in excess of recommended human doses) of norethisterone in the first year of life conceived normally and produced normal pups. Loss of fertility has been reported in mated animals as a result of pituitary inhibition, but fertility is rapidly restored at the end of the treatment period.

Reports of teratogenic effects in animals are uncommon, but masculinisation of foetuses, estimated by changes in the anogenital distance, has been reported at doses greater than 5 mg daily in rats. In the mouse with 1-10 mg daily from days 8 to 15 of pregnancy, there was no virilisation but some foetuses had cleft palates. Micronor HRT tablets are consequently not recommended during pregnancy.

Extensive carcinogenicity studies have been conducted with norethisterone but no tumourogenic potential was found.

In conclusion, the low toxicity of norethisterone together with the well established use of this active ingredient in oral contraceptives for the last 40 years, gives reassurance that Micronor HRT tablets at the proposed dose demonstrates acceptable level of safety.

6. PHARMACEUTICAL PARTICULARS

6.1 List of excipients
Anhydrous lactose

Pregelatinised starch

Magnesium stearate

6.2 Incompatibilities
None known.

6.3 Shelf life
3 years

6.4 Special precautions for storage
Protect from light. Store at room temperature (at or below 25°C).

6.5 Nature and contents of container
1 or 3 Aluminium/PVC blister strips containing 12 tablets packed in a cardboard carton.

Micronor HRT/norethisterone 1 mg tablets are also available in a combination pack as Evorel Pak. Evorel Pak contains 8 × Evorel 50 Patches (PL/0242/0223) and 12 × 1 mg Micronor HRT/norethisterone tablets (PL/0242/0241).

6.6 Instructions for use and handling
None stated.

Administrative Data

7. MARKETING AUTHORISATION HOLDER
Janssen-Cilag Ltd
Saunderton
High Wycombe
Buckinghamshire
HP14 4HJ
UK

8. MARKETING AUTHORISATION NUMBER(S)
PL 0242/0241

9. DATE OF FIRST AUTHORISATION/RENEWAL OF THE AUTHORISATION
1 October 1995

10. DATE OF REVISION OF THE TEXT
September 2001

11. Legal category
POM

Micronor Oral Contraceptive Tablets

(Janssen-Cilag Ltd)

1. NAME OF THE MEDICINAL PRODUCT
Micronor Oral Contraceptive Tablets

2. QUALITATIVE AND QUANTITATIVE COMPOSITION
Each tablet contains norethisterone 0.35 mg.

3. PHARMACEUTICAL FORM
Small, round, white tablet, engraved C035 on both faces.

4. CLINICAL PARTICULARS

4.1 Therapeutic indications
Oral contraceptive.

4.2 Posology and method of administration
For oral administration.

Adults:

Tablet intake from the first pack is started on the first day of menstruation; no extra contraceptive precautions are necessary.

One tablet is taken at the same time each day, every day of the year, whether menstruation occurs or not.

Elderly:

Not applicable.

Children:

Not recommended.

4.3 Contraindications

- Existing thrombophlebitis
- Existing thrombo-embolic disorders
- Cerebrovascular disease or a past history of this condition
- Myocardial infarction or a past history of this condition
- Markedly impaired liver function
- Known or suspected hormone dependent neoplasia
- Known or suspected carcinoma of the breast
- Undiagnosed abnormal genital tract bleeding
- Known or suspected pregnancy
- Cholestatic jaundice of pregnancy or jaundice with prior pill use
- Hepatic adenomas or carcinomas

4.4 Special warnings and special precautions for use
There is a general opinion, based on statistic evidence, that users of combined oral contraceptives (ie oestrogen plus progestogen) experience more often than non-users various disorders of the circulation of blood, including strokes (blood clots in, and haemorrhages from, the blood vessels of the brain), heart attacks (coronary thromboses) and blood clots obstructing the arteries of the lungs (pulmonary emboli). There may not be a full recovery from such disorders and it should be realised that in a few cases they may be fatal.

To date no association between these disorders and progestogen-only oral contraceptives (such as Micronor Oral Contraceptive Tablets) has been shown. However there is a risk that the users of such progestogen only oral contraceptives will (like users of the combined oral contraceptive) be exposed to an increased risk of suffering from these disorders.

Reasons for stopping oral contraceptives immediately

- Early manifestations of thrombotic or thrombo-embolic disorders, thrombophlebitis
- Cerebrovascular disorders (including haemorrhage)
- Myocardial infarction
- Pulmonary embolism
- Gradual or sudden, partial or complete loss of vision
- Proptosis or diplopia
- Onset or aggravation of migraine or development of headaches of a new pattern which are recurrent, persistent or severe
- Papilloedema or any evidence of retinal vascular lesions
- During periods of immobility (eg after accidents)
- Pregnancy
- Manifestations of liver tumours

Assessment of women prior to starting oral contraceptives (and at regular intervals thereafter) should include a personal and family medical history of each woman. Physical examination should be guided by this and by the contraindications (Section 4.3) and warnings (Section 4.4) for this product. The frequency and nature of these assessments should be based upon relevant guidelines and should be adapted to the individual woman, but should include measurement of blood pressure and, if judged appropriate by the clinician, breast, abdominal and pelvic examination including cervical cytology.

Because of a possible increased risk of post surgery thrombo-embolic complications in oral contraceptive users, therapy should be discontinued six weeks prior to elective surgery.

When Micronor is administered during the post-partum period, the increased risk of thrombo-embolic disease associated with the post-partum period must be considered.

The following are some of the medical conditions reported to be influenced by the combined pill, and may be affected by Micronor. The physician will have to exercise medical judgement to commence, continue or discontinue therapy as appropriate. The worsening or first appearance of any of these conditions may indicate that Micronor should be discontinued.

1. Pre-existing uterine fibromyomata may increase in size.
2. A decrease in glucose tolerance in a significant number of women.
3. An increase in blood pressure in a small but significant number of women.
4. Cholestatic jaundice. Patients with a history of cholestatic jaundice of pregnancy are more likely to develop cholestatic jaundice during oral contraceptive therapy.
5. Amenorrhoea during and after oral contraceptive therapy. Temporary infertility after discontinuation of treatment.
6. Depression.
7. Fluid retention. Conditions which might be influenced by this factor including epilepsy, migraine, asthma, cardiac or renal dysfunction.
8. Varicose veins.
9. Multiple sclerosis.
10. Porphyria.
11. Tetany.
12. Intolerance to contact lenses.

Or any condition that is prone to worsening during pregnancy.

Ectopic pregnancy

Pregnancies in progestogen-only pill (POP) users are more likely to be ectopic than are pregnancies occurring in the general population, since POPs offer less protection against ectopic pregnancy than against intra-uterine pregnancy.

Changing from another oral contraceptive

Start Micronor on the day following completion of the previous oral contraceptive pack without a break (or, in the case of the ED pill, omitting the inactive pills). No extra contraceptive precautions are required.

Post-partum administration

Micronor can be started on the 21st day after childbirth. This will ensure the patient is protected immediately. If there is any delay in taking the first dose, contraception may not be established until 7 days after the first tablet has been taken. In these circumstances, patients should be advised that extra contraceptive precautions (non-hormonal methods) are necessary.

After miscarriage or abortion

Patients can take Micronor on the day after miscarriage or abortion, in which case no additional contraceptive precautions are required.

Missed tablets

If a tablet is missed within 3 hours of the correct dosage time, then the missed tablet should be taken as soon as possible; this will ensure that contraceptive protection is maintained. If one (for longer than 3 hours) or more tablets are missed, it is recommended that the patient takes the last missed tablet as soon as possible and continues to take the rest of the tablets as usual. Additional means of contraception (non-hormonal) should be used for the next seven days.

If the patient does not have a period within 45 days of her last period, Micronor should be discontinued and pregnancy should be excluded.

Vomiting and diarrhoea

Additional contraceptive measures (non-hormonal) should be employed during the period of gastro-intestinal upset and for the next seven days.

Laboratory tests

The following laboratory determinations may be altered in patients using oral contraceptives.

Hepatic: increased BSP retention and other tests.

Coagulation: increased prothrombin, factors VII, VIII, IX and X, decreased antithrombin III, increased platelet aggregability.

Endocrine: increased PBI and butanol extractable protein-bound iodine and decreased T3 uptake, increased blood glucose levels.

Other: increased phospholipids and triglycerides, decreased serum folate values and disturbance in tryptophan metabolism, decreased pregnanediol excretion, reduced response to metapyrone test.

These tests usually return to pre-therapy values after discontinuing oral contraceptive use. However, the physician should be aware that these altered determinations may mask an underlying disease.

4.5 Interaction with other medicinal products and other forms of Interaction
Reduced efficacy and increased incidence of breakthrough bleeding have been associated with concomitant use of oral contraceptives and rifampicin. A similar association has been suggested with oral contraceptives and barbiturates, phenytoin sodium, ampicillin, tetracyclines and griseofulvin.

The herbal remedy St John's wort *(Hypericum perforatum)* should not be taken concomitantly with this medicine as this could potentially lead to a loss of contraceptive effect.

4.6 Pregnancy and lactation
Masculinisation of the female foetus has occurred when progesterones have been used in pregnant women, although this has been observed at doses much higher than that contained in Micronor. Pregnancy should be ruled out before continuing administration of Micronor to patients who have gone 45 days without a menstrual period.

A small fraction of the active ingredient in oral contraceptives has been identified in the milk of mothers receiving these drugs. The effects, if any, on the breast-fed child have not been determined. If possible the use of oral contraceptives should be deferred until the infant is weaned.

4.7 Effects on ability to drive and use machines
Not applicable

4.8 Undesirable effects
Side effects are usually self-limiting and of relatively short duration. Amongst the symptoms reported are:

- Headaches/migraine
- Nausea
- Vomiting
- Breast changes
- Change in weight
- Changes in libido
- Chloasma
- Breakthrough bleeding and spotting
- Rash
- Depression
- Irregular cycle length (particularly in early cycles of therapy). It is important that patients should be advised that whilst on Micronor therapy they may experience that variation in cycle length and that they should continue taking a tablet every day whether they have a period or not. However, patients should be advised to discontinue Micronor and to consult their doctor if they have gone 45 days without having a period.

Malignant hepatic tumours have been reported on rare occasions in long-term users of oral contraceptives. Benign hepatic tumours have also been associated with oral contraceptive use. A hepatic tumour should be considered in the differential diagnosis when upper abdominal pain, enlarged liver or signs of intra-abdominal haemorrhage occur.

A meta-analysis from 54 epidemiological studies reported that there is a slightly increased relative risk of having breast cancer diagnosed in women who are currently using oral contraceptives (OCs). The observed pattern of increased risk may be due to an earlier diagnosis of breast cancer in OC users, the biological effects of OCs or a combination of both. The additional breast cancers diagnosed in current users of OCs or in women who have used OCs in the last 10 years are more likely to be localised to the breast than those in women who have never used OCs.

Breast cancer is rare among women under 40 years of age whether or not they take OCs. Whilst the background risk increases with age, the excess number of breast cancer diagnoses in current and recent progesterone-only pill (POP) users is small in relation to the overall risk of breast cancer, possibly of similar magnitude to that associated with combined OCs. However, for POPs, the evidence is based on much smaller populations of users and so is less conclusive than that for combined OCs.

The most important risk factor for breast cancer in POP users is the age women discontinue the POP; the older the age at stopping, the more breast cancers are diagnosed. Duration of use is less important and the excess risk gradually disappears during the course of the 10 years after stopping POP use, such that by 10 years there appears to be no excess.

The evidence suggests that compared with never-users, among 10,000 women who use POPs for up to five years but stop by age 20, there would be much less than one extra case of breast cancer diagnosed up to 10 years afterwards. For those stopping by age 30 after 5 years use of the POP, there would be an estimated 2-3 extra cases (additional to the 44 cases of breast cancer per 10,000 women in this age group never exposed to oral contraceptives). For those stopping by age 40 after 5 years use, there would be an estimated 10 extra cases diagnosed up to 10 years afterwards (additional to the 160 cases of breast cancer per 10,000 never-exposed women in this age group).

It is important to inform patients that users of all contraceptive pills appear to have a small increase in the risk of being diagnosed with breast cancer, compared with non-users of oral contraceptives, but that this has to be weighed against the known benefits.

4.9 Overdose
Serious ill effects have not been reported following acute ingestion of large doses of oral contraceptives by young children. Overdosage may cause nausea and withdrawal bleeding may occur in females. An appropriate method of gastric emptying may be used if considered desirable.

5. PHARMACOLOGICAL PROPERTIES

5.1 Pharmacodynamic properties
Micronor Oral Contraceptive Tablets have a progestational effect on the endometrium and the cervical mucus.

5.2 Pharmacokinetic properties
Norethisterone is absorbed from the gastro-intestinal tract and metabolised in the liver. To obtain maximal contraceptive effectiveness, the tablets should be taken at the same time each day, every day.

5.3 Preclinical safety data
No relevant information additional to that contained elsewhere in the Summary of Product Characteristics.

6. PHARMACEUTICAL PARTICULARS

6.1 List of excipients
Lactose

Magnesium stearate

Pregelatinised starch

6.2 Incompatibilities
Not applicable.

6.3 Shelf life
36 months.

6.4 Special precautions for storage
Store at room temperature (below 25°C).

Protect from light.

6.5 Nature and contents of container
PVC/aluminium foil blister strips with or without a card wallet in cardboard carton, containing either 42, 2 × 42, 3 × 28, 1 × 28 or 100 × 28 tablets.

6.6 Instructions for use and handling
Not applicable.

7. MARKETING AUTHORISATION HOLDER
Janssen-Cilag Ltd

Saunderton

High Wycombe

Buckinghamshire

HP14 4HJ

UK

8. MARKETING AUTHORISATION NUMBER(S)
0242/0234

9. DATE OF FIRST AUTHORISATION/RENEWAL OF THE AUTHORISATION
Date of First Authorisation: 1 October 1995

10. DATE OF REVISION OF THE TEXT
11 July 2000

Legal category POM

Microval

(Wyeth Pharmaceuticals)

1. NAME OF THE MEDICINAL PRODUCT
MICROVAL®

2. QUALITATIVE AND QUANTITATIVE COMPOSITION
Each tablet contains 0.03mg levonorgestrel.

3. PHARMACEUTICAL FORM
White sugar coated tablets.

4. CLINICAL PARTICULARS

4.1 Therapeutic indications
Oral contraception.

4.2 Posology and method of administration
Adult Women Only:

The tablets are started on the first day of menstruation and taken daily without interruption for as long as contraception is desired. They should be taken at the same time each day, preferably after the evening meal or at bedtime so that the interval between tablets is always about 24 hours. Protection may be reduced when the interval increases beyond 27 hours.

During the first cycle additional contraceptive precautions should be taken for the first 14 days.

If a tablet is not taken at the usual time it should be taken as soon as possible and the next tablet taken at the usual time. If the interval between tablets is more than 27 hours protection may be impaired. The patient should take one tablet as soon as she remembers and thereafter one tablet daily as before but should use additional contraceptive measures until the tablets have been taken regularly for 14 days.

If vomiting occurs shortly after a tablet has been taken contraceptive protection can be maintained by taking another tablet, provided that it is taken within three hours of the normal time. The last tablet in the pack may be used for this purpose. If repeated vomiting or diarrhoea endanger absorption additional contraceptive precautions should be used for 14 days after the symptoms have disappeared.

Irregular spotting or bleeding may occur with a proportion of women initially but menstrual regularity is usually re-established after the first few cycles. Those patients whose menstrual patterns do not become reasonably regular after three to four cycles or who have prolonged bleeding or amenorrhoea lasting for two months should be instructed to return for advice.

Women who change from a combined oral contraceptive to MICROVAL should stop taking the previous product, leave seven clear days and take the first MICROVAL tablet on the eighth day, then continue to take 1 tablet daily. Additional contraceptive precautions should be taken until the fourteenth tablet has been taken.

MICROVAL does not diminish the yield of breast milk and can be used from the seventh post-partum day.

4.3 Contraindications
Patients with established hepatic disease or those in whom there is evidence of persistently abnormal liver function such as the Dubin-Johnson and rotor syndrome, or those who have a history during pregnancy of idiopathic jaundice or severe pruritus.

Patients with a history of infectious hepatitis until the liver function tests have returned to normal values.

Patients with abnormal vaginal bleeding of unknown aetiology.

Patients with suspected pregnancy.

Although the risk of thromboembolism has not been associated with progestogen-only contraceptives, it is at present required that a history of thromboembolic disorders should be regarded as a contraindication.

4.4 Special warnings and special precautions for use
Oral contraceptive medication should be discontinued if there is a gradual or sudden, partial or complete loss of vision, proptosis or diplopia, papilloedema or any evidence of retinal or vascular lesions.

Caution should be observed in prescribing oral contraceptives for any patients with a history of migraine, or if migraine is being treated with vasoconstrictor drugs. If migraine worsens or migraine or severe headache develops for the first time during treatment, medication should be discontinued immediately.

Women with hypertension who are taking MICROVAL require careful observation and their blood pressure should be monitored regularly.

A small fraction of the progestogen has been identified in the milk of mothers receiving the drug. The long-range effects to the nursing infant is currently unknown.

Assessment of women prior to starting oral contraceptives (and at regular intervals thereafter) should include a personal and family medical history of each woman. Physical examination should be guided by this and by the contraindications (section 4.3) and warnings (section 4.4) for this product. The frequency and nature of these assessments should be based upon relevant guidelines and should be adapted to the individual woman, but should include measurement of blood pressure and, if judged appropriate by the clinician, breast, abdominal and pelvic examination including cervical cytology.

Ectopic pregnancies appear to occur more frequently on progestogen-only oral contraceptives.

A meta-analysis of 54 epidemiological studies reported that there is a slightly increased relative risk of having breast cancer diagnosed in women who are currently using oral contraceptives (OC). The observed pattern of increased risk may be due to an earlier diagnosis of breast cancer in OC users, the biological effects of OCs or a combination of both. The additional breast cancers diagnosed in current users of OCs or in women who have used OCs in the last ten years are more likely to be localised to the breast than those in women who never used OCs.

Breast cancer is rare among women under 40 years of age whether or not they take OCs. Whilst the background risk increases with age, the excess number of breast cancer diagnoses in current and recent progestogen-only pill (POP) users is small in relation to the overall risk of breast cancer, possibly of similar magnitude to that associated with combined OCs. However, for POPs, the evidence is based on much smaller populations of users and so is less conclusive than that for combined OCs.

The most important risk factor for breast cancer in POP users is the age women discontinue the POP; the older the age at stopping, the more breast cancers are diagnosed. Duration of use is less important and the excess risk gradually disappears during the course of the 10 years after stopping POP use, such that by 10 years there appears to be no excess.

The evidence suggests that compared with never-users, among 10,000 women who use POPs for up to 5 years but stop by age 20, there would be much less than 1 extra case of breast cancer diagnosed up to 10 years afterwards. For those stopping by age 30 after 5 years use of the POP, there would be an estimated 2-3 extra cases (additional to the 44 cases of breast cancer per 10,000 women in this age group never exposed to oral contraceptives). For those stopping by age 40 after 5 years use, there would be an estimated 10 extra cases diagnosed up to 10 years afterwards (additional to the 160 cases of breast cancer per 10,000 never-exposed women in this age group).

It is important to inform patients that users of all contraceptive pills appear to have a small increase in the risk of being diagnosed with breast cancer, compared with non-users of oral contraceptives, but that this has to be weighed against the known benefits.

4.5 Interaction with other medicinal products and other forms of Interaction
Caution should be observed in prescribing oral contraceptives for patients taking other drugs since various interactions have been reported. Pregnancies have been reported in women taking oral contraceptives concurrently with rifampicin and other antibiotics, anti-epileptic drugs, barbiturates and other sedative drugs.

Steroids affect drug metabolism and the therapeutic or toxic effects of other drugs may be modified. Interactions have been reported between oral contraceptives and tricyclic antidepressants, anticoagulants and corticosteroids.

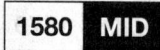

The herbal remedy St John's Wort (*Hypericum perforatum*) should not be taken concomitantly with this medicine as it could potentially lead to a loss of contraceptive effect.

4.6 Pregnancy and lactation
MICROVAL is contraindicated to patients with suspected pregnancy. A small fraction of the progestogen has been identified in the milk of mothers receiving the drug. The long-range effects to the nursing infant is currently unknown.

4.7 Effects on ability to drive and use machines
None known.

4.8 Undesirable effects
MICROVAL is well tolerated but certain endocrine effects which are also characteristic of ovulatory cycles may occur. Those noted are headache, depressive moods, slight weight gain, nausea, skin disorders, breast tenderness and spotting between periods. The incidence of such effects with MICROVAL is low and tends to decrease as treatment continues.

4.9 Overdose
No reports of serious ill-effects from overdosage with oral contraceptives have been reported. In general, therefore, treatment of overdosage is not necessary. If overdosage is however, discovered within one hour and is so large that treatment seems desirable, gastric lavage or a suitable dose of ipecacuanha can be used. There are no specific antidotes and further treatment should be symptomatic.

5. PHARMACOLOGICAL PROPERTIES

5.1 Pharmacodynamic properties
Only levonorgestrel is biologically active in the racemic mixture of d-l norgestrel. Levonorgestrel has the same potency as the racemic mixture at half the dosage. Levonorgestrel is a progestogen with some androgenic and anti-oestrogenic properties and no significant oestrogenic activity.

Levonorgestrel appears to exert its contraceptive effects by various methods. These include:

An effect on cervical mucus by which sperm do not penetrate through it easily and which appears to affect the capacitation phenomenon.

Inhibition of ovulation in some cases.

An effect on steroid biosynthesis in corpora lutea.

5.2 Pharmacokinetic properties
Studies with ^{14}C labelled norgestrel in man showed that 21% of the ingested dose was excreted in the urine on the day of administration and a further 20.5% during the following 5 days, after which urinary excretion fell to less than 1% daily, plasma levels of norgestrel were lower and decreased more quickly than those of norethisterone. After 24 hours only 1.2% of the administered dose was present in the plasma. Over 50% of the norgestrel excreted is in the form of the sulphate or glucuronide, the metabolites isolated from the urine are composed completely of the d-forms.

5.3 Preclinical safety data
Nothing of relevance to the prescriber.

6. PHARMACEUTICAL PARTICULARS

6.1 List of excipients
Tablet core: lactose, starch, poly-n-vinyl pyrrolidone 25, talc, magnesium stearate.

Coating: sucrose, poly-n-vinyl pyrrolidone K 90, calcium carbonate, polyethylene glycol 6000, talc, carnauba wax, white wax.

6.2 Incompatibilities
Not applicable.

6.3 Shelf life
5 years.

6.4 Special precautions for storage
Store at, or below 25°C.

6.5 Nature and contents of container
Single aluminium foil/PVC blisters containing 35 tablets.

6.6 Instructions for use and handling
Not applicable.

7. MARKETING AUTHORISATION HOLDER
John Wyeth and Brother Limited

Trading as Wyeth Laboratories

Huntercombe Lane South

Taplow

Maidenhead

Berkshire SL6 0PH

8. MARKETING AUTHORISATION NUMBER(S)
PL 0011/0040

9. DATE OF FIRST AUTHORISATION/RENEWAL OF THE AUTHORISATION
5 February 1973.

10. DATE OF REVISION OF THE TEXT
16 January 2001

˙ Trade Marks

Midazolam Injection BP 2mg/ml

(Wockhardt UK Ltd)

1. NAME OF THE MEDICINAL PRODUCT
Midazolam Injection BP 2mg/ml

2. QUALITATIVE AND QUANTITATIVE COMPOSITION
Midazolam 2mg/ml

Each 5ml ampoule contains 10mg midazolam.

3. PHARMACEUTICAL FORM
Solution for injection

4. CLINICAL PARTICULARS

4.1 Therapeutic indications
Midazolam may be used as an intravenous sedative before and during minor medical, dental and surgical procedures.

As an intravenous sedative, (either by continuous infusion or intermittent bolus injection) in critically ill patients in intensive care.

As an alternative intravenous agent for the induction of anaesthesia in high risk and elderly patients where cardiovascular stability is of particular importance. Induction is more reliable when heavy opiate medication has been administered or when midazolam injection is given with a narcotic analgesic such as fentanyl.

4.2 Posology and method of administration
Dosage depends on the individual response, age and weight. Midazolam 2mg/ml may be given by intramuscular, intravenous or slow intravenous injection.

Intravenous sedation

One or more intravenous injections to be administered over a single operating session.

Dosage should be titrated according to an individual's response, age and weight. The end-point of this titration is dependent on the procedure. Full sedation will be evident by drowsiness and slurred speech, although a response to commands will be maintained.

Adults	2mg, (1ml of 2mg/ml midazolam injection solution) over a period of 30 seconds initially
Elderly	1 to 1.5mg (0.5-0.75ml of 2mg/ml midazolam injection solution) over a period of 30 seconds initially.

If adequate sedation is not achieved after two minutes, incremental doses of 0.5-1mg, (0.25-0.5ml of 2mg/ml midazolam injection solution) should be given until the desired level of sedation is achieved, usually at a total dose of 2.5-7.5mg (about 70 micrograms/kg) in adults.

Children	Not recommended. Midazolam injection has not been evaluated as an intravenous sedative in children.

Combination therapy:-

If analgesia is provided by a narcotic analgesic, this should be administered first. The dose of midazolam injection should then be carefully titrated. Low total doses of 1-2mg may be adequate with lower total doses of 0.5-1mg in the elderly.

Mode of administration:-

For the administration of midazolam injection the patient should be placed in a supine position and remain there throughout the procedure. Resuscitation facilities should always be available and a second person, fully trained in the use of such equipment, always be present. It is recommended that patients should remain under medical supervision until at least one hour has elapsed from the time of injection. They should always be accompanied home by a responsible adult.

Patients who have received only midazolam injection for iv sedation prior to minor procedures, should be warned not to drive or operate machinery for 12 hours. Where midazolam injection is used concurrently with other central nervous system depressants (e.g. potent analgesics) recovery may be prolonged. Patients should therefore be assessed carefully before being allowed to go home or resume normal activities.

Sedation in the critically ill patient:-

Midazolam injection can be given intravenously by two methods for this purpose, either by continuous infusion or by intermittent bolus dose. Both have their own advantages and disadvantages and the appropriate method of giving midazolam injection will need to be determined for each patient.

The dose of midazolam injection needed to sedate critically ill patients varies considerably between patients. The dose should be titrated to the desired state of sedation. This will depend on clinical need, physical status, age and concomitant medication.

Midazolam injection can also be given in combination with an opioid. The opioid may be used for its analgesic effects or as an antitussive agent to help the patient tolerate the tracheal tube and ventilatory support.

Patients receiving midazolam injection for sedation in the intensive care situation should receive ventilatory support.

Safe use for midazolam for periods of over 14 days in duration has not been established in clinical trials.

Potential drug interactions:-

The critically ill patient is exposed to many drugs. Because of this, there is a potential for drug interactions. (See Interactions section under Contraindications, Warnings etc.)

After prolonged iv administration of midazolam injection, abrupt discontinuation may be accompanied by withdrawal symptoms, therefore a gradual reduction of the drug is recommended.

Midazolam injection is stable both physically and chemically for up to 24 hours at room temperature when mixed with infusion fluids containing 4% dextrose with 0.18% sodium chloride, 5% dextrose or 0.9% sodium chloride.

Sedation by intermittent bolus dose in intensive care

Midazolam injection only

The exact dose of midazolam needs to be titrated to the individual patient response. Small doses of midazolam 1.0-2.0mg can be given, and repeated, until the required degree of sedation is reached.

Midazolam injection and an opioid

When midazolam and an opioid are used together, the opioid should be administered first. Both drugs need to be titrated to the individual patient's response and to the level of sedation thought to be necessary.

Small doses of midazolam 1-2mg (0.5-1.0ml of 2mg/ml midazolam injection solution) can be given, and repeated, until the required degree of sedation is reached. In the elderly, smaller doses as little as 0.5-1.0mg (0.25-0.5ml of 2mg/ml midazolam injection solution) may be adequate.

The use of these two groups of drugs can increase the risk of respiratory depression. If the patient is being given ventilatory support using a mode that depends upon some spontaneous effort by the patient, then the minute volume may decrease.

Sedation by continuous infusion in intensive care

Midazolam injection only

Adults, Elderly and children

For patients already sedated or anaesthetised after an operation, a loading dose of midazolam is unnecessary.

In other situations a loading dose of 0.03-0.3mg/kg given over a five minute period is recommended, depending on the level of sedation required. The loading dose should be reduced or omitted in hypovolaemic, vasoconstricted or hypothermic patients.

Maintenance dose

A dose between 0.03-0.2mg/kg/hour is recommended, starting at the lower dose.

The dose should be reduced in hypovolaemic, vasoconstricted or hypothermic patients.

Midazolam injection and an opioid

When opioid analgesics are used, the rate of infusion of midazolam should be titrated carefully to the sedative needs of the patient. Low doses of midazolam 0.01 to 0.1mg/kg/hour may be used to start.

The use of these two groups of drugs can increase the risk of respiratory depression. If the patient is being given ventilatory support using a mode that depends upon some spontaneous effort by the patient, then the minute volume may decrease.

Whenever a continuous infusion of midazolam is used (with or without an opioid analgesic), its need should be assessed on a daily basis in order to reduce the risk of accumulation and prolonged recovery. Each day the infusion of midazolam should be stopped or its rate reduced and the patient seen to recover from its effect. If recovery is prolonged (>2 hours) a lower dose should be used when it is restarted. A sedation score should be used routinely.

When midazolam has been given for a number of days and then gradually withdrawn, patients may be awake but show signs of residual sedation for the next 12 to 24 hours. This can cause difficulties because patients may not cough and expectorate well if they are then weaned from ventilatory support. However, while recovering from the effects of midazolam, patients may not be sufficiently sedated to tolerate ventilatory support. In such circumstances sedation may be provided with a shorter acting agent while there is recovery from the effects of midazolam.

The recommended concentration of a solution for infusion in a critically ill adult patient is 1mg/ml.

Induction of anaesthesia by slow intravenous injection

One or more bolus intravenous injections should be administered over a single anaesthetic session.

Adults

The dose should be titrated against the individual response of the patient. Midazolam injection should be given by slow intravenous injection until there is a loss of eyelid reflex, response to commands and voluntary movements.

In anticipating the required dose of midazolam, both the premedication already given and the age of the patient are important. Young, fit unpremedicated patients may need at least 0.3mg/kg bodyweight, whereas patients premedicated with an opiate usually need only 0.2mg/kg bodyweight.

Use in the elderly

The elderly are more sensitive to the effects of benzodiazepines. Induction may be adequate with 0.1mg/kg body weight in premedicated patients and 0.2mg/kg body weight in unpremedicated patients.

Children over seven years

Midazolam injection has been shown to be an effective agent for induction of anaesthesia in children over seven years of age, at a dose of 0.15mg/kg body-weight.

4.3 Contraindications

Known hypersensitivity to benzodiazepines or any of the ingredients.

Myasthenia gravis

Severe respiratory insufficiency

4.4 Special warnings and special precautions for use

Midazolam injection should be used with caution in patients with renal or hepatic dysfunction, chronic pulmonary insufficiency, elderly or debilitated patients. During bolus sedation for operative procedures, patients with acute pulmonary insufficiency or respiratory depression should be treated with extreme caution.

Midazolam may enhance the effects of other CNS depressants and may result in severe respiratory or cardiovascular depression. Their concurrent use should be avoided.

The dependence potential of midazolam is low when limited to short term use. Due to the possibility of withdrawal symptoms, midazolam should be gradually reduced following a prolonged iv administration. Withdrawal symptoms may occur with benzodiazepines following normal use of therapeutic doses for only short periods and may be associated with physiological and psychological sequelae, including depression. This should be considered when treating patients for more than a few days.

As with other benzodiazepines, extreme caution should be used if prescribing midazolam for patients with personality disorders. The disinhibiting effects of benzodiazepines may be manifested as the precipitation of suicide in patients who are depressed or show aggressive behaviour towards self and others.

4.5 Interaction with other medicinal products and other forms of Interaction

Enhanced sedation or respiratory and cardiovascular depression may occur if midazolam is given with other drugs that have CNS depressant properties (e.g. antipsychotics, anxiolytics, sedatives, antidepressants, hypnotics, narcotic analgesics, anaesthetics, antiepileptics).

If such centrally acting depressant drugs are given parenterally in conjunction with intravenous midazolam, severe respiratory and cardiovascular depression may occur. When intravenous midazolam is to be administered concurrently with a narcotic analgesic agent (e.g. in dentistry), it is recommended that midazolam be given after the analgesic and that the dose be carefully titrated to meet the patient's needs.

The efficacy of cyclosporin and nifedipine may be potentiated when administered concurrently with midazolam.

Agents that interfere with metabolism by hepatic enzymes (e.g. isoniazid, disulfiram, cimetidine, omeprazole, ranitidine, erythromycin, diltiazem, verapamil, ketoconazole, itraconazole and possibly fluconazole, oral contraceptives) have been shown to reduce the clearance of benzodiazepines and may potentiate their actions, whilst known inducers of hepatic enzymes, for example, rifampicin, may increase the clearance of benzodiazepines.

Midazolam may interact with other hepatically metabolised drugs, causing inhibition (levodopa) or potentiation (phenytoin, muscle relaxants).

Alcohol should be avoided for at least eight hours before and after the administration of midazolam due to increased sedative effects.

4.6 Pregnancy and lactation

There is no evidence regarding the safety of midazolam in pregnancy. It should not be used, especially in the first and third trimesters, unless the benefit is considered to outweigh the risk.

If the product is prescribed to a woman of childbearing potential she should be warned to contact her physician regarding discontinuance of the product if she intends to become or suspects that she is pregnant.

If, for compelling medical reasons, the product is administered during the late phase of pregnancy, or during labour at high doses, effects on the neonate, such as hypothermia, hypotonia and moderate respiratory depression, can be expected, due to the pharmacological action of the compound. If midazolam is administered during the last trimester of pregnancy it may produce irregularities in the foetal heart rate, and poor suckling in the neonate.

Since benzodiazepines are found in the breast milk, benzodiazepines should not be given to breast-feeding mothers.

4.7 Effects on ability to drive and use machines

The concurrent use of midazolam with other central nervous system depressants, may result in a prolonged recovery. A careful assessment should be undertaken prior to allowing the patient to go home or resume normal activities.

Patients treated with midazolam injection should not drive or use machinery for twelve hours after receiving this medicine.

4.8 Undesirable effects

Midazolam can produce respiratory depression, apnoea and hypertension. Midazolam may cause decreases in cardiac output, stroke volume and systemic vascular resistance. These effects are important in those patients with a reduced myocardial oxygen delivery capacity or suffering hypovolaemia.

Midazolam may cause respiratory arrest following iv administration especially in the elderly with pre-existing respiratory insufficiency or when the dose is excessive or administered too rapidly.

Other side-effects are usually mild. The most common side effects are sedation, drowsiness, headaches, muscle weakness, dizziness (with risk of falls in the elderly), ataxia, confusion, slurred speech, tremor, numbed emotions, reduced alertness, fatigue, double vision, anterograde amnesia and a hangover effect. Elderly or debilitated patients are particularly susceptible to side effects and may require lower doses. Other effects which may occur rarely are dry mouth, increased appetite, gastrointestinal and visual disturbances, jaundice, urinary retention, bradycardia, changes in libido, menstrual disturbances, skin reactions, blood dyscrasias, laryngeal spasm and chest pain.

In susceptible patients, an unnoticed depression may become evident. Paradoxical reactions (restlessness, agitation, instability, rages, hallucinations) are known to occur with benzodiazepines and are more likely in children and the elderly.

Local pain on injection and thrombophlebitis may occur.

4.9 Overdose

a) Symptoms

The symptoms of mild overdose may include confusion, somnolence, paradoxical excitation, coma, ataxia, dysarthria, hypotension and muscular weakness. In severe overdose, depression of vital functions may occur, particularly the respiratory centre. As drug levels fall severe agitation may develop.

b) Treatment

Treatment is symptomatic. Respiration, heart rate, blood pressure and body temperature should be monitored and supportive measures taken to maintain cardiovascular function. Ventilation should be used to support respiratory function if appropriate. Anexate® is a specific antidote for use in midazolam overdosage, under hospital supervision.

5. PHARMACOLOGICAL PROPERTIES

5.1 Pharmacodynamic properties

Midazolam is a soluble benzodiazepine with marked properties of suppression of tension, agitation and anxiety as well as sedative and hypnotic effects. In addition, midazolam demonstrates muscle relaxant and anticonvulsive properties. In clinical use, the main action is sleep induction.

Midazolam binds to specific receptors in the central nervous system (CNS). The benzodiazepine receptors in the CNS have a close functional connection with receptors of the GABA-ergic transmitter system. After binding to the benzodiazepine receptor, midazolam augments the inhibitory effect of GABA-ergic transmission.

5.2 Pharmacokinetic properties

Midazolam is highly lipid soluble and crosses the blood brain barrier. These properties qualify it for intravenous use in short term anaesthetic procedures since it acts promptly on the brain, and its initial effects decrease rapidly as it is distributed into fat deposits and tissues. Following the administration of 150 micrograms/kg intravenously, plasma concentrations in the range 291-425 ng/ml are reached within five minutes.

Midazolam is almost completely absorbed following intramuscular injection, peak plasma levels being attained within 45 minutes.

Midazolam is extensively protein bound (94-98%). The volume of distribution is between 0.8 and 1.7 litres/kg. Midazolam crosses the placenta. It is not known whether midazolam enters breast milk, but this is likely as it is known to occur with other benzodiazepines.

Midazolam is extensively metabolised in the liver, involving the P450 IIIA enzymes. The principal metabolite, 1-hydroxy midazolam, appears in the urine as a glucuronide. The metabolite is less pharmacologically active than midazolam and has a shorter half-life of about one hour. Midazolam has a mean elimination half-life of two to three hours. The half-life is short compared with other benzodiazepines. Less than 1% midazolam is excreted unchanged via the kidneys and the drug is cleared virtually entirely by the liver. The half-life of midazolam is prolonged in neonates, in the elderly and patients with liver disorders.

5.3 Preclinical safety data

In vitro and *in vivo* microbial and mammalian test systems have revealed no evidence of mutagenicity. No evidence of carcinogenic potential was seen in rats or mice given oral midazolam maleate in doses up to 25 times the human recommended daily dose for two years.

In humans, the risk of congenital abnormalities from the ingestion of therapeutic doses of benzodiazepines is slight, although a few epidemiological studies have pointed to an increased risk of cleft palate. There are case reports of congenital abnormalities and mental retardation in prenatally exposed children following overdosage and intoxication with benzodiazepines.

6. PHARMACEUTICAL PARTICULARS

6.1 List of excipients

Sodium Chloride

Hydrochloric Acid Solution 3M

Sodium Hydroxide Solution 3M

Water for Injections

6.2 Incompatibilities

Midazolam is incompatible with alkaline solutions (due to reduced solubility) and some medicines.

Published data show that midazolam injection is incompatible with alkaline injections such as some antibiotic and steroid injections, bumetanide, frusemide, omeprazole sodium, sodium bicarbonate and thiopental sodium. It is also incompatible with albumin, clonidine, perphenazine, prochlorperazine, ranitidine and certain parenteral solutions.

Mixture or dilution with Hartmann's solution is not recommended, as the potency of midazolam decreases.

Compatibility must be checked before administration, if intended to be mixed with other drugs.

6.3 Shelf life

Two years.

6.4 Special precautions for storage

Do not store above 25°C. Keep container in outer carton.

6.5 Nature and contents of container

Neutral glass ampoules Type I Ph Eur 5ml packed in 5 or 10s in an outer printed carton

6.6 Instructions for use and handling

The injection is for single patient use and should be used immediately after opening. The injection should not be used if particles are present. Any unused portion should be discarded.

Midazolam for infusion may be prepared by dilution with infusion fluids containing 5% glucose, 4% glucose with 0.18% sodium chloride or 0.9% sodium chloride.

Chemical and physical in-use stability has been demonstrated for 24 hours at 25°C.

From a microbiological point of view, the product should be used immediately. If not used immediately, in-use storage times and conditions prior to use are the responsibility of the user and would normally not be longer than 24 hours at 2-8°C, unless dilution has taken place in controlled and validated aseptic conditions.

7. MARKETING AUTHORISATION HOLDER

CP Pharmaceuticals Ltd

Ash Road North

Wrexham

LL13 9UF

8. MARKETING AUTHORISATION NUMBER(S)

4543/0389

9. DATE OF FIRST AUTHORISATION/RENEWAL OF THE AUTHORISATION

25 August 1999

10. DATE OF REVISION OF THE TEXT

July 1999

Midazolam Injection BP 5mg/ml

(Wockhardt UK Ltd)

1. NAME OF THE MEDICINAL PRODUCT

Midazolam Injection BP 5mg/ml

2. QUALITATIVE AND QUANTITATIVE COMPOSITION

Midazolam 5mg/ml

Each 2ml ampoule contains 10mg midazolam

3. PHARMACEUTICAL FORM

Solution for injection

4. CLINICAL PARTICULARS

4.1 Therapeutic indications

As intravenous sedative cover before and during minor medical, dental and surgical procedures such as gastroscopy, endoscopy, cystoscopy, bronchoscopy and cardiac catheterisation.

For sedation by intravenous injection (either continuous infusion or intermittent bolus injection) in critically ill patients in intensive care.

As an intramuscular premedication for patients with physical status ASA I-IV who are to undergo surgical procedures.

As an alternative intravenous agent for the induction of anaesthesia in high risk and elderly patients, especially where cardiovascular stability is of particular importance. Induction is more reliable when heavy opiate premedication has been administered or when Midazolam Injection is given with a narcotic analgesic such as fentanyl.

4.2 Posology and method of administration

Dosage depends on the individual response, age and weight. Midazolam 5mg/ml may be given by intramuscular, intravenous or slow intravenous injection.

Intravenous sedation

One or more intravenous injections to be administered over a single operating session.

Dosage should be titrated according to an individual's response, age and weight. The end-point of this titration is dependent on the procedure. Full sedation will be evident by drowsiness and slurred speech, although a response to commands will be maintained.

Adults	2mg, (0.4ml of 5mg/ml midazolam injection solution) over a period of 30 seconds initially
Elderly	1 to 1.5mg (0.2-0.3ml of 5mg/ml midazolam injection solution) over a period of 30 seconds initially.

If adequate sedation is not achieved after two minutes, incremental doses of 0.5-1mg, (0.1-0.2ml of 5mg/ml midazolam injection solution) should be given until the desired level of sedation is achieved, usually at a total dose of 2.5-7.5mg (about 70 micrograms/kg) in adults.

Children	Not recommended. Midazolam injection has not been evaluated as an intravenous sedative in children.

Combination therapy:-

If analgesia is provided by a narcotic analgesic, this should be administered first. The dose of midazolam injection should then be carefully titrated. Low total doses of 1-2mg may be adequate with lower total doses of 0.5-1mg in the elderly.

Mode of administration:-

For the administration of midazolam injection the patient should be placed in a supine position and remain there throughout the procedure. Resuscitation facilities should always be available and a second person, fully trained in the use of such equipment, always be present. It is recommended that patients should remain under medical supervision until at least one hour has elapsed from the time of injection. They should always be accompanied home by a responsible adult.

Patients who have received only midazolam injection for iv sedation prior to minor procedures, should be warned not to drive or operate machinery for 12 hours. Where midazolam injection is used concurrently with other central nervous system depressants (e.g. potent analgesics) recovery may be prolonged. Patients should therefore be assessed carefully before being allowed to go home or resume normal activities.

Sedation in the critically ill patient:-

Midazolam injection can be given intravenously by two methods for this purpose, either by continuous infusion or by intermittent bolus dose. Both have their own advantages and disadvantages and the appropriate method of giving midazolam injection will need to be determined for each patient.

The dose of midazolam injection needed to sedate critically ill patients varies considerably between patients. The dose should be titrated to the desired state of sedation. This will depend on clinical need, physical status, age and concomitant medication.

Midazolam injection can also be given in combination with an opioid. The opioid may be used for its analgesic effects or as an antitussive agent to help the patient tolerate the tracheal tube and ventilatory support.

Patients receiving midazolam injection for sedation in the intensive care situation should receive ventilatory support.

Safe use for midazolam for periods of over 14 days in duration has not been established in clinical trials.

Potential drug interactions:-

The critically ill patient is exposed to many drugs. Because of this, there is a potential for drug interactions. (See Interactions section under Contraindications, Warnings etc.)

After prolonged iv administration of midazolam injection, abrupt discontinuation may be accompanied by withdrawal symptoms, therefore a gradual reduction of the drug is recommended.

Midazolam injection is stable both physically and chemically for up to 24 hours at room temperature when mixed with infusion fluids containing 4% dextrose with 0.18% sodium chloride, 5% dextrose or 0.9% sodium chloride.

Sedation by intermittent bolus dose in intensive care

Midazolam injection only

The exact dose of midazolam needs to be titrated to the individual patient response. Small doses of midazolam 1.0-2.0mg can be given, and repeated, until the required degree of sedation is reached.

Midazolam injection and an opioid

When midazolam and an opioid are used together, the opioid should be administered first. Both drugs need to be titrated to the individual patient's response and to the level of sedation thought to be necessary.

Small doses of midazolam 1-2mg (0.2-0.4ml of 5mg/ml midazolam injection solution) can be given, and repeated, until the required degree of sedation is reached. In the elderly, smaller doses as little as 0.5-1.0mg (0.1-0.2ml of 5mg/ml midazolam injection solution) may be adequate.

The use of these two groups of drugs can increase the risk of respiratory depression. If the patient is being given ventilatory support using a mode that depends upon some spontaneous effort by the patient, then the minute volume may decrease.

Sedation by continuous infusion in intensive care

Midazolam injection only

Adults, Elderly and children

For patients already sedated or anaesthetised after an operation, a loading dose of midazolam is unnecessary.

In other situations a loading dose of 0.03-0.3mg/kg given over a five minute period is recommended, depending on the level of sedation required. The loading dose should be reduced or omitted in hypovolaemic, vasoconstricted or hypothermic patients.

Maintenance dose

A dose between 0.03-0.2mg/kg/hour is recommended, starting at the lower dose.

The dose should be reduced in hypovolaemic, vasoconstricted or hypothermic patients.

Midazolam injection and an opioid

When opioid analgesics are used, the rate of infusion of midazolam should be titrated carefully to the sedative needs of the patient. Low doses of midazolam 0.01 to 0.1mg/kg/hour may be used to start.

The use of these two groups of drugs can increase the risk of respiratory depression. If the patient is being given ventilatory support using a mode that depends upon some spontaneous effort by the patient, then the minute volume may decrease.

Whenever a continuous infusion of midazolam is used (with or without an opioid analgesic), its need should be assessed on a daily basis in order to reduce the risk of accumulation and prolonged recovery. Each day the infusion of midazolam should be stopped or its rate reduced and the patient seen to recover from its effect. If recovery is prolonged (>2 hours) a lower dose should be used when it is restarted. A sedation score should be used routinely.

When midazolam has been given for a number of days and then gradually withdrawn, patients may be awake but show signs of residual sedation for the next 12 to 24 hours. This can cause difficulties because patients may not cough and expectorate well if they are then weaned from ventilatory support. However, while recovering from the effects of midazolam, patients may not be sufficiently sedated to tolerate ventilatory support. In such circumstances sedation may be provided with a shorter acting agent while there is recovery from the effects of midazolam.

The recommended concentration of a solution for infusion in a critically ill adult patient is 1mg/ml.

Pre-medication (by intramuscular injection)

Adults and elderly	70-100 micrograms/kg, 30-60 minutes before the operation. The usual dose is about 5mg (2.5mg in the elderly)
Children	Not recommended

Atropine or hyoscine hydrobromide may be given concomitantly, bearing in mind that hyoscine hydrobromide will enhance and prolong the sedative and amnesic effects of midazolam injection.

Midazolam injection can be combined with atropine or hyoscine hydrobromide in the same syringe to be given as a single intramuscular injection.

Induction of anaesthesia by slow intravenous injection

One or more bolus intravenous injections should be administered over a single anaesthetic session.

Adults

The dose should be titrated against the individual response of the patient. Midazolam injection should be given by slow intravenous injection until there is a loss of eyelid reflex, response to commands and voluntary movements.

In anticipating the required dose of midazolam, both the premedication already given and the age of the patient are important. Young, fit unpremedicated patients may need at least 0.3mg/kg bodyweight, whereas patients premedicated with an opiate usually need only 0.2mg/kg bodyweight.

Use in the elderly

The elderly are more sensitive to the effects of benzodiazepines. Induction may be adequate with 0.1mg/kg body weight in premedicated patients and 0.2mg/kg body weight in unpremedicated patients.

Children over seven years

Midazolam injection has been shown to be an effective agent for induction of anaesthesia in children over seven years of age, at a dose of 0.15mg/kg body-weight.

4.3 Contraindications

Known hypersensitivity to benzodiazepines or any of the ingredients.

Myasthenia gravis

Severe respiratory insufficiency

4.4 Special warnings and special precautions for use

Midazolam injection should be used with caution in patients with renal or hepatic dysfunction, chronic pulmonary insufficiency, elderly or debilitated patients. During bolus sedation for operative procedures, patients with acute pulmonary insufficiency or respiratory depression should be treated with extreme caution.

Midazolam may enhance the effects of other CNS depressants and may result in severe respiratory or cardiovascular depression. Their concurrent use should be avoided.

The dependence potential of midazolam is low when limited to short term use. Due to the possibility of withdrawal symptoms, midazolam should be gradually reduced following a prolonged iv administration. Withdrawal symptoms may occur with benzodiazepines following normal use of therapeutic doses for only short periods and may be associated with physiological and psychological sequelae, including depression. This should be considered when treating patients for more than a few days.

As with other benzodiazepines, extreme caution should be used if prescribing midazolam for patients with personality disorders. The disinhibiting effects of benzodiazepines may be manifested as the precipitation of suicide in patients who are depressed or show aggressive behaviour towards self and others.

4.5 Interaction with other medicinal products and other forms of Interaction

Enhanced sedation or respiratory and cardiovascular depression may occur if midazolam is given with other drugs that have CNS depressant properties (e.g. antipsychotics, anxiolytics, sedatives, antidepressants, hypnotics, narcotic analgesics, anaesthetics, antiepileptics).

If such centrally acting depressant drugs are given parenterally in conjunction with intravenous midazolam, severe respiratory and cardiovascular depression may occur. When intravenous midazolam is to be administered concurrently with a narcotic analgesic agent (e.g. in dentistry), it is recommended that midazolam be given after the analgesic and that the dose be carefully titrated to meet the patient's needs.

The efficacy of cyclosporin and nifedipine may be potentiated when administered concurrently with midazolam.

Agents that interfere with metabolism by hepatic enzymes (e.g. isoniazid, disulfiram, cimetidine, omeprazole, ranitidine, erythromycin, diltiazem, verapamil, ketoconazole, itraconazole and possibly fluconazole, oral contraceptives) have been shown to reduce the clearance of benzodiazepines and may potentiate their actions, whilst known inducers of hepatic enzymes, for example, rifampicin, may increase the clearance of benzodiazepines.

Midazolam may interact with other hepatically metabolised drugs, causing inhibition (levodopa) or potentiation (phenytoin, muscle relaxants).

Alcohol should be avoided for at least eight hours before and after the administration of midazolam due to increased sedative effects.

4.6 Pregnancy and lactation

There is no evidence regarding the safety of midazolam in pregnancy. It should not be used, especially in the first and third trimesters, unless the benefit is considered to outweigh the risk.

If the product is prescribed to a woman of childbearing potential she should be warned to contact her physician regarding discontinuance of the product if she intends to become or suspects that she is pregnant.

If, for compelling medical reasons, the product is administered during the late phase of pregnancy, or during labour at high doses, effects on the neonate, such as hypothermia, hypotonia and moderate respiratory depression, can be expected, due to the pharmacological action of the compound. If midazolam is administered during the last trimester of pregnancy it may produce irregularities in the foetal heart rate, and poor suckling in the neonate.

Since benzodiazepines are found in the breast milk, benzodiazepines should not be given to breast-feeding mothers.

4.7 Effects on ability to drive and use machines

The concurrent use of midazolam with other central nervous system depressants, may result in a prolonged recovery. A careful assessment should be undertaken prior to allowing the patient to go home or resume normal activities.

Patients treated with midazolam injection should not drive or use machinery for twelve hours after receiving this medicine.

4.8 Undesirable effects

Midazolam can produce respiratory depression, apnoea and hypertension. Midazolam may cause decreases in cardiac output, stroke volume and systemic vascular resistance. These effects are important in those patients with a reduced myocardial oxygen delivery capacity or suffering hypovolaemia.

Midazolam may cause respiratory arrest following iv administration especially in the elderly with pre-existing respiratory insufficiency or when the dose is excessive or administered too rapidly.

Other side-effects are usually mild. The most common side effects are sedation, drowsiness, headaches, muscle weakness, dizziness (with risk of falls in the elderly), ataxia, confusion, slurred speech, tremor, numbed emotions, reduced alertness, fatigue, double vision, anterograde amnesia and a hangover effect. Elderly or debilitated patients are particularly susceptible to side effects and may require lower doses. Other effects which may occur rarely are dry mouth, increased appetite, gastrointestinal and visual disturbances, jaundice, urinary retention, bradycardia, changes in libido, menstrual disturbances, skin reactions, blood dyscrasias, laryngeal spasm and chest pain.

In susceptible patients, an unnoticed depression may become evident. Paradoxical reactions (restlessness, agitation, instability, rages, hallucinations) are known to occur with benzodiazepines and are more likely in children and the elderly.

Local pain on injection and thrombophlebitis may occur.

4.9 Overdose

a) Symptoms

The symptoms of mild overdose may include confusion, somnolence, paradoxical excitation, coma, ataxia, dysarthria, hypotension and muscular weakness. In severe overdose, depression of vital functions may occur, particularly the respiratory centre. As drug levels fall severe agitation may develop.

b) Treatment

Treatment is symptomatic. Respiration, heart rate, blood pressure and body temperature should be monitored and supportive measures taken to maintain cardiovascular function. Ventilation should be used to support respiratory function if appropriate. Anexate® is a specific antidote for use in midazolam overdosage, under hospital supervision.

5. PHARMACOLOGICAL PROPERTIES

5.1 Pharmacodynamic properties

Midazolam is a soluble benzodiazepine with marked properties of suppression of tension, agitation and anxiety as well as sedative and hypnotic effects. In addition, midazolam demonstrates muscle relaxant and anticonvulsive properties. In clinical use, the main action is sleep induction.

Midazolam binds to specific receptors in the central nervous system (CNS). The benzodiazepine receptors in the CNS have a close functional connection with receptors of the GABA-ergic transmitter system. After binding to the benzodiazepine receptor, midazolam augments the inhibitory effect of GABA-ergic transmission.

5.2 Pharmacokinetic properties

Midazolam is highly lipid soluble and crosses the blood brain barrier. These properties qualify it for intravenous use in short term anaesthetic procedures since it acts promptly on the brain, and its initial effects decrease rapidly as it is distributed into fat deposits and tissues. Following the administration of 150 micrograms/kg intravenously, plasma concentrations in the range 291-425 ng/ml are reached within five minutes.

Midazolam is almost completely absorbed following intramuscular injection, peak plasma levels being attained within 45 minutes.

Midazolam is extensively protein bound (94-98%). The volume of distribution is between 0.8 and 1.7 litres/kg. Midazolam crosses the placenta. It is not known whether midazolam enters breast milk, but this is likely as it is known to occur with other benzodiazepines.

Midazolam is extensively metabolised in the liver, involving the P450 IIIA enzymes. The principal metabolite, 1-hydroxy midazolam, appears in the urine as a glucuronide. The metabolite is less pharmacologically active than midazolam and has a shorter half-life of about one hour. Midazolam has a mean elimination half-life of two to three hours. The half-life is short compared with other benzodiazepines. Less than 1% midazolam is excreted unchanged via the kidneys and the drug is cleared virtually entirely by the liver. The half-life of midazolam is prolonged in neonates, in the elderly and patients with liver disorders.

5.3 Preclinical safety data

In vitro and *in vivo* microbial and mammalian test systems have revealed no evidence of mutagenicity. No evidence of carcinogenic potential was seen in rats or mice given oral midazolam maleate in doses up to 25 times the human recommended daily dose for two years.

In humans, the risk of congenital abnormalities from the ingestion of therapeutic doses of benzodiazepines is slight, although a few epidemiological studies have pointed to an increased risk of cleft palate. There are case reports of congenital abnormalities and mental retardation in prenatally exposed children following overdosage and intoxication with benzodiazepines.

6. PHARMACEUTICAL PARTICULARS

6.1 List of excipients

Sodium Chloride

Hydrochloric Acid Solution 3M

Sodium Hydroxide Solution 3M

Water for Injections

6.2 Incompatibilities

Midazolam is incompatible with alkaline solutions (due to reduced solubility) and some medicines.

Published data show that midazolam injection is incompatible with alkaline injections such as some antibiotic and steroid injections, bumetanide, frusemide, omeprazole sodium, sodium bicarbonate and thiopental sodium. It is also incompatible with albumin, clonidine, perphenazine, prochlorperazine, ranitidine and certain parenteral solutions.

Mixture or dilution with Hartmann's solution is not recommended, as the potency of midazolam decreases.

Compatibility must be checked before administration, if intended to be mixed with other drugs.

6.3 Shelf life

Two years.

6.4 Special precautions for storage

Do not store above 25°C. Keep container in outer carton.

6.5 Nature and contents of container

Neutral glass ampoules Type I Ph Eur 2ml packed in 5 or 10s in an outer printed carton

6.6 Instructions for use and handling

The injection is for single patient use and should be used immediately after opening. The injection should not be used if particles are present. Any unused portion should be discarded.

Midazolam for infusion may be prepared by dilution with infusion fluids containing 5% glucose, 4% glucose with 0.18% sodium chloride or 0.9% sodium chloride.

Chemical and physical in-use stability has been demonstrated for 24 hours at 25°C.

From a microbiological point of view, the product should be used immediately. If not used immediately, in-use storage times and conditions prior to use are the responsibility of the user and would normally not be longer than 24 hours at 2-8°C, unless dilution has taken place in controlled and validated aseptic conditions.

7. MARKETING AUTHORISATION HOLDER

CP Pharmaceuticals Ltd

Ash Road North

Wrexham

LL13 9UF

8. MARKETING AUTHORISATION NUMBER(S)

4543/0390

9. DATE OF FIRST AUTHORISATION/RENEWAL OF THE AUTHORISATION

25 August 1999

10. DATE OF REVISION OF THE TEXT

July 1999

Mifegyne

(Exelgyn Laboratoires)

1. NAME OF THE MEDICINAL PRODUCT

Mifegyne

2. QUALITATIVE AND QUANTITATIVE COMPOSITION

Each tablet contains: Active Ingredient – Mifepristone 200mg

3. PHARMACEUTICAL FORM

Light yellow, cylindrical, bi-convex tablets

4. CLINICAL PARTICULARS

4.1 Therapeutic indications

(1) Medical termination of intra uterine pregnancy of up to 63 days gestation.

(2) Softening and dilatation of the cervix uteri prior to mechanical cervical dilatation for pregnancy termination.

(3) For use in combination with gemeprost for termination of pregnancy between 13 and 24 weeks gestation.

(4) Labour induction in fetal death in utero

For termination of pregnancy mifepristone may only be administered **in accordance with the Abortion Act 1967 as amended by The Human Fertilisation and Embryology Act 1990**.

As a consequence, when used for termination of pregnancy, mifepristone and any treatment necessary to effect complete termination of the pregnancy can only be prescribed by a medical doctor and administered in a NHS or non NHS hospital or centre (having approval to undertake termination of pregnancy). The product will be administered under the supervision of a medical practitioner.

4.2 Posology and method of administration

(1) Therapeutic termination of pregnancy of up to 63 days gestation.

600mg of mifepristone (3x200mg tablets) by mouth in a single dose. The dosage is independent of body weight.

Unless abortion has already been completed, gemeprost 1.0mg p.v should be given 36 – 48 hour later in the treatment centre.

(2) Softening and dilatation of the cervix

600mg mifepristone by mouth 36-48 hours prior to the planned operative procedure.

(3) For use in combination with gemeprost for termination of pregnancy between 13 – 24 weeks gestation

600mg mifepristone (3x200mg tablets) is taken by mouth 36-48 prior to scheduled prostaglandin termination of pregnancy

The patient must return to the treatment centre 36-48 hours later, the recommended procedure for therapeutic termination of pregnancy with gemeprost **must** then be followed. ***See gemeprost SPC***

(4) Labour induction for fetal death in utero

600 mg of mifepristone (200mg × 3 tablets) in a single oral daily dose for two consecutive days.

Labour should be induced by the usual methods if it has not started within 72 hours following the first administration of mifepristone.

If the patient vomits shortly after administration of the mifepristone she should inform the doctor.

When used in association with 1mg gemeprost pessaries for termination of pregnancy, a dose of 200mg mifepristone may also be effective.

4.3 Contraindications

Suspected ectopic pregnancy

Pregnancy not confirmed by ultrasound scan or biological tests

Chronic adrenal failure

Severe Asthma not controlled by therapy

Known allergy to mifepristone or any component of the product

Inherited porphyria

If gemeprost is used, any contraindication to gemeprost (see gemeprost product information).

4.4 Special warnings and special precautions for use

WARNINGS

In the absence of specific studies, mifepristone is not recommended in patients with:

Renal failure, hepatic failure or malnutrition.

Patients with prosthetic heart valves or who have had one previous episode of infective endocarditis should receive chemoprophylaxis according to the current UK recommendations.

1) Medical termination of pregnancy of up to 63 days gestation

The method requires active involvement of the woman who should be informed of the requirements of the methods:

- the necessity to combine treatment with prostaglandin to be administered at a second visit.

- The need for a follow up visit within 10 to 14 days after intake of mifepristone to check that abortion is complete.

- The possibility of failure of the method which may require termination by another method.

In the case of a pregnancy occurring with an intra-uterine device in situ, this device must be removed before administration of mifepristone.

The expulsion may take place before prostaglandin administration (in about 3% of cases). This does not preclude the follow up visit to check that the abortion is complete.

Risks related to the method

• Failures

The non-negligible risk of failure, makes the follow up visit mandatory to check that abortion is complete.

• Bleeding

The patient must be informed of the occurrence of prolonged vaginal bleeding (up to 12 days after intake of mifepristone) which may be heavy. Bleeding occurs in almost all cases and it not in any way proof of complete expulsion.

The patient should receive precise instructions on whom she should contact and where to go in the event of any problems, particularly in the case of very heavy vaginal bleeding.

A follow-up visit must take place within a period of 10 to 14 days after administration of mifepristone to verify by the appropriate means (clinical examination, ultrasound scan, and Beta-HCG measurement) that expulsion has been completed and that vaginal bleeding has stopped or substantially reduced. In case of persistent bleeding beyond the control visit, its disappearance should be checked within a few days.

If continuing pregnancy is suspected, a further ultrasound scan may be required to evaluate its viability.

Persistence of vaginal bleeding at this point could signify incomplete abortion, or an unnoticed extra-uterine pregnancy, and appropriate treatment should be considered.

In the event of continuing pregnancy diagnosed after the control visit, termination by another method will be proposed to the woman.

Since heavy bleeding requiring hemostatic curettage occurs in 0 to 1.4% of the cases during the medical method of pregnancy termination, special care should be given to patients with hemostatic disorders with hypocoagulability, or with anemia. The decision to use the medical or the surgical method should be decided with specialised consultants according to the type of hemostatic disorder and the level of anaemia.

2) Softening and dilatation of the cervix uteri prior to surgical pregnancy termination

For the full efficacy of therapy, the use of Mifepristone must be followed 36 to 48 hours later and not beyond, by surgical termination.

Risks related to the method

• Bleeding

The woman will be informed of the risk of vaginal bleeding which may be heavy, following intake of mifepristone. She should be informed of the risk of abortion prior to surgery (although minimal): she will be informed on where to go in order to check for the completeness of expulsion, or in any case of emergency.

Other risks

They are those of the surgical procedure.

3) For use with gemeprost for termination of pregnancy between 13 – 24 weeks.

For the full efficacy of therapy, Mifepristone must be followed, 36 to 48 hours later by initiation of gemeprost.

Risks related to the method

• Bleeding

The woman will be informed of the risk of vaginal bleeding following intake of mifepristone. She should be informed of the risk of abortion prior to administration of gemeprost (although minimal): she will be informed on where to go in case of emergency.

Other risks

They are those of gemeprost administration.

A follow-up visit is recommended at an appropriate interval after delivery of the fetus to verify that vaginal bleeding has stopped or has substantially reduced. Persistence of vaginal bleeding could signify incomplete abortion and appropriate investigation/treatment should be considered.

4) In all instances

The use of mifepristone requires rhesus determination and hence the prevention of rhesus allo-immunisation as well as other general measures taken usually during any termination of pregnancy.

During clinical trials, pregnancies occurred between embryo expulsion and the resumption of menses.

To avoid potential exposure of a subsequent pregnancy to mifepristone, it is recommended that conception be avoided during the next menstrual cycle. Reliable contraceptive precautions should therefore commence as early as possible after mifepristone administration.

PRECAUTIONS

1) In all instances

In case of suspected acute adrenal failure, dexamethasone administration is recommended. 1 mg of dexamethasone antagonises a dose of 400 mg of mifepristone.

Due to the antiglucocorticoid activity of mifepristone, the efficacy of long-term corticosteroid therapy, including inhaled corticosteroids in asthmatic patients, may be decreased during the 3 to 4 days following intake of mifepristone. Therapy should be adjusted.

A decrease of the efficacy of the method can theoretically occur due to the antiprostaglandin properties of non-steroidal anti-inflammatory drugs (NSAIDs) including aspirin (acetyl salicylic acid). Use non-NSAI analgesics.

2) Medical termination of intra-uterine pregnancy with mifepristone and gemeprost

Rare serious cardiovascular accidents have been reported following the intra muscular administration of the prostaglandin analogue sulprostone (withdrawn in 1992). No such cases have been reported since analogues of PGE_1 (gemeprost or misoprostol) have been used. For these reasons and as a special precautionary measure, the medical method is not recommended for use in women over 35 years of age and who smoke more than 10 cigarettes a day.

<u>Method of prostaglandin administration</u>

During administration and for a minimum of three hours following administration and in accordance with clinical judgement, the patients should be monitored in the treatment centre, which must be equipped with the appropriate equipment.

3) For the sequential use of mifepristone - prostaglandin, whatever the indication

The precautions related to the prostaglandin used should be followed where relevant.

The treatment procedure should be fully explained and completely understood by the patient. There is a Patient Information Leaflet available for each of the indications in the tablet carton. Prior to administration of mifepristone the appropriate leaflet should be given to the patient to read.

4.5 Interaction with other medicinal products and other forms of Interaction

In view of the single dose administration, no specific interactions have been studied. However, there could be interactions with drugs which modulate or inhibit prostaglandin synthesis and metabolism. See PRECAUTIONS above.

4.6 Pregnancy and lactation

In animals (see section 5.3 Pre-clinical safety data), the abortifacient effect of mifepristone precludes the proper assessment of any teratogenic effect of the molecule.

With subabortive doses, isolated cases of malformations observed in rabbits, but not in rats or mice were too few to be considered significant, or attributable to mifepristone.

In humans, the few reported cases of malformations do not allow a causality assessment for mifepristone alone or associated to prostaglandin. Therefore, data is too limited to determine whetherthe molecule is a human teratogen.

Consequently:

- Women should be informed, that due to the risk of failure of the medical method of pregnancy termination and to the unknown risk to the fetus, the control visit is mandatory (see Section 4.4 special warnings and special precautions for use).

- Should a failure of the method be diagnosed at the control visit (viable ongoing pregnancy), and should the patient still agree, pregnancy termination should be completed by another method.

- Should the patient wish to continue with her pregnancy, the available data is too limited to justify a systematic termination of an exposed pregnancy. In that event, careful ultra-sonographic monitoring of the pregnancy should be carried out.

<u>Lactation</u>

Mifepristone is a lipophilic compound and may theoretically be excreted in the mother's breast milk. However, no data is available. Consequently, mifepristone use should be avoided during breast-feeding.

4.7 Effects on ability to drive and use machines

None known.

4.8 Undesirable effects

<u>**Most frequently reported undesirable effects (mifepristone)**</u>

• Urogenital

- Bleeding

Heavy bleeding occurs in about 5% of the cases and may require hemostatic curettage in up to 0.7% of cases.

- Very common uterine contractions or cramping (10 to 45%) in the hours following prostaglandin intake.

- During induction of second trimester termination of uterine rupture has been uncommonly reported after prostaglandin intake. The reports occurred particularly in multiparous women or in women with a caesarean section scar.

• Gastrointestinal

- Cramping, light or moderate.

- Nausea, vomiting.

<u>**Other undesirable effects (mifepristone)**</u>

• Hypersensitivity and skin

- Hypersensitivity: uncommon incidences of skin rash, urticaria and facial oedema Single cases of erythroderma, erythema nodosum, epidermal necrolysis have also been reported.

• **Other Systems**

- Rare cases of headaches, malaise, vagal symptoms (hot flushes, dizziness, chills have been reported) and fever.

Undesirable effects (gemeprost)

- nausea, vomiting or diarrhoea, and rarely hypotension (0.25%)

4.9 Overdose

Tolerance studies have shown that administration of doses of mifepristone of up to 2g caused no unwanted reactions. Nevertheless, in the event of massive ingestion signs of adrenal failure might occur. Any suggestion of acute intoxication, therefore, requires treatment in a specialist environment.

5. PHARMACOLOGICAL PROPERTIES

5.1 Pharmacodynamic properties

Mifepristone is a synthetic steroid with an antiprogestational action as a result of competition with progesterone at the progesterone receptors.

At doses ranging from 3 to 10mg/kg orally, it inhibits the action of endogenous or exogenous progesterone in different animal species (rat, mouse, rabbit and monkey). This action is manifested in the form of pregnancy termination in rodents.

In women at doses of greater than or equal to 1mg/kg, mifepristone antagonises the endometrial and myometrial effects of progesterone. During pregnancy it sensitises the myometrium to the contraction inducing action of prostaglandins.

Mifepristone induces softening and dilatation of the cervix, softening and dilatation has been shown to be detectable from 24 hours after administration of mifepristone and increases to a maximum at approximately 36 – 48 hours after administration.

During the termination of pregnancy between 13 and 24 weeks gestation, mifepristone administered at a 600-mg dose, 36 to 48 hours prior to the first administration of prostaglandins, reduces the induction-abortion interval, and also decreases the dose of gemeprost required for the expulsion.

Mifepristone binds to the glucocorticoid receptor. In animals at doses of 10 to 25 mg/kg it inhibits the action of dexamethasone. In man the antiglucocorticoid action is manifested at a dose equal to or greater than 4.5 mg/kg by a compensatory elevation of ACTH and cortisol.

Mifepristone has a weak anti-androgenic action which only appears in animals during prolonged administration of very high doses.

5.2 Pharmacokinetic properties

After oral administration of a single dose of 600 mg mifepristone is rapidly absorbed. The peak concentration of 1.98 mg/l is reached after 1.30 hours (means of 10 subjects).

There is a non-linear dose response. After a distribution phase, elimination is at first slow, the concentration decreasing by a half between about 12 and 72 hours, and then more rapid, giving an elimination half-life of 18 hours. With radio receptor assay techniques, the terminal half-life is of up to 90 hours, including all metabolites of mifepristone able to bind to progesterone receptors.

After administration of low doses of mifepristone (20 mg orally or intravenously), the absolute bioavailability is 69%.

In plasma mifepristone is 98% bound to plasma proteins: albumin and principally alpha-1-acid glycoprotein (AAG), to which binding is saturable. Due to this specific binding, volume of distribution and plasma clearance of mifepristone are inversely proportional to the plasma concentration of AAG.

N-Demethylation and terminal hydroxylation of the 17-propynyl chain are primary metabolic pathways of hepatic oxidative metabolism.

Mifepristone is mainly excreted in faeces. After administration of a 600 mg labelled dose, 10% of the total radioactivity is eliminated in the urine and 90% in the faeces.

6. PHARMACEUTICAL PARTICULARS

6.1 List of excipients

Anhydrous colloidal silica 3mg, Maize Starch 102mg, Povidone 12mg, Microcrystaline cellulose 30mg, Magnesium Stearate 3mg.

6.2 Incompatibilities

None known.

6.3 Shelf life

Tablets - 36 months.

6.4 Special precautions for storage

None.

6.5 Nature and contents of container

Blister pack (PVC and Aluminium foil and carton) containing 3 tablets.

6.6 Instructions for use and handling

The treatment procedure should be fully explained and completely understood by the patient.

Administrative Data

7. MARKETING AUTHORISATION HOLDER

Exelgyn S.A.

6 rue Christophe Colomb

75008 Paris

France

8. MARKETING AUTHORISATION NUMBER(S)

Mifegyne Tablets 16152/0001

9. DATE OF FIRST AUTHORISATION/RENEWAL OF THE AUTHORISATION

Renewal February 2005

10. DATE OF REVISION OF THE TEXT

February 2005

Migard

(A. Menarini Pharma U.K. S.R.L.)

1. NAME OF THE MEDICINAL PRODUCT

MIGARD 2.5 mg film-coated tablets

2. QUALITATIVE AND QUANTITATIVE COMPOSITION

Each film-coated tablet contains 2.5 mg of frovatriptan (as succinate monohydrate)

For excipients see 6.1 List of excipients

3. PHARMACEUTICAL FORM

Film-coated tablet.

Round biconvex white film-coated tablet, debossed with "m" on one side and "2.5" on the other.

4. CLINICAL PARTICULARS

4.1 Therapeutic indications

Acute treatment of the headache phase of migraine attacks with or without aura.

4.2 Posology and method of administration

General

Frovatriptan should be taken as early as possible after the onset of a migraine attack but it is also effective when taken at a later stage. Frovatriptan should not be used prophylactically. The tablets should be swallowed whole with water.

If a patient does not respond to the first dose of frovatriptan, a second dose should not be taken for the same attack, since no benefit has been shown.

Frovatriptan may be used for subsequent migraine attacks.

Adults (18 to 65 years of age)

The recommended dose of frovatriptan is 2.5 mg.

If the migraine recurs after initial relief, a second dose may be taken, providing there is an interval of at least 2 hours between the two doses.

The total daily dose should not exceed 5 mg per day.

Children and adolescents (under 18 years)

There are no data of the use of frovatriptan in children and adolescents. Therefore, its use in this age group is not recommended.

Elderly (over 65 years)

Frovatriptan data in patients over 65 years remain limited. Therefore, its use in this category of patients is not recommended.

Renal impairment

No dosage adjustment is required in patients with renal impairment (see 5.2 Pharmacokinetic properties).

Hepatic impairment

No dosage adjustment is required in patients with mild to moderate hepatic impairment (see 5.2 Pharmacokinetic properties). Frovatriptan is contraindicated in patients with severe hepatic impairment (see 4.3 Contra-indications).

4.3 Contraindications

- hypersensitivity to frovatriptan or to any of the excipients.
- patients with a history of myocardial infarction, ischaemic heart disease, coronary vasospasm (e.g. Prinzmetal's angina), peripheral vascular disease, patients presenting with symptoms or signs compatible with ischaemic heart disease.
- Moderately severe or severe hypertension, uncontrolled mild hypertension.
- previous cerebrovascular accident (CVA) or transient ischaemic attack (TIA).
- severe hepatic impairment (Child-Pugh C).
- Concomitant administration of frovatriptan with ergotamine or ergotamine derivatives (including méthysergide) or other 5-hydroxytryptamine ($5\text{-}HT_1$) receptor agonists.

4.4 Special warnings and special precautions for use

Frovatriptan should only be used where a clear diagnosis of migraine has been established.

Frovatriptan is not indicated for the management of hemiplegic, basilar or ophthalmoplegic migraine.

As with other treatments of migraine attack, it is necessary to exclude other, potentially serious, neurological conditions before treating the headache of patients without a previous diagnosis of migraine, or migraine patients presenting with atypical symptoms. It should be noted that migraineurs present an increased risk of certain cerebral vascular events (eg CVA or TIA).

The safety and efficacy of frovatriptan administered during the aura phase, before the headache phase of migraine, has not been established.

As for other $5\text{-}HT_1$ receptor agonists, frovatriptan must not be administered to patients at risk of coronary artery disease (CAD, including heavy smokers or users of nicotine substitution therapy without a prior cardiovascular evaluation (see 4.3 Contra-indications). Specific attention should be given to post- menopausal women and men over 40 years of age presenting with these risk factors.

However, cardiac evaluations may not identify every patient who has cardiac disease. In very rare cases serious cardiac events have occurred in patients with no underlying cardio-vascular disease when taking $5\text{-}HT_1$ receptor agonists.

Frovatriptan administration can be associated with transient symptoms including chest pain or tightness which may be intense and involve the throat. (see 4.8 Undesirable effects).

Where such symptoms are thought to indicate ischaemic heart disease no further doses of frovatriptan should be taken and additional investigations should be carried out.

It is advised to wait 24 hours following the use of frovatriptan before administering an ergotamine- type medication. At least 24 hours should be elapse after administration of an ergotamine-containg preparation before frovatriptan is given (see 4.3 Contra-indications and 4.5 Interactions with other medicinal products and other forms of interactions).

In case of too frequent use (repeated administration several days in a row corresponding to a misuse of the product), the active substance can accumulate leading to an increase of the side-effects. In addition, excessive use of an anti-migraine medicinal product can lead to daily chronic headaches requiring a therapeutic window.

Do not exceed the recommended dose of frovatriptan.

Patients with rare hereditary problems of galactose intolerance, the Lapp lactase deficiency or glucose-galactose malabsorption should not take this medicine.

Undesirable effects may be more common during concomitant use of triptans (5HT agonists) and herbal preparations containing St John's Wort (Hypericum perforatum).

4.5 Interaction with other medicinal products and other forms of Interaction

CONCOMITANT USE CONTRA-INDICATED

Ergotamine and ergotamine derivatives (including méthysergide) and other 5 HT1 agonists

Risks of hypertension and coronary artery constriction due to additive vasospastic effects when used concomitantly for the same migraine attack (see 4.3 Contra-indications).

Effects can be additive. It is recommended to wait at least 24 hours after administration of ergotamine-type medication before administering frovatriptan. Conversely it is recommended to wait 24 hours after frovatriptan administration before administering an ergotamine-type medication (see 4.4 Special warnings and precautions for use).

CONCOMITANT USE NOT RECOMMENDED

Monoamine Oxidase Inhibitors

Frovatriptan is not a substrate for MAO-A, however a potential risk of serotonin syndrome or hypertension cannot be excluded (see 5.2 Pharmacokinetic Properties).

CONCOMITANT USE REQUIRING CAUTION

Selective serotonin-reuptake inhibitors (citalopram, fluoxetine, fluvoxamine, paroxetine, sertraline)

Potential risk of hypertension, coronary vasoconstriction or serotonin syndrome.

Strict adherence to the recommended dose is an essential factor to prevent this syndrome.

Methylergometrine

Risks of hypertension, coronary artery constriction.

Fluvoxamine

Fluvoxamine is a potent inhibitor of cytochrome CYP1A2 and has been shown to increase the blood levels of frovatriptan by 27-49%.

Oral contraceptives

In female subjects taking oral contraceptives, concentrations of frovatriptan were 30% higher than in females not taking oral contraceptives. No increased incidence in the adverse event profile was reported.

Hypericum perforatum (St. John wort) (oral route)

As with other triptans the risk of the occurence of serotonin syndrome may be increased.

4.6 Pregnancy and lactation

Pregnancy

The safety of frovatriptan in pregnant women has not been established.

Studies in animals have shown reproductive toxicity (see 5.3 Preclinical safety data). The potential risk for humans is unknown. Frovatriptan should not be used during pregnancy unless clearly necessary.

Lactation

Frovatriptan and/or its metabolites are excreted in the milk of lactating rats with the maximum concentration in milk being four-fold higher than maximum blood levels. Although it is not known whether frovatriptan or its metabolites are excreted in human breast milk, the administration of frovatriptan to women who are breastfeeding is not recommended, unless is clearly needed. In this case, a 24 hours interval must be observed.

4.7 Effects on ability to drive and use machines

No studies on the effects on the ability to drive and use machines have been performed.

Migraine or treatment with frovatriptan may cause somnolence. Patients should be advised to evaluate their ability to perform complex tasks such as driving during migraine attacks and following administration of frovatriptan.

4.8 Undesirable effects

Frovatriptan has been administered to over 2700 patients at the recommended dose of 2.5 mg and the most common side effects (< 10%) include dizziness, fatigue, paraesthesia, headache and vascularflushing. The undesirable effects reported in clinical trials with frovatriptan were transient, generally mild to moderate and resolved spontaneously. Some of the symptoms reported as undesirable effects may be associated symptoms of migraine.

The table below shows all the adverse reactions that are considered to be related to treatment with 2.5 mg frovatriptan and showed a greater incidence than with placebo in the 4 placebo controlled trials. They are listed in decreasing incidence by body-system.

(see Table 1 on next page)

In two open long-term clinical studies the observed effects were not different from those listed above.

4.9 Overdose

There is no direct experience of any patient taking an overdose of frovatriptan. The maximum single oral dose of frovatriptan given to male and female patients with migraine was 40 mg (16 times the recommended clinical dose of 2.5 mg) and the maximum single dose given to healthy male subjects was 100 mg (40 times the recommended clinical dose). Both were well-tolerated.

There is no specific antidote for frovatriptan. The elimination half-life of frovatriptan is approximately 26 hours (5.2. Pharmacokinetic properties).

The effects of haemodialysis or peritoneal dialysis on serum concentrations of frovatriptan are unknown.

Treatment

In case of overdose with frovatriptan, the patient should be monitored closely for at least 48 hours and be given any necessary supportive therapy.

5. PHARMACOLOGICAL PROPERTIES

5.1 Pharmacodynamic properties

Pharmacotherapeutic group: selective $5\text{-}HT_1$ receptor agonists (N: central nervous system)

ATC code: N02C C07

Frovatriptan is a selective agonist for 5-HT receptors, which shows high affinity for $5\text{-}HT_{1B}$ and $5\text{-}HT_{1D}$ binding sites in radioligand assays and exhibits potent agonist effects at $5\text{-}HT_{1B}$ and $5\text{-}HT_{1D}$ receptors in functional bioassays. It exhibits marked selectivity for $5\text{-}HT_{1B/1D}$ receptors and has no significant affinity for $5\text{-}HT_2$, $5\text{-}HT_3$, $5\text{-}HT_4$, $5\text{-}HT_6$, α- adrenoreceptors, or histamine receptors. Frovatriptan has no significant affinity for benzodiazepine binding sites.

Frovatriptan is believed to act selectively on extracerebral, intracranial arteries to inhibit the excessive dilatation of these vessels in migraine. At clinically relevant concentrations, frovatriptan produced constriction of human isolated cerebral arteries with little or no effect on isolated human coronary arteries.

The clinical efficacy of frovatriptan for treatment of migraine headache and accompanying symptoms was investigated in three multicenter placebo controlled studies. In these studies frovatriptan 2.5 mg was consistently superior to placebo in terms of headache response at 2 and 4 hours post-dosing and time to first response. Pain relief (reduction from moderate-or severe headache to no or mild pain) after 2 hours was 37-46% for frovatriptan and 21-27% for placebo.

Complete pain relief after 2 hours was 9-14% for frovatriptan and 2-3% for placebo. Maximum efficacy with frovatriptan is reached in 4 hours.

In a clinical study comparing frovatriptan 2.5 mg with sumatriptan 100 mg, the efficacy of frovatriptan 2.5 mg was slightly lower than that of sumatriptan 100 mg at 2 hours and 4 hours. The frequency of undesirable events was slightly lower with frovatriptan 2.5 mg compared to sumatriptan 100 mg. No study comparing frovatriptan 2.5 mg and sumatriptan 50 mg has been carried out.

In elderly subjects in good health, transient changes in systolic arterial pressure (within normal limits) have been observed in some subjects, following a single oral dose of frovatriptan 2.5 mg.

5.2 Pharmacokinetic properties

Absorption

After administration of a single oral 2.5 mg dose to healthy subjects, the mean maximum blood concentration of frovatriptan (C_{max}), reached between 2 and 4 hours, was 4.2 ng/mL in males and 7.0 ng/mL in females. The mean area under the curve (AUC) was 42.9 and 94.0 ng.h/mL for males and females respectively.

The oral bioavailability was 22% in males and 30% in females. The pharmacokinetics of frovatriptan were similar between healthy subjects and migraine patients and there was no difference in pharmacokinetic parameters in the patients during a migraine attack or between attacks.

Frovatriptan displayed generally linear pharmacokinetics over the dose range used in clinical studies (1 mg to 40 mg).

Food had no significant effect on the bioavailability of frovatriptan, but delayed t_{max} slightly by approximately 1 hour.

Distribution

The steady state volume of distribution of frovatriptan following intravenous administration of 0.8 mg was 4.2 L/kg in males and 3.0 L/kg in females.

Binding of frovatriptan to serum proteins was low (approximately 15%). Reversible binding to blood cells at steady state was approximately 60% with no difference between males and females. The blood: plasma ratio was about 2:1 at equilibrium.

Metabolism

Following oral administration of radiolabelled frovatriptan 2.5 mg to healthy male subjects, 32% of the dose was recovered in urine and 62% in faeces. Radiolabelled compounds excreted in urine were unchanged frovatriptan, hydroxy frovatriptan, N-acetyl desmethyl frovatriptan, hydroxy N-acetyl desmethyl frovatriptan, and desmethyl frovatriptan, together with several other minor metabolites. Desmethyl frovatriptan had about 3-fold lower affinity at 5-HT1 receptors than the parent compound. N-acetyl desmethyl frovatriptan had negligible affinity at 5-HT1 receptors. The activity of other metabolites has not been studied.

The results of in vitro studies have provided strong evidence that CYP1A2 is the cytochrome P450 isoenzyme primarily involved in the metabolism of frovatriptan. Frovatriptan does not inhibit or induce CYP1A2 in vitro.

Table 1

Organ system	Common >1/100 <1/10	Uncommon >1/1000 <1/100	Rare >1/10,000 <1/1000
Central and peripheral nervous system	Dizziness, paraesthesia, headache, somnolence, dysaesthesia, hypoaesthesia	Tremor, hyperaesthesia, vertigo, involuntary muscle contractions	Hypertonia, hypotonia, slowed reflexes, tongue paralysis
Gastro-intestinal system disorders	Nausea, dry-mouth, dyspepsia, abdominal pain	Diarrhoea, dysphagia, flatulence, constipation	cheilitis, eructation, gastrointestinal disorder NOS, gastroesophageal reflux, hiccup, oesophago-spasm, peptic ulcer, salivary gland pain, stomatitis, toothache
Body as a whole-general disorders	Fatigue, sensation of abnormal temperature, chest pain	Pain, asthaenia, fever	Leg pain
Psychiatric disorders		Anxiety, insomnia, confusion, nervousness, agitation, impaired concentration, euphoria, depression, abnormal thinking, depersonalisation	Amnesia, depression aggravated, abnormal dreaming, personality disorder
Vascular (extracardiac)	Flushing		
Respiratory	Throat tightness	Rhinitis, pharyngitis, sinusitis, laryngitis	Hyperventilation
Musculo-skeletal	Skeletal pain	Back pain, arthralgia, arthrosis, muscle weakness	
Vision disorders	Vision abnormal		
Skin and appendages	Increased sweating	Pruritis	Urticaria
Heart rate and rhythm	Palpitation	Tachycardia	Bradycardia
Hearing and vestibular disorders		Tinnitus, ear ache, ear disorder NOS	Hyperacusis
Special senses, other disorders		Taste perversion	
Metabolic and nutritional disorders		Thirst, dehydration	Hypocalcaemia, hypoglycaemia
Urinary system disorders		Micturition frequency, polyuria	Nocturia, renal pain, dark urine
Cardiovascular disorders general		Hypertension	
Platelet, bleeding and clotting disorders			Epistaxis, Purpura
Autonomic nervous system			Syncope
Liver and biliary system disorders			Bilirubinaemia
Secondary terms			Inflicted injury
White cell and res disorders			Lymphadenopathy

Frovatriptan is not an inhibitor of human monoamine oxidase (MAO) enzymes or cytochrome P450 isozymes and therefore has little potential for drug-drug interactions (see 4.5 Interactions with other medicinal products and other forms of interactions). Frovatriptan is not a substrate for MAO.

EliminationThe elimination of frovatriptan is biphasic with a distribution phase prevailing between 2 and 6 hours. Mean systemic clearance was 216 and 132 mL/min in males and females, respectively. Renal clearance accounted for 38% (82 mL/min) and 49% (65 mL/min) of total clearance in males and females, respectively. The terminal elimination half-life is approximately 26 hours, irrespective of the sex of the subjects, however the terminal elimination phase only becomes dominant after about 12 hours.

Gender

AUC and C_{max} values for frovatriptan are lower (by approximately 50%) in males than in females. This is due, at least in part, to the concomitant use of oral contraceptives. Based on the efficacy or safety of the 2.5 mg dose in clinical use, dosage adjustment with respect to gender is not necessary (See 4.2 Posology and method of administration).

Elderly

In healthy elderly subjects (65 to 77 years) AUC is increased by 73% in males and by 22% in females, compared to younger subjects (18 to 37 years). There was no difference in t_{max} or $t_{1/2}$ between the two populations (see 4.2 Posology and method of administration).

Renal impairment

Systemic exposure to frovatriptan and its $t_{1/2}$ were not significantly different in male and female subjects with renal impairment (creatinine clearance 16 - 73 mL/min), compared to that in healthy subjects.

Hepatic impairment

Following oral administration in male and female subjects aged 44 to 57, with mild or moderate hepatic impairment (Child-Pugh grades A and B), mean blood concentrations of frovatriptan were within the range observed in healthy young and elderly subjects. There is no pharmacokinetic or clinical experience with frovatriptan in subjects with severe hepatic impairment (See 4.3 Contra-indications).

5.3 Preclinical safety data

During toxicity studies after single or repeated administration, preclinical effects were only observed at exposure levels in excess of the maximum exposure level in man.

Standard genotoxicity studies did not reveal a clinically relevant genotoxic potential of frovatriptan.

Frovatriptan was foetotoxic in rats, but in rabbits foetotoxicity was observed only at maternally toxic dose levels.

Frovatriptan was not potentially carcinogenic in standard rodent carcinogenicity studies and in p53 (+/-) mouse studies at exposures considerably higher than anticipated in humans.

6. PHARMACEUTICAL PARTICULARS

6.1 List of excipients

Tablet core

Lactose, anhydrous

Microcrystalline cellulose

Silica, colloidal anhydrous

Sodium starch glycollate (Type A)

Magnesium stearate

Film Coat

Opadry white:

Hypromellose (E 464)

Titanium dioxide (E 171)

Lactose, anhydrous

Macrogol

Triacetin

6.2 Incompatibilities

Not applicable

6.3 Shelf life

Blister: 3 years

Bottle: 2 years

6.4 Special precautions for storage

Do not store above 30°C.

Blister: store in the original package.

Bottle: keep the container tightly closed.

6.5 Nature and contents of container

Child-proof HDPE bottles containing 30 tablets.

PVC/PE/ACLAR/Aluminium blister packs with 1, 2, 3, 4, 6 and 12 tablets.

Not all pack sizes may be marketed.

6.6 Instructions for use and handling

No special requirements.

7. MARKETING AUTHORISATION HOLDER

Menarini International Operations Luxembourg S.A.

1, Avenue de la Gare

L-1611, Luxembourg

8. MARKETING AUTHORISATION NUMBER(S)

PL 16239/0017

9. DATE OF FIRST AUTHORISATION/RENEWAL OF THE AUTHORISATION

7th October 2002

10. DATE OF REVISION OF THE TEXT

February 2005

Legal Category

POM

Migraleve

(Pfizer Consumer Healthcare)

1. NAME OF THE MEDICINAL PRODUCT

Migraleve

2. QUALITATIVE AND QUANTITATIVE COMPOSITION

Each Migraleve Pink tablet contains:

Paracetamol DC 96% 520 mg

(equivalent to Paracetamol 500 mg)

Codeine Phosphate 8 mg

Buclizine Hydrochloride 6.25 mg

Each Migraleve Yellow tablet contains:

Paracetamol DC 96% 520 mg

(equivalent to Paracetamol 500 mg)

Codeine Phosphate 8 mg

3. PHARMACEUTICAL FORM

Pink (Migraleve Pink) or yellow (Migraleve Yellow) aqueous film-coated tablets.

4. CLINICAL PARTICULARS

4.1 Therapeutic indications

For the treatment of migraine attacks which can include the symptoms of migraine headache, nausea and vomiting. Route of administration - oral.

4.2 Posology and method of administration

Adults and the elderly: Two Migraleve Pink tablets to be swallowed immediately it is known that a migraine attack has started or is imminent. If further treatment is required, two Migraleve Yellow tablets every 4 hours.

Maximum dose: 8 tablets (two Migraleve Pink and six Migraleve Yellow) in 24 hours.

Children 10 - 14 years: One Migraleve Pink tablet to be swallowed immediately it is known that a migraine attack has started or is imminent. If further treatment is required, one Migraleve Yellow tablet every 4 hours.

Maximum dose: 4 tablets (one Migraleve Pink and three Migraleve Yellow) in 24 hours.

Do not give to children under 10 years of age except under medical supervision.

4.3 Contraindications

Do not give to children under 10 years of age except under medical supervision. Hypersensitivity to any of the ingredients.

4.4 Special warnings and special precautions for use

Migraine should be medically diagnosed. Because some medicines do not combine, if you are already taking prescribed medicines please consult your doctor. If symptoms persist, consult your doctor. Migraleve tablets contain potent medicaments and should not be taken continuously for extended periods without the advice of a doctor. Do not exceed the stated dose. Migraleve Pink Tablets only: May cause drowsiness. If affected, do not drive or operate machinery. Avoid alcoholic drink. Should be used with caution in patients with severe renal disease or liver dysfunction.

4.5 Interaction with other medicinal products and other forms of Interaction

None known.

4.6 Pregnancy and lactation

Although experiments in some animal species gave rise to adverse effects following the administration of buclizine to pregnant animals e.g. foetal abnormalities and maternal deaths, these occurred at doses in excess of 120 times the human daily dose. Whilst there are no specific reasons for contra-indicating Migraleve during pregnancy, as with all drugs it is recommended that Migraleve be used in pregnancy only when the physician has considered the need in respect of the patients' welfare. Migraleve is not contra-indicated in breast-feeding mothers

4.7 Effects on ability to drive and use machines

Migraleve Pink Tablets only: May cause drowsiness. If affected do not drive or operate machinery. Avoid alcoholic drink.

4.8 Undesirable effects

Rare allergic reactions to paracetamol, such as skin rashes, hives or itching. Codeine may cause constipation. Buclizine hydrochloride may cause drowsiness.

4.9 Overdose

Paracetamol

Liver damage is possible in adults who have taken 10g or more of paracetamol Ingestion of 5g or more of paracetamol may lead to liver damage if the patient has risk factors (see below).

Risk Factors:

If the patient

§ Is on long term treatment with carbamazepine, phenobarbital, phenytoin, primidone, rifampicin, St John's Wort or other drugs that induce liver enzymes.

Or

§ Regularly consumes ethanol in excess of recommended amounts.

Or

§ Is likely to be glutathione deplete e.g. eating disorders, cystic fibrosis, HIV infection, starvation, cachexia.

Symptoms of paracetamol overdosage in the first 24 hours are pallor, nausea, vomiting, anorexia and abdominal pain. Liver damage may become apparent 12 to 48 hours after ingestion. Abnormalities of glucose metabolism and metabolic acidosis may occur. In severe poisoning, hepatic failure may progress to encephalopathy, haemorrhage, hypoglycaemia, cerebral oedema, and death. Acute renal failure with acute tubular necrosis, strongly suggested by loin pain, haematuria and proteinuria, may develop even in the absence of severe liver damage. Cardiac arrhythmias and pancreatitis have been reported.

Immediate treatment is essential in the management of paracetamol overdose. Despite a lack of significant early symptoms, patients should be referred to hospital urgently for immediate medical attention. Symptoms may be limited to nausea or vomiting and may not reflect the severity of overdose or the risk of organ damage. Management should be in accordance with established treatment guidelines, see BNF overdose section. Treatment with activated charcoal should be considered if the overdose has been taken within 1 hour. Plasma paracetamol concentration should be measured at 4 hours or later after ingestion (earlier concentrations are unreliable) but results should not delay initiation of treatment beyond 8 hours after ingestion, as the effectiveness of the antidote declines sharply after this time. If required the patient should be given intravenous N-acetylcysteine, in line with the established dosage schedule. If vomiting is not a problem, oral methionine may be a suitable alternative for remote areas, outside hospital.

Codeine

The effects in codeine overdosage will be potentiated by simultaneous ingestion of alcohol and psychotropic drugs. Codeine overdose associated with central nervous system depression, including respiratory depression, may develop but is unlikely to be severe unless other sedative agents have been co-ingested, including alcohol, or the overdose is very large. The pupils may be pin-point in size; nausea and vomiting are common. Hypotension and tachycardia are possible but unlikely.

Management of codeine overdose include general symptomatic and supportive measures including a clear airway and monitoring of vital signs until stable. Consider activated charcoal if an adult presents within one hour of ingestion of more than 350 mg or a child more than 5 mg/kg.

Give naloxone if coma or respiratory depression is present. Naloxone is a competitive antagonist and has a short half-life so large and repeated doses may be required in a seriously poisoned patient. Observe for at least four hours after ingestion, or eight hours if a sustained release preparation has been taken.

5. PHARMACOLOGICAL PROPERTIES

5.1 Pharmacodynamic properties

Paracetamol has analgesic, antipyretic and mild, acute anti-inflammatory properties. Paracetamol inhibits prostaglandin synthesis, especially in the CNS. Paracetamol does not inhibit chronic inflammatory reactions.

Codeine is an opioid analgesic. Codeine also has antitussive properties.

The combination of paracetamol and codeine has been shown to have hyperadditive analgesic effects in animals.

Buclizine is a piperazine derivative with the actions and uses of H_1-receptor antagonists. It has anti-muscarinic and central sedative properties. It is used mainly for its anti-emetic properties.

5.2 Pharmacokinetic properties

Paracetamol is rapidly absorbed from the upper G.I. tract after oral administration, with the small intestine being an important site of absorption. Peak blood levels of 15-20 mcg/ml after normal 1 g oral doses of paracetamol occur within 30 - 90 minutes. Depending upon dosage form, it is rapidly distributed throughout the body and is primarily metabolised in the liver with excretion via the kidney. Elimination half-life is about 2 hours after reaching a peak following a 1 g oral dose. Paracetamol crosses the placental barrier and is present in breast milk.

Codeine is absorbed from the gastro-intestinal tract and peak plasma concentrations occur after one hour. Codeine is metabolised by O- and N-demethylation in the liver to morphine, norcodeine and other metabolites. Codeine and its metabolites are excreted almost entirely by the kidney, mainly as conjugates with glucuronic acid. Codeine is not extensively bound to plasma proteins. The plasma half-life has been reported to be between 3 and 4 hours.

Buclizine hydrochloride is more slowly absorbed from the G.I. tract (T_{max} 3 hours). The elimination half-life is approximately 15 hours.

5.3 Preclinical safety data

No data presented.

6. PHARMACEUTICAL PARTICULARS

6.1 List of excipients

Migraleve Pink Tablets

Gelatin
Magnesium Stearate
Colloidal Anhydrous Silica
Stearic Acid
Pregelatinised Maize Starch
Colour Erythrosine Lake (E127)
Opadry Pink OY-1367 *
*Opadry Pink OY-1367 contains:
Hypromellose
Titanium Dioxide (E171)
Macrogol 400
Erythrosine Lake (E127)**
**consists of Erythrosine (E127) and Aluminium Oxide

Migraleve Yellow Tablets

Gelatin
Magnesium Stearate
Colloidal Anhydrous Silica
Stearic Acid
Pregelatinised Maize Starch
Opadry Yellow OY-6126 *
*Opadry Yellow OY-6126 contains:
Hypromellose
Titanium Dioxide (E171)
Macrogol 400
Iron Oxide Yellow (E172)
Quinoline Yellow Aluminium Lake (E104)**
**consists of Quinoline Yellow (E104) and Aluminium Oxide

6.2 Incompatibilities

None known.

6.3 Shelf life

36 months

6.4 Special precautions for storage

None.

6.5 Nature and contents of container

Packs of: 12 tablets (8 Migraleve Pink and 4 Migraleve Yellow)

Packs of: 24 tablets (16 Migraleve Pink and 8 Migraleve Yellow)

Packs of: 48 tablets (32 Migraleve Pink and 16 Migraleve Yellow)

Blister strips consist of clear amber PVC blister film and either:

Aluminium foil blister lidding

Or

Paper/aluminium foil child resistant blister lidding

6.6 Instructions for use and handling

None.

Administrative Data

7. MARKETING AUTHORISATION HOLDER

Pfizer Consumer Healthcare

Alternative Trading Style:

Warner-Lambert Consumer Healthcare
Walton Oaks
Dorking Road
Walton-on-the-Hill
Surrey KT20 7NS
United Kingdom

8. MARKETING AUTHORISATION NUMBER(S)

PL 15513/0105

9. DATE OF FIRST AUTHORISATION/RENEWAL OF THE AUTHORISATION

23 April 2001

10. DATE OF REVISION OF THE TEXT

May 2005

Legal Category

Packs of 12 and 24 tablets: P

Packs of 48 tablets: POM

MigraMax

(Zeneus Pharma Ltd)

1. NAME OF THE MEDICINAL PRODUCT

MIGRAMAX

2. QUALITATIVE AND QUANTITATIVE COMPOSITION

Active ingredientsPer sachet

DL-lysine acetylsalicylate 1,620mg

equivalent to acetylsalicylic acid 900mg

Metoclopramide (INN) hydrochloride EP 10.54mg

equivalent in terms of the anhydrous substance to: 10mg

3. PHARMACEUTICAL FORM

Sachet containing powder for oral solution

4. CLINICAL PARTICULARS

4.1 Therapeutic indications

MigraMax is indicated for the treatment of migraine-associated symptoms such as headache, nausea and vomiting.

4.2 Posology and method of administration

For oral administration only.

MigraMax must be dissolved completely in some water before taking.

Renal and hepatic insufficiency

Caution should be exercised in significant renal or hepatic impairment. Metoclopramide is metabolised in the liver and eliminated mainly via the kidney. A dose reduction may be necessary.

Adults (aged 20 years and older) and elderly : One sachet should be taken at the first warning of a migraine attack. A second sachet may be taken two hours later if the symptoms have not resolved. Do not exceed three sachets in a 24 hour period.

Migramax should not be given to patients under 20 years of age (see Section 4.4).

4.3 Contraindications

- Hypersensitivity to metoclopramide, salicylates or any of the components.
- Not recommended for patients under 20 years of age in view of the particular risk of dystonic reactions in young adults and children with metoclopramide.
- Active, chronic or recurrent gastric or duodenal ulcers.
- Congenital or acquired bleeding disorders; obstruction, haemorrhage or perforation of the GI tract.
- Known or suspected phaeochromocytoma.
- Third trimester of pregnancy.
- Metoclopramide should not be used in the immediate post-operative period (up to 3-4 days) following

pyloroplasty or gut anastomosis, as vigorous gastro-intestinal contractions may adversely affect healing.

4.4 Special warnings and special precautions for use

If vomiting persists the patient should be reassessed to exclude the possibility of an underlying disorder eg. cerebral irritation.

As salicylates may induce asthma attacks in susceptible individuals MigraMax should be avoided in patients at risk of developing sensitivity reactions. These include individuals with asthma or rhinitis, a history of atopy or nasal polyps, and also patients who have been sensitive to other salicylates or NSAIDs.

Use with caution in patients with a history of gastroduodenal ulcer or GI haemorrhage, or with significant hepatic impairment, gout, menorrhagia, or epilepsy. Care should be taken in patients using intra-uterine contraceptive devices and patients who have a high alcohol intake.

There is a possible association between aspirin and Reye's syndrome when given to children with a fever. Reye's syndrome is a very rare disease which affects the brain and liver, and can be fatal. For this reason aspirin should not be given to children under 12 years and should be avoided up to and including 16 years of age if feverish. MigraMax is contraindicated in patients under 20 years of age (see section 4.3).

As total clearance of metoclopramide is reduced and elimination prolonged in patients with renal failure use in patients with significant degrees of renal impairment should be approached with caution.

Metoclopramide may induce an acute hypertensive response in patients with phaeochromocytoma.

Young adults and the elderly should be treated with care as they are at increased risk of extrapyramidal reactions. Symptomatic treatment may be necessary (benzodiazepines or anticholinergic anti-parkinsonian drugs).

Neuroleptic Malignant Syndrome (NMS), a potentially fatal symptom complex with hyperthermia, muscle rigidity, extrapyramidal symptoms, altered mental status and autonomic dysfunction, may occur. The management of NMS should include 1) immediate discontinuation of the product, 2) intensive symptomatic treatment and medical monitoring, and 3) treatment of any concomitant serious medical problems for which specific treatments are available.

Methaemoglobinemia has been reported with metoclopramide. In case of methaemoglobinemia, MigraMax should be immediately and permanently discontinued and appropriate measures initiated.

Metoclopramide is not recommended in epileptic patients as benzamides may decrease the epileptic threshold.

4.5 Interaction with other medicinal products and other forms of Interaction

Metoclopramide-related interactions

Alcohol:

Alcohol potentiates the sedative effect of metoclopramide

Anticholinergics and morphine derivatives:

Anticholinergics and morphine derivatives antagonise the effects of metoclopramide on gastrointestinal motility.

CNS depressants (morphine derivatives, hypnotics, anxiolytics, sedative H1 antihistamines, sedative antidepressants, barbiturates, clonidine and related):

Combination of CNS depressants with metoclopramide may result in potentiation of sedative effects.

Antipsychotics:

Combination of antipsychotics with metoclopramide may result in potentiation of extrapyramidal effects.

Digoxin:

Metoclopramide decreased the gastric absorption of digoxin. Therefore, dose adjustment may be required.

Ciclosporin:

Metoclopramide increases ciclosporin bioavailability. Dose adjustment may be required. In one study, dosing requirements for ciclosporin were reported to be reduced by 20% when metoclopramide was administered concomitantly. To avoid toxicity, careful monitoring of ciclosporin plasma concentration is required.

Levodopa:

Levodopa and metoclopramide have a mutual antagonism. Concomitant use should be avoided.

Salicylate-related interactions

Anti-coagulants:

Salicylates may enhance the effects of anti-coagulants.

Oral anti-diabetic agents:

Salicylates may enhance the effects of oral anti-diabetic agents.

Anti-epileptics:

Salicylates may enhance the effects of phenytoin, sodium valproate.

Antimetabolites:

Salicylates may enhance the effects of methotrexate

Immunomodulating agents:

Salicylates may inhibit the action of alpha interferon

Salicylates may interact with other NSAIDs, antacids and glucorticosteroids, which may lower blood salicylate concentration during treatment and result in high levels when treatment is stopped.

The effects of diuretics and uricosurics may also be affected by salicylates.

Other anti-platelet drugs

Salicylates may increase risk of bleeding with clopidogrel and ticlopidine.

Leukotriene antagonists

Aspirin may increase plasma concentration of zafirlukast

Mifepristone

Based on theoretical grounds, mifepristone may interact with salicylates.

4.6 Pregnancy and lactation

Although teratogenic effects of acetylsalicylic acid have been recorded in animals, no such effects have been observed in humans. No teratogenic effects have been observed with metoclopramide.

In the third trimester, the use of prostaglandin synthesis inhibitors such as acetylsalicylic acid may expose the foetus to premature closure of the ductus arteriosus. MigraMax is therefore contra-indicated during the third trimester. During the first and second trimester MigraMax, like all drugs, should be used only if the physician believes the benefits outweigh the risks.

MigraMax is not recommended during lactation because acetylsalicylic acid and metoclopramide are excreted in breast milk.

4.7 Effects on ability to drive and use machines

MigraMax may cause drowsiness. This effect can be potentiated by CNS depressants or alcohol. If affected, patients should not drive or operate machinery.

4.8 Undesirable effects

Extrapyramidal symptoms may occur. Acute dystonia and dyskinesia, Parkinsonian syndrome, akathisia may occur even following administration of a single dose of the drug (see section 4.4 Special warnings and precautions for use).

Extrapyramidal reactions include spasm of the facial muscles, trismus, rhythmic protrusion of the tongue, a bulbar type of speech, spasm of extra-ocular muscles including oculogyric crises, unnatural positioning of the head and shoulders and opisthotonos. There may be a generalised increase in muscle tone. The majority of reactions occur within 36 hours of starting treatment and the effects usually disappear within 24 hours of withdrawal of the drug. Should treatment of a dystonic reaction be required, a benzodazepine or an anticholinergic anti-Parkinsonian drug may be used.

Tardive dyskinesia, particularly in elderly patients and during prolonged treatment.

Metoclopramide may cause drowsiness, lethargy, insomnia, dizziness

Depressive tendency

Restlessness, anxiety, confusion

Very rare cases of seizures and neuroleptic malignant syndrome have been reported (see 4.4 Special warnings and precautions for use).

Hyperprolactinaemia with amenorrhea, galactorrhea, gynaecomastia.

Very rare cases of methaemoglobinaemia which could be related to NADH cytochrome b5 reductase deficiency have been reported (see section 4.4 Special warnings and precautions for use).

Very rare cases of bradycardia and heart block have been reported with metoclopramide, particularly the intravenous formulation.

Diarrhoea, flatulence

The most common side effects occurring with therapeutic doses of salicylates are gastrointestinal disturbances such as gastric irritation with blood loss, nausea, dyspepsia, vomiting and gastric ulceration. The gastrointestinal haemorrhaging is occasionally severe but in most cases blood loss is not significant.

Aspirin may increase bleeding time, decrease platelet adhesiveness, and in large doses cause hypothrombinaemia. It may cause other blood disorders, including thrombocytopenia, iron deficiency or haemolytic anaemia and rarely agranulocytosis.

Salicylates may induce hypersensitivity especially in those individuals with asthma or rhinitis, and a history of atopy or nasal polyps. The observed hypersensitivity reactions include anaphylaxis, urticara and bronchospasm.

Tinnitus

Other reported effects of salicylates include urate kidney stones.

4.9 Overdose

In cases of overdose, toxic reactions are mainly ascribable to aspirin.

Salicylate poisoning is usually associated with plasma concentrations >350 mg/L

(2.5 mmol/L). Most adult deaths occur in patients whose concentrations exceed 700 mg/L (95.1 mmol/L). Single doses less than 100 mg/kg are unlikely to cause serious poisoning.

Symptoms

Common features include vomiting, dehydration, tinnitus, vertigo, deafness, sweating, warm extremities with bounding pulses, increased respiratory rate and hyperventilation. Some degree of acid-base disturbance is present in most cases.

A mixed respiratory alkalosis and metabolic acidosis with normal or high arterial pH (normal or reduced hydrogen ion concentration) is usual in adults and children over the age of 4 years. In children aged 4 years or less, a dominant metabolic acidosis with low arterial pH (raised hydrogen ion concentration) is common. Acidosis may increase salicylate transfer across the blood brain barrier.

Uncommon features include haematemesis, hyperpyrexia, hypoglycaemia, hypokalaemia, thrombocytopaenia, increased INR/PTR, intravascular coagulation, renal failure and non-cardiac pulmonary oedema.

Central nervous system features including confusion, disorientation, coma and convulsions are less common in adults than in children.

Management

Give activated charcoal if an adult presents within one hour of ingestion of more than 250 mg/kg. The plasma salicylate concentration should be measured, although the severity of poisoning cannot be determined from this alone and the clinical and biochemical features must be taken into account. Elimination is increased by urinary alkalisation, which is achieved by the administration of 1.26% sodium bicarbonate.

The urine pH should be monitored. Correct metabolic acidosis with intravenous 8.4% sodium bicarbonate (first check serum potassium). Forced diuresis should not be used since it does not enhance salicylate excretion and may cause pulmonary oedema.

Haemodialysis is the treatment of choice for severe poisoning and should be considered in patients with plasma salicylate concentrations >700 mg/L (5.1 mmol/L), or lower concentrations associated with severe clinical or metabolic features. Patients under 10 years or over 70 have increased risk of salicylate toxicity and may require dialysis at an earlier stage.

5. PHARMACOLOGICAL PROPERTIES

5.1 Pharmacodynamic properties

The pharmacological properties of this product are those of the two active ingredients i.e. an analgesic and an antiemetic.

Acetylsalcylic acid has analgesic, antipyretic and anti-inflammatory properties. It inhibits prostaglandin synthesis so that the prostaglandin-induced sensitivity of peripheral nerve endings to kinins and other mediators of pain and inflammation is reduced. Acetylsalicylic acid also exerts a powerful inhibition on platelet aggregation by blocking thromboxane A2 synthesis in the platelets.

Metoclopramide is an effective anti-emetic, although its exact mechanism(s) of action is not fully established. It is a cholinergic agonist acting peripherally to enhance the action of acetylcholine at muscarinic synapses and in the CNS by blocking dopamine receptors in the chemoreceptor trigger zone for vomiting.

Local effects include the promotion of gastric emptying and normal peristalsis, impairment of which are a common feature of migraine attacks.

5.2 Pharmacokinetic properties

Lysine acetylsalicylate

Absorption of lysine acetylsalicylate as a solution is rapid in healthy subjects. Lysine acetylsalicylate dissociates into lysine and acetylsalicylic acid which is rapidly hydrolysed to salicylic acid. The plasma peak of acetylsalicylic acid is achieved within 20 minutes.

Plasma salicylates are essentially bound to plasma proteins and are converted to inactive metabolites in the liver. Salicylic acid and its metabolites are excreted via the kidneys. Clearance increases with increasing urinary pH. The elimination half-life of salicylic acid is dose-dependent owing to the saturable nature of salicylic acid conjugation and ranges from as little as 2 hours after a single dose of 500 mg, lengthening to as long as 20 hours in overdosage.

Metoclopramide

The plasma peak of metoclopramide is reached within an average time of 40 minutes following oral administration. Peak plasma concentrations are 32 and 70 g/L for 10 and 20 mg doses.

Bioavailability is 80% following oral administration. Inter-individual variations are related to a 20% first-pass effect. Metoclopramide is rapidly and extensively distributed in tissues. The volume of distribution is 2.2 - 3.4 l/kg. Metoclopramide has a low degree of binding to plasma proteins (30%). The plasma elimination half-life of metoclopramide is 5 - 6 hours. Total clearance is 0.4 - 0.7 l/min.

Metoclopramide is only partially metabolised in humans; urinary excretion occurs essentially as the unchanged and sulphoconjugated compounds (50% of the dose administered).

Renal insufficiency significantly reduces the clearance of metoclopramide and increases the plasma elimination half-life.

Combination

When administered as an oral solution, lysine acetylsalicylate and metoclopramide are rapidly absorbed.

In subjects not suffering from migraine, plasma concentrations of total salicylates, acetylsalicylic acid and metoclopramide do not differ from those recorded following both drugs administered singly.

The elimination half-life of salicylates and metoclopramide is unaffected in subjects suffering from migraine receiving the two drugs in combination compared with normal subjects.

5.3 Preclinical safety data

No data of therapeutic relevance.

6. PHARMACEUTICAL PARTICULARS

6.1 List of excipients

Aspartame

Glycine

Lemon flavour (essential oil of lemon absorbed on a maltodextrin substrate)

6.2 Incompatibilities

No known major incompatibilities

6.3 Shelf life

24 Months

6.4 Special precautions for storage

Store at or below 25°C.

6.5 Nature and contents of container

Pack sizes: Carton containing 2 sachets

Carton containing 6 sachets

Carton containing 20 sachets

MigraMax is packaged in sachets made of a paper-polyethylene-aluminium complex, containing one unit dose and heat-sealed.

6.6 Instructions for use and handling

Consult the patient leaflet before use.

Do not use after the stated expiry date on the sachet or carton.

To be taken orally when the powder is completely dissolved.

7. MARKETING AUTHORISATION HOLDER

Sanofi-Synthelabo Limited

One Onslow Street

Guildford

Surrey

GU1 4YS

UK

Trading as Lorex Synthelabo or Sanofi-Synthelabo, PO Box 597, Guildford, Surrey

8. MARKETING AUTHORISATION NUMBER(S)

PL 11723/0310

9. DATE OF FIRST AUTHORISATION/RENEWAL OF THE AUTHORISATION

29 May 2001

10. DATE OF REVISION OF THE TEXT

June 2004

11. LEGAL CATEGORY

POM

Migril

(Wockhardt UK Ltd)

1. NAME OF THE MEDICINAL PRODUCT

Migril Tablets

2. QUALITATIVE AND QUANTITATIVE COMPOSITION

Ergotamine tartrate 2.0mg, cyclizine hydrochloride 50.0mg and caffeine equivalent to caffeine hydrate 100mg

For excipients, see 6.1.

3. PHARMACEUTICAL FORM

Tablet

White, round, biconvex compression-coated tablets with a pink core, scored and impressed 'CP A4A'.

4. CLINICAL PARTICULARS

4.1 Therapeutic indications

Migril is indicated for the relief of acute migraine attack.

4.2 Posology and method of administration

Adults: Migril should be taken as soon as possible after the first warning of an attack of migraine and repeated if necessary at the prescribed intervals.

The usual initial dose is one tablet.

Additional doses of a half to one tablet may then be required at half-hourly intervals.

No more than 3 tablets (6mg ergotamine) should be taken in any 24 hours or 4 tablets (8mg ergotamine) during any one attack.

The recommended minimum interval between successive courses is 4 days.

No more than 6 tablets (12mg ergotamine) should be given in any one week.

No more than two courses of treatment should be administered in a month.

Children: There is no absolute contra-indication to the use of Migril in children but its use is not recommended.

Use in the elderly: There are no absolute contra-indications to the use of Migril in the elderly, but see Section 4.3*'Contra-indications'* and Section 4.4 *'Precautions'*.

4.3 Contraindications

Co-administration of ergotamine with potent CYP 3A4 inhibitors (ritonavir, nelfinavir, indinavir, amprenavir, azithromycin, erythromycin, clarithromycin) has been associated with acute ergot toxicity (ergotism) characterised by vasospasm and ischaemia of the extremities, with some cases resulting in amputation. There have been rare reports of cerebral ischaemia in patients on protease inhibitor therapy when ergotamine was co-administered, at least one resulting in death. Due to the increased risk for ergotism and other serious vasopastic adverse events, ergotamine use is contraindicated with these drugs and other potent inhibitors of CYP 3A4 (e.g. ketoconazole, itraconazole).

Migril is contra-indicated during pregnancy because of a direct effect of ergotamine on the uterus. In animals, ergotamine has been reported to inhibit implantation, cause perinatal mortality and foetal retardation.

Migril is contra-indicated during lactation and breast-feeding, it may suppress milk production and may also be excreted in milk at levels high enough to cause pharmacological effects in breast-fed infants.

Migril is contra-indicated in pre-existing vascular disease including coronary disease, obliterative vascular disease, angina, claudication, peripheral ischaemia, Raynaud's syndrome and hypertension.

Migril should not be taken if there is a hypersensitivity to any of its constituents.

4.4 Special warnings and special precautions for use

Migril should not be used for migraine prophylaxis or taken regularly, even if the dosage recommendations above are adhered to, because of the risks of inducing ergotism or ergotamine dependence (see also Section 4.8, Undesirable Effects).

The use of ergotamine-containing compounds carries the risk of precipitating arterial constriction and other manifestations of ergotism. Co-administration of ergotamine with potent CYP3A4 inhibitors has been associated with serious adverse events (see Section 4.5 Interaction with medicinal products and other forms of interaction).

Use the minimum effective dosage of Migril necessary since individual sensitivity to the arterial effects of ergotamine varies considerably.

Discontinue the use of Migril if symptoms of arterial insufficiency develop, including coldness, numbness or tingling of the extremities.

Doses of ergotamine as small as 2mg have caused signs of arterial insufficiency but this is a very rare occurrence.

Migril should be used with caution in patients with infective hepatitis because of an increased risk of precipitating peripheral ischaemia.

Repeated doses of ergotamine have occasionally been associated with renal artery spasm and loss of renal function.

Alcohol and Migril should not be taken concurrently.

Ergotamine should be used with care when hyperthyroidism, sepsis or anaemia are present.

There have been a few reports of patients on ergotamine developing retroperitoneal and/or pleuropulmonary fibrosis. There have also been rare reports of fibrotic thickening of the aortic, mitral, tricuspid and/or pulmonary valves with long-term continuous use of ergotamine.

4.5 Interaction with other medicinal products and other forms of Interaction

Migril should not be administered with other vasoconstrictors. Nicotine may provoke vasoconstriction in some patients, predisposing to a greater ischemic response to ergot therapy. The concomitant use of alkaloids and beta-blocking agents increases the risks of peripheral vasoconstriction.

The blood levels of ergotamine-containing drugs are reported to be elevated by the concomitant administration of macrolide antibiotics (e.g. clarithromycin, erythromycin) and their concomitant use is contraindicated (see 4.3 Contraindications).

The concomitant use of certain HIV-protease inhibitors which are potent CYP 3A4 inhibitors (amprenavir, indinavir, nelfinavir, ritonavir) is also contraindicated, due to an increased risk of ergotism (see 4.3 Contraindications). Co-administration of ergotamine with potent CYP 3A4 inhibitors such as protease inhibitors or macrolide antibiotics has been associated with serious adverse events. For this reason, these drugs should not be given concomitantly with ergotamine (see 4.3 Contraindications). While these reactions have not been reported with less potent CYP 3A4 inhibitors, there is a potential risk for serious toxicity including vasospasm when these drugs are used with ergotamine. Examples of less potent CYP 3A4 inhibitors include: grapefruit juice, saquinavir, nefazodone, fluoxetine, fluvoxamine, metronidazole, fluconazole and clotrimazole. These lists are not exhaustive and the prescriber should consider the effects on CYP 3A4 of other agents being considered for concomitant use with ergotamine.

5-HT_1 agonists (increased risk of vasospasm): Ergotamine should be avoided for six hours after almotriptan, eletriptan, sumatriptan, rizatriptan and zolmitriptan. Almotriptan, eletriptan, sumatriptan, rizatriptan and zolmitriptan should be avoided for 24 hours after ergotamine.

Use with sympathomimetics (pressor agents) may cause extreme elevation of blood pressure.

4.6 Pregnancy and lactation

See Contra-indications (Section 4.3)

4.7 Effects on ability to drive and use machines

Cyclizine, in common with other anthistamines, may cause sedation; patients should be cautioned about driving or operating machinery.

4.8 Undesirable effects

Habitual use of ergotamine-containing preparations should be avoided (see 4.4 Special Warnings and Precautions for Use). Ergotamine dependence can develop insidiously when ergotamine tartrate is used for more than two days in a week, even if the total daily or weekly dosage recommendations are observed. Ergotamine dependence can produce a syndrome of daily or almost daily non-migrainous "analgesic-induced" or "rebound headaches", which are only relieved by ergotamine. An intensifying headache with autonomic disturbances occurs within 24-48 hours of ergotamine withdrawal and may continue for 72 hours or longer. Headache is also a recognised symptom of caffeine withdrawal.

Side-effects seen with Migril are usually due to the ergotamine components of the preparation and are more common if the dosage recommendations are exceeded. They include intermittent claudication, coldness and whiteness of the extremities, dysaethesia, paraesthsia, formication and precordial pain.

Other side-effects seen with ergotamine include muscle cramps, joint pains, raised blood pressure, pulselessness, cyanosis, thrombophlebitis, peripheral arterial thrombosis, gangrene, abdominal pain, coronary infarction, cerebral thrombosis, nausea, dyspnoea, decreased visual acuity, vertigo, diarrhoea, retroperitoneal and/or pleuropulmonary fibrosis or fibrotic thickening of the heart valves (see 4.4 Special Warnings and Precautions for Use). These effects have mostly occurred following habitual chronic use exceeding the recommended dose; they may occasionally occur however at the therapeutic dose.

Arterial vasospasm severe enough to threaten the viability of the limbs has been reported after routine therapy but it is more normally to be expected after prolonged overdosage.

4.9 Overdose

Acute overdosage: Symptoms: Acute overdosage with an ergotamine-containing preparation is characterised by nausea, vomiting, tachycardia, hypotonia and peripheral ischaemia. Blood pressure may be difficult to measure.

Treatment: If vomiting has not occurred, efforts should be made to clear the stomach contents. General supportive measures should be applied and intravenous vasodilators may be necessary to relieve vasospasm.

Peritoneal dialysis and forced diuresis may help to eliminate ergotamine from the body.

Chronic overdosage: Symptoms: Chronic overdosage with ergotamine-containing preparations usually presents as peripheral ischaemia threatening the viability of the affected limb.

Treatment: Withdraw Migril immediately.

Intravenous vasodilators such as nitroprusside and nitroglycerin may be used to re-establish normal blood flow. Captopril has also been used to reverse the effects of chronic overdosage with ergotamine.

Re-establishment of blood flow may be associated with intense burning sensations in the affected areas but these usually resolve after several weeks.

5. PHARMACOLOGICAL PROPERTIES

5.1 Pharmacodynamic properties

None stated

5.2 Pharmacokinetic properties

Pharmacokinetic interactions (increased blood levels of ergotamine) have been reported in patients treated orally with ergotamine and macrolide antibiotics (e.g. troleandomycin, clarithromycin, erythromycin), and in patients treated orally with ergotamine and protease inhibitors (e.g. ritonavir) presumably due to inhibition of cytochrome P450 3A metabolism of ergotamine. Ergotamine has also been shown to be an inhibitor of cytochrome P450 3A catalysed reactions. No pharmacokinetic interactions involving other cytochrome P450 isoenzymes are known.

5.3 Preclinical safety data

No additional data of relevance

6. PHARMACEUTICAL PARTICULARS

6.1 List of excipients

Maizestarch

Liquid glucose

Amaranth

Dicotyl sodium sulphsuccinate or docusate sodium

Magnesium stearate

Lactose

Glucose

Gelatin

Sodium metabisulphate.

Industrial methylated spirit or ethanol, purified water and sulphurous acid solution are all used in the manufacturing process but are not detected in the final formulation.

6.2 Incompatibilities

None stated

6.3 Shelf life

36 months

6.4 Special precautions for storage

Do not store above 25°C

Keep the container tightly closed

Store in the original container

6.5 Nature and contents of container

Amber glass bottles containing 100 tablets with low density polyethylene snap fit closures

6.6 Instructions for use and handling

None stated

Administrative Data

7. MARKETING AUTHORISATION HOLDER

CP Pharmaceuticals Ltd

Ash Road North

Wrexham

LL13 9UF

UK

8. MARKETING AUTHORISATION NUMBER(S)

PL 4543/0423

9. DATE OF FIRST AUTHORISATION/RENEWAL OF THE AUTHORISATION

2nd December 1999

10. DATE OF REVISION OF THE TEXT

August 2003

Mildison Lipocream

(Astellas Pharma Limited)

1. NAME OF THE MEDICINAL PRODUCT

MILDISON LIPOCREAM

2. QUALITATIVE AND QUANTITATIVE COMPOSITION

Contains 1% w/w hydrocortisone.

For excipients, see 6.1

3. PHARMACEUTICAL FORM

Cream.

White or practically white smooth cream.

4. CLINICAL PARTICULARS

4.1 Therapeutic indications

Eczema and dermatitis of all types including atopic eczema, otitis externa, primary irritant and allergic dermatitis, intertrigo, prurigo nodularis, seborrhoeic dermatitis, and insect bite reactions.

4.2 Posology and method of administration

For topical application.

For Adults, Children, and the Elderly:

Apply a small quantity only sufficient to cover the affected area two or three times a day. Due to the formulation of the base the product may be used both for dry scaly lesions and for moist or weeping lesions.

Children and infants: Long term treatment should be avoided. Courses should be limited to seven days where possible.

4.3 Contraindications

Hypersensitivity to hydrocortisone or to any of the ingredients of the cream.

This preparation is contraindicated in the presence of untreated viral or fungal infections, tubercular or syphilitic lesions, peri-oral dermatitis, acne vulgaris and rosacea and in bacterial infections unless used in connection with appropriate chemotherapy.

4.4 Special warnings and special precautions for use

Although generally regarded as safe even for long term administration in adults there is a potential for overdosage in infancy. Extreme caution is required in dermatoses of infancy including napkin eruption. In such patients courses of treatment should not normally exceed seven days.

As with all corticosteroids, application to the face, flexures and other areas of thin skin may cause skin atrophy and increased absorption and should be avoided.

Keep away from eyes.

4.5 Interaction with other medicinal products and other forms of Interaction

None known.

4.6 Pregnancy and lactation

There is inadequate evidence of safety in human pregnancy. Topical administration of corticosteroids to pregnant animals can cause abnormalities of foetal development including cleft palate and intra-uterine growth retardation. There may therefore be a very small risk of such effects in the human foetus. Theoretically, there is the possibility that if maternal systemic absorption occurred the infant's adrenal function could be affected.

The use of topical corticosteroids during lactation is unlikely to present a hazard to infants being breast-fed.

4.7 Effects on ability to drive and use machines

None known.

4.8 Undesirable effects

Local atrophic changes may occur, particularly in skin folds, intertriginous areas or in nappy areas in young children where moist conditions favour hydrocortisone absorption. Systemic absorption from such sites may be sufficient to produce hypercorticism and suppression of the pituitary adrenal axis after prolonged treatment. This effect is more likely to occur in infants and children and if occlusive dressings are used or large areas of skin treated. Napkins may act as occlusive dressings.

The cetostearyl alcohol may cause local skin reactions (e.g. contact dermatitis) and the methyl parahydroxybenzoate may cause allergic reactions which can be delayed.

4.9 Overdose

Excessive use, especially under occlusive dressings or over a long period of time, may produce adrenal suppression. No special procedures or antidote. Treat any adverse effects symptomatically

5. PHARMACOLOGICAL PROPERTIES

5.1 Pharmacodynamic properties

The active ingredient, hydrocortisone, is a well-established corticosteroid with the pharmacological actions of a corticosteroid classified as mildly potent.

5.2 Pharmacokinetic properties

In human in-vivo studies the potency of this formulation has been demonstrated as being of the same order as other widely available formulations of hydrocortisone 1%.

5.3 Preclinical safety data

No relevant pre-clinical safety data has been generated.

6. PHARMACEUTICAL PARTICULARS

6.1 List of excipients

Cetostearyl alcohol

Macrogol Cetostearyl Ether

Light Liquid paraffin

White soft paraffin

Methyl parahydroxybenzoate

Sodium citrate anhydrous

Citric acid anhydrous

Purified water

6.2 Incompatibilities

None stated.

6.3 Shelf life

Three years

6.4 Special precautions for storage

Do not store above 25°C.

6.5 Nature and contents of container

Collapsible membrane-necked internally coated aluminium tubes with a polyethylene screw cap containing 10 g, 15 g, 30 g, or 100 g.

6.6 Instructions for use and handling

No special requirements.

7. MARKETING AUTHORISATION HOLDER

Yamanouchi Pharma Ltd

Yamanouchi House

Pyrford Road

West Byfleet

Surrey

KT14 6RA

8. MARKETING AUTHORISATION NUMBER(S)

PL 0166/0131

9. DATE OF FIRST AUTHORISATION/RENEWAL OF THE AUTHORISATION

23 September 1987; renewed 30 September 1997

10. DATE OF REVISION OF THE TEXT

Date of revision = December 2004

11. LEGAL CATEGORY

POM

Minims Artificial Tears

(Chauvin Pharmaceuticals Ltd)

1. NAME OF THE MEDICINAL PRODUCT

Minims Artificial Tears

2. QUALITATIVE AND QUANTITATIVE COMPOSITION

Clear, colourless, sterile eye drops containing hydroxyethylcellulose 0.44% w/w BP and sodium chloride EP 0.35% w/w.

3. PHARMACEUTICAL FORM

Sterile single-use eye drop.

4. CLINICAL PARTICULARS

4.1 Therapeutic indications

For the relief of dry eye syndromes associated with deficient tear secretion.

4.2 Posology and method of administration

One or two drops instilled into the affected eye three or four times daily, or as often as is required.

4.3 Contraindications

None known.

4.4 Special warnings and special precautions for use

If irritation persists or worsens or continued redness occurs, discontinue use and consult a physician or ophthalmologist.

4.5 Interaction with other medicinal products and other forms of Interaction

None known.

4.6 Pregnancy and lactation

There is no evidence of safety of the drug in human pregnancy but it has been in wide use for many years without apparent ill consequence. If drug therapy is needed in pregnancy this preparation can be used if recommended by a physician and it is considered that the benefits outweigh the possible risks.

4.7 Effects on ability to drive and use machines

May cause transient blurring of vision on instillation. Do not drive or operate hazardous machinery unless vision is clear.

4.8 Undesirable effects

May cause transient mild stinging or temporarily blurred vision.

4.9 Overdose

Overdose would not be expected to produce symptoms.

5. PHARMACOLOGICAL PROPERTIES

5.1 Pharmacodynamic properties

The viscolising properties of hydroxyethylcellulose combined with sodium chloride have been shown to increase the tear break-up time in animal models, whilst also acting as a lubricating agent for dry eyes.

5.2 Pharmacokinetic properties

Not applicable.

5.3 Preclinical safety data

No adverse safety issues were detected during the development of this formulation. The active ingredients are well-established in clinical ophthalmology.

6. PHARMACEUTICAL PARTICULARS

6.1 List of excipients

Purified water

Borax

Boric acid

6.2 Incompatibilities

None known.

6.3 Shelf life

24 months.

6.4 Special precautions for storage

Store below 25°C. Do not freeze. Protect from light.

6.5 Nature and contents of container

A sealed conical shaped polypropylene container fitted with a twist and pull off cap. Each Minims unit is overwrapped in an individual polypropylene/paper pouch.

6.6 Instructions for use and handling

Each Minims unit should be discarded after a single use.

7. MARKETING AUTHORISATION HOLDER

Chauvin Pharmaceuticals Ltd

106 London Road

Kingston-upon-Thames

Surrey

KT2 6TN

8. MARKETING AUTHORISATION NUMBER(S)

PL 0033/0137

9. DATE OF FIRST AUTHORISATION/RENEWAL OF THE AUTHORISATION

11 January 1990

10. DATE OF REVISION OF THE TEXT

December 1996

August 2000

November 2002

Minims Atropine Sulphate

(Chauvin Pharmaceuticals Ltd)

1. NAME OF THE MEDICINAL PRODUCT

Minims Atropine Sulphate 1%.

2. QUALITATIVE AND QUANTITATIVE COMPOSITION

Clear, colourless, sterile eye drops containing Atropine Sulphate Ph Eur 1% w/v.

3. PHARMACEUTICAL FORM

Sterile, single-use eye drops.

4. CLINICAL PARTICULARS

4.1 Therapeutic indications

As a topical mydriatic and cycloplegic.

4.2 Posology and method of administration

Adults (including the elderly):

One drop to be instilled into the eye, or as required.

4.3 Contraindications

Hypersensitivity to any component of the preparation.

Due to the risk of precipitating an acute attack, do not use in cases of confirmed narrow-angle glaucoma or where latent narrow angle glaucoma is suspected. If in doubt it is recommended that an alternative preparation is used.

4.4 Special warnings and special precautions for use

The protracted mydriasis which is difficult to reverse, may be a disadvantage.

Systemic absorption may be reduced by compressing the lacrimal sac at the medial canthus for a minute during and following the instillation of the drops. (This blocks the passage of the drops via the naso-lacrimal duct to the wide absorptive area of the nasal and pharyngeal mucosa. It is especially advisable in children.)

4.5 Interaction with other medicinal products and other forms of Interaction

None known.

4.6 Pregnancy and lactation

The safety for use in pregnancy and lactation has not been established, therefore, use only when directed by a physician.

4.7 Effects on ability to drive and use machines

May cause transient blurring of vision on instillation. Warn patients not to drive or operate hazardous machinery until vision is clear.

4.8 Undesirable effects

Side effects rarely occur but include anticholinergic effects such as dry mouth and skin, flushing, increased body temperature, urinary symptoms, gastrointestinal symptoms and tachycardia. These effects are more likely to occur in infants and children.

4.9 Overdose

Systemic reactions to topical atropine are unlikely at normal doses. Symptoms which can occur following an overdose, however, include anticholinergic effects (as listed in section 4.8 above), cardiovascular changes (tachycardia, atrial arrhythmias, atrio-ventricular dissociation) and central nervous system effects (confusion, ataxia, restlessness, hallucination, convulsions). Treatment is supportive.

5. PHARMACOLOGICAL PROPERTIES

5.1 Pharmacodynamic properties

Atropine sulphate is a competitive antagonist of acetylcholine at postganglionic cholinergic (parasympathetic) nerve endings.

Atropine does not discriminate between the recently discovered muscarinic receptor sub types M1 (in parasympathetic ganglia of the submucous plexus, with high affinity for selecting antimuscarinic pirenzepine) and M2 (low affinity for pirenzepine and occurring predominantly in heart and smooth muscle).

5.2 Pharmacokinetic properties

Atropine is well absorbed from the small bowel and not at all from the stomach. Thus the effects of oral dosing are much slower in onset than after parenteral dosing. Atropine is also absorbed by mucous membranes but less readily from the eye and skin, although significant toxicity can sometimes occur through absorption of excessive eye drops.

Atropine has a volume of distribution of 1 - 6 L/kg. Protein binding is moderate, with approximately 50% of the drug bound in plasma. Its plasma clearance is 8ml/min/kg.

Only traces of atropine are found in breast milk. The drug readily crosses the blood-brain barrier and may cause confusion and delirium post-operatively. It crosses the placenta readily.

Atropine is metabolised by hepatic oxidation and conjugation to inactive metabolites, with about 2% undergoing hydrolysis to tropine and tropic acid. About 30% of the dose is excreted unchanged in the urine. Only trace amounts of the dose are eliminated in the faeces.

There is some evidence of prolonged elimination in elderly subjects.

5.3 Preclinical safety data

There are no preclinical data of relevance to the prescriber which are additional to that already included in other sections of the SPC.

6. PHARMACEUTICAL PARTICULARS

6.1 List of excipients

Hydrochloric acid

Purified water

6.2 Incompatibilities

None known.

6.3 Shelf life

15 months.

6.4 Special precautions for storage

Store below 25°C. Do not freeze. Protect from light.

6.5 Nature and contents of container

A sealed, conical shaped container fitted with a twist and pull-off cap. Each Minims unit is overwrapped in an individual polypropylene/paper pouch. Each container holds approximately 0.5ml of solution.

6.6 Instructions for use and handling

Each Minims unit should be discarded after a single use.

7. MARKETING AUTHORISATION HOLDER

Chauvin Pharmaceuticals Ltd

106 London Road

Kingston-upon-Thames

Surrey

KT2 6TN

8. MARKETING AUTHORISATION NUMBER(S)

PL 0033/5002R

9. DATE OF FIRST AUTHORISATION/RENEWAL OF THE AUTHORISATION

Date of first authorisation: 17 June 1987

Renewal of authorisation: 17 June 1992

10. DATE OF REVISION OF THE TEXT

August 1997.

November 2002

Minims Chloramphenicol

(Chauvin Pharmaceuticals Ltd)

1. NAME OF THE MEDICINAL PRODUCT

Minims Chloramphenicol 0.5%

2. QUALITATIVE AND QUANTITATIVE COMPOSITION

Clear, colourless, sterile eye drops containing Chloramphenicol PhEur 0.5% w/v.

3. PHARMACEUTICAL FORM

Sterile single use eye drop.

4. CLINICAL PARTICULARS

4.1 Therapeutic indications

Chloramphenicol is a broad spectrum bacteriostatic antibiotic. It is active against a wide variety of gram-negative and gram-positive organisms as well as rickettsiae and spirochaetes. It is indicated for use as a topical antibacterial in the treatment of superficial ocular infections.

4.2 Posology and method of administration

<u>Adults (including the Elderly) and Children</u>

One to two drops applied topically to each affected eye up to six times daily or more frequently if required. (Severe infections may require one to two drops every fifteen to twenty minutes initially, reducing the frequency of instillation gradually as the infection is controlled).

4.3 Contraindications

Hypersensitivity to chloramphenicol or any component of the preparation.

4.4 Special warnings and special precautions for use

In severe infections topical use of chloramphenicol should be supplemented with appropriate systemic treatment.

Aplastic anaemia has, rarely, followed topical use of chloramphenicol eye drops and, whilst this hazard is an uncommon one, it should be borne in mind when the benefits of the use of chloramphenicol are assessed.

Prolonged use should be avoided as it may increase the likelihood of sensitisation and the emergence of resistant organisms.

Contact lenses should be removed during the period of treatment.

Systemic absorption may be reduced by compressing the lacrimal sac at the medial canthus for a minute during and following the instillation of the drops. (This blocks the passage of the drops via the naso lacrimal duct to the wide absorptive area of the nasal and pharyngeal mucosa. It is especially advisable in children.)

4.5 Interaction with other medicinal products and other forms of Interaction

Chymotrypsin will be inhibited if given simultaneously with chloramphenicol.

4.6 Pregnancy and lactation

Safety for use in pregnancy and lactation has not been established, therefore, use only when considered essential by the physician.

4.7 Effects on ability to drive and use machines

May cause transient blurring of vision on installation. Warn patients not to drive or operate hazardous machinery unless vision is clear.

4.8 Undesirable effects

<u>Local</u>

Sensitivity reactions such as transient irritation, burning, stinging, itching and dermatitis, may occur.

<u>Systemic</u>

Rarely, cases of major adverse haematological events (bone marrow depression, aplastic anaemia and death) have been reported following ocular use of chloramphenicol.

4.9 Overdose

Not applicable.

5. PHARMACOLOGICAL PROPERTIES

5.1 Pharmacodynamic properties

Chloramphenicol is an antibiotic which is mainly bacteriostatic in action, but exerts a bactericidal effect against some strains of gram-positive cocci and against <u>Haemophilus influenzae</u> and <u>Neisseria</u>. It has a broad spectrum of action against both gram-positive and gram-negative bacteria, rickettsiae and chlamydia.

5.2 Pharmacokinetic properties

Chloramphenicol is rapidly absorbed after oral administration. In the liver, chloramphenicol is inactivated by conjugation with glucuronic acid or by reduction to inactive aryl amines. Excretion is mainly renal, though some bile excretion occurs following oral administration.

5.3 Preclinical safety data

There are no preclinical data of relevance to the prescriber which are additional to that already included in other sections of the SPC.

6. PHARMACEUTICAL PARTICULARS

6.1 List of excipients

Borax

Boric acid

Purified water

6.2 Incompatibilities

None known.

6.3 Shelf life

30 months.

6.4 Special precautions for storage

Store between 2° and 8°C. Do not freeze. Protect from light.

If necessary, the product may be stored at temperatures not exceeding 25°C for up to 1 month only.

6.5 Nature and contents of container

A sealed conical shaped polypropylene container fitted with a twist and pull off cap. Each Minims Chloramphenicol unit is overwrapped in an individual polyethylene sachet. 20 units each containing 0.5ml are packed into a suitable carton.

6.6 Instructions for use and handling

Each Minims unit should be discarded after a single use.

If the product is to be stored unrefrigerated at temperatures not exceeding 25°C, prior to supply of the product by the pharmacy the adhesive label provided in the carton should be completed and affixed over the bar code, by a pharmacist. An expiry date one month from the supply date, plus the pharmacist's initials should be written in the spaces provided on this label.

7. MARKETING AUTHORISATION HOLDER

Chauvin Pharmaceuticals Ltd

106 London Road

Kingston-upon-Thames

Surrey

KT2 6TN

8. MARKETING AUTHORISATION NUMBER(S)

PL 0033/0055R

9. DATE OF FIRST AUTHORISATION/RENEWAL OF THE AUTHORISATION

Date of Grant: 31.7.91

Date of Renewal: 23.4.97

10. DATE OF REVISION OF THE TEXT

November 2000

November 2002

11. LEGAL CATEGORY
POM

Minims Cyclopentolate Hydrochloride

(Chauvin Pharmaceuticals Ltd)

1. NAME OF THE MEDICINAL PRODUCT
Minims Cyclopentolate Hydrochloride

2. QUALITATIVE AND QUANTITATIVE COMPOSITION
Clear, colourless, sterile eye drops containing cyclopentolate hydrochloride BP Two strengths are available: Cyclopentolate Hydrochloride BP 0.5% and 1.0% w/v solutions.

3. PHARMACEUTICAL FORM
Single-use, sterile eye drops.

4. CLINICAL PARTICULARS

4.1 Therapeutic indications
As a topical mydriatic and cycloplegic.

4.2 Posology and method of administration
Adults (including the elderly):

Instil dropwise into eye according to the recommended dosage.

One or two drops as required. Maximum effect is induced in 30 - 60 minutes after instillation.

For refraction and examination of the back of the eye: 1 drop of solution, which may be repeated after five minutes, is usually sufficient.

For anterior and posterior uveitis (if associated with signs of anterior uveitis) and for the breakdown of posterior synechiae: 1 - 2 drops are instilled every 6 - 8 hours.

Resistance to cycloplegia can occur in young children, in patients with dark skin and/or patients with dark irides, therefore, the strength of cyclopentolate used should be adjusted accordingly.

Children

< 3 months: Not recommended

3 months - 12 years: 1 drop of a 1% solution to each eye.

12 years - adult: 1 drop of 0.5% solution to each eye repeated after 10 minutes if necessary.

Children should be observed for 45 minutes after instillation.

4.3 Contraindications
Do not use in patients with a known hypersensitivity to any component of the preparation.

Should not be used in neonates except where, on expert evaluation, the need is considered to be compelling.

Do not use in patients with confirmed or suspected narrow-angle glaucoma as an acute attack may be precipitated.

4.4 Special warnings and special precautions for use
Recovery of accommodation occurs within 24 hours.

Use with caution in very young children and other patients at special risk, such as debilitated or aged patients.

Caution is also advised in hyperaemia as increased systemic absorption may occur.

Systemic absorption may be reduced by compressing the lacrimal sac at the medial canthus for a minute during and following the instillation of the drops. (This blocks the passage of the drops via the naso lacrimal duct to the wide absorptive area of the nasal and pharyngeal mucosa. It is especially advisable in children.)

4.5 Interaction with other medicinal products and other forms of Interaction
None known.

4.6 Pregnancy and lactation
The safety for use in pregnancy and lactation has not been established, therefore, use only when considered essential by the physician.

4.7 Effects on ability to drive and use machines
May cause transient blurring of vision on instillation. Warn patients not to drive or operate hazardous machinery until vision is clear.

4.8 Undesirable effects
Local Effects

Local irritation may result following the use of this product. The frequency of this effect occurring is dependant on the concentration instilled.

Increased intraocular pressure may occur in predisposed patients.

Allergic reactions may rarely occur, manifesting as diffusely red eyes with lacrimation and stringy white mucus discharge.

Systemic Effects

Systemic cyclopentolate toxicity is dose-related and is uncommon following administration of 1% solution and would not be expected to occur following instillation of 0.5% solution. Children are, however, more susceptible to such reactions than adults. Toxicity is usually transient and is manifest mainly by CNS disturbances. Any CNS disturbances are characterised by signs and symptoms of cerebellar dysfunction and visual and tactile hallucinations.

Peripheral effects typical of anti-cholinergics, such as flushing or dryness of the skin and mucous membranes, have not been observed with topical cyclopentolate in children or adults. Temperature, pulse and blood pressure are not normally affected.

4.9 Overdose
Overdose is rare but symptoms can include those mentioned in Section 4.8 above. Treatment is supportive.

5. PHARMACOLOGICAL PROPERTIES

5.1 Pharmacodynamic properties
Cyclopentolate hydrochloride is a synthetic tertiary amine, antimuscarinic compound with actions similar to atropine.

5.2 Pharmacokinetic properties
As a group, the synthetic tertiary amine antimuscarinic compounds are well absorbed following oral administration. Cyclopentolate may be absorbed systemically either by transcorneal absorption, direct topical absorption through the skin or by absorption from the nasal or naso lacrimal system.

5.3 Preclinical safety data
There are no preclinical data of relevance to the prescriber which are additional to that already included in other sections of the SPC.

6. PHARMACEUTICAL PARTICULARS

6.1 List of excipients
Hydrochloric acid

Purified water

6.2 Incompatibilities
None known.

6.3 Shelf life
15 months.

6.4 Special precautions for storage
Store below 25°C. Do not freeze. Protect from light.

6.5 Nature and contents of container
A sealed, conical shaped container fitted with a twist and pull-off cap. Each Minims unit is overwrapped in an individual polypropylene/paper pouch. Each container holds approximately 0.5ml of solution.

6.6 Instructions for use and handling
Each Minims unit should be discarded after a single use.

7. MARKETING AUTHORISATION HOLDER
Chauvin Pharmaceuticals Ltd

106 London Road

Kingston-upon-Thames

Surrey

KT2 6TN

8. MARKETING AUTHORISATION NUMBER(S)
Minims Cyclopentolate Hydrochloride 0.5%: PL 0033/5005R

Minims Cyclopentolate Hydrochloride 1.0%: PL 0033/5006R

9. DATE OF FIRST AUTHORISATION/RENEWAL OF THE AUTHORISATION

Minims Cyclopentolate Hydrochloride 0.5%

Date of first Authorisation: 17 June 1987

Renewal of Authorisation: 13 July 2002

Minims Cyclopentolate Hydrochloride 1.0%

Date of first Authorisation: 17 June 1987

Renewal of Authorisation: 13 July 2002

10. DATE OF REVISION OF THE TEXT

Minims Cyclopentolate Hydrochloride 0.5%

July 1997.

November 2002

Minims Cyclopentolate Hydrochloride 1.0%

May 1997.

November 2002

Minims Dexamethasone

(Chauvin Pharmaceuticals Ltd)

1. NAME OF THE MEDICINAL PRODUCT
Minims Dexamethasone 0.1% w/v Eye Drops.

2. QUALITATIVE AND QUANTITATIVE COMPOSITION
Dexamethasone sodium phosphate Ph Eur 0.1% w/v.

3. PHARMACEUTICAL FORM
Single-use, sterile eye drops.

A colourless solution when examined under suitable conditions of visibility, practically clear and practically free from particles.

4. CLINICAL PARTICULARS

4.1 Therapeutic indications
Non-infected, steroid responsive, inflammatory conditions of the eye.

4.2 Posology and method of administration
Adults (including the elderly):

One or two drops should be applied topically to the eye up to six times a day. *Note:* In severe conditions the treatment may be initiated with 1 or 2 drops every hour, the dosage should then be gradually reduced as the inflammation subsides.

Children:

At the discretion of the physician.

4.3 Contraindications
Use is contra-indicated in herpes simplex and other viral diseases of the cornea and conjunctiva, fungal disease, ocular tuberculosis, untreated purulent infections and hypersensitivity to any component of the preparation.

In children, long-term, continuous corticosteroid therapy should be avoided due to possible adrenal suppression.

4.4 Special warnings and special precautions for use
Care should be taken to ensure that the eye is not infected before Minims Dexamethasone is used.

These drops should be used cautiously in patients with glaucoma and should be considered carefully in patients with a family history of this disease.

Topical corticosteroids should not be used for longer than one week except under ophthalmic supervision, as prolonged application to the eye of preparations containing corticosteroids has caused increased intraocular pressure. The dose of anti-glaucoma medication may need to be adjusted in these patients. Prolonged use may also increase the hazard of secondary ocular infections.

Contact lenses should not be worn during treatment with corticosteroid eye drops due to increased risk of infection.

Systemic absorption may be reduced by compressing the lacrimal sac at the medial canthus for a minute during and following the instillation of the drops. (This blocks the passage of drops via the naso-lacrimal duct to the wide absorptive area of the nasal and pharyngeal mucosa. It is especially advisable in children.)

4.5 Interaction with other medicinal products and other forms of Interaction
The risk of increased intraocular pressure associated with prolonged corticosteroid therapy may be more likely to occur with concomitant use of anticholinergics, especially atropine and related compounds, in patients predisposed to acute angle closure.

The following drug interactions are possible, but are unlikely to be of clinical significance, following the use of Minims Dexamethasone in the eye:

The therapeutic efficacy of dexamethasone may be reduced by phenytoin, phenobarbitone, ephedrine and rifampicin.

Glucocorticoids may increase the need for salicylates as plasma salicylate clearance is increased.

4.6 Pregnancy and lactation
Topically applied steroids can be absorbed systemically and have been shown to cause abnormalities of foetal development in pregnant animals. Although the relevance of this finding to human beings has not been established, the use of Minims Dexamethasone during pregnancy should be avoided.

Topically applied dexamethasone is not recommended in breastfeeding mothers, as it is possible that traces of dexamethasone may enter the breast milk.

4.7 Effects on ability to drive and use machines
Instillation of this eye drop may cause transient blurring of vision. Warn patients not to drive or operate hazardous machinery until vision is clear.

4.8 Undesirable effects
Administration of dexamethasone to the eye may rarely cause stinging, burning, redness or watering of the eyes.

Prolonged treatment with corticosteroids in high dosage is, rarely, associated with sub-capsular cataract. In diseases which cause thinning of the cornea or sclera, perforations of the globe have been known to occur. In addition, optic nerve damage and visual acuity and field defects may arise following long term use of this product.

The systemic effects of corticosteroids are possible with excessive use of steroid eye drops.

4.9 Overdose
As Minims are single-dose units, overdose is unlikely to occur.

5. PHARMACOLOGICAL PROPERTIES

5.1 Pharmacodynamic properties
Dexamethasone is a highly potent and long-acting glucocorticoid. It has an approximately 7 times greater anti-inflammatory potency than prednisolone, another commonly prescribed corticosteroid.

The actions of corticosteroids are mediated by the binding of the corticosteroid molecules to receptor molecules located within sensitive cells. Corticosteroid receptors are present in human trabecular meshwork cells and in rabbit iris ciliary body tissue.

Corticosteroids will inhibit phospholipase A2 thereby preventing the generation of substances which mediate inflammation, for example, prostaglandins. Corticosteroids also produce a marked, though transient, lymphocytopenia. This depletion is due to redistribution of the cells, the T lymphocytes being affected to a greater degree than the B lymphocytes. Lymphokine production is reduced, as is the sensitivity of macrophages to activation by lymphokines. Corticosteroids also retard epithelial regeneration, diminish post-inflammatory neo-vascularisation and reduce towards normal levels the excessive permeability of inflamed capillaries.

The actions of corticosteroids described above are exhibited by dexamethasone and they all contribute to its anti-inflammatory effect.

5.2 Pharmacokinetic properties

When given topically to the eye, dexamethasone is absorbed into the aqueous humour, cornea, iris, choroid, ciliary body and retina. Systemic absorption occurs but may be significant only at higher dosages or in extended paediatric therapy.

Up to 90% of dexamethasone is absorbed when given by mouth; peak plasma levels are reached between 1 and 2 hours after ingestion and show wide individual variations. Dexamethasone sodium phosphate is rapidly converted to dexamethasone within the circulation. Up to 77% of dexamethasone is bound to plasma proteins, mainly albumin. This percentage, unlike cortisol, remains practically unchanged with increasing steroid concentrations. The mean plasma half life of dexamethasone is 3.6 ± 0.9h.

Tissue distribution studies in animals show a high uptake of dexamethasone by the liver, kidney and adrenal glands; a volume of distribution has been quoted as 0.58 l/kg. In man, over 60% of circulating steroids are excreted in the urine within 24 hours, largely as unconjugated steroid.

Dexamethasone also appears to be cleared more rapidly from the circulation of the foetus and neonate than in the mother; plasma dexamethasone levels in the foetus and the mother have been found in the ratio of 0.32:1.

5.3 Preclinical safety data

The use of corticosteroids, including dexamethasone and its derivatives, in ophthalmology is well established. Little relevant toxicology has been reported, however, the breadth of clinical experience confirms its suitability as a topical ophthalmic agent.

6. PHARMACEUTICAL PARTICULARS

6.1 List of excipients

Anhydrous disodium hydrogen phosphate

Sodium dihydrogen phosphate ($2H_2O$)

Disodium edetate

Purified water

6.2 Incompatibilities

None known.

6.3 Shelf life

15 months.

6.4 Special precautions for storage

Store below 25°C. Do not freeze. Protect from light.

6.5 Nature and contents of container

A sealed conical shaped polypropylene container fitted with a twist and pull-off cap. Each Minims unit contains approximately 0.5 ml of solution. Each unit is overwrapped in a sachet. 20 units are packed into a suitable carton.

6.6 Instructions for use and handling

Each Minims unit should be discarded after a single use.

7. MARKETING AUTHORISATION HOLDER

Chauvin Pharmaceuticals Ltd

106 London Road

Kingston-upon-Thames

Surrey

KT2 6TN

8. MARKETING AUTHORISATION NUMBER(S)

PL 00033/0153

9. DATE OF FIRST AUTHORISATION/RENEWAL OF THE AUTHORISATION

6 November 1997

10. DATE OF REVISION OF THE TEXT

24 June 2002

November 2002

Minims Fluorescein Sodium

(Chauvin Pharmaceuticals Ltd)

1. NAME OF THE MEDICINAL PRODUCT

Minims Fluorescein Sodium

2. QUALITATIVE AND QUANTITATIVE COMPOSITION

Solution of Fluorescein Sodium BP. Two strengths are available: Fluorescein Sodium BP 1% and 2% w/v.

3. PHARMACEUTICAL FORM

Single-use, sterile eye drops.

4. CLINICAL PARTICULARS

4.1 Therapeutic indications

As a diagnostic stain.

Fluorescein does not stain a normal cornea but conjunctival abrasions are stained yellow or orange, corneal abrasions or ulcers are stained a bright green and foreign bodies are surrounded by a green ring.

Fluorescein can be used in diagnostic examinations including Goldmann tonometry and in the fitting of hard contact lenses.

4.2 Posology and method of administration

Adults, Children and the Elderly

Instil dropwise into the eye.

Sufficient solution should be applied to stain the damaged areas. Excess may be washed away with sterile saline solution.

4.3 Contraindications

Not to be used with soft contact lenses.

4.4 Special warnings and special precautions for use

Special care should be taken to avoid microbial contamination. *Pseudomonas aeruginosa* grows well in fluorescein solutions, therefore, a single dose solution is preferred. Each Minims unit should be discarded after a single use.

4.5 Interaction with other medicinal products and other forms of Interaction

None known.

4.6 Pregnancy and lactation

Safety for use in pregnancy and lactation has not been established, therefore use only when considered essential by the physician.

4.7 Effects on ability to drive and use machines

May cause transient blurring of vision on instillation. Warn patients not to drive or operate hazardous machinery until vision is clear.

4.8 Undesirable effects

None

4.9 Overdose

Overdose following the recommended use is unlikely.

5. PHARMACOLOGICAL PROPERTIES

5.1 Pharmacodynamic properties

Fluorescein acts as a diagnostic stain.

5.2 Pharmacokinetic properties

Fluorescein will resist penetration of a normal cornea and most excess solution will, therefore, be carried with the tear film away from the conjunctival sac. The majority will be lost through the naso-lacrimal ducts and absorbed via the gastro-intestinal tract from where it is converted rapidly to its glucuronide and excreted via the urine.

If fluorescein crosses the cornea it will enter the Bowman's membrane, stroma and possibly the anterior chamber. Aqueous flow and diffusion into the blood in the anterior chamber finally removes fluorescein from the eye and it is excreted unchanged in the urine.

5.3 Preclinical safety data

There are no preclinical data of relevance to the prescriber which are additional to that already included in other sections of this SPC.

6. PHARMACEUTICAL PARTICULARS

6.1 List of excipients

Purified Water

6.2 Incompatibilities

None known.

6.3 Shelf life

Unopened: 15 months.

6.4 Special precautions for storage

Store below 25°C. Do not freeze. Protect from light.

6.5 Nature and contents of container

A sealed conical shaped polypropylene container fitted with a twist and pull off cap. Each Minims unit contains approximately 0.5ml of solution. Each unit is overwrapped in a polypropylene/paper pouch. 20 units are packed into a suitable carton.

6.6 Instructions for use and handling

Each Minims unit should be discarded after use.

7. MARKETING AUTHORISATION HOLDER

Chauvin Pharmaceuticals Ltd

106 London Road

Kingston-upon-Thames

Surrey

KT2 6TN

8. MARKETING AUTHORISATION NUMBER(S)

Fluorescein Sodium 1% PL 0033/0079

Fluorescein Sodium 2% PL 0033/5008R

9. DATE OF FIRST AUTHORISATION/RENEWAL OF THE AUTHORISATION

Fluorescein Sodium 1% 07.01.80

Fluorescein Sodium 2% 23.04.87

10. DATE OF REVISION OF THE TEXT

Fluorescein Sodium 1% November 2002

Fluorescein Sodium 2% November 2002

Minims Gentamicin Sulphate

(Chauvin Pharmaceuticals Ltd)

1. NAME OF THE MEDICINAL PRODUCT

Minims Gentamicin Sulphate

2. QUALITATIVE AND QUANTITATIVE COMPOSITION

Clear, colourless, sterile eye drop solution of Gentamicin Sulphate BP equivalent to 0.3% w/v gentamicin base.

3. PHARMACEUTICAL FORM

Single-use eye drops.

4. CLINICAL PARTICULARS

4.1 Therapeutic indications

As a broad spectrum antibiotic for the topical treatment of ocular infections caused by both gram-positive and gram-negative organisms.

4.2 Posology and method of administration

Adults (including the elderly):

One drop as required.

Children:

At the discretion of the physician.

Route of administration: Topically to the eye

4.3 Contraindications

Gentamicin should not be used in patients with a known hypersensitivity to gentamicin or other aminoglycosides.

4.4 Special warnings and special precautions for use

Gentamicin should not be the first choice antibiotic for minor infections in order to minimise the possibility of bacterial resistance.

Systemic absorption may be reduced by compressing the lacrimal sac at the medial canthus for a minute during and following the instillation of the drops. (This blocks the passage of drops via the naso-lacrimal duct to the wide absorptive area of the nasal and pharyngeal mucosa. It is especially advisable in children.)

4.5 Interaction with other medicinal products and other forms of Interaction

The use of sulphacetamide with gentamicin in the treatment of eye infections is not recommended.

Concomitant administration of frusemide with gentamicin may reduce the renal clearance of gentamicin but this is unlikely to be of significance with topical use.

4.6 Pregnancy and lactation

The use of gentamicin during pregnancy is not recommended.

4.7 Effects on ability to drive and use machines

May cause blurred vision on instillation. If affected, do not drive until vision is restored.

4.8 Undesirable effects

Gentamicin has been used topically without any evidence of significant absorption of the drug to cause systemic reactions.

Gentamicin is well tolerated when applied topically to the eye.

4.9 Overdose

As Minims are single-dose units, overdose is unlikely to occur.

5. PHARMACOLOGICAL PROPERTIES

5.1 Pharmacodynamic properties

Gentamicin is an aminoglycoside which has a bactericidal action. It acts by inhibiting protein synthesis in susceptible bacteria. Gentamicin possesses a wide spectrum of activity being effective against both gram-positive and gram-negative organisms, including *Pseudomonas Aeruginosa*.

5.2 Pharmacokinetic properties

Gentamicin pharmacokinetics conform to a two-compartment model, in which the drug is rapidly eliminated from the tissue compartment. Its biological half-life is 1 - 4 hours.

With regard to ocular pharmacokinetics, gentamicin is not very lipid-soluble and thus it does not easily pass through the corneal epithelium. However, gentamicin 0.3% drops do penetrate into the aqueous humour of normal and inflamed eyes at significant therapeutic levels.

Only very low levels of gentamicin will be absorbed systemically. Gentamicin is 25 - 30% protein bound and is excreted in the urine.

5.3 Preclinical safety data

There are no preclinical data of relevance to the prescriber which are additional to that already included in other sections of the SPC.

6. PHARMACEUTICAL PARTICULARS

6.1 List of excipients

Purified Water

Sodium Chloride

Borax

Sodium Hydroxide

6.2 Incompatibilities

Gentamicin is incompatible with amphotericin, cephalosporins, erythromycin, heparin, penicillins, sodium bicarbonate and sulphadiazine sodium. This is unlikely to be relevant regarding topical use.

6.3 Shelf life
15 months.

6.4 Special precautions for storage
Store below 25°C. Do not freeze. Protect from light.

6.5 Nature and contents of container
A sealed, conical shaped container fitted with a twist and pull-off cap. Each Minims unit is overwrapped in an individual polypropylene/paper pouch. Each container holds approximately 0.5ml of solution.

6.6 Instructions for use and handling
Each Minims unit should be discarded after a single use.

7. MARKETING AUTHORISATION HOLDER
Chauvin Pharmaceuticals Ltd

106 London Road

Kingston-upon-Thames

Surrey

KT2 4TN

8. MARKETING AUTHORISATION NUMBER(S)
PL 0033/0094

9. DATE OF FIRST AUTHORISATION/RENEWAL OF THE AUTHORISATION
21.9.81

10. DATE OF REVISION OF THE TEXT
June 1997

November 2002

Minims Lidocaine & Fluorescein

(Chauvin Pharmaceuticals Ltd)

1. NAME OF THE MEDICINAL PRODUCT
Minims Lidocaine & Fluorescein.

2. QUALITATIVE AND QUANTITATIVE COMPOSITION
Clear, slightly yellow, slightly viscous eye drops containing Lidocaine Hydrochloride PhEur 4% w/v and Fluorescein Sodium BP 0.25% w/v.

3. PHARMACEUTICAL FORM
Single-use, sterile eye drops.

4. CLINICAL PARTICULARS
4.1 Therapeutic indications
As a diagnostic stain and topical anaesthetic combined Minims Lidocaine and Fluorescein can be used in the measurement of intraocular pressure by Goldmann tonometry.

4.2 Posology and method of administration
Adults (including the elderly):

One or more drops, as required.

Children:

As directed by the physician.

4.3 Contraindications
Do not use in patients with a known hypersensitivity to fluorescein or lidocaine and other amide-type local anaesthetics.

4.4 Special warnings and special precautions for use
The anaesthetised eye should be protected from foreign body contamination, particularly in elderly patients in whom the duration of anaesthesia may exceed 30 minutes.

Use with caution in an inflamed eye as hyperaemia greatly increases the rate of systemic absorption through the conjunctiva.

Systemic absorption may be reduced by compressing the lacrimal sac at the medial canthus for a minute during and following the instillation of the drops. (This blocks the passage of the drops via the naso-lacrimal duct to the wide absorptive area of the nasal and pharyngeal mucosa. It is especially advisable in children.)

4.5 Interaction with other medicinal products and other forms of Interaction
None known.

4.6 Pregnancy and lactation
This combination has been used for a number of years without apparent ill-consequence.

4.7 Effects on ability to drive and use machines
None known.

4.8 Undesirable effects
None known.

4.9 Overdose
Overdose is not expected to cause any adverse effects, however, overuse of local anaesthetics can cause keratitis, with loss of corneal epithelium and stromal opacity.

5. PHARMACOLOGICAL PROPERTIES
5.1 Pharmacodynamic properties
Lidocaine is an established topical anaesthetic which blocks the sensory nerve endings of the cornea.

The fluorescein moiety does not stain a normal cornea but conjunctival abrasions are stained yellow or orange, corneal abrasions or ulcers are stained a bright green and foreign bodies are surrounded by a green ring.

5.2 Pharmacokinetic properties
None relevant.

5.3 Preclinical safety data
There are no preclinical data of relevance to the prescriber which are additional to that already included in other sections of the SPC.

6. PHARMACEUTICAL PARTICULARS
6.1 List of excipients
Povidone

Hydrochloric Acid

Purified Water

6.2 Incompatibilities
None known.

6.3 Shelf life
15 months.

6.4 Special precautions for storage
Store below 25°C. Do not freeze. Protect from light.

6.5 Nature and contents of container
A sealed, conical shaped container fitted with a twist and pull-off cap. Each Minims unit is overwrapped in an individual polypropylene/paper pouch. Each container holds approximately 0.5ml of solution.

6.6 Instructions for use and handling
Each Minims unit should be discarded after a single use.

7. MARKETING AUTHORISATION HOLDER
Chauvin Pharmaceuticals Ltd

106 London Road

Kingston-upon-Thames

Surrey

KT2 6TN

8. MARKETING AUTHORISATION NUMBER(S)
PL 0033/0073

9. DATE OF FIRST AUTHORISATION/RENEWAL OF THE AUTHORISATION
Date of first Authorisation: 14.6.78

10. DATE OF REVISION OF THE TEXT
September 1999

July 1997

November 2002

January 2005

Minims Metipranolol 0.1% w/v

(Chauvin Pharmaceuticals Ltd)

1. NAME OF THE MEDICINAL PRODUCT
Minims Metipranolol 0.1%

2. QUALITATIVE AND QUANTITATIVE COMPOSITION
Clear, colourless, sterile eye drops containing Metipranolol 0.1% w/v.

3. PHARMACEUTICAL FORM
Sterile, single-use eye drops.

4. CLINICAL PARTICULARS
4.1 Therapeutic indications
Metipranolol is a beta-adrenoceptor blocking agent. Minims Metipranolol is an eyedrop for topical use which may be used for the treatment of raised intraocular pressure. It is particularly suitable for the treatment of patients who are hypersensitive to preservatives, for control of post operative increases of intraocular pressure and as an initial test for responsiveness to beta-blocker therapy.

4.2 Posology and method of administration
<u>Adults (including the Elderly)</u>

One drop instilled into the affected eye twice daily. In the treatment of post operative rises in intraocular pressure the dosage and frequency should be at the discretion of the physician.

<u>Children</u>

Treatment should be at the discretion of the physician.

4.3 Contraindications
Minims Metipranolol should not be used in patients with bronchial asthma, history of bronchial asthma, chronic obstructive airways disease, sinus bradycardia, second or third degree atrio-ventricular block, cardiac failure, cardiogenic shock or hypersensitivity to any of the components of the preparation.

4.4 Special warnings and special precautions for use
Ophthalmic solutions should only be used in patients with contact lenses at the discretion of the physician.

The use of Minims Metipranolol in patients with chronic glaucoma should be restricted only to those patients who are allergic to the preservatives commonly used in multidose preparations, or those patients wearing soft contact lenses in whom benzalkonium chloride should be avoided.

Systemic absorption may be reduced by compressing the lacrimal sac at the medial canthus for a minute during and following the instillation of the drops. (This blocks the passage of the drops via the naso-lacrimal duct to the wide absorptive area of the nasal and pharyngeal mucosa. It is especially advisable in children.)

As with other topically applied beta-blockers, systemic absorption may occur giving adverse reactions similar to those of orally admininstered beta-blockers.

Cardiac and respiratory reactions have been reported with topically applied beta-blockers including, rarely, death due to bronchospasm or cardiac failure.

Congestive cardiac failure should be adequately controlled before starting therapy with Minims Metipranolol. If the patient has a history of cardiac disease, pulse rate should be monitored.

Diabetic control should be monitored during Minims Metipranolol therapy in patients with labile diabetes.

4.5 Interaction with other medicinal products and other forms of Interaction
Beta-blockers should not be given with verapamil and neither drug should be administered within several days of discontinuing the other. As absorption into the circulation is possible, Minims Metipranolol should be used only with caution in patients already receiving similar drugs by mouth. In particular care should be taken in patients with sinus bradycardia and greater than first degree heart block.

4.6 Pregnancy and lactation
Although there is no evidence to suggest that metipranolol has teratogenic properties, its use in pregnancy should be avoided unless the potential benefits are considered to outweigh the possible hazards.

As β-blockers can pass into breast milk, consideration should be given to stopping breast feeding if Minims Metipranolol is considered necessary.

4.7 Effects on ability to drive and use machines
No such effects have been seen nor are anticipated.

4.8 Undesirable effects
Granulomatous anterior uveitis has been reported in association with the use of the multidose preparation of Metipranolol (Glauline) in patients with chronic glaucoma.

Transient burning or stinging on instillation, blurred vision and anterior uveitis have been reported.

Bradycardia and hypotension can occasionally occur following the systemic absorption of topically applied β-blockers.

Bronchospasm may occur, predominantly in patients with a history of reversible obstructive airways disease. Dyspnoea and respiratory failure have been reported with topically applied β-blockers.

Headache, ataxia, weakness and lethargy can occur.

Local manifestations of contact sensitivity can occur. Reactions around the eyes can involve skin rashes on the lower lids and cheeks and periorbital oedema.

4.9 Overdose
As Minims Metipranolol is a unit dose application, overdose is unlikely to occur.

5. PHARMACOLOGICAL PROPERTIES
5.1 Pharmacodynamic properties
Metipranolol is a beta-adrenoceptor blocking agent used to lower intraocular pressure. It has a non-selective action and hence will block both beta-1 and beta-2 receptor subtypes. There is no evidence to suggest that it possesses any intrinsic sympathomimetic activity. The resulting reduction in intraocular pressure is achieved primarily by a decrease in the production of aqueous humour.

5.2 Pharmacokinetic properties
Following topical administration of 0.6% metipranolol no desacetyl metipranolol, the principle metabolite, could be detected in the plasma of volunteers at a detection limit of 1ng/ml.

There are sufficient clinical data on the efficacy of topical metipranolol to obviate the need for the measurement of ocular pharmacokinetics.

5.3 Preclinical safety data
There are no preclinical data of relevance to the prescriber which are additional to that already included in other sections of the SPC.

6. PHARMACEUTICAL PARTICULARS
6.1 List of excipients
Hydrochloric acid BP

Sodium chloride PhEur

Sodium hydroxide

Purified water PhEur

6.2 Incompatibilities
Verapamil, as described in section 4.5.

6.3 Shelf life
18 months

6.4 Special precautions for storage
Store below 25°C. Do not freeze. Protect from light.

6.5 Nature and contents of container
A sealed, conical shaped container fitted with a twist and pull-off cap. Each Minims unit is overwrapped in an

individual polypropylene/paper pouch. Each container holds approximately 0.5ml of solution.

6.6 Instructions for use and handling
Each Minims unit should be discarded after a single use. Full instructions for use are provided on the enclosed leaflet.

7. MARKETING AUTHORISATION HOLDER
Chauvin Pharmaceuticals Ltd

106 London Road

Kingston-upon-Thames

Surrey

KT2 6TN

8. MARKETING AUTHORISATION NUMBER(S)
PL 0033/0121

9. DATE OF FIRST AUTHORISATION/RENEWAL OF THE AUTHORISATION
Date of first Authorisation: 16.12.87

Renewed on 08.07.1994

10. DATE OF REVISION OF THE TEXT
January 1999

November 2001

November 2002

Minims Metipranolol 0.3% w/v

(Chauvin Pharmaceuticals Ltd)

1. NAME OF THE MEDICINAL PRODUCT
Minims Metipranolol 0.3%

2. QUALITATIVE AND QUANTITATIVE COMPOSITION
Clear, colourless, sterile eye drops containing Metipranolol 0.3% w/v.

3. PHARMACEUTICAL FORM
Sterile, single-use eye drops.

4. CLINICAL PARTICULARS

4.1 Therapeutic indications
Metipranolol is a beta-adrenoceptor blocking agent. Minims Metipranolol is an eyedrop for topical use which may be used for the treatment of raised intraocular pressure. It is particularly suitable for the treatment of patients who are hypersensitive to preservatives, for control of post operative increases of intraocular pressure and as an initial test for responsiveness to beta-blocker therapy.

4.2 Posology and method of administration
Adults (including the Elderly)

One drop instilled into the affected eye twice daily. In the treatment of post operative rises in intraocular pressure the dosage and frequency should be at the discretion of the physician.

Children

Treatment should be at the discretion of the physician.

4.3 Contraindications
Minims Metipranolol should not be used in patients with bronchial asthma, history of bronchial asthma, chronic obstructive airways disease, sinus bradychardia, second or third degree atrio-ventricular block, cardiac failure, cardiogenic shock or hypersensitivity to any of the components of the preparation.

4.4 Special warnings and special precautions for use
Ophthalmic solutions should only be used in patients with contact lenses at the discretion of the physician.

The use of Minims Metipranolol in patients with chronic glaucoma should be restricted only to those patients who are allergic to the preservatives commonly used in multidose preparations, or those patients wearing soft contact lenses in whom benzalkonium chloride should be avoided.

Systemic absorption may be reduced by compressing the lacrimal sac at the medial canthus for a minute during and following the instillation of the drops. (This blocks the passage of the drops via the naso-lacrimal duct to the wide absorptive area of the nasal and pharyngeal mucosa. It is especially advisable in children.)

As with other topically applied beta-blockers, systemic absorption may occur giving adverse reactions similar to those of orally admininstered beta-blockers.

Cardiac and respiratory reactions have been reported with topically applied beta-blockers including, rarely, death due to bronchospasm or cardiac failure.

Congestive cardiac failure should be adequately controlled before starting therapy with Minims Metipranolol. If the patient has a history of cardiac disease, pulse rate should be monitored.

Diabetic control should be monitored during Minims Metiprannolol therapy in patients with labile diabetes.

4.5 Interaction with other medicinal products and other forms of Interaction
Beta-blockers should not be given with verapamil and neither drug should be administered within several days of discontinuing the other. As absorption into the circulation is possible, Minims Metipranolol should be used only with caution in patients already receiving similar drugs by mouth. In particular care should be taken in patients with sinus bradycardia and greater than first degree heart block.

4.6 Pregnancy and lactation
Although there is no evidence to suggest that metipranolol has teratogenic properties, its use in pregnancy should be avoided unless the potential benefits are considered to outweigh the possible hazards.

As β-blockers can pass into breast milk, consideration should be given to stopping breast feeding if Minims Metipranolol is considered necessary.

4.7 Effects on ability to drive and use machines
No such effects have been seen nor are anticipated.

4.8 Undesirable effects
Granulomatous anterior uveitis has been reported in association with the use of the multidose preparation of Metipranolol (Glauline) in patients with chronic glaucoma.

Transient burning or stinging on instillation, blurred vision and anterior uveitis have been reported.

Bradycardia and hypotension can occasionally occur following the systemic absorption of topically applied β-blockers.

Bronchospasm may occur, predominantly in patients with a history of reversible obstructive airways disease. Dyspnoea and respiratory failure have been reported with topically applied β-blockers.

Headache, ataxia, weakness and lethargy can occur.

Local manifestations of contact sensitivity can occur. Reactions around the eyes can involve skin rashes on the lower lids and cheeks and periorbital oedema.

4.9 Overdose
As Minims Metipranolol is a unit dose application, overdose is unlikely to occur.

5. PHARMACOLOGICAL PROPERTIES

5.1 Pharmacodynamic properties
Metipranolol is a beta-adrenoceptor blocking agent used to lower intraocular pressure. It has a non-selective action and hence will block both beta-1 and beta-2 receptor subtypes. There is no evidence to suggest that it possesses any intrinsic sympathomimetic activity. The resulting reduction in intraocular pressure is achieved primarily by a decrease in the production of aqueous humour.

5.2 Pharmacokinetic properties
Following topical administration of 0.6% metipranolol no desacetyl metipranolol, the principle metabolite, could be detected in the plasma of volunteers at a detection limit of 1ng/ml.

There are sufficient clinical data on the efficacy of topical metipranolol to obviate the need for the measurement of ocular pharmacokinetics.

5.3 Preclinical safety data
There are no preclinical data of relevance to the prescriber which are additional to that already included in other sections of the SPC.

6. PHARMACEUTICAL PARTICULARS

6.1 List of excipients
Hydrochloric acid BP

Sodium chloride PhEur

Sodium hydroxide

Purified water PhEur

6.2 Incompatibilities
Verapamil, as described in section 4.5.

6.3 Shelf life
18 months

6.4 Special precautions for storage
Store below 25°C. Do not freeze. Protect from light.

6.5 Nature and contents of container
A sealed, conical shaped container fitted with a twist and pull-off cap. Each Minims unit is overwrapped in an individual polypropylene/paper pouch. Each container holds approximately 0.5ml of solution.

6.6 Instructions for use and handling
Each Minims unit should be discarded after a single use. Full instructions for use are provided on the enclosed leaflet.

7. MARKETING AUTHORISATION HOLDER
Chauvin Pharmaceuticals Ltd

106 London Road

Kingston-upon-Thames

Surrey

KT2 6TN

8. MARKETING AUTHORISATION NUMBER(S)
PL 0033/0122

9. DATE OF FIRST AUTHORISATION/RENEWAL OF THE AUTHORISATION
Date of first Authorisation: 16.7.87

Renewed: 08.07.1999

10. DATE OF REVISION OF THE TEXT
January 1999

November 2001

November 2002

Minims Oxybuprocaine Hydrochloride 0.4% w/v

(Chauvin Pharmaceuticals Ltd)

1. NAME OF THE MEDICINAL PRODUCT
Minims Oxybuprocaine Hydrochloride 0.4% w/v.

2. QUALITATIVE AND QUANTITATIVE COMPOSITION
Single-use, clear, colourless, sterile eye drops, available as a 0.4% w/v solution of Oxybuprocaine Hydrochloride Ph.Eur.

3. PHARMACEUTICAL FORM
Single-use sterile eye drops

4. CLINICAL PARTICULARS

4.1 Therapeutic indications
As a topical ocular anaesthetic.

4.2 Posology and method of administration
Adults (including the Elderly) and Children

One drop is sufficient when dropped into the conjunctival sac to anaesthetise the surface of the eye to allow tonometry after one minute. A further drop after 90 seconds provides adequate anaesthesia for the fitting of contact lenses. Three drops at 90 second intervals provides sufficient anaesthesia for a foreign body to be removed from the corneal epithelium or for incision of a meibomian cyst through the conjunctiva. Corneal sensitivity is normal again after about one hour.

Instil dropwise into the eye according to the recommended dosage.

Each Minims unit should be discarded after use.

4.3 Contraindications
Not to be used in patients with a known hypersensitivity to the product.

4.4 Special warnings and special precautions for use
Transient stinging and blurring of vision may occur on instillation.

The anaesthetised eye should be protected from dust and bacterial contamination.

When applied to the conjunctiva, oxybuprocaine is less irritant than amethocaine in normal concentrations.

The cornea may be damaged by prolonged application of anaesthetic eye drops.

Systemic absorption may be reduced by compressing the lacrimal sac at the medial canthus for a minute during and following the instillation of the drops. (This blocks the passage of the drops via the naso-lacrimal duct to the wide absorptive area of the nasal and pharyngeal mucosa. It is especially advisable in children).

4.5 Interaction with other medicinal products and other forms of Interaction
None stated.

4.6 Pregnancy and lactation
This product should not be used in pregnancy or lactation, unless considered essential by the physician.

4.7 Effects on ability to drive and use machines
Patients should be advised not to drive or operate hazardous machinery until normal vision is restored.

4.8 Undesirable effects
See 4.4.

4.9 Overdose
Overdose following the recommended use is unlikely.

5. PHARMACOLOGICAL PROPERTIES

5.1 Pharmacodynamic properties
Oxybuprocaine hydrochloride is used as a local anaesthetic as it reversibly blocks the propagation and conduction of nerve impulses along nerve axons.

5.2 Pharmacokinetic properties
The rate of loss of local anaesthetics through tearflow is very high as they induce an initial stinging reaction which stimulates reflex lacrimation and leads to dilution of the drugs. It is thought that this is responsible for the very short duration of maximum effect of local anaesthetics. The non-ionised base of oxybuprocaine is rapidly absorbed from the pre-corneal tear film by the lipophilic corneal epithelium. The drug then passes into the corneal stroma and from there into the anterior chamber where it is carried away by the aqueous flow and diffuses into the blood circulation in the anterior uvea. As with other ester type local anaesthetics, oxybuprocaine is probably rapidly metabolised by plasma cholinesterases (and also by esterases in the liver).

5.3 Preclinical safety data
No adverse safety issues were detected during the development of this formulation. The active ingredient is well established in clinical ophthalmology.

6. PHARMACEUTICAL PARTICULARS

6.1 List of excipients

Hydrochloric Acid

Purified Water

6.2 Incompatibilities

None known

6.3 Shelf life

Unopened: 15 months

6.4 Special precautions for storage

Store below 25°C. Do not freeze. Protect from light.

6.5 Nature and contents of container

A sealed conical shaped polypropylene container fitted with a twist and pull off cap. Overwrapped in an individual polypropylene/paper pouch. Each container holds approximately 0.5ml of solution.

6.6 Instructions for use and handling

Each Minims unit should be discarded after use.

7. MARKETING AUTHORISATION HOLDER

Chauvin Pharmaceuticals Ltd

106 London Road

Kingston-upon-Thames

Surrey

KT2 6TN

8. MARKETING AUTHORISATION NUMBER(S)

PL 0033/5004R

9. DATE OF FIRST AUTHORISATION/RENEWAL OF THE AUTHORISATION

Date of first authorisation: 19 May 1987

Date of Renewal of Authorisation: 22 May 2002

10. DATE OF REVISION OF THE TEXT

December 1997

November 2002

January 2005

Minims Phenylephrine Hydrochloride

(Chauvin Pharmaceuticals Ltd)

1. NAME OF THE MEDICINAL PRODUCT

Minims Phenylephrine Hydrochloride

2. QUALITATIVE AND QUANTITATIVE COMPOSITION

Clear, colourless, sterile eye drops containing Phenylephrine Hydrochloride BP. There are two strengths 2.5% w/v Phenylephrine Hydrochloride and 10% w/v Phenylephrine Hydrochloride.

3. PHARMACEUTICAL FORM

Sterile, single-use eye drop

4. CLINICAL PARTICULARS

4.1 Therapeutic indications

Phenylephrine is a directly acting sympathomimetic agent used topically in the eye as a mydriatic. It may be indicated to dilate the pupil for diagnostic or therapeutic procedures.

4.2 Posology and method of administration

Adults

Apply one drop topically to each eye. If necessary, this dose may be repeated once only, at least one hour after the first drop.

The use of a drop of topical anaesthetic a few minutes before instillation of phenylephrine is recommended to prevent stinging.

Children and the Elderly

Apply one drop topically to the eye. It is not usually necessary to exceed this dose.

The use of phenylephrine 10% solution is contraindicated in these groups because of the increased risks of systemic toxicity.

4.3 Contraindications

Patients with cardiac disease, hypertension, aneurysms, thyrotoxicosis, long-standing insulin dependent diabetes mellitus and tachycardia.

Patients on monoamine oxidase inhibitors, tricyclic antidepressants and anti-hypertensive agents (including beta-blockers).

Patients with closed angle glaucoma (unless previously treated with iridectomy) and patients with a narrow angle prone to glaucoma precipitated by mydriatics.

Hypersensitivity to phenylephrine or any component of the preparation.

4.4 Special warnings and special precautions for use

Use with caution in the presence of diabetes, cerebral arteriosclerosis or long-standing bronchial asthma.

To reduce the risk of precipitating an attack of narrow angle glaucoma evaluate the anterior chamber angle before use.

Ocular hyperaemia can increase the absorption of phenylephrine given topically.

Corneal clouding may occur if phenylephrine 10% is instilled when the corneal epithelium has been denuded or damaged.

Systemic absorption may be minimised by compressing the lacrimal sac at the medial canthus for one minute during and after the instillation of the drops. (This blocks the passage of the drops via the naso-lacrimal duct to the wide absorptive area of the nasal and pharyngeal mucosa. It is especially advisable in children.)

4.5 Interaction with other medicinal products and other forms of Interaction

Anti-hypertensive Agents

Topical phenylephrine should not be used as it may reverse the action of many anti-hypertensive agents with possibly fatal consequences.

Monoamine Oxidase Inhibitors

There is an increased risk of adrenergic reactions when used simultaneously with, or up to three weeks after, the administration of MAOIs.

Tricyclic Antidepressants

The pressor response to adrenergic agents and the risk of cardiac arrythmia may be potentiated in patients receiving tricyclic antidepressants (or within several days of their discontinuation).

Halothane

Because of the increased risk of ventricular fibrillation, phenylephrine should be used with caution during general anaesthesia with anaesthetic agents which sensitise the myocardium to sympathomimetics.

Cardiac Glycosides or Quinidine

There is an increased risk of arrythmias.

4.6 Pregnancy and lactation

Safety for use during pregnancy and lactation has not been established. This product should only be used during pregnancy if it is considered by the physician to be essential.

4.7 Effects on ability to drive and use machines

May cause stinging and temporarily blurred vision. Warn patients not to drive or operate hazardous machinery until vision is clear.

4.8 Undesirable effects

Local

Eye pain and stinging on instillation (use of a drop of topical anaesthetic a few minutes before the instillation of phenylephrine is recommended), temporarily blurred vision and photophobia, conjunctival sensitisation and allergy may occur.

Systemic

Palpitations, tachycardia, extrasystoles, cardiac arrythmias and hypertension.

Serious cardiovascular reactions including coronary artery spasm, ventricular arrythmias and myocardial infarctions have occurred following topical use of 10% phenylephrine. These sometimes fatal reactions have usually occurred in patients with pre-existing cardiovascular disease.

4.9 Overdose

Because a severe toxic reaction to phenylephrine is of rapid onset and short duration, treatment is primarily supportive. Prompt injection of a rapidly acting alpha-adrenergic blocking agent such as phentolamine (dose 2 to 5mg iv) has been recommended.

5. PHARMACOLOGICAL PROPERTIES

5.1 Pharmacodynamic properties

Phenylephrine is a direct acting sympathomimetic agent. It causes mydriasis via the stimulation of alpha receptors. There is almost no cycloplegic effect.

Maximal mydriasis occurs in 60 - 90 minutes with recovery after 5 - 7 hours.

The mydriatic effects of phenylephrine can be reversed with thymoxamine.

5.2 Pharmacokinetic properties

Phenylephrine is a weak base at physiological pH. The extent of ocular penetration is determined by the condition of the cornea. A healthy cornea presents a physical barrier, in addition to which, some metabolic activity may occur. Where the corneal epithelium is damaged, the effect of the barrier and the extent of metabolism are reduced, leading to greater absorption.

5.3 Preclinical safety data

The use of phenylephrine in ophthalmology has been well established for many years. No unexpected adverse safety issues were identified during the development of the Minims format.

6. PHARMACEUTICAL PARTICULARS

6.1 List of excipients

Sodium metabisulphite

Disodium edetate

Purified water

6.2 Incompatibilities

None stated.

6.3 Shelf life

15 months.

6.4 Special precautions for storage

Store below 25°C. Do not freeze. Protect from light.

6.5 Nature and contents of container

A sealed conical shaped polypropylene container fitted with a twist and pull off cap. Each Minims unit is overwrapped in an individual polypropylene/paper pouch. Each container holds approximately 0.5ml of solution.

6.6 Instructions for use and handling

Each Minims unit should be discarded after a single use.

7. MARKETING AUTHORISATION HOLDER

Chauvin Pharmaceuticals Ltd

106 London Road

Kingston-upon-Thames

Surrey

KT2 6TN

8. MARKETING AUTHORISATION NUMBER(S)

Minims Phenylephrine Hydrochloride 2.5% PL 0033/0117

Minims Phenylephrine Hydrochloride 10% PL 0033/5021R

9. DATE OF FIRST AUTHORISATION/RENEWAL OF THE AUTHORISATION

Minims Phenylephrine Hydrochloride 2.5% 21.5.86

Minims Phenylephrine Hydrochloride 10% 09.1.90

10. DATE OF REVISION OF THE TEXT

Minims Phenylephrine Hydrochloride 2.5%

January 1996

November 2002

Minims Phenylephrine Hydrochloride 2.5%

January 1997

November 2002

11. LEGAL CATEGORY

Pharmacy

Minims Pilocarpine Nitrate 2% w/v

(Chauvin Pharmaceuticals Ltd)

1. NAME OF THE MEDICINAL PRODUCT

Minims Pilocarpine Nitrate 2%

2. QUALITATIVE AND QUANTITATIVE COMPOSITION

Clear, colourless, sterile eye drops containing Pilocarpine Nitrate PhEur 2.0% w/v.

3. PHARMACEUTICAL FORM

Sterile, single-use eye drops.

4. CLINICAL PARTICULARS

4.1 Therapeutic indications

Pilocarpine is used as a miotic, for reversing the action of weaker mydriatics and in the emergency treatment of glaucoma.

4.2 Posology and method of administration

Adults (including the elderly) and children:

Instil dropwise into the eye according to the recommended dosage.

To induce miosis, one or two drops should be used.

In cases of emergency treatment of acute narrow-angle glaucoma, one drop should be used every five minutes until miosis is achieved.

4.3 Contraindications

Conditions where pupillary constriction is undesirable e.g. acute iritis, anterior uveitis and some forms of secondary glaucoma.

Hypersensitivity to any component of the preparation.

Patients with soft contact lenses should not use this preparation.

4.4 Special warnings and special precautions for use

Systemic reactions rarely occur when treating chronic simple glaucoma at normal doses. However, in the treatment of acute closed-angle glaucoma the possibility of systemic reactions must be considered because of the higher doses given. Caution is particularly advised in patients with acute heart failure, bronchial asthma, peptic ulceration, hypertension, urinary tract obstruction, Parkinson's disease and corneal abrasions.

Retinal detachments have been caused in susceptible individuals and those with pre-existing retinal disease, therefore, fundus examination is advised in all patients prior to the initiation of therapy.

Patients with chronic glaucoma on long-term pilocarpine therapy should have regular monitoring of intraocular pressure and visual fields.

Systemic absorption may be reduced by compressing the lacrimal sac at the medial canthus for a minute during and following the instillation of the drops. (This blocks the passage of the drops via the naso-lacrimal duct to the wide absorptive area of the nasal and pharyngeal mucosa. It is especially advisable in children.)

4.5 Interaction with other medicinal products and other forms of Interaction

Although clinically not proven, the miotic effects of pilocarpine may be antagonised by long-term topical or systemic corticosteroid therapy, systemic anticholinergics, antihistamines, pethidine, sympathomimetics or tricyclic antidepressants.

Concomitant administration of two miotics is not recommended because of inter-drug antagonism and the risk that unresponsiveness may develop to both drugs.

4.6 Pregnancy and lactation
Safety for use in pregnancy and lactation has not been established, therefore, use only when clearly indicated.

4.7 Effects on ability to drive and use machines
Causes difficulty with dark adaptation, therefore, caution is necessary when night driving and when hazardous tasks are undertaken in poor illumination. May cause accommodation spasm. Patients should be advised not to drive or use machinery if vision is not clear.

4.8 Undesirable effects
Local
Burning, itching, smarting, blurring of vision, ciliary spasm, conjunctival vascular congestion, induced myopia, sensitisation of the lids and conjunctiva, reduced visual acuity in poor illumination, lens changes with chronic use, increased pupillary block, retinal detachments and vitreous haemorrhages.

CNS
Browache and headache (especially in younger patients who have recently started therapy).

Systemic
Systemic reactions rarely occur in the treatment of chronic simple glaucoma but they may include hypotension, bradycardia, bronchial spasm, pulmonary oedema, salivation, sweating, nausea, vomiting, diarrhoea and lacrimation.

4.9 Overdose
If accidentally ingested, induce emesis or perform gastric lavage. Observe for signs of toxicity (salivation, lacrimation, sweating, bronchial spasm, cyanosis, nausea, vomiting and diarrhoea).

5. PHARMACOLOGICAL PROPERTIES

5.1 Pharmacodynamic properties
Pilocarpine is a direct acting parasympathomimetic drug. It duplicates the muscarinic effect of acetyl choline, but not its nicotinic effects. Consequently, pilocarpine stimulates the smooth muscle and secretary glands but does not affect the striated muscle.

5.2 Pharmacokinetic properties
Pilocarpine has a low ocular bioavailability when topically applied and this has been attributed to extensive precorneal drug loss in conjunction with the resistance to normal corneal penetration. Further, pilocarpine appears to bind to the eye pigments from which it is gradually released to the muscles.

Inactivation of pilocarpine in the eye is thought to occur by a hydrolysing enzyme. The amount of this enzyme is not changed by the prolonged use of pilocarpine by glaucoma patients, nor is it changed in patients poorly controlled by glaucoma therapy.

5.3 Preclinical safety data
There are no preclinical data of relevance to the prescriber which are additional to that already included in other sections of the SPC.

6. PHARMACEUTICAL PARTICULARS

6.1 List of excipients
Purified water

6.2 Incompatibilities
None known.

6.3 Shelf life
24 Months.

6.4 Special precautions for storage
Store below 25°C. Do not freeze. Protect from light.

6.5 Nature and contents of container
A sealed, conical shaped container fitted with a twist and pull-off cap. Each Minims unit is overwrapped in an individual polypropylene/paper pouch. Each container holds approximately 0.5ml of solution.

6.6 Instructions for use and handling
Each Minims unit should be discarded after a single use.

7. MARKETING AUTHORISATION HOLDER
Chauvin Pharmaceuticals Ltd

106 London Road

Kingston-upon-Thames

Surrey

KT2 6TN

8. MARKETING AUTHORISATION NUMBER(S)
PL 0033/5014R

9. DATE OF FIRST AUTHORISATION/RENEWAL OF THE AUTHORISATION
Date of first Authorisation: 19 May 1987

Date of renewal: 19 May 1992

10. DATE OF REVISION OF THE TEXT
March 1999.

June 2000

November 2002

Minims Pilocarpine Nitrate 4% w/v

(Chauvin Pharmaceuticals Ltd)

1. NAME OF THE MEDICINAL PRODUCT
Minims Pilocarpine Nitrate 4%

2. QUALITATIVE AND QUANTITATIVE COMPOSITION
Clear, colourless, sterile eye drops containing Pilocarpine Nitrate PhEur 4.0% w/v.

3. PHARMACEUTICAL FORM
Sterile, single-use eye drops.

4. CLINICAL PARTICULARS

4.1 Therapeutic indications
Pilocarpine is used as a miotic, for reversing the action of weaker mydriatics and in the emergency treatment of glaucoma.

4.2 Posology and method of administration
Adults (including the elderly) and children:

Instil dropwise into the eye according to the recommended dosage.

To induce miosis, one or two drops should be used.

In cases of emergency treatment of acute narrow-angle glaucoma, one drop should be used every five minutes until miosis is achieved.

4.3 Contraindications
Conditions where pupillary constriction is undesirable e.g. acute iritis, anterior uveitis and some forms of secondary glaucoma.

Hypersensitivity to any component of the preparation.

Patients with soft contact lenses should not use this preparation.

4.4 Special warnings and special precautions for use
Systemic reactions rarely occur when treating chronic simple glaucoma at normal doses. However, in the treatment of acute closed-angle glaucoma the possibility of systemic reactions must be considered because of the higher doses given. Caution is particularly advised in patients with acute heart failure, bronchial asthma, peptic ulceration, hypertension, urinary tract obstruction, Parkinson's disease and corneal abrasions.

Retinal detachments have been caused in susceptible individuals and those with pre-existing retinal disease, therefore, fundus examination is advised in all patients prior to the initiation of therapy.

Patients with chronic glaucoma on long-term pilocarpine therapy should have regular monitoring of intraocular pressure and visual fields.

Systemic absorption may be reduced by compressing the lacrimal sac at the medial canthus for a minute during and following the instillation of the drops. (This blocks the passage of the drops via the naso-lacrimal duct to the wide absorptive area of the nasal and pharyngeal mucosa. It is especially advisable in children.)

4.5 Interaction with other medicinal products and other forms of Interaction
Although clinically not proven, the miotic effects of pilocarpine may be antagonised by long-term topical or systemic corticosteroid therapy, systemic anticholinergics, antihistamines, pethidine, sympathomimetics or tricyclic antidepressants.

Concomitant administration of two miotics is not recommended because of inter-drug antagonism and the risk that unresponsiveness may develop to both drugs.

4.6 Pregnancy and lactation
Safety for use in pregnancy and lactation has not been established, therefore, use only when clearly indicated.

4.7 Effects on ability to drive and use machines
Causes difficulty with dark adaptation, therefore, caution is necessary when night driving and when hazardous tasks are undertaken in poor illumination. May cause accommodation spasm. Patients should be advised not to drive or use machinery if vision is not clear.

4.8 Undesirable effects
Local
Burning, itching, smarting, blurring of vision, ciliary spasm, conjunctival vascular congestion, induced myopia, sensitisation of the lids and conjunctiva, reduced visual acuity in poor illumination, lens changes with chronic use, increased pupillary block, retinal detachments and vitreous haemorrhages.

CNS
Browache and headache (especially in younger patients who have recently started therapy).

Systemic
Systemic reactions rarely occur in the treatment of chronic simple glaucoma but they may include hypotension, bradycardia, bronchial spasm, pulmonary oedema, salivation, sweating, nausea, vomiting, diarrhoea and lacrimation.

4.9 Overdose
If accidentally ingested, induce emesis or perform gastric lavage. Observe for signs of toxicity (salivation, lacrimation, sweating, bronchial spasm, cyanosis, nausea, vomiting and diarrhoea).

5. PHARMACOLOGICAL PROPERTIES

5.1 Pharmacodynamic properties
Pilocarpine is a direct acting parasympathomimetic drug. It duplicates the muscarinic effect of acetyl choline, but not its nicotinic effects. Consequently, pilocarpine stimulates the smooth muscle and secretary glands but does not affect the striated muscle.

5.2 Pharmacokinetic properties
Pilocarpine has a low ocular bioavailability when topically applied and this has been attributed to extensive precorneal drug loss in conjunction with the resistance to normal corneal penetration. Further, pilocarpine appears to bind to the eye pigments from which it is gradually released to the muscles.

Inactivation of pilocarpine in the eye is thought to occur by a hydrolysing enzyme. The amount of this enzyme is not changed by the prolonged use of pilocarpine by glaucoma patients, nor is it changed in patients poorly controlled by glaucoma therapy.

5.3 Preclinical safety data
There are no preclinical data of relevance to the prescriber which are additional to that already included in other sections of the SPC.

6. PHARMACEUTICAL PARTICULARS

6.1 List of excipients
Purified water

6.2 Incompatibilities
None known.

6.3 Shelf life
24 months.

6.4 Special precautions for storage
Store below 25°C. Do not freeze. Protect from light.

6.5 Nature and contents of container
A sealed, conical shaped container fitted with a twist and pull-off cap. Each Minims unit is overwrapped in an individual polypropylene/paper pouch. Each container holds approximately 0.5ml of solution.

6.6 Instructions for use and handling
Each Minims unit should be discarded after a single use.

7. MARKETING AUTHORISATION HOLDER
Chauvin Pharmaceuticals Ltd

106 London Road

Kingston-upon-Thames

Surrey

KT2 6TN

8. MARKETING AUTHORISATION NUMBER(S)
PL 0033/5016R

9. DATE OF FIRST AUTHORISATION/RENEWAL OF THE AUTHORISATION
Date of first Authorisation: 21 May 1987

Date of renewal: 21 May 1992

10. DATE OF REVISION OF THE TEXT
May 1997

March 1999

June 2000

November 2002

Minims Prednisolone Sodium Phosphate

(Chauvin Pharmaceuticals Ltd)

1. NAME OF THE MEDICINAL PRODUCT
Minims Prednisolone Sodium Phosphate

2. QUALITATIVE AND QUANTITATIVE COMPOSITION
Clear, colourless, sterile eye drops containing Prednisolone Sodium Phosphate BP 0.5% w/v.

3. PHARMACEUTICAL FORM
Sterile single-use eye drop.

4. CLINICAL PARTICULARS

4.1 Therapeutic indications
Non-infected inflammatory conditions of the eye.

4.2 Posology and method of administration
Adults and the elderly

One or two drops applied topically to the eye as required.

Children

At the discretion of the physician.

4.3 Contraindications
Use is contraindicated in viral, fungal, tuberculous and other bacterial infections.

Prolonged application to the eye of preparations containing corticosteroids has caused increased intraocular pressure and therefore the drops should not be used in patients with glaucoma.

In children, long-term, continuous topical corticosteroid therapy should be avoided due to possible adrenal suppression.

4.4 Special warnings and special precautions for use
Care should be taken to ensure that the eye is not infected before Minims Prednisolone is used.

Systemic absorption may be reduced by compressing the lacrimal sac at the medial canthus for a minute during and following the instillation of the drops. (This blocks the passage of drops via the naso-lacrimal duct to the wide absorptive area of the nasal and pharyngeal mucosa. It is especially advisable in children.).

4.5 Interaction with other medicinal products and other forms of Interaction
Corticosteroids are known to increase the effects of barbiturates, sedative hypnotics and tricyclic antidepressants.

They will, however, decrease the effects of anticholinesterases, antiviral eye preparations and salicylates.

4.6 Pregnancy and lactation
Topical administration of corticosteroids to pregnant animals can cause abnormalities of foetal development and although the relevance of this finding to human beings has not been established, the use of Minims Prednisolone during pregnancy should be avoided.

4.7 Effects on ability to drive and use machines
None known.

4.8 Undesirable effects
Prolonged treatment with corticosteroids in high dosage is occasionally associated with cataract.

The systemic effects of steroids are possible following the use of Minims Prednisolone, but are, however, unlikely due to the reduced absorption of topical eye drops.

4.9 Overdose
As Minims are single dose units, overdose is unlikely to occur.

5. PHARMACOLOGICAL PROPERTIES

5.1 Pharmacodynamic properties
The actions of corticosteroids are mediated by the binding of the corticosteroid molecules to receptor molecules located within sensitive cells. Corticosteroid receptors are present in human trabecular meshwork cells and in rabbit iris ciliary body tissue.

Prednisolone, in common with other corticosteroids, will inhibit phospholipase A2 and thus decrease prostaglandin formation.

The activation and migration of leucocytes will be affected by prednisolone. A 1% solution of prednisolone has been demonstrated to cause a 5.1% reduction in polymorphonuclear leucocyte mobilisation to an inflamed cornea. Corticosteroids will also lyse and destroy lymphocytes. These actions of prednisolone all contribute to its anti-inflammatory effect.

5.2 Pharmacokinetic properties
The oral availability, distribution and excretion of prednisolone is well documented. A figure of 82 ± 13% has been quoted as the oral availability and 1.4 ± 0.3ml/min/kg as the clearance rate. A half life of 2.1 - 4.0 hours has been calculated.

With regard to ocular pharmacokinetics, prednisolone sodium phosphate is a highly water soluble compound and is almost lipid insoluble. Therefore, theoretically it should not penetrate the intact corneal epithelium. Nevertheless, 30 minutes after instillation of a drop of 1% drug, corneal concentrations of 10μg/g and aqueous levels of 0.5μg/g have been attained. When a 0.5% solution was instilled in rabbit eyes every 15 minutes for an hour, an aqueous concentration of 2.5μg/ml was measured. Considerable variance exists in the intraocular penetration of prednisolone depending on whether the cornea is normal or abraded.

It can be seen that only low levels of prednisolone will be absorbed systemically, particularly where the cornea is intact.

Any prednisolone which is absorbed will be highly protein-bound in common with other corticosteroids.

5.3 Preclinical safety data
The use of prednisolone in ophthalmology is well-established. Little specific toxicology work has been reported, however, the breadth of clinical experience confirms its suitability as a topical ophthalmic agent.

6. PHARMACEUTICAL PARTICULARS

6.1 List of excipients
Disodium edetate

Disodium dihydrogen phosphate

Sodium chloride

Sodium hydroxide for pH adjustment

Purified water

6.2 Incompatibilities
None known.

6.3 Shelf life
15 months

6.4 Special precautions for storage
Store below 25°C. Do not freeze. Protect from light.

6.5 Nature and contents of container
A sealed conical shaped polypropylene container fitted with a twist and pull off cap. Each Minims unit is overwrapped in an individual polypropylene/paper pouch. Each container holds approximately 0.5ml of solution.

6.6 Instructions for use and handling
Each Minims unit should be discarded after a single use.

7. MARKETING AUTHORISATION HOLDER
Chauvin Pharmaceuticals Ltd

106 London Road

Kingston-upon-Thames

Surrey

KT2 6TN

8. MARKETING AUTHORISATION NUMBER(S)
PL 0033/0091

Legal category: **POM**

9. DATE OF FIRST AUTHORISATION/RENEWAL OF THE AUTHORISATION
Date of Grant: 11.3.81

Date of Last Renewal: 03.09.02

10. DATE OF REVISION OF THE TEXT
December 1996

November 2002

Minims Proxymetacaine

(Chauvin Pharmaceuticals Ltd)

1. NAME OF THE MEDICINAL PRODUCT
Minims Proxymetacaine 0.5% w/v, Eye Drops.

2. QUALITATIVE AND QUANTITATIVE COMPOSITION
Proxymetacaine hydrochloride 0.5%w/v.

For excipients see section 6.1

3. PHARMACEUTICAL FORM
Eye drops, solution.

Clear, colourless to pale yellow solution

4. CLINICAL PARTICULARS

4.1 Therapeutic indications
To be used as a topical ocular anaesthetic.

4.2 Posology and method of administration
Adults (including the elderly) and children:

Deep anaesthesia: Instil 1 drop every 5 - 10 minutes for 5 - 7 applications.

Removal of sutures: Instil 1 or 2 drops 2 to 3 minutes before removal of stitches.

Removal of foreign bodies: Instil 1 or 2 drops prior to operating.

Tonometry: Instil 1 or 2 drops immediately before measurement.

Do not use if the solution is more than pale yellow in colour.

Each Minims unit should be discarded after a single use

A period of at least one minute should be allowed after administration of Minims Proxymetacaine 0.5%, before subsequent administration of other topical agents.

4.3 Contraindications
Do not use in patients with a known hypersensitivity to any component of the preparation.

In view of the immaturity of the enzyme system which metabolises the ester type local anaesthetics in premature babies, this product should be avoided in these patients.

4.4 Special warnings and special precautions for use
This product should be used cautiously and sparingly in patients with known allergies, cardiac disease or hyperthyroidism because of the increased risk of sensitivity reactions.

This product is not intended for long term use. Regular and prolonged use of topical ocular anaesthetics e.g. in conjunction with contact lens insertion, may cause softening and erosion of the corneal epithelium, which could produce corneal opacification with accompanying loss of vision.

Minims Proxymetacaine is not miscible with fluorescein, however, fluorescein can be added to the eye after it has been anaesthetised with Minims Proxymetacaine.

Protection of the eye from rubbing, irritating chemicals and foreign bodies during the period of anaesthesia is very important. Patients should be advised to avoid touching the eye until the anaesthesia has worn off.

Tonometers soaked in sterilising or detergent solutions should be thoroughly rinsed with sterile distilled water prior to use.

Systemic absorption may be reduced by compressing the lacrimal sac at the medial canthus for a minute during and following instillation of the drops. (This blocks the passage of the drops via the naso lacrimal duct to the wide absorptive area of the nasal and pharyngeal mucosa. It is especially advisable in children).

Use with caution in an inflamed eye as hyperaemia greatly increases the rates of systemic absorption through the conjunctiva.

4.5 Interaction with other medicinal products and other forms of Interaction
None stated.

4.6 Pregnancy and lactation
Safety for use in pregnancy and lactation has not been established, therefore, use only when considered essential by the physician.

4.7 Effects on ability to drive and use machines
May cause transient blurring of vision on instillation. Warn patients not to drive or operate hazardous machinery unless vision is clear.

4.8 Undesirable effects
Pupillary dilatation or cycloplegic effects have rarely been observed with proxymetacaine preparations. Irritation of the conjunctiva or other toxic reactions have occurred only rarely. A severe, immediate-type apparently hyperallergic corneal reaction may rarely occur. This includes acute, intense and diffuse epithelial keratitis; a grey ground-glass appearance; sloughing of large areas of necrotic epithelium; corneal filaments and sometimes, iritis with descemetitis.

4.9 Overdose
Not applicable.

5. PHARMACOLOGICAL PROPERTIES

5.1 Pharmacodynamic properties
Proxymetacaine, in common with other local anaesthetics, reversibly blocks the initiation and conduction of nerve impulses by decreasing the permeability of the neuronal membrane to sodium ions.

The delay to onset of effect, duration of effect and potency of proxymetacaine are similar to those of amethocaine.

5.2 Pharmacokinetic properties
Proxymetacaine is readily absorbed into the systemic circulation where, in common with other ester-type local anaesthetics, it is hydrolysed by plasma esterases. Proxymetacaine is also subject to hepatic metabolism.

5.3 Preclinical safety data
No adverse safety issues were identified during the development of this formulation. The ingredients are well established in clinical ophthalmology.

6. PHARMACEUTICAL PARTICULARS

6.1 List of excipients
Purified water

Hydrochloric acid

Sodium hydroxide

6.2 Incompatibilities
None known.

6.3 Shelf life
2 years.

6.4 Special precautions for storage
Store at 2 - 8°C. Do not freeze. Keep container in the outer carton.

If necessary, the product may be stored at temperatures not exceeding 25°C for up to 1 month only.

6.5 Nature and contents of container
A sealed conical shaped polypropylene container fitted with a twist and pull off cap. Each Minims unit contains approximately 0.5ml of solution. Each unit is overwrapped in a polyethylene sachet. 20 units are packed into a suitable carton.

6.6 Instructions for use and handling
Each Minims unit should be discarded after a single use

If the product is to be stored unrefrigerated at temperatures not exceeding 25°C, prior to supply of the product by the pharmacy the adhesive label provided in the carton should be completed and affixed over the bar code, by a pharmacist. An expiry date one month from the supply date, plus the pharmacist's initials, should be written in the spaces provided on this label.

Administrative Data

7. MARKETING AUTHORISATION HOLDER
Chauvin Pharmaceuticals Ltd

106 London Road

Kingston-upon-Thames

Surrey

KT2 6TN

8. MARKETING AUTHORISATION NUMBER(S)
PL 0033/0151

PA 118/46/01

Legal category: **POM**

9. DATE OF FIRST AUTHORISATION/RENEWAL OF THE AUTHORISATION
6 March 1996/6 March 2001

10. DATE OF REVISION OF THE TEXT
February 2002

November 2002

Minims Proxymetacaine and Fluorescein

(Chauvin Pharmaceuticals Ltd)

1. NAME OF THE MEDICINAL PRODUCT
Minims Proxymetacaine & Fluorescein

2. QUALITATIVE AND QUANTITATIVE COMPOSITION
Clear, yellow solution containing 0.5% w/v proxymetacaine hydrochloride BP and 0.25% w/v fluorescein sodium BP.

3. PHARMACEUTICAL FORM
Single-use, sterile eye drops.

4. CLINICAL PARTICULARS
4.1 Therapeutic indications
As a combined topical ocular anaesthetic and diagnostic stain. Uses include tonometry, removal of corneal foreign bodies and other corneal or conjunctival procedures of short duration.

4.2 Posology and method of administration
Adults (including the elderly) and children:
Instil one or two drops into the conjunctival sac prior to the procedure.

Each Minims unit should be discarded after a single use to avoid risk of cross infection.

4.3 Contraindications
Do not use in patients with a known hypersensitivity to any component of the preparation.

In view of the immaturity of the enzyme system which metabolises the ester type local anaesthetics in premature babies, this product should be avoided in these patients.

4.4 Special warnings and special precautions for use
This product should be used cautiously and sparingly in patients with known allergies, cardiac disease or hyperthyroidism because of the increased risk of sensitivity reactions.

This product is not intended for long term use. Regular and prolonged use of topical ocular anaesthetics e.g. in conjunction with contact lens insertion, may cause softening and erosion of the corneal epithelium, which could produce corneal opacification with accompanying loss of vision.

Protection of the eye from rubbing, irritating chemicals and foreign bodies during the period of anaesthesia is very important. Patients should be advised to avoid touching the eye until the anaesthesia has worn off.

Tonometers soaked in sterilising or detergent solutions should be thoroughly rinsed with sterile distilled water prior to use.

Systemic absorption may be reduced by compressing the lacrimal sac at the medial canthus for a minute during and following instillation of the drops. (This blocks the passage of the drops via the naso-lacrimal duct to the wide absorptive area of the nasal and pharyngeal mucosa. It is especially advisable in children.)

4.5 Interaction with other medicinal products and other forms of Interaction
None stated.

4.6 Pregnancy and lactation
Safety for use in pregnancy and lactation has not been established, therefore, use only when considered essential by the doctor or eye specialist.

4.7 Effects on ability to drive and use machines
May cause transient blurring of vision on instillation. Warn patients not to drive or operate hazardous machinery unless vision is clear.

4.8 Undesirable effects
Transient mild stinging or blurring of vision may occur immediately following the use of this product.

Pupillary dilatation or cycloplegic effects have been observed infrequently with proxymetacaine preparations. Irritation of the conjunctiva or other toxic reactions have occurred only rarely. A severe, immediate-type apparently hyperallergic corneal reaction may rarely occur. This includes acute, intense and diffuse epithelial keratitis; a grey ground-glass appearance; sloughing of large areas of necrotic epithelium; corneal filaments and sometimes, iritis with descemetitis.

4.9 Overdose
Not applicable.

5. PHARMACOLOGICAL PROPERTIES
5.1 Pharmacodynamic properties
Proxymetacaine, in common with other local anaesthetics, reversibly blocks the initiation and conduction of the nerve impulses by decreasing the permeability of the neuronal membrane to sodium ions.

The time to onset of effect, duration of effect and potency of proxymetacaine are similar to those of amethocaine.

Fluorescein does not stain a normal cornea but conjunctival abrasions are stained yellow or orange, corneal abrasions are stained a bright green and foreign bodies are surrounded by a green ring.

5.2 Pharmacokinetic properties
Proxymetacaine is readily absorbed into the systemic circulation where, in common with other ester-type local anaesthetics, it is hydrolysed by plasma esterases. Proxymetacaine is also subject to hepatic metabolism.

Fluorescein will resist penetration of a normal cornea and most will therefore be carried with the tear film away from the conjunctival sac. The majority will be lost through the naso-lacrimal ducts and absorbed via the gastro-intestinal tract from where it is converted rapidly to glucuronide and excreted via the urine.

If fluorescein crosses the cornea it will enter the Bowman's membrane, stroma and possibly the anterior chamber. Aqueous flow and diffusion into the blood in the anterior area finally remove fluorescein from the eye and it is excreted unchanged in the urine.

5.3 Preclinical safety data
No adverse safety issues were identified during the development of this formulation. The ingredients are well established in clinical ophthalmology.

6. PHARMACEUTICAL PARTICULARS
6.1 List of excipients
Purified water

Povidone K30

Hydrochloric acid

Sodium Hydroxide

6.2 Incompatibilities
None known.

6.3 Shelf life
24 months.

6.4 Special precautions for storage
The product should be transported in the original packaging. It should be stored at 2 - 8°C and prevented from freezing.

If necessary, the product may be stored at temperatures not exceeding 25°C for up to 1 month only.

6.5 Nature and contents of container
A sealed conical shaped polypropylene container fitted with a twist and pull-off cap. Each Minims unit contains approximately 0.5ml of solution. Each unit is overwrapped in a polyethylene sachet. 20 units are packed into a suitable carton.

6.6 Instructions for use and handling
Each Minims unit should be discarded after a single use.

Excess solution may be washed away with sterile saline solution.

If the product is to be stored unrefrigerated at temperatures not exceeding 25°C, the adhesive label provided in the carton should be completed and affixed over the bar code, by a pharmacist prior to supply of the product by the pharmacy. An expiry date one month from the supply date, plus the pharmacist's initials, should be written in the spaces provided on this label.

Administrative Data
7. MARKETING AUTHORISATION HOLDER
Chauvin Pharmaceuticals Ltd

106 London Road

Kingston-upon-Thames

Surrey

KT2 6TN

8. MARKETING AUTHORISATION NUMBER(S)
PL 0033/0152

Legal category: POM

9. DATE OF FIRST AUTHORISATION/RENEWAL OF THE AUTHORISATION
17 February 1997

10. DATE OF REVISION OF THE TEXT
January 1999.

May 2000

November 2002

Minims Rose Bengal

(Chauvin Pharmaceuticals Ltd)

1. NAME OF THE MEDICINAL PRODUCT
Minims Rose Bengal.

2. QUALITATIVE AND QUANTITATIVE COMPOSITION
1% w/v solution of rose bengal.

3. PHARMACEUTICAL FORM
Single-use, sterile eye drops.

4. CLINICAL PARTICULARS
4.1 Therapeutic indications
As a diagnostic stain.

Rose bengal solution stains degenerated conjunctival and corneal epithelial cells. It is particularly useful in demonstrating these changes in Sjögren's syndrome, where lack of tears has caused damage.

4.2 Posology and method of administration
Adults (including the elderly) and Children:

One or two drops to be instilled topically into the eye, as required.

4.3 Contraindications
Rose bengal can produce severe stinging in dry eyes, where it should be used with care.

4.4 Special warnings and special precautions for use
Rose bengal should not be instilled into the eye when the patient is wearing contact lenses.

4.5 Interaction with other medicinal products and other forms of Interaction
None known.

4.6 Pregnancy and lactation
The use of rose bengal over the last 15 years has not shown any adverse effects. In the absence of any teratology studies, however, rose bengal is not recommended in pregnancy unless the therapeutic benefit exceeds the potential risk.

4.7 Effects on ability to drive and use machines
May cause transient blurring of vision on instillation. Warn patients not to drive or operate hazardous machinery until vision is clear.

4.8 Undesirable effects
Rose bengal may discolour the eye lids and/or conjunctiva.

4.9 Overdose
As Minims are single-dose units, overdose is unlikely to occur.

5. PHARMACOLOGICAL PROPERTIES
5.1 Pharmacodynamic properties
Not applicable.

5.2 Pharmacokinetic properties
Rose bengal stains degenerated conjunctival and corneal epithelial cells. It will resist penetration through a normal cornea as it is virtually unable to pass through the membrane of live cells. Therefore, the majority of solution will be carried with the tear film away from the conjunctiva and lost via the naso-lacrimal ducts. In rabbits, this has been demonstrated to occur within a few minutes, but in humans with a normal function, this would seem to occur within 15 - 30 minutes. Rose bengal remains in the stained structure and does not diffuse further nor penetrate into the aqueous humour from a mucosal defect. Thus, the stain will remain in the damaged corneal cells and be removed together with these cells. Therefore, the concentration of rose bengal absorbed systemically is likely to be negligible.

5.3 Preclinical safety data
There are no preclinical data of relevance to the prescriber which are additional to that already included in other sections of the SPC.

6. PHARMACEUTICAL PARTICULARS
6.1 List of excipients
Sodium hydroxide BP

Purified water PhEur

6.2 Incompatibilities
None known.

6.3 Shelf life
15 months.

6.4 Special precautions for storage
Store below 25°C. Do not freeze. Protect from light.

6.5 Nature and contents of container
A sealed conical shaped polypropylene container fitted with a twist and pull-off cap. Overwrapped in an individual polypropylene/paper pouch. Each container holds approximately 0.5ml of solution. 20 units are packed into a suitable carton.

6.6 Instructions for use and handling
Each Minims unit should be discarded after a single use.

7. MARKETING AUTHORISATION HOLDER
Chauvin Pharmaceuticals Ltd

106 London Road

Kingston-upon-Thames

Surrey

KT2 6TN

8. MARKETING AUTHORISATION NUMBER(S)
PL 0033/0048R

9. DATE OF FIRST AUTHORISATION/RENEWAL OF THE AUTHORISATION
15.7.87/15.7.92

10. DATE OF REVISION OF THE TEXT
July 1997.

November 2002

Minims Saline

(Chauvin Pharmaceuticals Ltd)

1. NAME OF THE MEDICINAL PRODUCT
Minims Saline (Astromins, Ultra Saline Minims).

2. QUALITATIVE AND QUANTITATIVE COMPOSITION
A clear, colourless liquid containing Sodium Chloride PhEur 0.9% w/v.

3. PHARMACEUTICAL FORM
Single-use, sterile eye drops.

4. CLINICAL PARTICULARS
4.1 Therapeutic indications
As a topical ocular irrigating solution.

4.2 Posology and method of administration
Adults (including the elderly) and Children:
Adequate solution should be used to irrigate the eye.

4.3 Contraindications
None.

4.4 Special warnings and special precautions for use
None.

4.5 Interaction with other medicinal products and other forms of Interaction
None known.

4.6 Pregnancy and lactation
Not applicable.

4.7 Effects on ability to drive and use machines
None known.

4.8 Undesirable effects
None known.

4.9 Overdose
Not applicable.

5. PHARMACOLOGICAL PROPERTIES
5.1 Pharmacodynamic properties
Minims Saline is an isotonic solution of sodium chloride used for irrigation of the eye. There are no pharmacodynamic properties of relevance for this product.

5.2 Pharmacokinetic properties
There are no pharmacokinetic properties which are applicable for this product.

5.3 Preclinical safety data
There are no preclinical data of relevance to the prescriber which are additional to that already included in other sections of the SPC.

6. PHARMACEUTICAL PARTICULARS
6.1 List of excipients
Purified Water

6.2 Incompatibilities
None known.

6.3 Shelf life
15 months.

6.4 Special precautions for storage
Store below 25°C. Do not freeze. Protect from light.

6.5 Nature and contents of container
A sealed conical shaped container fitted with a twist and pull off cap overwrapped in an individual polypropylene/paper pouch. Each Minims unit contains approximately 0.5ml of solution.

6.6 Instructions for use and handling
Discard each unit after a single use.

7. MARKETING AUTHORISATION HOLDER
Chauvin Pharmaceuticals Ltd
106 London Road
Kingston-upon-Thames
Surrey
KT2 6TN

8. MARKETING AUTHORISATION NUMBER(S)
PL 0033/5017R

9. DATE OF FIRST AUTHORISATION/RENEWAL OF THE AUTHORISATION
Date of first Authorisation: 19.5.87.

10. DATE OF REVISION OF THE TEXT
June 1997
November 2002

Minims Tetracaine Hydrochloride 0.5%

(Chauvin Pharmaceuticals Ltd)

1. NAME OF THE MEDICINAL PRODUCT
Minims Tetracaine Hydrochloride 0.5% w/v

2. QUALITATIVE AND QUANTITATIVE COMPOSITION
Single-use, clear, colourless, sterile eye drops containing tetracaine hydrochloride Ph.Eur. 0.5% w/v solution.

3. PHARMACEUTICAL FORM
Single-use, sterile eye drops.

4. CLINICAL PARTICULARS
4.1 Therapeutic indications
Ocular anaesthetic for topical instillation into the conjunctival sac.

4.2 Posology and method of administration
Adults and children
One drop or as required. Each Minims unit should be discarded after use.

4.3 Contraindications
Not to be used in patients with a known hypersensitivity to the product.

Tetracaine is hydrolysed in the body to p-amino-benzoic acid and should not therefore be used in patients being treated with sulphonamides.

In view of the immaturity of the enzyme system which metabolises the ester type local anaesthetics in premature babies, tetracaine should be avoided in these patients.

4.4 Special warnings and special precautions for use
The anaesthetised eye should be protected from dust and bacterial contamination.

Tetracaine may give rise to dermatitis in hypersensitive patients.

On instillation an initial burning sensation may be experienced. This may last for up to 30 seconds.

The cornea may be damaged by prolonged application of anaesthetic eye drops.

Systemic absorption may be reduced by compressing the lacrimal sac at the medial canthus for a minute during and following the instillation of the drops. (This blocks the passage of the drops via the naso lacrimal duct to the wide absorptive area of the nasal and pharyngeal mucosa. It is especially advisable in children.)

4.5 Interaction with other medicinal products and other forms of Interaction
Tetracaineshould not be used in patients being treated with sulphonamides (see 4.3 above)

4.6 Pregnancy and lactation
Safety for use in pregnancy and lactation has not been established, therefore, use only when considered essential by the physician.

4.7 Effects on ability to drive and use machines
May cause transient blurring of vision on instillation. Warn patients not to drive or operate hazardous machinery unless vision is clear.

4.8 Undesirable effects
Not applicable.

4.9 Overdose
Not expected.

5. PHARMACOLOGICAL PROPERTIES
5.1 Pharmacodynamic properties
Tetracaine hydrochloride is used as a local anaesthetic which acts by reversibly blocking the propagation and conduction of nerve impulses along nerve axons. Tetracaine stabilises the nerve membrane, preventing the increase in sodium permeability necessary for the production of an action potential.

5.2 Pharmacokinetic properties
Tetracaine is a weak base (pK_a 8.5), therefore, significant changes in the rate of ionised lipid soluble drug uptake may occur with changes in the acid base balance.

In vitro studies have shown that tetracaine has a high affinity for melanin, therefore, differences in duration of action may be expected between deeply pigmented eyes and less pigmented eyes.

The primary site of metabolism for tetracaine is the plasma. Pseudocholinesterases in the plasma hydrolyse tetracaine to 4-aminobenzoic acid. Unmetabolised drug is excreted in the urine.

5.3 Preclinical safety data
No adverse safety issues were detected during the development of this formulation. The active ingredient is well established in clinical ophthalmology.

6. PHARMACEUTICAL PARTICULARS
6.1 List of excipients
Hydrochloric Acid
Purified Water

6.2 Incompatibilities
None known.

6.3 Shelf life
Unopened: 24 Months.

6.4 Special precautions for storage
Store below 25°C. Do not freeze. Protect from light.

6.5 Nature and contents of container
A sealed conical shaped polypropylene container fitted with a twist and pull off cap. Overwrapped in an individual polypropylene/paper pouch. Each container holds approximately 0.5ml of solution.

6.6 Instructions for use and handling
Each Minims unit should be discarded after use.

7. MARKETING AUTHORISATION HOLDER
Chauvin Pharmaceuticals Ltd
106 London Road
Kingston-upon-Thames
Surrey
KT2 6TN

8. MARKETING AUTHORISATION NUMBER(S)
PL 0033/5000R

9. DATE OF FIRST AUTHORISATION/RENEWAL OF THE AUTHORISATION
Date of first Authorisation: 1.5.87

10. DATE OF REVISION OF THE TEXT
December 1997
August2000
November 2002
January 2005

Minims Tetracaine Hydrochloride 1.0%

(Chauvin Pharmaceuticals Ltd)

1. NAME OF THE MEDICINAL PRODUCT
Minims Tetracaine Hydrochloride 1% w/v

2. QUALITATIVE AND QUANTITATIVE COMPOSITION
Single-use, clear, colourless, sterile eye drops tetracaine hydrochloride Ph.Eur. 1% w/v solution.

3. PHARMACEUTICAL FORM
Single-use, sterile eye drops.

4. CLINICAL PARTICULARS
4.1 Therapeutic indications
Ocular anaesthetic for topical instillation into the conjunctival sac.

4.2 Posology and method of administration
Adults and children
One drop or as required. Each Minims unit should be discarded after use.

4.3 Contraindications
Not to be used in patients with a known hypersensitivity to the product.

Tetracaine is hydrolysed in the body to p-amino-benzoic acid and should not therefore be used in patients being treated with sulphonamides.

In view of the immaturity of the enzyme system which metabolises the ester type local anaesthetics in premature babies, tetracaine should be avoided in these patients.

4.4 Special warnings and special precautions for use
The cornea may be damaged by prolonged application of anaesthetic eye drops.

The anaesthetised eye should be protected from dust and bacterial contamination.

Systemic absorption may be reduced by compressing the lacrimal sac at the medial canthus for a minute during and following the instillation of the drops. (This blocks the passage of the drops via the naso lacrimal duct to the wide absorptive area of the nasal and pharyngeal mucosa. It is especially advisable in children.)

4.5 Interaction with other medicinal products and other forms of Interaction
Tetracaine should not be used in patients being treated with sulphonamides (see 4.3 above)

4.6 Pregnancy and lactation
Safety for use in pregnancy and lactation has not been established, therefore, use only when considered essential by the physician.

4.7 Effects on ability to drive and use machines
May cause transient blurring of vision on instillation. Warn patients not to drive or operate hazardous machinery unless vision is clear.

4.8 Undesirable effects
Tetracaine may give rise to dermatitis in hypersensitive patients.

On instillation an initial burning sensation may be experienced. This may last for up to 30 seconds.

The cornea may be damaged by prolonged application of anaesthetic eye drops.

4.9 Overdose
Not expected.

5. PHARMACOLOGICAL PROPERTIES
5.1 Pharmacodynamic properties
Tetracaine hydrochloride is used as a local anaesthetic which acts by reversibly blocking the propagation and conduction of nerve impulses along nerve axons. Tetracaine stabilises the nerve membrane, preventing the increase in sodium permeability necessary for the production of an action potential.

5.2 Pharmacokinetic properties
Tetracaine is a weak base (pK_a 8.5), therefore, significant changes in the rate of ionised lipid soluble drug uptake may occur with changes in the acid base balance.

In vitro studies have shown that tetracaine has a high affinity for melanin, therefore, differences in duration of action may be expected between deeply pigmented eyes and less pigmented eyes.

The primary site of metabolism for tetracaine is the plasma. Pseudocholinesterases in the plasma hydrolyse tetracaine to 4-aminobenzoic acid. Unmetabolised drug is excreted in the urine.

5.3 Preclinical safety data
No adverse safety issues were detected during the development of this formulation. The active ingredient is well established in clinical ophthalmology.

6. PHARMACEUTICAL PARTICULARS

6.1 List of excipients
Hydrochloric Acid

Purified Water

6.2 Incompatibilities
None known.

6.3 Shelf life
Unopened: 24 months.

6.4 Special precautions for storage
Store below 25°C. Do not freeze. Protect from light.

6.5 Nature and contents of container
A sealed conical shaped polypropylene container fitted with a twist and pull off cap. Overwrapped in an individual polypropylene/paper pouch. Each container holds approximately 0.5ml of solution.

6.6 Instructions for use and handling
Each Minims unit should be discarded after use.

7. MARKETING AUTHORISATION HOLDER
Chauvin Pharmaceuticals Ltd

106 London Road

Kingston-upon-Thames

Surrey

KT2 6TN

8. MARKETING AUTHORISATION NUMBER(S)
PL 0033/5001R

9. DATE OF FIRST AUTHORISATION/RENEWAL OF THE AUTHORISATION
Date of first Authorisation: 5.3.87

Date of last renewal of Authorisation: 10.4.97

10. DATE OF REVISION OF THE TEXT
December 1997

August 2000

July 2002

November2002

January 2005

Minims Tropicamide 0.5% w/v

(Chauvin Pharmaceuticals Ltd)

1. NAME OF THE MEDICINAL PRODUCT
Minims Tropicamide 0.5 %.

2. QUALITATIVE AND QUANTITATIVE COMPOSITION
Clear, colourless, sterile eye drops containing tropicamide BP 0.5 % w/v.

3. PHARMACEUTICAL FORM
Single-use, sterile eye drops.

4. CLINICAL PARTICULARS

4.1 Therapeutic indications
As a topical mydriatic and cycloplegic.

4.2 Posology and method of administration
Adults (including the elderly):

2 drops at 5 minute intervals, with a further 1 to 2 drops after 30 minutes, if required.

Children:

At the discretion of the physician.

4.3 Contraindications
Do not use in patients with a known hypersensitivity to tropicamide.

Tropicamide is contraindicated in narrow angle glaucoma and in eyes where the filtration angle is narrow, as an acute attack of angle closure glaucoma may be precipitated.

4.4 Special warnings and special precautions for use
Use with caution in an inflamed eye, as hyperaemia greatly increases the rate of systemic absorption through the conjunctiva.

Care should be exercised in small children.

Systemic absorption may be reduced by compressing the lacrimal sac at the medial canthus for a minute during and following the instillation of the drops. (This blocks the passage of drops via the naso-lacrimal duct to the wide absorptive area of the nasal and pharyngeal mucosa. It is especially advisable in children.)

4.5 Interaction with other medicinal products and other forms of Interaction
None known.

4.6 Pregnancy and lactation
There is no evidence as to the drug's safety in human pregnancy, nor is there evidence from animal work that it is free from hazard. This product should only be used in pregnancy if considered essential by the physician.

4.7 Effects on ability to drive and use machines
Patient warning: Patients who receive a mydriatic may suffer from photophobia and this may impair their ability to drive under certain circumstances.

4.8 Undesirable effects
Transient stinging, dry mouth and blurred vision may occur following the use of this product.

4.9 Overdose
Systemic effects from Minims Tropicamide are not expected. Should an overdose occur causing local effects, e.g. sustained mydriasis, pilocarpine or 0.25% w/v physostigmine should be applied.

5. PHARMACOLOGICAL PROPERTIES

5.1 Pharmacodynamic properties
Tropicamide is a parasympatholytic agent, which acts by blocking the action of the parasympathetic nervous system. As acetylcholine is the neuro-humoral transmitter at the receptor site of the parasympathetic nervous system, tropicamide competes with acetylcholine for uptake at the receptor sites, thereby blocking its action. The results are mydriasis, due to unopposed action of the dilator pupillae, and cycloplegia.

5.2 Pharmacokinetic properties
No data on the pharmacokinetics of topical tropicamide are available.

5.3 Preclinical safety data
There are no preclinical data of relevance to the prescriber which are additional to that already included in other sections of the SPC.

6. PHARMACEUTICAL PARTICULARS

6.1 List of excipients
Sodium hydroxide

Hydrochloric acid

Purified water

6.2 Incompatibilities
None known.

6.3 Shelf life
15 months.

6.4 Special precautions for storage
Store below 25°C. Do not freeze. Protect from light.

6.5 Nature and contents of container
A sealed, conical shaped container fitted with a twist and pull-off cap. Each Minims unit is overwrapped in an individual polypropylene/paper pouch. Each container holds approximately 0.5ml of solution.

6.6 Instructions for use and handling
Each Minims unit should be discarded after a single use.

7. MARKETING AUTHORISATION HOLDER
Chauvin Pharmaceuticals Ltd

106 London Road

Kingston-upon-Thames

Surrey

KT2 6TN

England

8. MARKETING AUTHORISATION NUMBER(S)
PL 0033/0077

Legal category: POM

9. DATE OF FIRST AUTHORISATION/RENEWAL OF THE AUTHORISATION
Date of first Authorisation: 10.7.79

10. DATE OF REVISION OF THE TEXT
June 1997.

November 2002

Minims Tropicamide 1% w/v

(Chauvin Pharmaceuticals Ltd)

1. NAME OF THE MEDICINAL PRODUCT
Minims Tropicamide 1%.

2. QUALITATIVE AND QUANTITATIVE COMPOSITION
Clear, colourless, sterile eye drops containing tropicamide BP 1% w/v.

3. PHARMACEUTICAL FORM
Single-use, sterile eye drops.

4. CLINICAL PARTICULARS

4.1 Therapeutic indications
As a topical mydriatic and cycloplegic.

4.2 Posology and method of administration
Adults (including the elderly):

2 drops at 5 minute intervals, with a further 1 to 2 drops after 30 minutes, if required.

Children:

At the discretion of the physician.

4.3 Contraindications
Do not use in patients with a known hypersensitivity to tropicamide.

Tropicamide is contraindicated in narrow angle glaucoma and in eyes where the filtration angle is narrow, as an acute attack of angle closure glaucoma may be precipitated.

4.4 Special warnings and special precautions for use
Use with caution in an inflamed eye, as hyperaemia greatly increases the rate of systemic absorption through the conjunctiva.

Care should be exercised in small children.

Systemic absorption may be reduced by compressing the lacrimal sac at the medial canthus for a minute during and following the instillation of the drops. (This blocks the passage of drops via the naso-lacrimal duct to the wide absorptive area of the nasal and pharyngeal mucosa. It is especially advisable in children.)

4.5 Interaction with other medicinal products and other forms of Interaction
None known.

4.6 Pregnancy and lactation
There is no evidence as to the drug's safety in human pregnancy, nor is there evidence from animal work that it is free from hazard. This product should only be used in pregnancy if considered essential by the physician

4.7 Effects on ability to drive and use machines
Patient warning: Patients who receive a mydriatic may suffer from photophobia and this may impair their ability to drive under certain circumstances.

4.8 Undesirable effects
Transient stinging, dry mouth and blurred vision may occur following the use of this product.

4.9 Overdose
Systemic effects from Minims Tropicamide are not expected. Should an overdose occur causing local effects, e.g. sustained mydriasis, pilocarpine or 0.25% w/v physostigmine should be applied.

5. PHARMACOLOGICAL PROPERTIES

5.1 Pharmacodynamic properties
Tropicamide is a parasympatholytic agent, which acts by blocking the action of the parasympathetic nervous system. As acetylcholine is the neuro-humoral transmitter at the receptor site of the parasympathetic nervous system, tropicamide competes with acetylcholine for uptake at the receptor sites, thereby blocking its action. The results are mydriasis, due to unopposed action of the dilator pupillae, and cycloplegia.

5.2 Pharmacokinetic properties
No data on the pharmacokinetics of topical tropicamide are available.

5.3 Preclinical safety data
There are no preclinical data of relevance to the prescriber which are additional to that already included in other sections of the SPC.

6. PHARMACEUTICAL PARTICULARS

6.1 List of excipients
Sodium hydroxide

Hydrochloric acid

Purified water

6.2 Incompatibilities
None known.

6.3 Shelf life
15 months.

6.4 Special precautions for storage
Store below 25°C. Do not freeze. Protect from light.

6.5 Nature and contents of container
A sealed, conical shaped container fitted with a twist and pull-off cap. Each Minims unit is overwrapped in an individual polypropylene/paper **pouch. Each container holds approximately 0.5ml of solution.**

6.6 Instructions for use and handling
Each Minims unit should be discarded after a single use.

7. MARKETING AUTHORISATION HOLDER
Chauvin Pharmaceuticals Ltd

106 London Road

Kingston-upon-Thames

Surrey

KT2 6TN

England

8. MARKETING AUTHORISATION NUMBER(S)
PL 0033/0078

Legal category: POM

9. DATE OF FIRST AUTHORISATION/RENEWAL OF THE AUTHORISATION
Date of first Authorisation: 10.7.79

10. DATE OF REVISION OF THE TEXT
June 1997.

November 2002

Minitran 5, Minitran 10, Minitran 15

(3M Health Care Limited)

1. NAME OF THE MEDICINAL PRODUCT
Minitran 5

Minitran 10

Minitran 15

2. QUALITATIVE AND QUANTITATIVE COMPOSITION
Minitran 5 has a surface area of 6.7 sq cm and contains 18 mg of glyceryl trinitrate. The average amount delivered in 24 hours is 5 mg.

Minitran 10 has a surface area of 13.3 sq cm and contains 36 mg of glyceryl trinitrate. The average amount delivered in 24 hours is 10 mg.

Minitran 15 has a surface area of 20 sq cm and contains 54 mg of glyceryl trinitrate. The average amount delivered in 24 hours is 15 mg.

3. PHARMACEUTICAL FORM
Adhesive transdermal patch.

4. CLINICAL PARTICULARS
4.1 Therapeutic indications
Minitran 5, Minitran 10 and Miniitran 15 are indicated for:

1. Prophylaxis of angina pectoris either alone or in combination with other anti-anginal therapy.

Minitran 5 is also indicated for:

2. Maintenance of venous patency at peripheral infusion sites.

4.2 Posology and method of administration
ADULTS:

1. Prophylaxis of angina pectoris

The response to nitrates differs between individuals, and the minimum effective dose should be prescribed in each case. It is therefore recommended that treatment is started with one Minitran 5 patch per day, with upward dosage titration when necessary. Application can either be for a continuous period of 24 hours or intermittently, incorporating a patch free interval (usually at night). Attenuation of effect has occurred in some patients being treated with sustained release nitrate preparations. On the basis of current clinical studies it is recommended that in such cases Minitran should be applied daily with a patch free interval of 8 - 12 hours.

Each Minitran patch is contained in a sealed sachet. The adhesive layer is covered by a protective film, which should be removed before application. The Minitran patch should be applied to a clean, dry healthy area of skin on the torso or the arms.

Subsequent patches should not be applied to the same area of skin until several days have elapsed. The Minitran patch adheres easily to the skin, and also stays in place whilst bathing or during physical exercise.

2. Maintenance of Venous Patency

One Minitran 5 patch is applied distal and close to the site of intravenous cannulation at the time of venepuncture. The patch should be changed daily. Treatment with Minitran 5 should be discontinued when intravenous therapy is stopped.

ELDERLY: No specific information on use in the elderly is available, but there is no evidence to suggest that an alteration in dose is required.

CHILDREN: The safety and efficacy of Minitran in children has yet to be established, and therefore recommendations for its use cannot be made.

4.3 Contraindications
Sildenafil has been shown to potentiate the hypotensive effects of nitrates, and its co-administration with nitrates or nitric oxide donors is therefore contra-indicated.

The use of glyceryl trinitrate is contra-indicated in cases of known hypersensitivity to nitrates, severe anaemia, increased intra-ocular and intracranial pressure, and marked arterial hypotension. It is also contra-indicated in acute myocardial insufficiency due to obstruction as in aortic or mitral stenosis or of constrictive pericarditis.

4.4 Special warnings and special precautions for use
Minitran is not indicated for the treatment of acute angina attacks requiring rapid relief. Minitran should be used only under strict medical supervision in recent myocardial infarction or acute congestive cardiac insufficiency. Minitran should be used with caution in patients with hypoxaemia, severe anaemia or ventilation perfusion imbalance.

The appearance of cross-tolerance with other nitrates is possible.

The use of products for topical application, especially if prolonged, may give rise to sensitisation phenomena, in which case treatment should be suspended, and suitable therapeutic measures adopted.

Minitran does not contain any metal components, and therefore it is not considered necessary to remove the patch prior to diathermy or cardioversion.

4.5 Interaction with other medicinal products and other forms of Interaction
The hypotensive effects of nitrates are potentiated by concurrent administration of sildenafil. Concomitant use of Minitran and other vasodilatory agents, calcium antagonists, beta-blockers, ACE inhibitors, neuroleptics, diuretics, antihypertensives, tricyclic antidepressants, and alcohol may decrease blood pressure. The effect of Minitran may be weakened by acetylsalicylic acid or other NSAID's. There is a risk of coronary artery constriction with concurrent administration of dihydroergotamine.

4.6 Pregnancy and lactation
As with all drugs Minitran should not be prescribed during pregnancy, particularly during the first trimester, unless there are compelling reasons for doing so. It is not known whether the active substance passes into the breast milk. The benefits for the mother must be weighed against the risks for the child.

4.7 Effects on ability to drive and use machines
The product may give rise to postural hypotension, and it is therefore advisable to warn patients of this possibility, so that they avoid sudden positional changes at the start of treatment. Care should also be exercised when driving vehicles and operating machinery.

4.8 Undesirable effects
Central Nervous System: Glyceryl trinitrate is generally well tolerated. The most frequently encountered side effect is headache, particularly when high doses are used; this usually disappears after a few days, but in particularly intense cases, it may be necessary to reduce the dose or interrupt treatment.

Cardio-vascular: Other undesirable effects observed, especially at the start of treatment, are: arterial hypotension (especially postural), tachycardia, fainting, palpitations, hot flushes, dizziness.

Gastro-intestinal: Nausea and vomiting are rarely observed.

Skin: Reddening of the skin, with or without itching or a slight erythematous reaction is occasionally observed. These effects, however, generally disappear a few hours after removal of the patch without adopting other measures. The site of application should be altered daily to avoid local irritation.

4.9 Overdose
High doses of glyceryl trinitrate may sometimes induce too rapid a reduction in arterial pressure, causing collapse. Due to the controlled release of glyceryl trinitrate from Minitran, overdosage is likely to be rare. In cases of suspected overdosage the Minitran patch should be removed and any reduction of the arterial blood pressure and symptoms of collapse should be treated by appropriate measures.

5. PHARMACOLOGICAL PROPERTIES
5.1 Pharmacodynamic properties
Nitroglycerin, the active constituent of Minitran is a dilator of smooth muscle, producing relaxation by an unknown mechanism. It has no direct effects on the inotropic or chronotropic state of the heart. It affects cardiac output only as a consequence of its effect on venous capacitance and arteriolar resistance vessels. These effects on preload and afterload reduce myocardial oxygen consumption and are primarily responsible for the mechanism by which nitroglycerin relieves the symptoms of angina pectoris. The drug's principal side effects (headache, flushing, dizziness, postural hypotension and tachycardia) are also a result of its smooth muscle relaxing effects.

5.2 Pharmacokinetic properties
When Minitran is applied to the skin, nitroglycerin is absorbed continuously through the skin into the systemic circulation and thus reaches the target organs (heart, vascular system) before deactivation by the liver. Minitran gives continuous release of nitroglycerin over 24 hours maintaining constant plasma levels. Nitroglycerin is metabolised by hydrolysis to dinitrates and the mononitrate.

5.3 Preclinical safety data
Not applicable.

6. PHARMACEUTICAL PARTICULARS
6.1 List of excipients
Isooctyl Acrylate/Acrylamide Copolymer (93:7)

Ethyl Oleate BP

Glyceryl Monolaurate

Low Density Polyethylene Film

One Side Silicone Coated Polyester Film

6.2 Incompatibilities
None known.

6.3 Shelf life
3 years.

6.4 Special precautions for storage
Minitran must be stored at room temperature (below 25 °C) under exclusion of light and moisture.

6.5 Nature and contents of container
Each patch is individually packed in a heat sealed foil sachet. Cartons contain 30 patches.

6.6 Instructions for use and handling
The patch is covered by a protective polyester film, which is detached and discarded before use.

7. MARKETING AUTHORISATION HOLDER
3M Health Care Limited

3M House

Morley Street

Loughborough

Leics LE11 1EP

8. MARKETING AUTHORISATION NUMBER(S)
Minitran 5 00068/0182

Minitran 10 00068/0183

Minitran 15 00068/0184

9. DATE OF FIRST AUTHORISATION/RENEWAL OF THE AUTHORISATION
25 July 2001

10. DATE OF REVISION OF THE TEXT
03 January 2002

Minocin MR

(Wyeth Pharmaceuticals)

1. NAME OF THE MEDICINAL PRODUCT
MINOCIN MR Capsules 100mg.

2. QUALITATIVE AND QUANTITATIVE COMPOSITION
MINOCIN MR Capsules contain 100mg of the active ingredient minocycline hydrochloride.

For excipients see 6.1

3. PHARMACEUTICAL FORM
Modified release capsule.

Two piece capsule with an orange body and brown cap, printed "Lederle" and "8560" in white ink, containing a mixture of yellow and off- white round pellets.

4. CLINICAL PARTICULARS
4.1 Therapeutic indications
MINOCIN MR Capsules are indicated for the treatment of acne.

4.2 Posology and method of administration
Dosage:

Adults: One 100mg capsule every 24 hours.

Children over 12 years: One 100mg capsule every 24 hours.

Children under 12 years: MINOCIN is not recommended.

Elderly: No special dosing requirements.

Administration:

To reduce the risk of oesophageal irritation and ulceration, the capsules should be swallowed whole with plenty of fluid, while sitting or standing. Unlike earlier tetracyclines, absorption of Minocin MR is not significantly impaired by food or moderate amounts of milk.

Treatment of acne should be continued for a minimum of 6 weeks. If, after six months, there is no satisfactory response Minocin MR should be discontinued and other therapies considered. If Minocin MR is to be continued for longer than six months, patients should be monitored at least three monthly thereafter for signs and symptoms of hepatitis or SLE or unusual pigmentation (see Special Warnings and Precautions).

4.3 Contraindications
Known hypersensitivity to tetracyclines, or to any of the components of Minocin MR. Use in pregnancy, lactation, children under the age of 12 years, complete renal failure.

4.4 Special warnings and special precautions for use
Minocin MR should be used with caution in patients with hepatic dysfunction and in conjunction with alcohol and other hepatotoxic drugs. It is recommended that alcohol consumption should remain within the Government's recommended limits.

Rare cases of auto-immune hepatotoxicity and isolated cases of systemic lupus erythematosus (SLE) and also exacerbation of pre-existing SLE have been reported. If patients develop signs or symptoms of SLE or hepatotoxicity, or suffer exacerbation of pre-existing SLE, minocycline should be discontinued.

Clinical studies have shown that there is no significant drug accumulation in patients with renal impairment when they are treated with Minocin MR in the recommended doses. In cases of severe renal insufficiency, reduction of dosage and monitoring of renal function may be required. The anti-anabolic action of the tetracyclines may cause an increase in serum urea. In patients with significantly impaired renal function, higher serum levels of tetracyclines may lead to uraemia, hyperphosphataemia and acidosis. If renal impairment exists, even usual oral and parenteral doses may lead to excessive systemic accumulations of the drug and possible liver toxicity.

Caution is advised in patients with myasthenia gravis as tetracyclines can cause weak neuromuscular blockade.

Cross-resistance between tetracyclines may develop in micro-organisms and cross-sensitisation in patients. Minocin MR should be discontinued if there are signs/symptoms of overgrowth of resistant organisms, e.g. enteritis, glossitis, stomatitis, vaginitis, pruritus ani or Staphylococcal enteritis.

Patients taking oral contraceptives should be warned that if diarrhoea or breakthrough bleeding occur there is a possibility of contraceptive failure.

Minocycline may cause hyperpigmentation at various body sites (see Administration and 4.8 Undesirable Effects). Hyperpigmentation may present regardless of dose or duration of therapy but develops more commonly during long term treatment. Patients should be advised to report any unusual pigmentation without delay and Minocin should be discontinued.

If a photosensitivity reaction occurs, patients should be warned to avoid direct exposure to natural or artificial light and to discontinue therapy at the first signs of skin discomfort.

As with other tetracyclines, bulging fontanelleles in infants and benign intracranial hypertension in juveniles and adults have been reported. Presenting features were headache and visual disturbances including blurring of vision, scotoma and diplopia. Permanent vision loss has been reported. Treatment should cease if evidence of raised intracranial pressure develops.

Use in the elderly:

Dose selection for an elderly patient should be cautious, reflecting the greater frequency of decreased hepatic, renal, or cardiac function, and of concomitant disease or other drug therapy.

Use in children:

The use of tetracyclines during tooth development in children under the age of 12 years may cause permanent discolouration. Enamel hypoplasia has also been reported.

Laboratory monitoring:

Periodic laboratory evaluations of organ system function, including haematopoietic, renal and hepatic should be conducted.

4.5 Interaction with other medicinal products and other forms of Interaction

Tetracyclines depress plasma prothrombin activity and reduced doses of concomitant anticoagulants may be necessary.

Diuretics may aggravate nephrotoxicity by volume depletion.

Bacteriostatic drugs may interfere with the bactericidal action of penicillin. Avoid giving tetracycline-class drugs in conjunction with penicillin. Absorption of Minocin MR is impaired by the concomitant administration of antacids, iron, calcium, magnesium, aluminium bismuth and zinc salts (interactions with specific salts, antacids, bismuth containing ulcer – healing drugs, quinapril which contains a magnesium carbonate excipient). It is recommended that any indigestion remedies, vitamins, or other supplements containing these salts are taken at least 3 hours before or after a dose of Minocin MR. Unlike earlier tetracyclines, absorption of Minocin MR is not significantly impaired by food or moderate amounts of milk.

The concomitant use of tetracyclines may reduce the efficacy of oral contraceptives.

Administration of isotretinoin should be avoided shortly before, during and shortly after minocycline therapy. Each drug alone has been associated with pseudotumor cerebri (benign intracranial hypertension) (see 4.4 Special warnings and precautions).

Interference with laboratory and other diagnostic tests:

False elevations of urinary catecholamine levels may occur due to interference with the fluorescence test.

4.6 Pregnancy and lactation

Use in pregnancy:

Minocin MR should not be used in pregnancy unless considered essential.

Results of animal studies indicate that tetracyclines cross the placenta, are found in foetal tissues and can have toxic effects on the developing foetus (often related to retardation of skeletal development). Evidence of embryotoxicity has also been noted in animals treated early in pregnancy. Minocin MR therefore, should not be used in pregnancy unless considered essential.

In humans, Minocin, like other tetracycline-class antibiotics, crosses the placenta and may cause foetal harm when administered to a pregnant woman. In addition, there have been post marketing reports of congenital abnormalities including limb reduction. If Minocin is used during pregnancy or if the patient becomes pregnant while taking this drug, the patient should be informed of the potential hazard to the foetus.

The use of drugs of the tetracycline class during tooth development (last half of pregnancy) may cause permanent discolouration of the teeth (yellow-grey-brown). This adverse reaction is more common during long term use of the drugs but has been observed following repeated short term courses. Enamel hypoplasia has also been reported.

Tetracyclines administered during the last trimester form a stable calcium complex throughout the human skeleton. A decrease in fibula growth rate has been observed in premature human infants given oral tetracyclines in doses up to 25mg/kg every 6 hours. Changes in fibula growth rate were shown to be reversible when the drug was discontinued.

Use in lactation:

Tetracyclines have been found in the milk of lactating women who are taking a drug in this class. Permanent tooth discolouration may occur in the developing infant and enamel hypoplasia has been reported.

4.7 Effects on ability to drive and use machines

Headache, light-headedness, dizziness, tinnitus and vertigo (more common in women) and, rarely, impaired hearing have occurred with Minocin MR. Patients should be warned about the possible hazards of driving or operating machinery during treatment. These symptoms may disappear during therapy and usually disappear when the drug is discontinued.

4.8 Undesirable effects

Adverse reactions are listed in the Table in CIOMS frequency categories under MedDRA system/organ classes:

Common: $\geqslant$ 1%

Uncommon: $\geqslant$ 0.1% and $<$ 1%

Rare: $\geqslant$ 0.01% and $<$ 0.1%

Very Rare: $<$ 0.01%

Infections and Infestations

Very Rare: Oral and anogenital candidiasis, vulvovaginitis.

Blood and Lymphatic System Disorders

Rare: Eosinophilia, leucopenia, neutropenia, thrombocytopenia.

Very Rare: Haemolytic anaemia, pancytopenia.

There are also reports of: Agranulocytosis

Immune System Disorders

Rare: Anaphylaxis /anaphylactoid reaction (including shock), including fatalities.

There are also reports of: Hypersensitivity, pulmonary infiltrates, anaphylactoid purpura.

Endocrine Disorders

Very Rare: Abnormal thyroid function, brown-black discolouration of the thyroid.

Metabolism and Nutrition Disorders

Rare: Anorexia.

Nervous System Disorders

Common: Dizziness (lightheadedness).

Rare: Headache, hypaesthesia, paraesthesia, intracranial hypertension, vertigo.

Very Rare: Bulging fontanelle.

There are also reports of: convulsions, sedation.

Ear and Labyrinth Disorders

Rare: Impaired hearing, tinnitus.

Cardiac Disorders

Rare: Myocarditis, pericarditis.

Respiratory, Thoracic and Mediastinal Disorders

Rare: Cough, dyspnoea.

Very Rare: Bronchospasm, exacerbation of asthma, pulmonary eosinophilia.

There are also reports of: Pneumonitis.

Gastrointestinal Disorders

Rare: Diarrhoea, nausea, stomatitis, discolouration of teeth, vomiting.

Very Rare: Dyspepsia, dysphagia, enamel hypoplasia, enterocolitis, oesophagitis, oesophageal ulceration, glossitis, pancreatitis, pseudomembranous colitis.

Hepatobiliary Disorders

Rare: Increased liver enzymes, hepatitis, autoimmune hepatoxicity. (See Section 4.4 Special warnings and precautions for use).

Very Rare: Hepatic cholestatis, hepatic failure (including fatalities), hyperbilirubinaemia, jaundice.

Skin and Subcutaneous Tissue Disorders

Rare: Alopecia, erythema multiforme, erythema nodosum, fixed drug eruption, hyperpigmentation of skin, photosensitivity, pruritis, rash, urticaria, vasculitis.

Very Rare: Angioedema, exfoliative dermatitis, hyperpigmentation of nails, Stevens-Johnson Syndrome, toxic epidermal necrolysis.

Musculoskeletal, Connective Tissue and Bone Disorders

Rare: Arthralgia, lupus-like syndrome, myalgia.

Very Rare: Arthritis, bone discolouration, cases of or exacerbation of systemic lupus erythematosus (SLE) (See Section 4.4 Special warnings and Special precautions for use), joint stiffness, joint swelling.

Renal and Urinary Disorders

Rare: Increased serum urea, acute renal failure, interstitial nephritis.

Reproductive System and Breast Disorders

Very Rare: Balanitis.

General Disorders and Administration Site Conditions

Uncommon: Fever.

Very Rare: Discolouration of secretions.

The following syndromes have been reported. In some cases involving these syndromes, death has been reported. As with other serious adverse reactions, if any of these syndromes are recognised, the drug should be discontinued immediately:

- Hypersensitivity syndrome consisting of cutaneous reaction (such as rash or exfoliative dermatitis), eosinophilia, and one or more of the following: hepatitis, pneumonitis, nephritis, myocarditis, pericarditis. Fever and lymphadenopathy may be present.
- Lupus-like syndrome consisting of positive antinuclear antibody, arthralgia, arthritis, joint stiffness or joint swelling, and one or more of the following: fever, myalgia, hepatitis, rash, vasculitis.
- Serum sickness-like syndrome consisting of fever, urticaria or rash, and arthralgia, arthritis, joint stiffness or joint swelling. Eosinophilia may be present.

Hyperpigmentation of various body sites including the skin, nails, teeth, oral mucosa, bones, thyroid, eyes (including sclera and conjunctiva), breast milk, lacrimal secretions and perspiration has been reported. This blue/black/grey or muddy-brown discolouration may be localised or diffuse. The most frequently reported site is in the skin. Pigmentation is often reversible on discontinuation of the drug, although it may take several months or may persist in some cases. The generalised muddy-brown skin pigmentation may persist, particularly in areas exposed to the sun.

4.9 Overdose

Dizziness, nausea and vomiting are the adverse effects most commonly seen with overdose. There is no specific antidote. In cases of overdose, discontinue medication, treat symptomatically with gastric lavage and appropriate supportive measures. Minocin is not removed in significant quantities by haemodialysis or peritoneal dialysis.

5. PHARMACOLOGICAL PROPERTIES

5.1 Pharmacodynamic properties

MINOCIN MR Capsules contain the active ingredient minocycline as minocycline hydrochloride, a semi-synthetic derivative of tetracycline.

5.2 Pharmacokinetic properties

MINOCIN MR Capsules have been formulated as a "double pulse" delivery system in which a portion of the minocycline dose is delivered in the stomach, and a second portion of the dose is available for absorption in the duodenum and upper GI tract.

5.3 Preclinical safety data

None stated.

6. PHARMACEUTICAL PARTICULARS

6.1 List of excipients

Pellets:	Microcrystalline cellulose Croscarmellose sodium Hydroxypropylmethyl cellulose phthalate 50 Hydroxypropylmethyl cellulose Light mineral oil Opaspray K-1-7000 (white), (containing:	Titanium dioxide Hypropxypropylcellulose)
Capsule shells:	Titanium dioxide Iron oxide yellow Iron oxide red Iron oxide black Gelatin	
Printing ink:	Colorcon S-7020 containing Shellac Titanium dioxide Purified water Soya lecithin Simethicone	

6.2 Incompatibilities

None known.

6.3 Shelf life

18 months.

6.4 Special precautions for storage

Do not store above 25°C.

Blisters:	Store in the original package Keep the container in the outer carton
Bottles:	Store in the original container Keep the container tightly closed

6.5 Nature and contents of container

PVC/PVDC aluminium blister packs containing 2, 49 and 56 capsules.

Polypropylene bottle with urea cap containing 100 capsules.

6.6 Instructions for use and handling
Not applicable.

7. MARKETING AUTHORISATION HOLDER
John Wyeth & Brother Limited
Trading as Wyeth Pharmaceuticals
Huntercombe Lane South
Taplow
Maidenhead
Berks, SL6 0PH
UK

8. MARKETING AUTHORISATION NUMBER(S)
PL 00011/0278.

9. DATE OF FIRST AUTHORISATION/RENEWAL OF THE AUTHORISATION
14 February 2005

10. DATE OF REVISION OF THE TEXT
14 February 2005

* Trade marks.

Minodiab 2.5, Minodiab 5
(Pharmacia Limited)

1. NAME OF THE MEDICINAL PRODUCT
Minodiab 2.5
Minodiab 5

2. QUALITATIVE AND QUANTITATIVE COMPOSITION
Glipizide 2.5 mg
Glipizide 5.0 mg

3. PHARMACEUTICAL FORM
White biconvex tablets.

4. CLINICAL PARTICULARS

4.1 Therapeutic indications
As an adjunct to diet, in non-insulin-dependent diabetics (NIDDM), when proper dietary management alone has failed.

4.2 Posology and method of administration
Route of administration Oral

As for any hypoglycaemic agent, dosage must be adapted for each individual case.

Short term administration of glipizide may be sufficient during periods of transient loss of control in patients usually controlled well on diet.

In general, glipizide should be given shortly before a meal to achieve the greatest reduction in post-prandial hyperglycaemia.

Initial Dose
The recommended starting dose is 5 mg, given before breakfast or the midday meal. Mild diabetics, geriatric patients or those with liver disease may be started on 2.5 mg.

Titration
Dosage adjustments should ordinarily be in increments of 2.5 to 5 mg, as determined by blood glucose response. At least several days should elapse between titration steps. The maximum recommended single dose is 15 mg. If this is not sufficient, splitting the daily dosage may prove effective. Doses above 15 mg should ordinarily be divided.

Maintenance
Some patients may be effectively controlled on a once-a-day regimen. Total daily dosage above 15 mg should ordinarily be divided.

The maximum recommended daily dosage is 20 mg.

Use in Children
Safety and effectiveness in children have not been established.

Use in Elderly and in High Risk Patients
In elderly patients, debilitated or malnourished patients and patients with an impaired renal or hepatic function, the initial and maintenance dosing should be conservative to avoid hypoglycaemic reactions (see Initial Dose and Special Warnings and Special Precautions for Use sections).

Patients Receiving Other Oral Hypoglycaemic Agents
As with other sulphonylurea class hypoglycaemics, no transition period is necessary when transferring patients to glipizide. Patients should be observed carefully (1-2 weeks) for hypoglycaemia when being transferred from longer half-life sulphonylureas (e.g. chlorpropamide) to glipizide due to potential overlapping of drug effect.

4.3 Contraindications
Glipizide is contraindicated in patients with:

1. Hypersensitivity to glipizide, other sulphonylureas or sulphonamides, or any excipients in the tablets;

2. Insulin-dependent diabetes, diabetic ketoacidosis, diabetic coma;

3. Severe renal or hepatic insufficiency;

4. Patients treated with miconazole (see 4.5 Interactions);

5. Pregnancy and lactation

4.4 Special warnings and special precautions for use
Hypoglycaemia
All sulphonylurea drugs are capable of producing severe hypoglycaemia. Proper patient selection, dosage, and instructions are important to avoid hypoglycaemic episodes. Regular, timely carbohydrate intake is important to avoid hypoglycaemic events occurring when a meal is delayed or insufficient food is eaten or carbohydrate intake is unbalanced. Renal or hepatic insufficiency may cause elevated blood levels of glipizide and the latter may also diminish gluconeogenic capacity, both of which increase the risk of serious hypoglycaemic reactions. Elderly, debilitated or malnourished patients and those with adrenal or pituitary insufficiency are particularly susceptible to the hypoglycaemic action of glucose-lowering drugs.

Hypoglycaemia may be difficult to recognise in the elderly, and in people who are taking beta-adrenergic blocking drugs (see interactions). Hypoglycaemia is more likely to occur when caloric- intake is deficient, after severe or prolonged exercise, when alcohol is ingested, or when more than one glucose-lowering drug is used.

Loss of control of blood glucose
When a patient stabilised on a diabetic regimen is exposed to stress such as fever, trauma, infection, or surgery, a loss of control may occur. At such times, it may be necessary to discontinue glipizide and administer insulin.

The effectiveness of any oral hypoglycaemic drug, including glipizide, in lowering blood glucose to a desired level decreases in many patients over a period of time, which may be due to progression of the severity of diabetes or to diminished responsiveness to the drug. This phenomenon is known as secondary failure, to distinguish it from primary failure in which the drug is ineffective in an individual patient when first given. Adequate adjustment of dose and adherence to diet should be assessed before classifying a patient as a secondary failure.

Renal and Hepatic Disease
The pharmacokinetics and/or pharmacodynamics of glipizide may be affected in patients with impaired renal or hepatic function. If hypoglycaemia should occur in such patients, it may be prolonged and appropriate management should be instituted.

Information for Patients
Patients should be informed of the potential risks and advantages of glipizide and of alternative modes of therapy. They should also be informed about the importance of adherence to dietary instructions, of a regular exercise program, and of regular testing of urine and/or blood glucose.

The risks of hypoglycaemia, its symptoms and treatment, and conditions that predispose to its development should be explained to patients and responsible family members. Primary and secondary failure should also be explained.

Laboratory Tests
Blood and urine glucose should be monitored periodically. Measurement of glycosylated haemoglobin may be useful.

4.5 Interaction with other medicinal products and other forms of Interaction
- The following products are likely to increase the hypoglycaemic effect:

- **Contraindicated combinations**

Miconazole: increase in hypoglycaemic effect, possibly leading to symptoms of hypoglycaemia or even coma.

- **Inadvisable combinations**

Nonsteroidal anti-inflammatory agents (NSAIDS) e.g. phenylbutazone: increase in hypoglycaemic effect of sulphonylureas (displacement of sulphonylurea binding to plasma proteins and/or decrease in sulphonylurea elimination).

Alcohol: increase in hypoglycaemic reaction which can lead to hypoglycaemic coma.

- **Combinations requiring precaution**

Fluconazole: increase in the half-life of the sulphonylurea, possibly giving rise to symptoms of hypoglycaemia.

Salicylates (acetylsalicylic acid): increase in hypoglycaemic effect by high doses of acetylsalicylic acid (hypoglycaemic action of the acetylsalicylic acid).

Beta-blockers: all beta-blockers mask some of the symptoms of hypoglycaemia, i.e. palpitations and tachycardia. Most non cardioselective beta-blockers increase the incidence and severity of hypoglycaemia.

Angiotensin converting enzyme inhibitors: the use of angiotensin converting enzyme inhibitors may lead to an increased hypoglycaemic effect in diabetic patients treated with sulphonylureas.

Cimetidine: the use of cimetidine may be associated with a reduction in post prandial blood glucose in patients treated with glipizide.

The hypoglycaemic action of sulphonylureas in general may also be potentiated by monoamine oxidase inhibitors and drugs that are highly protein bound, such as sulfonamides, chloramphenicol, probenecid, coumarins and fibrates.

When such drugs are administered to (or withdrawn from) a patient receiving glipizide, the patient should be observed closely for hypoglycaemia (or loss of control).

The following products could lead to hyperglycaemia:

- **Inadvisable combinations**

Danazol: diabetogenic effect of danazol. If it cannot be avoided, warn the patient and step up self monitoring of blood glucose and urine. Possibly adjust the dosage of antidiabetic agent during treatment with danazol and after its discontinuation.

- **Combinations requiring precaution**

Phenothiazines (e.g. chlorpromazine) at high doses ≥ 100 mg per day of chlorpromazine): elevation in blood glucose (reduction in insulin release).

Corticosteroids: elevation in blood glucose.

Sympathomimetics (e.g. ritodrine, salbutamol, terbutaline): elevation in blood glucose due to beta-2-adrenoceptor stimulation.

Progestogens: diabetogenic effects of high-dose progestogens. Warn the patient and step up self-monitoring of blood glucose and urine. Possibly adjust the dosage of antidiabetic agent during treatment with the neuroleptics, corticoids or progestogen and after discontinuation.

Other drugs that may produce hyperglycaemia and lead to a loss of control include the thiazides and other diuretics, thyroid products, oestrogens, oral contraceptives, phenytoin, nicotinic acid, calcium channel blocking drugs, and isoniazid.

When such drugs are withdrawn from a patient receiving glipizide, the patient should be observed closely for hypoglycaemia.

4.6 Pregnancy and lactation
Pregnancy
Glipizide is contraindicated in pregnancy.

Glipizide was found to be mildly fetotoxic in rat reproductive studies. No teratogenic effects were found in rat or rabbit studies.

Prolonged severe hypoglycaemia (4 to 10 days) has been reported in neonates born to mothers who were receiving a sulphonylurea drug at the time of delivery.

Because recent information suggests that abnormal blood glucose levels during pregnancy are associated with a higher incidence of congenital abnormalities, many experts recommend that insulin be used during pregnancy to maintain blood glucose levels as close to normal as possible.

Lactation
No data are available on secretion into breast milk. Therefore glipizide is contraindicated in lactation.

4.7 Effects on ability to drive and use machines
The effect of glipizide on the ability to drive or operate machinery has not been studied. However, there is no evidence to suggest that glipizide may affect these abilities. Patients should be aware of the symptoms of hypoglycaemia and be careful about driving and the use of machinery, especially when optimum stabilisation has not been achieved, for example during the change-over from other medications or during irregular use.

4.8 Undesirable effects
The majority of side effects have been dose related, transient, and have responded to dose reduction or withdrawal of the medication. However, clinical experience thus far has shown that, as with other sulphonylureas, some side effects associated with hypersensitivity may be severe and deaths have been reported in some instances.

Hypoglycaemia
See Special Warnings and Special Precautions for Use and Overdose sections.

Gastrointestinal
Gastrointestinal complaints include nausea, diarrhoea, constipation and gastralgia. They appear to be dose related and usually disappear on division or reduction of dosage.

Dermatologic
Allergic skin reactions including erythema, morbilliform or maculopapular reactions, urticaria, pruritus and eczema have been reported. They frequently disappear with continued therapy. However, if they persist, the drug should be discontinued. As with other sulphonylureas, photosensitivity reactions have been reported.

Miscellaneous
Confusion, dizziness, drowsiness, headache, tremor, and visual disturbances have each been reported in patients treated with glipizide. They are usually transient and do not require discontinuance of therapy; however, they may also be symptoms of hypoglycaemia.

Laboratory Test
The pattern of laboratory test abnormalities observed with glipizide is similar to that for other sulphonylureas. Occasional mild to moderate elevations of SGOT, LDH, alkaline phosphatase, BUN and creatinine were noted. The relationship of these abnormalities to glipizide is uncertain, and they have rarely been associated with clinical symptoms.

Hepatic disorder
Cholestatic jaundice, impaired hepatic function, and hepatitis have been reported. Discontinue treatment if cholestatic jaundice occurs.

Haematologic Reactions

Leucopenia, agranulocytosis, thrombocytopenia, haemolytic anaemia, aplastic anaemia and pancytopenia have been reported.

Metabolic Reactions

Hepatic porphyria and porphyria cutanea tarda have been reported. Disulfiram-like reactions have been reported with other sulphonylureas.

Endocrine Reactions

Hyponatraemia has been reported.

4.9 Overdose

There is no well documented experience with glipizide overdosage.

Overdosage of sulphonylureas including glipizide can produce glycaemia. Mild hypoglycaemic symptoms without loss of consciousness or neurologic findings should be treated actively with oral glucose and adjustments in drug dosage and/or meal patterns. Close monitoring should continue until the physician is assured that the patient is out of danger. Severe hypoglycaemic reactions with coma, seizure, or other neurological impairment occur infrequently, but constitute medical emergencies requiring immediate hospitalisation. If hypoglycaemic coma is diagnosed or suspected, the patient should be given a rapid intravenous injection of concentrated (50%) glucose solution. This should be followed by a continuous infusion of a more dilute (10%) glucose solution at a rate that will maintain the blood glucose at a level above 100 mg/dL (5.55 mmol/L). Patients should be closely monitored for a minimum of 48 hours and depending on the status of the patient at this time the physician should decide whether further monitoring is required. Clearance of glipizide from plasma may be prolonged in persons with liver disease. Because of the extensive protein binding of glipizide, dialysis is unlikely to be of benefit.

5. PHARMACOLOGICAL PROPERTIES

5.1 Pharmacodynamic properties

Glipizide is an oral blood glucose lowering drug of the sulphonylurea class. The primary mode of action of glipizide is the stimulation of insulin secretion from the beta-cells of pancreatic islet tissue. Stimulation of insulin secretion by glipizide in response to a meal is of major importance. Fasting insulin levels are not elevated even on long-term glipizide administration, but the post-prandial insulin response continues to be enhanced after at least 6 months of treatment. The insulinotropic response to a meal occurs within 30 minutes after oral dose of glipizide in diabetic patients, but elevated insulin levels do not persist beyond the time of the meal challenge. There is also increasing evidence that extrapancreatic effects involving potentiation of insulin action form a significant component of the activity of glipizide.

Blood sugar control persists for up to 24 hours after a single dose of glipizide, even though plasma levels have declined to a small fraction of peak levels by that time (see "Pharmacokinetics" below).

5.2 Pharmacokinetic properties

Gastrointestinal absorption of glipizide in man is uniform, rapid and essentially complete. Peak plasma concentrations occur 1-3 hours after a single oral dose. The half-life of elimination ranges from 2-4 hours in normal subjects, whether given intravenously or orally. The metabolic and excretory patterns are similar with the two routes of administration, indicating that first-pass metabolism is not significant. Glipizide does not accumulate in plasma on repeated oral administration. Total absorption and disposition of an oral dose was unaffected by food in normal volunteers, but absorption was delayed by about 40 minutes. Thus, glipizide was more effective when administered about 30 minutes before, rather than with, a test meal in diabetic patients. Protein binding was studied in serum from volunteers who received either oral or intravenous glipizide and found to be 98-99% one hour after either route of administration. The apparent volume of distribution of glipizide after intravenous administration was 11 litres, indicative of localisation within the extracellular fluid compartment. In mice, no glipizide or metabolites were detectable autoradiographically in the brain or spinal cord of males or females, nor in the foetuses of pregnant females. In another study, however, very small amounts of radioactivity were detected in the foetuses of rats given labelled drug.

The metabolism of glipizide is extensive and occurs mainly in the liver. The primary metabolites are inactive hydroxylation products and polar conjugates and are excreted mainly in the urine. Less than 10% unchanged glipizide is found in urine.

5.3 Preclinical safety data

Acute toxicity studies showed no specific susceptibility. The acute oral toxicity of glipizide was extremely low in all species tested (LD50 greater than 4 g/kg). Chronic toxicity tests in rats and dogs at doses up to 8.0 mg/kg did not show any evidence of toxic effects.

A 20-month study in rats and an 18-month study in mice at doses up to 75 times the maximum human dose revealed no evidence of drug related carcinogenicity. Bacterial and in vivo mutagenicity tests were uniformly negative. Studies in rats of both sexes at doses up to 75 times the human dose showed no effects on fertility.

6. PHARMACEUTICAL PARTICULARS

6.1 List of excipients

Microcrystalline cellulose Ph. Eur.

Starch Ph. Eur.

Stearic acid HSE

Lactose Ph. Eur.

6.2 Incompatibilities

None stated.

6.3 Shelf life

12 months.

6.4 Special precautions for storage

None.

6.5 Nature and contents of container

Blister strips containing 28 or 60 tablets

6.6 Instructions for use and handling

None.

Administrative Data

7. MARKETING AUTHORISATION HOLDER

Pharmacia Limited

Davy Avenue

Milton Keynes

MK5 8PH

UK

8. MARKETING AUTHORISATION NUMBER(S)

Minodiab 2.5 - PL 00032/0318

Minodiab 5 - PL 00032/0319

9. DATE OF FIRST AUTHORISATION/RENEWAL OF THE AUTHORISATION

Minodiab 2.5 - 26th June 2002

Minodiab 5 - 5th April 2002

10. DATE OF REVISION OF THE TEXT

March 2003

Company Ref: MN 1_0

Mintec

(Shire Pharmaceuticals Limited)

1. NAME OF THE MEDICINAL PRODUCT

Mintec®

2. QUALITATIVE AND QUANTITATIVE COMPOSITION

Each capsule contains 0.2ml Peppermint Oil BP

3. PHARMACEUTICAL FORM

Enteric coated, soft gelatin capsule.

Oral, size no. 4, one half green, the other half ivory.

4. CLINICAL PARTICULARS

4.1 Therapeutic indications

Symptomatic relief of irritable bowel or spastic colon syndrome.

4.2 Posology and method of administration

Adults and elderly: one capsule orally three times a day, preferably before meals with a small quantity of water, but not immediately after food. The capsules must not be broken or chewed.

When symptoms are more severe, the dose may be increased to two capsules three times a day.

Mintec should be taken until symptoms resolve, but may be continued for up to 2 to 3 months.

Children: not recommended for children.

4.3 Contraindications

None known.

4.4 Special warnings and special precautions for use

If this is the first occurrence of these symptoms, a doctor should be consulted before self medication begins, to confirm the appropriateness of the treatment.

Before beginning self medication, a doctor should be consulted if:

The patient is over 40 years old and it is some time since the last attack, or the symptoms have changed; blood has been passed from the bowel; the patient has experienced nausea or vomiting, loss of appetite or loss of weight, paleness and tiredness, severe constipation, fever, abnormal vaginal bleeding or discharge, difficulty or pain in passing urine.

If the patient has recently travelled abroad, or is pregnant or possibly pregnant, they should consult their doctor prior to self medication.

If there are new symptoms or worsening of the condition or failure to improve over two weeks of treatment, the patient should consult their doctor.

In patients with pre-existing heartburn, symptoms may be exacerbated.

4.5 Interaction with other medicinal products and other forms of Interaction

None known.

4.6 Pregnancy and lactation

The usual precautions concerning the administration of any drug during pregnancy should be observed.

4.7 Effects on ability to drive and use machines

None known.

4.8 Undesirable effects

Heartburn, and rarely allergic reactions including erythematous skin rash, bradycardia, muscle tremor and ataxia, which may also occur in association with alcohol.

4.9 Overdose

Treatment consists of gastric lavage, together with symptomatic and supportive measures.

5. PHARMACOLOGICAL PROPERTIES

5.1 Pharmacodynamic properties

Mintec (peppermint oil) is an aromatic carminative which acts locally to relax gastro-intestinal smooth muscle and relieve gastro-intestinal flatulence and colic. The enteric coating of the capsules is designed to delay release of the peppermint oil beyond the stomach and upper small bowel.

5.2 Pharmacokinetic properties

An open cross-over study was conducted in eight healthy volunteers, to compare the excretion pattern of menthol (the major constituent of peppermint oil) from peppermint oil contained in enteric coated soft gelatin capsules (Mintec), and similar, uncoated capsules. In each leg of the study, each volunteer received 0.4 ml of peppermint oil as two capsules of one of the preparations. The excretion of the oil in the urine (as the glucuronide) was followed over a 24 hour period. Mintec capsules significantly delayed the rate of excretion of menthol compared with the non-coated capsules. The maximum amounts of menthol were excreted within 0 to 2 hours following administration of uncoated capsules and between 2 to 4 hours following Mintec administration. There were no significant differences between treatments in terms of the maximum or total amounts of menthol excreted over the 24 hour post-dose period.

5.3 Preclinical safety data

No additional data available.

6. PHARMACEUTICAL PARTICULARS

6.1 List of excipients

Capsule shell:

Gelatin

Glycerol

Titanium dioxide (E171)

Chlorophyll KK (E141)

Enteric coat:

Hydroxypropylmethyl cellulose phthalate

Dibutyl phthalate

6.2 Incompatibilities

Not applicable.

6.3 Shelf life

Thirty months.

6.4 Special precautions for storage

Store at a temperature not exceeding 25°C.

Protect from light.

6.5 Nature and contents of container

Aluminium/PVC/PVDC blister strips in packs of 84.

6.6 Instructions for use and handling

None.

7. MARKETING AUTHORISATION HOLDER

Monmouth Pharmaceuticals Limited

Hampshire International Business Park

Chineham

Basingstoke

Hampshire RG24 8EP

United Kingdom

8. MARKETING AUTHORISATION NUMBER(S)

PL 10536/0036

9. DATE OF FIRST AUTHORISATION/RENEWAL OF THE AUTHORISATION

21st July 1995

10. DATE OF REVISION OF THE TEXT

March 2001

LEGAL CATEGORY

GSL

MINULET*

(Wyeth Pharmaceuticals)

Presentation:

Each white sugar coated tablet contains 30 micrograms ethinyloestradiol and 75 micrograms gestodene.

Uses:

Oral contraception and the recognised gynaecological indications for such oestrogen-progestogen combinations.

The mode of action includes the inhibition of ovulation by suppression of the mid-cycle surge of luteinising hormone, the inspissation of cervical mucus so as to constitute a barrier to sperm, and the rendering of the endometrium unreceptive to implantation.

Dosage and administration:

First treatment cycle: 1 tablet daily for 21 days, starting with the tablet marked number 1, on the first day of the menstrual cycle. Additional contraception (barriers and spermicides) is not required.

Subsequent cycles: Each subsequent course is started when 7 tablet-free days have followed the preceding course. A withdrawal bleed should occur during the 7 tablet-free days.

Changing from another 21 day combined oral contraceptive: The first tablet of Minulet should be taken on the first day immediately after the end of the previous oral contraceptive course. Additional contraception is not required. A withdrawal bleed should not be expected until the end of the first pack of Minulet.

Changing from an Every Day (ED) 28 day combined oral contraceptive: The first tablet of Minulet should be taken on the day immediately after the day on which the last active pill in the ED pack has been taken. The remaining tablets in the ED pack should be discarded. Additional contraception is not required. A withdrawal bleed should not be expected until the end of the first pack of Minulet.

Changing from a Progestogen-only-Pill (POP): The first tablet of Minulet should be taken on the first day of menstruation even if the POP for that day has already been taken. The remaining tablets in the POP pack should be discarded. Additional contraception is not required.

Post-partum and post-abortum use: After pregnancy combined oral contraception can be started in non-lactating women 21 days after a vaginal delivery, provided that the patient is fully ambulant and there are no puerperal complications.

If the pill is started later than 21 days after delivery, then alternative contraception (barriers and spermicides) should be used until oral contraception is started and for the first 7 days of pill-taking. If unprotected intercourse has taken place after 21 days post partum, then oral contraception should not be started until the first menstrual bleed after childbirth. After a miscarriage or abortion oral contraception may be started immediately.

Special circumstances requiring additional contraception

Missed Pills: If a tablet is delayed it should be taken as soon as possible and if it is taken within 12 hours of the correct time, additional contraception is not needed. Further tablets should then be taken at the usual time. If the delay exceeds 12 hours, the last missed pill should be taken when remembered, the earlier missed pills left in the pack and normal pill-taking resumed. If one or more tablets are omitted from the 21 days of pill-taking, additional contraception (barriers and spermicides) should be used for the next 7 days of pill-taking. In addition, if one or more pills are missed during the last 7 days of pill-taking, the subsequent pill-free interval should be disregarded and the next pack started the day after taking the last tablet from the previous pack. In this case, a withdrawal bleed should not be expected until the end of the second pack. If the patient does not have a withdrawal bleed at the end of the second pack she must return to her doctor to exclude the possibility of pregnancy.

Gastro-intestinal upset: Vomiting or diarrhoea may reduce the efficacy by preventing full absorption. Additional contraception (barriers and spermicides) should be used during the upset and for the 7 days following the upset. If these 7 days overrun the end of a pack, the next pack should be started without a break. In this case, a withdrawal bleed should not be expected until the end of the second pack. If the patient does not have a withdrawal bleed at the end of the second pack she must return to her doctor to exclude the possibility of pregnancy.

Mild laxatives do not impair contraceptive action.

Interaction with other drugs: Some drugs accelerate the metabolism of oral contraceptives when taken concurrently and these include barbiturates, phenytoin, phenylbutazone and rifampicin. Other drugs suspected of having the capacity to reduce the efficacy of oral contraceptives include ampicillin and other antibiotics. It is, therefore, advisable to use non-hormonal methods of contraception (barriers and spermicides) in addition to the oral contraceptive as long as an extremely high degree of protection is required during treatment with such drugs. The additional contraception should be used while the concurrent medication continues and for 7 days afterwards. If these extra precautions overrun the end of the pack, the next pack should be started without a break. In this case, a withdrawal bleed should not be expected until the end of the second pack. If the patient does not have a withdrawal bleed at the end of the second pack she must return to her doctor to exclude the possibility of pregnancy.

The herbal remedy St John's Wort (*Hypericum perforatum*) should not be taken concomitantly with this medicine as it could potentially lead to a loss of contraceptive effect.

Contra-indications, warnings etc.

Contra-indications:

1. Suspected pregnancy.

2. History of confirmed venous thromboembolism (VTE). Family history of idiopathic VTE. Other known risk factors for VTE. Thrombotic disorders and a history of these conditions, sickle-cell anaemia, disorders of lipid metabolism and other conditions in which, in individual cases, there is known or suspected to be a much increased risk of thrombosis.

3. Acute or severe chronic liver diseases. Dubin-Johnson syndrome. Rotor syndrome. History, during pregnancy, of idiopathic jaundice or severe pruritus.

4. History of herpes gestationis.

5. Mammary or endometrial carcinoma, or a history of these conditions.

6. Abnormal vaginal bleeding of unknown cause.

7. Deterioration of otosclerosis during pregnancy.

Warnings:

1. **Venous and Arterial Thrombosis and Thromboembolism**

Use of COCs is associated with an increased risk of venous and arterial thrombotic and thromboembolic events.

Minimising exposure to oestrogens and progestogens is in keeping with good principles of therapeutics. For any particular oestrogen/progestogen combination, the dosage regimen prescribed should be one that contains the least amount of oestrogen and progestogen that is compatible with a low failure rate and the needs of the patient.

Unless clinically indicated otherwise, new users of COCs should be started on preparations containing less than 50ôçg of oestrogen.

Venous Thrombosis and Thromboembolism

Use of COCs increases the risk of venous thrombotic and thromboembolic events. Reported events include deep venous thrombosis and pulmonary embolism.

The use of any COC carries an increased risk of venous thrombotic and thromboembolic events compared with no use. The excess risk is highest during the first year a woman ever uses a combined oral contraceptive. This increased risk is less than the risk of venous thrombotic and thromboembolic events associated with pregnancy which is estimated as 60 cases per 100,000 woman-years. Venous thromboembolism is fatal in 1-2% of cases.

Some epidemiological studies have reported a greater risk of VTE for women using combined oral contraceptives containing desogestrel or gestodene (the so-called third generation pills) than for women using pills containing levonorgestrel (the so-called second generation pills).

The spontaneous incidence of VTE in healthy non-pregnant women (not taking any oral contraceptive) is about 5 cases per 100,000 women per year. The incidence in users of the second generation pills is about 15 per 100,000 women per year of use. The incidence in users of third generation pills (such as Minulet) is about 25 cases per 100,000 women per year of use; this excess incidence has not been satisfactorily explained by bias or confounding. The level of all these risks of VTE increases with age and is likely to be further increased in women with other known risk factors of VTE.

All this information should be taken into account when prescribing this COC. When counselling on the choice of contraceptive method(s) all of the above information should be considered.

The risk of venous thrombotic and thromboembolic events is further increased in women with conditions predisposing for venous thrombosis and thromboembolism. Caution must be exercised when prescribing COCs for such women.

Examples of predisposing conditions for venous thrombosis are:

- Certain inherited or acquired thrombophilias (the presence of an inherited thrombophilia may be indicated by a family history of venous thrombotic/thromboembolic events)
- Obesity (body mass index of 30kg/m^2 or over)
- Surgery or trauma with increased risk of thrombosis (see reasons for discontinuation)
- Recent delivery or second-trimester abortion
- Prolonged immobilisation
- Increasing age
- Systemic Lupus Erythematosus (SLE)

The relative risk of post-operative thromboembolic complications has been reported to be increased two- or fourfold with the use of COCs (see reasons for discontinuation).

Since the immediate post-partum period is associated with an increased risk of thromboembolism, COCs should be started no earlier than day 28 after delivery or second-trimester abortion.

Arterial Thrombosis and Thromboembolism

The use of COCs increases the risk or arterial thrombotic and thromboembolic events. Reported events include myocardial infarction and cerebrovascular events (ischaemic and haemorrhagic stroke).

The risk of arterial thrombotic and thromboembolic events is further increased in women with underlying risk factors.

Caution must be exercised when prescribing COCs for women with risk factors for arterial thrombotic and thromboembolic events.

Examples of risk factors for arterial thrombotic and thromboembolic events are:

- Smoking, especially over the age of 35
- Certain inherited and acquired thrombophilias
- Hypertension
- Dyslipoproteinaemias
- Thrombogenic valvular heart disease, atrial fibillation
- Obesity (body mass index of 30kg/m^2)
- Increasing age
- Diabetes
- Systemic Lupus Erythematosus (SLE)

COC users with migraine (particularly migraine with aura) may be at increased risk of stroke.

There is no consensus about the possible role of varicose veins and superficial thrombophlebitis in venous thromboembolism

The suitability of a combined oral contraceptive should be judged according to the severity of such conditions in the individual case, and should be discussed with the patient before she decides to take it.

2. The risk of arterial thrombosis associated with combined oral contraceptives increases with age, and this risk is aggravated by cigarette smoking. The use of combined oral contraceptives by women in the older age group, especially those who are cigarette smokers, should therefore be discouraged and alternative methods used.

3. The possibility cannot be ruled out that certain chronic diseases may occasionally deteriorate during the use of combined oral contraceptives. (See 'Precautions').

4. The combination of ethinyloestradiol and gestodene, like other contraceptive steroids, is associated with an increased incidence of neoplastic nodules in the rat liver, the relevance of which to man is unknown.

5. Malignant liver tumours have been reported on rare occasions in long-term users of oral contraceptives. Benign hepatic tumours have also been associated with oral contraceptive usage. A hepatic tumour should be considered in the differential diagnosis when upper abdominal pain, enlarged liver or signs of intra-abdominal haemorrhage occur.

6. Numerous epidemiological studies have been reported on the risks of ovarian, endometrial, cervical and breast cancer in women using combined oral contraceptives. The evidence is clear that combined oral contraceptives offer substantial protection against both ovarian and endometrial cancer.

An increased risk of cervical cancer in long term users of combined oral contraceptives has been reported in some studies, but there continues to be controversy about the extent to which this is attributable to the confounding effects of sexual behaviour and other factors.

A meta-analysis from 54 epidemiological studies reported that there is a slightly increased relative risk (RR = 1.24) of having breast cancer diagnosed in women who are currently using combined oral contraceptives (COCs). The observed pattern of increased risk may be due to an earlier diagnosis of breast cancer in COC users, the biological effects of COCs or a combination of both. The additional breast cancers diagnosed in current users of COCs or in women who have used COCs in the last ten years are more likely to be localised to the breast than those in women who never used COCs.

Breast cancer is rare among women under 40 years of age whether or not they take COCs. Whilst this background risk increases with age, the excess number of breast cancer diagnoses in current and recent COC users is small in relation to the overall risk of breast cancer (see bar chart).

(see Figure 1 on next page)

The most important risk factor for breast cancer in COC users is the age women discontinue the COC; the older the age at stopping, the more breast cancers are diagnosed. Duration of use is less important and the excess risk gradually disappears during the course of the 10 years after stopping COC use such that by 10 years there appears to be no excess.

The possible increase in risk of breast cancer should be discussed with the user and weighed against the benefits of COCs taking into account the evidence that they offer substantial protection against the risk of developing certain other cancers (e.g. ovarian and endometrial cancer).

Reasons for stopping oral contraception immediately:

1. Occurrence of migraine in patients who have never previously suffered from it. Exacerbation of pre-existing migraine. Any unusually frequent or unusually severe headaches.

2. Any kind of acute disturbance of vision.

3. Suspicion of thrombosis or infarction including symptoms such as unusual pains in or swelling of the legs, stabbing pains on breathing, persistent cough or coughing blood, pain or tightness in the chest.

Figure 1

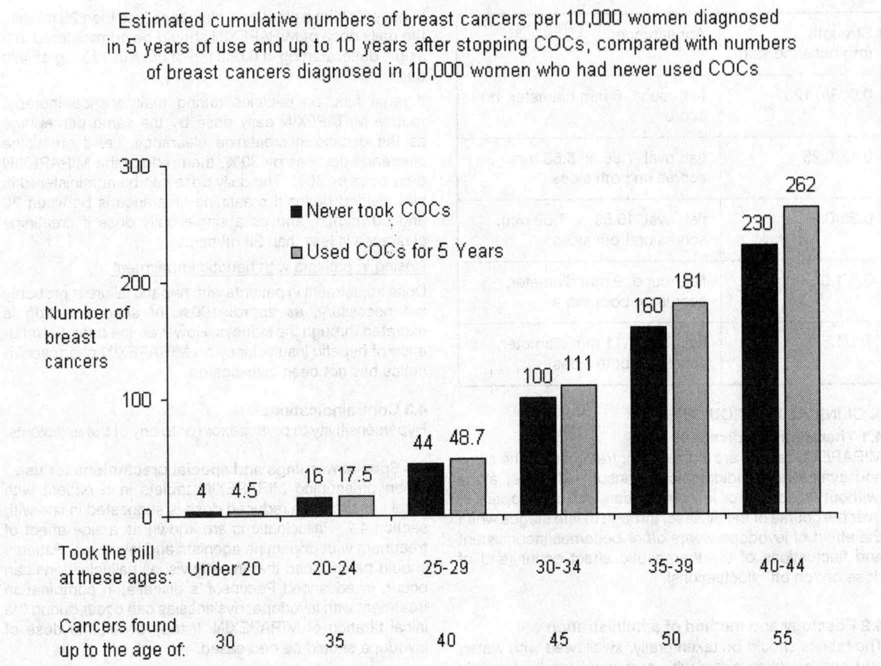

4. Six weeks before elective operations and during immobilisation, e.g. after accidents, etc.

5. Significant rise in blood-pressure.

6. Jaundice.

7. Clear exacerbation of conditions known to be capable of deteriorating during oral contraception or pregnancy.

8. Pregnancy is a reason for stopping immediately because it has been suggested by some investigations that oral contraceptives taken in early pregnancy may slightly increase the risk of foetal malformations. Other investigations have failed to support these findings. The possibility therefore cannot be excluded, but it is certain that if a risk exists at all, it is very small.

If oral contraception is stopped for any reason and pregnancy is not desired, it is recommended that alternative non-hormonal methods of contraception (such as barriers or spermicides) are used to ensure contraceptive protection is maintained.

Precautions:

1. Assessment of women prior to starting oral contraceptives (and at regular intervals thereafter) should include a personal and family medical history of each woman. Physical examination should be guided by this and by the Contraindications and Warnings for this product. The frequency and nature of these assessments should be based upon relevant guidelines and should be adapted to the individual woman, but should include measurement of blood pressure and, if judged appropriate by the clinician, breast, abdominal and pelvic examination including cervical cytology.

2. Before starting treatment, pregnancy must be excluded.

3. The following conditions require careful observation during medication: a history of severe depressive states, varicose veins, diabetes, hypertension, epilepsy, migraine, otosclerosis, multiple sclerosis, porphyria, tetany, disturbed liver function, gall-stones, cardiovascular diseases, renal diseases, chloasma, uterine fibroids, asthma, the wearing of contact lenses, or any disease that is prone to worsen during pregnancy. The first appearance or deterioration of any of these conditions may indicate that the oral contraceptive should be stopped.

4. The risk of the deterioration of chloasma, which is often not fully reversible, is reduced by the avoidance of excessive exposure to sunlight.

Side-effects:

See "Warnings and Precautions"

There is an increased risk of venous thromboembolism for all women using a combined oral contraceptive. For information on differences between oral contraceptives, see "Warnings".

Occasional side-effects may include nausea, vomiting, headaches, breast tenderness, changed body weight or libido, depressive moods and chloasma.

Menstrual changes:

1. Reduction of menstrual flow: This is not abnormal and it is to be expected in some patients. Indeed, it may be beneficial where heavy periods were previously experienced.

2. Missed menstruation: Occasionally, withdrawal bleeding may not occur at all. If the tablets have been taken correctly, pregnancy is very unlikely, but should be ruled out before a new course of tablets is started.

Intermenstrual bleeding: Very light 'spotting' or heavier 'breakthrough bleeding' may occur during tablet-taking, especially in the first few cycles. It appears to be generally of no significance, except where it indicates errors of tablet-taking, or where the possibility of interaction with other drugs exists (q.v.). However, if irregular bleeding is persistent, an organic cause should be considered.

Effect on adrenal and thyroid glands: Oral contraceptives have no significant influence on adrenocortical function. The ACTH function test for the adrenal cortex remains unchanged. The reduction in corticosteroid excretion and the elevation of plasma corticosteroids are due to an increased cortisol-binding capacity of the plasma proteins.

The response to metyrapone is less pronounced than in untreated women and is thus similar to that during pregnancy.

The radio-iodine uptake shows that thyroid function is unchanged. There is a rise in serum protein-bound iodine, similar to that in pregnancy and during the administration of oestrogens. This is due to the increased capacity of the plasma proteins for binding thyroid hormones, rather than to any change in glandular function. In women taking oral contraceptives, the content of protein-bound iodine in blood serum should therefore, not be used for evaluation of thyroid function.

Effect on blood chemistry: Oral contraceptives may accelerate erythrocyte sedimentation in the absence of any disease. This effect is due to a change in the proportion of the plasma protein fractions. Increases in plasma copper, iron and alkaline phosphatase have also been recorded.

Overdosage:

There have been no reports of serious ill-effects from overdosage, even when a considerable number of tablets have been taken by a small child. In general, it is, therefore, unnecessary to treat overdosage. However, if overdosage is discovered within two or three hours and is so large that treatment seems desirable, gastric lavage can be safely used.

There are no specific antidotes and further treatment should be symptomatic.

Pharmaceutical precautions:	Store in cool, dry conditions.
Shelf-Life:	Five years.
Legal category:	POM
Package quantities:	Individual packs containing 3 months' supply.
Further information:	NIL
Product Licence Number:	PL 0011/0135
Date of approval:	3rd March 2003

Further information may be obtained from:

Wyeth Pharmaceuticals

Huntercombe Lane South,

Taplow,

Maidenhead,

Berkshire SL6 0PH.

MIOCHOL-E

(Novartis Pharmaceuticals UK Ltd)

1. NAME OF THE MEDICINAL PRODUCT

Miochol-E®

2. QUALITATIVE AND QUANTITATIVE COMPOSITION

Lower Chamber Acetylcholine Chloride 20.0mg

2ml of the reconstituted solution contains 20mg of the active substance acetylcholine chloride (1:100).

3. PHARMACEUTICAL FORM

Intraocular irrigation, powder with solvent for solution.

4. CLINICAL PARTICULARS

4.1 Therapeutic indications

To obtain rapid and complete miosis after delivery of the lens in cataract surgery as well as in penetrating keratoplasty, iridectomy and other anterior segment surgery where rapid complete miosis is required.

4.2 Posology and method of administration

Miochol-E is for intraocular irrigation only. A freshly prepared 1% solution should be used in the anterior chamber of the eye during surgery.

Adults and Elderly

In most cases a satisfactory miosis, which will last for approximately 20 minutes, is produced in seconds by 0.5 - 2.0ml. A second application may be made at the discretion of the surgeon if prolonged miosis is required.

Children

Safety and effectiveness in children has not been established.

Route of administration: Intraocular irrigation during surgery.

4.3 Contraindications

Hypersensitivity to any of the ingredients.

4.4 Special warnings and special precautions for use

If miosis is to be obtained quickly and completely, obstructions to miosis such as anterior or posterior synechiae may require surgery prior to administration of Miochol-E. In cataract surgery Miochol-E should be used only after delivery of the lens.

If blister or paper backing is damaged or broken, sterility of the Miochol-E vial cannot be assured. The solvent should be in the upper chamber before use. If the centre rubber plug in the univial does not go down when the plunger-stopper is pressed or is already down, the vial should not be used.

Aqueous solutions of Miochol-E are unstable. The solution should therefore be prepared immediately before use. Any remainder should be discarded.

4.5 Interaction with other medicinal products and other forms of Interaction

Although clinical studies with acetylcholine chloride and animal studies with acetylcholine or carbachol revealed no interference, and there is no known pharmacological basis for an interaction, there have been reports that acetylcholine and carbachol have been ineffective when used in patients treated with topical non-steroidal anti-inflammatory agents.

4.6 Pregnancy and lactation

The safety and efficacy of Miochol-E in pregnancy and lactation have not been established. Miochol-E should not be used in pregnant or lactating patients.

4.7 Effects on ability to drive and use machines

Not applicable

4.8 Undesirable effects

Adverse reactions which are indicative of systemic absorption have been reported rarely in the literature. Symptoms include bradycardia, hypotension, flushing, breathing difficulties and sweating. Isolated cases of corneal oedema, corneal clouding and corneal decompensation have been reported with the use of Miochol-E, although a causal relationship has not been established.

4.9 Overdose

The symptoms of overdosage are likely to be effects resulting from systemic absorption, ie bradycardia, hypotension, flushing, breathing difficulties and sweating. Atropine sulphate (0.5 - 1mg) should be given intramuscularly or intravenously and should be readily available to counteract possible overdosage. Adrenaline (0.1 - 1mg subcutaneously) is also of value in overcoming severe cardiovascular or bronchoconstrictor responses.

5. PHARMACOLOGICAL PROPERTIES

5.1 Pharmacodynamic properties

Acetylcholine is a physiological neuromediator of postganglionic parasympathetic nerve fibres (muscarinic action), skeletal muscles and ganglia of the sympathetic system (nicotinic action).

The ocular parasympathetic receptors of the muscarinic type are very numerous and localised:

- at the level of the pupillary sphincter, whose contraction causes miosis
- at the level of the ciliary muscle, whose contraction allows accommodation and facilitates the flow of the aqueous

humor by opening of the trabecular meshwork. In addition, the acetylcholine can have an inhibitory effect on the aqueous secretion. These two last factors result in a decrease in the intraocular pressure.

• at the level of the lacrimal glands, whose stimulation causes tearing.

5.2 Pharmacokinetic properties
Topical: Not applicable.

5.3 Preclinical safety data
The pharmacology and toxicology of the active ingredient acetylcholine are well known. Miochol-E showed good local tolerability.

6. PHARMACEUTICAL PARTICULARS
6.1 List of excipients
Mannitol
Calcium chloride
Magnesium chloride
Potassium chloride
Sodium acetate
Water for injection

6.2 Incompatibilities
Acetylcholine is incompatible with solutions of acidic or alkaline pH but this is unlikely to be relevant during clinical use.

6.3 Shelf life
Unopened: 24 months
Opened: Use immediately after reconstitution

6.4 Special precautions for storage
Do not store above 25°C. Keep from freezing. Do not resterilise.

6.5 Nature and contents of container
Type 1 clear glass univial (2 chambered vial) with rubber closures.

6.6 Instructions for use and handling
• Inspect univial whilst inside unopened blister. Diluent must be in upper chamber.
• Peel open blister.
• Aseptically transfer univial to sterile field. Maintain sterility of outer container during preparation of solution.
• Immediately before use, give plunger-stopper a quarter turn and press to force diluent and centre plug into lower chamber.
• Shake gently to dissolve powder. Do not use unless a clear and colourless solution is produced.
• Draw the solution into a suitable syringe for intraocular irrigation.
• After use discard univial and any unused solution.

7. MARKETING AUTHORISATION HOLDER
Novartis Pharmaceutucals UK Ltd
Frimley Business Park
Frimley
Camberley
Surrey
GU16 7SR

8. MARKETING AUTHORISATION NUMBER(S)
PL 00101/0609

9. DATE OF FIRST AUTHORISATION/RENEWAL OF THE AUTHORISATION
1 May 2001

10. DATE OF REVISION OF THE TEXT
1 May 2001

Legal Category
POM

Mirapexin 0.088 mg tablets

(Boehringer Ingelheim Limited)

1. NAME OF THE MEDICINAL PRODUCT
MIRAPEXIN 0.088 mg tablets

2. QUALITATIVE AND QUANTITATIVE COMPOSITION
MIRAPEXIN 0.088 mg tablets contain 0.088 mg of pramipexole base (as 0.125 mg of pramipexole dihydrochloride monohydrate).

Please note:

Pramipexole doses as published in the literature refer to the salt form. Therefore, doses will be expressed in terms of both pramipexole base <u>and</u> pramipexole salt (in brackets).

For excipients, see 6.1.

3. PHARMACEUTICAL FORM
Tablets.

Tablet description: All tablets are white and have a code embossed.

Strength (mg base/mg salt)	Appearance
0.088/0.125	flat, round, 6 mm diameter, no score
0.18/0.25	flat, oval, 7.86 × 5.63 mm, scores on both sides
0.35/0.5	flat, oval, 10.59 × 7.59 mm, scores on both sides
0.7/1.0	flat, round, 9 mm diameter, scores on both sides
1.1/1.5	flat, round, 11 mm diameter, scores on both sides

4. CLINICAL PARTICULARS
4.1 Therapeutic indications
MIRAPEXIN tablets are indicated for treatment of the signs and symptoms of idiopathic Parkinson's disease, alone (without levodopa) or in combination with levodopa, i.e. over the course of the disease, through to late stages when the effect of levodopa wears off or becomes inconsistent and fluctuations of the therapeutic effect occur (end of dose or "on off" fluctuations).

4.2 Posology and method of administration
The tablets should be taken orally, swallowed with water, and can be taken either with or without food. The daily dosage is administered in equally divided doses 3 times a day.

<u>Initial treatment:</u>

Dosages should be increased gradually from a starting-dose of 0.264 mg of base (0.375 mg of salt) per day and then increased every 5 – 7 days. Providing patients do not experience intolerable side-effects, the dosage should be titrated to achieve a maximal therapeutic effect.

(see Table 1 below)

If a further dose increase is necessary the daily dose should be increased by 0.54 mg base (0.75 mg salt) at weekly intervals up to a maximum dose of 3.3 mg of base (4.5 mg of salt) per day.

However, it should be noted that the incidence of somnolence is increased at doses higher than 1.5 mg/day (see section 4.8).

<u>Maintenance treatment:</u>

The individual dose should be in the range of 0.264 mg of base (0.375 mg of salt) to a maximum of 3.3 mg of base (4.5 mg of salt) per day. During dose escalation in three pivotal studies, efficacy was observed starting at a daily dose of 1.1 mg of base (1.5 mg of salt). Further dose adjustments should be done based on the clinical response and tolerability. In clinical trials approximately 5 % of patients were treated at doses below 1.1 mg (1.5 mg of salt). In advanced Parkinson's disease, doses higher than 1.1 mg (1.5 mg of salt) per day can be useful in patients where a reduction of the levodopa therapy is intended. It is recommended that the dosage of levodopa is reduced during both the dose escalation and the maintenance treatment with MIRAPEXIN, depending on reactions in individual patients.

<u>Treatment discontinuation:</u>

Abrupt discontinuation of dopaminergic therapy can lead to the development of a neuroleptic malignant syndrome. Therefore, pramipexole should be tapered off at a rate of 0.54 mg of base (0.75 mg of salt) per day until the daily dose has been reduced to 0.54 mg of base (0.75 mg of salt). Thereafter the dose should be reduced by 0.264 mg of base (0.375 mg of salt) per day (see section 4.4).

<u>Dosing in patients with renal impairment:</u>

The elimination of pramipexole is dependent on renal function. The following dosage schedule is suggested for initiation of therapy:

Patients with a creatinine clearance above 50 ml/min require no reduction in daily dose.

In patients with a creatinine clearance between 20 and 50 ml/min, the initial daily dose of MIRAPEXIN should be administered in two divided doses, starting at 0.088 mg of base (0.125 mg of salt) twice a day (0.176 mg of base/ 0.25 mg of salt daily).

In patients with a creatinine clearance less than 20 ml/min, the daily dose of MIRAPEXIN should be administered in a single dose, starting at 0.088 mg of base (0.125 mg of salt) daily.

If renal function declines during maintenance therapy, reduce MIRAPEXIN daily dose by the same percentage as the decline in creatinine clearance, i.e. if creatinine clearance declines by 30%, then reduce the MIRAPEXIN daily dose by 30%. The daily dose can be administered in two divided doses if creatinine clearance is between 20 and 50 ml/min, and as a single daily dose if creatinine clearance is less than 20 ml/min.

<u>Dosing in patients with hepatic impairment</u>

Dose adjustment in patients with hepatic failure is probably not necessary, as approx. 90% of absorbed drug is excreted through the kidneys. However, the potential influence of hepatic insufficiency on MIRAPEXIN pharmacokinetics has not been investigated.

4.3 Contraindications
Hypersensitivity to pramipexole or to any of the excipients.

4.4 Special warnings and special precautions for use
When prescribing MIRAPEXIN tablets in a patient with renal impairment a reduced dose is suggested in line with section 4.2. Hallucinations are known as a side-effect of treatment with dopamine agonists and levodopa. Patients should be informed that (mostly visual) hallucinations can occur. In advanced Parkinson's disease, in combination treatment with levodopa, dyskinesias can occur during the initial titration of MIRAPEXIN. If they occur, the dose of levodopa should be decreased.

MIRAPEXIN has been associated with somnolence and episodes of sudden sleep onset, particularly in patients with Parkinson's disease. Sudden onset of sleep during daily activities, in some cases without awareness or warning signs, has been reported uncommonly. Patients must be informed of this and advised to exercise caution while driving or operating machines during treatment with MIRAPEXIN. Patients who have experienced somnolence and/ or an episode of sudden sleep onset must refrain from driving or operating machines. Furthermore a reduction of dosage or termination of therapy may be considered. Because of possible additive effects, caution should be advised when patients are taking other sedating medication or alcohol in combination with pramipexole (see section 4.7 and section 4.8).

Patients with psychotic disorders should only be treated with dopamine agonists if the potential benefits outweigh the risks.

Coadministration of antipsychotic drugs with pramipexole should be avoided (see section 4.5).

Ophthalmologic monitoring is recommended at regular intervals or if vision abnormalities occur.

In case of severe cardiovascular disease, care should be taken. It is recommended to monitor blood pressure, especially at the beginning of treatment, due to the general risk of postural hypotension associated with dopaminergic therapy.

Symptoms suggestive of neuroleptic malignant syndrome have been reported with abrupt withdrawal of dopaminergic therapy (See section 4.2).

4.5 Interaction with other medicinal products and other forms of Interaction
Pramipexole is bound to plasma proteins to a very low (< 20%) extent, and little biotransformation is seen in man. Therefore, interactions with other medications affecting plasma protein binding or elimination by biotransformation are unlikely. As anticholinergics are mainly eliminated by biotransformation, the potential for an interaction is limited, although an interaction with anticholinergics has not been investigated. There is no pharmacokinetic interaction with selegiline and levodopa.

Cimetidine reduced the renal clearance of pramipexole by approximately 34%, presumably by inhibition of the cationic secretory transport system of the renal tubules. Therefore, medications that are inhibitors of this active renal elimination pathway or are eliminated by this pathway, such as cimetidine and amantadine, may interact with pramipexole resulting in reduced clearance of either or both drugs. Reduction of the pramipexole dose should be considered when these drugs are administered concomitantly with MIRAPEXIN.

Table 1

Ascending – Dose Schedule of MIRAPEXIN				
Week	Dosage (mg of base)	Total Daily Dose (mg of base)	Dosage (mg of salt)	Total Daily Dose (mg of salt)
1	3 × 0.088	0.264	3 × 0.125	0.375
2	3 × 0.18	0.54	3 × 0.25	0.75
3	3 × 0.35	1.05	3 × 0.5	1.50

When MIRAPEXIN is given in combination with levodopa, it is recommended that the dosage of levodopa is reduced and the dosage of other anti-parkinsonian medication is kept constant while increasing the dose of MIRAPEXIN.

Because of possible additive effects, caution should be advised when patients are taking other sedating medication or alcohol in combination with pramipexole.

Coadministration of antipsychotic drugs with pramipexole should be avoided (see section 4.4).

4.6 Pregnancy and lactation

The effect on pregnancy and lactation has not been investigated in humans. Pramipexole was not teratogenic in rats and rabbits, but was embryotoxic in the rat at maternotoxic doses (see section 5.3). MIRAPEXIN should not be used during pregnancy unless clearly necessary, i.e. if the potential benefit justifies the potential risk to the foetus.

As MIRAPEXIN treatment inhibits secretion of prolactin in humans, inhibition of lactation is expected.

The excretion of MIRAPEXIN into breast milk has not been studied in women. In rats, the concentration of drug-related radioactivity was higher in breast milk than in plasma.

In the absence of human data, MIRAPEXIN should not be used during breast-feeding, if possible. However, if its use is unavoidable, breast-feeding should be discontinued.

4.7 Effects on ability to drive and use machines

Hallucinations or somnolence can occur.

Patients being treated with MIRAPEXIN and presenting with somnolence and/or sudden sleep episodes must be informed to refrain from driving or engaging in activities where impaired alertness may put themselves or others at risk of serious injury or death (e.g. operating machines) until such recurrent episodes and somnolence have resolved (see also Sections 4.4, 4.5 and 4.8).

4.8 Undesirable effects

Based on the analysis of pooled placebo-controlled trials, comprising a total of 1351 patients on MIRAPEXIN and 1131 patients on placebo, adverse experiences were frequently reported for both groups. 88% of patients on MIRAPEXIN and 83.6% of patients on placebo reported at least one adverse event.

The incidence of somnolence is increased at doses higher than 1.5 mg/day (see section 4.2). More frequent adverse reactions in combination with levodopa were dyskinesias. Constipation, nausea and dyskinesia tended to disappear with continued therapy. Hypotension may occur at the beginning of treatment, especially if MIRAPEXIN is titrated too fast.

The following adverse drug reactions have been observed in placebo-controlled clinical trials with MIRAPEXIN (figures have been calculated as excess incidences, compared with placebo):

Psychiatric disorders: Common (1% - 10%): Insomnia, hallucinations, confusion

Nervous system disorders: Common (1% - 10%): Dizziness, dyskinesia, somnolence (see below)

Vascular disorders: Uncommon (0.1% - 1%): Hypotension

Gastrointestinal disorders: Common (1% - 10%): Nausea, constipation

General disorders: Common (1% - 10%): Oedema peripheral

MIRAPEXIN is associated with somnolence and has been associated uncommonly with excessive daytime somnolence and sudden sleep onset episodes.

MIRAPEXIN may be associated with libido disorders (increase or decrease).

As described in literature for dopamine agonists used for treatment of Parkinson's disease, patients treated with Mirapexin, especially at high doses, have been reported as showing pathological gambling, generally reversible upon treatment discontinuation.

See also 4.4.

4.9 Overdose

There is no clinical experience with massive overdosage. The expected adverse events would be those related to the pharmacodynamic profile of a dopamine agonist, including nausea, vomiting, hyperkinesia, hallucinations, agitation and hypotension. There is no established antidote for overdosage of a dopamine agonist. If signs of central nervous system stimulation are present, a neuroleptic agent may be indicated. Management of the overdose may require general supportive measures, along with gastric lavage, intravenous fluids, and electrocardiogram monitoring.

5. PHARMACOLOGICAL PROPERTIES

5.1 Pharmacodynamic properties

Pharmacotherapeutic group: dopamine agonists, ATC code: N04B C

Pramipexole is a dopamine agonist that binds with high selectivity and specificity to the D2 subfamily of dopamine receptors of which it has a preferential affinity to D_3 receptors, and has full intrinsic activity.

Pramipexole alleviates Parkinsonian motor deficits by stimulation of dopamine receptors in the striatum. Animal studies have shown that pramipexole inhibits dopamine synthesis, release, and turnover.

In human volunteers, a dose-dependent decrease in prolactin was observed.

In patients MIRAPEXIN alleviates signs and symptoms of idiopathic Parkinson's disease.

Controlled clinical trials included approximately 2100 patients of Hoehn and Yahr stages I – IV. Out of these, approximately 900 were in more advanced stages, received concomitant levodopa therapy, and suffered from motor complications.

In early and advanced Parkinson's disease, efficacy of MIRAPEXIN in the controlled clinical trials was maintained for approximately six months. In open continuation trials lasting for more than three years there were no signs of decreasing efficacy. In a controlled double blind clinical trial of 2 year duration, initial treatment with pramipexole significantly delayed the onset of motor complications, and reduced their occurrence compared to initial treatment with levodopa. This delay in motor complications with pramipexole should be balanced against a greater improvement in motor function with levodopa (as measured by the mean change in UPDRS-score). The overall incidence of hallucinations and somnolence was generally higher in the escalation phase with the pramipexole group. However there was no significant difference during the maintenance phase. These points should be considered when initiating pramipexole treatment in patients with Parkinson's disease.

5.2 Pharmacokinetic properties

Pramipexole is rapidly and completely absorbed following oral administration. The absolute bioavailability is greater than 90% and the maximum plasma concentrations occur between 1 and 3 hours. Concomitant administration with food did not reduce the extent of pramipexole absorption, but the rate of absorption was reduced. Pramipexole shows linear kinetics and a small inter-patient variation of plasma levels.

In humans, the protein binding of pramipexole is very low (< 20%) and the volume of distribution is large (400 l). High brain tissue concentrations were observed in the rat (approx. 8-fold compared to plasma).

Pramipexole is metabolised in man only to a small extent.

Renal excretion of unchanged pramipexole is the major route of elimination. Approximately 90% of ^{14}C-labelled dose is excreted through the kidneys while less than 2% is found in the faeces. The total clearance of pramipexole is approximately 500 ml/min and the renal clearance is approximately 400 ml/min. The elimination half-life ($t^{1/2}$) varies from 8 hours in the young to 12 hours in the elderly.

5.3 Preclinical safety data

Repeated dose toxicity studies showed that pramipexole exerted functional effects, mainly involving the CNS and female reproductive system, and probably resulting from an exaggerated pharmacodynamic effect of pramipexole.

Decreases in diastolic and systolic pressure and heart rate were noted in the minipig, and a tendency to an hypotensive effect was discerned in the monkey.

The potential effects of pramipexole on reproductive function have been investigated in rats and rabbits. Pramipexole was not teratogenic in rats and rabbits but was embryotoxic in the rat at maternally toxic doses. Due to the selection of animal species and the limited parameters investigated, the adverse effects of pramipexole on pregnancy and male fertility have not been fully elucidated.

Pramipexole was not genotoxic. In a carcinogenicity study, male rats developed Leydig cell hyperplasia and adenomas, explained by the prolactin-inhibiting effect of pramipexole. This finding is not clinically relevant to man. The same study also showed that, at doses of 2 mg/kg (of salt) and higher, pramipexole was associated with retinal degeneration in albino rats. The latter finding was not observed in pigmented rats, nor in a 2-year albino mouse carcinogenicity study or in any other species investigated.

6. PHARMACEUTICAL PARTICULARS

6.1 List of excipients

Mannitol,

maize starch,

anhydrous colloidal silica,

povidone,

magnesium stearate

6.2 Incompatibilities

Not applicable

6.3 Shelf life

3 years

6.4 Special precautions for storage

Do not store above 30°C.

Store in the original package in order to protect from light.

6.5 Nature and contents of container

10 tablets per aluminium blister strips

Cartons containing 3 or 10 blister strips (30 or 100 tablets)

Not all pack sizes may be marketed.

6.6 Instructions for use and handling

No special requirements

7. MARKETING AUTHORISATION HOLDER

Boehringer Ingelheim International GmbH

D-55216 Ingelheim am Rhein

Germany

8. MARKETING AUTHORISATION NUMBER(S)

EU 1/97/051/001-002

9. DATE OF FIRST AUTHORISATION/RENEWAL OF THE AUTHORISATION

Date of first authorisation: 23 February 1998

Date of Renewal of the authorisation: 23 February 2003

10. DATE OF REVISION OF THE TEXT

29.3.2005

11. LEGAL CATEGORY

POM

M5(0.088)/B/SPC/3

Mirapexin 0.18 mg tablets

(Boehringer Ingelheim Limited)

1. NAME OF THE MEDICINAL PRODUCT

MIRAPEXIN 0.18 mg tablets

2. QUALITATIVE AND QUANTITATIVE COMPOSITION

MIRAPEXIN 0.18 mg tablets contain 0.18 mg of pramipexole base (as 0.25 mg of pramipexole dihydrochloride monohydrate).

Please note:

Pramipexole doses as published in the literature refer to the salt form. Therefore, doses will be expressed in terms of both pramipexole base and pramipexole salt (in brackets).

For excipients, see 6.1.

3. PHARMACEUTICAL FORM

Tablets.

Tablet description: All tablets are white and have a code embossed.

Strength (mg base/mg salt)	Appearance
0.088/0.125	flat, round, 6 mm diameter, no score
0.18/0.25	flat, oval, 7.86 × 5.63 mm, scores on both sides
0.35/0.5	flat, oval, 10.59 × 7.59 mm, scores on both sides
0.7/1.0	flat, round, 9 mm diameter, scores on both sides
1.1/1.5	flat, round, 11 mm diameter, scores on both sides

4. CLINICAL PARTICULARS

4.1 Therapeutic indications

MIRAPEXIN tablets are indicated for treatment of the signs and symptoms of idiopathic Parkinson's disease, alone (without levodopa) or in combination with levodopa, i.e. over the course of the disease, through to late stages when the effect of levodopa wears off or becomes inconsistent and fluctuations of the therapeutic effect occur (end of dose or "on off" fluctuations).

4.2 Posology and method of administration

The tablets should be taken orally, swallowed with water, and can be taken either with or without food. The daily dosage is administered in equally divided doses 3 times a day.

Initial treatment:

Dosages should be increased gradually from a starting-dose of 0.264 mg of base (0.375 mg of salt) per day and then increased every 5 – 7 days. Providing patients do not experience intolerable side-effects, the dosage should be titrated to achieve a maximal therapeutic effect.

(see Table 1 on next page)

If a further dose increase is necessary the daily dose should be increased by 0.54 mg base (0.75 mg salt) at weekly intervals up to a maximum dose of 3.3 mg of base (4.5 mg of salt) per day.

However, it should be noted that the incidence of somnolence is increased at doses higher than 1.5 mg/day (see section 4.8).

Maintenance treatment:

The individual dose should be in the range of 0.264 mg of base (0.375 mg of salt) to a maximum of 3.3 mg of base (4.5 mg of salt) per day. During dose escalation in three pivotal studies, efficacy was observed starting at a daily dose of 1.1 mg of base (1.5 mg of salt). Further dose adjustments should be done based on the clinical response and tolerability. In clinical trials approximately 5 % of patients were treated at doses below 1.1 mg (1.5 mg of salt). In advanced Parkinson's disease, doses higher

Table 1

Ascending – Dose Schedule of MIRAPEXIN				
Week	Dosage (mg of base)	Total Daily Dose (mg of base)	Dosage (mg of salt)	Total Daily Dose (mg of salt)
1	3 × 0.088	0.264	3 × 0.125	0.375
2	3 × 0.18	0.54	3 × 0.25	0.75
3	3 × 0.35	1.05	3 × 0.5	1.50

than 1.1 mg (1.5 mg of salt) per day can be useful in patients where a reduction of the levodopa therapy is intended. It is recommended that the dosage of levodopa is reduced during both the dose escalation and the maintenance treatment with MIRAPEXIN, depending on reactions in individual patients.

Treatment discontinuation:

Abrupt discontinuation of dopaminergic therapy can lead to the development of a neuroleptic malignant syndrome. Therefore, pramipexole should be tapered off at a rate of 0.54 mg of base (0.75 mg of salt) per day until the daily dose has been reduced to 0.54 mg of base (0.75 mg of salt). Thereafter the dose should be reduced by 0.264 mg of base (0.375 mg of salt) per day (see section 4.4).

Dosing in patients with renal impairment:

The elimination of pramipexole is dependent on renal function. The following dosage schedule is suggested for initiation of therapy:

Patients with a creatinine clearance above 50 ml/min require no reduction in daily dose.

In patients with a creatinine clearance between 20 and 50 ml/min, the initial daily dose of MIRAPEXIN should be administered in two divided doses, starting at 0.088 mg of base (0.125 mg of salt) twice a day (0.176 mg of base/ 0.25 mg of salt daily).

In patients with a creatinine clearance less than 20 ml/min, the daily dose of MIRAPEXIN should be administered in a single dose, starting at 0.088 mg of base (0.125 mg of salt) daily.

If renal function declines during maintenance therapy, reduce MIRAPEXIN daily dose by the same percentage as the decline in creatinine clearance, i.e. if creatinine clearance declines by 30%, then reduce the MIRAPEXIN daily dose by 30%. The daily dose can be administered in two divided doses if creatinine clearance is between 20 and 50 ml/min, and as a single daily dose if creatinine clearance is less than 20 ml/min.

Dosing in patients with hepatic impairment

Dose adjustment in patients with hepatic failure is probably not necessary, as approx. 90% of absorbed drug is excreted through the kidneys. However, the potential influence of hepatic insufficiency on MIRAPEXIN pharmacokinetics has not been investigated.

4.3 Contraindications

Hypersensitivity to pramipexole or to any of the excipients.

4.4 Special warnings and special precautions for use

When prescribing MIRAPEXIN tablets in a patient with renal impairment a reduced dose is suggested in line with section 4.2. Hallucinations are known as a side-effect of treatment with dopamine agonists and levodopa. Patients should be informed that (mostly visual) hallucinations can occur. In advanced Parkinson's disease, in combination treatment with levodopa, dyskinesias can occur during the initial titration of MIRAPEXIN. If they occur, the dose of levodopa should be decreased.

MIRAPEXIN has been associated with somnolence and episodes of sudden sleep onset, particularly in patients with Parkinson's disease. Sudden onset of sleep during daily activities, in some cases without awareness or warning signs, has been reported uncommonly. Patients must be informed of this and advised to exercise caution while driving or operating machines during treatment with MIRAPEXIN. Patients who have experienced somnolence and/ or an episode of sudden sleep onset must refrain from driving or operating machines. Furthermore a reduction of dosage or termination of therapy may be considered. Because of possible additive effects, caution should be advised when patients are taking other sedating medication or alcohol in combination with pramipexole (see section 4.7 and section 4.8).

Patients with psychotic disorders should only be treated with dopamine agonists if the potential benefits outweigh the risks.

Coadministration of antipsychotic drugs with pramipexole should be avoided (see section 4.5).

Ophthalmologic monitoring is recommended at regular intervals or if vision abnormalities occur.

In case of severe cardiovascular disease, care should be taken. It is recommended to monitor blood pressure, especially at the beginning of treatment, due to the general risk of postural hypotension associated with dopaminergic therapy.

Symptoms suggestive of neuroleptic malignant syndrome have been reported with abrupt withdrawal of dopaminergic therapy (See section 4.2).

4.5 Interaction with other medicinal products and other forms of Interaction

Pramipexole is bound to plasma proteins to a very low (< 20%) extent, and little biotransformation is seen in man. Therefore, interactions with other medications affecting plasma protein binding or elimination by biotransformation are unlikely. As anticholinergics are mainly eliminated by biotransformation, the potential for an interaction is limited, although an interaction with anticholinergics has not been investigated. There is no pharmacokinetic interaction with selegiline and levodopa.

Cimetidine reduced the renal clearance of pramipexole by approximately 34%, presumably by inhibition of the cationic secretory transport system of the renal tubules. Therefore, medications that are inhibitors of this active renal elimination pathway or are eliminated by this pathway, such as cimetidine and amantadine, may interact with pramipexole resulting in reduced clearance of either or both drugs. Reduction of the pramipexole dose should be considered when these drugs are administered concomitantly with MIRAPEXIN.

When MIRAPEXIN is given in combination with levodopa, it is recommended that the dosage of levodopa is reduced and the dosage of other anti-parkinsonian medication is kept constant while increasing the dose of MIRAPEXIN.

Because of possible additive effects, caution should be advised when patients are taking other sedating medication or alcohol in combination with pramipexole.

Coadministration of antipsychotic drugs with pramipexole should be avoided (see section 4.4).

4.6 Pregnancy and lactation

The effect on pregnancy and lactation has not been investigated in humans. Pramipexole was not teratogenic in rats and rabbits, but was embryotoxic in the rat at maternotoxic doses (see section 5.3). MIRAPEXIN should not be used during pregnancy unless clearly necessary, i.e. if the potential benefit justifies the potential risk to the foetus.

As MIRAPEXIN treatment inhibits secretion of prolactin in humans, inhibition of lactation is expected.

The excretion of MIRAPEXIN into breast milk has not been studied in women. In rats, the concentration of drug-related radioactivity was higher in breast milk than in plasma.

In the absence of human data, MIRAPEXIN should not be used during breast-feeding, if possible. However, if its use is unavoidable, breast-feeding should be discontinued.

4.7 Effects on ability to drive and use machines

Hallucinations or somnolence can occur.

Patients being treated with MIRAPEXIN and presenting with somnolence and/or sudden sleep episodes must be informed to refrain from driving or engaging in activities where impaired alertness may put themselves or others at risk of serious injury or death (e.g. operating machines) until such recurrent episodes and somnolence have resolved (see also Sections 4.4, 4.5 and 4.8).

4.8 Undesirable effects

Based on the analysis of pooled placebo-controlled trials, comprising a total of 1351 patients on MIRAPEXIN and 1131 patients on placebo, adverse experiences were frequently reported for both groups. 88% of patients on MIRAPEXIN and 83.6% of patients on placebo reported at least one adverse event.

The incidence of somnolence is increased at doses higher than 1.5 mg/day (see section 4.2). More frequent adverse reactions in combination with levodopa were dyskinesias. Constipation, nausea and dyskinesia tended to disappear with continued therapy. Hypotension may occur at the beginning of treatment, especially if MIRAPEXIN is titrated too fast.

The following adverse drug reactions have been observed in placebo-controlled clinical trials with MIRAPEXIN (figures have been calculated as excess incidences, compared with placebo):

Psychiatric disorders: Common (1% - 10%): Insomnia, hallucinations, confusion

Nervous system disorders: Common (1% - 10%): Dizziness, dyskinesia, somnolence (see below)

Vascular disorders: Uncommon (0.1% - 1%): Hypotension

Gastrointestinal disorders: Common (1% - 10%): Nausea, constipation

General disorders: Common (1% - 10%): Oedema peripheral

MIRAPEXIN is associated with somnolence and has been associated uncommonly with excessive daytime somnolence and sudden sleep onset episodes.

MIRAPEXIN may be associated with libido disorders (increase or decrease).

As described in literature for dopamine agonists used for treatment of Parkinson's disease, patients treated with Mirapexin, especially at high doses, have been reported as showing pathological gambling, generally reversible upon treatment discontinuation.

See also 4.4.

4.9 Overdose

There is no clinical experience with massive overdosage. The expected adverse events would be those related to the pharmacodynamic profile of a dopamine agonist, including nausea, vomiting, hyperkinesia, hallucinations, agitation and hypotension. There is no established antidote for overdosage of a dopamine agonist. If signs of central nervous system stimulation are present, a neuroleptic agent may be indicated. Management of the overdose may require general supportive measures, along with gastric lavage, intravenous fluids, and electrocardiogram monitoring.

5. PHARMACOLOGICAL PROPERTIES

5.1 Pharmacodynamic properties

Pharmacotherapeutic group: dopamine agonists, ATC code: N04B C

Pramipexole is a dopamine agonist that binds with high selectivity and specificity to the D2 subfamily of dopamine receptors of which it has a preferential affinity to D_3 receptors, and has full intrinsic activity.

Pramipexole alleviates Parkinsonian motor deficits by stimulation of dopamine receptors in the striatum. Animal studies have shown that pramipexole inhibits dopamine synthesis, release, and turnover.

In human volunteers, a dose-dependent decrease in prolactin was observed.

In patients MIRAPEXIN alleviates signs and symptoms of idiopathic Parkinson's disease.

Controlled clinical trials included approximately 2100 patients of Hoehn and Yahr stages I – IV. Out of these, approximately 900 were in more advanced stages, received concomitant levodopa therapy, and suffered from motor complications.

In early and advanced Parkinson's disease, efficacy of MIRAPEXIN in the controlled clinical trials was maintained for approximately six months. In open continuation trials lasting for more than three years there were no signs of decreasing efficacy. In a controlled double blind clinical trial of 2 year duration, initial treatment with pramipexole significantly delayed the onset of motor complications, and reduced their occurrence compared to initial treatment with levodopa. This delay in motor complications with pramipexole should be balanced against a greater improvement in motor function with levodopa (as measured by the mean change in UPDRS-score). The overall incidence of hallucinations and somnolence was generally higher in the escalation phase with the pramipexole group. However there was no significant difference during the maintenance phase. These points should be considered when initiating pramipexole treatment in patients with Parkinson's disease.

5.2 Pharmacokinetic properties

Pramipexole is rapidly and completely absorbed following oral administration. The absolute bioavailability is greater than 90% and the maximum plasma concentrations occur between 1 and 3 hours. Concomitant administration with food did not reduce the extent of pramipexole absorption, but the rate of absorption was reduced. Pramipexole shows linear kinetics and a small inter-patient variation of plasma levels.

In humans, the protein binding of pramipexole is very low (< 20%) and the volume of distribution is large (400 l). High brain tissue concentrations were observed in the rat (approx. 8-fold compared to plasma).

Pramipexole is metabolised in man only to a small extent.

Renal excretion of unchanged pramipexole is the major route of elimination. Approximately 90% of ^{14}C-labelled dose is excreted through the kidneys while less than 2% is found in the faeces. The total clearance of pramipexole is approximately 500 ml/min and the renal clearance is approximately 400 ml/min. The elimination half-life (t½) varies from 8 hours in the young to 12 hours in the elderly.

5.3 Preclinical safety data

Repeated dose toxicity studies showed that pramipexole exerted functional effects, mainly involving the CNS and female reproductive system, and probably resulting from an exaggerated pharmacodynamic effect of pramipexole.

Decreases in diastolic and systolic pressure and heart rate were noted in the minipig, and a tendency to an hypotensive effect was discerned in the monkey.

The potential effects of pramipexole on reproductive function have been investigated in rats and rabbits. Pramipexole was not teratogenic in rats and rabbits but was embryotoxic in the rat at maternally toxic doses. Due to the selection of animal species and the limited parameters investigated, the adverse effects of pramipexole on pregnancy and male fertility have not been fully elucidated.

Pramipexole was not genotoxic. In a carcinogenicity study, male rats developed Leydig cell hyperplasia and adenomas, explained by the prolactin-inhibiting effect of pramipexole. This finding is not clinically relevant to man. The same study also showed that, at doses of 2 mg/kg (of salt) and higher, pramipexole was associated with retinal degeneration in albino rats. The latter finding was not observed in pigmented rats, nor in a 2-year albino mouse carcinogenicity study or in any other species investigated.

6. PHARMACEUTICAL PARTICULARS

6.1 List of excipients

Mannitol,

maize starch,

anhydrous colloidal silica,

povidone,

magnesium stearate

6.2 Incompatibilities

Not applicable

6.3 Shelf life

3 years

6.4 Special precautions for storage

Do not store above 30°C.

Store in the original package in order to protect from light.

6.5 Nature and contents of container

10 tablets per aluminium blister strips

Cartons containing 3 or 10 blister strips (30 or 100 tablets)

Not all pack sizes may be marketed.

6.6 Instructions for use and handling

No special requirements

7. MARKETING AUTHORISATION HOLDER

Boehringer Ingelheim International GmbH

D-55216 Ingelheim am Rhein

Germany

8. MARKETING AUTHORISATION NUMBER(S)

EU 1/97/051/003-004

9. DATE OF FIRST AUTHORISATION/RENEWAL OF THE AUTHORISATION

Date of first authorisation: 23 February 1998

Date of Renewal of the authorisation: 23 February 2003

10. DATE OF REVISION OF THE TEXT

29.3.2005

11. LEGAL CATEGORY

POM

M5(0.18)/B/SPC/3

Mirapexin 0.7 mg tablets

(Boehringer Ingelheim Limited)

1. NAME OF THE MEDICINAL PRODUCT

MIRAPEXIN 0.7 mg tablets

2. QUALITATIVE AND QUANTITATIVE COMPOSITION

MIRAPEXIN 0.7 mg tablets contain 0.7 mg of pramipexole base (as 1.0 mg of pramipexole dihydrochloride monohydrate).

Please note:

Pramipexole doses as published in the literature refer to the salt form. Therefore, doses will be expressed in terms of both pramipexole base <u>and</u> pramipexole salt (in brackets).

For excipients, see 6.1.

3. PHARMACEUTICAL FORM

Tablets.

Tablet description: All tablets are white and have a code embossed.

Strength (mg base/mg salt)	Appearance
0.088/0.125	flat, round, 6 mm diameter, no score
0.18/0.25	flat, oval, 7.86 × 5.63 mm, scores on both sides
0.35/0.5	flat, oval, 10.59 × 7.59 mm, scores on both sides
0.7/1.0	flat, round, 9 mm diameter, scores on both sides
1.1/1.5	flat, round, 11 mm diameter, scores on both sides

Table 1

Ascending – Dose Schedule of MIRAPEXIN

Week	Dosage (mg of base)	Total Daily Dose (mg of base)	Dosage (mg of salt)	Total Daily Dose (mg of salt)
1	3 × 0.088	0.264	3 × 0.125	0.375
2	3 × 0.18	0.54	3 × 0.25	0.75
3	3 × 0.35	1.05	3 × 0.5	1.50

4. CLINICAL PARTICULARS

4.1 Therapeutic indications

MIRAPEXIN tablets are indicated for treatment of the signs and symptoms of idiopathic Parkinson's disease, alone (without levodopa) or in combination with levodopa, i.e. over the course of the disease, through to late stages when the effect of levodopa wears off or becomes inconsistent and fluctuations of the therapeutic effect occur (end of dose or "on off" fluctuations).

4.2 Posology and method of administration

The tablets should be taken orally, swallowed with water, and can be taken either with or without food. The daily dosage is administered in equally divided doses 3 times a day.

<u>Initial treatment:</u>

Dosages should be increased gradually from a starting-dose of 0.264 mg of base (0.375 mg of salt) per day and then increased every 5 – 7 days. Providing patients do not experience intolerable side-effects, the dosage should be titrated to achieve a maximal therapeutic effect.

(see Table 1 above)

If a further dose increase is necessary the daily dose should be increased by 0.54 mg base (0.75 mg salt) at weekly intervals up to a maximum dose of 3.3 mg of base (4.5 mg of salt) per day.

However, it should be noted that the incidence of somnolence is increased at doses higher than 1.5 mg/day (see section 4.8).

<u>Maintenance treatment:</u>

The individual dose should be in the range of 0.264 mg of base (0.375 mg of salt) to a maximum of 3.3 mg of base (4.5 mg of salt) per day. During dose escalation in three pivotal studies, efficacy was observed starting at a daily dose of 1.1 mg of base (1.5 mg of salt). Further dose adjustments should be done based on the clinical response and tolerability. In clinical trials approximately 5 % of patients were treated at doses below 1.1 mg (1.5 mg of salt). In advanced Parkinson's disease, doses higher than 1.1 mg (1.5 mg of salt) per day can be useful in patients where a reduction of the levodopa therapy is intended. It is recommended that the dosage of levodopa is reduced during both the dose escalation and the maintenance treatment with MIRAPEXIN, depending on reactions in individual patients.

<u>Treatment discontinuation:</u>

Abrupt discontinuation of dopaminergic therapy can lead to the development of a neuroleptic malignant syndrome. Therefore, pramipexole should be tapered off at a rate of 0.54 mg of base (0.75 mg of salt) per day until the daily dose has been reduced to 0.54 mg of base (0.75 mg of salt). Thereafter the dose should be reduced by 0.264 mg of base (0.375 mg of salt) per day (see section 4.4).

<u>Dosing in patients with renal impairment:</u>

The elimination of pramipexole is dependent on renal function. The following dosage schedule is suggested for initiation of therapy:

Patients with a creatinine clearance above 50 ml/min require no reduction in daily dose.

In patients with a creatinine clearance between 20 and 50 ml/min, the initial daily dose of MIRAPEXIN should be administered in two divided doses, starting at 0.088 mg of base (0.125 mg of salt) twice a day (0.176 mg of base/0.25 mg of salt daily).

In patients with a creatinine clearance less than 20 ml/min, the daily dose of MIRAPEXIN should be administered in a single dose, starting at 0.088 mg of base (0.125 mg of salt) daily.

If renal function declines during maintenance therapy, reduce MIRAPEXIN daily dose by the same percentage as the decline in creatinine clearance, i.e. if creatinine clearance declines by 30%, then reduce the MIRAPEXIN daily dose by 30%. The daily dose can be administered in two divided doses if creatinine clearance is between 20 and 50 ml/min, and as a single daily dose if creatinine clearance is less than 20 ml/min.

<u>Dosing in patients with hepatic impairment</u>

Dose adjustment in patients with hepatic failure is probably not necessary, as approx. 90% of absorbed drug is excreted through the kidneys. However, the potential influence of hepatic insufficiency on MIRAPEXIN pharmacokinetics has not been investigated.

4.3 Contraindications

Hypersensitivity to pramipexole or to any of the excipients.

4.4 Special warnings and special precautions for use

When prescribing MIRAPEXIN tablets in a patient with renal impairment a reduced dose is suggested in line with section 4.2. Hallucinations are known as a side-effect of treatment with dopamine agonists and levodopa. Patients should be informed that (mostly visual) hallucinations can occur. In advanced Parkinson's disease, in combination treatment with levodopa, dyskinesias can occur during the initial titration of MIRAPEXIN. If they occur, the dose of levodopa should be decreased.

MIRAPEXIN has been associated with somnolence and episodes of sudden sleep onset, particularly in patients with Parkinson's disease. Sudden onset of sleep during daily activities, in some cases without awareness or warning signs, has been reported uncommonly. Patients must be informed of this and advised to exercise caution while driving or operating machines during treatment with MIRAPEXIN. Patients who have experienced somnolence and/or an episode of sudden sleep onset must refrain from driving or operating machines. Furthermore a reduction of dosage or termination of therapy may be considered. Because of possible additive effects, caution should be advised when patients are taking other sedating medication or alcohol in combination with pramipexole (see section 4.7 and section 4.8).

Patients with psychotic disorders should only be treated with dopamine agonists if the potential benefits outweigh the risks.

Coadministration of antipsychotic drugs with pramipexole should be avoided (see section 4.5).

Ophthalmologic monitoring is recommended at regular intervals or if vision abnormalities occur.

In case of severe cardiovascular disease, care should be taken. It is recommended to monitor blood pressure, especially at the beginning of treatment, due to the general risk of postural hypotension associated with dopaminergic therapy.

Symptoms suggestive of neuroleptic malignant syndrome have been reported with abrupt withdrawal of dopaminergic therapy (See section 4.2).

4.5 Interaction with other medicinal products and other forms of Interaction

Pramipexole is bound to plasma proteins to a very low (< 20%) extent, and little biotransformation is seen in man. Therefore, interactions with other medications affecting plasma protein binding or elimination by biotransformation are unlikely. As anticholinergics are mainly eliminated by biotransformation, the potential for an interaction is limited, although an interaction with anticholinergics has not been investigated. There is no pharmacokinetic interaction with selegiline and levodopa.

Cimetidine reduced the renal clearance of pramipexole by approximately 34%, presumably by inhibition of the cationic secretory transport system of the renal tubules. Therefore, medications that are inhibitors of this active renal elimination pathway or are eliminated by this pathway, such as cimetidine and amantadine, may interact with pramipexole resulting in reduced clearance of either or both drugs. Reduction of the pramipexole dose should be considered when these drugs are administered concomitantly with MIRAPEXIN.

When MIRAPEXIN is given in combination with levodopa, it is recommended that the dosage of levodopa is reduced and the dosage of other anti-parkinsonian medication is kept constant while increasing the dose of MIRAPEXIN.

Because of possible additive effects, caution should be advised when patients are taking other sedating medication or alcohol in combination with pramipexole.

Coadministration of antipsychotic drugs with pramipexole should be avoided (see section 4.4).

4.6 Pregnancy and lactation

The effect on pregnancy and lactation has not been investigated in humans. Pramipexole was not teratogenic in rats and rabbits, but was embryotoxic in the rat at maternotoxic doses (see section 5.3). MIRAPEXIN should not be used during pregnancy unless clearly necessary, i.e. if the potential benefit justifies the potential risk to the foetus.

As MIRAPEXIN treatment inhibits secretion of prolactin in humans, inhibition of lactation is expected.

The excretion of MIRAPEXIN into breast milk has not been studied in women. In rats, the concentration of drug-related radioactivity was higher in breast milk than in plasma.

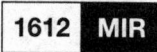

In the absence of human data, MIRAPEXIN should not be used during breast-feeding, if possible. However, if its use is unavoidable, breast-feeding should be discontinued.

4.7 Effects on ability to drive and use machines
Hallucinations or somnolence can occur.

Patients being treated with MIRAPEXIN and presenting with somnolence and/or sudden sleep episodes must be informed to refrain from driving or engaging in activities where impaired alertness may put themselves or others at risk of serious injury or death (e.g. operating machines) until such recurrent episodes and somnolence have resolved (see also Sections 4.4, 4.5 and 4.8).

4.8 Undesirable effects
Based on the analysis of pooled placebo-controlled trials, comprising a total of 1351 patients on MIRAPEXIN and 1131 patients on placebo, adverse experiences were frequently reported for both groups. 88% of patients on MIRAPEXIN and 83.6% of patients on placebo reported at least one adverse event.

The incidence of somnolence is increased at doses higher than 1.5 mg/day (see section 4.2). More frequent adverse reactions in combination with levodopa were dyskinesias. Constipation, nausea and dyskinesia tended to disappear with continued therapy. Hypotension may occur at the beginning of treatment, especially if MIRAPEXIN is titrated too fast.

The following adverse drug reactions have been observed in placebo-controlled clinical trials with MIRAPEXIN (figures have been calculated as excess incidences, compared with placebo):

Psychiatric disorders: Common (1% - 10%): Insomnia, hallucinations, confusion

Nervous system disorders: Common (1% - 10%): Dizziness, dyskinesia, somnolence (see below)

Vascular disorders: Uncommon (0.1% - 1%): Hypotension

Gastrointestinal disorders: Common (1% - 10%): Nausea, constipation

General disorders: Common (1% - 10%): Oedema peripheral

MIRAPEXIN is associated with somnolence and has been associated uncommonly with excessive daytime somnolence and sudden sleep onset episodes.

MIRAPEXIN may be associated with libido disorders (increase or decrease).

As described in literature for dopamine agonists used for treatment of Parkinson's disease, patients treated with Mirapexin, especially at high doses, have been reported as showing pathological gambling, generally reversible upon treatment discontinuation.

See also 4.4.

4.9 Overdose
There is no clinical experience with massive overdosage. The expected adverse events would be those related to the pharmacodynamic profile of a dopamine agonist, including nausea, vomiting, hyperkinesia, hallucinations, agitation and hypotension. There is no established antidote for overdosage of a dopamine agonist. If signs of central nervous system stimulation are present, a neuroleptic agent may be indicated. Management of the overdose may require general supportive measures, along with gastric lavage, intravenous fluids, and electrocardiogram monitoring.

5. PHARMACOLOGICAL PROPERTIES

5.1 Pharmacodynamic properties
Pharmacotherapeutic group: dopamine agonists, ATC code: N04B C

Pramipexole is a dopamine agonist that binds with high selectivity and specificity to the D2 subfamily of dopamine receptors of which it has a preferential affinity to D_3 receptors, and has full intrinsic activity.

Pramipexole alleviates Parkinsonian motor deficits by stimulation of dopamine recepters in the striatum. Animal studies have shown that pramipexole inhibits dopamine synthesis, release, and turnover.

In human volunteers, a dose-dependent decrease in prolactin was observed.

In patients MIRAPEXIN alleviates signs and symptoms of idiopathic Parkinson's disease.

Controlled clinical trials included approximately 2100 patients of Hoehn and Yahr stages I – IV. Out of these, approximately 900 were in more advanced stages, received concomitant levodopa therapy, and suffered from motor complications.

In early and advanced Parkinson's disease, efficacy of MIRAPEXIN in the controlled clinical trials was maintained for approximately six months. In open continuation trials lasting for more than three years there were no signs of decreasing efficacy. In a controlled double blind clinical trial of 2 year duration, initial treatment with pramipexole significantly delayed the onset of motor complications, and reduced their occurrence compared to initial treatment with levodopa. This delay in motor complications with pramipexole should be balanced against a greater improvement in motor function with levodopa (as measured by the mean change in UPDRS-score). The overall incidence of hallucinations and somnolence was generally higher in the escalation phase with the pramipexole group. However there was no significant difference during the maintenance phase. These points should be considered when initiating pramipexole treatment in patients with Parkinson's disease.

5.2 Pharmacokinetic properties
Pramipexole is rapidly and completely absorbed following oral administration. The absolute bioavailability is greater than 90% and the maximum plasma concentrations occur between 1 and 3 hours. Concomitant administration with food did not reduce the extent of pramipexole absorption, but the rate of absorption was reduced. Pramipexole shows linear kinetics and a small inter-patient variation of plasma levels.

In humans, the protein binding of pramipexole is very low (< 20%) and the volume of distribution is large (400 l). High brain tissue concentrations were observed in the rat (approx. 8-fold compared to plasma).

Pramipexole is metabolised in man only to a small extent.

Renal excretion of unchanged pramipexole is the major route of elimination. Approximately 90% of ^{14}C-labelled dose is excreted through the kidneys while less than 2% is found in the faeces. The total clearance of pramipexole is approximately 500 ml/min and the renal clearance is approximately 400 ml/min. The elimination half-life ($t_{1/2}$) varies from 8 hours in the young to 12 hours in the elderly.

5.3 Preclinical safety data
Repeated dose toxicity studies showed that pramipexole exerted functional effects, mainly involving the CNS and female reproductive system, and probably resulting from an exaggerated pharmacodynamic effect of pramipexole.

Decreases in diastolic and systolic pressure and heart rate were noted in the minipig, and a tendency to an hypotensive effect was discerned in the monkey.

The potential effects of pramipexole on reproductive function have been investigated in rats and rabbits. Pramipexole was not teratogenic in rats and rabbits but was embryotoxic in the rat at maternally toxic doses. Due to the selection of animal species and the limited parameters investigated, the adverse effects of pramipexole on pregnancy and male fertility have not been fully elucidated.

Pramipexole was not genotoxic. In a carcinogenicity study, male rats developed Leydig cell hyperplasia and adenomas, explained by the prolactin-inhibiting effect of pramipexole. This finding is not clinically relevant to man. The same study also showed that, at doses of 2 mg/kg (of salt) and higher, pramipexole was associated with retinal degeneration in albino rats. The latter finding was not observed in pigmented rats, nor in a 2-year albino mouse carcinogenicity study or in any other species investigated.

6. PHARMACEUTICAL PARTICULARS

6.1 List of excipients
Mannitol,

maize starch,

anhydrous colloidal silica,

povidone,

magnesium stearate

6.2 Incompatibilities
Not applicable

6.3 Shelf life
3 years

6.4 Special precautions for storage
Do not store above 30°C.

Store in the original package in order to protect from light.

6.5 Nature and contents of container
10 tablets per aluminium blister strips

Cartons containing 3 or 10 blister strips (30 or 100 tablets)

Not all pack sizes may be marketed.

6.6 Instructions for use and handling
No special requirements

7. MARKETING AUTHORISATION HOLDER
Boehringer Ingelheim International GmbH

D-55216 Ingelheim am Rhein

Germany

8. MARKETING AUTHORISATION NUMBER(S)
EU 1/97/051/005-006

9. DATE OF FIRST AUTHORISATION/RENEWAL OF THE AUTHORISATION
Date of first authorisation: 23 February 1998

Date of Renewal of the authorisation: 23 February 2003

10. DATE OF REVISION OF THE TEXT
29.3.2005

11. LEGAL CATEGORY
POM

M5(0.7)/B/SPC/3

Mirena

(Schering Health Care Limited)

1. NAME OF THE MEDICINAL PRODUCT
Mirena®

2. QUALITATIVE AND QUANTITATIVE COMPOSITION
Active ingredient: Levonorgestrel 52mg. The initial release rate is 20 micrograms/24hours

For excipients, see 6.1

3. PHARMACEUTICAL FORM
Levonorgestrel Intrauterine System (IUS).

The product consists of an inserter and levonorgestrel intrauterine system, which is loaded at the tip of the inserter. Inserter components are an insertion tube, plunger, flange, body and slider. The system consists of a white or almost white hormone-elastomer core, mounted on a T-body and covered in opaque tubing, which regulates the release of levonorgestrel. The T-body has a loop at one end and two arms at the other end. Removal threads are attached to the loop.

4. CLINICAL PARTICULARS

4.1 Therapeutic indications
Contraception.

Idiopathic menorrhagia. Mirena may be particularly useful in women with idiopathic menorrhagia requiring (reversible) contraception.

Protection from endometrial hyperplasia during oestrogen replacement therapy.

4.2 Posology and method of administration
The initial release of levonorgestrel is about 20 micrograms/24 hours.

Mirena is effective for five years in the indications for contraception and idiopathic menorrhagia.

In the indication for protection from endometrial hyperplasia during oestrogen replacement therapy, clinical data beyond 4 years of use are limited. Mirena should therefore be removed after 4 years.

Clinical trials were conducted in women of 18 years and over.

Before insertion, the patient must be informed of the efficacy, risks and side-effects of Mirena. A gynaecological examination, including examination of the breasts and exclusion of a pregnancy, should be performed. Cervical infection and sexually transmitted diseases should be excluded. The position of the uterus and the size of the uterine cavity should be determined. The instructions for insertion should be followed carefully. The patient should be re-examined six weeks after insertion and once a year thereafter, or more frequently if clinically indicated.

Special instructions for insertion are in the package.

Insertion:

In women of fertile age, Mirena is inserted into the uterine cavity within seven days of the onset of menstruation. It can be replaced by a new system at any time of the cycle.

Mirena can also be inserted immediately after the first trimester abortion by curettage.

Postpartum insertions should be postponed until six weeks after delivery.

In women under hormonal replacement therapy, Mirena can be used in combination with oral or transdermal oestrogen preparations without progestogens.

When used for endometrial protection during oestrogen replacement therapy, Mirena can be inserted at any time in an amenorrhoeic woman, or during the last days of menstruation or withdrawal bleeding.

Because irregular bleeding/spotting may occur during the first months of therapy, it is recommended to exclude endometrial pathology before insertion of Mirena. If the woman continues the use of Mirena inserted earlier for contraception, endometrial pathology has to be excluded if bleeding disturbances appear after commencing oestrogen replacement therapy. If bleeding irregularities develop during a prolonged treatment, appropriate diagnostic measures should also be taken.

Removal:

The system should be removed after five years in the indications for contraception and menorrhagia and after 4 years for endometrial protection. If the user wishes to continue using the same method, a new system can be inserted at the same time.

Mirena is removed by gently pulling on the threads with forceps. If the threads are not visible and the system is in the uterine cavity, it may be removed using a narrow tenaculum. This may require dilatation of the cervical canal.

If pregnancy is not desired, removal should be carried out during menstruation in women of fertile age, provided that there appears to be a menstrual cycle. If the system is removed mid-cycle and the woman has had intercourse within a week, she is at risk of pregnancy unless a new system is inserted immediately following removal.

4.3 Contraindications
Known or suspected pregnancy; undiagnosed abnormal genital bleeding; congenital or acquired abnormality of the

uterus including fibroids if they distort the uterine cavity; current genital infection; current or recurrent pelvic inflammatory disease; postpartum endometritis, infected abortion during the past three months; cervicitis; cervical dysplasia; uterine or cervical malignancy; past attack of bacterial endocarditis or of severe pelvic infection in a woman with an anatomical lesion of the heart or after any prosthetic valve replacement; active or previous severe arterial disease, such as stroke or myocardial infarction; liver tumour or other acute or severe liver disease; conditions associated with increased susceptibility to infections; acute malignancies affecting the blood or leukaemias except when in remission; recent trophoblastic disease while hCG levels remain elevated; hypersensitivity to the constituents of the preparation.

4.4 Special warnings and special precautions for use

Mirena may be used with caution after specialist consultation, or removal of the system should be considered, if any of the following conditions exist or arise for the first time:

- Migraine, crescendo migraine, focal migraine with asymmetrical visual loss or other symptoms indicating transient cerebral ischaemia
- Unusually severe or unusually frequent headache
- Jaundice
- Marked increase of blood pressure
- Confirmed or suspected hormone dependent neoplasia including breast cancer
- Malignancies affecting the blood or leukaemias in remission
- Use of chronic corticosteroid therapy
- Past history of symptomatic functional ovarian cysts
- Severe or multiple risk factors for arterial disease
- Thrombotic arterial or any current embolic disease
- Venous thromboembolism.

In general, women using hormonal contraception should be encouraged to give up smoking.

Menorrhagia: Mirena usually achieves a significant reduction in menstrual blood loss in 3 to 6 months of treatment. If significant reduction in blood loss is not achieved in these time-frames, alternative treatments should be considered.

Patients with congenital or acquired cardiac valve defects may be given antibiotic prophylaxis at the time of IUS insertion or removal to prevent endocarditis.

Ectopic pregnancy: Women with a previous history of ectopic pregnancy carry a higher risk of a further ectopic pregnancy. The possibility of ectopic pregnancy should be considered in the case of lower abdominal pain - especially in connection with missed periods or if an amenorrhoeic woman starts bleeding. The rate of ectopic pregnancy in users of Mirena is 0.06 per 100 woman-years. This rate is lower than the rate of 0.3-0.5 per 100 woman-years estimated for women not using any contraception. The corresponding figure for the copper IUD is 0.12 per 100 woman years.

Irregular bleeding may mask symptoms and signs of endometrial cancer.

Functional ovarian cysts have been diagnosed in about 10-12% of patients, and these are also common with progestogen-only contraception. In most cases, the enlarged follicles disappear spontaneously during two to three months' observation. Should this not happen, continued ultrasound monitoring and other diagnostic/therapeutic measures are recommended.

Use with caution in postmenopausal women with advanced uterine atrophy.

Low-dose levonorgestrel may affect glucose tolerance, and the blood glucose concentration should be monitored in diabetic users of Mirena.

Insertion and removal may be associated with some pain and bleeding. If the pain is unusually severe, or if bleeding continues, the possibility of perforation of the uterine corpus or cervix must be considered (see also special warnings and precautions for use '*Perforation*'). The procedure may precipitate fainting as a vasovagal reaction, or a seizure in an epileptic patient. In the event of early signs of a vasovagal attack, insertion may need to be abandoned or the system removed. The woman should be kept supine, the head lowered and the legs elevated to the vertical position if necessary in order to restore cerebral blood flow. A clear airway must be maintained; an airway should always be at hand. Persistent bradycardia may be controlled with intravenous atropine. If oxygen is available it may be administered.

The possibility of pregnancy should be considered if menstruation does not occur within six weeks of the onset of previous menstruation and expulsion should be excluded. A repeated pregnancy test is not necessary in amenorrhoeic subjects unless indicated by other symptoms.

Pelvic infection: Known risk factors for pelvic inflammatory disease are multiple sexual partners, frequent intercourse and young age. Mirena must be removed if the woman experiences recurrent endometritis or pelvic infection, or if an acute infection is severe or does not respond to treatment within a few days. Pelvic infection may have serious consequences as it may impair fertility and increase the risk of ectopic pregnancy.

Delayed follicular atresia: Since the contraceptive effect of Mirena is mainly due to its local effect, ovulatory cycles with follicular rupture usually occur in women of fertile age. Sometimes atresia of the follicle is delayed and folliculogenesis may continue. These enlarged follicles cannot be distinguished clinically from ovarian cysts. Enlarged follicles have been diagnosed in about 12% of the subjects using Mirena. Most of these follicles are asymptomatic, although some may be accompanied by pelvic pain or dyspareunia. In most cases, the enlarged follicles disappear spontaneously during two to three months' observation. Should this not happen, continued ultrasound monitoring and other diagnostic/therapeutic measures are recommended. Rarely, surgical intervention may be required.

Expulsion: Symptoms of the partial or complete expulsion of any IUS may include bleeding or pain. However, a system can be expelled from the uterine cavity without the woman noticing it. Partial expulsion may decrease the effectiveness of Mirena. As the system decreases menstrual flow, increase of menstrual flow may be indicative of an expulsion. A displaced Mirena should be removed and a new system inserted. The woman should be advised how to check the threads of Mirena.

Perforation: Perforation of the uterine corpus or cervix may occur, most commonly during insertion. This may be associated with severe pain and continued bleeding. If perforation is suspected the system should be removed as soon as possible.

Lost threads: If the retrieval threads are not visible at the cervix on follow-up examination - first exclude pregnancy. The threads may have been drawn up into the uterus or cervical canal and may reappear during the next menstrual period. If pregnancy has been excluded, the threads may usually be located by gently probing with a suitable instrument. If they cannot be found, they may have broken off, or the system may have been expelled. Ultrasound or X-ray may be used to locate Mirena.

Post-coital contraception: Limited experience suggests that Mirena is not suitable for use as a post-coital contraceptive.

4.5 Interaction with other medicinal products and other forms of Interaction

The effect of hormonal contraceptives may be impaired by drugs which induce liver enzymes, including barbiturates, primidone, phenytoin, carbamazepine, griseofulvin and rifampicin. The influence of these drugs on the contraceptive efficacy of Mirena has not been studied.

4.6 Pregnancy and lactation

Pregnancy: Mirena is not to be used during an existing or suspected pregnancy. In case of an accidental pregnancy with Mirena in situ, the system must be removed and termination of the pregnancy should be considered. Should these procedures not be possible, the woman should be informed about increased risk of spontaneous abortion or premature labour observed during the use of copper and plastic IUDs. Accordingly, such pregnancies should be closely monitored. Ectopic pregnancy should be excluded. The woman should be instructed to report all symptoms that suggest complications of the pregnancy, like cramping abdominal pain with fever.

Because of the intrauterine administration and the local exposure to the hormone, teratogenicity (especially virilisation) cannot be completely excluded. It can be expected that the systemic hormone exposure of the foetus through the maternal circulation is lower than with any other hormonal contraceptive method. Clinical experience of the outcomes of pregnancies with Mirena in situ is limited. However, the woman should be informed that, to date, there is no evidence of birth defects caused by Mirena use in cases where pregnancy continues to term with Mirena in place.

Lactation: Levonorgestrel has been identified in the breast milk, but it is not likely that there will be a risk for the child with the dose released from Mirena, when it is inserted in the uterine cavity.

There appears to be no deleterious effects on infant growth or development when using any progestogen-only method after six weeks postpartum. Progestogen-only methods do not appear to affect the quantity or quality of breast milk. Uterine bleeding has rarely been reported in women using Mirena during lactation.

4.7 Effects on ability to drive and use machines

There are no known effects on the ability to drive or use machines.

4.8 Undesirable effects

Undesirable effects are more common during the first months after the insertion, and subside during prolonged use. In addition to the adverse effects listed in section 4.4 "Special warnings and special precautions for use" the following undesirable effects have been reported in users of Mirena, although a causal relationship with Mirena could not always be confirmed.

Ectopic pregnancy in case of method failure should be ruled out (see section 4.4).

Very common undesirable effects (occurring in more than 10% of users) include bleeding changes and ovarian cysts.

Different kinds of bleeding changes (frequent, prolonged or heavy bleeding, spotting, oligomenorrhoea, amenorrhoea) are experienced by all users of Mirena. In fertile women the average number of spotting days/month decreases gradually from nine to four days during the first six months of use. The percentage of women with prolonged bleeding (more than eight days) decreases from 20% to 3% during the first three months of use. In clinical studies during the first year of use, 17% of women experienced amenorrhoea of at least three months duration.

Table 1

Organ system	Common undesirable effects > 1/100, < 1/10	Uncommon undesirable effects > 1/1000, < 1/100	Rare undesirable effects > 1/10000, < 1/1000
Infection		Genital infections including salpingitis and pelvic inflammatory disease	
Endocrine disorders	Oedema (peripheral or abdominal)		
Metabolism and nutrition disorders	Weight gain		
Psychiatric disorders	Depressive mood Nervousness Mood lability		Reduced libido
Nervous system disorders	Headache		Migraine
Gastrointestinal disorders	Abdominal pain Pelvic pain Nausea		Abdominal bloating
Skin and subcutaneous disorders	Acne	Hirsutism Hair loss Pruritus	Rash Urticaria Eczema
Musculoskeletal, connective tissue and bone disorders	Back pain		
Reproductive system and breast disorders	Dysmenorrhoea Vaginal discharge Cervicitis Breast tension Mastalgia		Uterine perforation
General disorders and administration site conditions	Expulsion		

When used in combination with oestrogen replacement therapy, perimenopausal users of Mirena may experience spotting and irregular bleeding during the first months of the treatment. The amount of bleeding becomes minimal during the first year, and 30-60% of users are totally free of bleedings.

The frequency of benign ovarian cysts depends on the diagnostic method used, and in clinical trials enlarged follicles have been diagnosed in 12% of the subjects using Mirena. Most of the follicles are asymptomatic and disappear within three months.

(see Table 1 on previous page)

4.9 Overdose
Not applicable

5. PHARMACOLOGICAL PROPERTIES

5.1 Pharmacodynamic properties
Levonorgestrel is a progestogen used in gynaecology in various ways: as the progestogen component in oral contraceptives, in hormonal replacement therapy or alone for contraception in minipills and subdermal implants. Levonorgestrel can also be administered directly into the uterine cavity as an intrauterine system. This allows a very low daily dosage, as the hormone is released directly into the target organ.

The contraceptive mechanism of action of Mirena is based on mainly hormonal effects producing the following changes:

- Prevention of proliferation of the endometrium
- Thickening of the cervical mucus thus inhibiting the passage of sperm
- Suppression of ovulation in some women.

The physical presence of the system in the uterus would also be expected to make a minor contribution to its contraceptive effect.

Studies on contraceptive efficacy have suggested a pregnancy rate (Pearl Index) of less than 1 per 100 woman-years.

Mirena may be particularly useful for contraception in patients with excessive menstrual bleeding, and can be successfully used in the treatment of idiopathic menorrhagia. The volume of menstrual bleeding was decreased by 88% in menorrhagic women by the end of three months of use. Menorrhagia caused by submucosal fibroids may respond less favourably. Reduced bleeding promotes the increase of blood haemoglobin in patients with menorrhagia.

In idiopathic menorrhagia, prevention of proliferation of the endometrium is the probable mechanism of action of Mirena in reducing blood loss.

The efficacy of Mirena in preventing endometrial hyperplasia during continuous oestrogen treatment is the same when oestrogen is administered orally or transdermally. The observed hyperplasia rate under oestrogen therapy alone is as high as 20%. In clinical studies with 201 perimenopausal and 259 postmenopausal users of Mirena, no cases of endometrial hyperplasia were reported in the postmenopausal group during the observation period up to 4 years.

5.2 Pharmacokinetic properties
The pharmacokinetics of levonorgestrel itself have been extensively investigated and reported in the literature. One key finding is that the bioavailability of levonorgestrel administered orally is almost 90 per cent. In postmenopausal users of Mirena, plasma levonorgestrel concentrations have been 184±54 pg/ml, 188±47 pg/ml and 134±30 pg/ml, respectively. A half life of 20 hours is considered the best estimate although some studies have reported values as short as 9 hours and others as long as 80 hours. Another important finding, although one in agreement with experience with other synthetic steroids, has been marked differences in metabolic clearance rates among individuals, even when administration was by the intravenous route. Levonorgestrel is extensively bound to proteins (mainly sex hormone binding globulin (SHBG) and extensively metabolised to a large number of inactive metabolites.

The initial release of levonorgestrel from Mirena is 20 micrograms/24 hours, delivered directly into the uterine cavity. Because of the low plasma concentrations, there are only minor effects on the metabolism.

5.3 Preclinical safety data
Levonorgestrel is a well established progestogen with anti-oestrogenic activity. The safety profile following systemic administration is well documented. A study in monkeys with intrauterine delivery of levonorgestrel for 12 months confirmed local pharmacological activity with good local tolerance and no signs of systemic toxicity. No embryotoxicity was seen in the rabbit following intrauterine administration of levonorgestrel.

6. PHARMACEUTICAL PARTICULARS

6.1 List of excipients
Polydimethylsiloxane elastomer, polydimethylsiloxane tubing, polyethylene, barium sulphate, iron oxide

6.2 Incompatibilities
None known

6.3 Shelf life
Three years

6.4 Special precautions for storage
Not applicable.

6.5 Nature and contents of container
The product is individually packed into a thermoformed blister package with a peelable lid.

6.6 Instructions for use and handling
As the insertion technique is different from intrauterine devices, special emphasis should be given to training in the correct insertion technique. Special instructions for insertion are in the package.

Mirena is supplied in a sterile pack which should not be opened until required for insertion. Each system should be handled with aseptic precautions. If the seal of the sterile envelope is broken, the system inside should be disposed of in accordance with the local guidelines for the handling of biohazardous waste. Likewise, a removed Mirena and inserter should be disposed of in this manner. The outer carton package and the inner blister package can be handled as household waste.

7. MARKETING AUTHORISATION HOLDER
Schering Health Care Limited
The Brow
Burgess Hill
West Sussex RH15 9NE

8. MARKETING AUTHORISATION NUMBER(S)
0053/0265

9. DATE OF FIRST AUTHORISATION/RENEWAL OF THE AUTHORISATION
22 February 1995

10. DATE OF REVISION OF THE TEXT
14th July 2004

Legal Category
POM

Mitomycin-C Kyowa

(Kyowa Hakko UK Ltd)

1. NAME OF THE MEDICINAL PRODUCT
Mitomycin-C Kyowa 2mg, 10mg, 20mg or 40 mg.

2. QUALITATIVE AND QUANTITATIVE COMPOSITION
Active Constituent Quantity per vial
Mitomycin-C 2 mg, 10 mg, 20 mg or 40 mg

3. PHARMACEUTICAL FORM
Sterile powder for injection.

4. CLINICAL PARTICULARS

4.1 Therapeutic indications
Antimitotic and Cytotoxic
Recommended for certain types of cancer in combination with other drugs or after primary therapy has failed. It has been successfully used to improve subjective and objective symptoms in a wide range of neoplastic conditions.

1. As a single agent in the treatment of superficial bladder cancer. In addition it has been shown that post-operative instillations of Mitomycin-C can reduce recurrence rates in newly diagnosed patients with superficial bladder cancer.

2. As a single agent and in combination with other drugs in metastatic breast cancer.

3. In combination with other agents in advanced squamous cell carcinoma of the uterine cervix.

4. It shows a degree of activity as part of combination therapy in carcinoma of the stomach, pancreas and lung (particularly non-small cell).

5. It shows a degree of activity as a single agent and in combination in liver cancer when given by the intra-arterial route.

6. It has a possible role in combination with other cytotoxic drugs in colo-rectal cancer.

7. It shows a degree of activity as a single agent or part of combination therapy in cancer of the head and neck.

8. It shows a degree of activity as a single agent in cancer of the prostate.

9. It has a possible role in skin cancer.

10. It has a degree of activity in leukaemia and non-solid tumours.

11. It has a possible role in sarcomas.

12. It has been successfully used in combination with surgery, pre-operatively (oesophageal squamous cell carcinoma) and post-operatively (gastric cancer).

13. It has shown to be effective when used in combination with radiotherapy.

4.2 Posology and method of administration
For parenteral use.
Intravenously, the dose should be given with great care in order to avoid extravasation. The usual dose is in the range of 4 – 10mg (0.06-0.15mg/kg) given at 1 – 6 weekly intervals depending on whether other drugs are given in combination and on bone marrow recovery. In a number of combination schedules, the dose is 10mg/m^2 of body surface area, the course being repeated at intervals for as long as required. A course ranging from 40-80mg (0.58 –1.2mg/kg) is often required for a satisfactory response when used alone or in combination. A higher dosage course may be given when used alone or as part of a particular combination schedule and total cumulative doses exceeding 2mg/kg have been given.

For administration into specific tissues, Mitomycin-C Kyowa can be given by the intra-arterial route directly into the tumours.

Because of cumulative myelosuppression, patients should be fully re-evaluated after each course and the dose reduced if the patient has experienced any toxic effects. Doses greater than 0.6mg/kg have not been shown to be more effective and are more toxic than lower doses.

Treatment of superficial bladder tumours: In the treatment of superficial bladder tumours the usual dose is 20-40mg dissolved in 20-40 of diluent, instilled into the bladder through a urethral catheter, weekly or three times a week for a total of 20 doses. The dose should be retained by the patient for a minimum of one hour. During this one-hour period the patient should be rotated every 15 minutes to ensure that the Mitomycin-C comes into contact with all areas of the bladder urthelium.

When the bladder is emptied in the voiding process, care must be taken to ensure that no contamination occurs locally in the groin and genitalia areas.

In the prevention of recurrent superficial bladder tumours, various doses have been used. These include 20mg in 20ml of diluent every two weeks and 40mg in 40ml of diluent monthly or three monthly. The dose is instilled into the bladder through a urethral catheter.

4.3 Contraindications
Patients who have demonstrated a hypersensitive or idiosyncratic reaction to Mitomycin-C Kyowa in the past. Thrombocytopenia, coagulation disorders and increased bleeding tendency.

4.4 Special warnings and special precautions for use
Mitomycin-C Kyowa should be administered under the supervision of a physician experienced in cytotoxic cancer chemotherapy. Local ulceration and cellulitis may be caused by tissue extravasation during intravenous injection and utmost care should be taken in administration.

If extravasation occurs, it is recommended that the area is immediately infiltrated with sodium bicarbonate 8.4% solution, followed by an injection of 4mg dexamethasone. A systemic injection of 200mg of Vitamin B6 may be of some value in promoting the regrowth of tissues that have been damaged.

Mitomycin-C Kyowa should not be allowed to come into contact with the skin. If it does, it should be washed several times with 8.4% sodium bicarbonate solution, followed by soap and water. Hand creams and emollients should not be used as they may assist the penetration of the drug into the epidermal tissue.

In the event of contact with the eye, it should be rinsed several times with 8.4% sodium bicarbonate solution. It should then be observed for several days for evidence of corneal damage. If necessary, appropriate treatment should be instituted.

4.5 Interaction with other medicinal products and other forms of Interaction
Not Known.

4.6 Pregnancy and lactation
Mitomycin-C Kyowa should not normally be administrated to patients who are pregnant or to mothers who are breast-feeding. Teratological changes have been noted in animal studies.

4.7 Effects on ability to drive and use machines
Generalised weakness and lethargy have been reported on rare occasions. If affected, patients should be advised not to drive or operate machinery.

4.8 Undesirable effects
Thrombocytopenia and leucopenia resulting from myelosuppression, which is delayed and cumulative. Patients should be monitored closely during each course of treatment, paying particular attention to peripheral blood count including platelet count. No repeat dose should be given unless the leucocyte count is above 3.0×10^9/L or more and the platelet count is 90×10^9/L or more. The nadir is usually around four weeks after treatment and toxicity is usually cumulative, with increasing risk after each course of treatment. If disease progression continues after two courses of treatment, the drug should be stopped since the chances of response are minimal. Severe renal toxicity has occasionally been reported after treatment and renal function should be monitored before starting treatment and again after each course. Nausea and vomiting are sometimes experienced immediately after treatment, but these are usually mild and of short duration. Pulmonary toxicity and fever have been reported. Skin toxicity may occur in a small proportion of patients, with side effects such as alopecia (although this is less frequent and less severe than with certain other cytotoxic agents). Bleeding, rashes and mouth ulcers have been reported. General weakness and lethargy have been reported on rare occasions. Other reported effects include anorexia, diarrhoea, stomatitis, interstitial pneumonitis, pulmonary fibrosis and microangiopathic haemolytic anaemia syndrome.

4.9 Overdose
In the unlikely event of accidental overdosage then an increase in the more common side effects should be expected, such as fever, nausea, vomiting and myelosuppression. Appropriate supportive measures should be instituted.

5. PHARMACOLOGICAL PROPERTIES
5.1 Pharmacodynamic properties
Mitomycin-C Kyowa is an antitumour antibiotic that is activated in the tissues to an alkylating agent which disrupts deoxyribonucleic acid (DNA) in cancer cells by forming a complex with DNA and also acts by inhibiting division of cancer cells by interfering with the biosynthesis of DNA.

5.2 Pharmacokinetic properties
In vivo
Mitomycin-C Kyowa is rapidly cleared from the serum after intravenous administration. The time required to reduce the serum concentration by 50% after a 30mg bolus injection is 17 minutes. After injection of 30mg, 20mg or 10mg intravenously, the maximal serum concentrations were 2.4 mcg/ml, 1.7 mcg/ml and 0.52mcg/ml respectively. Clearance is effected primarily by metabolism in the liver, but metabolism occurs in other tissues as well. The rate of clearance is inversely proportional to the maximal serum concentration because, it is thought, of saturation of the degradative pathways. Approximately 10% of a dose of Mitomycin-C Kyowa is excreted unchanged in the urine. Since metabolic pathways are saturated at relatively low doses, the percentage dose excreted in the urine increases with increasing dose. In children, the excretion of intravenously administered Mitomycin-C Kyowa is similar to that in adults.

5.3 Preclinical safety data
There are no preclinical data of relevance to the prescriber which are additional to that already included elsewhere in the SPC.

6. PHARMACEUTICAL PARTICULARS
6.1 List of excipients
Sodium Chloride Ph.Eur.

6.2 Incompatibilities
Not known

6.3 Shelf life
Four years from the date of manufacture.
After reconstitution, the solution is stable for 24 hours when protected from light and stored in a cool place. Do not refrigerate.

6.4 Special precautions for storage
None.

6.5 Nature and contents of container
Mitomycin-C Kyowa consists of a blue/purple crystalline powder, contained within a colourless, type I or III glass vial with a rubber stopper and an aluminium seal.
The vials are packaged into cardboard cartons containing 1, 5 or 10 vials.

6.6 Instructions for use and handling
The contents of the vial should be reconstituted with Water for Injections or saline solution, at least 5 ml for the 2 mg vial, at least 10 ml for the 10 mg vial, at least 20 ml for the 20 mg vial, and at least 40 ml for the 40 mg vial.

Administrative Data
7. MARKETING AUTHORISATION HOLDER
Kyowa Hakko (UK) Ltd
258 Bath Road
Slough
Berkshire
SL1 4DX

8. MARKETING AUTHORISATION NUMBER(S)
PL12196/0001/0002/0003

9. DATE OF FIRST AUTHORISATION/RENEWAL OF THE AUTHORISATION
26th November 1992

10. DATE OF REVISION OF THE TEXT
July 2003

Mitoxantrone 2mg/ml Sterile Concentrate
(Wockhardt UK Ltd)

1. NAME OF THE MEDICINAL PRODUCT
Mitoxantrone 2mg/ml Sterile Concentrate

2. QUALITATIVE AND QUANTITATIVE COMPOSITION
Each 1ml contains mitoxantrone hydrochloride equivalent to 2.0mg mitoxantrone. The vial contains 10mg in 5ml or 20mg in 10ml
For excipients, see section 6.1.

3. PHARMACEUTICAL FORM
Concentrate for solution for infusion
The concentrate is a dark blue, aqueous solution.

Table 1

Nadir after prior dose WBC(per mm^3)		Platelets (per mm^3)	Time to Recovery	Subsequent dose after adequate haematological recovery
>1,500	AND	>50,000	≤21 days	Repeat prior dose after recovery or increase by 2mg/m^2 if myelosuppression is not considered adequate.
>1,500	AND	>50,000	> 21 days	Withhold until recovery, then repeat prior dose.
<1,500	OR	<50,000	Any duration	Decrease by 2mg/m^2 from prior dose after recovery.
<1,000	OR	<25,000	Any duration	Decrease by 4mg/m^2 from prior dose after recovery.

4. CLINICAL PARTICULARS
4.1 Therapeutic indications
Mitoxantrone is indicated in the treatment of metastatic breast cancer, non-Hodgkin's lymphoma and adult acute non-lymphocytic leukaemia.
Mitoxantrone has also been used in the palliation of non-resectable primary hepatocellular carcinoma.

4.2 Posology and method of administration
Posology
Metastatic Breast Cancer, Non-Hodgkin's Lymphoma, Hepatoma:
(a) Single Agent Dosage
The recommended initial dosage of mitoxantrone used as a single agent is 14mg/m^2 of body surface area, given as a single intravenous dose which may be repeated at 21-day intervals. A lower initial dosage (12mg/m^2 or less) is recommended in patients with inadequate bone marrow reserves. e.g. due to prior chemotherapy or poor general condition.
Dosage modification and the timing of subsequent dosing should be determined by clinical judgement depending on the degree and duration of myelosuppression. For subsequent courses the prior dose can usually be repeated if white blood cell and platelet counts have returned to normal levels after 21 days. The following table is suggested as a guide to dosage adjustment, in the treatment of advanced breast cancer, non-Hodgkin's lymphoma and hepatoma according to the haematological nadir (which usually occurs about 10 days after dosing).

(see Table 1 above)

(b) Combination Therapy
Mitoxantrone has been given as part of combination therapy. In metastatic breast cancer, combinations of mitoxantrone with other cytotoxic agents including cyclophosphamide and 5-fluorouracil or methotrexate and mitomycin C have been shown to be effective. Reference should be made to the published literature for information on dosage modifications and administration. Mitoxantrone has also been used in various combinations for non-Hodgkin's lymphoma, however data are presently limited and specific regimens cannot be recommended.
As a guide, when mitoxantrone is used in combination chemotherapy with another myelosuppressive agent, the initial dose of mitoxantrone should be reduced by 2-4mg/m^2 below the doses recommended for single agent usage; subsequent dosing, as outlined in the table above, depends on the degree and duration of myelosuppression.

Acute Non-Lymphocytic Leukaemia
(a) Single Agent Dosage in Relapse
The recommended dosage for remission induction is 12mg/m^2 of body surface area, given as a single intravenous dose daily for five consecutive days (total of 60mg/m^2). In clinical studies with a dosage of 12mg/m^2 daily for 5 days, patients who achieved a complete remission did so as a result of the first induction course.

(b) Combination Therapy
Mitoxantrone has been used in combination regimens for the treatment of ANLL. Most clinical experience has been with mitoxantrone combined with cytosine arabinoside. This combination has been used successfully for primary treatment of ANLL as well as in relapse.
An effective regimen for induction in previously untreated patients has been mitoxantrone 10-12mg/m^2 IV for 3 days combined with cytosine arabinoside 100mg/m^2 IV for 7 days (by continuous infusion). This is followed by second induction and consolidation courses as thought appropriate by the treating clinician. In clinical studies, duration of therapy in induction and consolidation courses with mitoxantrone has been reduced to 2 days and that of cytosine arabinoside to 5 days. However, modification to the above regimen should be carried out by the treating clinician depending on individual patient factors.
Efficacy has also been demonstrated with mitoxantrone in combination with etoposide in patients who had relapsed or who were refractory to primary conventional chemotherapy. The use of mitoxantrone in combination with etoposide as with other cytotoxics may result in greater myelosuppression than with mitoxantrone alone.
Reference should be made to the published literature for information on specific dosage regimens. Mitoxantrone should be used by clinicians experienced in the use of chemotherapy regimens. Dosage adjustments should be made by the treating clinician as appropriate, taking into account toxicity, response and individual patient characteristics. As with other cytotoxic drugs, mitoxantrone should be used with caution in combination therapy until wider experience is available.

(c) Paediatric Leukaemia
As experience with mitoxantrone in paediatric leukaemia is limited, dosage recommendations in this patient population cannot at present be given.

Method of administration
Mitoxantrone should be given by intravenous infusion. **Not for intrathecal use.**
Syringes containing this product should be labelled "For intravenous use only".
Care should be taken to avoid contact of mitoxantrone with skin, mucous membranes or eyes; see section 6.6 Instructions for use and handling for further directions.

4.3 Contraindications
NOT FOR INTRATHECAL USE.
Demonstrated hypersensitivity tomitoxantrone or other anthracyclines.
Mitoxantrone Sterile Concentrate should not be used during pregnancy or lactation.

4.4 Special warnings and special precautions for use
There may be an increased risk of leukaemia when mitoxantrone is used as adjuvant treatment of non metastatic breast cancer. In the absence of sufficient efficacy data, mitoxantrone must not be used as adjuvant treatment of non metastatic breast cancer.
Mitoxantrone should be used with caution in patients with myelosuppression or poor general condition.
Cases of functional cardiac changes, including congestive heart failure and decreases in left ventricular ejection fraction have been reported. The majority of these cardiac events have occurred in patients who have had prior treatment with anthracyclines, prior mediastinal/thoracic radiotherapy, or with pre-existing heart disease. It is recommended that patients in these categories are treated with mitoxantrone at full cytotoxic dosage and schedule. However, added caution is required in these patients and careful regular cardiac examinations are recommended from the initiation of treatment.
As experience of prolonged treatment with mitoxantrone is presently limited, it is suggested that cardiac examinations also be performed in patients without identifiable risk factors during therapy exceeding a cumulative dose of 160mg/m^2.
Careful supervision is recommended when treating patients with severe hepatic insufficiency.
Mitoxantrone is mutagenic in vitro and in vivo in the rat. In the same species there was a possible association between administration of the drug and development of malignant neoplasia.
Topoisomerase II inhibitors, including mitoxantrone, when used concomitantly with other antineoplastic agents and/or radiotherapy, have been associated with the

development of Acute Myeloid leukaemia (AML) or Myelodysplastic Syndrome (MDS).

Mitoxantrone is not indicated for intra-arterial injection. There have been reports of local/regional neuropathy, some irreversible, following intra-arterial injection. Safety for intrathecal use has not been established. There have been reports of neuropathy, including paralysis and bowel and bladder dysfunction following intrathecal injection.

Sulphites can cause allergic-type reactions including anaphylactic symptoms and bronchospasm in susceptible people, especially those with a history of asthma or allergy.

Mitoxantrone is an active cytotoxic drug which should be used by clinicians familiar with the use of antineoplastic agents, and having the facilities for regular monitoring of clinical, haematological and biochemical parameters during and after treatment.

Full blood counts should be undertaken serially during a course of treatment. Dosage adjustments may be necessary based on these counts.

Immunisation may be ineffective when given during mitoxantrone therapy. Immunisation with live virus vaccines are generally not recommended.

This medicinal product contains 0.74mmol of sodium in each vial. To be taken into consideration by patients on a controlled sodium diet.

4.5 Interaction with other medicinal products and other forms of Interaction

Not applicable

4.6 Pregnancy and lactation

The effects of mitoxantrone on human fertility or pregnancy have not been established. As with other antineoplastic agents, patients and their partner should be advised to avoid conception for at least six months after cessation of therapy. Mitoxantrone should not normally be administered to patients who are pregnant.

Mitoxantrone is excreted in human milk and significant concentrations (18ng/ml) have been reported for 28 days after the last administration. Because of the potential for serious adverse reactions in infants, breast feeding should be discontinued before starting treatment.

4.7 Effects on ability to drive and use machines

Not applicable.

4.8 Undesirable effects

Some degree of leucopenia is to be expected following recommended doses of mitoxantrone. With a single dose every 21 days, suppression of WBC count below 1000/mm^3 is infrequent; leucopenia is usually transient, reaching its nadir at about 10 days after dosing, with recovery usually occurring by the 21st day. Thrombocytopenia can occur and anaemia occurs less frequently. Myelosuppression may be more severe and prolonged in patients who have had extensive prior chemotherapy or radiotherapy or in debilitated patients.

When mitoxantrone is used as a single injection given every 21 days in the treatment of metastatic breast cancer and lymphomas, the most commonly encountered side effects are nausea and vomiting, although in the majority of cases these are mild and transient. Alopecia may occur, but is most frequently of minimal severity and reversible on cessation of therapy.

Other side effects which have been occasionally been reported include skin rashes, allergic reactions, amenorrhoea, anorexia, constipation, diarrhoea, dysponea, fatigue and weakness, fever, gastrointestinal bleeding, stomatitis/mucositis/conjunctivitis and non-specific neurological side effects such as somnolence, confusion, anxiety and mild paraesthesia. Tissue necrosis following extravasation has been reported rarely. In patients with an increase in both frequency and severity, particularly of stomatitis and mucositis.

Changes in laboratory test values have been observed infrequently e.g. elevated serum creatinine and blood urea nitrogen levels, increased liver enzyme levels (with occasional reports of severe impairment of hepatic function in patients with leukaemia). Hyperuricaemia has also been reported.

Cardiovascular effects, which have occasionally been of clinical significance, include decreased left ventricular ejection fraction, ECG changes and acute arrhythmia. Congestive heart failure has been reported and has generally responded well to treatment with digitalis and/or diuretics. In patients with leukaemia, an increase in the frequency of adverse cardiac events has been observed; the direct role of mitoxantrone in these cases is difficult to assess as most patients had received prior therapy with anthracyclines and since the clinical course in leukaemic patients is often complicated by anaemia, fever, sepsis and intravenous fluid therapy.

Extravasation at the infusion site has been reported, which may result in erythema, swelling, pain, burning and/or blue discoloration of the skin. Extravasation can result in tissue necrosis with resultant need for debridement and skin grafting. Phlebitis has also been reported at the site of infusion.

Mitoxantrone may impart a blue-green coloration to the urine for 24 hours after administration and patients should be advised that this is to be expected. Blue discoloration of skin and nails has been reported occasionally. Nail dystrophy or reversible blue coloration of the sclerae may be seen rarely.

Topoisomerase II inhibitors, including mitoxantrone, when used concomitantly with other antineoplastic agents, and/or radiotherapy, have been associated with the development of Acute Myeloid leukaemia (AML) of Myelodysplastic Syndrome (MDS).

Rare reports of cardiomyopathy have been received.

4.9 Overdose

There is no known specific antidote for mitoxantrone. Haemopoietic, gastrointestinal, hepatic or renal toxicity may be seen depending on dosage given and the physical condition of the patient. In cases of overdosage the patient should be monitored closely and management should be symptomatic and supportive.

Fatalities have occurred on rare occasions as a result of severe leucopenia with infection in patients accidentally given single bolus injections of mitoxantrone at over ten times the recommended dosage. Mitoxantrone is extensively tissue-bound and peritoneal dialysis or haemodialysis is unlikely to be effective in managing overdose.

5. PHARMACOLOGICAL PROPERTIES

5.1 Pharmacodynamic properties

Pharmacotherapeutic group: Cytotoxic antibiotics and related substances/Anthracyclines and related substances, ATC Code: L01D B07.

Although its mechanism of action has not been determined, mitoxantrone is a DNA-reactive agent. It has a cytocidal effect on proliferating and non-proliferating cultured human cells, suggesting activity against rapidly proliferating and slow-growing neoplasms.

5.2 Pharmacokinetic properties

Pharmacokinetic studies in patients following intravenous administration of mitoxantrone demonstrated a triphasic plasma clearance. Distribution to tissues is rapid and extensive. Elimination of the drug is slow with a mean half-life of 12 days (range 5-18) and persistent tissue concentrations. Similar estimates of half-life were obtained from patients receiving a single dose of mitoxantrone every 21 days and patients dosed on 5 consecutive days every 21 days.

Mitoxantrone is excreted via the renal and hepatobiliary systems. Only 20-32% of the administered dose was excreted within the first five days after dosing (urine 6-11%, faeces 13-25%). Of the material recovered in the urine, 65% was unchanged mitoxantrone and the remaining 35% primarily comprised of two inactive metabolites and their glucuronide conjugates. Approximately two thirds of the excretion occurred during the first day.

5.3 Preclinical safety data

Animal pharmacokinetic studies in rats, dogs and monkeys given radiolabeled mitoxantrone indicate rapid, extensive dose proportional distribution into most tissues. Mitoxantrone does not cross the blood-brain barrier to any appreciable extent. Distribution into testes is relatively low. In pregnant rats the placenta is an effective barrier. Plasma concentrations decrease rapidly during the first two hours and slowly thereafter. Animal data established biliary excretion as the major route of elimination. In rats, tissue elimination half-life of radioactivity ranged from 20 days to 25 daysas compared with plasma half-life of 12 days. Mitoxantrone is not absorbed significantly in animals following oral administration.

6. PHARMACEUTICAL PARTICULARS

6.1 List of excipients

Sodium chloride

Sodium acetate

Acetic acid

Sodium sulphate

Water for injections

6.2 Incompatibilities

Mitoxantrone should not be mixed in the same infusion as heparin since a precipitate may form. Mitoxantrone should not be mixed in the same infusion as other drugs.

6.3 Shelf life

18 months

After dilution (see section 6.4) 24 hours.

6.4 Special precautions for storage

Do not store above 25°C.

Do not refrigerate or freeze

Mitoxantrone Sterile Concentrate does not contain an antimicrobial preservative.

After dilution

Chemical and physical in-use stability has been demonstrated for 24 hours at 25°C. From a microbiological point of view, the product should be used immediately. If not used immediately, in-use storage times and conditions prior to use are the responsibility of the user and would normally not be longer than 24 hours at 2 to 8°C, unless dilution has taken place in controlled and validated aseptic conditions.

6.5 Nature and contents of container

Colourless 5ml Type I glass vial with fluropolymer-coated chlorobutyl rubber stoppers and aluminium overseal.

Packs of 1 vial containing 5ml sterile concentrate.

Or

Colourless 10ml Type I glass vial with fluropolymer-coated chlorobutyl rubber stoppers and aluminium overseal.

Packs of 1 vial containing 10 ml sterile concentrate.

6.6 Instructions for use and handling

a) Instructions for use

Syringes containing this product should be labelled

" For intravenous use only"

Care should be taken to avoid contact of mitoxantrone with the skin, mucous membranes, or eyes: see 6.6 for further directions on handling. Vials should be dispensed in the upright position in order to prevent drops of mitoxantrone collecting in the stopper during preparation and leading to potential aerosolisation of the solution.

Dilute the required volume of Mitoxantrone Injection to at least 50 ml in the following intravenous infusion: Sodium Chloride 0.9% orGlucose 5%. Use Luer-lock fittings on all syringes and sets. Large bore needles are recommended to minimise pressure and the possible formation of aerosols. The latter may also be reduced by the use of a venting needle. Administer the resulting solution over not less than 3 minutes via the tubing of freely running intravenous infusion of one of the above fluids. Mitoxantrone should not be mixed with other drugs in the same infusion.

If extravasation occurs the administration should be stopped immediately and restarted in another vein.

b) Handling Cytotoxic drugs

Mitoxantrone, in common with other potentially hazardous cytotoxic drugs, should only be handled by adequately trained personnel. Pregnant staff should not be involved in the reconstitution or administration of mitoxantrone.

Care should be taken to avoid contact of mitoxantrone with the skin, mucous membranes, or eyes. The use of goggles, gloves and protective gowns is recommended during preparation, administration and disposal and the work surface should be covered with disposable plastic-backed absorbent paper.

Aerosol generation should be minimised. Mitoxantrone can cause staining. Skin accidentally exposed to mitoxantrone should be rinsed copiously with warm water and if the eyes are involved standard irrigation techniques should be used.

c) Spillage disposal

The following clean-up procedure is recommended if mitoxantrone is spilled on equipment or environmental surfaces. Prepare a 50% solution of fresh concentrated bleach (any recognised proprietary brand containing either sodium or calcium hypochlorite) in water. Wet absorbent tissues in the bleach solution and apply the wetted tissues to the spillage. The spillage is deactivated when the blue colour has been fully discharged. Collect up the tissues with dry tissues. Wash the area with water and soak up the water with dry tissues. Appropriate protective equipment should be worn during the clean-up procedure.

All mitoxantrone contaminated items (eg, syringes, needles, tissues, etc) should be treated as toxic waste and disposed of accordingly. Incineration is recommended.

7. MARKETING AUTHORISATION HOLDER

CP Pharmaceuticals Ltd

Ash Road North

Wrexham

LL13 9UF

UK

8. MARKETING AUTHORISATION NUMBER(S)

PL 4543/0445 (10mg in 5ml)

PL 4543/0463 (20mg in 20ml)

9. DATE OF FIRST AUTHORISATION/RENEWAL OF THE AUTHORISATION

28th October 2004

10. DATE OF REVISION OF THE TEXT

4th October 2004

Mivacron Injection

(GlaxoSmithKline UK)

1. NAME OF THE MEDICINAL PRODUCT

Mivacron Injection 2mg/ml

2. QUALITATIVE AND QUANTITATIVE COMPOSITION

Mivacurium chloride 2.14mg in each 1ml of product

3. PHARMACEUTICAL FORM

Liquid for injection

4. CLINICAL PARTICULARS

4.1 Therapeutic indications

Mivacron is a highly selective, short-acting, non-depolarising neuromuscular blocking agent with a fast recovery profile. Mivacron is used as an adjunct to general anaesthesia to relax skeletal muscles and to facilitate tracheal intubation and mechanical ventilation.

This formulation contains no antimicrobial preservative and is intended for single patient use.

4.2 Posology and method of administration

Use By Injection In Adults

Mivacron is administered by intravenous injection. The mean dose required to produce 95% suppression of the adductor pollicis single twitch response to ulnar nerve stimulations (ED_{95}) is 0.07 mg/kg (range 0.06 to 0.09) in adults receiving narcotic anaesthesia.

The recommended bolus dose range for healthy adults is 0.07-0.25 mg/kg. The duration of neuromuscular blockade is related to the dose. Doses of 0.07, 0.15, 0.20 and 0.25 mg/kg produce clinically effective block for approximately 13, 16, 20 and 23 minutes respectively.

Doses of up to 0.15 mg/kg may be administered over 5 to 15 seconds. Higher doses should be administered over 30 seconds in order to minimise the possibility of occurrence of cardiovascular effects.

The following dose regimens are recommended for tracheal intubation:

I A dose of 0.2 mg/kg, administered over 30 seconds, produces good to excellent conditions for tracheal intubation within 2 to 2.5 minutes.

II A dose of 0.25 mg/kg administered as a divided dose (0.15 mg/kg followed 30 seconds later by 0.1 mg/kg) produces good to excellent conditions for tracheal intubation within 1.5 to 2.0 minutes of completion of administration of the first dose portion.

With Mivacron, significant train-of-four fade is not seen during onset. It is often possible to intubate the trachea before complete abolition of the train-of-four response of the adductor pollicis muscle has occurred.

Full block can be prolonged by maintenance doses of Mivacron. Doses of 0.1 mg/kg administered during narcotic anaesthesia each provide approximately 15 minutes of additional clinically effective block. Successive supplementary doses do not give rise to accumulation of neuromuscular blocking effect.

The neuromuscular blocking action of Mivacron is potentiated by isoflurane or enflurane anaesthesia. If steady-state anaesthesia with isoflurane or enflurane has been established, the recommended initial Mivacron dose should be reduced by up to 25%. Halothane appears to have only a minimal potentiating effect on Mivacron and dose reduction of Mivacron is probably not necessary.

Once spontaneous recovery is underway it is complete in approximately 15 minutes and is independent of the dose of Mivacron administered.

The neuromuscular block produced by Mivacron can be reversed with standard doses of anticholinesterase agents. However, because spontaneous recovery after Mivacron is rapid, a reversal may not be routinely required as it shortens recovery time by only 5-6 minutes.

Use as an Infusion in Adults

Continuous infusion of Mivacron may be used to maintain neuromuscular block. Upon early evidence of spontaneous recovery from an initial Mivacron dose, an infusion rate of 8 to 10 micrograms/kg/min (0.5 to 0.6 mg/kg/hr) is recommended.

The initial infusion rate should be adjusted according to the patient's response to peripheral nerve stimulation and clinical criteria. Adjustments of the infusion rate should be made and should be increments of approximately 1 microgram/kg/min (0.06 mg/kg/hr). In general, a given rate should be maintained for at least 3 minutes before a rate change is made. On average, an infusion rate of 6 to 7 micrograms/kg/minute will maintain neuromuscular block within the range of 89% to 99% for extended periods in adults receiving narcotic anaesthesia. During steady-state isoflurane or enflurane anaesthesia, reduction in the infusion rate by up to 40% should be considered. A study has shown that the mivacurium infusion rate requirement should be reduced by up to 50% with sevoflurane. With halothane, smaller reductions in infusion rate may be required.

Spontaneous recovery after Mivacron infusion is independent of the duration of infusion and comparable to recovery reported for single doses.

Continuous infusion of Mivacron has not been associated with the development of tachyphylaxis or cumulative neuromuscular blockade.

Mivacron (2 mg/ml) may be used undiluted for infusion.

Mivacron is compatible with the following infusion fluids.

Sodium chloride intravenous infusion (0.9% w/v)

Glucose intravenous infusion (5% w/v)

Sodium chloride (0.18% w/v) and glucose (4% w/v) intravenous infusion

Lactated Ringer's Injection USP

When diluted with the listed infusion solutions in the proportion of 1 plus 3 (i.e. to give 0.5 mg/ml) Mivacron injection has been shown to be chemically and physically stable for at least 48 hours at 30°C. However, since the product contains no antimicrobial preservative, dilution should be carried out immediately prior to use, administration should commence as soon as possible thereafter, and any remaining solution should be discarded.

Doses in Infants and Children Aged 2 Months - 12 Years

Mivacron has a faster onset, shorter clinically effective duration of action and more rapid spontaneous recovery profile in infants and children than in adults.

The ED_{95} in infants aged 2 to 6 months is approximately 0.07 mg/kg; and in infants and children aged 7 months to 12 years is approximately 0.1 mg/kg.

Pharmacodynamic data for recommended initial doses in infants and children are summarised in the following table:

(see Table 1 below)

Since maximum block is usually achieved within 2 minutes following administration of these doses, tracheal intubation should be possible within this time.

Infants and children generally require more frequent maintenance doses and higher infusion rate than adults. Pharmacodynamic data for maintenance doses are summarised in the table below together with recommended infusion rates:

(see Table 2 below)

The neuromuscular blocking action of mivacurium is potentiated by inhalational agents. A study has shown that the mivacurium infusion rate requirement should be reduced by up to 70% with sevoflurane in children aged 2 – 12 years.

Once spontaneous recovery is underway, it is complete in approximately 10 minutes.

Dose in Neonates and Infants Under 2 Months of Age

No dose recommendation for neonates and infants under 2 months of age can be made until further information becomes available.

Dose in the Elderly

In elderly patients receiving single bolus doses of Mivacron, the onset time, duration of action and recovery rate may be extended relative to younger patients by 20 to 30%. Elderly patients may also require decreased infusion rates or smaller or less frequent maintenance bolus doses.

Dose in Patients with Cardiovascular Disease

In patients with clinically significant cardiovascular disease, the initial dose of Mivacron should be administered over 60 seconds. Mivacron has been administered in this way with minimal haemodynamic effects to patients undergoing cardiac surgery.

Dose in Patients with Reduced Renal Function

In patients with end-stage renal failure the clinically effective duration of block produced by 0.15 mg/kg is approximately 1.5 times longer than in patients with normal renal function. Subsequently, dosage should be adjusted according to individual clinical response.

Dose in Patients with Reduced Hepatic Function

In patients with end-stage liver failure the clinically effective duration of block produced by 0.15 mg/kg is approximately three times longer than in patients with normal hepatic function. This prolongation is related to the markedly reduced plasma cholinesterase activity seen in these patients. Subsequently, dosage should be adjusted according to individual clinical response.

Dose in Patients with Reduced Plasma Cholinesterase Activity

Mivacurium is metabolised by plasma cholinesterase. Plasma cholinesterase activity may be diminished in the presence of genetic abnormalities of plasma cholinesterase (e.g. patients heterozygous or homozygous for the atypical plasma cholinesterase gene), in various pathological conditions and by the administration of certain drugs (see interactions with other medicaments). The possibility of prolonged neuromuscular block following administration of Mivacron must be considered in patients with reduced plasma cholinesterase activity. Mild reductions (i.e. within 20% of the lower limit of the normal range) are not associated with clinically significant effects on duration. In patients heterozygous for the atypical plasma cholinesterase gene, the clinically effective duration of block of 0.15 mg/kg Mivacron is approximately 10 minutes longer than in control patients.

Dose in Obese Patients

In obese patients (those weighing 30% or more above their ideal bodyweight for height), the initial dose of Mivacron should be based upon ideal bodyweight and not actual bodyweight.

Instructions to open the ampoule

Ampoules are equipped with the OPC (One Point Cut) opening system and must be opened following the below instructions:

1. hold with the hand the bottom part of the ampoule as indicated in picture 1

2. put the other hand on the top of the ampoule positioning the thumb above the coloured point and press as indicated in picture 2

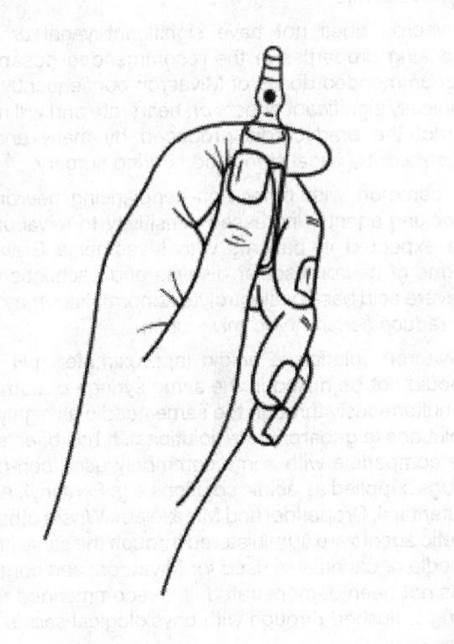

Picture 1

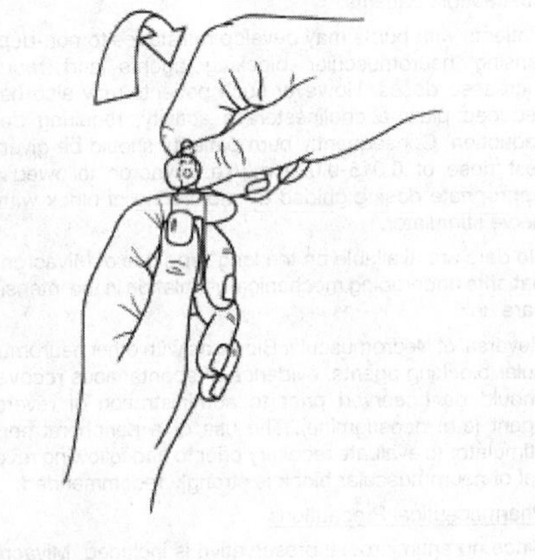

Picture 2

Monitoring

In common with all neuromuscular blocking agents, monitoring of neuromuscular function is recommended during the use of Mivacron in order to individualise dosage requirements.

4.3 Contraindications

Mivacron should not be administered to patients known to have allergic hypersensitivity to the drug.

Mivacron is contraindicated in pregnancy since there is no information on the use of Mivacron in pregnant women.

Table 1

Age	Dose for Tracheal Intubation	Time to Maximum Neuromuscular Block (min)	Duration of Clinically Effective Block (min)
2 - 6 months[A]	0.15 mg/kg	1.4	9
7 months - 12 years[B]	0.2 mg/kg	1.7	9

[A]Data obtained during halothane anaesthesia.

[B]Data obtained during halothane or narcotic anaesthesia.

Table 2

Age	Maintenance Dose	Duration of Clinically Effective Block (min)	Average Infusion Rate Required to Maintain 89-99% Neuromuscular Block
2 months - 12 years[A]	0.1 mg/kg	6 - 9	11 – 14 μg/kg/min (0.7 - 0.9 mg/kg/hr)

[A]Data obtained during halothane or narcotic anaesthesia.

Mivacron is contraindicated in patients known or suspected of being homozygous for the atypical plasma cholinesterase gene (see "special warnings and precautions for use" section).

4.4 Special warnings and special precautions for use

In common with all the other neuromuscular blocking agents, Mivacron paralyses the respiratory muscles as well as the other skeletal muscles but has no effect on consciousness. Mivacron should be administered only by or under close supervision of an experienced anaesthetist with adequate facilities for endotracheal intubation and artificial ventilation.

In common with suxamethonium/succinylcholine, adult and paediatric patients homozygous for the atypical plasma cholinesterase gene (1 in 2500 patients) are extremely sensitive to the neuromuscular blocking effect of Mivacurium. In three such adults patients, a small dose of 0.03 mg/kg (approximately the ED_{10-20} in genotypically normal patients) produced complete neuromuscular block for 26 to 128 minutes. Once spontaneous recovery had begun, neuromuscular block in these patients was antagonised with conventional doses of neostigmine.

In adults, doses of Mivacron $\geq$ 0.2 mg/kg ($\geq 3 \times ED_{95}$) have been associated with histamine release when administered by rapid bolus injection. However, the slower administration of the 0.2 mg/kg Mivacron dose and the divided administration of the 0.25 mg/kg Mivacron dose minimised the cardiovascular effects of these doses. Cardiovascular safety did not appear to be compromised in children given a rapid bolus dose of 0.2 mg/kg in clinical studies.

Caution should be exercised in administering Mivacron to patients with a history suggestive of an increased sensitivity to the effects of histamine e.g. asthma. If Mivacron is used in this group of patients it should be administered over 60 seconds.

Mivacron should be administered over a period of 60 seconds to patients who may be unusually sensitive to falls in arterial blood pressure, for example those who are hypovolaemic.

Mivacron does not have significant vagal or ganglion blocking properties in the recommended dosage range. Recommended doses of Mivacron consequently have no clinically significant effects on heart rate and will not counteract the bradycardia produced by many anaesthetic agents or by vagal stimulation during surgery.

In common with other non-depolarising neuromuscular blocking agents, increased sensitivity to mivacurium can be expected in patients with Myasthenia Gravis, other forms of neuromuscular disease and cachectic patients. Severe acid base or electrolyte abnormalities may increase or reduce sensitivity to mivacurium.

Mivacron solution is acidic (approximately pH 4.5) and should not be mixed in the same syringe or administered simultaneously through the same needle as highly alkaline solutions (e.g. barbiturate solutions). It has been shown to be compatible with some commonly used peri-operative drugs supplied as acidic solutions e.g. Fentanyl, Alfentanil, Sufentanil, Droperidol and Midazolam. Where other anaesthetic agents are administered through the same indwelling needle or cannula as used for Mivacron, and compatibility has not been demonstrated, it is recommended that each drug is flushed through with physiological saline.

Studies in malignant hyperthermia-susceptible pigs, indicated that Mivacron does not trigger this syndrome. Mivacron has not been studied in malignant hyperthermia-susceptible patients.

Patients with burns may develop resistance to non-depolarising neuromuscular blocking agents and require increased doses. However such patients may also have reduced plasma cholinesterase activity, requiring dose reduction. Consequently burn patients should be given a test dose of 0.015-0.020 mg/kg Mivacron followed by appropriate dosing guided by monitoring of block with a nerve stimulator.

No data are available on the long-term use of Mivacron in patients undergoing mechanical ventilation in the intensive care unit.

Reversal of Neuromuscular Block: as with other neuromuscular blocking agents, evidence of spontaneous recovery should be observed prior to administration of reversal agent (e.g. neostigmine). The use of a peripheral nerve stimulator to evaluate recovery prior to and following reversal of neuromuscular block is strongly recommended.

Pharmaceutical Precautions

Since no antimicrobial preservative is included, Mivacron must be used under full aseptic conditions and any dilution carried out immediately before use. Any unused solution in open ampoules should be discarded.

Mivacron injection is acidic (approximately pH 4.5) and should not be mixed with highly alkaline solutions (e.g. barbiturates). Mivacron has been shown to be compatible with some commonly used peri-operative drugs supplied as acidic solutions. Where such agents are administered through the same indwelling needle or cannula as used for Mivacron injection, and compatibility has not been demonstrated, it is recommended that each drug is flushed through with physiological saline.

The pack will contain the following statements:

Store below 25°C.

Do not freeze.

Protect from light.

Any portion of the contents remaining after use should be discarded.

Keep out of reach of children.

4.5 Interaction with other medicinal products and other forms of Interaction

The neuromuscular block produced by Mivacron may be increased by the concomitant use of inhalational anaesthetics such as enflurane, isoflurane, sevoflurane and halothane.

Mivacron has been safely administered following succinylcholine facilitated intubation. Evidence of spontaneous recovery from succinylcholine should be observed prior to administration of Mivacron.

In common with all non-depolarising neuromuscular blocking agents, the magnitude and/or duration of non-depolarising neuromuscular block may be increased and infusion requirements may be reduced as a result of interaction with; antibiotics, including the aminoglycosides, polymyxins, Spectinomycin, tetracyclines, Lincomycin and Clindamycin; anti-arrhythmic drugs: Propranolol, calcium channel blockers, Lignocaine, Procainamide and Quinidine, diuretics: Frusemide and possibly thiazides, Mannitol and Acetazolamide, magnesium salts, ketamine, lithium salts, ganglion blocking drugs: Trimetaphan, Hexamethonium.

Drugs that may reduce plasma cholinesterase activity may also prolong the neuromuscular blocking action of Mivacron. These include anti-mitotic drugs, monoamine oxidase inhibitors, ecothiophate iodine, pancuronium, organophosphates, anticholinesterases, certain hormones, bambuterol.

Rarely, certain drugs may aggravate or unmask latent Myasthenia Gravis or actually induce a Myasthenic syndrome: increased sensitivity to Mivacron would be consequent on such a development. Such drugs include various antibiotics, beta-blockers. (Propranolol, Oxprenolol), anti-arrhythmic drugs (Procainamide, Quinidine), antirheumatic drugs (Chloroquine, D-Pencillamine), Trimetaphan, Chlorpromazine, Steroids, Phenytoin and Lithium.

The administration of combinations of non-depolarising neuromuscular blocking agents in conjunction with Mivacron may produce a degree of neuromuscular blockade in excess of that which might be expected from an equipotent total dose of Mivacron. Any synergistic effect may vary between different drug combinations.

A depolarising muscle relaxant such as suxamethonium chloride should not be administered to prolong the neuromuscular blocking effects of non-depolarising agents, as this may result in a prolonged and complex block which can be difficult to reverse with anticholinesterase drugs.

4.6 Pregnancy and lactation

Plasma cholinesterase levels decrease during pregnancy. Mivacurium has been used to maintain neuromuscular block during Caesarean section, but due to the reduced levels of plasma cholinesterase, dosage adjustments to the infusion rate were necessary. A further reduction in the infusion rate may also be required during Caesarean section in patients pre-treated with $MgSO_4$, due to the potentiating effects of Mg^{2+}.

It is not known whether mivacurium is excreted in human milk.

4.7 Effects on ability to drive and use machines

Not applicable.

4.8 Undesirable effects

Associated with the use of Mivacron there have been reports of skin flushing, erythema, urticaria, hypotension, transient tachycardia or bronchospasm which have been attributed to histamine release. These effects are dose related and more common following initial doses of $\geq$0.2 mg/kg or more when given rapidly and are reduced if Mivacron is injected over 30 to 60 seconds or in divided doses over 30 seconds.

Very rarely, severe anaphylactic or anaphylactoid reactions have been reported in patients receiving Mivacron in conjunction with one or more anaesthetic agents.

4.9 Overdose

Prolonged muscle paralysis and its consequences are the main signs of overdosage with neuromuscular blocking agents. However, the risk of haemodynamic side-effects especially decreases in blood pressure, may be increased.

It is essential to maintain a patent airway together with assisted positive pressure ventilation until spontaneous respiration is adequate. Full sedation will be required since consciousness is not impaired. Recovery may be hastened by the administration of anticholinesterase agents accompanied by atropine or glycopyrrolate, once evidence of spontaneous recovery is present. Cardiovascular support may be provided by proper positioning of the patient and administration of fluids or vasopressor agents as required.

5. PHARMACOLOGICAL PROPERTIES

5.1 Pharmacodynamic properties

Mivacurium is a short-acting, non-depolarising skeletal muscle relaxant which is hydrolysed by plasma cholinesterase. Mivacurium binds competitively with cholinergic receptors on the motor end-plate to prevent the action of acetylcholine, resulting in a blockade of neuromuscular transmission. This is rapidly reversed by the administration of the cholinesterase inhibitors, neostigmine and edrophonium.

5.2 Pharmacokinetic properties

Mivacurium chloride is a mixture of three stereoisomers, the trans-trans and cis-trans stereoisomers comprise 92% to 96% of mivacurium chloride and when studied in cats their neuromuscular blocking potencies are not significantly different from each other or from mivacurium chloride. The cis-cis isomer has been estimated from studies in cats to have one-tenth of the neuromuscular blocking potency of the other two stereoisomers. Enzymatic hydrolysis by plasma cholinesterase is the primary mechanism for inactivation of mivacurium and yields a quaternary alcohol and a quaternary monoester metabolite. Pharmacological studies in cats and dogs have shown that metabolites possess insignificant neuromuscular, autonomic or cardiovascular activity at concentrations higher than seen in man.

5.3 Preclinical safety data

Mivacurium has been evaluated in four short term mutagenicity tests. Mivacurium was non-mutagenic in the Ames salmonella assay, the mouse lymphoma assay, the human lymphocyte assay and the *in vivo* rat bone marrow cytogenetic assay.

There is no information available on whether Mivacurium has carcinogenic potential.

Fertility studies have not been performed.

Animal studies have indicated that mivacurium has no adverse effect on foetal development.

6. PHARMACEUTICAL PARTICULARS

6.1 List of excipients

Hydrochloric Acid EP

Water for Injections EP

6.2 Incompatibilities

None known

6.3 Shelf life

18 months

6.4 Special precautions for storage

Store below 25°C. Do not freeze. Protect from light.

6.5 Nature and contents of container

Neutral glass ampoules containing 5ml or 10ml of product.

6.6 Instructions for use and handling

No special instructions are required.

Administrative Data

7. MARKETING AUTHORISATION HOLDER

The Wellcome Foundation Ltd:

Berkeley Avenue

Greenford

Middlesex UB6 0NN

Trading as

Glaxo Wellcome and/or GlaxoSmithKline UK

Stockley Park West

Uxbridge

Middlesex UB11 1BT

8. MARKETING AUTHORISATION NUMBER(S)

PL 00003/0325

9. DATE OF FIRST AUTHORISATION/RENEWAL OF THE AUTHORISATION

29th October 1997

10. DATE OF REVISION OF THE TEXT

31 July 2003

11. Legal Status

POM

Mixtard 10 Penfill 100 IU/ml, Mixtard 10 NovoLet 100 IU/ml

(Novo Nordisk Limited)

1. NAME OF THE MEDICINAL PRODUCT

Mixtard 10 Penfill 100 IU/ml

Suspension for injection in a cartridge

Mixtard 10 NovoLet 100 IU/ml

Suspension for injection in a pre-filled pen

2. QUALITATIVE AND QUANTITATIVE COMPOSITION

Insulin human, rDNA (produced by recombinant DNA technology in *Saccharomyces cerevisiae*).

1 ml contains 100 IU of insulin human

1 cartridge contains 3 ml equivalent to 300 IU

1 pre-filled pen contains 3 ml equivalent to 300 IU

One IU (International Unit) corresponds to 0.035 mg of anhydrous human insulin.

Mixtard is a mixture of dissolved insulin and isophane (NPH) insulin.

Mixtard 10 consists of 10% dissolved insulin and 90% isophane insulin.

For excipients, see Section 6.1 List of excipients.

3. PHARMACEUTICAL FORM

Suspension for injection in a cartridge.

Suspension for injection in a pre-filled pen.

Mixtard is a cloudy, white, aqueous suspension.

4. CLINICAL PARTICULARS

4.1 Therapeutic indications

Treatment of diabetes mellitus.

4.2 Posology and method of administration

Mixtard is a dual-acting insulin. It is a biphasic formulation containing fast-acting and long-acting insulin.

Premixed insulins are usually given once or twice daily when a rapid initial effect together with a more prolonged effect is desired.

Dosage

Dosage is individual and determined in accordance with the needs of the patient. The individual insulin requirement is usually between 0.3 and 1.0 IU/kg/day. The daily insulin requirement may be higher in patients with insulin resistance (e.g. during puberty or due to obesity) and lower in patients with residual, endogenous insulin production.

In patients with diabetes mellitus optimised glycaemic control delays the onset of late diabetic complications. Close blood glucose monitoring is recommended.

An injection should be followed within 30 minutes by a meal or snack containing carbohydrates.

Dosage adjustment

Concomitant illness, especially infections and feverish conditions, usually increases the patient's insulin requirement.

Renal or hepatic impairment may reduce insulin requirement.

Adjustment of dosage may also be necessary if patients change physical activity or their usual diet.

Dosage adjustment may be necessary when transferring patients from one insulin preparation to another (see section 4.4 Special warnings and special precautions for use).

Administration

For subcutaneous use.

Mixtard is usually administered subcutaneously in the thigh or abdominal wall. If convenient, the gluteal region or the deltoid region may also be used.

Subcutaneous injection into the abdominal wall ensures a faster absorption than from other injection sites.

Injection into a lifted skin fold minimises the risk of unintended intramuscular injection.

Keep the needle under the skin for at least 6 seconds to make sure the entire dose is injected.

Injection sites should be rotated within an anatomic region in order to avoid lipodystrophy.

Insulin suspensions are never to be administered intravenously.

Mixtard is accompanied by a package leaflet with detailed instruction for use to be followed.

The cartridges are designed to be used with Novo Nordisk delivery systems (durable devices for repeated use) and NovoFine needles. Detailed instruction accompanying the delivery system must be followed.

Mixtard NovoLet is designed to be used with NovoFine needles.

NovoLet delivers 2-78 units in increments of 2 units.

The pens should be primed before injection so that the dose selector returns to zero and a drop of insulin appears at the needle tip.

The dose is set by turning the selector, which returns to zero during the injection.

4.3 Contraindications

Hypoglycaemia

Hypersensitivity to human insulin or to any of the excipients (see section 6.1 List of excipients).

4.4 Special warnings and special precautions for use

Inadequate dosage or discontinuation of treatment, especially in type 1 diabetes, may lead to **hyperglycaemia**.

Usually the first symptoms of hyperglycaemia set in gradually, over a period of hours or days. They include thirst, increased frequency of urination, nausea, vomiting, drowsiness, flushed dry skin, dry mouth, loss of appetite as well as acetone odour of breath.

In type 1 diabetes, untreated hyperglycaemic events eventually lead to diabetic ketoacidosis, which is potentially lethal.

Hypoglycaemia may occur if the insulin dose is too high in relation to the insulin requirement (see section 4.8 and 4.9).

Omission of a meal or unplanned, strenuous physical exercise may lead to hypoglycaemia.

Patients whose blood glucose control is greatly improved e.g. by intensified insulin therapy, may experience a change in their usual warning symptoms of hypoglycaemia and should be advised accordingly.

Usual warning symptoms may disappear in patients with long-standing diabetes.

Transferring a patient to another type or brand of insulin should be done under strict medical supervision. Changes in strength, brand (manufacturer), type (fast-, dual-, long-acting insulin etc.), origin (animal, human or analogue insulin) and/or method of manufacture (recombinant DNA versus animal source insulin) may result in a need for a change in dosage.

If an adjustment is needed when switching the patients to Mixtard, it may occur with the first dose or during the first several weeks or months.

A few patients who have experienced hypoglycaemic reactions after transfer from animal source insulin have reported that early warning symptoms of hypoglycaemia were less pronounced or different from those experienced with their previous insulin.

Before travelling between different time zones, the patient should be advised to consult the doctor, since this may mean that the patient has to take insulin and meals at different times.

Insulin suspensions are not to be used in insulin infusion pumps.

Mixtard contains metacresol, which may cause allergic reactions.

4.5 Interaction with other medicinal products and other forms of Interaction

A number of medicinal products are known to interact with glucose metabolism. The physician must therefore take possible interactions into account and should always ask their patients about any medicinal products they take.

The following substances may reduce insulin requirement:

Oral hypoglycaemic agents (OHA), monoamine oxidase inhibitors (MAOI), non-selective beta-blocking agents, angiotensin converting enzyme (ACE) inhibitors, salicylates and alcohol.

The following substances may increase insulin requirement:

Thiazides, glucocorticoids, thyroid hormones and beta-sympathomimetics, growth hormone and danazol.

Beta-blocking agents may mask the symptoms of hypoglycaemia and delay recovery from hypoglycaemia.

Octreotide/lanreotide may both decrease and increase insulin requirement.

Alcohol may intensify and prolong the hypoglycaemic effect of insulin.

4.6 Pregnancy and lactation

There are no restrictions on treatment of diabetes with insulin during pregnancy, as insulin does not pass the placental barrier.

Both hypoglycaemia and hyperglycaemia, which can occur in inadequately controlled diabetes therapy, increase the risk of malformations and death *in utero*. Intensified control in the treatment of pregnant women with diabetes is therefore recommended throughout pregnancy and when contemplating pregnancy.

Insulin requirements usually fall in the first trimester and increase subsequently during the second and third trimesters.

After delivery, insulin requirements return rapidly to pre-pregnancy values.

Insulin treatment of the nursing mother presents no risk to the baby. However, the Mixtard dosage may need to be adjusted.

4.7 Effects on ability to drive and use machines

The patient's ability to concentrate and react may be impaired as a result of hypoglycaemia. This may constitute a risk in situations where these abilities are of special importance (e.g. driving a car or operating machinery).

Patients should be advised to take precautions to avoid hypoglycaemia whilst driving. This is particularly important in those who have reduced or absent awareness of the warning signs of hypoglycaemia or have frequent episodes of hypoglycaemia. The advisability of driving should be considered in these circumstances.

4.8 Undesirable effects

As for other insulin products, hypoglycaemia, in general is the most frequently occurring undesirable effect. It may occur if the insulin dose is too high in relation to the insulin requirement. In clinical trials and during marketed use the frequency varies with patient population and dose regimens. Therefore, no specific frequency can be presented. Severe hypoglycaemia may lead to unconsciousness and/or convulsions and may result in temporary or permanent impairment of brain function or even death.

Frequencies of adverse drug reactions from clinical trials, that are considered related to Mixtard are listed below. The frequencies are defined as: Uncommon $>1/1000$, $<1/100$). Isolated spontaneous cases are presented as very rare defined as $<1/10{,}000$.

Immune system disorders

Uncommon – Urticaria, rash

Very rare – Anaphylactic reactions

Symptoms of generalized hypersensitivity may include generalized skin rash, itching, sweating, gastrointestinal upset, angioneurotic oedema, difficulties in breathing, palpitation, reduction in blood pressure and fainting/loss of consciousness. Generalised hypersensitivity reactions are potentially life threatening.

Nervous system disorders

Uncommon – Peripheral neuropathy

Fast improvement in blood glucose control may be associated with a condition termed "acute painful neuropathy", which is usually reversible.

Eye disorders

Very rare – Refraction disorders

Refraction anomalies may occur upon initiation of insulin therapy. These symptoms are usually of transitory nature.

Uncommon – Diabetic retinopathy

Long-term improved glycaemic control decreases the risk of progression of diabetic retinopathy. However, intensification of insulin therapy with abrupt improvement in glycaemic control may be associated with temporary worsening of diabetic retinopathy.

Skin and subcutaneous tissue disorders

Uncommon – Lipodystrophy

Lipodystrophy may occur at the injection site as a consequence of failure to rotate injection sites within an area.

General disorders and administration site conditions

Uncommon – Injection site reactions

Injection site reactions (redness, swelling, itching, pain and haematoma at the injection site) may occur during treatment with insulin. Most reactions are transitory and disappear during continued treatment.

Uncommon – Oedema

Oedema may occur upon initiation of insulin therapy. These symptoms are usually of transitory nature.

4.9 Overdose

A specific overdose of insulin cannot be defined. However, hypoglycaemia may develop over sequential stages:

- Mild hypoglycaemic episodes can be treated by oral administration of glucose or sugary products. It is therefore recommended that the diabetic patients carry some sugar lumps, sweets, biscuits or sugary fruit juice.
- Severe hypoglycaemic episodes, where the patient has become unconscious, can be treated by glucagon (0.5 to 1 mg) given intramuscularly or subcutaneously by a person who has received appropriate instruction, or by glucose given intravenously by a medical professional. Glucose must also be given intravenously, if the patient does not respond to glucagon within 10 to 15 minutes.

Upon regaining consciousness, administration of oral carbohydrate is recommended for the patient in order to prevent relapse.

5. PHARMACOLOGICAL PROPERTIES

5.1 Pharmacodynamic properties

Pharmacotherapeutic group: Insulins and analogues, intermediate-acting combined with fast-acting, insulin (human). ATC code: A10A D01.

The blood glucose lowering effect of insulin is due to the facilitated uptake of glucose following binding of insulin to receptors on muscle and fat cells and to the simultaneous inhibition of glucose output from the liver.

Mixtard is a dual-acting insulin.

Onset of action is within ½ hour, reaches a maximum effect within 2-8 hours and the entire duration of action is up to 24 hours.

5.2 Pharmacokinetic properties

Insulin in the blood stream has a half-life of a few minutes. Consequently, the time-action profile of an insulin preparation are determined solely by its absorption characteristics.

This process is influenced by several factors (e.g. insulin dosage, injection route and site, thickness of subcutaneous fat, type of diabetes). The pharmacokinetics of insulins is therefore affected by significant intra- and inter-individual variation.

Absorption

The absorption profile is due to the product being a mixture of insulins with fast and protracted absorption respectively. The maximum plasma concentration of Mixtard is reached within 1.5-2.5 hours after subcutaneous administration.

Distribution

No profound binding to plasma proteins, except circulating insulin antibodies (if present) has been observed.

Metabolism

Human insulin is reported to be degraded by insulin protease or insulin-degrading enzymes and possibly protein disulfide isomerase. A number of cleavage (hydrolysis) sites on the human insulin molecule have been proposed; none of the metabolites formed following the cleavage are active.

Elimination

The terminal half-life is determined by the rate of absorption from the subcutaneous tissue. The terminal half-life ($t_{1/2}$) is therefore a measure of the absorption rather than of the elimination per se of insulin from plasma (insulin in the blood stream has a $t_{1/2}$ of a few minutes). Trials have indicated a $t_{1/2}$ of about 5-10 hours.

5.3 Preclinical safety data

Preclinical data reveal no special hazard for humans based on conventional studies of safety pharmacology, repeated dose toxicity, genotoxicity, carcinogenic potential, toxicity to reproduction.

6. PHARMACEUTICAL PARTICULARS

6.1 List of excipients

Zinc chloride

Glycerol

Metacresol

Phenol

Disodium phosphate dihydrate

Sodium hydroxide or/and hydrochloric acid (for pH adjustment)

Protamine sulphate

Water for injections

6.2 Incompatibilities

Insulin suspensions should not be added to infusion fluids.

6.3 Shelf life

30 months.

After first opening: 6 weeks.

6.4 Special precautions for storage

Store in a refrigerator (2°C - 8°C).

Do not freeze.

Mixtard 10 Penfill:

Keep the cartridge in the outer carton in order to protect from light.

During use: do not refrigerate. Do not store above 30°C.

Mixtard 10 NovoLet:

During use: do not refrigerate. Do not store above 30°C.

Keep the pen cap on in order to protect the insulin from light.

Protect from excessive heat and sunlight.

6.5 Nature and contents of container

Glass cartridge (type 1) with a bromobutyl rubber plunger and a bromobutyl/polyisoprene rubber stopper. The cartridge contains a glass ball to facilitate the re-suspension.

Pack size: 5 cartridges × 3 ml.

Pre-filled pen (multidose disposable pen) comprising a pen injector with a cartridge (3 ml). The cartridge is made of glass (type 1), containing a bromobutyl rubber plunger and a bromobutyl/polyisoprene rubber stopper. The cartridge contains a glass ball to facilitate the re-suspension. The pen injector is made of plastic.

Pack size: 5 pre-filled pens × 3 ml.

6.6 Instructions for use and handling

Cartridges and pens should only be used in combination with products that are compatible with them and allow the cartridge and pen to function safely and effectively.

Mixtard Penfill and Mixtard NovoLet are for single person use only. The container must not be refilled.

Insulin preparations, which have been frozen, must not be used.

Insulin suspensions should not be used if they do not appear uniformly white and cloudy after re-suspension.

7. MARKETING AUTHORISATION HOLDER

Novo Nordisk A/S

Novo Allé

DK-2880 Bagsværd

Denmark

8. MARKETING AUTHORISATION NUMBER(S)

Mixtard 10 Penfill 100 IU/ml: EU/1/02/231/006

Mixtard 10 NovoLet 100 IU/ml: EU/1/02/231/020

9. DATE OF FIRST AUTHORISATION/RENEWAL OF THE AUTHORISATION

October 2002

10. DATE OF REVISION OF THE TEXT

2 August 2004

Legal Status

POM

Mixtard 20 Penfill 100 IU/ml, Mixtard 20 NovoLet 100 IU/ml

(Novo Nordisk Limited)

1. NAME OF THE MEDICINAL PRODUCT

Mixtard 20 Penfill 100 IU/ml

Suspension for injection in a cartridge

Mixtard 20 NovoLet 100 IU/ml

Suspension for injection in a pre-filled pen

2. QUALITATIVE AND QUANTITATIVE COMPOSITION

Insulin human, rDNA (produced by recombinant DNA technology in *Saccharomyces cerevisiae*).

1 ml contains 100 IU of insulin human

1 cartridge contains 3 ml equivalent to 300 IU

1 pre-filled pen contains 3 ml equivalent to 300 IU

One IU (International Unit) corresponds to 0.035 mg of anhydrous human insulin.

Mixtard is a mixture of dissolved insulin and isophane (NPH) insulin.

Mixtard 20 consists of 20% dissolved insulin and 80% isophane insulin.

For excipients, see Section 6.1 List of excipients.

3. PHARMACEUTICAL FORM

Suspension for injection in a cartridge.

Suspension for injection in a pre-filled pen.

Mixtard is a cloudy, white, aqueous suspension.

4. CLINICAL PARTICULARS

4.1 Therapeutic indications

Treatment of diabetes mellitus.

4.2 Posology and method of administration

Mixtard is a dual-acting insulin. It is a biphasic formulation containing fast-acting and long-acting insulin.

Premixed insulins are usually given once or twice daily when a rapid initial effect together with a more prolonged effect is desired.

Dosage

Dosage is individual and determined in accordance with the needs of the patient.

The individual insulin requirement is usually between 0.3 and 1.0 IU/kg/day. The daily insulin requirement may be higher in patients with insulin resistance (e.g. during puberty or due to obesity) and lower in patients with residual, endogenous insulin production.

In patients with diabetes mellitus optimised glycaemic control delays the onset of late diabetic complications. Close blood glucose monitoring is recommended.

An injection should be followed within 30 minutes by a meal or snack containing carbohydrates.

Dosage adjustment

Concomitant illness, especially infections and feverish conditions, usually increases the patient's insulin requirement.

Renal or hepatic impairment may reduce insulin requirement.

Adjustment of dosage may also be necessary if patients change physical activity or their usual diet.

Dosage adjustment may be necessary when transferring patients from one insulin preparation to another (see section 4.4 Special warnings and special precautions for use).

Administration

For subcutaneous use.

Mixtard is usually administered subcutaneously in the thigh or abdominal wall. If convenient, the gluteal region or the deltoid region may also be used.

Subcutaneous injection into the abdominal wall ensures a faster absorption than from other injection sites.

Injection into a lifted skin fold minimises the risk of unintended intramuscular injection.

Keep the needle under the skin for at least 6 seconds to make sure the entire dose is injected.

Injection sites should be rotated within an anatomic region in order to avoid lipodystrophy.

Insulin suspensions are never to be administered intravenously.

Mixtard is accompanied by a package leaflet with detailed instruction for use to be followed.

The cartridges are designed to be used with Novo Nordisk delivery systems (durable devices for repeated use) and NovoFine needles. Detailed instruction accompanying the delivery system must be followed.

Mixtard NovoLet is designed to be used with NovoFine needles.

NovoLet delivers 2-78 units in increments of 2 units.

The pens should be primed before injection so that the dose selector returns to zero and a drop of insulin appears at the needle tip.

The dose is set by turning the selector, which returns to zero during the injection.

4.3 Contraindications

Hypoglycaemia

Hypersensitivity to human insulin or to any of the excipients (see section 6.1 List of excipients).

4.4 Special warnings and special precautions for use

Inadequate dosage or discontinuation of treatment, especially in type 1 diabetes, may lead to **hyperglycaemia**.

Usually the first symptoms of hyperglycaemia set in gradually, over a period of hours or days. They include thirst, increased frequency of urination, nausea, vomiting, drowsiness, flushed dry skin, dry mouth, loss of appetite as well as acetone odour of breath.

In type 1 diabetes, untreated hyperglycaemic events eventually lead to diabetic ketoacidosis, which is potentially lethal.

Hypoglycaemia may occur if the insulin dose is too high in relation to the insulin requirement (see section 4.8 and 4.9).

Omission of a meal or unplanned, strenuous physical exercise may lead to hypoglycaemia.

Patients whose blood glucose control is greatly improved e.g. by intensified insulin therapy, may experience a change in their usual warning symptoms of hypoglycaemia and should be advised accordingly.

Usual warning symptoms may disappear in patients with long-standing diabetes.

Transferring a patient to another type or brand of insulin should be done under strict medical supervision. Changes in strength, brand (manufacturer), type (fast-, dual-, long-acting insulin etc.), origin (animal, human or analogue insulin) and/or method of manufacture (recombinant DNA versus animal source insulin) may result in a need for a change in dosage.

If an adjustment is needed when switching the patients to Mixtard, it may occur with the first dose or during the first several weeks or months.

A few patients who have experienced hypoglycaemic reactions after transfer from animal source insulin have reported that early warning symptoms of hypoglycaemia were less pronounced or different from those experienced with their previous insulin.

Before travelling between different time zones, the patient should be advised to consult the doctor, since this may mean that the patient has to take insulin and meals at different times.

Insulin suspensions are not to be used in insulin infusion pumps.

Mixtard contains metacresol, which may cause allergic reactions.

4.5 Interaction with other medicinal products and other forms of Interaction

A number of medicinal products are known to interact with glucose metabolism. The physician must therefore take possible interactions into account and should always ask their patients about any medicinal products they take.

The following substances may reduce insulin requirement:

Oral hypoglycaemic agents (OHA), monoamine oxidase inhibitors (MAOI), non-selective beta-blocking agents, angiotensin converting enzyme (ACE) inhibitors, salicylates and alcohol.

The following substances may increase insulin requirement:

Thiazides, glucocorticoids, thyroid hormones and beta-sympathomimetics, growth hormone and danazol.

Beta-blocking agents may mask the symptoms of hypoglycaemia and delay recovery from hypoglycaemia.

Octreotide/lanreotide may both decrease and increase insulin requirement.

Alcohol may intensify and prolong the hypoglycaemic effect of insulin.

4.6 Pregnancy and lactation

There are no restrictions on treatment of diabetes with insulin during pregnancy, as insulin does not pass the placental barrier.

Both hypoglycaemia and hyperglycaemia, which can occur in inadequately controlled diabetes therapy, increase the risk of malformations and death *in utero*. Intensified control in the treatment of pregnant women with diabetes is therefore recommended throughout pregnancy and when contemplating pregnancy.

Insulin requirements usually fall in the first trimester and increase subsequently during the second and third trimesters.

After delivery, insulin requirements return rapidly to pre-pregnancy values.

Insulin treatment of the nursing mother presents no risk to the baby. However, the Mixtard dosage may need to be adjusted.

4.7 Effects on ability to drive and use machines

The patient's ability to concentrate and react may be impaired as a result of hypoglycaemia. This may constitute a risk in situations where these abilities are of special importance (e.g. driving a car or operating machinery).

Patients should be advised to take precautions to avoid hypoglycaemia whilst driving. This is particularly important in those who have reduced or absent awareness of the warning signs of hypoglycaemia or have frequent episodes of hypoglycaemia. The advisability of driving should be considered in these circumstances.

4.8 Undesirable effects

As for other insulin products, hypoglycaemia, in general is the most frequently occurring undesirable effect. It may occur if the insulin dose is too high in relation to the insulin requirement. In clinical trials and during marketed use the frequency varies with patient population and dose regimens. Therefore, no specific frequency can be presented. Severe hypoglycaemia may lead to unconsciousness and/or convulsions and may result in temporary or permanent impairment of brain function or even death.

Frequencies of adverse drug reactions from clinical trials, that are considered related to Mixtard are listed below. The frequencies are defined as: Uncommon > 1/1000, < 1/100). Isolated spontaneous cases are presented as very rare defined as < 1/10,000.

Immune system disorders

Uncommon – Urticaria, rash

Very rare – Anaphylactic reactions

Symptoms of generalized hypersensitivity may include generalized skin rash, itching, sweating, gastrointestinal upset, angioneurotic oedema, difficulties in breathing, palpitation, reduction in blood pressure and fainting/loss of consciousness. Generalised hypersensitivity reactions are potentially life threatening.

Nervous system disorders

Uncommon – Peripheral neuropathy

Fast improvement in blood glucose control may be associated with a condition termed "acute painful neuropathy", which is usually reversible.

Eye disorders

Very rare – Refraction disorders

Refraction anomalies may occur upon initiation of insulin therapy. These symptoms are usually of transitory nature.

Uncommon – Diabetic retinopathy

Long-term improved glycaemic control decreases the risk of progression of diabetic retinopathy. However, intensification of insulin therapy with abrupt improvement in glycaemic control may be associated with temporary worsening of diabetic retinopathy.

Skin and subcutaneous tissue disorders

Uncommon – Lipodystrophy

Lipodystrophy may occur at the injection site as a consequence of failure to rotate injection sites within an area.

General disorders and administration site conditions

Uncommon – Injection site reactions

Injection site reactions (redness, swelling, itching, pain and haematoma at the injection site) may occur during treatment with insulin. Most reactions are transitory and disappear during continued treatment.

Uncommon – Oedema

Oedema may occur upon initiation of insulin therapy. These symptoms are usually of transitory nature.

4.9 Overdose

A specific overdose of insulin cannot be defined. However, hypoglycaemia may develop over sequential stages:

- Mild hypoglycaemic episodes can be treated by oral administration of glucose or sugary products. It is therefore recommended that the diabetic patients carry some sugar lumps, sweets, biscuits or sugary fruit juice.
- Severe hypoglycaemic episodes, where the patient has become unconscious, can be treated by glucagon (0.5 to 1 mg) given intramuscularly or subcutaneously by a person who has received appropriate instruction, or by glucose given intravenously by a medical professional. Glucose must also be given intravenously, if the patient does not respond to glucagon within 10 to 15 minutes.

Upon regaining consciousness, administration of oral carbohydrate is recommended for the patient in order to prevent relapse.

5. PHARMACOLOGICAL PROPERTIES

5.1 Pharmacodynamic properties

Pharmacotherapeutic group: Insulins and analogues, intermediate-acting combined with fast-acting, insulin (human). ATC code: A10A D01.

The blood glucose lowering effect of insulin is due to the facilitated uptake of glucose following binding of insulin to receptors on muscle and fat cells and to the simultaneous inhibition of glucose output from the liver.

Mixtard is a dual-acting insulin.

Onset of action is within ½ hour, reaches a maximum effect within 2-8 hours and the entire duration of action is up to 24 hours.

5.2 Pharmacokinetic properties

Insulin in the blood stream has a half-life of a few minutes. Consequently, the time-action profile of an insulin preparation is determined solely by its absorption characteristics.

This process is influenced by several factors (e.g. insulin dosage, injection route and site, thickness of subcutaneous fat, type of diabetes). The pharmacokinetics of insulins are therefore affected by significant intra- and inter-individual variation.

Absorption

The absorption profile is due to the product being a mixture of insulins with fast and protracted absorption respectively. The maximum plasma concentration of Mixtard is reached within 1.5-2.5 hours after subcutaneous administration.

Distribution

No profound binding to plasma proteins, except circulating insulin antibodies (if present) has been observed.

Metabolism

Human insulin is reported to be degraded by insulin protease or insulin-degrading enzymes and possibly protein disulfide isomerase. A number of cleavage (hydrolysis) sites on the human insulin molecule have been proposed; none of the metabolites formed following the cleavage are active.

Elimination

The terminal half-life is determined by the rate of absorption from the subcutaneous tissue. The terminal half-life ($t_{½}$) is therefore a measure of the absorption rather than of the elimination per se of insulin from plasma (insulin in the blood stream has a $t_{½}$ of a few minutes). Trials have indicated a $t_{½}$ of about 5-10 hours.

5.3 Preclinical safety data

Preclinical data reveal no special hazard for humans based on conventional studies of safety pharmacology, repeated dose toxicity, genotoxicity, carcinogenic potential, toxicity to reproduction.

6. PHARMACEUTICAL PARTICULARS

6.1 List of excipients

Zinc chloride

Glycerol

Metacresol

Phenol

Disodium phosphate dihydrate

Sodium hydroxide or/and hydrochloric acid (for pH adjustment)

Protamine sulphate

Water for injections

6.2 Incompatibilities

Insulin suspensions should not be added to infusion fluids.

6.3 Shelf life

30 months.

After first opening: 6 weeks.

6.4 Special precautions for storage

Store in a refrigerator (2°C - 8°C).

Do not freeze.

Mixtard 20 Penfill:

Keep the cartridge in the outer carton in order to protect from light.

During use: do not refrigerate. Do not store above 30°C.

Mixtard 20 NovoLet:

During use: do not refrigerate. Do not store above 30°C.

Keep the pen cap on in order to protect the insulin from light.

Protect from excessive heat and sunlight.

6.5 Nature and contents of container

Glass cartridge (type 1) with a bromobutyl rubber plunger and a bromobutyl/polyisoprene rubber stopper. The cartridge contains a glass ball to facilitate the re-suspension.

Pack size: 5 cartridges × 3 ml.

Pre-filled pen (multidose disposable pen) comprising a pen injector with a cartridge (3 ml). The cartridge is made of glass (type 1), containing a bromobutyl rubber plunger and a bromobutyl/polyisoprene rubber stopper. The cartridge contains a glass ball to facilitate the re-suspension. The pen injector is made of plastic.

Pack size: 5 pre-filled pens × 3 ml.

6.6 Instructions for use and handling

Cartridges and pens should only be used in combination with products that are compatible with them and allow the cartridge and pen to function safely and effectively.

Mixtard Penfill and Mixtard NovoLet are for single person use only. The container must not be refilled.

Insulin preparations, which have been frozen, must not be used.

Insulin suspensions should not be used if they do not appear uniformly white and cloudy after re-suspension.

7. MARKETING AUTHORISATION HOLDER

Novo Nordisk A/S

Novo Allé

DK-2880 Bagsværd

Denmark

8. MARKETING AUTHORISATION NUMBER(S)

Mixtard 20 Penfill 100 IU/ml: EU/1/02/231/009

Mixtard 20 NovoLet 100 IU/ml: EU/1/02/231/022

9. DATE OF FIRST AUTHORISATION/RENEWAL OF THE AUTHORISATION

October 2002

10. DATE OF REVISION OF THE TEXT

2 August 2004

Legal Status

POM

Mixtard 30 100 IU/ml, Mixtard 30 Penfill 100 IU/ml, Mixtard 30 NovoLet 100 IU/ml, Mixtard 30 InnoLet 100 IU/ml

(Novo Nordisk Limited)

1. NAME OF THE MEDICINAL PRODUCT

Mixtard 30 100 IU/ml

Suspension for injection in a vial

Mixtard 30 Penfill 100 IU/ml

Suspension for injection in a cartridge

Mixtard 30 NovoLet 100 IU/ml

Suspension for injection in a pre-filled pen

Mixtard 30 InnoLet 100 IU/ml

Suspension for injection in a pre-filled pen

2. QUALITATIVE AND QUANTITATIVE COMPOSITION

Insulin human, rDNA (produced by recombinant DNA technology in *Saccharomyces cerevisiae*).

1 ml contains 100 IU of insulin human

1 vial contains 10 ml equivalent to 1000 IU

1 cartridge contains 3 ml equivalent to 300 IU

1 pre-filled pen contains 3 ml equivalent to 300 IU

One IU (International Unit) corresponds to 0.035 mg of anhydrous human insulin.

Mixtard is a mixture of dissolved insulin and isophane (NPH) insulin.

Mixtard 30 consists of 30% dissolved insulin and 70% isophane insulin.

For excipients, see Section 6.1 List of excipients.

3. PHARMACEUTICAL FORM

Suspension for injection in a vial.

Suspension for injection in a cartridge.

Suspension for injection in a pre-filled pen.

Mixtard is a cloudy, white, aqueous suspension.

4. CLINICAL PARTICULARS

4.1 Therapeutic indications

Treatment of diabetes mellitus.

4.2 Posology and method of administration

Mixtard is a dual-acting insulin. It is a biphasic formulation containing fast-acting and long-acting insulin.

Premixed insulins are usually given once or twice daily when a rapid initial effect together with a more prolonged effect is desired.

Dosage

Dosage is individual and determined in accordance with the needs of the patient. The individual insulin requirement is usually between 0.3 and 1.0 IU/kg/day. The daily insulin requirement may be higher in patients with insulin resistance (e.g. during puberty or due to obesity) and lower in patients with residual, endogenous insulin production.

In patients with diabetes mellitus optimised glycaemic control delays the onset of late diabetic complications. Close blood glucose monitoring is recommended.

An injection should be followed within 30 minutes by a meal or snack containing carbohydrates.

Dosage adjustment

Concomitant illness, especially infections and feverish conditions, usually increases the patient's insulin requirement.

Renal or hepatic impairment may reduce insulin requirement.

Adjustment of dosage may also be necessary if patients change physical activity or their usual diet.

Dosage adjustment may be necessary when transferring patients from one insulin preparation to another (see section 4.4 Special warnings and special precautions for use).

Administration

For subcutaneous use.

Mixtard is usually administered subcutaneously in the thigh or abdominal wall. If convenient, the gluteal region or the deltoid region may also be used.

Subcutaneous injection into the abdominal wall ensures a faster absorption than from other injection sites.

Injection into a lifted skin fold minimises the risk of unintended intramuscular injection.

Keep the needle under the skin for at least 6 seconds to make sure the entire dose is injected.

Injection sites should be rotated within an anatomic region in order to avoid lipodystrophy.

Insulin suspensions are never to be administered intravenously.

Mixtard is accompanied by a package leaflet with detailed instruction for use to be followed.

The vials are for use with insulin syringes with a corresponding unit scale.

The cartridges are designed to be used with Novo Nordisk delivery systems (durable devices for repeated use) and NovoFine needles. Detailed instruction accompanying the delivery system must be followed.

Mixtard NovoLet is designed to be used with NovoFine needles.

NovoLet delivers 2-78 units in increments of 2 units.

Mixtard InnoLet is designed to be used with NovoFine short cap needles of 8 mm or shorter in length. The needle box is marked with an **S.**

InnoLet delivers 1-50 units in increments of 1 unit.

The pens should be primed before injection so that the dose selector returns to zero and a drop of insulin appears at the needle tip.

The dose is set by turning the selector, which returns to zero during the injection.

4.3 Contraindications

Hypoglycaemia

Hypersensitivity to human insulin or to any of the excipients (see section 6.1 List of excipients).

4.4 Special warnings and special precautions for use

Inadequate dosage or discontinuation of treatment, especially in type 1 diabetes, may lead to **hyperglycaemia**.

Usually the first symptoms of hyperglycaemia set in gradually, over a period of hours or days. They include thirst, increased frequency of urination, nausea, vomiting, drowsiness, flushed dry skin, dry mouth, loss of appetite as well as acetone odour of breath.

In type 1 diabetes, untreated hyperglycaemic events eventually lead to diabetic ketoacidosis, which is potentially lethal.

Hypoglycaemia may occur if the insulin dose is too high in relation to the insulin requirement (see section 4.8 and 4.9).

Omission of a meal or unplanned, strenuous physical exercise may lead to hypoglycaemia.

Patients whose blood glucose control is greatly improved e.g. by intensified insulin therapy, may experience a change in their usual warning symptoms of hypoglycaemia and should be advised accordingly.

Usual warning symptoms may disappear in patients with long-standing diabetes.

Transferring a patient to another type or brand of insulin should be done under strict medical supervision. Changes in strength, brand (manufacturer), type (fast-, dual-, long-acting insulin etc.), origin (animal, human or analogue insulin) and/or method of manufacture (recombinant DNA versus animal source insulin) may result in a need for a change in dosage.

If an adjustment is needed when switching the patients to Mixtard, it may occur with the first dose or during the first several weeks or months.

A few patients who have experienced hypoglycaemic reactions after transfer from animal source insulin have reported that early warning symptoms of hypoglycaemia were less pronounced or different from those experienced with their previous insulin.

Before travelling between different time zones, the patient should be advised to consult the doctor, since this may mean that the patient has to take insulin and meals at different times.

Insulin suspensions are not to be used in insulin infusion pumps.

Mixtard contains metacresol, which may cause allergic reactions.

4.5 Interaction with other medicinal products and other forms of Interaction

A number of medicinal products are known to interact with glucose metabolism. The physician must therefore take possible interactions into account and should always ask their patients about any medicinal products they take.

The following substances may reduce insulin requirement:

Oral hypoglycaemic agents (OHA), monoamine oxidase inhibitors (MAOI), non-selective beta-blocking agents, angiotensin converting enzyme (ACE) inhibitors, salicylates and alcohol.

The following substances may increase insulin requirement:

Thiazides, glucocorticoids, thyroid hormones and beta-sympathomimetics, growth hormone and danazol.

Beta-blocking agents may mask the symptoms of hypoglycaemia and delay recovery from hypoglycaemia.

Octreotide/lanreotide may both decrease and increase insulin requirement.

Alcohol may intensify and prolong the hypoglycaemic effect of insulin.

4.6 Pregnancy and lactation

There are no restrictions on treatment of diabetes with insulin during pregnancy, as insulin does not pass the placental barrier.

Both hypoglycaemia and hyperglycaemia, which can occur in inadequately controlled diabetes therapy, increase the risk of malformations and death *in utero*. Intensified control in the treatment of pregnant women with diabetes is therefore recommended throughout pregnancy and when contemplating pregnancy.

Insulin requirements usually fall in the first trimester and increase subsequently during the second and third trimesters.

After delivery, insulin requirements return rapidly to pre-pregnancy values.

Insulin treatment of the nursing mother presents no risk to the baby. However, the Mixtard dosage may need to be adjusted.

4.7 Effects on ability to drive and use machines

The patient's ability to concentrate and react may be impaired as a result of hypoglycaemia. This may constitute a risk in situations where these abilities are of special importance (e.g. driving a car or operating machinery).

Patients should be advised to take precautions to avoid hypoglycaemia whilst driving. This is particularly important in those who have reduced or absent awareness of the warning signs of hypoglycaemia or have frequent episodes of hypoglycaemia. The advisability of driving should be considered in these circumstances.

4.8 Undesirable effects

As for other insulin products, hypoglycaemia, in general is the most frequently occurring undesirable effect. It may occur if the insulin dose is too high in relation to the insulin requirement. In clinical trials and during marketed use the frequency varies with patient population and dose regimens. Therefore, no specific frequency can be presented. Severe hypoglycaemia may lead to unconsciousness and/ or convulsions and may result in temporary or permanent impairment of brain function or even death.

Frequencies of adverse drug reactions from clinical trials, that are considered related to Mixtard are listed below. The frequencies are defined as: Uncommon $>1/1000$, $<1/100$). Isolated spontaneous cases are presented as very rare defined as $<1/10{,}000$.

Immune system disorders

Uncommon – Urticaria, rash

Very rare – Anaphylactic reactions

Symptoms of generalized hypersensitivity may include generalized skin rash, itching, sweating, gastrointestinal upset, angioneurotic oedema, difficulties in breathing, palpitation, reduction in blood pressure and fainting/loss of consciousness. Generalised hypersensitivity reactions are potentially life threatening.

Nervous system disorders

Uncommon – Peripheral neuropathy

Fast improvement in blood glucose control may be associated with a condition termed "acute painful neuropathy", which is usually reversible.

Eye disorders

Very rare – Refraction disorders

Refraction anomalies may occur upon initiation of insulin therapy. These symptoms are usually of transitory nature.

Uncommon – Diabetic retinopathy

Long-term improved glycaemic control decreases the risk of progression of diabetic retinopathy. However, intensification of insulin therapy with abrupt improvement in glycaemic control may be associated with temporary worsening of diabetic retinopathy.

Skin and subcutaneous tissue disorders

Uncommon – Lipodystrophy

Lipodystrophy may occur at the injection site as a consequence of failure to rotate injection sites within an area.

General disorders and administration site conditions

Uncommon – Injection site reactions

Injection site reactions (redness, swelling, itching, pain and haematoma at the injection site) may occur during treatment with insulin. Most reactions are transitory and disappear during continued treatment.

Uncommon – Oedema

Oedema may occur upon initiation of insulin therapy. These symptoms are usually of transitory nature.

4.9 Overdose

A specific overdose of insulin cannot be defined. However, hypoglycaemia may develop over sequential stages:

- Mild hypoglycaemic episodes can be treated by oral administration of glucose or sugary products. It is therefore recommended that the diabetic patients carry some sugar lumps, sweets, biscuits or sugary fruit juice.
- Severe hypoglycaemic episodes, where the patient has become unconscious, can be treated by glucagon (0.5 to 1 mg) given intramuscularly or subcutaneously by a person who has received appropriate instruction, or by glucose given intravenously by a medical professional. Glucose must also be given intravenously, if the patient does not respond to glucagon within 10 to 15 minutes.

Upon regaining consciousness, administration of oral carbohydrate is recommended for the patient in order to prevent relapse.

5. PHARMACOLOGICAL PROPERTIES

5.1 Pharmacodynamic properties

Pharmacotherapeutic group: Insulins and analogues, intermediate-acting combined with fast-acting, insulin (human). ATC code: A10A D01.

The blood glucose lowering effect of insulin is due to the facilitated uptake of glucose following binding of insulin to receptors on muscle and fat cells and to the simultaneous inhibition of glucose output from the liver.

Mixtard is a dual-acting insulin.

Onset of action is within ½ hour, reaches a maximum effect within 2-8 hours and the entire time of duration is up to 24 hours.

5.2 Pharmacokinetic properties

Insulin in the blood stream has a half-life of a few minutes. Consequently, the time-action profile of an insulin preparation is determined solely by its absorption characteristics.

This process is influenced by several factors (e.g. insulin dosage, injection route and site, thickness of subcutaneous fat, type of diabetes). The pharmacokinetics of insulins is therefore affected by significant intra- and inter-individual variation.

Absorption

The absorption profile is due to the product being a mixture of insulins with fast and protracted absorption respectively. The maximum plasma concentration of Mixtard is reached within 1.5-2.5 hours after subcutaneous administration.

Distribution

No profound binding to plasma proteins, except circulating insulin antibodies (if present) has been observed.

Metabolism

Human insulin is reported to be degraded by insulin protease or insulin-degrading enzymes and possibly protein disulfide isomerase. A number of cleavage (hydrolysis) sites on the human insulin molecule have been proposed; none of the metabolites formed following the cleavage are active.

Elimination

The terminal half-life is determined by the rate of absorption from the subcutaneous tissue. The terminal half-life ($t_{½}$) is therefore a measure of the absorption rather than of the elimination per se of insulin from plasma (insulin in the blood stream has a $t_{½}$ of a few minutes). Trials have indicated a $t_{½}$ of about 5-10 hours.

5.3 Preclinical safety data

Preclinical data reveal no special hazard for humans based on conventional studies of safety pharmacology, repeated dose toxicity, genotoxicity, carcinogenic potential, toxicity to reproduction.

6. PHARMACEUTICAL PARTICULARS

6.1 List of excipients

Zinc chloride

Glycerol

Metacresol

Phenol

Disodium phosphate dihydrate

Sodium hydroxide or/and hydrochloric acid (for pH adjustment)

Protamine sulphate

Water for injections

6.2 Incompatibilities

Insulin suspensions should not be added to infusion fluids.

6.3 Shelf life

30 months.

After first opening: 6 weeks.

6.4 Special precautions for storage

Store in a refrigerator (2°C - 8°C).

Do not freeze.

Mixtard 30:

Keep the vial in the outer carton in order to protect from light.

During use: do not refrigerate. Do not store above 25°C.

Mixtard 30 Penfill:

Keep the cartridge in the outer carton in order to protect from light.

During use: do not refrigerate. Do not store above 30°C.

Mixtard 30 NovoLet and Mixtard 30 InnoLet

During use: do not refrigerate. Do not store above 30°C.

Keep the pen cap on in order to protect the insulin from light.

Protect from excessive heat and sunlight.

6.5 Nature and contents of container

Glass vial (type 1) closed with a bromobutyl/polyisoprene rubber stopper and a protective tamper-proof cap.

Pack size: 1 vial × 10 ml.

Glass cartridge (type 1) with a bromobutyl rubber plunger and a bromobutyl/polyisoprene rubber stopper. The cartridge contains a glass ball to facilitate the re-suspension.

Pack size: 5 cartridges × 3 ml.

Pre-filled pen (multidose disposable pen) comprising a pen injector with a cartridge (3 ml). The cartridge is made of glass (type 1), containing a bromobutyl rubber plunger and a bromobutyl/polyisoprene rubber stopper. The cartridge contains a glass ball to facilitate the re-suspension. The pen injector is made of plastic.

Pack size: 5 pre-filled pens × 3 ml.

6.6 Instructions for use and handling
Cartridges and pens should only be used in combination with products that are compatible with them and allow the cartridge and pen to function safely and effectively.

Mixtard Penfill, Mixtard NovoLet and Mixtard InnoLet are for single person use only. The container must not be refilled.

Insulin preparations, which have been frozen, must not be used.

Insulin suspensions should not be used if they do not appear uniformly white and cloudy after re-suspension.

7. MARKETING AUTHORISATION HOLDER
Novo Nordisk A/S

Novo Allé

DK-2880 Bagsværd

Denmark

8. MARKETING AUTHORISATION NUMBER(S)
Mixtard 30 100 IU/ml: EU/1/02/231/003

Mixtard 30 Penfill 100 IU/ml: EU/1/02/231/012

Mixtard 30 NovoLet 100 IU/ml: EU/1/02/231/024

Mixtard 30 InnoLet 100 IU/ml: EU/1/02/231/031

9. DATE OF FIRST AUTHORISATION/RENEWAL OF THE AUTHORISATION
October 2002

10. DATE OF REVISION OF THE TEXT
2 August 2004

Legal Status
POM

Mixtard 40 Penfill 100 IU/ml, Mixtard 40 NovoLet 100 IU/ml

(Novo Nordisk Limited)

1. NAME OF THE MEDICINAL PRODUCT
Mixtard 40 Penfill 100 IU/ml

Suspension for injection in a cartridge

Mixtard 40 NovoLet 100 IU/ml

Suspension for injection in a pre-filled pen

2. QUALITATIVE AND QUANTITATIVE COMPOSITION
Insulin human, rDNA (produced by recombinant DNA technology in *Saccharomyces cerevisiae*).

1 ml contains 100 IU of insulin human

1 cartridge contains 3 ml equivalent to 300 IU

1 pre-filled pen contains 3 ml equivalent to 300 IU

One IU (International Unit) corresponds to 0.035 mg of anhydrous human insulin.

Mixtard is a mixture of dissolved insulin and isophane (NPH) insulin.

Mixtard 40 consists of 40% dissolved insulin and 60% isophane insulin.

For excipients, see Section 6.1 List of excipients.

3. PHARMACEUTICAL FORM
Suspension for injection in a cartridge.

Suspension for injection in a pre-filled pen.

Mixtard is a cloudy, white, aqueous suspension.

4. CLINICAL PARTICULARS

4.1 Therapeutic indications
Treatment of diabetes mellitus.

4.2 Posology and method of administration
Mixtard is a dual-acting insulin. It is a biphasic formulation containing fast-acting and long-acting insulin.

Premixed insulins are usually given once or twice daily when a rapid initial effect together with a more prolonged effect is desired.

Dosage
Dosage is individual and determined in accordance with the needs of the patient. The individual insulin requirement is usually between 0.3 and 1.0 IU/kg/day. The daily insulin requirement may be higher in patients with insulin resistance (e.g. during puberty or due to obesity) and lower in patients with residual, endogenous insulin production.

In patients with diabetes mellitus optimised glycaemic control delays the onset of late diabetic complications. Close blood glucose monitoring is recommended.

An injection should be followed within 30 minutes by a meal or snack containing carbohydrates.

Dosage adjustment
Concomitant illness, especially infections and feverish conditions, usually increases the patient's insulin requirement.

Renal or hepatic impairment may reduce insulin requirement.

Adjustment of dosage may also be necessary if patients change physical activity or their usual diet.

Dosage adjustment may be necessary when transferring patients from one insulin preparation to another (see section 4.4 Special warnings and special precautions for use).

Administration
For subcutaneous use.

Mixtard is usually administered subcutaneously in the thigh or abdominal wall. If convenient, the gluteal region or the deltoid region may also be used.

Subcutaneous injection into the abdominal wall ensures a faster absorption than from other injection sites.

Injection into a lifted skin fold minimises the risk of unintended intramuscular injection.

Keep the needle under the skin for at least 6 seconds to make sure the entire dose is injected.

Injection sites should be rotated within an anatomic region in order to avoid lipodystrophy.

Insulin suspensions are never to be administered intravenously.

Mixtard is accompanied by a package leaflet with detailed instruction for use to be followed.

The cartridges are designed to be used with Novo Nordisk delivery systems (durable devices for repeated use) and NovoFine needles. Detailed instruction accompanying the delivery system must be followed.

Mixtard NovoLet is designed to be used with NovoFine needles.

NovoLet delivers 2-78 units in increments of 2 units.

The pens should be primed before injection so that the dose selector returns to zero and a drop of insulin appears at the needle tip.

The dose is set by turning the selector, which returns to zero during the injection.

4.3 Contraindications
Hypoglycaemia

Hypersensitivity to human insulin or to any of the excipients (see section 6.1 List of excipients).

4.4 Special warnings and special precautions for use
Inadequate dosage or discontinuation of treatment, especially in type 1 diabetes, may lead to **hyperglycaemia**.

Usually the first symptoms of hyperglycaemia set in gradually, over a period of hours or days. They include thirst, increased frequency of urination, nausea, vomiting, drowsiness, flushed dry skin, dry mouth, loss of appetite as well as acetone odour of breath.

In type 1 diabetes, untreated hyperglycaemic events eventually lead to diabetic ketoacidosis, which is potentially lethal.

Hypoglycaemia may occur if the insulin dose is too high in relation to the insulin requirement (see section 4.8 and 4.9).

Omission of a meal or unplanned, strenuous physical exercise may lead to hypoglycaemia.

Patients whose blood glucose control is greatly improved e.g. by intensified insulin therapy, may experience a change in their usual warning symptoms of hypoglycaemia and should be advised accordingly.

Usual warning symptoms may disappear in patients with long-standing diabetes.

Transferring a patient to another type or brand of insulin should be done under strict medical supervision. Changes in strength, brand (manufacturer), type (fast-, dual-, long-acting insulin etc.), origin (animal, human or analogue insulin) and/or method of manufacture (recombinant DNA versus animal source insulin) may result in a need for a change in dosage.

If an adjustment is needed when switching the patients to Mixtard, it may occur with the first dose or during the first several weeks or months.

A few patients who have experienced hypoglycaemic reactions after transfer from animal source insulin have reported that early warning symptoms of hypoglycaemia were less pronounced or different from those experienced with their previous insulin.

Before travelling between different time zones, the patient should be advised to consult the doctor, since this may mean that the patient has to take insulin and meals at different times.

Insulin suspensions are not to be used in insulin infusion pumps.

Mixtard contains metacresol, which may cause allergic reactions.

4.5 Interaction with other medicinal products and other forms of Interaction
A number of medicinal products are known to interact with glucose metabolism. The physician must therefore take possible interactions into account and should always ask their patients about any medicinal products they take.

The following substances may reduce insulin requirement:
Oral hypoglycaemic agents (OHA), monoamine oxidase inhibitors (MAOI), non-selective beta-blocking agents, angiotensin converting enzyme (ACE) inhibitors, salicylates and alcohol.

The following substances may increase insulin requirement:
Thiazides, glucocorticoids, thyroid hormones and beta-sympathomimetics, growth hormone and danazol.

Beta-blocking agents may mask the symptoms of hypoglycaemia and delay recovery from hypoglycaemia.

Octreotide/lanreotide may both decrease and increase insulin requirement.

Alcohol may intensify and prolong the hypoglycaemic effect of insulin.

4.6 Pregnancy and lactation
There are no restrictions on treatment of diabetes with insulin during pregnancy, as insulin does not pass the placental barrier.

Both hypoglycaemia and hyperglycaemia, which can occur in inadequately controlled diabetes therapy, increase the risk of malformations and death *in utero*. Intensified control in the treatment of pregnant women with diabetes is therefore recommended throughout pregnancy and when contemplating pregnancy.

Insulin requirements usually fall in the first trimester and increase subsequently during the second and third trimesters.

After delivery, insulin requirements return rapidly to pre-pregnancy values.

Insulin treatment of the nursing mother presents no risk to the baby. However, the Mixtard dosage may need to be adjusted.

4.7 Effects on ability to drive and use machines
The patient's ability to concentrate and react may be impaired as a result of hypoglycaemia. This may constitute a risk in situations where these abilities are of special importance (e.g. driving a car or operating machinery).

Patients should be advised to take precautions to avoid hypoglycaemia whilst driving. This is particularly important in those who have reduced or absent awareness of the warning signs of hypoglycaemia or have frequent episodes of hypoglycaemia. The advisability of driving should be considered in these circumstances.

4.8 Undesirable effects
As for other insulin products, hypoglycaemia, in general is the most frequently occurring undesirable effect. It may occur if the insulin dose is too high in relation to the insulin requirement. In clinical trials and during marketed use the frequency varies with patient population and dose regimens. Therefore, no specific frequency can be presented. Severe hypoglycaemia may lead to unconsciousness and/or convulsions and may result in temporary or permanent impairment of brain function or even death.

Frequencies of adverse drug reactions from clinical trials, that are considered related to Mixtard are listed below. The frequencies are defined as: Uncommon $>1/1000$, $<1/100$). Isolated spontaneous cases are presented as very rare defined as $<1/10{,}000$.

Immune system disorders

Uncommon – Urticaria, rash

Very rare – Anaphylactic reactions

Symptoms of generalized hypersensitivity may include generalized skin rash, itching, sweating, gastrointestinal upset, angioneurotic oedema, difficulties in breathing, palpitation, reduction in blood pressure and fainting/loss of consciousness. Generalised hypersensitivity reactions are potentially life threatening.

Nervous system disorders

Uncommon – Peripheral neuropathy

Fast improvement in blood glucose control may be associated with a condition termed "acute painful neuropathy", which is usually reversible.

Eye disorders

Very rare – Refraction disorders

Refraction anomalies may occur upon initiation of insulin therapy. These symptoms are usually of transitory nature.

Uncommon – Diabetic retinopathy

Long-term improved glycaemic control decreases the risk of progression of diabetic retinopathy. However, intensification of insulin therapy with abrupt improvement in glycaemic control may be associated with temporary worsening of diabetic retinopathy.

Skin and subcutaneous tissue disorders

Uncommon – Lipodystrophy

Lipodystrophy may occur at the injection site as a consequence of failure to rotate injection sites within an area.

General disorders and administration site conditions

Uncommon – Injection site reactions

Injection site reactions (redness, swelling, itching, pain and haematoma at the injection site) may occur during treatment with insulin. Most reactions are transitory and disappear during continued treatment.

Uncommon – Oedema

Oedema may occur upon initiation of insulin therapy. These symptoms are usually of transitory nature.

4.9 Overdose
A specific overdose of insulin cannot be defined. However, hypoglycaemia may develop over sequential stages:

• Mild hypoglycaemic episodes can be treated by oral administration of glucose or sugary products. It is therefore recommended that the diabetic patients carry some sugar lumps, sweets, biscuits or sugary fruit juice.

• Severe hypoglycaemic episodes, where the patient has become unconscious, can be treated by glucagon (0.5 to 1 mg) given intramuscularly or subcutaneously by a person who has received appropriate instruction, or by glucose given intravenously by a medical professional. Glucose must also be given intravenously, if the patient does not respond to glucagon within 10 to 15 minutes.

Upon regaining consciousness, administration of oral carbohydrate is recommended for the patient in order to prevent relapse.

5. PHARMACOLOGICAL PROPERTIES

5.1 Pharmacodynamic properties
Pharmacotherapeutic group: Insulins and analogues, intermediate-acting combined with fast-acting, insulin (human). ATC code: A10A D01.

The blood glucose lowering effect of insulin is due to the facilitated uptake of glucose following binding of insulin to receptors on muscle and fat cells and to the simultaneous inhibition of glucose output from the liver.

Mixtard is a dual-acting insulin.

Onset of action is within ½ hour, reaches a maximum effect within 2-8 hours and the entire duration of action is up to 24 hours.

5.2 Pharmacokinetic properties
Insulin in the blood stream has a half-life of a few minutes. Consequently, the time-action profile of an insulin preparation is determined solely by its absorption characteristics.

This process is influenced by several factors (e.g. insulin dosage, injection route and site, thickness of subcutaneous fat, type of diabetes). The pharmacokinetics of insulins are therefore affected by significant intra- and inter-individual variation.

Absorption

The absorption profile is due to the product being a mixture of insulins with fast and protracted absorption respectively. The maximum plasma concentration of Mixtard is reached within 1.5-2.5 hours after subcutaneous administration.

Distribution

No profound binding to plasma proteins, except circulating insulin antibodies (if present) has been observed.

Metabolism

Human insulin is reported to be degraded by insulin protease or insulin-degrading enzymes and possibly protein disulfide isomerase. A number of cleavage (hydrolysis) sites on the human insulin molecule have been proposed; none of the metabolites formed following the cleavage are active.

Elimination

The terminal half-life is determined by the rate of absorption from the subcutaneous tissue. The terminal half-life ($t_{1/2}$) is therefore a measure of the absorption rather than of the elimination per se of insulin from plasma (insulin in the blood stream has a $t_{1/2}$ of a few minutes). Trials have indicated a $t_{1/2}$ of about 5-10 hours.

5.3 Preclinical safety data
Preclinical data reveal no special hazard for humans based on conventional studies of safety pharmacology, repeated dose toxicity, genotoxicity, carcinogenic potential, toxicity to reproduction.

6. PHARMACEUTICAL PARTICULARS

6.1 List of excipients
Zinc chloride

Glycerol

Metacresol

Phenol

Disodium phosphate dihydrate

Sodium hydroxide or/and hydrochloric acid (for pH adjustment)

Protamine sulphate

Water for injections

6.2 Incompatibilities
Insulin suspensions should not be added to infusion fluids.

6.3 Shelf life
30 months.

After first opening: 6 weeks.

6.4 Special precautions for storage
Store in a refrigerator (2°C - 8°C).

Do not freeze.

Mixtard 40 Penfill:

Keep the cartridge in the outer carton in order to protect from light.

During use: do not refrigerate. Do not store above 30°C.

Mixtard 40 NovoLet:

During use: do not refrigerate. Do not store above 30°C.

Keep the pen cap on in order to protect the insulin from light.

Protect from excessive heat and sunlight.

6.5 Nature and contents of container
Glass cartridge (type 1) with a bromobutyl rubber plunger and a bromobutyl/polyisoprene rubber stopper. The cartridge contains a glass ball to facilitate the re-suspension.
Pack size: 5 cartridges × 3 ml.

Pre-filled pen (multidose disposable pen) comprising a pen injector with a cartridge (3 ml). The cartridge is made of glass (type 1), containing a bromobutyl rubber plunger and a bromobutyl/polyisoprene rubber stopper. The cartridge contains a glass ball to facilitate the re-suspension. The pen injector is made of plastic.

Pack size: 5 pre-filled pens × 3 ml.

6.6 Instructions for use and handling
Cartridges and pens should only be used in combination with products that are compatible with them and allow the cartridge and pen to function safely and effectively.

Mixtard Penfill and Mixtard NovoLet are for single person use only. The container must not be refilled.

Insulin preparations, which have been frozen, must not be used.

Insulin suspensions should not be used if they do not appear uniformly white and cloudy after re-suspension.

7. MARKETING AUTHORISATION HOLDER
Novo Nordisk A/S

Novo Allé

DK-2880 Bagsværd

Denmark

8. MARKETING AUTHORISATION NUMBER(S)
Mixtard 40 Penfill 100 IU/ml: EU/1/02/231/015

Mixtard 40 NovoLet 100 IU/ml: EU/1/02/231/026

9. DATE OF FIRST AUTHORISATION/RENEWAL OF THE AUTHORISATION
October 2002

10. DATE OF REVISION OF THE TEXT
2 August 2004

Legal Status
POM

Mixtard 50 Penfill 100 IU/ml, Mixtard 50 NovoLet 100 IU/ml

(Novo Nordisk Limited)

1. NAME OF THE MEDICINAL PRODUCT
Mixtard 50 Penfill 100 IU/ml

Suspension for injection in a cartridge

Mixtard 50 NovoLet 100 IU/ml

Suspension for injection in a pre-filled pen

2. QUALITATIVE AND QUANTITATIVE COMPOSITION
Insulin human, rDNA (produced by recombinant DNA technology in *Saccharomyces cerevisiae*).

1 ml contains 100 IU of insulin human

1 cartridge contains 3 ml equivalent to 300 IU

1 pre-filled pen contains 3 ml equivalent to 300 IU

One IU (International Unit) corresponds to 0.035 mg of anhydrous human insulin.

Mixtard is a mixture of dissolved insulin and isophane (NPH) insulin.

Mixtard 50 consists of 50% dissolved insulin and 50% isophane insulin.

For excipients, see Section 6.1 List of excipients.

3. PHARMACEUTICAL FORM
Suspension for injection in a cartridge.

Suspension for injection in a pre-filled pen.

Mixtard is a cloudy, white, aqueous suspension.

4. CLINICAL PARTICULARS

4.1 Therapeutic indications
Treatment of diabetes mellitus.

4.2 Posology and method of administration
Mixtard is a dual-acting insulin. It is biphasic formulation containing fast-acting and long-acting insulin.

Premixed insulins are usually given once or twice daily when a rapid initial effect together with a more prolonged effect is desired.

Dosage

Dosage is individual and determined in accordance with the needs of the patient. The individual insulin requirement is usually between 0.3 and 1.0 IU/kg/day. The daily insulin requirement may be higher in patients with insulin resistance (e.g. during puberty or due to obesity) and lower in patients with residual, endogenous insulin production.

In patients with diabetes mellitus optimised glycaemic control delays the onset of late diabetic complications. Close blood glucose monitoring is recommended.

An injection should be followed within 30 minutes by a meal or snack containing carbohydrates.

Dosage adjustment

Concomitant illness, especially infections and feverish conditions, usually increases the patient's insulin requirement.

Renal or hepatic impairment may reduce insulin requirement.

Adjustment of dosage may also be necessary if patients change physical activity or their usual diet.

Dosage adjustment may be necessary when transferring patients from one insulin preparation to another (see section 4.4 Special warnings and special precautions for use).

Administration

For subcutaneous use.

Mixtard is usually administered subcutaneously in the thigh or abdominal wall. If convenient, the gluteal region or the deltoid region may also be used.

Subcutaneous injection into the abdominal wall ensures a faster absorption than from other injection sites.

Injection into a lifted skin fold minimises the risk of unintended intramuscular injection.

Keep the needle under the skin for at least 6 seconds to make sure the entire dose is injected.

Injection sites should be rotated within an anatomic region in order to avoid lipodystrophy.

Insulin suspensions are never to be administered intravenously.

Mixtard is accompanied by a package leaflet with detailed instruction for use to be followed.

The cartridges are designed to be used with Novo Nordisk delivery systems (durable devices for repeated use) and NovoFine needles. Detailed instruction accompanying the delivery system must be followed.

Mixtard NovoLet is designed to be used with NovoFine needles.

NovoLet delivers 2-78 units in increments of 2 units.

The pens should be primed before injection so that the dose selector returns to zero and a drop of insulin appears at the needle tip.

The dose is set by turning the selector, which returns to zero during the injection.

4.3 Contraindications
Hypoglycaemia

Hypersensitivity to human insulin or to any of the excipients (see section 6.1 List of excipients).

4.4 Special warnings and special precautions for use
Inadequate dosage or discontinuation of treatment, especially in type 1 diabetes, may lead to **hyperglycaemia**.

Usually the first symptoms of hyperglycaemia set in gradually, over a period of hours or days. They include thirst, increased frequency of urination, nausea, vomiting, drowsiness, flushed dry skin, dry mouth, loss of appetite as well as acetone odour of breath.

In type 1 diabetes, untreated hyperglycaemic events eventually lead to diabetic ketoacidosis, which is potentially lethal.

Hypoglycaemia may occur if the insulin dose is too high in relation to the insulin requirement (see section 4.8 and 4.9).

Omission of a meal or unplanned, strenuous physical exercise may lead to hypoglycaemia.

Patients whose blood glucose control is greatly improved e.g. by intensified insulin therapy, may experience a change in their usual warning symptoms of hypoglycaemia and should be advised accordingly.

Usual warning symptoms may disappear in patients with long-standing diabetes.

Transferring a patient to another type or brand of insulin should be done under strict medical supervision. Changes in strength, brand (manufacturer), type (fast-, dual-, long-acting insulin etc.), origin (animal, human or analogue insulin) and/or method of manufacture (recombinant DNA versus animal source insulin) may result in a need for a change in dosage.

If an adjustment is needed when switching the patients to Mixtard, it may occur with the first dose or during the first several weeks or months.

A few patients who have experienced hypoglycaemic reactions after transfer from animal source insulin have reported that early warning symptoms of hypoglycaemia were less pronounced or different from those experienced with their previous insulin.

Before travelling between different time zones, the patient should be advised to consult the doctor, since this may mean that the patient has to take insulin and meals at different times.

Insulin suspensions are not to be used in insulin infusion pumps.

Mixtard contains metacresol, which may cause allergic reactions.

4.5 Interaction with other medicinal products and other forms of Interaction

A number of medicinal products are known to interact with glucose metabolism. The physician must therefore take possible interactions into account and should always ask their patients about any medicinal products they take.

The following substances may reduce insulin requirement:

Oral hypoglycaemic agents (OHA), monoamine oxidase inhibitors (MAOI), non-selective beta-blocking agents, angiotensin converting enzyme (ACE) inhibitors, salicylates and alcohol.

The following substances may increase insulin requirement:

Thiazides, glucocorticoids, thyroid hormones and beta-sympathomimetics, growth hormone and danazol.

Beta-blocking agents may mask the symptoms of hypoglycaemia and delay recovery from hypoglycaemia.

Octreotide/lanreotide may both decrease and increase insulin requirement.

Alcohol may intensify and prolong the hypoglycaemic effect of insulin.

4.6 Pregnancy and lactation

There are no restrictions on treatment of diabetes with insulin during pregnancy, as insulin does not pass the placental barrier.

Both hypoglycaemia and hyperglycaemia, which can occur in inadequately controlled diabetes therapy, increase the risk of malformations and death *in utero*. Intensified control in the treatment of pregnant women with diabetes is therefore recommended throughout pregnancy and when contemplating pregnancy.

Insulin requirements usually fall in the first trimester and increase subsequently during the second and third trimesters.

After delivery, insulin requirements return rapidly to pre-pregnancy values.

Insulin treatment of the nursing mother presents no risk to the baby. However, the Mixtard dosage may need to be adjusted.

4.7 Effects on ability to drive and use machines

The patient's ability to concentrate and react may be impaired as a result of hypoglycaemia. This may constitute a risk in situations where these abilities are of special importance (e.g. driving a car or operating machinery).

Patients should be advised to take precautions to avoid hypoglycaemia whilst driving. This is particularly important in those who have reduced or absent awareness of the warning signs of hypoglycaemia or have frequent episodes of hypoglycaemia. The advisability of driving should be considered in these circumstances.

4.8 Undesirable effects

As for other insulin products, hypoglycaemia, in general is the most frequently occurring undesirable effect. It may occur if the insulin dose is too high in relation to the insulin requirement. In clinical trials and during marketed use the frequency varies with patient population and dose regimens. Therefore, no specific frequency can be presented. Severe hypoglycaemia may lead to unconsciousness and/or convulsions and may result in temporary or permanent impairment of brain function or even death.

Frequencies of adverse drug reactions from clinical trials, that are considered related to Mixtard are listed below. The frequencies are defined as: Uncommon >1/1000, < 1/100). Isolated spontaneous cases are presented as very rare defined as < 1/10,000.

Immune system disorders

Uncommon – Urticaria, rash

Very rare – Anaphylactic reactions

Symptoms of generalized hypersensitivity may include generalized skin rash, itching, sweating, gastrointestinal upset, angioneurotic oedema, difficulties in breathing, palpitation, reduction in blood pressure and fainting/loss of consciousness. Generalised hypersensitivity reactions are potentially life threatening.

Nervous system disorders

Uncommon – Peripheral neuropathy

Fast improvement in blood glucose control may be associated with a condition termed "acute painful neuropathy", which is usually reversible.

Eye disorders

Very rare – Refraction disorders

Refraction anomalies may occur upon initiation of insulin therapy. These symptoms are usually of transitory nature.

Uncommon – Diabetic retinopathy

Long-term improved glycaemic control decreases the risk of progression of diabetic retinopathy. However, intensification of insulin therapy with abrupt improvement in glycaemic control may be associated with temporary worsening of diabetic retinopathy.

Skin and subcutaneous tissue disorders

Uncommon – Lipodystrophy

Lipodystrophy may occur at the injection site as a consequence of failure to rotate injection sites within an area.

General disorders and administration site conditions

Uncommon – Injection site reactions

Injection site reactions (redness, swelling, itching, pain and haematoma at the injection site) may occur during treatment with insulin. Most reactions are transitory and disappear during continued treatment.

Uncommon – Oedema

Oedema may occur upon initiation of insulin therapy. These symptoms are usually of transitory nature.

4.9 Overdose

A specific overdose of insulin cannot be defined. However, hypoglycaemia may develop over sequential stages:

- Mild hypoglycaemic episodes can be treated by oral administration of glucose or sugary products. It is therefore recommended that the diabetic patients carry some sugar lumps, sweets, biscuits or sugary fruit juice.
- Severe hypoglycaemic episodes, where the patient has become unconscious, can be treated by glucagon (0.5 to 1 mg) given intramuscularly or subcutaneously by a person who has received appropriate instruction, or by glucose given intravenously by a medical professional. Glucose must also be given intravenously, if the patient does not respond to glucagon within 10 to 15 minutes.

Upon regaining consciousness, administration of oral carbohydrate is recommended for the patient in order to prevent relapse.

5. PHARMACOLOGICAL PROPERTIES

5.1 Pharmacodynamic properties

Pharmacotherapeutic group: Insulins and analogues, intermediate-acting combined with fast-acting, insulin (human). ATC code: A10A D01.

The blood glucose lowering effect of insulin is due to the facilitated uptake of glucose following binding of insulin to receptors on muscle and fat cells and to the simultaneous inhibition of glucose output from the liver.

Mixtard is a dual-acting insulin.

Onset of action is within ½ hour, reaches a maximum effect within 2-8 hours and the entire duration of action is up to 24 hours.

5.2 Pharmacokinetic properties

Insulin in the blood stream has a half-life of a few minutes. Consequently, the time-action profile of an insulin preparation is determined solely by its absorption characteristics.

This process is influenced by several factors (e.g. insulin dosage, injection route and site, thickness of subcutaneous fat, type of diabetes). The pharmacokinetics of insulins are therefore affected by significant intra- and inter-individual variation.

Absorption

The absorption profile is due to the product being a mixture of insulins with fast and protracted absorption respectively. The maximum plasma concentration of Mixtard is reached within 1.5-2.5 hours after subcutaneous administration.

Distribution

No profound binding to plasma proteins, except circulating insulin antibodies (if present) has been observed.

Metabolism

Human insulin is reported to be degraded by insulin protease or insulin-degrading enzymes and possibly protein disulfide isomerase. A number of cleavage (hydrolysis) sites on the human insulin molecule have been proposed; none of the metabolites formed following the cleavage are active.

Elimination

The terminal half-life is determined by the rate of absorption from the subcutaneous tissue. The terminal half-life ($t_{½}$) is therefore a measure of the absorption rather than of the elimination per se of insulin from plasma (insulin in the blood stream has a $t_{½}$ of a few minutes). Trials have indicated a $t_{½}$ of about 5-10 hours.

5.3 Preclinical safety data

Preclinical data reveal no special hazard for humans based on conventional studies of safety pharmacology, repeated dose toxicity, genotoxicity, carcinogenic potential, toxicity to reproduction.

6. PHARMACEUTICAL PARTICULARS

6.1 List of excipients

Zinc chloride

Glycerol

Metacresol

Phenol

Disodium phosphate dihydrate

Sodium hydroxide or/and hydrochloric acid (for pH adjustment)

Protamine sulphate

Water for injections

6.2 Incompatibilities

Insulin suspensions should not be added to infusion fluids.

6.3 Shelf life

30 months.

After first opening: 6 weeks.

6.4 Special precautions for storage

Store in a refrigerator (2°C - 8°C).

Do not freeze.

Mixtard 50 Penfill:

Keep the cartridge in the outer carton in order to protect from light.

During use: do not refrigerate. Do not store above 30°C.

Mixtard 50 NovoLet:

During use: do not refrigerate. Do not store above 30°C.

Keep the pen cap on in order to protect the insulin from light.

Protect from excessive heat and sunlight.

6.5 Nature and contents of container

Glass cartridge (type 1) with a bromobutyl rubber plunger and a bromobutyl/polyisoprene rubber stopper. The cartridge contains a glass ball to facilitate the re-suspension.

Pack size: 5 cartridges × 3 ml.

Pre-filled pen (multidose disposable pen) comprising a pen injector with a cartridge (3 ml). The cartridge is made of glass (type 1), containing a bromobutyl rubber plunger and a bromobutyl/polyisoprene rubber stopper. The cartridge contains a glass ball to facilitate the re-suspension. The pen injector is made of plastic.

Pack size: 5 pre-filled pens × 3 ml.

6.6 Instructions for use and handling

Cartridges and pens should only be used in combination with products that are compatible with them and allow the cartridge and pen to function safely and effectively.

Mixtard Penfill and Mixtard NovoLet are for single person use only. The container must not be refilled.

Insulin preparations, which have been frozen, must not be used.

Insulin suspensions should not be used if they do not appear uniformly white and cloudy after re-suspension.

7. MARKETING AUTHORISATION HOLDER

Novo Nordisk A/S

Novo Allé

DK-2880 Bagsværd

Denmark

8. MARKETING AUTHORISATION NUMBER(S)

Mixtard 50 Penfill 100 IU/ml: EU/1/02/231/018

Mixtard 50 NovoLet 100 IU/ml: EU/1/02/231/028

9. DATE OF FIRST AUTHORISATION/RENEWAL OF THE AUTHORISATION

October 2002

10. DATE OF REVISION OF THE TEXT

2 August 2004

Legal Status

POM

Mizollen 10mg modified release tablet

(SCHWARZ PHARMA Limited)

1. NAME OF THE MEDICINAL PRODUCT

Mizollen 10mg modified release tablet

2. QUALITATIVE AND QUANTITATIVE COMPOSITION

Mizolastine (INN) 10mg per tablet.

For excipients, see 6.1.

3. PHARMACEUTICAL FORM

Film-coated modified release tablets.

Oblong, white tablets with a scored line on one side and a mark "MZI 10" on the reverse side.

4. CLINICAL PARTICULARS

4.1 Therapeutic indications

Mizolastine is a long-lasting H_1 –antihistamine indicated for the symptomatic relief of seasonal allergic rhinoconjunctivitis (hay fever), perennial allergic rhinoconjunctivitis and urticaria.

4.2 Posology and method of administration

Adults, including the elderly, and children 12 years of age and over.

The recommended daily dose is one 10mg tablet.

4.3 Contraindications

Hypersensitivity to the active ingredient or to any of the excipients.

Concomitant administration with macrolide antibiotics or systemic imidazole antifungals.

Significantly impaired hepatic function.

Clinically significant cardiac disease or a history of symptomatic arrhythmias.

Patients with known or suspected QT prolongation or with electrolyte imbalance, in particular hypokalaemia.

Clinically significant bradycardia.

Drugs known to prolong the QT interval, such as Class I and III anti-arrhythmics.

4.4 Special warnings and special precautions for use
Mizolastine has a weak potential to prolong the QT interval in a few individuals. The degree of prolongation is modest and has not been associated with cardiac arrhythmias.

The elderly may be particularly susceptible to the sedative effects of mizolastine and the potential effects of the drug on cardiac repolarisation.

4.5 Interaction with other medicinal products and other forms of Interaction
Although the bioavailability of mizolastine is high and the drug is principally metabolised by glucuronidation, systemically administered ketoconazole and erythromycin moderately increase the plasma concentration of mizolastine and their concurrent use is contraindicated.

Concurrent use of other potent inhibitors or substrates of hepatic oxidation (cytochrome P_{450} 3A4) with mizolastine should be approached with caution. These would include cimetidine, cyclosporin, and nifedipine.

Alcohol: In studies with mizolastine, no potentiation of the sedation and the alteration in performance caused by alcohol has been observed.

4.6 Pregnancy and lactation
The safety of mizolastine for use in human pregnancy has not been established. The evaluation of experimental animal studies does not indicate direct or indirect harmful effects with respect to the development of the embryo or foetus, the course of gestation and peri- and post-natal development. However, as with all drugs, mizolastine should be avoided in pregnancy, particularly during the first trimester.

Mizolastine is excreted into breast milk, therefore its use by lactating women is not recommended.

4.7 Effects on ability to drive and use machines
Most patients taking mizolastine may drive or perform tasks requiring concentration. However, in order to identify sensitive people who have unusual reactions to drugs, it is advisable to check the individual response before driving or performing complicated tasks.

4.8 Undesirable effects
- **Gastro-intestinal disorders:**

Common: dry mouth, diarrhoea, abdominal pain (including dyspepsia), nausea.

- **Central nervous system disorders, and psychiatric disorders:**

Common: drowsiness often transient, headache, dizziness

Uncommon: anxiety and depression

- **Liver disorders:**

Uncommon: raised liver enzymes

- **Haematological disorders:**

Very rare: low neutrophil count

- **Body as a whole:**

Common: asthenia often transient, increased appetite associated with weight gain.

Very rare: allergic reactions including anaphylaxis, angioedema, generalised rash/urticaria, pruritus and hypotension

- **Cardiovascular disorders:**

Uncommon: hypotension, tachycardia, palpitations

Very rare: vasovagal attack

- **Musculoskeletal disorders:**

Uncommon: arthralgia and myalgia

There were reports of bronchospasm and aggravation of asthma but in view of the high frequency of asthma in the patient population being treated, a causal relationship remains uncertain.

Treatment with certain antihistamines has been associated with QT interval prolongation increasing the risk of serious cardiac arrhythmias in susceptible subjects.

Minor changes in blood sugar and electrolytes have been observed rarely. The clinical significance of these changes in otherwise healthy individuals remains unclear. Patients at risk (diabetics, those susceptible to electrolyte imbalance and cardiac arrhythmias) should be monitored periodically.

4.9 Overdose
In cases of overdosage, general symptomatic surveillance with cardiac monitoring including QT interval and cardiac rhythm for at least 24 hours is recommended, along with standard measures to remove any unabsorbed drug.

Studies in patients with renal insufficiency suggest that haemodialysis does not increase clearance of the drug.

5. PHARMACOLOGICAL PROPERTIES
5.1 Pharmacodynamic properties
Antihistamine H_1 (ATC code: R06AX25)

Mizolastine possesses antihistamine and antiallergic properties due to a specific and selective antagonism of peripheral histamine H_1 receptors. It has also been shown to inhibit histamine release from mast cells (at 0.3 mg/kg orally) and the migration of neutrophils (at 3 mg/kg orally) in animal models of allergic reactions.

In man, histamine-induced wheal and flare studies have shown that mizolastine 10mg is a rapid, potent (80% inhibition after 4 hrs) and sustained (24hr) antihistamine. No tachyphylaxis occurred after long-term administration.

In both preclinical and clinical studies, no anticholinergic effect has been demonstrated.

5.2 Pharmacokinetic properties
Following oral administration mizolastine is rapidly absorbed. Peak plasma concentration is reached at a median time of 1.5 hours.

Bioavailability is 65% and linear kinetics have been demonstrated.

The mean elimination half-life is 13.0 hours with plasma protein binding of 98.4%.

In hepatic insufficiency the absorption of mizolastine is slower and the distribution phase longer, with a resulting moderate increase in AUC of 50%.

The principal metabolic pathway is glucuronidation of the parent compound. The cytochrome P_{450} 3A4 enzyme system is involved in one of the additional metabolic pathways with formation of the hydroxylated metabolites of mizolastine. None of the identified metabolites contribute to the pharmacological activity of mizolastine.

An increase in mizolastine plasma levels, observed with systemic ketoconazole and erythromycin, led to concentrations equivalent to those obtained after a 15 to 20mg dose of mizolastine alone.

In studies carried out in healthy volunteers, no clinically significant interaction has been recorded with food, warfarin, digoxin, theophylline, lorazepam, or diltiazem.

5.3 Preclinical safety data
Pharmacological studies in several species have shown an effect of cardiac repolarisation at doses in excess of 10-20 times the therapeutic dose. In conscious dogs, mizolastine has shown pharmacological interactions with ketoconazole at the electrocardiographic level at 70 times the therapeutic dose.

6. PHARMACEUTICAL PARTICULARS
6.1 List of excipients
Core:

Hydrogenated castor oil

Lactose monohydrate

Microcrystalline cellulose

Tartaric acid

Povidone

Anhydrous colloidal silica

Magnesium stearate.

Film-coating:

Hypromellose

Titanium dioxide (E171)

Propylene glycol.

6.2 Incompatibilities
Not applicable.

6.3 Shelf life
2 years in blisters.

3 years in securitainers.

6.4 Special precautions for storage
Do not store above 25°C. Store in the original package in order to protect from moisture.

6.5 Nature and contents of container
Aluminium/ (oPA/ Aluminium/PVC) blisters:

Packs of 4, 7, 10, 15, 20, 30, 50 or 100.

Aluminium/PVC blisters Packs of 4, 7, 10, 15, 20, 30, 50 or 100 tablets.

Polypropylene tubes with polyethylene caps

Packs of 4, 7, 10, 15, 20, 30, 50 or 100 tablets.

6.6 Instructions for use and handling
The tablets should not be taken if they become discoloured.

7. MARKETING AUTHORISATION HOLDER
Sanofi Synthelabo

PO Box 597

Guildford

Surrey

8. MARKETING AUTHORISATION NUMBER(S)
PL 11723/0318

9. DATE OF FIRST AUTHORISATION/RENEWAL OF THE AUTHORISATION
5 October 2001

10. DATE OF REVISION OF THE TEXT
October 2003

For further information, contact SCHWARZ PHARMA Limited, Schwarz House, East Street, Chesham, Bucks, HP5 1DG, England.

Code: Miz 2723

M-M-R II

(Sanofi Pasteur MSD)

1. NAME OF THE MEDICINAL PRODUCT
M-M-R㊉ II

Measles, Mumps and Rubella Vaccine, Live, Attenuated

2. QUALITATIVE AND QUANTITATIVE COMPOSITION
Each 0.5 millilitre dose when reconstituted contains not less than equivalent of:

1,000 TCID50 *of Measles Virus Live

(the more attenuated Enders Line of the Edmonston strain).

20,000 TCID50 of Mumps Virus Live (Jeryl Lynn® Level B strain).

1,000 TCID50 of Rubella Virus Live (Wistar, RA 27/3 Strain).

*Tissue Culture Infectious Dose

3. PHARMACEUTICAL FORM
Powder for injection.

4. CLINICAL PARTICULARS
4.1 Therapeutic indications
For simultaneous immunisation against measles, mumps and rubella in the following groups:

Children: Recommended for both primary and booster immunisation of both boys and girls 12 months of age or older.

Non-Pregnant Adolescent and Adult Females: Immunisation of susceptible non-pregnant adolescent and adult females of childbearing age is indicated when the potential vaccinee agrees not to become pregnant for the next 3 months after vaccination and is informed of the reason, (this also applies to women in the immediate post-partum period when it may be found most convenient to vaccinate, see also 4.6 Pregnancy and Lactation), and is told of the frequent occurrence of generally self-limiting arthralgia and/or arthritis beginning 2-4 weeks after vaccination.

International Travellers: Individuals planning travel abroad who are known to be susceptible to one or more of these diseases can receive either a single antigen vaccine (measles, mumps or rubella), if available, or a combined antigen vaccine as appropriate. A combined measles, mumps and rubella vaccine is preferred for persons likely to be susceptible to mumps and rubella as well as measles.

4.2 Posology and method of administration
The vaccine is administered by deep subcutaneous or intramuscular injection preferably into the outer aspect of the arm.

Children who suffered ITP within six weeks of the first dose of MMR (or its component vaccines), should have serological status evaluated at the time the second dose was due. If serology testing suggests that a child is not fully immune against measles, mumps and rubella then a second dose of MMR is recommended (see 4.4)

Adults and children: After suitably cleansing the injection site, 0.5 millilitre of reconstituted vaccine should be injected. M-M-R㊉ II must not be given intravenously.

Do not give immunoglobulin with M-M-R㊉ II.

Warning: A sterile syringe and epinephrine (adrenaline) injection should be available for immediate use should an anaphylactic reaction occur.

Elderly: No special comment.

Revaccination: A second dose of measles, mumps and rubella vaccine is recommended in the national immunisation schedule (see 4.4).

Children receiving their first dose of measles, mumps and rubella vaccine younger than 12 months of age should be revaccinated at 15 months of age. They may still receive a further dose at the time indicated in the national immunisation schedule, (M-M-R㊉ II is not recommended for infants under 12 months of age.)

Use with other vaccines: Vaccines containing diphtheria, tetanus and pertussis antigens and/or oral poliomyelitis vaccine can be administered at the same time as M-M-R㊉ II. For concurrent parenteral vaccination, separate syringes and separate sites for injection should be used.

M-M-R㊉ II should not be given less than one month before or after immunisation with other live viral vaccines.

4.3 Contraindications
Do not give M-M-R㊉ II to pregnant females; the possible effects of the vaccine on foetal development are unknown at this time. Pregnancy must be avoided for three months following vaccination of post-pubertal females.

Anaphylactic or anaphylactoid reactions to a previous dose of vaccine or to neomycin or any other vaccine constituent. (Each dose of reconstituted vaccine contains approximately 25 micrograms neomycin.)

Any febrile respiratory illness, or other active or suspected infection.

Those with impaired immune responsiveness, whether occurring naturally or as a result of therapy with steroids, radiotherapy, cytotoxic or other agents. This contra-indication does not apply to patients receiving corticosteroids as replacement therapy, e.g. for Addisons's disease.

Patients with active untreated tuberculosis, blood dyscrasias such as thrombocytopenia, leukaemia, malignant disease including lymphomas of any type or other malignant neoplasms affecting the bone marrow or lymphatic systems.

Primary and acquired immunodeficiency states, including patients who are immunosuppressed in association with AIDS or other clinical manifestations with human immunodeficiency viruses; cellular immune deficiencies; and hypogammaglobulinaemic and dysgammaglobulinaemic states. Fatal cases of measles inclusion body encephalitis (MIBE) and pneumonitis as a direct consequence of disseminated measles vaccine virus infection have been reported in severely immunocompromised individuals vaccinated with measles-containing vaccine. Those patients with a family history of congenital hereditary immunodeficiency until their immune competence has been demonstrated.

Children below 12 months of age: Children below 12 months of age should not normally be given M-M-R® II unless they are at special risk, since the presence of maternal antibody may interfere with their ability to respond. They may be given human normal immunoglobulin. However, where immunisation below the age of 12 months is deemed necessary, a second dose of vaccine should be given at 15 months of age and a further dose may still be given at the usual time.

4.4 Special warnings and special precautions for use

As with all vaccines, facilities for the management of anaphylaxis, including epinephrine (adrenaline), should always be available during vaccination.

Hypersensitivity to eggs: There is increasing evidence that M-M-R® II can be given safely to children even if they have previously had an anaphylactic reaction (generalised urticaria, swelling of the mouth and throat, difficulty in breathing, hypotension or shock) following food containing egg. Nevertheless, caution should be observed and if there is concern, paediatric advice should be sought with a view to immunisation under controlled conditions such as admission to hospital as a day case.

M-M-R® II should be given with caution to those with an individual or family history of cerebral injury or any other condition in which stress due to fever should be avoided. The physician should be alert to the rise in temperature that may follow vaccination.

Children and young adults who are known to be infected with, or have a history of immunodeficiency viruses, but without overt clinical manifestations of immunosuppression, may be vaccinated; however, the vaccinees should be closely monitored for exposure to vaccine-preventable diseases because immunisation may be less effective than for uninfected persons. In selected cases, confirmation of circulating antibody levels may be indicated to help guide appropriate protective measures, including immunoprophylaxis if immunity has waned to non-protective levels.

Children who suffered ITP within 6 weeks of the first dose of MMR (or its component vaccines) should have serological status evaluated at the time the second dose was due. If serology testing suggests that a child is not fully immune against measles, mumps and rubella then a second dose of MMR is recommended.

Excretion of small amounts of live attenuated rubella virus from the nose and throat has occurred in the majority of susceptible individuals 7-28 days after vaccination. There is no definite evidence to indicate that such a virus is transmitted to susceptible persons who are in contact with vaccinated individuals. Consequently, transmission, while accepted as a theoretical possibility, has not been regarded as a significant risk. However, transmission of the vaccine virus via breast milk has been documented.

There are no reports of transmission of live attenuated measles or mumps viruses from vaccinees to susceptible contacts.

Children under treatment for tuberculosis have not experienced exacerbation of the disease when immunised with live measles virus vaccine; no studies have been reported to date of the effect of measles virus vaccines on untreated tuberculous children.

Parents of children with a personal or family history of convulsions or idiopathic epilepsy should be advised that such children have a small increased risk of seizures following vaccination and be informed in advance of procedures for their management.

As for any vaccine, vaccination with M-M-R ®II may not result in protection in 100% of vaccinees.

4.5 Interaction with other medicinal products and other forms of Interaction

Vaccination should be deferred for at least three months following blood or plasma transfusions or administration of any human immune serum globulin. If any of these substances has been used near to the time of vaccination with M-M-R® II, a test should subsequently be made to confirm successful seroconversions.

Where anti-Rho (D) globulin (human) and rubella vaccine are required in the immediate post-partum period, rubella vaccine alone and not M-M-R® II should be used.

It has been reported that live attenuated measles, mumps and rubella vaccine may temporarily depress tuberculin skin sensitivity. If a tuberculin test is to be done, it should be administered before or simultaneously with M-M-R® II.

4.6 Pregnancy and lactation

Pregnant females: Pregnant females must NOT be given M-M-R® II. Furthermore, pregnancy should be avoided for three months following vaccination (see 'Contra-indications').

Animal reproduction studies have not been conducted with M-M-R® II. It is also not known whether M-M-R® II can cause foetal harm when given to pregnant women or affect reproductive capacity.

If a woman is inadvertently vaccinated or if she becomes pregnant within three months of vaccination, she should be counselled by her physician. It has been established that:

1) in a ten-year study involving 700 pregnant women who received rubella vaccination within three months of conception, none of their new-born infants had abnormalities compatible with a congenital rubella syndrome;

2) although mumps virus is capable of infecting the placenta and foetus, there is no good evidence that it causes congenital malformations in humans. Mumps vaccine virus has also been shown to affect the placenta, but the virus has not been isolated from foetal tissues taken from susceptible women who were vaccinated and underwent elective abortions; and

3) reports indicate that contracting natural measles during pregnancy increases the rates of spontaneous abortion, stillbirth, congenital defects and prematurity. Although there are no adequate studies on the attenuated (vaccine) strain in pregnancy, it would be prudent to assume that the strain of the virus in the vaccine is also capable of inducing adverse foetal effects.

Breast-feeding mothers: Caution should be exercised when M-M-R® II is given to a breast-feeding mother. Although it is not known whether measles or mumps vaccine virus is secreted in human milk, studies have shown that breast-feeding mothers immunised with live attenuated RA 27/3 strain rubella vaccine transmit the virus via breast milk. In those babies with serological evidence of rubella, none showed clinical disease.

4.7 Effects on ability to drive and use machines

The use of M-M-R®II generally does not interfere with the ability to drive or operate machinery.

4.8 Undesirable effects

Adverse reactions: Adverse reactions associated with M-M-R® II are similar to those to be expected from the administration of monovalent vaccines given separately.

The following adverse reactions occur commonly:

Burning and/or stinging at the injection site for a short period.

The following adverse reactions occur occasionally:

Body as a whole: Fever (+38.3°C (+101°F) or higher).

Skin: Rash, usually minimal but may be generalised.

Generally, fever, rash or both, appear between the 5th and the 12th days.

Mild, local reactions such as erythema; induration and tenderness.

The following adverse reactions occur rarely:

Body as a whole: Sore throat, malaise, atypical measles, syncope, irritability

Digestive: Parotitis, nausea, vomiting, diarrhoea.

Haematologic/lymphatic: Regional lymphadenopathy, thrombocytopenia, purpura.

Hypersensitivity: Allergic reactions such as wheal and flare at injection site, anaphylaxis and anaphylactoid reactions, as well as related phenomena such as angioneurotic oedema (including peripheral or facial oedema) and brochial spasm, urticaria in individuals with or without an allergic history.

Musculoskeletal: Arthralgia and/or arthritis (usually transient and rarely chronic), myalgia.

Nervous/Psychiatric: Febrile convulsions in children, afebrile convulsion or seizures, headache, dizziness, paraesthesia, polyneuritis, polyneuropathy, Guillain-Barré syndrome, ataxia, measles inclusion body encephalitis (MIBE) (see 4.3) Encephalitis/encephalopathy have been reported approximately once for every 3 million doses. In no cases has it been shown that reactions were actually caused by vaccine. The risk of such serious neurological disorders following live measles virus vaccine administered remains far less than that for encephalitis and encephalopathy with natural measles (1 per 2000 reported cases).

Respiratory System: Pneumonitis (see 4.3) cough, rhinitis

Skin: Erythema multiforme, Stevens-Johnson syndrome, vesiculation at injection site, swelling

Special senses: Forms of optic neuritis, including retrobulbar neuritis, papillitis, and retinitis; ocular palsies, otitis media, nerve deafness, conjunctivitis.

Urogenital: Orchitis.

There have been reports of subacute sclerosing panencephalitis (SSPE) in children who did not have a history of natural measles but did receive measles vaccine. Some of these cases may have resulted from unrecognised measles in the first year of life or possibly from the measles vaccination. Based on the estimated nationwide measles vaccine distribution in the USA, the association of SSPE cases to measles vaccination is about one case per million vaccine doses distributed. This is far less than the association with natural measles: 6-22 cases of SSPE per million cases of measles.

A study suggests that the overall effect of measles vaccine has been to protect against SSPE by preventing measles with its inherent higher risk of SSPE.

Local reactions characterised by marked swelling, redness and vesiculation at the injection site of attenuated live measles virus vaccines and systemic reations including atypical measles have occurred in vaccinees who had previously received killed measles vaccine. Rarely, there have been reports of more severe reactions, including prolonged high fevers and extensive local reactions requiring hospitalisation. Panniculitis has also been reported rarely following vaccination with measles vaccine.

Arthralgia or arthritis, or both, are usually transient and rarely chronic features of natural rubella. Like polyneuritis that is also a feature of natural infection, their frequency and severity vary with age and sex, being greatest in adult females and least in prepubertal children.

The chronic arthritis associated with natural rubella has been related to virus and/or viral antigen found in body tissues. Only rarely have vaccinees developed chronic joint symptoms.

Following vaccination in children, reactions in joints are uncommon and generally of brief duration. In women, incidence rates for arthritis and arthralgia are generally higher than those seen in children (children; 0-3%; women: 12-20%) and the reactions tend to be more marked and of longer duration. Symptoms may persist for a matter of months or, on rare occasions, for years. In adolescent girls, the reactions appear to be intermediate in incidence between those seen in children and in adult women. Even in older women (35-45 years) these reactions are generally well tolerated and rarely interfere with normal activities. Such reactions occur much less frequently after revaccination than primary vaccination.

4.9 Overdose

Poisoning is unlikely. Swallowing M-M-R® II would render the live attenuated vaccine benign, and the content of the neomycin (25 micrograms/0.5 millilitre) is not likely to cause toxicity. Overdose has been reported rarely and was not associated with any serious adverse events.

5. PHARMACOLOGICAL PROPERTIES

5.1 Pharmacodynamic properties

M-M-R® II vaccine is a mixture of live attenuated measles, mumps and rubella viruses to provide active immunisation against these diseases.

Clinical studies in 279 triple seronegative children aged 11 months to 7 years, showed that M-M-R® II is highly immunogenic and generally well-tolerated. In these studies, a single injection of the vaccine induced measles haemagglutination-inhibition (HI) antibodies in 95%, mumps neutralising antibodies in 96%, and rubella HI antibodies in 99% of susceptible persons.

Based on available evidence a second dose of measles, mumps and rubella vaccine in the national immunisation schedule has the potential to prevent epidemics of measles and overall is as well-tolerated as primary immunisation.

Vaccine induced antibody levels following administration of M-M-R® II have been shown to persist for over 11 years.

5.2 Pharmacokinetic properties

Not applicable.

5.3 Preclinical safety data

No further information available.

6. PHARMACEUTICAL PARTICULARS

6.1 List of excipients

Human Albumin Solution (which contains sodium caprylate and sodium N-acetyltryptophanate)

Sodium Phosphate, Monobasic

Sodium Phosphate, Dibasic

Sodium Hydrogen Carbonate

Medium 199*

Minimum Essential Medium, Eagle**

Neomycin Sulphate

Phenol Red

Sorbitol

Potassium Phosphate, Monobasic

Potassium Phosphate, Dibasic

Gelatin (Porcine) Hydrolyzed

Sucrose

Monosodium L-Glutamate

*Medium 199 is a complex mixture of amino acids (including phenylalanine), mineral salts, vitamins and other components (including glucose).

**a mixture of amino acids, mineral salts, vitamins and other components.

Diluent

Sterile Water.

6.2 Incompatibilities

None known.

6.3 Shelf life
18 months.

6.4 Special precautions for storage
Store between +2°C and +8°C. Protect from light.

6.5 Nature and contents of container
Lyophilised Vaccine:

3 millilitres type 1 glass tubing vials with 13 millimetres (West Co gray butyl 1816) lyophilisation stoppers and 13 millimetres 1 piece flip-off aluminium seal with plastic cap.

Diluent:

3 millilitres type I glass tubing vials with a West Co. 1082 chlorobutyl rubber stopper sealed with a roll-on aluminium collar with a grey plastic 'flip-off' top.

1 millilitre type 1 borosillicate glass pre-filled syringe with cholorobutyl rubber stopper and tip cap.

6.6 Instructions for use and handling
To reconstitute the vaccine, all the diluent provided should be injected into a vial of lyophilised vaccine, and this agitated to ensure thorough mixing. All the reconstituted vaccine is then drawn into the syringe and injected subcutaneously or intramuscularly.

Only the diluent supplied should be used for reconstitution, since it is free of preservatives and other antiviral substances that may inactivate the vaccine

A separate sterile disposable needle and syringe should be used for each vaccinee.

It is good practice to record title, dose and batch number of all vaccines and dates of administration.

When reconstituted, the vaccine is yellow. It is acceptable for use only when clear and free from particulate matter.

The vaccine should be used immediately after reconstitution. Protect from light at all times, since exposure may inactivate the virus.

7. MARKETING AUTHORISATION HOLDER
Sanofi Pasteur MSD Limited

Mallards Reach

Bridge Avenue

Maidenhead

Berkshire

SL6 1QP

8. MARKETING AUTHORISATION NUMBER(S)
PL 6745/0076 (lyophilised vaccine)

PL 6745/0078 (diluent)

9. DATE OF FIRST AUTHORISATION/RENEWAL OF THE AUTHORISATION
01 March 1995

10. DATE OF REVISION OF THE TEXT
April 2005

Mobic 7.5mg Suppositories

(Boehringer Ingelheim Limited)

1. NAME OF THE MEDICINAL PRODUCT
MOBIC 7.5 mg suppositories.

2. QUALITATIVE AND QUANTITATIVE COMPOSITION
Meloxicam 7.50 mg

For excipients see 6.1.

3. PHARMACEUTICAL FORM
Suppository.

Yellowish-green suppositories

4. CLINICAL PARTICULARS

4.1 Therapeutic indications
- Short term symptomatic treatment of exacerbations of osteoarthrosis.

- Long term symptomatic treatment of rheumatoid arthritis.

4.2 Posology and method of administration
Rectal use: exacerbations of osteoarthrosis: 7.5 mg/day, (one 7.5 mg suppository). If necessary, in the absence of improvement, the dose may be increased to 15 mg/day, (one 15 mg suppository).

Rheumatoid arthritis: 15 mg a day, (one 15 mg suppository). (See also 'special populations'). According to the therapeutic response, the dose may be reduced to 7.5 mg/day (one 7.5 mg suppository).

DO NOT EXCEED THE DOSE OF 15 MG/DAY.

Rectal administration should be used for the shortest time possible, in view of the risk of local toxicity added to the risks of oral administration.

Special populations

Elderly patients and patients with increased risks for adverse reaction (see section 5.): The recommended dose for long term treatment of rheumatoid arthritis in elderly patients is 7.5 mg per day. Patients with increased risks for adverse reactions should start treatment with 7.5 mg per day (see section 4.4).

Renal impairment (see section 5.2): In dialysis patients with severe renal failure, the dose should not exceed 7.5 mg per day. No dose reduction is required in patients with mild to moderate renal impairment (i.e. patients with a creatinine clearance of greater than 25 ml/min). (For patients with non-dialysed severe renal failure, see section 4.3).

Hepatic impairment (see section 5.2): No dose reduction is required in patients with mild to moderate hepatic impairment (For patients with severely impaired liver function, see section 4.3).

Children: Mobic should not be used in children aged under 15. This medicinal product exists in other dosages, which may be more appropriate.

4.3 Contraindications
This medicinal product is contra-indicated in the following situations:

- pregnancy and lactation (See section 4.6 Pregnancy and lactation)

- hypersensitivity to meloxicam or to one of the excipients or hypersensitivity to substances with a similar action, e.g. NSAIDs, aspirin. Mobic should not be given to patients who have developed signs of asthma, nasal polyps, angioneurotic oedema or urticaria following the administration of aspirin or other NSAIDs.

- active gastro-intestinal ulcer or history of recurrent gastro-intestinal ulcer;

- severely impaired liver function;

- non-dialysed severe renal failure;

- past history of proctitis or rectal bleeding;

- gastrointestinal bleeding, cerebrovascular bleeding or other bleeding disorders;

- severe uncontrolled heart failure.

4.4 Special warnings and special precautions for use
- Any history of oesophagitis, gastritis and/or peptic ulcer must be sought in order to ensure their total cure before starting treatment with meloxicam. Attention should routinely be paid to the possible onset of a recurrence in patients treated with meloxicam and with a past history of this type.

- Patients with gastrointestinal symptoms or history of gastrointestinal disease (i.e ulcerative colitis, Crohn's disease) should be monitored for digestive disturbances, especially for gastrointestinal bleeding.

- As with other NSAIDs, gastrointestinal bleeding or ulceration/perforation, in rare cases fatal, have been reported with meloxicam at any time during treatment, with or without warning symptoms or a previous history of serious gastrointestinal events. Gastrointestinal bleeding or ulceration/perforation have in general more serious consequences in the elderly (see section 4.8).

- If gastrointestinal bleeding or ulceration occurs in patients receiving meloxicam, the drug should be withdrawn.

- The possible occurrence of severe skin reactions and serious life threatening hypersensitivity reactions (i.e. anaphylactic reactions) is known to occur with NSAIDs including oxicams. In those cases, meloxicam should be withdrawn immediately and careful observation is necessary.

- In rare instances NSAIDs may be the cause of interstitial nephritis, glomerulonephritis, renal medullary necrosis or nephrotic syndrome.

- As with most NSAIDs, occasional increases in serum transaminase levels, increases in serum bilirubin or other liver function parameters, as well as increases in serum creatinine and blood urea nitrogen as well as other laboratory disturbances, have been reported. The majority of these instances involved transitory and slight abnormalities. Should any such abnormality prove significant or persistent, the administration of meloxicam should be stopped and appropriate investigations undertaken.

- Induction of sodium, potassium and water retention and interference with the natriuretic effects of diuretics and consequently possible exacerbations of the condition of patients with cardiac failure or hypertension may occur with NSAIDs (see sections 4.2 and 4.3).

- NSAIDs inhibit the synthesis of renal prostaglandins involved in the maintenance of renal perfusion, in patients with decreased renal blood flow and blood volume. Administration of NSAIDs in such situations may result in the decompensation of latent renal failure. However, renal function returns to its initial status when treatment is withdrawn. This risk concerns all elderly individuals, patients with congestive cardiac failure, cirrhosis, nephrotic syndrome or renal failure as well as patients on diuretics or having undergone major surgery leading to hypovolemia. Careful monitoring of diuresis and renal function during treatment is necessary in such patients (see sections 4.2 and 4.3).

- Adverse reactions are often less well tolerated in elderly, fragile or weakened individuals, who therefore require careful monitoring. As with other NSAIDs, particular caution is required in the elderly, in whom renal, hepatic and cardiac functions are frequently impaired.

- The recommended maximum daily dose should not be exceeded in case of insufficient therapeutic effect, nor should an additional NSAID be added to the therapy because this may increase the toxicity while therapeutic advantage has not been proven. In the absence of improvement after several days, the clinical benefit of the treatment should be reassessed.

- Meloxicam, as any other NSAID may mask symptoms of an underlying infectious disease.

- The use of meloxicam, as with any drug known to inhibit cyclooxygenase / prostaglandin synthesis, may impair fertility and is not recommended in women attempting to conceive. In women who have difficulties conceiving, or who are undergoing investigation of infertility, withdrawal of meloxicam should be considered.

4.5 Interaction with other medicinal products and other forms of Interaction

Pharmacodynamic Interactions:

Other NSAIDs, including salicylates (acetylsalicylic acid ⩾ 3 g/d): Administration of several NSAIDs together may increase the risk of gastrointestinal ulcers and bleeding, via a synergistic effect. The concomitant use of meloxicam with other NSAIDs is not recommended (see section 4.4).

Diuretics: Treatment with NSAIDs is associated with potential for acute renal failure, notably in dehydrated patients. Patients receiving meloxicam and diuretics should be adequately hydrated and be monitored for renal function prior to initiating treatment (see section 4.4).

Oral anticoagulants: Increased risk of bleeding, via inhibition of platelet function and damage to the gastroduodenal mucosa. The concomitant use of NSAIDs and oral anticoagulants is not recommended (see section 4.4).

Careful monitoring of the INR is required if it proves impossible to avoid such combination.

Thrombolytics and antiplatelet drugs: Increased risk of bleeding, via inhibition of platelet function and damage to the gastroduodenal mucosa.

ACE inhibitors and angiotensin II receptor antagonists: NSAIDs (including acetylsalicylic acid at doses ⩾ 3g/d) and angiotensin-II receptor antagonists exert a synergistic effect on the decrease of glomerular filtration, which may be exacerbated when renal function is altered. When given to the elderly and/or dehydrated patients, this combination can lead to acute renal failure by acting directly on glomerular filtration. Monitoring of renal function at the beginning of the treatment is recommended as well as regular hydration of the patient. Additionally, concomitant treatment can reduce antihypertensive effect of ACE inhibitors and angiotensin II receptor antagonists, leading to partial loss of efficacy (due to inhibition of prostaglandins with vasodilatory effect).

Other antihypertensive drugs (e.g. Beta-blockers): As for the latter, a decrease of the antihypertensive effect of beta-blockers (due to inhibition of prostaglandins with vasodilatory effect) can occur.

Cyclosporin: Nephrotoxicity of cyclosporin may be enhanced by NSAIDs via renal prostaglandin mediated effects. During combined treatment renal function is to be measured. A careful monitoring of the renal function is recommended, especially in the elderly.

Intrauterine devices: NSAIDs have been reported to decrease the efficacy of intrauterine devices. A decrease of the efficacy of intrauterine devices by NSAIDs has been previously reported but needs further confirmation.

Pharmacokinetic Interactions (Effect of meloxicam on the pharmacokinetics of other drugs)

Lithium: NSAIDs have been reported to increase blood lithium levels (via decreased renal excretion of lithium), which may reach toxic values. The concomitant use of lithium and NSAIDs is not recommended (see section 4.4). If this combination appears necessary, lithium plasma concentrations should be monitored carefully during the initiation, adjustment and withdrawal of meloxicam treatment.

Methotrexate: NSAIDs can reduce the tubular secretion of methotrexate thereby increasing the plasma concentrations of methotrexate. For this reason, for patients on high dosages of methotrexate (more than 15 mg/week) the concomitant use of NSAIDs is not recommended (see section 4.4).

The risk of an interaction between NSAID preparations and methotrexate, should be considered also in patients on low dosage of methotrexate, especially in patients with impaired renal function. In case combination treatment is necessary blood cell count and the renal function should be monitored. Caution should be taken in case both NSAID and methotrexate are given within 3 days, in which case the plasma level of methotrexate may increase and cause increased toxicity.

Although the pharmacokinetics of methotrexate (15mg/week) were not relevantly affected by concomitant meloxicam treatment, it should be considered that the haematological toxicity of methotrexate can be amplified by treatment with NSAID drugs (see above). (See section 4.8).

Pharmacokinetic Interactions (Effect of other drugs on the pharmacokinetics of meloxicam)

Cholestyramine: Cholestyramine accelerates the elimination of meloxicam by interrupting the enterohepatic circulation so that clearance for meloxicam increases by 50% and the half-life decreases to 13±3 hrs. This interaction is of clinical significance.

No clinically relevant pharmacokinetic drug-drug interactions were detected with respect to the concomitant administration of antacids, cimetidine and digoxin.

4.6 Pregnancy and lactation

Pregnancy

– In animals, lethal effects on the embryo have been reported at doses higher than those used clinically.

– It is advisable to avoid the administration of meloxicam during the first two trimesters of pregnancy.

– During the final three months, all prostaglandin synthesis inhibitors may expose the fetus to cardiopulmonary (pulmonary hypertension with premature closure of the ductus arteriosus) and renal toxicity or inhibit the contraction of the uterus. This effect on the uterus has been associated with an increase in the incidence of dystocia and delayed parturition in animals. Thus all NSAIDs are absolutely contra-indicated during the final three months.

Lactation

NSAIDs pass into mothers milk. Administration should therefore be avoided, as a precautionary measure, in women who are breast feeding.

4.7 Effects on ability to drive and use machines

There are no specific studies on the ability to drive and use machinery. However, on the basis of the pharmacodynamic profile and reported adverse drug reactions, meloxicam is likely to have no or negligible influence on these abilities. However, when visual disturbances or drowsiness, vertigo or other central nervous system disturbances occur, it is advisable to refrain from driving and operating machinery.

4.8 Undesirable effects

a) General Description

The following adverse events, which may be causally related to the administration of meloxicam, have been reported. The frequencies given below are based on corresponding occurrences in clinical trials, regardless of any causal relationship. The information is based on clinical trials involving 3750 patients who have been treated with daily oral doses of 7.5 or 15 mg meloxicam tablets or capsules over a period of up to 18 months (mean duration of treatment 127 days).

Adverse events which may be causally related to the administration of meloxicam that have come to light as a result of reports received in relation to administration of the marketed product are included.

Adverse reactions have been ranked under headings of frequency using the following convention:

Very common ($\geq$ 1/10); common ($\geq$ 1/100, < 1/10); uncommon ($\geq$ 1/1000, < 1/100); rare ($\geq$ 1/10000, < 1/1000); very rare (< 1/10000)

b) Table of adverse reactions

Blood and the lymphatic system disorders

Common: Anaemia

Uncommon: Disturbances of blood count: leucocytopenia; thrombocytopenia; agranulocytosis (see section c)

Immune system disorders

Rare: Anaphylactic/anaphylactoid reactions

Psychiatric disorders

Rare: Mood disorders, insomnia and nightmares

Nervous system disorders

Common: Lightheadedness, headache

Uncommon: Vertigo, tinnitus, drowsiness

Rare: Confusion

Eye disorders

Rare: Visual disturbances including blurred vision

Cardiac disorders

Uncommon: Palpitations

Vascular disorders

Uncommon: Increase in blood pressure (see section 4.4), flushes

Respiratory, thoracic and mediastinal disorders

Rare: Onset of asthma attacks in certain individuals allergic to aspirin or other NSAIDs

Gastrointestinal disorders

Common: Dyspepsia, nausea and vomiting symptoms, abdominal pain, constipation, flatulence, diarrhoea

Uncommon: Gastrointestinal bleeding, peptic ulcers, oesophagitis, stomatitis

Rare: Gastrointestinal perforation, gastritis, colitis

The peptic ulcers, perforation or gastrointestinal bleeding, that may occur can be sometimes severe, especially in elderly (see section 4.4).

Hepato-biliary disorders

Uncommon: Transitory disturbance of liver function test (e.g. raised transaminases or bilirubin)

Rare: Hepatitis

Skin and subcutaneous tissue disorders

Common: Pruritus, rash

Uncommon: Urticaria

Rare: Stevens-Johnson Syndrome and toxic epidermal necrolysis, angioedema, bullous reactions such as erythema multiforme, photosensitivity reactions

Renal and urinary disorders

Uncommon: Disturbances of laboratory tests investigating renal function (e.g. raised creatinine or urea)

Rare: Renal failure (see section 4.4)

General disorders and administration site conditions

Common: Oedema including oedema of the lower limbs

c) Information Characterising Individual Serious and/or Frequently Occurring Adverse Reactions

Isolated cases of agranulocytosis have been reported in patients treated with meloxicam and other potentially myelotoxic drugs (see section 4.5).

Adverse effects related to route of administration: risk of local toxicity all the more frequent and severe when treatment is for a long period and the number of daily doses and dosage are high (see 4.2 and 4.4).

4.9 Overdose

Symptoms following acute NSAID overdose are usually limited to lethargy, drowsiness, nausea, vomiting and epigastric pain, which are generally reversible with supportive care. Gastrointestinal bleeding can occur. Severe poisoning may result in hypertension, acute renal failure, hepatic dysfunction, respiratory depression, coma, convulsions, cardiovascular collapse and cardiac arrest. Anaphylactoid reactions have been reported with therapeutic ingestion of NSAIDs and may occur following an overdose.

Patients should be managed with symptomatic and supportive care following an NSAID overdose. Accelerated removal of meloxicam by 4 g oral doses of cholestyramine given three times a day was demonstrated in a clinical trial.

5. PHARMACOLOGICAL PROPERTIES

5.1 Pharmacodynamic properties

Pharmacotherapeutic group: Non Steroidal Anti-Inflammatory agent, Oxicams. ATC Code: M01AC06.

Meloxicam is a non-steroidal anti-inflammatory drug (NSAID) of the oxicam family, with anti-inflammatory, analgesic and antipyretic properties.

The anti-inflammatory activity of meloxicam has been proven in classical models of inflammation. As with other NSAIDs, its precise mechanism of action remains unknown. However, there is at least one common mode of action shared by all NSAIDs (including meloxicam): inhibition of the biosynthesis of prostaglandins, known inflammation mediators.

5.2 Pharmacokinetic properties

Absorption

Suppositories were shown to be bioequivalent to capsules. Maximum plasma concentrations at steady state following administration of the suppositories are achieved at about five hours postdose. The peak-trough fluctuations are similar to those observed with oral dosage forms.

Distribution

Meloxicam is very strongly bound to plasma proteins, essentially albumin (99%). Meloxicam penetrates into synovial fluid to give concentrations approximately half of those in plasma.

Volume of distribution is low, on average 11 L. Interindividual variation is the order of 30-40%.

Biotransformation

Meloxicam undergoes extensive hepatic biotransformation. Four different metabolites of meloxicam were identified in urine, which are all pharmacodynamically inactive. The major metabolite, 5'-carboxymeloxicam (60% of dose), is formed by oxidation of an intermediate metabolite 5'- hydroxymethylmeloxicam, which is also excreted to a lesser extent (9% of dose). In vitro studies suggest that CYP 2C9 plays an important role in this metabolic pathway, with a minor contribution from the CYP 3A4 isoenzyme. The patient's peroxidase activity is probably responsible for the other two metabolites, which account for 16% and 4% of the administered dose respectively.

Elimination

Meloxicam is excreted predominantly in the form of metabolites and occurs to equal extents in urine and faeces. Less than 5% of the daily dose is excreted unchanged in faeces, while only traces of the parent compound are excreted in urine.

The mean elimination half-life is about 20 hours. Total plasma clearance amounts on average 8 mL/min.

Linearity/non-linearity

Meloxicam demonstrates linear pharmacokinetics in the therapeutic dose range of 7.5 mg 15 mg following per oral or intramuscular administration.

Special populations

Hepatic/renal Insufficiency: Neither hepatic, mild nor moderate renal insufficiency have a substantial effect on meloxicam pharmacokinetics. In terminal renal failure, the increase in the volume of distribution may result in higher free meloxicam concentrations, and a daily dose of 7.5 mg must not be exceeded (see section 4.2).

Elderly: Mean plasma clearance at steady state in elderly subjects was slightly lower than that reported for younger subjects.

5.3 Preclinical safety data

The toxicological profile of meloxicam has been found in preclinical studies to be identical to that of NSAIDs: gastrointestinal ulcers and erosions, renal papillary necrosis at high doses during chronic administration in two animal species.

Oral reproductive studies in the rat have shown a decrease of ovulations and inhibition of implantations and embryotoxic effects (increase of resorptions) at maternotoxic dose levels at 1mg/kg and higher.

The affected dose levels exceeded the clinical dose (7.5-15 mg) by a factor of 10 to 5-fold on a mg/kg dose basis (75 kg person). Fetotoxic effects at the end of gestation, shared by all prostaglandin synthesis inhibitors, have been described. No evidence has been found of any mutagenic effect, either in vitro or in vivo. No carcinogenic risk has been found in the rat and mouse at doses far higher than those used clinically.

6. PHARMACEUTICAL PARTICULARS

6.1 List of excipients

Hard fat (type Suppocire BP)

Macrogolglycerolhydroxystearate 40

6.2 Incompatibilities

Not applicable

6.3 Shelf life

3 years

6.4 Special precautions for storage

Should be stored at a temperature not exceeding 30°C.

6.5 Nature and contents of container

Aluminium blister, boxes of 6, 7, 10, 12, 20, 30, 50, 60, 120, or 500 (10 × 50) suppositories.

Not all pack sizes may be marketed.

6.6 Instructions for use and handling

No special requirements

7. MARKETING AUTHORISATION HOLDER

Boehringer Ingelheim International GmbH

D-55216 Ingelheim am Rhein

Germany

8. MARKETING AUTHORISATION NUMBER(S)

PL 14598/0007

9. DATE OF FIRST AUTHORISATION/RENEWAL OF THE AUTHORISATION

31 July 1997

10. DATE OF REVISION OF THE TEXT

August 2003

11. Legal Category

POM

M2b7.5/UK/SPC 12

Mobic 7.5mg Tablets

(Boehringer Ingelheim Limited)

1. NAME OF THE MEDICINAL PRODUCT

MOBIC 7.5 mg tablets.

2. QUALITATIVE AND QUANTITATIVE COMPOSITION

Meloxicam 7.50 mg

For excipients see 6.1.

3. PHARMACEUTICAL FORM

Tablet

Light yellow round tablet with the logotype of the company on one side and a score with 59D/59D on the other side

4. CLINICAL PARTICULARS

4.1 Therapeutic indications

- Short-term symptomatic treatment of exacerbations of osteoarthrosis.

- Long term symptomatic treatment of rheumatoid arthritis or ankylosing spondylitis.

4.2 Posology and method of administration

Oral use

- Exacerbations of osteoarthrosis: 7.5 mg/day (one 7.5 mg tablet). If necessary, in the absence of improvement, the dose may be increased to 15 mg/day (two 7.5 mg tablets).

- Rheumatoid arthritis, ankylosing spondylitis: 15 mg/day (two 7.5 mg tablets).

(See also 'special populations')

According to the therapeutic response, the dose may be reduced to 7.5 mg/day (one 7.5 mg tablet).

DO NOT EXCEED THE DOSE OF 15 MG/DAY.

The total daily amount should be taken as a single dose, with water or another liquid, during a meal.

Special populations

Elderly patients and patients with increased risks for adverse reaction (see section 5.2):

The recommended dose for long term treatment of rheumatoid arthritis and ankylosing spondylitis in elderly patients is 7.5 mg per day. Patients with increased risks for adverse reactions should start treatment with 7.5 mg per day (see section 4.4).

Renal impairment (see section 5.2):

In dialysis patients with severe renal failure, the dose should not exceed 7.5 mg per day.

No dose reduction is required in patients with mild to moderate renal impairment (i.e. patients with a creatinine clearance of greater than 25 ml/min). (For patients with non-dialysed severe renal failure, see section 4.3).

Hepatic impairment (see section 5.2):

No dose reduction is required in patients with mild to moderate hepatic impairment (For patients with severely impaired liver function, see section 4.3).

Children:

Mobic should not be used in children aged under 15.

This medicinal product exists in other dosages, which may be more appropriate.

4.3 Contraindications

This medicinal product is contra-indicated in the following situations:

- pregnancy and lactation (See section 4.6 Pregnancy and lactation)

- hypersensitivity to meloxicam or to one of the excipients or hypersensitivity to substances with a similar action, e.g. NSAIDs, aspirin. Mobic should not be given to patients who have developed signs of asthma, nasal polyps, angioneurotic oedema or urticaria following the administration of aspirin or other NSAIDs.

- active gastro-intestinal ulcer or history of recurrent gastro-intestinal ulcer;

- severely impaired liver function;

- non-dialysed severe renal failure;

- gastrointestinal bleeding, cerebrovascular bleeding or other bleeding disorders;

- severe uncontrolled heart failure.

4.4 Special warnings and special precautions for use

- Any history of oesophagitis, gastritis and/or peptic ulcer must be sought in order to ensure their total cure before starting treatment with meloxicam. Attention should routinely be paid to the possible onset of a recurrence in patients treated with meloxicam and with a past history of this type.

- Patients with gastrointestinal symptoms or history of gastrointestinal disease (i.e. ulcerative colitis, Crohn's disease) should be monitored for digestive disturbances, especially for gastrointestinal bleeding.

- As with other NSAIDs, gastrointestinal bleeding or ulceration/perforation, in rare cases fatal, have been reported with meloxicam at any time during treatment, with or without warning symptoms or a previous history of serious gastrointestinal events. Gastrointestinal bleeding or ulceration/perforation have in general more serious consequences in the elderly (see section 4.8).

- If gastrointestinal bleeding or ulceration occurs in patients receiving Meloxicam, the drug should be withdrawn.

- The possible occurrence of severe skin reactions and serious life threatening hypersensitivity reactions (i.e. anaphylactic reactions) is known to occur with NSAIDs including oxicams. In those cases, Meloxicam should be withdrawn immediately and careful observation is necessary.

- In rare instances NSAIDs may be the cause of interstitial nephritis, glomerulonephritis, renal medullary necrosis or nephrotic syndrome.

- As with most NSAIDs, occasional increases in serum transaminase levels, increases in serum bilirubin or other liver function parameters, as well as increases in serum creatinine and blood urea nitrogen as well as other laboratory disturbances, have been reported. The majority of these instances involved transitory and slight abnormalities. Should any such abnormality prove significant or persistent, the administration of Meloxicam should be stopped and appropriate investigations undertaken.

- Induction of sodium, potassium and water retention and interference with the natriuretic effects of diuretics and consequently possible exacerbations of the condition of patients with cardiac failure or hypertension may occur with NSAIDs (see sections 4.2 and 4.3).

- NSAIDs inhibit the synthesis of renal prostaglandins involved in the maintenance of renal perfusion, in patients with decreased renal blood flow and blood volume. Administration of NSAIDs in such situations may result in the decompensation of latent renal failure. However, renal function returns to its initial status when treatment is withdrawn. This risk concerns all elderly individuals, patients with congestive cardiac failure, cirrhosis, nephrotic syndrome or renal failure as well as patients on diuretics or having undergone major surgery leading to hypovolemia. Careful monitoring of diuresis and renal function during treatment is necessary in such patients (see sections 4.2 and 4.3).

- Adverse reactions are often less well tolerated in elderly, fragile or weakened individuals, who therefore require careful monitoring. As with other NSAIDs, particular caution is required in the elderly, in whom renal, hepatic and cardiac functions are frequently impaired.

- The recommended maximum daily dose should not be exceeded in case of insufficient therapeutic effect, nor should an additional NSAID be added to the therapy because this may increase the toxicity while therapeutic advantage has not been proven. In the absence of improvement after several days, the clinical benefit of the treatment should be reassessed.

- Meloxicam, as any other NSAID, may mask symptoms of an underlying infectious disease.

- The use of Meloxicam, as with any drug known to inhibit cyclooxygenase/prostaglandin synthesis, may impair fertility and is not recommended in women attempting to conceive. In women who have difficulties conceiving, or who are undergoing investigation of infertility, withdrawal of Meloxicam should be considered.

4.5 Interaction with other medicinal products and other forms of Interaction

Pharmacodynamic Interactions:

Other NSAIDs, including salicylates (acetylsalicylic acid ⩾ 3 g/d):

Administration of several NSAIDs together may increase the risk of gastrointestinal ulcers and bleeding, via a synergistic effect. The concomitant use of meloxicam with other NSAIDs is not recommended (see section 4.4).

Diuretics:

Treatment with NSAIDs is associated with potential for acute renal failure, notably in dehydrated patients. Patients receiving meloxicam and diuretics should be adequately hydrated and be monitored for renal function prior to initiating treatment (see section 4.4).

Oral anticoagulants:

Increased risk of bleeding, via inhibition of platelet function and damage to the gastroduodenal mucosa. The concomitant use of NSAIDs and oral anticoagulants is not recommended (see section 4.4).

Careful monitoring of the INR is required if it proves impossible to avoid such combination.

Thrombolytics and antiplatelet drugs:

Increased risk of bleeding, via inhibition of platelet function and damage to the gastroduodenal mucosa.

ACE inhibitors and angiotensin II receptor antagonists:

NSAIDs (including acetylsalicylic acid at doses ≥ 3g/d) and angiotensin-II receptor antagonists exert a synergistic effect on the decrease of glomerular filtration, which may be exacerbated when renal function is altered. When given to the elderly and/or dehydrated patients, this combination can lead to acute renal failure by acting directly on glomerular filtration. Monitoring of renal function at the beginning of the treatment is recommended as well as regular hydration of the patient. Additionally, concomitant treatment can reduce antihypertensive effect of ACE inhibitors and angiotensin II receptor antagonists, leading to partial loss of efficacy (due to inhibition of prostaglandins with vasodilatory effect).

Other antihypertensive drugs (e.g. Beta-blockers):

As for the latter, a decrease of the antihypertensive effect of beta-blockers (due to inhibition of prostaglandins with vasodilatory effect) can occur.

Cyclosporin:

Nephrotoxicity of cyclosporin may be enhanced by NSAIDs via renal prostaglandin mediated effects. During combined treatment renal function is to be measured. A careful monitoring of the renal function is recommended, especially in the elderly.

Intrauterine devices:

NSAIDs have been reported to decrease the efficacy of intrauterine devices.

A decrease of the efficacy of intrauterine devices by NSAIDs has been previously reported but needs further confirmation.

Pharmacokinetic Interactions (Effect of meloxicam on the pharmacokinetics of other drugs)

Lithium:

NSAIDs have been reported to increase blood lithium levels (via decreased renal excretion of lithium), which may reach toxic values. The concomitant use of lithium and NSAIDs is not recommended (see section 4.4). If this combination appears necessary, lithium plasma concentrations should be monitored carefully during the initiation, adjustment and withdrawal of meloxicam treatment.

Methotrexate:

NSAIDs can reduce the tubular secretion of methotrexate thereby increasing the plasma concentrations of methotrexate. For this reason, for patients on high dosages of methotrexate (more than 15 mg/week) the concomitant use of NSAIDs is not recommended (see section 4.4).

The risk of an interaction between NSAID preparations and methotrexate, should be considered also in patients on low dosage of methotrexate, especially in patients with impaired renal function. In case combination treatment is necessary blood cell count and the renal function should be monitored. Caution should be taken in case both NSAID and methotrexate are given within 3 days, in which case the plasma level of methotrexate may increase and cause increased toxicity.

Although the pharmacokinetics of methotrexate (15mg/week) were not relevantly affected by concomitant meloxicam treatment, it should be considered that the haematological toxicity of methotrexate can be amplified by treatment with NSAID drugs (see above). (See section 4.8).

Pharmacokinetic Interactions (Effect of other drugs on the pharmacokinetics of meloxicam)

Cholestyramine:

Cholestyramine accelerates the elimination of meloxicam by interrupting the enterohepatic circulation so that clearance for meloxicam increases by 50% and the half-life decreases to 13±3 hrs. This interaction is of clinical significance.

No clinically relevant pharmacokinetic drug-drug interactions were detected with respect to the concomitant administration of antacids, cimetidine and digoxin.

4.6 Pregnancy and lactation

-Pregnancy

- In animals, lethal effects on the embryo have been reported at doses higher than those used clinically.

- It is advisable to avoid the administration of meloxicam during the first two trimesters of pregnancy.

- During the final three months, all prostaglandin synthesis inhibitors may expose the fetus to cardiopulmonary (pulmonary hypertension with premature closure of the ductus arteriosus) and renal toxicity or inhibit the contraction of the uterus. This effect on the uterus has been associated with an increase in the incidence of dystocia and delayed parturition in animals. Thus all NSAIDs are absolutely contra-indicated during the final three months.

Lactation

NSAIDs pass into mothers milk. Administration should therefore be avoided, as a precautionary measure, in women who are breast feeding.

4.7 Effects on ability to drive and use machines

There are no specific studies on the ability to drive and use machinery. However, on the basis of the pharmacodynamic profile and reported adverse drug reactions, meloxicam is likely to have no or negligible influence on these abilities. However, when visual disturbances or drowsiness, vertigo or other central nervous system disturbances occur, it is advisable to refrain from driving and operating machinery.

4.8 Undesirable effects

a) General Description

The following adverse events, which may be causally related to the administration of meloxicam, have been reported. The frequencies given below are based on corresponding occurrences in clinical trials, regardless of any causal relationship. The information is based on clinical trials involving 3750 patients who have been treated with daily oral doses of 7.5 or 15 mg meloxicam tablets or capsules over a period of up to 18 months (mean duration of treatment 127 days).

Adverse events which may be causally related to the administration of meloxicam that have come to light as a result of reports received in relation to administration of the marketed product are included.

Adverse reactions have been ranked under headings of frequency using the following convention:

Very common (≥ 1/10); common (≥ 1/100, < 1/10); uncommon (≥ 1/1000, < 1/100); rare (≥ 1/10000, < 1/1000); very rare (< 1/10000)

b) Table of adverse reactions

Blood and the lymphatic system disorders

Common: Anaemia

Uncommon: Disturbances of blood count: leucocytopenia; thrombocytopenia; agranulocytosis (see section c)

Immune system disorders

Rare: Anaphylactic / anaphylactoid reactions

Psychiatric disorders

Rare: Mood disorders, insomnia and nightmares

Nervous system disorders

Common: Lightheadedness, headache

Uncommon: Vertigo, tinnitus, drowsiness

Rare: Confusion

Eye disorders

Rare: Visual disturbances including blurred vision

Cardiac disorders

Uncommon: Palpitations

Vascular disorders

Uncommon: Increase in blood pressure (see section 4.4), flushes

Respiratory, thoracic and mediastinal disorders

Rare: Onset of asthma attacks in certain individuals allergic to aspirin or other NSAIDs

Gastrointestinal disorders

Common: Dyspepsia, nausea and vomiting symptoms, abdominal pain, constipation, flatulence, diarrhoea

Uncommon: Gastrointestinal bleeding, peptic ulcers, oesophagitis, stomatitis

Rare: Gastrointestinal perforation, gastritis, colitis

The peptic ulcers, perforation or gastrointestinal bleeding, that may occur can be sometimes severe, especially in elderly (see section 4.4).

Hepato-biliary disorders

Uncommon: Transitory disturbance of liver function test (e.g. raised transaminases or bilirubin)

Rare: Hepatitis

Skin and subcutaneous tissue disorders

Common: Pruritus, rash

Uncommon: Urticaria

Rare: Stevens-Johnson Syndrome and toxic epidermal necrolysis, angioedema, bullous reactions such as erythema multiforme, photosensitivity reactions

Renal and urinary disorders

Uncommon: Disturbances of laboratory tests investigating renal function (e.g. raised creatinine or urea)

Rare: Renal failure (see section 4.4)

General disorders and administration site conditions

Common: Oedema including oedema of the lower limbs

c) Information Characterising Individual Serious and/or Frequently Occurring Adverse Reactions

Isolated cases of agranulocytosis have been reported in patients treated with meloxicam and other potentially myelotoxic drugs (see section 4.5).

4.9 Overdose

Symptoms following acute NSAID overdose are usually limited to lethargy, drowsiness, nausea, vomiting and epigastric pain, which are generally reversible with supportive care. Gastrointestinal bleeding can occur. Severe poisoning may result in hypertension, acute renal failure, hepatic dysfunction, respiratory depression, coma, convulsions, cardiovascular collapse and cardiac arrest. Anaphylactoid reactions have been reported with therapeutic ingestion of NSAIDs and may occur following an overdose.

Patients should be managed with symptomatic and supportive care following an NSAID overdose. Accelerated removal of meloxicam by 4 g oral doses of cholestyramine given three times a day was demonstrated in a clinical trial.

5. PHARMACOLOGICAL PROPERTIES

5.1 Pharmacodynamic properties

Pharmacotherapeutic group: Non Steroidal Anti-Inflammatory agent, Oxicams

ATC Code: M01AC06

Meloxicam is a non-steroidal anti-inflammatory drug (NSAID) of the oxicam family, with anti-inflammatory, analgesic and antipyretic properties.

The anti-inflammatory activity of meloxicam has been proven in classical models of inflammation. As with other NSAIDs, its precise mechanism of action remains unknown. However, there is at least one common mode of action shared by all NSAIDs (including Meloxicam): inhibition of the biosynthesis of prostaglandins, known inflammation mediators.

5.2 Pharmacokinetic properties

Absorption

Meloxicam is well absorbed from the gastrointestinal tract, which is reflected by a high absolute bioavailability of 89% following oral administration (capsule). Tablets, oral suspension and capsules were shown to be bioequivalent.

Following single dose administration of meloxicam, mean maximum plasma concentrations are achieved within 2 hours for the suspension and within 5-6 hours with solid oral dosage forms (capsules and tablets).

With multiple dosing, steady state conditions were reached within 3 to 5 days. Once daily dosing leads to drug plasma concentrations with a relatively small peak-trough fluctuation in the range of 0.4 - 1.0 μg/mL for 7.5 mg doses and 0.8 - 2.0 μg/mL for 15 mg doses, respectively (C_{min} and C_{max} at steady state, respectively). Maximum plasma concentrations of meloxicam at steady state, are achieved within five to six hours for the tablet, capsule and the oral suspension, respectively. Continuous treatment for periods of more than one year results in similar drug concentrations to those seen once steady state is first achieved. Extent of absorption for meloxicam following oral administration is not altered by concomitant food intake.

Distribution

Meloxicam is very strongly bound to plasma proteins, essentially albumin (99%). Meloxicam penetrates into synovial fluid to give concentrations approximately half of those in plasma.

Volume of distribution is low, on average 11 L. Interindividual variation is the order of 30-40%.

Biotransformation

Meloxicam undergoes extensive hepatic biotransformation. Four different metabolites of meloxicam were identified in urine, which are all pharmacodynamically inactive. The major metabolite, 5'-carboxymeloxicam (60% of dose), is formed by oxidation of an intermediate metabolite 5'- hydroxymethylmeloxicam, which is also excreted to a lesser extent (9% of dose). In vitro studies suggest that CYP 2C9 plays an important role in this metabolic pathway, with a minor contribution from the CYP 3A4 isoenzyme. The patient's peroxidase activity is probably responsible for the other two metabolites, which account for 16% and 4% of the administered dose respectively.

Elimination

Meloxicam is excreted predominantly in the form of metabolites and occurs to equal extents in urine and faeces. Less than 5% of the daily dose is excreted unchanged in faeces, while only traces of the parent compound are excreted in urine.

The mean elimination half-life is about 20 hours. Total plasma clearance amounts on average 8 mL/min.

Linearity/non-linearity

Meloxicam demonstrates linear pharmacokinetics in the therapeutic dose range of 7.5 mg 15 mg following per oral or intramuscular administration.

Special populations

Hepatic/renal Insufficiency:

Neither hepatic, mild nor moderate renal insufficiency have a substantial effect on meloxicam pharmacokinetics. In terminal renal failure, the increase in the volume of distribution may result in higher free meloxicam concentrations, and a daily dose of 7.5 mg must not be exceeded (see section 4.2).

Elderly:

Mean plasma clearance at steady state in elderly subjects was slightly lower than that reported for younger subjects.

5.3 Preclinical safety data

The toxicological profile of Meloxicam has been found in preclinical studies to be identical to that of NSAIDs: gastrointestinal ulcers and erosions, renal papillary necrosis at high doses during chronic administration in two animal species.

Oral reproductive studies in the rat have shown a decrease of ovulations and inhibition of implantations and embryotoxic effects (increase of resorptions) at maternotoxic dose levels at 1 mg/kg and higher.

The affected dose levels exceeded the clinical dose (7.5-15 mg) by a factor of 10 to 5-fold on a mg/kg dose basis (75 kg person). Fetotoxic effects at the end of gestation, shared by all prostaglandin synthesis inhibitors, have been described. No evidence has been found of any mutagenic effect, either in vitro or in vivo. No carcinogenic risk has been found in the rat and mouse at doses far higher than those used clinically.

6. PHARMACEUTICAL PARTICULARS

6.1 List of excipients

Sodium citrate

Lactose monohydrate

Microcrystalline cellulose

Povidone

Anhydrous colloidal silica

Crospovidone

Magnesium stearate

6.2 Incompatibilities

Not applicable

6.3 Shelf life

5 years

6.4 Special precautions for storage

Blister sheets should be protected from moisture.

6.5 Nature and contents of container

PVC/PVDC/Aluminium blister, boxes of 1, 2, 7, 10, 14, 15, 20, 28, 30, 50, 60, 100, 140, 280, 300, 500, or 1000 tablets. Not all pack sizes may be marketed.

6.6 Instructions for use and handling

No special requirements

7. MARKETING AUTHORISATION HOLDER

Boehringer Ingelheim International GmbH

D-55216 Ingelheim am Rhein

Germany

8. MARKETING AUTHORISATION NUMBER(S)

PL 14598/0002

9. DATE OF FIRST AUTHORISATION/RENEWAL OF THE AUTHORISATION

21 February 1996

10. DATE OF REVISION OF THE TEXT

December 2004

11. Legal Category

POM

M2c7.5/UK/SPC/16

Mobiflex

(Roche Products Limited)

1. NAME OF THE MEDICINAL PRODUCT

Mobiflex Tablets 20mg.

2. QUALITATIVE AND QUANTITATIVE COMPOSITION

Each tablet contains 20mg tenoxicam.

For excipients, see *6.1*.

3. PHARMACEUTICAL FORM

Film-coated tablet.

A greyish-yellow, film-coated oval tablet imprinted "Roche" on one face with a break line on the other.

4. CLINICAL PARTICULARS

4.1 Therapeutic indications

Mobiflex is indicated for the relief of pain and inflammation in osteoarthritis and rheumatoid arthritis. It is also indicated for the short term management of acute musculoskeletal disorders including strains, sprains and other soft-tissue injuries. IV, IM tenoxicam is also available for these indications in those patients considered unable to take oral tenoxicam.

4.2 Posology and method of administration

Adults

A single daily dose of 20mg Mobiflex should be taken orally, at the same time each day. Mobiflex Tablets are for oral administration with water or other fluid.

Higher doses should be avoided as they do not usually achieve significantly greater therapeutic effect but may be associated with a higher risk of adverse events.

In acute musculoskeletal disorders treatment should not normally be required for more than 7 days, but in severe cases it may be continued up to a maximum of 14 days.

Elderly

As with other non-steroidal anti-inflammatory drugs, Mobiflex should be used with special caution in elderly patients since they may be less able to tolerate side-effects than younger patients. They are also more likely to be receiving concomitant medication or to have impaired hepatic, renal or cardiovascular function. The lowest dose should be used in elderly patients and the patient should be monitored for GI bleeding for 4 weeks following initiation of NSAID therapy.

Children

There are insufficient data to make a recommendation for administration of Mobiflex to children.

Use in renal and hepatic insufficiency

Creatinine clearance	Dosage regimen
Greater than 25ml/min	Usual dosage but monitor patients carefully (see *Special warnings and special precautions for use)*
Less than 25ml/min	Insufficient data to make dosage recommendations

Because of the high plasma protein-binding of tenoxicam, caution is required when plasma albumin concentrations are markedly reduced (e.g. in nephrotic syndrome) or when bilirubin concentrations are high.

There is insufficient information to make dosage recommendations for Mobiflex in patients with pre-existing hepatic impairment.

4.3 Contraindications

1. Active peptic ulceration and a past history of peptic ulceration, gastro-intestinal bleeding (melaena, haematemesis) or severe gastritis.

2. Hypersensitivity to Mobiflex. Mobiflex should also be avoided in cases where the patient has suffered a hypersensitivity reaction (symptoms of asthma, rhinitis, angioedema or urticaria) to other non-steroidal anti-inflammatory drugs, including aspirin, as the potential exists for cross-sensitivity to Mobiflex.

4.4 Special warnings and special precautions for use

NSAIDs should only be given with care to patients with a history of gastrointestinal disease.

Any patient being treated with Mobiflex who presents with symptoms of gastro-intestinal disease should be closely monitored. If peptic ulceration or gastro-intestinal bleeding occurs, Mobiflex should be withdrawn immediately.

In rare cases, non-steroidal anti-inflammatory drugs may cause interstitial nephritis, glomerulonephritis, papillary necrosis and the nephrotic syndrome. Such agents inhibit the synthesis of renal prostaglandin which plays a supportive role in the maintenance of renal perfusion in patients whose renal blood flow and blood volume are decreased. In these patients, administration of a non-steroidal anti-inflammatory drug may precipitate overt renal decompensation, which returns to the pre-treatment state upon withdrawal of the drug. Patients at greatest risk of such a reaction are those with pre-existing renal disease (including diabetics with impaired renal function), nephrotic syndrome, volume depletion, hepatic disease, congestive cardiac failure and those patients receiving concomitant therapy with diuretics or potentially nephrotoxic drugs. Such patients should have their renal, hepatic and cardiac functions carefully monitored, and the dose should be kept as low as possible in patients with renal, hepatic or cardiac impairment. NSAIDs should be given with care to patients with a history of heart failure or hypertension since oedema has been reported in association with ibuprofen administration.

Caution is required if administered to patients suffering from, or with a previous history of bronchial asthma since ibuprofen has been reported to cause bronchospasm in such patients.

Occasional elevations of serum transaminases or other indicators of liver function have been reported. In most cases these have been small and transient increases above the normal range. If the abnormality is significant or persistent, Mobiflex should be stopped and follow-up tests carried out. Particular care is required in patients with pre-existing hepatic disease.

Mobiflex reduces platelet aggregation and may prolong bleeding time. This should be borne in mind for patients who undergo major surgery (e.g. joint replacement) and when bleeding time needs to be determined.

Particular care should be taken to regularly monitor elderly patients to detect possible interactions with concomitant therapy and to review renal, hepatic and cardiovascular function which may be potentially influenced by non-steroidal anti-inflammatory drugs.

Adverse eye findings have been reported with non-steroidal anti-inflammatory drugs, therefore it is recommended that patients who develop visual disturbances during treatment with Mobiflex have ophthalmic evaluation.

4.5 Interaction with other medicinal products and other forms of Interaction

Antacids may reduce the rate, but not the extent, of absorption of Mobiflex. The differences are not likely to be of clinical significance. No interaction has been found with concomitantly administered cimetidine. In healthy subjects no clinically relevant interaction between Mobiflex and low molecular weight heparin has been observed.

Tenoxicam is highly bound to serum albumin, and can, as with all NSAIDs, enhance the anticoagulant effect of warfarin and other anticoagulants. Close monitoring of the effects of anticoagulants and oral glycaemic agents is advised, especially during the initial stages of treatment with Mobiflex. No interaction with digoxin has been observed.

Mobiflex and other NSAIDs can reduce the effects of anti-hypertensive drugs. NSAIDs may exacerbate cardiac failure, reduce GFR and increase plasma cardiac glycoside levels when co-administered with cardiac glycosides.

As with all NSAIDs caution is advised when cyclosporin is co-administered because of the increased risk of nephrotoxicity.

Concomitant use of two or more NSAIDs should be avoided.

Patients taking quinolones may have an increased risk of developing convulsions.

Salicylates can displace tenoxicam from protein-binding sites and so increase the clearance and volume of distribution of Mobiflex. Concurrent treatment with salicylates or other non-steroidal anti-inflammatory drugs should therefore be avoided because of the increased risk of adverse reactions (particularly gastro-intestinal).

Non-steroidal anti-inflammatory drugs have been reported to decrease elimination of lithium. If tenoxicam is prescribed for a patient receiving lithium therapy, the frequency of lithium monitoring should be increased, the patient warned to maintain fluid intake and to be aware of symptoms of lithium intoxication.

Non-steroidal anti-inflammatory drugs may cause sodium, potassium and fluid retention and may interfere with the natriuretic action of diuretic agents, which can increase the risk of nephrotoxicity of NSAIDs. These properties should be kept in mind when treating patients with compromised cardiac function or hypertension since they may be responsible for a worsening of those conditions.

No clinically relevant interaction was found in small numbers of patients receiving treatment with penicillamine or parenteral gold.

Caution is advised where methotrexate is given concurrently because of possible enhancement of its toxicity, since NSAIDs have been reported to decrease elimination of methotrexate.

NSAIDs should not be used for 8 – 12 days after mifepristone administration as NSAIDs can reduce the effects of mifepristone.

As with all NSAIDs, caution should be taken when co-administering cortico-steroids because of the increased risk of GI bleeding.

4.6 Pregnancy and lactation

The safety of Mobiflex during pregnancy and lactation has not been established and the drug should therefore not be given in these conditions. Congenital abnormalities have been reported in association with ibuprofen administration in man; however, these are low in frequency and do not appear to follow any discernible pattern.

Although no teratogenic effects were seen in animal studies, Mobiflex, like other non-steroidal anti-inflammatory drugs, is associated with prolonged and delayed parturition and an adverse influence on neonatal viability when administered to animals in late pregnancy. Non-steroidal anti-inflammatory agents are also known to induce closure of the ductus arteriosus in infants, therefore use in late pregnancy should be particularly avoided.

In the limited studies available so far, ibuprofen appears in the breast milk in very low concentrations and is unlikely to adversely affect the breast fed infant.

No information is available on penetration of Mobiflex into milk in humans; animal studies indicate that significant levels may be achieved.

4.7 Effects on ability to drive and use machines

None.

4.8 Undesirable effects

For most patients, any side-effects are transient and resolve without discontinuation of treatment.

The most common side-effects relate to the gastro-intestinal tract. They include dyspepsia, nausea, abdominal pain and discomfort, constipation, diarrhoea, flatulence, indigestion, epigastric distress, stomatitis and anorexia. As with other non-steroidal anti-inflammatory drugs, there is a risk of peptic ulceration and gastro-intestinal bleeding, both of which have been reported with Mobiflex. Should this occur, Mobiflex is to be discontinued immediately and appropriate treatment instituted.

As with other non-steroidal anti-inflammatory drugs, peripheral oedema of mild or moderate degree and without clinical sequelae occurred in a small proportion of patients and the possibility of precipitating congestive cardiac failure in elderly patients or those with compromised cardiac function should therefore be borne in mind.

Central nervous system reactions of headache and dizziness have been reported in a small number of patients. Somnolence, insomnia, depression, nervousness, dream abnormalities, mental confusion, paraesthesias and vertigo have been reported rarely.

Hypersensitivity reactions have been reported following treatment with NSAIDs, these include:

a) Non specific allergic reactions and anaphylaxis.

b) Respiratory tract reactivity comprising asthma, aggravated asthma, bronchospasm or dyspnoea or

c) Skin reactions of rash, angioedema and pruritus have been reported. Nail disorders, alopecia, erythema, urticaria and photosensitivity reactions have been reported rarely. As with other non-steroidal anti-inflammatory drugs, Lyell's syndrome and Stevens-Johnson syndrome may develop in rare instances. Vesiculo-bullous reactions and vasculitis have also been reported rarely. Reversible elevations of blood urea nitrogen and creatinine have been reported (see *Special warnings and special precautions for use*).

Decreases in haemoglobin, unrelated to gastro-intestinal bleeding, have occurred. Anaemia, aplastic anaemia, haemolytic anaemia, thrombocytopenia and non-thrombocytopenic purpura, leucopenia and eosinophilia have been reported. Epistaxis has been reported infrequently. Rare cases of agranulocytosis have been reported.

As with most other non-steroidal anti-inflammatory drugs, changes in various liver function parameters have been observed. Some patients may develop raised serum transaminase levels during treatment. Although such reactions are rare, if abnormal liver function tests persist or worsen, if clinical signs and symptoms consistent with liver disease develop or if systemic manifestations occur (e.g. eosinophilia, rash), Mobiflex should be discontinued. Hepatitis and jaundice have also been reported.

Palpitations and dyspnoea have also been reported rarely. Metabolic abnormalities, such as weight decrease or increase and hyperglycaemia, have occurred rarely.

Swollen eyes, blurred vision and eye irritation have been reported. Ophthalmoscopy and slit-lamp examination have revealed no evidence of ocular changes. Malaise and tinnitus may occur.

Nephrotoxicity has been reported in various forms, including interstitial nephritis, nephrotic syndrome and renal failure.

4.9 Overdose

There is no reported experience of serious overdosage with Mobiflex. No specific measures are available; administration of H2-antagonist drugs may be of benefit. Gastric lavage should be carried out as soon as possible after drug ingestion and the patient should be closely observed and general supportive measures taken as necessary.

5. PHARMACOLOGICAL PROPERTIES

5.1 Pharmacodynamic properties

Mobiflex is a non-steroidal anti-inflammatory drug which has marked anti-inflammatory and analgesic activity and some antipyretic activity. As with other non-steroidal anti-inflammatory drugs, the precise mode of action is unknown, though it is probably multifactorial, involving inhibition of prostaglandin biosynthesis and reduction of leucocyte accumulation at the inflammatory site.

5.2 Pharmacokinetic properties

Mobiflex is long-acting; a single daily dose is effective.

After oral administration, Mobiflex is rapidly and completely absorbed as unchanged drug. Concomitant food reduces the rate, but not the extent, of absorption of Mobiflex. Tenoxicam penetrates well into synovial fluid to give concentrations approximately half those in plasma. The mean plasma elimination half-life is approximately 72 hours.

With the recommended dosage regimen of 20mg once daily, steady-state plasma concentrations are reached within 10 - 15 days, with no unexpected accumulation.

Mobiflex is strongly bound to plasma proteins.

Mobiflex is cleared from the body almost exclusively by metabolism. Approximately two-thirds of the administered dose is excreted in the urine, mainly as the pharmacologically inactive 5-hydroxypyridyl metabolite, and the remainder in the bile, much of it as glucuronide conjugates of hydroxy-metabolites.

No age-specific changes in the pharmacokinetics of Mobiflex have been found although inter-individual variation tends to be higher in elderly persons.

5.3 Preclinical safety data

None stated.

6. PHARMACEUTICAL PARTICULARS

6.1 List of excipients

Lactose

Maize starch

Magnesium stearate

Talc

Hypromellose

Titanium dioxide E171

Yellow iron oxide E172.

6.2 Incompatibilities

Not applicable.

6.3 Shelf life

5 years.

6.4 Special precautions for storage

Do not store above 30°C.

6.5 Nature and contents of container

PVC/Aluminium foil blister pack containing 30 tablets.

6.6 Instructions for use and handling

No special requirements.

7. MARKETING AUTHORISATION HOLDER

Roche Products Limited, 40 Broadwater Road, Welwyn Garden City, Hertfordshire, AL7 3AY.

8. MARKETING AUTHORISATION NUMBER(S)

PL 0031/0200

9. DATE OF FIRST AUTHORISATION/RENEWAL OF THE AUTHORISATION

August 1988

10. DATE OF REVISION OF THE TEXT

December 2003

Mobiflex is a registered trade mark

P999758/104

Mobiflex Vials 20mg

(Roche Products Limited)

1. NAME OF THE MEDICINAL PRODUCT

Mobiflex Vials 20mg

2. QUALITATIVE AND QUANTITATIVE COMPOSITION

Mobiflex Vials containing 20mg tenoxicam as lyophilised sterile powder for reconstitution. Ampoules with 2ml sterile Water for Injections Ph. Eur.

Tenoxicam is 4-hydroxy-2-methyl-N-2-pyridyl-2H-thieno-[2,3-e]-1,2-thiazine-3-carboxamide-1, 1-dioxide, a non steroidal anti-inflammatory agent.

3. PHARMACEUTICAL FORM

Vials for IV or IM administration.

4. CLINICAL PARTICULARS

4.1 Therapeutic indications

Mobiflex is indicated for the relief of pain and inflammation in osteoarthritis and rheumatoid arthritis. It is also indicated for the short term management of acute musculoskeletal disorders including strains, sprains and other soft-tissue injuries. IV, IM tenoxicam can be used for these indications in those patients considered unable to take oral tenoxicam.

4.2 Posology and method of administration

Adults

Mobiflex Vials should be given IV or IM. A single daily dose of 20mg for one to two days initially to be continued with the oral form, with administration at the same time each day. The lyophilisate should be dissolved in 2 ml of the solvent provided (2ml sterile water for injections). This reconstituted solution should be used immediately.

Higher doses should be avoided as they do not usually achieve significantly greater therapeutic effect but may be associated with a higher risk of adverse events.

In acute musculoskeletal disorders treatment should not normally be required for more than 7 days, but in severe cases it may be continued up to a maximum of 14 days.

Elderly

As with other non-steroidal anti-inflammatory drugs, Mobiflex should be used with special caution in elderly patients since they may be less able to tolerate side-effects than younger patients. They are also more likely to be receiving concomitant medication or to have impaired hepatic, renal or cardiovascular function. The lowest dose should be used in elderly patients and the patient should be monitored for GI bleeding for 4 weeks following initiation of NSAID therapy.

Children

There are insufficient data to make a recommendation for administration of Mobiflex to children.

Use in renal and hepatic insufficiency

Creatinine clearance	Dosage regimen
Greater than 25ml/min	Usual dosage but monitor patients carefully (see *Special warnings and special precautions for use*)
Less than 25ml/min	Insufficient data to make dosage recommendations

Because of the high plasma protein-binding of tenoxicam, caution is required when plasma albumin concentrations are markedly reduced (e.g. in nephrotic syndrome) or when bilirubin concentrations are high.

There is insufficient information to make dosage recommendations for Mobiflex in patients with pre-existing hepatic impairment.

4.3 Contraindications

1. Active peptic ulceration and a past history of peptic ulceration, gastro-intestinal bleeding (melaena, haematemesis) or severe gastritis.

2. Hypersensitivity to Mobiflex. Mobiflex should also be avoided in cases where the patient has suffered a hypersensitivity reaction (symptoms of asthma, rhinitis, angioedema or urticaria) to other non-steroidal anti-inflammatory drugs, including aspirin, as the potential exists for cross-sensitivity to Mobiflex.

4.4 Special warnings and special precautions for use

NSAIDs should only be given with care to patients with a history of gastrointestinal disease.

Any patient being treated with Mobiflex who presents with symptoms of gastro-intestinal disease should be closely monitored. If peptic ulceration or gastro-intestinal bleeding occurs, Mobiflex should be withdrawn immediately.

In rare cases, non-steroidal anti-inflammatory drugs may cause interstitial nephritis, glomerulonephritis, papillary necrosis and the nephrotic syndrome. Such agents inhibit the synthesis of renal prostaglandin which plays a supportive role in the maintenance of renal perfusion in patients whose renal blood flow and blood volume are decreased. In these patients, administration of a non-steroidal anti-inflammatory drug may precipitate overt renal decompensation, which returns to the pre-treatment state upon withdrawal of the drug. Patients at greatest risk of such a reaction are those with pre-existing renal disease (including diabetics with impaired renal function), nephrotic syndrome, volume depletion, hepatic disease, congestive cardiac failure and those patients receiving concomitant therapy with diuretics or potentially nephrotoxic drugs. Such patients should have their renal, hepatic and cardiac functions carefully monitored, and the dose should be kept as low as possible in patients with renal, hepatic or cardiac impairment. NSAIDs should be given with care to patients with a history of heart failure or hypertension since oedema has been reported in association with ibuprofen administration.

Caution is required if administered to patients suffering from, or with a previous history of bronchial asthma, since ibuprofen has been reported to cause bronchospasm in such patients.

Occasional elevations of serum transaminases or other indicators of liver function have been reported. In most cases these have been small and transient increases above the normal range. If the abnormality is significant or persistent, Mobiflex should be stopped and follow-up tests carried out. Particular care is required in patients with pre-existing hepatic disease.

Mobiflex reduces platelet aggregation and may prolong bleeding time. This should be borne in mind for patients who undergo major surgery (e.g. joint replacement) and when bleeding time needs to be determined.

Particular care should be taken to regularly monitor elderly patients to detect possible interactions with concomitant therapy and to review renal, hepatic and cardiovascular function which may be potentially influenced by non-steroidal anti-inflammatory drugs.

Adverse eye findings have been reported with non-steroidal anti-inflammatory drugs, therefore it is recommended that patients who develop visual disturbances during treatment with Mobiflex have ophthalmic evaluation.

4.5 Interaction with other medicinal products and other forms of Interaction

Antacids may reduce the rate, but not the extent, of absorption of Mobiflex. The differences are not likely to be of clinical significance. No interaction has been found with concomitantly administered cimetidine. In healthy subjects no clinically relevant interaction between Mobiflex and low molecular weight heparin has been observed.

Tenoxicam is highly bound to serum albumin, and can, as with all NSAIDs, enhance the anticoagulant effect of warfarin and other anticoagulants. Close monitoring of the effects of anticoagulants and oral glycaemic agents is advised, especially during the initial stages of treatment with Mobiflex. No interaction with digoxin has been observed.

Mobiflex and other NSAIDs can reduce the effects of antihypertensive drugs. NSAIDs may exacerbate cardiac failure, reduce GFR and increase plasma cardiac glycoside levels when co-administered with cardiac glycosides.

As with all NSAIDs caution is advised when cyclosporin is co-administered because of the increased risk of nephrotoxicity.

Concomitant use of two or more NSAIDs should be avoided.

Patients taking quinolones may have an increased risk of developing convulsions.

Salicylates can displace tenoxicam from protein-binding sites and so increase the clearance and volume of distribution of Mobiflex. Concurrent treatment with salicylates or other non-steroidal anti-inflammatory drugs should therefore be avoided because of the increased risk of adverse reactions (particularly gastro-intestinal).

Non-steroidal anti-inflammatory drugs have been reported to decrease elimination of lithium. If tenoxicam is prescribed for a patient receiving lithium therapy, the frequency of lithium monitoring should be increased, the patient warned to maintain fluid intake and to be aware of symptoms of lithium intoxication.

Non-steroidal anti-inflammatory drugs may cause sodium, potassium and fluid retention and may interfere with the natriuretic action of diuretic agents, which can increase the risk of nephrotoxicity of NSAIDs. These properties should be kept in mind when treating patients with compromised cardiac function or hypertension since they may be responsible for a worsening of those conditions.

No clinically relevant interaction was found in small numbers of patients receiving treatment with penicillamine or parenteral gold.

Caution is advised where methotrexate is given concurrently because of possible enhancement of its toxicity, since NSAIDs have been reported to decrease elimination of methotrexate.

NSAIDs should not be used for 8 — 12 days after mifepristone administration as NSAIDs can reduce the effects of mifepristone.

As with all NSAIDs, caution should be taken when co-administering cortico-steroids because of the increased risk of GI bleeding.

4.6 Pregnancy and lactation

The safety of Mobiflex during pregnancy and lactation has not been established and the drug should therefore not be given in these conditions. Congenital abnormalities have been reported in association with ibuprofen administration in man; however, these are low in frequency and do not appear to follow any discernible pattern.

Although no teratogenic effects were seen in animal studies, Mobiflex, like other non-steroidal anti-inflammatory drugs, is associated with prolonged and delayed parturition and an adverse influence on neonatal viability when administered to animals in late pregnancy. Non-steroidal anti-inflammatory agents are also known to induce closure of the ductus arteriosus in infants, therefore use in late pregnancy should be particularly avoided.

In the limited studies available so far, ibuprofen appears in the breast milk in very low concentrations and is unlikely to adversely affect the breast fed infant.

No information is available on penetration of Mobiflex into milk in humans; animal studies indicate that significant levels may be achieved.

4.7 Effects on ability to drive and use machines

Patients experiencing adverse events that might affect driving or using machines such as vertigo, dizziness or visual disturbances should refrain from driving or using machines.

4.8 Undesirable effects

For most patients, any side-effects are transient and resolve without discontinuation of treatment.

The most common side-effects relate to the gastro-intestinal tract. They include dyspepsia, nausea, abdominal pain and discomfort, constipation, diarrhoea, flatulence, indigestion, epigastric distress, stomatitis and anorexia. As with other non-steroidal anti-inflammatory drugs, there is a risk of peptic ulceration and gastro-intestinal bleeding, both of which have been reported with Mobiflex. Should this occur, Mobiflex is to be discontinued immediately and appropriate treatment instituted.

As with other non-steroidal anti-inflammatory drugs, peripheral oedema of mild or moderate degree and without clinical sequelae occurred in a small proportion of patients and the possibility of precipitating congestive cardiac failure in elderly patients or those with compromised cardiac function should therefore be borne in mind.

Central nervous system reactions of headache and dizziness have been reported in a small number of patients. Somnolence, insomnia, depression, nervousness, dream abnormalities, mental confusion, paraesthesias and vertigo have been reported rarely.

Hypersensitivity reactions have been reported following treatment with NSAIDs, these include:

a) Non specific allergic reactions and anaphylaxis

b) Respiratory tract reactivity comprising asthma, aggravated asthma, bronchospasm or dyspnoea or

c) Skin reactions of rash, angioedema and pruritus have been reported. Nail disorders, alopecia, erythema, urticaria and photosensitivity reactions have been reported rarely. As with other non-steroidal anti-inflammatory drugs, Lyell's syndrome and Stevens-Johnson syndrome may develop in rare instances. Vesiculo-bullous reactions and vasculitis have also been reported rarely. Reversible elevations of blood urea nitrogen and creatinine have been reported (see *Special warnings and special precautions for use*).

Decreases in haemoglobin, unrelated to gastro-intestinal bleeding, have occurred. Anaemia, aplastic anaemia, haemolytic anaemia, thrombocytopenia and non-thrombocytopenic purpura, leucopenia and eosinophilia have been reported. Epistaxis has been reported infrequently. Rare cases of agranulocytosis have been reported.

As with most other non-steroidal anti-inflammatory drugs, changes in various liver function parameters have been observed. Some patients may develop raised serum transaminase levels during treatment. Although such reactions are rare, if abnormal liver function tests persist or worsen, if clinical signs and symptoms consistent with liver disease develop or if systemic manifestations occur (e.g. eosinophilia, rash), Mobiflex should be discontinued. Hepatitis and jaundice have also been reported.

Palpitations and dyspnoea have also been reported rarely. Metabolic abnormalities, such as weight decrease or increase and hyperglycaemia, have occurred rarely.

Swollen eyes, blurred vision and eye irritation have been reported. Ophthalmoscopy and slit-lamp examination have revealed no evidence of ocular changes. Malaise and tinnitus may occur.

Nephrotoxicity has been reported in various forms, including interstitial nephritis, nephrotic syndrome and renal failure.

4.9 Overdose

There is no reported experience of serious overdosage with Mobiflex. No specific measures are available; administration of H2-antagonist drugs may be of benefit. Gastric lavage should be carried out as soon as possible after drug ingestion and the patient should be closely observed and general supportive measures taken as necessary.

5. PHARMACOLOGICAL PROPERTIES

5.1 Pharmacodynamic properties

Mobiflex is a non-steroidal anti-inflammatory drug which has marked anti-inflammatory and analgesic activity and some antipyretic activity. As with other non-steroidal anti-inflammatory drugs, the precise mode of action is unknown, though it is probably multifactorial, involving inhibition of prostaglandin biosynthesis and reduction of leucocyte accumulation at the inflammatory site.

5.2 Pharmacokinetic properties

Mobiflex is long-acting; a single daily dose is effective.

After oral administration, Mobiflex is rapidly and completely absorbed as unchanged drug. Tenoxicam penetrates well into synovial fluid to give concentrations approximately half those in plasma. The mean plasma elimination half-life is approximately 72 hours.

Following intravenous administration of 20mg tenoxicam, plasma levels of the drug decline rapidly during the first two hours mainly due to distribution processes. After this short period, no difference in plasma concentrations between intravenous and oral dosing is seen. Following intramuscular injection levels at or above 90% of the maximally achieved concentrations are reached as early as 15 minutes after a dose, i.e. earlier than after oral dosing. However, again the difference in blood levels between the two routes of administration is restricted to the first two hours after a dose. The bioavailability after an intramuscular dose is complete and indistinguishable from that determined after oral dosing.

With the recommended dosage regimen of 20mg once daily, steady-state plasma concentrations are reached within 10 - 15 days, with no unexpected accumulation.

Mobiflex is strongly bound to plasma proteins.

Mobiflex is cleared from the body almost exclusively by metabolism. Approximately two-thirds of the administered dose is excreted in the urine, mainly as the pharmacologically inactive 5-hydroxypyridyl metabolite, and the remainder in the bile, much of it as glucuronide conjugates of hydroxy-metabolites.

No age-specific changes in the pharmacokinetics of Mobiflex have been found although inter-individual variation tends to be higher in elderly persons.

5.3 Preclinical safety data

None Stated.

6. PHARMACEUTICAL PARTICULARS

6.1 List of excipients

Mannitol, ascorbic acid, disodium edatate, sodium hydroxide, tromethamine and hydrochloric acid as a lyophilised powder for dissolving in solvent. The solvent in the ampoule contains water for injection.

6.2 Incompatibilities
None known.

6.3 Shelf life
3 years unopened

24 hours after reconstitution

6.4 Special precautions for storage
The pack should be stored at a temperature below 25°C. Do not freeze as the water ampoule may burst.

6.5 Nature and contents of container
Mobiflex Vials 20mg are in packs of 5 vials together with 5 ampoules containing 2ml of sterile Water for Injections Ph. Eur. as diluent.

6.6 Instructions for use and handling
Not Applicable.

7. MARKETING AUTHORISATION HOLDER
Roche Products Limited, 40 Broadwater Road, Welwyn Garden City, Hertfordshire, AL7 3AY.

8. MARKETING AUTHORISATION NUMBER(S)
PL 0031/0330 (vials 20mg)

PL 0031/0284 (Ampoules Water for Injections)

9. DATE OF FIRST AUTHORISATION/RENEWAL OF THE AUTHORISATION
August 1993

10. DATE OF REVISION OF THE TEXT
December 1998

Mobiflex is a registered trade mark

P999590/1199

Modalim Tablets 100mg

(sanofi-aventis)

1. NAME OF THE MEDICINAL PRODUCT
Modalim Tablets 100 mg

2. QUALITATIVE AND QUANTITATIVE COMPOSITION
Each tablet contains 100mg ciprofibrate as the active ingredient.

For excipients, see 6.1

3. PHARMACEUTICAL FORM
Tablet.

4. CLINICAL PARTICULARS

4.1 Therapeutic indications
Modalim tablets are recommended for the treatment of primary dyslipoproteinaemias, including types IIa, IIb, III and IV (hypercholesterolaemia, hypertriglyceridaemia and combined forms) - refractory to appropriate dietary treatment.

Dietary measures should be continued during therapy.

4.2 Posology and method of administration

Adults

The recommended dosage is one tablet (100mg ciprofibrate) per day. This dose should not be exceeded (see Precautions).

Elderly Patients

As for adults, but see Precautions and Warnings.

Use in Case of Impaired Renal Function

In moderate renal impairment it is recommended that dosage be reduced to one tablet every other day. Patients should be carefully monitored. Modalim should not be used in severe renal impairment.

Use in Children

Not recommended since safety and efficacy in children has not been established.

Modalim tablets are for oral administration only.

4.3 Contraindications
Severe hepatic impairment.

Severe renal impairment.

Pregnancy and lactation.

Concurrent use with another fibrate.

Hypersensitivity to the active substance or to any component of the product.

4.4 Special warnings and special precautions for use

4.4.1 **Special warnings**

Patients with rare hereditary problems of galactose intolerance, the Lapp lactose deficiency or glucose-galactose malabsorption should not take this medicine.

-Myalgia/myopathy:

- Patients should be advised to report unexplained muscle pain, tenderness or weakness immediately.

CPK levels should be assessed immediately in patients reporting these symptoms. Treatment should be discontinued if CPK levels are greater than ten times the upper limit of the normal range, if levels rise progressively or if there is other evidence of myopathy.

- Doses of 200mg Modalim per day or greater have been associated with a high risk of rhabdomyolysis. Therefore the daily dose should not exceed 100mg.

- Impaired renal function and any situation of hypoalbuminaemia such as nephrotic syndrome, high alcohol intake or hypothyroidism may increase the risk of myopathy.

- As with other fibrates, the risk of rhabdomyolysis and myoglobinuria may be increased if ciprofibrate is used in combination with other fibrates or HMG CoA reductase inhibitors *(see section 4.3 Contraindications and section 4.5 Interaction with other Medicinal Products and Other Forms of Interaction).*

Use with caution in patients with impaired hepatic function.

Periodic hepatic function tests are recommended. Modalim treatment should be discontinued if significant transaminases abnormalities persist or if cholestatic liver injury is evidenced.

Secondary causes of dyslipidaemia, such as hypothyroidism, should be excluded or corrected prior to commencing any lipid lowering drug treatment.

4.4.2 **Special precautions for use**

Association with oral anticoagulant therapy: concomitant oral anticoagulant therapy should be given at reduced dosage and adjusted according to INR *(see section 4.5 Interaction with Other Medicinal Products and Other Forms of Interaction).*

If after a period of administration lasting several months, a satisfactory reduction in serum lipid concentrations has not been obtained, additional or different therapeutic measures must be considered.

4.5 Interaction with other medicinal products and other forms of Interaction

• **Contra-indicated combination**

Other fibrates: As with other fibrates, the risk of rhabdomyolysis and myoglobinuria may be increased if ciprofibrate is used in combination with other fibrates *(see section 4.3 Contra-indications and section 4.4.1 Special warnings).*

• **Not recommended combinations**

HMG CoA reductase inhibitors: As with other fibrates, the risk of rhabdomyolysis and myoglobinuria may be increased if ciprofibrate is used in combination with HMG CoA reductase inhibitors *(see section 4.4.1 Special warnings).*

• **Combination requiring caution**

Oral anticoagulant therapy: Ciprofibrate is highly protein bound and therefore likely to displace other drugs from plasma protein binding sites. Ciprofibrate has been shown to potentiate the effect of warfarin, indicating that concomitant oral anticoagulant therapy should be given at reduced dosage and adjusted according to INR *(see section 4.4.2 Special precautions for use).*

• **Combination to be taken into account**

Oral hypoglycaemics: A possible interaction should be considered.

Oestrogens: Oestrogens can raise lipid levels. Although a pharmacodynamic interaction may be suggested, no clinical data are currently available.

4.6 Pregnancy and lactation
There is no evidence that ciprofibrate is teratogenic but signs of embryotoxicity were observed at high doses in animals. Ciprofibrate is excreted in the breast milk of lactating rats. There are no data on the use of the drug in human pregnancy or lactation. Therefore the use of ciprofibrate is contraindicated during pregnancy and in nursing mothers.

4.7 Effects on ability to drive and use machines
Dizziness, drowsiness, and tiredness have only rarely been reported in association with ciprofibrate. Patients should be warned that if they are affected they should not drive or operate machinery.

4.8 Undesirable effects

Cutaneous disorders:

Cutaneous reactions mainly allergic have been reported: rashes, urticaria and pruritus, and very rarely photosensitivity.

As with other drugs in this class, a low occurrence of alopecia has been reported.

Muscular disorders:

As with other fibrates, elevation of serum creatine phosphokinase (CPK), myalgia and myopathy including myositis and rare cases of rhabdomyolysis have been reported. In the majority of cases muscle toxicity is reversible when treatment is withdrawn *(see section 4.4 Special Warnings and Special Precautions for Use).*

Neurological disorders:

Occasional reports of headache, vertigo.

Dizziness, drowsiness have only rarely been reported in association with ciprofibrate.

As with other drugs of this class, a low occurrence of impotence has been reported.

Gastro-intestinal disorders:

There have been occasional reports of gastrointestinal symptoms including nausea, vomiting, diarrhoea, dyspepsia, and abdominal pain. Generally, these side effects were mild to moderate in nature and occurred early on, becoming less frequent as treatment progressed.

Hepato-biliary disorders:

As with other fibrates, abnormal liver function tests have been observed occasionally. Very rare cases of cholestasis or cytolysis have been reported *(see section 4.4 Special Warnings and Special Precautions for Use).* Exceptional cases with chronic evolution have been observed.

Pulmonary disorders:

Isolated cases of pneumonitis or pulmonary fibrosis have been reported.

General disorders:

Tiredness has only rarely been reported in association with ciprofibrate.

4.9 Overdose
Overdosage with ciprofibrate has been rarely reported. Associated adverse events reflect those seen in routine use. There are no specific antidotes to ciprofibrate. Treatment of overdosage should be symptomatic. Gastric lavage and appropriate supportive care may be instituted if necessary. Ciprofibrate is non-dialysable.

5. PHARMACOLOGICAL PROPERTIES

5.1 Pharmacodynamic properties
ATC Code: C10A B08

Pharmacotherapeutic group: Serum lipid reducing agents - fibrates.

Ciprofibrate is a new derivative of phenoxyisobutyric acid which has a marked hypolipidaemic action. It reduces both LDL and VLDL and hence the levels of triglyceride and cholesterol associated with these lipoprotein fractions. It also increases levels of HDL cholesterol.

Ciprofibrate is effective in the treatment of hyperlipidaemia associated with high plasma concentrations of LDL and VLDL (types IIa, IIb, III and IV according to the Fredrickson Classification). In clinical studies ciprofibrate has been shown to be effective in complementing the dietary treatment of such conditions.

5.2 Pharmacokinetic properties
Ciprofibrate is readily absorbed in man, with maximum plasma concentrations occurring mainly between one and four hours following an oral dose. Following a single dose of 100mg, in volunteers, maximum plasma concentration of ciprofibrate was between 21 and 36μg/ml. In patients on chronic therapy, maximum levels from 53 to 165μg/ml have been measured.

Terminal elimination half-life in patients on long term therapy varies from 38 to 86 hours. The elimination half-life in subjects with moderate renal insufficiency was slightly increased compared with normal subjects (116.7h compared with 81.1h). In subjects with severe renal impairment, a significant increase was noted (171.9h).

Approximately 30-75% of a single dose administered to volunteers was excreted in the urine in 72 hours, either as unchanged ciprofibrate (20-25% of the total excreted) or as a conjugate. Subjects with moderate renal impairment excreted on average 7.0% of a single dose as unchanged ciprofibrate over 96 hours, compared with 6.9% in normal subjects. In subjects with severe insufficiency this was reduced to 4.7%.

5.3 Preclinical safety data
There are no preclinical data of relevance to the prescriber which are additional to that already included in other sections of the SPC.

6. PHARMACEUTICAL PARTICULARS

6.1 List of excipients
Maize starch, Lactose monohydrate, Microcrystalline cellulose, Hypromellose, Powdered vegetable stearine, Sodium lauryl sulphate.

6.2 Incompatibilities
Not applicable.

6.3 Shelf life
5 years

6.4 Special precautions for storage
There are no special storage precautions.

6.5 Nature and contents of container
Clear PVC / Aluminium blister strips in packs of 28 tablets.

6.6 Instructions for use and handling
None stated.

7. MARKETING AUTHORISATION HOLDER
Sanofi-Synthelabo

PO Box 597

Guildford

Surrey

8. MARKETING AUTHORISATION NUMBER(S)
PL 11723/0050

9. DATE OF FIRST AUTHORISATION/RENEWAL OF THE AUTHORISATION
13 June 2002

10. DATE OF REVISION OF THE TEXT
May 2005

Legal category: POM

Modecate Concentrate Injection 100mg/ml

(sanofi-aventis)

1. NAME OF THE MEDICINAL PRODUCT

Modecate Concentrate Injection 100mg/ml.

2. QUALITATIVE AND QUANTITATIVE COMPOSITION

The product contains Fluphenazine Decanoate BP 100mg/ml.

3. PHARMACEUTICAL FORM

Intramuscular injection for administration to human beings.

4. CLINICAL PARTICULARS

4.1 Therapeutic indications

For the treatment and maintenance of schizophrenic patients and those with paranoid psychoses.

While Modecate concentrate injection has been shown to be effective in acute states, it is particularly useful in the maintenance treatment of chronic patients who are unreliable at taking their oral medication, and also of those who do not absorb their oral phenothiazine adequately.

4.2 Posology and method of administration

Dosage and Administration

Adults

It is recommended that patients be stabilised on the injection in hospital.

Recommended dosage regimes for all indications:

A. Patients without previous exposure to a depot fluphenazine formulation:

Initially 0.125ml ie. 12.5mg (0.0625ml ie 6.25mg for patients over 60) by deep intramuscular injection into the gluteal region.

The onset of action generally appears between 24 and 72 hours after injection and the effects of the drug on psychotic symptoms become significant within 48 to 96 hours. Subsequent injections and the dosage interval are determined in accordance with the patient's response. When administered as maintenance therapy, a single injection may be effective in controlling schizophrenic symptoms for up to four weeks or longer.

It is desirable to maintain as much flexibility in the dose as possible to achieve the best therapeutic response with the least side-effects; most patients are successfully maintained within the dose range 0.125ml (12.5mg) to 1ml (100mg) given at a dose interval of 2 to 5 weeks.

Patients previously maintained on oral fluphenazine:

It is not possible to predict the equivalent dose of depot formulation in view of the wide variability of individual response.

B. Patients previously maintained on depot fluphenazine:

Patients who have suffered a relapse following cessation of depot fluphenazine therapy may be restarted on the same dose (as they were receiving formerly), although the frequency of injections may need to be increased in the early weeks of treatment until satisfactory control is obtained.

Elderly:

Elderly patients may be particularly susceptible to extrapyramidal reactions. Therefore reduced maintenance dosage may be required and a smaller initial dose (See above).

Children:

Not recommended for children.

* Where a very small volume/low concentration of fluphenazine is required patients may be transferred to the equivalent dose of Modecate Injection 25mg/ml on the basis that 1ml Modecate Concentrate (100mg/ml) is equivalent to 4ml Modecate Injection.

Note

The dosage should not be increased without close supervision and it should be noted that there is a variability in individual response.

The response to antipsychotic drug treatment may be delayed. If drugs are withdrawn, recurrence of symptoms may not become apparent for several weeks or months.

Route of administration: Intramuscular.

4.3 Contraindications

The product is contraindicated in the following cases:

Comatose states

Marked cerebral atherosclerosis

Phaeochromocytoma

Renal failure

Liver failure

Severe cardiac insufficiency

Severely depressed states

Existing blood dyscrasias

History of hypersensitivity to any of the ingredients

4.4 Special warnings and special precautions for use

Caution should be exercised with the following:

Liver disease

Renal impairment

Cardiac arrhythmias, cardiac disease

Thyrotoxicosis

Severe respiratory disease

Epilepsy, conditions predisposing to epilepsy (eg. alcohol withdrawal or brain damage)

Parkinson's disease

Patients who have shown hypersensitivity to other phenothiazines

Personal or family history of narrow angle glaucoma

In very hot weather

The elderly, particularly if frail or at risk of hypothermia

Hypothyroidism

Myasthenia gravis

Prostatic hypertrophy

Patients with known or with a family history of cardiovascular disease should receive ECG screening, and monitoring and correction of electrolyte balance prior to treatment with fluphenazine.

Acute withdrawal symptoms, including nausea, vomiting, sweating and insomnia have been described after abrupt cessation of antipsychotic drugs. Recurrence of psychotic symptoms may also occur, and the emergence of involuntary movement disorders (such as akathisia, dystonia and dyskinesia) has been reported. Therefore, gradual withdrawal is advisable.

Psychotic patients on large doses of phenothiazines who are undergoing surgery should be watched carefully for hypotension. Reduced amounts of anaesthetics or central nervous system depressants may be necessary.

Fluphenazine should be used with caution in patients exposed to organophosphorus insecticides

Neuroleptic drugs elevate prolactin levels, and an increase in mammary neoplasms has been found in rodents after chronic administration. However, studies to date have not shown an association between chronic administration of these drugs and human mammary tumours.

As with any phenothiazine, the physician should be alert to the possibility of "silent pneumonias" in patients receiving long-term fluphenazine.

4.5 Interaction with other medicinal products and other forms of Interaction

The possibility should be borne in mind that phenothiazines may:

1. Increase the central nervous system depression produced by drugs such as alcohol, general anaesthetics, hypnotics, sedatives or strong analgesics.

2. Antagonise the action of adrenaline and other sympathomimetic agents and reverse the blood-pressure lowering effects of adrenergic-blocking agents such as guanethidine and clonidine.

3. Impair: the anti-parkinsonian effect of L-dopa; the effect of anti-convulsants; metabolism of tricyclic antidepressants; the control of diabetes.

4. Increase the effect of anticoagulants and antidepressants.

5. Interact with lithium.

Anticholinergic effects may be enhanced by anti-parkinsonian or other anticholinergic drugs.

Phenothiazines may enhance: the absorption of corticosteroids, digoxin, and neuromuscular blocking agents.

Fluphenazine is metabolised by P450 2D6 and is itself an inhibitor of this drug metabolising enzyme. The plasma concentrations and the effects of fluphenazine may therefore be increased and prolonged by drugs that are either the substrates or inhibitors of this P450 isoform, possibly resulting in severe hypotension, cardiac arrhythmias or CNS side effects. Examples of drugs which are substrates or inhibitors of cytochrome P450 2D6 include anti-arrhythmics, certain antidepressants including SSRIs and tricyclics, certain antipsychotics, β-blockers, protease inhibitors, opiates, cimetidine and ecstasy (MDMA). This list is not exhaustive.

Concomitant use of barbiturates with phenothiazines may result in reduced serum levels of both drugs, and an increased response if one of the drugs is withdrawn.

The effect of fluphenazine on the QT interval is likely to be potentiated by concurrent use of other drugs that also prolong the QT interval. Therefore, concurrent use of these drugs and fluphenazine is contraindicated. Examples include certain anti-arrhythmics, such as those of Class 1A (such as quinidine, disopyramide and procainamide) and Class III (such as amiodarone and sotalol), tricyclic antidepressants (such as amitriptyline); certain tetracyclic antidepressants (such as maprotiline); certain antipsychotic medications (such as phenothiazines and pimozide); certain antihistamines (such as terfenadine); lithium, quinine, pentamidine and sparfloxacin. This list is not exhaustive.

Electrolyte imbalance, particularly hypokalaemia, greatly increases the risk of QT interval prolongation. Therefore, concurrent use of drugs that cause electrolyte imbalance should be avoided.

Concurrent use of MAO inhibitors may increase sedation, constipation, dry mouth and hypotension.

Owing to their adrenolytic action, phenothiazines may reduce the pressor effect of adrenergic vasoconstrictors (i.e. ephedrine, phenylephrine).

Phenylpropanolamine has been reported to interact with phenothiazines and cause ventricular arrhythmias.

Concurrent use of phenothiazines and ACE inhibitors or angiotensin II antagonists may result in severe postural hypotension.

Concurrent use of thiazide diuretics may cause hypotension. Diuretic-induced hypokalaemia may potentiate phenothiazine-induced cardiotoxicity.

Clonidine may decrease the antipsychotic activity of phenothiazines.

Methyldopa increases the risk of extrapyramidal side effects with phenothiazines.

The hypotensive effect of calcium channel blockers is enhanced by concurrent use of antipsychotic drugs.

Phenothiazines may predispose to metrizamide-induced seizures.

Concurrent use of phenothiazines and amphetamine/anorectic agents may produce antagonistic pharmacological effects.

Concurrent use of phenothiazines and cocaine may increase the risk of acute dystonia.

There have been rare reports of acute Parkinsonism when an SSRI has been used in combination with a phenothiazine.

Phenothiazines may impair the action of anti-convulsants. Serum levels of phenytoin may be increased or decreased.

Phenothiazines inhibit glucose uptake into cells, and hence may affect the interpretation of PET studies using labelled glucose.

4.6 Pregnancy and lactation

Use in pregnancy: The safety for the use of this drug during pregnancy has not been established; therefore, the possible hazards should be weighed against the potential benefits when administering this drug to pregnant patients.

Nursing mothers: Breast feeding is not recommended during treatment with depot fluphenazines, owing to the possibility that fluphenazine is excreted in the breast milk.

4.7 Effects on ability to drive and use machines

The use of this drug may impair the mental and physical abilities required for driving a car or operating heavy machinery.

4.8 Undesirable effects

Side effects: Acute dystonic reactions occur infrequently, as a rule within the first 24-48 hours, although delayed reactions may occur. In susceptible individuals they may occur after only small doses. These may include such dramatic manifestations as oculogyric crises and opisthotonos. They are rapidly relieved by intravenous administration of an anti-parkinsonian agent such as procyclidine.

Parkinsonian-like states may occur particularly between the second and fifth days after each injection, but often decrease with subsequent injection. These reactions may be reduced by using smaller doses more frequently, or by the concomitant use of anti-parkinsonian drugs such as benzhexol, benztropine or procyclidine. Anti-parkinsonian drugs should not be prescribed routinely, because of the possible risks of aggravating anti-cholinergic side effects or precipitating toxic confusional states, or of impairing therapeutic efficacy.

With careful monitoring of the dose the number of patients requiring anti-parkinsonian drugs can be minimised.

Tardive Dyskinesia: As with all antipsychotic agents, tardive dyskinesia may appear in some patients on long term therapy or may occur after drug therapy has been discontinued. The risk seems to be greater in elderly patients on high dose therapy, especially females. The symptoms are persistent and in some patients appear to be irreversible.

The syndrome is characterised by rhythmical involuntary movements of the tongue, face, mouth or jaw (eg. protrusion of tongue, puffing of cheeks, puckering of mouth, chewing movements). Sometimes these may be accompanied by involuntary movements of the extremities. There is no known effective treatment for tardive dyskinesia: anti-parkinsonian agents usually do not alleviate the symptoms of this syndrome. It is suggested that all antipsychotic agents be discontinued if these symptoms appear. Should it be necessary to reinstitute treatment, or increase the dosage of the agent, or switch to a different antipsychotic agent, the syndrome may be masked. It has been reported that fine vermicular movements of the tongue may be an early sign of the syndrome and if the medication is stopped at that time, the syndrome may not develop.

Other Undesirable Effects: As with other phenothiazines, drowsiness, lethargy, blurred vision, dryness of the mouth, constipation, urinary hesitancy or incontinence, mild hypotension, impairment of judgement and mental skills, and epileptiform attacks are occasionally seen.

Headache, nasal congestion, vomiting, agitation, excitement and insomnia, and hyponatraemia have also been observed during phenothiazine therapy.

Blood dyscrasias have rarely been reported with phenothiazine derivatives. Blood counts should be performed if the patient develops signs of persistent infection. Transient leucopenia and thrombocytopenia have been reported. Antinuclear antibodies and SLE have been reported very rarely.

Jaundice has rarely been reported. Transient abnormalities of liver function tests may occur in the absence of jaundice.

A transient rise in serum cholesterol has been reported rarely in patients on oral fluphenazine.

Abnormal skin pigmentation and lens opacities have sometimes been seen following long-term administration of high doses of phenothiazines.

Phenothiazines are known to cause photosensitivity reactions but this has not been reported for fluphenazine. Skin rashes, hypersensitivity and anaphylactic reactions have occasionally been reported.

Elderly patients may be more susceptible to the sedative and hypotensive effects.

The effects of phenothiazines on the heart are dose-related. ECG changes with prolongation of the QT interval and T-Wave changes have been reported commonly in patients treated with moderate to high dosage; they have been reported to precede serious arrhythmias, including ventricular tachycardia and fibrillation, which have also occurred after overdosage. Sudden, unexpected and unexplained deaths have been reported in hospitalised psychotic patients receiving phenothiazines.

Phenothiazines may impair body temperature regulation. Elderly or hypothyroid patients may be particularly susceptible to hypothermia. The hazard of hyperpyrexia may be increased by especially hot or humid weather, or by drugs such as anti-parkinsonian agents, which impair sweating.

Rare occurrences of neuroleptic malignant syndrome (NMS) have been reported in patients on neuroleptic therapy. The syndrome is characterised by hyperthermia, together with some or all of the following: muscular rigidity, autonomic instability (labile blood pressure, tachycardia, diaphoresis), akinesia, and altered consciousness, sometimes progressing to stupor or coma. Leucocytosis, elevated CPK, liver function abnormalities, and acute renal failure may also occur. Neuroleptic therapy should be discontinued immediately and vigorous symptomatic treatment implemented since the syndrome is potentially fatal.

Hormonal effects of phenothiazines include hyperprolactinaemia, which may cause galactorrhoea, gynaecomastia and oligomenorrhoea or amenorrhoea. Sexual function may be impaired, and false results may be observed with pregnancy tests. Syndrome of inappropriate anti-diuretic hormone secretion has also been observed.

Oedema has been reported with phenothiazine medication.

4.9 Overdose
Overdosage should be treated symptomatically and supportively, extrapyramidal reactions will respond to oral or parenteral anti-parkinsonian drugs such as procyclidine or benztropine. In cases of severe hypotension, all procedures for the management of circulatory shock should be instituted, eg. vasoconstrictors and/or intravenous fluids. However, only the vasoconstrictors metaraminol or noradrenaline should be used, as adrenaline may further lower the blood pressure through interaction with the phenothiazine.

5. PHARMACOLOGICAL PROPERTIES

5.1 Pharmacodynamic properties
Fluphenazine decanoate is an ester of the potent neuroleptic fluphenazine, a phenothiazine derivative of the piperazine type. The ester is slowly absorbed from the intramuscular site of injection and is then hydrolysed in the plasma to the active therapeutic agent, fluphenazine.

Extrapyramidal reactions are not uncommon, but fluphenazine does not have marked sedative or hypotensive properties.

5.2 Pharmacokinetic properties
Plasma level profiles of fluphenazine following intramuscular injection have shown half-lives of plasma clearance ranging from 2.5 - 16 weeks, emphasising the importance of adjusting dose and interval to the individual requirements of each patient. The slow decline of plasma levels in most patients means that a reasonably stable plasma level can usually be achieved with injections spaced at 2 - 4 week intervals.

5.3 Preclinical safety data
Not applicable.

6. PHARMACEUTICAL PARTICULARS

6.1 List of excipients
Benzyl alcohol and sesame oil.

6.2 Incompatibilities
None.

6.3 Shelf life
24 months.

6.4 Special precautions for storage
Store below 25°C. Protect from direct sunlight.

6.5 Nature and contents of container
Clear type I glass ampoules containing 0.5ml (packs of 10) and 1ml

(packs of 5).

6.6 Instructions for use and handling
For intramuscular administration only.

7. MARKETING AUTHORISATION HOLDER
Sanofi-Synthelabo
PO Box 597
Guildford
Surrey

8. MARKETING AUTHORISATION NUMBER(S)
PL 11723/0104.

9. DATE OF FIRST AUTHORISATION/RENEWAL OF THE AUTHORISATION
23 September 2002.

10. DATE OF REVISION OF THE TEXT
September 2002.

Modecate Injection 25mg/ml

(sanofi-aventis)

1. NAME OF THE MEDICINAL PRODUCT
Modecate Injection 25mg/ml.

2. QUALITATIVE AND QUANTITATIVE COMPOSITION
The product contains Fluphenazine Decanoate BP 25mg/ml.

3. PHARMACEUTICAL FORM
Intramuscular injection for administration to human beings.

4. CLINICAL PARTICULARS

4.1 Therapeutic indications
For the treatment and maintenance of schizophrenic patients and those with paranoid psychoses.

While Modecate injection has been shown to be effective in acute states, it is particularly useful in the maintenance treatment of chronic patients who are unreliable at taking their oral medication, and also of those who do not absorb their oral phenothiazine adequately.

4.2 Posology and method of administration
Dosage and Administration

Adults

It is recommended that patients be stabilised on the injection in hospital.

Recommended dosage regimes for all indications:

A. Patients without previous exposure to a depot fluphenazine formulation:

Initially 0.5ml ie 12.5mg (0.25 ml ie 6.25mg for patients over 60) by deep intramuscular injection into the gluteal region.

The onset of action generally appears between 24 and 72 hours after injection and the effects of the drug on psychotic symptoms become significant within 48 to 96 hours. Subsequent injections and the dosage interval are determined in accordance with the patient's response. When administered as maintenance therapy, a single injection may be effective in controlling schizophrenic symptoms for up to four weeks or longer.

It is desirable to maintain as much flexibility in the dose as possible to achieve the best therapeutic response with the least side-effects; most patients are successfully maintained within the dose range 0.5ml (12.5mg) to 4.0ml (100mg) given at a dose interval of 2 to 5 weeks.

Patients previously maintained on oral fluphenazine:

It is not possible to predict the equivalent dose of depot formulation in view of the wide variability of individual response.

B. Patients previously maintained on depot fluphenazine:

Patients who have suffered a relapse following cessation of depot fluphenazine therapy may be restarted on the same dose, although the frequency of injections may need to be increased in the early weeks of treatment until satisfactory control is obtained.

Elderly:

Elderly patients may be particularly susceptible to extrapyramidal reactions, sedative and hypotensive effects. In order to avoid this, a reduced maintenance dosage may be required and a smaller initial dose (see above).

Children:

Not recommended for children.

* Where a smaller volume of injection is desirable, patients may be transferred directly to the equivalent dose of Modecate Concentrate injection on the basis that 1ml Modecate Concentrate injection is equivalent to 4ml Modecate injection.

Note

The dosage should not be increased without close supervision and it should be noted that there is a variability in individual response.

The response to antipsychotic drug treatment may be delayed. If drugs are withdrawn, recurrence of symptoms may not become apparent for several weeks or months.

Route of administration: Intramuscular.

4.3 Contraindications
The product is contraindicated in the following cases.

Comatose states

Marked cerebral atherosclerosis

Phaeochromocytoma

Renal failure

Liver failure

Severe cardiac insufficiency

Severely depressed states

Existing blood dyscrasias

History of hypersensitivity to any of the ingredients.

4.4 Special warnings and special precautions for use
Caution should be exercised with the following:

Liver disease

Renal impairment

Cardiac arrhythmias, cardiac disease

Thyrotoxicosis

Severe respiratory disease

Epilepsy, conditions predisposing to epilepsy (eg. alcohol withdrawal or brain damage)

Parkinson's disease

Patients who have shown hypersensitivity to other phenothiazines

Personal or family history of narrow angle glaucoma

In very hot weather

The elderly, particularly if frail or at risk of hypothermia

Hypothyroidism

Myasthenia gravis

Prostatic hypertrophy.

Patients with known or with a family history of cardiovascular disease should receive ECG screening, and monitoring and correction of electrolyte balance prior to treatment with fluphenazine.

Acute withdrawal symptoms, including nausea, vomiting, sweating and insomnia have been described after abrupt cessation of antipsychotic drugs. Recurrence of psychotic symptoms may also occur, and the emergence of involuntary movement disorders (such as akathisia, dystonia and dyskinesia) has been reported. Therefore, gradual withdrawal is advisable.

Psychotic patients on large doses of phenothiazines who are undergoing surgery should be watched carefully for hypotension. Reduced amounts of anaesthetics or central nervous system depressants may be necessary.

Fluphenazine should be used with caution in patients exposed to organophosphorus insecticides

Neuroleptic drugs elevate prolactin levels, and an increase in mammary neoplasms has been found in rodents after chronic administration. However, studies to date have not shown an association between chronic administration of these drugs and human mammary tumours.

As with any phenothiazine, the physician should be alert to the possibility of "silent pneumonias" in patients receiving long-term fluphenazine.

4.5 Interaction with other medicinal products and other forms of Interaction
The possibility should be borne in mind that phenothiazines may:

1 Increase the central nervous system depression produced by drugs such as alcohol, general anaesthetics, hypnotics, sedatives or strong analgesics.

2 Antagonise the action of adrenaline and other sympathomimetic agents and reverse the blood-pressure lowering effects of adrenergic-blocking agents such as guanethidine and clonidine.

3 Impair: the anti-parkinsonian effect of L-dopa; the effect of anti-convulsants; metabolism of tricyclic antidepressants; the control of diabetes.

4 Increase the effect of anticoagulants and antidepressants.

5 Interact with lithium.

Anticholinergic effects may be enhanced by anti-parkinsonian or other anticholinergic drugs.

Phenothiazines may enhance: the absorption of corticosteroids, digoxin, and neuromuscular blocking agents.

Fluphenazine is metabolised by P450 2D6 and is itself an inhibitor of this drug metabolising enzyme. The plasma concentrations and the effects of fluphenazine may therefore be increased and prolonged by drugs that are either the substrates or inhibitors of this P450 isoform, possibly resulting in severe hypotension, cardiac arrhythmias or CNS side effects. Examples of drugs which are substrates or inhibitors of cytochrome P450 2D6 include anti-arrhythmics, certain antidepressants including SSRIs and tricyclics, certain antipsychotics, β-blockers, protease inhibitors, opiates, cimetidine and ecstasy (MDMA). This list is not exhaustive.

Concomitant use of barbiturates with phenothiazines may result in reduced serum levels of both drugs, and an increased response if one of the drugs is withdrawn.

The effect of fluphenazine on the QT interval is likely to be potentiated by concurrent use of other drugs that also prolong the QT interval. Therefore, concurrent use of these drugs and fluphenazine is contraindicated. Examples include certain anti-arrhythmics, such as those of Class 1A (such as quinidine, disopyramide and procainamide) and Class III (such as amiodarone and sotalol), tricyclic antidepressants (such as amitriptyline); certain tetracyclic antidepressants (such as maprotiline); certain antipsychotic medications (such as phenothiazines and pimozide); certain antihistamines (such as terfenadine); lithium, quinine, pentamidine and sparfloxacin. This list is not exhaustive.

Electrolyte imbalance, particularly hypokalaemia, greatly increases the risk of QT interval prolongation. Therefore, concurrent use of drugs that cause electrolyte imbalance should be avoided.

Concurrent use of MAO inhibitors may increase sedation, constipation, dry mouth and hypotension.

Owing to their adrenolytic action, phenothiazines may reduce the pressor effect of adrenergic vasoconstrictors (i.e. ephedrine, phenylephrine).

Phenylpropanolamine has been reported to interact with phenothiazines and cause ventricular arrhythmias.

Concurrent use of phenothiazines and ACE inhibitors or angiotensin II antagonists may result in severe postural hypotension.

Concurrent use of thiazide diuretics may cause hypotension. Diuretic-induced hypokalaemia may potentiate phenothiazine-induced cardiotoxicity.

Clonidine may decrease the antipsychotic activity of phenothiazines.

Methyldopa increases the risk of extrapyramidal side effects with phenothiazines.

The hypotensive effect of calcium channel blockers is enhanced by concurrent use of antipsychotic drugs.

Phenothiazines may predispose to metrizamide-induced seizures.

Concurrent use of phenothiazines and amphetamine/anorectic agents may produce antagonistic pharmacological effects.

Concurrent use of phenothiazines and cocaine may increase the risk of acute dystonia.

There have been rare reports of acute Parkinsonism when an SSRI has been used in combination with a phenothiazine.

Phenothiazines may impair the action of anti-convulsants. Serum levels of phenytoin may be increased or decreased.

Phenothiazines inhibit glucose uptake into cells, and hence may affect the interpretation of PET studies using labelled glucose.

4.6 Pregnancy and lactation

Use in pregnancy: The safety for the use of this drug during pregnancy has not been established; therefore, the possible hazards should be weighed against the potential benefits when administering this drug to pregnant patients.

Nursing mothers: Breast feeding is not recommended during treatment with depot fluphenazines, owing to the possibility that fluphenazine may be excreted in the breast milk.

4.7 Effects on ability to drive and use machines

The use of this drug may impair the mental and physical abilities required for driving a car or operating heavy machinery.

4.8 Undesirable effects

Side Effects: Acute dystonic reactions occur infrequently, as a rule within the first 24-48 hours, although delayed reactions may occur. In susceptible individuals they may occur after only small doses. These may include such dramatic manifestations as oculogyric crises and opisthotonos. They are rapidly relieved by intravenous administration of an anti-parkinsonian agent such as procyclidine.

Parkinsonian-like states may occur particularly between the second and fifth days after each injection, but often decrease with subsequent injection. These reactions may be reduced by using smaller doses more frequently, or by the concomitant use of anti-parkinsonian drugs such as benzhexol, benztropine or procyclidine. Anti-parkinsonian drugs should not be prescribed routinely, because of the possible risks of aggravating anti-cholinergic side effects or precipitating toxic confusional states, or of impairing therapeutic efficacy.

With careful monitoring of the dose the number of patients requiring anti-parkinsonian drugs can be minimised.

Tardive Dyskinesia: As with all antipsychotic agents, tardive dyskinesia may appear in some patients on long term therapy or may occur after drug therapy has been discontinued. The risk seems to be greater in elderly patients on high dose therapy, especially females. The symptoms are persistent and in some patients appear to be irreversible. The syndrome is characterised by rhythmical involuntary movements of the tongue, face, mouth or jaw (eg protrusion of tongue, puffing of cheeks, puckering of mouth, chewing movements). Sometimes these may be accompanied by involuntary movements of the extremities. There is no known effective treatment for tardive dyskinesia: anti-parkinsonian agents usually do not alleviate the symptoms of this syndrome. It is suggested that all antipsychotic agents be discontinued if these symptoms appear. Should it be necessary to reinstitute treatment, or increase the dosage of the agent, or switch to a different antipsychotic agent, the syndrome may be masked. It has been reported that fine vermicular movements of the tongue may be an early sign of the syndrome and if the medication is stopped at that time, the syndrome may not develop.

Other Undesirable Effects: As with other phenothiazines, drowsiness, lethargy, blurred vision, dryness of the mouth, constipation, urinary hesitancy or incontinence, mild hypotension, impairment of judgement and mental skills, and epileptiform attacks are occasionally seen.

Headache, nasal congestion, vomiting, agitation, excitement, insomnia and hyponatraemia have also been observed during phenothiazine therapy.

Blood dyscrasias have rarely been reported with phenothiazine derivatives. Blood counts should be performed if the patient develops signs of persistent infection. Transient leucopenia and thrombocytopenia have been reported. Antinuclear antibodies and SLE have been reported very rarely.

Jaundice has rarely been reported. Transient abnormalities of liver function tests may occur in the absence of jaundice.

A transient rise in serum cholesterol has been reported rarely in patients on oral fluphenazine.

Abnormal skin pigmentation and lens opacities have sometimes been seen following long-term administration of high doses of phenothiazines.

Phenothiazines are known to cause photosensitivity reactions but this has not been reported for fluphenazine. Skin rashes, hypersensitivity and anaphylactic reactions have occasionally been reported.

Elderly patients may be more susceptible to the sedative and hypotensive effects.

The effects of phenothiazines on the heart are dose-related. ECG changes with prolongation of the QT interval and T-Wave changes have been reported commonly in patients treated with moderate to high dosage; they have been reported to precede serious arrhythmias, including ventricular tachycardia and fibrillation, which have also occurred after overdosage. Sudden, unexpected and unexplained deaths have been reported in hospitalised psychotic patients receiving phenothiazines.

Phenothiazines may impair body temperature regulation. Elderly or hypothyroid patients may be particularly susceptible to hypothermia. The hazard of hyperpyrexia may be increased by especially hot or humid weather, or by drugs such as anti-parkinsonian agents, which impair sweating.

Rare occurrences of neuroleptic malignant syndrome (NMS) have been reported in patients on neuroleptic therapy. The syndrome is characterised by hyperthermia, together with some or all of the following: muscular rigidity, autonomic instability (labile blood pressure, tachycardia, diaphoresis), akinesia, and altered consciousness, sometimes progressing to stupor or coma. Leucocytosis, elevated CPK, liver function abnormalities, and acute renal failure may also occur. Neuroleptic therapy should be discontinued immediately and vigorous symptomatic treatment implemented since the syndrome is potentially fatal.

Hormonal effects of phenothiazines include hyperprolactinaemia, which may cause galactorrhoea, gynaecomastia and oligomenorrhoea or amenorrhoea. Sexual function may be impaired, and false results may be observed with pregnancy tests. Syndrome of inappropriate anti-diuretic hormone secretion has also been observed.

Oedema has been reported with phenothiazine medication.

4.9 Overdose

Overdosage should be treated symptomatically and supportively, extrapyramidal reactions will respond to oral or parenteral anti-parkinsonian drugs such as procyclidine or benztropine. In cases of severe hypotension, all procedures for the management of circulatory shock should be instituted, eg vasoconstrictors and/or intravenous fluids. However, only the vasoconstrictors metaraminol or noradrenaline should be used, as adrenaline may further lower the blood pressure through interaction with the phenothiazine.

5. PHARMACOLOGICAL PROPERTIES

5.1 Pharmacodynamic properties

Fluphenazine decanoate is an ester of the potent neuroleptic fluphenazine, a phenothiazine derivative of the piperazine type. The ester is slowly absorbed from the intramuscular site of injection and is then hydrolysed in the plasma to the active therapeutic agent, fluphenazine.

Extrapyramidal reactions are not uncommon, but fluphenazine does not have marked sedative or hypotensive properties.

5.2 Pharmacokinetic properties

Plasma level profiles of fluphenazine following intramuscular injection have shown half-lives of plasma clearance ranging from 2.5-16 weeks, emphasising the importance of adjusting dose and interval to the individual requirements of each patient. The slow decline of plasma levels in most patients means that a reasonably stable plasma level can usually be achieved with injections spaced at 2-4 week intervals.

5.3 Preclinical safety data

Not applicable.

6. PHARMACEUTICAL PARTICULARS

6.1 List of excipients

Benzyl alcohol and sesame oil.

6.2 Incompatibilities

None.

6.3 Shelf life

24 months.

The inuse shelf life for the 10ml vial is 28 days.

6.4 Special precautions for storage

Store below 25°C. Protect from direct sunlight.

6.5 Nature and contents of container

Type I Glass ampoules containing 0.5, 1 and 2ml.

6.6 Instructions for use and handling

For intramuscular administration only.

7. MARKETING AUTHORISATION HOLDER

Sanofi-Synthelabo
PO Box 597
Guildford
Surrey

8. MARKETING AUTHORISATION NUMBER(S)

PL 11723/0103

9. DATE OF FIRST AUTHORISATION/RENEWAL OF THE AUTHORISATION

23 September 2002

10. DATE OF REVISION OF THE TEXT

September 2002

Legal category POM

Moditen Tablets 1mg

(sanofi-aventis)

1. NAME OF THE MEDICINAL PRODUCT

Moditen Tablets 1.0mg

2. QUALITATIVE AND QUANTITATIVE COMPOSITION

Each 1mg tablet contains Fluphenazine Hydrochloride BP 1.0mg.

3. PHARMACEUTICAL FORM

Round biconvex coated tablets.

4. CLINICAL PARTICULARS

4.1 Therapeutic indications

As an adjunct to the short-term management of anxiety, severe psychomotor agitation, excitement, violent or dangerously impulsive behaviour.

In schizophrenia; treatment of symptoms and prevention of relapse.

In other psychoses, especially paranoid.

In mania and hypomania.

4.2 Posology and method of administration

Adults

Anxiety and other non-psychotic behavioural disturbances: Initially 1mg twice daily rising to 2mg twice daily, if necessary, according to response.

Schizophrenia, mania, hypomania and other psychoses: Initially 2.5-10mg daily divided into 2 or 3 doses, depending on the severity and duration of symptoms, rising to 20mg daily, as necessary. Doses exceeding 20mg daily (10mg in the elderly) should be used with caution.

Elderly

Elderly patients may be extra susceptible to extrapyramidal reactions. Dosage at the lower end of the range is likely to be sufficient for elderly patients.

Children

Not recommended for children.

Note: The dosage should not be increased without close supervision and it should be noted that there is a variability in individual response.

The response to antipsychotic drug treatment may be delayed. If drugs are withdrawn, recurrence of symptoms may not become apparent for several weeks or months.

Method of Administration: Oral.

4.3 Contraindications

The product is contraindicated in the following cases:

Comatose states
Marked cerebral atherosclerosis
Phaeochromocytoma
Renal failure
Liver failure
Severe cardiac insufficiency
Severely depressed states
Existing blood dyscrasias
History of hypersensitivity to any of the ingredients.

4.4 Special warnings and special precautions for use
Caution should be exercised in patients with the following conditions:

Liver disease

Renal impairment

Cardiac arrhythmias, cardiac disease

Thyrotoxicosis

Severe respiratory disease

Epilepsy, conditions predisposing to epilepsy (e.g. alcohol withdrawal or brain damage)

Parkinson's disease

Patients who have shown hypersensitivity to other phenothiazines

Personal or family history of narrow angle glaucoma

In very hot weather

The elderly, particularly if frail or at risk of hypothermia

Hypothyroidism

Myasthenia gravis

Prostatic hypertrophy.

Patients with known or with a family history of cardiovascular disease should receive ECG screening, and monitoring and correction of electrolyte balance prior to treatment with fluphenazine.

Acute withdrawal symptoms, including nausea, vomiting, sweating and insomnia have been described after abrupt cessation of antipsychotic drugs. Recurrence of psychotic symptoms may also occur, and the emergence of involuntary movement disorders (such as akathisia, dystonia and dyskinesia) has been reported. Therefore, gradual withdrawal is advisable.

Psychotic patients on large doses of phenothiazines who are undergoing surgery should be watched carefully for hypotension. Reduced amounts of anaesthetics or central nervous system depressants may be necessary.

Fluphenazine should be used with caution in patients exposed to organophosphorus insecticides

Neuroleptic drugs elevate prolactin levels, and an increase in mammary neoplasms has been found in rodents after chronic administration. However, studies to date have not shown an association between chronic administration of these drugs and human mammary tumours.

As with any phenothiazine, the physician should be alert to the possibility of "silent pneumonias" in patients receiving long-term fluphenazine.

4.5 Interaction with other medicinal products and other forms of Interaction
The possibility should be borne in mind that phenothiazines may:

1 Increase the central nervous system depression produced by drugs such as alcohol, general anaesthetics, hypnotics, sedatives or strong analgesics.

2 Antagonise the action of adrenaline and other sympathomimetic agents and reverse the blood pressure-lowering effects of adrenergic-blocking agents such as guanethidine and clonidine.

3 Impair: The anti-parkinsonian effect of L-dopa; the effect of anti-convulsants; metabolism of tricyclic antidepressants; the control of diabetes.

4 Increase the effect of anticoagulants and antidepressants.

5 Interact with lithium.

Antacids may impair absorption.

Anticholinergic effects may be enhanced by anti-parkinsonian or other anticholinergic drugs.

Phenothiazines may enhance: the absorption of corticosteroids, digoxin, and neuromuscular blocking agents.

Fluphenazine is metabolised by P450 2D6 and is itself an inhibitor of this drug metabolising enzyme. The plasma concentrations and the effects of fluphenazine may therefore be increased and prolonged by drugs that are either the substrates or inhibitors of this P450 isoform, possibly resulting in severe hypotension, cardiac arrhythmias or CNS side effects. Examples of drugs which are substrates or inhibitors of cytochrome P450 2D6 include anti-arrhythmics, certain antidepressants including SSRIs and tricyclics, certain antipsychotics, β-blockers, protease inhibitors, opiates, cimetidine and ecstasy (MDMA). This list is not exhaustive.

Concomitant use of barbiturates with phenothiazines may result in reduced serum levels of both drugs, and an increased response if one of the drugs is withdrawn.

The effect of fluphenazine on the QT interval is likely to be potentiated by concurrent use of other drugs that also prolong the QT interval. Therefore, concurrent use of these drugs and fluphenazine is contraindicated. Examples include certain anti-arrhythmics, such as those of Class 1A (such as quinidine, disopyramide and procainamide) and Class III (such as amiodarone and sotalol), tricyclic antidepressants (such as amitriptyline); certain tetracyclic antidepressants (such as maprotiline); certain antipsychotic medications (such as phenothiazines and pimozide); certain antihistamines (such as terfenadine); lithium, quinine, pentamidine and sparfloxacin. This list is not exhaustive.

Electrolyte imbalance, particularly hypokalaemia, greatly increases the risk of QT interval prolongation. Therefore, concurrent use of drugs that cause electrolyte imbalance should be avoided.

Concurrent use of MAO inhibitors may increase sedation, constipation, dry mouth and hypotension.

Owing to their adrenolytic action, phenothiazines may reduce the pressor effect of adrenergic vasoconstrictors (i.e. ephedrine, phenylephrine).

Phenylpropanolamine has been reported to interact with phenothiazines and cause ventricular arrhythmias.

Concurrent use of phenothiazines and ACE inhibitors or angiotensin II antagonists may result in severe postural hypotension.

Concurrent use of thiazide diuretics may cause hypotension. Diuretic-induced hypokalaemia may potentiate phenothiazine-induced cardiotoxicity.

Clonidine may decrease the antipsychotic activity of phenothiazines.

Methyldopa increases the risk of extrapyramidal side effects with phenothiazines.

The hypotensive effect of calcium channel blockers is enhanced by concurrent use of antipsychotic drugs.

Phenothiazines may predispose to metrizamide-induced seizures.

Concurrent use of phenothiazines and amphetamine/anorectic agents may produce antagonistic pharmacological effects.

Concurrent use of phenothiazines and cocaine may increase the risk of acute dystonia.

There have been rare reports of acute Parkinsonism when an SSRI has been used in combination with a phenothiazine.

Phenothiazines may impair the action of anti-convulsants. Serum levels of phenytoin may be increased or decreased. Phenothiazines inhibit glucose uptake into cells, and hence may affect the interpretation of PET studies using labelled glucose.

4.6 Pregnancy and lactation
Use in pregnancy: The safety for the use of this drug during pregnancy has not been established; therefore, the possible hazards should be weighed against the potential benefits when administering this drug to pregnant patients.

Nursing mothers: Breast feeding is not recommended during treatment with fluphenazine, owing to the possibility that fluphenazine is excreted in the breast milk.

4.7 Effects on ability to drive and use machines
The use of this drug may impair the mental and physical abilities required for driving a car or operating heavy machinery.

4.8 Undesirable effects
Acute dystonic reactions occur infrequently, as a rule within the first 24-48 hours, although delayed reactions may occur. In susceptible individuals they may occur after only small doses. These may include such dramatic manifestations as oculogyric crises and opisthotonos. They are rapidly relieved by intravenous administration of an anti-parkinsonian agent such as procyclidine.

Parkinsonian-like states may occur. These reactions may be reduced by using smaller doses more frequently, or by the concomitant use of anti-parkinsonian drugs such as benzhexol, benztropine or procyclidine. Anti-parkinsonian drugs should not be prescribed routinely, because of the possible risks of aggravating anti-cholinergic side effects or precipitating toxic confusional states, or of impairing therapeutic efficacy.

With careful monitoring of the dose the number of patients requiring anti-parkinsonian drugs can be minimised.

Tardive dyskinesia: As with all antipsychotic agents, tardive dyskinesia may appear in some patients on long term therapy or may occur after drug therapy has been discontinued. The risk seems to be greater in elderly patients on high dose therapy, especially females. The symptoms are persistent and in some patients appear to be irreversible.

The syndrome is characterised by rhythmical involuntary movements of the tongue, face, mouth or jaw (eg protrusion of tongue, puffing of cheeks, puckering of mouth, chewing movements). Sometimes these may be accompanied by involuntary movements of the extremities. There is no known effective treatment for tardive dyskinesia: anti-parkinsonian agents usually do not alleviate the symptoms of this syndrome. It is suggested that all antipsychotic agents be discontinued if these symptoms appear. Should it be necessary to reinstitute treatment, or increase the dosage of the agent, or switch to a different antipsychotic agent, the syndrome may be masked. It has been reported that fine vermicular movements of the tongue may be an early sign of the syndrome and if the medication is stopped at that time, the syndrome may not develop.

Other Undesirable Effects: As with other phenothiazines, drowsiness, lethargy, blurred vision, dryness of the mouth, constipation, urinary hesitancy or incontinence, mild hypotension, impairment of judgement and mental skills and epileptiform attacks are occasionally seen.

Headache, nasal congestion, vomiting, agitation, excitement and insomnia, and hyponatraemia have also been observed during phenothiazine therapy.

Blood dyscrasias have rarely been reported with phenothiazine derivatives. Blood counts should be performed if the patient develops signs of persistent infection. Transient leucopenia and thrombocytopenia have been reported. Antinuclear antibodies and SLE have been reported very rarely.

Jaundice has rarely been reported. Transient abnormalities of liver function tests may occur in the absence of jaundice.

A transient rise in serum cholesterol has been reported rarely in patients on oral fluphenazine.

Abnormal skin pigmentation and lens opacities have sometimes been seen following long-term administration of high doses of phenothiazines.

Phenothiazines are known to cause photosensitivity reactions but this has not been reported for fluphenazine. Skin rashes, hypersensitivity and anaphylactic reactions have occasionally been reported.

Elderly patients may be more susceptible to the sedative and hypotensive effects.

The effects of phenothiazines on the heart are dose-related. ECG changes with prolongation of the QT interval and T-Wave changes have been reported commonly in patients treated with moderate to high dosage; they have been reported to precede serious arrhythmias, including ventricular tachycardia and fibrillation, which have also occurred after overdosage. Sudden, unexpected and unexplained deaths have been reported in hospitalised psychotic patients receiving phenothiazines.

Phenothiazines may impair body temperature regulation. Elderly or hypothyroid patients may be particularly susceptible to hypothermia. The hazard of hyperpyrexia may be increased by especially hot or humid weather, or by drugs such as anti-parkinsonian agents, which impair sweating.

Rare occurrences of neuroleptic malignant syndrome (NMS) have been reported in patients on neuroleptic therapy. The syndrome is characterised by hyperthermia, together with some or all of the following: muscular rigidity, autonomic instability (labile blood pressure, tachycardia, diaphoresis), akinesia, and altered consciousness, sometimes progressing to stupor or coma. Leucocytosis, elevated CPK, liver function abnormalities, and acute renal failure may also occur. Neuroleptic therapy should be discontinued immediately and vigorous symptomatic treatment implemented since the syndrome is potentially fatal.

Hormonal effects of phenothiazines include hyperprolactinaemia, which may cause galactorrhoea, gynaecomastia and oligomenorrhoea or amenorrhoea. Sexual function may be impaired, and false results may be observed with pregnancy tests. Syndrome of inappropriate anti-diuretic hormone secretion has also been observed.

Oedema has been reported with phenothiazine medication.

4.9 Overdose
Overdosage should be treated symptomatically and supportively. Extrapyramidal reactions will respond to oral or parenteral anti-parkinsonian drugs such as procyclidine or benztropine. In cases of severe hypotension, all procedures for the management of circulatory shock should be instituted e.g. vasoconstrictors and/or intravenous fluids. However, only the vasoconstrictors metaraminol or noradrenaline should be used, as adrenaline may further lower the blood pressure through interaction with the phenothiazine.

5. PHARMACOLOGICAL PROPERTIES

5.1 Pharmacodynamic properties
Fluphenazine hydrochloride is a salt of the potent neuroleptic fluphenazine, a phenothiazine derivative of the piperazine type. Extrapyramidal reactions are not uncommon but fluphenazine does not have marked sedative or hypotensive properties.

5.2 Pharmacokinetic properties
The plasma half-life of fluphenazine in patients given the hydrochloride by mouth has been shown to be approximately 14.7 hours.

5.3 Preclinical safety data
There are no preclinical data of relevance to the prescriber which are additional to that already included in other sections of the SPC.

6. PHARMACEUTICAL PARTICULARS

6.1 List of excipients
The core tablets also contain: Corn starch, lactose, talc, sodium benzoate, acacia powder, magnesium stearate. The coating solution is comprised of Shellac solution, castor oil, talc, polyvidone, chalk, sucrose, erythrosine, titanium dioxide, sodium benzoate, beeswax, carnauba wax, polysorbate and sorbic acid.

6.2 Incompatibilities
None.

6.3 Shelf life
60 months.

6.4 Special precautions for storage
Store below 25°C.

6.5 Nature and contents of container

Amber glass bottles containing 100 tablets with one of the following closures:

Wadless polypropylene cap; tin plate cap with pulpboard wad and waxed aluminium facing; black phenolic cap with composition cork wad and tinfoil / melinex lining; roll-on pilfer-proof aluminium cap with polyethylene liner; child-resistant polypropylene cap of the clic-lok type lined with expanded polyethylene with PVDC (saran) facing.

6.6 Instructions for use and handling

Not applicable.

7. MARKETING AUTHORISATION HOLDER

Sanofi-Synthelabo

PO Box 597

Guildford

Surrey

8. MARKETING AUTHORISATION NUMBER(S)

Moditen 1.0mg: PL 11723/0105

9. DATE OF FIRST AUTHORISATION/RENEWAL OF THE AUTHORISATION

2 November 1995

10. DATE OF REVISION OF THE TEXT

June 2004

Legal Category: POM

Modrasone Cream, Ointment

(Pliva Pharma Ltd)

1. NAME OF THE MEDICINAL PRODUCT

Modrasone Cream

Modrasone Ointment

2. QUALITATIVE AND QUANTITATIVE COMPOSITION

Alclometasone Dipropionate 0.05% w/w

3. PHARMACEUTICAL FORM

Cream/Ointment for topical use.

4. CLINICAL PARTICULARS

4.1 Therapeutic indications

Alclometasone dipropionate is a non-fluorinated topically active synthetic corticosteroid. Modrasone is indicated for the treatment of inflammatory and pruritic manifestations of corticosteroid responsive dermatoses.

4.2 Posology and method of administration

Adult and Children:

A thin film of Modrasone should be applied to the affected area two or three times daily or as directed by the physician. Massage gently into the skin until the medication disappears.

4.3 Contraindications

Hypersensitivity to any of the ingredients; rosacea; acne and perioral dermatitis; tuberculous and viral lesions of the skin, particularly Herpes Simplex; vaccinia; varicella.

Modrasone should not be used in fungal or bacterial skin infections.

4.4 Special warnings and special precautions for use

As with all topical steroids, long term continuous therapy should be avoided where possible, particularly in infants and children as adrenal suppression may occur even without occlusion. In infants the napkin may act as an occlusive dressing and thus increase absorption.

4.5 Interaction with other medicinal products and other forms of Interaction

None known.

4.6 Pregnancy and lactation

Topical administration of corticosteroids to pregnant animals can cause abnormalities in foetal development. The relevance of this finding to human beings has not been established; however, topical steroids should not be used extensively in pregnancy i.e. in large amounts or for long periods.

It is not known whether topical administration of corticosteroids could result in sufficient systemic absorption to produce detectable quantities in breast milk. Modrasone should be administered to nursing mothers only after careful consideration of the benefit/risk relationship.

4.7 Effects on ability to drive and use machines

Not applicable.

4.8 Undesirable effects

Excessive prolonged use may result in local atrophy of the skin, striae and superficial vascular dilation, particularly on the face.

4.9 Overdose

Excessive prolonged use of topical corticosteroids can suppress pituitary-adrenal function resulting in secondary adrenal insufficiency which is usually reversible. In such cases appropriate symptomatic treatment is indicated. In cases of chronic toxicity, corticosteroids should be withdrawn.

The steroid content is so low as to have little or no effect in the unlikely event of accidental oral ingestion.

5. PHARMACOLOGICAL PROPERTIES

5.1 Pharmacodynamic properties

Alclometasone dipropionate is a non-fluorinated, topically active synthetic corticosteroid. Alclometasone dipropionate suppresses local inflammation at doses producing minimal systemic effects. Studies have shown alclometasone dipropionate to be approximately 2/3 as potent as betamethasone valerate and 60 × as potent as hydrocortisone.

5.2 Pharmacokinetic properties

Not applicable in view of topical action and application.

5.3 Preclinical safety data

Modrasone appears to be a relatively non-toxic and non-irritating drug product that produces no unusual or unexpected teratologic effects in laboratory animals. A wide margin of safety was demonstrated in all species studied. Acute oral and intraperitoneal doses more than 3,000 times the proposed topical human dose were without any toxicologically significant effects.

6. PHARMACEUTICAL PARTICULARS

6.1 List of excipients

Cream:

Propylene Glycol Ph Eur

White Soft Paraffin BP

Cetostearyl Alcohol BP

Glyceryl stearate PEG 100 stearate

Polyoxyethylene (20) cetyl ether

Sodium dihydrogenium phosphate dihydrate

4-Chloro-M-Cresol BP

Phosphoric Acid Ph Eur

Purified Water Ph Eur

Ointment:

Hexylene glycol

Propylene glycol monostearate

White Beeswax BP

White Soft Paraffin BP

6.2 Incompatibilities

None known

6.3 Shelf life

Cream and Ointment: 60 months

6.4 Special precautions for storage

Store below 25°C

6.5 Nature and contents of container

Cream and Ointment: Aluminium tubes with white LDPE caps. Pack size: 50g

6.6 Instructions for use and handling

Not applicable

Administrative Data

7. MARKETING AUTHORISATION HOLDER

Schering-Plough Ltd

Shire Park

Welwyn Garden City

Hertfordshire

AL7 1TW

8. MARKETING AUTHORISATION NUMBER(S)

Cream: PL 0201/0060

Ointment: PL 0201/0061

9. DATE OF FIRST AUTHORISATION/RENEWAL OF THE AUTHORISATION

26 March 1995

10. DATE OF REVISION OF THE TEXT

5 March 1996

Legal Category POM

Distributed in the UK by: PLIVA Pharma Ltd., Vision House, Bedford Road, Petersfield,

Hampshire GU32 3QB

Moducren

(Merck Sharp & Dohme Limited)

1. NAME OF THE MEDICINAL PRODUCT

MODUCREN® Tablets

2. QUALITATIVE AND QUANTITATIVE COMPOSITION

'Moducren' contains the following active ingredients: 25 mg hydrochlorothiazide, 2.5 mg amiloride hydrochloride, and 10 mg timolol maleate.

3. PHARMACEUTICAL FORM

'Moducren' is supplied as light-blue coloured, square, compressed tablets with rounded corners; one side flat with bevelled edges and scored, the other side convex and imprinted 'MSD 17'.

4. CLINICAL PARTICULARS

4.1 Therapeutic indications

'Moducren' is indicated for the treatment of mild to moderate hypertension.

4.2 Posology and method of administration

1 to 2 tablets once a day, taken orally.

Use in the elderly: 'Moducren' has been shown to be as well tolerated in the elderly as in younger patients. The recommended starting dose is 1 tablet daily.

Children: Because the safety and efficacy of 'Moducren' have not been established in children, 'Moducren' is not recommended for paediatric use.

4.3 Contraindications

Patients with bronchial asthma or with a history of bronchial asthma, severe chronic obstructive pulmonary disease, sinus bradycardia, second- or third-degree AV block, overt cardiac failure, right ventricular failure secondary to pulmonary hypertension, significant cardiomegaly and cardiogenic shock. Hyperkalaemia (plasma potassium over 5.5 mmol/l). Anuria, acute and chronic renal insufficiency, severe progressive renal disease, and diabetic nephropathy. Patients with blood urea over 10 mmol/l or serum creatinine over 130 mmol/l or diabetes mellitus should not receive 'Moducren' without careful and frequent serum urea and serum electrolyte monitoring.

Anaesthetic agents causing myocardial depression, hypersensitivity to any component of 'Moducren' or other sulphonamide-derived drugs. Use with other potassium-conserving agents. Use with potassium-rich foods and potassium supplements except in severe and/or refractory cases of hypokalaemia when careful monitoring of the serum potassium level is necessary.

The packaging carries the warning: 'Do not take this medicine if you have a history of wheezing or asthma'.

See also *Children*, under 4.2 'Posology and method of administration'; *Breast-feeding mothers*, and *Pregnancy*, under 4.4 'Special warnings and precautions for use'.

4.4 Special warnings and special precautions for use

Congestive cardiac failure: Care should be exercised before and during treatment of patients with cardiomegaly or history of cardiac failure.

Cardiac arrhythmias: patients at risk of congestive heart failure should be carefully observed for bradycardia, AV block and respiratory distress. If congestive cardiac failure persists, 'Moducren' should be withdrawn. Beta-adrenergic blocking agents should be used with caution in patients with cerebrovascular insufficiency. If signs or symptoms suggesting reduced cerebral blood flow are observed, consideration should be given to discontinuing these agents.

Exacerbation of ischaemic heart disease following abrupt withdrawal: exacerbation of angina and, in some cases, myocardial infarction have occurred after abrupt withdrawal of beta-blocker therapy. Therefore, it is recommended that if 'Moducren' is to be withdrawn, dosage should be gradually reduced.

Elective or emergency surgery: 'Moducren' should also be gradually withdrawn prior to elective surgery of anginal patients. Agonists such as isoprenaline, dopamine, dobutamine or noradrenaline may be used to counter the effects of beta-blockade in emergency surgery.

Renal and hepatic disease and electrolyte disturbances: 'Moducren' should be used with caution in patients with renal or hepatic disease and in those patients in whom fluid and electrolyte balance is critical. When creatinine clearance falls below 30 ml/min, thiazide diuretics are ineffective. Azotaemia may be precipitated or increased by hydrochlorothiazide. Cumulative effects of the drug may develop in patients with impaired renal function. If increasing azotaemia and oliguria occur during treatment of renal disease, the diuretic should be discontinued. Metabolic or respiratory acidosis: acid-base balance should be monitored frequently in severely ill patients at risk of respiratory or metabolic acidosis.

Electrolyte and fluid balance: serum and urine electrolyte determinations should be made in patients vomiting excessively or receiving parenteral fluids. Dilutional hyponatraemia may occur in oedematous patients in hot weather, which calls for appropriate therapy; hypochloraemia requires specific treatment only under exceptional circumstances. Hyponatraemia, hypochloraemic alkalosis, hypokalaemia, hyperkalaemia or hypomagnesaemia may occur. If hyperkalaemia occurs, 'Moducren' should be discontinued immediately and, if necessary, active measures taken to reduce the plasma potassium level. The degree of thiazide-induced hypomagnesaemia is reduced.

Diabetes mellitus, hypoglycaemia: 'Moducren' should be given with caution to diabetic patients and to patients subject to spontaneous hypoglycaemia, as the symptoms and signs of acute hypoglycaemia may be masked. To minimise the risk of hyperkalaemia in diabetic or suspected diabetic patients, the status of the renal function should be known before initiating therapy with 'Moducren'. Therapy should be discontinued at least three days prior to glucose tolerance testing. Thiazide therapy may impair glucose tolerance. Dosage adjustments of antidiabetic agents, including insulin, may be required.

Skin and sensitivity reactions: there have been reports of skin rashes and/or dry eyes associated with the use of beta-adrenergic blocking drugs. The reported incidence is small and in most cases the symptoms have cleared when treatment was withdrawn. Discontinuation of the drug should be considered if any such reaction is not otherwise explicable. Withdrawal should be gradual. Sensitivity reactions to 'Moducren' may occur with or without a history of allergy or bronchial asthma. Possible exacerbation or activation of systemic lupus erythematosus reactions have been reported with thiazide diuretics.

Metabolic and endocrine: beta-adrenergic blocking agents may mask the signs of hyperthyroidism. Patients suspected of developing thyrotoxicosis should be managed carefully to avoid abrupt withdrawal of beta blockade which might precipitate a thyroid storm. Hypercalcaemia and hypophosphataemia have been reported with thiazide diuretics. 'Moducren' should be discontinued in patients prior to testing for parathyroid function. Increases in cholesterol and triglyceride levels may be associated with thiazide diuretic therapy. Hyperuricaemia or acute gout may be precipitated in some patients.

Musculoskeletal: beta-blockers have been reported to induce myasthenic symptoms such as diplopia, ptosis, and generalised weakness.

4.5 Interaction with other medicinal products and other forms of Interaction

'Moducren' may potentiate other antihypertensive agents, such as reserpine or guanethidine. The antihypertensive effect of beta-blockers may be reduced by NSAIDs. NSAIDs may reduce the diuretic, natriuretic and antihypertensive effects of diuretics. The effect of 'Moducren' may be enhanced in the post-sympathectomy patient.

Oral calcium antagonists may be combined with 'Moducren' only when heart function is normal. When the heart function is impaired, combination of beta-blockers with dihydropyridine derivatives such as nifedipine may lead to hypotension; and combination with verapamil or diltiazem may cause AV conduction disturbances or left ventricular failure. Intravenous calcium antagonists and 'Moducren' should only be used together with caution. Concomitant beta-blockers and digitalis with either diltiazem or verapamil may further prolong the AV conduction time.

When 'Moducren' (which contains amiloride HCl) is administered concomitantly with an angiotensin-converting enzyme inhibitor, the risk of hyperkalaemia may be increased. Therefore, if concomitant use of these agents is indicated because of demonstrated hypokalaemia, they should be used with caution and with frequent monitoring of serum potassium.

When given concomitantly, the following drugs may interact with thiazide diuretics:

Alcohol, barbiturates or narcotics: co-administration may potentiate orthostatic hypotension.

Oral and parenteral antidiabetic drugs may require adjustment of dosage with concurrent use.

Corticosteroids or ACTH may intensify any thiazide-induced electrolyte depletion, particularly hypokalaemia.

Pressor amines such as adrenaline may show decreased arterial responsiveness when used with 'Moducren', but this reaction is not enough to preclude their therapeutic usefulness.

Non-depolarising muscle relaxants such as tubocurarine may possibly interact with 'Moducren' to increase muscle relaxation. Lithium should not generally be given with diuretics, because they reduce its renal clearance and add a high risk of *lithium* toxicity.

Drug/laboratory test interactions: because thiazides may affect calcium metabolism, 'Moducren' may interfere with tests for parathyroid function (see 'Special warnings and precautions for use').

4.6 Pregnancy and lactation

Breast-feeding mothers: Thiazides appear in breast milk, but it is not known whether timolol maleate or amiloride are also excreted. If the use of 'Moducren' is deemed essential, the mother should stop breast-feeding.

Pregnancy: 'Moducren' is not recommended for use during pregnancy. The use of any drug in women of child-bearing age requires that the anticipated benefit be weighed against possible hazards, which include fetal or neonatal jaundice, thrombocytopenia, and possibly other adverse reactions which have occurred in the adult.

4.7 Effects on ability to drive and use machines

None stated.

4.8 Undesirable effects

'Moducren' is usually well tolerated, with significant side effects only infrequently reported.

Most common effects experienced are dizziness, asthenia, fatigue, and bradycardia. Other clinical adverse reactions reported are:

Body as a whole: asthenia, fatigue, headache.

Cardiovascular: bradycardia, peripheral vascular disorder (cold extremities), hypotension, syncope, arrhythmia, angina pectoris.

Respiratory: dyspnoea, wheezing.

Digestive: nausea, dyspepsia, constipation, diarrhoea, vomiting, GI pain, anorexia, thirst, dry mouth, stomatitis.

Urogenital: impotence.

Nervous: dizziness, vertigo, paraesthesiae, tremors.

Integumentary: sweating.

Musculoskeletal: muscle cramps.

Psychiatric: insomnia, nervousness, depression, somnolence, abnormal dreaming, sleep disturbance.

Special senses: visual disturbances.

Other side effects that have been reported with the individual components may be considered as potential adverse effects of 'Moducren'.

Amiloride-related effects

Digestive: abnormal liver function, activation or probable pre-existing peptic ulcer, jaundice.

Integumentary: dry mouth, alopecia.

Haematological: aplastic anaemia, neutropenia.

Cardiovascular: one patient with partial heart block developed complete heart block, palpitation.

Psychiatric: decreased libido.

Respiratory: cough.

Special senses: tinnitus, increased intra-ocular pressure.

Urogenital: polyuria, urinary frequency, bladder spasm.

Hydrochlorothiazide-related effects

Body as a whole: anaphylactic reaction, fever.

Cardiovascular: necrotising angiitis (vasculitis, cutaneous vasculitis).

Digestive: jaundice (intrahepatic cholestatic jaundice), pancreatitis, cramping, gastric irritation.

Integumentary: photosensitivity.

Endocrine/metabolic: glycosuria, hypoglycaemia, hyperglycaemia, hyperuricaemia, sialadenitis, urticaria.

Psychiatric: restlessness.

Renal: renal dysfunction, interstitial nephritis, renal failure.

Respiratory: respiratory distresses including, pneumonitis, pulmonary oedema.

Special senses: transient blurred vision, xanthopsia.

Haematological: agranulocytosis, aplastic anaemia, haemolytic anaemia, leucopenia, purpura, thrombocytopenia.

Timolol maleate-related effects

Body as a whole: chest pain, extremity pain, decreased exercise tolerance, weight loss.

Cardiovascular: cardiac arrest, cerebral vascular accident, palpitation, second- or third-degree AV block, sino-atrial block, oedema and pulmonary oedema, cardiac failure, Raynaud's phenomenon, claudication, worsening of arterial insufficiency and angina pectoris, vasodilatation.

Digestive: diarrhoea, hepatomegaly.

Endocrine: hypoglycaemia, hyperglycaemia.

Integumentary: rash, pruritus, skin irritation, increased pigmentation, exfoliative dermatitis (one case).

Musculoskeletal: arthralgia.

Nervous system: local weakness.

Psychiatric: diminished concentration, hallucination, decreased libido. *Haematological:* non-thrombocytopenic purpura. *Respiratory*: bronchial spasm, rales, cough.

Special senses: tinnitus, visual disturbances, diplopia, ptosis, eye irritation, dry eyes.

Urogenital: micturition difficulties.

Clinical laboratory tests: Clinically important changes in standard laboratory tests associated with timolol maleate are rare. Slight increases in blood urea, serum potassium and serum uric acid, and slight decreases in haemoglobin and haematocrit occurred but were not progressive or associated with clinical manifestations.

4.9 Overdose

No specific data are available regarding symptoms or the treatment of overdosage with 'Moducren', and no antidote is available. Little is known about dialysability of its components; a study of patients with renal failure showed that timolol did not readily dialyse. Treatment is symptomatic and supportive.

Therapy with 'Moducren' should be stopped and emesis and/or gastric lavage induced.

Hydrochlorothiazide and amiloride hydrochloride: The signs and symptoms most likely are dehydration and electrolyte imbalance. If hyperkalaemia occurs, active measures should be taken to reduce plasma potassium levels.

Timolol maleate: The most common signs and symptoms to be expected following overdosage with a beta-adrenergic receptor blocking agent are symptomatic bradycardia, hypotension, bronchospasm, acute cardiac failure and heart block.

If overdosage occurs, the following measures are recommended:

1. *Gastric lavage.*

2. *For symptomatic bradycardia:* atropine sulphate, 0.25 to 2 mg intravenously, should be used to induce vagal blockade. If bradycardia persists, intravenous isoprenaline hydrochloride should be administered cautiously. In refractory cases, the use of a cardiac pacemaker may be considered.

3. *For hypotension:* a sympathomimetic pressor agent such as dopamine, dobutamine or noradrenaline should be used. In refractory cases, the use of glucagon has been reported to be useful.

4. *For bronchospasm:* isoprenaline hydrochloride should be used. Additional therapy with aminophylline may be considered.

5. *For acute cardiac failure:* conventional therapy with digitalis, diuretics, and oxygen should be instituted immediately. In refractory cases, the use of intravenous aminophylline is suggested. This may be followed, if necessary, by glucagon which has been reported useful.

6. *For heart block:* isoprenaline hydrochloride or a transvenous cardiac pacemaker should be used.

The components of 'Moducren' have, respectively, plasma half-lives of: hydrochlorothiazide at 5.6 hours with a longer terminal phase; amiloride at about 6 hours; and timolol at about 4 hours.

5. PHARMACOLOGICAL PROPERTIES

5.1 Pharmacodynamic properties

In the doses studied, 'Moducren' was more effective in reducing blood pressure than was timolol maleate alone or a combination of hydrochlorothiazide and amiloride hydrochloride. 'Moducren' was shown to be well tolerated, and effective in lowering blood pressure in a large proportion of the patients studied.

5.2 Pharmacokinetic properties

The three components of 'Moducren' have similar dosage schedules, and study data have shown that the bioavailabilities of each component are the same when given singly as when the three agents are given together in the combination tablet.

Amiloride hydrochloride is not bound to plasma proteins and has a half-life of about 6-9 hours. It is excreted unchanged by the kidneys.

Hydrochlorothiazide has been estimated to have a plasma half-life of about 5.6 hours with a subsequent longer terminal phase; its biological half-life is up to about 15 hours. It is excreted unchanged in the urine.

Peak plasma concentrations of timolol maleate occur about 1 to 2 hours after a dose, with a plasma half-life of about 4 hours. It is extensively metabolised in the liver, the metabolites being excreted in the urine together with some unchanged timolol. Protein binding is reported to be low.

5.3 Preclinical safety data

No further information provided.

6. PHARMACEUTICAL PARTICULARS

6.1 List of excipients

'Moducren' Tablets contain the following inactive ingredients:

Indigo Carmine E132

Microcrystalline Cellulose

Pregelatinised Maize Starch

Magnesium Stearate

6.2 Incompatibilities

None known.

6.3 Shelf life

Opacified PVC blister packs of 28 tablets - 36 months.

Amber glass bottles, with Ropp or Jay-Cap seals, of 100 tablets - 36 months.

Aluminum/polyethylene strips of 14 tablets - 60 months.

6.4 Special precautions for storage

Store in a dry place below 25°C, protected from light.

6.5 Nature and contents of container

Opacified PVC blisters lidded with aluminum foil, in packs of 28 tablets.

Amber glass bottles, with Ropp or Jay-Cap seals, in packs of 100 tablets.

Aluminum/polyethylene strip packaging in packs of 14 tablets.

6.6 Instructions for use and handling

None.

7. MARKETING AUTHORISATION HOLDER

Merck Sharp & Dohme Limited

Hertford Road, Hoddesdon, Hertfordshire EN11 9BU

8. MARKETING AUTHORISATION NUMBER(S)

PL 0025/0141

9. DATE OF FIRST AUTHORISATION/RENEWAL OF THE AUTHORISATION

Renewal date 16 September 1999

Date of grant April 1980

10. DATE OF REVISION OF THE TEXT

February 2000

LEGAL CATEGORY

POM

® denotes registered trademark of Merck & Co., Inc., Whitehouse Station, NJ, USA.

SPC.MUE.024.GB(MUC-001).

24 February 2000

Moduretic

(Bristol-Myers Squibb Pharmaceuticals Ltd)

1. NAME OF THE MEDICINAL PRODUCT
MODURETIC® Tablets

2. QUALITATIVE AND QUANTITATIVE COMPOSITION
Amiloride hydrochloride equivalent to 5 mg anhydrous amiloride hydrochloride and 50 mg hydrochlorothiazide.

3. PHARMACEUTICAL FORM
Tablets.

Peach-coloured, half-scored, diamond shaped tablet, marked 'MSD 917'.

4. CLINICAL PARTICULARS
4.1 Therapeutic indications
Potassium-conserving diuretic and antihypertensive.

'Moduretic' is indicated in patients with: hypertension, congestive heart failure, hepatic cirrhosis with ascites and oedema. In hypertension, 'Moduretic' may be used alone or in conjunction with other antihypertensive agents.

'Moduretic' is intended for the treatment of patients in whom potassium depletion might be suspected or anticipated. The presence of amiloride hydrochloride minimises the likelihood of potassium loss during vigorous diuresis for long-term maintenance therapy. The combination is thus indicated especially in conditions where potassium balance is particularly important.

4.2 Posology and method of administration
Hypertension: Initially half a 'Moduretic' tablet given once a day. If necessary, increase to one 'Moduretic' tablet given once a day or in divided doses.

Congestive heart failure: Initially half a 'Moduretic' tablet a day, subsequently adjusted if required, but not exceeding two 'Moduretic' tablets a day. Optimal dosage is determined by the diuretic response and the plasma potassium level. Once an initial diuresis has been achieved, reduction in dosage may be attempted for maintenance therapy. Maintenance therapy may be on an intermittent basis.

Hepatic cirrhosis with ascites: Initiate therapy with a low dose. A single daily dose of one 'Moduretic' tablet may be increased gradually until there is an effective diuresis. Dosage should not exceed two 'Moduretic' tablets a day. Maintenance dosages may be lower than those required to initiate diuresis; dosage reduction should therefore be attempted when the patient's weight is stabilised. A gradual weight reduction is especially desirable in cirrhotic patients to reduce the likelihood of untoward reactions associated with diuretic therapy.

Paediatric use: 'Moduretic' is not recommended for children under 18 years as safety and efficacy have not been established (see 4.3 'Contra-indications').

Use in the elderly: Particular caution is needed in the elderly because of their susceptibility to electrolyte imbalance; the dosage should be carefully adjusted to renal function and clinical response.

4.3 Contraindications
Hyperkalaemia (plasma potassium over 5.5 mmol/l); other potassium-conserving diuretics. Potassium supplements or potassium-rich food (except in severe and/or refractory cases of hypokalaemia under careful monitoring); concomitant use with spironolactone or triamterene; anuria; acute renal failure, severe progressive renal disease, severe hepatic failure, precoma associated with hepatic cirrhosis, Addison's disease, hypercalcaemia, concurrent lithium therapy, diabetic nephropathy; patients with blood urea over 10 mmol/l, patients with diabetes mellitus, or those with serum creatinine over 130 μmol/l in whom serum electrolyte and blood urea levels cannot be monitored carefully and frequently. Prior hypersensitivity to amiloride hydrochloride, hydrochlorothiazide or other sulphonamide-derived drugs. Because the safety of amiloride hydrochloride for use in children has not been established, 'Moduretic' is not recommended for children under 18 years of age. For use in pregnancy and breast-feeding mothers, 4.6 'Pregnancy and lactation'.

4.4 Special warnings and special precautions for use
Hyperkalaemia has been observed in patients receiving amiloride hydrochloride, either alone or with other diuretics, particularly in the aged or in hospital patients with hepatic cirrhosis or congestive heart failure with renal involvement, who were seriously ill, or were undergoing vigorous diuretic therapy. Such patients should be carefully observed for clinical, laboratory, and ECG evidence of hyperkalaemia (not always associated with an abnormal ECG).

Neither potassium supplements nor a potassium-rich diet should be used with 'Moduretic' except under careful monitoring in severe and/or refractory cases of hypokalaemia.

Some deaths have been reported in this group of patients.

Treatment of hyperkalaemia: Should hyperkalaemia develop, discontinue treatment immediately and, if necessary, take active measures to reduce the plasma potassium to normal.

Impaired renal function: Renal function should be monitored because the use of 'Moduretic' in impaired renal function may result in the rapid development of hyperkalaemia. Thiazide diuretics become ineffective when creatinine levels fall below 30 ml/min.

Electrolyte imbalance: Although the likelihood of electrolyte imbalance is reduced by 'Moduretic', careful check should be kept for such signs of fluid and electrolyte imbalance as hyponatraemia, hypochloraemic alkalosis, hypokalaemia and hypomagnesaemia. It is particularly important to make serum and urine electrolyte determinations when the patient is vomiting excessively or receiving parenteral fluids. Warning signs or symptoms of fluid or electrolyte imbalance include: dryness of the mouth, weakness, lethargy, drowsiness, restlessness, seizures, confusion, muscle pains or cramps, muscular fatigue, hypotension, oliguria, tachycardia, and gastro-intestinal disturbances such as nausea and vomiting.

Hypokalaemia may develop, especially as a result of brisk diuresis, after prolonged therapy or when severe cirrhosis is present. Hypokalaemia can sensitise or exaggerate the response of the heart to the toxic effects of digitalis (e.g. increased ventricular irritability).

Diuretic-induced hyponatraemia is usually mild and asymptomatic. It may become severe and symptomatic in a few patients who will then require immediate attention and appropriate treatment.

Thiazides may decrease urinary calcium excretion. Thiazides may cause intermittent and slight elevation of serum calcium in the absence of known disorders of calcium metabolism. Therapy should be discontinued before carrying out tests for parathyroid function.

Azotaemia may be precipitated or increased by hydrochlorothiazide. Cumulative effects of the drug may develop in patients with impaired renal function. If increasing azotaemia and oliguria develop during treatment of renal disease, 'Moduretic' should be discontinued.

Hepatic disease: Thiazides should be used with caution in patients with impaired hepatic function or progressive liver disease (see 4.3 'Contra-indications'), since minor alterations of fluid and electrolyte balance may precipitate hepatic coma.

Metabolic*:* Hyperuricaemia may occur, or gout may be precipitated or aggravated, in certain patients receiving thiazides. Thiazides may impair glucose tolerance. Diabetes mellitus may be precipitated or aggravated by therapy with 'Moduretic' (see 4.3 'Contra-indications'). Dosage adjustment of antidiabetic agents, including insulin, may be required.

Increases in cholesterol and triglyceride levels may be associated with thiazide diuretic therapy.

To minimise the risk of hyperkalaemia in diabetic or suspected diabetic patients, the status of renal function should be determined before initiating therapy with 'Moduretic'. Therapy should be discontinued at least three days before giving a glucose tolerance test. Potassium-conserving therapy should be initiated only with caution in severely ill patients in whom metabolic or respiratory acidosis may occur, e.g. patients with cardiopulmonary disease or patients with inadequately controlled diabetes.

Shifts in acid-base balance alter the balance of extracellular/intracellular potassium, and the development of acidosis may be associated with rapid increases in plasma potassium.

Sensitivity reactions: The possibility that thiazides may activate or exacerbate systemic lupus erythematosus has been reported.

4.5 Interaction with other medicinal products and other forms of Interaction
Lithium generally should not be given with diuretics. Diuretic agents reduce the renal clearance of lithium and add a high risk of lithium toxicity. Refer to the prescribing information for lithium preparations before use of such preparations.

Non-Steroidal Anti-inflammatory Drugs: In some patients the administration of a non-steroidal anti-inflammatory agent can reduce the diuretic, natriuretic and antihypertensive effects of diuretics. Concomitant administration of non-steroidal anti-inflammatory drugs (NSAIDs) and potassium-sparing agents, including amiloride hydrochloride, may cause hyperkalaemia and renal failure, particularly in elderly patients. Therefore, when amiloride hydrochloride is used concomitantly with NSAIDs, renal function and serum potassium levels should be carefully monitored.

Amiloride Hydrochloride
When amiloride hydrochloride is administered concomitantly with an angiotensin-converting enzyme inhibitor, angiotensin II receptor antagonist, trilostane, cyclosporin or tacrolimus, the risk of hyperkalaemia may be increased. Therefore, if concomitant use of these agents is indicated because of demonstrated hypokalaemia, they should be used with caution and with frequent monitoring of serum potassium.

Hydrochlorothiazide
When given concurrently, the following drugs may interact with thiazide diuretics:

Alcohol, barbiturates or narcotics: Co-administration may potentiate orthostatic hypotension. **Oral and parenteral antidiabetic drugs** may require adjustment of dosage with concurrent use. 'Moduretic' can act synergistically with chlorpropamide to increase the risk of hyponatraemia. **Other antihypertensive drugs** may have an additive effect. Therefore the dosage of these agents, especially adrenergic-blockers, may need to be reduced when 'Moduretic' is added to the regimen. Diuretic therapy should be discontinued for 2-3 days prior to initiation of therapy with an ACE inhibitor to reduce the likelihood of first dose hypotension. **Cholestyramine and colestipol resins:** absorption of hydrochlorothiazide is impaired in the presence of anionic exchange resins. Single doses of either cholestyramine or colestipol resins bind the hydrochlorothiazide and reduce its absorption from the gastrointestinal tract by up to 85 and 43 percent, respectively. When cholestyramine is given 4 hours after the hydrochlorothiazide, the absorption of hydrochlorothiazide is reduced by 30 to 35 percent. **Corticosteroids or ACTH** may intensify any thiazide-induced electrolyte depletion, particularly hypokalaemia. **Pressor amines such as epinephrine (adrenaline)** may show decreased arterial responsiveness when used with 'Moduretic' but this reaction is not enough to preclude their therapeutic usefulness. **Non-depolarising muscle relaxants such as tubocurarine** may possibly interact with 'Moduretic' to increase muscle relaxation.

Drug/laboratory tests: Because thiazides may affect calcium metabolism, 'Moduretic' may interfere with tests for parathyroid function.

4.6 Pregnancy and lactation
Use in pregnancy: The routine use of diuretics in otherwise healthy pregnant women with or without mild oedema is not indicated, because they may be associated with hypovolaemia, increased blood viscosity, and decreased placental perfusion. Diuretics do not prevent the development of toxaemia of pregnancy and there is no satisfactory evidence that they are useful for its treatment.

Since thiazides cross the placental barrier and appear in cord blood, use where pregnancy is present or suspected requires that the benefits of the drug be weighed against possible hazards to the foetus. These hazards include foetal or neonatal jaundice, thrombocytopenia, bone marrow depression, and possibly other side effects that have occurred in the adult.

Use in breast-feeding mothers: Although it is not known whether amiloride hydrochloride is excreted in human milk, it is known that thiazides do appear in breast milk. If use of the drug combination is deemed essential, the patient should stop breast-feeding.

4.7 Effects on ability to drive and use machines
Infrequently, patients may experience weakness, fatigue, dizziness, stupor and vertigo. Should any of these occur, the patient should be cautioned not to drive or operate machinery.

4.8 Undesirable effects
Although minor side effects are relatively common, significant side effects are infrequent.

Reported side effects are generally associated with diuresis, thiazide therapy, or with the underlying disease.

No increase in the risk of adverse reactions has been seen over those of the individual components.

The following side effects have been reported with 'Moduretic':

Body as a whole: headache, weakness, fatigue, malaise, chest pain, back pain, syncope.

Cardiovascular: arrhythmias, tachycardia, digitalis toxicity, orthostatic hypotension, angina pectoris.

Digestive: anorexia, nausea, vomiting, diarrhoea, constipation, abdominal pain, GI bleeding, appetite changes, abdominal fullness, flatulence, thirst, hiccups.

Metabolic: elevated plasma potassium levels (above 5.5 mmol/l), electrolyte imbalance, hyponatraemia (see 'Special warnings and special precautions for use'), gout, dehydration, symptomatic hyponatraemia.

Integumentary: rash, pruritus, flushing, diaphoresis.

Musculoskeletal: leg ache, muscle cramps, joint pain.

Nervous: dizziness, vertigo, paraesthesiae, stupor.

Psychiatric: insomnia, nervousness, mental confusion, depression, sleepiness.

Respiratory: dyspnoea.

Special senses: bad taste, visual disturbance, nasal congestion.

Urogenital: impotence, dysuria, nocturia, incontinence, renal dysfunction including renal failure.

Additional side effects that have been reported with the individual components and may be potential side effects of 'Moduretic' are listed below:

Amiloride:

Body as a whole: neck/shoulder ache, pain in extremities.

Digestive: abnormal liver function, activation of probable pre-existing peptic ulcer, dyspepsia, jaundice.

Integumentary: dry mouth, alopecia.

Nervous: tremors, encephalopathy.

Haematological: aplastic anaemia, neutropenia.

Cardiovascular: one patient with partial heart block developed complete heart block, palpitation.

Psychiatric: decreased libido, somnolence.

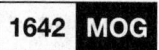

Respiratory: cough.

Special senses: tinnitus, increased intra-ocular pressure.

Urogenital: polyuria, urinary frequency, bladder spasm.

Hydrochlorothiazide:

Body as a whole: anaphylactic reaction, fever.

Cardiovascular: necrotising angiitis (vasculitis, cutaneous vasculitis.)

Digestive: jaundice (intrahepatic cholestatic jaundice), pancreatitis, cramping, gastric irritation.

Endocrine/Metabolic: glycosuria, hyperglycaemia, hyperuricaemia, hypokalaemia.

Integumentary: photosensitivity, sialadenitis, urticaria, toxic epidermal necrolysis.

Haematological: agranulocytosis, aplastic anaemia, haemolytic anaemia, leucopenia, purpura, thrombocytopenia.

Psychiatric: restlessness.

Renal: interstitial nephritis.

Respiratory: respiratory distress, including pneumonitis, pulmonary oedema.

Special senses: transient blurred vision, xanthopsia.

4.9 Overdose
No specific data are available on overdosage with 'Moduretic'. No specific antidote is available, and it is not known whether the drug is dialysable.

Treatment should be symptomatic and supportive. Therapy should be discontinued and the patient watched closely. Emesis should be induced and/or gastric lavage performed. The most common signs and symptoms of overdosage with amiloride hydrochloride are dehydration and electrolyte imbalance. Blood pressure should be monitored and corrected where necessary. If hyperkalaemia occurs, active measures should be taken to reduce the plasma potassium levels.

Electrolyte depletion (hypokalaemia, hypochloraemia, hyponatraemia) and dehydration are the most common signs and symptoms of hydrochlorothiazide overdosage. If digitalis has been administered, hypokalaemia may accentuate cardiac arrhythmias.

5. PHARMACOLOGICAL PROPERTIES

5.1 Pharmacodynamic properties
Hydrochlorothiazide is a diuretic with antihypertensive properties. It acts by inhibiting the renal tubular reabsorption of sodium and chloride ions, which are excreted with an accompanying volume of water. Potassium excretion is also promoted.

Amiloride hydrochloride is a potassium-sparing diuretic. It also promotes the excretion of sodium and chloride, but it reduces the excretion of potassium.

5.2 Pharmacokinetic properties
About 70% of an oral dose of hydrochlorothiazide is absorbed. It has a plasma half life of 5.6 to 14.8 hours. It is excreted unchanged in the urine. It crosses the placental barrier and is secreted in breast milk.

About 50% of an oral dose of amiloride hydrochloride is absorbed. It has a plasma half life of about 6 to 9 hours, but its effects may persist for up to 48 hours after a single dose. It is excreted unchanged in the urine and faeces.

5.3 Preclinical safety data
No relevant data.

6. PHARMACEUTICAL PARTICULARS

6.1 List of excipients
Calcium hydrogen phosphate

Guar gum

Lactose

Magnesium stearate

Maize starch

Pregelatinised maize starch

Sunset yellow aluminium lake E110

6.2 Incompatibilities
None known.

6.3 Shelf life
3 years.

6.4 Special precautions for storage
Store in a dry place below 25°C.

6.5 Nature and contents of container
PVC blister packs, lidded with aluminium foil containing 28 tablets.

6.6 Instructions for use and handling
None.

7. MARKETING AUTHORISATION HOLDER
Merck Sharp & Dohme Limited

Hertford Road, Hoddesdon, Hertfordshire EN11 9BU, UK

Distributed in the UK by:

Bristol-Myers Squibb Pharmaceuticals Ltd

Hounslow

TW3 3JA

UK

8. MARKETING AUTHORISATION NUMBER(S)
PL 0025/5016R

9. DATE OF FIRST AUTHORISATION/RENEWAL OF THE AUTHORISATION
6 November 1989

10. DATE OF REVISION OF THE TEXT
October 2003

***11. LEGAL CATEGORY** Prescription only medicine*

Mogadon 5 mg Tablets

(Valeant Pharmaceuticals Ltd)

1. NAME OF THE MEDICINAL PRODUCT
Mogadon 5 mg Tablets

2. QUALITATIVE AND QUANTITATIVE COMPOSITION
Round, white tablets with ICN marked on one face and single break bar on the other, containing 5 mg of nitrazepam.

3. PHARMACEUTICAL FORM
Tablets

4. CLINICAL PARTICULARS

4.1 Therapeutic indications
Short-term treatment of insomnia when it is severe, disabling or subjecting the individual to unacceptable distress, where daytime sedation is acceptable.

An underlying cause for insomnia should be sought before deciding upon the use of benzodiazepines for symptomatic relief.

Benzodiazepines are not recommended for the primary treatment of psychotic illness.

4.2 Posology and method of administration
Adults

5 mg before retiring. This dose may, if necessary, be increased to 10mg.

Elderly

Elderly or debilitated patients: the elderly or patients with impaired renal and/or hepatic function will be particularly susceptible to the adverse effects of Mogadon. Doses should not exceed half those normally recommended.

If organic brain changes are present, the dosage of Mogadon should not exceed 5mg in these patients.

In patients with chronic pulmonary insufficiency and in patients with chronic renal or hepatic disease, dosage may need to be reduced.

Children

Mogadon tablets are contraindicated for use in children.

Dosage should be adjusted on an individual basis. Treatment should, if possible, be on an intermittent basis.

Treatment should be as short as possible and should be started with the lowest recommended dose. The maximum dose should not be exceeded. Generally the duration of treatment varies from a few days to two weeks with a maximum of four weeks; including the tapering off process. Patients who have taken benzodiazepines for a prolonged time may require a longer period during which doses are reduced. Specialist help may be appropriate. Little is known regarding the efficacy or safety of benzodiazepines in long-term use.

In certain cases, extension beyond the maximum treatment period may be necessary; if so, it should not take place without re-evaluation of the patient's status. Long-term chronic use is not recommended. It may be useful to inform the patient when treatment is started that it will be of limited duration and to explain precisely how the dosage will be decreased. Moreover, it is important that the patient should be aware of the possibility of rebound phenomena (see *Undesirable Effects*) thereby minimising anxiety over such symptoms should they occur while the medicinal product is being discontinued. Mogadon therapy should not be stopped abruptly, but the dose tapered off.

The product should be taken just before going to bed.

In addition, for long acting benzodiazepines, it must be stated that the patient should be checked regularly at the start of treatment in order to decrease, if necessary, the dose or frequency of administration to prevent overdose due to accumulation.

Mogadon tablets are for oral administration.

4.3 Contraindications
Patients with known hypersensitivity to benzodiazepines or any of the excipients. Hypersensitivity reactions with the benzodiazepines including rash, angioedema and hypertension have been reported on rare occasions in susceptible patients.

Use of this drug is also contraindicated in patients with acute pulmonary insufficiency; respiratory depression; phobic or obsessional states; chronic psychosis; myasthenia gravis; sleep apnoea syndrome; severe hepatic insufficiency; use in children.

4.4 Special warnings and special precautions for use
In patients with chronic pulmonary insufficiency, and in patients with chronic renal or hepatic disease, dosage may need to be reduced. Benzodiazepines are contraindicated in patients with severe hepatic insufficiency.

Mogadon should not be used alone to treat depression or anxiety associated with depression, since suicide may be precipitated in such patients. Benzodiazepines should be used with extreme caution in patients with a history of alcohol or drug abuse. Benzodiazepines are not recommended for the primary treatment of psychotic illness.

If the patient is awoken during the period of maximum drug activity, recall may be impaired.

In cases of loss or bereavement, psychological adjustment may be inhibited by benzodiazepines.

Use of benzodiazepines may lead to the development of physical and psychological dependence upon these products. The risk of dependence increases when high doses are used, especially when given over long periods. This is particularly so in patients with a history of alcoholism or drug abuse or in patients with marked personality disorders. Regular monitoring in such patients is essential; routine repeat prescriptions should be avoided and treatment should be withdrawn gradually. Symptoms such as depression, headaches, muscle weakness, nervousness, extreme anxiety, tension, restlessness, confusion, mood changes, rebound insomnia, irritability, sweating, and diarrhoea have been reported following abrupt cessation of treatment in patients receiving even normal therapeutic doses for short periods of time.

When benzodiazepines with a long duration of action are being used it is important to warn against changing to a benzodiazepine with a short duration of action, as withdrawal symptoms may develop.

In severe cases the following symptoms may occur: derealisation, depersonalisation, hyperacusis, numbness and tingling of the extremities, hypersensitivity to light, noise and physical contact and hallucinations or epileptic seizures. In rare instances, withdrawal following excessive dosages may produce confusional states and psychotic manifestations and convulsions. Abuse of the benzodiazepines has been reported.

Some loss of efficacy to the hypnotic effects of short-acting benzodiazepines may develop after repeated use for a few weeks.

Abnormal psychological reactions to benzodiazepines have been reported. Rare behavioural effects include paradoxical aggressive outbursts, excitement, confusion, restlessness, agitation, irritability, delusion, rages, nightmares, hallucinations, psychoses, inappropriate behavior and the uncovering of depression with suicidal tendencies. Extreme caution should therefore be used in prescribing benzodiazepines to patients with personality disorders. If any of these reactions occur, use of the drug should be discontinued. These reactions may be quite severe and are more likely to occur in the elderly.

Benzodiazepines may induce anterograde amnesia. The condition usually occurs 1 to 2 hours after ingesting the product and may last up to several hours. Therefore, to reduce the risk, patients should ensure that they will be able to have an uninterrupted sleep of 7 to 8 hours.

4.5 Interaction with other medicinal products and other forms of Interaction
Enhancement of the central depressive effect may occur if benzodiazepines are combined with centrally-acting drugs such as neuroleptics, tranquillisers, antidepressants, hypnotics, analgesics and anesthetics, anti-epileptics and sedative antihistamines. In the case of narcotic analgesics, enhancement of the euphoria may also occur, leading to an increase in psychological dependence. The elderly require special supervision.

When Mogadon is used in conjunction with anti-epileptic drugs, side-effects and toxicity may be more evident, particularly with hydantoins or barbiturates or combinations including them. This requires extra care in adjusting dosage in the initial stages of treatment.

Known inhibitors of hepatic enzymes, particularly cythochrome P450 have been shown to reduce the clearance of benzodiazepines and may potentiate their action and known inducers of hepatic enzymes, e.g. rifampicin, may increase the clearance of benzodiazepines.

Concomitant intake with alcohol should be avoided. The sedative effect may be enhanced when the product is used in combination with alcohol. This adversely affects the ability to drive or use machines.

4.6 Pregnancy and lactation
There is no evidence as to drug safety in human pregnancy, nor is there evidence from animal work that it is free from hazard. Do not use during pregnancy, especially during the first and last trimesters, unless there are compelling reasons.

If the product is prescribed to a woman of childbearing potential, she should be warned to contact her physician regarding discontinuance of the product if she intends to become or suspects that she is pregnant.

Administration of benzodiazepines in the last trimester of pregnancy or during labour has been reported to produce irregularities in the foetal heart rate, and hypotonia, poor sucking, hypothermia and moderate respiratory depression in the neonate.

Infants born to mothers who took benzodiazepines chronically in the latter stages of pregnancy may have developed physical dependence and may be at some risk of developing withdrawal symptoms in the postnatal period.

Since benzodiazepines are found in the breast milk, the use of Mogadon in mothers who are breast-feeding should be avoided.

4.7 Effects on ability to drive and use machines

Patients should be advised that, like all medicaments of this type, Mogadon may modify patients' performance at skilled tasks. Sedation, amnesia, impaired concentration and impaired muscle function may adversely affect the ability to drive or use machinery. If insufficient sleep duration occurs, the likelihood of impaired alertness may be increased. Patients should further be advised that alcohol may intensify any impairment, and should, therefore, be avoided during treatment.

4.8 Undesirable effects

Common adverse effects include drowsiness during the day, numbed emotions reduced alertness, confusion, fatigue, headache, dizziness, muscle weakness, ataxia and double vision. These phenomena are dose related and occur predominantly at the start of therapy, they usually disappear with repeated administration. The elderly are particularly sensitive to the effects of centrally-depressant drugs.

Anterograde amnesia may occur at therapeutic dosages, the risk increasing at higher dosages. Amnesia effects may be associated with inappropriate behaviour.

Pre-existing depression may be unmasked during benzodiazepine use.

Other adverse effects are rare and include vertigo, hypotension, gastro-intestinal upsets, skin rashes, visual disturbances, changes in libido, and urinary retention. Isolated cases of blood dyscrasias and jaundice have also been reported.

Use (even at therapeutic doses) may lead to the development of physical and psychological dependence: discontinuation of the therapy may result in withdrawal or rebound phenomena, a transient syndrome whereby the symptoms that led to treatment with benzodiazepine or benzodiazepine-like agent recur in an enhanced form. It may be accompanied by other reactions including mood changes, anxiety and restlessness. Since the risk of withdrawal phenomena/rebound phenomena is greater after abrupt discontinuation of treatment, it is recommended that the dosage be decreased gradually.

Abuse of benzodiazepines has been reported.

4.9 Overdose

When taken alone in overdosage Mogadon presents few problems in management and should not present a threat to life unless combined with other CNS depressants (including alcohol).

In the management of overdose with any medicinal product, it should be borne in mind that multiple agents may have been taken.

Following overdose with oral benzodiazepines, vomiting should be induced (within one hour) if the patient is conscious or gastric lavage undertaken with the airway protected if the patient is unconscious. If there is no advantage in emptying the stomach, activated charcoal should be given to reduce absorption.

Special attention should be paid to respiratory and cardiovascular functions in intensive care. Overdosage of benzodiazepines is usually manifested by degrees of central nervous system depression ranging from drowsiness to coma. In mild cases, symptoms include drowsiness, mental confusion, dysarthria and lethargy; in more serious cases, symptoms may include ataxia, hypotonia, hypotension, respiratory depression, rarely coma and very rarely death.

The value of dialysis has not been determined. Anexate is a specific IV antidote for use in emergency situations. Patients requiring such intervention should be monitored closely in hospital (see separate prescribing information). The benzodiazepine antagonist Anexate® (active ingredients; flumazenil) is not indicated in patients with epilepsy who have been treated with benzodiazepines. Antagonism of the benzodiazepine effect in such patients may trigger seizures.

If excitation occurs, barbiturates should not be used.

5. PHARMACOLOGICAL PROPERTIES

5.1 Pharmacodynamic properties

Mogadon is a benzodiazepine compound with sedative properties. It acts in 30 to 60 minutes to produce sleep lasting 6 to 8 hours.

5.2 Pharmacokinetic properties

The drug is well absorbed form the GI tract with peak blood levels being achieved within 2 hours of administration. Two hours after administration, the concentration of nitrazepam in the cerebrospinal fluid is about 8% and after 36 hours approximately 16% of the concentration in the plasma. The cerebrospinal fluid concentration thus corresponds to the non-protein-bound fraction of active ingredient in the plasma. The half-life is, on average, 24 hours. Steady-state levels are achieved within 5 days. Nitrazepam undergoes biotransformation to a number of metabolites, none of which possess significant clinical activity. About 5% is excreted unchanged in the urine together with less than 10% each of the 7-amino- and 7-acetylamino- metabolites in the first 48 hours. In younger persons the volume of distribution is 2L/kg, in elderly patients the volume of distribution is greater and the mean elimination half-life rises to 40 hours.

No clear correlation has been demonstrated between the blood levels of Mogadon and its clinical effects.

5.3 Preclinical safety data

None stated.

6. PHARMACEUTICAL PARTICULARS

6.1 List of excipients

Each 5 mg tablet contains the following excipients: lactose, starch maize white and magnesium stearate.

6.2 Incompatibilities

None stated.

6.3 Shelf life

HDPE or glass bottles:5 years.

PVDC blister packs, clic-loc containers and polypropylene mini kegs:2 years.

6.4 Special precautions for storage

The recommended maximum storage temperature for Mogadon tablets is 25°C.

All packs should be protected from light and the blister packs should be protected from moisture i.e. stored in a dry place.

6.5 Nature and contents of container

HDPE or glass bottles, in packs of 30 or 100.

PVDC blister packs, containing 50 tablets.

Clic-loc containers, in pack of 10.

Polypropylene mini-kegs, containing 5000 tablets.

6.6 Instructions for use and handling

None.

7. MARKETING AUTHORISATION HOLDER

Valeant Pharmaceuticals Limited

Cedarwood

Chineham Business Park

Crockford Lane

Basingstoke

Hants

RG24 8WD

8. MARKETING AUTHORISATION NUMBER(S)

PL 15142/0018

9. DATE OF FIRST AUTHORISATION/RENEWAL OF THE AUTHORISATION

3 May 1999

10. DATE OF REVISION OF THE TEXT

December 2004

Molipaxin 50mg and 100mg Capsules

(sanofi-aventis)

1. NAME OF THE MEDICINAL PRODUCT

Molipaxin 50mg Capsules

Molipaxin 100mg Capsules

2. QUALITATIVE AND QUANTITATIVE COMPOSITION

Trazodone hydrochloride 50mg or 100mg per capsule.

For excipients, see 6.1.

3. PHARMACEUTICAL FORM

Capsules.

4. CLINICAL PARTICULARS

4.1 Therapeutic indications

Anxiety, depression, mixed anxiety and depression.

4.2 Posology and method of administration

Route of administration: Oral.

DEPRESSION:

Adults:

Initially 150mg/day in divided doses after food or as a single dose on retiring.

This may be increased up to 300mg/day in a single or divided doses. The major portion of a divided dose to be taken on retiring. The dose may be further increased to 600mg/day in divided doses in hospitalised patients.

Elderly:

For very elderly or frail patients initially 100mg/day in divided doses or as a single night-time dose. This may be increased, under supervision, according to efficacy and tolerance. It is unlikely that 300mg/day will be exceeded.

Children:

There are insufficient data to recommend the use of Molipaxin in children.

DEPRESSION ACCOMPANIED BY ANXIETY:

As for depression.

ANXIETY:

75mg/day increasing to 300mg/day as necessary.

Tolerability may be improved by taking Molipaxin after food.

4.3 Contraindications

Known sensitivity to trazodone or to any of the excipients.

4.4 Special warnings and special precautions for use

Care should be exercised when administering Molipaxin to patients suffering epilepsy, avoiding in particular, abrupt increases or decreases in dosage.

Molipaxin should be administered with care in patients with severe hepatic, renal or cardiac disease.

Potent CYP3A4 inhibitors may lead to increases in trazodone serum levels. See section 4.5 for further information.

4.5 Interaction with other medicinal products and other forms of Interaction

In vitro drug metabolism studies suggest that there is a potential for drug interactions when Molipaxin is given with potent CYP3A4 inhibitors such as erythromycin, ketoconazole, itraconazole, ritonavir, indinavir, and nefazodone. It is likely that potent CYP3A4 inhibitors may lead to substantial increases in trazodone plasma concentrations with the potential for adverse effects. Exposure to ritonavir during initiation or resumption of treatment in patients receiving Molipaxin will increase the potential for excessive sedation, cardiovascular, and gastrointestinal effects. If Molipaxin is used with a potent CYP3A4 inhibitor, a lower dose of Molipaxin should be considered. However, the co-administration of Molipaxin and potent CYP3A4 inhibitors should be avoided where possible.

Carbamazepine reduced plasma concentrations of trazodone when coadministered. Patients should be closely monitored to see if there is a need for an increased dose of Molipaxin when taken with carbamazepine.

Although no untoward effects have been reported, Molipaxin may enhance the effects of muscle relaxants and volatile anaesthetics. Similar considerations apply to combined administration with sedative and anti-depressant drugs, including alcohol. Molipaxin has been well tolerated in depressed schizophrenic patients receiving standard phenothiazine therapy and also in depressed parkinsonian patients receiving therapy with levodopa.

Possible interactions with monoamine oxidase inhibitors have occasionally been reported. Although some clinicians do give both concurrently, we do not recommend concurrent administration with MAOIs, or within two weeks of stopping treatment with these compounds. Nor do we recommend giving MAOIs within one week of stopping Molipaxin.

Since Molipaxin is only a very weak inhibitor of noradrenaline re-uptake and does not modify the blood pressure response to tyramine, interference with the hypotensive action of guanethidine-like compounds is unlikely. However, studies in laboratory animals suggest that Molipaxin may inhibit most of the acute actions of clonidine. In the case of other types of antihypertensive drug, although no clinical interactions have been reported, the possibility of potentiation should be considered.

Concurrent use with Molipaxin may result in elevated serum levels of digoxin or phenytoin. Monitoring of serum levels should be considered in these patients.

4.6 Pregnancy and lactation

Although studies in animals have not shown any direct teratogenic effect, the safety of Molipaxin in human pregnancy has not been established. On basic principles, therefore, its use during the first trimester should be avoided.

The possibility of Molipaxin being excreted in the milk should also be considered in nursing mothers.

4.7 Effects on ability to drive and use machines

As with all other drugs acting on the central nervous system, patients should be warned against the risk of handling machinery and driving.

4.8 Undesirable effects

Molipaxin is a sedative antidepressant and drowsiness, sometimes experienced during the first days of treatment, usually disappears on continued therapy.

Anticholinergic-like symptoms do occur but the incidence is similar to placebo.

The following symptoms, most of which are commonly reported in cases of untreated depression, have also been recorded in small numbers of patients receiving Molipaxin therapy: dizziness, headache, nausea and vomiting, weakness, decreased alertness, weight loss, tremor, dry mouth, bradycardia, tachycardia, postural hypotension, oedema, constipation, diarrhoea, blurred vision, restlessness, confusional states, insomnia and skin rash.

Blood dyscrasias, including agranulocytosis, thrombocytopenia and anaemia, have been reported on rare occasions. Adverse effects on hepatic function, including jaundice and hepatocellular damage, sometimes severe, have been rarely reported. Should such effects occur, Molipaxin should be discontinued immediately.

As with other drugs with alpha-adrenolytic activity, Molipaxin has very rarely been associated with priapism. This may be treated with an intracavernosum injection of an alpha-adrenergic agent such as adrenaline or

metaraminol. However there are reports of trazodone-induced priapism which have required surgical intervention or led to permanent sexual dysfunction. Patients developing this suspected adverse reaction should cease Molipaxin immediately.

In contrast to the tricyclic antidepressants, Molipaxin is devoid of anticholinergic activity. Consequently, troublesome side effects such as dry mouth, blurred vision and urinary hesitancy have occurred no more frequently than in patients receiving placebo therapy. This may be of importance when treating depressed patients who are at risk from conditions such as glaucoma, urinary retention and prostatic hypertrophy.

Studies in animals have shown that Molipaxin is less cardiotoxic than the tricyclic antidepressants, and clinical studies suggest that the drug may be less likely to cause cardiac arrhythmias in man. Clinical studies in patients with pre-existing cardiac disease indicate that trazodone may be arrhythmogenic in some patients in that population. Arrhythmias identified include isolated premature ventricular contractions, ventricular couplets, and short episodes (3-4 beats) of ventricular tachycardia.

There have been occasional reports of serotonin syndrome and convulsions associated with the use of Molipaxin hydrochloride, especially when associated with other psychotropic drugs. Neuroleptic malignant syndrome may, very rarely, arise in the course of treatment with Molipaxin.

Molipaxin has had no effect on arterial blood pCO_2 or pO_2 levels in patients with severe respiratory insufficiency due to chronic bronchial or pulmonary disease.

4.9 Overdose

FEATURES OF TOXICITY

The most frequently reported reactions to overdose have included drowsiness, dizziness, nausea and vomiting. In more serious cases coma, tachycardia, hypotension, hyponatraemia, convulsions and respiratory failure have been reported. Cardiac features may include bradycardia, QT prolongation and torsade de pointes. Symptoms may appear 24 hours or more after overdose.

Overdoses of Molipaxin in combination with other antidepressants may cause serotonin syndrome.

MANAGEMENT

There is no specific antidote to trazodone. Activated charcoal should be considered in adults who have ingested more than 1 g trazodone, or in children who have ingested more than 150 mg trazodone within 1 hour of presentation. Alternatively, in adults, gastric lavage may be considered within 1 hour of ingestion of a potentially life-threatening overdose.

Observe for at least 6 hours after ingestion (or 12 hours if a sustained release preparation has been taken). Monitor BP, pulse and GCS. Monitor oxygen if GCS is reduced. Cardiac monitoring is appropriate in symptomatic patients.

Single brief convulsions do not require treatment. Control frequent or prolonged convulsions with intravenous diazepam (0.1-0.3 mg/kg body weight) or lorazepam (4 mg in an adult and 0.05 mg/kg in a child). If these measures do not control the fits, an intravenous infusion of phenytoin may be useful. Give oxygen and correct acid base and metabolic disturbances as required.

Treatment should be symptomatic and supportive in the case of hypotension and excessive sedation. If severe hypotension persists consider use of inotropes, eg dopamine or dobutamine.

5. PHARMACOLOGICAL PROPERTIES

5.1 Pharmacodynamic properties

ATC code: N06A X05. Other antidepressants.

Molipaxin is a potent antidepressant. It also has anxiety reducing activity. Molipaxin is a triazolopyridine derivative chemically unrelated to known tricyclic, tetracyclic and other antidepressant agents. It has negligible effect on noradrenaline re-uptake mechanisms. Whilst the mode of action of Molipaxin is not known precisely, its antidepressant activity may concern noradrenergic potentiation by mechanisms other than uptake blockade. A central anti-serotonin effect may account for the drug's anxiety reducing properties.

5.2 Pharmacokinetic properties

Trazodone is rapidly absorbed from the gastro-intestinal tract and extensively metabolised. Paths of metabolism of Trazodone include n-oxidation and hydroxylation. The metabolic m-chlorophenylpiperazine is active. Trazodone is excreted in the urine almost entirely in the form of its metabolites, either in free or in conjugated form. The elimination of Trazodone is biphasic, with a terminal elimination half-life of 5 to 13 hours. Trazodone is excreted in breast milk.

There was an approximate two-fold increase in terminal phase half-life and significantly higher plasma concentrations of Trazodone in 10 subjects aged 65 to 74 years compared with 12 subjects aged 23 to 30 years following a 100mg dose of Trazodone. It was suggested that there is an age-related reduction in the hepatic metabolism of Trazodone.

In vitro studies in human liver microsomes show that trazodone is metabolised by cytochrome P4503A4 (CYP3A4) to form m-chlorophenylpiperazine. Whilst significant, the role of this pathway in the total clearance of trazodone in vivo has not been fully determined.

5.3 Preclinical safety data

None stated.

6. PHARMACEUTICAL PARTICULARS

6.1 List of excipients

Lactose

Magnesium stearate

Gelatin

Titanium dioxide E171

Erythrosine E127

Indigo Carmine E132

Yellow iron oxide E172

Red iron oxide E172 (100mg capsules only)

6.2 Incompatibilities

None stated.

6.3 Shelf life

60 months.

6.4 Special precautions for storage

Blister packs: Store below 30°C in a dry place.

6.5 Nature and contents of container

50mg: PVdC coated 250μm PVC blisters sealed with 20μm aluminium foil: contents 84 capsules.

100mg: PVdC coated 250μm PVC blisters sealed with 20μm aluminium foil: contents 56 capsules.

6.6 Instructions for use and handling

Not applicable.

7. MARKETING AUTHORISATION HOLDER

Aventis Pharma

50 Kings Hill Avenue

Kings Hill

West Malling

Kent ME19 4AH

8. MARKETING AUTHORISATION NUMBER(S)

50mg: PL 00109/0045

100mg: PL 00109/0046

9. DATE OF FIRST AUTHORISATION/RENEWAL OF THE AUTHORISATION

13 May 1999

10. DATE OF REVISION OF THE TEXT

13 July 2005

LEGAL CLASSIFICATION: POM

Molipaxin Liquid 50mg/5ml

(sanofi-aventis)

1. NAME OF THE MEDICINAL PRODUCT

Molipaxin™ Liquid (50mg/5ml)

2. QUALITATIVE AND QUANTITATIVE COMPOSITION

Each 5ml contains 50mg of Trazodone hydrochloride.

For excipients, see 6.1.

3. PHARMACEUTICAL FORM

Clear, colourless solution with an orange odour and taste.

4. CLINICAL PARTICULARS

4.1 Therapeutic indications

Relief of symptoms in all types of depression including depression accompanied by anxiety.

Symptoms of depression likely to respond in the first week of treatment include depressed mood, insomnia, anxiety, somatic symptoms and hypochondriasis.

4.2 Posology and method of administration

Route of administration: Oral.

Adults:

Starting dose is 150mg/day in divided doses after food or as a single dose before retiring. This may be increased to 300mg/day, the major portion of which is preferably taken on retiring. In hospitalised patients dosage may be further increased to 600mg/day.

Children:

There are insufficient data to recommend the use of Molipaxin in children.

Elderly or Frail:

For elderly or very frail patients initial starting dose 100mg/day in divided doses or as a single night-time dose. This may be increased, under supervision, according to efficacy and tolerance. Doses above 300mg/day are unlikely to be required.

Tolerability may be improved by taking Molipaxin after food.

In conformity with current psychiatric opinion, it is suggested that Molipaxin be continued for several months after remission. Cessation of Molipaxin treatment should be gradual.

4.3 Contraindications

Known sensitivity to trazodone or to any of the excipients.

4.4 Special warnings and special precautions for use

Molipaxin should be administered with care in patients with severe hepatic, renal or cardiac disease.

Care should be exercised when administering Molipaxin to patients suffering epilepsy, avoiding in particular, abrupt increases or decreases in dosage.

Potent CYP3A4 inhibitors may lead to increases in trazodone serum levels. See section 4.5 for further information.

4.5 Interaction with other medicinal products and other forms of Interaction

In vitro drug metabolism studies suggest that there is a potential for drug interactions when Molipaxin is given with potent CYP3A4 inhibitors such as erythromycin, ketoconazole, itraconazole, ritonavir, indinavir, and nefazodone. It is likely that potent CYP3A4 inhibitors may lead to substantial increases in trazodone plasma concentrations with the potential for adverse effects. Exposure to ritonavir during initiation or resumption of treatment in patients receiving Molipaxin will increase the potential for excessive sedation, cardiovascular, and gastrointestinal effects. If Molipaxin is used with a potent CYP3A4 inhibitor, a lower dose of Molipaxin should be considered. However, the co-administration of Molipaxin and potent CYP3A4 inhibitors should be avoided where possible.

Carbamazepine reduced plasma concentrations of trazodone when coadministered. Patients should be closely monitored to see if there is a need for an increased dose of Molipaxin when taken with carbamazepine.

Although no untoward effects have been reported, Molipaxin may enhance the effects of muscle relaxants and volatile anaesthetics. Similar considerations apply to combined administration with sedative and anti-depressant drugs, including alcohol.

Molipaxin has been well tolerated in depressed schizophrenic patients receiving standard phenothiazine therapy and also in depressed parkinsonian patients receiving therapy with levodopa.

Possible interactions with monoamine oxidase inhibitors have occasionally been reported. Although some clinicians do give both concurrently, we do not recommend concurrent administration with MAOIs, or within two weeks of stopping treatment with these compounds. Nor do we recommend giving MAOIs within one week of stopping Molipaxin.

Since Molipaxin is only a very weak inhibitor of noradrenaline re-uptake and does not modify the blood pressure response to tyramine, interference with the hypotensive action of guanethidine-like compounds is unlikely. However, studies in laboratory animals suggest that Molipaxin may inhibit most of the acute actions of clonidine. In the case of other types of antihypertensive drug, although no clinical interactions have been reported, the possibility of potentiation should be considered.

Concurrent use with Molipaxin may result in elevated serum levels of digoxin or phenytoin. Monitoring of serum levels should be considered in these patients.

Molipaxin has had no effect on arterial blood pCO_2 or pO_2 levels in patients with severe respiratory insufficiency due to chronic bronchial or pulmonary disease.

4.6 Pregnancy and lactation

Although studies in animals have not shown any direct teratogenic effect, the safety of Molipaxin in human pregnancy has not been established. On basic principles, therefore, its use during the first trimester should be avoided.

The possibility of Molipaxin being excreted in the milk should also be considered in nursing mothers.

Molipaxin should only be administered during pregnancy and lactation if considered essential by the physician.

4.7 Effects on ability to drive and use machines

As with all other drugs acting on the central nervous system, patients should be warned against the risk of handling machinery and driving.

4.8 Undesirable effects

Molipaxin is a sedative antidepressant and drowsiness, sometimes experienced during the first days of treatment, usually disappears on continued therapy.

Anticholinergic-like symptoms do occur but the incidence is similar to placebo.

The following symptoms, most of which are commonly reported in cases of untreated depression, have also been recorded in small numbers of patients receiving Molipaxin therapy: dizziness, headache, nausea and vomiting, weakness, decreased alertness, weight loss, tremor, dry mouth, bradycardia, tachycardia, postural hypotension, oedema, constipation, diarrhoea, blurred vision, restlessness, confusional states, insomnia and skin rash.

Blood dyscrasias, including agranulocytosis, thrombocytopenia and anaemia, have been reported on rare occasions. Adverse effects on hepatic function, including jaundice and hepatocellular damage, sometimes severe, have been rarely reported. Should such effects occur, Molipaxin should be discontinued immediately.

As with other drugs with alpha-adrenolytic activity, Molipaxin has very rarely been associated with priapism. This may be treated with an intracavernosum injection of an alpha-adrenergic agent such as adrenaline or

metaraminol. However there are reports of Trazodone-induced priapism which have required surgical intervention or led to permanent sexual dysfunction. Patients developing this suspected adverse reaction should cease Molipaxin immediately.

In contrast to the tricyclic antidepressants, Molipaxin is devoid of anticholinergic activity. Consequently, troublesome side effects such as dry mouth, blurred vision and urinary hesitancy have occurred no more frequently than in patients receiving placebo therapy. This may be of importance when treating depressed patients who are at risk from conditions such as glaucoma, urinary retention and prostatic hypertrophy.

Studies in animals have shown that Molipaxin is less cardiotoxic than the tricyclic antidepressants, and clinical studies suggest that the drug may be less likely to cause cardiac arrhythmias in man. Clinical studies in patients with pre-existing cardiac disease indicate that Molipaxin may be arrhythmogenic in some patients in that population. Arrhythmias identified include isolated premature ventricular contractions, ventricular couplets, and short episodes (3-4 beats) of ventricular tachycardia.

There have been occasional reports of serotonin syndrome and convulsions associated with the use of Molipaxin, especially when associated with other psychotropic drugs. Neuroleptic malignant syndrome may, very rarely, arise in the course of treatment with Molipaxin.

Molipaxin has had no effect on arterial blood pCO_2 or pO_2 levels in patients with severe respiratory insufficiency due to chronic bronchial or pulmonary disease.

4.9 Overdose

FEATURES OF TOXICITY

The most frequently reported reactions to overdose have included drowsiness, dizziness, nausea and vomiting. In more serious cases coma, tachycardia, hypotension, hyponatraemia, convulsions and respiratory failure have been reported. Cardiac features may include bradycardia, QT prolongation and torsade de pointes. Symptoms may appear 24 hours or more after overdose.

Overdoses of Molipaxin/Trazodone in combination with other antidepressants may cause serotonin syndrome.

MANAGEMENT

There is no specific antidote to trazodone. Activated charcoal should be considered in adults who have ingested more than 1 g trazodone, or in children who have ingested more than 150 mg trazodone within 1 hour of presentation. Alternatively, in adults, gastric lavage may be considered within 1 hour of ingestion of a potentially life-threatening overdose.

Observe for at least 6 hours after ingestion (or 12 hours if a sustained release preparation has been taken). Monitor BP, pulse and GCS. Monitor oxygen saturation if GCS is reduced. Cardiac monitoring is appropriate in symptomatic patients.

Single brief convulsions do not require treatment. Control frequent or prolonged convulsions with intravenous diazepam (0.1-0.3 mg/kg body weight) or lorazepam (4 mg in an adult and 0.05 mg/kg in a child). If these measures do not control the fits, an intravenous infusion of phenytoin may be useful. Give oxygen and correct acid base and metabolic disturbances as required.

Treatment should be symptomatic and supportive in the case of hypotension and excessive sedation. If severe hypotension persists consider use of inotropes, eg dopamine or dobutamine

5. PHARMACOLOGICAL PROPERTIES

5.1 Pharmacodynamic properties

ATC code: N06A X05. Other antidepressants.

Trazodone is a triazolopyridine derivative which differs chemically from other currently available antidepressants. Although Trazodone bears some resemblance to the benzodiazepines, phenothiazines and tricyclic antidepressants, its pharmacological profile differs from each of these classes of drugs. The basic idea for the development of Trazodone was the hypothesis that depression involves an imbalance of the mechanism responsible for the emotional integration of unpleasant experiences. Consequently, new animal models of depression consisting of responses to unpleasant or noxious stimuli, instead of the current tests related to the aminergic theory of depression, were used in studying the drug. Trazodone inhibits serotonin uptake into rat brain synaptosomes and by rat platelets at relatively high concentrations and inhibits brain uptake of noradrenaline *in vitro* only at very high concentrations. It possesses antiserotonin-adrenergic blocking and analgesic effects. The anticholinergic activity of Trazodone is less than that of the tricyclic antidepressants in animal studies and this has been confirmed in therapeutic trials in depressed patients.

The electroencephalographic profile of Trazodone in humans is distinct from that of the tricyclic antidepressants or the benzodiazepines, although bearing some resemblance to these agents in its effect in certain wavebands. Studies of the cardiovascular effects of Trazodone in humans, His bundle and surface electrocardiograms in dogs, and experience with overdosage in man indicate that Trazodone is less liable than imipramine to cause important adverse effects on the heart. However, studies in depressed patients with significant cardiac impairment suggest that Trazodone may aggravate existing ventricular arrhythmias in a small undefined subgroup of such patients.

5.2 Pharmacokinetic properties

Peak plasma concentrations are attained about 1.5 hours after oral administration of Trazodone. Absorption is delayed and somewhat enhanced by food. The area under the plasma concentration-time curve is directly proportional to dosage after oral administration of 25 to 100mg. Trazodone is extensively metabolised, less than 1% of an oral dose being excreted unchanged in the urine. The main route of elimination is via the kidneys with 70 to 75% of an oral dose being recovered in the urine within the first 72 hours of ingestion. The elimination half-life for unchanged drug has been reported to be about 7 hours.

In vitro studies in human liver microsomes show that trazodone is metabolised by cytochrome P4503A4 (CYP3A4) to form m-chlorophenylpiperazine. Whilst significant, the role of this pathway in the total clearance of trazodone in vivo has not been fully determined.

5.3 Preclinical safety data

None stated.

6. PHARMACEUTICAL PARTICULARS

6.1 List of excipients

Glycerol, sorbitol, benzoic acid, saccharin sodium, orange flavour FC 901775, sodium hydroxide solution 1N, purified water and nitrogen.

6.2 Incompatibilities

None stated.

6.3 Shelf life

18 Months

6.4 Special precautions for storage

Store below 25°C and protect from light.

6.5 Nature and contents of container

Type III PhEur, 125ml amber glass bottle, sealed with a polyethylene screw cap with polypropylene seal and tamper evident closure, containing 120ml of solution.

6.6 Instructions for use and handling

None.

7. MARKETING AUTHORISATION HOLDER

Roussel Laboratories Ltd.

Broadwater Park

Denham

Uxbridge

Middlesex UB9 5HP

8. MARKETING AUTHORISATION NUMBER(S)

PL 00109/0117

9. DATE OF FIRST AUTHORISATION/RENEWAL OF THE AUTHORISATION

18 September 1998

10. DATE OF REVISION OF THE TEXT

13 July 2005

Legal classification: POM

Molipaxin Tablets 150mg

(sanofi-aventis)

1. NAME OF THE MEDICINAL PRODUCT

Molipaxin 150mg Tablets

2. QUALITATIVE AND QUANTITATIVE COMPOSITION

Tablet containing 150mg of Trazodone Hydrochloride.

For excipients, see 6.1

3. PHARMACEUTICAL FORM

Tablets.

4. CLINICAL PARTICULARS

4.1 Therapeutic indications

Relief of symptoms in all types of depression including depression accompanied by anxiety.

4.2 Posology and method of administration

Route of administration: Oral.

Depression:

a) Adults:

Initially 150mg/day in divided doses after food or as a single dose on retiring.

This may be increased up to 300mg/day in a single or divided doses. The major portion of a divided dose to be taken on retiring. The dose may be further increased to 600mg/day in divided doses in hospitalised patients.

b) Elderly:

For very elderly or frail patients initially 100mg/day in divided doses or as a single night-time dose. This may be increased, under supervision, according to efficacy and tolerance. It is unlikely that 300mg/day will be exceeded.

Depression accompanied by anxiety:

As for depression.

Anxiety:

75mg/day increasing to 300mg/day as necessary.

Tolerability may be improved by taking Molipaxin after food.

4.3 Contraindications

Known sensitivity to trazodone and any of the excipients.

4.4 Special warnings and special precautions for use

Care should be exercised when administering Molipaxin to patients suffering epilepsy, avoiding in particular, abrupt increases or decreases in dosage.

Molipaxin should be administered with care in patients with severe hepatic, renal or cardiac disease.

Potent CYP3A4 inhibitors may lead to increases in trazodone serum levels. See section 4.5 for further information.

4.5 Interaction with other medicinal products and other forms of Interaction

In vitro drug metabolism studies suggest that there is a potential for drug interactions when Molipaxin is given with potent CYP3A4 inhibitors such as erythromycin, ketoconazole, itraconazole, ritonavir, indinavir, and nefazodone. It is likely that potent CYP3A4 inhibitors may lead to substantial increases in trazodone plasma concentrations with the potential for adverse effects. Exposure to ritonavir during initiation or resumption of treatment in patients receiving Molipaxin will increase the potential for excessive sedation, cardiovascular, and gastrointestinal effects. If Molipaxin is used with a potent CYP3A4 inhibitor, a lower dose of Molipaxin should be considered. However, the co-administration of Molipaxin and potent CYP3A4 inhibitors should be avoided where possible.

Carbamazepine reduced plasma concentrations of trazodone when coadministered. Patients should be closely monitored to see if there is a need for an increased dose of Molipaxin when taken with carbamazepine.

Although no untoward effects have been reported, Molipaxin may enhance the effects of muscle relaxants and volatile anaesthetics. Similar considerations apply to combined administration with sedative and anti-depressant drugs, including alcohol. Molipaxin has been well tolerated in depressed schizophrenic patients receiving standard phenothiazine therapy and also in depressed parkinsonian patients receiving therapy with levodopa.

Possible interactions with monoamine oxidase inhibitors have occasionally been reported. Although some clinicians do give both concurrently, we do not recommend concurrent administration with MAOIs, or within two weeks of stopping treatment with these compounds. Nor do we recommend giving MAOIs within one week of stopping Molipaxin.

Since Molipaxin is only a very weak inhibitor of noradrenaline re-uptake and does not modify the blood pressure response to tyramine, interference with the hypotensive action of guanethidine-like compounds is unlikely. However, studies in laboratory animals suggest that Molipaxin may inhibit most of the acute actions of clonidine. In the case of other types of antihypertensive drug, although no clinical interactions have been reported, the possibility of potentiation should be considered.

Concurrent use with Molipaxin may result in elevated serum levels of digoxin or phenytoin. Monitoring of serum levels should be considered in these patients.

4.6 Pregnancy and lactation

Although studies in animals have not shown any direct teratogenic effect, the safety of Molipaxin in human pregnancy has not been established. On basic principles, therefore, its use during the first trimester should be avoided.

The possibility of Molipaxin being excreted in the milk should also be considered in nursing mothers.

4.7 Effects on ability to drive and use machines

As with all other drugs acting on the central nervous system, patients should be warned against the risk of handling machinery and driving.

4.8 Undesirable effects

Molipaxin is a sedative antidepressant and drowsiness, sometimes experienced during the first days of treatment, usually disappears on continued therapy.

Anticholinergic-like symptoms do occur but the incidence is similar to placebo.

The following symptoms, most of which are commonly reported in cases of untreated depression, have also been recorded in small numbers of patients receiving Molipaxin therapy: dizziness, headache, nausea and vomiting, weakness, decreased alertness, weight loss, tremor, dry mouth, bradycardia, tachycardia, postural hypotension, oedema, constipation, diarrhoea, blurred vision, restlessness, confusional states, insomnia and skin rash.

Blood dyscrasias, including agranulocytosis, thrombocytopenia and anaemia, have been reported on rare occasions. Adverse effects on hepatic function, including jaundice and hepatocellular damage, sometimes severe, have been rarely reported. Should such effects occur, Molipaxin should be discontinued immediately.

As with other drugs with alpha-adrenolytic activity, Molipaxin has very rarely been associated with priapism. This may be treated with an intracavernosum injection of an alpha-adrenergic agent such as adrenaline or

metaraminol. However there are reports of Trazodone-induced priapism which have required surgical intervention or led to permanent sexual dysfunction. Patients developing this suspected adverse reaction should cease Molipaxin immediately.

In contrast to the tricyclic antidepressants, Molipaxin is devoid of anticholinergic activity. Consequently, troublesome side effects such as dry mouth, blurred vision and urinary hesitancy have occurred no more frequently than in patients receiving placebo therapy. This may be of importance when treating depressed patients who are at risk from conditions such as glaucoma, urinary retention and prostatic hypertrophy.

Studies in animals have shown that Molipaxin is less cardiotoxic than the tricyclic antidepressants, and clinical studies suggest that the drug may be less likely to cause cardiac arrhythmias in man. Clinical studies in patients with pre-existing cardiac disease indicate that trazodone may be arrhythmogenic in some patients in that population. Arrhythmias identified include isolated premature ventricular contractions, ventricular couplets, and short episodes (3-4 beats) of ventricular tachycardia.

There have been occasional reports of serotonin syndrome and convulsions associated with the use of Molipaxin, especially when associated with other psychotropic drugs. Neuroleptic malignant syndrome may, very rarely, arise in the course of treatment with Molipaxin.

Molipaxin has had no effect on arterial blood pCO_2 or pO_2 levels in patients with severe respiratory insufficiency due to chronic bronchial or pulmonary disease.

4.9 Overdose

FEATURES OF TOXICITY

The most frequently reported reactions to overdose have included drowsiness, dizziness, nausea and vomiting. In more serious cases coma, tachycardia, hypotension, hyponatraemia, convulsions and respiratory failure have been reported. Cardiac features may include bradycardia, QT prolongation and torsade de pointes. Symptoms may appear 24 hours or more after overdose.

Overdoses of Molipaxin in combination with other antidepressants may cause serotonin syndrome.

MANAGEMENT

There is no specific antidote to trazodone. Activated charcoal should be considered in adults who have ingested more than 1 g trazodone, or in children who have ingested more than 150 mg trazodone within 1 hour of presentation. Alternatively, in adults, gastric lavage may be considered within 1 hour of ingestion of a potentially life-threatening overdose.

Observe for at least 6 hours after ingestion (or 12 hours if a sustained release preparation has been taken). Monitor BP, pulse and GCS. Monitor oxygen saturation if GCS is reduced. Cardiac monitoring is appropriate in symptomatic patients.

Single brief convulsions do not require treatment. Control frequent or prolonged convulsions with intravenous diazepam (0.1-0.3 mg/kg body weight) or lorazepam (4 mg in an adult and 0.05 mg/kg in a child). If these measures do not control the fits, an intravenous infusion of phenytoin may be useful. Give oxygen and correct acid base and metabolic disturbances as required.

Treatment should be symptomatic and supportive in the case of hypotension and excessive sedation. If severe hypotension persists consider use of inotropes, eg dopamine or dobutamine

5. PHARMACOLOGICAL PROPERTIES

5.1 Pharmacodynamic properties

ATC code: N06A X05. Other antidepressants.

Molipaxin is a potent antidepressant. It also has anxiety reducing activity. Molipaxin is a triazolopyridine derivative chemically unrelated to known tricyclic, tetracyclic and other antidepressant agents. It has negligible effect on noradrenaline re-uptake mechanisms. Whilst the mode of action of Molipaxin is not known precisely, its antidepressant activity may concern noradrenergic potentiation by mechanisms other than uptake blockade. A central antiserotonin effect may account for the drug's anxiety reducing properties.

5.2 Pharmacokinetic properties

Trazodone is rapidly absorbed from the gastro-intestinal tract and extensively metabolised. Paths of metabolism of trazodone include n-oxidation and hydroxylation. The metabolic m-chlorophenylpiperazine is active. Trazodone is excreted in the urine almost entirely in the form of its metabolites, either in free or in conjugated form. The elimination of trazodone is biphasic, with a terminal elimination half-life of 5 to 13 hours. Trazodone is excreted in breast milk.

There was an approximate two-fold increase in terminal phase half-life and significantly higher plasma concentrations of trazodone in 10 subjects aged 65 to 74 years compared with 12 subjects aged 23 to 30 years following a 100mg dose of trazodone. It was suggested that there is an age-related reduction in the hepatic metabolism of Trazodone.

In vitro studies in human liver microsomes show that trazodone is metabolised by cytochrome P4503A4 (CYP3A4) to form m-chlorophenylpiperazine. Whilst significant, the role of this pathway in the total clearance of trazodone in vivo has not been fully determined.

5.3 Preclinical safety data

None stated.

6. PHARMACEUTICAL PARTICULARS

6.1 List of excipients

The tablets also contain lactose, calcium hydrogen phosphate, microcrystalline cellulose, maize starch, sodium starch glycollate, povidone and magnesium stearate. The film coating contains hydroxypropyl methyl cellulose, propylene glycol, red iron oxide E172 and titanium dioxide.

6.2 Incompatibilities

None stated.

6.3 Shelf life

36 months.

6.4 Special precautions for storage

Blister packs: Store in a dry place below 30°C.

6.5 Nature and contents of container

Blister packs: pack size 28.

6.6 Instructions for use and handling

None.

7. MARKETING AUTHORISATION HOLDER

Aventis Pharma
50 Kings Hill Avenue
Kings Hill
West Malling
Kent
ME19 4AH

8. MARKETING AUTHORISATION NUMBER(S)

PL 00109/0133

9. DATE OF FIRST AUTHORISATION/RENEWAL OF THE AUTHORISATION

16 April 1997

10. DATE OF REVISION OF THE TEXT

13 July 2005

Legal classification: POM

Monocor Tablets

(Wyeth Pharmaceuticals)

1. NAME OF THE MEDICINAL PRODUCT

MONOCOR* Tablets 5mg.
MONOCOR* Tablets 10mg

2. QUALITATIVE AND QUANTITATIVE COMPOSITION

Monocor Tablets 5mg:

Bisoprolol fumarate (2:1) 5mg, equivalent to 4.2mg bisoprolol.

Monocor Tablets 10mg:

Bisoprolol fumarate (2:1) 10mg, equivalent to 8.4mg bisoprolol

For excipients, see 6.1.

3. PHARMACEUTICAL FORM

Film-coated tablet.

Monocor Tablets 5mg:

Pink, round, biconvex film-coated tablet marked 'LL' on one face and '5' on the other face.

Monocor Tablets 10mg:

White, round, biconvex, film-coated tablet marked with 'LL' on one face and '10' on the other face.

4. CLINICAL PARTICULARS

4.1 Therapeutic indications

1. The management of hypertension.
2. The management of angina pectoris.

4.2 Posology and method of administration

For the management of hypertension and angina pectoris:

Adults

The usual adult dose is 10mg once daily with a maximum recommended dose of 20mg per day. In some patients, 5mg per day may be adequate.

It is not necessary to alter the dose in patients with mild to moderate hepatic or renal dysfunction. In patients with severe renal failure (creatinine clearance less than 20ml/min) or in patients with severe hepatic dysfunction, the dosage should not exceed 10mg Monocor once daily.

Experience of use of Monocor in renal dialysis patients is limited. It is thought that bisoprolol fumarate cannot be dialysed.

Elderly

No dosage adjustment is normally required but 5mg per day may be adequate in some elderly patients; as for other adults, the dosage may have to be reduced in cases of severe renal or hepatic dysfunction.

Children

There is no paediatric experience with bisoprolol, therefore its use cannot be recommended for children.

4.3 Contraindications

Patients with:

- untreated cardiac failure.
- cardiogenic shock.
- sinoatrial block.
- second or third degree AV block.
- marked bradycardia.
- severe asthma.
- sick sinus syndrome.
- hypotension.
- severe peripheral circulatory disturbances.
- hypersensitivity to any of the ingredients in Monocor (either bisoprolol or any of the excipients listed in Section 6.1).

4.4 Special warnings and special precautions for use

Bisoprolol should be used with care in patients with a prolonged PR conduction interval, poor cardiac reserve and peripheral circulatory disease such as Raynaud's phenomena, since aggravation of these disorders may occur. Treatment should not be discontinued abruptly. As with other beta-blockers, gradual dosage reduction over 1-2 weeks is recommended, particularly in patients with ischaemic heart disease. If necessary, replacement therapy should be initiated at the same time to prevent exacerbation of angina pectoris.

Bisoprolol does not impair carbohydrate metabolism but in diabetic patients, the symptoms of hypoglycaemia may be masked.

In the event of a precipitous drop in pulse rate and/or blood pressure, treatment with Monocor should be discontinued. See also Section 4.9 'Overdose'.

In patients with phaeochromocytoma, bisoprolol must not be administered until after alpha-receptor blockade.

Bisoprolol should be used with caution in patients with metabolic acidosis.

Beta-blockers should generally be avoided in patients with a history of asthma or chronic obstructive airway disease. However, if there is no alternative, a cardio-selective beta-blocker such as Monocor may be used with extreme caution under specialist supervision. In some asthmatic patients, some increase in airway resistance may occur, and this may be regarded as a signal to discontinue therapy. Bronchospasm can usually be reversed by commonly used bronchodilators such as salbutamol. As a warning to patients, both the label and patient information leaflet for Monocor advise patients not to take Monocor, but to talk to their doctor if they have ever suffered from wheezing or asthma.

Beta adrenergic blockade may mask clinical signs of hyperthyroidism.

Due to their negative effect on conduction time, beta-blockers should only be given with caution to patients with first degree heart block.

Beta-blockers may increase the number and duration of angina attacks in patients with Prinzmetal's angina due to unopposed alpha-receptor mediated coronary artery vasoconstriction. Therefore, Monocor should be used with great care in these patients.

Patients with psoriasis in their personal or family history should only be prescribed beta-blockers after carefully balancing the benefits against the risks.

Beta-blockers may increase both the sensitivity towards allergens and the seriousness of anaphylactic reactions.

Caution should be exercised when using anaesthetic agents with Monocor. The anaesthetist should be informed if the patient is taking Monocor, and anaesthetic agents causing myocardial depression, such as cyclopropane or trichloroethylene, are best avoided. In cases of severe ischaemic heart disease, the risk/benefit of continuing treatment should be carefully evaluated. If withdrawal of Monocor is desired, this should be completed at least 24 hours prior to anaesthesia. Continuation of beta-blockade reduces the risk of arrhythmias during induction and intubation, but may result in attenuation of reflex tachycardia and increase the risk of hypotension. The patient may be protected against vagal reactions by intravenous administration of atropine.

4.5 Interaction with other medicinal products and other forms of Interaction

Combinations not recommended:

Calcium antagonists: Monocor should be used with care when myocardial depressants or inhibitors of AV conduction such as verapamil and diltiazem, because of their negative inotropic effects on contractility and atrioventricular conduction.

Clonidine: May cause an exaggerated decrease in heart rate. In particular, if clonidine is to be discontinued this should not be done until Monocor treatment has been discontinued for several days.

Digitalis glycosides: May increase atrioventricular conduction time and induce a negative inotropic effect when used in combination with beta-blockers.

MAO inhibitors (except MAO-B inhibitors): May enhance the hypotensive effect of beta-blockers. There is also a risk of hypertensive crisis.

Precaution for use:

Class I antidysrhythmic agents, such as disopyramide and quinodine, may have a potentiating effect on atrial-conduction time and induce a negative inotropic effect when given concomitantly with beta-blockers.

Class III antidysrhythmic agents, such as amiodarone, may potentiate the effect of beta-blockers on atrial conduction time.

Insulin and oral anti-diabetic drugs: The use of beta-blockers may intensify the blood sugar lowering effects of these drugs. Beta-blockers may also mask signs of hypoglycaemia, such as tachycardia.

Anaesthetic drugs: Please refer to Section 4.4 'Special Warnings and Precautions for Use'.

Alcohol may potentiate the hypotensive effects of beta-blockers.

Take into account:

Dihydropyridines, such as nifedipine, may increase the risk of hypotension. Cardiac failure may occur in patients with latent cardiac insufficiency.

Prostaglandin synthetase inhibitors, such as indometacin, may decrease the antihypertensive effect of beta-blockers.

Sympathomimetic agents, such as adrenaline, may decrease the antihypertensive effect of beta-blockers.

Other anti-hypertensive drugs: concomitant Monocor may potentiate the effects of these. Concomitant treatment of Monocor with reserpine and alpha-methyldopa may cause an exaggerated decrease in heart rate.

Drugs with secondary hypotensive effects, such as tricyclic antidepressants, barbiturates and phenothiazines, may also potentiate the anti-hypertensive effect of Monocor.

Rifampicin can reduce the elimination half-life of Monocor, although an increase in the dose of Monocor is, generally, not necessary.

4.6 Pregnancy and lactation

Beta-blockers reduce placental perfusion, which may result in immature neonates or premature deliveries. Further adverse effects (especially hypoglycaemia and bradycardia) may occur in the foetus or neonate, and there is an increased risk of cardiac and pulmonary complications in the neonate during the postnatal period.

In order to avoid complications in the neonate in the postnatal period (e.g. hypoglycaemia and bradycardia), the beta-blocker therapy should be discontinued 72 hours before the calculated term of delivery. If this is not possible, the neonate must be closely monitored. Symptoms of hypoglycaemia are generally expected within the first 3 days.

Small amounts of bisoprolol (2% of the dose) have been detected in the milk of lactating rats. It is not known whether this drug is excreted in human milk. Because many drugs are excreted in human milk, breast-feeding is not recommended during administration of bisoprolol.

4.7 Effects on ability to drive and use machines

As bisoprolol can cause drowsiness, dizziness and fatigue as side effects, these may affect the patient's ability to drive or operate machinery.

4.8 Undesirable effects

Monocor is usually well tolerated. The reported side effects are generally attributable to the pharmacological activity. These include lassitude, fatigue, dizziness, mild headache, muscle and joint ache, perspiration, aggravation of intermittent claudication or Raynaud's disease, paraesthesia, coldness and cyanosis of the extremities, bronchospasm, oedema and occasional gastrointestinal side effects such as nausea, vomiting and diarrhoea. A marked decrease in blood pressure and pulse rate or slowed AV conduction may be observed occasionally. As with other beta-blockers, there have been rare reports of heart block and exacerbation of heart failure.

As with other beta-blockers, skin rashes, pruritus, dry eyes have been reported, although the incidence is low. Sleep disturbances (including vivid dreams), have been reported occasionally. Discontinuation of the drug is recommended if any such reaction is not otherwise explicable.

Other adverse events seen infrequently with Monocor, include impaired vision, hallucinations, confusion, psychosis, nightmares, depression, anxiety and impotence.

Beta-blockers may mask the symptoms of thyrotoxicosis or hypoglycaemia.

4.9 Overdose

If overdose occurs, bisoprolol treatment should be stopped. Supportive therapy and symptomatic treatment should be provided. Limited data suggest bisoprolol fumarate cannot be dialysed.

Symptoms of overdose with a beta-blocker may include bradycardia, hypotension, bronchospasm and acute cardiac insufficiency. Based on the expected pharmacological actions and recommendations for other beta-blockers, the following general measures should be considered when clinically warranted:

Bradycardia or extensive vagal reactions may be countered by atropine.

Hypotension and shock may be treated with intravenous fluids, and, if necessary, catecholamines. The beta-blocking effect may be counteracted by slow intravenous administration of isopranaline or dobutamine. In refractory cases, isopranaline may be combined with dopamine. If this does not produce the desired effect, intravenous glucagon may be considered. The administration of calcium ions, or the use of a cardiac pacemaker may also be considered.

AV block (second or third degree): Patients should be carefully monitored and treated with isoprenaline or cardiac pacemaker insertion, as appropriate.

Acute worsening of heart failure: Administration of intravenous diuretics and inotropic agents should be considered.

Bronchospasm can usually be reversed by intravenous bronchodilators.

5. PHARMACOLOGICAL PROPERTIES

5.1 Pharmacodynamic properties

Pharmacotherapeutic Group: Beta Blocking Agents, Selective

ATC Code: C07AB07

Bisoprolol is a potent, highly cardioselective β_1-adrenoreceptor blocking agent devoid of intrinsic sympathomimetic activity and without relevant membrane stabilising activity.

As with other beta-blocking agents, the mode of action in hypertension is not clear but it is known that bisoprolol reduces the heart rate and depresses plasma rennin activity.

In patients with angina, blocking of cardiac β_1-receptors causes a diminished cardiac oxygen demand because of the resulting reduced heart action. This makes bisoprolol effective in eliminating or reducing the symptoms.

5.2 Pharmacokinetic properties

Bisoprolol is absorbed almost completely from the gastrointestinal tract. Together with the very small first pass effect in the liver, this results in a high bioavailability of approximately 90%. The drug is cleared equally by the liver and kidneys.

The long plasma half-life (10-12 hours) provides 24-hour efficacy following a once daily dosage. About 95% of the drug substance is excreted through the kidneys, 50% of a dose as unchanged bisoprolol. There are no active metabolites in man.

5.3 Preclinical safety data

Nothing of note to the prescriber.

6. PHARMACEUTICAL PARTICULARS

6.1 List of excipients

Tablet cores:

Colloidal anhydrous silica, magnesium stearate, povidone, microcrystalline cellulose, maize starch and dicalcium phosphate anhydrous.

Film-coating:Monocor Tablets 5mg:

Opadry OY-S-6952 (Methocel E5 Premium, Methocel E3 Premium, titanium dioxide (E171), polyethylene glycol 400, iron oxide red (E172), polysorbate 80, iron oxide yellow (E172), polyethylene glycol 4000 micro, purified water, talc).

Film-coating: Monocor Tablets 10mg:

Opadry OY-S-7390 (Methocel E5 Premium, Methocel E3 Premium, titanium dioxide (E171), polyethylene glycol 400, polysorbate 80, polyethylene glycol 4000 micro, purified water, talc).

6.2 Incompatibilities

Not applicable.

6.3 Shelf life

36 months.

6.4 Special precautions for storage

No special precautions for storage.

6.5 Nature and contents of container

Blister packs of aluminium foil and PVC or PVDC in cartons (pack size: 28).

Polypropylene bottles fitted with white lined urea caps (pack size: 100).

6.6 Instructions for use and handling

Not applicable.

7. MARKETING AUTHORISATION HOLDER

John Wyeth & Brother Limited

Trading as Wyeth Pharmaceuticals

Huntercombe Lane South

Taplow

Maidenhead

Berkshire SL6 0PH

United Kingdom

8. MARKETING AUTHORISATION NUMBER(S)

Monocor Tablets 5mg: PL 00011/0268

Monocor Tablets 10mg: PL 00011/0269

9. DATE OF FIRST AUTHORISATION/RENEWAL OF THE AUTHORISATION

30 April 2004

10. DATE OF REVISION OF THE TEXT

30 June 2005

* Trade marks.

Monoparin 1,000 iu/ml

(Wockhardt UK Ltd)

1. NAME OF THE MEDICINAL PRODUCT

Monoparin 1,000 I.U./ml

2. QUALITATIVE AND QUANTITATIVE COMPOSITION

Heparin sodium (mucous) 1,000 I.U./ml

For excipients see 6.1

3. PHARMACEUTICAL FORM

Solution for injection

A colourless or straw-coloured liquid, free from turbidity and from matter that deposits on standing.

4. CLINICAL PARTICULARS

4.1 Therapeutic indications

Treatment of deep vein thrombosis, pulmonary embolism, unstable angina pectoris and acute peripheral arterial occlusion.

In extracorporeal circulation and haemodialysis.

4.2 Posology and method of administration

Route of administration

By continuous intravenous infusion in 5% glucose or 0.9% sodium chloride or by intermittent intravenous injection.

As the effects of heparin are short-lived, administration by intravenous infusion is preferable to intermittent intravenous injections.

Recommended dosage

Treatment of deep vein thrombosis, pulmonary embolism, unstable angina pectoris, acute peripheral arterial occlusion:

Adults:

Loading dose:	5,000 units intravenously (10,000 units may be required in severe pulmonary embolism)
Maintenance:	1,000-2,000 units/hour by intravenous infusion, or 5,000-10,000 units 4-hourly by intravenous injection.

Elderly:

Dosage reduction may be advisable.

Children and small adults:

Loading dose:	50 units/kg intravenously
Maintenance:	15-25 units/kg/hour by intravenous infusion, or 100 units/kg 4-hourly by intravenous injection

Daily laboratory monitoring (ideally at the same time each day, starting 4-6 hours after initiation of treatment) is essential during full-dose heparin treatment, with adjustment of dosage to maintain an APTT value 1.5-2.5 × mid-point of normal range or control value.

In extracorporeal circulation and haemodialysis

Adults:

Cardiopulmonary bypass:

Initially 300 units/kg intravenously, adjusted thereafter to maintain the activated clotting time (ACT) in the range 400-500 seconds.

Haemodialysis and haemofiltration:

Initially 1,000-5,000 units,

Maintenance: 1,000-2,000 units/hour, adjusted to maintain clotting time >40 minutes.

4.3 Contraindications

Patients who consume large amounts of alcohol, who are sensitive to the drug, who are actively bleeding or who have haemophilia or other bleeding disorders, severe liver disease (including oesophageal varices), purpura, severe hypertension, active tuberculosis or increased capillary permeability.

Patients with present or previous thrombocytopenia. The rare occurrence of skin necrosis in patients receiving heparin contra-indicates the further use of heparin either by subcutaneous or intravenous routes because of the risk of thrombocytopenia. Because of the special hazard of post-operative haemorrhage heparin is contra-indicated during surgery of the brain, spinal cord and eye, and in patients undergoing lumbar puncture or regional anaesthetic block.

The relative risks and benefits of heparin should be carefully assessed in patients with a bleeding tendency or those patients with an actual or potential bleeding site eg. hiatus hernia, peptic ulcer, neoplasm, bacterial endocarditis, retinopathy, bleeding haemorrhoids, suspected intracranial haemorrhage, cerebral thrombosis or threatened abortion.

Menstruation is not a contra-indication.

4.4 Special warnings and special precautions for use

Platelet counts should be measured in patients receiving heparin treatment for longer than 5 days and the treatment should be stopped immediately in those who develop thrombocytopenia.

In patients with advanced renal or hepatic disease, a reduction in dosage may be necessary. The risk of bleeding is increased with severe renal impairment and in women over 60 years of age.

Although heparin hypersensitivity is rare, it is advisable to give a trial dose of 1,000 I.U. in patients with a history of allergy. Caution should be exercised in patients with known hypersensitivity to low molecular weight heparins.

In most patients, the recommended low-dose regimen produces no alteration in clotting time. However, patients show an individual response to heparin, and it is therefore essential that the effect of therapy on coagulation time should be monitored in patients undergoing major surgery.

Caution is recommended in spinal or epidural anaesthesia (risk of spinal haematoma).

Heparin can suppress adrenal secretion of aldosterone leading to hyperkalemia, particularly in patients such as those with diabetes mellitus, chronic renal failure, pre-existing metabolic acidosis, a raised plasma potassium, or taking potassium sparing drugs. The risk of hyperkalemia appears to increase with duration of therapy but is usually reversible. Plasma potassium should be measured in patients at risk before starting heparin therapy and in all patients treated for more than 7 days.

4.5 Interaction with other medicinal products and other forms of Interaction

Drugs that interfere with platelet aggregation eg. aspirin and other NSAIDs, dextran solutions, dipyridamole or any other drug which may interfere with coagulation, should be used with care.

Hyperkalaemia may occur with concomitant ACE inhibitors.

Reduced activity of heparin has been reported with simultaneous intravenous glyceryl trinitrate infusion.

Interference with diagnostic tests may be associated with pseudo-hypocalcaemia (in haemodialysis patients), artefactual increases in total thyroxine and triiodothyronine, simulated metabolic acidosis and inhibition of the chromogenic lysate assay for endotoxin. Heparin may interfere with the determination of aminoglycosides by immunoassays.

4.6 Pregnancy and lactation

Heparin is not contraindicated in pregnancy. Heparin does not cross the placenta or appear in breast milk. The decision to use heparin in pregnancy should be taken after evaluation of the risk/benefit in any particular circumstances.

Reduced bone density has been reported with prolonged heparin treatment during pregnancy.

Haemorrhage may be a problem during pregnancy or after delivery.

4.7 Effects on ability to drive and use machines

None stated.

4.8 Undesirable effects

Haemorrhage (see also Special Warnings and Precautions and Overdosage Information).

Thrombocytopenia has been observed occasionally (see also Special Precautions and Warnings). Two types of heparin-induced thrombocytopenia have been defined. Type I is frequent, mild (usually $>50 \times 10^9$/L) and transient, occurring within 1-5 days of heparin administration. Type II is less frequent but often associated with severe thrombocytopenia (usually $<50 \times 10^9$/L). It is immune-mediated and occurs after a week or more (earlier in patients previously exposed to heparin). It is associated with the production of a platelet-aggregating antibody and thromboembolic complications which may precede the onset of thrombocytopenia. Heparin should be discontinued immediately.

There is some evidence that prolonged dosing with heparin (ie. over many months) may cause alopecia and osteoporosis. Significant bone demineralisation has been reported in women taking more than 10,000 I.U. per day of heparin for at least 6 months.

Heparin products can cause hypoaldosteronism which may result in an increase in plasma potassium. Rarely, clinically significant hyperkalemia may occur particularly in patients with chronic renal failure and diabetes mellitus (see Warnings and Precautions).

Hypersensitivity reactions to heparin are rare. They include urticaria, conjunctivitis, rhinitis, asthma, cyanosis, tachypnoea, feeling of oppression, fever, chills, angioneurotic oedema and anaphylactic shock.

Local irritation and skin necrosis may occur but are rare.

Priapism has been reported. Increased serum transaminase values may occur but usually resolve on discontinuation of heparin. Heparin administration is associated with release of lipoprotein lipase into the plasma; rebound hyperlipidaemia may follow heparin withdrawal.

4.9 Overdose

A potential hazard of heparin therapy is haemorrhage, but this is usually due to overdosage and the risk is minimised by strict laboratory control. Slight haemorrhage can usually be treated by withdrawing the drug. If bleeding is more severe, clotting time and platelet count should be determined. Prolonged clotting time will indicate the presence of an excessive anticoagulant effect requiring neutralisation by intravenous protamine sulphate, at a dosage of 1 mg for every 100 I.U. of heparin to be neutralised. The bolus dose of protamine sulphate should be given slowly over about 10 minutes and not exceed 50 mg. If more than 15 minutes have elapsed since the injection of heparin, lower doses of protamine will be necessary.

5. PHARMACOLOGICAL PROPERTIES

5.1 Pharmacodynamic properties

Heparin is an anticoagulant and acts by inhibiting thrombin and by potentiating the naturally occurring inhibitors of activated Factor X (Xa).

5.2 Pharmacokinetic properties

As heparin is not absorbed from the gastrointestinal tract and sublingual sites it is administered by injection. After injection heparin extensively binds to plasma proteins.

Heparin is metabolised in the liver and the inactive metabolic products are excreted in the urine.

The half life of heparin is dependent on the dose.

5.3 Preclinical safety data

There are no pre-clinical data of relevance to the prescriber which are additional to those already included in other sections.

6. PHARMACEUTICAL PARTICULARS

6.1 List of excipients

Water for injections

Sodium hydroxide solution 3M

Hydrochloric acid 3M

6.2 Incompatibilities

Heparin is incompatible with many injectable preparations e.g. some antibiotics, opioid analgesics and antihistamines.

Dobutamine hydrochloride and heparin should not be mixed or infused through the same intravenous line, as this causes precipitation.

Heparin and reteplase are incompatible when combined in solution.

If reteplase and heparin are to be given through the same line this, together with any Y-lines, must be thoroughly flushed with a 0.9% saline or a 5% glucose solution prior to and following the reteplase injection.

6.3 Shelf life

Unopened - 36 months

From a microbiological point of view, unless the method of opening precludes the risk of microbial contamination, the product should be used immediately.

If not used immediately, in-use storage times and conditions are the responsibility of the user.

6.4 Special precautions for storage

Monoparin should not be stored above 25°C

Store in the original package

6.5 Nature and contents of container

Neutral glass ampoules (Type I Ph Eur) of 1ml, 5ml, 10ml and 20ml capacity containing 1ml, 5ml, 10ml and 20ml of solution respectively. Cartons contain 10 ampoules.

6.6 Instructions for use and handling

Not applicable

Administrative Data

7. MARKETING AUTHORISATION HOLDER

CP Pharmaceuticals Ltd

Ash Road North

Wrexham

LL13 9UF

UK.

8. MARKETING AUTHORISATION NUMBER(S)

PL 4543/0221

9. DATE OF FIRST AUTHORISATION/RENEWAL OF THE AUTHORISATION

Date of first authorisation - 5 July 1991

Date of renewal - 21 November 1996

10. DATE OF REVISION OF THE TEXT

August 2001

Monoparin 25,000 iu/ml

(Wockhardt UK Ltd)

1. NAME OF THE MEDICINAL PRODUCT

Monoparin 25,000 I.U./ml Solution for injection or concentrate for solution for injection

2. QUALITATIVE AND QUANTITATIVE COMPOSITION

Heparin sodium (mucous) 25,000 I.U./ml (5,000 I.U. in 0.2ml, 12,500 I.U.in 0.5ml, 25,000 I.U. in 1ml, 125,000 I.U. in 5ml)

For excipients see 6.1

3. PHARMACEUTICAL FORM

Solution for injection or concentrate for solution for injection

A colourless or straw-coloured liquid, free from turbidity and from matter that deposits on standing.

4. CLINICAL PARTICULARS

4.1 Therapeutic indications

Prophylaxis of deep vein thrombosis and pulmonary embolism

Treatment of deep vein thrombosis, pulmonary embolism, unstable angina pectoris and acute peripheral arterial occlusion.

Prophylaxis of mural thrombosis following myocardial infarction.

In extracorporeal circulation and haemodialysis.

4.2 Posology and method of administration

Route of administration

By continuous intravenous infusion in 5% glucose or 0.9% sodium chloride or by intermittent intravenous injection, or by subcutaneous injection.

As the effects of heparin are short-lived, administration by intravenous infusion or subcutaneous injection is preferable to intermittent intravenous injections.

Recommended dosage

Prophylaxis of deep vein thrombosis and pulmonary embolism

Adults:

2 hours pre-operatively:	5,000 units subcutaneously
followed by:	5,000 units subcutaneously every 8-12 hours, for 7-10 days or until the patient is fully ambulant.

No laboratory monitoring should be necessary during low dose heparin prophylaxis. If monitoring is considered desirable, anti-Xa assays should be used as the activated partial thromboplastin time (APTT) is not significantly prolonged.

During pregnancy:	5,000 - 10,000 units every 12 hours, subcutaneously, adjusted according to APTT or anti-Xa assay.

Elderly:

Dosage reduction and monitoring of APTT may be advisable.

Children:

No dosage recommendations.

Treatment of deep vein thrombosis, pulmonary embolism, unstable angina pectoris, acute peripheral arterial occlusion:

Adults:

Loading dose:	5,000 units intravenously (10,000 units may be required in severe pulmonary embolism)
Maintenance:	1,000-2,000 units/hour by intravenous infusion, or 10,000-20,000 units 12 hourly subcutaneously, or 5,000-10,000 units 4-hourly by intravenous injection.

Elderly:

Dosage reduction may be advisable.

Children and small adults:

Loading dose:	50 units/kg intravenously
Maintenance:	15-25 units/kg/hour by intravenous infusion, or 250 units/kg 12 hourly subcutaneously or 100 units/kg 4-hourly by intravenous injection

Daily laboratory monitoring (ideally at the same time each day, starting 4-6 hours after initiation of treatment) is essential during full-dose heparin treatment, with adjustment of dosage to maintain an APTT value 1.5-2.5 × mid-point of normal range or control value.

Prophylaxis of mural thrombosis following myocardial infarction

Adults:

12,500 units 12 hourly subcutaneously for at least 10 days.

Elderly:

Dosage reduction may be advisable

In extracorporeal circulation and haemodialysis

Adults:

Cardiopulmonary bypass:

Initially 300 units/kg intravenously, adjusted thereafter to maintain the activated clotting time (ACT) in the range 400-500 seconds.

Haemodialysis and haemofiltration:

Initially 1,000-5,000 units,

Maintenance: 1,000-2,000 units/hour, adjusted to maintain clotting time >40 minutes.

4.3 Contraindications

Patients who consume large amounts of alcohol, who are sensitive to the drug, who are actively bleeding or who have haemophilia or other bleeding disorders, severe liver disease (including oesophageal varices), purpura, severe hypertension, active tuberculosis or increased capillary permeability.

Patients with present or previous thrombocytopenia. The rare occurrence of skin necrosis in patients receiving heparin contra-indicates the further use of heparin either by subcutaneous or intravenous routes because of the risk of thrombocytopenia. Because of the special hazard of post-operative haemorrhage heparin is contra-indicated during surgery of the brain, spinal cord and eye, and in patients undergoing lumbar puncture or regional anaesthetic block.

The relative risks and benefits of heparin should be carefully assessed in patients with a bleeding tendency or those patients with an actual or potential bleeding site eg. hiatus hernia, peptic ulcer, neoplasm, bacterial endocarditis, retinopathy, bleeding haemorrhoids, suspected intracranial haemorrhage, cerebral thrombosis or threatened abortion.

Menstruation is not a contra-indication.

4.4 Special warnings and special precautions for use

Platelet counts should be measured in patients receiving heparin treatment for longer than 5 days and the treatment should be stopped immediately in those who develop thrombocytopenia.

In patients with advanced renal or hepatic disease, a reduction in dosage may be necessary. The risk of bleeding is increased with severe renal impairment and in women over 60 years of age.

Although heparin hypersensitivity is rare, it is advisable to give a trial dose of 1,000 I.U. in patients with a history of allergy. Caution should be exercised in patients with known hypersensitivity to low molecular weight heparins.

In most patients, the recommended low-dose regimen produces no alteration in clotting time. However, patients show an individual response to heparin, and it is therefore essential that the effect of therapy on coagulation time should be monitored in patients undergoing major surgery.

Caution is recommended in spinal or epidural anaesthesia (risk of spinal haematoma).

Heparin can suppress adrenal secretion of aldosterone leading to hyperkalemia, particularly in patients such as those with diabetes mellitus, chronic renal failure, pre-existing metabolic acidosis, a raised plasma potassium, or taking potassium sparing drugs. The risk of hyperkalemia appears to increase with duration of therapy but is usually reversible. Plasma potassium should be measured in patients at risk before starting heparin therapy and in all patients treated for more than 7 days.

4.5 Interaction with other medicinal products and other forms of Interaction

Drugs that interfere with platelet aggregation eg. aspirin and other NSAIDs, dextran solutions, dipyridamole or any other drug which may interfere with coagulation, should be used with care.

Hyperkalaemia may occur with concomitant ACE inhibitors.

Reduced activity of heparin has been reported with simultaneous intravenous glyceryl trinitrate infusion.

Interference with diagnostic tests may be associated with pseudo-hypocalcaemia (in haemodialysis patients), artefactual increases in total thyroxine and triiodothyronine, simulated metabolic acidosis and inhibition of the chromogenic lysate assay for endotoxin. Heparin may interfere with the determination of aminoglycosides by immunoassays.

4.6 Pregnancy and lactation

Heparin is not contraindicated in pregnancy. Heparin does not cross the placenta or appear in breast milk. The decision to use heparin in pregnancy should be taken after evaluation of the risk/benefit in any particular circumstances.

Reduced bone density has been reported with prolonged heparin treatment during pregnancy.

Haemorrhage may be a problem during pregnancy or after delivery.

4.7 Effects on ability to drive and use machines

None stated.

4.8 Undesirable effects

Haemorrhage (see also Special Warnings and Precautions and Overdosage Information).

Thrombocytopenia has been observed occasionally (see also Special Precautions and Warnings). Two types of heparin-induced thrombocytopenia have been defined. Type I is frequent, mild (usually $>50 \times 10^9$/L) and transient, occurring within 1-5 days of heparin administration. Type II is less frequent but often associated with severe thrombocytopenia (usually $<50 \times 10^9$/L). It is immune-mediated and occurs after a week or more (earlier in patients previously exposed to heparin). It is associated with the production of a platelet-aggregating antibody and thromboembolic complications which may precede the onset of thrombocytopenia. Heparin should be discontinued immediately.

There is some evidence that prolonged dosing with heparin (ie. over many months) may cause alopecia and osteoporosis. Significant bone demineralisation has been reported in women taking more than 10,000 I.U. per day of heparin for at least 6 months.

Heparin products can cause hypoaldosteronism which may result in an increase in plasma potassium. Rarely, clinically significant hyperkalemia may occur particularly in patients with chronic renal failure and diabetes mellitus (see Warnings and Precautions).

Hypersensitivity reactions to heparin are rare. They include urticaria, conjunctivitis, rhinitis, asthma, cyanosis, tachypnoea, feeling of oppression, fever, chills, angioneurotic oedema and anaphylactic shock.

Local irritation and skin necrosis may occur but are rare. Erythematous nodules, or infiltrated and sometimes eczema-like plaques, at the site of subcutaneous injections are common, occurring 3-21 days after starting heparin treatment.

Priapism has been reported. Increased serum transaminase values may occur but usually resolve on discontinuation of heparin. Heparin administration is associated with release of lipoprotein lipase into the plasma; rebound hyperlipidaemia may follow heparin withdrawal.

4.9 Overdose

A potential hazard of heparin therapy is haemorrhage, but this is usually due to overdosage and the risk is minimised by strict laboratory control. Slight haemorrhage can usually be treated by withdrawing the drug. If bleeding is more severe, clotting time and platelet count should be determined. Prolonged clotting time will indicate the presence of an excessive anticoagulant effect requiring neutralisation by intravenous protamine sulphate, at a dosage of 1 mg for every 100 I.U. of heparin to be neutralised. The bolus dose of protamine sulphate should be given slowly over about 10 minutes and not exceed 50 mg. If more than 15 minutes have elapsed since the injection of heparin, lower doses of protamine will be necessary.

5. PHARMACOLOGICAL PROPERTIES

5.1 Pharmacodynamic properties

Heparin is an anticoagulant and acts by inhibiting thrombin and by potentiating the naturally occurring inhibitors of activated Factor X (Xa).

5.2 Pharmacokinetic properties

As heparin is not absorbed from the gastrointestinal tract and sublingual sites it is administered by injection. After injection heparin extensively binds to plasma proteins.

Heparin is metabolised in the liver and the inactive metabolic products are excreted in the urine.

The half life of heparin is dependent on the dose.

5.3 Preclinical safety data

There are no pre-clinical data of relevance to the prescriber which are additional to those already included in other sections.

6. PHARMACEUTICAL PARTICULARS

6.1 List of excipients

Water for injections

Sodium hydroxide solution 3M

Hydrochloric acid 3M

6.2 Incompatibilities

Heparin is incompatible with many injectable preparations e.g. some antibiotics, opioid analgesics and antihistamines.

Dobutamine hydrochloride and heparin should not be mixed or infused through the same intravenous line, as this causes precipitation.

Heparin and reteplase are incompatible when combined in solution.

If reteplase and heparin are to be given through the same line this, together with any Y-lines, must be thoroughly flushed with a 0.9% saline or a 5% glucose solution prior to and following the reteplase injection.

6.3 Shelf life

Unopened - 36 months

From a microbiological point of view, unless the method of opening precludes the risk of microbial contamination, the product should be used immediately.

If not used immediately, in-use storage times and conditions are the responsibility of the user.

6.4 Special precautions for storage

Monoparin should not be stored above 25°C

Store in the original package

6.5 Nature and contents of container

Neutral glass ampoules (Type I Ph Eur) of 1ml capacity containing 0.2ml, 0.5ml and 1ml of solution respectively and 5ml ampoules containing 5ml of solution. Cartons contain 10, 15 or 50 ampoules.

6.6 Instructions for use and handling

Not applicable

Administrative Data

7. MARKETING AUTHORISATION HOLDER

CP Pharmaceuticals Ltd
Ash Road North
Wrexham
LL13 9UF
UK.

8. MARKETING AUTHORISATION NUMBER(S)

PL 4543/0210

9. DATE OF FIRST AUTHORISATION/RENEWAL OF THE AUTHORISATION

Date of first authorisation - 18 June 1991

Date of renewal - 29 May 2002

10. DATE OF REVISION OF THE TEXT

November 2002

Monoparin 5,000 iu/ml

(Wockhardt UK Ltd)

1. NAME OF THE MEDICINAL PRODUCT

Monoparin 5,000 I.U./ml Solution for injection or concentrate for solution for infusion

2. QUALITATIVE AND QUANTITATIVE COMPOSITION

Heparin sodium (mucous) 5,000 I.U./ml (5,000 I.U. in 1ml, 25,000 I.U. in 5ml)

For excipients see 6.1

3. PHARMACEUTICAL FORM

Solution for injection or concentrate for solution for infusion

A colourless or straw-coloured liquid, free from turbidity and from matter that deposits on standing.

4. CLINICAL PARTICULARS

4.1 Therapeutic indications

Prophylaxis of deep vein thrombosis and pulmonary embolism

Treatment of deep vein thrombosis, pulmonary embolism, unstable angina pectoris and acute peripheral arterial occlusion.

Prophylaxis of mural thrombosis following myocardial infarction.

In extracorporeal circulation and haemodialysis.

4.2 Posology and method of administration

Route of administration

By continuous intravenous infusion in 5% glucose or 0.9% sodium chloride or by intermittent intravenous injection, or by subcutaneous injection.

As the effects of heparin are short-lived, administration by intravenous infusion or subcutaneous injection is preferable to intermittent intravenous injections.

Recommended dosage

Prophylaxis of deep vein thrombosis and pulmonary embolism

Adults:

2 hours pre-operatively:	5,000 units subcutaneously
followed by:	5,000 units subcutaneously every 8-12 hours, for 7-10 days or until the patient is fully ambulant.

No laboratory monitoring should be necessary during low dose heparin prophylaxis. If monitoring is considered desirable, anti-Xa assays should be used as the activated partial thromboplastin time (APTT) is not significantly prolonged.

During pregnancy:	5,000 - 10,000 units every 12 hours, subcutaneously, adjusted according to APTT or anti-Xa assay.

Elderly:

Dosage reduction and monitoring of APTT may be advisable.

Children:

No dosage recommendations.

Treatment of deep vein thrombosis, pulmonary embolism, unstable angina pectoris, acute peripheral arterial occlusion:

Adults:

Loading dose:	5,000 units intravenously (10,000 units may be required in severe pulmonary embolism)

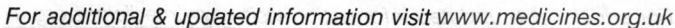

Maintenance: 1,000-2,000 units/hour by intravenous infusion,

or

10,000-20,000 units 12 hourly subcutaneously,

or

5,000-10,000 units 4-hourly by intravenous injection.

Elderly:

Dosage reduction may be advisable.

Children and small adults:

Loading dose: 50 units/kg intravenously

Maintenance: 15-25 units/kg/hour by intravenous infusion,

or

250 units/kg 12 hourly subcutaneously

or

100 units/kg 4-hourly by intravenous injection

Daily laboratory monitoring (ideally at the same time each day, starting 4-6 hours after initiation of treatment) is essential during full-dose heparin treatment, with adjustment of dosage to maintain an APTT value 1.5-2.5 × mid-point of normal range or control value.

Prophylaxis of mural thrombosis following myocardial infarction

Adults:

12,500 units 12 hourly subcutaneously for at least 10 days.

Elderly:

Dosage reduction may be advisable

In extracorporeal circulation and haemodialysis

Adults:

Cardiopulmonary bypass:

Initially 300 units/kg intravenously, adjusted thereafter to maintain the activated clotting time (ACT) in the range 400-500 seconds.

Haemodialysis and haemofiltration:

Initially 1,000-5,000 units,

Maintenance: 1,000-2,000 units/hour, adjusted to maintain clotting time >40 minutes.

4.3 Contraindications

Patients who consume large amounts of alcohol, who are sensitive to the drug, who are actively bleeding or who have haemophilia or other bleeding disorders, severe liver disease (including oesophageal varices), purpura, severe hypertension, active tuberculosis or increased capillary permeability.

Patients with present or previous thrombocytopenia. The rare occurrence of skin necrosis in patients receiving heparin contra-indicates the further use of heparin either by subcutaneous or intravenous routes because of the risk of thrombocytopenia. Because of the special hazard of post-operative haemorrhage heparin is contra-indicated during surgery of the brain, spinal cord and eye, and in patients undergoing lumbar puncture or regional anaesthetic block.

The relative risks and benefits of heparin should be carefully assessed in patients with a bleeding tendency or those patients with an actual or potential bleeding site eg. hiatus hernia, peptic ulcer, neoplasm, bacterial endocarditis, retinopathy, bleeding haemorrhoids, suspected intracranial haemorrhage, cerebral thrombosis or threatened abortion.

Menstruation is not a contra-indication.

4.4 Special warnings and special precautions for use

Platelet counts should be measured in patients receiving heparin treatment for longer than 5 days and the treatment should be stopped immediately in those who develop thrombocytopenia.

In patients with advanced renal or hepatic disease, a reduction in dosage may be necessary. The risk of bleeding is increased with severe renal impairment and in women over 60 years of age.

Although heparin hypersensitivity is rare, it is advisable to give a trial dose of 1,000 I.U. in patients with a history of allergy. Caution should be exercised in patients with known hypersensitivity to low molecular weight heparins.

In most patients, the recommended low-dose regimen produces no alteration in clotting time. However, patients show an individual response to heparin, and it is therefore essential that the effect of therapy on coagulation time should be monitored in patients undergoing major surgery.

Caution is recommended in spinal or epidural anaesthesia (risk of spinal haematoma).

Heparin can suppress adrenal secretion of aldosterone leading to hyperkalemia, particularly in patients such as those with diabetes mellitus, chronic renal failure, pre-existing metabolic acidosis, a raised plasma potassium, or taking potassium sparing drugs. The risk of hyperkalemia appears to increase with duration of therapy but is usually reversible. Plasma potassium should be measured in patients at risk before starting heparin therapy and in all patients treated for more than 7 days.

4.5 Interaction with other medicinal products and other forms of Interaction

Drugs that interfere with platelet aggregation eg. aspirin and other NSAIDs, dextran solutions, dipyridamole or any other drug which may interfere with coagulation, should be used with care.

Hyperkalaemia may occur with concomitant ACE inhibitors.

Reduced activity of heparin has been reported with simultaneous intravenous glyceryl trinitrate infusion.

Interference with diagnostic tests may be associated with pseudo-hypocalcaemia (in haemodialysis patients), artefactual increases in total thyroxine and triiodothyronine, simulated metabolic acidosis and inhibition of the chromogenic lysate assay for endotoxin. Heparin may interfere with the determination of aminoglycosides by immunoassays.

4.6 Pregnancy and lactation

Heparin is not contraindicated in pregnancy. Heparin does not cross the placenta or appear in breast milk. The decision to use heparin in pregnancy should be taken after evaluation of the risk/benefit in any particular circumstances.

Reduced bone density has been reported with prolonged heparin treatment during pregnancy.

Haemorrhage may be a problem during pregnancy or after delivery.

4.7 Effects on ability to drive and use machines

None stated.

4.8 Undesirable effects

Haemorrhage (see also Special Warnings and Precautions and Overdosage Information).

Thrombocytopenia has been observed occasionally (see also Special Precautions and Warnings). Two types of heparin-induced thrombocytopenia have been defined. Type I is frequent, mild (usually $>50 \times 10^9$/L) and transient, occurring within 1-5 days of heparin administration. Type II is less frequent but often associated with severe thrombocytopenia (usually $<50 \times 10^9$/L). It is immune-mediated and occurs after a week or more (earlier in patients previously exposed to heparin). It is associated with the production of a platelet-aggregating antibody and thromboembolic complications which may precede the onset of thrombocytopenia. Heparin should be discontinued immediately.

There is some evidence that prolonged dosing with heparin (ie. over many months) may cause alopecia and osteoporosis. Significant bone demineralisation has been reported in women taking more than 10,000 I.U. per day of heparin for at least 6 months.

Heparin products can cause hypoaldosteronism which may result in an increase in plasma potassium. Rarely, clinically significant hyperkalemia may occur particularly in patients with chronic renal failure and diabetes mellitus (see Warnings and Precautions).

Hypersensitivity reactions to heparin are rare. They include urticaria, conjunctivitis, rhinitis, asthma, cyanosis, tachypnoea, feeling of oppression, fever, chills, angioneurotic oedema and anaphylactic shock.

Local irritation and skin necrosis may occur but are rare. Erythematous nodules, or infiltrated and sometimes eczema-like plaques, at the site of subcutaneous injections are common, occurring 3-21 days after starting heparin treatment.

Priapism has been reported. Increased serum transaminase values may occur but usually resolve on discontinuation of heparin. Heparin administration is associated with release of lipoprotein lipase into the plasma; rebound hyperlipidaemia may follow heparin withdrawal.

4.9 Overdose

A potential hazard of heparin therapy is haemorrhage, but this is usually due to overdosage and the risk is minimised by strict laboratory control. Slight haemorrhage can usually be treated by withdrawing the drug. If bleeding is more severe, clotting time and platelet count should be determined. Prolonged clotting time will indicate the presence of an excessive anticoagulant effect requiring neutralisation by intravenous protamine sulphate, at a dosage of 1 mg for every 100 I.U. of heparin to be neutralised. The bolus dose of protamine sulphate should be given slowly over about 10 minutes and not exceed 50 mg. If more than 15 minutes have elapsed since the injection of heparin, lower doses of protamine will be necessary.

5. PHARMACOLOGICAL PROPERTIES

5.1 Pharmacodynamic properties

Heparin is an anticoagulant and acts by inhibiting thrombin and by potentiating the naturally occurring inhibitors of activated Factor X (Xa).

5.2 Pharmacokinetic properties

As heparin is not absorbed from the gastrointestinal tract and sublingual sites it is administered by injection. After injection heparin extensively binds to plasma proteins.

Heparin is metabolised in the liver and the inactive metabolic products are excreted in the urine.

The half life of heparin is dependent on the dose.

5.3 Preclinical safety data

There are no pre-clinical data of relevance to the prescriber which are additional to those already included in other sections.

6. PHARMACEUTICAL PARTICULARS

6.1 List of excipients

Water for injections

Sodium hydroxide solution 3M

Hydrochloric acid 3M

6.2 Incompatibilities

Heparin is incompatible with many injectable preparations e.g. some antibiotics, opioid analgesics and antihistamines.

Dobutamine hydrochloride and heparin should not be mixed or infused through the same intravenous line, as this causes precipitation.

Heparin and reteplase are incompatible when combined in solution.

If reteplase and heparin are to be given through the same line this, together with any Y-lines, must be thoroughly flushed with a 0.9% saline or a 5% glucose solution prior to and following the reteplase injection.

6.3 Shelf life

Unopened - 36 months

From a microbiological point of view, unless the method of opening precludes the risk of microbial contamination, the product should be used immediately.

If not used immediately, in-use storage times and conditions are the responsibility of the user.

6.4 Special precautions for storage

Monoparin should not be stored above 25°C

Store in the original package

6.5 Nature and contents of container

Neutral glass ampoules (Type I Ph Eur) of 1ml and 5ml capacity containing 1ml and 5ml of solution respectively. Cartons contain 10 ampoules.

6.6 Instructions for use and handling

Not applicable

Administrative Data

7. MARKETING AUTHORISATION HOLDER

CP Pharmaceuticals Ltd

Ash Road North

Wrexham

LL13 9UF

UK.

8. MARKETING AUTHORISATION NUMBER(S)

PL 4543/0208

9. DATE OF FIRST AUTHORISATION/RENEWAL OF THE AUTHORISATION

Date of first authorisation - 18 June 1991

Date of renewal - 29 May 2002

10. DATE OF REVISION OF THE TEXT

November 2002

Monphytol

(Laboratories for Applied Biology Limited)

1. NAME OF THE MEDICINAL PRODUCT

Monphytol Paint

2. QUALITATIVE AND QUANTITATIVE COMPOSITION

Active Constituents

Chlorobutanol	3 % w/v
Methyl Undecenoate	5 % w/v
Propyl Undecenoate	0.7% w/v
Salicylic Acid	3 % w/v
Methyl Salicylate	25 % w/v
Propyl Salicylate	5 % w/v

3. PHARMACEUTICAL FORM

Cutaneous solution. A colourless paint supplied with a brush.

4. CLINICAL PARTICULARS

4.1 Therapeutic indications

Erosio interdigitalis, intertrigo, tinea circinata, tinea pedis, tinea unguium.

4.2 Posology and method of administration

Adults and children over 12: Twice daily (4 times daily for fingers) moisten brush with Monphytol and apply to the affected parts, reaching gently into the folds of the skin. Treatment should be repeated from time to time after the condition has subsided to prevent reinfection.

Children under 12, pregnant and lactating women: The safety of this product has not been demonstrated for these groups. Its use must be at the physician's discretion.

4.3 Contraindications
Monphytol should not be used on bleeding areas.

4.4 Special warnings and special precautions for use
Monphytol may sting sensitive weeping areas of acutely inflamed skin. Other treatment (to reduce inflammation and exudation) may first be necessary. Monphytol should not be used on bleeding areas.

4.5 Interaction with other medicinal products and other forms of Interaction
None known.

4.6 Pregnancy and lactation
The safety of this product has not been demonstrated for pregnant or lactating women. Its use must be at the physician's discretion.

4.7 Effects on ability to drive and use machines
None known

4.8 Undesirable effects
Monphytol may sting sensitive areas.

4.9 Overdose
As Monphytol is applied topically, this is not applicable.

5. PHARMACOLOGICAL PROPERTIES

5.1 Pharmacodynamic properties
Pharmacological Group: Antifungal Skin Preparation (BNF 13.10.2)

Chlorobutanol has antibacterial and antifungal properties - Martindale 30th Edition.

Salicylic acid and the Salicylates have antifungal properties. The esters are used for the relief of pain. - Martindale 30th Edition.

Undecenoic acid and its salts are active against some pathogenic fungi. - Martindale 30th Edition. The esters are thought to be similarly active, but their increased solubility in the medium increases their efficacy.

5.2 Pharmacokinetic properties
The product is applied topically, so normal pharmacokinetic criteria do not apply.

5.3 Preclinical safety data
None stated.

6. PHARMACEUTICAL PARTICULARS

6.1 List of excipients

Methanol	50 % v/v
Propanol	15 % v/v

6.2 Incompatibilities
Major: None known

6.3 Shelf life
3 years

6.4 Special precautions for storage
No special precautions are necessary

6.5 Nature and contents of container
Amber glass (type III) winchester, containing 18 ml

6.6 Instructions for use and handling
No special precautions.

7. MARKETING AUTHORISATION HOLDER
Laboratories for Applied Biology Ltd
91 Amhurst Park
London N16 5 DR
United Kingdom

8. MARKETING AUTHORISATION NUMBER(S)
UK PL 0118/5010 R

9. DATE OF FIRST AUTHORISATION/RENEWAL OF THE AUTHORISATION
First granted: 22.04.87
Renewed: 09.03.98

10. DATE OF REVISION OF THE TEXT
27.03.98

Morphgesic SR Tablets

(Amdipharm)

1. NAME OF THE MEDICINAL PRODUCT
Morphgesic® SR 10mg Tablets
Morphgesic® SR 30mg Tablets
Morphgesic® SR 60mg Tablets
Morphgesic® SR 100mg Tablets

2. QUALITATIVE AND QUANTITATIVE COMPOSITION
Morphgesic® SR 10mg Tablets contain 10mg Morphine Sulphate.

Morphgesic® SR 30mg Tablets contain 30mg Morphine Sulphate.

Morphgesic® SR 60mg Tablets contain 60mg Morphine Sulphate.

Morphgesic® SR 100mg Tablets contain 100mg Morphine Sulphate.

Each tablet is a biconvex round film coated tablet.

10mg is buff coloured, 30mg is violet coloured, 60mg is orange coloured and

100mg is grey coloured.

3. PHARMACEUTICAL FORM
Controlled release tablets

4. CLINICAL PARTICULARS

4.1 Therapeutic indications
For the prolonged relief of severe pain.

4.2 Posology and method of administration
Route of administration: Oral

Morphgesic® SR tablets should be swallowed whole and not chewed.

Adults:

The dosage is dependant upon the severity of the pain and the patient's previous history of analgesic requirements. The tablets should normally be administered twice daily at 12 hourly intervals. One or two 10mg tablets (10mg) twice daily is the recommended starting dosage for a patient presenting with severe pain. With increasing severity of pain it is recommended that the dosage of morphine be increased to achieve the desired relief. The dosage may be varied by choosing combinations of available strengths (10, 30, 60, and 100mg) or by using higher strength tablets alone.

It is recommended that a patient transferred from another oral morphine preparation, having similar bioavailability to oral morphine liquid, should receive the same total morphine dose in one 24-hour period. This total dose should be divided between the morning and evening administration. Dosage titration and clinical assessment may be appropriate.

Where a patient had previously received parenteral morphine prior to being transferred to Morphgesic® SR tablets, a higher dosage of morphine may be required. Individual dosage adjustment will be necessary to compensate for any reduction in analgesic effect associated with oral administration.

When Morphgesic® SR is to be given for the relief of post-operative pain, it is not advisable to administer it during the first 24 hours. Following this initial period, the dosage should be at the physician's discretion.

Some patients may require supplemental parenteral morphine which is perfectly acceptable.

Careful attention should be paid to the total morphine dosage however, and the prolonged effects of morphine in the Morphgesic® SR formulation should also be borne in mind.

Morphgesic® SR tablets should be used with caution post-operatively (as with all morphine preparations) but especially in cases of 'acute abdomen' and following abdominal surgery.

Gastric motility should have returned and be maintained.

Children:

Morphgesic® SR tablets are not recommended for paediatric use.

4.3 Contraindications
Respiratory depression, paralytic ileus, delayed gastric emptying, obstructive airways disease, known morphine sensitivity or acute hepatic disease. It is also contraindicated in the presence of hypersensitivity to any of the constituents, acute alcoholism, head injuries and conditions in which intracranial pressure is raised. Neither should it be given during an attack of bronchial asthma nor heart failure secondary to chronic lung disease.

Not recommended for pre-operative use or for the first 24 hours post-operatively.

Not recommended during pregnancy and lactation.

Concurrent administration of monoamine oxidase inhibitors (MAOIs) or within two weeks of discontinuation of their use.

4.4 Special warnings and special precautions for use
Morphgesic® SR tablets should be given with caution or in reduced doses to patients with hypothyroidism, adrenocortical insufficiency, impaired kidney or liver function, prostatic hypertrophy or shock. It should be used with caution in patients with either obstructive bowel disorders or myasthenia gravis.

Caution in patients with convulsive disorders, hypotension with hypovolaemia, the elderly, opioid dependent patients, diseases of the biliary tract, pancreatitis and inflammatory bowel disorders.

Should not be used where there is a possibility of paralytic ileus occurring. Should paralytic ileus be suspected to occur during use, treatment should be discontinued immediately.

As with all morphine preparations, patients who are to undergo cordotomy or other pain relieving surgical procedures should not receive Morphgesic® SR tablets for 24 hours prior to surgery. If further treatment is then indicated, the dosage should be adjusted to the new post-operative requirement.

It is not possible to ensure bio-equivalence between different brands of controlled release morphine products. Therefore, it should be emphasised that patients, once titrated to an effective dose should not be changed from Morphgesic® SR tablets to other slow, sustained or controlled release morphine or other potent narcotic analgesic preparations without re-titration and clinical assessment.

4.5 Interaction with other medicinal products and other forms of Interaction
Morphgesic® SR should not be concurrently administered with monoamine oxidase inhibitors (MAOIs) or used within two weeks of discontinuation of MAOI use. The depressant effects of morphine are enhanced by depressants of the central nervous system such as alcohol, anaesthetics, hypnotics and sedatives, tricyclic antidepressants and phenothiazines. The action of morphine may in turn affect the activities of other compounds, for example its gastro-intestinal effects may delay absorption as with mexilitine or may be counteractive as with metoclopramide.

Cimetidine inhibits the metabolism of morphine.

Morphine potentiates the effects of tranquillisers, muscle relaxants and anti-hypertensives.

Mixed agonist/antagonist opioid analgesics (e.g. Buprenorphine, nalbuphine, pentazocine) should not be administered to a patient who has received a course of therapy with a pure opioid agonist analgesic.

4.6 Pregnancy and lactation
Morphgesic® SR tablets are contraindicated during pregnancy and lactation.

4.7 Effects on ability to drive and use machines
Patients taking Morphgesic® SR should not operate machines.

4.8 Undesirable effects
The commonest side-effects of morphine when administered at normal doses are nausea, vomiting, constipation, drowsiness and confusion. Micturition may be difficult and there may be ureteric or biliary spasm. There is also an antidiuretic effect. Dry mouth, sweating, facial flushing, vertigo, bradycardia, palpitations, orthostatic hypothermia, restlessness, changes of mood and miosis also occur. These effects occur more commonly in ambulant patients than in those at rest in bed. Raised intracranial pressure occurs in some patients. Larger doses of morphine produce respiratory depression and hypotension with circulatory failure and deepening coma. Death may occur from respiratory failure. Toxic doses vary considerably with the individual. Tolerance and dependence may occur.

Paralytic ileus may be associated with opioid usage. Other effects include bronchospasm, headache, disorientation, hallucinations, rash, myoclonus, decreased libido and colic.

Morphine has histamine releasing effects which may be responsible in part for reactions such as urticaria and pruritus.

4.9 Overdose
In acute poisoning by Morphgesic® SR the stomach should be emptied by aspiration and lavage. A laxative may be given to aid peristalsis. Signs of morphine toxicity and overdose are likely to consist of pin-point pupils, respiratory depression and hypotension. Circulatory failure and deepening coma may occur in more severe cases.

Treatment of respiratory failure and shock may require intensive supportive therapy. In addition to this the specific antagonist naloxone hydrochloride should be administered at a dose of 0.4 to 2 mg IV. This dose should be repeated at intervals of 2 to 3 minutes if required, up to a total dose of 10mg.

The physician should be aware that Morphgesic® SR tablets remaining in the intestine will continue to release morphine sulphate for a period of hours.

Rhabdomyolysis progressing to renal failure has been reported in opioid overdosage.

5. PHARMACOLOGICAL PROPERTIES

5.1 Pharmacodynamic properties
Morphine is an opioid analgesic. It acts mainly on the central nervous system and on smooth muscle. Although morphine is predominantly a central nervous system depressant it has some central stimulant actions which results in nausea and vomiting and miosis. Morphine generally increases smooth muscle tone, especially the sphincters of the gastro-intestinal tract.

Morphine and related analgesics may produce both physical and psychological dependence and should therefore be used with discrimination. Tolerance may also develop.

Morphine is an analgesic used for the symptomatic relief of moderate to severe pain, especially that associated with neoplastic disease, myocardial infarction and surgery. When pain is likely to be short of duration, a short-acting analgesic is usually preferred in addition to relieving pain, morphine also alleviates the anxiety associated with severe pain. It is useful as a hypnotic where sleeplessness is due to pain and may also relieve the pain of biliary or renal colic, although an antispasmodic may also be required since morphine may increase smooth muscle tone.

Morphine reduces intestinal motility and is used in the symptomatic treatment of diarrhoea.

It also relieves the dyspnoea of left ventricular failure and of pulmonary oedema. It is effective for the suppression of cough, but codeine is usually preferred as there is less risk of dependence. Morphine has been used pre-operatively as an adjunct to anaesthesia for pain relief and to allay anxiety. It has also been used in high doses as a general anaesthetic in specialised procedures. Morphine is usually administered as the sulphate, although the hydrochloride and the tartrate are used in similar doses; the acetate has also been used.

Routes of administration include the oral, subcutaneous, intramuscular, intravenous, intraspinal and rectal routes. Parenteral doses may be intermittent injections or continuous or intermittent infusions adjusted according to individual analgesic requirements.

5.2 Pharmacokinetic properties

Morphine has a plasma half life of about 2 to 3 hours and, if given IV, must be administered frequently. Morphgesic® SR, being a sustained release preparation of morphine, has the advantage that it is only administered twice daily.

A summary of the morphine pharmacokinetic parameters is given below:

a. Half life; plasma half life; about 2-3 hours

b. Volume of distribution; about 3-5 litre/kg

c. Clearance; plasma clearance; about 15 to 20ml/min/kg

d. Protein binding; in plasma 20-35%

Pharmacokinetic parameters pertinent to Morphgesic® SR are summarized in the following table:

Parameters	Morphgesic® SR Fasting (A)	Morphgesic® SR Food (B)
$AUC_{(0\text{-}t)}$ (ng.h/ml)	46.02 ± 18.85	59.88 ± 20.52
C_{max} (ng/ml)	9.2 ± 3.6	13.6 ± 4.6
T_{max} (hours)	2.5 ± 1.7	3.9 ± 1.6

5.3 Preclinical safety data

No preclinical safety data are available which are additional to the experience gained in man with morphine over many years.

6. PHARMACEUTICAL PARTICULARS

6.1 List of excipients

Lactose, Hydroxyethylcellulose, Hypromellose (E464), Povidone, Talc, Magnesium Stearate, Macrogol and Industrial Methylated Spirits 99% BP.

Morphgesic® SR tablets contain the colourants listed below:

10mg: Titanium Dioxide (E171), Iron Oxide Yellow (172), Iron Oxide Red (E172).

30mg: Erythrosine Lake (E127), Titanium Dioxide (E171), FD&C Blue #2/Indigo Carmine Lake (E132), FD&C Yellow #6/Sunset Yellow FCF Lake (E110).

60mg: Titanium Dioxide (E171), FD&C Yellow #6/ Sunset Yellow FCF Lake (E110).

100mg: Titanium Dioxide (E171), Iron Oxide Black (172).

6.2 Incompatibilities

None.

6.3 Shelf life

36 Months.

6.4 Special precautions for storage

Do not store above 25°C. Store in the original package.

6.5 Nature and contents of container

Each pack contains 60 tablets in PVC blister packs with aluminium foil lidding.

6.6 Instructions for use and handling

None.

7. MARKETING AUTHORISATION HOLDER

Waymade plc, Sovereign House, Miles Gray Road, Basildon, Essex SS14 3FR, United Kingdom.

Trading as:

Amdipharm, Regency House, Miles Gray Road, Basildon, Essex SS14 3AF, United Kingdom.

8. MARKETING AUTHORISATION NUMBER(S)

10mg: PL 06464/1651.

30mg: PL 06464/1652.

60mg: PL 06464/1653.

100mg: PL 06464/1654.

9. DATE OF FIRST AUTHORISATION/RENEWAL OF THE AUTHORISATION

28th June 2002.

10. DATE OF REVISION OF THE TEXT

January 2003.

Morphine Sulphate Injection BP 10mg in 1ml, 15mg in 1ml & 30mg in 1ml

(UCB Pharma Limited)

1. NAME OF THE MEDICINAL PRODUCT

Morphine Sulphate Injection BP 10mg, 15mg or 30mg in 1ml.

2. QUALITATIVE AND QUANTITATIVE COMPOSITION

Morphine Sulphate Injection BP 10mg, 15mg or 30mg in 1ml.

3. PHARMACEUTICAL FORM

Sterile aqueous solution for parenteral administration to human beings.

4. CLINICAL PARTICULARS

4.1 Therapeutic indications

Morphine is used for the symptomatic relief of severe pain; relief of dyspnoea of left ventricular failure and pulmonary oedema; pre-operative use.

4.2 Posology and method of administration

The injection may be given by the intravenous, intramuscular or subcutaneous route.

Adults: The dosage should be based on the severity of the pain and the response and tolerance of the patient. The usual adult subcutaneous or intramuscular dose is 10mg every 4 hours if necessary, but may range from 5mg to 20mg.

The usual adult intravenous dose is 2.5mg to 15mg not more than 4 hourly, where necessary, but dosage and dosing interval must be titrated against the patient's response and adjustments made until analgesia is achieved.

Elderly: Because of the depressant effect on respiration, caution is necessary when giving morphine to the elderly and reduced doses may be required.

Children: Use in children is not recommended.

4.3 Contraindications

Respiratory depression, obstructive airways disease, concurrent treatment with monoamine oxidase inhibitors or within two weeks of their discontinuation of treatment with them.

Known morphine sensitivity, or sensitivity to any of the ingredients. Cerebral oedema, head injuries, coma, convulsive disorders and raised intracranial pressure, biliary colic and acute alcoholism.

Administration of morphine is contra-indicated in patients with phaeochromocytoma or those at risk of paralytic ileus.

4.4 Special warnings and special precautions for use

Morphine should be administered with care to patients with hypotension, asthma, hypothyroidism, decreased respiratory reserve, hepatic and renal impairment, adrenocortical insufficiency, prostatic hypertrophy, shock, inflammatory or obstructive bowel disease or myasthenia gravis, and to patients with a history of drug abuse.

4.5 Interaction with other medicinal products and other forms of Interaction

Concurrent administration of other CNS depressants, including hypnotics and anxiolytics, may potentiate the sedative effects.

Morphine should not be administered to patients receiving monoamine oxidase inhibitors (see section 4.3).

Anticholinergic agents such as atropine antagonise morphine-induced respiratory depression and can partially reverse biliary spasm but are additive to the gastro-intestinal and urinary tract effects. Consequently, severe constipation and urinary retention may occur during intensive anticholinergic-analgesic therapy.

Morphine sulphate should not be used for premedication when ciprofloxacin is given for surgical prophylaxis as serum levels of ciprofloxacin are reduced and adequate cover may not be obtained during surgery.

4.6 Pregnancy and lactation

Pregnancy: Since morphine rapidly crosses the placental barrier, it is not advised to administer morphine during labour because of the risk of respiratory depression in the new born infant.

As with all drugs it is not advisable to administer morphine during pregnancy.

Lactation: Only small amounts of morphine are secreted in breast milk and the quantity that may reach the neonate via breast milk is probably insufficient to cause major problems of dependence or adverse effects. However, caution is advised on the use of morphine in breast-feeding patient and the benefit must outweigh the risk to the infant. If breast feeding is continued, the infant should be observed for possible adverse effects.

4.7 Effects on ability to drive and use machines

Morphine may cause drowsiness. If this occurs the patient should not be allowed to drive or operate machinery.

4.8 Undesirable effects

Morphine may cause nausea, vomiting, constipation, drowsiness, confusion, dry mouth, sweating, facial flushing, vertigo, bradycardia, palpitations, tachycardia, orthostatic hypotension, hypothermia, restlessness, hallucinations, headache, changes of mood and miosis, muscle rigidity with high doses, decreased libido or potency. Micturition may be difficult and there may be ureteric or biliary spasm. There is also an antidiuretic effect. These effects are more likely to occur in ambulant patients.

Raised intracranial pressure occurs in some patients. Morphine has been reported to increase liver enzymes as a result of spasm of the sphincter of Oddi.

Allergic reactions including urticaria, pruritus, rash, contact dermatitis, bronchospasm, angioedema and anaphylactic reactions may occasionally occur. Pain and irritation may occur on injection.

Larger doses of morphine may produce respiratory depression and hypotension with circulatory failure and deepening coma. Death may occur from respiratory failure.

Morphine may produce physical and psychological dependence.

4.9 Overdose

Symptoms of serious overdose include respiratory depression and hypotension with circulatory failure, deepening coma, hypothermia, convulsions especially in infants and children and rhabdomyolysis progressing to renal failure.

Treatment with specific antidote Naloxone is used to rapidly counteract the severe respiratory depression and coma produced by excessive doses of morphine.

5. PHARMACOLOGICAL PROPERTIES

5.1 Pharmacodynamic properties

Morphine is a narcotic analgesic obtained from opium, which acts mainly on the central nervous system and smooth muscle.

5.2 Pharmacokinetic properties

Absorption:Variably absorbed after oral administration; rapidly absorbed after subcutaneous or intramuscular administration.

Blood concentration: After an oral dose of 10mg as the sulphate, peak serum concentrations of free morphine of about 10ng/ml are attained in 15 to 60 minutes; after an intramuscular does of 10mg, peak serum concentrations of 70 to 80ng/ml are attained in 10 to 20 minutes; after an intravenous does of 10mg, serum concentrations of about 60ng/ml are obtained in 15 minutes falling to 30ng/ml after 30 minutes and to 10ng/ml after 3 hours; subcutaneous doses give similar concentrations to intramuscular doses at 15 minutes but remain slightly higher during the following 3 hours; serum concentrations measured soon after administration correlate closely with the ages of the subjects studied and are increased in the aged.

Half life: Serum half life in the period 10 minutes to 6 hours following intravenous administration, 2 to 3 hours; serum half life in the period 6 hours onwards, 10 to 44 hours.

Distribution: Widely distributed throughout the body, mainly in the kidneys, liver, lungs and spleen; lower concentrations appear in the brain and muscles; morphine crosses the placenta and traces are secreted in sweat and milk; protein binding, about 35% bound to albumin and to immunoglobulins at concentrations within the therapeutic range.

Metabolic reactions: Mainly glucuronic acid conjugation to form morphine-3 and

6-glucuronides, with sulphate conjugation. N-demethylation, 0-methylation and N-oxide glucuronide formation occurs in the intestinal mucosa and liver; N-demethylation occurs to a greater extent after oral than parenteral administration; the 0-methylation pathway to form codeine has been challenged and codeine and norcodeine metabolites in urine may be formed from codeine impurities in the morphine sample studied.

Excretion: After an oral dose, about 60% is excreted in the urine in 24 hours, with about 3% excreted as free morphine in 48 hours; after parenteral dose, about 90% is excreted in 24 hours, with about 10% as free morphine, 65 to 70% as conjugated morphine, 1% as normorphine and 3% as normorphine glucuronide; after administration of large doses to addicts about 0.1% of a dose is excreted as norcodeine; urinary excretion of morphine appears to be pH dependent to some extent: as the urine becomes more acid more free morphine is excreted and as the urine becomes more alkaline more of the glucuronide conjugate is excreted; up to 10% of a dose may be excreted in the bile.

5.3 Preclinical safety data

None available.

6. PHARMACEUTICAL PARTICULARS

6.1 List of excipients

Sodium metabisulphite BP

Sodium hydroxide (as in solution) BP

Sulphuric acid (as in solution) BP

Water for injection

6.2 Incompatibilities

Morphine salts may be precipitated in alkaline solution.

6.3 Shelf life

3 years.

6.4 Special precautions for storage

Store below 25°C and protect from light.

6.5 Nature and contents of container

Ceramically printed, ring snap ampoule manufactured from white neutral glass type 1, conforming to European Pharmacopoeia test for hydrolytic resistance containing morphine sulphate injection 10mg in 1ml, packed in cartons of 5 ampoules or 15mg in 1ml, packed in cartons of 5 ampoules or 30mg in 1ml and 60mg in 2ml, packed in cartons of 5 ampoules.

Ring snap ampoule manufactured from white neutral glass type 1 conforming to European Pharmacopoeia test for hydrolytic resistance to which will be attached an adhesive vinyl label after filling containing morphine sulphate injection 10mg in 1ml, packed in cartons of 5 ampoules, 15mg in 1ml, packed in a carton of 5 ampoules, or 300mg in 10ml, packed in a carton of 1 ampoule.

6.6 Instructions for use and handling

None.

7. MARKETING AUTHORISATION HOLDER

UCB Pharma Limited

208 Bath Road

Slough

Berkshire

SL1 3WE

UK

8. MARKETING AUTHORISATION NUMBER(S)

PL 00039/5682R

9. DATE OF FIRST AUTHORISATION/RENEWAL OF THE AUTHORISATION

17 May 1982 / 20 August 1997

10. DATE OF REVISION OF THE TEXT

June 2005

POM

Morphine Sulphate Injection BP 10mg/ml

(Wockhardt UK Ltd)

1. NAME OF THE MEDICINAL PRODUCT

Morphine Sulphate Injection BP 10mg/ml

2. QUALITATIVE AND QUANTITATIVE COMPOSITION

Morphine Sulphate 10mg/ml

3. PHARMACEUTICAL FORM

Solution for injection

4. CLINICAL PARTICULARS

4.1 Therapeutic indications

The symptomatic relief of severe pain; relief of dyspnoea of left ventricular failure and pulmonary oedema; pre-operative use.

4.2 Posology and method of administration

Morphine Sulphate may be given by the subcutaneous, intramuscular or intravenous route. The subcutaneous route is not suitable for oedematous patients. The dosage should be based on the severity of the pain and the response and tolerance of the individual patient. The epidural or intrathecal routes must not be used as the product contains a preservative.

Adults:

Subcutaneous or intramuscular injection:

10mg every four hours if necessary (the dose may vary from 5-20mg depending on the individual patient).

Slow intravenous injection (2mg/minute):

Quarter to half of corresponding intramuscular dose not more than four hourly.

Elderly: The dose should be reduced because of the depressant effect on respiration. Caution is required.

Children: Use in children is not recommended.

4.3 Contraindications

Respiratory depression, known morphine sensitivity, biliary colic, obstructive airways disease, acute alcoholism, concurrent treatment with MAOIs or within two weeks of discontinuing them, convulsive disorders, head injuries, acute abdomen, phaeochromocytoma (due to the risk of pressor response to histamine release), conditions in which intracranial pressure is raised and comatose patients.

4.4 Special warnings and special precautions for use

Opioid analgesics in general should be given with caution or in reduced doses to patients with hypothyroidism, adrenocortical insufficiency, asthma, decreased respiratory reserve, prostatic hypertrophy, hypotension, shock, inflammatory or obstructive bowel disorders, or myasthenia gravis and patients with a history of drug abuse.

Morphine can cause an increase in intrabiliary pressure as a result of effects on the sphincter of Oddi. Therefore in patients with biliary colic or other biliary tract disorders morphine may exacerbate pain. In patients given morphine after cholecystectomy, biliary pain has been induced.

Caution is advised when giving morphine to patients with impaired liver function due to its hepatic metabolism.

Severe and prolonged respiratory depression has occurred in patients with renal impairment who have been given morphine.

Dependence can develop rapidly with regular abuse of opioids but is less of a problem with therapeutic use. Abrupt withdrawal from persons physically dependent on them precipitates a withdrawal syndrome, the severity of which depends on the individual, the drug used, the size and frequency of the dose and the duration of drug use.

Dosage should be reduced in elderly and debilitated patients.

4.5 Interaction with other medicinal products and other forms of Interaction

The sedative effects of morphine (opioid analgesics) are enhanced when used with depressants of the central nervous system such as alcohol, anaesthetics, hypnotics, sedatives, anxiolytics, tricyclic antidepressants and phenothiazines.

Hypotensive effects of sedatives (including alcohol), antipsychotic and other hypotensive drugs may be increased.

Anticholinergic agents such as atropine antagonise morphine-induced respiratory depression and can partially reverse biliary spasm but are additive to the gastrointestinal and urinary tract effects. Consequently, severe constipation and urinary retention may occur during intensive anticholinergic-analgesic therapy.

Opioid analgesics reduce plasma ciprofloxacin concentration. The manufacturer advises that premedication with opioid analgesics be avoided.

There may be antagonism of the gastrointestinal effects of cisapride, metoclopramide and domperidone.

Hyperpyrexia and CNS toxicity have been reported with the dopaminergic, selegiline.

There may be delayed absorption of mexiletine.

Cimetidine, a histamine H_2 antagonist, may inhibit the metabolism of opioid analgesics, notably pethidine (increased plasma concentration).

4.6 Pregnancy and lactation

Morphine sulphate should only be used when benefit is known to outweigh risk. As with all drugs it is not advisable to administer morphine during pregnancy.

Morphine crosses the placental barrier. Administration during labour may cause respiratory depression in the new born infant. Therefore, it is not advisable to administer morphine during labour.

Babies born to opioid-dependent mothers may suffer withdrawal symptoms including CNS hyperirritability, gastrointestinal dysfunction, respiratory distress and vague autonomic symptoms including yawning, sneezing, mottling and fever.

While morphine can suppress lactation, the quantity from therapeutic doses that may reach the neonate via breast milk is probably insufficient to cause major problems of dependence or adverse effects.

4.7 Effects on ability to drive and use machines

Morphine causes drowsiness so patients should avoid driving or operating machinery.

4.8 Undesirable effects

In normal doses the commonest side-effects of morphine are nausea, vomiting, constipation, drowsiness and confusion. Tolerance generally develops with long term use, but not to constipation. Micturition may be difficult and there may be ureteric or biliary spasm and also an antidiuretic effect. Dry mouth, sweating, facial flushing, vertigo, bradycardia, palpitations, orthostatic hypotension, hypothermia, restlessness, mood changes, hallucinations and miosis also occur. These effects are more common in ambulant patients than in those at rest in bed, and in those without severe pain. Raised intracranial pressure occurs in some patients. Muscle rigidity has been reported following high doses.

The euphoric activity of morphine has led to its abuse and physical and psychological dependence may occur.

Morphine has a dose-related histamine-releasing effect, which may be responsible in part for reactions such as urticaria and pruritus as well as hypotension and flushing. Contact dermatitis has been reported and pain and irritation may occur on injection. Anaphylactic reactions following intravenous injection have been reported rarely.

4.9 Overdose

Toxic doses vary considerably with the individual, and regular users may tolerate large doses.

Symptoms: in mild overdose, symptoms include nausea and vomiting, tremor, miosis, dysphoria, confusion and sedation. In more severe cases, respiratory failure, hypothermia, hypotension, pulmonary oedema, circulatory failure and deepening coma may occur. Dilation of the pupils occurs as hypoxia develops. Death may occur from respiratory failure. Rhabdomyolysis progressing to renal failure has been reported in overdosage.

Treatment: The medical management of overdose involves prompt intravenous administration of naloxone. Both respiratory and cardiovascular support should be given where necessary.

5. PHARMACOLOGICAL PROPERTIES

5.1 Pharmacodynamic properties

Morphine is obtained from opium, which acts mainly on the CNS and smooth muscle.

Morphine is a potent analgesic with competitive agonist actions at the μ-receptor, which is thought to mediate many of its other actions of respiratory depression, euphoria, inhibition of gut motility and physical dependence. It is possible that analgesia, euphoria and dependence may be due to the effects of morphine on a μ-1 receptor subtype, while respiratory depression and inhibition of gut motility may be due to actions on a μ-2 receptor subtype. Morphine is also a competitive agonist at the κ-receptor that mediates spinal analgesia, miosis and sedation. Morphine has no significant actions at the other two major opioid receptors, the δ- and the σ-receptors.

Morphine directly suppresses cough by an effect on the cough centre in the medulla. Morphine also produces nausea and vomiting by directly stimulating the chemoreceptor trigger zone in the area postrema of the medulla. Morphine provokes the release of histamine.

5.2 Pharmacokinetic properties

Absorption:	Variably absorbed after oral administration; rapidly absorbed after subcutaneous or intramuscular administration.
Blood concentration:	After an oral dose of 10mg as the sulphate, peak serum concentrations of free morphine of about 10ng/ml are attained in 15 to 60 minutes.
	After an intramuscular dose of 10mg, peak serum concentrations of 70 to 80ng/ml are attained in 10 to 20 minutes.
	After an intravenous dose of 10mg, serum concentrations of about 60ng/ml are obtained in 15 minutes falling to 30ng/ml after 30 minutes and to 10ng/ml after three hours.
	Subcutaneous doses give similar concentrations to intramuscular doses at 15 minutes but remain slightly higher during the following three hours; serum concentrations measured soon after administration correlate closely with the ages of the subjects studied and are increased in the elderly.
Half-life	Serum half-life in the period ten minutes to six hours following intravenous administration-two to three hours; serum half-life in the period six hours onwards-10 to 44 hours.
Distribution:	Widely distributed throughout the body, mainly in the kidneys, liver, lungs and spleen; lower concentrations appear in the brain and muscles.
	Morphine crosses the placenta and traces are secreted in sweat and milk.
	Protein binding-about 35% bound to albumin and to immunoglobulins at concentrations within the therapeutic range.
Metabolic reactions:	Mainly glucuronic acid conjugation to form morphine-3 and 6-glucuronides. N-demethylation, O-methylation and N-oxide glucuronide formation occurs in the intestinal mucosa and liver; N-demethylation occurs to a greater extent after oral than parental administration; the O-methylation pathway to form codeine has been challenged and codeine and norcodeine metabolites in urine may be formed from codeine impurities in the morphine sample studied.
Excretion:	After an oral dose, about 60% is excreted in the urine in 24 hours, with about 3% excreted as free morphine in 48 hours.
	After a parental dose, about 90% is excreted in 24 hours, with about 10% as free morphine, 65 to 70% as conjugated morphine, 1% as normorphine and 3% as normorphine glucuronide.
	After administration of large doses to addicts about 0.1% of a dose is excreted as norcodeine.
	Urinary excretion of morphine appears to be pH dependent to some extent; as the urine becomes more acidic more free morphine is excreted and as the urine becomes more alkaline more of the glucuronide conjugate is excreted.
	Up to 10% of a dose may be excreted in the bile.

5.3 Preclinical safety data

There are no pre-clinical data of relevance to the prescriber, which are additional to those included in other sections.

6. PHARMACEUTICAL PARTICULARS

6.1 List of excipients

Water for injections

Sodium metabisulphite

Sodium hydroxide

Hydrochloric acid

6.2 Incompatibilities

Morphine salts are sensitive to changes in pH and morphine is liable to be precipitated out of solution in an alkaline environment. Compounds incompatible with morphine salts include aminophylline and sodium salts of barbiturates and phenytoin. Other incompatibilities (sometimes attributed to particular formulations) have included aciclovir sodium, chlorpromazine hydrochloride injection, frusemide, heparin sodium, pethidine hydrochloride, promethazine hydrochloride and tetracyclines.

6.3 Shelf life

36 months

6.4 Special precautions for storage

Do not store above 25°C. Keep container in the outer carton.

6.5 Nature and contents of container

5 × 1ml Type I glass ampoules

10 × 1ml Type I glass ampoules

6.6 Instructions for use and handling

None

Administrative Data

7. MARKETING AUTHORISATION HOLDER

CP Pharmaceuticals Ltd

Ash Road North

Wrexham

LL13 9UF

8. MARKETING AUTHORISATION NUMBER(S)

Morphine Sulphate Injection BP 10mg/ml – PL 4543/0406

9. DATE OF FIRST AUTHORISATION/RENEWAL OF THE AUTHORISATION

N/A

10. DATE OF REVISION OF THE TEXT

August 2001

Morphine Sulphate Injection BP 15mg/ml

(Wockhardt UK Ltd)

1. NAME OF THE MEDICINAL PRODUCT

Morphine Sulphate Injection BP 15mg/ml

2. QUALITATIVE AND QUANTITATIVE COMPOSITION

Morphine Sulphate 15mg/ml

3. PHARMACEUTICAL FORM

Solution for injection

4. CLINICAL PARTICULARS

4.1 Therapeutic indications

The symptomatic relief of severe pain; relief of dyspnoea of left ventricular failure and pulmonary oedema; pre-operative use.

4.2 Posology and method of administration

Morphine Sulphate may be given by the subcutaneous, intramuscular or intravenous route. The subcutaneous route is not suitable for oedematous patients. The dosage should be based on the severity of the pain and the response and tolerance of the individual patient. The epidural or intrathecal routes must not be used as the product contains a preservative.

Adults:

Subcutaneous or intramuscular injection:

10mg every four hours if necessary (the dose may vary from 5-20mg depending on the individual patient).

Slow intravenous injection (2mg/minute):

Quarter to half of corresponding intramuscular dose not more than four hourly.

Elderly: The dose should be reduced because of the depressant effect on respiration. Caution is required.

Children: Use in children is not recommended.

4.3 Contraindications

Respiratory depression, known morphine sensitivity, biliary colic, obstructive airways disease, acute alcoholism, concurrent treatment with MAOIs or within two weeks of discontinuing them, convulsive disorders, head injuries, acute abdomen, phaeochromocytoma (due to the risk of pressor response to histamine release), conditions in which intracranial pressure is raised and comatose patients.

4.4 Special warnings and special precautions for use

Opioid analgesics in general should be given with caution or in reduced doses to patients with hypothyroidism, adrenocortical insufficiency, asthma, decreased respiratory reserve, prostatic hypertrophy, hypotension, shock, inflammatory or obstructive bowel disorders, or myasthenia gravis and patients with a history of drug abuse.

Morphine can cause an increase in intrabiliary pressure as a result of effects on the sphincter of Oddi. Therefore in patients with biliary colic or other biliary tract disorders morphine may exacerbate pain. In patients given morphine after cholecystectomy, biliary pain has been induced.

Caution is advised when giving morphine to patients with impaired liver function due to its hepatic metabolism.

Severe and prolonged respiratory depression has occurred in patients with renal impairment who have been given morphine.

Dependence can develop rapidly with regular abuse of opioids but is less of a problem with therapeutic use. Abrupt withdrawal from persons physically dependent on them precipitates a withdrawal syndrome, the severity of which depends on the individual, the drug used, the size and frequency of the dose and the duration of drug use.

Dosage should be reduced in elderly and debilitated patients.

4.5 Interaction with other medicinal products and other forms of Interaction

The sedative effects of morphine (opioid analgesics) are enhanced when used with depressants of the central nervous system such as alcohol, anaesthetics, hypnotics, sedatives, anxiolytics, tricyclic antidepressants and phenothiazines.

Hypotensive effects of sedatives (including alcohol), antipsychotic and other hypotensive drugs may be increased.

Anticholinergic agents such as atropine antagonise morphine-induced respiratory depression and can partially reverse biliary spasm but are additive to the gastrointestinal and urinary tract effects. Consequently, severe constipation and urinary retention may occur during intensive anticholinergic-analgesic therapy.

Opioid analgesics reduce plasma ciprofloxacin concentration. The manufacturer advises that premedication with opioid analgesics be avoided.

There may be antagonism of the gastrointestinal effects of cisapride, metoclopramide and domperidone.

Hyperpyrexia and CNS toxicity have been reported with the dopaminergic, selegiline.

There may be delayed absorption of mexiletine.

Cimetidine, a histamine H_2 antagonist, may inhibit the metabolism of opioid analgesics, notably pethidine (increased plasma concentration).

4.6 Pregnancy and lactation

Morphine sulphate should only be used when benefit is known to outweigh risk. As with all drugs it is not advisable to administer morphine during pregnancy.

Morphine crosses the placental barrier. Administration during labour may cause respiratory depression in the new born infant. Therefore, it is not advisable to administer morphine during labour.

Babies born to opioid-dependent mothers may suffer withdrawal symptoms including CNS hyperirritability, gastrointestinal dysfunction, respiratory distress and vague autonomic symptoms including yawning, sneezing, mottling and fever.

While morphine can suppress lactation, the quantity from therapeutic doses that may reach the neonate via breast milk is probably insufficient to cause major problems of dependence or adverse effects.

4.7 Effects on ability to drive and use machines

Morphine causes drowsiness so patients should avoid driving or operating machinery.

4.8 Undesirable effects

The commonest side-effects of morphine are nausea, vomiting, constipation, drowsiness and confusion. Tolerance generally develops with long term use, but not to constipation. Micturition may be difficult and there may be ureteric or biliary spasm and also an antidiuretic effect. Dry mouth, sweating, facial flushing, vertigo, bradycardia, palpitations, orthostatic hypotension, hypothermia, restlessness, mood changes, hallucinations and miosis also occur. These effects are more common in ambulant patients than in those at rest in bed, and in those without severe pain. Raised intracranial pressure occurs in some patients. Muscle rigidity has been reported following high doses.

The euphoric activity of morphine has led to its abuse and physical and psychological dependence may occur.

Morphine has a dose-related histamine-releasing effect, which may be responsible in part for reactions such as urticaria and pruritus as well as hypotension and flushing. Contact dermatitis has been reported and pain and irritation may occur on injection. Anaphylactic reactions following intravenous injection have been reported rarely.

4.9 Overdose

Toxic doses vary considerably with the individual, and regular users may tolerate large doses.

Symptoms: in mild overdose, symptoms include nausea and vomiting, tremor, miosis, dysphoria, confusion and sedation. In more severe cases, respiratory failure, hypothermia, hypotension, pulmonary oedema, circulatory failure and deepening coma may occur. Dilation of the pupils occurs as hypoxia develops. Death may occur from respiratory failure. Rhabdomyolysis progressing to renal failure has been reported in overdosage.

Treatment: The medical management of overdose involves prompt intravenous administration of naloxone. Both respiratory and cardiovascular support should be given where necessary.

5. PHARMACOLOGICAL PROPERTIES

5.1 Pharmacodynamic properties

Morphine is obtained from opium, which acts mainly on the CNS and smooth muscle.

Morphine is a potent analgesic with competitive agonist actions at the μ-receptor, which is thought to mediate many of its other actions of respiratory depression, euphoria, inhibition of gut motility and physical dependence. It is possible that analgesia, euphoria and dependence may be due to the effects of morphine on a μ-1 receptor subtype, while respiratory depression and inhibition of gut motility may be due to actions on a μ-2 receptor subtype. Morphine is also a competitive agonist at the κ-receptor that mediates spinal analgesia, miosis and sedation. Morphine has no significant actions at the other two major opioid receptors, the δ- and the σ-receptors.

Morphine directly suppresses cough by an effect on the cough centre in the medulla. Morphine also produces nausea and vomiting by directly stimulating the chemoreceptor trigger zone in the area postrema of the medulla. Morphine provokes the release of histamine.

5.2 Pharmacokinetic properties

Absorption:	Variably absorbed after oral administration; rapidly absorbed after subcutaneous or intramuscular administration.
Blood concentration:	After an oral dose of 10mg as the sulphate, peak serum concentrations of free morphine of about 10ng/ml are attained in 15 to 60 minutes.
	After an intramuscular dose of 10mg, peak serum concentrations of 70 to 80ng/ml are attained in 10 to 20 minutes.
	After an intravenous dose of 10mg, serum concentrations of about 60ng/ml are obtained in 15 minutes falling to 30ng/ml after 30 minutes and to 10ng/ml after three hours.
	Subcutaneous doses give similar concentrations to intramuscular doses at 15 minutes but remain slightly higher during the following three hours; serum concentrations measured soon after administration correlate closely with the ages of the subjects studied and are increased in the elderly.
Half-life	Serum half-life in the period ten minutes to six hours following intravenous administration-two to three hours; serum half-life in the period six hours onwards-10 to 44 hours.
Distribution:	Widely distributed throughout the body, mainly in the kidneys, liver, lungs and spleen; lower concentrations appear in the brain and muscles.
	Morphine crosses the placenta and traces are secreted in sweat and milk.
	Protein binding-about 35% bound to albumin and to immunoglobulins at concentrations within the therapeutic range.
Metabolic reactions:	Mainly glucuronic acid conjugation to form morphine-3 and 6-glucuronides. N-demethylation, O-methylation and N-oxide glucuronide formation occurs in the intestinal mucosa and liver; N-demethylation occurs to a greater extent after oral than parental administration; the O-methylation pathway to form codeine has been challenged and codeine and norcodeine metabolites in urine may be formed from codeine impurities in the morphine sample studied.
Excretion:	After an oral dose, about 60% is excreted in the urine in 24 hours, with about 3% excreted as free morphine in 48 hours.
	After a parental dose, about 90% is excreted in 24 hours, with about 10% as free morphine, 65 to 70% as conjugated morphine, 1% as normorphine and 3% as normorphine glucuronide.
	After administration of large doses to addicts about 0.1% of a dose is excreted as norcodeine.
	Urinary excretion of morphine appears to be pH dependent to some extent; as the urine becomes more acidic more free morphine is excreted and as the urine becomes more alkaline more of the glucuronide conjugate is excreted.
	Up to 10% of a dose may be excreted in the bile.

5.3 Preclinical safety data
There are no pre-clinical data of relevance to the prescriber, which are additional to those included in other sections.

6. PHARMACEUTICAL PARTICULARS
6.1 List of excipients
Water for injections
Sodium metabisulphite
Sodium hydroxide
Hydrochloric acid

6.2 Incompatibilities
Morphine salts are sensitive to changes in pH and morphine is liable to be precipitated out of solution in an alkaline environment. Compounds incompatible with morphine salts include aminophylline and sodium salts of barbiturates and phenytoin. Other incompatibilities (sometimes attributed to particular formulations) have included aciclovir sodium, chlorpromazine hydrochloride injection, frusemide, heparin sodium, pethidine hydrochloride, promethazine hydrochloride and tetracyclines.

6.3 Shelf life
36 months

6.4 Special precautions for storage
Do not store above 25°C. Keep container in the outer carton.

6.5 Nature and contents of container
5 × 1ml glass ampoules
10 × 1ml glass ampoules

6.6 Instructions for use and handling
None

Administrative Data
7. MARKETING AUTHORISATION HOLDER
CP Pharmaceuticals Ltd
Ash Road North
Wrexham
LL13 9UF

8. MARKETING AUTHORISATION NUMBER(S)
Morphine Sulphate Injection BP 15mg/ml – PL 4543/0411

9. DATE OF FIRST AUTHORISATION/RENEWAL OF THE AUTHORISATION
N/A

10. DATE OF REVISION OF THE TEXT
October 2001

Morphine Sulphate Injection BP 30mg/ml

(Wockhardt UK Ltd)

1. NAME OF THE MEDICINAL PRODUCT
Morphine Sulphate Injection BP 30mg/ml

2. QUALITATIVE AND QUANTITATIVE COMPOSITION
Morphine Sulphate 30mg/ml

3. PHARMACEUTICAL FORM
Solution for injection

4. CLINICAL PARTICULARS
4.1 Therapeutic indications
The symptomatic relief of severe pain; relief of dyspnoea of left ventricular failure and pulmonary oedema; pre-operative use.

4.2 Posology and method of administration
Morphine Sulphate may be given by the subcutaneous, intramuscular or intravenous route. The subcutaneous route is not suitable for oedematous patients. The dosage should be based on the severity of the pain and the response and tolerance of the individual patient. The epidural or intrathecal routes must not be used as the product contains a preservative.

Adults:

Subcutaneous or intramuscular injection:

10mg every four hours if necessary (the dose may vary from 5-20mg depending on the individual patient).

Slow intravenous injection (2mg/minute):

Quarter to half of corresponding intramuscular dose not more than four hourly.

Elderly: The dose should be reduced because of the depressant effect on respiration. Caution is required.

Children: Use in children is not recommended.

4.3 Contraindications
Respiratory depression, known morphine sensitivity, biliary colic, obstructive airways disease, acute alcoholism, concurrent treatment with MAOIs or within two weeks of discontinuing them, convulsive disorders, head injuries, acute abdomen, phaeochromocytoma (due to the risk of pressor response to histamine release), conditions in which intracranial pressure is raised and comatose patients.

4.4 Special warnings and special precautions for use
Opioid analgesics in general should be given with caution or in reduced doses to patients with hypothyroidism, adrenocortical insufficiency, asthma, decreased respiratory reserve, prostatic hypertrophy, hypotension, shock, inflammatory or obstructive bowel disorders, or myasthenia gravis and patients with a history of drug abuse.

Morphine can cause an increase in intrabiliary pressure as a result of effects on the sphincter of Oddi. Therefore in patients with biliary colic or other biliary tract disorders morphine may exacerbate pain. In patients given morphine after cholecystectomy, biliary pain has been induced.

Caution is advised when giving morphine to patients with impaired liver function due to its hepatic metabolism.

Severe and prolonged respiratory depression has occurred in patients with renal impairment who have been given morphine.

Dependence can develop rapidly with regular abuse of opioids but is less of a problem with therapeutic use. Abrupt withdrawal from persons physically dependent on them precipitates a withdrawal syndrome, the severity of which depends on the individual, the drug used, the size and frequency of the dose and the duration of drug use.

Dosage should be reduced in elderly and debilitated patients.

4.5 Interaction with other medicinal products and other forms of Interaction
The sedative effects of morphine (opioid analgesics) are enhanced when used with depressants of the central nervous system such as alcohol, anaesthetics, hypnotics, sedatives, anxiolytics, tricyclic antidepressants and phenothiazines.

Hypotensive effects of sedatives (including alcohol), antipsychotic and other hypotensive drugs may be increased.

Anticholinergic agents such as atropine antagonise morphine-induced respiratory depression and can partially reverse biliary spasm but are additive to the gastrointestinal and urinary tract effects. Consequently, severe constipation and urinary retention may occur during intensive anticholinergic-analgesic therapy.

Opioid analgesics reduce plasma ciprofloxacin concentration. The manufacturer advises that premedication with opioid analgesics be avoided.

There may be antagonism of the gastrointestinal effects of cisapride, metoclopramide and domperidone.

Hyperpyrexia and CNS toxicity have been reported with the dopaminergic, selegiline.

There may be delayed absorption of mexiletine.

Cimetidine, a histamine H_2 antagonist, may inhibit the metabolism of opioid analgesics, notably pethidine (increased plasma concentration).

4.6 Pregnancy and lactation
Morphine sulphate should only be used when benefit is known to outweigh risk. As with all drugs it is not advisable to administer morphine during pregnancy.

Morphine crosses the placental barrier. Administration during labour may cause respiratory depression in the new born infant. Therefore, it is not advisable to administer morphine during labour.

Babies born to opioid-dependent mothers may suffer withdrawal symptoms including CNS hyperirritability, gastrointestinal dysfunction, respiratory distress and vague autonomic symptoms including yawning, sneezing, mottling and fever.

While morphine can suppress lactation, the quantity from therapeutic doses that may reach the neonate via breast milk is probably insufficient to cause major problems of dependence or adverse effects.

4.7 Effects on ability to drive and use machines
Morphine causes drowsiness so patients should avoid driving or operating machinery.

4.8 Undesirable effects
The commonest side-effects of morphine are nausea, vomiting, constipation, drowsiness and confusion. Tolerance generally develops with long term use, but not to constipation. Micturition may be difficult and there may be ureteric or biliary spasm and also an antidiuretic effect. Dry mouth, sweating, facial flushing, vertigo, bradycardia, palpitations, orthostatic hypotension, hypothermia, restlessness, mood changes, hallucinations and miosis also occur. These effects are more common in ambulant patients than in those at rest in bed, and in those without severe pain. Raised intracranial pressure occurs in some patients. Muscle rigidity has been reported following high doses.

The euphoric activity of morphine has led to its abuse and physical and psychological dependence may occur.

Morphine has a dose-related histamine-releasing effect, which may be responsible in part for reactions such as urticaria and pruritus as well as hypotension and flushing. Contact dermatitis has been reported and pain and irritation may occur on injection. Anaphylactic reactions following intravenous injection have been reported rarely.

4.9 Overdose
Toxic doses vary considerably with the individual, and regular users may tolerate large doses.

Symptoms: in mild overdose, symptoms include nausea and vomiting, tremor, miosis, dysphoria, confusion and sedation. In more severe cases, respiratory failure, hypothermia, hypotension, pulmonary oedema, circulatory failure and deepening coma may occur. Dilation of the pupils occurs as hypoxia develops. Death may occur from respiratory failure. Rhabdomyolysis progressing to renal failure has been reported in overdosage.

Treatment: The medical management of overdose involves prompt intravenous administration of naloxone. Both respiratory and cardiovascular support should be given where necessary.

5. PHARMACOLOGICAL PROPERTIES
5.1 Pharmacodynamic properties
Morphine is obtained from opium, which acts mainly on the CNS and smooth muscle.

Morphine is a potent analgesic with competitive agonist actions at the μ-receptor, which is thought to mediate many of its other actions of respiratory depression, euphoria, inhibition of gut motility and physical dependence. It is possible that analgesia, euphoria and dependence may be due to the effects of morphine on a μ-1 receptor subtype, while respiratory depression and inhibition of gut motility may be due to actions on a μ-2 receptor subtype. Morphine is also a competitive agonist at the κ-receptor that mediates spinal analgesia, miosis and sedation. Morphine has no significant actions at the other two major opioid receptors, the δ- and the σ-receptors.

Morphine directly suppresses cough by an effect on the cough centre in the medulla. Morphine also produces nausea and vomiting by directly stimulating the chemoreceptor trigger zone in the area postrema of the medulla. Morphine provokes the release of histamine.

5.2 Pharmacokinetic properties

Absorption:	Variably absorbed after oral administration; rapidly absorbed after subcutaneous or intramuscular administration.
Blood concentration:	After an oral dose of 10mg as the sulphate, peak serum concentrations of free morphine of about 10ng/ml are attained in 15 to 60 minutes.
	After an intramuscular dose of 10mg, peak serum concentrations of 70 to 80ng/ml are attained in 10 to 20 minutes.
	After an intravenous dose of 10mg, serum concentrations of about 60ng/ml are obtained in 15 minutes falling to 30ng/ml after 30 minutes and to 10ng/ml after three hours.
	Subcutaneous doses give similar concentrations to intramuscular doses at 15 minutes but remain slightly higher during the following three hours; serum concentrations measured soon after administration correlate closely with the ages of the subjects studied and are increased in the elderly.
Half-life	Serum half-life in the period ten minutes to six hours following intravenous administration-two to three hours; serum half-life in the period six hours onwards-10 to 44 hours.
Distribution:	Widely distributed throughout the body, mainly in the kidneys, liver, lungs and spleen; lower concentrations appear in the brain and muscles.
	Morphine crosses the placenta and traces are secreted in sweat and milk.
	Protein binding-about 35% bound to albumin and to immunoglobulins at concentrations within the therapeutic range.
Metabolic reactions:	Mainly glucuronic acid conjugation to form morphine-3 and 6-glucuronides. N-demethylation, O-methylation and N-oxide glucuronide formation occurs in the intestinal mucosa and liver; N-demethylation occurs to a greater extent after oral than parental administration; the O-methylation pathway to form codeine has been challenged and codeine and norcodeine metabolites in urine may be formed from codeine impurities in the morphine sample studied.
Excretion:	After an oral dose, about 60% is excreted in the urine in 24 hours, with about 3% excreted as free morphine in 48 hours.
	After a parental dose, about 90% is excreted in 24 hours, with about 10% as free morphine, 65 to 70% as conjugated morphine, 1% as normorphine and 3% as normorphine glucuronide.

After administration of large doses to addicts about 0.1% of a dose is excreted as norcodeine.

Urinary excretion of morphine appears to be pH dependent to some extent; as the urine becomes more acidic more free morphine is excreted and as the urine becomes more alkaline more of the glucuronide conjugate is excreted.

Up to 10% of a dose may be excreted in the bile.

5.3 Preclinical safety data

There are no pre-clinical data of relevance to the prescriber, which are additional to those included in other sections.

6. PHARMACEUTICAL PARTICULARS

6.1 List of excipients

Water for injections

Sodium metabisulphite

Sodium hydroxide

Hydrochloric acid

6.2 Incompatibilities

Morphine salts are sensitive to changes in pH and morphine is liable to be precipitated out of solution in an alkaline environment. Compounds incompatible with morphine salts include aminophylline and sodium salts of barbiturates and phenytoin. Other incompatibilities (sometimes attributed to particular formulations) have included aciclovir sodium, chlorpromazine hydrochloride injection, frusemide, heparin sodium, pethidine hydrochloride, promethazine hydrochloride and tetracyclines.

6.3 Shelf life

36 months

6.4 Special precautions for storage

Do not store above 25°C. Keep container in the outer carton.

6.5 Nature and contents of container

5 × 1ml Type I glass ampoules

10 × 1ml Type I glass ampoules

5 × 2ml Type I glass ampoules

6.6 Instructions for use and handling

None

Administrative Data

7. MARKETING AUTHORISATION HOLDER

CP Pharmaceuticals Ltd

Ash Road North

Wrexham

LL13 9UF

8. MARKETING AUTHORISATION NUMBER(S)

Morphine Sulphate Injection BP 30mg/ml – PL 4543/0407

9. DATE OF FIRST AUTHORISATION/RENEWAL OF THE AUTHORISATION

N/A

10. DATE OF REVISION OF THE TEXT

August 2001

Morphine Sulphate Injection BP Minijet 1mg/ml

(International Medication Systems (UK) Ltd)

1. NAME OF THE MEDICINAL PRODUCT

Morphine Sulphate Injection BP Minijet™

Morphine Sulphate Injection BP Rapiject®

2. QUALITATIVE AND QUANTITATIVE COMPOSITION

Morphine Sulphate 1 mg/ml

For excipients, see 6.1.

3. PHARMACEUTICAL FORM

Sterile aqueous solution for intravenous, intramuscular or subcutaneous injection.

4. CLINICAL PARTICULARS

4.1 Therapeutic indications

For intravenous, intramuscular or subcutaneous injection.

For the relief of moderate to severe pain such as in myocardial infarction, severe injuries, neoplastic disease, surgery, renal colic, terminal disease and other conditions where non-narcotic analgesia has failed.

Morphine is effective in the control of post-operative pain and anxiety.

Morphine may be used for its sedative effect in the management of the severe dyspnoea in terminal lung cancer or other terminal respiratory disease.

Morphine should be used as a sedative or hypnotic generally only when pain relief and sedation are required. It is used in pre-anaesthetic medication for surgery, where it reduces anxiety and also the amount of anaesthetic required.

For open-heart surgery, especially in high risk patients with cardiac disease, morphine may be used to produce anaesthesia.

4.2 Posology and method of administration

The dose and dosing regimen should be tailored to the individual patient's needs.

Adults and children over 12 years:

Intramuscular or subcutaneous administration

5-20 mg every 4 hours as necessary, dependent upon the patient's response and cause of pain.

For the relief of pain and as pre-anaesthetic, the usual dose is 10mg every 4 hours depending on the severity of the condition and the patient's response. The usual individual dose range is 5-15mg. The usual daily dose range is 12-120mg.

Intravenous administration

Acute pain:

2 to 15mg by slow intravenous injection.

or

Loading dose as above, followed by 2.5 - 5mg every hour by infusion. If using Patient Controlled Analgesia (PCA), bolus doses of 1 - 2mg may be given with a lock out of 5 - 20 minutes. A commonly applied dose limit used in PCA is 30mg in 4 hours, although some patients may require higher doses.

or

Frequent small doses (eg 1 -3 mg every 5 minutes) reaching a maximum cumulative dose of 2 - 3mg/kg. (This is the preferred regimen for patients with myocardial infarction.)

Chronic pain:

Loading doses of 15mg or more. Maintenance doses for infusion are in the range 0.8 - 80mg/hour, although higher maintenance doses of 150-200mg/hour may be required.

Similar doses have been given by subcutaneous infusion.

Open heart surgery

Large doses (0.5 - 3mg/kg) may be administered intravenously by slow continuous infusion as the sole anaesthetic agent.

Elderly:

Morphine should be administered with caution in the elderly and a reduced starting dose titrated to provide optimal pain relief.

Children under 12 years:

Intramuscular or subcutaneous administration:

Up to 1 month: 150mcg/kg every 4 hours

1-12 months: 200mcg/kg every 4 hours

1-5 years: 2.5-5mg every 4 hours

6-12 years: 5-10mg every 4 hours

Slow intravenous infusion:

Up to 6 months: up to 10mcg/kg/hour with respiratory support. Bolus injection to be avoided.

6 months - 12 years: 10-30mcg/kg/hour. A loading dose of 100-200mcg/kg may be given initially with bolus top-up doses of 50-100mcg/kg every 4 hours.

Subcutaneous infusion:

6 months - 12 years: 30-60mcg/kg/hour. For the relief of pain in terminal disease.

4.3 Contraindications

Morphine is contraindicated in patients with obstructive airways disease; respiratory depression; known morphine sensitivity; head injuries; coma; convulsive disorders and raised intracranial pressure; biliary colic; poor coronary perfusion; acute alcoholism.

4.4 Special warnings and special precautions for use

Morphine is a potent medicine but with considerable potential for harmful effect, including addiction. It should be used only if other drugs with fewer hazards are inadequate, and with the recognition that it may possibly mask significant manifestations of disease which should be identified for proper diagnosis and treatment. Dependence may occur after 1-2 weeks of treatment.

Morphine should be given with caution where there is a reduced respiratory reserve as in emphysema, chronic cor pulmonale, kyphoscoliosis and excessive obesity. Opiates should also be used cautiously in patients with cardiac arrhythmias, myasthenia gravis or inflammatory or obstructive bowel disorders.

Morphine should be administered with caution or in reduced doses to patients with hypothyroidism, adrenocortical insufficiency, impaired kidney or liver function, prostatic hypertrophy or shock.

Morphine should be given with great care to infants, especially neonates. Dosage should be reduced in elderly and debilitated patients.

4.5 Interaction with other medicinal products and other forms of Interaction

Monoamine oxidase inhibitors markedly potentiate the action of morphine; morphine should not be concurrently administered with MAO inhibitors or used within two weeks of discontinuation of MAOI use.

The depressant effects of morphine may be potentiated and prolonged by central nervous system depressants such as alcohol, anaesthetics, analgesics, antihistamines, barbiturates, narcotics, phenothiazines, sedatives, hypnotics and tricyclic antidepressants.

Chlorpromazine and some other phenothiazines appear to enhance the sedative action but diminish the analgesic effect of morphine. The use of tricyclic antidepressants, dexamphetamine, aspirin and other NSAIDs may increase the extent of pain relief of morphine. They also increase the risks of adverse effects.

Anticholinergic agents such as atropine antagonise morphine-induced respiratory depression and can partially reverse biliary spasm but are additive to the gastro-intestinal and urinary tract effects. Consequently, severe constipation and urinary retention may occur during intensive anticholinergic-analgesic therapy.

4.6 Pregnancy and lactation

There is inadequate evidence of safety in human pregnancy and lactation. Care should be taken if morphine is given during labour. It may reduce uterine contractions, cause respiratory depression in the foetus and neonate, and may have significant effects on the foetal heart rate. Morphine is known to cross the placenta and is excreted in breast milk. It may cause respiratory depression by this route.

4.7 Effects on ability to drive and use machines

Morphine may cause drowsiness. Patients receiving morphine should not drive or operate machinery.

4.8 Undesirable effects

The commonest side effects are nausea, vomiting, constipation, drowsiness and confusion. Psychological and physical dependence may occur. Other side effects include asthma, elevated liver enzymes, urinary retention, ureteric or biliary spasm, dry mouth, sweating, rash, facial flushing, vertigo, tachycardia, bradycardia, palpitations, orthostatic hypotension, hypothermia, restlessness, mood change, hallucinations, seizures (adults and children) and miosis, headache and allergic reactions (including anaphylaxis) and decreased libido or potency. Raised intracranial pressure occurs in some patients. Muscle rigidity may occur with high doses.

Large doses can produce respiratory depression, hypotension with circulatory failure and coma. Convulsions may occur in children and infants. Rhabdomyolysis may progress to renal failure. Death may occur from respiratory depression or from pulmonary oedema after overdose.

Urticaria, pruritus, hypotension and flushing may be caused by a morphine dose-related histamine release. Contact dermatitis may occur. Pain at the site of the injection has been reported.

4.9 Overdose

Symptoms: respiratory depression, pin-point pupils and coma. In addition, shock, reduced body temperature and hypotension may occur. In mild overdose, symptoms include nausea and vomiting, tremor, miosis, dysphoria, hypothermia, hypotension, confusion and sedation. In acute poisoning, respiratory collapse and death may occur.

Treatment: the patient must be given respiratory support and the specific antagonist, naloxone, should be administered at a dose of 0.4-2.0 mg intravenously. This dose should be repeated at 2-3 minute intervals if improvement is not achieved, up to a total of 10 mg. Fluid and electrolyte levels should be maintained.

5. PHARMACOLOGICAL PROPERTIES

5.1 Pharmacodynamic properties

ATC Code: N02A A01

Morphine is the principle alkaloid of opium and is a potent analgesic. It exerts its primary effects on the central nervous system and smooth muscle. Pharmacological effects include analgesia, drowsiness, alteration in mood, reduction in body temperature, dose-related respiratory depression, interference with adrenocortical response to stress (at high doses) and a reduction in peripheral resistance with little or no effect on cardiac index and miosis. Morphine, as other opioids, acts as an agonist interacting with stereo-specific and saturable binding sites/receptors in the brain, spinal cord and other tissues.

Morphine acts on the cough centre to suppress coughing and also directly stimulates the chemoreceptor trigger zone in the medulla to produce nausea and vomiting. Morphine provokes the release of histamine.

5.2 Pharmacokinetic properties

After subcutaneous or intramuscular injection, morphine is readily absorbed into the blood. Peak analgesia occurs 50-90 minutes after SC injection, 30-60 minutes after IM and 20 minutes after IV infusion. The effect persists for up to 4-5 hours.

Most of the morphine dose is conjugated with glucoronide in the liver (first pass effect), resulting in morphine-3-glucoronide (inactive) and morphine-6-glucuronide (active). Other active metabolites are formed in small amounts.

About 35% of the dose is protein bound. Morphine can cross the placenta and blood-brain barrier and its metabolites have been detected in the cerebrospinal fluid. Morphine is distributed throughout the body, mainly into skeletal muscle, kidneys, liver, intestinal tract, lungs and spleen.

The mean plasma elimination half life for morphine is 1.5-2.0 hours and for the 3-glucuronide ranges from 2.5-7.0 hours.

Approximately 90% of a parenteral dose of morphine appears in the urine within 24 hours, primarily as the product of glucuronide conjugation with only a small amount as the unchanged drug. 7-10% is excreted in the bile and eliminated in the faeces.

5.3 Preclinical safety data
Not applicable, since morphine sulphate has been used in clinical practice for many years and its effects on man are well known.

6. PHARMACEUTICAL PARTICULARS

6.1 List of excipients
Disodium edetate

Sodium metabisulphite

Water for Injection

6.2 Incompatibilities
Morphine salts may be precipitated in alkaline solution. Compatibility should be checked before admixture with other drugs.

6.3 Shelf life
24 months.

6.4 Special precautions for storage
Store at controlled room temperature (15 to 30°C). Protect from light.

6.5 Nature and contents of container
The solution is contained in a Type I USP glass vial with a rubber closure which meets all the relevant USP specifications for elastomeric closures.

The following volumes are available:

Morphine Sulphate Injection 1mg/ml: 2ml (Minijet™)

10ml (Minijet™)

50ml (Rapiject®)

6.6 Instructions for use and handling
The 2ml and 10ml containers are designed for use with the IMS Minijet™ injector. The 50ml container is designed for use with a syringe driver.

7. MARKETING AUTHORISATION HOLDER
International Medication Systems (UK) Ltd

208 Bath Road

Slough

Berkshire

SL1 3WE

UK

8. MARKETING AUTHORISATION NUMBER(S)
PL 03265/0037

9. DATE OF FIRST AUTHORISATION/RENEWAL OF THE AUTHORISATION
Date first granted: 14 March 1978

Date renewed: 12 October 2002

10. DATE OF REVISION OF THE TEXT
March 2003

POM

Motens Tablets 2mg

(Boehringer Ingelheim Limited)

1. NAME OF THE MEDICINAL PRODUCT
Motens® 2 mg Tablets.

2. QUALITATIVE AND QUANTITATIVE COMPOSITION
Tablets containing lacidipine 2 mg.

For excipients, see 6.1.

3. PHARMACEUTICAL FORM
Film coated tablets.

4. CLINICAL PARTICULARS

4.1 Therapeutic indications
MOTENS is indicated for the treatment of hypertension either alone or in combination with other antihypertensive agents, including β-adrenoceptor antagonists, diuretics, and ACE-inhibitors.

4.2 Posology and method of administration
Adults:

The treatment of hypertension should be adapted to the severity of the condition, and according to the individual response.

The recommended initial dose is 2 mg once daily. The dose may be increased to 4 mg (and then, if necessary, to 6 mg) after adequate time has been allowed for the full pharmacological effect to occur. In practice, this should not be less than 3 to 4 weeks. Daily doses above 6 mg have not been shown to be significantly more effective.

MOTENS should be taken at the same time each day, preferably in the morning.

Treatment with MOTENS may be continued indefinitely.

Patients with kidney disease:

As MOTENS is not cleared by the kidneys, the dose does not require modification in patients with kidney disease.

Use in children:

No experience has been gained with MOTENS in children.

4.3 Contraindications
MOTENS tablets are contra-indicated in patients with known hypersensitivity to any ingredient of the preparation. MOTENS should only be used with great care in patients with a previous allergic reaction to another dihydropyridine because there is a theoretical risk of cross-reactivity.

As with other calcium antagonists, MOTENS should be discontinued in patients who develop cardiogenic shock. In addition, dihydropyridines have been shown to reduce coronary arterial blood-flow in patients with aortic stenosis and in such patients MOTENS is contra-indicated.

MOTENS should not be used during or within one month of a myocardial infarction.

4.4 Special warnings and special precautions for use
In specialised studies MOTENS has been shown neither to affect the spontaneous function of the sinoatrial (SA) node nor to cause prolonged conduction within the atrioventricular (AV) node. However, the theoretical potential for a calcium antagonist to affect the activity of the SA and AV nodes should be noted, and care should be taken in patients with pre-existing abnormalities. As has been reported with certain dihydropyridine calcium channel antagonists, MOTENS should be used with caution in patients with congenital or documented acquired QT prolongation. MOTENS should also be used with caution in patients treated concomitantly with medications known to prolong the QT interval such as class I and III antiarrhythmics, tricyclic antidepressants, certain antipsychotics, antibiotics and antihistaminic agents.

There is no evidence that MOTENS is useful for secondary prevention of myocardial infarction.

In healthy volunteers, patients and pre-clinical studies, MOTENS did not inhibit myocardial contractility. But as with other calcium antagonists, MOTENS should be used with caution in patients with poor cardiac reserve.

The efficacy and safety of MOTENS in the treatment of malignant hypertension has not been established.

Caution should be exercised in patients with hepatic impairment because the antihypertensive effect may be increased.

There is no evidence that MOTENS impairs glucose tolerance or alters diabetic control.

4.5 Interaction with other medicinal products and other forms of Interaction
Concomitant administration of MOTENS with other antihypertensive agents e.g. diuretics, β-adrenoceptor antagonists or ACE-inhibitors may have an additive hypotensive effect.

The plasma concentration of MOTENS may be increased by simultaneous administration of cimetidine.

As with other dihydropyridines, MOTENS should not be taken with grapefruit juice as bioavailability may be altered.

MOTENS is highly protein-bound (>95%) to albumin and α_1-acid glycoprotein. No specific pharmacodynamic interaction problems have been identified in studies with common antihypertensive agents e.g. β-adrenoceptor antagonists and diuretics, or with digoxin, tolbutamide or warfarin.

4.6 Pregnancy and lactation
Although some dihydropyridine compounds have been found to be teratogenic in animals, data in the rat and rabbit for MOTENS provide no evidence of a teratogenic effect. Using doses far above the therapeutic range, in animals MOTENS shows evidence of maternal toxicity resulting in increased pre- and post-implantation losses and possibly delayed ossification. Evidence from experimental animals has indicated that administration of Motens results in prolongation of gestational period and prolonged and difficult labour as a consequence of relaxation of uterine muscle. Milk transfer studies in animals have shown that lacidipine (or its metabolites) are likely to be excreted into breast milk. There is, however, no clinical experience of MOTENS in pregnancy and lactation. Accordingly, MOTENS should not be used during pregnancy or lactation.

4.7 Effects on ability to drive and use machines
None reported.

4.8 Undesirable effects
MOTENS is generally well tolerated. Some individuals may experience minor side effects which are related to its known pharmacological action of peripheral vasodilation. The most common of these are headache, flushing, oedema, dizziness and palpitations. Such effects are usually transient and usually disappear with continued administration of MOTENS at the same dosage.

Asthenia, skin rash (including erythema and itching), gastric upset, nausea, gingival hyperplasia, polyuria, muscle cramps and disturbances of mood have also been reported rarely.

As with other dihydropyridines aggravation of underlying angina has been reported in a small number of individuals, especially after the start of treatment. This is more likely to happen in patients with symptomatic ischaemic heart disease. MOTENS should be discontinued under medical supervision in patients who develop unstable angina

Transient and reversible increases in alkaline phosphatase have been noted on rare occasions.

4.9 Overdose
Symptoms:

There have been no recorded cases of MOTENS overdosage. The expected symptoms could comprise prolonged peripheral vasodilation associated with hypotension and tachycardia. Bradycardia or prolonged AV conduction could occur.

Therapy:

Symptomatic treatment is warranted. There is no specific antidote.

5. PHARMACOLOGICAL PROPERTIES

5.1 Pharmacodynamic properties
MOTENS is a specific and potent calcium antagonist with a predominant selectivity for calcium channels in the vascular smooth muscle. Its main action is to dilate peripheral arterioles, reducing peripheral vascular resistance and lowering blood pressure.

In a study of ten patients with a renal transplant, MOTENS has been shown to prevent an acute decrease in renal plasma flow and glomerular filtration rate about six hours after administering oral cyclosporin. During the trough phase of cyclosporin treatment, there was no difference in renal plasma flow and glomerular filtration rate between patients with or without MOTENS.

Following the oral administration of 4 mg lacidipine to volunteer subjects, a minimal prolongation of QTc interval has been observed (mean QTcF increase between 3.44 and 9.60 ms in young and elderly volunteers). This was not associated with any adverse clinical effects or cardiac arrhythmias on monitoring.

5.2 Pharmacokinetic properties
MOTENS is a highly lipophilic compound; it is rapidly absorbed from the gastrointestinal tract following oral dosing. Absolute bioavailability averages about 10% due to extensive first-pass metabolism in the liver.

Peak plasma concentrations are reached between 30 and 150 minutes. The drug is eliminated primarily by hepatic metabolism. There is no evidence that MOTENS causes either induction or inhibition of hepatic enzymes.

The principal metabolites possess little, if any, pharmacodynamic activity.

Approximately 70% of the administered dose is eliminated as metabolites in the faeces and the remainder as metabolites in the urine.

The average terminal half-life of MOTENS ranges from between 13 and 19 hours at steady state.

5.3 Preclinical safety data
In acute toxicity studies, MOTENS has shown a wide safety margin.

In repeated dose toxicological studies, findings in animals, related to the safety profile of MOTENS in man, were reversible and reflected the pharmacodynamic effect of MOTENS.

No data of clinical relevance have been gained from *in vivo* and *in vitro* studies on reproduction toxicity, genetic toxicity or oncogenicity.

6. PHARMACEUTICAL PARTICULARS

6.1 List of excipients
Tablet core:

Lactose (monohydrate)

Lactose (spray-dried)

Povidone K30

Magnesium stearate

Film coating:

Titanium Dioxide (E 171)

Methylhydroxypropylcellulose

6.2 Incompatibilities
None known.

6.3 Shelf life
24 months

6.4 Special precautions for storage
Do not store above 30°C.

MOTENS is light sensitive. MOTENS tablets should, therefore, be stored in the original container and should not be removed from their foil pack until required for administration.

Keep out of the reach of children.

6.5 Nature and contents of container
Cartons containing 7, 14 and 28 tablets packed in blister strips.

[The 7 tablet pack is not currently marketed.]

6.6 Instructions for use and handling
Do not remove from foil pack until required for administration.

7. MARKETING AUTHORISATION HOLDER

Boehringer Ingelheim Limited
Ellesfield Avenue
Bracknell
Berkshire
RG12 8YS
United Kingdom

8. MARKETING AUTHORISATION NUMBER(S)

PL 00015/0188

9. DATE OF FIRST AUTHORISATION/RENEWAL OF THE AUTHORISATION

29 April 1993

10. DATE OF REVISION OF THE TEXT

July 2003

Legal category

POM

M9/2mg/UK/SPC/4

Motifene 75mg

(Sankyo Pharma UK Limited)

1. NAME OF THE MEDICINAL PRODUCT

Motifene

2. QUALITATIVE AND QUANTITATIVE COMPOSITION

Capsules containing 75 mg diclofenac sodium. Each capsule contains 25 mg diclofenac as enteric coated pellets and 50 mg diclofenac as sustained release pellets.

3. PHARMACEUTICAL FORM

Hard gelatin capsules (size 2) with light blue opaque cap and colourless transparent body marked in white print "D75M".

4. CLINICAL PARTICULARS

4.1 Therapeutic indications

Motifene is indicated for the treatment of rheumatoid arthritis; osteoarthrosis; low back pain; acute musculo-skeletal disorders and trauma such as periarthritis (especially frozen shoulder), tendinitis, tenosynovitis, bursitis, sprains, strains and dislocations; relief of pain in fractures; ankylosing spondylitis; acute gout; control of pain and inflammation in orthopaedic, dental and other minor surgery.

4.2 Posology and method of administration

For oral administration

The capsules should be swallowed whole with a liberal quantity of liquid.

To be taken preferably with or after food.

Adults:

One capsule daily. Dose may be increased to two capsules daily if necessary. The first dose should be taken in the morning before breakfast and the second if required 8-12 hours later.

Children:

Not for use in children.

Elderly:

The elderly are at increased risk of the serious consequences of adverse reactions. If an NSAID is considered necessary, the lowest effective dose should be used and for the shortest possible duration. The patient should be monitored regularly for GI bleeding during NSAID therapy.

4.3 Contraindications

- Hypersensitivity to any of the constituents.
- Previous hypersensitivity reactions (eg asthma, urticaria, angioedema or rhinitis) in response to ibuprofen, aspirin or other non-steroidal anti-inflammatory drugs.
- Severe hepatic, renal and cardiac failure (See section 4.4 – Special warnings and precautions for use).
- During the last trimester of pregnancy (See section 4.6 – Pregnancy and lactation).
- Active or previous peptic ulcer.
- History of upper gastrointestinal bleeding or perforation, related to previous NSAID therapy.
- Use with concomitant NSAIDs including cyclooxygenase-2 specific inhibitors (See section 4.5 - Interactions).

4.4 Special warnings and special precautions for use

In all patients:

Undesirable effects may be minimised by using the minimum effective dose for the shortest possible duration.

Elderly:

The elderly have an increased frequency of adverse reactions to NSAIDs especially gastrointestinal bleeding and perforation which may be fatal (See section 4.2 – Posology and administration).

Respiratory disorders:

Caution is required if administered to patients suffering from, or with a previous history of, bronchial asthma since NSAIDs have been reported to precipitate bronchospasm in such patients.

Cardiovascular, Renal and Hepatic Impairment:

The administration of an NSAID may cause a dose dependent reduction in prostaglandin formation and precipitate renal failure. Patients at greatest risk of this reaction are those with impaired renal function, cardiac impairment, liver dysfunction, those taking diuretics and the elderly. Renal function should be monitored in these patients (See section 4.3 – Contraindications).

Caution in patients with a history of hypertension and/or heart failure as fluid retention and oedema have been reported in association with NSAID therapy.

Gastrointestinal bleeding, ulceration and perforation:

GI bleeding, ulceration or perforation, which can be fatal, has been reported with all NSAIDs at any time during treatment, with or without warning symptoms or a previous history of serious GI events.

Patients with a history of GI toxicity, particularly when elderly, should report any unusual abdominal symptoms (especially GI bleeding) particularly in the initial stages of treatment.

Caution should be advised in patients receiving concomitant medications which could increase the risk of gastrotoxicity or bleeding, such as corticosteroids, or anticoagulants such as warfarin or anti-platelet agents such as aspirin (See section 4.5 – Interactions).

When GI bleeding or ulceration occurs in patients receiving Motifene, the treatment should be withdrawn.

NSAIDs should be given with care to patients with a history of gastrointestinal disease (ulcerative colitis, Crohn's disease) as these conditions may be exacerbated (See section 4.8 – Undesirable effects).

SLE and mixed connective tissue disease:

In patients with systemic lupus erythematosus (SLE) and mixed connective tissue disorders there may be an increased risk of aseptic meningitis (See section 4.8 – Undesirable effects).

Female fertility:

The use of Motifene may impair female fertility and is not recommended in women attempting to conceive. In women who have difficulties conceiving or who are undergoing investigation of infertility, withdrawal of Motifene should be considered.

Motifene, in common with other NSAIDs, can reversibly inhibit platelet aggregation.

4.5 Interaction with other medicinal products and other forms of Interaction

Other analgesics: Avoid concomitant use of two or more NSAIDs (including aspirin) as this may increase the risk of adverse effects (See section 4.3 – Contraindications).

Anti-hypertensives: Reduced anti-hypertensive effect.

Diuretics: Reduced diuretic effect. Diuretics can increase the risk of nephrotoxicity of NSAIDs. Concomitant treatment with potassium-sparing diuretics may be associated with increased serum potassium levels, hence serum potassium should be monitored.

Cardiac glycosides: NSAIDs may exacerbate cardiac failure, reduced GFR (Glomerular Filtration Rate) and increase plasma glycoside levels.

Lithium: Decreased elimination of lithium.

Methotrexate: Decreased elimination of methotrexate.

Caution should be exercised if NSAIDs and methotrexate are administered within 24 hours of each other.

Ciclosporin: Increased risk of nephrotoxicity.

Mifepristone: NSAIDs should not be used for 8-12 days after mifepristone administration as NSAIDs can reduce the effect of mifepristone.

Corticosteroids: Increased risk of GI bleeding (See section 4.4 – Special warnings and precautions for use).

Anti-coagulants: NSAIDs may enhance the effects of anti-coagulants, such as warfarin (See section 4.4 – Special warnings and precautions for use).

Quinolone antibiotics: Animal data indicate that NSAIDs can increase the risk of convulsions associated with quinolone antibiotics. Patients taking NSAIDs and quinolones may have an increased risk of developing convulsions.

Tacrolimus: Possible increased risk of nephrotoxicity when NSAIDs are given with tacrolimus.

Pharmacodynamic studies have shown no potentiation of oral hypoglycaemic drugs, but caution and adequate monitoring are nevertheless advised.

4.6 Pregnancy and lactation

Pregnancy:

Congenital abnormalities have been reported in association with NSAID administration in man, however these are low in frequency and do not appear to follow any discernible pattern.

In view of the known effects of NSAIDs on the foetal cardiovascular system (risk of closure of the ductus arteriosus), use in the last trimester of pregnancy is contra-indicated.

The onset of labour may be delayed and the duration increased with an increased bleeding tendency in both mother and child (See section 4.3 – Contraindications).

NSAIDs should not be used during the first two trimesters of pregnancy or labour unless the potential benefit to the patient outweighs the potential risk to the foetus.

Lactation:

Following oral doses of 50mg every 8 hours, traces of active substance have been detected in breast milk. Motifene should therefore be avoided in patients who are breast-feeding.

4.7 Effects on ability to drive and use machines

Patients who experience dizziness, drowsiness, fatigue and visual disturbances while taking NSAIDs should not drive or operate machinery.

4.8 Undesirable effects

If serious side-effects occur, Motifene should be withdrawn.

Gastrointestinal tract: The most commonly observed adverse events are gastrointestinal in nature. Peptic ulcers, perforation or GI bleeding (sometimes fatal, particularly in the elderly) may occur (See section 4.4 – Special warnings and precautions for use).

Nausea, vomiting, diarrhoea, flatulence, constipation, dyspepsia, abdominal pain, melaena, haematemesis, ulcerative stomatitis, exacerbation of colitis and Crohn's disease (See section 4.4 – Special warnings and precautions for use) have been reported following administration. Less frequently, gastritis has been observed.

Hypersensitivity: Hypersensitivity reactions have been reported following treatment with NSAIDs. These may consist of:

(a) non-specific allergic reactions and anaphylaxis

(b) respiratory reactivity comprising asthma, aggravated asthma, bronchospasm or dyspnoea

(c) assorted skin disorders, including rashes of various types, pruritus, urticaria, purpura, angiodema and, more rarely, exfoliative and bullous dermatoses (including epidermal necrolysis and erythema multiforme).

Cardiovascular: Oedema has been reported in association with NSAID treatment.

Other adverse events reported less commonly include:

Renal: Nephrotoxicity in various forms, including interstitial nephritis, nephrotic syndrome, renal failure and urinary abnormalities (e.g. haemuturia).

Hepatic: Abnormal liver function, hepatitis (in isolated cases fulminant) and jaundice.

Neurological and special senses: Disturbances of vision (blurred vision, diplopia), optic neuritis, headache, paraesthesia, reports of aseptic meningitis (especially in patients with existing auto-immune disorders, such as lupus erythematosus, mixed connective tissue disease) with symptoms such as stiff neck, headache, nausea, vomiting, fever or disorientation (See section 4.4), depression, confusion, hallucinations, tinnitus, dizziness, vertigo, malaise, fatigue and drowsiness.

Isolated cases of memory disturbance, disorientation, impaired hearing, insomnia, irritability, convulsions, anxiety, nightmares, tremor, psychotic reactions.

Dermatological: Photosensitivity reactions, rashes, skin eruptions, urticaria.

Isolated cases of bullous eruptions, eczema, erythema multiforme, Stevens-Johnson syndrome, Lyell's syndrome, loss of hair.

Haematological: Thrombocytopenia, neutropenia, leucopenia, agranulocytosis, haemolytic anaemia, aplastic anaemia.

4.9 Overdose

Symptoms:

Symptoms include headache, nausea, vomiting, epigastric pain, gastrointestinal bleeding, rarely diarrhoea, disorientation, excitation, coma, drowsiness, dizziness, tinnitus, fainting and occasionally convulsions. In cases of significant poisoning, acute renal failure and liver damage are possible.

Treatment:

Management of acute poisoning with NSAIDs essentially consists of supportive and symptomatic measures.

Within one hour of ingestion of a potentially toxic amount, activated charcoal should be considered. Alternatively, in adults, gastric lavage should be considered within on hour of ingestion of a potentially life-threatening overdose.

Good urine output should be ensured.

Renal and liver function should be closely monitored.

Patients should be closely monitored for at least four hours after ingestion of potentially toxic amounts.

Frequent or prolonged convulsions should be treated with intravenous diazepam.

Other measures may be indicated by the patient's clinical condition. Specific therapies such as forced diureses; dialysis or haemoperfusion are probably of no help in eliminating NSAIDs due to their high rate of protein binding and extensive metabolism.

5. PHARMACOLOGICAL PROPERTIES

5.1 Pharmacodynamic properties

Motifene is a non-steroidal agent with marked analgesic/anti-inflammatory properties.

It is an inhibitor of prostaglandin synthetase (cyclo-oxygenase).

5.2 Pharmacokinetic properties
Diclofenac sodium is rapidly absorbed from the gut and is subject to first-pass metabolism. Therapeutic plasma concentrations occur about ½ hour after administration of Motifene. The active substance is 99.7% protein bound and the plasma half-life for the terminal elimination phase is 1-2 hours. Approximately 60% of the administered dose is excreted via the kidneys in the form of metabolites and less than 1% in unchanged form. The remainder of the dose is excreted via the bile in metabolised form.

Following rapid gastric passage, the enteric coated pellet component of Motifene ensures quick availability of the active component in the blood stream. The sustained release pellets cause a delayed release of the active component, which means one single daily dose is usually sufficient.

5.3 Preclinical safety data
Not applicable

6. PHARMACEUTICAL PARTICULARS

6.1 List of excipients

Enteric Coated Pellets:

Microcrystalline cellulose, polyvidone, collodial anhydrous silica, methacrylic acid copolymer type C, sodium hydroxide, propylene glycol, talc, isopropanol, purified water.

Sustained Release Pellets:

Microcrystalline cellulose, polyvidone, colloidal anhydrous silica, poly (ethyl acrylate, methyl methacrylate, trimethylammonio, ethyl methacrylate choloride), dibutyl phthalate, talc, isopropanol, acetone.

Capsule Shell:

Indigotine E132, titanium dioxide E171, purified water, gelatin.

Capsule Body:

Gelatin, ink: containing shellac (USP/NF), soy lecithin (food grade) (USP), antifoam DC 1510, titanium dioxide E171, industrial methylated spirit, purified water, N-butyl alcohol.

6.2 Incompatibilities
None known

6.3 Shelf life
5 years

6.4 Special precautions for storage
Store below 25°C

6.5 Nature and contents of container
The capsules are blister packed in PVC/PDVC and aluminium foil and are packed into folding cardboard cartons.

Motifene is available in 2, 4, 28, 56s.

6.6 Instructions for use and handling
Not applicable.

Administrative Data

7. MARKETING AUTHORISATION HOLDER
Sankyo Pharma (UK) Ltd

Sankyo House

Repton Place

White Lion Road

Amersham

Bucks HP7 9LP

8. MARKETING AUTHORISATION NUMBER(S)
PL 8265/0003

9. DATE OF FIRST AUTHORISATION/RENEWAL OF THE AUTHORISATION
5th August 1994

9th September 1999

10. DATE OF REVISION OF THE TEXT
November 2004

Motilium 30 mg suppositories

(sanofi-aventis)

1. NAME OF THE MEDICINAL PRODUCT
Motilium 30 mg suppositories

2. QUALITATIVE AND QUANTITATIVE COMPOSITION
One suppository contains domperidone 30 mg.

For excipients, see 6.1.

3. PHARMACEUTICAL FORM
Suppositories - white to slightly yellow suppositories.

4. CLINICAL PARTICULARS

4.1 Therapeutic indications

Adults

• The relief of the symptoms of nausea and vomiting, epigastric sense of fullness, upper abdominal discomfort and regurgitation of gastric contents.

Children

• The relief of the symptoms of nausea and vomiting.

4.2 Posology and method of administration
Adults and adolescents (over 12 years and weighing 35 kg or more)

The initial duration of treatment is four weeks. Patients should be re-evaluated after four weeks and the need for continued treatment re-assessed.

60 mg suppositories two times per day.

Infants and children

The total daily dose is dependent on the child's weight:

For a child weighing more than 15 kg: 30 mg suppositories two times per day.

30 mg suppositories are unsuitable for use in children weighing less than 15 kg.

4.3 Contraindications
Motilium is contraindicated in the following situations:

• Known hypersensitivity to domperidone or any of the excipients

• Prolactin-releasing pituitary tumour (prolactinoma).

Motilium should not be used when stimulation of the gastric motility could be harmful: gastro-intestinal haemorrhage, mechanical obstruction or perforation.

4.4 Special warnings and special precautions for use

Precautions for use

Use during lactation:

The total amount of domperidone excreted in human breast milk is expected to be less than 7μg per day at the highest recommended dosing regimen. It is not known whether this is harmful to the newborn. Therefore breast-feeding is not recommended for mothers who are taking Motilium.

Use in infants:

Neurological side effects are rare (see "Undesirable effects" section). Since metabolic functions and the blood-brain barrier are not fully developed in the first months of life the risk of neurological side effects is higher in young children. Therefore, it is recommended that the dose be determined accurately and followed strictly in neonates, infants, toddlers and small children.

Overdosing may cause extrapyramidal symptoms in children, but other causes should be taken into consideration.

Use in liver disorders:

Since domperidone is highly metabolised in the liver, Motilium should not be used in patients with hepatic impairment.

Renal insufficiency:

In patients with severe renal insufficiency (serum creatinine > 6 mg/100 ml, i.e. > 0.6 m mol/l) the elimination half-life of domperidone was increased from 7.4 to 20.8 hours, but plasma drug levels were lower than in healthy volunteers. Since very little unchanged drug is excreted via the kidneys, it is unlikely that the dose of a single administration needs to be adjusted in patients with renal insufficiency. However, on repeated administration, the dosing frequency should be reduced to once or twice daily depending on the severity of the impairment, and the dose may need to be reduced. Such patients on prolonged therapy should be reviewed regularly.

Use with ketoconazole:

A slight increase of QT interval (mean less than 10msec) was reported in a drug-drug interaction study with *oral* ketoconazole. Even if the significance of this study is not fully clear, alternative therapeutic options should be considered if antifungal treatment is required. (see also section 4.5).

4.5 Interaction with other medicinal products and other forms of Interaction
The main metabolic pathway of domperidone is through CYP3A4. *In vitro* data suggest that the concomitant use of drugs that significantly inhibit this enzyme may result in increased plasma levels of domperidone. *In vivo* interaction studies with ketoconazole revealed a marked inhibition of domperidone's CYP3A4 mediated first pass metabolism by ketoconazole.

A pharmacokinetic study has demonstrated that the AUC and the peak plasma concentration of domperidone is increased by a factor 3 when oral ketoconazole is administered concomitantly (at steady state). A slight QT prolonging effect (mean less than 10msec) of this combination was detected, which was greater than the one seen with ketoconazole alone. A QT prolonging effect could not be detected when domperidone was given alone in patients with no co-morbidity, even at high oral doses (up to 160mg/day).

The results of this interaction study should be taken into account when prescribing domperidone concomitantly with strong CYP3A4 inhibitors: for example: ketoconazole, ritonavir and erythromycin (see also section 5.2).

4.6 Pregnancy and lactation
There are limited post-marketing data on the use of domperidone in pregnant women. A study in rats has shown reproductive toxicity at a high, maternally toxic dose. The potential risk for humans is unknown. Therefore, Motilium should only be used during pregnancy when justified by the anticipated therapeutic benefit.

The drug is excreted in breast milk of lactating rats (mostly as metabolites: peak concentration of 40 and 800 ng/ml after oral and i.v. administration of 2.5 mg/kg respectively). Domperidone concentrations in breast milk of lactating women are 10 to 50% of the corresponding plasma concentrations and expected not to exceed 10ng/ml. The total amount of domperidone excreted in human breast milk is expected to be less than 7μg per day at the highest recommended dosing regimen. It is not known whether this is harmful to the newborn. Therefore breast-feeding is not recommended for mothers who are taking Motilium.

4.7 Effects on ability to drive and use machines
Motilium has no or negligible influence on the ability to drive and use machines

4.8 Undesirable effects

• *Immune System Disorder:* Very rare; Allergic reaction

• *Endocrine disorder:* Rare; increased prolactin levels

• *Nervous system disorders:* Very rare; extrapyramidal side effects

• *Gastrointestinal disorders:* Rare; gastro-intestinal disorders, including very rare transient intestinal cramps

• *Skin and subcutaneous tissue disorders:* Very rare; urticaria

• *Reproductive system and breast disorders:* Rare; galactorrhoea, gynaecomastia, amenorrhoea.

As the hypophysis is outside the blood brain barrier, domperidone may cause an increase in prolactin levels. In rare cases this hyperprolactinaemia may lead to neuro-endocrinological side effects such as galactorrhoea, gynaecomastia and amenorrhoea.

Extrapyramidal side effects are very rare in neonates and infants, and exceptional in adults. These side effects reverse spontaneously and completely as soon as the treatment is stopped.

4.9 Overdose

Symptoms

Symptoms of overdosage may include drowsiness, disorientation and extrapyramidal reactions, especially in children.

Treatment

There is no specific antidote to domperidone, but in the event of overdose, gastric lavage as well as the administration of activated charcoal, may be useful. Close medical supervision and supportive therapy is recommended.

Anticholinergic, anti-parkinson drugs may be helpful in controlling the extrapyramidal reactions.

5. PHARMACOLOGICAL PROPERTIES

5.1 Pharmacodynamic properties
Pharmacotherapeutic group: Propulsives, ATC code: A03F A 03

Domperidone is a dopamine antagonist with anti-emetic properties. Domperidone does not readily cross the blood-brain barrier. In domperidone users, especially in adults, extrapyramidal side effects are very rare, but domperidone promotes the release of prolactin from the pituitary. Its anti-emetic effect may be due to a combination of peripheral (gastrokinetic) effects and antagonism of dopamine receptors in the chemoreceptor trigger zone, which lies outside the blood-brain barrier in the area postrema. Animal studies, together with the low concentrations found in the brain, indicate a predominantly peripheral effect of domperidone on dopamine receptors.

Studies in man have shown oral domperidone to increase lower oesophageal pressure, improve antroduodenal motility and accelerate gastric emptying. There is no effect on gastric secretion.

5.2 Pharmacokinetic properties

Absorption

In fasting subjects, domperidone is rapidly absorbed after oral administration, with peak plasma concentrations at 30 to 60 minutes. The low absolute bioavailability of oral domperidone (approximately 15%) is due to an extensive first-pass metabolism in the gut wall and liver. Although domperidone's bioavailability is enhanced in normal subjects when taken after a meal, patients with gastro-intestinal complaints should take domperidone 15-30 minutes before a meal. Reduced gastric acidity impairs the absorption of domperidone. Oral bioavailability is decreased by prior concomitant administration of cimetidine and sodium bicarbonate. The time of peak absorption is slightly delayed and the AUC somewhat increased when the oral drug is taken after a meal.

After rectal administration of 60mg domperidone suppositories, a plateau is attained with domperidone plasma concentrations of about 20ng/ml lasting from 1 to 5 hours after administration. Although peak plasma levels are only about one third of that of an oral dose, the mean rectal bioavailability of 12.4% is quite similar to that after oral administration.

Distribution

Oral domperidone does not appear to accumulate or induce its own metabolism; a peak plasma level after 90 minutes of 21 ng/ml after two weeks oral administration of 30 mg per day was almost the same as that of 18 ng/ml after the first dose. Domperidone is 91-93% bound to plasma proteins. Distribution studies with radiolabelled drug in animals have shown wide tissue distribution, but low brain concentration. Small amounts of drug cross the placenta in rats.

Metabolism

Domperidone undergoes rapid and extensive hepatic metabolism by hydroxylation and N-dealkylation. *In vitro* metabolism experiments with diagnostic inhibitors revealed that CYP3A4 is a major form of cytochrome P-450 involved in the N-dealkylation of domperidone, whereas CYP3A4, CYP1A2 and CYP2E1 are involved in domperidone aromatic hydroxylation.

Excretion

Urinary and faecal excretions amount to 31 and 66% of the oral dose respectively. The proportion of the drug excreted unchanged is small (10% of faecal excretion and approximately 1% of urinary excretion). The plasma half-life after a single oral dose is 7-9 hours in healthy subjects but is prolonged in patients with severe renal insufficiency.

5.3 Preclinical safety data

Electrophysiological *in vitro* and *in vivo* studies indicate an overall moderate risk of domperidone to prolong the QT interval in humans. In *in vitro* experiments on isolated cells transfected with HERG and on isolated guinea pig myocytes, ratios were about 10, based on IC50 values inhibiting currents through ion channels in comparison to the free plasma concentrations in humans after administration of the maximum daily dose of 20mg (q.i.d.). However, safety margins in *in vitro* experiments on isolated cardiac tissues in *in vivo* models (dog, guinea pig, rabbits sensitised for torsades de pointes) exceeded the free plasma concentrations in humans at maximum daily dose (20mg q.i.d.) by more than 50-fold. In the presence of inhibition of the metabolism via CYP3A4 free plasma concentrations of domperidone can rise up to 10-fold.

At a high, maternally toxic dose (more than 40 times the recommended human dose), teratogenic effects were seen in the rat. No teratogenicity was observed in mice and rabbits.

6. PHARMACEUTICAL PARTICULARS

6.1 List of excipients

Macrogol 4000

Macrogol 400

Macrogol 1000

Tartaric acid

Butylhydroxyanisole.

6.2 Incompatibilities

Not applicable.

6.3 Shelf life

5 years.

6.4 Special precautions for storage

Do not store above 25°C.

6.5 Nature and contents of container

PVC-PE strips enclosed in cardboard cartons.

Pack size of 10 suppositories.

6.6 Instructions for use and handling

No special requirements.

7. MARKETING AUTHORISATION HOLDER

Sanofi-Synthelabo

PO Box 597

Guildford

Surrey

8. MARKETING AUTHORISATION NUMBER(S)

PL 11723/0051

9. DATE OF FIRST AUTHORISATION/RENEWAL OF THE AUTHORISATION

16th June 2002

10. DATE OF REVISION OF THE TEXT

June 2004

Legal category: POM

Motilium Suspension 1mg/ml

(sanofi-aventis)

1. NAME OF THE MEDICINAL PRODUCT

Motilium 1 mg/ml suspension

2. QUALITATIVE AND QUANTITATIVE COMPOSITION

The oral suspension contains domperidone 1 mg per ml.

For excipients, see 6.1.

3. PHARMACEUTICAL FORM

Oral suspension - white homogenous suspension.

4. CLINICAL PARTICULARS

4.1 Therapeutic indications

Adults

- The relief of the symptoms of nausea and vomiting, epigastric sense of fullness, upper abdominal discomfort and regurgitation of gastric contents.

Children

- The relief of the symptoms of nausea and vomiting.

4.2 Posology and method of administration

It is recommended to take oral Motilium before meals. If taken after meals, absorption of the drug is somewhat delayed.

Adults and adolescents (over 12 years and weighing 35 kg or more)

The initial duration of treatment is four weeks. Patients should be re-evaluated after four weeks and the need for continued treatment re-assessed.

10 ml to 20 ml (of oral suspension containing domperidone 1mg per ml) three to four times per day with a maximum daily dose of 80 ml.

Infants and children

0.25 – 0.5 mg/kg three to four times per day with a maximum daily dose of 2.4 mg/kg (but do not exceed 80 mg per day).

4.3 Contraindications

Motilium is contraindicated in the following situations:

- Known hypersensitivity to domperidone or any of the excipients
- Prolactin-releasing pituitary tumour (prolactinoma).

Motilium should not be used when stimulation of the gastric motility could be harmful:

gastro-intestinal haemorrhage, mechanical obstruction or perforation.

4.4 Special warnings and special precautions for use

Precautions for use

The oral suspension contains sorbitol and may be unsuitable for patients with sorbitol intolerance.

Use during lactation

The total amount of domperidone excreted in human breast milk is expected to be less than 7μg per day at the highest recommended dosing regimen. It is not known whether this is harmful to the newborn. Therefore breast-feeding is not recommended for mothers who are taking Motilium.

Use in infants:

Neurological side effects are rare (see "Undesirable effects" section). Since metabolic functions and the blood-brain barrier are not fully developed in the first months of life the risk of neurological side effects is higher in young children. Therefore, it is recommended that the dose be determined accurately and followed strictly in neonates, infants, toddlers and small children.

Overdosing may cause extrapyramidal symptoms in children, but other causes should be taken into consideration.

Use in liver disorders:

Since domperidone is highly metabolised in the liver, Motilium should be not be used in patients with hepatic impairment.

Renal insufficiency:

In patients with severe renal insufficiency (serum creatinine > 6 mg/100 ml, i.e. > 0.6 m mol/l) the elimination half-life of domperidone was increased from 7.4 to 20.8 hours, but plasma drug levels were lower than in healthy volunteers. Since very little unchanged drug is excreted via the kidneys, it is unlikely that the dose of a single administration needs to be adjusted in patients with renal insufficiency. However, on repeated administration, the dosing frequency should be reduced to once or twice daily depending on the severity of the impairment, and the dose may need to be reduced. Such patients on prolonged therapy should be reviewed regularly.

Use with ketoconazole:

A slight increase of QT interval (mean less than 10msec) was reported in a drug-drug interaction study with *oral* ketoconazole. Even if the significance of this study is not fully clear, alternative therapeutic options should be considered if antifungal treatment is required. (see also section 4.5).

4.5 Interaction with other medicinal products and other forms of Interaction

The main metabolic pathway of domperidone is through CYP3A4. *In vitro* data suggest that the concomitant use of drugs that significantly inhibit this enzyme may result in increased plasma levels of domperidone. *In vivo* interaction studies with ketoconazole revealed a marked inhibition of domperidone's CYP3A4 mediated first pass metabolism by ketoconazole.

A pharmacokinetic study has demonstrated that the AUC and the peak plasma concentration of domperidone is increased by a factor 3 when oral ketoconazole is administered concomitantly (at steady state). A slight QT prolonging effect (mean less than 10msec) of this combination was detected, which was greater than the one seen with ketoconazole alone. A QT prolonging effect could not be detected when domperidone was given alone in patients with no co-morbidity, even at high oral doses (up to 160mg/day).

The results of this interaction study should be taken into account when prescribing domperidone concomitantly with strong CYP3A4 inhibitors: for example: ketoconazole, ritonavir and erythromycin (see also section 5.2).

4.6 Pregnancy and lactation

There are limited post-marketing data on the use of domperidone in pregnant women. A study in rats has shown reproductive toxicity at a high, maternally toxic dose. The potential risk for humans is unknown. Therefore, Motilium should only be used during pregnancy when justified by the anticipated therapeutic benefit.

The drug is excreted in breast milk of lactating rats (mostly as metabolites: peak concentration of 40 and 800 ng/mL after oral and i.v. administration of 2.5 mg/kg respectively). Domperidone concentrations in breast milk of lactating women are 10 to 50% of the corresponding plasma concentrations and expected not to exceed 10ng/ml. The total amount of domperidone excreted in human breast milk is expected to be less than 7μg per day at the highest recommended dosing regimen. It is not known whether this is harmful to the newborn. Therefore breast-feeding is not recommended for mothers who are taking Motilium.

4.7 Effects on ability to drive and use machines

Motilium has no or negligible influence on the ability to drive and use machines.

4.8 Undesirable effects

- *Immune System Disorder:* Very rare; Allergic reaction
- *Endocrine disorder:* Rare; increased prolactin levels
- *Nervous system disorders:* Very rare; extrapyramidal side effects
- *Gastrointestinal disorders:* Rare; gastro-intestinal disorders, including very rare transient intestinal cramps
- *Skin and subcutaneous tissue disorders:* Very rare; urticaria
- *Reproductive system and breast disorders:* Rare; galactorrhoea, gynaecomastia, amenorrhoea.

As the hypophysis is outside the blood brain barrier, domperidone may cause an increase in prolactin levels. In rare cases this hyperprolactinaemia may lead to neuro-endocrinological side effects such as galactorrhoea, gynaecomastia and amenorrhoea.

Extrapyramidal side effects are very rare in neonates and infants, and exceptional in adults. These side effects reverse spontaneously and completely as soon as the treatment is stopped.

4.9 Overdose

Symptoms

Symptoms of overdosage may include drowsiness, disorientation and extrapyramidal reactions, especially in children.

Treatment

There is no specific antidote to domperidone, but in the event of overdose, gastric lavage as well as the administration of activated charcoal, may be useful. Close medical supervision and supportive therapy is recommended.

Anticholinergic, anti-parkinson drugs may be helpful in controlling the extrapyramidal reactions.

5. PHARMACOLOGICAL PROPERTIES

5.1 Pharmacodynamic properties

Pharmacotherapeutic group: Propulsives, ATC code: A03F A 03

Domperidone is a dopamine antagonist with anti-emetic properties. Domperidone does not readily cross the blood-brain barrier. In domperidone users, especially in adults, extrapyramidal side effects are very rare, but domperidone promotes the release of prolactin from the pituitary. Its anti-emetic effect may be due to a combination of peripheral (gastrokinetic) effects and antagonism of dopamine receptors in the chemoreceptor trigger zone, which lies outside the blood-brain barrier in the area postrema. Animal studies, together with the low concentrations found in the brain, indicate a predominantly peripheral effect of domperidone on dopamine receptors.

Studies in man have shown oral domperidone to increase lower oesophageal pressure, improve antroduodenal motility and accelerate gastric emptying. There is no effect on gastric secretion.

5.2 Pharmacokinetic properties

Absorption

In fasting subjects, domperidone is rapidly absorbed after oral administration, with peak plasma concentrations at 30 to 60 minutes. The low absolute bioavailability of oral domperidone (approximately 15%) is due to an extensive first-pass metabolism in the gut wall and liver. Although domperidone's bioavailability is enhanced in normal subjects when taken after a meal, patients with gastro-intestinal complaints should take domperidone 15-30 minutes before a meal. Reduced gastric acidity impairs the absorption of domperidone. Oral bioavailability is decreased by prior concomitant administration of cimetidine and sodium bicarbonate. The time of peak absorption is slightly delayed and the AUC somewhat increased when the oral drug is taken after a meal.

Distribution

Oral domperidone does not appear to accumulate or induce its own metabolism; a peak plasma level after 90 minutes of 21 ng/ml after two weeks oral administration of 30 mg per day was almost the same as that of 18 ng/ml after the first dose. Domperidone is 91-93% bound to plasma proteins. Distribution studies with radiolabelled drug in animals have shown wide tissue distribution, but low brain concentration. Small amounts of drug cross the placenta in rats.

Metabolism

Domperidone undergoes rapid and extensive hepatic metabolism by hydroxylation and N-dealkylation. *In vitro* metabolism experiments with diagnostic inhibitors revealed that CYP3A4 is a major form of cytochrome P-450 involved in the N-dealkylation of domperidone, whereas CYP3A4, CYP1A2 and CYP2E1 are involved in domperidone aromatic hydroxylation.

Excretion

Urinary and faecal excretions amount to 31 and 66% of the oral dose respectively. The proportion of the drug excreted unchanged is small (10% of faecal excretion and approximately 1% of urinary excretion). The plasma half-life after a single oral dose is 7-9 hours in healthy subjects but is prolonged in patients with severe renal insufficiency.

5.3 Preclinical safety data

Electrophysiological *in vitro* and *in vivo* studies indicate an overall moderate risk of domperidone to prolong the QT interval in humans. In *in vitro* experiments on isolated cells transfected with HERG and on isolated guinea pig myocytes, ratios were about 10, based on IC50 values inhibiting currents through ion channels in comparison to the free plasma concentrations in humans after administration of the maximum daily dose of 20mg (q.i.d.). However, safety margins in *in vitro* experiments on isolated cardiac tissues in *in vivo* models (dog, guinea pig, rabbits sensitised for torsades de pointes) exceeded the free plasma concentrations in humans at maximum daily dose (20mg q.i.d.) by more than 50-fold. In the presence of inhibition of the metabolism via CYP3A4 free plasma concentrations of domperidone can rise up to 10-fold.

At a high, maternally toxic dose (more than 40 times the recommended human dose), teratogenic effects were seen in the rat. No teratogenicity was observed in mice and rabbits.

6. PHARMACEUTICAL PARTICULARS

6.1 List of excipients

Sorbitol solution 70% non crystallizable

Dispersible cellulose (contains microcrystalline cellulose and carmellose sodium)

Methyl p-hydroxybenzoate

Propyl p-hydroxybenzoate

Sodium saccharin

Polysorbate 20

Sodium hydroxide

Purified water.

6.2 Incompatibilities

Not applicable.

6.3 Shelf life

3 years.

6.4 Special precautions for storage

No special requirements.

6.5 Nature and contents of container

Amber glass bottles with tamper-proof aluminium screw caps or tamper-evident polyethylene screw caps and graduated polypropylene measuring cap.

Bottle size of 200 ml.

6.6 Instructions for use and handling

No special requirements.

7. MARKETING AUTHORISATION HOLDER

Sanofi-Synthelabo

PO Box 597

Guildford

Surrey

8. MARKETING AUTHORISATION NUMBER(S)

11723/0054

9. DATE OF FIRST AUTHORISATION/RENEWAL OF THE AUTHORISATION

16th June 2002

10. DATE OF REVISION OF THE TEXT

June 2004

Legal category: POM

Motilium Tablets 10mg

(sanofi-aventis)

1. NAME OF THE MEDICINAL PRODUCT

Motilium

2. QUALITATIVE AND QUANTITATIVE COMPOSITION

One film-coated tablet contains domperidone maleate 12.72 mg equivalent to domperidone 10 mg.

For excipients, see 6.1.

3. PHARMACEUTICAL FORM

Film-coated tablets - white to faintly cream coloured, circular, biconvex tablets.

4. CLINICAL PARTICULARS

4.1 Therapeutic indications

Adults

- The relief of the symptoms of nausea and vomiting, epigastric sense of fullness, upper abdominal discomfort and regurgitation of gastric contents.

Children

- The relief of the symptoms of nausea and vomiting.

4.2 Posology and method of administration

It is recommended to take oral Motilium before meals. If taken after meals, absorption of the drug is somewhat delayed.

Adults and adolescents (over 12 years and weighing 35 kg or more)

The initial duration of treatment is four weeks. Patients should be re-evaluated after four weeks and the need for continued treatment re-assessed.

1 to 2 of the 10mg tablets three to four times per day with a maximum daily dose of 80 mg.

Infants and children

0.25 – 0.5 mg/kg three to four times per day with a maximum daily dose of 2.4 mg/kg (but do not exceed 80 mg per day).

Tablets are unsuitable for use in children weighing less than 35 kg.

4.3 Contraindications

Motilium is contraindicated in the following situations:

- Known hypersensitivity to domperidone or any of the excipients
- Prolactin-releasing pituitary tumour (prolactinoma).

Motilium should not be used when stimulation of the gastric motility could be harmful:

gastro-intestinal haemorrhage, mechanical obstruction or perforation.

4.4 Special warnings and special precautions for use

Precautions for use

The film-coated tablets contain lactose and may be unsuitable for patients with lactose intolerance, galactosaemia or glucose/galactose malabsorption.

Use during lactation:

The total amount of domperidone excreted in human breast milk is expected to be less than 7μg per day at the highest recommended dosing regimen. It is not known whether this is harmful to the newborn. Therefore breast-feeding is not recommended for mothers who are taking Motilium.

Use in infants:

Neurological side effects are rare (see "Undesirable effects" section). Since metabolic functions and the blood-brain barrier are not fully developed in the first months of life the risk of neurological side effects is higher in young children. Therefore, it is recommended that the dose be determined accurately and followed strictly in neonates, infants, toddlers and small children.

Overdosing may cause extrapyramidal symptoms in children, but other causes should be taken into consideration.

Use in liver disorders:

Since domperidone is highly metabolised in the liver, Motilium should be not be used in patients with hepatic impairment.

Renal insufficiency:

In patients with severe renal insufficiency (serum creatinine > 6 mg/100 ml, i.e. > 0.6 m mol/l) the elimination half-life of domperidone was increased from 7.4 to 20.8 hours, but plasma drug levels were lower than in healthy volunteers. Since very little unchanged drug is excreted via the kidneys, it is unlikely that the dose of a single administration needs to be adjusted in patients with renal insufficiency. However, on repeated administration, the dosing frequency should be reduced to once or twice daily depending on the severity of the impairment, and the dose may need to be reduced. Such patients on prolonged therapy should be reviewed regularly.

Use with ketoconazole:

A slight increase of QT interval (mean less than 10msec) was reported in a drug-drug interaction study with *oral* ketoconazole. Even if the significance of this study is not fully clear, alternative therapeutic options should be considered if antifungal treatment is required. (see also section 4.5).

4.5 Interaction with other medicinal products and other forms of Interaction

The main metabolic pathway of domperidone is through CYP3A4. *In vitro* data suggest that the concomitant use of drugs that significantly inhibit this enzyme may result in increased plasma levels of domperidone. *In vivo* interaction studies with ketoconazole revealed a marked inhibition of domperidone's CYP3A4 mediated first pass metabolism by ketoconazole.

A pharmacokinetic study has demonstrated that the AUC and the peak plasma concentration of domperidone is increased by a factor 3 when oral ketoconazole is administered concomitantly (at steady state). A slight QT prolonging effect (mean less than 10msec) of this combination was detected, which was greater than the one seen with ketoconazole alone. A QT prolonging effect could not be detected when domperidone was given alone in patients with no co-morbidity, even at high oral doses (up to 160mg/day).

The results of this interaction study should be taken into account when prescribing domperidone concomitantly with strong CYP3A4 inhibitors: for example: ketoconazole, ritonavir and erythromycin (see also section 5.2).

4.6 Pregnancy and lactation

There are limited post-marketing data on the use of domperidone in pregnant women. A study in rats has shown reproductive toxicity at a high, maternally toxic dose. The potential risk for humans is unknown. Therefore, Motilium should only be used during pregnancy when justified by the anticipated therapeutic benefit.

The drug is excreted in breast milk of lactating rats (mostly as metabolites: peak concentration of 40 and 800 ng/ml after oral and i.v. administration of 2.5 mg/kg respectively). Domperidone concentrations in breast milk of lactating women are 10 to 50% of the corresponding plasma concentrations and expected not to exceed 10ng/ml. The total amount of domperidone excreted in human breast milk is expected to be less than 7μg per day at the highest recommended dosing regimen. It is not known whether this is harmful to the newborn. Therefore breast-feeding is not recommended for mothers who are taking Motilium.

4.7 Effects on ability to drive and use machines

Motilium has no or negligible influence on the ability to drive and use machines.

4.8 Undesirable effects

- *Immune System Disorder:* Very rare; Allergic reaction
- *Endocrine disorder:* Rare; increased prolactin levels
- *Nervous system disorders:* Very rare; extrapyramidal side effects
- *Gastrointestinal disorders:* Rare; gastro-intestinal disorders, including very rare transient intestinal cramps
- *Skin and subcutaneous tissue disorders:* Very rare; urticaria
- *Reproductive system and breast disorders:* Rare; galactorrhoea, gynaecomastia, amenorrhoea.

As the hypophysis is outside the blood brain barrier, domperidone may cause an increase in prolactin levels. In rare cases this hyperprolactinaemia may lead to neuro-endocrinological side effects such as galactorrhoea, gynaecomastia and amenorrhoea.

Extrapyramidal side effects are very rare in neonates and infants, and exceptional in adults. These side effects reverse spontaneously and completely as soon as the treatment is stopped.

4.9 Overdose

Symptoms

Symptoms of overdosage may include drowsiness, disorientation and extrapyramidal reactions, especially in children.

Treatment

There is no specific antidote to domperidone, but in the event of overdose, gastric lavage as well as the administration of activated charcoal, may be useful. Close medical supervision and supportive therapy is recommended.

Anticholinergic, anti-parkinson drugs may be helpful in controlling the extrapyramidal reactions.

5. PHARMACOLOGICAL PROPERTIES

5.1 Pharmacodynamic properties

Pharmacotherapeutic group: Propulsives, ATC code: A03F A 03

Domperidone is a dopamine antagonist with anti-emetic properties, Domperidone does not readily cross the blood-brain barrier. In domperidone users, especially in adults, extrapyramidal side effects are very rare, but domperidone promotes the release of prolactin from the pituitary. Its anti-emetic effect may be due to a combination of peripheral (gastrokinetic) effects and antagonism of dopamine receptors in the chemoreceptor trigger zone, which lies outside the blood-brain barrier in the area postrema. Animal studies, together with the low concentrations found in the brain, indicate a predominantly peripheral effect of domperidone on dopamine receptors.

Studies in man have shown oral domperidone to increase lower oesophageal pressure, improve antroduodenal motility and accelerate gastric emptying. There is no effect on gastric secretion.

5.2 Pharmacokinetic properties

Absorption

In fasting subjects, domperidone is rapidly absorbed after oral administration, with peak plasma concentrations at 30 to 60 minutes. The low absolute bioavailability of oral domperidone (approximately 15%) is due to an extensive first-pass metabolism in the gut wall and liver. Although domperidone's bioavailability is enhanced in normal subjects when taken after a meal, patients with gastro-intestinal complaints should take domperidone 15-30 minutes before a meal. Reduced gastric acidity impairs the absorption of domperidone. Oral bioavailability is decreased by prior concomitant administration of cimetidine and sodium bicarbonate. The time of peak absorption is slightly delayed and the AUC somewhat increased when the oral drug is taken after a meal.

Distribution

Oral domperidone does not appear to accumulate or induce its own metabolism; a peak plasma level after 90 minutes of 21 ng/ml after two weeks oral administration of 30 mg per day was almost the same as that of 18 ng/ml after the first dose. Domperidone is 91-93% bound to plasma proteins. Distribution studies with radiolabelled drug in animals have shown wide tissue distribution, but low brain concentration. Small amounts of drug cross the placenta in rats.

Metabolism

Domperidone undergoes rapid and extensive hepatic metabolism by hydroxylation and N-dealkylation. In vitro metabolism experiments with diagnostic inhibitors revealed that CYP3A4 is a major form of cytochrome P-450 involved in the N-dealkylation of domperidone, whereas CYP3A4, CYP1A2 and CYP2E1 are involved in domperidone aromatic hydroxylation.

Excretion

Urinary and faecal excretions amount to 31 and 66% of the oral dose respectively. The proportion of the drug excreted unchanged is small (10% of faecal excretion and approximately 1% of urinary excretion). The plasma half-life after a single oral dose is 7-9 hours in healthy subjects but is prolonged in patients with severe renal insufficiency.

5.3 Preclinical safety data

Electrophysiological *in vitro* and *in vivo* studies indicate an overall moderate risk of domperidone to prolong the QT interval in humans. In *in vitro* experiments on isolated cells transfected with HERG and on isolated guinea pig myocytes, ratios were about 10, based on IC50 values inhibiting currents through ion channels in comparison to the free plasma concentrations in humans after administration of the maximum daily dose of 20mg (q.i.d.). However, safety margins in *in vitro* experiments on isolated cardiac tissues in *in vivo* models (dog, guinea pig, rabbits sensitised for torsades de pointes) exceeded the free plasma concentrations in humans at maximum daily dose (20mg q.i.d.) by more than 50-fold. In the presence of inhibition of the metabolism via CYP3A4 free plasma concentrations of domperidone can rise up to 10-fold.

At a high, maternally toxic dose (more than 40 times the recommended human dose), teratogenic effects were seen in the rat. No teratogenicity was observed in mice and rabbits.

6. PHARMACEUTICAL PARTICULARS

6.1 List of excipients

Lactose monohydrate

Maize starch

Microcrystalline cellulose

Pregelatinised starch

Povidone K90

Magnesium stearate

Silicon dioxide

Polysorbate 20

Hypromellose

Propylene glycol.

6.2 Incompatibilities

Not applicable.

6.3 Shelf life

5 years.

6.4 Special precautions for storage

Do not store above 25°C.

6.5 Nature and contents of container

Blister packs consisting of aluminium foil and PVC genotherm clear glass.

Pack sizes of 30 and 100 tablets.

6.6 Instructions for use and handling

No special requirements.

7. MARKETING AUTHORISATION HOLDER

Sanofi-Synthelabo

PO Box 597

Guildford

Surrey

8. MARKETING AUTHORISATION NUMBER(S)

11723/0055

9. DATE OF FIRST AUTHORISATION/RENEWAL OF THE AUTHORISATION

16th June 2002

10. DATE OF REVISION OF THE TEXT

June 2004

Legal category: POM

Motival Tablets

(sanofi-aventis)

1. NAME OF THE MEDICINAL PRODUCT

Motival Tablets

2. QUALITATIVE AND QUANTITATIVE COMPOSITION

Fluphenazine hydrochloride BP 0.5mg

Nortriptyline hydrochloride BP 11.40mg (equivalent to 10.0mg nortriptyline base)

3. PHARMACEUTICAL FORM

Triangular biconvex tablet.

4. CLINICAL PARTICULARS

4.1 Therapeutic indications

The treatment of patients suffering from mild to moderate mixed anxiety depressive states.

4.2 Posology and method of administration

Adults

One tablet three times daily.

The course of treatment should be limited to three months. If the patient does not respond after four weeks, an alternative treatment should be given.

Children

Not indicated for the treatment of children.

Elderly

Elderly patients should be started on one tablet twice daily.

Motival tablets are for oral administration.

4.3 Contraindications

The product is contraindicated in the following cases.

Comatose states

Marked cerebral atherosclerosis

Phaeochromocytoma

Renal failure

Liver failure

Severe cardiac insufficiency

Severely depressed states

Existing blood dyscrasias

History of hypersensitivity to any of the ingredients.

4.4 Special warnings and special precautions for use

Caution should be exercised with the following:

Liver disease

Renal impairment

Cardiac arrhythmias, cardiac disease

Thyrotoxicosis

Severe respiratory disease

Epilepsy, conditions predisposing to epilepsy (e.g. alcohol withdrawal or brain damage)

Parkinson's disease

Patients who have shown hypersensitivity to other phenothiazines

Personal or family history of narrow angle glaucoma

In very hot weather

The elderly, particularly if frail or at risk of hypothermia

Hypothyroidism

Myasthenia gravis

Prostatic hypertrophy

History of urinary retention.

Patients with known or with a family history of cardiovascular disease should receive ECG screening, and monitoring and correction of electrolyte balance prior to treatment with fluphenazine.

Acute withdrawal symptoms, including nausea, vomiting, sweating and insomnia have been described after abrupt cessation of antipsychotic drugs. Recurrence of psychotic symptoms may also occur, and the emergence of involuntary movement disorders (such as akathisia, dystonia and dyskinesia) has been reported. Therefore, gradual withdrawal is advisable.

Psychotic patients on large doses of phenothiazines who are undergoing surgery should be watched carefully for hypotension. Reduced amounts of anaesthetics or central nervous system depressants may be necessary.

Fluphenazine should be used with caution in patients exposed to organophosphorus insecticides

Neuroleptic drugs elevate prolactin levels, and an increase in mammary neoplasms has been found in rodents after chronic administration. However, studies to date have not shown an association between chronic administration of these drugs and human mammary tumours.

As with any phenothiazine, the physician should be alert to the possibility of "silent pneumonias" in patients receiving long-term fluphenazine.

4.5 Interaction with other medicinal products and other forms of Interaction

The possibility should be borne in mind that phenothiazines may:

1 Increase the central nervous system depression produced by drugs such as alcohol, general anaesthetics, hypnotics, sedatives or strong analgesics.

2 Antagonise the action of adrenaline and other sympathomimetic agents and reverse the blood-pressure lowering effects of adrenergic-blocking agents such as guanethidine and clonidine.

3 Impair: the anti-parkinsonian effect of L-dopa; the effect of anti-convulsants; metabolism of tricyclic antidepressants; the control of diabetes.

4 Increase the effect of anticoagulants and antidepressants.

5 Interact with lithium.

Anticholinergic effects may be enhanced by anti-parkinsonian or other anticholinergic drugs.

Phenothiazines may enhance: the absorption of corticosteroids, digoxin, and neuromuscular blocking agents.

Fluphenazine is metabolised by P450 2D6 and is itself an inhibitor of this drug metabolising enzyme. The plasma concentrations and the effects of fluphenazine may therefore be increased and prolonged by drugs that are either the substrates or inhibitors of this P450 isoform, possibly resulting in severe hypotension, cardiac arrhythmias or CNS side effects. Examples of drugs which are substrates or inhibitors of cytochrome P450 2D6 include anti-arrhythmics, certain antidepressants including SSRIs and tricyclics, certain antipsychotics, β-blockers, protease inhibitors, opiates, cimetidine and ecstasy (MDMA). This list is not exhaustive.

Concomitant use of barbiturates with phenothiazines may result in reduced serum levels of both drugs, and an increased response if one of the drugs is withdrawn.

The effect of fluphenazine on the QT interval is likely to be potentiated by concurrent use of other drugs that also prolong the QT interval. Therefore, concurrent use of these drugs and fluphenazine is contraindicated. Examples include certain anti-arrhythmics, such as those of Class 1A (such as quinidine, disopyramide and procainamide) and Class III (such as amiodarone and sotalol), tricyclic antidepressants (such as amitriptyline); certain tetracyclic antidepressants (such as maprotiline); certain antipsychotic medications (such as phenothiazines and pimozide); certain antihistamines (such as terfenadine); lithium, quinine, pentamidine and sparfloxacin. This list is not exhaustive.

Electrolyte imbalance, particularly hypokalaemia, greatly increases the risk of QT interval prolongation. Therefore, concurrent use of drugs that cause electrolyte imbalance should be avoided.

Concurrent use of MAO inhibitors may increase sedation, constipation, dry mouth and hypotension.

Owing to their adrenolytic action, phenothiazines may reduce the pressor effect of adrenergic vasoconstrictors (i.e. ephedrine, phenylephrine).

Phenylpropanolamine has been reported to interact with phenothiazines and cause ventricular arrhythmias.

Concurrent use of phenothiazines and ACE inhibitors or angiotensin II antagonists may result in severe postural hypotension.

Concurrent use of thiazide diuretics may cause hypotension. Diuretic-induced hypokalaemia may potentiate phenothiazine-induced cardiotoxicity.

Clonidine may decrease the antipsychotic activity of phenothiazines.

Methyldopa increases the risk of extrapyramidal side effects with phenothiazines.

The hypotensive effect of calcium channel blockers is enhanced by concurrent use of antipsychotic drugs.

Phenothiazines may predispose to metrizamide-induced seizures.

Concurrent use of phenothiazines and amphetamine/anorectic agents may produce antagonistic pharmacological effects.

Concurrent use of phenothiazines and cocaine may increase the risk of acute dystonia.

There have been rare reports of acute Parkinsonism when an SSRI has been used in combination with a phenothiazine.

Phenothiazines may impair the action of anti-convulsants. Serum levels of phenytoin may be increased or decreased.

Phenothiazines inhibit glucose uptake into cells, and hence may affect the interpretation of PET studies using labelled glucose.

4.6 Pregnancy and lactation

Use in pregnancy: The safety for the use of this drug during pregnancy has not been established; therefore, the possible hazards should be weighed against the potential benefits when administering this drug to pregnant patients.

Nursing mothers: Breast feeding is not recommended during treatment with fluphenazine, owing to the possibility that fluphenazine is excreted in the breast milk.

4.7 Effects on ability to drive and use machines
The use of this drug may impair the mental and physical abilities required for driving a car or operating heavy machinery.

4.8 Undesirable effects
Acute dystonic reactions occur infrequently, as a rule within the first 24-48 hours, although delayed reactions may occur. In susceptible individuals they may occur after only small doses. These may include such dramatic manifestations as oculogyric crises and opisthotonos. They are rapidly relieved by intravenous administration of an anti-parkinsonian agent such as procyclidine.

Parkinsonian-like states may occur. These reactions may be reduced by using smaller doses more frequently, or by the concomitant use of anti-parkinsonian drugs such as benzhexol, benztropine or procyclidine. Anti-parkinsonian drugs should not be prescribed routinely, because of the possible risks of aggravating anti-cholinergic side effects or precipitating toxic confusional states, or impairing therapeutic efficacy.

With careful monitoring of the dose the number of patients requiring anti-parkinsonian drugs can be minimised.

Tardive Dyskinesia: As with all antipsychotic agents, tardive dyskinesia may appear in some patients on long term therapy or may occur after drug therapy has been discontinued. The risk seems to be greater in elderly patients on high dose therapy, especially females. The symptoms are persistent and in some patients appear to be irreversible.

The syndrome is characterised by rhythmical involuntary movements of the tongue, face, mouth or jaw (e.g. protrusion of tongue, puffing of cheeks, puckering of mouth, chewing movements). Sometimes these may be accompanied by involuntary movements of the extremities. There is no known effective treatment for tardive dyskinesia: anti-parkinsonian agents usually do not alleviate the symptoms of this syndrome. It is suggested that all antipsychotic agents be discontinued if these symptoms appear. Should it be necessary to reinstitute treatment, or increase the dosage of the agent, or switch to a different antipsychotic agent, the syndrome may be masked. It has been reported that fine vermicular movements of the tongue may be an early sign of the syndrome and if the medication is stopped at that time, the syndrome may not develop.

Other Undesirable Effects: As with other phenothiazines, drowsiness, faintness, lethargy, blurred vision, dryness of the mouth, constipation, urinary hesitancy or incontinence, mild hypotension, impairment of judgement and mental skills, and epileptiform attacks are occasionally seen.

Headache, nasal congestion, vomiting, agitation, excitement and insomnia, and hyponatraemia have also been observed during phenothiazine therapy.

Extrapyramidal reactions are unlikely to occur with this dose of fluphenazine alone, and it probable that the anticholinergic activity of nortriptyline affords protection against such effects.

Blood dyscrasias have rarely been reported with phenothiazine derivatives. Blood counts should be performed if the patient develops signs of persistent infection. Transient leucopenia and thrombocytopenia have been reported. Antinuclear antibodies and SLE have been reported very rarely.

Jaundice has rarely been reported. Transient abnormalities of liver function tests may occur in the absence of jaundice.

A transient rise in serum cholesterol has been reported rarely in patients on oral fluphenazine.

Abnormal skin pigmentation and lens opacities have sometimes been seen following long-term administration of high doses of phenothiazines.

Phenothiazines are known to cause photosensitivity reactions but this has not been reported for fluphenazine. Skin rashes, hypersensitivity and anaphylactic reactions have occasionally been reported.

Elderly patients may be more susceptible to the sedative and hypotensive effects.

The effects of phenothiazines on the heart are dose-related. ECG changes with prolongation of the QT interval and T-Wave changes have been reported commonly in patients treated with moderate to high dosage; they have been reported to precede serious arrhythmias, including ventricular tachycardia and fibrillation, which have also occurred after overdosage. Sudden, unexpected and unexplained deaths have been reported in hospitalised psychotic patients receiving phenothiazines.

Phenothiazines may impair body temperature regulation. Elderly or hypothyroid patients may be particularly susceptible to hypothermia. The hazard of hyperpyrexia may be increased by especially hot or humid weather, or by drugs such as anti-parkinsonian agents, which impair sweating.

Rare occurrences of neuroleptic malignant syndrome (NMS) have been reported in patients on neuroleptic therapy. The syndrome is characterised by hyperthermia, together with some or all of the following: muscular rigidity, autonomic instability (labile blood pressure, tachycardia, diaphoresis), akinesia, and altered consciousness, sometimes progressing to stupor or coma. Leucocytosis, elevated CPK, liver function abnormalities, and acute renal failure may also occur. Neuroleptic therapy should be discontinued immediately and vigorous symptomatic treatment implemented since the syndrome is potentially fatal.

Hormonal effects of phenothiazines include hyperprolactinaemia, which may cause galactorrhoea, gynaecomastia and oligomenorrhoea or amenorrhoea. Sexual function may be impaired, and false results may be observed with pregnancy tests. Syndrome of inappropriate anti-diuretic hormone secretion has also been observed.

Oedema has been reported with phenothiazine medication.

4.9 Overdose
Overdosage should be treated symptomatically and supportively, extrapyramidal reactionswill respond to oral or parenteral anti-parkinsonian drugs such as procyclidine or benztropine. In cases of severe hypotension, all procedures for the management of circulatory shock should be instituted, e.g.vasoconstrictors and/or intravenous fluids. However, only the vasoconstrictors metaraminol or noradrenaline should be used, as adrenalinemay further lower the blood pressure through interaction with the phenothiazine.

5. PHARMACOLOGICAL PROPERTIES

5.1 Pharmacodynamic properties
Nortriptyline hydrochloride is a tricyclic antidepressant.

Fluphenazine hydrochloride is a tranquilliser of the phenothiazine type with a piperazine side chain.

5.2 Pharmacokinetic properties
Due to the nature of the two active constituents and the large inter and intra-subject variability seen in trials, accurate and consistent pharmacokinetic data are not available. This can be illustrated by the fact that studies of nortriptyline hydrochloride have produced half-life values ranging from 16 to 38 hours. In the case of fluphenazine hydrochloride these values have been 10 to 16 hours.

5.3 Preclinical safety data
There are no preclinical data of relevance to the prescriber which are additional to that already included in other sections of the SPC.

6. PHARMACEUTICAL PARTICULARS

6.1 List of excipients
Tablet core: Lactose, dicalcium phosphate, corn starch, gelatin, magnesium stearate. Coating solutions: Shellac, castor oil, talc, polyvidone, sugar granular, chalk, erythrosine, curcumin, sucrose, titanium dioxide, sodium benzoate, beeswax, carnauba wax, polysorbate and sorbic acid.

6.2 Incompatibilities
None known.

6.3 Shelf life
24 months.

6.4 Special precautions for storage
Store below 25°C.

6.5 Nature and contents of container
Packs of 100 tablets supplied in amber glass bottles with one of the following closures:

Wadless polypropylene cap; tin plate cap with pulpboard wad and waxed aluminium facing; black phenolic cap with composition cork wad and tinfoil / melinex lining; child resistant polypropylene cap of the clik-lock type lined with expanded polyethylene with PVDC (saran) facing.

6.6 Instructions for use and handling
None stated.

7. MARKETING AUTHORISATION HOLDER
Sanofi-Synthelabo

PO Box 597

Guildford

Surrey

8. MARKETING AUTHORISATION NUMBER(S)
PL 11723/0108

9. DATE OF FIRST AUTHORISATION/RENEWAL OF THE AUTHORISATION
10 November 1995

10. DATE OF REVISION OF THE TEXT
June 2004

Legal Category: POM

Motrin Tablets 800mg

(Pharmacia Limited)

1. NAME OF THE MEDICINAL PRODUCT
Motrin® Tablets 800 mg

2. QUALITATIVE AND QUANTITATIVE COMPOSITION
Ibuprofen BP 800 mg

3. PHARMACEUTICAL FORM
Film coated tablet

4. CLINICAL PARTICULARS

4.1 Therapeutic indications
Non-steroidal, anti-inflammatory agent with analgesic and antipyretic properties. Motrin is indicated for the relief of the signs and symptoms of rheumatoid arthritis (including Still's disease), osteo-arthritis, ankylosing spondylitis and seronegative (non-rheumatoid) arthropathies. It may also be used in non-articular rheumatic conditions and soft tissue injuries; these include low back pain, capsulitis, bursitis, tenosynovitis, sprains and strains.

4.2 Posology and method of administration
Route of administration: Oral

Adults:

1200 - 1800 mg daily in three divided doses; up to 2400 mg daily may be given in severe conditions.

Children:

20 mg/kg daily in divided doses. In juvenile rheumatoid arthritis, up to 40 mg/kg daily in divided doses may be taken. In those children weighing less than 30 kg, the total dose in 24 hours should not exceed 500 mg.

If gastro-intestinal complaints occur, administer Motrin with food or milk.

Elderly patients: The elderly are at increased risk of the serious consequences of adverse reactions. If Motrin is considered necessary, the lowest dose should be used.

4.3 Contraindications
Active peptic ulceration. Motrin tablets should not be given to patients who have previously shown hypersensitivity to the drug, or to those patients in whom aspirin, Motrin or other non-steroidal anti-inflammatory drugs induce the syndrome of nasal polyps, bronchospastic reactivity or angioedema. Fatal asthmatic and anaphylactoid reactions have occurred in such patients.

4.4 Special warnings and special precautions for use
Warnings

Use with extreme caution in those patients with asthma. Fatal asthmatic and anaphylactoid reactions have been reported.

Serious gastro-intestinal toxicity such as bleeding, ulceration and perforation of the stomach, small intestine or large intestine, have been reported in patients receiving ibuprofen. Motrin should be given under close supervision to patients with a history of upper gastro-intestinal tract disease.

Treatment should be discontinued in patients reporting blurred or diminished vision, scotomata and/or changes in colour vision.

Precautions

Pre-existing asthma: about 10% of patients with asthma may have aspirin-sensitive asthma. The use of aspirin in patients with aspirin-sensitive asthma has been associated with severe bronchospasm which can be fatal. Since cross-reactivity, including bronchospasm, between aspirin and other non-steroidal anti-inflammatory drugs has been reported in such aspirin-sensitive patients, Motrin tablets should not be administered to patients with this form of aspirin-sensitivity and should be used with caution in all patients with pre-existing asthma.

Fluid retention and oedema have been reported in association with Motrin; therefore, the drug should be used with caution in patients with a history of cardiac decompensation or hypertension.

As with other non-steroidal anti-inflammatory drugs, long-term administration of ibuprofen to animals has resulted in renal papillary necrosis and other abnormal renal pathology. In humans, there have been reports of acute interstitial nephritis with haematuria, proteinuria and occasionally nephrotic syndrome.

A second form of renal toxicity has been seen in patients with prerenal conditions leading to a reduction in renal blood flow or blood volume, where the renal prostaglandins have a supportive role in the maintenance of renal perfusion. In these patients, administration of a non-steroidal anti-inflammatory drug may cause a dose dependent reduction in prostaglandin formation and may precipitate overt renal decompensation. Patients at greatest risk of this reaction are those with impaired renal function, heart failure, liver dysfunction, those taking diuretics and the elderly. Discontinuation of non-steroidal anti-inflammatory drug therapy is typically followed by recovery to the pre-treatment state.

Since ibuprofen is eliminated primarily by the kidneys, patients with significantly impaired renal function should be closely monitored and a reduction in dosage should be anticipated to avoid drug accumulation.

Those patients at high risk of developing renal dysfunction during long-term treatment should have renal function monitored periodically.

Ibuprofen, like other non-steroidal anti-inflammatory drugs, can inhibit platelet aggregation, but the effect is quantitatively less and of shorter duration than that seen with aspirin. Motrin has been shown to prolong bleeding time (but within the normal range) in normal subjects. Because this prolonged bleeding effect may be exaggerated in patients with underlying haemostatic defects, Motrin should be used with caution in persons with intrinsic coagulation defects and those on anticoagulant therapy.

Patients on Motrin should report to their physicians signs or symptoms of gastro-intestinal ulceration or bleeding, blurred vision or other eye symptoms, skin rash, weight gain or oedema.

The antipyretic and anti-inflammatory activity of ibuprofen may reduce fever and inflammation, thus diminishing their utility as diagnostic signs in detecting complications of presumed non-infectious, non-inflammatory painful conditions.

4.5 Interaction with other medicinal products and other forms of Interaction

Care should be taken in patients treated with any of the following drugs, as interactions have been reported in some patients.

Anti-hypertensives: Reduced anti-hypertensive effect.

Diuretics: Reduced diuretic effect. Diuretics can increase the risk of nephrotoxicity of NSAIDs.

Cardiac glycosides: NSAIDs may exacerbate cardiac failure, reduce GFR and increase plasma levels of cardiac glycosides.

Lithium: Decreased elimination of lithium.

Methotrexate: Decreased elimination of methotrexate.

Cyclosporin: Increased risk of nephrotoxicity.

Mifepristone: NSAIDs should not be used for 8-12 days after mifepristone administration as NSAIDs can reduce the effect of mifepristone.

Other analgesics: Avoid concomitant use of two or more NSAIDs.

Corticosteroids: Increased risk of G.I. bleeding

Anticoagulants: Enhanced anti-coagulant effect.

Quinolone antibiotics: Animal data indicate that NSAIDs can increase the risk of convulsions associated with quinolone antibiotics. Patients taking NSAIDs and quinolones may have an increased risk of developing convulsions.

4.6 Pregnancy and lactation

Administration of Motrin is not recommended during pregnancy. Reproductive studies conducted in rats and rabbits at doses somewhat less than the clinical maximum dose did not demonstrate any evidence of developmental abnormalities, however, whilst no teratogenic effects have been demonstrated in animal toxicity studies, the use of ibuprofen during pregnancy should if possible be avoided. Congenital abnormalities have been reported in association with ibuprofen administration in man, however, these are low in frequency and do not appear to follow any discernible pattern. Because of the known effects of non-steroidal anti-inflammatory drugs on the foetal cardiovascular system (closure of ductus arteriosus), use in late pregnancy should be avoided. As with other drugs known to inhibit prostaglandin synthesis, an increased incidence of dystocia and delayed parturition occurred in rats.

In the limited studies so far available, ibuprofen appears in the breastmilk in very low concentrations and is unlikely to adversely affect the breast-fed infants.

4.7 Effects on ability to drive and use machines

None stated.

4.8 Undesirable effects

A decrease in haemoglobin content of 1 gram or more has been observed in 20% of patients.

Gastrointestinal: The most commonly-observed adverse events are gastrointestinal in nature. Nausea, vomiting, diarrhoea, dyspepsia, abdominal pain, melaena, haematemesis, ulcerative stomatitis and gastrointestinal haemorrhage have been reported following administration. Less frequently, gastritis, duodenal ulcer, gastric ulcer, gastrointestinal perforation, colitis, exacerbation of inflammatory bowel disease, perforations of the colon, inflammation of the small intestine with loss of blood and protein, collagenous colitis, ulcer or stricture, complications of colonic diverticula (perforation, fistula), have been observed. Epidemiological data indicate that of the most widely-used oral, non-aspirin NSAIDs, ibuprofen presents the lowest risk of upper gastrointestinal toxicity.

Cardiovascular: Oedema has been reported in association with ibuprofen treatment.

Other adverse events reported less commonly for which causality has not necessarily been established include:

Renal: Nephrotoxicity in various forms, including interstitial nephritis, nephrotic syndrome and renal failure.

Hepatic: Abnormal liver function, hepatitis and jaundice.

Neurological & special senses: Visual disturbances, optic neuritis, headaches, paraesthesia, depression, confusion, hallucinations, tinnitus, vertigo, dizziness, malaise, fatigue and drowsiness.

Haematological: Thrombocytopenia, neutropenia, agranulocytosis, aplastic anaemia and haemolytic anaemia.

Dermatological: Photosensitivity

The following rarely occurring adverse reactions have been reported in patients taking Motrin tablets:, lupus erythematosus syndrome with aseptic meningitis. Aseptic meningitis is probably more common in patients with systemic lupus erythematosus and related connective tissue diseases.

4.9 Overdose

The treatment of overdosage: gastric lavage. No specific antidote. It is theoretically advantageous to administer alkali and induce diuresis as the drug is acidic and excreted in the urine.

5. PHARMACOLOGICAL PROPERTIES

5.1 Pharmacodynamic properties

Ibuprofen has the pharmacological action of a non-steroidal anti-inflammatory compound.

5.2 Pharmacokinetic properties

Ibuprofen is absorbed from the gastro-intestinal tract and peak plasma concentrations occur about 1-2 hours after ingestion. Ibuprofen is extensively bound to plasma proteins and has a half-life of about 2 hours. It is rapidly excreted in the urine mainly as metabolites and their conjugates. About 1% is excreted in the urine as unchanged ibuprofen and about 14% as conjugated ibuprofen.

5.3 Preclinical safety data

Reproductive studies conducted in rats and rabbits at doses somewhat less than the clinical maximum dose did not demonstrate any evidence of developmental abnormalities. As there are no adequate and well-controlled studies in pregnant women, this drug should be used during pregnancy only if clearly needed. Because of the known effect of non-steroidal anti-inflammatory drugs in the foetal cardiovascular system (closure of the ductus arteriosus), use during late pregnancy should be avoided. As with other drugs known to inhibit prostaglandin synthesis an increased incidence of dystocia and delayed parturition occurred in rats.

6. PHARMACEUTICAL PARTICULARS

6.1 List of excipients

Colloidal silicon dioxide Ph. Eur.

Croscarmellose sodium NF

Magnesium stearate Ph. Eur.

Microcrysalline cellulose Ph. Eur.

Lactose Ph. Eur.

Opadry YS-1-7000E Hse

Carnauba wax Ph. Eur.

Purified water Ph. Eur.

6.2 Incompatibilities

None known.

6.3 Shelf life

36 months

6.4 Special precautions for storage

Store below 25°C.

6.5 Nature and contents of container

High density polyethylene bottle containing 90 or 100 tablets or blister packs, blister - 250 microns, opaque, unplasticized PVC, sealed to 20-25 micron hard temper aluminium foil containing 10 or 90 tablets per pack.

6.6 Instructions for use and handling

None

7. MARKETING AUTHORISATION HOLDER

Pharmacia Limited

Davy Avenue

Milton Keynes

MK5 8PH

UK

8. MARKETING AUTHORISATION NUMBER(S)

PL 0032/0134

9. DATE OF FIRST AUTHORISATION/RENEWAL OF THE AUTHORISATION

3 July 1986/9 February 1999

10. DATE OF REVISION OF THE TEXT

April 2001

LEGAL CATEGORY

POM.

Movicol

(Norgine Limited)

1. NAME OF THE MEDICINAL PRODUCT

MOVICOL 13.8g sachet, powder for oral solution

2. QUALITATIVE AND QUANTITATIVE COMPOSITION

Each sachet of MOVICOL contains the following active ingredients:

Macrogol (Polyethylene Glycol) 3350	13.125 g
Sodium Chloride	350.7 mg
Sodium Bicarbonate	178.5 mg
Potassium Chloride	46.6 mg

The content of electrolyte ions per sachet when made up to 125 ml of solution is as follows:

Sodium	65 mmol/l
Chloride	53 mmol/l
Potassium	5.4 mmol/l
Bicarbonate	17 mmol/l

For excipients, see 6.1.

3. PHARMACEUTICAL FORM

Powder for oral solution.

Free flowing white powder.

4. CLINICAL PARTICULARS

4.1 Therapeutic indications

For the treatment of chronic constipation. MOVICOL is also effective in resolving faecal impaction, defined as refractory constipation with faecal loading of the rectum and/or colon confirmed by physical examination of the abdomen and rectum.

4.2 Posology and method of administration

Chronic Constipation

A course of treatment for constipation with MOVICOL does not normally exceed two weeks, although this can be repeated if required.

As for all laxatives, prolonged use is not usually recommended. Extended use may be necessary in the care of patients with severe chronic or resistant constipation, secondary to multiple sclerosis or Parkinson's Disease, or induced by regular constipating medication, in particular opioids and antimuscarinics.

Adults, adolescents and elderly: 1-3 sachets daily in divided doses, according to individual response.

For extended use, the dose can be adjusted down to 1 or 2 sachets daily.

Children (below 12 years old): Not recommended.

Faecal impaction

A course of treatment for faecal impaction with MOVICOL does not normally exceed 3 days.

Adults, adolescents and the elderly: 8 sachets daily, all of which should be consumed within a 6 hour period.

Children (below 12 years old): Not recommended.

Patients with impaired cardiovascular function: For the treatment of faecal impaction the dose should be divided so that no more than two sachets are taken in any one hour.

Patients with renal insufficiency: No dosage change is necessary for treatment of either constipation or faecal impaction.

Administration

Each sachet should be dissolved in 125ml water. For use in faecal impaction 8 sachets may be dissolved in 1 litre water.

4.3 Contraindications

Intestinal perforation or obstruction due to structural or functional disorder of the gut wall, ileus, severe inflammatory conditions of the intestinal tract, such as Crohn's disease and ulcerative colitis and toxic megacolon.

Known hypersensitivity to any of the active substances or to any of the excipients.

4.4 Special warnings and special precautions for use

Mild adverse drug reactions are possible as indicated in Section 4.8. If patients develop any symptoms indicating shifts of fluid/electrolytes (e.g. oedema, shortness of breath, increasing fatigue, dehydration, cardiac failure) MOVICOL should be stopped immediately and electrolytes measured, and any abnormality should be treated appropriately.

There is no clinical trial data on the use of MOVICOL in children, therefore it is not recommended.

4.5 Interaction with other medicinal products and other forms of Interaction

No clinical interactions with other medicinal products have been reported. Macrogol raises the solubility of drugs that are soluble in alcohol and relatively insoluble in water. There is therefore a theoretical possibility that the absorption of such drugs could be transiently reduced.

4.6 Pregnancy and lactation

There is no experience of the use of MOVICOL during pregnancy and lactation and it should only be used if considered essential by the physician.

4.7 Effects on ability to drive and use machines

There is no effect on the ability to drive and use machines.

4.8 Undesirable effects

Abdominal distension and pain, borborygmi and nausea, attributable to the expansion of the contents of the intestinal tract can occur. Mild diarrhoea which usually responds to dose reduction. Allergic reactions are a possibility.

4.9 Overdose

Severe pain or distension can be treated by nasogastric aspiration. Extensive fluid loss by diarrhoea or vomiting may require correction of electrolyte disturbances.

5. PHARMACOLOGICAL PROPERTIES

5.1 Pharmacodynamic properties

ATC code: A06A D

Macrogol 3350 acts by virtue of its osmotic action in the gut, which induces a laxative effect. The electrolytes also present in the formulation ensure that there is virtually no net gain or loss of sodium, potassium or water. The laxative action of macrogol 3350 has a time course which will vary according to the severity of the constipation or faecal impaction being treated.

For the indication of faecal impaction controlled comparative studies have not been performed with other treatments (e.g. enemas). In a non-comparative study in 27 adult patients, MOVICOL cleared the faecal impaction in 12/27 (44%) after 1 day's treatment; 23/27 (85%) after 2 days' treatment and 24/27 (89%) at the end of 3 days.

Clinical studies in the use of Movicol in chronic constipation have shown that the dose needed to produce normal formed stools tends to reduce over time. Many patients respond to between 1 and 2 sachets a day, but this dose should be adjusted depending on individual response.

5.2 Pharmacokinetic properties

Macrogol 3350 is unchanged along the gut. It is virtually unabsorbed from the gastro-intestinal tract and has no known pharmacological activity. Any macrogol 3350 that is absorbed is excreted via the urine.

5.3 Preclinical safety data

Preclinical studies provide evidence that macrogol 3350 has no significant systemic toxicity potential, although no tests of its effects on reproduction or genotoxicity have been conducted.

There are no long-term animal toxicity or carcinogenicity studies involving macrogol 3350, although there are toxicity studies using high levels of orally administered high molecular macrogols that provide evidence of safety at the recommended therapeutic dose.

6. PHARMACEUTICAL PARTICULARS

6.1 List of excipients

Acesulfame K (E950)

Lime and Lemon Flavour

6.2 Incompatibilities

None are known.

6.3 Shelf life

The shelf life of the sachets is 3 years.

Discard any solution not used within 6 hours.

6.4 Special precautions for storage

Sachet: Do not store above 25°C.

Solution:Store at 2-8°C (in a refrigerator and covered)

6.5 Nature and contents of container

13.8g sachets contained in boxes of 2, 6, 8, 10, 20, 30, 50, 60 or 100 sachets.

6.6 Instructions for use and handling

None.

7. MARKETING AUTHORISATION HOLDER

Norgine Limited

Chaplin House

Widewater Place

Moorhall Road

Harefield

UXBRIDGE

Middlesex UB9 6NS

United Kingdom

8. MARKETING AUTHORISATION NUMBER(S)

PL 00322/0070

9. DATE OF FIRST AUTHORISATION/RENEWAL OF THE AUTHORISATION

March 2001

10. DATE OF REVISION OF THE TEXT

August 2002

Legal Category: **P**

Movicol Paediatric Plain

(Norgine Limited)

1. NAME OF THE MEDICINAL PRODUCT

Movicol® Paediatric Plain 6.9 g sachet, powder for oral solution.

2. QUALITATIVE AND QUANTITATIVE COMPOSITION

Each sachet of Movicol Paediatric Plain contains the following active ingredients:

Macrogol 3350	6.563 g
Sodium Chloride	175.4 mg
Sodium Bicarbonate	89.3 mg
Potassium Chloride	25.1 mg

The content of electrolyte ions per sachet when made up to 62.5 ml of solution is as follows:

Sodium	65 mmol/l
Chloride	53 mmol/l
Potassium	5.4 mmol/l
Bicarbonate	17 mmol/l

3. PHARMACEUTICAL FORM

Powder for oral solution.

Free flowing white powder.

4. CLINICAL PARTICULARS

4.1 Therapeutic indications

For the treatment of chronic constipation in children 2 to 11 years of age.

For the treatment of faecal impaction in children from the age of five years, defined as refractory constipation with faecal loading of the rectum and/or colon confirmed by physical or radiological examination of the abdomen and rectum.

For the prevention of the recurrence of faecal impaction in children.

4.2 Posology and method of administration

Chronic constipation and prevention of re-impaction

The usual starting dose is 1 sachet daily for children aged 2 to 6 years, and 2 sachets daily for children aged 7 – 11 years. The dose should be adjusted up or down as required to produce regular soft stools. The maximum dose needed does not normally exceed 4 sachets a day.

Faecal impaction

A course of treatment for faecal impaction with Movicol Paediatric Plain is for up to 7 days as follows:

Daily dosage regimen:

(see Table 1 below)

The daily number of sachets should be taken in divided doses, all consumed within a 12 hour period. The above dosage regimen should be stopped once disimpaction has occurred. An indicator of disimpaction is the passage of a large volume of stools. After disimpaction it is recommended that the child follows an appropriate bowel management program to prevent reimpaction.

The dosage regimen for faecal impaction is based on one clinical trial.

Movicol Paediatric Plain is not recommended for children below five years of age for the treatment of faecal impaction, or in children below two years of age for the treatment of chronic constipation. For patients of 12 years and older it is recommended to use Movicol.

Patients with impaired cardiovascular function:

There are no clinical data for this group of patients. Therefore Movicol Paediatric Plain is not recommended for treating faecal impaction in children with impaired cardiovascular function.

Patients with renal insufficiency:

There are no clinical data for this group of patients. Therefore Movicol Paediatric Plain is not recommended for treating faecal impaction in children with impaired renal function.

Administration

Each sachet should be dissolved in 62.5 ml (quarter of a glass) of water. The correct number of sachets may be reconstituted in advance and kept covered and refrigerated for up to 24 hours. For example, for use in faecal impaction, 12 sachets can be made up into 750 ml of water.

4.3 Contraindications

Intestinal perforation or obstruction due to structural or functional disorder of the gut wall, ileus, severe inflammatory conditions of the intestinal tract, such as Crohn's disease and ulcerative colitis and toxic megacolon.

Known hypersensitivity to any of the ingredients.

4.4 Special warnings and special precautions for use

Mild adverse drug reactions are possible as indicated in Section 4.8. Rarely symptoms indicating shifts of fluid/electrolytes e.g. oedema, shortness of breath, increasing fatigue, dehydration and cardiac failure have been reported in adults when using preparations containing macrogol. If this occurs Movicol Paediatric Plain should be stopped immediately, electrolytes measured, and any abnormality should be treated appropriately.

4.5 Interaction with other medicinal products and other forms of Interaction

Medication in solid dose form taken within one hour of administration of large volumes of macrogol preparations (as used when treating faecal impaction) may be flushed from the gastrointestinal tract and not absorbed.

No clinical interactions with other medicaments have been reported. Macrogol raises the solubility of drugs that are soluble in alcohol and relatively insoluble in water. There is therefore a theoretical possibility that the absorption of such drugs could be transiently altered.

4.6 Pregnancy and lactation

There are no data on the use of Movicol Paediatric Plain during pregnancy and lactation and it should only be used if considered essential by the physician.

4.7 Effects on ability to drive and use machines

There is no effect on the ability to drive and use machines.

4.8 Undesirable effects

Abdominal distension and pain, borborygmi and nausea can occur. Diarrhoea or loose stools usually respond to reduction in dose. In children who are being treated for faecal impaction, mild vomiting is very common (approximately 20%) and this may be resolved if the subsequent dose is reduced or delayed. Other reported undesirable effects include perianal inflammation and soreness. Allergic reactions are a possibility.

4.9 Overdose

Severe abdominal pain or distension can be treated by nasogastric aspiration. Extensive fluid loss by diarrhoea or vomiting may require correction of electrolyte disturbances.

5. PHARMACOLOGICAL PROPERTIES

5.1 Pharmacodynamic properties

ATC code: A06A D

Macrogol 3350 acts by virtue of its osmotic action in the gut, which induces a laxative effect. The electrolytes also present in the formulation ensure that there is virtually no net gain or loss of sodium, potassium or water. The laxative action of macrogol 3350 has a time course, which will vary according to the severity of the faecal impaction being treated.

In an open study of Movicol (Paediatric Plain) in chronic constipation, weekly defaecation frequency was increased from 1.3 at baseline to 7.7, 7.2 and 7.1 at weeks 2, 4 and 12 respectively. In a study comparing Movicol (Paediatric Plain) and lactulose as maintenance therapy after disimpaction, weekly stool frequency at the last visit was 9.4 (SD 4.46) in the Movicol group compared with 5.9 (SD 4.29). In the lactulose group 7 children re-impacted (23%) compared with no children in the Movicol group.

For the indication of faecal impaction comparative studies have not been performed with other treatments (e.g. enemas). In a non-comparative study in 63 children, Movicol (Paediatric) cleared the faecal impaction in the majority of patients within 3 - 7 days of treatment. For the 5 -11 years age group the average total number of sachets of Movicol Paediatric required was 47.2.

5.2 Pharmacokinetic properties

Macrogol 3350 is unchanged along the gut. It is virtually unabsorbed from the gastro-intestinal tract and has no known pharmacological activity. Any macrogol 3350 that is absorbed is excreted via the urine.

5.3 Preclinical safety data

Preclinical studies provide evidence that macrogol 3350 has no significant systemic toxicity potential, although no tests of its effects on reproduction or genotoxicity have been conducted.

There are no long-term animal toxicity or carcinogenicity studies involving macrogol 3350, although there are toxicity studies using high levels of orally administered high molecular macrogols that provide evidence of safety at the recommended therapeutic dose.

6. PHARMACEUTICAL PARTICULARS

6.1 List of excipients

None

6.2 Incompatibilities

None are known.

6.3 Shelf life

The shelf life of the sachets is 3 years.

Discard any solution not used within 24 hours.

6.4 Special precautions for storage

Sachet: Do not store above 25°C.

Solution: Store at 2 - 8° C (refrigerated and covered)

6.5 Nature and contents of container

6.9g sachets contained in boxes of 6, 8, 10, 20, 30, 40, 50, 60 or 100 sachets.

6.6 Instructions for use and handling

None.

7. MARKETING AUTHORISATION HOLDER

Norgine Limited

Chaplin House

Widewater Place

Moorhall Road, Harefield

UXBRIDGE, Middlesex

UB9 6NS, United Kingdom

8. MARKETING AUTHORISATION NUMBER(S)

PL 00322/0083

9. DATE OF FIRST AUTHORISATION/RENEWAL OF THE AUTHORISATION

24 September 2003

Table 1 Daily dosage regimen

Number of MOVICOL Paediatric Plain sachets							
Age (years)	**Day 1**	**Day 2**	**Day 3**	**Day 4**	**Day 5**	**Day 6**	**Day 7**
5 - 11	**4**	**6**	**8**	**10**	**12**	**12**	**12**

10. DATE OF REVISION OF THE TEXT
Approved: 30th March 2005.

Legal Category: **POM**

MOVICOL-Half

(Norgine Limited)

1. NAME OF THE MEDICINAL PRODUCT
MOVICOL-Half 6.9g sachet, powder for oral solution

2. QUALITATIVE AND QUANTITATIVE COMPOSITION
Each sachet of MOVICOL-Half contains the following active ingredients:

Macrogol 3350	6.563g
Sodium Chloride	175.4 mg
Sodium Bicarbonate	89.3 mg
Potassium Chloride	23.3 mg

The content of electrolyte ions per sachet when made up to 62.5 ml of solution is as follows:

Sodium	65 mmol/l
Chloride	53 mmol/l
Potassium	5.4 mmol/l
Bicarbonate	17 mmol/l

For excipients, see 6.1.

3. PHARMACEUTICAL FORM
Powder for oral solution.

Free flowing white powder.

4. CLINICAL PARTICULARS
4.1 Therapeutic indications
Chronic Constipation

For the treatment of chronic constipation in adults, adolescents and the elderly.

Faecal Impaction

For resolving faecal impaction in adults, adolescents, and the elderly. Faecal impaction is defined as refractory constipation with faecal loading of the rectum and/or colon confirmed by physical or radiological examination of the abdomen and rectum.

4.2 Posology and method of administration
Chronic Constipation

A course of treatment for constipation with MOVICOL-Half does not normally exceed two weeks, although this can be repeated if required.

As for all laxatives, prolonged use is not usually recommended. Extended use may be necessary in the care of patients with severe chronic or resistant constipation, secondary to multiple sclerosis or Parkinson's Disease, or induced by regular constipating medication, in particular opioids and antimuscarinics.

Adults, adolescents and elderly

2 - 6 sachets daily in divided doses, according to individual response.

For extended use, the dose can be adjusted down to 2 - 4 sachets daily.

Faecal Impaction

Adults, adolescents and elderly

A course of treatment for faecal impaction with MOVICOL-Half does not normally exceed 3 days.

Dosage is 16 sachets daily, all of which should be consumed within a

6 hour period.

The above dosage regimen should be stopped once disimpaction has occurred. An indicator of disimpaction is the passage of a large volume of stools. After disimpaction it is recommended that the patient follow an appropriate bowel management programme to prevent reimpaction.

This dosage regimen is based on one clinical trial.

Children (below 12 years of age): Not recommended.

Patients with impaired cardiovascular function

For the treatment of faecal impaction the dose should be divided so that no more than four sachets are taken in any one hour.

Patients with renal insufficiency

No dosage change is necessary for treatment of either constipation or faecal impaction.

Administration

Each sachet should be dissolved in 62.5ml water. For use in faecal impaction the correct number of sachets can be reconstituted in advance and kept covered and refrigerated for up to 6 hours. For example 16 sachets can be made up into one litre of water.

4.3 Contraindications
Intestinal perforation or obstruction due to structural or functional disorder of the gut wall, ileus, severe inflammatory conditions of the intestinal tract, such as Crohn's disease and ulcerative colitis and toxic megacolon.

Known hypersensitivity to any of the active substances or excipients.

4.4 Special warnings and special precautions for use
Mild adverse drug reactions are possible as indicated in Section 4.8. If patients develop any symptoms indicating shifts of fluid/electrolytes (e.g. oedema, shortness of breath, increasing fatigue, dehydration, cardiac failure) MOVICOL-Half should be stopped immediately and electrolytes measured, and any abnormality should be treated appropriately.

4.5 Interaction with other medicinal products and other forms of Interaction
Medication in solid dose form taken within one hour of administration of large volumes of macrogol preparations may be flushed from the gastrointestinal tract and not absorbed.

No clinical interactions with other medicaments have been reported. Macrogol raises the solubility of drugs that are soluble in alcohol and relatively insoluble in water. There is therefore a theoretical possibility that the absorption of such drugs could be transiently altered.

4.6 Pregnancy and lactation
There is no experience of the use of MOVICOL-Half during pregnancy and lactation and it should only be used if considered essential by the physician.

4.7 Effects on ability to drive and use machines
There is no effect on the ability to drive and use machines.

4.8 Undesirable effects
Abdominal distension and pain, borborygmi and nausea and mild vomiting attributable to the expansion of the contents of the intestinal tract can occur. There may be mild diarrhoea, which usually responds to dose reduction. Allergic reactions are a possibility.

4.9 Overdose
Severe pain or distension can be treated by nasogastric aspiration. Extensive fluid loss by diarrhoea or vomiting may require correction of electrolyte disturbances.

5. PHARMACOLOGICAL PROPERTIES
5.1 Pharmacodynamic properties
ATC code: A06A D

Macrogol 3350 acts by virtue of its osmotic action in the gut, which induces a laxative effect. The electrolytes also present in the formulation ensure that there is virtually no net gain or loss of sodium, potassium or water. The laxative action of macrogol 3350 has a time course which will vary according to the severity of the constipation or faecal impaction being treated.

For the indication of faecal impaction comparative studies have not been performed with other treatments (e.g. enemas). In a non-comparative study in 27 adult patients, MOVICOL 13.8g cleared the faecal impaction in 12/27 (44%) after 1 day's treatment; 23/27 (85%) after 2 days' treatment and 24/27 (89%) at the end of 3 days.

Clinical studies in the use of MOVICOL in chronic constipation have shown that the dose needed to produce normal formed stools tends to reduce over time. Many patients respond to between 2-4 sachets of MOVICOL-Half per day, but this dose should be adjusted depending on individual response.

5.2 Pharmacokinetic properties
Macrogol 3350 is unchanged along the gut. It is virtually unabsorbed from the gastro-intestinal tract and has no known pharmacological activity. Any macrogol 3350 that is absorbed is excreted via the urine.

5.3 Preclinical safety data
Preclinical studies provide evidence that macrogol 3350 has no significant systemic toxicity potential, although no tests of its effects on reproduction or genotoxicity have been conducted.

There are no long-term animal toxicity or carcinogenicity studies involving macrogol 3350, although there are toxicity studies using high levels of orally administered high molecular macrogols that provide evidence of safety at the recommended therapeutic dose.

6. PHARMACEUTICAL PARTICULARS
6.1 List of excipients
Acesulfame K (E950)

Lime and Lemon Flavour

6.2 Incompatibilities
None are known.

6.3 Shelf life
The shelf life of the sachets is 3 years.

Discard any solution not used within 6 hours.

6.4 Special precautions for storage
Sachet: Do not store above 25°C.

Solution: Store at 2 - 8°C (refrigerated and covered)

6.5 Nature and contents of container
6.9g sachets contained in boxes of 6, 8, 10, 20, 30, 40, 50, 60 or 100 sachets.

6.6 Instructions for use and handling
None.

7. MARKETING AUTHORISATION HOLDER
Norgine Limited
Chaplin House
Widewater Place
Moorhall Road, Harefield
UXBRIDGE, Middlesex
UB9 6NS, United Kingdom

8. MARKETING AUTHORISATION NUMBER(S)
PL 00322/0080

9. DATE OF FIRST AUTHORISATION/RENEWAL OF THE AUTHORISATION
16th October 2002

10. DATE OF REVISION OF THE TEXT
16th June 2004

Legal Category: **P**

MST Continus suspensions 20, 30, 60, 100 and 200 mg

(Napp Pharmaceuticals Limited)

1. NAME OF THE MEDICINAL PRODUCT
MST® CONTINUS® suspension 20, 30, 60, 100 and 200 mg.

2. QUALITATIVE AND QUANTITATIVE COMPOSITION
Morphine equivalent to Morphine Sulphate PhEur 20, 30, 60, 100 and 200 mg.

For excipients see 6.1.

3. PHARMACEUTICAL FORM
Prolonged release granules for oral suspension.

4. CLINICAL PARTICULARS
4.1 Therapeutic indications
For the prolonged relief of severe and intractable pain.

4.2 Posology and method of administration
Route of administration

Oral.

20, 30 & 60 mg strengths: The contents of one sachet should be mixed with at least 10 ml water or sprinkled on to soft food, for example yogurt.

100 mg strength: The contents of one sachet should be mixed with at least 20 ml water or sprinkled on to soft food, for example yogurt.

200 mg strength: The contents of one sachet should be mixed with at least 30 ml water or sprinkled on to soft food, for example yogurt.

MST CONTINUS suspension should be used at 12-hourly intervals. The dosage is dependent upon the severity of the pain, the patient's age and previous history of analgesic requirements.

Adults:

A patient presenting with severe pain, uncontrolled by weaker opioids (e.g. dihydrocodeine) should normally be started on 30 mg 12-hourly. Patients previously on normal release oral morphine should be given the same total daily dose as MST CONTINUS suspension but in divided doses at 12-hourly intervals.

Increasing severity of pain will require an increased dosage of the suspension. Higher doses should be made, where possible in 30-50% increments as required. The correct dosage for any individual patient is that which is sufficient to control pain with no, or tolerable, side effects for a full 12 hours. It is recommended that the 200 mg strength is reserved for patients who have already been titrated to a stable analgesic dose using lower strengths of morphine or other opioid preparations.

Patients receiving MST CONTINUS suspension in place of parenteral morphine should be given a sufficiently increased dosage to compensate for any reduction in analgesic effects associated with oral administration. Usually such increased requirement is of the order of 100%. In such patients individual dose adjustments are required.

Children:

The use of MST CONTINUS suspension in children has not been extensively evaluated. For children with severe cancer pain, a starting dose in the range of 0.2 to 0.8 mg morphine per kg bodyweight 12-hourly is recommended. Doses should then be titrated as for adults.

Post-operative pain

MST CONTINUS suspension is not recommended in the first 24 hours post-operatively or until normal bowel function has returned; thereafter it is suggested that the following dosage schedule be observed at the physician's discretion:

(a) MST CONTINUS suspension 20 mg 12-hourly to patients under 70 kg

(b) MST CONTINUS suspension 30 mg 12-hourly to patients over 70 kg

(c) Elderly - a reduction in dosage may be advisable in the elderly

(d) Children - not recommended

Supplemental parenteral morphine may be given if required but with careful attention to the total dosages of morphine, and bearing in mind the prolonged effects of morphine in this controlled release formulation.

4.3 Contraindications

Hypersensitivity to any of the constituents. Respiratory depression, head injury, paralytic ileus, 'acute abdomen', delayed gastric emptying, obstructive airways disease, known morphine sensitivity, acute hepatic disease, concurrent administration of monoamine oxidase inhibitors or within two weeks of discontinuation of their use. Children under one year of age. Pre-operative administration of MST CONTINUS suspension is not recommended.

4.4 Special warnings and special precautions for use

As with all narcotics a reduction in dosage may be advisable in the elderly, in hypothyroidism and in patients with significantly impaired renal or hepatic function. Use with caution in opiate dependent patients and in patients with raised intracranial pressure, hypotension with hypovolaemia, diseases of the biliary tract, pancreatitis, inflammatory bowel disorders, prostatic hypertrophy and adrenocortical insufficiency.

Should paralytic ileus be suspected or occur during use, MST CONTINUS suspension should be discontinued immediately. As with all morphine preparations, patients who are to undergo cordotomy or other pain relieving surgical procedures should not receive MST CONTINUS suspension for 24 hours prior to surgery. If further treatment with MST CONTINUS suspension is then indicated, the dosage should be adjusted to the new post-operative requirement.

As with all oral morphine preparations, MST CONTINUS suspension should be used with caution post-operatively and following abdominal surgery, as morphine impairs intestinal motility and should not be used until the physician is assured of normal bowel function.

It is not possible to ensure bioequivalence between different brands of controlled release morphine products. Therefore, it should be emphasised that patients, once titrated to an effective dose, should not be changed from MST CONTINUS preparations to other slow, sustained or controlled release morphine or other potent narcotic analgesic preparations without retitration and clinical assessment.

4.5 Interaction with other medicinal products and other forms of Interaction

Morphine potentiates the effects of tranquillisers, anaesthetics, hypnotics, sedatives, alcohol, muscle relaxants and antihypertensives. Concurrent administration of antacids may result in a more rapid release of morphine than otherwise expected; dosing should therefore be separated by a minimum of two hours. Cimetidine inhibits the metabolism of morphine. Monoamine oxidase inhibitors are known to interact with narcotic analgesics producing CNS excitation or depression with hyper- or hypotensive crisis.

4.6 Pregnancy and lactation

MST CONTINUS suspension is not recommended during pregnancy and labour due to the risk of neonatal respiratory depression. Administration to nursing mothers is not recommended as morphine is excreted in breast milk. Withdrawal symptoms may be observed in the newborn of mothers undergoing chronic treatment.

4.7 Effects on ability to drive and use machines

Morphine may modify the patient's reactions to a varying extent depending on the dosage and susceptibility. If affected, patients should not drive or operate machinery.

4.8 Undesirable effects

In normal doses, the commonest side effects of morphine are nausea, vomiting, constipation and drowsiness. With chronic therapy, nausea and vomiting are unusual with MST CONTINUS suspension but should they occur the suspension can be readily combined with an anti-emetic if required. Constipation may be treated with appropriate laxatives.

Other adverse reactions include:

Cardiovascular: Palpitations and rarely, clinically relevant reductions in blood pressure and heart rate have been observed.

Central Nervous System: Headache, disorientation, vertigo, mood changes, hallucinations and myoclonus. Overdose may induce respiratory depression.

Respiratory: Bronchospasm.

Gastrointestinal: Dry mouth, biliary spasm and colic may occur in a few patients. Paralytic ileus may be associated with opioid usage.

Genitourinary: Decreased libido, ureteric spasm and micturition may be difficult.

Dermatological: Rash, morphine has histamine releasing effects which may be responsible for reactions such as urticaria and pruritus.

General: Sweating, facial flushing and miosis.

The effects of morphine have led to its abuse and dependence may develop with regular, inappropriate use. This is not a major concern in the treatment of patients with severe pain.

4.9 Overdose

Signs of morphine toxicity and overdosage are pin-point pupils, respiratory depression and hypotension. Circulatory failure and deepening coma may occur in more severe cases. Rhabdomyolysis progressing to renal failure has been reported in opioid overdosage.

Treatment of morphine overdosage

Primary attention should be given to the establishment of a patent airway and institution of assisted or controlled ventilation.

In the case of massive overdosage, administer naloxone 0.8 mg intravenously. Repeat at 2-3 minute intervals as necessary, or by an infusion of 2 mg in 500 ml of normal saline or 5% dextrose (0.004 mg/ml).

The infusion should be run at a rate related to the previous bolus doses administered and should be in accordance with the patient's response. However, because the duration of action of naloxone is relatively short, the patient must be carefully monitored until spontaneous respiration is reliably re-established. MST CONTINUS suspension will continue to release and add to the morphine load for up to 12 hours after administration and the management of morphine overdosage should be modified accordingly.

For less severe overdosage, administer naloxone 0.2 mg intravenously followed by increments of 0.1 mg every 2 minutes if required.

Naloxone should not be administered in the absence of clinically significant respiratory or circulatory depression secondary to morphine overdosage. Naloxone should be administered cautiously to persons who are known, or suspected, to be physically dependent on morphine. In such cases, an abrupt or complete reversal of opioid effects may precipitate an acute withdrawal syndrome.

Gastric contents may need to be emptied as this can be useful in removing unabsorbed drug, particularly when a prolonged release formulation has been taken.

5. PHARMACOLOGICAL PROPERTIES

5.1 Pharmacodynamic properties

Pharmacotherapeutic group: Natural opium alkaloid.

ATC Code: N02A 01

Morphine acts as an agonist at opiate receptors in the CNS, particularly mu and, to a lesser extent, kappa receptors. Mu receptors are thought to mediate supraspinal analgesia, respiratory depression and euphoria, and kappa receptors, spinal analgesia, miosis and sedation. Morphine also has a direct action on the bowel wall nerve plexuses, causing constipation.

5.2 Pharmacokinetic properties

Morphine is bound to a cationic exchange resin and drug release is effected when morphine is displaced by ions in the gastrointestinal tract. Morphine is well absorbed and adequate plasma morphine levels are achieved following the recommended dosage regimen. However, first-pass metabolism occurs in the liver. In a single-dose study in healthy volunteers, the systemic availability of morphine from MST CONTINUS suspension 30 mg was equivalent to that from an immediate release solution 30 mg (mean 91%, 95% CI 81-102%) and from MST CONTINUS tablet 30 mg (mean 101%, 95% CI 93-109%). The suspension provided a retarded plasma profile which was comparable to that of the MST CONTINUS tablet.

5.3 Preclinical safety data

There are no pre-clinical data of relevance to the prescriber which are additional to that already included in other sections of the SPC.

6. PHARMACEUTICAL PARTICULARS

6.1 List of excipients

Dowex 50WX8 100-200 mesh cationic exchange resin

Xylitol

Xanthan gum

Raspberry flavour

Ponceau 4R (E124)

6.2 Incompatibilities

None known.

6.3 Shelf life

2 years.

6.4 Special precautions for storage

Do not store above 25°C.

6.5 Nature and contents of container

Pack type: Surlyn lined, laminated aluminium foil sachets coated with polyethylene and clay coated Kraft paper.

Pack size: Boxboard cartons of 30 sachets.

6.6 Instructions for use and handling

The contents of the sachet should be added to water or sprinkled onto soft food, e.g. yogurt (see 4.2 Posology and method of administration).

Administrative Data

7. MARKETING AUTHORISATION HOLDER

Napp Pharmaceuticals Limited
Cambridge Science Park
Milton Road
Cambridge
CB4 0GW
United Kingdom

8. MARKETING AUTHORISATION NUMBER(S)

PL 16950/0030-0034

9. DATE OF FIRST AUTHORISATION/RENEWAL OF THE AUTHORISATION

14 January 1994/19 November 2001

10. DATE OF REVISION OF THE TEXT

October 2001

11. Legal Category

CD (Sch 2), POM

MST Continus tablets 5 mg, 10 mg, 15 mg, 30 mg, 60 mg, 100 mg, 200 mg

(Napp Pharmaceuticals Limited)

1. NAME OF THE MEDICINAL PRODUCT

MST® CONTINUS® tablets 5 mg, 10 mg, 15 mg, 30 mg, 60 mg, 100 mg, 200 mg.

2. QUALITATIVE AND QUANTITATIVE COMPOSITION

Tablets containing Morphine Sulphate PhEur 5 mg, 10 mg, 15 mg, 30 mg, 60 mg, 100 mg, 200 mg.

3. PHARMACEUTICAL FORM

Prolonged release, film-coated, biconvex tablets marked with the NAPP logo on one side and the strength of the preparation on the other.

MST CONTINUS tablets 5 mg are white.

MST CONTINUS tablets 10 mg are golden brown.

MST CONTINUS tablets 15 mg are green.

MST CONTINUS tablets 30 mg are purple.

MST CONTINUS tablets 60 mg are orange.

MST CONTINUS tablets 100 mg are grey.

MST CONTINUS tablets 200 mg are teal green.

4. CLINICAL PARTICULARS

4.1 Therapeutic indications

For the prolonged relief of severe and intractable pain. MST CONTINUS tablets 5 mg, 10 mg, 15 mg and 30 mg are additionally indicated for the relief of post-operative pain.

4.2 Posology and method of administration

Route of administration:

Oral.

MST CONTINUS tablets should be swallowed whole and not chewed.

MST CONTINUS tablets should be used at 12-hourly intervals. The dosage is dependent upon the severity of the pain, the patient's age and previous history of analgesic requirements.

Adults:

A patient presenting with severe pain, uncontrolled by weaker opioids (e.g. dihydrocodeine) should normally be started on 30 mg 12-hourly. Patients previously on normal release oral morphine should be given the same total daily dose as MST CONTINUS tablets but in divided doses at 12-hourly intervals.

Increasing severity of pain will require an increased dosage of the tablets. Higher doses should be made, where possible in 30-50% increments as required. The correct dosage for any individual patient is that which is sufficient to control pain with no, or tolerable, side effects for a full 12 hours. It is recommended that the 200 mg strength is reserved for patients who have already been titrated to a stable analgesic dose using lower strengths of morphine or other opioid preparations.

Patients receiving MST CONTINUS tablets in place of parenteral morphine should be given a sufficiently increased dosage to compensate for any reduction in analgesic effects associated with oral administration. Usually such increased requirement is of the order of 100%. In such patients individual dose adjustments are required.

Children:

For children with severe cancer pain, a starting dose in the range of 0.2 to 0.8 mg morphine per kg bodyweight 12-hourly is recommended. Doses should then be titrated as for adults.

Post-operative pain:

MST CONTINUS tablets are not recommended in the first 24 hours post-operatively or until normal bowel function has returned; thereafter it is suggested that the following dosage schedule be observed at the physician's discretion:

(a) MST CONTINUS tablets 20 mg 12-hourly to patients under 70 kg

(b) MST CONTINUS tablets 30 mg 12-hourly to patients over 70 kg

(c) Elderly - a reduction in dosage may be advisable in the elderly

(d) Children - not recommended.

Supplemental parenteral morphine may be given if required but with careful attention to the total dosages of morphine, and bearing in mind the prolonged effects of morphine in this prolonged release formulation.

4.3 Contraindications

Respiratory depression, head injury, paralytic ileus, 'acute abdomen', delayed gastric emptying, obstructive airways disease, known morphine sensitivity, acute hepatic disease, concurrent administration of monoamine oxidase inhibitors or within two weeks of discontinuation of their use. Children under one year of age.

Not recommended for pre-operative use or for the first 24 hours post-operatively.

4.4 Special warnings and special precautions for use

As with all narcotics a reduction in dosage may be advisable in the elderly, in hypothyroidism and in patients with significantly impaired renal or hepatic function. Use with caution in opiate dependent patients and in patients with raised intracranial pressure, hypotension with hypovolaemia, diseases of the biliary tract, pancreatitis, inflammatory bowel disorders, prostatic hypertrophy and adrenocortical insufficiency.

Should paralytic ileus be suspected or occur during use, MST CONTINUS tablets should be discontinued immediately. As with all morphine preparations, patients who are to undergo cordotomy or other pain relieving surgical procedures should not receive MST CONTINUS tablets for 24 hours prior to surgery. If further treatment with MST CONTINUS tablets is then indicated, the dosage should be adjusted to the new post-operative requirement.

As with all oral morphine preparations, MST CONTINUS tablets should be used with caution post-operatively and following abdominal surgery, as morphine impairs intestinal motility and should not be used until the physician is assured of normal bowel function.

It is not possible to ensure bioequivalence between different brands of prolonged release morphine products. Therefore, it should be emphasised that patients, once titrated to an effective dose, should not be changed from MST CONTINUS preparations to other slow, sustained or prolonged release morphine or other potent narcotic analgesic preparations without retitration and clinical assessment.

4.5 Interaction with other medicinal products and other forms of Interaction

Morphine potentiates the effects of tranquillisers, anaesthetics, hypnotics, sedatives, alcohol, muscle relaxants and antihypertensives. Cimetidine inhibits the metabolism of morphine. Monoamine oxidase inhibitors are known to interact with narcotic analgesics producing CNS excitation or depression with hyper- or hypotensive crisis.

4.6 Pregnancy and lactation

MST CONTINUS tablets are not recommended during pregnancy and labour due to the risk of neonatal respiratory depression. Administration to nursing mothers is not recommended as morphine is excreted in breast milk. Withdrawal symptoms may be observed in the newborn of mothers undergoing chronic treatment.

4.7 Effects on ability to drive and use machines

Morphine may modify the patient's reactions to a varying extent depending on the dosage and susceptibility. If affected, patients should not drive or operate machinery.

4.8 Undesirable effects

In normal doses, the commonest side effects of morphine are nausea, vomiting, constipation and drowsiness. With chronic therapy, nausea and vomiting are unusual with MST CONTINUS tablets but should they occur the tablets can be readily combined with an anti-emetic if required. Constipation may be treated with appropriate laxatives. Dry mouth, sweating, vertigo, headache, disorientation, facial flushing, mood changes, palpitations, hallucinations, bronchospasm and colic may occur in a few patients. Micturition may be difficult and there may be biliary or ureteric spasm. Overdose may produce respiratory depression. Rarely, clinically relevant reductions in blood pressure and heart rate have been observed. Morphine has histamine-releasing effects which may be responsible in part for reactions such as urticaria and pruritus.

The effects of morphine have led to its abuse and dependence may develop with regular, inappropriate use. This is not a major concern in the treatment of patients with severe pain.

4.9 Overdose

Signs of morphine toxicity and overdosage are pin-point pupils, respiratory depression and hypotension. Circulatory failure and deepening coma may occur in more severe cases.

Treatment of morphine overdosage:

Primary attention should be given to the establishment of a patent airway and institution of assisted or controlled ventilation.

In the case of massive overdosage, administer naloxone 0.8 mg intravenously. Repeat at 2-3 minute intervals as necessary, or by an infusion of 2 mg in 500 ml of normal saline or 5% dextrose (0.004 mg/ml).

The infusion should be run at a rate related to the previous bolus doses administered and should be in accordance with the patient's response. However, because the duration of action of naloxone is relatively short, the patient must be carefully monitored until spontaneous respiration is reliably re-established. MST CONTINUS tablets will continue to release and add to the morphine load for up to 12 hours after administration and the management of morphine overdosage should be modified accordingly.

For less severe overdosage, administer naloxone 0.2 mg intravenously followed by increments of 0.1 mg every 2 minutes if required.

Naloxone should not be administered in the absence of clinically significant respiratory or circulatory depression secondary to morphine overdosage. Naloxone should be administered cautiously to persons who are known, or suspected, to be physically dependent on morphine. In such cases, an abrupt or complete reversal of opioid effects may precipitate an acute withdrawal syndrome.

Gastric contents may need to be emptied as this can be useful in removing unabsorbed drug, particularly when a prolonged release formulation has been taken.

5. PHARMACOLOGICAL PROPERTIES

5.1 Pharmacodynamic properties

Morphine acts as an agonist at opiate receptors in the CNS, particularly mu and, to a lesser extent, kappa receptors. Mu receptors are thought to mediate supraspinal analgesia, respiratory depression and euphoria, and kappa receptors, spinal analgesia, miosis and sedation. Morphine also has a direct action on the bowel wall nerve plexus, causing constipation.

5.2 Pharmacokinetic properties

Morphine is well absorbed from MST CONTINUS tablets and, in general, peak plasma concentrations are achieved 1-5 hours following administration. The availability is complete when compared to an equivalent dose of immediate release oral solution. Morphine is subject to a significant first-pass effect which results in a lower bioavailability when compared to an equivalent intravenous dose.

The major metabolic transformation of morphine is glucuronidation to morphine-3-glucuronide and morphine-6-glucuronide which then undergo renal excretion. These metabolites are excreted in bile and may be subject to hydrolysis and subsequent re-absorption.

Patients are titrated to appropriate pain control using the wide range of strengths of MST CONTINUS tablets. Consequently, there is a large inter-patient variation in required dosage, the minimum dosage being 5 mg 12-hourly, and a dose of 5.6 g 12-hourly has been recorded.

5.3 Preclinical safety data

There are no pre-clinical data of relevance to the prescriber which are additional to that already included in other sections of the SPC.

6. PHARMACEUTICAL PARTICULARS

6.1 List of excipients

Tablet core:

Hydroxyethylcellulose

Purified Water

Cetostearyl Alcohol

Magnesium Stearate

Purified Talc

Lactose Anhydrous (except for 100 mg and 200 mg tablets)

Hypromellose (E464)

Macrogol

Titanium dioxide (E171)

The following tablets have the colourants listed below:

10 mg - Iron oxide (E172)

15 mg - Iron oxide (E172), brilliant blue (E133), quinoline yellow (E104), indigo carmine (E132)

30 mg - Erythrosine (E127), indigo carmine (E132), sunset yellow (E110)

60 mg - Erythrosine (E127), quinoline yellow (E104), sunset yellow (E110)

100 mg - Iron oxide (E172), indigo carmine (E132)

200 mg - Brilliant blue (E133), quinoline yellow (E104).

6.2 Incompatibilities

None stated.

6.3 Shelf life

Five years.

6.4 Special precautions for storage

Do not store above 25°C.

6.5 Nature and contents of container

Aluminium foil-backed PVdC/PVC blister packs. Pack size 60 tablets.

6.6 Instructions for use and handling

None.

Administrative Data

7. MARKETING AUTHORISATION HOLDER

Napp Pharmaceuticals Ltd
Cambridge Science Park
Milton Road
Cambridge CB4 0GW

8. MARKETING AUTHORISATION NUMBER(S)

PL 16950/0035-0041

9. DATE OF FIRST AUTHORISATION/RENEWAL OF THE AUTHORISATION

1 May 1999

10. DATE OF REVISION OF THE TEXT

June 2001

11. Legal Category

CD (Sch 2), POM

® MST, MST CONTINUS, CONTINUS, NAPP and the NAPP devices are Registered Trade Marks.

Mucodyne Capsules, Syrup and Paediatric Syrup

(sanofi-aventis)

1. NAME OF THE MEDICINAL PRODUCT

Mucodyne Capsules 375 mg

Mucodyne Syrup 250 mg/5 ml

Mucodyne Paediatric Syrup 125 mg

2. QUALITATIVE AND QUANTITATIVE COMPOSITION

Mucodyne Capsules: Carbocisteine 375 mg

Mucodyne Syrup: Carbocisteine 250 mg/5 ml.

Mucodyne Paediatric Syrup: Carbocisteine 125 mg/5 ml.

3. PHARMACEUTICAL FORM

Mucodyne Capsules: Size 1, yellow capsules printed 'Mucodyne 375' in black.

Mucodyne Syrup: A clear amber syrup smelling of rum and slightly of cinnamon.

Mucodyne Paediatric Syrup: Clear, red syrup.

4. CLINICAL PARTICULARS

4.1 Therapeutic indications

Mucodyne Capsules and Syrup

Carbocisteine is a mucolytic agent for the adjunctive therapy of respiratory tract disorders characterised by excessive, viscous mucus, including chronic obstructive airways disease.

Mucodyne Paediatric Syrup

Carbocisteine is a mucolytic agent for the adjunctive therapy of respiratory tract disorders characterised by excessive or viscous mucus.

4.2 Posology and method of administration

Mucodyne Capsules and Syrup

Adults including the elderly:

Dosage is based upon an initial daily dosage of 2250 mg carbocisteine in divided doses, reducing to 1500 mg daily in divided doses when a satisfactory response is obtained e.g. for normal syrup 15ml tds. reducing to 10ml tds.

Children:

These formulations are not recommended for children. The normal daily dosage is 20 mg/kg bodyweight in divided doses. It is recommended that this is achieved with Mucodyne Paediatric Syrup.

Mucodyne Paediatric Syrup

Children 5 - 12 years: 10 ml three times daily.

Children 2 - 5 years: 2.5 - 5 ml four times daily.

Mucodyne Capsules, Syrup and Paediatric Syrup are for oral administration.

4.3 Contraindications

Mucodyne Capsules and Syrup

Active peptic ulceration.

Mucodyne Paediatric Syrup

None

4.4 Special warnings and special precautions for use

None stated.

4.5 Interaction with other medicinal products and other forms of Interaction

None stated.

4.6 Pregnancy and lactation

Although tests in mammalian species have revealed no teratogenic effects, Mucodyne is not recommended during the first trimester of pregnancy.

Use in lactation: Effects not known.

4.7 Effects on ability to drive and use machines

None.

4.8 Undesirable effects

Mucodyne Capsules and Syrup

There have been rare reports of skin rashes or gastrointestinal bleeding occurring during treatment with Mucodyne.

Mucodyne Paediatric Syrup

None stated

4.9 Overdose

Gastric lavage may be beneficial, followed by observation. Gastrointestinal disturbance is the most likely symptom of Mucodyne overdosage.

5. PHARMACOLOGICAL PROPERTIES

5.1 Pharmacodynamic properties

Carbocisteine (5-carboxymethyl L-cysteine) has been shown in normal and bronchitic animal models to affect the nature and amount of mucus glycoprotein which is secreted by the respiratory tract. An increase in the acid:-neutral glycoprotein ratio of the mucus and a transformation of serous cells to mucus cells is known to be the initial response to irritation and will normally be followed by hypersecretion. The administration of carbocisteine to animals exposed to irritants indicates that the glycoprotein that is secreted remains normal; administration after exposure indicates that return to the normal state is accelerated. Studies in humans have demonstrated that carbocisteine reduces goblet cell hyperplasia. Carbocisteine can therefore be demonstrated to have a role in the management of disorders characterised by abnormal mucus.

5.2 Pharmacokinetic properties

Carbocisteine is rapidly absorbed from the GI tract. In an 'in-house' study, at steady state (7 days) Mucodyne capsules 375mg given as 2 capsules t.d.s. to healthy volunteers gave the following pharmacokinetic parameters:

Plasma Determinations	Mean	Range
T Max (Hr)	2.0	1.0-3.0
T½ (Hr)	1.87	1.4-2.5
K_{EL} (Hr^{-1})	0.387	0.28-0.50
$AUC_{0-7.5}$ ($mcg.Hr.ml^{-1}$)	39.26	26.0-62.4

Derived Pharmacokinetic Parameters		
*CL_S ($L.Hr^{-1}$)	20.2	-
CL_S ($ml.min^{-1}$)	331	-
V_D (L)	105.2	-
V_D($L.Kg^{-1}$)	1/75	-

*Calculated from dose for day 7 of study

5.3 Preclinical safety data

No additional data of relevance to the prescriber.

6. PHARMACEUTICAL PARTICULARS

6.1 List of excipients

Mucodyne Capsules: Magnesium stearate (E572) BP, Silica, anhydrous collodial (E551) Ph. Eur., Lactose (spray dried) BP, Sodium lauryl sulphate BP, Size 1 yellow opaque gelatin capsules.

Mucodyne Syrup: Nipagin in sodium BP, Sucrose (granulated sugar) BP, Caramel liquid (E150), Rum flavour A662, Cinnamon flavour no. 1 NA, Sodium hydroxide solution 32% w/v (E524), Hydrochloric acid (E507) BP, Deionised water.

Mucodyne Paediatric Syrup: Sucrose BP, Sodium methylhydroxybenzoate BP, Vanillin BP, Raspberry flavour, Cherry flavour, Red Ponceau 4R (E124), Sodium hydroxide solution 32% w/w (E524), Hydrochloric acid (E507) BP, Distilled water.

6.2 Incompatibilities

Mixture of Mucodyne Syrup with linctus of pholcodine causes precipitation of carbocisteine from solution.

6.3 Shelf life

36 months.

6.4 Special precautions for storage

Do not store above 25°C. Dilution of Mucodyne Syrup and Mucodyne Paediatric Syrup may be effected with unpreserved syrup BP but diluted preparations should not be kept for more than 14 days.

6.5 Nature and contents of container

Mucodyne Capsules: Grey HDPE tampertainer bottles with white LDPE cap or child resistant cap, or grey polypropylene securitainer bottles with white LDPE cap, containing 30 capsules.

Mucodyne Syrup: Clear PVC bottle with white polypropylene cap containing 300 ml (with measuring beaker).

Mucodyne Paediatric Syrup: Clear PVC bottle with white polypropylene cap containing 300 ml (with measuring beaker).

6.6 Instructions for use and handling

None stated

7. MARKETING AUTHORISATION HOLDER

Aventis Pharma Ltd
50 Kings Hill Avenue
Kings Hill
West Malling
Kent ME19 4AH
United Kingdom

8. MARKETING AUTHORISATION NUMBER(S)

MUCODYNE Capsules: PL 00012/0238

Mucodyne Syrup: PL 04425/0204

Mucodyne Paediatric Syrup: PL 04425/0205

9. DATE OF FIRST AUTHORISATION/RENEWAL OF THE AUTHORISATION

Mucodyne Capsules: June 2002

Mucodyne Syrup: 30 April 2003

Mucodyne Paediatric Syrup: 23 February 2004

10. DATE OF REVISION OF THE TEXT

Mucodyne Capsules: June 2002

Mucodyne Syrup: April 2003

Mucodyne Paediatric Syrup: 23 February 2004

Legal category: POM

Mucogel Suspension

(Forest Laboratories UK Limited)

1. NAME OF THE MEDICINAL PRODUCT

MUCOGEL SUSPENSION

2. QUALITATIVE AND QUANTITATIVE COMPOSITION

Each 5ml dose contains:

Aluminium Hydroxide Gel BP 220mg

Magnesium Hydroxide BP 195mg

3. PHARMACEUTICAL FORM

Antacid suspension for oral administration

4. CLINICAL PARTICULARS

4.1 Therapeutic indications

Antacid therapy in gastric and duodenal ulcer, gastritis, heartburn, gastric hyperacidity. Treatment of indigestion. Relief of symptoms of heartburn and dyspepsia associated with gastric reflux in hiatus hernia, reflux oesophagitis and similar conditions.

4.2 Posology and method of administration

Adults, elderly and children over 12 years of age:

10-20ml three times daily 20 minutes to one hour after meals, and at bedtime, or as required.

Children under 12 years of age:

Not recommended.

4.3 Contraindications

Should not be used in patients who are severely debilitated or suffering from kidney failure.

4.4 Special warnings and special precautions for use

None stated

4.5 Interaction with other medicinal products and other forms of Interaction

Antacids inhibit the absorption of tetracyclines and vitamins and should not be taken concomitantly.

4.6 Pregnancy and lactation

For Mucogel Suspension no clinical data on exposed pregnancies are available.

Animal studies do not indicate direct or indirect harmful effects with respect to pregnancy, embryonal/foetal development, parturition or postnatal development.

Caution should be exercised when prescribing to pregnant women.

4.7 Effects on ability to drive and use machines

None stated

4.8 Undesirable effects

Gastrointestinal side-effects are uncommon. This formulation minimises the problems of diarrhoea and constipation.

4.9 Overdose

Serious symptoms are unlikely to follow overdosage.

5. PHARMACOLOGICAL PROPERTIES

5.1 Pharmacodynamic properties

The product contains two established antacids, magnesium and aluminium hydroxides with an acid neutralising capacity in excess of 25ml of 0.1N HCl consumed, per gram of suspension.

5.2 Pharmacokinetic properties

Not applicable

5.3 Preclinical safety data

There are no preclinical data of relevance to the prescriber which are additional to that already included in other sections of the SPC.

6. PHARMACEUTICAL PARTICULARS

6.1 List of excipients

Sorbitol solution 70%

Mannitol

Hydrochloric acid

Methyl P-hydroxybenzoate

Propyl P-hydroxybenzoate

Citric acid

Simethicone emulsion 30%

Saccharin sodium

Hydrogen peroxide 35% solution

Peppermint oil

Strong sodium hypochlorite solution.

Purified Water

6.2 Incompatibilities

None stated

6.3 Shelf life

Unopened - 2 years

Opened - 28 days

6.4 Special precautions for storage

Store below 25°C. Do not freeze.

6.5 Nature and contents of container

High-density polyethylene bottle with a polypropylene closure fitted with a tamper evident ring.

Pack sizes: 100ml, 300ml and 500ml

6.6 Instructions for use and handling

None

7. MARKETING AUTHORISATION HOLDER

Forest Laboratories UK Limited
Bourne Road
Bexley
Kent DA5 1NX

8. MARKETING AUTHORISATION NUMBER(S)

PL 0108/0074

9. DATE OF FIRST AUTHORISATION/RENEWAL OF THE AUTHORISATION

6 December 1982 / 15 January 1999

10. DATE OF REVISION OF THE TEXT

February 2004

11. Legal Category

GSL

Multi-Action Actifed Chesty Coughs

(Pfizer Consumer Healthcare)

1. NAME OF THE MEDICINAL PRODUCT

Multi-Action ACTIFED Chesty Coughs

2. QUALITATIVE AND QUANTITATIVE COMPOSITION

TRIPROLIDINE HYDROCHLORIDE	1.25 mg
PSEUDOEPHEDRINE HYDROCHLORIDE	30.0 mg
GUAIFENESIN	100.0 mg

3. PHARMACEUTICAL FORM

Oral solution

4. CLINICAL PARTICULARS

4.1 Therapeutic indications

Multi-Action ACTIFED Chesty Coughs is indicated for the symptomatic relief of upper respiratory tract disorders accompanied by productive cough, which are benefited by the combination of a histamine H_1-receptor antagonist, a decongestant of the mucous membranes of the upper respiratory tract, especially the nasal mucosa and sinuses, and an expectorant.

4.2 Posology and method of administration

Adults and children over 12 years:

Oral. 10 ml every 4-6 hours up to 4 times a day

Children

6 -12 Years

Oral. 5 ml every 4-6 hours up to 4 times a day

2 -5 Years

Oral. 2.5 ml every 4-6 hours up to 4 times a day

Multi-Action ACTIFED Chesty Coughs may be diluted 1:1 (1 in 2) or 1:3 (1 in 4) with unpreserved syrup BP. These dilutions have a shelf life of 4 weeks if stored at 25C.

Use in the Elderly

No specific studies have been carried out in the elderly. Experience has indicated that normal adult dosage is appropriate.

Hepatic Dysfunction

Caution should be exercised when administering Multi-Action ACTIFED Chesty Coughs to patients with severe hepatic impairment.

Renal Dysfunction

Caution should be exercised when administering Multi-Action ACTIFED Chesty Coughs to patients with moderate to severe renal impairment.

4.3 Contraindications

Multi-Action ACTIFED Chesty Coughs is contraindicated in individuals with known hypersensitivity to the product, any of its components, or acrivastine.

Multi-Action ACTIFED Chesty Coughs is contraindicated in individuals with severe hypertension or severe coronary artery disease.

Multi-Action ACTIFED Chesty Coughs is contraindicated in individuals who are taking, or have taken, monoamine oxidase inhibitors within the preceding two weeks. The concomitant use of pseudoephedrine and this type of product may occasionally cause a rise in blood pressure.

4.4 Special warnings and special precautions for use

Although pseudoephedrine has virtually no pressor effects in normotensive patients, Multi-Action ACTIFED Chesty Coughs should be used with caution in individuals suffering mild to moderate hypertension.

As with other sympathomimetic agents, Multi-Action ACTIFED Chesty Coughs should be used with caution in individuals with heart disease, hyperthyroidism, diabetes, elevated intra-ocular pressure or prostatic enlargement.

Multi-Action ACTIFED Chesty Coughs should not be used for persistent or chronic cough, such as occurs with asthma, or where cough is accompanied by excessive secretions, unless directed by a physician.

Multi-Action ACTIFED Chesty Coughs may cause drowsiness and impair performance in tests of auditory vigilance. There is individual variation in response to antihistamines.

Caution should be exercised when using the product in the presence of severe hepatic impairment or moderate to severe renal impairment (particularly if accompanied by cardiovascular disease).

4.5 Interaction with other medicinal products and other forms of Interaction

Although there are no objective data, users of Multi-Action ACTIFED Chesty Coughs should avoid concomitant use of alcohol or other centrally acting sedatives.

Concomitant use of Multi-Action ACTIFED Chesty Coughs with tricyclic antidepressants, sympathomimetic agents (such as decongestants, appetite suppressants and amfetamine-like psychostiumulants) or with monoamine oxidase inhibitors, which interfere with the catabolism of sympathomimetic amines, may occasionally cause a rise in blood pressure.

Because of its pseudoephedrine content, Multi-Action ACTIFED Chesty Coughs may partially reverse the hypotensive action of drugs which interfere with sympathetic activity including bretylium, bethanidine, guanethidine, debrisoquine, methyldopa, alpha-and beta-adrenergic blocking agents.

If urine is collected within 24 hours of a dose of Multi-Action ACTIFED Chesty Coughs, a metabolite of guaifenesin may cause a colour interference with laboratory determinations of urinary 5-hydroxyindoleacetic acid

(5-HIAA) and vanillylmandelic acid (VMA).

4.6 Pregnancy and lactation

Insufficient information is available on the effects of administration of Multi-Action ACTIFED Chesty Coughs during human pregnancy. Like most medicines, it should not be used during pregnancy unless the potential benefit of treatment to the mother outweighs any possible risk to the developing foetus.

Pseudoephedrine and triprolidine are excreted in breast milk in small amounts but the effect of this on breast-fed infants is not known. It has been estimated that, following the ingestion of a single dose of Multi-Action ACTIFED Tablets/Syrup (2.5 mg triprolidine + 60 mg pseudoephedrine) by a nursing mother, approximately 0.4 to 0.7% of pseudoephedrine and 0.06% to 0.2% triprolidine in the dose will be excreted in the breast milk over 24 hours.

Guaifenesin is excreted in breast milk in small amounts with no effect expected on the infant.

4.7 Effects on ability to drive and use machines

It is recommended that patients are advised not to engage in activities requiring mental alertness, such as driving a car or operating machinery, until they have established their own response to the drug this medicine.

4.8 Undesirable effects

PSEUDOEPHEDRINE - serious adverse effects associated with the use of pseudoephedrine are extremely rare. Symptoms of central nervous system excitation may occur including sleep disturbance and, rarely, hallucinations. Skin rashes with or without irritation and tachycardia have occasionally been reported with pseudoephedrine. Urinary retention has been reported in men receiving pseudoephedrine; prostatic enlargement could have been a predisposing factor

TRIPROLIDINE - triprolidine may cause drowsiness. Skin rashes, with or without irritation have occasionally been reported. Dryness of the mouth, nose and throat may occur.

GUAIFENESIN - side effects resulting from guaifenesin administration are very rare.

4.9 Overdose

Signs and symptoms - the effects of acute toxicity from Multi-Action ACTIFED Chesty Coughs may include drowsiness, irritability, restlessness, lethargy, dizziness, gastro-intestinal discomfort, nausea, vomiting, difficulty with micturition, dryness of the skin and mucous membranes, ataxia, weakness, hypotonicity, respiratory depression, hyperpyrexia, hyperactivity, convulsions, tremor, tachycardia, palpitations, hypertension.

Treatment

Necessary measures should be taken to maintain and support respiration and control convulsions. Gastric lavage may be undertaken if indicated. Catheterisation of the bladder may be necessary. Acid diuresis can accelerate the elimination of pseudoephedrine, although the potential therapeutic gain of this procedure is now in dispute. The value of dialysis in overdose is not known, although four hours of haemodialysis removed approximately 20% of the total body load of pseudoephedrine in a combination product containing 60mg pseudoephedrine and 8mg acrivastine.

5. PHARMACOLOGICAL PROPERTIES

5.1 Pharmacodynamic properties

PSEUDOEPHEDRINE - pseudoephedrine has direct and indirect sympathomimetic activity and is an effective upper respiratory decongestant. Pseudoephedrine is less potent than ephedrine in producing both tachycardia and elevation of systolic blood pressure and is also less potent in causing stimulation of the central nervous system. Pseudoephedrine produces its decongestant effect within 30 minutes, persisting for at least 4 hours.

TRIPROLIDINE - triprolidine is a potent, competitive H_1-receptor antagonist. Being an alkylamine the drug possesses minimal anticholinergic activity. Triprolidine provides symptomatic relief in conditions believed to depend wholly, or partly, upon the triggered release of histamine. After oral administration of a single dose of 2.5 mg triprolidine to adults, the onset of action, as determined by the ability to antagonise histamine-induced wheals and flares in the skin, was within 1 to 2 hours. Peak effects occurred after 3 hours, and although activity declines thereafter, significant inhibition of histamine-induced wheals and flares still occurred 8 hours after a single dose.

GUAIFENESIN - guaifenesin is though to exert its pharmacological action by stimulating receptors in the gastric mucosa. This increases the output from secretory glands of the gastrointestinal system and reflexly increases the flow of fluids from glands lining the respiratory tract. The result is an increase in volume and decrease in viscosity of bronchial secretions. Other actions may include stimulating vagal nerve endings in bronchial secretory glands and stimulating certain centres in the brain which in turn enhance respiratory fluid flow. Guaifenesin produces its expectorant action within 24 hours.

5.2 Pharmacokinetic properties

ABSORPTION

Pseudoephedrine and triprolidine are well absorbed from the gut follwing oral administration. After the administration of one Multi-Action ACTIFED Tablet or 10 ml Multi-Action ACTIFED Syrup (each containing 2.5 mg triprolidine and 60 mg pseudoephedrine) to healthy adult volunteers, the following pharmacokinetic values were found;

PSEUDOEPHEDRINE - the C_{max} of pseudoephedrine was approximately 180 ng/ml for both the tablet and syrup with t_{max} occurring at approximately 2.0 hours for the tablet and 1.5 hours for the syrup after drug administration.

TRIPROLIDINE - the peak plasma concentration (C_{max}) of triprolidine was approximately 5.5 ng/ml-6.0 ng/ml, occurring at about 2.0 hours (t_{max}) for the tablet and 1.5 hours for the syrup after drug administration.

GUAIFENESIN - guaifenesin is well absorbed from the gastro-intestinal tract following oral administration, although limited information is available on its pharmacokinetics. After the administration of 600 mg guaifenesin to healthy volunteers, the C_{max} was approximately 1.4 μg/ml, with t_{max} occurring approximately 15 minutes after drug administration.

DISTRIBUTION

The apparent volume of distribution of pseudoephedrine (Vd/F) was approximately 2.8 l/kg. The apparent volume of distribution of triprolidine was approximately 6.5 l/kg for the tablet formulation and 7.5 l/kg for the syrup. No information is available on the distribution of guaifenesin in humans.

METABOLISM AND ELIMINATION

PSEUDOEPHEDRINE - the $t_{½}$ was approximately 5.5 hours. Pseudoephedrine is partly metabolised in the liver by N-demethylation to norpseudoephedrine, an active metabolite. Pseudoephedrine and its metabolite are excreted in the urine; 55% to 90% of a dose is excreted unchanged. The apparent total body clearance of pseudoephedrine (C1/F) was approximately 7.5 ml/min/kg. The elimination rate constant (K_{el}) was approximately 0.13 h^{-1}. The rate of urinary elimination is accelerated when the urine is acidified. Conversely, as the urine pH increases, the rate of urinary elimination is slowed.

TRIPROLIDINE - the plasma half-life ($t_{½}$) of triprolidine was approximately 3.2 hours. Animal hepatic microsomal enzyme studies have revealed the presence of several triprolidine metabolites with an oxidised product of the toluene methyl group predominating. In man, it has been reported that only about 1% of an administered dose is eliminated as unchanged triprolidine over a 24-hour period. The apparent total body clearance of triprolidine (Cl/F) was approximately 30-37 ml/min/kg. The elimination rate constant (K_{el}) was approximately 0.26 h^{-1}.

GUAIFENESIN - guaifenesin appears to undergo both oxidation and demethylation. Following an oral dose of 600 mg guaifenesin to 3 healthy male volunteers, the $t_{½}$ was approximately 1 hour and the drug was not detectable in the blood after approximately 8 hours.

PHARMACOKINETICS IN RENAL IMPAIRMENT

Following the administration of a single dose of DUACT CAPSULES (8mg acrivastine + 60 mg pseudoephedrine) to patients with varying degrees of renal impairment, the C_{max} for pseudoephedrine increased approximately 1.5 fold in patients with moderate to severe renal impairment when compared to the C_{max} in healthy volunteers. The t_{max} was not affected by renal impairment. The $t_{½}$ increased 3 to 12 fold in patients with mild to severe renal impairment respectively, when compared to the $t_{½}$ in healthy volunteers.

There have been no specific studies of Multi-Action ACTIFED Chesty Coughs, triprolidine or guaifenesin in renally impaired patients.

PHARMACOKINETICS IN HEPATIC IMPAIRMENT

There have been no specific studies of Multi-Action ACTIFED Chesty Coughs, triprolidine, pseudoephedrine or guaifenesin in hepatic impairment.

PHARMACOKINETICS IN THE ELDERLY

In elderly volunteers, following the administration of DUACT Capsules (8 mg acrivastine + 60 mg pseudoephedrine), the $t_{½}$ for pseudoephedrine was 1.4 fold that seen in healthy volunteers. The apparent Cl/F was 0.8 fold that seen in healthy volunteers, and the Vd/F was essentially unchanged. There have been no specific studies of Multi-Action ACTIFED Chesty Coughs, triprolidine or guaifenesin in the elderly.

5.3 Preclinical safety data

There is insufficient information available to determine whether some of the active ingredients have mutagenic, carcinogenic, teratogenic potential, or the potential to impair fertility.

6. PHARMACEUTICAL PARTICULARS

6.1 List of excipients

Sorbitol solution

Sucrose

Sodium benzoate

Methyl hydroxybenzoate

F D and C yellow No 6 (E 110)

Ethanol (96 per cent)

Flavoured compound FC 900853

Menthol

Purified water

6.2 Incompatibilities

None known

6.3 Shelf life

36 months

6.4 Special precautions for storage

Do not store above 25°C. Do not refrigerate. Store in the original container to protect from light.

6.5 Nature and contents of container

30ml, 40ml, 50ml, 100ml, 200ml or 1000ml amber glass bottles fitted with a metal roll on closure or polypropylene screw cap with Saran or Steran faced wad or polyethylene/expanded polyethylene laminated wad.

OR

Amber glass bottles with a 3 piece plastic child resistant, tamper evident closure fitted with a polyvinylidene chloride (PVDC) wad or polyethylene/expanded polyethylene laminated wad.

A spoon with a 5ml and a 2.5ml measure is supplied with the 30ml, 40ml, 50ml, 100ml and 200ml bottles.

6.6 Instructions for use and handling

None applicable.

7. MARKETING AUTHORISATION HOLDER

Pfizer Consumer Healthcare

Alternative Trading Style

Warner Lambert Consumer Healthcare

Dorking Road

Walton Oaks

Walton-on-the-Hill

Surrey KT20 7NS

United Kingdom

8. MARKETING AUTHORISATION NUMBER(S)

15513/0011

9. DATE OF FIRST AUTHORISATION/RENEWAL OF THE AUTHORISATION
29 October 1998

10. DATE OF REVISION OF THE TEXT
February 2004

Multi-Action Actifed Dry Coughs

(Pfizer Consumer Healthcare)

1. NAME OF THE MEDICINAL PRODUCT
Multi-Action ACTIFED Dry Coughs

2. QUALITATIVE AND QUANTITATIVE COMPOSITION
Multi-Action ACTIFED Dry Coughs contains 1.25 mg triprolidine hydrochloride, 30 mg pseudoephedrine hydrochloride and 10 mg dextromethorphan hydrobromide in each 5 ml.

3. PHARMACEUTICAL FORM
Liquid

4. CLINICAL PARTICULARS

4.1 Therapeutic indications
Multi-Action ACTIFED Dry Coughs is indicated for the symptomatic relief of upper respiratory tract disorders which are benefited by the combination of a nasal decongestant, a histamine H_1-receptor antagonist, and an antitussive.

4.2 Posology and method of administration
Adults and children over 12 years old:

Oral. 10 ml every 4 -6 hours up to four times a day

Children aged 6 to 12 years:

Oral. 5 ml every 4 -6 hours up to four times a day

Children aged 2 years to 5 years:

Oral. 2.5 ml every 4 - 6 hours up to four times a day

Children under 2 years old:

Not recommended.

Multi-Action ACTIFED Dry Coughs may be diluted 1:1 (1 in 2) or 1:3 (1 in 4) with unpreserved Syrup BP. These dilutions have a shelf life of 4 weeks if stored at 25°C.

The Elderly:

There have been no specific studies of Multi-Action ACTIFED Dry Coughs in the elderly. Experience has indicated that normal adult dosage is appropriate.

Hepatic dysfunction:

Caution should be exercised when administering Multi-Action ACTIFED Dry Coughs to patients with severe hepatic impairment.

Renal dysfunction:

Caution should be exercised when administering Multi-Action ACTIFED Dry Coughs to patients with moderate to severe renal impairment.

4.3 Contraindications
Multi-Action ACTIFED Dry Coughs is contraindicated in individuals who have previously exhibited intolerance to it or to any of its constituents.

Multi-Action ACTIFED Dry Coughs is contraindicated in patients with severe hypertension or severe coronary artery disease.

Multi-Action ACTIFED Dry Coughs is contraindicated in individuals who are taking, or have taken, monoamine oxidase inhibitors within the preceding two weeks. The concomitant use of pseudoephedrine and this type of product may occasionally cause a rise in blood pressure.

The antibacterial agent, furazolidone, is known to cause a dose-related inhibition of monoamine oxidase. Although there are no reports of hypertensive crises caused by the concurrent administration of Multi-Action ACTIFED Dry Coughs and furazolidone they should not be taken together.

Multi-Action ACTIFED Dry Coughs should not be administered to patients where cough is associated with asthma or where cough is accompanied by excessive secretions.

Dextromethorphan, in common with other centrally acting antitussive agents, should not be given to patients in, or at risk of developing respiratory failure.

4.4 Special warnings and special precautions for use
Multi-Action ACTIFED Dry Coughs may cause drowsiness, and impair performance in tests of auditory vigilance. Patients should not drive or operate machinery until they have determined their own response.

Although there are no objective data, users of Multi-Action ACTIFED Dry Coughs should avoid the concomitant use of alcohol or other centrally acting sedatives.

Although pseudoephedrine has virtually no pressor effects in patients with normal blood pressure, Multi-Action ACTIFED Dry Coughs should be used with caution in patients taking antihypertensive agents, tricyclic antidepressants, other sympathomimetic agents such as decongestants, appetite suppressants and amfetamine-like psychostimulants. The effects of a single dose of Multi-Action ACTIFED Dry Coughs on the blood pressure of these patients should be observed before recommending repeated or unsupervised treatment.

As with other sympathomimetic agents, caution should be exercised in patients with hypertension, heart disease, diabetes, hyperthyroidism, elevated intra-ocular pressure or prostatic enlargement.

There have been no specific studies of Multi-Action ACTIFED Dry Coughs in patients with hepatic and/or renal dysfunction Multi-Action ACTIFED Dry Coughs should be used with caution in patients with liver disease.

There have been a few reports of abuse of dextromethorphan but there is no evidence of drug dependence at therapeutic dosages.

The packs carry the following statements

Warning: May cause drowsiness. If affected do not drive or operate machinery. Avoid alcoholic drink.

If you are pregnant or currently taking any other medicine, consult your doctor or pharmacist before taking this product.

If symptoms persist consult your doctor.

4.5 Interaction with other medicinal products and other forms of Interaction
Concomitant use of Multi-Action ACTIFED Dry Coughs with sympathomimetic agents such as decongestants, tricyclic antidepressants, appetite suppressants and amphetamine-like psychostimulants or with monoamine oxidase inhibitors, which interfere with the catabolism of sympathomimetic amines, may occasionally cause a rise in blood pressure, [See Contraindications and Special warnings and precautions for use].

Because of its pseudoephedrine content, Multi-Action ACTIFED Dry Coughs may partially reverse the hypotensive action of drugs which interfere with sympathetic activity including bretylium, betanidine, guanethidine, debrisoquine, methyldopa, alpha- and beta- adrenergic blocking agents, [See Special warnings and precautions for use].

4.6 Pregnancy and lactation
Although pseudoephedrine, triprolidine and dextromethorphan have been in widespread use for many years without apparent ill consequence, there are no specific data on their use during pregnancy. Caution should therefore be exercised by balancing the potential benefit of treatment to the mother against any possible hazards to the developing foetus.

Pseudoephedrine and triprolidine are excreted in breast milk in small amounts but the effect of this on breast-fed infants is not known. It has been estimated that 0.5 to 0.7% of a single dose of pseudoephedrine ingested by a mother will be excreted in the breast milk over 24 hours.

It is not known whether dextromethorphan or its metabolites are excreted in breast milk.

No studies have been conducted in animals to determine whether triprolidine, pseudoephedrine or dextromethorphan have potential to impair fertility. There is no experience of the effect of Multi-Action ACTIFED Dry Coughs on human fertility.

In rats and rabbits, systemic administration of triprolidine up to 75 times the human daily dosage did not produce teratogenic effects.

Systemic administration of pseudoephedrine, up to 50 times the human daily dosage in rats and up to 35 times the human daily dosage in rabbits, did not produce teratogenic effects.

There is insufficient information available to determine whether dextromethorphan has teratogenic potential.

4.7 Effects on ability to drive and use machines
Triprolidine may cause drowsiness and patients should not drive or operate machinery until they have determined their own response.

4.8 Undesirable effects
Central nervous system depression or excitation may occur, drowsiness being reported most frequently. Sleep disturbance and rarely, hallucinations have been reported.

Skin rashes, with or without irritation, tachycardia, dryness of mouth nose and throat have occasionally been reported. Urinary retention has been reported occasionally in male patients in whom prostatic enlargement could be an important predisposing factor.

Side effects attributed to dextromethorphan are uncommon; occasionally nausea, vomiting or gastro-intestinal disturbance may occur.

4.9 Overdose
The signs of acute toxicity from Multi-Action ACTIFED Dry Coughs may include drowsiness, lethargy, dizziness, ataxia, weakness, hypotonicity, respiratory depression, dryness of the skin and mucous membranes, tachycardia, hypertension, hyperpyrexia, hyperactivity, irritability, convulsions, difficulty with micturition, nausea and vomiting.

Necessary measures should be taken to maintain and support respiration and control convulsions. Gastric lavage may be undertaken if indicated. Catheterisation of the bladder may be necessary. If desired, the elimination of pseudoephedrine can be accelerated by acid diuresis or by dialysis.

Naloxone has been used successfully as a specific antagonist to dextromethorphan toxicity in children.

5. PHARMACOLOGICAL PROPERTIES

5.1 Pharmacodynamic properties
Triprolidine provides symptomatic relief in conditions believed to depend wholly or partially upon the triggered release of histamine. It is a potent competitive histamine H_1-receptor antagonist of the pyrrolidine class with mild central nervous system depressant properties which may cause drowsiness. Pseudoephedrine has a direct and indirect sympathomimetic activity and is an effective upper respiratory decongestant. Pseudoephedrine is substantially less potent than ephedrine in producing both tachycardia and elevation of systolic blood pressure and considerably less potent in causing stimulation of the central nervous system. Dextromethorphan has an antitussive action. It controls coughs by depressing the medullary cough centre.

After oral administration of a single dose of 2.5 mg triprolidine to adults, the onset of action as determined by the ability to antagonise histamine-induced weals and flares in the skin is within 1 to 2 hours. Peak effects occur at about 3 hours and, although activity declines thereafter, significant inhibition of histamine-induced weals and flares still occurs 8 hours after the dose. Pseudoephedrine produces its decongestant effect within 30 minutes, persisting for at least 4 hours.

A single oral dose of 10 - 20 mg dextromethorphan produces its antitussive action within 1 hour and lasts for at least 4 hours.

5.2 Pharmacokinetic properties
After the administration of 2.5 mg triprolidine hydrochloride and 60 mg pseudoephedrine hydrochloride to healthy adult volunteers, the peak plasma concentration (C_{max}) of triprolidine is approximately 5.5 ng/ml - 6.0 ng/ml occurring at about 1.5 - 2.0 hours (T_{max}) after drug administration. Its plasma half-life is approximately 3.2 hours. The C_{max} of pseudoephedrine is approximately 180 ng/ml with T_{max} approximately 1.5 - 2.0 hours after drug administration. The plasma half-life is approximately 5.5 hours (urine pH maintained between 5.0 - 7.0). The plasma half-life of pseudoephedrine is markedly decreased by acidification of urine and increased by alkalinisation. Genetically controlled O-demethylation is the main determinant of dextromethorphan pharmacokinetics in human volunteers. It appears that there are two distinct phenotypes for this oxidation process resulting in highly variable pharmacokinetics between subjects.

5.3 Preclinical safety data
The active ingredients of Multi-Action ACTIFED Dry Coughs are well-known constituents of medicinal products and their safety profiles are well documented. The results of pre-clinical studies do not add anything of relevance for therapeutic purposes.

6. PHARMACEUTICAL PARTICULARS

6.1 List of excipients
Sorbitol solution (70 %)

Sucrose

Sodium benzoate

Methyl hydroxybenzoate

Ponceau 4R

Ethanol (96%)

Blackberry 72.385E

Levomenthol

Vanillin

Purified water

6.2 Incompatibilities
None known

6.3 Shelf life
36 months

6.4 Special precautions for storage
Do not store above 25°C. Store in the original container to protect from light.

6.5 Nature and contents of container
30 ml, 40 ml, 50 ml, 100 ml or 200 ml amber glass bottles with metal roll on closures or plastic screw caps with Saran or Steran faced wads or polyethylene/expanded polyethylene laminated wads.

30 ml, 40 ml, 50 ml, 100 ml or 200 ml amber glass bottles with a 3 piece plastic child resistant, tamper evident closure fitted with a polyvinylidene chloride (PVDC) faced wad or polyethylene/expanded polyethylene laminated wad.

A spoon with a 5ml and 2.5ml measure is supplied with this product.

6.6 Instructions for use and handling
None applicable.

Administrative Data

7. MARKETING AUTHORISATION HOLDER
Pfizer Consumer Healthcare

Alternative Trading Style

Warner Lambert Consumer Healthcare

Walton Oaks

Dorking Road

Walton-on-the-Hill

Surrey KT20 7NS

United Kingdom

8. MARKETING AUTHORISATION NUMBER(S)

PL 15513/0010

9. DATE OF FIRST AUTHORISATION/RENEWAL OF THE AUTHORISATION

28 October 1998

10. DATE OF REVISION OF THE TEXT

February 2004

Multi-Action Actifed Syrup

(Pfizer Consumer Healthcare)

1. NAME OF THE MEDICINAL PRODUCT

Multi-Action ACTIFED Syrup

2. QUALITATIVE AND QUANTITATIVE COMPOSITION

TRIPROLIDINE HYDROCHLORIDE	1.25mg
PSEUDOEPHEDRINE HYDROCHLORIDE	30 mg

3. PHARMACEUTICAL FORM

Oral solution

4. CLINICAL PARTICULARS

4.1 Therapeutic indications

Multi-Action ACTIFED Syrup is for the symptomatic relief of upper respiratory tract disorders which are benefited by a combination of a nasal decongestant and histamine H_1-receptor antagonist, for example:

Allergic Rhinitis

Vasomotor Rhinitis

The Common Cold and Influenza.

4.2 Posology and method of administration

Route of administration: oral

Adults and children over 12 years

10 ml every 4-6 hours up to 4 times a day

Children

6 -12 Years

5 ml every 4-6 hours up to 4 times a day

2 -5 Years

2.5 ml every 4-6 hours up to 4 times a day

Multi-Action ACTIFED Syrup may be diluted 1:1 (1 in 2) or 1:3 (1 in 4) with syrup BP. These dilutions have a shelf life of 4 weeks if stored at 25°C.

Use in the Elderly

No specific studies have been carried out in the elderly, but triprolidine and pseudoephedrine have been widely used in older people.

Hepatic Dysfunction

Caution should be exercised when administering Multi-Action ACTIFED Syrup to patients with severe hepatic impairment.

Renal Dysfunction

Caution should be exercised when administering Multi-Action ACTIFED Syrup to patients with moderate to severe renal impairment.

4.3 Contraindications

Multi-Action ACTIFED Syrup is contraindicated in individuals who have previously exhibited intolerance to it or to pseudoephedrine or triprolidine.

Multi-Action ACTIFED Syrup is contra-indicated in patients who are taking or have taken monoamine oxidase inhibitors within the preceding two weeks. The concomitant use of pseudoephedrine and this type of product may occasionally cause a rise in blood pressure.

Multi-Action ACTIFED Syrup is contra-indicated in patients with severe hypertension or severe coronary artery disease.

The antibacterial agent furazolidone is known to cause a dose-related inhibition of monoamine oxidase. Although there are no reports of hypertensive crises caused by the concurrent administration of Multi-Action ACTIFED Syrup and furazolidone they should not be taken together.

4.4 Special warnings and special precautions for use

Multi-Action ACTIFED Syrup may cause drowsiness and impair performance in tests of auditory vigilance. Patients should not drive or operate machinery until they have determined their own response.

Although there are no objective data, users of Multi-Action ACTIFED Syrup should avoid the concomitant use of alcohol or other centrally acting sedatives.

Although pseudoephedrine has virtually no pressor effect in normotensive patients, Multi-Action ACTIFED Syrup should be used with caution in patients taking anti-hypertensive agents, tricyclic antidepressants or other sympathomimetic agents, such as decongestants, appetite suppressants and amfetamine-like psychostimulants. The effects of a single dose of Multi-Action ACTIFED Syrup on the blood pressure of these patients should be observed before recommending repeated or unsupervised treatment.

As with other sympathomimetic agents Multi-Action ACTIFED Syrup should be used with caution in patients with hypertension, heart disease, diabetes, hyperthyroidism, elevated intraocular pressure and prostatic enlargement.

There have been no specific studies of Multi-Action ACTIFED Syrup in patients with hepatic and/or renal dysfunction. Caution should be exercised in the presence of severe renal or hepatic impairment.

There is insufficient information available to determine whether triprolidine or pseudoephedrine have mutagenic or carcinogenic potential.

4.5 Interaction with other medicinal products and other forms of Interaction

Concomitant use of Multi-Action ACTIFED Syrup with other sympathomimetic agents, such as decongestants, tricyclic antidepressants, appetite suppressants and amfetamine-like psychostimulants, or with monoamine oxidase inhibitors which interfere with the catabolism of sympathomimetic amines, may occasionally cause a rise in blood pressure.

Because of its pseudoephedrine content, Multi-Action ACTIFED Syrup may partially reverse the hypotensive action of drugs which interfere with sympathetic activity including bretylium, betanidine, guanethidine, debrisoquine, methyldopa, alpha- and beta-adrenergic blocking agents.

4.6 Pregnancy and lactation

Although pseudoephedrine and triprolidine have been in widespread use for many years without apparent ill consequence, there are no specific data on their use during pregnancy. Caution should therefore be exercised by balancing the potential benefit of treatment to the mother against any possible hazards to the developing foetus.

Systemic administration of triprolidine in rats and rabbits up to 75 times the human dose did not produce teratogenic effects.

Systemic administration of pseudoephedrine, up to 50 times the human daily dosage in rats and up to 35 times the human daily dosage in rabbits, did not produce teratogenic effects.

Pseudoephedrine and triprolidine are excreted in breast-milk in small amounts but the effect of this on breast-fed infants is not known. It has been estimated that approximately 0.4 to 0.7% and 0.06 to 0.2% of a single dose of pseudoephedrine and triprolidine respectively ingested by a mother will be excreted in the breast milk over 24 hours.

4.7 Effects on ability to drive and use machines

Multi-Action ACTIFED Syrup may cause drowsiness and impair performance in tests of auditory vigilance. Patients should not drive or operate machinery until they have determined their own response.

4.8 Undesirable effects

Central nervous system depression or excitation may occur, drowsiness being reported most frequently. Sleep disturbance and, rarely, hallucinations have been reported.

Skin rashes, with or without irritation, tachycardia, dryness of mouth, nose and throat, have occasionally been reported.

Urinary retention has been reported occasionally in men receiving pseudoephedrine; prostatic enlargement could have been an important predisposing factor.

4.9 Overdose

The effects of acute toxicity from Multi-Action ACTIFED Syrup may include drowsiness, lethargy, dizziness, ataxia, weakness, hypotonicity, respiratory depression, dryness of the skin and mucous membranes, tachycardia, hypertension, hyperpyrexia, hyperactivity, irritability, convulsions and difficulty with micturition.

Necessary measures should be taken to maintain and support respiration and control convulsions. Gastric lavage should be performed up to 3 hours after ingestion if indicated. Catheterisation of the bladder may be necessary. If desired the elimination of pseudoephedrine can be accelerated by acid diuresis or by dialysis.

5. PHARMACOLOGICAL PROPERTIES

5.1 Pharmacodynamic properties

Triprolidine provides symptomatic relief in conditions believed to depend wholly or partly upon the triggered release of histamine. It is a potent competitive histamine H_1-receptor antagonist of the pyrrolidine class with mild central nervous system depressant properties which may cause drowsiness. Pseudoephedrine has direct and indirect sympathomimetic activity and is an effective upper respiratory tract decongestant. Pseudoephedrine is substantially less potent than ephedrine in producing both tachycardia and elevation of systolic blood pressure and considerably less potent in causing stimulation of the central nervous system.

After oral administration of a single dose of 2.5 mg triprolidine to adults the onset of action, as determined by the ability to antagonise histamine-induced weals and flares in the skin, is within 1 to 2 hours. Peak effects occur at about 3 hours, and although activity declines thereafter, significant inhibition of histamine-induced weals and flares still occurs 8 hours after dose. Pseudoephedrine produces its decongestant effect within 30 minutes, persisting for at least 4 hours.

5.2 Pharmacokinetic properties

After the administration of 10 ml Multi-Action ACTIFED Syrup (containing 2.5 mg triprolidine hydrochloride and 60 mg pseudoephedrine hydrochloride) in healthy adult volunteers, the peak plasma concentration (C_{max}) of triprolidine is approximately 5.5 ng/ml - 6.0 ng/ml, occurring at about 1.5 hours (T_{max}) after drug administration. The plasma half-life of triprolidine is approximately 3.2 hours. The C_{max} of pseudoephedrine is approximately 180 ng/ml with T_{max} approximately 1.5 hours after drug administration. The plasma half-life of pseudoephedrine is approximately 5.5 hours (urine pH maintained between 5.0-7.0). The plasma half-life of pseudoephedrine is markedly decreased by acidification of urine and increased by alkalinisation.

5.3 Preclinical safety data

The active ingredients of Multi-Action ACTIFED Syrup are well known constituents of medicinal products and their safety profiles are well documented. The results of preclinical studies do not add anything of relevance for therapeutic purposes.

6. PHARMACEUTICAL PARTICULARS

6.1 List of excipients

Sucrose

Glycerol

Methyl hydroxybenzoate

Sodium benzoate

Quinoline yellow, E104

Sunset yellow, E110/FD & C yellow no 6

Purified water

6.2 Incompatibilities

None known

6.3 Shelf life

36 months (unopened)

6.4 Special precautions for storage

Below 25°C

Protect From Light

6.5 Nature and contents of container

100.000 ml amber glass bottles capped with metal roll-on closures or plastic screw caps. Each cap type containing PVDC-lined wads or polyethylene/expanded polyethylene laminated wad.

closure fitted with a polyvinylidene chloride (PVDC) faced wad or polyethylene/expanded polyethylene laminated wad.

A spoon with a 5ml and a 2.5ml measure is supplied with this product.

6.6 Instructions for use and handling

Not applicable

Administrative Data

7. MARKETING AUTHORISATION HOLDER

Pfizer Consumer Healthcare

Alternative Trading Style

Warner Lambert Consumer Healthcare

Walton Oaks

Dorking Road

Walton-on-the-Hill

Surrey KT20 7NS

United Kingdom

8. MARKETING AUTHORISATION NUMBER(S)

15513/0013

9. DATE OF FIRST AUTHORISATION/RENEWAL OF THE AUTHORISATION

11/04/2000

10. DATE OF REVISION OF THE TEXT

January 2004

Multi-Action Actifed Tablets

(Pfizer Consumer Healthcare)

1. NAME OF THE MEDICINAL PRODUCT

Multi-Action ACTIFED Tablets

2. QUALITATIVE AND QUANTITATIVE COMPOSITION

Each tablet contains:-

Triprolidine hydrochloride 2.5 mg

Pseudoephedrine hydrochloride 60.0 mg

3. PHARMACEUTICAL FORM

Tablets for oral administration.

4. CLINICAL PARTICULARS

4.1 Therapeutic indications

For the symptomatic relief of upper respiratory tract disorders which are benefited by a combination of a nasal decongestant and histamine H_1-receptor antagonist, for example:

Allergic Rhinitis

Vasomotor Rhinitis

The Common Cold and Influenza

4.2 Posology and method of administration

Adults and children over 12 years

One tablet every 4-6 hours up to 4 times a day

Use in the Elderly

No specific studies have been carried out in the elderly, but triprolidine and pseudoephedrine have been widely used in older people.

Hepatic Dysfunction

Caution should be exercised when administering Multi-Action ACTIFED Tablets to patients with severe hepatic impairment.

Renal Dysfunction

Caution should be exercised when administering Multi-Action ACTIFED Tablets to patients with moderate to severe renal impairment.

4.3 Contraindications

Multi-Action ACTIFED is contraindicated in individuals who have previously exhibited intolerance to it or to pseudoephedrine or triprolidine.

Multi-Action ACTIFED is contraindicated in patients who are taking or have taken monoamine oxidase inhibitors within the preceding two weeks. The concomitant use of pseudoephedrine and this type of product may occasionally cause a rise in blood pressure.

Multi-Action ACTIFED is contraindicated in patients with severe hypertension or severe coronary artery disease.

The antibacterial agent furazolidone, is known to cause a dose-related inhibition of monoamine oxidase. Although there are no reports of hypertensive crises caused by the concurrent administration of Multi-Action ACTIFED Tablets and furazolidone they should not be taken together.

4.4 Special warnings and special precautions for use

Multi-Action ACTIFED Tablets may cause drowsiness and impair performance in tests of auditory vigilance. Patients should not drive or operate machinery until they have determined their own response.

Although there are no objective data, users of Multi-Action ACTIFED Tablets should avoid the concomitant use of alcohol or other centrally acting sedatives.

Although pseudoephedrine has virtually no pressor effect in normotensive patients, Multi-Action ACTIFED Tablets should be used with caution in patients taking anti-hypertensive agents, tricyclic antidepressants or other sympathomimetic agents, such as decongestants, appetite suppressants and amfetamine-like psychostimulants. The effects of a single dose of Multi-Action ACTIFED Tablets on the blood pressure of these patients should be observed before recommending repeated or unsupervised treatment.

As with other sympathomimetic agents Multi-Action ACTIFED Tablets should be used with caution in patients with hypertension, heart disease, diabetes, hyperthyroidism, elevated intraocular pressure and prostatic enlargement.

There have been no specific studies of Multi-Action ACTIFED Tablets in patients with hepatic and/or renal dysfunction. Caution should be exercised in the presence of severe renal or hepatic impairment.

There is insufficient information available to determine whether triprolidine or pseudoephedrine have mutagenic or carcinogenic potential.

Systemic administration of pseudoephedrine in rats, up to 7 times the human daily dosage in females and 35 times the human daily dosage in males, did not impair fertility nor alter foetal morphological development and survival.

No studies have been conducted in animals to determine if triprolidine has the potential to impair fertility.

There is no information on the effects of Multi-Action ACTIFED on human fertility.

The packs carry the following statements:-

Store below 25°C

Keep dry

Protect from light

Keep out of the reach of children

Warnings, may cause drowsiness. If affected do not drive or operate machinery. Avoid alcoholic drink.

The 12 tablet pack carries the additional statements:-

If symptoms persist consult your doctor.

Do not exceed the stated dose.

As with all medicines if you are pregnant, or currently taking any other medicine, consult your doctor or pharmacist before taking this product.

4.5 Interaction with other medicinal products and other forms of Interaction

Concomitant use of Multi-Action ACTIFED Tablets with sympathomimetic agents, such as decongestants, tricyclic antidepressants, appetite suppressants and amfetamine-like psychostimulants, or with monoamine oxidase inhibitors which interfere with the catabolism of sympathomimetic amines, may occasionally cause a rise in blood pressure.

Because of its pseudoephedrine content, Multi-Action ACTIFED may partially reverse the hypotensive action of drugs which interfere with sympathetic activity including bretylium, betanidine, guanethidine, debrisoquine, methyldopa, alpha-and beta-adrenergic blocking agents.

4.6 Pregnancy and lactation

Although pseudoephedrine, and triprolidine have been in widespread use for many years without apparent ill consequence, there are no specific data on their use during pregnancy. Caution should therefore be exercised by balancing the potential benefit of treatment to the mother against any possible hazards to the developing foetus.

Systemic administration of triprolidine in rats and rabbits up to 75 times the human dose did not produce teratogenic effects.

Systemic administration of pseudoephedrine, up to 50 times the human daily dosage in rats and up to 35 times the human daily dosage in rabbits, did not produce teratogenic effects.

Pseudoephedrine and triprolidine are excreted in breast-milk in small amounts but the effect of this on breast-fed infants is not known. It has been estimated that approximately 0.5 to 0.7% of a single dose of pseudoephedrine ingested by a mother will be excreted in the breast-milk over 24 hours.

4.7 Effects on ability to drive and use machines

Multi-Action ACTIFED may cause drowsiness and impair performance in tests of auditory vigilance. Patients should not drive or operate machinery until they have determined their own response.

4.8 Undesirable effects

Central nervous system depression or excitation may occur, drowsiness being reported most frequently. Sleep disturbance and, rarely, hallucinations have been reported.

Skin rashes, with or without irritation, tachycardia, dryness of mouth, nose and throat, have occasionally been reported.

Urinary retention has been reported occasionally in men receiving pseudoephedrine; prostatic enlargement could have been an important predisposing factor.

4.9 Overdose

The effects of acute toxicity from Multi-Action ACTIFED may include drowsiness, lethargy, dizziness, ataxia, weakness, hypotonicity, respiratory depression, dryness of the skin and mucous membranes, tachycardia, hypertension, hyperpyrexia, hyperactivity, irritability, convulsions, and difficulty with micturition.

Necessary measures should be taken to maintain and support respiration and control convulsions. Gastric lavage should be performed up to 3 hours after ingestion if indicated. Catheterisation of the bladder may be necessary. If desired, the elimination of pseudoephedrine can be accelerated by acid diuresis or by dialysis.

5. PHARMACOLOGICAL PROPERTIES

5.1 Pharmacodynamic properties

Triprolidine provides symptomatic relief in conditions believed to depend wholly or partly upon the triggered release of histamine. It is a potent competitive histamine H_1-receptor antagonist of the pyrrolidine class with mild central nervous system depressant properties which may cause drowsiness. Pseudoephedrine has direct and indirect sympathomimetic activity and is an effective upper respiratory tract decongestant. Pseudoephedrine is substantially less potent than ephedrine in producing both tachycardia and elevation of systolic blood pressure and considerably less potent in causing stimulation of the central nervous system.

After oral administration of a single dose of 2.5mg triprolidine to adults the onset of action, as determined by the ability to antagonise histamine-induced weals and flares in the skin, is within 1 to 2 hours. Peak effects occur at about 3 hours and, although activity declines thereafter, significant inhibition of histamine-induced weals and flares still occurs 8 hours after the dose. Pseudoephedrine produces its decongestant effect within 30 minutes, persisting for at least 4 hours.

5.2 Pharmacokinetic properties

After the administration of one Multi-Action ACTIFED Tablet (containing 2.5 mg triprolidine hydrochloride and 60 mg pseudoephedrine hydrochloride) in healthy adult volunteers, the peak plasma concentration (C_{max}) of triprolidine is approximately 5.5 ng/ml - 6.0 ng/nl, occurring at about 2.0 hours (T_{max}) after drug administration. The plasma half life of triprolidine is approximately 3.2 hours. The C_{max} of pseudoephedrine is approximately 180 ng/ml with T_{max} approximately 2.0 hours after drug administration. The plasma half life of pseudoephedrine is approximately 5.5 hours (urine pH maintained between 5.0-7.0). The plasma half life of pseudoephedrine is markedly decreased by acidification of urine and increased by alkalinisation.

5.3 Preclinical safety data

6. PHARMACEUTICAL PARTICULARS

6.1 List of excipients

Lactose

Maize starch

Povidone

Magnesium stearate

6.2 Incompatibilities

None known

6.3 Shelf life

36 months

6.4 Special precautions for storage

Below 25°C

Keep Dry

Protect From Light

6.5 Nature and contents of container

12 pack pvc/pvdc/aluminium foil blister packs.

500 tablets in polypropylene containers with polyethylene snap-on lids.

500 tablets in amber glass bottles with low density polyethylene snap-fit closures.

6.6 Instructions for use and handling

None

Administrative Data

7. MARKETING AUTHORISATION HOLDER

Pfizer Consumer Healthcare

Alternative Trading Style

Warner Lambert Consumer Healthcare

Walton Oaks

Dorking Road

Walton-on-the-Hill

Surrey KT20 7NS

United Kingdom

8. MARKETING AUTHORISATION NUMBER(S)

PL 15513/0014

9. DATE OF FIRST AUTHORISATION/RENEWAL OF THE AUTHORISATION

28 February 1997 / 25 July 2001

10. DATE OF REVISION OF THE TEXT

January 2004

Multiparin 1,000 iu/ml

(Wockhardt UK Ltd)

1. NAME OF THE MEDICINAL PRODUCT

Multiparin 1,000 I.U./ml solution for injection or concentrate for solution for infusion

2. QUALITATIVE AND QUANTITATIVE COMPOSITION

Heparin sodium (mucous) 1,000 I.U./ml (5,000 I.U. in 5ml)

For excipients see 6.1

3. PHARMACEUTICAL FORM

Solution for injection or concentrate for solution for infusion

A colourless or straw-coloured liquid, free from turbidity and from matter that deposits on standing.

4. CLINICAL PARTICULARS

4.1 Therapeutic indications

Treatment of deep vein thrombosis, pulmonary embolism, unstable angina pectoris and acute peripheral arterial occlusion.

In extracorporeal circulation and haemodialysis.

4.2 Posology and method of administration

Route of Administration

By continuous intravenous infusion in 5% glucose or 0.9% sodium chloride or by intermittent intravenous injection.

The intravenous injection volume of Multiparin should not exceed 15ml.

As the effects of heparin are short-lived, administration by intravenous infusion is preferable to intermittent intravenous injections.

Recommended dosage

Treatment of deep vein thrombosis, pulmonary embolism, unstable angina pectoris, acute peripheral arterial occlusion:

Adults:

Loading dose:	5,000 units intravenously (10,000 units may be required in severe pulmonary embolism)
Maintenance:	1,000-2,000 units/hour by intravenous infusion, or 5,000-10,000 units 4-hourly by intravenous injection.

Elderly:

Dosage reduction may be advisable.

Children and small adults:

Loading dose:	50 units/kg intravenously
Maintenance:	15-25 units/kg/hour by intravenous infusion, or 100 units/kg 4-hourly by intravenous injection

Daily laboratory monitoring (ideally at the same time each day, starting 4-6 hours after initiation of treatment) is essential during full-dose heparin treatment, with adjustment of dosage to maintain an APTT value 1.5-2.5 × mid-point of normal range or control value.

In extracorporeal circulation and haemodialysis

Adults:

Cardiopulmonary bypass:

Initially 300 units/kg intravenously, adjusted thereafter to maintain the activated clotting time (ACT) in the range 400-500 seconds.

Haemodialysis and haemofiltration:

Initially 1,000-5,000 units,

Maintenance: 1,000-2,000 units/hour, adjusted to maintain clotting time >40 minutes.

4.3 Contraindications

Known hypersensitivity to heparin or any of the other ingredients.

Patients who consume large amounts of alcohol, who are sensitive to the drug, who are actively bleeding or who have haemophilia or other bleeding disorders, severe liver disease (including oesophageal varices), purpura, severe hypertension, active tuberculosis or increased capillary permeability.

Patients with present or previous thrombocytopenia. The rare occurrence of skin necrosis in patients receiving heparin contra-indicates the further use of heparin either by subcutaneous or intravenous routes because of the risk of thrombocytopenia. Because of the special hazard of post-operative haemorrhage heparin is contra-indicated during surgery of the brain, spinal cord and eye, and in patients undergoing lumbar puncture or regional anaesthetic block.

The relative risks and benefits of heparin should be carefully assessed in patients with a bleeding tendency or those patients with an actual or potential bleeding site eg. hiatus hernia, peptic ulcer, neoplasm, bacterial endocarditis, retinopathy, bleeding haemorrhoids, suspected intracranial haemorrhage, cerebral thrombosis or threatened abortion.

Menstruation is not a contra-indication.

4.4 Special warnings and special precautions for use

Platelet counts should be measured in patients receiving heparin treatment for longer than 5 days and the treatment should be stopped immediately in those who develop thrombocytopenia.

In patients with advanced renal or hepatic disease, a reduction in dosage may be necessary. The risk of bleeding is increased with severe renal impairment and in women over 60 years of age.

Although heparin hypersensitivity is rare, it is advisable to give a trial dose of 1,000 I.U. in patients with a history of allergy. Caution should be exercised in patients with known hypersensitivity to low molecular weight heparins. Multiparin contains benzyl alcohol and methyl parahydroxybenzoate as preservatives. Caution should be used if prescribing Multiparin to susceptible patients as benzyl alcohol may increase the risk of jaundice in neonates and cause toxic reactions in infants and children up to three years old. Methyl parahydroxybenzoate may cause allergic reactions (possibly delayed).

In most patients, the recommended low-dose regimen produces no alteration in clotting time. However, patients show an individual response to heparin, and it is therefore essential that the effect of therapy on coagulation time should be monitored in patients undergoing major surgery.

Caution is recommended in spinal or epidural anaesthesia (risk of spinal haematoma).

Heparin can suppress adrenal secretion of aldosterone leading to hyperkalemia, particularly in patients such as those with diabetes mellitus, chronic renal failure, pre-existing metabolic acidosis, a raised plasma potassium, or taking potassium sparing drugs. The risk of hyperkalemia appears to increase with duration of therapy but is usually reversible. Plasma potassium should be measured in patients at risk before starting heparin therapy and in all patients treated for more than 7 days.

4.5 Interaction with other medicinal products and other forms of Interaction

Drugs that interfere with platelet aggregation eg. aspirin and other NSAIDs, dextran solutions, dipyridamole or any other drug which may interfere with coagulation, should be used with care.

Hyperkalaemia may occur with concomitant ACE inhibitors.

Reduced activity of heparin has been reported with simultaneous intravenous glyceryl trinitrate infusion.

Interference with diagnostic tests may be associated with pseudo-hypocalcaemia (in haemodialysis patients), artefactual increases in total thyroxine and triiodothyronine, simulated metabolic acidosis and inhibition of the chromogenic lysate assay for endotoxin. Heparin may interfere with the determination of aminoglycosides by immunoassays.

4.6 Pregnancy and lactation

Heparin is not contraindicated in pregnancy. Heparin does not cross the placenta or appear in breast milk. The decision to use heparin in pregnancy should be taken after evaluation of the risk/benefit in any particular circumstances.

Reduced bone density has been reported with prolonged heparin treatment during pregnancy.

Haemorrhage may be a problem during pregnancy or after delivery.

4.7 Effects on ability to drive and use machines

None stated.

4.8 Undesirable effects

Haemorrhage (see also Special Warnings and Precautions and Overdosage Information).

Thrombocytopenia has been observed occasionally (see also Special Precautions and Warnings). Two types of heparin-induced thrombocytopenia have been defined. Type I is frequent, mild (usually $>50 \times 10^9$/L) and transient, occurring within 1-5 days of heparin administration. Type II is less frequent but often associated with severe thrombocytopenia (usually $<50 \times 10^9$/L). It is immune-mediated and occurs after a week or more (earlier in patients previously exposed to heparin). It is associated with the production of a platelet-aggregating antibody and thromboembolic complications which may precede the onset of thrombocytopenia. Heparin should be discontinued immediately.

There is some evidence that prolonged dosing with heparin (ie. over many months) may cause alopecia and osteoporosis. Significant bone demineralisation has been reported in women taking more than 10,000 I.U. per day of heparin for at least 6 months.

Heparin products can cause hypoaldosteronism which may result in an increase in plasma potassium. Rarely, clinically significant hyperkalemia may occur particularly in patients with chronic renal failure and diabetes mellitus (see Warnings and Precautions).

Hypersensitivity reactions to heparin are rare. They include urticaria, conjunctivitis, rhinitis, asthma, cyanosis, tachypnoea, feeling of oppression, fever, chills, angioneurotic oedema and anaphylactic shock. In some instances the precipitating agent will prove to be the preservative rather than the heparin itself.

Local irritation and skin necrosis may occur but are rare.

Priapism has been reported. Increased serum transaminase values may occur but usually resolve on discontinuation of heparin. Heparin administration is associated with release of lipoprotein lipase into the plasma; rebound hyperlipidaemia may follow heparin withdrawal.

4.9 Overdose

A potential hazard of heparin therapy is haemorrhage, but this is usually due to overdosage and the risk is minimised by strict laboratory control. Slight haemorrhage can usually be treated by withdrawing the drug. If bleeding is more severe, clotting time and platelet count should be determined. Prolonged clotting time will indicate the presence of an excessive anticoagulant effect requiring neutralisation by intravenous protamine sulphate, at a dosage of 1 mg for every 100 I.U. of heparin to be neutralised. The bolus dose of protamine sulphate should be given slowly over about 10 minutes and not exceed 50 mg. If more than 15 minutes have elapsed since the injection of heparin, lower doses of protamine will be necessary.

5. PHARMACOLOGICAL PROPERTIES

5.1 Pharmacodynamic properties

Heparin is an anticoagulant and acts by inhibiting thrombin and by potentiating the naturally occurring inhibitors of activated Factor X (Xa).

5.2 Pharmacokinetic properties

As heparin is not absorbed from the gastrointestinal tract and sublingual sites it is administered by injection. After injection heparin extensively binds to plasma proteins.

Heparin is metabolised in the liver and the inactive metabolic products are excreted in the urine.

The half life of heparin is dependent on the dose.

5.3 Preclinical safety data

There are no pre-clinical data of relevance to the prescriber which are additional to those already included in other sections.

6. PHARMACEUTICAL PARTICULARS

6.1 List of excipients

Benzyl alcohol

Methyl parahydroxybenzoate (E218)

Water for injections

Sodium hydroxide solution

Hydrochloric acid

6.2 Incompatibilities

Heparin is incompatible with many injectable preparations e.g. some antibiotics, opioid analgesics and antihistamines.

Dobutamine hydrochloride and heparin should not be mixed or infused through the same intravenous line, as this causes precipitation.

Heparin and reteplase are incompatible when combined in solution.

If reteplase and heparin are to be given through the same line this, together with any Y-lines, must be thoroughly flushed with a 0.9% saline or a 5% glucose solution prior to and following the reteplase injection.

6.3 Shelf life

18 months

6.4 Special precautions for storage

Do not store above 25°C

Store in the original package

6.5 Nature and contents of container

5ml multidose neutral glass (Type 1, Ph Eur) vial. Carton contains 10 vials.

6.6 Instructions for use and handling

Each multidose vial should be restricted to use in a single patient.

Administrative Data

7. MARKETING AUTHORISATION HOLDER

CP Pharmaceuticals Ltd
Ash Road North
Wrexham
LL13 9UF
UK.

8. MARKETING AUTHORISATION NUMBER(S)

4543/0218

9. DATE OF FIRST AUTHORISATION/RENEWAL OF THE AUTHORISATION

Date of first authorisation - 1 July 1991

Date of renewal – 29 May 2002

10. DATE OF REVISION OF THE TEXT

January 2003

Multiparin 25,000 iu/ml

(Wockhardt UK Ltd)

1. NAME OF THE MEDICINAL PRODUCT

Multiparin 25,000 I.U./ml solution for injection or concentrate for solution for infusion

2. QUALITATIVE AND QUANTITATIVE COMPOSITION

Heparin sodium (mucous) 25,000 I.U./ml (125,000 I.U. in 5ml)

For excipients see 6.1

3. PHARMACEUTICAL FORM

Solution for injection or concentrate for solution for infusion

A colourless or straw-coloured liquid, free from turbidity and from matter that deposits on standing.

4. CLINICAL PARTICULARS

4.1 Therapeutic indications

Prophylaxis of deep vein thrombosis and pulmonary embolism

Treatment of deep vein thrombosis, pulmonary embolism, unstable angina pectoris and acute peripheral arterial occlusion.

Prophylaxis of mural thrombosis following myocardial infarction.

In extracorporeal circulation and haemodialysis.

4.2 Posology and method of administration

Route of administration

By continuous intravenous infusion in 5% glucose or 0.9% sodium chloride or by intermittent intravenous injection, or by subcutaneous injection.

The intravenous injection volume of Multiparin should not exceed 15ml.

As the effects of heparin are short-lived, administration by intravenous infusion or subcutaneous injection is preferable to intermittent intravenous injections.

Recommended dosage

Prophylaxis of deep vein thrombosis and pulmonary embolism:

Adults:

2 hours pre-operatively:	5,000 units subcutaneously
followed by:	5,000 units subcutaneously every 8-12 hours, for 7-10 days or until the patient is fully ambulant.

No laboratory monitoring should be necessary during low dose heparin prophylaxis. If monitoring is considered desirable, anti-Xa assays should be used as the activated partial thromboplastin time (APTT) is not significantly prolonged.

During pregnancy: 5,000 - 10,000 units every 12 hours, subcutaneously, adjusted according to APTT or anti-Xa assay.

Elderly:

Dosage reduction and monitoring of APTT may be advisable.

Children:

No dosage recommendations.

Treatment of deep vein thrombosis, pulmonary embolism, unstable angina pectoris, acute peripheral arterial occlusion:

Adults:

Loading dose: 5,000 units intravenously (10,000 units may be required in severe pulmonary embolism)

Maintenance: 1,000-2,000 units/hour by intravenous infusion,

<u>or</u>

10,000-20,000 units 12 hourly subcutaneously,

<u>or</u>

5,000-10,000 units 4-hourly by intravenous injection.

Elderly:

Dosage reduction may be advisable.

Children and small adults:

Loading dose: 50 units/kg intravenously

Maintenance: 15-25 units/kg/hour by intravenous infusion,

<u>or</u>

250 units/kg 12 hourly subcutaneously

<u>or</u>

100 units/kg 4-hourly by intravenous injection

Daily laboratory monitoring (ideally at the same time each day, starting 4-6 hours after initiation of treatment) is essential during full-dose heparin treatment, with adjustment of dosage to maintain an APTT value 1.5-2.5 × mid-point of normal range or control value.

Prophylaxis of mural thrombosis following myocardial infarction

Adults:

12,500 units 12 hourly subcutaneously for at least 10 days.

Elderly:

Dosage reduction may be advisable

In extracorporeal circulation and haemodialysis

Adults:

Cardiopulmonary bypass:

Initially 300 units/kg intravenously, adjusted thereafter to maintain the activated clotting time (ACT) in the range 400-500 seconds.

Haemodialysis and haemofiltration:

Initially 1-5,000 units,

Maintenance: 1-2,000 units/hour, adjusted to maintain clotting time >40 minutes.

4.3 Contraindications

Known hypersensitivity to heparin or any of the other ingredients.

Patients who consume large amounts of alcohol, who are sensitive to the drug, who are actively bleeding or who have haemophilia or other bleeding disorders, severe liver disease (including oesophageal varices), purpura, severe hypertension, active tuberculosis or increased capillary permeability.

Patients with present or previous thrombocytopenia. The rare occurrence of skin necrosis in patients receiving heparin contra-indicates the further use of heparin either by subcutaneous or intravenous routes because of the risk of thrombocytopenia. Because of the special hazard of post-operative haemorrhage heparin is contra-indicated during surgery of the brain, spinal cord and eye, and in patients undergoing lumbar puncture or regional anaesthetic block.

The relative risks and benefits of heparin should be carefully assessed in patients with a bleeding tendency or those patients with an actual or potential bleeding site eg. hiatus hernia, peptic ulcer, neoplasm, bacterial endocarditis, retinopathy, bleeding haemorrhoids, suspected intracranial haemorrhage, cerebral thrombosis or threatened abortion.

Menstruation is not a contra-indication.

4.4 Special warnings and special precautions for use

Platelet counts should be measured in patients receiving heparin treatment for longer than 5 days and the treatment should be stopped immediately in those who develop thrombocytopenia.

In patients with advanced renal or hepatic disease, a reduction in dosage may be necessary. The risk of bleeding is increased with severe renal impairment and in women over 60 years of age.

Although heparin hypersensitivity is rare, it is advisable to give a trial dose of 1,000 I.U. in patients with a history of allergy. Caution should be exercised in patients with known hypersensitivity to low molecular weight heparins. Multiparin contains benzyl alcohol and methyl parahydroxybenzoate as preservatives. Caution should be used if prescribing Multiparin to susceptible patients as benzyl alcohol may increase the risk of jaundice in neonates and cause toxic reactions in infants and children up to three years old. Methyl parahydroxybenzoate may cause allergic reactions (possibly delayed).

In most patients, the recommended low-dose regimen produces no alteration in clotting time. However, patients show an individual response to heparin, and it is therefore essential that the effect of therapy on coagulation time should be monitored in patients undergoing major surgery.

Caution is recommended in spinal or epidural anaesthesia (risk of spinal haematoma).

Heparin can suppress adrenal secretion of aldosterone leading to hyperkalemia, particularly in patients such as those with diabetes mellitus, chronic renal failure, pre-existing metabolic acidosis, a raised plasma potassium, or taking potassium sparing drugs. The risk of hyperkalemia appears to increase with duration of therapy but is usually reversible. Plasma potassium should be measured in patients at risk before starting heparin therapy and in all patients treated for more than 7 days.

4.5 Interaction with other medicinal products and other forms of Interaction

Drugs that interfere with platelet aggregation eg. aspirin and other NSAIDs, dextran solutions, dipyridamole or any other drug which may interfere with coagulation, should be used with care.

Hyperkalaemia may occur with concomitant ACE inhibitors.

Reduced activity of heparin has been reported with simultaneous intravenous glyceryl trinitrate infusion.

Interference with diagnostic tests may be associated with pseudo-hypocalcaemia (in haemodialysis patients), artefactual increases in total thyroxine and triiodothyronine, simulated metabolic acidosis and inhibition of the chromogenic lysate assay for endotoxin. Heparin may interfere with the determination of aminoglycosides by immunoassays.

4.6 Pregnancy and lactation

Heparin is not contraindicated in pregnancy. Heparin does not cross the placenta or appear in breast milk. The decision to use heparin in pregnancy should be taken after evaluation of the risk/benefit in any particular circumstances.

Reduced bone density has been reported with prolonged heparin treatment during pregnancy.

Haemorrhage may be a problem during pregnancy or after delivery.

4.7 Effects on ability to drive and use machines

None stated.

4.8 Undesirable effects

Haemorrhage (see also Special Warnings and Precautions and Overdosage Information).

Thrombocytopenia has been observed occasionally (see also Special Precautions and Warnings). Two types of heparin-induced thrombocytopenia have been defined. Type I is frequent, mild (usually $>50 \times 10^9/L$) and transient, occurring within 1-5 days of heparin administration. Type II is less frequent but often associated with severe thrombocytopenia (usually $<50 \times 10^9/L$). It is immune-mediated and occurs after a week or more (earlier in patients previously exposed to heparin). It is associated with the production of a platelet-aggregating antibody and thromboembolic complications which may precede the onset of thrombocytopenia. Heparin should be discontinued immediately.

There is some evidence that prolonged dosing with heparin (ie. over many months) may cause alopecia and osteoporosis. Significant bone demineralisation has been reported in women taking more than 10,000 I.U. per day of heparin for at least 6 months.

Heparin products can cause hypoaldosteronism which may result in an increase in plasma potassium. Rarely, clinically significant hyperkalemia may occur particularly in patients with chronic renal failure and diabetes mellitus (see Warnings and Precautions).

Hypersensitivity reactions to heparin are rare. They include urticaria, conjunctivitis, rhinitis, asthma, cyanosis, tachypnoea, feeling of oppression, fever, chills, angioneurotic oedema and anaphylactic shock. In some instances the precipitating agent will prove to be the preservative rather than the heparin itself.

Local irritation and skin necrosis may occur but are rare. Erythematous nodules, or infiltrated and sometimes eczema-like plaques, at the site of subcutaneous injections are common, occurring 3-21 days after starting heparin treatment.

Priapism has been reported. Increased serum transaminase values may occur but usually resolve on discontinuation of heparin. Heparin administration is associated with release of lipoprotein lipase into the plasma; rebound hyperlipidaemia may follow heparin withdrawal.

4.9 Overdose

A potential hazard of heparin therapy is haemorrhage, but this is usually due to overdosage and the risk is minimised by strict laboratory control. Slight haemorrhage can usually be treated by withdrawing the drug. If bleeding is more severe, clotting time and platelet count should be determined. Prolonged clotting time will indicate the presence of an excessive anticoagulant effect requiring neutralisation by intravenous protamine sulphate, at a dosage of 1 mg for every 100 I.U. of heparin to be neutralised. The bolus dose of protamine sulphate should be given slowly over about 10 minutes and not exceed 50 mg. If more than 15 minutes have elapsed since the injection of heparin, lower doses of protamine will be necessary.

5. PHARMACOLOGICAL PROPERTIES

5.1 Pharmacodynamic properties

Heparin is an anticoagulant and acts by inhibiting thrombin and by potentiating the naturally occurring inhibitors of activated Factor X (Xa).

5.2 Pharmacokinetic properties

As heparin is not absorbed from the gastrointestinal tract and sublingual sites it is administered by injection. After injection heparin extensively binds to plasma proteins.

Heparin is metabolised in the liver and the inactive metabolic products are excreted in the urine.

The half life of heparin is dependent on the dose.

5.3 Preclinical safety data

There are no pre-clinical data of relevance to the prescriber which are additional to those already included in other sections.

6. PHARMACEUTICAL PARTICULARS

6.1 List of excipients

Benzyl alcohol

Methyl parahydroxybenzoate (E218)

Water for injections

Sodium hydroxide solution

Hydrochloric acid

6.2 Incompatibilities

Heparin is incompatible with many injectable preparations e.g. some antibiotics, opioid analgesics and antihistamines.

Dobutamine hydrochloride and heparin should not be mixed or infused through the same intravenous line, as this causes precipitation.

Heparin and reteplase are incompatible when combined in solution.

If reteplase and heparin are to be given through the same line this, together with any Y-lines, must be thoroughly flushed with a 0.9% saline or a 5% glucose solution prior to and following the reteplase injection.

6.3 Shelf life

18 months

6.4 Special precautions for storage

Do not store above 25°C

Store in the original package

6.5 Nature and contents of container

5ml multidose neutral glass (Type 1, Ph Eur) vial. Carton containing 10 vials.

6.6 Instructions for use and handling

Each multidose vial should be restricted to use in a single patient.

Administrative Data

7. MARKETING AUTHORISATION HOLDER

CP Pharmaceuticals Ltd

Ash Road North

Wrexham

LL13 9UF

UK.

8. MARKETING AUTHORISATION NUMBER(S)

PL 4543/0220

9. DATE OF FIRST AUTHORISATION/RENEWAL OF THE AUTHORISATION

Date of first authorisation - 1 July 1991

Date of renewal – 29 May 2002

10. DATE OF REVISION OF THE TEXT

January 2003

Multiparin 5,000 iu/ml

(Wockhardt UK Ltd)

1. NAME OF THE MEDICINAL PRODUCT

Multiparin 5,000 I.U./ml solution for injection or concentrate for solution for infusion

2. QUALITATIVE AND QUANTITATIVE COMPOSITION

Heparin sodium (mucous) 5,000 I.U./ml (25,000 I.U. in 5ml)

For excipients see 6.1

3. PHARMACEUTICAL FORM

Solution for injection or concentrate for solution for infusion

A colourless or straw-coloured liquid, free from turbidity and from matter that deposits on standing.

4. CLINICAL PARTICULARS

4.1 Therapeutic indications

Prophylaxis of deep vein thrombosis and pulmonary embolism

Treatment of deep vein thrombosis, pulmonary embolism, unstable angina pectoris and acute peripheral arterial occlusion.

Prophylaxis of mural thrombosis following myocardial infarction.

In extracorporeal circulation and haemodialysis.

4.2 Posology and method of administration

Route of administration

By continuous intravenous infusion in 5% glucose or 0.9% sodium chloride or by intermittent intravenous injection, or by subcutaneous injection.

The intravenous injection volume of Multiparin should not exceed 15ml.

As the effects of heparin are short-lived, administration by intravenous infusion or subcutaneous injection is preferable to intermittent intravenous injections.

Recommended dosage

Prophylaxis of deep vein thrombosis and pulmonary embolism:

Adults:

2 hours pre-operatively:	5,000 units subcutaneously
followed by:	5,000 units subcutaneously every 8-12 hours, for 7-10 days or until the patient is fully ambulant.

No laboratory monitoring should be necessary during low dose heparin prophylaxis. If monitoring is considered desirable, anti-Xa assays should be used as the activated partial thromboplastin time (APTT) is not significantly prolonged.

During pregnancy:	5,000 - 10,000 units every 12 hours, subcutaneously, adjusted according to APTT or anti-Xa assay.

Elderly:

Dosage reduction and monitoring of APTT may be advisable.

Children:

No dosage recommendations.

Treatment of deep vein thrombosis, pulmonary embolism, unstable angina pectoris, acute peripheral arterial occlusion:

Adults:

Loading dose:	5,000 units intravenously (10,000 units may be required in severe pulmonary embolism)
Maintenance:	1,000-2,000 units/hour by intravenous infusion, or 10,000-20,000 units 12 hourly subcutaneously, or 5,000-10,000 units 4-hourly by intravenous injection.

Elderly:

Dosage reduction may be advisable.

Children and small adults:

Loading dose:	50 units/kg intravenously
Maintenance:	15-25 units/kg/hour by intravenous infusion, or 250 units/kg 12 hourly subcutaneously or 100 units/kg 4-hourly by intravenous injection

Daily laboratory monitoring (ideally at the same time each day, starting 4-6 hours after initiation of treatment) is essential during full-dose heparin treatment, with adjustment of dosage to maintain an APTT value 1.5-2.5 × midpoint of normal range or control value.

Prophylaxis of mural thrombosis following myocardial infarction

Adults:

12,500 units 12 hourly subcutaneously for at least 10 days.

Elderly:

Dosage reduction may be advisable

In extracorporeal circulation and haemodialysis

Adults:

Cardiopulmonary bypass:

Initially 300 units/kg intravenously, adjusted thereafter to maintain the activated clotting time (ACT) in the range 400-500 seconds.

Haemodialysis and haemofiltration:

Initially 1-5,000 units,

Maintenance: 1-2,000 units/hour, adjusted to maintain clotting time >40 minutes.

4.3 Contraindications

Known hypersensitivity to heparin or any of the other ingredients.

Patients who consume large amounts of alcohol, who are sensitive to the drug, who are actively bleeding or who have haemophilia or other bleeding disorders, severe liver disease (including oesophageal varices), purpura, severe hypertension, active tuberculosis or increased capillary permeability.

Patients with present or previous thrombocytopenia. The rare occurrence of skin necrosis in patients receiving heparin contra-indicates the further use of heparin either by subcutaneous or intravenous routes because of the risk of thrombocytopenia. Because of the special hazard of post-operative haemorrhage heparin is contra-indicated during surgery of the brain, spinal cord and eye, and in patients undergoing lumbar puncture or regional anaesthetic block.

The relative risks and benefits of heparin should be carefully assessed in patients with a bleeding tendency or those patients with an actual or potential bleeding site eg. hiatus hernia, peptic ulcer, neoplasm, bacterial endocarditis, retinopathy, bleeding haemorrhoids, suspected intracranial haemorrhage, cerebral thrombosis or threatened abortion. Menstruation is not a contra-indication.

4.4 Special warnings and special precautions for use

Platelet counts should be measured in patients receiving heparin treatment for longer than 5 days and the treatment should be stopped immediately in those who develop thrombocytopenia.

In patients with advanced renal or hepatic disease, a reduction in dosage may be necessary. The risk of bleeding is increased with severe renal impairment and in women over 60 years of age.

Although heparin hypersensitivity is rare, it is advisable to give a trial dose of 1,000 I.U. in patients with a history of allergy. Caution should be exercised in patients with known hypersensitivity to low molecular weight heparins. Multiparin contains benzyl alcohol and methyl parahydroxybenzoate as preservatives. Caution should be used if prescribing Multiparin to susceptible patients as benzyl alcohol may increase the risk of jaundice in neonates and cause toxic reactions in infants and children up to three years old. Methyl parahydroxybenzoate may cause allergic reactions (possibly delayed).

In most patients, the recommended low-dose regimen produces no alteration in clotting time. However, patients show an individual response to heparin, and it is therefore essential that the effect of therapy on coagulation time should be monitored in patients undergoing major surgery.

Caution is recommended in spinal or epidural anaesthesia (risk of spinal haematoma).

Heparin can suppress adrenal secretion of aldosterone leading to hyperkalemia, particularly in patients such as those with diabetes mellitus, chronic renal failure, pre-existing metabolic acidosis, a raised plasma potassium, or taking potassium sparing drugs. The risk of hyperkalemia appears to increase with duration of therapy but is usually reversible. Plasma potassium should be measured in patients at risk before starting heparin therapy and in all patients treated for more than 7 days.

4.5 Interaction with other medicinal products and other forms of Interaction

Drugs that interfere with platelet aggregation eg. aspirin and other NSAIDs, dextran solutions, dipyridamole or any other drug which may interfere with coagulation, should be used with care.

Hyperkalaemia may occur with concomitant ACE inhibitors.

Reduced activity of heparin has been reported with simultaneous intravenous glyceryl trinitrate infusion.

Interference with diagnostic tests may be associated with pseudo-hypocalcaemia (in haemodialysis patients), artefactual increases in total thyroxine and triiodothyronine, simulated metabolic acidosis and inhibition of the chromogenic lysate assay for endotoxin. Heparin may interfere with the determination of aminoglycosides by immunoassays.

4.6 Pregnancy and lactation

Heparin is not contraindicated in pregnancy. Heparin does not cross the placenta or appear in breast milk. The decision to use heparin in pregnancy should be taken after evaluation of the risk/benefit in any particular circumstances.

Reduced bone density has been reported with prolonged heparin treatment during pregnancy.

Haemorrhage may be a problem during pregnancy or after delivery.

4.7 Effects on ability to drive and use machines

None stated.

4.8 Undesirable effects

Haemorrhage (see also Special Warnings and Precautions and Overdosage Information).

Thrombocytopenia has been observed occasionally (see also Special Precautions and Warnings). Two types of heparin-induced thrombocytopenia have been defined. Type I is frequent, mild (usually >50 × 109/L) and transient, occurring within 1-5 days of heparin administration. Type II is less frequent but often associated with severe thrombocytopenia (usually <50 × 109/L). It is immune-mediated and occurs after a week or more (earlier in patients previously exposed to heparin). It is associated with the production of a platelet-aggregating antibody and thromboembolic complications which may precede the onset of thrombocytopenia. Heparin should be discontinued immediately.

There is some evidence that prolonged dosing with heparin (ie. over many months) may cause alopecia and osteoporosis. Significant bone demineralisation has been reported in women taking more than 10,000 I.U. per day of heparin for at least 6 months.

Heparin products can cause hypoaldosteronism which may result in an increase in plasma potassium. Rarely, clinically significant hyperkalemia may occur particularly in patients with chronic renal failure and diabetes mellitus (see Warnings and Precautions).

Hypersensitivity reactions to heparin are rare. They include urticaria, conjunctivitis, rhinitis, asthma, cyanosis, tachypnoea, feeling of oppression, fever, chills, angioneurotic oedema and anaphylactic shock. In some instances the precipitating agent will prove to be the preservative rather than the heparin itself.

Local irritation and skin necrosis may occur but are rare. Erythematous nodules, or infiltrated and sometimes eczema-like plaques, at the site of subcutaneous injections are common, occurring 3-21 days after starting heparin treatment.

Priapism has been reported. Increased serum transaminase values may occur but usually resolve on discontinuation of heparin. Heparin administration is associated with release of lipoprotein lipase into the plasma; rebound hyperlipidaemia may follow heparin withdrawal.

4.9 Overdose

A potential hazard of heparin therapy is haemorrhage, but this is usually due to overdosage and the risk is minimised by strict laboratory control. Slight haemorrhage can usually be treated by withdrawing the drug. If bleeding is more severe, clotting time and platelet count should be determined. Prolonged clotting time will indicate the presence of an excessive anticoagulant effect requiring neutralisation by intravenous protamine sulphate, at a dosage of 1 mg for every 100 I.U. of heparin to be neutralised. The bolus dose of protamine sulphate should be given slowly over about 10 minutes and not exceed 50 mg. If more than 15 minutes have elapsed since the injection of heparin, lower doses of protamine will be necessary.

5. PHARMACOLOGICAL PROPERTIES

5.1 Pharmacodynamic properties

Heparin is an anticoagulant and acts by inhibiting thrombin and by potentiating the naturally occurring inhibitors of activated Factor X (Xa).

5.2 Pharmacokinetic properties

As heparin is not absorbed from the gastrointestinal tract and sublingual sites it is administered by injection. After injection heparin extensively binds to plasma proteins.

Heparin is metabolised in the liver and the inactive metabolic products are excreted in the urine.

The half life of heparin is dependent on the dose.

5.3 Preclinical safety data

There are no pre-clinical data of relevance to the prescriber which are additional to those already included in other sections.

6. PHARMACEUTICAL PARTICULARS

6.1 List of excipients

Benzyl alcohol

Methyl parahydroxybenzoate (E218)

Water for injections

Sodium hydroxide solution

Hydrochloric acid

6.2 Incompatibilities

Heparin is incompatible with many injectable preparations e.g. some antibiotics, opioid analgesics and antihistamines.

Dobutamine hydrochloride and heparin should not be mixed or infused through the same intravenous line, as this causes precipitation.

Heparin and reteplase are incompatible when combined in solution.

If reteplase and heparin are to be given through the same line this, together with any Y-lines, must be thoroughly flushed with a 0.9% saline or a 5% glucose solution prior to and following the reteplase injection.

6.3 Shelf life

18 months

6.4 Special precautions for storage

Do not store above 25°C

Store in the original package

6.5 Nature and contents of container

5ml multidose neutral glass (Type 1, Ph Eur) vial. Carton containing 10 vials.

6.6 Instructions for use and handling

Each multidose vial should be restricted to use in a single patient.

Administrative Data

7. MARKETING AUTHORISATION HOLDER

CP Pharmaceuticals Ltd
Ash Road North
Wrexham
LL13 9UF
UK.

8. MARKETING AUTHORISATION NUMBER(S)

PL 4543/0219

9. DATE OF FIRST AUTHORISATION/RENEWAL OF THE AUTHORISATION

Date of first authorisation - 1 July 1991

Date of renewal - 29 May 2002

10. DATE OF REVISION OF THE TEXT

January 2003

MUSE 125 microgram, 250 micrograms, 500 micrograms or 1000 micrograms urethral stick.

(Meda Pharmaceuticals)

1. NAME OF THE MEDICINAL PRODUCT

MUSE 125 microgram, 250 micrograms, 500 micrograms or 1000 micrograms urethral stick.

2. QUALITATIVE AND QUANTITATIVE COMPOSITION

Each urethral stick contains 125 micrograms, 250 micrograms, 500 micrograms or 1000 micrograms alprostadil. For excipients, see 6.1.

3. PHARMACEUTICAL FORM

Urethral Stick.

MUSE is a sterile, single-use transurethral system for the delivery of alprostadil to the male urethra. Alprostadil is suspended in macrogol and is formed into a urethral stick (1.4mm in diameter by 3mm or 6mm in length), which is contained in the tip of the polypropylene applicator.

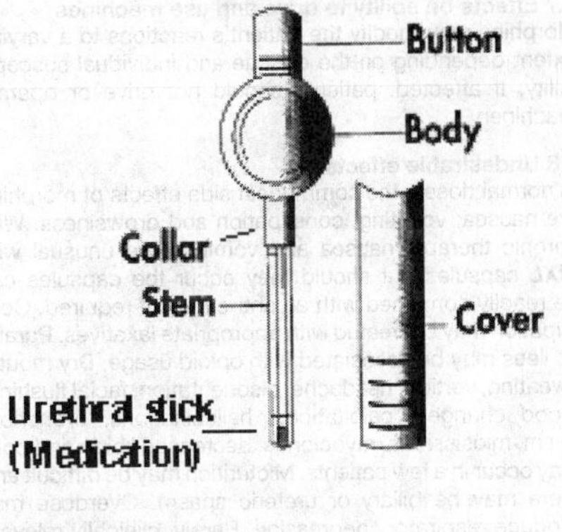

4. CLINICAL PARTICULARS

4.1 Therapeutic indications

Treatment of erectile dysfunction of primarily organic etiology.

Adjunct to other tests in the diagnosis and management of erectile dysfunction.

4.2 Posology and method of administration

Use in adults

Treatment of erectile dysfunction

Initiation of therapy: a medical professional should instruct each patient on the correct use of MUSE. The recommended starting dose is 250 micrograms.

Dosage may be increased in a stepwise manner (from 500 to 1000 micrograms), or decreased (to 125 micrograms) under medical supervision until the patient achieves a satisfactory response. After an assessment of the patient's skill and competence with the procedure, the chosen dose may then be prescribed for home use.

It is important for the patient to urinate before administration since a moist urethra makes administration of MUSE easier and is essential to dissolve the drug. To administer MUSE, remove the protective cover from the MUSE applicator, stretch the penis upward to its full length, and insert the applicator stem into the urethra. Depress the applicator button to release the medication from the applicator and remove the applicator from the urethra, (rocking the applicator gently prior to removal will ensure that the medication is separated from the applicator stem). Roll the penis between the hands for at least 10 seconds to ensure that the medication is adequately distributed along the wall of the urethra. If the patient feels a burning sensation it may help to roll the penis for an additional 30 to 60 seconds or until the burning subsides. The erection will develop within 5-10 minutes after administration and lasts approximately 30-60 minutes. After administration of MUSE, it is important to sit, or preferably, stand or walk for about 10 minutes while the erection is developing. More detailed information is given in the patient information leaflet. During home use, periodic checks of efficacy and safety are recommended.

Not more than 2 doses are recommended to be used in any 24-hour period, and not more than 7 doses are recommended to be used in a 7-day period. The prescribed dosage should not be exceeded.

Adjunct to other tests in the diagnosis and management of erectile dysfunction.

MUSE can be used as an adjunct in evaluating penile vascular function using Doppler duplex ultrasonography. It has been shown that a 500 microgram dose of MUSE has a comparable effect on penile arterial dilatation and peak systolic velocity flow to 10 microgram of alprostadil given by intracavernosal injection. At the time of discharge from the clinic, the erection should have subsided.

Use in the elderly

No adjustment for age is required.

4.3 Contraindications

MUSE is contraindicated in men with any of the following conditions:

Hypersensitivity to the active substance or to any of the excipients.

Abnormal penile anatomy (stenosis of the distal urethra, severe hypospadia or severe curvature), balanitis, acute or chronic urethritis.

Conditions with an increased risk of priapism (sickle cell anaemia or trait, thrombocythaemia, polycythaemia, multiple myeloma; predisposition to venous thrombosis), or a history of recurrent priapism.

MUSE should not be used in men for whom sexual activity is inadvisable, as in men with unstable cardiovascular or unstable cerebrovascular conditions.

MUSE should not be used if the female partner is or may be pregnant unless the couple uses a condom barrier.

MUSE is contraindicated in women and children.

4.4 Special warnings and special precautions for use

Underlying treatable medical causes of erectile dysfunction should be diagnosed and treated prior to initiation of treatment with MUSE.

Incorrect insertion of MUSE may cause urethral abrasion and minor urethral bleeding. Patients on anticoagulants or with bleeding disorders may have an increased risk of urethral bleeding.

Patients should be asked to report promptly to their treating physician any erections lasting 4 hours or longer. For treatment: see 4.9. Overdose. In clinical trials of MUSE, priapism (rigid erections lasting ⩾6 hours) and prolonged erection (rigid erection lasting 4 hours and <6 hours) were reported infrequently (<0.1% and 0.3% of patients, respectively). Nevertheless, these events are a potential risk of pharmacologic therapy. It may be necessary to reduce the dose or discontinue treatment in any patient who develops priapism.

Patients and their partners should be advised that MUSE offers no protection from transmission of sexually transmitted diseases. They should be counselled about the protective measures that are necessary to guard against the spread of sexually transmitted agents, including the human immunodeficiency virus (HIV). The use of MUSE will not affect the integrity of condoms. Since MUSE may add small amounts of alprostadil to the naturally occurring PGE_1 already present in the semen, it is recommended that adequate contraception is used if the woman is of child-bearing potential.

4.5 Interaction with other medicinal products and other forms of Interaction

Systemic interactions are unlikely because of the low levels of alprostadil in the peripheral venous circulation, however the presence of medication affecting erectile function may influence the response to MUSE. Decongestants and appetite suppressants may diminish the effect of MUSE. Patients on anticoagulants or with bleeding disorders may have an increased risk of urethral bleeding. Insufficient data exists concerning the concomitant use of MUSE with vasoactive medications. There is the potential that this combination may increase the risk of hypotensive symptoms; this effect may be more common in the elderly.

There is limited information available in the literature concerning the concomitant use of MUSE and sildenafil for the treatment of erectile dysfunction. No conclusions can be drawn, however, regarding the safety or efficacy of this combination.

The use of MUSE in patients with penile implants has been reported in a limited number of cases in the literature. However no conclusions can be drawn regarding the safety or efficacy of this combination.

4.6 Pregnancy and lactation

MUSE may add small amounts of alprostadil to the naturally occurring PGE_1 already present in the semen. A condom barrier should therefore be used during sexual intercourse if the female partner is pregnant to avoid irritation of the vagina and guard against any risk to the foetus.

4.7 Effects on ability to drive and use machines

Patients should be cautioned to avoid activities, such as driving or hazardous tasks, where injury could result if hypotension or syncope were to occur after MUSE administration. In patients experiencing hypotension and/or syncope, these events have usually occurred during initial titration and within one hour of drug administration.

4.8 Undesirable effects

The most frequently reported adverse events in treatment with MUSE are presented in the table below. (Very common > 1/10; Common > 1/100, < 1/10; Uncommon > 1/1000, < 1/100; Rare > 1/10000, < 1/1000; Very rare < 1/10000)

System Organ Class	Frequency	Adverse Reaction
Nervous system disorders	Common	Headache, dizziness
	Uncommon	Syncope
Vascular disorders	Common	Symptomatic hypotension
Skin and subcutaneous disorders	Uncommon	Swelling of the leg veins
	Very rare	Rash, urticaria
Musculoskeletal, connective tissue and bone disorders	Uncommon	Leg pain
Renal and urinary disorders	Rare	Urinary tract infection
	Very common	Urethral burning
	Common	Minor urethral bleeding
Reproductive system	Very common	Penile pain
	Common	Testicular pain, vaginal burning/itching (in partners)
	Uncommon	Perineal pain
	Rare	Prolonged erection/priapism, penile disorders (e.g. fibrotic complications)
Investigations	Uncommon	Rapid pulse

Vaginal burning/itching was reported by approximately 6% of partners of patients on active treatment. This may be due to resuming sexual intercourse or due to the use of MUSE.

4.9 Overdose

Overdosage has not been reported with MUSE.

Symptomatic hypotension, persistent penile pain and in rare instances, priapism may occur with alprostadil overdosage. Patients should be kept under medical supervision until systemic or local symptoms have resolved.

Should a prolonged erection lasting 4 or more hours occur, the patient should be advised to seek medical help. The following actions can be taken:

- The patient should be supine or lying on his side. Apply an ice pack alternately for two minutes to each upper inner thigh (this may cause a reflex opening of the venous valves). If there is no response after 10 minutes, discontinue treatment.

- If this treatment is ineffective and a rigid erection has lasted for more than 6 hours, penile aspiration should be performed. Using aseptic technique, insert a 19-21 gauge butterfly needle into the corpus cavernosum and aspirate 20-50 ml of blood. This may detumesce the penis. If necessary, the procedure may be repeated on the opposite side of the penis.

- If still unsuccessful, intracavernous injection of α-adrenergic medication is recommended. Although the usual contraindication to intrapenile administration of a vasoconstrictor does not apply in the treatment of priapism, caution is advised when this option is exercised. Blood pressure and pulse should be continuously monitored during the procedure. Extreme caution is required in patients with coronary heart disease, uncontrolled hypertension, cerebral ischaemia, and in subjects taking monoamine oxidase inhibitors. In the latter case, facilities should be available to manage a hypertensive crisis.

- A 200 microgram/ml solution of phenylephrine should be prepared, and 0.5 to 1.0 ml of the solution injected every 5-10 minutes. Alternatively, a 20 microgram/ml solution of adrenaline should be used. If necessary, this may be followed by further aspiration of blood through the same butterfly needle. The maximum dose of phenylephrine should be 1 mg, or adrenaline 100 micrograms (5ml of the solution).

- As an alternative metaraminol may be used, but it should be noted that fatal hypertensive crises have been reported. If this still fails to resolve the priapism, the patient should immediately be referred for surgical management.

5. PHARMACOLOGICAL PROPERTIES

5.1 Pharmacodynamic properties

ATC Code: G04B E01 (Drugs used in erectile dysfunction).

Alprostadil is chemically identical to prostaglandin E_1, the actions of which include vasodilatation of blood vessels in the erectile tissues of the corpora cavernosa and increase in cavernosal artery blood flow, causing penile rigidity.

5.2 Pharmacokinetic properties

Approximately 80% of the alprostadil delivered by MUSE is absorbed through the urethral mucosa within 10 minutes. The half-life is less than 10 minutes and peripheral venous plasma concentrations are low or undetectable. Alprostadil is rapidly metabolised, both locally and in the pulmonary capillary bed; metabolites are excreted in the urine (90% within 24 hours) and the faeces. There is no evidence of tissue retention of alprostadil or its metabolites.

5.3 Preclinical safety data

In rats, high doses of prostaglandin E_1 increased foetal resorption, presumably due to maternal stress. High concentrations of alprostadil (400 microgram/ml) had no effect on human sperm motility or viability *in vitro*. In rabbits, there was no foetal damage or effect on reproductive function at the maximum tested intravaginal dose of 4mg.

In the majority of *in vitro* and *in vivo* genotoxicity test systems in which alprostadil has been evaluated it produced negative results. These tests include the bacterial reversion test using *Salmonella typhimurium*, unscheduled DNA synthesis in rat primary hepatocytes, forward mutation assay at the *hprt* locus in cultured ovary cells from Chinese hamsters, alkaline elution test, sister chromatid exchange assay (all *in vitro* tests) and the micronucleus test in both mice and rats (*in vivo* tests). In two other *in vitro* tests, the mouse lymphoma forward mutation assay and the Chinese hamster ovary chromosomal aberration assay, alprostadil produced borderline positive and positive evidence, respectively, for chromosomal damage. In view of the number of negative *in vitro* results and the lack of evidence for genotoxicity in two *in vivo* tests, it is considered that the positive results obtained in these two *in vitro* tests are of doubtful biological significance. Overall the presently available evidence cannot fully exclude the risk of genotoxic activity in humans.

6. PHARMACEUTICAL PARTICULARS

6.1 List of excipients

Macrogol 1450.

6.2 Incompatibilities

Not applicable.

6.3 Shelf life

2 years.

From a microbiological point of view, the product should be used immediately after opening the foil pouch.

6.4 Special precautions for storage

Store at 2°- 8°C (in a refrigerator). Store in the original package.

Unopened pouches may be kept out of the refrigerator by the patient, at a temperature below 30°C, for up to 14 days prior to use.

6.5 Nature and contents of container

MUSE is supplied as cartons of 1, 2, 3, 6 or 10 foil pouches, with each pouch containing one delivery system. Not all pack sizes may be marketed.

The pouches are composed of aluminium foil/laminate. The applicators are made from radiation-resistant medical-grade polypropylene.

6.6 Instructions for use and handling

Not applicable.

7. MARKETING AUTHORISATION HOLDER

Meda Pharmaceuticals Ltd

Sherwood House

7 Gregory Boulevard

Nottingham

NG7 6LB

UK

Trading as:

Meda Pharmaceuticals

Regus House

Herald Way

Pegasus Business Park

Castle Donington

DE74 2TZ

UK

8. MARKETING AUTHORISATION NUMBER(S)

MUSE® 125 micrograms PL 19477/0005

MUSE® 250 micrograms PL 19477/0006

MUSE® 500 micrograms PL 19477/0007

MUSE® 1000 micrograms PL 19477/0008

9. DATE OF FIRST AUTHORISATION/RENEWAL OF THE AUTHORISATION

24th November 1997/ 25th November 2002.

10. DATE OF REVISION OF THE TEXT

22nd June 2004.

11. LEGAL STATUS

POM.

MXL capsules

(Napp Pharmaceuticals Limited)

1. NAME OF THE MEDICINAL PRODUCT

MXL® capsules 30 mg, 60 mg, 90 mg, 120 mg, 150 mg, 200 mg.

2. QUALITATIVE AND QUANTITATIVE COMPOSITION

Capsules containing Morphine Sulphate PhEur 30 mg, 60 mg, 90 mg, 120 mg,

150 mg, 200 mg.

3. PHARMACEUTICAL FORM

Capsules, prolonged release.

Hard gelatin capsules containing white to off white multi-particulates.

MXL capsules 30 mg are size 4, light blue capsules marked MS OD30.

MXL capsules 60 mg are size 3, brown capsules marked MS OD60.

MXL capsules 90 mg are size 2, pink capsules marked MS OD90.

MXL capsules 120 mg are size 1, olive capsules marked MS OD120.

MXL capsules 150 mg are size 1, blue capsules marked MS OD150.

MXL capsules 200 mg are size 0, rust capsules marked MS OD200.

4. CLINICAL PARTICULARS

4.1 Therapeutic indications

The prolonged relief of severe and intractable pain.

4.2 Posology and method of administration

Route of administration

Oral.

The capsules may be swallowed whole or opened and the contents sprinkled on to soft cold food. The capsules and contents should not be crushed or chewed. ***MXL*** capsules should be used at 24-hourly intervals. The dosage is dependent upon the severity of the pain, the patient's age and previous history of analgesic requirements.

Adults and elderly

Patients presenting with severe uncontrolled pain, who are not currently receiving opioids, should have their dose requirements calculated through the use of immediate release morphine, where possible, before conversion to ***MXL*** capsules.

Patients presenting in pain, who are currently receiving weaker opioids should be started on:

a) 60 mg ***MXL*** capsule once-daily if they weigh over 70 kg.

b) 30 mg ***MXL*** capsule once-daily if they weigh under 70 kg, are frail or elderly.

Increasing severity of pain will require an increased dosage of ***MXL*** capsules using 30 mg, 60 mg, 90 mg, 120 mg, 150 mg or 200 mg alone or in combination to achieve pain relief. Higher doses should be made, where appropriate in 30% - 50% increments as required. The correct dosage for any individual patient is that which controls the pain with no or tolerable side effects for a full 24 hours.

Patients receiving ***MXL*** capsules in place of parenteral morphine should be given a sufficiently increased dosage to compensate for any reduction in analgesic effects associated with oral administration. Usually such increased requirement is of the order of 100%. In such patients individual dose adjustments are required.

Children aged 1 year and above

The use of ***MXL*** capsules in children has not been extensively evaluated.

For severe and intractable pain in cancer a starting dose in the range of 0.4 to 1.6 mg morphine per kg bodyweight daily is recommended. Doses should be titrated in the normal way as for adults.

4.3 Contraindications

Hypersensitivity to any of the constituents.

Respiratory depression, head injury, paralytic ileus, acute abdomen, delayed gastric emptying, obstructive airways disease, known morphine sensitivity, acute hepatic disease, concurrent administration of monoamine oxidase inhibitors (MAOIs) or within two weeks of discontinuation of their use. Not recommended during pregnancy or for pre-operative use or for the first 24 hours post-operatively. Children under one year of age.

4.4 Special warnings and special precautions for use

As with all narcotics, a reduction in dosage may be advisable in the elderly, in hypothyroidism, in renal and chronic hepatic disease. Use with caution in patients with convulsive disorders, raised intracranial pressure, hypotension with hypovolaemia, opioid dependent patients, diseases of the biliary tract, pancreatitis, inflammatory bowel disorders, prostatic hypertrophy and adrenocortical insufficiency.***MXL*** capsules should not be used where there is a possibility of paralytic ileus occurring. Should paralytic ileus be suspected or occur during use, ***MXL*** capsules should be discontinued immediately. As with all morphine preparations, patients who are to undergo cordotomy or other pain relieving surgical procedures should not receive ***MXL*** capsules for 24 hours prior to surgery. If further treatment with ***MXL*** capsules is then indicated the dosage should be adjusted to the new post-operative requirement.

It is not possible to ensure bio-equivalence between different brands of controlled release morphine products. Therefore, it should be emphasised that patients, once titrated to an effective dose should not be changed from ***MXL*** capsules to other slow, sustained or controlled release morphine or other potent narcotic analgesic preparations without retitration and clinical assessment.

4.5 Interaction with other medicinal products and other forms of Interaction

Monoamine oxidase inhibitors have been reported to react with narcotic analgesics, producing CNS excitation or depression with hyper- or hypotensive crisis. Morphine potentiates the effects of tranquillisers, anaesthetics, hypnotics and sedatives, alcohol, muscle relaxants and antihypertensives. Cimetidine inhibits the metabolism of morphine. Mixed agonist/antagonist opioid analgesics (e.g. buprenorphine, nalbuphine, pentazocine) should not be administered to a patient who has received a course of therapy with a pure opioid agonist analgesic.

4.6 Pregnancy and lactation

MXL capsules are not recommended for use in pregnancy and labour due to the risk of neonatal respiratory depression. Administration to nursing mothers is not recommended as morphine is excreted in breast milk. Withdrawal symptoms may be observed in the newborn of mothers undergoing chronic treatment.

4.7 Effects on ability to drive and use machines

Morphine may modify the patient's reactions to a varying extent depending on the dosage and individual susceptibility. If affected, patients should not drive or operate machinery.

4.8 Undesirable effects

In normal doses, the commonest side effects of morphine are nausea, vomiting, constipation and drowsiness. With chronic therapy, nausea and vomiting are unusual with ***MXL*** capsules but should they occur the capsules can be readily combined with an anti-emetic if required. Constipation may be treated with appropriate laxatives. Paralytic ileus may be associated with opioid usage. Dry mouth, sweating, vertigo, headache, disorientation, facial flushing, mood changes, palpitations, hallucinations, bronchospasm, miosis, rash, myoclonus, decreased libido and colic may occur in a few patients. Micturition may be difficult and there may be biliary or ureteric spasm. Overdose may produce respiratory depression. Rarely, clinically relevant reductions in blood pressure and heart rate have been observed. Morphine has histamine releasing effects which may be responsible in part for reactions such as urticaria and pruritus.

The effects of morphine have led to its abuse and dependence may develop with regular, inappropriate use. This is not a major concern in the treatment of patients with severe pain.

4.9 Overdose

Signs of morphine toxicity and overdosage are drowsiness, pin-point pupils, respiratory depression and hypotension. Circulatory failure and deepening coma may occur in more severe cases. Rhabdomyolysis progressing to renal failure has been reported in opioid overdosage.

Treatment of morphine overdosage:

Primary attention should be given to the establishment of a patent airway and institution of assisted or controlled ventilation.

In the case of massive overdosage, administer naloxone 0.8 mg intravenously. Repeat at 2-3 minute intervals as necessary, or by an infusion of 2 mg in 500 ml of normal saline or 5% dextrose (0.004 mg/ml).

The infusion should be run at a rate related to the previous bolus doses administered and should be in accordance with the patient's response. However, because the duration of action of naloxone is relatively short, the patient must be carefully monitored until spontaneous respiration is reliably re-established. MXL capsules will continue to release and add to the morphine load for up to 24 hours after administration and the management of morphine overdosage should be modified accordingly.

For less severe overdosage, administer naloxone 0.2 mg intravenously followed by increments of 0.1 mg every 2 minutes if required.

Naloxone should not be administered in the absence of clinically significant respiratory or circulatory depression secondary to morphine overdosage. Naloxone should be administered cautiously to persons who are known, or suspected, to be physically dependent on morphine. In such cases, an abrupt or complete reversal of opioid effects may precipitate an acute withdrawal syndrome.

Gastric contents may need to be emptied as this can be useful in removing unabsorbed drug, particularly when a modified release formulation has been taken.

5. PHARMACOLOGICAL PROPERTIES

5.1 Pharmacodynamic properties

Morphine acts as an agonist at opiate receptors in the CNS particularly mu and to a lesser extent kappa receptors. mu receptors are thought to mediate supraspinal analgesia, respiratory depression and euphoria and kappa receptors, spinal analgesia, miosis and sedation. Morphine has also a direct action on the bowel wall nerve plexuses causing constipation.

5.2 Pharmacokinetic properties

Morphine is well absorbed from the capsules and, in general, peak plasma concentrations are achieved 2-6 hours following administration. The availability is complete when compared to an immediate release oral solution or MST® CONTINUS® tablets. The pharmacokinetics of morphine are linear across a very wide dose range. Morphine is subject to a significant first-pass effect which results in a lower bioavailability when compared to an equivalent intravenous or intramuscular dose.

The major metabolic transformation of morphine is glucuronidation to morphine-3-glucuronide and morphine-6-glucuronide which then undergo renal excretion. These metabolites are excreted in bile and may be subject to hydrolysis and subsequent reabsorption.

Because of the high inter-patient variation in morphine pharmacokinetics, and in analgesic requirements, the daily dosage in individual patients must be titrated to achieve appropriate pain control. Daily doses of up to 11.2 g have been recorded from 12-hourly MST CONTINUS tablets. For this reason the capsules have been formulated in strengths of 30 mg, 60 mg, 90 mg, 120 mg, 150 mg and 200 mg.

5.3 Preclinical safety data

There are no pre-clinical data of relevance to the prescriber which are additional to that already included in other sections of the SPC.

6. PHARMACEUTICAL PARTICULARS

6.1 List of excipients

Hydrogenated Vegetable Oil

Macrogol 6000

Talc

Magnesium Stearate

Capsule shells

Gelatin (containing sodium dodecylsulphate)

The following colours are also present:

30 mg: indigo carmine (E132), titanium dioxide (E171);

60 mg: indigo carmine (E132), titanium dioxide (E171), iron oxide (E172);

90 mg: erythrosine (E127), titanium dioxide (E171), iron oxide (E172);

120 mg: indigo carmine (E132), titanium dioxide (E171), iron oxide (E172);

150 mg: erythrosine (E127), indigo carmine (E132), titanium dioxide (E171), iron oxide (E172);

200 mg: titanium dioxide (E171), iron oxide (E172).

Printing ink

Shellac DAB 10

Iron oxide, black (E172)

Soya lecithin

Dimethylpolysiloxane

6.2 Incompatibilities

None known.

6.3 Shelf life

3 years.

6.4 Special precautions for storage

Do not store above 25°C.

6.5 Nature and contents of container

PVdC (⩾ 40 gsm) coated PVC (250 μm) blister strip with aluminium backing foil. The blister strips will be enclosed in a cardboard box. Each box contains 28 capsules.

6.6 Instructions for use and handling

None.

Administrative Data

7. MARKETING AUTHORISATION HOLDER

Napp Pharmaceuticals Ltd

Cambridge Science Park

Milton Road

Cambridge CB4 0GW

8. MARKETING AUTHORISATION NUMBER(S)

PL 16950/0042-47

9. DATE OF FIRST AUTHORISATION/RENEWAL OF THE AUTHORISATION

29 March 1996/ 28 March 2001

10. DATE OF REVISION OF THE TEXT

May 2002

11. Legal Category

CD (Sch 2), POM

MXL capsules are the subject of European Patent Application Numbers: 94304144.2, 94308493.9, 94115465.0 and 94109655.4

® ***MXL*** and the NAPP device are Registered Trade Marks.

Mycobutin

(Pharmacia Limited)

1. NAME OF THE MEDICINAL PRODUCT

Mycobutin®

2. QUALITATIVE AND QUANTITATIVE COMPOSITION

Rifabutin INN 150.0 mg

3. PHARMACEUTICAL FORM

Opaque, red-brown, hard gelatin capsules Size N°. 0 containing 150 mg rifabutin in transparent PVC/Al blisters or in amber glass bottles.

The capsules are for oral administration.

4. CLINICAL PARTICULARS

4.1 Therapeutic indications

Mycobutin is indicated for:

- the prophylaxis of *M. avium intracellulare complex* (MAC) infections in patients with HIV disease with CD4 counts lower than 75 cells/mcl.

- the treatment of non-tuberculous mycobacterial disease (such as that caused by MAC and M. xenopi).

- pulmonary tuberculosis.

4.2 Posology and method of administration

Mycobutin can be administered as a single, daily, oral dose at any time independently of meals.

-Adults

- prophylaxis of *M. avium intracellulare complex* (MAC) infections in patients with HIV disease with CD4 counts lower than 75 cells/mcl.:

300 mg (2 capsules) as a single agent.

- treatment of non-tuberculous mycobaterial disease:

450 - 600 mg (3 - 4 capsules) in combination regimens for up to 6 months after negative cultures are obtained.

When Mycobutin is given in association with clarithromycin (or other macrolides) and/or fluconazole (or related compounds) the Mycobutin dosage may need to be reduced to 300 mg (see Section 4.5).

- treatment of pulmonary tuberculosis:

150 - 450 mg (1 - 3 capsules) in combination regimens for at least 6 months.

In accordance with the commonly accepted criteria for the treatment of mycobacterial infections, Mycobutin should always be given in combination with other anti-mycobacterial drugs not belonging to the family of rifamycins.

Children

There are inadequate data to support the use of Mycobutin in children at the present time.

Elderly

No specific recommendations for dosage alterations in the elderly are suggested.

4.3 Contraindications

Mycobutin is contra-indicated in patients with a history of hypersensitivity to rifabutin or other rifamycins (eg rifampicin).

Due to insufficient clinical experience in pregnant and breast-feeding women and in children, Mycobutin should not be used in these patients.

4.4 Special warnings and special precautions for use

Before starting Mycobutin prophylaxis, patients should be assessed to ensure that they do not have active disease caused by pulmonary tuberculosis or other mycobacteria.

Prophylaxis against MAC infection may need to be continued throughout the patient's lifetime.

Mycobutin may impart a red-orange colour to the urine and possibly to skin and body secretions. Contact lenses, especially soft, may be permanently stained.

Mild hepatic impairment does not require a dose modification. Mycobutin should be used with caution in cases of severe liver insufficiency. Mild to moderate renal impairment does not require any dosage adjustment.

Severe renal impairment (creatinine clearance below 30 ml/min) requires a dosage reduction of 50%.

It is recommended that white blood cell and platelet counts and liver enzymes be monitored periodically during treatment.

Because of the possibility of occurrence of uveitis, patients should be carefully monitored when rifabutin is given in combination with clarithromycin (or other macrolides) and/or fluconazole (and related compounds). If such an event occurs, the patient should be referred to an ophthalmologist and, if considered necessary, Mycobutin treatment should be suspended.

Uveitis associated with Mycobutin must be distinguished from other ocular complications of HIV.

4.5 Interaction with other medicinal products and other forms of Interaction

Rifabutin has been shown to induce the enzymes of the cytochrome P450 3A subfamily and therefore may affect the pharmacokinetic behaviour of drugs metabolised by the enzymes belonging to this subfamily. Upward adjustment of the dosage of such drugs may be required when administered with Mycobutin.

Similarly, Mycobutin might reduce the activity of analgesics, anticoagulants, corticosteroids, cyclosporin, digitalis (although not digoxin), oral hypoglycaemics, narcotics, phenytoin and quinidine.

Clinical studies have shown that Mycobutin does not affect the pharmacokinetics of didanosine (DDI), and isoniazid (however, for the latter refer also to undesirable effects). On the basis of the above metabolic considerations no significant interaction may be expected with ethambutol, theophylline, sulphonamides, pyrazinamide and zalcitabine (DDC).

As p-aminosalicylic acid has been shown to impede GI absorption of rifamycins it is recommended that when it and Mycobutin are both to be administered they be given with an interval of 8 - 12 hours.

The following table provides details of the possible effects of co-administration, on rifabutin and the co-administered drug, and risk-benefit statement.

(see Table 1 on next page)

4.6 Pregnancy and lactation

Due to lack of data in pregnant women, as a precautionary measure, Mycobutin should not be administered to pregnant women or those breast-feeding children even though in experimental animal studies the drug was not teratogenic.

Mycobutin may interact with oral contraceptives (see Section 4.5).

4.7 Effects on ability to drive and use machines

There have been no reports of adverse effects on ability to drive and use machines.

4.8 Undesirable effects

The tolerability of Mycobutin in multiple drug regimens, was assessed in both immunocompetent and immunocompromised patients, suffering from tuberculosis and non-tuberculous mycobacteriosis in long term studies with daily dosages up to 600 mg.

Bearing in mind that Mycobutin was often given in these studies as part of a multidrug regimen it is not possible to define with certainty a drug-event relationship. Treatment discontinuation was necessary only in a very few cases. The most commonly reported adverse events, were primarily related to:

- the gastro-intestinal system, such as nausea, vomiting, increase of liver enzymes, jaundice;
- the blood and lymphatic system, such as leucopenia, neutropenia, thrombocytopenia and anemia, where the frequency and severity of haematologic reactions could be increased by combined administration of isoniazid;
- the musculo-skeletal system: arthralgia and myalgia.

Table 1

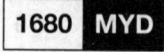

Coadministered drugs	Effect on rifabutin	Effect on co-administered drug	Comments
ANTIVIRALS			
Indinavir	20% increase in AUC.	32% decrease in AUC.	
Saquinavir	No data.	40% decrease in AUC.	
Ritonavir	4-fold increase in AUC, 2.5-fold increase in Cmax	No data	Due to this multifold increase in rifabutin concentrations and the subsequent risk of side effects, patients requiring both rifabutin and a protease inhibitor, other protease inhibitors should be considered.
Zidovudine	No significant change in kinetics	Approx. 32% decrease in Cmax and AUC.	A large clinical study has shown that these changes are of no clinical relevance.
ANTIFUNGALS			
Fluconazole	82% increase in AUC.	No significant change in steady-state plasma concentrations	
Itraconazole	No data.	70-75% decrease in Cmax and AUC.	A case report indicates an increase in rifabutin serum levels in the presence of itraconazole.
Ketoconazole/ miconazole	No data.	No data.	Co-administered medications, such as ketoconazole, that competitively inhibit the Cyt P450IIIA activity may increase circulating drug levels of rifabutin.
ANTI-PCP (Pneumocystis carinii pneumonia)			
Dapsone	No data.	Approximately 27%-40% decrease in AUC.	Study conducted in HIV infected patients (rapid and slow acetylators)
Sulfamethoxazole-Trimethoprim	No significant change in Cmax and AUC.	Approx. 15-20% decrease in AUC.	In another study, only trimethoprim (not sulfamethoxazole) had 14% decrease in AUC and 6% in Cmax but were not considered clinically significant.
ANTI-MAC (Mycobacterium avium intracellulare complex)			
Clarithromycin	Approx. 77% increase in AUC.	Approx. 50% decrease in AUC.	Study conducted in HIV infected patients
OTHER			
Methadone	No data.	No significant effect.	No apparent effect of rifabutin on either peak levels of methadone or systemic exposure based upon AUC. Rifabutin kinetics not evaluated.
Oral contraceptives	No data.	No data.	Contraceptive cover may not be adequate during concomitant therapy with rifabutin, therefore, patients should be advised to use other methods of contraception.
Tacrolimus	No data.	No data.	Rifabutin decreases tacrolimus trough blood levels.

Also, fever, rash and rarely other hypersensitivity reactions such as eosinophilia, bronchospasm and shock might occur as has been seen with other antibiotics.

In addition, mild to severe, reversible uveitis has been reported. The risk appears to be low, when Mycobutin is used at 300 mg as monotherapy in MAC prophylaxis, but increases when Mycobutin is administered at higher doses in combination with clarithromycin (or other macrolides) for MAC treatment (see Section 4.4). The possible role of fluconazole (and related compounds) has not been established yet.

Asymptomatic corneal opacities have been reported after long term therapy.

Pseudojaundice (yellow skin discolouration with normal plasma bilirubin) has been reported with high doses of rifabutin. Flu-like syndrome, chest pressure or pain with dyspnoea and rarely hepatitis and haemolysis. Clostridium difficile diarrhoea has been reported rarely.

4.9 Overdose

Gastric lavage and diuretic treatment should be carried out. Supportive care and symptomatic treatment should be administered.

5. PHARMACOLOGICAL PROPERTIES

5.1 Pharmacodynamic properties

In vitro activity of rifabutin against laboratory strains and clinical isolates of *M. tuberculosis* has been shown to be very high. *In vitro* studies carried out so far have shown that from one-third to half of *M.tuberculosis* strains resistant to rifampicin are susceptible to rifabutin, indicating that cross-resistance between the two antibiotics is incomplete.

The *in vivo* activity of rifabutin on experimental infections caused by *M. tuberculosis* was about 10 times greater than that of rifampicin in agreement with the *in vitro* findings.

Rifabutin was seen to be active against non-tuberculous (atypical) mycobacteria including *M. avium-intracellulare* (MAC), *in vitro* as well as in experimental infections caused by these pathogens in mice with induced immuno-deficiency.

5.2 Pharmacokinetic properties

In man, rifabutin is rapidly absorbed and maximum plasma concentrations are reached around 2-4 hours after oral administration. The pharmacokinetics of rifabutin is linear after single administration of 300, 450, and 600 mg to healthy volunteers. With these doses, C max is in the range of 0.4-0.7 μg/ml. Plasma concentrations are maintained above the MIC values for *M. tuberculosis* up to about 30 hours from administration.

Rifabutin is widely distributed in various animal organs with the exception of the brain. In particular, in human lung tissue the concentrations measured up to 24 hours after dosing were about 5-10 times higher than the plasma levels.

The intracellular penetration of rifabutin is very high as demonstrated by intracellular/extracellular concentration ratios which ranged from 9 in neutrophils to 15 in monocytes, both obtained from human sources.

The high intracellular concentration is likely to play a crucial role in sustaining the efficacy of rifabutin against intracellular pathogens such as mycobacteria.

Rifabutin and its metabolites are eliminated mainly by the urinary route. The $t_{1/2}$ of rifabutin in man is approximately 35-40 hours.

5.3 Preclinical safety data

Preclinical safety studies of rifabutin indicate a good safety margin in rodents and in monkeys.

In repeated dose studies, target organs were identified at doses producing blood levels higher than those achieved with recommended doses for human therapy. The main target organs are liver and, to a lesser degree, erythrocytes.

Rifabutin did not show any teratogenic, mutagenic or carcinogenic potential.

6. PHARMACEUTICAL PARTICULARS

6.1 List of excipients

Microcrystalline cellulose

Sodium lauryl sulphate

Magnesium stearate

Silica gel

6.2 Incompatibilities

None known.

6.3 Shelf life

24 months at room temperature.

6.4 Special precautions for storage

None.

6.5 Nature and contents of container

Transparent PVC/Al blisters in cardboard cartons containing 30 capsules or amber glass bottles containing 30 or 100 capsules.

6.6 Instructions for use and handling

There are no special instructions for handling.

Administrative Data

7. MARKETING AUTHORISATION HOLDER

Pharmacia Limited

Davy Avenue

Milton Keynes

MK5 8PH

United Kingdom

8. MARKETING AUTHORISATION NUMBER(S)

PL 00032/0320

9. DATE OF FIRST AUTHORISATION/RENEWAL OF THE AUTHORISATION

15th January 2003.

10. DATE OF REVISION OF THE TEXT

Legal Category

POM

Mydrilate 0.5% Eye Drops

(Intrapharm Laboratories Ltd)

1. NAME OF THE MEDICINAL PRODUCT

Mydrilate 0.5 % Eye Drops.

2. QUALITATIVE AND QUANTITATIVE COMPOSITION

Cyclopentolate Hydrochloride BP 0.5 % w/v.

3. PHARMACEUTICAL FORM

Eye drops.

4. CLINICAL PARTICULARS

4.1 Therapeutic indications

(i) Diagnostic purposes for fundoscopy and cycloplegic refraction.

(ii) Dilating the pupil in inflammatory conditions of the iris and uveal tract.

4.2 Posology and method of administration

(i) Refraction / Fundoscopy

Adults (and the elderly):

One drop of 0.5 % solution instilled into the eye, repeated after 15 minutes if necessary, approximately 40 minutes before examination.

Deeply pigmented eyes may require the use of a 1 % solution.

NB: Maximum effect is reached after 30-60 minutes.

Children 6-16 years:

One drop of 1 % solution instilled into the eye, repeated after 15 minutes if necessary, approximately 40 minutes before examination.

Children under 6 years:

One or two drops of 1 % solution instilled into the eye, repeated after 15 minutes if necessary, approximately 40 minutes before examination.

(ii) For Uveitis, Iritis and Iridocyclitis:

Adults and the elderly:

One or two drops of 0.5 % solution instilled into the eye up to 4 times daily or as required.

Deeply pigmented eyes may require the use of a 1 % solution.

Children:

At the discretion of the physician

Do not use during the first three months of life due to possible association between the cycloplegia produced and the development of amblyopia and also the increased risks of systemic toxicity in neonates.

Cycloplegia following administration is quick in onset and short-lived. Maximal cycloplegia is achieved within 15 - 45 minutes of instillation and lasts on average about 20 minutes. Recovery normally takes place in about 4 hours, but very occasionally some effect persists for up to 24 hours.

Mydriasis is produced very rapidly and an average pupil diameter of 7 mm is usually reached 15 - 30 minutes after instillation of one drop of 0.5 % solution. Complete recovery from the mydriatic effect generally occurs spontaneously in not more than 20 hours.

No specific information on the use of this product in the elderly is available. Clinical trials have included patients over 65 years and no adverse reactions specific to this age group have been reported.

4.3 Contraindications

(i) Use in narrow-angle glaucoma or those with a tendency towards glaucoma e.g. patients with a shallow anterior chamber.

(ii) Hypersensitivity to cyclopentolate hydrochloride, benzalkonium chloride or any other components of the formulation.

(iii) This preparation contains benzalkonium chloride and should not be used whilst soft contact lenses are being worn.

(iv) Use in patients with paralytic ileus.

(v) Use in children with organic brain syndromes, including congenital or neuro-developmental abnormalities, particularly those predisposing to epileptic seizures.

4.4 Special warnings and special precautions for use

Because of the risk of precipitating angle-closure glaucoma in the elderly and others prone to raised intraocular pressure, an estimate of the depth of the anterior chamber should be made before use, particularly if therapy is likely to be intense or protracted.

Caution should be observed when drugs of this group are administered to patients with prostatic enlargement, coronary insufficiency or cardiac failure, or ataxia. Atropine-like effects have been reported as side-effects.

Extreme caution is advised for use in children and individuals susceptible to belladonna alkaloids because of the increased risk of systemic toxicity.

Patients should be warned of the oral toxicity of this preparation, and advised to wash their hands after use. If accidentally swallowed, patients should be advised to seek medical attention.

Use with caution in an inflamed eye as the hyperaemia greatly increases the rate of systemic absorption through the conjunctiva.

To reduce systemic absorption the lacrimal sac should be compressed at the medial canthus by digital pressure for at least two minutes after instillation of the drops.

4.5 Interaction with other medicinal products and other forms of Interaction

The effects of anti-muscarinic agents may be enhanced by the concomitant administration of other drugs with anti-muscarinic properties such as some antihistamines, butyrophenones, phenothiazines, tricyclic antidepressants and amantadine.

4.6 Pregnancy and lactation

There is insufficient evidence as to drug safety in pregnancy and lactation. This product should not be used during pregnancy unless it is considered essential by a physician.

4.7 Effects on ability to drive and use machines

May cause blurred vision, difficulty in focusing and sensitivity to light. Patients should be warned not to drive or engage in other hazardous activities (including climbing ladders and scaffolding) unless vision is clear. Complete recovery from the effects of Mydrilate Eye Drops may take up to 24 hours.

4.8 Undesirable effects

(i) Local:

Increased intraocular pressure, transient stinging, and sensitivity to light secondary to pupillary dilation. Prolonged administration may lead to local irritation, hyperaemia, oedema and conjunctivitis.

(ii) Systemic:

Systemic anticholinergic toxicity is manifested by dryness of the mouth, flushing, dryness of the skin, bradycardia followed by tachycardia with palpitations and arrhythmias, urinary urgency, difficulty and retention, reduction in the tone and motility of the gastrointestinal tract leading to constipation.

(iii) Vomiting, giddiness and staggering may occur, a rash may be present in children, abdominal distension in infants. Psychotic reactions, behavioural disturbances and cardio-respiratory collapse may occur in children.

4.9 Overdose

Systemic toxicity may occur following topical use, particularly in children. It is manifested by flushing and dryness of the skin (a rash may be present in children), blurred vision, a rapid and irregular pulse, fever, abdominal distension in infants, convulsions and hallucinations and the loss of neuromuscular co-ordination.

Treatment is supportive (there is no evidence that physostigmine is superior to supportive management). In infants and small children the body surface must be kept moist. If accidentally ingested, induce emesis or perform gastric lavage.

5. PHARMACOLOGICAL PROPERTIES

5.1 Pharmacodynamic properties

Cyclopentolate is an anti-muscarinic agent used topically in the eye as a mydriatic and cycloplegic. The effects are similar to those of atropine, but with a more rapid onset and a shorter duration of action.

5.2 Pharmacokinetic properties

None stated.

5.3 Preclinical safety data

None stated.

6. PHARMACEUTICAL PARTICULARS

6.1 List of excipients

Boric acid

Potassium chloride

Benzalkonium chloride solution

Purified water.

6.2 Incompatibilities

None stated.

6.3 Shelf life

2 years.

6.4 Special precautions for storage

Store at 2-8 C. Refrigerate, do not freeze. Protect from light.

Do not dilute or dispense from any container other than the original bottle. Discard one month after opening.

6.5 Nature and contents of container

5 ml dropper bottle of 0.5 % solution.

Bottle: LE 6601 PH (LDPE)

Natural colour

Cap Melochem ™

White colour

6.6 Instructions for use and handling

When using the product for the first time, screw down firmly to pierce the seal at the tip of the plastic nozzle.

7. MARKETING AUTHORISATION HOLDER

Intrapharm Laboratories Ltd

60 Boughton Lane

Maidstone

Kent

ME15 9QS

United Kingdom

8. MARKETING AUTHORISATION NUMBER(S)

17509/0007

9. DATE OF FIRST AUTHORISATION/RENEWAL OF THE AUTHORISATION

17 December 1999

10. DATE OF REVISION OF THE TEXT

June 2002

11. Legal category

POM

Mydrilate 1.0% Eye Drops

(Intrapharm Laboratories Ltd)

1. NAME OF THE MEDICINAL PRODUCT

Mydrilate 1.0 % Eye Drops

2. QUALITATIVE AND QUANTITATIVE COMPOSITION

Cyclopentolate Hydrochloride BP 1.0 % w/v.

3. PHARMACEUTICAL FORM

Eye drops.

4. CLINICAL PARTICULARS

4.1 Therapeutic indications

(i) Diagnostic purposes for fundoscopy and cycloplegic refraction.

(ii) Dilating the pupil in inflammatory conditions of the iris and uveal tract.

4.2 Posology and method of administration

(i) Refraction / Fundoscopy

Adults (and the elderly):

One drop of 0.5 % solution instilled into the eye, repeated after 15 minutes if necessary, approximately 40 minutes before examination.

Deeply pigmented eyes may require the use of a 1 % solution.

NB: Maximum effect is reached after 30-60 minutes.

Children 6-16 years:

One drop of 1 % solution instilled into the eye, repeated after 15 minutes if necessary, approximately 40 minutes before examination.

Children under 6 years:

One or two drops of 1 % solution instilled into the eye, repeated after 15 minutes if necessary, approximately 40 minutes before examination.

(ii) For Uveitis, Iritis and Iridocyclitis:

Adults and the elderly:

One or two drops of 0.5 % solution instilled into the eye up to 4 times daily or as required.

Deeply pigmented eyes may require the use of a 1 % solution.

Children:

At the discretion of the physician

Do not use during the first three months of life due to possible association between the cycloplegia produced and the development of amblyopia and also the increased risks of systemic toxicity in neonates.

Cycloplegia following administration is quick in onset and short-lived. Maximal cycloplegia is achieved within 15 - 45 minutes of instillation and lasts on average about 20 minutes. Recovery normally takes place in about 4 hours, but very occasionally some effect persists for up to 24 hours.

Mydriasis is produced very rapidly and an average pupil diameter of 7 mm is usually reached 15 - 30 minutes after instillation of one drop of 0.5 % solution. Complete recovery from the mydriatic effect generally occurs spontaneously in not more than 20 hours.

No specific information on the use of this product in the elderly is available. Clinical trials have included patients over 65 years and no adverse reactions specific to this age group have been reported.

4.3 Contraindications

(i) Use in narrow-angle glaucoma or those with a tendency towards glaucoma e.g. patients with a shallow anterior chamber.

(ii) Hypersensitivity to cyclopentolate hydrochloride, benzalkonium chloride or any other components of the formulation.

(iii) This preparation contains benzalkonium chloride and should not be used whilst soft contact lenses are being worn.

(iv) Use in patients with paralytic ileus.

(v) Use in children with organic brain syndromes, including congenital or neuro-developmental abnormalities, particularly those predisposing to epileptic seizures.

4.4 Special warnings and special precautions for use

Because of the risk of precipitating angle-closure glaucoma in the elderly and others prone to raised intraocular pressure, an estimate of the depth of the anterior chamber should be made before use, particularly if therapy is likely to be intense or protracted.

Caution should be observed when drugs of this group are administered to patients with prostatic enlargement, coronary insufficiency or cardiac failure, or ataxia. Atropine-like effects have been reported as side-effects.

Extreme caution is advised for use in children and individuals susceptible to belladonna alkaloids because of the increased risk of systemic toxicity.

Patients should be warned of the oral toxicity of this preparation, and advised to wash their hands after use. If accidentally swallowed, patients should be advised to seek medical attention.

Use with caution in an inflamed eye as the hyperaemia greatly increases the rate of systemic absorption through the conjunctiva.

To reduce systemic absorption the lacrimal sac should be compressed at the medial canthus by digital pressure for at least two minutes after instillation of the drops.

4.5 Interaction with other medicinal products and other forms of Interaction

The effects of anti-muscarinic agents may be enhanced by the concomitant administration of other drugs with anti-muscarinic properties such as some antihistamines, butyrophenones, phenothiazines, tricyclic antidepressants and amantadine.

4.6 Pregnancy and lactation

There is insufficient evidence as to drug safety in pregnancy and lactation. This product should not be used during pregnancy unless it is considered essential by a physician.

4.7 Effects on ability to drive and use machines
May cause blurred vision, difficulty in focusing and sensitivity to light. Patients should be warned not to drive or engage in other hazardous activities (including climbing ladders and scaffolding) unless vision is clear. Complete recovery from the effects of Mydrilate Eye Drops may take up to 24 hours.

4.8 Undesirable effects

(i) Local:

Increased intraocular pressure, transient stinging, and sensitivity to light secondary to pupillary dilation. Prolonged administration may lead to local irritation, hyperaemia, oedema and conjunctivitis.

(ii) Systemic:

Systemic anticholinergic toxicity is manifested by dryness of the mouth, flushing, dryness of the skin, bradycardia followed by tachycardia with palpitations and arrhythmias, urinary urgency, difficulty and retention, reduction in the tone and motility of the gastrointestinal tract leading to constipation.

(iii) Vomiting, giddiness and staggering may occur, a rash may be present in children, abdominal distension in infants. Psychotic reactions, behavioural disturbances and cardio-respiratory collapse may occur in children.

4.9 Overdose
Systemic toxicity may occur following topical use, particularly in children. It is manifested by flushing and dryness of the skin (a rash may be present in children), blurred vision, a rapid and irregular pulse, fever, abdominal distension in infants, convulsions and hallucinations and the loss of neuromuscular co-ordination.

Treatment is supportive (there is no evidence that physostigmine is superior to supportive management). In infants and small children the body surface must be kept moist. If accidentally ingested, induce emesis or perform gastric lavage.

5. PHARMACOLOGICAL PROPERTIES

5.1 Pharmacodynamic properties
Cyclopentolate is an anti-muscarinic agent used topically in the eye as a mydriatic and cycloplegic. The effects are similar to those of atropine, but with a more rapid onset and a shorter duration of action.

5.2 Pharmacokinetic properties
None stated.

5.3 Preclinical safety data
None stated.

6. PHARMACEUTICAL PARTICULARS

6.1 List of excipients
Boric acid

Potassium chloride

Benzalkonium chloride solution

Purified water.

6.2 Incompatibilities
None stated.

6.3 Shelf life
2 years.

6.4 Special precautions for storage
Store at 2-8 C. Refrigerate, do not freeze. Protect from light. Do not dilute or dispense from any container other than the original bottle. Discard one month after opening.

6.5 Nature and contents of container
5 ml dropper bottle of 1.0 % solution.

Bottle: LE 6601 PH (LDPE)

Natural colour

Cap: Melochem

White colour

6.6 Instructions for use and handling
When using the product for the first time, screw down the cap firmly on the bottle to pierce the seal at the tip of the plastic nozzle and unscrew the cap for use.

7. MARKETING AUTHORISATION HOLDER
Intrapharm Laboratories Ltd

60 Boughton Lane

Maidstone

Kent

ME15 9QS

United Kingdom

8. MARKETING AUTHORISATION NUMBER(S)
PL 17509/0008

9. DATE OF FIRST AUTHORISATION/RENEWAL OF THE AUTHORISATION
8 August 2001

10. DATE OF REVISION OF THE TEXT
June 2002

11. Legal category
POM

MYFORTIC film-coated gastro-resistant tablets

(Novartis Pharmaceuticals UK Ltd)

1. NAME OF THE MEDICINAL PRODUCT
Myfortic® 180 mg film-coated gastro-resistant tablet

Myfortic® 360 mg film-coated gastro-resistant tablet.

2. QUALITATIVE AND QUANTITATIVE COMPOSITION
Each film-coated gastro-resistant tablet contains 180mg or 360 mg mycophenolic acid (as mycophenolate sodium).

For excipients, see Section 6.1.

3. PHARMACEUTICAL FORM
Film-coated gastro-resistant tablet.

180mg: Lime green, film-coated round tablet, with bevelled edges and the imprint (debossing) "C" on one side.

360mg: Pale orange red film-coated ovaloid tablets with imprint (debossing) 'CT' on one side.

4. CLINICAL PARTICULARS

4.1 Therapeutic indications
Myfortic is indicated in combination with ciclosporin and corticosteroids for the prophylaxis of acute transplant rejection in adult patients receiving allogeneic renal transplants.

4.2 Posology and method of administration
Treatment with Myfortic should be initiated and maintained by appropriately qualified transplant specialists.

The recommended dose is 720 mg administered twice daily (1440 mg daily dose). This dose of mycophenolate sodium corresponds to 1g mycophenolate mofetil administered twice daily (2 g daily dose) in terms of mycophenolic acid (MPA) content.

For additional information about the corresponding therapeutic doses of mycophenolate sodium and mycophenolate mofetil, see Sections 4.4 and 5.2.

In *de novo* patients, Myfortic should be initiated within 72 hours following transplantation.

Myfortic can be taken with or without food. Patients may select either option but must adhere to their selected option (see Section 5.2).

In order to retain the integrity of the enteric coating, Myfortic tablets should not be crushed.

Children and adolescents:

Insufficient data are available to support the efficacy and safety of Myfortic in children and adolescents. Limited pharmacokinetic data are available for paediatric renal transplant patients (see Section 5.2).

Elderly:

The recommended dose in elderly patients is 720 mg twice daily.

Patients with renal impairment:

In patients experiencing delayed renal graft function post-operatively, no dose adjustments are needed (see Section 5.2).

Patients with severe renal impairment (glomerular filtration rate < 25 ml·min^{-1}·1.73 m^{-2}) should be carefully monitored and the daily dose of Myfortic should not exceed 1440 mg.

Patients with hepatic impairment:

No dose adjustments are needed for renal transplant patients with severe hepatic impairment.

Treatment during rejection episodes:

Renal transplant rejection does not lead to changes in mycophenolic acid (MPA) pharmacokinetics; dosage modification or interruption of Myfortic is not required.

4.3 Contraindications
Hypersensitivity to mycophenolate sodium, mycophenolic acid or mycophenolate mofetil or to any of the excipients (see Section 6.1).

For information on use in pregnancy and lactation and contraceptive requirements, see Section 4.6.

4.4 Special warnings and special precautions for use
Patients receiving immunosuppressive regimens involving combinations of drugs, including Myfortic, are at increased risk of developing lymphomas and other malignancies, particularly of the skin (see Section 4.8). The risk appears to be related to the intensity and duration of immunosuppression rather than to the use of any specific agent. As general advice to minimise the risk for skin cancer, exposure to sunlight and UV light should be limited by wearing protective clothing and using a sunscreen with a high protection factor.

Patients receiving Myfortic should be instructed to immediately report any evidence of infection, unexpected bruising, bleeding or any other manifestation of bone marrow depression. Oversuppression of the immune system increases the susceptibility to infection including opportunistic infections, fatal infections and sepsis (see Section 4.8).

Patients receiving Myfortic should be monitored for neutropenia, which may be related to MPA itself, concomitant medications, viral infections, or some combination of these causes. Patients taking MPA should have complete blood counts weekly during the first month, twice monthly for the second and third months of treatment, then monthly through the first year. If neutropenia develops (absolute neutrophil count $<1.5 \times 10^3/\mu l$) it may be appropriate to interrupt or discontinue Myfortic.

Patients should be advised that during treatment with MPA vaccinations may be less effective and the use of live attenuated vaccines should be avoided (see Section 4.5). Influenza vaccination may be of value. Prescribers should refer to national guidelines for influenza vaccination.

Because MPA derivatives have been associated with an increased incidence of digestive system adverse events, including infrequent cases of gastrointestinal tract ulceration and haemorrhage and perforation, MPA should be administered with caution in patients with active serious digestive system disease.

It is recommended that Myfortic not be administered concomitantly with azathioprine because concomitant administration of these drugs has not been evaluated.

Mycophenolate sodium and mycophenolate mofetil should not be indiscriminately interchanged or substituted because of their different pharmacokinetic profiles. Myfortic has been administered in combination with corticosteroids and ciclosporin. There is limited experience with its concomitant use with induction therapies such as anti-lymphocyte globulin or basiliximab. The efficacy and safety of the use of Myfortic with other immunosuppressive agents (for example, tacrolimus) have not been studied.

Myfortic contains lactose and patients with rare hereditary problems of galactose intolerance, Lapp lactase deficiency or glucose-galactose malabsorption should not take this medicine.

The concomitant administration of Myfortic and drugs which interfere with enterohepatic circulation, for example colestyramine or activated charcoal, may result in sub-therapeutic systemic MPA exposure and reduced efficacy.

Myfortic is an IMPDH (inosine monophosphate dehydrogenase) inhibitor. Therefore, it should be avoided in patients with rare hereditary deficiency of hypoxanthine-guanine phosphoribosyl-transferase (HGPRT) such as Lesch-Nyhan and Kelley-Seegmiller syndrome.

4.5 Interaction with other medicinal products and other forms of Interaction
The following interactions have been reported between MPA and other medicinal products.

Aciclovir and Ganciclovir: The potential for myelosuppression in patients receiving both Myfortic and Aciclovir or Ganciclovir has not been studied. Increased levels of MPAG and aciclovir/ganciclovir may be expected when aciclovir/ganciclovir and Myfortic are administered concomitantly, possibly as a result of competition for the tubular secretion pathway. The changes in MPAG pharmacokinetics are unlikely to be of clinical significance in patients with adequate renal function. In the presence of renal impairment, the potential exists for increases in plasma MPAG and aciclovir/ganciclovir concentrations; dose recommendations for aciclovir/ganciclovir should be followed and patients carefully observed.

Magnesium-aluminium containing antacids: MPA AUC and Cmax has been shown to decrease by approximately 37% and 25%, respectively, when a single dose of magnesium-aluminium containing antacids was given concomitantly with Myfortic. Magnesium aluminium-containing antacids may be used intermittently for the treatment of occasional dyspepsia. However the chronic, daily use of magnesium-aluminium containing antacids with Myfortic is not recommended due to the potential for decreased mycophenolic acid exposure and reduced efficacy.

Oral contraceptives: Interaction studies between MMF and oral contraceptives indicate no interaction. Given the metabolic profile of MPA, no interactions would be expected for Myfortic and oral contraceptives.

Colestyramine and drugs that bind bile acids: Caution should be used when co-administering drugs or therapies that may bind bile acids, for example bile acid sequestrates or oral activated charcoal, because of the potential to decrease MPA exposure and thus reduce the efficacy of Myfortic.

Ciclosporin : When studied in stable renal transplant patients, ciclosporin pharmacokinetics were unaffected by steady state dosing of Myfortic. When co-administered with mycophenolate mofetil, ciclosporin is known to decrease the exposure of MPA. When co-administered with Myfortic, ciclosporin may decrease the concentration of MPA as well (by approximately 20%, extrapolated from mycophenolate mofetil data), but the exact extent of this decrease is unknown because such an interaction has not been studied. However, as efficacy studies were conducted in combination with ciclosporin, this interaction does not modify the recommended posology of Myfortic. In case of interruption or discontinuation of ciclosporin, Myfortic dosage should be re-evaluated depending on the immunosuppressive regimen.

Live attenuated vaccines: Live vaccines should not be given to patients with an impaired immune response. The antibody response to other vaccines may be diminished.

4.6 Pregnancy and lactation

Pregnancy

It is recommended that Myfortic therapy should not be initiated until a negative pregnancy test has been obtained.

Effective contraception must be used before beginning Myfortic therapy, during Myfortic therapy and for six weeks after discontinuing therapy. Patients should be instructed to consult their physician immediately should pregnancy occur.

The use of Myfortic is not recommended during pregnancy and should be reserved for cases where no alternative treatment is available. Myfortic should be used in pregnant women only if the potential benefit outweighs the potential risk to the foetus. While there are no adequate clinical data in pregnant women, animal studies have shown a teratogenic potential (CNS) (see Section 5.3).

Lactation

MPA is excreted in milk in lactating rats. It is not known whether this drug is excreted in human milk. Because of the potential for serious adverse reactions to MPA in breast-fed infants, Myfortic is contra-indicated in women who are breast-feeding.

4.7 Effects on ability to drive and use machines

No studies on the effects on the ability to drive and use machines have been performed. The mechanism of action and pharmacodynamic profile and the reported adverse reactions indicate that an effect is unlikely.

4.8 Undesirable effects

The following undesirable effects cover adverse drug reactions from clinical trials:

Malignancies:

Patients receiving immunosuppressive regimens involving combinations of drugs, including MPA, are at increased risk of developing lymphomas and other malignancies, particularly of the skin (see Section 4.4). Lymphoproliferative disease or lymphoma developed in 0.3.% of patients receiving Myfortic for up to 1 year. Non-melanoma skin carcinomas occurred in 0.8% of patients receiving Myfortic for up to 1 year; no other types of malignancy occurred.

Opportunistic infections:

All transplant patients are at increased risk of opportunistic infections; the risk increased with total immunosuppressive load (see Section 4.4). The most common opportunistic infections in *de novo* renal transplant patients receiving Myfortic with other immunosuppressants in controlled clinical trials of renal transplant patients followed for 1 year were CMV, candidiasis and herpes simplex. CMV infections (serology, viraemia or disease) was reported in 21.6% of *de novo* and in 1.9% of maintenance renal transplant patients.

Elderly patients:

Elderly patients may generally be at increased risk of adverse drug reactions due to immunosuppression.

Other Adverse Drug Reactions:

The table below contains adverse drug reactions possibly or probably related to Myfortic reported in the two phase III randomised, double blind, controlled, multi-centre trials: 1 in *de novo* kidney transplant patients and 1 maintenance kidney transplant patients, in which Myfortic® was administered at a dose of 1440 mg /day for 12 months together with ciclosporin microemulsion and corticosteroids. It is compiled according to MedDRA standard organ class.

Adverse reactions are listed according to the following categories:

Very common ⩾10 % (⩾1/10)

Common ⩾1 % and <10 % (⩾1/100 and <1/10)

Uncommon ⩾0.1 % and <1 % (⩾1/1,000 and <1/100)

Rare ⩾0.01 and <0.1 % (<1/1,000)

Very rare (<1/10,000)

(see Table 1)

The following additional adverse reactions are attributed to mycophenolic acid compounds (including MMF) as a class effect:

Gastrointestinal: Colitis, CMV gastritis, intestinal perforation, gastric ulcers, duodenal ulcers.

Disorders related to immunosuppression: Serious, sometimes life-threatening infections, including meningitis, infectious endocarditis, tuberculosis, and atypical mycobacterial infection.

Hematological: Neutropenia, pancytopenia

4.9 Overdose

There has been no reported experience of overdosage of Myfortic in humans.

Although dialysis may be used to remove the inactive metabolite MPAG, it would not be expected to remove clinically significant amounts of the active moiety MPA. This is in large part due to the very high plasma protein binding of MPA, 97%. By interfering with enterohepatic circulation of MPA, bile acid sequestrants, such as colestyramine, may reduce the systemic MPA exposure.

5. PHARMACOLOGICAL PROPERTIES

5.1 Pharmacodynamic properties

Pharmacotherapeutic group: immunosuppressant.

ATC code: L04 AA06.

MPA is a potent, selective, uncompetitive and reversible inhibitor of inosine monophosphate dehydrogenase, and therefore inhibits the *de novo* pathway of guanosine nucleotide synthesis without incorporation into DNA. Because T- and B-lymphocytes are critically dependent for their proliferation on *de novo* synthesis of purines whereas other cell types can utilize salvage pathways, MPA has more potent cytostatic effects on lymphocytes than on other cells.

5.2 Pharmacokinetic properties

Absorption: Following oral administration, mycophenolate sodium is extensively absorbed. Consistent with its enteric coated design, the time to maximal concentration (Tmax) of MPA was approximately 1.5-2 hours. Approximately 10% of all morning pharmacokinetic profiles showed a delayed Tmax, sometimes up to several hours, without any expected impact on 24 hour/daily MPA exposure.

In stable renal transplant patients on ciclosporin based immunosuppression, the gastrointestinal absorption of MPA was 93% and the absolute bioavailability was 72%. Myfortic pharmacokinetics are dose proportional and linear over the studied dose range of 180 to 2160 mg.

Compared to the fasting state, administration of a single dose of Myfortic 720 mg with a high fat meal (55g fat, 1000 calories) had no effect on the systemic exposure of MPA (AUC), which is the most relevant pharmacokinetic parameter linked to efficacy. However there was a 33% decrease in the maximal concentration of MPA (Cmax). Moreover, T_{lag} and T_{max} were on average 3-5 hours delayed, with several patients having a tmax of > 15 hours. The effect of food on Myfortic may lead to an absorption overlap from one dose interval to another. However, this effect was not shown to be clinically significant.

Distribution: The volume of distribution at steady state for MPA is 50 litres. Both mycophenolic acid and mycophenolic acid glucuronide are highly protein bound, 97% and 82%, respectively. The free MPA concentration may increase under conditions of decreased protein binding sites (uremia, hepatic failure, hypoalbuminemia, concomitant use of drugs with high protein binding). This may put patients at increased risk of MPA-related adverse effects.

Elimination: The half life of MPA is approximately 12 hours and the clearance is 8.6 L/hr.

Metabolism: MPA is metabolized principally by glucuronyl transferase to form the phenolic glucuronide of MPA, mycophenolic acid glucuronide (MPAG). MPAG is the predominant metabolite of MPA and does not manifest biologic activity. In stable renal transplant patients on ciclosporin based immunosuppression, approximately 28% of the oral Myfortic dose is converted to MPAG by presystemic metabolism. The half life of MPAG is longer

Table 1

Body system	Incidence	Adverse reaction
Infections and infestations	Common	Viral, bacterial and fungal infections
	Uncommon	Wound infection, sepsis*, osteomyelitis*
Blood and lymphatic system disorders	Very common	Leukopenia
	Common	Anaemia, thrombocytopenia
	Uncommon	lymphocele*, lymphopenia*, neutropenia*, lymphadenopathy*
Nervous system disorders	Common	Headache
	Uncommon	Tremor, insomnia*
Respiratory, thoracic and mediastinal disorders	Common	Cough
	Uncommon	Pulmonary congestion*, wheezing*
Gastrointestinal disorders	Very common	Diarrhoea
	Common	Abdominal distension, abdominal pain, abdominal tenderness, constipation, dyspepsia, flatulence, gastritis, loose stools, nausea, vomiting
	Uncommon	Pancreatitis, Eructation*, halitosis*, ileus*, oesophagitis*, peptic ulcer*, subileus*, tongue discolouration*, gastrointestinal haemorrhage*, dry mouth*, gastro-oesophageal reflux disease*, gingival hyperplasia*, peritonitis*
General disorders and administration site conditions	Common	Fatigue, pyrexia
	Uncommon	Influenza like illness, Oedema* lower limb, pain*, weakness*
Metabolism and nutrition disorders	Uncommon	Anorexia, hyperlipidaemia, Diabetes mellitus*, hypercholesterolaemia*, hypophosphataemia *
Skin and subcutaneous tissue disorders	Uncommon	Alopecia, Contusion*
Hepato-biliary disorders	Common	Hepatic function tests abnormal
Cardiac disorders	Uncommon	Tachycardia, pulmonary oedema*, ventricular extrasystoles*
Eye disorders	Uncommon	Conjunctivitis*, vision blurred*
Musculoskeletal, connective tissue and bone disorders	Uncommon	Arthritis*
Neoplasms benign and malignant	Uncommon	Skin papilloma Basal cell carcinoma*, Kaposi's sarcoma*, lymphoproliferative disorder*, squamous cell carcinoma*
Renal and urinary disorders	Common	Increased blood creatinine
	Uncommon	Renal tubular necrosis*, urethral stricture*
Reproductive system and breast disorders	Uncommon	Impotence *

* event reported in a single patient (out of 362) only.

Note:

Renal transplant patients were treated with 1440 mg Myfortic daily up to one year. A similar profile was seen in the *de-novo* and maintenance transplant population although the incidence tended to be lower in the maintenance patients.

Table 2 Mean (SD) Pharmacokinetic Parameters for MPA Following Oral Administration of Myfortic to Renal Transplant Patients on Ciclosporin-based Immunosuppression

Adult chronic, multiple dosing 720 mg BID **(Study ERLB 301)** n=48	**Dose**	**Tmax* (hr)**	**Cmax (μ g/mL)**	**AUC 0-12 (μ g × hr/mL)**
14 days post-transplant	720 mg	2	13.9 (8.6)	29.1 (10.4)
3 months post -transplant	720 mg	2	24.6 (13.2)	50.7 (17.3)
6 months post-transplant	720 mg	2	23.0 (10.1)	55.7 (14.6)
Adult chronic, multiple dosing 720 mg BID 18 months post-transplant	**Dose**	**Tmax* (hr)**	**Cmax (μ g/mL)**	**AUC 0-12 (μ g × hr/mL)**
(Study ERLB 302) n=18	720 mg	1.5	18.9 (7.9)	57.4 (15.0)
Paediatric 450 mg/m^2 single dose **(Study ERL 0106)**	**Dose**	**Tmax* (hr)**	**Cmax (μ g/mL)**	**AUC 0- ∞ (μ g × hr/mL)**
n=16	450 mg/m^2	2.5	31.9 (18.2)	74.5 (28.3)

* median values

than that of MPA, approximately 16 hours and its clearance is 0.45 L/hr.

Excretion: Although negligible amounts of MPA are present in the urine (<1.0%), the majority of MPA is eliminated in the urine as MPAG. MPAG secreted in the bile is available for deconjugation by gut flora. The MPA resulting from this deconjugation may then be reabsorbed. Approximately 6-8 hours after Myfortic dosing a second peak of MPA concentration can be measured, consistent with reabsorption of the deconjugated MPA.

Pharmacokinetics in Renal Transplant Patients on ciclosporin based immunosuppression: Shown in the following table are mean pharmacokinetic parameters for MPA following the administration of Myfortic. In the early post transplant period, mean MPA AUC and mean MPA Cmax were approximately one-half of that measured six months post transplant.

Mean (SD) Pharmacokinetic Parameters for MPA Following Oral Administration of Myfortic to Renal Transplant Patients on Ciclosporin-based Immuno-suppression

(see Table 2 above)

Renal Impairment: MPA pharmacokinetic appeared to be unchanged over the range of normal to absent renal function. In contrast, MPAG exposure increased with decreased renal function; MPAG exposure being approximately 8 fold higher in the setting of anuria. Clearance of either MPA or MPAG was unaffected by haemodialysis. Free MPA may also significantly increase in the setting of renal failure. This may be due to decreased plasma protein binding of MPA in the presence of high blood urea concentration.

Hepatic Impairment: In volunteers with alcoholic cirrhosis, hepatic MPA glucuronidation processes were relatively unaffected by hepatic parenchymal disease. Effects of hepatic disease on this process probably depend on the particular disease. However, hepatic disease with predominantly biliary damage, such as primary biliary cirrhosis, may show a different effect.

Children and adolescents: Limited data are available on the use of Myfortic in children and adolescents. In the table above the mean (SD) MPA pharmacokinetics are shown for stable paediatric renal transplant patients (aged 5-16 years) on ciclosporin-based immuno-suppression. Mean MPA AUC at a dose of 450 mg/m^2 was similar to that measured in adults receiving 720 mg Myfortic. The mean apparent clearance of MPA was approximately 6.7 L/hr/m^2.

Gender: There are no clinically significant gender differences in Myfortic pharmacokinetics.

Elderly: Pharmacokinetics in the elderly have not formally been studied. MPA exposure does not appear to vary to a clinically significant degree by age.

5.3 Preclinical safety data

The haematopoetic and lymphoid system were the primary organs affected in repeated-dose toxicity studies conducted with mycophenolate sodium in rats and mice. These effects occurred at systemic exposure levels which are equivalent to or less than the clinical exposure at the recommended dose of 1.44g/day of Myfortic in renal transplant patients. Gastrointestinal effects were observed in the dog at systemic exposure levels equivalent to or less than the clinical exposure at the recommended doses. The nonclinical toxicity profile of mycophenolate sodium appears to be consistent with adverse events observed in human clinical trials which now provide safety data of more relevance to the patient population (see Section 4.8).

Three genotoxicity assays (in vitro mouse lymphoma assay, micronucleus test in V79 Chinese hamster cells and in vivo mouse bone marrow micronucleus test) showed a potential of mycophenolic acid to cause chromosomal aberrations. These effects can be related to the pharmacodynamic mode of action, i.e. inhibition of nucleotide synthesis in sensitive cells. Other in vitro tests for detection of gene mutation did not demonstrate genotoxic activity.

Mycophenolate sodium was not tumourigenic in rats and mice. The highest dose tested in the animal carcinogenicity studies resulted in approximately 0.6 - 5 times the systemic exposure (AUC or C_{max}) observed in renal transplant patients at the recommended clinical dose of 1.44 g/day.

Mycophenolate sodium had no effect on fertility of male or female rats up to dose levels at which general toxicity and embryotoxicity were observed.

In a teratology study performed with mycophenolate sodium in rats, at a dose as low as 1 mg/kg, malformations in the offspring were observed, including anophthalmia, exencephaly and umbilical hernia. The systemic exposure at this dose represents 0.05 times the clinical exposure at the dose of 1.44 g/day of Myfortic (see Section 4.6).

6. PHARMACEUTICAL PARTICULARS

6.1 List of excipients

Maize starch

Povidone

Crospovidone

Lactose, anhydrous

Silica, colloidal anhydrous

Magnesium stearate.

Coating:

Hypromellose phthalate

Titanium dioxide (E 171)

Iron oxide yellow (E 172)

Indigo Carmine (E 132) (180mg only)

Iron oxide red (E 172) (360mg only)

6.2 Incompatibilities

Not applicable.

6.3 Shelf life

30 months.

6.4 Special precautions for storage

Do not store above 30°C.

Store in the original package in order to protect from moisture and light.

6.5 Nature and contents of container

The tablets are packed in Polyamide/Aluminium/PVC blister packs of 10 tablets per blister in quantities of 20, (180mg only), 50,100, 120 and 250 tablets per carton.

6.6 Instructions for use and handling

Myfortic tablets should not be crushed in order to retain the integrity of the enteric coating because mycophenolic acid has demonstrated teratogenic effects in rats and rabbits.

7. MARKETING AUTHORISATION HOLDER

Novartis Pharmaceuticals UK Limited

Frimley Business Park

Frimley

Camberley

Surrey

GU16 7SR

United Kingdom

8. MARKETING AUTHORISATION NUMBER(S)

Myfortic 180mg film-coated gastro-resistant tablets: PL 00101/0664

Myfortic 360mg film-coated gastro-resistant tablets: PL 00101/0665

9. DATE OF FIRST AUTHORISATION/RENEWAL OF THE AUTHORISATION

5 July 2004

10. DATE OF REVISION OF THE TEXT

LEGAL CATEGORY

POM

Myleran film coated tablets 2mg

(GlaxoSmithKline UK)

1. NAME OF THE MEDICINAL PRODUCT

Myleran film coated tablets 2 mg

2. QUALITATIVE AND QUANTITATIVE COMPOSITION

Each 2 mg tablet contains 2 mg of the active substance busulfan

3. PHARMACEUTICAL FORM

Film coated tablet

Myleran 2 mg tablets are white, film-coated, round, biconvex tablets engraved "GXEF3" on one side and "M" on the other.

4. CLINICAL PARTICULARS

4.1 Therapeutic indications

Myleran is indicated for the palliative treatment of the chronic phase of chronic granulocytic leukaemia.

Myleran is effective in producing prolonged remission in polycythaemia vera, particularly in cases with marked thrombocytosis.

Myleran may be useful in selected cases of essential thrombocythaemia and myelofibrosis.

4.2 Posology and method of administration

General:

Myleran tablets are usually given in courses or administered continuously. The dose must be adjusted for the individual patient under close clinical and haematological control. Should a patient require an average daily dose of less than the content of the available Myleran tablets, this can be achieved byintroducing one or more busulfan free days between treatment days. The tablets should not be divided (see 6.6 Instructions for Use/Handling).

The relevant literature should be consulted for full details of treatment schedules.

Chronic granulocytic leukaemia

Induction in Adults

Treatment is usually initiated as soon as the condition is diagnosed. The dose is 0.06 mg/kg/day, with an initial daily maximum of 4 mg, which may be given as a single dose.

There is individual variation in the response to Myleran and in a small proportion of patients the bone marrow may be extremely sensitive. (See 4.4 Special Warnings and Precautions for Use).

The blood count must be monitored at least weekly during the induction phase and it may be helpful to plot counts on semilog graph paper.

The dose should be increased only if the response is inadequate after three weeks.

Treatment should be continued until the total leucocyte count has fallen to between 15 and 25 × 10^9 per litre (typically 12 to 20 weeks). Treatment may then be interrupted, following which a further fall in the leucocyte count may occur over the next two weeks. Continued treatment at the induction dose after this point or following depression of the platelet count to below 100 × 10^9 per litre is associated with a significant risk of prolonged and possibly irreversible bone marrow aplasia.

Maintenance in adults:

Control of the leukaemia may be achieved for long periods without further Myleran treatment; further courses are usually given when the leucocyte count rises to 50 × 10^9 per litre, or symptoms return.

Some clinicians prefer to give continuous maintenance therapy. Continuous treatment is more practical when the duration of unmaintained remissions is short.

The aim is to maintain a leucocyte count of 10 to 15 × 10^9 per litre and blood counts must be performed at least every 4 weeks. The usual maintenance dosage is on average 0.5 to 2 mg/day, but individual requirements may be much less. Should a patient require an average daily dose of less than the content of one tablet, the maintenance dose may be adjusted by introducing one or more busulfan free days between treatment days.

Note: Lower doses of Myleran should be used if it is administered in conjunction with other cytotoxic agents. (See also 4.8 Undesirable Effects and 4.5 Interactions with other Medicaments and other forms of Interaction).

Children:

Chronic granulocytic leukaemia is rare in the paediatric age group. Busulfan may be used to treat Philadelphia chromosome positive (Ph' positive) disease, but the Ph' negative juvenile variant responds poorly.

Polycythaemia vera

The usual dose is 4 to 6 mg daily, continued for 4 to 6 weeks, with careful monitoring of the blood count, particularly the platelet count.

Further courses are given when relapse occurs; alternatively, maintenance therapy may be given using approximately half the induction dose.

If the polycythaemia is controlled primarily by venesection, short courses of Myleran may be given solely to control the platelet count.

Myelofibrosis

The usual initial dose is 2 to 4 mg daily.

Very careful haematological control is required because of the extreme sensitivity of the bone marrow in this condition.

Essential thrombocythaemia

The usual dose is 2 to 4 mg per day.

Treatment should be interrupted if the total leucocyte count falls below 5×10^9 per litre or the platelet count below 500×10^9 per litre.

4.3 Contraindications

Myleran should not be used in patients whose disease has demonstrated resistance to busulfan.

Myleran should not be given to patients who have previously suffered a hypersensitivity reaction to the busulfan or any other component of the preparation.

4.4 Special warnings and special precautions for use

Myleran is an active cytotoxic agent for use only under the direction of physicians experienced in the administration of such agents.

Myleran should be discontinued if lung toxicity develops (See 4.8 Undesirable Effects).

Myleran should not generally be given in conjunction with or soon after radiotherapy.

Myleran is ineffective once blast transformation has occurred.

If anaesthesia is required in patients with possible pulmonary toxicity, the concentration of inspired oxygen should be kept as low as safely as possible and careful attention given to post-operative respiratory care.

Hyperuricaemia and/or hyperuricosuria are not uncommon in patients with chronic granulocytic leukaemia and should be corrected before starting treatment with Myleran. During treatment, hyperuricaemia and the risk of uric acid nephropathy should be prevented by adequate prophylaxis, including adequate hydration and the use of allopurinol.

Very careful consideration should be given to the use of Myleran for the treatment of polycythaemia vera and essential thrombocythaemia in view of the drug's carcinogenic potential. The use of Myleran for these indications should be avoided in younger or asymptomatic patients. If the drug is considered necessary treatment courses should be kept as short as possible.

Patients co-prescribed systemic itraconazole with Myleran should be monitored for signs of busulfan toxicity (see 4.5 Interactions with other Medicaments and other forms of Interaction).

Monitoring:

Careful attention must be paid to monitoring the blood counts throughout treatment to avoid the possibility of excessive myelosuppression and the risk of irreversible bone marrow aplasia (see also 4.8 Undesirable Effects).

High-dose Treatment:

If high-dose Myleran is prescribed (see 4.9 Overdose), patients should be given prophylactic anticonvulsant therapy, preferably with a benzodiazepine rather than phenytoin.

A reduced incidence of hepatic veno-occlusive disease and other regimen-related toxicities have been observed in patients treated with high-dose Myleran and cyclophosphamide when the first dose of cyclophosphamide has been delayed for > 24 hours after the last dose of busulfan.

Safe Handling of Myleran Tablets:

See 6.6 Instructions for Use/Handling

Myleran is genotoxic in non-clinical studies (see Section 5.3 Preclinical Safety Data).

Mutagenicity:

Various chromosome aberrations have been noted in cells from patients receiving busulfan.

Carcinogenicity:

On the basis of human studies, Myleran was considered by the International Agency for Research on cancer to show sufficient evidence for carcinogenicity. The World Health Association has concluded that there is a causal relationship between Myleran exposure and cancer.

Widespread epithelial dysplasia has been observed in patients treated with long-term Myleran, with some of the changes resembling precancerous lesions.

A number of malignant tumours have been reported in patients who have received Myleran treatment.

The evidence is growing that Myleran, in common with other alkylating agents, is leukaemogenic. In a controlled prospective study in which 2 years' Myleran treatment was given as an adjuvant to surgery for lung cancer, long-term follow-up showed an increased incidence of acute leukaemia compared with the placebo-treated group. The incidence of solid tumours was not increased.

Although acute leukaemia is probably part of the natural history of polycythaemia vera, prolonged alkylating agent therapy may increase the incidence.

4.5 Interaction with other medicinal products and other forms of Interaction

The combination of Myleran and tioguanine has resulted in the development of nodular regenerative hyperplasia, portal hypertension and oesophageal varices.

The effects of other cytotoxics producing pulmonary toxicity may be additive.

The administration of phenytoin to patients receiving high-dose Myleran (see 4.9 Overdose) may result in a decrease in the myeloblative effect.

The concomitant systemic administration of itraconazole to patients receiving high-dose Myleran may result in reduced busulfan clearance.

A reduced incidence of hepatic veno-occlusive disease and other regimen-related toxicities have been observed in patients treated with high-dose Myleran and cyclophosphamide when the first dose of cyclophosphamide has been delayed for > 24 hours after the last dose of busulfan.

4.6 Pregnancy and lactation

Pregnancy:

As with all cytotoxic chemotherapy, adequate contraceptive precautions should be advised when either partner is receiving Myleran.

The use of Myleran should be avoided during pregnancy whenever possible. In animal studies (see section 5.3 Preclinical Safety Data) it has the potential for teratogenic effects, whilst exposure during the latter half of pregnancy resulted in impairment of fertility in offspring. In every individual case the expected benefit of treatment to the mother must be weighed against the possible risk to the foetus.

A few cases of congenital abnormalities, not necessarily attributable to busulfan, have been reported and third trimester exposure may be associated with impaired intra-uterine growth. However, there have also been many reported cases of apparently normal children born after exposure to Myleran *in utero*, even during the first trimester.

Lactation:

It is not known whether Myleran or its metabolites are excreted in human breast milk. Mothers receiving Myleran should not breast-feed their infants.

4.7 Effects on ability to drive and use machines

There are no data on the effect of busulfan on driving performance or the ability to operate machinery. A detrimental effect on these activities cannot be predicted from the pharmacology of the drug.

4.8 Undesirable effects

Haematological effects:

The main adverse reaction of Myleran treatment is dose-related bone marrow depression, manifest as leucopoenia and particularly thrombocytopenia.

Aplastic anaemia (often irreversible) has been reported rarely, often following long-term conventional doses and also high doses of Myleran.

Gastro-intestinal effects:

Gastro-intestinal effects such as nausea, vomiting and diarrhoea have been reported rarely at normal therapeutic doses and may possibly be ameliorated by using divided doses.

Effects on reproduction:

Ovarian suppression and amenorrhoea with menopausal symptoms commonly occur in pre-menopausal patients. In very rare cases, recovery of ovarian function has been reported with continuing treatment.

Treatment with high-dose Myleran has been associated with severe and persistent ovarian failure, including failure to achieve puberty after administration to young girls and pre-adolescents.

There have been clinical reports of sterility, azoospermia and testicular atrophy in male patients receiving busulfan.

Studies of busulfan treatment in animals have shown reproductive toxicity (see 5.3 Preclinical Safety Data).

Pulmonary effects:

Diffuse interstitial pulmonary fibrosis, with progressive dyspnoea and a persistent, non-productive cough has occurred rarely, usually after prolonged treatment over a number of years. Histological features include atypical changes of the alveolar and bronchiolar epithelium and the presence of giant cells with large hyperchromatic nuclei. Once pulmonary toxicity is established the prognosis is poor despite Myleran withdrawal and there is little evidence that corticosteroids are helpful. The onset is usually insidious but may also be acute. The lung pathology may be complicated by superimposed infections. Pulmonary ossification and dystrophic calcification have also been reported. It is possible that subsequent radiotherapy can augment subclinical lung injury caused by Myleran. Other cytotoxic agents may cause additive lung toxicity.

Dermatological effects:

Hyperpigmentation is the most common skin reaction and occurs in 5 to 10% of patients, particularly those with a dark complexion. It is often most marked on the neck, upper trunk, nipples, abdomen and palmar creases. In a few cases following prolonged Myleran therapy, hyperpigmentation occurs as a part of a clinical syndrome resembling adrenal insufficiency (Addison's disease). It is characterised by weakness, severe fatigue, anorexia, weight loss, nausea and vomiting and hyperpigmentation of the skin, but without biochemical evidence of adrenal impairment or mucous membrane hyperpigmentation or hair loss. The syndrome has sometimes resolved when Myleran has been withdrawn.

Other rare skin reactions include urticaria, erythema multiforme, erythema nodosum, alopecia, porphyria cutanea tarda, an "allopurinol-type" rash and excessive dryness and fragility of the skin with complete anhydrosis, dryness of the oral mucous membranes and cheilosis. Sjogren's syndrome has also been reported.

An increased cutaneous radiation effect has been observed in patients receiving radiotherapy soon after high-dose Myleran (see 4.9 Overdose).

Hepatic effects:

There have been occasional reports of cholestatic jaundice and liver function abnormalities, but Myleran is not generally considered to be significantly hepatotoxic at normal therapeutic doses. However, retrospective review of post-mortem reports of patients who had been treated with low-dose Myleran for at least two years for chronic granulocytic leukaemia showed evidence of centrilobular sinusoidal fibrosis.

The combination of Myleran and tioguanine is associated with significant hepatotoxicity (see 4.5 Interactions with other Medicaments and other forms of Interaction).

Hyperbilirubinaemia, jaundice, hepatic veno-occlusive disease (see 4.4 Special Warnings and Precautions for Use and 4.5 Interaction with Other Medicinal Products and Other Forms of Interaction) and centrilobular sinusoidal fibrosis with hepatocellular atrophy and necrosis have been observed after high-dose Myleran treatment (see 4.9 Overdose).

Ophthalmic effects:

Lens changes and cataracts, which may be bilateral, have been reported during Myleran therapy. Corneal thinning has been reported after bone marrow transplantation preceded by high-dose Myleran treatment (see 4.9 Overdose).

Miscellaneous effects:

Convulsions have been observed in patients who have received high-dose Myleran (see 4.9 Overdose, 4.5 Interactions with other Medicaments and other forms of Interaction, and 4.4 Special Warnings and Precautions for Use).

Cardiac tamponade has been reported in a small number of patients with thalassaemia who received high-dose Myleran (see 4.9 Overdose).

Gynaecomastia has been reported as a side effect of Myleran, as have myasthenia gravis and haemorrhagic cystitis.

Many histological and cytological changes have been observed in patients treated with Myleran, including widespread dysplasia affecting uterine cervical, bronchial and other epithelia. Most reports relate to long-term treatment but transient epithelial abnormalities have been observed following short-term, high-dose treatment (see 4.9 Overdose).

4.9 Overdose

Symptoms and signs:

The acute dose-limiting toxicity of Myleran in man is myelosuppression (see 4.8 Undesirable Effects).

The main effect of chronic overdose is bone marrow depression and pancytopenia. If high-dose Myleran is used in association with bone marrow transplantation (The usual total dose of Myleran, given in combination with other agents is 14 to 16 mg/kg given orally over 4 consecutive days [3.5 to 4 mg/kg/day in divided doses]), gastro-intestinal toxicity becomes dose-limiting, with mucositis, nausea, vomiting, diarrhoea and anorexia.

Treatment:

There is no known antidote to Myleran. Haemoialysis should be considered in the management of overdose as there is one report of successful haemodialysis of busulfan.

Appropriate supportive treatment should be given during the period of haematological toxicity.

5. PHARMACOLOGICAL PROPERTIES

5.1 Pharmacodynamic properties

Busulfan (1,4-butanediol dimethanesulfonate) is a bifunctional alkylating agent. Binding to DNA is believed to play a role in its mode of action and di-guanyl derivaties have been isolated but interstrand crosslinking has not been conclusively demonstrated.

The basis for the uniquely selective effect of busulfan on granulocytopoiesis is not fully understood. Although not curative, Myleran is very effective in reducing the total granulocyte mass, relieving the symptoms of disease and improving the clinical state of the patient. Myleran has been shown to be superior to splenic irradiation when judged by survival times and maintenance of haemoglobin levels and is as effective in controlling spleen size.

5.2 Pharmacokinetic properties

Absorption:

Early studies were carried out with radioactively labelled busulfan. More recently, gas liquid chromatography with selected ion monitoring has been used to quantitate busulfan in biological fluids. Absorption of busulfan shows intra-individual variation. Both zero and first-order absorption, one compartment open models have been fitted to the pharmacokinetic data. The mean half-life for drug elimination was 2.57 hours.

The bioavailability of oral busulfan shows large intra-individual variations ranging from 22% to 120% in adults and children.

High-dose Treatment:

The pharmacokinetics of busulfan have also been studied in patients following high-dose administration (1 mg/kg every 6 hours for 4 days). Drug was assayed either using gas liquid chromatography with electron capture detection or by high-performance liquid chromatography (HPLC). Using the former technique, the mean elimination half-life was 2.3 hours after the final busulfan dose and 3.4 hours after the first dose.

The mean steady-state plasma concentration was 1.1 microgram/ml after 2 to 3 doses 6 hours apart. Due to the variable absorption kinetics observed, it was not possible to evaluate the order of kinetics.

Using HPLC, steady-state plasma levels of busulfan ranged from 2 to 8 microM (approximately 0.5 to 2 microgram/ml, respectively) with 4 doses 6 hours apart.

Peak plasma levels ranged from 3.1 to 5.9 microgram/ml in a patient treated with total dose of 16 mg/kg, or from 3.8 to 9.7 microgram/ml in two patients treated with a total of 20 mg/kg.

Distribution:

Busulfan given in high doses has recently been shown to enter the cerebrospinal fluid (CSF) in concentrations comparable to those found in plasma, with a mean CSF:plasma ration of 1.3:1. The saliva:plasma distribution of busulfan was 1.1:1.

The level of busulfan bound reversibly to plasma proteins has been variably reported to be insignificant or approximately 55%. Irreversible binding of drug to blood cells and plasma proteins has been reported to be 47% and 32%, respectively.

Metabolism and Excretion:

The urinary metabolites of busulfan have been identified as 3-hydroxysulpholane, tetrahydrothiophene 1-oxide and sulpholane, in patients treated with high-dose busulfan. Very little busulfane is excreted unchanged in the urine.

5.3 Preclinical safety data

Busulfan has been shown to be mutagenic in various experimental systems, including bacteria, fungi, *Drosophila* and cultured mouse lymphoma cells.

In vivo cytogenetic studies in rodents have shown an increased incidence of chromosome aberrations in both germ cells and somatic cells after busulfan treatment.

Carcinogenicity:

There is limited evidence from preclinical studies that Myleran is carcinogenic in animals (see 4.4 Special Warnings and Precautions for Use).

Teratogenicity:

There is evidence form animal studies that busulfan produces foetal abnormalities and adverse effects on off-spring, including defects of the musculo-skeletal system, reduced body weight and size, impairment of gonad development and effects on fertility.

Fertility:

Busulfan interferes with spermatogenesis in experimental animals. Limited studies in female animals indicate busulfan has a marked and irreversible effect on fertility through oocyte depletion.

6. PHARMACEUTICAL PARTICULARS

6.1 List of excipients

2 mg Tablets:

Tablet core: Anhydrous lactose

Pregelatinised starch

Magnesium stearate

Tablet coating: Hypromellose

Titanium dioxide

Triacetin

6.2 Incompatibilities

None known

6.3 Shelf life

3 years

6.4 Special precautions for storage

Do not store above25°C

6.5 Nature and contents of container

Myleran tablets are supplied in amber glass bottles with a child resistant closure containing 25 or 100 tablets.

6.6 Instructions for use and handling

Safe handling of Myleran tablets:

The tablets should not be divided and provided the outer coating is intact, there is no risk in handling Myleran tablets.

Handlers of Myleran tablets should follow guidelines for the handling of cytotoxic drugs.

Disposal:

Myleran tablets surplus to requirements should be destroyed in a manner appropriate for the destruction of dangerous substances.

Administrative Data

7. MARKETING AUTHORISATION HOLDER

The Wellcome Foundation Ltd trading as GlaxoSmithKline UK

Glaxo Wellcome House Stockley Park West

Berkeley Avenue Uxbridge

Greenford Middlesex UB11 1BT

Middlesex UB6 ONN

8. MARKETING AUTHORISATION NUMBER(S)

PL0003/5112R

9. DATE OF FIRST AUTHORISATION/RENEWAL OF THE AUTHORISATION

23 January 2003

10. DATE OF REVISION OF THE TEXT

19 January 2005

Myocet

(Zeneus Pharma Ltd)

1. NAME OF THE MEDICINAL PRODUCT

Myocet▼ 50 mg powder and pre-admixtures for concentrate for liposomal dispersion for infusion

2. QUALITATIVE AND QUANTITATIVE COMPOSITION

Liposome-encapsulated doxorubicin–citrate complex corresponding to 50 mg doxorubicin HCl.

For excipients, see 6.1.

3. PHARMACEUTICAL FORM

Powder and pre-admixtures for concentrate for liposomal dispersion for infusion

Myocet is supplied as a three-vial system:

Myocet doxorubicin HCl (a red lyophilised powder),

Myocet liposomes (a white to off-white, opaque and homogeneous solution),

Myocet buffer (a clear colourless solution).

4. CLINICAL PARTICULARS

4.1 Therapeutic indications

Myocet, in combination with cyclophosphamide, is indicated for the first line treatment of metastatic breast cancer in women.

4.2 Posology and method of administration

The use of Myocet should be confined to units specialised in the administration of cytotoxic chemotherapy and should only be administered under the supervision of a physician experienced in the use of chemotherapy.

Dosage

When Myocet is administered in combination with cyclophosphamide (600 mg/m^2) the initial recommended dose of Myocet is 60-75 mg/m^2 every three weeks.

Administration

Myocet must be reconstituted and further diluted prior to administration (see 6.6). A final concentration of between 0.4 to 1.2 mg/ml doxorubicin HCl, is required. Myocet is administered by intravenous infusion over a period of 1 hour.

Myocet must not be administered by the intramuscular or subcutaneous route or as a bolus injection.

Paediatric patients

The safety and efficacy of Myocet has not yet been established in paediatric patients (below 18 years of age).

Elderly patients

Safety and efficacy of Myocet have been assessed in 61 patients with metastatic breast cancer, age 65 and over. Data from randomised controlled clinical trials show that the efficacy and cardiac safety of Myocet in this population was comparable to that observed in patients less than 65 years old.

Use in patients with impaired hepatic function

As metabolism and excretion of doxorubicin occurs primarily by the hepatobiliary route, evaluation of hepatobiliary function should be performed before and during therapy with Myocet. No specific studies that can form the basis for dose recommendations have been performed with Myocet in patients with impaired hepatic function. Thus, dose reduction of Myocet may be considered based upon dosing recommendations for conventional doxorubicin, as follows:

Serum bilirubin = 20.3 – 50.8μmol (1.2 – 3.0 mg/dl) = 50% dose reduction

Serum bilirubin > 50.8 μmol (3.0 mg/dl) = 75% dose reduction

For dose reductions due to other toxicity, see 4.4.

Use in patients with impaired renal function

Doxorubicin is metabolised largely by the liver and excreted in the bile. Therefore dose modification is not required for patients with renal function impairment.

4.3 Contraindications

Hypersensitivity to the active substance, to the pre-admixtures or to any of the ingredients.

4.4 Special warnings and special precautions for use

Myelosuppression

Therapy with Myocet causes myelosuppression. Myocet should not be administered to individuals with absolute neutrophil counts (ANC) lower than 1,500 cells/μl or platelets less than 100,000/μl prior to the next cycle. Careful haematological monitoring (including white blood cell and platelet count, and haemoglobin) should be performed during therapy with Myocet.

Haematological as well as other toxicity may require dose reductions or delays. The following dosage modifications are recommended during therapy and should be performed in parallel for both Myocet and cyclophosphamide. Dosing subsequent to a dose reduction is left to the discretion of the physician in charge of the patient.

(see Table 1 on next page)

If myelotoxicity delays treatment to greater than 35 days after the first dose of the previous cycle, then consideration should be given to stopping treatment.

Mucositis		
Grade	Symptoms	Modification
1	Painless ulcers, erythema, or mild soreness.	None
2	Painful erythema, oedema or ulcers but can eat.	Wait one week and if the symptoms improve redose at 100% dose
3	Painful erythema, oedema or ulcers and cannot eat	Wait one week and if symptoms improve redose at 25% dose reduction
4	Requires parenteral or enteral support	Wait one week and if symptoms improve redose at 50% dose reduction

For dose reduction of Myocet due to liver function impairment, see 4.2.

Cardiac toxicity

Doxorubicin and other anthracyclines can cause cardiotoxicity. The risk of toxicity rises with increasing cumulative doses of those medicinal products and is higher in individuals with a history of cardiomyopathy, or mediastinal irradiation or pre-existing cardiac disease.

Analyses of cardiotoxicity in clinical trials have shown a statistically significant reduction in cardiac events in patients treated with Myocet compared to patients treated with conventional doxorubicin at the same dose in mg. The full clinical relevance of these findings is currently unclear.

In a phase III study in combination with cyclophosphamide (CPA) comparing Myocet (60 mg/m^2) + CPA (600 mg/m^2) versus doxorubicin (60 mg/m^2) + CPA (600 mg/m^2), 6% versus 21% of patients, respectively, developed a significant decrease in left ventricular ejection fraction (LVEF). In a phase III study comparing single-agent Myocet (75 mg/m^2) versus single-agent doxorubicin (75 mg/m^2), 12% versus 27% of patients, respectively developed a significant decrease in LVEF. The corresponding figures for congestive heart failure (CHF), which was less accurately assessed, were 0% for Myocet + CPA versus 3% for doxorubicin + CPA, and 2% for Myocet versus 8% for doxorubicin. The median lifetime cumulative dose of Myocet in combination with CPA to a cardiac event was > 1260 mg/m^2, compared to 480 mg/m^2 for doxorubicin combination with CPA.

There is no experience with Myocet in patients with a history of cardiovascular disease, e.g. myocardial infarction within 6 months prior to treatment. Thus, caution should be exercised in patients with impaired cardiac function, and the total dose of Myocet should also take into account any previous, or concomitant, therapy with other cardiotoxic compounds, including anthracyclines and anthraquinones.

Before initiation of Myocet therapy a measurement of left ventricular ejection fraction (LVEF) is routinely recommended, either by Multiple Gated Arteriography (MUGA) or by echocardiography. These methods should also be applied routinely during Myocet treatment. The evaluation of left ventricular function is considered mandatory before

Table 1

Haematological Toxicity			
Grade	**Nadir ANC** (cells/μl)	**Nadir Platelet Count** (cells/μl)	Modification
1	1500 – 1900	75,000 – 150,000	None
2	1000 – Less than 1500	50,000 – Less than 75,000	None
3	500 – 999	25,000 – Less than 50,000	Wait until ANC 1500 or more and/or platelets
4	Less than 500	Less than 25,000	Wait until ANC 1500 and/or platelets 100,000 or more then redose at 50% dose reduction

each additional administration of Myocet once a patient exceeds a lifetime cumulative anthracycline dose of 550 mg/m^2 or whenever cardiomyopathy is suspected. If LVEF has decreased substantially from baseline e.g. by > 20 points to a final value > 50% or by > 10 points to a final value of < 50%, the benefit of continued therapy must be carefully evaluated against the risk of producing irreversible cardiac damage. However, the most definitive test for anthracycline myocardial injury, i.e., endomyocardial biopsy, should be considered.

All patients receiving Myocet should also routinely undergo ECG monitoring. Transient ECG changes such as T-wave flattening, S-T segment depression and benign arrhythmias are not considered mandatory indications for the cessation of Myocet therapy.

Congestive heart failure due to cardiomyopathy may occur suddenly, and may also be encountered after discontinuation of therapy.

Injection site reactions

Myocet should be considered an irritant and precautions should be taken to avoid extravasation. If extravasation occurs, the infusion should be immediately terminated. Ice may be applied to the affected area for approximately 30 minutes. Subsequently, the Myocet infusion should be restarted in a different vein than that in which the extravasation has occurred. Note that Myocet may be administered through a central or peripheral vein. In the clinical program, there were nine cases of accidental extravasation of Myocet, none of which were associated with severe skin damage, ulceration or necrosis.

Infusion associated reactions

When infused rapidly acute reactions associated with liposomal infusions have been reported. Reported symptoms have included flushing, dyspnoea, fever, facial swelling, headache, back pain, chills, tightness in the chest and throat, and/or hypotension. These acute phenomena may be avoided by using a 1-hour infusion time.

Other

For precautions regarding the use of Myocet with other medicinal products, see 4.5.

Efficacy and safety of Myocet in the adjuvant treatment of breast cancer have not been determined. The importance of apparent differences in tissue distribution between Myocet and conventional doxorubicin has not been elucidated with respect to long-term antitumour efficacy.

4.5 Interaction with other medicinal products and other forms of Interaction

Specific drug compatibility studies have not been performed with Myocet. Myocet is likely to interact with substances that are known to interact with conventional doxorubicin. Plasma levels of doxorubicin and its metabolite, doxorubicinol, may be increased when doxorubicin is administered with cyclosporin, verapamil, paclitaxel or other agents that inhibit P-glycoprotein (P-Gp). Interactions with doxorubicin have also been reported for streptozocin, phenobarbital, phenytoin and warfarin. Studies of the effect of Myocet on other substances are also lacking. However, doxorubicin may potentiate the toxicity of other antineoplastic agents. Concomitant treatment with other substances reported to be cardiotoxic or with cardiologically active substances (e.g. calcium antagonists) may increase the risk for cardiotoxicity. Concomitant therapy with other liposomal or lipid-complexed substances or intravenous fat emulsions could change the pharmacokinetic profile of Myocet.

4.6 Pregnancy and lactation

Due to the known cytotoxic, mutagenic and embryotoxic properties of doxorubicin, Myocet should not be used during pregnancy unless clearly necessary. Women of childbearing potential should use an effective contraceptive during treatment with Myocet and up to 6 months following discontinuation of therapy. Women receiving Myocet should not breastfeed.

4.7 Effects on ability to drive and use machines

Myocet has been reported to cause dizziness. Patients who suffer from this should avoid driving and operating machinery.

4.8 Undesirable effects

The safety database is composed of data from 716 patients who were treated with Myocet. Data in Tables 1 and 2 are based on the experience of 323 patients with metastatic breast cancer in three randomised phase III trials of Myocet as a single agent and in combination with cyclophosphamide (CPA). Treatment cycles were every three weeks in each trial and G-CSF was used in 38-56% of the cycles.

Table 2

Haematological adverse events[c]

(see Table 2 below)

Table 3

Non-haematological adverse events[c]

(see Table 3 on next page)

The following grade ¾ adverse reactions with an incidence of < 5% were also observed (utilising the database from 16 clinical studies in 647 patients with solid tumours). AIDS patients with Kaposi's sarcoma were not included.

Incidence less than 5% (Grade 3 or 4, possibly, probably, or definitely related):

Body As a Whole: fever, rigors, hot flushes, pain, headache, dizziness, dehydration, weight loss, sepsis

Cardiovascular: arrhythmia, chest pain, hypotension, pericardial effusion

Gastrointestinal: constipation, gastric ulcer, increased hepatic transaminases, increased alkaline phosphatase, increased serum bilirubin, jaundice

Haematological: purpura, lymphopenia

Metabolic/ Nutritional: hypokalaemia, hyperglycaemia

Musculoskeletal: back pain, muscle weakness, myalgia

Nervous System: abnormal gait, dysphonia

Psychiatric: anorexia, insomnia, agitation, somnolence

Respiratory: dyspnoea, pharyngitis, epistaxis, pneumonitis, haemoptysis

Skin and Appendages: nail disorder, injection site reaction, injection site infection, pruritus, folliculitis, Herpes Zoster

Urogenital: oliguria, haemorrhagic cystitis

4.9 Overdose

Acute overdose with Myocet will worsen toxic side effects. Treatment of acute overdose should focus on supportive care for expected toxicity and may include hospitalisation, antibiotics, platelet and granulocyte transfusions and symptomatic treatment of mucositis.

5. PHARMACOLOGICAL PROPERTIES

5.1 Pharmacodynamic properties

Pharmaco-therapeutic group: Cytotoxic agents (anthracyclines and related substances), ATC code: L01DB

The active substance in Myocet is doxorubicin HCl. Doxorubicin may exert its antitumour and toxic effects by a number of mechanisms including inhibition of topoisomerase II, intercalation with DNA and RNA polymerases, free radical formation and membrane binding. Liposomal-encapsulated compared with conventional doxorubicin was not found more active in doxorubicin resistant cell lines *in vitro.* In animals, liposome-encapsulated doxorubicin reduced the distribution to heart and gastrointestinal mucosa compared with conventional doxorubicin, while antitumoural efficacy in experimental tumours was maintained.

Myocet (60 mg/m^2) + CPA (600 mg/m^2) was compared with conventional doxorubicin + CPA (at the same doses) and Myocet (75 mg/m^2) + CPA (600 mg/m^2) was compared to epirubicin + CPA (at the same doses). In a third trial, Myocet (75 mg/m^2) monotherapy was compared with conventional doxorubicin monotherapy (at the same dose). Findings regarding response rate and progression-free survival are provided in Table 4.

Table 4

Antitumour efficacy summary for combination and single-agent studies

(see Table 4 on next page)

5.2 Pharmacokinetic properties

The plasma pharmacokinetics for total doxorubicin in patients receiving Myocet shows a high degree of interpatient variability. In general however, the plasma levels of total doxorubicin are substantially higher with Myocet than with conventional doxorubicin, while the data indicate that peak plasma levels of free (not liposome-encapsulated) doxorubicin are lower with Myocet than with conventional doxorubicin. Available pharmacokinetic data preclude conclusions regarding the relationship between plasma levels of total/free doxorubicin and its influence on the efficacy/safety of Myocet. The clearance of total doxorubicin was 5.1 ± 4.8 l/h and the volume of distribution at steady state (V_d) was 56.6 ± 61.5 l whereas after conventional doxorubicin, clearance and V_d were 46.7 ± 9.6 l/h and 1,451 ± 258 l, respectively. The major circulating metabolite of doxorubicin, doxorubicinol, is formed via aldo-keto-reductase. The peak levels of doxorubicinol occur in the plasma later with Myocet than with conventional doxorubicin.

The pharmacokinetics of Myocet have not been specifically studied in patients with renal or hepatic insufficiency. Doxorubicin is known to be eliminated in large part by the liver. Thus, dose reduction of Myocet may be considered in patients with impaired hepatic function (see also 4.2).

Substances that inhibit P-glycoprotein (P-Gp) have been shown to alter the disposition of doxorubicin and doxorubicinol (see also 4.5).

5.3 Preclinical safety data

Studies of genotoxicity, carcinogenicity and reproductive toxicity of Myocet have not been performed but doxorubicin is known to be both mutagenic and carcinogenic and may cause toxicity to reproduction.

Table 2 Haematological adverse events[c]

	Myocet /CPA (60/600 mg/m^2) (n = 142)[a] %	Myocet /CPA (75/600 mg/m^2) (n = 76)[b] %	Myocet (75 mg/m^2) (n = 105) %
Neutropenia <2000/μl	96	100 87	87
<500/μl	61	25	50
<500/μl for ⩾ 7 days	1		0
Thrombocytopenia			
<100,000/μl	51	54	83
<20,000/μl	4	4	13
Anaemia			
<11 g/dl	88	96	85
<8 g/dl	23	25	22
Infection			
All Grades	53	22	36
Grade ⩾3	11	7	5
Neutropenic Fever			
ANC<500 & fever>38°C	10	8	14
ANC>500 & fever> 38°C with IV antibiotics and/or hospitalisation	9	5	11

[a] From doxorubicin-controlled study

[b] From epirubicin-controlled study

[c] Regardless of causality

Table 3 Non-haematological adverse events[c]

	Myocet /CPA (60/600 mg/m^2) (n = 142)[a] %	Myocet /CPA (75/600 mg/m^2) (n = 76)[b] %	Myocet (75 mg/m^2) (n = 105) %
Nausea/Vomiting All Grades Grade ≥ 3	80 13	84 21	90 13
Stomatitis/Mucositis All Grades Grade ≥3	40 4	36 7	56 9
Fatigue/Malaise/Asthenia All Grades Grade ≥ 3	42 6	33 0	70 14
Diarrhoea All Grades Grade ≥ 3	28 3	21 1	26 1
Cutaneous All Grades Grade ≥ 3	11 0	4 0	16 1
Injection site toxicity All Grades Grade ≥ 3	5 1	1 0	15 0
Alopecia Pronounced	91	82	84

[a] From doxorubicin-controlled study
[b] From epirubicin-controlled study
[c] Regardless of causality

Table 4 Antitumour efficacy summary for combination and single-agent studies

	Myocet/CPA (60/600 mg/m^2) (n=142)	Dox 60/CPA (60/600 mg/m^2) (n=155)	Myocet/CPA (75/600 mg/m^2) (n=80)	Epi/CPA (75/600 mg/m^2) (n=80)	Myocet (75 mg/m^2) (n=108)	Dox (75 mg/m^2) (n=116)
Tumour response rate	43%	43%	46%	39%	26%	26%
Relative Risk (95% C.I.)	1.01 (0.78-1.31)		1.19 (0.83-1.72)		1.00 (0.64-1.56)	
Median PFS (months)[a]	5.1	5.5	7.7	5.6	2.9	3.2
Risk Ratio (95% C.I.)	1.03 (0.80-1.34)		1.52 (1.06-2.20)		0.87 (0.66-1.16)	

Abbreviations: PFS, progression-free survival; Dox, doxorubicin; Epi, epirubicin; Relative Risk, comparator taken as reference; Risk Ratio, Myocet taken as reference
[a] Secondary endpoint

6. PHARMACEUTICAL PARTICULARS

6.1 List of excipients

Myocet doxorubicin HCl
• lactose

Myocet liposomes
• egg phosphatidylcholine
• cholesterol
• citric acid
• sodium chloride
• water for injections

Myocet buffer
• sodium carbonate
• water for injections

6.2 Incompatibilities

This medicinal product must not be mixed with other medicinal products except those mentioned in 6.6.

6.3 Shelf life

18 months

Chemical and physical in-use stability after reconstitution has been demonstrated for up to 8 hours at 25°C, and for up to 5 days at 2°C – 8°C.

From a microbiological point of view, the product should be used immediately. If not used immediately, in-use storage times and conditions prior to use are the responsibility of the user and would normally not be longer than 24 hours at 2°C – 8°C, unless reconstitution and dilution has taken place in controlled and validated aseptic conditions.

6.4 Special precautions for storage

Store at 2°C – 8°C (in a refrigerator).

6.5 Nature and contents of container

Myocet is available in cartons containing 2 sets of the three constituents. Sodium chloride for injection 0.9%, needed to dissolve doxorubicin HCl, is not provided in the package.

Myocet doxorubicin HCl

Type I glass vials containing 50 mg of doxorubicin HCl lyophilised powder, sealed with grey butyl rubber stoppers and orange flip-off aluminium seals.

Myocet liposomes

Type I flint glass tubing vials containing not less than 1.9 ml of liposomes, sealed with siliconised grey stopper and green flip-off aluminium seals.

Myocet buffer

Glass vials containing not less than 3 ml of buffer, sealed with siliconised grey stopper and blue aluminium flip-off seals.

6.6 Instructions for use and handling

Preparation of Myocet

ASEPTIC TECHNIQUE MUST BE STRICTLY OBSERVED THROUGHOUT HANDLING OF MYOCET SINCE NO PRESERVATIVE IS PRESENT.

Caution should be exercised in the handling and preparation of Myocet. The use of gloves is required

Step 1. Set up

Two alternative heating methods can be used: a Techne DB-3 Dri Block heater or a water bath:

• Turn on the Techne DB-3 Dri Block heater and set the controller to 75-76°C. Verify the temperature set point by checking the thermometer(s) on each heat block insert.

• If using a water bath, turn on the water bath and allow it to equilibrate at 58°C (55-60°C). Verify the temperature set point by checking the thermometer.

(Please note that whilst the control settings on the water bath and heat block are set to different levels the temperature of the vial contents are in the same range (55-60°C)).

Remove the carton of Myocet constituents from the refrigerator.

Step 2. Reconstitute doxorubicin HCl

• Withdraw 20 ml sodium chloride for injection (0.9%), *preservative free*, (not provided in the package), and inject into each Myocet doxorubicin HCl, intended for preparation.

• Shake well in the inverted position to ensure doxorubicin is fully dissolved.

Step 3. Heat in water bath or dry heat block

• Heat the reconstituted Myocet doxorubicin HCl vial in the Techne Dri Block heater with the thermometer in the block reading (75-76°C) for 10 minutes (not to exceed 15 minutes). If using the water bath heat the Myocet doxorubicin HCl vial with the thermometer temperature reading 55-60°C for 10 minutes (not to exceed 15 minutes).

• While heating proceed to step 4

Step 4. Adjust Ph of liposomes

• Withdraw 1.9 ml of Myocet liposomes. Inject into Myocet buffer vial to adjust the Ph of liposomes. *Pressure build-up may require venting.*

• Shake well.

Step 5. Add Ph-adjusted liposomes to doxorubicin

• Using syringe, withdraw the entire vial contents of Ph-adjusted liposomes from the Myocet buffer vial.

• Remove the reconstituted Myocet doxorubicin HCl vial from the water bath or dry heat block. SHAKE VIGOROUSLY. Carefully insert a pressure-venting device equipped with a hydrophobic filter. Then IMMEDIATELY (within 2 minutes) inject Ph-adjusted liposomes into vial of heated reconstituted Myocet doxorubicin HCl. Remove venting device.

• SHAKE VIGOROUSLY.

• WAIT FOR A MINIMUM OF 10 MINUTES BEFORE USING, KEEPING THE MEDICINE AT ROOM TEMPERATURE.

The Techne DB3 Dri Block Heater is fully validated for use in the constitution of Myocet. Three inserts, each with two 43.7mm openings per insert must be used. To ensure correct temperature control the use of a 35mm immersion thermometer is recommended.

The resulting reconstituted preparation of Myocet contains 50 mg of doxorubicin HCl/25 ml of liposomal dispersion (2 mg/ml).

After reconstitution the finished product must be further diluted in 0.9% (w/v) sodium chloride for injection, or 5% (w/v) glucose for injection to a final volume of 40 ml to 120 ml per 50 mg reconstituted Myocet so that a final concentration of 0.4 to 1.2 mg/ml doxorubicin is obtained.

Once constituted, the liposomal dispersion for infusion containing liposome-encapsulated doxorubicin should be a red orange opaque homogeneous dispersion. All parenteral solutions should be inspected visually for particulate matter and discoloration prior to administration. Do not use the preparation if foreign particulate matter is present.

Procedure for proper disposal

Any unused product or waste material should be disposed of in accordance with local requirements.

7. MARKETING AUTHORISATION HOLDER

Elan Pharma International Limited
WIL House
Shannon Business Park
Shannon, County Clare
Ireland

8. MARKETING AUTHORISATION NUMBER(S)

EU/1/00/141/001

9. DATE OF FIRST AUTHORISATION/RENEWAL OF THE AUTHORISATION

13-07-2000

10. DATE OF REVISION OF THE TEXT

17-07-2002

11. LEGAL CATEGORY

POM

Myocrisin

(sanofi-aventis)

1. NAME OF THE MEDICINAL PRODUCT

MYOCRISIN

2. QUALITATIVE AND QUANTITATIVE COMPOSITION

Sodium Aurothiomalate BP 10 mg in 0.5 ml (2.0% w/v)

Sodium Aurothiomalate BP 20 mg in 0.5 ml (4.0% w/v)

Sodium Aurothiomalate BP 50 mg in 0.5 ml (10.0% w/v)

3. PHARMACEUTICAL FORM

Injection

4. CLINICAL PARTICULARS

4.1 Therapeutic indications

Myocrisin is used in the management of active progressive rheumatoid arthritis and progressive juvenile chronic arthritis especially if polyarticular or seropositive.

4.2 Posology and method of administration

Do not use a darkened solution (more than pale yellow).

Myocrisin should be administered only by deep intramuscular injection followed by gentle massage of the area. The patient should remain under medical observation for a period of 30 minutes after drug administration.

Adults

An initial test dose of 10 mg should be given in the first week followed by weekly doses of 50 mg until signs of remission occur. At this point 50 mg doses should be given at two week intervals until full remission occurs. With full remission the interval between injections should be increased progressively to three, four and then, after 18 months to 2 years, to six weeks.

If after reaching a total dose of 1 g (excluding the test dose), no major improvement has occurred and the patient has not shown any signs of gold toxicity, six 100 mg injections may be administered at weekly intervals. If no sign of remission occurs after this time other forms of treatment are to be considered.

Elderly

There are no specific dosage recommendations. Elderly patients should be monitored with extra caution

Children: Progressive juvenile chronic arthritis:

Weekly doses of 1 mg/kg should be given but not exceeding a maximum weekly dose of 50 mg. Depending on urgency, this dose may be preceded by a smaller test dose such as 1/10 or 1/5 of the full dose for 2-3 weeks. Continue weekly doses until signs of remission appear then increase the intervals between injections to two weeks. With full remission increase the interval to three then four weeks. In the absence of signs of remission after twenty weeks consider raising the dose slightly or changing to another therapy.

Treatment should be continued for six months. Response can be expected at the 300-500 mg level. If patients respond, maintenance therapy should be continued with the dosage administered over the previous 2-4 weeks, for 1-5 years.

4.3 Contraindications

Pregnancy (see section 4.6)

Myocrisin is contraindicated in patients with gross renal or hepatic disease, a history of blood dyscrasias, exfoliative dermatitis or systemic lupus erythematosus.

The absolute contraindications should be positively excluded before considering gold therapy.

4.4 Special warnings and special precautions for use

As with other gold preparations, reactions which resemble anaphylactoid effects have been reported. These effects may occur after any course of therapy within the first ten minutes following drug administration (see administration). If anaphylactoid effects are observed, treatment with Myocrisin should be discontinued (see section 4.8).

Myocrisin should be administered with extra caution in the elderly and in patients with a history of urticaria, eczema or colitis. Extra caution should also be exercised if phenylbutazone or oxyphenbutazone are administered concurrently.

Before starting treatment and again before each injection, the urine should be tested for protein, the skin inspected for rash and a full blood count performed, including a numerical platelet count (not an estimate) and the readings plotted. Blood dyscrasias are most likely to occur when between 400 mg and 1 g of gold have been given, or between the 10th and 20th week of treatment, but can also occur with much lower doses or after only 2-4 weeks of therapy (see section 4.8).

The presence of albuminuria, pruritus or rash, or an eosinophilia, are indications of developing toxicity (see section 4.8). The Myocrisin should be withheld for one or two weeks until all signs have disappeared when the course may be restarted on a test dose followed by a decreased frequency of gold injections.

A complaint of sore throat, glossitis, buccal ulceration and/or easy bruising or bleeding, demands an immediate blood count, followed if indicated, by appropriate treatment for agrananulocytosis, aplastic anaemia and/or thrombocytopenia (see section 4.8). Every patient treated with Myocrisin should be warned to report immediately the appearance of pruritus, metallic taste, sore throat or tongue, buccal ulceration or easy bruising, purpura, epistaxis, bleeding gums, menorrhagia or diarrhoea (see section 4.8).

4.5 Interaction with other medicinal products and other forms of Interaction

Concurrent gold administration may exacerbate aspirin-induced hepatic dysfunction. Caution should be exercised if phenylbutazone or oxyphenbutazone are administered concurrently.

Caution is needed in patients treated concomitantly with sodium aurothiomalate and angiotensin-converting enzyme inhibitors due to an increased risk of severe anaphylactoid reaction in these patients.

4.6 Pregnancy and lactation

The safety of Myocrisin in the foetus and the newborn has not been established. Female patients receiving Myocrisin should be instructed to avoid pregnancy. Pregnant patients should not be treated with Myocrisin. Lactating mothers under treatment with Myocrisin excrete significant amounts of gold in their breast milk and should not breast feed their infants.

4.7 Effects on ability to drive and use machines

None

4.8 Undesirable effects

Blood dyscrasias including thrombocytopenia, pancytopenia, agranulocytosis, aplastic anaemia, leucopenia & neutropenia have been reported (see section 4.4).

Anaphylactic/Anaphylactoid reactions have been reported, symptoms of which may include weakness, flushing, hypotension, tachycardia, dyspnoea, palpitations, abdominal pain, shock and possibly collapse (see section 4.4).

Hepatotoxicity with cholestatic jaundic is a rare complication which may occur early in the course of treatment. It subsides on withdrawing Myocrisin. A rare but severe form of enterocolitis has been described.

Diffuse unilateral or bilateral pulmonary fibrosis very rarely occurs. This progressive condition usually responds to drug withdrawal and steroid therapy. An annual x-ray is recommended and attention should be paid to unexplained breathlessness and dry cough.

Side effects may be largly avoided by the indicated careful titration of dosage. Minor reactions, usually manifest as skin rashes and pruritus are the most frequent and commonly benign, but as such reactions may be the forerunners of severe gold toxicity they must never be treated lightly. Other indicators of developing toxicity could be the presence of albuminuria or an eosophilia (see section 4.4)

Severe skin reactions that have been reported include exfoliative dermatitis and bullous eruptions. Irreversible skin pigmentation (chrysiasis) can occur in sun-exposed areas after prolonged treatment with Myocrisin. Rare reports of alopecia exist. Nephrotic syndrome has been rarely reported.

Neurological manifestations of gold toxicity including very rare cases of peripheral neuropathy, Guillain-Barré syndrome and encephalopathy have been observed

4.9 Overdose

Minor side effects resolve spontaneously on withdrawal of Myocrisin. Symptomatic treatment of pruritus with antihistamines may be helpful. Major skin lesions and serious blood dyscrasias demand hospital admission when dimercaprol or penacillamine may be used to enhance gold excretion. Fresh blood and/or platelet transfusions, corticosteroids and androgenic steroids may be required in the management of severe blood dyscasias.

5. PHARMACOLOGICAL PROPERTIES

5.1 Pharmacodynamic properties

The precise mode of action of sodium aurothiomalate is not yet known. Treatment with gold has been shown to be accompanied by a fall in ESR and C-reactive protein, an increase in serum histidine and sulphydryl levels and a reduction in serum immunoglobulins, rheumatoid factor titres and Clq-binding activity.

Numerous experimental observations have been recorded including physico-chemical changes in collagen and interference with complement activation, gammaglobulin aggregation, prostaglandin biosythesis, inhibition of cathepsin and production of superoxide radicals by activated polymophonuclear leucocytes.

5.2 Pharmacokinetic properties

Sodium aurothiomalate is absorbed readily after intramuscular injection and becomes bound to plasma proteins. With doses of 50 mg weekly the steady-state serum concentration of gold is about 3 to 5 microgram per ml. It is widely distributed and accumulates in the body. Concentrations in synovial fluid have been shown to be similar or slightly less than those in plasma. Sodium aurothiomalate is mainly excreted in the urine with smaller amounts in the faeces. The serum half-life of gold clearance is about 5 or 6 days but after a course of treatment, gold may be found in the urine for up to a year or more owing to its presence in deep body compartments. Gold has been detected in the foetus following administration of sodium aurothiomalate to the mother. Gold has been detected in the breast fed child where the mother has received sodium aurothiomalate.

5.3 Preclinical safety data

No additional pre-clinical data of relevance to the prescriber.

6. PHARMACEUTICAL PARTICULARS

6.1 List of excipients

Phenylmercuric nitrate BP

Water for Injections BP

6.2 Incompatibilities

None stated

6.3 Shelf life

36 months

6.4 Special precautions for storage

Store below 25°C. Protect from light

6.5 Nature and contents of container

Carton containing 10 sealed glass ampoules each containing 0.5ml injection solution.

6.6 Instructions for use and handling

None stated

7. MARKETING AUTHORISATION HOLDER

JHC Healthcare Ltd

5 Lower Merrion Street

Dublin 2

Eire

8. MARKETING AUTHORISATION NUMBER(S)

Injection 10mg 16186/0007

Injection 20mg 16186/0008

Injection 50mg 16186/0009

9. DATE OF FIRST AUTHORISATION/RENEWAL OF THE AUTHORISATION

1 September 1997

10. DATE OF REVISION OF THE TEXT

September 2002

11. LEGAL CLASSIFICATION

POM

Myotonine

(Glenwood Laboratories Ltd)

1. NAME OF THE MEDICINAL PRODUCT

Myotonine ® (bethanechol chloride).

2. QUALITATIVE AND QUANTITATIVE COMPOSITION

Each 10mg tablet weighs 400mg; total active ingredient 10mg bethanechol chloride USPXXIV

The 25mg tablet weighs 450mg; total active ingredient 25mg bethanechol chloride USPXXIV

3. PHARMACEUTICAL FORM

Each 25mg tablet is white, flat with bevelled edge and cross score.

Each 10mg tablet is white, flat with bevelled edge and with a single score.

4. CLINICAL PARTICULARS

4.1 Therapeutic indications

Urinary retention -indicated for the treatment of acute postoperative and postpartum non-obstructive (functional) urinary retention and neurogenic atony of the urinary bladder with retention.

Reflux oesophagitis; treatment of reflux associated with decreased pressure of the lower oesophageal sphincter or delayed gastric emptying.

4.2 Posology and method of administration

Administration orally by tablets.

Adults: 10mg –25mg three or four times daily, taken half an hour before food. Occasionally it may be necessary to initiate therapy with a 50mg dose.

Children: The experience with children is limited therefore no recommended dose is given.

4.3 Contraindications

Intestinal or urinary obstruction, recent myocardial infarction, recent intestinal anastomosis.

4.4 Special warnings and special precautions for use

A severe cholinergic reaction is likely if bethanechol chloride is administered IV or IM. This reaction has also rarely occurred in cases of hypersensitivity or overdose.

4.5 Interaction with other medicinal products and other forms of Interaction

Cholinergics, other, especially cholinesterase inhibitors.

Ganglionic blocking agents such as mecamylamine, pentolinium and trimethaphan.

Procainamide or quniidine.

4.6 Pregnancy and lactation

Should not be used during pregnancy or lactation.

4.7 Effects on ability to drive and use machines

In some cases the ability to drive and operate machinery may be impaired.

4.8 Undesirable effects

Nausea, vomiting, sweating and intestinal colic.

4.9 Overdose

The symptoms of overdose include nausea, salivation, lachrymation, eructation, involuntary defecation and urination, transient dyspnoea, palpitation, bradycardia and peripheral vasodilation leading to hypertension, transient heart block and a feeling of constriction under the sternum.

Procedure: The stomach should be emptied by aspiration or lavage. Give atropine sulphate 1-2mg intravenously, intramuscularly or subcutaneously to control muscarinic effects. The dose may be repeated every 2-4 hours as necessary.

Supportive treatment includes intravenous administration of diazepam 5-10mg: muscle twitching may be controlled by small doses of tubocararine (together with assisted respiration): oxygen may be required.

5. PHARMACOLOGICAL PROPERTIES

5.1 Pharmacodynamic properties

Bethanechol is a synthetic choline ester of carbamic acid which possesses a significant acetylcholine-like activity. It is active after oral administration. As a consequence of the very slow hydrolysation by acetylcholinesterase bethanechol has a prolonged action as has been demonstrated in the urinary tract.[1] The onset of action occurs after oral administration within an hour.[2,3]

The major pharmacological effects of bethanechol result from interaction of the drug with muscarinic receptor sites of smooth muscles, especially those of the urinary bladder and gastrointestinal tract.[1,4,5]

In addition, minor but important nicotinic effects have been noted. In usual therapeutic doses, bethanechol does not cross the blood brain barrier.[6]

5.2 Pharmacokinetic properties

Studies not available.

5.3 Preclinical safety data

N/A

6. PHARMACEUTICAL PARTICULARS

6.1 List of excipients

Calcium sulphate dihydrate BP.

Maize starch BP.

Talc BP(iron free)

Magnesium stearate BP.

6.2 Incompatibilities

Major –none known.

6.3 Shelf life

The shelf life of Myotonine tablets is currently two years from date of manufacture.

6.4 Special precautions for storage

Keep out of reach of children and away from direct heat or light sources.

Store below 25 °C.

6.5 Nature and contents of container

The container is of polypropylene with a tamper-evident polyethylene cap and closure. A filla may be inserted to reduce the risk of tablet breakage due to ullage.

Each container is filled with 100 tablets.

6.6 Instructions for use and handling

7. MARKETING AUTHORISATION HOLDER

Glenwood Laboratories UK Ltd.

Jenkins Dale

Chatham

Kent

ME4 5RD

8. MARKETING AUTHORISATION NUMBER(S)

Myotonine 10mg 00245/5009R

Myotonine 25mg 00245/5010R.

9. DATE OF FIRST AUTHORISATION/RENEWAL OF THE AUTHORISATION

November 1996

10. DATE OF REVISION OF THE TEXT

February 2000, April 1996, July 1995.

References

1. Draper JW, Zorgniotta AW. The effects of banthine and similar agents on the urinary tract. N.Y. State J.Med 1954: 54;77

2. Boas E.Comarr AE. Neurological Urology. Baltimore, University Park Press 1971; 215

3. Lapides J., Friend CR, Ajemian EP, Sonda LP. Comparison of action of oral and parenteral bethanechol chloride upon the urinary bladder. Invest.Urol 1963: 1:94

4. Paul DA, Icardi JA, Parkman HP, Ryan JP. Development changes in gastric fundus smooth muscle contractility and involvement of extra cellular calcium in foetal and adult guinea pigs. Paediatr. Res. 1994:36:642-646

5. Ursillo RC. Rationale for drug therapy in bladder dysfunction. In. Boyarsk S. The Neurogenic Bladder, Baltimore, The Williams and Wilkins Co. 1967;187

6. Goodman Gilman. The Pharmacological basis of Therapeutics. Editors: Goodman, Gilman A: Rale T.W., Nies AS, Taylor P., New York. Pergamon Press. 8th Edition 1991.

Myotonine 10 mg (Bethanechol Chloride)

(Glenwood Laboratories Ltd)

1. NAME OF THE MEDICINAL PRODUCT

Myotonine ®(bethanechol chloride).

2. QUALITATIVE AND QUANTITATIVE COMPOSITION

Each 10mg tablet weighs 400mg; total active ingredient 10mg bethanechol chloride USPXXIV

3. PHARMACEUTICAL FORM

Each 10mg tablet is white, flat with bevelled edge with a single score and embossed "MYO10"

4. CLINICAL PARTICULARS

4.1 Therapeutic indications

Urinary retention -indicated for the treatment of acute postoperative and postpartum non-obstructive (functional) urinary retention and neurogenic atony of the urinary bladder with retention.

Reflux oesophagitis; treatment of reflux associated with decreased pressure of the lower oesophageal sphincter or delayed gastric emptying.

4.2 Posology and method of administration

Administration orally by tablets.

Adults: 10mg –25mg three or four times daily, taken half an hour before food. Occasionally it may be necessary to initiate therapy with a 50mg dose.

Children: The experience with children is limited therefore no recommended dose is given.

4.3 Contraindications

Intestinal or urinary obstruction, recent myocardial infarction, recent intestinal anastomosis.

4.4 Special warnings and special precautions for use

A severe cholinergic reaction is likely if bethanechol chloride is administered IV or IM. This reaction has also rarely occurred in cases of hypersensitivity or overdose.

4.5 Interaction with other medicinal products and other forms of Interaction

Cholinergics, other, especially cholinesterase inhibitors.

Ganglionic blocking agents such as mecamylamine, pentolinium and trimethaphan.

Procainamide or quinidine.

4.6 Pregnancy and lactation

Should not be used during pregnancy or lactation.

4.7 Effects on ability to drive and use machines

In some cases the ability to drive and operate machinery may be impaired.

4.8 Undesirable effects

Nausea, vomiting, sweating and intestinal colic.

4.9 Overdose

The symptoms of overdose include nausea, salivation, lachrymation, eructation, involuntary defecation and urination, transient dyspnoea, palpitation, bradycardia and peripheral vasodilation leading to hypertension, transient heart block and a feeling of constriction under the sternum.

Procedure: The stomach should be emptied by aspiration or lavage. Give atropine sulphate 1-2mg intravenously, intramuscularly or subcutaneously to control muscarinic effects. The dose may be repeated every 2-4 hours as necessary.

Supportive treatment includes intravenous administration of diazepam 5-10mg: muscle twitching may be controlled by small doses of tubocararine (together with assisted respiration): oxygen may be required.

5. PHARMACOLOGICAL PROPERTIES

5.1 Pharmacodynamic properties

Bethanechol is a synthetic choline ester of carbamic acid which possesses a significant acetylcholine-like activity. It is active after oral administration. As a consequence of the very slow hydrolysation by acetylcholinesterase bethanechol has a prolonged action as has been demonstrated in the urinary tract.[1] The onset of action occurs after oral administration within an hour.[2,3]

The major pharmacological effects of bethanechol result from interaction of the drug with muscarinic receptor sites of smooth muscles, especially those of the urinary bladder and gastrointestinal tract.[1,4,5]

In addition, minor but important nicotinic effects have been noted. In usual therapeutic doses, bethanechol does not cross the blood brain barrier.[6]

5.2 Pharmacokinetic properties

Studies not available.

5.3 Preclinical safety data

N/A

6. PHARMACEUTICAL PARTICULARS

6.1 List of excipients

Calcium sulphate dihydrate BP.

Maize starch BP.

Talc BP(iron free)

6.2 Incompatibilities

Major –none known.

6.3 Shelf life

The shelf life of Myotonine tablets is currently two years from date of manufacture.

6.4 Special precautions for storage

Keep out of reach of children and away from direct heat or light **sources.**

Store below 25EC.

6.5 Nature and contents of container

The container is of polypropylene with a tamper-evident polyethylene cap and closure. A filla may be inserted to reduce the risk of tablet breakage due to ullage.

Each container is filled with 100 tablets.

6.6 Instructions for use and handling

7. MARKETING AUTHORISATION HOLDER

Glenwood Laboratories UK Ltd.

Jenkins Dale

Chatham

Kent

ME4 5RD

8. MARKETING AUTHORISATION NUMBER(S)

Myotonine 10mg 00245/5009R

9. DATE OF FIRST AUTHORISATION/RENEWAL OF THE AUTHORISATION

November 1996

10. DATE OF REVISION OF THE TEXT

February 2002, Feb 2000, April 1996, July 1995.

References

1. Draper JW, Zorgniotta AW. The effects of banthine and similar agents on the urinary tract. N.Y. State J.Med 1954: 54;77

2. Boas E.Comarr AE. Neurological Urology. Baltimore, University Park Press 1971; 215

3. Lapides J., Friend CR, Ajemian EP, Sonda LP. Comparison of action of oral and parenteral bethanechol chloride upon the urinary bladder. Invest.Urol 1963: 1:94

4. Paul DA, Icardi JA, Parkman HP, Ryan JP. Development changes in gastric fundus smooth muscle contractility and involvement of extra cellular calcium in foetal and adult guinea pigs. Paediatr. Res. 1994:36:642-646

5. Ursillo RC. Rationale for drug therapy in bladder dysfunction. In. Boyarsk S. The Neurogenic Bladder, Baltimore, The Williams and Wilkins Co. 1967;187

6. Goodman Gilman. The Pharmacological basis of Therapeutics. Editors: Goodman, Gilman A: Rale T.W., Nies AS, Taylor P., New York. Pergamon Press. 8th Edition 1991.

Myotonine 25 mg (Bethanechol Chloride)

(Glenwood Laboratories Ltd)

1. NAME OF THE MEDICINAL PRODUCT

Myotonine ®(bethanechol chloride).

2. QUALITATIVE AND QUANTITATIVE COMPOSITION

Each 25mg tablet weighs 440mg; total active ingredient 25mg bethanechol chloride USPXXIV

3. PHARMACEUTICAL FORM

Each 25mg tablet is white, flat with bevelled edge and with a cross score and the embossment "MY25"

4. CLINICAL PARTICULARS

4.1 Therapeutic indications

Urinary retention -indicated for the treatment of acute postoperative and postpartum non-obstructive (functional) urinary retention and neurogenic atony of the urinary bladder with retention.

Reflux oesophagitis; treatment of reflux associated with decreased pressure of the lower oesophageal sphincter or delayed gastric emptying.

4.2 Posology and method of administration

Administration orally by tablets.

Adults: 10mg –25mg three or four times daily, taken half an hour before food. Occasionally it may be necessary to initiate therapy with a 50mg dose.

Children: The experience with children is limited therefore no recommended dose is given.

4.3 Contraindications

Intestinal or urinary obstruction, recent myocardial infarction, recent intestinal anastomosis.

4.4 Special warnings and special precautions for use

A severe cholinergic reaction is likely if bethanechol chloride is administered IV or IM. This reaction has also rarely occurred in cases of hypersensitivity or overdose.

4.5 Interaction with other medicinal products and other forms of Interaction

Cholinergics, other, especially cholinesterase inhibitors.

Ganglionic blocking agents such as mecamylamine, pentolinium and trimethaphan.

Procainamide or quinidine.

4.6 Pregnancy and lactation

Should not be used during pregnancy or lactation.

4.7 Effects on ability to drive and use machines

In some cases the ability to drive and operate machinery may be impaired.

4.8 Undesirable effects

Nausea, vomiting, sweating and intestinal colic.

4.9 Overdose

The symptoms of overdose include nausea, salivation, lachrymation, eructation, involuntary defecation and urination, transient dyspnoea, palpitation, bradycardia and peripheral vasodilation leading to hypertension, transient heart block and a feeling of constriction under the sternum.

Procedure: The stomach should be emptied by aspiration or lavage. Give atropine sulphate 1-2mg intravenously, intramuscularly or subcutaneously to control muscarinic effects. The dose may be repeated every 2-4 hours as necessary.

Supportive treatment includes intravenous administration of diazepam 5-10mg: muscle twitching may be controlled by small doses of tubocararine (together with assisted respiration): oxygen may be required.

5. PHARMACOLOGICAL PROPERTIES

5.1 Pharmacodynamic properties

Bethanechol is a synthetic choline ester of carbamic acid which possesses a significant acetylcholine-like activity. It is active after oral administration. As a consequence of the very slow hydrolysation by acetylcholinesterase bethanechol has a prolonged action as has been demonstrated in the urinary tract.[1] The onset of action occurs after oral administration within an hour.[2,3]

The major pharmacological effects of bethanechol result from interaction of the drug with muscarinic receptor sites of smooth muscles, especially those of the urinary bladder and gastrointestinal tract.[1,4,5]

In addition, minor but important nicotinic effects have been noted. In usual therapeutic doses, bethanechol does not cross the blood brain barrier.[6]

5.2 Pharmacokinetic properties

Studies not available.

5.3 Preclinical safety data

N/A

6. PHARMACEUTICAL PARTICULARS

6.1 List of excipients

Calcium sulphate dihydrate BP.

Maize starch BP.

Talc BP(iron free)

6.2 Incompatibilities

Major –none known.

6.3 Shelf life

The shelf life of Myotonine tablets is currently two years from date of manufacture.

6.4 Special precautions for storage

Keep out of reach of children and away from direct heat or light sources.

Store below 25EC.

6.5 Nature and contents of container

The container is of polypropylene with a tamper-evident polyethylene cap and closure. A filla may be inserted to reduce the risk of tablet breakage due to ullage.

Each container is filled with 100 tablets.

6.6 Instructions for use and handling

7. MARKETING AUTHORISATION HOLDER

Glenwood Laboratories UK Ltd.

Jenkins Dale

Chatham

Kent

ME4 5RD

8. MARKETING AUTHORISATION NUMBER(S)

Myotonine 25mg 00245/5010R

9. DATE OF FIRST AUTHORISATION/RENEWAL OF THE AUTHORISATION

November 1996

10. DATE OF REVISION OF THE TEXT

February 2002, 2000, April 1996, July 1995.

References

1. Draper JW, Zorgniotta AW. The effects of banthine and similar agents on the urinary tract. N.Y. State J.Med 1954: 54;77

2. Boas E.Comarr AE. Neurological Urology. Baltimore, University Park Press 1971; 215

3. Lapides J., Friend CR, Ajemian EP, Sonda LP. Comparison of action of oral and parenteral bethanechol chloride upon the urinary bladder. Invest.Urol 1963: 1:94

4. Paul DA, Icardi JA, Parkman HP, Ryan JP. Development changes in gastric fundus smooth muscle contractility and involvement of extra cellular calcium in foetal and adult guinea pigs. Paediatr. Res. 1994:36:642-646

5. Ursillo RC. Rationale for drug therapy in bladder dysfunction. In. Boyarsk S. The Neurogenic Bladder, Baltimore, The Williams and Wilkins Co. 1967;187

6. Goodman Gilman. The Pharmacological basis of Therapeutics. Editors: Goodman, Gilman A: Rale T.W., Nies AS, Taylor P., New York. Pergamon Press. 8th Edition 1991.

Nabilone Capsules

(Cambridge Laboratories)

1. NAME OF THE MEDICINAL PRODUCT
Nabilone Capsules

2. QUALITATIVE AND QUANTITATIVE COMPOSITION
Nabilone Capsules contain 1.0mg Nabilone per capsule.

3. PHARMACEUTICAL FORM
Blue and white capsules imprinted "CL 3101".

4. CLINICAL PARTICULARS

4.1 Therapeutic indications
Nabilone is indicated for the control of nausea and vomiting, caused by chemotherapeutic agents used in the treatment of cancer, in patients who have failed to respond adequately to conventional antiemetic treatments.

4.2 Posology and method of administration
Nabilone is for administration to adults only. It is not recommended for use in children younger than 18 years of age as safety and efficacy have not been established.

The usual adult dosage is 1mg or 2mg twice a day. To minimise side-effects, it is recommended that the lower starting dose is used and that the dose is increased as necessary. The first dose should be administered the night before initiation of chemotherapy, and the second dose should be given one to three hours before the first dose of the oncolytic agent is administered.

The maximum daily dose should not exceed 6mg, given in three divided doses.

Nabilone may be administered throughout each cycle of chemotherapy and, if necessary, for 48 hours after the last dose of each cycle. Data on the chronic use of nabilone are not available.

The elderly: as for adults (see 'precautions').

4.3 Contraindications
Nabilone is contra-indicated in patients with a known allergy to cannabinoid agents and when the nausea and vomiting arises from any cause other than cancer chemotherapy.

4.4 Special warnings and special precautions for use
As nabilone is excreted primarily by the biliary route, the drug is not recommended for use in patients with severe liver dysfunction.

Patients receiving Nabilone should be closely observed, if possible, within an inpatient setting. This is especially important during the treatment of naive patients. However, even patients experienced with cannabinoid agents may have serious untoward responses not predicted by prior uneventful exposures. Patients should be made aware of possible changes of mood and other adverse behavioural effects of the drug.

Since Nabilone can elevate supine and standing heart rates and cause postural hypotension, it should be used with caution in the elderly and in patients with hypertension and heart disease.

4.5 Interaction with other medicinal products and other forms of Interaction
Nabilone should be administered with caution to patients who are taking other psychoactive drugs or CNS depressants, including alcohol, barbiturates and narcotic analgesics, or to those with a history of psychiatric disorder (including manic-depressive illness and schizophrenia). Nabilone has been shown to have an additive CNS depressant effect when given with either diazepam, secobarbitone sodium, alcohol or codeine.

4.6 Pregnancy and lactation
Usage in pregnancy: Laboratory studies have so far shown no evidence of teratogenicity. There are no adequate and well controlled studies in pregnant women. Nabilone should be used during pregnancy only if clearly needed.

Reproduction studies performed in rats at 150 times the human dose and rabbits at 40 times the human dose revealed a dose-related reduction in litter size, an increase in the incidence of foetal resorptions, and an increase in the incidence of stillborn pups. The number of implantations was unaffected by treatment. These effects appear related to the dose-dependent reduction in maternal food intake and gain in body weight induced by Nabilone. At 150 times the maximum recommended human dose, Nabilone produced a reduction in neonatal survival that may be related to reduced milk production by mothers. Nabilone is known to have an inhibitory effect on prolactin release, which could contribute to the observed reduction in milk production. Hypothermia was also reported in the offspring of high-dose groups of female rats, which may have also contributed to reduced neonatal survival.

Nursing mothers: It is not known whether this drug is excreted in breast milk. It is not recommended that Nabilone be given to nursing mothers.

4.7 Effects on ability to drive and use machines
Nabilone may impair the mental and/or physical abilities required for the performance of potentially hazardous tasks such as operating machinery or driving a car; therefore the patient should be advised accordingly. The effects of Nabilone may persist for a variable and unpredictable period of time following its oral administration. Adverse psychiatric reactions can persist for 48 to 72 hours following cessation of treatment.

4.8 Undesirable effects
During controlled clinical trials of nabilone, virtually all patients experienced at least one adverse reaction. These included pyschotomimetic reactions.

In these trials, the commonest statistically significant adverse events (in decreasing order of incidence) were: drowsiness, vertigo/dizziness, euphoria (high), dry mouth, ataxia, visual disturbance, concentration difficulties, sleep disturbance, dysphoria, hypotension, headache and nausea.

Other reported events include confusion, disorientation, hallucinations, psychosis, depression, decreased co-ordination, tremors, tachycardia, decreased appetite and abdominal pain.

Tolerance to such CNS effects as relaxation, drowsiness and euphoria develops rapidly and is readily reversible.

D rug abuse and dependence: Nabilone is an abusable substance, capable of producing subjective side-effects, such as euphoria or "high", at therapeutic doses. Prescriptions should be limited to the amount necessary for a single cycle of chemotherapy (ie., a few days). The physical dependence capability of Nabilone is unknown. Patients who participated in clinical trials, up to 5 days duration, showed no withdrawal symptoms on cessation of dosing.

4.9 Overdose
Signs and symptoms are an extension of the psychotomimetic and physiological effects of nabilone. Overdosage may be considered to have occurred, even at prescribed dosages, if disturbing psychiatric symptoms are present. Subsequent doses should be withheld until patients have returned to their baseline mental status; routine dosing, possibly at a lower dose, may then be resumed if clinically indicated. In controlled clinical trials, alterations in mental status, related to the use of nabilone, resolved within 72 hours without specific medical therapy. Vital signs should be monitored, since hypertension, hypotension and tachycardia have occurred.

No cases of overdosage with more than 10mg/day of Nabilone have been reported during clinical trials. Signs and symptoms to be anticipated in large overdose situations are psychotic episodes, including hallucinations and anxiety reactions, respiratory depression and coma.

Treatment: Conservative management, if possible (ie. verbal support and comfort). In more severe cases, antipsychotic drugs may be useful, although they have not been systematically evaluated. Such patients should be closely monitored because of the potential for drug interactions (eg., additive CNS depressant effects due to Nabilone and chlorpromazine).

General supportive care is recommended. Consider giving activated charcoal to decrease absorption from the gastrointestinal tract. The use of forced diuresis, peritoneal dialysis, haemodialysis, charcoal haemoperfusion, or cholestyramine, has not been reported. Most of a dose of Nabilone is eliminated through the biliary system.

Treatment for respiratory depression and comatose state consists of symptomatic and supportive therapy. Attention should be paid to the occurrence of hypothermia. Consider fluids, inotropes and/or vasopressors for hypotension.

5. PHARMACOLOGICAL PROPERTIES

5.1 Pharmacodynamic properties
Nabilone is a synthetic cannabinoid which has been shown to have significant anti-emetic activity in patients undergoing chemotherapy for malignant neoplasms. The mode of action of Nabilone has been studied in cats and dogs. Although its anti-emetic action is not yet fully understood, it is apparent that there are a number of points in the control systems of the body at which Nabilone could block the emetic mechanism.

5.2 Pharmacokinetic properties
Absorption
Two fasted subjects were given an oral dose of 2mg ^{14}C-nabilone. Nabilone was readily absorbed from the gastrointestinal tract. Pharmacokinetic comparison between the oral and intravenous routes of administration suggested that most of the drug was available after oral dosage. Similarly, the percentages of radioactivity in the faeces and urine were approximately sixty per cent and twenty-four per cent respectively whichever route was employed, supporting the view that most of the oral dose was absorbed.

Half-life
The plasma half-life of unchanged Nabilone in these volunteers was approximately two hours. The estimated half-life of the carbinol metabolite was somewhat longer at between five and ten hours. Total radioactivity had a half-life of approximately thirty-five hours.

Transport
The rapid disappearance of absorbed drug from the plasma has been related to extensive tissue distribution and to rapid metabolism and excretion.

Metabolism
Two metabolic pathways have been suggested. The major pathway probably involves the direct oxidation of Nabilone to produce hydroxylic and carboxylic analogues. These compounds are thought to account for the remaining plasma radioactivity when carbinol metabolites have been extracted.

Excretion
When 2mg of ^{14}C-nabilone was administered orally, over sixty per cent of the total radioactivity was eliminated in the faeces and about twenty five per cent in the urine. The discrepancy is probably due to additive analytical errors, since respiratory $^{14}C\ CO_2$ did not account for the remaining fifteen per cent. Comparison with intravenous administration indicated no significant differences in the excretion pattern suggesting the biliary system to be the major excretory pathway.

5.3 Preclinical safety data
Monkeys treated with Nabilone at doses as high as 2mg/kg/day for a year experienced no significant adverse events. This result contrasts with the finding in a planned 1-year dog study that was prematurely terminated because of deaths associated with convulsions in dogs receiving as little as 0.5mg/kg/day. The earliest deaths, however, occurred at 56 days in dogs receiving 2mg/kg/day. The unusual vulnerability of the dog is not understood; it is hypothesised, however, that the explanation lies in the fact that the dog differs markedly from other species (including humans) in its metabolism of Nabilone.

Carcinogenesis, Mutagenesis, Impairment of Fertility: Carcinogenicity studies have not been performed with Nabilone. The influence on fertility and reproduction at doses of 150 and 40 times the maximum recommended human dose was evaluated in rats and rabbits, respectively. In these studies there was no evidence of teratogenicity due to Nabilone. In high dose groups, however, Nabilone produced a slight decrease in mean litter size, although the number of implantations was unaffected by treatment.

6. PHARMACEUTICAL PARTICULARS

6.1 List of excipients
Povidone

Starch flowable

Indigo carmine

Red iron oxide

Titanium dioxide

Gelatin

Edible black ink

6.2 Incompatibilities
None known.

6.3 Shelf life
Three years.

6.4 Special precautions for storage
Bottles: Keep tightly closed. Store at 15° - 25°C.

Blisters: Store at 15° - 25°C.

6.5 Nature and contents of container
High density polyethylene bottles with screw caps or blister packs, each containing 20 capsules.

6.6 Instructions for use and handling
None.

7. MARKETING AUTHORISATION HOLDER
Cambridge Laboratories Limited

Deltic House

Kingfisher Way

Silverlink Business Park

Wallsend

Tyne & Wear

NE28 9NX

8. MARKETING AUTHORISATION NUMBER(S)
PL 12070/0013

9. DATE OF FIRST AUTHORISATION/RENEWAL OF THE AUTHORISATION
Not Applicable.

10. DATE OF REVISION OF THE TEXT
March 2000

Nalcrom

(sanofi-aventis)

1. NAME OF THE MEDICINAL PRODUCT
Nalcrom™

2. QUALITATIVE AND QUANTITATIVE COMPOSITION
in terms of the active ingredient (INN) name

The active component per capsule is:

Sodium Cromoglicate 100.0mg

3. PHARMACEUTICAL FORM
Nalcrom is presented as a hard gelatin capsule with a colourless, transparent cap and body, printed in black 'SODIUM CROMOGLICATE 100 mg' and containing a white powder.

4. CLINICAL PARTICULARS

4.1 Therapeutic indications
Nalcrom is indicated for food allergy (where adequate investigations have been performed to determine sensitivity to one or more ingested allergens) in conjunction with restriction of main causative allergens.

4.2 Posology and method of administration
Nalcrom must be administered orally

Adults (including the elderly)

Initial dose: 2 capsules four times daily before meals

Children (2 - 14 years)

Initial dose: 1 capsule four times daily before meals

For adults (including the elderly) and children, if satisfactory control is not achieved within two to three weeks, the dosage may be doubled but should not exceed 40 mg/Kg/day.

Maintenance dose: Once a therapeutic response has been achieved, the dose may be reduced to the minimum required to maintain the patient free from symptoms.

4.3 Contraindications
Nalcrom is contraindicated in patients with a known sensitivity to sodium cromoglicate.

4.4 Special warnings and special precautions for use
None stated

4.5 Interaction with other medicinal products and other forms of Interaction
None known.

4.6 Pregnancy and lactation
As with all medication caution should be exercised especially during the first trimester of pregnancy. Cumulative experience with sodium cromoglicate suggests that it has no adverse effects on foetal development. It should only be used in pregnancy where there is a clear need.

It is not known whether sodium cromoglicate is excreted in the breast milk but on the basis of its physico-chemical properties this is considered unlikely. There is no information to suggest that the use of sodium cromoglicate has any undesirable effects on the baby.

4.7 Effects on ability to drive and use machines
None known.

4.8 Undesirable effects
Nausea, skin rashes and joint pains have been reported in a few cases.

4.9 Overdose
As Nalcrom is only absorbed to a minimum extent, no action other than medical supervision should be necessary.

5. PHARMACOLOGICAL PROPERTIES

5.1 Pharmacodynamic properties
Sodium cromoglicate inhibits the release from mast cells of mediators of the allergic reaction. In gastrointestinal allergy the release of mediators can result in gastrointestinal symptoms or may allow absorption of antigenic material leading to systemic allergic reactions.

5.2 Pharmacokinetic properties
Not applicable

5.3 Preclinical safety data
Animal studies have shown that sodium cromoglicate has a very low order of local or systemic toxicity.

6. PHARMACEUTICAL PARTICULARS

6.1 List of excipients
Purified Water, No 2 hard gelatin capsules.

6.2 Incompatibilities
None stated.

6.3 Shelf life
60 months

6.4 Special precautions for storage
Store in a dry place.

6.5 Nature and contents of container
An aluminium can with aluminium screw cap containing 100 capsules or an HDPE bottle with screw cap containing 100 capsules.

6.6 Instructions for use and handling
Instructions for use are supplied with each pack.

7. MARKETING AUTHORISATION HOLDER
Aventis Pharma Ltd
50 Kings Hill Avenue
West Malling
Kent
ME19 4AH
United Kingdom

8. MARKETING AUTHORISATION NUMBER(S)
PL 04425/0370

9. DATE OF FIRST AUTHORISATION/RENEWAL OF THE AUTHORISATION
1st May 2005

10. DATE OF REVISION OF THE TEXT

11. LEGAL CATEGORY
POM

Nalorex

(Bristol-Myers Squibb Pharmaceuticals Ltd)

1. NAME OF THE MEDICINAL PRODUCT
NALOREX®

2. QUALITATIVE AND QUANTITATIVE COMPOSITION
Naltrexone hydrochloride 50 mg per tablet.

3. PHARMACEUTICAL FORM
Pale yellow, film coated, capsule-shaped tablet debossed on one side with 'R11' and scored and debossed with '50' on the other side.

4. CLINICAL PARTICULARS

4.1 Therapeutic indications
Nalorex is indicated as an adjunctive prophylactic therapy in the maintenance of detoxified, formerly opioid-dependent patients.

4.2 Posology and method of administration
Route of administration - oral.

Nalorex treatment should be initiated in a drug addiction centre and supervised by suitably qualified physicians.

The initial dose of Nalorex should be 25 mg (half a tablet) followed by 50 mg (one tablet) daily.

A three-times-a-week dosing schedule may be considered if it is likely to result in better compliance e.g. 100 mg on Monday, 100 mg on Wednesday and 150 mg on Friday.

Treatment with Nalorex should be considered only in patients who have remained opioid-free for a minimum of 7-10 days.

Narcan® (Naloxone hydrochloride) challenge is recommended to minimise the chance of a prolonged withdrawal syndrome precipitated by Nalorex (see also Warnings).

As Nalorex is an adjunctive therapy and full recovery from opioid dependence is variable, no standard duration of treatment can be recommended; an initial period of three months should be considered. However, prolonged administration may be necessary.

Use in Children
Safe use in children has not been established.

Use in Elderly
There is no experience of use in the elderly.

4.3 Contraindications
Nalorex should not be given to patients with acute hepatitis or liver failure.

Nalorex should not be given to patients currently dependent on opioids since an acute withdrawal syndrome may ensue.

Nalorex should not be used in conjunction with an opioid-containing medication.

Nalorex should not be given to patients who are hypersensitive to it.

4.4 Special warnings and special precautions for use
It is not uncommon for opioid abusing individuals to have impaired liver function.

Liver function test abnormalities have been reported in obese and elderly patients taking naltrexone who have no history of drug abuse. Liver function tests should be carried out both before and during treatment.

Since NALOREX is extensively metabolised by the liver and excreted predominantly in the urine, caution should be observed in administering the drug to patients with impaired hepatic or renal function. Liver function tests should be carried out both before and during treatment.

A withdrawal syndrome may be precipitated by NALOREX in opioid dependent patients; signs and symptoms may develop within 5 minutes and last up to 48 hours. Treatment should be symptomatic and may include opioid administration.

Narcan (Naloxone Hydrochloride) challenge is recommended to screen for presence of opioid use; a withdrawal syndrome precipitated by Narcan will be of shorter duration than one precipitated by Nalorex.

The recommended procedure is as follows:

- i.v. injection of 0.2 mg Narcan
- if after 30 seconds no adverse reactions occur, a further i.v. injection of 0.6 mg Narcan may be administered
- continue to observe the patient for withdrawal effects for a further 30 minutes.

If doubt exists that the patient is opioid-free, the challenge may be repeated with a Narcan dose of 1.6 mg.

If there is no evidence of a reaction, Nalorex administration may be initiated with 25 mg by mouth (half a tablet).

4.5 Interaction with other medicinal products and other forms of Interaction
Concomitant administration of Nalorex with an opioid-containing medication should be avoided. Patients should be warned that attempts to overcome the blockade may result in acute opioid intoxication which may be life threatening. In an emergency requiring opioid analgesia an increased dose of opioid may be required to control pain. The patient should be closely monitored for evidence of respiratory depression or other adverse symptoms and signs.

4.6 Pregnancy and lactation
Animal studies do not suggest a teratogenic effect. Because of absence of documented clinical experience Nalorex should only be given to pregnant or breast-feeding women when, in the judgement of the attending physician, the potential benefits outweigh the possible risks.

4.7 Effects on ability to drive and use machines
Nalorex may impair the mental and/or physical abilities required for performance of potentially hazardous tasks such as driving a car or operating machinery.

4.8 Undesirable effects
The following adverse reactions have been reported before and during naltrexone medication:

- an incidence of more than 10% in detoxified opioid abusers: difficulty sleeping, anxiety, nervousness, abdominal pain/cramps, nausea and/or vomiting, low energy, joint and muscle pain, and headache;
- an incidence of less than 10%: loss of appetite, diarrhoea, constipation, increased thirst, increased energy, feeling down, irritability, dizziness, skin rash, delayed ejaculation, decreased potency, chills, chest pain, increased sweating and increased lacrimation.

Occasional liver function abnormalities have also been reported. One case of reversible idiopathic thrombocytopenic purpura has occurred in a patient taking Nalorex.

4.9 Overdose
There is no clinical experience with NALOREX overdose in patients. There was no evidence of toxicity in volunteers receiving 800 mg/day for seven days, however, in case of overdose, patients should be monitored and treated symptomatically in a closely supervised environment.

5. PHARMACOLOGICAL PROPERTIES

5.1 Pharmacodynamic properties
Naltrexone is a specific, high affinity, long acting competitive antagonist at opioid receptors. It has negligible opioid agonist activity. Tolerance does not develop with prolonged use.

5.2 Pharmacokinetic properties
Naltrexone is rapidly absorbed after oral administration. It is metabolised by the liver and excreted primarily in the urine, less than 5% is excreted in the faeces. Naltrexone has an elimination half-life of four hours. The major metabolite 6-beta-naltrexol has an elimination half-life of 12.9 hours.

5.3 Preclinical safety data
Nalorex is well established in medical use. Preclinical data is broadly consistent with clinical experience.

6. PHARMACEUTICAL PARTICULARS

6.1 List of excipients
Lactose Monohydrate

Microcrystalline Cellulose

Crospovidone

Silica, Colloidal Anhydrous

Magnesium Stearate

Pale Yellow Opadry

Pale Yellow Opadry contains hypromellose, macrogol, polysorbate 80 and colouring agents titanium dioxide (E171) and yellow and red iron oxides (E172).

6.2 Incompatibilities
Not applicable

6.3 Shelf life
36 months

6.4 Special precautions for storage
No special precautions for storage

6.5 Nature and contents of container
White opaque PVC/PE/Aclar blister with aluminium foil in packs of 28 tablets.

6.6 Instructions for use and handling
Not applicable.

7. MARKETING AUTHORISATION HOLDER
Bristol-Myers Squibb Pharmaceuticals Limited

Uxbridge Business park

Sanderson Road

Uxbridge

Middlesex, UB8 1DH

8. MARKETING AUTHORISATION NUMBER(S)
PL 11184/0104

9. DATE OF FIRST AUTHORISATION/RENEWAL OF THE AUTHORISATION
31 July 1992 / 15 July 1999

10. DATE OF REVISION OF THE TEXT
June 2005

Naloxone Hydrochloride Injection, Minijet.

(International Medication Systems (UK) Ltd)

1. NAME OF THE MEDICINAL PRODUCT
Naloxone Hydrochloride Injection, Minijet™

2. QUALITATIVE AND QUANTITATIVE COMPOSITION
Naloxone hydrochloride USP (as dihydrate) 0.4mg/ml in 1ml, 2ml, or 5ml Minijet™ prefilled syringes.

3. PHARMACEUTICAL FORM
Sterile aqueous solution for injection.

4. CLINICAL PARTICULARS

4.1 Therapeutic indications
Naloxone is indicated for the treatment of respiratory depression induced by natural and synthetic opioids, such as codeine, diamorphine, levorphanol, methadone, morphine, concentrated opium alkaloid hydrochlorides and propoxyphene. It is also useful for the treatment of respiratory depression caused by opioid agonist/ antagonists nalbuphine and pentazocine. Naloxone is also used for the diagnosis of suspected acute opioid overdose.

4.2 Posology and method of administration
Naloxone hydrochloride may be administered by IV, IM or SC injection or IV infusion.

Adults:

Naloxone may be diluted for intravenous infusion in normal saline or 5% dextrose solutions. The addition of 2 mg of naloxone in 500 ml of either solution provides a concentration of 4 μg /ml. Infusion should be commenced as soon as practicable after preparation of the mixture in order to reduce microbiological hazards. Preparations not used within 24 hours should be discarded. The rate of administration should be titrated in accordance with the patient's response. Parenteral drug products should be inspected visually for particulate matter and discolouration prior to administration whenever solution and container permit.

Naloxone hydrochloride may be used postoperatively to reverse central depression resulting from the use of opioids during surgery. The usual dosage is 100 - 200 μg IV given at 2 to 3 minute intervals to obtain optimum respiratory response while maintaining adequate analgesia. Additional doses may be necessary at one to two hour intervals depending on the response of the patient and the dosage and duration of action of the opioid administered.

For the treatment of known opioid overdosage or as an aid in the diagnosis of suspected opioid overdosage, the usual initial adult dosage of naloxone hydrochloride is 400 - 2000 μg IV, administered at 2 to 3 minute intervals if necessary. If no response is observed after a total of 10 mg of the drug has been administered, the depressive condition may be caused by a drug or disease process not responsive to naloxone. When the IV route cannot be used, the drug may be administered by IM or SC injection.

Children:

The usual initial dose in children is 10 μg / kg bodyweight given IV. If the dose does not result in the desired degree of clinical improvement, a subsequent dose of 100 μg / kg body weight may be administered. If the IV route of administration is not available, naloxone may be administered IM or SC in divided doses. If necessary naloxone can be diluted with sterile water for injection.

Opioid - induced depression in neonates resulting from the administration of opioid analgesics to the mother during labour may be reversed by administering naloxone hydrochloride 10 μg / kg body weight to the infant by IM, IV or SC injections, repeated at intervals of 2 to 3 minutes if necessary. Alternatively, a single IM dose of about 60 μg / kg may be given at birth for a more prolonged action.

Elderly:

In elderly patients with pre-existing cardiovascular disease or in those receiving potentially cardiotoxic drugs, naloxone should be used with caution since serious adverse cardiovascular effects such as ventricular tachycardia and fibrillation have occurred in postoperative patients following administration of naloxone.

4.3 Contraindications
Naloxone is contraindicated in patients with known hypersensitivity to the drug.

4.4 Special warnings and special precautions for use
It should be administered with caution to patients who have received large doses of opioids or to those physically dependent on opioids since too rapid reversal may precipitate an acute withdrawal syndrome in such patients. When naloxone hydrochloride is used in the management of acute opioid overdosage, other resuscitation measures should be readily available. A withdrawal syndrome may also be precipitated in newborn infants of opioid-dependent mothers.

Following the use of opioids during surgery, excessive dosage of naloxone hydrochloride should be avoided, because it may cause excitement, increase in blood pressure and clinically important reversal of analgesia. A reversal of opioid effects achieved too rapidly may induce nausea, vomiting, sweating or tachycardia.

Naloxone should be also used with caution in patients with preexisting cardiovascular disease or in those receiving potentially cardiotoxic drugs, since serious adverse cardiovascular effects such as ventricular tachycardia and fibrillation have occurred in postoperative patients following administration of naloxone.

Patients who have responded to naloxone should be carefully monitored, since the duration of action of some opioids may exceed that of naloxone.

4.5 Interaction with other medicinal products and other forms of Interaction
No drug or chemical agent should be added to naloxone unless its effect on the chemical and physical stability of the solution has first been established.

4.6 Pregnancy and lactation
Reproductive studies in mice and rats using naloxone hydrochloride dosage up to 1000 times the usual human dosage have not revealed evidence of impaired fertility or harm to the foetus. There are no adequate and controlled studies using the drug in pregnant women. Naloxone hydrochloride should be used only when clearly needed. Since it is not known whether naloxone hydrochloride is distributed into breast milk, the drug should be used with caution in nursing women.

4.7 Effects on ability to drive and use machines
Not applicable.

4.8 Undesirable effects
Abrupt reversal of narcotic depression may result in nausea, vomiting, sweating, tachycardia, hyperventilation, increased blood pressure and tremulousness.

In postoperative patients, larger than necessary dosages of naloxone may result in significant reversal of analgesia and in excitement.

Hypotension, hypertension, ventricular tachycardia and fibrillation, hyperventilation and pulmonary oedema have been associated with the use of naloxone postoperatively. Seizures have occurred on rare occasions following the administration of naloxone, but a causal relationship to the drug has not been established.

4.9 Overdose
There have been no reports of acute overdosage due to naloxone hydrochloride.

5. PHARMACOLOGICAL PROPERTIES

5.1 Pharmacodynamic properties
Naloxone hydrochloride is a semisynthetic (N-allylnoroxymorphine hydrochloride) opioid antagonist which is derived from thebaine. When administered in usual doses to patients who have not recently received opioids, naloxone exerts little or no pharmacologic effect. Even extremely high doses of the drug (10 times the usual therapeutic dose) produces insignificant analgesia, only slight drowsiness and no respiratory depression, psychotomimetic effects, circulatory changes or miosis.

In patients who have received large doses of diamorphine or other analgesic drugs with morphine-like effects, naloxone antagonises most of the effects of the opioid. There is an increase in respiratory rate and minute volume, arterial CO_2 decreases toward normal and blood pressure returns to normal if depressed. Naloxone antagonises mild respiratory depression cause by small doses of opioids. Because the duration of action of naloxone is generally shorter than that of the opioid, the effects of the opioid may return as the effects of naloxone dissipates. Naloxone antagonises opioid-induced sedation or sleep. Reports are conflicting on whether or not the drug modifies opioid-induced excitement or siezures.

Naloxone does not produce tolerance or physical or psychological dependence. However, 0.4 mg of naloxone hydrochloride administered SC will precipitate potentially severe withdrawal symptoms in patients physically dependent on opioids or pentazocine. The precise mechanism of action of the opioid antagonist effects of naloxone is not known. Naloxone is thought to act as a competitive antagonist at μ, K or σ opioid receptors in the central nervous system. It is thought that the drug has the highest affinity for the μ receptor.

5.2 Pharmacokinetic properties
Naloxone has an onset of action within 1 to 2 minutes following IV administration and within 2 to 5 minutes following SC or IM administration. The duration of action depends on the dose and route of administration and is more prolonged following IM administration than after IV administration. In one study, the duration of action was 45 minutes following IV administration of naloxone hydrochloride 0.4 mg/70 kg.

Following administration of 35 or 70 μg of naloxone hydrochloride in the umbilical vein in neonates in one study, peak plasma naloxone concentrations occurred within 40 minutes and were 4 - 5.4 ng/ml and 9.2 - 20.2 ng/ml, respectively. After IM administration of 0.2 mg to neonates in the same study, peak plasma naloxone concentrations of 11.3 - 34.7 ng/ml occurred within 0.5 - 2 hours.

Following parenteral administration, naloxone is rapidly distributed into body tissues and fluids. In rats, high concentrations are observed in the brain, kidney, spleen, lungs, heart and skeletal muscles. In humans, the drug readily crosses the placenta. It is not known whether naloxone is distributed into milk.

The plasma half-life of naloxone has been reported to be 60 to 90 minutes in adults and about 3 hours in neonates.

Naloxone is rapidly metabolised in the liver, principally by conjugation with glucuronic acid. The major metabolite is naloxone-3-glucuronide. Naloxone also undergoes N-dealkylation and reduction of the 6-keto group followed by conjugation. Limited studies with radiolabeled naloxone indicated that 25 - 40% IV doses of the drug is excreted as metabolites in urine in 6 hours, about 50% in 24 hours and 60 - 70% in 72 hours.

5.3 Preclinical safety data
Not applicable since naloxone has been used in clinical practice for many years and its effects in man are well known.

6. PHARMACEUTICAL PARTICULARS

6.1 List of excipients
Sodium Chloride USP

Hydrochloric Acid NF

Water for Injection USP

6.2 Incompatibilities
Naloxone should not be mixed with preparations containing bisulphite, metabisulphite, long-chain or high molecular anions or any solution having an alkaline pH.

6.3 Shelf life
2 years

6.4 Special precautions for storage
Store below 25°C.

6.5 Nature and contents of container
The solution is contained in a Type I USP glass vial with a rubber closure which meets all the relevent USP specifications for elastomeric closures. The product is available as 1ml, 2ml or 5ml.

6.6 Instructions for use and handling
The container is specially designed for use with the IMS Minijet™ injector.

Administrative Data

7. MARKETING AUTHORISATION HOLDER
International Medication Systems (UK) Ltd

208 Bath Road

Slough

Berkshire

SL1 3WE

UK

8. MARKETING AUTHORISATION NUMBER(S)
PL 3265/0071

9. DATE OF FIRST AUTHORISATION/RENEWAL OF THE AUTHORISATION
Date first granted: 29 September 1986

Date renewed: 24 June 1999

10. DATE OF REVISION OF THE TEXT
April 2001

POM

Napratec OP

(Pharmacia Limited)

1. NAME OF THE MEDICINAL PRODUCT
NAPRATEC® OP

2. QUALITATIVE AND QUANTITATIVE COMPOSITION
Napratec is a combination pack containing 56 Naproxen 500mg tablets and 56 Cytotec (misoprostol) 200mcg tablets.

For excipients, see 6.1

3. PHARMACEUTICAL FORM
Tablet

Naproxen 500mg tablets are yellow, oblong and engraved SEARLE N500 with a breakline on one side.

Cytotec is a white/off-white hexagonal tablet, scored on both sides, engraved SEARLE 1461 on one side.

4. CLINICAL PARTICULARS

4.1 Therapeutic indications

Napratec combination pack is indicated for patients who require Naproxen 500mg twice daily and Cytotec 200mcg twice daily.

Naproxen is indicated for the treatment of rheumatoid arthritis, osteoarthritis (degenerative arthritis) and ankylosing spondylitis.

Cytotec is indicated for the prophylaxis of nonsteroidal anti-inflammatory drug (NSAID)-induced gastroduodenal ulceration.

4.2 Posology and method of administration

Adults

1 tablet of Naproxen and 1 tablet of Cytotec taken together twice daily with food.

Elderly

Studies indicate that although total plasma concentration of naproxen is unchanged, the unbound plasma fraction of naproxen is increased in the elderly.

With Cytotec the usual dosage may be used in the elderly.

Napratec should only be used in those patients for whom 500mg naproxen twice daily is appropriate and in whom no reduction of naproxen dosage is necessary (see also sections on renal and hepatic impairment).

Renal Impairment

As the final pathway for the elimination of naproxen metabolites is largely (95%) by urinary excretion via glomerular filtration it should be used with great caution in patients with impaired renal function and the monitoring of serum creatinine and/or creatinine clearance is advised in these patients. Naproxen is not recommended in patients having a baseline creatinine clearance of less than 20ml/minute.

Certain patients, specifically those whose renal blood flow is compromised, such as in extracellular volume depletion, cirrhosis of the liver, sodium restriction, congestive heart failure, and pre-existing renal disease, should have renal function assessed before and during naproxen therapy. Some elderly patients in whom impaired renal function may be expected could also fall within this category. Where there is a possibility of accumulation of naproxen metabolites, such patients may not be suitable to receive naproxen 500mg twice daily.

With Cytotec no dosage alteration is necessary in patients with impaired renal function.

Hepatic Impairment

Chronic alcoholic liver disease and probably also other forms of cirrhosis reduce the total plasma concentration of naproxen, but the plasma concentration of unbound naproxen is increased.

With Cytotec no dosage alteration is necessary in patients with impaired hepatic function.

Children

Napratec is not recommended.

4.3 Contraindications

Use in Pregnancy and Lactation

Napratec is contraindicated in pregnancy and lactation (see 4.6)

This medicine is also contraindicated in patients planning to become pregnant.

Napratec is contraindicated in patients with a known allergy to any of the constituents.

As the potential exists with naproxen for cross-sensitivity to aspirin and other nonsteroidal anti-inflammatory drugs, Napratec should not be administered to patients in whom aspirin and other NSAIDs induce asthma, rhinitis, urticaria or angioedema.

As Napratec is a "prevention pack" it should not be used for treating arthritis in patients with active gastric or duodenal ulceration. Such patients may be treated with a healing dose of Cytotec, 800 micrograms daily in divided doses with meals, and the NSAID continued or discontinued at the physician's discretion.

Use in pre-menopausal women

Napratec should not be used in pre-menopausal women unless the patient is at high risk of complications from NSAID-induced ulceration. In such patients it is advised that Napratec should only be used if the patient:

- takes effective contraceptive measures

- has been advised of the risks of taking the product if pregnant

4.4 Special warnings and special precautions for use

Precautions

Naproxen, in common with other NSAIDs, decreases platelet aggregation and prolongs bleeding time. This effect should be considered when bleeding times are determined.

Naproxen may precipitate bronchospasm in patients suffering from, or with a history of, bronchial asthma or allergic disease.

Mild peripheral oedema has been observed in a few patients receiving naproxen. Although sodium retention has not been reported in metabolic studies, it is possible that patients with questionable or compromised cardiac function may be at a greater risk when taking naproxen.

In patients with renal, cardiac or hepatic impairment caution is required since the use of NSAIDs may result in deterioration of renal function.

Sporadic abnormalities in laboratory tests (e.g. liver function tests) have occurred in patients on naproxen, but no definite trend was seen in any test indicating toxicity.

Cytotec should be used with caution in disease states where hypotension might precipitate severe complications, e.g. cerebrovascular disease, coronary artery disease or severe peripheral vascular disease including hypertension.

Patients with rare hereditary problems of galactose intolerance, the Lapp lactase deficiency or glucose-galactose malabsorption should not take this medicine.

4.5 Interaction with other medicinal products and other forms of Interaction

Drug Interactions

Due to the high plasma protein binding of naproxen, patients simultaneously receiving hydantoins, anti-coagulants or a highly protein-bound sulphonamide should be observed for signs of over dosage of these drugs. No interactions have been observed in clinical studies with naproxen and anti-coagulants or sulphonylureas, but caution is nevertheless advised since interaction has been seen with other non-steroidal agents of this class.

NSAIDs may attenuate the natriuretic efficacy of diuretics due to inhibition of intrarenal synthesis of prostaglandins.

Because of their effect on renal prostaglandins, cyclo-oxygenase inhibitors such as naproxen can increase the nephrotoxicity of cyclosporin.

NSAID including naproxen have been reported to increase steady state plasma lithium levels. It is recommended that these are monitored whenever initiating, adjusting or discontinuing naproxen products.

Concomitant administration of Naproxen with cardiac glycosides may exacerbate cardiac failure, reduce GFR and increase plasma glycoside levels.

Concomitant administration of naproxen with beta-blockers may reduce their antihypertensive effect.

Concomitant use with other NSAIDs or with corticosteroids may increase the frequency of side effects generally.

Animal data indicate that NSAIDs can increase the risk of convulsions associated with quinolone antibiotics. Patients taking NSAIDs and quinolones may have an increased risk of developing convulsions.

Probenecid given concurrently increases naproxen plasma levels and extends it plasma half-life considerably.

Caution is advised when methotrexate is administered concurrently because of possible enhancement of its toxicity since naproxen, among other NSAIDs, has been reported to induce the tubular secretion of methotrexate in an animal model.

Naproxen therapy should be temporarily withdrawn before adrenal function tests are performed as it may artificially interfere with some tests for 17-ketogenic steroids. Similarly, naproxen may interfere with some assays of urinary 5-hydroxyindoleacetic acid.

Cytotec is predominantly metabolised via fatty acid oxidising systems and has shown no adverse effect on the hepatic microsomal mixed function oxidase (P450) enzyme system. No drug interactions have been attributed to Cytotec, and in specific studies, no clinically significant pharmacokinetic or pharmacodynamic interaction has been demonstrated with antipyrine, diazepam, propranolol or NSAIDs.

4.6 Pregnancy and lactation

Napratec is contraindicated in pregnancy. This is on the basis that Cytotec is contraindicated in pregnancy or women planning a pregnancy as it increases uterine tone and contractions in pregnancy which may cause partial or complete expulsion of the products of conception.

Teratology studies with naproxen in rats and rabbits at dose levels equivalent on a human multiple basis to those which have produced foetal abnormality with certain other NSAIDs, e.g. aspirin, have not produced evidence of foetal damage with naproxen. As with other drugs of this type, naproxen delays parturition in animals (the relevance of this finding to human patients is unknown) and also affects the human foetal cardiovascular system (closure of the ductus arteriosus).

4.7 Effects on ability to drive and use machines

Dizziness, drowsiness, visual disturbances or headaches are possible undesirable effects after taking NSAIDs, if affected, patients should not drive or operate machinery.

4.8 Undesirable effects

Naproxen:

Gastrointestinal: The more frequent reactions are nausea, vomiting, abdominal discomfort and epigastric distress. The more serious reaction, colitis, may occasionally occur.

Naproxen also causes gastrointestinal bleeding and gastric and duodenal ulceration, the consequences of which may be haemorrhage and perforation. The inclusion of Cytotec in the combination pack is to prevent naproxen-induced gastric and duodenal ulceration.

Dermatological/Hypersensitivity: Non-specific allergic reactions, respiratory tract reactivity comprising asthma, aggravated asthma, bronchospasm or dyspnoea, skin rashes, purpura, urticaria, angio-oedema. Anaphylactic reactions to naproxen and naproxen sodium formulations, eosinophilic pneumonitis, alopecia, erythema multiforme, Stevens Johnson syndrome, epidermal necrolysis, photosensitivity reactions, pseudoporphyria and epidermolysis bullosa may occur rarely.

Central Nervous System: Headache, paraesthesia, depression, confusion, hallucinations, dizziness, malaise, fatigue, drowsiness, optic neuritis, insomnia, inability to concentrate and cognitive dysfunction have been reported.

Renal: As a class NSAIDs have been associated with renal pathology including papillary necrosis, interstitial nephritis, nephrotic syndrome and renal failure.

Haematological: Thrombocytopenia, granulocytopenia, agranulocytosis, aplastic anaemia and haemolytic anaemia may occur rarely.

Other: Tinnitus, hearing impairment, vertigo, mild peripheral oedema. Jaundice, fatal hepatitis, nephropathy, haematuria, visual disturbances, vasculitis, aseptic meningitis and ulcerative stomatitis have been reported rarely.

Cytotec:

Gastrointestinal: Diarrhoea has been reported and is occasionally severe and prolonged, and may require withdrawal of the drug. It can be minimised by taking Cytotec with food and by avoiding the use of predominantly magnesium-containing antacids when an antacid is required. Abdominal pain with or without associated dyspepsia can follow Cytotec therapy. Other gastrointestinal adverse effects reported include dyspepsia, flatulence, nausea and vomiting.

Female Reproductive System: Menorrhagia, vaginal bleeding and intermenstrual bleeding have been reported in both pre- and post-menopausal women.

Other Adverse Effects: Skin rashes have been reported. Dizziness has been infrequently reported.

4.9 Overdose

Naproxen:

Significant overdosage of the drug may be characterised by drowsiness, heartburn, indigestion, nausea or vomiting. A few patients have experienced seizures, but it is not clear whether these were naproxen-related or not. It is not known what dose of the drug would be life-threatening.

In the event of overdosage with naproxen, the stomach may be emptied and usual supportive measures employed. Animal studies indicate that the prompt administration of activated charcoal in adequate amounts would tend to reduce markedly the absorption of the drug.

Haemodialysis does not decrease the plasma concentration of naproxen because of the high degree of protein binding. However, haemodialysis may still be appropriate in a patient with renal failure who has taken naproxen.

Cytotec:

Intensification of pharmacological and adverse effects may occur with overdose. In the event of overdosage with Cytotec, symptomatic and supportive therapy should be given as appropriate.

5. PHARMACOLOGICAL PROPERTIES

5.1 Pharmacodynamic properties

Naproxen is a non-steroidal anti-inflammatory drug with well-documented properties, i.e. analgesic, antipyretic and anti-inflammatory.

Misoprostol is a synthetic prostaglandin E_1 analogue which enhances several of the factors that maintain gastroduodenal mucosal integrity.

5.2 Pharmacokinetic properties

Naproxen is readily absorbed from the GI tract. Peak plasma concentrations are obtained 2-4 hours after ingestion. At therapeutic concentrations, naproxen is more than 98% bound to plasma proteins and has an elimination half-life of between 12-15 hours.

Misoprostol is rapidly absorbed following oral administration with peak plasma levels of the active metabolite (misoprostol acid) occurring after about 30 minutes. The plasma elimination half-life of misoprostol acid is 20-40 minutes.

Increases in C_{max} and AUC for misoprostol acid have been observed when co-administered with naproxen in a single dose study. These changes are not thought to be clinically significant since the higher values are still well within the variation seen after 200 micrograms misoprostol in other studies. No accumulation of misoprostol acid in plasma occurs after repeated dosing of 400 micrograms twice daily.

5.3 Preclinical safety data

Naproxen causes gastric erosions when given orally or subcutaneously to fasting rats. There is no evidence of mutagenicity or carcinogenicity when administered to rats in studies of two years duration. There is no evidence of teratogenicity in mice, rats or rabbits.

Misoprostol in multiples of the recommended therapeutic dose in animals has produced gastric mucosal hyperplasia. This characteristic response to E-series prostaglandins reverts to normal on discontinuation of the compound.

6. PHARMACEUTICAL PARTICULARS

6.1 List of excipients

Naproxen 500mg tablets contain: Lactose, maize starch, povidone, sodium starch glycolate, magnesium stearate, yellow lake CLF 3076 (E104 and E172).

Cytotec 200mcg tablets contain: microcrystalline cellulose, sodium starch glycolate, hydrogenated castor oil and hypromellose.

6.2 Incompatibilities

Not applicable.

6.3 Shelf life

3 years

6.4 Special precautions for storage

Do not store above 30°C. Store in the original package.

6.5 Nature and contents of container

Combination pack containing 4 × 7 day treatment wallets each containing 56 Naproxen 500mg tablets in PVC/foil blisters and 56 Cytotec 200mcg tablets in cold-formed aluminium blisters.

6.6 Instructions for use and handling

No special requirements.

7. MARKETING AUTHORISATION HOLDER

Pharmacia Limited

Ramsgate Road

Sandwich

Kent, CT13 9NJ

United Kingdom

8. MARKETING AUTHORISATION NUMBER(S)

PL 00032/0486

9. DATE OF FIRST AUTHORISATION/RENEWAL OF THE AUTHORISATION

26 June 2002

10. DATE OF REVISION OF THE TEXT

July 2004

11. LEGAL CATEGORY

POM

Ref: NA1_2 UK

Naprosyn

(Roche Products Limited)

1. NAME OF THE MEDICINAL PRODUCT

Naprosyn

2. QUALITATIVE AND QUANTITATIVE COMPOSITION

Naproxen BP 250mg.

Naproxen BP 500mg.

3. PHARMACEUTICAL FORM

Naproxen 250

Round, buff, uncoated tablet embossed "NPR LE 250" on one face and with a breakline on the other.

Naproxen 500

Oval, buff, uncoated tablet embossed "NPR LE 500" on one face with a breakline on the other.

4. CLINICAL PARTICULARS

4.1 Therapeutic indications

Treatment of rheumatoid arthritis, osteoarthrosis (degenerative arthritis), ankylosing spondylitis, juvenile rheumatoid arthritis, acute gout, acute musculoskeletal disorders and dysmenorrhoea.

4.2 Posology and method of administration

Route of administration

Oral.

Adults

Rheumatoid arthritis, osteoarthritis and ankylosing spondylitis

500mg to 1g taken in 2 doses at 12-hour intervals or alternatively, as a single administration. In the following cases a loading dose of 750mg or 1g per day for the acute phase is recommended:

a) In patients reporting severe night-time pain/or morning stiffness.

b) In patients being switched to Naprosyn from a high dose of another anti-rheumatic compound.

c) In osteoarthrosis where pain is the predominant symptom.

Acute gout

750mg at once then 250mg every 8 hours until the attack has passed.

Acute musculoskeletal disorders and dysmenorrhoea

500mg initially followed by 250mg at 6 - 8 hour intervals as needed, with a maximum daily dose after the first day of 1250mg.

Elderly

Studies indicate that although total plasma concentration of naproxen is unchanged, the unbound plasma fraction of naproxen is increased in the elderly. The implication of this finding for Naprosyn dosing is unknown. As with other drugs used in the elderly it is prudent to use the lowest effective dose. For the effect of reduced elimination in the elderly refer to *Special warnings and special precautions for use*.

Children (over 5 years)

For juvenile rheumatoid arthritis: 10mg/kg/day taken in 2 doses at 12-hour intervals.

4.3 Contraindications

Active peptic ulceration or active gastrointestinal bleeding. Hypersensitivity to naproxen or naproxen sodium formulations. Since the potential exists for cross-sensitivity reactions, Naprosyn should not be given to patients in whom aspirin or other non-steroidal anti-inflammatory/analgesic drugs induce the syndrome of asthma, rhinitis or urticaria.

4.4 Special warnings and special precautions for use

Episodes of gastro-intestinal bleeding have been reported in patients with naproxen therapy. Naprosyn should be given under close supervision to patients with a history of gastro-intestinal disease.

Serious gastro-intestinal adverse reactions, can occur at any time in patients on therapy with non-steroidal anti-inflammatory drugs. The risk of occurrence does not seem to change with duration of therapy. Studies to date have not identified any subset of patients not at risk of developing peptic ulcer and bleeding. However, elderly and debilitated patients tolerate gastro-intestinal ulceration or bleeding less well than others. Most of the serious gastro-intestinal events associated with non-steroidal anti-inflammatory drugs occurred in this patient population.

The antipyretic and anti-inflammatory activities of Naprosyn may reduce fever and inflammation, thereby diminishing their utility as diagnostic signs.

Bronchospasm may be precipitated in patients suffering from, or with a history of, bronchial asthma or allergic disease.

Sporadic abnormalities in laboratory tests (e.g. liver function tests) have occurred in patients on naproxen therapy, but no definite trend was seen in any test indicating toxicity.

Naproxen decreases platelet aggregation and prolongs bleeding time. This effect should be kept in mind when bleeding times are determined.

Mild peripheral oedema has been observed in a few patients receiving naproxen. Although sodium retention has not been reported in metabolic studies, it is possible that patients with questionable or compromised cardiac function may be at a greater risk when taking Naprosyn.

Use in patients with impaired renal function

As naproxen is eliminated to a large extent (95%) by urinary excretion via glomerular filtration, it should be used with great caution in patients with impaired renal function and the monitoring of serum creatinine and/or creatinine clearance is advised in these patients. Naprosyn is not recommended in patients having a baseline creatinine clearance of less than 20ml/minute.

Certain patients, specifically those whose renal blood flow is compromised, such as in extracellular volume depletion, cirrhosis of the liver, sodium restriction, congestive heart failure, and pre-existing renal disease, should have renal function assessed before and during Naprosyn therapy. Some elderly patients in whom impaired renal function may be expected, as well as patients using diuretics, may also fall within this category. A reduction in daily dosage should be considered to avoid the possibility of excessive accumulation of naproxen metabolites in these patients.

Use in patients with impaired liver function

Chronic alcoholic liver disease and probably also other forms of cirrhosis reduce the total plasma concentration of naproxen, but the plasma concentration of unbound naproxen is increased. The implication of this finding for Naprosyn dosing is unknown but it is prudent to use the lowest effective dose.

Haematological

Patients who have coagulation disorders or are receiving drug therapy that interferes with haemostasis should be carefully observed if naproxen-containing products are administered.

Patients at high risk of bleeding or those on full anti-coagulation therapy (e.g. dicoumarol derivatives) may be at increased risk of bleeding if given naproxen-containing products concurrently.

Anaphylactic (anaphylactoid) reactions

Hypersensitivity reactions may occur in susceptible individuals. Anaphylactic (anaphylactoid) reactions may occur both in patients with and without a history of hypersensitivity or exposure to aspirin, other non-steroidal anti-inflammatory drugs or naproxen-containing products. They may also occur in individuals with a history of angioedema, bronchospastic reactivity (e.g. asthma), rhinitis and nasal polyps.

Anaphylactoid reactions, like anaphylaxis, may have a fatal outcome.

Steroids

If steroid dosage is reduced or eliminated during therapy, the steroid dosage should be reduced slowly and the patients must be observed closely for any evidence of adverse effects, including adrenal insufficiency and exacerbation of symptoms of arthritis.

Ocular effects

Studies have not shown changes in the eye attributable to naproxen administration. In rare cases, adverse ocular disorders including papillitis, retrobulbar optic neuritis and papilloedema, have been reported in users of NSAIDs including naproxen, although a cause-and-effect relationship cannot be established; accordingly, patients who develop visual disturbances during treatment with naproxen-containing products should have an ophthalmological examination.

Combination with other NSAIDs

The combination of naproxen-containing products and other NSAIDs is not recommended, because of the cumulative risks of inducing serious NSAID-related adverse events.

4.5 Interaction with other medicinal products and other forms of Interaction

Concomitant administration of antacid or cholestyramine can delay the absorption of naproxen but does not affect its extent. Concomitant administration of food can delay the absorption of naproxen, but does not affect its extent.

Due to the high plasma protein binding of naproxen, patients simultaneously receiving hydantoins, anticoagulants or a highly protein-bound sulphonamide should be observed for signs of overdosage of these drugs. No interactions have been observed in clinical studies with naproxen and anticoagulants or sulphonylureas, but caution is nevertheless advised since interaction has been seen with other non-steroidal agents of this class.

The natriuretic effect of frusemide has been reported to be inhibited by some drugs of this class.

Inhibition of renal lithium clearance leading to increases in plasma lithium concentrations has also been reported.

Naproxen and other non-steroidal anti-inflammatory drugs can reduce the antihypertensive effect of propranolol and other beta-blockers and may increase the risk of renal impairment associated with the use of ACE inhibitors.

Probenecid given concurrently increases naproxen plasma levels and extends its half-life considerably.

Caution is advised where methotrexate is given concurrently because of possible enhancement of its toxicity, since naproxen, among other non-steroidal anti-inflammatory drugs, has been reported to reduce the tubular secretion of methotrexate in an animal model.

NSAIDs may exacerbate cardiac failure, reduce GFR and increase plasma cardiac glycoside levels when co-administered with cardiac glycosides.

As with all NSAIDs caution is advised when cyclosporin is co-administered because of the increased risk of nephrotoxicity.

NSAIDs should not be used for 8 - 12 days after mifepristone administration as NSAIDs can reduce the effects of mifepristone.

As with all NSAIDs, caution should be taken when co-administering with cortico-steroids because of the increased risk of bleeding.

Patients taking quinolones may have an increased risk of developing convulsions.

It is suggested that Naprosyn therapy be temporarily discontinued 48 hours before adrenal function tests are performed, because naproxen may artifactually interfere with some tests for 17-ketogenic steroids. Similarly, naproxen may interfere with some assays of urinary 5-hydroxyindoleacetic acid.

4.6 Pregnancy and lactation

Teratology studies in rats and rabbits at dose levels equivalent on a human multiple basis to those which have produced foetal abnormality with certain other non-steroidal anti-inflammatory agents, e.g. aspirin, have not produced evidence of foetal damage with naproxen. As with other drugs of this type naproxen delays parturition in animals (the relevance of this finding to human patients is unknown) and also affects the human foetal cardiovascular system (closure of the ductus arteriosus). Good medical practice indicates minimal drug usage in pregnancy, and the use of this class of therapeutic agent requires cautious balancing of possible benefit against potential risk to the mother and foetus, especially in the first and third trimesters.

The use of Naprosyn should be avoided in patients who are breast-feeding.

4.7 Effects on ability to drive and use machines

Some patients may experience drowsiness, dizziness, vertigo, insomnia or depression with the use of Naprosyn. If patients experience these or similar undesirable effects, they should exercise caution in carrying out activities that require alertness.

4.8 Undesirable effects

Gastro-intestinal: The more frequent reactions are nausea, vomiting, abdominal discomfort and epigastric distress. More serious reactions which may occur occasionally are gastro-intestinal bleeding, peptic ulceration (sometimes with haemorrhage and perforation), non-peptic gastro-intestinal ulceration and colitis.

Dermatological: Skin rashes, urticaria, angio-oedema. Alopecia, erythema multiforme, Stevens Johnson syndrome, epidermal necrolysis and photosensitivity reactions (including cases in which the skin resembles porphyria cutanea tarda, "pseudoporphyria") or epidermolysis bullosa may occur rarely.

Renal: Including but not limited to glomerular nephritis, interstitial nephritis, nephrotic syndrome, haematuria, renal papillary necrosis and renal failure.

CNS: Convulsions, headache, insomnia, inability to concentrate and cognitive dysfunction have been reported.

Haematological: Thrombocytopenia, granulocytopenia including agranulocytosis, aplastic anaemia and haemolytic anaemia may occur rarely.

Other: Tinnitus, hearing impairment, vertigo, mild peripheral oedema. Anaphylactic reactions to naproxen and naproxen sodium formulations have been reported in patients with, or without, a history of previous sensitivity reactions to NSAIDs. Jaundice, fatal hepatitis, visual disturbances, eosinophilic pneumonitis, vasculitis, hyperkalaemia, aseptic meningitis and ulcerative stomatitis have been reported rarely.

4.9 Overdose

Significant overdosage of the drug may be characterised by drowsiness, heartburn, indigestion, nausea or vomiting. A few patients have experienced seizures, but it is not known whether these were naproxen-related or not. It is not known what dose of the drug would be life-threatening.

Should a patient ingest a large amount of Naprosyn accidentally or purposefully, the stomach may be emptied and usual supportive measures employed. Animal studies indicate that the prompt administration of activated charcoal in adequate amounts would tend to reduce markedly the absorption of the drug.

Haemodialysis does not decrease the plasma concentration of naproxen because of the high degree of protein binding. However, haemodialysis may still be appropriate in a patient with renal failure who has taken naproxen.

5. PHARMACOLOGICAL PROPERTIES

5.1 Pharmacodynamic properties

Naproxen is a non-steroidal anti-inflammatory analgesic compound with antipyretic properties as has been demonstrated in classical animal test systems. Naproxen exhibits its anti-inflammatory effect even in adrenalectomised animals, indicating that its action is not mediated through the pituitary-adrenal axis.

Naproxen inhibits prostaglandin synthetase (as do other NSAIDs). As with other NSAIDs, however, the exact mechanism of its anti-inflammatory action is not known.

5.2 Pharmacokinetic properties

Naproxen is completely absorbed from the gastro-intestinal tract, and peak plasma levels are reached in 2 to 4 hours. Naproxen is present in the blood mainly as unchanged drug, extensively bound to plasma proteins. The plasma half-life is between 12 and 15 hours, enabling a steady state to be achieved within 3 days of initiation of therapy on a twice daily dose regimen. The degree of absorption is not significantly affected by either foods or most antacids. Excretion is almost entirely via the urine, mainly as conjugated naproxen, with some unchanged drug. Metabolism in children is similar to that in adults. Chronic alcoholic liver disease reduces the total plasma concentration of naproxen but the concentration of unbound naproxen increases. In the elderly, the unbound plasma concentration of naproxen is increased although total plasma concentration is unchanged.

5.3 Preclinical safety data

None stated.

6. PHARMACEUTICAL PARTICULARS

6.1 List of excipients

Povidone, croscarmellose sodium, magnesium stearate, iron oxide E 172, purified water.

6.2 Incompatibilities

None stated.

6.3 Shelf life

60 months.

6.4 Special precautions for storage

Store below 30°C. Protect from light.

6.5 Nature and contents of container

Naproxen 250 and 500 are supplied in polypropylene securitainers with LDPE closures or polypropylene bottles with induction seals and polypropylene screw closures or amber glass bottles with metal closures fitted with an expanded polythene wad, containing 50, 60, 120, 250 and 500 tablets.

Clear or opaque PVC blister packaging with aluminium lidding in cartons, containing 2, 4, 56, 60 and 112 Naproxen 250, or 2, 4, 56, 60 Naproxen 500 tablets.

6.6 Instructions for use and handling

None given.

7. MARKETING AUTHORISATION HOLDER

Roche Products Limited, 40 Broadwater Road, Welwyn Garden City, Hertfordshire, AL7 3AY.

8. MARKETING AUTHORISATION NUMBER(S)

Naproxen 250: PL 0031/0471

Naproxen 500: PL 0031/0484

9. DATE OF FIRST AUTHORISATION/RENEWAL OF THE AUTHORISATION

Naproxen 250: 26 April 1996

Naproxen 500: 31 May 1994

10. DATE OF REVISION OF THE TEXT

March 1999

Naprosyn is a registered trade mark

P575071/300

Naprosyn EC

(Roche Products Limited)

1. NAME OF THE MEDICINAL PRODUCT

Naprosyn EC.

2. QUALITATIVE AND QUANTITATIVE COMPOSITION

Naproxen Ph. Eur. 250mg/tablet.

Naproxen Ph. Eur. 375mg/tablet.

Naproxen Ph. Eur. 500mg/tablet.

3. PHARMACEUTICAL FORM

Enteric film-coated tablets.

4. CLINICAL PARTICULARS

4.1 Therapeutic indications

Naprosyn EC is indicated for the treatment of rheumatoid arthritis, osteoarthrosis (degenerative arthritis), ankylosing spondylitis, juvenile rheumatoid arthritis, acute gout, acute musculoskeletal disorders (such as sprains and strains, direct trauma, lumbosacral pain, cervical spondylitis, tenosynovitis and fibrositis) and dysmenorrhoea.

4.2 Posology and method of administration

Adults

Naprosyn EC tablets should be swallowed whole and not broken or crushed.

Therapy should be started at the lowest recommended dose, especially in the elderly.

Rheumatoid arthritis, osteoarthritis and ankylosing spondylitis

The usual dose is 500mg to 1g daily taken in 2 doses at 12-hour intervals. Where 1g per day is needed either one 500mg tablet twice daily or two 500mg tablets in a single administration (morning or evening) is recommended. In the following cases a loading dose of 750mg or 1g per day for the acute phase is recommended:

a) In patients reporting severe night-time pain/or morning stiffness.

b) In patients being switched to Naprosyn from a high dose of another anti-rheumatic compound.

c) In osteoarthrosis where pain is the predominant symptom.

Acute gout

750mg once, then 250mg every 8 hours until the attack has passed.

Acute musculoskeletal disorders and dysmenorrhoea

500mg initially followed by 250mg at 6 - 8 hour intervals as needed, with a maximum daily dose after the first day of 1250mg.

Elderly

Studies indicate that although total plasma concentration of naproxen is unchanged, the unbound plasma fraction of naproxen is increased in the elderly. The implication of this finding for Naprosyn EC dosing is unknown. As with other drugs used in the elderly it is prudent to use the lowest effective dose. For the effect of reduced elimination in the elderly see section *Use in patients with impaired renal function*.

Children

Naprosyn EC is effective in the treatment of juvenile rheumatoid arthritis in children over 5 years of age at a dose of 10mg/kg/day taken in 2 doses at 12-hour intervals. Naprosyn EC is not recommended for use in any other indication in children under 16 years of age.

4.3 Contraindications

Active or history of peptic ulceration or active gastrointestinal bleeding. Hypersensitivity to naproxen and naproxen sodium formulations. Since the potential exists for cross-sensitivity reactions, Naprosyn EC should not be given to patients in whom aspirin or other non-steroidal anti-inflammatory/analgesic drugs induce asthma, rhinitis or urticaria.

4.4 Special warnings and special precautions for use

Episodes of gastro-intestinal bleeding have been reported in patients with naproxen therapy. Naprosyn EC should be given under close supervision to patients with a history of gastro-intestinal disease.

Serious gastro-intestinal adverse reactions, can occur at any time in patients on therapy with non-steroidal anti-inflammatory drugs. The risk of occurrence does not seem to change with duration of therapy. Studies to date have not identified any subset of patients not at risk of developing peptic ulcer and bleeding. However, elderly and debilitated patients tolerate gastro-intestinal ulceration or bleeding less well than others. Most of the serious gastro-intestinal events associated with non-steroidal anti-inflammatory drugs occurred in this patient population.

The antipyretic and anti-inflammatory activities of Naprosyn EC may reduce fever and inflammation, thereby diminishing their utility as diagnostic signs.

Bronchospasm may be precipitated in patients suffering from, or with a history of, bronchial asthma or allergic disease.

Sporadic abnormalities in laboratory tests (e.g. liver function tests) have occurred in patients on naproxen therapy, but no definite trend indicating toxicity was seen in any test.

Naproxen decreases platelet aggregation and prolongs bleeding time. This effect should be kept in mind when bleeding times are determined.

Mild peripheral oedema has been observed in a few patients receiving naproxen. Although sodium retention has not been reported in metabolic studies, it is possible that patients with questionable or compromised cardiac function may be at a greater risk when taking Naprosyn EC.

Use in patients with impaired renal function

As naproxen is eliminated to a large extent (95%) by urinary excretion via glomerular filtration, it should be used with great caution in patients with impaired renal function and the monitoring of serum creatinine and/or creatinine clearance is advised in these patients. Naprosyn EC is not recommended in patients having a baseline creatinine clearance of less than 20ml/minute.

Certain patients, specifically those whose renal blood flow is compromised, because of extracellular volume depletion, cirrhosis of the liver, sodium restriction, congestive heart failure, and pre-existing renal disease, should have renal function assessed before and during Naprosyn EC therapy. Some elderly patients in whom impaired renal function may be expected, as well as patients using diuretics, may also fall within this category. A reduction in daily dosage should be considered to avoid the possibility of excessive accumulation of naproxen metabolites in these patients.

Use in patients with impaired liver function

Chronic alcoholic liver disease and probably also other forms of cirrhosis reduce the total plasma concentration of naproxen, but the plasma concentration of unbound naproxen is increased. The implication of this finding for Naprosyn EC dosing is unknown but it is prudent to use the lowest effective dose.

Haematological

Patients who have coagulation disorders or are receiving drug therapy that interferes with haemostasis should be carefully observed if naproxen-containing products are administered.

Patients at high risk of bleeding or those on full anti-coagulation therapy (e.g. dicoumarol derivatives) may be at increased risk of bleeding if given naproxen-containing products.

Anaphylactic (anaphylactoid) reactions

Hypersensitivity reactions may occur in susceptible individuals. Anaphylactic (anaphylactoid) reactions may occur both in patients with and without a history of hypersensitivity or exposure to aspirin, other non-steroidal anti-inflammatory drugs or naproxen-containing products. They may also occur in individuals with a history of angioedema, bronchospastic reactivity (e.g. asthma), rhinitis and nasal polyps.

Anaphylactoid reactions, like anaphylaxis, may have a fatal outcome.

Steroids

If steroid dosage is reduced or eliminated during therapy, the steroid dosage should be reduced slowly and the patients must be observed closely for any evidence of adverse effects, including adrenal insufficiency and exacerbation of symptoms of arthritis.

Ocular effects

Studies have not shown changes in the eye attributable to naproxen administration. In rare cases, adverse ocular disorders including papillitis, retrobulbar optic neuritis and papilloedema, have been reported in users of NSAIDs including naproxen, although a cause-and-effect relationship cannot be established; accordingly, patients who develop visual disturbances during treatment with naproxen-containing products should have an ophthalmological examination.

Combination with other NSAIDs

The combination of naproxen-containing products and other NSAIDs is not recommended, because of the cumulative risks of inducing serious NSAID-related adverse events.

4.5 Interaction with other medicinal products and other forms of Interaction

Concomitant administration of antacid or cholestyramine can delay the absorption of naproxen but does not affect its extent. Concomitant administration of food can delay the absorption of naproxen, but does not affect its extent.

Due to the high plasma protein binding of naproxen, patients simultaneously receiving hydantoins, anticoagulants or a highly protein-bound sulphonamide should be observed for signs of overdosage of these drugs. No interactions have been observed in clinical studies with naproxen and anticoagulants or sulphonylureas, but caution is nevertheless advised since interaction has been seen with other non-steroidal agents of this class.

The natriuretic effect of frusemide has been reported to be inhibited by some drugs of this class.

Inhibition of renal lithium clearance leading to increases in plasma lithium concentrations has also been reported.

Naproxen and other non-steroidal anti-inflammatory drugs can reduce the antihypertensive effect of propranolol and other beta-blockers and may increase the risk of renal impairment associated with the use of ACE-inhibitors.

Probenecid given concurrently increases naproxen plasma levels and extends its half-life considerably.

Caution is advised where methotrexate is administered concurrently because of possible enhancement of its toxicity, since naproxen, in common with other non-steroidal anti-inflammatory drugs, has been reported to reduce the tubular secretion of methotrexate in an animal model.

NSAIDs may exacerbate cardiac failure, reduce GFR and increase plasma cardiac glycoside levels when co-administered with cardiac glycosides.

As with all NSAIDs caution is advised when cyclosporin is co-administered because of the increased risk of nephrotoxicity.

NSAIDs should not be used for 8 - 12 days after mifepristone administration as NSAIDs can reduce the effects of mifepristone.

As with all NSAIDs, caution should be taken when co-administering with corticosteroids because of the increased risk of bleeding.

Patients taking quinolones may have an increased risk of developing convulsions.

It is suggested that Naprosyn EC therapy be temporarily discontinued 48 hours before adrenal function tests are performed, because naproxen may artifactually interfere with some tests for 17-ketogenic steroids. Similarly, naproxen may interfere with some assays of urinary 5-hydroxyindoleacetic acid.

4.6 Pregnancy and lactation

Teratology studies in rats and rabbits at dose levels equivalent on a human multiple basis to those which have produced foetal abnormality with certain other non-steroidal anti-inflammatory agents, e.g. aspirin, have not produced evidence of foetal damage with naproxen. As with other drugs of this type naproxen delays parturition in animals (the relevance of this finding to human patients is unknown) and also affects the human foetal cardiovascular system (closure of the ductus arteriosus). Good medical practice indicates minimal drug usage in pregnancy, and the use of this class of therapeutic agent requires cautious balancing of possible benefit against potential risk to the mother and foetus, especially in the first and third trimesters.

Naproxen has been found in the milk of lactating mothers. The use of Naprosyn EC should therefore be avoided in patients who are breast-feeding.

4.7 Effects on ability to drive and use machines

Some patients may experience drowsiness, dizziness, vertigo, insomnia or depression with the use of Naprosyn. If patients experience these or similar undesirable effects, they should exercise caution in carrying out activities that require alertness.

4.8 Undesirable effects

Gastro-intestinal: The more frequent reactions are nausea, vomiting, abdominal discomfort and epigastric distress. More serious reactions which may occur occasionally are gastro-intestinal bleeding, peptic ulceration (sometimes with haemorrhage and perforation), non-peptic gastro-intestinal ulceration and colitis.

Dermatological: Skin rashes, urticaria, angioedema. Alopecia, erythema multiforme, Stevens Johnson syndrome, epidermal necrolysis and photosensitivity reactions (including cases in which the skin resembles porphyria cutanea tarda, "pseudoporphyria") or epidermolysis bullosa may occur rarely.

Renal: Including but not limited to glomerular nephritis, interstitial nephritis, nephrotic syndrome, haematuria, renal papillary necrosis and renal failure.

CNS: Convulsions, headache, insomnia, inability to concentrate and cognitive dysfunction have been reported.

Haematological: Thrombocytopenia, granulocytopenia including agranulocytosis, aplastic anaemia and haemolytic anaemia may occur rarely.

Other: Tinnitus, hearing impairment, vertigo, mild peripheral oedema. Anaphylactic reactions to naproxen and naproxen sodium formulations have been reported in patients with, or without, a history of previous hypersensitivity reactions to NSAIDs. Jaundice, fatal hepatitis, visual disturbances, eosinophilic pneumonitis, vasculitis, hyperkalaemia, aseptic meningitis and ulcerative stomatitis have been reported rarely.

4.9 Overdose

Significant overdosage of the drug may be characterised by drowsiness, heartburn, indigestion, nausea or vomiting. A few patients have experienced seizures, but it is not known whether these were naproxen-related or not. It is not known what dose of the drug would be life-threatening.

Should a patient ingest a large amount of Naprosyn EC accidentally or purposefully, the stomach may be emptied and usual supportive measures employed. Animal studies indicate that the prompt administration of activated charcoal in adequate amounts would tend to reduce markedly the absorption of the drug.

Haemodialysis does not decrease the plasma concentration of naproxen because of the high degree of protein binding. However, haemodialysis may still be appropriate in a patient with renal failure who has taken naproxen.

5. PHARMACOLOGICAL PROPERTIES

5.1 Pharmacodynamic properties

Naproxen has been shown to have anti-inflammatory, analgesic and antipyretic properties when tested in classical animal test systems. It exhibits its anti-inflammatory effect even in adrenalectomised animals, indicating that its action is not mediated through the pituitary-adrenal axis. It inhibits prostaglandin synthetase, as do other non-steroidal anti-inflammatory agents. As with other agents, however, the exact mechanism of its anti-inflammatory action is not known.

5.2 Pharmacokinetic properties

Naproxen is completely absorbed from the gastro-intestinal tract, and peak plasma levels are reached in 2 to 4 hours. Naproxen is present in the blood mainly as unchanged drug, extensively bound to plasma proteins. The plasma half-life is between 12 and 15 hours, enabling a steady state to be achieved within 3 days of initiation of therapy on a twice daily dose regimen. The degree of absorption is not significantly affected by either foods or most antacids. Excretion is almost entirely via the urine, mainly as conjugated naproxen, with some unchanged drug. Metabolism in children is similar to that in adults. Chronic alcoholic liver disease reduces the total plasma concentration of naproxen but the concentration of unbound naproxen increases. In the elderly, the unbound plasma concentration of naproxen is increased although total plasma concentration is unchanged.

When naproxen is administered in the enteric-coated form, the peak plasma levels are delayed compared to those seen with standard tablets. However, the mean areas under the plasma concentration-time curves, and hence bioavailability, are equivalent. The tablets, therefore, perform as one would anticipate for a drug which does not disintegrate until it reaches the small intestine, where dissolution is rapid and complete.

5.3 Preclinical safety data

No evidence of carcinogenicity was found in rats. Reproduction studies performed in rats, rabbits and mice at doses up to 6 times the human dose revealed no evidence of impaired fertility or harm to the foetus. As with other drugs known to inhibit prostaglandin synthesis, an increased incidence of dystocia and delayed parturition occurred in rats.

6. PHARMACEUTICAL PARTICULARS

6.1 List of excipients

The tablets also contain povidone EP, croscarmellose sodium NF, magnesium stearate EP, purified water EP, methacrylic acid copolymer NF, purified talc EP, sodium hydroxide EP, triethyl citrate NF, simethicone emulsion USP and opacode S-1-8106.

6.2 Incompatibilities

None known.

6.3 Shelf life

36 months.

6.4 Special precautions for storage

Protect from light and store below 30°C.

6.5 Nature and contents of container

Polypropylene, polyethylene or glass bottles containing 50, 60, 100 or 250 tablets.

Clear or opaque PVC blister with aluminium lidding in cartons containing 2, 4 or 56 tablets.

6.6 Instructions for use and handling

None applicable.

7. MARKETING AUTHORISATION HOLDER

Roche Products Limited, 40 Broadwater Road, Welwyn Garden City, Hertfordshire, AL7 3AY.

8. MARKETING AUTHORISATION NUMBER(S)

Naprosyn EC 250: PL 0031/0467

Naprosyn EC 375: PL 0031/0468

Naprosyn EC 500: PL 0031/0469

9. DATE OF FIRST AUTHORISATION/RENEWAL OF THE AUTHORISATION

12 July 1991

10. DATE OF REVISION OF THE TEXT

March 1999

Naprosyn is a registered trade mark P575070/300

Naramig Tablets 2.5mg

(GlaxoSmithKline UK)

1. NAME OF THE MEDICINAL PRODUCT

Naramig Tablets 2.5mg

2. QUALITATIVE AND QUANTITATIVE COMPOSITION

Tablets containing 2.5mg of naratriptan as naratriptan hydrochloride.

3. PHARMACEUTICAL FORM

Tablets

4. CLINICAL PARTICULARS

4.1 Therapeutic indications

Naramig Tablets are indicated for the acute treatment of migraine attacks with or without aura.

4.2 Posology and method of administration

Naramig Tablets are recommended as monotherapy for the acute treatment of a migraine attack.

Naramig Tablets should not be used prophylactically.

Naramig Tablets should be swallowed whole with water.

Adults (18-65 years of age)

The recommended dose of Naramig Tablets is a single 2.5mg tablet.

The total dose should not exceed two 2.5mg tablets in any 24 hour period.

If symptoms of migraine should recur, following an initial response, a second dose may be taken provided that there is a minimum interval of four hours between the two doses.

If a patient does not respond to a first dose of Naramig Tablets a second dose should not be taken for the same attack, as it is unlikely to be of benefit. However Naramig Tablets may be used for subsequent migraine attacks.

Adolescents (12-17 years of age)

Efficacy of Naramig Tablets at single doses of 0.25, 1.0 and 2.5mg was not demonstrated to be greater than placebo in a placebo-controlled study in adolescents (12 to 17 years). Therefore, the use of Naramig Tablets in patients under 18 years of age is not recommended.

Children (under 12 years of age)

There are no data available on the use of naratriptan in children under 12 years of age therefore its use in this age group is not recommended.

Elderly (over 65 years of age)

The safety and effectiveness of naratriptan in individuals over age 65 have not been evaluated and therefore, its use in this age group can not be recommended. There is a moderate decrease in clearance with age (see Pharmacokinetics).

Renal Impairment

Naramig should be used with caution in patients with renal impairment. The maximum dose in any 24 hour treatment period is a single 2.5mg tablet. The use of Naramig is contraindicated in patients with severe renal impairment (creatinine clearance < 15mL/min)

(See Contraindications and Pharmacokinetics).

Hepatic Impairment

Naramig should be used with caution in patients with hepatic impairment. The maximum dose in any 24 hour treatment period is a single 2.5mg tablet. The use of Naramig is contraindicated in patients with severe hepatic impairment (Child-Pugh grade C)

(See Contraindications and Pharmacokinetics).

4.3 Contraindications

Hypersensitivity to any component of the preparation.

As with other 5-hydroxytryptamine1 (5-HT1) receptor agonists naratriptan should not be used in patients who have had a myocardial infarction or have ischaemic heart disease, or Prinzmetal's angina/coronary vasospasm, peripheral vascular disease or patients who have symptoms or signs consistent with ischaemic heart disease.

Naratriptan should not be administered to patients with a history of cerebrovascular accident (CVA) or transient ischaemic attack (TIA).

The use of naratriptan in patients with uncontrolled hypertension is contraindicated.

As with other 5-HT1 receptor agonists the concomitant use of naratriptan and other 5HT1 agonists is contraindicated.

Naratriptan is contraindicated in patients with severely impaired renal or hepatic function.

4.4 Special warnings and special precautions for use

Naratriptan should only be used where there is a clear diagnosis of migraine.

Naratriptan is not indicated for use in the management of hemiplegic, basilar or ophthalmoplegic migraine.

As with other acute migraine therapies, before treating headaches in patients not previously diagnosed as migraineurs, and in migraineurs who present with atypical symptoms, care should be taken to exclude other potentially serious neurological conditions. It should be noted that migraineurs may be at risk of certain cerebrovascular events (eg. CVA or TIA).

As with other 5-HT1 receptor agonists, naratriptan should not be given to patients in whom unrecognised cardiac disease is likely without a prior evaluation for underlying cardiovascular disease. Such patients include postmenopausal women, males over 40 and patients with risk factors for coronary artery disease.

If symptoms consistent with ischaemic heart disease occur appropriate evaluation should be carried out.

The concomitant administration of ergotamine and derivatives of ergotamine (including methysergide) with naratriptan is not recommended.

Naratriptan contains a sulphonamide component therefore there is a theoretical risk of a hypersensitivity reaction in patients with known hypersensitivity to sulphonamides.

The recommended dose of naratriptan should not be exceeded.

Undesirable effects may be more common during concomitant use of triptans and herbal preparations containing St John's Wort (*Hypericum perforatum*).

4.5 Interaction with other medicinal products and other forms of Interaction

There is no evidence of interactions with β-blockers, tricyclic antidepressants, selective serotonin reuptake inhibitors, alcohol or food.

Co-administration of naratriptan with ergotamine, dihydroergotamine, or sumatriptan did not result in clinically significant effects on blood pressure, heart rate or ECG or affect naratriptan exposure.

Naratriptan does not inhibit monoamine oxidase enzymes; therefore interactions with monoamine oxidase inhibitors are not anticipated. In addition, the limited metabolism of naratriptan and the wide range of cytochrome P450 isoenzymes involved suggest that significant drug interactions with naratriptan are unlikely (see Pharmacokinetics).

4.6 Pregnancy and lactation

The safe use of naratriptan in pregnant women has not been established. Evaluation of experimental animal studies does not indicate any direct teratogenic effects or harmful effects on peri- and postnatal development.

Because animal reproduction studies are not always predictive of human response administration of naratriptan should only be considered if the expected benefit to the mother is greater than any possible risk to the foetus.

Naratriptan and/or drug related metabolites are secreted into the milk of lactating rats. Caution should be exercised when considering administration of naratriptan to nursing women.

4.7 Effects on ability to drive and use machines

Caution is recommended in patients performing skilled tasks (e.g. driving or operating machinery) as drowsiness may occur as a result of migraine. Drowsiness was no more apparent with naratriptan than with placebo in clinical trials.

4.8 Undesirable effects

At therapeutic doses of naratriptan the incidence of side effects reported in clinical trials was similar to placebo. Some of the symptoms may be part of the migraine attack.

Undesirable effects are ranked under headings of frequency using the following convention: Very common ($\geq$1/10), common ($\geq$1/100 and $<$1/10), uncommon ($\geq$1/1,000 and $<$1/100), rare ($\geq$1/10,000 and $<$1/1,000) and very rare ($<$1/10,000).

Immune system disorders

Rare: Hypersensitivity reactions ranging from cutaneous hypersensitivity to rare cases of anaphylaxis.

Nervous system disorders

Common: Tingling. This is usually of short duration, may be severe and may affect any part of the body including the chest or throat. Dizziness and drowsiness.

Eye disorders

Uncommon: Visual disturbance.

Cardiac disorders

Uncommon: Bradycardia, tachycardia, palpitations.

Rare: Coronary artery vasospasm and transient ischaemic ECG changes have been reported rarely (see Contraindications and Warnings and Precautions).

Vascular disorders

Very rare: Peripheral vascular ischaemia.

Gastrointestinal

Common: Nausea and vomiting.

Rare: Ischaemic colitis.

General disorders and administration site conditions:

The following symptoms are usually of short duration, may be severe and may affect any part of the body including the chest or throat:

Common: Pain, sensations of heat. Malaise/fatigue.

Uncommon: Sensations of heaviness, pressure or tightness.

4.9 Overdose

There is limited experience of accidental overdosage with naratriptan. However, there is no evidence to suggest that overdose is associated with adverse events other than those described above (see section 4.8 Undesirable Effects).

It is unknown what effect haemodialysis or peritoneal dialysis has on the plasma concentrations of naratriptan.

Treatment

If overdosage with naratriptan occurs, the patient should be monitored for at least 24 hours and standard supportive treatment applied as required.

5. PHARMACOLOGICAL PROPERTIES

5.1 Pharmacodynamic properties

Naratriptan has been shown to be a selective agonist for 5 hydroxytryptamine1 (5-HT_1) receptors mediating vascular contraction. This receptor is found predominantly in intracranial (cerebral and dural) blood vessels. Naratriptan has high affinity for human cloned 5-HT_{1B} and 5-HT_{1D} receptors, the human 5-HT_{1B} receptor is thought to correspond to the vascular 5-HT_1 receptor mediating contraction of intracranial blood vessels. Naratriptan has little or no effect at other 5-HT receptor (5-HT_2, 5-HT_3, 5-HT_4 and 5-HT_7) subtypes.

In animals, naratriptan selectively constricts the carotid arterial circulation. This circulation supplies blood to the extracranial and intracranial tissues such as the meninges, and dilatation and/or oedema formation in these vessels is thought to be the underlying mechanism of migraine in man. In addition, experimental evidence suggests that naratriptan inhibits trigeminal nerve activity. Both these actions may contribute to the anti-migraine action of naratriptan in humans.

In man, a meta-analysis of BP recordings in 15 studies showed that the population average maximum increases in systolic and diastolic blood pressure after a 2.5mg dose of naratriptan tablets would be less than 5mmHg and 3mmHg respectively. The blood pressure response was unaffected by age, weight, hepatic or renal impairment.

5.2 Pharmacokinetic properties

Absorption, distribution, metabolism and elimination

Following oral administration, naratriptan is rapidly absorbed with maximum plasma concentrations observed at 2-3 hours. After administration of a 2.5mg naratriptan tablet Cmax is approximately 8.3ng/mL (95% CI: 6.5 to 10.5ng/mL) in women and 5.4ng/mL (95% CI: 4.7 to 6.1ng/mL) in men.

The oral bioavailability is 74% in women and 63% in men with no differences in efficacy and tolerability in clinical use. Therefore a gender related dose adjustment is not required.

Naratriptan is distributed in a volume of 170L. Plasma protein binding is low (29%).

The mean elimination half-life ($t_{1/2}$) is 6 hours.

Mean clearance after intravenous administration was 470mL/min in men and 380mL/min in women. Renal clearance is similar in men and women at 220mL/min and is higher than the glomerular filtration rate suggesting that naratriptan is actively secreted in the renal tubules. Naratriptan is predominantly excreted in the urine with 50% of the dose recovered as unchanged naratriptan and 30% recovered as inactive metabolites. In vitro naratriptan was metabolised by a wide range of cytochrome P450 isoenzymes. Consequently significant metabolic drug interactions with naratriptan are not anticipated (see Interactions).

Special Patient Populations

Elderly

In healthy elderly subjects (n=12), clearance was decreased by 26% when compared to healthy young subjects (n=12) in the same study (See Posology and method of administration).

Gender

The naratriptan AUC and Cmax were approximately 35% lower in males compared to females however, with no differences in efficacy and tolerability in clinical use.

Therefore a gender related dose adjustment is not required (see Posology and method of administration).

Renal Impairment

Renal excretion is the major route for the elimination of naratriptan. Accordingly exposure to naratriptan may be increased in patients with renal disease.

In a study in male and female renally impaired patients (creatinine clearance 18 to 115mL/min; n=15) matched for sex, age and weight with healthy subjects (n=8), renally impaired patients had an approximately 80% increase in $t_{1/2}$ and an approximately 50% reduction in clearance (See Posology and method of administration).

Hepatic Impairment

The liver plays a lesser role in the clearance of orally administered naratriptan. In a study in male and female hepatically impaired patients (Child-Pugh grade A or B n=8) matched for sex, age and weight with healthy subjects who received oral naratriptan, hepatically impaired patients had an approximately 40% increase in $t_{1/2}$ and an approximately 30% reduction in clearance (See Posology and method of administration).

5.3 Preclinical safety data

No clinically relevant findings were observed in preclinical studies.

6. PHARMACEUTICAL PARTICULARS

6.1 List of excipients

Tablet core

Microcrystalline cellulose

Anhydrous lactose

Croscarmellose sodium

Magnesium stearate

Film coat

Methylhydroxypropylcellulose

Titanium dioxide (E171)

Triacetin

Iron oxide yellow (E172)

Indigo carmine aluminium lake (E132)

6.2 Incompatibilities

None reported

6.3 Shelf life

36 months

6.4 Special precautions for storage

Store below 30°C.

6.5 Nature and contents of container

2, 4, 6 or 12 tablets in a double foil blister pack

Not all pack sizes may be marketed

6.6 Instructions for use and handling

None

Administrative Data

7. MARKETING AUTHORISATION HOLDER

Glaxo Wellcome UK Ltd, trading as GlaxoSmithKline UK

Stockley Park West,

Uxbridge,

Middlesex. UB11 1BT

8. MARKETING AUTHORISATION NUMBER(S)

PL 10949/0273

9. DATE OF FIRST AUTHORISATION/RENEWAL OF THE AUTHORISATION

28 April 2002

10. DATE OF REVISION OF THE TEXT

13 July 2004

11. Legal Status

POM

Naropin 10 mg/ml solution for injection

(AstraZeneca UK Limited)

1. NAME OF THE MEDICINAL PRODUCT

Naropin® 10 mg/ml solution for injection

2. QUALITATIVE AND QUANTITATIVE COMPOSITION

Naropin 10 mg/ml: 10 mg/ml ropivacaine hydrochloride

For excipients, see 6.1

3. PHARMACEUTICAL FORM

Solution for injection for perineural and epidural administration (10-20 ml).

4. CLINICAL PARTICULARS

4.1 Therapeutic indications

Naropin is indicated for:

1. Surgical anaesthesia:

- Epidural blocks for surgery, including Caesarean section.
- Major nerve blocks.
- Field blocks.

2. Acute pain management

- Continuous epidural infusion or intermittent bolus administration during postoperative or labour pain.
- Field blocks.

4.2 Posology and method of administration

Naropin should only be used by, or under the supervision of, clinicians experienced in regional anaesthesia.

Posology

The following table is a guide to dosage for the more commonly used blocks. The smallest dose required to produce an effective block should be used. The clinician's experience and knowledge of the patient's physical status are of importance when deciding the dose.

(see Table 1 on next page)

In general, surgical anaesthesia (e.g. epidural administration) requires the use of the higher concentrations and doses. Naropin 10 mg/ml is recommended for epidural anaesthesia in which a complete motor block is essential for surgery. For analgesia (e.g. epidural administration for acute pain management) the lower concentrations and doses are recommended.

Method of administration

Careful aspiration before and during injection is recommended to prevent intravascular injection. When a large dose is to be injected, a test dose of 3-5 ml lidocaine (lignocaine) with adrenaline (Xylocaine® 2% with Adrenaline 1:200,000) is recommended. An inadvertent intravascular

Table 1

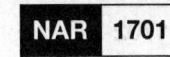

	Conc.	Volume	Dose	Onset	Duration
	mg/ml	ml	mg	minutes	hours
SURGICAL ANAESTHESIA					
Lumbar Epidural Administration					
Surgery	7.5	15-25	113-188	10-20	3-5
	10	15-20	150-200	10-20	4-6
Caesarean Section	7.5	15-20	113-150(1)	10-20	3-5
Thoracic Epidural Administration					
To establish block for post-operative pain relief	7.5	5-15 (depending on the level of injection)	38-113	10-20	n/a(2)
Major Nerve Block*					
Brachial plexus block	7.5	30-40	225-300	10-25	6-10
Field Block (e.g. minor nerve blocks and infiltration)	7.5	1-30	7.5-225	1-15	2-6
ACUTE PAIN MANAGEMENT					
Lumbar Epidural Administration					
Bolus	2	10-20	20-40	10-15	0.5-1.5
Intermittent injections (top up)	2	10-15	20-30		
(e.g. labour pain management)		(minimum interval 30 minutes)			
Continuous infusion e.g.					
Labour pain	2	6-10 ml/h	12-20 mg/h	n/a(2)	n/a(2)
Postoperative pain management	2	6-14 ml/h	12-28 mg/h	n/a(2)	n/a(2)
Thoracic Epidural Administration Continuous infusion (postoperative pain management)	2	6-14 ml/h	12-28 mg/h	n/a(2)	n/a(2)
Field Block					
(e.g. minor nerve blocks and infiltration)	2	1-100	2-200	1-5	2-6

The doses in the table are those considered to be necessary to produce a successful block and should be regarded as guidelines for use in adults. Individual variations in onset and duration occur. The figures in the column 'Dose' reflect the expected average dose range needed. Standard textbooks should be consulted for both factors affecting specific block techniques and individual patient requirements.

* With regard to major nerve block, only for brachial plexus block a dose recommendation can be given. For other major nerve blocks lower doses may be required. However, there is presently no experience of specific dose recommendations for other blocks.

(1) Incremental dosing should be applied, the starting dose of about 100 mg (97.5 mg = 13 ml; 105 mg = 14 ml) to be given over 3-5 minutes. Two additional doses, each of 25 mg, may be administered as needed. The total administered dose should not exceed 150 mg.

(2) n/a = not applicable

injection may be recognised by a temporary increase in heart rate and an accidental intrathecal injection by signs of a spinal block.

Aspiration should be repeated prior to and during administration of the main dose, which should be injected slowly or in incremental doses, at a rate of 25-50 mg/min, while closely observing the patient's vital functions and maintaining verbal contact. If toxic symptoms occur, the injection should be stopped immediately.

In epidural block for surgery, single doses of up to 250 mg ropivacaine have been used and well tolerated.

In brachial plexus block a single dose of 300 mg has been used in a limited number of patients and was well tolerated.

When prolonged blocks are used, either through continuous epidural infusion or through repeated bolus administration, the risks of reaching a toxic plasma concentration or inducing local neural injury must be considered. Cumulative doses up to 675 mg ropivacaine for surgery and postoperative analgesia administered over 24 hours were well tolerated in adults, as were postoperative continuous epidural infusions at rates up to 28 mg/hour for 72 hours. In a limited number of patients, higher doses of up to 800 mg/day have been administered with relatively few adverse reactions.

For treatment of postoperative pain, the following technique can be recommended: Unless preoperatively instituted, an epidural block with Naropin 7.5 mg/ml is induced via an epidural catheter. Analgesia is maintained with Naropin 2 mg/ml infusion. Infusion rates of 6-14 ml (12-28 mg) per hour provide adequate analgesia with only slight and non-progressive motor block in most cases of moderate to severe postoperative pain. The maximum duration of epidural block is 3 days.

However, close monitoring of analgesic effect should be performed in order to remove the catheter as soon as the pain condition allows it.

With this technique a significant reduction in the need for opioids has been observed.

Concentrations above 7.5 mg/ml Naropin have not been documented for Caesarean section.

Naropin cannot be recommended for use in children below the age of 12 years as there is no data with regard to efficacy and safety in this group of patients.

4.3 Contraindications

Naropin solutions are contraindicated in patients with known hypersensitivity to anaesthetics of the amide type.

General contraindications related to epidural anaesthesia, regardless of the local anaesthetic used, should be taken into account.

Intravenous regional anaesthesia.

Obstetric paracervical anaesthesia.

Hypovolaemia.

4.4 Special warnings and special precautions for use

Regional anaesthetic procedures should always be performed in a properly equipped and staffed area. Equipment and drugs necessary for monitoring and emergency resuscitation should be immediately available. For emergency medication, patients receiving major blocks or high doses should have an intravenous line inserted before the blocking procedure. The clinician responsible should be appropriately trained and familiar with diagnosis and treatment of side effects, systemic toxicity and other complications such as inadvertent subarachnoid injection which may produce a high spinal block with apnoea and hypotension. Convulsions have occurred most often after brachial plexus block and epidural block. This is likely to be the result of either accidental intravascular injection or rapid absorption from the injection site.

Certain local anaesthetic procedures, such as injections in the head and neck regions, may be associated with a higher frequency of serious adverse reactions, regardless of the local anaesthetic used. Caution is required to prevent injections in inflamed areas.

Patients in poor general condition due to ageing or other compromising factors such as partial or complete heart conduction block, advanced liver disease or severe renal dysfunction require special attention, although regional anaesthesia is frequently indicated in these patients.

Ropivacaine is metabolised in the liver and should therefore be used with caution in patients with severe liver disease. Repeated doses may need to be reduced due to delayed elimination. Normally there is no need to modify the dose in patients with impaired renal function when used for single dose or short term treatment. Acidosis and reduced plasma protein concentration, frequently seen in patients with chronic renal failure, may increase the risk of systemic toxicity.

Patients with hypovolaemia due to any cause can develop sudden and severe hypotension during epidural anaesthesia, regardless of the local anaesthetic used.

Prolonged administration of ropivacaine should be avoided in patients concomitantly treated with strong CYP1A2 inhibitors, such as fluvoxamine and enoxacin, see 4.5.

A possible cross-hypersensitivity with other amide-type local anaesthetics should be taken into account.

4.5 Interaction with other medicinal products and other forms of Interaction

Naropin should be used with caution in patients receiving other local anaesthetics or agents structurally related to amide-type local anaesthetics, e.g. certain antiarrhythmics, since the toxic effects are additive. Simultaneous use of Naropin with general anaesthetics or opioids may potentiate each others (adverse) effects.

Cytochrome P450 (CYP) 1A2 is involved in the formation of 3-hydroxy-ropivacaine, the major metabolite. *In vivo*, the plasma clearance of ropivacaine was reduced by 70% during coadministration of fluvoxamine, a selective and potent CYP1A2 inhibitor. Thus strong inhibitors of CYP1A2, such as fluvoxamine and enoxacin, given concomitantly during prolonged administration of Naropin, can interact with Naropin. Prolonged administration of ropivacaine should be avoided in patients concomitantly treated with strong CYP1A2 inhibitors, see also 4.4.

In vivo, the plasma clearance of ropivacaine was reduced by 15% during coadministration of ketoconazole, a selective and potent inhibitor of CYP3A4. However, the inhibition of this isozyme is not likely to have clinical relevance.

In vitro, ropivacaine is a competitive inhibitor of CYP2D6 but does not seem to inhibit this isozyme at clinically attained plasma concentrations.

4.6 Pregnancy and lactation

Pregnancy

Apart from obstetrical use, there are no adequate data on the use of ropivacaine in pregnancy. Animal studies do not indicate direct or indirect harmful effects with respect to pregnancy, embryonal/foetal development, parturition or postnatal development (see section 5.3).

Lactation

There is no data available concerning the excretion of ropivacaine into human milk.

4.7 Effects on ability to drive and use machines

No data is available. Depending on the dose, local anaesthetics may have a minor influence on mental function and co-ordination even in the absence of overt CNS toxicity and may temporarily impair locomotion and alertness.

4.8 Undesirable effects

General

The adverse reaction profile for Naropin is similar to those for other long acting local anaesthetics of the amide type. Adverse drug reactions should be distinguished from the physiological effects of the nerve block itself e.g. a decrease in blood pressure and bradycardia during spinal/epidural block.

The percentage of patients that can be expected to experience adverse reactions varies with the route of administration of Naropin. Systemic and localised adverse reactions of Naropin usually occur because of excessive dosage, rapid absorption, or inadvertent intravascular injection. The most frequently reported adverse reactions, nausea and hypotension, are very frequent during anaesthesia and surgery in general and it is not possible to distinguish those caused by the clinical situation from those caused by the drug or the block.

Table of adverse drug reactions

Within each system organ class, the ADRs have been ranked under the headings of frequency, most frequent reactions first.

Very common (>1/10)	*Vascular Disorders:* Hypotension
	Gastrointestinal Disorders: Nausea
Common (>1/100)	*Nervous System Disorders:* Headache, Paraesthesia, Dizziness
	Cardiac Disorders: Bradycardia, Tachycardia
	Vascular Disorders: Hypertension
	Gastrointestinal Disorders: Vomiting
	Renal and Urinary Disorders: Urinary retention
	General Disorder and Administration Site Conditions: Temperature Elevation, Rigors
Uncommon (>1/1,000)	*Nervous system disorders:* Hypoaesthesia
Rare (>1/10,000)	*Psychiatric Disorders:* Anxiety
	Nervous System Disorders: Convulsions

Class-related adverse drug reactions

Allergic reactions

Allergic reactions (in the most severe instances anaphylactic shock) to local anaesthetics of the amide type are rare.

Neurological complications

Neuropathy and spinal cord dysfunction (e.g. anterior spinal artery syndrome, arachnoiditis, cauda equina), which may result in rare cases of permanent sequelae, have been associated with regional anaesthesia, regardless of the local anaesthetic used.

Acute systemic toxicity

Naropin may cause acute toxic effects following high doses or if very rapidly rising blood levels occur due to accidental intravascular injection or overdose. (See 4.9 "Overdose").

4.9 Overdose

Symptoms

Acute systemic toxicity

Accidental intravascular injections of local anaesthetics may cause immediate toxic effects. In the event of overdose, peak plasma concentrations may not be reached for one to two hours, depending on the site of the injection, and signs of toxicity may thus be delayed. Systemic toxic reactions may involve the central nervous system and the cardiovascular system.

Central nervous system

Central nervous system toxicity is a graded response with symptoms and signs of escalating severity. Initially symptoms such as visual or hearing disturbances, perioral numbness, dizziness, light-headedness, tingling and paraesthesia are seen. Dysarthria, muscular rigidity and muscular twitching are more serious and may precede the onset of generalised convulsions. These signs must not be mistaken for neurotic behaviour. Unconsciousness and grand mal convulsions may follow, which may last from a few seconds to several minutes. Hypoxia and hypercarbia occur rapidly during convulsions due to the increased muscular activity, together with the interference with respiration. In severe cases even apnoea may occur. The respiratory and metabolic acidosis increases and extends the toxic effects of local anaesthetics.

Recovery follows the redistribution of the local anaesthetic drug from the central nervous system and subsequent metabolism and excretion. Recovery may be rapid unless large amounts of the drug have been injected.

Cardiovascular toxicity

Cardiovascular toxicity indicates a more severe situation. Hypotension, bradycardia, arrhythmia and even cardiac arrest may occur as a result of high systemic concentrations of local anaesthetics. In volunteers the intravenous infusion of ropivacaine resulted in signs of depression of conductivity and contractility.

Cardiovascular toxicity effects are generally preceded by signs of toxicity in the central nervous system, unless the patient is receiving a general anaesthetic or is heavily sedated with drugs such as benzodiazepines or barbiturates.

Treatment of acute toxicity

Equipment and drugs necessary for monitoring and emergency resuscitation should be immediately available. If signs of acute systemic toxicity appear, injection of the local anaesthetic should be stopped immediately.

In the event of convulsions, treatment will be required. The objectives of treatment are to maintain oxygenation, stop the convulsions and support the circulation. Oxygen must be given and ventilation assisted, when necessary (mask and bag). An anticonvulsant should be given intravenously if the convulsions do not stop spontaneously in 15-20 seconds. Thiopentone sodium 1-3 mg/kg intravenously will abort the convulsions rapidly. Alternatively diazepam 0.1 mg/kg intravenously may be used, although its action is slower. Suxamethonium will stop the muscle convulsions rapidly, but the patient will require controlled ventilation and tracheal intubation.

If cardiovascular depression is evident (hypotension, bradycardia), ephedrine 5-10 mg intravenously should be given and repeated, if necessary, after 2-3 minutes.

Should circulatory arrest occur, immediate cardiopulmonary resuscitation should be instituted. Optimal oxygenation and ventilation and circulatory support as well as treatment of acidosis are of vital importance.

5. PHARMACOLOGICAL PROPERTIES

5.1 Pharmacodynamic properties

Pharmacotherapeutic group (ATC code): N01B B09

Ropivacaine is a long-acting amide-type local anaesthetic with both anaesthetic and analgesic effects. At high doses it produces surgical anaesthesia, while at lower doses it produces sensory block with limited and non-progressive motor block.

The mechanism is a reversible reduction of the membrane permeability of the nerve fibre to sodium ions. Consequently the depolarisation velocity is decreased and the excitable threshold increased, resulting in a local blockade of nerve impulses.

The most characteristic property of ropivacaine is the long duration of action. Onset and duration of the local anaesthetic efficacy are dependent upon the administration site and dose, but are not influenced by the presence of a vasoconstrictor (e.g. adrenaline). For details concerning the onset and duration of action, see table under "Posology and method of administration".

Healthy volunteers exposed to intravenous infusions tolerated ropivacaine well at low doses and with expected CNS symptoms at the maximum tolerated dose. The clinical experience with this drug indicates a good margin of safety when adequately used in recommended doses.

5.2 Pharmacokinetic properties

Ropivacaine has a chiral center and is available as the pure S-(-)-enantiomer. It is highly lipid-soluble. All metabolites have a local anaesthetic effect but of considerably lower potency and shorter duration than that of ropivacaine.

The plasma concentration of ropivacaine depends upon the dose, the route of administration and the vascularity of the injection site. Ropivacaine follows linear pharmacokinetics and the C_{max} is proportional to the dose.

Ropivacaine shows complete and biphasic absorption from the epidural space with half-lives of the two phases of the order of 14 min and 4 h in adults. The slow absorption is the rate -limiting factor in the elimination of ropivacaine, which explains why the apparent elimination half-life is longer after epidural than after intravenous administration.

Ropivacaine has a mean total plasma clearance in the order of 440 ml/min, a renal clearance of 1 ml/min, a volume of distribution at steady state of 47 litres and a terminal half-life of 1.8 h after iv administration. Ropivacaine has an intermediate hepatic extraction ratio of about 0.4. It is mainly bound to α_1- acid glycoprotein in plasma with an unbound fraction of about 6%.

An increase in total plasma concentrations during continuous epidural infusion has been observed, related to a postoperative increase of α_1- acid glycoprotein.

Variations in unbound, i.e. pharmacologically active, concentration have been much less than in total plasma concentration.

Ropivacaine readily crosses the placenta and equilibrium in regard to unbound concentration will be rapidly reached. The degree of plasma protein binding in the foetus is less than in the mother, which results in lower total plasma concentrations in the foetus than in the mother.

Ropivacaine is extensively metabolised, predominantly by aromatic hydroxylation. In total, 86% of the dose is excreted in the urine after intravenous administration, of which only about 1% relates to unchanged drug. The major metabolite is 3-hydroxy-ropivacaine, about 37% of which is excreted in the urine, mainly conjugated. Urinary excretion of 4-hydroxy-ropivacaine, the N-dealkylated metabolite and the 4-hydroxy-dealkylated accounts for 1-3%. Conjugated+unconjugated 3-hydroxy-ropivacaine shows only detectable concentrations in plasma.

There is no evidence of *in vivo* racemisation of ropivacaine.

5.3 Preclinical safety data

Based on conventional studies of safety pharmacology, single and repeated dose toxicity, reproduction toxicity, mutagenic potential and local toxicity, no hazards for humans were identified other than those which can be expected on the basis of the pharmacodynamic action of high doses of ropivacaine (e.g. CNS signs, including convulsions, and cardiotoxicity).

6. PHARMACEUTICAL PARTICULARS

6.1 List of excipients

Sodium chloride

Hydrochloric acid

Sodium hydroxide

Water for injection

6.2 Incompatibilities

In alkaline solutions precipitation may occur as ropivacaine shows poor solubility at pH > 6.0.

6.3 Shelf life

3 years.

6.4 Special precautions for storage

Do not store above 30°C. Do not freeze.

6.5 Nature and contents of container

10 ml polypropylene ampoules (Polyamp) in packs of 5 and 10

10 ml polypropylene ampoules (Polyamp) in sterile blister packs of 5 and 10

20 ml polypropylene ampoules (Polyamp) in packs of 5 and 10

20 ml polypropylene ampoules (Polyamp) in sterile blister packs of 5 and 10

The polypropylene ampoules (Polyamp) are specially designed to fit Luer lock and Luer fit syringes.

6.6 Instructions for use and handling

Naropin products are preservative free and are intended for single use only. Discard any unused solution.

The intact container must not be re-autoclaved. A blistered container should be chosen when a sterile outside is required.

7. MARKETING AUTHORISATION HOLDER

AstraZeneca UK Ltd.,

600 Capability Green,

Luton, LU1 3LU, UK.

8. MARKETING AUTHORISATION NUMBER(S)

PL 17901/0150

9. DATE OF FIRST AUTHORISATION/RENEWAL OF THE AUTHORISATION

15th September 2000

10. DATE OF REVISION OF THE TEXT

22 March 2004

Trademarks herein are the property of the AstraZeneca group

Naropin 2 mg/ml solution for injection

(AstraZeneca UK Limited)

1. NAME OF THE MEDICINAL PRODUCT

Naropin® 2 mg/ml solution for injection

2. QUALITATIVE AND QUANTITATIVE COMPOSITION

Naropin 2 mg/ml: 2 mg/ml ropivacaine hydrochloride

For excipients, see 6.1

3. PHARMACEUTICAL FORM

Solution for injection for perineural and epidural administration (10-20 ml).

4. CLINICAL PARTICULARS

4.1 Therapeutic indications

Naropin is indicated for:

1. Surgical anaesthesia:

- Epidural blocks for surgery, including Caesarean section.
- Major nerve blocks.
- Field blocks.

2. Acute pain management

- Continuous epidural infusion or intermittent bolus administration during postoperative or labour pain.
- Field blocks.
- Continuous peripheral nerve block via a continuous infusion or intermittent bolus injections, e.g. postoperative pain management

3. Acute pain management in paediatrics:

- Caudal epidural block for pre- and post-operative pain management.

4.2 Posology and method of administration

Naropin should only be used by, or under the supervision of, clinicians experienced in regional anaesthesia.

Posology

The following table is a guide to dosage for the more commonly used blocks. The smallest dose required to produce an effective block should be used. The clinician's experience and knowledge of the patient's physical status are of importance when deciding the dose.

(see Table 1)

In general, surgical anaesthesia (e.g. epidural administration) requires the use of the higher concentrations and doses. Naropin 10 mg/ml is recommended for epidural anaesthesia in which a complete motor block is essential for surgery. For analgesia (e.g. epidural administration for acute pain management) the lower concentrations and doses are recommended.

Method of administration

Careful aspiration before and during injection is recommended to prevent intravascular injection. When a large dose is to be injected, a test dose of 3-5 ml lidocaine (lignocaine) with adrenaline (Xylocaine® 2% with Adrenaline 1:200,000) is recommended. An inadvertent intravascular injection may be recognised by a temporary increase in heart rate and an accidental intrathecal injection by signs of a spinal block.

Aspiration should be repeated prior to and during administration of the main dose, which should be injected slowly or in incremental doses, at a rate of 25-50 mg/min, while closely observing the patient's vital functions and maintaining verbal contact. If toxic symptoms occur, the injection should be stopped immediately.

In epidural block for surgery, single doses of up to 250 mg ropivacaine have been used and well tolerated.

In brachial plexus block a single dose of 300 mg has been used in a limited number of patients and was well tolerated.

When prolonged blocks are used, either through continuous epidural infusion or through repeated bolus administration, the risks of reaching a toxic plasma concentration or inducing local neural injury must be considered. Cumulative doses up to 675 mg ropivacaine for surgery and postoperative analgesia administered over 24 hours were well tolerated in adults, as were postoperative continuous epidural infusions at rates up to 28 mg/hour for 72 hours. In a limited number of patients, higher doses of up to 800 mg/day have been administered with relatively few adverse reactions.

For treatment of postoperative pain, the following technique can be recommended: Unless preoperatively instituted, an epidural block with Naropin 7.5 mg/ml is induced via an epidural catheter. Analgesia is maintained with Naropin 2 mg/ml infusion. Infusion rates of 6-14 ml (12-28 mg) per hour provide adequate analgesia with only slight and non-progressive motor block in most cases of moderate to severe postoperative pain. The maximum duration of epidural block is 3 days.

However, close monitoring of analgesic effect should be performed in order to remove the catheter as soon as the pain condition allows it.

With this technique a significant reduction in the need for opioids has been observed.

When prolonged peripheral nerve blocks are applied, either through continuous infusion or through repeated injections, the risks of reaching a toxic plasma concentration or inducing local neural injury must be considered. In clinical studies, femoral nerve block was established with 300mg Naropin 7.5 mg/ml and interscalene block with 225mg Naropin 7.5mg/ml, respectively, before surgery. Analgesia was then maintained with Naropin 2mg/ml. Infusion rates or intermittent injections of 10-20mg per hour fro 48 hours provided adequate analgesia and were well tolerated.

Concentrations above 7.5 mg/ml Naropin have not been documented for Caesarean section.

Paediatric patients 1 to 12 years of age:

(see Table 2 on next page)

Method of Administration

Careful aspiration before and during injection is recommended to prevent intravascular injection. The patient's vital functions should be observed closely during the injection. If toxic symptoms occur, the injection should be stopped immediately.

A single caudal epidural injection of ropivacaine 2 mg/ml produces adequate postoperative analgesia below T12 in the majority of patients when a dose of 2 mg/kg is used in a volume of 1 ml/kg. The volume of the caudal epidural injection may be adjusted to achieve a different distribution of sensory block, as recommended in standard textbooks. Doses up to 3 mg/kg of a concentration of ropivacaine 3 mg/ml have been studied. However, this concentration is associated with a higher incidence of motor block.

Fractionation of the calculated local anaesthetic dose is recommended, whatever the route of administration.

Until further experience has been gained, Naropin cannot be recommended for use in children below the age of one year.

4.3 Contraindications

Naropin solutions are contraindicated in patients with known hypersensitivity to anaesthetics of the amide type.

Table 1

	Conc.	Volume	Dose	Onset	Duration
	mg/ml	ml	mg	minutes	hours
SURGICAL ANAESTHESIA					
Lumbar Epidural Administration					
Surgery	7.5	15-25	113-188	10-20	3-5
	10	15-20	150-200	10-20	4-6
Caesarean Section	7.5	15-20	113-150(1)	10-20	3-5
Thoracic Epidural Administration					
To establish block for post-operative pain relief	7.5	5-15 (depending on the level of injection)	38-113	10-20	n/a(2)
Major Nerve Block*					
Brachial plexus block	7.5	30-40	225-300	10-25	6-10
Field Block	7.5	1-30	7.5-225	1-15	2-6
(e.g. minor nerve blocks and infiltration)					
ACUTE PAIN MANAGEMENT					
Lumbar Epidural Administration					
Bolus	2	10-20	20-40	10-15	0.5-1.5
Intermittent injections (top up)	2	10-15	20-30		
(e.g. labour pain management)		(minimum interval 30 minutes)			
Continuous infusion e.g.					
Labour pain	2	6-10 ml/h	12-20 mg/h	n/a(2)	n/a(2)
Postoperative pain management	2	6-14 ml/h	12-28 mg/h	n/a(2)	n/a(2)
Thoracic Epidural Administration					
Continuous infusion (postoperative pain management)	2	6-14 ml/h	12-28 mg/h	n/a(2)	n/a(2)
Field Block					
(e.g. minor nerve blocks and infiltration)	2	1-100	2-200	1-5	2-6
Peripheral nerve block					
(Femoral or interscalene block)					
Continuous infusion or intermittent	2	5-10 ml/h	10-20 mg/h	n/a	n/a
injections					
(e.g. postoperative pain management)					

The doses in the table are those considered to be necessary to produce a successful block and should be regarded as guidelines for use in adults. Individual variations in onset and duration occur. The figures in the column 'Dose' reflect the expected average dose range needed. Standard textbooks should be consulted for both factors affecting specific block techniques and individual patient requirements.

* With regard to major nerve block, only for brachial plexus block a dose recommendation can be given. For other major nerve blocks lower doses may be required. However, there is presently no experience of specific dose recommendations for other blocks.

(1) Incremental dosing should be applied, the starting dose of about 100 mg (97.5 mg = 13 ml; 105 mg = 14 ml) to be given over 3-5 minutes. Two additional doses, each of 25 mg, may be administered as needed. The total administered dose should not exceed 150 mg.

(2) n/a = not applicable

General contraindications related to epidural anaesthesia, regardless of the local anaesthetic used, should be taken into account.

Intravenous regional anaesthesia.

Obstetric paracervical anaesthesia.

Hypovolaemia.

4.4 Special warnings and special precautions for use

Regional anaesthetic procedures should always be performed in a properly equipped and staffed area. Equipment and drugs necessary for monitoring and emergency resuscitation should be immediately available. For emergency medication, patients receiving major blocks or high doses should have an intravenous line inserted before the blocking procedure. The clinician responsible should be appropriately trained and familiar with diagnosis and treatment of side effects, systemic toxicity and other complications such as inadvertent subarachnoid injection which may produce a high spinal block with apnoea and hypotension. Convulsions have occurred most often after brachial plexus block and epidural block. This is likely to be the result of either accidental intravascular injection or rapid absorption from the injection site.

Certain local anaesthetic procedures, such as injections in the head and neck regions, may be associated with a higher frequency of serious adverse reactions, regardless of the local anaesthetic used. Care should be taken to avoid injections in infected areas.

Until further experience has been gained, Naropin cannot be recommended for use in children below the age of one year.

Patients in poor general condition due to ageing or other compromising factors such as partial or complete heart

Table 2 Paediatric patients 1 to 12 years of age

	Conc.	Volume	Dose
	mg/ml	ml/kg	mg/kg
ACUTE PAIN MANAGEMENT			
(pre- and post-operative)			
Caudal Epidural Administration Single injection	2.0	1	2
Blocks below T12, in children with a body weight up to 25kg			

The dose in the table should be regarded as guidelines for use in paediatrics. Individual variations occur. In children with a high body weight a gradual reduction of the dosage is often necessary and should be based on the ideal body weight. Standard textbooks should be consulted for factors affecting specific block techniques and for individual patient requirements.

conduction block, advanced liver disease or severe renal dysfunction require special attention, although regional anaesthesia is frequently indicated in these patients.

Ropivacaine is metabolised in the liver and should therefore be used with caution in patients with severe liver disease. Repeated doses may need to be reduced due to delayed elimination. Normally there is no need to modify the dose in patients with impaired renal function when used for single dose or short term treatment. Acidosis and reduced plasma protein concentration, frequently seen in patients with chronic renal failure, may increase the risk of systemic toxicity.

Patients with hypovolaemia due to any cause can develop sudden and severe hypotension during epidural anaesthesia, regardless of the local anaesthetic used.

Prolonged administration of ropivacaine should be avoided in patients concomitantly treated with strong CYP1A2 inhibitors, such as fluvoxamine and enoxacin, see 4.5.

A possible cross-hypersensitivity with other amide-type local anaesthetics should be taken into account.

4.5 Interaction with other medicinal products and other forms of Interaction

Naropin should be used with caution in patients receiving other local anaesthetics or agents structurally related to amide-type local anaesthetics, e.g. certain antiarrhythmics, since the toxic effects are additive. Simultaneous use of Naropin with general anaesthetics or opioids may potentiate each others (adverse) effects.

Cytochrome P450 (CYP) 1A2 is involved in the formation of 3-hydroxy-ropivacaine, the major metabolite. *In vivo*, the plasma clearance of ropivacaine was reduced by 70% during coadministration of fluvoxamine, a selective and potent CYP1A2 inhibitor. Thus strong inhibitors of CYP1A2, such as fluvoxamine and enoxacin given concomitantly during prolonged administration of Naropin, can interact with Naropin. Prolonged administration of ropivacaine should be avoided in patients concomitantly treated with strong CYP1A2 inhibitors, see also 4.4.

In vivo, the plasma clearance of ropivacaine was reduced by 15% during coadministration of ketoconazole, a selective and potent inhibitor of CYP3A4. However, the inhibition of this isozyme is not likely to have clinical relevance.

In vitro, ropivacaine is a competitive inhibitor of CYP2D6 but does not seem to inhibit this isozyme at clinically attained plasma concentrations.

4.6 Pregnancy and lactation

Pregnancy

Apart from obstetrical use, there are no adequate data on the use of ropivacaine in pregnancy. Animal studies do not indicate direct or indirect harmful effects with respect to pregnancy, embryonal/foetal development, parturition or postnatal development (see section 5.3)

Lactation

There is no data available concerning the excretion of ropivacaine into human milk.

4.7 Effects on ability to drive and use machines

No data is available. Depending on the dose, local anaesthetics may have a minor influence on mental function and co-ordination even in the absence of overt CNS toxicity and may temporarily impair locomotion and alertness.

4.8 Undesirable effects

General

The adverse reaction profile for Naropin is similar to those for other long acting local anaesthetics of the amide type. Adverse drug reactions should be distinguished from the physiological effects of the nerve block itself e.g. a decrease in blood pressure and bradycardia during spinal/epidural block.

The percentage of patients that can be expected to experience adverse reactions varies with the route of administration of Naropin. Systemic and localised adverse reactions of Naropin usually occur because of excessive dosage, rapid absorption, or inadvertent intravascular injection. The most frequently reported adverse reactions, nausea and hypotension, are very frequent during anaesthesia and surgery in general and it is not possible to distinguish those caused by the clinical situation from those caused by the drug or the block.

Table of adverse drug reactions

Within each system organ class, the ADRs have been ranked under the headings of frequency, most frequent reactions first.

Very common (>1/10)	*Vascular Disorders*: Hypotension *Gastrointestinal Disorders:* Nausea
Common (>1/100)	*Nervous System Disorders:* Headache, Paraesthesia, Dizziness *Cardiac Disorders:* Bradycardia, Tachycardia *Vascular Disorders:* Hypertension *Gastrointestinal Disorders:* Vomiting *Renal and Urinary Disorders:* Urinary retention *General Disorder and Administration Site Conditions:* Temperature Elevation, Rigors
Uncommon (>1/1,000)	*Nervous system disorders:* Hypoaesthesia
Rare (>1/10,000)	*Psychiatric Disorders:* Anxiety *Nervous System Disorders:* Convulsions

In children, the most commonly reported adverse events of clinical importance are vomiting, nausea, pruritus and urinary retention.

Class-related adverse drug reactions

Allergic reactions

Allergic reactions (in the most severe instances anaphylactic shock) to local anaesthetics of the amide type are rare.

Neurological complications

Neuropathy and spinal cord dysfunction (e.g. anterior spinal artery syndrome, arachnoiditis, cauda equina), which may result in rare cases of permanent sequelae, have been associated with regional anaesthesia, regardless of the local anaesthetic used.

Acute systemic toxicity

Naropin may cause acute toxic effects following high doses or if very rapidly rising blood levels occur due to accidental intravascular injection or overdose. (See 4.9 "Overdose").

4.9 Overdose

Symptoms

Acute systemic toxicity

Accidental intravascular injections of local anaesthetics may cause immediate toxic effects. In the event of overdose, peak plasma concentrations may not be reached for one to two hours, depending on the site of the injection, and signs of toxicity may thus be delayed. Systemic toxic reactions may involve the central nervous system and the cardiovascular system.

In children, early signs of local anaesthetic toxicity may be difficult to detect in cases where the block is given during general anaesthesia.

Central nervous system

Central nervous system toxicity is a graded response with symptoms and signs of escalating severity. Initially symptoms such as visual or hearing disturbances, perioral numbness, dizziness, light-headedness, tingling and paraesthesia are seen. Dysarthria, muscular rigidity and muscular twitching are more serious and may precede the onset of generalised convulsions. These signs must not be mistaken for neurotic behaviour. Unconsciousness and grand mal convulsions may follow, which may last from a few seconds to several minutes. Hypoxia and hypercarbia occur rapidly during convulsions due to the increased muscular activity, together with the interference with respiration. In severe cases even apnoea may occur. The respiratory and metabolic acidosis increases and extends the toxic effects of local anaesthetics.

Recovery follows the redistribution of the local anaesthetic drug from the central nervous system and subsequent metabolism and excretion. Recovery may be rapid unless large amounts of the drug have been injected.

Cardiovascular toxicity

Cardiovascular toxicity indicates a more severe situation. Hypotension, bradycardia, arrhythmia and even cardiac arrest may occur as a result of high systemic concentrations of local anaesthetics. In volunteers the intravenous infusion of ropivacaine resulted in signs of depression of conductivity and contractility.

Cardiovascular toxicity effects are generally preceded by signs of toxicity in the central nervous system, unless the patient is receiving a general anaesthetic or is heavily sedated with drugs such as benzodiazepines or barbiturates.

Treatment of acute toxicity

Equipment and drugs necessary for monitoring and emergency resuscitation should be immediately available. If signs of acute systemic toxicity appear, injection of the local anaesthetic should be stopped immediately.

In the event of convulsions, treatment will be required. The objectives of treatment are to maintain oxygenation, stop the convulsions and support the circulation. Oxygen must be given and ventilation assisted, when necessary (mask and bag). An anticonvulsant should be given intravenously if the convulsions do not stop spontaneously in 15-20 seconds. Thiopentone sodium 1-3 mg/kg intravenously will abort the convulsions rapidly. Alternatively diazepam 0.1 mg/kg intravenously may be used, although its action is slower. Suxamethonium will stop the muscle convulsions rapidly, but the patient will require controlled ventilation and tracheal intubation.

If cardiovascular depression is evident (hypotension, bradycardia), ephedrine 5-10 mg intravenously should be given and repeated, if necessary, after 2-3 minutes. Children should be given ephedrine doses commensurate with their age and weight.

Should circulatory arrest occur, immediate cardiopulmonary resuscitation should be instituted. Optimal oxygenation and ventilation and circulatory support as well as treatment of acidosis are of vital importance.

5. PHARMACOLOGICAL PROPERTIES

5.1 Pharmacodynamic properties

Pharmacotherapeutic group (ATC code): N01B B09

Ropivacaine is a long-acting amide-type local anaesthetic with both anaesthetic and analgesic effects. At high doses it produces surgical anaesthesia, while at lower doses it produces sensory block with limited and non-progressive motor block.

The mechanism is a reversible reduction of the membrane permeability of the nerve fibre to sodium ions. Consequently the depolarisation velocity is decreased and the excitable threshold increased, resulting in a local blockade of nerve impulses.

The most characteristic property of ropivacaine is the long duration of action. Onset and duration of the local anaesthetic efficacy are dependent upon the administration site and dose, but are not influenced by the presence of a vasoconstrictor (e.g. adrenaline). For details concerning the onset and duration of action, see table under "Posology and method of administration".

Healthy volunteers exposed to intravenous infusions tolerated ropivacaine well at low doses and with expected CNS symptoms at the maximum tolerated dose. The clinical experience with this drug indicates a good margin of safety when adequately used in recommended doses.

Hypotension and bradycardia are uncommon after caudal epidural block in children.

5.2 Pharmacokinetic properties

Ropivacaine has a chiral center and is available as the pure S-(-)-enantiomer. It is highly lipid-soluble. All metabolites have a local anaesthetic effect but of considerably lower potency and shorter duration than that of ropivacaine.

The plasma concentration of ropivacaine depends upon the dose, the route of administration and the vascularity of the injection site. Ropivacaine follows linear pharmacokinetics and the C_{max} is proportional to the dose.

Ropivacaine shows complete and biphasic absorption from the epidural space with half-lives of the two phases of the order of 14 min and 4 h in adults. The slow absorption is the rate -limiting factor in the elimination of ropivacaine, which explains why the apparent elimination half-life is longer after epidural than after intravenous administration.

Ropivacaine has a mean total plasma clearance in the order of 440 ml/min, a renal clearance of 1 ml/min, a volume of distribution at steady state of 47 litres and a terminal half-life of 1.8 h after iv administration. Ropivacaine has an intermediate hepatic extraction ratio of about 0.4. It is mainly bound to α_1- acid glycoprotein in plasma with an unbound fraction of about 6%.

An increase in total plasma concentrations during continuous epidural and interscalene infusion has been observed, related to a postoperative increase of α_1- acid glycoprotein.

Variations in unbound, i.e. pharmacologically active, concentration have been much less than in total plasma concentration.

In children, aged between 1 and 12 years, ropivacaine pharmacokinetics after regional anaesthesia has been shown to be unrelated to age. In this group ropivacaine has a total plasma clearance in the order of 7.5 ml/min kg, an unbound plasma clearance of 0.15 l/min kg, a volume of distribution at steady state of 2.4 l/kg, an unbound fraction of 5% and a terminal half-life of 3 hours. Ropivacaine shows biphasic absorption from the caudal space. The clearance related to body weight in this age group is similar to that in adults.

Ropivacaine readily crosses the placenta and equilibrium in regard to unbound concentration will be rapidly reached. The degree of plasma protein binding in the foetus is less than in the mother, which results in lower total plasma concentrations in the foetus than in the mother.

Ropivacaine is extensively metabolised, predominantly by aromatic hydroxylation. In total, 86% of the dose is excreted in the urine after intravenous administration, of which only about 1% relates to unchanged drug. The major metabolite is 3-hydroxy-ropivacaine, about 37% of which is excreted in the urine, mainly conjugated. Urinary excretion of 4-hydroxy-ropivacaine, the N-dealkylated metabolite and the 4-hydroxy-dealkylated accounts for 1-3%. Conjugated+unconjugated 3-hydroxy-ropivacaine shows only detectable concentrations in plasma.

A similar pattern of metabolites has been found in children above one year.

There is no evidence of *in vivo* racemisation of ropivacaine.

5.3 Preclinical safety data

Based on conventional studies of safety pharmacology, single and repeated dose toxicity, reproduction toxicity, mutagenic potential and local toxicity, no hazards for humans were identified other than those which can be expected on the basis of the pharmacodynamic action of high doses of ropivacaine (e.g. CNS signs, including convulsions, and cardiotoxicity).

6. PHARMACEUTICAL PARTICULARS

6.1 List of excipients

Sodium chloride

Hydrochloric acid

Sodium hydroxide

Water for injection

6.2 Incompatibilities

In alkaline solutions precipitation may occur as ropivacaine shows poor solubility at pH > 6.0.

6.3 Shelf life

3 years.

6.4 Special precautions for storage

Do not store above 30°C. Do not freeze.

6.5 Nature and contents of container

10 ml polypropylene ampoules (Polyamp) in packs of 5 and 10

10 ml polypropylene ampoules (Polyamp) in sterile blister packs of 5 and 10

20 ml polypropylene ampoules (Polyamp) in packs of 5 and 10

20 ml polypropylene ampoules (Polyamp) in sterile blister packs of 5 and 10

The polypropylene ampoules (Polyamp) are specially designed to fit Luer lock and Luer fit syringes.

6.6 Instructions for use and handling

Naropin products are preservative free and are intended for single use only. Discard any unused solution.

The intact container must not be re-autoclaved. A blistered container should be chosen when a sterile outside is required.

7. MARKETING AUTHORISATION HOLDER

AstraZeneca UK Ltd.,

600 Capability Green,

Luton, LU1 3LU, UK

8. MARKETING AUTHORISATION NUMBER(S)

PL 17901/0151

9. DATE OF FIRST AUTHORISATION/RENEWAL OF THE AUTHORISATION

18th August 2002

10. DATE OF REVISION OF THE TEXT

8th October 2003

Trademarks herein are the property of the AstraZeneca group

Naropin 2 mg/ml solution for infusion

(AstraZeneca UK Limited)

1. NAME OF THE MEDICINAL PRODUCT

Naropin® 2 mg/ml solution for infusion

2. QUALITATIVE AND QUANTITATIVE COMPOSITION

Naropin 2 mg/ml: 2 mg/ml ropivacaine hydrochloride

For excipients, see 6.1

3. PHARMACEUTICAL FORM

Solution for infusion for perineural and epidural administration (100 and 200 ml)

4. CLINICAL PARTICULARS

4.1 Therapeutic indications

Naropin is indicated for:

1. Surgical anaesthesia:

- Epidural blocks for surgery, including Caesarean section.
- Major nerve blocks.
- Field blocks.

2. Acute pain management

- Continuous epidural infusion or intermittent bolus administration during postoperative or labour pain.
- Field blocks.
- Continuous peripheral nerve block via a continuous infusion or intermittent bolus injections, e.g. postoperative pain management.

4.2 Posology and method of administration

Naropin should only be used by, or under the supervision of, clinicians experienced in regional anaesthesia.

Posology

The following table is a guide to dosage for the more commonly used blocks. The smallest dose required to produce an effective block should be used. The clinician's experience and knowledge of the patient's physical status are of importance when deciding the dose.

(see Table 1 below)

In general, surgical anaesthesia (e.g. epidural administration) requires the use of the higher concentrations and doses. Naropin 10 mg/ml is recommended for epidural anaesthesia in which a profound motor block is essential for surgery. For analgesia (e.g. epidural administration for acute pain management) the lower concentrations and doses are recommended.

Method of administration

Careful aspiration before and during injection is recommended to prevent intravascular injection. When a large dose is to be injected, a test dose of 3-5 ml lidocaine (lignocaine) with adrenaline (Xylocaine® 2% with Adrenaline

Table 1

	Conc. mg/ml	Volume ml	Dose mg	Onset minutes	Duration hours
SURGICAL ANAESTHESIA					
Lumbar Epidural Administration					
Surgery	7.5	15-25	113-188	10-20	3-5
	10	15-20	150-200	10-20	4-6
Caesarean Section	7.5	15-20	113-150(1)	10-20	3-5
Thoracic Epidural Administration					
To establish block for post-operative pain relief	7.5	5-15 (depending on the level of injection)	38-113	10-20	n/a(2)
Major Nerve Block*					
Brachial plexus block	7.5	30-40	225-300	10-25	6-10
Field Block (e.g. minor nerve blocks and infiltration)	7.5	1-30	7.5-225	1-15	2-6
ACUTE PAIN MANAGEMENT					
Lumbar Epidural Administration					
Bolus	2	10-20	20-40	10-15	0.5-1.5
Intermittent injections (top up)	2	10-15	20-30		
(e.g. labour pain management)		(minimum interval 30 minutes)			
Continuous infusion e.g.					
Labour pain	2	6-10 ml/h	12-20 mg/h	n/a(2)	n/a(2)
Postoperative pain management	2	6-14 ml/h	12-28 mg/h	n/a(2)	n/a(2)
Thoracic Epidural Administration					
Continuous infusion (postoperative pain management)	2	6-14 ml/h	12-28 mg/h	n/a(2)	n/a(2)
Field Block					
(e.g. minor nerve blocks and infiltration)	2	1-100	2-200	1-5	2-6
Peripheral nerve block (Femoral or interscalene block)					
Continuous infusion or intermittent injections (e.g. postoperative pain management)	2.0	5-10 ml/h	10-20 mg/h	n/a	n/a

The doses in the table are those considered to be necessary to produce a successful block and should be regarded as guidelines for use in adults. Individual variations in onset and duration occur. The figures in the column 'Dose' reflect the expected average dose range needed. Standard textbooks should be consulted for both factors affecting specific block techniques and individual patient requirements.

* With regard to major nerve block, a dose recommendation can only be given for brachial plexus block. For other major nerve blocks lower doses may be required. However, there is presently no experience of specific dose recommendations for other blocks.

(1) Incremental dosing should be applied, the starting dose of about 100 mg (97.5 mg = 13 ml; 105 mg = 14 ml) to be given over 3-5 minutes. Two additional doses, each of 25 mg, may be administered as needed. The total administered dose should not exceed 150 mg.

(2) n/a = not applicable

1:200,000) is recommended. An inadvertent intravascular injection may be recognised by a temporary increase in heart rate and an accidental intrathecal injection by signs of a spinal block.

Aspiration should be repeated prior to and during administration of the main dose, which should be injected slowly or in incremental doses, at a rate of 25-50 mg/min, while closely observing the patient's vital functions and maintaining verbal contact. If toxic symptoms occur, the injection should be stopped immediately.

In epidural block for surgery, single doses of up to 250 mg ropivacaine have been used and well tolerated.

In brachial plexus block a single dose of 300 mg has been used in a limited number of patients and was well tolerated.

When prolonged blocks are used, either through continuous epidural infusion or through repeated bolus administration, the risks of reaching a toxic plasma concentration or inducing local neural injury must be considered. Cumulative doses up to 675 mg ropivacaine for surgery and postoperative analgesia administered over 24 hours were well tolerated in adults, as were postoperative continuous epidural infusions at rates up to 28 mg/hour for 72 hours. In a limited number of patients, higher doses of up to 800 mg/day have been administered with relatively few adverse reactions.

For treatment of postoperative pain, the following technique can be recommended: Unless preoperatively instituted, an epidural block with Naropin 7.5 mg/ml is induced via an epidural catheter. Analgesia is maintained with Naropin 2 mg/ml infusion. Infusion rates of 6-14 ml (12-28 mg) per hour provide adequate analgesia with only slight and non-progressive motor block in most cases of moderate to severe postoperative pain. The maximum duration of epidural block is 3 days. However, close monitoring of analgesic effect should be performed in order to remove the catheter as soon as the pain condition allows it.

With this technique a significant reduction in the need for opioids has been observed.

In clinical studies an epidural infusion of Naropin 2mg/ml alone or mixed with fentanyl 1-4 mcg/ml has been given for postoperative pain management for up to 72 hours. The combination of Naropin and fentanyl provided improved pain relief but caused opioid side effects. The combination of Naropin and fentanyl has been investigated only for Naropin 2 mg/ml.

When prolonged peripheral nerve blocks are applied, either through continuous infusion or through repeated injections, the risks of reaching a toxic plasma concentration or inducing local neural injury must be considered. In clinical studies, femoral nerve block was established with 300 mg Naropin 7.5 mg/ml and interscalene block with 225 mg Naropin 7.5 mg/ml, respectively, before surgery. Analgesia was then maintained with Naropin 2 mg/ml. Infusion rates or intermittent injections of 10-20 mg per hour for 48 hours provided adequate analgesia and were well tolerated.

Concentrations above 7.5 mg/ml Naropin have not been documented for Caesarean section.

Naropin cannot be recommended for use in children below the age of 12 years as there is no data with regard to efficacy and safety in this group of patients.

4.3 Contraindications

Naropin solutions are contraindicated in patients with known hypersensitivity to anaesthetics of the amide type.

General contraindications related to epidural anaesthesia, regardless of the local anaesthetic used, should be taken into account.

Intravenous regional anaesthesia.

Obstetric paracervical anaesthesia.

Hypovolaemia.

4.4 Special warnings and special precautions for use

Regional anaesthetic procedures should always be performed in a properly equipped and staffed area. Equipment and drugs necessary for monitoring and emergency resuscitation should be immediately available. For emergency medication, patients receiving major blocks or high doses should have an intravenous line inserted before the blocking procedure. The clinician responsible should be appropriately trained and familiar with diagnosis and treatment of side effects, systemic toxicity and other complications such as inadvertent subarachnoid injection which may produce a high spinal block with apnoea and hypotension. Convulsions have occurred most often after brachial plexus block and epidural block. This is likely to be the result of either accidental intravascular injection or rapid absorption from the injection site.

Certain local anaesthetic procedures, such as injections in the head and neck regions, may be associated with a higher frequency of serious adverse reactions, regardless of the local anaesthetic used. Care should be taken to avoid injections in infected areas.

Patients in poor general condition due to ageing or other compromising factors such as partial or complete heart conduction block, advanced liver disease or severe renal dysfunction require special attention, although regional anaesthesia is frequently indicated in these patients.

Ropivacaine is metabolised in the liver and should therefore be used with caution in patients with severe liver disease. Repeated doses may need to be reduced due to delayed elimination. Normally there is no need to modify the dose in patients with impaired renal function when used for single dose or short term treatment. Acidosis and reduced plasma protein concentration, frequently seen in patients with chronic renal failure, may increase the risk of systemic toxicity.

Patients with hypovolaemia due to any cause can develop sudden and severe hypotension during epidural anaesthesia, regardless of the local anaesthetic used.

Prolonged administration of ropivacaine should be avoided in patients concomitantly treated with strong CYP1A2 inhibitors, such as fluvoxamine and enoxacin, see 4.5.

A possible cross-hypersensitivity with other amide-type local anaesthetics should be taken into account.

4.5 Interaction with other medicinal products and other forms of Interaction

Naropin should be used with caution in patients receiving other local anaesthetics or agents structurally related to amide-type local anaesthetics, e.g. certain antiarrhythmics, since the toxic effects are additive. Simultaneous use of Naropin with general anaesthetics or opioids may potentiate each others (adverse) effects.

Cytochrome P450 (CYP) 1A2 is involved in the formation of 3-hydroxy-ropivacaine, the major metabolite. *In vivo*, the plasma clearance of ropivacaine was reduced by 70% during coadministration of fluvoxamine, a selective and potent CYP1A2 inhibitor. Thus strong inhibitors of CYP1A2, such as fluvoxamine and enoxacin, given concomitantly during prolonged administration of Naropin, can interact with Naropin. Prolonged administration of ropivacaine should be avoided in patients concomitantly treated with strong CYP1A2 inhibitors, see also 4.4.

In vivo, the plasma clearance of ropivacaine was reduced by 15% during coadministration of ketoconazole, a selective and potent inhibitor of CYP3A4. However, the inhibition of this isozyme is not likely to have clinical relevance.

In vitro, ropivacaine is a competitive inhibitor of CYP2D6 but does not seem to inhibit this isozyme at clinically attained plasma concentrations.

4.6 Pregnancy and lactation

Pregnancy

Apart from obstetrical use, there are no adequate data on the use of ropivacaine in pregnancy. Animal studies do not indicate direct or indirect harmful effects with respect to pregnancy, embryonal/foetal development, parturition or postnatal development (see section 5.3).

Lactation

There is no data available concerning the excretion of ropivacaine into human milk.

4.7 Effects on ability to drive and use machines

No data is available. Depending on the dose, local anaesthetics may have a minor influence on mental function and co-ordination even in the absence of overt CNS toxicity and may temporarily impair locomotion and alertness.

4.8 Undesirable effects

General

The adverse reaction profile for Naropin is similar to those for other long acting local anaesthetics of the amide type. Adverse drug reactions should be distinguished from the physiological effects of the nerve block itself e.g. a decrease in blood pressure and bradycardia during spinal/epidural block.

The percentage of patients that can be expected to experience adverse reactions varies with the route of administration of Naropin. Systemic and localised adverse reactions of Naropin usually occur because of excessive dosage, rapid absorption, or inadvertent intravascular injection. The most frequently reported adverse reactions, nausea and hypotension, are very frequent during anaesthesia and surgery in general and it is not possible to distinguish those caused by the clinical situation from those caused by the drug or the block.

Table of adverse drug reactions

Within each system organ class, the ADRs have been ranked under the headings of frequency, most frequent reactions first.

Very common (>1/10)	*Vascular Disorders:* Hypotension
	Gastrointestinal Disorders: Nausea
Common (>1/100)	*Nervous System Disorders:* Headache, Paraesthesia, Dizziness
	Cardiac Disorders: Bradycardia, Tachycardia
	Vascular Disorders: Hypertension
	Gastrointestinal Disorders: Vomiting
	Renal and Urinary Disorders: Urinary retention
	General Disorder and Administration Site Conditions: Temperature Elevation, Rigors
Uncommon (>1/1,000)	*Nervous system disorders:* Hypoaesthesia
Rare (>1/10,000)	*Psychiatric Disorders:* Anxiety
	Nervous System Disorders: Convulsions

Class-related adverse drug reactions

Allergic reactions

Allergic reactions (in the most severe instances anaphylactic shock) to local anaesthetics of the amide type are rare.

Neurological complications

Neuropathy and spinal cord dysfunction (e.g. anterior spinal artery syndrome, arachnoiditis, cauda equina), which may result in rare cases of permanent sequelae, have been associated with regional anaesthesia, regardless of the local anaesthetic used.

Acute systemic toxicity

Naropin may cause acute toxic effects following high doses or if very rapidly rising blood levels occur due to accidental intravascular injection or overdose. (See 4.9 "Overdose").

4.9 Overdose

Symptoms

Acute systemic toxicity

Accidental intravascular injections of local anaesthetics may cause immediate toxic effects. In the event of overdose, peak plasma concentrations may not be reached for one to two hours, depending on the site of the injection, and signs of toxicity may thus be delayed. Systemic toxic reactions may involve the central nervous system and the cardiovascular system.

Central nervous system

Central nervous system toxicity is a graded response with symptoms and signs of escalating severity. Initially symptoms such as visual or hearing disturbances, perioral numbness, dizziness, light-headedness, tingling and paraesthesia are seen. Dysarthria, muscular rigidity and muscular twitching are more serious and may precede the onset of generalised convulsions. These signs must not be mistaken for neurotic behaviour. Unconsciousness and grand mal convulsions may follow, which may last from a few seconds to several minutes. Hypoxia and hypercarbia occur rapidly during convulsions due to the increased muscular activity, together with the interference with respiration. In severe cases even apnoea may occur. The respiratory and metabolic acidosis increases and extends the toxic effects of local anaesthetics.

Recovery follows the redistribution of the local anaesthetic drug from the central nervous system and subsequent metabolism and excretion. Recovery may be rapid unless large amounts of the drug have been injected.

Cardiovascular toxicity

Cardiovascular toxicity indicates a more severe situation. Hypotension, bradycardia, arrhythmia and even cardiac arrest may occur as a result of high systemic concentrations of local anaesthetics. In volunteers the intravenous infusion of ropivacaine resulted in signs of depression of conductivity and contractility.

Cardiovascular toxicity effects are generally preceded by signs of toxicity in the central nervous system, unless the patient is receiving a general anaesthetic or is heavily sedated with drugs such as benzodiazepines or barbiturates.

Treatment of acute toxicity

Equipment and drugs necessary for monitoring and emergency resuscitation should be immediately available. If signs of acute systemic toxicity appear, injection of the local anaesthetic should be stopped immediately.

In the event of convulsions, treatment will be required. The objectives of treatment are to maintain oxygenation, stop the convulsions and support the circulation. Oxygen must be given and ventilation assisted, when necessary (mask and bag). An anticonvulsant should be given intravenously if the convulsions do not stop spontaneously in 15-20 seconds. Thiopentone sodium 1-3 mg/kg intravenously will abort the convulsions rapidly. Alternatively diazepam 0.1 mg/kg intravenously may be used, although its action is slower. Suxamethonium will stop the muscle convulsions rapidly, but the patient will require controlled ventilation and tracheal intubation.

If cardiovascular depression is evident (hypotension, bradycardia), ephedrine 5-10 mg intravenously should be given and repeated, if necessary, after 2-3 minutes.

Should circulatory arrest occur, immediate cardiopulmonary resuscitation should be instituted. Optimal oxygenation and ventilation and circulatory support as well as treatment of acidosis are of vital importance.

5. PHARMACOLOGICAL PROPERTIES

5.1 Pharmacodynamic properties

Pharmacotherapeutic group (ATC code): N01B B09

Ropivacaine is a long-acting amide-type local anaesthetic with both anaesthetic and analgesic effects. At high doses it produces surgical anaesthesia, while at lower doses it produces sensory block with limited and non-progressive motor block.

The mechanism is a reversible reduction of the membrane permeability of the nerve fibre to sodium ions. Consequently the depolarisation velocity is decreased and the excitable threshold increased, resulting in a local blockade of nerve impulses.

The most characteristic property of ropivacaine is the long duration of action. Onset and duration of the local anaesthetic efficacy are dependent upon the administration site and dose, but are not influenced by the presence of a vasoconstrictor (e.g. adrenaline). For details concerning the onset and duration of action, see table under "Posology and method of administration".

Healthy volunteers exposed to intravenous infusions tolerated ropivacaine well at low doses and with expected CNS symptoms at the maximum tolerated dose. The clinical experience with this drug indicates a good margin of safety when adequately used in recommended doses.

5.2 Pharmacokinetic properties

Ropivacaine has a chiral center and is available as the pure S-(-)-enantiomer. It is highly lipid-soluble. All metabolites have a local anaesthetic effect but of considerably lower potency and shorter duration than that of ropivacaine.

The plasma concentration of ropivacaine depends upon the dose, the route of administration and the vascularity of the injection site. Ropivacaine follows linear pharmacokinetics and the C_{max} is proportional to the dose.

Ropivacaine shows complete and biphasic absorption from the epidural space with half-lives of the two phases of the order of 14 min and 4 h in adults. The slow absorption is the rate -limiting factor in the elimination of ropivacaine, which explains why the apparent elimination half-life is longer after epidural than after intravenous administration.

Ropivacaine has a mean total plasma clearance in the order of 440 ml/min, a renal clearance of 1 ml/min, a volume of distribution at steady state of 47 litres and a terminal half-life of 1.8 h after iv administration. Ropivacaine has an intermediate hepatic extraction ratio of about 0.4. It is mainly bound to α_1- acid glycoprotein in plasma with an unbound fraction of about 6%.

An increase in total plasma concentrations during continuous epidural and interscalene infusion has been observed, related to a postoperative increase of α_1- acid glycoprotein.

Variations in unbound, i.e. pharmacologically active, concentration have been much less than in total plasma concentration.

Ropivacaine readily crosses the placenta and equilibrium in regard to unbound concentration will be rapidly reached. The degree of plasma protein binding in the foetus is less than in the mother, which results in lower total plasma concentrations in the foetus than in the mother.

Ropivacaine is extensively metabolised, predominantly by aromatic hydroxylation. In total, 86% of the dose is excreted in the urine after intravenous administration, of which only about 1% relates to unchanged drug. The major metabolite is 3-hydroxy-ropivacaine, about 37% of which is excreted in the urine, mainly conjugated. Urinary excretion of 4-hydroxy-ropivacaine, the N-dealkylated metabolite and the 4-hydroxy-dealkylated accounts for 1-3%. Conjugated+unconjugated 3-hydroxy-ropivacaine shows only detectable concentrations in plasma.

There is no evidence of *in vivo* racemisation of ropivacaine.

5.3 Preclinical safety data

Based on conventional studies of safety pharmacology, single and repeated dose toxicity, reproduction toxicity, mutagenic potential and local toxicity, no hazards for humans were identified other than those which can be expected on the basis of the pharmacodynamic action of high doses of ropivacaine (e.g. CNS signs, including convulsions, and cardiotoxicity).

6. PHARMACEUTICAL PARTICULARS

6.1 List of excipients

Sodium chloride

Hydrochloric acid

Sodium hydroxide

Water for injection

6.2 Incompatibilities

Compatibilities with other solutions than those mentioned in section 6.6 have not been investigated. In alkaline solutions precipitation may occur as ropivacaine shows poor solubility at pH > 6.0.

6.3 Shelf life

2 years.

6.4 Special precautions for storage

Do not store above 30°C. Do not freeze.

6.5 Nature and contents of container

100 ml polypropylene bags (Polybag) in sterile blister packs of 5

200 ml polypropylene bags (Polybag) in sterile blister packs of 5

6.6 Instructions for use and handling

Naropin products are preservative free and are intended for single use only. Discard any unused solution.

The intact container must not be re-autoclaved. A blistered container should be chosen when a sterile outside is required.

Naropin solution for infusion in plastic infusion bags (Polybag) is chemically and physically compatible with the following drugs:

Concentration of Naropin: 1-2 mg/ml	
Additive	**Concentration***
Fentanyl citrate	1.0 – 10.0 microgram/ml
Sufentanil citrate	0.4 – 4.0 microgram/ml
Morphine sulphate	20.0 – 100 microgram/ml
Clonidine hydrochloride	5.0 – 50.0 microgram/ml

* The concentration ranges stated in the table are wider than those used in clinical practice. Epidural infusions of Naropin/sufentanil citrate, Naropin/morphine sulphate and Naropin/clonidine hydrochloride have not been evaluated in clinical studies.

The mixtures are chemically and physically stable for 30 days at 20 to 30°C. From a microbiological point of view, the mixtures should be used immediately. If not used immediately, in-use storage times and conditions prior to use are the responsibility of the user and would normally not be longer than 24 hours at 2 to 8°C.

7. MARKETING AUTHORISATION HOLDER

AstraZeneca UK Ltd.,

600 Capability Green,

Luton, LU1 3LU, UK.

8. MARKETING AUTHORISATION NUMBER(S)

PL 17901/0149

9. DATE OF FIRST AUTHORISATION/RENEWAL OF THE AUTHORISATION

15th September 2000

10. DATE OF REVISION OF THE TEXT

22 March 2004

Naropin 7.5 mg/ml solution for injection

(AstraZeneca UK Limited)

1. NAME OF THE MEDICINAL PRODUCT

Naropin® 7.5 mg/ml solution for injection

2. QUALITATIVE AND QUANTITATIVE COMPOSITION

Naropin 7.5 mg/ml: 7.5 mg/ml ropivacaine hydrochloride

For excipients, see 6.1

3. PHARMACEUTICAL FORM

Solution for injection for perineural and epidural administration (10-20 ml).

4. CLINICAL PARTICULARS

4.1 Therapeutic indications

Naropin is indicated for:

1. Surgical anaesthesia:

- Epidural blocks for surgery, including Caesarean section.

- Major nerve blocks.

- Field blocks.

2. Acute pain management

- Continuous epidural infusion or intermittent bolus administration during postoperative or labour pain.

- Field blocks.

4.2 Posology and method of administration

Naropin should only be used by, or under the supervision of, clinicians experienced in regional anaesthesia.

Posology

The following table is a guide to dosage for the more commonly used blocks. The smallest dose required to produce an effective block should be used. The clinician's experience and knowledge of the patient's physical status are of importance when deciding the dose.

(see Table 1 on next page)

In general, surgical anaesthesia (e.g. epidural administration) requires the use of the higher concentrations and doses. Naropin 10 mg/ml is recommended for epidural anaesthesia in which a complete motor block is essential for surgery. For analgesia (e.g. epidural administration for acute pain management) the lower concentrations and doses are recommended.

Method of administration

Careful aspiration before and during injection is recommended to prevent intravascular injection. When a large dose is to be injected, a test dose of 3-5 ml lidocaine (lignocaine) with adrenaline (Xylocaine® 2% with Adrenaline 1:200,000) is recommended. An inadvertent intravascular injection may be recognised by a temporary increase in heart rate and an accidental intrathecal injection by signs of a spinal block.

Aspiration should be repeated prior to and during administration of the main dose, which should be injected slowly or in incremental doses, at a rate of 25-50 mg/min, while closely observing the patient's vital functions and maintaining verbal contact. If toxic symptoms occur, the injection should be stopped immediately.

In epidural block for surgery, single doses of up to 250 mg ropivacaine have been used and well tolerated.

In brachial plexus block a single dose of 300 mg has been used in a limited number of patients and was well tolerated.

When prolonged blocks are used, either through continuous epidural infusion or through repeated bolus administration, the risks of reaching a toxic plasma concentration or inducing local neural injury must be considered. Cumulative doses up to 675 mg ropivacaine for surgery and postoperative analgesia administered over 24 hours were well tolerated in adults, as were postoperative continuous epidural infusions at rates up to 28 mg/hour for 72 hours. In a limited number of patients, higher doses of up to 800 mg/day have been administered with relatively few adverse reactions.

For treatment of postoperative pain, the following technique can be recommended: Unless preoperatively instituted, an epidural block with Naropin 7.5 mg/ml is induced via an epidural catheter. Analgesia is maintained with Naropin 2 mg/ml infusion. Infusion rates of 6-14 ml (12-28 mg) per hour provide adequate analgesia with only slight and non-progressive motor block in most cases of moderate to severe postoperative pain. The maximum duration of epidural block is 3 days.

However, close monitoring of analgesic effect should be performed in order to remove the catheter as soon as the pain condition allows it.

With this technique a significant reduction in the need for opioids has been observed.

Concentrations above 7.5 mg/ml Naropin have not been documented for Caesarean section.

Naropin cannot be recommended for use in children below the age of 12 years as there is no data with regard to efficacy and safety in this group of patients.

4.3 Contraindications

Naropin solutions are contraindicated in patients with known hypersensitivity to anaesthetics of the amide type.

General contraindications related to epidural anaesthesia, regardless of the local anaesthetic used, should be taken into account.

Intravenous regional anaesthesia.

Obstetric paracervical anaesthesia.

Hypovolaemia.

4.4 Special warnings and special precautions for use

Regional anaesthetic procedures should always be performed in a properly equipped and staffed area. Equipment and drugs necessary for monitoring and emergency resuscitation should be immediately available. For emergency medication, patients receiving major blocks or high doses should have an intravenous line inserted before the blocking procedure. The clinician responsible should be appropriately trained and familiar with diagnosis and treatment of side effects, systemic toxicity and other complications such as inadvertent subarachnoid injection which may produce a high spinal block with apnoea and hypotension. Convulsions have occurred most often after brachial plexus block and epidural block. This is likely to be the result of either accidental intravascular injection or rapid absorption from the injection site.

Certain local anaesthetic procedures, such as injections in the head and neck regions, may be associated with a higher frequency of serious adverse reactions, regardless of the local anaesthetic used. Caution is required to prevent injections in inflamed areas.

Patients in poor general condition due to ageing or other compromising factors such as partial or complete heart conduction block, advanced liver disease or severe renal dysfunction require special attention, although regional anaesthesia is frequently indicated in these patients.

Ropivacaine is metabolised in the liver and should therefore be used with caution in patients with severe liver disease. Repeated doses may need to be reduced due to delayed elimination. Normally there is no need to modify the dose in patients with impaired renal function when used for single dose or short term treatment. Acidosis and reduced plasma protein concentration, frequently seen in patients with chronic renal failure, may increase the risk of systemic toxicity.

Patients with hypovolaemia due to any cause can develop sudden and severe hypotension during epidural anaesthesia, regardless of the local anaesthetic used.

Prolonged administration of ropivacaine should be avoided in patients concomitantly treated with strong CYP1A2 inhibitors, such as fluvoxamine and enoxacin, see 4.5.

A possible cross-hypersensitivity with other amide-type local anaesthetics should be taken into account.

Table 1

	Conc.	Volume	Dose	Onset	Duration
	mg/ml	ml	mg	minutes	hours
SURGICAL ANAESTHESIA					
Lumbar Epidural Administration					
Surgery	7.5	15-25	113-188	10-20	3-5
	10	15-20	150-200	10-20	4-6
Caesarean Section	7.5	15-20	113-150(1)	10-20	3-5
Thoracic Epidural Administration					
To establish block for post-operative pain relief	7.5	5-15 (depending on the level of injection)	38-113	10-20	n/a(2)
Major Nerve Block*					
Brachial plexus block	7.5	30-40	225-300	10-25	6-10
Field Block (e.g. minor nerve blocks and infiltration)	7.5	1-30	7.5-225	1-15	2-6
ACUTE PAIN MANAGEMENT					
Lumbar Epidural Administration					
Bolus	2	10-20	20-40	10-15	0.5-1.5
Intermittent injections (top up)	2	10-15	20-30		
(e.g. labour pain management)		(minimum interval 30 minutes)			
Continuous infusion e.g.					
Labour pain	2	6-10 ml/h	12-20 mg/h	n/a(2)	n/a(2)
Postoperative pain management	2	6-14 ml/h	12-28 mg/h	n/a(2)	n/a(2)
Thoracic Epidural Administration Continuous infusion (postoperative pain management)	2	6-14 ml/h	12-28 mg/h	n/a(2)	n/a(2)
Field Block					
(e.g. minor nerve blocks and infiltration)	2	1-100	2-200	1-5	2-6

The doses in the table are those considered to be necessary to produce a successful block and should be regarded as guidelines for use in adults. Individual variations in onset and duration occur. The figures in the column 'Dose' reflect the expected average dose range needed. Standard textbooks should be consulted for both factors affecting specific block techniques and individual patient requirements.

* With regard to major nerve block, only for brachial plexus block a dose recommendation can be given. For other major nerve blocks lower doses may be required. However, there is presently no experience of specific dose recommendations for other blocks.

(1) Incremental dosing should be applied, the starting dose of about 100 mg (97.5 mg = 13 ml; 105 mg = 14 ml) to be given over 3-5 minutes. Two additional doses, each of 25 mg, may be administered as needed. The total administered dose should not exceed 150 mg.

(2) n/a = not applicable

4.5 Interaction with other medicinal products and other forms of Interaction

Naropin should be used with caution in patients receiving other local anaesthetics or agents structurally related to amide-type local anaesthetics, e.g. certain antiarrhythmics, since the toxic effects are additive. Simultaneous use of Naropin with general anaesthetics or opioids may potentiate each others (adverse) effects.

Cytochrome P450 (CYP) 1A2 is involved in the formation of 3-hydroxy-ropivacaine, the major metabolite. *In vivo*, the plasma clearance of ropivacaine was reduced by 70% during coadministration of fluvoxamine, a selective and potent CYP1A2 inhibitor. Thus strong inhibitors of CYP1A2, such as fluvoxamine and enoxacin, given concomitantly during prolonged administration of Naropin, can interact with Naropin. Prolonged administration of ropivacaine should be avoided in patients concomitantly treated with strong CYP1A2 inhibitors, see also 4.4.

In vivo, the plasma clearance of ropivacaine was reduced by 15% during coadministration of ketoconazole, a selective and potent inhibitor of CYP3A4. However, the inhibition of this isozyme is not likely to have clinical relevance.

In vitro, ropivacaine is a competitive inhibitor of CYP2D6 but does not seem to inhibit this isozyme at clinically attained plasma concentrations.

4.6 Pregnancy and lactation

Pregnancy

Apart from obstetrical use, there are no adequate data on the use of ropivacaine in pregnancy. Animal studies do not indicate direct or indirect harmful effects with respect to pregnancy, embryonal/foetal development, parturition or postnatal development (see section 5.3).

Lactation

There is no data available concerning the excretion of ropivacaine into human milk.

4.7 Effects on ability to drive and use machines

No data is available. Depending on the dose, local anaesthetics may have a minor influence on mental function and co-ordination even in the absence of overt CNS toxicity and may temporarily impair locomotion and alertness.

4.8 Undesirable effects

General

The adverse reaction profile for Naropin is similar to those for other long acting local anaesthetics of the amide type. Adverse drug reactions should be distinguished from the physiological effects of the nerve block itself e.g. a decrease in blood pressure and bradycardia during spinal/epidural block.

The percentage of patients that can be expected to experience adverse reactions varies with the route of administration of Naropin. Systemic and localised adverse reactions of Naropin usually occur because of excessive dosage, rapid absorption, or inadvertent intravascular injection. The most frequently reported adverse reactions, nausea and hypotension, are very frequent during anaesthesia and surgery in general and it is not possible to distinguish those caused by the clinical situation from those caused by the drug or the block.

Table of adverse drug reactions

Within each system organ class, the ADRs have been ranked under the headings of frequency, most frequent reactions first.

Very common (>1/10)	*Vascular Disorders:* Hypotension
	Gastrointestinal Disorders: Nausea
Common (1/100)	*Nervous System Disorders:* Headache, Paraesthesia, Dizziness
	Cardiac Disorders: Bradycardia, Tachycardia
	Vascular Disorders: Hypertension
	Gastrointestinal Disorders: Vomiting
	Renal and Urinary Disorders: Urinary retention
	General Disorder and Administration Site Conditions: Temperature Elevation, Rigors
Uncommon (>1/1,000)	*Nervous system disorders:* Hypoaesthesia
Rare (>1/10,000)	*Psychiatric Disorders:* Anxiety
	Nervous System Disorders: Convulsions

Class-related adverse drug reactions

Allergic reactions

Allergic reactions (in the most severe instances anaphylactic shock) to local anaesthetics of the amide type are rare.

Neurological complications

Neuropathy and spinal cord dysfunction (e.g. anterior spinal artery syndrome, arachnoiditis, cauda equina), which may result in rare cases of permanent sequelae, have been associated with regional anaesthesia, regardless of the local anaesthetic used.

Acute systemic toxicity

Naropin may cause acute toxic effects following high doses or if very rapidly rising blood levels occur due to accidental intravascular injection or overdose. (See 4.9 "Overdose").

4.9 Overdose

Symptoms

Acute systemic toxicity

Accidental intravascular injections of local anaesthetics may cause immediate toxic effects. In the event of overdose, peak plasma concentrations may not be reached for one to two hours, depending on the site of the injection, and signs of toxicity may thus be delayed. Systemic toxic reactions may involve the central nervous system and the cardiovascular system.

Central nervous system

Central nervous system toxicity is a graded response with symptoms and signs of escalating severity. Initially symptoms such as visual or hearing disturbances, perioral numbness, dizziness, light-headedness, tingling and paraesthesia are seen. Dysarthria, muscular rigidity and muscular twitching are more serious and may precede the onset of generalised convulsions. These signs must not be mistaken for neurotic behaviour. Unconsciousness and grand mal convulsions may follow, which may last from a few seconds to several minutes. Hypoxia and hypercarbia occur rapidly during convulsions due to the increased muscular activity, together with the interference with respiration. In severe cases even apnoea may occur. The respiratory and metabolic acidosis increases and extends the toxic effects of local anaesthetics.

Recovery follows the redistribution of the local anaesthetic drug from the central nervous system and subsequent metabolism and excretion. Recovery may be rapid unless large amounts of the drug have been injected.

Cardiovascular toxicity

Cardiovascular toxicity indicates a more severe situation. Hypotension, bradycardia, arrhythmia and even cardiac arrest may occur as a result of high systemic concentrations of local anaesthetics. In volunteers the intravenous infusion of ropivacaine resulted in signs of depression of conductivity and contractility.

Cardiovascular toxicity effects are generally preceded by signs of toxicity in the central nervous system, unless the patient is receiving a general anaesthetic or is heavily sedated with drugs such as benzodiazepines or barbiturates.

Treatment of acute toxicity

Equipment and drugs necessary for monitoring and emergency resuscitation should be immediately available. If signs of acute systemic toxicity appear, injection of the local anaesthetic should be stopped immediately.

In the event of convulsions, treatment will be required. The objectives of treatment are to maintain oxygenation, stop the convulsions and support the circulation. Oxygen must be given and ventilation assisted, when necessary (mask and bag). An anticonvulsant should be given intravenously if the convulsions do not stop spontaneously in 15-20 seconds. Thiopentone sodium 1-3 mg/kg intravenously will abort the convulsions rapidly. Alternatively diazepam 0.1 mg/kg intravenously may be used, although its action is slower. Suxamethonium will stop the muscle convulsions rapidly, but the patient will require controlled ventilation and tracheal intubation.

If cardiovascular depression is evident (hypotension, bradycardia), ephedrine 5-10 mg intravenously should be given and repeated, if necessary, after 2-3 minutes.

Should circulatory arrest occur, immediate cardiopulmonary resuscitation should be instituted. Optimal oxygenation and ventilation and circulatory support as well as treatment of acidosis are of vital importance.

5. PHARMACOLOGICAL PROPERTIES

5.1 Pharmacodynamic properties

Pharmacotherapeutic group (ATC code): N01B B09

Ropivacaine is a long-acting amide-type local anaesthetic with both anaesthetic and analgesic effects. At high doses it produces surgical anaesthesia, while at lower doses it produces sensory block with limited and non-progressive motor block.

The mechanism is a reversible reduction of the membrane permeability of the nerve fibre to sodium ions. Consequently the depolarisation velocity is decreased and the excitable threshold increased, resulting in a local blockade of nerve impulses.

The most characteristic property of ropivacaine is the long duration of action. Onset and duration of the local anaesthetic efficacy are dependent upon the administration site and dose, but are not influenced by the presence of a vasoconstrictor (e.g. adrenaline). For details concerning the onset and duration of action, see table under "Posology and method of administration".

Healthy volunteers exposed to intravenous infusions tolerated ropivacaine well at low doses and with expected CNS symptoms at the maximum tolerated dose. The clinical experience with this drug indicates a good margin of safety when adequately used in recommended doses.

5.2 Pharmacokinetic properties

Ropivacaine has a chiral center and is available as the pure S-(-)-enantiomer. It is highly lipid-soluble. All metabolites have a local anaesthetic effect but of considerably lower potency and shorter duration than that of ropivacaine.

The plasma concentration of ropivacaine depends upon the dose, the route of administration and the vascularity of the injection site. Ropivacaine follows linear pharmacokinetics and the C_{max} is proportional to the dose.

Ropivacaine shows complete and biphasic absorption from the epidural space with half-lives of the two phases of the order of 14 min and 4 h in adults. The slow absorption is the rate -limiting factor in the elimination of ropivacaine, which explains why the apparent elimination half-life is longer after epidural than after intravenous administration.

Ropivacaine has a mean total plasma clearance in the order of 440 ml/min, a renal clearance of 1 ml/min, a volume of distribution at steady state of 47 litres and a terminal half-life of 1.8 h after iv administration. Ropivacaine has an intermediate hepatic extraction ratio of about 0.4. It is mainly bound to α_1- acid glycoprotein in plasma with an unbound fraction of about 6%.

An increase in total plasma concentrations during continuous epidural infusion has been observed, related to a postoperative increase of α_1- acid glycoprotein.

Variations in unbound, i.e. pharmacologically active, concentration have been much less than in total plasma concentration.

Ropivacaine readily crosses the placenta and equilibrium in regard to unbound concentration will be rapidly reached. The degree of plasma protein binding in the foetus is less than in the mother, which results in lower total plasma concentrations in the foetus than in the mother.

Ropivacaine is extensively metabolised, predominantly by aromatic hydroxylation. In total, 86% of the dose is excreted in the urine after intravenous administration, of which only about 1% relates to unchanged drug. The major metabolite is 3-hydroxy-ropivacaine, about 37% of which is excreted in the urine, mainly conjugated. Urinary excretion of 4-hydroxy-ropivacaine, the N-dealkylated metabolite and the 4-hydroxy-dealkylated accounts for 1-3%. Conjugated+unconjugated 3-hydroxy-ropivacaine shows only detectable concentrations in plasma.

There is no evidence of *in vivo* racemisation of ropivacaine.

5.3 Preclinical safety data

Based on conventional studies of safety pharmacology, single and repeated dose toxicity, reproduction toxicity, mutagenic potential and local toxicity, no hazards for humans were identified other than those which can be expected on the basis of the pharmacodynamic action of high doses of ropivacaine (e.g. CNS signs, including convulsions, and cardiotoxicity).

6. PHARMACEUTICAL PARTICULARS

6.1 List of excipients

Sodium chloride

Hydrochloric acid

Sodium hydroxide

Water for injection

6.2 Incompatibilities

In alkaline solutions precipitation may occur as ropivacaine shows poor solubility at pH > 6.0.

6.3 Shelf life

3 years.

6.4 Special precautions for storage

Do not store above 30°C. Do not freeze.

6.5 Nature and contents of container

10 ml polypropylene ampoules (Polyamp) in packs of 5 and 10

10 ml polypropylene ampoules (Polyamp) in sterile blister packs of 5 and 10

20 ml polypropylene ampoules (Polyamp) in packs of 5 and 10

20 ml polypropylene ampoules (Polyamp) in sterile blister packs of 5 and 10

The polypropylene ampoules (Polyamp) are specially designed to fit Luer lock and Luer fit syringes.

6.6 Instructions for use and handling

Naropin products are preservative free and are intended for single use only. Discard any unused solution.

The intact container must not be re-autoclaved. A blistered container should be chosen when a sterile outside is required.

7. MARKETING AUTHORISATION HOLDER

AstraZeneca UK Ltd.,

600 Capability Green,

Luton, LU1 3LU, UK

8. MARKETING AUTHORISATION NUMBER(S)

PL 17901/0152

9. DATE OF FIRST AUTHORISATION/RENEWAL OF THE AUTHORISATION

15th September 2000

10. DATE OF REVISION OF THE TEXT

22 March 2004

Trademarks herein are the property of the AstraZeneca group

Nasacort Nasal Spray

(sanofi-aventis)

1. NAME OF THE MEDICINAL PRODUCT

NASACORT 55 micrograms/dose, nasal spray, suspension.

2. QUALITATIVE AND QUANTITATIVE COMPOSITION

Triamcinolone acetonide

Bottles of NASACORT contain 16.5 g of suspension (with 9.075 mg triamcinolone acetonide). Each actuation delivers 55 micrograms triamcinolone acetonide.

For excipients, see 6.1.

3. PHARMACEUTICAL FORM

Nasal spray, suspension.

It is an unscented, thixotropic suspension of microcrystalline triamcinolone acetonide in an aqueous medium.

4. CLINICAL PARTICULARS

4.1 Therapeutic indications

NASACORT is indicated for the treatment of symptoms of seasonal and perennial allergic rhinitis.

4.2 Posology and method of administration

NASACORT is for nasal use only.

Patients aged 12 years and over:

The recommended starting dose is 220 micrograms as 2 sprays in each nostril once daily. Once symptoms are controlled patients can be maintained on 110 micrograms (1 spray in each nostril once daily).

Paediatric patients aged 6 to 12 years:

The recommended dose is 110 micrograms as 1 spray in each nostril once daily. In patients with more severe symptoms, a dose of 220 micrograms may be used. But once symptoms are controlled, patients should be maintained on the lowest effective dose.

Until further evidence is available, continuous use beyond 3 months in children under 12 years is not recommended.

4.3 Contraindications

Hypersensitivity to the active substance or to any of the excipients.

4.4 Special warnings and special precautions for use

If there is any reason to suppose that adrenal function is impaired, care must be taken while transferring patients from systemic steroid treatment to NASACORT.

In clinical studies with NASACORT administered intranasally, the development of localised infections of the nose and pharynx with *Candida albicans* has rarely occurred. When such an infection develops it may require treatment with appropriate local therapy and temporary discontinuance of treatment with NASACORT.

Because of the inhibitory effect of corticosteroids on wound healing in patients who have experienced recent nasal septal ulcers, nasal surgery or trauma, NASACORT should be used with caution until healing has occurred.

Systemic effects of nasal corticosteroids may occur, particularly at high doses prescribed for prolonged periods. Treatment with higher than recommended doses may result in clinically significant adrenal suppression. If there is evidence for higher than recommended doses being used then additional systemic corticosteroid cover should be considered during periods of stress or elective surgery.

As experience with NASACORT in children under 6 years of age is limited, use in this age group is not recommended.

Growth retardation has been reported in children receiving nasal corticosteroids at licensed doses.

It is recommended that the height of children receiving prolonged treatment with nasal corticosteroids is regularly monitored. If growth is slowed, therapy should be reviewed with the aim of reducing the dose of nasal corticosteroid, if possible, to the lowest dose at which effective control of symptoms is maintained. In addition, consideration should be given to referring the patient to a paediatric specialist.

4.5 Interaction with other medicinal products and other forms of Interaction

No interactions with other medicaments are known.

4.6 Pregnancy and lactation

Clinical experience in pregnant women is limited. In animal studies, corticosteroids have been shown to induce teratogenic effects. Triamcinolone acetonide may pass into human breast milk. Triamcinolone acetonide should not be administered during pregnancy or lactation unless the therapeutic benefit to the mother is considered to outweigh the potential risk to the foetus/baby.

4.7 Effects on ability to drive and use machines

NASACORT has no known effect on the ability to drive and operate machines.

4.8 Undesirable effects

The most commonly reported adverse reactions are rhinitis, headache and pharyngitis.

Respiratory disorders: epistaxis, nasal irritation, dry mucous membrane, naso-sinus congestion and sneezing; rarely, nasal septal perforations

In clinical trials, these adverse reactions with the exception of epistaxis, were reported at approximately the same or lower incidence as placebo treated patients.

Skin or subcutaneous disorders: rarely allergic reactions including rash, urticaria, pruritus and facial oedema.

Systemic effects of nasal corticosteroids may occur, particularly when prescribed at high doses for prolonged periods.

4.9 Overdose

Like any other nasally administered corticosteroid, acute overdosing with NASACORT is unlikely in view of the total amount of active ingredient present. In the event that the entire contents of the bottle were administered all at once, via either oral or nasal application, clinically significant systemic adverse events would most likely not result. The patient may experience some gastrointestinal upset if taken orally.

5. PHARMACOLOGICAL PROPERTIES

5.1 Pharmacodynamic properties

Pharmacotherapeutic group: nasal corticosteroid, ATC code: R 01 AD.

Triamcinolone acetonide is a more potent derivative of triamcinolone and is approximately 8 times more potent than prednisone. Although the precise mechanism of corticosteroid antiallergic action is unknown, corticosteroids are very effective in the treatment of allergic diseases in man.

NASACORT does not have an immediate effect on allergic signs and symptoms. An improvement in some patient symptoms may be seen within the first day of treatment with NASACORT and relief may be expected in 3 to 4 days. When NASACORT is prematurely discontinued symptoms may not recur for several days.

In clinical studies performed in adults and children at doses up to 440 mcg/day intranasally, no suppression of the Hypothalamic-Pituitary-Adrenal (HPA) axis has been observed.

5.2 Pharmacokinetic properties

Single dose intranasal administration of 220 micrograms of NASACORT in normal adult subjects and in adult patients with allergic rhinitis demonstrated low absorption of triamcinolone acetonide. The mean peak plasma concentration was approximately 0.5 ng/ml (range 0.1 to 1 ng/ml) and occurred at 1.5 hours post dose. The mean plasma drug concentration was less than 0.06 ng/ml at 12 hours and below the assay detection limit at 24 hours. The average terminal half life was 3.1 hours. Dose proportionality was demonstrated in normal subjects and in patients following a single intranasal dose of 110 micrograms or 220 micrograms NASACORT. Following multiple doses in paediatric patients, plasma drug concentrations, AUC, C_{max} and T_{max} were similar to those values observed in adult patients.

5.3 Preclinical safety data

In preclinical studies, only effects typical of glucocorticoids were observed.

Like other corticosteroids, triamcinolone acetonide (administered by inhalation or other routes) has been shown to be teratogenic in rats and rabbits, resulting in cleft palate and/or internal hydrocephaly and axial skeletal defects. Teratogenic effects, including CNS and cranial malformations, have also been observed in non-human primates.

No evidence of mutagenicity was detected in *in vitro* gene mutation tests.

Carcinogenicity assays in rodents show no increase in the incidence of individual tumour types.

6. PHARMACEUTICAL PARTICULARS

6.1 List of excipients

Microcrystalline cellulose and carmellose sodium (Avicel CL-611), polysorbate 80, purified water, glucose anhydrous, benzalkonium chloride and edetate disodium. Hydrochloric acid or sodium hydroxide (for adjustment of pH).

6.2 Incompatibilities

None known.

6.3 Shelf life

The shelf life of NASACORT is 2 years.

The shelf life after the bottle is first opened is 2 months.

6.4 Special precautions for storage

Do not store above 25°C.

6.5 Nature and contents of container

NASACORT is contained in a 20 ml high density polyethylene (HDPE) bottle fitted with a metered-dose spray pump unit. Bottles of NASACORT contain 16.5 g of suspension, providing 120 actuations.

6.6 Instructions for use and handling

It is important to shake the bottle gently before each use.

Each actuation delivers 55 micrograms triamcinolone acetonide from the nose piece to the patient (estimated from *in vitro* testing) after an initial priming of 5 sprays until a fine mist is achieved. NASACORT will remain adequately primed for 2 weeks. If the product is unused for more than 2 weeks, then it can be adequately reprimed with one spray. The nozzle should be pointed away from you while you are doing this.

After using the spray: Wipe the nozzle carefully with a clean tissue or handkerchief, and replace the dust-cap.

If the spray does not work and it may be blocked, clean it as follows. NEVER try to unblock it or enlarge the tiny spray hole with a pin or other sharp object because this will destroy the spray mechanism.

The nasal spray should be cleaned at least once a week or more often if it gets blocked.

TO CLEAN THE SPRAY

1. Remove the dust-cap and the spray nozzle only* (pull off).
2. Soak the dust-cap and spray nozzle in warm water for a few minutes, and then rinse under cold running tap water.
3. Shake or tap off the excess water and allow to air-dry.
4. Re-fit the spray nozzle.
5. Prime the unit as necessary until a fine mist is produced and use as normal.

* Part as indicated on diagram below,

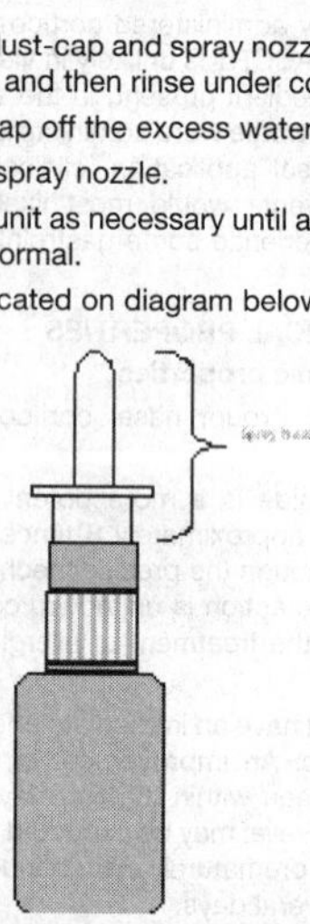

Also, the bottle should be discarded after 120 actuations or within 2 months of starting treatment. Do not transfer any remaining suspension to another bottle.

7. MARKETING AUTHORISATION HOLDER

Aventis Pharma Ltd
Aventis House
50 Kings Hill Avenue
Kings Hill
West Malling
Kent
ME19 4AH

8. MARKETING AUTHORISATION NUMBER(S)

PL 04425/0287

9. DATE OF FIRST AUTHORISATION/RENEWAL OF THE AUTHORISATION

26 September 2002

10. DATE OF REVISION OF THE TEXT

November 2002

11. Legal Category

POM

Naseptin Nasal Cream

(Alliance Pharmaceuticals)

1. NAME OF THE MEDICINAL PRODUCT

Naseptin Nasal Cream

2. QUALITATIVE AND QUANTITATIVE COMPOSITION

Chlorhexidine hydrochloride PhEur 0.1% w/w and neomycin sulphate PhEur 0.5% w/w.

3. PHARMACEUTICAL FORM

A smooth white cream with a fatty odour.

4. CLINICAL PARTICULARS

4.1 Therapeutic indications

Eradication of nasal infection with, and carriage of, Staphylococci.

4.2 Posology and method of administration

For nasal application only.

A small amount of Naseptin is placed on the little finger and applied to the inside of each nostril.

For prophylaxis: Naseptin is applied as above, twice daily, to prevent patients from becoming carriers and to inhibit the dispersion of Staphylococci.

For eradication of infection: Naseptin is applied four times daily for 10 days to eliminate organisms from the nares.

Children and elderly patients: There are no special dosage recommendations for either children or elderly patients.

4.3 Contraindications

Patients who have previously shown a hypersensitivity reaction to neomycin or chlorhexidine, although such reactions are extremely rare.

4.4 Special warnings and special precautions for use

For nasal application only. Keep out of the eyes and ears.

Naseptin contains Arachis oil (peanut oil) and should not be taken/applied by patients known to be allergic to peanut. As there is a possible relationship between allergy to peanut and allergy to Soya, patients with Soya allergy should also avoid Naseptin.

Irritative skin reactions can occasionally occur. Prolonged use of neomycin can lead to skin sensitisation, ototoxicity and nephrotoxicity.

4.5 Interaction with other medicinal products and other forms of Interaction

None known.

4.6 Pregnancy and lactation

Chlorhexidine and neomycin cannot be detected in the blood following application of Naseptin and its use is unlikely to have any effect on the foetus or on breast feeding.

4.7 Effects on ability to drive and use machines

None known.

4.8 Undesirable effects

Irritative skin reactions can occasionally occur.

Topical application of neomycin preparations can lead to skin sensitisation in a small number of patients. Prolonged use of neomycin can lead to ototoxicity and nephrotoxicity. Therefore, use with caution in children, elderly patients and patients with impaired hearing.

4.9 Overdose

Accidental ingestion of the contents of a Naseptin tube is unlikely to have any adverse effects on the patient.

5. PHARMACOLOGICAL PROPERTIES

5.1 Pharmacodynamic properties

Chlorhexidine is effective against a wide range of Gram negative and Gram positive vegetative bacteria, yeasts, dermatophyte fungi and lipophilic viruses. It is inactive against bacterial spores except at elevated temperatures.

Neomycin is a rapidly bactericidal aminoglycoside antibiotic effective against Gram positive organisms including staphylococci and a wide range of Gram negative organisms. Strains of *Pseudomonas aeruginosa* are resistant to neomycin, as are fungi and viruses.

5.2 Pharmacokinetic properties

Because of its cationic nature, chlorhexidine binds strongly to the skin, mucosa and other tissues and is thus very poorly absorbed. No detectable blood levels have been found in man following oral use and percutaneous absorption, if it occurs at all, is insignificant.

Neomycin is either not absorbed or is absorbed only minimally through intact skin. Any neomycin which is absorbed will be rapidly excreted by the kidneys in an unchanged state.

5.3 Preclinical safety data

There are no pre-clinical data of relevance to the prescriber which are additional to those already included in other sections of the Summary of Product Characteristics.

6. PHARMACEUTICAL PARTICULARS

6.1 List of excipients

Arachis oil, cetostearyl alcohol, cetostearyl alcohol/ethylene oxide condensate, purified water.

6.2 Incompatibilities

Hypochlorite bleaches may cause brown stains to develop in fabrics which have previously been in contact with preparations containing chlorhexidine.

Chlorhexidine is incompatible with soap and other anionic agents.

6.3 Shelf life

3 years.

6.4 Special precautions for storage

Store below 30°C.

6.5 Nature and contents of container

Collapsible, internally lacquered aluminium tubes of 15g with white food-grade polypropylene screw caps.

6.6 Instructions for use and handling

For nasal application only.

Administrative Data

7. MARKETING AUTHORISATION HOLDER

Alliance Pharmaceuticals Ltd
Avonbridge House
Bath Road
Chippenham
Wiltshire
SN15 2BB

8. MARKETING AUTHORISATION NUMBER(S)

PL16853/0024

9. DATE OF FIRST AUTHORISATION/RENEWAL OF THE AUTHORISATION

August 1999

10. DATE OF REVISION OF THE TEXT

March 2003

11. Legal Status

POM

Alliance, Alliance Pharmaceuticals and associated devices are registered Trademarks of Alliance Pharmaceuticals Ltd.

Nasonex 50 micrograms/actuation Nasal Spray, Suspension

(Schering-Plough Ltd)

1. NAME OF THE MEDICINAL PRODUCT

NASONEX 50 micrograms/actuation Nasal Spray, Suspension

2. QUALITATIVE AND QUANTITATIVE COMPOSITION

Mometasone furoate (as the monohydrate) 50 micrograms/actuation.

For excipients, see 6.1.

3. PHARMACEUTICAL FORM

Nasal Spray, Suspension.

White to off-white opaque suspension.

4. CLINICAL PARTICULARS

4.1 Therapeutic indications

NASONEX Nasal Spray is indicated for use in adults and children 12 years of age and older to treat the symptoms of seasonal allergic or perennial rhinitis.

NASONEX Nasal Spray is also indicated for use in children 6 to 11 years of age to treat the symptoms of seasonal allergic or perennial allergic rhinitis.

In patients who have a history of moderate to severe symptoms of seasonal allergic rhinitis, prophylactic treatment with NASONEX Nasal Spray may be initiated up to four weeks prior to the anticipated start of the pollen season.

NASONEX Nasal Spray is indicated for the treatment of nasal polyps in adults 18 years of age and older.

4.2 Posology and method of administration

After initial priming of the NASONEX Nasal Spray pump (usually 6 or 7 actuations, until a uniform spray is observed), each actuation delivers approximately 100 mg of mometasone furoate suspension, containing mometasone furoate monohydrate equivalent to 50 micrograms mometasone furoate. If the spray pump has not been used for 14 days or longer, it should be reprimed before next use.

Seasonal or Perennial Allergic Rhinitis

Adults (including geriatric patients) and children 12 years of age and older: The usual recommended dose is two actuations (50 micrograms/actuation) in each nostril once daily (total dose 200 micrograms). Once symptoms are controlled, dose reduction to one actuation in each nostril (total dose 100 micrograms) may be effective for maintenance.

If symptoms are inadequately controlled, the dose may be increased to a maximum daily dose of four actuations in each nostril once daily (total dose 400 micrograms). Dose reduction is recommended following control of symptoms.

Children between the ages of 6 and 11 years: The usual recommended dose is one actuation (50 micrograms/actuation) in each nostril once daily (total dose 100 micrograms).

NASONEX Nasal Spray demonstrated a clinically significant onset of action within 12 hours after the first dose in some patients with seasonal allergic rhinitis; however, full benefit of treatment may not be achieved in the first 48 hours. Therefore, the patient should continue regular use to achieve full therapeutic benefit.

Nasal Polyposis

The usual recommended starting dose for polyposis is two actuations (50 micrograms/actuation) in each nostril once daily (total daily dose of 200 micrograms). If after 5 to 6 weeks symptoms are inadequately controlled, the dose may be increased to a daily dose of two sprays in each nostril twice daily (total daily dose of 400 micrograms). The dose should be reduced following control of symptoms. If no improvement in symptoms is seen after 5 to 6 weeks of twice daily administration, alternative therapies should be considered.

Efficacy and Safety studies of NASONEX Nasal Spray for the treatment of nasal polyposis were four months in duration.

Prior to administration of the first dose shake container well, and actuate pump 6 or 7 times (until a uniform spray is obtained). If pump is not used for 14 days or longer, reprime the pump as before. Shake container well before each use. The bottle should be discarded after the labelled number of actuations or within 2 months of first use.

4.3 Contraindications

Hypersensitivity to any ingredients of NASONEX Nasal Spray.

NASONEX Nasal Spray should not be used in the presence of untreated localised infection involving the nasal mucosa.

Because of the inhibitory effect of corticosteroids on wound healing, patients who have experienced recent nasal surgery or trauma should not use a nasal corticosteroid until healing has occurred.

4.4 Special warnings and special precautions for use

NASONEX Nasal Spray should be used with caution, if at all, in patients with active or quiescent tuberculous infections of the respiratory tract, or in untreated fungal, bacterial, systemic viral infections or ocular herpes simplex.

Following 12 months of treatment with NASONEX Nasal Spray there was no evidence of atrophy of the nasal mucosa; also, mometasone furoate tended to reverse the nasal mucosa closer to a normal histologic phenotype. As with any long-term treatment, patients using NASONEX Nasal Spray over several months or longer should be examined periodically for possible changes in the nasal mucosa. If localised fungal infection of the nose or pharynx develops, discontinuance of NASONEX Nasal Spray therapy or appropriate treatment may be required. Persistence of nasopharyngeal irritation may be an indication for discontinuing NASONEX Nasal Spray.

Although NASONEX will control the nasal symptoms in most patients, the concomitant use of appropriate additional therapy may provide additional relief of other symptoms, particularly ocular symptoms.

There is no evidence of hypothalamic-pituitary-adrenal (HPA) axis suppression following prolonged treatment with NASONEX Nasal Spray. However, patients who are transferred from long-term administration of systemically active corticosteroids to NASONEX Nasal Spray require careful attention. Systemic corticosteroid withdrawal in such patients may result in adrenal insufficiency for a number of months until recovery of HPA axis function. If these patients exhibit signs and symptoms of adrenal insufficiency, systemic corticosteroid administration should be resumed and other modes of therapy and appropriate measures instituted.

During transfer from systemic corticosteroids to NASONEX Nasal Spray some patients may experience symptoms of withdrawal from systemically active corticosteroids (e.g., joint and/or muscular pain, lassitude, and depression initially) despite relief from nasal symptoms and will require encouragement to continue NASONEX Nasal Spray therapy. Such transfer may also unmask pre-existing allergic conditions, such as allergic conjunctivitis and eczema, previously suppressed by systemic corticosteroid therapy.

The safety and efficacy of Nasonex has not been studied for use in the treatment of unilateral polyps, polyps associated with cystic fibrosis, or polyps that completely obstruct the nasal cavities.

Unilateral polyps that are unusual or irregular in appearance, especially if ulcerating or bleeding, should be further evaluated.

Patients receiving corticosteroids who are potentially immunosuppressed should be warned of the risk of exposure to certain infections (e.g., chickenpox, measles) and of the importance of obtaining medical advice if such exposure occurs.

Following the use of intranasal corticosteroids, instances of nasal septum perforation or increased intraocular pressure have been reported very rarely.

Safety and efficacy of NASONEX Nasal Spray for the treatment of nasal polyposis in children and adolescents under 18 years of age have not been studied.

Systemic effects of nasal corticosteroids may occur, particularly at high doses prescribed for prolonged periods. Growth retardation has been reported in children receiving nasal corticosteroids at licensed doses.

It is recommended that the height of children receiving prolonged treatment with nasal corticosteroids is regularly monitored. If growth is slowed, therapy should be reviewed with the aim of reducing the dose of nasal corticosteroid if possible, to the lowest dose at which effective control of symptoms is maintained. In addition, consideration should be given to referring the patient to a paediatric specialist.

Treatment with higher than recommended doses may result in clinically significant adrenal suppression. If there is evidence for higher than recommended doses being used, then additional systemic corticosteroid cover should be considered during periods of stress or elective surgery

4.5 Interaction with other medicinal products and other forms of Interaction

(See 4.4 Special warnings and special precautions for use with systemic corticosteroids)

A clinical interaction study was conducted with loratadine. No interactions were observed.

4.6 Pregnancy and lactation

There are no adequate or well-controlled studies in pregnant women. Following intranasal administration of the maximal recommended clinical dose, mometasone plasma concentrations are not measurable; thus foetal exposure is expected to be negligible and the potential for reproductive toxicity, very low. As with other nasal corticosteroid preparations, NASONEX Nasal Spray should not be used in pregnancy or lactation unless the potential benefit to the mother justifies any potential risk to the mother, foetus or infant. Infants born of mothers who received corticosteroids during pregnancy should be observed carefully for hypoadrenalism.

4.7 Effects on ability to drive and use machines

None known.

4.8 Undesirable effects

Treatment-related adverse events reported in clinical studies for allergic rhinitis in adult and adolescent patients are shown below (Table 1).

Table 1: *Allergic Rhinitis* - Treatment Related Undesirable Effects for Nasonex Nasal Spray
very common > 1/10); common > 1/100, < 1/10); uncommon > 1/1000, < 1/100); rare > 1/10,000, < 1/1000); very rare (< 1/10,000)

Respiratory, thoracic and mediastinal disorders	
Common:	Epistaxis, pharyngitis, nasal burning, nasal irritation, nasal ulceration
General disorders and administration site conditions	
Common:	Headache

Epistaxis was generally self-limiting and mild in severity, and occurred at a higher incidence compared to placebo (5%), but at a comparable or lower incidence when compared to the active control nasal corticosteroids studied (up to 15%). The incidence of all other effects was comparable with that of placebo.

In the paediatric population, the incidence of adverse events, e.g., epistaxis (6%), headache (3%), nasal irritation (2%) and sneezing (2%) was comparable to placebo.

In patients treated for nasal polyposis, the overall incidence of adverse events was comparable to placebo and similar to that observed for patients with allergic rhinitis. Treatment-related adverse events reported in ⩾ 1% of patients in clinical studies for polyposis are shown below (Table 2)

Table 2: *Polyposis* - Treatment Related Undesirable Effects ⩾ 1% for Nasonex Nasal Spray
very common > 1/10); common > 1/100, < 1/10); uncommon > 1/1000, < 1/100); rare > 1/10,000, < 1/1000); very rare (< 1/10,000)

	(200 mcg once a day)	(200 mcg twice a day)
Respiratory, thoracic and mediastinal disorders		
Upper respiratory tract infection	common	uncommon
Epistaxis	common	very common
Gastrointestinal disorders		
Throat irritation	—	common
General disorders and administration site conditions		
Headache	common	common

Rarely, immediate hypersensitivity reactions, including bronchospasm and dyspnoea, may occur after intranasal administration of mometasone furoate monohydrate. Very rarely, anaphylaxis and angioedema have been reported.

Disturbances of taste and smell have been reported very rarely.

Systemic effects of nasal corticosteroids may occur, particularly when prescribed at high doses for prolonged periods.

4.9 Overdose

Because of the negligible (≤0.1%) systemic bioavailability of NASONEX, overdose is unlikely to require any therapy other than observation, followed by initiation of the appropriate prescribed dosage. Inhalation or oral administration of excessive doses of corticosteroids may lead to suppression of HPA axis function.

5. PHARMACOLOGICAL PROPERTIES

5.1 Pharmacodynamic properties

Pharmacotherapeutic group: Decongestants and Other Nasal Preparations for Topical Use-Corticosteroids, ATC code: R01A D09

Mometasone furoate is a topical glucocorticosteroid with local anti-inflammatory properties at doses that are not systemically active.

It is likely that much of the mechanism for the anti-allergic and anti-inflammatory effects of mometasone furoate lies in its ability to inhibit the release of mediators of allergic reactions. Mometasone furoate significantly inhibits the release of leukotrienes from leucocytes of allergic patients.

In cell culture, mometasone furoate demonstrated high potency in inhibition of synthesis and release of IL-1, IL-5, IL-6 and TNFα; it is also a potent inhibitor of leukotriene production. In addition, it is an extremely potent inhibitor of the production of the Th2 cytokines, IL-4 and IL-5, from human CD4+ T-cells.

In studies utilising nasal antigen challenge, NASONEX Nasal Spray has shown anti-inflammatory activity in both the early- and late- phase allergic responses. This has been demonstrated by decreases (vs placebo) in histamine and eosinophil activity and reductions (vs baseline) in eosinophils, neutrophils, and epithelial cell adhesion proteins.

In 28% of the patients with seasonal allergic rhinitis, NASONEX Nasal Spray demonstrated a clinically significant onset of action within 12 hours after the first dose. The median (50%) onset time of relief was 35.9 hours.

In a placebo-controlled clinical trial in which paediatric patients (n=49/group) were administered NASONEX 100 micrograms daily for one year, no reduction in growth velocity was observed.

There are limited data available on the safety and efficacy of NASONEX in the paediatric population aged 3 to 5 years, and an appropriate dosage range cannot be established. In a study involving 48 children aged 3 to 5 years treated with intranasal mometasone furoate 50, 100 or 200 μg/day for 14 days, there was no significant differences from placebo in the mean change in plasma cortisol level in response to the tetracosactrin stimulation test.

5.2 Pharmacokinetic properties

Mometasone furoate, administered as an aqueous nasal spray, has a negligible (≤0.1%) systemic bioavailability and is generally undetectable in plasma, despite the use of a sensitive assay with a lower quantitation limit of 50 pg/ml; thus, there are no relevant pharmacokinetic data for this dosage form. Mometasone furoate suspension is very poorly absorbed from the gastrointestinal tract, and the small amount that may be swallowed and absorbed undergoes extensive first-pass hepatic metabolism prior to excretion in urine and bile.

5.3 Preclinical safety data

No toxicological effects unique to mometasone furoate exposure were demonstrated. All observed effects are typical of this class of compounds and are related to exaggerated pharmacologic effects of glucocorticoids.

Preclinical studies demonstrate that mometasone furoate is devoid of androgenic, antiandrogenic, estrogenic or antiestrogenic activity but, like other glucocorticoids, it exhibits some antiuterotrophic activity and delays vaginal opening in animal models at high oral doses of 56 mg/kg/day and 280 mg/kg/day.

Like other glucocorticoids, mometasone furoate showed a clastogenic potential in-vitro at high concentrations. However, no mutagenic effects can be expected at therapeutically relevant doses.

In studies of reproductive function, subcutaneous mometasone furoate, at 15 micrograms/kg prolonged gestation and prolonged and difficult labour occurred with a reduction in offspring survival and body weight or body weight gain. There was no effect on fertility.

Like other glucocorticoids, mometasone furoate is a teratogen in rodents and rabbits. Effects noted were umbilical hernia in rats, cleft palate in mice and gallbladder agenesis, umbilical hernia, and flexed front paws in rabbits. There were also reductions in maternal body weight gains, effects on foetal growth (lower foetal body weight and/or delayed ossification) in rats, rabbits and mice, and reduced offspring survival in mice.

The carcinogenicity potential of inhaled mometasone furoate (aerosol with CFC propellant and surfactant) at concentrations of 0.25 to 2.0 micrograms/l was investigated in 24-month studies in mice and rats. Typical glucocorticoid-related effects, including several non-neoplastic lesions, were observed. No statistically significant dose-response relationship was detected for any of the tumour types.

6. PHARMACEUTICAL PARTICULARS

6.1 List of excipients

Dispersable cellulose BP 65 cps (microcrystalline cellulose and carmellose sodium), glycerol, sodium citrate dihydrate, citric acid monohy-drate, Polysorbate 80, benzalkonium chloride, phenylethyl alcohol, purified water

6.2 Incompatibilities

Not applicable

6.3 Shelf life

2 years

Use within 2 months of first use.

6.4 Special precautions for storage

Do not store above 30°C. Do not freeze.

6.5 Nature and contents of container

NASONEX Nasal Spray is contained in a white, high density polyethylene bottle, that contains 10 g (60 actuations) or 18 g (140 actuations) of product formulation, supplied with a metered-dose, manual polypropylene spray pump actuator. Each package contains one bottle.

6.6 Instructions for use and handling

No special requirements

7. MARKETING AUTHORISATION HOLDER

Schering-Plough Ltd

Shire Park

Welwyn Garden City

Hertfordshire AL7 1TW

UK

8. MARKETING AUTHORISATION NUMBER(S)

PL 0201/0216 (UK)

PA 277/77/1 (Ireland)

9. DATE OF FIRST AUTHORISATION/RENEWAL OF THE AUTHORISATION

10 April 1997 / 10 May 2002 (UK)

23 January 1998 / 10 May 2002 (Ireland)

10. DATE OF REVISION OF THE TEXT

24th November 2004

Legal Category

Prescription Only Medicine

Nasonex/11-04/9

Natrilix

(Servier Laboratories Limited)

1. NAME OF THE MEDICINAL PRODUCT

NATRILIX®

2. QUALITATIVE AND QUANTITATIVE COMPOSITION

Indapamide hemihydrate, 2.5 mg

3. PHARMACEUTICAL FORM

White, round, biconvex, film-coated tablets.

4. CLINICAL PARTICULARS

4.1 Therapeutic indications

For the treatment of essential hypertension. Natrilix® may be used as sole therapy or combined with other antihypertensive agents.

4.2 Posology and method of administration

Adults:

The dosage is one tablet, containing 2.5 mg indapamide hemihydrate, daily, to be taken in the morning. The action of Natrilix® is progressive and the reduction in blood pressure may continue and not reach a maximum until several months after the start of therapy. A larger dose than 2.5 mg Natrilix® daily is not recommended as there is no appreciable additional antihypertensive effect but a diuretic effect may become apparent. If a single daily tablet of Natrilix® does not achieve a sufficient reduction in blood pressure, another antihypertensive agent may be added; those which have been used in combination with Natrilix® include beta-blockers, ACE inhibitors, methyldopa, clonidine and other adrenergic blocking agents. The co-administration of Natrilix® with diuretics which may cause hypokalaemia is not recommended.

There is no evidence of rebound hypertension on withdrawal of Natrilix®.

Elderly:

There are no significant changes in the pharmacokinetics of indapamide in the elderly. Numerous clinical studies have shown that it can be used without problems, and, indeed has a particular benefit on systolic blood pressure in the elderly.

Children:

There is no experience of the use of this drug in children.

4.3 Contraindications

Natrilix® is not recommended in patients with:

- severe hepatic failure,
- a known history of allergy to sulphonamide derivatives.

4.4 Special warnings and special precautions for use

- Blood potassium and urate levels should be closely monitored in patients predisposed or sensitive to hypokalaemia (cardiac patients treated with glycosides, elderly, or patients suffering from hyperaldosteronism); and in patients suffering from gout.
- In case of an aggravation of pre-existing renal insufficiency, it is recommended to interrupt the treatment with Natrilix®.
- In patients with hyperparathyroidism, the treatment with Natrilix® should be interrupted on the occurrence of hypercalcaemia.
- Studies in functionally anephric patients for one month undergoing chronic haemodialysis, have not shown evidence of drug accumulation despite the fact that indapamide is not dialysable.
- Although indapamide 2.5 mg daily (one tablet) can be safely administered to hypertensive patients with impaired renal function, the treatment should be discontinued if there are signs of increasing renal insufficiency.
- As with all antihypertensive agents, care should be taken in patients in whom excessive hypotension could result in a myocardial infarction or cerebrovascular accident.

4.5 Interaction with other medicinal products and other forms of Interaction

The concomitant administration of the following medicaments with Natrilix is not recommended:

- Diuretics (risk of electrolyte imbalance)
- Antiarrhythmics such as quinidine derivatives, cardiac glycosides, corticoids or laxatives in case of hypokalaemia
- Lithium (increase in blood levels due to a diminished urinary excretion of lithium)

4.6 Pregnancy and lactation

Pregnancy: no teratological effects have been seen in animals but because animal reproduction studies are not always predictive of human response, Natrilix® should be used during pregnancy only if clearly needed.

Lactation: It is not known if Natrilix® is excreted in human milk.

Because most drugs are excreted in human milk, if use of Natrilix® is deemed essential, the patient should stop nursing.

4.7 Effects on ability to drive and use machines

There is no evidence of any adverse effect on mental alertness.

4.8 Undesirable effects

- Hypokalaemia, headache, dizziness, fatigue, muscular cramps, nausea, anorexia, diarrhoea, constipation, dyspepsia and cutaneous rash may occur as a result of treatment with Natrilix®.
- There have been some rare reports of orthostatic hypotension, palpitations, increase in liver enzymes, blood dyscrasias including thrombocytopenia, hyponatraemia, metabolic alkaloses, hyperglycaemia, increase in blood urate levels, paraesthesiae, erythema multiforme, epidermal necrolysis, photosensitivity, impotence, renal insufficiency and reversible acute myopia.
- At the dosage recommended for hypertension, indapamide does not usually adversely influence plasma triglycerides, LDL cholesterol or the LDL-HDL cholesterol ratio. Indapamide does not appear to adversely affect glucose tolerance when used in patients with diabetes and also in non diabetics.

4.9 Overdose

Symptoms of overdosage would be those associated with a diuretic effect: electrolyte disturbances, hypotension and muscular weakness.

Treatment would be symptomatic, directed at correcting the electrolyte abnormalities and gastric lavage or emesis should be considered.

5. PHARMACOLOGICAL PROPERTIES

5.1 Pharmacodynamic properties

Natrilix® (indapamide) is a non-thiazide sulphonamide with an indole ring, belonging to the diuretic family. At the dose of 2.5 mg per day Natrilix® exerts a prolonged antihypertensive activity in hypertensive human subjects.

Dose-effect studies have demonstrated that, at the dose of 2.5 mg per day, the antihypertensive effect is maximal and the diuretic effect is sub-clinical.

At this antihypertensive dose of 2.5 mg per day, Natrilix® reduces vascular hyperreactivity to noradrenaline in hypertensive patients and decreases total peripheral resistance and arteriolar resistance.

The implication of an extrarenal mechanism of action in the antihypertensive effect is demonstrated by maintenance of its antihypertensive efficacy in functionally anephric hypertensive patients.

The vascular mechanism of action of Natrilix® involves:

- a reduction in the contractility of vascular smooth muscle due to a modification of transmembrane ion exchanges, essentially calcium;
- vasodilatation due to stimulation of the synthesis of prostaglandin PGE_2 and the vasodilator and platelet anti-aggregant prostacyclin PGI_2;
- potentiation of the vasodilator action of bradykinin.

It has also been demonstrated that in the short-, medium- and long-term, in hypertensive patients, Natrilix®:

- reduces left ventricular hypertropy;
- does not appear to alter lipid metabolism: triglycerides, LDL-cholesterol and HDL-cholesterol;
- does not appear to alter glucose metabolism, even in diabetic hypertensive patients. Normalisation of blood pressure and a significant reduction in microalbuminuria have been observed after prolonged administration of Natrilix® in diabetic hypertensive subjects.

Lastly, the co-prescription of Natrilix® with other antihypertensives (beta-blockers, calcium channel blockers, angiotensin converting enzyme inhibitors) results in an improved control of hypertension with an increased percentage of responders compared to that observed with single-agent therapy.

5.2 Pharmacokinetic properties

Indapamide is rapidly and completely absorbed after oral administration. Peak blood levels are obtained after 1 to 2 hours.

Indapamide is concentrated in the erythrocytes and is 79% bound to plasma protein and to erythrocytes. It is taken up by the vascular wall in smooth vascular muscle according to its high lipid solubility. 70% of a single oral dose is eliminated by the kidneys and 23% by the gastrointestinal tract. Indapamide is metabolised to a marked degree with 7% of the unchanged product found in the urine during the 48 hours following administration. Elimination half-life (β phase) of indapamide is approximately 15 - 18 hours.

5.3 Preclinical safety data

No findings in the preclinical testing which could be of relevance for the prescriber.

6. PHARMACEUTICAL PARTICULARS

6.1 List of excipients

Lactose, maize starch, magnesium stearate, talc, povidone.

Tablet Coating: glycerol, white beeswax, sodium lauryl sulphate, methylhydroxypropylcellulose, polyoxyethylene glycol 6000, magnesium stearate, titanium dioxide.

6.2 Incompatibilities

None stated.

6.3 Shelf life

5 years.

6.4 Special precautions for storage

None.

6.5 Nature and contents of container

30 tablet pack: 1 blister strip (PVC / Aluminium) of 30 tablets in a carton.

60 tablet pack: 2 blister strips (PVC / Aluminium) of 30 tablets in a carton.

6.6 Instructions for use and handling

Not applicable.

7. MARKETING AUTHORISATION HOLDER

Servier Laboratories Ltd

Gallions, Wexham Springs

Framewood Road, Wexham

Slough

SL3 6RJ

8. MARKETING AUTHORISATION NUMBER(S)

PL 0093/0022

9. DATE OF FIRST AUTHORISATION/RENEWAL OF THE AUTHORISATION

20 December 1977

10. DATE OF REVISION OF THE TEXT

July 2005

Natrilix SR

(Servier Laboratories Limited)

1. NAME OF THE MEDICINAL PRODUCT

NATRILIX® SR, prolonged-release film-coated tablets.

2. QUALITATIVE AND QUANTITATIVE COMPOSITION

Indapamide, 1.5 mg per prolonged-release film-coated tablet.

For excipients, see 6.1.

3. PHARMACEUTICAL FORM

Prolonged-release tablet.

White, round, film-coated tablet.

4. CLINICAL PARTICULARS

4.1 Therapeutic indications

Essential hypertension.

4.2 Posology and method of administration

Oral administration.

One tablet per 24 hours, preferably in the morning, to be swallowed whole with water and not chewed.

At higher doses the antihypertensive action of indapamide is not enhanced but the saluretic effect is increased.

4.3 Contraindications

- Hypersensitivity to sulphonamides.

- Severe renal failure.

- Hepatic encephalopathy or severe impairment of liver function.

- Hypokalaemia.

4.4 Special warnings and special precautions for use

Special Warnings

When liver function is impaired, thiazide-related diuretics may cause hepatic encephalopathy. Administration of the diuretic must be stopped immediately if this occurs.

Special precautions for use

Water and electrolyte balance:

Plasma sodium:

This must be measured before starting treatment, then at regular intervals subsequently. Any diuretic treatment may cause hyponatraemia, sometimes with very serious consequences. The fall in plasma sodium may be asymptomatic initially and regular monitoring is therefore essential, and should be even more frequent in the elderly and cirrhotic patients (see Undesirable Effects and Overdose sections).

Plasma potassium:

Potassium depletion with hypokalaemia is the major risk of thiazide and related diuretics. The risk of onset of hypokalaemia (< 3.4 mmol/l) must be prevented in certain high risk populations, *i.e.* the elderly, malnourished and/or polymedicated, cirrhotic patients with oedema and ascites, coronary artery disease and cardiac failure patients. In this situation, hypokalaemia increases the cardiac toxicity of digitalis preparations and the risks of arrhythmias.

Individuals with a long QT interval are also at risk, whether the origin is congenital or iatrogenic. Hypokalaemia, as well as bradycardia, is then a predisposing factor to the onset of severe arrhythmias, in particular, potentially fatal *torsades de pointes*.

More frequent monitoring of plasma potassium is required in all the situations indicated above. The first measurement of plasma potassium should be obtained during the first week following the start of treatment.

Detection of hypokalaemia requires its correction.

Plasma calcium:

Thiazide and related diuretics may decrease urinary calcium excretion and cause a slight and transitory rise in plasma calcium. Frank hypercalcaemia may be due to previously unrecognised hyperparathyroidism. Treatment should be withdrawn before the investigation of parathyroid function.

Blood glucose:

Monitoring of blood glucose is important in diabetics, in particular in the presence of hypokalaemia.

Uric acid:

Tendency to gout attacks may be increased in hyperuricaemic patients.

Renal function and diuretics:

Thiazide and related diuretics are fully effective only when renal function is normal or only minimally impaired (plasma creatinine below levels of the order of 25 mg/l, *i.e.* 220 μmol/l in an adult). In the elderly, this plasma creatinine must be adjusted in relation to age, weight and gender.

Hypovolaemia, secondary to the loss of water and sodium induced by the diuretic at the start of treatment causes a reduction in glomerular filtration. This may lead to an increase in blood urea and plasma creatinine. This transitory functional renal insufficiency is of no consequence in individuals with normal renal function but may worsen preexisting renal insufficiency.

Athletes:

The attention of athletes is drawn to the fact that this drug contains an active ingredient which may give a positive reaction in doping tests.

4.5 Interaction with other medicinal products and other forms of Interaction

Combinations that are not recommended

Lithium:

Increased plasma lithium with signs of overdosage, as with a salt-free diet (decreased urinary lithium excretion). However, if the use of diuretics is necessary, careful monitoring of plasma lithium and dose adjustment are required.

Combinations requiring precautions for use

Torsades de pointes-inducing drugs:

– class Ia antiarrhythmics (quinidine, hydroquinidine, disopyramide),

– class III antiarrhythmics (amiodarone, sotalol, dofetilide, ibutilide),

– some antipsychotics: phenothiazines (chlorpromazine, cyamemazine, levomepromazine, thioridazine, trifluoperazine),

– benzamides (amisulpride, sulpiride, sultopride, tiapride),

– butyrophenones (droperidol, haloperidol);

– others: bepridil, cisapride, diphemanil, erythromycin IV, halofantrine, mizolastine, pentamidine, sparfloxacin, moxifloxacin, vincamine IV.

Increased risk of ventricular arrhythmias, particularly *torsades de pointes* (hypokalaemia is a risk factor). Monitor for hypokalaemia and correct, if required, before introducing this combination. Clinical, plasma electrolytes and ECG monitoring. *Use substances which do not have the disadvantage of causing torsades de pointes in the presence of hypokalaemia.*

N.S.A.I.Ds. (systemic route) including COX-2 selective inhibitors, high dose salicylic acid (≥ 3 g/day):

Possible reduction in the antihypertensive effect of indapamide. Risk of acute renal failure in dehydrated patients (decreased glomerular filtration). Hydrate the patient; monitor renal function at the start of treatment.

Angiotensin converting enzyme (A.C.E.) inhibitors:

Risk of sudden hypotension and/or acute renal failure when treatment with an A.C.E. inhibitor is initiated in the presence of preexisting sodium depletion (particularly in patients with renal artery stenosis).

In hypertension, when prior diuretic treatment may have caused sodium depletion, it is necessary:

– either to stop the diuretic 3 days before starting treatment with the A.C.E. inhibitor, and restart a hypokalaemic diuretic if necessary;

– or give low initial doses of the A.C.E. inhibitor and increase the dose gradually.

In congestive heart failure, start with a very low dose of A.C.E. inhibitor, possibly after a reduction in the dose of the concomitant hypokalaemic diuretic.

In all cases, monitor renal function (plasma creatinine) during the first weeks of treatment with an A.C.E. inhibitor.

Other compounds causing hypokalaemia: amphotericin B (IV), gluco- and mineralo-corticoids (systemic route), tetracosactide, stimulant laxatives:

Increased risk of hypokalaemia (additive effect). Monitoring of plasma potassium and correction if required. Must be particularly borne in mind in case of concomitant digitalis treatment. Use non-stimulant laxatives.

Baclofen:

Increased antihypertensive effect. Hydrate the patient; monitor renal function at the start of treatment.

Digitalis preparations:

Hypokalaemia predisposing to the toxic effects of digitalis. Monitoring of plasma potassium and ECG and, if necessary, adjust the treatment.

Combinations to be taken into consideration:

Potassium-sparing diuretics (amiloride, spironolactone, triamterene):

Whilst rational combinations are useful in some patients, hypokalaemia or hyperkalaemia (particularly in patients with renal failure or diabetes) may still occur. Plasma potassium and ECG should be monitored and, if necessary, treatment reviewed.

Metformin:

Increased risk of metformin induced lactic acidosis due to the possibility of functional renal failure associated with diuretics and more particularly with loop diuretics. Do not use metformin when plasma creatinine exceeds 15 mg/l (135 μmol/l) in men and 12 mg/l (110 μmol/l) in women.

Iodinated contrast media:

In the presence of dehydration caused by diuretics, increased risk of acute renal failure, in particular when large doses of iodinated contrast media are used. Rehydration before administration of the iodinated compound.

Imipramine-like antidepressants, neuroleptics:

Antihypertensive effect and increased risk of orthostatic hypotension increased (additive effect).

Calcium (salts):

Risk of hypercalcaemia resulting from decreased urinary elimination of calcium.

Cyclosporin, tacrolimus:

Risk of increased plasma creatinine without any change in circulating cyclosporin levels, even in the absence of water/sodium depletion.

Corticosteroids, tetracosactide (systemic route):

Decreased antihypertensive effect (water/sodium retention due to corticosteroids).

4.6 Pregnancy and lactation

Pregnancy

As a general rule, the administration of diuretics should be avoided in pregnant women and should never be used to treat physiological oedema of pregnancy. Diuretics can cause foetoplacental ischaemia, with a risk of impaired foetal growth.

Lactation

Breast-feeding is inadvisable (Indapamide is excreted in human milk).

4.7 Effects on ability to drive and use machines

Indapamide does not affect vigilance but different reactions in relation with the decrease in blood pressure may occur in individual cases, especially at the start of the treatment or when another antihypertensive agent is added. As a result the ability to drive vehicles or to operate machinery may be impaired.

4.8 Undesirable effects

The majority of adverse effects concerning clinical or laboratory parameters are dose-dependent. Thiazide-related diuretics, including indapamide, may cause:

Blood and the lymphatic system disorders:

Very rare: thrombocytopenia, leucopenia, agranulocytosis, aplastic anaemia, haemolytic anaemia

Nervous system disorders:

Rare: vertigo, fatigue, headache, paresthesia.

Cardiac disorders:

Very rare: arrhythmia, hypotension.

Gastrointestinal disorders:

Rare: nausea, constipation, dry mouth.

Very rare: pancreatitis.

Hepato-biliary disorders:

In case of hepatic insufficiency, there is a possibility of onset of hepatic encephalopathy (See Contra-indications and special warnings).

Very rare: abnormal hepatic function.

Skin and subcutaneous tissue disorders:

Hypersensitivity reactions, mainly dermatological (common: maculopapular rashes; uncommon: purpura) in subjects with a predisposition to allergic and asthmatic reactions

Possible worsening of pre-existing acute disseminated lupus erythematosus

Laboratory parameters:

During clinical trials, hypokalaemia (plasma potassium <3.4 mmol/l) was seen in 10 % of patients and < 3.2 mmol/l in 4 % of patients after 4 to 6 weeks treatment. After 12 weeks treatment, the mean fall in plasma potassium was 0.23 mmol/l.

Potassium depletion with hypokalaemia, particularly serious in certain high risk populations (see Special Warnings and Special Precautions for Use).

Hyponatraemia with hypovolaemia responsible for dehydration and orthostatic hypotension. Concomitant loss of chloride ions may lead to secondary compensatory metabolic alkalosis: the incidence and degree of this effect are slight.

Increase in plasma uric acid and blood glucose during treatment: appropriateness of these diuretics must be very carefully weighed in patients with gout or diabetes.

Very rare: Hypercalcaemia.

4.9 Overdose

Indapamide has been found free of toxicity at up to 40 mg, *i.e.* 27 times the therapeutic dose. Signs of acute poisoning take the form above all of water/electrolyte disturbances (hyponatraemia, hypokalaemia). Clinically, possibility of nausea, vomiting, hypotension, cramps, vertigo, drowsiness, confusion, polyuria or oliguria possibly to the point of anuria (by hypovolaemia). Initial measures involve the rapid elimination of the ingested substance(s) by gastric wash-out and/or administration of activated charcoal, followed by restoration of water/electrolyte balance to normal in a specialised centre.

5. PHARMACOLOGICAL PROPERTIES

5.1 Pharmacodynamic properties

ANTIHYPERTENSIVE DIURETICS

ATC code: C 03 BA 11

Indapamide is a sulphonamide derivative with an indole ring, pharmacologically related to thiazide diuretics, which acts by inhibiting the reabsorption of sodium in the cortical dilution segment. It increases the urinary excretion of sodium and chlorides and, to a lesser extent, the excretion of potassium and magnesium, thereby increasing urine output and having an antihypertensive action.

Phase II and III studies using monotherapy have demonstrated an antihypertensive effect lasting 24 hours. This was present at doses where the diuretic effect was of mild intensity.

The antihypertensive activity of indapamide is related to an improvement in arterial compliance and a reduction in arteriolar and total peripheral resistance.

Indapamide reduces left ventricular hypertrophy.

Thiazide and related diuretics have a plateau therapeutic effect beyond a certain dose, while adverse effects continue to increase. The dose should not be increased if treatment is ineffective.

It has also been shown, in the short-, mid- and long-term in hypertensive patients, that indapamide:

- does not interfere with lipid metabolism: triglycerides, LDL-cholesterol and HDL-cholesterol;

- does not interfere with carbohydrate metabolism, even in diabetic hypertensive patients.

5.2 Pharmacokinetic properties

Indapamide 1.5 mg is supplied in a prolonged release dosage based on a matrix system in which the active ingredient is dispersed within a support which allows sustained release of indapamide.

Absorption

The fraction of indapamide released is rapidly and totally absorbed via the gastrointestinal digestive tract. Eating slightly increases the rapidity of absorption but has no influence on the amount of the drug absorbed. Peak serum level following a single dose occurs about 12 hours after ingestion, repeated administration reduces the variation in serum levels between 2 doses. Intra-individual variability exists.

Distribution

Binding of indapamide to plasma proteins is 79%. The plasma elimination half-life is 14 to 24 hours (mean 18 hours). Steady state is achieved after 7 days. Repeated administration does not lead to accumulation.

Metabolism

Elimination is essentially urinary (70% of the dose) and faecal (22%) in the form of inactive metabolites.

High risk individuals

Pharmacokinetic parameters are unchanged in renal failure patients.

5.3 Preclinical safety data

The highest doses administered orally to different animal species (40 to 8000 times the therapeutic dose) have shown an exacerbation of the diuretic properties of indapamide. The major symptoms of poisoning during acute toxicity studies with indapamide administered intravenously or intraperitoneally were related to the pharmacological action of indapamide, *i.e.* bradypnoea and peripheral vasodilation. Indapamide has been tested negative concerning mutagenic and carcinogenic properties.

6. PHARMACEUTICAL PARTICULARS

6.1 List of excipients

Tablet: silica, colloidal anhydrous; hypromellose, lactose monohydrate, magnesium stearate, povidone.

Film-coating: glycerol, hypromellose, macrogol 6000, magnesium stearate, titanium dioxide.

6.2 Incompatibilities

Not applicable.

6.3 Shelf life

2 years.

6.4 Special precautions for storage

No special precautions for storage.

6.5 Nature and contents of container

10, 14, 15, 20, 30, 50, 60, 90, 100 tablets in blisters (PVC/aluminium). Not all pack sizes may be marketed.

6.6 Instructions for use and handling

No special requirements.

7. MARKETING AUTHORISATION HOLDER

LES LABORATOIRES SERVIER, 22 rue Garnier, 9200 Neuilly-sur-Seine, France

8. MARKETING AUTHORISATION NUMBER(S)

PL 05815/0010

9. DATE OF FIRST AUTHORISATION/RENEWAL OF THE AUTHORISATION

25th February 2001

10. DATE OF REVISION OF THE TEXT

March 2003

Navelbine

(Pierre Fabre Limited)

1. NAME OF THE MEDICINAL PRODUCT

NAVELBINE® 10mg/ml

Concentrate for solution for infusion

2. QUALITATIVE AND QUANTITATIVE COMPOSITION

(see Table 1 below)

3. PHARMACEUTICAL FORM

Concentrate for solution for infusion

4. CLINICAL PARTICULARS

4.1 Therapeutic indications

• As a single agent or in combination for the first line treatment of stage 3 or 4 non small cell lung cancer.

• Treatment of advanced breast cancer stage 3 and 4 relapsing after or refractory to an anthracycline containing regimen.

4.2 Posology and method of administration

Strictly by intravenous injection through an infusion line.

The use of intrathecal route is contra-indicated.

In adults:

• NAVELBINE® is usually given at 25-30mg/m^2 weekly.

• NAVELBINE® may be administered by slow bolus (5-10 minutes) after dilution in 20-50 ml of normal saline solution or by a short infusion (20-30 minutes) after dilution in 125 ml of normal saline solution. Administration should always be followed by a normal saline infusion to flush the vein.

Dose modifications:

Vinorelbine metabolism and clearance are mostly hepatic: only 18.5% is excreted unchanged in the urine. No prospective study relating altered metabolism of the drug to its pharmacodynamic effects is available in order to establish guidelines for Vinorelbine dose reduction in patients with impaired liver or kidney function.

However, in breast cancer patients, Vinorelbine clearance is not altered in presence of moderate liver metastases (i.e. ≤75% of liver volume replaced by the tumour). In these patients, there is no pharmacokinetic rationale for reducing Vinorelbine doses.

In patients with massive liver metastases (i.e. >75% of liver volume replaced by the tumour), it is empirically suggested that the dose be reduced by 1/3 and the haematological toxicity closely followed-up.

There is no pharmacokinetic rationale for reducing Vinorelbine dose in patients with impaired kidney function.

The dose limiting toxicity of Vinorelbine is mainly neutropenia. This usually occurs between day 8 and day 12 after drug administration, is short-lived, and is not cumulative. If the neutrophil count is <2000/mm^3 and/or platelet number is <75000/mm^3, then the treatment should be delayed until recovery. Drug administration is expected to be delayed by 1 week in about 35% of treatment courses.

The maximum tolerated dose per administration: 35.4mg/m^2

The maximum total dose per administration: 60 mg

4.3 Contraindications

• Pregnancy

• Lactation

• Severe hepatic insufficiency not related to the tumoural process.

4.4 Special warnings and special precautions for use

• NAVELBINE® must only be administered by the intravenous route. **The use of intrathecal route is contra-indicated.** Administration should always be followed by a normal saline infusion to flush the vein.

• Treatment should be undertaken with close haematological monitoring (determination of hemoglobin level and number of leucocytes, granulocytes and platelets before each new injection); if the neutrophil count is <2000/mm^3, treatment should be delayed until recovery and the patient should be observed.

• If the patient presents signs or symptoms suggestive of infection, a prompt investigation should be carried out.

• If there is significant hepatic impairment the dose should be reduced.

• In case of renal impairment, because of the low level of renal excretion, no dose modification is necessary.

• NAVELBINE® should not be given concomitantly with radiotherapy if the treatment field includes the liver.

• All contact with the eye should be strictly avoided: risk of severe irritation and even corneal ulceration if the drug is sprayed under pressure. Immediate liberal washing of the eye with normal saline solution should be undertaken if any contact occurs.

4.5 Interaction with other medicinal products and other forms of Interaction

The combination Vinorelbine-Cisplatin shows no interaction on the pharmacokinetic parameters.

4.6 Pregnancy and lactation

In animal reproductive studies NAVELBINE® was embryo- and feto-lethal and teratogenic.

Women should not become pregnant during treatment with NAVELBINE®.

This product should not be used during pregnancy.

If pregnancy should occur during the treatment, the possibility of genetic counselling should be used.

It is not known whether NAVELBINE® passes into the breast milk. Lactation must therefore be discontinued before treatment with this medicine.

4.7 Effects on ability to drive and use machines

Not applicable.

4.8 Undesirable effects

Haematological tolerance

• The limiting toxicity is neutropenia (G1: 9.7%; G2: 15.2%; G3: 24.3%; G4: 27.8%) which is rapidly reversible (5 to 7 days) and non-cumulative; it is maximal between 5 and 7 days after administration. Further treatment may be given after recovery of the granulocyte count.

• Anaemia (G1-2: 61.2%; G3-4: 7.4%) and thrombocytopenia (G1-2: 5.1%; G3-4: 2.5%) are seldom severe.

Neurological tolerance

• Peripheral

This is generally limited to loss of deep tendon reflexes; severe paraesthesiae are uncommon (G1: 17.2%; G2: 3.6%; G3: 2.6%; G4: 0.1%). The effects are dose dependent but reversible when treatment is discontinued.

• Autonomic neuropathy

The main symptom is intestinal paresis causing constipation (G1: 16.9%; G2: 4.9%) which rarely progresses to paralytic ileus (G3: 2%; G4: 0.7%). Treatment may be resumed after recovery of normal bowel mobility.

Gastrointestinal tolerance

• Constipation (see autonomic neuropathy)

• Diarrhoea (G1: 7.6%; G2: 3.6%; G3: 0.7%; G4: 0.1%): severe diarrhoea is uncommon.

• Nausea-vomiting (G1: 19.9%; G2: 8.3%; G3: 1.9%; G4: 0.3%): severe nausea and vomiting may occasionally occur. Conventional anti-emetic therapy reduces these undesirable effects.

Allergic reactions

As with other vinca alkaloids, NAVELBINE® may occasionally produce dyspnoea and bronchospasm and more rarely local or generalised cutaneous reactions.

Venous tolerance

Burning pain at the injection site and local phlebitis (G1: 12.3%; G2: 8.2%; G3: 3.6%; G4: 0.1%) may be observed with repeated injections of NAVELBINE®.

Bolus injection followed by liberal flushing of the vein can limit this effect. Insertion of a central venous line may be necessary.

Other undesirable effects

• Alopecia is mild and may appear progressively with extended courses of treatment (G1-2: 21%; G3-4: 4.1%)

• Jaw pain has occasionally been reported.

• Any extravasation may induce local reactions which rarely progress to necrosis (see 4.2. posology and method of administration).

4.9 Overdose

• Studies of acute toxicity in animals:

The symptoms of overdose are pilo erection, behaviour abnormalities (lethargy, prostration), pulmonary lesions,

Table 1

ACTIVE INGREDIENT	FORMULATION		
	10 mg / 1 ml	40 mg / 4 ml	50 mg / 5 ml
vinorelbine tartrate (mg)	13.85	55.40	69.25
equivalent to vinorelbine (INN) base (mg)	10.00	40.00	50.00

Table 2

EXCIPIENTS	FORMULATION		
	10 mg / 1 ml	40 mg / 4 ml	50 mg / 5 ml
Water for injections (ml) qs	1.00	4.00	5.00
nitrogen qs	inert filling	inert filling	inert filling

weight loss and bone marrow hypoplasia more or less severe in animals sacrificed during the course of the study.

• Accidental overdosages have been reported in humans: they may produce a period of bone marrow aplasia sometimes associated with fever, infection and possibly paralytic ileus. Management of the infectious complications is by broad-spectrum antibiotic therapy and the paralytic ileus is managed by naso-gastric aspiration.

5. PHARMACOLOGICAL PROPERTIES

5.1 Pharmacodynamic properties

NAVELBINE® is a cytostatic antineoplastic drug of the vinca alkaloid family with a molecular action on the dynamic equilibrium of tubulin in the microtubular apparatus of the cell. It inhibits tubulin polymerisation and binds preferentially to mitotic microtubules, only affecting axonal microtubules at high concentration. The induction of tubulin spiralization is less than that produced by vincristine. NAVELBINE® blocks mitosis at G2-M, causing cell death in interphase or at the following mitosis.

5.2 Pharmacokinetic properties

After intravenous administration of NAVELBINE® 30mg/m^2 in patients, the plasma concentration of the active ingredient is characterised by a three exponential elimination curve. The end-elimination phase reflects a long half-life greater than 40 hours. Total clearance of vinorelbine is high (1.3 l/h/kg) with excretion occurring mainly by the biliary route; renal excretion is minimal (18.5% of label is recovered in urine).

The active ingredient is widely distributed in the body with a volume of distribution greater than 40 l/kg. There is moderate binding to plasma proteins (13.5%), but strong binding to platelets (78%). Penetration of vinorelbine into pulmonary tissue is significant with tissue/plasma concentration ratios of greater than 300 in a study involving surgical biopsy.

Small concentrations of deacetyl vinorelbine have been recovered in humans, but vinorelbine is principally detected as the parent compound in urine.

5.3 Preclinical safety data

• Mutagenic and carcinogenic potential

The interaction of NAVELBINE® with the spindle apparatus during mitosis can cause an incorrect distribution of chromosomes. In animal studies NAVELBINE® induced aneuploidy and polyploidy. It is therefore to be assumed that NAVELBINE® can also cause mutagenic effects (induction of aneuploidy) in man.

The carcinogenicity studies, in which NAVELBINE® was administered only once every two weeks in order to avoid the toxic effects of the drug, are negative.

• Reproductive toxicity

In animal reproductive studies NAVELBINE® was embryo- and feto-lethal and teratogenic.

The NOEL in the rat was 0.26 mg/kg every 3 days.

Following peri/postnatal administration in the rat at doses of 1.0 mg/kg every 3 days i.v., retarded weight gain was found in the offspring up to the 7th week of life.

• Safety pharmacology

Bibliographic review concerning the tolerance of vinca alkaloids on the cardiovascular system shows the occurrence of some cardiac events (such as angina, myocardial infarction), but the incidence of these is low.

Haemodynamic and electrocardiographic studies on animals have been carried out by Pierre Fabre Médicament Laboratories; no haemodynamic effects have been found using a maximal tolerated dose in dogs, however only some non significant disturbances of repolarization were found for all vinca alkaloids tested. No effect on the cardiovascular system has been detected using repeated doses (study 39 weeks) of NAVELBINE® on primates.

6. PHARMACEUTICAL PARTICULARS

6.1 List of excipients

(see Table 2 above)

6.2 Incompatibilities

• NAVELBINE® solution (10mg/ml) may be diluted in a solution for infusion of normal saline or 5% dextrose.

• The volume of dilution depends on the mode of administration:

Bolus = 20-50 ml

Infusion = 125 ml

• NAVELBINE® should not be diluted in alkaline solutions (risk of precipitate)

• In case of polychemotherapy, NAVELBINE® should not be mixed with other agents.

• NAVELBINE® is not absorbed to or affected by either PVC or clear neutral glass.

6.3 Shelf life

• The product is stable for 3 years.

• After diluting NAVELBINE® in normal saline solution or dextrose solution, the product should be used either immediately or it can be stored in the clear glass vials or in the PVC perfusion bags during 24 hours in a refrigerator (+2°C to +8°C).

6.4 Special precautions for storage

Store at 2°C - 8°C (in a refrigerator). Store in the original container in order to protect from light.

6.5 Nature and contents of container

The drug is distributed in glass vials (type I) of appropriated volume closed by a butyl or chlorobutyl stopper. The stopper is covered with a crimped-on aluminium cap equipped with a polypropylene seal. Vials of 1, 4 and 5 ml.

6.6 Instructions for use and handling

NAVELBINE® has a more or less yellow colouration which does not affect the quality of the product.

Handling guidelines: the preparation and administration of NAVELBINE® should be carried out only by trained staff and as with all cytotoxic agents, precautions should be taken to avoid exposing staff during pregnancy.

Preparation of solution for administration should be carried out in a designated handling area and working over a washable tray or disposable plastic-backed absorbent paper.

Suitable eye protection, disposable gloves, face mask and disposable apron should be worn.

Syringes and infusion sets should be assembled carefully to avoid leakage (use of Luer lock fittings is recommended).

Eventual spillage or leakage should be mopped up wearing protective gloves.

All contact with the eye should be strictly avoided: risk of severe irritation and even corneal ulceration if the drug is sprayed under pressure. Immediate liberal washing of the eye with normal saline solution should be undertaken if any contact occurs.

On completion, any exposed surface should be thoroughly cleaned and hands and face washed.

NAVELBINE® may be administered by slow bolus (5-10 minutes) after dilution in 20-50 ml of normal saline solution or by a short infusion (20-30 minutes) after dilution in 125 ml of normal saline solution. Administration should always be followed by a normal saline infusion to flush the vein.

NAVELBINE® must be given strictly intravenously: it is very important to make sure that the cannula is accurately placed in the vein before starting to infuse NAVELBINE®.

If the drug extravasates during intravenous administration, a substantial local reaction may occur. In this case, the injection should be stopped and the rest of the dose should be administered in another vein.

Disposal guidelines: all sharps should be placed in an appropriate container and all other disposable items and cleaning materials in a sealed plastic bag which should be incinerated with other clinical waste.

Waste material may be disposed of by incineration.

7. MARKETING AUTHORISATION HOLDER

PIERRE FABRE LIMITED Hyde Abbey House, 23 Hyde Street, Winchester, Hants SO23 7DR

UNITED KINGDOM Tel 01962 856956

8. MARKETING AUTHORISATION NUMBER(S)

PL 00603 / 0028

9. DATE OF FIRST AUTHORISATION/RENEWAL OF THE AUTHORISATION

10 May 1996

10. DATE OF REVISION OF THE TEXT

July 2001

Navelbine 20mg soft capsule

(Pierre Fabre Limited)

1. NAME OF THE MEDICINAL PRODUCT

NAVELBINE 20 mg soft capsule▼

2. QUALITATIVE AND QUANTITATIVE COMPOSITION

20 mg vinorelbine (as tartrate)

For excipients, see 6.1.

3. PHARMACEUTICAL FORM

Soft capsule

Light brown soft capsule printed N20

4. CLINICAL PARTICULARS

4.1 Therapeutic indications

As a single agent or in combination for the first line treatment of stage 3 or 4 non small cell lung cancer.

4.2 Posology and method of administration

For oral use only.

Navelbine® soft capsules should be swallowed with water without chewing or sucking the capsule. It is recommended to take the capsule with some food.

As a single agent, the recommended regimen is:

First three administrations

60mg/m^2 of body surface area, administered once weekly.

Subsequent administrations

Beyond the third administration, it is recommended to increase the dose of Navelbine® soft capsules to 80mg/m^2 once weekly **except** in those patients for whom the neutrophil count dropped once below 500/mm^3, or more than once between 500 and 1000/mm^3 during the first three administrations at 60mg/m^2.

(see Table 1 on next page)

For any administration planned to be given at 80mg/m^2, if the neutrophil count is below 500/mm^3 or more than once between 500 and 1000 / mm^3, the administration should be delayed until recovery and the dose reduced from 80 to 60mg/m^2 per week during the 3 following administrations.

(see Table 2 on next page)

It is possible to reescalate the dose from 60 to 80 mg/m^2 per week if the neutrophil count did not drop below 500/mm^3, or more than once between 500 and 1000/mm^3 during 3 administrations given at 60 mg/m^2 according to the rules previously defined for the first 3 administrations.

If the neutrophil count is below 1500 /mm^3 and/or the platelet count is between 75000 and 100000/mm^3, then the treatment should be delayed until recovery.

Based on clinical studies, the oral dose of 80 mg/m^2 was demonstrated to correspond to 30 mg/m^2 of the iv form and 60 mg/m^2 to 25 mg/m^2.

This has been the base for combination regimens alternating iv and oral forms improving patient's convenience.

For combination regimens, the dose and schedule will be adapted to the treatment protocol.

Capsules of different strengths (20, 30, 40, 80 mg) are available in order to choose the adequate combination for the right dosage.

The following table gives the dose required for appropriate ranges of body surface area (BSA).

	60 mg/m^2	80 mg/m^2
BSA (m^2)	Dose (mg)	Dose (mg)
0.95 to 1.	60	80
1.05 to 1.14	70	90
1.15 to 1.24	70	100
1.25 to 1.34	80	100
1.35 to 1.44	80	110
1.45 to 1.54	90	120
1.55 to 1.64	100	130
1.65 to 1.74	100	140
1.75 to 1.84	110	140
1.85 to 1.94	110	150
⩾ 1.95	120	160

Even for patients with BSA ⩾ 2 m^2 the total dose should never exceed 160 mg per week.

Clinical experience has not identified relevant differences in responses in the elderly or younger patients but greater sensitivity of some older individuals cannot be ruled out.

Safety and effectiveness in children have not been established.

Dosage adjustment in specific patient groups: refer to section 4.4.: Special warnings and special precautions for use.

Instruction for use / handling: refer to section 6.6

4.3 Contraindications

• Patients with current or recent (within 2 weeks) history of infection

• Patients requiring long-term oxygen therapy

• Known hypersensitivity to vinorelbine or other vinca alkaloids

• Disease significantly affecting absorption

• Previous significant surgical resection of stomach or small bowel

• Neutrophil count < 1500/mm^3 or severe infection due to neutropenia

• Severe hepatic insufficiency not related to the tumoural process

• Pregnancy

• Lactation.

Table 1

Neutrophil count during the first 3 administrations of 60 mg/m²/week	Neutrophils > 1000	Neutrophils ⩾ 500 and < 1000 (1 episode)	Neutrophils ⩾ 500 and < 1000 (2 episodes)	Neutrophils < 500
Recommended dose starting with the 4th administration	80	80	60	60

Table 2

Neutrophil count beyond the 4th administration of 80 mg/m²/week	Neutrophils > 1000	Neutrophils ⩾ 500 and < 1000 (1 episode)	Neutrophils ⩾ 500 and < 1000 (2 episodes)	Neutrophils < 500
Recommended dose for the next administration	80	60		

4.4 Special warnings and special precautions for use

It is recommended that Navelbine® soft capsules be given under the supervision of a qualified doctor who is experienced in the use of chemotherapy.

If the patient chews or sucks the capsule by error, proceed to mouth rinses with water or preferably a normal saline solution.

In the event of the capsule has being cut or damaged, the liquid content is an irritant, and so may cause damage if in contact with skin, mucosa or eyes. Damaged capsules should not be swallowed and should be returned to the pharmacy or to the doctor in order to be properly destroyed. If any contact occurs, immediate thorough washing with water or preferably with normal saline solution should be undertaken.

In the case of vomiting within a few hours after drug intake, never repeat the administration of this dose. Supportive treatment (such as metoclopramide) may reduce the occurrence of this.

Dosing should be determined by haematological status.

Close haematological monitoring should be undertaken during treatment (determination of haemoglobin level and the leucocyte, neutrophil and platelet counts on the day of each new administration).

During clinical trials where treatments were initiated at 80 mg/m², a few patients developed excessive neutropenia complications. Therefore it is recommended that the starting dose should be 60 mg/m² escalating to 80 mg/m² if the dose is tolerated as described in section 4.2: Posology and Method of administration.

If patients present signs or symptoms suggestive of infection, a prompt investigation should be carried out.

Because of the presence of Sorbitol, patients with rare hereditary problems of fructose intolerance should not take this medicine.

Special care should be taken when prescribing for patients with history of ischemic cardiac disease.

In patients with impaired liver or kidney function no prospective study is available in order to establish guidelines for the Navelbine® soft capsules dose reduction.

However, if there is significant hepatic impairment the dose of Navelbine® soft capsules should be reduced. In patients with massive liver metastases (i.e.> 75% of liver volume replaced by the tumour) it is empirically suggested that the dose be reduced by 25 % and the haematological parameters closely monitored.

Navelbine® soft capsules should not be given concomitantly with radiotherapy if the treatment field includes the liver.

As there is a low level of renal excretion there is no pharmacokinetic rationale for reducing Navelbine® soft capsules dose in patients with impaired kidney function.

4.5 Interaction with other medicinal products and other forms of Interaction

The combination of Navelbine® soft capsules with other drugs with known bone marrow toxicity is likely to exacerbate the myelosuppressive adverse effects.

Previous studies of iv Navelbine® associated with cisplatin show no interaction on pharmacokinetic parameters. However the incidence of granulocytopenia associated with Navelbine in combination with cisplatin was higher than the one associated with Navelbine single agent.

As isoform CYP3A4 of cytochrome P450 is likely to be mainly involved in the metabolism of vinorelbine, combination with inducers or inhibitors of this isoenzyme may alter its pharmacokinetics. Omeprazole and fluoxetine (norfluoxetine), inhibitors for CYP3A4, were both found to moderately inhibit the metabolism of vinorelbine, although the clinical relevance of this inhibition is not known.

Food interaction: a simultaneous food intake does not modify the exposure to vinorelbine.

4.6 Pregnancy and lactation

In animal reproductive studies Navelbine® was embryo-foeto-lethal and teratogenic. Therefore, Navelbine® soft capsules should not be used during pregnancy. If pregnancy occurs during treatment genetic counselling should be offered.

It is not known whether Navelbine® passes into the breast milk.

Breast-feeding must be discontinued prior to starting Navelbine® soft capsules treatment.

4.7 Effects on ability to drive and use machines

Navelbine® soft capsules are unlikely to impair the ability of patients to drive or to operate machinery. However, patients should be advised that their ability to drive or operate machinery may be affected.

4.8 Undesirable effects

The overall reported incidence of undesirable effects was determined from clinical studies in 138 patients (76 patients with non small cell lung cancer and 62 patients with breast cancer) who received the recommended regimen of Navelbine® soft capsules (first three administrations at 60mg/m²/week followed by 80mg/m²/week).

The most common undesirable effects are gastro-intestinal.

-Haematopoietic system

- Neutropenia is the dose limiting toxicity. Grade 1-2 neutropenia was seen in 21 % of patients. Grade 3 neutropenia (neutrophil count between 1000 and 500/mm³) was observed in 18.8 % of patients. Grade 4 neutropenia (< 500/mm³) was reported in 23.2 % of patients and was associated with fever over 38°C in 3.0 % of patients. Infections were observed in 15.9 % of patients but were severe in only 5.8 % of them.

- Anaemia was very common but usually mild to moderate (72.5 % of patients with grade 1 or 2, 4.3 % with grade 3, 0.7 % with grade 4).

- Thrombocytopenia might occur but was seldom severe (8 % of patients with grade 1-2).

Gastro-intestinal System

Gastrointestinal adverse events were reported and included: nausea (71 % grade 1-2, 8.1 % grade 3, 0.6 % grade 4), vomiting (55.8 % grade 1-2, 4.3 % grade 3, 2.9 % grade 4) and diarrhoea (44.2 % grade1-2), 2.9 % grade 3, 2.2 % grade 4) and anorexia (29.7 % with grade 1-2, 6.5 % with grade 3, 1.5 % with grade 4). Symptoms of severe intensity were infrequently observed.

Supportive treatment (such as metoclopramide) may reduce their occurrence.

Stomatitis usually mild to moderate occurred in 8.7 % (grade 1-2) of patients.

Oesophagitis was seen in 4.3 % of patients (grade 3 in 0.7 %).

Peripheral and Central Nervous System

• Peripheral:

Neurosensory disorders were generally limited to loss of tendon reflexes in 8 % (grade 1-2) of patients and infrequently severe. One patient presented partially reversible grade 3 ataxia.

Neuromotor disorders were seen in 8 % of patients (2.2 % of patients with grade 3).

• Gastro-intestinal autonomic nervous system:

Neuroconstipation was seen in 9.4 % of patients (8 % grade 1-2) and rarely progressed to paralytic ileus (1.4 %). One episode of fatal paralytic ileus was reported. Prescription of laxatives may be appropriate in patients with prior history of constipation and/or who received concomitant treatment with morphine or morphinomimetics.

Skin

Alopecia may appear progressively with an extended course of treatment.

Alopecia, usually mild in nature, may occur in 25.4 % of patients (24 % grade 1-2, 1.4 % grade 3).

Other adverse effects

Fatigue (19.5 % of patients with grade 1-2, 6.7 % with grade 3), fever (9.4 % with grade 1-2), arthralgia including jaw pain/ myalgia (10.7 % with grade 1-2), pain including pain at the tumour site (5.8 % with grade 1-2) have been experienced by patients receiving Navelbine® soft capsules.

In addition, it cannot be ruled out that the following effects may be observed with the use of oral vinorelbine as with other vinca alkaloids:

Cardiovascular System

There have been rare reports of ischemic cardiac disease (angina pectoris, myocardial infarction).

Liver

Transient elevations of liver function tests without clinical symptoms were reported.

Respiratory system

As with other vinca alkaloids, the intravenous administration of Navelbine® has been associated with dyspnea, bronchospasm and rare cases of interstitial pneumopathy in particular in patients treated with Navelbine® injectable solution in combination with mitomycin.

Skin

Rarely vincaalkaloids may produce generalized cutaneous reactions.

4.9 Overdose

• Human experience

No case of overdosage with Navelbine® soft capsules has been reported, however, overdosage with Navelbine® soft capsules could result in bone marrow hypoplasia sometimes associated with infection, fever and paralytic ileus.

• Management of overdose in man

General supportive measures together with blood transfusion, growth factors, and broad spectrum antibiotic therapy should be instituted as deemed necessary by the doctor. There is no known antidote for overdosage of Navelbine® soft capsules.

5. PHARMACOLOGICAL PROPERTIES

Pharmacotherapeutic group: L01CA04 (ATC Code)

5.1 Pharmacodynamic properties

Navelbine® is a cytostatic antineoplastic drug of the vinca alkaloid family but unlike all the other vinca alkaloids, the catharantine moiety of vinorelbine has been structurally modified. At the molecular level, it acts on the dynamic equilibrium of tubulin in the microtubular apparatus of the cell. It inhibits tubulin polymerization and binds preferentially to mitotic microtubules, affecting axonal microtubules at high concentrations only. The induction of tubulin spiralization is less than that produced by vincristine.

Navelbine® blocks mitosis at G2-M, causing cell death in interphase or at the following mitosis.

5.2 Pharmacokinetic properties

After oral administration, Navelbine® is promptly absorbed and the T_{max} is reached between 1.5 to 3 h with a blood concentration peak (C_{max}) of approximately 130 ng/ml after dosing at 80 mg/m².

The absolute bioavailability is about 40% and a simultaneous food intake does not modify the exposure to vinorelbine.

Oral vinorelbine 60 and 80 mg/m² leads to comparable blood exposure to that obtained from 25 and 30 mg/m² of the iv form respectively.

Interindividual variability of the exposure is similar after administration by iv and oral routes.

There is a proportional increase between the blood exposure and the dose.

There is moderate binding to plasma proteins (13.5 %) but strong binding to platelets (78 %).

Vinorelbine is widely distributed in the body and steady-state volume of distribution is large, ranging 11-21 l.kg-1 after iv administration, which indicates an extensive tissue uptake.

There is a significant uptake of vinorelbine in lungs, as assessed by pulmonary surgical biopsies showing a mean ratio of tissue/plasma concentration greater than 300.

Elimination half-life of vinorelbine is 35 to 40 h.

Oral Navelbine is mainly excreted through biliary route and weakly eliminated in urine.

Unchanged vinorelbine is the major compound recovered in both urine and faeces.

4-O-deacetyl-vinorelbine is an active metabolite detected in blood and eliminated in bile.

Glucoro or sulfo conjugation is not involved in vinorelbine metabolism.

5.3 Preclinical safety data

Preclinical data reveal no special hazard for humans based on conventional studies of repeated dose toxicity and carcinogenic potential.

It is assumed that Navelbine® can cause mutagenic effects (induction of aneuploidy) in man.

In animal reproductive studies, Navelbine® was embryo-foeto-lethal and teratogenic.

No haemodynamic effects were found in dogs receiving vinorelbine at maximal tolerated dose; only some minor, non significant disturbances of repolarisation were found as with other vinca alkaloids tested. No effect on the cardiovascular system was observed in primates receiving repeated doses of vinorelbine over 39 weeks.

6. PHARMACEUTICAL PARTICULARS

6.1 List of excipients

Fill solution:

Ethanol, anhydrous

Water, purified

Glycerol

Macrogol 400

Shell capsule:

Gelatin

Glycerol 85 %

Sorbitol / Sorbitan (Anidrisorb 85/70)

Yellow iron oxide E172

Titanium dioxide E171

Triglycerides, medium chain

Phosal 53 MCT (Phosphatidylcholine; Glycerides; Ethanol, anhydrous)

Edible printing ink:

Cochineal extract E120

Hypromellose

Propylene glycol

6.2 Incompatibilities

Not applicable

6.3 Shelf life

The product is stable for 30 months

6.4 Special precautions for storage

Store between 2° C and 8° C (in a refrigerator). Store in the original container.

6.5 Nature and contents of container

PVC/PVDC/child resistant aluminium blister.

Pack size: 1 capsule

6.6 Instructions for use and handling

For safety reason any unused capsule must be returned to doctor or pharmacy for destruction according to local standard procedure for cytotoxics.

To open the child resistant packaging:

1. Cut the blister along the black dotted line
2. Peel the soft plastic foil off
3. Push the capsule through the aluminium foil

For precautions of use refer to section 4.4: Special warnings and special precautions for use.

7. MARKETING AUTHORISATION HOLDER

PIERRE FABRE Limited

Hyde Abbey House

23 Hyde Street

Winchester Hampshire S023 7DR

United Kingdom

8. MARKETING AUTHORISATION NUMBER(S)

PL 00603/0029

9. DATE OF FIRST AUTHORISATION/RENEWAL OF THE AUTHORISATION

31st March 2005

10. DATE OF REVISION OF THE TEXT

20th June 2005

Navelbine 30mg soft capsule

(Pierre Fabre Limited)

1. NAME OF THE MEDICINAL PRODUCT

NAVELBINE 30 mg soft capsule▼

2. QUALITATIVE AND QUANTITATIVE COMPOSITION

30 mg vinorelbine (as tartrate)

For excipients, see 6.1.

3. PHARMACEUTICAL FORM

Soft capsule

Pink soft capsule printed N30

4. CLINICAL PARTICULARS

4.1 Therapeutic indications

As a single agent or in combination for the first line treatment of stage 3 or 4 non small cell lung cancer.

4.2 Posology and method of administration

For oral use only.

Navelbine® soft capsules should be swallowed with water without chewing or sucking the capsule. It is recommended to take the capsule with some food.

As a single agent, the recommended regimen is:

First three administrations

60mg/m² of body surface area, administered once weekly.

Subsequent administrations

Beyond the third administration, it is recommended to increase the dose of Navelbine® soft capsules to 80mg/m² once weekly **except** in those patients for whom the neutrophil count dropped once below 500/mm³, or more than once between 500 and 1000/mm³ during the first three administrations at 60mg/m².

Table 1

Neutrophil count during the first 3 administrations of 60 mg/m²/week	Neutrophils > 1000	Neutrophils ⩾ 500 and < 1000 (1 episode)	Neutrophils ⩾ 500 and < 1000 (2 episodes)	Neutrophils < 500
Recommended dose starting with the 4th administration	80	80	60	60

Table 2

Neutrophil count beyond the 4th administration of 80 mg/m²/week	Neutrophils > 1000	Neutrophils ⩾ 500 and < 1000 (1 episode)	Neutrophils ⩾ 500 and < 1000 (2 episodes)	Neutrophils < 500
Recommended dose for the next administration	80		60	

(see Table 1 above)

For any administration planned to be given at 80mg/m², if the neutrophil count is below 500/mm³ or more than once between 500 and 1000 / mm³, the administration should be delayed until recovery and the dose reduced from 80 to 60mg/m² per week during the 3 following administrations.

(see Table 2 above)

It is possible to reescalate the dose from 60 to 80 mg/m² per week if the neutrophil count did not drop below 500/mm³, or more than once between 500 and 1000/mm³ during 3 administrations given at 60 mg/m² according to the rules previously defined for the first 3 administrations.

If the neutrophil count is below 1500 /mm³ and/or the platelet count is between 75000 and 100000/mm³, then the treatment should be delayed until recovery.

Based on clinical studies, the oral dose of 80 mg/m² was demonstrated to correspond to 30 mg/m² of the iv form and 60 mg/m² to 25 mg/m².

This has been the base for combination regimens alternating iv and oral forms improving patient's convenience.

For combination regimens, the dose and schedule will be adapted to the treatment protocol.

Capsules of different strengths (20, 30, 40, 80 mg) are available in order to choose the adequate combination for the right dosage.

The following table gives the dose required for appropriate ranges of body surface area (BSA).

BSA (m²)	60 mg/m² Dose (mg)	80 mg/m² Dose (mg)
0.95 to 1.	60	80
1.05 to 1.14	70	90
1.15 to 1.24	70	100
1.25 to 1.34	80	100
1.35 to 1.44	80	110
1.45 to 1.54	90	120
1.55 to 1.64	100	130
1.65 to 1.74	100	140
1.75 to 1.84	110	140
1.85 to 1.94	110	150
⩾ 1.95	120	160

Even for patients with BSA ⩾ 2 m² the total dose should never exceed 160 mg per week.

Clinical experience has not identified relevant differences in responses in the elderly or younger patients but greater sensitivity of some older individuals cannot be ruled out.

Safety and effectiveness in children have not been established.

Dosage adjustment in specific patient groups: refer to section 4.4.: Special warnings and special precautions for use.

Instruction for use / handling: refer to section 6.6

4.3 Contraindications

- Patients with current or recent (within 2 weeks) history of infection
- Patients requiring long-term oxygen therapy
- Known hypersensitivity to vinorelbine or other vinca alkaloids
- Disease significantly affecting absorption
- Previous significant surgical resection of stomach or small bowel
- Neutrophil count < 1500/mm³ or severe infection due to neutropenia
- Severe hepatic insufficiency not related to the tumoural process
- Pregnancy
- Lactation.

4.4 Special warnings and special precautions for use

It is recommended that Navelbine® soft capsules be given under the supervision of a qualified doctor who is experienced in the use of chemotherapy.

If the patient chews or sucks the capsule by error, proceed to mouth rinses with water or preferably a normal saline solution.

In the event of the capsule has being cut or damaged, the liquid content is an irritant, and so may cause damage if in contact with skin, mucosa or eyes. Damaged capsules should not be swallowed and should be returned to the pharmacy or to the doctor in order to be properly destroyed. If any contact occurs, immediate thorough washing with water or preferably with normal saline solution should be undertaken.

In the case of vomiting within a few hours after drug intake, never repeat the administration of this dose. Supportive treatment (such as metoclopramide) may reduce the occurrence of this.

Dosing should be determined by haematological status.

Close haematological monitoring should be undertaken during treatment (determination of haemoglobin level and the leucocyte, neutrophil and platelet counts on the day of each new administration).

During clinical trials where treatments were initiated at 80 mg/m², a few patients developed excessive neutropenia complications. Therefore it is recommended that the starting dose should be 60 mg/m² escalating to 80 mg/m² if the dose is tolerated as described in section 4.2: Posology and Method of administration.

If patients present signs or symptoms suggestive of infection, a prompt investigation should be carried out.

Because of the presence of Sorbitol, patients with rare hereditary problems of fructose intolerance should not take this medicine.

Special care should be taken when prescribing for patients with history of ischemic cardiac disease.

In patients with impaired liver or kidney function no prospective study is available in order to establish guidelines for the Navelbine® soft capsules dose reduction.

However, if there is significant hepatic impairment the dose of Navelbine® soft capsules should be reduced. In patients with massive liver metastases (i.e.> 75% of liver volume replaced by the tumour) it is empirically suggested that the dose be reduced by 25 % and the haematological parameters closely monitored.

Navelbine® soft capsules should not be given concomitantly with radiotherapy if the treatment field includes the liver.

As there is a low level of renal excretion there is no pharmacokinetic rationale for reducing Navelbine® soft capsules dose in patients with impaired kidney function.

4.5 Interaction with other medicinal products and other forms of Interaction

The combination of Navelbine® soft capsules with other drugs with known bone marrow toxicity is likely to exacerbate the myelosuppressive adverse effects.

Previous studies of iv Navelbine® associated with cisplatin show no interaction on pharmacokinetic parameters. However the incidence of granulocytopenia associated with Navelbine in combination with cisplatin was higher than the one associated with Navelbine single agent.

As isoform CYP3A4 of cytochrome P450 is likely to be mainly involved in the metabolism of vinorelbine, combination with inducers or inhibitors of this isoenzyme may alter its pharmacokinetics. Omeprazole and fluoxetine (norfluoxetine), inhibitors for CYP3A4, were both found to moderately inhibit the metabolism of vinorelbine, although the clinical relevance of this inhibition is not known.

Food interaction: a simultaneous food intake does not modify the exposure to vinorelbine.

4.6 Pregnancy and lactation

In animal reproductive studies Navelbine® was embryo-feto-lethal and teratogenic. Therefore, Navelbine® soft capsules should not be used during pregnancy. If pregnancy occurs during treatment genetic counselling should be offered.

It is not known whether Navelbine® passes into the breast milk.

Breast-feeding must be discontinued prior to starting Navelbine® soft capsules treatment.

4.7 Effects on ability to drive and use machines

Navelbine® soft capsules are unlikely to impair the ability of patients to drive or to operate machinery. However, patients should be advised that their ability to drive or operate machinery may be affected.

4.8 Undesirable effects

The overall reported incidence of undesirable effects was determined from clinical studies in 138 patients (76 patients with non small cell lung cancer and 62 patients with breast cancer) who received the recommended regimen of Navelbine® soft capsules (first three administrations at $60mg/m^2$/week followed by $80mg/m^2$/week).

The most common undesirable effects are gastro-intestinal.

-Haematopoietic system

- Neutropenia is the dose limiting toxicity. Grade 1-2 neutropenia was seen in 21 % of patients. Grade 3 neutropenia (neutrophil count between 1000 and $500/mm^3$) was observed in 18.8 % of patients. Grade 4 neutropenia ($< 500/mm^3$) was reported in 23.2 % of patients and was associated with fever over 38°C in 3.0 % of patients. Infections were observed in 15.9 % of patients but were severe in only 5.8 % of them.

- Anaemia was very common but usually mild to moderate (72.5 % of patients with grade 1 or 2, 4.3 % with grade 3, 0.7 % with grade 4).

- Thrombocytopenia might occur but was seldom severe (8 % of patients with grade 1-2).

Gastro-intestinal System

Gastrointestinal adverse events were reported and included: nausea (71 % grade 1-2, 8.1 % grade 3, 0.6 % grade 4), vomiting (55.8 % grade 1-2, 4.3 % grade 3, 2.9 % grade 4) and diarrhoea (44.2 % grade1-2), 2.9 % grade 3, 2.2 % grade 4) and anorexia (29.7 % with grade 1-2, 6.5 % with grade 3, 1.5 % with grade 4). Symptoms of severe intensity were infrequently observed.

Supportive treatment (such as metoclopramide) may reduce their occurrence.

Stomatitis usually mild to moderate occurred in 8.7 % (grade 1-2) of patients.

Oesophagitis was seen in 4.3 % of patients (grade 3 in 0.7 %).

Peripheral and Central Nervous System

• Peripheral:

Neurosensory disorders were generally limited to loss of tendon reflexes in 8 % (grade 1-2) of patients and infrequently severe. One patient presented partially reversible grade 3 ataxia.

Neuromotor disorders were seen in 8 % of patients (2.2 % of patients with grade 3).

• Gastro-intestinal autonomic nervous system:

Neuroconstipation was seen in 9.4 % of patients (8 % grade 1-2) and rarely progressed to paralytic ileus (1.4 %). One episode of fatal paralytic ileus was reported. Prescription of laxatives may be appropriate in patients with prior history of constipation and/or who received concomitant treatment with morphine or morphinomimetics.

Skin

Alopecia may appear progressively with an extended course of treatment.

Alopecia, usually mild in nature, may occur in 25.4 % of patients (24 % grade 1-2, 1.4 % grade 3).

Other adverse effects

Fatigue (19.5 % of patients with grade 1-2, 6.7 % with grade 3), fever (9.4 % with grade 1-2), arthralgia including jaw pain/ myalgia (10.7 % with grade 1-2), pain including pain at the tumour site (5.8 % with grade 1-2) have been experienced by patients receiving Navelbine® soft capsules.

In addition, it cannot be ruled out that the following effects may be observed with the use of oral vinorelbine as with other vinca alkaloids:

Cardiovascular System

There have been rare reports of ischemic cardiac disease (angina pectoris, myocardial infarction).

Liver

Transient elevations of liver function tests without clinical symptoms were reported.

Respiratory system

As with other vinca alkaloids, the intravenous administration of Navelbine® has been associated with dyspnea, bronchospasm and rare cases of interstitial pneumopathy in particular in patients treated with Navelbine® injectable solution in combination with mitomycin.

Skin

Rarely vincaalkaloids may produce generalized cutaneous reactions.

4.9 Overdose

• Human experience

No case of overdosage with Navelbine® soft capsules has been reported, however, overdosage with Navelbine® soft capsules could result in bone marrow hypoplasia sometimes associated with infection, fever and paralytic ileus.

• Management of overdose in man

General supportive measures together with blood transfusion, growth factors, and broad spectrum antibiotic therapy should be instituted as deemed necessary by the doctor. There is no known antidote for overdosage of Navelbine® soft capsules.

5. PHARMACOLOGICAL PROPERTIES

Pharmacotherapeutic group: L01CA04 (ATC Code)

5.1 Pharmacodynamic properties

Navelbine® is a cytostatic antineoplastic drug of the vinca alkaloid family but unlike all the other vinca alkaloids, the catharantine moiety of vinorelbine has been structurally modified. At the molecular level, it acts on the dynamic equilibrium of tubulin in the microtubular apparatus of the cell. It inhibits tubulin polymerization and binds preferentially to mitotic microtubules, affecting axonal microtubules at high concentrations only. The induction of tubulin spiralization is less than that produced by vincristine.

Navelbine® blocks mitosis at G2-M, causing cell death in interphase or at the following mitosis.

5.2 Pharmacokinetic properties

After oral administration, Navelbine® is promptly absorbed and the T_{max} is reached between 1.5 to 3 h with a blood concentration peak (C_{max}) of approximately 130 ng/ml after dosing at 80 mg/m^2.

The absolute bioavailability is about 40% and a simultaneous food intake does not modify the exposure to vinorelbine.

Oral vinorelbine 60 and 80 mg/m^2 leads to comparable blood exposure to that obtained from 25 and 30 mg/m^2 of the iv form respectively.

Interindividual variability of the exposure is similar after administration by iv and oral routes.

There is a proportional increase between the blood exposure and the dose.

There is moderate binding to plasma proteins (13.5 %) but strong binding to platelets (78 %).

Vinorelbine is widely distributed in the body and steady-state volume of distribution is large, ranging 11-21 l.kg-1 after iv administration, which indicates an extensive tissue uptake.

There is a significant uptake of vinorelbine in lungs, as assessed by pulmonary surgical biopsies showing a mean ratio of tissue/plasma concentration greater than 300.

Elimination half-life of vinorelbine is 35 to 40 h.

Oral Navelbine is mainly excreted through biliary route and weakly eliminated in urine.

Unchanged vinorelbine is the major compound recovered in both urine and faeces.

4-O-deacetyl-vinorelbine is an active metabolite detected in blood and eliminated in bile.

Glucoro or sulfo conjugation is not involved in vinorelbine metabolism.

5.3 Preclinical safety data

Preclinical data reveal no special hazard for humans based on conventional studies of repeated dose toxicity and carcinogenic potential.

It is assumed that Navelbine® can cause mutagenic effects (induction of aneuploidy) in man.

In animal reproductive studies, Navelbine® was embryo-foeto-lethal and teratogenic.

No haemodynamic effects were found in dogs receiving vinorelbine at maximal tolerated dose; only some minor, non significant disturbances of repolarisation were found as with other vinca alkaloids tested. No effect on the cardiovascular system was observed in primates receiving repeated doses of vinorelbine over 39 weeks.

6. PHARMACEUTICAL PARTICULARS

6.1 List of excipients

Fill solution:

Ethanol, anhydrous

Water, purified

Glycerol

Macrogol 400

Shell capsule:

Gelatin

Glycerol 85 %

Sorbitol / Sorbitan (Anidrisorb 85/70)

Red iron oxide E172

Titanium dioxide E171

Triglycerides, medium chain

Phosal 53 MCT (Phosphatidylcholine; Glycerides; Ethanol, anhydrous)

Edible printing ink:

Cochineal extract E120

Hypromellose

Propylene glycol

6.2 Incompatibilities

Not applicable

6.3 Shelf life

The product is stable for 30 months

6.4 Special precautions for storage

Store between 2° C and 8° C (in a refrigerator). Store in the original container.

6.5 Nature and contents of container

PVC/PVDC/child resistant aluminium blister.

Pack size: 1 capsule

6.6 Instructions for use and handling

For safety reason any unused capsule must be returned to doctor or pharmacy for destruction according to local standard procedure for cytotoxics.

To open the child resistant packaging:

1. Cut the blister along the black dotted line
2. Peel the soft plastic foil off
3. Push the capsule through the aluminium foil

For precautions of use refer to section 4.4: Special warnings and special precautions for use.

7. MARKETING AUTHORISATION HOLDER

PIERRE FABRE Limited

Hyde Abbey House

23 Hyde Street

Winchester Hampshire S023 7DR

United Kingdom

8. MARKETING AUTHORISATION NUMBER(S)

PL 00603/0030

9. DATE OF FIRST AUTHORISATION/RENEWAL OF THE AUTHORISATION

31st March 2005

10. DATE OF REVISION OF THE TEXT

20th June 2005

Navoban Ampoules 2mg/2ml

(Novartis Pharmaceuticals UK Ltd)

1. NAME OF THE MEDICINAL PRODUCT

NAVOBAN Ampoules 2mg/2ml.

2. QUALITATIVE AND QUANTITATIVE COMPOSITION

2mg/2ml ampoules. Uncoloured glass ampoules containing clear, colourless or very faintly brown-yellow solution. Each ampoule contains 2.26mg of tropisetron hydrochloride (corresponding to 2mg of tropisetron base) in 2ml.

3. PHARMACEUTICAL FORM

Glass ampoules containing an aqueous solution for intravenous administration.

4. CLINICAL PARTICULARS

4.1 Therapeutic indications

Adults

Treatment of post-operative nausea and vomiting.

Prevention of post-operative nausea and vomiting in patients at high risk of developing post-operative nausea and vomiting.

Children

Prevention of cancer chemotherapy-induced nausea and vomiting.

4.2 Posology and method of administration

Post-operative nausea and vomiting in adults

navoban is recommended as a single 2mg dose given intravenously either as an infusion (diluted in a common infusion fluid such as normal saline, Ringer's solution, glucose 5% or fructose 5%) administered over 15 minutes, or as a slow injection (not less than 30 seconds).

In the case of treatment of post-operative nausea and vomiting, NAVOBAN has been shown to be effective when given within two hours of the end of anaesthesia prior to patients being moved from the operating theatre recovery area.

In the case of prevention of post-operative nausea and vomiting, NAVOBAN should be administered shortly before the induction of anaesthesia.

Cancer chemotherapy-induced nausea and vomiting in children

In children, the efficacy and safety of tropisetron 0.2mg/kg/day (maximum 5mg/day) has only been investigated in open label, non-comparative studies which have included 164 children aged 2 years and over.

The recommended dose for NAVOBAN in children over two years of age is 0.2mg/kg, up to a maximum dose of 5mg per day. On day one, shortly before chemotherapy commences, NAVOBAN should be given by intravenous administration as a slow injection (not less than 1 minute) or as an injection into a running infusion. For intravenous infusion, NAVOBAN should be diluted (1mg tropisetron per 20ml diluent) in sodium chloride 0.9% w/v (physiological saline). Alternative diluents are Ringer's solution, glucose 5% and fructose 5%; diluents other than those recommended should not be used.

For children weighing less than 25kg, NAVOBAN should be given once daily by intravenous administration on days 2 up to 5 dependent upon the chemotherapy regimen. For children weighing 25kg and above, NAVOBAN (5mg) should be given once daily by oral administration on days 2 up to 6. If oral administration is problematic NAVOBAN (5mg) can be given by intravenous administration.

4.3 Contraindications

Hypersensitivity to tropisetron, or other 5-HT_3 receptor antagonists. NAVOBAN must not be given to pregnant women, unless termination of early pregnancy is part of the surgical procedure.

4.4 Special warnings and special precautions for use

Use in poor metabolisers of sparteine/debrisoquine

In patients belonging to this group (about 8% of the Caucasian population) the elimination half-life of tropisetron is prolonged (4 to 5 times longer than in extensive metabolisers), however, studies indicate that for 7 day courses in patients with poor metabolism, the usual dose of 2mg does not need to be reduced.

Use in patients with impaired hepatic or renal function

No change in the pharmacokinetics of tropisetron occurs in patients with acute hepatitis or fatty liver disease. In contrast, patients with liver cirrhosis or impaired kidney function may have plasma concentrations up to 50% higher than those found in healthy volunteers belonging to the group of extensive metabolisers of sparteine/debrisoquine. Nevertheless, no dosage reduction is necessary in such patients when the recommended 2mg dose is given.

Use in children

NAVOBAN is not recommended for the treatment or prevention of post-operative nausea and vomiting in children.

Use in the elderly

There is no evidence that elderly patients require different dosages or experience side effects different from those in younger patients.

Use in adults

When used for the prevention of cancer chemotherapy-induced nausea and vomiting in adults, NAVOBAN capsules 5mg and NAVOBAN ampoules 5mg/5ml should be used. Use of NAVOBAN ampoules 2mg/2ml for this indication is reserved for children.

Use in cardiac patients

Prolongation of the QTc interval, which was not clinically significant, has been observed after high (up to 80mg) doses of IV tropisetron. Therefore caution should be exercised in patients with cardiac rhythm or conduction disturbances, or in patients treated with anti-arrhythmic agents or beta-adrenergic blocking agents.

Preclinical safety studies

In several *in vitro* and *in vivo* tests, NAVOBAN has been shown to have no mutagenic potential. In 2-year carcinogenicity studies in rats and mice, the incidence of liver adenomas was increased only in male mice receiving 30 and 90mg/kg/day, with no effects seen at 10mg/kg/day Additional *in vitro* and *in vivo* investigative studies suggested that the observed effects in the livers of male mice were probably both species- and sex-specific.

4.5 Interaction with other medicinal products and other forms of Interaction

Concomitant administration of NAVOBAN with therapeutic agents known to induce hepatic metabolic enzymes (e.g. rifampicin, phenobarbital) results in lower plasma concentrations of tropisetron and therefore requires an increase in dosage in extensive metabolisers (but not in poor metabolisers). The effects of cytochrome P450 enzyme inhibitors such as cimetidine on tropisetron plasma levels are negligible and do not require dose adjustment.

Care should be taken when other drugs that are likely to prolong QT interval are used concomitantly with tropisetron.

4.6 Pregnancy and lactation

NAVOBAN must not be given to pregnant women, unless termination of early pregnancy is part of the surgical procedure. There is no experience of NAVOBAN in human pregnancy. In animal studies, no teratogenic effects occurred at doses which were not toxic to dams, but effects on female reproductive capacity were observed.

Nursing mothers

In the rat, after administration of radiolabelled tropisetron, radioactivity was excreted in the milk. Breast-feeding patients should not be given NAVOBAN.

4.7 Effects on ability to drive and use machines

No data exist on the effect of this drug on the ability to drive. The occurrence of dizziness and fatigue as side effects should be taken into account. Not relevant in the context of general anaesthesia.

4.8 Undesirable effects

The undesirable effects are transient at the recommended dose. Most frequently reported at the recommended 2mg dose was headache, whereas at higher doses constipation and, less frequently, dizziness, fatigue and gastrointestinal disorders such as abdominal pain and diarrhoea were observed as well.

As with other 5-HT_3 receptor antagonists, hypersensitivity reactions ('type I-reactions') with one or more of the following symptoms have rarely been observed: facial flushing and/or generalised urticaria, chest tightness, dyspnoea, acute bronchospasm, hypotension. In very rare instances when NAVOBAN has been used to prevent chemotherapy-induced nausea and vomiting, collapse, syncope or cardiovascular arrest have been reported. The relationship to NAVOBAN has not been established and these effects may have been caused by the concomitant therapy or the underlying disease.

4.9 Overdose

At very high repeated doses (100mg for 5 days), visual hallucinations have been observed. In patients with pre-existing hypertension, an increase in blood pressure has been observed at cumulative doses of 27 to 80mg NAVOBAN. Symptomatic treatment with frequent monitoring of vital signs and close observation of the patient is indicated.

5. PHARMACOLOGICAL PROPERTIES

5.1 Pharmacodynamic properties

Tropisetron is a highly potent and selective competitive antagonist of the 5-HT_3 receptor, a subclass of serotonin receptors located on peripheral neurons and within the CNS.

Surgery and treatment with certain substances, including some chemotherapeutic agents, may trigger the release of serotonin (5 HT) from enterochromaffin-like cells in the visceral mucosa and initiate the emesis reflex and its accompanying feeling of nausea. Tropisetron selectively blocks the excitation of the presynaptic 5-HT_3 receptors of the peripheral neurons in this reflex, and may exert additional direct actions within the CNS on 5-HT_3 receptors mediating the actions of vagal input to the area postrema. These effects are considered to be the underlying mechanism of action of the anti-emetic effect of tropisetron.

5.2 Pharmacokinetic properties

Absorption of NAVOBAN from the gastrointestinal tract is rapid (mean half-life of about 20 minutes) and extensive (more than 95%). The peak plasma concentration is attained within 3 hours.

Tropisetron is 71% bound to plasma proteins (particularly a_1-glycoproteins) in a non-specific manner. The volume of distribution in adults is 400 to 600L. The volume of distribution was found to be reduced in children younger than 6 (145L) and 15 (265L) years of age.

The metabolism of tropisetron occurs by hydroxylation at the 5, 6 or 7 position of its indole ring, followed by a conjugation reaction to form the glucuronide or sulphate and excretion in the urine or bile (urine to faeces ratio 5:1). The metabolites have a greatly reduced potency for the 5-HT_3 receptor and do not contribute to the pharmacological action of the drug. The metabolism of tropisetron is linked to the genetically determined sparteine/debrisoquine polymorphism. About 8% of the Caucasian population are known to be poor metabolisers for the sparteine/debrisoquine pathway. The absolute bioavailability and terminal half-life in children was similar to those in healthy volunteers.

The elimination half-life (b-phase) is about 8 hours in extensive metabolisers; in poor metabolisers this could be extended to 45 hours (see special warnings and special precautions for use). The total clearance of tropisetron is about 1L/min, with the renal clearance contributing approximately 10%. In patients who are poor metabolisers, the total clearance is reduced to 0.1 to 0.2L/min although the renal clearance remains unchanged. This reduction in non-renal clearance results in an approximately 4 to 5-fold longer elimination half-life and in 5 to 7-fold higher AUC values. C_{max} and volume of distribution are not different when compared to extensive metabolisers. In poor metabolisers, a greater proportion of unchanged tropisetron is excreted in the urine than in extensive metabolisers.

5.3 Preclinical safety data

In several *in vitro* and *in vivo* tests, NAVOBAN has been shown to have no mutagenic potential. In 2-year carcinogenicity studies in rats and mice, the incidence of liver adenomas was increased in male mice receiving 30 and 90mg/kg/day, with no effects at 10mg/kg/day Additional *in vitro* and *in vivo* investigative studies suggested that the observed effects in the livers of male mice were probably both species- and sex-specific. The result is therefore not considered relevant for patients when NAVOBAN is used as recommended.

6. PHARMACEUTICAL PARTICULARS

6.1 List of excipients

Acetic acid, glacial EP; sodium acetate trihydrate EP; sodium chloride EP; water for injection EP.

6.2 Incompatibilities

navoban glass ampoules contain a 1mg/ml aqueous solution to be used for i.v. administration. Ampoule solutions are compatible with the following solutions for injection: glucose 5% (w/v); Ringer's solution; sodium chloride 0.9% (w/v) and fructose 5% (w/v), in concentrations of 5mg in 100ml solution. Diluents other than those listed should not be used. The diluted solutions are physically and chemically stable for at least 24 hours. However, considering the risk of microbial contamination during the preparation of the infusion, the solution must be used within 8 hours of preparation. The solutions are also compatible with the usual types of containers (glass, PVC) and their infusion sets.

6.3 Shelf life

5 years.

6.4 Special precautions for storage

No special precautions.

6.5 Nature and contents of container

navoban ampoules 2mg/2ml are made of uncoloured glass, and are coded with two blue colour rings. They are available in packs of five.

6.6 Instructions for use and handling

None.

7. MARKETING AUTHORISATION HOLDER

Novartis Pharmaceuticals UK Ltd

Trading as "Sandoz Pharmaceuticals"

Frimley Business Park

Frimley

Camberley

Surrey,

GU16 7SR

8. MARKETING AUTHORISATION NUMBER(S)

PL 0101/0413

9. DATE OF FIRST AUTHORISATION/RENEWAL OF THE AUTHORISATION

12 June 2002

10. DATE OF REVISION OF THE TEXT

13 September 2002

Legal Category:

POM

Navoban Capsules 5mg Navoban Ampoules 5mg/5ml

(Novartis Pharmaceuticals UK Ltd)

1. NAME OF THE MEDICINAL PRODUCT

NAVOBAN Capsules 5mg

NAVOBAN Ampoules 5mg/5ml

2. QUALITATIVE AND QUANTITATIVE COMPOSITION

Capsule: opaque yellow and white, hard gelatin capsule, 16mm in length and 6mm in diameter. Each capsule contains 5mg tropisetron base (equivalent to tropisetron hydrochloride 5.64mg) and is marked with NAVOBAN 5mg in red print.

Ampoule: uncoloured glass ampoules containing clear, colourless or very faintly brown-yellow solution. Each ampoule contains 5.64mg of tropisetron hydrochloride (corresponding to 5mg of tropisetron base) in 5ml.

3. PHARMACEUTICAL FORM

Capsule: hard gelatin capsule for oral administration.

Ampoule: glass ampoule containing an aqueous solution for intravenous administration.

4. CLINICAL PARTICULARS

4.1 Therapeutic indications

Prevention of cancer chemotherapy-induced nausea and vomiting.

4.2 Posology and method of administration

Adults

NAVOBAN is recommended as six-day courses of 5mg per day.

On day one, shortly before chemotherapy commences, 5mg NAVOBAN should be given by intravenous administration as a slow injection or as an injection into a running infusion. For intravenous administration, one NAVOBAN ampoule should be diluted in 100ml of sodium chloride 0.9% w/v (physiological saline). Alternatively, diluents are Ringer's solution, glucose 5% and fructose 5%; diluents other than those specified should not be used.

On days two to six, one NAVOBAN capsule 5mg should be taken with water each morning upon rising at least one hour before food.

Children

In children, the efficacy and safety of tropisetron 0.2mg/kg/day (maximum 5mg/day) has only been investigated in open label, non-comparative studies which have included 164 children aged 2 years and over.

The recommended dose for NAVOBAN in children over two years of age is 0.2mg/kg up to a maximum dose of 5mg per day. On day one, shortly before chemotherapy commences, NAVOBAN should be given by intravenous administration as a slow injection (not less than 1 minute) or an injection into a running infusion. For intravenous infusion, NAVOBAN should be diluted (1mg tropisetron per 20ml diluent) in sodium chloride 0.9% w/v (physiological saline). Alternative diluents are Ringer's solution, glucose 5% and fructose 5%; diluents other than those recommended should not be used.

For children weighing less than 25kg, NAVOBAN should be given once daily by intravenous administration on days 2 up to 5 dependent on the chemotherapy regimen.

For children weighing 25kg and above, NAVOBAN (5mg) should be given once daily by oral administration on days 2 up to 6. If oral administration is problematic NAVOBAN (5mg) can be given by intravenous administration.

Elderly

There is no evidence that a special dosing schedule is needed in this patient group. 5mg NAVOBAN daily for six days is recommended.

Poor metabolisers of sparteine/debrisoquine

In patients belonging to this group (about 8% of the Caucasian population) the elimination half-life of tropisetron is prolonged (4-5 times longer than in extensive metabolisers). However, no dosage reduction is necessary in such patients. The recommended dosage is, therefore, 5mg daily for 6 successive days.

Patients with impaired hepatic or renal function

No change in pharmacokinetics of tropisetron occurs in patients with acute hepatitis or fatty liver disease. In contrast, patients with liver cirrhosis or impaired kidney function may have plasma concentrations up to 50% higher than those found in healthy volunteers belonging to the group of extensive metabolisers of sparteine/debrisoquine. Never-the-less, no dosage reduction is necessary in such patients when the recommended 6-day courses of 5mg NAVOBAN per day are given.

Use in patients with uncontrolled hypertension

In patients with uncontrolled hypertension, it is important not to exceed the recommended daily dose since higher dosages, particularly when administered after intravenous prehydration therapy, have been reported to aggravate this condition.

Method of Administration

Capsule: oral

Ampoule: intravenous

4.3 Contraindications

Hypersensitivity to tropisetron or other 5-HT_3 receptor antagonists. NAVOBAN must not be given to pregnant women.

4.4 Special warnings and special precautions for use

In patients with uncontrolled hypertension, it is important not to exceed the recommended daily dose since higher doses, particularly when administered after intravenous prehydration therapy have been reported to aggravate this condition.

Use in cardiac patients

Prolongation of the QTc interval, which was not clinically significant, has been observed after high (up to 80mg) doses of i.v. tropisetron. Therefore caution should be exercised in patients with cardiac rhythm or conduction disturbances, or in patients treated with anti-arrhythmic agents or beta-adrenergic blocking agents.

Preclinical safety studies

In several *in vitro* and *in vivo* tests, NAVOBAN has been shown to have no mutagenic potential. In 2-year carcinogenicity studies in rats and mice, the incidence of liver adenomas was increased only in male mice receiving 30 and 90mg/kg/day, with no effects seen at 10mg/kg/day. Additional *in vitro* and *in vivo* investigative studies suggested that the observed effects in the livers of male mice were probably both species- and sex-specific.

4.5 Interaction with other medicinal products and other forms of Interaction

Concomitant administration of NAVOBAN with therapeutic agents known to induce hepatic enzymes may result in lower tropisetron plasma concentrations, particularly in extensive metabolisers. Conversely the effects of the agents which characteristically inhibit these enzyme systems may lead to enhanced plasma concentrations. Such changes are unlikely to be of practical importance provided the dosage regime of 5mg daily for six days is followed.

Ingestion of the capsule with food has no relevant influence on the bioavailability but may slightly delay the absorption of NAVOBAN.

Care should be taken when other drugs that are likely to prolong QT interval are used concomitantly with tropisetron.

4.6 Pregnancy and lactation

NAVOBAN must not be given to pregnant women. There is no experience with NAVOBAN in human pregnancy. In animal studies, no teratogenic effects occurred at doses which were not toxic to the dams, but effects on reproductive capacity were observed. Therefore, women should not try to conceive when on NAVOBAN therapy.

It has not been established whether tropisetron is excreted into human milk. Patients taking NAVOBAN should not therefore breast-feed.

4.7 Effects on ability to drive and use machines

Patients should be cautioned against driving or operating machinery until it is established that they do not become dizzy or drowsy whilst receiving NAVOBAN.

4.8 Undesirable effects

The most frequently reported adverse reactions are headache, constipation, dizziness, fatigue and gastrointestinal disorders such as abdominal pain and diarrhoea. In very rare incidences, collapse, syncope, bradycardia or cardiovascular arrest have been reported with NAVOBAN. However, as with other 5-HT_3 receptor antagonists, the relationship to NAVOBAN has not been established. Some of these reactions could be attributed to concomitant chemotherapy or the underlying disease. As with other 5-HT_3 receptor antagonists, hypersensitivity reactions (Type 1 reactions) with one or more of the following symptoms have rarely been observed: Facial flushing and/or generalised urticaria, chest tightness, dyspnoea, acute bronchospasm, hypotension.

4.9 Overdose

At very high repeated doses, visual hallucinations and in patients with pre-existing hypertension, an increase in blood pressure may have been observed. Seizure threshold may also be lowered in susceptible patients. Symptomatic treatment with frequent monitoring of vital signs and close observation of the patient is indicated.

5. PHARMACOLOGICAL PROPERTIES

5.1 Pharmacodynamic properties

NAVOBAN is a highly potent and selective competitive antagonist of the 5-HT_3 receptor, a subclass of serotonin receptors located on peripheral neurons and within the CNS. Certain substances including some chemotherapeutic agents are believed to trigger the release of serotonin (5-HT) from enterochromaffin-like cells in the visceral mucosa and initiate the emesis reflex and its accompanying feeling of nausea. NAVOBAN selectively blocks the excitation of the pre-synaptic 5-HT_3 receptors of the peripheral neurons in this reflex, and may exert additional direct actions within the CNS on 5-HT_3 receptors mediating the actions of vagal input to the area postrema.

NAVOBAN has a 24 hour duration of action which allows once-a-day administration. In studies where NAVOBAN has been administered over multiple chemotherapy cycles, treatment has remained effective. NAVOBAN prevents nausea and vomiting induced by cancer chemotherapy without causing extrapyramidal side-effects.

5.2 Pharmacokinetic properties

Absorption of NAVOBAN from the gastro-intestinal tract is rapid (mean half-life of about 20 minutes) and extensive (more than 95%). The peak plasma concentration is attained within 3 hours. Owing to a saturable metabolic pathway, the absolute bioavailability is dose-dependent. The absolute bioavailability and terminal half-life in children was similar to those in healthy volunteers. Tropisetron is 71% bound to plasma protein in a non-specific manner. The volume of distribution in adults is 400-600L. The volume of distribution was found to be reduced in children younger than 6 (145L) and 15 (265L) years of age.

The metabolism of tropisetron is linked to the genetically determined sparteine/debrisoquine pathway.

The elimination half-life (β-phase) is about 8 hours in extensive metabolisers, and 30 hours after i.v. administration or 42 hours after oral administration in poor metabolisers. In extensive metabolisers, about 8% of tropisetron is excreted in the urine as unchanged drug, 70% as metabolites; 15% is excreted in the faeces, almost entirely as metabolites. The metabolites of tropisetron do not contribute to its pharmacological action. In poor metabolisers, a greater proportion of unchanged tropisetron is excreted in the urine than in extensive metabolisers.

5.3 Preclinical safety data

In several *in vitro* and *in vivo* tests, NAVOBAN has been shown to have no mutagenic potential. In 2-year carcinogenicity studies in rats and mice, the incidence of liver adenomas was increased only in male mice receiving 30 and 90mg/kg/day, with no effects seen at 10mg/kg/day. Additional *in vitro* and *in vivo* investigative studies suggested that the observed effects in the livers of male mice were probably both species- and sex-specific. The result if therefore not considered relevant for patients when NAVOBAN is used as recommended.

6. PHARMACEUTICAL PARTICULARS

6.1 List of excipients

Capsule:

Contents

Silica, colloidal anhydrous

Magnesium stearate

Maize starch

Lactose

Shell

Iron oxide, yellow (E172)

Titanium dioxide (E171)

Gelatin

Imprint

Shellac

Iron oxide, red (E172)

Ampoule:

Acetic acid, glacial EP; sodium acetate trihydrate EP; sodium chloride EP; water for injection EP

6.2 Incompatibilities

None

6.3 Shelf life

60 months

6.4 Special precautions for storage

Capsule: Do not store above 30°C.

Ampoule: No special precautions (see 6.6)

6.5 Nature and contents of container

NAVOBAN 5mg Capsules are available commercially in PVC/PVDC blister strips containing 5 capsules in boxes of 1 or 10. Capsules are number 3 size hard gelatin capsules with an opaque yellow upper part with a Sandoz triangle imprinted in red, and an opaque white lower part with NAVOBAN (or the code EA in NL and B) and the dose strength of 5mg imprinted in red.

NAVOBAN 5mg/5ml Ampoules are clear glass 5ml ampoules with a rupture ring in pack sizes of 1 and 10 ampoules.

6.6 Instructions for use and handling

Capsule: for oral administration.

Ampoule: ampoule solution may be diluted with specified diluents (see 4.2 for diluents). Diluted solution should be used immediately or stored between 2 and 8°C for no more than 24 hours.

7. MARKETING AUTHORISATION HOLDER

Novartis Pharmaceuticals UK Limited

Trading as Sandoz Pharmaceuticals

Frimley Business Park

Frimley

Camberley

Surrey

GU16 7SR

8. MARKETING AUTHORISATION NUMBER(S)

Capsule: 0101/0345

Ampoule: 0101/0344

9. DATE OF FIRST AUTHORISATION/RENEWAL OF THE AUTHORISATION

28 October 1997

10. DATE OF REVISION OF THE TEXT

13 September 2002

LEGAL CATEGORY:

POM

Nebido 1000mg/4ml, solution for injection

(Schering Health Care Limited)

1. NAME OF THE MEDICINAL PRODUCT

Nebido▼ 1000 mg/4ml, solution for injection

2. QUALITATIVE AND QUANTITATIVE COMPOSITION

Each ml solution for injection contains 250 mg testosterone undecanoate corresponding to 157.9 mg testosterone.

Each ampoule with 4 ml solution for injection contains 1000 mg testosterone undecanoate.

For excipients, see 6.1.

3. PHARMACEUTICAL FORM

Solution for injection.

Clear, yellowish oily solution.

4. CLINICAL PARTICULARS

4.1 Therapeutic indications

Testosterone replacement therapy for male hypogonadism when testosterone deficiency has been confirmed by clinical features and biochemical tests (see section 4.4 Special warnings and precautions for use).

4.2 Posology and method of administration

For intramuscular use.

Adults and Elderly men

One ampoule of Nebido (corresponding to 1000 mg testosterone undecanoate) is injected every 10 to 14 weeks. Injections with this frequency are capable of maintaining sufficient testosterone levels and do not lead to accumulation.

The injections must be administered very slowly. Care should be taken to inject Nebido deeply into the gluteal muscle following the usual precautions for intramuscular administration. Special care must be given to avoid intravasal injection. The contents of an ampoule are to be injected intramuscularly immediately after opening the ampoule.

- Start of treatment

Serum testosterone levels should be measured before start and during initiation of treatment. Depending on serum testosterone levels and clinical symptoms, the first injection interval may be reduced to a minimum of 6 weeks as compared to the recommended range of 10 to 14 weeks for maintenance. With this loading dose, sufficient steady state testosterone levels may be achieved more rapidly.

- Maintenance and individualisation of treatment

The injection interval should be within the recommended range of 10 to 14 weeks. Careful monitoring of serum testosterone levels is required during maintenance of treatment. It is advisable to measure testosterone serum levels regularly. Measurements should be performed at the end of an injection interval and clinical symptoms considered. These serum levels should be within the lower third of the normal range. Serum levels below normal range would indicate the need for a shorter injection interval. In case of high serum levels an extension of the injection interval may be considered.

Children and Adolescents

Nebido is not indicated for use in children and adolescents and it has not been evaluated clinically in males under 18 years of age.

4.3 Contraindications

The use of Nebido is contraindicated in androgen-dependent carcinoma of the prostate or of the male mammary gland; past or present liver tumours; hypersensitivity to the active substance or to any of the excipients.

4.4 Special warnings and special precautions for use

Nebido is not recommended for use in children and adolescents.

Nebido should be used only if hypogonadism (hyper- and hypogonadotrophic) has been demonstrated and if other aetiology, responsible for the symptoms, has been excluded before treatment is started. Testosterone insufficiency should be clearly demonstrated by clinical features (regression of secondary sexual characteristics, change in body composition, asthenia, reduced libido, erectile dysfunction etc.) and confirmed by two separate blood testosterone measurements.

There is limited experience of the use of Nebido in elderly patients over 65 years of age. Currently, there is no consensus about age specific testosterone reference values. However, it should be taken into account that physiologically testosterone serum levels are lower with increasing age.

Medical examination

Prior to testosterone initiation, all patients must undergo a detailed examination in order to exclude a risk of pre-existing prostatic cancer. Careful and regular monitoring of the prostate gland and breast must be performed in accordance with recommended methods (digital rectal examination and estimation of serum PSA) in patients receiving testosterone therapy at least once yearly and twice yearly in elderly patients and at risk patients (those with clinical or familial factors).

Besides laboratory tests of the testosterone concentrations in patients on long-term androgen therapy the following laboratory parameters should be checked periodically: haemoglobin, haematocrit and liver function tests.

Due to variability in laboratory values, all measures of testosterone should be carried out in the same laboratory.

Tumours

Androgens may accelerate the progression of sub-clinical prostatic cancer and benign prostatic hyperplasia.

Nebido should be used with caution in cancer patients at risk of hypercalcaemia (and associated hypercalcuria), due to bone metastases. Regular monitoring of serum calcium concentrations is recommended in these patients.

Rarely, benign and malignant liver tumours have been reported in patients receiving testosterone replacement therapy.

Other conditions

In patients suffering from severe cardiac, hepatic or renal insufficiency or ischaemic heart disease, treatment with testosterone may cause severe complications characterised by oedema with or without congestive cardiac failure. In such cases, treatment must be stopped immediately. There are no studies undertaken to demonstrate the efficacy and safety of this medicinal product in patients with renal or hepatic impairment. Therefore, testosterone replacement therapy should be used with caution in these patients.

As a general rule, the limitations of using intramuscular injections in patients with acquired or inherited blood clotting irregularities always have to be observed.

Nebido should be used with caution in patients with epilepsy and migraine, as the conditions may be aggravated.

Improved insulin sensitivity may occur in patients treated with androgens who achieve normal testosterone plasma concentrations following replacement therapy.

Certain clinical signs: irritability, nervousness, weight gain, prolonged or frequent erections may indicate excessive androgen exposure requiring dosage adjustment.

Pre-existing sleep apnoea may be potentiated.

Athletes treated for testosterone replacement in primary and secondary male hypogonadism should be advised that the medicinal product contains an active substance which may produce a positive reaction in anti-doping tests.

Androgens are not suitable for enhancing muscular development in healthy individuals or for increasing physical ability.

Nebido should be permanently withdrawn if symptoms of excessive androgen exposure persist or reappear during treatment with the recommended dosage regimen.

Application

Nebido must be injected intramuscularly. Experience shows that the short-lasting reactions (urge to cough, coughing fits, respiratory distress) which occur in rare cases during or immediately after the injection of oily solutions can be avoided by injecting the solution extremely slowly.

4.5 Interaction with other medicinal products and other forms of Interaction

Oral anti-coagulants

Testosterone and derivatives have been reported to increase the activity of oral anti-coagulants. Patients receiving oral anti-coagulants require close monitoring, especially at the beginning or end of androgen therapy. Increased monitoring of the prothrombin time, and INR determinations, are recommended.

Other interactions

The concurrent administration of testosterone with ACTH or corticosteroids may enhance oedema formation; thus these active substancesshould be administered cautiously, particularly in patients with cardiac or hepatic disease or in patients predisposed to oedema.

Laboratory Test Interactions: Androgens may decrease levels of thyroxine-binding globulin resulting in decreased total T4 serum levels and increased resin uptake of T3 and T4. Free thyroid hormone levels remain unchanged, however, and there is no clinical evidence of thyroid dysfunction.

4.6 Pregnancy and lactation

Nebido is not indicated for use in women and must not be used in pregnant or breast-feeding women.

4.7 Effects on ability to drive and use machines

Nebido has no influence on the ability to drive and use machines.

4.8 Undesirable effects

The most frequently observed adverse reaction was injection site pain (10%).

The following adverse reactionswere reported in clinical trials with a suspected relationship to Nebido (according to the HARTS Body System and Dictionary Term system):

Body System	Common* ($>1/100$, $<1/10$)
Digestive	Diarrhoea
Musculoskeletal system	Leg pain, arthralgia
Nervous system	Dizziness, increased sweating, headache
Respiratory system	Respiratory disorder
Skin and appendages	Acne, breast pain, gynaecomastia, pruritus, skin disorder
Urogenital	Testicular pain, prostate disorder
General disorders and administration site conditions	Subcutaneous haematoma at the injection site

*) Due to the small sample size of the studies, the frequency of each reported adverse event with a suggested causal relationship falls at least into the category common ($>1/100$).

In the literature the following adverse reactions from testosterone containing preparations have been reported:

Body System	Adverse reactions
Blood and the lymphatic system disorders	Rare cases of polycythaemia (erythrocytosis)
Metabolism and nutrition disorders	Weight gain, electrolyte changes (retention of sodium, chloride, potassium, calcium, inorganic phosphate and water) during high dose and/ or prolonged treatment
Musculoskeletal system	Muscle cramps
Nervous system	Nervousness, hostility, depression
Respiratory system	Sleep apnoea
Hepatobiliary disorders	In very rare cases jaundice and liver function test abnormalities
Skin and appendages	Various skin reactions may occur including acne, seborrhoea and balding (alopecia)
Reproductive system and breast disorders	Libido changes, increased frequency of erections; therapy with high doses of testosterone preparations commonly reversibly interrupts or reduces spermatogenesis, thereby reducing the size of the testicles; testosterone replacement therapy of hypogonadism can in rare cases cause persistent, painful erections (priapism), prostate abnormalities, prostate cancer**, urinary obstruction
General disorders and administration site conditions	High-dose or long-term administration of testosterone occasionally increases the occurrences of water retention and oedema; hypersensitivity reactions may occur

**) Data on prostate cancer risk in association with testosterone therapy are inconclusive.

4.9 Overdose

No special therapeutic measure apart from termination of therapy with the medicinal product or dose reduction is necessary after overdose.

5. PHARMACOLOGICAL PROPERTIES

5.1 Pharmacodynamic properties

Pharmacotherapeutic group: Androgens, 3-oxoandrosten (4) derivatives

ATC code: G03B A03

Testosterone undecanoate is an ester of the naturally occurring androgen, testosterone. The active form, testosterone, is formed by cleavage of the side chain.

Testosterone is the most important androgen of the male, mainly synthesised in the testicles, and to a small extent in the adrenal cortex.

Testosterone is responsible for the expression of masculine characteristics during foetal, early childhood and pubertal development and thereafter for maintaining the masculine phenotype and androgen-dependent functions (e.g. spermatogenesis, accessory sexual glands). It also performs functions, e.g. in the skin, muscles, skeleton, kidney, liver, bone marrow and CNS.

Dependent on the target organ, the spectrum of activities of testosterone is mainly androgenic (e.g. prostate, seminal vesicles, epididymis) or protein-anabolic (muscle, bone, haematopoiesis, kidney, liver).

The effects of testosterone in some organs arise after peripheral conversion of testosterone to estradiol, which then binds to oestrogen receptors in the target cell nucleus e.g. the pituitary, fat, brain, bone and testicular Leydig cells.

5.2 Pharmacokinetic properties

• *Absorption*

Nebido is an intramuscularly administered depot preparation of testosterone undecanoate and thus circumvents the first-pass effect. Following intramuscular injection of testosterone undecanoate as an oily solution, the compound is gradually released from the depot and is almost completely cleaved by serum esterases into testosterone and undecanoic acid. An increase inserum levels of testosterone above basal values may be seen one day after administration.

• *Steady-state conditions*

After the 1st intramuscular injection of 1000 mg testosterone undecanoate to hypogonadal men, mean Cmax values of 38 nmol/l (11 ng/ml) were obtained after 7 days. The second dose was administered 6 weeks after the 1st injection and maximum testosterone concentrations of about 50 nmol/l (15 ng/ml) were reached. A constant dosing interval of 10 weeks was maintained during the following 3 administrations and steady-state conditions were achieved between the 3rd and the 5th administration. Mean Cmax and Cmin values of testosterone at steady-state were about 37 (11 ng/ml) and 16 nmol/l (5 ng/ml), respectively. The median intra- and inter-individual variability (coefficient of variation, %) of Cmin values was 22 % (range: 9-28%) and 34% (range: 25-48%), respectively.

• *Distribution*

In serum of men, about 98% of the circulating testosterone is bound to sex hormone binding globulin(SHBG) and albumin. Only the free fraction of testosterone is considered as biologically active. Following intravenous infusion of testosterone to elderly men, the elimination half-life of testosterone was approximately one hour and an apparent volume of distribution of about 1.0 l/kg was determined.

• *Metabolism*

Testosterone which is generated by ester cleavage from testosterone undecanoate is metabolised and excreted the same way as endogenous testosterone. The undecanoic acid is metabolised by β-oxidation in the same way as other aliphatic carboxylic acids. The major active metabolites of testosterone are estradiol and dihydrotestosterone.

• *Elimination*

Testosterone undergoes extensive hepatic and extrahepatic metabolism. After the administration of radiolabelled testosterone, about 90% of the radioactivity appears in the urine as glucuronic and sulphuric acid conjugates and 6% appears in the faeces after undergoing enterohepatic circulation. Urinary medicinal products include androsterone and etiocholanolone. Following intramuscular administration of this depot formulation the release rateis characterised by a half life of 90±40 days.

5.3 Preclinical safety data

Toxicological studies have not revealed other effects than those which can be explained based on the hormone profile of Nebido.

Testosterone has been found to be non-mutagenic in vitro using the reverse mutation model (Ames test) or hamster ovary cells. A relationship between androgen treatment and certain cancers has been found in studies on laboratory animals. Experimental data in rats have shown increased incidences of prostate cancer after treatment with testosterone.

Sex hormones are known to facilitate the development of certain tumours induced by known carcinogenic agents. The clinical relevance of the latter observation is not known.

Fertility studies in rodents and primates have shown that treatment with testosterone can impair fertility by suppressing spermatogenesis in a dose dependent manner.

6. PHARMACEUTICAL PARTICULARS

6.1 List of excipients

Benzyl benzoate, castor oil, refined

6.2 Incompatibilities

In the absence of compatibility studies, this medicinal product must not be mixed with other medicinal products.

6.3 Shelf life

3 years

The medicinal product must be used immediately after first opening.

6.4 Special precautions for storage

This medicinal product does not require any special storage conditions.

6.5 Nature and contents of container

5 ml amber glass (type I) ampoules, containing a fill volume of 4 ml.

Pack size: 1 × 4 ml

6.6 Instructions for use and handling

The solution for intramuscular injection is to be visually inspected prior to use and only clear solutions free from particles should be used.

The medicinal product is for single use only and any unused solution should be discarded.

7. MARKETING AUTHORISATION HOLDER

Schering Health Care Limited

The Brow

Burgess Hill

West Sussex RH15 9NE

8. MARKETING AUTHORISATION NUMBER(S)

PL/0053/0350

9. DATE OF FIRST AUTHORISATION/RENEWAL OF THE AUTHORISATION

20th October 2004

10. DATE OF REVISION OF THE TEXT

LEGAL CATEGORY

POM

Nebilet

(A. Menarini Pharma U.K. S.R.L.)

1. NAME OF THE MEDICINAL PRODUCT

NEBILET® 5 mg tablets

2. QUALITATIVE AND QUANTITATIVE COMPOSITION

Each Nebilet tablet contains 5 mg of nebivolol (as nebivolol hydrochloride).

For excipients, see section 6.1.

3. PHARMACEUTICAL FORM

Tablets.

White, round, scored tablets.

4. CLINICAL PARTICULARS

4.1 Therapeutic indications

Treatment of essential hypertension.

4.2 Posology and method of administration

Adults

The dose is one tablet (5 mg) daily, preferably at the same time of the day. Tablets may be taken with meals.

The blood pressure lowering effect becomes evident after 1-2 weeks of treatment. Occasionally, the optimal effect is reached only after 4 weeks.

Combination with other antihypertensive agents

Beta-blockers can be used alone or concomitantly with other antihypertensive agents. Till date, an additional antihypertensive effect has been observed only when Nebilet 5 mg is combined with hydrochlorothiazide 12.5-25 mg.

Patients with renal insufficiency

In patients with renal insufficiency, the recommended starting dose is 2.5 mg daily. If needed, the daily dose may be increased to 5 mg.

Patients with hepatic insufficiency

Data in patients with hepatic insufficiency or impaired liver function are limited. Therefore the use of Nebilet in these patients is contra-indicated.

Elderly

In patients over 65 years, the recommended starting dose is 2.5 mg daily. If needed, the daily dose may be increased to 5 mg. However, in view of the limited experience in patients above 75 years, caution must be exercised and these patients monitored closely.

Childrenand adolescents

No studies have been conducted in children and adolescents. Therefore, use in children and adolescents is not recommended.

4.3 Contraindications

Hypersensitivity to the active substance or to any of the excipients.

Liver insufficiency or liver function impairment.

Pregnancy and lactation.

Beta-adrenergic antagonists are contra-indicated in:

- cardiogenic shock.
- uncontrolled heart failure.
- sick sinus syndrome, including sino-atrial block.
- second and third degree heart block.
- history of bronchospasm and bronchial asthma.
- untreated phaeochromocytoma.
- metabolic acidosis.
- bradycardia (heart rate < 50 bpm).
- hypotension.
- severe peripheral circulatory disturbances.

4.4 Special warnings and special precautions for use

The following warnings and precautions apply to beta-adrenergic antagonists in general.

See also 4.8 Undesirable effects

Anaesthesia:

Continuation of beta blockade reduces the risk of arrhythmias during induction and intubation. If beta blockade is interrupted in preparation for surgery, the beta-adrenergic antagonist should be discontinued at least 24 hours beforehand.

Caution should be observed with certain anaesthetics that cause myocardial depression, such as cyclopropane, ether or trichlorethylene. The patient can be protected against vagal reactions by intravenous administration of atropine.

Cardiovascular

In general, beta-adrenergic antagonists should not be used in patients with untreated congestive heart failure (CHF), unless their condition has been stabilised.

In patients with ischaemic heart disease, treatment with a beta-adrenergic antagonist should be discontinued gradually, i.e. over 1-2 weeks. If necessary replacement therapy should be initiated at the same time, to prevent exacerbation of angina pectoris.

Beta-adrenergic antagonists may induce bradycardia: if the pulse rate drops below 50-55 bpm at rest and/or the patient experiences symptoms are suggestive of bradycardia, the dosage should be reduced.

Beta-adrenergic antagonists should be used with caution:

in patients with peripheral circulatory disorders (Raynaud's disease or syndrome, intermittent claudication), as aggravation of these disorders may occur;

in patients with first degree heart block, because of the negative effect of beta-blockers on conduction time;

in patients with Prinzmetal's angina due to unopposed alphareceptor mediated coronary artery vasoconstriction: beta-adrenergic antagonists may increase the number and duration of anginal attacks.

Metabolic/Endocrinological

Nebilet does not affect glucose levels in diabetic patients. Care should be taken in diabetic patients however, as nebivolol may mask certain symptoms of hypoglycaemia (tachycardia, palpitations).

Beta-adrenergic blocking agents may mask tachycardic symptoms in hyperthyroidism. Abrupt withdrawal may intensify symptoms.

Respiratory

In patients with chronic obstructive pulmonary disorders, beta-adrenergic antagonists should be used with caution as airway constriction may be aggravated.

Other

Patients with a history of psoriasis should take beta-adrenergic antagonists only after careful consideration.

Beta-adrenergic antagonists may increase the sensitivity to allergens and the severity of anaphylactic reactions.

Use in children is not recommended.

4.5 Interaction with other medicinal products and other forms of Interaction

The following interactions apply to beta-adrenergic antagonists in general.

Calcium antagonists:

Care should be exercised when administering beta-adrenergic antagonists with calcium antagonists of the verapamil or diltiazem type, because of their negative effect on contractility and atrio-ventricular conduction. Intravenous verapamil is contra-indicated in patients on Nebilet.

Anti-arrhythmics:

Caution should be exercised when administering beta-adrenergic antagonists in association with Class I antiarrhythmic drugs and amiodarone, as their effect on atrial conduction time and their negative inotropic effect may be potentiated.

Clonidine:

Beta-adrenergic antagonists increase the risk of rebound hypertension after sudden withdrawal of chronic clonidine treatment.

Digitalis:

Digitalis glycosides associated with beta-adrenergic antagonists may increase atrio-ventricular conduction time. Clinical trials with nebivolol have not shown any clinical evidence of an interaction. Nebivolol does not influence the kinetics of digoxin.

Insulin and oral antidiabetic drugs:

Although Nebilet does not affect glucose levels, certain symptoms of hypoglycaemia (palpitations, tachycardia) may be masked.

Anaesthetics:

Concomitant use of beta-adrenergic antagonists and anaesthetics may attenuate reflex tachycardia and increase the risk of hypotension. The anaesthesiologist should be informed when the patient is receiving Nebilet.

Other:

Concomitant use of NSAID's had no effect on the blood pressure lowering effect of Nebilet.

Co-administration of cimetidine increased the plasma levels of nebivolol, without changing the clinical effect. Co-administration of ranitidine did not affect the pharmacokinetics of nebivolol. Provided Nebilet is taken with the meal, and an antacid between meals, the two treatments can be co-prescribed.

Combining nebivolol with nicardipine slightly increased the plasma levels of both drugs, without changing the clinical effect. Co-administration of alcohol, furosemide or hydrochlorothiazide did not affect the pharmacokinetics of nebivolol. Nebivolol does not affect the pharmacokinetics and pharmacodynamics of warfarin.

Sympathicomimetic agents may counteract the effect of beta-adrenergic antagonists. Beta-adrenergic agents may lead to unopposed alpha-adrenergic activity of sympathicomimetic agents with both alpha- and beta-adrenergic effects (risk of hypertension, severe bradycardia and heart block).

Concomitant administration of tricyclic antidepressants, barbiturates and phenothiazines may increase the blood pressure lowering effect.

As nebivolol metabolism involves the CYP2D6 isoenzyme, concomitant administration of serotonin reuptake inhibitors, dextrometorphan or other compounds predominantly metabolised via this pathway, may make extensive metabolisers resemble poor metabolisers.

4.6 Pregnancy and lactation

Use in pregnancy

Insufficient data exist on the use of Nebilet in human pregnancy to determine its potential harmfulness. Animal studies have not shown any indication of harmful effects, other than on the basis of its pharmacological properties. Beta-blockers reduce placental perfusion, which may result in intrauterine fetal death and in immature and premature delivery. In addition, adverse effects (hypoglycaemia and bradycardia) may occur in the fetus and the neonate. There is an increased risk of cardiac and pulmonary complications in the neonate in the postnatal period. Therefore, Nebilet should not be used during pregnancy.

Use in lactation

Most beta-blockers, particularly lipophilic compounds like nebivolol and its active metabolites, pass into breast milk although to a variable extent. Since it is not known whether nebivolol is excreted into human milk, the use of Nebilet when breast feeding is contra-indicated. Animal studies have shown that nebivolol is excreted in breast milk.

4.7 Effects on ability to drive and use machines
No studies on the effects on the ability to drive and use machine have been performed. Pharmacodynamic studies have shown that Nebilet 5 mg does not affect psychomotor function. When driving vehicles or operating machines it should be taken into account that dizziness and fatigue may occasionally occur.

4.8 Undesirable effects
The adverse reactions reported, which are in most of the cases of mild to moderate intensity, are tabulated below, classified by system organ class and ordered by frequency:

SYSTEM ORGAN CLASS	Common (1-10%)	Uncommon (0,1-1%)
Nervous system disorders	headache, dizziness, paraesthesia	nightmares
Eye disorders		impaired vision
Cardiac disorders		bradycardia, heart failure, slowed AV conduction/ AV-block
Vascular disorders		hypotension, (increase of) intermittent claudication
Respiratory, thoracic and mediastinal disorders	dyspnoea	bronchospasm
Gastrointestinal disorders	constipation, nausea, diarrhoea	dyspepsia, flatulence, vomiting
Skin and subcutaneous tissue disorders		pruritus, rash erythematous
Reproductive system and breast disorders		impotence
General disorders and administration site conditions	tiredness, oedema	depression

The following adverse reactions have also been reported with some beta adrenergic antagonists: hallucinations, psychoses, confusion, cold/cyanotic extremities, Raynaud phenomenon, dry eyes, and oculo-mucocutaneous toxicity of the practolol-type.

4.9 Overdose
No data are available on overdosage with Nebilet.

Symptoms
Symptoms of overdosage with beta-blockers are: bradycardia, hypotension, bronchospasm and acute cardiac insufficiency.

Treatment
In case of overdosage or hypersensitivity, the patient should be kept under close supervision and be treated in an intensive care ward. Blood glucose levels should be checked. Absorption of any drug residues still present in the gastro-intestinal tract can be prevented by gastric lavage and the administration of activated charcoal and a laxative. Artificial respiration may be required. Bradycardia or extensive vagal reactions should be treated by administering atropine or methylatropine. Hypotension and shock should be treated with plasma/plasma substitutes and, if necessary, catecholamines. The beta-blocking effect can be counteracted by slow intravenous administration of isoprenaline hydrochloride, starting with a dose of approximately 5 μg/minute, or dobutamine, starting with a dose of 2.5 μg/minute, until the required effect has been obtained. In refractory cases isoprenaline can be combined with dopamine. If this does not produce the desired effect either, intravenous administration of glucagon 50-100 μg/kg i.v. may be considered. If required, the injection should be repeated within one hour, to be followed -if required- by an i.v. infusion of glucagon 70 μg/kg/h. In extreme cases of treatment-resistant bradycardia, a pacemaker may be inserted.

5. PHARMACOLOGICAL PROPERTIES

5.1 Pharmacodynamic properties
Pharmacotherapeutic group: Beta blocking agent, selective.

ATC code: C07AB12

Nebivolol is a racemate of two enantiomers, SRRR-nebivolol (or d-nebivolol) and RSSS-nebivolol (or l-nebivolol). It combines two pharmacological activities:

- It is a competitive and selective beta-receptor antagonist: this effect is attributed to the SRRR-enatiomer (d-enantiomer).
- It has mild vasodilating properties, due to an interaction with the L-arginine/nitric oxide pathway.

Single and repeated doses of nebivolol reduce heart rate and blood pressure at rest and during exercise, both in normotensive subjects and in hypertensive patients. The antihypertensive effect is mantained during chronic treatment.

At therapeutic doses, nebivolol is devoid of alpha-adrenergic antagonism.

During acute and chronic treatment with nebivolol in hypertensive patients systemic vascular resistance is decreased. Despite heart rate reduction, reduction in cardiac output during rest and exercise may be limited due to an increase in stroke volume. The clinical relevance of these haemodynamic differences as compared to other beta1 receptor antagonists has not been fully established.

In hypertensive patients, nebivolol increases the NO-mediated vascular response to acetylcholine (ACh) which is reduced in patients with endothelial dysfunction.

In vitro and in vivo experiments in animals showed that Nebivolol has no intrinsic sympathicomimetic activity.

In vitro and in vivo experiments in animals showed that at pharmacological doses nebivolol has no membrane stabilising action.

In healthy volunteers, nebivolol has no significant effect on maximal exercise capacity or endurance.

5.2 Pharmacokinetic properties
Both nebivolol enantiomers are rapidly absorbed after oral administration. The absorption of nebivolol is not affected by food; nebivolol can be given with or without meals.

Nebivolol is extensively metabolised, partly to active hydroxy-metabolites. Nebivol is metabolised via alicyclic and aromatic hydroxylation, N-dealkylation and glucuronidation; in addition, glucuronides of the hydroxy-metabolites are formed. The methabolism of nebivolol by aromatic hydroxylation is subject to the CYP2D6 dependent genetic oxidative polymorphism. The oral bioavailability of nebivolol averages 12% in fast metabolisers and is virtually complete in slow metabolisers. At steady state and at the same dose level, the peak plasma concentration of unchanged nebivolol is about 23 times higher in poor metabolisers than in extensive metabolisers. When unchanged drug plus active metabolites are considered, the difference in peak plasma concentrations is 1.3 to 1.4 fold. Because of the variation in rates of metabolism, the dose of Nebilet should always be adjusted to the individual requirements of the patient: poor metabolisers therefore may require lower doses.

In fast metabolisers, elimination half-lives of the nebivolol enantiomers average 10 hours. In slow metabolisers, they are 3-5 times longer. In fast metabolisers, plasma levels of the RSSS-enantiomer are slightly higher than for the SRRR-enantiomer. In slow metabolisers, this difference is larger. In fast metabolisers, elimination half-lives of the hydroxymetabolites of both enantiomers average 24 hours, and are about twice as long in slow metabolisers.

Steady-state plasma levels in most subjects (fast metabolisers) are reached within 24 hours for nebivolol and within a few days for the hydroxy-metabolites.

Plasma concentrations are dose-proportional between 1 and 30 mg. The pharmacokinetics of nebivolol are not affected by age.

In plasma, both nebivolol enantiomers are predominantly bound to albumin.

Plasma protein binding is 98.1% for SRRR-nebivolol and 97.9% for RSSS-nebivolol.

One week after administration, 38% of the dose is excreted in the urine and 48% in the faeces. Urinary excretion of unchanged nebivolol is less than 0.5% of the dose.

5.3 Preclinical safety data
No particulars.

6. PHARMACEUTICAL PARTICULARS

6.1 List of excipients
Polysorbate 80, hypromellose, lactose monohydrate, maize starch, croscarmellose sodium, microcristalline cellulose, colloidal anhydrous silica, magnesium stearate

6.2 Incompatibilities
Not applicable

6.3 Shelf life
3 years.

6.4 Special precautions for storage
No special precautions for storage

6.5 Nature and contents of container
Tablets are provided in blister packs (PVC/aluminium blister).

7, 14, 28, 30, 50, 56, 100, 500 tablets

(Not all pack sizes may be marketed)

6.6 Instructions for use and handling
No special requirements.

7. MARKETING AUTHORISATION HOLDER
Menarini International Operations Luxembourg S.A.

1, Avenue de la Gare,

L-1611 Luxembourg

8. MARKETING AUTHORISATION NUMBER(S)
PL 16239/0013

9. DATE OF FIRST AUTHORISATION/RENEWAL OF THE AUTHORISATION
18 October 2000

10. DATE OF REVISION OF THE TEXT
October 2003

Legal category
POM

Negram 500mg Tablets
(sanofi-aventis)

1. NAME OF THE MEDICINAL PRODUCT
Negram 500mg Tablets.

2. QUALITATIVE AND QUANTITATIVE COMPOSITION
Nalidixic Acid Ph. Eur. 500.0mg.

3. PHARMACEUTICAL FORM
Tablet.

4. CLINICAL PARTICULARS

4.1 Therapeutic indications
Negram is recommended for the treatment of acute or chronic infections, especially those of the urinary tract caused by gram-negative organisms, other than Pseudomonas species, sensitive to nalidixic acid. It may also be used for the treatment of gastrointestinal gram-negative infections sensitive to nalidixic acid where appropriate, though relapse rate and treatment failure in gastrointestinal infection may be more common.

4.2 Posology and method of administration
For oral administration only. Nalidixic acid should be taken on an empty stomach, preferably one hour before a meal.

Adults: For acute infections 1g four times daily for at least seven days, reducing to 0.5g four times a day for chronic infections.

Children: For those over the age of three months, the maximum recommended dose is 50mg/kg body weight per day in divided doses. When prolonged treatment is necessary it may be possible to reduce the dose to 30mg/kg body weight without loss of therapeutic benefit.

Patients with renal failure: The normal dose of nalidixic acid may be employed in patients with creatinine clearance of more than 20 ml/minute. Dosage should be halved in patients with creatinine clearance of 20 ml/minute or less.

4.3 Contraindications
Negram is contraindicated for patients with a history of convulsive disorders, porphyria or hypersensitivity to nalidixic acid or related compounds.

Nalidixic acid should not be administered to infants less than three months of age.

4.4 Special warnings and special precautions for use
Nalidixic acid is mainly metabolised by the liver and should therefore be used with caution in patients with liver disease.

Caution should be observed in patients with severe cerebral arteriosclerosis or glucose-6-phosphate dehydrogenase deficiency (see 4.8 Undesirable Effects) as well as in patients with severe renal failure, in whom the dosage may be reduced (see 4.2 Posology and Method of Administration).

Although care should be exercised in treating patients with renal failure, the full dosage of nalidixic acid may be administered in patients with creatinine clearance of more than 20ml/min and half the normal dosage in patients with creatinine clearance less than this.

Particular caution is advised in patients with a known allergic disposition.

Patients taking nalidixic acid should avoid excessive exposure to sunlight (including sunbathing) and therapy should be discontinued if photosensitivity occurs.

When nalidixic acid is given to patients on anticoagulant therapy, it may be necessary to reduce the anticoagulant dosage.

Nalidixic acid has been shown to induce lesions in weight-bearing joints of young animals. The relevance of this to man is unknown. The possible risk of late degenerative joint changes in young patients receiving nalidixic acid preparations should therefore be considered. If symptoms of arthralgia occur, treatment with nalidixic acid should be stopped.

Caution should be observed and therapy discontinued if patients develop signs or symptoms suggestive of an increase in intracranial pressure, psychosis or other toxic manifestations.

Blood count, renal and liver function should be monitored periodically if treatment is continued for more than two weeks.

If the clinical response is unsatisfactory or if relapse occurs, therapy should be reviewed in the light of appropriate culture and sensitivity tests. If bacterial resistance to nalidixic acid develops, it does so usually within 48 hours. Cross-resistance between nalidixic acid and other quinolone derivatives such as oxolinic acid and cinoxacin have been observed.

4.5 Interaction with other medicinal products and other forms of Interaction

Nalidixic acid may interact with oralanticoagulants such as warfarin due to competition for protein binding sites and it may therefore be necessary to reduce the anticoagulant dosage. Appropriate monitoring of prothrombin time or international normalised ratio (INR) and adjustment of anticoagulant dosage should therefore be observed.

There have been reports of serious gastro-intestinal toxicity following the concomitant use of nalidixic acid and melphalan.

Nalidixic acid in therapeutic doses can interfere with the estimation of urinary 17-ketosteroids and may cause high results in the assay of the urinary vanillylmandelic -acid (Pisano method).

When testing for glycosuria in patients receiving nalidixic acid, glucose-specific methods based on glucose oxidase should be used because copper reduction methods, such as Benedict's or Fehling's solution, may give false-positive results.

Active proliferation of the organisms is a necessary condition for the antibacterial activity of nalidixic acid: the action of nalidixic acid may therefore be inhibited by the presence of other antibacterial substances especially bacteriostatic agents such as tetracycline, chloroamphenicol, and nitrofurantoin which are antagonistic to nalidixic acid in vitro.

Nalidixic acid also interacts with probenecid, which inhibits the tubular secretion of nalidixic acid. This may reduce the efficacy of the product in the treatment of urinary tract infections.

It is possible that there will be an increased risk of nephrotoxicity with cyclosporin.

It is recognised that convulsions may occur due to an interaction between quinolones and non steroidal anti-inflammatory drugs. This has not however been observed so far with nalidixic acid.

4.6 Pregnancy and lactation

The safety of nalidixic acid during pregnancy has not been established. Therefore, it should be used during pregnancy only if the potential benefits outweigh the potential risks, especially during the first trimester (nalidixic acid crosses the placental barrier and has been shown to be taken up by growing cartilage in several animal species) and during the last month of pregnancy because of the potential risk for the neonate. Exposure to maternal nalidixic acid in utero may lead to significant blood levels of nalidixic acid in the neonate immediately after birth.

Since nalidixic acid is excreted in breast milk, it is contra-indicated during lactation.

4.7 Effects on ability to drive and use machines

Adverse reactions such as drowsiness, weakness and dizziness may occur. Patients should be advised not to drive or operate machinery if these reactions are experienced.

4.8 Undesirable effects

Reactions reported after oral administration of Negram include:

CNS side effects: Drowsiness, weakness, headache and dizziness and vertigo. Reversible subjective visual disturbances without objective findings have occurred infrequently (generally with each dose during the first few days of treatment). These reactions include overbrightness of lights, change in colour perception, difficulty in focusing, decrease in visual acuity, and double vision. They usually disappear promptly when dosage is reduced or therapy is discontinued.

Toxic psychosis or brief convulsions have been reported rarely, usually following excessive doses. In general, the convulsions have occurred in patients with predisposing factors such as epilepsy or cerebral arteriosclerosis.

In infants and children receiving therapeutic doses of Negram, increased intracranial pressure with bulging anterior fontanelle, papilloedema and headache have occasionally been observed. A few cases of 6th cranial nerve palsy have been reported. Although the mechanisms of these reactions are unknown, the signs and symptoms usually disappear rapidly with no sequelae when treatment is discontinued.

Gastrointestinal: Abdominal pain, nausea, vomiting and diarrhoea.

Allergic: Rash, pruritus, urticaria, angio-oedema, eosinophilia, arthralgia with joint stiffness and swelling, and rarely, anaphylactic shock and anaphylactoid reaction. Photosensitivity reactions consisting of erythema and bullae on exposed skin surfaces usually resolve completely in 2 weeks to 2 months after Negram is discontinued; however, bullae may continue to appear with successive exposures to sunlight or with mild skin trauma for up to 3 months after discontinuation of the drug. (See Warnings).

Other: Rarely cholestasis, paraesthesia, metabolic acidosis, thrombocytopenia, leukopenia, or haemolytic anaemia, sometimes associated with glucose-6-phosphate dehydrogenase deficiency.

4.9 Overdose

In adults, symptoms of overdose have been noted following single doses of 20g and 25g. These have included toxic psychosis, convulsions and increased intracranial pressure. Occasional reports of metabolic acidosis have occurred in association with overdosage, use in infants under the age of three months, or overdose with concurrent use of probenecid. Vomiting, nausea and lethargy may also occur following overdosage. Reactions are likely to be short-lived because nalidixic acid is normally excreted rapidly.

If systemic absorption has occurred, fluid intake should be promoted, supportive measures such as oxygen and means of artificial respiration should be available. Anticonvulsant therapy may be indicated in a severe case, although it has not been used in the few instances of overdosage that have been reported.

5. PHARMACOLOGICAL PROPERTIES

5.1 Pharmacodynamic properties

Nalidixic acid is particularly active against gram-negative organisms most commonly encountered in infections of the urinary and intestinal tracts, particularly Escherichia and Proteus species, and members of the typhoid-dysentery group. Nalidixic acid acts by selectively inhibiting bacterial DNA synthesis.

5.2 Pharmacokinetic properties

Nalidixic acid is well absorbed following oral administration. Almost all of the drug is excreted by the kidneys, about 80% being recoverable from the urine. Effective antibacterial concentrations of nalidixic acid are readily obtainable in urine. In human volunteers, single 0.5 and 1g oral doses produce peak urine levels of biologically active drug varying from 25 to 250μg/ml. Although high urine levels of nalidixic acid may be expected, serum levels are unpredictable and tend to be significant only at higher dosage levels.

5.3 Preclinical safety data

There are no pre-clinical data of relevance to the prescriber which are additional to that already in other sections of the SPC.

6. PHARMACEUTICAL PARTICULARS

6.1 List of excipients

Sodium lauryl sulphate, Microcrystalline cellulose (Avicel Ph.102), Brown iron oxide (E172), Methylcellulose, Hydrogenated vegetable oil, Purified water *

* Not detected in final formulation

6.2 Incompatibilities

None.

6.3 Shelf life

36 months.

6.4 Special precautions for storage

None.

6.5 Nature and contents of container

Clear PVC blister packs of 56 tablets. Amber glass bottles of 500 tablets.

6.6 Instructions for use and handling

Not applicable.

7. MARKETING AUTHORISATION HOLDER

Sanofi-Synthelabo

PO Box 597

Guildford

Surrey

8. MARKETING AUTHORISATION NUMBER(S)

PL 11723/0059

9. DATE OF FIRST AUTHORISATION/RENEWAL OF THE AUTHORISATION

15th September 2005

10. DATE OF REVISION OF THE TEXT

15th September 2005

Legal category: POM

Neoclarityn 0.5 mg/ml syrup

(Schering-Plough Ltd)

1. NAME OF THE MEDICINAL PRODUCT

Neoclarityn▼ 0.5 mg/ml syrup

2. QUALITATIVE AND QUANTITATIVE COMPOSITION

Each ml of syrup contains 0.5 mg desloratadine.

For excipients, see section 6.1.

3. PHARMACEUTICAL FORM

Syrup

4. CLINICAL PARTICULARS

4.1 Therapeutic indications

Neoclarityn is indicated for the relief of symptoms associated with:

- allergic rhinitis (AR)
- chronic idiopathic urticaria (CIU)

4.2 Posology and method of administration

Neoclarityn may be taken without regard to mealtime.

The prescriber should be aware that most cases of rhinitis below 2 years of age are of infectious origin (see section 4.4) and there are no data supporting the treatment of infection rhinitis with Neoclarityn.

Children 1 through 5 years of age: 2.5 ml (1.25 mg) Neoclarityn syrup once a day.

Children 6 through 11 years of age: 5 ml (2.5 mg) Neoclarityn syrup once a day.

In adults and adolescents (12 years of age and over): 10 ml (5 mg) Neoclarityn syrup once a day.

4.3 Contraindications

Hypersensitivity to the active substance or to any of the excipients, or to loratadine.

4.4 Special warnings and special precautions for use

Efficacy and safety of Neoclarityn syrup in children under 1 year of age have not been established.

In children below 2 years of age, the diagnosis of AR is particularly difficult to distinguish from other forms of rhinitis. The absence of upper respiratory tract infection or structural abnormalities, as well as patient history, physical examinations, and appropriate laboratory and skin tests should be considered.

Approximately 6 % of adults and children 2- to 11-year old are phenotypic poor metabolisers of desloratadine and exhibit a higher exposure (see section 5.2). The safety of Neoclarityn syrup in children 2- to 11-years of age who are poor metabolisers is the same as in children who are normal metabolisers. The effects of Neoclarityn syrup in poor metabolisers < 2 years of age have not been studied.

In the case of severe renal insufficiency, Neoclarityn should be used with caution (see section 5.2).

This medicinal product contains sucrose and sorbitol; thus, patients with rare hereditary problems of fructose intolerance, glucose-galactose malabsorption or sucrase-isomaltase insufficiency should not take this medicine.

4.5 Interaction with other medicinal products and other forms of Interaction

No clinically relevant interactions were observed in clinical trials with Neoclarityn tablets in which erythromycin or ketoconazole were co-administered (see section 5.1).

In a clinical pharmacology trial, Neoclarityn tablets taken concomitantly with alcohol did not potentiate the performance impairing effects of alcohol (see 5.1).

4.6 Pregnancy and lactation

Desloratadine was not teratogenic in animal studies. The safe use of the medicinal product during pregnancy has not been established. The use of Neoclarityn during pregnancy is therefore not recommended.

Desloratadine is excreted into breast milk, therefore the use of Neoclarityn is not recommended in breastfeeding women.

4.7 Effects on ability to drive and use machines

In clinical trials that assessed the driving ability, no impairment occurred in patients receiving desloratadine. However, patients should be informed that very rarely some people experience drowsiness, which may affect their ability to drive or use machines.

4.8 Undesirable effects

In clinical trials in a paediatric population, Neoclarityn syrup was administered to a total of 246 children aged 6 months through 11 years. The overall incidence of adverse events in children 2 through 11 years of age was similar for the Neoclarityn syrup and the placebo groups. In infants and toddlers aged 6 to 23 months, the most frequent adverse events reported in excess of placebo were diarrhoea (3.7 %), fever (2.3 %) and insomnia (2.3 %).

At the recommended dose, in clinical trials involving adults and adolescents in a range of indications including AR and CIU, undesirable effects with Neoclarityn were reported in 3 % of patients in excess of those treated with placebo. The most frequent of the adverse events reported in excess of placebo were fatigue (1.2 %), dry mouth (0.8 %) and headache (0.6 %). Other undesirable effects reported very rarely during the post-marketing period are listed in the following table.

Nervous system disorders	Dizziness, somnolence, insomnia
Cardiac disorders	Tachycardia, palpitations
Gastrointestinal disorders	Abdominal pain, nausea, vomiting, dyspepsia, diarrhea
Hepato-biliary disorders	Elevations of liver enzymes, increased bilirubin, hepatitis
Musculoskeletal and connective tissue disorders	Myalgia

General disorders	Hypersensitivity reactions (such as anaphylaxis, angioedema, dyspnoea, pruritus, rash, and urticaria)

4.9 Overdose

In the event of overdose, consider standard measures to remove unabsorbed active substance.

Symptomatic and supportive treatment is recommended.

Based on a multiple dose clinical trial in adults and adolescents, in which up to 45 mg of desloratadine was administered (nine times the clinical dose), no clinically relevant effects were observed.

Desloratadine is not eliminated by haemodialysis; it is not known if it is eliminated by peritoneal dialysis.

5. PHARMACOLOGICAL PROPERTIES

5.1 Pharmacodynamic properties

Pharmacotherapeutic group: antihistamines – H_1 antagonist, ATC code: R06A X27

Desloratadine is a non-sedating, long-acting histamine antagonist with selective peripheral H_1-receptor antagonist activity. After oral administration, desloratadine selectively blocks peripheral histamine H_1-receptors because the substance is excluded from entry to the central nervous system.

Desloratadine has demonstrated antiallergic properties from *in vitro* studies. These include inhibiting the release of proinflammatory cytokines such as IL-4, IL-6, IL-8, and IL-13 from human mast cells/basophils, as well as inhibition of the expression of the adhesion molecule P-selectin on endothelial cells. The clinical relevance of these observations remains to be confirmed.

Efficacy of Neoclarityn syrup has not been investigated in separate paediatric trials. Safety of Neoclarityn syrup was demonstrated in three paediatric trials. Children, 1-11 years of age, who were candidates for antihistamine therapy received a daily desloratadine dose of 1.25 mg (1 through 5 years of age) or 2.5 mg (6 through 11 years of age). Treatment was well tolerated as documented by clinical laboratory tests, vital signs, and ECG interval data, including QTc. When given at the recommended doses, the plasma concentrations of desloratadine (see section 5.2) were comparable in the paediatric and adult populations. Thus, since the course of AR/CIU and the profile of desloratadine are similar in adults and paediatric patients, desloratadine efficacy data in adults can be extrapolated to the paediatric population.

In a multiple dose clinical trial, in adults and adolescents, in which up to 20 mg of desloratadine was administered daily for 14 days, no statistically or clinically relevant cardiovascular effect was observed. In a clinical pharmacology trial, in adults and adolescents, in which desloratadine was administered to adults at a dose of 45 mg daily (nine times the clinical dose) for ten days, no prolongation of QTc interval was seen.

Desloratadine does not readily penetrate the central nervous system. In controlled clinical trials, at the recommended dose of 5 mg daily for adults and adolescents, there was no excess incidence of somnolence as compared to placebo. Neoclarityn tablets given at a single daily dose of 7.5 mg to adults and adolescents did not affect psychomotor performance in clinical trials. In a single dose study performed in adults, desloratadine 5 mg did not affect standard measures of flight performance including exacerbation of subjective sleepiness or tasks related to flying.

In clinical pharmacology trials in adults, co-administration with alcohol did not increase the alcohol-induced impairment in performance or increase in sleepiness. No significant differences were found in the psychomotor test results between desloratadine and placebo groups, whether administered alone or with alcohol.

No clinically relevant changes in desloratadine plasma concentrations were observed in multiple-dose ketoconazole and erythromycin interaction trials.

In adult and adolescent patients with AR, Neoclarityn tablets were effective in relieving symptoms such as sneezing, nasal discharge and itching, as well as ocular itching, tearing and redness, and itching of palate. Neoclarityn effectively controlled symptoms for 24 hours. Efficacy has not been clearly demonstrated in patients 1 through 17 years of age.

In two placebo-controlled six week trials in patients with CIU, Neoclarityn was effective in relieving pruritus and decreasing the size and number of hives by the end of the first dosing interval. In each trial, the effects were sustained over the 24 hour dosing interval. As with other antihistamine trials in CIU, the minority of patients who were identified as non-responsive to antihistamines was excluded. An improvement in pruritus of more than 50 % was observed in 55 % of patients treated with desloratadine compared with 19 % of patients treated with placebo. Treatment with Neoclarityn also significantly reduced interference with sleep and daytime function, as measured by a four-point scale used to assess these variables.

Neoclarityn tablets were effective in alleviating the burden of seasonal allergic rhinitis (SAR) as shown by the total score of the rhino-conjunctivitis quality of life questionnaire. The greatest amelioration was seen in the domains of practical problems and daily activities limited by symptoms.

5.2 Pharmacokinetic properties

Desloratadine plasma concentrations can be detected within 30 minutes of desloratadine administration in adults and adolescents. Desloratadine is well absorbed with maximum concentration achieved after approximately 3 hours; the terminal phase half-life is approximately 27 hours. The degree of accumulation of desloratadine was consistent with its half-life (approximately 27 hours) and a once daily dosing frequency. The bioavailability of desloratadine was dose proportional over the range of 5 mg to 20 mg.

In a series of pharmacokinetic and clinical trials, 6 % of the subjects reached a higher concentration of desloratadine. The prevalence of this poor metaboliser phenotype was comparable for adult (6 %) and paediatric subjects 2- to 11-year old (6 %), and greater among Blacks (18 % adult, 16 % paediatric) than Caucasians (2 % adult, 3 % paediatric) in both populations.

In a multiple-dose pharmacokinetic study conducted with the tablet formulation in healthy adult subjects, four subjects were found to be poor metabolisers of desloratadine. These subjects had a C_{max} concentration about 3-fold higher at approximately 7 hours with a terminal phase half-life of approximately 89 hours.

Similar pharmacokinetic parameters were observed in a multiple-dose pharmacokinetic study conducted with the syrup formulation in paediatric poor metaboliser subjects 2- to 11-year old diagnosed with allergic rhinitis. The exposure (AUC) to desloratadine was about 6-fold higher and the C_{max} was about 3 to 4 fold higher at 3-6 hours with a terminal half-life of approximately 120 hours. Exposure was the same in adult and paediatric poor metabolisers when treated with age-appropriate doses. The overall safety profile of these subjects was not different from that of the general population. The effects of Neoclarityn syrup in poor metabolizers < 2 years of age have not been studied.

Desloratadine is moderately bound (83 % - 87 %) to plasma proteins. There is no evidence of clinically relevant active substance accumulation following once daily adult and adolescent dosing of desloratadine (5 mg to 20 mg) for 14 days.

In a single dose, crossover study of desloratadine, the tablet and the syrup formulations were found to be bioequivalent.

In separate single dose studies, at the recommended doses, paediatric patients had comparable AUC and C_{max} values of desloratadine to those in adults who received a 5 mg dose of desloratadine syrup.

The enzyme responsible for the metabolism of desloratadine has not been identified yet, and therefore, some interactions with other medicinal products can not be fully excluded. Desloratadine does not inhibit CYP3A4 *in vivo*, and *in vitro* studies have shown that the drug does not inhibit CYP2D6 and is neither a substrate nor an inhibitor of P-glycoprotein.

In a single dose trial using a 7.5 mg dose of desloratadine, there was no effect of food (high-fat, high caloric breakfast) on the disposition of desloratadine. In another study, grapefruit juice had no effect on the disposition of desloratadine.

5.3 Preclinical safety data

Desloratadine is the primary active metabolite of loratadine. Preclinical studies conducted with desloratadine and loratadine demonstrated that there are no qualitative or quantitative differences in the toxicity profile of desloratadine and loratadine at comparable levels of exposure to desloratadine.

Preclinical data with desloratadine reveal no special hazard for humans based on conventional studies of safety pharmacology, repeated dose toxicity, genotoxicity, and toxicity to reproduction. The lack of carcinogenic potential was demonstrated in studies conducted with loratadine.

6. PHARMACEUTICAL PARTICULARS

6.1 List of excipients

Propylene glycol,

sorbitol,

citric acid anhydrous,

sodium citrate,

sodium benzoate,

disodium edetate,

purified water,

sucrose,

natural and artificial flavour (bubblegum),

orange colour E110.

6.2 Incompatibilities

Not applicable.

6.3 Shelf life

2 years

6.4 Special precautions for storage

Do not store above 30°C. Store in the original package.

6.5 Nature and contents of container

Neoclarityn syrup is supplied in bottles of 30, 50, 60, 100, 120, 150, 225, and 300 ml in type III amber glass bottles closed with a childproof polypropylene cap. The caps have a liner made of Low Density Polyethylene (LDPE), polyethylene foam, ethylenevinylacetate (EVA), and polyvinylidene chloride (PvDC). LDPE is the product contact surface.

Supplied with a rigid, transparent, polystyrene measuring spoon, calibrated at 2.5 ml and 5 ml.

Not all pack sizes may be marketed.

6.6 Instructions for use and handling

No special requirements.

7. MARKETING AUTHORISATION HOLDER

SP Europe

Rue de Stalle 73

B-1180 Brussels

Belgium

8. MARKETING AUTHORISATION NUMBER(S)

EU1/00/161/014-21

9. DATE OF FIRST AUTHORISATION/RENEWAL OF THE AUTHORISATION

16th April 2002

10. DATE OF REVISION OF THE TEXT

10th January 2005

11. LEGAL CATEGORY

Prescription Only Medicine

Neoclarityn Syrup/01-05/8

Neoclarityn 5 mg film-coated tablets

(Schering-Plough Ltd)

1. NAME OF THE MEDICINAL PRODUCT

Neoclarityn▼ 5 mg film-coated tablets

2. QUALITATIVE AND QUANTITATIVE COMPOSITION

Each tablet contains 5 mg desloratadine.

For excipients, see section 6.1.

3. PHARMACEUTICAL FORM

Film-coated tablets

4. CLINICAL PARTICULARS

4.1 Therapeutic indications

Neoclarityn is indicated for the relief of symptoms associated with:

- allergic rhinitis (AR)
- chronic idiopathic urticaria (CIU)

4.2 Posology and method of administration

Adults and adolescents (12 years of age and over): one tablet once a day, with or without a meal.

4.3 Contraindications

Hypersensitivity to the active substance, to any of the excipients, or to loratadine.

4.4 Special warnings and special precautions for use

Efficacy and safety of Neoclarityn tablets in children under 12 years of age have not been established.

In the case of severe renal insufficiency, Neoclarityn should be used with caution (see section 5.2).

4.5 Interaction with other medicinal products and other forms of Interaction

No clinically relevant interactions were observed in clinical trials with desloratadine tablets in which erythromycin or ketoconazole were co-administered (see section 5.1).

In a clinical pharmacology trial Neoclarityn taken concomitantly with alcohol did not potentiate the performance impairing effects of alcohol (see section 5.1).

4.6 Pregnancy and lactation

Desloratadine was not teratogenic in animal studies. The safe use of the drug during pregnancy has not been established. The use of Neoclarityn during pregnancy is therefore not recommended.

Desloratadine is excreted into breast milk, therefore the use of Neoclarityn is not recommended in breast-feeding women.

4.7 Effects on ability to drive and use machines

In clinical trials that assessed the driving ability, no impairment occurred in patients receiving desloratadine. However, patients should be informed that very rarely some people experience drowsiness, which may affect their ability to drive or use machines.

4.8 Undesirable effects

In clinical trials in a range of indications including AR and CIU, at the recommended dose of 5 mg daily, undesirable effects with Neoclarityn were reported in 3 % of patients in excess of those treated with placebo. The most frequent of adverse events reported in excess of placebo were fatigue (1.2 %), dry mouth (0.8 %) and headache (0.6 %). Other undesirable effects reported very rarely during the post-marketing period are listed in the following table.

Nervous system disorders	Dizziness, somnolence, insomnia
Cardiac disorders	Tachycardia, palpitations

Gastrointestinal disorders	Abdominal pain, nausea, vomiting, dyspepsia, diarrhoea
Hepato-biliary disorders	Elevations of liver enzymes, increased bilirubin, hepatitis
Musculoskeletal and connective tissue disorders	Myalgia
General disorders	Hypersensitivity reactions (such as anaphylaxis, angioedema, dyspnoea, pruritus, rash, and urticaria)

4.9 Overdose
In the event of overdose, consider standard measures to remove unabsorbed active substance. Symptomatic and supportive treatment is recommended.

Based on a multiple dose clinical trial, in which up to 45 mg of desloratadine was administered (nine times the clinical dose), no clinically relevant effects were observed.

Desloratadine is not eliminated by haemodialysis; it is not known if it is eliminated by peritoneal dialysis.

5. PHARMACOLOGICAL PROPERTIES
5.1 Pharmacodynamic properties
Pharmacotherapeutic group: antihistamines – H_1 antagonist, ATC code: R06A X27

Desloratadine is a non-sedating, long-acting histamine antagonist with selective peripheral H_1-receptor antagonist activity. After oral administration, desloratadine selectively blocks peripheral histamine H_1-receptors because the substance is excluded from entry to the central nervous system.

Desloratadine has demonstrated antiallergic properties from *in vitro* studies. These include inhibiting the release of proinflammatory cytokines such as IL-4, IL-6, IL-8, and IL-13 from human mast cells/basophils, as well as inhibition of the expression of the adhesion molecule P-selectin on endothelial cells. The clinical relevance of these observations remains to be confirmed.

In a multiple dose clinical trial, in which up to 20 mg of desloratadine was administered daily for 14 days, no statistically or clinically relevant cardiovascular effect was observed. In a clinical pharmacology trial, in which desloratadine was administered at a dose of 45 mg daily (nine times the clinical dose) for ten days, no prolongation of QTc interval was seen.

No clinically relevant changes in desloratadine plasma concentrations were observed in multiple-dose ketoconazole and erythromycin interaction trials.

Desloratadine does not readily penetrate the central nervous system. In controlled clinical trials, at the recommended dose of 5 mg daily, there was no excess incidence of somnolence as compared to placebo. Neoclarityn given at a single daily dose of 7.5 mg did not affect psychomotor performance in clinical trials. In a single dose study performed in adults, desloratadine 5 mg did not affect standard measures of flight performance including exacerbation of subjective sleepiness or tasks related to flying.

In clinical pharmacology trials, co-administration with alcohol did not increase the alcohol-induced impairment in performance or increase in sleepiness. No significant differences were found in the psychomotor test results between desloratadine and placebo groups, whether administered alone or with alcohol.

In patients with AR, Neoclarityn was effective in relieving symptoms such as sneezing, nasal discharge and itching, as well as ocular itching, tearing and redness, and itching of palate. Neoclarityn effectively controlled symptoms for 24 hours. Efficacy has not been clearly demonstrated in patients 12–17 years of age.

In two placebo-controlled six week trials in patients with CIU, Neoclarityn was effective in relieving pruritus and decreasing the size and number of hives by the end of the first dosing interval. In each trial, the effects were sustained over the 24 hour dosing interval. As with other antihistamine trials in CIU, the minority of patients who were identified as non-responsive to antihistamines was excluded. An improvement in pruritus of more than 50 % was observed in 55 % of patients treated with desloratadine compared with 19 % of patients treated with placebo. Treatment with Neoclarityn also significantly reduced interference with sleep and daytime function, as measured by a four-point scale used to assess these variables.

Neoclarityn was effective in alleviating the burden of seasonal allergic rhinitis (SAR) as shown by the total score of the rhino-conjunctivitis quality of life questionnaire. The greatest amelioration was seen in the domains of practical problems and daily activities limited by symptoms.

5.2 Pharmacokinetic properties
Desloratadine plasma concentrations can be detected within 30 minutes of administration. Desloratadine is well absorbed with maximum concentration achieved after approximately 3 hours; the terminal phase half-life is approximately 27 hours. The degree of accumulation of desloratadine was consistent with its half-life (approximately 27 hours) and a once daily dosing frequency. The bioavailability of desloratadine was dose proportional over the range of 5 mg to 20 mg.

In a pharmacokinetic trial in which patient demographics were comparable to those of the general SAR population, 4 % of the subjects achieved a higher concentration of desloratadine. This percentage may vary according to ethnic background. Maximum desloratadine concentration was about 3-fold higher at approximately 7 hours with a terminal phase half-life of approximately 89 hours. The safety profile of these subjects was not different from that of the general population.

Desloratadine is moderately bound (83 % - 87 %) to plasma proteins. There is no evidence of clinically relevant drug accumulation following once daily dosing of desloratadine (5 mg to 20 mg) for 14 days.

The enzyme responsible for the metabolism of desloratadine has not been identified yet, and therefore, some interactions with other drugs can not be fully excluded. Desloratadine does not inhibit CYP3A4 *in vivo,* and *in vitro* studies have shown that the drug does not inhibit CYP2D6 and is neither a substrate nor an inhibitor of P-glycoprotein.

In a single dose trial using a 7.5 mg dose of desloratadine, there was no effect of food (high-fat, high caloric breakfast) on the disposition of desloratadine. In another study, grapefruit juice had no effect on the disposition of desloratadine.

5.3 Preclinical safety data
Desloratadine is the primary active metabolite of loratadine. Preclinical studies conducted with desloratadine and loratadine demonstrated that there are no qualitative or quantitative differences in the toxicity profile of desloratadine and loratadine at comparable levels of exposure to desloratadine.

Preclinical data with desloratadine reveal no special hazard for humans based on conventional studies of safety pharmacology, repeated dose toxicity, genotoxicity, and toxicity to reproduction. The lack of carcinogenic potential was demonstrated in studies conducted with loratadine.

6. PHARMACEUTICAL PARTICULARS
6.1 List of excipients
Tablet core: calcium hydrogen phosphate dihydrate, microcrystalline cellulose, maize starch, talc.

Tablet coating: film coat (containing lactose monohydrate, hypromellose, titanium dioxide, macrogol 400, indigotin (E132)), clear coat (containing hypromellose, macrogol 400), carnauba wax, white wax.

6.2 Incompatibilities
Not applicable.

6.3 Shelf life
2 years

6.4 Special precautions for storage
Do not store above 30°C.

Store in the original package.

6.5 Nature and contents of container
Neoclarityn is supplied in unit dose blisters comprised of laminant blister film with foil lidding.

The materials of the blister consist of a polychlorotrifluoroethylene (PCTFE)/Polyvinyl Chloride (PVC) film (product contact surface) with an aluminium foil lidding coated with a vinyl heat seal coat (product contact surface) which is heat sealed.

Packs of 1, 2, 3, 5, 7, 10, 14, 15, 20, 21, 30, 50, 100 tablets.

Not all pack sizes may be marketed.

6.6 Instructions for use and handling
No special requirements.

7. MARKETING AUTHORISATION HOLDER
SP Europe

Rue de Stalle 73

B-1180 Brussels

Belgium

8. MARKETING AUTHORISATION NUMBER(S)
EU/1/00/161/001-013

9. DATE OF FIRST AUTHORISATION/RENEWAL OF THE AUTHORISATION
15 January 2001

10. DATE OF REVISION OF THE TEXT
10 January 2005

11. LEGAL CATEGORY
Prescription Only Medicine

Neoclarityn/1-05/8

Neo-Cytamen Injection 1000mcg

(UCB Pharma Limited)

1. NAME OF THE MEDICINAL PRODUCT
Neo-Cytamen Injection 1000mcg

2. QUALITATIVE AND QUANTITATIVE COMPOSITION
Hydroxocobalamin chloride 1.027mg equivalent to 1.0 mg Hydroxocobalamin.

For excipients, see 6.1

3. PHARMACEUTICAL FORM
Solution for injection.

4. CLINICAL PARTICULARS
4.1 Therapeutic indications
Addisonian pernicious anaemia.

Prophylaxis and treatment of other macrocytic anaemias associated with vitamin B_{12} deficiency.

Tobacco amblyopia and Leber's optic atrophy.

4.2 Posology and method of administration
Route of administration: Intramuscular.

Adults and Children

Addisonian pernicious anaemia and other macrocytic anaemias without neurological involvement:

Initially: 250 to 1000mcg intramuscularly on alternate days for one to two weeks, then 250mcg weekly until the blood count is normal.

Maintenance: 1000mcg every two to three months.

Addisonian pernicious anaemia and other macrocytic anaemias with neurological involvement:

Initially: 1000mcg on alternate days as long as improvement is occurring.

Maintenance: 1000mcg every two months.

Prophylaxis of macrocytic anaemia associated with vitamin B_{12} deficiency resulting from gastrectomy, some malabsorption syndromes and strict vegetarianism:

1000mcg every two to three months.

Tobacco amblyopia and Leber's optic atrophy:

Initially: 1000mcg or more daily by intramuscular injection for two weeks. Then twice weekly as long as improvement is occurring.

Maintenance: 1000mcg monthly.

4.3 Contraindications
Hypersensitivity to any ingredient of the preparation.

Hydroxocobalamin should not be used for treatment of megaloblastic anaemia of pregnancy unless vitamin B12 deficiency has been demonstrated.

4.4 Special warnings and special precautions for use
Precautions:

The dosage schemes given above are usually satisfactory, but regular examination of the blood is advisable. If megaloblastic anaemia fails to respond to hydroxocobalamin, folate metabolism should be investigated. Doses in excess of 10mcg daily may produce a haematological response in patients with folate deficiency. Indiscriminate administration may mask the true diagnosis. The haematological and neurological state should be monitored regularly to ensure adequacy of therapy. Cardiac arrhythmias secondary to hypokalaemia during initial therapy have been reported. Plasma potassium should therefore be monitored during this period.

4.5 Interaction with other medicinal products and other forms of Interaction
Chloramphenicol-treated patients may respond poorly to hydroxocobalamin. Serum concentrations of hydroxocobalamin may be lowered by oral contraceptives but this interaction is unlikely to have clinical significance. Antimetabolites and most antibiotics invalidate vitamin B_{12} assays by microbiological techniques.

4.6 Pregnancy and lactation
Hydroxocobalamin should not be used for the treatment of megaloblastic anaemia of pregnancy unless vitamin B_{12} deficiency has been demonstrated. Hydroxocobalamin is secreted into breast milk but this is unlikely to harm the infant, and may be beneficial if the mother and infant are vitamin B_{12} deficient.

4.7 Effects on ability to drive and use machines
None stated.

4.8 Undesirable effects
The following effects have been reported and are listed below by body system:

Cardiovascular disorders:

Arrhythmias secondary to hypokalaemia.

Disorders of the immune system:

Hypersensitivity reactions including skin reactions (e.g. rash, itching) and exceptionally anaphylaxis.

Gastro intestinal disorders:

Nausea, vomiting, diarrhoea.

General disorders:

Fever, chills, hot flushing, dizziness, malaise, pain including pain at injection site.

Neurological disorders:

Headache, sensory abnormalities such as paraesthesiae.

Skin and subcutaneous tissue disorders:

Acneiform and bullous eruptions.

4.9 Overdose
Treatment is unlikely to be needed in cases of overdosage.

5. PHARMACOLOGICAL PROPERTIES

5.1 Pharmacodynamic properties
Hydroxocobalamin isone of the forms of vitamin B_{12}.

5.2 Pharmacokinetic properties
An intramuscular injection of hydroxocobalamin produces higher serum levels than the same dose of cyanocobalamin, and these levels are well maintained.

After injection of hydroxocobalamin, 90% of a 100 microgram dose and 30% of a 1000 microgram dose are retained. Vitamin B12 is extensively bound to specific plasma proteins called transcobalamins; transcobalamin II appears to be involved in the rapid transport of the cobalamins to tissues. Vitamin B12 is stored in the liver, excreted in the bile, and undergoes extensive enterohepatic recycling; part of an administered dose is excreted in the urine, most of it in the first 8 hours; urinary excretion, however, accounts for only a small fraction in the reduction of total body stores acquired by dietary means. Vitamin B12 diffuses across the placenta and also appears in breast milk.

5.3 Preclinical safety data
None stated.

6. PHARMACEUTICAL PARTICULARS

6.1 List of excipients
Sodium chloride, acetic acid, Water for Injections.

6.2 Incompatibilities
None.

6.3 Shelf life
36 months.

6.4 Special precautions for storage
Protect from light. Do not store above 25°C.

6.5 Nature and contents of container
1ml glass ampoules in packs of 5.

6.6 Instructions for use and handling
Not applicable.

7. MARKETING AUTHORISATION HOLDER
UCB Pharma Limited
208 Bath Road
Slough
Berkshire
SL1 3WE
UK

8. MARKETING AUTHORISATION NUMBER(S)
PL 00039/0405

9. DATE OF FIRST AUTHORISATION/RENEWAL OF THE AUTHORISATION
14 October 1992 / October 1997/October 2002

10. DATE OF REVISION OF THE TEXT
June 2005

POM

NeoMercazole 5 and NeoMercazole 20
(Amdipharm)

1. NAME OF THE MEDICINAL PRODUCT
NeoMercazole® 5 and NeoMercazole 20

2. QUALITATIVE AND QUANTITATIVE COMPOSITION
Each NeoMercazole 5 tablet contains carbimazole Ph. Eur. 5mg and each NeoMercazole 20 tablet contains carbimazole Ph.Eur. 20mg.

3. PHARMACEUTICAL FORM
Tablet

Pink, circular biconvex tablet, imprinted with Neo/5 on the obverse and plain on the reverse.

Pink, circular biconvex tablet, imprinted with Neo/20 on the obverse and plain on the reverse.

4. CLINICAL PARTICULARS

4.1 Therapeutic indications
NeoMercazole is an anti-thyroid agent. It is indicated in all conditions where reduction of thyroid function is required.

1. Hyperthyroidism.
2. Preparation for thyroidectomy in hyperthyroidism.
3. Preparation for, and as concomitant therapy with, radio-iodine treatment.

4.2 Posology and method of administration
Adults

The initial dose is in the range 20 - 60mg, taken as two to three divided doses. This is continued until the patient is euthyroid. Subsequent therapy may then be administered in one of two ways.

Maintenance regimen: Dosage is gradually reduced so as to maintain a euthyroid state. Final dosage is usually in the range 5 - 15mg per day, which may be taken as a single daily dose. Therapy should be continued for at least six, and up to eighteen months.

Blocking-replacement regimen: Dosage is maintained at the initial level, i.e. 20 - 60mg per day, and supplemental l-thyroxine, 50 - 150mcg per day, is administered concomitantly, in order to prevent hypothyroidism. Therapy should be continued for at least six months, and up to eighteen months.

Where a single dosage of less than 20mg is recommended, it is intended that NeoMercazole 5 should be taken.

Elderly
No special dosage regimen is required, but care should be taken to observe the contra-indications and warnings.

Children
The usual initial daily dose is 15mg per day.

4.3 Contraindications
NeoMercazole is contra-indicated in patients with a previous history of adverse reactions to carbimazole.

4.4 Special warnings and special precautions for use
Patients should be warned about the onset of sore throats, mouth ulcers, pyrexia, or other symptoms which might suggest the early development of bone marrow depression. In such cases it is important that drug treatment is stopped and medical advice sought immediately. In such patients, blood cell counts should be performed, particularly where there is any clinical evidence of infection. Early withdrawal of the drug will increase the chance of complete recovery.

NeoMercazole should be used with caution in patients with liver disorders.

NeoMercazole should be stopped temporarily at the time of administration of radio-iodine.

The use of carbimazole in non-pregnant women of childbearing potential should be based on individual risk/benefit assessment (see section *4.6*).

4.5 Interaction with other medicinal products and other forms of Interaction
None.

4.6 Pregnancy and lactation
Carbimazole crosses the placenta but, provided the mother's dose is within the standard range, and her thyroid status is monitored, there is no evidence of neonatal thyroid abnormalities. Studies have shown that the incidence of congenital malformations is greater in the children of mothers whose hyperthyroidism has remained untreated than in those to whom treatment with carbimazole has been given. However, very rare cases of congenital malformations have been observed following the use of carbimazole or its active metabolite methimazole during pregnancy. A causal relationship of these malformations, especially choanal atresia and aplasia cutis congenita, to transplacental exposure to carbimazole and methimazole cannot be excluded. Therefore, the use of carbimazole in non-pregnant women of childbearing potential should be based on individual risk/benefit assessment (see section *4.4*). The dose of NeoMercazole must be regulated by the patient's clinical condition. The lowest dose possible should be used, and this can often be discontinued three to four weeks before term, in order to reduce the risk of neonatal complications. The blocking-replacement regimen should not be used during pregnancy since very little thyroxine crosses the placenta in the last trimester.

NeoMercazole is secreted in breast milk and, if treatment is continued during lactation, the patient should not continue to breast-feed her baby.

4.7 Effects on ability to drive and use machines
None.

4.8 Undesirable effects
Adverse reactions usually occur in the first eight weeks of treatment. The most frequently occurring reactions are nausea, headache, arthralgia, mild gastric distress, skin rashes and pruritus. These reactions are usually self-limiting and may not require withdrawal of the drug.

Blood and lymphatic system disorders

Bone marrow depression has been reported and can lead to agranulocytosis. Rare cases of pancytopenia/aplastic anaemia and isolated thrombocytopenia have also been reported. Additionally, very rare cases of haemolytic anaemia have been reported.

Patients should always be instructed to recognise symptoms which may suggest bone marrow depression, to stop the drug and to seek medical advice immediately. In such patients, blood cell counts should be performed, particularly where there is any clinical evidence of infection.

Nervous system disorders

Headache.

Gastro-intestinal system disorders

Nausea, mild gastric distress.

Hepato-biliary system disorders

Hepatic disorders, most commonly jaundice, have been reported; in these cases carbimazole should be withdrawn.

Skin and subcutaneous tissue disorders

Skin rashes, pruritus, urticaria. Hair loss has been occasionally reported.

Musculoskeletal system disorders

Isolated cases of myopathy have been reported. Patients experiencing myalgia after the intake of NeoMercazole should have their creatine phosphokinase levels monitored.

4.9 Overdose
No symptoms are likely from a single large dose, and so no specific treatment is indicated.

5. PHARMACOLOGICAL PROPERTIES

5.1 Pharmacodynamic properties
Carbimazole is a thyroid reducing agent.

5.2 Pharmacokinetic properties
Carbimazole is rapidly metabolised to methimazole. The mean peak plasma concentration of methimazole is reported to occur one hour after a single dose of carbimazole. The apparent plasma half-life of methimazole is reported as 6.4 hours.

5.3 Preclinical safety data
Not relevant.

6. PHARMACEUTICAL PARTICULARS

6.1 List of excipients
Lactose, Starch Maize, Gelatin, Magnesium Stearate, Sucrose, Acacia, Talc, Red Iron Oxide (E172). Microcrystalline Cellulose (NeoMercazole 20 only).

6.2 Incompatibilities
None known.

6.3 Shelf life
5 years.

6.4 Special precautions for storage
Do not store above 25°C. Store in the original container.

6.5 Nature and contents of container
NeoMercazole tablets are available in HDPE bottles with a low density polyethylene tamper evident snap-fit closure. Each bottle contains 100 tablets.

6.6 Instructions for use and handling
No special requirements.

7. MARKETING AUTHORISATION HOLDER
Amdipharm Plc
Regency House
Miles Gray Road
Basildon
Essex
SS14 3AF
United Kingdom

8. MARKETING AUTHORISATION NUMBER(S)
NeoMercazole 5: PL 20072/0013
NeoMercazole 20: PL 20072/0014

9. DATE OF FIRST AUTHORISATION/RENEWAL OF THE AUTHORISATION
NeoMercazole 5: 31 May 2004
NeoMercazole 20: 31 May 2004

10. DATE OF REVISION OF THE TEXT

Neoral Soft Gelatin Capsules, Neoral Oral Solution
(Novartis Pharmaceuticals UK Ltd)

1. NAME OF THE MEDICINAL PRODUCT
NEORAL® Soft Gelatin Capsules and NEORAL Oral Solution (ciclosporin*, also known as ciclosporin A) - Immunosuppressive agent

*INN rec.

2. QUALITATIVE AND QUANTITATIVE COMPOSITION
NEORAL Soft Gelatin Capsules containing 10, 25, 50, or 100mg ciclosporin.

NEORAL Oral Solution containing 100mg ciclosporin/mL

3. PHARMACEUTICAL FORM
NEORAL Soft Gelatin Capsules and NEORAL Oral Solution are for oral administration.

NEORAL is an improved pharmaceutical form of the active ingredient ciclosporin. NEORAL is a pre-concentrate formulation of ciclosporin which undergoes a microemulsification process in the presence of water, either in the form of a beverage or in the form of the gastrointestinal fluid. NEORAL reduces the intra-patient variability of pharmacokinetic parameters, with a more consistent absorption profile and less influence of concomitant food intake and the presence of bile. In pharmacokinetic and clinical studies it has been demonstrated that the correlation between trough concentration (Cmin) and total exposure (AUC) is significantly stronger when ciclosporin is given as NEORAL than when it is given as SANDIMMUN. NEORAL therefore allows greater predictability and consistency of ciclosporin exposure.

4. CLINICAL PARTICULARS

4.1 Therapeutic indications

Transplantation indications

Organ transplantation

Prevention of graft rejection following kidney, liver, heart, combined heart-lung, lung or pancreas transplants.

Treatment of transplant rejection in patients previously receiving other immunosuppressive agents.

Bone marrow transplantation

Prevention of graft rejection following bone marrow transplantation and prophylaxis of graft-versus-host disease (GVHD).

Treatment of established graft-versus-host disease (GVHD).

Non-transplantation indications

Psoriasis

NEORAL Soft Gelatin Capsules and NEORAL Oral Solution are indicated in patients with severe psoriasis in whom conventional therapy is ineffective or inappropriate.

Atopic dermatitis

NEORAL Soft Gelatin Capsules and NEORAL Oral Solution are indicated for the short term treatment (8 weeks) of patients with severe atopic dermatitis in whom conventional therapy is ineffective or inappropriate.

Rheumatoid arthritis

NEORAL Soft Gelatin Capsules and NEORAL Oral Solution are indicated for the treatment of severe, active rheumatoid arthritis in patients in whom classical, slow-acting anti-rheumatic agents are inappropriate or ineffective.

Nephrotic syndrome

NEORAL Soft Gelatin Capsules and NEORAL Oral Solution are indicated for the treatment of steroid dependent or steroid resistant nephrotic syndrome (associated with adverse prognostic features) due to minimal change glomerulonephritis, focal segmental glomerulosclerosis or membranous glomerulonephritis in both adults and children.

4.2 Posology and method of administration

Dosage

Following initiation of treatment with NEORAL, due to the different bioavailabilities of the different oral ciclosporin formulations, patients should not be transferred to any other oral formulation of ciclosporin without appropriate monitoring of ciclosporin blood concentrations, serum creatinine levels and blood pressure. This does not apply to the conversion between NEORAL Soft Gelatin Capsules and NEORAL Oral Solution as these two forms are bioequivalent.

Due to the differences in bioavailability between different oral formulations of ciclosporin, it is important that prescribers, pharmacists and patients be aware that substitution of NEORAL with any other oral formulation of ciclosporin is not recommended as this may lead to alterations in ciclosporin blood levels. For this reason it may be appropriate to prescribe by brand.

Transplantation indications

Organ transplantation

Treatment with NEORAL Soft Gelatin Capsules or NEORAL Oral Solution should be initiated within 12 hours before transplantation at a dose of 10 to 15mg/kg body weight given in two divided doses.

As a general rule, treatment should continue at a dose of 10 to 15mg/kg per day given in two divided doses for one to two weeks post-operatively. Dosage should then be gradually reduced until a maintenance dose of about 2 to 6mg/kg per day is reached. This total daily dose should be given in two divided doses. Dosage should be adjusted by monitoring ciclosporin trough levels and kidney function (see **ADMINISTRATION AND PRECAUTIONS**).

When NEORAL is given with other immunosuppressants (e.g. with corticosteroids or as part of a triple or quadruple drug therapy), lower doses (e.g. 3 to 6mg/kg per day given orally in two divided doses) may be used for the initial treatment. For trough level monitoring, whole blood is preferred, measured by a specific analytical method. Target trough concentration ranges depend on organ type, time after transplantation and immunosuppressive regimen.

The use of SANDIMMUN Concentrate for Intravenous Infusion is recommended only in organ transplant patients who are unable to take SANDIMMUN/NEORAL orally (e.g. shortly after surgery) or in whom the absorption of the oral forms might be impaired such as during episodes of gastrointestinal disturbances. It is recommended, however, that patients be transferred to NEORAL therapy as soon as the given circumstances allow (please refer to SANDIMMUN data sheet/SmPC for prescribing information on SANDIMMUN Concentrate for I.V. Infusion).

Bone marrow transplantation/prevention and treatment of graft-versus-host-disease (GVHD)

SANDIMMUN Concentrate for Intravenous Infusion is usually preferred for initiation of therapy, although NEORAL Soft Gelatin Capsules or NEORAL Oral Solution may be used (please refer to SANDIMMUN data sheet/SmPC for prescribing information on SANDIMMUN Concentrate for I.V. Infusion).

Maintenance treatment should continue using NEORAL Soft Gelatin Capsules or NEORAL Oral Solution at a dosage of 12.5mg/kg per day, given in two divided doses, for at least three and preferably six months before tailing off to zero. In some cases it may not be possible to withdraw NEORAL until a year after bone marrow transplantation. Higher doses of NEORAL or the use of SANDIMMUN Concentrate for Intravenous Infusion may be necessary in the presence of gastro-intestinal disturbances which might decrease absorption.

If NEORAL Soft Gelatin Capsules or NEORAL Oral Solution are used to initiate therapy, the recommended dose is 12.5 to 15mg/kg per day, given in two divided doses, starting on the day before transplantation.

If GVHD develops after NEORAL is withdrawn it should respond to reinstitution of therapy. Low doses of NEORAL should be used for mild, chronic GVHD.

Non-transplantation indications

Psoriasis

*(Refer also to **Additional precautions in psoriasis and atopic dermatitis section**)*

Due to the variability of this condition, treatment must be individualised. To induce remission, the recommended initial dose of NEORAL is 2.5mg/kg a day given orally in two divided doses. If there is no improvement after 1 month, the daily dose may be gradually increased, but should not exceed 5mg/kg. Treatment should be discontinued if sufficient response is not achieved within 6 weeks on a daily basis of 5mg/kg per day, or if the effective dose is not compatible with the safety guidelines given below (see **PRECAUTIONS**). Initial doses of 5mg/kg per day of NEORAL are justified in patients whose condition requires rapid improvement.

For *maintenance treatment*, NEORAL dosage must be individually titrated to the lowest effective level, and the dosage should not exceed 5mg/kg per day, given orally in two divided doses. Some clinical data are available which provide evidence that once satisfactory response is achieved, NEORAL may be discontinued and subsequent relapse managed with re-introduction of NEORAL at the previous effective dose. In some patients continuous maintenance therapy may be necessary.

Atopic dermatitis

*(Refer also to **Additional precautions in atopic dermatitis section**)*

The recommended dose range for NEORAL is 2.5-5mg/kg per day given orally in two divided doses for a maximum of 8 weeks. If a starting dose of 2.5mg/kg/day does not achieve a good initial response within 2 weeks the dose may be rapidly increased to a maximum of 5mg/kg per day. In very severe cases rapid and adequate control of disease is more likely with a starting dose of 5mg/kg per day, given orally in two divided doses.

Rheumatoid arthritis

*(Refer also to **Additional precautions in rheumatoid arthritis section**)*

It is recommended that initiation of NEORAL therapy should take place over a period of 12 weeks. For the first 6 weeks of treatment, the recommended dose is 2.5mg/kg per day, given orally in two divided doses. If the clinical effect is considered insufficient, the daily dose may be increased gradually as tolerability permits, but should not exceed 4mg/kg per day.

If, after 3 months of treatment at the maximum permitted or tolerable dose the response is considered inadequate, treatment should be discontinued.

For maintenance treatment the dose has to be titrated individually according to tolerability.

NEORAL can be given in combination with low-dose corticosteroids. Pharmacodynamic interactions can occur between ciclosporin and NSAIDs and therefore this combination should be used with care (see ***Additional precautions in rheumatoid arthritis section*** and **INTERACTIONS WITH OTHER MEDICAMENTS AND OTHER FORMS OF INTERACTIONS section**).

Long-term data on the use of ciclosporin in the treatment of rheumatoid arthritis are still limited. Therefore, it is recommended that patients are re-evaluated after 6 months of maintenance treatment and therapy only continued if the benefits of treatment outweigh the risks.

Nephrotic syndrome

*(Refer also to **Additional precautions in nephrotic syndrome section**)*

To induce remission, the recommended dose is 5mg/kg per day given orally in two divided doses for adults and 6mg/kg per day given orally in two divided doses for children if, with the exception of proteinuria, renal function is normal. In patients with impaired renal function, the initial dose should not exceed 2.5mg/kg per day orally.

In focal segmental glomerulosclerosis, the combination of NEORAL and low dose corticosteroids may be of benefit.

In the absence of efficacy after 3 months treatment for minimal change glomerulonephritis and focal segmental glomerulosclerosis or 6 months treatment for membranous glomerulonephritis, NEORAL therapy should be discontinued.

For maintenance treatment the maximum recommended dose is 5mg/kg per day orally in adults or 6mg/kg per day orally in children. The doses need to be slowly reduced individually according to efficacy (proteinuria) and safety (primarily serum creatinine), to the lowest effective level.

Long-term data of ciclosporin in the treatment of nephrotic syndrome are limited. However, in clinical trials patients have received treatment for 1 to 2 years. Long-term treatment may be considered if there has been a significant reduction in proteinuria with preservation of creatinine clearance and provided adequate precautions are taken (see ***Additional precautions in nephrotic syndrome section***).

Conversion of transplant patients from SANDIMMUN Soft Gelatin Capsules or Oral Solution to NEORAL

Ciclosporin absorption from SANDIMMUN oral formulations is highly variable and the relationship between SANDIMMUN dose and ciclosporin exposure (AUC) is non-linear. In contrast with NEORAL the absorption of ciclosporin is less variable and the correlation between ciclosporin trough concentrations and exposure is much stronger than with SANDIMMUN.

For converting patients from SANDIMMUN to NEORAL an initial mg for mg conversion from SANDIMMUN to NEORAL is recommended with subsequent dose titration if required. Available data confirm that following this initial mg for mg conversion, comparable trough concentrations of ciclosporin in whole blood are achieved, maintaining adequate immunosuppression. In many patients, higher peak concentrations (Cmax) and an increased exposure to the drug (AUC) may occur. In a small proportion of patients headache and paresthesia may occur during transfer from SANDIMMUN to NEORAL, presumably related to higher exposure to ciclosporin. No additional adverse events, including renal dysfunction, however, were observed due to these changes in pharmacokinetic parameters during long-term treatment. In a small percentage of patients, these changes may be more marked and of clinical significance. Their magnitude depends largely on the individual ability to absorb ciclosporin from the originally used SANDIMMUN. In these patients, dose reduction should be undertaken to achieve the appropriate trough concentration range.

Long-term clinical data in renal transplant patients have demonstrated that a large proportion of patients previously on SANDIMMUN therapy can be maintained at the same dose of NEORAL as with SANDIMMUN.

All patients should be monitored according to the following recommendations:

a) Preconversion (ie on SANDIMMUN): Measure ciclosporin trough concentration, serum creatinine and blood pressure.

b) Day 1: Convert the patient to the same daily dose of NEORAL as was previously used with oral SANDIMMUN (ie on a mg to mg basis).

c) Day 4-7 post conversion: Follow-up visit to measure ciclosporin trough concentration, serum creatinine and blood pressure.

d) Subsequent follow-up: Depending on the findings on review at day 4-7, subsequent follow-up visits may need to be arranged (e.g. week 2 and week 4) in the first 12 week period after conversion to NEORAL. During these visits, ciclosporin trough concentrations, serum creatinine and blood pressure should be measured and dependent on these measurements the dose of NEORAL adjusted accordingly.

Further information on conversion can be obtained via the NEORAL Helpline (01276 698494)

Conversion of non-transplant (i.e. psoriasis, atopic dermatitis, rheumatoid arthritis, nephrotic syndrome) patients from SANDIMMUN Soft Gelatin Capsules or Oral Solution to NEORAL

Ciclosporin absorption from SANDIMMUN oral formulations is highly variable and the relationship between SANDIMMUN dose and ciclosporin exposure (AUC) is non-linear. In contrast with NEORAL the absorption of ciclosporin is less variable.

With equivalent doses following conversion from SANDIMMUN to NEORAL, higher peak concentrations (Cmax) and an increased exposure to the drug (AUC) may occur. In a small percentage of patients, these changes may be more marked and of clinical significance. Their magnitude depends largely on the individual ability to absorb ciclosporin from the originally used SANDIMMUN. Therefore, the clinical status of each patient should be assessed prior to initiating NEORAL therapy.

It is recommended that where any potential loss of efficacy results in considerable risk to the patients (eg. rheumatoid arthritis), conversion from SANDIMMUN to NEORAL is on a mg for mg basis. In other patients, the lowest recommended starting dose of NEORAL is recommended initially with appropriate dose titration according to clinical response, serum creatinine and blood pressure levels.

All patients converting on a mg for mg basis should be monitored according to the following recommendations:-

a) Preconversion (i.e. on SANDIMMUN): Measure serum creatinine and blood pressure.

b) Day 1: Start the patient with the same daily dose of NEORAL as was previously used with oral SANDIMMUN (i.e. on a mg for mg basis).

c) Week 2: Measure serum creatinine and blood pressure and consider reducing the dose of NEORAL if either parameter significantly exceeds the preconversion level.

d) Week 4: Measure serum creatinine and blood pressure and consider reducing the dose of NEORAL if either parameter significantly exceeds the preconversion level.

e) Week 8: Measure serum creatinine and blood pressure and consider reducing the dose of NEORAL if either parameter significantly exceeds the preconversion level.

f) Week 12: Measure serum creatinine and blood pressure and consider reducing the dose of NEORAL if either parameter significantly exceeds the preconversion level.

If, on more than one measurement, the serum creatinine increases more than 30% above the pre-SANDIMMUN baseline, the dose of NEORAL should be decreased (see ***Additional precautions for psoriasis, atopic dermatitis, rheumatoid arthritis and nephrotic syndrome sections***).

Administration

The total daily dosage of NEORAL Soft Gelatin Capsules or NEORAL Oral Solution should always be given in two divided doses. NEORAL Soft Gelatin Capsules should be taken with a mouthful of water and should then be swallowed whole.

NEORAL Oral Solution should be diluted immediately before being taken. For improved taste the solution can be diluted with orange juice or squash or apple juice. However, it may also be taken with water if preferred. It should be stirred well.

NEORAL Oral Solution has a characteristic taste which is distinct to that of SANDIMMUN Oral Solution.

The measuring device should not come into contact with the diluent. The measuring device should not be rinsed with water, alcohol or any other liquid. If it is necessary to clean the measuring device, the outside should be wiped with a dry tissue.

Owing to its possible interference with the P450-dependent enzyme system, grapefruit or grapefruit juice should not be ingested for 1 hour prior to dose administration, and grapefruit juice should not be used as a diluent for the Oral Solution.

Use In The Elderly

There is currently no experience with NEORAL in the elderly. However, no particular problems have been reported following the use of ciclosporin at the recommended dose. However, factors sometimes associated with ageing, in particular impaired renal function, make careful supervision essential and may necessitate dosage adjustment.

Use In Children

There is currently no experience with NEORAL in young children. However, transplant recipients from three months of age have received ciclosporin at the recommended dosage with no particular problems although at dosages above the upper end of the recommended range children seem to be more susceptible to fluid retention, convulsions and hypertension. This responds to dosage reduction.

4.3 Contraindications

Known hypersensitivity to ciclosporin.

NEORAL is contra-indicated in psoriatic and atopic dermatitis patients with abnormal renal function, uncontrolled hypertension, uncontrolled infections or any kind of malignancy other than that of the skin (see **PRECAUTIONS**).

NEORAL is contra-indicated in rheumatoid arthritis patients with abnormal renal function, uncontrolled hypertension, uncontrolled infections or any kind of malignancy.

NEORAL should not be used to treat rheumatoid arthritis in patients under the age of 18 years.

NEORAL is contra-indicated in nephrotic syndrome patients with uncontrolled hypertension, uncontrolled infections, or any kind of malignancy.

Concomitant use of tacrolimus is specifically contra-indicated.

4.4 Special warnings and special precautions for use

Precautions

Ciclosporin can impair renal function. Close monitoring of serum creatinine and urea is required and dosage adjustment may be necessary. Increases in serum creatinine and urea occurring during the first few weeks of ciclosporin therapy are generally dose-dependent and reversible and usually respond to dosage reduction. During long-term treatment, some patients may develop structural changes in the kidney (e.g. interstitial fibrosis) which, in renal transplant recipients, must be distinguished from chronic rejection.

Ciclosporin may also affect liver function and dosage adjustment, based on the results of bilirubin and liver enzyme monitoring, may be necessary.

Ciclosporin enhances the risk of hyperkalaemia, especially in patients with renal dysfunction. Caution is also required when ciclosporin is co-administered with potassium sparing diuretics, angiotensin converting enzyme inhibitors, angiotensin II receptor antagonists and potassium containing drugs as well as in patients on a potassium rich diet. Control of potassium levels in these situations is advisable.

Ciclosporin enhances the clearance of magnesium. This can lead to symptomatic hypomagnesaemia, especially in the peri-transplant period. Control of serum magnesium levels is therefore recommended in the peri-transplant period, particularly in the presence of neurological symptom/signs. If considered necessary, magnesium supplementation should be given.

Caution is required in treating patients with hyperuricaemia.

Ciclosporin increases the risk of malignancies including lymphomas, skin and other tumours. The increased risk appears to be related to the degree and duration of immunosuppression rather than to the specific use of ciclosporin. Hence a treatment regimen containing immunosuppressants should be used with caution as this could lead to lymphoproliferative disorders and solid organ tumours, some with reported fatalities.

Ciclosporin predisposes patients to infection with a variety of pathogens including bacteria, parasites, viruses and other opportunistic pathogens. This appears to be related to the degree and duration of immunosuppression rather than to the specific use of ciclosporin. As this can lead to a fatal outcome, effective pre-emptive and therapeutic strategies should be employed particularly in patients on multiple long-term immunosuppressive therapy.

There are differences in bioavailability between different oral formulations of ciclosporin, however NEORAL Soft Gelatin Capsules are bioequivalent to NEORAL Oral Solution.

Regular monitoring of blood pressure is required during treatment with ciclosporin. If hypertension develops, appropriate anti-hypertensive treatment must be instituted.

Ciclosporin can induce a reversible increase in blood lipids. It is therefore advisable to perform lipid determinations before treatment and thereafter as appropriate.

Ciclosporin may increase the risk of Benign Intracranial Hypertension. Patients presenting with signs of raised intracranial pressure should be investigated and if Benign Intracranial Hypertension is diagnosed, ciclosporin should be withdrawn due to the possible risk of permanent visual loss.

Additional precautions in psoriasis and atopic dermatitis *(see also section 4.2 Posology and Method of Administration)*

Careful dermatological and physical examinations, including measurements of blood pressure and renal function on at least two occasions prior to starting therapy should be performed to establish an accurate baseline status.

Development of malignancies (particularly of the skin) have been reported in psoriatic patients treated with ciclosporin as well as during treatment with conventional therapy. A search for all forms of pre-existing tumours, including those of the skin and cervix should be carried out. Skin lesions which are not typical for psoriasis should be biopsied before starting NEORAL treatment to exclude skin cancers, mycosis fungoides or other pre-malignant disorders. Patients with malignant or pre-malignant alterations of the skin should be treated with NEORAL only after appropriate treatment of such lesions and only if no other option for successful therapy exists.

Because of the possibility of renal dysfunction or renal structural changes, serum creatinine should be measured at two weekly intervals during the first three months of therapy. Thereafter, if creatinine remains stable, measurements should be made at monthly intervals. If serum creatinine increases and remains increased to more than 30% above baseline at more than one measurement, NEORAL dosage must be reduced by 25 to 50%. These recommendations apply even if the patient's values still lie within the laboratory's normal range. If dosage reduction is not successful in reducing levels within one month, NEORAL treatment should be discontinued.

In atopic dermatitis patients serum creatinine should be measured at two weekly intervals throughout the treatment period.

If hypertension develops which cannot be controlled by NEORAL dosage reduction or appropriate antihypertensive therapy, discontinuation of NEORAL is recommended.

NEORAL treatment and its monitoring should be carried out under the supervision of a dermatologist experienced in the management of severe skin diseases.

In view of the potential risk of skin malignancy, patients on NEORAL should be warned to avoid excessive unprotected sun exposure and should not receive concomitant therapeutic ultraviolet B irradiation or PUVA photochemotherapy.

Additional precautions in atopic dermatitis *(see also section 4.2 Posology and Method of Administration)*

Active Herpes simplex infections should be allowed to clear before initiating treatment with NEORAL but are not necessarily a reason for drug withdrawal if they occur during treatment unless infection is severe.

Skin infections with *Staphylococcus aureus* are not an absolute contra-indication for NEORAL therapy but should be controlled with appropriate antibacterial agents. Oral erythromycin, known to have the potential to increase the blood concentration of ciclosporin (see **INTERACTIONS WITH OTHER MEDICAMENTS AND OTHER FORMS OF INTERACTIONS**) should be avoided or, if there is no alternative, its concomitant use must be accompanied by close monitoring of the blood levels of ciclosporin.

There is currently no experience with NEORAL in children with atopic dermatitis. Its use in patients under 16 years of age cannot therefore be recommended.

Additional precautions in rheumatoid arthritis *(see also section 4.2 Posology and Method of Administration)*

Since ciclosporin can impair renal function, a reliable baseline level of serum creatinine should be established by at least two measurements prior to treatment, and serum creatinine should be monitored at 2 weekly intervals during the first 3 months of therapy. Thereafter, measurements can be made every 4 weeks, but more frequent checks are necessary when the NEORAL dose is increased or concomitant treatment with a non-steroidal anti-inflammatory drug is initiated or its dosage increased. Because the pharmacodynamic interaction between ciclosporin and NSAIDs may adversely affect renal function, caution should be exercised if NSAID therapy is to be continued.

If the serum creatinine remains increased by more than 30% above baseline at more than one measurement, the dosage of NEORAL should be reduced. If the serum creatinine increases by more than 50%, a dosage reduction by 50% is mandatory. These recommendations apply even if the patient's values still lie within the laboratory normal range. If dosage reduction is not successful in reducing levels within one month, NEORAL treatment should be discontinued.

Discontinuation of the drug may also become necessary if hypertension developing during NEORAL therapy cannot be controlled by appropriate antihypertensive therapy.

The combination of non-steroidal anti-inflammatory drugs and ciclosporin should be used with caution in patients with rheumatoid arthritis and should be accompanied by particularly close monitoring of renal function as detailed above. (Please also see **INTERACTIONS WITH OTHER MEDICAMENTS AND OTHER FORMS OF INTERACTIONS**).

As hepatotoxicity is a potential side effect of non-steroidal anti-inflammatory drugs, regular monitoring of hepatic function is advised when NEORAL is co-administered with these drugs in rheumatoid arthritis patients.

The use of ciclosporin therapy for the treatment of patients with rheumatoid arthritis requires careful monitoring and follow-up. NEORAL should only be used provided that the necessary expertise and adequate equipment, laboratory and supportive medical resources are available.

Patients with rheumatoid arthritis have an increased incidence of malignancies compared to the general population. Use of disease modifying drugs increases the risk of malignancy further. The use of ciclosporin in the treatment of rheumatoid arthritis has not been shown to increase the incidence of malignancies more than other disease-modifying drugs.

Additional precautions in nephrotic syndrome *(see also section 4.2 Posology and Method of Administration)*

Development of malignancies, (including Hodgkin's lymphoma) has occasionally been reported in nephrotic syndrome patients treated with ciclosporin, as well as during treatment with other immunosuppressive agents. However, malignancy may be related to the pathogenesis of the disease.

Since ciclosporin can impair renal function, it is necessary to assess renal function frequently and if the serum creatinine remains increased by more than 30% above baseline at more than one measurement, to reduce the dosage of NEORAL by 25-50%. Patients with abnormal baseline renal function are at higher risk. They should initially be treated with 2.5mg/kg per day orally and must be monitored very carefully.

In some patients it may be difficult to detect NEORAL-induced renal dysfunction because of changes in renal function related to the underlying renal disease. If NEORAL is indicated for more than one year in the long-term management, then renal biopsies should be performed at 1 yearly intervals to assess the progression of the renal disease and the extent of any NEORAL-associated changes in the renal morphology that may co-exist.

The use of NEORAL therapy for the treatment of patients with nephrotic syndrome requires careful monitoring and follow-up. NEORAL should only be used provided that the necessary expertise and adequate equipment, laboratory and supporting medical resources are available.

4.5 Interaction with other medicinal products and other forms of Interaction

Food interactions

The concomitant intake of grapefruit juice has been reported to increase the bioavailability of ciclosporin.

Drug interactions

Of the many drugs reported to interact with ciclosporin, those for which the interactions are adequately substantiated and considered to have clinical implications are listed below.

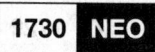

Various agents are known to either increase or decrease plasma or whole blood ciclosporin levels usually by inhibition or induction of enzymes involved in the metabolism of ciclosporin, in particular cytochrome P450.

Drugs that decrease ciclosporin levels:

Barbiturates, carbamazepine, phenytoin; rifampicin; octreotide; orlistat; hypericum perforatum (St John's Wort); ticlopidine.

Drugs that increase ciclosporin levels:

Macrolide antibiotics (mainly erythromycin and clarithromycin); ketoconazole, fluconazole, itraconazole; diltiazem, nicardipine, verapamil; metoclopramide; oral contraceptives; danazol; methylprednisolone (high dose); allopurinol; amiodarone; ursodeoxycholic acid; protease inhibitors.

Other relevant drug interactions

Care should be taken when using ciclosporin together with other drugs that exhibit nephrotoxic synergy: aminoglycosides (including gentamicin, tobramycin), amphotericin B, ciprofloxacin, vancomycin, trimethoprim (+ sulfamethoxazole); non-steroidal anti-inflammatory drugs (including diclofenac, naproxen, sulindac); melphalan.

During treatment with ciclosporin, vaccination may be less effective; the use of live-attenuated vaccines should be avoided.

The concurrent administration of nifedipine with ciclosporin may result in an increased rate of gingival hyperplasia compared with that observed when ciclosporin is given alone.

The concomitant use of diclofenac and ciclosporin has been found to result in a significant increase in the bioavailability of diclofenac, with the possible consequence of reversible renal function impairment. The increase in the bioavailability of diclofenac is most probably caused by a reduction of its first-pass effect. If non-steroidal anti-inflammatory drugs with a low first-pass effect (e.g. acetylsalicylic acid) are given together with ciclosporin, no increase in their bioavailability is to be expected.

Ciclosporin may also reduce the clearance of digoxin thereby causing digoxin toxicity.

Ciclosporin has also been reported to reduce the clearance of prednisolone.

Administration of ciclosporin may enhance the potential of HMG-CoA reductase inhibitors and colchicine to induce muscular toxicity eg muscle pain and weakness, myositis and occasionally rhabdomyolysis.

Recommendations

If the concomitant use of drug known to interact with ciclosporin cannot be avoided, the following basic recommendations should be observed.

During the concomitant use of a drug that may exhibit nephrotoxic synergy, close monitoring of renal function (in particular serum creatinine) should be performed. If a significant impairment of renal function occurs, the dosage of the co-administered drug should be reduced or alternative treatment considered.

Drugs known to reduce or increase the bioavailability of ciclosporin: in transplant patients frequent measurement of ciclosporin levels and, if necessary, ciclosporin dosage adjustment are required, particularly during the introduction or withdrawal of the co-administered drug. In non-transplant patients the value of ciclosporin blood level monitoring is questionable, as in these patients the relationship between blood level and clinical effect is less well established. If drugs known to increase ciclosporin levels are given concomitantly, frequent assessment of renal function and careful monitoring for ciclosporin related side-effects may be more appropriate than blood level measurement.

The concomitant use of nifedipine should be avoided in patients in whom gingival hyperplasia develops as a side effect of ciclosporin.

Non-steroidal anti-inflammatory drugs known to undergo strong first-pass metabolism (e.g. diclofenac) should be given at doses lower than than those that would be used in patients not receiving ciclosporin. When diclofenac is given concomitantly with ciclosporin the dose of diclofenac should be reduced by approximately half(see section 4.2 Posology & Administration).

If digoxin, colchicine or HMG-CoA reductase inhibitors are used concurrently with ciclosporin, close clinical observation is required in order to enable early detection of toxic manifestations of the drug, followed by reduction of its dosage or its withdrawal.

4.6 Pregnancy and lactation

Ciclosporin is not teratogenic in animals. There is currently no clinical experience with NEORAL and experience with SANDIMMUN is still limited. However data available from organ transplant recipients indicate that, compared with other immunosuppressive agents, ciclosporin treatment imposes no increased risk of adverse effects on the course and outcome of pregnancy. However there are no adequate and well controlled studies in pregnant women, therefore ciclosporin should be used during pregnancy only if the potential benefit justifies the potential risk to the foetus.

Ciclosporin passes into breast milk. Mothers receiving treatment with ciclosporin should not therefore breast-feed their infants.

4.7 Effects on ability to drive and use machines

No data exists on the effects of NEORAL on the ability to drive and use machines.

4.8 Undesirable effects

Many side effects associated with ciclosporin therapy are dose-dependent and responsive to dose reduction. In the various indications the overall spectrum of side effects is essentially the same; there are, however, differences in incidence and severity. As a consequence of the higher initial doses and longer maintenance therapy required after transplantation, side effects are more frequent and usually more severe in transplant patients than in patients treated for other indications.

Frequency estimate: very common ⩾10%, common ⩾ 1% to <10%,

Uncommon ⩾ 0.1% to <1%, rare ⩾ 0.01% to <0.1%, very rare <0.01%.

Blood and the lymphatic system disorders:

Uncommon: anaemia, thrombocytopenia

Rare: micro-angiopathic haemolytic anaemia, haemolytic uraemic syndrome

Endocrine disorders:

Rare: menstrual disturbances, gynaecomastia

Metabolism and nutrition disorders:

Very common: hyperlipidaemia

Common: hyperuricaemia, hyperkalaemia, hypomagnesaemia

Rare: hyperglycaemia

Nervous system disorders:

Very common: tremor, headache

Common: paraesthesia

Uncommon: signs of encephalopathy or demyelination, especially in liver transplant patients, such as convulsions, confusion, disorientation, decreased responsiveness, agitation, insomnia, visual disturbances, cortical blindness, coma, paresis, cerebellar ataxia.

Rare: motor polyneuropathy

Very rare: optic disc oedema including papilloedema with possible visual impairment secondary to Benign Intracranial Hypertension.

Cardiovascular disorders:

Very common: hypertension

Gastrointestinal disorders:

Common: anorexia, nausea, vomiting, abdominal pain, diarrhoea, gingival hyperplasia,

Hepato-biliary disorders:

Common: hepatic dysfunction

Rare: pancreatitis.

Skin and subcutaneous tissue disorders:

Common: hypertrichosis

Uncommon: allergic rashes

Musculoskeletal, connective tissue and bone disorders:

Common: muscle cramps, myalgia

Rare: muscle weakness, myopathy

Renal and urinary disorders:

Very common: renal dysfunction (see 4.4 'Special Warnings and special precautions for use')

General disorders and administration site conditions:

Common: fatigue

Uncommon: oedema, weight increase

The increased risk of developing malignancies and lymphoproliferative disorders appears to be related to the degree and duration of immunosuppression rather than to the use of specific agents (refer to Section 4.4 "Special Warnings and Precautions").

4.9 Overdose

No experience of acute overdosage with NEORAL is available and little experience is available with regards to overdosage with SANDIMMUN. Symptomatic treatment and general supportive measures should be followed in all cases of overdosage. Forced emesis could be of value within the first few hours after intake. Signs of nephrotoxicity might occur which should be expected to resolve following drug withdrawal. Ciclosporin is not dialysable to any great extent nor is it well cleared by charcoal haemoperfusion. Hypertension and convulsions have been reported in some patients receiving ciclosporin therapy at doses above the recommended range and in others with high trough blood levels of ciclosporin. This might therefore, be expected as a feature of overdosage.

5. PHARMACOLOGICAL PROPERTIES

5.1 Pharmacodynamic properties

Pharmacotherapeutic group: Selective immunosuppressive agents (ATC code L04A A01).

Ciclosporin (also known as ciclosporin A) is a cyclic polypeptide consisting of 11 amino acids. It is a potent immunosuppressive agent which prolongs survival of allogeneic transplants involving skin, heart, kidney, pancreas, cornea, bone marrow, small intestine and lung in animals.

Successful solid organ and bone marrow allogeneic transplants have been performed in man, using ciclosporin to prevent and treat rejection and GVHD. Marked beneficial effects of ciclosporin therapy have also been shown in patients with severe psoriasis, atopic dermatitis, rheumatoid arthritis and nephrotic syndrome, conditions that may be considered to have an immunological mechanism.

Studies in animals suggest that ciclosporin inhibits the development of cell mediated reactions. It appears to block the resting lymphocytes in the G_O or early G_1 phase of the cell cycle, and also inhibits lymphokine production and release, including interleukin 2 (T cell growth factor, TCGF). The available evidence suggests that ciclosporin acts specifically and reversibly on lymphocytes. It does not depress haemopoiesis and has no effect on the function of phagocytic cells.

5.2 Pharmacokinetic properties

NEORAL is an improved pharmaceutical form of the active ingredient ciclosporin. NEORAL is a pre-concentrate formulation of ciclosporin which undergoes a microemulsification process in the presence of water, either in the form of a beverage or in the form of the gastrointestinal fluid. NEORAL reduces the intra-patient variability of pharmacokinetic parameters, with a more consistent absorption profile and less influence of concomitant food intake and the presence of bile. In pharmacokinetic and clinical studies it has been demonstrated that the correlation between trough concentration (Cmin) and total exposure (AUC) is significantly stronger when ciclosporin is given as NEORAL than when it is given as SANDIMMUN. NEORAL therefore allows greater predictability and consistency of ciclosporin exposure.

The data available indicate that following a 1:1 conversion from SANDIMMUN Soft Gelatin Capsules and SANDIMMUN Oral Solution to NEORAL, trough concentrations in whole blood are comparable, thereby remaining in the desired therapeutic trough level range. Compared to oral administration of SANDIMMUN (with which peak blood concentrations are achieved within 1 to 6 hours), NEORAL is more quickly absorbed (resulting in a 1 hour earlier mean t_{max} and a 59% higher mean C_{max}) and exhibits, on average, a 29% higher bioavailability. In a clinical trial involving maintained renal transplant patients the correlation (r^2) between trough concentration (C_{min}) and exposure (AUC) was good (0.8).

Ciclosporin is distributed largely outside the blood volume. In the blood, 33-47% is present in plasma, 4-9% in lymphocytes, 5-12% in granulocytes, and 41-58% in erythrocytes. In plasma, approximately 90% is bound to proteins, mostly lipoproteins.

Ciclosporin is extensively biotransformed to approximately 15 metabolites. There is no single major metabolic pathway. Elimination is primarily biliary, with only 6% of the oral dose excreted in the urine, only 0.1% is excreted in the urine as unchanged drug.

There is a high variability in the data reported on the terminal half-life of ciclosporin depending on the assay applied and the target population. The terminal half-life ranged from 6.3 hours in healthy volunteers to 20.4 hours in patients with severe liver disease.

5.3 Preclinical safety data

Ciclosporin gave no evidence of mutagenic or teratogenic effects in appropriate test systems. Only at dose levels toxic to dams were adverse effects seen in reproduction studies in rats. At toxic doses (rats at 30mg/kg and rabbits at 100mg/kg a day orally), ciclosporin was embryo- and fetotoxic as indicated by increased prenatal and post-natal mortality and reduced fetal weight together with related skeletal retardation. In the well-tolerated dose range (rats up to 17mg/kg and rabbits up to 30mg/kg a day orally), ciclosporin proved to be without any embryolethal or teratogenic effects.

Carcinogenicity studies were carried out in male and female rats and mice. In the 78-week mouse study, at doses of 1, 4, and 16mg/kg a day, evidence of a statistically significant trend was found for lymphocytic lymphomas in females, and the incidence of hepatocellular carcinomas in mid-dose males significantly exceeded the control value. In the 24-month rat study conducted at 0.5, 2 and 8mg/kg a day, pancreatic islet cell adenomas significantly exceeded the control rate at the low dose level. The hepatocellular carcinomas and pancreatic islet cell adenomas were not dose-related.

No impairment in fertility was demonstrated in studies in male and female rats.

Ciclosporin has not been found mutagenic/genotoxic in the Ames test, the V79-HGPRT test, the micronucleus test in mice and Chinese hamsters, the chromosome-aberration tests in Chinese hamster bone marrow, the mouse dominant lethal assay, and the DNA repair test in sperm from treated mice. A study analysing sister chromatid exchange (SCE) induction by ciclosporin using human lymphocytes *in vitro* gave indication of a positive effect (i.e. induction of SCE) at high concentrations in this system.

An increased incidence of malignancy is a recognised complication of immunosuppression in recipients of organ transplants. The most common forms of neoplasms are non-Hodgkin's lymphoma and carcinomas of the skin. The risk of malignancies during ciclosporin treatment is higher than in the normal, healthy population, but similar to that in patients receiving other immunosuppressive therapies. It has been reported that reduction or discontinuance of immunosuppression may cause lesions to regress.

6. PHARMACEUTICAL PARTICULARS

6.1 List of excipients

Soft gelatin capsules

DL-α-tocopherol, absolute ethanol, propylene glycol, corn oil-mono-di-triglycerides, polyoxyl 40 hydrogenated castor oil.

Capsule shell

Iron oxide black (25- and 100-mg capsules), titanium dioxide, glycerol 85%, propylene glycol, gelatin.

Solution

DL-α-tocopherol, absolute ethanol, propylene glycol, corn oil-mono-di-triglycerides, polyoxyl 40 hydrogenated castor oil.

6.2 Incompatibilities

None known.

6.3 Shelf life

Soft gelatin capsules 36 months

Solution 36 months

6.4 Special precautions for storage

NEORAL Soft Gelatin Capsules should be stored below 25°C.

NEORAL Soft Gelatin Capsules should be left in the blister pack until required for use. When a blister is opened, a characteristic smell is noticeable.

NEORAL Oral Solution should be stored below 30°C (preferably not below 15°C, as it contains oily components of natural origin which tend to solidify at low temperatures). A jelly-like formation may occur below 20°C which is however reversible at temperatures up to 30°C. Minor flakes or a slight sediment may still be observed. These phenomena do not affect the efficacy and safety of the product, and the dosing by means of the measuring device remains accurate.

6.5 Nature and contents of container

NEORAL Soft Gelatin Capsules are available in 6 × 5 and 10 × 6 (10mg only) blister packs of double-sided aluminium consisting of an aluminium bottom foil and an aluminium covering foil.

NEORAL Oral Solution is available in 50mL amber glass bottles with an aluminium cap and rubber stopper. A dispenser set is also provided.

6.6 Instructions for use and handling

Initial use of NEORAL Oral Solution

1. Raise the plastic cap.
2. Tear off the sealing ring completely.
3. Remove the black stopper and throw it away.
4. Push the tube unit with the white stopper firmly into the neck of the bottle
5. Insert the syringe into the white stopper
6. Draw up prescribed volume of solution
7. Expel any *large* bubbles by depressing and withdrawing plunger a few times before removing syringe containing prescribed dose from bottle. The presence of a few tiny bubbles is of no importance and will not affect the dose in any way.
8. After use, wipe syringe *on outside only* with a *dry* tissue and replace in its case. Dispose of the tissue carefully. White stopper and tube should remain in bottle. Close bottle with cap provided.

Subsequent use

Commence at point 5.

7. MARKETING AUTHORISATION HOLDER

Novartis Pharmaceuticals UK Ltd

Trading as Sandoz Pharmaceuticals

Frimley Business Park

Frimley

Camberley

Surrey

GU16 7SR

8. MARKETING AUTHORISATION NUMBER(S)

NEORAL Soft Gelatin Capsules 10mg: PL 00101/0483

NEORAL Soft Gelatin Capsules 25mg, 50mg and 100mg: PL 00101/0387-0389

NEORAL Oral Solution: PL 00101/0390

9. DATE OF FIRST AUTHORISATION/RENEWAL OF THE AUTHORISATION

PL 00101/0483. 3 April 1998

PL 00101/0387 27 March 1995 / 27 June 2001

PL 00101/0388 27 March 1995/ 27 June 2001

PL 00101/0389 27 March 1995 / 27 June 2001

PL 00101/0390. 27 March 1995 / 24 July 2001.

10. DATE OF REVISION OF THE TEXT

18 December 2004

Legal Category

POM

Neorecormon Multidose Powder and Solvent for Solution for Injection

(Roche Products Limited)

1. NAME OF THE MEDICINAL PRODUCT

NeoRecormon Multidose Powder and solvent for solution for injection.

2. QUALITATIVE AND QUANTITATIVE COMPOSITION

NeoRecormon Multidose 50,000 Powder and solvent for solution for injection:

1 vial contains 50,000 international units (IU) corresponding to 415 micrograms epoetin beta* (recombinant human erythropoietin).

1 ampoule contains 10ml solvent (water for injection with benzyl alcohol and benzalkonium chloride as preservatives).

1ml of reconstituted solution contains 5000 IU epoetin beta.

*Produced by recombinant DNA technology in CHO cell line.

NeoRecormon Multidose 100,000 Powder and solvent for solution for injection:

1 vial contains 100,000 international units (IU) corresponding to 830 micrograms epoetin beta* (recombinant human erythropoietin).

1 ampoule contains 5ml solvent (water for injection with benzyl alcohol and benzalkonium chloride as preservatives).

1ml of reconstituted solution contains 20,000 IU epoetin beta.

*Produced by recombinant DNA technology in CHO cell line.

For excipients, see *6.1*.

3. PHARMACEUTICAL FORM

Powder and solvent for solution for injection.

Appearance: White powder (lyophilisate) and clear colourless to slightly opalescent solution.

4. CLINICAL PARTICULARS

4.1 Therapeutic indications

Treatment of anaemia associated with chronic renal failure (renal anaemia) in patients on dialysis.

Treatment of symptomatic renal anaemia in patients not yet undergoing dialysis.

Treatment of symptomatic anaemia in adult patients with solid tumours receiving chemotherapy.

Treatment of symptomatic anaemia in adult patients with multiple myeloma, low grade non-Hodgkin's lymphoma or chronic lymphocytic leukaemia, who have a relative erythropoietin deficiency and are receiving anti-tumour therapy. Deficiency is defined as an inappropriately low serum erythropoietin level in relation to the degree of anaemia.

Increasing the yield of autologous blood from patients in a pre-donation programme.

Its use in this indication must be balanced against the reported increased risk of thromboembolic events. Treatment should only be given to patients with moderate anaemia (Hb 10 – 13 g/dl [6.21 - 8.07 mmol/l], no iron deficiency) if blood conserving procedures are not available or insufficient when the scheduled major elective surgery requires a large volume of blood (4 or more units of blood for females or 5 or more units for males).

4.2 Posology and method of administration

Therapy with NeoRecormon should be initiated by physicians experienced in the above mentioned indications. As anaphylactoid reactions were observed in isolated cases, it is recommended that the first dose be administered under medical supervision.

This multidose preparation can be used for several patients. To avoid the risk of cross-infection always follow aseptic techniques and use disposable sterile syringes and needles for each administration. Please check that only one vial of NeoRecormon Multidose is in use (i.e. reconstituted) at any one time.

Treatment of anaemic patients with chronic renal failure

The reconstituted solution can be administered subcutaneously or intravenously. In case of intravenous administration, the solution should be injected over approx. 2 minutes, e.g. in haemodialysis patients via the arterio-venous fistula at the end of dialysis.

For non-haemodialysed patients, subcutaneous administration should always be preferred in order to avoid puncture of peripheral veins.

The aim of treatment is to increase the packed cell volume to 30 - 35% where the weekly increase should be at least 0.5 vol%. A value of 35% should not be exceeded.

In the presence of hypertension or existing cardiovascular, cerebrovascular or peripheral vascular diseases, the weekly increase in the PCV and the target PCV should be determined individually taking into account the clinical picture. In some patients the optimum PCV may be below 30%.

Treatment with NeoRecormon is divided into two stages.

<u>1. Correction phase</u>

Subcutaneous administration:

The initial dosage is 3 × 20 IU/kg body weight per week. The dosage may be increased every 4 weeks by 3 × 20 IU/kg per week if the increase of packed cell volume is not adequate (< 0.5% per week).

The weekly dose can also be divided into daily doses.

Intravenous administration:

The initial dosage is 3 × 40 IU/kg per week. The dosage may be raised after 4 weeks to 80 IU/kg - three times per week - and by further increments of 20 IU/kg if needed, three times per week, at monthly intervals.

For both routes of administration, the maximum dose should not exceed 720 IU/kg per week.

<u>2. Maintenance phase</u>

To maintain a packed cell volume of between 30 and 35%, the dosage is initially reduced to half of the previously administered amount. Subsequently, the dose is adjusted at intervals of one or two weeks individually for the patient (maintenance dose).

In the case of subcutaneous administration, the weekly dose can be given as one injection per week or in divided doses three or seven times per week. Patients who are stable on a once weekly dosing regimen may be switched to once every two weeks administration. In this case dose increases may be necessary.

Results of clinical studies in children have shown that, on average, the younger the patients, the higher the NeoRecormon doses required. Nevertheless, the recommended dosing schedule should be followed as the individual response cannot be predicted.

Treatment with NeoRecormon is normally a long-term therapy. It can, however, be interrupted, if necessary, at any time. Data on the once weekly dosing schedule are based on clinical studies with a treatment duration of 24 weeks.

Treatment of symptomatic anaemia in patients with solid tumours

The reconstituted solution is administered subcutaneously; the weekly dose can be divided into 3 to 7 single doses.

NeoRecormon treatment is indicated if the haemoglobin value is ⩽ 11g/dl (6.83 mmol/l). The recommended initial dose is 450 IU/kg body weight per week.

Haemoglobin level should not exceed 13 g/dl (8.07 mmol/l) (see section 5.1).

If, after 4 weeks, a patient does not show a satisfactory response in terms of haemoglobin values, then the dose should be doubled. The therapy should be continued for up to 3 weeks after the end of chemotherapy.

If haemoglobin falls by more than 1 g/dl (0.62 mmol/l) in the first cycle of chemotherapy despite concomitant NeoRecormon therapy, further therapy may not be effective.

Once the therapeutic objective for an individual patient has been achieved, the dose should be reduced by 25 to 50 % in order to maintain haemoglobin at that level. If required, further dose reduction may be instituted to ensure that haemoglobin level does not exceed 13 g/dl.

If the rise in haemoglobin is greater than 2 g/dl (1.3 mmol/l) in 4 weeks, the dose should be reduced by 25 to 50 %.

Treatment of symptomatic anaemia in patients with multiple myeloma, low-grade non-Hodgkin's lymphoma or chronic lymphocytic leukaemia

Patients with multiple myeloma, non-Hodgkin's lymphoma or chronic lymphocytic leukaemia should have a relative erythropoietin deficiency. Deficiency is defined as an inappropriately low serum erythropoietin level in relation to the degree of anaemia:

serum erythropoietin level of ⩽ 100mU/ml at a haemoglobin of > 9 to < 10g/dl (> 5.58 to < 6.21 mmol/l)

serum erythropoietin level of ⩽ 180mU/ml at a haemoglobin of > 8 to ⩽ 9g/dl (> 4.96 to 5.58 mmol/l)

serum erythropoietin level of ⩽ 300mU/ml at a haemoglobin of ⩽ 8g/dl (⩽ 4.96 mmol/l)

The above values should be measured at least 7 days after the last blood transfusion and the last cycle of cytotoxic chemotherapy.

The reconstituted solution is administered subcutaneously; the weekly dose can be given as one injection per week or in divided doses 3 to 7 times per week.

The recommended initial dose is 450 IU/kg body weight per week.

Haemoglobin level should not exceed 13 g/dl (8.07 mmol/l) (see section 5.1).

If, after 4 weeks of therapy, the haemoglobin value has increased by at least 1 g/dl (0.62 mmol/l), the current dose should be continued. If the haemoglobin value has not increased by at least 1 g/dl (0.62 mmol/l), a dose increase to 900 IU/kg body weight, given in divided doses 2 to 7 times per week, may be considered. If, after 8 weeks of therapy, the haemoglobin value has not increased by at least 1 g/dl (0.62 mmol/l), response is unlikely and treatment should be discontinued.

Clinical studies have shown that response to epoetin beta treatment is delayed by about 2 weeks in chronic lymphocytic leukaemia patients, as compared with patients with multiple myeloma, non-Hodgkin's lymphoma and solid tumours. The therapy should be continued up to 4 weeks after the end of chemotherapy.

The maximum dose should not exceed 900 IU/kg body weight per week.

Once the therapeutic objective for an individual patient has been achieved, the dose should be reduced by 25 to 50 % in order to maintain haemoglobin at that level. If required, further dose reduction may be instituted to ensure that haemoglobin level does not exceed 13 g/dl.

If the rise in haemoglobin is greater than 2 g/dl (1.3 mmol/l) in 4 weeks, the dose should be reduced by 25 to 50 %.

Therapy should only be reintroduced if the erythropoietin deficiency is the most likely cause of the anaemia.

Treatment for increasing the amount of autologous blood

The reconstituted solution is administered intravenously over approx. 2 minutes or subcutaneously. NeoRecormon is administered twice weekly over 4 weeks. On those occasions where the patient's PCV allows blood donation, i.e. PCV ⩾ 33%, NeoRecormon is administered at the end of blood donation.

During the entire treatment period, a PCV of 48% should not be exceeded.

The dosage must be determined by the surgical team individually for each patient as a function of the required amount of pre-donated blood and the endogenous red cell reserve:

1. The required amount of pre-donated blood depends on the anticipated blood loss, use of blood conserving procedures and the physical condition of the patient.

This amount should be that quantity which is expected to be sufficient to avoid homologous blood transfusions.

The required amount of pre-donated blood is expressed in units whereby one unit in the nomogram is equivalent to 180ml red cells.

2. The ability to donate blood depends predominantly on the patient's blood volume and baseline PCV. Both variables determine the endogenous red cell reserve, which can be calculated according to the following formula.

Endogenous red cell reserve = blood volume [ml] × (PCV - 33) ÷ 100

Women: blood volume [ml] = 41 [ml/kg] × body weight [kg] + 1200 [ml]

Men: blood volume [ml] = 44 [ml/kg] × body weight [kg] + 1600 [ml]

(body weight ⩾ 45kg)

The indication for NeoRecormon treatment and, if given, the single dose should be determined from the required amount of pre-donated blood and the endogenous red cell reserve according to the following graphs.

(see Figure 1 below)

The single dose thus determined is administered twice weekly over 4 weeks. The maximum dose should not exceed 1600 IU/kg body weight per week for intravenous or 1200 IU/kg per week for subcutaneous administration.

4.3 Contraindications

NeoRecormon must not be used in the presence of poorly controlled hypertension and known hypersensitivity to the active substance or to any of the excipients of NeoRecormon Multidose or benzoic acid, a metabolite of benzyl alcohol.

In the indication "increasing the yield of autologous blood", NeoRecormon must not be used in patients who, in the month preceding treatment, have suffered a myocardial infarction or stroke, patients with unstable angina pectoris, or patients who are at risk of deep venous thrombosis such as those with a history of venous thromboembolic disease.

NeoRecormon Multidose contains benzyl alcohol as a preservative and must therefore not be used in infants or young children up to three years old.

4.4 Special warnings and special precautions for use

NeoRecormon should be used with caution in the presence of refractory anaemia with excess blasts in transformation, epilepsy, thrombocytosis, and chronic liver failure. Folic acid and vitamin B_{12} deficiencies should be ruled out as they reduce the effectiveness of NeoRecormon.

Severe aluminium overload due to treatment of renal failure may compromise the effectiveness of NeoRecormon.

The indication for NeoRecormon treatment of nephrosclerotic patients not yet undergoing dialysis should be defined individually, as a possible acceleration of progression of renal failure cannot be ruled out with certainty.

Patients who have developed anti-erythropoietin antibodies and pure red cell aplasia under treatment with another erythropoietic substance should not be switched to NeoRecormon due to possible cross-reactivity of antibodies to all erythropoietic substances.

In *chronic renal failure* patients there may be a moderate dose-dependent rise in the platelet count within the normal range during treatment with NeoRecormon, especially after intravenous administration. This regresses during the course of continued therapy. It is recommended that the platelet count be monitored regularly during the first 8 weeks of therapy.

Effect on tumour growth

Epoetins are growth factors that primarily stimulate red blood cell production. Erythropoietin receptors may be expressed on the surface of a variety of tumour cells. As with all growth factors, there is a concern that epoetins could stimulate the growth of any type of malignancy. Two controlled clinical studies in which epoetins were administered to patients with various cancers including head and neck cancer, and breast cancer, have shown an unexplained excess mortality.

Platelet counts and haemoglobin level should also be monitored at regular intervals in cancer patients.

In patients in an *autologous blood predonation programme* there may be an increase in platelet count, mostly within the normal range. Therefore, it is recommended that the platelet count be determined at least once a week in these patients. If there is an increase in platelets of more than 150 × 10^9/l or if platelets rise above the normal range, treatment with NeoRecormon should be discontinued.

In chronic renal failure patients an increase in heparin dose during haemodialysis is frequently required during the course of therapy with NeoRecormon as a result of the increased packed cell volume. Occlusion of the dialysis system is possible if heparinisation is not optimum.

Early shunt revision and thrombosis prophylaxis by administration of acetylsalicylic acid, for example, should be considered in chronic renal failure patients at risk of shunt thrombosis.

Serum potassium levels should be monitored regularly during NeoRecormon therapy. Potassium elevation has been reported in a few uraemic patients receiving NeoRecormon, though causality has not been established. If an elevated or rising potassium level is observed then consideration should be given to ceasing NeoRecormon administration until the level has been corrected.

For use of NeoRecormon in an autologous predonation programme, the official guidelines on principles of blood donation must be considered, in particular:

– only patients with a PCV ⩾ 33% (haemoglobin ⩾ 11g/dl [6.83 mmol/l]) should donate;

– special care should be taken with patients below 50kg weight;

– the single volume drawn should not exceed approx. 12% of the patient's estimated blood volume.

Treatment should be reserved for patients in whom it is considered of particular importance to avoid homologous blood transfusion taking into consideration the risk/benefit assessment for homologous transfusions.

Misuse by healthy persons may lead to an excessive increase in packed cell volume. This may be associated with life-threatening complications of the cardiovascular system.

NeoRecormon Multidose contains up to 5.0mg phenylalanine/vial as an excipient. Therefore this should be taken into consideration in patients affected with severe forms of phenylketonuria.

4.5 Interaction with other medicinal products and other forms of Interaction

The clinical results obtained so far do not indicate any interaction of NeoRecormon with other substances.

Animal experiments revealed that epoetin beta does not increase the myelotoxicity of cytostatic drugs like etoposide, cisplatin, cyclophosphamide, and fluorouracil.

4.6 Pregnancy and lactation

Animal experiments have yielded no indications of teratogenic effects of epoetin beta in dosing regimens that do not lead to an unphysiologically high PCV. No adequate experience in human pregnancy and lactation has been gained, but a potential risk appears to be minimal under therapeutic conditions.

4.7 Effects on ability to drive and use machines

No effects on ability to drive and use machines have been observed.

4.8 Undesirable effects

Based on results from clinical trials including 1725 patients approximately 8% of patients treated with NeoRecormon are expected to experience adverse reactions. Undesirable effects during treatment with NeoRecormon are observed predominantly in patients with chronic renal failure or underlying malignancies and are most commonly an increase in blood pressure or aggravation of existing hypertension and headache.

• Cardiovascular system

<u>Anaemic patients with chronic renal failure</u>

The most frequent undesirable effect during treatment with NeoRecormon is an increase in blood pressure or aggravation of existing hypertension, especially in cases of rapid PCV increase. These increases in blood pressure can be treated with medicinal products. If blood pressure rises cannot be controlled by drug therapy, a transient interruption of NeoRecormon therapy is recommended. Particularly at the beginning of therapy, regular monitoring of the blood pressure is recommended, including between dialyses. Hypertensive crisis with encephalopathy-like symptoms (e.g. headaches and confused state, sensorimotor disorders - such as speech disturbance or impaired gait - up to tonoclonic seizures) may also occur in individual patients with otherwise normal or low blood pressure. This requires the immediate attention of a physician and intensive medical care. Particular attention should be paid to sudden stabbing migraine-like headaches as a possible warning sign.

<u>Patients with solid tumours, multiple myeloma, non-Hodgkin's lymphoma or chronic lymphocytic leukaemia</u>

Occasionally there may be an increase in blood pressure which can be treated with drugs. It is therefore recommended to monitor blood pressure, in particular in the initial treatment phase. Headache may also occur occasionally.

• Blood

<u>Anaemic patients with chronic renal failure</u>

Shunt thromboses may occur, especially in patients who have a tendency to hypotension or whose arteriovenous fistulae exhibit complications (e.g. stenoses, aneurisms), see section 4.4. In most cases, a fall in serum ferritin values simultaneous with a rise in packed cell volume is observed. Therefore, oral iron substitution of 200 - 300mg Fe^{2+}/day is recommended in all patients with serum ferritin values below 100 micrograms/l or transferrin saturation below 20%. In addition, transient increases in serum potassium and phosphate levels have been observed in isolated cases. These parameters should be monitored regularly.

In very rare cases, neutralising anti-erythropoietin antibodies with or without pure red cell aplasia (PRCA) occurred during rHuEPO therapy. In case PRCA is diagnosed, therapy with erythropoietin must be discontinued and patients should not be switched to another erythropoietic substance.

<u>Patients with solid tumours, multiple myeloma, non-Hodgkin's lymphoma or chronic lymphocytic leukaemia</u>

In some patients, a fall in serum iron parameters is observed. Therefore, oral iron substitution of 200 - 300mg Fe^{2+}/day is recommended in all patients with serum ferritin values below 100 micrograms/l or transferrin saturation below 20%. In patients with multiple myeloma, non-Hodgkin's lymphoma or chronic lymphocytic leukaemia

Figure 1

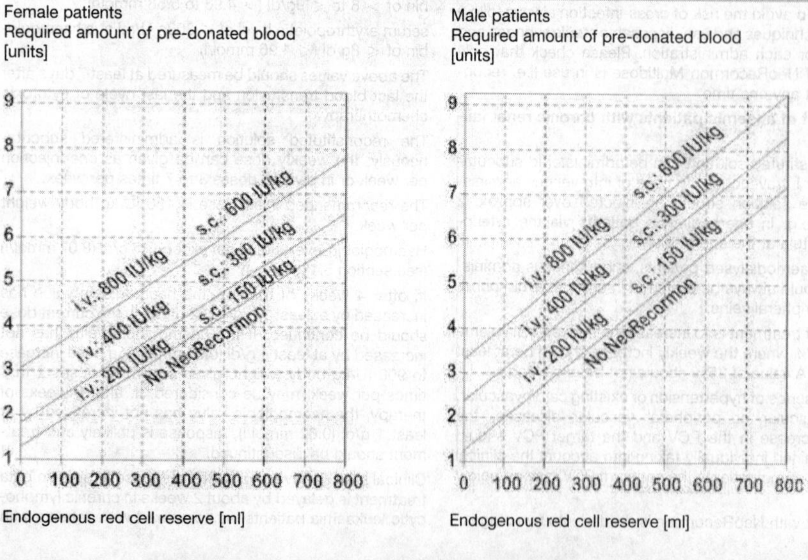

with transferrin saturation below 25%, 100mg intravenous Fe^{3+}/week has also been used.

Clinical studies have shown a higher frequency of thromboembolic events in cancer patients treated with NeoRecormon compared to untreated controls or placebo. In patients treated with NeoRecormon, this incidence is 5.9 % compared to 4.2 % in controls; this is not associated with any increase in thromboembolic mortality compared with controls.

Patients in an autologous blood predonation programme

Patients in an autologous blood predonation programme have been reported to show a slightly higher frequency of thromboembolic events. However, a causal relationship with treatment with NeoRecormon could not be established.

As there are indications of a temporary iron deficiency all patients should be treated orally with 300mg Fe^{2+}/day from start of NeoRecormon treatment up to normalisation of ferritin values. If, despite oral iron substitution, iron deficiency (ferritin below or equal to 20 micrograms/l or transferrin saturation below 20%) develops, the additional intravenous administration of iron should be considered.

• **Others**

Rarely, skin reactions such as rash, pruritus, urticaria or injection site reactions may occur. In isolated cases anaphylactoid reactions have been reported. However, in controlled clinical studies no increased incidence of hypersensitivity reactions was found.

In isolated cases, particularly when starting treatment, flu-like symptoms such as fever, chills, headaches, pain in the limbs, malaise and/or bone pain have been reported. These reactions were mild or moderate in nature and subsided after a couple of hours or days.

The following incidences of undesirable effects in clinical trials, considered related to treatment with NeoRecormon and classified by indication area are:

(see Table 1 below)

4.9 Overdose

The therapeutic margin of NeoRecormon is very wide. Even at very high serum levels no symptoms of poisoning have been observed.

5. PHARMACOLOGICAL PROPERTIES

5.1 Pharmacodynamic properties

Pharmacotherapeutic group: antianaemic; ATC code: B03XA

Epoetin beta is identical in its amino acid and carbohydrate composition to erythropoietin that has been isolated from the urine of anaemic patients.

Erythropoietin is a glycoprotein that stimulates the formation of erythrocytes from its committed progenitors. It acts as a mitosis stimulating factor and differentiation hormone.

The biological efficacy of epoetin beta has been demonstrated after intravenous and subcutaneous administration in various animal models *in vivo* (normal and uraemic rats, polycythaemic mice, dogs). After administration of epoetin beta, the number of erythrocytes, the Hb values and reticulocyte counts increase as well as the ^{59}Fe-incorporation rate.

An increased ^{3}H-thymidine incorporation in the erythroid nucleated spleen cells has been found *in vitro* (mouse spleen cell culture) after incubation with epoetin beta.

Investigations in cell cultures of human bone marrow cells showed that epoetin beta stimulates erythropoiesis specifically and does not affect leucopoiesis. Cytotoxic actions of epoetin beta on bone marrow or on human skin cells were not detected.

After single dose administration of epoetin beta no effects on behaviour or locomotor activity of mice and circulatory or respiratory function of dogs were observed.

Erythropoietin is a growth factor that primarily stimulates red cell production. Erythropoietin receptors may be expressed on the surface of a variety of tumour cells. There is insufficient information to establish whether the use of epoetin products have an adverse effect on time to tumour progression or progression free survival.

Two studies explored the effect of epoetins on survival and/or tumour progression with higher haemoglobin targets.

In a randomised placebo-controlled study using epoetin alfa in 939 metastatic breast cancer patients, study drug was administered to attempt to maintain haemoglobin levels between 12 and 14 g/dL. At four months, death attributed to disease progression was higher (6 % vs. 3 %) in women receiving epoetin alfa. The overall mortality was significantly higher in the epoetin alfa arm.

In another placebo-controlled study using epoetin beta in 351 patients with head and neck cancer, study drug was administered to maintain the haemoglobin levels of 14 g/dL in women and 15 g/dL in men. Locoregional progression free survival was significantly shorter in patients receiving epoetin beta. The results of this study were confounded by imbalances between the treatment groups, especially with regard to tumour localisation, smoking status and the heterogeneity of the study population.

In addition, several other studies have shown a tendency to improved survival suggesting that epoetin has no negative effect on tumour progression.

In very rare cases, neutralising anti-erythropoietin antibodies with or without pure red cell aplasia (PRCA) occurred during rHuEPO therapy.

5.2 Pharmacokinetic properties

Pharmacokinetic investigations in healthy volunteers and uraemic patients show that the half-life of intravenously administered epoetin beta is between 4 and 12 hours and that the distribution volume corresponds to one to two times the plasma volume. Analogous results have been found in animal experiments in uraemic and normal rats.

After subcutaneous administration of epoetin beta to uraemic patients, the protracted absorption results in a serum concentration plateau, whereby the maximum concentration is reached after an average of 12 - 28 hours. The terminal half-life is higher than after intravenous administration, with an average of 13 - 28 hours.

Bioavailability of epoetin beta after subcutaneous administration is between 23 and 42% as compared with intravenous administration.

5.3 Preclinical safety data

Acute toxicity

The single intravenous administration of 6000 IU/kg b.w. epoetin beta in the dog and in doses of 3; 30; 300; 3000 or 30,000 IU/kg b.w. in the rat did not lead to any detectable toxic damage.

Chronic toxicity

Toxic signs were not observed in 3-month toxicity studies in rats with doses of up to 10,000 IU/kg b.w. or in dogs with doses of up to 3000 IU/kg b.w. administered daily either subcutaneously or intravenously, with the exception of fibrotic changes of the bone marrow which occurred if PCV values exceeded 80%. A further study in dogs revealed that the myelofibrosis does not occur if the packed cell volume is kept below 60%. The observation of myelofibrosis is therefore irrelevant to the clinical situation in man.

Table 1

Indication Area	Body System	Adverse Drug Reaction	Incidence
Renal anaemia			
	Vascular disorders	Hypertension	Common (>1%, <10%)
	Vascular disorders	Hypertensive crisis	Uncommon (>0.1%, <1%)
	Nervous system disorders	Headache	Common (>1%, <10%)
	Blood and the lymphatic system disorders	Thrombocytosis	Very rare (< 0.01%)
	Blood and the lymphatic system disorders	Shunt thrombosis	Rare (>0.01%, <0.1%)
Anaemia in oncology			
	Vascular disorders	Hypertension	Common (>1%, <10%)
	Nervous system disorders	Headache	Uncommon (>0.1%, <1%)
	Blood and the lymphatic system disorders	Thromboembolic event	Common (>1%, <10%)
Autologous blood predonation programme			
	Nervous system disorders	Headache	Common (>1%, <10%)

Carcinogenicity

A carcinogenicity study with homologous erythropoietin in mice did not reveal any signs of proliferative or tumourigenic potential.

Mutagenicity

Epoetin beta did not reveal any genotoxic potential in the Ames test, in the micronucleus test, in the *in vitro* HGPRT test or in a chromosomal aberration test in cultured human lymphocytes.

Reproduction toxicology

Studies on rats and rabbits showed no relevant evidence of embryotoxic, foetotoxic or teratogenic properties. No alteration of fertility was detected. A peri-postnatal toxicity study revealed no adverse effects in pregnant/lactating females and on the development of conceptus and offspring.

Safety of preservatives

Subchronic and chronic toxicity studies have demonstrated a wide safety margin of the selected preservatives.

6. PHARMACEUTICAL PARTICULARS

6.1 List of excipients

Powder*:* urea, sodium chloride, polysorbate 20, sodium dihydrogen phosphate, sodium monohydrogen phosphate, calcium chloride, glycine, leucine, isoleucine, threonine, glutamic acid, and phenylalanine.

Solvent*:* benzyl alcohol, benzalkonium chloride and water for injections.

6.2 Incompatibilities

This medicinal product should be used only with the solvent provided and not mixed with other medicinal products.

6.3 Shelf life

3 years.

The reconstituted solution remains stable for one month if stored in a refrigerator.

6.4 Special precautions for storage

Store at 2°C - 8°C (in a refrigerator).

Keep the container in the outer carton, in order to protect from light.

For the purpose of ambulatory use the patient may remove the unreconstituted product from the refrigerator and store it at room temperature (not above 25°C) for one single period of up to 5 days.

Leaving the reconstituted solution outside the refrigerator should be limited to the time necessary for preparing the injections.

6.5 Nature and contents of container

1 vial with powder for injection and 1 ampoule with preserved solvent, 1 reconstitution and withdrawal device, 1 needle 21G2, 1 disposable syringe (10ml).

Vials and ampoules are made of glass type I. The stopper is made of teflonised rubber material.

6.6 Instructions for use and handling

NeoRecormon Multidose is supplied as a powder for solution for injection in vials. This is dissolved with the contents of the accompanying solvent ampoule by means of a reconstitution and withdrawal device according to the instructions given below. Only solutions which are clear or slightly opalescent, colourless and practically free of visible particles may be injected. Do not use glass materials for injection, use only plastic materials.

This is a multidose preparation from which different single doses can be withdrawn over a period of 1 month after dissolution. To avoid the risk of contamination of the contents always observe aseptic techniques (i.e. use disposable sterile syringes and needles to administer each dose) and strictly follow the handling instructions below. Before withdrawing each dose disinfect the rubber seal of the withdrawal device with alcohol to prevent contamination of the contents by repeated needle insertions.

Preparation of NeoRecormon Multidose solution

(1) Take the vial with the freeze-dried substance out of the package. Write the date of reconstitution and expiry on the label (expiry is 1 month after reconstitution).

(2) Remove the plastic cap from the vial.

(3) Disinfect the rubber seal with alcohol.

(4) Take the reconstitution and withdrawal device (which allows sterile air exchange) out of the blister and remove the protective cover from the spike.

(5) Attach the device to the vial until the snap lock clicks home.

(6) Put the green needle on the syringe contained in the package and remove the needle cover.

(7) Hold the OPC (One-Point-Cut) ampoule with the blue point upwards. Shake or tap the ampoule to get any fluid in the stem into the body of the ampoule. Take hold of the stem and snap off away from you. Withdraw all the solvent into the syringe. Disinfect the rubber seal of the device with alcohol.

(8) Penetrate the seal with the needle to a depth of about 1cm and slowly inject the solvent into the vial. Then disconnect the syringe (with needle) from the device.

(9) Swirl the vial gently until the powder has dissolved. Do not shake. Check that the solution is clear, colourless and

practically free from particles. Put the protective cap on the top of the device.

(10) Before and after reconstitution NeoRecormon Multidose must be stored at +2° to +8°C (refrigerator).

Preparation of a single injection

(1) Before withdrawing each dose disinfect the rubber seal of the device with alcohol.

(2) Place a 26G needle onto an appropriate single-use syringe (max. 1ml).

(3) Remove the needle cover and insert the needle through the rubber seal of the device. Withdraw NeoRecormon solution into the syringe, expel air from the syringe into the vial and adjust the amount of NeoRecormon solution in the syringe to the dose prescribed. Then disconnect the syringe (with needle) from the device.

(4) Replace the needle with a new one (the new needle should have the size which you normally use for injections).

(5) Remove the needle cover and carefully expel air from the needle by holding the syringe vertically and gently pressing the plunger upwards until a bead of liquid appears at the needle tip.

For subcutaneous injection, clean the skin at the site of injection using an alcohol wipe. Form a skin fold by pinching the skin between the thumb and the forefinger. Hold the syringe near to the needle and insert the needle into the skin with a quick, firm action. Inject NeoRecormon solution. Withdraw the needle quickly and apply pressure over the injection site with a dry, sterile pad.

Any unused product or waste material should be disposed of in accordance with local requirements.

7. MARKETING AUTHORISATION HOLDER

Roche Registration Limited, 40 Broadwater Road, Welwyn Garden City, Hertfordshire, AL7 3AY, United Kingdom.

8. MARKETING AUTHORISATION NUMBER(S)

NeoRecormon Multidose 50,000 Powder and solvent for solution for injection:

EU/1/97/031/019

NeoRecormon Multidose 100,000 Powder and solvent for solution for injection:

EU/1/97/031/020

9. DATE OF FIRST AUTHORISATION/RENEWAL OF THE AUTHORISATION

22 August 2002

10. DATE OF REVISION OF THE TEXT

13 July 2005

NeoRecormon is a registered trade mark

NeoRecormon Powder and Solvent for Solution for Injection in Cartridge

(Roche Products Limited)

1. NAME OF THE MEDICINAL PRODUCT

NeoRecormon® Powder and solvent for solution for injection in cartridge.

2. QUALITATIVE AND QUANTITATIVE COMPOSITION

1 cartridge contains 10,000 international units (IU) corresponding to 83 micrograms epoetin beta* (recombinant human erythropoietin) and 1ml solvent (water for injection with benzyl alcohol and benzalkonium chloride as preservatives).

1 cartridge contains 20,000 international units (IU) corresponding to 166 micrograms epoetin beta* (recombinant human erythropoietin) and 1ml solvent (water for injection with benzyl alcohol and benzalkonium chloride as preservatives).

1 cartridge contains 60,000 international units (IU) corresponding to 498 micrograms epoetin beta* (recombinant human erythropoietin) and 1ml solvent (water for injection with benzyl alcohol and benzalkonium chloride as preservatives).

*Produced by recombinant DNA technology in CHO cell line.

For excipients, see 6.1.

3. PHARMACEUTICAL FORM

Powder and solvent for solution for injection.

Appearance: White powder (lyophilisate) and clear colourless to slightly opalescent solution.

4. CLINICAL PARTICULARS

4.1 Therapeutic indications

Treatment of anaemia associated with chronic renal failure (renal anaemia) in patients on dialysis.

Treatment of symptomatic renal anaemia in patients not yet undergoing dialysis.

Treatment of symptomatic anaemia in adult patients with solid tumours receiving chemotherapy.

Treatment of symptomatic anaemia in adult patients with multiple myeloma, low grade non-Hodgkin's lymphoma or chronic lymphocytic leukaemia, who have a relative erythropoietin deficiency and are receiving anti-tumour therapy. Deficiency is defined as an inappropriately low serum erythropoietin level in relation to the degree of anaemia.

Increasing the yield of autologous blood from patients in a pre-donation programme.

Its use in this indication must be balanced against the reported increased risk of thromboembolic events. Treatment should only be given to patients with moderate anaemia (Hb 10 - 13g/dl [6.21 - 8.07 mmol/l], no iron deficiency) if blood conserving procedures are not available or insufficient when the scheduled major elective surgery requires a large volume of blood (4 or more units of blood for females or 5 or more units for males).

4.2 Posology and method of administration

Therapy with NeoRecormon should be initiated by physicians experienced in the above mentioned indications. As anaphylactoid reactions were observed in isolated cases, it is recommended that the first dose be administered under medical supervision.

The prepared solution is administered subcutaneously.

Treatment of anaemic patients with chronic renal failure

The aim of treatment is to increase the packed cell volume to 30 - 35% where the weekly increase should be at least 0.5 vol%. A value of 35% should not be exceeded.

In the presence of hypertension or existing cardiovascular, cerebrovascular or peripheral vascular diseases, the weekly increase in the PCV and the target PCV should be determined individually taking into account the clinical picture. In some patients the optimum PCV may be below 30%.

Treatment with NeoRecormon is divided into two stages.

1. Correction phase

The initial dosage is 3 × 20 IU/kg body weight per week. The dosage may be increased every 4 weeks by 3 × 20 IU/kg per week if the increase of packed cell volume is not adequate (< 0.5% per week).

The weekly dose can also be divided into daily doses.

The maximum dose should not exceed 720 IU/kg per week.

2. Maintenance phase

To maintain a packed cell volume of between 30 and 35%, the dosage is initially reduced to half of the previously administered amount. Subsequently, the dose is adjusted at intervals of one or two weeks individually for the patient (maintenance dose).

The weekly dose can be given as one injection per week or in divided doses three or seven times per week. Patients who are stable on a once weekly dosing regimen may be switched to once every two weeks administration. In this case dose increases may be necessary.

Results of clinical studies in children have shown that, on average, the younger the patients, the higher the NeoRecormon doses required. Nevertheless, the recommended dosing schedule should be followed as the individual response cannot be predicted.

Treatment with NeoRecormon is normally a long-term therapy. It can, however, be interrupted, if necessary, at any time. Data on the once weekly dosing schedule are based on clinical studies with a treatment duration of 24 weeks.

Treatment of symptomatic anaemia in patients with solid tumours

The reconstituted solution is administered subcutaneously; the weekly dose can be divided into 3 to 7 single doses.

NeoRecormon treatment is indicated if the haemoglobin value is ⩽ 11 g/dl (6.83 mmol/l).

The recommended initial dose is 450 IU/kg body weight per week.

Haemoglobin level should not exceed 13 g/dl (8.07 mmol/l) (see section 5.1).

If, after 4 weeks, a patient does not show a satisfactory response in terms of haemoglobin values, then the dose should be doubled. The therapy should be continued for up to 3 weeks after the end of chemotherapy.

If haemoglobin falls by more than 1 g/dl (0.62mmol/l) in the first cycle of chemotherapy despite concomitant NeoRecormon therapy, further therapy may not be effective.

Once the therapeutic objective for an individual patient has been achieved, the dose should be reduced by 25 to 50 % in order to maintain haemoglobin at that level. If required, further dose reduction may be instituted to ensure that haemoglobin level does not exceed 13 g/dl.

If the rise in haemoglobin is greater than 2 g/dl (1.3 mmol/l) in 4 weeks, the dose should be reduced by 25 to 50 %.

Treatment of symptomatic anaemia in patients with multiple myeloma, low-grade non-Hodgkin's lymphoma or chronic lymphocytic leukaemia

Patients with multiple myeloma, non-Hodgkin's lymphoma or chronic lymphocytic leukaemia should have a relative erythropoietin deficiency. Deficiency is defined as an inappropriately low serum erythropoietin level in relation to the degree of anaemia:

serum erythropoietin level of ⩽ 100mU/ml at a haemoglobin of > 9 to < 10g/dl (> 5.58 to < 6.21 mmol/l)

serum erythropoietin level of ⩽ 180mU/ml at a haemoglobin of > 8 to ⩽ 9 g/dl (> 4.96 to 5.58 mmol/l)

serum erythropoietin level of ⩽ 300mU/ml at a haemoglobin of ⩽ 8 g/dl (⩽ 4.96 mmol/l)

The above values should be measured at least 7 days after the last blood transfusion and the last cycle of cytotoxic chemotherapy.

The reconstituted solution is administered subcutaneously; the weekly dose can be given as one injection per week or in divided doses 3 to 7 times per week.

The recommended initial dose is 450 IU/kg body weight per week.

Haemoglobin level should not exceed 13 g/dl (8.07 mmol/l) (see section 5.1).

If, after 4 weeks of therapy, the haemoglobin value has increased by at least 1 g/dl (0.62 mmol/l), the current dose should be continued. If the haemoglobin value has not increased by at least 1 g/dl (0.62 mmol/l), a dose increase to 900 IU/kg body weight, given in divided doses 2 to 7 times per week, may be considered. If, after 8 weeks of therapy, the haemoglobin value has not increased by at least 1 g/dl (0.62 mmol/l), response is unlikely and treatment should be discontinued.

Clinical studies have shown that response to epoetin beta treatment is delayed by about 2 weeks in chronic lymphocytic leukaemia patients, as compared with patients with multiple myeloma, non-Hodgkin's lymphoma and solid tumours. The therapy should be continued up to 4 weeks after the end of chemotherapy.

The maximum dose should not exceed 900 IU/kg body weight per week.

Once the therapeutic objective for an individual patient has been achieved, the dose should be reduced by 25 to 50 % in order to maintain haemoglobin at that level. If required, further dose reduction may be instituted to ensure that haemoglobin level does not exceed 13 g/dl.

If the rise in haemoglobin is greater than 2 g/dl (1.3 mmol/l) in 4 weeks, the dose should be reduced by 25 to 50 %.

Therapy should only be reintroduced if the erythropoietin deficiency is the most likely cause of the anaemia.

Treatment for increasing the amount of autologous blood

NeoRecormon is administered twice weekly over 4 weeks. On those occasions where the patient's PCV allows blood donation, i.e. PCV ⩾ 33%, NeoRecormon is administered at the end of blood donation.

During the entire treatment period, a PCV of 48% should not be exceeded.

The dosage must be determined by the surgical team individually for each patient as a function of the required amount of pre-donated blood and the endogenous red cell reserve:

1. The required amount of pre-donated blood depends on the anticipated blood loss, use of blood conserving procedures and the physical condition of the patient.

This amount should be that quantity which is expected to be sufficient to avoid homologous blood transfusions. The required amount of pre-donated blood is expressed in units whereby one unit in the nomogram is equivalent to 180ml red cells.

2. The ability to donate blood depends predominantly on the patient's blood volume and baseline PCV. Both variables determine the endogenous red cell reserve, which can be calculated according to the following formula.

Endogenous red cell reserve = blood volume [ml] × (PCV - 33) ÷ 100

Women:	blood volume [ml] = 41 [ml/kg] × body weight [kg] + 1200 [ml]
Men:	blood volume [ml] = 44 [ml/kg] × body weight [kg] + 1600 [ml]
	(body weight ⩾ 45kg)

The indication for NeoRecormon treatment and, if given, the single dose should be determined from the required amount of pre-donated blood and the endogenous red cell reserve according to the following graphs.

(see Figure 1 on next page)

The single dose thus determined is administered twice weekly over 4 weeks. The maximum dose should not exceed 1200 IU/kg body weight per week.

4.3 Contraindications

NeoRecormon must not be used in the presence of poorly controlled hypertension and known hypersensitivity to the active substances to any of the excipients of NeoRecormon in cartridge or benzoic acid, a metabolite of benzyl alcohol.

In the indication "increasing the yield of autologous blood", NeoRecormon must not be used in patients who, in the month preceding treatment, have suffered a myocardial infarction or stroke, patients with unstable angina pectoris, or patients who are at risk of deep venous thrombosis such as those with a history of venous thromboembolic disease.

NeoRecormon in cartridge contains benzyl alcohol as a preservative and must therefore not be used in infants or young children up to three years old.

Figure 1

Female patients

Required amount of pre-donated blood

[units]

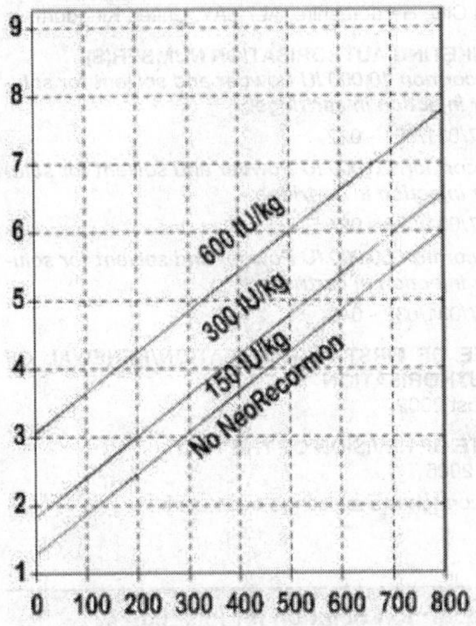

Endogenous red cell reserve [ml]

Male patients

Required amount of pre-donated blood

[units]

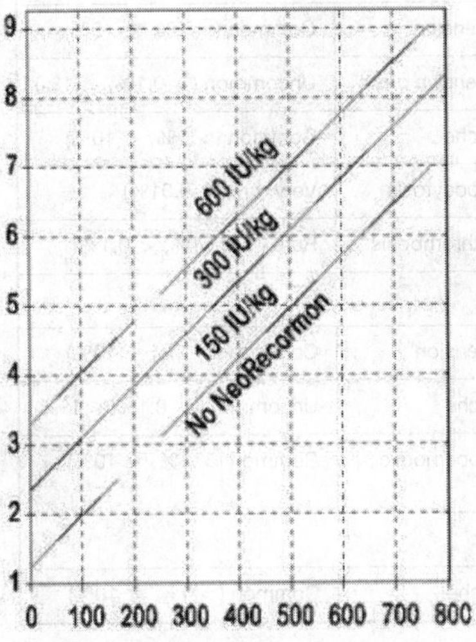

Endogenous red cell reserve [ml]

4.4 Special warnings and special precautions for use

NeoRecormon should be used with caution in the presence of refractory anaemia with excess blasts in transformation, epilepsy, thrombocytosis, and chronic liver failure. Folic acid and vitamin B_{12} deficiencies should be ruled out as they reduce the effectiveness of NeoRecormon.

Severe aluminium overload due to treatment of renal failure may compromise the effectiveness of NeoRecormon.

The indication for NeoRecormon treatment of nephrosclerotic patients not yet undergoing dialysis should be defined individually, as a possible acceleration of progression of renal failure cannot be ruled out with certainty.

Patients who have developed anti-erythropoietin antibodies and pure red cell aplasia under treatment with another erythropoietic substance should not be switched to NeoRecormon due to possible cross-reactivity of antibodies to all erythropoietic substances.

In *chronic renal failure* patients there may be a moderate dose-dependent rise in the platelet count within the normal range during treatment with NeoRecormon, especially after intravenous administration. This regresses during the course of continued therapy. It is recommended that the platelet count be monitored regularly during the first 8 weeks of therapy.

Effect on tumour growth

Epoetins are growth factors that primarily stimulate red blood cell production. Erythropoietin receptors may be expressed on the surface of a variety of tumour cells. As with all growth factors, there is a concern that epoetins could stimulate the growth of any type of malignancy. Two controlled clinical studies in which epoetins were administered to patients with various cancers including head and neck cancer, and breast cancer, have shown an unexplained excess mortality.

Platelet counts and haemoglobin level should also be monitored at regular intervals in cancer patients.

In patients in an *autologous blood predonation programme* there may be an increase in platelet count, mostly within the normal range. Therefore, it is recommended that the platelet count be determined at least once a week in these patients. If there is an increase in platelets of more than 150×10^9/l or if platelets rise above the normal range, treatment with NeoRecormon should be discontinued.

In chronic renal failure patients an increase in heparin dose during haemodialysis is frequently required during the course of therapy with NeoRecormon as a result of the increased packed cell volume. Occlusion of the dialysis system is possible if heparinisation is not optimum.

Early shunt revision and thrombosis prophylaxis by administration of acetylsalicylic acid, for example, should be considered in chronic renal failure patients at risk of shunt thrombosis.

Serum potassium levels should be monitored regularly during NeoRecormon therapy. Potassium elevation has been reported in a few uraemic patients receiving NeoRecormon, though causality has not been established. If an elevated or rising potassium level is observed then consideration should be given to ceasing NeoRecormon administration until the level has been corrected.

For use of NeoRecormon in an autologous predonation programme, the official guidelines on principles of blood donation must be considered, in particular:

- only patients with a PCV $\geqslant$ 33% (haemoglobin $\geqslant$ 11 g/dl [6.83 mmol/l]) should donate;
- special care should be taken with patients below 50kg weight;
- the single volume drawn should not exceed approx. 12% of the patient's estimated blood volume.

Treatment should be reserved for patients in whom it is considered of particular importance to avoid homologous blood transfusion taking into consideration the risk/benefit assessment for homologous transfusions.

Misuse by healthy persons may lead to an excessive increase in packed cell volume. This may be associated with life-threatening complications of the cardiovascular system.

NeoRecormon in cartridge contains up to 0.5mg phenylalanine/cartridge as an excipient. Therefore, this should be taken into consideration in patients affected with severe forms of phenylketonuria.

4.5 Interaction with other medicinal products and other forms of Interaction

The clinical results obtained so far do not indicate any interaction of NeoRecormon with other substances.

Animal experiments revealed that epoetin beta does not increase the myelotoxicity of cytostatic drugs like etoposide, cisplatin, cyclophosphamide, and fluorouracil.

4.6 Pregnancy and lactation

Animal experiments have yielded no indications of teratogenic effects of epoetin beta in dosing regimens that do not lead to an unphysiologically high PCV. No adequate experience in human pregnancy and lactation has been gained, but a potential risk appears to be minimal under therapeutic conditions.

4.7 Effects on ability to drive and use machines

No effects on ability to drive and use machines have been observed.

4.8 Undesirable effects

Based on results from clinical trials including 1725 patients approximately 8% of patients treated with NeoRecormon are expected to experience adverse reaction. Undesirable effects during treatment with NeoRecormon are observed predominantly in patients with chronic renal failure or underlying malignancies and are most commonly an increase in blood pressure or aggravation of existing hypertension and headache.

• Cardiovascular system

Anaemic patients with chronic renal failure

The most frequent undesirable effect during treatment with NeoRecormon is an increase in blood pressure or aggravation of existing hypertension, especially in cases of rapid PCV increase. These increases in blood pressure can be treated with medicinal products. If blood pressure rises cannot be controlled by drug therapy, a transient interruption of NeoRecormon therapy is recommended. Particularly at beginning of therapy, regular monitoring of the blood pressure is recommended, including between dialyses. Hypertensive crisis with encephalopathy-like symptoms (e.g. headaches and confused state, sensorimotor disorders - such as speech disturbance and impaired gait - up to tonoclonic seizures) may also occur in individual patients with otherwise normal or low blood pressure. This requires the immediate attention of a physician and intensive medical care. Particular attention should be paid to sudden stabbing migraine-like headaches as a possible warning sign.

Patients with solid tumours, multiple myeloma, non-Hodgkin's lymphoma or chronic lymphocytic leukaemia

Occasionally there may be an increase in blood pressure which can be treated with drugs. It is therefore recommended to monitor blood pressure, in particular in the initial treatment phase. Headache may also occur occasionally.

• Blood

Anaemic patients with chronic renal failure

Shunt thromboses may occur, especially in patients who have a tendency to hypotension or whose arteriovenous fistulae exhibit complications (e.g. stenoses, aneurisms), see section 4.4. In most cases, a fall in serum ferritin values simultaneous with a rise in packed cell volume is observed. Therefore, oral iron substitution of 200 - 300mg Fe^{2+}/day is recommended in all patients with serum ferritin values below 100 micrograms/l or transferrin saturation below 20%. In addition, transient increases in serum potassium and phosphate levels have been observed in isolated cases. These parameters should be monitored regularly.

In very rare cases, neutralising anti-erythropoietin antibodies with or without pure red cell aplasia (PRCA) occurred during rHuEPO therapy. In case PRCA is diagnosed, therapy with erythropoietin must be discontinued and patients should not be switched to another erythropoietic substance.

Patients with solid tumours, multiple myeloma, non-Hodgkin's lymphoma or chronic lymphocytic leukaemia

In some patients, a fall in serum iron parameters is observed. Therefore, oral iron substitution of 200 - 300mg Fe^{2+}/day is recommended in all patients with serum ferritin values below 100 micrograms/l or transferrin saturation below 20%. In patients with multiple myeloma, non-Hodgkin's lymphoma or chronic lymphocytic leukaemia, with transferrin saturation below 25%, 100mg intravenous Fe^{3+}/week has also been used.

Clinical studies have shown a higher frequency of thromboembolic events in cancer patients treated with NeoRecormon compared to untreated controls or placebo. In patients treated with NeoRecormon, this incidence is 5.9 % compared to 4.2 % in controls; this is not associated with any increase in thromboembolic mortality compared with controls.

Patients in an autologous blood predonation programme

Patients in an autologous blood predonation programme have been reported to show a slightly higher frequency of thromboembolic events. However, a causal relationship with treatment with NeoRecormon could not be established.

As there are indications of a temporary iron deficiency all patients should be treated orally with 300mg Fe^{2+}/day from start of NeoRecormon treatment up to normalisation of ferritin values. If, despite oral iron substitution, iron deficiency (ferritin below or equal to 20 micrograms/l or transferrin saturation below 20%) develops, the additional intravenous administration of iron should be considered.

• Others

Rarely, skin reactions such as rash, pruritus, urticaria or injection site reactions may occur. In isolated cases anaphylactoid reactions have been reported. However, in controlled clinical studies no increased incidence of hypersensitivity reactions was found.

In isolated cases, particularly when starting treatment, flu-like symptoms such as fever, chills, headaches, pain in the limbs, malaise and/or bone pain have been reported. These reactions were mild or moderate in nature and subsided after a couple of hours or days.

The following incidences of undesirable effects in clinical trials, considered related to treatment with NeoRecormon and classified by indication area are:

(see Table 1 on next page)

4.9 Overdose

The therapeutic margin of NeoRecormon is very wide. Even at very high serum levels no symptoms of poisoning have been observed.

5. PHARMACOLOGICAL PROPERTIES

5.1 Pharmacodynamic properties

Pharmacotherapeutic group: antianaemic; ATC code: B03XA

Epoetin beta is identical in its amino acid and carbohydrate composition to erythropoietin that has been isolated from the urine of anaemic patients.

Erythropoietin is a glycoprotein that stimulates the formation of erythrocytes from its committed progenitors. It acts as a mitosis stimulating factor and differentiation hormone.

The biological efficacy of epoetin beta has been demonstrated after intravenous and subcutaneous administration in various animal models *in vivo* (normal and uraemic rats, polycythaemic mice, dogs). After administration of epoetin beta, the number of erythrocytes, the Hb values and reticulocyte counts increase as well as the ^{59}Fe-incorporation rate.

An increased ^{3}H-thymidine incorporation in the erythroid nucleated spleen cells has been found *in vitro* (mouse spleen cell culture) after incubation with epoetin beta.

Investigations in cell cultures of human bone marrow cells showed that epoetin beta stimulates erythropoiesis

Table 1

Indication Area	Body System	Adverse Drug Reaction	Incidence
Renal anaemia			
	Vascular disorders	Hypertension	Common (> 1%, < 10%)
	Vascular disorders	Hypertensive crisis	Uncommon (> 0.1%, < 1%)
	Nervous system disorders	Headache	Common (> 1%, < 10%)
	Blood and the lymphatic system disorders	Thrombocytosis	Very rare (< 0.01%)
	Blood and the lymphatic system disorders	Shunt thrombosis	Rare (> 0.01%, < 0.1%)
Anaemia in oncology			
	Vascular disorders	Hypertension	Common (> 1%, < 10%)
	Nervous system disorders	Headache	Uncommon (> 0.1%, <1%)
	Blood and the lymphatic system disorders	Thromboembolic event	Common (> 1%, < 10%)
Autologous blood predonation programme			
	Nervous system disorders	Headache	Common (> 1%, < 10%)

specifically and does not affect leucopoiesis. Cytotoxic actions of epoetin beta on bone marrow or on human skin cells were not detected.

After single dose administration of epoetin beta no effects on behaviour or locomotor activity of mice and circulatory or respiratory function of dogs were observed.

Erythropoietin is a growth factor that primarily stimulates red cell production. Erythropoietin receptors may be expressed on the surface of a variety of tumour cells. There is insufficient information to establish whether the use of epoetin products have an adverse effect on time to tumour progression or progression free survival.

Two studies explored the effect of epoetins on survival and/or tumour progression with higher haemoglobin targets.

In a randomised placebo-controlled study using epoetin alfa in 939 metastatic breast cancer patients, study drug was administered to attempt to maintain haemoglobin levels between 12 and 14 g/dL. At four months, death attributed to disease progression was higher (6 % vs. 3 %) in women receiving epoetin alfa. The overall mortality was significantly higher in the epoetin alfa arm.

In another placebo-controlled study using epoetin beta in 351 patients with head and neck cancer, study drug was administered to maintain the haemoglobin levels of 14 g/dL in women and 15 g/dL in men. Locoregional progression free survival was significantly shorter in patients receiving epoetin beta. The results of this study were confounded by imbalances between the treatment groups, especially with regard to tumour localisation, smoking status and the heterogeneity of the study population.

In addition, several other studies have shown a tendency to improved survival suggesting that epoetin has no negative effect on tumour progression.

In very rare cases, neutralising anti-erythropoietin antibodies with or without pure red cell aplasia (PRCA) occurred during rHuEPO therapy.

5.2 Pharmacokinetic properties
Pharmacokinetic investigations in healthy volunteers and uraemic patients show that the half-life of intravenously administered epoetin beta is between 4 and 12 hours and that the distribution volume corresponds to one to two times the plasma volume. Analogous results have been found in animal experiments in uraemic and normal rats.

After subcutaneous administration of epoetin beta to uraemic patients, the protracted absorption results in a serum concentration plateau, whereby the maximum concentration is reached after an average of 12 - 28 hours. The terminal half-life is higher than after intravenous administration, with an average of 13 - 28 hours.

Bioavailability of epoetin beta after subcutaneous administration is between 23 and 42% as compared with intravenous administration.

5.3 Preclinical safety data
Acute toxicity
The single intravenous administration of 6000 IU/kg b.w. epoetin beta in the dog and in doses of 3; 30; 300; 3000 or 30,000 IU/kg b.w. in the rat did not lead to any detectable toxic damage.

Chronic toxicity
Toxic signs were not observed in 3-month toxicity studies in rats with doses of up to 10,000 IU/kg b.w. or in dogs with doses of up to 3000 IU/kg b.w. administered daily either subcutaneously or intravenously, with the exception of fibrotic changes of the bone marrow which occurred if PCV values exceeded 80%. A further study in dogs revealed that the myelofibrosis does not occur if the packed cell volume is kept below 60%. The observation of myelofibrosis is therefore irrelevant to the clinical situation in man.

Carcinogenicity
A carcinogenicity study with homologous erythropoietin in mice did not reveal any signs of proliferative or tumourigenic potential.

Mutagenicity
Epoetin beta did not reveal any genotoxic potential in the Ames test, in the micronucleus test, in the *in vitro* HGPRT test or in a chromosomal aberration test in cultured human lymphocytes.

Reproduction toxicology
Studies on rats and rabbits showed no relevant evidence of embryotoxic, foetotoxic or teratogenic properties. No alteration of fertility was detected. A peri-postnatal toxicity study revealed no adverse effects in pregnant/lactating females and on the development of conceptus and offspring.

Safety of preservatives
Subchronic and chronic toxicity studies have demonstrated a wide safety margin of the selected preservatives.

6. PHARMACEUTICAL PARTICULARS
6.1 List of excipients
Powder: urea, sodium chloride, polysorbate 20, sodium dihydrogen phosphate, sodium monohydrogen phosphate, calcium chloride, glycine, leucine, isoleucine, threonine, glutamic acid, and phenylalanine.

Solvent: benzyl alcohol, benzalkonium chloride, and water for injections.

6.2 Incompatibilities
NeoRecormon in cartridge should only be used with the Reco-Pen.

6.3 Shelf life
2 years.

The reconstituted solution remains stable for one month if stored in a refrigerator.

6.4 Special precautions for storage
Store at 2°C - 8°C (in a refrigerator).

Keep the container in the outer carton, in order to protect from light.

For the purpose of ambulatory use, the patient may remove the cartridge not yet inserted into the Reco-Pen from the refrigerator and store it at room temperature (not above 25°C) for one single period of up to 5 days.

After insertion into the Reco-Pen, the cooling chain may only be interrupted for administration of the product.

6.5 Nature and contents of container
This NeoRecormon presentation is available in packages containing 1 or 3 two-chamber cartridges for Reco-Pen which are made of glass type I. The front disk is made of rubber material and the stoppers of teflonised rubber material.

Not all pack sizes may be marketed.

6.6 Instructions for use and handling
This NeoRecormon presentation is a two-chamber cartridge containing powder for solution for injection and preserved solution. The ready-to-use solution is prepared by inserting the cartridge into the Reco-Pen. Prior to this a needle should be attached to the Reco-Pen. Only solutions which are clear or slightly opalescent, colourless and practically free of visible particles may be injected.

Please observe the instructions for use which are delivered with the Reco-Pen.

Any unused product or waste material should be disposed of in accordance with local requirements.

7. MARKETING AUTHORISATION HOLDER
Roche Registration Limited, 40 Broadwater Road, Welwyn Garden City, Hertfordshire, AL7 3AY, United Kingdom.

8. MARKETING AUTHORISATION NUMBER(S)
***NeoRecormon 10,000 IU Powder and solvent for solution for injection in cartridge*:**
EU/1/97/031/021 - 022

***NeoRecormon 20,000 IU Powder and solvent for solution for injection in cartridge*:**
EU/1/97/031/023 - 024

***NeoRecormon 60,000 IU Powder and solvent for solution for injection in cartridge*:**
EU/1/97/031/039 - 040.

9. DATE OF FIRST AUTHORISATION/RENEWAL OF THE AUTHORISATION
22 August 2002.

10. DATE OF REVISION OF THE TEXT
13 July 2005

NeoRecormon is a registered trade mark

Neorecormon Solution for Injection in Pre-Filled Syringe

(Roche Products Limited)

1. NAME OF THE MEDICINAL PRODUCT
NeoRecormon® Solution for injection in pre-filled syringe.

2. QUALITATIVE AND QUANTITATIVE COMPOSITION
1 pre-filled syringe with 0.3ml solution for injection contains **500** international units (IU) corresponding to 4.15 micrograms epoetin beta* (recombinant human erythropoietin).

1 pre-filled syringe with 0.3ml solution for injection contains **1000** international units (IU) corresponding to 8.3 micrograms epoetin beta* (recombinant human erythropoietin).

1 pre-filled syringe with 0.3ml solution for injection contains **2000** international units (IU) corresponding to 16.6 micrograms epoetin beta* (recombinant human erythropoietin).

1 pre-filled syringe with 0.3ml solution for injection contains **3000** international units (IU) corresponding to 24.9 micrograms epoetin beta* (recombinant human erythropoietin).

1 pre-filled syringe with 0.3ml solution for injection contains **4000** international units (IU) corresponding to 33.2 micrograms epoetin beta* (recombinant human erythropoietin).

1 pre-filled syringe with 0.3ml solution for injection contains **5000** international units (IU) corresponding to 41.5 micrograms epoetin beta* (recombinant human erythropoietin).

1 pre-filled syringe with 0.3ml solution for injection contains **6000** international units (IU) corresponding to 49.8 micrograms epoetin beta* (recombinant human erythropoietin).

1 pre-filled syringe with 0.6ml solution for injection contains **10,000** international units (IU) corresponding to 83 micrograms epoetin beta* (recombinant human erythropoietin).

1 pre-filled syringe with 0.6ml solution for injection contains **20,000** international units (IU) corresponding to 166 micrograms epoetin beta* (recombinant human erythropoietin).

1 pre-filled syringe with 0.6ml solution for injection contains **30,000** international units (IU) corresponding to 250 micrograms epoetin beta* (recombinant human erythropoietin).

*Produced by recombinant DNA technology in CHO cell line.

For excipients, see 6.1.

3. PHARMACEUTICAL FORM
Solution for injection.

Appearance: Clear colourless to slightly opalescent solution.

4. CLINICAL PARTICULARS
4.1 Therapeutic indications
– Treatment of anaemia associated with chronic renal failure (renal anaemia) in patients on dialysis.

– Treatment of symptomatic renal anaemia in patients not yet undergoing dialysis.

– Prevention of anaemia of prematurity in infants with a birth weight of 750 to 1500g and a gestational age of less than 34 weeks.

– Treatment of symptomatic anaemia in adult patients with solid tumours receiving chemotherapy.

– Treatment of symptomatic anaemia in adult patients with multiple myeloma, low grade non-Hodgkin's lymphoma or chronic lymphocytic leukaemia, who have a relative erythropoietin deficiency and are receiving anti-tumour therapy. Deficiency is defined as an inappropriately low serum erythropoietin level in relation to the degree of anaemia.

– Increasing the yield of autologous blood from patients in a pre-donation programme.

Its use in this indication must be balanced against the reported increased risk of thromboembolic events.

Treatment should only be given to patients with moderate anaemia (Hb 10 – 13 g/dl [6.21 - 8.07 mmol/l], no iron deficiency) if blood conserving procedures are not available or insufficient when the scheduled major elective surgery requires a large volume of blood (4 or more units of blood for females or 5 or more units for males).

4.2 Posology and method of administration

Therapy with NeoRecormon should be initiated by physicians experienced in the above mentioned indications. As anaphylactoid reactions were observed in isolated cases, it is recommended that the first dose be administered under medical supervision.

The NeoRecormon pre-filled syringe is ready for use. Only solutions which are clear or slightly opalescent, colourless and practically free of visible particles may be injected.

NeoRecormon in pre-filled syringe is a sterile but unpreserved product. Under no circumstances should more than one dose be administered per syringe.

Treatment of anaemic patients with chronic renal failure

The solution can be administered subcutaneously or intravenously. In case of intravenous administration, the solution should be injected over approx. 2 minutes, e.g. in haemodialysis patients via the arterio-venous fistula at the end of dialysis.

For non-haemodialysed patients, subcutaneous administration should always be preferred in order to avoid puncture of peripheral veins.

The aim of treatment is to increase the packed cell volume to 30 - 35% whereby the weekly increase should be at least 0.5 vol%. A value of 35% should not be exceeded.

In the presence of hypertension or existing cardiovascular, cerebrovascular or peripheral vascular diseases, the weekly increase in the PCV and the target PCV should be determined individually taking into account the clinical picture. In some patients the optimum PCV may be below 30%.

Treatment with NeoRecormon is divided into two stages.

1. Correction phase

Subcutaneous administration:

The initial dosage is 3 × 20 IU/kg body weight per week. The dosage may be increased every 4 weeks by 3 × 20 IU/kg per week if the increase of packed cell volume is not adequate (< 0.5% per week).

The weekly dose can also be divided into daily doses.

Intravenous administration:

The initial dosage is 3 × 40 IU/kg per week. The dosage may be raised after 4 weeks to 80 IU/kg - three times per week - and by further increments of 20 IU/kg if needed, three times per week, at monthly intervals.

For both routes of administration, the maximum dose should not exceed 720 IU/kg per week.

2. Maintenance phase

To maintain a packed cell volume of between 30 and 35%, the dosage is initially reduced to half of the previously administered amount. Subsequently, the dose is adjusted at intervals of one or two weeks individually for the patient (maintenance dose).

In the case of subcutaneous administration, the weekly dose can be given as one injection per week or in divided doses three or seven times per week. Patients who are stable on a once weekly dosing regimen may be switched to once every two weeks administration. In this case dose increases may be necessary.

Results of clinical studies in children have shown that, on average, the younger the patients, the higher the NeoRecormon doses required. Nevertheless, the recommended dosing schedule should be followed as the individual response cannot be predicted.

Treatment with NeoRecormon is normally a long-term therapy. It can, however, be interrupted, if necessary, at any time. Data on the once weekly dosing schedule are based on clinical studies with a treatment duration of 24 weeks.

Prevention of anaemia of prematurity

The solution is administered subcutaneously at a dose of 3 × 250 IU/kg b.w. per week. Treatment with NeoRecormon should start as early as possible, preferably by day 3 of life. Premature infants who have already been transfused by the start of treatment with NeoRecormon are not likely to benefit as much as untransfused infants. The treatment should last for 6 weeks.

Treatment of symptomatic anaemia in patients with solid tumours

The solution is administered subcutaneously; the weekly dose can be divided into 3 to 7 single doses.

NeoRecormon treatment is indicated if the haemoglobin value is ⩽ 11 g/dl (6.83 mmol/l).

The recommended initial dose is 450 IU/kg body weight per week.

Haemoglobin level should not exceed 13 g/dl (8.07 mmol/l) (see section 5.1).

If, after 4 weeks, a patient does not show a satisfactory response in terms of haemoglobin values, then the dose should be doubled. The therapy should be continued for up to 3 weeks after the end of chemotherapy.

Figure 1

Female patients

Required amount of predonated blood

[units]

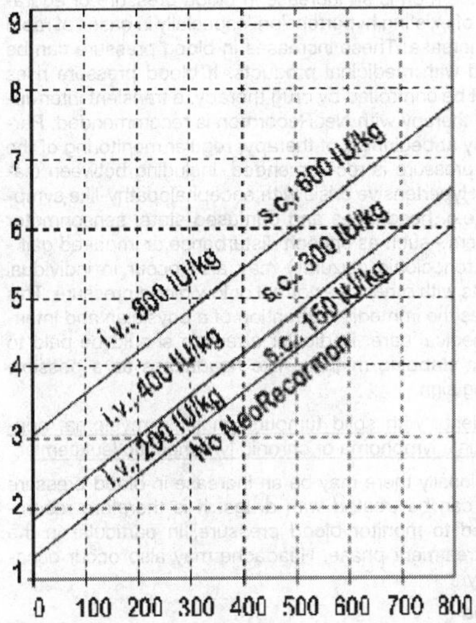

Endogenous red cell reserve [ml]

Male patients

Required amount of predonated blood

[units]

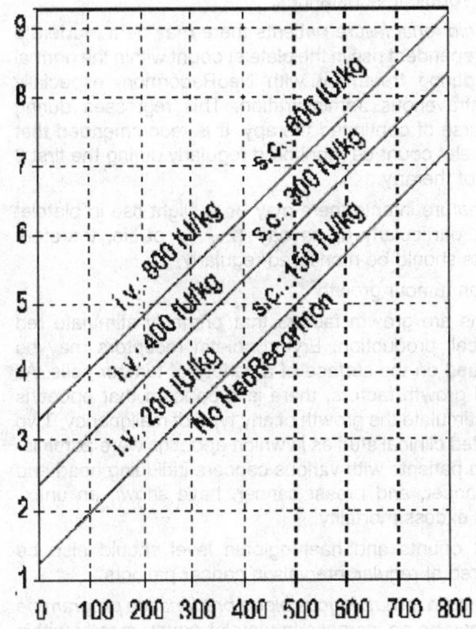

Endogenous red cell reserve [ml]

If haemoglobin falls by more than 1 g/dl (0.62 mmol/l) in the first cycle of chemotherapy despite concomitant NeoRecormon therapy, further therapy may not be effective.

Once the therapeutic objective for an individual patient has been achieved, the dose should be reduced by 25 to 50 % in order to maintain haemoglobin at that level. If required, further dose reduction may be instituted to ensure that haemoglobin level does not exceed 13 g/dl.

If the rise in haemoglobin is greater than 2 g/dl (1.3 mmol/l) in 4 weeks, the dose should be reduced by 25 to 50 %.

Treatment of symptomatic anaemia in patients with multiple myeloma, low-grade non-Hodgkin's lymphoma or chronic lymphocytic leukaemia

Patients with multiple myeloma, non-Hodgkin's lymphoma or chronic lymphocytic leukaemia should have a relative erythropoietin deficiency. Deficiency is defined as an inappropriately low serum erythropoietin level in relation to the degree of anaemia:

serum erythropoietin level of ⩽ 100mU/ml at a haemoglobin of > 9 to < 10 g/dl (> 5.58 to < 6.21 mmol/l)

serum erythropoietin level of ⩽ 180mU/ml at a haemoglobin of > 8 to ⩽ 9 g/dl (> 4.96 to 5.58 mmol/l)

serum erythropoietin level of ⩽ 300mU/ml at a haemoglobin of ⩽ 8 g/dl (⩽ 4.96 mmol/l)

The above values should be measured at least 7 days after the last blood transfusion and the last cycle of cytotoxic chemotherapy.

The solution is administered subcutaneously; the weekly dose can be given as one injection per week or in divided doses 3 to 7 times per week.

The recommended initial dose is 450 IU/kg body weight per week.

Haemoglobin level should not exceed 13 g/dl (8.07 mmol/l) (see section 5.1).

If, after 4 weeks of therapy, the haemoglobin value has increased by at least 1 g/dl (0.62 mmol/l), the current dose should be continued. If the haemoglobin value has not increased by at least 1 g/dl (0.62 mmol/l), a dose increase to 900 IU/kg body weight, given in divided doses 2 to 7 times per week, may be considered. If, after 8 weeks of therapy, the haemoglobin value has not increased by at least 1 g/dl (0.62 mmol/l), response is unlikely and treatment should be discontinued.

Clinical studies have shown that response to epoetin beta treatment is delayed by about 2 weeks in chronic lymphocytic leukaemia patients, as compared with patients with multiple myeloma, non-Hodgkin's lymphoma and solid tumours. The therapy should be continued up to 4 weeks after the end of chemotherapy.

The maximum dose should not exceed 900 IU/kg body weight per week.

Once the therapeutic objective for an individual patient has been achieved, the dose should be reduced by 25 to 50 % in order to maintain haemoglobin at that level. If required, further dose reduction may be instituted to ensure that haemoglobin level does not exceed 13 g/dl.

If the rise in haemoglobin is greater than 2 g/dl (1.3 mmol/l) in 4 weeks, the dose should be reduced by 25 to 50 %.

Therapy should only be reintroduced if the erythropoietin deficiency is the most likely cause of the anaemia.

Treatment for increasing the amount of autologous blood

The solution is administered intravenously over approx. 2 minutes or subcutaneously.

NeoRecormon is administered twice weekly over 4 weeks. On those occasions where the patient's PCV allows blood donation, i.e. PCV ⩾ 33%, NeoRecormon is administered at the end of blood donation.

During the entire treatment period, a PCV of 48% should not be exceeded.

The dosage must be determined by the surgical team individually for each patient as a function of the required amount of pre-donated blood and the endogenous red cell reserve:

1. The required amount of pre-donated blood depends on the anticipated blood loss, use of blood conserving procedures and the physical condition of the patient.

This amount should be that quantity which is expected to be sufficient to avoid homologous blood transfusions.

The required amount of pre-donated blood is expressed in units whereby one unit in the nomogram is equivalent to 180ml red cells.

2. The ability to donate blood depends predominantly on the patient's blood volume and baseline PCV. Both variables determine the endogenous red cell reserve, which can be calculated according to the following formula.

Endogenous red cell reserve = blood volume [ml] × (PCV - 33) ÷ 100

Women: blood volume [ml] = 41 [ml/kg] × body weight [kg] + 1200 [ml]

Men: blood volume [ml] = 44 [ml/kg] × body weight [kg] + 1600 [ml]

(body weight ⩾ 45 kg)

The indication for treatment with NeoRecormon and, if given, the single dose should be determined from the required amount of pre-donated blood and the endogenous red cell reserve according to the following graphs.

(see Figure 1 above)

The single dose thus determined is administered twice weekly over 4 weeks. The maximum dose should not exceed 1600 IU/kg body weight per week for intravenous or 1200 IU/kg per week for subcutaneous administration.

4.3 Contraindications

NeoRecormon must not be used in the presence of poorly controlled hypertension and known hypersensitivity to the active substance or to any of the excipients.

In the indication "increasing the yield of autologous blood", NeoRecormon must not be used in patients who, in the month preceding treatment, have suffered a myocardial infarction or stroke, patients with unstable angina pectoris, or patients who are at risk of deep venous thrombosis such as those with a history of venous thromboembolic disease.

4.4 Special warnings and special precautions for use

NeoRecormon should be used with caution in the presence of refractory anaemia with excess blasts in transformation, epilepsy, thrombocytosis, and chronic liver failure. Folic acid and vitamin B_{12} deficiencies should be ruled out as they reduce the effectiveness of NeoRecormon.

Severe aluminium overload due to treatment of renal failure may compromise the effectiveness of NeoRecormon.

The indication for treatment with NeoRecormon of nephrosclerotic patients not yet undergoing dialysis should be defined individually, as a possible acceleration of progression of renal failure cannot be ruled out with certainty.

Patients who have developed anti-erythropoietin antibodies and pure red cell aplasia under treatment with another erythropoietic substance should not be switched to NeoRecormon due to possible cross-reactivity of antibodies to all erythropoietic substances.

In *chronic renal failure* patients there may be a moderate dose-dependent rise in the platelet count within the normal range during treatment with NeoRecormon, especially after intravenous administration. This regresses during the course of continued therapy. It is recommended that the platelet count be monitored regularly during the first 8 weeks of therapy.

In premature infants there may be a slight rise in platelet counts, particularly up to day 12 - 14 of life, therefore platelets should be monitored regularly.

Effect on tumour growth

Epoetins are growth factors that primarily stimulate red blood cell production. Erythropoietin receptors may be expressed on the surface of a variety of tumour cells. As with all growth factors, there is a concern that epoetins could stimulate the growth of any type of malignancy. Two controlled clinical studies in which epoetins were administered to patients with various cancers including head and neck cancer, and breast cancer, have shown an unexplained excess mortality.

Platelet counts and haemoglobin level should also be monitored at regular intervals in cancer patients.

In patients in an *autologous blood predonation programme* there may be an increase in platelet count, mostly within the normal range. Therefore, it is recommended that the platelet count be determined at least once a week in these patients. If there is an increase in platelets of more than 150×10^9/l or if platelets rise above the normal range, treatment with NeoRecormon should be discontinued.

In *chronic renal failure* patients an increase in heparin dose during haemodialysis is frequently required during the course of therapy with NeoRecormon as a result of the increased packed cell volume. Occlusion of the dialysis system is possible if heparinisation is not optimum.

Early shunt revision and thrombosis prophylaxis by administration of acetylsalicylic acid, for example, should be considered in chronic renal failure patients at risk of shunt thrombosis.

Serum potassium levels should be monitored regularly during therapy with NeoRecormon. Potassium elevation has been reported in a few uraemic patients receiving NeoRecormon, though causality has not been established. If an elevated or rising potassium level is observed then consideration should be given to ceasing administration of NeoRecormon until the level has been corrected.

For use of NeoRecormon in an autologous predonation programme, the official guidelines on principles of blood donation must be considered, in particular:

– only patients with a PCV ≥ 33% (haemoglobin ≥ 11 g/dl [6.83 mmol/l]) should donate;

– special care should be taken with patients below 50 kg weight;

– the single volume drawn should not exceed approx. 12% of the patient's estimated blood volume.

Treatment should be reserved for patients in whom it is considered of particular importance to avoid homologous blood transfusion taking into consideration the risk/benefit assessment for homologous transfusions.

Misuse by healthy persons may lead to an excessive increase in packed cell volume. This may be associated with life-threatening complications of the cardiovascular system.

NeoRecormon in pre-filled syringe contains up to 0.3mg phenylalanine/syringe as an excipient. Therefore this should be taken into consideration in patients affected with severe forms of phenylketonuria.

4.5 Interaction with other medicinal products and other forms of Interaction

The clinical results obtained so far do not indicate any interaction of NeoRecormon with other substances.

Animal experiments revealed that epoetin beta does not increase the myelotoxicity of cytostatic drugs like etoposide, cisplatin, cyclophosphamide, and fluorouracil.

4.6 Pregnancy and lactation

Animal experiments have yielded no indications of teratogenic effects of epoetin beta in dosing regimens that do not lead to an unphysiologically high PCV. No adequate experience in human pregnancy and lactation has been gained, but a potential risk appears to be minimal under therapeutic conditions.

4.7 Effects on ability to drive and use machines

No effects on ability to drive or use machines have been observed.

4.8 Undesirable effects

Based on results from clinical trials including 1725 patients approximately 8% of patients treated with NeoRecormon are expected to experience adverse reactions. Undesirable effects during treatment with NeoRecormon are observed predominantly in patients with chronic renal failure or underlying malignancies and are most commonly an increase in blood pressure or aggravation of existing hypertension and headache.

• Cardiovascular system

– Anaemic patients with chronic renal failure

The most frequent undesirable effect during treatment with NeoRecormon is an increase in blood pressure or aggravation of existing hypertension, especially in cases of rapid PCV increase. These increases in blood pressure can be treated with medicinal products. If blood pressure rises cannot be controlled by drug therapy, a transient interruption of therapy with NeoRecormon is recommended. Particularly at beginning of therapy, regular monitoring of the blood pressure is recommended, including between dialyses. Hypertensive crisis with encephalopathy-like symptoms (e.g. headaches and confused state, sensorimotor disorders - such as speech disturbance or impaired gait - up to tonoclonic seizures) may also occur in individual patients with otherwise normal or low blood pressure. This requires the immediate attention of a physician and intensive medical care. Particular attention should be paid to sudden stabbing migraine-like headaches as a possible warning sign.

– Patients with solid tumours, multiple myeloma, non-Hodgkin's lymphoma or chronic lymphocytic leukaemia

Occasionally there may be an increase in blood pressure which can be treated with drugs. It is therefore recommended to monitor blood pressure, in particular in the initial treatment phase. Headache may also occur occasionally.

• Blood

– Anaemic patients with chronic renal failure

Shunt thromboses may occur, especially in patients who have a tendency to hypotension or whose arteriovenous fistulae exhibit complications (e.g. stenoses, aneurisms), see section 4.4. In most cases, a fall in serum ferritin values simultaneous with a rise in packed cell volume is observed. Therefore, oral iron substitution of 200 - 300mg Fe^{2+}/day is recommended in all patients with serum ferritin values below 100 micrograms/l or transferrin saturation below 20%. In addition, transient increases in serum potassium and phosphate levels have been observed in isolated cases. These parameters should be monitored regularly.

In very rare cases, neutralising anti-erythropoietin antibodies with or without pure red cell aplasia (PRCA) occurred during rHuEPO therapy. In case PRCA is diagnosed, therapy with erythropoietin must be discontinued and patients should not be switched to another erythropoietic substance.

– Premature infants

In most cases, a fall in serum ferritin values is observed. Therefore, oral iron treatment should begin as early as possible (by day 14 of life at the latest) with 2mg Fe^{2+}/day. Iron dosing should be modified according to the serum ferritin level. If serum ferritin is below 100 micrograms/l or if there are other signs of iron deficiency, Fe^{2+} administration should be increased to 5 - 10mg Fe^{2+} per day. Iron therapy should be continued until signs of iron deficiency disappear.

– Patients with solid tumours, multiple myeloma, non-Hodgkin's lymphoma or chronic lymphocytic leukaemia

In some patients, a fall in serum iron parameters is observed. Therefore, oral iron substitution of 200 - 300mg Fe^{2+}/day is recommended in all patients with serum ferritin values below 100 micrograms/l or transferrin saturation below 20%. In patients with multiple myeloma, non-Hodgkin's lymphoma or chronic lymphocytic leukaemia, with transferrin saturation below 25%, 100mg intravenous Fe^{3+}/week has also been used.

Clinical studies have shown a higher frequency of thromboembolic events in cancer patients treated with NeoRecormon compared to untreated controls or placebo. In patients treated with NeoRecormon, this incidence is 5.9 % compared to 4.2 % in controls; this is not associated with any increase in thromboembolic mortality compared with controls.

– Patients in an autologous blood predonation programme

Patients in an autologous blood predonation programme have been reported to show a slightly higher frequency of thromboembolic events. However, a causal relationship with treatment with NeoRecormon could not be established.

As there are indications of a temporary iron deficiency all patients should be treated orally with 300mg Fe^{2+}/day from start of treatment with NeoRecormon up to normalisation of ferritin values. If, despite oral iron substitution, iron deficiency (ferritin below or equal to 20 micrograms/l or transferrin saturation below 20%) develops, the additional intravenous administration of iron should be considered.

• Others

Rarely, skin reactions such as rash, pruritus, urticaria or injection site reactions may occur. In isolated cases anaphylactoid reactions have been reported. However, in controlled clinical studies no increased incidence of hypersensitivity reactions was found.

In isolated cases, particularly when starting treatment, flu-like symptoms such as fever, chills, headaches, pain in the limbs, malaise and/or bone pain have been reported. These reactions were mild or moderate in nature and subsided after a couple of hours or days.

The following incidences of undesirable effects in clinical trials, considered related to treatment with NeoRecormon and classified by indication area are:

(see Table 1 below)

4.9 Overdose

The therapeutic margin of NeoRecormon is very wide. Even at very high serum levels no symptoms of poisoning have been observed.

5. PHARMACOLOGICAL PROPERTIES

5.1 Pharmacodynamic properties

Pharmacotherapeutic group: antianaemic, ATC code: B03XA

Epoetin beta is identical in its amino acid and carbohydrate composition to erythropoietin that has been isolated from the urine of anaemic patients.

Erythropoietin is a glycoprotein that stimulates the formation of erythrocytes from its committed progenitors. It acts as a mitosis stimulating factor and differentiation hormone.

The biological efficacy of epoetin beta has been demonstrated after intravenous and subcutaneous administration in various animal models *in vivo* (normal and uraemic rats, polycythaemic mice, dogs). After administration of epoetin beta, the number of erythrocytes, the Hb values and reticulocyte counts increase as well as the ^{59}Fe-incorporation rate.

An increased ^{3}H-thymidine incorporation in the erythroid nucleated spleen cells has been found *in vitro* (mouse spleen cell culture) after incubation with epoetin beta.

Investigations in cell cultures of human bone marrow cells showed that epoetin beta stimulates erythropoiesis specifically and does not affect leucopoiesis. Cytotoxic actions of epoetin beta on bone marrow or on human skin cells were not detected.

Table 1

Indication Area	Body System	Adverse Drug Reaction	Incidence
Renal anaemia			
	Vascular disorders	Hypertension	Common (> 1%, < 10%)
	Vascular disorders	Hypertensive crisis	Uncommon (> 0.1%, < 1%)
	Nervous system disorders	Headache	Common (> 1%, < 10%)
	Blood and the lymphatic system disorders	Thrombocytosis	Very rare (< 0.01%)
	Blood and the lymphatic system disorders	Shunt thrombosis	Rare (> 0.01%, < 0.1%)
Anaemia in oncology			
	Vascular disorders	Hypertension	Common (> 1%, < 10%)
	Nervous system disorders	Headache	Uncommon (> 0.1%, <1%)
	Blood and the lymphatic system disorders	Thromboembolic event	Common (> 1%, < 10%)
Autologous blood predonation programme			
	Nervous system disorders	Headache	Common (> 1%, < 10%)

After single dose administration of epoetin beta no effects on behaviour or locomotor activity of mice and circulatory or respiratory function of dogs were observed.

Erythropoietin is a growth factor that primarily stimulates red cell production. Erythropoietin receptors may be expressed on the surface of a variety of tumour cells. There is insufficient information to establish whether the use of epoetin products have an adverse effect on time to tumour progression or progression free survival.

Two studies explored the effect of epoetins on survival and/or tumour progression with higher haemoglobin targets.

In a randomised placebo-controlled study using epoetin alfa in 939 metastatic breast cancer patients, study drug was administered to attempt to maintain haemoglobin levels between 12 and 14 g/dL. At four months, death attributed to disease progression was higher (6 % vs. 3 %) in women receiving epoetin alfa. The overall mortality was significantly higher in the epoetin alfa arm.

In another placebo-controlled study using epoetin beta in 351 patients with head and neck cancer, study drug was administered to maintain the haemoglobin levels of 14 g/dL in women and 15 g/dL in men. Locoregional progression free survival was significantly shorter in patients receiving epoetin beta. The results of this study were confounded by imbalances between the treatment groups, especially with regard to tumour localisation, smoking status and the heterogeneity of the study population.

In addition, several other studies have shown a tendency to improved survival suggesting that epoetin has no negative effect on tumour progression.

In very rare cases, neutralising anti-erythropoietin antibodies with or without pure red cell aplasia (PRCA) occurred during rHuEPO therapy.

5.2 Pharmacokinetic properties

Pharmacokinetic investigations in healthy volunteers and uraemic patients show that the half-life of intravenously administered epoetin beta is between 4 and 12 hours and that the distribution volume corresponds to one to two times the plasma volume. Analogous results have been found in animal experiments in uraemic and normal rats.

After subcutaneous administration of epoetin beta to uraemic patients, the protracted absorption results in a serum concentration plateau, whereby the maximum concentration is reached after an average of 12 - 28 hours. The terminal half-life is higher than after intravenous administration, with an average of 13 - 28 hours.

Bioavailability of epoetin beta after subcutaneous administration is between 23 and 42% as compared with intravenous administration.

5.3 Preclinical safety data

Acute toxicity

The single intravenous administration of 6000 IU/kg b.w. epoetin beta in the dog and in doses of 3; 30; 300; 3000 or 30,000 IU/kg b.w. in the rat did not lead to any detectable toxic damage.

Chronic toxicity

Toxic signs were not observed in 3-month toxicity studies in rats with doses of up to 10,000 IU/kg b.w. or in dogs with doses of up to 3000 IU/kg b.w. administered daily either subcutaneously or intravenously, with the exception of fibrotic changes of the bone marrow which occurred if PCV values exceeded 80%. A further study in dogs revealed that the myelofibrosis does not occur if the packed cell volume is kept below 60%. The observation of myelofibrosis is therefore irrelevant to the clinical situation in man.

Carcinogenicity

A carcinogenicity study with homologous erythropoietin in mice did not reveal any signs of proliferative or tumourigenic potential.

Mutagenicity

Epoetin beta did not reveal any genotoxic potential in the Ames test, in the micronucleus test, in the *in vitro* HGPRT test or in a chromosomal aberration test in cultured human lymphocytes.

Reproduction toxicology

Studies on rats and rabbits showed no relevant evidence of embryotoxic, foetotoxic or teratogenic properties. No alteration of fertility was detected. A peri-postnatal toxicity study revealed no adverse effects in pregnant/lactating females and on the development of conceptus and offspring.

6. PHARMACEUTICAL PARTICULARS

6.1 List of excipients

Urea, sodium chloride, polysorbate 20, sodium dihydrogen phosphate, sodium monohydrogen phosphate, calcium chloride, glycine, leucine, isoleucine, threonine, glutamic acid, phenylalanine, and water for injections.

6.2 Incompatibilities

This medicinal product must not be mixed with other medicinal products.

6.3 Shelf life

2 years.

6.4 Special precautions for storage

Store at 2°C - 8°C (in a refrigerator).

Keep the container in the outer carton, in order to protect from light.

For the purpose of ambulatory use, the patient may remove the product from the refrigerator and store it at room temperature (not above 25°C) for one single period of up to 3 days.

6.5 Nature and contents of container

One pack contains 1 or 6 prefilled syringes and 1 or 6 needles 27G1/2.

The syringes are made of glass type I and the tip cap and plunger stopper of rubber material.

Not all pack sizes may be marketed.

6.6 Instructions for use and handling

First wash your hands!

1. Remove one syringe from the pack and check that the solution is clear, colourless and practically free from visible particles. Remove the cap from the syringe.

2. Remove one needle from the pack, fix it on the syringe and remove the protective cap from the needle.

3. Expel air from the syringe and needle by holding the syringe vertically and gently pressing the plunger upwards. Keep pressing the plunger until the amount of NeoRecormon in the syringe is as prescribed.

4. Clean the skin at the site of injection using an alcohol wipe. Form a skin fold by pinching the skin between thumb and forefinger. Hold the syringe barrel near to the needle, and insert the needle into the skin fold with a quick, firm action. Inject the NeoRecormon solution. Withdraw the needle quickly and apply pressure over the injection site with a dry, sterile pad.

Any unused product or waste material should be disposed of in accordance with local requirements.

7. MARKETING AUTHORISATION HOLDER

Roche Registration Limited, 40 Broadwater Road, Welwyn Garden City, Hertfordshire, AL7 3AY, United Kingdom.

8. MARKETING AUTHORISATION NUMBER(S)

NeoRecormon 500 IU solution for injection in pre-filled syringe:

EU/1/97/031/026

NeoRecormon 1000 IU solution for injection in pre-filled syringe:

EU/1/97/031/028

NeoRecormon 2000 IU solution for injection in pre-filled syringe:

EU/1/97/031/030

NeoRecormon 3000 IU solution for injection in pre-filled syringe:

EU/1/97/031/032

NeoRecormon 4000 IU solution for injection in pre-filled syringe:

EU/1/97/031/042

NeoRecormon 5000 IU solution for injection in pre-filled syringe:

EU/1/97/031/034

NeoRecormon 6000 IU solution for injection in pre-filled syringe:

EU/1/97/031/044

NeoRecormon 10,000 IU solution for injection in pre-filled syringe:

EU/1/97/031/036

NeoRecormon 20,000 IU solution for injection in pre-filled syringe:

EU/1/97/031/038

NeoRecormon 30,000 IU solution for injection in pre-filled syringe:

EU/1/97/031/046

9. DATE OF FIRST AUTHORISATION/RENEWAL OF THE AUTHORISATION

NeoRecormon 500-20,000 IU solution for injection in pre-filled syringe:

22 August 2002

NeoRecormon 30,000 IU solution for injection in pre-filled syringe:

February 2004

10. DATE OF REVISION OF THE TEXT

13 July 2005

NeoRecormon is a registered trade mark

Neosporin Eye Drops

(Pliva Pharma Ltd)

1. NAME OF THE MEDICINAL PRODUCT

Neosporin Eye Drops

2. QUALITATIVE AND QUANTITATIVE COMPOSITION

Polymyxin B Sulphate E.P.	5,000 IU
Neomycin Sulphate E.P.	1,700 IU
Gramicidin	25 IU

(IU = International units)

3. PHARMACEUTICAL FORM

Topical Antibacterial Agent

4. CLINICAL PARTICULARS

4.1 Therapeutic indications

For the prophylaxis and treatment of external bacterial infections of the eye.

Prophylactically, it is useful following removal of foreign bodies, and before and after ophthalmic surgery, to help provide and maintain a sterile field.

4.2 Posology and method of administration

Dosage in Adults (over 18 years of age)

1 or 2 drops in the affected eye, two to four times daily or more frequently as required. In severe infections therapy should be started with 1 or 2 drops every 15 to 30 minutes, reducing the frequency of instillation gradually as the infection is controlled.

Treatment should be continued for at least 2 days after the condition has resolved, but treatment should not be continued for more than 7 days without medical supervision, and therefore patients should be advised to return to their doctor if their condition has not improved after 7 days.

Dosage in Children (over 2 years to 18 years of age)

As for adults.

Dosage in Infants under 2 years of age

Contra-indicated

Dosage in Elderly

As for adults. Caution should be exercised in cases where a decrease in renal function exists and significant systemic absorption of neomycin sulphate may occur (see 4.4 Special Warnings and Special Precautions for Use).

Dosage in renal impairment

Dosage should be reduced in patients with reduced renal function (see 4.4 Special Warnings and Special Precautions for Use).

4.3 Contraindications

The use of Neosporin Eye Drops is contra-indicated in patients who have demonstrated allergic hypersensitivity to the product or any of its constituents, or to cross-sensitizing substances such as framycetin, kanamycin, gentamicin and other related antibiotics.

The use of Neosporin Eye Drops is contra-indicated in circumstances where the product could gain access to intra-ocular fluids (see 4.4 Special Warnings and Special Precautions for Use).

Due to the known ototoxic and nephrotoxic potential of neomycin sulphate, the use of Neosporin in large quantities or on large areas for prolonged periods of time is not recommended in circumstances where significant absorption may occur.

A possibility of increased absorption exists in very young children, thus Neosporin Eye Drops are contra-indicated for use in neonates and infants (up to 2 years of age).

In neonates and infants, absorption by immature skin may be enhanced and renal function may be immature.

Due to the risk of adsorption of the preservative (benzalkonium chloride), contact lenses should not be worn when using Neosporin Eye Drops.

4.4 Special warnings and special precautions for use

Following significant systemic absorption, aminoglycosides such as neomycin can cause irreversible ototoxicity; neomycin and polymyxin B sulphate have nephrotoxic potential and polymyxin B sulphate has neurotoxic potential.

Neomycin eye drops should not be used during surgical procedures nor before surgery in circumstances where access of the product to intra-ocular fluids could occur (see 4.3 Contra-Indications).

In renal impairment the plasma clearance of neomycin is reduced (see 4.2 Dosage in Renal Impairment).

4.5 Interaction with other medicinal products and other forms of Interaction

Following significant systemic absorption, both neomycin sulphate and polymyxin B sulphate can intensify and prolong the respiratory depressant effects of neuromuscular blocking agents.

4.6 Pregnancy and lactation

There is little information to demonstrate the possible effect of topically applied neomycin in pregnancy and lactation. No information is available regarding the excretion of the active ingredients or their metabolites in human breast milk. However, neomycin present in maternal blood can cross the placenta and may give rise to a small potential risk of foetal toxicity, thus the use of Neosporin Eye Drops is not recommended in pregnancy or lactation.

4.7 Effects on ability to drive and use machines

None known.

4.8 Undesirable effects

Allergic reactions following the topical application of Neomycin have been reported in the literature, but such reactions following the application of Polymyxin B and Gramicidin are rare events.

As with all antibacterial preparations prolonged use may result in the overgrowth of non-susceptible organisms including fungi.

4.9 Overdose

Symptoms and signs:

No specific symptoms or signs have been associated with excessive use of Neosporin Eye Drops. However, consideration should be given to significant systemic absorption (see 4.4 Special Warnings and Special Precautions for Use).

Following accidental ingestion, minimal absorption is expected.

Management:

Use of the product should be stopped and the patient's general status, hearing acuity, renal and neuromuscular functions should be monitored. Plasma levels of neomycin may be reduced by haemodialysis.

5. PHARMACOLOGICAL PROPERTIES

5.1 Pharmacodynamic properties

Neomycin is an aminoglycoside antibiotic isolated from cultures of *Streptomyces fradiae* and is active against many Gram-negative bacteria. It diffuses through the channels formed by porin-proteins in the outer membrane of the bacteria. Transport across the inner membrane is energy-dependant and is blocked by the presence of calcium ions or in acidic conditions.

Neomycin inhibits protein synthesis by binding to subunits of the bacterial ribosome thus disrupting the normal cycle of ribosomal function. It leads to a misreading of the genetic code of the messenger RNA template resulting in the incorporation of incorrect amino acids. Neomycin may inhibit the bacterial DNA polymerase.

Polymyxin B is one of a family of polypeptide antibiotics produced by various *Bacillus polymyxa* strains. It is bactericidal for a variety of Gram-negative bacteria.

Polymixin B sulphate is a cationic cyclic decapeptide that is surface active. It intercalates into the bacterial cell membrane binding to the lipid A region of lipopolysaccharides, in particular to phosphatidylethanolamine, and renders the osmotic barrier ineffective. This leads to loss of cell contents and bacterial cell death.

Gramicidin is a polypeptide antibiotic produced by the growth of *Bacillus brevis*. It is effective against many Gram-positive organisms.

Gramicidin increases the permeability of cell membranes and uncouples oxidative phosphorylation in the bacterial cell wall with a temporary stimulation of oxygen consumption.

5.2 Pharmacokinetic properties

Not applicable.

5.3 Preclinical safety data

A. Mutagenicity

There is insufficient information available to determine whether the active ingredients have mutagenic potential.

B. Carcinogenicity

There is insufficient information available to determine whether the active ingredients have carcinogenic potential.

C. Teratogenicity

There is insufficient information available to determine whether the active ingredients have teratogenic potential.

Neomycin present in maternal blood can cross the placenta and may give rise to a theoretical risk of foetal ototoxicity.

D. Fertility

There is insufficient information available to determine whether any of the active ingredients can affect fertility

6. PHARMACEUTICAL PARTICULARS

6.1 List of excipients

Ethanol (96%)

Propylene Glycol

Poloxamer 188

Benzalkonium chloride

Sodium Chloride

Sulphuric Acid 0.1M

Sodium Hydroxide 1M

Water for Injections

6.2 Incompatibilities

None known.

6.3 Shelf life

2 years.

Use within one month of first opening.

6.4 Special precautions for storage

Do not store above 25 °C.

Keep the bottle tightly closed.

Keep the bottle in the outer carton.

6.5 Nature and contents of container

Polypropylene bottle with integral nozzle and pilfer proof cap containing 5ml.

6.6 Instructions for use and handling

No special instructions.

Adminstrative Date

7. MARKETING AUTHORISATION HOLDER

The Wellcome Foundation Ltd

Glaxo Wellcome House

Berkeley Avenue

Greenford

Middlesex UB6 0NN

Trading as

GlaxoSmithKline UK

Stockley Park West,

Uxbridge, Middlesex,

UB11 1BT

United Kingdom

8. MARKETING AUTHORISATION NUMBER(S)

PL 0003/5108R

9. DATE OF FIRST AUTHORISATION/RENEWAL OF THE AUTHORISATION

13 January 2004

10. DATE OF REVISION OF THE TEXT

18 February 2005

11. Legal Status

POM

Neostigmine Bromide Tablets

(Cambridge Laboratories)

1. NAME OF THE MEDICINAL PRODUCT

Neostigmine Bromide Tablets

2. QUALITATIVE AND QUANTITATIVE COMPOSITION

Each tablet contains 15 mg Neostigmine Bromide Ph.Eur.

3. PHARMACEUTICAL FORM

Tablets

4. CLINICAL PARTICULARS

4.1 Therapeutic indications

Myasthenia gravis; paralytic ileus; post-operative urinary retention.

4.2 Posology and method of administration

Neostigmine bromide has a slower onset of effect when given orally than when given parenterally, but the duration of action is longer and the intensity of action more uniform.

To facilitate change of treatment from one route of administration to another, the following doses are approximately equivalent in effect:

0.5 mg intravenously = 1-1.5 mg intramuscularly or subcutaneously = 15 mg orally.

Myasthenia gravis

Adults: Doses of 15 to 30 mg by mouth are given at intervals throughout the day when maximum strength is needed (for example, on rising and before mealtimes). The usual duration of action of a dose is two to four hours.

The total daily dose is usually in the range of 5-20 tablets but doses higher than these may be needed by some patients.

Newborn infants: Neostigmine bromide ampoules are recommended.

Older children: Children under 6 years old should receive an initial dose of half a tablet (7.5 mg) of Neostigmine Bromide; children 6-12 years old should receive one tablet (15 mg). Dosage requirements should be adjusted according to the response but are usually in the range of 15-90 mg orally per day.

The requirement for Neostigmine Bromide is usually markedly decreased after thymectomy, or when additional therapy (steroids, immunosuppressant drugs) is given.

When relatively large doses of Neostigmine Bromide are taken by myasthenic patients, it may be necessary to give atropine or other anticholinergic drugs to counteract the muscarinic effects. It should be noted that the slower gastro-intestinal motility caused by these drugs may affect the absorption of oral Neostigmine Bromide.

In all patients the possibility of 'cholinergic crisis', due to overdosage of Neostigmine Bromide, and its differentiation from 'myasthenic crisis', due to increased severity of disease, must be borne in mind. Both types of crisis are manifested by increased muscle weakness, but whereas myasthenic crisis may require more intensive anticholinesterase treatment, cholinergic crisis calls for immediate discontinuation of this treatment and institution of appropriate supportive measures, including respiratory assistance.

Other indications

Adults: The usual dose is 1 to 2 tablets orally.

Children: 2.5-15 mg orally.

The frequency of these doses may be varied according to the needs of the patient.

The elderly: There are no specific dosage recommendations for Neostigmine Bromide in elderly patients.

4.3 Contraindications

Neostigmine Bromide should not be given to patients with mechanical gastro-intestinal or urinary obstruction.

Neostigmine Bromide is contra-indicated in patients with known hypersensitivity to the drug and to bromides.

Neostigmine Bromide should not be used in conjunction with depolarising muscle relaxants such as suxamethonium as neuromuscular blockade may be potentiated and prolonged apnoea may result.

4.4 Special warnings and special precautions for use

Extreme caution is required when administering Neostigmine Bromide to patients with bronchial asthma.

Care should also be taken in patients with bradycardia, recent coronary occlusion, hypotension, peptic ulcer, vagotonia, epilepsy or Parkinsonism.

4.5 Interaction with other medicinal products and other forms of Interaction

Neostigmine Bromide should not be given during cyclopropane or halothane anaesthesia; however, it may be used after withdrawal of these agents.

4.6 Pregnancy and lactation

The safety of Neostigmine Bromide during pregnancy or lactation has not been established. Although the possible hazards to mother and child must therefore be weighed against the potential benefits in every case, experience with Neostigmine Bromide in pregnant patients with myasthenia gravis has revealed no untoward effect of the drug on the course of pregnancy.

As the severity of myasthenia gravis often fluctuates considerably, particular care is required to avoid cholinergic crisis, due to overdosage of the drug, but otherwise management is no different from that in non-pregnant patients.

Observations indicate that only negligible amounts of Neostigmine Bromide are excreted in breast milk; nevertheless due regard should be paid to possible effects on the breast-feeding infant.

4.7 Effects on ability to drive and use machines

Not known.

4.8 Undesirable effects

There is no evidence to suggest that Neostigmine Bromide has any special effects in the elderly, however, elderly patients may be more susceptible to dysrhythmias than the younger adult.

Side-effects and adverse reactions may include nausea and vomiting, increased salivation, diarrhoea and abdominal cramps.

4.9 Overdose

Signs of overdose due to muscarinic effects may include abdominal cramps, increased peristalsis, diarrhoea, nausea and vomiting, increased bronchial secretions, salivation, diaphoresis and miosis. Nicotinic effects consist of muscular cramps, fasciculations and general weakness. Bradycardia and hypotension may also occur.

Artificial ventilation should be instituted if respiration is severely depressed. Atropine sulphate 1 to 2 mg intravenously is an antidote to the muscarinic effects.

5. PHARMACOLOGICAL PROPERTIES

5.1 Pharmacodynamic properties

Neostigmine Bromide is an antagonist to cholinesterase, the enzyme which normally destroys acetylcholine. The action of Neostigmine Bromide can briefly be described, therefore, as the potentiation of naturally occurring acetylcholine.

5.2 Pharmacokinetic properties

Neostigmine Bromide is a quaternary ammonium compound and is poorly absorbed from the gastro-intestinal tract. Following parenteral administration as the methylsulphate, neostigmine is rapidly eliminated with a plasma half-life of 50-90 minutes and is excreted in the urine both as unchanged drug and metabolites. It is metabolised partly by hydrolysis of the ester linkage.

5.3 Preclinical safety data

Neostigmine has not been reported to have mutagenic or carcinogenic potential. In rats, acute and chronic exposure causes changes in the fine structure at the end-plate region of muscle.

6. PHARMACEUTICAL PARTICULARS

6.1 List of excipients

Lactose

Maize starch

Talc

Magnesium stearate

6.2 Incompatibilities

None known.

6.3 Shelf life

Five years

6.4 Special precautions for storage

The recommended maximum storage temperature is 30°C. The tablets should be protected from light.

6.5 Nature and contents of container

White pigmented HDPE bottles with plastic snap-on caps, each containing 140 tablets.

6.6 Instructions for use and handling
None.

7. MARKETING AUTHORISATION HOLDER
Lifehealth Limited
23 Winkfield Road
Windsor
Berkshire
SL4 4BA.

8. MARKETING AUTHORISATION NUMBER(S)
PL 14576/0004

9. DATE OF FIRST AUTHORISATION/RENEWAL OF THE AUTHORISATION
23rd October 1995

10. DATE OF REVISION OF THE TEXT
January 2001

Neotigason

(Roche Products Limited)

1. NAME OF THE MEDICINAL PRODUCT
Neotigason 10mg capsules and Neotigason 25mg capsules

2. QUALITATIVE AND QUANTITATIVE COMPOSITION
Capsules with brown cap and white body with ROCHE printed in black on both cap and body, containing 10mg acitretin.

Capsules with brown cap and yellow body with ROCHE printed in black on both cap and body, containing 25mg acitretin.

3. PHARMACEUTICAL FORM
Capsules for oral administration.

4. CLINICAL PARTICULARS
4.1 Therapeutic indications
Severe extensive psoriasis which is resistant to other forms of therapy.

Palmo-plantar pustular psoriasis.

Severe congenital ichthyosis.

Severe Darier's disease (keratosis follicularis).

4.2 Posology and method of administration
It is recommended that Neotigason be given only by, or under supervision of, a dermatological specialist.

Neotigason capsules are for oral administration.

The capsules should be taken once daily with meals or with milk.

There is a wide variation in the absorption and rate of metabolism of Neotigason. This necessitates individual adjustment of dosage. For this reason the following dosage recommendations can serve only as a guide.

Adults

Initial daily dose should be 25mg or 30mg for 2 to 4 weeks. After this initial treatment period the involved areas of the skin should show a marked response and/or side-effects should be apparent. Following assessment of the initial treatment period, titration of the dose upwards or downwards may be necessary to achieve the desired therapeutic response with the minimum of side-effects. In general, a daily dosage of 25 - 50mg taken for a further 6 to 8 weeks achieves optimal therapeutic results. However, it may be necessary in some cases to increase the dose up to a maximum of 75mg/day.

In patients with Darier's disease a starting dose of 10mg may be appropriate. The dose should be increased cautiously as isomorphic reactions may occur.

Therapy can be discontinued in patients with psoriasis whose lesions have improved sufficiently. Relapses should be treated as described above.

Patients with severe congenital ichthyosis and severe Darier's disease may require therapy beyond 3 months. The lowest effective dosage, not exceeding 50mg/day, should be given.

Continuous use beyond 6 months is contra-indicated as only limited clinical data are available on patients treated beyond this length of time.

Elderly

Dosage recommendations are the same as for other adults.

Children

In view of possible severe side-effects associated with long-term treatment, Neotigason is contra-indicated in children unless, in the opinion of the physician, the benefits significantly outweigh the risks.

The dosage should be established according to bodyweight. The daily dosage is about 0.5mg/kg. Higher doses (up to 1mg/kg daily) may be necessary in some cases for limited periods, but only up to a maximum of 35mg/day. The maintenance dose should be kept as low as possible in view of possible long-term side-effects.

Combination therapy

Other dermatological therapy, particularly with keratolytics, should normally be stopped before administration of Neotigason. However, the use of topical corticosteroids or bland emollient ointment may be continued if indicated.

When Neotigason is used in combination with other types of therapy, it may be possible, depending on the individual patient's response, to reduce the dosage of Neotigason.

4.3 Contraindications
Neotigason is highly teratogenic. Its use is contra-indicated in pregnant women and women who might become pregnant during or within 2 years of the cessation of treatment (see section *4.4 Special warnings and special precautions for use*).

The use of Neotigason is contra-indicated in women who are breast feeding.

Neotigason is contra-indicated in patients with hepatic or renal impairment and in patients with chronic abnormally elevated blood lipid values.

Rare cases of benign intracranial hypertension have been reported after Neotigason and after tetracyclines. Supplementary treatment with antibiotics such as tetracyclines is therefore contra-indicated.

An increased risk of hepatitis has been reported following the concomitant use of methotrexate and etretinate. Consequently, the concomitant use of methotrexate and Neotigason should be avoided.

Concomitant administration of Neotigason with other retinoids or preparations containing high doses of Vitamin A, (i.e. more than the recommended dietary allowance of 4,000 - 5,000 i.u. per day) is contra-indicated due to the risk of hypervitaminosis A.

Neotigason is contra-indicated in cases of hypersensitivity to the preparation (acitretin or excipients) or to other retinoids.

4.4 Special warnings and special precautions for use
Neotigason should only be prescribed by physicians who are experienced in the use of systemic retinoids and understand the risk of teratogenicity associated with acitretin therapy.

Neotigason is highly teratogenic. The risk of giving birth to a deformed child is exceptionally high if Neotigason is taken before or during pregnancy, no matter for how long or at what dosage. Foetal exposure to Neotigason always involves a risk of congenital malformation.

Neotigason is contra-indicated in women of childbearing potential unless the following criteria are met:

1. Pregnancy has been excluded before instituting therapy with Neotigason (negative pregnancy test within 2 weeks prior to therapy). Whenever practicable a monthly repetition of the pregnancy test is recommended during therapy.

2. She starts Neotigason therapy only on the second or third day of the next menstrual cycle.

3. Having excluded pregnancy, any woman of childbearing potential who is receiving Neotigason must practice effective contraception for at least one month before treatment, during the treatment period and for at least 2 years following its cessation.

Even female patients who normally do not practice contraception because of a history of infertility should be advised to do so, while taking Neotigason.

4. The same effective and uninterrupted contraceptive measures must also be taken every time therapy is repeated, however long the intervening period may have been, and must be continued for 2 years afterwards.

5. Any pregnancy occurring during treatment with Neotigason, or in the 2 years following its cessation, carries a high risk of severe foetal malformation. Therefore, before instituting Neotigason the treating physician must explain clearly and in detail what precautions must be taken. This should include the risks involved and the possible consequences of pregnancy occurring during Neotigason treatment or in the 2 years following its cessation.

6. She is reliable and capable of understanding the risk and complying with effective contraception, and confirms that she has understood the warnings.

In view of the importance of the above precautions, Neotigason Patient Information Leaflets are available to doctors and it is strongly recommended that these be given to all patients.

If oral contraception is chosen as the most appropriate contraceptive method for women undergoing retinoid treatment, then a combined oestrogen-progestogen formulation is recommended.

Patients should not donate blood either during or for at least one year following discontinuation of therapy with Neotigason. Theoretically there would be a small risk to a woman in the first trimester of pregnancy who received blood donated by a patient on Neotigason therapy.

Acitretin has been shown to affect diaphyseal and spongy bone adversely in animals at high doses in excess of those recommended for use in man. Since skeletal hyperostosis and extraosseous calcification have been reported following long-term treatment with etretinate in man, this effect should be expected with acitretin therapy.

Since there have been occasional reports of bone changes in children, including premature epiphyseal closure, skeletal hyperostosis and extraosseous calcification after long-term treatment with etretinate, these effects may be expected with acitretin. Neotigason therapy in children is not, therefore, recommended. If, in exceptional circumstances, such therapy is undertaken the child should be carefully monitored for any abnormalities of musculo-skeletal development.

In adults receiving long-term treatment with Neotigason, appropriate examinations should be periodically performed in view of possible ossification abnormalities (see section *4.8 Undesirable effects*). Any patients complaining of atypical musculo-skeletal symptoms on treatment with Neotigason should be promptly and fully investigated to exclude possible acitretin-induced bone changes. If clinically significant bone or joint changes are found, Neotigason therapy should be discontinued.

The effects of UV light are enhanced by retinoid therapy, therefore patients should avoid excessive exposure to sunlight and the unsupervised use of sun lamps.

Hepatic function should be checked before starting treatment with Neotigason, every 1 - 2 weeks for the first 2 months after commencement and then every 3 months during treatment. If abnormal results are obtained, weekly checks should be instituted. If hepatic function fails to return to normal or deteriorates further, Neotigason must be withdrawn. In such cases it is advisable to continue monitoring hepatic function for at least 3 months.

Serum cholesterol and serum triglycerides (fasting values) must be monitored, especially in high-risk patients (disturbances of lipid metabolism, diabetes mellitus, obesity, alcoholism) and during long-term treatment.

In diabetic patients, retinoids can alter glucose tolerance. Blood sugar levels should therefore be checked more frequently than usual at the beginning of the treatment period.

Patients should be warned of the possibility of alopecia occurring (see section *4.8 Undesirable effects*).

4.5 Interaction with other medicinal products and other forms of Interaction
Existing data suggests that concurrent intake of acitretin with ethanol led to the formation of etretinate. However, etretinate formation without concurrent alcohol intake cannot be excluded. Therefore, since the elimination half-life of etretinate is 120 days the post-therapy contraception period in women of childbearing potential must be 2 years (see section *4.4 Special warnings and precautions for use).*

An increased risk of hepatitis has been reported following the concomitant use of methotrexate and etretinate. Consequently, the concomitant use of methotrexate and Neotigason should be avoided (see section *4.3 Contraindications).*

In concurrent treatment with phenytoin, it must be remembered that Neotigason partially reduces the protein binding of phenytoin. The clinical significance of this is as yet unknown.

Interaction studies show acitretin does not interfere with the anti-ovulatory action of the combined oral contraceptives.

Interactions between Neotigason and other substances (e.g. digoxin, cimetidine) have not been observed to date.

4.6 Pregnancy and lactation
Neotigason is contra-indicated during pregnancy as it is a known human teratogen.

The use of Neotigason is contra-indicated in women who are breast feeding. It is also contra-indicated in women of childbearing potential unless specific criteria are met, (see section *4.4 Special warnings and special precautions for use*).

4.7 Effects on ability to drive and use machines
Decreased night vision has been reported with Neotigason therapy. Patients should be advised of this potential problem and warned to be cautious when driving or operating any vehicle at night. Visual problems should be carefully monitored (see section *4.8 Undesirable effects*).

4.8 Undesirable effects
Most of the clinical side-effects of Neotigason are dose-related and are usually well-tolerated at the recommended dosages. However, the toxic dose of Neotigason is close to the therapeutic dose and most patients experience some side-effects during the initial period whilst dosage is being adjusted. They are usually reversible with reduction of dosage or discontinuation of therapy.

The skin and mucous membranes are most commonly affected, and it is recommended that patients should be so advised before treatment is commenced.

Skin: Dryness of the skin may be associated with scaling, thinning, erythema (especially of the face) and pruritus. Palmar and plantar exfoliation may occur. Sticky skin and dermatitis occur frequently. Epidermal fragility, nail fragility and paronychia have been observed.

Occasionally bullous eruptions and abnormal hair texture have been reported. Hair thinning and frank alopecia may occur, usually noted 4 to 8 weeks after starting therapy, and are reversible following discontinuation of Neotigason. Full recovery usually occurs within 6 months of stopping treatment in the majority of patients.

Granulomatous lesions have occasionally been observed.

Sweating has been reported infrequently.

Rarely, patients may experience photosensitivity reactions.

Mucous membranes: Dryness of mucous membranes, sometimes with erosion, involving the lips, mouth, conjunctivae and nasal mucosa have been reported. Corneal ulcerations have been observed rarely.

Dryness of the conjunctivae may lead to mild-to-moderate conjunctivitis or xerophthalmia and result in intolerance of contact lenses; it may be alleviated by lubrication with artificial tears or topical antibiotics.

Cheilitis, rhagades of the corner of the mouth, dry mouth and thirst have occurred. Occasionally stomatitis, gingivitis and taste disturbance have been reported.

Rhinitis and epistaxis have been observed.

Central nervous system: Headache has occurred infrequently. Benign intracranial hypertension has been reported. Patients with severe headache, nausea, vomiting and visual disturbance should discontinue Neotigason immediately and be referred for neurological evaluation and care.

Neuro-sensory system: Blurred or decreased night vision has been reported occasionally.

Musculo-skeletal system: Myalgia and arthralgia may occur and be associated with reduced tolerance to exercise. Bone pain has also been reported.

Maintenance treatment may result in hyperostosis and extraskeletal calcification, as observed in long-term systemic treatment with other retinoids.

Gastrointestinal tract: Nausea has been reported infrequently. Vomiting, diarrhoea and abdominal pain have been observed rarely.

Liver and biliary system disorders: Transient, usually reversible elevation of serum levels of liver enzymes may occur. When significant, dosage reduction or discontinuation of therapy may be necessary. Jaundice and hepatitis have occurred rarely.

Metabolic: Elevation of serum triglycerides above the normal range has been observed, especially where predisposing factors such as a family history of lipid disorders, obesity, alcohol abuse, diabetes mellitus or smoking are present. The changes are dose-related and may be controlled by dietary means (including restriction of alcohol intake) and/or by reduction of dosage of Neotigason. Increases in serum cholesterol have occurred.

Cardiovascular system: Occasionally peripheral oedema and flushing have been reported.

Miscellaneous reactions: Increased incidence of vulvovaginitis due to Candida albicans has been noted during treatment with acitretin. Malaise and drowsiness have been infrequently reported.

4.9 Overdose

Manifestations of acute Vitamin A toxicity include severe headache, nausea or vomiting, drowsiness, irritability and pruritus. Signs and symptoms of accidental or deliberate overdosage with Neotigason would probably be similar. They would be expected to subside without need for treatment.

Because of the variable absorption of the drug, gastric lavage may be worthwhile within the first few hours after ingestion.

5. PHARMACOLOGICAL PROPERTIES

5.1 Pharmacodynamic properties

Retinol (Vitamin A) is known to be essential for normal epithelial growth and differentiation, though the mode of this effect is not yet established. Both retinol and retinoic acid are capable of reversing hyperkeratotic and metaplastic skin changes. However, these effects are generally only obtained at dosages associated with considerable local or systemic toxicity. Acitretin, a synthetic aromatic derivative of retinoic acid, has a favourable therapeutic ratio, with a greater and more specific inhibitory effect on psoriasis and disorders of epithelial keratinisation. The usual therapeutic response to acitretin consists of desquamation (with or without erythema) followed by more normal re-epithelialisation.

Acitretin is the main active metabolite of etretinate.

5.2 Pharmacokinetic properties

Absorption

Acitretin reaches peak plasma concentration 1 - 4 hours after ingestion of the drug. Bioavailability of orally administered acitretin is enhanced by food. Bioavailability of a single dose is approximately 60%, but inter-patient variability is considerable (36 - 95%).

Distribution

Acitretin is highly lipophilic and penetrates readily into body tissues. Protein binding of acitretin exceeds 99%. In animal studies, acitretin passed the placental barrier in quantities sufficient to produce foetal malformations. Due to its lipophilic nature, it can be assumed that acitretin passes into breast milk in considerable quantities.

Metabolism

Acitretin is metabolised by isomerization into its 13-cis isomer (*cis* acitretin), by glucuronidation and cleavage of the side chain.

Elimination

Multiple-dose studies in patients aged 21 - 70 years showed an elimination half-life of approximately 50 hours for acitretin and 60 hours for its main metabolite in plasma, *cis* acitretin, which is also a teratogen. From the longest elimination half-life observed in these patients for acitretin (96 hours) and *cis* acitretin (123 hours), and assuming linear kinetics, it can be predicted that more than 99% of the drug is eliminated within 36 days after cessation of long-term therapy. Furthermore, plasma concentrations of acitretin and *cis* acitretin dropped below the sensitivity limit of the assay (< 6ng/ml) within 36 days following cessation of treatment. Acitretin is excreted entirely in the form of its metabolites, in approximately equal parts via the kidneys and the bile.

5.3 Preclinical safety data

None stated.

6. PHARMACEUTICAL PARTICULARS

6.1 List of excipients

Maltodextrin, sodium ascorbate, gelatin, purified water, microcrystalline cellulose, iron oxide black (E172), iron oxide yellow (E172), iron oxide red (E172), titanium dioxide (E171).

6.2 Incompatibilities

None.

6.3 Shelf life

Neotigason capsules have a shelf-life of 3 years.

6.4 Special precautions for storage

Store in the original package. Do not store above 25°C.

6.5 Nature and contents of container

All aluminium blisters containing 56 capsules.

PVC/PE/PVDC (Triplex) blisters with aluminium cover foil containing 56 or 60 capsules.

Amber glass bottles with metal screw caps containing 30 or 100 capsules.

6.6 Instructions for use and handling

None.

7. MARKETING AUTHORISATION HOLDER

Roche Products Limited, 40 Broadwater Road, Welwyn Garden City, Hertfordshire, AL7 3AY.

8. MARKETING AUTHORISATION NUMBER(S)

PL 0031/0262

PL 0031/0263

9. DATE OF FIRST AUTHORISATION/RENEWAL OF THE AUTHORISATION

8 June 1992

10. DATE OF REVISION OF THE TEXT

August 2004

Neotigason is a registered trade mark

Item Code

Neulactil Forte

(sanofi-aventis)

1. NAME OF THE MEDICINAL PRODUCT

Neulactil Forte Syrup

2. QUALITATIVE AND QUANTITATIVE COMPOSITION

Pericyazine 10mg/5ml

3. PHARMACEUTICAL FORM

Clear orange brown syrupy liquid

4. CLINICAL PARTICULARS

4.1 Therapeutic indications

a) In adults with schizophrenia or other psychoses, for the treatment of symptoms or prevention of relapse.

b) In anxiety, psychomotor agitation, violent or dangerously impulsive behaviour. Neulactil is used as an adjunct to the short-term management of these conditions.

c) In children with behaviour disorders or schizophrenia

4.2 Posology and method of administration

Route of administration: oral.

Dosage requirement varies with the individual and the severity of the condition being treated. Initial dosage should be low with progressive increases until the desired response is obtained, after which dosage should be adjusted to maintain control of the symptoms.

Severe conditions

Schizophrenia and other psychoses

Adults: Initially 75 mg per day in divided doses. Dosage should be increased by 25 mg per day at weekly intervals until the optimum effect is achieved. Maintenance therapy would not normally be expected to exceed 300 mg per day.

Elderly: Initially 15-30 mg per day in divided doses. If this is well tolerated the dosage may be increased if necessary for optimum control of behaviour.

Children: The initial daily dose should be calculated on bodyweight. A child weighing 10kg should receive 0.5 milligram and this initial dose should be increased by 1mg for each additional 5kg of bodyweight up to a total daily dose of 10mg daily. This dosage may be gradually increased until the desired effect is achieved, but the maintenance dose should not exceed twice the initial amount.

Neulactil is not recommended for use in children below 1 year of age.

Mild or moderate conditions

Anxiety, psychomotor agitation, violent or dangerously impulsive behaviour.

Adults: Initially 15-30 mg daily, divided into two portions with a larger dose being given in the evening.

Elderly: 5-10 mg per day is suggested as a starting dose. It may be divided so that a larger portion is given in the evening. Half or quarter the normal adult dose may be sufficient for maintenance therapy.

Children: Not recommended for children.

4.3 Contraindications

Known hypersensitivity to pericyazine or to any of the other ingredients.

4.4 Special warnings and special precautions for use

Neuroleptics should be avoided in patients with liver or renal dysfunction, Parkinson's disease, hypothyroidism, cardiac failure, phaeochromocytoma, myasthenia gravis, prostrate hypertrophy. It should be avoided in patients known to be hypersensitive to phenothiazines or with a history of narrow angle glaucoma or agranulocytosis. It should be used with caution in the elderly, particularly during very hot or very cold weather (risk of hyper-hypothermia).

Close monitoring is required in patients with epilepsy or a history of seizures, as phenothiazines may lower the seizure threshold.

As agranulocytosis may occur rarely, regular monitoring of the complete blood count is recommended.

It is imperative that treatment be discontinued in the event of unexplained fever, as this may be a sign of neuroleptic malignant syndrome (pallor, hyperthermia, autonomic dysfunction, altered consciousness, muscle rigidity). Signs of autonomic dysfunction, such as sweating and arterial instability, may precede the onset of hyperthermia and serve as early warning signs. Although neuroleptic malignant syndrome may be idiosyncratic in origin, dehydration and organic brain disease are predisposing factors.

The occurrence of unexplained infections or fever may be evidence of blood dyscrasia (see section 4.8 below), and requires immediate haematological investigation.

Acute withdrawal symptoms, including nausea, vomiting and insomnia, have very rarely been reported following the abrupt cessation of high doses of neuroleptics. Relapse may also occur, and the emergence of extrapyramidal reactions has been reported. Therefore, gradual withdrawal is advisable.

In schizophrenia, the response to neuroleptic treatment may be delayed. If treatment is withdrawn, the recurrence of symptoms may not become apparent for some time.

As with other neuroleptics, cases of QT interval prolongation have been reported with pericyazine very rarely (see section 4.8, below). The risk-benefit should be fully assessed before Neulactil treatment is commenced, and patients with predisposing factors for ventricular arrhythmias, (e.g. cardiac disease; metabolic abnormalities such as hypokalaemia, hypocalcaemia or hypomagnesaemia; starvation; alcohol abuse; concomitant therapy with other drugs known to prolong the QT interval) should be carefully monitored (biochemical status and ECG), particularly during the initial phase of treatment.

As with all antipsychotic drugs, Neulactil should not be used alone where depression is predominant. However, it may be combined with antidepressant therapy to treat those conditions in which depression and psychosis coexist.

Because of the risk of photosensitisation, patients should be advised to avoid exposure to direct sunlight.

In those frequently handling preparations of phenothiazines, the greatest care must be taken to avoid contact of the drug with the skin, since contact skin sensitisation occurs rarely.

4.5 Interaction with other medicinal products and other forms of Interaction

The CNS depressant actions of neuroleptic agents may be intensified (additively) by alcohol, barbiturates and other sedatives. Respiratory depression may occur.

The hypotensive effect of most antihypertensive drugs, especially alpha adrenoceptor blocking agents may be exaggerated by neuroleptics.

There is an increased risk of arrhythmias when neuroleptics are used concurrently with drugs which prolong the QT interval, including certain antiarrhythmics, antidepressants, and other antipsychotics (see section 4.8, below).

The mild anticholinergic effect of neuroleptics may be enhanced by other anticholinergic drugs, possibly leading to constipation, heat stroke, etc.

The action of some drugs may be opposed by neuroleptics; these include amphetamine, levodopa, clonidine, guanethidine, adrenaline.

Where treatment for neuroleptic-induced extrapyramidal symptoms is required, anticholinergic antiparkinsonian agents should be used in preference to levodopa, since neuroleptics antagonise the antiparkinsonian action of dopaminergics.

Anticholinergic agents may reduce the antipsychotic effect of neuroleptics.

Some drugs interfere with absorption of neuroleptic agents: antacids, anti-Parkinson drugs, lithium. Increases or decreases in the plasma concentrations of a number of drugs, e.g: propranolol, phenobarbitone have been observed but were not of clinical significance.

High doses of neuroleptics may reduce the response to hypoglycaemic agents the dosage of which might have to be raised.

In patients treated concurrently with neuroleptics and lithium, there have been rare reports of neurotoxicity.

Adrenaline must not be used in patients overdosed with neuroleptics.

Simultaneous administration of desferrioxamine and prochlorperazine has been observed to induce a transient metabolic encephalopathy characterised by loss of consciousness for 48-72 hours. It is possible this may occur with Neulactil since it shares many of the pharmacological properties of prochlorperazine.

There is an increased risk of agranulocytosis when neuroleptics are used concurrently with drugs with myelosuppressive potential, such as carbamazepine or certain antibiotics and cytotoxics.

4.6 Pregnancy and lactation

There is inadequate evidence of the safety of Neulactil in human. There is evidence with some neuroleptics of harmful effects in animals. Like other drugs Neulactil should be avoided in pregnancy unless the physician considers it essential. It may occasionally prolong labour and at such a time should be withheld until the cervix is dilated 3-4 cm. Possible adverse effects on the foetus include lethargy or paradoxical hyperexcitability, tremor and low Apgar score.

Phenothiazines may be excreted in milk, therefore breastfeeding should be suspended during treatment.

4.7 Effects on ability to drive and use machines

Patients should be warned about drowsiness during early days of treatment, and advised not to drive or operate machinery. The elderly are particularly susceptible to postural hypotension.

4.8 Undesirable effects

Liver function: jaundice occurs in a very small percentage of patients taking neuroleptics. A premonitory sign may be a sudden onset of fever after one to three weeks of treatment followed by the development of jaundice. Neuroleptic jaundice has the biochemical and other characteristics of obstructive jaundice and is associated with obstruction of the canaliculi by bile thrombi; the frequent presence of an accompanying eosinophilia indicates the allergic nature of this phenomenon. Treatment should be withheld on the development of jaundice.

Cardiorespiratory: hypotension, usually postural, commonly occurs. Elderly or volume depleted subjects are particularly susceptible.

Cardiac arrhythmias, including atrial arrhythmia, A-V block, ventricular tachycardia and fibrillation have been reported during neuroleptic therapy, possibly related to dosage. Pre-existing cardiac disease, old age, hypokalaemia and concurrent tricyclic anti-depressants may predispose. ECG changes, usually benign, include widened QT interval, ST depression, U-waves and T-wave changes (see section 4.4, above).

Respiratory depression is possible in susceptible patients.

Blood picture: a mild leukopenia occurs in up to 30% of patients on prolonged high dosage of neuroleptics; agranulocytosis may occur rarely; it is not dose-related.

Extrapyramidal: acute dystonias or dyskinesias, usually transitory are commoner in children and young adults, and usually occur within the first four days of treatment or after dosage increases.

Akathisia characteristically occurs after large initial doses.

Parkinsonism is commoner in adults and the elderly. It usually develops after weeks or months of treatment. One or more of the following may be seen: tremor, rigidity, akinesia, or other features of Parkinsonism. Commonly just tremor.

Tardive dyskinesia: if this occurs it is usually, but not necessarily after prolonged or high dosage. It can even occur after treatment has been stopped. Dosage should therefore be kept low whenever possible.

Skin and eyes: contact skin sensitisation may occur rarelyin those frequently handling preparations of phenothiazines (see section 4.4, above. Skin rashes of various kinds may also be seen in patients treated with the drug. Patients on high dosage should be warned that they may develop photosensitivity in sunny weather and should avoid exposure to direct sunlight.

Endocrine: hyperprolactinaemia which may result in galactorrhoea, gynaecomastia, amenorrhoea; impotence.

Priapism has very rarely been reported in patients treated with peryciazine

Neuroleptic malignant syndrome (hyperthermia, rigidity autonomic dysfunction and altered consciousness) may occur with any neuroleptic.

Minor side effects are nasal stuffiness, dry mouth, insomnia, agitation

4.9 Overdose

Symptoms of neuroleptic overdosage include drowsiness or loss of consciousness, hypotension, tachycardia, ECG changes, ventricular arrhythmias and hypothermia. Severe extrapyramidal dyskinesias may occur.

If the patient is seen sufficiently soon (up to 6 hours) after ingestion of a toxic dose, gastric lavage may be attempted. Pharmacological induction of emesis is unlikely to be of any use. Activated charcoal should be given. There is no specific antidote. Treatment is supportive.

Generalised vasodilatation may result in circulatory collapse; raising the patient's legs may suffice; in severe cases, volume expansion by intravenous fluids may be needed; infusion fluids should be warmed before administration in order not to aggravate hypothermia.

Positive inotropic agents such as dopamine may be tried if fluid replacement is insufficient to correct the circulatory collapse. Peripheral vasoconstrictor agents are not generally recommended; avoid the use of adrenaline.

Ventricular or supraventricular tachy-arrhythmias usually respond to restoration of normal body temperature and correction of circulatory or metabolic disturbances. If persistent or life threatening, appropriate anti-arrhythmic therapy may be considered. Avoid lignocaine, and as far as possible long acting, anti-arrhythmic drugs.

Pronounced central nervous system depression requires airway maintenance or, in extreme circumstances, assisted respiration. Severe dystonic reactions usually respond to procyclidine (5-10 mg) or orphenedrine (20-40 mg) administered intramuscularly or intravenously. Convulsions should be treated with intravenous diazepam.

Neuroleptic malignant syndrome should be treated with cooling. Dantrolene sodium may be tried.

5. PHARMACOLOGICAL PROPERTIES

5.1 Pharmacodynamic properties

Pericyazine is a neuroleptic with cardiovascular and antihistamine effects similar to those of chlorpromazine, but it has a stronger antiserotonin effect and a powerful central sedative effect.

5.2 Pharmacokinetic properties

Kinetics: there is little information about plasma concentrations, distribution and excretion in humans. The rate of metabolism and excretion of phenothiazines decreases in old age.

5.3 Preclinical safety data

There are no preclinical data of relevance to the prescriber which are additional to that already included in other sections of the SPC.

6. PHARMACEUTICAL PARTICULARS

6.1 List of excipients

Sugar, Caramel Flavour, Spearmint Oil BP, Peppermint Oil, Fruit cup 868,

'Tween' 20 (Polysorbate 20) BP, Citric acid anhydrous BP, Sodium citrate gran. BP

Sodium sulphite anhydrous BP, Sodium metabisulphite Powder BP

L(+) Ascorbic acid BP, Sodium benzoate BP, Demineralised water BP

6.2 Incompatibilities

None known.

6.3 Shelf life

24 months unopened, 1 month after opening

6.4 Special precautions for storage

Protect from light.

6.5 Nature and contents of container

Amber glass bottle containing 1000ml or 100ml. HDPE/polypropylene child resistant cap with tamper evident band. or rolled on pilfer proof aluminium cap and a PVDC emulsion coated wad.

6.6 Instructions for use and handling

Care must be taken to avoid contact of the drug with the skin. Contact skin sensitisation is a serious but rare complication in those frequently handling preparations of phenothiazines.

7. MARKETING AUTHORISATION HOLDER

JHC Healthcare Ltd

5 Lower Merrion Street

Dublin 2

Eire

8. MARKETING AUTHORISATION NUMBER(S)

PL 16186/0005

9. DATE OF FIRST AUTHORISATION/RENEWAL OF THE AUTHORISATION

1 September 1997

10. DATE OF REVISION OF THE TEXT

March 2002

11. Legal Classification

POM

Neulactil Tablets

(sanofi-aventis)

1. NAME OF THE MEDICINAL PRODUCT

NEULACTIL TABLETS

2. QUALITATIVE AND QUANTITATIVE COMPOSITION

Pericyazine 2.5 mg

Pericyazine 10 mg

3. PHARMACEUTICAL FORM

2.5mg - Circular, very pale lime-yellow tablet, with one face impressed Neulactil just inside the perimeter. Break-line on reverse.

10mg - Circular, very pale lime-yellow tablet, with one face impressed Neulactil just inside the perimeter around a central 10. Break-line on reverse.

4. CLINICAL PARTICULARS

4.1 Therapeutic indications

a) In adults with schizophrenia or other psychoses, for the treatment of symptoms or prevention of relapse.

b) In anxiety, psychomotor agitation, violent or dangerously impulsive behaviour. Neulactil is used as an adjunct to the short-term management of these conditions.

4.2 Posology and method of administration

Route of administration: oral.

Dosage requirement varies with the individual and the severity of the condition being treated. Initial dosage should be low with progressive increases until the desired response is obtained, after which dosage should be adjusted to maintain control of the symptoms.

Severe conditions

Indication (a)

Adults: Initially 75 mg per day in divided doses. Dosage should be increased by 25 mg per day at weekly intervals until the optimum effect is achieved. Maintenance therapy would not normally be expected to exceed 300 mg per day.

Elderly: Initially 15-30 mg per day in divided doses. If this is well tolerated the dosage may be increased if necessary for optimum control of behaviour.

Mild or moderate conditions

Indication (b)

Adults: Initially 15-30 mg daily, divided into two portions with a larger dose being given in the evening.

Elderly: 5-10 mg per day is suggested as a starting dose. It may be divided so that a larger portion is given in the evening. Half or quarter the normal adult dose may be sufficient for maintenance therapy.

Neulactil tablets are not recommended for children.

4.3 Contraindications

See use in pregnancy below. Known hypersensitivity to pericyazine or to any of the other ingredients.

4.4 Special warnings and special precautions for use

Neuroleptics should be avoided in patients with liver or renal dysfunction, Parkinson's disease, hypothyroidism, cardiac failure, phaeochromocytoma, myasthenia gravis, prostrate hypertrophy. It should be avoided in patients known to be hypersensitive to phenothiazines or with a history of narrow angle glaucoma or agranulocytosis. It should be used with caution in the elderly, particularly during very hot or very cold weather (risk of hyperhypothermia).

Close monitoring is required in patients with epilepsy or a history of seizures, as phenothiazines may lower the seizure threshold.

As agranulocytosis may occur rarely, regular monitoring of the complete blood count is recommended.

It is imperative that treatment be discontinued in the event of unexplained fever, as this may be a sign of neuroleptic malignant syndrome (pallor, hyperthermia, autonomic dysfunction, altered consciousness, muscle rigidity). Signs of autonomic dysfunction, such as sweating and arterial instability, may precede the onset of hyperthermia and serve as early warning signs. Although neuroleptic malignant syndrome may be idiosyncratic in origin, dehydration and organic brain disease are predisposing factors.

The occurrence of unexplained infections or fever may be evidence of blood dyscrasia (see section 4.8 below), and requires immediate haematological investigation.

Acute withdrawal symptoms, including nausea, vomiting and insomnia, have very rarely been reported following the abrupt cessation of high doses of neuroleptics. Relapse may also occur, and the emergence of extrapyramidal reactions has been reported. Therefore, gradual withdrawal is advisable.

In schizophrenia, the response to neuroleptic treatment may be delayed. If treatment is withdrawn, the recurrence of symptoms may not become apparent for some time.

As with other neuroleptics, cases of QT interval prolongation have been reported with pericyazine very rarely (see section 4.8, below). The risk-benefit should be fully assessed before Neulactil treatment is commenced, and patients with predisposing factors for ventricular arrhythmias, (e.g. cardiac disease; metabolic abnormalities such as hypokalaemia, hypocalcaemia or hypomagnesaemia; starvation; alcohol abuse; concomitant therapy with other drugs known to prolong the QT interval) should be carefully monitored (biochemical status and ECG), particularly during the initial phase of treatment.

As with all antipsychotic drugs, Neulactil should not be used alone where depression is predominant. However, it may be combined with antidepressant therapy to treat those conditions in which depression and psychosis coexist.

Because of the risk of photosensitisation, patients should be advised to avoid exposure to direct sunlight.

In those frequently handling preparations of phenothiazines, the greatest care must be taken to avoid contact of the drug with the skin, since contact skin sensitisation occurs rarely.

4.5 Interaction with other medicinal products and other forms of Interaction

Interactions of phenothiazine neuroleptics:

The CNS depressant actions of neuroleptic agents may be intensified (additively) by alcohol, barbiturates and other sedatives. Respiratory depression may occur.

The hypotensive effect of most antihypertensive drugs, especially alpha adrenoceptor blocking agents may be exaggerated by neuroleptics.

There is an increased risk of arrhythmias when neuroleptics are used concurrently with drugs which prolong the QT interval, including certain antiarrhythmics, antidepressants, and other antipsychotics (see section 4.8, below).

The mild anticholinergic effect of neuroleptics may be enhanced by other anticholinergic drugs, possibly leading to constipation, heat stroke, etc.

The action of some drugs may be opposed by neuroleptics; these include amphetamine, levodopa, clonidine, guanethidine, adrenaline.

Where treatment for neuroleptic-induced extrapyramidal symptoms is required, anticholinergic antiparkinsonian agents should be used in preference to levodopa, since neuroleptics antagonise the antiparkinsonian action of dopaminergics.

Anticholinergic agents may reduce the antipsychotic effect of neuroleptics.

Some drugs interfere with absorption of neuroleptic agents: antacids, anti-Parkinson drugs, lithium. Increases or decreases in the plasma concentrations of a number of drugs, e.g: propranolol, phenobarbitone have been observed but were not of clinical significance. High doses of neuroleptics may reduce the response to hypoglycaemic agents the dosage of which might have to be raised.

In patients treated concurrently with neuroleptics and lithium, there have been rare reports of neurotoxicity.

Adrenaline must not be used in patients overdosed with neuroleptics.

Simultaneous administration of desferrioxamine and prochlorperazine has been observed to induce a transient metabolic encephalopathy characterised by loss of consciousness for 48-72 hours. It is possible this may occur with Neulactil since it shares many of the pharmacological properties of prochlorperazine.

There is an increased risk of agranulocytosis when neuroleptics are used concurrently with drugs with myelosuppressive potential, such as carbamazepine or certain antibiotics and cytotoxics.

4.6 Pregnancy and lactation

There is inadequate evidence of the safety of Neulactil in human. There is evidence with some neuroleptics of harmful effects in animals. Like other drugs Neulactil should be avoided in pregnancy unless the physician considers it essential. It may occasionally prolong labour and at such a time should be withheld until the cervix is dilated 3-4 cm. Possible adverse effects on the foetus include lethargy or paradoxical hyperexcitability, tremor and low Apgar score.

Phenothiazines may be excreted in milk, therefore breast-feeding should be suspended during treatment.

4.7 Effects on ability to drive and use machines

Patients should be warned about drowsiness during early days of treatment, and advised not to drive or operate machinery. The elderly are particularly susceptible to postural hypotension.

4.8 Undesirable effects

Liver function: jaundice occurs in a very small percentage of patients taking neuroleptics. A premonitory sign may be a sudden onset of fever after one to three weeks of treatment followed by the development of jaundice. Neuroleptic jaundice has the biochemical and other characteristics of obstructive jaundice and is associated with obstruction of the canaliculi by bile thrombi; the frequent presence of an accompanying eosinophilia indicates the allergic nature of this phenomenon. Treatment should be withheld on the development of jaundice.

Cardiorespiratory: hypotension, usually postural, commonly occurs. Elderly or volume depleted subjects are particularly susceptible.

Cardiac arrhythmias, including atrial arrhythmia, A-V block, ventricular tachycardia and fibrillation have been reported during neuroleptic therapy, possibly related to dosage. Pre-existing cardiac disease, old age, hypokalaemia and concurrent tricyclic anti-depressants may predispose. ECG changes, usually benign, include widened QT interval, ST depression, U-waves and T-wave changes (see section 4.4, above).

Respiratory depression is possible in susceptible patients.

Blood picture: a mild leukopenia occurs in up to 30% of patients on prolonged high dosage of neuroleptics; agranulocytosis may occur rarely; it is not dose-related.

Extrapyramidal: acute dystonias or dyskinesias, usually transitory are commoner in children and young adults, and usually occur within the first four days of treatment or after dosage increases.

Akathisia characteristically occurs after large initial doses.

Parkinsonism is commoner in adults and the elderly. It usually develops after weeks or months of treatment. One or more of the following may be seen: tremor, rigidity, akinesia, or other features of Parkinsonism. Commonly just tremor.

Tardive dyskinesia: if this occurs it is usually, but not necessarily after prolonged or high dosage. It can even occur after treatment has been stopped. Dosage should therefore be kept low whenever possible.

Skin and eyes: contact skin sensitisation may occur rarelyin those frequently handling preparations of phenothiazines (see section 4.4, above). Skin rashes of various kinds may also be seen in patients treated with the drug. Patients on high dosage should be warned that they may develop photosensitivity in sunny weather and should avoid exposure to direct sunlight.

Endocrine: hyperprolactinaemia which may result in galactorrhoea, gynaecomastia, amenorrhoea; impotence.

Neuroleptic malignant syndrome (hyperthermia, rigidity autonomic dysfunction and altered consciousness) may occur with any neuroleptic.

Minor side effects are nasal stuffiness, dry mouth, insomnia, agitation

4.9 Overdose

Symptoms of neuroleptic overdosage include drowsiness or loss of consciousness, hypotension, tachycardia, ECG changes, ventricular arrhythmias and hypothermia. Severe extrapyramidal dyskinesias may occur.

If the patient is seen sufficiently soon (up to 6 hours) after ingestion of a toxic dose, gastric lavage may be attempted. Pharmacological induction of emesis is unlikely to be of any use. Activated charcoal should be given. There is no specific antidote. Treatment is supportive.

Generalised vasodilatation may result in circulatory collapse; raising the patient's legs may suffice; in severe cases, volume expansion by intravenous fluids may be needed; infusion fluids should be warmed before administration in order not to aggravate hypothermia.

Positive inotropic agents such as dopamine may be tried if fluid replacement is insufficient to correct the circulatory collapse. Peripheral vasoconstrictor agents are not generally recommended; avoid the use of adrenaline.

Ventricular or supraventricular tachy-arrhythmias usually respond to restoration of normal body temperature and correction of circulatory or metabolic disturbances. If persistent or life threatening, appropriate anti-arrhythmic therapy may be considered. Avoid lignocaine, and as far as possible long acting, anti-arrhythmic drugs.

Pronounced central nervous system depression requires airway maintenance or, in extreme circumstances, assisted respiration. Severe dystonic reactions usually respond to procyclidine (5-10 mg) or orphenedrine (20-40 mg) administered intramuscularly or intravenously. Convulsions should be treated with intravenous diazepam.

Neuroleptic malignant syndrome should be treated with cooling. Dantrolene sodium may be tried.

5. PHARMACOLOGICAL PROPERTIES

5.1 Pharmacodynamic properties

Pericyazine is a neuroleptic with cardiovascular and antihistamine effects similar to those of chlorpromazine, but it has a stronger antiserotonin effect and a powerful central sedative effect.

5.2 Pharmacokinetic properties

Kinetics: there is little information about plasma concentrations, distribution and excretion in humans. The rate of metabolism and excretion of phenothiazines decreases in old age.

5.3 Preclinical safety data

There are no preclinical data of relevance to the prescriber which are additional to that already included in other sections of the SPC.

6. PHARMACEUTICAL PARTICULARS

6.1 List of excipients

2.5mg - Lactose anhydrous USP, Avicel, Sodium starch glycollate, Magnesium stearate BP, Aerosil, Methyl hydroxybenzoate BP.

10mg - Lactose anhydrous USP, Microcrystalline cellulose (E460), Sodium starch glycollate, Magnesium stearate BP, Colloidal silicon dioxide (E551), Methyl hydroxybenzoate BP (E218).

6.2 Incompatibilities

None known.

6.3 Shelf life

60 months.

6.4 Special precautions for storage

Protect from light.

6.5 Nature and contents of container

Securitainer or HDPE bottle containing 500 tablets.

PVDC coated UPVC aluminium foil blister containing 84 tablets.

6.6 Instructions for use and handling

None stated.

7. MARKETING AUTHORISATION HOLDER

JHC Healthcare Ltd

5 Lower Merrion Street

Dublin 2

Eire

8. MARKETING AUTHORISATION NUMBER(S)

Tablets 2.5mg PL 16186/0003

Tablets 10mg PL 16186/0004

9. DATE OF FIRST AUTHORISATION/RENEWAL OF THE AUTHORISATION

1 September 1997

10. DATE OF REVISION OF THE TEXT

March 2002

11. Legal Classification

POM

Neurontin

(Parke Davis)

1. NAME OF THE MEDICINAL PRODUCT

Neurontin Capsules 100 mg

Neurontin Capsules 300 mg

Neurontin Capsules 400 mg

Neurontin Tablets 600 mg

Neurontin Tablets 800 mg

2. QUALITATIVE AND QUANTITATIVE COMPOSITION

Neurontin Capsules 100 mg contain 100 mg gabapentin per capsule.

Neurontin Capsules 300 mg contain 300 mg gabapentin per capsule.

Neurontin Capsules 400 mg contain 400 mg gabapentin per capsule.

Neurontin Tablets 600 mg contain 600 mg gabapentin per tablet.

Neurontin Tablets 800 mg contain 800 mg gabapentin per tablet.

Refer to Section 6.1 for details of inactive ingredients.

3. PHARMACEUTICAL FORM

Neurontin Capsules

Capsule, hard

Neurontin Capsules 100 mg:	A two-piece, white opaque hard gelatin capsule, imprinted with 'Neurontin 100 mg' and the Parke Davis company logo, containing a white to off-white powder.
Neurontin Capsules 300 mg:	A two-piece, yellow opaque hard gelatin capsule, imprinted with 'Neurontin 300 mg' and the Parke Davis company logo, containing a white to off-white powder.
Neurontin Capsules 400 mg:	A two-piece, orange opaque hard gelatin capsule, imprinted with 'Neurontin 400 mg' and the Parke Davis company logo, containing a white to off-white powder.

Neurontin Tablets

Neurontin Tablets 600 mg:	White, film coated elliptical tablets, imprinted in black ink.
Neurontin Tablets 800 mg:	White, film coated elliptical tablets, imprinted in orange ink.

For oral administration.

4. CLINICAL PARTICULARS

4.1 Therapeutic indications

Neuropathic Pain

Neurontin is indicated for the treatment of neuropathic pain.

Epilepsy

Adults and children over 12 years of age

Neurontin is an anti-epileptic drug indicated as add-on therapy for partial seizures and partial seizures with

Table 1 DOSING CHART - INITIAL TITRATION

Dose	Day 1	Day 2	Day 3
900 mg	300 mg once a day	300 mg two times a day	300 mg three times a day

secondary generalisation in patients who have not achieved satisfactory control with or who are intolerant to standard anticonvulsants used alone or in combination.

Children 6-12 years of age

Neurontin may be used as add-on therapy for partial seizures and partial seizures with secondary generalisation, in children aged between 6-12 years, who have not achieved satisfactory control with, or who are intolerant to, standard anticonvulsants used alone or in combination, if the benefit: risk is considered favourable. Neurontin should be initiated and supervised by a neurological specialist.

Children under 6 years of age

There are inadequate data in this age group and therefore the use of Neurontin is not recommended.

4.2 Posology and method of administration

Neuropathic Pain

Adults (over the age of 18)

Neurontin should be titrated to a maximum dose of 1800 mg per day.

Titration to an effective dose can progress rapidly and can be accomplished over a few days by administering 300 mg once a day on day 1, 300 mg twice a day on day 2 and 300 mg three times a day on day 3, as described in Table 1.

(see Table 1 above)

Thereafter, the dose can be increased using increments of 300 mg per day given in three divided doses to a maximum of 1800 mg per day. It is not necessary to divide the doses equally when titrating Neurontin.

It is not necessary to monitor Neurontin plasma concentrations to optimise Neurontin therapy.

The maximum time between doses in a three times daily schedule should not exceed 12 hours. Gabapentin may be given orally with or without food.

If Neurontin is discontinued, or the dose reduced or substituted with an alternative medication, this should be done gradually over a minimum of one week.

Neurontin Titration Pack:

The Neurontin Titration Pack is available for the convenience of prescribers, for the treatment of neuropathic pain. The titration pack contains all capsules and tablets required to reach 1800 mg per day, over 15 days of treatment, with 1800 mg per day reached on day 13. It starts with 1 × 300 mg capsule on day one and finishes with 3 × 600 mg tablets on days 13-15, carefully packed in sequence to ensure correct usage.

Elderly

Elderly patients may require dosage adjustment because of declining renal function with age (see Table 2).

Epilepsy

Adults and Children aged over 12

The anti-epileptic effect of Neurontin generally occurs at 900 to 1200 mg/day.

It is not necessary to monitor Neurontin plasma concentrations to optimise Neurontin therapy.

Titration to an effective dose can progress rapidly and can be accomplished over a few days by administering 300 mg once a day on day 1, 300 mg twice day on day 2 and 300 mg three times a day on day 3, as described in Table 1.

Thereafter, the dose can be increased using increments of 300 mg per day given in three equally divided doses to a maximum dose of 2400 mg per day.

The maximum time between doses in a three times daily schedule should not exceed 12 hours. Gabapentin may be given orally with or without food.

If Neurontin is discontinued and/or an alternate anticonvulsant medication is added to the therapy, this should be done gradually over a minimum of one week.

Elderly

Elderly patients may require dosage adjustment because of declining renal function with age (see table 2).

Children 6-12 years of age

The recommended dose of Neurontin is 25 to 35 mg/kg/day given in divided doses (3 times a day). Titration to an effective dose can take place over 3 days by giving 10 mg/kg/day on Day 1, 20 mg/kg/day on Day 2 and 25 to 35 mg/kg/day on Day 3.

The following maintenance dosing schedule is suggested:

Weight Range kg	Total mg Dose/Day
26-36	900
37-50	1200

Dosage Adjustment in Patients with Compromised Renal Function or those Undergoing Haemodialysis

Dosage adjustment is recommended in patients with compromised renal function as described in Table 2, or those undergoing haemodialysis.

Patients with Compromised Renal Function:

(see Table 2 below)

Patients Undergoing Haemodialysis:

For patients undergoing haemodialysis who have never received gabapentin, a loading dose of 300 to 400 mg is recommended then 200 to 300 mg of gabapentin following each 4 hours of haemodialysis.

4.3 Contraindications

Neurontin is contra-indicated in patients who are hypersensitive to Neurontin or to the product's components.

4.4 Special warnings and special precautions for use

Although there is no evidence of rebound seizures with Neurontin, abrupt withdrawal of anticonvulsant agents in epileptic patients may precipitate status epilepticus. When, in the judgement of the clinician, there is a need for dose reduction, discontinuation or substitution of alternative anticonvulsant medication, this should be done gradually over a minimum of one week.

Neurontin is not generally considered effective in the treatment of absence seizures.

Patients who require concomitant treatment with morphine may experience increases in gabapentin concentrations. Patients should be carefully observed for signs of CNS depression, such as somnolence, and the dose of gabapentin or morphine should be reduced appropriately. (See Section **4.5 – Interactions with Other Medicaments and Other Forms of Interaction**)

Patients taking Neurontin can be the subject of mood and behavioural disturbances. Such reports have been noted in patients on Neurontin although a causal link has not been established.

Caution is recommended in patients with a history of psychotic illness. On commencing Neurontin therapy, psychotic episodes have been reported in some patients with, and rarely without, a history of psychotic illness. Most of these events resolved when Neurontin was discontinued or the dosage was reduced.

4.5 Interaction with other medicinal products and other forms of Interaction

Morphine: In a study involving healthy volunteers (N=12), when a 60-mg controlled-release morphine capsule was administered 2 hours prior to a 600-mg gabapentin capsule, mean gabapentin AUC increased by 44% compared to gabapentin administered without morphine. Morphine pharmacokinetic parameter values were not affected by administration of gabapentin 2 hours after morphine. The magnitude of interaction at other doses of gabapentin and / or morphine is not known. (See Section **4.4 – Special Warnings and Special Precautions for Use**)

Table 2 MAINTENANCE DOSAGE OF NEURONTIN IN ADULTS WITH REDUCED RENAL FUNCTION

Renal function Creatinine Clearance (ml/minute)	Total Daily Dose[a] mg/day NORMAL DOSAGE		
≥ 80	900	1200	2400
50-79	600	600	1200
30-49	300	300	600
15-29	150[b]	300	300
<15	150[b]	150[b]	150[b]

[a] Total daily dose should be administered as a tid regimen. Doses used to treat patients with normal renal function (creatinine clearance >80 ml/min) range from 900 to 2400 mg/day. Reduced dosages are for patients with renal impairment (creatinine clearance <79 ml/min).

[b] To be administered as 300 mg every other day.

Neurontin may be used in combination with other anti-epileptic drugs without concern for alteration of the plasma concentrations of Neurontin or serum concentrations of other anti-epileptic drugs.

There is no interaction between Neurontin and phenytoin, valproic acid, carbamazepine or phenobarbitone. Neurontin steady-state pharmacokinetics are similar for healthy subjects and patients with epilepsy receiving anti-epileptic agents.

Co-administration of Neurontin with oral contraceptives including norethisterone and/or ethinyl oestradiol does not influence the steady-state pharmacokinetics of either component.

In a clinical study where Neurontin and an aluminium and magnesium containing antacid when given at the same time, Neurontin's bioavailability was reduced by up to 24%. It is recommended that Neurontin is taken about two hours following any such antacid administration. The slight decrease in renal excretion of Neurontin observed when co-administered with cimetidine is not expected to be of clinical importance.

Renal excretion of Neurontin is unaltered by probenecid.

Food has no effect on Neurontin pharmacokinetics.

Because false positive readings were reported with the Ames N-Multistix SG® dipstick test when Neurontin was added to other anticonvulsant drugs, the more specific sulphosalicylic acid precipitation procedure is recommended to determine urinary protein.

4.6 Pregnancy and lactation

Safe use in human pregnancy has not been established. Reproduction studies in mice, rats or rabbits at doses up to 50, 30 and 25 times respectively, the daily human dose of 3600 mg revealed no evidence of impaired fertility or harm to the foetus due to Neurontin administration. However, because animal reproduction studies are not always predictive of human response, this drug should be used in pregnancy only if clearly needed.

Neurontin is excreted in human milk but the effect on the nursing infant is unknown. Because many drugs are excreted in human milk, and because of the potential for serious adverse reactions in nursing infants from Neurontin, a decision should be made whether to discontinue nursing or to discontinue the drug, taking into account the importance of the drug to the mother.

4.7 Effects on ability to drive and use machines

Neurontin acts on the central nervous system and may produce drowsiness, dizziness, or other related symptoms. These otherwise mild or moderate adverse events could be potentially dangerous in patients driving or operating machinery, particularly until such time as the individual patient's experience with the drug is established.

4.8 Undesirable effects

Neuropathic Pain

Based on placebo-controlled studies, the most common possible side-effects (> 1/10) associated with treating neuropathic pain with Neurontin are: dizziness and somnolence.

Common possible side-effects (between 1/10 and 1/100) are: diarrhoea, dry mouth, peripheral oedema, weight gain, abnormal gait, amnesia, ataxia, abnormal thinking, rash and amblyopia.

Uncommon possible side-effects (between 1/100 and 1/1000) are: accidental injury, asthenia, back pain, constipation, flatulence, nausea, confusion, hypesthesia, vertigo, dyspnea and pharyngitis.

Epilepsy (Adults)

Since Neurontin has most often been administered in combination with other anti-epileptic agents, it is not possible to determine which agents, if any are associated with adverse events. However, based on placebo-controlled, double blind studies, the most common possible side-effects (> 1/10) are: somnolence and dizziness.

Common possible side-effects (between 1/10 and 1/100) are: ataxia, fatigue, nystagmus, tremor, diplopia, amblyopia, abnormal vision most often described as a visual disturbance, dysarthria, amnesia, asthenia, paraesthesia, arthralgia, purpura, dyspepsia, anxiety, weight increase, urinary tract infection and pharyngitis.

Uncommon possible side-effects (between 1/100 and 1/1000) are: leucopenia, nervousness, rhinitis and male sexual dysfunction (impotence).

As with the other AEDs there have been rare reports of urinary incontinence, pancreatitis, elevated liver function tests, erythema multiforme and Stevens Johnson Syndrome where a causal relationship to treatment has not been established. Rarely confusion, depression, emotional lability, hostility, abnormal thinking and psychoses/hallucinations have been reported. Blood glucose fluctuations in patients with diabetes, myalgia, headache, nausea and/or vomiting have also been reported.

Epilepsy (Children)

In children aged 3-12 years in placebo controlled and long term trials, the most common (> 10%) side-effects were emotional lability, nervousness and thinking abnormally. All reports of these events were rated as mild or moderate and discontinuation or dose reduction were infrequent.

In children aged 3-12 years in controlled add-on trials, side-effects that occurred with an incidence of 2% or greater than placebo were: somnolence, fatigue, weight increase, hostility, emotional lability, dizziness, hyperkinesia, nausea/vomiting, viral infection, fever, bronchitis, respiratory infection. Some of these side-effects could be attributed to common viral childhood illness.

Additional Post-Marketing Adverse Events

Additional post-marketing adverse events (associated with treating epilepsy and/or neuropathic pain) include acute kidney failure, allergic reaction including urticaria, alopecia, angioedema, chest pain, hepatitis, jaundice, hallucinations, movement disorders such as choreoathetosis, dyskinesia and dystonia, palpitation, thrombocytopenia, and tinnitus.

Adverse events following the abrupt discontinuation of gabapentin have also been reported. The most frequently reported events are anxiety, insomnia, nausea, pain and sweating.

4.9 Overdose

Acute, life-threatening toxicity has not been observed with Neurontin overdoses of up to 49 grams. Symptoms of the overdoses included dizziness, double vision, slurred speech, drowsiness, lethargy and mild diarrhoea. All patients recovered fully with supportive care. Reduced absorption of Neurontin at higher doses may limit drug absorption at the time of overdosing and, hence, minimise toxicity from overdoses.

Although Neurontin can be removed by haemodialysis it is not usually required. However, in patients with renal impairment, haemodialysis may be indicated.

5. PHARMACOLOGICAL PROPERTIES

5.1 Pharmacodynamic properties

Neurontin is structurally related to the neurotransmitter gamma-aminobutyric acid (GABA) but its mechanism of action is different from that of several drugs that interact with GABA synapses. The identification and function of the gabapentin binding site remains to be elucidated and the relevance of its various actions to the anticonvulsant effect to be established. Analgesic activity has been shown in animal models of inflammatory and neuropathic pain.

One placebo controlled randomised trial was undertaken in 247 children aged 3-12 years with refractory seizures. Participants received 25-35 mg/kg/day or placebo as add-on therapy. Efficacy was not established in children under 6 years of age.

5.2 Pharmacokinetic properties

Mean plasma gabapentin concentrations (Cmax) occurred approximately 3 hours (Tmax) following single oral doses of Neurontin regardless of dose size or formulation. Mean Tmax values following multiple dose administration were approximately 1 hour shorter than the values following single-dose administration.

Mean Cmax and AUC values increased with increasing dose; however, the increase was less than dose proportional. Deviation from linearity was very slight up to 600 mg for both parameters and thus should be minimal at doses of 300 mg to 400 mg three times daily where the anti-epileptic effect generally occurs.

Following repeated Neurontin administration, steady state was achieved within 1 to 2 days after the start of the multiple dosing and was maintained throughout the dosing regime.

Plasma gabapentin concentration-time profiles were similar between gabapentin solution and capsule formulations following single doses of 300 and 400 mg. Absolute bioavailability of a 300 mg oral dose of Neurontin was approximately 60%. At doses of 300 mg and 400 mg, Neurontin bioavailability was unchanged following multiple-dose administration.

Based on results of bioavailability studies performed with Neurontin Tablets, the 600 and 800 mg tablets are bioequivalent to marketed Neurontin Capsules. The 600 mg tablets were found to be bioequivalent to 2 × 300 mg marketed capsules based on similar rate and extent of drug absorption. Likewise, 800 mg tablets were found to be bioequivalent to 2 × 400 mg marketed capsules based on a similar rate and extent of drug absorption.

The presence of food did not influence the bioavailability of Neurontin.

Gabapentin is not metabolised in humans and does not induce hepatic mixed function oxidase enzymes.

Gabapentin elimination from plasma following IV administration was best described by linear pharmacokinetics. Elimination half-life (T½) of gabapentin ranged from 5 to 7 hours. Gabapentin elimination parameters, apparent plasma T½ and renal clearance (CL_R) were independent of dose and remained unchanged following repeated administration. Renal clearance was the sole elimination pathway for gabapentin. Since gabapentin is not metabolised in humans, the amount of drug recovered in urine is indicative of gabapentin bioavailability. Following a single 200 mg oral dose of [C_{14}]gabapentin recovery of radioactivity was essentially complete with approximately 80% and 20% of the dose recovered in urine and faeces, respectively.

As renal function (as determined by creatinine clearance) decreases with increasing age, gabapentin oral clearance, renal clearance and elimination-rate constant decrease proportionally.

Gabapentin pharmacokinetics were determined in a single dose study and a population study in paediatric subjects aged between 1 month and 13 years.

Clearance of gabapentin based on body weight in children above 4 years of age is similar to that in adults. Children between 2-4 years appear to have higher clearances per body weight. Below 2 years the clearance of gabapentin is highly variable.

5.3 Preclinical safety data

Gabapentin was given in the diet to mice at 200, 600, and 2000 mg/kg/day and to rats at 250, 1000, and 2000 mg/kg/day for two years. A statistically significant increase in the incidence of pancreatic acinar cell tumours was found only in male rats at the highest dose. Peak plasma drug concentrations and areas under the concentration time curve in rats at 2000 mg/kg is 10 times higher than plasma concentrations in humans given 3600 mg/day.

The pancreatic acinar cell tumours in male rats are low-grade malignancies, did not affect survival, did not metastasise or invade surrounding tissue, and were similar to those seen in concurrent controls. The relevance of these pancreatic acinar cell tumours in male rats to carcinogenic risk in humans is therefore of uncertain significance.

Gabapentin has no genotoxic potential. It was not mutagenic in the Ames bacterial plate incorporation assay or at the HGPRT locus in mammalian cells in the presence or absence of metabolic activation. Gabapentin did not induce structural chromosome aberrations in mammalian cells *in vitro* or *in vivo*, and did not induce micronucleus formation in the bone marrow of hamsters.

6. PHARMACEUTICAL PARTICULARS

6.1 List of excipients

Neurontin Capsules

Each capsule contains the following excipients: lactose, maize starch, talc, gelatin, water and sodium lauryl sulphate.

The 100 mg capsules contain the colouring E171 (titanium dioxide), the 300 mg capsules contain the colourings E171 (titanium dioxide) and E172 (yellow iron oxide) and the 400 mg capsules contain the colourings E171 (titanium dioxide) and E172 (red and yellow iron oxide).

The printing ink used on all capsules contains: shellac, E171 (titanium dioxide), E132 (indigo carmine).

Neurontin Tablets

Each tablet contains the following excipients: poloxamer 407 (ethylene oxide and propylene oxide), copolyvidone, corn starch, magnesium stearate, opadry white YS-1-18111 (talc and hydroxypropyl cellulose), candelilla wax, talc.

The printing ink used on the 600 mg tablet is: black monogram ink (n-butyl alcohol, black iron oxide E172, shellac glaze, pharmaceutical shellac in n-butyl alcohol, propylene glycol, ammonium hydroxide and isopropyl alcohol).

The printing ink used on the 800 mg tablet is: opacode orange (purified water, iron oxide yellow E172, propylene glycol, methanol, hydroxypropyl methylcellulose, iron oxide red E172 and isopropyl alcohol).

6.2 Incompatibilities

None

6.3 Shelf life

Neurontin Capsules: Three years

Neurontin Tablets: Two years

6.4 Special precautions for storage

Neurontin Capsules: Do not store above 30°C.

Neurontin Tablets: Do not store above 25°C.

6.5 Nature and contents of container

Neurontin Capsules: PVC/PVDC blister pack with vinyl heat seal/aluminium-coating backing. Supplied in packs of 84 or 100 capsules.

Neurontin Tablets: PVC/PE/PVDC blister pack with vinyl heat seal/aluminium-coating backing. Supplied in packs of 84 or100 tablets.

Also supplied as a titration pack for treatment of neuropathic pain containing 40 × 300 mg capsules and 10 × 600 mg tablets.

6.6 Instructions for use and handling

No special instructions needed.

7. MARKETING AUTHORISATION HOLDER

Warner Lambert (UK) Ltd trading as Parke Davis, Lambert Court, Chestnut Avenue, Eastleigh, Hampshire, SO53 3ZQ, United Kingdom.

8. MARKETING AUTHORISATION NUMBER(S)

Neurontin 100 mg capsules PL 0019/0172

Neurontin 300 mg capsules PL 0019/0173

Neurontin 400 mg capsules PL 0019/0174

Neurontin 600 mg tablets PL 0019/0192

Neurontin 800 mg tablets PL 0019/0193

9. DATE OF FIRST AUTHORISATION/RENEWAL OF THE AUTHORISATION

Neurontin Capsules: 31 December 1997

Neurontin Tablets: 26 November 1999

10. DATE OF REVISION OF THE TEXT

March 2005

LEGAL CATEGORY

POM

Neurontin is a registered trademark

Company reference NN 11_1

Nexium 20mg, 40mg Tablets

(AstraZeneca UK Limited)

1. NAME OF THE MEDICINAL PRODUCT

NEXIUM® 20 mg Tablets

NEXIUM® 40 mg Tablets

2. QUALITATIVE AND QUANTITATIVE COMPOSITION

Each tablet contains: 20mg esomeprazole (as magnesium trihydrate).

Each tablet contains: 40mg esomeprazole (as magnesium trihydrate).

For excipients see 6.1.

3. PHARMACEUTICAL FORM

Gastro-resistant tablet

20 mg: A light pink, oblong, biconvex, film-coated tablet engraved 20 mg on one side and A/EH on the other side.

40 mg: A pink, oblong, biconvex, film-coated tablet engraved 40 mg on one side and A/EI on the other side.

4. CLINICAL PARTICULARS

4.1 Therapeutic indications

NEXIUM tablets are indicated for:

- Gastro-Oesophageal Reflux Disease (GORD)

- treatment of erosive reflux oesophagitis

- long-term management of patients with healed oesophagitis to prevent relapse

- symptomatic treatment of gastro-oesophageal reflux disease (GORD)

In combination with an appropriate antibacterial therapeutic regimen for the eradication of *Helicobacter pylori* and

- healing of *Helicobacter pylori* associated duodenal ulcer and

- prevention of relapse of peptic ulcers in patients with *Helicobacter pylori* associated ulcers.

Patients requiring continued NSAID therapy

Healing of gastric ulcers associated with NSAID therapy.

Prevention of gastric and duodenal ulcers associated with NSAID therapy, in patients at risk.

4.2 Posology and method of administration

The tablets should be swallowed whole with liquid. The tablets should not be chewed or crushed. For patients who have difficulty in swallowing, the tablets can also be dispersed in half a glass of non-carbonated water. No other liquids should be used as the enteric coat may be dissolved. Stir until the tablets disintegrate and drink the liquid with the pellets immediately or within 30 minutes. Rinse the glass with half a glass of water and drink. The pellets must not be chewed or crushed.

For patients who cannot swallow, the tablets can be dispersed in non-carbonated water and administered through a gastric tube. It is important that the appropriateness of the selected syringe and tube is carefully tested.

For preparation and administration instructions see section 6.6.

- Gastro-Oesophageal Reflux Disease (GORD)

- treatment of erosive reflux oesophagitis

40 mg once daily for 4 weeks.

An additional 4 weeks treatment is recommended for patients in whom oesophagitis has not healed or who have persistent symptoms.

- long-term management of patients with healed oesophagitis to prevent relapse

20 mg once daily.

- symptomatic treatment of gastro-oesophageal reflux disease (GORD)

20 mg once daily in patients without oesophagitis. If symptom control has not been achieved after four weeks, the patient should be further investigated. Once symptoms have resolved, subsequent symptom control can be achieved using an on-demand regimen taking 20 mg once daily, when needed.

In combination with an appropriate antibacterial therapeutic regimen for the eradication of *Helicobacter pylori* and

- healing of *Helicobacter pylori* associated duodenal ulcer and

- prevention of relapse of peptic ulcers in patients with *Helicobacter pylori* associated ulcers.

20 mg NEXIUM with 1 g amoxicillin and 500 mg clarithromycin, all twice daily for 7 days.

Patients requiring continued NSAID therapy

Healing of gastric ulcers associated with NSAID therapy:

The usual dose is 20 mg once daily. The treatment duration is 4-8 weeks.

Prevention of gastric and duodenal ulcers associated with NSAID therapy in patients at risk:

20 mg once daily.

Children and adolescents

NEXIUM should not be used in children since no data is available.

Impaired renal function

Dose adjustment is not required in patients with impaired renal function. Due to limited experience in patients with severe renal insufficiency, such patients should be treated with caution, (see section 5.2).

Impaired hepatic function

Dose adjustment is not required in patients with mild to moderate liver impairment. For patients with severe liver impairment, a maximum dose of 20 mg NEXIUM should not be exceeded, (see section 5.2).

Elderly

Dose adjustment is not required in the elderly.

4.3 Contraindications

Known hypersensitivity to esomeprazole, substituted benzimidazoles or any other constituents of the formulation.

4.4 Special warnings and special precautions for use

In the presence of any alarm symptom (e.g. significant unintentional weight loss, recurrent vomiting, dysphagia, haematemesis or melaena) and when gastric ulcer is suspected or present, malignancy should be excluded, as treatment with NEXIUM may alleviate symptoms and delay diagnosis.

Patients on long-term treatment (particularly those treated for more than a year) should be kept under regular surveillance.

Patients on on-demand treatment should be instructed to contact their physician if their symptoms change in character. When prescribing esomeprazole for on-demand therapy, the implications for interactions with other pharmaceuticals, due to fluctuating plasma concentrations of esomeprazole should be considered, see section 4.5.

When prescribing esomeprazole for eradication of *Helicobacter pylori* possible drug interactions for all components in the triple therapy should be considered. Clarithromycin is a potent inhibitor of CYP3A4 and hence contraindications and interactions for clarithromycin should be considered when the triple therapy is used in patients concurrently taking other drugs metabolised via CYP3A4 such as cisapride.

Patients with rare hereditary problems of fructose intolerance, glucose-galactose malabsorption or sucrase-isomaltase insufficiency should not take this medicine.

4.5 Interaction with other medicinal products and other forms of Interaction

Effects of esomeprazole on the pharmacokinetics of other drugs

The decreased intragastric acidity during treatment with esomeprazole, might increase or decrease the absorption of drugs if the mechanism of absorption is influenced by gastric acidity. In common with the use of other inhibitors of acid secretion or antacids, the absorption of ketoconazole and itraconazole can decrease during treatment with esomeprazole.

Esomeprazole inhibits CYP2C19, the major esomeprazole metabolising enzyme. Thus, when esomeprazole is combined with drugs metabolised by CYP2C19, such as diazepam, citalopram, imipramine, clomipramine, phenytoin etc., the plasma concentrations of these drugs may be increased and a dose reduction could be needed. This should be considered especially when prescribing esomeprazole for on-demand therapy. Concomitant administration of 30 mg esomeprazole resulted in a 45% decrease in clearance of the CYP2C19 substrate diazepam. Concomitant administration of 40 mg esomeprazole resulted in a 13% increase in trough plasma levels of phenytoin in epileptic patients. It is recommended to monitor the plasma concentrations of phenytoin when treatment with esomeprazole is introduced or withdrawn. Concomitant administration of 40mg esomeprazole to warfarin-treated patients in a clinical trial showed that coagulation times were within the accepted range. However, post-marketing, a few isolated cases of elevated INR of clinical significance have been reported during concomitant treatment. Monitoring is recommended when initiating and ending concomitant treatment.

In healthy volunteers, concomitant administration of 40 mg esomeprazole resulted in a 32% increase in area under the plasma concentration-time curve (AUC) and a 31% prolongation of elimination half-life($t_{1/2}$) but no significant increase in peak plasma levels of cisapride. The slightly prolonged QTc interval observed after administration of cisapride alone, was not further prolonged when cisapride was given in combination with esomeprazole (see also section 4.4).

Esomeprazole has been shown to have no clinically relevant effects on the pharmacokinetics of amoxicillin or quinidine.

Studies evaluating concomitant administration of esomeprazole and either naproxen or rofecoxib did not identify any clinically relevant pharmacokinetic interactions during short-term studies.

Effects of other drugs on the pharmacokinetics of esomeprazole

Esomeprazole is metabolised by CYP2C19 and CYP3A4. Concomitant administration of esomeprazole and a CYP3A4 inhibitor, clarithromycin (500 mg b.i.d.), resulted in a doubling of the exposure (AUC) to esomeprazole. Dose adjustment of esomeprazole is not required.

4.6 Pregnancy and lactation

For Nexium, clinical data on exposed pregnancies are insufficient. With the racemic mixture omeprazole data on a larger number of exposed pregnancies stemmed from epidemiological studies indicate no malformative nor foetotoxic effects. Animal studies with esomeprazole do not indicate direct or indirect harmful effects with respect to embryonal/fetal development. Animal studies with the racemic mixture do not indicate direct or indirect harmful effects with respect to pregnancy, parturition or postnatal development. Caution should be exercised when prescribing to pregnant women.

It is not known whether esomeprazole is excreted in human breast milk. No studies in lactating women have been performed. Therefore NEXIUM should not be used during breast-feeding.

4.7 Effects on ability to drive and use machines

No effects have been observed.

4.8 Undesirable effects

The following adverse drug reactions have been identified or suspected in the clinical trials programme for esomeprazole and post-marketing. None was found to be dose-related.

Common (>1/100, <1/10)	Headache, abdominal pain, diarrhoea, flatulence, nausea/ vomiting, constipation.
Uncommon (>1/1,000, <1/100)	Dermatitis, pruritus, urticaria, dizziness, dry mouth
Rare (>1/10,000, 1<1,000)	Hypersensitivity reactions e.g. angioedema, anaphylactic reaction, increased liver enzymes, blurred vision, Stevens Johnson syndrome, erythema multiforme, myalgia

The following adverse drug reactions have been observed for the racemate (omeprazole) and may occur with esomeprazole:

Central and peripheral nervous system

Paraesthesia, somnolence, insomnia, vertigo. Reversible mental confusion, agitation, aggression, depression and hallucinations, predominantly in severely ill patients.

Endocrine

Gynaecomastia.

Gastrointestinal

Stomatitis and gastrointestinal candidiasis.

Haematological

Leukopenia, thrombocytopenia, agranulocytosis and pancytopenia.

Hepatic

Encephalopathy in patients with pre-existing severe liver disease; hepatitis with or without jaundice, hepatic failure.

Musculoskeletal

Arthralgia and muscular weakness.

Skin

Rash, photosensitivity, toxic epidermal necrolysis (TEN), alopecia.

Other

Malaise. Hypersensitivity reactions e.g. fever, bronchospasm, interstitial nephritis. Increased sweating, peripheral oedema, taste disturbance and hyponatraemia.

4.9 Overdose

There is very limited experience to date with deliberate overdose. The symptoms described in connection with 280mg were gastrointestinal symptoms and weakness. Single doses of 80 mg esomeprazole were uneventful. No specific antidote is known. Esomeprazole is extensively plasma protein bound and is therefore not readily dialyzable. As in any case of overdose, treatment should be symptomatic and general supportive measures should be utilised.

5. PHARMACOLOGICAL PROPERTIES

5.1 Pharmacodynamic properties

Pharmacotherapeutic group: Proton Pump Inhibitor

ATC Code: A02B C05.

Esomeprazole is the *S*-isomer of omeprazole and reduces gastric acid secretion through a specific targeted mechanism of action. It is a specific inhibitor of the acid pump in the parietal cell. Both the R- and S-isomer of omeprazole have similar pharmacodynamic activity.

Site and mechanism of action

Esomeprazole is a weak base and is concentrated and converted to the active form in the highly acidic environment of the secretory canaliculi of the parietal cell, where it inhibits the enzyme H^+K^+-ATPase – the acid pump and inhibits both basal and stimulated acid secretion.

Effect on gastric acid secretion

After oral dosing with esomeprazole 20 mg and 40 mg the onset of effect occurs within one hour. After repeated administration with 20 mg esomeprazole once daily for five days, mean peak acid output after pentagastrin stimulation is decreased 90% when measured 6 – 7 hours after dosing on day five.

After five days of oral dosing with 20 mg and 40 mg of esomeprazole, intragastric pH above 4 was maintained for a mean time of 13 hours and 17 hours, respectively over 24 hours in symptomatic GORD patients. The proportion of patients maintaining an intragastric pH above 4 for at least 8, 12 and 16 hours respectively were for esomeprazole 20 mg 76%, 54% and 24%. Corresponding proportions for esomeprazole 40 mg were 97%, 92% and 56%.

Using AUC as a surrogate parameter for plasma concentration, a relationship between inhibition of acid secretion and exposure has been shown.

Therapeutic effects of acid inhibition

Healing of reflux oesophagitis with esomeprazole 40 mg occurs in approximately 78% of patients after four weeks, and in 93% after eight weeks.

One week treatment with esomeprazole 20 mg b.i.d. and appropriate antibiotics, results in successful eradication of *H. pylori* in approximately 90% of patients.

After eradication treatment for one week there is no need for subsequent monotherapy with antisecretory drugs for effective ulcer healing and symptom resolution in uncomplicated duodenal ulcers.

Other effects related to acid inhibition

During treatment with antisecretory drugs serum gastrin increases in response to the decreased acid secretion.

An increased number of ECL cells possibly related to the increased serum gastrin levels, have been observed in some patients during long-term treatment with esomeprazole.

During long-term treatment with antisecretory drugs gastric glandular cysts have been reported to occur at a somewhat increased frequency. These changes are a physiological consequence of pronounced inhibition of acid secretion, are benign and appear to be reversible.

In two studies with ranitidine as an active comparator, Nexium showed better effect in healing of gastric ulcers in patients using NSAIDs, including COX-2 selective NSAIDs.

In two studies with placebo as comparator, Nexium showed better effect in the prevention of gastric and duodenal ulcers in patients using NSAIDs (aged >60 and/or with previous ulcer), including COX-2 selective NSAIDs.

5.2 Pharmacokinetic properties

Absorption and distribution

Esomeprazole is acid labile and is administered orally as enteric-coated granules. *In vivo* conversion to the R-isomer is negligible. Absorption of esomeprazole is rapid, with peak plasma levels occurring approximately 1-2 hours after dose. The absolute bioavailability is 64% after a single dose of 40mg and increases to 89% after repeated once-daily administration. For 20mg esomeprazole the corresponding values are 50% and 68%, respectively. The apparent volume of distribution at steady state in healthy subjects is approximately 0.22 L/kg body weight. Esomeprazole is 97% plasma protein bound.

Food intake both delays and decreases the absorption of esomeprazole although this has no significant influence on the effect of esomeprazole on intragastric acidity.

Metabolism and excretion

Esomeprazole is completely metabolised by the cytochrome P450 system (CYP). The major part of the metabolism of esomeprazole is dependent on the polymorphic CYP2C19, responsible for the formation of the hydroxy- and desmethyl metabolites of esomeprazole. The remaining part is dependent on another specific isoform, CYP3A4, responsible for the formation of esomeprazole sulphone, the main metabolite in plasma.

The parameters below reflect mainly the pharmacokinetics in individuals with a functional CYP2C19 enzyme, extensive metabolisers.

Total plasma clearance is about 17 L/h after a single dose and about 9 L/h after repeated administration. The plasma elimination half-life is about 1.3 hours after repeated once-daily dosing. The area under the plasma concentration-time curve increases with repeated administration of esomeprazole. This increase is dose-dependent and results in a non-linear dose-AUC relationship after repeated administration. This time - and dose-dependency is due to a decrease of first pass metabolism and systemic clearance probably caused by an inhibition of the CYP2C19 enzyme by esomeprazole and/or its sulphone metabolite. Esomeprazole is completely eliminated from plasma between doses with no tendency for accumulation during once-daily administration.

The major metabolites of esomeprazole have no effect on gastric acid secretion. Almost 80% of an oral dose of esomeprazole is excreted as metabolites in the urine, the remainder in the faeces. Less than 1% of the parent drug is found in urine.

Special patient populations

Approximately 1-2% of the population lack a functional CYP2C19 enzyme and are called poor metabolisers. In these individuals the metabolism of esomeprazole is probably mainly catalysed by CYP3A4. After repeated once-daily administration of 40 mg esomeprazole, the mean area under the plasma concentration-time curve was approximately 100% higher in poor metabolisers than in subjects having a functional CYP2C19 enzyme (extensive metabolisers). Mean peak plasma concentrations were increased by about 60%. These findings have no implications for the posology of esomeprazole.

The metabolism of esomeprazole is not significantly changed in elderly subjects (71-80 years of age).

Following a single dose of 40mg esomeprazole the mean area under the plasma concentration-time curve is approximately 30% higher in females than in males. No gender difference is seen after repeated once-daily administration. These findings have no implications for the posology of esomeprazole.

The metabolism of esomeprazole in patients with mild to moderate liver dysfunction may be impaired. The metabolic rate is decreased in patients with severe liver dysfunction resulting in a doubling of the area under the plasma concentration-time curve of esomeprazole. Therefore, a maximum of 20mg should not be exceeded in patients with severe dysfunction. Esomeprazole or its major metabolites do not show any tendency to accumulate with once-daily dosing.

No studies have been performed in patients with decreased renal function. Since the kidney is responsible for the excretion of the metabolites of esomeprazole but not for the elimination of the parent compound, the metabolism of esomeprazole is not expected to be changed in patients with impaired renal function.

5.3 Preclinical safety data

Preclinical bridging studies reveal no particular hazard for humans based on conventional studies of repeated dose toxicity, genotoxicity, and toxicity to reproduction. Carcinogenicity studies in the rat with the racemic mixture have shown gastric ECL-cell hyperplasia and carcinoids. These gastric effects in the rat are the result of sustained, pronounced hypergastrinaemia secondary to reduced production of gastric acid and are observed after long-term treatment in the rat with inhibitors of gastric acid secretion.

6. PHARMACEUTICAL PARTICULARS

6.1 List of excipients

Glycerol monostearate 40-55

hydroxypropyl cellulose

hypromellose

iron oxide (reddish-brown, yellow) (E 172)

magnesium stearate

methacrylic acid ethyl acrylate copolymer (1:1) dispersion 30 per cent

cellulose microcrystalline

synthetic paraffin

macrogol

polysorbate 80

crospovidone

sodium stearyl fumarate

sugar spheres (sucrose and maize starch)

talc

titanium dioxide (E 171)

triethyl citrate.

6.2 Incompatibilities

Not applicable

6.3 Shelf life

3 years

2 years in climate zones III-IV

6.4 Special precautions for storage

Do not store above 30°C

Keep the container tightly closed (bottle). Store in the original package (blister).

6.5 Nature and contents of container

- Polyethylene bottle with a tamper proof, polypropylene screw cap equipped with a desiccant capsule.
- Aluminium blister package.

20 mg, 40 mg: Bottles of 2, 5, 7, 14, 15, 28, 30, 56, 60, 100, 140(5x28) tablets.

20 mg, 40 mg: Blister packs in wallet and/or carton of 3, 7, 7x1, 14, 15, 25x1, 28, 30, 50x1, 56, 60, 90, 98, 100x1, 140 tablets

6.6 Instructions for use and handling

Administration through gastric tube

Put the tablet into an appropriate syringe and fill the syringe with approximately 25 mL water and approximately 5 mL air. For some tubes, dispersion in 50 mL water is needed to prevent the pellets from clogging the tube. Immediately shake the syringe for approximately 2 minutes to disperse the tablet. Hold the syringe with the tip up and check that the tip has not clogged. Attach the syringe to the tube whilst maintaining the above position. Shake the syringe and position it with the tip pointing down. Immediately inject 5-10 mL into the tube. Invert the syringe after injection and shake (the syringe must be held with the tip pointing up to avoid clogging of the tip). Turn the syringe with the tip down and immediately inject another 5-10 mL into the tube. Repeat this procedure until the syringe is empty. Fill the syringe with 25 mL of water and 5 mL of air and repeat step 5 if necessary to wash down any sediment left in the syringe. For some tubes, 50 mL water is needed.

7. MARKETING AUTHORISATION HOLDER

AstraZeneca UK Limited
600 Capability Green
Luton, LU1 3LU, UK

8. MARKETING AUTHORISATION NUMBER(S)

PL 17901/0068

PL 17901/0069

9. DATE OF FIRST AUTHORISATION/RENEWAL OF THE AUTHORISATION

27th July 2000

10. DATE OF REVISION OF THE TEXT

15th October 2004

Nexium I.V. 40mg Powder for solution for injection/infusion

(AstraZeneca UK Limited)

1. NAME OF THE MEDICINAL PRODUCT

Nexium I.V.▼40 mg Powder for solution for injection/infusion

2. QUALITATIVE AND QUANTITATIVE COMPOSITION

Each vial contains esomeprazole sodium 42.5 mg, equivalent to esomeprazole 40 mg.

For excipients see 6.1.

3. PHARMACEUTICAL FORM

Powder for solution for injection/infusion

White to off-white porous cake or powder

4. CLINICAL PARTICULARS

4.1 Therapeutic indications

Nexium I.V. is indicated for gastroesophageal reflux disease in patients with oesophagitis and/or severe symptoms of reflux as an alternative to oral therapy when oral intake is not appropriate.

4.2 Posology and method of administration

Patients who cannot take oral medication may be treated parenterally with 20-40 mg once daily. Patients with reflux oesophagitis should be treated with 40 mg once daily. Patients treated symptomatically for reflux disease should be treated with 20 mg once daily. Usually the iv treatment duration is short and transfer to oral treatment should be made as soon as possible.

Method of administration

Injection

40 mg dose

The reconstituted solution should be given as an intravenous injection over a period of at least 3 minutes.

20 mg dose

Half of the reconstituted solution should be given as an intravenous injection over a period of approximately 3 minutes. Any unused solution should be discarded.

Infusion

40 mg dose

The reconstituted solution should be given as an intravenous infusion over a period of 10 to 30 minutes.

20 mg dose

Half of the reconstituted solution should be given as an intravenous infusion over a period of 10 to 30 minutes. Any unused solution should be discarded.

Children and adolescents

Nexium I.V. should not be used in children since no data is available.

Impaired renal function

Dose adjustment is not required in patients with impaired renal function. Due to limited experience in patients with severe renal insufficiency, such patients should be treated with caution. (See section 5.2).

Impaired hepatic function

Dose adjustment is not required in patients with mild to moderate liver impairment. For patients with severe liver impairment, a maximum daily dose of 20 mg Nexium I.V. should not be exceeded. (See section 5.2).

Elderly

Dose adjustment is not required in the elderly.

4.3 Contraindications

Hypersensitivity to the active substance esomeprazole or to other substituted benzimidazoles or to any of the excipients of this medicinal product.

4.4 Special warnings and special precautions for use

In the presence of any alarm symptom (e.g. significant unintentional weight loss, recurrent vomiting, dysphagia, haematemesis or melaena) and when gastric ulcer is suspected or present, malignancy should be excluded, as treatment with Nexium I.V. may alleviate symptoms and delay diagnosis.

4.5 Interaction with other medicinal products and other forms of Interaction

Effects of esomeprazole on the pharmacokinetics of other drugs

The decreased intragastric acidity during treatment with Nexium I.V. might increase or decrease the absorption of drugs if the mechanism of absorption is influenced by gastric acidity. In common with the use of other inhibitors of acid secretion or antacids, the absorption of ketoconazole and itraconazole can decrease during treatment with Nexium I.V.

Esomeprazole inhibits CYP2C19, the major esomeprazole metabolising enzyme. Thus, when esomeprazole is combined with drugs metabolised by CYP2C19, such as diazepam, citalopram, imipramine, clomipramine, phenytoin etc., the plasma concentrations of these drugs may be increased and a dose reduction could be needed. Concomitant oral administration of 30 mg esomeprazole resulted in a 45% decrease in clearance of the CYP2C19 substrate diazepam. Concomitant oral administration of 40 mg esomeprazole and phenytoin resulted in a 13% increase in trough plasma levels of phenytoin in epileptic patients. It is recommended to monitor the plasma concentrations of phenytoin when treatment with esomeprazole is introduced or withdrawn.

Concomitant oral administration of 40 mg esomeprazole to warfarin-treated patients in a clinical trial showed that coagulation times were within the accepted range. However, post-marketing of oral esomeprazole, a few isolated cases of elevated INR of clinical significance have been reported during concomitant treatment. Monitoring is recommended when initiating and ending concomitant treatment.

In healthy volunteers, concomitant oral administration of 40 mg esomeprazole and cisapride resulted in a 32% increase in area under the plasma concentration-time curve (AUC) and a 31% prolongation of elimination half-life($t_{1/2}$) but no significant increase in peak plasma levels of cisapride. The slightly prolonged QTc interval observed after administration of cisapride alone, was not further prolonged when cisapride was given in combination with esomeprazole.

Esomeprazole has been shown to have no clinically relevant effects on the pharmacokinetics of amoxicillin or quinidine.

Effects of other drugs on the pharmacokinetics of esomeprazole

Esomeprazole is metabolised by CYP2C19 and CYP3A4. Concomitant oral administration of esomeprazole and a CYP3A4 inhibitor, clarithromycin (500 mg b.i.d.), resulted in a doubling of the exposure (AUC) to esomeprazole. Dose adjustment of esomeprazole is not required.

4.6 Pregnancy and lactation

For esomeprazole limited data on exposed pregnancies are available. Animal studies with esomeprazole do not indicate direct or indirect harmful effects with respect to embryonal/foetal development. Animal studies with the racemic mixture do not indicate direct or indirect harmful effects with respect to pregnancy, parturition or postnatal development. Caution should be exercised when prescribing Nexium I.V. to pregnant women.

It is not known whether esomeprazole is excreted in human breast milk. No studies in lactating women have been performed. Therefore Nexium I.V. should not be used during breast-feeding.

4.7 Effects on ability to drive and use machines

Nexium I.V. is not likely to affect the ability to drive or use machines.

4.8 Undesirable effects

The following adverse drug reactions have been identified or suspected in the clinical trials programme for esomeprazole administered orally or intravenously and post-marketing when administered orally.

Common (>1/100, <1/10)	Headache, abdominal pain, diarrhoea, flatulence, nausea/vomiting, constipation
Uncommon (>1/1000, <1/100)	Dermatitis, pruritus, urticaria, dizziness, dry mouth, blurred vision

Rare (>1/10000, <1/1000)	Hypersensitivity reactions e.g. angioedema, anaphylactic reaction. Increased liver enzymes. Stevens Johnson syndrome, erythema multiforme, myalgia.

The following adverse drug reactions have been observed for the racemate (omeprazole) and may occur with esomeprazole:

Central and peripheral nervous system

Paraesthesia, somnolence, insomnia, vertigo. Reversible mental confusion, agitation, aggression, depression and hallucinations, predominantly in severely ill patients.

Endocrine

Gynaecomastia.

Gastrointestinal

Stomatitis and gastrointestinal candidiasis.

Haematological

Leukopenia, thrombocytopenia, agranulocytosis and pancytopenia.

Hepatic

Encephalopathy in patients with pre-existing severe liver disease; hepatitis with or without jaundice, hepatic failure.

Musculoskeletal

Arthralgia and muscular weakness.

Skin

Rash, photosensitivity, toxic epidermal necrolysis (TEN), alopecia.

Other

Malaise. Hypersensitivity reactions e.g. fever, bronchospasm and interstitial nephritis. Increased sweating, peripheral oedema, taste disturbance and hyponatraemia.

Irreversible visual impairment has been reported in isolated cases of critically ill patients who have received omeprazole intravenous injection, especially at high doses, but no causal relationship has been established.

4.9 Overdose

There is very limited experience to date with deliberate overdose. The symptoms described in connection with an oral dose of 280 mg were gastrointestinal symptoms and weakness. Single oral doses of 80 mg esomeprazole and intravenous doses of 100 mg were uneventful. No specific antidote is known. Esomeprazole is extensively plasmaprotein bound and is therefore not readily dialyzable. As in any case of overdose, treatment should be symptomatic and general supportive measures should be utilised.

5. PHARMACOLOGICAL PROPERTIES

5.1 Pharmacodynamic properties

Pharmacotherapeutic group: Proton pump inhibitor

ATC Code: A02B C05

Esomeprazole isthe S-isomer of omeprazole and reduces gastric acid secretion through a specific targeted mechanism of action. It is a specific inhibitor of the acid pump in the parietal cell. Both the R- and S-isomer of omeprazole have similar pharmacodynamic activity.

Site and mechanism of action

Esomeprazole is a weak base and is concentrated and converted to the active form in the highly acidic environment of the secretory canaliculi of the parietal cell, where it inhibits the enzyme H^+K^+-ATPase – the acid pump and inhibits both basal and stimulated acid secretion.

Effect on gastric acid secretion

After 5 days of oral dosing with 20 mg and 40 mg of esomeprazole, intragastric pH above 4 was maintained for a mean time of 13 hours and 17 hours, respectively over 24 hours in symptomatic GORD patients. The effect is similar irrespective of whether esomeprazole is administered orally or intravenously.

Using AUC as a surrogate parameter for plasma concentration, a relationship between inhibition of acid secretion and exposure has been shown after oral administration of esomeprazole.

Therapeutic effects of acid inhibition

Healing of reflux oesophagitis with esomeprazole 40 mg occurs in approximately 78% of patients after 4 weeks, and in 93% after 8 weeks of oral treatment.

Other effects related to acid inhibition

During treatment with antisecretory drugs serum gastrin increases in response to the decreased acid secretion.

An increased number of ECL cells possibly related to the increased serum gastrin levels, have been observed in some patients during long term treatment with orally administered esomeprazole.

During long-term oral treatment with antisecretory drugs gastric glandular cysts have been reported to occur at a somewhat increased frequency. These changes are a physiological consequence of pronounced inhibition of acid secretion, are benign and appear to be reversible.

5.2 Pharmacokinetic properties

Distribution

The apparent volume of distribution at steady state in healthy subjects is approximately 0.22 L/kg body weight. Esomeprazole is 97% plasma protein bound.

Metabolism and excretion

Esomeprazole is completely metabolised by the cytochrome P450 system (CYP). The major part of the metabolism of esomeprazole is dependent on the polymorphic CYP2C19, responsible for the formation of the hydroxy- and desmethyl metabolites of esomeprazole. The remaining part is dependent on another specific isoform, CYP3A4, responsible for the formation of esomeprazole sulphone, the main metabolite in plasma.

The parameters below reflect mainly the pharmacokinetics in individuals with a functional CYP2C19 enzyme, extensive metabolisers.

Total plasma clearance is about 17 L/h after a single dose and about 9 L/h after repeated administration. The plasma elimination half-life is about 1.3 hours after repeated once-daily dosing. Total exposure (AUC) increases with repeated administration of esomeprazole. This increase is dose-dependent and results in a non-linear dose-AUC relationship after repeated administration. This time - and dose-dependency is due to a decrease of first pass metabolism and systemic clearance probably caused by inhibition of the CYP2C19 enzyme by esomeprazole and/or its sulphone metabolite. Esomeprazole is completely eliminated from plasma between doses with no tendency for accumulation during once-daily administration.

Following repeated doses of 40 mg administered as intravenous injections, the mean peak plasma concentration is approx. 13.6 micromol/L. The mean peak plasma concentration after corresponding oral doses is approx. 4.6 micromol/L. A smaller increase (of approx 30%) can be seen in total exposure after intravenous administration compared to oral administration.

The major metabolites of esomeprazole have no effect on gastric acid secretion. Almost 80% of an oral dose of esomeprazole is excreted as metabolites in the urine, the remainder in the faeces. Less than 1% of the parent drug is found in urine.

Special patient populations

Approximately 1-2% of the population lack a functional CYP2C19 enzyme and are called poor metabolisers. In these individuals the metabolism of esomeprazole is probably mainly catalysed by CYP3A4. After repeated once-daily administration of 40 mg oral esomeprazole, the mean total exposure was approximately 100% higher in poor metabolisers than in subjects with a functional CYP2C19 enzyme (extensive metabolisers). Mean peak plasma concentrations were increased by about 60%. Similar differences have been seen for intravenous administration of esomeprazole. These findings have no implications for the posology of esomeprazole.

The metabolism of esomeprazole is not significantly changed in elderly subjects (71-80 years of age).

Following a single oral dose of 40 mg esomeprazole the mean total exposure is approximately 30% higher in females than in males. No gender difference is seen after repeated once-daily administration. Similar differences have been observed for intravenous administration of esomeprazole. These findings have no implications for the posology of esomeprazole.

The metabolism of esomeprazole in patients with mild to moderate liver dysfunction may be impaired. The metabolic rate is decreased in patients with severe liver dysfunction resulting in a doubling of the total exposure of esomeprazole. Therefore, a maximum dose of 20 mg should not be exceededin patients with severe dysfunction. Esomeprazole or its major metabolites do not show any tendency to accumulate with once-daily dosing.

No studies have been performed in patients with decreased renal function. Since the kidney is responsible for the excretion of the metabolites of esomeprazole but not for the elimination of the parent compound, the metabolism of esomeprazole is not expected to be changed in patients with impaired renal function.

5.3 Preclinical safety data

Preclinical studies reveal no particular hazard for humans, based on conventional studies of single and repeated dose toxicity, embryo-foetal toxicity and mutagenicity. Oral carcinogenicity studies in the rat with the racemic mixture have shown gastric ECL-cell hyperplasia and carcinoids. These gastric effects are the result of sustained, pronounced hypergastrinaemia secondary to reduced production of gastric acid, and are observed after long-term treatment in the rat with inhibitors of gastric acid secretion.

6. PHARMACEUTICAL PARTICULARS

6.1 List of excipients

Disodium edetate dihydrate

Sodium hydroxide

6.2 Incompatibilities

This medicinal product should not be used with other medicinal products except those mentioned in section 6.6.

6.3 Shelf life

2 years in all climate zones

Shelf-life after reconstitution

Chemical and physical in-use stability has been demonstrated for 12 hours at 25°C. From a microbiological point of view, the product should be used immediately.

6.4 Special precautions for storage

Store in the original package, in order to protect from light. Vials can however be stored exposed to normal in-door light outside the box for up to 24 hours. Do not store above 30°C.

6.5 Nature and contents of container

5 mL vial made of colourless borosilicate glass, type I. Stopper made of bromobutyl latex-free rubber, cap made of aluminium and a plastic flip-off seal.

Pack sizes: 1 vial, 1x10 vials.

Not all pack sizes may be marketed.

6.6 Instructions for use and handling

The reconstituted solution should be inspected visually for particulate matter and discoloration prior to administration. Only clear solution should be used. For single use only.

When administering a 20 mg dose only half of the reconstituted solution should be used. Any unused solution should be discarded.

Injection

A solution for injection is prepared by adding 5 mL of 0.9% sodium chloride for intravenous use to the vial with esomeprazole.

The reconstituted solution for injection is clear and colourless to very slightly yellow.

Infusion

A solution for infusion is prepared by dissolving the content of one vial with esomeprazole in up to 100 mL 0.9% sodium chloride for intravenous use.

The reconstituted solution for infusion is clear and colourless to very slightly yellow.

7. MARKETING AUTHORISATION HOLDER

AstraZeneca UK Limited

600 Capability Green

Luton

LU1 3LU

United Kingdom

8. MARKETING AUTHORISATION NUMBER(S)

PL 17901/0221

9. DATE OF FIRST AUTHORISATION/RENEWAL OF THE AUTHORISATION

28th January 2004

10. DATE OF REVISION OF THE TEXT

Niaspan Prolonged Release Tablets

(Merck Pharmaceuticals)

1. NAME OF THE MEDICINAL PRODUCT

Niaspan Prolonged-Release Tablets Starter Pack

Niaspan 500 mg Prolonged-Release Tablets

Niaspan 750 mg Prolonged-Release Tablets

Niaspan 1000 mg Prolonged-Release Tablets

2. QUALITATIVE AND QUANTITATIVE COMPOSITION

The Starter Pack contains 7 tablets each of Niaspan 375mg, Niaspan 500mg and Niaspan 750mg Prolonged-Release Tablets.

Each Niaspan 375 mg prolonged-release tablet contains 375 mg nicotinic acid.

Each Niaspan 500 mg prolonged-release tablet contains 500 mg nicotinic acid.

Each Niaspan 750 mg prolonged-release tablet contains 750 mg nicotinic acid.

Each Niaspan 1000 mg prolonged-release tablet contains 1000 mg nicotinic acid.

For excipients, see section 6.1.

3. PHARMACEUTICAL FORM

Prolonged-release tablet

White to off-white capsule-shaped tablet. Each tablet is embossed with the tablet strength on one side.

4. CLINICAL PARTICULARS

4.1 Therapeutic indications

Treatment of dyslipidaemia, particularly in patients with combined mixed dyslipidaemia, characterised by elevated levels of LDL-cholesterol and triglycerides and low HDL-cholesterol, and in patients with primary hypercholesterolaemia. Niaspan should be used in patients in combination with HMG-CoA reductase inhibitors (statins), when the cholesterol lowering effect of HMG-CoA reductase inhibitor monotherapy is inadequate. Niaspan can be used as monotherapy only in patients who do not tolerate HMG-CoA reductase inhibitors. Diet and other non-pharmacological treatments (e.g. exercise, weight reduction) should be continued during therapy with Niaspan.

4.2 Posology and method of administration

Niaspan should be taken at bedtime, after a low-fat snack (e.g. an apple, low fat yoghurt, slice of bread) and doses should be individualised according to the patient's response.

Initial dose

Therapy with Niaspan must be initiated with a low dose and increased gradually. The recommended dose escalation schedule is shown below in Table 1:

Table 1: Dose escalation schedule

(see Table 1 below)

Maintenance dose

The recommended maintenance dose is 1000mg (two 500mg tablets) to 2000mg (two 1000mg tablets) once daily at bedtime depending on the patient's response and tolerance. If the response to 1000mg daily is inadequate, the dose may be increased to 1500mg daily and subsequently to 2000mg daily.

The daily dosage of Niaspan should not be increased by more than 500mg in any four-week period after the initial titration to 1000mg. The maximum dose is 2000mg per day.

The different Niaspan tablet strengths have different bioavailability and are therefore not interchangeable.

Niaspan must not be replaced with other nicotinic acid preparations, see section 4.4.

In patients previously treated with other nicotinic acid products, Niaspan treatment must be initiated with the recommended Niaspan dose escalation schedule. The maintenance dose should subsequently be individualised according to the patient's response.

If Niaspan therapy is discontinued for an extended period, re-institution of therapy must include a dose escalation.

Niaspan tablets must not be broken, crushed or chewed before swallowing.

Renal impairment

No studies have been performed in patients with impaired renal function, Niaspan must be used with caution in patients with renal disease.

Hepatic impairment

No studies have been performed in patients with impaired hepatic function. Niaspan must be used with caution in patients with a history of liver disease and who consume substantial quantities of alcohol, see section 4.4. Niaspan is contraindicated in patients with significant hepatic dysfunction, see section 4.3.

Elderly

No dose adjustment necessary.

Children

The safety and efficacy of nicotinic acid therapy in children and adolescents has not been established. Use in children and adolescents is not recommended.

4.3 Contraindications

Niaspan is contraindicated in patients with

- hypersensitivity to nicotinic acid or to any of the excipients, see section 6.1,
- significant hepatic dysfunction,
- active peptic ulcer disease,
- arterial bleeding.

4.4 Special warnings and special precautions for use

Niaspan must not be replaced with other nicotinic acid preparations. When switching from other nicotinic acid preparations to Niaspan, therapy with Niaspan must be initiated with the recommended dose escalation schedule, see section 4.2.

Liver

Nicotinic acid preparations have been associated with abnormal liver tests. Severe hepatic toxicity, including fulminant hepatic necrosis, has occurred in patients who have taken long-acting nicotinic acid products in place of immediate-release nicotinic acid. Since the pharmacokinetics of Niaspan are different to other nicotinic acid preparations, Niaspan must not be replaced with other preparations. The prescribing information of the HMG-CoA reductase inhibitor should also be consulted for warnings and precautions for use.

Caution is advised when Niaspan is used in patients who consume substantial quantities of alcohol and/or have a past history of liver disease.

Elevated liver transaminases have been observed with Niaspan therapy. However, transaminase elevations were reversible upon discontinuation of Niaspan.

Liver tests including AST and ALT must be performed periodically in all patients during therapy with Niaspan and prior to treatment in case of history and/or symptoms of hepatic dysfunction (e.g. jaundice, nausea, fever, and/or malaise). If the transaminase levels show evidence of progression, particularly if they rise to three times the upper limit of normal, the drug must be discontinued.

Skeletal muscle

Single reports on rhabdomyolysis in patients on combined therapy with Niaspan and HMG-CoA reductase inhibitors have been received from spontaneous reporting. Physicians contemplating combined therapy with HMG-CoA reductase inhibitors and Niaspan should carefully weigh the potential benefits and risks and should carefully monitor patients for any symptoms of rhabdomyolysis e.g. muscle pain, tenderness or weakness, particularly during the initial months of therapy and during any periods of upward dosage titration of either drug. Periodic serum creatine phosphokinase (CPK) and potassium determinations should be considered in such situations.

A CPK level should be measured before starting such a combination in patients with pre-disposing factors for rhabdomyolysis, as follows:

- renal impairment
- hypothyroidism
- alcohol abuse
- age > 70 years
- personal or family history of hereditary muscular disorders
- previous history of muscular toxicity with fibrate or HMG-CoA reductase inhibitor

Muscle damage must be considered in any patient presenting with diffuse myalgia, muscle tenderness and/or marked increase in muscle CK levels (>5 × ULN); under these conditions treatment must be discontinued.

The prescribing information of the HMG-CoA reductase inhibitors should be consulted.

Glucose Intolerance

Diabetic or potentially diabetic patients should be observed closely since there may be a dose-related increase in glucose intolerance. Adjustment of diet and/or oral antidiabetics and/or insulin therapy may become necessary.

Unstable angina and acute myocardial infarction

Caution is advised when Niaspan is used in patients with unstable angina or in the acute phase of myocardial infarction, particularly when such patients are also receiving vasoactive drugs such as nitrates, calcium channel blockers, or adrenergic blocking agents.

Uric acid

Elevated uric acid levels have occurred with Niaspan therapy. Monitoring of patients predisposed to gout is recommended.

Coagulation

Niaspan may affect platelet count and prothrombin time, see section 4.5. Patients undergoing surgery should be carefully evaluated. Caution is also advised when Niaspan is administered concomitantly with anti-coagulants; patients receiving anti-coagulants must be monitored closely for prothrombin time and platelet count.

Hypophosphataemia

Niaspan has been associated with reductions in phosphorous levels. Although these reductions were transient, monitoring of phosphorous levels is recommended in patients at risk of hypophosphataemia.

Other

Patients with a history of jaundice, hepatobiliary disease, or peptic ulcer should be observed closely during Niaspan therapy.

4.5 Interaction with other medicinal products and other forms of Interaction

Concomitant alcohol or hot drinks may increase undesirable flushing and pruritus and should be avoided around the time of Niaspan ingestion.

Niaspan has been associated with small but statistically significant dose-related reductions in platelet count (mean of -11% with 2000mg). In addition, Niaspan has been associated with small but statistically significant increases in prothrombin time (mean of approximately +4%). When Niaspan is administered concomitantly with anti-coagulants, prothrombin time and platelet counts must be monitored closely.

Nicotinic acid may potentiate the blood-pressure lowering effect of ganglionic blocking agents e.g. transdermal nicotine or vasoactive drugs such as nitrates, calcium channel blockers or adrenergic blocking agents.

Bile acid sequestrants bind to other orally administered medicinal products and should be taken separately, see also prescribing information of the concerned product.

Nicotinic acid may produce false elevations in some fluorometric determinations of plasma or urinary catecholamines. Nicotinic acid may also give false-positive reactions with cupric sulphate solution (Benedict's reagent) in urine glucose tests.

For combined use of Niaspan and HMG-CoA reductase inhibitors (statins) see section 4.4 *(this refers to liver and skeletal muscle).*

4.6 Pregnancy and lactation

Pregnancy

It is not known whether nicotinic acid at doses typically used for lipid disorders can cause foetal harm when administered to pregnant women or whether it can affect reproductive capacity. Animal studies are incomplete, see section 5.3.

Niaspan should not be prescribed to pregnant women unless strictly necessary.

Lactation

Nicotinic acid has been reported to appear in breast milk. Because of the potential for serious adverse reactions in nursing infants from lipid-altering doses of nicotinic acid, a decision should be made whether to discontinue nursing or to discontinue the drug, taking into account the importance of the drug to the mother. No studies have been conducted with Niaspan in nursing mothers.

4.7 Effects on ability to drive and use machines

Niaspan has no or negligible influence on the ability to drive and use machines.

4.8 Undesirable effects

Flush

In the placebo-controlled clinical trials, flushing episodes (i.e. warmth, redness, itching and/or tingling) were the most common treatment-emergent adverse events for Niaspan (reported by 88% of patients). In these studies fewer than 6% of Niaspan patients discontinued due to flushing.

In comparisons of immediate-release (IR) nicotinic acid and Niaspan, although the number of patients who flushed was similar, fewer flushing episodes were reported by patients who received Niaspan. Following four weeks of maintenance therapy with Niaspan at daily doses of 1500mg, the frequency of flushing over the four week period averaged 1.88 events per patient.

Flushing reactions generally occur during early treatment and the dose titration phase. They are thought to be mediated by the release of prostaglandin D2 and tolerance to flushing usually develops over the course of several weeks.

Spontaneous reports suggest that in rare cases, flushing may be more severe and accompanied by symptoms of dizziness, tachycardia, palpitations, dyspnoea, sweating, chills and/or oedema which in rare cases may lead to syncope. Medical treatment should be administered as necessary.

Hypersensitivity reactions

Hypersensitivity reactions have been reported very rarely. These may be characterised by symptoms such as generalised exanthema, flush, urticaria, vesiculobullous rash, angioedema, laryngospasm, dyspnoea, hypotension, and circulatory collapse. Medical treatment should be administered as necessary.

The following adverse reactions have been observed in clinical studies or in routine patient management, in patients receiving the recommended daily maintenance doses (1000, 1500, and 2000mg) of Niaspan. They are presented by system organ class and frequency grouping (very common >1/10; common >1/100, <1/10; uncommon >1/1,000, <1/100; rare >1/10,000, <1/1,000; very rare <1/10,000, including isolated reports). In general, the incidence of adverse reactions was higher in women compared to men. (Please refer to Table 2 below).

Table 1 Dose escalation schedule

	Week(s)	Dosage	Daily nicotinic acid dose		
↑	1	Niaspan 375mg	1 tablet at bedtime	375mg	↑
INITIAL TITRATION SCHEDULE	2	Niaspan 500mg	1 tablet at bedtime	500mg	TITRATION STARTER PACK
	3	Niaspan 750mg	1 tablet at bedtime	750mg	↓
↓	4-7	Niaspan 500mg	2 tablets at bedtime	1000mg	
		Niaspan 750mg	2 tablets at bedtime	1500mg	
		Niaspan 1000mg	2 tablets at bedtime	2000mg	

Table 2: Adverse reactions

(see Table 2)

4.9 Overdose

Information on acute overdose with Niaspan in humans is limited. The signs and symptoms of an acute overdose are anticipated to be those of excessive pharmacological effect: severe flushing, nausea/vomiting, diarrhoea, dyspepsia, dizziness, syncope, hypotension, potential cardiac arrhythmias and clinical laboratory abnormalities including elevations in liver function tests. The patient should be carefully observed and given supportive treatment. Insufficient information is available on the dialysis potential of nicotinic acid.

5. PHARMACOLOGICAL PROPERTIES

5.1 Pharmacodynamic properties

Pharmacotherapeutic group: nicotinic acid, ATC code: C10AD02

Nicotinic acid is a water-soluble B-complex vitamin which is a naturally occurring constituent of foods. The human body is not entirely dependent on dietary sources of nicotinic acid, since it may also be synthesised from tryptophan.

The mechanism of action by which nicotinic acid modifies lipid profiles is not fully elucidated. However, it is recognised that nicotinic acid inhibits the release of free fatty acids from adipose tissue resulting in less free fatty acids being presented to the liver. Since fewer fatty acids are being transported to the liver, fewer are esterified to triglycerides and then incorporated into VLDL. This may lead to a decrease in LDL generation. By increasing lipoprotein lipase activity, nicotinic acid may increase the rate of chylomicron triglycerides removal from plasma. Thus, nicotinic acid decreases the rate of hepatic synthesis of VLDL and subsequently LDL. It does not appear to affect faecal excretion of fats, sterols, or bile acids.

At the recommended maintenance dose, Niaspan (but not nicotinamide) resulted in a clinical reduction in total cholesterol to HDL ratio (-17, to -27%), LDL (-8 to -16%), triglycerides (-14 to -35%) with an increase in HDL (16% to 26%). In addition to the above mentioned reduction in LDL levels, nicotinic acid causes a shift in LDL composition from the small dense LDL particles (major atherogenic lipoprotein) to the larger, more buoyant LDL particles (less atherogenic). The increase in HDL is also associated with a shift in the distribution of HDL sub-fractions including an increase in the HDL2 to HDL3 ratio, the protective effect of HDL being mainly due to HDL2. Moreover, nicotinic acid increases serum levels of apolipoprotein A1 (Apo 1), one of the two major lipoproteins of HDL, while decreases concentrations of apolipoprotein B-100 (Apo B), the major protein component of the very low-density lipoprotein (VLDL) and LDL fractions known to play important roles in atherogenesis. The serum levels of lipoprotein a, (Lp (a)), which present great homology with LDL but considered as an independent risk factor for coronary heart disease, are also significantly reduced by Niaspan.

Data from clinical trials suggest that women have a greater hypolipidaemic response than men at equivalent doses of Niaspan.

There are no specific studies of the combination of Niaspan with statins.

The beneficial effect of Niaspan on morbidity and mortality has not been directly assessed. However, relevant clinical data are available with immediate release (IR) nicotinic acid.

5.2 Pharmacokinetic properties

Absorption

Nicotinic acid is rapidly and extensively absorbed when administered orally (at least 60-76% of dose).

Peak steady-state nicotinic acid concentrations were 0.6, 4.9, and 15.5 microgram/ml after doses of 1000, 1500, and 2000mg Niaspan once daily (given as two 500mg, two 750mg, and two 1000mg tablets, respectively).

Single-dose bioavailability studies have demonstrated that Niaspan tablet strengths are not interchangeable.

Distribution

Studies using radiolabelled nicotinic acid in mice show that nicotinic acid and its metabolites concentrate in the liver, kidney and adipose tissue.

Metabolism

The pharmacokinetic profile of nicotinic acid is complicated due to rapid and extensive first-pass metabolism which is species and dose-rate specific. In humans, one pathway (Pathway 1) is through a simple conjugation step with glycine to form nicotinuric acid (NUA). NUA is then excreted in the urine, although there may be a small amount of reversible metabolism back to nicotinic acid. There is evidence to suggest that nicotinic acid metabolism along this pathway leads to flush. The other pathway (Pathway 2) results in the formation of nicotinamide adenine dinucleotide (NAD). A predominance of metabolism down Pathway 2 may lead to hepatotoxicity. It is unclear whether nicotinamide is formed as a precursor to, or following the synthesis of, NAD. Nicotinamide is further metabolised to at least N-methylnicotinamide (MNA) and nicotinamide N-oxide (NNO). MNA is further metabolised to two other compounds, N-methyl-2-pyridone-5-carboxamide (2PY) and N-methyl-4-pyridone-5-carboxamide (4PY). The formation of 2PY appears to predominate over 4PY in humans. At the doses used to treat hyperlipidaemia, these metabolic pathways are saturable, which explains the non-linear relationship between nicotinic acid dose and plasma concentrations following multiple dose Niaspan administration.

Nicotinamide does not have hypolipidaemic activity; the activity of the other metabolites is unknown.

Elimination

Nicotinic acid and its metabolites are rapidly eliminated in the urine. Following single and multiple doses, approximately 60-76% of the dose administered as Niaspan was recovered in the urine as nicotinic acid and metabolites; up to 12% was recovered as unchanged nicotinic acid after multiple dosing. The ratio of metabolites recovered in the urine was dependent on the dose administered.

Gender differences

Steady state plasma concentrations of nicotinic acid and metabolites after administration of Niaspan are generally higher in women than in men, with the magnitude of difference varying with dose and metabolite. Recovery of nicotinic acid and metabolites in urine, however, is generally similar for men and women, indicating the absorption is similar for both genders. The gender differences observed in plasma levels of nicotinic acid and its metabolites may be due to gender-specific differences in metabolic rate or volume of distribution.

5.3 Preclinical safety data

Nicotinic acid has been shown to be of low toxicity in customary animal studies.

Female rabbits have been dosed with 0.3g nicotinic acid per day from pre-conception to lactation, and gave birth to offspring without teratogenic effects. Further specific animal reproduction studies have not been conducted with nicotinic acid or with Niaspan.

In a life-time study in mice, high dose levels of nicotinic acid showed no treatment-related carcinogenic effects and no effects on survival rates.

6. PHARMACEUTICAL PARTICULARS

6.1 List of excipients

Povidone

Hypromellose

Stearic Acid

6.2 Incompatibilities

Not applicable

6.3 Shelf life

3 years

6.4 Special precautions for storage

Do not store above 25°C

Store in the original package to protect from moisture

Table 2 Adverse reactions

Organ Class	Very common >1/10	Common >1/100, <1/10	Uncommon >1/1,000, <1/100	Rare >1/10,000, <1/1,000	Very rare <1/10,000, including isolated reports
Immune system disorders					Hypersensitivity reaction
Metabolism and nutrition disorders				Decreased glucose tolerance	Anorexia, gout
Psychiatric disorders				Insomnia, nervousness	
Nervous system disorders			Headache, dizziness	Syncope, paraesthesia	Migraine
Eye disorders				Visual disturbance	Toxic amblyopia, cystoid macular oedema
Cardiac disorders			Tachycardia, palpitations		Atrial fibrillation, other cardiac dysrhythmias
Vascular disorders	Flushing episodes (warmth, redness, itching, tingling)			Hypotension, postural hypotension	Collapse
Respiratory, thoracic and mediastinal disorders			Dyspnoea	Rhinitis	
Gastrointestinal disorders		Diarrhoea, nausea, vomiting, abdominal pain, dyspepsia			Activation of peptic ulcers, peptic ulceration
Hepatobiliary disorders					Jaundice
Skin and subcutaneous tissue disorders		Pruritus, rash	Sweating, generalised exanthema, urticaria, dry skin	Face oedema, vesiculobullous rash, maculopapular rash	Hyperpigmentation, acanthosis nigricans
Musculoskeletal, connective tissue and bone disorders				Leg cramps, myalgia, myopathy, myasthenia	
General disorders and administration site conditions			Pain, asthenia, chills, peripheral oedema	Chest pain	
Investigations			Elevations in serum transaminases (AST, ALT), alkaline phosphatase, total bilirubin, LDH, amylase, fasting glucose, uric acid; slight reduction in platelet counts, prolongation of prothrombin time, reduction in phosphorus, CK increase		

6.5 Nature and contents of container
Niaspan prolonged-release tablets are packed in individually sealed strips (PVC/Chlortrifluoroethylene/PE/Aluminium).

Starter packs: Niaspan Prolonged Release Tablets Starter Pack is presented in a 21 tablet starter pack containing three weeks supply of medication packed in three individually sealed strips as follows:

Week 1: seven Niaspan 375mg Prolonged Release Tablets

Week 2: seven Niaspan 500mg Prolonged Release Tablets

Week 3: seven Niaspan 750mg Prolonged Release Tablets

500mg, 750mg, 1000mg: Blister (aluminium foil blisters) packs of 56 tablets.

6.6 Instructions for use and handling
No special requirements

7. MARKETING AUTHORISATION HOLDER
Merck KGaA

Frankfurter Straβe 250

64293 Darmstadt

Germany

8. MARKETING AUTHORISATION NUMBER(S)
Starter Pack:

PL 04691/0003

500 mg, 750mg, 1000mg:

PL 04961/0005-7

9. DATE OF FIRST AUTHORISATION/RENEWAL OF THE AUTHORISATION
23rd December 2004

10. DATE OF REVISION OF THE TEXT
22nd June 2005

Legal category
POM

Nicam Gel

(Dermal Laboratories Limited)

1. NAME OF THE MEDICINAL PRODUCT
NICAM™ GEL

2. QUALITATIVE AND QUANTITATIVE COMPOSITION
Nicotinamide 4% w/w.

3. PHARMACEUTICAL FORM
Topical gel.

4. CLINICAL PARTICULARS

4.1 Therapeutic indications
For the topical treatment of mild to moderate inflammatory acne vulgaris.

4.2 Posology and method of administration
Apply to the affected area twice daily after the skin has been thoroughly washed with warm water and soap. Enough gel should be used to cover the affected area.

No difference in dose or dose schedule is recommended for adults, children or the elderly.

For topical administration only.

4.3 Contraindications
Contraindicated in persons who have shown hypersensitivity to any of its components.

4.4 Special warnings and special precautions for use
For external use only and to be kept away from the eyes and mucous membranes, including those of the nose and mouth. If excessive dryness, irritation or peeling occurs reduce the dosage to one application per day or every other day.

4.5 Interaction with other medicinal products and other forms of Interaction
None known.

4.6 Pregnancy and lactation
Vitamin B derivative requirements such as nicotinamide, are increased during pregnancy and infancy. Nicotinamide is excreted in breast milk. As with all medicines, care should be exercised during the first trimester of pregnancy.

4.7 Effects on ability to drive and use machines
None known.

4.8 Undesirable effects
The most frequently encountered adverse effect is dryness of the skin. Other less frequent adverse effects include pruritus, erythema, burning sensation and irritation.

4.9 Overdose
Not applicable.

5. PHARMACOLOGICAL PROPERTIES

5.1 Pharmacodynamic properties
Niacin (nicotinic acid) is an essential B complex Vitamin (B_3), whose deficiency results in the clinical syndrome known as pellagra. Nicotinic acid is converted in the body to nicotinamide adenine dinucleotide (NAD) or nicotinamide adenine dinucleotide phosphate (NADP), which function as coenzymes for a wide variety of vital oxidation-reduction reactions. Nicotinamide (niacinamide), the active ingredient, is the physiologically active form of niacin and is the chemical form of Vitamin B_3 found in virtually all multivitamin products. Though nicotinic acid and nicotinamide are so closely related chemically, they differ somewhat in pharmacological properties. Nicotinic acid products exhibit moderately intense cutaneous vasodilation, resulting frequently in mild headaches and flushing or tingling of the skin, but such reactions have not been observed with nicotinamide. Nicotinic acid has also been used for its effect to lower plasma cholesterol, again a property not shared by nicotinamide.

Nicotinamide has demonstrated beneficial effects on inflammatory acne. It is considered that these effects are related to its significant anti-inflammatory activity.

5.2 Pharmacokinetic properties
Following oral administration, nicotinamide is readily absorbed from the gastro-intestinal tract and widely distributed in the body tissues. The main route of metabolism is the conversion to N-methylnicotinamide and the 2-pyridone and 4-pyridone derivatives; nicotinuric acid is also formed. Small amounts of nicotinamide are excreted unchanged in the urine; this amount increases with larger doses.

5.3 Preclinical safety data
Nicotinic acid amide (nicotinamide) has been recognised since 1937 as an essential B complex vitamin whose deficiency results in the clinical syndrome known as pellagra. It is widely available, in tablets and in sterile solution in water for intravenous administration, for the prophylaxis and treatment of pellagra and nutritional deficiency.

In the United States, nicotinamide is included in the Food and Drug Administration's listing of nutritional agents which are Generally Recognised As Safe (GRAS).

6. PHARMACEUTICAL PARTICULARS

6.1 List of excipients
Aluminium Magnesium Silicate; Hydroxypropylmethylcellulose; Citric Acid; Polyoxyethylene Lauryl Ether; Ethanol; Purified Water.

6.2 Incompatibilities
None known.

6.3 Shelf life
36 months.

6.4 Special precautions for storage
Do not store above 25°C.

6.5 Nature and contents of container
60g LDPE tube with white polypropylene cap. This is supplied as an original pack (OP).

6.6 Instructions for use and handling
None stated.

7. MARKETING AUTHORISATION HOLDER
Dermal Laboratories

Tatmore Place, Gosmore

Hitchin, Herts SG4 7QR, UK.

8. MARKETING AUTHORISATION NUMBER(S)
0173/0166.

9. DATE OF FIRST AUTHORISATION/RENEWAL OF THE AUTHORISATION
10 September 2002.

10. DATE OF REVISION OF THE TEXT
February 2003.

Nicorette 10 mg Patch

(Pharmacia Ltd - (Consumer Products))

1. NAME OF THE MEDICINAL PRODUCT
Nicorette 10mg Patch or Boots NicAssist 10 mg patch.

2. QUALITATIVE AND QUANTITATIVE COMPOSITION
Nicotine, 10mg released over 16 hours use. Each patch is 20 sq.cm, containing nicotine 0.83mg/sq.cm.

3. PHARMACEUTICAL FORM
Transdermal Patch

4. CLINICAL PARTICULARS

4.1 Therapeutic indications
The treatment of nicotine dependence and for the relief of withdrawal symptoms associated with smoking cessation

4.2 Posology and method of administration
Adults:
The recommended treatment programme for Nicorette Patch should occupy 3 months. Nicorette Patch should not be used concurrently with any other nicotine products and patients must stop smoking completely when starting treatment.

The daily dose is one patch delivering 15mg, 10mg or 5mg nicotine as appropriate, with application limited to 16 hours in a 24 hour period in each case.

Daily treatment commences with one 15mg ($30cm^2$) patch, applied on waking (usually in the morning) and removed 16 hours later (usually at bedtime). Treatment should continue at this dose for an initial period of 8 weeks. Patients who have successfully abstained from smoking during this 8 week period should be supported through a further 4 week weaning period, using the lower strength patches. Downward titration of dose is achieved by applying one 10mg ($20cm^2$) patch daily for 2 weeks followed by one 5mg ($10cm^2$) patch daily for a further 2 weeks.

If abstinence has not been achieved, further courses of treatment may be recommended if it is considered to be of benefit to the patient

Nicorette Patch should be applied to clean, dry intact areas of hairless skin, for example on the hip, upper arm, or chest. These areas should be varied each day and the same site should not be used on consecutive days.

There is no clinically significant difference in bioavailability of nicotine when the patch is applied to either the hip, upper arm or chest.

After removal, used patches should be disposed of carefully (see warnings).

Experience with the treatment of nicotine dependence shows that success rates are improved if patients also receive supportive therapy and counselling.

Children:
Not for use by persons under 18 except on the advice of a doctor.

4.3 Contraindications
Nicorette Patches should not be administered to non-tobacco users, or administered to patients with known hypersensitivity to nicotine or any component of the patch.

Nicotine in any form is contraindicated in pregnancy and lactation (see section 4.6).

4.4 Special warnings and special precautions for use
Due to the cardiovascular effects of nicotine, Nicorette Patch should be used with caution in patients with a history of angina, recent myocardial infarction, or cerebrovascular accident, serious cardiac arrythmias, systemic hypertension or peripheral vascular disease. Nicorette Patch should be used with caution in patients with a history of peptic ulcer.

Nicotine can stimulate production of adrenaline; Nicorette Patch should be used with caution in patients with diabetes mellitus, hyperthyroidism or phaeochromocytoma.

Patients with chronic generalised dermatological disorders such as psoriasis, chronic dermatitis or urticaria should not use Nicorette Patch.

Erythema may occur. If it is severe or persistent, treatment should be discontinued.

After removal, the patch should be folded in half, adhesive side innermost, and placed inside the opened sachet, or in a piece of aluminium foil. The used patch should then be disposed of carefully, away from the reach of children or animals.

The label will state "Not for use by persons under the age of 18 except on the advice of a doctor)

"If you need advice before starting to use nicotine patches, talk to your pharmacist or doctor."

4.5 Interaction with other medicinal products and other forms of Interaction
Smoking cessation with or without nicotine replacement, may alter the pharmacokinetics of certain concomitant medications.

May require a decrease in dose at cessation of smoking	Possible mechanism
Paracetamol, caffeine, imipramine, oxazepam, pentazocine, propranolol, theophylline, warfarin, oestrogens, lignocaine, phenacetin	Deinduction of hepatic enzymes on smoking cessation
Insulin	Increase of subcutaneous insulin absorption with smoking cessation
Adrenergic antagonists (e.g. prazosin, labetalol)	Decrease in circulating catecholamines with smoking cessation
May require an increase in dose at cessation of smoking	**Possible mechanism**
Adrenergic agonists (e.g. isoprenaline, phenylephrine)	Decrease in circulating catecholamines with smoking cessation

Other effects, associated with smoking, include reduced analgesic efficacy with propoxyphene, reduced diuretic response to frusemide and reduced rates of ulcer healing with H_2 antagonists.

4.6 Pregnancy and lactation
Nicotine crosses the placenta and is excreted in breast milk; thus it may be a hazard to the foetus or infant. Patients should be advised to try to give up smoking without the use of nicotine replacement therapy. Should this fail a medical assessment of the risk/benefit ratio of NRT use should be made.

4.7 Effects on ability to drive and use machines
No effects

4.8 Undesirable effects

Nicorette Patch may cause adverse reactions similar to those associated with nicotine administered by other means.

During controlled clinical studies, the following adverse events were reported at an incidence of greater than 1% and more frequently with active than with placebo treatment.

Application site reactions (eg erythema and itching),

Headache

Dizziness

Nausea

Palpitations

Dyspepsia and

Myalgia

Other subjective sensations associated with smoking cessation may occur, such as impaired concentration, fatigue, anxiety, irritability and increased appetite.

Concurrent smoking may be associated with symptoms of nicotine overdose.

4.9 Overdose

Overdosage with nicotine can occur if many patches are used simultaneously, or if the patient has very low nicotine dependence or uses other forms of nicotine concomitantly. Should Nicorette Patch be swallowed, the risk of poisoning is small due to slow release of nicotine and high first pass metabolism.

Symptoms of overdosage are those of acute nicotine poisoning and include nausea, salivation, abdominal pain, diarrhoea, sweating, headache, dizziness, disturbed hearing and marked weakness. In extreme cases, these symptoms may be followed by hypotension, rapid, weak irregular pulse, breathing difficulties, prostration, circulatory collapse and terminal convulsions.

The acute minimum lethal oral dose of nicotine in man is believed to be 40-60mg.

Treatment of Overdosage

All nicotine patches should be removed and the patient should be treated symptomatically. Artificial respiration with oxygen should be instituted if necessary.

5. PHARMACOLOGICAL PROPERTIES

5.1 Pharmacodynamic properties

Nicotine has no therapeutic uses except as replacement therapy for the relief of abstinence symptoms in nicotine-dependent smokers.

Owing to its many actions, the overall effects of nicotine are complex. A wide variety of stimulant and depressant effects are observed that involve the central and peripheral nervous, cardiovascular, endocrine, gastro-intestinal and skeletal motor systems. Nicotine acts on specific binding sites or receptors throughout the nervous system.

5.2 Pharmacokinetic properties

Taking into account the residual concentration of nicotine in the transdermal system, the nicotine released from the system is efficiently absorbed: a bioavailability of between 80-100% has been reported. There is no clinically significant difference in bioavailability of nicotine when the patch is applied to either the hip, upper arm or chest.

Steady state concentrations of plasma nicotine in volunteers were examined during a study period of six days. Although nicotine was detectable 24 hours after the first dose, the data did not indicate any accumulation.

Tmax of nicotine after application of a 30cm^2 nicotine transdermal system has been shown to vary between 6 ± 2 and 9 ± 3 hours: Cmax has been shown to vary between 13 ± 3 and 16 ± 5 ng/ml. No differences in these pharmacokinetic parameters have been observed between males and females.

All Nicorette Patches are labelled by the average amount of nicotine absorbed by the patient over 16 hours.

5.3 Preclinical safety data

Preclinical data indicate that nicotine is neither mutagenic nor genotoxic.

There are no other findings derived from preclinical testing of relevance to the prescriber in determining the safety of the product which have not been considered in other relevant sections of this Summary of Product Characteristics.

6. PHARMACEUTICAL PARTICULARS

6.1 List of excipients

Medium molecular weight polyisobutylene

Low molecular weight polyisobutylene

Polybutylene

Polyester non- woven

Backing film

Siliconised polyester release liner

6.2 Incompatibilities

Not applicable

6.3 Shelf life

36 months

6.4 Special precautions for storage

Do not store at above 30°C.

6.5 Nature and contents of container

Heat sealed multilaminate pouch containing one patch. Cartons of 1, 2, 3, 7*, 14 and 28 pouches (*pack presently marketed).

6.6 Instructions for use and handling

Cut open the pouch with scissors along the line, as indicated. A clean, dry intact area of skin is selected which is hairless, such as the hip, upper arm or chest. The transparent plastic backing is peeled away and the patch pressed carefully onto the skin. The fingers should be rubbed firmly round the edge to ensure that the patch sticks properly. The patch will normally resist bathing, showering, or swimming, but if it does come off it should be replaced with a new one. Use of skin oils or talc can prevent proper adhesion of the patch.

It is intended that the patch is worn through the waking hours (approximately 16 hours) being applied on waking and removed at bedtime. Nicotine residues in the used patches may present a hazard to children and pets, thus used patches should be folded, sticky sides together, put back in an empty pouch and placed in household rubbish.

7. MARKETING AUTHORISATION HOLDER

Pharmacia Ltd.

Ramsgate Road

Sandwich

Kent CT13 9NJ

8. MARKETING AUTHORISATION NUMBER(S)

PL 0032/0293

9. DATE OF FIRST AUTHORISATION/RENEWAL OF THE AUTHORISATION

1 May 2001/ 1st January 2002

10. DATE OF REVISION OF THE TEXT

2 April 2005

Nicorette 15mg Patch

(Pharmacia Ltd - (Consumer Products))

1. NAME OF THE MEDICINAL PRODUCT

Nicorette 15mg Patch or Boots NicAssist 15 mg patch.

2. QUALITATIVE AND QUANTITATIVE COMPOSITION

Nicotine, 15mg released over 16 hours use. Each patch is 30 sq.cm, containing nicotine 0.83mg/sq.cm.

3. PHARMACEUTICAL FORM

Transdermal Patch

4. CLINICAL PARTICULARS

4.1 Therapeutic indications

The treatment of nicotine dependence and for the relief of withdrawal symptoms associated with smoking cessation

4.2 Posology and method of administration

Adults:

The recommended treatment programme for Nicorette Patch should occupy 3 months. Nicorette Patch should not be used concurrently with any other nicotine products and patients must stop smoking completely when starting treatment.

The daily dose is one patch delivering 15mg, 10mg or 5mg nicotine as appropriate, with application limited to 16 hours in a 24 hour period in each case.

Daily treatment commences with one 15mg (30cm^2) patch, applied on waking (usually in the morning) and removed 16 hours later (usually at bedtime). Treatment should continue at this dose for an initial period of 8 weeks. Patients who have successfully abstained from smoking during this 8 week period should be supported through a further 4 week weaning period, using the lower strength patches. Downward titration of dose is achieved by applying one 10mg (20cm^2) patch daily for 2 weeks followed by one 5mg (10cm^2) patch daily for a further 2 weeks.

If abstinence has not been achieved, further courses of treatment may be recommended if it is considered to be of benefit to the patient

Nicorette Patch should be applied to clean, dry intact areas of hairless skin, for example on the hip, upper arm, or chest. These areas should be varied each day and the same site should not be used on consecutive days.

There is no clinically significant difference in bioavailability of nicotine when the patch is applied to either the hip, upper arm or chest.

After removal, used patches should be disposed of carefully (see warnings).

Experience with the treatment of nicotine dependence shows that success rates are improved if patients also receive supportive therapy and counselling.

Children:

Not for use by persons under 18 except on the advice of a doctor.

4.3 Contraindications

Nicorette Patches should not be administered to non-tobacco users, or administered to patients with known hypersensitivity to nicotine or any component of the patch.

Nicotine in any for is contraindicated in pregnancy and lactation (see section 4,6)

4.4 Special warnings and special precautions for use

Due to the cardiovascular effects of nicotine, Nicorette Patch should be used with caution in patients with a history of angina, recent myocardial infarction, or cerebrovascular accident, serious cardiac arrythmias, systemic hypertension or peripheral vascular disease. Nicorette Patch should be used with caution in patients with a history of peptic ulcer.

Nicotine can stimulate production of adrenaline; Nicorette Patch should be used with caution in patients with diabetes mellitus, hyperthyroidism or phaeochromocytoma.

Patients with chronic generalised dermatological disorders such as psoriasis, chronic dermatitis or urticaria should not use Nicorette Patch.

Erythema may occur. If it is severe or persistent, treatment should be discontinued.

After removal, the patch should be folded in half, adhesive side innermost, and placed inside the opened sachet, or in a piece of aluminium foil. The used patch should then be disposed of carefully, away from the reach of children or animals.

The label will state "Not for use by persons under the age of 18 except on the advice of a doctor. You should not use if you are pregnant or breast feeding unless recommended by your doctor".

"If you need advice before starting to use nicotine patches, talk to your pharmacist or doctor".

4.5 Interaction with other medicinal products and other forms of Interaction

Smoking cessation with or without nicotine replacement, may alter the pharmacokinetics of certain concomitant medications.

May require a decrease in dose at cessation of smoking	Possible mechanism
Paracetamol, caffeine, imipramine, oxazepam, pentazocine, propranolol, theophylline, warfarin, oestrogens, lignocaine, phenacetin	Deinduction of hepatic enzymes on smoking cessation
Insulin	Increase of subcutaneous insulin absorption with smoking cessation
Adrenergic antagonists (e.g. prazosin, labetalol)	Decrease in circulating catecholamines with smoking cessation

May require an increase in dose at cessation of smoking	Possible mechanism
Adrenergic agonists (e.g. isoprenaline, phenylephrine)	Decrease in circulating catecholamines with smoking cessation

Other effects, associated with smoking, include reduced analgesic efficacy with propoxyphene, reduced diuretic response to frusemide and reduced rates of ulcer healing with H_2 antagonists.

4.6 Pregnancy and lactation

Nicotine crosses the placenta and is excreted in breast milk; thus it may be a hazard to the foetus or infant. Patients should be advised to try to give up smoking without the use of nicotine replacement therapy. Should this fail, a medical assessment of the risk/benefit ratio of NRT use should be made.

4.7 Effects on ability to drive and use machines

No Effects

4.8 Undesirable effects

Nicorette Patch may cause adverse reactions similar to those associated with nicotine administered by other means.

During controlled clinical studies, the following adverse events were reported at an incidence of greater than 1% and more frequently with active than with placebo treatment.

Application site reactions (eg erythema and itching),

Headache

Dizziness

Nausea

Palpitations

Dyspepsia and

Myalgia

Other subjective sensations associated with smoking cessation may occur, such as impaired concentration, fatigue, anxiety, irritability and increased appetite.

Concurrent smoking may be associated with symptoms of nicotine overdose.

4.9 Overdose
Overdosage with nicotine can occur if many patches are used simultaneously, or if the patient has very low nicotine dependence or uses other forms of nicotine concomitantly. Should Nicorette Patch be swallowed, the risk of poisoning is small due to slow release of nicotine and high first pass metabolism.

Symptoms of overdosage are those of acute nicotine poisoning and include nausea, salivation, abdominal pain, diarrhoea, sweating, headache, dizziness, disturbed hearing and marked weakness. In extreme cases, these symptoms may be followed by hypotension, rapid, weak irregular pulse, breathing difficulties, prostration, circulatory collapse and terminal convulsions.

The acute minimum lethal oral dose of nicotine in man is believed to be 40-60mg.

Treatment of Overdosage
All nicotine patches should be removed and the patient should be treated symptomatically. Artificial respiration with oxygen should be instituted if necessary.

5. PHARMACOLOGICAL PROPERTIES
5.1 Pharmacodynamic properties
Nicotine has no therapeutic uses except as replacement therapy for the relief of abstinence symptoms in nicotine-dependent smokers.

Owing to its many actions, the overall effects of nicotine are complex. A wide variety of stimulant and depressant effects are observed that involve the central and peripheral nervous, cardiovascular, endocrine, gastro-intestinal and skeletal motor systems. Nicotine acts on specific binding sites or receptors throughout the nervous system.

5.2 Pharmacokinetic properties
Taking into account the residual concentration of nicotine in the transdermal system, the nicotine released from the system is efficiently absorbed: a bioavailability of between 80-100% has been reported. There is no clinically significant difference in bioavailability of nicotine when the patch is applied to either the hip, upper arm or chest.

Steady state concentrations of plasma nicotine in volunteers were examined during a study period of six days. Although nicotine was detectable 24 hours after the first dose, the data did not indicate any accumulation.

Tmax of nicotine after application of a 30cm^2 nicotine transdermal system has been shown to vary between 6 ± 2 and 9 ± 3 hours: Cmax has been shown to vary between 13 ± 3 and 16 ± 5 ng/ml. No differences in these pharmacokinetic parameters have been observed between males and females.

All Nicorette Patches are labelled by the average amount of nicotine absorbed by the patient over 16 hours.

5.3 Preclinical safety data
Preclinical data indicate that nicotine is neither mutagenic nor genotoxic.

There are no other findings derived from preclinical testing of relevance to the prescriber in determining the safety of the product which have not been considered in other relevant sections of this Summary of Product Characteristics.

6. PHARMACEUTICAL PARTICULARS
6.1 List of excipients
Medium molecular weight polyisobutylene

Low molecular weight polyisobutylene

Polybutylene

Polyester non-woven backing film

Siliconised polyester release liner

6.2 Incompatibilities
Not applicable

6.3 Shelf life
36 months

6.4 Special precautions for storage
Do not store at above 30°C.

6.5 Nature and contents of container
Heat sealed multilaminate pouch containing one patch. Cartons of 1, 2, 3, 7*, 14* and 28 pouches (*pack presently marketed).

6.6 Instructions for use and handling
Cut open the pouch with scissors along the line, as indicated. A clean, dry intact area of skin is selected which is hairless, such as the hip, upper arm or chest. The transparent plastic backing is peeled away and the patch pressed carefully onto the skin. The fingers should be rubbed firmly round the edge to ensure that the patch sticks properly. The patch will normally resist bathing, showering, or swimming, but if it does come off it should be replaced with a new one. Use of skin oils or talc can prevent proper adhesion of the patch.

It is intended that the patch is worn through the waking hours (approximately 16 hours) being applied on waking and removed at bedtime. Nicotine residues in the used patches may present a hazard to children and pets, thus used patches should be folded, sticky sides together, put back in an empty pouch and placed in household rubbish.

Administrative Data
7. MARKETING AUTHORISATION HOLDER
Pharmacia Ltd.

Ramsgate Road

Sandwich

Kent CT13 9NJ

8. MARKETING AUTHORISATION NUMBER(S)
PL 0032/0294

9. DATE OF FIRST AUTHORISATION/RENEWAL OF THE AUTHORISATION
1 May 2001

10. DATE OF REVISION OF THE TEXT
2 April 2005

Nicorette 2mg Gum

(Pharmacia Ltd - (Consumer Products))

1. NAME OF THE MEDICINAL PRODUCT
Nicorette 2mg Gum

2. QUALITATIVE AND QUANTITATIVE COMPOSITION
Chewing Gum containing 2mg nicotine

3. PHARMACEUTICAL FORM
Chewing Gum

4. CLINICAL PARTICULARS
4.1 Therapeutic indications
Nicorette 2mg Gum is for the relief of nicotine withdrawal symptoms as an aid to smoking cessation in smokers ready to stop smoking.

In smokers currently unable or not ready to stop smoking abruptly, the gum may also be used as part of a programme to reduce smoking prior to stopping completely.

4.2 Posology and method of administration
Nicorette 2mg Gum should be chewed slowly according to the instructions.

Adults

The strength of gum to be used will depend on the smoking habits of the individual. In general, if the patient smokes 20 or less cigarettes a day, 2mg nicotine gum is indicated. If more that 20 cigarettes per day are smoked, 4mg nicotine gum will be needed to meet the withdrawal of the high serum nicotine levels from heavy smoking.

The chewing gums should be used whenever there is an urge to smoke according to the "chew and rest" technique described on the pack. After about 30 minutes of such use, the gum will be exhausted. Not more than 15 pieces of the chewing gum may be used each day. Absorption of nicotine is through the buccal mucosa, any nicotine which is swallowed being destroyed by the liver.

Advice and support normally improve the success rate.

Smoking cessation

Use the gum whenever there is an urge to smoke to maintain complete abstinence from smoking. Sufficient gums should be used, usually 8-12, up to a maximum of 15.

Continue use for up to three months to break the habit of smoking, then gradually reduce gum use. When daily use is 1-2 gums, use should be stopped. Any spare gum should be retained, as craving may suddenly return.

For those using 4 mg nicotine gum, the 2 mg nicotine gum will be helpful during withdrawal from treatment.

Smoking reduction

Use the gum between smoking episodes to manage the urge to smoke, to prolong smoke-free intervals and with the intention to reduce smoking as much as possible. If a reduction in number of cigarettes per day has not been achieved after 6 weeks, professional advice should be sought.

A quit attempt should be made as soon as the smoker feels ready, but not later than 6 months after start of treatment. If a quit attempt cannot be made within 9 months after starting treatment, professional advice should be sought.

When making a quit attempt the smoking cessation instructions above, can be followed

Children:

Not for use by persons under age 18 except on the advice of a doctor.

4.3 Contraindications
Hypersensitivity to nicotine or to any component of the chewing gum.

4.4 Special warnings and special precautions for use
Smokers who wear dentures may experience difficulty in chewing Nicorette 2mg Gum.

Transferred dependence is rare and is both less harmful and easier to break than smoking dependence.

Swallowed nicotine may exacerbate symptoms in patients suffering from gastritis or peptic ulcers.

Allergic reactions such as angioedema and urticaria and ulcerative stomatitis have been reported.

In general Nicorette 2mg Gum presents a lesser hazard than continuing to smoke in those with stable cardiovascular disease. However those with unstable cardiovascular disease from any cause should be encouraged to stop smoking with non-pharmacological interventions. This includes patients who are unstable following myocardial infarction or stroke, and patients with unstable angina or unstable cardiac dysrhythmias. If encouragement to stop smoking with non-pharmacological interventions fails, Nicorette 2mg Gum may be considered, but as data on safety in this patient group are limited, initiation should only be under close medical supervision.

Renal and or hepatic impairment

Nicorette 2mg Gum should be used with caution in patients with moderate to severe hepatic impairment and/or severe renal impairment as the clearance of nicotine or its metabolites may be decreased with the potential for increased adverse effects (see section 4.8).

Nicotine gum should be used with caution in patients with diabetes mellitus, hyperthyroidism or pheochromocytoma, since nicotine causes the release of catecholamines from the adrenal medulla.

The label will state "Not for use by persons under age 18 except on the advice of a doctor".

4.5 Interaction with other medicinal products and other forms of Interaction
None Known

4.6 Pregnancy and lactation
Pregnancy

Smoking can seriously harm the fetus and infant and pregnant smokers should be given every support and encouragement to completely stop with non-pharmacological means. However, nicotine passes to the fetus affecting breathing movements and having a dose dependent effect on placental/fetal circulation. As risks for the fetus are not fully known, pregnant smokers should only use Nicorette 2mg Gum after consulting a healthcare professional.

Breastfeeding

Nicotine passes into breast milk in small quantities that may affect the infant, even at low doses. Breastfeeding smokers should only use Nicorette 2mg Gum after consulting a healthcare professional. To reduce the risk of exposure to the child, whenever possible, Nicorette 2mg Gum should be used just after breastfeeding.

4.7 Effects on ability to drive and use machines
Not applicable.

4.8 Undesirable effects
Nicorette 2mg Gum in the recommended dose has not been found to cause any serious adverse effects. Nicotine from the gum may sometimes cause a slight irritation of the throat at the start of treatment and may also cause increased salivation. Excessive swallowing of dissolved nicotine may, at first, cause hiccuping.

Excessive consumption of Nicorette 2mg Gum by those who have not been in the habit of inhaling tobacco smoke could possibly lead to nausea, faintness or headaches (as may be experienced by such a patient if tobacco smoke is inhaled).

Common

>1/100) CNS: Dizziness, headache

Gastro-Intestinal: Nausea, gastro-intestinal discomfort, hiccups

Local: Sore mouth or throat. Jaw-muscle ache. The gum may stick to, and may, in rare cases damage dentures.

Uncommon

(1/100 – 1/1000) Circulatory: Palpitation

Dermatological: Erythema, urticaria.

Local: Stomatitis

Rare

(<1/1000) Cardiovascular: Atrial fibrillation

Other: Allergic reactions such as angioedema

Some symptoms, such as dizziness, headache and sleep disturbances may be related to withdrawal symptoms associated with abstinence from smoking. Increased frequency of aphthous ulcer may occur after abstinence from smoking.

Those who are prone to indigestion may suffer initially from minor degrees of indigestion or heartburn if the 4mg nicotine gum is used; slower chewing and the use of the 2mg nicotine gum (if necessary more frequently) will usually overcome this problem.

4.9 Overdose
Overdosage can occur if many gums are taken simultaneously or in rapid succession. The consequences of an overdose are most likely to be minimised by the early nausea and vomiting known to occur with excessive nicotine intake. Nicotine is also subject to a significant first-pass metabolism.

Symptoms of overdosage are those of acute nicotine poisoning and include nausea, salivation, abdominal pain, diarrhoea, sweating headache, dizziness, disturbed hearing and marked weakness. In extreme cases, these symptoms may be followed by hypotension, rapid or weak or irregular pulse, breathing difficulties, prostration, circulatory collapse and terminal convulsions.

The minimum lethal dose of nicotine in a non-tolerant man has been estimated to be 40 to 60mg.

Management of an overdose

All nicotine intake should cease immediately and the patient should be treated symptomatically. Artificial respiration with oxygen should be instituted if necessary.

5. PHARMACOLOGICAL PROPERTIES

5.1 Pharmacodynamic properties

The pharmacological effects of nicotine are well documented. Those resulting from chewing Nicorette 2mg Gum are comparatively small. The response at any one time represents a summation of stimulant and depressant actions from direct, reflex and chemical mediator influences on several organs. The main pharmacological actions are central stimulation and/or depression; transient hyperpnoea; peripheral vasoconstriction (usually associated with a rise in systolic pressure); suppression of appetite and stimulation of peristalsis.

5.2 Pharmacokinetic properties

Nicotine administered in chewing gums is readily absorbed from the buccal mucous membranes. Demonstrable blood levels are obtained within 5 – 7 minutes and reach a maximum about 30 minutes after the start of chewing. Blood levels are roughly proportional to the amount of nicotine chewed and have been shown never to exceed those obtained from smoking cigarettes.

5.3 Preclinical safety data

Preclinical data indicate that nicotine is neither mutagenic nor genotoxic.

There are no other findings derived from preclinical testing of relevance to the prescriber in determining the safety of the product which have not been considered in other relevant sections of this Summary of Product Characteristics.

6. PHARMACEUTICAL PARTICULARS

6.1 List of excipients

Polacrilin

Chewing gum base, containing butylated hydroxy toluene (E321)

Sorbitol

Sodium carbonate, anhydrous

Sodium bicarbonate

Flavour for smoker

Haverstroo flavour

Glycerol

Talcum

6.2 Incompatibilities

None relevant

6.3 Shelf life

30 months

6.4 Special precautions for storage

Do not store above 25°C

6.5 Nature and contents of container

PVC/PVDC/Al Blister packed strips each containing 15 pieces supplied in packs of 15 (not marketed), 30 and 105 pieces. Pack containing blister strip of 6 pieces (not marketed)

6.6 Instructions for use and handling

See section 4.2

Administrative Data

7. MARKETING AUTHORISATION HOLDER

Pharmacia Limited

Ramsgate Road

Sandwich

Kent CT13 9NJ

United Kingdom

8. MARKETING AUTHORISATION NUMBER(S)

PL 00032/0248

9. DATE OF FIRST AUTHORISATION/RENEWAL OF THE AUTHORISATION

27 April, 1999 / 1st January 2002

10. DATE OF REVISION OF THE TEXT

15 August 2005

Nicorette 4mg Gum

(Pharmacia Ltd - (Consumer Products))

1. NAME OF THE MEDICINAL PRODUCT

Nicorette 4 mg Gum

2. QUALITATIVE AND QUANTITATIVE COMPOSITION

Chewing Gum containing 4 mg nicotine

3. PHARMACEUTICAL FORM

Chewing Gum

4. CLINICAL PARTICULARS

4.1 Therapeutic indications

Nicorette 4 mg Gum is for the relief of nicotine withdrawal symptoms as an aid to smoking cessation in smokers ready to stop smoking.

In smokers currently unable or not ready to stop smoking abruptly, the gum may also be used as part of a programme to reduce smoking prior to stopping completely.

4.2 Posology and method of administration

Nicorette 4 mg Gum should be chewed slowly according to the instructions.

Adults

The strength of gum to be used will depend on the smoking habits of the individual. In general, if the patient smokes 20 or less cigarettes a day, 2mg nicotine gum is indicated. If more that 20 cigarettes per day are smoked, 4mg nicotine gum will be needed to meet the withdrawal of the high serum nicotine levels from heavy smoking.

The chewing gums should be used whenever there is an urge to smoke according to the "chew and rest" technique described on the pack. After about 30 minutes of such use, the gum will be exhausted. Not more than 15 pieces of the chewing gum may be used each day. Absorption of nicotine is through the buccal mucosa, any nicotine which is swallowed being destroyed by the liver.

Advice and support normally improve the success rate.

Smoking cessation

Use the gum whenever there is an urge to smoke to maintain complete abstinence from smoking. Sufficient gums should be used, usually 8-12, up to a maximum of 15.

Continue use for up to three months to break the habit of smoking, then gradually reduce gum use. When daily use is 1-2 gums, use should be stopped. Any spare gum should be retained, as craving may suddenly return.

For those using 4 mg nicotine gum, the 2 mg nicotine gum will be helpful during withdrawal from treatment.

Smoking reduction

Use the gum between smoking episodes to manage the urge to smoke, to prolong smoke-free intervals and with the intention to reduce smoking as much as possible. If a reduction in number of cigarettes per day has not been achieved after 6 weeks, professional advice should be sought.

A quit attempt should be made as soon as the smoker feels ready, but not later than 6 months after start of treatment. If a quit attempt cannot be made within 9 months after starting treatment, professional advice should be sought.

When making a quit attempt the smoking cessation instructions above, can be followed.

Children:

Not for use by persons under age 18 except on the advice of a doctor.

4.3 Contraindications

Hypersensitivity to nicotine or to any component of the chewing gum.

4.4 Special warnings and special precautions for use

Smokers who wear dentures may experience difficulty in chewing Nicorette 4 mg Gum.

Transferred dependence is rare and is both less harmful and easier to break than smoking dependence.

Swallowed nicotine may exacerbate symptoms in patients suffering from gastritis or peptic ulcers.

Allergic reactions such as angioedema and urticaria and ulcerative stomatitis have been reported.

In general Nicorette 4mg Gum presents a lesser hazard than continuing to smoke in those with stable cardiovascular disease. However those with unstable cardiovascular disease from any cause should be encouraged to stop smoking with non-pharmacological interventions. This includes patients who are unstable following myocardial infarction or stroke, and patients with unstable angina or unstable cardiac dysrhythmias. If encouragement to stop smoking with non-pharmacological interventions fails, Nicorette 4mg Gum may be considered, but as data on safety in this patient group are limited, initiation should only be under close medical supervision.

Renal and or hepatic impairment

Nicorette 4mg Gum should be used with caution in patients with moderate to severe hepatic impairment and/or severe renal impairment as the clearance of nicotine or its metabolites may be decreased with the potential for increased adverse effects (see section 4.8).

Nicotine gum should be used with caution in patients with diabetes mellitus, hyperthyroidism or pheochromocytoma, since nicotine causes the release of catecholamines from the adrenal medulla.

The label will state "Not for use by persons under age 18 except on the advice of a doctor".

4.5 Interaction with other medicinal products and other forms of Interaction

None Known

4.6 Pregnancy and lactation

Pregnancy

Smoking can seriously harm the fetus and infant and pregnant smokers should be given every support and encouragement to completely stop with non-pharmacological means. However, nicotine passes to the fetus affecting breathing movements and having a dose dependent effect on placental/fetal circulation. As risks for the fetus are not fully known, pregnant smokers should only use Nicorette 4mg Gum after consulting a healthcare professional.

Breastfeeding

Nicotine passes into breast milk in small quantities that may affect the infant, even at low doses. Breastfeeding smokers should only use Nicorette 4mg Gum after consulting a healthcare professional. To reduce the risk of exposure to the child, whenever possible, Nicorette 4mg Gum should be used just after breastfeeding.

4.7 Effects on ability to drive and use machines

Not applicable.

4.8 Undesirable effects

Nicorette 4 mg Gum in the recommended dose has not been found to cause any serious adverse effects. Nicotine from the gum may sometimes cause a slight irritation of the throat at the start of treatment and may also cause increased salivation. Excessive swallowing of dissolved nicotine may, at first, cause hiccuping.

Excessive consumption of Nicorette 4 mg Gum by those who have not been in the habit of inhaling tobacco smoke could possibly lead to nausea, faintness or headaches (as may be experienced by such a patient if tobacco smoke is inhaled).

Common >1/100	CNS:	Dizziness, headache
	Gastro-Intestinal:	Nausea, gastro-intestinal discomfort, hiccups
	Local:	Sore mouth or throat. Jaw-muscle ache. The gum may stick to, and may, in rare cases damage dentures.
Uncommon (1/100 – 1/1000)	Circulatory:	Palpitation
	Dermatological:	Erythema, urticaria.
	Local:	Stomatitis
Rare (<1/1000)	Cardiovascular:	Atrial fibrillation
	Other:	Allergic reactions such as angioedema

Some symptoms, such as dizziness, headache and sleep disturbances may be related to withdrawal symptoms associated with abstinence from smoking. Increased frequency of aphthous ulcer may occur after abstinence from smoking.

Those who are prone to indigestion may suffer initially from minor degrees of indigestion or heartburn if the 4mg nicotine gum is used; slower chewing and the use of the 2mg nicotine gum (if necessary more frequently) will usually overcome this problem.

4.9 Overdose

Overdosage can occur if many gums are taken simultaneously or in rapid succession. The consequences of an overdose are most likely to be minimised by the early nausea and vomiting known to occur with excessive nicotine intake. Nicotine is also subject to a significant first-pass metabolism.

Symptoms of overdosage are those of acute nicotine poisoning and include nausea, salivation, abdominal pain, diarrhoea, sweating headache, dizziness, disturbed hearing and marked weakness. In extreme cases, these symptoms may be followed by hypotension, rapid or weak or irregular pulse, breathing difficulties, prostration, circulatory collapse and terminal convulsions.

The minimum lethal dose of nicotine in a non-tolerant man has been estimated to be 40 to 60mg.

Management of an overdose

All nicotine intake should cease immediately and the patient should be treated symptomatically. Artificial respiration with oxygen should be instituted if necessary.

5. PHARMACOLOGICAL PROPERTIES

5.1 Pharmacodynamic properties

The pharmacological effects of nicotine as well documented. Those resulting from chewing Nicorette 4 mg Gum are comparatively small. The response at any one time represents a summation of stimulant and depressant actions from direct, reflex and chemical mediator influences on several organs. The main pharmacological actions are central stimulation and/or depression; transient hyperpnoea; peripheral vasoconstriction (usually associated with a rise in systolic pressure); suppression of appetite and stimulation of peristalsis.

5.2 Pharmacokinetic properties

Nicotine administered in chewing gums is readily absorbed from the buccal mucous membranes. Demonstrable blood levels are obtained within 5 – 7 minutes and reach a maximum about 30 minutes after the start of chewing. Blood levels are roughly proportional to the amount of nicotine chewed and have been shown never to exceed those obtained from smoking cigarettes.

5.3 Preclinical safety data

Preclinical data indicate that nicotine is neither mutagenic nor genotoxic.

There are no other findings derived from preclinical testing of relevance to the prescriber in determining the safety of the product which have not been considered in other relevant sections of this Summary of Product Characteristics.

6. PHARMACEUTICAL PARTICULARS

6.1 List of excipients

Polacrilin

Chewing gum base, containing butylated hydroxy toluene (E321)

Sorbitol powder

Sorbitol 70%

Flavour for smoker

Haverstroo flavour

Sodium carbonate anhydrous

Quinoline Yellow

Glycerol 85%

Talc

6.2 Incompatibilities

None relevant

6.3 Shelf life

24 months

6.4 Special precautions for storage

Do not store above $25^{\circ}C$

6.5 Nature and contents of container

PVC/PVDC/Al Blister packed strips each containing 15, 30 and 105 pieces supplied in a pack of 30 pieces.

6.6 Instructions for use and handling

See section 4.2

Administrative Data

7. MARKETING AUTHORISATION HOLDER

Pharmacia Limited

Ramsgate Road

Sandwich

Kent CT13 9NJ

United Kingdom

8. MARKETING AUTHORISATION NUMBER(S)

00032/0249

9. DATE OF FIRST AUTHORISATION/RENEWAL OF THE AUTHORISATION

26 April 1999 / 1st January 2002

10. DATE OF REVISION OF THE TEXT

15 August 2005

Nicorette 5mg Patch

(Pharmacia Ltd - (Consumer Products))

1. NAME OF THE MEDICINAL PRODUCT

Nicorette 5mg Patch or Boots NicAssist 5 mg Patch.

2. QUALITATIVE AND QUANTITATIVE COMPOSITION

Nicotine, 5mg released over 16 hours use. Each patch is 10 sq.cm, containing nicotine 0.83mg/sq.cm.

3. PHARMACEUTICAL FORM

Transdermal Patch

4. CLINICAL PARTICULARS

4.1 Therapeutic indications

The treatment of nicotine dependence and for the relief of withdrawal symptoms associated with smoking cessation

4.2 Posology and method of administration

Adults:

The recommended treatment programme for Nicorette Patch should occupy 3 months. Nicorette Patch should not be used concurrently with any other nicotine products and patients must stop smoking completely when starting treatment.

The daily dose is one patch delivering 15mg, 10mg or 5mg nicotine as appropriate, with application limited to 16 hours in a 24 hour period in each case.

Daily treatment commences with one 15mg ($30cm^2$) patch, applied on waking (usually in the morning) and removed 16 hours later (usually at bedtime). Treatment should continue at this dose for an initial period of 8 weeks. Patients who have successfully abstained from smoking during this 8 week period should be supported through a further 4 week weaning period, using the lower strength patches. Downward titration of dose is achieved by applying one 10mg ($20cm^2$) patch daily for 2 weeks followed by one 5mg ($10cm^2$) patch daily for a further 2 weeks.

If abstinence has not been achieved, further courses of treatment may be recommended if it is considered to be of benefit to the patient

Nicorette Patch should be applied to clean, dry intact areas of hairless skin, for example on the hip, upper arm, or chest. These areas should be varied each day and the same site should not be used on consecutive days.

There is no clinically significant difference in bioavailability of nicotine when the patch is applied to either the hip, upper arm or chest.

After removal, used patches should be disposed of carefully (see warnings).

Experience with the treatment of nicotine dependence shows that success rates are improved if patients also receive supportive therapy and counselling.

Children:

Not for use by persons under 18 except on the advice of a doctor.

4.3 Contraindications

Nicorette Patches should not be administered to non-tobacco users, or administered to patients with known hypersensitivity to nicotine or any component of the patch.

Nicotine in any form is contraindicated in pregnancy and lactation (see section 4.6)

4.4 Special warnings and special precautions for use

Due to the cardiovascular effects of nicotine, Nicorette Patch should be used with caution in patients with a history of angina, recent myocardial infarction, or cerebrovascular accident, serious cardiac arythmias, systemic hypertension or peripheral vascular disease. Nicorette Patch should be used with caution in patients with a history of peptic ulcer.

Nicotine can stimulate production of adrenaline; Nicorette Patch should be used with caution in patients with diabetes mellitus, hyperthyroidism or phaeochromocytoma.

Patients with chronic generalised dermatological disorders such as psoriasis, chronic dermatitis or urticaria should not use Nicorette Patch.

Erythema may occur. If it is severe or persistent, treatment should be discontinued.

After removal, the patch should be folded in half, adhesive side innermost, and placed inside the opened sachet, or in a piece of aluminium foil. The used patch should then be disposed of carefully, away from the reach of children or animals.

The label will state "Not for use by persons under the age of 18 except on the advice of a doctor). You should not use if you are pregnant or breast feeding unless recommended by a doctor".

"If you need advice before starting to use nicotine patches, talk to your pharmacist or doctor."

4.5 Interaction with other medicinal products and other forms of Interaction

Smoking cessation with or without nicotine replacement, may alter the pharmacokinetics of certain concomitant medications.

May require a decrease in dose at cessation of smoking	Possible mechanism
Paracetamol, caffeine, imipramine, oxazepam, pentazocine, propranolol, theophylline, warfarin, oestrogens, lignocaine, phenacetin	Deinduction of hepatic enzymes on smoking cessation
Insulin	Increase of subcutaneous insulin absorption with smoking cessation
Adrenergic antagonists (e.g. prazosin, labetalol)	Decrease in circulating catecholamines with smoking cessation

May require an increase in dose at cessation of smoking	Possible mechanism
Adrenergic agonists (e.g. isoprenaline, phenylephrine)	Decrease in circulating catecholamines with smoking cessation

Other effects, associated with smoking, include reduced analgesic efficacy with propoxyphene, reduced diuretic response to frusemide and reduced rates of ulcer healing with H_2 antagonists.

4.6 Pregnancy and lactation

Nicotine crosses the placenta and is excreted in breast milk; thus it may be a hazard to the foetus or infant. Patients should be advised to try to give up smoking without the use of nicotine replacement therapy. Should this fail, a medical assessment of the risk/benefit ratio of NRT use should be made.

4.7 Effects on ability to drive and use machines

No Effects

4.8 Undesirable effects

Nicorette Patch may cause adverse reactions similar to those associated with nicotine administered by other means.

During controlled clinical studies, the following adverse events were reported at an incidence of greater than 1% and more frequently with active than with placebo treatment.

Application site reactions (eg erythema and itching),

Headache

Dizziness

Nausea

Palpitations

Dyspepsia and

Myalgia

Other subjective sensations associated with smoking cessation may occur, such as impaired concentration, fatigue, anxiety, irritability and increased appetite.

Concurrent smoking may be associated with symptoms of nicotine overdose.

4.9 Overdose

Overdosage with nicotine can occur if many patches are used simultaneously, or if the patient has very low nicotine dependence or uses other forms of nicotine concomitantly. Should Nicorette Patch be swallowed, the risk of poisoning is small due to slow release of nicotine and high first pass metabolism.

Symptoms of overdosage are those of acute nicotine poisoning and include nausea, salivation, abdominal pain, diarrhoea, sweating, headache, dizziness, disturbed hearing and marked weakness. In extreme cases, these symptoms may be followed by hypotension, rapid, weak irregular pulse, breathing difficulties, prostration, circulatory collapse and terminal convulsions.

The acute minimum lethal oral dose of nicotine in man is believed to be 40-60mg.

Treatment of Overdosage

All nicotine patches should be removed and the patient should be treated symptomatically. Artificial respiration with oxygen should be instituted if necessary.

5. PHARMACOLOGICAL PROPERTIES

5.1 Pharmacodynamic properties

Nicotine has no therapeutic uses except as replacement therapy for the relief of abstinence symptoms in nicotine-dependent smokers.

Owing to its many actions, the overall effects of nicotine are complex. A wide variety of stimulant and depressant effects are observed that involve the central and peripheral nervous, cardiovascular, endocrine, gastro-intestinal and skeletal motor systems. Nicotine acts on specific binding sites or receptors throughout the nervous system.

5.2 Pharmacokinetic properties

Taking into account the residual concentration of nicotine in the transdermal system, the nicotine released from the system is efficiently absorbed: a bioavailability of between 80-100% has been reported. There is no clinically significant difference in bioavailability of nicotine when the patch is applied to either the hip, upper arm or chest.

Steady state concentrations of plasma nicotine in volunteers were examined during a study period of six days. Although nicotine was detectable 24 hours after the first dose, the data did not indicate any accumulation.

Tmax of nicotine after application of a $30cm^2$ nicotine transdermal system has been shown to vary between 6 ± 2 and 9 ± 3 hours: Cmax has been shown to vary between 13 ± 3 and 16 ± 5 ng/ml. No differences in these pharmacokinetic parameters have been observed between males and females.

All Nicorette Patches are labelled by the average amount of nicotine absorbed by the patient over 16 hours.

5.3 Preclinical safety data

Preclinical data indicate that nicotine is neither mutagenic nor genotoxic.

There are no other findings derived from preclinical testing of relevance to the prescriber in determining the safety of the product which have not been considered in other relevant sections of this Summary of Product Characteristics.

6. PHARMACEUTICAL PARTICULARS

6.1 List of excipients

Medium molecular weight polyisobutylene

Low molecular weight polyisobutylene

Polybutylene

Polyester non-woven backing film

Siliconised polyester release liner

6.2 Incompatibilities

Not applicable

6.3 Shelf life
36 months

6.4 Special precautions for storage
Do not store at above 30°C.

6.5 Nature and contents of container
Heat sealed multilaminate pouch containing one patch. Cartons of 1, 2, 3, 7*, 14 and 28 pouches (*pack presently marketed).

6.6 Instructions for use and handling
Cut open the pouch with scissors along the line, as indicated. A clean, dry intact area of skin is selected which is hairless, such as the hip, upper arm or chest. The transparent plastic backing is peeled away and the patch pressed carefully onto the skin. The fingers should be rubbed firmly round the edge to ensure that the patch sticks properly. The patch will normally resist bathing, showering, or swimming, but if it does come off it should be replaced with a new one. Use of skin oils or talc can prevent proper adhesion of the patch.

It is intended that the patch is worn through the waking hours (approximately 16 hours) being applied on waking and removed at bedtime. Nicotine residues in the used patches may present a hazard to children and pets, thus used patches should be folded, sticky sides together, put back in an empty pouch and placed in household rubbish.

Administrative Data

7. MARKETING AUTHORISATION HOLDER
Pharmacia Ltd.
Ramsgate Road
Sandwich
Kent CT13 9NJ

8. MARKETING AUTHORISATION NUMBER(S)
PL 0032/0292

9. DATE OF FIRST AUTHORISATION/RENEWAL OF THE AUTHORISATION
1 May 2001/ 1st January 2002

10. DATE OF REVISION OF THE TEXT
2 April 2005

Nicorette Freshmint 2mg Gum

(Pharmacia Ltd - (Consumer Products))

1. NAME OF THE MEDICINAL PRODUCT
Nicorette Freshmint 2mg Gum or Boots NicAssist 2 mg Minty Fresh Gum

2. QUALITATIVE AND QUANTITATIVE COMPOSITION
Chewing Gum containing 2mg nicotine

For excipients, see 6.1.

3. PHARMACEUTICAL FORM
Medicated Chewing Gum

4. CLINICAL PARTICULARS

4.1 Therapeutic indications
Nicorette Freshmint 2mg Gum is for the relief of nicotine withdrawal symptoms as an aid to smoking cessation in smokers ready to stop smoking.

In smokers currently unable or not ready to stop smoking abruptly, the gum may also be used as part of a programme to reduce smoking prior to stopping completely.

4.2 Posology and method of administration
Nicorette Freshmint 2mg Gum should be chewed slowly according to the instructions.

Adults

The strength of gum to be used will depend on the smoking habits of the individual. In general, if the patient smokes 20 or less cigarettes a day, 2mg nicotine gum is indicated. If more that 20 cigarettes per day are smoked, 4mg nicotine gum will be needed to meet the withdrawal of the high serum nicotine levels from heavy smoking.

The chewing gums should be used whenever there is an urge to smoke according to the "chew and rest" technique described on the pack. After about 30 minutes of such use, the gum will be exhausted. Not more than 15 pieces of the chewing gum may be used each day. Absorption of nicotine is through the buccal mucosa, any nicotine which is swallowed being destroyed by the liver.

Advice and support normally improve the success rate.

Smoking cessation:

Use the gum whenever there is an urge to smoke to maintain complete abstinence from smoking. Sufficient gums should be used, usually 8-12, up to a maximum of 15.

Continue use for up to three months to break the habit of smoking, then gradually reduce gum use. When daily use is 1-2 gums, use should be stopped. Any spare gum should be retained, as craving may suddenly return.

For those using 4 mg nicotine gum, the 2 mg nicotine gum will be helpful during withdrawal from treatment.

Smoking reduction:

Use the gum between smoking episodes to manage the urge to smoke, to prolong smoke-free intervals and with the intention to reduce smoking as much as possible. If a reduction in number of cigarettes per day has not been achieved after 6 weeks, professional advice should be sought.

A quit attempt should be made as soon as the smoker feels ready, but not later than 6 months after start of treatment. If a quit attempt cannot be made within 9 months after starting treatment, professional advice should be sought.

When making a quit attempt the smoking cessation instructions above, can be followed.

Children:

Not for use by persons under age 18 except on the advice of a doctor.

4.3 Contraindications
Hypersensitivity to nicotine or to any component of the chewing gum.

4.4 Special warnings and special precautions for use
Smokers who wear dentures may experience difficulty in chewing Nicorette Freshmint 2mg Gum.

Transferred dependence is rare and is both less harmful and easier to break than smoking dependence.

Swallowed nicotine may exacerbate symptoms in patients suffering from gastritis or peptic ulcers.

Allergic reactions such as angioedema, urticaria and ulcerative stomatitis have been reported.

In general Nicorette Freshmint 2mg Gum presents a lesser hazard than continuing to smoke in those with stable cardiovascular disease. However those with unstable cardiovascular disease from any cause should be encouraged to stop smoking with non-pharmacological interventions. This includes patients who are unstable following myocardial infarction or stroke, and patients with unstable angina or unstable cardiac dysrhythmias. If encouragement to stop smoking with non-pharmacological interventions fails, Nicorette Freshmint 2mg Gum may be considered, but as data on safety in this patient group are limited, initiation should only be under close medical supervision.

Renal and or hepatic impairment

Nicorette Freshmint 2mg Gum should be used with caution in patients with moderate to severe hepatic impairment and/or severe renal impairment as the clearance of nicotine or its metabolites may be decreased with the potential for increased adverse effects (see section 4.8).

Nicotine gum should be used with caution in patients with diabetes mellitus, hyperthyroidism or pheochromocytoma, since nicotine causes the release of catecholamines from the adrenal medulla.

The label will state "Not for use by persons under age 18 except on the advice of a doctor".

4.5 Interaction with other medicinal products and other forms of Interaction
None Known

4.6 Pregnancy and lactation

Pregnancy

Smoking can seriously harm the fetus and infant and pregnant smokers should be given every support and encouragement to completely stop with non-pharmacological means. However, nicotine passes to the fetus affecting breathing movements and having a dose dependent effect on placental/fetal circulation. As risks for the fetus are not fully known, pregnant smokers should only use Nicorette Freshmint 2mg Gum after consulting a healthcare professional.

Breastfeeding

Nicotine passes into breast milk in small quantities that may affect the infant, even at low doses. Breastfeeding smokers should only use Nicorette Freshmint 2mg Gum after consulting a healthcare professional. To reduce the risk of exposure to the child, whenever possible, Nicorette Freshmint 2mg Gum should be used just after breastfeeding.

4.7 Effects on ability to drive and use machines
Not applicable.

4.8 Undesirable effects
Nicorette Freshmint 2mg Gum in the recommended dose has not been found to cause any serious adverse effects. Nicotine from the gum may sometimes cause a slight irritation of the throat at the start of treatment and may also cause increased salivation. Excessive swallowing of dissolved nicotine may, at first, cause hiccuping.

Excessive consumption of Nicorette Freshmint 2mg Gum by those who have not been in the habit of inhaling tobacco smoke could possibly lead to nausea, faintness or headaches (as may be experienced by such a patient if tobacco smoke is inhaled).

Common

(>1/100) CNS: Dizziness, headache

Gastro-Intestinal: Nausea, gastro-intestinal discomfort, hiccups

Local: Sore mouth or throat. Jaw-muscle ache. The gum may stick to, and may, in rare cases damage dentures.

Uncommon

(1/100 – 1/1000) Circulatory: Palpitation

Dermatological: Erythema, urticaria.

Local: Stomatitis

Rare

(<1/1000) Cardiovascular: Atrial fibrillation

Other: Allergic reactions such as angioedema

Some symptoms, such as dizziness, headache and sleep disturbances may be related to withdrawal symptoms associated with abstinence from smoking. Increased frequency of aphthous ulcer may occur after abstinence from smoking.

Those who are prone to indigestion may suffer initially from minor degrees of indigestion or heartburn if the 4mg nicotine gum is used; slower chewing and the use of the 2mg nicotine gum (if necessary more frequently) will usually overcome this problem.

4.9 Overdose
Overdosage can occur if many gums are taken simultaneously or in rapid succession. The consequences of an overdose are most likely to be minimised by the early nausea and vomiting known to occur with excessive nicotine intake. Nicotine is also subject to a significant first-pass metabolism.

Symptoms of overdosage are those of acute nicotine poisoning and include nausea, salivation, abdominal pain, diarrhoea, sweating headache, dizziness, disturbed hearing and marked weakness. In extreme cases, these symptoms may be followed by hypotension, rapid or weak or irregular pulse, breathing difficulties, prostration, circulatory collapse and terminal convulsions.

The minimum lethal dose of nicotine in a non-tolerant man has been estimated to be 40 to 60mg.

Management of an overdose

All nicotine intake should cease immediately and the patient should be treated symptomatically. Artificial respiration with oxygen should be instituted if necessary.

5. PHARMACOLOGICAL PROPERTIES

5.1 Pharmacodynamic properties
Pharmacotherapeutic group: Drugs used in nicotine dependence

ATC code: N07B A01

The pharmacological effects of nicotine are well documented. Those resulting from chewing Nicorette Freshmint 2mg Gum are comparatively small. The response at any one time represents a summation of stimulant and depressant actions from direct, reflex and chemical mediator influences on several organs. The main pharmacological actions are central stimulation and/or depression; transient hyperpnoea; peripheral vasoconstriction (usually associated with a rise in systolic pressure); suppression of appetite and stimulation of peristalsis.

5.2 Pharmacokinetic properties
Nicotine administered in chewing gums is readily absorbed from the buccal mucous membranes. Demonstrable blood levels are obtained within 5 – 7 minutes and reach a maximum about 30 minutes after the start of chewing. Blood levels are roughly proportional to the amount of nicotine chewed and have been shown never to exceed those obtained from smoking cigarettes.

5.3 Preclinical safety data
Preclinical data indicate that nicotine is neither mutagenic nor genotoxic.

There are no other findings derived from preclinical testing of relevance to the prescriber in determining the safety of the product which have not been considered in other relevant sections of this Summary of Product Characteristics.

6. PHARMACEUTICAL PARTICULARS

6.1 List of excipients

Core Gum

Polacrilin

Chewing gum base, containing butylated hydroxy toluene (E321)

Xylitol

Peppermint oil

Sodium carbonate, anhydrous

Sodium bicarbonate

Acesulfame Potassium

Levomenthol

Magnesium oxide, light

Talcum

Nitrogen, food grade

Coating

Xylitol

Peppermint oil

Acacia

Titanium dioxide (E171)

Carnauba wax

6.2 Incompatibilities
None relevant

6.3 Shelf life
2 Years

6.4 Special precautions for storage
Do not store above 25°C

6.5 Nature and contents of container

PVC/PVDC/Al Blister packed strips each containing 15 pieces supplied in packs of 15, 30 and 105 pieces.

Blister packed strips each containing 6 pieces supplied in packs of 12 pieces.

Not all pack sizes may be marketed.

6.6 Instructions for use and handling

See section 4.2

Administrative Data

7. MARKETING AUTHORISATION HOLDER

Pharmacia Limited

Ramsgate Road

Sandwich

Kent CT13 9NJ

United Kingdom

8. MARKETING AUTHORISATION NUMBER(S)

PL 00032/0283

9. DATE OF FIRST AUTHORISATION/RENEWAL OF THE AUTHORISATION

31 July 2000 / 1st January 2002

10. DATE OF REVISION OF THE TEXT

15 August 2005

Nicorette Freshmint 4 mg Gum

(Pharmacia Ltd - (Consumer Products))

1. NAME OF THE MEDICINAL PRODUCT

Nicorette Freshmint 4 mg Gum or Boots NicAssist 4 mg Minty Fresh Gum

2. QUALITATIVE AND QUANTITATIVE COMPOSITION

Chewing Gum containing 4 mg nicotine

For excipients, see 6.1

3. PHARMACEUTICAL FORM

Medicated Chewing Gum

4. CLINICAL PARTICULARS

4.1 Therapeutic indications

Nicorette Freshmint 4 mg Gum is for the relief of nicotine withdrawal symptoms as an aid to smoking cessation in smokers ready to stop smoking.

In smokers currently unable or not ready to stop smoking abruptly, the gum may also be used as part of a programme to reduce smoking prior to stopping completely.

4.2 Posology and method of administration

Nicorette Freshmint 4 mg Gum should be chewed slowly according to the instructions.

Adults

The strength of gum to be used will depend on the smoking habits of the individual. In general, if the patient smokes 20 or less cigarettes a day, 2mg nicotine gum is indicated. If more that 20 cigarettes per day are smoked, 4mg nicotine gum will be needed to meet the withdrawal of the high serum nicotine levels from heavy smoking.

The chewing gums should be used whenever there is an urge to smoke according to the "chew and rest" technique described on the pack. After about 30 minutes of such use, the gum will be exhausted. Not more than 15 pieces of the chewing gum may be used each day. Absorption of nicotine is through the buccal mucosa, any nicotine which is swallowed being destroyed by the liver.

Advice and support normally improve the success rate.

Smoking cessation

Use the gum whenever there is an urge to smoke to maintain complete abstinence from smoking. Sufficient gums should be used, usually 8-12, up to a maximum of 15.

Continue use for up to three months to break the habit of smoking, then gradually reduce gum use. When daily use is 1-2 gums, use should be stopped. Any spare gum should be retained, as craving may suddenly return.

For those using 4 mg nicotine gum, the 2 mg nicotine gum will be helpful during withdrawal from treatment.

Smoking reduction

Use the gum between smoking episodes to manage the urge to smoke, to prolong smoke-free intervals and with the intention to reduce smoking as much as possible. If a reduction in number of cigarettes per day has not been achieved after 6 weeks, professional advice should be sought.

A quit attempt should be made as soon as the smoker feels ready, but not later than 6 months after start of treatment. If a quit attempt cannot be made within 9 months after starting treatment, professional advice should be sought.

When making a quit attempt the smoking cessation instructions above, can be followed.

Children:

Not for use by persons under age 18 except on the advice of a doctor.

4.3 Contraindications

Hypersensitivity to nicotine or to any component of the chewing gum.

4.4 Special warnings and special precautions for use

Smokers who wear dentures may experience difficulty in chewing Nicorette Freshmint 4 mg Gum.

Transferred dependence is rare and is both less harmful and easier to break than smoking dependence.

Swallowed nicotine may exacerbate symptoms in patients suffering from gastritis or peptic ulcers.

Allergic reactions such as angioedema, urticaria and ulcerative stomatitis have been reported.

In general Nicorette Freshmint 4mg Gum presents a lesser hazard than continuing to smoke in those with stable cardiovascular disease. However those with unstable cardiovascular disease from any cause should be encouraged to stop smoking with non-pharmacological interventions. This includes patients who are unstable following myocardial infarction or stroke, and patients with unstable angina or unstable cardiac dysrhythmias. If encouragement to stop smoking with non-pharmacological interventions fails, Nicorette Freshmint 4mg Gum may be considered, but as data on safety in this patient group are limited, initiation should only be under close medical supervision.

Renal and or hepatic impairment

Nicorette Freshmint 4mg Gum should be used with caution in patients with moderate to severe hepatic impairment and/or severe renal impairment as the clearance of nicotine or its metabolites may be decreased with the potential for increased adverse effects (see section 4.8).

Nicotine gum should be used with caution in patients with diabetes mellitus, hyperthyroidism or pheochromocytoma, since nicotine causes the release of catecholamines from the adrenal medulla.

The label will state 'Not for use by persons under age 18 except on the advice of a doctor'.

4.5 Interaction with other medicinal products and other forms of Interaction

None known

4.6 Pregnancy and lactation

Pregnancy

Smoking can seriously harm the fetus and infant and pregnant smokers should be given every support and encouragement to completely stop with non-pharmacological means. However, nicotine passes to the fetus affecting breathing movements and having a dose dependent effect on placental/fetal circulation. As risks for the fetus are not fully known, pregnant smokers should only use Nicorette Freshmint 4mg Gum after consulting a healthcare professional.

Breastfeeding

Nicotine passes into breast milk in small quantities that may affect the infant, even at low doses. Breastfeeding smokers should only use Nicorette Freshmint 4mg Gum after consulting a healthcare professional. To reduce the risk of exposure to the child, whenever possible, Nicorette Freshmint 4mg Gum should be used just after breastfeeding.

4.7 Effects on ability to drive and use machines

Not applicable.

4.8 Undesirable effects

Nicorette Freshmint 4 mg Gum in the recommended dose has not been found to cause any serious adverse effects. Nicotine from the gum may sometimes cause a slight irritation of the throat at the start of treatment and may also cause increased salivation. Excessive swallowing of dissolved nicotine may, at first, cause hiccuping.

Excessive consumption of Nicorette Freshmint 4 mg Gum by patients who have not been in the habit of inhaling tobacco smoke could possibly lead to nausea, faintness or headaches (as may be experienced by such a patient if tobacco is inhaled).

Common > 1/100)	CNS:	Dizziness, headache
	Gastro-intestinal:	Nausea, gastro-intestinal discomfort, hiccups
	Local:	Sore mouth or throat. Jaw muscle ache. The gum may stick to, and may, in rare cases damage dentures
Uncommon (1/100 – 1/1000)	Circulatory:	Palpitation
	Dermatological:	Erythema, urticaria
	Local:	Stomatitis
Rare (<1/1000	Cardiovascular:	Atrial fibrillation
	Other:	Allergic reactions such as angioedema

Some symptoms, such as dizziness, headache and sleep disturbances may be related to withdrawal symptoms associated with abstinence from smoking. Increased frequency of aphthous ulcer may occur after abstinence from smoking.

Those with a tendency to indigestion may suffer initially from minor degrees of indigestion or heartburn if the 4 mg nicotine gum is used; slower chewing and the use of the 2 mg nicotine gum (if necessary more frequently) will usually overcome this problem.

4.9 Overdose

Overdosage may occur if many gums are taken simultaneously or in rapid succession. The consequences of an overdose are most likely to be minimised by the early nausea and vomiting known to occur with excessive nicotine intake. Nicotine is also subject to a significant first-pass metabolism.

Symptoms of overdosage are those of acute nicotine poisoning and include nausea, salivation, abdominal pain, diarrhoea, sweating, headache, dizziness, disturbed hearing and marked weakness. In extreme cases, these symptoms may be followed by hypotension, rapid or weak or irregular pulse, breathing difficulties, prostration, circulatory collapse and terminal convulsions. The minimum lethal dose of nicotine in a non-tolerant man has been estimated to be 40 to 60 mg.

Management of an overdose

All nicotine intake should cease immediately and the patient should be treated symptomatically. Artificial respiration with oxygen should be instituted if necessary.

5. PHARMACOLOGICAL PROPERTIES

5.1 Pharmacodynamic properties

Pharmacotherapeutic group: Drugs used in nicotine dependence

ATC code: N07B A01

The pharmacological effects of nicotine are well documented. Those resulting from chewing Nicorette Freshmint 4 mg Gum are comparatively small. The response at any one time represents a summation of stimulant and depressant actions from direct, reflex and chemical mediator influences on several organs. The main pharmacological actions are central stimulation and/or depression; transient hyperpnoea; peripheral vasoconstriction (usually associated with a rise in systolic pressure); suppression of appetite and stimulation of peristalsis.

5.2 Pharmacokinetic properties

Nicotine administered in chewing gums is readily absorbed from the buccal mucous membranes. Demonstrable blood levels are obtained within 5 – 7 minutes and reach a maximum about 30 minutes after the start of chewing. Blood levels are roughly proportional to the amount of nicotine chewed and have been shown never to exceed those obtained from smoking cigarettes.

5.3 Preclinical safety data

Preclinical data indicate that nicotine is neither mutagenic nor genotoxic.

There are no other findings derived from preclinical testing of relevance to the prescriber in determining the safety of the product which have not been considered in other relevant sections of this Summary of Product Characteristics.

6. PHARMACEUTICAL PARTICULARS

6.1 List of excipients

Core Gum

Polacrilin

Chewing gum base, containing butylated hydroxyl toluene (E321)

Xylitol

Peppermint oil

Sodium carbonate, anhydrous

Acesulfame Potassium

Levomenthol

Magnesium oxide, light

Quinoline yellow Al lake (E104)

Talcum

Nitrogen, food grade

Coating

Xylitol

Peppermint oil

Acacia

Titanium dioxide (E171)

Carnauba wax

Quinoline yellow Al lake (E104)

6.2 Incompatibilities

None known

6.3 Shelf life

2 Years

6.4 Special precautions for storage

Do not store above 25°C

6.5 Nature and contents of container

Blister packed strips each containing 15 pieces supplied in packs of 15, 30 and 105 pieces.

Blister packed strips each containing 6 pieces supplied in packs of 12 pieces.

Not all pack sizes may be marketed.

6.6 Instructions for use and handling
See section 4.2

Administrative Data

7. MARKETING AUTHORISATION HOLDER
Pharmacia Limited.
Ramsgate Road
Sandwich
Kent CT13 9NJ
United Kingdom

8. MARKETING AUTHORISATION NUMBER(S)
PL 00032/0295

9. DATE OF FIRST AUTHORISATION/RENEWAL OF THE AUTHORISATION
1 May 2001 / 1st January 2002

10. DATE OF REVISION OF THE TEXT
15 August 2005

Nicorette Inhalator

(Pharmacia Ltd - (Consumer Products))

1. NAME OF THE MEDICINAL PRODUCT
Nicorette® Inhalator / Boots NicAssist 10 mg inhalator

2. QUALITATIVE AND QUANTITATIVE COMPOSITION
Nicotine 10mg per cartridge.

3. PHARMACEUTICAL FORM
Inhalation cartridge for oromucosal use.

4. CLINICAL PARTICULARS

4.1 Therapeutic indications
The treatment of nicotine dependence and for the relief of withdrawal symptoms associated with smoking cessation in smokers ready to stop smoking.

In smokers currently unable or not ready to stop smoking abruptly, the inhalator may also be used as part of a programme to reduce smoking prior to stopping completely.

4.2 Posology and method of administration
Adults (including elderly)

As air is inhaled through the cartridge the nicotine is vaporized and absorbed in the mouth.

Nicorette Inhalator should be used whenever the urge to smoke is felt, up to a maximum usage of 12 cartridges per day. The more the subject is able to use the inhalator, the easier it will be to stay smoke-free. Each cartridge can be used for approximately 4 sessions, with each one lasting approximately 20 minutes.

Advice and support normally improve the success rate.

Any spare cartridges should be retained, as craving may suddenly occur.

Smoking cessation

In the treatment of nicotine dependence, a course not exceeding three months is suggested, the patient stopping smoking completely at the start of the course.

a) For up to 8 weeks the patient uses not less than six and not more than 12 cartridges each day, to relieve craving.

b) Over the following two weeks the aim is to reduce the number of cartridges used by half, and over the next two weeks to reduce the number to zero by the last day.

c) Patients who revert to smoking during or upon completion of the course should see a doctor before attempting a new course. Similarly, where a course extends into chronic use because of inability to cut down use of the Inhalator, medical advice should be sought.

Smoking reduction

Use the Inhalator between smoking episodes to prolong smoke-free intervals and with the intention to reduce smoking as much as possible. If a reduction in number of cigarettes per day has not been achieved after 6 weeks, professional advice should be sought.

A quit attempt should be made as soon the smoker feels ready, but not later than 6 months after start of treatment. If a quit attempt cannot be made within 9 months after starting treatment, professional advice should be sought.

When making a quit attempt the smoking cessation instructions above, can be followed.

Method of administration

The cartridge is inserted into the mouthpiece according to the instructions. The patient draws air into the mouth through the mouthpiece: there is a greater effort needed than with a cigarette. The patient may find deep drawing or short sucks on the mouthpiece most effective – patients soon find a favoured technique, Nicotine vapour passing through the mouth is absorbed by the buccal mucosa: little reaches the lungs. After about 20 minutes of intense use the maximal dose is achieved and it is about then that the nicotine amounts released from the cartridge begin the fall away, such that the cartridge is rejected by the user.

The actual time that the cartridge is active depends on the intensity of use.

Children

Nicorette Inhalator should not be administered to individuals under 18 years of age, except on the advice of a doctor.

Lung Disease

Patients with obstructive lung disease may find use of the Inhalator difficult. Nicotine Gum, Patch, Nasal Spray or Sublingual tablet may be preferred in such cases.

4.3 Contraindications
The product should not be administered to non tobacco users or to patients hypersensitive to nicotine or to any component of the inhalator.

4.4 Special warnings and special precautions for use
Patients who continue smoking or use other sources of nicotine when using the Nicorette Inhalator may experience adverse effects due to peak nicotine levels being higher than those experienced from smoking alone.

Nicorette Inhalator is best used at room temperature. Low temperature (below 15°C) may depress the release of nicotine, whilst high temperature (above 30°C) may increase release. Patient should avoid use in high temperatures or make fewer inhalations.

In general Nicorette Inhalator presents a lesser hazard than continuing to smoke in those with stable cardiovascular disease. However those with unstable cardiovascular disease from any cause should be encouraged to stop smoking with non-pharmacological interventions. This includes patients who are unstable following myocardial infarction or stroke, and patients with unstable angina or unstable cardiac dysrhythmias. If encouragement to stop smoking with non-pharmacological interventions fails, Nicorette Inhalator may be considered, but as data on safety in this patient group are limited, initiation should only be under close medical supervision.

Renal and or hepatic impairment

Nicorette Inhalator should be used with caution in patients with moderate to severe hepatic impairment and/or severe renal impairment as the clearance of nicotine or its metabolites may be decreased with the potential for increased adverse effects (see section 4.8). In patients smoking and undergoing haemodialysis, elevated nicotine levels have been seen.

Nicorette Inhalator should be used with caution in patients with gastritis or peptic ulcers.

Nicotine can stimulate production of adrenaline. Nicorette Inhalator should be used with caution in patients with diabetes mellitus, hyperthyroidism or phaeochromocytoma.

The label will state "Not for use by persons under age 18 except on the advice of a doctor".

4.5 Interaction with other medicinal products and other forms of Interaction
Smoking is associated with increase in CYP1A2 activity. After cessation of smoking, reduced clearance of substrates for this enzyme may occur. This may lead to an increase in plasma levels for some medicinal products of potential clinical importance for products with a narrow therapeutic window, e.g. theophylline, tacrine and clozapine.

The plasma concentration of other drugs metabolised in part by CYP1A2, e.g. imipramine, olanzapine, clomipramine and fluvoxamine may also increase on cessation of smoking, although data to support this are lacking and the possible clinical significance of this effect for these drugs is unknown.

Limited data indicate that the metabolism of flecainide and pentazocine may also be induced by smoking.

4.6 Pregnancy and lactation
Pregnancy

Smoking can seriously harm the fetus and infant and pregnant smokers should be given every support and encouragement to completely stop with non-pharmacological means. However, nicotine passes to the fetus affecting breathing movements and having a dose dependent effect on placental/fetal circulation. As risks for the fetus are not fully known, pregnant smokers should only use Nicorette Inhalator after consulting a healthcare professional.

Breastfeeding

Nicotine passes into breast milk in small quantities that may affect the infant, even at low doses. Breastfeeding smokers should only use Nicorette Inhalator after consulting a healthcare professional. To reduce the risk of exposure to the child, whenever possible, Nicorette Inhalator should be used just after breastfeeding.

4.7 Effects on ability to drive and use machines
None

4.8 Undesirable effects
The most frequently reported adverse events are local, i.e. cough and irritation in mouth and throat. During controlled clinical trials the following events were reported at an incidence of greater than 1% in the active than with placebo treatment:

§ Cough 27%
§ Headache 26%
§ Throat irritation 24%
§ Rhinitis 18%
§ Pharyngitis 15%
§ Stomatitis 15%
§ Dyspepsia 14%
§ Anxiety 13%
§ Nausea 10%
§ Sinusitis 8%
§ Dry mouth 7%
§ Chest pain 5%
§ Skeletal pain 5%
§ Diarrhoea 4%
§ Flatulence 4%
§ Local paraesthesia 4%
§ Allergy 3%
§ Depression 3%
§ Vomiting 2%
§ Dyspnoea 2%
§ Thirst 2%
§ Gingival irritation 2%
§ Hiccup 2%

In addition, palpitations have been reported infrequently. Some symptoms, such as dizziness, headache and sleeplessness, may be related to withdrawal symptoms associated with smoking cessation. Increased frequency of aphthous ulcer may occur after smoking cessation. The causality is unclear. Maintained nicotine dependence may occur.

4.9 Overdose
Overdosage with nicotine can occur if the patient has very low nicotine dependence or uses other forms of nicotine concomitantly. During non-clinical forced inhalation techniques, maximum plasma levels produced were in the range found when smoking.

Symptoms of overdosage are those of acute nicotine poisoning and include nausea, salivation, abdominal pain, diarrhoea, sweating, headache, dizziness, disturbed hearing and marked weakness. In extreme cases, these symptoms may be followed by hypotension, rapid, weak, irregular pulse, breathing difficulties, prostration, circulatory collapse and terminal convulsions.

The minimum acute lethal dose of nicotine in man is believed to be 40-60mg.

Management of overdosage

All nicotine intake should cease immediately and the patient should be treated symptomatically. Artificial respiration with oxygen should be instituted if necessary.

5. PHARMACOLOGICAL PROPERTIES

5.1 Pharmacodynamic properties
Nicorette Inhalator facilitates uptake of nicotine through the buccal mucosa into the venous circulation. The amount taken up alleviates the craving symptoms caused by the absence of nicotine from smoking.

5.2 Pharmacokinetic properties
Nicotine given i.v. has a volume of the distribution of 2 or 3 l/kg with a half life of 1-2 hours. Average plasma clearance is about 1-2 l/min mainly in the liver. More than 20 metabolites are known, all less active than nicotine: cotinine, with a half life of 15-20 hours and concentrations ten times that of nicotine is the main one.

Plasma binding of nicotine below 5% means significant displacement of drugs or nicotine are unlikely. Nicotine is excreted in the urine principally as cotinine (15%), 3-hydroxycotinine (45%), nicotine (10%).

Most inhaled nicotine is absorbed via the buccal mucosa. Forced rapid inhalation over 20 minutes will remove 40% of the nicotine from the cartridge. Uptake is slow and free of the peaks resultant from cigarette smoking. In normal use, plasma levels of 6-8ng/ml nicotine are obtained – about one third that from smoking, and equivalent to an hourly 2mg nicotine chewing gum.

Peak plasma levels occur within 15 minutes after the end of inhalation. Forced rapid inhalation for 20 minutes per hour for 12 hours achieved steady state plasma levels of 20-25ng/ml.

Ambient temperature affects volatilisation of nicotine, the biologically available dose rising by 35% for each 10°C above 20°C. Use below 15°C is not recommended.

Because the pattern of use if decided by the patient up to a limit of 12 cartridges per day to relieve craving, therapeutic levels of nicotine are individual, dictated by the level of dependence.

5.3 Preclinical safety data
None stated.

6. PHARMACEUTICAL PARTICULARS

6.1 List of excipients
Levomenthol and porous plug.

6.2 Incompatibilities
None relevant.

6.3 Shelf life
Two years.

6.4 Special precautions for storage
Store below 30°C.

6.5 Nature and contents of container
Aluminium foil sealed plastic cartridge.

6.6 Instructions for use and handling
1. Remove the sealed tray and the mouthpiece from the carton box.
2. Peel back the foil from the tray.
3. Separate the mouthpiece by twisting the two halves until the two marks line up. The mouthpiece can now be pulled apart.
4. Take a cartridge and push it firmly into the bottom of the mouthpiece until the seal breaks.
5. Push the other part of the mouthpiece back into place over the cartridge. Line up the marks and push the top and bottom together firmly to break the top seal of the cartridge.
6. Twist to lock: the product is ready for use.
7. Grip the mouthpiece with the lips.

As air is inhaled, the nicotine is vaporised and absorbed in the mouth.

Disposal Instructions

Because of residual nicotine, used cartridges may be a hazard to children, animals and fish and so should never be thrown away or left lying around. They should be kept in the case and disposed of with household rubbish.

Cleaning of mouthpiece

The empty mouthpiece should be rinsed in water several times a week.

Nicorette Inhalator should be used when the patient has the urge for a cigarette or feels the onset of other withdrawal symptoms, up to a maximum of twelve cartridges per day.

The number, frequency, puffing/inhalation time and technique vary individually. Studies show that different inhalation techniques give similar effects: deep inhalation (the cigarette smoker's way) or shallow puffing (the pipe smoker's way). The amount of nicotine from a puff is less than that from a cigarette.

To compensate for less nicotine delivery from a puff it is necessary to inhale more often than when smoking a cigarette, i.e. use the Nicorette Inhalator for longer periods at a time. After using a few cartridges the patient will have found a method that suits him/her and gives the best effect.

This product works best at room temperature. In cold conditions (below 15°C) the nicotine evaporates less readily and it will be necessary to inhale more frequently, whilst in warm conditions (above 30°C) nicotine will evaporate more readily and inhalation should be less frequent to avoid overdose.

Administrative Data

7. MARKETING AUTHORISATION HOLDER
Pharmacia Limited
Ramsgate Road
Sandwich
Kent CT13 9NJ
United Kingdom.

8. MARKETING AUTHORISATION NUMBER(S)
PL 00032/0280

9. DATE OF FIRST AUTHORISATION/RENEWAL OF THE AUTHORISATION
15 August 2000 / 1st January 2002

10. DATE OF REVISION OF THE TEXT
15 August 2005

Nicorette Mint 2mg Gum

(Pharmacia Ltd - (Consumer Products))

1. NAME OF THE MEDICINAL PRODUCT
Nicorette Mint 2mg Gum (or Boots NicAssist 2 mg mint gum)

2. QUALITATIVE AND QUANTITATIVE COMPOSITION
Chewing Gum containing 2mg nicotine

3. PHARMACEUTICAL FORM
Chewing Gum

4. CLINICAL PARTICULARS

4.1 Therapeutic indications
Nicorette Mint 2mg Gum is for the relief of nicotine withdrawal symptoms as an aid to smoking cessation in smokers ready to stop smoking.

In smokers currently unable or not ready to stop smoking abruptly, the gum may also be used as part of a programme to reduce smoking prior to stopping completely.

4.2 Posology and method of administration
Nicorette Mint 2mg Gum should be chewed slowly according to the instructions.

Adults

The strength of gum to be used will depend on the smoking habits of the individual. In general, if the patient smokes 20 or less cigarettes a day, 2mg nicotine gum is indicated. If more that 20 cigarettes per day are smoked, 4mg nicotine gum will be needed to meet the withdrawal of the high serum nicotine levels from heavy smoking.

The chewing gums should be used whenever there is an urge to smoke according to the "chew and rest" technique described on the pack. After about 30 minutes of such use, the gum will be exhausted. Not more than 15 pieces of the chewing gum may be used each day. Absorption of nicotine is through the buccal mucosa, any nicotine which is swallowed being destroyed by the liver.

Advice and support normally improve the success rate.

Smoking cessation

Use the gum whenever there is an urge to smoke to maintain complete abstinence from smoking. Sufficient gums should be used, usually 8-12, up to a maximum of 15.

Continue use for up to three months to break the habit of smoking, then gradually reduce gum use. When daily use is 1-2 gums, use should be stopped. Any spare gum should be retained, as craving may suddenly return.

For those using 4 mg nicotine gum, the 2 mg nicotine gum will be helpful during withdrawal from treatment.

Smoking reduction

Use the gum between smoking episodes to manage the urge to smoke, to prolong smoke-free intervals and with the intention to reduce smoking as much as possible. If a reduction in number of cigarettes per day has not been achieved after 6 weeks, professional advice should be sought.

A quit attempt should be made as soon as the smoker feels ready, but not later than 6 months after start of treatment. If a quit attempt cannot be made within 9 months after starting treatment, professional advice should be sought.

When making a quit attempt the smoking cessation instructions above, can be followed.

Children:

Not for use by persons under age 18 except on the advice of a doctor.

4.3 Contraindications
Hypersensitivity to nicotine or to any component of the chewing gum

4.4 Special warnings and special precautions for use
Smokers who wear dentures may experience difficulty in chewing Nicorette Mint 2mg Gum.

Transferred dependence is rare and is both less harmful and easier to break than smoking dependence.

Swallowed nicotine may exacerbate symptoms in patients suffering from gastritis or peptic ulcers.

Allergic reactions such as angioedema and urticaria and ulcerative stomatitis have been reported.

In general Nicorette Mint 2mg Gum presents a lesser hazard than continuing to smoke in those with stable cardiovascular disease. However those with unstable cardiovascular disease from any cause should be encouraged to stop smoking with non-pharmacological interventions. This includes patients who are unstable following myocardial infarction or stroke, and patients with unstable angina or unstable cardiac dysrhythmias. If encouragement to stop smoking with non-pharmacological interventions fails, Nicorette Mint 2mg Gum may be considered, but as data on safety in this patient group are limited, initiation should only be under close medical supervision.

Renal and or hepatic impairment:

Nicorette Mint 2mg Gum should be used with caution in patients with moderate to severe hepatic impairment and/or severe renal impairment as the clearance of nicotine or its metabolites may be decreased with the potential for increased adverse effects (see section 4.8).

Nicotine gum should be used with caution in patients with diabetes mellitus, hyperthyroidism or pheochromocytoma, since nicotine causes the release of catecholamines from the adrenal medulla.

The label will state "Not for use by persons under age 18 except on the advice of a doctor".

4.5 Interaction with other medicinal products and other forms of Interaction
None Known

4.6 Pregnancy and lactation
Pregnancy

Smoking can seriously harm the fetus and infant and pregnant smokers should be given every support and encouragement to completely stop with non-pharmacological means. However, nicotine passes to the fetus affecting breathing movements and having a dose dependent effect on placental/fetal circulation. As risks for the fetus are not fully known, pregnant smokers should only use Nicorette Mint 2mg Gum after consulting a healthcare professional.

Breastfeeding

Nicotine passes into breast milk in small quantities that may affect the infant, even at low doses. Breastfeeding smokers should only use Nicorette Mint 2mg Gum after consulting a healthcare professional. To reduce the risk of exposure to the child, whenever possible, Nicorette Mint 2mg Gum should be used just after breastfeeding.

4.7 Effects on ability to drive and use machines
Not applicable.

4.8 Undesirable effects
Nicorette Mint 2mg Gum in the recommended dose has not been found to cause any serious adverse effects. Nicotine from the gum may sometimes cause a slight irritation of the throat at the start of treatment and may also cause increased salivation. Excessive swallowing of dissolved nicotine may, at first, cause hiccuping.

Excessive consumption of Nicorette Mint 2mg Gum by those who have not been in the habit of inhaling tobacco smoke could possibly lead to nausea, faintness or headaches (as may be experienced by such a patient if tobacco smoke is inhaled).

Common

(>1/100) CNS: Dizziness, headache

Gastro-Intestinal: Nausea, gastro-intestinal discomfort, hiccups

Local: Sore mouth or throat. Jaw-muscle ache. The gum may stick to, and may, in rare cases damage dentures.

Uncommon

(1/100 – 1/1000) Circulatory: Palpitation

Dermatological: Erythema, urticaria.

Local: Stomatitis

Rare

(<1/1000) Cardiovascular: Atrial fibrillation

Other: Allergic reactions such as angioedema

Some symptoms, such as dizziness, headache and sleep disturbances may be related to withdrawal symptoms associated with abstinence from smoking. Increased frequency of aphthous ulcer may occur after abstinence from smoking.

Those who are prone to indigestion may suffer initially from minor degrees of indigestion or heartburn if the 4mg nicotine gum is used; slower chewing and the use of the 2mg nicotine gum (if necessary more frequently) will usually overcome this problem.

4.9 Overdose
Overdosage can occur if many gums are taken simultaneously or in rapid succession. The consequences of an overdose are most likely to be minimised by the early nausea and vomiting known to occur with excessive nicotine intake. Nicotine is also subject to a significant first-pass metabolism.

Symptoms of overdosage are those of acute nicotine poisoning and include nausea, salivation, abdominal pain, diarrhoea, sweating headache, dizziness, disturbed hearing and marked weakness. In extreme cases, these symptoms may be followed by hypotension, rapid or weak or irregular pulse, breathing difficulties, prostration, circulatory collapse and terminal convulsions.

The minimum lethal dose of nicotine in a non-tolerant man has been estimated to be 40 to 60mg.

Management of an overdose

All nicotine intake should cease immediately and the patient should be treated symptomatically. Artificial respiration with oxygen should be instituted if necessary.

5. PHARMACOLOGICAL PROPERTIES

5.1 Pharmacodynamic properties
The pharmacological effects of nicotine are well documented. Those resulting from chewing Nicorette Mint 2mg Gum are comparatively small. The response at any one time represents a summation of stimulant and depressant actions from direct, reflex and chemical mediator influences on several organs. The main pharmacological actions are central stimulation and/or depression; transient hyperpnoea; peripheral vasoconstriction (usually associated with a rise in systolic pressure); suppression of appetite and stimulation of peristalsis.

5.2 Pharmacokinetic properties
Nicotine administered in chewing gums is readily absorbed from the buccal mucous membranes. Demonstrable blood levels are obtained within 5 – 7 minutes and reach a maximum about 30 minutes after the start of chewing. Blood levels are roughly proportional to the amount of nicotine chewed and have been shown never to exceed those obtained from smoking cigarettes.

5.3 Preclinical safety data
Preclinical data indicate that nicotine is neither mutagenic nor genotoxic.

There are no other findings derived from preclinical testing of relevance to the prescriber in determining the safety of the product which have not been considered in other relevant sections of this Summary of Product Characteristics.

6. PHARMACEUTICAL PARTICULARS

6.1 List of excipients

Polacrilin

Chewing gum base, containing butylated hydroxy toluene (E321)

Xylitol

Sodium carbonate, anhydrous

Sodium bicarbonate

Peppermint oil

Menthol

Magnesium oxide, light

Talcum

Nitrogen, food grade

6.2 Incompatibilities

None relevant

6.3 Shelf life

30 months

6.4 Special precautions for storage

Do not store above 25°C

6.5 Nature and contents of container

PVC/PVDC/Al Blister packed strips each containing 15 pieces supplied in packs of 15, 30 and 105 pieces. Packs containing a blister strip of 6 pieces (not marketed).

6.6 Instructions for use and handling

See section 4.2

Administrative Data

7. MARKETING AUTHORISATION HOLDER

Pharmacia Limited

Ramsgate Road

Sandwich

Kent CT13 9NJ

United Kingdom

8. MARKETING AUTHORISATION NUMBER(S)

PL 00032/0250

9. DATE OF FIRST AUTHORISATION/RENEWAL OF THE AUTHORISATION

27 April, 1999 / 1st January 2002

10. DATE OF REVISION OF THE TEXT

15 August 2005

Nicorette Mint 4mg Gum

(Pharmacia Ltd - (Consumer Products))

1. NAME OF THE MEDICINAL PRODUCT

Nicorette Mint 4 mg Gum / Boots NicAssist 4 mg mint gum

2. QUALITATIVE AND QUANTITATIVE COMPOSITION

Chewing Gum containing 4 mg nicotine

3. PHARMACEUTICAL FORM

Chewing Gum

4. CLINICAL PARTICULARS

4.1 Therapeutic indications

Nicorette Mint 4 mg Gum is for the relief of nicotine withdrawal symptoms as an aid to smoking cessation in smokers ready to stop smoking.

In smokers currently unable or not ready to stop smoking abruptly, the gum may also be used as part of a programme to reduce smoking prior to stopping completely.

4.2 Posology and method of administration

Nicorette Mint 4 mg Gum should be chewed slowly according to the instructions.

Adults

The strength of gum to be used will depend on the smoking habits of the individual. In general, if the patient smokes 20 or less cigarettes a day, 2mg nicotine gum is indicated. If more that 20 cigarettes per day are smoked, 4mg nicotine gum will be needed to meet the withdrawal of the high serum nicotine levels from heavy smoking.

The chewing gums should be used whenever there is an urge to smoke according to the "chew and rest" technique described on the pack. After about 30 minutes of such use, the gum will be exhausted. Not more than 15 pieces of the chewing gum may be used each day. Absorption of nicotine is through the buccal mucosa, any nicotine which is swallowed being destroyed by the liver.

Advice and support normally improve the success rate.

Smoking cessation

Use the gum whenever there is an urge to smoke to maintain complete abstinence from smoking. Sufficient gums should be used, usually 8-12, up to a maximum of 15.

Continue use for up to three months to break the habit of smoking, then gradually reduce gum use. When daily use is 1-2 gums, use should be stopped. Any spare gum should be retained, as craving may suddenly return.

For those using 4 mg nicotine gum, the 2 mg nicotine gum will be helpful during withdrawal from treatment.

Smoking reduction

Use the gum between smoking episodes to manage the urge to smoke, to prolong smoke-free intervals and with the intention to reduce smoking as much as possible. If a reduction in number of cigarettes per day has not been achieved after 6 weeks, professional advice should be sought.

A quit attempt should be made as soon as the smoker feels ready, but not later than 6 months after start of treatment. If a quit attempt cannot be made within 9 months after starting treatment, professional advice should be sought.

When making a quit attempt the smoking cessation instructions above, can be followed.

Children:

Not for use by persons under age 18 except on the advice of a doctor.

4.3 Contraindications

Hypersensitivity to nicotine or to any component of the chewing gum.

4.4 Special warnings and special precautions for use

Smokers who wear dentures may experience difficulty in chewing Nicorette Mint 4 mg Gum.

Transferred dependence is rare and is both less harmful and easier to break than smoking dependence.

Swallowed nicotine may exacerbate symptoms in patients suffering from gastritis or peptic ulcers.

Allergic reactions such as angioedema and urticaria and ulcerative stomatitis have been reported.

In general Nicorette Mint 4mg Gum presents a lesser hazard than continuing to smoke in those with stable cardiovascular disease. However those with unstable cardiovascular disease from any cause should be encouraged to stop smoking with non-pharmacological interventions. This includes patients who are unstable following myocardial infarction or stroke, and patients with unstable angina or unstable cardiac dysrhythmias. If encouragement to stop smoking with non-pharmacological interventions fails, Nicorette Mint 4mg Gum may be considered, but as data on safety in this patient group are limited, initiation should only be under close medical supervision.

Renal and or hepatic impairment

Nicorette Mint 4mg Gum should be used with caution in patients with moderate to severe hepatic impairment and/ or severe renal impairment as the clearance of nicotine or its metabolites may be decreased with the potential for increased adverse effects (see section 4.8).

Nicotine gum should be used with caution in patients with diabetes mellitus, hyperthyroidism or pheochromocytoma, since nicotine causes the release of catecholamines from the adrenal medulla.

The label will state "Not for use by persons under age 18 except on the advice of a doctor".

4.5 Interaction with other medicinal products and other forms of Interaction

None Known

4.6 Pregnancy and lactation

Pregnancy

Smoking can seriously harm the fetus and infant and pregnant smokers should be given every support and encouragement to completely stop with non-pharmacological means. However, nicotine passes to the fetus affecting breathing movements and having a dose dependent effect on placental/fetal circulation. As risks for the fetus are not fully known, pregnant smokers should only use Nicorette Mint 4mg Gum after consulting a healthcare professional.

Breastfeeding

Nicotine passes into breast milk in small quantities that may affect the infant, even at low doses. Breastfeeding smokers should only use Nicorette Mint 4mg Gum after consulting a healthcare professional. To reduce the risk of exposure to the child, whenever possible, Nicorette Mint 4mg Gum should be used just after breastfeeding.

4.7 Effects on ability to drive and use machines

Not applicable.

4.8 Undesirable effects

Nicorette Mint 4 mg Gum in the recommended dose has not been found to cause any serious adverse effects. Nicotine from the gum may sometimes cause a slight irritation of the throat at the start of treatment and may also cause increased salivation. Excessive swallowing of dissolved nicotine may, at first, cause hiccuping.

Excessive consumption of Nicorette Mint 4 mg Gum by those who have not been in the habit of inhaling tobacco smoke could possibly lead to nausea, faintness or headaches (as may be experienced by such a patient if tobacco smoke is inhaled).

Common (>1/100)	CNS:	Dizziness, headache
	Gastro-Intestinal:	Nausea, gastro-intestinal discomfort, hiccups
	Local:	Sore mouth or throat. Jaw-muscle ache. The gum may stick to, and may, in rare cases damage dentures.
Uncommon (1/100 – 1/1000)	Circulatory:	Palpitation
	Dermatological:	Erythema, urticaria.
	Local:	Stomatitis
Rare (<1/1000)	Cardiovascular:	Atrial fibrillation
	Other:	Allergic reactions such as angioedema

Some symptoms, such as dizziness, headache and sleep disturbances may be related to withdrawal symptoms associated with abstinence from smoking. Increased frequency of aphthous ulcer may occur after abstinence from smoking.

Those who are prone to indigestion may suffer initially from minor degrees of indigestion or heartburn if the 4mg nicotine gum is used; slower chewing and the use of the 2mg nicotine gum (if necessary more frequently) will usually overcome this problem.

4.9 Overdose

Overdosage can occur if many gums are taken simultaneously or in rapid succession. The consequences of an overdose are most likely to be minimised by the early nausea and vomiting known to occur with excessive nicotine intake. Nicotine is also subject to a significant first-pass metabolism.

Symptoms of overdosage are those of acute nicotine poisoning and include nausea, salivation, abdominal pain, diarrhoea, sweating headache, dizziness, disturbed hearing and marked weakness. In extreme cases, these symptoms may be followed by hypotension, rapid or weak or irregular pulse, breathing difficulties, prostration, circulatory collapse and terminal convulsions.

The minimum lethal dose of nicotine in a non-tolerant man has been estimated to be 40 to 60mg.

Management of an overdose

All nicotine intake should cease immediately and the patient should be treated symptomatically. Artificial respiration with oxygen should be instituted if necessary.

5. PHARMACOLOGICAL PROPERTIES

5.1 Pharmacodynamic properties

The pharmacological effects of nicotine as well documented. Those resulting from chewing Nicorette Mint 4 mg Gum are comparatively small. The response at any one time represents a summation of stimulant and depressant actions from direct, reflex and chemical mediator influences on several organs. The main pharmacological actions are central stimulation and/or depression; transient hyperpnoea; peripheral vasoconstriction (usually associated with a rise in systolic pressure); suppression of appetite and stimulation of peristalsis.

5.2 Pharmacokinetic properties

Nicotine administered in chewing gums is readily absorbed from the buccal mucous membranes. Demonstrable blood levels are obtained within 5 – 7 minutes and reach a maximum about 30 minutes after the start of chewing. Blood levels are roughly proportional to the amount of nicotine chewed and have been shown never to exceed those obtained from smoking cigarettes.

5.3 Preclinical safety data

Preclinical data indicate that nicotine is neither mutagenic nor genotoxic.

There are no other findings derived from preclinical testing of relevance to the prescriber in determining the safety of the product which have not been considered in other relevant sections of this Summary of Product Characteristics.

6. PHARMACEUTICAL PARTICULARS

6.1 List of excipients

Polacrilin

Chewing gum base, containing butylated hydroxy toluene (E321)

Xylitol

Peppermint oil

Menthol

Sodium carbonate anhydrous

Quinoline Yellow Al-lake (E104)

Magnesium oxide, light

Talc

6.2 Incompatibilities

None relevant

6.3 Shelf life

24 months

6.4 Special precautions for storage

Do not store above 25°C

6.5 Nature and contents of container

PVC/PVDC/Al Blister packed strips each containing 15 pieces supplied in a pack of 15, 30 or 105 pieces. Packs containing a blister strip of 6 pieces (not marketed).

6.6 Instructions for use and handling

See section 4.2

Administrative Data

7. MARKETING AUTHORISATION HOLDER

Pharmacia Limited

Ramsgate Road

Sandwich

Kent CT13 9NJ

United Kingdom

8. MARKETING AUTHORISATION NUMBER(S)

PL 00032/0251

9. DATE OF FIRST AUTHORISATION/RENEWAL OF THE AUTHORISATION

26 April 1999 / 1st January 2002

10. DATE OF REVISION OF THE TEXT

15 August 2005

Nicorette Nasal Spray

(Pharmacia Ltd - (Consumer Products))

1. NAME OF THE MEDICINAL PRODUCT

Nicorette Nasal Spray

2. QUALITATIVE AND QUANTITATIVE COMPOSITION

Nicotine 10 mg/ml. Each spray of 50 μl delivers 0.5 mg nicotine.

3. PHARMACEUTICAL FORM

Nasal Spray, solution.

4. CLINICAL PARTICULARS

4.1 Therapeutic indications

Nicorette Nasal Spray is for the treatment of nicotine dependence and the rapid relief of withdrawal symptoms which may occur during smoking cessation. It may be of particular benefit to the most heavily dependent smokers.

4.2 Posology and method of administration

Adults and elderly

1. The frequency of use depends on the previous smoking habit of the individual and the level of their nicotine dependence.

2. On commencing treatment the patient uses the spray to treat craving as required, subject to a limit of one spray to each nostril twice an hour.

3. A 50 μl dose of solution is sprayed into the nostril when the unit is activated. This is described as a "spray" and dosage is described using this term. Each spray delivers 0.5 mg of nicotine, about half of which is absorbed.

4. The daily limit of use is 32mg of nicotine (64 sprays) which is the equivalent of two sprays to each nostril every hour for 16 hours.

5. The method of use of the spray should be according to the instructions.

6. The 3 month course should take the following pattern:-

a. For 8 weeks the patient uses the spray as required, subject to the maxima described above, to relieve craving.

b. After this period the patient reduces usage until after 4 more weeks treatment has ended. It is suggested that after 2 weeks into this period usage will have been reduced by a half and usage be zero by the last day. Spraying into a single nostril during this period may be helpful in achieving this.

c. In order to avoid substituted dependence, treatment should be limited to three months. No other nicotine containing drugs, or tobacco products should be used during the treatment. The patient should understand the aim of decreasing the use of the spray to make a final break with nicotine at the end of the course, and also accept that for the first few days of the course nasal irritation may be unpleasant.

Children and young adults

The product is not for use by any person under the age of 18 years.

4.3 Contraindications

i. The product should not be administered to non-tobacco users or to patients known to be allergic to components of the spray.

ii. Nicotine in any form should be avoided during pregnancy and lactation.

iii. Nicorette Nasal Spray is contraindicated in persons up to 18 years of age.

iv. Other nicotine-containing preparations or tobacco products must not be used during the Nicorette Nasal Spray treatment.

4.4 Special warnings and special precautions for use

The patient should stop smoking completely when initiating therapy with the product. Patients who continue smoking or use other nicotine products when using the spray may experience adverse effects due to peak nicotine levels higher than those experienced from smoking alone.

The cardiovascular effects of nicotine may be deleterious to patients with a history of angina pectoris. Nicorette Nasal Spray should be used with caution in patients with a history of gastritis or peptic ulcer and chronic nasal disorders (polyposis, vasomotor rhinitis, perennial rhinitis), recent myocardial infarction, serious cardiac arrhythmias, systemic hypertension, peripheral vascular disease or severe renal disease. Any worsening of the nasal disorders should be reported to the patient's physician.

Nicotine can stimulate production of adrenaline; Nicorette Nasal Spray should be used with caution in patients with diabetes mellitus, hyperthyroidism or pheochromocytoma.

4.5 Interaction with other medicinal products and other forms of Interaction

Smoking is associated with increase in CYP1A2 activity. After cessation of smoking, reduced clearance of substrates for this enzyme may occur. This may lead to an increase in plasma levels for some medicinal products of potential clinical importance for products with a narrow therapeutic window, e.g. theophylline, tacrine and clozapine.

The plasma concentration of other drugs metabolised in part by CYP1A2, e.g. imipramine, olanzapine, clomipramine and fluvoxamine may also increase on cessation of smoking, although data to support this are lacking and the possible clinical significance of this effect for these drugs is unknown.

Limited data indicate that the metabolism of flecainide and pentazocine may also be induced by smoking.

4.6 Pregnancy and lactation

Nicotine in any form is contraindicated in pregnancy. As nicotine passes into breast milk, it should also be avoided by nursing mothers.

4.7 Effects on ability to drive and use machines

The nasal spray should not be used whilst the user is driving or operating machinery as sneezing and watering eyes could contribute to accidents.

4.8 Undesirable effects

Nicorette Nasal Spray may cause adverse reactions similar to those produced by nicotine given by other means, including smoking.

Principal adverse effects

These occur commonly at the start of therapy but usually decline within the first few days of treatment.

Local: Nasal irritation (sneezing, running nose), watering eyes and throat irritation.

Systemic: Nausea, headache and dizziness (some symptoms such as dizziness and headache may be related to withdrawal symptoms associated with smoking cessation).

Other

Additionally an incidence greater that 1% compared with placebo was noted in clinical studies for the following:-

Sore nose, ear sensations, increased urination, tingling or burning sensation in the head, nose bleed, dyspepsia.

4.9 Overdose

Overdosage with nicotine can only occur, if the patient has very low nicotine dependence or uses other forms of nicotine concomitantly. Should Nicorette Nasal Spray be used orally, the risk of poisoning is small due to high first pass metabolism. Due to the nature of the container it is not possible to take the product without using the spraying device.

Symptoms of overdosage are those of acute nicotine poisoning and include nausea, salivation, abdominal pain, diarrhoea, sweating, headache, dizziness, disturbed hearing and marked weakness. In extreme cases, these symptoms may be followed by hypotension, rapid weak irregular pulse, breathing difficulties, prostration, circulatory collapse and terminal convulsions.

The acute minimum lethal oral dose of nicotine in man is believed to be 40-60 mg.

Management of overdosage

All nicotine intake should cease immediately and the patient should be treated symptomatically. Artificial respiration with oxygen should be instituted if necessary.

5. PHARMACOLOGICAL PROPERTIES

5.1 Pharmacodynamic properties

Through rapid uptake of nicotine through the nasal membranes Nicorette Nasal Spray provides early relief of nicotine withdrawal symptoms. Clinical studies have shown that the nicotine containing products can help people give up smoking.

5.2 Pharmacokinetic properties

Following administration of one dose Nicorette Nasal Spray approximately 56% of the nicotine enters the systemic circulation.

The volume of distribution following i.v. administration of nicotine is approximately (2 to) 3 l/kg and the half-life ranges from 1 to 2 hours. The major eliminating organ is the liver, and average plasma clearance is about 1.2 l/min; the kidney and lung also metabolise nicotine. More than 20 metabolites of nicotine have been identified, all of which are believed to be less active than the parent compound. The primary metabolite of nicotine in plasma, cotinine, has a half-life of 15 to 20 hours and concentrations that exceed nicotine by 10-fold.

Plasma protein binding of nicotine is <5%. Therefore, changes in nicotine binding from use of concomitant drugs or alterations of plasma proteins by disease states would not be expected to have a significant effect on the nicotine kinetics.

The primary urinary metabolites are cotinine (15% of dose) and trans-3-hydroxycotinine (45% of the dose). Usually about 10% of nicotine is excreted unchanged in the urine. As much as 30% may be excreted in the urine with high urine flow rates and acidification below pH5.

Plasma levels of nicotine obtained with Nicorette Nasal Spray rise rapidly, reaching a maximum level – mean – after approximately 10-15 minutes. The mean peak plasma level of nicotine – after steady –state is achieved – given 1 dose/hour, 2 doses/hour and 3 doses/hour approximately 10, 19 and 28 ng/ml respectively.

After repeated administration of the Nicorette Nasal Spray the AUC was significantly higher during the last dosing interval as compared to the first giving an accumulation ratio of 3.1. No dose-dependency has been shown for the doses 0.5 mg and 1 mg nicotine.

The therapeutic blood concentrations of nicotine, (i.e. the blood levels which relieve craving) are individually based on the patient's nicotine dependence.

5.3 Preclinical safety data

No further information.

6. PHARMACEUTICAL PARTICULARS

6.1 List of excipients

Disodium phosphate dodecahydrate

Sodium dihydrogen phosphate dihydrate

Anhydrous citric acid

Sodium chloride

Polysorbate 80

NNS aroma DZ-03226 (B-ionone)

Methyl parahyroxybenzoate

Propyl parahydroxybenzoate

Disodium edetate

Purified water

6.2 Incompatibilities

None relevant.

6.3 Shelf life

Two years.

6.4 Special precautions for storage

No special temperature conditions. Should be stored protected from light.

6.5 Nature and contents of container

The solution is filled in a glass container equipped with a spray pump and a nosepiece.

6.6 Instructions for use and handling

1) Remove the protective cap.

2) Prime Nicorette Nasal Spray by placing the nozzle between first and second finger with the thumb on the bottom of the bottle. Press several times firmly and quickly until a fine spray appears (up to 7-8 strokes).

Important: Point the spray safely away when priming it. Do not prime it near children or pets.

3) Insert the spray tip into one nostril, pointing the top towards the back of the nose.

Press firmly and quickly. Give a spray into the other nostril.

4) Put on the protective cap.

Administrative Data

7. MARKETING AUTHORISATION HOLDER

Pharmacia Limited

Ramsgate Road

Sandwich

Kent CT13 9NJ

8. MARKETING AUTHORISATION NUMBER(S)

PL 00032/0255

9. DATE OF FIRST AUTHORISATION/RENEWAL OF THE AUTHORISATION

30 August 1999 / 1st January 2002.

10. DATE OF REVISION OF THE TEXT

2 April 2005

Nicotinell Chewing Gums

(Novartis Consumer Health)

1. NAME OF THE MEDICINAL PRODUCT

NICOTINELL® Fruit 2 mg & 4 mg chewing gum.

NICOTINELL® Mint 2 mg & 4 mg chewing gum.

NICOTINELL® Liquorice 2 mg & 4 mg chewing gum.

2. QUALITATIVE AND QUANTITATIVE COMPOSITION

Nicotine 2 mg or 4 mg per gum, (as 10mg nicotine polacrilin (1:4) for the 2 mg gum or as 20 mg nicotine polacrilin (1:6) for the 4 mg gum, available in a fruit, mint or liquorice flavour

(For excipients see section 6.1)

3. PHARMACEUTICAL FORM
Medicated chewing gum.

Each piece of coated chewing-gum is off-white in colour and rectangular in shape.

4. CLINICAL PARTICULARS

4.1 Therapeutic indications
Nicotinell treatment is indicated for the relief of nicotine withdrawal symptoms, in nicotine dependency as an aid to smoking cessation. Nicotinell 4 mg gums are used when severe withdrawal symptoms are experienced.

4.2 Posology and method of administration
Adults and elderly:

Users should stop smoking completely during treatment with Nicotinell gum. One piece of Nicotinell gum to be chewed when the user feels the urge to smoke.

Normally, 8-12 pieces per day, up to a maximum of 25 pieces per day of the 2 mg gum or 15 pieces per day of the 4 mg gum.

The 2 mg chewing-gum may not be well suited to smokers with a strong or very strong nicotine dependency. The 4 mg gum is intended to be used by smokers with a strong or very strong nicotine dependency and those who have previously failed to stop smoking with the aid of nicotine replacement therapy.

The characteristics of chewing gum as a pharmaceutical form are such that individually different nicotine levels can result in the blood. Therefore, dosage frequency should be adjusted according to individual requirements within the stated maximum limit.

Directions for use:

1. One piece of gum should be chewed until the taste becomes strong.

2. The chewing gum should be rested between the gum and cheek.

3. When the taste fades, chewing should commence again.

4. The chewing routine should be repeated for 30 minutes.

The treatment time is individual. Normally, treatment should continue for at least 3 months. After three months, the user should gradually cut down the number of pieces chewed each day until they have stopped using the product. Treatment should be discontinued when the dose has been reduced to 1-2 pieces of gum per day. Use of nicotine products like Nicotinell gums beyond 6 months is generally not recommended. Some ex-smokers may need treatment with the gum for longer to avoid returning to smoking.

Children & Young Adults:

Nicotinell gums should not be used by people under 18 years of age without recommendation from a physician. There is no experience in treating adolescents under the age of 18 years with Nicotinell gums.

Concomitant use of acidic beverages such as coffee or soda may interfere with the buccal absorption of nicotine. Acidic beverages should be avoided for 15 minutes prior to chewing the gum.

4.3 Contraindications
Hypersensitivity to any excipients of the gum.

Liquorice gums are contra-indicated in pregnancy and lactation due to the presence of liquorice (glycyrrhizin). When use of nicotine replacement therapy is recommended the use of other flavoured gums (e.g. fruit or mint) may be considered (see section 4.6).

Nicotinell gum should not be used by non-smokers.

Use is contra-indicated in patients during the immediate post-infarction period, unstable or worsening angina pectoris (including Prinzmetal's angina), severe cardiac arrhythmias, and recent cerebrovascular accident.

4.4 Special warnings and special precautions for use
Swallowed nicotine may exacerbate symptoms in subjects suffering from active oesophagitis, oral or pharyngeal inflammation, gastritis or peptic ulcer.

Use with caution in patients with hypertension, stable angina pectoris, cerebrovascular disease, occlusive peripheral arterial disease, heart failure, hyperthyroidism, diabetes mellitus, fructose intolerance (Please see section 6.1), pheochromocytoma and renal or hepatic impairment.

To improve the chance of successfully quitting smoking, the use of the medicated gum should be accompanied by cessation of smoking. Counselling may help smokers to quit.

Doses of nicotine that are tolerated by adult smokers during treatment may produce severe symptoms of poisoning in small children and may prove fatal (please see Section 4.9).

If denture wearers experience difficulty in chewing the gum it is recommended that they use a different pharmaceutical form of nicotine replacement therapy

4.5 Interaction with other medicinal products and other forms of Interaction
Drug Interactions: No information is available on interactions between Nicotinell gum and other drugs.

Smoking Cessation:

This is different in the case of smoking where interactions with other medications may occur due to a multitude of other substances contained in the smoke. Presumably due to the polycyclic aromatic hydrocarbons contained in the smoke, the metabolism of different medicinal products may be speeded up by enzyme induction: e.g. caffeine, theophylline, paracetamol, phenazone, phenylbutazone, pentazocine, lidocaine, benzodiazepines, imipramine, warfarin, oestrogen and vitamin B12.

Upon smoking cessation it may be expected that the hitherto increased metabolism of these medicinal products is slowed down or normalised. Unaltered dosage of the products may result in an increase in their blood concentration.

Therefore when prescribing Nicotinell a possible dose adjustment should be considered in patients treated with the above mentioned medicinal products.

Other reported effects of smoking include reduction of the analgesic effects of propoxyphene, reduced diuretic response to furosemide (frusemide), change in the pharmacological effect of propranolol and altered responder rates in ulcer healing with H_2-antagonists.

Smoking and nicotine may raise the blood levels of cortisol and catecholamines. Dose adjustment of nifedipine, adrenergic agonists or adrenergic antagonists may be necessary.

Increased subcutaneous absorption of insulin which occurs upon smoking cessation may necessitate a reduction in insulin dose.

4.6 Pregnancy and lactation
There is no adequate data from the use of preparations containing glycyrrhizin in pregnant or lactating women. Nicotinell Liquorice gum should therefore not be used during pregnancy and lactation. When use of nicotine replacement therapy is recommended (see below) the use of other flavoured gums (e.g. fruit or mint) may be considered.

Pregnancy:

In the pregnant smoker the aim should be to achieve complete cessation of smoking before the third trimester of pregnancy due to the perinatal risk. Smoking continued during the third trimester may lead to intra-uterine growth retardation or even premature birth or stillbirth, depending on the daily amount of tobacco.

Consequently,

- in pregnant women complete cessation of tobacco smoking should always be recommended without nicotine replacement therapy;
- nevertheless, in the case of failure in highly dependent pregnant smokers, tobacco withdrawal via nicotine replacement therapy may be recommended. Indeed, fetal risk is probably lower than that expected with tobacco smoking, due to:
- lower maximal plasma nicotine concentration than with inhaled nicotine
- no additional exposure to polycyclic hydrocarbons and carbon monoxide
- improved chances of quitting smoking by the third trimester

Tobacco withdrawal with or without nicotine replacement therapy should not be undertaken alone but as part of a medically supervised smoking cessation program.

In the third trimester nicotine has haemodynamic effects (e.g. changes in fetal heart rate) which could affect the foetus close to delivery. Therefore, after the sixth month of pregnancy, the gum should only be used under medical supervision in pregnant smokers who have failed to stop smoking by the third trimester.

Lactation:

Nicotine is excreted in breast milk in quantities that may affect the child even in therapeutic doses. The gum, like smoking itself, should therefore be avoided during breast feeding. Should smoking withdrawal not be achieved, use of the gum by breast feeding smokers should only be initiated after advice from a physician. Where nicotine replacement therapy is used whilst breast-feeding, the gum should be taken just after breast feeding and not during the two hours before breast feeding.

4.7 Effects on ability to drive and use machines
There is no evidence of any risks associated with driving or operating machinery when the gum is used following the recommended dose. Nevertheless one should take into consideration that smoking cessation can cause behavioural changes.

4.8 Undesirable effects
In principle, Nicotinell gum can cause adverse reactions similar to those associated with nicotine administered by smoking.

Common
CNS: headache, dizziness

GI: hiccups, gastric symptoms e.g. nausea, vomiting, indigestion, heartburn,

Local: increased salivation, irritation or sore mouth or throat, jaw muscle ache, the gum may stick to and in rare cases damage dentures and dental appliances.

Less Common
Cardiovascular: palpitations

Skin: erythema, urticaria

Rare
Cardiovascular: cardiac arrhythmias (e.g. atrial fibrillation)

Others: allergic reactions

4.9 Overdose
In overdose, symptoms corresponding to heavy smoking may be seen.

The acute lethal oral dose of nicotine is about 0.5 - 0.75 mg per kg bodyweight, corresponding in an adult to 40 - 60 mg. Even small quantities of nicotine are dangerous in children, and may result in severe symptoms of poisoning which may prove fatal. If poisoning is suspected in a child, a doctor must be consulted immediately.

Overdose with Nicotinell gum may only occur if many pieces are chewed simultaneously. Risk of overdose is small as nausea or vomiting usually occurs at an early stage. Risk of poisoning by swallowing the gum is small. Since the release of nicotine from the gum is slow, very little nicotine is absorbed from the stomach and intestine, and if any is, it will be inactivated in the liver.

General symptoms of nicotine poisoning include: weakness, perspiration, salivation, throat burn, nausea, vomiting, diarrhoea, abdominal pain, hearing and visual disturbances, headache, tachycardia and cardiac arrhythmia, dyspnoea, prostration, circulatory collapse, coma and terminal convulsions.

Treatment of overdosage:

In the event of overdosage, vomiting should be induced with syrup of ipecacuanha or gastric lavage carried out (wide bore tube). A suspension of activated charcoal should then be passed through the tube and left in the stomach. Artificial respiration with oxygen should be instituted if needed and continued for as long as necessary. Other therapy, including treatment of shock, is purely symptomatic.

5. PHARMACOLOGICAL PROPERTIES

5.1 Pharmacodynamic properties
Therapeutic classification

ATC code N07B A01

Nicotine gum mimics the pharmacological effects of nicotine from smoking, and may therefore be used to help provide relief from nicotine withdrawal symptoms. In addition to effects on the central nervous system, nicotine produces haemodynamic effects such as increased heart rate and systolic blood pressure.

5.2 Pharmacokinetic properties
When the gum is chewed, nicotine is steadily released into the mouth and is rapidly absorbed through the buccal mucosa. A proportion, by the swallowing of nicotine containing saliva, reaches the stomach and intestine where it is inactivated.

The nicotine peak plasma mean concentration after a single dose of the 2mg coatedgum is approximately 6.4 ng/ml (after 45 minutes) and approximately 9.3 ng/ml (after approximately 60 minutes) with the 4 mg gum (average plasma concentration of nicotine when smoking a cigarette is 15-30 ng/ml).

Nicotine is eliminated mainly via hepatic metabolism; small amounts of nicotine are eliminated in unchanged form via the kidneys. The plasma half-life is approximately three hours. Nicotine crosses the blood-brain barrier, the placenta and is detectable in breast milk.

5.3 Preclinical safety data
No animal studies have been undertaken on Nicotinell chewing gum.

The toxicity of nicotine as a constituent of tobacco has been well documented. Acute toxic effects include convulsions, cardiac insufficiency, and paralysis of the respiratory system.

At high doses in cats and dogs, nicotine has been shown to potentiate histamine-induced peptic ulcer.

Nicotine has no genotoxic activity in most of the mutagenicity test systems. The well-known carcinogenicity of tobacco smoking is mainly caused by pyrolysis products. Application of nicotine chewing gum, however, avoids the high temperature required for the formation of these carcinogenic products.

6. PHARMACEUTICAL PARTICULARS

6.1 List of excipients
Gum base (containing butylated hydroxytoluene), calcium carbonate, sorbitol*, sodium carbonate anhydrous, sodium hydrogen carbonate, polacrilin, glycerol, purified water, levomenthol, saccharin, sodium saccharin, acesulfame potassium, xylitol, mannitol, gelatin, titanium dioxide, carnauba wax and talc.

Nicotinell Fruit contains fruit flavouring, Nicotinell Mint contains peppermint and eucalyptus oils and Nicotinell Liquorice contains annis oil, glycyrrhizae soluble and eycalyptus oil.

*Nicotinell Fruit and Mint 2 mg and 4 mg and Nicotinell Liquorice 2 mg chewing gums contains sorbitol (E420) 0.2 g per chewing-gum, a source of 0.04 g fructose. Nicotinell

Liquorice 4 mg contains (E420) 0.2 g per chewing-gum, a source of 0.03 g fructose.

Calorific value 1.0 kcal/piece of chewing-gum.

Nicotinell gums contains sodium 11.5 mg per piece.

6.2 Incompatibilities
Not applicable

6.3 Shelf life
Nicotinell Fruit and Mint and Nicotinell Liquorice 4 mg chewing gums:- 2 years

Nicotinell Liquorice 2 mg chewing gum:- 30 months

6.4 Special precautions for storage
Do not store above 25°C

6.5 Nature and contents of container
The chewing gum is packed in PVC/aluminium blister packs each containing 12 pieces of gum.

The blisters are packed in boxes containing 12, 24 and 96 pieces of gum for the Fruit and Mint gums and 24 and 96 pieces of gum for the Liquorice gums.

6.6 Instructions for use and handling
No special requirements.

7. MARKETING AUTHORISATION HOLDER
Novartis Consumer Health

Wimblehurst Road

Horsham

West Sussex RH12 5AB

8. MARKETING AUTHORISATION NUMBER(S)
PL 0030/0162 Nicotinell Fruit 2 mg

PL 0030/0164 Nicotinell Mint 2 mg

PL 0030/0166 Nicotinell Liquorice 2 mg

PL 0030/0167 Nicotinell Liquorice 4 mg

9. DATE OF FIRST AUTHORISATION/RENEWAL OF THE AUTHORISATION
22 August 2000

10. DATE OF REVISION OF THE TEXT
Nicotinell Fruit and Mint 2 mg and 4 mg:-13 August 2002.

Nicotinell Liquorice 2 mg and 4 mg:- 15 May 2002

Legal category:
For general sale (GSL)

Nicotinell Classic Gum

(Novartis Consumer Health)

1. NAME OF THE MEDICINAL PRODUCT
Nicotinell® Classic 2 mg & 4 mg, medicated chewing-gum.

2. QUALITATIVE AND QUANTITATIVE COMPOSITION
One piece of medicated chewing-gum contains 2mg nicotine (as 10 mg nicotine – polacrilin (1:4)) or 4mg nicotine (as 20 mg nicotine – polacrilin (1:4)).

For excipients, see Section 6.1

3. PHARMACEUTICAL FORM
Medicated chewing-gum.

Each piece of coated chewing-gum is off-white in colour and rectangular in shape.

4. CLINICAL PARTICULARS
4.1 Therapeutic indications
Nicotinell treatment is indicated for the relief of nicotine withdrawal symptoms, in nicotine dependency as an aid to smoking cessation. NicotinellClassic 4mg is for use when severe withdrawal symptoms are experienced.

Advice and support normally improve the success rate.

4.2 Posology and method of administration
Adults and elderly

Nicotinell Classic medicated chewing-gum is a gum with reduced amount of flavouring. It is more appropriate for smokers who prefer the classic nicotine taste.

Users should stop smoking completely during treatment withNicotinell gum.

One piece of Nicotinell gum to be chewed when the user feels the urge to smoke.

Normally, 8-12 pieces per day, up to a maximum of 25 pieces of 2 mg gum or 15 pieces per day of 4 mg gum.

The 2mg chewing-gum may not be well suited to smokers with a strong or very strong nicotine dependency. Recommended for people smoking less than 20 cigarettes per day.

The 4mg chewing-gum is intended to be used by smokers with a strong or very strong nicotine dependency (e.g. smokers smoking more than 20 cigarettes per day) and those who have previously failed to stop smoking with the aid of nicotine replacement therapy.

The characteristics of chewing-gum as a pharmaceutical form are such that individually different nicotine levels can result in the blood. Therefore, dosage frequency should be adjusted according to individual requirements within the stated maximum limit.

Directions for use:

1. One piece of gum should be chewed until the taste becomes strong.

2. The chewing-gum should be rested between the gum and cheek.

3. When the taste fades, chewing should commence again.

4. The chewing routine should be repeated for 30 minutes.

The treatment time is individual. Normally, treatment should continue for at least 3 months.

After three months, the user should gradually cut down the number of pieces chewed each day until they have stopped using the product.

Treatment should be discontinued when the dose has been reduced to 1-2 pieces of gum per day. Use of nicotine products like Nicotinell gum beyond 6 months is generally not recommended. Some ex-smokers may need treatment with the gum for longer to avoid returning to smoking.

Counselling may help smokers to quit.

Nicotinell gum is sugar free.

Children and young adults

Nicotinell gum should not be used by people under 18 years of age without recommendation from a physician. There is no experience in treating adolescents under the age of 18 years with Nicotinell gum.

Concomitant use of acidic beverages such as coffee or soda may interfere with the buccal absorption of nicotine. Acidic beverages should be avoided for 15 minutes prior to chewing the gum.

4.3 Contraindications
Hypersensitivity to any excipients of the gum.

Nicotinell gum should not be used by non-smokers.

Use is contra-indicated in patients during the immediate post-infarction period, unstable or worsening angina pectoris (including Prinzmetal's angina), severe cardiac arrhythmias, and recent cerebrovascular accident.

4.4 Special warnings and special precautions for use
Swallowed nicotine may exacerbate symptoms in subjects suffering from active oesophagitis, oral or pharyngeal inflammation, gastritis or peptic ulcer.

Use with caution in patients with hypertension, stable angina pectoris, cerebrovascular disease, occlusive peripheral arterial disease, heart failure, hyperthyroidism, pheochromocytoma, diabetes mellitus and severe hepatic and/or renal impairment.

Doses of nicotine that are tolerated by adult smokers during treatment may produce severe symptoms of poisoning in small children and may prove fatal (please see Section 4.9).

If denture wearers experience difficulty in chewing the gum, it is recommended that they use a different pharmaceutical form of nicotine replacement therapy.

Patients with rare hereditary problems of fructose intolerance should not take this medicine.

Nicotinell Classic 2mg and 4mg coated chewing-gum contains sorbitol (E420) 0.2 g per chewing-gum and maltitol liquid 0.03 g per chewing-gum, a source of 0.04 g fructose. Calorific value 1.2 kcal/piece of chewing-gum.

Nicotinell Classic 2mg and 4mg coated chewing-gum contains sodium 11.50 mg per piece.

4.5 Interaction with other medicinal products and other forms of Interaction
Drug Interactions: No information is available on interactions between Nicotinell gum and other medicinal products.

Smoking Cessation: This is different in the case of smoking where interactions with other medications may occur due to a multitude of other substances contained in the smoke. Smoking is associated with increase in CYP1A2 activity. After cessation of smoking, reduced clearance of substrates for this enzyme may occur. Presumably due to the polycyclic aromatic hydrocarbons contained in the smoke, the metabolism of different medicinal products may be speeded up by enzyme induction: eg caffeine, theophylline, paracetamol, phenazone, phenylbutazone, pentazocine, lidocaine, benzodiazepines, olanzapine,, warfarin, oestrogen and vitamin B12.

Upon smoking cessation it may be expected that the hitherto increased metabolism of these medicinal products is slowed down or normalised. Unaltered dosage of the medicinal products may result in an increase in their blood concentration.

Therefore when using Nicotinell a possible dose reduction should be considered in patients treated with the above mentioned medicinal products.

Other reported effects of smoking include a reduction of the analgesic effects of propoxyphene, reduced diuretic response to furosemide (frusemide), change in the pharmacological effect of propranolol and altered responder rates in ulcer healing with H2-antagonists.

Smoking and nicotine may raise the blood levels of cortisol and catecholamines. Dose adjustment of nifedipine, adrenergic agonists or adrenergic antagonists may be necessary.

Increased subcutaneous absorption of insulin which occurs upon smoking cessation may necessitate a reduction in insulin dose.

4.6 Pregnancy and lactation
Pregnancy

In pregnant women complete cessation of tobacco smoking should always be recommended without nicotine replacement therapy;

Nevertheless, in the case of failure in highly dependent pregnant smokers, tobacco withdrawal via nicotine replacement therapy may be recommended. Indeed, fetal risk is probably lower than that expected with tobacco smoking, due to:

• lower maximal plasma nicotine concentration than with inhaled nicotine

• no additional exposure to polycyclic hydrocarbons and carbon monoxide

• improved chances of quitting smoking by the third trimester

Smoking continued during the third trimester may lead to intra-uterine growth retardation or even premature birth or stillbirth, depending on the daily amount of tobacco.

Tobacco withdrawal with or without nicotine replacement therapy should not be undertaken alone but as part of a medically supervised smoking cessation program.

In the third trimester nicotine has haemodynamic effects (e.g. changes in fetal heart rate) which could affect the fetus close to delivery. Therefore, after the sixth month of pregnancy, the gum should only be used under medical supervision in pregnant smokers who have failed to stop smoking by the third trimester.

Lactation

Nicotine is excreted in breast milk in quantities that may affect the child even in therapeutic doses. Nicotinell gum, like smoking itself, should therefore be avoided during breast-feeding. Should smoking withdrawal not be achieved, use of the gum by breast-feeding smokers should only be initiated after advice from a physician. Where nicotine replacement therapy is used whilst breast-feeding, the gum should be taken just after breast-feeding and not during the two hours before breast-feeding.

4.7 Effects on ability to drive and use machines
There is no evidence of any risks associated with driving or operating machinery when the gum is used following the recommended dose. Nevertheless one should take into consideration that smoking cessation can cause behavioural changes.

4.8 Undesirable effects
Nicotinell gum can cause adverse reactions similar to those associated with nicotine administered by smoking. These can be attributed to the pharmacological effects of nicotine, which are dose-dependent.

Most of the side effects which are reported by patients occur generally during the first 3-4 weeks after initiation of therapy.

Nicotine from gums may sometimes cause a slight irritation of the throat and increase salivation at the start of the treatment.

The gum may stick to and in rare cases damage dentures and dental appliances.

Common $\geq 1/100$, $<1/10$).

Nervous system disorders: headache, dizziness

Gastrointestinal disorders: hiccups, gastric symptoms e.g. nausea, vomiting, indigestion, heartburn, increased salivation, irritation or sore mouth or throat

Musculoskeletal, connective and bone disorders: jaw muscle ache.

Uncommon $\geq 1/1,000$, $<1/100$)

Cardiac disorders: palpitations

Skin and subcutaneous tissue disorders: erythema, urticaria

Rare ($<1/10,000$, $<1/1,000$).

Immune system disorders: allergic reactions

Cardiac disorders: cardiac arrhythmias (e.g. atrial fibrillation)

4.9 Overdose
In overdose, symptoms corresponding to heavy smoking may be seen.

The acute lethal oral dose of nicotine is about 0.5 - 0.75 mg per kg bodyweight, corresponding in an adult to 40 - 60 mg. Even small quantities of nicotine are dangerous in children, and may result in severe symptoms of poisoning which may prove fatal. If poisoning is suspected in a child, a doctor must be consulted immediately.

Overdose with Nicotinell gum may only occur if many pieces are chewed simultaneously. Risk of overdose is small as nausea or vomiting usually occurs at an early stage. Risk of poisoning by swallowing the gum is small. Since the release of nicotine from the gum is slow, very little nicotine is absorbed from the stomach and intestine, and if any is, it will be inactivated in the liver.

General symptoms of nicotine poisoning include: weakness, perspiration, salivation, throat burn, nausea, vomiting, diarrhoea, abdominal pain, hearing and visual disturbances, headache, tachycardia and cardiac arrhythmia, dyspnoea, prostration, circulatory collapse, coma and terminal convulsions.

Treatment of overdosage:

In the event of overdosage, vomiting should be induced with syrup of ipecacuanha or gastric lavage carried out (wide bore tube). A suspension of activated charcoal should then be passed through the tube and left in the stomach. Artificial respiration with oxygen should be instituted if needed and continued for as long as necessary. Other therapy, including treatment of shock, is purely symptomatic.

5. PHARMACOLOGICAL PROPERTIES

5.1 Pharmacodynamic properties

ATC Code N07B A01

Pharmacotherapeutic group: Drugs used in nicotine dependence

Nicotine, the primary alkaloid in tobacco products and a naturally occurring autonomous substance, is a nicotine receptor agonist in the peripheral and central nervous systems and has pronounced CNS and cardiovascular effects. On consumption of tobacco products, nicotine has proven to be addictive, resulting in craving and other withdrawal symptoms when administration is stopped. This craving and these withdrawal symptoms include a strong urge to smoke, dysphoria, insomnia, irritability, frustration or anger, anxiety, concentration difficulties agitation and increased appetite or weight gain. The gum replaces part of the nicotine that would have been administrated via tobacco and reduces the intensity of the withdrawal symptoms and smoking urge.

5.2 Pharmacokinetic properties

When the gum is chewed, nicotine is steadily released into the mouth and is rapidly absorbed through the buccal mucosa. A proportion, by the swallowing of nicotine containing saliva, reaches the stomach and intestine where it is inactivated.

The nicotine peak plasma mean concentration after a single dose of the 2mg coatedgum is approximately 6.4 ng/ml (after 45 minutes) and approximately 9.3 nanograms per ml (after approximately 60 minutes) with the 4 mg gum (average plasma concentration of nicotine when smoking a cigarette is 15-30 nanograms per ml).

Nicotine is eliminated mainly via hepatic metabolism; small amounts of nicotine are eliminated in unchanged form via the kidneys. The plasma half-life is approximately three hours. Nicotine crosses the blood-brain barrier, the placenta and is detectable in breast milk.

5.3 Preclinical safety data

There are no pre-clinical data on the safety of nicotine gums.

Nicotine was positive in some in vitro genotoxicity tests but there are also negative results with the same test systems. Nicotine was negative in in vivo tests.

Animal experiments have shown that nicotine induces post-implantation loss and reduces the growth of fetuses.

The results of carcinogenicity assays did not provide any clear evidence of a tumorigenic effect of nicotine.

6. PHARMACEUTICAL PARTICULARS

6.1 List of excipients

Gum base (containing butylated hydroxytoluene), calcium carbonate, sorbitol (E420), maltitol liquid, sodium carbonate anhydrous, sodium hydrogen carbonate, polacrilin, glycerol (E422), purified water, levomenthol, tutti flavour, xylitol, mannitol, gelatin, titanium dioxide (E171), carnauba wax and talc.

6.2 Incompatibilities

Not applicable

6.3 Shelf life

2 years

6.4 Special precautions for storage

Do not store above 25°C.

6.5 Nature and contents of container

The chewing-gum is packed in PVC/PVdC/aluminium blisters each containing 12 pieces of gum. The blisters are packed in boxes containing 24, and 96 pieces of gum.

6.6 Instructions for use and handling

No special requirements.

7. MARKETING AUTHORISATION HOLDER

Novartis Consumer Health UK Ltd

Trading as Novartis Consumer Health

Wimblehurst Road

Horsham

West Sussex

RH12 5AB

8. MARKETING AUTHORISATION NUMBER(S)

Nicotinell® Classic 2 mg, medicated chewing-gum PL 00030/0207

Nicotinell® Classic 4 mg, medicated chewing-gum PL 00030/0208

9. DATE OF FIRST AUTHORISATION/RENEWAL OF THE AUTHORISATION

15 April 2003

10. DATE OF REVISION OF THE TEXT

August 16, 2004

Scheduling status GSL

Nicotinell Lozenges

(Novartis Consumer Health)

1. NAME OF THE MEDICINAL PRODUCT

Nicotinell® Mint 1 mg Lozenge

Nicotinell® Mint 2 mg Lozenge

2. QUALITATIVE AND QUANTITATIVE COMPOSITION

Each lozenge contains either 1 mg nicotine or 2 mg nicotine corresponding to 3.072 mg or 6.144 mg nicotine bitartrate dehydrate respectively)

(For excipients see section 6.1)

3. PHARMACEUTICAL FORM

Lozenge

White, mint flavoured, round biconvex lozenge

4. CLINICAL PARTICULARS

4.1 Therapeutic indications

Relief of nicotine withdrawal symptoms, in nicotine dependency as an aid to smoking cessation.

Advice and support normally improve the success rate.

4.2 Posology and method of administration

Nicotinell® Mint 2 mg lozenge is intended to be used by smokers with a strong nicotine dependency (e.g. smokers smoking more than 30 cigarettes per day)or those who have previously failed to stop smoking with the aid of Nicotinell Mint 1 mg lozenge.

In medium nicotine dependency it is recommended to use the 1 mg lozenge.

Simultaneous use of coffee, acid drinks or soft drinks may decrease the absorption of nicotine in the oral cavity. These drinks should be avoided for 15 minutes prior to sucking the lozenge.

Children and young adults

Nicotinell® Lozenges should not be administered to persons under 18 years of age without recommendation from a physician. There is no experience in treating adolescents under the age of 18 with Nicotinell Lozenges.

Adults and elderly

The initial dosage should be individualised on the basis of the patient's nicotine dependence. One lozenge to be sucked when the user feels the urge to smoke.

Initially, 1 lozenge should be taken every 1-2 hours. The usual dosage is 8-12 lozenges per day. The maximum daily dose is 30 of the 1 mg lozenges or 15 of the 2 mg lozenges.

Smokers are advised to quit smoking when they start using Nicotinell Lozenge.

Directions for use:

1. One lozenge to be sucked until the taste becomes strong.
2. The lozenge should then be lodged between the gum and cheek.
3. When the taste fades, sucking of the lozenge should commence again
4. The sucking routine will be adapted individually and should be repeated until the lozenge dissolves completely (about 30 minutes)

The treatment time is individual. Normally, treatment should continue for at least 3 months. After 3 months, the user should gradually reduce the number of lozenges or alternatively the user is taking the 2 mg lozenge they should switch to 1 mg lozenges and then gradually reduce the number of lozenges per day.

Treatment should be discontinued when the dose has been reduced to 1-2 lozenges per day. Use of nicotine products, like Nicotinell Lozenge, beyond 6 months is generally not recommended. Some ex-smokers may need treatment with the lozenge longer to avoid returning to smoking.

Nicotinell Mint Lozenges are sugar-free.

4.3 Contraindications

Hypersensitivity to any excipients of the lozenge.

Nicotinell Mint Lozenge should not be used by non-smokers.

Use is contraindicated in patients during the immediate post-infarction period, unstable or worsening angina pectoris (including Prinzmetal's angina), severe cardiac arrhythmias and recent cerebrovascular accident.

4.4 Special warnings and special precautions for use

Nicotine can stimulate the production of adrenaline. Nicotinell® Mint Lozenge should be used with caution in patients with uncontrolled hypertension, stable angina pectoris, cerebrovascular disease, occlusive peripheral arterial disease, heart failure, diabetes mellitus, hyperthyroidism or phaeochromocytoma and severe hepatic and/or renal impairment.

Swallowed nicotine may exacerbate symptoms in patients suffering from active oesophagitis, oral and pharyngeal inflammation, gastritis or peptic ulcer.

Nicotinell Mint lozenge contains aspartame which metabolises to phenylalanine, equivalent to 5 mg/dose, which is of relevance for patients with phenylketonuria.

4.5 Interaction with other medicinal products and other forms of Interaction

Smoking is associated with increase in CYP1A2 activity. After cessation of smoking, reduced clearance of substrates for this enzyme may occur. This may lead to an increase in plasma levels for some medicinal products of potential clinical importance for products with a narrow therapeutic window, e.g. theophylline, tacrine and clozapine.

The plasma concentration of other drugs metabolised in part by CYP1A2 e.g. imipramine, olanzapine, clomipramine and fluvoxamine may also increase on cessation of smoking, although data to support this are lacking and the possible clinical significance of this effect for these drugs is unknown.

Limited data indicate that the metabolism of flecainide and pentazocine may also be induced by smoking.

4.6 Pregnancy and lactation

Pregnancy

In the pregnant smoker the aim should be to achieve complete cessation of smoking before the third trimester of pregnancy due to the perinatal risk. Smoking continued during the third trimester may lead to intra-uterine growth retardation or even premature birth or stillbirth, depending on the daily amount of tobacco.

Consequently,

- in pregnant women complete cessation of tobacco smoking should always be recommended without nicotine replacement therapy;
- nevertheless, in the case of failure in highly dependent pregnant smokers, tobacco withdrawal via nicotine replacement therapy may be recommended. Indeed, fetal risk is probably lower than that expected with tobacco smoking, due to:
- lower maximal plasma nicotine concentration than with inhaled nicotine
- no additional exposure to polycyclic hydrocarbons and carbon monoxide
- improved chances of quitting smoking by the third trimester

Tobacco withdrawal with or without nicotine replacement therapy should not be undertaken alone but as part of a medically supervised smoking cessation program.

In the third trimester nicotine has haemodynamic effects (e.g. changes in fetal heart rate) which could affect the foetus close to delivery. In view of this, the lozenge should only be used after the sixth month of pregnancy under medical supervision in pregnant smokers who have failed to stop smoking by the third trimester.

Lactation:

Nicotine is excreted in breast milk in quantities that may affect the child even in therapeutic doses. The lozenge, like smoking itself, should therefore be avoided during breast feeding. Should smoking withdrawal not be achieved, use of the lozenge by breast feeding smokers should only be initiated after advice from a physician. Where nicotine replacement therapy is used whilst breast-feeding, the lozenge should be taken just after breast feeding and not during the two hours before breast feeding.

4.7 Effects on ability to drive and use machines

Smoking cessation can cause behavioural changes. There is no evidence of any risks associated with driving or operating machinery when the lozenge is used following the recommended dose.

4.8 Undesirable effects

Nicotinell Mint Lozenge can cause adverse reactions similar to those associated with nicotine administered in other ways. These can be attributed to the pharmacological effects of nicotine, which are dose-dependent.

Most of the side effects which are reported by patients occur generally during the first 3-4 weeks after initiation of therapy.

Nicotine from lozenges may sometimes cause a slight irritation of the throat and increase salivation at the start of the treatment. Excessive swallowing of nicotine which is released in the saliva may, at first, cause hiccups. Those with a tendency to indigestion may suffer initially from slight dyspepsia or heartburn.

Slower sucking will usually overcome this problem.

Excessive consumption of lozenges by subjects who have not been in the habit of inhaling tobacco smoke, could possibly lead to nausea, faintness and headache.

Common (>1/100)

General: Dizziness, headache

GI: Nausea, flatulence, hiccups, epigastritis, dryness of the mouth and irritation of the oral cavity and oesophagus.

Less common (1/100-1/1000)

Circ.: Palpitation

Rare (<1/1000)

Circ: Atrium arrhythmia.

Certain symptoms which have been reported such as dizziness, headache and insomnia may be ascribed to withdrawal symptoms in connection with smoking cessation and may be due to insufficient administration of nicotine.

Cold sores may develop in connection with smoking cessation, but any relation with the nicotine treatment is unclear. The patient may still experience nicotine dependence after smoking cessation.

4.9 Overdose

In overdose, symptoms corresponding to heavy smoking may be seen.

The acute lethal oral dose of nicotine is about 0.5 - 0.75 mg per kg body weight, corresponding in an adult to 40 - 60 mg. Even small quantities of nicotine are dangerous in children, and may result in severe symptoms of poisoning which may prove fatal. If poisoning is suspected in a child, a doctor must be consulted immediately.

Overdose with Nicotinell Mint Lozenges may only occur if many pieces are sucked simultaneously. Risk of overdose is small as nausea or vomiting usually occurs at an early stage.

General symptoms of nicotine poisoning include: weakness, perspiration, salivation, throat burn, nausea, vomiting, diarrhoea, abdominal pain, hearing and visual disturbances, headache, tachycardia and cardiac arrhythmia, dyspnoea, prostration, circulatory collapse, coma and terminal convulsions.

Treatment of overdosage:

In the event of overdosage, vomiting should be induced with syrup of ipecacuanha or gastric lavage carried out (wide bore tube). A suspension of activated charcoal should then be passed through the tube and left in the stomach. Artificial respiration with oxygen should be instituted if needed and continued for as long as necessary. Other therapy, including treatment of shock, is purely symptomatic.

5. PHARMACOLOGICAL PROPERTIES

5.1 Pharmacodynamic properties

Therapeutic classification

ATC code: N07B A01

Nicotinell Mint Lozenges mimics the pharmacological effects of nicotine from smoking. Clinical studies have shown that nicotine replacement products can help smokers abstain from smoking by relieving these withdrawal symptoms.

5.2 Pharmacokinetic properties

The absorbed amount of nicotine depends on the amount released into the mouth and absorbed through the buccal mucosa.

The main part of nicotine in Nicotinell Mint Lozenge is absorbed through the buccal mucosa. A proportion, by the swallowing of nicotine containing saliva, reaches the stomach and intestine where it is inactivated. Due to the first-pass effect in the liver, the systemic bioavailability of nicotine is low. Consequently, in the treatment with Nicotinell Mint Lozenge the high and quick systemic nicotine concentration, as seen when smoking, is rarely obtained.

Distribution volume after i.v. administration of nicotine is approximately (2-)3 l/kg and the half-life is 2 hours. Nicotine is metabolised principally in the liver and the plasma clearance is reached within approximately 1.2 l/min; nicotine also metabolises in the kidney and lungs. Nicotine crosses the blood-brain barrier.

More than 20 metabolites have been identified, all believed to be less active than nicotine. The main metabolite is cotinine which has a half-life of 15-20 hours and with approximately 10 times higher plasma concentration than nicotine. Nicotine's plasma-protein binding is less than 5%. Changes in nicotine binding from the use of concomitant drugs or due to altered disease state are not expected to have significant effect on nicotine kinetics. The main metabolite in urine is cotinine (15% of the dose) and trans-3-hydroxy cotinine (45% of the dose).

About 10% of the nicotine is excreted unchanged. Up to 30% may be excreted with urine in increased diuresis and the acidity under pH 5.

The peak value for the plasma concentration of 1 mg lozenge after a single dose is approximately 4 nanogram per ml and the maximal concentration at steady state is approximately 10.6 nanogram per ml (average plasma concentration of nicotine after smoking one cigarette is 15-30 nanogram per ml). Peak plasma concentration is reached after about 45 minutes following sucking of a single lozenge and after about 30 minutes at steady state.

The peak value for the plasma concentration of 2 mg lozenge after a single dose is approximately 7.0 nanogram per ml and the maximal concentration at steady state (one 2 mg lozenge/hour for 12 hours)is approximately 22.5 nanogram per ml (average plasma concentration of nicotine after smoking one cigarette is 15-30 nanogram per ml). Peak plasma concentration is reached after about 48 minutes following sucking of a single lozenge and after about 30 minutes at steady state.

Studies have demonstrated that there is a linear dose-concentration proportionality between the 1mg and 2 mg Nicotinell Mint lozenges for both C_{max} and AUC. The T_{max} are similar for both strengths.

5.3 Preclinical safety data

There are no pre-clinical data on the safety of nicotine lozenges.

Although most of the genotoxic tests carried out showed negative results, some of them were positive so, no definite conclusion can be drawn on the genotoxic activity of nicotine.

Epidemiological studies have shown a certain correlation between smoking and a reduced growth and development of the foetus. Animal experiments have identified the nicotine in tobacco smoke to be mainly responsible for these effects, as it induces post-implantation loss and reduces the growth of foetuses.

The results of carcinogenicity assays did not provide any clear evidence of a tumorigenic effect of nicotine.

6. PHARMACEUTICAL PARTICULARS

6.1 List of excipients

Maltitol, sodium carbonate, sodium hydrogen carbonate, polyacrylate dispersion 30%, xanthan gum, colloidal anhydrous silica, levomenthol, peppermint oil, aspartame, magnesium stearate.

6.2 Incompatibilities

Not applicable

6.3 Shelf life

36 months

6.4 Special precautions for storage

Do not store above 25°C. Store in the original package.

6.5 Nature and contents of container

12, 36, 96 lozenges inopaque blister packs.

6.6 Instructions for use and handling

Not applicable

7. MARKETING AUTHORISATION HOLDER

Novartis Consumer Health UK Ltd

Trading as Novartis Consumer Health

Wimblehurst Road

Horsham

West Sussex RH12 5AB

8. MARKETING AUTHORISATION NUMBER(S)

Nicotinell Mint 1 mg Lozenge:- PL 0030/0146

Nicotinell Mint 2 mg Lozenge:- PL 0030/0202

9. DATE OF FIRST AUTHORISATION/RENEWAL OF THE AUTHORISATION

Nicotinell Mint 1 mg Lozenge:- 20 July 1999

Nicotinell Mint 2 mg Lozenge:- 9 April 2003

10. DATE OF REVISION OF THE TEXT

Nicotinell Mint 1 mg Lozenge:- 26 March 2002

Legal category:

General Sales List

Nicotinell Patches

(Novartis Consumer Health)

1. NAME OF THE MEDICINAL PRODUCT

Nicotinell TTS 10

Nicotinell TTS 20

Nicotinell TTS 30

2. QUALITATIVE AND QUANTITATIVE COMPOSITION

Each Nicotinell TTS 10 patch contains S(-)-nicotine 17.5 mg; each Nicotinell TTS 20 patch contains S(-)-nicotine 35 mg; each Nicotinell TTS 30 patch contains S(-)-nicotine 52.5 mg.

3. PHARMACEUTICAL FORM

Transdermal patch.

Nicotinell is a transdermal therapeutic system, consisting of a round, flat, matrix-type self-adhesive, yellowish-ochre coloured patch. It is protected by a rectangular metallic release liner backing to be discarded before application.

Nicotinell TTS 10 has a drug releasing area of 10 cm^2 and is printed CG CWC on the patch surface. Nicotinell TTS 20 has a drug releasing area of 20 cm^2 and is printed CG FEF on the patch surface. Nicotinell TTS 30 has a drug releasing area of 30 cm^2 and is printed CG EME on the patch surface.

4. CLINICAL PARTICULARS

4.1 Therapeutic indications

The treatment of nicotine dependence, as an aid to smoking cessation.

Route of administration: transdermal.

4.2 Posology and method of administration

Adults: Users should stop smoking completely during treatment with Nicotinell TTS.

For individuals smoking 20 cigarettes or more a day, it is recommended that treatment be started with Nicotinell TTS 30 (Step 1) once daily, applied to a dry non-hairy area of the skin on the trunk or upper arm. Those smoking less than this are recommended to start with Nicotinell TTS 20 (Step 2). Sizes of $30cm^2$, $20cm^2$ and $10cm^2$ are available to permit gradual withdrawal of nicotine replacement, using treatment periods of 3-4 weeks (for each size). The size of patch may be adjusted according to individual response, maintaining or increasing the dose if abstinence is not achieved or if withdrawal symptoms are experienced. Total treatment periods of more than 3 months and daily doses above $30cm^2$ have not been evaluated. The treatment is designed to be used continuously for 3 months but not beyond. However, if abstinence is not achieved at the end of the 3 month treatment period, further treatments may be recommended following a re-evaluation of the patient's motivation by the doctor.

The dosage must not be adjusted by cutting a patch.

Nicotinell TTS should be used as soon as it has been removed from the child-resistant pouch. Following removal of the metallic backing, the Nicotinell TTS patch should be applied to the skin and held in position for 10-20 seconds with the palm of the hand. Each patch should be removed after 24 hours and disposed of safely (see "Warnings"). A different site of application should be chosen each day and several days should be allowed to elapse before a new patch is applied to the same area of skin.

Children & young adults:

Nicotinell TTS should not be administered to persons under 18 years of age without recommendation from a physician. There is no experience in treating adolescents under the age of 18 with Nicotinell TTS.

Elderly:

Experience in the use of Nicotinell TTS in smokers over the age of 65 years is limited. Nicotinell TTS does not appear to pose safety problems in this age group.

Potential for abuse and dependence:

Transdermal nicotine is likely to have a very low abuse potential because of its slow onset of action, low fluctuations in blood concentrations, inability to produce high blood concentrations of nicotine, and the infrequent (once daily) use. Moreover, gradual weaning from Nicotinell TTS is instituted within the treatment schedule, and the risk of dependence after therapy is minimal. The effects of abrupt withdrawal from Nicotinell TTS are likely to be similar to those observed with tobacco withdrawal from comparable nicotine concentrations.

4.3 Contraindications

Nicotinell TTS should not be administered to non-smokers or occasional smokers. The system is also contra-indicated in acute myocardial infarction, unstable or worsening angina pectoris, severe cardiac arrhythmias, recent cerebrovascular accident, diseases of the skin which may complicate patch therapy, and known hypersensitivity to nicotine or any of the components of the patch.

4.4 Special warnings and special precautions for use

Warnings: Nicotine is a toxic drug and milligram doses are potentially fatal if rapidly absorbed. Treatment with Nicotinell TTS should be discontinued if symptoms of nicotine overdosage appear. Mild intoxication produces nausea, vomiting, abdominal pain, diarrhoea, headache, sweating and pallor (see 'Overdosage').

Doses of nicotine that are tolerated by adult smokers during treatment can produce severe symptoms of poisoning in small children and may prove fatal. Both before and after use, Nicotinell TTS contains a significant amount of nicotine. Subjects must be cautioned that the patches must not be handled casually or left where they might be inadvertently misused or consumed by children. Used patches must be disposed of with care by folding them in half with the adhesive sides inwards, and ensuring that they do not fall into the hands of children under any circumstances.

Precautions: Users should stop smoking completely during therapy with Nicotinell TTS. They should be informed that if they continue to smoke while using Nicotinell TTS, they may experience increased adverse effects due to the hazards of smoking, including cardiovascular effects.

In subjects with the conditions listed below, Nicotinell TTS should only be used following a careful risk-benefit assessment, and only in cases where subjects have found it impossible to stop smoking without use of Nicotinell TTS: hypertension, stable angina pectoris, cerebrovascular disease, occlusive peripheral arterial disease, heart failure, hyperthyroidism, diabetes mellitus, renal or hepatic impairment and peptic ulcer.

Discontinuation of treatment may be advisable in cases of severe or persistent skin reactions.

Contact sensitisation was reported in a few patients using transdermal nicotine in clinical trials. Patients who develop contact sensitisation to nicotine should be cautioned that a severe reaction could occur from smoking or exposure to other nicotine containing products.

4.5 Interaction with other medicinal products and other forms of Interaction

No information is available on interactions between Nicotinell TTS and other drugs.

Cessation of smoking, with or without nicotine replacement, may alter the individual's response to concomitant medication and may require adjustment of dose. Smoking is thought to increase the metabolism through enzyme induction and thus to lower the blood concentrations of drugs such as antipyrine, caffeine, oestrogens, desmethyldiazepam, imipramine, lignocaine, oxazepam, pentazocine, phenacetin, theophylline, and warfarin. Cessation of smoking may result in increased concentrations of these drugs.

Other reported effects of smoking include reduced analgesic efficacy of propoxyphene, reduced diuretic response to frusemide and reduced pharmacological response to propranolol, as well as reduced rates of ulcer healing with H_2-antagonists.

Both smoking and nicotine can increase levels of circulating cortisol and catecholamines. Dosages of nifedipine, adrenergic agonists, or adrenergic blocking agents may need to be adjusted.

4.6 Pregnancy and lactation

Patients should be advised to give up smoking without the use of nicotine replacement therapy. Should this fail, a medical assessment of the risk benefit of Nicotinell TTS should be made.

Teratogenicity studies with nicotine in several animal species have demonstrated non-specific retardation of foetal growth. Studies in pregnant rats have indicated the presence of behavioural disorders in the offspring, and in the mouse the unborn offspring of animals treated with approximately 120 times the human transdermal dose showed skeletal defects in the peripheral parts of the limbs. Embryo implantation in rats and rabbits may be inhibited or delayed by nicotine. Overall, there are no clear cut grounds for believing that nicotine at the concentrations reached by treatment with Nicotinell TTS has any teratogenic potential and/or inhibitory effects on fertility.

4.7 Effects on ability to drive and use machines

When Nicotinell TTS is used as recommended, there are minimal risks for driving vehicles or operating machinery.

4.8 Undesirable effects

In principle, Nicotinell TTS can cause adverse reactions similar to those associated with nicotine administered by smoking. Since the maximum plasma concentrations of nicotine that are produced by Nicotinell TTS are lower than those produced by smoking and fluctuate less, nicotine-related adverse reactions occurring during treatment with Nicotinell TTS can be expected to be less marked than during smoking.

Some of the symptoms listed below are hard to differentiate from recognised tobacco withdrawal symptoms when comparison with placebo is made. The placebo used contained about 13% of the nicotine of a matching Nicotinell TTS (to match colour and odour for blinding purposes).

The main unwanted effect of Nicotinell TTS is application site reaction. This led to premature discontinuation of Nicotinell TTS in about 6% of clinical trial participants. Skin reactions consisted of erythema or pruritus at the patch site. Oedema, burning sensation, blisters, rash, or pinching sensation at the application site was also noted. The majority of these reactions were mild. Most of the skin reactions resolved within 48 hours, but in more severe cases the erythema and infiltration lasted from 1 to 3 weeks. The time of onset of important skin reactions was between 3 and 8 weeks from the start of therapy. In isolated cases the skin reactions extended beyond the application sites. Isolated cases of urticaria, angioneurotic oedema and dyspnoea were reported.

The following are the adverse events/withdrawal symptoms most commonly reported in three double-blind clinical trials <u>irrespective of causal association to study drug</u>.

	Nicotinell TTS (N=401)	Placebo (N=391)
Application site reaction	34.9%	17.6%
Headache	29.7%	29.2%
Cold and flu-like symptoms	12.0%	8.4%
Dysmenorrhoea (% of female subjects)	6.6%	8.8%
Insomnia	6.5%	5.4%
Nausea	6.2%	4.6%
Myalgia	6.0%	4.1%
Dizziness	6.0%	5.9%

Other unwanted experiences reported (irrespective of causal association with Nicotinell TTS) with an incidence of 1% - 5.9% and more frequently than placebo, included: abdominal pain, vomiting, dyspepsia, allergy, motor dysfunction, chest pain, vivid dreams, blood pressure changes, generalised rash, somnolence, impaired concentration and fatigue.

4.9 Overdose

The toxicity of nicotine cannot be directly compared with that of smoking, because tobacco smoke contains additional toxic substances (e.g. carbon monoxide, and tar).

Chronic smokers can tolerate doses of nicotine that, in a non-smoker, would be more toxic, because of the development of tolerance.

Application of several Nicotinell TTS patches could result in serious overdosage. Slower absorption after cutaneous exposure to nicotine favours the development of tolerance to toxic effects.

Rapid systemic delivery of nicotine from Nicotinell TTS would not be expected on chewing and swallowing, owing to the slow release of nicotine from the patch and first-pass metabolism.

Acute toxic effects*:* Signs and symptoms of overdosage would be the same as those of acute nicotine poisoning. In non-smoking children and adults, these include pallor, sweating, nausea, salivation, vomiting, abdominal cramps, diarrhoea, headache, dizziness, hearing and vision disturbances, tremor, mental confusion, muscle weakness, convulsions, prostration, absence of neurological reaction, and respiratory failure. Lethal doses may produce convulsions, and death follows as a result of peripheral or central respiratory paralysis, or, less frequently, cardiac failure.

The acute lethal oral dose of nicotine in non-smoking adults is approximately 60mg.

Management: If the patient shows signs of overdosage, Nicotinell TTS should be removed immediately. The skin surface may be washed with water and dried (no soap should be used). The skin will continue to deliver nicotine into the blood stream for several hours after removal of the system, possibly because of a depot of nicotine in the skin.

Other treatment measures for acute nicotine poisoning include artificial respiration in the case of respiratory paralysis, maintaining normal body temperature, and treatment of hypotension and cardiovascular collapse.

Each Nicotinell TTS patch is sealed in a child-resistant sachet and the product must be kept out of the reach of children at all times (see "Warnings"). Even doses of nicotine which are tolerated by adults during treatment with Nicotinell TTS could produce severe symptoms of poisoning in small children following accidental application, and may prove fatal.

5. PHARMACOLOGICAL PROPERTIES

5.1 Pharmacodynamic properties

S(-)-nicotine is the most pharmacologically active form of nicotine, the major alkaloid of tobacco. S(-)-nicotine acts primarily on cholinergic receptors of the nicotinic type in the peripheral and central nervous system. For many effects, low doses of S(-)-nicotine have a stimulant action, and high doses a depressant effect. Intermittent administration of S(-)-nicotine affects neurohormonal pathways, and results in the release of acetylcholine, noradrenaline, dopamine, serotinin, vasopressin, beta-endorphin, growth hormone, cortisol and ACTH. These neuroregulators may be involved in the reported behavioural and subjective effects of smoking.

Nicotine replacement is an established therapy as an aid to smoking cessation. Nicotinell TTS provides for a convenient once daily administration by exploiting the fact that S(-)-nicotine is readily absorbed through the skin into the systemic circulation. Placebo-controlled, double-blind studies have shown that nicotine replacement with Nicotinell TTS produces smoking abstinence rates statistically significantly better than placebo, with or without group support. There was also a strong trend towards reduction of withdrawal symptoms.

Application of Nicotinell TTS 20 to smokers abstinent overnight resulted in small increases in mean heart rate and systolic blood pressure and a decrease in stroke volume. The effects were smaller in magnitude than those produced by cigarette smoking.

5.2 Pharmacokinetic properties

Following single application of Nicotinell TTS to the skin of healthy abstinent smokers there is an initial 1-2 hours delay followed by a progressive rise in nicotine plasma concentrations, with a plateau attained at about 8-10 hours after application.

In the majority of subjects the area under the plasma concentration curve (AUC 0-24 hours) varies approximately in proportion to the drug releasing area of the patch. Nicotinell TTS is designed to deliver approximately 0.7mg/cm^2/24 hours. In comparison with an i.v. infusion, 76.8% of the nicotine released from Nicotinell TTS is systemically available. Steady state plasma concentrations after repeated daily administration are within the range observed during moderate cigarette smoking.

Absorption of nicotine over 24 hours varies by a factor of two between different individuals; however within-individual variability is small indicating consistent performance of the transdermal system.

S(-)-nicotine is distributed widely in the body with a volume of distribution of approximately 180 litres. It crosses the blood-brain barrier, placenta and is detectable in breast milk. Plasma protein binding is only 5%. Total plasma clearance of nicotine ranges from 0.92 to 2.43 litres/min. It is eliminated mainly via hepatic metabolism. Only small amounts of nicotine are eliminated in unchanged form via the kidneys, a process which is pH dependent, being negligible under alkaline conditions.

5.3 Preclinical safety data

No additional data.

6. PHARMACEUTICAL PARTICULARS

6.1 List of excipients

Pad

Polyester film

Acrylate esters vinylacetate co-polymers

Fractionated coconut oil

Methacrylic acid esters co-polymers.

Aluminised polyester backing film

Aluminised and siliconised polyester film release liner

6.2 Incompatibilities

None known.

6.3 Shelf life

24 months.

6.4 Special precautions for storage

Do not store above 25°C.

6.5 Nature and contents of container

Heat-seal paper/aluminium/polyamide/polyacrylnitrile pouches (child-resistant) enclosed in a cardboard carton.

Pack sizes:

Nicotinell TTS 10: 7 day supply

Nicotinell TTS 20: 2 and 7 day supply

Nicotinell TTS 30: 2, 7 and 21 day supply

6.6 Instructions for use and handling

Keep all medicines out of the reach of children.

7. MARKETING AUTHORISATION HOLDER

Novartis Consumer Health

Wimblehurst Road

Horsham

West Sussex

RH12 5AB

8. MARKETING AUTHORISATION NUMBER(S)

Nicotinell TTS 10: PL 00030/0107

Nicotinell TTS 20: PL 00030/0108

Nicotinell TTS 30: PL 00030/0109

9. DATE OF FIRST AUTHORISATION/RENEWAL OF THE AUTHORISATION

Original grant date: 1 August 1997

Renewed: 11 February 2003

10. DATE OF REVISION OF THE TEXT

Legal category:

General Sales List

Nimbex Forte Injection 5mg/ml

(GlaxoSmithKline UK)

1. NAME OF THE MEDICINAL PRODUCT

NIMBEX® FORTE 5mg/ml, solution for injection.

2. QUALITATIVE AND QUANTITATIVE COMPOSITION

Cisatracurium 5mg as cisatracurium besilate 6.70mg per 1ml

One vial of 30ml contains 150mg of cisatracurium

For excipients, see Section 6.1.

3. PHARMACEUTICAL FORM

Solution for Injection.

4. CLINICAL PARTICULARS

NIMBEX is an intermediate-duration, non-depolarising neuromuscular blocking agent for intravenous administration.

4.1 Therapeutic indications

NIMBEX is indicated for use during surgical and other procedures and in intensive care. NIMBEX can be used as an adjunct to general anaesthesia, or sedation in the Intensive Care Unit (ICU) to relax skeletal muscles, and to facilitate tracheal intubation and mechanical ventilation.

4.2 Posology and method of administration

Please note that NIMBEX should not be mixed in the same syringe or administered simultaneously through the same needle as propofol injectable emulsion or with alkaline solutions such as sodium thiopentone. (Please refer to section 6.2 for details of incompatibilities).

NIMBEX contains no antimicrobial preservative and is intended for single patient use.

4.2.1 Monitoring advice

As with other neuromuscular blocking agents, monitoring of neuromuscular function is recommended during the use of NIMBEX in order to individualise dosage requirements.

4.2.2 Use by intravenous bolus injection

4.2.2.1 Dosage in adults

Tracheal Intubation. The recommended intubation dose of NIMBEX for adults is 0.15mg/kg (body weight). This dose produced good to excellent conditions for tracheal intubation 120 seconds after administration of NIMBEX, following induction of anaesthesia with propofol.

Higher doses will shorten the time to onset of neuromuscular block.

Table 1

Initial NIMBEX Dose mg/kg (body weight)	Anaesthetic Background	Time to 90% T1* Suppression (min)	Time to Maximum T1* Suppression (min)	Time to 25% Spontaneous T1* Recovery (min)
0.1	Opioid	3.4	4.8	45
0.15	Propofol	2.6	3.5	55
0.2	Opioid	2.4	2.9	65
0.4	Opioid	1.5	1.9	91

* T_1 Single twitch response as well as the first component of the Train-of-four response of the adductor pollicis muscle following supramaximal electrical stimulation of the ulnar nerve.

The following table summarises mean pharmacodynamic data when NIMBEX was administered at doses of 0.1 to 0.4mg/kg (body weight) to healthy adult patients during opioid (thiopentone/fentanyl/midazolam) or propofol anaesthesia.

(see Table 1 above)

Enflurane or isoflurane anaesthesia may extend the clinically effective duration of an initial dose of NIMBEX by as much as 15%.

Maintenance. Neuromuscular block can be extended with maintenance doses of NIMBEX. A dose of 0.03 mg/kg (body weight) provides approximately 20 minutes of additional clinically effective neuromuscular block during opioid or propofol anaesthesia.

Consecutive maintenance doses do not result in progressive prolongation of effect.

Spontaneous Recovery. Once spontaneous recovery from neuromuscular block is underway, the rate is independent of the NIMBEX dose administered. During opioid or propofol anaesthesia, the median times from 25 to 75% and from 5 to 95% recovery are approximately 13 and 30 minutes, respectively.

Reversal. Neuromuscular block following NIMBEX administration is readily reversible with standard doses of anticholinesterase agents. The mean times from 25 to 75% recovery and to full clinical recovery (T_4:T_1 ratio ≥ 0.7) are approximately 4 and 9 minutes respectively, following administration of the reversal agent at an average of 10% T_1 recovery.

4.2.2.2 Dosage in paediatric patients

Tracheal Intubation (paediatric patients aged 1 month to 12 years): As in adults, the recommended intubation dose of NIMBEX is 0.15 mg/kg (body weight) administered rapidly over 5 to 10 seconds. This dose produces good to excellent conditions for tracheal intubation 120 seconds following injection of NIMBEX. Pharmacodynamic data for this dose are presented in the tables below.

NIMBEX has not been studied for intubation in ASA Class III-IV paediatric patients. There are limited data on the use of NIMBEX in paediatric patients under 2 years of age undergoing prolonged or major surgery.

In paediatric patients aged 1 month to 12 years, NIMBEX has a shorter clinically effective duration and a faster spontaneous recovery profile than those observed in adults under similar anaesthetic conditions. Small differences in the pharmacodynamic profile were observed between the age ranges 1 to 11 months and 1 to 12 years which are summarised in the tables below.

Paediatric Patients aged 1 to 11 months

(see Table 2 below)

Paediatric Patients aged 1 to 12 years

(see Table 3 below)

When NIMBEX is not required for intubation: A dose of less than 0.15mg/kg can be used. Pharmacodynamic data for doses of 0.08 and 0.1 mg/kg for paediatric patients aged 2 to 12 years are presented in the table below:

(see Table 4 below)

Administration of NIMBEX following suxamethonium has not been studied in paediatric patients (see section 4.5 Interaction with Other Medicaments and Other Forms of Interaction).

Halothane may be expected to extend the clinically effective duration of a dose of NIMBEX by up to 20%. No information is available on the use of NIMBEX in children during anaesthesia with other halogenated fluorocarbon anaesthetic agents, but these agents may also be expected to extend the clinically effective duration of a dose of NIMBEX.

Maintenance (paediatric patients aged 2-12 years). Neuromuscular block can be extended with maintenance doses of NIMBEX. In paediatric patients aged 2 to 12 years, a dose of 0.02 mg/kg (body weight) provides approximately 9 minutes of additional clinically effective neuromuscular block during halothane anaesthesia. Consecutive maintenance doses do not result in progressive prolongation of effect.

There are insufficient data to make a specific recommendation for maintenance dosing in paediatric patients under 2 years of age. However, very limited data from clinical studies in paediatric patients under 2 years of age suggest that a maintenance dose of 0.03mg/kg may extend clinically effective neuromuscular block for a period of up to 25 minutes during opioid anaesthesia.

Spontaneous Recovery. Once recovery from neuromuscular block is underway, the rate is independent of the NIMBEX dose administered. During opioid or halothane anaesthesia, the median times from 25 to 75% and from 5 to 95% recovery are approximately 11 and 28 minutes, respectively.

Reversal. Neuromuscular block following NIMBEX administration is readily reversible with standard doses of anticholinesterase agents. The mean times from 25 to 75% recovery and to full clinical recovery (T_4:T_1 ratio ≥ 0.7) are approximately 2 and 5 minutes respectively, following administration of the reversal agent at an average of 13% T_1 recovery.

4.2.3 Use by intravenous infusion

4.2.3.1 Dosage in adults and children aged 2 to 12 years

Maintenance of neuromuscular block may be achieved by infusion of NIMBEX. An initial infusion rate of 3 μg/kg (body weight)/min (0.18 mg/kg/hr) is recommended to restore 89 to 99% T_1 suppression following evidence of spontaneous recovery. After an initial period of stabilisation of neuromuscular block, a rate of 1 to 2 μg/kg (body weight)/min (0.06 to 0.12 mg/kg/hr) should be adequate to maintain block in this range in most patients.

Reduction of the infusion rate by up to 40% may be required when NIMBEX is administered during isoflurane or enflurane anaesthesia.(See Section 4.5).

The infusion rate will depend upon the concentration of cisatracurium in the infusion solution, the desired degree of neuromuscular block, and the patient's weight. The following table provides guidelines for delivery of undiluted NIMBEX.

Infusion Delivery Rate of NIMBEX injection 2mg/ml

(see Table 5)

Steady rate continuous infusion of NIMBEX is not associated with a progressive increase or decrease in neuromuscular blocking effect.

Following discontinuation of infusion of NIMBEX, spontaneous recovery from neuromuscular block proceeds at a rate comparable to that following administration of a single bolus.

4.2.4 Dosage in neonates (aged less than 1 month)

The use of NIMBEX in neonates is not recommended as it has not been studied in this patient population.

4.2.5 Dosage in elderly patients

No dosing alterations are required in elderly patients. In these patients NIMBEX has a similar pharmacodynamic profile to that observed in young adult patients but, as with other neuromuscular blocking agents, it may have a slightly slower onset.

4.2.6 Dosage in patients with renal impairment

No dosing alterations are required in patients with renal failure.

In these patients NIMBEX has a similar pharmacodynamic profile to that observed in patients with normal renal function but it may have a slightly slower onset.

4.2.7 Dosage in patients with hepatic impairment

No dosing alterations are required in patients with end-stage liver disease. In these patients NIMBEX has a similar pharmacodynamic profile to that observed in patients with normal hepatic function but it may have a slightly faster onset.

4.2.8 Dosage in patients with cardiovascular disease

When administered by rapid bolus injection (over 5 to 10 seconds) to adult patients with serious cardiovascular disease (New York Heart Association Class I-III) undergoing coronary artery bypass graft (CABG) surgery, NIMBEX has not been associated with clinically significant cardiovascular effects at any dose studied (up to and including 0.4 mg/kg (8x ED_{95}). However, there are limited data for doses above 0.3 mg/kg in this patient population).

NIMBEX has not been studied in children undergoing cardiac surgery.

4.2.9 Dosage in Intensive Care Unit (ICU) patients

NIMBEX may be administered by bolus dose and/or infusion to adult patients in the ICU.

An initial infusion rate of NIMBEX of 3 μg/kg (body weight)/min (0.18 mg/kg/hr) is recommended for adult ICU patients. There may be wide interpatient variation in dosage requirements and these may increase or decrease

Table 2 Paediatric Patients aged 1 to 11 months

NIMBEX Dose mg/kg (body weight)	Anaesthetic Background	Time to 90% Suppression (min)	Time to Maximum Suppression (min)	Time to 25% Spontaneous T1 Recovery (min)
0.15	Halothane	1.4	2.0	52
0.15	Opioid	1.4	1.9	47

Table 3 Paediatric Patients aged 1 to 12 years

NIMBEX Dose mg/kg (body weight)	Anaesthetic Background	Time to 90% Suppression (min)	Time to Maximum Suppression (min)	Time to 25% Spontaneous T1 Recovery (min)
0.15	Halothane	2.3	3.0	43
0.15	Opioid	2.6	3.6	38

Table 4

NIMBEX Dose mg/kg (body weight)	Anaesthetic Background	Time to 90% Suppression (min)	Time to Maximum Suppression (min)	Time to 25% Spontaneous T1 Recovery (min)
0.08	Halothane	1.7	2.5	31
0.1	Opioid	1.7	2.8	28

Table 5 Infusion Delivery Rate of NIMBEX injection 2mg/ml

Patient (body weight)	Dose (μg/kg/min)				Infusion Rate
(kg)	1.0	1.5	2.0	3.0	
20	0.6	0.9	1.2	1.8	mL/hr
70	2.1	3.2	4.2	6.3	mL/hr
100	3.0	4.5	6.0	9.0	mL/hr

Table 6 Infusion Delivery Rate of NIMBEX FORTE injection 5mg/ml

Patient (body weight)	Dose (mg/kg/min)				Infusion Rate
(kg)	1.0	1.5	2.0	3.0	
70	0.8	1.2	1.7	2.5	mL/hr
100	1.2	1.8	2.4	3.6	mL/hr

with time. In clinical studies the average infusion rate was 3 μg/kg/min [range 0.5 to 10.2 μg/kg (body weight)/min (0.03 to 0.6mg/kg/hr)]

The median time to full spontaneous recovery following long-term (up to 6 days) infusion of NIMBEX in ICU patients was approximately 50 minutes.

Infusion Delivery Rate of NIMBEX FORTE injection 5mg/ml

(see Table 6 above)

The recovery profile after infusions of NIMBEX to ICU patients is independent of duration of infusion.

4.3 Contraindications

NIMBEX is contra-indicated in patients known to be hypersensitive to cisatracurium, atracurium, or benzenesulfonic acid.

4.4 Special warnings and special precautions for use

4.4.1 Product specific topics

Cisatracurium paralyses the respiratory muscles as well as other skeletal muscles but has no known effect on consciousness or pain threshold. NIMBEX should be only administered by or under the supervision of anaesthetists or other clinicians who are familiar with the use and action of neuromuscular blocking agents. Facilities for tracheal intubation, and maintenance of pulmonary ventilation and adequate arterial oxygenation have to be available.

Great caution should be exercised when administering NIMBEX to patients who have shown allergic hypersensitivity to other neuromuscular blocking agents since cross-reactivity between neuromuscular blocking agents has been reported.

Cisatracurium does not have significant vagolytic or ganglion- blocking properties. Consequently, NIMBEX has no clinically significant effect on heart rate and will not counteract the bradycardia produced by many anaesthetic agents or by vagal stimulation during surgery.

Patients with myasthenia gravis and other forms of neuromuscular disease have shown greatly increased sensitivity to non-depolarising blocking agents. An initial dose of not more than 0.02 mg/kg NIMBEX is recommended in these patients.

Severe acid-base and/or serum electrolyte abnormalities may increase or decrease the sensitivity of patients to neuromuscular blocking agents.

There is no information on the use of NIMBEX in pregnant women since it has not been studied in this patient population (see section 4.6 Pregnancy and Lactation).

There is no information on the use of NIMBEX in neonates aged less than one month since it has not been studied in this patient population.

Cisatracurium has not been studied in patients with a history of malignant hyperthermia. Studies in malignant hyperthermia- susceptible pigs indicated that cisatracurium does not trigger this syndrome.

There have been no studies of cisatracurium in patients undergoing surgery with induced hypothermia (25 to 28°C). As with other neuromuscular blocking agents the rate of infusion required to maintain adequate surgical relaxation under these conditions may be expected to be significantly reduced.

Cisatracurium has not been studied in patients with burns; however, as with other non-depolarising neuromuscular blocking agents, the possibility of increased dosing requirements and shortened duration of action must be considered if NIMBEX injection is administered to these patients.

NIMBEX is hypotonic and must not be applied into the infusion line of a blood transfusion.

Intensive Care Unit (ICU) Patients: -

When administered to laboratory animals in high doses, laudanosine, a metabolite of cisatracurium and atracurium, has been associated with transient hypotension and in some species, cerebral excitatory effects. In the most sensitive animal species, these effects occurred at laudanosine plasma concentrations similar to those that have been observed in some ICU patients following prolonged infusion of atracurium.

Consistent with the decreased infusion rate requirements of cisatracurium, plasma laudanosine concentrations are approximately one third those following atracurium infusion.

There have been rare reports of seizures in ICU patients who have received atracurium and other agents. These patients usually had one or more medical conditions predisposing to seizures (eg. cranial trauma, hypoxic encephalopathy, cerebral oedema, viral encephalitis, uraemia). A causal relationship to laudanosine has not been established.

4.5 Interaction with other medicinal products and other forms of Interaction

Many drugs have been shown to influence the magnitude and/or duration of action of non-depolarising neuromuscular blocking agents, including the following:-

Increased Effect:

By anaesthetic agents such as enflurane, isoflurane, halothane (see Posology and Method of Administration) and ketamine, by other non- depolarising neuromuscular blocking agents or by other drugs such as antibiotics (including the aminoglycosides, polymyxins, spectinomycin, tetracyclines, lincomycin and clindamycin), anti-arrhythmic drugs (including propranolol, calcium channel blockers, lignocaine, procainamide and quinidine), diuretics, (including frusemide and possibly thiazides, mannitol and acetazolamide), magnesium and lithium salts and ganglion blocking drugs (trimetaphan, hexamethonium).

A decreased effect is seen after prior chronic administration of phenytoin or carbamazepine.

Prior administration of suxamethonium has no effect on the duration of neuromuscular block following bolus doses of NIMBEX or on infusion rate requirements.

Administration of suxamethonium to prolong the effects of non- depolarising neuromuscular blocking agents may result in a prolonged and complex block which can be difficult to reverse with anticholinesterases.

Rarely, certain drugs may aggravate or unmask latent myasthenia gravis or actually induce a myasthenic syndrome; increased sensitivity to non-depolarising neuromuscular blocking agents might result. Such drugs include various antibiotics, β-blockers (propranolol, oxprenolol), anti-arrhythmic drugs (procainamide, quinidine), anti-rheumatic drugs (chloroquine, D-penicillamine), trimetaphan, chlorpromazine, steroids, phenytoin and lithium.

4.6 Pregnancy and lactation

NIMBEX is contra-indicated in pregnancy since there is no information on the use of NIMBEX in pregnant women. Fertility studies have not been performed. Reproduction studies in rats have not revealed any adverse effects on foetal development of cisatracurium. The relevance of these studies is limited due to species differences in metabolism and low systemic exposure levels.

It is not known whether cisatracurium or its metabolites are excreted in human milk.

4.7 Effects on ability to drive and use machines

This precaution is not relevant to the use of NIMBEX. However the usual precautions relating to performance of tasks following general anaesthesia still apply.

4.8 Undesirable effects

Adverse effects recorded following administration of NIMBEX were cutaneous flushing or rash, bradycardia, hypotension and bronchospasm (See Sections 4.2.8 and 5.1).

Anaphylactic reactions of varying degrees of severity have been observed after the administration of neuromuscular blocking agents. Very rarely, severe anaphylactic reactions have been reported in patients receiving NIMBEX in conjunction with one or more anaesthetic agents.

There have been some reports of muscle weakness and/or myopathy following prolonged use of muscle relaxants in severely ill patients in the ICU. Most patients were receiving concomitant corticosteroids. These events have been reported infrequently in association with NIMBEX and a causal relationship has not been established.

4.9 Overdose

4.9.1 Symptoms and signs

Prolonged muscle paralysis and its consequences are expected to be the main signs of overdosage with NIMBEX.

4.9.2 Management

It is essential to maintain pulmonary ventilation and arterial oxygenation until adequate spontaneous respiration returns. Full sedation will be required since consciousness is not impaired by NIMBEX. Recovery may be accelerated by the administration of anti- cholinesterase agents once evidence of spontaneous recovery is present.

5. PHARMACOLOGICAL PROPERTIES

5.1 Pharmacodynamic properties

Cisatracurium is a neuromuscular blocking agent, ATC code: M03A C11.

Cisatracurium is an intermediate-duration, non-depolarising benzylisoquinolinium skeletal muscle relaxant.

Clinical studies in man indicated that NIMBEX is not associated with dose dependent histamine release even at doses up to and including 8 × ED_{95}.

5.1.1 Mode of action

Cisatracurium binds to cholinergic receptors on the motor end-plate to antagonise the action of acetylcholine, resulting in a competitive block of neuromuscular transmission. This action is readily reversed by anti-cholinesterase agents such as neostigmine or edrophonium.

The ED_{95} (dose required to produce 95% depression of the twitch response of the adductor pollicis muscle to stimulation of the ulnar nerve) of cisatracurium is estimated to be 0.05 mg/kg bodyweight during opioid anaesthesia (thiopentone/fentanyl/midazolam).

The ED_{95} of cisatracurium in children during halothane anaesthesia is 0.04 mg/kg.

5.2 Pharmacokinetic properties

Cisatracurium undergoes degradation in the body at physiological pH and temperature by Hofmann elimination (a chemical process) to form laudanosine and the monoquaternary acrylate metabolite. The monoquaternary acrylate undergoes hydrolysis by non-specific plasma esterases to form the monoquaternary alcohol metabolite. Elimination of cisatracurium is largely organ independent but the liver and kidneys are primary pathways for the clearance of its metabolites.

These metabolites do not possess neuromuscular blocking activity.

5.2.1 Pharmacokinetics in adult patients

Non-compartmental pharmacokinetics of cisatracurium are independent of dose in the range studied (0.1 to 0.2 mg/kg, i.e. 2 to 4 × ED_{95}).

Population pharmacokinetic modelling confirms and extends these findings up to 0.4 mg/kg (8 × ED_{95}). Pharmacokinetic parameters after doses of 0.1 and 0.2 mg/kg NIMBEX administered to healthy adult surgical patients are summarised in the table below:

Parameter	Range of Mean Values
Clearance	4.7 to 5.7 mL/min/kg
Volume of distribution at steady state	121 to 161 mL/kg
Elimination half-life	22 to 29 min

5.2.2 Pharmacokinetics in elderly patients

There are no clinically important differences in the pharmacokinetics of cisatracurium in elderly and young adult patients. The recovery profile is also unchanged.

5.2.3 Pharmacokinetics in patients with renal/hepatic impairment

There are no clinically important differences in the pharmacokinetics of cisatracurium in patients with end-stage renal failure or end stage liver disease and in healthy adult patients. Their recovery profiles are also unchanged.

5.2.4 Pharmacokinetics during infusions

The pharmacokinetics of cisatracurium after infusions of NIMBEX are similar to those after single bolus injection. The recovery profile after infusion of NIMBEX is independent of duration of infusion and is similar to that after single bolus injection.

5.2.5 Pharmacokinetics in Intensive Care Unit (ICU) patients

The pharmacokinetics of cisatracurium in ICU patients receiving prolonged infusions are similar to those in healthy surgical adults receiving infusions or single bolus injections. The recovery profile after infusions of NIMBEX in ICU patients is independent of duration of infusion.

Concentrations of metabolites are higher in ICU patients with abnormal renal and/or hepatic function (see Section 4.4 Special Warnings and Special Precautions for Use). These metabolites do not contribute to neuromuscular block.

5.3 Preclinical safety data

5.3.1 Acute toxicity

Meaningful acute studies with cisatracurium could not be performed.

For symptoms of toxicity see "Overdosage"

Subacute Toxicity:

Studies with repeated administration for three weeks in dogs and monkeys showed no compound specific toxic signs.

5.3.2 Mutagenicity

Cisatracurium was not mutagenic in an in vitro microbial mutagenicity test at concentrations up to 5000μg/plate.

In an in vivo cytogenetic study in rats, no significant chromosomal abnormalities were seen at s.c doses up to 4mg/kg.

Cisatracurium was mutagenic in an in vitro mouse lymphoma cell mutagenicity assay, at concentrations of 40μg/ml and higher.

A single positive mutagenic response for a drug used infrequently and/or briefly is of questionable clinical relevance.

5.3.3 Carcinogenicity

Carcinogenicity studies have not been performed.

5.3.4 Local tolerance

The result of an intra-arterial study in rabbits showed that NIMBEX injection is well tolerated and no drug related changes were seen.

6. PHARMACEUTICAL PARTICULARS

6.1 List of excipients

Benzene sulfonic acid solution 32% w/v, water for injections.

6.2 Incompatibilities

Degradation of cisatracurium besilate has been demonstrated to occur more rapidly in lactated Ringer's Injection and 5% Dextrose and lactated Ringer's Injection than in the infusion fluids listed under Section 6.6.

Therefore it is recommended that lactated Ringer's Injection and 5% Dextrose and lactated Ringer's Injection are not used as the diluent in preparing solutions of NIMBEX for infusion.

Since NIMBEX is stable only in acidic solutions it should not be mixed in the same syringe or administered simultaneously through the same needle with alkaline solutions, e.g., sodium thiopentone. It is not compatible with ketorolac trometamol or propofol injectable emulsion.

6.3 Shelf life

Shelf-life before dilution: 2 years.

Shelf-life after dilution: The product should be used immediately on dilution, or failing this the aseptically prepared dilution should be stored at 2-8°C for no more than 24 hours, after which time unused solution should be discarded.

The pack is designed for use on a single occasion, injected or diluted immediately after opening, any remaining solution should be discarded.

6.4 Special precautions for storage

Store at 2-8°C. Do not freeze. Keep vial in the outer carton.

Protect from light.

6.5 Nature and contents of container

NIMBEX 5mg/ml, solution for injection

30ml in vial (glass): box of 1

Type I, clear, neutral glass vial with a polymeric coated synthetic bromobutyl rubber stopper and aluminium collar with plastic flip-top cover.

6.6 Instructions for use and handling

Use only clear and almost colourless up to slightly yellow/greenish yellow coloured solutions.

Diluted NIMBEX is physically and chemically stable for at least 24 hours at 5°C and 25°C at concentrations between 0.1 and 2 mg/mL in the following infusion fluids, in either polyvinyl chloride or polypropylene containers.

Sodium Chloride (0.9% w/v) Intravenous Infusion.

Glucose (5% w/v) Intravenous Infusion.

Sodium Chloride (0.18% w/v) and Glucose (4% w/v) Intravenous Infusion.

Sodium Chloride (0.45% w/v) and Glucose (2.5% w/v) Intravenous Infusion.

However, since the product contains no antimicrobial preservative, dilution should be carried out immediately prior to use, or failing this be stored as directed under section 6.3.

NIMBEX has been shown to be compatible with the following commonly used peri-operative drugs, when mixed in conditions simulating administration into a running intravenous infusion via a Y-site injection port: alfentanil hydrochloride, droperidol, fentanyl citrate, midazolam hydrochloride and sufentanil citrate. Where other drugs are administered through the same indwelling needle or cannula as NIMBEX, it is recommended that each drug be flushed through with an adequate volume of a suitable intravenous fluid, e.g., Sodium Chloride Intravenous Infusion (0.9% w/v).

As with other drugs administered intravenously, when a small vein is selected as the injection site, NIMBEX should be flushed through the vein with a suitable intravenous fluid, e.g., sodium chloride intravenous infusion (0.9% w/v).

7. MARKETING AUTHORISATION HOLDER

The Wellcome Foundation Limited

Trading as GlaxoSmithKline UK, Stockley Park West, Uxbridge, Middlesex, UB11 1BT

8. MARKETING AUTHORISATION NUMBER(S)

PL 00003/0365

9. DATE OF FIRST AUTHORISATION/RENEWAL OF THE AUTHORISATION

Country	Name	Date
UK	NIMBEX 5mg/ml, solution for injection	07/08/1995

10. DATE OF REVISION OF THE TEXT

21st May 2002

11. Legal Status

POM

Nimbex Injection 2mg/ml

(GlaxoSmithKline UK)

1. NAME OF THE MEDICINAL PRODUCT

Nimbex® 2mg/ml, solution for injection.

2. QUALITATIVE AND QUANTITATIVE COMPOSITION

Cisatracurium 2mg as cisatracurium besilate 2.68mg per 1ml

one ampoule of 2.5ml contains 5mg of cisatracurium

one ampoule of 5ml contains 10mg of cisatracurium

one ampoule of 10ml contains 20mg of cisatracurium

one ampoule of 25ml contains 50mg of cisatracurium

For excipients, see Section 6.1.

3. PHARMACEUTICAL FORM

Solution for Injection.

4. CLINICAL PARTICULARS

Nimbex is an intermediate-duration, non-depolarising neuromuscular blocking agent for intravenous administration.

4.1 Therapeutic indications

Nimbex is indicated for use during surgical and other procedures and in intensive care. Nimbex can be used as an adjunct to general anaesthesia, or sedation in the Intensive Care Unit (ICU) to relax skeletal muscles, and to facilitate tracheal intubation and mechanical ventilation.

4.2 Posology and method of administration

Please note that Nimbex should not be mixed in the same syringe or administered simultaneously through the same needle as propofol injectable emulsion or with alkaline solutions such as sodium thiopentone. (Please refer to section 6.2 for details of incompatibilities).

Nimbex contains no antimicrobial preservative and is intended for single patient use.

Monitoring advice

As with other neuromuscular blocking agents, monitoring of neuromuscular function is recommended during the use of Nimbex in order to individualise dosage requirements.

Use by intravenous bolus injection

Dosage in adults

Tracheal Intubation. The recommended intubation dose of Nimbex for adults is 0.15mg/kg (body weight). This dose produced good to excellent conditions for tracheal intubation 120 seconds after administration of Nimbex, following induction of anaesthesia with propofol.

Higher doses will shorten the time to onset of neuromuscular block.

The following table summarises mean pharmacodynamic data when Nimbex was administered at doses of 0.1 to 0.4mg/kg (body weight) to healthy adult patients during opioid (thiopentone/fentanyl/midazolam) or propofol anaesthesia.

(see Table 1 below)

Enflurane or isoflurane anaesthesia may extend the clinically effective duration of an initial dose of Nimbex by as much as 15%.

Maintenance. Neuromuscular block can be extended with maintenance doses of Nimbex. A dose of 0.03 mg/kg (body weight) provides approximately 20 minutes of additional clinically effective neuromuscular block during opioid or propofol anaesthesia.

Consecutive maintenance doses do not result in progressive prolongation of effect.

Spontaneous Recovery. Once spontaneous recovery from neuromuscular block is underway, the rate is independent of the NIMBEX dose administered. During opioid or propofol anaesthesia, the median times from 25 to 75% and from 5 to 95% recovery are approximately 13 and 30 minutes, respectively.

Reversal. Neuromuscular block following NIMBEX administration is readily reversible with standard doses of anticholinesterase agents. The mean times from 25 to 75% recovery and to full clinical recovery (T_4:T_1 ratio $\geqslant$ 0.7) are approximately 4 and 9 minutes respectively, following administration of the reversal agent at an average of 10% T_1 recovery.

Dosage in paediatric patients

Tracheal Intubation (paediatric patients aged 1 month to 12 years): As in adults, the recommended intubation dose of Nimbex is 0.15 mg/kg (body weight) administered rapidly over 5 to 10 seconds. This dose produces good to excellent conditions for tracheal intubation 120 seconds following injection of Nimbex. Pharmacodynamic data for this dose are presented in the tables below.

Nimbex has not been studied for intubation in ASA Class III-IV paediatric patients. There are limited data on the use of Nimbex in paediatric patients under 2 years of age undergoing prolonged or major surgery.

In paediatric patients aged 1 month to 12 years, Nimbex has a shorter clinically effective duration and a faster spontaneous recovery profile than those observed in adults under similar anaesthetic conditions. Small differences in the pharmacodynamic profile were observed between the age ranges 1 to 11 months and 1 to 12 years which are summarised in the tables below.

Paediatric Patients aged 1 to 11 months

(see Table 2 below)

Paediatric Patients aged 1 to 12 years

(see Table 3 below)

When Nimbex is not required for intubation: A dose of less than 0.15mg/kg can be used. Pharmacodynamic data for doses of 0.08 and 0.1 mg/kg for paediatric patients aged 2 to 12 years are presented in the table below:

(see Table 4 on next page)

Administration of Nimbex following suxamethonium has not been studied in paediatric patients (see section 4.5

Table 1

Initial Nimbex Dose mg/kg (body weight)	Anaesthetic Background	Time to 90% T1* Suppression (min)	Time to Maximum T1* Suppression (min)	Time to 25% Spontaneous T1* Recovery (min)
0.1	Opioid	3.4	4.8	45
0.15	Propofol	2.6	3.5	55
0.2	Opioid	2.4	2.9	65
0.4	Opioid	1.5	1.9	91

* T_1 Single twitch response as well as the first component of the Train-of-four response of the adductor pollicis muscle following supramaximal electrical stimulation of the ulnar nerve.

Table 2 Paediatric Patients aged 1 to 11 months

Nimbex Dose mg/kg (body weight)	Anaesthetic Background	Time to 90% Suppression (min)	Time to Maximum Suppression (min)	Time to 25% Spontaneous T1 Recovery (min)
0.15	Halothane	1.4	2.0	52
0.15	Opioid	1.4	1.9	47

Table 3 Paediatric Patients aged 1 to 12 years

Nimbex Dose mg/kg (body weight)	Anaesthetic Background	Time to 90% Suppression (min)	Time to Maximum Suppression (min)	Time to 25% Spontaneous T1 Recovery (min)
0.15	Halothane	2.3	3.0	43
0.15	Opioid	2.6	3.6	38

Table 4

Nimbex Dose mg/kg (body weight)	Anaesthetic Background	Time to 90% Suppression (min)	Time to Maximum Suppression (min)	Time to 25% Spontaneous T1 Recovery (min)
0.08	Halothane	1.7	2.5	31
0.1	Opioid	1.7	2.8	28

Table 5 Infusion Delivery Rate of Nimbex injection 2mg/ml

Patient (body weight) (kg)	Dose (μg/kg/min)				Infusion Rate
	1.0	1.5	2.0	3.0	
20	0.6	0.9	1.2	1.8	mL/hr
70	2.1	3.2	4.2	6.3	mL/hr
100	3.0	4.5	6.0	9.0	mL/hr

Table 6 Infusion Delivery Rate of Nimbex Forte injection 5mg/ml

Patient (body weight) (kg)	Dose (μg/kg/min)				Infusion Rate
	1.0	1.5	2.0	3.0	
70	0.8	1.2	1.7	2.5	mL/hr
100	1.2	1.8	2.4	3.6	mL/hr

Interaction with Other Medicaments and Other Forms of Interaction).

Halothane may be expected to extend the clinically effective duration of a dose of Nimbex by up to 20%. No information is available on the use of Nimbex in children during anaesthesia with other halogenated fluorocarbon anaesthetic agents, but these agents may also be expected to extend the clinically effective duration of a dose of Nimbex.

Maintenance (paediatric patients aged 2-12 years). Neuromuscular block can be extended with maintenance doses of Nimbex. In paediatric patients aged 2 to 12 years, a dose of 0.02 mg/kg (body weight) provides approximately 9 minutes of additional clinically effective neuromuscular block during halothane anaesthesia. Consecutive maintenance doses do not result in progressive prolongation of effect.

There are insufficient data to make a specific recommendation for maintenance dosing in paediatric patients under 2 years of age. However, very limited data from clinical studies in paediatric patients under 2 years of age suggest that a maintenance dose of 0.03mg/kg may extend clinically effective neuromuscular block for a period of up to 25 minutes during opioid anaesthesia.

Spontaneous Recovery. Once recovery from neuromuscular block is underway, the rate is independent of the Nimbex dose administered. During opioid or halothane anaesthesia, the median times from 25 to 75% and from 5 to 95% recovery are approximately 11 and 28 minutes, respectively.

Reversal. Neuromuscular block following Nimbex administration is readily reversible with standard doses of anticholinesterase agents. The mean times from 25 to 75% recovery and to full clinical recovery (T_4:T_1 ratio $\geqslant$ 0.7) are approximately 2 and 5 minutes respectively, following administration of the reversal agent at an average of 13% T_1 recovery.

Use by intravenous infusion

Dosage in adults and children aged 2 to 12 years

Maintenance of neuromuscular block may be achieved by infusion of Nimbex. An initial infusion rate of 3 μg/kg (body weight)/min (0.18 mg/kg/hr) is recommended to restore 89 to 99% T_1 suppression following evidence of spontaneous recovery. After an initial period of stabilisation of neuromuscular block, a rate of 1 to 2 μg/kg (body weight)/min (0.06 to 0.12 mg/kg/hr) should be adequate to maintain block in this range in most patients.

Reduction of the infusion rate by up to 40% may be required when Nimbex is administered during isoflurane or enflurane anaesthesia.(See Section 4.5).

The infusion rate will depend upon the concentration of cisatracurium in the infusion solution, the desired degree of neuromuscular block, and the patient's weight. The following table provides guidelines for delivery of undiluted Nimbex.

Infusion Delivery Rate of Nimbex injection 2mg/ml

(see Table 5 above)

Steady rate continuous infusion of Nimbex is not associated with a progressive increase or decrease in neuromuscular blocking effect.

Following discontinuation of infusion of Nimbex, spontaneous recovery from neuromuscular block proceeds at a rate comparable to that following administration of a single bolus.

Dosage in neonates (aged less than 1 month)

The use of Nimbex in neonates is not recommended as it has not been studied in this patient population.

Dosage in elderly patients

No dosing alterations are required in elderly patients. In these patients Nimbex has a similar pharmacodynamic profile to that observed in young adult patients but, as with other neuromuscular blocking agents, it may have a slightly slower onset.

Dosage in patients with renal impairment

No dosing alterations are required in patients with renal failure.

In these patients Nimbex has a similar pharmacodynamic profile to that observed in patients with normal renal function but it may have a slightly slower onset.

Dosage in patients with hepatic impairment

No dosing alterations are required in patients with end-stage liver disease. In these patients Nimbex has a similar pharmacodynamic profile to that observed in patients with normal hepatic function but it may have a slightly faster onset.

Dosage in patients with cardiovascular disease

When administered by rapid bolus injection (over 5 to 10 seconds) to adult patients with serious cardiovascular disease (New York Heart Association Class I-III) undergoing coronary artery bypass graft (CABG) surgery, Nimbex has not been associated with clinically significant cardiovascular effects at any dose studied (up to and including 0.4 mg/kg (8x ED_{95}). However, there are limited data for doses above 0.3 mg/kg in this patient population).

Nimbex has not been studied in children undergoing cardiac surgery.

Dosage in Intensive Care Unit (ICU) patients

Nimbex may be administered by bolus dose and/or infusion to adult patients in the ICU.

An initial infusion rate of Nimbex of 3 μg/kg (body weight)/min (0.18 mg/kg/hr) is recommended for adult ICU patients. There may be wide interpatient variation in dosage requirements and these may increase or decrease with time. In clinical studies the average infusion rate was 3 μg/kg/min [range 0.5 to 10.2 μg/kg (body weight)/min (0.03 to 0.6mg/kg/hr)]

The median time to full spontaneous recovery following long-term (up to 6 days) infusion of Nimbex in ICU patients was approximately 50 minutes.

Infusion Delivery Rate of Nimbex Forte injection 5mg/ml

(see Table 6 above)

The recovery profile after infusions of Nimbex to ICU patients is independent of duration of infusion.

4.3 Contraindications

Nimbex is contra-indicated in patients known to be hypersensitive to cisatracurium, atracurium, or benzenesulfonic acid.

4.4 Special warnings and special precautions for use

Product specific topics

Cisatracurium paralyses the respiratory muscles as well as other skeletal muscles but has no known effect on consciousness or pain threshold. Nimbex should be only administered by or under the supervision of anaesthetists or other clinicians who are familiar with the use and action of neuromuscular blocking agents. Facilities for tracheal intubation, and maintenance of pulmonary ventilation and adequate arterial oxygenation have to be available.

Great caution should be exercised when administering Nimbex to patients who have shown allergic hypersensitivity to other neuromuscular blocking agents since cross-reactivity between neuromuscular blocking agents has been reported.

Cisatracurium does not have significant vagolytic or ganglion- blocking properties. Consequently, Nimbex has no clinically significant effect on heart rate and will not counteract the bradycardia produced by many anaesthetic agents or by vagal stimulation during surgery.

Patients with myasthenia gravis and other forms of neuromuscular disease have shown greatly increased sensitivity to non-depolarising blocking agents. An initial dose of not more than 0.02 mg/kg Nimbex is recommended in these patients.

Severe acid-base and/or serum electrolyte abnormalities may increase or decrease the sensitivity of patients to neuromuscular blocking agents.

There is no information on the use of Nimbex in pregnant women since it has not been studied in this patient population (see section 4.6 Pregnancy and Lactation).

There is no information on the use of Nimbex in neonates aged less than one month since it has not been studied in this patient population.

Cisatracurium has not been studied in patients with a history of malignant hyperthermia. Studies in malignant hyperthermia- susceptible pigs indicated that cisatracurium does not trigger this syndrome.

There have been no studies of cisatracurium in patients undergoing surgery with induced hypothermia (25 to 28°C). As with other neuromuscular blocking agents the rate of infusion required to maintain adequate surgical relaxation under these conditions may be expected to be significantly reduced.

Cisatracurium has not been studied in patients with burns; however, as with other non-depolarising neuromuscular blocking agents, the possibility of increased dosing requirements and shortened duration of action must be considered if Nimbex injection is administered to these patients.

Nimbex is hypotonic and must not be applied into the infusion line of a blood transfusion.

Intensive Care Unit (ICU) Patients: -

When administered to laboratory animals in high doses, laudanosine, a metabolite of cisatracurium and atracurium, has been associated with transient hypotension and in some species, cerebral excitatory effects. In the most sensitive animal species, these effects occurred at laudanosine plasma concentrations similar to those that have been observed in some ICU patients following prolonged infusion of atracurium.

Consistent with the decreased infusion rate requirements of cisatracurium, plasma laudanosine concentrations are approximately one third those following atracurium infusion.

There have been rare reports of seizures in ICU patients who have received atracurium and other agents. These patients usually had one or more medical conditions predisposing to seizures (eg. cranial trauma, hypoxic encephalopathy, cerebral oedema, viral encephalitis, uraemia). A causal relationship to laudanosine has not been established.

4.5 Interaction with other medicinal products and other forms of Interaction

Many drugs have been shown to influence the magnitude and/or duration of action of non-depolarising neuromuscular blocking agents, including the following:-

Increased Effect:

By anaesthetic agents such as enflurane, isoflurane, halothane (see Posology and Method of Administration) and ketamine, by other non- depolarising neuromuscular blocking agents or by other drugs such as antibiotics (including the aminoglycosides, polymyxins, spectinomycin, tetracyclines, lincomycin and clindamycin), anti-arrhythmic drugs (including propranolol, calcium channel blockers, lignocaine, procainamide and quinidine), diuretics, (including frusemide and possibly thiazides, mannitol and acetazolamide), magnesium and lithium salts and ganglion blocking drugs (trimetaphan, hexamethonium).

A decreased effect is seen after prior chronic administration of phenytoin or carbamazepine.

Prior administration of suxamethonium has no effect on the duration of neuromuscular block following bolus doses of Nimbex or on infusion rate requirements.

Administration of suxamethonium to prolong the effects of non- depolarising neuromuscular blocking agents may result in a prolonged and complex block which can be difficult to reverse with anticholinesterases.

Rarely, certain drugs may aggravate or unmask latent myasthenia gravis or actually induce a myasthenic syndrome; increased sensitivity to non-depolarising neuromuscular blocking agents might result. Such drugs include various antibiotics, b-blockers (propranolol, oxprenolol), anti-arrhythmic drugs (procainamide, quinidine), anti-rheumatic drugs (chloroquine, D-penicillamine), trimetaphan, chlorpromazine, steroids, phenytoin and lithium.

4.6 Pregnancy and lactation

Nimbex is contra-indicated in pregnancy since there is no information on the use of Nimbex in pregnant women. Fertility studies have not been performed. Reproduction studies in rats have not revealed any adverse effects on foetal development of cisatracurium. The relevance of these studies is limited due to species differences in metabolism and low systemic exposure levels.

It is not known whether cisatracurium or its metabolites are excreted in human milk.

4.7 Effects on ability to drive and use machines

This precaution is not relevant to the use of Nimbex. However the usual precautions relating to performance of tasks following general anaesthesia still apply.

4.8 Undesirable effects

Adverse effects recorded following administration of Nimbex were cutaneous flushing or rash, bradycardia, hypotension and bronchospasm (See Sections 4.2.8 and 5.1).

Anaphylactic reactions of varying degrees of severity have been observed after the administration of neuromuscular blocking agents. Very rarely, severe anaphylactic reactions have been reported in patients receiving Nimbex in conjunction with one or more anaesthetic agents.

There have been some reports of muscle weakness and/or myopathy following prolonged use of muscle relaxants in severely ill patients in the ICU. Most patients were receiving concomitant corticosteroids. These events have been reported infrequently in association with Nimbex and a causal relationship has not been established.

4.9 Overdose

4.9.1 Symptoms and signs

Prolonged muscle paralysis and its consequences are expected to be the main signs of overdosage with Nimbex.

Management

It is essential to maintain pulmonary ventilation and arterial oxygenation until adequate spontaneous respiration returns. Full sedation will be required since consciousness is not impaired by Nimbex. Recovery may be accelerated by the administration of anti- cholinesterase agents once evidence of spontaneous recovery is present.

5. PHARMACOLOGICAL PROPERTIES

5.1 Pharmacodynamic properties

Cisatracurium is a neuromuscular blocking agent, ATC code: M03A C11.

Cisatracurium is an intermediate-duration, non-depolarising benzylisoquinolinium skeletal muscle relaxant.

Clinical studies in man indicated that Nimbex is not associated with dose dependent histamine release even at doses up to and including 8 × ED_{95}.

Mode of action

Cisatracurium binds to cholinergic receptors on the motor end-plate to antagonise the action of acetylcholine, resulting in a competitive block of neuromuscular transmission. This action is readily reversed by anti-cholinesterase agents such as neostigmine or edrophonium.

The ED_{95} (dose required to produce 95% depression of the twitch response of the adductor pollicis muscle to stimulation of the ulnar nerve) of cisatracurium is estimated to be 0.05 mg/kg bodyweight during opioid anaesthesia (thiopentone/fentanyl/midazolam).

The ED_{95} of cisatracurium in children during halothane anaesthesia is 0.04 mg/kg.

5.2 Pharmacokinetic properties

Cisatracurium undergoes degradation in the body at physiological pH and temperature by Hofmann elimination (a chemical process) to form laudanosine and the monoquaternary acrylate metabolite. The monoquaternary acrylate undergoes hydrolysis by non-specific plasma esterases to form the monoquaternary alcohol metabolite. Elimination of cisatracurium is largely organ independent but the liver and kidneys are primary pathways for the clearance of its metabolites.

These metabolites do not possess neuromuscular blocking activity.

Pharmacokinetics in adult patients

Non-compartmental pharmacokinetics of cisatracurium are independent of dose in the range studied (0.1 to 0.2 mg/kg, i.e. 2 to 4 × ED_{95}).

Population pharmacokinetic modelling confirms and extends these findings up to 0.4 mg/kg (8 × ED_{95}). Pharmacokinetic parameters after doses of 0.1 and 0.2 mg/kg Nimbex administered to healthy adult surgical patients are summarised in the table below:

Parameter	Range of Mean Values
Clearance	4.7 to 5.7 mL/min/kg
Volume of distribution at steady state	121 to 161 mL/kg
Elimination half-life	22 to 29 min

Pharmacokinetics in elderly patients

There are no clinically important differences in the pharmacokinetics of cisatracurium in elderly and young adult patients. The recovery profile is also unchanged.

Pharmacokinetics in patients with renal/hepatic impairment

There are no clinically important differences in the pharmacokinetics of cisatracurium in patients with end-stage renal failure or end stage liver disease and in healthy adult patients. Their recovery profiles are also unchanged.

Pharmacokinetics during infusions

The pharmacokinetics of cisatracurium after infusions of Nimbex are similar to those after single bolus injection. The recovery profile after infusion of Nimbex is independent of duration of infusion and is similar to that after single bolus injection.

Pharmacokinetics in Intensive Care Unit (ICU) patients

The pharmacokinetics of cisatracurium in ICU patients receiving prolonged infusions are similar to those in healthy surgical adults receiving infusions or single bolus injections. The recovery profile after infusions of Nimbex in ICU patients is independent of duration of infusion.

Concentrations of metabolites are higher in ICU patients with abnormal renal and/or hepatic function (see Section 4.4 Special Warnings and Special Precautions for Use). These metabolites do not contribute to neuromuscular block.

5.3 Preclinical safety data

Acute toxicity

Meaningful acute studies with cisatracurium could not be performed.

For symptoms of toxicity see "Overdosage"

Subacute Toxicity:

Studies with repeated administration for three weeks in dogs and monkeys showed no compound specific toxic signs.

Mutagenicity

Cisatracurium was not mutagenic in an in vitro microbial mutagenicity test at concentrations up to 5000μg/plate.

In an in vivo cytogenetic study in rats, no significant chromosomal abnormalities were seen at s.c doses up to 4mg/kg.

Cisatracurium was mutagenic in an in vitro mouse lymphoma cell mutagenicity assay, at concentrations of 40μg/ml and higher.

A single positive mutagenic response for a drug used infrequently and/or briefly is of questionable clinical relevance.

Carcinogenicity

Carcinogenicity studies have not been performed.

Local tolerance

The result of an intra-arterial study in rabbits showed that Nimbex injection is well tolerated and no drug related changes were seen.

6. PHARMACEUTICAL PARTICULARS

6.1 List of excipients

Benzene sulfonic acid solution 32% w/v, water for injections.

6.2 Incompatibilities

Degradation of cisatracurium besilate has been demonstrated to occur more rapidly in lactated Ringer's Injection and 5% Dextrose and lactated Ringer's Injection than in the infusion fluids listed under Section 6.6.

Therefore it is recommended that lactated Ringer's Injection and 5% Dextrose and lactated Ringer's Injection are not used as the diluent in preparing solutions of Nimbex for infusion.

Since Nimbex is stable only in acidic solutions it should not be mixed in the same syringe or administered simultaneously through the same needle with alkaline solutions, e.g., sodium thiopentone. It is not compatible with ketorolac trometamol or propofol injectable emulsion.

6.3 Shelf life

Shelf life before dilution: 2 years.

Shelf-life after dilution: The product should be used immediately on dilution, or failing this the aseptically prepared dilution should be stored at 2-8°C for no more than 24 hours, after which time unused solution should be discarded.

The pack is designed for use on a single occasion, injected or diluted immediately after opening, any remaining solution should be discarded.

6.4 Special precautions for storage

Store at 2-8°C. Do not freeze. Keep ampoules in the outer carton.

Protect from light.

6.5 Nature and contents of container

Nimbex 2mg/ml, solution for injection

2.5ml in ampoule (glass): box of 5

5ml in ampoule (glass): box of 5

10ml in ampoule (glass): box of 5

25ml in ampoule (glass: box of 2

Type I, clear, neutral glass ampoules.

6.6 Instructions for use and handling

Use only clear and almost colourless up to slightly yellow/greenish yellow coloured solutions.

Diluted Nimbex is physically and chemically stable for at least 24 hours at 5°C and 25°C at concentrations between 0.1 and 2 mg/mL in the following infusion fluids, in either polyvinyl chloride or polypropylene containers.

Sodium Chloride (0.9% w/v) Intravenous Infusion.

Glucose (5% w/v) Intravenous Infusion.

Sodium Chloride (0.18% w/v) and Glucose (4% w/v) Intravenous Infusion.

Sodium Chloride (0.45% w/v) and Glucose (2.5% w/v) Intravenous Infusion.

However, since the product contains no antimicrobial preservative, dilution should be carried out immediately prior to use, or failing this be stored as directed under section 6.3.

Nimbex has been shown to be compatible with the following commonly used peri-operative drugs, when mixed in conditions simulating administration into a running intravenous infusion via a Y-site injection port: alfentanil hydrochloride, droperidol, fentanyl citrate, midazolam hydrochloride and sufentanil citrate. Where other drugs are administered through the same indwelling needle or cannula as Nimbex, it is recommended that each drug be flushed through with an adequate volume of a suitable intravenous fluid, e.g., Sodium Chloride Intravenous Infusion (0.9% w/v).

As with other drugs administered intravenously, when a small vein is selected as the injection site, Nimbex should be flushed through the vein with a suitable intravenous fluid, e.g., sodium chloride intravenous infusion (0.9% w/v).

Instructions to open the ampoule (only applicable to 2mg/ml ampoule)

Ampoules are equipped with the OPC (One Point Cut) opening system and must be opened following the below instructions:

- Hold with the hand the bottom part of the ampoule as indicated in picture 1
- Put the other hand on the top of the ampoule positioning the thumb above the coloured point and press as indicated in picture 2

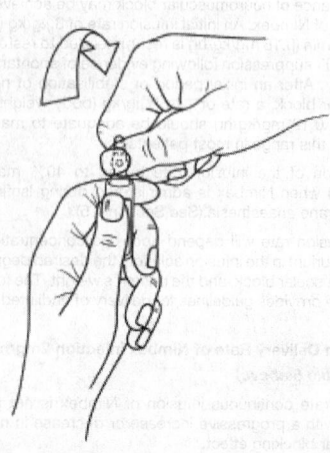

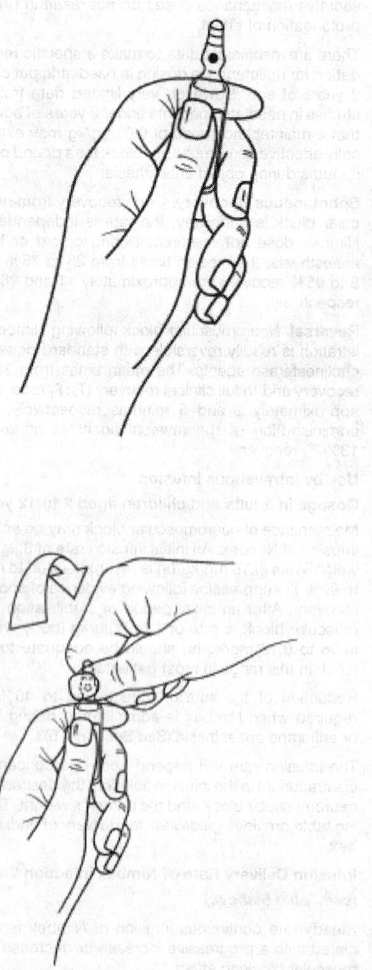

Picture 1

Picture 2

Administrative Data

7. MARKETING AUTHORISATION HOLDER
The Wellcome Foundation Limited
Trading as GlaxoSmithKline UK, Stockley Park West, Uxbridge, Middlesex, UB11 1BT

8. MARKETING AUTHORISATION NUMBER(S)
PL 00003/0364

9. DATE OF FIRST AUTHORISATION/RENEWAL OF THE AUTHORISATION

Country	Name	Date
UK	NIMBEX 2mg/ml, solution for injection	07/08/1995

10. DATE OF REVISION OF THE TEXT
21st May 2002

11. Legal Status
POM

Nimotop 0.02% Solution

(Bayer plc)

1. NAME OF THE MEDICINAL PRODUCT
Nimotop 0.02% Solution for Infusion

2. QUALITATIVE AND QUANTITATIVE COMPOSITION
A sterile solution containing 10 mg nimodipine in 50 ml vials or 50 mg nimodipine in 250 ml bottles of aqueous alcoholic solvent (0.02%).

3. PHARMACEUTICAL FORM
Clear yellow sterile solution for intravenous use.

4. CLINICAL PARTICULARS

4.1 Therapeutic indications
Nimodipine is indicated for the treatment of ischaemic neurological deficits following aneurysmal subarachnoid haemorrhage.

4.2 Posology and method of administration
Recommended dose - Aneurysmal Subarachnoid Haemorrhage

For the first two hours of treatment 1 mg of nimodipine, i.e. 5 ml Nimotop solution, (about 15 μg/kg bw/h), should be infused each hour via a central catheter. The dose should be increased after two hours to 2 mg nimodipine, i.e. 10 ml Nimotop solution per hour (about 30 μg/kg bw/h), providing no severe decrease in blood pressure is observed.

Patients of body weight less than 70 kg or with unstable blood pressure should be started on a dose of 0.5 mg nimodipine per hour (2.5 ml of Nimotop solution), or less if necessary.

Duration of treatment

Aneurysmal subarachnoid haemorrhage

Intravenous treatment should begin as early as possible after neurological deficit occurs due to arterial spasm, post subarachnoid haemorrhage. This should continue for at least five days up to a maximum of 14 days.

In the event of surgical intervention during treatment, administration of nimodipine should be continued (dose as above) for at least five days.

Nimotop solution may be used with or without pre-treatment with Nimotop tablets. In the event of Nimotop tablets and Nimotop solution being administered sequentially the total duration of treatment should not exceed 21 days. Nimotop solution should not be administered for longer than 14 days. Nimotop solution and tablets should not be used concomitantly.

Traumatic subarachnoid haemorrhage

Not recommended as a positive benefit to risk ratio has not been established (see Section 4.4).

Route of administration

For administration, Nimotop solution must be drawn up into a 50ml syringe and connected to a three-way stopcock using the infusion line provided. (The stopcock must allow for concomitant flow of the Nimotop solution and a co-infusion solution.) Nimotop solution must be administered with a co-infusion running at a rate of 40 ml/hr of either sodium chloride 0.9%, glucose 5%, Ringer's lactate solution, dextran 40, human albumin 5% or mannitol 10% which is connected to the second port of the three-way stopcock prior to its connection with the central line catheter.

Nimotop solution must not be added to an infusion bag or bottle and must not be mixed with other drugs.

Nimotop solution may be used during anaesthesia or surgical procedures.

4.3 Contraindications
Nimodipine should not be administered to patients during or/within one month of a myocardial infarction or an episode of unstable angina.

4.4 Special warnings and special precautions for use
Nimotop should not be used in patients with traumatic subarachnoid haemorrhage as a positive benefit to risk ratio has not been established and the specific patient groups that might benefit cannot be identified for this indication.

Nimotop solution should be used with care when cerebral oedema or severely raised intracranial pressure are present.

Nimotop solution must be used with caution in hypotensive patients.

Decreased drug clearance may occur in cirrhotic patients receiving Nimotop and, therefore, close monitoring of blood pressure is recommended in these patients.

Patients with known renal disease and/or receiving nephrotoxic drugs, should have renal function monitored closely during intravenous treatment with Nimotop solution.

4.5 Interaction with other medicinal products and other forms of Interaction
Nimotop tablets should not be administered concomitantly with Nimotop solution.

Nimodipine may potentiate the hypotensive effect of antihypertensives. Where concomitant administration of other calcium channel blockers, (e.g. nifedipine, diltiazem, verapamil), α-methyldopa or beta-blockers is necessary blood pressure must be monitored, and careful dose titration of nimodipine should be undertaken with possible reduction or discontinuation of the antihypertensive agent.

Concurrent twice daily administration of 30mg nimodipine and daily administration of 20mg of the antidepressant fluoxetine to elderly patients resulted in an increase in nimodipine plasma levels, a reduction in fluoxetine levels and a trend towards increased norfluoxetine levels. The daily dose used in patients with subarachnoid haemorrhage is four times the daily dose used in this trial, and as a steady state norfluoxetine level was not achieved, the clinical significance of this interaction in the treatment of aneurysmal subarachnoid haemorrhage (aSAH) is uncertain.

Concurrent three times daily administration of 30mg nimodipine and three times daily administration of 10mg of the antidepressant nortriptyline to elderly patients resulted in a slight decrease in nimodipine plasma levels with no effect on nortriptyline plasma levels. The daily dose used in patients with subarachnoid haemorrhage is four times the daily dose used in this trial, thus the clinical significance of this interaction in the treatment of aneurysmal subarachnoid haemorrhage (aSAH) is uncertain.

The simultaneous administration of cimetidine or sodium valproate may lead to an increase in the plasma nimodipine concentration.

Animal studies have shown that when nimodipine and zidovudine are administered concomitantly, the AUC for zidovudine was increased, and the volume of distribution and clearance rate decreased. The clinical relevance of this interaction is unknown, but since the side-effect profile of zidovudine is known to be dose related, this interaction should be considered in patients receiving nimodipine and zidovudine concomitantly.

Nimodipine is metabolised via the cytochrome P450 3A4 system located in both the intestinal mucosa and in the liver. Drugs that are known to either inhibit or to induce this enzyme system may therefore alter the first pass metabolism or clearance of nimodipine. The concomitant administration of nimodipine and potent CYP 3A4 inhibitors, e.g. macrolide antibiotics (e.g. erythromycin), azole antimycotics (e.g. ketoconazole, itraconazole, fluconazole) and anti-HIV protease inhibitors (e.g. indinavir, ritonavir, nelfinavir, saquinavir), may lead to substantially increased plasma concentrations of nimodipine, with the possible development of hypotension and should be avoided. If co-administration of nimodipine and one of these drugs is unavoidable then the patient's blood pressure should be carefully monitored.

Nimotop solution should not be administered concomitantly with drugs which induce the CYP 3A4 system such as the anti-epileptics phenobarbitone, phenytoin and carbamazepine since this markedly reduces the bioavailability of nimodipine. The same is also true for rifampicin.

A study examining the effects of 90mg nimodipine (in divided doses) on elderly patients receiving haloperidol did not show evidence of potential interactions. It is unclear whether this study is relevant to use in subarachnoid haemorrhage because of the higher dose of nimodipine used.

The intake of grapefruit juice is not recommended in combination with nimodipine as it can result in increased plasma nimodipine concentrations due to the inhibition of the oxidative metabolism of dihydropyridines.

Since Nimotop infusion solution contains 20% ethanol, patients should be monitored for any possible interactions with alcohol-incompatible drugs.

4.6 Pregnancy and lactation
No reproductive toxicology studies following parenteral administration are available. Reproductive toxicology studies in animals after oral administration showed no teratogenic effect. Nimotop solution should be used with caution in pregnant women, and only when the benefit of treatment is considered to outweigh the risk.

4.7 Effects on ability to drive and use machines
In theory, the possibility of the occurrence of the side-effect dizziness may impair the patient's ability to drive or operate machinery. However, this is unlikely to be of clinical relevance in patients receiving Nimotop Solution.

4.8 Undesirable effects
The following have been reported: decrease in blood pressure, slight increase or decrease in heart rate, flushing, headache, dizziness, gastro-intestinal disorders, nausea, sweating and feeling of warmth. Very rarely thrombocytopenia and ileus have been reported. A transient rise in liver enzymes may occur during intravenous administration; this usually reverts to normal on completion of treatment. The infusion contains 20% ethanol and 17% macrogol 400; this should be taken into account during treatment.

Phlebitis may occur at the site of infusion if the solution is administered undiluted. The solution should always be administered alongside a compatible co-infusion product (see Section 4.2 Posology and method of administration under section headed Route of administration).

4.9 Overdose
If overdosage occurs, treatment should be discontinued immediately. If there is a large drop in blood pressure an intravenous injection of dopamine or noradrenaline may be indicated.

5. PHARMACOLOGICAL PROPERTIES

5.1 Pharmacodynamic properties
Nimodipine is a calcium channel blocker of the dihydropyridine group with preferential activity on cerebral vessels. Nimodipine increases cerebral perfusion, particularly in poorly perfused areas, by arterial dilatation, an effect which is proportionately greater in smaller than in larger vessels.

5.2 Pharmacokinetic properties
The intravenous Nimotop solution is 100% available to the tissues as the peripheral venous blood takes the drug to the lungs and heart and from there to all organs. The drug circulates in the plasma, bound to protein (97 - 99%) having an equal distribution between red cells and plasma proteins.

Nimodipine is eliminated as metabolites, mainly by dehydrogenation of the dihydropyridine ring and oxidative O-demethylation. Oxidative ester cleavage, hydroxylation of the 2- and 6-methyl groups, and glucuronidation as a conjugation reaction are other important metabolic steps. The three primary metabolites occurring in plasma show no or only therapeutically negligible residual activity.

Effects on liver enzymes by induction or inhibition are unknown. In humans the metabolites are excreted about 50 % renally and 30 % in the bile.

The elimination kinetics are linear. The half-life for nimodipine is between 1.1 and 1.7 h. The terminal half-life is 5-10 h, and is not relevant for establishing the recommended dosing interval for the medicinal product.

5.3 Preclinical safety data
One preclinical finding may be of relevance to the prescribing physician. In chronic repeat dose toxicity studies in dogs, doses of 1 and 2.5 mg/kg/day were shown to be tolerated without adverse effect. However, at the higher dose of 6.25 mg/kg/day significant changes in ECG's were noted due to disturbances in myocardial blood flow, but there was no indication of histopathological damage to the heart.

6. PHARMACEUTICAL PARTICULARS

6.1 List of excipients
Nimodipine 0.02% solution contains the following excipients:

Ethanol 96%, Macrogol 400, sodium citrate, citric acid, Water for Injections Ph. Eur.

6.2 Incompatibilities
Nimotop solution reacts with polyvinylchloride (PVC) and should not be allowed to come in contact with PVC. Nimotop solution must not be added to an infusion bag or bottle and must not be mixed with other drugs.

6.3 Shelf life
Shelf-life of the product as packaged for sale:

(see Table 1 below)

Table 1

	Shelf-life		Pack size
	A	B	(ml)
Primary packaging material			
Brown glass type II infusion vials	48m	N/A	50
Brown glass type II infusion bottles	48m	N/A	250

A = Unopened
B = After reconstitution or when the container is opened for the first time, if appropriate.

6.4 Special precautions for storage

Nimotop solution is light sensitive and therefore should be stored in the manufacturer's light-protective container within the cardboard carton at a temperature not exceeding 25°C.

6.5 Nature and contents of container

Brown glass type II infusion vials containing 50 ml of solution; or brown glass type II infusion bottles containing 250 ml solution, with grey chlorobutyl stopper laminated with fluoropolymer.

6.6 Instructions for use and handling

The only plastic materials suitable for use are polyethylene or polypropylene. Nimotop solution is compatible with glass infusion bottles and infusion packs made of polyethylene (e.g. Polyfusor, Boots).

The solution when in the syringe must be protected from direct sunlight during administration, but it is stable in diffuse daylight and artificial light for up to 10 hours. Nimotop solution should be infused using a glass or rigid plastic (polyethylene or polypropylene) syringe and giving set (Gillette Sabre syringe; BD plastipak syringe; Monoject disposable syringe, Sherwood Medical Ltd; Combidyn tubes, Braun; Nitrocassette giving set, Imed Ltd.). Nimotop solution is incompatible with infusion bags and any giving sets made of PVC (e.g. Viaflex, Travenol; Steriflex, Boots).

Nimotop solution 250 ml bottles are for single use and the rubber stopper should be pierced only once. One 250 ml bottle is sufficient for 24 hours administration at the maximum recommended dose with a safety margin of one hour. A single bottle should not be used for longer than 25 hours regardless of whether all the solution has been used.

The 250 ml bottle should be protected from direct sunlight at all times. If appropriate, infusion pumps and tubing should be protected with opaque covering, or black, brown, yellow, or red infusion lines (Braun) can be used. If a peristaltic pump is used for administration, polyethylene or polypropylene lines should be used. If a volumetric pump, e.g. Imed, is used for administration, then Nitrocassette cartridges that are polyethylene lined should be used.

7. MARKETING AUTHORISATION HOLDER

Bayer plc

Bayer House

Strawberry Hill

Newbury, Berkshire

RG14 1JA

Also trading as Bayer plc, Pharmaceutical Division or BAYPHARM or BAYMET

8. MARKETING AUTHORISATION NUMBER(S)

PL 00010/0138

9. DATE OF FIRST AUTHORISATION/RENEWAL OF THE AUTHORISATION

21 January 1988/ 24 November 1998

10. DATE OF REVISION OF THE TEXT

Date of revision: June 2002

Nimotop 30mg Tablets

(Bayer plc)

1. NAME OF THE MEDICINAL PRODUCT

Nimotop 30mg Tablets

2. QUALITATIVE AND QUANTITATIVE COMPOSITION

Each film-coated tablet contains 30mg nimodipine.

3. PHARMACEUTICAL FORM

Yellow film-coated tablet.

4. CLINICAL PARTICULARS

4.1 Therapeutic indications

Nimodipine is indicated for the prevention of ischaemic neurological deficits following aneurysmal subarachnoid haemorrhage.

4.2 Posology and method of administration

Adults:

Aneurysmal subarachnoid haemorrhage:

Prophylactic administration

The recommended dose is two tablets at 4-hourly intervals (total daily dose 360mg) to be taken with water. Prophylactic administration should commence within four days of onset of subarachnoid haemorrhage and should be continued for 21 days.

In the event of surgical intervention, administration of Nimotop tablets should be continued (dosage as above) to complete the 21 days treatment period.

Traumatic subarachnoid haemorrhage:

Not recommended as a positive benefit to risk ratio has not been established (see Section 4.4)

Elderly: There are no special dosage requirements for use in the elderly.

Children: Paediatric dosage has not been established.

4.3 Contraindications

Nimodipine should not be administered to patients during or within one month of a myocardial infarction or an episode of unstable angina.

4.4 Special warnings and special precautions for use

Nimotop should not be used in patients with traumatic subarachnoid haemorrhage as a positive benefit to risk ratio has not been established and the specific patient groups that might benefit cannot be identified for this indication.

Nimotop tablets should be used with care when cerebral oedema or severely raised intracranial pressure are present.

Decreased drug clearance may occur in cirrhotic patients receiving Nimotop and, therefore, close monitoring of blood pressure is recommended in these patients.

4.5 Interaction with other medicinal products and other forms of Interaction

Nimotop tablets should not be administered concomitantly with Nimotop solution.

Nimodipine may potentiate the hypotensive effect of antihypertensives. Where concomitant administration of other calcium channel blockers (e.g. nifedipine, diltiazem, verapamil), α-methyldopa or beta-blockers is necessary, blood pressure must be monitored, and careful dose titration of nimodipine should be undertaken with possible reduction or discontinuation of the antihypertensive agent.

Concurrent twice daily administration of 30mg nimodipine and daily administration of 20mg of the antidepressant fluoxetine to elderly patients resulted in an increase in nimodipine plasma levels, a reduction in fluoxetine levels and a trend towards increased norfluoxetine levels. The daily dose used in patients with subarachnoid haemorrhage is four times the daily dose used in this trial, and as a steady state norfluoxetine level was not achieved, the clinical significance of this interaction in the treatment of aneurysmal subarachnoid haemorrhage (aSAH) is uncertain.

Concurrent three times daily administration of 30mg nimodipine and three times daily administration of 10mg of the antidepressant nortriptyline to elderly patients resulted in a slight decrease in nimodipine plasma levels with no effect on nortriptyline plasma levels. The daily dose used in patients with subarachnoid haemorrhage is four times the daily dose used in this trial, thus the clinical significance of this interaction in the treatment of aneurysmal subarachnoid haemorrhage (aSAH) is uncertain.

The simultaneous administration of cimetidine or sodium valproate may lead to an increase in the plasma nimodipine concentration.

Animal studies have shown that when nimodipine and zidovudine are administered concomitantly, the AUC for zidovudine was increased, and the volume of distribution and clearance rate decreased. The clinical relevance of this interaction is unknown, but since the side-effects profile of zidovudine is known to be dose-related, this interaction should be considered in patients receiving nimodipine and zidovudine concomitantly.

Nimodipine is metabolised via the cytochrome P450 3A4 system located in both the intestinal mucosa and in the liver. Drugs that are known to either inhibit or to induce this enzyme system may therefore alter the first pass metabolism or clearance of nimodipine. The concomitant administration of nimodipine and potent CYP 3A4 inhibitors, e.g. macrolide antibiotics (e.g. erythromycin), azole antimycotics (e.g. ketoconazole, itraconazole, fluconazole) and anti-HIV protease inhibitors (e.g. indinavir, ritonavir, nelfinavir, saquinavir), may lead to substantially increased plasma concentrations of nimodipine and should be avoided. If co-administration of nimodipine and one of these drugs is unavoidable then the patient's blood pressure should be carefully monitored.

Nimotop tablets should not be administered concomitantly with drugs which induce the CYP 3A4 system such as the anti-epileptics phenobarbitone, phenytoin and carbamazepine since this markedly reduces the bioavailability of nimodipine. The same is also true for rifampicin.

A study examining the effects of 90mg nimodipine (in divided doses) on elderly patients receiving haloperidol did not show evidence of potential interactions. It is unclear whether this study is relevant to use in subarachnoid haemorrhage because of the higher dose of nimodipine used.

The intake of grapefruit juice is not recommended in combination with nimodipine as it can result in increased plasma nimodipine concentrations due to the inhibition of the oxidative metabolism of dihydropyridines.

4.6 Pregnancy and lactation

Reproductive toxicology studies in animals using oral administration showed no teratogenic effect. Nimotop tablets should be used with caution in pregnant women, and only when the benefit of treatment is considered to outweigh the risk.

4.7 Effects on ability to drive and use machines

In theory, the possibility of the occurrence of the side-effect dizziness may impair the patient's ability to drive or operate machinery.

4.8 Undesirable effects

The following side-effects have been reported: decrease in blood pressure, slight increase or decrease in heart rate, flushing, headache, dizziness, gastro-intestinal disorders, nausea, sweating and feeling of warmth. Very rarely, thrombocytopenia and ileus have been reported.

4.9 Overdose

If overdosage occurs, gastric lavage should be carried out and activated charcoal administered. If blood pressure is low, a vasopressor should be administered.

5. PHARMACOLOGICAL PROPERTIES

5.1 Pharmacodynamic properties

Nimodipine is a calcium channel blocker of the dihydropyridine group with preferential activity on cerebral vessels. Nimodipine increases cerebral perfusion, particularly in poorly perfused areas, by arterial dilatation, an effect which is proportionately greater in smaller than in larger vessels.

5.2 Pharmacokinetic properties

After oral ingestion, absorption is rapid; peak plasma concentrations are observed 30 to 60 minutes following administration. Nimodipine has a high first-pass metabolism resulting in a low bioavailability of approximately 10%.

Protein binding in the plasma is approximately 98%.

Nimodipine is eliminated as metabolites, mainly by dehydrogenation of the dihydropyridine ring and oxidative O-demethylation. Oxidative ester cleavage, hydroxylation of the 2- and 6-methyl groups, and glucuronidation as a conjugation reaction are other important metabolic steps. The three primary metabolites occurring in plasma show no or only therapeutically negligible residual activity.

Effects on liver enzymes by induction or inhibition are unknown. In humans the metabolites are excreted about 50% renally and 30% in the bile.

The elimination kinetics are linear. The half-life for nimodipine is between 1.1 and 1.7h. The terminal half-life is 5-10h, and is not relevant for establishing the recommended dosing interval for the medicinal product.

5.3 Preclinical safety data

One preclinical finding may be of relevance to the prescribing physician. In chronic repeat dose toxicity studies in dogs, doses of 1 and 2.5 mg/kg/day were shown to be tolerated without adverse effect. However, at the higher dose of 6.25 mg/kg/day significant changes in ECGs were noted due to disturbances in myocardial blood flow, but there was no indication of histopathological damage to the heart.

6. PHARMACEUTICAL PARTICULARS

6.1 List of excipients

Microcrystalline cellulose, maize starch, povidone, crospovidone, magnesium stearate, hypromellose, macrogol 4000, titanium dioxide E171, iron oxide yellow E172.

6.2 Incompatibilities

None known.

6.3 Shelf life

5 years.

6.4 Special precautions for storage

Do not store above 30°C.

6.5 Nature and contents of container

PVC/PVDC/aluminium, or PP/aluminium blister packs contained in cardboard outer, containing 100 × 30mg tablets, or 20 × 30mg tablets (professional sample pack).

6.6 Instructions for use and handling

Not applicable.

7. MARKETING AUTHORISATION HOLDER

Bayer plc

Bayer House

Strawberry Hill

Newbury, Berkshire

RG14 1JA

Trading as Bayer plc, Pharmaceutical Division, or BAYPHARM or BAYMET

8. MARKETING AUTHORISATION NUMBER(S)

PL 0010/0137

9. DATE OF FIRST AUTHORISATION/RENEWAL OF THE AUTHORISATION

23 February 1989/11 July 2000

10. DATE OF REVISION OF THE TEXT

June 2002

Nipent

(Wyeth Pharmaceuticals)

1. NAME OF THE MEDICINAL PRODUCT

NIPENT™ 10 mg powder for solution for injection, powder for solution for infusion.

2. QUALITATIVE AND QUANTITATIVE COMPOSITION

One vial contains 10 mg Pentostatin.

For excipients see Section 6.1.

When reconstituted (see Section 6.6), the resulting solution contains pentostatin 2 mg/ml.

3. PHARMACEUTICAL FORM

Powder for solution for injection, powder for solution for infusion.

The vials contain a solid white to off-white cake or powder.

4. CLINICAL PARTICULARS

4.1 Therapeutic indications

Pentostatin is indicated as single agent therapy in the treatment of adult patients with hairy cell leukaemia.

4.2 Posology and method of administration

Pentostatin is indicated for adult patients.

Administration to Patient

It is recommended that patients receive hydration with 500 to 1,000 ml of 5% glucose only or 5% glucose in 0.18% or 0.9% saline or glucose 3.3% in 0.3% saline or 2.5% glucose in 0.45% saline or equivalent before pentostatin administration. An additional 500 ml of 5% glucose only or 5% glucose in 0.18% or 0.9% saline or 2.5% glucose in 0.45% saline or equivalent should be administered after pentostatin is given.

The recommended dosage of pentostatin for the treatment of hairy cell leukaemia is 4 mg/m^2 in a single administration every other week. Pentostatin may be given intravenously by bolus injection or diluted in a larger volume and given over 20 to 30 minutes. (See Instruction for use and handling [6.6].)

Higher doses are not recommended.

No extravasation injuries were reported in clinical studies.

The optimal duration of treatment has not been determined. In the absence of major toxicity and with observed continuing improvement, the patient should be treated until a complete response has been achieved. Although not established as required, the administration of two additional doses has been recommended following the achievement of a complete response.

All patients receiving pentostatin at 6 months should be assessed for response to treatment. If the patient has not achieved a complete or partial response, treatment with pentostatin should be discontinued.

If the patient has achieved a partial response, pentostatin treatment should be continued in an effort to achieve a complete response. At any time thereafter that a complete response is achieved, two additional doses of pentostatin are recommended. Pentostatin treatment should then be stopped. If the best response to treatment at the end of 12 months is a partial response, it is recommended that treatment with pentostatin be stopped.

Withholding or discontinuation of individual doses may be needed when severe adverse reactions occur. Drug treatment should be withheld in patients with severe rash, and withheld or discontinued in patients showing evidence of nervous system toxicity.

Pentostatin treatment should be withheld in patients with active infection occurring during the treatment but may be resumed when the infection is controlled.

Dosage in Patients with Cytopenias

No dosage reduction is recommended at the start of therapy with pentostatin in patients with anaemia, neutropenia, or thrombocytopenia. In addition, dosage reductions are not recommended during treatment in patients with anaemia and thrombocytopenia. Pentostatin should be temporarily withheld if the absolute neutrophil count during treatment falls below 200 cells/mm^3 in a patient who had an initial neutrophil count greater than 500 cells/mm^3 and may be resumed when the count returns to predose levels.

Renal Insufficiency

There is limited experience in patients with impaired renal function (creatinine clearance <60 ml/min). Two patients with impaired renal function (creatinine clearances 50 to 60 ml/min) achieved complete response without unusual adverse events when treated with 2 mg/m^2. However, given this limited experience, pentostatin is contraindicated in patients whose creatinine clearance is <60 ml/min.

Liver Impairment

Because of limited experience treating patients with abnormal liver function, treatment of such patients should be done with caution.

Administration to Elderly Patients

The recommended dosage of pentostatin for the treatment of hairy cell leukaemia in the elderly is 4 mg/m^2 in a single administration every other week. Clinical trials have included patients over 65 years old and no adverse reactions specific to this age group have been reported.

Paediatric Use

Hairy cell leukaemia is a disease affecting adults, most commonly in the sixth decade of life. Safety and effectiveness of Nipent in children have not been established.

4.3 Contraindications

Pentostatin is contraindicated in patients who have demonstrated hypersensitivity to the active ingredients or to any of the excipients.

Pentostatin is contraindicated in patients with impaired renal function (Creatinine clearance <60 ml/min).

Pentostatin is contraindicated in patients with active infection.

Pentostatin is contraindicated in pregnancy.

4.4 Special warnings and special precautions for use

Warnings

Pentostatin should be administered under the supervision of a physician qualified and experienced in the use of cancer chemotherapeutic agents. The use of doses higher than those specified (see Administration to Patient [4.2]) is not recommended. Dose-limiting severe renal, liver, pulmonary, and CNS toxicities occurred in Phase 1 studies that used pentostatin at a higher dose (20-50 mg/m^2/course) than recommended.

In a clinical investigation in patients with refractory chronic lymphocytic leukaemia using pentostatin at the recommended dose in combination with fludarabine phosphate, four of six patients entered on the study had severe or fatal pulmonary toxicity. The use of pentostatin in combination with fludarabine phosphate is not recommended.

Biochemical studies have demonstrated that pentostatin enhances the effects of vidarabine, a purine nucleoside with antiviral activity. The combined use of vidarabine and pentostatin may result in an increase in adverse reactions associated with each drug. The therapeutic benefit of the drug combination has not been established.

Patients with hairy cell leukaemia may experience myelosuppression primarily during the first few courses of treatment. Patients with infections prior to pentostatin treatment have in some cases developed worsening of their condition leading to death; whereas others have achieved complete response. Patients with infection should be treated only when the potential benefit of treatment justifies the potential risk to the patient. Efforts should be made to control the infection before treatment is initiated or resumed.

In patients with progressive hairy cell leukaemia, the initial courses of pentostatin treatment were associated with worsening of neutropaenia. Therefore, frequent monitoring of complete blood counts during this time is necessary. If severe neutropenia continues beyond the initial cycles, patient should be evaluated for disease status, including a bone marrow examination.

Pentostatin might have harmful effects on the genotype. Therefore, it is recommended that men undergoing treatment with pentostatin should not father a child during treatment up to 6 months thereafter. Contraception is to be guaranteed for women of childbearing age. Should a pregnancy occur during treatment, the possibility of a genetic consultation is to be considered.

Bone Marrow Transplant Regimen with high dose cyclophosphamide

Acute pulmonary oedema and hypotension leading to death, have been reported in the literature in patients treated with pentostatin in combination with carmustine, etoposide and high dose cyclophosphamide as part of an ablative regimen for bone marrow transplant. The combination of pentostatin and high dose cyclophosphamide is not recommended.

Elevations in liver function tests occurred during treatment with pentostatin and were generally reversible.

Renal toxicity was observed at higher doses in early studies; however, in patients treated at the recommended dose, elevations in serum creatinine were usually minor and reversible. There were some patients who began treatment with normal renal function who had evidence of mild to moderate toxicity at a final assessment. (See Administration to Patient [4.2].)

Rashes, occasionally severe, were commonly reported and may worsen with continued treatment. Withholding of treatment may be required. (See Administration to Patient [4.2]).

Extra care should be taken in treating patients beginning therapy with poor performance.

Precautions

Therapy with pentostatin requires regular patient observation and monitoring of haematologic parameters and blood chemistry values. If severe adverse reactions occur, the drug should be withheld (see Administration to Patient [4.2]) and appropriate corrective measures should be taken according to the clinical judgement of the physician.

Pentostatin treatment should be withheld or discontinued in patients showing evidence of nervous system toxicity.

Prior to initiating therapy with pentostatin, renal function should be assessed with a serum creatinine and/or a creatinine clearance assay. (See Pharmacokinetic properties [5.2], Administration to Patient [4.2].) Complete blood counts, serum creatinine, and BUN should be performed before each dose of pentostatin and at appropriate periods during therapy. Severe neutropenia has been observed following the early courses of treatment with pentostatin and therefore frequent monitoring of complete blood counts is recommended during this time. If haematologic parameters do not improve with subsequent courses, patients should be evaluated for disease status, including a bone marrow examination. Periodic monitoring of the peripheral blood for hairy cells should be performed to assess the response to treatment.

In addition, bone marrow aspirates and biopsies may be required at 2 to 3 month intervals to assess the response to treatment.

4.5 Interaction with other medicinal products and other forms of Interaction

Allopurinol

Allopurinol and pentostatin are both associated with skin rashes. Based on clinical studies in 25 refractory patients who received both pentostatin and allopurinol, the combined use of pentostatin and allopurinol did not appear to produce a higher incidence of skin rashes than observed with pentostatin alone. There has been a report of one patient who received both drugs and experienced a hypersensitivity vasculitis that resulted in death. It was unclear whether this adverse event and subsequent death resulted from the drug combination.

Vidarabine

Biochemical studies have demonstrated that pentostatin enhances the effects of vidarabine, a purine nucleoside with antiviral activity. The combined use of vidarabine and pentostatin may result in an increase in adverse reactions associated with each drug. The therapeutic benefit of the drug combination has not been established.

Fludarabine

The combined use of pentostatin and fludarabine phosphate is not recommended because it has been associated with an increased risk of fatal pulmonary toxicity. (See WARNINGS.)

Bone Marrow Transplant Regimen with high dose cyclophosphamide

Acute pulmonary oedema and hypotension leading to death, have been reported in the literature in patients treated with pentostatin in combination with carmustine, etoposide and high dose cyclophosphamide as part of an ablative regimen for bone marrow transplant. The combination of pentostatin and high dose cyclophosphamide is not recommended.

4.6 Pregnancy and lactation

Pentostatin must not be used during pregnancy. Women of childbearing potential receiving pentostatin should be advised not to become pregnant.

No fertility studies have been conducted in animals. Incompletely reversible seminiferous tubular atrophy and degeneration in rats and in dogs may be indicative of potential effects on male fertility. The possible adverse effects on human fertility have not been determined.

Pentostatin is teratogenic in mice and rats. There are no adequate and well-controlled studies in pregnant women. If the patient becomes pregnant while receiving this drug, the patient should be apprised of the potential hazards to the foetus.

It is not known whether pentostatin is excreted in human milk. Because many drugs are excreted in human milk and because of the potential for serious adverse reactions from pentostatin in nursing infants, nursing is not recommended.

4.7 Effects on ability to drive and use machines

On the basis of the reported adverse event profile pentostatin is likely to produce minor or moderate adverse effects. Patients should be advised to use caution in driving or using machinery following drug administration.

4.8 Undesirable effects

Pentostatin is lymphotoxic. Aside from myelosuppression, pentostatin is immunosuppressive in particular by suppression of the CD_4+ lymphocyte subset. CD_4+ counts smaller than 200 per μl are usually seen during treatment with pentostatin and CD_4+ count suppression can outlast the end of treatment by more than 6 months. With the exception of frequent herpes zoster infections the clinical consequences of the suppression of CD_4+ counts in hairy cell leukaemia are not well understood yet. Long term consequences are not predictable, but currently there is no evidence for higher frequency of secondary malignancies of opportunistic infections.

The following adverse events were reported during clinical studies in patients with hairy cell leukaemia who were refractory to alpha-interferon or were treated as front-line therapy. Most patients experienced an adverse event. Twelve percent of patients withdrew from treatment due to an adverse event. Many hairy cell leukaemia patients experience adverse events while under therapy with pentostatin. Given the natural history of the disease and the pharmacological properties of the drug it may be difficult in certain cases to discriminate between drug-related and disease-related adverse events.

Adverse Events Occurring in over 10% of Patients Treated with Pentostatin in Front-line Therapy for Hairy Cell Leukaemia

Body as a Whole

Abdominal pain, Asthenia, Chills, Fatigue, Fever, Headache, Infection, Pain

Digestive System

Anorexia, Diarrhoea, Liver damage, Nausea, Vomiting

Haemic and Lymphatic System

Anaemia, Blood dyscrasia, Leucopenia, Thrombocytopenia

Metabolic and Nutritional System

Peripheral oedema

Nervous System

Somnolence

Respiratory System

Cough/ increased coughing, Lung disorder, Pneumonia, Respiratory disorder

Skin and Appendages

Dry skin, Herpes simplex, Maculopapular rash, Pruritus, Rash, Skin disorder

Special Senses

Conjunctivitis

Adverse Events Occurring in 3 to 10% of Patients Treated with Pentostatin in Front-line Therapy for Hairy Cell Leukaemia

Body as a Whole

Abscess, Allergic reaction, Back pain, Cellulitis, Chest pain, Cyst, Death, Facial oedema, Flu syndrome, Malaise, Moniliasis, Neoplasm, Photosensitivity reaction, Sepsis

Cardiovascular System

Atrial fibrillation, Cardiovascular disorder, Congestive heart failure, Flushing, Haemorrhage, Shock

Digestive System

Constipation, Dyspepsia, Dysphagia, Flatulence, Gastrointestinal disorder, Gum haemorrhage, Jaundice, LFTs abnormal, Mouth ulceration, Oral moniliasis, Rectal disorder, Rectal haemorrhage

Haemic and Lymphatic System

Eosinophilia, Hypochromic anaemia, Pancytopenia, Petechia, Splenomegaly

Metabolic and Nutritional System

Bilirubinemia, BUN increased, Creatinine increased, Oedema, Hyperglycaemia, SGOT increased, SGPT increased, Weight gain, Weight loss

Musculoskeletal System

Arthralgia, Bone disorder, Joint disorder, Myalgia

Nervous System

Abnormal thinking, Anxiety, Confusion, Depersonalisation, Depression, Dizziness, Dry Mouth, Hypaesthesia, Insomnia, Nervousness, Neurologic disorder PNS, Tremor, Twitching

Respiratory System

Asthma, Dyspnoea, Lung oedema, Pharyngitis, Rhinitis, Sinusitis, Upper respiratory infection

Skin and Appendages

Acne, Alopecia, Exfoliative dermatitis, Herpes zoster, Skin carcinoma, Skin discoloration, Sweating/sweating increased, Vesiculobullous rash

Special Senses

Ear pain, Eye disorder, Photophobia, Taste perversion

Urogenital System

Dysuria, Genitourinary disorder, Urinary retention

Adverse Events Occurring in over 10% of Alpha-Interferon Refractory Patients Treated with Pentostatin

Body as a Whole

Allergic reaction, Chills, Fatigue, Fever, Headache, Infection, Pain

Digestive System

Anorexia, Diarrhoea, Elevated LFTs, Nausea, Nausea and vomiting

Haemic and Lymphatic System

Anaemia, Leucopenia, Thrombocytopenia

Musculoskeletal System

Myalgia

Nervous System

Neurologic disorder CNS

Respiratory System

Cough increased/coughing, Lung disorder, Upper respiratory infection

Skin and Appendages

Rash, Skin disorder

Urogenital System

Genitourinary disorder

Adverse Events Occurring in 3 to 10% of Alpha-Interferon Refractory Patients Treated with Pentostatin

Body as a Whole

Abdominal pain, Asthaenia, Back pain, Chest pain, Death, Flu syndrome, Malaise, Neoplasm, Sepsis

Cardiovascular System

Abnormal electrocardiogram, Arrhythmia, Haemorrhage, Thrombophlebitis

Digestive System

Constipation, Flatulence, Stomatitis

Haemic and Lymphatic System

Ecchymosis, Lymphadenopathy, Petechia

Metabolic and Nutritional System

BUN increased, Creatinine increased, LDH increased, Peripheral oedema, Weight loss.

Musculoskeletal System

Arthralgia

Nervous System

Abnormal thinking, Anxiety, Confusion, Depression, Dizziness, Insomnia, Nervousness, Paraesthesia, Somnolence

Respiratory System

Bronchitis, Dyspnoea, Epistaxis, Lung oedema, Pharyngitis, Pneumonia, Rhinitis, Sinusitis

Skin and Appendages

Dry skin, Eczema, Herpes simplex, Herpes zoster, Maculopapular rash, Pruritus, Seborrhoea, Skin discoloration, Sweating/sweating increased, Vesiculobullous rash

Special Senses

Abnormal vision, Conjunctivitis, Ear pain, Eye pain

Urogenital System

Dysuria, Haematuria

4.9 Overdose

No specific antidote for pentostatin overdose is known. Pentostatin administered at higher doses (20-50 mg/m2/ course) than recommended was associated with deaths due to severe renal, hepatic, pulmonary, and CNS toxicity. In case of overdose, management would include general supportive measures through any period of toxicity that occurs.

5. PHARMACOLOGICAL PROPERTIES

5.1 Pharmacodynamic properties

LO1X X08

Pharmacotherapeutic Group

Pentostatin is an adenosine deaminase (ADA) inhibitor.

Mechanism of Action

Pentostatin is a potent transition state inhibitor of the enzyme adenosine deaminase. The greatest activity of ADA is found in cells of the lymphoid system with T-cells having higher activity than B- cells and T-cell malignancies higher ADA activity than B-cell malignancies. Pentostatin inhibition of ADA, as well as direct inhibition of RNA synthesis and increased DNA damage, may contribute to the overall cytotoxic effect of pentostatin. The precise mechanism of pentostatin's antitumour effect, however, in hairy cell leukaemia is not known.

Pentostatin has been shown to have activity against a variety of lymphoid malignancies, but is most active against indolent cancers with lower ADA concentration, such as hairy cell leukaemia.

5.2 Pharmacokinetic properties

In man, pentostatin pharmacokinetics are linear with plasma concentrations increasing proportionately with dose. Following a single dose of 4 mg/m^2 of pentostatin infused over 5 minutes, the distribution half-life was 11 minutes and the mean terminal half-life was 5.7 hours, with a range of 2.6 to 10 hours; the mean plasma clearance was 68 ml/min/m^2, and approximately 90% of the dose was excreted in the urine as unchanged pentostatin and/or metabolites as measured by adenosine deaminase inhibitory activity. The plasma protein binding of pentostatin is low, approximately 4%.

A positive correlation was observed between pentostatin clearance and creatinine clearance (CrCl) in patients with creatinine clearance values ranging from 60 ml/min to 130 ml/min. Pentostatin half-life in patients with renal impairment (CrCl $<$50 ml/min, n = 2) was 18 hours, which was much longer than that observed in patients with normal renal function (CrCl $>$60 ml/min, n = 14), about 6 hours.

A tissue distribution and whole-body autoradiography study in the rat revealed that radioactivity concentrations were highest in the kidneys with very little central nervous system penetration.

Pentostatin penetrates the blood-brain barrier leading to measurable concentrations in the cerebrospinal fluid (CSF).

5.3 Preclinical safety data

Acute Toxicity

The combined-sex intravenous LD_{10}, LD_{50} and LD_{90} values in mice given formulated pentostatin were 129, 300 and 697 mg/kg (387, 900, and 2091 mg/m^2), respectively.

Signs of acute toxicity in rodents and dogs were hypoactivity, dehydration, and emaciation. Lymphoid tissue was a principal target of pentostatin in rats and dogs; thymic atrophy and liver damage occurred in mice. There were no gonadal effects in rodents or dogs.

Multidose Toxicity

Five daily dose IV combined-sex LD_{10}, LD_{50} and LD_{90} values in mice administered bulk pentostatin were 4.9, 6.4, and 8.3 mg/kg (14.8, 19.1, and 24.8 mg/m^2), respectively.

Regardless of route or duration of treatment, lymphoid tissue was the primary target of pentostatin in all species examined in toxicology studies. This is consistent with pentostatin's antineoplastic activity in hairy cell leukaemia. Effects of lymphoid tissue may be related to adenosine deaminase inhibition, the major pharmacologic action of pentostatin. Increased serum hepatic enzymes and liver changes in rodents and dogs indicate that the liver is also a target organ at high doses. Testicular changes in rats and dogs may be indicative of potential effects on male fertility. Effects on lymphoid tissue, liver, and testes did not resolve completely during observation periods after drug withdrawal. Target organ effects occurring only in rats included alveolar duct metaplasia and/or goblet cell hyperplasia of the bronchioles, lymphoplasmacytic thyroiditis, and an increased incidence of spontaneous glomerulonephritis. Published studies, not conducted by the sponsor, indicate that pentostatin has immunosuppressive properties in mice and rats given multiple doses.

Mutagenesis

Pentostatin was not mutagenic in Salmonella typhimurium at concentrations up to 10000 μg/plate or in V79 Chinese hamster lung cells at concentrations up to 3000 μg/ml, in the presence or absence of metabolic activation. Pentostatin was not clastogenic in V79 Chinese hamster lung cells in vitro at concentrations up to 3000 μg/ml. However, pentostatin did increase the frequency of micronucleus formation in mice administered single intravenous injections of formulated pentostatin at 60, 360, and 720 mg/m^2. The relevance of the positive mouse micronucleus test for man is not known.

Carcinogenicity

The carcinogenic potential of pentostatin has not been evaluated. The possibility that Nipent causes tumours cannot be ruled out.

6. PHARMACEUTICAL PARTICULARS

6.1 List of excipients

Mannitol

Sodium hydroxide or Hydrochloric acid

6.2 Incompatibilities

Acidic solutions should be avoided (the pH of the reconstituted powder is 7.0 to 8.2).

6.3 Shelf life

2 years

The reconstituted solution for injection or reconstituted and further diluted solution for infusion should be used within 8 hours. Immediate administration after reconstitution is recommended.

6.4 Special precautions for storage

Store at 2°C to 8°C (in a refrigerator).

After reconstitution the solution should not be stored above 25°C.

6.5 Nature and contents of container

NIPENT is supplied in single-dose, 10-mg vials packaged in individual cartons (packs of 1).

Vials are made from Type I glass and siliconised stoppers.

6.6 Instructions for use and handling

Procedures for proper handling and disposal of anticancer drugs should be followed.

1. Reconstitution of Nipent should only be carried out by trained personnel in a cytotoxic-designated area.

2. Adequate protective gloves should be worn.

3. The cytotoxic preparation should not be handled by pregnant staff.

4. Adequate care and precautions should be taken in the disposal of items syringes, needles etc. used to reconstitute cytotoxic drugs.

5. Contaminated surfaces should be washed with copious amounts of water.

6. Any remaining solution should be discarded.

Prescribers should refer to national or recognised guidelines on handling cytotoxic agents.

Transfer 5 ml of Sterile Water for Injection to the vial containing NIPENT and mix thoroughly to obtain complete dissolutionThe solution should be colourless to pale yellow and yield 2 mg/ml. Parenteral drug products should be inspected visually for particulate matter and discoloration prior to administration.

NIPENT may be given intravenously by bolus injection or diluted in a larger volume (25 to 50 ml) with 5% Dextrose Injection (5% glucose solution) or 0.9% Sodium Chloride Injection (0.9% saline solution). Dilution of the entire contents of a reconstituted vial with 25 ml or 50 ml provides a pentostatin concentration of 0.33 mg/ml or 0.18 mg/ml, respectively, for the diluted solutions.

NIPENT solution when diluted for infusion with 5% Dextrose Injection (5% glucose solution) or 0.9% Sodium Chloride Injection (0.9% saline solution) does not interact with PVC infusion containers or administration sets at concentrations of 0.18 mg/ml to 0.33 mg/ml.

7. MARKETING AUTHORISATION HOLDER

Warner Lambert (UK) Ltd
trading as Parke Davis
Lambert Court
Chestnut Avenue
Eastleigh
Hampshire
SO53 3ZQ
United Kingdom

8. MARKETING AUTHORISATION NUMBER(S)
PL 0019/0176

9. DATE OF FIRST AUTHORISATION/RENEWAL OF THE AUTHORISATION
20 November 1998

10. DATE OF REVISION OF THE TEXT
November 2003

Nitrocine

(SCHWARZ PHARMA Limited)

1. NAME OF THE MEDICINAL PRODUCT
Nitrocine

2. QUALITATIVE AND QUANTITATIVE COMPOSITION
Ampoules containing 10mg glyceryl trinitrate in 10 ml, or as glass bottles containing 50mg glyceryl trinitrate in 50ml.

For excipients see 6.1.

3. PHARMACEUTICAL FORM
Isotonic sterile solution for infusion

4. CLINICAL PARTICULARS
4.1 Therapeutic indications
Surgery:

Nitrocine is indicated for:

1. the rapid control of hypertension during cardiac surgery.

2. reducing blood pressure and maintaining controlled hypotension during surgical procedures.

3. controlling myocardial ischaemia during and after cardiovascular surgery.

Unresponsive congestive heart failure:

Nitrocine may be used to treat unresponsive congestive heart failure secondary to acute myocardial infarction.

Unstable angina:

Nitrocine may be used to treat unstable angina, which is refractory to treatment with beta blockers and sublingual nitrates.

4.2 Posology and method of administration
Adults and Elderly
The dose of Nitrocine should be adjusted to meet the individual needs of the patient.

The recommended dosage range is 10 - 200 mcg/min but up to 400 mcg/min may be necessary during some surgical procedures.

Children:

The safety and efficacy of Nitrocine has not yet been established in children.

Surgery:

A starting dose of 25 mcg/min is recommended for the control of hypertension, or to produce hypotension during surgery. This may be increased by increments of 25 mcg/min at 5 minute intervals until the blood pressure is stabilized. Doses between 10 - 200 mcg/min are usually sufficient during surgery, although doses of up to 400 mcg/min have been required in some cases.

The treatment of perioperative myocardial ischaemia may be started with a dose of 15 - 20 mcg/min, with subsequent increments of 10 - 15 mcg/min until the required effect is obtained.

Unresponsive congestive heart failure:

The recommended starting dose is 20 - 25 mcg/min. This may be decreased to 10 mcg/min, or increased in steps of 20-25 mcg/min every 15 - 30 minutes until the desired effect is obtained.

Unstable angina:

An initial dose of 10 mcg/min is recommended with increments of 10mcg/min being made at approximately 30 minute intervals according to the needs of the patient.

Administration
Nitrocine can be administered undiluted by slow intravenous infusion using a syringe pump incorporating a glass or rigid plastic syringe.

Alternatively, Nitrocine may be administered intravenously as an admixture using a suitable vehicle such as Sodium Chloride Injection B.P. or Dextrose Injection B.P.

Prepared admixtures should be given by intravenous infusion or with the aid of a syringe pump to ensure a constant rate of infusion.

During Nitrocine administration there should be close haemodynamic monitoring of the patient.

Example of admixture preparation
To obtain an admixture of GTN at a concentration of 100 mcg/ml, add 50ml Nitrocine solution (containing 50mg glyceryl trinitrate) to 450ml of infusion vehicle to give a final volume of 500ml.

A dosage of 100 mcg/min. can be obtained by giving 60ml of the admixture per hour. This is equivalent to a drip rate of 60 paediatric microdrops per minute or 20 standard drops per minute. At this drip rate the admixture provides enough solution for an infusion time of 8 hours 20 minutes.

For full details it is advisable to consult the dosage chart on the package insert.

Bottles of Nitrocine are for single use only and should not be regarded as multi-dose containers.

4.3 Contraindications
Nitrocine should not be used in the following cases:

Known hypersensitivity to nitrates, marked anaemia, severe cerebral haemorrhage, head trauma, uncorrected hypovolaemia or severe hypotension.

As the safety of Nitrocine during pregnancy and lactation has not yet been established, it should not be used unless considered absolutely essential.

Sildenafil has been shown to potentiate the hypotensive effects of nitrates, and its co-administration with nitrates or nitric oxide donors is therefore contraindicated.

4.4 Special warnings and special precautions for use
Close attention to pulse and blood pressure is necessary during the administration of Nitrocine infusions.

Nitrocine should be used with caution in patients suffering from hypothyroidism, severe liver or renal disease, hypothermia and malnutrition.

4.5 Interaction with other medicinal products and other forms of Interaction
Concurrent intake of drugs with blood pressure lowering properties e.g. beta blockers, calcium antagonists, vasodilators etc. and/or alcohol may potentiate the hypotensive effect of Nitrocine. The hypotensive effect of nitrates are potentiated by concurrent administration of sildenafil (Viagra®). This might also occur with neuroleptics and tricyclic antidepressants.

4.6 Pregnancy and lactation
There is no, or inadequate, evidence of safety of the drug in human pregnancy or lactation, but it has been in widespread use for many years without apparent ill consequence, animal studies having shown no hazard. If drug therapy is needed in pregnancy, this product can be used if there is no safer alternative.

4.7 Effects on ability to drive and use machines
None stated.

4.8 Undesirable effects
In common with other nitrates, headaches and nausea may occur during administration. Other possible adverse reactions include hypotension, tachycardia, retching, diaphoresis, apprehension, restlessness, muscle twitching, retrosternal discomfort, palpitations, dizziness and abdominal pain. Paradoxical bradycardia has also been observed.

4.9 Overdose
Mild overdose usually results in hypotension and tachycardia. If arterial systolic blood pressure drops below 90 mmHg and if heart rate increases 10% above its initial value, the infusion should be discontinued to allow a return to pre-treatment levels. If hypotension persists, or in more severe cases, this may be reversed by elevating the legs and/or treatment with hypertensive agents.

5. PHARMACOLOGICAL PROPERTIES
5.1 Pharmacodynamic properties
ATC Code: C01DA 02 – Organic Nitrates

Glyceryl trinitrate reduces the tone of vascular smooth muscle. This action is more marked on the venous capacitance vessels than the arterial vessels. There is a reduction in venous return to the heart and a lowering of elevated filling pressure. This lowering of filling pressure reduces the left ventricular end diastolic volume and preload. The net effect is a lowering of myocardial oxygen consumption.

Systemic vascular resistance, pulmonary vascular pressure and arterial pressure are also reduced by glyceryl trinitrate and there is a net reduction in the afterload.

By reducing the preload and afterload, glyceryl trinitrate reduces the workload on the heart.

Glyceryl trinitrate affects oxygen supply by redistributing blood flow along collateral channels from the epicardial to endocardial regions.

5.2 Pharmacokinetic properties
As with all commonly used organic nitrates the metabolic degradation of glyceryl trinitrate occurs via denitration and glucuronidation. The less active metabolites resulting from this biotransformation can be recovered from the urine within 24 hours.

Glyceryl trinitrate is eliminated from plasma with a short half-life of about 2-3 minutes. This rapid disappearance from plasma is consistent with the high systemic clearance values for this drug (up to 3270 L/hour)

5.3 Preclinical safety data
None stated

6. PHARMACEUTICAL PARTICULARS
6.1 List of excipients
Glucose

Propylene glycol

Water for injection.

Hydrochloric acid (for pH adjustment)

6.2 Incompatibilities
Nitrocine contains glyceryl trinitrate in isotonic sterile solution and is compatible with commonly employed infusion solutions. No incompatibilities have so far been demonstrated.

Nitrocine is compatible with glass infusion bottles and with rigid infusion packs made of polyethylene. Nitrocine may also be infused slowly using a syringe pump with a glass or plastic syringe.

Nitrocine is incompatible with polyvinylchloride (PVC) and severe losses of glyceryl trinitrate (over 40%) may occur if this material is used. Contact with polyvinylchloride bags should be avoided. Polyurethane also induces a loss of the active ingredient.

6.3 Shelf life
Glass ampoules 5 years

Glass vials 36 months

For admixture shelf life, refer to section 6.4.

6.4 Special precautions for storage
Chemical and physical in-use stability of the admixture has been demonstrated for 24 hours at 25°C in suitable containers.

From a microbiological point of view, in-use storage times and conditions prior to use are the responsibility of the user and would normally not be longer than 24 hours at 2 to 8°C, unless dilution has taken place in controlled and validated aseptic conditions.

6.5 Nature and contents of container
Glass ampoules 10ml (Type I glass)

Glass, rubber stoppered vials 50ml (Type II glass)

6.6 Instructions for use and handling
Bottles of Nitrocine are for single use only and should not be regarded as multi-dose containers.

Admixtures are prepared by replacing a given volume of infusion vehicle with an equal volume of the product to produce the final infusion solution. For admixture storage, refer to section 6.4.

7. MARKETING AUTHORISATION HOLDER
Schwarz Pharma Ltd

Schwarz House

East Street

Chesham

Bucks. HP5 1DG

England

8. MARKETING AUTHORISATION NUMBER(S)
PL 04438/0006

9. DATE OF FIRST AUTHORISATION/RENEWAL OF THE AUTHORISATION
09 September 1997

10. DATE OF REVISION OF THE TEXT
April 2002

Nitro-Dur 0.2mg/h; 0.4mg/h and 0.6mg/h Transdermal Patch

(Schering-Plough Ltd)

1. NAME OF THE MEDICINAL PRODUCT
Nitro-Dur 0.2mg/h; 0.4mg/h and 0.6mg/h Transdermal Patch

2. QUALITATIVE AND QUANTITATIVE COMPOSITION
Glyceryl trinitrate 37.4 % w/w

For excipients, see 6.1.

3. PHARMACEUTICAL FORM
Transdermal Patch

4. CLINICAL PARTICULARS
4.1 Therapeutic indications
For prophylaxis of angina pectoris either alone or in combination with other anti-anginal therapy.

4.2 Posology and method of administration
Adults, including elderly patients:

The recommended initial dose is one 0.2mg/h Nitro-Dur patch daily. In some patients dose titration to higher or lower doses may be necessary to achieve optimum therapeutic effect.

Maximum dose: 15 mg in 24 hours.

Nitro-Dur is suitable for continuous or intermittent use. Patients already receiving continuous 24-hour nitrate therapy without signs of nitrate tolerance may continue on this regimen provided clinical response is maintained. Attenuation of effect has however occurred in some patients being treated with sustained release nitrate preparations. In such patients intermittent therapy may be more appropriate. Under these circumstances Nitro-Dur is applied daily for a period of approximately 12 hours. The patch is then removed to provide a nitrate-free interval of 12 hours which may be varied between 8-12 hours to suit individual patients (see section 4.4).

Patients experiencing nocturnal angina may benefit from overnight treatment with a nitrate-free interval during the day. In this patient group additional anti-anginal therapy may be needed during the day.

Patients with severe angina may need additional anti-anginal therapy during nitrate-free intervals.

Nitro-Dur Transdermal patches may be applied to any convenient skin area; the recommended site is the chest or outer upper arm. Application sites should be rotated and suitable areas may be shaved if necessary. Nitro-Dur patches should not be applied to the distal part of the extremities.

Children:

Not recommended.

4.3 Contraindications
Contra-indicated in patients hypersensitive to nitrates and in patients with marked anaemia. Use is also contra-indicated in severe hypotension, increased cranial pressure, cerebral haemorrhage, head trauma and myocardial insufficiency due to valvular or left ventricular outflow tract obstruction, hypertrophic obstructive cardiomyopathy, cardiac tamponade, constrictive pericarditis as well as closed-angle glaucoma.

Phosphodiesterase inhibitors, e.g. sildenafil, tadalafil, vardenafil have been shown to potentiate the hypotensive effects of nitrates and their co-administration with nitrates or nitric oxide donors is therefore contra-indicated.

4.4 Special warnings and special precautions for use
Nitro-Dur should only be used under careful clinical and/or haemodynamic monitoring in patients with acute myocardial infarction or congestive heart failure. Nitro-Dur is not indicated for the immediate treatment of acute anginal attacks.

Nitro-Dur should be removed before attempting defibrillation or cardioversion, to avoid possibility of electrical arcing, and before diathermy.

The possibility of increased frequency of angina during patch-off periods should be considered. In such cases, the use of concomitant anti-anginal therapy is desirable.

In some patients severe hypotension may occur particularly with upright posture, even with small doses of glyceryl trinitrate. Thus Nitro-Dur should be used with caution in patients who may have volume depletion from diuretic therapy and in patients who have low systolic blood pressure (e.g. below 90mm Hg).

Paradoxical bradycardia and increased angina may accompany glyceryl-trinitrate-induced hypotension.

Caution should be exercised in patients with arterial hypoxaemia, due to severe anaemia and patients with hypoxaemia and a ventilation/perfusion imbalance due to lung disease or ischaemic heart failure, where biotransformation of GTN may be reduced.

The lowest effect dose should be used.

Attenuation of effect has occurred in some patients being treated with sustained release preparations. In such patients intermittent therapy may be more appropriate (see section 4.2).

Caution should be exercised in patients suffering from hypothyroidism, malnutrition, severe renal or hepatic impairment, hypothermia and recent history of myocardial infarction.

Severe postural hypotension with light-headedness and dizziness is frequently observed after the consumption of alcohol.

4.5 Interaction with other medicinal products and other forms of Interaction
Concomitant use of Nitro-Dur with other vasodilating agents, alcohol, anti-hypertensive agents, beta-adrenergic blocking agents, ACE inhibitors, phenothiazines or calcium channel blocking agents may cause additive hypotensive effects.

The hypotensive effect of nitrates are potentiated by concurrent administration of phosphodiesterase inhibitors, e.g. sildenafil, tadalafil, vardenafil (see section 4.3).

4.6 Pregnancy and lactation
It is not known whether glyceryl trinitrate in transdermal form can affect reproductive capacity or cause foetal harm. Thus Nitro-Dur should only be administered to pregnant women if the potential benefit to the mother clearly outweighs the potential hazard to the foetus. It is not known whether glyceryl trinitrate is excreted in human milk. Caution should therefore be exercised when Nitro-Dur is administered to nursing mothers.

4.7 Effects on ability to drive and use machines
Nitrates may cause dizziness and blurred vision, which may affect ability to drive and operate machines.

4.8 Undesirable effects
Headache is the most common side-effect, especially at higher doses. Transient episodes of dizziness and light-headedness which may be related to blood pressure change may also occur. Hypotension occurs infrequently but may be severe enough to warrant discontinuation of therapy. Syncope and reflex tachycardia have been reported but are uncommon. Application site reactions (including erythema, rash, burning and purpura may occur but are rarely severe. Contact dermatitis has been reported. Hypersensitivity reactions may occur.

4.9 Overdose
High doses of glyceryl trinitrate may produce severe hypotension, syncope and methaemoglobinaemia. Increased intracranial pressure with associated cerebral symptoms may occur. Treatment is by removal of the patch or reduction of dose, depending on severity. Thorough scrubbing of underlying skin may reduce absorption more quickly after removal. Intravenous infusion of normal saline or similar fluid may be necessary to increase the central fluid volume. Any fall in blood pressure or signs of collapse that may occur may be managed by general supportive or resuscitative measures. Adrenaline and related products are ineffective in reversing the severe hypotensive events associated with overdose.

5. PHARMACOLOGICAL PROPERTIES

5.1 Pharmacodynamic properties
Glyceryl trinitrate, (as other organic nitrates), is a potent dilator of vascular smooth muscle. The effect on veins predominates over that on arteries resulting in decreased cardiac preload. Systemic vascular resistance is relatively unaffected, heart rate is unchanged or slightly increased and pulmonary vascular resistance is consistently reduced.

In normal individuals or those with coronary artery disease (in the absence of heart failure) glyceryl trinitrate decreases cardiac output slightly. Doses which do not alter systemic arterial pressure often product arteriolar dilatation in the face and neck resulting in flushing. Dilatation of the meningeal arterioles may explain the headache which is often reported. Rapid administration of high doses of glyceryl trinitrate decreases blood pressure and cardiac output resulting in pallor, weakness, dizziness and activation of compensatory sympathetic reflexes. A marked hypotensive effect may occasionally occur especially in the upright position.

5.2 Pharmacokinetic properties
Glyceryl trinitrate is rapidly hydrolysed by liver enzymes which are a major factor in bioavailability. Orally administered glyceryl trinitrate is ineffective as a therapeutic agent due to first-pass metabolism and administration has therefore routinely been via the sub-lingual route thus bypassing the hepatic circulation initially. Peak concentrations of glyceryl trinitrate following sub-lingual administration occur within 4 minutes in man with a half-life of 1 to 3 minutes. Transdermal administration, initially with ointment preparations but more recently with sustained-release delivery systems provide an alternative route to bypass the hepatic circulation with longer term concentrations of approximately 200pg/ml are achieved within approximately 2h or application of Nitro-Dur and are maintained for 24 h. Rate of absorption is controlled by the skin.

5.3 Preclinical safety data
There are no pre-clinical data of relevance to the prescriber which are additional to that already included in other sections of the SPC.

6. PHARMACEUTICAL PARTICULARS

6.1 List of excipients
Butylacrylate Polymer (Polymer C);

Butylacrylate Polymer (Polymer D);

Sodium Polyacrylate (Polymer A);

Melamine Formaldehyde Resin (Polymer B);

Purified Water.

Coated onto tan-coloured Saranex® 2014 extruded thermoplastic film

Adhesive layer covered by PVC Release Liner.

6.2 Incompatibilities
None known

6.3 Shelf life
24 months

6.4 Special precautions for storage
Store below 30°C. Do not refrigerate.

6.5 Nature and contents of container
Sealed pouches consisting of paper lined with polyethylene/foil laminate enclosing individual transdermal patches; 28 patches are contained in a cardboard carton.

6.6 Instructions for use and handling
Nitro-Dur patches are applied after removal from the protective pouch. With the brown lines on the backing cover facing the user, edges are bent away to break open the cover along the brown line. The halves of the cover are peeled off and the patch applied firmly to the skin. Hands should be washed thoroughly after application.

Patients should be advised to dispose of patches carefully to avoid accidental application or use.

Administrative Data

7. MARKETING AUTHORISATION HOLDER
Schering-Plough Ltd

Shire Park

Welwyn Garden City

Hertfordshire

AL7 1TW

UK

8. MARKETING AUTHORISATION NUMBER(S)
Nitro-Dur 0.2mg/h: PL 0201/0158

Nitro-Dur 0.4mg/h: PL 0201/0159

Nitro-Dur 0.6mg/h: PL 0201/0160

9. DATE OF FIRST AUTHORISATION/RENEWAL OF THE AUTHORISATION
22 October 1991 / 09 February 2002

10. DATE OF REVISION OF THE TEXT
January 2005

Legal Category
P

N-Dur/UK/1-05/4

Nitrolingual Pump Spray

(Merck Pharmaceuticals)

1. NAME OF THE MEDICINAL PRODUCT
Nitrolingual Pumpspray

2. QUALITATIVE AND QUANTITATIVE COMPOSITION
Each metered dose contains 400 micrograms glyceryl trinitrate.

3. PHARMACEUTICAL FORM
Sublingual spray.

4. CLINICAL PARTICULARS

4.1 Therapeutic indications
For the treatment and prophylaxis of angina pectoris and the treatment of variant angina.

4.2 Posology and method of administration
Adults and the Elderly:

At the onset of an attack or prior to a precipitating event: one or two 400 microgram metered doses sprayed under the tongue. It is recommended that no more than three metered-doses are taken at any one time and that there should be a minimum interval of 15 minutes between consecutive treatments.

For the prevention of exercise induced angina or in other precipitating conditions: one or two 400 microgram metered doses sprayed under the tongue immediately prior to the event.

Children:

Nitrolingual Pumpspray is not recommended for use.

Administration:

The bottle should be held vertically with the valve head uppermost. If the pump is new, or has not been used for a week or more, the first actuation should be released into the air. The spray orifice should then be placed as close to the mouth as possible. The dose should be sprayed under the tongue and the mouth should be closed immediately after each dose. The spray should not be inhaled. Patients should be instructed to familiarise themselves with the position of the spray orifice, which can be identified by the finger rest on the top of the valve, in order to facilitate orientation for administration at night. During application the patient should rest, ideally in the sitting position.

4.3 Contraindications
Hypersensitivity to nitrates or any constituent of the formulation. Hypotension, hypovolaemia, severe anaemia, cerebral haemorrhage and brain trauma, mitral stenosis and angina caused by hypertrophic obstructive cardiomyopathy. Concomitant administration with sildenafil (see section 4.5).

4.4 Special warnings and special precautions for use
Any lack of effect may be an indicator of early myocardial infarction.

As with all glyceryl trinitrate preparations, use in patients with incipient glaucoma should be avoided.

4.5 Interaction with other medicinal products and other forms of Interaction
Tolerance to this drug and cross tolerance to other nitrates may occur. Alcohol may potentiate any hypotensive effect.

The hypotensive effects of nitrates are potentiated by concurrent administration of sildenafil. A severe and possibly dangerous fall in blood pressure may occur. This can result in collapse, unconsciousness and may be fatal. Such use is therefore contra-indicated (see section 4.3)

4.6 Pregnancy and lactation
Nitrolingual Pump spray is not generally recommended and should be used only if its potential benefit justifies any potential risk to the foetus or neonate.

4.7 Effects on ability to drive and use machines
Only as a result of hypotension.

4.8 Undesirable effects
Headache, dizziness, postural hypotension, flushing, tachycardia and paradoxical bradycardia have been reported.

4.9 Overdose
Signs and symptoms:

Flushing, severe headache, a feeling of suffocation, hypotension, fainting, restlessness, blurred vision, impairment of respiration, bradycardia and rarely, cyanosis and methaemoglobinaemia may occur. In a few patients there may be a reaction comparable to shock with nausea, vomiting, weakness, sweating and syncope.

Treatment:

Recovery often occurs without special treatment. Hypotension may be corrected by elevation of the legs to promote venous return. Methaemoglobinaemia should be treated by intravenous methylene blue.

Symptomatic treatment should be given for respiratory and circulatory defects in more serious cases.

5. PHARMACOLOGICAL PROPERTIES

5.1 Pharmacodynamic properties

Glyceryl trinitrate relieves angina pectoris by reduction of cardiac work and dilation of the coronary arteries. In this way, not only is there a lessening in arterial oxygen requirement but the amount of oxygenated blood reaching the ischaemic heart is increased.

5.2 Pharmacokinetic properties

The pharmacokinetics of glyceryl trinitrate are complex; venous plasma levels of the drug show wide and variable fluctuations and are not predictive of clinical effect. In a human pharmacodynamic study, pharmacological activity had commenced one minute after dosing and was obvious by two minutes.

5.3 Preclinical safety data

None stated.

6. PHARMACEUTICAL PARTICULARS

6.1 List of excipients

Fractionated coconut oil, ethanol, medium chain partial glycerides, peppermint oil.

6.2 Incompatibilities

None known.

6.3 Shelf life

3 years.

6.4 Special precautions for storage

Do not store above 25 degree C.

6.5 Nature and contents of container

Red plastic coated glass bottle fitted with metering pump. Each bottle contains 4.9, 11.2 or 14.2g solution (equivalent to about 75, 200 or 250 doses). Nitrolingual Pumpspray Duo pack contains a 4.9g and a 14.2g bottle.

6.6 Instructions for use and handling

See 'Administration' section.

7. MARKETING AUTHORISATION HOLDER

Lipha Pharmaceuticals Limited

Harrier House

High Street

West Drayton

Middlesex

UB7 7QG

United Kingdom

8. MARKETING AUTHORISATION NUMBER(S)

PL 03759/0042

9. DATE OF FIRST AUTHORISATION/RENEWAL OF THE AUTHORISATION

19 April 1995/12 July 2000

10. DATE OF REVISION OF THE TEXT

27 March 2003.

LEGAL CATEGORY Pharmacy

Nitronal

(Merck Pharmaceuticals)

1. NAME OF THE MEDICINAL PRODUCT

Nitronal®

2. QUALITATIVE AND QUANTITATIVE COMPOSITION

Glyceryl trinitrate 1 mg/ml.

3. PHARMACEUTICAL FORM

Solution for infusion.

4. CLINICAL PARTICULARS

4.1 Therapeutic indications

(1) Unresponsive congestive heart failure, including that secondary to acute myocardial infarction.

(2) Refractory unstable angina pectoris and coronary insufficiency, including Prinzmetal's angina.

(3) Control of hypertensive episodes and / or myocardial ischaemia during and after cardiac surgery. For the induction of controlled hypotension for surgery.

4.2 Posology and method of administration

For intravenous use. Nitronal® should be administered by means of a micro-drip set infusion pump or similar device which permits maintenance of constant infusion rate.

Adults and the elderly - the dose should be titrated against the individual clinical response.

(1) Unresponsive congestive heart failure. The normal dose range is 10-100 micrograms / minute administered as a continuous intravenous infusion with frequent monitoring of blood pressure and heart rate. The infusion should be started at the lower rate and increased cautiously until the desired clinical response is achieved. Other haemodynamic measurements are extremely important in monitoring response to the drug: These may include pulmonary capillary wedge pressure, cardiac output and precordial electrocardiogram depending on the clinical picture.

(2) Refractory unstable angina pectoris. An initial infusion rate of 10-15 micrograms / minute is recommended; this may be increased cautiously in increments of 5-10 micrograms until either relief of angina is achieved, headache prevents further increase in dose, or the mean arterial pressure falls by more than 20 mm Hg.

(3) Use in surgery. An initial infusion rate of 25 micrograms / minute is recommended; this should be increased gradually until the desired systolic arterial pressure is attained. The usual dose is 25-200 micrograms / minute.

Children - Not recommended for use in children.

4.3 Contraindications

Hypersensitivity to nitrates. Hypotensive shock, severe anaemia, cerebral haemorrhage, arterial hypoxaemia, uncorrected hypovolaemia and angina caused by hypertrophic obstructive cardiomyopathy. Concomitant administration of sildenafil (section 4.5).

4.4 Special warnings and special precautions for use

Caution should be exercised in patients with severe liver or renal disease, hypothermia, hypothyroidism.

Nitronal® should not be given by bolus injection.

4.5 Interaction with other medicinal products and other forms of Interaction

Glyceryl trinitrate may potentiate the action of other hypotensive drugs, and the hypotensive and anticholinergic effects of tricyclic anti-depressants; it may also slow the metabolism of morphine-like analgesics.

The hypotensive effects of nitrates are potentiated by concurrent administration of sildenafil. A severe and possibly dangerous fall in blood pressure may occur. This can result in collapse, unconsciousness and may be fatal. Such use is therefore contra-indicated (section 4.3).

4.6 Pregnancy and lactation

This product should not be used in pregnancy or in women who are breast feeding infants unless considered essential by the physician.

4.7 Effects on ability to drive and use machines

No information available.

4.8 Undesirable effects

Nitronal® is generally well tolerated because a minimum dose is administered in unit time. Headache, dizziness, flushing, hypotension and tachycardia may be encountered, particularly if the infusion is administered too rapidly. Nausea, diaphoresis, restlessness, retrosternal discomfort, abdominal pain and paradoxical bradycardia have been reported. These symptoms should be readily reversible on reducing the rate of infusion or, if necessary, discontinuing treatment.

4.9 Overdose

Signs and symptoms: Vomiting, restlessness, hypotension, syncope, cyanosis, coldness of the skin, impairment of respiration, bradycardia, psychosis and methaemoglobinaemia may occur.

Treatment: The symptoms may be readily reversed by discontinuing treatment; if hypotension persists, raising the foot of the bed and the use of vasoconstrictors such as intravenous methoxamine or phenylephrine are recommended. Methaemoglobinaemia should be treated by intravenous methylene blue. Oxygen and assisted respiration may be required.

5. PHARMACOLOGICAL PROPERTIES

5.1 Pharmacodynamic properties

Glyceryl trinitrate exerts a spasmolytic action on smooth muscle, particularly in the vascular system. The predominant effect is an increase in venous capacitance resulting in marked diminution of both the left ventricular filling pressure and volume (preload). There is also a reduction in afterload due to moderate dilation of the arteriolar resistance vessels. These haemodynamic changes lower the myocardial oxygen demand. By direct action and through the reduction of myocardial wall tension glyceryl trinitrate also lowers the resistance to flow in the coronary collateral channels and allows re-distribution of blood flow to ischaemic areas of the myocardium.

Administration of Nitronal® by intravenous infusion to patients with congestive heart failure results in a marked improvement in haemodynamics, reduction of elevated left ventricular filling pressure and systolic wall tension, and an increase in the depressed cardiac output. It reduces the imbalance that exists between myocardial oxygen demand and delivery, thereby diminishing myocardial ischaemia and controlling ischaemia-induced ventricular arrhythmias.

5.2 Pharmacokinetic properties

It is important that the dose of Nitronal® be titrated against the individual clinical response.

After intravenous administration, glyceryl trinitrate is widely distributed in the body with an estimated apparent volume of distribution of approximately 200 litres, and is rapidly metabolised to dinitrate and mononitrate with an estimated half life of 1 to 4 minutes, resulting in plasma levels of less than 1 microgram / ml.

5.3 Preclinical safety data

None, of relevance to the prescriber, which are not given elsewhere in this document.

6. PHARMACEUTICAL PARTICULARS

6.1 List of excipients

Glucose, water for injections, hydrochloric acid.

6.2 Incompatibilities

Glyceryl trinitrate is adsorbed onto administration systems composed of polyvinyl chloride, - see 6.6.

6.3 Shelf life

Ampoules: 4 years

Vial: 2 years

The diluted solution should be administered as soon as possible; it is stable for up to 24 hours in the recommended infusion system.

6.4 Special precautions for storage

Do not store above 25°C. Store in the original container.

6.5 Nature and contents of container

Cartons of 10 ampoules or single vials.

Amber glass ampoule (containing 5ml or 25ml).

Clear glass vial (containing 50ml).

6.6 Instructions for use and handling

Nitronal® need not be diluted before use but can be diluted with Dextrose Injection BP, Sodium Chloride and Dextrose Injection BP, 0.9% Sodium Chloride Injection BP or other protein-free infusion solution, if required.

The solution, whether or not diluted, should be infused slowly (see dosage section) and not given by bolus injection.

To ensure a constant infusion rate of glyceryl trinitrate it is recommended that Nitronal® be administered by means of a syringe pump or polyethylene infusion bag with a counter, or with a glass or rigid polyethylene syringe and polyethylene tubing. Systems made of polyvinyl chloride may absorb up to 50% of the glyceryl trinitrate from the solution, thus reducing the efficacy of the infusion. If the recommended type of system is unavailable, a 1:10 dilution of Nitronal® should be used and the infusion rate modified according to the haemodynamic response of the patient, until the required parameters are attained.

7. MARKETING AUTHORISATION HOLDER

Lipha Pharmaceuticals Limited

Harrier House

High Street

West Drayton

Middlesex

UB7 7QG

8. MARKETING AUTHORISATION NUMBER(S)

PL 03759 / 0025

9. DATE OF FIRST AUTHORISATION/RENEWAL OF THE AUTHORISATION

30 January 2000

10. DATE OF REVISION OF THE TEXT

18 December 2003

Legal Category POM

Nivaquine Tablets and Syrup

(sanofi-aventis)

1. NAME OF THE MEDICINAL PRODUCT

Nivaquine Tablets

Nivaquine Syrup

2. QUALITATIVE AND QUANTITATIVE COMPOSITION

Chloroquine Sulphate BP 200 mg.

Chloroquine Sulphate BP 68 mg/5 ml.

3. PHARMACEUTICAL FORM

Tablet.

Syrup.

4. CLINICAL PARTICULARS

4.1 Therapeutic indications

Nivaquine is a 4-aminoquinoline compound which has a high degree of activity against the asexual erythrocytic forms of all species of malaria parasites. It is indicated for the suppression and clinical cure of all forms of malaria and, in addition, produces radical cure of falciparum malaria.

Nivaquine also exerts a beneficial effect in certain collagen diseases and protects against the effects of solar radiation. It is employed in the treatment of rheumatoid arthritis, juvenile arthritis, discoid and systemic lupus erythematosus and skin conditions aggravated by sunlight.

Nivaquine is also active against *Entamoeba histolytica* and *Giardia lamblia* and when Flagyl (metronidazole) is not available it may be used in hepatic amoebiasis and giardiasis.

Packs for supply directly to the public: For the prevention of malaria.

4.2 Posology and method of administration

Rheumatoid arthritis

Adults: One Nivaquine tablet or 3 × 5 ml Nivaquine Syrup (150 mg chloroquine base) daily.

Children: 3 mg/kg bodyweight daily. Treatment should be discontinued if no improvement has occurred after 6 months.

Systemic lupus erythematosus

Adults: One Nivaquine tablet or 3 × 5 ml Nivaquine Syrup (150 mg chloroquine base) daily until maximum improvement is obtained followed by smaller maintenance dosage.

Children: 3 mg/kg bodyweight daily. Treatment should be discontinued if no improvement has occurred after 6 months.

Light sensitive skin eruptions

Adults: One or two Nivaquine tablets or 3 to 6 × 5 ml Nivaquine Syrup (150 mg to 300 mg chloroquine base) daily during the period of maximum light exposure.

Children: 3 mg/kg body weight daily. Treatment should be discontinued if no improvement has occurred after 6 months.

Suppression of malaria

Adults: Two Nivaquine tablets or 6 × 5 ml Nivaquine Syrup (300 mg chloroquine base) to be taken once a week on the same day each week.

Infants and children up to 12 years:

5 mg chloroquine base per kg bodyweight to be taken once a week on the same day each week.

It is advisable to start taking Nivaquine 1 week before entering an endemic area and to continue for 4 weeks after leaving.

Treatment of malaria

1. Partially immune adults

A single dose of four Nivaquine tablets or 12 × 5 ml Nivaquine Syrup (600 mg chloroquine base) will provide a safe and effective course of treatment.

2. Non-immune adults

Day 1: Four Nivaquine tablets or 12 × 5 ml Nivaquine Syrup (600 mg chloroquine base) in one dose followed by a further two tablets or 6 × 5 ml syrup (300 mg chloroquine base) six hours later.

Day 2: Two Nivaquine tablets or 6 × 5 ml Nivaquine Syrup (300 mg chloroquine base).

Day 3: Two Nivaquine tablets or 6 × 5 ml Nivaquine Syrup (300 mg chloroquine base).

The above dosage is intended as a guide in the treatment of *Plasmodium falciparum* malaria. However, due to a variation in the strain sensitivity, it may sometimes be necessary to increase the duration of treatment by administering two Nivaquine tablets or 6 × 5 ml Nivaquine Syrup (300 mg chloroquine base) daily on days 4 to 7.

3. Non-immune or partially immune infants and children

Nivaquine Syrup can be conveniently used in patients in this age group to permit flexibility of dosage.

Day 1: 10 mg chloroquine base/kg bodyweight (maximum 600 mg base) followed by 5 mg chloroquine base/kg bodyweight (maximum 300 mg base) six hours later.

Day 2: 5 mg chloroquine base/kg bodyweight (maximum 300 mg base).

Day 3: 5 mg chloroquine base/kg bodyweight (maximum 300 mg base).

Route of administration is oral.

4.3 Contraindications

The use of chloroquine is contraindicated in patients with known hypersensitivity to 4-aminoquinoline compounds.

Nivaquine is generally contraindicated in pregnancy. However, clinicians may decide to administer Nivaquine to pregnant women for the prevention or treatment of malaria. Ocular or inner ear damage may occur in infants born of mothers who receive high doses of chloroquine throughout pregnancy.

4.4 Special warnings and special precautions for use

Nivaquine should be used with care in patients with a history of epilepsy as it has been reported to provoke seizures. Caution is advised in cases of porphyria (precipitated disease may be especially apparent in patients with a high alcohol intake), hepatic disease (particularly cirrhosis) or renal disease, severe gastrointestinal, neurological and blood disorders and in patients receiving anticoagulant therapy.

Nivaquine should be used with care in patients with psoriasis as the condition may be exacerbated.

Although Nivaquine may have a temporary effect on visual accommodation during short term treatment, irreversible retinal damage may occur with prolonged treatment (see sections 4.7 and 4.8, below). Therefore, patients should be advised to discontinue the medication and seek immediate medical advice if they notice any deterioration in their vision which persists for more than 48 hours. Ophthalmological examination should always be carried out before and regularly (3-6 monthly intervals) during prolonged treatment. Retinal damage is particularly likely to occur if treatment has been given for longer than one year, or if the total dosage has exceeded 1.6 g/kg bodyweight. These precautions also apply to patients receiving chloroquine continuously at weekly intervals as a prophylactic against malarial attack for more than three years.

Bone marrow depression, including aplastic anaemia occurs rarely. Full blood counts should therefore be carried out regularly during extended treatment. Caution is required if drugs known to induce blood disorders are used concurrently.

Resistance of Plasmodium falciparum to chloroquine is well documented. When used as malaria prophylaxis official guidelines and local information on prevalence of resistance to anti-malarial drugs should be taken into consideration.

4.5 Interaction with other medicinal products and other forms of Interaction

Concomitant administration of chloroquine with magnesium-containing antacids or kaolin may result in reduced absorption of chloroquine. Chloroquine should, therefore, be administered at least two hours apart from antacids or kaolin.

Concomitant use of cimetidine and chloroquine may result in an increased half-life and a decreased clearance of chloroquine.

Chloroquine and mefloquine can lower the convulsive threshold. Co-administration of chloroquine and mefloquine may increase the risk of convulsions. Also, the activity of antiepileptic drugs might be impaired if co-administered with chloroquine.

There have been isolated case reports of an increased plasma ciclosporin level when ciclosporin and chloroquine were co-administered.

Chloroquine may affect the antibody response to rabies vaccine (HDCV).

Caution is advised in patients receiving anticoagulant therapy.

Co-administration of chloroquine and other drugs that have arrhythmogenic potential (e.g. amiodarone) may increase the risk of cardiac arrhythmias.

Concomitant administration of chloroquine and digoxin may increase plasma concentrations of digoxin.

Concomitant use of chloroquine with neostigmine or pyridostigmine has the potential to increase the symptoms of myasthenia gravis and thus diminish the effects of neostigmine and pyridostigmine.

4.6 Pregnancy and lactation

Nivaquine is generally contraindicated in pregnancy. However, clinicians may decide to administer Nivaquine to pregnant women for the prevention or treatment of malaria. Ocular or inner ear damage may occur in infants born of mothers who receive high doses of chloroquine throughout pregnancy.

Although chloroquine is excreted in breast milk, the amount is insufficient to confer any benefit on the infant. Separate chemoprophylaxis for the infant is required.

When used for rheumatoid disease breast feeding is not recommended.

4.7 Effects on ability to drive and use machines

Nivaquine has a temporary effect on visual accommodation and patients should be warned that they should not drive or operate machinery if they are affected.

4.8 Undesirable effects

Cardiovascular

- cardiomyopathy has been reported during long term therapy at high doses,

- cardiac dysrhythmias at high doses can occur,

- hypotension.

Central Nervous System (See Section 4.4)

- seizures,

- convulsions have been reported rarely (these may result from cerebral malaria. Such patients should receive an injections of phenobarbitone to prevent seizures, in a dose of 3.5mg/kg in addition to intravenous administration of Nivaquine),

- psychiatric disorders such as anxiety, confusion, hallucinations, delirium.

Eye disorders (See Sections 4.4 and 4.7)

- transient blurred vision and reversible corneal opacity,

- cases of retinopathy as well as cases of irreversible retinal damage have damage have been reported during long term, high dose therapy.

- Macular defects of colour vision, optic atrophy, scotomas, field defects, blindness and pigmented deposits, difficult in focusing, diplopia.

Gastro-intestinal

- gastrointestinal disturbances such as nausea, vomiting, diarrhoea, abdominal cramps.

General

- headache.

Haematological (See Section 4.4)

- bone marrow depression, including aplastic anaemia, agranulocytosis, thrombocytopenia, neutropenia occurs rarely.

Hepatic

- changes in liver function, including hepatitis and abnormal liver function tests, have been reported rarely.

Hypersensitivity

- allergic and anaphylactic reactions, urticaria and angiodema have occurred rarely.

Hearing disorders

- ototoxicity such as tinnitus, reduced hearing, nerve deafness.

Muscular

- neuropathy, myopathy.

Skin (See Section 4.4)

- skin eruptions, pruritis, depigmentation, loss of hair, exacerbation of psoriasis, photosensitivity, pigmentation of the nails and mucosae (long term use).

- Rare reports of erythema multiforme, Stevens-Johnson syndrome, toxic epidermal necrolysis, exfoliative dermatitis and similar desquamation-type events.

4.9 Overdose

Chloroquine is highly toxic in overdosage; children are particularly susceptible to toxic doses of chloroquine. The chief symptoms of overdose include circulatory collapse due to a potent cardiotoxic effect, respiratory arrest and coma. Symptoms may progress rapidly after initial headache, drowsiness, visual disturbancesnausea and vomiting. Death may result from circulatory or respiratory failure or cardiac dysrhythmia.

Gastric lavage should be carried out urgently, first protecting the airways and instituting artificial ventilation where necessary. There is a risk of cardiac arrest following aspiration of gastric contents in more serious cases. Activated charcoal left in the stomach may reduce absorption of any remaining chloroquine from the gut. Circulatory status (with central venous pressure measurement), respiration, plasma electrolytes and blood gases should be monitored, with correction of hypokalaemia and acidosis if indicated. Cardiac arrhythmias should not be treated unless life threatening; drugs with quinidine-like effects should be avoided.

Early administration of the following has been shown to improve survival in cases of serious poisoning:

1) Adrenaline infusion (0.25 micrograms/kg/min initially, with increments of 0.25 micrograms/kg/min until adequate systolic blood pressure (more than 100 mm mercury) is restored; adrenaline reduces the effects of chloroquine on the heart through its inotropic and vasoconstrictor effects.

2) Diazepam infusion (2 mg/kg over 30 minutes as a loading dose, followed by 1-2 mg/kg/day for up to 2-4 days). Diazepam may minimise cardiotoxicity.

Acidification of the urine, haemodialysis, peritoneal dialysis or exchange transfusions have not been shown to be of value in treating chloroquine poisoning. Chloroquine is excreted very slowly, therefore symptomatic cases merit observation for several days.

5. PHARMACOLOGICAL PROPERTIES

5.1 Pharmacodynamic properties

Chloroquine is used for the suppression and treatment of malaria. It has rapid schizonticidal effect and appears to affect cell growth by interfering with DNA; its activity also seems to depend on preferential accumulation in the infected erythrocyte. Chloroquine kills the erythrocytic forms of malaria parasites at all stages of development. In addition to its antimalarial properties, it possesses other pharmacological properties. Its anti-inflammatory properties enable Nivaquine to be used in certain collagen diseases and it protects against the effects of solar radiation. Nivaquine is also active against *Entamoeba histolytica* and *Giardia lamblia*. It may be used in hepatic amoebiasis and giardiasis.

5.2 Pharmacokinetic properties

Chloroquine is readily absorbed from the gastro-intestinal tract and about 55% in the circulation is bound to plasma proteins. It accumulates in high concentrations in some tissues, such as kidneys, liver, lungs and spleen and is strongly bound in melanin containing cells such as those in the eyes and the skin; it is also bound to double stranded DNA, present in red blood cells containing schizonts. Chloroquine is eliminated very slowly from the body and it may persist in tissues for a long period. Up to 70% of a dose may be excreted unchanged in urine and up to 25% may be excreted also in the urine as the desethyl metabolite. The rate of urinary excretion of chloroquine is increased at low pH values.

5.3 Preclinical safety data

No additional preclinical data of relevance to the prescriber.

6. PHARMACEUTICAL PARTICULARS

6.1 List of excipients

Nivaquine Tablets: Microcrystalline cellulose (E460) BP, Glucose BP, Acacia powder BP, Magnesium stearate BP, Sodium starch glycollate BP, Hydroxypropylmethyl Cellulose (Pharmacoat 606), Polyethylene glycol 400, Yellow opaspray K-1-3040.

Nivaquine Syrup: Liquid sugar gran. liquors, Sodium L glutamate, Saccharin sodium BP, Propylene glycol BP, Methyl hydroxybenzoate BP, Propyl hydroxybenzoate

BP, Oil peppermint (Chinese), Witham pineapple flavour (F), Caramel HT, Demineralised water BP.

6.2 Incompatibilities

None known.

6.3 Shelf life

36 months.

6.4 Special precautions for storage

Nivaquine Tablets: protect from light.

Nivaquine Syrup should be stored below 25°C, protected from light.

6.5 Nature and contents of container

Cartons containing blister packs of 28 tablets.

Amber glass bottle containing 100 ml. Either with rolled on pilfer proof aluminium cap and PVDC emulsion coated wad, or HDPE/polypropylene child resistant cap with a tamper evident band.

6.6 Instructions for use and handling

None stated.

7. MARKETING AUTHORISATION HOLDER

Nivaquine Tablets: Rhône-Poulenc Rorer

Nivaquine Syrup: Aventis Pharma

50 Kings Hill Avenue

Kings Hill

West Malling

Kent ME19 4AH

8. MARKETING AUTHORISATION NUMBER(S)

Nivaquine tablets: PL 00012/5260R

Nivaquine syrup: PL 04425/0329

9. DATE OF FIRST AUTHORISATION/RENEWAL OF THE AUTHORISATION

Nivaquine Tablets: 12 February 1999

Nivaquine Syrup: 06 March 2003

10. DATE OF REVISION OF THE TEXT

January 2005

Legal classification: POM

When used solely for the prevention of malaria: Pharmacy Medicine.

Nivemycin Tablets 500mg

(Sovereign Medical)

1. NAME OF THE MEDICINAL PRODUCT

Nivemycin Tablets 500mg

2. QUALITATIVE AND QUANTITATIVE COMPOSITION

Neomycin sulphate Ph Eur.

an amount equivalent to 550mg of material having a potency of 700 units per mg.

3. PHARMACEUTICAL FORM

Tablets.

4. CLINICAL PARTICULARS

4.1 Therapeutic indications

Nivemycin (Neomycin sulphate BP) is indicated for pre-operative sterilisation of the bowel and maybe useful in the treatment of impending hepatic coma, including portal systemic encephalopathy.

For oral administration.

4.2 Posology and method of administration

Pre-operative sterilisation of the bowel.

Adults: 2 tablets every hour for 4 hours; then 2 tablets every 4 hours for two or three days before the operation.

Children over 12 years: 2 tablets every 4 hours for 2 or 3 days before the operation.

Children from 6 to 12 years: ½ to 1 tablet every 4 hours for 2 or 3 days before the operation.

For practical reasons, use of the tablets in children under 6 years is not recommended.

In hepatic coma, the adult dose is 4-12 gm/day in divided doses for a period of 5-7 days, whilst for children, 50-100mg/kg/day in divided doses appears appropriate. Chronic hepatic insufficiency may require up to 4gm/day over an indefinite period.

The elderly dose is the same as for adults.

4.3 Contraindications

Nivemycin should not be given when intestinal obstruction is present.

Hypersensitivity to aminoglycosides.

Infants under 1 year.

Myasthenia gravis.

4.4 Special warnings and special precautions for use

The absorption of neomycin is poor from the alimentary tract, with about 97% of an orally administered dose being excreted unchanged in the faeces. Impaired G.I. motility however may increase absorption of the drug and it is therefore possible, as with other broad spectrum antibiotics, that prolonged therapy could result in ototoxicity and nephrotoxicity, particularly in patients with a degree of renal failure. In such patients, and infants and the elderly, it is generally desirable to determine dosage requirements of aminoglycosides by individual monitoring. Some authorities consider that monitoring is also important in obese patients and those with cystic fibrosis.

Impaired hepatic function or auditory function, bacteraemia, fever, and possibly exposure to loud noises have been reported to increase the risk of ototoxicity, while volume depletion or hypotension, liver disease, or female sex have reported as additional risk factors for nephrotoxicity. Regular assessment of auditory, vestibular and renal function is particularly necessary in patients with additional risk factors.

When used as an adjunct in the management of hepatic coma, care should be taken that administration is of the minimal period necessary, since prolonged exposure to the drug may result in malabsorption.

Neomycin should be used with caution in patients with neuromuscular disorders and Parkinsonism.

There is almost complete cross-resistance between neomycin, kanamycin, paromomycin and framycetin. Cross-resistance with gentamicin has also been reported.

Since prolonged therapy may result in the overgrowth of non-sensitive organisms, treatment should not be continued longer than necessary to prevent superinfection due to the over growth of non-sensitive organisms.

4.5 Interaction with other medicinal products and other forms of Interaction

Neomycin may impair absorption of other drugs including phenoxymethylpenicillin, digoxin, methotrexate and some vitamins. Aminoglycosides exhibit synergistic activity with a number of beta lactams, but aminoglycoside activity was reported to be diminished in a few patients with severe renal impairment.

Care should be taken when considering the use of neomycin concurrently with drugs with a potential to cause nephrotoxicity (including other aminoglycosides, some of the cephalosporins, amphotericin, ciclosporin, capreomycin, polymixins, platinum compounds, teicoplanin and vancomycin) or ototoxicity (including loop diuretics, capreomycin, teicoplanin, vancomycin and possibly platinum compounds).

The effect of non-depolarising muscle relaxants may be enhanced by aminoglycosides. Care is required if other drugs with a neuromuscular blocking action, including botulinum toxic, are given concomitantly. Care is required when patients being treated with aminoglycosides are to receive a general anaesthetic or opioids in order to avoid the possible neuromuscular side-effects provoking severe respiratory depression.

The effect of the parasympathomimetic drugs neostigmine and pyridostigmine, may be antagonised by aminoglycosides.

The hypoglycaemic effect of acarbose may be enhanced by neomycin and the severity of gastrointestinal side effects increased.

Aminoglycosides may increase the risk of hypocalcaemia in patients receiving bisphosphonates.

Experience in anticoagulant clinics suggests that INR (International Normalised Ratio) may be altered by antibacterials such as neomycin given for local action on the gut.

The efficacy of oral contraceptives may be reduced with broad spectrum antibiotics.

Oral typhoid vaccine is inactivated by concomitant antibiotic administration.

4.6 Pregnancy and lactation

The use of neomycin in pregnancy is not recommended unless the benefits outweigh the potential risks.

There are no reports linking the use of neomycin to congenital defects. However, small amounts of the drug are absorbed when given orally and neomycin and other aminoglycosides may have harmful effects on the foetus following oral absorption during pregnancy.

In some circumstances neomycin may enter the breast milk of lactating mothers. There is little risk of ototoxicity in the infant, but abnormal development of the gut flora may occur. The use of neomycin in lactating mothers is not recommended unless the benefits outweigh the potential risks.

4.7 Effects on ability to drive and use machines

Not applicable.

4.8 Undesirable effects

Nausea, vomiting, diarrhoea, increased salivation, stomatitis, nephrotoxicity, ototoxicity, rise in serum levels of hepatic enzymes and bilirubin, blood dyscrasias, haemolytic anaemia, confusion, paraesthesia, disorientation, nystagmus, hypersensitivity reactions including dermatitis, pruritus, drug fever and anaphylaxis.

Cross-sensitivity with other aminoglycosides may occur.

Malabsorption syndrome with steatorrhoea an diarrhoea, which can be severe, may be caused by prolonged oral therapy.

Superinfection may occur, especialy with prolonged treatment.

Electrolyte disturbances (notably hypomagnesaemia but also hypocalcaemia and hypokalaemia) have occurred with other aminoglycosides.

4.9 Overdose

In overdose, exacerbation of the adverse events reported for neomycin (nausea, diarrhoea nephrotoxicity, ototoxicity etc.) is expected.

Monitor renal and auditory function. If these are impaired, haemodialysis is indicated.

Prolonged assisted ventilation may also be required.

5. PHARMACOLOGICAL PROPERTIES

5.1 Pharmacodynamic properties

Neomycin is an aminoglycoside antibiotic.

Neomycin acts by binding to polysomes, inhibiting protein synthesis and generating errors in the transcription of the genetic code.

5.2 Pharmacokinetic properties

The absorption of neomycin from the alimentary tract is poor: Only 3% of an oral dose is absorbed, neomycin is rapidly excreted by the kidneys in the unchanged form. The plasma half-life in healthy adults is approximately 2-3 hours. Oral doses of 3g produce peak plasma concentrations of up to 4 μg/ml.

5.3 Preclinical safety data

Not applicable.

6. PHARMACEUTICAL PARTICULARS

6.1 List of excipients

Plasdone K29-32

Isopropyl alcohol

Calcium stearate.

6.2 Incompatibilities

Not applicable.

6.3 Shelf life

3 years.

6.4 Special precautions for storage

Store below 30°C in a dry place – protect from light.

6.5 Nature and contents of container

An amber glass bottle having a tin-plate screw cap with a waxed aluminium-faced pulpboard liner. The ullage is filled with cotton wool.

Pack size: 100 tablets.

6.6 Instructions for use and handling

Not applicable.

Administrative Data

7. MARKETING AUTHORISATION HOLDER

Waymade Plc.

Trading as Sovereign Medical

Sovereign House

Miles Gray Road

Basildon

Essex SS14 3FR.

8. MARKETING AUTHORISATION NUMBER(S)

PL 06464/0710.

9. DATE OF FIRST AUTHORISATION/RENEWAL OF THE AUTHORISATION

11 January 1999.

10. DATE OF REVISION OF THE TEXT

July 2003.

Nizoral Cream

(Janssen-Cilag Ltd)

1. NAME OF THE MEDICINAL PRODUCT

POM: Nizoral Cream

P: Daktarin Gold

2. QUALITATIVE AND QUANTITATIVE COMPOSITION

Ketoconazole Ph.Eur 2% w/w.

3. PHARMACEUTICAL FORM

Cream

4. CLINICAL PARTICULARS

4.1 Therapeutic indications

POM

For topical application in the treatment of dermatophyte infections of the skin such as tinea corporis, tinea cruris, tinea manus and tinea pedis infections due to Trichophyton spp, Microsporon spp and Epidermophyton spp. Nizoral cream is also indicated for the treatment of cutaneous candidosis (including vulvitis), pityriasis versicolor and seborrhoeic dermatitis caused by Pityrosporum spp.

P

For the treatment of the following mycotic infections of the skin: tinea pedis, tinea cruris and candidal intertrigo.

4.2 Posology and method of administration
POM

Tinea pedis:

Nizoral cream should be applied to the affected areas twice daily. The usual duration of treatment for mild infections is 1 week. For more severe or extensive infections (eg involving the sole or sides of the feet) treatment should be continued until a few days after all signs and symptoms have disappeared in order to prevent relapse.

For other infections:

Nizoral cream should be applied to the affected areas once or twice daily, depending on the severity of the infection.

The treatment should be continued until a few days after the disappearance of all signs and symptoms. The usual duration of treatment is: pityriasis versicolor 2–3 weeks, tinea corporis 3–4 weeks.

The diagnosis should be reconsidered if no clinical improvement is noted after 4 weeks. General measures in regard to hygiene should be observed to control sources of infection or reinfection.

Seborrhoeic dermatitis is a chronic condition and relapse is highly likely.

If a potent topical corticosteroid has been used previously in the treatment of seborrhoeic dermatitis, a recovery period of 2 weeks should be allowed before using Nizoral cream, as an increased incidence of steroid induced skin sensitisation has been reported when no recovery period is allowed.

P

For the treatment of tinea pedis (athlete's foot) and tinea cruris (dhobie itch) and candidal intertrigo (sweat rash).

For tinea pedis, Daktarin Gold cream should be applied to the affected areas twice daily. The usual duration of treatment for mild infections is 1 week. For more severe or extensive infections (eg involving the sole or sides of the feet) treatment should be continued for 2–3 days after all signs of infection have disappeared to prevent relapse.

For tinea cruris and candidal intertrigo, apply cream to the affected areas once or twice daily until 2-3 days after all signs of infection have disappeared to prevent relapse. Treatment for up to 6 weeks may be necessary. If no improvement in symptoms is experienced after 4 weeks treatment, a doctor should be consulted.

Method of administration: Topical administration.

4.3 Contraindications
Ketoconazole cream is contra-indicated in patients who have shown hypersensitivity to any of the ingredients or to ketoconazole itself.

4.4 Special warnings and special precautions for use
Not for ophthalmic use.

4.5 Interaction with other medicinal products and other forms of Interaction
None known except possible corticosteroid interaction (see POM dosage section).

4.6 Pregnancy and lactation
After topical application, ketoconazole cream is not systematically absorbed and does not produce detectable plasma concentrations. However, as with any medication, ketoconazole cream should only be used in pregnant women if its use is considered essential by a doctor. Since no ketoconazole is detected in plasma following topical administration, use of ketoconazole cream is not contra-indicated for breast feeding women.

4.7 Effects on ability to drive and use machines
None.

4.8 Undesirable effects
A few instances of irritation, dermatitis and burning sensation have been observed during treatment with ketoconazole cream.

4.9 Overdose
If accidental ingestion of ketoconazole cream occurs, an appropriate method of gastric emptying may be used if considered appropriate.

5. PHARMACOLOGICAL PROPERTIES
5.1 Pharmacodynamic properties
Ketoconazole has a potent antimycotic action against dermatophytes and yeasts. Ketoconazole cream acts rapidly on the pruritus, which is commonly seen in dermatophyte and yeast infections. This symptomatic improvement often occurs before the first signs of healing are observed.

5.2 Pharmacokinetic properties
After topical application, ketoconazole is not systematically absorbed and does not produce detectable plasma concentrations.

5.3 Preclinical safety data
Since ketoconazole administered topically as a cream is not systemically absorbed and does not produce detectable plasma concentrations, there is no specific relevant information. However, oral administration of high doses >80mg/kg) of ketoconazole to pregnant rats has been shown to cause abnormalities of foetal development. The relevance of this finding to humans has not been established and it is not of practical relevance to ketoconazole cream which is for external use only.

6. PHARMACEUTICAL PARTICULARS
6.1 List of excipients
Propylene Glycol

Stearyl Alcohol

Cetyl Alcohol

Sorbitan Stearate

Polysorbate 60

Isopropyl Myristate

Sodium Sulphite Anhydrous

Polysorbate 80

Purified Water

6.2 Incompatibilities
Not applicable.

6.3 Shelf life
60 months.

6.4 Special precautions for storage
Do not store above 25°C.

6.5 Nature and contents of container
Tube made of 99.7% aluminum, lined on inner side with heat polymerised epoxyphenol resin with a latex coldseal ring at the end of the tube. The cap is made of 60% polypropylene, 30% calcium carbonate and 10% glyceryl monostearate.

Tubes of 5, 15 and 30g.

6.6 Instructions for use and handling
Not applicable.

7. MARKETING AUTHORISATION HOLDER
Janssen-Cilag Ltd

Saunderton

High Wycombe

Bucks

HP14 4HJ

UK

8. MARKETING AUTHORISATION NUMBER(S)
PL 00242/0107

9. DATE OF FIRST AUTHORISATION/RENEWAL OF THE AUTHORISATION
Renewed 25 April 1996

10. DATE OF REVISION OF THE TEXT
December 2002

Legal Category
POM: Nizoral Cream

P: Daktarin Gold

Nizoral Dandruff Shampoo & Nizoral Anti-Dandruff Shampoo

(Janssen-Cilag Ltd)

1. NAME OF THE MEDICINAL PRODUCT
1A P-supply

Nizoral® Dandruff Shampoo

1B GSL-supply

Nizoral® anti-dandruff Shampoo

2. QUALITATIVE AND QUANTITATIVE COMPOSITION
Ketoconazole 2% w/w.

3. PHARMACEUTICAL FORM
Pink viscous shampoo.

4. CLINICAL PARTICULARS
4.1 Therapeutic indications
4.1A P-supply

In the prevention and treatment of the scalp conditions dandruff and seborrhoeic dermatitis.

4.1B GSL-supply

In the prevention and treatment of the scalp condition dandruff.

4.2 Posology and method of administration
For topical administration.

Adults, elderly and children:

Wash affected areas and leave for 3 to 5 minutes before rinsing.

Treatment:

Wash the hair every 3 or 4 days for 2 to 4 weeks.

Prophylaxis:

Use once, every 1 to 2 weeks.

Do not use more often than directed.

4.3 Contraindications
Patients showing hypersensitivity to any of the ingredients.

4.4 Special warnings and special precautions for use
Keep out of the eyes. If the shampoo should get into the eyes, they should be bathed with water.

Seborrhoeic dermatitis and dandruff have been associated with increased hair shedding and this has also been reported, although rarely, with the use of Nizoral Dandruff or anti-dandruff Shampoo.

If the scalp has not cleared within 4 weeks, a doctor or pharmacist should be consulted.

4.5 Interaction with other medicinal products and other forms of Interaction
To prevent a rebound effect after stopping a prolonged treatment with topical corticosteroids, it is recommended to continue applying the topical corticosteroid together with Nizoral Dandruff or anti-dandruff Shampoo and to subsequently and gradually withdraw the steroid therapy over a period of 2-3 weeks.

4.6 Pregnancy and lactation
Since no ketoconazole is detected in plasma following topical administration, pregnancy and lactation are not a contra-indication for the use of ketoconazole shampoo.

4.7 Effects on ability to drive and use machines
None likely.

4.8 Undesirable effects
Topical treatment with Nizoral Dandruff or anti-dandruff Shampoo is generally well tolerated.

As with other shampoos, a local burning sensation, itching, or contact dermatitis (due to irritation or allergy) may occur on exposed areas. Oily and dry hair have been reported rarely with the use of Nizoral Dandruff or anti-dandruff Shampoo.

In rare instances, mainly in patients with chemically damaged hair or grey hair, a discolouration of the hair has been observed.

4.9 Overdose
In the event of accidental ingestion, only supportive measures should be carried out. In order to avoid aspiration, neither emesis nor gastric lavage should be instigated.

5. PHARMACOLOGICAL PROPERTIES
5.1 Pharmacodynamic properties
Ketoconazole is a synthetic imidazole dioxolane antimycotic active against yeasts, including *Malassezia*,, and dermatophytes. Its broad spectrum of activity is already well known.

Ketoconazole also has a direct anti-inflammatory action independent from its antifungal activity which may contribute to symptom relief in dandruff and seborrhoeic dermatitis.

5.2 Pharmacokinetic properties
Ketoconazole is not detectable in blood stream (assay limit 2 ng/ml) after topical administration of the shampoo.

5.3 Preclinical safety data
Not applicable.

6. PHARMACEUTICAL PARTICULARS
6.1 List of excipients
Sodium lauryl ether sulphate

Disodium monolauryl ether sulphosuccinate

Coconut fatty acid diethanolamide

Laurdimonium hydrolysed animal collagen

Macrogol 120 methyl glucose dioleate

Sodium chloride

Concentrated hydrochloric acid

Imidurea

Sodium hydroxide

Erythrosine sodium (E127)

Purified water

6.2 Incompatibilities
None known.

6.3 Shelf life
3 years.

6.4 Special precautions for storage
Store at or below 25°C.

6.5 Nature and contents of container
P-supply:

1. High-density polyethylene bottle containing 60 ml, 100 ml or 120ml Nizoral Dandruff Shampoo.

2. 7.5 ml aluminium sachet in pack sizes of 2, 4, 6 or 12.

GSL supply:

1. High-density polyethylene bottle containing 60 ml or 100 ml Nizoral anti-dandruff Shampoo.

2. 7.5 ml aluminium sachet in pack sizes of 4.

6.6 Instructions for use and handling
Not applicable.

7. MARKETING AUTHORISATION HOLDER
Janssen-Cilag Limited

Saunderton

High Wycombe

Buckinghamshire

HP14 4HJ

England

8. MARKETING AUTHORISATION NUMBER(S)
PL 00242/0140

9. DATE OF FIRST AUTHORISATION/RENEWAL OF THE AUTHORISATION

Date of First Authorisation: 18 April 1988

Date of Renewal of Authorisation: 14 July 2000

10. DATE OF REVISION OF THE TEXT

November 2002

Legal category: P: Dandruff and Seborrhoeic dermatitis

GSL: Dandruff

Nizoral Shampoo

(Janssen-Cilag Ltd)

1. NAME OF THE MEDICINAL PRODUCT

Nizoral® Shampoo

2. QUALITATIVE AND QUANTITATIVE COMPOSITION

Ketoconazole 2% w/w.

3. PHARMACEUTICAL FORM

Pink viscous liquid.

4. CLINICAL PARTICULARS

4.1 Therapeutic indications

Prevention and treatment of infections in which the yeast *Pityrosporum* is likely to be involved, such as dandruff, seborrhoeic dermatitis and pityriasis versicolor.

4.2 Posology and method of administration

For topical administration.

Adults, Elderly and Children:

Wash affected areas and leave for 3-5 minutes before rinsing.

Treatment:

Dandruff and seborrhoeic dermatitis: Wash hair twice weekly for 2-4 weeks.

Pityriasis versicolor: Once daily for a maximum of 5 days.

Prophylaxis:

Dandruff and seborrhoeic dermatitis: Use once every 1-2 weeks.

Pityriasis versicolor: Once daily for a maximum of 3 days before exposure to sunshine.

4.3 Contraindications

Patients showing hypersensitivity to any of the ingredients.

4.4 Special warnings and special precautions for use

Seborrhoeic dermatitis and dandruff are often associated with increased hair shedding and this has also been reported, although rarely, with the use of Nizoral Shampoo.

Keep out of the eyes. If the shampoo should get into the eyes, they should be bathed with water.

4.5 Interaction with other medicinal products and other forms of Interaction

To prevent a rebound effect after stopping prolonged treatment with topical corticosteroids, it is recommended to continue applying the topical corticosteroid together with Nizoral Shampoo and to subsequently and gradually withdraw the steroid therapy over a period of 2 -3 weeks.

4.6 Pregnancy and lactation

Since no ketoconazole is detected in plasma following topical administration, pregnancy and lactation are not a contra-indication for the use of ketoconazole shampoo.

4.7 Effects on ability to drive and use machines

None likely.

4.8 Undesirable effects

As with other shampoos, a local burning sensation, itching, or contact dermatitis (due to irritation or allergy) may occur on exposed areas. Oily and dry hair have been reported rarely with the use of Nizoral shampoo.

In rare instances, mainly in patients with chemically damaged hair or grey hair, a discolouration of the hair has been observed.

4.9 Overdose

In the event of accidental ingestion, only supportive measures should be carried out. In order to avoid aspiration, neither emesis nor gastric lavage should be instigated.

5. PHARMACOLOGICAL PROPERTIES

5.1 Pharmacodynamic properties

Ketoconazole is an imidazole-dioxolane antimycotic, active against yeasts, including *Pityrosporum*, and dermatophytes. Its broad spectrum of activity is already well known.

5.2 Pharmacokinetic properties

Ketoconazole is not detectable in the blood stream (assay limit 2 ng/ml) after topical administration of the shampoo.

5.3 Preclinical safety data

No relevant information additional to that contained elsewhere in the Summary of Product Characteristics.

6. PHARMACEUTICAL PARTICULARS

6.1 List of excipients

Sodium lauryl ether sulphate

Disodium monolauryl ether sulphosuccinate

Coconut fatty acid diethanolamide

Laurdimonium hydrolysed animal collagen

Macrogol 120 methyl glucose dioleate

Sodium chloride

Concentrated hydrochloric acid

Imidurea

Sodium hydroxide

Erythrosine sodium

Purified water

6.2 Incompatibilities

None known.

6.3 Shelf life

36 months.

6.4 Special precautions for storage

Store at 25°C or below.

6.5 Nature and contents of container

Aluminium sachet lined with polyethylene, containing 7.5 ml shampoo.

Boxes of 2, 6 and 12 sachets.

High density polyethylene bottles, containing 120 ml shampoo.

6.6 Instructions for use and handling

Not applicable.

7. MARKETING AUTHORISATION HOLDER

Janssen-Cilag Ltd

Saunderton

High Wycombe

Buckinghamshire

HP14 4HJ

UK

8. MARKETING AUTHORISATION NUMBER(S)

0242/0139

9. DATE OF FIRST AUTHORISATION/RENEWAL OF THE AUTHORISATION

Date of Renewal of Authorisation: 24 June 1993

10. DATE OF REVISION OF THE TEXT

May 2000

Legal category POM

Nizoral Tablets

(Janssen-Cilag Ltd)

1. NAME OF THE MEDICINAL PRODUCT

Nizoral®

2. QUALITATIVE AND QUANTITATIVE COMPOSITION

200 mg ketoconazole.

3. PHARMACEUTICAL FORM

Tablet.

4. CLINICAL PARTICULARS

4.1 Therapeutic indications

Systemic mycoses, eg systemic candidosis, paracoccidioidomycosis, coccidioidomycosis, histoplasmosis.

Serious chronic mucocutaneous candidosis (including exceptionally disabling paronychia) not responsive to other therapy or when the organism is resistant to other therapy.

Serious mycoses of the gastrointestinal tract not responsive to other therapy or when organisms are resistant to other therapy.

Chronic vaginal candidosis not responsive to other therapy.

Prophylactic treatment to prevent mycotic infection in patients with reduced immune responses, e.g. in cancer, during treatment with immunosuppressive medication, or with burns.

Culturally determined dermatophyte infections of skin or finger nails which have failed to respond to adequate dose regimes of conventional anti-dermatophyte agents (excluding fungal infection of toe nails). Nizoral is not indicated for pityriasis versicolor, usually an asymptomatic skin rash.

4.2 Posology and method of administration

Nizoral tablets should be taken orally with meals to ensure maximum absorption.

Adults:

Mycoses and dermatophyte infections (except vaginal infections)

One tablet once daily, usually for 14 days.

If an adequate response has not been achieved after 14 days, treatment can be continued until at least one week after symptoms have cleared and cultures have become negative. The dose may also be increased to 400 mg once daily if necessary.

As nail infections always require long term therapy, they should only be treated when a clinical rather than a purely cosmetic problem exists and only after alternative treatment has failed.

Prophylaxis and maintenance treatment:

One tablet daily.

Chronic vaginal candidosis:

Two tablets once daily for 5 days.

Children:

Dosage should be reduced to 50 or 100 mg depending on body weight (i.e. approximately 3 mg/kg), for example:

Age 1-4 years: 50 mg

Age 5-12 years: 100 mg

Elderly:

In the absence of specific data, chronic vaginal candidosis - as for adults;

All other indications - 200 mg daily.

Method of administration:

Oral.

4.3 Contraindications

Nizoral should not be used in patients with a known hypersensitivity to ketoconazole, to any of the other ingredients, or to any other imidazole antifungal.

Since it cannot be excluded that patients with pre-existing liver disease may be at greater risk of developing hepatic damage, oral ketoconazole treatment is contra-indicated in these patients. In patients suspected of having pre-existing liver disease, liver function tests should be performed prior to treatment and ketoconazole should not be used if significant abnormalities are observed.

Astemizole, mizolastine, terfenadine, cisapride, dofetilide, quinidine, pimozide, CYP3A4 metabolised HMG-CoA reductase inhibitors such as simvastatin and lovastatin, oral midazolam and triazolam should not be given concurrently with oral ketoconazole (see Section 4.5 Interactions).

4.4 Special warnings and special precautions for use

Ketoconazole does not penetrate well into the CNS. Therefore, fungal meningitis should not be treated with oral ketoconazole.

Absorption is impaired when gastric acidity is decreased. Acid neutralising medicines (e.g. aluminium hydroxide), should not be administered for at least 2 hours after the intake of Nizoral Tablets. In patients with achlorhydria, such as certain AIDS patients and patients on acid secretion suppressors (eg H_2-antagonists, proton pump inhibitors), it is advisable to administer Nizoral Tablets with a cola beverage.

Patients on chronic Nizoral treatment must be made aware of symptoms of liver disease such as abnormal fatigue, fever, dark urine, pale stools or jaundice. The risk factors for the development of hepatitis include: age over 50 (especially women); known drug intolerance or concomitant administration of potentially hepatotoxic agents; history of liver disease.

The risk of developing hepatitis is greater in patients on long term treatment >14 days). In patients receiving long term treatment, the benefits must be weighed against the possible risks and liver function tests (LFTs) should be performed prior to starting treatment.

Asymptomatic elevations in serum transaminase can occur early during treatment with ketoconazole. These may either be insignificant and transient, or can represent early evidence of hepatotoxicity. Patients should therefore be monitored clinically and biochemically with serum transaminase determinations after the first 2 weeks of treatment, at 4 weeks and at monthly intervals thereafter. If significantly elevated levels are observed, liver function tests (LFTs) should be performed at weekly intervals until transaminase levels return to normal. If significant progressive elevation occurs or the patient develops symptoms of hepatitis (malaise, fever, dark urine, pale stools or jaundice), treatment with ketoconazole should be stopped immediately. The patient should then be monitored both clinically and biochemically for at least 2 months or until enzyme levels return to normal. Patients should also be told to consult their doctor if any of the above symptoms develop.

Hepatic damage has usually been reversible on discontinuation of treatment. Rarely, however, fatalities have been reported following ketoconazole treatment, usually where therapy has been continued despite development of symptoms of hepatitis.

Patients with impaired adrenal function, or who may be under periods of stress (eg major surgery, intensive care, etc) should have their adrenal function monitored.

A risk/benefit evaluation should be made before ketoconazole is used in cases of non-life threatening diseases requiring long treatment periods.

4.5 Interaction with other medicinal products and other forms of Interaction

1. Drugs affecting the metabolism of ketoconazole

Enzyme-inducing drugs such as rifampicin, rifabutin, carbamazepine, isoniazid and phenytoin significantly reduce the bioavailability of ketoconazole. As plasma levels are lower than those expected if ketoconazole is used alone (no co-medication), it is not really necessary to monitor plasma levels.

Drugs affecting gastric acidity (see Section 4.4)

Ritonavir increases the bioavailability of ketoconazole. Therefore, when it is given concomitantly, a dose reduction of ketoconazole should be considered.

2. Effect of ketoconazole on the metabolism of other drugs

Ketoconazole can inhibit the metabolism of drugs metabolised by certain hepatic P450 enzymes, especially of the CYP3A family. This can result in an increase and/or prolongation of their effects including side effects.

Concurrent treatment with astemizole, mizolastine, terfenadine, cisapride, dofetilide, quinidine, pimozide, oral midazolam, triazolam and CYP3A4 metabolised HMG-CoA reductase inhibitors such as simvastatin and lovastatin, is contra-indicated.

Plasma levels, effects or side effects should be monitored, and dosage reduced if necessary, when ketoconazole and the following drugs are co-administered:

- Oral anticoagulants.
- HIV Protease Inhibitors such as indinavir, saquinavir.
- Certain Antineoplastic Agents such as vinca alkaloids, busulphan and docetaxel.
- CYP3A4 metabolised Calcium Channel Blockers such as dihydropyridines and probably verapamil.
- Certain Immunosuppressive Agents: cyclosporin, tacrolimus, sirolimus (= rapamycin)
- Others: digoxin, carbamazepine, buspirone, alfentanil, sildenafil, alprazolam, brotizolam, intravenous midazolam, rifabutin, methyl prednisolone, trimetrexate, ebastine and reboxetine

Exceptional cases of a disulfiram-like reaction to alcohol, characterised by flushing, rash, peripheral oedema, nausea and headache, have been reported. All symptoms resolved completely within a few hours.

4.6 Pregnancy and lactation

Nizoral Tablets are contra-indicated in pregnancy. Although any relevance to humans has not been established, when administered in high doses >80 mg/kg) to pregnant rats, ketoconazole has been shown to cause abnormalities of foetal development.

Ketoconazole is excreted in breast milk and therefore it is not advisable to breast feed whilst being treated with Nizoral Tablets.

4.7 Effects on ability to drive and use machines

None known.

4.8 Undesirable effects

Alterations in liver function tests have occurred in patients on ketoconazole; these changes may be transient. Cases of hepatitis have been reported (see Section 4.4.). Such side effect is usually reversible if the treatment is promptly discontinued.

In rare cases, anaphylactoid reactions have been reported after the first dose. Hypersensitivity reactions including urticaria and angio- oedema have also been reported.

The most commonly observed side effects are gastric upsets (dyspepsia, nausea, vomiting, abdominal pain and diarrhoea), rash, urticaria, pruritus and headache. Less frequently reported adverse effects include menstrual irregularities (including when co-administered with oral contraceptives), dizziness, photophobia and paraesthesia. Thrombocytopenia, alopecia, impotence, and reversible increased intracranial pressure (e.g. papilloedema, bulging fontanelle in infants) have been reported very rarely.

Ketoconazole, 200 mg once daily, produces a transient decrease in plasma testosterone levels during the first 4-6 hours after intake of the drug. During long-term therapy at this dose, testosterone levels are usually not significantly different from controls.

In rare instances, at doses higher than the recommended dose, reversible gynaecomastia and oligospermia have been reported.

Although impaired response of plasma cortisol to ACTH has been described, clinically significant symptoms of adrenal insufficiency are unlikely to occur at recommended doses (see Section 4.4).

4.9 Overdose

In the event of overdosage cases should be treated symptomatically with supportive measures. Within the first hour after ingestion gastric lavage may be performed. Activated charcoal may be given if considered appropriate.

5. PHARMACOLOGICAL PROPERTIES

5.1 Pharmacodynamic properties

Ketoconazole is an imidazole-dioxolane anti-mycotic which is effective after oral administration and has a broad spectrum of activity against dermatophytes, yeasts and other pathogenic fungi.

5.2 Pharmacokinetic properties

Ketoconazole is incompletely absorbed by the gastro-intestinal tract; absorption is reduced when gastric acidity is reduced. Peak plasma levels are obtained 2 hours after oral administration.

Ketoconazole is extensively bound to plasma proteins. Penetration into cerebrospinal fluid is poor. Ketoconazole is extensively metabolised in the body and is excreted in the urine as inactive metabolites and unchanged drug. It is also excreted in the faeces.

5.3 Preclinical safety data

Not applicable.

6. PHARMACEUTICAL PARTICULARS

6.1 List of excipients

Maize starch

Lactose

Polyvidone K90

Microcrystalline cellulose

Colloidal anhydrous silica

Magnesium stearate

6.2 Incompatibilities

None known.

6.3 Shelf life

Five years.

6.4 Special precautions for storage

Store in a dry place between 15°C and 30°C.

6.5 Nature and contents of container

PVC/aluminium blister packs containing 30 tablets

6.6 Instructions for use and handling

Not applicable.

7. MARKETING AUTHORISATION HOLDER

Janssen-Cilag Ltd
Saunderton
High Wycombe
Buckinghamshire
HP14 4HJ
UK

8. MARKETING AUTHORISATION NUMBER(S)

PL 0242/0083

9. DATE OF FIRST AUTHORISATION/RENEWAL OF THE AUTHORISATION

Date of First Authorisation: 22 December 1980

10. DATE OF REVISION OF THE TEXT

May 2001

Legal category POM.

Nocutil Desmopressin 0.1 mg/ml Nasal Spray

(Norgine Limited)

1. NAME OF THE MEDICINAL PRODUCT

Nocutil Desmopressin 0.1 mg/ml Nasal Spray

2. QUALITATIVE AND QUANTITATIVE COMPOSITION

1ml nasal spray solution contains 0.1mg desmopressin acetate

(corresponding to 0.089 mg desmopressin).

One spray delivers 10μg desmopressin acetate.

For excipients, see 6.1.

3. PHARMACEUTICAL FORM

Nasal spray, solution

4. CLINICAL PARTICULARS

4.1 Therapeutic indications

For the treatment of nocturnal enuresis in children (from 5 years of age) following exclusion of organic causes:

- as part of a global therapeutic management (e.g. if other, non-pharmaceutical treatment measures have failed)
- caused by nocturnal ADH deficiency.

For the treatment of vasopressin - sensitive cranial diabetes insipidus.

4.2 Posology and method of administration

For nasal use.

Before application blow the nose. Place nozzle just inside the nostril and press once. One spray delivers a dose of 10 μg. If higher doses are prescribed use alternating nostrils. While spraying breathe in slightly. Replace the protective cap after use.

Nocturnal enuresis:

The dosage should be adjusted within the range of 10 - 40 μg daily.

The usual initial dose in children from 5 years of age is 20 μg at bedtime. The efficacy can be enhanced by restricted fluid intake before bedtime.

In the event of non-response to the lowest dose, the following scheme for incremental dosing is recommended: after starting with 20 μg for 1-2 weeks, increase to 30 μg in the 3rd week and if necessary to 40 μg no earlier than the 4th week. If a single bedtime dose of 20μg is effective, a dose reduction to a single spray (10μg) can be assessed.

The need for continued treatment should be reassessed after 3 months by means of a period of at least 1 week without treatment.

Diabetes insipidus:

The dosage should be adjusted individually according to need.

In children: the average daily dose is 10μg.

In adults: the average daily dose ranges between 10 and 20μg, once or twice daily.

The voided volume and the osmolality of urine should be determined in order to titrate the optimal dose.

4.3 Contraindications

Due to the dose of 10 μg desmopressin acetate delivered per spray, Nocutil is not indicated for use in infants and small children.

Desmopressin must not be used in cases of:

- hypersensitivity to the active substance or to any of the excipients,
- toxaemia of pregnancy,
- primary and psychogenic polydipsia or polydipsia in alcoholics,
- von Willebrand's disease (subtype II),
- cardiac insufficiency and other conditions requiring treatment with diuretic agents,
- hyponatremia.

4.4 Special warnings and special precautions for use

Care should be taken in cases of cystic fibrosis, coronary heart disease, hypertension and chronic renal disease.

When used to control primary nocturnal enuresis, desmopressin should only be used in patients with normal blood pressure.

Patients and their parents should be warned to avoid fluid overload (including during swimming) and to stop desmopressin during an episode of vomiting or diarrhoea until fluid balance is normal. The risk of hyponatraemia convulsions can also be minimised by keeping to the recommended starting doses and by avoiding concomitant use of substances which increase secretion of vasopressin (see Section 4.5).

As a precautionary measure to prevent hyperhydration and hyponatraemia, fluid intake should be reduced, especially in very young and elderly patients, in conditions characterised by fluid and electrolyte imbalance and by increased intracranial pressure.

During the treatment of nocturnal enuresis fluid intake should be limited to a minimum and only to satisfy thirst from 1 hour before to 8 hours following administration.

Absorption may be irregular in patients with oedema, scarring or other abnormal conditions of the nasal mucosa.

Fluid retention can be monitored by weighing the patient or by the measurement of plasma sodium or osmolality.

An increase in body weight may bedue to overdosage or more often due to increased fluid intake.

Desmopressin therapy without concomitant adjustment of fluid intake may lead to fluid retention and hyponatraemia, accompanied by symptoms such as weight gain, headache, nausea and oedema. In severe cases cerebral oedema, convulsions and coma may occur.

Cerebral oedema was repeatedly reported in otherwise healthy children and young adults treated with desmopressin for nocturnal enuresis.

4.5 Interaction with other medicinal products and other forms of Interaction

Indomethacin (and possibly other NSAIDs), clofibrate and oxytocin may augment the antidiuretic effect of desmopressin.

Substances, which are known to release antidiuretic hormone, for example, tricyclic antidepressants, selective serotonin re-uptake inhibitors, chlorpromazine and carbamazepine, may cause an additive antidiuretic effect and increase the risk of water retention.

Glibenclamide and lithiummay diminish the antidiuretic effect.

If hypo- or hypertensive drugs are used concurrently blood pressure, plasma sodium levels and excretion of urine should be monitored.

4.6 Pregnancy and lactation

Preliminary clinical experience with the use of nasal desmopressin during pregnancy and lactation did not indicate any harmful effects to mothers or infants. The dosage of desmopressin to treat diabetes insipidus during pregnancy has to be adjusted to the needs of the individual patient, as this might change during pregnancy. Blood pressure monitoring is recommended.

Desmopressin is excreted in breast milk in minimal amounts without reported adverse effects to infants.

4.7 Effects on ability to drive and use machines

No studies on the effect of the ability to drive and use machines have been performed

4.8 Undesirable effects

The following undesirable effects have been observed with the use of desmopressin. Adverse reactions are listed according to the following categories:

Very common:	⩾ 10%
Common:	⩾ 1% and < 10%
Uncommon:	⩾ 0.1% and < 1%

Rare:	> 0.01% and < 0.1%
Very rare:	< 0.01%

Respiratory, thoracic and mediastinal disorders:

Uncommon: nasal congestion, epistaxis, rhinitis

Eye disorders:

Common: conjunctivitis

Gastrointestinal disorders:

Uncommon: nausea, abdominal cramps, vomiting

Nervous system disorders:

Uncommon: headache

Rare: cerebral oedema, hyponatremic seizures

Skin/General disorders:

Common: asthenia

Very rare: allergic and hypersensitivity reactions (e.g. pruritus, exanthema, fever, bronchospasms, anaphylaxis) as reported with peptides in general. On the other hand, these may represent hypersensitivity to the preservative benzalkonium chloride.

Cardiac / vascular disorders

Due to increased water reabsorption blood pressure may rise and in some cases hypertension may develop. In patients with coronary heart disease angina pectoris may occur.

These adverse effects, except for allergic reactions, may be prevented or disappear if the desmopressin dose is reduced.

4.9 Overdose

An overdose increases the risk of hyperhydration. Therefore symptoms such as slight hypertension, tachycardia, flush, headache, convulsions, nausea and abdominal cramps are to be expected.

Treatment should be discontinued and fluid intake restricted until serum sodium is normalised. Subsequently, the dose should be reduced.

In cases of massive overdose with the risk of water intoxication the administration of furosemide should be considered.

All cases of suspected cerebral oedema require immediate admission for intensive care measures.

5. PHARMACOLOGICAL PROPERTIES

5.1 Pharmacodynamic properties

Variations in plasma half-life of 2.5 - 4.5 hours.

Systemic bioavailability of nasal desmopressin is about 10%.

Desmopressin is a synthetic polypeptide that represents a structural analogue of the native posterior pituitary hormone arginine vasopressin. It has considerably longer antidiuretic action and at the same time diminished vasopressor activity.

Action sets in within 1 hour of application and lasts between 8 and 12 hours.

5.2 Pharmacokinetic properties

Intranasal absorption of desmopressin is fast, but incomplete. Interindividual differences regarding the rate of absorption from the nasal mucosa and the duration of the presence of the active ingredient in the plasma result in variations in plasma half-life of 2.5 - 4.5 hours.

Systemic bioavailability of nasal desmopressin is about 10%.

5.3 Preclinical safety data

Preclinical effects, e.g. nephrotoxicity, were observed only at exposures considered sufficiently in excess of the maximum human exposure indicating little relevance to clinical use. Studies on carcinogenicity and mutagenicity (except one negative Ames-Test) are not available.

6. PHARMACEUTICAL PARTICULARS

6.1 List of excipients

Benzalkonium chloride, malic acid, sodium hydroxide, sodium chloride, purified water.

6.2 Incompatibilities

Not applicable.

6.3 Shelf life

3 years.

After first opening 56 days.

6.4 Special precautions for storage

Do not store above 25°C.

Keep container in outer carton and store in an upright position.

6.5 Nature and contents of container

Package sizes of: 5ml and 6ml – amber, transparent glass bottle.

The following sizes are not marketed in the UK:

2.5ml, 3.5ml, 7ml and 8.4ml.

Closure: Spray head with metered-dose valve, applicator and protective cap.

6.6 Instructions for use and handling

Before first use:

Remove the protective cap and prime the spray several times until the first consistent spray is seen. Spray is now ready for use.

7. MARKETING AUTHORISATION HOLDER

Gebro Pharma GmbH, 6391 Fieberbrunn, Austria

8. MARKETING AUTHORISATION NUMBER(S)

PL 04536/0004

9. DATE OF FIRST AUTHORISATION/RENEWAL OF THE AUTHORISATION

18 January 2004

10. DATE OF REVISION OF THE TEXT

June 2004

Nolvadex

(AstraZeneca UK Limited)

1. NAME OF THE MEDICINAL PRODUCT

'Nolvadex'

2. QUALITATIVE AND QUANTITATIVE COMPOSITION

Tamoxifen Citrate Ph. Eur. 15.2 mg (equivalent to 10 mg tamoxifen).

3. PHARMACEUTICAL FORM

Tablet.

4. CLINICAL PARTICULARS

4.1 Therapeutic indications

'Nolvadex' is indicated for:

1. The treatment of breast cancer.

2. The treatment of anovulatory infertility.

4.2 Posology and method of administration

Route of administration: ORAL

1. **Breast Cancer**

Adults

The recommended daily dose of tamoxifen is normally 20 mg. No additional benefit, in terms of delayed recurrence or improved survival in patients, has been demonstrated with higher doses. Substantive evidence supporting the use of treatment with 30 - 40 mg per day is not available, although these doses have been used in some patients with advanced disease.

Elderly patients

Similar dosing regimens of 'Nolvadex' have been used in elderly patients with breast cancer and in some of these patients it has been used as sole therapy.

2. **Anovulatory Infertility**

Before commencing any course of treatment, whether initial or subsequent, the possibility of pregnancy must be excluded. In women who are menstruating regularly, but with anovular cycles, the initial course of treatment consists of 20 mg given daily on the second, third, fourth and fifth days of the menstrual cycle. If unsatisfactory basal temperature records or poor pre-ovulatory cervical mucus indicate that this initial course of treatment has been unsuccessful, further courses may be given during subsequent menstrual periods, increasing the dosage to 40 mg and then to 80 mg daily.

In women who are not menstruating regularly, the initial course may begin on any day. If no signs of ovulation are demonstrable, then a subsequent course of treatment may start 45 days later, with dosage increased as above. If a patient responds with menstruation, then the next course of treatment is commenced on the second day of the cycle.

4.3 Contraindications

'Nolvadex' must not be given during pregnancy. Premenopausal patients must be carefully examined before treatment for breast cancer or infertility to exclude the possibility of pregnancy (see also Section 4.6).

'Nolvadex' should not be given to patients who have experienced hypersensitivity to the product or any of its ingredients.

Treatment for infertility: Patients with a personal or family history of confirmed idiopathic venous thromboembolic events or a known genetic defect.

4.4 Special warnings and special precautions for use

Menstruation is suppressed in a proportion of pre-menopausal women receiving 'Nolvadex' for the treatment of breast cancer.

An increased incidence of endometrial changes including hyperplasia, polyps, cancer and uterine sarcoma (mostly malignant mixed Mullerian tumours), has been reported in association with 'Nolvadex' treatment. The underlying mechanism is unknown but may be related to the oestrogen-like effect of 'Nolvadex'. Any patient receiving or having previously received 'Nolvadex' who report abnormal gynaecological symptoms, especially vaginal bleeding, or who presents with menstrual irregularities, vaginal discharge and symptoms such as pelvic pain or pressure should be promptly investigated.

A number of second primary tumours, occurring at sites other than the endometrium and the opposite breast, have been reported in clinical trials, following the treatment of breast cancer patients with tamoxifen. No causal link has been established and the clinical significance of these observations remains unclear.

Venous thromboembolism

• A 2-3-fold increase in the risk for VTE has been demonstrated in healthy tamoxifen-treated women (see section 4.8).

• In patients with *breast cancer*, prescribers should obtain careful histories with respect to the patient's personal and family history of VTE. If suggestive of a prothrombotic risk, patients should be screened for thrombophilic factors. Patients who test positive should be counselled regarding their thrombotic risk. The decision to use tamoxifen in these patients should be based on the overall risk to the patient. In selected patients, the use of tamoxifen with prophylactic anticoagulation may be justified (cross-reference section 4.5)

• The risk of VTE is further increased by severe obesity, increasing age and all other risk factors for VTE. The risks and benefits should be carefully considered for *all* patients before treatment with tamoxifen. In patients with *breast cancer*, this risk is also increased by concomitant chemotherapy (see section 4.5). Long-term anti-coagulant prophylaxis may be justified for some patients with *breast cancer* who have multiple risk factors for VTE.

• Surgery and immobility: For patients being treated for *infertility*, tamoxifen should be stopped at least 6 weeks before surgery or long-term immobility (when possible) and re-started only when the patient is fully mobile. For patients with *breast cancer*, tamoxifen treatment should only be stopped if the risk of tamoxifen-induced thrombosis clearly outweighs the risks associated with interrupting treatment. All patients should receive appropriate thrombosis prophylactic measures and should include graduated compression stockings for the period of hospitalisation, early ambulation, if possible, and anti-coagulant treatment.

• If *any* patient presents with VTE, tamoxifen should be stopped immediately and appropriate anti-thrombosis measures initiated. In patients being treated for *infertility*, tamoxifen should not be re-started unless there is a compelling alternative explanation for their thrombotic event. In patients receiving tamoxifen for *breast cancer*, the decision to re-start tamoxifen should be made with respect to the overall risk for the patient. In selected patients with *breast cancer*, the continued use of tamoxifen with prophylactic anticoagulation may be justified.

• *All* patients should be advised to contact their doctors immediately if they become aware of any symptoms of VTE.

4.5 Interaction with other medicinal products and other forms of Interaction

When 'Nolvadex' is used in combination with coumarin-type anticoagulants, a significant increase in anticoagulant effect may occur. Where such co-administration is initiated, careful monitoring of the patient is recommended.

When 'Nolvadex' is used in combination with cytotoxic agents for the treatment of breast cancer, there is increased risk of thromboembolic events occurring. (See also Sections 4.4 and 4.8). Because of this increase in risk of VTE, thrombosis prophylaxis should be considered for these patients for the period of concomitant chemotherapy.

As 'Nolvadex' is metabolised by cytochrome P450 3A4, care is required when co-administering with drugs, such as rifampicin, known to induce this enzyme as tamoxifen levels may be reduced. The clinical relevance of this reduction is unknown.

4.6 Pregnancy and lactation

Pregnancy

'Nolvadex' must not be administered during pregnancy. There have been a small number of reports of spontaneous abortions, birth defects and foetal deaths after women have taken 'Nolvadex', although no causal relationship has been established.

Reproductive toxicology studies in rats, rabbits and monkeys have shown no teratogenic potential.

In rodent models of foetal reproductive tract development, tamoxifen was associated with changes similar to those caused by oestradiol, ethynyloestradiol, clomiphene and diethylstilboestrol (DES). Although the clinical relevance of these changes is unknown, some of them, especially vaginal adenosis, are similar to those seen in young women who were exposed to DES in-utero and who have a 1 in 1000 risk of developing clear-cell carcinoma of the vagina or cervix. Only a small number of pregnant women have been exposed to tamoxifen. Such exposure has not been reported to cause subsequent vaginal adenosis or clear-cell carcinoma of the vagina or cervix in young women exposed in utero to tamoxifen.

Women should be advised not to become pregnant whilst taking 'Nolvadex' and should use barrier or other non-hormonal contraceptive methods if sexually active. Pre-menopausal patients must be carefully examined before treatment to exclude pregnancy. Women should be informed of the potential risks to the foetus, should they become pregnant whilst taking 'Nolvadex' or within two months of cessation of therapy.

Lactation

It is not known if 'Nolvadex' is excreted in human milk and therefore the drug is not recommended during lactation.

The decision either to discontinue nursing or discontinue 'Nolvadex' should take into account the importance of the drug to the mother.

4.7 Effects on ability to drive and use machines

There is no evidence that 'Nolvadex' results in impairment of these activities.

4.8 Undesirable effects

Side effects can be classified as either due to the pharmacological action of the drug, e.g. hot flushes, vaginal bleeding, vaginal discharge, pruritus vulvae and tumour flare, or as more general side effects, e.g. gastro-intestinal intolerance, headache, light-headedness and occasionally, fluid retention and alopecia.

When side effects are severe, it may be possible to control them by a simple reduction of dosage (to not less than 20 mg/day) without loss of control of the disease. If side effects do not respond to this measure, it may be necessary to stop the treatment.

Skin rashes (including isolated reports of erythema multiforme, Stevens-Johnson syndrome and bullous pemphigoid) and rare hypersensitivity reactions including angioedema have been reported.

A small number of patients with bony metastases have developed hypercalcaemia on initiation of therapy.

Falls in platelet count, usually to 80,000 to 90,000 per cu mm but occasionally lower, have been reported in patients taking tamoxifen for breast cancer.

A number of cases of visual disturbance including reports of corneal changes and retinopathy have been described in patients receiving 'Nolvadex'. An increased incidence of cataracts has been reported in association with the administration of 'Nolvadex'.

Uterine fibroids, endometriosis and other endometrial changes including hyperplasia and polyps have been reported.

Cystic ovarian swellings have occasionally been observed in pre-menopausal women receiving 'Nolvadex'.

Leucopenia has been observed following the administration of 'Nolvadex', sometimes in association with anaemia and/or thrombocytopenia. Neutropenia has been reported on rare occasions; this can sometimes be severe.

Cases of deep vein thrombosis and pulmonary embolism have been reported during tamoxifen therapy (see sections 4.3, 4.4 and 4.5. When 'Nolvadex' is used in combination with cytotoxic agents, there is an increased risk of thrombo-embolic events.

Very rarely, cases of interstitial pneumonitis have been reported.

'Nolvadex' has been associated with changes in liver enzyme levels and on rare occasions with a spectrum of more severe liver abnormalities including fatty liver, cholestasis and hepatitis.

Rarely, elevation of serum triglyceride levels, in some cases with pancreatitis, may be associated with the use of 'Nolvadex'.

An increased incidence of endometrial cancer and uterine sarcoma (mostly malignant mixed Mullerian tumours) has been reported in association with 'Nolvadex' treatment.

4.9 Overdose

On theoretical grounds, an overdosage would be expected to cause enhancement of the pharmacological side effects mentioned above. Observations in animals show that extreme overdosage (100 - 200 times recommended daily dose) may produce oestrogenic effects.

There have been reports in the literature that 'Nolvadex' given at several times the standard dose may be associated with prolongation of the QT interval of the ECG.

There is no specific antidote to overdosage, and treatment must be symptomatic.

5. PHARMACOLOGICAL PROPERTIES

5.1 Pharmacodynamic properties

'Nolvadex' (tamoxifen) is a non-steroidal, triphenylethylene-based drug which displays a complex spectrum of oestrogen antagonist and oestrogen agonist-like pharmacological effects in different tissues. In breast cancer patients, at the tumour level, tamoxifen acts primarily as an antioestrogen, preventing oestrogen binding to the oestrogen receptor. However, clinical studies have shown some benefit in oestrogen receptor negative tumours which may indicate other mechanisms of action. In the clinical situation, it is recognised that tamoxifen leads to reductions in levels of blood total cholesterol and low density lipoproteins in postmenopausal women of the order of 10 - 20%. Tamoxifen does not adversely affect bone mineral density.

5.2 Pharmacokinetic properties

After oral administration, tamoxifen is absorbed rapidly with maximum serum concentrations attained within 4 - 7 hours. Steady state concentrations (about 300 ng/ml) are achieved after four weeks treatment with 40 mg daily. The drug is highly protein bound to serum albumin (>99%). Metabolism is by hydroxylation, demethylation and conjugation, giving rise to several metabolites which have a similar pharmacological profile to the parent compound and thus contribute to the therapeutic effect. Excretion occurs primarily via the faeces and an elimination half-life of approximately seven days has been calculated for the drug itself, whereas that for N-desmethyltamoxifen, the principal circulating metabolite, is 14 days.

5.3 Preclinical safety data

Tamoxifen was not mutagenic in a range of in-vitro and in-vivo mutagenicity tests. Tamoxifen was genotoxic in some in-vitro and in-vivo genotoxicity tests in rodents. Gonadal tumours in mice and liver tumours in rats receiving tamoxifen have been reported in long-term studies. The clinical relevance of these findings has not been established.

Tamoxifen is a drug on which extensive clinical experience has been obtained. Relevant information for the prescriber is provided elsewhere in the Summary of Product Characteristics.

6. PHARMACEUTICAL PARTICULARS

6.1 List of excipients

Croscarmellose Sodium USNF

Gelatin Ph. Eur

Lactose Ph. Eur

Macrogol 300 B.P.

Magnesium Stearate Ph. Eur

Maize Starch Ph. Eur

Methylhydroxypropylcellulose Ph. Eur

Titanium Dioxide Ph. Eur (E171)

6.2 Incompatibilities

None known.

6.3 Shelf life

5 years.

6.4 Special precautions for storage

Do not store above 30°C. Store in the original container.

6.5 Nature and contents of container

Aluminium blister pack containing 30 or 250 tablets.

HDPE bottles containing 30 or 250 tablets.

6.6 Instructions for use and handling

Use as directed by the prescriber.

7. MARKETING AUTHORISATION HOLDER

AstraZeneca UK Limited,

600 Capability Green,

Luton, LU1 3LU, UK.

8. MARKETING AUTHORISATION NUMBER(S)

PL 17901/0033

9. DATE OF FIRST AUTHORISATION/RENEWAL OF THE AUTHORISATION

11th June 2000/19th September 2001

10. DATE OF REVISION OF THE TEXT

29th January 2004

Nolvadex D

(AstraZeneca UK Limited)

1. NAME OF THE MEDICINAL PRODUCT

Nolvadex D

2. QUALITATIVE AND QUANTITATIVE COMPOSITION

Tamoxifen Citrate Ph. Eur. 30.4 mg (equivalent to 20 mg tamoxifen).

3. PHARMACEUTICAL FORM

Tablet.

4. CLINICAL PARTICULARS

4.1 Therapeutic indications

Nolvadex is indicated for:

1. The treatment of breast cancer.

2. The treatment of anovulatory infertility.

4.2 Posology and method of administration

Route of administration: Oral

1. Breast Cancer

Adults

The recommended daily dose of tamoxifen is normally 20 mg. No additional benefit, in terms of delayed recurrence or improved survival in patients, has been demonstrated with higher doses. Substantive evidence supporting the use of treatment with 30–40 mg per day is not available, although these doses have been used in some patients with advanced disease.

Elderly patients

Similar dosing regimens of Nolvadex have been used in elderly patients with breast cancer and in some of these patients it has been used as sole therapy.

2. Anovulatory Infertility

Before commencing any course of treatment, whether initial or subsequent, the possibility of pregnancy must be excluded. In women who are menstruating regularly, but with anovular cycles, the initial course of treatment consists of 20 mg given daily on the second, third, fourth and fifth days of the menstrual cycle. If unsatisfactory basal temperature records or poor pre-ovulatory cervical mucus indicate that this initial course of treatment has been unsuccessful, further courses may be given during subsequent menstrual periods, increasing the dosage to 40 mg and then to 80 mg daily.

In women who are not menstruating regularly, the initial course may begin on any day. If no signs of ovulation are demonstrable, then a subsequent course of treatment may start 45 days later, with dosage increased as above. If a patient responds with menstruation, then the next course of treatment is commenced on the second day of the cycle.

Use in children

The use of Nolvadex is not recommended in children, as safety and efficacy have not been established (see sections 5.1 and 5.2).

4.3 Contraindications

Nolvadex must not be given during pregnancy. Premenopausal patients must be carefully examined before treatment for breast cancer or infertility to exclude the possibility of pregnancy (see also section 4.6).

'Nolvadex' should not be given to patients who have experienced hypersensitivity to the product or any of its ingredients.

Treatment for infertility: Patients with a personal or family history of confirmed idiopathic venous thromboembolic events or a known genetic defect.

4.4 Special warnings and special precautions for use

Menstruation is suppressed in a proportion of premenopausal women receiving Nolvadex for the treatment of breast cancer.

An increased incidence of endometrial changes including hyperplasia, polyps, cancer and uterine sarcoma (mostly malignant mixed Mullerian tumours), has been reported in association with Nolvadex treatment. The underlying mechanism is unknown but may be related to the oestrogen-like effect of Nolvadex. Any patient receiving or having previously received Nolvadex who report abnormal gynaecological symptoms, especially vaginal bleeding, or who presents with menstrual irregularities, vaginal discharge and symptoms such as pelvic pain or pressure should be promptly investigated.

A number of second primary tumours, occurring at sites other than the endometrium and the opposite breast, have been reported in clinical trials, following the treatment of breast cancer patients with tamoxifen. No causal link has been established and the clinical significance of these observations remains unclear.

Venous thromboembolism

- A 2–3-fold increase in the risk for VTE has been demonstrated in healthy tamoxifen-treated women (see section 4.8).
- In patients with *breast cancer*, prescribers should obtain careful histories with respect to the patient's personal and family history of VTE. If suggestive of a prothrombotic risk, patients should be screened for thrombophilic factors. Patients who test positive should be counselled regarding their thrombotic risk. The decision to use tamoxifen in these patients should be based on the overall risk to the patient. In selected patients, the use of tamoxifen with prophylactic anticoagulation may be justified (cross-reference section 4.5).
- The risk of VTE is further increased by severe obesity, increasing age and all other risk factors for VTE. The risks and benefits should be carefully considered for *all* patients before treatment with tamoxifen. In patients with *breast cancer*, this risk is also increased by concomitant chemotherapy (see section 4.5). Long-term anticoagulant prophylaxis may be justified for some patients with *breast cancer* who have multiple risk factors for VTE.
- Surgery and immobility: For patients being treated for *infertility*, tamoxifen should be stopped at least 6 weeks before surgery or long-term immobility (when possible) and re-started only when the patient is fully mobile. For patients with *breast cancer*, tamoxifen treatment should only be stopped if the risk of tamoxifen-induced thrombosis clearly outweighs the risks associated with interrupting treatment. All patients should receive appropriate thrombosis prophylactic measures and should include graduated compression stockings for the period of hospitalisation, early ambulation, if possible, and anticoagulant treatment.
- If *any* patient presents with VTE, tamoxifen should be stopped immediately and appropriate anti-thrombosis measures initiated. In patients being treated for *infertility*, tamoxifen should not be re-started unless there is a compelling alternative explanation for their thrombotic event. In patients receiving tamoxifen for *breast cancer*, the decision to re-start tamoxifen should be made with respect to the overall risk for the patient. In selected patients with *breast cancer*, the continued use of tamoxifen with prophylactic anticoagulation may be justified.
- *All* patients should be advised to contact their doctors immediately if they become aware of any symptoms of VTE.

In an uncontrolled trial in 28 girls aged 2–10 years with McCune Albright Syndrome (MAS), who received 20 mg once a day for up to 12 months duration, mean uterine volume increased after 6 months of treatment and doubled at the end of the one-year study. While this finding is in line with the pharmacodynamic properties of tamoxifen, a causal relationship has not been established(see section 5.1).

4.5 Interaction with other medicinal products and other forms of Interaction

When Nolvadex is used in combination with coumarin-type anticoagulants, a significant increase in anticoagulant effect may occur. Where such co-administration is initiated, careful monitoring of the patient is recommended.

When Nolvadex is used in combination with cytotoxic agents for the treatment of breast cancer, there is increased risk of thromboembolic events occurring. (See also sections 4.4 and 4.8). Because of this increase in risk of VTE, thrombosis prophylaxis should be considered for these patients for the period of concomitant chemotherapy.

As Nolvadex is metabolised by cytochrome P450 3A4, care is required when co-administering with drugs, such as rifampicin, known to induce this enzyme as tamoxifen levels may be reduced. The clinical relevance of this reduction is unknown.

4.6 Pregnancy and lactation

Pregnancy

Nolvadex must not be administered during pregnancy. There have been a small number of reports of spontaneous abortions, birth defects and foetal deaths after women have taken Nolvadex, although no causal relationship has been established.

Reproductive toxicology studies in rats, rabbits and monkeys have shown no teratogenic potential.

In rodent models of foetal reproductive tract development, tamoxifen was associated with changes similar to those caused by estradiol, ethinylestradiol, clomiphene and diethylstilboestrol (DES). Although the clinical relevance of these changes is unknown, some of them, especially vaginal adenosis, are similar to those seen in young women who were exposed to DES *in utero* and who have a 1 in 1000 risk of developing clear-cell carcinoma of the vagina or cervix. Only a small number of pregnant women have been exposed to tamoxifen. Such exposure has not been reported to cause subsequent vaginal adenosis or clear-cell carcinoma of the vagina or cervix in young women exposed *in utero* to tamoxifen.

Women should be advised not to become pregnant whilst taking Nolvadex and should use barrier or other non-hormonal contraceptive methods if sexually active. Premenopausal patients must be carefully examined before treatment to exclude pregnancy. Women should be informed of the potential risks to the foetus, should they become pregnant whilst taking Nolvadex or within two months of cessation of therapy.

Lactation

It is not known if Nolvadex is excreted in human milk and therefore the drug is not recommended during lactation. The decision either to discontinue nursing or discontinue Nolvadex should take into account the importance of the drug to the mother.

4.7 Effects on ability to drive and use machines

There is no evidence that Nolvadex results in impairment of these activities.

4.8 Undesirable effects

Side effects can be classified as either due to the pharmacological action of the drug, e.g. hot flushes, vaginal bleeding, vaginal discharge, pruritus vulvae and tumour flare, or as more general side effects, e.g. gastrointestinal intolerance, headache, light-headedness and occasionally, fluid retention and alopecia.

When side effects are severe, it may be possible to control them by a simple reduction of dosage (to not less than 20 mg/day) without loss of control of the disease. If side effects do not respond to this measure, it may be necessary to stop the treatment.

Skin rashes (including isolated reports of erythema multiforme, Stevens-Johnson syndrome and bullous pemphigoid) and rare hypersensitivity reactions including angioedema have been reported.

A small number of patients with bony metastases have developed hypercalcaemia on initiation of therapy.

Falls in platelet count, usually to 80,000 to 90,000 per cu mm but occasionally lower, have been reported in patients taking tamoxifen for breast cancer.

A number of cases of visual disturbance including reports of corneal changes and retinopathy have been described in patients receiving Nolvadex. An increased incidence of cataracts has been reported in association with the administration of Nolvadex.

Uterine fibroids, endometriosis and other endometrial changes including hyperplasia and polyps have been reported.

Cystic ovarian swellings have occasionally been observed in premenopausal women receiving Nolvadex.

Leucopenia has been observed following the administration of Nolvadex, sometimes in association with anaemia and/or thrombocytopenia. Neutropenia has been reported on rare occasions; this can sometimes be severe.

Cases of deep vein thrombosis and pulmonary embolism have been reported during tamoxifen therapy (see sections 4.3, 4.4 and 4.5). When Nolvadex is used in combination with cytotoxic agents, there is an increased risk of thromboembolic events.

Very rarely, cases of interstitial pneumonitis have been reported.

Nolvadex has been associated with changes in liver enzyme levels and on rare occasions with a spectrum of more severe liver abnormalities including fatty liver, cholestasis and hepatitis.

Rarely, elevation of serum triglyceride levels, in some cases with pancreatitis, may be associated with the use of Nolvadex.

An increased incidence of endometrial cancer and uterine sarcoma (mostly malignant mixed Mullerian tumours) has been reported in association with Nolvadex treatment.

4.9 Overdose

On theoretical grounds, an overdosage would be expected to cause enhancement of the pharmacological side effects mentioned above. Observations in animals show that extreme overdosage (100–200 times recommended daily dose) may produce oestrogenic effects.

There have been reports in the literature that Nolvadex given at several times the standard dose may be associated with prolongation of the QT interval of the ECG.

There is no specific antidote to overdosage, and treatment must be symptomatic.

5. PHARMACOLOGICAL PROPERTIES

5.1 Pharmacodynamic properties

Nolvadex (tamoxifen) is a non-steroidal, triphenylethylene-based drug which displays a complex spectrum of oestrogen antagonist and oestrogen agonist-like pharmacological effects in different tissues. In breast cancer patients, at the tumour level, tamoxifen acts primarily as an antioestrogen, preventing oestrogen binding to the oestrogen receptor. However, clinical studies have shown some benefit in oestrogen receptor negative tumours which may indicate other mechanisms of action. In the clinical situation, it is recognised that tamoxifen leads to reductions in levels of blood total cholesterol and low density lipoproteins in postmenopausal women of the order of 10–20%. Tamoxifen does not adversely affect bone mineral density.

An uncontrolled trial was undertaken in a heterogenous group of 28 girls aged 2 to 10 years with McCune Albright Syndrome (MAS), who received 20 mg once a day for up to 12 months duration. Among the patients who reported vaginal bleeding during the pre-study period, 62% (13 out of 21 patients) reported no bleeding for a 6-month period and 33% (7 out of 21 patients) reported no vaginal bleeding for the duration of the trial. Mean uterine volume increased after 6 months of treatment and doubled at the end of the one-year study. While this finding is in line with the pharmacodynamic properties of tamoxifen, a causal relationship has not been established(see section 4.4). There are no long-term safety data in children. In particular, the long-term effects of tamoxifen on growth, puberty and general development have not been studied.

5.2 Pharmacokinetic properties

After oral administration, tamoxifen is absorbed rapidly with maximum serum concentrations attained within 4–7 hours. Steady state concentrations (about 300 ng/ml) are achieved after four weeks treatment with 40 mg daily. The drug is highly protein bound to serum albumin (>99%). Metabolism is by hydroxylation, demethylation and conjugation, giving rise to several metabolites which have a similar pharmacological profile to the parent compound and thus contribute to the therapeutic effect. Excretion occurs primarily via the faeces and an elimination half-life of approximately seven days has been calculated for the drug itself, whereas that for N-desmethyltamoxifen, the principal circulating metabolite, is 14 days.

In a clinical study where girls between 2 and 10 years with McCune Albright Syndrome (MAS) received 20 mg tamoxifen once a day for up to 12 months duration, there was an age-dependent decrease in clearance and an increase in exposure (AUC), (with values up to 50% higher in the youngest patients) compared with adults.

5.3 Preclinical safety data

Tamoxifen was not mutagenic in a range of *in vitro* and *in vivo* mutagenicity tests. Tamoxifen was genotoxic in some *in vitro* and *in vivo* genotoxicity tests in rodents. Gonadal tumours in mice and liver tumours in rats receiving tamoxifen have been reported in long-term studies. The clinical relevance of these findings has not been established.

Tamoxifen is a drug on which extensive clinical experience has been obtained. Relevant information for the prescriber is provided elsewhere in the Summary of Product Characteristics.

6. PHARMACEUTICAL PARTICULARS

6.1 List of excipients

Croscarmellose Sodium USNF

Gelatin BP

Lactose Ph. Eur.

Macrogol 300 B.P.

Magnesium Stearate Ph. Eur.

Maize Starch Ph. Eur.

Hydroxypropylmethylcellulose USP

Titanium Dioxide Ph. Eur. (E171)

6.2 Incompatibilities

None known.

6.3 Shelf life

5 years.

6.4 Special precautions for storage

Do not store above 30°C. Store in the original container.

6.5 Nature and contents of container

Aluminium blister pack containing 30 or 250 tablets.

HDPE bottles containing 30 or 250 tablets.

6.6 Instructions for use and handling

Use as directed by the prescriber.

7. MARKETING AUTHORISATION HOLDER

AstraZeneca UK Limited,

600 Capability Green,

Luton, LU1 3LU, UK.

8. MARKETING AUTHORISATION NUMBER(S)

PL 17901/0034

9. DATE OF FIRST AUTHORISATION/RENEWAL OF THE AUTHORISATION

11th June 2000

10. DATE OF REVISION OF THE TEXT

4th July 2005

Non Drowsy Sudafed Congestion Relief Capsules

(Pfizer Consumer Healthcare)

1. NAME OF THE MEDICINAL PRODUCT

Non-Drowsy Sudafed Congestion Relief Capsules

Strength: 12mg

2. QUALITATIVE AND QUANTITATIVE COMPOSITION

Active ingredient	mg/cap
Phenylephrine hydrochloride	12.00

3. PHARMACEUTICAL FORM

Capsule, hard.

Capsules description: A yellow cap and body printed 'Sudafed 0593' in black.

4. CLINICAL PARTICULARS

4.1 Therapeutic indications

For the relief of nasal congestion associated with colds and hay fever.

4.2 Posology and method of administration

Adults and children over 12 years: One capsule if necessary, up to four times daily.

Children under 12 years: Not recommended.

Elderly: There is no need for dosage reduction in the elderly.

4.3 Contraindications

Hypersensitivity to any of the ingredients. Avoid in patients with cardiovascular disease, diabetes mellitus, closed angle glaucoma, hyperthyroidism, prostatic enlargement and phaeochromocytoma.

4.4 Special warnings and special precautions for use

This medicine should be used with caution in patients with occlusive vascular disease including Raynaud's Phenomenon.

Do not take for longer than 7 days, unless your doctor agrees.

If symptoms do not go away talk to your doctor.

Keep all medicines out of the reach of children.

Warning: Do not exceed the stated dose.

4.5 Interaction with other medicinal products and other forms of Interaction

Should not be given to patients being treated with monoamine oxidase inhibitors or within 14 days of stopping such treatment. May enhance the effects of anticholinergic drugs such as tricyclic antidepressants. May increase the possibility of arrhythmias in digitalised patients. May enhance the cardiovascular effects of other sympathomimetic amines (e.g. decongestants).

This medicine should not be taken together with vasodilators, beta-blockers or enzyme inducers such as alcohol.

4.6 Pregnancy and lactation

The safety of this medicine during pregnancy and lactation has not been established but in view of a possible association of foetal abnormalities with first trimester exposure to phenylephrine, the use of the product during pregnancy should be avoided. In addition, because phenylephrine may educe placental perfusion, the product should not be used in patients with a history of pre-eclampsia. In view of the lack of data on the use of phenylephrine during lactation, this medicine should not be used during breast-feeding.

4.7 Effects on ability to drive and use machines

No adverse effects known.

4.8 Undesirable effects

Adverse effects may include tachycardia, cardiac arrhythmias, palpitations, hypertension, nausea, vomiting, headache and occasionally urinary retention in males.

4.9 Overdose

Symptoms of overdosage include irritability, restlessness, palpitations, hypertension, difficulty in micturition, nausea, vomiting, thirst and convulsions. In severe overdosage gastric lavage and aspiration should be performed. Symptomatic and supportive measures should be undertaken, particularly with regard to cardiovascular and respiratory systems. Convulsions should be controlled with intravenous diazepam. Chlorpromazine may be used to control marked excitement and hallucinations. Severe hypertension may need to be treated with an alpha-adrenoreceptor blocking drug, such as phentolamine. A beta blocker may be required to control cardiac arrhythmias.

5. PHARMACOLOGICAL PROPERTIES

5.1 Pharmacodynamic properties

Phenylephrine is a sympathomimetic agent with mainly direct effects on adrenergic receptors. It has predominantly alpha adrenergic activity and is without stimulating effects on the central nervous system. The sympathomimetic effect of phenylephrine produces vasoconstriction which in turn relieves nasal congestion.

5.2 Pharmacokinetic properties

Phenylephrine is readily absorbed after oral administration but is subject to extensive presystemic metabolism, much of which occurs in the enterocytes. As a consequence, systemic bioavailability is only about 40%. Following oral administration, peak plasma concentrations are achieved in 1-2 hours. The mean plasma half life is in the range 2-3 hours. Penetration into the brain appears to be minimal.

Following absorption, the drug is extensively metabolised in the liver. Both phenylephrine and its metabolites are excreted in the urine.

The volume of distribution is between 200 and 500 litres, but there are no data on the extent of plasma protein binding.

5.3 Preclinical safety data

There are no preclinical data of relevance to the prescriber which are additional to that already included in other sections of the SPC.

6. PHARMACEUTICAL PARTICULARS

6.1 List of excipients

Pregelatinised maize starch

Dried maize starch

Lactose monohydrate

Magnesium stearate

Hard Gelatin Capsule (Gelatin, Quinoline yellow E104, Titanium dioxide E171)

Ink (Black iron oxide E172, Shellac, Soya lecithin, Silicone)

6.2 Incompatibilities

Not applicable.

6.3 Shelf life

36 months.

6.4 Special precautions for storage

Do not store above 25°C. Store in the original package.

6.5 Nature and contents of container

Blister pack of pigmented 250 micron PVC coated with 40gsm PVdC and 20 micron aluminium foil.

Pack sizes: 5, 6, 7, 10, 12, 14, 18, 20, 21, 24, 25, 28, 30, 36, 48, 50.

6.6 Instructions for use and handling

Not applicable.

7. MARKETING AUTHORISATION HOLDER

Pfizer Consumer Healthcare

Walton Oaks

Dorking Road

Walton-on-the-Hill

Surrey

KT20 7NS

8. MARKETING AUTHORISATION NUMBER(S)

PL 15513/0125

9. DATE OF FIRST AUTHORISATION/RENEWAL OF THE AUTHORISATION

8 June 2004

10. DATE OF REVISION OF THE TEXT

Non Drowsy Sudafed Decongestant Elixir

(Pfizer Consumer Healthcare)

1. NAME OF THE MEDICINAL PRODUCT

NON-DROWSY SUDAFED DECONGESTANT ELIXIR

NON-DROWSY SUDAFED CHILDREN'S SYRUP*

2. QUALITATIVE AND QUANTITATIVE COMPOSITION

NON-DROWSY SUDAFED DECONGESTANT ELIXIR contains -

Pseudoephedrine Hydrochloride 30.0 mg per 5 ml

3. PHARMACEUTICAL FORM

Liquid for oral administration.

4. CLINICAL PARTICULARS

4.1 Therapeutic indications

NON-DROWSY SUDAFED DECONGESTANT ELIXIR is a decongestant of the mucous membranes of the upper respiratory tract, especially the nasal mucosa and sinuses and is indicated for the symptomatic relief of conditions such as allergic rhinitis, vasomotor rhinitis, the common cold and influenza.

4.2 Posology and method of administration

Oral

Adults and Children over 12 years

10 ml elixir every 4-6 hours up to 4 times a day.

Children 6 - 12 years

5 ml elixir every 4-6 hours up to 4 times a day.

Children 2-5 years

2.5 ml elixir every 4-6 hours up to 4 times a day.

NON-DROWSY SUDAFED DECONGESTANT ELIXIR may be diluted 1:1 (1 in 2) or 1:3 (1 in 4) with syrup BP. These dilutions are stable for 4 weeks if stored at 25°C.

Use in the Elderly

There have been no specific studies of NON-DROWSY SUDAFED DECONGESTANT ELIXIRin the elderly, experience has indicated that normal adult dosage is appropriate.

Hepatic Dysfunction

Caution should be exercised when administering NON-DROWSY SUDAFED DECONGESTANT ELIXIR to patients with severe hepatic impairment.

Renal Dysfunction

Caution should be exercised when administering NON-DROWSY SUDAFED DECONGESTANT ELIXIR to patients with moderate to severe renal impairment.

4.3 Contraindications

NON-DROWSY SUDAFED DECONGESTANT ELIXIR is contraindicated in individuals with known hypersensitivity to the product or any of its components.

NON-DROWSY SUDAFED DECONGESTANT ELIXIR is contraindicated in individuals with severe hypertension or coronary artery disease.

NON-DROWSY SUDAFED DECONGESTANT ELIXIR is contraindicated in individuals who are taking or have taken monoamine oxidase inhibitors within the preceding two weeks. The concomitant use of pseudoephedrine and this type of product may occasionally cause a rise in blood pressure.

4.4 Special warnings and special precautions for use

Although pseudoephedrine has virtually no pressor effects in normotensive patients, NON-DROWSY SUDAFED DECONGESTANT ELIXIR should be used with caution in patients suffering mild to moderate hypertension. As with other sympathomimetic agents, NON-DROWSY SUDAFED DECONGESTANT ELIXIR should be used with caution in patients with hypertension, heart disease, diabetes, hyperthyroidism, elevated intraocular pressure and prostatic enlargement.

Caution should be exercised when using the product in the presence of severe hepatic impairment or moderate to severe renal impairment (particularly if accompanied by cardiovascular disease).

The following statements will appear on packs of this product:-

- Store below 25C.
- Protect from light.
- Warning: do not exceed the stated dose.
- Keep out of reach of children.
- As with all medicines, if you are pregnant or currently taking any other medicine, consult your doctor or pharmacist before taking this product.
- If symptoms persist consult your doctor.
- Causes no drowsiness.

4.5 Interaction with other medicinal products and other forms of Interaction

Concomitant use of NON-DROWSY SUDAFED DECONGESTANT ELIXIR with tricylclic antidepressants, sympathomimetic agents (such as decongestants, appetite suppressants and amfetamine-like psychostimulants) or with monoamine oxidase inhibitors, which interferes with the catabolism of sympathomimetic amines, may occasionally cause a rise in blood pressure.

Because of its pseudoephedrine content, NON-DROWSY SUDAFED DECONGESTANT ELIXIR may partially reverse the hypotensive action of drugs which interfere with sympathetic activity including bretylium betanidine, guanethedine, debrisoquine, methyldopa, alpha- and beta-adrenergic blocking agents.

4.6 Pregnancy and lactation

Although pseudoephedrine has been in widespread use for many years without apparent ill consequence, there are no specific data on its use during pregnancy. Caution should therefore be exercised by balancing the potential benefit of treatment to the mother against any possible hazards to the developing foetus.

Systemic administration of pseudoephedrine, up to 50 times the human daily dose in rats and up to 35 times the human daily dosage in rabbits did not produce teratogenic effects. Pseudoephedrine is excreted in breast milk in small amounts, but the effect of this on breast-fed infants is not known. It has been estimated that 0.5 - 0.7% of a single dose of pseudoephedrine ingested by a mother will be excreted in the breast milk over 24 hours.

4.7 Effects on ability to drive and use machines

None known.

4.8 Undesirable effects

Serious side effects associated with the use of pseudoephedrine are rare. Symptoms of central nervous system excitation may occur, including sleep disturbance and, rarely hallucination.

Skin rashes, with or without irritation, have occasionally been reported with pseudoephedrine. Urinary retention has been reported occasionally in men receiving pseudoephedrine. Prostatic enlargement could have been an important predisposing factor.

4.9 Overdose

As with other sympathomimetic agents, symptoms of overdose include irritability, restlessness, tremor, convulsions, palpitations, hypertension and difficulty in micturition.

Necessary measures should be taken to maintain and support respiration and control convulsions. Gastric lavage should be performed if indicated. Catheterisation of the bladder may be necessary. If desired, the elimination of pseudoephedrine can be accelerated by acid diuresis or by dialysis.

5. PHARMACOLOGICAL PROPERTIES

5.1 Pharmacodynamic properties

Psuedoephedrine has direct and indirect sympathlomimetic activity and is an orally effective upper respiratory tract decongestant. Psuedoephedrine is substantially less potent than ephedrine in producing both tachycardia and elevation in systolic blood pressure and considerably less potent in causing stimulation of the central nervous system.

5.2 Pharmacokinetic properties

Pseudoephedrine is rapidly and completely absorbed after oral administration. After an oral dose of 180 mg to man, peak plasma concentrations of 500-900 ng/ml were obtained about 2 hours post dose. The plasma half life was about 5.5 hours and was increased in subjects with alkaline urine and decreased in subjects with acid urine. The only metabolism was n-demethylation which occurred to a small extent. Excretion was mainly via the urine.

5.3 Preclinical safety data

None stated.

6. PHARMACEUTICAL PARTICULARS

6.1 List of excipients

Citric Acid Monohydrate

Sucrose

Glycerol

Methyl Hydroxybenzoate

Sodium Benzoate

Ponceau 4R, E124

Flavour, Raspberry Essence No 1NA

Purified Water

6.2 Incompatibilities

None known

6.3 Shelf life

36 months unopened

6.4 Special precautions for storage

Store below 25°C.

Protect from light.

6.5 Nature and contents of container

30 ml, *100 ml and 1000 ml amber glass bottles with metal roll on closures or plastic screw caps, each cap containing a PVDC-lined wad or polyethylene/expanded polyethylene laminated wad.

Amber glass bottles with a 3 piece plastic child resistant, tamper evident closure fitted with a polyvinylidene chloride (PVDC) faced wad or polyethylene/expanded polyethylene laminated wad.

The 30 ml bottle is a sample pack.

*A spoon with a 5 ml and a 2.5 ml measure is supplied with this pack.

6.6 Instructions for use and handling

Not applicable

7. MARKETING AUTHORISATION HOLDER

Pfizer Consumer Healthcare

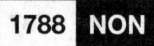

Alternative Trading Style:
Warner-Lambert Consumer Healthcare
Walton Oaks
Dorking Road
Walton-on-the-Hill
Surrey, KT20 7NS
United Kingdon

8. MARKETING AUTHORISATION NUMBER(S)
PL 15513/0023

9. DATE OF FIRST AUTHORISATION/RENEWAL OF THE AUTHORISATION
28 March 1997

10. DATE OF REVISION OF THE TEXT
November 2004

* Non-Drowsy Sudafed Decongestant Elixir is an alternative name for this product. Please read Non-Drowsy Sudafed Children's Syrup as an alternative where Non-Drowsy Sudafed Decongestant Elixir appears

Non-Drowsy Sinutab

(Pfizer Consumer Healthcare)

1. NAME OF THE MEDICINAL PRODUCT
NON-DROWSY SINUTAB
SUDAFED SINUS*

2. QUALITATIVE AND QUANTITATIVE COMPOSITION
NON-DROWSY SINUTAB tablets contain 30 mg Pseudoephedrine hydrochloride and 500 mg Paracetamol.

3. PHARMACEUTICAL FORM
Tablets

4. CLINICAL PARTICULARS

4.1 Therapeutic indications
NON-DROWSY SINUTAB is indicated for the symptomatic relief of conditions where congestion of the mucous membranes of the upper respiratory tract, especially nasal mucosa and sinuses, is accompanied by mild to moderate pain or pyrexia, e.g: the common cold and influenza, sinusitis, nasopharyngitis, allergic rhinitis and vasomotor rhinitis.

4.2 Posology and method of administration

Adults and children 12 years and over:
Oral. Two tablets every four to six hours, up to four times a day. Maximum daily dose: 8 tablets (i.e. 240 mg pseudoephedrine hydrochloride, 4 g paracetamol).

Children aged 6 to 12 years:
Oral. One tablet every four to six hours, up to four times a day. Maximum daily dose: 4 tablets (120 mg pseudoephedrine hydrochloride, 2 g paracetamol).

Children under 6 years:
NON-DROWSY SINUTAB is not suitable for administration to children under 6 years of age, except on the advice of a physician.

The Elderly:
There have been no specific studies of NON-DROWSY SINUTAB in the elderly. Experience has indicated that normal adult dosage is appropriate.

In the elderly the rate and extent of paracetamol absorption is normal but plasma half life is longer and paracetamol clearance is lower than in young adults.

Hepatic dysfunction
Caution should be exercised when administering NON-DROWSY SINUTAB to patients with severe hepatic impairment.

Renal dysfunction:
Caution should be exercised when administering NON-DROWSY SINUTAB to patients with moderate to severe renal impairment.

4.3 Contraindications
NON-DROWSY SINUTAB is contraindicated in individuals with known hypersensitivity to the product or any of its components.

NON-DROWSY SINUTAB is contraindicated in patients with severe hypertension or coronary artery disease.

NON-DROWSY SINUTAB is contraindicated in patients who are taking or have taken monoamine oxidase inhibitors within the preceding two weeks. The concomitant use of pseudoephedrine and this type of product may occasionally cause a rise in blood pressure.

4.4 Special warnings and special precautions for use
Although pseudoephedrine has virtually no pressor effects in normotensive patients, NON-DROWSY SINUTAB should be used with caution in patients suffering from mild to moderate hypertension.

As with other sympathomimetic agents NON-DROWSY SINUTAB should be used with caution in patients with hypertension, heart disease, diabetes, hyperthyroidism, elevated intraocular pressure and prostatic enlargement.

Care is advised in the administration of paracetamol to patients with severe renal or severe hepatic impairment.

The hazards of overdose are greater in those with alcoholic liver disease.

The following statements will appear on packs of this product.

Do not store above 25°C. Store in the original packaging.

Warning: Do not exceed the recommended dose.

Keep out of the reach of children.

If symptoms persist consult your doctor.

Contains paracetamol.

Causes no drowsiness.

'Immediate medical advice should be sought in the event of an overdose, even if you feel well. (label).

Immediate medical advice should be sought in the event of an overdose, even if you feel well, because of the risk of delayed, serious liver damage.' (leaflet)

Do not take with any other paracetamol-containing products.'

As with all medicines, if you are pregnant or currently taking any other medicine, consult your doctor or pharmacist before taking this product.

4.5 Interaction with other medicinal products and other forms of Interaction
Concomitant use of NON-DROWSY SINUTAB with tricyclic antidepressants, sympathomimetic agents (such as decongestants, appetite suppressants and amfetamine-like psychostimulants) or with monoamine oxidase inhibitors, which interferes with the catabolism of sympathomimetic amines, may occasionally cause a rise in blood pressure, [See Contraindications].

Because of the pseudoephedrine content, NON-DROWSY SINUTAB may partially reverse the hypotensive action of drugs which interfere with sympathetic activity including bretylium, betanidine, guanethedine, debrisoquine, methyldopa, alpha- and beta-adrenergic blocking agents,[See Special warnings and precautions for use].

Patients who have taken barbiturates, tricyclic antidepressants and alcohol may show diminished ability to metabolise large doses of paracetamol, the plasma half-life of which can be prolonged. Alcohol can increase the hepatotoxicity of paracetamol overdose and may have contributed to the acute pancreatitis reported in one patient who had taken an overdose of paracetamol.

Chronic ingestion of anticonvulsants or oral steroid contraceptives induce liver enzymes and may prevent attainment of therapeutic paracetamol levels by increasing first pass metabolism or clearance.

The speed of absorption of paracetamol may be increased by metoclopramide or domperidone and absorption reduced by colestyramine.

The anticoagulant effect of warfarin and other coumarins may be enhanced by prolonged regular use of paracetamol with increased risk of bleeding; occasional doses have no significant effect.

4.6 Pregnancy and lactation

Pseudoephedrine
Although pseudoephedrine has been in widespread use for many years without apparent ill consequence, there are no specific data on its use during pregnancy.

Caution should therefore be exercised by balancing the potential benefit of treatment to the mother against any possible hazards to the developing foetus.

Systemic administration of pseudoephedrine, up to 50 times the human daily dosage in rats and up to 35 times the human daily dosage in rabbits, did not produce teratogenic effects.

Pseudoephedrine is excreted in breast milk in small amounts but the effect of this on breast-fed infants is not known. It has been estimated that 0.5 to 0.7% of a single dose of pseudoephedrine ingested by a mother will be excreted in the breast milk over 24 hours.

No studies have been conducted in animals to determine whether pseudoephedrine has the potential to impair fertility. There is no information of the effect of NON-DROWSY SINUTAB on fertility.

Paracetamol
Epidemiological studies in human pregnancy have shown no ill effects due to paracetamol used in the recommended dosage, but patients should follow the advice of their doctor regarding its use.

Paracetamol is excreted in breast milk but not in a clinically significant amount. Available published data do not contra-indicate breast feeding.

4.7 Effects on ability to drive and use machines
None known.

4.8 Undesirable effects

Pseudoephedrine
Serious side effects associated with the use of pseudoephedrine are rare. Symptoms of central nervous system excitation may occur, including sleep disturbance and, rarely, hallucinations.

Skin rashes, with or without irritation, have occasionally been reported with pseudoephedrine.

Urinary retention has been reported occasionally in men receiving pseudoephedrine: prostatic enlargement could have been an important predisposing factor.

Paracetamol
Paracetamol has been widely used and, when taken at the usual recommended dosage, side effects are mild and infrequent and reports of adverse reactions are rare. Skin rash and other allergic reactions occur rarely.

Most reports of adverse reactions to paracetamol relate to overdose with the drug.

There have been reports of blood dyscrasias including thrombocytopenia and agranulocytosis, but these were not necessarily causality related to paracetamol.

Chronic hepatic necrosis has been reported in a patient who took daily therapeutic dosages of paracetamol for about a year and liver damage has been reported after daily ingestion of excessive amounts for shorter periods. A review of a group of patients with chronic active hepatitis failed to reveal differences in the abnormalities of liver function in those who were long-term users of paracetamol nor was the control of their disease improved after paracetamol withdrawal.

Nephrotoxic effects following therapeutic dosages of paracetamol are uncommon. Papillary necrosis has been reported after prolonged administration.

4.9 Overdose

Pseudoephedrine
As with other sympathomimetic agents, symptoms and signs of pseudoephedrine overdose include irritability, restlessness, tremor, convulsions, palpitations, hypertension and difficulty with micturition.

Measures should be taken to maintain and support respiration and control convulsions. Gastric lavage should be performed if indicated. Catheterisation of the bladder may be necessary. If desired, the elimination of pseudoephedrine can be accelerated by acid diuresis or by dialysis.

Paracetamol
Symptoms of paracetamol overdose in the first 24 hours are pallor, nausea, vomiting, anorexia and abdominal pain. Liver damage may become apparent 12 to 48 hours after ingestion. Abnormalities of glucose metabolism and metabolic acidosis may occur. In severe poisoning, hepatic failure may progress to encephalopathy, coma and death. Acute renal failure with acute tubular necrosis may develop even in the absence of severe liver damage. Cardiac arrhythmias and pancreatitis have been reported.

Liver damage is likely in adults who have taken 10 g or more of paracetamol. It is considered that excess quantities of a toxic metabolite (usually adequately detoxified by glutathione when normal doses of paracetamol are ingested), become irreversibly bound to liver tissue.

Immediate treatment is essential in the management of paracetamol overdose. Despite a lack of significant early symptoms, patients should be referred to hospital urgently for immediate medical attention and any patient who had ingested around 7.5 g or more of paracetamol in the preceding 4 hours should undergo gastric lavage. Administration of oral methionine or intravenous N-acetylcysteine which may have a beneficial effect up to at least 48 hours after the overdose, may be required. General supportive measures must be available.

5. PHARMACOLOGICAL PROPERTIES

5.1 Pharmacodynamic properties

Pseudoephedrine
Pseudoephedrine has direct and indirect sympathomimetic activity and is an effective upper respiratory tract decongestant. Pseudoephedrine is substantially less potent than ephedrine in producing both tachycardia and elevation of systolic blood pressure and considerably less potent in causing stimulation of the central nervous system.

Paracetamol
Paracetamol has analgesic and antipyretic actions but only weak anti-inflammatory properties. This may be explained by presence of cellular peroxides at sites of inflammation which prevent inhibition of cyclo-oxygenase by paracetamol. At other sites associated with low levels of cellular perioxides, e.g. pain, fever, paracetamol can successfully inhibit prostaglandin biosynthesis.

5.2 Pharmacokinetic properties

Pseudoephedrine
Pseudoephedrine is partly metabolised in the liver by N-demethylation to norpseudoephedrine, an active metabolite. Pseudoephedrine and its metabolite are excreted in the urine: 55% to 75% of a dose is excreted unchanged. The rate of urinary excretion of pseudoephedrine is accelerated when the urine is acidified. Conversely as the urine pH increases, the rate of urinary excretion is slowed.

Paracetamol
Peak plasma paracetamol concentration usually occurs between 30 and 90 minutes after oral ingestion. Paracetamol is distributed uniformly throughout most body fluids and is only 15 to 25 per cent bound to plasma proteins. The plasma half life of paracetamol after therapeutic doses is in the range of 1 to 3 hours.

5.3 Preclinical safety data

The active ingredients of NON-DROWSY SINUTAB are well known constituents of medicinal products and their safety profile is well documented. The results of pre-clinical studies do not add anything of relevance for therapeutic purposes.

6. PHARMACEUTICAL PARTICULARS

6.1 List of excipients

(contained in Compressible Paracetamol 90%)

Pregelatinised Maize Starch

Crospovidone

Povidone K30

Stearic Acid

Other ingredients

Microcrystalline Cellulose

Sodium Starch Glycollate

Magnesium Stearate

6.2 Incompatibilities

None known

6.3 Shelf life

24 months

6.4 Special precautions for storage

Do not store above 25°C. Store in the original packaging.

6.5 Nature and contents of container

Carton containing 4, 12, 15, 24 or 30 tablets.

Each blister strip consists of a white, opaque PVC/PVdC film and either:

Aluminium foil blister lidding

Or

Paper/aluminium foil child resistant blister lidding

6.6 Instructions for use and handling

None applicable.

7. MARKETING AUTHORISATION HOLDER

Pfizer Consumer Healthcare

Alternative Trading Style:

Warner-Lambert Consumer Healthcare

Walton Oaks

Dorking Road

Walton-on-the-Hill

Surrey KT20 7NS

United Kingdom

8. MARKETING AUTHORISATION NUMBER(S)

PL 15513/0027

9. DATE OF FIRST AUTHORISATION/RENEWAL OF THE AUTHORISATION

28/3/97

10. DATE OF REVISION OF THE TEXT

December 2004

* Sudafed Sinus is an alternative name for this product. Please read Sudafed Sinus as an alternative where Non-Drowsy Sinutab appears.

Non-Drowsy Sudafed 12 Hour Relief

(Pfizer Consumer Healthcare)

1. NAME OF THE MEDICINAL PRODUCT

Non-Drowsy SUDAFED 12 Hour Relief

2. QUALITATIVE AND QUANTITATIVE COMPOSITION

Non-Drowsy SUDAFED 12 Hour Relief tablets each contain 120 mg pseudoephedrine hydrochloride in a modified-release formulation.

3. PHARMACEUTICAL FORM

Modified-release tablet.

4. CLINICAL PARTICULARS

4.1 Therapeutic indications

Non-Drowsy SUDAFED 12 Hour Relief tablets are indicated for the symptomatic relief of conditions such as allergic rhinitis, vasomotor rhinitis, the common cold and influenza.

4.2 Posology and method of administration

Posology

Adults and children 12 years and over:

Oral: One tablet (120 mg pseudoephedrine hydrochloride) every 12 hours.

Maximum daily dose: 2 tablets (240 mg pseudoephedrine hydrochloride).

Non-Drowsy SUDAFED 12 Hour Relief tablets should be swallowed whole without chewing.

Children under 12 years:

Non-Drowsy SUDAFED 12 Hour Relief tablets are not suitable for administration to children under 12 years of age.

The Elderly:

Normal adult dosage is appropriate (See Pharamacokinetics in Elderly).

Hepatic Dysfunction:

Experience with the use of the product suggests that normal adult dosage is appropriate, although it may be prudent to exercise caution in the presence of severe hepatic impairment (See Pharmacokinetics).

Renal Dysfunction:

Caution should be exercised when administering Non-Drowsy SUDAFED 12 Hour Relief tablets to patients with moderate to severe renal impairment, particularly if accompanied by cardiovascular disease (See Pharmacokinetics in Renal Impairment).

4.3 Contraindications

Non-Drowsy SUDAFED 12 Hour Relief tablets are contraindicated in individuals with known hypersensitivity to the product or any of its components.

Non-Drowsy SUDAFED 12 Hour Relief tablets are contraindicated in patients with severe hypertension or severe coronary artery disease.

Non-Drowsy SUDAFED 12 Hour Relief tablets are contraindicated in patients who are taking, or have taken, monoamine oxidase inhibitors and the antibacterial agent furazolidone within the preceding two weeks.

4.4 Special warnings and special precautions for use

Although pseudoephedrine has virtually no pressor effects in normotensive patients Non-Drowsy SUDAFED 12 Hour Relief tablets should be used with caution in patients suffering from mild to moderate hypertension.

As with other sympathomimetic agents, Non-Drowsy SUDAFED 12 Hour Relief tablets should be used with caution in patients with heart disease, diabetes, hyperthyroidism, elevated intra-ocular pressure or prostatic enlargement.

Caution should be exercised when using the product in the presence of severe hepatic impairment or moderate to severe renal impairment (particularly if accompanied by cardiovascular disease (See Pharmacokinetics).

4.5 Interaction with other medicinal products and other forms of Interaction

Concomitant use of Non-Drowsy SUDAFED 12 Hour Relief tablets with other pseudoephedrine-containing products, tricyclic antidepressants, monoamine oxidase inhibitors and furazolidone, which interfere with the catabolism of sympathomimetics amines, may occasionally cause a rise in blood pressure.

A rise in blood pressure may also occur with the concomitant use of other sympathomimetic agents such as decongestants, appetite suppressants and amfetamine-like psychostimulants.

Because of their pseudoephedrine content, Non-Drowsy SUDAFED 12 Hour Relief tablets may partially reverse the hypotensive action of drugs which interfere with sympathetic activity including bretylium, betanidine, guanethidine, debrisoquine, methyldopa, alpha- and beta-adrenergic blocking agents (See Special Warnings and Precautions for Use).

4.6 Pregnancy and lactation

Insufficient information is available on the effects of administration of Non-Drowsy SUDAFED 12 Hour Relief tablets during human pregnancy.

Pseudoephedrine is excreted in breast milk in small amounts but the effect of this on breast-fed infants is not known. It has been estimated that approximately 0.4 to 0.7% of a single 60 mg (non-controlled release) dose of pseudoephedrine ingested by a nursing mother will be excreted in the breast milk over 24 hours.

Non-Drowsy SUDAFED 12 Hour Relief tablets, like most medicines, should not be used during pregnancy and lactation unless the potential benefit of treatment to the mother outweighs any possible risk.

4.7 Effects on ability to drive and use machines

No special comment.

4.8 Undesirable effects

Serious adverse effects associated with the use of pseudoephedrine are extremely rare. Symptoms of central nervous system excitation may occur including sleep disturbance and, rarely, hallucinations.

Skin rashes, with or without irritation, have occasionally been reported with pseudoephedrine.

Urinary retention has been reported occasionally in men receiving pseudoephedrine; prostatic enlargement could have been an important predisposing factor.

4.9 Overdose

Symptoms and Signs

As with other sympathomimetic-containing products, symptoms and signs of overdose may include irritability, restlessness, tremor, convulsions, palpitations, hypertension and difficulty with micturition.

Treatment

Necessary measures should be taken to maintain and support respiration and control convulsions. Gastric lavage may be undertaken if indicated. Catheterisation of the bladder may be necessary. Acid diuresis can accelerate the elimination of pseudoephedrine although the potential therapeutic gain of this procedure is now in dispute. The value of dialysis in overdose is not known, although four hours of haemodialysis removed approximately 20% of the total body load of pseudoephedrine in an instant-release combination product containing 60 mg pseudoephedrine and 8 mg acrivastine.

5. PHARMACOLOGICAL PROPERTIES

5.1 Pharmacodynamic properties

Pseudoephedrine has direct and indirect sympathomimetic activity and is an effective upper respiratory decongestant. Pseudoephedrine is less potent than ephedrine in producing both tachycardia and elevation of systolic blood pressure and is also less potent in causing stimulation of the central nervous system.

Pseudoephedrine in a bioequivalent controlled-release formulation has been shown to produce its decongestant effect within 1 hour of dosing, persisting for up to 12 hours.

5.2 Pharmacokinetic properties

Bioequivalence between Non-Drowsy SUDAFED 12 Hour Relief tablets and instant release Sudafed Elixir has been demonstrated.

Absorption

After the administration of one tablet of Non-Drowsy SUDAFED 12 Hour Relief (containing 120 mg pseudoephedrine) to healthy adult volunteers, the C_{max} for pseudoephedrine was approximately 293 ng/ml irrespective of whether the tablet was taken with or without food. The t_{max} occurred at about 5.5 hours when the tablet was taken by fasting subjects or at approximately 5.9 hours when taken with food.

At steady state, following multiple dosing for Non-Drowsy SUDAFED 12 Hour Relief tablets, the C_{max} and C_{min} for pseudoephedrine have been estimated to be 459 ng/ml and 243 ng/ml respectively.

Distribution

The volume of distribution for Non-Drowsy SUDAFED 12 Hour Relief tablets has not been identified. However, the apparent volume of distribution of immediate-release pseudoephedrine (Vd/F) is approximately 2.8 1/kg.

Metabolism and Elimination

Pseudoephedrine is partly metabolised in the liver by N-demethylation to norpseudoephedrine, an active metabolite. Pseudoephedrine and its metabolite are excreted in the urine; 55% to 90% of a dose is excreted unchanged.

Following administration of 1 tablet of Non-Drowsy SUDAFED 12 Hour Relief to fasted healthy volunteers, the elimination t½ was approximately 6.3 hours, or 5.78 hours when taken with food. The rate of urinary excretion is accelerated when the urine is acidified. Conversely, as the urine pH increases, the rate of urinary elimination is slowed.

Pharamacokinetics in Renal Impairment

There have been no specific studies of Non-Drowsy SUDAFED 12 Hour Relief in renal impairment.

Following the administration of a single dose on instant-release DUACT capsules (8 mg acrivastine + 60 mg pseudoephedrine) to patients with varying degrees of renal impairment, the C_{max} for pseudoephedrine increased approximately 1.5 fold in patients with moderate to severe renal impairment when compared to the C_{max} in healthy volunteers. The t_{max} was not affected by renal impairment. The t½ increased 3 -12 fold in patients with mild to severe renal impairment respectively, when compared to the t½ in healthy volunteers.

Pharmacokinetics in Hepatic Impairment

There have been no specific studies of Non-Drowsy SUDAFED 12 Hour Relief or pseudoephedrine in hepatic impairment.

Pharamcokinetics in the Elderly

There have been no specific studies of Non-Drowsy SUDAFED 12 Hour Relief in the elderly. In elderly volunteers, following the administration of instant-release DUACT capsules (8 mg acrivastine + 60 mg pseudoephedrine), the t½ for pseudoephedrine was 1.4 - fold that seen in healthy volunteers. The apparent C1/F was 0.8 - fold that seen in healthy volunteers, and the Vd/F was essentially unchanged.

5.3 Preclinical safety data

Mutagenicity

The results of a wide range of tests indicate that pseudoephedrine does not pose a mutagenic risk to man.

Carcinogenicity

There is insufficient information available to determine whether pseudoephedrine has carcinogenic potential.

Teratogenicity

Systemic administration of pseudoephedrine up to 50 times the human daily dosage in rats and up to 35 times the human daily dosage in rabbits did not produce teratogenic effects.

Fertility

Systemic administration of pseudoephedrine to rats, up to 7 times the human daily dosage in females and 35 times the human daily dosage in males, did not impair fertility or alter foetal morphological development and survival.

There is insufficient information relating to the effect of SUDAFED 12 hour tablets on human fertility.

6. PHARMACEUTICAL PARTICULARS

6.1 List of excipients

Hydroxypropyl Methylcellulose

Magnesium Stearate

Microcrystalline Cellulose

Povidone

Titanium Dioxide

Polyethylene Glycol

Candelilla Wax

Purified Water

6.2 Incompatibilities

None known

6.3 Shelf life

3 years

6.4 Special precautions for storage

Do not store above 25°C. Keep dry. Protect from light.

6.5 Nature and contents of container

6, 10, 12, 20 or 24 tablets presented in a PVC or PVC/PVdC blister card backed with aluminium foil.

6.6 Instructions for use and handling

Not applicable

Administrative Data

7. MARKETING AUTHORISATION HOLDER

Pfizer Consumer Healthcare

Alternative trading style:

Warner-Lambert Consumer Healthcare

Walton Oaks

Dorking Road

Walton-on-the-Hill

Surrey KT20 7NS

United Kingdom

8. MARKETING AUTHORISATION NUMBER(S)

PL 15513/0034

9. DATE OF FIRST AUTHORISATION/RENEWAL OF THE AUTHORISATION

31 October 2001

10. DATE OF REVISION OF THE TEXT

March 2004

Non-Drowsy Sudafed Congestion, Cold & Flu Tablets

(Pfizer Consumer Healthcare)

1. NAME OF THE MEDICINAL PRODUCT

Non-Drowsy Sudafed Congestion, Cold & Flu Tablets

2. QUALITATIVE AND QUANTITATIVE COMPOSITION

Non-Drowsy Sudafed Congestion, Cold & Flu Tablets contain 60 mg Pseudoephedrine hydrochloride and 500 mg Paracetamol.

3. PHARMACEUTICAL FORM

Tablets

4. CLINICAL PARTICULARS

4.1 Therapeutic indications

Non-Drowsy Sudafed Congestion, Cold & Flu Tablets is indicated for the symptomatic relief of conditions where congestion of the mucous membranes of the upper respiratory tract, is accompanied by pain or pyrexia, e.g. the common cold and influenza, sinusitis, nasopharyngitis.

4.2 Posology and method of administration

Adults and children 12 years and over:

Oral. One tablet every 4-6 hours up to four times a day

Maximum daily dose: 4 tablets (240 mg pseudoephedrine and 2 g paracetamol).

Children aged 6 to 12 years:

Oral. Half a tablet every 4-6 hours up to four times a day.

Maximum daily dose: 2 tablets (120 mg pseudoephedrine and 1 g paracetamol).

Children under 6 years:

Non-Drowsy Sudafed Congestion, Cold & Flu Tablets is not suitable for administration to children under 6 years of age.

The Elderly:

There have been no specific studies of Non-Drowsy Sudafed Congestion, Cold & Flu Tablets in the elderly. Experience has shown that normal adult dosage is appropriate.

In the elderly the rate and extent of paracetamol absorption is normal but plasma half-life is longer and paracetamol clearance is lower than in young adults.

Hepatic dysfunction:

Caution should be exercised when administering Non-Drowsy Sudafed Congestion, Cold & Flu Tablets to patients with severe hepatic impairment (See Pharmacokinetics in Hepatic Impairment).

Renal dysfunction:

Caution should be exercised when administering Non-Drowsy Sudafed Congestion, Cold & Flu Tablets to patients with moderate to severe renal impairment, particularly if accompanied by cardiovascular disease (See Pharmacokinetics in Renal Impairment).

4.3 Contraindications

Non-Drowsy Sudafed Congestion, Cold & Flu Tablets is contraindicated in individuals with known hypersensitivity to paracetamol or any other constituents of the product.

Non-Drowsy Sudafed Congestion, Cold & Flu Tablets is contraindicated in patients with severe hypertension or coronary artery disease.

Non-Drowsy Sudafed Congestion, Cold & Flu Tablets is contraindicated in patients who are taking or have taken monoamine oxidase inhibitors within the preceding two weeks. The concomitant use of pseudoephedrine and this type of product may occasionally cause a rise in blood pressure.

4.4 Special warnings and special precautions for use

Although pseudoephedrine has virtually no pressor effects in normotensive patients, Non-Drowsy Sudafed Congestion, Cold & Flu Tablets should be used with caution in patients suffering from mild to moderate hypertension.

As with other sympathomimetic agents Non-Drowsy Sudafed Congestion, Cold & Flu Tablets should be used with caution in patients with heart disease, diabetes, hyperthyroidism, elevated intraocular pressure or prostatic enlargement.

Caution should be exercised in the administration of Non-Drowsy Sudafed Congestion, Cold & Flu Tablets to patients with severe hepatic impairment or moderate to severe renal impairment, (particularly if accompanied by cardiovascular disease) (See Pharmacokinetics). The hazards of overdose are greater in those with non-cirrhotic alcoholic liver disease.

Concomitant use of other products containing paracetamol or decongestants with Non-Drowsy Sudafed Congestion, Cold & Flu Tablets could lead to overdose and therefore should be avoided.

The following statements will appear on packs of this product:

Keep out of the reach and sight of children.

As with all medicines, if you are pregnant or currently taking any other medicine, consult your doctor or pharmacist before taking this product.

If symptoms persist consult your doctor.

Store below 25°C. Keep dry. Protect from light.

Warning: Do not exceed the stated dose.

Causes no drowsiness.

Contains paracetamol.

The label contains the following additional statements:

Immediate medical advice should be sought in the event of an overdose, even if you feel well.

Do not take with any other paracetamol-containing products.

Immediate medical advice should be sought in the event of an overdose, even if you feel well, because of the risk of delayed, serious liver damage (leaflet).

4.5 Interaction with other medicinal products and other forms of Interaction

Concomitant use of Non-Drowsy Sudafed Congestion, Cold & Flu Tablets with tricyclic antidepressants, sympathomimetic agents (such as decongestants, appetite suppressants and amfetamine-like psychostimulants) or with monoamine oxidase inhibitors, which interfere with the catabolism of sympathomimetic amines, may occasionally cause a rise in blood pressure (See Contraindications).

Because of the pseudoephedrine content, Non-Drowsy Sudafed Congestion, Cold & Flu Tablets may partially reverse the hypotensive action of drugs which interfere with sympathetic activity including bretylium, betanidine, guanethidine, debrisoquine, methyldopa, alpha- and beta-adrenergic blocking agents (See Special warnings and precautions for use).

The use of drugs which induce hepatic microsomal enzymes, such as anticonvulsants and oral contraceptive steroids, may increase the extent of metabolism of paracetamol, resulting in reduced plasma concentrations of the drug and a faster elimination rate.

The speed of absorption of paracetamol may be increased by metoclopramide or domperidone and absorption reduced by colestyramine.

The anticoagulant effect of warfarin and other coumarins may be enhanced by prolonged regular use of paracetamol with increased risk of bleeding; occasional doses have no significant effect.

4.6 Pregnancy and lactation

Non-Drowsy Sudafed Congestion, Cold & Flu Tablets, like most medicines, should not be used during pregnancy unless the potential benefit of treatment to the mother outweighs any possible risk to the developing foetus.

Pseudoephedrine and paracetamol have been in widespread use for many years without apparent ill consequence. Epidemiological studies in human pregnancy have shown no ill effects due to paracetamol used in the recommended dosage, but patients should follow the advice of their doctor regarding its use. The safety of pseudoephedrine during pregnancy has not been directly established.

Pseudoephedrine is excreted in breast milk in small amounts but the effect of this on breast-fed infants is not known. It has been estimated that approximately 0.4 to 0.7% of a single 60 mg dose of pseudoephedrine ingested by a nursing mother will be excreted in the breast milk over 24 hours.

Paracetamol is excreted in breast milk but not in a clinically significant amount. Available published data do not contra-indicate breast feeding. A pharmacokinetic study of paracetamol in 12 nursing mothers revealed that less than 1% of a 650 mg oral dose of paracetamol appeared in the breast milk. Similar findings have been reported in other studies, therefore maternal ingestion of therapeutic doses of paracetamol does not appear to present a risk to the neonate/infant.

4.7 Effects on ability to drive and use machines

No special comment - unlikely to produce an effect.

4.8 Undesirable effects

Pseudoephedrine

Serious side effects associated with the use of pseudoephedrine are extremely rare. Symptoms of central nervous system excitation may occur, including sleep disturbance and, rarely, hallucinations.

Skin rashes, with or without irritation, have occasionally been reported with pseudoephedrine.

Urinary retention has been reported occasionally in men receiving pseudoephedrine: prostatic enlargement could have been an important predisposing factor.

Paracetamol

Adverse effects of paracetamol are rare but hypersensitivity including skin rash may occur. There have been reports of blood dyscrasias including thrombocytopenia and agranulocytosis, but these were not necessarily causality related to paracetamol.

4.9 Overdose

Pseudoephedrine

Symptoms

As with other sympathomimetic agents, symptoms and signs of pseudoephedrine overdose include irritability, restlessness, tremor, convulsions, palpitations, hypertension and difficulty with micturition.

Management

Necessary measures should be taken to maintain and support respiration and control convulsions. Gastric lavage should be performed if indicated. Catheterisation of the bladder may be necessary. Acid diuresis can accelerate the elimination of pseudoephedrine, although the potential therapeutic gain of this procedure is now in dispute. The value of dialysis in overdose is not known, although four hours of haemodialysis removed approximately 20 % of the total body load of pseudoephedrine in a combination product containing 60 mg pseudoephedrine and 8 mg acrivastine.

Paracetamol

Liver damage is possible in adults who have taken 10g or more of paracetamol. Ingestion of 5g or more of paracetamol may lead to liver damage if the patient has risk factors (see below).

Risk Factors:

If the patient:

Is on long term treatment with carbamazepine, phenobarbital, phenytoin, primidone, rifampicin, St John's Wort or other drugs that induce liver enzymes.

Or

Regularly consumes ethanol in excess of recommended amounts.

Or

Is likely to be glutathione deplete e.g. eating disorders, cystic fibrosis, HIV infection, starvation, cachexia.

Symptoms:

Symptoms of paracetamol overdosage in the first 24 hours are pallor, nausea, vomiting, anorexia and abdominal pain. Liver damage may become apparent 12 to 48 hours after ingestion. Abnormalities of glucose metabolism and metabolic acidosis may occur. In severe poisoning, hepatic failure may progress to encephalopathy, haemorrhage, hypoglycaemia, cerebral oedema, and death. Acute renal failure with acute tubular necrosis, strongly suggested by loin pain, haematuria and proteinuria, may develop even in the absence of severe liver damage. Cardiac arrhythmias and pancreatitis have been reported.

Management:

Immediate treatment is essential in the management of paracetamol overdose. Despite a lack of significant early symptoms, patients should be referred to hospital urgently for immediate medical attention. Symptoms may be limited to nausea or vomiting and may not reflect the severity of overdose or the risk of organ damage. Management should be in accordance with established treatment guidelines, see BNF overdose section.

Treatment with activated charcoal should be considered if the overdose has been taken within 1 hour. Plasma paracetamol concentration should be measured at 4 hours or later after ingestion (earlier concentrations unreliable). Treatment with N-acetylcysteine may be used up to 24 hours after ingestion of paracetamol, however the maximum protective effect is obtained up to 8 hours post-ingestion. The effectiveness of the antidote declines sharply after this time. If required the patient should be given intravenous N-acetylcysteine, in line with the established dosage schedule. If vomiting is not a problem, oral methionine may be a suitable alternative for remote areas, outside hospital. Management of patients who present with serious hepatic dysfunction beyond 24h from ingestion should be discussed with the NPIS or a liver unit.

5. PHARMACOLOGICAL PROPERTIES

5.1 Pharmacodynamic properties

Paracetamol:

Paracetamol is an analgesic and antipyretic. The therapeutic effects of paracetamol are thought to be related to inhibition of prostaglandin synthesis, as a result of inhibition of cyclo-oxygenase. There is some evidence that it is a more effective inhibitor of central as opposed to peripheral cyclo-oxygenase. Paracetamol has only weak anti-inflammatory properties. This may be explained by the concept that inflammatory tissues have higher levels of cellular peroxides than other tissues and that cellular peroxides prevent inhibition of cyclo-oxygenase by paracetamol.

Pseudoephedrine

Pseudoephedrine has direct and indirect sympathomimetic activity and is an effective upper respiratory decongestant. Pseudoephedrine is less potent than ephedrine in producing both tachycardia and elevation of systolic blood pressure and is also less potent in causing stimulation of the central nervous system. Pseudoephedrine produces its decongestant effect within 30 minutes persisting for at least 4 hours.

5.2 Pharmacokinetic properties

Absorption:

Paracetamol

Absorption of paracetamol occurs mainly by passive transfer from the small intestine. Gastric emptying is the rate-limiting step in the absorption of orally administered paracetamol. Any drug, disease or other condition, which alters the rate of gastric emptying, will therefore influence the rate of paracetamol absorption.

Peak plasma paracetamol concentration usually occurs between 30 and 90 minutes after oral ingestion, depending on the formulation. Mean maximum plasma concentrations of paracetamol of 12.84 ug/ml were determined following the administration of Calpol Six Plus suspension (containing 1g paracetamol) to adults.

Paracetamol is incompletely available to the systemic circulation after oral administration since a variable proportion is lost through first-pass metabolism. Oral bioavailability in adults appears to depend on the amount of paracetamol administered, increasing from 63% of the administered dose after 500mg to nearly 90% of the dose after 1 or 2 g (in tablet form).

Pseudoephedrine

Pseudoephedrine is well absorbed from the gut following oral administration. After the administration of one 60 mg pseudoephedrine tablet to healthy adult volunteers, the Cmax for pseudoephedrine was approximately 180 ng/ml, with tmax occurring at approximately 1.5-2.0 hours.

Distribution:

Paracetamol

Paracetamol is distributed uniformly throughout most body fluids, with an estimated volume of distribution of 0.95 l/kg. Following therapeutic doses, paracetamol is not appreciably bound to plasma proteins.

Pseudoephedrine

The apparent volume of distribution of pseudoephedrine (Vd/F) was approximately 2.8 l/kg.

Metabolism and elimination:

Paracetamol

The plasma half-life of paracetamol after therapeutic doses is in the range 1.5-2.5 hours. Paracetamol is metabolised by the liver and several metabolites of paracetamol have been identified in man. The two major metabolites excreted in the urine are the glucuronide and sulphate conjugates. About 10 % of administered paracetamol is converted, via a minor pathway, by a cytochrome P-450 mixed function oxidase system to a reactive metabolite, acetamidoquinone. This metabolite is rapidly conjugated with reduced glutathione and excreted as cysteine and mercapturic acid conjugates. When large amounts of paracetamol are taken, hepatic glutathione may become depleted causing excessive accumulation within the hepatocyte of acetamidoquinone, which binds covalently to vital hepatocellular macromolecules. In overdose, this can lead to hepatic necrosis. Total body clearance of paracetamol following a single dose (1000 mg i.v) is approximately 5 ml/min/kg.

Renal excretion of paracetamol involves glomerular filtration and passive reabsorption, and the sulphate and glucuronide conjugates are subject to active renal tubular secretion. Renal clearance of paracetamol depends on urine flow rate, but not pH.

Less than 4 % of the administered drug is excreted as unchanged paracetamol. In healthy subjects, approximately 85-95% of a therapeutic dose is excreted in the urine within 24 hours.

Pseudoephedrine

The plasma t½ was approximately 5.5 hours. Pseudoephedrine is partly metabolised in the liver by N demethylation to norpseudoephedrine, an active metabolite. Pseudoephedrine and its metabolite are excreted in the urine; 55% to 90% of a dose is excreted unchanged. The apparent total body clearance of pseudoephedrine (Cl/F) was 6 - 6.5 ml/min/kg. The elimination rate constant (Kel) was approximately 0.13 hr-1. The rate of urinary elimination is accelerated when the urine is acidified. Conversely, as the urine pH increases, the rate of urinary elimination is slowed.

Pharmacokinetics in Renal Impairment:

Paracetamol

The mean plasma half-life of paracetamol is similar in normal and renally impaired subjects between 2-8hrs, but from 8-24hrs paracetamol is eliminated less rapidly. Marked accumulation of the glucuronide and sulphate conjugates occurs in chronic renal failure.

There may be some extra renal elimination of retained paracetamol conjugates in patients with chronic renal failure, with limited regeneration of the parent compound. An increase in the interval between doses of paracetamol has been recommended for adults with chronic renal failure. Haemodialysis may result in reduced plasma levels of paracetamol. Supplementary doses of paracetamol may be necessary in order to maintain therapeutic blood levels.

Pseudoephedrine

Following the administration of a single dose of Duact Capsules (60 mg pseudoephedrine + 8 mg acrivastine) to patients with varying degrees of renal impairment, the Cmax for pseudoephedrine increased approximately 1.5 fold in patients with moderate to severe renal impairment when compared to the Cmax in healthy volunteers. The tmax was not affected by renal impairment. The t½ increased 3 -12 fold in patients with mild to severe renal impairment respectively, when compared to the t½ in healthy volunteers.

Pharmacokinetics in Hepatic Impairment:

Paracetamol

The mean plasma paracetamol half-life is similar in normal subjects and those with mild liver disease, but is significantly prolonged (approximately 75%) in patients with severe liver disease. However, the clinical significance of the increase in half-life is unclear, since there is no evidence of drug accumulation or hepatotoxicity in patients with liver disease, and glutathione conjugation is not impaired. The administration of 4g paracetamol daily for 13 days to 20 subjects with chronic stable liver disease, resulted in no deterioration of liver function, and in mild liver disease, there is no evidence that paracetamol is harmful when taken at recommended doses. However, in severe liver disease, the plasma paracetamol half-life is significantly prolonged.

Pseudoephedrine

There have been no specific studies of pseudoephedrine in hepatic impairment.

Pharmacokinetics in the Elderly:

Paracetamol

Differences in pharmacokinetic parameters observed between fit young and fit elderly subjects are not thought to be of clinical significance. However, there is some evidence to suggest that serum paracetamol half-life is markedly increased (by approximately 84%) and clearance of paracetamol is decreased (by approximately 47%) in frail, immobile, elderly subjects when compared to fit young subjects.

Pseudoephedrine

In elderly volunteers, following the administration of Duact Capsules (60 mg pseudoephedrine + 8 mg acrivastine) the t½ for pseudoephedrine was 1.4 fold that seen in healthy volunteers. The apparent Cl/F was 0.8 fold that seen in healthy volunteers, and the Vd/F was essentially unchanged.

5.3 Preclinical safety data

Mutagenicity:

Paracetamol

In vivo mutagenicity tests of paracetamol in mammals are limited and show conflicting results. Therefore, there is insufficient information to determine whether paracetamol poses a mutagenic risk to man.

Paracetamol has been found to be non-mutagenic in bacterial mutagenicity assays, although a clear clastogenic effect has been observed in mammalian cells in vitro following exposure to paracetamol (3 and 10 mM for 2 hr).

Pseudoephedrine

The results of a wide range of tests indicate that pseudoephedrine does not pose a mutagenic risk to man.

Carcinogenicity:

Paracetamol

There is inadequate evidence to determine the carcinogenic potential of paracetamol in humans. A positive association between the use of paracetamol and cancer of the urethra (but not of other sites in the urinary tract) was observed in a case-control study in which approximate lifetime consumption of paracetamol (whether acute or chronic) was estimated. However, other similar studies have failed to demonstrate a statistically significant association between paracetamol and cancer of the urinary tract, or paracetamol and renal cell carcinoma.

There is limited evidence for the carcinogenicity of paracetamol in experimental animals. Liver cell tumours can be detected in mice and liver and bladder carcinomas can be detected in rats, following chronic feeding of 500mg/kg/day paracetamol.

Pseudoephedrine

There is insufficient information available to determine whether pseudoephedrine has carcinogenic potential.

Teratogenicity:

Paracetamol

There is no information relating to the teratogenic potential of paracetamol. In humans, paracetamol crosses the placenta and attains concentrations in the foetal circulation similar to those in the maternal circulation. Intermittent maternal ingestion of therapeutic doses of paracetamol is not associated with teratogenic effects in humans.

Paracetamol has been found to be fetotoxic to cultured rat embryos.

Pseudoephedrine

Systemic administration of pseudoephedrine, up to 50 times the human daily dosage in rats and up to 35 times the human daily dosage in rabbits did not produce teratogenic effects.

Fertility:

Paracetamol

There is no information relating to the effects of paracetamol on human fertility. A significant decrease in testicular weight was observed when male Sprague-Dawley rats were given daily high doses of paracetamol (500 mg/kg body weight/day) orally for 70 days.

Pseudoephedrine

Systemic administration of pseudoephedrine to rats, up to 7 times the human daily dosage in females and 35 times the human daily dosage in males, did not impair fertility or alter foetal morphological development and survival.

6. PHARMACEUTICAL PARTICULARS

6.1 List of excipients

Pregelatinised maize starch

Povidone

Crospovidone

Stearic acid

Microcrystalline cellulose

Croscarmellose sodium

Magnesium stearate

6.2 Incompatibilities

None known.

6.3 Shelf life

36 months.

6.4 Special precautions for storage

Store below 25°C. Keep dry and protect from light

6.5 Nature and contents of container

Amber glass bottles with polyethylene snap-fit closures (100 tablets).

or

Blister packs (12 and 24 tablets) consisting of a white, opaque PVC/PVdC film and either:

Aluminium foil blister lidding

Or

Paper/aluminium foil child resistant blister lidding

6.6 Instructions for use and handling

None applicable.

Administrative Data

7. MARKETING AUTHORISATION HOLDER

Pfizer Consumer Healthcare

Alternative trading style:

Warner-Lambert Consumer Healthcare

Walton Oaks

Dorking Road

Walton-on-the-Hill

Surrey

KT20 7NS

United Kingdom

8. MARKETING AUTHORISATION NUMBER(S)

PL 15513/0025

9. DATE OF FIRST AUTHORISATION/RENEWAL OF THE AUTHORISATION

28th October 1997

10. DATE OF REVISION OF THE TEXT

April 2005

Non-Drowsy Sudafed Decongestant Nasal Spray

(Pfizer Consumer Healthcare)

1. NAME OF THE MEDICINAL PRODUCT
Non-Drowsy Sudafed Decongestant Nasal Spray

2. QUALITATIVE AND QUANTITATIVE COMPOSITION
Non-Drowsy Sudafed Decongestant Nasal Spray is an aqueous solution of Xylometazoline Hydrochloride 0.1% w/v presented in a metered-dose pack, delivering 0.14 ml per actuation.

For excipients see 6.1.

3. PHARMACEUTICAL FORM
Aqueous solution

4. CLINICAL PARTICULARS
4.1 Therapeutic indications
Non-Drowsy Sudafed Decongestant Nasal Spray is indicated for the symptomatic relief of nasal congestion associated with the common cold, influenza, sinusitis, allergic and non-allergic rhinitis, and other upper respiratory tract allergies.

4.2 Posology and method of administration
Adults and children 12 years and over:

Nasal. One spray to be expressed into each nostril 2-3 times daily, as necessary.

Maximum daily dose: 3 sprays.

Use for more than seven consecutive days is not recommended, [See Undesirable effects].

Children under 12 years:

Non-Drowsy Sudafed Decongestant Nasal Spray is not recommended for children under 12 years of age.

The Elderly

Experience has indicated that normal adult dosage is appropriate, [See Pharmacokinetics in the elderly].

Hepatic/renal dysfunction

Normal adult dosage is appropriate, [See Pharmacokinetic properties].

4.3 Contraindications
Non-Drowsy Sudafed Decongestant Nasal Spray is contraindicated in individuals with known hypersensitivity to the product or any of its constituents.

Non-Drowsy Sudafed Decongestant Nasal Spray is contraindicated in individuals who are taking or have taken, monoamine oxidase inhibitors within the preceding two weeks.

Non-Drowsy Sudafed Decongestant Nasal Spray is contraindicated in individuals with hypophysectomy or surgery exposing dura mater.

4.4 Special warnings and special precautions for use
There is minimal systemic absorption with topically applied imidazoline sympathomimetics such as xylometazoline, however, Non-Drowsy Sudafed Decongestant Nasal Spray should be used with caution in patients suffering coronary artery disease, hypertension, hyperthyroidism or diabetes mellitus.

4.5 Interaction with other medicinal products and other forms of Interaction
Due to the low systemic absorption of xylometazoline when administered intra-nasally, interaction with drugs administered via other routes is considered unlikely.

4.6 Pregnancy and lactation
No foetal toxicity or fertility studies have been carried out in animals. In view of its potential vasoconstrictor effect, it is advisable to take the precaution of not using Non-Drowsy Sudafed Decongestant Nasal Spray during pregnancy.

4.7 Effects on ability to drive and use machines
No special comment - unlikely to produce an effect.

4.8 Undesirable effects
Xylometazoline nasal preparations are generally well tolerated following short-term use and local side effects are mild and infrequent. Localised burning, stinging, itching, soreness, dryness or irritation and sneezing may occur occasionally. Rarely, nausea and headache may occur.

Rebound congestion has been reported occasionally, particularly following longer-term use of xylometazoline.

4.9 Overdose
Symptoms and signs

Systemic action is unlikely when applied nasally due to the local vasoconstriction that inhibits absorption. If systemic absorption does occur xylometazoline as an α_2-adrenergic agonist could be expected to produce effects similar to those of clonidine with a short lived rise in blood pressure, followed by more prolonged hypotension and sedation.

Treatment

Treatment of overdose should be supportive.

5. PHARMACOLOGICAL PROPERTIES
5.1 Pharmacodynamic properties
Xylometazoline is a sympathomimetic amine of the imidazoline class.

It act directly on α-adrenoreceptors but does not act on β-receptors. When used topically as a nasal decongestant, xylometazoline acts rapidly and provides long-lasting relief. Onset of action is within minutes, the decongestant effect being prolonged and lasting for up to 10 hours.

5.2 Pharmacokinetic properties
Absorption, Distribution, Metabolism and Elimination

Little information is available concerning the absorption, distribution, metabolism and elimination of xylometazoline in man. Absorption into the nasal mucosal tissues is rapid.

Pharmacokinetics inRenal/Hepatic Impairment

There have been no specific studies of Non-Drowsy Sudafed Decongestant Nasal Spray or xylometazoline in hepatic or renal impairment.

Pharmacokinetics in the Elderly

There have been no specific clinical studies of Non-Drowsy Sudafed Decongestant Nasal Spray or xylometazoline in the elderly.

5.3 Preclinical safety data
Mutagenicity

There is insufficient information available to determine whether xylometazoline has mutagenic potential.

Carcinogenicity

There is insufficient information available to determine whether xylometazoline has carcinogenic potential.

Teratogenicity

There is insufficient information available to determine whether xylometazoline has teratogenic potential.

Fertility

No studies have been conducted in animals to determine whether xylometazoline has the potential to impair fertility. There is no information on the effects of Non-Drowsy Sudafed Decongestant Nasal Spray on fertility.

6. PHARMACEUTICAL PARTICULARS
6.1 List of excipients
Benzalkonium chloride solution

Disodium edetate

Sodium dihydrogen phosphate dihydrate

Sodium monohydrogen phosphate dihydrate

Sodium chloride

Sorbitol solution, 70% (Non crystalline)

Purified water

6.2 Incompatibilities
None known

6.3 Shelf life
3 years.

6.4 Special precautions for storage
Do not store above 25°C.

6.5 Nature and contents of container
Amber glass bottle of either 10 ml or 15 ml nominal fill volume.

The bottle is sealed with an integral snap-on metered 0.14 ml pump consisting of a white plastic (composed of polyethylene, polypropylene, polyoxymethylene parts and polyethylene seal) actuator and natural polyethylene pull-off overcap.

6.6 Instructions for use and handling
None applicable.

7. MARKETING AUTHORISATION HOLDER
Pfizer Consumer Healthcare

<u>Alternative Trading Style:</u>

Warner-Lambert Consumer Healthcare

Walton Oaks

Dorking Road

Walton-on-the-Hill

Surrey

KT20 7NS

United Kingdom.

8. MARKETING AUTHORISATION NUMBER(S)
PL 15513/0074

9. DATE OF FIRST AUTHORISATION/RENEWAL OF THE AUTHORISATION
21/04/99

10. DATE OF REVISION OF THE TEXT
April 2004

Non-Drowsy Sudafed Decongestant Tablets

(Pfizer Consumer Healthcare)

1. NAME OF THE MEDICINAL PRODUCT
Non-Drowsy Sudafed Decongestant Tablets

2. QUALITATIVE AND QUANTITATIVE COMPOSITION
Non-Drowsy Sudafed Decongestant Tablets contain:

Pseudoephedrine Hydrochloride 60.00 mg

3. PHARMACEUTICAL FORM
Film-coated tablets.

4. CLINICAL PARTICULARS
4.1 Therapeutic indications
Non-Drowsy Sudafed Decongestant Tablets is a decongestant of the mucous membranes of the upper respiratory tract, especially the nasal mucosa and sinuses and is indicated for the symptomatic relief of conditions such as allergic rhinitis, vasomotor rhinitis, the common cold and influenza.

4.2 Posology and method of administration
Adults and Children over 12 years

1 tablet every 4 - 6 hours up to 4 times a day.

Use in the Elderly

There have been no specific studies of Non-Drowsy Sudafed Decongestant Tablets in the elderly. Experience has indicated that normal adult dosage is appropriate.

Hepatic Dysfunction

Caution should be exercised when administering Non-Drowsy Sudafed Decongestant Tablets to patients with severe hepatic impairment.

Renal Dysfunction

Caution should be exercised when administering Non-Drowsy Sudafed Decongestant Tablets to patients with moderate to severe renal impairment.

4.3 Contraindications
Non-Drowsy Sudafed Decongestant Tablets is contraindicated in individuals with known hypersensitivity to the product or any of its components.

Non-Drowsy Sudafed Decongestant Tablets is contraindicated in individuals with severe hypertension or coronary artery disease.

Non-Drowsy Sudafed Decongestant Tablets is contraindicated in individuals who are taking or have taken monoamine oxidase inhibitors within the preceding two weeks. The concomitant use of pseudoephedrine and this type of product may occasionally cause a rise in blood pressure.

4.4 Special warnings and special precautions for use
Although pseudoephedrine has virtually no pressor effects in normotensive patients, Non-Drowsy Sudafed Decongestant Tablets should be used with caution in patients suffering mild to moderate hypertension. As with other sympathomimetic agents, Non-Drowsy Sudafed Decongestant Tablets should be used with caution in patients with hypertension, heart disease, diabetes, hyperthyroidism, elevated intraocular pressure and prostatic enlargement.

Caution should be exercised when using the product in the presence of severe hepatic impairment or moderate to severe renal impairment (particularly if accompanied by cardiovascular disease).

The following statements will appear on packs of this product:

Store below 30°C.

Keep Dry.

Warning: Do not exceed stated dose.

Keep out of reach of children.

As with all medicines, if you are pregnant or currently taking any other medicine, consult your doctor or pharmacist before taking this product.

If symptoms persist consult your doctor.

Causes no drowsiness.

4.5 Interaction with other medicinal products and other forms of Interaction
Concomitant use of Non-Drowsy Sudafed Decongestant Tablets with tricyclic antidepressants, sympathomimetic agents (such as decongestants, appetite suppressants and amfetamine-like psychostimulants) or with monoamine oxidase inhibitors, which interferes with the catabolism of sympathomimetic amines, may occasionally cause a rise in blood pressure.

Because of its pseudoephedrine contents, Non-Drowsy Sudafed Decongestant Tablets may partially reverse the hypotensive action of drugs which interfere with sympathetic activity including bretylium, betanidine, guanethedine, debrisoquine, methyldopa, alpha- and beta-adrenergic blocking agents

4.6 Pregnancy and lactation
Although pseudoephedrine has been in widespread use for many years without apparent ill consequence, there are no specific data on its use during pregnancy. Caution should therefore be exercised by balancing the potential benefit of treatment to the mother against any possible hazards to the developing foetus.

Systemic administration of pseudoephedrine, up to 50 times the human daily dosage in rats and up to 35 times the human daily dosage in rabbits, did not produce teratogenic effects.

Pseudoephedrine is excreted in breast milk in small amounts but the effect of this on breast-fed infants is not known. It has been estimated that 0.5 - 07% of a single dose of pseudoephedrine ingested by a mother will be excreted in the breast milk over 24 hours.

4.7 Effects on ability to drive and use machines
None known.

4.8 Undesirable effects
Serious adverse effects associated with the use of pseudoephedrine are rare. Symptoms of central nervous system excitation may occur, including sleep disturbances and rarely hallucinations have been reported.

Skin rashes with or without irritation have occasionally been reported. Urinary retention has been reported occasionally in men receiving pseudoephedrine, prostatic enlargement could have been an important predisposing factor.

4.9 Overdose
As with other sympathomimetic agents. Symptoms of overdose include irritability, restlessness, tremor, convulsions, palpitations, hypertension and difficulty in micturition.

Necessary measures should be taken to maintain the support respiration and control convulsions. Gastric lavage should be performed if indicated. Catheterisation of the bladder may be necessary. If desired, the elimination of pseudoephedrine can be accelerated by acid diuresis or by dialysis.

5. PHARMACOLOGICAL PROPERTIES

5.1 Pharmacodynamic properties
Pseudoephedrine has direct and indirect sympathomimetic activity and is an orally effective upper respiratory tract decongestant.

Pseudoephedrine is substantially less potent than ephedrine in producing both tachycardia and elevation in systolic blood pressure and considerably less potent in causing stimulation of the central nervous system.

5.2 Pharmacokinetic properties
Pseudoephedrine is rapidly and completely absorbed after oral administration. After an oral dose of 180 mg to man, peak plasma concentrations of 500-900 ng/ml were obtained about 2 hours post dose. The plasma half-life was about 5.5 hours and was increased in subjects with alkaline urine and decreased in subjects with acid urine. The only metabolism was N-demethylation which occurred to a small extent. Excretion was mainly via the urine.

5.3 Preclinical safety data
The active ingredient of Non-Drowsy Sudafed Decongestant Tablets is a well- known constituent of medicinal products and its safety is well documented. The results of pre-clinical studies do not add anything of relevance for therapeutic purposes.

6. PHARMACEUTICAL PARTICULARS

6.1 List of excipients
Lactose monohydrate

Pregelatinised maize starch

Cellulose microcrystalline

Magnesium Stearate

Silica colloidal

Film Coat:

Opadry OY-S-9473

Opadry OY-S-9473 contains:

Hypomellose

Red iron oxide (E172)

Talc

Polyethylene glycol 400

6.2 Incompatibilities
None known.

6.3 Shelf life
24 months unopened.

6.4 Special precautions for storage
Store below 30°C.

Keep dry.

6.5 Nature and contents of container
12 and 24 - PVC/PVDC/Aluminium foil blister packs

100 – High density polyethylene containers with low density polyethylene tamper-evident snap-on lids.

6.6 Instructions for use and handling
Not applicable.

Administrative Data

7. MARKETING AUTHORISATION HOLDER
Pfizer Consumer Healthcare

Alternative Trading Style:

Warner-Lambert Consumer Healthcare

Walton Oaks

Dorking Road

Walton-on-the-Hill

Surrey, KT20 7NS

United Kingdom

8. MARKETING AUTHORISATION NUMBER(S)
PL 15513/0024

9. DATE OF FIRST AUTHORISATION/RENEWAL OF THE AUTHORISATION
29th September 1998

10. DATE OF REVISION OF THE TEXT
April 2004

Non-Drowsy Sudafed Dual Relief

(Pfizer Consumer Healthcare)

1. NAME OF THE MEDICINAL PRODUCT
Cold Relief Capsules

Paramed Cold Relief Capsules

Superdrug Paracetamol Cold Relief with Decongestant

Non-Drowsy Sudafed Dual Relief.

Non-Drowsy Decongestant with Paracetamol

Paramed Non-Drowsy Decongestant with Paracetamol

Benylin Cold & Flu Multi Action Caps

WILKO Non-Drowsy Decongestant with Paracetamol

2. QUALITATIVE AND QUANTITATIVE COMPOSITION
INGREDIENT / QTY / UNIT / DOSE

Paracetamol 300 mg Capsule

Caffeine 25 mg Capsule

Phenylephrine Hydrochloride 5 mg Capsule

3. PHARMACEUTICAL FORM
Capsule.

4. CLINICAL PARTICULARS

4.1 Therapeutic indications
For the relief of the symptoms of colds and flu, including headache, feverishness, nasal and sinus congestion and its associated pressure and pain, catarrh, aches and pains.

4.2 Posology and method of administration
Route of administration: Oral

Adults, the elderly and children over 12 years of age:-

2 capsules every 4 to 6 hours as required, up to a maximum of 12 capsules in any 24 hour period.

Children 6 – 12 years:-

1 capsule every 4 to 6 hours as required, up to a maximum of 4 capsules in any 24 hour period.

Children under 6 years:-

Not recommended.

4.3 Contraindications
Hypersensitivity to paracetamol and/or other constituents.

Concurrent administration of monoamine oxidase inhibitors and tricyclic antidepressants, severe hypertension, myocardial infarction, hyperthyroidism and pregnancy.

4.4 Special warnings and special precautions for use
PARACETAMOL

Paracetamol should be used with caution in patients with hepatic or renal impairment and alcohol dependence as the hazards of overdose are greater in those with non-cirrhotic alcoholic liver disease.

The following warnings will appear on the pack:-

CONTAINS PARACETAMOL

- If symptoms persist consult your doctor.

- Do not exceed the stated dose.

- Keep all medicines out of the reach and sight of children.

- The pack shall also say "Do not take with any other paracetamol-containing products" and "Immediate medical advice should be sought in the event of an overdose, even if you feel well".

- Care is advised in the administration of paracetamol to patients with severe renal or hepatic impairment. The hazards of overdose are greater in those with non-cirrhotic alcoholic liver disease.

The leaflet shall say "Immediate medical advice should be sought in the event of an overdose, even if you feel well, because of the risk of delayed, serious liver damage".

4.5 Interaction with other medicinal products and other forms of Interaction
PARACETAMOL

The speed of absorption of paracetamol may be increased by metoclopramide or domperidone. Colestyramine may reduce the speed of absorption of paracetamol.

The anticoagulant effect of warfarin and other coumarins may be enhanced by prolonged regular use of paracetamol with increased risk of bleeding; occasional doses have no significant effect.

PHENYLEPHRINE HYDROCHLORIDE

Phenylephrine Hydrochloride may cause hypertension, sometimes severe, where used concurrently with both monoamine oxidase, and tricyclic type antidepressants, ganglion blocking agents, adrenergic blocking drugs, and methyldopa.

4.6 Pregnancy and lactation
PREGNANCY

Although epidemiological studies in human pregnancy have shown no ill effects due to paracetamol used in the recommended doses, patients should follow the advice of their doctor regarding the use of paracetamol during pregnancy.

Paracetamol is excreted in breast milk, but not in a clinically significant amount. Available published data do not contra indicate breast feeding.

PHENYLEPHRINE HYDROCHLORIDE

The safety of phenylephrine hydrochloride in pregnancy has not been established and unless advised medically its use should be avoided.

Although excreted in breast milk, provided maternal intake is not excessive, no harm should come to the neonate during lactation.

4.7 Effects on ability to drive and use machines
None stated.

4.8 Undesirable effects
PARACETAMOL

Adverse effects of paracetamol are rare but hypersensitivity including skin rash may occur. There have been reports of blood dyscrasias including thrombocytopenia and agranulocytosis, but these were not necessarily causally related to paracetamol.

CAFFEINE

Nausea and insomnia have been noted.

PHENYLEPHRINE HYDROCHLORIDE

Rarely phenylephrine hydrochloride may elevate blood pressure with headache, palpitation and vomiting; tachycardia or reflex bradycardia; tingling and coolness of the skin.

4.9 Overdose
PARACETAMOL

Liver damage is possible in adults who have taken 10g or more of paracetamol. Ingestion of 5g or more of paracetamol may lead to liver damage if the patient has risk factors (see below).

Risk factors

If the patient

a, Is on long term treatment with carbamazepine, phenobarbitone, phenytoin, primidone, rifampicin, St John's Wort or other drugs that induce liver enzymes.

Or

b, Regularly consumes ethanol in excess of recommended amounts.

Or

c, Is likely to be glutathione deplete e.g. eating disorders, cystic fibrosis, HIV infection, starvation, cachexia.

Symptoms

Symptoms of paracetamol overdosage in the first 24 hours are pallor, nausea, vomiting, anorexia and abdominal pain. Liver damage may become apparent 12 to 48 hours after ingestion. Abnormalities of glucose metabolism and metabolic acidosis may occur. In severe poisoning, hepatic failure may progress to encephalopathy, haemorrhage, hypoglycaemia, cerebral oedema, and death. Acute renal failure with acute tubular necrosis, strongly suggested by loin pain, haematuria and proteinuria, may develop even in the absence of severe liver damage. Cardiac arrhythmias and pancreatitis have been reported.

Management

Immediate treatment is essential in the management of paracetamol overdose. Despite a lack of significant early symptoms, patients should be referred to hospital urgently for immediate medical attention. Symptoms may be limited to nausea or vomiting and may not reflect the severity of overdose or the risk of organ damage. Management should be in accordance with established treatment guidelines, see BNF overdose section.

Treatment with activated charcoal should be considered if the overdose has been taken within 1 hour. Plasma paracetamol concentration should be measured at 4 hours or later after ingestion (earlier concentrations are unreliable). Treatment with N-acetylcysteine may be used up to 24 hours after ingestion of paracetamol, however, the maximum protective effect is obtained up to 8 hours post-ingestion. The effectiveness of the antidote declines sharply after this time. If required the patient should be given intravenous N-acetylcysteine, in line with the established dosage schedule. If vomiting is not a problem, oral methionine may be a suitable alternative for remote areas, outside hospital. Management of patients who present with serious hepatic dysfunction beyond 24h from ingestion should be discussed with the NPIS or a liver unit.

CAFFEINE

Doses over 1g are probably necessary to induce toxicity, 2 – 5g to produce severe toxicity and 5 – 10g is likely to be lethal.

Symptoms include: epigastric pain, vomiting, diuresis, tachycardia, CNS stimulation (insomnia, restlessness, excitement, agitation, jitteriness, tremors, convulsions).

No specific antidote is available, reduce or stop dosage and avoid excessive intake of coffee or tea.

PHENYLEPHRINE HYDROCHLORIDE

Severe overdosage may produce hypertension and associated reflex bradycardia. Treatment measures include early gastric lavage and symptomatic and supportive Measures. The hypertensive effects may be treated with an alpha-receptor blocking agent (such as phentolamine mesilate 6 – 10 mg) given intravenously, and the bradycardia treated with atropine, preferable only after the pressure has been controlled.

5. PHARMACOLOGICAL PROPERTIES

5.1 Pharmacodynamic properties

PARACETAMOL

Analgesic:

The mechanism of analgesic action has not been fully determined. Paracetamol may act predominantly by inhibiting a prostaglandin synthesis in the central nervous system (CNS) and to a lesser extent through a peripheral action by blocking pain-impulse generation. The peripheral action may also be due to inhibition of prostaglandin synthesis or to inhibition of the synthesis or actions of other substances that sensitise pain receptors to mechanical or chemical stimulation.

Antipyretic:

Paracetamol probably produces antipyresis by acting on the hypothalamic heat-regulating center to produce peripheral vasodilation resulting in increased blood flow through the skin, sweating and heat loss. The central action probably involves inhibition of prostaglandin synthesis in the hypothalamus.

CAFFEINE

Central nervous system stimulant – Caffeine stimulates all levels of the CNS, although its cortical effects are milder and of shorter duration than those of amphetamines.

Analgesia Adjunct:

Caffeine constricts cerebral vasculature with an accompanying decrease in cerebral blood flow and in the oxygen tension of the brain. It is believed that caffeine helps to relieve headache by providing a more rapid onset of action and/or enhanced pain relief with lower doses of analgesic. Recent studies with ergotamine indicate that the enhancement of effect by the addition of caffeine may also be due to improved gastrointestinal absorption of ergotamine when administered with caffeine.

PHENYLEPHRINE HYDROCHLORIDE

Sympathomimetic amines, such as phenylephrine, act on alpha-adrenergic receptors of the respiratory tract to produce vasoconstriction, which temporarily reduces the swelling associated with inflammation of the mucous membranes lining the nasal and sinus passages. This allows the free drainage of the sinusoidal fluid from the sinuses.

In addition to reducing mucosal lining swelling, decongestants also suppress the production of mucus, therefore preventing a build up of fluid within the cavities which could otherwise lead to pressure and pain.

5.2 Pharmacokinetic properties

PARACETAMOL

Absorption and Fate

Paracetamol is rapidly absorbed from the gastro-intestinal tract, with peak plasma concentrations occurring between 10 and 120 minutes after oral administration. It is metabolised in the liver and excreted in the urine mainly as the glucuronide and sulphate conjugates. Less than 5% is excreted as unchanged paracetamol. The elimination half-life varies from about 1 to 4 hours.

Plasma-protein binding is negligible at usual therapeutic concentrations but increases with increasing concentrations.

A minor hydroxylated metabolite which is usually produced in very small amounts by mixed-function oxidases in the liver and which is usually detoxified by conjugation with liver glutathione may accumulate following paracetamol overdose and cause liver damage.

CAFFEINE

Absorption and Fate

Caffeine is absorbed readily after oral administration and is widely distributed throughout the body. Caffeine is metabolised almost completely via oxidation, demethylation, and acetylation, and is excreted in the urine as 1-methyluric acid, 1-methylxanthine, 7-methylxanthine, 1,7-dimethylxanthine (paraxanthine), 5-acetylamino-6-formylamino-3-methyluracil (AFMU), and other metabolites with only about 1% unchanged.

PHENYLEPHRINE HYDROCHLORIDE

Absorption and Fate

Phenylephrine has reduced bioavailability from the gastro-intestinal tract owing to irregular absorption and first-pass metabolism by monoamine oxidase in the gut and liver.

5.3 Preclinical safety data

There are no preclinical data of relevance to the prescriber additional to that already covered in other sections of the SPC.

6. PHARMACEUTICAL PARTICULARS

6.1 List of excipients

Capsule contents:

Maize Starch

Croscarmellose Sodium

Sodium Lauryl Sulphate

Magnesium Stearate

Capsule:

Gelatin

Titanium Dioxide (E171)

Iron Oxide Yellow (E172)

Patent Blue V (E131)

Quinoline Yellow (E104)

6.2 Incompatibilities

None other than those listed in 4.3 and 4.5.

6.3 Shelf life

3 years.

6.4 Special precautions for storage

None.

6.5 Nature and contents of container

White opaque UPVC/aluminium foil blisters in cartons of 8, 12, 16, 24, 32 and 48.

6.6 Instructions for use and handling

None.

7. MARKETING AUTHORISATION HOLDER

Wrafton Laboratories Limited

Wrafton

Braunton

North Devon EX33 2DL

8. MARKETING AUTHORISATION NUMBER(S)

PL 12063/0003

9. DATE OF FIRST AUTHORISATION/RENEWAL OF THE AUTHORISATION

First Authorisation 5 July 1993

10. DATE OF REVISION OF THE TEXT

April 2005

Non-Drowsy Sudafed Dual Relief Max

(Pfizer Consumer Healthcare)

1. NAME OF THE MEDICINAL PRODUCT

Non-Drowsy Sudafed Dual Relief Max

2. QUALITATIVE AND QUANTITATIVE COMPOSITION

Active Ingredientsmg/tablet

Ibuprofen Ph Eur 200

Pseudoephedrine hydrochloride BP 30

3. PHARMACEUTICAL FORM

Tablet for oral administration.

4. CLINICAL PARTICULARS

4.1 Therapeutic indications

For symptomatic relief in conditions where both the decongestant action of Pseudoephedrine hydrochloride and the analgesic and/or anti-inflammatory action of Ibuprofen are required e.g. nasal and/or sinus congestion with headache, pain, fever and other symptoms of the common cold or influenza.

4.2 Posology and method of administration

Adults, the elderly and young persons over 12 years: 1 or 2 tablets every 4 – 6 hours to a maximum of 6 tablets in 24 hours.

Not to be given to children under the age of 12.

The minimum effective dose should be used for the shortest time necessary to relieve symptoms. If the product is required for more than 10 days, the patient should consult a doctor.

4.3 Contraindications

Hypersensitivity to any of the ingredients. Patients suffering from heart disease, circulatory problems, kidney disease, peptic ulcers, hypertension, diabetes, phaeochromocytoma, or closed angle glaucoma. This product is contraindicated in patients who have previously shown hypersensitivity reactions (e.g. asthma, rhinitis, or urticaria) in response to aspirin or other non-steroidal anti-inflammatory drugs. Active or previous peptic ulcer. History of upper gastrointestinal bleeding or perforation, related to previous NSAIDs therapy. Use with concomitant NSAIDs including cyclo-oxygenase specific inhibitors. Patients taking other painkillers or decongestants. Patients receiving tricyclic antidepressants. Patients currently receiving, or have had within the last two weeks received, monoamine oxidase inhibitors.

4.4 Special warnings and special precautions for use

Patients suffering from asthma, hypertension, heart disease, diabetes, thyroid disease or prostatic hypertrophy should consult their doctor before using this product. Non-Drowsy Sudafed Dual Relief Max should not be taken with other decongestants or analgesics.

Bronchospasm may be precipitated in patients suffering from or with a previous history of bronchial asthma or allergic disease.

Undesirable effects may be minimised by using the minimum effective dose for the shortest possible duration.

The elderly are at increased risk of the serious consequences of adverse reactions.

Caution is required in patients with renal, cardiac, or hepatic impairment since renal function may deteriorate. Renal function should be monitored in such patients.

There is some evidence that drugs which inhibit cyclo-oxygenase / prostaglandin synthesis may cause impairment of female fertility by an effect on ovulation. This is reversible of withdrawal of treatment.

GI bleeding, ulceration or perforation, which can be fatal, has been reported with all NSAIDs at anytime during treatment, with or without warning symptoms or a previous history of serious GI events.

Patients with a history of GI toxicity, particularly when elderly, should report any unusual abdominal symptoms (especially GI bleeding) particularly in the early stages of treatment.

Caution should be advised in patients receiving concomitant medications which could increase the risk of gastrotoxicity or bleeding, such as corticosteroids, or anticoagulants such as warfarin or anti-platelet agents such as aspirin (see Section 4.5).

Where GI bleeding or ulceration occurs in patients receiving ibuprofen, the treatment should be withdrawn.

The label will state; Do not use if you have had or are suffering from stomach ulcers. If you are taking any other pain relieving medication. If you are allergic or ibuprofen or any of the other ingredients, aspirin or any other painkillers. Do not use if you have ever had stomach bleeding or perforation after taking a non-steroidal anti-inflammatory medicine. Consult your doctor if you are asthmatic or are pregnant. Keep out of the reach of children. If symptoms persist consult your doctor. Do not exceed the stated dose.

4.5 Interaction with other medicinal products and other forms of Interaction

NSAIDs may interact with the actions of oral anticoagulants, such as warfarin, and diminish the effect of anti-hypertensives – or diuretics. Concurrent aspirin or other NSAIDs may result in an increased incidence of adverse reactions. Corticosteroids may increase the risk of adverse reactions in the gastrointestinal tract. Pseudoephedrine may interact with the actions of other sympathomimetic drugs and the antibacterial agent furazolidine. The action of Pseudoephedrine may be reduced by guanethidine, reserpine or methyldopa and may be reduced or enhanced by tricyclic antidepressants. Pseudoephedrine may reduce the action of guanethidine and may increase the possibility or arrhythmias in patients taking digitalis, quinidine or tricyclic antidepressants.

4.6 Pregnancy and lactation

There have been reports of foetal maldevelopment in animals following the use of Pseudoephedrine. Whilst no teratogenic effects have been demonstrated in animal studies Ibuprofen should be avoided during pregnancy. The onset of labour may be delayed and duration of labour increased. Both Pseudoephedrine and to a lesser degree Ibuprofen pass into breast milk. The product should therefore not be used during pregnancy, or during lactation except under the supervision of a doctor.

4.7 Effects on ability to drive and use machines

None.

4.8 Undesirable effects

Gastrointestinal: abdominal pain, nausea and dyspepsia. Rarely peptic ulcer, perforation or gastrointestinal haemorrhage, sometimes fatal, particularly in the elderly, may occur (see Section 4.4).

Haematological: thrombocytopenia.

Renal: papillary necrosis which can lead to renal failure.

Hypersensitivity reactions have been reported following treatment with NSAIDs. These may consist of:

a) Non-specific allergic reactions and anaphylaxis.

b) Respiratory tract reactivity comprising of asthma, aggravated asthma, bronchospasm or dyspnoea.

c) Assorted skin disorders, including rashes of various types, pruritis, urticaria, purpura, angioedema, more rarely bullous dermatoses (including epidermal necrolysis and erythema multiforme).

Insomnia, dizziness, excitability, anxiety, tremor, palpitations, dry mouth, nausea, dyspepsia, GI bleeding, loss of appetite, thirst, chest pains. Less frequently: difficulty in micturition, muscle weakness and hallucinations.

Others: rarely hepatic dysfunction, headache, hearing disturbances, exacerbation of colitis, aseptic meningitis.

4.9 Overdose

Overdosage may result in nervousness, dizziness, insomnia, headache, vomiting, drowsiness and hypotension.

Due to the rapid absorption of the two active ingredients from the gastro-intestinal tract, emetics and gastric lavage must be instituted within 4 hours of overdosage to be effective. Charcoal is effective only if given within one hour. Cardiac status should be monitored and the serum electrolytes measured.

If there are signs of cardiac toxicity, propranolol may be administered intravenously. A slow infusion of a dilute solution of potassium chloride should be initiated in the event of a drop in the serum potassium level. Despite hypokalaemia, the patient is unlikely to be potassium depleted, therefore overload must be avoided. Continued monitoring of the serum potassium is advisable for several hours after administration of the salt. For delirium or convulsions, intravenous administration of diazepam is indicated.

5. PHARMACOLOGICAL PROPERTIES

5.1 Pharmacodynamic properties

Ibuprofen is a non-steroidal anti-inflammatory agent belonging to the Propionic Acid class of drugs. It has analgesic, antipyretic and anti-inflammatory properties. Ibuprofen inhibits prostaglandin synthesis. Pseudoephedrine hydrochloride is a sympathomimetic agent which causes vasoconstriction of nasal mucosa, thereby reducing rhinorrhoea and nasal congestion.

5.2 Pharmacokinetic properties

Ibuprofen is rapidly absorbed from the gastrointestinal tract with peak concentrations being achieved 45-90 minutes later. It is over 90% plasma protein bound in the circulation and has a short elimination half-life of 0.9 – 2.5 hours. Ibuprofen is primarily metabolised in the liver to 2-Hydrocyibuprofen and 2-Carboxyibuprofen. These are excreted in the urine along with approximately 9% of unchanged drug.

Pseudoephedrine hydrochloride is rapidly absorbed from the gastro-intestinal tract with peak plasma levels at 1 – 3 hours. It is partly metabolised in the liver like most sympathomimetics, but is mainly excreted unchanged in the urine.

5.3 Preclinical safety data

None stated.

6. PHARMACEUTICAL PARTICULARS

6.1 List of excipients

Sucrose Ph Eur

Starch Ph Eur

Pregelatinised starch NF

Croscarmellose sodium NF

Microcrystalline cellulose Ph Eur

Opalux butterscotch AS-3739*

Stearic acid TP fine powder NF

Colloidal anyhydrous silica Ph Eur

Opaglos GS-2-0310 (solids)*

Sodium lauryl sulphate Ph Eur

Carnauba wax No. yellow powder NF

*The colouring agents contain shellac, iron oxide (yellow, red), acetylated monoglyceride, povidone, sucrose, titanium dioxide, sodium hydroxide, propyl hydroxybenzoate, methyl hydroxybenzoate.

6.2 Incompatibilities

None known.

6.3 Shelf life

3 years.

6.4 Special precautions for storage

No special precautions required.

6.5 Nature and contents of container

a) PVC/PE/PVDC/Aluminium blister packs in cardboard cartons containing 10, 12, 20, 24, 48 or 96 tablets.

b) UPVC/Aluminium blister packs in cardboard cartons containing 10, 12, 20, 24, 48 or 96 tablets.

6.6 Instructions for use and handling

Not applicable.

7. MARKETING AUTHORISATION HOLDER

Pfizer Consumer Healthcare

Walton Oaks

Dorking Road

Walton-on-the-Hill

Surrey

KT20 7NS

8. MARKETING AUTHORISATION NUMBER(S)

PL 15513/0126

9. DATE OF FIRST AUTHORISATION/RENEWAL OF THE AUTHORISATION

13th August 2004

10. DATE OF REVISION OF THE TEXT

Non-Drowsy Sudafed Expectorant

(Pfizer Consumer Healthcare)

1. NAME OF THE MEDICINAL PRODUCT

Non-Drowsy SUDAFED Expectorant

2. QUALITATIVE AND QUANTITATIVE COMPOSITION

Non-Drowsy SUDAFED Expectorant contains 30 mg pseudoephedrine hydrochloride and 100 mg guaifenesin in each 5 ml.

For excipients see 6.1.

3. PHARMACEUTICAL FORM

Liquid

4. CLINICAL PARTICULARS

4.1 Therapeutic indications

Non-Drowsy SUDAFED Expectorant is indicated for the symptomatic relief of upper respiratory tract disorders accompanied by productive cough, which are benefited by the combination of a decongestant of the mucous membranes of the upper respiratory tract, especially the nasal mucosa and sinuses, and an expectorant.

4.2 Posology and method of administration

Adults and children over 12 years:

Oral. 10 ml syrup every 4 - 6 hours up to 4 times a day.

Maximum daily dose: 40 ml

Children aged 6 to 12 years:

Oral. 5 ml syrup every 4 - 6 hours up to 4 times a day.

Maximum daily dose: 20 ml

Children aged 2years to 5 years:

Oral. 2.5 ml syrup every 4 - 6 hours up to 4 times a day.

Maximum daily dose: 10 ml

Children under 2 years:

Non-Drowsy SUDAFED Expectorant is not recommended for administration to children under 2 years of age.

Theelderly:

Normal adult dosage is appropriate, [See Pharmacokinetics in the elderly].

Hepatic dysfunction:

Experience with the use of the product suggests normal adult dosage is appropriate, although it may be prudent to exercise caution in the presence of severe hepatic impairment, [See Pharmacokinetics in the elderly].

Renal dysfunction:

Caution should be exercised when administering Non-Drowsy SUDAFED Expectorant to patients with moderate to severe renal impairment, particularly if accompanied by cardiovascular disease, [See Pharmacokinetics in Renal Impairment].

4.3 Contraindications

Non-Drowsy SUDAFED Expectorant is contraindicated in individuals with known hypersensitivity to the product, or any of its components.

Non-Drowsy SUDAFED Expectorant is contraindicated in individuals with severe hypertension or severe coronary artery disease.

Non-Drowsy SUDAFED Expectorant is contraindicated in individuals who are taking, or have taken, monoamine oxidase inhibitors within the preceding two weeks. The concomitant use of pseudoephedrine and this type of product may occasionally cause a rise in blood pressure.

4.4 Special warnings and special precautions for use

Although pseudoephedrine has virtually no pressor effects in normotensive patients, Non-Drowsy SUDAFED Expectorant should be used with caution in individuals suffering from mild to moderate hypertension, [See Contraindications and interactions with other medicinal products].

As with other sympathomimetic agents, Non-Drowsy SUDAFED Expectorant should be used with caution in individuals with heart disease, diabetes, hyperthyroidism, elevated intra-ocular pressure or prostatic enlargement.

Non-Drowsy SUDAFED Expectorant should be not used for persistent or chronic cough, such as occurs with asthma, or emphysema where cough is accompanied by excessive secretions, unless directed by a physician.

Caution should be exercised when using the product in the presence of severe hepatic impairment or renal impairment (particularly if accompanied by cardiovascular disease), [See Pharmacokinetics].

4.5 Interaction with other medicinal products and other forms of Interaction

Concomitant use of Non-Drowsy SUDAFED Expectorant with anti-hypertensive agents, tricyclic antidepressants, sympathomimetic agents (such as decongestants, appetite suppressants and amfetamine-like psychostimulants) or with monoamine oxidase inhibitors, which interfere with the catabolism of sympathomimetic amines, may occasionally cause a rise in blood pressure. [See Contra-indications].

Because of its pseudoephedrine content, Non-Drowsy SUDAFED Expectorant may partially reverse the hypotensive action of drugs which interfere with sympathetic activity including bretylium, betanidine, guanethidine, debrisoquine, methyldopa, alpha- and beta- adrenergic blocking agents, [See Special Warnings and Special Precautions for Use].

4.6 Pregnancy and lactation

Insufficient information is available on the effects of administration of Non-Drowsy SUDAFED Expectorant during human pregnancy. Non-Drowsy SUDAFED Expectorant, like most medicines, should not be used during pregnancy unless the potential benefit of treatment to the mother outweighs the possible risks to the developing foetus.

Pseudoephedrine is excreted in breast milk in small amounts but the effect of this on breast-fed infants is not known. It has been estimated that approximately 0.5 to 0.7 % of a single 60 mg dose of pseudoephedrine ingested by a nursing mother will be excreted in the breast milk over 24 hours.

Guaifenesin is excreted in breast milk in small amounts with no effect expected on the infant.

4.7 Effects on ability to drive and use machines

No special comment - unlikely to produce an effect.

4.8 Undesirable effects

Serious adverse effects associated with the use of pseudoephedrine are extremely rare. Symptoms of central nervous system excitation may occur, including sleep disturbance and, rarely, hallucinations.

Skin rashes, with or without irritation, have occasionally been reported with pseudoephedrine.

Urinary retention has been reported occasionally in men receiving pseudoephedrine; prostatic enlargement could have been an important factor.

Side effects resulting from guaifenesin administration are very rare.

4.9 Overdose

Symptoms and signs

The effects of acute toxicity from Non-Drowsy SUDAFED Expectorant may include drowsiness, irritability, restlessness, tremor, palpitations, convulsions, hypertension, difficulty with micturition, gastro-intestinal discomfort, nausea and vomiting.

Treatment

Necessary measures should be taken to maintain and support respiration and control convulsions. Gastric lavage may be undertaken if indicated. Catheterisation of the bladder may be necessary. Acid diuresis can accelerate the elimination of pseudoephedrine, although the potential therapeutic gain of this procedure is now in dispute. The value of dialysis in overdose is not known, although four hours of haemodialysis removed approximately 20 % of the total body load of pseudoephedrine in a combination product containing 60 mg pseudoephedrine and 8 mg acrivastine.

5. PHARMACOLOGICAL PROPERTIES

5.1 Pharmacodynamic properties

Pseudoephedrine has direct and indirect sympathomimetic activity and is an orally effective upper respiratory decongestant. Pseudoephedrine is substantially less potent than ephedrine in producing both tachycardia and elevation of systolic blood pressure and considerably less potent in causing stimulation of the central nervous system. Pseudoephedrine produces its decongestant effect within 30 minutes, persisting for at least 4 hours.

Guaifenesin is thought to exert its pharmacological action by stimulating receptors in the gastric mucosa. This increases the output from secretory glands of the gastrointestinal system and reflexly increases the flow of fluids from glands lining the respiratory tract. The result is an increase in volume and decrease in viscosity of bronchial secretions. Other actions may include stimulating vagal nerve endings in bronchial secretory glands and stimulating certain centres in the brain which in mm enhance respiratory fluid flow. Guaifenesin produces its expectorant action within 24 hours.

5.2 Pharmacokinetic properties

Absorption

Pseudoephedrine

Pseudoephedrine is well absorbed from the gut following oral administration. After the administration of one 60 mg pseudoephedrine tablet to healthy adult volunteers, the Cmax for pseudoephedrine was approximately 180 ng/ml with tmax occurring at approximately 1.5 - 2.0 hours.

Guaifenesin

Guaifenesin is well absorbed from the gastro-intestinal tract following oral administration, although limited information is available on its pharmacokinetics. After the administration of 600 mg guaifenesin to healthy adult volunteers, the Cmax was approximately 1.4 micrograms/ml, with tmax occurring approximately 15 minutes after drug administration.

Distribution

The apparent volume of distribution of pseudoephedrine (Vd/F) was approximately 2.8 l/kg. No information is available on the distribution of guaifenesin in humans.

Metabolism and elimination

Pseudoephedrine

The $t_{1/2}$ was approximately 5.5 hours. Pseudoephedrine is partly metabolised in the liver by N-demethylation to norpseudoephedrine, an active metabolite. Pseudoephedrine and its metabolite are excreted in the urine; 55 % to 90 % of a dose is excreted unchanged. The apparent total body clearance of pseudoephedrine (Cl/F) was approximately 6 - -6.5 ml/min/kg. The rate of urinary elimination is accelerated when the urine is acidified. Conversely, as the urine pH increases, the rate of urinary elimination is slowed.

Guaifenesin

Guaifenesin appears to undergo both oxidation and demethylation. Following an oral dose of 600 mg guaifenesin to 3 healthy male volunteers, the $t_{1/2}$ was approximately 1 hour and the drug was not detectable in the blood after approximately 8 hours.

Pharmacokinetics in Renal Impairment

Following the administration of a pseudoephedrine-containing product (8 mg acrivastine + 60 mg pseudoephedrine) to patients with varying degrees of renal impairment, the Cmax for pseudoephedrine increased approximately 1.5 fold in patients with moderate to severe renal impairment when compared to the Cmax in healthy volunteers. The tmax was not affected by renal impairment. The t½ increased 3 to 12 fold in patients with mild to severe renal impairment respectively, when compared to the t½ in healthy volunteers.

There have been no specific studies of Non-Drowsy SUDAFED Expectorant, or guaifenesin in renally impaired patients.

Pharmacokinetics in Hepatic Impairment

There have been no specific studies of Non-Drowsy SUDAFED Expectorant, guaifenesin or pseudoephedrine in hepatic impairment.

Pharmacokinetics in the Elderly

After the administration of a pseudoephedrine-containing product (8 mg acrivastine + 60 mg pseudoephedrine) to elderly volunteers, the t½ for pseudoephedrine was 1.4 fold that seen in younger healthy volunteers. The apparent Cl/F was 0.8 fold that seen in younger healthy volunteers, and the Vd/F was essentially unchanged.

There have been no specific studies of Non-Drowsy SUDAFED Expectorant, pseudoephedrine or guaifenesin in the elderly.

5.3 Preclinical safety data

The active ingredients of Non-Drowsy SUDAFED Expectorant are well known constituents of medicinal products and their safety profiles are well documented. The results of pre-clinical studies do not add anything of relevance for therapeutic purposes.

6. PHARMACEUTICAL PARTICULARS

6.1 List of excipients

Sucrose

Glycerol

Methyl Hydroxybenzoate

Propyl Hydroxybenzoate

Menthol

Ethanol 96 %v/v

Wild Cherry flavour

Ponceau 4R (E 124)

Sunset Yellow (El 10)

Purified Water

6.2 Incompatibilities

None known

6.3 Shelf life

36 months

6.4 Special precautions for storage

Do not store above 25°C. Keep container in the outer carton. Do not refrigerate.

6.5 Nature and contents of container

Non-Drowsy SUDAFED Expectorant is stored in 30, 40, 50, 100 and 1000 ml amber glass bottles fitted with metal roll-on closures, plastic screw caps fitted with PVDC faced wads or polyethylene/expanded polyethylene laminated wad.

or

Non-Drowsy SUDAFED Expectorant is stored in 30, 40, 50, 100 and 1000 ml amber glass bottles fitted with a 3 piece plastic child resistant, tamper evident closure fitted with a PVDC faced wad or polyethylene/expanded polyethylene laminated wad.

6.6 Instructions for use and handling

None applicable

7. MARKETING AUTHORISATION HOLDER

Pfizer Consumer Healthcare Alternative Trading Style:

Warner-Lambert Consumer Healthcare

Walton Oaks

Dorking Road

Walton-on-the-Hill

Surrey

KT20 7NS

United Kingdom

8. MARKETING AUTHORISATION NUMBER(S)

PL 15513/0022

9. DATE OF FIRST AUTHORISATION/RENEWAL OF THE AUTHORISATION

27.09.1997

10. DATE OF REVISION OF THE TEXT

October 2004

Non-Drowsy Sudafed Linctus

(Pfizer Consumer Healthcare)

1. NAME OF THE MEDICINAL PRODUCT

Non-Drowsy Sudafed Linctus

2. QUALITATIVE AND QUANTITATIVE COMPOSITION

Each 5 ml of Non-Drowsy Sudafed Linctus contains:

Pseudoephedrine hydrochloride 30.00 mg

Dextromethorphan hydrobromide 10.00 mg

3. PHARMACEUTICAL FORM

Liquid for oral administration.

4. CLINICAL PARTICULARS

4.1 Therapeutic indications

For the symptomatic relief of upper respiratory tract disorders which may benefit from a combination of a nasal decongestant and an antitussive.

4.2 Posology and method of administration

Adults and Children over 12 years

Oral. 10 ml every 4 - 6 hours up to 4 times a day.

Children 6 - 12 years

Oral. 5 ml every 4 - 6 hours up to 4 times a day.

Children 2 - 5 years

Oral. 2.5 ml every 4 - 6 hours up to 4 times a day.

Use in the Elderly

There have been no specific studies of Sudafed in the elderly. Experience has indicated that normal adult dosage is appropriate.

Hepatic Dysfunction

Caution should be exercised when administering Non-Drowsy Sudafed Linctus to patients with severe hepatic impairment.

Renal Dysfunction

Caution should be exercised when administering Non-Drowsy Sudafed Linctus to patients with moderate to severe renal impairment.

4.3 Contraindications

Non-Drowsy Sudafed Linctus is contraindicated in individuals with known hypersensitivity to the product or any of its components. Non-Drowsy Sudafed Linctus is contraindicated in individuals with severe hypertension or coronary artery disease.

Non-Drowsy Sudafed Linctus is contraindicated in individuals who are taking or have taken monoamine oxidase inhibitors within the preceding two weeks. The concomitant use of pseudoephedrine and this type of product may occasionally cause a rise in blood pressure.

Non-Drowsy Sudafed Linctus is not intended for use in chronic or persistent cough as occurs with asthma or where cough is accompanied by excessive secretions. Dextromethorphan, in common with other centrally acting antitussive agents should not be given to patients with or at risk of developing respiratory failure.

4.4 Special warnings and special precautions for use

Although pseudoephedrine has virtually no pressor effects in normotensive patients, Non-Drowsy Sudafed Linctus should be used with caution in patients suffering mild to moderate hypertension. As with other sympathomimetic agents, Non-Drowsy Sudafed Linctus should be used with caution in patients with hypertension, heart disease, diabetes, hyperthyroidism, elevated intraocular pressure and prostatic enlargement.

Caution should be exercised when using the product in the presence of severe hepatic impairment or moderate to severe renal impairment (particularly if accompanied by cardiovascular disease).

There have been a few reports of abuse of dextromethorphan but there is no evidence of drug dependance at therapeutic doses.

The pack carries the following statements:

Store below 25°C. Protect from light.

Keep out of the reach of children.

'Warning: do not exceed stated dose.'

Avoid alcoholic drink.

As with all medicines if you are pregnant, or currently taking any other medicine, consult your doctor or pharmacist before taking this product.

If symptoms persist consult your doctor.

Causes no drowsiness.

4.5 Interaction with other medicinal products and other forms of Interaction

Concomitant use of Non-Drowsy Sudafed Linctus with tricyclic antidepressants, sympathomimetic agents (such as decongestants, appetite suppressants and amfetamine-like psychostimulants) or with monoamine oxidase inhibitors, which interfere with the catabolism of sympathomimetic amines, may occasionally cause a rise in blood pressure.

Because of its pseudoephedrine content, Non-Drowsy Sudafed Linctus may partially reverse the hypotensive action of drugs which interfere with sympathetic activity including bretylium, betanidine, guanethedine, debrisoquine, methyldopa, alpha and beta-adrenergic blocking agents.

4.6 Pregnancy and lactation

Although pseudoephedrine and dextromethorphan have been in widespread use for many years without apparent ill consequence, there are no specific data on their use during pregnancy. Caution should therefore be exercised by balancing the potential benefit of treatment to the mother against any possible hazards to the developing foetus.

Systemic administration of pseudoephedrine, up to 50 times the human daily dosage in rats and up to 35 times the human daily dosage in rabbits, did not produce teratogenic effects. There is insufficient information available to determine whether or not dextromethorphan has teratogenic potential.

Pseudoephedrine is excreted in breast milk in small amounts but the effect of this on breast fed infants is not known. It has been estimated that 0.5 - 0.7% of a single dose of pseudoephedrine ingested by a mother will be excreted in the breast milk over 24 hours. It is not known whether dextromethorphan or its metabolites are excreted in breast milk.

4.7 Effects on ability to drive and use machines

None known.

4.8 Undesirable effects

Serious adverse effects associated with the use of pseudoephedrine are rare. Symptoms of central nervous system excitation may occur including sleep disturbance and rarely, hallucinations. Skin rashes; with or without irritation have occasionally been reported.

Urinary retention has been reported occasionally in men receiving pseudoephedrine; prostatic enlargement could have been an important predisposing factor.

Side effects attributed to dextromethorphan are uncommon; occasionally nausea, vomiting or gastro-intestinal disturbance may occur.

4.9 Overdose

The effects of acute toxicity from Non-Drowsy Sudafed Linctus may include nystagmus, hypertension, irritability, restlessness, tremor, convulsions, palpitations, difficulty with micturition, depression, nausea and vomiting.

Necessary measures should be taken to maintain and support respiration and control convulsions. Gastric lavage should be performed if indicated. Catherisation of the bladder may be necessary. If desired, the elimination of pseudoephedrine can be accelerated by acid diuresis or by dialysis.

Naloxone has been used successfully as a specific antagonist to dextromethorphan toxicity in a child.

5. PHARMACOLOGICAL PROPERTIES

5.1 Pharmacodynamic properties

Pseudoephedrine has direct and indirect sympathomimetic activity and is an effective upper respiratory tract decongestant. Pseudoephedrine is substantially less potent than ephedrine in producing both tachycardia and elevation of systolic blood pressure and is considerably less potent in causing stimulation of the central nervous system.

Dextromethorphan provides antitussive activity by acting on the medullary cough centre.

5.2 Pharmacokinetic properties

Pseudoephedrine is rapidly and completely absorbed after oral administration. After an oral dose of 180 mg to man, peak plasma concentrations of 500-900 ng/ml were obtained about 2 hours post dose. The plasma half-life was approximately 5.5 hours and was increased in subjects with alkaline urine and decreased in subjects with acid urine. The only metabolism was n-demethylation which occurred to a small extent. Excretion was mainly via the urine.

Dextromethorphan is well absorbed following oral administration with peak plasma levels (30 mg dose) being seen 2 hours post dose. It is metabolised in the liver by n- and o-demethylation followed by sulphate or glucuronic acid conjugation. It is excreted unchanged and as metabolites in the urine (up to 56 per cent of dose).

5.3 Preclinical safety data

There are no preclinical data of relevance to the prescriber which are additional to that already included in other sections of the SPC.

6. PHARMACEUTICAL PARTICULARS

6.1 List of excipients

Sucrose

Sorbitol solution

Sodium benzoate

Methyl hydroxybenzoate

Ethanol (96 %)

Flavour, blackcurrant

L-menthol

Ponceau 4R (E124)

Purified water

6.2 Incompatibilities

None known.

6.3 Shelf life
36 months unopened.

6.4 Special precautions for storage
Store below 25°C.

Protect from light.

6.5 Nature and contents of container
Container:

30 ml, 40 ml, 50 ml and 100 ml amber glass bottles with metal roll on closures or plastic screw caps with saran or steran faced wad or polyethylene/expanded polyethylene laminated wad.

Amber glass bottles with a 3 piece plastic child resistant, tamper evident closure fitted with a polyvinylidene chloride (PVDC) faced wad or polyethylene/expanded polyethylene laminated wad.

A spoon with a 5ml and a 2.5ml measure is supplied with this product.

6.6 Instructions for use and handling
Not applicable.

7. MARKETING AUTHORISATION HOLDER
Pfizer Consumer Healthcare

Alternative Trading Style:

Warner-Lambert Consumer Healthcare

Walton Oaks

Dorking Road

Walton-on-the-Hill

Surrey, KT20 7NS

United Kingdom

8. MARKETING AUTHORISATION NUMBER(S)
PL 15513/0028

9. DATE OF FIRST AUTHORISATION/RENEWAL OF THE AUTHORISATION
28th March 1997

10. DATE OF REVISION OF THE TEXT
October 2004

Nootropil 800mg & 1200mgTablets and Solution

(UCB Pharma Limited)

1. NAME OF THE MEDICINAL PRODUCT
NOOTROPIL TABLETS 1200 MG.

NOOTROPIL TABLETS 800 MG.

NOOTROPIL SOLUTION 33%

2. QUALITATIVE AND QUANTITATIVE COMPOSITION
Piracetam - 1200 mg per tablet

Piracetam - 800 mg per tablet

Piracetam – 33% w/v

3. PHARMACEUTICAL FORM
Tablet for oral administration.

Solution for oral administration.

4. CLINICAL PARTICULARS

4.1 Therapeutic indications
NOOTROPIL is indicated for patients suffering from myoclonus of cortical origin, irrespective of aetiology, and should be used in combination with other anti-myoclonic therapies.

4.2 Posology and method of administration
Adults:

The dosage regime shows important interindividual variability, requiring an individualised dose finding approach. A reasonable protocol would be to introduce piracetam at a dosage of 7.2 g/day, increasing by 4.8 g/day every 3 to 4 days up to a maximum of 20g/day, given in either 2 or 3 divided doses while keeping other antimyoclonic drugs unchanged at their optimal dosage. If possible, depending on clinical benefit, an attempt should be made to subsequently reduce the dosage of other antimyoclonic drugs.

4.3 Contraindications
Piracetam is contra-indicated in patients with severe renal impairment (renal creatinine clearance of less than 20 ml per minute), hepatic impairment and to those under 16 years of age. It is also contraindicated in patients with cerebral haemorrhage and in those with hypersensitivity to piracetam, other pyrrolidone derivatives or any of the excipients.

4.4 Special warnings and special precautions for use
Due to the effect of piracetam on platelet aggregation (see section 5.1. Pharmacodynamic Properties), caution is recommended in patients with underlying disorders of haemostasis, major surgery or severe haemorrhage.

Abrupt discontinuation of treatment should be avoided as this may induce myoclonic or generalised seizures in some myoclonic patients.

As piracetam is almost exclusively excreted by the kidneys caution should be exercised in treating patients with known renal impairment. In renally impaired and elderly patients an increase in terminal half-life is directly related to renal function as measured by creatinine clearance. Dosage adjustment is therefore required in those with mild to moderate renal impairment and elderly patients with diminished renal function.

The daily dose must be individualized according to renal function. Refer to the following table and adjust the dose as indicated. To use this dosing table, an estimate of the patient's creatinine clearance (CLcr) in ml/min is needed. The CLcr in ml/min may be estimated from serum creatinine (mg/dl) determination using the following formula:

$$CLcr = \frac{[140 - age\ (years)] \times weight\ (kg)}{72 \times serum\ creatinine\ (mg/dl)} (\times 0.85\ for\ women)$$

Group	Creatinine clearance (ml/min)	Posology and frequency
Normal	> 80	usual daily dose, 2 to 4 sub-doses
Mild	50-79	2/3 usual daily dose, 2 or 3 sub-doses
Moderate	30-49	1/3 usual daily dose, 2 sub-doses
Severe	< 30	1/6 usual daily dose, 1 single intake
	< 20	contraindicated

4.5 Interaction with other medicinal products and other forms of Interaction
In a single case, confusion, irritability and sleep disorders were reported in concomitant use with thyroid extract (T3 + T4). At present although based on a small number of patients, no interaction has been found with the following anti-epileptic medications: clonazepam, carbamazepine, phenytoin, phenobarbitone and sodium valproate.

In a published single-blind study on patients with severe recurrent venous thrombosis, piracetam 9.6 g/d did not modify the doses of acenocoumarol necessary to reach INR 2.5 to 3.5, but compared with the effects of acenocoumarol alone, the addition of piracetam 9.6 g/d significantly decreased platelet aggregation, β-thromboglobulin release, levels of fibrinogen and von Willebrand's factors (VIII: C; VIII: vW: Ag; VIII: vW: RCo) and whole blood and plasma viscosity.

To date, there are no known interactions with other drugs.

4.6 Pregnancy and lactation
In animal studies piracetam was not teratogenic and had no effect on fertility at the maximal tested dose of 2.7 /g/kg/day for the rabbit and 4.8 g/kg/day for rats and mice.

Piracetam readily crosses the placental barrier. Since the safety of use in human pregnancy is not established, piracetam is to be avoided during pregnancy.

Piracetam is excreted in human breast milk. Therefore, piracetam should be avoided during breastfeeding or breastfeeding should be discontinued, while receiving treatment with piracetam.

Young women using the product should be taking adequate contraceptive precautions.

4.7 Effects on ability to drive and use machines
In clinical studies, at dosages between 1.6 - 15 grams per day, hyperkinesia, somnolence, nervousness and depression were reported more frequently in patients on piracetam than on placebo. There is no experience on driving ability in dosages between 15 and 20 grams daily. Caution should therefore be exercised by patients intending to drive or use machinery whilst taking piracetam.

4.8 Undesirable effects
A. Clinical studies

Double-blind placebo-controlled clinical or pharmacoclinical trials, of which quantified safety data are available (extracted from the UCB Documentation Data Bank on June 1997), included more than 3000 subjects receiving piracetam, regardless of indication, dosage form, daily dosage or population characteristics.

When adverse events are grouped together according to WHO System Organ Classes, the following classes were found to be related to a statistically significantly higher occurrence under treatment with piracetam: psychiatric disorders, central and peripheral nervous system disorders, metabolic and nutritional disorders, body as a whole - general disorders.

Following adverse experiences were reported for piracetam with a statistically significantly higher incidence than placebo. Incidences are given for piracetam versus placebo treated patients.

WHO System Organ Class	Common > 1 %, ⩽ 10 %)	Uncommon > 0.1 %, ⩽ 1 %)
Central and peripheral nervous system disorders	Hyperkinesia (1.72 versus 0.42 %)	
Metabolic and nutritional disorders	Weight increase (1.29 versus 0.39 %)	
Psychiatric disorders	Nervousness (1.13 versus 0.25 %)	Somnolence (0.96 versus 0.25 %) Depression (0.83 versus 0.21 %)
Body as a whole - general disorders		Asthenia (0.23 versus 0.00 %)

B. Post-marketing experience

From the post-marketing experience, the following adverse drug reactions have been reported (sorted according to MedDRA System Organ Classes). Data are insufficient to support an estimate of their incidence in the population to be treated.

- Ear and labyrinth disorders:

vertigo

- Gastrointestinal disorders:

abdominal pain, abdominal pain upper, diarrhoea, nausea, vomiting

- Immune system disorders:

anaphylactoid reaction, hypersensitivity

- Nervous system disorders:

ataxia, balance impaired, epilepsy aggravated, headache, insomnia, somnolence

- Psychiatric disorders:

agitation, anxiety, confusion, hallucination

- Skin and subcutaneous tissue disorders:

angioneurotic oedema, dermatitis, pruritus, urticaria, rash

4.9 Overdose
Acute toxicological studies in animals showed lethal doses were obtained in mice (18.2 g/kg and higher) but not in rats and dogs dosed respectively at 21 g/kg or 10 g/kg.

No specific measure is indicated. The patient's general condition should be closely monitored. Close attention should be given to keeping the patient well hydrated and monitoring the urine flow.

5. PHARMACOLOGICAL PROPERTIES

5.1 Pharmacodynamic properties
Piracetam's mode of action in cortical myoclonus is as yet unknown.

Piracetam exerts its haemorrheological effects on the platelets, red blood cells, and vessel walls by increasing erythrocyte deformability and by decreasing platelet aggregation, erythrocyte adhesion to vessel walls and capillary vasospasm.

- Effects on the red blood cells:

In patients with sickle cell anemia, piracetam improves the deformability of the erythrocyte membrane, decreases blood viscosity, and prevents rouleaux formation.

- Effects on platelets:

In open studies in healthy volunteers and in patients with Raynaud's phenomenon, increasing doses of piracetam up to 12 g was associated with a dose-dependent reduction in platelet functions compared with pre-treatment values (tests of aggregation induced by ADP, collagen, epinephrine and βTG release), without significant change in platelet count. In these studies, piracetam prolonged bleeding time.

- Effects on blood vessels:

In animal studies, piracetam inhibited vasospasm and counteracted the effects of various spasmogenic agents. It lacked any vasodilatory action and did not induce "steal" phenomenon, nor low or no reflow, nor hypotensive effects.

In healthy volunteers, piracetam reduced the adhesion of RBCs to vascular endothelium and possessed also a direct stimulant effect on prostacycline synthesis in healthy endothelium.

- Effects on coagulation factors:

In healthy volunteers, compared with pre-treatment values, piracetam up to 9.6 g reduced plasma levels of fibrinogen and von Willebrand's factors (VIII: C; VIII R: AG; VIII R: vW) by 30 to 40 %, and increased bleeding time.

In patients with both primary and secondary Raynaud phenomenon, compared with pre-treatment values, piracetam 8 g/d during 6 months reduced plasma levels of fibrinogen and von Willebrand's factors (VIII: C; VIII R: AG; VIII R: vW (RCF)) by 30 to 40 %, reduced plasma viscosity, and increased bleeding time.

5.2 Pharmacokinetic properties
Piracetam is rapidly and almost completely absorbed. Peak plasma levels are reached within 1.5 hours after administration. The extent of oral bioavailability, assessed from the Area Under Curve (AUC), is close to 100% for capsules, tablets and solution. Peak levels and AUC are proportional to the dose given. The volume of distribution

of piracetam is 0.7 L/kg, and the plasma half-life is 5.0 hours, in young adult men. Piracetam crosses the blood-brain and the placental barrier and diffuses across membranes used in renal dialysis. Up to now, no metabolite of piracetam has been found. Piracetam is excreted almost completely in urine and the fraction of the dose excreted in urine is independent of the dose given. Excretion half-life values are consistent with those calculated from plasma / blood data. Clearance of the compound is dependent on the renal creatinine clearance and would be expected to diminish with renal insufficiency.

5.3 Preclinical safety data
Single doses of piracetam yielded LD 50 values at 26 g/kg in mice but LD 50 values were not reached in rats. In dogs, clinical signs after acute oral dosing were mild and lethality was not observed at the maximum tested dose of 10 g/kg.

Repeated oral treatment for up to 1 year in dogs (10 g/kg) and 6 months in rats (2 g/kg) was very well tolerated: no target organ toxicity or signs of (irreversible) toxicity were clearly demonstrated. Safe dose levels represent a multiple of the maximum intended human daily dose of 0.4 g/kg.

In terms of exposure (C max) safe levels obtained in the rat and the dog represent respectively 8 fold and 50 fold of the maximum human therapeutic level. AUC levels obtained in the same animals were a multiple of the human AUC level at the maximum intended daily dose.

The only change which might eventually be attributed to chronic treatment in male, but not in female, rats was an increase of the incidence over control animals of progressive glomerulonephrosis at the dose of 2.4 g/k/day given for 112 weeks.

Although piracetam crosses the placenta into the foetal circulation, no teratogenic effects were observed at dose levels up to 4.8 g/kg/day (mice, rats) and 2.7 g/kg/day (rabbits). Furthermore, the compound affects neither fertility nor the peri- or postnatal development of the pregnancy at doses up to 2.7 g/kg/day.

Piracetam was found to be devoid of any mutagenic or clastogenic activity and does not represent any genotoxic or carcinogenic risk to man.

6. PHARMACEUTICAL PARTICULARS

6.1 List of excipients
Nootropil 800 and 1200 mg Tablets:

Polyethylene glycol 6000

Colloidal anhydrous silica

Magnesium stearate

Methocel

Titanium dioxide (E171)

Polyethylene glycol 400

Nootropil Solution 33%:

Glycerol

Methy parahydroxybenzoate

Propyl parahydroxybenzoate

Sodium acetate

Acetic acid

Purified water

6.2 Incompatibilities
None known.

6.3 Shelf life
Nootropil 800 and 1200 mg Tablets:

Four (4) years.

Nootropil Solution 33%:

Five (5) years.

6.4 Special precautions for storage
None.

6.5 Nature and contents of container
Nootropil 800 mg Tablets - Blister pack in an outer cardboard carton (90 tablets per carton).

Nootropil 1200 mg Tablets – Blister pack in an outer cardboard carton (60 tablets per carton).

Nootropil Solution 33% - Glass bottle containing 125 ml or 300 ml solution.

6.6 Instructions for use and handling
Tablets – None.

Solution – Do not store above 25°C.

7. MARKETING AUTHORISATION HOLDER
UCB Pharma Ltd.,

UCB House,

3, George Street,

WATFORD,

Herts WD18 0UH.

8. MARKETING AUTHORISATION NUMBER(S)
Nootropil Tablets 800 mg: PL 08972/0011

Nootropil Tablets 1200 mg: PL 08972/0012

Nootropil Solution 33%: PL 08972/0013

9. DATE OF FIRST AUTHORISATION/RENEWAL OF THE AUTHORISATION
14 December 1992.

10. DATE OF REVISION OF THE TEXT
May 2005.

Norditropin Simplexx 5 mg/1.5 ml, Norditropin Simplexx 10 mg/1.5 ml, Norditropin Simplexx 15 mg/1.5 ml

(Novo Nordisk Limited)

1. NAME OF THE MEDICINAL PRODUCT
Norditropin® SimpleXx® 5 mg/1.5 ml, solution for injection.

Norditropin® SimpleXx® 10 mg/1.5 ml, solution for injection.

Norditropin® SimpleXx® 15 mg/1.5 ml, solution for injection.

2. QUALITATIVE AND QUANTITATIVE COMPOSITION
Norditropin SimpleXx:

Somatropin 5 mg/1.5 ml (3.3 mg/ml), 10 mg/1.5 ml (6.7 mg/ml) and 15 mg/1.5 ml (10 mg/ml).

Somatropin (epr).

1 mg of somatropin corresponds to 3 IU (International Unit) of somatropin.

3. PHARMACEUTICAL FORM
Solution for injection.

4. CLINICAL PARTICULARS

4.1 Therapeutic indications
Children:

Growth failure due to growth hormone insufficiency.

Growth failure in girls due to gonadal dysgenesis (Turner's Syndrome).

Growth retardation in prepubertal children due to chronic renal disease.

Growth disturbance (current height SDS < -2.5 and parental adjusted height SDS < -1) in short children born small for gestational age (SGA), with a birth weight and/or length below -2 SD, who failed to show catch-up growth (HV SDS < 0 during the last year) by 4 years of age or later.

Adults:

Pronounced growth hormone deficiency in known hypothalamic-pituitary disease (one other deficient axis, other than prolactin), demonstrated by two provocative tests after institution of adequate replacement therapy for any other deficient axis.

Childhood onset growth hormone insufficiency, reconfirmed by two provocative tests.

In adults, the insulin tolerance test is the provocative test of choice. When the insulin tolerance test is contraindicated, alternative provocative tests must be used. The combined arginine-growth hormone releasing hormone is recommended. An arginine or the glucagon test may also be considered; however these tests have less established diagnostic value than the insulin tolerance test.

4.2 Posology and method of administration
The dosage is individual and must always be adjusted in accordance with the individual's response to therapy.

Prescription only.

Norditropin should only be prescribed by doctors with special knowledge of the therapeutic indication of use.

Generally, daily subcutaneous administration in the evening is recommended. The injection site should be varied to prevent lipoatrophy.

Generally recommended dosages:

Children:

Growth hormone insufficiency

25-35 μg/kg/day or 0.7-1.0 mg/m²/day

Equal to: 0.07-0.1 IU/kg/day (2-3 IU/m²/day)

Turner's syndrome

50 μg/kg/day or 1.4 mg/m²/day

Equal to: 0.14 IU/kg/day (4.3 IU/m²/day)

Chronic Renal Disease

50 μg/kg/day or 1.4 mg/m²/day

Equal to: 0.14 IU/kg/day (4.3 IU/m²/day)

Small for Gestational Age

35 μg/kg/day or 1 mg/m²/day

Equal to: 0.1 IU/kg/day (3 IU/m²/day)

A dose of 0.035 mg/kg/day is usually recommended until final height is reached. (See section 5.1).

Treatment should be discontinued after the first year of treatment, if the height velocity SDS is below +1.

Treatment should be discontinued if height velocity is < 2 cm/year and, if confirmation is required, bone age is > 14 years (girls) or > 16 years (boys), corresponding to closure of the epiphyseal growth plates.

Adults:

Replacement therapy in adults

The dosage must be adjusted to the need of the individual patient. It is recommended to start treatment with a low dose 0.15-0.3 mg/day (equal to 0.45-0.9 IU/day). It is recommended to increase the dosage gradually at monthly intervals based on the clinical response and the patient's experience of adverse events. Serum insulin-like growth factor I (IGF-I) can be used as guidance for the dose titration.

Dose requirements decline with age. Maintenance dosage varies considerably from person to person, but seldom exceeds 1.0 mg/day (equal to 3 IU/day).

4.3 Contraindications
Any evidence of active malignant tumours.

Intracranial neoplasm must be inactive and anti-tumour therapy should be completed prior to institution of therapy.

Pregnancy and lactation. Please refer to Section 4.6.

Hypersensitivity to somatropin or to any of the excipients.

In the children with chronic renal disease treatment with Norditropin SimpleXx should be discontinued at renal transplantation.

4.4 Special warnings and special precautions for use
Children treated with Norditropin SimpleXx should be regularly assessed by a specialist in child growth. Norditropin SimpleXx treatment should always be instigated by a physician with special knowledge of growth hormone insufficiency and its treatment. This is true also for the management of Turner's syndrome and chronic renal disease and SGA. Data of final adult height following the use of Norditropin for children with chronic renal disease are not available.

The stimulation of skeletal growth in children can only be expected until the epiphysial discs are closed.

The dosage in children with chronic renal disease is individual and must be adjusted according to the individual response to therapy. The growth disturbance should be clearly established before Norditropin SimpleXx treatment by following growth on optimal treatment for renal disease over one year. Conservative management of uraemia with customary medication and if needed dialysis should be maintained during Norditropin SimpleXx therapy.

Patients with chronic renal disease normally experience a decline in renal function as part of the natural course of their illness. However, as a precautionary measure during Norditropin SimpleXx treatment renal function should be monitored for an excessive decline, or increase in the glomerular filtration rate (which could imply hyperfiltration).

In short children born SGA other medical reasons or treatments that could explain growth disturbance should be ruled out before starting treatment.

In SGA children it is recommended to measure fasting insulin and blood glucose before start of treatment and annually thereafter. In patients with increased risk for diabetes mellitus (e.g. familial history of diabetes, obesity, severe insulin resistance, acanthosis nigricans) oral glucose tolerance testing (OGTT) should be performed. If overt diabetes occurs, growth hormone should not be administered.

In SGA children it is recommended to measure the IGF-I level before start of treatment and twice a year thereafter. If on repeated measurements IGF-I levels exceed +2 SD compared to references for age and pubertal status, the IGF-I / IGFBP-3 ratio could be taken into account to consider dose adjustment.

Experience in initiating treatment in SGA patients near onset of puberty is limited. It is therefore not recommended to initiate treatment near onset of puberty.

Experience with patients with Silver-Russell syndrome is limited.

Some of the height gain obtained with treating short children born SGA with growth hormone may be lost if treatment is stopped before final height is reached.

Somatropin has been found to influence carbohydrate metabolism, therefore, patients should be observed for evidence of glucose intolerance.

Serum thyroxine levels may fall during treatment with Norditropin SimpleXx due to the increased peripheral deiodination of T4 to T3.

In patients with a pituitary disease in progression, hypothyroidism may develop.

Patients with Turner's syndrome have an increased risk of developing primary hypothyroidism associated with anti-thyroid antibodies.

As hypothyroidism interferes with the response to Norditropin SimpleXx therapy patients should have their thyroid function tested regularly, and should receive replacement therapy with thyroid hormone when indicated.

In insulin treated patients adjustment of insulin dose may be needed after initiation of Norditropin SimpleXx treatment.

Patients with growth hormone deficiency secondary to an intracranial lesion should be examined frequently for progression or recurrence of the underlying disease process.

Leukaemia has been reported in a small number of growth hormone deficient patients some of whom have been treated with somatropin. Based on 10 years global assessment there is no increased risk of development of leukaemia during somatropin treatment. In patients in complete remission from tumours or malignant disease, growth hormone therapy has not been associated with an increased relapse rate. Nevertheless, patients who have achieved complete remission of malignant disease should be followed closely for relapse after commencement of Norditropin SimpleXx therapy.

Slipped capital femoral epiphysis may occur more frequently in patients with endocrine disorders and

Legg-Calvé-Perthes disease may occur more frequently in patients with short stature. These diseases may present as the development of a limp or complaints of hip or knee pain and physicians and parents should be alerted to this possibility.

Scoliosis may progress in any child during rapid growth. Signs of scoliosis should be monitored during treatment. However, growth hormone treatment has not been shown to increase the incidence or severity of scoliosis.

In the event of severe or recurrent headache, visual problems, nausea, and/or vomiting, a funduscopy for papilloedema is recommended. If papilloedema is confirmed, a diagnosis of benign intracranial hypertension should be considered and if appropriate the growth hormone treatment should be discontinued.

At present there is insufficient evidence to guide clinical decision making in patients with resolved intracranial hypertension. If growth hormone treatment is restarted, careful monitoring for symptoms of intracranial hypertension is necessary.

Growth hormone deficiency in adults is a lifelong disease and needs to be treated accordingly, however, experience in patients older than 60 years and in patients with more than five years of treatment in adult growth hormone deficiency is still limited.

4.5 Interaction with other medicinal products and other forms of Interaction

Concomitant glucocorticoid therapy may inhibit growth and thereby oppose the growth promoting effect of Norditropin SimpleXx. The effect of growth hormone on final height can also be influenced by additional therapy with other hormones, e.g. gonadotrophin, anabolic steroids, estrogen and thyroid hormone.

4.6 Pregnancy and lactation

Currently there is insufficient evidence of safety of somatropin therapy during pregnancy. The possibility that somatropin is secreted in breast milk cannot be discounted.

4.7 Effects on ability to drive and use machines

No effects.

4.8 Undesirable effects

Fluid retention with peripheral oedema may occur and especially in adults carpal tunnel syndrome may be seen. The symptoms are usually transient and dose dependent, but may require dose reduction. Mild arthralgia, muscle pain, paresthesia may also occur in adults, but is usually self-limiting.

Adverse reactions in children are rare. The integrated Norditropin database comprises data from children being treated for up to eight years. Headache has been reported with an incidence of 0.04 per patient year.

Formation of antibodies directed against somatropin has rarely been observed during Norditropin therapy. The titres and binding capacities of these antibodies have been very low and have not interfered with the growth response to Norditropin administration.

During treatment with Norditropin SimpleXx local injection site reactions may occur.

Some rare cases of benign intracranial hypertension have been reported.

4.9 Overdose

Information on overdose and poisoning is lacking.

Acute overdosage can lead to low blood glucose levels initially, followed by high blood glucose levels. These decreased glucose levels have been detected biochemically, but without clinical signs of hypoglycaemia. Long-term overdosage could result in signs and symptoms consistent with the known effects of human growth hormone excess.

5. PHARMACOLOGICAL PROPERTIES

5.1 Pharmacodynamic properties

ATC:H 01 AC 01.

Norditropin SimpleXx contains somatropin, which is human growth hormone produced by recombinant DNA-technology. It is an anabolic peptide of 191 amino acids stabilised by two disulphide bridges with a molecular weight of approximately 22,000 Daltons.

The major effects of Norditropin SimpleXx are stimulation of skeletal and somatic growth and pronounced influence on the body's metabolic processes.

When growth hormone deficiency is treated a normalisation of body composition takes place resulting in an increase in lean body mass and a decrease in fat mass. Somatropin exerts most of its actions through insulin-like growth factor I (IGF-I), which are produced in tissues throughout the body, but predominantly by the liver.

More than 90% of IGF-I is bound to binding proteins (IGFBPs) of which IGFBP-3 is the most important.

A lipolytic and protein sparing effect of the hormone becomes of particular importance during stress.

Somatropin also increases bone turnover indicated by an increase in plasma levels of biochemical bone markers. In adults bone mass is slightly decreased during the initial months of treatment due to more pronounced bone resorption, however, bone mass increases with prolonged treatment.

In clinical trials in short children born SGA doses of 0.033 and 0.067 mg/kg/day have been used for treatment until final height. In 56 patients who were continuously treated and have reached (near) final height, the mean change from height at start of treatment was +1.90 SDS (0.033 mg/kg/day) and +2.19 SDS (0.067 mg/kg/day). Literature data from untreated SGA children without early spontaneous catch-up suggest a late growth of 0.5 SDS. Long-term safety data are still limited.

5.2 Pharmacokinetic properties

I.v. infusion of Norditropin (33 ng/kg/min for 3 hours) to nine growth hormone deficient patients, gave the following results: serum half-time of 21.1 ± 1.7 min., metabolic clearance rate of 2.33 ± 0.58 ml/kg/min. and a distribution space of 67.6 ± 14.6 ml/kg.

S.c. injection of Norditropin SimpleXx (2.5 mg/m^2) to 31 healthy subjects (with endogenous somatropin suppressed by continuous infusion of somastatin) gave the following results:

Maximal concentration of human growth hormone (42-46 ng/ml) after approximately 4 hours. Thereafter human growth hormone declined with a half life of approximately 2.6 hours.

In addition the different strengths of Norditropin SimpleXx were demonstrated to be bioequivalent to each other and to conventional Norditropin after subcutaneous injection to healthy subjects.

5.3 Preclinical safety data

The general pharmacological effects on the CNS, cardiovascular and respiratory systems following administration of Norditropin SimpleXx with and without forced degradation were investigated in mice and rats; renal function was also evaluated. The degraded product showed no difference in effect when compared with Norditropin SimpleXx and Norditropin. All three preparations showed the expected dose dependent decrease in urine volume and retention of sodium and chloride ions.

In rats, similar pharmacokinetics has been demonstrated between Norditropin SimpleXx and Norditropin. Degraded Norditropin SimpleXx has also been demonstrated to be bioequivalent with Norditropin SimpleXx.

Single and repeated dose toxicity and local tolerance studies of Norditropin SimpleXx or the degraded product did not reveal any toxic effect or damage to the muscle tissue.

The toxicity of Poloxamer 188 has been tested in mice, rats, rabbits and dogs and no findings of toxicological relevance were revealed.

Poloxamer 188 was rapidly absorbed from the injection site with no significant retention of the dose at the site of injection. Poloxamer 188 was excreted primarily via the urine.

6. PHARMACEUTICAL PARTICULARS

6.1 List of excipients

Mannitol, Histidine, Poloxamer 188, Phenol, Water for Injections.

6.2 Incompatibilities

In the absence of compatibility studies, the medicinal product must not be mixed with other medicinal products.

6.3 Shelf life

Norditropin SimpleXx 5 mg/1.5 ml and 10 mg/1.5 ml:

The shelf life is 2 years.

After first opening: store for a maximum of 28 days at + 2°C - + 8°C.

Alternatively, the medicinal product may be stored for a maximum of 21 days not above +25°C.

Norditropin SimpleXx 15 mg/1.5 ml

The shelf life is 2 years.

After first opening: store for a maximum of 28 days at + 2°C - + 8°C.

6.4 Special precautions for storage

Norditropin SimpleXx 5 mg/1.5 ml and 10 mg/1.5 ml:

Before use: Store at + 2°C - + 8°C in the outer carton. Do not freeze.

Once opened, the product may be stored for a maximum of 28 days at + 2°C - + 8°C, *alternatively* stored not above + 25°C for a maximum of 21 days. Store in the pen (NordiPen®) during use. Do not freeze.

Norditropin SimpleXx 15 mg/1.5 ml

Before use: Store at + 2°C - + 8°C in the outer carton. Do not freeze.

Once opened, the product may be stored for a maximum of 28 days at + 2°C - + 8°C. Store in the pen (NordiPen®) during use. Do not freeze.

6.5 Nature and contents of container

Norditropin SimpleXx is contained in a colourless cartridge made of type I glass. The cartridge is closed at the bottom with a rubber stopper shaped as a plunger and at the top with a laminated rubber stopper shaped as a disc and sealed with an aluminium cap. The aluminium cap is finally sealed with a coloured cap (5 mg/1.5 ml (yellow), 10 mg/1.5 ml (blue), 15 mg/1.5 ml (green)).

The cartridge is contained in a blister packed in a carton.

Pack sizes: Norditropin SimpleXx 1 × 5mg/1.5ml

Norditropin SimpleXx 1 × 10mg/1.5ml

Norditropin SimpleXx 1 × 15 mg/1.5ml

6.6 Instructions for use and handling

Patients should be reminded to wash their hands thoroughly with soap and water and/or disinfectant prior to any contact with Norditropin. Norditropin should not be shaken vigorously at any time.

Norditropin SimpleXx 5 mg/1.5 ml, 10 mg/1.5 ml and 15 mg/1.5 ml should only be prescribed for use with the matching NordiPen® (NordiPen® 5, 10 and 15 respectively). Instructions for use of Norditropin SimpleXx in NordiPen® are provided within the respective packs. Patients should be advised to read these instructions very carefully.

Do not use Norditropin SimpleXx if it does not appear water clear and colourless.

7. MARKETING AUTHORISATION HOLDER

Novo Nordisk Limited

Broadfield Park, Brighton Road

Crawley, West Sussex

RH11 9RT

8. MARKETING AUTHORISATION NUMBER(S)

Norditropin® SimpleXx® 5 mg/1.5 ml - PL 03132/0131

Norditropin® SimpleXx® 10 mg/1.5 ml - PL 03132/0132

Norditropin® SimpleXx® 15 mg/1.5 ml - PL 03132/0133

9. DATE OF FIRST AUTHORISATION/RENEWAL OF THE AUTHORISATION

October 1999.

10. DATE OF REVISION OF THE TEXT

16 January 2002, 22 April 2002, 7 August 2003.

Legal Status

POM (Prescription Only Medicine), CD (Sch. 4).

Norethisterone Tablets

(Wockhardt UK Ltd)

1. NAME OF THE MEDICINAL PRODUCT

Norethisterone Tablets BP 5mg.

2. QUALITATIVE AND QUANTITATIVE COMPOSITION

Norethisterone 5.0mg.

3. PHARMACEUTICAL FORM

Tablet.

Norethisterone Tablets BP 5mg are 6.5mm, round, white, uncoated tablets with "NE 5" on one side and a break line on the other.

4. CLINICAL PARTICULARS

4.1 Therapeutic indications

Norethisterone has the following clinical indications:

At low dose:

Metropathia haemorrhagica

Pre-menstrual syndrome

Postponement of menstruation

Dysmenorrhoea

Endometriosis

Menorrhagia

At high dose:

Disseminated carcinoma of the breast.

4.2 Posology and method of administration

For oral administration

Low dose

1. Metropathia haemorrhagica (dysfunctional uterine bleeding): 5mg three times daily for ten days. Bleeding is arrested usually within one to three days. A withdrawal bleeding resembling normal menstruation occurs within two to four days after discontinuing treatment.

Prophylaxis of recurrence of dysfunctional bleeding: if there are no signs of resumption of normal ovarian function (no rise of morning temperature in the second half of the cycle), recurrence must be anticipated. Cyclical bleeding can be established with 5mg twice daily from the 19th to the 26th day of the cycle.

2. Pre-menstrual syndrome (including pre-menstrual mastalgia): Pre-menstrual symptoms such as headache, migraine, breast discomfort, water retention, tachycardia and psychic disturbances may be relieved by the administration of 10 – 15mg daily from the 19th to the 26th day of the cycle. Treatment should be repeated for several cycles. When treatment is stopped, the patient may remain symptom free for a number of months.

3. Postponement of menstruation: In cases of too frequent menstrual bleeding, and in special circumstances (e.g. operations, travel, sports) 5mg three times daily, starting three days before the expected onset of menstruation. A normal period should occur two to three days after the patient has stopped taking tablets.

4. Dysmenorrhoea: Functional or primary dysmenorrhoea is almost invariably relieved by the suppression of ovulation. 5mg three times daily for 20 days, starting on the fifth day of the cycle (the first day of menstruation counting as day one). Treatment should be maintained for three to four cycles followed by treatment-free cycles. A further course of therapy may be employed if symptoms return.

5. Endometriosis (pseudo-pregnancy therapy): long-term treatment is commenced on the fifth day of the cycle with 10mg daily for the first few weeks. In the event of spotting, the dosage is increased to 20mg and, if necessary, 25mg daily.

After bleeding has ceased, the initial dose is usually sufficient. Duration of treatment: four to six months continuously, or longer if necessary.

6. Menorrhagia (hypermenorrhoea): 5mg two to three times a day from the 19th to the 26th day of the cycle (counting the first day of menstruation as day one).

High dose

For disseminated breast carcinoma the starting dose is 8 tablets (40mg) per day increasing to 12 tablets (60mg) if no regression is noted.

Not for use in children.

Not for elderly patients.

4.3 Contraindications

Pregnancy. Hepatic impairment or hepatic disease. Dubin-Johnson and Rotor syndromes. History during pregnancy of: idiopathic jaundice, severe pruritus, pemphigoid gestationis or herpes gestationis. Undiagnosed vaginal bleeding. History or current high risk of arterial disease. Breast or genital tract carcinoma, unless norethisterone is being used as part of the management of these conditions. Porphyria.

4.4 Special warnings and special precautions for use

Alterations in liver function have been reported. In common with other steroids, norethisterone should be given with care to patients with:

- Liver disturbances
- History of depression
- Epilepsy
- Asthma
- Migraine
- Diabetes mellitus
- Hypertension
- Cardiac or renal disease
- Other conditions which may be aggravated by fluid retention.

4.5 Interaction with other medicinal products and other forms of Interaction

The effects of norethisterone will be altered if other sex hormones are prescribed simultaneously.

Cyclosporin metabolism is inhibited by progestogens.

Rifamycins and nevirapine may accelerate metabolism of progestogens.

4.6 Pregnancy and lactation

Norethisterone is contraindicated in pregnancy, and should be avoided during lactation, as it is present in breast milk.

4.7 Effects on ability to drive and use machines

None.

4.8 Undesirable effects

Side-effects rarely occur with doses of 15mg daily.

The commonest side-effect is breakthrough bleeding, particularly when treatment is continuous over a long period. Other reported side effects are nausea, vomiting, acne, oedema, changes in appetite or weight, fluid retention, melasma or chloasma, allergic skin rashes and urticaria. Breast changes, including discomfort, headache and depression, changes in libido, hair loss, fatigue, drowsiness or insomnia, fever, pre-menstrual syndrome like symptoms. Androgenic effects with deepening of the voice and hirsutism and oestrogenic effects have been reported after prolonged therapy.

Anaphylaxis or anaphylactoid reactions may occur rarely. Alterations in liver function have been reported and jaundice has been reported rarely. Virilisation of female foetuses have been reported. Exacerbation of epilepsy and migraine.

Intolerance to contact lenses and deterioration in vision in patients who are short sighted has been reported with the use of the combined oral contraceptive pill and may be applicable to this product.

4.9 Overdose

There are no reports of ill-effects from overdose.

5. PHARMACOLOGICAL PROPERTIES

5.1 Pharmacodynamic properties

Norethisterone is a synthetic, potent, orally active progestogen which, by virtue of its progestogenic effects, produces secretory effects on oestrogen-primed genital tissue, has a sedative effect on uterine muscle and a styptic effect on uterine haemorrhage.

Norethisterone also has some androgenic effects and some weak oestrogenic activity.

5.2 Pharmacokinetic properties

Norethisterone when given orally is well absorbed from the gastrointestinal tract, with peak plasma concentrations (which may be dose dependent) generally occurring within one to two and a half-hours.

Bioavailability of norethisterone is variable, probably due to first pass effects in gut wall or liver, which may be influenced by many factors including hormonal status, diet and exercise.

Plasma half-life after a dose of 5mg is of the order of five hours. After 24 hours plasma levels are generally about 1% of peak concentration.

5.3 Preclinical safety data

There are no pre-clinical data of any relevance to the prescriber which are additional to those already included in other sections.

6. PHARMACEUTICAL PARTICULARS

6.1 List of excipients

Lactose

Maize starch

Magnesium stearate

6.2 Incompatibilities

None.

6.3 Shelf life

Five years.

6.4 Special precautions for storage

Do not store above 25°C.

Store in the original package.

6.5 Nature and contents of container

Opaque plastic tablet containers with press-on tamper evident lid containing 100 and 500 tablets.

Blister pack of PVC and aluminium foil containing 30, 72 and 180 tablets.

6.6 Instructions for use and handling

None.

Administrative Data

7. MARKETING AUTHORISATION HOLDER

CP Pharmaceuticals Ltd

Ash Road North

Wrexham

LL13 9UF

UK

8. MARKETING AUTHORISATION NUMBER(S)

4543/0409

9. DATE OF FIRST AUTHORISATION/RENEWAL OF THE AUTHORISATION

15th September 1998

10. DATE OF REVISION OF THE TEXT

August 2002

Norgalax

(Norgine Limited)

1. NAME OF THE MEDICINAL PRODUCT

NORGALAX

2. QUALITATIVE AND QUANTITATIVE COMPOSITION

Norgalax contains the active ingredient Docusate Sodium 0.12 g in each 10 g micro-enema:

3. PHARMACEUTICAL FORM

Rectal gel.

4. CLINICAL PARTICULARS

4.1 Therapeutic indications

For the symptomatic treatment of constipation whenever an enema is required and for the preparation of the colon and rectum for endoscopic examination.

4.2 Posology and method of administration

Adults: use one micro-enema. If required, a second micro-enema may be used on the same or the next day.

Children: not recommended for children under 12 years old.

Norgalax is to be administered rectally. Remove the protective cap and insert the applicator into the rectum, squeezing gently until the tube is empty. A drop of the gel may be used as a lubricant if required.

4.3 Contraindications

Haemorrhoids, anal fissures, rectocolitis, bleeding, abdominal pain, intestinal obstruction, nausea, vomiting and inflammatory bowel disease.

4.4 Special warnings and special precautions for use

As with all laxatives, Norgalax should not be administered chronically. Prolonged use can precipitate the onset of an atonic non-functioning colon and hypokalaemia.

4.5 Interaction with other medicinal products and other forms of Interaction

Norgalax may increase the resorption of medicines and is not to be used in combination with hepatotoxic agents.

4.6 Pregnancy and lactation

Norgalax may be used during pregnancy and lactation.

4.7 Effects on ability to drive and use machines

None known.

4.8 Undesirable effects

Anal or rectal burning and pain, usually short lasting diarrhoea, congestion of the rectal mucosa and rectal bleeding may occur occasionally. Hepatotoxicity has been reported especially when used in association with other laxatives.

4.9 Overdose

Overdose will lead to excessive purgation which should be treated symptomatically.

5. PHARMACOLOGICAL PROPERTIES

Docusate sodium is an anionic surfactant and used as a faecal softening agent. It is considered to ease constipation by increasing the penetration of fluid into the faeces thereby causing them to soften. Norgalax is usually effective in 5 to 20 minutes.

5.1 Pharmacodynamic properties

Not applicable.

5.2 Pharmacokinetic properties

Not applicable.

5.3 Preclinical safety data

Not applicable.

6. PHARMACEUTICAL PARTICULARS

6.1 List of excipients

Glycerol

Sodium carboxymethyl cellulose

Purified Water

6.2 Incompatibilities

None known

6.3 Shelf life

The shelf life is 4 years.

6.4 Special precautions for storage

Do not store above 25°C.

6.5 Nature and contents of container

A polyethylene tube with fixed applicator and a cap closure, containing 10g of gel in pack sizes of 6 and 100 tubes.

6.6 Instructions for use and handling

None.

7. MARKETING AUTHORISATION HOLDER

Norgine Limited

Chaplin House

Widewater Place

Moorhall Road

Harefield

UXBRIDGE

Middlesex UB9 6NS

United Kingdom

8. MARKETING AUTHORISATION NUMBER(S)

PL 0322/0065.

9. DATE OF FIRST AUTHORISATION/RENEWAL OF THE AUTHORISATION

February 1999

10. DATE OF REVISION OF THE TEXT

January 1999

Norgeston

(Schering Health Care Limited)

1. NAME OF THE MEDICINAL PRODUCT

Norgeston®

2. QUALITATIVE AND QUANTITATIVE COMPOSITION

Each tablet contains 30 micrograms levonorgestrel.

3. PHARMACEUTICAL FORM

Sugar-coated tablets

4. CLINICAL PARTICULARS

4.1 Therapeutic indications

Oral contraception

4.2 Posology and method of administration

First treatment cycle:

One tablet daily, starting on the first day of the menstrual cycle, at a time of day chosen by the patient. All subsequent tablets must then be taken at this time. The contraceptive effect is likely to be reduced if a tablet is delayed by more than three hours. Additional non-hormonal methods of contraception (except the rhythm or temperature methods) must be used until the first 14 tablets have been taken.

Subsequent cycles:

The tablets are taken daily and pack follows pack without interruption, and without regard to bleeding.

Changing from other hormonal contraceptives:

The first tablet of Norgeston should be taken on the first day immediately after the end of the previous oral contraceptive course. Additional, non-hormonal contraceptive methods (except the rhythm or temperature methods) should be used for the first 14 days of tablet-taking.

Post-partum and post-abortum use:

After pregnancy, Norgeston can be started 7 days after a vaginal delivery provided that the patient is fully ambulant and there are no puerperal complications. After a first trimester abortion, Norgeston may be started immediately. Additional contraceptive precautions will be required for the first 14 days of pill-taking.

Special circumstances requiring additional contraception:

Incorrect administration:

If a tablet is taken late (i.e. if it is more than 27 hours since the last tablet was taken) or if a tablet is missed, protection against conception may be impaired. Therefore, when such incidents occur, additional, non-hormonal contraceptive methods (except the rhythm or temperature methods) must be employed until 14 consecutive tablets have been taken in the correct manner.

Gastro-intestinal upsets:

Vomiting or diarrhoea may reduce the effectiveness of the tablets by preventing them from being fully absorbed. If the user vomits shortly after taking her daily Norgeston tablet, she can maintain protection against contraception by taking a second tablet within 3 hours of the normal time - provided she does not vomit again. For this second intake, the last tablet in the pack should be used.

In the case of repeated vomiting or prolonged diarrhoea, additional, non-hormonal contraceptive methods (except the rhythm or temperature method) should be continued for a further 14 days after the symptoms have subsided. If the condition reducing the efficacy of the preparation is protracted, other methods of contraception should be considered.

4.3 Contraindications

1. Pregnancy
2. Severe disturbances of liver function
3. Jaundice or persistent itching during a previous pregnancy
4. Dubin-Johnson syndrome
5. Rotor syndrome
6. Previous or existing liver tumours
7. A history of herpes of pregnancy
8. Mammary carcinoma or a history of this condition
9. Undiagnosed abnormal vaginal bleeding
10. History of or existing thromboembolic processes (e.g. stroke, myocardial infarction)
11. Severe diabetes with vascular changes
12. Sickle-cell anaemia
13. Hypersensitivity to any of the components of Norgeston

4.4 Special warnings and special precautions for use

Diabetes mellitus or tendency towards diabetes mellitus require careful medical supervision.

There is a general opinion, based on statistical evidence, that users of hormonal contraceptives experience, more often than non-users, venous thromboembolism, arterial thrombosis, including cerebral and myocardial infarction, and subarachnoid haemorrhage. Full recovery from such disorders does not always occur, and it should be realised that in a few cases they are fatal.

According to the present state of knowledge, an association between the use of hormonal contraceptives and an increased risk of venous and arterial thromboembolic diseases cannot be ruled out.

The relative risk of arterial thrombosis (e.g. stroke, myocardial infarction) appears to increase further when heavy smoking, increasing age and the use of hormonal contraceptives coincide.

A meta-analysis from 54 epidemiological studies reported that there is a slightly increased relative risk of having breast cancer diagnosed in women who are currently using oral contraceptives (OC). The observed pattern of increased risk may be due to an earlier diagnosis of breast cancer in OC users, the biological effects of OCs or a combination of both. The additional breast cancers diagnosed in current users of OCs or in women who have used OCs in the last 10 years are more likely to be localised to the breast than those in women who never used OCs.

Breast cancer is rare among women under 40 years of age whether or not they take OCs. Whilst the background risk increases with age, the excess number of breast cancer diagnoses in current and recent progestogen-only pill (POP) users is small in relation to the overall risk of breast cancer, possibly of similar magnitude to that associated with combined OCs. However, for POPs, the evidence is based on much smaller populations of users and so is less conclusive than that for combined OCs.

The most important risk factor for breast cancer in POP users is the age women discontinue the POP; the older the age at stopping, the more breast cancers are diagnosed. Duration of use is less important and the excess risk gradually disappears during the course of the 10 years after stopping POP use, such that by 10 years there appears to be no excess.

The evidence suggests that compared with never-users, among 10,000 women who use POPs for up to 5 years but stop by age 20, there would be much less than 1 extra case of breast cancer diagnosed up to 10 years afterwards. For those stopping by age 30 after 5 years use of the POP, there would be an estimated 2-3 extra cases (additional to the 44 cases of breast cancer per 10,000 women in this age group never exposed to oral contraceptives). For those stopping by age 40 after 5 years use, there would be an estimated 10 extra cases diagnosed up to 10 years afterwards (additional to the 160 cases of breast cancer per 10,000 never-exposed women in this age group).

It is important to inform patients that users of all contraceptive pills appear to have a small increase in the risk of being diagnosed with breast cancer, compared with non-users of oral contraceptives, but that this has to be weighed against the known benefits.

If there is a history of ectopic pregnancy or one Fallopian tube is missing, the use of Norgeston should be decided on only after carefully weighing the benefits against the risks.

If obscure lower abdominal complaints occur together with an irregular cycle pattern (above all amenorrhoea followed by persistent irregular bleeding), an extrauterine pregnancy must be considered.

In rare cases benign, and in even rarer cases, malignant liver tumours leading in isolated cases to life-threatening intra-abdominal haemorrhage have been observed after the use of hormonal substances such as the one contained in Norgeston. If severe upper abdominal complaints, liver enlargement or signs of intra-abdominal haemorrhage occur, a liver tumour should be included in the differential diagnostic considerations.

Reasons for stopping Norgeston immediately

1. Occurrence for the first time, or exacerbation, of migrainous headaches or unusually frequent or unusually severe headaches
2. Sudden disturbances of vision or hearing or other perceptual disorders
3. First signs of thrombophlebitis or thromboembolic symptoms (for example, unusual pains in or swelling of the legs, stabbing pains on breathing or coughing for no apparent reason), feeling of pain and tightness in the chest.
4. Six weeks before an elective major operation (e.g. abdominal, orthopaedic) any surgery to the legs, medical treatment for varicose veins or prolonged immobilisation e.g. after accidents or surgery. Do not restart until 2 weeks after full ambulation. In case of emergency surgery, thrombotic prophylaxis is usually indicated e.g. subcutaneous heparin.
5. Onset of jaundice, hepatitis, itching of the whole body
6. Significant rise in blood pressure
7. Clear exacerbation of conditions known to be capable of deteriorating during oral contraception or pregnancy
8. Pregnancy

Pregnancy is a reason for stopping immediately because it has been suggested by some investigations that oral contraceptives taken in early pregnancy may slightly increase the risk of foetal malformations. Other investigations have failed to support these findings. The possibility therefore cannot be excluded, but it is certain that if a risk exists at all it is very small.

Assessment of women prior to starting oral contraceptives (and at regular intervals thereafter) should include a personal and family medical history of each woman. Physical examination should be guided by this and by the contraindications (section 4.3) and warnings (section 4.4) for this product. The frequency and nature of these assessments should be based upon relevant guidelines and should be adapted to the individual woman, but should include measurement of blood pressure and, if judged appropriate by the clinician, breast, abdominal and pelvic examination including cervical cytology.

4.5 Interaction with other medicinal products and other forms of Interaction

Hepatic enzyme inducers such as barbiturates, primidone, phenobarbitone, phenytoin, phenylbutazone, rifampicin, carbamazepine and griseofulvin can impair the efficacy of Norgeston. For women receiving long-term therapy with hepatic enzyme inducers, another method of contraception should be used. The use of antibiotics may also reduce the efficacy of Norgeston, possibly by altering the intestinal flora.

Women receiving short courses of enzyme inducers or broad spectrum antibiotics should take additional non-hormonal (except rhythm or temperature methods) contraceptive precautions during the time of concurrent medication and for 14 days afterwards. With rifampicin, additional contraceptive precautions should be continued for 4 weeks after treatment stops, even if only a short course was administered.

The requirement for oral antidiabetics or insulin can change as a result of an effect on glucose tolerance in diabetes mellitus.

The herbal remedy St John's wort (Hypericum perforatum) should not be taken concomitantly with Norgeston as this could potentially lead to a loss of contraceptive effect.

4.6 Pregnancy and lactation

The administration of Norgeston during pregnancy is contraindicated.

If pregnancy occurs during medication with Norgeston the preparation is to be withdrawn immediately.

There is no evidence that Norgeston diminishes the yield of breast milk. However, minute amounts of the active substance are excreted with the milk.

4.7 Effects on ability to drive and use machines

None known.

4.8 Undesirable effects

In rare cases, nausea, vomiting, dizziness, headaches, migraine, depressive moods, changes in body weight and libido and allergic reactions can occur. Amenorrhoea and changes in the pattern of the menstrual cycle have also been observed.

Menstrual changes:

A usual, feature of all progestogen-only oral contraceptives is that they can produce an initial irregularity of the bleeding pattern, but such irregularity tends to decrease with time. Some women may experience amenorrhoea.

For these reasons the possibility of such changes in menstrual rhythm should, as a precaution, be pointed out to the patient before the start of tablet-taking.

Missed menstruation:

If no menstrual bleeding has occurred within 6 weeks after the last menstrual bleeding, pregnancy must be excluded before tablet-taking is continued. If pregnancy has been excluded and the amenorrhoea lasts longer than 3 months or recurs repeatedly, Norgeston should be withheld until normal menstrual bleeding has been restored.

Procedure in the event of irregular bleeding:

Irregular bleeding is not a medical reason for stopping tablet-taking, as long as organic causes for such bleeding and pregnancy can be ruled out provided it is ensured that the patient is fully compliant.

It is extremely inadvisable to attempt to influence cycle disturbances by the additional administration of an oestrogen. This would only serve to reverse the changes brought about by Norgeston in the cervical mucus, thereby seriously reducing the contraceptive effect.

Effect on blood chemistry:

The use of oral contraceptives may influence the results of certain laboratory tests including biochemical parameters of liver, thyroid, adrenal and renal function, plasma levels of carrier proteins and lipid/lipoprotein fractions, parameters of carbohydrate metabolism and parameters of coagulation and fibrinolysis. Laboratory staff should therefore be informed about oral contraceptive use when laboratory tests are requested.

4.9 Overdose

Acute toxicity studies did not indicate a risk of acute adverse effects in case of inadvertent intake of a multiple of the daily contraceptive dose. In general it is therefore unnecessary to treat overdosage. There are no specific antidotes and further treatment should be symptomatic.

5. PHARMACOLOGICAL PROPERTIES

5.1 Pharmacodynamic properties

The contraceptive action of Norgeston may be explained as follows: it changes the cervical mucus so that a barrier is formed against the migration of sperm into the uterine cavity; nidation is impeded because of changes in the structure of the endometrium. As a rule there is no inhibition of ovulation. Evidence suggests that a reduction in corpus luteum function may also contribute to the contraceptive action.

5.2 Pharmacokinetic properties

As is known from a series of studies comprising various preparations and dosages, levonorgestrel is rapidly and completely absorbed after oral administration. Following ingestion of Norgeston, maximum serum levels of about 0.8 ng/ml were determined at 1 hour. Thereafter, drug serum levels declined biphasically with half-lives of 0.2 - 0.4 hours and 20 hours. Metabolic clearance rate from serum or plasma accounts for 1.0 to 1.5 ml/min/kg. Levonorgestrel is not excreted in unchanged form but as metabolites, which are eliminated with a half-life of about 1 day. Almost equal dose parts are excreted via the kidney and the liver. The biotransformation follows the known pathways of steroid metabolism. No pharmacologically active metabolites are known.

Levonorgestrel is bound to serum albumin and to SHBG. Only about 1.5% of the respective total serum drug levels are present as free steroid, but about 65% are specifically bound to SHBG. The relative portions (free, albumin-bound, SHBG-bound) depend on the SHBG serum concentrations. Following induction of the carrier protein, the SHBG-bound portion increases while the unbound and albumin-bound portions decrease.

Following daily repeated administration, levonorgestrel accumulates by a factor of approx. 2. Steady-state conditions are reached after about 3 - 4 days. Levonorgestrel pharmacokinetics is influenced by SHBG serum levels.

Under Norgeston treatment, a slight decline of the SHBG serum levels could occur. The daily ingestion of 0.15 mg levonorgestrel (corresponding to the 5 fold daily dose of Norgeston) led to a 50% decrease in the SHBG serum levels and thus to a 40% reduction in levonorgestrel through levels after 2 - 3 weeks. A similarly directed effect of Norgeston should account, however, for a decrease of only about 10% in the two parameters. The absolute bioavailability of levonorgestrel from Norgeston was determined to 82% of the dose. About 0.1% of the maternal dose can be transferred to a newborn via milk.

5.3 Preclinical safety data
There are no preclinical safety data which could be of relevance to the prescriber and which are not already included in other relevant sections of the SPC.

6. PHARMACEUTICAL PARTICULARS

6.1 List of excipients
lactose
maize starch
povidone
talc
magnesium stearate [E572]
sucrose
polyethylene glycol 6000
calcium carbonate [E170]
montan glycol wax

6.2 Incompatibilities
None known

6.3 Shelf life
5 years

6.4 Special precautions for storage
Not applicable.

6.5 Nature and contents of container
Norgeston tablets are contained in aluminium foil and PVC blister packs.

These calendar-packs contain 35 tablets.

6.6 Instructions for use and handling
Keep out of the reach of children.

7. MARKETING AUTHORISATION HOLDER
Schering Health Care Limited
The Brow
Burgess Hill
West Sussex RH15 9NE

8. MARKETING AUTHORISATION NUMBER(S)
0053/0068

9. DATE OF FIRST AUTHORISATION/RENEWAL OF THE AUTHORISATION
5 February 1973/ 21 April 1998

10. DATE OF REVISION OF THE TEXT
2 May 2000

LEGAL CATEGORY
POM

Noriday Tablets

(Pharmacia Limited)

1. NAME OF THE MEDICINAL PRODUCT
Noriday®

2. QUALITATIVE AND QUANTITATIVE COMPOSITION
Each tablet contains 350 micrograms norethisterone.

3. PHARMACEUTICAL FORM
White, flat, circular, bevel-edged tablet inscribed 'SEARLE' on one side and

'NY' on the other side.

4. CLINICAL PARTICULARS

4.1 Therapeutic indications
Noriday is a progestogen-only oral contraceptive. It is particularly useful for women for whom oestrogens may not be appropriate.

4.2 Posology and method of administration
Oral Administration
Starting on the first day of menstruation, one pill every day without a break in medication for as long as contraception is required. Additional contraceptive precautions (such as a condom) should be taken for the first 7 days of the first pack. Pills should be taken at the same time each day.

Missed Pills

If a pill is missed within 3 hours of the correct dosage time then the missed pill should be taken as soon as possible; this will ensure that contraceptive protection is maintained. If a pill is taken 3 or more hours late it is recommended that the woman takes the last missed pill as soon as possible and then continues to take the rest of the pills in the normal manner. However, to provide continued contraceptive protection it is recommended that an alternative method of contraception, such as a condom, is used for the next 7 days.

Changing from another oral contraceptive

In order to ensure that contraception is maintained it is advised that the first pill is taken on the day immediately after the patient has finished the previous pack.

Use after childbirth, miscarriage or abortion

The first pill should be taken on the 21st day after childbirth. This will ensure the patient is protected immediately. If there is any delay in taking the first pill, contraception may not be established until 7 days after the first pill has been taken. In these circumstances women should be advised that extra contraceptive methods will be necessary.

After a miscarriage or abortion patients can take the first pill on the next day; in this way they will be protected immediately.

Vomiting and diarrhoea

Gastrointestinal upsets, such as vomiting and diarrhoea, may interfere with the absorption of the pill leading to a reduction in contraceptive efficacy. Women should continue to take Noriday, but they should also be advised to use another contraceptive method during the period of gastrointestinal upset and for the next 7 days.

4.3 Contraindications
The contraindications for progestogen-only oral contraceptives are:

(i) known, suspected, or a past history of breast, genital or hormone dependent cancer;

(ii) acute or severe chronic liver diseases including past or present liver tumours, Dubin-Johnson or Rotor syndrome;

(iii) active liver disease;

(iv) history during pregnancy of idiopathic jaundice or severe pruritus;

(v) disorders of lipid metabolism;

(vi) undiagnosed abnormal vaginal bleeding;

(vii) known or suspected pregnancy;

(viii) hypersensitivity to any component.

Combined oestrogen/progestogen preparations have been associated with an increase in the risk of thromboembolic and thrombotic disease. Risk has been reported to be related to both oestrogenic and progestogenic activity. In the absence of long term epidemiological studies with progestogen-only oral contraceptives, it is required that the existence, or history of thrombophlebitis, thromboembolic disorders, cerebral vascular disease, myocardial infarction, angina, or coronary artery disease be described as a contraindication to Noriday as it is to oestrogen containing oral contraceptives.

4.4 Special warnings and special precautions for use
Assessment of women prior to starting oral contraceptives (and at regular intervals thereafter) should include a personal and family medical history of each woman. Physical examination should be guided by this and by the contraindications (section 4.3) and warnings (section 4.4) for this product. The frequency and nature of these assessments should be based upon relevant guidelines and should be adapted to the individual woman, but should include measurement of blood pressure and, if judged appropriate by the clinician, breast, abdominal and pelvic examination including cervical cytology.

Malignant hepatic tumours have been reported on rare occasions in long-term users of contraceptives. Benign hepatic tumours have also been associated with oral contraceptive usage. A hepatic tumour should be considered in the differential diagnosis when upper abdominal pain, enlarged liver or signs of intra-abdominal haemorrhage occur.

A statistical association between the use of oral contraceptives and the occurrence of thrombosis, embolism or haemorrhage has been reported. Patients receiving oral contraceptives should be kept under regular surveillance, in view of the possibility of development of conditions such as thrombo-embolism.

The risk of coronary artery disease in women taking oral contraceptives is increased by the presence ofother predisposing factors such as cigarette smoking, hypercholesterolaemia, obesity, diabetes, history of pre-eclamptic toxaemia and increasing age. After the age of thirty-five years, the patient and physician should carefully re-assess the risk/benefit ratio of using oral contraceptives as opposed to alternative methods of contraception.

Noriday should be discontinued at least 4 weeks before elective surgery or during periods of prolonged immobilisation. It would be reasonable to resume Noriday 2 weeks after surgery provided the woman is ambulant. However, every woman should be considered individually with regard to the nature of the operation, the extent of immobilisation, the presence of additional risk factors and the chance of unwanted conception.

Noriday should be discontinued if there is a gradual or sudden, partial or complete loss of vision or any evidence of ocular changes, onset or aggravation of migraine or development of headache of a new kind which is recurrent, persistent or severe, suspicion of thrombosis or infarction, significant rise in blood pressure or if jaundice occurs.

Caution should be exercised where there is the possibility of an interaction between a pre-existing disorder and a known or suspected side effect. The use of Noriday in women suffering from epilepsy, or with a history of migraine or cardiac or renal dysfunction may result in exacerbation of these disorders because of fluid retention. Caution should also be observed in women who wear contact lenses, women with impaired carbohydrate tolerance, depression, gallstones, a past history of liver disease, varicose veins, hypertension, asthma or any disease that is prone to worsen during pregnancy (e.g. multiple sclerosis, porphyria, tetany and otosclerosis).

An increased risk of congenital abnormalities, including heart defects and limb defects, has been reported following the use of sex hormones, including oral contraceptives, in pregnancy. If the patient does not adhere to the prescribed schedule, the possibility of pregnancy should be considered at the time of the first missed period and further use of oral contraceptives should be withheld until pregnancy has been ruled out. It is recommended that for any patient who has missed two consecutive periods, pregnancy should be ruled out before continuing the contraceptive regimen. If pregnancy is confirmed the patient should be advised of the potential risks to the foetus and the advisability of continuing the pregnancy should be discussed in the light of these risks. It is advisable to discontinue Noriday three months before a planned pregnancy.

Progestogen-only oral contraceptives may offer less protection against ectopic pregnancy, than against intrauterine pregnancy.

A meta-analysis from 54 epidemiological studies reported that there is a slightly increased relative risk of having breast cancer diagnosed in women who are currently using oral contraceptives (OC). The observed pattern of increased risk may be due to an earlier diagnosis of breast cancer in OC users, the biological effects of OCs or a combination of both. The additional breast cancers diagnosed in current users of OCs or in women who have used OCs in the last ten years are more likely to be localised to the breast than those in women who never used OCs.

Breast cancer is rare among women under 40 years of age whether or not they take OCs. Whilst the background risk increases with age, the excess number of breast cancer diagnoses in current and recent progesterone-only pill (POP) users is small in relation to the overall risk of breast cancer, possibly of similar magnitude to that associated with combined OCs. However, for POPs, the evidence is based on much smaller populations of users and so is less conclusive than that for combined OCs.

The most important risk factor for breast cancer in POP users is the age women discontinue the POP; the older the age at stopping, the more breast cancers are diagnosed. Duration of use is less important and the excess risk gradually disappears during the course of the 10 years after stopping POP use, such that by 10 years there appears to be no excess.

The evidence suggests that compared with never-users, among 10,000 women who use POPs for up to 5 years but stop by age 20, there would be much less than 1 extra case of breast cancer diagnosed up to 10 years afterwards. For those stopping by age 30 after 5 years use of the POP, there would be an estimated 2-3 extra cases (additional to the 44 cases of breast cancer per 10,000 women in this age group never exposed to oral contraceptives). For those stopping by age 40 after 5 years use, there would be an estimated 10 extra cases diagnosed up to 10 years afterwards (additional to the 160 cases of breast cancer per 10,000 never-exposed women in this age group).

It is important to inform patients that users of all contraceptive pills appear to have a small increase in the risk of being diagnosed with breast cancer, compared with non-users of oral contraceptives, but this has to be weighed against the known benefits.

4.5 Interaction with other medicinal products and other forms of Interaction
The herbal remedy St John's wort (*Hypericum perforatum*) should not be taken concomitantly with this medicine as this could potentially lead to a loss of contraceptive effect.

Some drugs may modify the metabolism of Noriday reducing its effectiveness; these include certain sedatives, antibiotics, and antiepileptics. During the time such agents are used concurrently, it is advised that an alternative method of contraception, such as a condom, is also used.

The serum levels of prednisone, prednisolone, cloprednol and possibly other corticosteroids are considerably increased in those taking oral contraceptives. Both the therapeutic and toxic effects may be expected to increase accordingly.

4.6 Pregnancy and lactation
Noriday is contraindicated in women with suspected pregnancy. Several reports suggest an association between foetal exposure to female sex hormones, including oral contraceptives, and congenital anomalies.

There is no evidence that Noriday tablets diminish the yield of breast milk. Small amounts of steroid materials appear in the milk; their effect on the breast-fed child has not been determined.

4.7 Effects on ability to drive and use machines
None known.

4.8 Undesirable effects
The incidence of side effects in clinical trials was lower than that experienced with oestrogen-containing oral contraceptives. Side effects which did occur included some cycle irregularity during the first few months of therapy, spotting or breakthrough bleeding, amenorrhoea, breast discomfort, gastrointestinal symptoms, rash, headaches, migraine, depression, fatigue, nervousness, disturbance of appetite and changes in weight and libido.

Hypertension, which is usually reversible on discontinuing treatment, has occurred in a small percentage of women taking oral contraceptives.

Menstrual pattern: Women taking Noriday for the first time should be informed that they may initially experience menstrual irregularity. This may include amenorrhoea, prolonged bleeding and/or spotting but such irregularity tends to decrease with time. If a woman misses two consecutive periods, pregnancy should be ruled out before continuing the contraceptive regimen.

4.9 Overdose

Serious ill effects have not been reported following acute ingestion of large doses of oral contraceptives by young children. Overdosage may be manifested by nausea, vomiting, breast enlargement and vaginal bleeding. There is no specific antidote and treatment should be symptomatic. Gastric lavage may be employed if the overdose is large and the patient is seen sufficiently early (within four hours).

5. PHARMACOLOGICAL PROPERTIES

5.1 Pharmacodynamic properties

Norethisterone administration increases the protein and sialic acid content of cervical mucus which prevents penetration of the mucus by spermatozoa. It causes changes in the structure of the endometrium such that implantation of blastocysts is impaired. It also reduces numbers and height of cilia on cells lining the fallopian tube, which could delay tubal transport of ova.

5.2 Pharmacokinetic properties

Norethisterone is rapidly and completely absorbed after oral administration, peak plasma concentrations occurring in the majority of subjects between 1 and 3 hours. Due to first-pass metabolism, blood levels after oral administration are 60% of those after i.v. administration. The half life of elimination varies from 5 to 12 hours, with a mean of 7.6 hours. Norethisterone is metabolised mainly in the liver. Approximately 60% of the administered dose is excreted as metabolites in urine and faeces.

5.3 Preclinical safety data

The toxicity of norethisterone is very low. Reports of teratogenic effects in animals are uncommon. No carcinogenic effects have been found even in long-term studies. In subacute and chronic studies only minimal differences between treated and control animals are observed.

6. PHARMACEUTICAL PARTICULARS

6.1 List of excipients

Noriday tablets contain:

Maize starch, polyvidone, magnesium stearate and lactose.

6.2 Incompatibilities

None known.

6.3 Shelf life

The shelf life of Noriday tablets is 5 years.

6.4 Special precautions for storage

Store in a cool, dry place away from direct sunlight.

6.5 Nature and contents of container

Noriday tablets are supplied in pvc/foil blister packs of 28 and 84 tablets.

Blister packaging consists of 250 micron PVC and 20 micron aluminium foil.

6.6 Instructions for use and handling

None

7. MARKETING AUTHORISATION HOLDER

Pharmacia Limited

Ramsgate Road

Sandwich

Kent, CT13 9NJ

United Kingdom

8. MARKETING AUTHORISATION NUMBER(S)

PL. 00032/0410

9. DATE OF FIRST AUTHORISATION/RENEWAL OF THE AUTHORISATION

26th July 2002

10. DATE OF REVISION OF THE TEXT

March 2004

11. LEGAL CATEGORY

POM

Norimin Tablets

(Pharmacia Limited)

1. NAME OF THE MEDICINAL PRODUCT

Norimin.

2. QUALITATIVE AND QUANTITATIVE COMPOSITION

Each tablet contains 1 milligram norethisterone and 35 micrograms ethinylestradiol.

3. PHARMACEUTICAL FORM

White round flat tablets with bevel-edged tablet inscribed 'SEARLE' on one side and 'BX' on the other.

4. CLINICAL PARTICULARS

4.1 Therapeutic indications

Norimin is indicated for oral contraception, with the benefit of a low intake of oestrogen.

4.2 Posology and method of administration

Oral Administration: The dosage of Norimin for the initial cycle of therapy is 1 tablet taken at the same time each day from the first day of the menstrual cycle. For subsequent cycles, no tablets are taken for 7 days, then a new course is started of 1 tablet daily for the next 21 days. This sequence of 21 days on treatment, seven days off treatment is repeated for as long as contraception is required.

Patients unable to start taking Norimin tablets on the first day of the menstrual cycle may start treatment on any day up to and including the 5th day of the menstrual cycle.

Patients starting on day 1 of their period will be protected at once. Those patients delaying therapy up to day 5 may not be protected immediately and it is recommended that another method of contraception is used for the first 7 days of tablet-taking. Suitable methods are condoms, caps plus spermicides and intra-uterine devices. The rhythm, temperature and cervical-mucus methods should not be relied upon.

Tablet omissions

Tablets must be taken daily in order to maintain adequate hormone levels and contraceptive efficacy.

If a tablet is missed within 12 hours of the correct dosage time then the missed tablet should be taken as soon as possible, even if this means taking 2 tablets on the same day, this will ensure that contraceptive protection is maintained. If one or more tablets are missed for more than 12 hours from the correct dosage time it is recommended that the patient takes the last missed tablet as soon as possible and then continues to take the rest of the tablets in the normal manner. In addition, it is recommended that extra contraceptive protection, such as a condom, is used for the next 7 days.

Patients who have missed one or more of the last 7 tablets in a pack should be advised to start the next pack of tablets as soon as the present one has finished (i.e. without the normal seven day gap between treatments). This reduces the risk of contraceptive failure resulting from tablets being missed close to a 7 day tablet free period.

Changing from another oral contraceptive

In order to ensure that contraception is maintained it is advised that the first dose of Norimin tablets is taken on the day immediately after the patient has finished the previous pack of tablets.

Use after childbirth, miscarriage or abortion

Providing the patient is not breast feeding the first dose of Norimin tablets should be taken on the 21st day after childbirth. This will ensure the patient is protected immediately. If there is any delay in taking the first dose, contraception may not be established until 7 days after the first tablet has been taken. In these circumstances patients should be advised that extra contraceptive methods will be necessary.

After a miscarriage or abortion patients can take the first dose of Norimin tablets on the next day; in this way they will be protected immediately.

4.3 Contraindications

As with all combined progestogen/oestrogen oral contraceptives, the following conditions should be regarded as contra-indications:

i. History of confirmed venous thromboembolic disease (VTE), family history of idiopathic VTE and other known risk factors of VTE

ii. Thrombophlebitis, cerebrovascular disorders, coronary artery disease, myocardial infarction, angina, hyperlipidaemia or a history of these conditions.

iii. Acute or severe chronic liver disease, including liver tumours, Dubin-Johnson or Rotor syndrome.

iv. History during pregnancy of idiopathic jaundice, severe pruritus or pemphigoid gestationis.

v. Known or suspected breast or genital cancer.

vi. Known or suspected oestrogen-dependent neoplasia.

vii. Undiagnosed abnormal vaginal bleeding.

viii. A history of migraines classified as classical focal or crescendo.

ix. Pregnancy.

4.4 Special warnings and special precautions for use

Assessment of women prior to starting oral contraceptives (and at regular intervals thereafter) should include a personal and family medical history of each woman. Physical examination should be guided by this and by the contraindications (section 4.3) and warnings (section 4.4) for this product. The frequency and nature of these assessments should be based upon relevant guidelines and should be adapted to the individual woman, but should include measurement of blood pressure and, if judged appropriate by the clinician, breast, abdominal and pelvic examination including cervical cytology.

Women taking oral contraceptives require careful observation if they have or have had any of the following conditions: breast nodules; fibrocystic disease of the breast or an abnormal mammogram; uterine fibroids; a history of severe depressive states; varicose veins; sickle-cell anaemia; diabetes; hypertension; cardiovascular disease; migraine; epilepsy; asthma; otosclerosis; multiple sclerosis; porphyria; tetany; disturbed liver functions; gallstones; kidney disease; chloasma; any condition that is likely to worsen during pregnancy. The worsening or first appearance of any of these conditions may indicate that the oral contraceptive should be stopped. Discontinue treatment if there is a gradual or sudden, partial or complete loss of vision or any evidence of ocular changes, onset or aggravation of migraine or development of headache of a new kind which is recurrent, persistent or severe.

Gastro-intestinal upsets, such as vomiting and diarrhoea, may interfere with the absorption of the tablets leading to a reduction in contraceptive efficacy. Patients should continue to take Norimin, but they should also be encouraged to use another contraceptive method during the period of gastro-intestinal upset and for the next 7 days.

Progestogen oestrogen preparations should be used with caution in patients with a history of hepatic dysfunction or hypertension.

An increased risk of venous thromboembolic disease (VTE) associated with the use of oral contraceptives is well established but is smaller than that associated with pregnancy, which has been estimated at 60 cases per 100,000 pregnancies. Some epidemiological studies have reported a greater risk of VTE for women using combined oral contraceptives containing desogestrel or gestodene (the so-called 'third generation' pills) than for women using pills containing levonorgestrel or norethisterone (the so-called 'second generation' pills

The spontaneous incidence of VTE in healthy non-pregnant women (not taking any oral contraceptive) is about 5 cases per 100,000 per year. The incidence in users of second generation pills is about 15 per 100,000 women per year of use. The incidence in users of third generation pills is about 25 cases per 100,000 women per year of use; this excess incidence has not been satisfactorily explained by bias or confounding. The level of all of these risks of VTE increases with age and is likely to be further increased in women with other known risk factors for VTE such as obesity. The excess risk of VTE is highest during the first year a woman ever uses a combined oral contraceptive.

Patients receiving oral contraceptives should be kept under regular surveillance, in view of the possibility of developments such as thromboembolism.

The risk of coronary artery disease in women taking oral contraceptives is increased by the presence of other predisposing factors such as cigarette smoking, hypercholesterolaemia, obesity, diabetes, history of pre-eclamptic toxaemia and increasing age. After the age of thirty-five years, the patient and physician should carefully re-assess the risk/benefit ratio of using combined oral contraceptives as opposed to alternative methods of contraception.

Norimin should be discontinued at least four weeks before, and for two weeks following, elective operations and during immobilisation. Patients undergoing injection treatment for varicose veins should not resume taking Norimin until 3 months after the last injection.

Benign and malignant liver tumours have been associated with oral contraceptive use. The relationship between occurrence of liver tumours and use of female sex hormones is not known at present. These tumours may rupture causing intra-abdominal bleeding. If the patient presents with a mass or tenderness in the right upper quadrant or an acute abdomen, the possible presence of a tumour should be considered.

An increased risk of congenital abnormalities, including heart defects and limb defects, has been reported following the use of sex hormones, including oral contraceptives, in pregnancy. If the patient does not adhere to the prescribed schedule, the possibility of pregnancy should be considered at the time of the first missed period and further use of oral contraceptives should be withheld until pregnancy has been ruled out. It is recommended that for any patient who has missed two consecutive periods, pregnancy should be ruled out before continuing the contraceptive regimen. If pregnancy is confirmed the patient should be advised of the potential risks to the foetus and the advisability of continuing the pregnancy should be discussed in the light of these risks. It is advisable to discontinue Norimin three months before a planned pregnancy.

The risk of arterial thrombosis associated with combined oral contraceptives increases with age, and this risk is aggravated by cigarette smoking. The use of combined oral contraceptives by women in the older age group, especially those who are cigarette smokers, should therefore be discouraged and alternative methods advised.

The use of this product in patients suffering from epilepsy, migraine, asthma or cardiac dysfunction may result in exacerbation of these disorders because of fluid retention. Caution should also be observed in patients who wear contact lenses.

Decreased glucose tolerance may occur in diabetic patients on this treatment, and their control must be carefully supervised.

The use of oral contraceptives has also been associated with a possible increased incidence of gall bladder disease.

Figure 1 Estimated cumulative numbers of breast cancers per 10,000 women diagnosed in 5 years of use and up to 10 years after stopping COCs, compared with numbers of breast cancers diagnosed in 10,000 women who had never used COCs

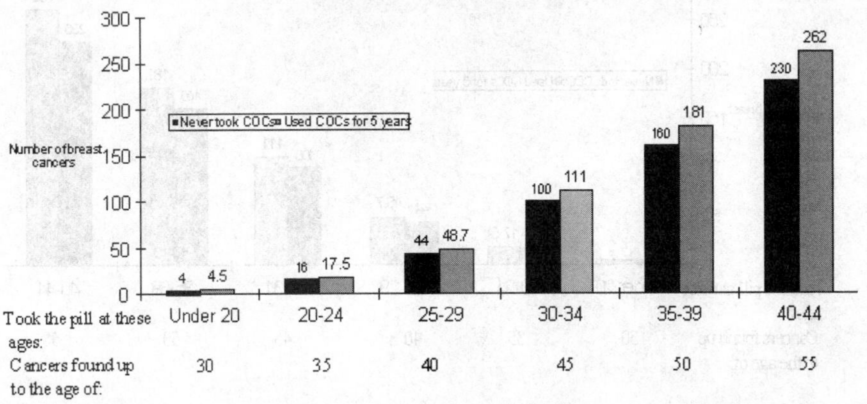

Women with a history of oligomenorrhoea or secondary amenorrhoea or young women without regular cycles may have a tendency to remain anovulatory or to become amenorrhoeic after discontinuation of oral contraceptives. Women with these pre-existing problems should be advised of this possibility and encouraged to use other contraceptive methods.

Numerous epidemiological studies have been reported on the risks of ovarian, endometrial, cervical and breast cancer in women using combined oral contraceptives. The evidence is clear that combined oral contraceptives offer substantial protection against both ovarian and endometrial cancer.

An increased risk of cervical cancer in long-term users of combined oral contraceptives has been reported in some studies, but there continues to be controversy about the extent to which this is attributable to the confounding effects of sexual behaviour and other factors.

A meta-analysis from 54 epidemiological studies reported that there is a slightly increased relative risk (RR = 1.24) of having breast cancer diagnosed in women who are currently using combined oral contraceptives (COCs). The observed pattern of increased risk may be due to an earlier diagnosis of breast cancer in COC users, the biological effects of COCs or a combination of both. The additional breast cancers diagnosed in current users of COCs or in women who have used COCs in the last ten years are more likely to be localised to the breast than those in women who never used COCs.

Breast cancer is rare among women under 40 years of age whether or not they take COCs. Whilst this background risk increases with age, the excess number of breast cancer diagnoses in current and recent COC users is small in relation to the overall risk of breast cancer (see bar chart).

The most important risk factor for breast cancer in COC users is the age women discontinue the COC; the older the age at stopping, the more breast cancers are diagnosed. Duration of use is less important and the excess risk gradually disappears during the course of the 10 years after stopping COC use such that by 10 years there appears to be no excess.

The possible increase in risk of breast cancer should be discussed with the user and weighed against the benefits of COCs taking into account the evidence that they offer substantial protection against the risk of developing certain other cancers (e.g. ovarian and endometrial cancer).

Estimated cumulative numbers of breast cancers per 10,000 women diagnosed in 5 years of use and up to 10 years after stopping COCs, compared with numbers of breast cancers diagnosed in 10,000 women who had never used COCs.

(see Figure 1 above)

4.5 Interaction with other medicinal products and other forms of Interaction

The herbal remedy St John's wort (*Hypericum perforatum*) should not be taken concomitantly with this medicine as this could potentially lead to a loss of contraceptive effect.

Some drugs may modify the metabolism of Norimin reducing its effectiveness; these include certain sedatives, antibiotics, anti-epileptic and anti-arthritic drugs. During the time such agents are used concurrently, it is advised that mechanical contraceptives also be used.

The results of a large number of laboratory tests have been shown to be influenced by the use of oestrogen containing oral contraceptives, which may limit their diagnostic value. Among these are: biochemical markers of thyroid and liver function; plasma levels of carrier proteins, triglycerides, coagulation and fibrinolysis factors.

4.6 Pregnancy and lactation

Contra-indicated in pregnancy.

Patients who are fully breast-feeding should not take Norimin tablets since, in common with other combined oral contraceptives, the oestrogen component may reduce the amount of milk produced. In addition, active ingredients or their metabolites have been detected in the milk of mothers taking oral contraceptives. The effect of Norimin on breast-fed infants has not been determined.

4.7 Effects on ability to drive and use machines

Not applicable.

4.8 Undesirable effects

As with all oral contraceptives, there may be slight nausea at first, weight gain or breast discomfort, which soon disappear.

Other side-effects known or suspected to occur with oral contraceptives include gastro-intestinal symptoms, changes in libido and appetite, headache, exacerbation of existing uterine fibroid disease, depression, and changes in carbohydrate, lipid and vitamin metabolism.

Spotting or bleeding may occur during the first few cycles. Usually menstrual bleeding becomes light and occasionally there may be no bleeding during the tablet-free days.

Hypertension, which is usually reversible on discontinuing treatment, has occurred in a small percentage of women taking oral contraceptives.

4.9 Overdose

Overdosage may be manifested by nausea, vomiting, breast enlargement and vaginal bleeding. There is no specific antidote and treatment should be symptomatic. Gastric lavage may be employed if the overdose is large and the patient is seen sufficiently early (within four hours).

5. PHARMACOLOGICAL PROPERTIES

5.1 Pharmacodynamic properties

The mode of action of Norimin is similar to that of other progestogen/oestrogen oral contraceptives and includes the inhibition of ovulation, the thickening of cervical mucus so as to constitute a barrier to sperm and the rendering of the endometrium unreceptive to implantation. Such activity is exerted through a combined effect on one or more of the following: hypothalamus, anterior pituitary, ovary, endometrium and cervical mucus.

5.2 Pharmacokinetic properties

Norethisterone is rapidly and completely absorbed after oral administration, peak plasma concentrations occurring in the majority of subjects between 1 and 3 hours. Due to first-pass metabolism, blood levels after oral administration are 60% of those after i.v. administration. The half life of elimination varies from 5 to 12 hours, with a mean of 7.6 hours. Norethisterone is metabolised mainly in the liver. Approximately 60% of the administered dose is excreted as metabolites in urine and faeces.

Ethinylestradiol is rapidly and well absorbed from the gastro-intestinal tract but is subject to some first-pass metabolism in the gut-wall. Compared to many other oestrogens it is only slowly metabolised in the liver. Excretion is via the kidneys with some appearing also in the faeces.

5.3 Preclinical safety data

The toxicity of norethisterone is very low. Reports of teratogenic effects in animals are uncommon. No carcinogenic effects have been found even in long-term studies.

Long-term continuous administration of oestrogens in some animals increases the frequency of carcinoma of the breast, cervix, vagina and liver.

6. PHARMACEUTICAL PARTICULARS

6.1 List of excipients

Norimin tablets contain:

Maize starch, polyvidone, magnesium stearate and lactose.

6.2 Incompatibilities

None stated.

6.3 Shelf life

The shelf life of Norimin tablets is 5 years.

6.4 Special precautions for storage

Store in a dry place, below 25°C, away from direct sunlight.

6.5 Nature and contents of container

Norimin tablets are supplied in pvc/foil blister packs of 21 and 63 tablets.

6.6 Instructions for use and handling

None.

7. MARKETING AUTHORISATION HOLDER

Pharmacia Limited
Davy Avenue
Milton Keynes
Buckinghamshire
MK5 8PH
United Kingdom

8. MARKETING AUTHORISATION NUMBER(S)

PL 00032/0411.

9. DATE OF FIRST AUTHORISATION/RENEWAL OF THE AUTHORISATION

8 July 2002

10. DATE OF REVISION OF THE TEXT

December 2004

Norinyl-1 Tablets

(Pharmacia Limited)

1. NAME OF THE MEDICINAL PRODUCT

Norinyl-1®

2. QUALITATIVE AND QUANTITATIVE COMPOSITION

Each tablet contains 1 milligram norethisterone and 50 micrograms mestranol.

3. PHARMACEUTICAL FORM

White, flat, circular, bevel-edged tablet inscribed 'SEARLE' on one side and '1' on the other side.

4. CLINICAL PARTICULARS

4.1 Therapeutic indications

Norinyl-1 is indicated for oral contraception.

4.2 Posology and method of administration

Oral Administration: The dosage of Norinyl-1 for the initial cycle of therapy is 1 tablet taken at the same time each day from the first day of the menstrual cycle. For subsequent cycles, no tablets are taken for 7 days, then a new course is started of 1 tablet daily for the next 21 days. This sequence of 21 days on treatment, seven days off treatment is repeated for as long as contraception is required.

Patients unable to start taking Norinyl-1 tablets on the first day of the menstrual cycle may start treatment on any day up to and including the 5th day of the menstrual cycle.

Patients starting on day 1 of their period will be protected at once. Those patients delaying therapy up to day 5 may not be protected immediately and it is recommended that another method of contraception is used for the first 7 days of tablet-taking. Suitable methods are condoms, caps plus spermicides and intra-uterine devices. The rhythm, temperature and cervical-mucus methods should not be relied upon.

Tablet omissions

Tablets must be taken daily in order to maintain adequate hormone levels and contraceptive efficacy.

If a tablet is missed within 12 hours of the correct dosage time then the missed tablet should be taken as soon as possible, even if this means taking 2 tablets on the same day, this will ensure that contraceptive protection is maintained. If one or more tablets are missed for more than 12 hours from the correct dosage time it is recommended that the patient takes the last missed tablet as soon as possible and then continues to take the rest of the tablets in the normal manner. In addition, it is recommended that extra contraceptive protection, such as a condom, is used for the next 7 days.

Patients who have missed one or more of the last 7 tablets in a pack should be advised to start the next pack of tablets as soon as the present one has finished (i.e. without the normal seven day gap between treatments). This reduces the risk of contraceptive failure resulting from tablets being missed close to a 7 day tablet free period.

Changing from another oral contraceptive

In order to ensure that contraception is maintained it is advised that the first dose of Norinyl-1 tablets is taken on the day immediately after the patient has finished the previous pack of tablets.

Use after childbirth, miscarriage or abortion

Providing the patient is not breast feeding the first dose of Norinyl-1 tablets should be taken on the 21st day after childbirth. This will ensure the patient is protected immediately. If there is any delay in taking the first dose, contraception may not be established until 7 days after the first tablet has been taken. In these circumstances patients should be advised that extra contraceptive methods will be necessary.

After a miscarriage or abortion patients can take the first dose of Norinyl-1 tablets on the next day; in this way they will be protected immediately.

4.3 Contraindications

As with all combined progestogen/oestrogen oral contraceptives, the following conditions should be regarded as contra-indications:

i. History of confirmed venous thromboembolic disease (VTE), family history of idiopathic VTE and other known risk factors of VTE

ii. Thrombophlebitis, cerebrovascular disorders, coronary artery disease, myocardial infarction, angina, hyperlipidaemia or a history of these conditions.

iii. Acute or severe chronic liver disease, including liver tumours, Dubin-Johnson or Rotor syndrome.

iv. History during pregnancy of idiopathic jaundice, severe pruritus or pemphigoid gestationis.

v. Known or suspected breast or genital cancer

vi. Known or suspected oestrogen-dependent neoplasia.

vii. Undiagnosed abnormal vaginal bleeding.

viii. A history of migraines classified as classical focal or crescendo.

ix. Pregnancy.

4.4 Special warnings and special precautions for use

Assessment of women prior to starting oral contraceptives (and at regular intervals thereafter) should include a personal and family medical history of each woman. Physical examination should be guided by this and by the contra-indications (section 4.3) and warnings (section 4.4) for this product. The frequency and nature of these assessments should be based upon relevant guidelines and should be adapted to the individual woman, but should include measurement of blood pressure and, if judged appropriate by the clinician, breast, abdominal and pelvic examination including cervical cytology.

Women taking oral contraceptives require careful observation if they have or have had any of the following conditions: breast nodules; fibrocystic disease of the breast or an abnormal mammogram; uterine fibroids; a history of severe depressive states; varicose veins; sickle-cell anaemia; diabetes; hypertension; cardiovascular disease; migraine; epilepsy; asthma; otosclerosis; multiple sclerosis; porphyria; tetany; disturbed liver functions; gallstones; kidney disease; chloasma; any condition that is likely to worsen during pregnancy. The worsening or first appearance of any of these conditions may indicate that the oral contraceptive should be stopped. Discontinue treatment if there is a gradual or sudden, partial or complete loss of vision or any evidence of ocular changes, onset or aggravation of migraine or development of headache of a new kind which is recurrent, persistent or severe.

Gastro-intestinal upsets, such as vomiting and diarrhoea, may interfere with the absorption of the tablets leading to a reduction in contraceptive efficacy. Patients should continue to take Norinyl-1, but they should also be encouraged to use another contraceptive method during the period of gastro-intestinal upset and for the next 7 days.

Progestogen oestrogen preparations should be used with caution in patients with a history of hepatic dysfunction or hypertension.

An increased risk of venous thromboembolic disease (VTE) associated with the use of oral contraceptives is well established but is smaller than that associated with pregnancy, which has been estimated at 60 cases per 100,000 pregnancies. Some epidemiological studies have reported a greater risk of VTE for women using combined oral contraceptives containing desogestrel or gestodene (the so-called 'third generation' pills) than for women using pills containing levonorgestrel or norethisterone (the so-called 'second generation' pills).

The spontaneous incidence of VTE in healthy non-pregnant women (not taking any oral contraceptive) is about 5 cases per 100,000 per year. The incidence in users of second generation pills is about 15 per 100,000 women per year of use. The incidence in users of third generation pills is about 25 cases per 100,000 women per year of use; this excess incidence has not been satisfactorily explained by bias or confounding. The level of all of these risks of VTE increases with age and is likely to be further increased in women with other known risk factors for VTE such as obesity). The excess risk of VTE is highest during the first year a woman ever uses a combined oral contraceptive.

Patients receiving oral contraceptives should be kept under regular surveillance, in view of the possibility of development of such conditions as thromboembolism.

The risk of coronary artery disease in women taking oral contraceptives is increased by the presence of other predisposing factors such as cigarette smoking, hypercholesterolaemia, obesity, diabetes, history of pre-eclamptic toxaemia and increasing age. After the age of thirty-five years, the patient and physician should carefully re-assess the risk/benefit ratio of using combined oral contraceptives as opposed to alternative methods of contraception.

Norinyl-1 should be discontinued at least four weeks before, and for two weeks following, elective operations and during immobilisation. Patients undergoing injection treatment for varicose veins should not resume taking Norinyl-1 until 3 months after the last injection.

Benign and malignant liver tumours have been associated with oral contraceptive use. The relationship between occurrence of liver tumours and use of female sex hormones is not known at present. These tumours may rupture causing intra-abdominal bleeding. If the patient presents with a mass or tenderness in the right upper quadrant or an acute abdomen, the possible presence of a tumour should be considered.

An increased risk of congenital abnormalities, including heart defects and limb defects, has been reported following the use of sex hormones, including oral contraceptives, in pregnancy. If the patient does not adhere to the prescribed schedule, the possibility of pregnancy should be considered at the time of the first missed period and further use of oral contraceptives should be withheld until pregnancy has been ruled out. It is recommended that for any patient who has missed two consecutive periods, pregnancy should be ruled out before continuing the contraceptive regimen. If pregnancy is confirmed the patient should be advised of the potential risks to the foetus and the advisability of continuing the pregnancy should be discussed in the light of these risks. It is advisable to discontinue Norinyl-1 three months before a planned pregnancy.

The risk of arterial thrombosis associated with combined oral contraceptives increases with age, and this risk is aggravated by cigarette smoking. The use of combined oral contraceptives by women in the older age group, especially those who are cigarette smokers, should therefore be discouraged and alternative methods advised.

The use of this product in patients suffering from epilepsy, migraine, asthma or cardiac dysfunction may result in exacerbation of these disorders because of fluid retention. Caution should also be observed in patients who wear contact lenses.

Decreased glucose tolerance may occur in diabetic patients on this treatment, and their control must be carefully supervised.

The use of oral contraceptives has also been associated with a possible increased incidence of gall bladder disease.

Women with a history of oligomenorrhoea or secondary amenorrhoea or young women without regular cycles may have a tendency to remain anovulatory or to become amenorrhoeic after discontinuation of oral contraceptives. Women with these pre-existing problems should be advised of this possibility and encouraged to use other contraceptive methods.

Numerous epidemiological studies have been reported on the risks of ovarian, endometrial, cervical and breast cancer in women using combined oral contraceptives. The evidence is clear that combined oral contraceptives offer substantial protection against both ovarian and endometrial cancer.

An increased risk of cervical cancer in long-term users of combined oral contraceptives has been reported in some studies, but there continues to be controversy about the extent to which this is attributable to the confounding effects of sexual behaviour and other factors.

A meta-analysis from 54 epidemiological studies reported that there is a slightly increased relative risk (RR = 1.24) of having breast cancer diagnosed in women who are currently using combined oral contraceptives (COCs). The observed pattern of increased risk may be due to an earlier diagnosis of breast cancer in COC users, the biological effects of COCs or a combination of both. The additional breast cancers diagnosed in current users of COCs or in women who have used COCs in the last ten years are more likely to be localised to the breast than those in women who never used COCs.

Breast cancer is rare among women under 40 years of age whether or not they take COCs. Whilst this background risk increases with age, the excess number of breast cancer diagnoses in current and recent COC users is small in relation to the overall risk of breast cancer (see bar chart).

The most important risk factor for breast cancer in COC users is the age women discontinue the COC; the older the age at stopping, the more breast cancers are diagnosed. Duration of use is less important and the excess risk gradually disappears during the course of the 10 years after stopping COC use such that by 10 years there appears to be no excess.

The possible increase in risk of breast cancer should be discussed with the user and weighed against the benefits of COCs taking into account the evidence that they offer substantial protection against the risk of developing certain other cancers (e.g. ovarian and endometrial cancer).

Estimated cumulative numbers of breast cancers per 10,000 women diagnosed in 5 years of use and up to 10 years after stopping COCs, compared with numbers of breast cancers diagnosed in 10,000 women who had never used COCs.

(see Figure 1 above)

Figure 1

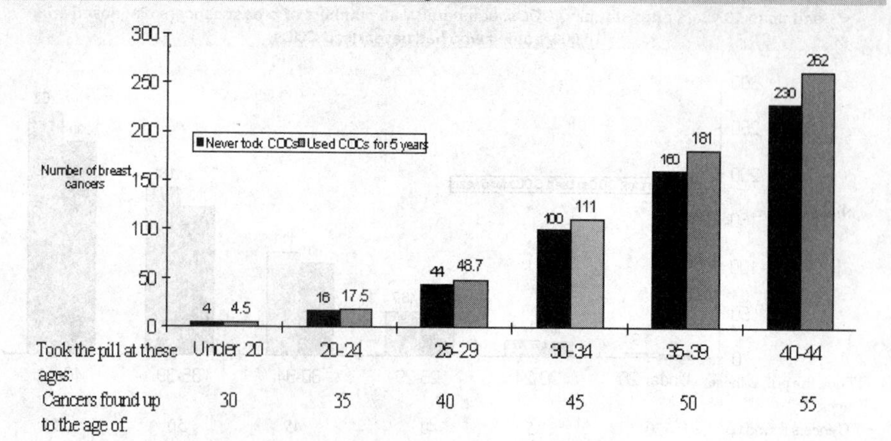

4.5 Interaction with other medicinal products and other forms of Interaction

The herbal remedy St John's wort (*Hypericum perforatum*) should not be taken concomitantly with this medicine as this could potentially lead to a loss of contraceptive effect.

Some drugs may modify the metabolism of Norinyl-1 reducing its effectiveness; these include certain sedatives, antibiotics, anti-epileptic and anti-arthritic drugs. During the time such agents are used concurrently, it is advised that mechanical contraceptives also be used.

The results of a large number of laboratory tests have been shown to be influenced by the use of oestrogen containing oral contraceptives, which may limit their diagnostic value. Among these are: biochemical markers of thyroid and liver function; plasma levels of carrier proteins, triglycerides, coagulation and fibrinolysis factors.

4.6 Pregnancy and lactation

Contra-indicated in pregnancy.

Patients who are fully breast-feeding should not take Norinyl-1 tablets since, in common with other combined oral contraceptives, the oestrogen component may reduce the amount of milk produced. In addition, active ingredients or their metabolites have been detected in the milk of mothers taking oral contraceptives. The effect of Norinyl-1 on breast-fed infants has not been determined.

4.7 Effects on ability to drive and use machines

Not applicable.

4.8 Undesirable effects

As with all oral contraceptives, there may be slight nausea at first, weight gain or breast discomfort, which soon disappear.

Other side-effects known or suspected to occur with oral contraceptives include gastro-intestinal symptoms, changes in libido and appetite, headache, exacerbation of existing uterine fibroid disease, depression, and changes in carbohydrate, lipid and vitamin metabolism.

Spotting or bleeding may occur during the first few cycles. Usually menstrual bleeding becomes light and occasionally there may be no bleeding during the tablet-free days.

Hypertension, which is usually reversible on discontinuing treatment, has occurred in a small percentage of women taking oral contraceptives.

4.9 Overdose

Overdosage may be manifested by nausea, vomiting, breast enlargement and vaginal bleeding. There is no specific antidote and treatment should be symptomatic. Gastric lavage may be employed if the overdose is large and the patient is seen sufficiently early (within four hours).

5. PHARMACOLOGICAL PROPERTIES

5.1 Pharmacodynamic properties

The mode of action of Norinyl-1 is similar to that of other progestogen/oestrogen oral contraceptives and includes the inhibition of ovulation, the thickening of cervical mucus so as to constitute a barrier to sperm and the rendering of the endometrium unreceptive to implantation. Such activity is exerted through a combined effect on one or more of the following: hypothalamus, anterior pituitary, ovary, endometrium and cervical mucus.

5.2 Pharmacokinetic properties

Norethisterone is rapidly and completely absorbed after oral administration, peak plasma concentrations occurring in the majority of subjects between 1 and 3 hours. Due to first-pass metabolism, blood levels after oral administration are 60% of those after i.v. administration. The half life of elimination varies from 5 to 12 hours, with a mean of 7.6 hours. Norethisterone is metabolised mainly in the liver. Approximately 60% of the administered dose is excreted as metabolites in urine and faeces.

Mestranol is rapidly absorbed and extensively metabolised to ethinyloestradiol. Ethinyloestradiol is rapidly and well absorbed from the gastro-intestinal tract but is subject to some first-pass metabolism in the gut-wall. Compared to many other oestrogens it is only slowly metabolised in the liver. Excretion is via the kidneys with some appearing also in the faeces.

5.3 Preclinical safety data

The toxicity of norethisterone is very low. Reports of teratogenic effects in animals are uncommon. No carcinogenic effects have been found even in long-term studies.

Long-term continuous administration of oestrogens in some animals increases the frequency of carcinoma of the breast, cervix, vagina and liver.

6. PHARMACEUTICAL PARTICULARS

6.1 List of excipients

Norinyl-1 tablets contain:

Maize starch, polyvidone, magnesium stearate and lactose.

6.2 Incompatibilities

None stated.

6.3 Shelf life

The shelf life of Norinyl-1 tablets is 5 years.

6.4 Special precautions for storage

Store in a dry place below 25°C away from direct sunlight.

6.5 Nature and contents of container

Norinyl-1 tablets are supplied in pvc/foil blister packs of 21 and 63 tablets.

6.6 Instructions for use and handling

None.

7. MARKETING AUTHORISATION HOLDER

Pharmacia Limited

Davy Avenue

Milton Keynes

Buckinghamshire

MK5 8PH

UK

8. MARKETING AUTHORISATION NUMBER(S)

PL 00032/0412

9. DATE OF FIRST AUTHORISATION/RENEWAL OF THE AUTHORISATION

May 16th 1996

10. DATE OF REVISION OF THE TEXT

February 1998

January 2000

April 2000

December 2000

August 2002

Legal Category

POM

Normacol

(Norgine Limited)

1. NAME OF THE MEDICINAL PRODUCT

NORMACOL

2. QUALITATIVE AND QUANTITATIVE COMPOSITION

The active ingredient is Sterculia 62% w/w.

3. PHARMACEUTICAL FORM

Oral granules.

4. CLINICAL PARTICULARS

4.1 Therapeutic indications

The treatment of constipation, particularly simple or idiopathic constipation and constipation during pregnancy.

Management of colostomies and ileostomies.

The 'High Residue Diet' management of diverticular disease of the colon and other conditions requiring a high fibre regimen.

The initiation and maintenance of bowel action after rectal and anal surgery.

Administration after ingestion of sharp foreign bodies to provide a coating and reduce the possibility of intestinal damage during transit.

4.2 Posology and method of administration

Adults: 1 or 2 sachets or 1-2 heaped 5ml spoonfuls, once or twice daily after meals.

Elderly: As adult dose.

Children: (6-12 years): one half the above amount.

The granules should be placed dry on the tongue and without chewing or crushing, swallowed immediately with plenty of water or a cool drink. Prior to drinking they may also be sprinkled onto and taken with soft food such as yoghurt.

4.3 Contraindications

Intestinal obstruction, faecal impaction, and total atony of the colon.

4.4 Special warnings and special precautions for use

Not to be taken immediately before retiring, especially in the elderly. Adequate fluid should be maintained. Caution should be exercised in cases of ulcerative colitis. Not to be taken for more than 4 days if there has been no movement of the bowels.

4.5 Interaction with other medicinal products and other forms of Interaction

None known.

4.6 Pregnancy and lactation

NORMACOL may be recommended during pregnancy or lactation.

4.7 Effects on ability to drive and use machines

None known.

4.8 Undesirable effects

Occasionally mild abdominal distension may occur. Oesophageal obstruction is possible if the product is taken in overdosage or if it is not adequately washed down with fluid.

4.9 Overdose

Intestinal obstruction is possible in overdosage particularly in combination with inadequate fluid intake. Management is as for intestinal obstruction from other causes.

5. PHARMACOLOGICAL PROPERTIES

5.1 Pharmacodynamic properties

Sterculia acts in the colon by forming a soft bulky stool and inducing a laxative effect.

5.2 Pharmacokinetic properties

Sterculia is not absorbed or digested in the gastrointestinal tract and its laxative action is normally effective within 12 hours of oral administration.

5.3 Preclinical safety data

There is no evidence that Sterculia has a significant systemic toxicity potential.

6. PHARMACEUTICAL PARTICULARS

6.1 List of excipients

Sodium bicarbonate

Sucrose

Talc

Paraffin wax

Titanium dioxide

Vanillin

6.2 Incompatibilities

None known.

6.3 Shelf life

The shelf life is 3 years.

6.4 Special precautions for storage

Store in a dry place below 25°C.

6.5 Nature and contents of container

Sachet containing 7 g of white granules in boxes of 2, 7, 30 or 60 sachets.

Lined box of 100 g or 500 g of white granules.

6.6 Instructions for use and handling

None.

7. MARKETING AUTHORISATION HOLDER

Norgine Limited

Chaplin House

Widewater Place

Moorhall Road

Harefield

UXBRIDGE

Middlesex UB9 6NS

United Kingdom

8. MARKETING AUTHORISATION NUMBER(S)

PL 0322/5010R

9. DATE OF FIRST AUTHORISATION/RENEWAL OF THE AUTHORISATION

January 1991

10. DATE OF REVISION OF THE TEXT

September 1997

Normacol Plus

(Norgine Limited)

1. NAME OF THE MEDICINAL PRODUCT

NORMACOL PLUS.

2. QUALITATIVE AND QUANTITATIVE COMPOSITION

The active ingredients are 62% Sterculia and 8.0% Frangula.

3. PHARMACEUTICAL FORM

Brown granules.

4. CLINICAL PARTICULARS

4.1 Therapeutic indications

The treatment of constipation, particularly hypertonic or slow transit constipation, resistant to bulk alone.

The initiation and maintenance of bowel action after rectal surgery and after haemorrhoidectomy.

4.2 Posology and method of administration

Adults (including the elderly): 1 or 2 sachets or 1-2 heaped 5ml spoonfuls, once or twice daily after meals.

Children: (6-12 years): A reduced amount may be given at the discretion of the physician.

The granules should be placed dry on the tongue and, without chewing or crushing, swallowed immediately with plenty of water or a cool drink. Prior to drinking they may also be sprinkled on, and taken with, soft food such as yoghurt.

4.3 Contraindications

Intestinal obstruction, faecal impaction, and total atony of the colon.

4.4 Special warnings and special precautions for use

Caution should be exercised in the use of NORMACOL PLUS in cases of ulcerative colitis. Patients should be advised to maintain an adequate fluid intake, to avoid taking NORMACOL PLUS immediately before going to bed (especially if they are elderly), and to suspend treatment if bowel movements do not occur within four days.

4.5 Interaction with other medicinal products and other forms of Interaction

None known.

4.6 Pregnancy and lactation

Pregnancy: No teratogenic effects have been reported, but caution should be exercised during the first trimester.

Lactation: There is no evidence to suggest that NORMACOL PLUS is unsuitable for use.

NORMACOL (Sterculia alone) is available if required in pregnancy and lactation.

4.7 Effects on ability to drive and use machines

None known.

4.8 Undesirable effects

Abdominal distension may occur. Oesophageal obstruction is possible if the product is not adequately washed down with fluid.

4.9 Overdose

Intestinal obstruction is possible in overdosage particularly in combination with inadequate fluid intake. Management is as for intestinal obstruction from other causes.

5. PHARMACOLOGICAL PROPERTIES

5.1 Pharmacodynamic properties

Sterculia acts in the colon by forming a soft bulky stool and inducing a laxative effect. Frangula acts as a mild peristaltic stimulant and aids the evacuation of the softened faecal mass.

5.2 Pharmacokinetic properties

Sterculia is not absorbed in the gastrointestinal tract; Frangula acts locally on the wall of the intestinal tract. The laxative action of NORMACOL PLUS is normally effective within 12 hours of oral administration.

5.3 Preclinical safety data

There are no preclinical data of relevance to the prescriber except as already included in the SPC.

6. PHARMACEUTICAL PARTICULARS

6.1 List of excipients

Sucrose

Talc

Sodium bicarbonate

Paraffin wax

Peppermint flavouring

Colourings: E110, E127 and E132

The sugar provides 7-14 calories per dose (1.7 to 3.4g carbohydrate per dose). The sodium content is 1.25 to 2.5 mmol per dose. NORMACOL PLUS is gluten free.

6.2 Incompatibilities

None known.

6.3 Shelf life

The shelf life of the sachet is 3 years, and the lined cartons 4 years.

6.4 Special precautions for storage

Store in a dry place below 25°C.

6.5 Nature and contents of container

Sachet containing 7g of granules in cartons of 2, 7, 10, 30 or 60 sachets.

Lined carton of 200 g or 500 g of granules.

6.6 Instructions for use and handling

None.

7. MARKETING AUTHORISATION HOLDER
Norgine Limited
Chaplin House
Widewater Place
Moorhall Road
Harefield
UXBRIDGE
Middlesex UB9 6NS
United Kingdom

8. MARKETING AUTHORISATION NUMBER(S)
PL 00322/5011R

9. DATE OF FIRST AUTHORISATION/RENEWAL OF THE AUTHORISATION
1 May 1986/1 May 1991

10. DATE OF REVISION OF THE TEXT
January 1996.

Legal category: GSL

Normax Capsules or Co-danthrusate Capsules

(UCB Pharma Limited)

1. NAME OF THE MEDICINAL PRODUCT
Co-danthrusate Capsules
Normax Capsules

2. QUALITATIVE AND QUANTITATIVE COMPOSITION
Docusate Sodium 60mg
Dantron 50mg
For excipients, see 6.1.

3. PHARMACEUTICAL FORM
Capsule for oral administration

4. CLINICAL PARTICULARS
4.1 Therapeutic indications
Constipation in terminally ill patients.

4.2 Posology and method of administration
Adults (including elderly): One to three capsules at bedtime.

Children (6-12 years): One capsule at bedtime.

4.3 Contraindications
In common with all laxatives, Co-danthrusate is contraindicated in cases of non-specific abdominal pain and when intestinal obstruction is suspected.

4.4 Special warnings and special precautions for use
In experimental animals, dantron has been associated with adenocarcinomas in the bowel and tumours in the liver. A theoretical risk of similar effects in humans cannot be excluded.

Dantron is excreted in the urine and metabolised dantron in the faeces. There is evidence that these may cause perineal erythema in patients with urinary and/or faecal incontinence. It is recommended therefore that Co-danthrusate should be used with caution in all incontinent patients.

As with all laxatives, prolonged use is not recommended.

4.5 Interaction with other medicinal products and other forms of Interaction
Docusate may enhance the gastrointestinal or hepatic cell uptake of mineral oil and quinidine potentiating their activity and possibly increasing their toxicity.

4.6 Pregnancy and lactation
Co-danthrusate should not be used in pregnancy or lactation.

4.7 Effects on ability to drive and use machines
None known.

4.8 Undesirable effects
Occasionally an orange tint in the urine may be observed due to the dantron component. Skin rash may occur and reports of skin irritation, skin discolouration and superficial sloughing of the perianal skin have been reported after prolonged use of Co-danthrusate.

4.9 Overdose
The patient should be encouraged to drink fluids. An anticholinergic preparation may be used to ease excessive intestinal motility if necessary.

5. PHARMACOLOGICAL PROPERTIES
5.1 Pharmacodynamic properties
Dantron is a mild peristaltic stimulant acting on the lower bowel to encourage normal bowel movement without causing irritation. Docusate sodium is a softening agent which prevents excessive colonic dehydration and hardening of stools.

5.2 Pharmacokinetic properties
None available.

5.3 Preclinical safety data
In experimental animals, dantron has been associated with adenocarcinomas in the bowel and tumours in the liver.

6. PHARMACEUTICAL PARTICULARS
6.1 List of excipients
Lactose
Sodium benzoate (intra and extragranular)
Povidone
Colloidal silicon dioxide
Magnesium stearate
Capsule Shell:
Gelatin
Black iron oxide
Red iron oxide
Titanium dioxide
Yellow iron oxide
Printing Ink:
Titanium dioxide
Shellac glaze-45%
Soya lethicin
Antifoam DC 1510

6.2 Incompatibilities
None known.

6.3 Shelf life
5 years for blister packs and aluminium canisters.
3 years for securitainers.

6.4 Special precautions for storage
Do not store above 25°C.
Store in a dry place.

6.5 Nature and contents of container
Blister pack containing 3 (professional sample pack), 21 or 63 capsules.
Aluminium canisters containing 12, 30 or 250 capsules.
Securitainers containing 30 or 250 capsules
Not all pack sizes may be marketed.

6.6 Instructions for use and handling
None.

7. MARKETING AUTHORISATION HOLDER
UCB Pharma Limited
208 Bath Road
Slough
Berkshire
SL1 3WE
UK

8. MARKETING AUTHORISATION NUMBER(S)
PL 00039/0380

9. DATE OF FIRST AUTHORISATION/RENEWAL OF THE AUTHORISATION
26 November 1991 / 12 November 1998 / November 2003

10. DATE OF REVISION OF THE TEXT
June 2005

11. LEGAL CATEGORY

POM

Normax Suspension or Co-danthrusate Suspension

(UCB Pharma Limited)

1. NAME OF THE MEDICINAL PRODUCT
'Normax' Suspension or Co-danthrusate Suspension

2. QUALITATIVE AND QUANTITATIVE COMPOSITION
Each 5 ml containing 60 mg Sodium Docusate BP and 50 mg Danthron BP

3. PHARMACEUTICAL FORM
Suspension

4. CLINICAL PARTICULARS
4.1 Therapeutic indications
Constipation in terminally ill patients of all ages.

4.2 Posology and method of administration
Adults: One to three 5ml doses at bedtime
Children One 5ml dose at bedtime
Method of Administration: Oral

4.3 Contraindications
In common with all laxatives, 'Normax' or Co-danthrusate is contraindicated in cases of non-specific abdominal pain and when intestinal obstruction is suspected.

4.4 Special warnings and special precautions for use
In experimental animals, Danthron has been associated with adenocarcinomas in the bowel and tumours in the liver. A theoretical risk of similar effects in humans cannot be excluded.

Danthron is excreted in the urine and metabolised danthron in the faeces. There is evidence that these may cause perineal erythema in patients with urinary and or faecal incontinence. It is recommended therefore that co-danthrusate should be used with caution in all incontinent patients.

Prolonged use is not recommended.

4.5 Interaction with other medicinal products and other forms of Interaction
None known.

4.6 Pregnancy and lactation
Co-danthrusate should not be used in pregnancy or lactation.

4.7 Effects on ability to drive and use machines
None known.

4.8 Undesirable effects
Occasionally an orange tint in the urine may be observed due to the Danthron component.

4.9 Overdose
The patient should be encouraged to drink fluids. An anticholinergic preparation may be used to ease excessive intestinal motility if necessary.

5. PHARMACOLOGICAL PROPERTIES
5.1 Pharmacodynamic properties
Danthron is a mild peristaltic stimulant acting on the lower bowel to encourage normal bowel movement without causing irritation. Docusate sodium is a softening agent which prevents excessive colonic dehydration and hardening of stools.

5.2 Pharmacokinetic properties
Not available

5.3 Preclinical safety data
No further information

6. PHARMACEUTICAL PARTICULARS
6.1 List of excipients
Methylcellulose BP
Xanthan Gum NF
Glycerol BP
Propyl Parahydroxybenzoate BP
Methyl Parahydroxybenzoate BP
Sorbitol Powder (E200) BP
Saccharin Sodium BP
Disodium Hydrogen Orthophosphate HSE (Anhydrous)
Sodium Dihydrogen Orthophosphate BP
Peppermint Oil BP
Purified Water BP

6.2 Incompatibilities
Not known

6.3 Shelf life
36 month (200 ml)
24 month (30 ml)

6.4 Special precautions for storage
Store at a temperature not exceeding 25°C in carton and protect from light.

6.5 Nature and contents of container
Amber glass bottle with either roll-on pilfer proof aluminium cap with 'steran' faced wad or plastic cap with 'saranex' faced wad. The 30ml volume is for promotional purposes only. The 200ml volume is for prescription.

6.6 Instructions for use and handling
None

7. MARKETING AUTHORISATION HOLDER
UCB Pharma Limited
208 Bath Road
Slough
Berkshire
SL1 3WE
UK

8. MARKETING AUTHORISATION NUMBER(S)
PL 00039/0381

9. DATE OF FIRST AUTHORISATION/RENEWAL OF THE AUTHORISATION
8 June 1994 / 8 June 1999

10. DATE OF REVISION OF THE TEXT
June 2005

POM

Norprolac Tablets 25, 50 and 75 micrograms.

(Ferring Pharmaceuticals Ltd)

1. NAME OF THE MEDICINAL PRODUCT
NORPROLAC® Tablets 25 micrograms
NORPROLAC® Tablets 50 micrograms
NORPROLAC® Tablets 75 micrograms

2. QUALITATIVE AND QUANTITATIVE COMPOSITION

Quinagolide, as the hydrochloride, 25, 50 or 75 micrograms

3. PHARMACEUTICAL FORM

Tablet for oral administration

4. CLINICAL PARTICULARS

4.1 Therapeutic indications

Hyperprolactinaemia (idiopathic or originating from a prolactin-secreting pituitary microadenoma or macroadenoma).

4.2 Posology and method of administration

Since dopaminergic stimulation may lead to symptoms of orthostatic hypotension, the dosage of NORPROLAC should be initiated gradually with the aid of the 'starter pack', and given only at bedtime.

Adults

The optimal dose must be titrated individually on the basis of the prolactin-lowering effect and tolerability.

With the 'starter pack' treatment begins with 25 micrograms/day for the first 3 days, followed by 50 micrograms/day for a further 3 days. From day 7 onwards, the recommended dose is 75 micrograms/day.

If necessary, the daily dose may then be increased stepwise until the optimal individual response is attained. The usual maintenance dosage is 75 to 150 micrograms/day.

Daily doses of 300 micrograms or higher doses are required in less than one-third of the patients.

In such cases, the daily dosage may be increased in steps of 75 to 150 micrograms at intervals not shorter than 4 weeks until satisfactory therapeutic effectiveness is achieved or reduced tolerability, requiring the discontinuation of treatment, occurs.

Elderly

Experience with the use of NORPROLAC in elderly patients is not available.

Children

Experience with the use of NORPROLAC in children is not available.

Method of Administration

NORPROLAC should be taken once a day with some food at bedtime.

4.3 Contraindications

Hypersensitivity to the drug

Impaired hepatic or renal function

For procedure during pregnancy, (see section 4.6 Pregnancy and lactation).

4.4 Special warnings and special precautions for use

Fertility may be restored by treatment with NORPROLAC. Women of child-bearing age who do not wish to conceive should therefore be advised to practice a reliable method of contraception.

Since orthostatic hypotension may result in syncope, it is recommended to check blood pressure both lying and standing during the first days of therapy and following dosage increases.

In a few cases, including patients with no previous history of mental illness, treatment with NORPROLAC has been associated with the occurrence of acute psychosis, usually reversible upon discontinuation. Particular caution is required in patients who have had psychotic episodes in their previous history.

To date no data is available with the use of NORPROLAC in patients with impaired renal or hepatic function (see Section 4.3 Contraindications).

NORPROLAC has been associated with somnolence. Other dopamine agonists can be associated with sudden sleep onset episodes, particularly in patients with Parkinson's disease. Patients must be informed of this and advised to exercise caution whilst driving or operating machines during treatment with NORPROLAC.

Patients who have experienced somnolence must not drive or operate machines. Furthermore, a reduction of dosage or termination of therapy may be considered (see Section 4.7 Effects on the ability to drive and use machines).

NORPROLAC should be kept out of the reach and sight of children.

4.5 Interaction with other medicinal products and other forms of Interaction

No interactions between NORPROLAC and other drugs have so far been reported. On theoretical grounds, a reduction of the prolactin-lowering effect could be expected when drugs (e.g. neuroleptic agents) with strong dopamine antagonistic properties are used concomitantly. As the potency of NORPROLAC for 5-HT_1 and 5-HT_2 receptors is some 100 times lower than that for D_2 receptors, an interaction between NORPROLAC and 5-HT_{1a} receptors is unlikely. However, care should be taken when using these medicaments concomitantly.

The tolerability of NORPROLAC may be reduced by alcohol.

4.6 Pregnancy and lactation

Pregnancy

Animal data provide no evidence that NORPROLAC has any embryotoxic or teratogenic potential, but experience in pregnant women is still limited. In patients wishing to conceive, NORPROLAC should be discontinued when pregnancy is confirmed, unless there is a medical reason for continuing therapy. No increased incidence of abortion has been observed following withdrawal of the drug at this point.

If pregnancy occurs in the presence of a pituitary adenoma and NORPROLAC treatment has been stopped, close supervision throughout pregnancy is essential.

Lactation

Breast-feeding is usually not possible since NORPROLAC suppresses lactation. If lactation should continue during treatment, breast-feeding cannot be recommended because it is not known whether quinagolide passes into human breast milk.

4.7 Effects on ability to drive and use machines

Since, especially during the first days of treatment, hypotensive reactions may occasionally occur and result in reduced alertness, patients should be cautious when driving a vehicle or operating machinery.

Patients being treated with NORPROLAC and presenting with somnolence must be advised not to drive or engage in activities where impaired alertness may put themselves or others at risk of serious injury or death (e.g. operating machines) unless patients have overcome such experiences of somnolence (see Section 4.4 Special warnings and precautions for use).

4.8 Undesirable effects

Frequency estimate: very common $\geqslant$10%, common $\geqslant$1% to <10%, uncommon $\geqslant$0.1% to <1%, rare $\geqslant$0.01% to <0.1%, very rare <0.01%.

The adverse reactions reported with the use of NORPROLAC are characteristic for dopamine receptor agonist therapy. They are usually not sufficiently serious to require discontinuation of treatment and tend to disappear when treatment is continued.

Very common undesirable effects are nausea, vomiting, headache, dizziness and fatigue. They occur predominantly during the first few days of the initial treatment or, as a mostly transient event, following dosage increase. If necessary, nausea and vomiting may be prevented by the intake of a peripheral dopaminergic antagonist, such as domperidone, for a few days, at least 1 hour before ingestion of NORPROLAC.

Common undesirable effects include anorexia, abdominal pain, constipation or diarrhoea, insomnia, oedema, flushing, nasal congestion and hypotension. Orthostatic hypotension may result in faintness or syncope (see 4.4 Special warnings and precautions for use).

Rarely NORPROLAC has been associated with somnolence.

In very rare cases, treatment with NORPROLAC has been associated with the occurrence of acute psychosis, reversible upon discontinuation.

4.9 Overdose

Symptoms

Acute overdosage with NORPROLAC Tablets has not been reported. It would be expected to cause severe nausea, vomiting, headache, dizziness, drowsiness, hypotension and possibly collapse. Hallucinations could also occur.

Treatment

Should be symptomatic.

5. PHARMACOLOGICAL PROPERTIES

5.1 Pharmacodynamic properties

Pharmacotherapeutic group: prolactin inhibitors (ATC code G02C B04).

Quinagolide, the active ingredient of NORPROLAC, is a selective dopamine D_2-receptor agonist not belonging to the chemical classes of ergot or ergoline compounds. Owing to its dopaminergic action, the drug exerts a strong inhibitory effect on the secretion of the anterior pituitary hormone prolactin, but does not reduce normal levels of other pituitary hormones. In some patients the reduction of prolactin secretion may be accompanied by short-lasting, small increases in plasma growth hormone levels, the clinical significance of which is unknown.

As a specific inhibitor of prolactin secretion with a prolonged duration of action, NORPROLAC has been shown to be effective and suitable for once-a-day oral treatment of patients presenting with hyperprolactinaemia and its clinical manifestations such as galactorrhoea, oligomenorrhoea, amenorrhoea, infertility and reduced libido.

5.2 Pharmacokinetic properties

After oral administration of radiolabelled drug, quinagolide is rapidly and well absorbed. Plasma concentration values obtained by a non-selective radio-immunoassay (RIA), measuring quinagolide together with some of its metabolites, were close to the limit of quantification and gave no reliable information.

The apparent volume of distribution of quinagolide after single oral administration of radiolabelled compound was calculated to be approx. 100L. For the parent drug, a terminal half-life of 11.5 hours has been calculated under single dose conditions, and of 17 hours at steady state.

Quinagolide is extensively metabolised during its first pass. Studies performed with ^{3}H-labelled quinagolide revealed that more than 95% of the drug is excreted as metabolites. About equal amounts of total radioactivity are found in faeces and urine.

In blood, quinagolide and its N-desethyl analogue are the biologically active but minor components. Their inactive sulphate or glucuronide conjugates represent the major circulating metabolites. In urine, the main metabolites are the glucuronide and sulphate conjugates of quinagolide and the N-desethyl, N,N-didesethyl analogues. In the faeces the unconjugated forms of the three components were found.

The protein binding of quinagolide is approximately 90% and is non-specific.

The results, obtained in pharmacodynamic studies, indicate that with the recommended therapeutic dosage a clinically significant prolactin-lowering effect occurs within 2 hours after ingestion, reaches a maximum of 4 to 6 hours and is maintained for about 24 hours.

A definite dose-response relationship could be established for the duration, but not for the magnitude of the prolactin-lowering effect which, with a single oral dose of 50 micrograms was close to maximum. Higher doses did not result in a considerably greater effect but prolonged its duration.

5.3 Preclinical safety data

Acute toxicity

The LD_{50} of quinagolide was determined for several species after single oral administration: mice 357 to > 500mg/kg; rats > 500mg/kg; rabbits > 150mg/kg.

Chronic toxicity

Decreased cholesterol levels of treated female rats suggest that quinagolide influences lipid metabolism. Since similar observations have been made with other dopaminergic drugs, a causal relationship with low prolactin levels is assumed. In several chronic studies with rats, enlarged ovaries resulting from an increased number of corpora lutea and, additionally, hydrometra and endometritis were observed. These changes were reversible and reflect the pharmacodynamic effect of quinagolide: suppression of prolactin secretion inhibits luteolysis in rats and thus influences the normal sexual cycle. In humans, however, prolactin is not involved in luteolysis.

Carcinogenic and mutagenic potential

In comprehensive *in vitro* and *in vivo* mutagenic studies there was no evidence of a mutagenic effect.

The changes which were observed in carcinogenicity studies reflect the pharmacodynamic activity of quinagolide. The drug modulates the prolactin level as well as, especially in male rats, the level of luteinising hormone and, in female rodents, the ratio of progesterone to oestrogen.

Long-term studies with high doses of quinagolide revealed Leydig cell tumours in rats and mesenchymal uterine tumours in mice. The incidence of Leydig cell tumours in a carcinogenicity study in rats was increased even at low doses (0.01mg/kg). These results were without relevance for the therapeutic application in humans since there are fundamental differences between humans and rodents in the regulation of the endocrine system.

Reproductive toxicity

Animal studies in rats and rabbits showed no evidence for embryotoxic or teratogenic effects. The prolactin inhibiting effect led to a decrease of milk production in rats, which was associated with an increased loss of rat pups. Possible post-natal effects of exposure during fetal development (2nd and 3rd trimester) and effects on female fertility are not sufficiently investigated.

6. PHARMACEUTICAL PARTICULARS

6.1 List of excipients

Silica, colloidal anhydrous; magnesium stearate; methylhydroxypropylcellulose; maize starch; cellulose, microcrystalline; lactose.

Colourings

25 micrograms: Iron oxide, red

50 micrograms: Indigotin lake

6.2 Incompatibilities

Not applicable

6.3 Shelf life

The shelf life is 5 years. The expiry date is printed on the box. On the blister the expiry date is marked with the letters EXP.

6.4 Special precautions for storage

The expiry date refers to original unopened boxes, which were stored below 25°C. No special warning with respect to light sensitivity or humidity is necessary because the tablets are protected by the packaging.

6.5 Nature and contents of container

The 'starter pack' (NORPROLAC 25/50) consists of 3 tablets of 25 micrograms and 3 tablets of 50 micrograms. These tablets are packed in an aluminium PVC/PVDC blister which is sealed in a moisture-proof aluminium bag.

The 75 micrograms tablets are in packs of 30 tablets (3 times 10 tablets) in aluminium blisters.

6.6 Instructions for use and handling

None

7. MARKETING AUTHORISATION HOLDER

Ferring Pharmaceuticals Ltd., The Courtyard, Waterside Drive, Langley, Berkshire SL3 6EZ.

8. MARKETING AUTHORISATION NUMBER(S)
NORPROLAC 25 micrograms PL 03194/0096

NORPROLAC 50 micrograms PL 03194/0097

NORPROLAC 75 micrograms PL 03194/0098

9. DATE OF FIRST AUTHORISATION/RENEWAL OF THE AUTHORISATION
15th December 2004

10. DATE OF REVISION OF THE TEXT
-

11. LEGAL CATEGORY
POM

Norvir Oral Solution

(Abbott Laboratories Limited)

1. NAME OF THE MEDICINAL PRODUCT
Norvir 80 mg/ml oral solution

2. QUALITATIVE AND QUANTITATIVE COMPOSITION
Norvir oral solution contains 80 mg of ritonavir per ml.

For excipients, see section 6.1

3. PHARMACEUTICAL FORM
Oral solution.

4. CLINICAL PARTICULARS

4.1 Therapeutic indications
Norvir is indicated in combination with other antiretroviral agents for the treatment of HIV-1 infected patients (adults and children of 2 years of age and older).

In protease inhibitor experienced patients the choice of ritonavir should be based on individual viral resistance testing and treatment history of patients.

4.2 Posology and method of administration
Adult use: Norvir solution is administered orally and should preferably be ingested with food. The recommended dosage of Norvir solution is 600 mg (7.5 ml) twice daily by mouth.

Gradually increasing the dose of ritonavir when initiating therapy may help to improve tolerance.

Single Protease Inhibitor (PI) containing combination regimen for adults: Treatment should be initiated at 300 mg (3.75 ml) twice daily for a period of three days and increased by 100 mg (1.25 ml) twice daily increments up to 600 mg twice daily over a period of no longer than 14 days. Patients should not remain on 300 mg twice daily for more than 3 days.

Dual PI containing combination regimens: Clinical experience with dual therapy including therapeutic doses of ritonavir with another protease inhibitor is limited. Ritonavir extensively inhibits the metabolism of most available protease inhibitors. Hence, any consideration of dual therapy with ritonavir should take into account the pharmacokinetic interaction and safety data of involved agents. There is extensive cross-resistance in this class of agents. The combination of two PIs with the least overlapping patterns of resistance should be considered. The use of ritonavir in such regimens should be guided by these factors.

Ritonavir as a pharmacokinetic enhancer for other PIs: In clinical practice ritonavir is frequently used as a pharmacokinetic enhancer (at low doses of 100 – 200 mg once or twice daily) to boost the plasma concentrations of other PIs in HIV-infected adult patients. For further specific information, refer to the Summary of Product Characteristics of the concerned PIs. See also section 4.5.

For the use of ritonavir with saquinavir a cautious titration of the dose has been used by initiating ritonavir dosing at 300 mg twice daily.

For the use of ritonavir with indinavir a cautious titration of the dose has been used by initiating ritonavir dosing at 200 mg twice daily increasing by 100 mg twice daily reaching 400 mg twice daily within 2 weeks.

Paediatric use (2 years of age and above): the recommended dosage of Norvir solution in children is 350 mg/m^2 by mouth twice daily and should not exceed 600 mg twice daily. Norvir should be started at 250 mg/m^2 and increased at 2 to 3 day intervals by 50 mg/m^2 twice daily.

When possible, dose should be administered using a calibrated dosing syringe.

The bitter taste of Norvir solution may be lessened if mixed with chocolate milk.

Paediatric Dosage Guidelines

(see Table 1 below)

Doses for intermediate body surface areas not included in the above table can be calculated using the following equations:

To calculate the volume to be administered (in ml) the body surface area should be multiplied by a factor of: 3.1 for a dose of 250 mg/m^2; 3.8 for one of 300 mg/m^2; and by 4.4 for 350 mg/m^2.

Renal impairment: currently, there are no data specific to this patient population and therefore specific dosage recommendations cannot be made. Because ritonavir is highly protein bound it is unlikely that it will be significantly removed by haemodialysis or peritoneal dialysis.

Hepatic impairment: ritonaviris principally metabolised and eliminated by the liver. Pharmacokinetic data indicate that no dose adjustment seems necessary in patients with mild to moderate hepatic impairment (see section 5.2). Norvir should not be given to patients with severe hepatic impairment (see section 4.3).

Ritonavir should be administered by physicians who are experienced in the treatment of HIV infection.

4.3 Contraindications
Patients with known hypersensitivity to ritonavir or any of its excipients. Patients with severe hepatic impairment.

In vitro and *in vivo* studies have demonstrated that ritonavir is a potent inhibitor of CYP3A- and CYP2D6- mediated biotransformations. Based primarily on literature review, ritonavir is expected to produce large increases in the plasma concentrations of the following medicines: amiodarone, astemizole, bepridil, bupropion, cisapride, clozapine, dihydroergotamine, encainide, ergotamine, flecainide, meperidine, pimozide, piroxicam, propafenone, propoxyphene, quinidine, and terfenadine. These agents have recognised risks of arrhythmias, haematologic abnormalities, seizures, or other potentially serious adverse effects. Additionally, acute ergot toxicity characterised by peripheral vasospasm and ischaemia has been associated with co-administration of ritonavir and ergotamine or dihydroergotamine. These medicines should not be co-administered with ritonavir. Ritonavir in addition is likely to produce large increases in these highly metabolised sedatives and hypnotics: clorazepate, diazepam, estazolam, flurazepam, midazolam and triazolam. Due to the potential for extreme sedation and respiratory depression from these agents, they should not be co-administered with ritonavir.

Concomitant use of ritonavir and rifabutin is contraindicated because of clinical consequences such as uveitis resulting from a multifold increase of rifabutin serum concentrations.

Herbal preparations containing St John's wort (*Hypericum perforatum)* must not be used while taking ritonavir due to the risk of decreased plasma concentrations and reduced clinical effects of ritonavir. (See section 4.5).

4.4 Special warnings and special precautions for use
Patients with pre-existing conditions:

Renal disease: there are no data on the pharmacokinetics and safety of ritonavir in patients with significant renal dysfunction.

Liver disease: the safety and efficacy of Norvir has not been established in patients with significant underlying liver disorders. Norvir is contraindicated in patients with severe hepatic impairment (see section 4.3). Patients with chronic hepatitis B or C and treated with combination antiretroviral therapy are at an increased risk for severe and potentially fatal hepatic adverse events. In case of concomitant antiviral therapy for hepatitis B or C, please refer to the relevant product information for these medicinal products.

Patients with pre-existing liver dysfunction including chronic active hepatitis have an increased frequency of liver function abnormalities during combination antiretroviral therapy and should be monitored according to standard practice. If there is evidence of worsening liver disease in such patients, interruption or discontinuation of treatment must be considered.

Haemophilia: there have been reports of increased bleeding, including spontaneous skin haematomas and haemarthroses, in haemophiliac patients type A and B treated with protease inhibitors. In some patients additional factor VIII was given. In more than a half of the reported cases, treatment with protease inhibitors was continued or reintroduced if treatment had been discontinued. A causal relationship has been evoked, although the mechanism of action has not been elucidated. Haemophiliac patients should therefore be made aware of the possibility of increased bleeding.

Immune Reactivation Syndrome: in HIV-infected patients with severe immune deficiency at the time of institution of combination antiretroviral therapy (CART), an inflammatory reaction to asymtomatic or residual opportunistic pathogens may arise and cause serious clinical conditions, or aggravation of symptoms. Typically, such reactions have been observed within the first few weeks or months of initiation of CART. Relevant examples are cytomegalovirus retinitis, generalised and/or focal mycobacterial infections, and Pneumocystis carinii pneumonia. Any inflammatory symptoms should be evaluated and treatment instituted when necessary.

The safety and efficacy of ritonavir in children below the age of 2 years have not been established.

Human pharmacokinetic data for combination of ritonavir with antiretroviral medicinal products other than zidovudine and didanosine (ddI) are not yet available. Although the clinical use of combinations with zalcitabine (ddC) and stavudine (d4T) in a relatively limited number of patients did not seem to be associated with unfavourable effects, the use of combinations of ritonavir with other nucleoside analogues should be guided by cautious therapeutic and safety monitoring.

Extra monitoring is recommended when diarrhoea occurs. The relatively high frequency of diarrhoea during treatment with ritonavir may compromise the absorption and efficacy (due to decreased compliance) of ritonavir or other concurrent medications. Serious persistent vomiting and/or diarrhoea associated with ritonavir use might also compromise renal function. It is advisable to monitor renal function in patients with renal function impairment.

A pharmacokinetic study demonstrated that ritonavir extensively inhibits the metabolism of saquinavir resulting in greatly increased saquinavir plasma concentrations (see section 4.5). Doses greater than 400 mg twice daily of either medicine were associated with an increased incidence of adverse events.

Norvir oral solution contains alcohol (43% v/v), therefore concomitant administration of Norvir with disulfiram or medicines with disulfiram-like reactions (eg, metronidazole) should be avoided.

New onset diabetes mellitus, hyperglycaemia or exacerbation of existing diabetes mellitus has been reported in patients receiving protease inhibitors. In some of these the hyperglycaemia was severe and in some cases also associated with ketoacidosis. Many patients had confounding medical conditions, some of which required therapy with agents that have been associated with the development of diabetes mellitus or hyperglycaemia.

Combination antiretroviral therapy has been associated with redistribution of body fat (lipodystrophy) in HIV patients. The long-term consequences of these events are currently unknown. Knowledge about the mechanism is incomplete. A connection between visceral lipomatosis and PIs and lipoatrophy and nucleoside reverse transcriptase inhibitors (NRTIs) has been hypothesised. A higher risk of lipodystrophy has been associated with individual factors such as older age, and with drug related factors such as longer duration of antiretroviral treatment and associated metabolic disturbances. Clinical examination should include evaluation for physical signs of fat redistribution. Consideration should be given to measurement of fasting serum lipids and blood glucose. Lipid disorders should be managed as clinically appropriate (see section 4.8).

Particular caution should be used when prescribing sildenafil in patients receiving ritonavir. Co-administration of ritonavir with sildenafil is expected to substantially increase sildenafil concentrations (11-fold increase in AUC) and may result in sildenafil-associated adverse events, including hypotension, syncope, visual changes and prolonged erection (see also section 4.5).

The HMG-CoA reductase inhibitors simvastatin and lovastatin are highly dependent on CYP3A for metabolism, thus concomitant use of Norvir with simvastatin or lovastatin is not recommended due to an increased risk of myopathy including rhabdomyolysis. Caution must also be exercised and reduced doses should be considered if Norvir is used concurrently with atorvastatin, which is metabolised to a lesser extent by CYP3A. If treatment with an HMG-CoA reductase inhibitor is indicated, pravastatin or fluvastatin is recommended (see section 4.5).

Concomitant use of ritonavir (including low-dose) and fluticasone propionate significantly increased fluticasone propionate plasma concentrations and reduced serum cortisol concentrations in a clinical study. Concomitant use of ritonavir (including low-dose) and fluticasone is

Table 1 Paediatric Dosage Guidelines

Body Surface area* (m^2)	Twice daily dose 250 mg/m^2	Twice daily dose 300 mg/m^2	Twice daily dose 350 mg/m^2
0.25	0.8 ml (62.5 mg)	0.9 ml (75 mg)	1.1 ml (87.5 mg)
0.50	1.6 ml (125 mg)	1.9 ml (150 mg)	2.2 ml (175 mg)
1.00	3.1 ml (250 mg)	3.8 ml (300 mg)	4.4 ml (350 mg)
1.25	3.9 ml (312.5 mg)	4.7 ml (375 mg)	5.5 ml (437.5 mg)
1.50	4.7 ml (375 mg)	5.6 ml (450 mg)	6.6 ml (525 mg)

* Body surface area can be calculated with the following equation

BSA (m^2) = $\sqrt{}$(Height (cm) X Weight (kg) / 3600)

therefore not recommended unless the potential benefit of treatment outweighs the risk of systemic corticosteroid effects. Systemic corticosteroid effects including Cushing's syndrome and adrenal suppression have been reported when ritonavir has been co-administered with inhaled or intranasal administered fluticasone propionate (see section 4.5).

4.5 Interaction with other medicinal products and other forms of Interaction

Refer also to Contraindications (section 4.3)

Ritonavir has a high affinity for several cytochrome P450 (CYP) isoforms with the following ranked order: CYP3A > CYP2D6 > CYP2C9. In addition to the medicines listed in the Contraindications section, the following medicines or drug classes are known or suspected to be metabolised by these same cytochrome P450 isozymes: immunosuppressants (eg, cyclosporine, tacrolimus), macrolide antibiotics (eg, erythromycin), various steroids (eg, dexamethasone, prednisolone), other HIV-protease inhibitors, delavirdine, nonsedating antihistamines (eg, loratidine), buspirone, calcium channel antagonists, several tricyclic antidepressants (eg, desipramine, imipramine, amitriptyline, nortriptyline), other antidepressants (eg, fluoxetine, paroxetine, sertraline), neuroleptics (eg, haloperidol, risperidone, thioridazine), antifungals (eg, itraconazole), morphinomimetics (eg, fentanyl), carbamazepine, tolbutamide, amphetamine and amphetamine derivatives. Due to the potential for significant elevation of serum levels of these medicines they should not be used concomitantly with ritonavir without a careful assessment of the potential risks and benefits. Careful monitoring of therapeutic and adverse effects is recommended when these medicines are concomitantly administered with ritonavir.

Warfarin oral anticoagulant concentrations may be affected, and notably decreased, when co-administered with ritonavir. This frequently leads to reduced anticoagulation, therefore it is recommended that anticoagulation parameters are monitored.

Serum levels of ritonavir can be reduced by concomitant use of the herbal preparation St John's wort (*Hypericum perforatum).* This is due to the induction of drug metabolising enzymes by St John's wort. Herbal preparations containing St John's wort should therefore not be combined with ritonavir. If a patient is already taking St John's wort, stop St John's wort and if possible check viral levels. Ritonavir levels may increase on stopping St John's wort. The dose of ritonavir may need adjusting. The inducing effect may persist for at least 2 weeks after cessation of treatment with St John's wort.

There are no pharmacokinetic data available on the concomitant use of morphine with ritonavir. On the basis of the metabolism of morphine (glucuronidation) lower levels of morphine may be expected.

Norvir INCREASES the AUCs (area under the curve) of the following medicines when administered concomitantly:

Clarithromycin: because of the large therapeutic window for clarithromycin, no dosage reduction should be necessary in patients with normal renal function. For patients with renal impairment the following dosage adjustment should be considered: for creatinine clearance (CL_{CR}) of 30 to 60 ml/min the clarithromycin dose should be reduced by 50%, for $CL_{CR} < 30$ ml/min the clarithromycin dose should be reduced by 75%. Doses of clarithromycin > 1 g/day should not be co-administered with Norvir.

Desipramine: dosage reduction of desipramine should be considered in patients taking the combination.

Rifabutin and its active metabolite 25-O-desacetyl rifabutin: concomitant use with ritonavir has resulted in a multifold increase in the AUC of rifabutin and its active metabolite 25-O-desacetyl rifabutin with clinical consequences. Therefore, the concomitant use of ritonavir and rifabutin is contraindicated (see section 4.3).

Saquinavir: data from pharmacokinetic studies in patients indicate that co-administration of ritonavir 400 mg twice daily produce multifold increases in saquinavir steady state blood levels (AUC, 17 fold; C_{max}, 14 fold increase). Doses greater than 400 mg twice daily of either medicine were associated with an increased incidence of adverse events.

In HIV-infected patients, Invirase and Fortovase in combination with ritonavir at doses of 1000/100 mg twice daily provide saquinavir systemic exposure over a 24 hour period greater than those achieved with Fortovase 1200 mg three times daily. For further information, physicians should refer to the Invirase and Fortovase Summary of Product Characteristics.

Indinavir: ritonavir inhibits the CYP3A-mediated metabolism of indinavir. In healthy subjects, 200 mg to 400 mg of ritonavir twice daily given with a single 400 mg to 600 mg indinavir dose increased the indinavir AUC by 185% to 475%, C_{max} 21% to 110%, and C_{8h} 11 to 33-fold, relative to 400 mg to 600 mg indinavir given alone. Concomitant administration of 400 mg ritonavir and 400 mg indinavir twice daily with a meal yielded a similar indinavir AUC, a 4 fold increase in C_{min} and a 50% to 60% decrease in C_{max} as compared to those resulting from administration of indinavir 800 mg three times daily under fasting conditions. Co-administration of ritonavir with indinavir will result in increased indinavir serum concentrations. There are limited safety or efficacy data available on the use of this combination in patients. The risk of nephrolithiasis may be increased when doses of indinavir equal to or greater than 800 mg twice daily are given with ritonavir. Adequate hydration and monitoring of the patients is warranted.

Nelfinavir: interactions between ritonavir and nelfinavir are likely to involve both Cytochrome P450 inhibition and induction. Concurrent ritonavir 400 mg twice daily significantly increases the concentrations of M8 (the major active metabolite of nelfinavir), and results in a smaller increase in nelfinavir concentrations. In a study in 10 patients, nelfinavir 750 mg and ritonavir 400 mg twice daily yielded slightly higher nelfinavir AUC (160%), C_{max} (121%) and C_{trough} (123%) than historical data for nelfinavir 750 mg three times daily monotherapy. The AUC of M8 was increased by 347%.

Amprenavir: concentrations of amprenavir are increased when co-administered with ritonavirdue to inhibition of the metabolism of amprenavir mediated by Cytochrome P450 isoenzymes. Booster doses of ritonavir given together with amprenavir result in clinically significant increases in amprenavir AUC and C_{min} with variable effects on maximum concentration. When given in combination in adults, reduced doses of both medicinal products (amprenavir 600 mg twice daily and ritonavir 100 mg twice daily) should be used. For further information, physicians should refer to the Agenerase Summary of Product Characteristics.

Efavirenz: in healthy volunteers receiving 500 mg ritonavir twice daily with efavirenz 600 mg once daily, the steady state AUC of efavirenz was increased by 21%. An associated increase in the AUC of ritonavir of 17% was observed. Patients using this dose regimen have experienced a higher frequency of adverse events (eg, dizziness, nausea, paraesthesia) and laboratory abnormalities (elevated liver enzymes).

Nevirapine: co-administration of ritonavir at therapeutic dose levels does not lead to clinically relevant changes in ritonavir or nevirapine plasma levels. For further information physicians should refer to the Nevirapine Summary of Product Characteristics.

Delavirdine: delavirdine is an inhibitor of CYP3A-mediated metabolism. In a published study, concurrent administration of clinical doses of delavirdine 400 mg three times daily with ritonavir 600 mg twice daily (n = 12 HIV-infected patients) was reported to increase steady-state ritonavir C_{max} and AUC by approximately 50% and C_{min} by about 75%. Based on comparison to historical data, the pharmacokinetics of delavirdine did not appear to be affected by ritonavir. When used in combination with delavirdine, a dose reduction of ritonavir should be considered.

Sildenafil: co-administration of sildenafil 100 mg single dose with ritonavir 500 mg twice daily at steady state resulted in a 300% (4-fold) increase in sildenafil c_{max} and a 1000% (11-fold) increase in sildenafil plasma AUC. At 24 hours after sildenafil dosing, plasma sildenafil concentrations were approximately 200 ng/ml, compared to 5 ng/ml when sildenafil was administered alone.

Sildenafil had no effect on the pharmacokinetics of ritonavir. On the basis of these data, concomitant use of sildenafil with ritonavir is not recommended and in no case should sildenafil doses exceed 25 mg within 48 hours (see also section 4.4).

Ketoconazole: concomitant administration of ritonavir and ketoconazole resulted in markedly elevated ketoconazole plasma levels: mean AUC_{0-24} increased 3.4 fold and C_{max} increased 1.6 fold. The mean half-life of ketoconazole increased from 2.7 to 13.2 h. Because of the large increases in the two agents, doses of ketoconazole 200 mg/day or greater should not be used concomitantly with ritonavir without assessing the risk and benefits. This interaction can have serious gastrointestinal and hepatic consequences.

Alprazolam: after 10 days of ritonavir given at doses titrated up to 500 mg twice daily, the AUC of alprazolam was not significantly affected during co-administration. In a published study, administration of short-term ritonavir (200 mg twice daily for 2 days) resulted in a 2.5 fold increase in the AUC of alprazolam. Alprazolam can be co-administered during chronic therapy with ritonavir > 10 days). Caution is warranted regarding alprazolam co-administration during the first several days after initiating ritonavir therapy, before induction of alprazolam metabolism has occurred.

Triazolam: in a published study, co-administration of short-term ritonavir and triazolam resulted in a very large > 20 fold) increase in the AUC of triazolam. These data support that triazolam and ritonavir should not be co-administered (see section 4.3).

Zolpidem: in a published study, co-administration of short-term ritonavir and zolpidem resulted in a small (< 30%) increase in the AUC of zolpidem. These data support that zolpidem and ritonavir may be co-administered with careful monitoring for excessive sedative effects.

F usidic acid: co-administration of ritonavir with fusidic acid is expected to significantly increase fusidic acid and ritonavir concentrations in plasma.

HMG-CoA reductase inhibitors: HMG-CoA reductase inhibitors which are highly dependent on CYP3A metabolism, such as lovastatin and simvastatin, are expected to have markedly increased plasma concentrations when co-administered with Norvir. Since increased concentrations of HMG-CoA reductase inhibitors may cause myopathy, including rhabdomyolysis, the combination of these medicinal products with Norvir is not recommended. Atorvastatin is less dependent on CYP3A for metabolism. When used with Norvir, the lowest possible doses of atorvastatin should be administered. The metabolism of pravastatin and fluvastatin is not dependent on CYP3A, and interactions are not expected with Norvir. If treatment with an HMG-CoA reductase inhibitor is indicated, pravastatin or fluvastatin is recommended.

Buspirone: ritonavir has been associated with increase in the risk of adverse events to buspirone (such as neurological or psychiatric disorders) when these medicines were co-administered. This may be explained by clinically relevant elevations of buspirone levels due to inhibition of CYP3A-dependent metabolism of buspirone by ritonavir. Caution and clinical monitoring should be exercised when ritonavir is concomitantly used with buspirone.

Norvir DECREASES the AUCs of the following medicines when administered concomitantly:

Zidovudine (AZT) and ddI: zidovudine and ddI have little if any effect on ritonavir pharmacokinetics. Ritonavir decreased the mean zidovudine AUC by approximately 25% in a study, which has not been of sufficient duration to reach steady state for ritonavir. Ritonavir resulted in a reduction of the mean ddI AUC by 13% when given 2.5 hours apart from ritonavir. Dose alteration of AZT or ddI during concomitant Norvir therapy should usually not be necessary. However, dosing of ritonavir and ddI should be separated by 2.5 hours to avoid formulation incompatibilities. Human pharmacokinetic data for combination with antiretroviral medicines other than zidovudine and ddI are not yet available (see also section 4.4).

Ethinyl oestradiol: because concomitant administration of ritonavir with a fixed combination oral contraceptive resulted in a reduction of the ethinyl oestradiol mean AUC by 41%, increased doses of oral contraceptives containing ethinyl oestradiol, or alternate methods of contraception should be considered.

Theophylline: an increased dosage of theophylline may be required, as concomitant use with ritonavir caused an approximately 45% decrease in the AUC of theophylline.

Fixed combination of sulfamethoxazole/trimethoprim: the concomitant administration of Norvir and sulfamethoxazole/trimethoprim resulted in a 20% reduction of the sulfamethoxazole AUC and a 20% increase of the trimethoprim AUC. Dose alteration of sulfamethoxazole/trimethoprim during concomitant Norvir therapy should not be necessary.

Methadone: concomitant administration of ritonavir and methadone resulted in a reduction of the mean methadone AUC by 36%. An increased methadone dose may be necessary when concomitantly administered with ritonavir, depending on the patient's response.

Meperidine: co-administration of multiple-dose ritonavir with single dose oral meperidine resulted in a 62% decrease in meperidine AUC and a 47% increase in normeperidine AUC. Dosage increase and long term use of meperidine and ritonavir are not recommended due to the increased concentrations of the metabolite, normeperidine, which has both analgesic and CNS stimulant activity (eg, seizures).

Fluticasone propionate: in a clinical study where ritonavir 100 mg capsules twice daily were co – administered with 50 μg intranasal fluticasone propionate (4 times daily) for seven days in healthy subjects, the fluticasone propionate plasma levels increased significantly, whereas the intrinsic cortisol levels decreased by approximately 86% (90% confidence interval 82 – 89%). Greater effects may be expected when fluticasone propionate is inhaled. Systemic corticosteroid effects including Cushing's syndrome and adrenal suppression have been reported when ritonavir has been co – administered with inhaled or intranasally administered fluticasone propionate; this could also occur with other corticosteroids eg budesonide. Consequently, concomitant administration of Norvir (including low dose of ritonavir) and inhaled or intranasally administered glucocorticoids is not recommended unless the potential benefit of treatment outweighs the risk of systemic corticosteroid effects. A dose reduction of the glucocorticoid should be considered with close monitoring. Moreover, in case of withdrawal of glucocorticoids progressive dose reduction may have to be performed over a longer period. The effects of high fluticasone systemic exposure on ritonavir plasma levels is yet unknown (see section 4.4).

Because ritonavir is highly protein bound, the possibility of increased therapeutic and toxic effects due to protein binding displacement of concomitant medications should be considered.

Cardiac and neurologic events have been reported when ritonavir has been co-administered with disopyramide, mexiletine, nefazadone, or fluoxetine. The possibility of drug interaction cannot be excluded.

4.6 Pregnancy and lactation

No treatment-related malformations were observed with ritonavir in either rats or rabbits. Developmental toxicity observed in rats (embryolethality, decreased foetal body weight and ossification delays and visceral changes, including delayed testicular descent) occurred mainly at a maternally toxic dosage. Developmental toxicity in rabbits (embryolethality, decreased litter size and decreased foetal weights) occurred at a maternally toxic dosage.

There are no studies in pregnant women. This medicine should be used during pregnancy only if the potential benefits clearly outweigh the potential risks.

It is not known whether this medicine is excreted in human milk. Milk excretion has not been measured in the animal studies, however a study in rats showed some effects on offspring development during lactation which are compatible with excretion of ritonavir in milk in that species. HIV infected women should not breast-feed their infants under any circumstances to avoid transmission of HIV.

4.7 Effects on ability to drive and use machines

Norvir has not specifically been tested for its possible effects on the ability to drive a car or operate machines. As somnolence and dizziness are known undesirable effects, this should be taken into account when driving or using machinery.

Norvir oral solution contains alcohol (43%).

4.8 Undesirable effects

In clinical studies (Phase II/III), the following adverse events with possible, probable or unknown relationship to ritonavir have been reported in ⩾ 2% of 1033 patients:

Classification of expected frequencies:

Very common	> 1/10)
Common	> 1/100, < 1/10)
Uncommon	> 1/1,000, < 1/100)
Rare	> 1/10,000, < 1/1,000)

Nausea, diarrhoea, vomiting, asthenia, taste perversion, circumoral and peripheral paraesthesia were very common and are felt to be clearly related to ritonavir.

Nervous system disorders: Dizziness, paraesthesia, hyperaesthesia, somnolence, insomnia and anxiety were commonly reported.

Cardiovascular disorders: Vasodilation was commonly reported.

Respiratory system disorders: Pharyngitis and cough increased were commonly reported.

Gastrointestinal disorders: Very common events reported were abdominal pain. Dyspepsia, anorexia, local throat irritation, flatulence, dry mouth, eructation and mouth ulcer were commonly reported.

Musculoskeletal system disorders: Increased CPK and myalgia were commonly reported. Myositis was reported rarely. Rarely, rhabdomyolysis has been reported with protease inhibitors, particularly in combination with nucleoside analogues.

Skin and subcutaneous tissue disorders: Rash, pruritus and sweating were commonly reported.

Allergic reactions including urticaria, mild skin eruptions, bronchospasm, and angioedema have been reported. Rare cases of anaphylaxis and Stevens-Johnson syndrome have been reported

Other disorders: Very common events reported were headache. Fever, pain and weight loss were commonly reported.

There have been spontaneous reports of thrombocytopenia, seizure and menorrhagia.

Dehydration usually associated with gastrointestinal symptoms, and sometimes resulting in hypotension, syncope, or renal insufficiency has been reported. Syncope, orthostatic hypotension and renal insufficiency have also been reported without known dehydration.

Hepatic transaminase elevations exceeding five times the upper limit or normal, clinical hepatitis, and jaundice have occurred in patients receiving ritonavir alone or in combination with other antiretrovirals.

Combination antiretroviral therapy has been associated with redistribution of body fat (lipodystrophy) in HIV patients including the loss of peripheral and facial subcutaneous fat, increased intra-abdominal and visceral fat, breast hypertrophy and dorsocervical fat accumulation (buffalo hump).

Combination antiretroviral therapy has been associated with metabolic abnormalities such as hypertriglyceridaemia, hypercholesterolaemia, insulin resistance, hyperglycaemia and hyperlactataemia (see section 4.4).

In HIV-infected patients with severe immune deficiency at the time of initiation of combination antiretroviral therapy (CART), an inflammatory reaction to asymptomatic or residual opportunistic infections may arise (see section 4.4).

Hyperglycaemia has been reported in individuals with and without a known history of diabetes. Cause and effect relationship has not been established.

Hypertriglyceridaemia, hypercholesterolaemia and hyperuricaemia were clearly related to ritonavir therapy.

Pancreatitis has been observed in patients receiving Norvir therapy, including those who developed hypertriglyceridemia. In some cases fatalities have been observed. Patients with advanced HIV disease may be at risk of elevated triglycerides and pancreatitis.

Pancreatitis should be considered if clinical symptoms (nausea, vomiting, abdominal pain) or abnormalities in laboratory values (such as increased serum lipase or amylase values) suggestive of pancreatitis should occur. Patients who exhibit these signs or symptoms should be evaluated and Norvir therapy should be discontinued if a diagnosis of pancreatitis is made.

Clinical chemistry:

High gamma-glutamyl transpeptidase (GGT), high creatine phosphokinase (CPK), high triglycerides, high alanine transaminase (SGPT); high aspartate transaminase (SGOT), high amylase, high uric acid, low potassium and decrease of free and total thyroxin (T_4) values were commonly reported. Uncommon events were high glucose, low total calcium, high magnesium, high total bilirubin, high alkaline phosphatase.

Haematology:

Low white blood cell (WBC), low haemoglobin, low neutrophils and high eosinophils were commonly reported. Uncommon events were high WBC, high neutrophils and high prothrombin time.

4.9 Overdose

Human experience of acute overdose with ritonavir is limited. One patient in clinical trials took ritonavir 1500 mg/day for two days and reported paraesthesia, which resolved after the dose was decreased. A case of renal failure with eosinophilia has been reported.

The signs of toxicity observed in animals (mice and rats) included decreased activity, ataxia, dyspnoea and tremors.

There is no specific antidote for overdose with ritonavir. Treatment of overdose with ritonavir should consist of general supportive measures including monitoring of vital signs and observation of the clinical status of the patient. Due to the solubility characteristics and possibility of transintestinal elimination, it is proposed that management of overdose could entail gastric lavage and administration of activated charcoal. Since ritonavir is extensively metabolised by the liver and is highly protein bound, dialysis is unlikely to be beneficial in significant removal of the medicine.

5. PHARMACOLOGICAL PROPERTIES

5.1 Pharmacodynamic properties

Pharmaco-therapeutic group: antiviral for systemic use, ATC code: J05A E03

Ritonavir is an orally active peptidomimetic inhibitor of the HIV-1 and HIV-2 aspartyl proteases. Inhibition of HIV protease renders the enzyme incapable of processing the *gag-pol* polyprotein precursor which leads to the production of HIV particles with immature morphology that are unable to initiate new rounds of infection. Ritonavir has selective affinity for the HIV protease and has little inhibitory activity against human aspartyl proteases.

In vitro data indicates that ritonavir is active against all strains of HIV tested in a variety of transformed and primary human cell lines. The concentration of ritonavir that inhibits 50% and 90% of viral replication *in vitro* is approximately 0.02 μM and 0.11 μM, respectively. Similar potencies were found with both AZT-sensitive and AZT-resistant strains of HIV. Studies which measured direct cell toxicity of ritonavir on several cell lines showed no direct toxicity at concentrations up to 25 μM, with a resulting *in vitro* therapeutic index of at least 1000.

Resistance

Ritonavir-resistant isolates of HIV-1 have been selected *in vitro*. The resistant isolates showed reduced susceptibility to ritonavir and genotypic analysis showed that the resistance was attributable primarily to specific amino acid substitutions in the HIV-1 protease at codons 82 and 84.

Susceptibility of clinical isolates to ritonavir was monitored in controlled clinical trials. Some patients receiving ritonavir monotherapy developed HIV strains with decreased susceptibility to ritonavir. Serial genotypic and phenotypic analysis indicated that susceptibility to ritonavir declined in an ordered and stepwise fashion. Initial mutations occurred at position 82 from wildtype valine to usually alanine or phenylalanine (V82A/F). Viral strains isolated *in vivo* without a change at codon 82 did not have decreased susceptibility to ritonavir.

Cross-resistance to other antiretrovirals

Serial HIV isolates obtained from six patients during ritonavir therapy showed a decrease in ritonavir susceptibility *in vitro* but did not demonstrate a concordant decrease in susceptibility to saquinavir *in vitro* when compared to matched baseline isolates. However, isolates from two of these patients demonstrated decrease susceptibility to indinavir *in vitro* (8-fold). Cross-resistance between ritonavir and reverse transcriptase inhibitors is unlikely because of the different enzyme targets involved. One AZT-resistant HIV isolate tested *in vitro* retained full susceptibility to ritonavir.

Clinical pharmacodynamic data

The effects of ritonavir (alone or combined with other antiretroviral agents) on biological markers of disease activity such as CD4 cell count and viral RNA were evaluated in several studies involving HIV-1 infected patients. The following studies are the most important.

Adult Use

A controlled study with ritonavir as add-on therapy in HIV-1 infected patients extensively pre-treated with nucleoside analogues and baseline CD4 cell counts ⩽ 100 cells/μl showed a reduction in mortality and AIDS defining events. The mean average change from baseline over 16 weeks for HIV RNA levels was -0.79 $\log_{10}$ (maximum mean decrease: 1.29 $\log_{10}$) in the ritonavir group versus-0.01 $\log_{10}$ in the control group. The most frequently used nucleosides in this study were zidovudine, stavudine, didanosine and zalcitabine.

In a study recruiting less advanced HIV-1 infected patients (CD4 200-500 cells/μl) without previous antiretroviral therapy, ritonavir in combination with zidovudine or alone reduced viral load in plasma and increased CD4 count. The effects of ritonavir monotherapy seemed unexpectedly to be at least as large as the combination therapy, a finding which has not been explained adequately. The mean average change from baseline over 48 weeks for HIV RNA levels was -0.88 $\log_{10}$ in the ritonavir group versus -0.66 $\log_{10}$ in the ritonavir + zidovudine group versus -0.42 $\log_{10}$ in the zidovudine group.

The continuation of ritonavir therapy should be evaluated by viral load because of the possibility of the emergence of resistance as described under section 4.1 Therapeutic indications.

In an open label trial in 32 antiretroviral naive HIV-1 infected patients the combination of ritonavir with zidovudine and zalcitabine decreased the viral load (mean decrease at week 20 of -1.76 $\log_{10}$).

Paediatric Use

In an open label trial in HIV infected, clinically stable children there was a significant difference (p = 0.03) in the detectable RNA levels in favour of a triple regimen (ritonavir, zidovudine and lamivudine) following 48 weeks treatment.

Studies investigating optimal combinations and the long term efficacy and safety of ritonavir are ongoing.

5.2 Pharmacokinetic properties

There is no parenteral formulation of ritonavir, therefore the extent of absorption and absolute bioavailability have not been determined. The pharmacokinetics of ritonavir during multiple dose regimens were studied in non-fasting HIV positive adult volunteers. Upon multiple dosing, ritonavir accumulation is slightly less than predicted from a single dose due to a time and dose-related increase in apparent clearance (Cl/F). Trough concentrations of ritonavir were observed to decrease over time, possibly due to enzyme induction, but appeared to stabilise by the end of 2 weeks. At steady state with a 600 mg twice daily dose, maximal concentration (C_{max}) and trough concentration (C_{trough}) values of 11.2 ± 3.6 and 3.7 ± 2.6 μg/ml (mean ± SD) were observed, respectively. Over a 12 hour dosing interval, the AUC_{12h} was 77.5 +/- 31.5 μg·h/ml. The half life ($t_{1/2}$) of ritonavir was approximately 3 to 5 hours. The steady-state apparent clearance in patients treated with 600 mg bid has averaged 8.8 ± 3.2 l/h. Renal clearance averaged less than 0.1 l/h and was relatively constant throughout the dosage range. The time to maximum concentration (T_{max}) remained constant at approximately 4 hours with increasing dose.

The pharmacokinetics of ritonavir are dose-dependent: more than proportional increases in the AUC and C_{max} were reported with increasing dose. Ingestion with food results in higher ritonavir exposure than ingestion in the fasted state.

No clinically significant differences in AUC or C_{max} were noted between males and females. Ritonavir pharmacokinetic parameters were not statistically significantly associated with body weight or lean body mass.

Patients with impaired liver function: after multiple dosing of ritonavir to healthy volunteers (500 mg twice daily) and subjects with mild to moderate hepatic impairment (400 mg twice daily) exposure to ritonavir after dose normalisation was not significantly different between the two groups.

The apparent volume of distribution (V_B/F) of ritonavir is approximately 20 - 40 l after a single 600 mg dose. The protein binding of ritonavir in human plasma was noted to be approximately 98 - 99%. Ritonavir binds to both human alpha 1-acid glycoprotein (AAG) and human serum albumin (HSA) with comparable affinities. Plasma protein binding is constant over the concentration range of 0.1 – 100 μg /ml.

Tissue distribution studies with ^{14}C-labelled ritonavir in rats showed the liver, adrenals, pancreas, kidneys and thyroid to have the highest concentrations of ritonavir. Tissue to plasma ratios of approximately 1 measured in rat lymph nodes suggests that ritonavir distributes into lymphatic tissues. Ritonavir penetrates minimally into the brain.

Ritonavir was noted to be extensively metabolised by the hepatic cytochrome P450 system, primarily isozyme CYP3A4 and to a lesser extent CYP2D6. Animal studies as well as *in vitro* experiments with human hepatic microsomes indicated that ritonavir primarily underwent oxidative metabolism. Four ritonavir metabolites have been identified in man. The isopropylthiazole oxidation metabolite (M-2) is the major metabolite and has antiviral activity similar to that of parent drug. However, the AUC of the M-2 metabolite was approximately 3% of the AUC of parent drug.

Human studies with radiolabelled ritonavir demonstrated that the elimination of ritonavir was primarily via the hepatobiliary system; approximately 86% of radiolabel was recovered from stool, part of which is expected to be unabsorbed ritonavir. In these studies renal elimination was not found to be a major route of elimination of ritonavir.

This was consistent with the observations in animal studies.

Steady-state pharmacokinetics were evaluated in HIV infected children above 2 years of age receiving doses ranging from 250 mg/m^2 twice daily to 400 mg/m^2 twice daily. Ritonavir concentrations obtained after 350 to 400 mg/m^2 twice daily in paediatric patients were comparable to those obtained in adults receiving 600 mg (approximately 330 mg/m^2) twice daily.

5.3 Preclinical safety data

Repeated dose toxicity studies in animals identified major target organs as the liver, retina, thyroid gland and kidney. Hepatic changes involved hepatocellular, biliary and phagocytic elements and were accompanied by increases in hepatic enzymes. Hyperplasia of the retinal pigment epithelium (RPE) and retinal degeneration have been seen in all of the rodent studies conducted with ritonavir, but have not been seen in dogs. Ultrastructural evidence suggests that these retinal changes may be secondary to phospholipidosis. However, clinical trials revealed no evidence of drug-induced ocular changes in humans. All thyroid changes were reversible upon discontinuation of ritonavir. Clinical investigation in humans has revealed no clinically significant alteration in thyroid function tests. Renal changes including tubular degeneration, chronic inflammation and proteinurea were noted in rats and are felt to be attributable to species-specific spontaneous disease. Furthermore, no clinically significant renal abnormalities were noted in clinical trials.

Ritonavir was not found to be mutagenic or clastogenic in a battery of *in vitro* and *in vivo* assays including the Ames bacterial reverse mutation assay using *S. typhimurium* and *E. coli*, the mouse lymphoma assay, the mouse micronucleus test and chromosomal aberration assays in human lymphocytes.

Long term carcinogenicity studies of ritonavir in mice and rats revealed tumourigenic potential specific for these species, but are regarded as of no relevance for humans.

6. PHARMACEUTICAL PARTICULARS

6.1 List of excipients

Norvir oral solution contains: alcohol, purified water, polyoxyl 35 castor oil, propylene glycol, anhydrous citric acid, saccharin sodium, peppermint oil, creamy caramel flavour, and dye E110.

6.2 Incompatibilities

Norvir should not be diluted with water.

6.3 Shelf life

6 months

6.4 Special precautions for storage

Norvir oral solution should be stored below 25°C and should be used within the expiry date shown on the bottle. Do not refrigerate or freeze. Shake well before each use. If, after shaking, particles or precipitate can be seen in the solution, the patient should take the next dose and see their doctor about a fresh supply.

Avoid exposure to excessive heat.

6.5 Nature and contents of container

Norvir oral solution is supplied in amber coloured multiple-dose polyethylene terephthalate (PET) bottles in a 90 ml size. Each pack contains 5 bottles of 90 ml (450 ml). A dosage cup containing graduations at 3.75 ml (300 mg dose), 5 ml (400 mg dose), 6.25 ml (500 mg dose) and 7.5 ml (600 mg dose) is provided.

6.6 Instructions for use and handling

The dosage cup or oral syringe should be cleaned immediately with hot water and dish soap after use. When cleaned immediately, drug residue is removed. The device **must** be dry prior to use

7. MARKETING AUTHORISATION HOLDER

Abbott Laboratories Limited

Queenborough

Kent ME11 5EL

United Kingdom

8. MARKETING AUTHORISATION NUMBER(S)

EU/1/96/016/001

9. DATE OF FIRST AUTHORISATION/RENEWAL OF THE AUTHORISATION

Date of first authorisation: 26 August 1996

Date of last renewal: 27 August 2001

10. DATE OF REVISION OF THE TEXT

20th January 2005

Norvir Soft Capsules

(Abbott Laboratories Limited)

1. NAME OF THE MEDICINAL PRODUCT

Norvir 100 mg soft capsules

2. QUALITATIVE AND QUANTITATIVE COMPOSITION

Each soft capsule of Norvir contains 100 mg ritonavir.

For excipients, see section 6.1

3. PHARMACEUTICAL FORM

SoftCapsule.

4. CLINICAL PARTICULARS

4.1 Therapeutic indications

Norvir is indicated in combination with other antiretroviral agents for the treatment of HIV-1 infected patients (adults and children of 2 years of age and older).

In protease inhibitor experienced patients the choice of ritonavir should be based on individual viral resistance testing and treatment history of patients.

4.2 Posology and method of administration

Adult use: Norvir softcapsules are administered orally and should preferably be ingested with food. The recommended dosage of Norvir soft capsules is 600 mg (6 capsules) twice daily by mouth.

Gradually increasing the dose of ritonavir when initiating therapy may help to improve tolerance.

Single Protease Inhibitor (PI) containing combination regimen for adults: Treatment should be initiated at 300 mg (3 capsules) twice daily for a period of three days and increased by 100 mg (1 capsule) twice daily increments up to 600 mg twice daily over a period of no longer than 14 days. Patients should not remain on 300 mg twice daily for more than 3 days.

Dual PI containing combination regimens: Clinical experience with dual therapy including therapeutic doses of ritonavir with another protease inhibitor is limited. Ritonavir extensively inhibits the metabolism of most available protease inhibitors. Hence, any consideration of dual therapy with ritonavir should take into account the pharmacokinetic interaction and safety data of involved agents. There is extensive cross-resistance in this class of agents. The combination of two PIs with the least overlapping patterns of resistance should be considered. The use of ritonavir in such regimens should be guided by these factors.

Ritonavir as a pharmacokinetic enhancer for other PIs: In clinical practice ritonavir is frequently used as a pharmacokinetic enhancer (at low doses of 100 – 200 mg once or twice daily) to boost the plasma concentrations of other PIs in HIV-infected adult patients. For further specific information, refer to the Summary of Product Characteristics of the concerned PIs. See also section 4.5.

For the use of ritonavir with saquinavir a cautious titration of the dose has been used by initiating ritonavir dosing at 300 mg twice daily.

For the use of ritonavir with indinavir a cautious titration of the dose has been used by initiating ritonavir dosing at 200 mg twice daily increasing by 100 mg twice daily reaching 400 mg twice daily within 2 weeks.

Paediatric use (2 years of age and above): the recommended dosage of Norvir in children is 350 mg/m^2 by mouth twice daily and should not exceed 600 mg twice daily. Norvir should be started at 250 mg/m^2 and increased at 2 to 3 day intervals by 50 mg/m^2 twice daily (please refer to the Norvir 80 mg/ml oral solution Summary of Product Characteristics)

For older children it may be feasible to substitute soft capsules for the maintenance dose of the oral solution.

Dosage conversion from oral solution to soft capsules for children

Oral solution dose	Capsule dose
175 mg (2.2 ml) twice daily	200 mg in the morning and 200 mg in the evening
350 mg (4.4 ml) twice daily	400 mg in the morning and 300 mg in the evening
437.5 mg (5.5 ml) twice daily	500 mg in the morning and 400 mg in the evening
525 mg (6.6 ml) twice daily	500 mg in the morning and 500 mg in the evening

The safety and efficacy of ritonavir in children under the age of 2 have not been established.

Renal impairment: currently, there are no data specific to this patient population and therefore specific dosage recommendations cannot be made. Because ritonavir is highly protein bound it is unlikely that it will be significantly removed by haemodialysis or peritoneal dialysis.

Hepatic impairment: ritonavir is principally metabolised and eliminated by the liver. Pharmacokinetic data indicate that no dose adjustment seems necessary in patients with mild to moderate hepatic impairment (see section 5.2). Norvir should not be given to patients with severe hepatic impairment (see section 4.3).

Ritonavir should be administered by physicians who are experienced in the treatment of HIV infection.

4.3 Contraindications

Patients with known hypersensitivity to ritonavir or any of its excipients. Patients with severe hepatic impairment.

In vitro and *in vivo* studies have demonstrated that ritonavir is a potent inhibitor of CYP3A- and CYP2D6- mediated biotransformations. Based primarily on literature review, ritonavir is expected to produce large increases in the plasma concentrations of the following medicines: amiodarone, astemizole, bepridil, bupropion, cisapride, clozapine, dihydroergotamine, encainide, ergotamine, flecainide, meperidine, pimozide, piroxicam, propafenone, propoxyphene, quinidine, and terfenadine. These agents have recognised risks of arrhythmias, haematologic abnormalities, seizures, or other potentially serious adverse effects. Additionally, acute ergot toxicity characterised by peripheral vasospasm and ischaemia has been associated with co-administration of ritonavir and ergotamine or dihydroergotamine. These medicines should not be co-administered with ritonavir. Ritonavir in addition is likely to produce large increases in these highly metabolised sedatives and hypnotics: clorazepate, diazepam, estazolam, flurazepam, midazolam and triazolam. Due to the potential for extreme sedation and respiratory depression from these agents, they should not be co-administered with ritonavir.

Concomitant use of ritonavir and rifabutin is contraindicated because of clinical consequences such as uveitis resulting from a multifold increase of rifabutin serum concentrations.

Herbal preparations containing St John's wort (*Hypericum perforatum)* must not be used while taking ritonavir due to the risk of decreased plasma concentrations and reduced clinical effects of ritonavir. (See section 4.5).

4.4 Special warnings and special precautions for use

Patients with pre-existing conditions

Renal disease: there are no data on the pharmacokinetics and safety of ritonavir in patients with significant renal dysfunction.

Liver disease: the safety and efficacy of Norvir has not been established in patients with significant underlying liver disorders. Norvir is contraindicated in patients with severe hepatic impairment (see section 4.3). Patients with chronic hepatitis B or C and treated with combination antiretroviral therapy are at an increased risk for severe and potentially fatal hepatic adverse events. In case of concomitant antiviral therapy for hepatitis B or C, please refer to the relevant product information for these medicinal products.

Patients with pre-existing liver dysfunction including chronic active hepatitis have an increased frequency of liver function abnormalities during combination antiretroviral therapy and should be monitored according to standard practice. If there is evidence of worsening liver disease in such patients, interruption or discontinuation of treatment must be considered.

Haemophilia: there have been reports of increased bleeding, including spontaneous skin haematomas and haemarthroses, in haemophiliac patients type A and B treated with protease inhibitors. In some patients additional factor VIII was given. In more than a half of the reported cases, treatment with protease inhibitors was continued or reintroduced if treatment had been discontinued. A causal relationship has been evoked, although the mechanism of action has not been elucidated. Haemophiliac patients should therefore be made aware of the possibility of increased bleeding.

Immune Reactivation Syndrome: in HIV-infected patients with severe immune deficiency at the time of institution of combination antiretroviral therapy (CART), an inflammatory reaction to asymptomatic or residual opportunistic pathogens may arise and cause serious clinical conditions, or aggravation of symptoms. Typically, such reactions have been observed within the first few weeks or months of initiation of CART. Relevant examples are cytomegalovirus retinitis, generalised and/or focal mycobacterial infections, and Pneumocystis carinii pneumonia. Any inflammatory symptoms should be evaluated and treatment instituted when necessary.

The safety and efficacy of ritonavir in children below the age of 2 years have not been established.

Human pharmacokinetic data for combination of ritonavir with antiretroviral medicinal products other than zidovudine and didanosine (ddI) are not yet available. Although the clinical use of combinations with zalcitabine (ddC) and stavudine (d4T) in a relatively limited number of patients did not seem to be associated with unfavourable effects, the use of combinations of ritonavir with other nucleoside analogues should be guided by cautious therapeutic and safety monitoring.

Extra monitoring is recommended when diarrhoea occurs. The relatively high frequency of diarrhoea during treatment with ritonavir may compromise the absorption and efficacy (due to decreased compliance) of ritonavir or other concurrent medications. Serious persistent vomiting and/or diarrhoea associated with ritonavir use might also compromise renal function. It is advisable to monitor renal function in patients with renal function impairment.

A pharmacokinetic study demonstrated that ritonavir extensively inhibits the metabolism of saquinavir resulting in greatly increased saquinavir plasma concentrations (see section 4.5). Doses greater than 400 mg twice daily of either medicine were associated with an increased incidence of adverse events.

Norvir soft capsules contain alcohol (12% w/w), therefore concomitant administration of Norvir with disulfiram or medicines with disulfiram-like reactions (eg, metronidazole) should be avoided.

New onset diabetes mellitus, hyperglycaemia or exacerbation of existing diabetes mellitus has been reported in patients receiving protease inhibitors. In some of these the hyperglycaemia was severe and in some cases also associated with ketoacidosis. Many patients had confounding medical conditions, some of which required therapy with agents that have been associated with the development of diabetes mellitus or hyperglycaemia.

Combination antiretroviral therapy has been associated with redistribution of body fat (lipodystrophy) in HIV patients. The long-term consequences of these events are currently unknown. Knowledge about the mechanism is incomplete. A connection between visceral lipomatosis and PIs and lipoatrophy and reverse transcriptase inhibitors (NRTIs) has been hypothesised. A higher risk of lipodystrophy has been associated with individual factors such as older age, and with drug related factors such as longer duration of antiretroviral treatment and associated metabolic disturbances. Clinical examination should include evaluation for physical signs of fat redistribution. Consideration should be given to measurement of fasting serum lipids and blood glucose. Lipid disorders should be managed as clinically appropriate (see section 4.8).

Particular caution should be used when prescribing sildenafil in patients receiving ritonavir. Co-administration of ritonavir with sildenafil is expected to substantially increase sildenafil concentrations (11-fold increase in AUC) and may result in sildenafil-associated adverse events, including hypotension, syncope, visual changes and prolonged erection (see also section 4.5).

The HMG-CoA reductase inhibitors simvastatin and lovastatin are highly dependent on CYP3A for metabolism, thus concomitant use of Norvir with simvastatin or lovastatin is not recommended due to an increased risk of myopathy including rhabdomyolysis. Caution must also be exercised and reduced doses should be considered if Norvir is used concurrently with atorvastatin, which is metabolised to a lesser extent by CYP3A. If treatment with an HMG-CoA reductase inhibitor is indicated, pravastatin or fluvastatin is recommended (see section 4.5).

Concomitant use of ritonavir (including low-dose) and fluticasone propionate significantly increased fluticasone propionate plasma concentrations and reduced serum cortisol concentrations in a clinical study. Concomitant use of ritonavir (including low-dose) and fluticasone is therefore not recommended unless the potential benefit of treatment outweighs the risk of systemic corticosteroid effects. Systemic corticosteroid effects including Cushing's syndrome and adrenal suppression have been reported when ritonavir has been co-administered with inhaled or intranasal administered fluticasone propionate (see section 4.5).

4.5 Interaction with other medicinal products and other forms of Interaction

Refer also to Contraindications (section 4.3)

Ritonavir has a high affinity for several cytochrome P450 (CYP) isoforms with the following ranked order: CYP3A> CYP2D6> CYP2C9. In addition to the medicines listed in the Contraindications section, the following medicines or drug classes are known or suspected to be metabolised by these same cytochrome P450 isozymes: immunosuppressants (eg, cyclosporine, tacrolimus), macrolide antibiotics (eg, erythromycin), various steroids (eg, dexamethasone, prednisolone), other HIV-protease inhibitors, delavirdine, nonsedating antihistamines (eg, loratidine), buspirone, calcium channel antagonists, several tricyclic antidepressants (eg, desipramine, imipramine, amitriptyline, nortriptyline), other antidepressants (eg, fluoxetine, paroxetine, sertraline), neuroleptics (eg, haloperidol, risperidone, thioridazine), antifungals (eg, itraconazole), morphinomimetics (eg, fentanyl), carbamazepine, tolbutamide, amphetamine and amphetamine derivatives. Due to the potential for significant elevation of serum levels of these medicines they should not be used concomitantly with ritonavir without a careful assessment of the potential risks and benefits. Careful monitoring of therapeutic and adverse effects is recommended when these medicines are concomitantly administered with ritonavir.

Warfarin oral anticoagulant concentrations may be affected, and notably decreased, when co-administered with ritonavir. This frequently leads to reduced anticoagulation, therefore it is recommended that anticoagulation parameters are monitored.

Serum levels of ritonavir can be reduced by concomitant use of the herbal preparation St John's wort (*Hypericum perforatum*). This is due to the induction of drug metabolising enzymes by St John's wort. Herbal preparations containing St John's wort should therefore not be combined with ritonavir. If a patient is already taking St John's wort, stop St John's wort and if possible check viral levels. Ritonavir levels may increase on stopping St John's wort. The dose of ritonavir may need adjusting. The inducing effect may persist for at least 2 weeks after cessation of treatment with St John's wort.

There are no pharmacokinetic data available on the concomitant use of morphine with ritonavir. On the basis of the metabolism of morphine (glucuronidation) lower levels of morphine may be expected.

Norvir INCREASES the AUCs (area under the curve) of the following medicines when administered concomitantly:

Clarithromycin: because of the large therapeutic window for clarithromycin, no dosage reduction should be necessary in patients with normal renal function. For patients with renal impairment the following dosage adjustment should be considered: for creatinine clearance (CL_{CR}) of 30 to 60 ml/min the clarithromycin dose should be reduced by 50%, for CL_{CR} < 30 ml/min the clarithromycin dose should be reduced by 75%. Doses of clarithromycin > 1 g/day should not be co-administered with Norvir.

Desipramine: dosage reduction of desipramine should be considered in patients taking the combination.

Rifabutin and its active metabolite 25-O-desacetyl rifabutin: concomitant use with ritonavir has resulted in a multi-fold increase in the AUC of rifabutin and its active metabolite 25-O-desacetyl rifabutin with clinical consequences. Therefore, the concomitant use of ritonavir and rifabutin is contraindicated (see section 4.3).

Saquinavir: data from pharmacokinetic studies in patients indicate that co-administration of ritonavir 400 mg twice daily produce multifold increases in saquinavir steady state blood levels (AUC, 17 fold; C_{max}, 14 fold increase). Doses greater than 400 mg twice daily of either medicine were associated with an increased incidence of adverse events.

In HIV-infected patients, Invirase and Fortovase in combination with ritonavir at doses of 1000/100 mg twice daily provide saquinavir systemic exposure over a 24 hour period greater than those achieved with Fortovase 1200 mg three times daily. For further information, physicians should refer to the Invirase and Fortovase Summary of Product Characteristics.

Indinavir: ritonavir inhibits the CYP3A-mediated metabolism of indinavir. In healthy subjects, 200 mg to 400 mg of ritonavir twice daily given with a single 400 mg to 600 mg indinavir dose increased the indinavir AUC by 185% to 475%, C_{max} 21% to 110%, and C_{8h} 11 to 33-fold, relative to 400 mg to 600 mg indinavir given alone. Concomitant administration of 400 mg ritonavir and 400 mg indinavir twice daily with a meal yielded a similar indinavir AUC, a 4 fold increase in C_{min} and a 50% to 60% decrease in C_{max} as compared to those resulting from administration of indinavir 800 mg three times daily under fasting conditions. Co-administration of ritonavir with indinavir will result in increased indinavir serum concentrations. There are limited safety or efficacy data available on the use of this combination in patients. The risk of nephrolithiasis may be increased when doses of indinavir equal to or greater than 800 mg twice daily are given with ritonavir. Adequate hydration and monitoring of the patients is warranted.

Nelfinavir: interactions between ritonavir and nelfinavir are likely to involve both Cytochrome P450 inhibition and induction. Concurrent ritonavir 400 mg twice daily significantly increases the concentrations of M8 (the major active metabolite of nelfinavir), and results in a smaller increase in nelfinavir concentrations. In a study in 10 patients, nelfinavir 750 mg and ritonavir 400 mg twice daily yielded slightly higher nelfinavir AUC (160%), C_{max} (121%) and C_{trough} (123%) than historical data for nelfinavir 750 mg three times daily monotherapy. The AUC of M8 was increased by 347%.

Amprenavir: concentrations of amprenavir, are increased when co-administered with ritonavir due to inhibition of the metabolism of amprenavir mediated by Cytochrome P450 isoenzymes. Booster doses of ritonavir given together with amprenavir result in clinically significant increases in amprenavir AUC and C_{min} with variable effects on maximum concentration. When given in combination in adults, reduced doses of both medicinal products (amprenavir 600 mg twice daily and ritonavir 100 mg twice daily) should be used. For further information, physicians should refer to the Agenerase Summary of Product Characteristics.

Efavirenz: in healthy volunteers receiving 500 mg ritonavir twice daily with efavirenz 600 mg once daily, the steady state AUC of efavirenz was increased by 21%. An associated increase in the AUC of ritonavir of 17% was observed. Patients using this dose regimen have experienced a higher frequency of adverse events (eg, dizziness, nausea, paraesthesia) and laboratory abnormalities (elevated liver enzymes).

Nevirapine: co-administration of ritonavir at therapeutic dose levels does not lead to clinically relevant changes in ritonavir or nevirapine plasma levels. For further information physicians should refer to the Nevirapine Summary of Product Characteristics.

Delavirdine: delavirdine is an inhibitor of CYP3A-mediated metabolism. In a published study, concurrent administration of clinical doses of delavirdine 400 mg three times daily with ritonavir 600 mg twice daily (n = 12 HIV-infected patients) was reported to increase steady-state ritonavir C_{max} and AUC by approximately 50% and C_{min} by about 75%. Based on comparison to historical data, the pharmacokinetics of delavirdine did not appear to be affected by ritonavir. When used in combination with delavirdine, a dose reduction of ritonavir should be considered.

Sildenafil: co-administration of sildenafil 100 mg single dose with ritonavir 500 mg twice daily at steady state resulted in a 300% (4-fold) increase in sildenafil C_{max} and a 1000% (11-fold) increase in sildenafil plasma AUC. At 24 hours after sildenafil dosing, plasma sildenafil concentrations were approximately 200 ng/ml, compared to 5 ng/ml when sildenafil was administered alone.

Sildenafil had no effect on the pharmacokinetics of ritonavir. On the basis of these data, concomitant use of sildenafil with ritonavir is not recommended and in no case should sildenafil doses exceed 25 mg within 48 hours (see also section 4.4).

Ketoconazole: concomitant administration of ritonavir and ketoconazole resulted in markedly elevated ketoconazole plasma levels: mean AUC_{0-24} increased 3.4 fold and C_{max} increased 1.6 fold. The mean half-life of ketoconazole increased from 2.7 to 13.2 h. Because of the large increases in the two agents, doses of ketoconazole 200 mg/day or greater should not be used concomitantly with ritonavir without assessing the risk and benefits. This interaction can have serious gastrointestinal and hepatic consequences.

Alprazolam: after 10 days of ritonavir given at doses titrated up to 500 mg twice daily, the AUC of alprazolam was not significantly affected during co-administration. In a published study, administration of short-term ritonavir (200 mg twice daily for 2 days) resulted in a 2.5 fold increase in the AUC of alprazolam. Alprazolam can be co-administered during chronic therapy with ritonavir > 10 days). Caution is warranted regarding alprazolam co-administration during the first several days after initiating ritonavir therapy, before induction of alprazolam metabolism has occurred.

Triazolam: in a published study, co-administration of short-term ritonavir and triazolam resulted in a very large > 20 fold) increase in the AUC of triazolam. These data support that triazolam and ritonavir should not be co-administered (see section 4.3).

Zolpidem: in a published study, co-administration of short-term ritonavir and zolpidem resulted in a small (< 30%) increase in the AUC of zolpidem. These data support that zolpidem and ritonavir may be co-administered with careful monitoring for excessive sedative effects.

Fusidic acid: co-administration of ritonavir with fusidic acid is expected to significantly increase fusidic acid and ritonavir concentrations in plasma.

HMG-CoA reductase inhibitors: HMG-CoA reductase inhibitors which are highly dependent on CYP3A metabolism, such as lovastatin and simvastatin, are expected to have markedly increased plasma concentrations when co-administered with Norvir. Since increased concentrations of HMG-CoA reductase inhibitors may cause myopathy, including rhabdomyolysis, the combination of these medicinal products with Norvir is not recommended. Atorvastatin is less dependent on CYP3A for metabolism. When used with Norvir, the lowest possible doses of atorvastatin should be administered. The metabolism of pravastatin and fluvastatin is not dependent on CYP3A, and interactions are not expected with Norvir. If treatment with an HMG-CoA reductase inhibitor is indicated, pravastatin or fluvastatin is recommended.

Buspirone: ritonavir has been associated with increase in the risk of adverse events to buspirone (such as neurological or psychiatric disorders) when these medicines were co-administered. This may be explained by clinically relevant elevations of buspirone levels due to inhibition of CYP3A-dependent metabolism of buspirone by ritonavir. Caution and clinical monitoring should be exercised when ritonavir is concomitantly used with buspirone.

Norvir DECREASES the AUCs of the following medicines when administered concomitantly:

Zidovudine (AZT) and ddI: zidovudine and ddI have little if any effect on ritonavir pharmacokinetics. Ritonavir decreased the mean zidovudine AUC by approximately 25% in a study, which has not been of sufficient duration to reach steady state for ritonavir. Ritonavir resulted in a reduction of the mean ddI AUC by 13% when given 2.5 hours apart from ritonavir. Dose alteration of AZT or ddI during concomitant Norvir therapy should usually not be necessary. However, dosing of ritonavir and ddI should be separated by 2.5 hours to avoid formulation incompatibilities. Human pharmacokinetic data for combination with antiretroviral medicines other than zidovudine and ddI are not yet available (see also section 4.4).

Ethinyl oestradiol: because concomitant administration of ritonavir with a fixed combination oral contraceptive resulted in a reduction of the ethinyl oestradiol mean AUC by 41%, increased doses of oral contraceptives containing ethinyl oestradiol, or alternate methods of contraception should be considered.

Theophylline: an increased dosage of theophylline may be required, as concomitant use with ritonavir caused an approximately 45% decrease in the AUC of theophylline.

Fixed combination of sulfamethoxazole/trimethoprim: the concomitant administration of Norvir and sulfamethoxazole/trimethoprim resulted in a 20% reduction of the sulfamethoxazole AUC and a 20% increase of the trimethoprim AUC. Dose alteration of sulfamethoxazole/trimethoprim during concomitant Norvir therapy should not be necessary.

Methadone: concomitant administration of ritonavir and methadone resulted in a reduction of the mean methadone AUC by 36%. An increased methadone dose may be necessary when concomitantly administered with ritonavir, depending on the patient's response.

Meperidine: co-administration of multiple-dose ritonavir with single dose oral meperidine resulted in a 62% decrease in meperidine AUC and a 47% increase in normeperidine AUC. Dosage increase and long term use of meperidine and ritonavir are not recommended due to the increased concentrations of the metabolite, normeperidine, which has both analgesic and CNS stimulant activity (eg, seizures).

Fluticasone propionate: in a clinical study where ritonavir 100 mg capsules twice daily were co – administered with 50 μg intranasal fluticasone propionate (4 times daily) for seven days in healthy subjects, the fluticasone propionate plasma levels increased significantly, whereas the intrinsic cortisol levels decreased by approximately 86% (90% confidence interval 82 – 89%). Greater effects may be expected when fluticasone propionate is inhaled. Systemic corticosteroid effects including Cushing's syndrome and adrenal suppression have been reported when ritonavir has been co – administered with inhaled or intranasally administered fluticasone propionate; this could also occur with other corticosteroids eg budesonide. Consequently, concomitant administration of Norvir (including low dose of ritonavir) and inhaled or intranasally administered glucocorticoids is not recommended unless the potential benefit of treatment outweighs the risk of systemic corticosteroid effects. A dose reduction of the glucocorticoid should be considered with close monitoring. Moreover, in case of withdrawal of glucocorticoids progressive dose reduction may have to be performed over a longer period. The effects of high fluticasone systemic exposure on ritonavir plasma levels is yet unknown (see section 4.4).

Because ritonavir is highly protein bound, the possibility of increased therapeutic and toxic effects due to protein binding displacement of concomitant medications should be considered.

Cardiac and neurologic events have been reported when ritonavir has been co-administered with disopyramide, mexiletine, nefazadone, or fluoxetine. The possibility of drug interaction cannot be excluded.

4.6 Pregnancy and lactation

No treatment-related malformations were observed with ritonavir in either rats or rabbits. Developmental toxicity observed in rats (embryolethality, decreased foetal body weight and ossification delays and visceral changes, including delayed testicular descent) occurred mainly at a maternally toxic dosage. Developmental toxicity in rabbits (embryolethality, decreased litter size and decreased foetal weights) occurred at a maternally toxic dosage. There are no studies in pregnant women. This medicine should be used during pregnancy only if the potential benefits clearly outweigh the potential risks.

It is not known whether this medicine is excreted in human milk. Milk excretion has not been measured in the animal studies, however a study in rats showed some effects on offspring development during lactation which are compatible with excretion of ritonavir in milk in that species. HIV infected women should not breast-feed their infants under any circumstances to avoid transmission of HIV.

4.7 Effects on ability to drive and use machines

Norvir has not specifically been tested for its possible effects on the ability to drive a car or operate machines. As somnolence and dizziness are known undesirable effects, this should be taken into account when driving or using machinery.

4.8 Undesirable effects

In clinical studies (Phase II/III), the following adverse events with possible, probable or unknown relationship to ritonavir have been reported in ⩾ 2% of 1033 patients:

Classification of expected frequencies:

Very common	> 1/10)
Common	> 1/100, < 1/10)
Uncommon	> 1/1,000, < 1/100)
Rare	> 1/10,000, < 1/1,000)

Nausea, diarrhoea, vomiting, asthenia, taste perversion, circumoral and peripheral paraesthesia were very common and are felt to be clearly related to ritonavir.

Nervous system disorders: Dizziness, paraesthesia, hyperaesthesia, somnolence, insomnia and anxiety were commonly reported.

Cardiovascular disorders: Vasodilation was commonly reported.

Respiratory system disorders: Pharyngitis and cough increased were commonly reported.

Gastrointestinal disorders: Very common events reported were abdominal pain. Dyspepsia, anorexia, local throat irritation flatulence, dry mouth, eructation and mouth ulcer were commonly reported.

Musculoskeletal system disorders: Increased CPK and myalgia were commonly reported. Myositis was reported rarely. Rarely, rhabdomyolysis has been reported with protease inhibitors, particularly in combination with nucleoside analogues.

Skin and subcutaneous tissue disorders: Rash, pruritus and sweating were commonly reported.

Allergic reactions including urticaria, mild skin eruptions, bronchospasm, and angioedema have been reported. Rare cases of anaphylaxis and Stevens-Johnson syndrome have been reported

Other disorders: Very common events reported were headache. Fever, pain and weight loss were commonly reported.

There have been spontaneous reports of thrombocytopenia, seizure and menorrhagia.

Dehydration usually associated with gastrointestinal symptoms, and sometimes resulting in hypotension, syncope, or renal insufficiency has been reported. Syncope, orthostatic hypotension and renal insufficiency have also been reported without known dehydration.

Hepatic transaminase elevations exceeding five times the upper limit or normal, clinical hepatitis, and jaundice have occurred in patients receiving ritonavir alone or in combination with other antiretrovirals.

Combination antiretroviral therapy has been associated with redistribution of body fat (lipodystrophy) in HIV patients including the loss of peripheral and facial subcutaneous fat, increased intra-abdominal and visceral fat, breast hypertrophy and dorsocervical fat accumulation (buffalo hump).

Combination antiretroviral therapy has been associated with metabolic abnormalities such as hypertriglyceridaemia, hypercholesterolaemia, insulin resistance, hyperglycaemia and hyperlactataemia (see section 4.4).

In HIV-infected patients with severe immune deficiency at the time of initiation of combination antiretroviral therapy (CART), an inflammatory reaction to asymptomatic or residual opportunistic infections may arise (see section 4.4).

Hyperglycaemia has been reported in individuals with and without a known history of diabetes. Cause and effect relationship has not been established.

Hypertriglyceridaemia, hypercholesterolaemia and hyperuricaemia were clearly related to ritonavir therapy.

Pancreatitis has been observed in patients receiving Norvir therapy, including those who developed hypertriglyceridemia. In some cases fatalities have been observed. Patients with advanced HIV disease may be at risk of elevated triglycerides and pancreatitis.

Pancreatitis should be considered if clinical symptoms (nausea, vomiting, abdominal pain) or abnormalities in laboratory values (such as increased serum lipase or amylase values) suggestive of pancreatitis should occur. Patients who exhibit these signs or symptoms should be evaluated and Norvir therapy should be discontinued if a diagnosis of pancreatitis is made.

Clinical chemistry:

High gamma-glutamyl transpeptidase (GGT), high creatine phosphokinase (CPK), high triglycerides, high alanine transaminase (SGPT); high aspartate transaminase (SGOT), high amylase, high uric acid low potassium and decrease of free and total thyroxin (T_4) values were commonly reported. Uncommon events were high glucose, low total calcium, high magnesium, high total bilirubin, high alkaline phosphatase.

Haematology:

Low white blood cell (WBC), low haemoglobin, low neutrophils and high eosinophils were commonly reported. Uncommon events were high WBC, high neutrophils and high prothrombin time.

4.9 Overdose

Human experience of acute overdose with ritonavir is limited. One patient in clinical trials took ritonavir 1500 mg/day for two days and reported paraesthesia, which resolved after the dose was decreased. A case of renal failure with eosinophilia has been reported.

The signs of toxicity observed in animals (mice and rats) included decreased activity, ataxia, dyspnoea and tremors.

There is no specific antidote for overdose with ritonavir. Treatment of overdose with ritonavir should consist of general supportive measures including monitoring of vital signs and observation of the clinical status of the patient. Due to the solubility characteristics and possibility of transintestinal elimination, it is proposed that management of overdose could entail gastric lavage and administration of activated charcoal. Since ritonavir is extensively metabolised by the liver and is highly protein bound, dialysis is unlikely to be beneficial in significant removal of the medicine.

5. PHARMACOLOGICAL PROPERTIES

5.1 Pharmacodynamic properties

Pharmacotherapeutic group: antiviral for systemic use, ATC code: J05A E03

Ritonavir is an orally active peptidomimetic inhibitor of the HIV-1 and HIV-2 aspartyl proteases. Inhibition of HIV protease renders the enzyme incapable of processing the *gag-pol* polyprotein precursor which leads to the production of HIV particles with immature morphology that are unable to initiate new rounds of infection. Ritonavir has selective affinity for the HIV protease and has little inhibitory activity against human aspartyl proteases.

In vitro data indicates that ritonavir is active against all strains of HIV tested in a variety of transformed and primary human cell lines. The concentration of ritonavir that inhibits 50% and 90% of viral replication *in vitro* is approximately 0.02 μM and 0.11 μM, respectively. Similar potencies were found with both AZT-sensitive and AZT-resistant strains of HIV. Studies which measured direct cell toxicity of ritonavir on several cell lines showed no direct toxicity at concentrations up to 25 μM, with a resulting *in vitro* therapeutic index of at least 1000.

Resistance

Ritonavir-resistant isolates of HIV-1 have been selected *in vitro*. The resistant isolates showed reduced susceptibility to ritonavir and genotypic analysis showed that the resistance was attributable primarily to specific amino acid substitutions in the HIV-1 protease at codons 82 and 84.

Susceptibility of clinical isolates to ritonavir was monitored in controlled clinical trials. Some patients receiving ritonavir monotherapy developed HIV strains with decreased susceptibility to ritonavir. Serial genotypic and phenotypic analysis indicated that susceptibility to ritonavir declined in an ordered and stepwise fashion. Initial mutations occurred at position 82 from wildtype valine to usually alanine or phenylalanine (V82A/F). Viral strains isolated *in vivo* without a change at codon 82 did not have decreased susceptibility to ritonavir.

Cross-resistance to other antiretrovirals

Serial HIV isolates obtained from six patients during ritonavir therapy showed a decrease in ritonavir susceptibility *in vitro* but did not demonstrate a concordant decrease in susceptibility to saquinavir *in vitro* when compared to matched baseline isolates. However, isolates from two of these patients demonstrated decrease susceptibility to indinavir *in vitro* (8-fold). Cross-resistance between ritonavir and reverse transcriptase inhibitors is unlikely because of the different enzyme targets involved. One AZT-resistant HIV isolate tested *in vitro* retained full susceptibility to ritonavir.

Clinical pharmacodynamic data

The effects of ritonavir (alone or combined with other antiretroviral agents) on biological markers of disease activity such as CD4 cell count and viral RNA were evaluated in several studies involving HIV-1 infected patients. The following studies are the most important.

Adult Use

A controlled study with ritonavir as add-on therapy in HIV-1 infected patients extensively pre-treated with nucleoside analogues and baseline CD4 cell counts ⩽ 100 cells/μl showed a reduction in mortality and AIDS defining events. The mean average change from baseline over 16 weeks for HIV RNA levels was -0.79 $\log_{10}$ (maximum mean decrease: 1.29 $\log_{10}$) in the ritonavir group versus -0.01 $\log_{10}$ in the control group. The most frequently used nucleosides in this study were zidovudine, stavudine, didanosine and zalcitabine.

In a study recruiting less advanced HIV-1 infected patients (CD4 200-500 cells/μl) without previous antiretroviral therapy, ritonavir in combination with zidovudine or alone reduced viral load in plasma and increased CD4 count. The effects of ritonavir monotherapy seemed unexpectedly to be at least as large as the combination therapy, a finding which has not been explained adequately. The mean average change from baseline over 48 weeks for HIV RNA levels was -0.88 $\log_{10}$ in the ritonavir group versus -0.66 $\log_{10}$ in the ritonavir + zidovudine group versus -0.42 $\log_{10}$ in the zidovudine group.

The continuation of ritonavir therapy should be evaluated by viral load because of the possibility of the emergence of resistance as described under section 4.1 Therapeutic indications.

In an open label trial in 32 antiretroviral naive HIV-1 infected patients the combination of ritonavir with zidovudine and zalcitabine decreased the viral load (mean decrease at week 20 of -1.76 $\log_{10}$).

Paediatric Use

In an open label trial in HIV infected, clinically stable children there was a significant difference (p = 0.03) in the detectable RNA levels in favour of a triple regimen (ritonavir, zidovudine and lamivudine) following 48 weeks treatment.

Studies investigating optimal combinations and the long term efficacy and safety of ritonavir are ongoing.

5.2 Pharmacokinetic properties

There is no parenteral formulation of ritonavir, therefore the extent of absorption and absolute bioavailability have not been determined. The pharmacokinetics of ritonavir during multiple dose regimens were studied in non-fasting HIV positive adult volunteers. Upon multiple dosing, ritonavir accumulation is slightly less than predicted from a single dose due to a time and dose-related increase in apparent clearance (Cl/F). Trough concentrations of ritonavir were observed to decrease over time, possibly due to enzyme induction, but appeared to stabilise by the end of 2 weeks. At steady state with a 600 mg twice daily dose, maximal concentration (C_{max}) and trough concentration (C_{trough}) values of 11.2 ± 3.6 and 3.7 ± 2.6 μg/ml (mean ± SD) were observed, respectively. Over a 12 hour dosing interval, the AUC_{12h} was 77.5 +/- 31.5 μg·h/ml. The half life ($t_{1/2}$) of ritonavir was approximately 3 to 5 hours. The steady-state apparent clearance in patients treated with 600 mg twice daily has averaged 8.8 ± 3.2 l/h. Renal clearance averaged less than 0.1 l/h and was relatively constant throughout the dosage range. The time to maximum concentration (T_{max}) remained constant at approximately 4 hours with increasing dose.

The pharmacokinetics of ritonavir are dose-dependent: more than proportional increases in the AUC and C_{max} were reported with increasing dose. Ingestion with food results in higher ritonavir exposure than ingestion in the fasted state.

No clinically significant differences in AUC or C_{max} were noted between males and females. Ritonavir pharmacokinetic parameters were not statistically significantly associated with body weight or lean body mass.

Patients with impaired liver function: after multiple dosing of ritonavir to healthy volunteers (500 mg twice daily) and subjects with mild to moderate hepatic impairment (400 mg twice daily) exposure to ritonavir after dose normalisation was not significantly different between the two groups.

The apparent volume of distribution (V_B/F) of ritonavir is approximately 20-40 l after a single 600 mg dose. The protein binding of ritonavir in human plasma was noted to be approximately 98 - 99%. Ritonavir binds to both human alpha 1-acid glycoprotein (AAG) and human serum albumin (HSA) with comparable affinities. Plasma protein binding is constant over the concentration range of 0.1-100 μg/ml.

Tissue distribution studies with ^{14}C-labelled ritonavir in rats showed the liver, adrenals, pancreas, kidneys and thyroid to have the highest concentrations of ritonavir. Tissue to plasma ratios of approximately 1 measured in rat lymph nodes suggests that ritonavir distributes into lymphatic tissues. Ritonavir penetrates minimally into the brain.

Ritonavir was noted to be extensively metabolised by the hepatic cytochrome P450 system, primarily isozyme CYP3A4 and to a lesser extent CYP2D6. Animal studies as well as *in vitro* experiments with human hepatic microsomes indicated that ritonavir primarily underwent oxidative metabolism. Four ritonavir metabolites have been identified in man. The isopropylthiazole oxidation metabolite (M-2) is the major metabolite and has antiviral activity similar to that of parent drug. However, the AUC of the M-2 metabolite was approximately 3% of the AUC of parent drug.

Human studies with radiolabelled ritonavir demonstrated that the elimination of ritonavir was primarily via the hepatobiliary system; approximately 86% of radiolabel was recovered from stool, part of which is expected to be unabsorbed ritonavir. In these studies renal elimination was not found to be a major route of elimination of ritonavir. This was consistent with the observations in animal studies.

Steady-state pharmacokinetics were evaluated in HIV infected children above 2 years of age receiving doses ranging from 250 mg/m^2 twice daily to 400 mg/m^2 twice daily. Ritonavir concentrations obtained after 350 to 400 mg/m^2 twice daily in paediatric patients were comparable to those obtained in adults receiving 600 mg (approximately 330 mg/m^2) twice daily.

5.3 Preclinical safety data

Repeated dose toxicity studies in animals identified major target organs as the liver, retina, thyroid gland and kidney. Hepatic changes involved hepatocellular, biliary and phagocytic elements and were accompanied by increases in hepatic enzymes. Hyperplasia of the retinal pigment epithelium (RPE) and retinal degeneration have been seen in all of the rodent studies conducted with ritonavir, but have not been seen in dogs. Ultrastructural evidence suggests that these retinal changes may be secondary to phospholipidosis. However, clinical trials revealed no evidence of drug-induced ocular changes in humans. All thyroid changes were reversible upon discontinuation of ritonavir. Clinical investigation in humans has revealed no clinically significant alteration in thyroid function tests. Renal changes including tubular degeneration, chronic inflammation and proteinurea were noted in rats and are felt to be attributable to species-specific spontaneous disease. Furthermore, no clinically significant renal abnormalities were noted in clinical trials.

Ritonavir was not found to be mutagenic or clastogenic in a battery of *in vitro* and *in vivo* assays including the Ames bacterial reverse mutation assay using *S. typhimurium* and *E. coli*, the mouse lymphoma assay, the mouse micronucleus test and chromosomal aberration assays in human lymphocytes.

Long term carcinogenicity studies of ritonavir in mice and rats revealed tumourigenic potential specific for these species, but are regarded as of no relevance for humans.

6. PHARMACEUTICAL PARTICULARS

6.1 List of excipients

Norvir soft capsules contain: alcohol, butylated hydroxytoluene (E321), oleic acid and polyoxyl 35 castor oil. The capsule shell components are: gelatine, "sorbitol special" (ie sorbitol sorbitolanhydrides and mannitol), glycerine, titanium dioxide (white colour), medium chain triglycerides, lecithin and black ink containing: propylene glycol, black iron oxide, polyvinyl acetate phthalate, polyethylene glycol 400 and ammonium hydroxide.

6.2 Incompatibilities

None known

6.3 Shelf life

2 years

6.4 Special precautions for storage

Norvir soft capsules should be stored in a refrigerator (2° - 8°C) until they are dispensed to the patient. Refrigeration by the patient is not required if used within 30 days and stored below 25°C.

Avoid exposure to freezing and excessive heat.

6.5 Nature and contents of container

Norvir soft capsules are supplied in white high density polyethylene (HDPE) bottles closed with polypropylene caps containing 84 capsules. Each pack contains 4 bottles of 84 capsules (336 capsules).

6.6 Instructions for use and handling

No special requirements

7. MARKETING AUTHORISATION HOLDER

Abbott Laboratories Limited

Queenborough

Kent ME11 5EL

United Kingdom

8. MARKETING AUTHORISATION NUMBER(S)

EU/1/96/016/003

9. DATE OF FIRST AUTHORISATION/RENEWAL OF THE AUTHORISATION

Date of first authorisation: 26 August 1996

Date of last renewal: 27 August 2001

10. DATE OF REVISION OF THE TEXT

20th January 2005

NOVA T™ 380 Copper Containing Intrauterine Contraceptive Device

(Schering Health Care Limited)

INFORMATION FOR HEALTH CARE PROFESSIONAL

NOVA T 380 is supplied sterile, sterilized by irradiation. For single use only. Do not use if the pouch is damaged or open. Do not resterilise. Use before the date shown on the pouch label. To be inserted by a qualified health care professional. Store at 15-30°C protected from direct sunlight and moisture.

1. NAME OF THE PRODUCT

NOVA T™ 380

2. COMPOSITION

Intrauterine device made of polyethylene and wound with copper wire with silver core. The surface area of copper is 380 mm2.

3. PHARMACEUTICAL FORM

Intrauterine device (IUD)

4. CLINICAL PARTICULARS

4.1. Therapeutic indications

Contraception

4.2. Posology and administration

NOVA T 380 is inserted into the uterine cavity. It is effective for five years.

4.3. Contraindications

Known or suspected pregnancy; current or recurrent pelvic inflammatory disease; lower genital tract infection; postpartum endometritis, infected abortion during the past three months; untreated cervicitis; untreated cervical dysplasia; untreated uterine or cervical malignancy; undiagnosed abnormal uterine bleeding; congenital or acquired uterine anomaly including fibroids if they distort the uterine cavity; copper allergy; Wilson's disease; coagulation disturbances; conditions associated with increased susceptibility to infections.

4.4. Special warnings and special precautions

Copper IUDs may increase menstrual blood loss and dysmenorrhea. NOVA T 380 may not be the method of first choice for women with excessive menstrual bleeding, anemia, dysmenorrhea, or for women receiving anticoagulants. If these conditions develop during use of NOVA T 380, removal of the device should be considered.

NOVA T 380 may be used with caution in women who have congenital heart disease or valvular heart disease at risk of infective endocarditis. Antibiotic prophylaxis should be administered to these patients when inserting or removing the IUD.

NOVA T 380 is not the method of first choice for young nulligravid women. In this group, the pregnancy rates and removal rates for expulsion, bleeding and/or pain, and for infection have been reported higher than in other users.

Insertion and removal/replacement

Before insertion, the woman must be informed on the efficacy, risks and side effects of NOVA T 380. A physical examination including pelvic examination and a cervical smear should be performed. Pregnancy, genital infection and sexually transmitted diseases should be excluded. The position of the uterus and the size of the uterine cavity should be determined. The instructions for insertion should be followed carefully. The woman should be re-examined 4 to 12 weeks after insertion and once a year thereafter, or more frequently if clinically indicated.

Insertion is recommended during or shortly following menstruation. If pregnancy is excluded, NOVA T 380 may be inserted at any time of the cycle. The small diameter of the insertion tube, which is easy to introduce, makes dilatation usually unnecessary. It can be replaced by a new device at any time in the cycle. NOVA T 380 can also be inserted immediately after first trimester abortion. Postpartum insertions should be postponed until six weeks after delivery as they are associated with high rates of perforation and expulsion.

NOVA T 380 is removed by gently pulling on the threads with a forceps. If the threads are not visible and the device is in the uterine cavity, removal should be postponed until after the next menstrual bleeding since the threads usually become visible immediately after menstruation. If they are still not visible, the device may be removed using a narrow tenaculum. This may require dilatation of the cervical canal.

NOVA T 380 should be removed after five years. If the woman wishes to continue using the method, a new device can be inserted at the same time.

If pregnancy is not desired, the removal should be carried out during the menstruation. If the device is removed in the mid-cycle and the woman has had an intercourse within a week, she is at a risk of pregnancy unless a new device is inserted immediately following removal.

Insertion and removal may be associated with some pain and bleeding. The procedure may precipitate fainting as a vasovagal reaction, and a seizure in an epileptic patient.

Pelvic infection

The insertion tube protects NOVA T 380 from contamination with micro-organisms during the insertion. In users of copper IUDs, the highest rate of pelvic infections occurs during the first month after insertion and decreases later. Known risk factors for pelvic inflammatory disease are multiple sexual partners, frequent intercourse and young age. Pelvic infection may impair fertility and increase the risk of ectopic pregnancy.

If the woman experiences recurrent endometritis or pelvic infections, or if an acute infection does not respond to treatment within a few days, NOVA T 380 must be removed.

Bacteriological examinations are indicated and monitoring is recommended, even with discrete symptoms indicative of infection, such as pathologic discharge.

Expulsion

Symptoms of the partial or complete expulsion of any IUD may include bleeding or pain. However, a device can be expelled from the uterine cavity without the woman noticing it. Partial expulsion may decrease the effectiveness of NOVA T 380. A displaced device should be removed and a new device inserted.

The woman should be advised how to check the threads of the IUD.

Perforation

Perforation or penetration of the uterine corpus or cervix by the IUD may occur, most often during insertion. The risk is increased during the postpartum period. Such a device must be removed as soon as possible.

Ectopic pregnancy

Even though ectopic pregnancies may occur when IUDs are used, current data indicate that copper IUD users do not have a higher overall risk of ectopic pregnancy than women using no contraception. However, a pregnancy with an IUD in place is more likely to be ectopic than if pregnancy occurs without an IUD in situ. Women with a previous ectopic pregnancy, pelvic surgery or pelvic infection carry a higher risk of ectopic pregnancy. The possibility of ectopic pregnancy should be considered in the case of lower abdominal pain - especially in connection with missed periods or if an amenorrheic woman starts bleeding.

Lost threads

If the retrieval threads are not visible at the cervix on follow-up examinations, pregnancy must be excluded. The threads may have been drawn up into the uterus or cervical canal and may reappear during the next menstrual period. If pregnancy has been excluded, the threads may usually be located by gently probing with a suitable instrument. If they cannot be found, the device may have been expelled. Ultrasound diagnosis may be used to ascertain the position of the IUD. If ultrasound is not available or successful, X-ray may be used to locate NOVA T 380.

4.5 Drug interactions

The available experience with NOVA T 380 indicates that drug effects interfering with Nova T's contraceptive efficacy are highly unlikely. The evidence from published reports of such interactions with non-steroidal anti-inflammatory drugs and corticoids does not justify general precautions.

4.6 Use in pregnancy and lactation
Pregnancy.

The Nova T 380 is not to be used during an existing or suspected pregnancy. If the woman becomes pregnant when using NOVA T 380 removal of the device is recommended, since the IUD left in situ may increase the risk of abortion and preterm labor. Removal of the IUD or probing of the uterus may result in spontaneous abortion. If the device cannot be gently removed, termination of the pregnancy may be considered. If the woman wishes to continue the pregnancy and the device cannot be withdrawn, she should be informed about these risks and the possible consequence of premature birth to the infant. In addition, ectopic pregnancy should be excluded and the course of such a pregnancy should be closely monitored. The women should be instructed to report all symptoms that suggest complications of the pregnancy, like cramping abdominal pain with fever. She should be informed that, to date there is no evidence of birth defects in cases where a pregnancy continues to term with the IUD in place.

Lactation. NOVA T 380 does not interfere with lactation.

4.7 Effects on ability to drive and use machines
There are no known effects on the ability to drive or use machines.

4.8 Adverse reactions
Increased menstrual bleeding; spotting; dysmenorrhea; lower abdominal or back pain; anemia. Pregnancy in the case of the method failure may be ectopic. Pelvic inflammatory disease may occur during the use of the IUD. The IUD or parts of it may perforate or penetrate the uterine wall. Allergic skin reaction may occur.

4.9 Overdose
Not applicable.

5. PHARMACOLOGICAL PROPERTIES
5.1 Pharmacodynamic properties
Copper IUDs prevent pregnancy by preventing fertilization. This is based on the inhibition of sperm and egg transport and/or the capacity of sperm to fertilize eggs. This happens through cytotoxic and phagocytic effects before the egg reaches the uterine cavity. After removal of IUD fertility is promptly restored.

The pregnancy rate with NOVA T 380 has been 0.6 per 100 woman-years.

5.2 Pharmacokinetic properties
Not applicable.

5.3 Preclinical safety data
The preclinical safety of intrauterine copper is well-established. No teratogenicity was found in animal studies. The studies did not indicate any particular risk for human use.

6. PHARMACEUTICAL PARTICULARS
6.1 List of excipients
Copper

Silver

Polyethylene

Barium sulphate

Iron oxide

6.2 Incompatibilities
None known.

6.3 Shelf-life
Three years.

6.4 Special precautions for storage
Store at 15-30 °C protected from direct sunlight and moisture.

6.5 Nature and contents of container
The device with accessories has been packed in a heat-sealed sterilization pouch of polyester/polyethylene/polyamide.

6.6 Instructions for use/handling
NOVA T 380 is supplied sterile, sterilized by irradiation. For single use only. Do not resterilize. Do not use if the pouch is damaged or open. Insert the device before the expiry date shown on the pouch label. Each device should be handled with aseptic precautions. Special instructions for insertion are in the package. After removal, NOVA T 380 should be disposed of in accordance with the local guidelines for the handling of biohazardous waste.

MANUFACTURER

Schering Oy

Pansiontie 47

(P.O. Box 415, 20101 Turku)

20210 Turku

Finland

DISTRIBUTED BY

Schering Health Care Ltd

The Brow, Burgess Hill,

West Sussex RH15 9NE

CE 0344

EXPLANATIONS OF THE SYMBOLS

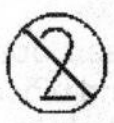
= Symbol for "DO NOT REUSE"

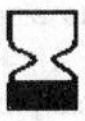

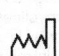
= Symbol for "USE BY"

LOT = Symbol for "BATCH CODE"

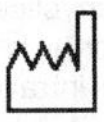
= Symbol for "DATE OF MANUFACTURE"

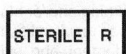

STERILE R = Symbol for method of sterilization using irradiation

= Symbol for "ATTENTION, SEE INSTRUCTIONS FOR USE"

DATE OF REVISION OF THE LEAFLET
13.5.2003

Novantrone Injection

(Wyeth Pharmaceuticals)

1. NAME OF THE MEDICINAL PRODUCT
Novantrone 2mg/ml. Concentrate for Solution for Injection or Infusion.

2. QUALITATIVE AND QUANTITATIVE COMPOSITION
Each ml of Novantrone 2mg/ml Concentrate for solution for injection or infusion contains 2mg Mitoxantrone as Mitoxantrone hydrochloride.

3. PHARMACEUTICAL FORM
Concentrate for solution for injection or infusion. Novantrone is a dark blue aqueous isotonic concentrate for solution for injection or infusion packaged in Type I glass vials.

4. CLINICAL PARTICULARS
4.1 Therapeutic indications
Novantrone is indicated in the treatment of metastatic breast cancer, non-Hodgkin's lymphoma and adult acute non-lymphocytic leukaemia.

Novantrone has also been used in the palliation of non-resectable primary hepatocellular carcinoma.

4.2 Posology and method of administration
Novantrone should be given by intravenous infusion. **NOT FOR INTRATHECAL USE.**

Syringes containing this product should be labelled

" NOVANTRONE NOT FOR INTRATHECAL USE "

Metastatic Breast Cancer, Non-Hodgkin's Lymphoma, Hepatoma:

(a) **Single Agent Dosage**

The recommended initial dosage of Novantrone used as a single agent is $14mg/m^2$ of body surface area, given as a single intravenous dose which may be repeated at 21-day intervals. A lower initial dosage ($12mg/m^2$ or less) is recommended in patients with inadequate bone marrow reserves. e.g. due to prior chemotherapy or poor general condition.

Dosage modification and the timing of subsequent dosing should be determined by clinical judgement depending on the degree and duration of myelosuppression. For subsequent courses the prior dose can usually be repeated if white blood cell and platelet counts have returned to normal levels after 21 days. The following table is suggested as a guide to dosage adjustment, in the treatment of metastatic breast cancer, non-Hodgkin's lymphoma and hepatoma according to haematological nadir (which usually occurs about 10 days after dosing).

(see Table 1 below)

(b) **Combination Therapy**

Novantrone has been given as part of combination therapy. In metastatic breast cancer, combinations of Novantrone with other cytotoxic agents including cyclophosphamide and 5-fluorouracil or methotrexate and mitomycin C have been shown to be effective. Reference should be made to the published literature for information on dosage modifications and administration. Novantrone has also been used in various combinations for non-Hodgkin's lymphoma, however data are presently limited and specific regimens cannot be recommended.

As a guide, when Novantrone is used in combination chemotherapy with another myelosuppressive agent, the initial dose of Novantrone should be reduced by $2\text{-}4mg/m^2$ below the doses recommended for single agent usage; subsequent dosing, as outlined in the table above, depends on the degree and duration of myelosuppression.

Acute Non-Lymphocytic Leukaemia

(a) **Single Agent Dosage in Relapse**

The recommended dosage for remission induction is $12mg/m^2$ of body surface area, given as a single intravenous dose daily for five consecutive days (total of $60mg/m^2$). In clinical studies with a dosage of $12mg/m^2$ daily for 5 days, patients who achieved a complete remission did so as a result of the first induction course.

(b) **Combination Therapy**

Novantrone has been used in combination regimens for the treatment of ANLL. Most clinical experience has been with Novantrone combined with cytosine arabinoside. This combination has been used successfully for primary treatment of ANLL as well as in relapse.

An effective regimen for induction in previously untreated patients has been Novantrone $10\text{-}12mg/m^2$ IV for 3 days combined with cytosine arabinoside $100mg/m^2$ IV for 7 days (by continuous infusion). This is followed by second induction and consolidation courses as thought appropriate by the treating clinician. In clinical studies, duration of therapy in induction and consolidation courses with Novantrone have been reduced to 2 days and that of cytosine arabinoside to 5 days. However, modification to the above regimen should be carried out by the treating clinician depending on individual patient factors.

Efficacy has also been demonstrated with Novantrone in combination with Etoposide in patients who had relapsed or who were refractory to primary conventional chemotherapy. The use of Novantrone in combination with Etoposide as with other cytotoxics may result in greater myelosuppression than with Novantrone alone.

Reference should be made to the published literature for information on specific dosage regimens. Novantrone should be used by clinicians experienced in the use of chemotherapy regimens. Dosage adjustments should be made by the treating clinician as appropriate, taking into account toxicity, response and individual patient characteristics. As with other cytotoxic drugs, Novantrone should be used with caution in combination therapy until wider experience is available.

(c) **Paediatric Leukaemia**

As experience with Novantrone in paediatric leukaemia is limited, dosage recommendations in this patient population cannot at present be given.

4.3 Contraindications
Not for Intrathecal Use

Demonstrated hypersensitivity to the drug or any of its components.

4.4 Special warnings and special precautions for use
There may be an increased risk of leukaemia when mitoxantrone is used as adjuvant treatment of non metastatic

Table 1 Nadir after Prior Dose

WBC (per mm^3)		Platelets (per mm^3)	Time to Recovery	Subsequent dose after adequate haematological recovery
> 1,500	AND	> 50,000	⩽ 21 days	Repeat prior dose after recovery or increase by $2mg/m^2$ if myelosuppression is not considered adequate
> 1,500	AND	> 50,000	> 21 days	Withhold until recovery then repeat prior dose
< 1,500	OR	< 50,000	Any duration	Decrease by $2mg/m^2$ from prior dose after recovery
< 1,000	OR	< 25,000	Any duration	Decrease by $4mg/m^2$ from prior dose after recovery

breast cancer. In the absence of sufficient efficacy data, mitoxantrone must not be used as adjuvant treatment of non metastatic breast cancer.

Novantrone should be used with caution in patients with myelosuppression or poor general condition.

Cases of functional cardiac changes, including congestive heart failure and decreases in left ventricular ejection fraction have been reported. The majority of these cardiac events have occurred in patients who have had prior treatment with anthracyclines, prior mediastinal/thoracic radiotherapy, or with pre-existing heart disease. It is recommended that patients in these categories are treated with Novantrone at full cytotoxic dosage and schedule. However, added caution is required in these patients and careful regular cardiac examinations are recommended from the initiation of treatment.

As experience of prolonged treatment with Novantrone is presently limited, it is suggested that cardiac examinations also be performed in patients without identifiable risk factors during therapy exceeding a cumulative dose of 160mg/m^2.

Careful supervision is recommended when treating patients with severe hepatic insufficiency.

Novantrone is mutagenic in vitro and in vivo in the rat. In the same species there was a possible association between administration of the drug and development of malignant neoplasia.

Topoisomerase II inhibitors, including Novantrone, when used concomitantly with other antineoplastic agents and/ or radiotherapy, have been associated with the development of Acute Myeloid leukaemia (AML) or Myelodysplastic Syndrome (MDS).

Novantrone is not indicated for intra-arterial injection. There have been reports of local/regional neuropathy, some irreversible, following intra-arterial injection. Safety for intrathecal use has not been established. There have been reports of neuropathy, including paralysis and bowel and bladder dysfunction following intrathecal injection.

Sulphites can cause allergic-type reactions including anaphylactic symptoms and bronchospasm in susceptible people, especially those with a history of asthma or allergy.

Novantrone is an active cytotoxic drug which should be used by clinicians familiar with the use of antineoplastic agents, and having the facilities for regular monitoring of clinical, haematological and biochemical parameters during and after treatment.

Full blood counts should be undertaken serially during a course of treatment. Dosage adjustments may be necessary based on these counts.

Immunisation may be ineffective when given during Novantrone therapy. Immunisation with live virus vaccines are generally not recommended.

4.5 Interaction with other medicinal products and other forms of Interaction
Not applicable.

4.6 Pregnancy and lactation
The effects of Novantrone on human fertility or pregnancy have not been established. As with other antineoplastic agents, patients and their partners should be advised to avoid conception for at least six months after cessation of therapy. Novantrone should not normally be administered to patients who are pregnant.

Novantrone is excreted in human milk and significant concentrations (18ng/ml) have been reported for 28 days after the last administration. Because of the potential for serious adverse reactions in infants, breast-feeding should be discontinued before starting treatment.

4.7 Effects on ability to drive and use machines
Not applicable.

4.8 Undesirable effects
Some degree of leucopenia is to be expected following recommended doses of Novantrone. With the single dose every 21 days, suppression of WBC count below 1000/ mm^3 is infrequent; leucopenia is usually transient reaching its nadir at about 10 days after dosing with recovery usually occurring by the 21st day. Thrombocytopenia can occur and anaemia occurs less frequently. Myelosuppression may be more severe and prolonged in patients having had extensive prior chemotherapy or radiotherapy or in debilitated patients.

When Novantrone is used as a single injection given every 21 days in the treatment of metastatic breast cancer and lymphomas, the most commonly encountered side effects are nausea and vomiting, although in the majority of cases these are mild and transient. Alopecia may occur, but is most frequently of minimal severity and reversible on cessation of therapy.

Other side effects which have occasionally been reported include skin rashes, anaphylactic/anapylactoid reactions (including shock), amenorrhoea, anorexia, constipation, diarrhoea, dyspnoea, fatigue and weakness, fever, gastrointestinal bleeding, stomatitis/mucositis/conjunctivitis and non-specific neurological side effects such as somnolence, confusion, anxiety and mild paraesthesia. Tissue necrosis following extravasation has been reported rarely. In patients with leukaemia, the pattern of side effects is generally similar, although there is an increase in both frequency and severity, particularly of stomatitis and mucositis.

Changes in laboratory test values have been observed infrequently e.g. elevated serum creatinine and blood urea nitrogen levels, increased liver enzyme levels (with occasional reports of severe impairment of hepatic function in patients with leukaemia). Hyperuricaemia has also been reported.

Cardiovascular effects, which have occasionally been of clinical significance, include decreased left ventricular ejection fraction, ECG changes and acute arrhythmia. Congestive heart failure has been reported and has generally responded well to treatment with digitalis and/or diuretics. In patients with leukaemia an increase in the frequency of adverse cardiac events has been observed; the direct role of Novantrone in these cases is difficult to assess as most patients had received prior therapy with anthracyclines and since the clinical course in leukaemic patients is often complicated by anaemia, fever, sepsis and intravenous fluid therapy.

Extravasation at the infusion site has been reported, which may result in erythema, swelling, pain, burning and/or blue discolouration of the skin. Extravasation can result in tissue necrosis with resultant need for debridement and skin grafting. Phlebitis has also been reported at the site of infusion.

Novantrone may impart a blue-green coloration to the urine for 24 hours after administration and patients should be advised that this is to be expected. Blue discoloration of skin and nails has been reported occasionally. Nail dystrophy or reversible blue coloration of the sclerae may be seen very rarely.

Topoisomerase II inhibitors, including Novantrone, when used concomitantly with other antineoplastic agents, and/ or radiotherapy, have been associated with the development of Acute Myeloid leukaemia (AML) or Myelodysplastic Syndrome (MDS).

Rare reports of cardiomyopathy have been received.

4.9 Overdose
There is no known specific antidote for Novantrone. Haemopoietic, gastrointestinal, hepatic or renal toxicity may be seen depending on dosage given and the physical condition of the patient. In cases of overdosage the patient should be monitored closely and management should be symptomatic and supportive.

Fatalities have occurred on rare occasions as a result of severe leucopenia with infection in patients accidentally given single bolus injections of mitoxantrone at over ten times the recommended dosage. Novantrone is extensively tissue-bound and peritoneal dialysis or haemodialysis is unlikely to be effective in managing overdose.

5. PHARMACOLOGICAL PROPERTIES

5.1 Pharmacodynamic properties
Although its mechanism of action has not been determined, Novantrone is a DNA-reactive agent. It has a cytocidal effect on proliferating and non-proliferating cultured human cells, suggesting activity against rapidly proliferating and slow-growing neoplasms.

5.2 Pharmacokinetic properties
Animal pharmacokinetic studies in rats, dogs and monkeys given radiolabelled Novantrone indicate rapid, extensive dose proportional distribution into most tissues. Novantrone does not cross the blood-brain barrier to any appreciable extent. Distribution into testes is relatively low. In pregnant rats the placenta is an effective barrier. Plasma concentrations decrease rapidly during the first two hours and slowly thereafter. Animal data established biliary excretion as the major route of elimination. In rats, tissue elimination half-life of radioactivity ranged from 20 days to 25 days as compared with plasma half-life of 12 days. Novantrone is not absorbed significantly in animals following oral administration.

Pharmacokinetic studies in patients following intravenous administration of Novantrone demonstrated a triphasic plasma clearance. Distribution to tissues is rapid and extensive. Elimination of the drug is slow with a mean half-life of 12 days (range 5-18) and persistent tissue concentrations. Similar estimates of half-life were obtained from patients receiving a single dose of Novantrone every 21 days and patients dosed on 5 consecutive days every 21 days.

Novantrone is excreted via the renal and hepatobiliary systems. Only 20-32% of the administered dose was excreted within the first five days after dosing (urine 6-11%, faeces 13-25%). Of the material recovered in the urine 65% was unchanged mitoxantrone and the remaining 35% is primarily comprised of two inactive metabolites and their glucuronide conjugates. Approximately two thirds of the excretion occurred during the first day.

5.3 Preclinical safety data
Nothing of note to the prescriber

6. PHARMACEUTICAL PARTICULARS

6.1 List of excipients
Sodium chloride
Sodium acetate
Acetic acid
Sodium metabisulphite
Water for injections

6.2 Incompatibilities
Novantrone must not be mixed in the same infusion as heparin since a precipitate may form.

Because specific compatibility data are not available, it is recommended that Novantrone should not be mixed in the same infusion with other drugs.

6.3 Shelf life
3 years.

6.4 Special precautions for storage
Do not store above 25°C. Do not freeze.

Chemical and physical in use stability has been demonstrated for 24 hours at 15-25°C.

From a microbiological point of view, the product should be used immediately. If not used immediately, in-use storage times and conditions prior to use are the responsibility of the user and would normally not be longer than 24 hours at 2-8°C, unless dilution has taken place in controlled and validated aseptic conditions.

Unused solution should be discarded.

6.5 Nature and contents of container
2, 5, 7.5, 10, 12.5 or 15ml Type I Glass vial with a grey butyl rubber stopper, aluminium seal and plastic flip-off cap. Contents 2ml, 5ml, 7.5ml, 10ml, 12.5ml or 15ml. Novantrone is presented in packs of 1 vial.

6.6 Instructions for use and handling
a) Instructions for use
Syringes containing this product should be labelled 'NOVANTRONE NOT FOR INTRATHECAL USE'

Care should be taken to avoid contact of Novantrone with the skin, mucous membranes, or eyes. Vials should be dispensed in the upright position in order to prevent drops of Novantrone collecting in the stopper during preparation and leading to potential aerosolisation of the solution.

Dilute the required volume of Novantrone injection to at least 50 ml in either of the following intravenous infusions: Sodium Chloride 0.9%, Glucose 5%, or Sodium Chloride 0.18% and Glucose 4%. Use Luer-lock fittings on all syringes and sets. Large bore needles are recommended to minimise pressure and the possible formation of aerosols. The latter may also be reduced by the use of a venting needle. Administer the resulting solution over not less than 3 minutes via the tubing of freely running intravenous infusion of the above fluids. Novantrone should not be mixed with other drugs in the same infusion.

If extravasation occurs the administration should be stopped immediately and restarted in another vein.

b) Handling Cytotoxic drugs
Novantrone, in common with other potentially hazardous cytotoxic drugs, should only be handled by adequately trained personnel. Pregnant staff should not be involved in the reconstitution or administration of Novantrone.

Care should be taken to avoid contact of Novantrone with the skin, mucous membranes, or eyes. The use of goggles, gloves and protective gowns is recommended during preparation, administration and disposal and the work surface should be covered with disposable plastic-backed absorbent paper.

Aerosol generation should be minimised. Novantrone can cause staining. Skin accidentally exposed to Novantrone should be rinsed copiously with warm water and if the eyes are involved standard irrigation techniques should be used.

c) Spillage disposal
The following clean-up procedure is recommended if Novantrone is spilled on equipment or environmental surfaces. Prepare a 50% solution of fresh concentrated bleach (any recognised proprietary brand containing either sodium or calcium hypochlorite) in water. Wet absorbent tissues in the bleach solution and apply the wetted tissues to the spillage. The spillage is deactivated when the blue colour has been fully discharged. Collect up the tissues with dry tissues. Appropriate protective equipment should be worn during the clean-up procedure.

All Novantrone contaminated items (eg, syringes, needles, tissues, etc) should be treated as toxic waste and disposed of accordingly. Incineration is recommended.

7. MARKETING AUTHORISATION HOLDER
John Wyeth & Brother Limited
Trading as Wyeth Pharmaceuticals
Huntercombe Lane South
Taplow
Maidenhead
Berkshire
SL6 0PH
UK

8. MARKETING AUTHORISATION NUMBER(S)
PL 00011/0276

9. DATE OF FIRST AUTHORISATION/RENEWAL OF THE AUTHORISATION
21 July 2003

10. DATE OF REVISION OF THE TEXT
7 October 2004

Novofem film-coated tablets.

(Novo Nordisk Limited)

1. NAME OF THE MEDICINAL PRODUCT

Novofem® film-coated tablet

2. QUALITATIVE AND QUANTITATIVE COMPOSITION

One red film-coated tablet contains:

Estradiol 1 mg (as estradiol hemihydrate)

One white film-coated tablet contains:

Estradiol 1 mg (as estradiol hemihydrate) and norethisterone acetate 1 mg

For excipients see 6.1.

3. PHARMACEUTICAL FORM

Film-coated tablet

Red film-coated, biconvex tablets engraved with NOVO 282. Diameter: 6mm.

White film-coated, biconvex tablets engraved with NOVO 283. Diameter: 6mm.

4. CLINICAL PARTICULARS

4.1 Therapeutic indications

Hormone Replacement Therapy (HRT) for oestrogen deficiency symptoms in postmenopausal women with an intact uterus.

Prevention of osteoporosis in postmenopausal women at high risk of future fractures who are intolerant of, or contraindicated for, other medicinal products approved for the prevention of osteoporosis.

The experience of treating women older than 65 years is limited.

4.2 Posology and method of administration

Novofem is a continuous sequential preparation for hormone replacement therapy. The oestrogen is dosed continuously. The progestogen is added for 12 days of every 28 day cycle in a sequential manner.

One tablet is taken daily in the following order: oestrogen therapy (red film-coated tablet) over 16 days, followed by 12 days of oestrogen/progestogen therapy (white film-coated tablet).

After intake of the last white tablet, treatment is continued with the first red tablet of a new pack on the next day. A menstruation-like bleeding usually occurs at the beginning of a new treatment cycle.

In women who are not taking HRT or women transferring from a continuous combined HRT product, treatment may be started on any convenient day. In women transferring from a sequential HRT regimen, treatment should begin the day following completion of the prior regimen.

For initiation and continuation of treatment of postmenopausal symptoms, the lowest effective dose for the shortest duration (see also section 4.4) should be used.

A switch to a higher dose combination product could be indicated if the response after three months is insufficient for satisfactory symptom relief.

If the patient has forgotten to take one tablet, the forgotten tablet is to be discarded. Forgetting a dose may increase the likelihood of breakthrough bleeding and spotting.

4.3 Contraindications

- Known, past or suspected breast cancer
- Known or suspected oestrogen-dependent malignant tumours (e.g. endometrial cancer)
- Undiagnosed genital bleeding
- Untreated endometrial hyperplasia
- Previous idiopathic or current venous thromboembolism (deep venous thrombosis, pulmonary embolism)
- Active or recent arterial thromboembolic disease (e.g. angina, myocardial infarction)
- Acute liver disease or a history of liver disease, as long as liver function tests have failed to return to normal
- Known hypersensitivity to the active substances or to any of the excipients
- Porphyria

4.4 Special warnings and special precautions for use

For the treatment of postmenopausal symptoms, HRT should only be initiated for symptoms that adversely affect quality of life. In all cases, a careful appraisal of the risks and benefits should be undertaken at least annually and HRT should only be continued as long as the benefit outweighs the risk.

Medical examination/follow-up

Before initiating or reinstituting HRT, a complete personal and family medical history should be taken. Physical (including pelvic and breast) examination should be guided by this and by the contraindications and warnings for use. During treatment, periodic check-ups are recommended of a frequency and nature adapted to the individual woman. Women should be advised what changes in their breasts should be reported to their doctor or nurse (see 'Breast cancer' below). Investigations, including mammography, should be carried out in accordance with currently accepted screening practices, modified to the clinical needs of the individual.

Conditions which need supervision:

If any of the following conditions are present, have occurred previously and/or have been aggravated during pregnancy or previous hormone treatment, the patient should be closely supervised. It should be taken into account that these conditions may recur or be aggravated during treatment with Novofem, in particular:

- Leiomyoma (uterine fibroids) or endometriosis
- A history of or risk factors for thromboembolic disorders (see below)
- Risk factors for oestrogen dependent tumours, e.g. 1st degree heredity for breast cancer
- Hypertension
- Liver disorders (e.g. liver adenoma)
- Diabetes mellitus with or without vascular involvement
- Cholelithiasis
- Migraine or (severe) headache
- Systemic lupus erythematosus
- A history of endometrial hyperplasia (see below)
- Epilepsy
- Asthma
- Otosclerosis

Reasons for immediate withdrawal of therapy:

Therapy should be discontinued in case a contraindication is discovered and in the following situations:

- Jaundice or deterioration in liver function
- Significant increase in blood pressure
- New onset of migraine-type headache
- Pregnancy

Endometrial hyperplasia

The risk of endometrial hyperplasia and carcinoma is increased when oestrogens are administered alone for prolonged periods (see section 4.8). The addition of a progestogen, for at least 12 days per cycle in non-hysterectomised women greatly reduces this risk.

Breakthrough bleeding and spotting may occur during the first months of treatment. If breakthrough bleeding or spotting appears after some time on therapy, or continues after treatment has been discontinued, the reason should be investigated, which may include endometrial biopsy to exclude endometrial malignancy.

Breast Cancer

A randomised placebo-controlled trial, the Women's Health Initiative study (WHI), and epidemiological studies, including the Million Women Study (MWS), have reported an increased risk of breast cancer in women taking oestrogens, oestrogen-progestogen combinations or tibolone for HRT for several years (see section 4.8).

For all HRT, an excess risk becomes apparent within a few years of use and increases with duration of intake but returns to baseline within a few (at most five) years after stopping treatment.

In the MWS, the relative risk of breast cancer with conjugated equine oestrogens (CEE) or estradiol (E2) was greater when a progestogen was added, either sequentially or continuously, and regardless of type of progestogen. There was no evidence of a difference in risk between the different routes of administration.

In the WHI study, the continuous combined conjugated equine oestrogen and medroxyprogesterone acetate (CEE + MPA) product used was associated with breast cancers that were slightly larger in size and more frequently had local lymph node metastases compared to placebo.

HRT, especially oestrogen-progestogen combined treatment, increases the density of mammographic images which may adversely affect the radiological detection of breast cancer.

Venous thromboembolism

HRT is associated with a higher relative risk of developing venous thromboembolism (VTE), i.e. deep vein thrombosis or pulmonary embolism. One randomised controlled trial and epidemiological studies found a two- to three-fold higher risk for users compared with non-users. For non-users it is estimated that the number of cases of VTE that will occur over a 5 year period is about 3 per 1000 women aged 50-59 years and 8 per 1000 women aged between 60-69 years. It is estimated that in healthy women who use HRT for 5 years, the number of additional cases of VTE over a 5 year period will be between 2 and 6 (best estimate =4) per 1000 women aged 50-59 years and between 5 and 15 (best estimate =9) per 1000 women aged 60-69 years. The occurrence of such an event is more likely in the first year of HRT than later.

Generally recognised risk factors for VTE include a personal history or family history, severe obesity (BM > 30 kg/m^2) and systemic lupus erythematosus (SLE). There is no consensus about the possible role of varicose veins in VTE.

Patients with a history of VTE or known thrombophilic states have an increased risk of VTE. HRT may add to this risk. Personal or strong family history of thromboembolism, or recurrent spontaneous abortion, should be investigated in order to exclude a thrombophilic predisposition. Until a thorough evaluation of thrombophilic factors has been made or anticoagulant treatment initiated, use of HRT in such patients should be viewed as contraindicated. Those women already on anticoagulant treatment require careful consideration of the benefit-risk of use of HRT.

The risk of VTE may be temporarily increased with prolonged immobilisation, major trauma or major surgery. As in all postoperative patients, scrupulous attention should be given to prophylactic measures to prevent VTE following surgery. Where prolonged immobilisation is liable to follow elective surgery, particularly abdominal or orthopaedic surgery to the lower limbs, consideration should be given to temporarily stopping HRT four to six weeks earlier, if possible. Treatment should not be restarted until the woman is completely mobilised.

If VTE develops after initiating therapy, the drug should be discontinued. Patients should be told to contact their doctors immediately when they are aware of a potential thromboembolic symptom (e.g., painful swelling of a leg, sudden pain in the chest, dyspnea).

Coronary artery disease (CAD)

There is no evidence from randomised controlled trials of cardiovascular benefit with continuous combined conjugated oestrogens and medroxyprogesterone acetate (MPA). Two large clinical trials (WHI and HERS i.e. Heart and Estrogen/progestin Replacement Study) showed a possible increased risk of cardiovascular morbidity in the first year of use and no overall benefit. For other HRT products there are only limited data from randomised controlled trials examining effects in cardiovascular morbidity or mortality. Therefore, it is uncertain whether these findings also extend to other HRT products.

Stroke

One large randomised clinical trial (WHI-trial) found, as a secondary outcome, an increased risk of ischaemic stroke in healthy women during treatment with continuous combined conjugated oestrogens and MPA. For women who do not use HRT, it is estimated that the number of cases of stroke that will occur over a 5 year period is about 3 per 1000 women aged 50-59 years and 11 per 1000 women aged 60-69 years. It is estimated that for women who use conjugated oestrogens and MPA for 5 years, the number of additional cases will be between 0 and 3 (best estimate = 1) per 1000 users aged 50-59 years and between 1 and 9 (best estimate = 4) per 1000 users aged 60-69 years. It is unknown whether the increased risk also extends to other HRT products.

Ovarian cancer

Long-term (at least 5-10 years) use of oestrogen-only HRT products in hysterectomised women has been associated with an increased risk of ovarian cancer in some epidemiological studies. It is uncertain whether long-term use of combined HRT confers a different risk than oestrogen-only products.

Other conditions

Oestrogens may cause fluid retention and, therefore patients with cardiac or renal dysfunction should be carefully observed. Patients with terminal renal insufficiency should be closely observed since it is expected that the level of circulating active ingredients in Novofem will increase.

Women with pre-existing hypertriglyceridemia should be followed closely during oestrogen replacement or hormone replacement therapy, since rare cases of large increases of plasma triglycerides leading to pancreatitis have been reported with oestrogen therapy in this condition.

Oestrogens increase thyroid binding globulin (TBG), leading to increased circulating total thyroid hormone, as measured by protein-bound iodine (PBI), T4 levels (by column or by radio-immunoassay) or T3 levels (by radio-immunoassay). T3 resin uptake is decreased, reflecting the elevated TBG. Free T4 and free T3 concentrations are unaltered. Other binding proteins may be elevated in serum, i.e. corticoid binding globulin (CBG), sex-hormone-binding globulin (SHBG) leading to increased circulating corticosteroids and sex steroids, respectively. Free or biological active hormone concentrations are unchanged. Other plasma proteins may be increased (angiotensinogen/renin substrate, alpha-I-antitrypsin, ceruloplasmin).

There is no conclusive evidence for improvement of cognitive function. There is some evidence from the WHI trial of increased risk of probable dementia in women who start using continuous combined CEE and MPA after the age of 65. It is unknown whether the findings apply to younger post-menopausal women or other HRT products.

4.5 Interaction with other medicinal products and other forms of Interaction

The metabolism of oestrogens and protestogens may be increased at concomitant use of substances known to induce drug-metabolising enzymes, specifically cytochrome P450 enzymes such as anticonvulsants (e.g. phenobarbital, phenytoin, carbamezapin) and anti-infectives (e.g. rifampicin, rifabutin, nevirapine, efavirenz). Ritonavir and nelfinavir, although known as strong inhibitors, by contrast exhibit inducing properties when used concomitantly with steroid hormones. Herbal preparations containing St John's Wort (*Hypericum perforatum*) may induce the metabolism of oestrogens and progestogens.

Clinically, an increased metabolism of oestrogens and progestogens may lead to decreased effect and changes in the uterine bleeding profile.

Table 1

System organ class	Very common>1/10	Common >1/100; <1/10	Uncommon >1/1,000; <1/100	Rare >1/10,000; <1/1,000
Infections and infestations		Vaginal candidiasis		
Immune system disorders				Allergic reaction
Psychiatric disorders				Nervousness
Nervous system disorders	Headache	Dizziness Insomnia Depression	Migraine Libido disorder NOS (not otherwise specified	Vertigo
Vascular disorders		Increased blood pressure Aggravated hypertension	Peripheral embolism and thrombosis	
Gastrointestinal disorders		Dyspepsia Abdominal pain Flatulence Nausea	Vomiting	Diarrhoea Bloating
Hepatobiliary disorders			Gallbladder disease Gallstones	
Skin and subcutaneous tissue disorders		Rash Pruritus	Alopecia	Acne
Musculoskeletal and connective tissue disorders			Muscle cramps	
Reproductive system and breast disorders	Breast tenderness	Vaginal haemorrhage Uterine fibroids aggravated		Uterine fibroid
General disorders and administration site conditions		Oedema		
Investigations		Weight increased		

Reduced estradiol levels have been observed under the simultaneous use of antibiotics e.g. penicillins and tetracycline.

Oestrogens can enhance the effects and side effects of imipramine.

If cyclosporin is given concomitantly, there may be increased blood levels of cyclosporin, creatinine and transaminases due to the decreased hepatic excretion of cyclosporin.

The requirement of treatment with oral antidiabetic drugs or with insulin may change due to the oestrogen effect on glucose tolerance (will be decreased) and the response to insulin, i.e. the requirement of insulin or oral antidiabetics can be increased as a consequence of a reduced glucose tolerance.

4.6 Pregnancy and lactation

Novofem is not indicated during pregnancy.

If pregnancy occurs during medication with Novofem, treatment should be withdrawn immediately.

Data on a limited number of exposed pregnancies indicate adverse effects of norethisterone on the foetus. At doses higher than normally used in OC and HRT formulations masculinisation of female foetuses was observed.

The results of most epidemiological studies to date relevant to inadvertent foetal exposure to combinations of oestrogens and progestogens indicate no teratogenic or foetotoxic effect.

Lactation

Novofem is not indicated during lactation.

4.7 Effects on ability to drive and use machines

No effects known.

4.8 Undesirable effects

The most frequently reported adverse event during treatment in clinical trials conducted with an HRT product similar to Novofem is breast tenderness and headache >1/10).

The adverse events listed below may occur during oestrogen-progestogen treatment. The frequencies are derived from clinical trials conducted with an HRT product similar to Novofem and from a Post Marketing Surveillance study on Novofem.

(see Table 1 above)

Breast cancer

According to evidence from a large number of epidemiological studies and one randomised placebo-controlled trial, the Women's Health Initiative (WHI), the overall risk of breast cancer increases with increasing duration of HRT use in current or recent HRT users.

For *oestrogen-only* HRT, estimates of relative risk (RR) from a reanalysis of original data from 51 epidemiological studies (in which >80% of HRT use was oestrogen-only HRT) and from the epidemiological Million Women Study (MWS) are similar at 1.35 (95% CI: 1.21-1.49) and 1.30 (95% CI: 1.21-1.40), respectively.

For *oestrogen plus progestogen* combined HRT, several epidemiological studies have reported an overall higher risk for breast cancer than with oestrogens alone.

The MWS reported that, compared to never users, the use of various types of oestrogen-progestogen combined HRT was associated with a higher risk of breast cancer (RR = 2.00, 95% CI: 1.88-2.12) than use of oestrogens alone (RR = 1.30, 95% CI: 1.21-1.40) or use of tibolone (RR = 1.45, 95% CI: 1.25-1.68).

The WHI trial reported a risk estimate of 1.24 (95% CI: 1.01-1.54) after 5.6 years of use of oestrogen-progestogen combined HRT (CEE + MPA) in all users compared with placebo.

The absolute risks calculated from the MWS and the WHI trial are presented below:

The MWS has estimated, from the known average incidence of breast cancer in developed countries, that:

- For women not using HRT, about 32 in every 1000 are expected to have breast cancer diagnosed between the ages of 50 and 64 years.
- For 1000 current or recent users of HRT, the number of *additional* cases during the corresponding period will be
- For users of *oestrogen-only* replacement therapy,

- between 0 and 3 (best estimate = 1.5) for 5 years' use

- between 3 and 7 (best estimate = 5) for 10 years' use.

- For users of *oestrogen plus progestogen* combined HRT,

- between 5 and 7 (best estimate = 6) for 5 years' use

- between 18 and 20 (best estimate = 19 for 10 years use.

The WHI trial estimated that after 5.6 years of follow-up of women between the ages of 50 and 79 years, an *additional* 8 cases of invasive breast cancer would be due to *oestrogen-progestogen combined* HRT (CEE + MPA) per 10,000 women years. According to calculations from the trial data, it is estimated that:

- For 1000 women in the placebo group,

- about 16 cases of invasive breast cancer would be diagnosed in 5 years.

- For 1000 women who used oestrogen + progestogen combined HRT (CEE +

MPA), the number of additional cases would be

- between 0 an 9 (best estimate = 4) for 5 years' use.

The number of additional cases of breast cancer in women who use HRT is broadly similar for women who start HRT irrespective of age at start of use (between the ages of 45-65) (see section 4.4).

Endometrial cancer

In women with an intact uterus, the risk of endometrial hyperplasia and endometrial cancer increases with increasing duration of use of unopposed oestrogens. According to data from epidemiological studies, the best estimate of the risk is that for women not using HRT, about 5 in every 1000 are expected to have endometrial cancer diagnosed between the ages of 50 and 65. Depending on the duration of treatment and oestrogen dose, the reported increase in endometrial cancer risk among unopposed oestrogen users varies from 2- to 12-fold greater compared with non-users. Adding a progestogen to oestrogen-only therapy greatly reduces this increased risk.

Post-marketing experience:

In addition to the above mentioned adverse drug reactions, those presented below have been spontaneously reported, and are by an overall judgment considered possibly related to Novofem treatment. The reporting rate of these spontaneous adverse drug reactions is very rare: (<1/10,000 patient years). Post-marketing experience is subject to underreporting especially with regard to trivial and well known adverse drug reactions. The presented frequencies should be interpreted in that light:

Reproductive system and breast disorders: Hyperplasia of endometrium (for further information see section 4.4)

Skin and subcutaneous tissue disorders: Hirsutism.

Other adverse reactions have been reported in association with oestrogen/progestogen treatment:

- Oestrogen-dependent neoplasms benign and malignant, e.g. endometrial cancer.

- Venous thromboembolism, i.e. deep leg or pelvic venous thrombosis and pulmonary embolism, is more frequent among hormone replacement therapy users than among non-users. For further information, see sections 4.3 Contraindications and 4.4 Special warnings and precautions for use.

- Myocardial infarction and stroke

- Skin and subcutaneous disorders: chloasma, erythema multiforme, erythema nodosum, haemorrhagic eruption, vascular purpura.

- Probable dementia (see section 4.4)

- Gallbladder disease.

4.9 Overdose

Overdose may be manifested by nausea and vomiting. Treatment should be symptomatic.

5. PHARMACOLOGICAL PROPERTIES

5.1 Pharmacodynamic properties

ATC Code G03F B05

Oestrogen and progestogen, sequential combination for continuous treatment.

Estradiol: The active ingredient, synthetic 17β-estradiol, is chemically and biologically identical to endogenous human estradiol. It substitutes for the loss of oestrogen production in menopausal women, and alleviates menopausal symptoms.

Oestrogens prevent bone loss following menopause or ovariectomy.

Norethisterone acetate: As oestrogens promote the growth of the endometrium, unopposed oestrogens increase the risk of endometrial hyperplasia and cancer. The addition of a progestogen greatly reduces the oestrogen-induced risk of endometrial hyperplasia in non-hysterectomised women.

Relief of menopausal symptoms is achieved during the first few weeks of treatment.

In a PMS study regular withdrawal bleeding with a mean duration of 3-4 days occurred in 91% of women, who took Novofem over 6 month. Withdrawal bleeding usually started a few days after the last tablet of the progestogen phase.

Oestrogen deficiency at menopause is associated with an increasing bone turnover and decline in bone mass. The effect of oestrogens on the bone mineral density is dose-dependent. Protection appears to be effective for as long as treatment is continued. After discontinuation of HRT, bone mass is lost at a rate similar to that in untreated women.

Evidence from the WHI trial and meta-analysed trials shows that current use of HRT, alone or in combination with a progestogen – given to predominantly healthy women – reduces the risk of hip, vertebral, and other osteoporotic fractures. HRT may also prevent fractures in women with low bone density and/or established osteoporosis, but the evidence for that is limited.

Randomised, double-blind, placebo-controlled studies showed that 1 mg estradiol prevents the postmenopausal loss of bone minerals and increases the bone mineral density. The responses in the spine, femoral neck and trochanter were 2.8%, 1.6% and 2.5%, respectively, over 2 years with 1mg 17β-estradiol unopposed.

5.2 Pharmacokinetic properties

Following oral administration of 17β-estradiol in micronised form, rapid absorption from the gastrointestinal tract occurs. It undergoes extensive first-pass metabolism in the liver and other enteric organs, and a peak plasma concentration of approximately 28 pg/ml (range 13-40 pg/ml) occurs within 6 hours after intake of 1 mg. The area under the curve (AUC_{0-tz}) = 629 h $\times$ pg/ml. The half-life of 17β-estradiol is about 25 hours. It circulates bound to SHBG (37%) and to albumin (61%), while only approximately 1-2% is unbound. Metabolism of 17β-estradiol occurs mainly in the liver and gut but also in target organs, and involves the formation of less active or inactive metabolites, including oestrone, catecholoestrogens and several oestrogen sulphates and glucuronides. Oestrogens are partly excreted with the bile, hydrolysed and reabsorbed (enterohepatic circulation), and mainly eliminated in urine in biologically inactive form.

After oral administration, norethisterone acetate is rapidly absorbed and transformed to norethisterone (NET). It undergoes first-pass metabolism in the liver and other enteric organs, and a peak plasma concentration of approximately 9 ng/ml (range 6-11 ng/ml) occurs within 1 hour after intake of 1 mg. The area under the curve (AUC_{0-tz}) = 29 h $\times$ pg/ml. The terminal half-life of NET is about 10 hours. NET binds to SHBG (36%) and to albumin (61%). The most important metabolites are isomers of 5α-dihydro-NET and of tetrahydro-NET, which are excreted mainly in the urine as sulphate or glucuronide conjugates. The pharmacokinetics in the elderly have not been studied.

5.3 Preclinical safety data

Animal studies with estradiol and norethisterone acetate have shown expected oestrogenic and progestogenic effects. Both compounds induced adverse effects in preclinical reproductive toxicity studies, in particular embryotoxic effects and anomalies in urogenital tract development. Concerning other preclinic effects, the toxicity profiles of estradiol and norethisterone acetate are well known and reveal no particular human risks beyond those discussed in other sections of the SPC and which generally apply to hormone substitution therapy.

6. PHARMACEUTICAL PARTICULARS

6.1 List of excipients

Both the white and the red tablets contain:

Lactose monohydrate

Maize starch

Gelatin

Talc

Magnesium stearate

Film-coating

White film-coated tablet:

Hypromellose, triacetin, talc

Red film-coated tablet:

Hypromellose, red iron oxide (E 172), titanium dioxide (E 171), propylene glycol and talc

6.2 Incompatibilities

Not applicable.

6.3 Shelf life

3 years.

6.4 Special precautions for storage

Do not store above 25°C. Do not refrigerate. Keep the container in the outer carton.

6.5 Nature and contents of container

1 $\times$ 28 tablets or 3 $\times$ 28 tablets in calendar dial packs.

The calendar dial pack with 28 tablets consists of the following 3 parts:

- The base made of coloured non-transparent polypropylene,

- The ring-shaped lid made of transparent polystyrene,

- The centre-dial made of coloured non-transparent polystyrene.

Not all pack sizes may be marketed.

6.6 Instructions for use and handling

No special requirements.

7. MARKETING AUTHORISATION HOLDER

Novo Nordisk Limited

Broadfield Park, Brighton Road,

Crawley, West Sussex, RH11 9RT

8. MARKETING AUTHORISATION NUMBER(S)

PL 03132/0141

9. DATE OF FIRST AUTHORISATION/RENEWAL OF THE AUTHORISATION

May 2002

10. DATE OF REVISION OF THE TEXT

9 March 2004

LEGAL STATUS

POM (Prescription only medicine)

Novolizer Budesonide 200 micrograms Inhalation Powder

(Viatris Pharmaceuticals Ltd)

1. NAME OF THE MEDICINAL PRODUCT

Novolizer® Budesonide 200 micrograms inhalation powder ▼

2. QUALITATIVE AND QUANTITATIVE COMPOSITION

One metered dose contains 200 micrograms of budesonide.

For excipients, see 6.1

3. PHARMACEUTICAL FORM

Inhalation powder

White powder

4. CLINICAL PARTICULARS

4.1 Therapeutic indications

Treatment of persistent asthma

4.2 Posology and method of administration

For inhalation use

Steroid naive patients and patients previously controlled on inhaled steroids:

Adults (including the elderly) and children/adolescents over 12 years of age:

Initial recommended dose: 200 - 400 micrograms once or twice daily

Maximum recommended dose: 800 micrograms twice daily

Children 6 - 12 years:

Initial recommended dose: 200 micrograms twice or 200 - 400 micrograms once daily

Maximum recommended dose: 400 micrograms twice daily

The dose should be adapted to the requirements of each individual, the severity of the disease and the clinical response of the patient. The dose should be adjusted until control is achieved and then should be titrated to the lowest dose at which effective control of asthma is maintained.

If a patient is switched from another inhalation system to Novolizer Budesonide 200 micrograms the dose should be re-adjusted on an individual basis. The drug, dose regimen and method of delivery should be considered.

Posology limits:

Adults (including the elderly) and children/adolescents over 12 years of age: 200 - 1600 micrograms daily

Children 6 - 12 years: 200 - 800 micrograms daily

Twice daily dosing in adults, including the elderly should be used when starting treatment, during periods of severe asthma and while reducing or discontinuing oral glucocorticosteroids.

Once daily dosing up to 800 micrograms may be used in adults, including the elderly with mild to moderate asthma and already controlled on inhaled glucocorticosteroids (either budesonide or beclometasone dipropionate) administered twice daily.

If a patient is transferred from twice daily dosing to once daily dosing this should be at the same equivalent total daily dose (with consideration of the drug and the method of delivery) and this dose should then be reduced to the minimum dose needed to maintain effective control of asthma. The once daily regimen can be considered only when asthma symptoms are controlled.

In case of once daily dosing this dose should be taken in the evening.

In case of deterioration of asthma control (recognised by e.g. persistent respiratory symptoms, increased use of an inhaled bronchodilator) the dose of inhaled steroids should be increased. Those patients receiving the once daily dose regimen, should be advised to double their dose of inhaled corticosteroid, such that a once daily dose would be administered twice daily. In any case of deterioration of asthma control the patient should seek advice from a medical doctor as soon as possible.

A short acting inhaled β-2-agonist should be available for the relief of acute symptoms of asthma at all times.

Mode and duration of treatment:

Novolizer Budesonide 200 micrograms is intended for long-term therapy and as such also for prophylactic therapy. It should be administered regularly according to the recommended schedule even when asymptomatic.

The improvement in the control of asthma can appear in 24 hours, although 1 - 2 weeks additional treatment period may be necessary to reach a maximum benefit.

In order to ensure that the active substance optimally reaches the intended site of action it is necessary to inhale steadily and as vigorously, deeply and rapidly as possible (up to the maximum inhalation depth). Novolizer Budesonide 200 microgramsindicates that inhalation has been performed correctly by a clearly audible click and a colour change in the control window from green to red.

This multiple feedback mechanism of NovolizerBudesonide 200 microgramsindicates that inhalation has been performed correctly. If the Novolizer Budesonide 200 microgramsdoes not indicate that inhalation has been performed correctly, inhalation should be repeated. The inhaler remains blocked until inhalation is performed correctly.

To reduce the risk of oral candidiasis and hoarseness it is recommended that inhalation be performed before meals and that the mouth is rinsed with water or the teeth brushed after each inhalation.

Usage and handling of the Novolizer Device

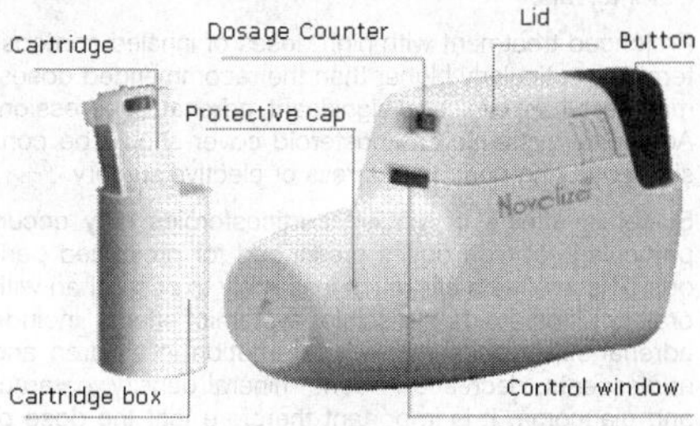

Refilling

1. Lightly press together the ribbed surfaces on both sides of the lid, move the lid forwards and lift off.

2. Remove the protective aluminium foil from the cartridge box and take out the new cartridge.

3. Insert the cartridge into the Novolizer with the dosage counter facing the mouthpiece.

4. Replace the lid into the side guides from above and push down flat towards the button until it snaps into place. The cartridge can be left in the Novolizer until it has been used up, or for up to 6 months after insertion.

Note: Novolizer Budesonide 200 micrograms cartridges may only be used in the Novolizer powder inhaler

Usage

1. When using the Novolizer always keep it horizontal. First remove the protective cap.

2. Completely depress the coloured button. A loud double click will be heard and the colour of the control window (lower) will change from red to green. Then release the coloured button. The colour green in the window indicates that the Novolizer is ready for use.

3. Exhale (but not into the powder inhaler).

4. Put the lips around the mouthpiece. Inhale the powder with a deep breath. During this breath a loud click should be heard, indicating correct inhalation. Hold the breath for a few seconds and then continue with normal breathing.

Note: If the patient needs to take more than 1 actuation at a time, steps 2 - 4 should be repeated.

5. Replace the protective cap on the mouth piece - the dosing procedure is now complete.

6. The number in the top window indicates the number of inhalations left.

Note: The coloured button should onlybe pressed immediately before inhalation.

A double inhalation in error is not possible with the Novolizer. The click sound and the change of colour in the control window indicate that inhalation has been performed correctly. If the colour of the control window does not change then inhalation should be repeated. If inhalation is not completed correctly after several attempts, then the patient should consult the doctor/physician.

Cleaning

The Novolizer should be cleaned at regular intervals, but at least every time the cartridge is changed. Instructions on how to clean the device can be found in the operating instructions attached.

Note: In order to ensure correct use of the inhaler, patients should receive thorough instructions on how to use the device. Children should only use this product under the supervision of an adult.

4.3 Contraindications

Novolizer Budesonide 200 micrograms is contraindicated in patients with hypersensitivity to budesonide or lactose.

4.4 Special warnings and special precautions for use

Novolizer Budesonide 200 micrograms is not indicated for treatment of acute dyspnoea or status asthmaticus. These conditions should be treated in the normal way.

Treatment of acute exacerbations of asthma and asthma symptoms may need an increase in the dose of Novolizer Budesonide 200 micrograms. The patient should be advised to use a short-acting inhaled bronchodilator as rescue medication to relieve acute asthma symptoms.

Close observation and special care is needed in patients with both active and quiescent pulmonary tuberculosis. Patients with active pulmonary tuberculosis may use Novolizer Budesonide 200 micrograms only if they are treated simultaneously with effective tuberculostatics.

Similarly patients with fungal, viral or other infections of the airways require close observation and special care and should use Novolizer Budesonide 200 micrograms only if they are also receiving adequate treatment for such infections.

Patients who repeatedly fail to perform the inhalation correctly should consult their doctor.

In patients with severe hepatic dysfunction treatment with Novolizer Budesonide 200 micrograms - similar to treatment with other glucocorticosteroids - may lead to a reduced elimination rate and an increase in systemic availability. Attention is to be paid to possible systemic effects. Therefore the hypothalamic pituitary adrenocortical (HPA) axis function of these patients should be checked at regular intervals.

Prolonged treatment with high doses of inhaled corticosteroids, particularly higher than the recommended doses, may result in clinically significant adrenal suppression. Additional systemic corticosteroid cover should be considered during periods of stress or elective surgery.

Systemic effects of inhaled corticosteroids may occur, particularly at high doses prescribed for prolonged periods. These effects are much less likely to occur than with oral corticosteroids. Possible systemic effects include adrenal suppression, growth retardation in children and adolescents, decrease in bone mineral density, cataract and glaucoma. It is important therefore that the dose of inhaled corticosteroid is titrated to the lowest dose at which effective control of asthma is maintained.

It is recommended that the height of children receiving prolonged treatment with inhaled corticosteroids is regularly monitored. If growth is slowed, therapy should be reviewed with the aim of reducing the dose of inhaled corticosteroid, if possible, to the lowest dose at which effective control of asthma is maintained. In addition, consideration should be given to referring the patient to a paediatric respiratory specialist.

Precautions for patients not previously treated with corticosteroids:

When Novolizer Budesonide 200 micrograms is used regularly as directed, patients who have previously never or only occasionally received brief treatment with corticosteroids, should experience an improvement in breathing after approximately 1 - 2 weeks. However, extreme mucous congestion and inflammatory processes may obstruct the bronchial passages to such an extent that budesonide cannot fully exert its local effects. In such cases, inhaled therapy with Novolizer Budesonide 200 micrograms should be supplemented with a short course of systemic corticosteroids (starting with 40 - 60 mg of prednisolone equivalent daily). Inhalation doses are continued after gradually reducing the dose of systemic corticosteroids.

Precautions for switching patients from systemically active corticosteroids to inhalation treatment:

Patients receiving systemic treatment with corticosteroids should be switched to Novolizer Budesonide 200 micrograms at a time when their symptoms are under control. In these patients, whose adrenocortical function is usually impaired, systemic treatment with corticosteroids must not be stopped abruptly. At the beginning of the switchover, a high dose of Novolizer Budesonide 200 micrograms should be given in addition to the systemic corticosteroids for about 7 to 10 days. Then, depending on the patient's response and depending on the original dose of the systemic steroid, the daily dose of the systemic corticosteroid can be reduced gradually (e.g. 1 milligram prednisolone or the equivalent each week or 2.5 milligram prednisolone or the equivalent each month). The oral steroid should be reduced to the lowest possible level and it may be possible to completely replace the oral steroid with inhaled budesonide.

Within the first few months of switching patients from systemic administration of corticosteroids to inhalation treatment, it may be necessary to resume systemic administration of corticosteroids during periods of stress or in the case of emergencies (e.g. severe infections, injuries, surgery). This applies also to patients who have received prolonged treatment with high doses of inhaled corticosteroids. They may also have impaired adrenocortical function and may need systemic corticosteroid cover during periods of stress.

Recovery from impaired adrenal function may take some considerable time. Hypothalamic pituitary adrenocortical axis function should be monitored regularly.

The patient might feel generally unwell in a non specific way during the withdrawal of systemic corticosteroids despite maintenance or even improvement in respiratory function. The patient should be encouraged to continue with inhaled budesonide and withdrawal of oral steroids unless there are clinical signs which might indicate adrenal insufficiency.

After the patient has been switched to inhalation treatment, symptoms may become manifest that had been suppressed by the previous systemic treatment with glucocorticosteroids, e.g. allergic rhinitis, allergic eczema, muscle and joint pain. Suitable drugs should be co-administered to treat these symptoms.

Inhaled budesonide should not be stopped abruptly.

Exacerbation of clinical symptoms due to acute respiratory tract infections:

If clinical symptoms become exacerbated by acute respiratory tract infections, treatment with appropriate antibiotics should be considered. The dose of Novolizer Budesonide 200 micrograms can be adjusted as required and, in certain situations, systemic treatment with glucocorticosteroids may be indicated.

Patients with rare hereditary problems of galactose intolerance, the Lapp lactase deficiency or glucose-galactose malabsorbtion should not take this medicine.

4.5 Interaction with other medicinal products and other forms of Interaction

Ketoconazole 200 mg once daily increased plasma levels of concomitantly administered oral budesonide (single dose of 3 mg) on average six-fold. When ketoconazole was administered 12 hours after budesonide the concentration was on average increased three-fold. Information about this interaction is lacking for inhaled budesonide, but marked increases in plasma levels could be expected. Since data to give dosage recommendations are lacking, the combination should be avoided. If this is not possible the time interval between administration of ketoconazole and budesonide should be as long as possible. A reduction in the dose of budesonide should also be considered. Other potent inhibitors of CYP3A4 (e.g. ritonavir) are also likely to markedly increase plasma levels of budesonide.

4.6 Pregnancy and lactation

The need for use during pregnancy has to be considered with special care. Although there is no indication according to the experience in pregnant women up to now, that the teratogenic effects of budesonide, which did occur in animal experiments (see 5.3), are of any relevance in humans, other types of adverse effects (e.g. intrauterine growth retardation, atrophy of the adrenal cortex, cardiovascular disease in adulthood) which have been shown in animal studies cannot be ruled out. There is suspicion, that especially synthetic glucocorticosteroids, which can only be inactivated insufficiently by the placenta, may contribute to cardiovascular diseases in later age by an in utero programming of the fetus.

Novolizer Budesonide 200 micrograms should only be used when the expected benefit outweighs the potential risks. The lowest effective dose of budesonide needed to maintain adequate asthma control should be used.

It is not known whether budesonide passes into human breast milk. However, even though the systemic exposure to budesonide after inhalation therapy is low, administration of Novolizer Budesonide 200 micrograms to women who are breastfeeding should only be considered if the expected benefit to the mother is greater than any possible risk to the child.

4.7 Effects on ability to drive and use machines

Novolizer Budesonide 200 micrograms has no effect on the ability to drive or use machines.

4.8 Undesirable effects

The table below presents possible adverse drug reactions in system organ class order and sorted by frequency.

(see Table 1 below)

Mild mucosal irritations accompanied by difficulty in swallowing, hoarseness and cough may commonly occur.

Treatment with inhaled budesonide may result in candida infections in the oropharynx. Experience has shown that candida infection occurs less often when inhalation is performed before meals and/or when the mouth is rinsed after inhalation. In most cases this condition responds to topical anti-fungal therapy without discontinuing treatment with inhaled budesonide.

As with other inhalation therapies, in rare cases paradoxical bronchospasm may occur, manifest by an immediate increase in wheezing after dosing. Paradoxical bronchospasm responds to a fast acting inhaled bronchodilator and should be treated straightaway. Budesonide should be discontinued immediately, the patient should be assessed and, if necessary, alternative treatment instituted.

In rare cases hypersensitivity with skin reactions such as urticaria, rash, dermatitis, pruritus and erythema were observed. There have been rare reports of angioneurotic oedema (oedema of the face, lips, eyes and throat) following inhaled budesonide. In rare cases skin bruising may occur.

In very rare cases restlessness, abnormal behaviour and increased motor activity may result.

Systemic effects of inhaled corticosteroids may occur, particularly at high doses prescribed for prolonged periods. These may include adrenal suppression, growth retardation in children and adolescents, decrease in bone mineral density, cataract and glaucoma. In long-term treatment growth in children should be monitored regularly.

The susceptibility to infection can be increased. The ability to adapt to stress can be impaired.

4.9 Overdose

Symptoms of overdose

An acute overdose of Novolizer Budesonide 200 micrograms requiring counter-measures is virtually impossible. In the longer term, atrophy of the adrenal cortex can occur.

Table 1

Organ system	Very common (> 1/10)	Common (> 1/100, < 1/10)	Uncommon (> 1/1000, < 1/100)	Rare (> 1/10000, < 1/1000)	Very rare including isolated case < 1/10000
INFECTIONS AND INFESTATIONS		– Oropharyngeal candidiasis			
IMMUNE SYSTEM DISORDERS				– Hypersensitivity – Angioneurotic oedema	
ENDOCRINE DISORDERS					– Adrenal suppression
PSYCHIATRIC DISORDERS					– Restlessness – Nervousness – Depression – Abnormal behaviour
NERVOUS SYSTEM DISORDERS					– Psychomotor hyperactivity
EYE DISORDERS					– Cataract – Glaucoma
RESPIRATORY, THORACIC AND MEDIASTINAL DISORDERS		– Hoarseness – Cough		– Bronchospasm paradoxical	
GASTROINTESTINAL DISORDERS		– Oral mucosal irritation – Swallowing difficult			
SKIN AND SUBCUTANEOUS TISSUE DISORDERS				– Skin reactions – Urticaria – Rash – Dermatitis – Pruritus – Erythema – Bruising	
MUSCULOSKELETAL, CONNECTIVE TISSUE AND BONE DISORDERS				– Growth retardation	– Bone density decreased

The effects which are usual for glucocorticosteroids, e.g. increased susceptibility to infection, can occur. The ability to adapt to stress can be impaired.

Therapeutic management of overdose

In general, no special emergency treatment is required for acute overdosage. When inhalation treatment is continued at the prescribed dosage, the function of the hypothalamic pituitary adrenocortical axis should normalise within about 1 - 2 days.

In stress situations, it may be necessary to administer corticosteroids as a precaution (e.g. high doses of hydrocortisone).

Patients with adrenocortical atrophy are regarded as being steroid-dependent and must be adjusted to the adequate maintenance therapy of a systemic steroid until the condition has stabilised.

5. PHARMACOLOGICAL PROPERTIES

5.1 Pharmacodynamic properties

Topically applied glucocorticoid

ATC-Code: R03BA02

Budesonide is a synthetic glucocorticoid. After oral inhalation, it has a local anti-inflammatory effect on the bronchial mucosa.

Budesonide penetrates cellular membranes and binds to a cytoplasmic receptor protein. This complex enters the nucleus and induces there the biosynthesis of specific proteins, like macrocortin (lipocortin). The hormone-like effects occur after a certain latency period (30-60 min) and result in an inhibition of phospholipase A2. It is also possible that therapeutically effective doses of budesonide (like other anti-inflammatory glucocorticosteroids) suppress cytokine-induced COX-2 expression.

Clinically, the anti-inflammatory effect results, e.g. in improvement of the symptoms, such as dyspnoea. The hyperresponsiveness of the bronchial tract to exogenic challenges is reduced.

5.2 Pharmacokinetic properties

Peak plasma levels appear approximately 30 minutes after inhalation.

Systemic bioavailability after inhalation is 73% and the concentration in human plasma after inhalation of a single dose of 1600 micrograms is 0.63 nmol/L. Plasma protein binding is 85- 90% and the volume of distribution around 3 l/kg. The elimination half-life from plasma is approximately 2.8 h in adults and markedly lower in children (1.5 h).

The trigger threshold of the Novolizer which must be overcome for successful inhalation is to be found at inspiratory flows through the inhaler of at least 35 - 50 l/min. The respirable fraction measured in vitro in the clinically relevant range is approximately 25 – 50 %. In healthy subjects, approximately 20 – 30 % of the administered dose of budesonide passes into the lungs, based on the declared dose. The remainder deposits in mouth, nose and throat and a large part of it is swallowed. The swallowed portion is subject to a high first-pass effect in the liver. Budesonide is essentially metabolised in the liver via oxidation, catalysed mainlyby the enzyme CYP3A4.

The main metabolites are 6β-hydroxybudesonide and 16α-hydroxyprednisolone which show much less pharmacological activity. This limits systemic bioavailability and toxicity.

5.3 Preclinical safety data

Preclinical data revealed no special hazard for humans at therapeutic doses based on studies of chronic toxicity, genotoxicity and carcinogenicity.

Glucocorticosteroids, including budesonide, have produced teratogenic effects in animals, including cleft palate and skeletal abnormalities. Similar effects are considered unlikely to occur in humans at therapeutic doses.

6. PHARMACEUTICAL PARTICULARS

6.1 List of excipients

Lactose monohydrate

6.2 Incompatibilities

Not applicable

6.3 Shelf life

• Novolizer Budesonide 200 micrograms inhalation powder

Shelf life before opening the package

3 years

Shelf life after first opening the container

6 months

• Novolizer device

Shelf life before first use

3 years

In-use shelf life

1 year

To note: The functioning of the Novolizer has been demonstrated in tests for 2000 metered doses. Therefore a maximum of 10 cartridges containing 200 metered doses or 20 cartridges containing 100 metered doses can be used with this device (within a single year) prior to replacement.

Novolizer Budesonide 200 micrograms should not be used after the expiry date.

6.4 Special precautions for storage

Store in the original package.

When in use, Novolizer Budesonide 200 micrograms should be stored protected from moisture.

6.5 Nature and contents of container

Original sales packs:

1 cartridge 100 metered doses (polystyrene / polypropylene) packed in a polypropylene tube sealed by aluminium foil and 1 powder inhaler (mouthpiece in polycarbonate and device in acrylnitrilbutadienestyrol copolymer, polyoxymethylene).

1 cartridge 200 metered doses (polystyrene / polypropylene) packed in a polypropylene tube sealed by aluminium foil and 1 powder inhaler (mouthpiece in polycarbonate and device in acrylnitrilbutadienestyrol copolymer, polyoxymethylene).

2 cartridges 200 metered doses each (polystyrene / polypropylene) packed in a polypropylene tube sealed by aluminium foil and 1 powder inhaler (mouthpiece in polycarbonate and device in acrylnitrilbutadienestyrol copolymer, polyoxymethylene).

Refill packs:

1 cartridge 100 metered doses (polystyrene / polypropylene) packed in a polypropylene tube sealed by aluminium foil

1 cartridge 200 metered doses (polystyrene / polypropylene) packed in a polypropylene tube sealed by aluminium foil

2 cartridges 200 metered doses (polystyrene / polypropylene) packed in a polypropylene tube sealed by aluminium foil

Hospital pack:

1 cartridge 100 metered doses (polystyrene / polypropylene) packed in a polypropylene tube sealed by aluminium foil and 1 powder inhaler (mouthpiece in polycarbonate and device in acrylnitrilbutadienestyrol copolymer, polyoxymethylene).

Pack of 10

Samples:

1 cartridge 100 metered doses (polystyrene / polypropylene) packed in a polypropylene tube sealed by aluminium foil and 1 powder inhaler (mouthpiece in polycarbonate and device in acrylnitrilbutadienestyrol copolymer, polyoxymethylene).

1 cartridge 200 metered doses (polystyrene / polypropylene) packed in a polypropylene tube sealed by aluminium foil and 1 powder inhaler (mouthpiece in polycarbonate and device in acrylnitrilbutadienestyrol copolymer, polyoxymethylene).

"Not all pack sizes may be marketed"

6.6 Instructions for use and handling

Please see 4.2.

7. MARKETING AUTHORISATION HOLDER

VIATRIS Pharmaceuticals Ltd

Building 2000, Beach Drive

Cambridge Research Park

Waterbeach, Cambridge

CB5 9PD UK

8. MARKETING AUTHORISATION NUMBER(S)

PL 19166/0037

PA 1058/6/1

9. DATE OF FIRST AUTHORISATION/RENEWAL OF THE AUTHORISATION

9 March 2004

10. DATE OF REVISION OF THE TEXT

November 2004.

NovoMix 30 Penfill 100 U/ml, NovoMix 30 FlexPen 100 U/ml

(Novo Nordisk Limited)

1. NAME OF THE MEDICINAL PRODUCT

NovoMix 30 Penfill 100 U/ml, suspension for injection in cartridge.

NovoMix 30 FlexPen 100 U/ml, suspension for injection in a pre-filled pen.

2. QUALITATIVE AND QUANTITATIVE COMPOSITION

Soluble insulin aspart*/protamine-crystallised insulin aspart* .... 100 U/ml in the ratio of 30/70

* produced by recombinant DNA technology in *Saccharomyces cerevisiae*.

One unit of insulin aspart corresponds to 6 nmol, 0.035 mg salt-free anhydrous insulin aspart.

For excipients, see 6.1.

3. PHARMACEUTICAL FORM

Suspension for injection.

White suspension of 30% soluble insulin aspart and 70% insulin aspart protamine crystals.

4. CLINICAL PARTICULARS

4.1 Therapeutic indications

Treatment of patients with diabetes mellitus.

4.2 Posology and method of administration

Dosage of NovoMix 30 is individual and determined in accordance with the needs of the patient. NovoMix 30 has a faster onset of action than biphasic human insulin and should generally be given immediately before a meal. When necessary, NovoMix 30 can be given soon after a meal.

The individual insulin requirement is usually between 0.5 and 1.0 Units/kg/day and this may be fully or partially supplied with NovoMix 30. The daily insulin requirement may be higher in patients with insulin resistance (e.g. due to obesity), and lower in patients with residual endogenous insulin production.

NovoMix 30 is administered subcutaneously in the thigh or in the abdominal wall. If convenient, the gluteal or deltoid region may be used. Injection sites should be rotated within the same region. As with all insulins the duration of action will vary according to the dose, injection site, blood flow, temperature and level of physical activity. The influence of different injection sites on the absorption of NovoMix 30 has not been investigated.

In patients with type 2 diabetes, NovoMix 30 can be given in monotherapy or in combination with metformin, when the blood glucose is inadequately controlled with metformin alone. The recommended starting dose of NovoMix 30 in combination with metformin is 0.2 Units/kg/day and should be adjusted depending on individual requirement based on blood glucose response.

Renal or hepatic impairment may reduce the patient's insulin requirements.

No studies have been performed with NovoMix 30 in children and adolescents under the age of 18 years.

NovoMix 30 should never be administered intravenously.

4.3 Contraindications

Hypoglycaemia.

Hypersensitivity to insulin aspart or any of the excipients.

4.4 Special warnings and special precautions for use

The use of dosages which are inadequate or discontinuation of treatment, especially in insulin-dependent diabetics, may lead to hyperglycaemia and diabetic ketoacidosis; conditions which are potentially lethal.

Patients whose blood glucose control is greatly improved, e.g. by intensified insulin therapy, may experience a change in their usual warning symptoms of hypoglycaemia, and should be advised accordingly.

NovoMix 30 should be administered in immediate relation to a meal. The fast onset of action should therefore be considered in patients with concomitant diseases or medication where a delayed absorption of food might be expected.

Concomitant illness, especially infections, usually increases the patient's insulin requirements.

When patients are transferred between different types of insulin products the early warning symptoms of hypoglycaemia may change or become less pronounced than those experienced with their previous insulin.

Transferring a patient to a new type or brand of insulin should be done under strict medical supervision. Changes in strength, brand, type, species (animal, human, human insulin analogue), and/or method of manufacture may result in the need for a change in dosage. Patients taking NovoMix 30 may need a change in dosage from that used with their usual insulins. If an adjustment is needed, it may be done with the first dose or during the first few weeks or months.

Omission of a meal or unplanned, strenuous physical exercise may lead to hypoglycaemia (see Sections 4.8 and 4.9). Compared with biphasic human insulin, NovoMix 30 may have a stronger hypoglycaemic effect up to 6 hours after injection. This may have to be compensated for in the individual patient, through adjustment of insulin dose and/or food intake.

Adjustment of dosage may also be necessary if patients undertake increased physical activity or change their usual diet. Exercise taken immediately after a meal may increase the risk of hypoglycaemia.

Insulin suspensions are not to be used in insulin infusion pumps.

4.5 Interaction with other medicinal products and other forms of Interaction

A number of medicinal products are known to interact with glucose metabolism.

The following substances may reduce the patient's insulin requirements:

Oral hypoglycaemic agents (OHAs), octreotide, monoamine oxidase inhibitors (MAOIs), non-selective beta-adrenergic blocking agents, angiotensin converting enzyme (ACE) inhibitors, salicylates, alcohol, anabolic steroids and sulphonamides.

The following substances may increase the patient's insulin requirements:

Oral contraceptives, thiazides, glucocorticoids, thyroid hormones, sympathomimetics and danazol.

Beta-blocking agents may mask the symptoms of hypoglycaemia.

Alcohol may intensify and prolong the hypoglycaemic effect of insulin.

4.6 Pregnancy and lactation

There is limited clinical experience with insulin aspart in pregnancy.

Animal reproduction studies have not revealed any differences between insulin aspart and human insulin regarding embryotoxicity or teratogenicity.

Intensified blood glucose control and monitoring of pregnant women with diabetes are recommended throughout pregnancy and when contemplating pregnancy. Insulin requirements usually fall in the first trimester and increase subsequently during the second and third trimesters. After delivery, insulin requirements return rapidly to pre-pregnancy levels.

There are no restrictions on treatment with NovoMix 30 during lactation. Insulin treatment of the nursing mother presents no risk to the baby. However, the NovoMix 30 dosage may need to be adjusted.

4.7 Effects on ability to drive and use machines

The patient's ability to concentrate and react may be impaired as a result of hypoglycaemia. This may constitute a risk in situations where these abilities are of special importance (e.g. driving a car or operating machinery).

Patients should be advised to take precautions in order to avoid hypoglycaemia whilst driving. This is particularly important in those who have reduced or absent awareness of the warning signs of hypoglycaemia or have frequent episodes of hypoglycaemia. The advisability of driving should be considered in these circumstances.

4.8 Undesirable effects

Adverse drug reactions observed in patients using NovoMix 30 are mainly dose-dependent and due to the pharmacological effect of insulin. As for other insulin products, hypoglycaemia, in general is the most frequently occurring undesirable effect. It may occur if the insulin dose is too high in relation to the insulin requirement. Severe hypoglycaemia may lead to unconsciousness and/or convulsions and may result in temporary or permanent impairment of brain function or even death.

In clinical trials and during marketed use the frequency varies with patient population and dose regimen therefore no specific frequency can be presented.

During clinical trials the overall rates of hypoglycaemia did not differ between patients treated with insulin aspart compared to human insulin.

Frequencies of adverse drug reactions from clinical trials, which by an overall judgement are considered related to insulin aspart are listed below. The frequencies are defined as: Uncommon (>1/1,000, <1/100) and rare (>1/10,000, <1/1,000). Isolated spontaneous cases are presented as very rare defined as (<1/10,000).

Immune system disorders

Uncommon – Urticaria, rash, eruptions

Very rare – Anaphylactic reactions

Symptoms of generalised hypersensitivity may include generalised skin rash, itching, sweating, gastrointestinal upset, angioneurotic oedema, difficulties in breathing, palpitation and reduction in blood pressure. Generalised hypersensitivity reactions are potentially life threatening.

Nervous system disorders

Rare – peripheral neuropathy

Fast improvement in blood glucose control may be associated with a condition termed acute painful neuropathy, which is usually reversible.

Eye disorders

Uncommon – Refraction disorder

Refraction anomalies may occur upon initiation of insulin therapy. These symptoms are usually of transitory nature.

Uncommon – Diabetic retinopathy

Long-term improved glycaemic control decreases the risk of progression of diabetic retinopathy. However, intensification of insulin therapy with abrupt improvement in glycaemic control may be associated with worsening of diabetic retinopathy.

Skin and subcutaneous tissue disorders

Uncommon – Lipodystrophy

Lipodystrophy may occur at the injection site as a consequence of failure to rotate injections within an area.

Uncommon – Local hypersensitivity

Local hypersensitivity reactions (redness, swelling and itching at the injection site) may occur during treatment with insulin. These reactions are usually transitory and normally they disappear during continued treatment.

General disorders and administration site conditions

Uncommon – Oedema

Oedema may occur upon initiation of insulin therapy. These symptoms are usually of transitory nature.

4.9 Overdose

A specific overdose for insulin cannot be defined, however, hypoglycaemia may develop over sequential stages if too high doses relative to the patient's requirements are administered:

- Mild hypoglycaemic episodes can be treated by oral administration of glucose or sugary products. It is therefore recommended that the diabetic patient constantly carries some sugar-containing products.
- Severe hypoglycaemic episodes, where the patient has become unconscious, can be treated by glucagon (0.5 to 1 mg) given intramuscularly or subcutaneously by a trained person, or glucose given intravenously by a medical professional. Glucose must also be given intravenously if the patient does not respond to glucagon within 10 to 15 minutes. Upon regaining consciousness administration of oral carbohydrate is recommended for the patient in order to prevent relapse.

Figure 1 Activity profile of NovoMix 30 (—) and biphasic human insulin 30 (—) in healthy subjects

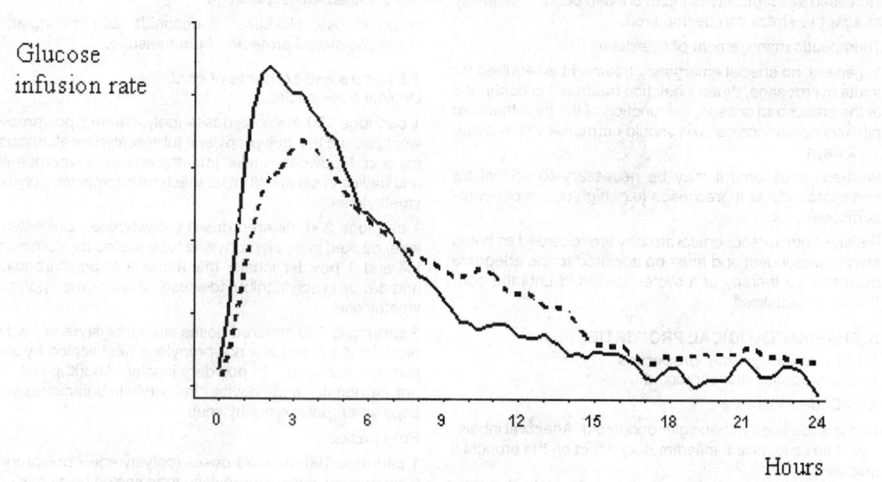

5. PHARMACOLOGICAL PROPERTIES

5.1 Pharmacodynamic properties

Pharmacotherapeutic group: Antidiabetic agent. ATC code A10A D05. NovoMix 30 is a biphasic suspension of insulin aspart (rapid-acting human insulin analogue) and insulin aspart protamine (intermediate-acting human insulin analogue).

The blood glucose lowering effect of insulin occurs when the molecules facilitate the uptake of glucose by binding to insulin receptors on muscle and fat cells - and simultaneously inhibit the output of glucose from the liver.

NovoMix 30 is a biphasic insulin, which contains 30% soluble insulin aspart. This has a rapid onset of action, thus allowing it to be given closer to a meal (within zero to 10 minutes of the meal) when compared to soluble human insulin. The crystalline phase (70%) consists of insulin aspart protamine, which has an activity profile that is similar to that of human NPH insulin (Figure 1).

When NovoMix 30 is injected subcutaneously, the onset of action will occur within 10 to 20 minutes of injection. The maximum effect is exerted between 1 and 4 hours after injection. The duration of action is up to 24 hours.

Figure 1: Activity profile of NovoMix 30 (—) and biphasic human insulin 30 (—) in healthy subjects.

(see Figure 1 above)

In a 3 month trial in patients with Type 1 and Type 2 diabetes NovoMix 30 showed equal control of glycosylated haemoglobin compared to treatment with biphasic human insulin 30. Insulin aspart is equipotent to human insulin on a molar basis.

In one study, 341 patients with type II diabetes were randomised to treatment with NovoMix 30 either alone or in combination with metformin, or to metformin together with sulfonylurea. The primary efficacy variable – HbA_{1c} after 16 weeks of treatment – did not differ between patients with NovoMix 30 combined with metformin and patients with metformin plus sulfonylurea. In this trial 57% of the patients had baseline HbA_{1c} above 9%; in these patients treatment with NovoMix 30 in combination with metformin resulted in significantly lower HbA_{1c} than metformin in combination with sulfonylurea.

5.2 Pharmacokinetic properties

In insulin aspart substitution of amino acid proline with aspartic acid at position B28 reduces the tendency to form hexamers in the soluble fraction of NovoMix 30, as compared with soluble human insulin. The insulin aspart in the soluble phase of NovoMix 30 comprises 30% of the total insulin: this is absorbed more rapidly from the subcutaneous layer than the soluble insulin component of biphasic human insulin. The remaining 70% is in crystalline form as insulin aspart protamine; this has a prolonged absorption profile similar to human NPH insulin.

The maximum serum insulin concentration is, on average, 50% higher with NovoMix 30 than with biphasic human insulin 30. The time to maximum concentration is, on average, half of that for biphasic human insulin 30. In healthy volunteers a mean maximum serum concentration of 140 ± 32 pmol/l was reached about 60 minutes after a subcutaneous dose of 0.20 U/kg body weight. The mean half life ($t_{1/2}$) of NovoMix 30, reflecting the absorption rate of the protamine bound fraction, was about 8-9 hours. Serum insulin levels returned to baseline 15-18 hours after a subcutaneous dose. In Type 2 diabetic patients, the maximum concentration was reached about 95 minutes after dosing, and concentrations well above zero for not less than 14 hours post-dosing were measured.

The pharmacokinetics of NovoMix 30 have not been investigated in the elderly, children or patients with impaired renal or liver function.

5.3 Preclinical safety data

In *in vitro* tests, including binding to insulin and IGF-1 receptor sites and effects on cell growth, insulin aspart behaved in a manner that closely resembled human insulin. Studies also demonstrate that the dissociation of binding to the insulin receptor of insulin aspart is equivalent to human insulin. Acute, one month and twelve months toxicity studies with insulin aspart produced no toxicity findings of clinical relevance.

6. PHARMACEUTICAL PARTICULARS

6.1 List of excipients

Mannitol

Phenol

Metacresol

Zinc (as chloride)

Sodium chloride

Disodium phosphate dihydrate

Protamine sulphate

Sodium hydroxide

Hydrochloric acid

Water for injections

6.2 Incompatibilities

NovoMix 30 should not be added to infusion fluids.

6.3 Shelf life

2 years

The in-use shelf life is 4 weeks (not above 30°C).

6.4 Special precautions for storage

Store at 2°C – 8°C. Do not freeze.

NovoMix 30 Penfill cartridges and NovoMix 30 FlexPen in use or carried as a spare: Do not refrigerate. Do not store above 30°C. in order to protect from light keep the container (Penfill cartridge) in the outer carton or keep the cap on when NovoMix 30 FlexPen is not in use.

6.5 Nature and contents of container

NovoMix 30 Penfill:

A glass (Type 1) cartridge which is closed with a rubber piston at one end and a latex-free rubber closure at the other, and containing 3ml of suspension. The cartridge contains a glass ball to facilitate resuspension.

Cartons of 5 or 10 cartridges.

NovoMix 30 FlexPen:

A glass (Type 1) cartridge which is closed with a rubber piston at one end and a latex-free rubber closure at the other, and containing 3ml suspension in a multidose disposable pre-filled pen with a pen injector. The cartridge contains a glass ball to facilitate resuspension.

Cartons of 5 or 10 pre-filled pens.

Not all pack sizes may be marketed.

6.6 Instructions for use and handling

The carton contains a package leaflet with instructions for use and handling. The necessity of resuspending the NovoMix 30 suspension immediately before use is to be stressed to the patient. The resuspended liquid must appear uniformly white and cloudy.

For use by one person only. NovoMix 30 Penfill and FlexPen must not be refilled.

NovoMix 30 Penfill is designed to be used with the Novo Nordisk insulin delivery system and NovoFine needles. NovoFine **S** needles are designed to be used with FlexPen.

7. MARKETING AUTHORISATION HOLDER
Novo Nordisk A/S

Novo Allé

DK-2880 Bagsværd

Denmark

8. MARKETING AUTHORISATION NUMBER(S)
NovoMix 30 Penfill EU/1/00/142/004-005

NovoMix 30 FlexPen EU/1/00/142/009-010

9. DATE OF FIRST AUTHORISATION/RENEWAL OF THE AUTHORISATION
1 August 2000.

10. DATE OF REVISION OF THE TEXT
7 July 2004

LEGAL CATEGORY
POM (Prescription Only Medicine)

NovoNorm 0.5 mg, 1 mg and 2 mg tablets

(Novo Nordisk Limited)

1. NAME OF THE MEDICINAL PRODUCT
NovoNorm 0.5 mg tablets

NovoNorm 1 mg tablets

NovoNorm 2 mg tablets

2. QUALITATIVE AND QUANTITATIVE COMPOSITION
Each tablet contains:

Repaglinide 0.5 mg or Repaglinide 1 mg or Repaglinide 2 mg, respectively.

For excipients, see 6.1

3. PHARMACEUTICAL FORM
Tablet

Repaglinide tablets are white (0.5 mg), yellow (1 mg), or peach-coloured (2 mg), round and convex and engraved with Novo Nordisk logo (Apis bull).

4. CLINICAL PARTICULARS
4.1 Therapeutic indications
Repaglinide is indicated in patients with Type 2 diabetes (Non Insulin-Dependent Diabetes Mellitus (NIDDM)) whose hyperglycaemia can no longer be controlled satisfactorily by diet, weight reduction and exercise. Repaglinide is also indicated in combination with metformin in Type 2 diabetes patients who are not satisfactorily controlled on metformin alone.

Treatment should be initiated as an adjunct to diet and exercise to lower the blood glucose in relation to meals.

4.2 Posology and method of administration
Repaglinide is given preprandially and is titrated individually to optimise the glycaemic control. In addition to the usual self-monitoring by the patient of blood and/or urinary glucose, the patient's blood glucose must be monitored periodically by the physician to determine the minimum effective dose for the patient. Glycosylated haemoglobin levels are also of value in monitoring the patient's response to therapy. Periodic monitoring is necessary to detect inadequate lowering of blood glucose at the recommended maximum dose level (i.e. primary failure) and to detect loss of adequate blood-glucose-lowering response after an initial period of effectiveness (i.e. secondary failure).

Short-term administration of repaglinide may be sufficient during periods of transient loss of control in Type 2 diabetic patients usually controlled well on diet.

Repaglinide should be taken before main meals (i.e. preprandially).

Initial dose
The dosage should be determined by the physician, according to the patient's requirements.

The recommended starting dose is 0.5 mg. One to two weeks should elapse between titration steps (as determined by blood glucose response).

If patients are transferred from another oral hypoglycaemic agent the recommended starting dose is 1 mg.

Maintenance
The recommended maximum single dose is 4 mg taken with main meals.

The total maximum daily dose should not exceed 16 mg.

Specific patient groups
Repaglinide is primarily excreted via the bile and excretion is therefore not affected by renal disorders.

Only 8% of one dose of repaglinide is excreted through the kidneys and total plasma clearance of the product is decreased in patients with renal impairment. As insulin sensitivity is increased in diabetic patients with renal impairment, caution is advised when titrating these patients.

No clinical studies have been conducted in patients >75 years of age or in patients with hepatic insufficiency. Please be referred to section 4.4.

In debilitated or malnourished patients the initial and maintenance dosage should be conservative and careful dose titration is required to avoid hypoglycaemic reactions.

Patients receiving other oral hypoglycaemic agents (OHAs)
Patients can be transferred directly from other oral hypoglycaemic agents to repaglinide. However, no exact dosage relationship exists between repaglinide and the other oral hypoglycaemic agents. The recommended maximum starting dose of patients transferred to repaglinide is 1 mg given before main meals.

Repaglinide can be given in combination with metformin, when the blood glucose is insufficiently controlled with metformin alone. In this case, the dosage of metformin should be maintained and repaglinide administered concomitantly. The starting dose of repaglinide is 0.5 mg, taken before main meals; titration is according to blood glucose response as for monotherapy.

4.3 Contraindications
- Hypersensitivity to repaglinide or to any of the excipients in NovoNorm
- Type 1 diabetes (Insulin-Dependent Diabetes Mellitus: IDDM), C-peptide negative
- Diabetic ketoacidosis, with or without coma
- Pregnancy and lactation (Section 4.6)
- Children <12 years of age
- Severe hepatic function disorder
- Concomitant use of gemfibrozil (see section 4.5 Interaction with other medicinal products and other forms of interaction)

4.4 Special warnings and special precautions for use
General
Repaglinide should only be prescribed if poor blood glucose control and symptoms of diabetes persist despite adequate attempts at dieting, exercise and weight reduction.

Repaglinide like other insulin secretagogues, is capable of producing hypoglycaemia.

The blood glucose lowering effect of oral hypoglycaemic agents decreases in many patients over time. This may be due to progression of the severity of the diabetes or to diminished responsiveness to the product. This phenomenon is known as secondary failure, to distinguish it from primary failure, where the drug is ineffective in an individual patient when first given. Adjustment of dose and adherence to diet and exercise should be assessed before classifying a patient as a secondary failure.

Repaglinide acts through a distinct binding site with a short action on the β-cells. Use of repaglinide in case of secondary failure to insulin secretagogues has not been investigated in clinical trials.

Trials investigating the combination with other insulin secretagogues and acarbose have not been performed.

No trials of combination therapy with insulin or thiazolidinediones have been performed.

Combination treatment with metformin is associated with an increased risk of hypoglycaemia.

When a patient stabilised on any oral hypoglycaemic agent is exposed to stress such as fever, trauma, infection or surgery, a loss of glycaemic control may occur. At such times, it may be necessary to discontinue repaglinide and treat with insulin on a temporary basis.

Concomitant use
Concomitant use of trimethoprim with repaglinide should be avoided as the safety of this combination has not been established with doses higher than 0.25 mg for repaglinide and 320 mg for trimethoprim (see section 4.5). If concomitant use is necessary, careful monitoring of blood glucose and close clinical monitoring should be performed.

NovoNorm should be used with caution during concomitant administration of CYP2C8 inducers (e.g. rifampicin and St John's wort). Upon concomitant use of rifampicin and repaglinide, the repaglinide dose should be adjusted based on carefully monitored blood glucose concentrations at both initiation of rifampicin treatment (acute inhibition), following dosing (mixed inhibition and induction), withdrawal (induction alone) and up to approximately two weeks after withdrawal of rifampicin where the inductive effect of rifampicin is no longer present (see section 4.5).

Specific patient groups
No clinical studies have been conducted in patients with impaired hepatic function. No clinical studies have been performed in children and adolescents <18 years of age or in patients >75 years of age. Therefore, treatment is not recommended in these patient groups.

4.5 Interaction with other medicinal products and other forms of Interaction
A number of drugs are known to influence glucose metabolism, possible interactions should therefore be taken into account by the physician:

In vitro data indicate that repaglinide is metabolised predominantly by CYP2C8, but also by CYP3A4. Clinical data in healthy volunteers support CYP2C8 as being the most important enzyme involved in repaglinide metabolism with CYP3A4 playing a minor role, but the relative contribution of CYP3A4 can be increased if CYP2C8 is inhibited. Consequently metabolism, and by that clearance of repaglinide, may be altered by drugs which influence these cytochrome P-450 enzymes via inhibition or induction. Special care should be taken when both inhibitors of CYP2C8 and 3A4 are co-administered simultaneously with repaglinide.

The following substances may enhance and/or prolong the hypoglycaemic effect of repaglinide: Gemfibrozil, clarithromycin, itraconazole, ketoconazole, trimethoprim, other antidiabetic agents, monoamine oxidase inhibitors (MAOI), non selective beta blocking agents, angiotensin converting enzyme (ACE)-inhibitors, salicylates, NSAIDs, octreotide, alcohol, and anabolic steroids.

Co-administration of gemfibrozil, (600 mg twice daily), an inhibitor of CYP2C8, and repaglinide (a single dose of 0.25 mg) increased the repaglinide AUC 8.1-fold and C_{max} 2.4-fold in healthy volunteers. Half-life was prolonged from 1.3 hr to 3.7 hr, resulting in possibly enhanced and prolonged blood glucose-lowering effect of repaglinide, and plasma repaglinide concentration at 7 hr was increased 28.6-fold by gemfibrozil. The concomitant use of gemfibrozil and repaglinide is contraindicated (see section 4.3 Contraindications).

Co-administration of trimethoprim (160 mg twice daily), a moderate CYP2C8 inhibitor, and repaglinide (a single dose of 0.25 mg) increased the repaglinide AUC, C_{max} and $t_{½}$ (1.6-fold, 1.4-fold and 1.2-fold respectively) with no statistically significant effects on the blood glucose levels. This lack of pharmacodynamic effect was observed with a subtherapeutic dose of repaglinide. Since the safety profile of this combination has not been established with dosages higher than 0.25 mg for repaglinide and 320 mg for trimethoprim, the concomitant use of trimethoprim with repaglinide should be avoided. If concomitant use is necessary, careful monitoring of blood glucose and close clinical monitoring should be performed (see section 4.4).

Rifampicin, a potent inducer of CYP3A4, but also CYP2C8, acts both as an inducer and inhibitor of the metabolism of repaglinide. Seven days pre-treatment with rifampicin (600 mg) followed by co-administration of repaglinide (a single dose of 4 mg) at day seven resulted in a 50% lower AUC (effect of combined induction and inhibition). When repaglinide was given 24 hours after the last rifampicin dose, an 80% reduction of the repaglinide AUC was observed (effect of induction alone). Concomitant use of rifampicin and repaglinide might therefore induce a need for repaglinide dose adjustment which should be based on carefully monitored glucose concentrations at both initiation of rifampicin treatment (acute inhibition), following dosing (mixed inhibition and induction), withdrawal (induction alone) and up to approximately two weeks after withdrawal of rifampicin where the inductive effect of rifampicin is no longer present. It cannot be excluded that other inducers, e.g. phenytoin, carbamazepine, phenobarbital, St John's wort, may have a similar effect.

The effect of ketoconazole, a prototype of potent and competitive inhibitors of CYP3A4, on the pharmacokinetics of repaglinide has been studied in healthy subjects. Co-administration of 200 mg ketoconazole increased the repaglinide (AUC and C_{max}) by 1.2-fold with profiles of blood glucose concentrations altered by les than 8% when administered concomitantly (a single dose of 4 mg repaglinide). Co-administration of 100mg itraconazole, an inhibitor of CYP3A4, has also been studied in healthy volunteers, and increased the AUC by 1.4-fold. No significant effect on the glucose level in healthy volunteers was observed. In an interaction study in healthy volunteers, co-administration of 250 mg clarithromycin, a potent mechanism-based inhibitor of CYP3A4, slightly increased the repaglinide (AUC) by 1.4-fold and C_{max} by 1.7-fold and increased the mean incremental AUC of serum insulin by 1.5-fold and the maximum concentration by 1.6-fold. The exact mechanism of this interaction is not clear.

β-blocking agents may mask the symptoms of hypoglycaemia.

Co-administration of cimetidine, nifedipine, oestrogen, or simvastatin with repaglinide, all CYP3A4 substrates, did not significantly alter the pharmacokinetic parameters of repaglinide.

Repaglinide had no clinically relevant effect on the pharmacokinetic properties of digoxin, theophylline or warfarin at steady state, when administered to healthy volunteers. Dosage adjustment of these compounds when co-administered with repaglinide is therefore not necessary.

The following substances may reduce the hypoglycaemic effect of repaglinide:

Oral contraceptives, rifampicin, barbiturates, carbamazepine, thiazides, corticosteroids, danazol, thyroid hormones and sympathomimetics.

When these medications are administered to or withdrawn from a patient receiving repaglinide, the patient should be observed closely for changes in glycaemic control.

When repaglinide is used together with other drugs that are mainly secreted by the bile, like repaglinide, any potential interaction should be considered.

4.6 Pregnancy and lactation

There are no studies of repaglinide in pregnant or lactating women. Therefore the safety of repaglinide in pregnant women cannot be assessed. Up to now repaglinide showed not to be teratogenic in animals studies. Embryotoxicity, abnormal limb development in foetuses and new born pups, was observed in rats exposed to high doses in the last stage of pregnancy and during the lactation period. Repaglinide is detected in the milk of experimental animals. For that reason repaglinide should be avoided during pregnancy and should not be used in lactating women.

4.7 Effects on ability to drive and use machines

Patients should be advised to take precautions to avoid hypoglycaemia whilst driving. This is particularly important in those who have reduced or absent awareness of the warning signs of hypoglycaemia or have frequent episodes of hypoglycaemia. The advisability of driving should be considered in these circumstances

4.8 Undesirable effects

Based on the experience with repaglinide and with other hypoglycaemic agents the following side effects have been seen: Frequencies are defined as: rare (>1/10,000, < 1/1000) and very rare (<1/10,000)

Metabolism and nutrition disorders

Rare: Hypoglycaemia

As with other hypoglycaemic agents, hypoglycaemic reactions have been observed after administration of repaglinide. These reactions are mostly mild and easily handled through intake of carbohydrates. If severe, requiring third party assistance, infusion of glucose may be necessary. The occurrence of such reactions depends, as for every diabetes therapy, on individual factors, such as dietary habits, dosage, exercise and stress (see further under 4.4 "Special warnings and special precautions for use"). During post marketing experience, cases of hypoglycaemia have been reported in patients treated in combination with metformin or thiazolidinedione.

Gastro-intestinal disorders

Rare: Abdominal pain and nausea

Very rare: Diarrhoea, vomiting and constipation

Gastro-intestinal complaints such as abdominal pain, diarrhoea, nausea, vomiting and constipation have been reported in clinical trials. The rate and severity of these symptoms did not differ from that seen with other oral insulin secretagogues.

Skin and subcutaneous tissue disorders

Rare: Allergy

Hypersensitivity reactions of the skin may occur as itching, rashes and urticaria. There is no reason to suspect cross-allergenicity with sulphonylurea drugs due to the difference of the chemical structure.

Generalised hypersensitivity reactions, or immunological reactions such as vasculitis, may occur very rarely.

Eye disorders

Very rare: Visual disturbances

Changes in blood glucose levels have been known to result in transient visual disturbances, especially at the commencement of treatment. Such disturbances have only been reported in very few cases after initiation of repaglinide treatment. No such cases have led to discontinuation of repaglinide treatment in clinical trials.

Liver disorders

Very rare: Increased liver enzymes

Isolated cases of increase in liver enzymes have been reported during treatment with repaglinide. Most cases were mild and transient, and very few patients discontinued treatment due to increase in liver enzymes. In very rare cases, severe hepatic dysfunction has been reported.

4.9 Overdose

Repaglinide has been given with weekly escalating doses from 4 - 20 mg four times daily in a 6 week period. No safety concerns were raised. As hypoglycaemia in this study was avoided through increased calorie intake, a relative overdose may result in an exaggerated glucose lowering effect with development of hypoglycaemic symptoms (dizziness, sweating, tremor, headache etc.). Should these symptoms occur, adequate action should be taken to correct the low blood glucose (oral carbohydrates). More severe hypoglycaemia with seizure, loss of consciousness or coma should be treated with i.v. glucose.

5. PHARMACOLOGICAL PROPERTIES

5.1 Pharmacodynamic properties

Pharmaco-therapeutic group: Carbamoylmethyl benzoic acid derivative

(ATC code: A 10 B X02)

Repaglinide is a novel short-acting oral secretagogue. Repaglinide lowers the blood glucose levels acutely by stimulating the release of insulin from the pancreas, an effect dependent upon functioning β-cells in the pancreatic islets.

Repaglinide closes ATP-dependent potassium channels in the β-cell membrane via a target protein different from other secretagogues. This depolarises the β-cell and leads to an opening of the calcium channels. The resulting increased calcium influx induces insulin secretion from the β-cell.

In Type 2 diabetic patients, the insulinotropic response to a meal occurred within 30 minutes after an oral dose of repaglinide. This resulted in a blood glucose-lowering effect throughout the meal period. The elevated insulin levels did not persist beyond the time of the meal challenge. Plasma repaglinide levels decreased rapidly, and low drug concentrations were seen in the plasma of Type 2 diabetic patients 4 hours post-administration.

A dose-dependent decrease in blood glucose was demonstrated in Type 2 diabetic patients when administered in doses from 0.5 to 4 mg repaglinide.

Clinical study results have shown that repaglinide is optimally dosed in relation to main meals (preprandial dosing).

Doses are usually taken within 15 minutes of the meal, but time may vary from immediately preceding the meal to as long as 30 minutes before the meal.

5.2 Pharmacokinetic properties

Repaglinide is rapidly absorbed from the gastrointestinal tract, which leads to a rapid increase in the plasma concentration of the drug. The peak plasma level occurs within one hour post administration. After reaching a maximum, the plasma level decreases rapidly, and repaglinide is eliminated within 4 - 6 hours. The plasma elimination half-life is approximately one hour.

Repaglinide pharmacokinetics are characterised by a mean absolute bioavailability of 63% (CV 11%), low volume of distribution, 30 L (consistent with distribution into intracellular fluid), and rapid elimination from the blood.

A high interindividual variability (60%) in repaglinide plasma concentrations has been detected in the clinical trials. Intraindividual variability is low to moderate (35%) and as repaglinide should be titrated against the clinical response, efficacy is not affected by interindividual variability.

Repaglinide exposure is increased in patients with hepatic insufficiency and in the elderly Type 2 diabetic patients. The AUC (SD) after 2 mg single dose exposure (4 mg in patients with hepatic insufficiency) was 31.4 ng/ml × hr (28.3) in healthy volunteers, 304.9 ng/ml × hr (228.0) in patients with hepatic insufficiency, and 117.9 ng/ml × hr (83.8) in the elderly Type 2 diabetic patients.

After a 5-day treatment of repaglinide (2mg × 3/day) in patients with a severe impaired renal function (creatinine clearance: 20 - 39 ml/min), the results showed a significant 2-fold increase of the exposure (AUC) and half-life ($t_{½}$) as compared to subjects with normal renal function.

Repaglinide is highly bound to plasma proteins in humans (greater than 98%).

No clinically relevant differences were seen in the pharmacokinetics of repaglinide, when repaglinide was administered 0, 15 or 30 minutes before a meal or in fasting state.

Repaglinide is almost completely metabolised, and no metabolites with clinically relevant hypoglycaemic effect have been identified. Repaglinide and its metabolites are excreted primarily via the bile. A small fraction (less than 8%) of the administered dose appears in the urine, primarily as metabolites. Less than 1% of the parent drug is recovered in faeces.

5.3 Preclinical safety data

Preclinical data revealed no special hazard for humans based on conventional studies of safety pharmacology, repeated dose toxicity, genotoxicity and carcinogenic potential.

6. PHARMACEUTICAL PARTICULARS

6.1 List of excipients

Microcrystalline cellulose (E460)

Calcium hydrogen phosphate, anhydrous

Maize starch

Amberlite (Polacrilin potassium)

Povidone (Polyvidone)

Glycerol 85%

Magnesium stearate

Meglumine

Poloxamer

Iron oxide, yellow (1 mg tablets only) (E172)

Iron oxide, red (2 mg tablets only) (E172)

6.2 Incompatibilities

Not applicable.

6.3 Shelf life

5 years

6.4 Special precautions for storage

Store in the original package.

6.5 Nature and contents of container

The blister pack (aluminium/aluminium) contains 30, 90, 120 or 360 tablets respectively.

Not all pack sizes may be marketed.

6.6 Instructions for use and handling

No special requirements.

7. MARKETING AUTHORISATION HOLDER

Novo Nordisk A/S

Novo Alle

DK-2880 Bagsværd

Denmark

8. MARKETING AUTHORISATION NUMBER(S)

EU/1/98/076/001-002, EU/1/98/076/004-007

9. DATE OF FIRST AUTHORISATION/RENEWAL OF THE AUTHORISATION

1 August 2003

10. DATE OF REVISION OF THE TEXT

2 February 2005

LEGAL CATEGORY

Prescription only medicine (POM).

NovoRapid 100 U/ml, NovoRapid Penfill 100 U/ml, NovoRapid FlexPen 100 U/ml

(Novo Nordisk Limited)

1. NAME OF THE MEDICINAL PRODUCT

NovoRapid 100 U/ml, solution for injection in a vial.

NovoRapid Penfill 100 U/ml, solution for injection in a cartridge.

NovoRapid FlexPen 100 U/ml, solution for injection in a pre-filled pen.

2. QUALITATIVE AND QUANTITATIVE COMPOSITION

Insulin aspart* 100 U/ml

*produced by recombinant DNA technology in *Saccharomyces cerevisiae*.

One unit of insulin aspart corresponds to 6 nmol, 0.035 mg salt-free anhydrous insulin aspart.

For excipients, see section 6.1.

3. PHARMACEUTICAL FORM

Solution for injection.

Clear, colourless, aqueous, solution.

4. CLINICAL PARTICULARS

4.1 Therapeutic indications

Treatment of patients with diabetes mellitus.

4.2 Posology and method of administration

NovoRapid has a faster onset and a shorter duration of action than soluble human insulin. Due to the faster onset of action, NovoRapid should generally be given immediately before the meal. When necessary NovoRapid can be given soon after the meal.

Dosage of NovoRapid is individual and determined on the basis of the physician's advice in accordance with the needs of the patient. It should normally be used in combination with intermediate-acting or long-acting insulin given at least once a day.

The individual insulin requirement is usually between 0.5 and 1.0 U/kg/day. In a meal-related treatment 50–70% of this requirement may be provided by NovoRapid and the remainder by intermediate-acting or long-acting insulin.

NovoRapid is administered subcutaneously by injection in the abdominal wall, the thigh, the deltoid region or the gluteal region. Injection sites should be rotated within the same region. When injected subcutaneously into the abdominal wall, the onset of action will occur within 10–20 minutes of injection. The maximum effect is exerted between 1 and 3 hours after the injection. The duration of action is 3 to 5 hours. As with all insulins, the duration of action will vary according to the dose, injection site, blood flow, temperature and level of physical activity. As with all insulins, subcutaneous injection in the abdominal wall ensures a faster absorption than other injection sites. However, the faster onset of action compared to soluble human insulin is maintained regardless of injection site.

If necessary, NovoRapid may also be administered intravenously (see section 6.6) which should be carried out by health care professionals.

NovoRapid may be used for Continuous Subcutaneous Insulin Infusion (CSII) in pump systems suitable for insulin infusion. CSII should be administered in the abdominal wall. Infusion sites should be rotated.

When used with an insulin infusion pump NovoRapid should not be mixed with any other insulin.

Patients using CSII should be comprehensively instructed in the use of the pump system, and use the correct reservoir and tubing for the pump (see section 6.6).

The infusion set (tubing and cannula) should be changed in accordance with the instructions in the product information supplied with the infusion set.

Patients administering NovoRapid by CSII must have alternative insulin available in case of pump system failure.

Renal or hepatic impairment may reduce the patient's insulin requirements.

No studies have been performed in children under the age of 2 years.

NovoRapid can be used in children in preference to soluble insulin human when a rapid onset of action might be beneficial. For example in the timing of injections in relation to meals.

FlexPen are prefilled pens designed to be used with NovoFine short cap needles. The needle box is marked with an **S.** FlexPen delivers 1-60 units in increments of 1 unit.

Detailed instruction accompanying the device must be followed.

4.3 Contraindications

- Hypoglycaemia
- Hypersensitivity to insulin aspart or to any of the excipients

4.4 Special warnings and special precautions for use

The use of dosages which are inadequate or discontinuation of treatment, especially in insulin-dependent diabetics, may lead to hyperglycaemia and diabetic ketoacidosis; conditions which are potentially lethal.

Patients whose blood glucose control is greatly improved, e.g. by intensified insulin therapy, may experience a change in their usual warning symptoms of hypoglycaemia, and should be advised accordingly.

A consequence of the pharmacodynamics of rapid-acting insulin analogues is that if hypoglycaemia occurs, it may occur earlier after an injection when compared with soluble human insulin.

NovoRapid should be administered in immediate relation to a meal. The rapid onset of action should therefore be considered in patients with concomitant diseases or medication where a delayed absorption of food might be expected.

Concomitant illness, especially infections, usually increases the patient's insulin requirements.

When patients are transferred between different types of insulin products, the early warning symptoms of hypoglycaemia may change or become less pronounced than those experienced with their previous insulin.

Transferring a patient to a new type or brand of insulin should be done under strict medical supervision. Changes in strength, brand, type, species (animal, human, human insulin analogue) and/or method of manufacture may result in a change in dosage. Patients taking NovoRapid may require an increased number of daily injections or a change in dosage from that used with their usual insulins. If an adjustment is needed, it may occur with the first dose or during the first several weeks or months.

Omission of a meal or unplanned, strenuous physical exercise may lead to hypoglycaemia.

Adjustment of dosage may also be necessary if patients undertake increased physical activity or change their usual diet. Exercise taken immediately after a meal may increase the risk of hypoglycaemia.

NovoRapid contains metacresol, which in rare cases may cause allergic reactions.

4.5 Interaction with other medicinal products and other forms of Interaction

A number of medicinal products are known to interact with glucose metabolism.

The following substances may reduce the patient's insulin requirements: Oral hypoglycaemic agents (OHAs), octreotide, monoamine oxidase inhibitors (MAOIs), non-selective beta-adrenergic blocking agents, angiotensin converting enzyme (ACE) inhibitors, salicylates, alcohol, anabolic steroids and sulphonamides.

The following substances may increase the patient's insulin requirements:

Oral contraceptives, thiazides, glucocorticoids, thyroid hormones, sympathomimetics and danazol.

Beta-blocking agents may mask the symptoms of hypoglycaemia.

Alcohol may intensify and prolong the hypoglycaemic effect of insulin.

4.6 Pregnancy and lactation

There is limited clinical experience with NovoRapid in pregnancy.

Animal reproduction studies have not revealed any differences between NovoRapid and human insulin regarding embryotoxicity or teratogenicity.

Intensified monitoring of pregnant women with diabetes is recommended throughout pregnancy and when contemplating pregnancy. Insulin requirements usually fall in the first trimester and increase subsequently during the second and third trimesters.

There are no restrictions on treatment with NovoRapid during lactation. Insulin treatment of the nursing mother presents no risk to the baby. However, the NovoRapid dosage may need to be adjusted.

4.7 Effects on ability to drive and use machines

The patient's ability to concentrate and react may be impaired as a result of hypoglycaemia. This may constitute a risk in situations where these abilities are of special importance (e.g. driving a car or operating machinery).

Patients should be advised to take precautions in order to avoid hypoglycaemia whilst driving, this is particularly important in those who have reduced or absent awareness of the warning signs of hypoglycaemia or have frequent episodes of hypoglycaemia. The advisability of driving should be considered in these circumstances.

4.8 Undesirable effects

Adverse drug reactions observed in patients using NovoRapid are mainly dose-dependent and due to the pharmacological effect of insulin. As for other insulin products, hypoglycaemia, in general is the most frequently occurring undesirable effect. It may occur if the insulin dose is too high in relation to the insulin requirement. Severe hypoglycaemia may lead to unconsciousness and/or convulsions and may result in temporary or permanent impairment of brain function or even death.

In clinical trials and during marketed use the frequency varies with patient population and dose regimens therefore no specific frequency can be presented. During clinical trials the overall rates of hypoglycaemia did not differ between patients treated with insulin aspart compared to human insulin.

Frequencies of adverse drug reactions from clinical trials, which by an overall judgement are considered related to insulin aspart are listed below. The frequencies are defined as: Uncommon $>1/1,000$, $<1/100$) and rare $>1/10,000$, $<1/1,000$). Isolated spontaneous cases are presented as very rare defined as ($<1/10,000$).

Immune system disorders

Uncommon – Urticaria, rash, eruptions

Very rare – Anaphylactic reactions

Symptoms of generalised hypersensitivity may include generalised skin rash, itching, sweating, gastrointestinal upset, angioneurotic oedema, difficulties in breathing, palpitation and reduction in blood pressure. Generalised hypersensitivity reactions are potentially life threatening.

Nervous system disorders

Rare – Peripheral neuropathy

Fast improvement in blood glucose control may be associated with a condition termed acute painful neuropathy, which is usually reversible.

Eye disorders

Uncommon – Refraction disorder

Refraction anomalies may occur upon initiation of insulin therapy. These symptoms are usually of transitory nature.

Uncommon – Diabetic retinopathy

Long-term improved glycaemic control decreases the risk of progression of diabetic retinopathy. However, intensification of insulin therapy with abrupt improvement in glycaemic control may be associated with worsening of diabetic retinopathy.

Skin and subcutaneous tissue disorders

Uncommon – Lipodystrophy

Lipodystrophy may occur at the injection site as a consequence of failure to rotate injection sites within an area.

Uncommon – Local hypersensitivity

Local hypersensitivity reactions (redness, swelling and itching at the injection site) may occur during treatment with insulin. These reactions are usually transitory and normally they disappear during continued treatment.

General disorders and administration site conditions

Uncommon – Oedema

Oedema may occur upon initiation of insulin therapy. These symptoms are usually of transitory nature.

4.9 Overdose

A specific overdose for insulin cannot be defined, however hypoglycaemia may develop over sequential stages if too high doses relative to the patient's requirements are administered:

- Mild hypoglycaemic episodes can be treated by oral administration of glucose or sugary products. It is therefore recommended that the diabetic patient constantly carries some sugar-containing products.
- Severe hypoglycaemic episodes, where the patient has become unconscious, can be treated by glucagon (0.5 to 1 mg) given intramuscularly or subcutaneously by a trained person, or glucose given intravenously by a medical professional. Glucose must also be given intravenously if the patient does not respond to glucagon within 10 to 15 minutes. Upon regaining consciousness, administration of oral carbohydrate is recommended for the patient in order to prevent relapse.

Figure 1

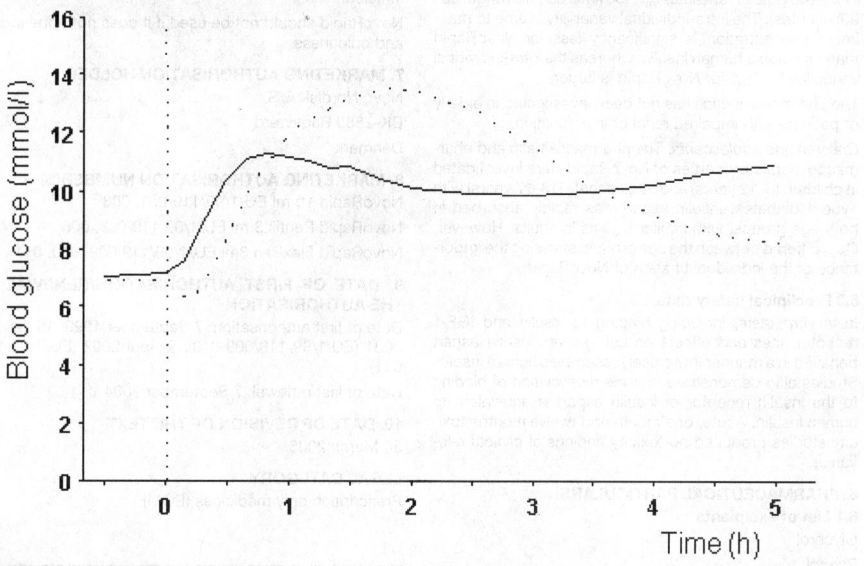

5. PHARMACOLOGICAL PROPERTIES

5.1 Pharmacodynamic properties

Pharmacotherapeutic group: insulin and analogues, fast acting. ATC code A10A B05.

The blood glucose lowering effect of insulin occurs when the molecules facilitate the uptake of glucose by binding to insulin receptors on muscle and fat cells - and simultaneously inhibit the output of glucose from the liver.

NovoRapid produces a more rapid onset of action compared to soluble human insulin, together with a lower glucose concentration, as assessed within the first four hours after a meal. NovoRapid has a shorter duration of action compared to soluble human insulin after subcutaneous injection.

Fig. I. Blood glucose concentrations following a single premeal dose of NovoRapid injected immediately before a meal (solid curve) or soluble human insulin administered 30 minutes before a meal (hatched curve) in patients with Type 1 diabetes mellitus.

(see Figure 1 above)

When NovoRapid is injected subcutaneously, the onset of action will occur within 10 to 20 minutes of injection. The maximum effect is exerted between 1 and 3 hours after injection. The duration of action is 3 to 5 hours.

Adults: Clinical trials in patients with Type 1 diabetes have demonstrated a lower postprandial blood glucose with NovoRapid compared to soluble human insulin (Fig. I). In two long-term open label trials in patients with Type 1 diabetes comprising 1070 and 884 patients, respectively, NovoRapid reduced glycosylated haemoglobin by 0.12 [95% C.I. 0.03; 0.22] percentage points and by 0.15 [95% C.I. 0.05; 0.26] percentage points compared to human insulin; a difference of doubtful clinical significance.

Children and adolescents: A clinical trial comparing preprandial soluble human insulin with postprandial insulin aspart was performed in small children (20 patients aged 2 to less than 6 years, studied for 12 weeks, among these four were younger than 4 years old) and a single PK/PD trial was performed in children (6-12 years) and adolescents (13-17 years). The pharmacodynamic profile of insulin aspart in children was similar to that in adults.

Clinical trials in patients with Type 1 diabetes have demonstrated a reduced risk of nocturnal hypoglycaemia with insulin aspart compared with soluble human insulin. The risk of daytime hypoglycaemia was not significantly increased.

Insulin aspart is equipotent to soluble human insulin on a molar basis.

5.2 Pharmacokinetic properties

In NovoRapid substitution of the amino acid proline with aspartic acid at position B28 reduces the tendency to form hexamers as observed with soluble human insulin.

NovoRapid is therefore more rapidly absorbed from the subcutaneous layer compared to soluble human insulin.

The time to maximum concentration is, on average, half of that for soluble human insulin. A mean maximum plasma concentration of 492±256 pmol/1 was reached 40 (interquartile range: 30–40) minutes after a subcutaneous dose of 0.15 U/kg bodyweight in Type 1 diabetic patients. The insulin concentrations returned to baseline about 4 to 6 hours after dose. The absorption rate was somewhat slower in Type 2 diabetic patients, resulting in a lower C_{max} (352±240 pmol/1) and later t_{max} (60 (interquartile range: 50–90) minutes). The intra-individual variability in time to maximum concentration is significantly less for NovoRapid than for soluble human insulin, whereas the intra-individual variability in C_{max} for NovoRapid is larger.

The pharmacokinetics has not been investigated in elderly or patients with impaired renal or liver function.

Children and adolescents. The pharmacokinetic and pharmacodynamic properties of NovoRapid were investigated in children (6–12 years) and adolescents (13–17 years) with Type 1 diabetes. Insulin aspart was rapidly absorbed in both age groups, with similar t_{max} as in adults. However, C_{max} differed between the age groups, stressing the importance of the individual titration of NovoRapid.

5.3 Preclinical safety data

In *in vitro* tests, including binding to insulin and IGF-1 receptor sites and effects on cell growth, insulin aspart behaved in a manner that closely resembled human insulin. Studies also demonstrate that the dissociation of binding to the insulin receptor of insulin aspart is equivalent to human insulin. Acute, one month and twelve months toxicity studies produced no toxicity findings of clinical relevance.

6. PHARMACEUTICAL PARTICULARS

6.1 List of excipients

Glycerol

Phenol

Metacresol

Zinc chloride

Disodium phosphate dihydrate

Sodium chloride

Hydrochloric acid and/or Sodium hydroxide (for pH adjustment)

Water for injections

6.2 Incompatibilities

Substances added to the insulin may cause degradation of the insulin, e.g. if the medicinal product contains thiol or sulphites.

6.3 Shelf life

30 months.

The in-use shelf life is 4 weeks.

6.4 Special precautions for storage

Store in a refrigerator (2°C – 8°C). Do not freeze.

In order to protect from light keep the container (vial, cartridge) in the outer carton or keep the cap on when NovoRapid FlexPen is not in use.

Vials, cartridges, and FlexPen pens in use or carried as a spare: Do not refrigerate. Do not store above 30°C.

6.5 Nature and contents of container

NovoRapid 100 U/ml, 10 ml vial

Glass vial (Type I) closed with a disc (bromobutyl/polyisoprene rubber) and a protective tamper-proof plastic cap containing 10 ml of solution.

Cartons of 1 or 5 vials.

NovoRapid Penfill 100 U/ml

A glass (Type I) cartridge which contains a piston (bromobutyl rubber) and is closed with a disc (bromobutyl/polyisoprene rubber) containing 3 ml of solution.

Cartons of 5 or 10 cartridges.

NovoRapid FlexPen 100 U/ml

A glass (Type I) cartridge which contains a piston (bromobutyl rubber) and is closed with a disc (bromobutyl/polyisoprene rubber) containing 3 ml solution in a multidose disposable pre-filled pen with a pen injector (plastic).

Cartons of 1, 5 or 10 pre-filled pens.

Not all packs may be marketed.

6.6 Instructions for use and handling

NovoRapid vials are for use with insulin syringes with the corresponding unit scale.

Cartridges and pens should only be used in combination with products that are compatible with them and allow the cartridges and pens to function safely and effectively.

NovoRapid Penfill and NovoRapid FlexPen are for use by one person only. The container must not be refilled.

NovoRapid Penfill is designed to be used with the Novo Nordisk insulin delivery system and NovoFine needles.

NovoFine **S** needles are designed to be used with NovoRapid FlexPen.

NovoRapid may be used in an infusion pump system (CSII) as described in section 4.2. Tubings in which the inner surface materials are made of polyethylene or polyolefin have been evaluated and found compatible with pump use.

For intravenous use, infusion systems with NovoRapid 100 U/ml at concentrations from 0.05 U/ml to 1.0 U/ml insulin aspart in the infusion fluids 0.9% sodium chloride, 5% dextrose or 10% dextrose inclusive 40 mmol/l potassium chloride using polypropylene infusion bags are stable at room temperature for 24 hours.

Although stable over time, a certain amount of insulin will be initially adsorbed to the material of the infusion bag. Monitoring of blood glucose is necessary during insulin infusion.

NovoRapid should not be used if it does not appear clear and colourless.

7. MARKETING AUTHORISATION HOLDER

Novo Nordisk A/S

DK-2880 Bagsværd

Denmark

8. MARKETING AUTHORISATION NUMBER(S)

NovoRapid 10 ml EU/1/99/119/001, 008

NovoRapid Penfill 3 ml EU/1/99/119/003, 006

NovoRapid FlexPen 3ml EU/1/99/119/009, 010, 011

9. DATE OF FIRST AUTHORISATION/RENEWAL OF THE AUTHORISATION

Date of first authorisation: 7 September 1999, 15 January 2001 (EU/1/99/119/009-010), 2 April 2002 (EU/1/99/119/011)

Date of last renewal: 7 September 2004

10. DATE OF REVISION OF THE TEXT

30 March 2005

LEGAL CATEGORY

Prescription only medicines (POM)

Novoseven 1.2 mg (60 KIU),2.4 mg (120 KIU), 4.8 mg (240 KIU).

(Novo Nordisk Limited)

1. NAME OF THE MEDICINAL PRODUCT

NovoSeven® 1.2 mg (60 KIU) – powder and solvent for solution for injection

NovoSeven® 2.4 mg (120 KIU) – powder and solvent for solution for injection

NovoSeven® 4.8 mg (240 KIU) – powder and solvent for solution for injection

2. QUALITATIVE AND QUANTITATIVE COMPOSITION

eptacog alfa (activated) 1.2 mg/vial (corresponds to 60 KIU/vial)

eptacog alfa (activated) 2.4 mg/vial (corresponds to 120 KIU/vial)

eptacog alfa (activated) 4.8 mg/vial (corresponds to 240 KIU/vial)

1 KIU equals 1000 IU (International Units)

eptacog alfa (activated) is recombinant coagulation factor VIIa with a molecular mass of approximately 50,000 Dalton produced by genetic engineering from baby hamster kidney cells (BHK Cells).

After reconstitution 1 ml solution contains 0.6 mg eptacog alfa (activated).

For excipients see 6.1.

3. PHARMACEUTICAL FORM

Powder and solvent for solution for injection.

4. CLINICAL PARTICULARS

4.1 Therapeutic indications

NovoSeven is indicated for the treatment of bleeding episodes and for the prevention of bleeding in those undergoing surgery or invasive procedures in the following patient groups

- in patients with congenital haemophilia with inhibitors to coagulation factors VIII or IX> 5 BU

- in patients with congenital haemophilia who are expected to have a high anamnestic response to factor VIII or factor IX administration

- in patients with acquired haemophilia

- in patients with congenital FVII deficiency

- in patients with Glanzmann's thrombasthenia with antibodies to GP IIb-IIIa and/or HLA, and with past or present refractoriness to platelet transfusions.

4.2 Posology and method of administration

4.2.1 Dosage

Haemophilia A or B with inhibitors or acquired haemophilia

Dose:

NovoSeven should be given as early as possible after the start of a bleeding episode. The recommended initial dose, administered by intravenous bolus injection, is 90 μg per kg body weight.

Following the initial dose of NovoSeven further injections may be repeated. The duration of treatment and the interval between injections will vary with the severity of the haemorrhage, the invasive procedures or surgery being performed.

Dose interval:

Initially 2-3 hours to obtain haemostasis.

If continued therapy is needed, the dose interval can be increased successively once effective haemostasis is achieved to every 4, 6, 8 or 12 hours for as long as treatment is judged as being indicated.

Mild to moderate bleeding episodes (including ambulatory treatment)

Early intervention in the ambulatory treatment setting with a dose of 90 μg per kg body weight has been efficacious in treating mild to moderate joint, muscle and mucocutaneous bleeds. One to three doses were administered at three-hour intervals to achieve haemostasis and one additional dose was given to maintain haemostasis. The duration of ambulatory treatment should not exceed 24 hours.

Serious bleeding episodes

An initial dose of 90 μg per kg body weight is recommended and could be administered on the way to the hospital where the patient is usually treated. The following dose varies according to the type and severity of the haemorrhage. Dosing frequency should initially be every second hour until clinical improvement is observed. If continued therapy is indicated, the dose interval can then be increased to 3 hours for 1-2 days. Thereafter, the dose interval can be increased successively to every 4, 6, 8 or 12 hours for as long as treatment is judged as being indicated. A major bleeding episode may be treated for 2-3 weeks but can be extended beyond this if clinically warranted.

Invasive procedure/surgery

An initial dose of 90 μg per kg body weight should be given immediately before the intervention. The dose should be repeated after 2 hours and then at 2-3 hour intervals for the first 24-48 hours depending on the intervention performed and the clinical status of the patient. In major surgery, the dose should be continued at 2-4 hour intervals for 6-7 days. The dose interval may then be increased to 6-8 hours for another 2 weeks of treatment. Patients undergoing major surgery may be treated for up to 2-3 weeks until healing has occurred.

Factor VII deficiency

Dose, dose range and dose interval

The recommended dose range for treatment of bleeding episodes in patients undergoing surgery or invasive procedures is 15-30 μg per kg body weight every 4-6 hours until haemostasis is achieved. Dose and frequency of injections should be adapted to each individual.

Glanzmann's thrombasthenia

Dose, dose range and dose interval

The recommended dose for treatment of bleeding episodes and for the prevention of bleeding in patients undergoing surgery or invasive procedures is 90 μg (range 80-120 μg) per kg body weight at intervals of two hours (1.5 - 2.5 hours). At least three doses should be administered to secure effective haemostasis. The recommended route of administration is bolus injection as lack of efficacy may appear in connection with continuous infusion.

For those patients who are not refractory, platelets are the first line treatment for Glanzmann's thrombasthenia.

4.2.2 Administration

Reconstitute the preparation as described under 6.6 and administer as an intravenous bolus injection over 2-5 minutes.

NovoSeven should not be mixed with infusion solutions or be given in a drip.

4.2.3 Monitoring of treatment – Laboratory Tests

There is no requirement for monitoring of NovoSeven therapy. Severity of bleeding condition and clinical response to NovoSeven administration must guide dosing requirements.

After administration of NovoSeven, prothrombin time (PT) and activated partial thromboplastin time (aPTT) have been shown to shorten, however no correlation has been demonstrated between PT and aPTT and clinical efficacy of NovoSeven.

4.3 Contraindications

Known hypersensitivity to the active substance, the excipients, or to mouse, hamster or bovine protein may be a contraindication to the use of NovoSeven.

4.4 Special warnings and special precautions for use

In pathological conditions in which tissue factor may be expressed more extensively than considered normal, there may be a potential risk of development of thrombotic events or induction of Disseminated Intravascular Coagulation (DIC) in association with NovoSeven treatment. Such situations may include patients with advanced atherosclerotic disease, crush injury, septicaemia or DIC.

As recombinant coagulation factor VIIa NovoSeven may contain trace amounts of mouse IgG, bovine IgG and other residual culture proteins (hamster and bovine serum proteins), the remote possibility exists that patients treated with the product may develop hypersensitivity to these proteins.

In case of severe bleeds the product should be administered in hospitals preferably specialised in treatment of haemophilia patients with coagulation factor VIII or IX inhibitors, or if not possible in close collaboration with a physician specialised in haemophilia treatment.

The duration of the ambulatory treatment should not exceed 24 hours. If bleeding is not kept under control hospital care is mandatory. Patients/carers should inform the physician/supervising hospital at the earliest possible opportunity about all usages of NovoSeven.

Factor VII deficient patients should be monitored for prothrombin time and factor VII coagulant activity before and after administration of NovoSeven. In case the factor VIIa activity fails to reach the expected level or bleeding is not controlled after treatment with the recommended doses, antibody formation may be suspected and analysis for antibodies should be performed. The risk of thrombosis in factor VII deficient patients treated with NovoSeven is unknown.

4.5 Interaction with other medicinal products and other forms of Interaction

The risk of a potential interaction between NovoSeven and coagulation factor concentrates is unknown. Simultaneous use of prothrombin complex concentrates, activated or not, should be avoided.

Anti-fibrinolytics have been reported to reduce blood loss in association with surgery in haemophilia patients, especially in orthopaedic surgery and surgery in regions rich in fibrinolytic activity, such as the oral cavity. Experience with concomitant administration of anti-fibrinolytics and NovoSeven treatment is however limited.

4.6 Pregnancy and lactation

From animal reproduction studies it was concluded that intravenous administration of NovoSeven had no effect upon foetal development, fertility or reproductive performance. It is not known whether NovoSeven can cause foetal harm when administered to a pregnant woman or can affect reproduction capacity. NovoSeven should only be given to pregnant women if clearly needed.

Use during lactation: It is not known whether NovoSeven is excreted in human milk. Caution should be exercised when NovoSeven is administered to lactating women.

4.7 Effects on ability to drive and use machines

None known.

4.8 Undesirable effects

Based on post-marketing experience adverse drug reactions are rare (<1 per 1,000 standard doses). When analysed by system organ classes, the reporting rates of adverse drug reactions during the post-marketing period, including both serious and non-serious reactions, are as indicated in the table below:

Blood and lymphatic disorders

Very rare (<1/10,000)

Few cases of coagulopathic disorders such as increased D-dimer and consumptive coagulopathy have been reported. Patients at increased risk of disseminated intravascular coagulation as described in 4.4 "Special warnings and special precautions" should be carefully monitored.

Cardiac disorders

Very rare (<1/10,000)

Myocardial infarction: Described below under 'serious thrombotic adverse reactions during the post-marketing period'.

Gastrointestinal disorders

Very rare (<1/10,000)

Few cases of nausea have been reported.

General disorders and administration site conditions

Rare (>1/10,000, <1/1,000)

Lack of efficacy (therapeutic response decreased) has been reported. It is important that the dosage regimen of NovoSeven is compliant with the recommended dosage as stated in 4.2.1 "Dosage".

Very rare (<1/10,000)

Fever may occur. Pain, especially at injection site may also occur on rare occasions.

Investigations

Very rare (<1/10,000)

Increase of alanine aminotransferase, alkaline phosphatase, lactate dehydrogenase and prothrombin levels have been reported.

Nervous system disorders

Very rare (<1/10,000)

Cerebrovascular disorders including cerebral infarction and cerebral ischaemia have been reported: Described below under 'serious thrombotic adverse reactions during the post-marketing period'.

Skin and subcutaneous tissue disorders

Very rare (<1/10,000)

Skin rashes may occur.

Vascular disorders

Very rare (<1/10,000)

Venous thrombotic events have been reported: Described below under 'serious thrombotic adverse reactions during the post-marketing period'.

Incidents of haemorrhage have been reported. NovoSeven is not expected to precipitate haemorrhage, but pre-existing haemorrhage may continue in case of insufficient efficacy or sub-optimal dosage regimen.

Serious adverse reactions reported during the post-marketing period include:

• Arterial thrombotic events such as myocardial infarctions or ischaemia, cerebrovascular disorders and bowel infarction. In the vast majority of cases the patients were predisposed to arterial thrombotic disorders either due to underlying disease, age, atherosclerotic or current medical conditions as described in 4.4 "Special warnings and special precautions".

• Venous thrombotic events such as thrombophlebitis, deep vein thrombosis and hereto related pulmonary embolism. In the vast majority of cases the patients were predisposed to venous thrombotic events due to concurrent risk factors. Patients at increased risk of venous thrombotic disorders either due to concurrent conditions, previous history of thrombotic events, post surgery immobilisation or venous catheterisation should be carefully monitored.

Anaphylactic reactions have not been reported spontaneously during the post-marketing period but patients with a history of allergic reactions should be carefully monitored.

There have been no reports of antibodies against factor VII in haemophilia A or B patients. Isolated cases of factor VII deficient patients developing antibodies against factor VII have been reported after treatment with NovoSeven. These patients have previously been treated with human plasma and/or plasma-derived factor VII. In two patients the antibodies showed inhibitory effect *in vitro*. Patients with factor VII deficiency should be monitored for factor VII antibodies.

One case of angioneurotic oedema has been reported spontaneously in a patient with Glanzmann's thrombasthenia after administration of NovoSeven.

4.9 Overdose

From human use no thrombotic complications to overdose have been reported, even after accidental administration of 800 μg per kg body weight.

5. PHARMACOLOGICAL PROPERTIES

5.1 Pharmacodynamic properties

Pharmacotherapeutic group: Coagulation factors, ATC code B02B D08.

NovoSeven contains activated recombinant coagulation factor VII. The mechanism of action includes the binding of factor VIIa to exposed tissue factor. This complex activates factor IX into factor IXa and factor X into factor Xa, leading to the initial conversion of small amounts of prothrombin into thrombin. Thrombin leads to the activation of platelets and factors V and VIII at the site of injury and to the formation of the haemostatic plug by converting fibrinogen into fibrin. Pharmacological doses of NovoSeven activate factor X directly on the surface of activated platelets, localised to the site of injury, independently of tissue factor. This results in the conversion of prothrombin into large amounts of thrombin independently of tissue factor. Accordingly, the pharmacodynamic effect of factor VIIa gives rise to an increased local formation of factor Xa, thrombin and fibrin.

A theoretical risk for the development of systemic activation of the coagulation system in patients suffering from underlying diseases predisposing them to DIC cannot be totally excluded although clinical post-marketing experience to-date has not resulted in reporting of this as a significant adverse drug reaction.

5.2 Pharmacokinetic properties

Haemophilia A and B with inhibitors

Using a factor VII clot assay, the pharmacokinetic properties of NovoSeven were investigated in 25 non-bleeding and in 5 bleeding study episodes.

Factor VII clotting activities measured in plasma drawn prior to and during a 24-hour period after NovoSeven administration were analysed. Single dose pharmacokinetics of NovoSeven, 17.5, 35 and 70 μg per kg body weight exhibited linear behaviour. The median apparent volumes of distribution at steady state and at elimination were 106 and 122 ml/kg respectively in non-bleeding episodes and 103 and 121 ml/kg, respectively in bleeding episodes. Median clearance was 31.0 ml/h × kg and 32.6 ml/h × kg respectively in the two groups. The drug elimination was described by mean residence time and half-life. The figures were 3.44 h and 2.89 h (median values), respectively in non-bleeding episodes and 2.97 h and 2.30 h (median values), respectively in bleeding episodes.

The median *in vivo* plasma recovery was 45.6% in patients with non-bleeding episodes and 43.5% in patients with bleeding episodes.

Factor VII deficiency

Single dose pharmacokinetics of NovoSeven, 15 and 30 μg per kg body weight, showed no significant difference between the two doses used with regard to dose-independent parameters: total body clearance (70.8-79.1 ml/h × kg), volume of distribution at steady state (280-290 ml/kg), mean residence time (3.75-3.80 h), and half-life (2.82-3.11 h). The mean *in vivo* plasma recovery was approximately 20%.

Glanzmann's thrombasthenia

Pharmacokinetics of NovoSeven in patients with Glanzmann's thrombasthenia has not been investigated, but is expected to be similar to the pharmacokinetics in haemophilia A and B patients.

5.3 Preclinical safety data

All findings in the pre-clinical safety programme were related to the pharmacological effect of NovoSeven.

6. PHARMACEUTICAL PARTICULARS

6.1 List of excipients

Sodium chloride

Calcium chloride dihydrate

Glycylglycine

Polysorbate 80

Mannitol

Water for injection

6.2 Incompatibilities

NovoSeven must not be mixed with infusion solutions or be given in a drip.

6.3 Shelf life

The shelf life is 3 years for the product packed for sale.

After reconstitution, chemical and physical stability has been demonstrated for 24 hours at 25°C. From a microbiological point of view, the product should be used immediately. If not used immediately, storage time and storage conditions prior to use are the responsibility of the user, and would normally not be longer than 24 hours at 2°C-8°C, unless reconstitution has taken place in controlled and validated aseptic conditions.

6.4 Special precautions for storage

- Store NovoSeven at 2°C-8°C (in a refrigerator).
- Store in original package in order to protect from light.
- Do not freeze to prevent damage to the solvent vial.

6.5 Nature and contents of container

The NovoSeven package contains:

- 1 vial with white powder (NovoSeven) for solution for injection
- 1 vial with solvent (Water for injections) for reconstitution
- 1 sterile needle for reconstitution (transfer needle)
- 1 sterile disposable syringe for reconstitution and administration
- 1 sterile infusion set
- 2 alcohol swabs for cleansing the rubber stoppers on the vials
- Package leaflet with instructions for use.

Vials for NovoSeven

Glass, closed with a bromobutyl rubber stopper covered with an aluminium cap. The closed vials are equipped with a tamper-evident snap-off cap which is made of polypropylene.

Vials for solvent

Glass, closed with a bromobutyl rubber disc with teflon, covered with an aluminium cap. The closed vials are equipped with a tamper-evident snap-off cap which is made of polypropylene.

Syringe for reconstitution and administration

The disposable syringe is made of polypropylene.

6.6 Instructions for use and handling

Always use an aseptic technique.

6.6.1 Reconstitution

- Bring NovoSeven (powder) and solvent (water) vials to room temperature (but not above 37°C). You can do that by holding them in your hands.
- Remove the protective plastic caps from powder vial and water vial so that you can see the central part of a rubber stopper on each vial. If the cap is loose or missing, do not use the vial.
- Clean the rubber stoppers with alcohol swabs. Allow them to dry before use.
- Take the transfer needle out of its package and take the syringe out of its package. Screw the transfer needle onto the syringe, making sure that the needle is tightly fastened. Carefully remove the needle cap.
- Draw air into the syringe by pulling the plunger right back to the same volume as there is in the water vial (ml equals cc on the syringe).
- Push the transfer needle into the water vial through the centre of the rubber stopper. Inject the air into the vial until you notice a clear resistance. Then, holding the vial upside down, draw all the water into the syringe. You need to keep the needle tip in the water to do this.
- Push the transfer needle into the powder vial through the centre of the rubber stopper. Aim the needle at the side of the vial and then gently inject all the water.

You must aim the stream of liquid at the glass wall, not directly at the powder. This prevents the mixture from "foaming". Keep the transfer needle in the vial.

- Gently swirl the vial until everything is dissolved, and you cannot see any more powder. Do not shake the vial, as this will cause "foaming". Still keep the transfer needle in the vial.

NovoSeven reconstituted solution should be inspected visually for particulate matter and discolouration prior to administration.

The enclosed disposable syringe is compatible with the reconstituted preparation, but **do not** store reconstituted NovoSeven in plastic syringes.

It is recommended to use NovoSeven immediately after reconstitution.

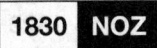

6.6.2 Administration

- Then holding the vial upside down, draw all the injection solution into the syringe. You need to keep the needle tip in the solution to do this.

- Remove the transfer needle from the vial. Replace the needle cap. Then twist the needle off the syringe.

- Take the infusion set out of its package and remove the cap. Attach the infusion set to the syringe. Remove the sheath from the needle of the infusion set. Locate a suitable site, and slowly inject NovoSeven into a vein over a period of 2-5 minutes without removing the needle from the injection site.

- Dispose of the syringe, needle and the infusion set safely.

Any unused product or waste material should be disposed of in accordance

with local requirements.

7. MARKETING AUTHORISATION HOLDER

Novo Nordisk A/S

DK-2880 Bagsvaerd

Denmark

8. MARKETING AUTHORISATION NUMBER(S)

NovoSeven® 60 KIU EU/1/96/006/001

NovoSeven® 120 KIU EU/1/96/006/002

NovoSeven® 240 KIU EU/1/96/006/003

9. DATE OF FIRST AUTHORISATION/RENEWAL OF THE AUTHORISATION

23 February 2001

10. DATE OF REVISION OF THE TEXT

27 January 2004

Legal Category

POM

Nozinan injection

(Link Pharmaceuticals Ltd)

1. NAME OF THE MEDICINAL PRODUCT

Nozinan injection.

2. QUALITATIVE AND QUANTITATIVE COMPOSITION

Levomepromazine INN (methotrimeprazine BAN) hydrochloride 25mg per ml.

3. PHARMACEUTICAL FORM

Solution for injection.

4. CLINICAL PARTICULARS

4.1 Therapeutic indications

Management of the terminally ill patient. Levomepromazine resembles chlorpromazine and promethazine in the pattern of its pharmacology. It possesses anti-emetic, antihistamine and anti-adrenaline activity and exhibits a strong sedative effect.

Nozinan potentiates the action of other central nervous system depressants but may be given in conjunction with appropriately modified doses of narcotic analgesics in the management of severe pain. Nozinan does not significantly depress respiration and is particularly useful where pulmonary reserve is low.

Nozinan is indicated in the management of pain and accompanying restlessness or distress in the terminally ill patient.

4.2 Posology and method of administration

Intramuscular and intravenous injection

Dosage varies with the condition and individual response of the patient. Nozinan injection may be administered by intramuscular injection or intravenous injection after dilution with an equal volume of normal saline.

The usual dose for adults and the elderly is 12.5mg to 25mg (0.5ml to 1ml) by intramuscular injection, or by the intravenous route after dilution with an equal volume of normal saline immediately before use. In cases of severe agitation, up to 50mg (2ml) may be used, repeated every 6 to 8 hours.

Continuous subcutaneous infusion

Nozinan injection may be administered over a 24 hour period via a syringe driver. The required dose of Nozinan injection (25mg to 200mg per day) should be diluted with the calculated volume of normal saline. Diamorphine hydrochloride is compatible with this solution and may be added if greater analgesia is required.

Nozinan tablets 25mg may be substituted for the injection if oral therapy is more convenient.

Children

Clinical experience with parenteral levomepromazine in children is limited. Where indicated, doses of 0.35mg/kg/day to 3.0mg/kg/day are recommended.

4.3 Contraindications

Safety in pregnancy has not been established. There are no absolute contraindications to the use of Nozinan in terminal care.

4.4 Special warnings and special precautions for use

The drug should be avoided, or used with caution, in patients with liver dysfunction or cardiac disease.

The hypotensive effects of Nozinan should be taken into account when it is administered to patients with cardiac disease and the elderly or debilitated. Patients receiving large initial doses should be kept in bed.

As with other neuroleptics, cases of QT interval prolongation have been reported with levomepromazine very rarely. Consequently, and if the clinical situation permits, absence of the following risk factors for onset of this type of arrhythmia should be verified prior to administration:

- Bradycardia or 2nd or 3rd degree heart block.
- Metabolic abnormalities such as hypokalaemia, hypocalcaemia or hypomagnesaemia.
- Starvation or alcohol abuse.
- A history of QT interval prolongation, ventricular arrhythmias or Torsades de Pointes.
- A family history of QT interval prolongation.
- Ongoing treatment with another drug liable to induce marked bradycardia, hypokalaemia, slowed intracardiac conduction or prolonged QT interval.

It is recommended, as part of the initial evaluation in patients to be treated with levomepromazine, that an ECG is performed with measurement of serum calcium, magnesium and potassium levels. Periodic serum electrolyte levels should be monitored and corrected especially when long-term chronic usage is anticipated. An ECG should be repeated to assess the QT interval whenever dose escalation is proposed and when the maximum therapeutic dose is reached.

4.5 Interaction with other medicinal products and other forms of Interaction

Cytochrome P450 2D6 Metabolism: Levomepromazine and its non-hydroxylated metabolites are reported to be potent inhibitors of cytochrome P450 2D6. Co-administration of levomepromazine and drugs primarily metabolised by the cytochrome P450 2D6 enzyme system may result in increased plasma concentrations of the drugs that could increase or prolong both therapeutic or adverse effects of those drugs.

There is an increased risk of arrhythmias when neuroleptics are used with drugs that prolong the QT interval such as certain anti-arrhythmics, antidepressants and other antipsychotics. If these drugs are co-administered this should be done with ECG monitoring.

The anticholinergic effect of neuroleptics may be enhanced by other anticholinergic drugs.

Simultaneous administration of desferrioxamine and prochlorperazine has been observed to induce a transient metabolic encephalopathy, characterised by loss of consciousness for 48 to 72 hours. It is possible that this may occur with Nozinan, since it shares many of the pharmacological activities of prochlorperazine. Adrenaline (epinephrine) must not be used in patients overdosed with neuroleptics. Alcohol should be avoided.

4.6 Pregnancy and lactation

Safety in pregnancy has not been established.

4.7 Effects on ability to drive and use machines

Nozinan can cause drowsiness, disorientation, confusion or excessive hypotension, which may affect the patient's ability to drive or operate machinery.

4.8 Undesirable effects

Somnolence and asthenia are frequent side effects. Dry mouth is encountered occasionally. Hypotension may occur, especially in elderly patients. A raised ESR may occasionally be encountered. Agranulocytosis has been reported, as have photosensitivity and allergic skin reactions.

Parkinsonian-like reactions may occur in patients receiving prolonged high dosage. Jaundice is a rare side effect. Other adverse effects common to phenothiazine neuroleptics may be seen, such as heat stroke in hot and humid conditions, constipation that may become severe leading to paralytic ileus, neuroleptic malignant syndrome and rare cases of cardiac rhythm disturbances and prolongation of the QT interval.

Very rarely cases of Torsades de Pointes have been reported, treatment of which should include discontinuation of levomepromazine and correction of hypoxia, electrolyte abnormalities and acid base disturbances.

Necrotizing enterocolitis which can be fatal, has been very rarely reported in patients treated with levomepromazine. Priapism has also been very rarely reported.

4.9 Overdose

Symptoms of levomepromazine overdosage include drowsiness or loss of consciousness, hypotension, tachycardia, ECG changes, ventricular arrhythmias and hypothermia. Severe extrapyramidal dyskinesias may occur.

General vasodilatation may result in circulatory collapse; raising the patient's legs may suffice but, in severe cases, volume expansion by intravenous fluids may be needed; infusion fluids should be warmed before administration in order not to aggravate hypothermia.

Positive inotropic agents such as dopamine may be tried if fluid replacement is insufficient to correct the circulatory collapse. Peripheral vasoconstrictor agents are not generally recommended; avoid use of adrenaline (epinephrine).

Ventricular or supraventricular tachy-arrhythmias usually respond to restoration of normal body temperature and correction of circulatory or metabolic disturbances. If persistent or life-threatening, appropriate anti-arrhythmic therapy may be considered. Avoid lidocaine (lignocaine) and, as far as possible, long acting anti-arrhythmic drugs.

Pronounced central nervous system depression requires airway maintenance or, in extreme circumstances, assisted respiration. Severe dystonic reactions usually respond to procyclidine (5mg to 10mg) or orphenadrine (20mg to 40mg) administered intramuscularly or intravenously. Convulsions should be treated with intravenous diazepam. Neuroleptic malignant syndrome should be treated with cooling. Dantrolene sodium may be tried.

5. PHARMACOLOGICAL PROPERTIES

5.1 Pharmacodynamic properties

Levomepromazine resembles chlorpromazine and promethazine in the pattern of its pharmacology. It possesses anti-emetic, antihistamine and anti-adrenaline activity and exhibits a strong sedative effect.

5.2 Pharmacokinetic properties

Maximum serum concentrations are achieved in 2 to 3 hours depending on the route of administration. Excretion is slow, with a half-life of about 30 hours. It is eliminated via urine and faeces.

5.3 Preclinical safety data

There are no pre-clinical safety data of relevance to the prescriber which are additional to those already included in other sections of the Summary of Product Characteristics.

6. PHARMACEUTICAL PARTICULARS

6.1 List of excipients

Ascorbic acid, sodium sulphite, sodium chloride, Water for Injections.

6.2 Incompatibilities

Incompatible with alkaline solutions.

6.3 Shelf life

60 months.

6.4 Special precautions for storage

Protect from light.

6.5 Nature and contents of container

Colourless type I glass ampoule. Each pack contains 10 ampoules.

6.6 Instructions for use and handling

Nozinan may be administered by intramuscular injection or intravenous injection after dilution with an equal volume of normal saline, or by continuous subcutaneous infusion with an appropriate volume of normal saline.

Diamorphine hydrochloride is compatible with this solution.

7. MARKETING AUTHORISATION HOLDER

Link Pharmaceuticals Limited, Bishops Weald House, Albion Way, Horsham, West Sussex, RH12 1AH, United Kingdom

8. MARKETING AUTHORISATION NUMBER(S)

PL 12406/0006

9. DATE OF FIRST AUTHORISATION/RENEWAL OF THE AUTHORISATION

12th May 1999 / 11 May 2004

10. DATE OF REVISION OF THE TEXT

February 2004

11. Legal Category

POM

® Nozinan is a registered trade mark

SPC0405

Nozinan tablets

(Link Pharmaceuticals Ltd)

1. NAME OF THE MEDICINAL PRODUCT

Nozinan tablets.

2. QUALITATIVE AND QUANTITATIVE COMPOSITION

Levomepromazine maleate INN (methotrimeprazine maleate BAN) 25mg per tablet.

3. PHARMACEUTICAL FORM

Tablets.

4. CLINICAL PARTICULARS

4.1 Therapeutic indications

Nozinan is a neuroleptic with indications in psychiatry and general medicine, particularly in terminal illness. Clinically it is more sedative and more potent than chlorpromazine in the management of psychotic conditions and in the relief of severe chronic pain.

Psychiatry

As an alternative to chlorpromazine in schizophrenia especially when it is desirable to reduce psychomotor activity.

General medicine

Alone, or together with appropriately modified doses of analgesics and narcotics, in the relief of severe pain and accompanying anxiety and distress.

4.2 Posology and method of administration

Dosage varies with the condition under treatment and the individual response of the patient.

1. Terminal illness

Nozinan tablets 25mg may be substituted for the injection if oral therapy is more convenient, the dosage being 12.5mg to 50mg every 4 to 8 hours.

Elderly

No specific dosage recommendations.

2. Psychiatric conditions

Adults

Ambulant patients: initially the total daily oral dose should not exceed 25mg to 50mg usually divided into 3 doses; a larger portion of the dosage may be taken at bedtime to minimise diurnal sedation. The dosage is then gradually increased to the most effective level compatible with sedation and other side effects.

Bed patients: initially the total daily oral dosage may be 100mg to 200mg, usually divided into 3 doses, gradually increased to 1g daily if necessary. When the patient is stable attempts should be made to reduce the dosage to an adequate maintenance level.

Children

Children are very susceptible to the hypotensive and soporific effects of levomepromazine. It is advised that a total daily oral dosage of 1½ tablets should not be exceeded. The average effective daily intake for a ten year old is ½ to 1 tablet.

Elderly patients

It is not advised to give levomepromazine to ambulant patients over 50 years of age unless the risk of a hypotensive reaction has been assessed.

4.3 Contraindications

Safety in pregnancy has not been established.

There are no absolute contraindications to the use of Nozinan in terminal care.

4.4 Special warnings and special precautions for use

The drug should be avoided, or used with caution, in patients with liver dysfunction or cardiac disease.

The hypotensive effects of Nozinan should be taken into account when it is administered to patients with cardiac disease and the elderly or debilitated. Patients receiving large initial doses should be kept in bed.

As with other neuroleptics, cases of QT interval prolongation have been reported with levomepromazine very rarely. Consequently, and if the clinical situation permits, absence of the following risk factors for onset of this type of arrhythmia should be verified prior to administration:

- Bradycardia or 2nd or 3rd degree heart block.
- Metabolic abnormalities such as hypokalaemia, hypocalcaemia or hypomagnesaemia.
- Starvation or alcohol abuse.
- A history of QT interval prolongation, ventricular arrhythmias or Torsades de Pointes.
- A family history of QT interval prolongation.
- Ongoing treatment with another drug liable to induce marked bradycardia, hypokalaemia, slowed intracardiac conduction or prolonged QT interval.

It is recommended, as part of the initial evaluation in patients to be treated with levomepromazine, that an ECG is performed with measurement of serum calcium, magnesium and potassium levels. Periodic serum electrolyte levels should be monitored and corrected especially when long-term chronic usage is anticipated. An ECG should be repeated to assess the QT interval whenever dose escalation is proposed and when the maximum therapeutic dose is reached.

4.5 Interaction with other medicinal products and other forms of Interaction

Cytochrome P450 2D6 Metabolism: Levomepromazine and its non-hydroxylated metabolites are reported to be potent inhibitors of cytochrome P450 2D6. Co-administration of levomepromazine and drugs primarily metabolised by the cytochrome P450 2D6 enzyme system may result in increased plasma concentrations of the drugs that could increase or prolong both therapeutic or adverse effects of those drugs.

There is an increased risk of arrhythmias when neuroleptics are used with drugs that prolong the QT interval such as certain antiarrhythmics, antidepressants and other antipsychotics. If these drugs are co-administered this should be done with ECG monitoring.

The anticholinergic effect of neuroleptics may be enhanced by other anticholinergic drugs.

Simultaneous administration of desferrioxamine and prochlorperazine has been observed to induce a transient metabolic encephalopathy, characterised by loss of consciousness for 48 to 72 hours. It is possible that this may occur with Nozinan since it shares many of the pharmacological activities of prochlorperazine. Adrenaline (epinephrine) must not be used in patients overdosed with neuroleptics. Alcohol should be avoided.

4.6 Pregnancy and lactation

Safety in pregnancy has not been established.

4.7 Effects on ability to drive and use machines

Nozinan can cause drowsiness, disorientation, confusion or excessive hypotension, which may affect the patient's ability to drive or operate machinery.

4.8 Undesirable effects

Somnolence and asthenia are frequent side effects. Dry mouth is encountered occasionally. Hypotension may occur, especially in elderly patients. A raised ESR may occasionally be encountered. Agranulocytosis has been reported, as have photosensitivity and allergic skin reactions.

Parkinsonian-like reactions may occur in patients receiving prolonged high dosage. Jaundice is a rare side effect. Other adverse effects common to phenothiazine neuroleptics may be seen, such as heat stroke in hot and humid conditions, constipation that may become severe leading to paralytic ileus, neuroleptic malignant syndrome and rare cases of cardiac rhythm disturbances and prolongation of the QT interval.

Very rarely cases of Torsades de Pointes have been reported, treatment of which should include discontinuation of levomepromazine and correction of hypoxia, electrolyte abnormalities and acid base disturbances.

Necrotizing enterocolitis which can be fatal, has been very rarely reported in patients treated with levomepromazine. Priapism has also been very rarely reported.

4.9 Overdose

Symptoms of levomepromazine overdosage include drowsiness or loss of consciousness, hypotension, tachycardia, ECG changes, ventricular arrhythmias and hypothermia. Severe extrapyramidal dyskinesias may occur.

If the patient is seen sufficiently soon (up to 6 hours) after ingestion of a toxic dose, gastric lavage may be attempted. Pharmacological induction of emesis is unlikely to be of any use. Activated charcoal should be given. There is no specific antidote. Treatment is supportive.

Generalised vasodilatation may result in circulatory collapse; raising the patient's legs may suffice but, in severe cases, volume expansion by intravenous fluids may be needed; infusion fluids should be warmed before administration in order not to aggravate hypothermia.

Positive inotropic agents such as dopamine may be tried if fluid replacement is insufficient to correct the circulatory collapse. Peripheral vasoconstrictor agents are not generally recommended; avoid use of adrenaline (epinephrine).

Ventricular or supraventricular tachy-arrhythmias usually respond to restoration of normal body temperature and correction of circulatory or metabolic disturbances. If persistent or life-threatening, appropriate anti-arrhythmic therapy may be considered. Avoid lidocaine (lignocaine) and, as far as possible, long acting anti-arrhythmic drugs.

Pronounced central nervous system depression requires airway maintenance or, in extreme circumstances, assisted respiration. Severe dystonic reactions usually respond to procyclidine (5mg to 10mg) or orphenadrine (20mg to 40mg) administered intramuscularly or intravenously. Convulsions should be treated with intravenous diazepam.

Neuroleptic malignant syndrome should be treated with cooling. Dantrolene sodium may be tried.

5. PHARMACOLOGICAL PROPERTIES

5.1 Pharmacodynamic properties

Levomepromazine resembles chlorpromazine and promethazine in the pattern of its pharmacology. It possesses anti-emetic, antihistamine and anti-adrenaline activity and exhibits a strong sedative effect.

5.2 Pharmacokinetic properties

Maximum serum concentrations are achieved in 2 to 3 hours depending on the route of administration. Excretion is slow, with a half-life of about 30 hours. It is eliminated via urine and faeces.

5.3 Preclinical safety data

There are no pre-clinical safety data of relevance to the prescriber which are additional to those already included in other sections of the Summary of Product Characteristics.

6. PHARMACEUTICAL PARTICULARS

6.1 List of excipients

Potato starch, calcium hydrogen phosphate, magnesium stearate, sodium lauryl sulphate.

6.2 Incompatibilities

Not applicable.

6.3 Shelf life

36 months for blister pack.

60 months for polyethylene or polypropylene containers.

Not all pack sizes may be marketed

6.4 Special precautions for storage

Protect from light.

6.5 Nature and contents of container

PVC/PVdC/aluminium foil blister pack containing 84 tablets.

OR

High density polyethylene bottle with flip cap or polypropylene tablet container. Each pack contains 500 tablets.

Not all pack sizes may be marketed

6.6 Instructions for use and handling

None.

7. MARKETING AUTHORISATION HOLDER

Link Pharmaceuticals Limited, Bishops Weald House, Albion Way, Horsham, West Sussex, RH12 1AH, United Kingdom

8. MARKETING AUTHORISATION NUMBER(S)

PL 12406/0007

9. DATE OF FIRST AUTHORISATION/RENEWAL OF THE AUTHORISATION

12th May 1999 / 11 May 2004

10. DATE OF REVISION OF THE TEXT

February 2004

11. Legal Category

POM

® Nozinan is a registered trade mark

SPC0405

Nuelin Liquid

(3M Health Care Limited)

1. NAME OF THE MEDICINAL PRODUCT

'Nuelin' Liquid

2. QUALITATIVE AND QUANTITATIVE COMPOSITION

Each 5 ml dose of Nuelin Liquid contains the equivalent of 60 mg theophylline hydrate BP as the sodium glycinate salt.

3. PHARMACEUTICAL FORM

Clear, light brown, pleasantly flavoured syrup.

4. CLINICAL PARTICULARS

4.1 Therapeutic indications

Nuelin Liquid is indicated for the prophylaxis and treatment of reversible bronchospasm associated with asthma and chronic obstructive pulmonary disease.

4.2 Posology and method of administration

Adults: 10 to 20 ml three or four times daily, preferably after food.

Children 7 to 12 years: 7.5 to 10 ml three to four times daily, preferably after food.

2 to 6 years: 5 to 7.5 ml three or four times daily, preferably after food.

Nuelin Liquid is not recommended for children under 2 years of age.

Elderly: Elderly patients may require lower doses due to reduced theophylline clearance.

The dosage should be titrated for each individual and adjusted with caution. Serum theophylline levels should be monitored to ensure that they remain within the therapeutic range.

4.3 Contraindications

- Porphyria
- Hypersensitivity to any constituent or to xanthines.
- Concomitant use with ephedrine in children.

4.4 Special warnings and special precautions for use

The patients response to therapy should be carefully monitored. Worsening of asthma symptoms requires urgent medical attention.

Use with caution in patients with cardiac arrhythmias, peptic ulcer, hyperthyroidism and severe hypertension.

Smoking and alcohol consumption may increase theophylline clearance and increased doses of theophylline are therefore required. In patients with cardiac failure, hepatic dysfunction/disease and fever the reverse is true and these patients may require a reduced dosage.

Alternative bronchodilator therapy should be used in patients with a history of seizures.

It is not recommended that the product be used concurrently with other preparations containing xanthine derivatives.

Xanthines can potentiate hypokalaemia resulting from beta-2-agonist therapy, steroids, diuretics and hypoxia. Particular caution is advised in severe asthma. It is recommended that serum potassium levels are monitored in such situations.

4.5 Interaction with other medicinal products and other forms of Interaction

Cimetidine, allopurinol, corticosteroids, frusemide, isoprenaline, oral contraceptives, thiobendazole, ciprofloxacin, erythromycin or other macrolide antibiotics and the calcium channel blockers, diltiazem, verapamil, nizatidine, norfloxacin, isoniazid, fluconazole, carbimazole, mexiletine, propafenone, oxpentifylline, disulfiram, interferon alfa, and influenza vaccine increase plasma theophylline concentrations. A reduction of the theophylline dosage is recommended.

Phenytoin, carbamazepine, barbiturates, lithium, rifampicin, sulphinpyrazone, ritonavir and aminoglutethimide may reduce plasma theophylline concentrations and therefore the theophylline dosage may need to be increased.

The concomitant use of theophylline and fluvoxamine should usually be avoided. Where this is not posssible, patients should have their theophylline dose halved and plasma theophylline should be monitored closely.

Plasma concentrations of theophylline can be reduced by concomitant use of the herbal remedy St John's wort (Hypericum perforatum).

Other interactions:

- β-Blockers: antagonism of bronchodilation.
- Ketamine: reduced convulsive threshold.
- Doxapram: increased CNS stimulation.

4.6 Pregnancy and lactation

Administration of theophylline drugs during pregnancy should only be considered if there is no safe alternative and the benefits of treatment outweigh the risks.

Theophylline is excreted in breast milk and should not therefore be routinely administered to nursing mothers.

4.7 Effects on ability to drive and use machines

No effect.

4.8 Undesirable effects

Nausea or other gastric distress may occur rarely. Palpitations, tachycardia, arrhythmias, convulsions, headache, CNS stimulation and insomnia have been reported occasionally.

4.9 Overdose

Symptoms:

Nausea, vomiting, electrolyte imbalance and gastro-intestinal irritation. Tachycardia and convulsions may also occur.

Treatment:

Gastric lavage and general supportive measures (eg to maintain circulation, respiration and fluid and electrolyte balance) are recommended. Oral activated charcoal may reduce serum theophylline levels, whilst in severe cases charcoal haemoperfusion may be required.

5. PHARMACOLOGICAL PROPERTIES

5.1 Pharmacodynamic properties

Theophylline directly relaxes smooth muscle thus acting mainly as a bronchodilator and vasodilator. The drug also possesses other actions typical of the xanthine derivatives; coronary vasodilator, diuretic, cardiac stimulant, cerebral stimulant and skeletal muscle stimulant.

5.2 Pharmacokinetic properties

It has been established that the xanthines, which include theophylline, are readily absorbed after oral, rectal or parenteral administration and this fact is well documented in published literature.

Theophylline is excreted in the urine as metabolites, mainly 1,3-dimethyluric acid and 3-methylxanthine and about 10% is excreted unchanged.

Plasma half-lives ranging from 3-9 hours and therapeutic plasma concentrations from about 5-20 μg per ml have been reported.

5.3 Preclinical safety data

No remarks

6. PHARMACEUTICAL PARTICULARS

6.1 List of excipients

Glycerol, sucrose, propylene glycol, sodium butyl hydroxybenzoate, apricot essence No. 1 NS, banana flavour (50/211A), caramel (2 stars), purified water.

6.2 Incompatibilities

None known.

6.3 Shelf life

3 years.

6.4 Special precautions for storage

Do not store above 25° C. Do not freeze.

6.5 Nature and contents of container

Bottles of 200 ml, 300 ml and 500 ml.

6.6 Instructions for use and handling

None.

7. MARKETING AUTHORISATION HOLDER

3M Health Care Limited, 3M House, Morley Street, Loughborough, Leics, LE11 1EP

8. MARKETING AUTHORISATION NUMBER(S)

PL 00068/0084

9. DATE OF FIRST AUTHORISATION/RENEWAL OF THE AUTHORISATION

21 February 1978/21 May 1999

10. DATE OF REVISION OF THE TEXT

June 2000

Nuelin SA 175 mg Tablets

(3M Health Care Limited)

1. NAME OF THE MEDICINAL PRODUCT

Nuelin SA 175 mg Tablets

2. QUALITATIVE AND QUANTITATIVE COMPOSITION

Theophylline 175mg

3. PHARMACEUTICAL FORM

Prolonged release tablet

4. CLINICAL PARTICULARS

4.1 Therapeutic indications

Nuelin SA are indicated for the prophylaxis and treatment of reversible bronchospasm associated with asthma and chronic obstructive pulmonary disease.

Because effective plasma levels are maintained for up to twelve hours from a single dose, less frequent dosing is required than with conventional theophylline preparations.

4.2 Posology and method of administration

ADULTS: One tablet twice daily, preferably after food, increasing to two tablets twice daily, if necessary.

CHILDREN: 6 TO 12 YEARS: One tablet twice daily, preferably after food.

ELDERLY: Elderly patients may require lower doses due to reduced theophylline clearance.

Nuelin SA and tablets are not recommended for children under six years.

Nuelin SA tablets should be swallowed whole and not crushed or chewed.

The dosage should be titrated for each individual and adjusted with caution. Serum theophylline levels should be monitored to ensure that they remain within the therapeutic range.

4.3 Contraindications

Porphyria

Hypersensitivity to any constituent or to xanthines.

Concomitant use with ephedrine in children.

4.4 Special warnings and special precautions for use

The patients response to therapy should be carefully monitored. Worsening of asthma symptoms requires urgent medical attention.

Use with caution in patients with cardiac arrhythmias, peptic ulcer, hyperthyroidism, severe hypertension, acute porphyria, hepatic dysfunction, chronic alcoholism, acute febrile illness and chronic lung disease.

Smoking and alcohol consumption may increase theophylline clearance and increased doses of theophylline are therefore required. In patients with cardiac failure, hepatic dysfunction/disease and fever the reverse is true and these patients may require a reduced dosage.

Alternative bronchodilator therapy should be used in patients with a history of seizures.

It is not recommended that the product be used concurrently with other preparations containing xanthine derivatives.

WARNINGS: Xanthines can potentiate hypokalaemia resulting from beta-2-agonist therapy steroids, diuretics and hypoxia. Particular caution is advised in severe asthma. It is recommended that serum potassium levels are monitored in such situations.

PRECAUTIONS: In the case of an acute asthmatic attack in a patient receiving a sustained action theophylline preparation, great caution should be taken when administering intravenous aminophylline. Half the recommended loading dose of aminophylline (generally 6 mg/kg) should be given, i.e. 3 mg/kg, cautiously.

4.5 Interaction with other medicinal products and other forms of Interaction

Cimetidine, allopurinol, corticosteroids, frusemide, isoprenaline, oral contraceptives, thiobendazole, ciprofloxacin, erythromycin or other macrolide antibiotics and the calcium channel blockers, diltiazem and verapamil, nizatidine, norfloxacin, isoniazid, fluconazole, carbimazole, mexiletine, propafenone, oxpentifylline, disulfiram, viloxazine, interferon alfa, and influenza vaccine increase plasma theophylline concentrations. A reduction of the theophylline dosage is recommended.

Phenytoin, carbamazepine, barbiturates, lithium, rifampicin, sulphinpyrazone, ritonavir, primidone and aminoglutethimide may reduce plasma theophylline concentrations and therefore the theophylline dosage may need to be increased.

The concomitant use of theophylline and fluvoxamine should usually be avoided. Where this is not possible, patients should have their theophylline dose halved and plasma theophylline should be monitored closely.

Warnings about the concurrent use of xanthines and xanthine derivatives are shown in Section 4, Special Warnings.

Plasma concentrations of theophylline can be reduced by concomitant use of the herbal remedy St John's wort (Hypericum perforatum).

Other interactions:

β-Blockers: antagonism of bronchodilation.

Ketamine: reduced convulsive threshold.

Doxapram: increased CNS stimulation.

Also see Warnings.

4.6 Pregnancy and lactation

Administration of theophylline drugs during pregnancy should only be considered if there is no safe alternative and the benefits of treatment outweigh the risks.

Theophylline is excreted in breast milk and should not therefore be routinely administered to nursing mothers.

4.7 Effects on ability to drive and use machines

No effect.

4.8 Undesirable effects

The side-effects commonly associated with xanthine derivatives such as nausea, gastric irritation, palpitations, tachycardia, arrhythmias, convulsions, headache, CNS stimulation and insomnia are much diminished when a sustained action preparation such as Nuelin SA is used. These side-effects are mild and infrequent when the plasma concentration is maintained at less than 20 microgrammes/ml.

4.9 Overdose

Over 3 g could be serious in an adult (40 mg/kg in a child). The fatal dose may be as little as 4.5 g in an adult (60 mg/kg in a child), but is generally higher.

Symptoms

Warning: Serious features may develop as long as 12 hours after overdosage with sustained release formulations.

Alimentary features:

Nausea, vomiting (which is often severe), epigastric pain and haematemesis. Consider pancreatitis if abdominal pain persists.

Neurological features:

Restlessness, hypertonia, exaggerated limb reflexes and convulsions. Coma may develop in very severe cases.

Cardiovascular features:

Sinus tachycardia is common. Ectopic beats and supraventricular and ventricular tachycardia may follow.

Metabolic features:

Hypokalaemia due to shift of potassium from plasma into cells is common, can develop rapidly and may be severe. Hyperglycaemia, hypomagnesaemia and metabolic acidosis may also occur. Rhabdomyolysis may also occur.

Management

Activated charcoal or gastric lavage should be considered if a significant overdose has been ingested within 1-2 hours. Repeated doses of activated charcoal given by mouth can enhance theophylline elimination. Measure the plasma potassium concentration urgently, repeat frequently and correct hypokalaemia. BEWARE! If large amounts of potassium have been given, serious hyperkalaemia may develop during recovery. If plasma potassium is low then the plasma magnesium concentration should be measured as soon as possible.

In the treatment of ventricular arrhythmias, proconvulsant antiarrhythmic agents such as lignocaine (lidocaine) should be avoided because of the risk of causing or exacerbating seizures.

Measure the plasma theophylline concentration regularly when severe poisoning is suspected, until concentrations are falling. Vomiting should be treated with an antiemetic such as metoclopramide or ondansetron.

Tachycardia with an adequate cardiac output is best left untreated. Beta-blockers may be given in extreme cases but not if the patient is asthmatic. Control isolated convulsions with intravenous diazepam. Exclude hypokalaemia as a cause.

5. PHARMACOLOGICAL PROPERTIES

5.1 Pharmacodynamic properties

Theophylline directly relaxes smooth muscle thus acting mainly as a bronchodilator and vasodilator. The drug also possesses other action typical of the xanthines derivatives - coronary vasodilator, diuretic, cardiac stimulant, cerebral stimulant and skeletal muscle stimulant.

5.2 Pharmacokinetic properties

It has been established that the xanthines, which include theophylline, are readily absorbed after oral, rectal or parenteral administration and this is well documented in published literature.

Theophylline is excreted in the urine as metabolites, mainly 1,3-dimethyluric acid and 3-methylxanthine, and about 10% is excreted unchanged.

Plasma half-lives ranging from3 to 9 hours and therapeutic plasma concentrations from about 5 to 20 μg per ml have been reported.

5.3 Preclinical safety data

Not applicable

6. PHARMACEUTICAL PARTICULARS

6.1 List of excipients

Lactose Ph Eur

Cellulose Acetate Phthalate Ph Eur

Magnesium Stearate Ph Eur

6.2 Incompatibilities

None known

6.3 Shelf life

3 Years

6.4 Special precautions for storage

Store below 30°C.

6.5 Nature and contents of container

Bottle or Blister packs of 60

6.6 Instructions for use and handling
None

7. MARKETING AUTHORISATION HOLDER
3M Health Care Limited

3M House

Morley Street

Loughborough

Leics

LE11 1EP

8. MARKETING AUTHORISATION NUMBER(S)
00068/0092

9. DATE OF FIRST AUTHORISATION/RENEWAL OF THE AUTHORISATION
22 January 1980/9 March 1995

10. DATE OF REVISION OF THE TEXT
March 2004

Nuelin SA 250 mg Tablets

(3M Health Care Limited)

1. NAME OF THE MEDICINAL PRODUCT
Nuelin SA 250 mg Tablets

2. QUALITATIVE AND QUANTITATIVE COMPOSITION
Theophylline 250mg

3. PHARMACEUTICAL FORM
Prolonged release tablet

4. CLINICAL PARTICULARS

4.1 Therapeutic indications
Nuelin SA are indicated for the prophylaxis and treatment of reversible bronchospasm associated with asthma and chronic obstructive pulmonary disease.

Because effective plasma levels are maintained for up to twelve hours from a single dose, less frequent dosing is required than with conventional theophylline preparations.

4.2 Posology and method of administration
ADULTS: One tablet twice daily, preferably after food, increasing to two tablets twice daily, if necessary.

CHILDREN: 6 TO 12 YEARS: Half to one tablet twice daily, preferably after food.

ELDERLY: Elderly patients may require lower doses due to reduced theophylline clearance.

Nuelin SA-250 are not recommended for children under six years.

Nuelin SA-250 tablets are scored and may be halved but should not be crushed or chewed.

The dosage should be titrated for each individual and adjusted with caution. Serum theophylline levels should be monitored to ensure that they remain within the therapeutic range.

4.3 Contraindications
Porphyria

Hypersensitivity to any constituent or to xanthines.

Concomitant use with ephedrine in children.

4.4 Special warnings and special precautions for use
The patients response to therapy should be carefully monitored. Worsening of asthma symptoms requires urgent medical attention.

Use with caution in patients with cardiac arrhythmias, peptic ulcer, hyperthyroidism, severe hypertension, acute porphyria, hepatic dysfunction, chronic alcoholism, acute febrile illness and chronic lung disease.

Smoking and alcohol consumption may increase theophylline clearance and increased doses of theophylline are therefore required. In patients with cardiac failure, hepatic dysfunction/disease and fever the reverse is true and these patients may require a reduced dosage.

Alternative bronchodilator therapy should be used in patients with a history of seizures.

It is not recommended that the product be used concurrently with other preparations containing xanthine derivatives.

WARNINGS: Xanthines can potentiate hypokalaemia resulting from beta-2-agonist therapy steroids, diuretics and hypoxia. Particular caution is advised in severe asthma. It is recommended that serum potassium levels are monitored in such situations.

PRECAUTIONS: In the case of an acute asthmatic attack in a patient receiving a sustained action theophylline preparation, great caution should be taken when administering intravenous aminophylline. Half the recommended loading dose of aminophylline (generally 6 mg/kg) should be given, ie. 3 mg/kg, cautiously.

4.5 Interaction with other medicinal products and other forms of Interaction
Cimetidine, allopurinol, corticosteroids, frusemide, isoprenaline, oral contraceptives, thiobendazole, ciprofloxacin, erythromycin or other macrolide antibiotics and the calcium channel blockers, diltiazem and verapamil, nizatidine, norfloxacin, isoniazid, fluconazole, carbimazole, mexiletine, propafenone, oxpentifylline, disulfiram, viloxazine, interferon alfa, and influenza vaccine increase plasma theophylline concentrations. A reduction of the theophylline dosage is recommended.

Phenytoin, carbamazepine, barbiturates, lithium, rifampicin, sulphinpyrazone, ritonavir, primidone and aminoglutethimide may reduce plasma theophylline concentrations and therefore the theophylline dosage may need to be increased.

The concomitant use of theophylline and fluvoxamine should usually be avoided. Where this is not possible, patients should have their theophylline dose halved and plasma theophylline should be monitored closely.

Warnings about the concurrent use of xanthines and xanthine derivatives are shown in Section 4, Special Warnings.

Plasma concentrations of theophylline can be reduced by concomitant use of the herbal remedy St John's wort (Hypericum perforatum).

Other interactions:

β-Blockers: antagonism of bronchodilation.

Ketamine: reduced convulsive threshold.

Doxapram: increased CNS stimulation.

Also see Warnings.

4.6 Pregnancy and lactation
Administration of theophylline drugs during pregnancy should only be considered if there is no safe alternative and the benefits of treatment outweigh the risks.

Theophylline is excreted in breast milk and should not therefore be routinely administered to nursing mothers.

4.7 Effects on ability to drive and use machines
No effect.

4.8 Undesirable effects
The side-effects commonly associated with xanthine derivatives such as nausea, gastric irritation, palpitations, tachycardia, arrhythmias, convulsions, headache, CNS stimulation and insomnia are much diminished when a sustained action preparation such as Nuelin SA is used. These side-effects are mild and infrequent when the plasma concentration is maintained at less than 20 microgrammes/ml.

4.9 Overdose
Over 3 g could be serious in an adult (40 mg/kg in a child). The fatal dose may be as little as 4.5 g in an adult (60 mg/kg in a child), but is generally higher.

Symptoms
Warning: Serious features may develop as long as 12 hours after overdosage with sustained release formulations.

Alimentary features:

Nausea, vomiting (which is often severe), epigastric pain and haematemesis. Consider pancreatitis if abdominal pain persists.

Neurological features:

Restlessness, hypertonia, exaggerated limb reflexes and convulsions. Coma may develop in very severe cases.

Cardiovascular features:

Sinus tachycardia is common. Ectopic beats and supraventricular and ventricular tachycardia may follow.

Metabolic features:

Hypokalaemia due to shift of potassium from plasma into cells is common, can develop rapidly and may be severe. Hyperglycaemia, hypomagnesaemia and metabolic acidosis may also occur. Rhabdomyolysis may also occur.

Management
Activated charcoal or gastric lavage should be considered if a significant overdose has been ingested within 1-2 hours. Repeated doses of activated charcoal given by mouth can enhance theophylline elimination. Measure the plasma potassium concentration urgently, repeat frequently and correct hypokalaemia. BEWARE! If large amounts of potassium have been given, serious hyperkalaemia may develop during recovery. If plasma potassium is low then the plasma magnesium concentration should be measured as soon as possible.

In the treatment of ventricular arrhythmias, proconvulsant antiarrhythmic agents such as lignocaine (lidocaine) should be avoided because of the risk of causing or exacerbating seizures.

Measure the plasma theophylline concentration regularly when severe poisoning is suspected, until concentrations are falling. Vomiting should be treated with an antiemetic such as metoclopramide or ondansetron.

Tachycardia with an adequate cardiac output is best left untreated. Beta-blockers may be given in extreme cases but not if the patient is asthmatic. Control isolated convulsions with intravenous diazepam. Exclude hypokalaemia as a cause.

5. PHARMACOLOGICAL PROPERTIES

5.1 Pharmacodynamic properties
Theophylline directly relaxes smooth muscle thus acting mainly as a bronchodilator and vasodilator. The drug also possesses other action typical of the xanthines derivatives - coronary vasodilator, diuretic, cardiac stimulant, cerebral stimulant and skeletal muscle stimulant.

5.2 Pharmacokinetic properties
It has been established that the xanthines, which include theophylline, are readily absorbed after oral, rectal or parenteral administration and this is well documented in published literature.

Theophylline is excreted in the urine as metabolites, mainly 1,3-dimethyluric acid and 3-methylxanthine, and about 10% is excreted unchanged.

Plasma half-lives ranging from3 to 9 hours and therapeutic plasma concentrations from about 5 to 20 μg per ml have been reported.

5.3 Preclinical safety data
Not applicable

6. PHARMACEUTICAL PARTICULARS

6.1 List of excipients
Lactose Ph Eur

Cellulose Acetate Phthalate Ph Eur

Magnesium Stearate Ph Eur

6.2 Incompatibilities
None known

6.3 Shelf life
3 Years

6.4 Special precautions for storage
Store below 30°C.

6.5 Nature and contents of container
Bottle or Blister packs of 60

6.6 Instructions for use and handling
None

7. MARKETING AUTHORISATION HOLDER
3M Health Care Limited

3M House

Morley Street

Loughborough

Leics

LE11 1EP

8. MARKETING AUTHORISATION NUMBER(S)
00068/0093

9. DATE OF FIRST AUTHORISATION/RENEWAL OF THE AUTHORISATION
22 January 1980/9 March 1995

10. DATE OF REVISION OF THE TEXT
March 2004

Nu-Seals 300

(Alliance Pharmaceuticals)

1. NAME OF THE MEDICINAL PRODUCT
Nu-Seals 300

Aspirin 300mg Enteric Coated

2. QUALITATIVE AND QUANTITATIVE COMPOSITION
Acetylsalicylic Acid 300mg

3. PHARMACEUTICAL FORM
White, enteric coated tablets, coded "300" in red or "GP" in black

4. CLINICAL PARTICULARS

4.1 Therapeutic indications
Aspirin has analgesic, antipyretic and anti-inflammatory actions. It can also be used for the secondary prevention of thrombotic cerebrovascular or cardiovascular disease and following by-pass surgery (see below).

Aspirin has an anti-thrombotic action, mediated through inhibition of platelet activation, which has been shown to be useful in secondary prophylaxis following myocardial infarction, and in patients with unstable angina or ischaemic stroke including cerebral transient attacks.

Nu-Seals 300 is indicated wherever high and prolonged dosage of aspirin is required. The special coating resists dissolution in gastric juice, but will dissolve readily in the relatively less acid environment of the duo-denum. Owing to the delay that the coating imposes on the release of the active ingredient, Nu-Seals 300 is unsuitable for the short-term relief of pain.

4.2 Posology and method of administration
Nu-Seals 300 is for oral administration to adults only.

Analgesic, antipyretic and anti-inflammatory actions: The usual dose of aspirin is 300-900mg repeated three to four times daily according to clinical needs. In acute rheumatic disorders the dose is in the range of 4-8 g daily, taken in divided doses.

Antithrombotic action: Patients should seek the advice of a doctor before commencing therapy for the first time. The usual dosage, for long-term use following myocardial infarction, transient ischaemic attack, or in patients with unstable angina, is 75-150mg once daily. In some circumstances a higher dose may be appropriate, especially in the short term, and up to 300mg a day may be used on the advice of a doctor.

The elderly: *Analgesic, antipyretic and anti-inflammatory actions*: As for adults. The elderly are more likely to experience gastric side-effects and tinnitus. *Antithrombotic action:* The risk-benefit ratio has not been fully established.

Children: Do not give to children aged under 16 years, unless specifically indicated (e.g. for Kawasaki's disease). See 'Special Warnings and Special Precautions for Use'.

4.3 Contraindications
Hypersensitivity to aspirin. Hypoprothrombinaemia, haemophilia and active peptic ulceration or a history of peptic ulceration.

4.4 Special warnings and special precautions for use
There is a possible association between aspirin and Reye's syndrome when given to children. Reye's syndrome is a very rare disease, which affects the brain and liver, and can be fatal. For this reason aspirin should not be given to children aged under 16 years unless specifically indicated (e.g. for Kawasaki's disease).

Before commencing long-term aspirin therapy for the management of cerebrovascular or cardiovascular disease patients should consult their doctor who can advise on the relative benefits versus the risks for the individual patient.

Salicylates should be used with caution in patients with a history of peptic ulceration or coagulation abnormalities. They may also induce gastro-intestinal haemorrhage, occasionally major.

They may also precipitate bronchospasm or induce attacks of asthma in susceptible subjects.

Aspirin should be used with caution in patients with impaired renal function (avoid if severe), or in patients who are dehydrated.

Patients with hypertension should be carefully monitored.

4.5 Interaction with other medicinal products and other forms of Interaction
Salicylates may enhance the effect of anticoagulants, oral hypoglycaemic agents, phenytoin and sodium valproate. They inhibit the uricosuric effect of probenecid and may increase the toxicity of sulphonamides.

In large doses, salicylates may also decrease insulin requirements.

Patients using enteric coated aspirin should be advised against ingesting antacids simultaneously to avoid premature drug release.

4.6 Pregnancy and lactation
Usage in pregnancy: Aspirin does not appear to have teratogenic effects. However, prolonged pregnancy and labour, with increased bleeding before and after delivery, decreased birth weight and increased rate of stillbirth were reported with high blood salicylate levels. Aspirin should be avoided during the last 3 months of pregnancy.

Usage in nursing mothers: As aspirin is excreted in breast milk, Nu-Seals 300 should not be taken by patients who are breast-feeding.

4.7 Effects on ability to drive and use machines
None known.

4.8 Undesirable effects
Salicylates may induce hypersensitivity, asthma, bronchospasm, urate kidney stones, chronic gastro-intestinal blood loss, tinnitus, nausea and vomiting. The special coating of Nu-Seals 300 helps to reduce the incidence of side-effects resulting from gastric irritation.

4.9 Overdose
Overdosage produces dizziness, tinnitus, sweating, nausea and vomiting, confusion and hyperventilation. Gross overdosage may lead to CNS depres-sion with coma, cardiovascular collapse and respiratory depression. If overdosage is suspected, the patient should be kept under observation for at least 24 hours, as symptoms and salicylate blood levels may not become apparent for several hours. Treatment of overdosage consists of gastric lavage and forced alkaline diuresis. Haemodialysis may be necessary in severe cases.

5. PHARMACOLOGICAL PROPERTIES

5.1 Pharmacodynamic properties
Aspirin has analgesic, antipyretic and anti-inflammatory actions.

It also has antithrombotic action, which is mediated through inhibition of platelet activation.

Nu-Seals 300 tablets have an enteric coat sandwiched between a sealing coat and a top coat. The enteric coat is intended to resist gastric fluid whilst allowing disintegration in the intestinal fluid.

Owing to the delay that the coating imposes on the release of the active ingredient, Nu-Seals 300 is unsuitable for the short-term relief of pain.

5.2 Pharmacokinetic properties
In a bioequivalence study comparing the pharmacokinetics of the 300mg product with 4 × 75mg presentation in human volunteers, measures such as terminal phase half-life, area-under-the curve and peak plasma concentrations were recorded on days 1 and 4. On day 1 salicylate reached a peak plasma concentration of between 10.34 and 31.57 mcg/ml and between 11.76 and 27.47mcg/ml for the 300mg and 75mg tablets respectively. Time to peak concentration ranged from 4 to 8 hours and from 3 to 6 hours respectively. AUC ranged from 54.0 to 131.2 and from 64.3 to 137.6 h.mcg/ml respectively. The terminal phase half-life ranged from 1.33 to 2.63 hours and from 1.47 to 2.59 hours respectively. On day 4 C_{max} varied from 15.01 to 48.97 mcg/ml for the 300mg tablet and from 11.26 to 60.21 mcg/ml for 4 × 75mg tablets. T_{max} ranged from 4 to 8 hours and from 3 to 8 hours, whilst AUC ranged from 89.8 to 297.4 h.mcg/ml and from 61.5 to 293.4 h.mcg/ml respectively.

5.3 Preclinical safety data
There are no pre-clinical data of relevance to the prescriber in addition to that summarised in other sections of the Summary of Product Characteristics.

6. PHARMACEUTICAL PARTICULARS

6.1 List of excipients
Maize Starch

Hypromellose

Talc

Methacrylic acid – ethyl acrylate (1:1) copolymer dispersion 30 per cent

Polyethylene Glycol 3350

Propylene Glycol

Benzyl Alcohol

Emulsion silicone

Edible Printing Ink – containing either: E124 Red and Shellac or: E172 Black, Shellac and E322 Lecithin

6.2 Incompatibilities
None

6.3 Shelf life
2 years

6.4 Special precautions for storage
Do not store above 25°C. Keep containers tightly closed.

6.5 Nature and contents of container
HDPE bottles with screw caps containing 14, 56, 100 or 500 tablets.

6.6 Instructions for use and handling
None

7. MARKETING AUTHORISATION HOLDER
Alliance Pharmaceuticals Ltd

Avonbridge House

Bath Road

Chippenham

Wiltshire

SN15 2BB

8. MARKETING AUTHORISATION NUMBER(S)
PL 16853/0063

9. DATE OF FIRST AUTHORISATION/RENEWAL OF THE AUTHORISATION
Date of first authorisation:22 May 1973

Date of last renewal of authorisation: 04 April 2000

10. DATE OF REVISION OF THE TEXT
November 2003

Nu-Seals 75

(Alliance Pharmaceuticals)

1. NAME OF THE MEDICINAL PRODUCT
Nu-Seals 75, Aspirin 75mg Enteric Coated Tablets, PostMI 75EC, Nu-seals Cardio 75

2. QUALITATIVE AND QUANTITATIVE COMPOSITION
Acetylsalicylic Acid 75mg

3. PHARMACEUTICAL FORM
White, enteric coated tablets, coded "75" or "GP".

4. CLINICAL PARTICULARS

4.1 Therapeutic indications
For the secondary prevention of thrombotic cerebrovascular or cardiovascular disease and following by-pass surgery (see below).

Aspirin has an antithrombotic action, mediated through inhibition of platelet activation, which has been shown to be useful in secondary prophylaxis following myocardial infarction and in patients with unstable angina or ischaemic stroke including cerebral transient attacks.

Nuseals 75 is indicated when prolonged dosage of aspirin is required. The special coating resists dissolution in gastric juice, but will dissolve readily in the relatively less acid environment of the duodenum. Owing to the delay that the coating imposes on the release of the active ingredient, Nuseals 75 is unsuitable for the short-term relief of pain.

4.2 Posology and method of administration
Nuseals 75 is for oral administration to adults only.

Patients should seek the advice of a doctor before commencing therapy for the first time.

The usual dosage, for long-term use, is 75-150mg once daily. In some circumstances a higher dose may be appropriate, especially in the short term, and up to 300mg a day may be used on the advice of a doctor.

Antithrombotic action: 150mg at diagnosis and 75mg daily thereafter. Tablets taken at diagnosis should be chewed in order to gain rapid absorption.

The elderly: The risk-benefit ratio of the antithrombotic action of aspirin has not been fully established.

Children:

Do not give to children aged under 16 years, unless specifically indicated (e.g. for Kawasaki's disease). See 'Special Warnings and Special Precautions for Use'.

4.3 Contraindications
Hypersensitivity to aspirin. Hypoprothrombinaemia, haemophilia and active peptic ulceration or a history of peptic ulceration.

4.4 Special warnings and special precautions for use
There is a possible association between aspirin and Reye's syndrome when given to children. Reye's syndrome is a very rare disease, which affects the brain and liver, and can be fatal. For this reason aspirin should not be given to children aged under 16 years unless specifically indicated (e.g. for Kawasaki's disease).

Before commencing long-term aspirin therapy for the management of cerebrovascular or cardiovascular disease patients should consult their doctor who can advise on the relative benefits versus the risks for the individual patient.

Salicylates should be used with caution in patients with a history of peptic ulceration or coagulation abnormalities. They may also induce gastro-intestinal haemorrhage, occasionally major.

They may also precipitate bronchospasm or induce attacks of asthma in susceptible subjects.

Aspirin should be used with caution in patients with impaired renal function (avoid if severe), or in patients who are dehydrated.

Patients with hypertension should be carefully monitored.

4.5 Interaction with other medicinal products and other forms of Interaction
Salicylates may enhance the effect of anticoagulants, oral hypoglycaemic agents, phenytoin and sodium valproate. They inhibit the uricosuric effect of probenecid and may increase the toxicity of sulphonamides.

In large doses, salicylates may also decrease insulin requirements.

Patients using enteric coated aspirin should be advised against ingesting antacids simultaneously to avoid premature drug release.

4.6 Pregnancy and lactation
Usage in pregnancy: Aspirin does not appear to have teratogenic effects. However, prolonged pregnancy and labour, with increased bleeding before and after delivery, decreased birth weight and increased rate of stillbirth were reported with high blood salicylate levels. Aspirin should be avoided during the last 3 months of pregnancy.

Usage in nursing mothers: As aspirin is excreted in breast milk, Nu-Seals 75 should not be taken by patients who are breast-feeding.

4.7 Effects on ability to drive and use machines
None known.

4.8 Undesirable effects
Salicylates may induce hypersensitivity, asthma, bronchospasm, urate kidney stones, chronic gastro-intestinal blood loss, tinnitus, nausea and vomiting.

4.9 Overdose
Overdosage produces dizziness, tinnitus, sweating, nausea and vomiting, confusion and hyperventilation. Gross overdosage may lead to CNS depres-sion with coma, cardiovascular collapse and respiratory depression. If overdosage is suspected, the patient should be kept under observation for at least 24 hours, as symptoms and salicylate blood levels may not become apparent for several hours. Treatment of overdosage consists of gastric lavage and forced alkaline diuresis. Haemodialysis may be necessary in severe cases.

5. PHARMACOLOGICAL PROPERTIES

5.1 Pharmacodynamic properties
Aspirin has analgesic, antipyretic and anti-inflammatory actions.

It also has antithrombotic action which is mediated through inhibition of platelet activation.

Nu-Seals 75 tablets have an enteric coat sandwiched between a sealing coat and a top coat. The enteric coat is intended to resist gastric fluid whilst allowing disintegration in the intestinal fluid.

Owing to the delay that the coating imposes on the release of the active ingredient, Nu-Seals 75 is unsuitable for the short-term relief of pain.

5.2 Pharmacokinetic properties
In a bioequivalence study comparing the pharmacokinetics of the 300mg product with 4 × 75mg presentation in human volunteers, measures such as terminal phase half-life, area-under-the curve and peak plasma concentrations were recorded on days 1 and 4. On day 1 salicylate reached a peak plasma concentration of between 10.34

and 31.57 mcg/ml and between 11.76 and 27.47mcg/ml for the 300mg and 75mg tablets respectively. Time to peak concentration ranged from 4 to 8 hours and from 3 to 6 hours respectively. AUC ranged from 54.0 to 131.2 and from 64.3 to 137.6 h.mcg/ml respectively. The terminal phase half-life ranged from 1.33 to 2.63 hours and from 1.47 to 2.59 hours respectively. On day 4 C_{max} varied from 15.01 to 48.97 mcg/ml for the 300mg tablet and from 11.26 to 60.21 mcg/ml for 4 × 75mg tablets. T_{max} ranged from 4 to 8 hours and from 3 to 8 hours, whilst AUC ranged from 89.8 to 297.4 h.mcg/ml and from 61.5 to 293.4 h.mcg/ml respectively.

5.3 Preclinical safety data
There are no pre-clinical data of relevance to the prescriber in addition to that summarised in other sections of the Summary of Product Characteristics.

6. PHARMACEUTICAL PARTICULARS

6.1 List of excipients
Maize Starch

Hypromellose

Talc

Methacrylic acid – ethyl acrylate (1:1) copolymer dispersion 30 per cent

Polyethylene Glycol 3350

Propylene Glycol

Benzyl Alcohol

Emulsion silicone

Edible Printing Ink - containing either: E124 Red and Shellac or: E172 Black, Shellac and E322 Lecithin

6.2 Incompatibilities
None known.

6.3 Shelf life
2 years.

6.4 Special precautions for storage
Do not store above 25°C. Keep containers tightly closed.

6.5 Nature and contents of container
Blisters comprising of UPVC on one side and aluminium foil on the other containing 14, 28, 56 or 84 tablets. HDPE bottles with screw caps containing 500 tablets.

6.6 Instructions for use and handling
None.

7. MARKETING AUTHORISATION HOLDER
Alliance Pharmaceuticals Ltd

Avonbridge House

Bath Road

Chippenham

Wiltshire

SN15 2BB

8. MARKETING AUTHORISATION NUMBER(S)
PL 16853/0062

9. DATE OF FIRST AUTHORISATION/RENEWAL OF THE AUTHORISATION
Date of first authorisation: 21 April 1994

Date of last renewal of authorisation: 05 April 2000

10. DATE OF REVISION OF THE TEXT
February 2004.

Nutraplus Cream

(Galderma (U.K.) Ltd)

1. NAME OF THE MEDICINAL PRODUCT
Nutraplus Cream

2. QUALITATIVE AND QUANTITATIVE COMPOSITION
Urea 10% w/w

For excipients see section 6.1

3. PHARMACEUTICAL FORM
Cream

Smooth white, almost odourless cream (water in oil emulsion).

4. CLINICAL PARTICULARS

4.1 Therapeutic indications
An emollient, moisturising and protective cream for the treatment of dry or damaged skin.

4.2 Posology and method of administration
Adults, elderly and children

Apply evenly to the dry skin areas two to three times daily, or as directed by the physician or pharmacist.

4.3 Contraindications
None

4.4 Special warnings and special precautions for use
Avoid contact with the eyes. If irritation occurs, discontinue use temporarily.

4.5 Interaction with other medicinal products and other forms of Interaction
None known

4.6 Pregnancy and lactation
No known effects. Use at the discretion of the physician or pharmacist.

4.7 Effects on ability to drive and use machines
Not applicable.

4.8 Undesirable effects
None known.

4.9 Overdose
Not applicable

5. PHARMACOLOGICAL PROPERTIES

5.1 Pharmacodynamic properties
Urea is a recognised hydrating agent that has been widely used topically to treat dry or damaged skin.

5.2 Pharmacokinetic properties
Not applicable. Nutraplus is a topical (cutaneous) preparation.

5.3 Preclinical safety data
No specific information is presented given the widespread use of topically applied urea on humans over many years.

6. PHARMACEUTICAL PARTICULARS

6.1 List of excipients
Glycerol monostearate

Octyl palmitate

Myristyl lactate

Mineral oil

Promulgen D (contains Cetearyl alcohol and ceteareth-20)

Propylene glycol

Propyl parahydroxybenzoate (E216)

Methyl parahydroxybenzoate (E218)

Purified water

6.2 Incompatibilities
None known.

6.3 Shelf life
Thirty six months.

6.4 Special precautions for storage
Do not store above 25°C.

As with all medicines, Nutraplus Cream should be stored out of the sight and reach of children.

6.5 Nature and contents of container
White, polyethylene tube with a white polypropylene screw cap as the closure.

Pack size: 100g

6.6 Instructions for use and handling
No special instructions.

7. MARKETING AUTHORISATION HOLDER
Galderma (UK) Limited

Galderma House

Church Lane

Kings Langley

Hertfordshire, WD4 8JP

England

8. MARKETING AUTHORISATION NUMBER(S)
PL 10590/0002

9. DATE OF FIRST AUTHORISATION/RENEWAL OF THE AUTHORISATION
4 June 1991

10. DATE OF REVISION OF THE TEXT
September 2001

Nutrizym 10

(Merck Pharmaceuticals)

1. NAME OF THE MEDICINAL PRODUCT
Nutrizym 10

2. QUALITATIVE AND QUANTITATIVE COMPOSITION
Each capsule contains Pancreatin BP 155mg with not less than the following activities. Lipase 10,000 BP Units, Protease 500 BP Units and Amylase 9000 BP Units.

3. PHARMACEUTICAL FORM
Hard gelatin capsule containing enteric coated pancreatin minitablets for oral administration.

4. CLINICAL PARTICULARS

4.1 Therapeutic indications
For the symptomatic relief of pancreatic exocrine insufficiency such as in fibrocystic disease of the pancreas and chronic pancreatitis.

4.2 Posology and method of administration
Adults (including the elderly) and children:

1-2 capsules with meals and 1 capsule with snacks.

Since the individual response to pancreatin supplements is variable, the number of capsules taken may need to be titrated to the individual according to symptoms and at the discretion of the physician. Dose increase, if required should be added slowly with careful monitoring of response and symptomatology.

Colonic damage has been reported in patients with cystic fibrosis taking in excess of 10,000 units of lipase/kg/day. The dose of Nutrizym 10 should usually not exceed this dose.

Capsules should be swallowed whole with water. Where swallowing of capsules proves to be difficult, the minitablets may be removed and taken with water or mixed with a small amount of soft food and swallowed immediately without chewing.

Adequate patient hydration should be ensured at all times whilst treating with Nutrizym 10.

4.3 Contraindications
Known hypersensitivity to the active ingredient (porcine pancreatin) or any of the excipients.

4.4 Special warnings and special precautions for use
Hyperuricaemia and hyperuricosuria have been reported to occur in cystic fibrosis patients; pancreatin extracts contain a small amount of purine which might, in high doses, contribute to this condition.

4.5 Interaction with other medicinal products and other forms of Interaction
None known.

4.6 Pregnancy and lactation
Safety has not been established and animal toxicological studies are lacking, therefore the use of Nutrizym 10 capsules is not recommended.

4.7 Effects on ability to drive and use machines
Not known.

4.8 Undesirable effects
Hypersensitivity reactions may occur. As with any pancreatin extract, high doses may cause buccal and perianal irritation, in some cases resulting in inflammation.

Stricture of the ileo-caecum and large bowel, and colitis have been reported in children with cystic fibrosis taking pancreatic enzymes. Abdominal symptoms (those not usually experienced by the patient) or changes in abdominal symptoms should be reviewed to exclude the possibility of colonic damage - especially if the patient is taking in excess of 10,000 units of lipase/kg/day.

4.9 Overdose
Inappropriately large doses could result in abdominal discomfort, nausea, vomiting and perianal irritation or inflammation.

5. PHARMACOLOGICAL PROPERTIES

5.1 Pharmacodynamic properties
The active ingredient is a preparation of porcine pancreas with lipase, amylase and protease activity. Lipase enzymes hydrolyse fats to glycerol and fatty acids. Amylase converts starch into dextrins and sugars and protease enzymes change proteins into proteoses and derived substances.

5.2 Pharmacokinetic properties
The active ingredient of Nutrizym 10 is pancreatin which is a substance involved in the digestive process. During the enzymatic degradation of food substances the enzymes themselves are degraded. Any breakdown products are those that would be expected to appear following normal digestion.

5.3 Preclinical safety data
Preclinical data are not available.

6. PHARMACEUTICAL PARTICULARS

6.1 List of excipients
Uncoated minitablets:

Castor Oil (hydrogenated)

Silicon dioxide, colloidal

Magnesium stearate

Sodium carboxymethylcellulose

Microcrystalline cellulose

Minitablet coating:

Simethicone emulsion

Methacrylic acid copolymer, type C (Eudragit L30D)

Talc

Triethyl citrate

Gelatin capsules:

Titanium dioxide

Iron oxide, red

Iron oxide, yellow

Gelatin

6.2 Incompatibilities
Not known.

6.3 Shelf life
Two years.

6.4 Special precautions for storage
Store below 25 degree C in tightly closed containers.

6.5 Nature and contents of container
Polyethylene or polypropylene containers with polyethylene tamper evident closures containing 50, 100, 200 or 500 capsules.

6.6 Instructions for use and handling
Not relevant.

7. MARKETING AUTHORISATION HOLDER
E Merck Ltd trading as

Merck Pharmaceuticals

(A Division of Merck Ltd)

Harrier House

High Street

West Drayton

Middlesex

UB7 7QG

8. MARKETING AUTHORISATION NUMBER(S)
PL 00493/0157

9. DATE OF FIRST AUTHORISATION/RENEWAL OF THE AUTHORISATION
17 August 1992

10. DATE OF REVISION OF THE TEXT
16 July 1997

LEGAL CATEGORY
P

Nutrizym 22

(Merck Pharmaceuticals)

1. NAME OF THE MEDICINAL PRODUCT
Nutrizym 22

2. QUALITATIVE AND QUANTITATIVE COMPOSITION
Each capsule contains Pancreatin BP 340mg with not less than the following activities. Lipase 22,000 BP Units, Protease 1,100 BP Units and Amylase 19,800 BP Units.

3. PHARMACEUTICAL FORM
Hard gelatin capsule containing enteric coated pancreatin minitablets for oral administration.

4. CLINICAL PARTICULARS

4.1 Therapeutic indications
For the symptomatic relief of pancreatic exocrine insufficiency such as in fibrocystic disease of the pancreas and chronic pancreatitis.

4.2 Posology and method of administration
Adults (including the elderly) and children:

1-2 capsules with meals and 1 capsule with snacks.

Since the individual response to pancreatin supplements is variable, the number of capsules taken may need to be titrated to the individual according to symptoms and at the discretion of the physician. Dose increase, if required should be added slowly with careful monitoring of response and symptomatology.

Colonic damage has been reported in patients with cystic fibrosis taking in excess of 10,000 units of lipase/kg/day. The dose of Nutrizym 22 should usually not exceed this dose.

Where a patient is already receiving a lower unit dose enteric coated pancreatic supplement, then Nutrizym 22 may be substituted at 1/2 of the number of capsules normally consumed with the previous preparation.

Capsules should be swallowed whole with water. Where swallowing of capsules proves to be difficult, the minitablets may be removed and taken with water or mixed with a small amount of soft food and swallowed immediately without chewing.

Adequate patient hydration should be ensured at all times whilst treating with Nutrizym 22.

4.3 Contraindications
In children aged 15 years and under with cystic fibrosis. Known hypersensitivity to the active ingredient (porcine pancreatin) or any of the excipients.

4.4 Special warnings and special precautions for use
Hyperuricaemia and hyperuricosuria have been reported to occur in cystic fibrosis patients; pancreatin extracts contain a small amount of purine which might, in high doses, contribute to this condition.

4.5 Interaction with other medicinal products and other forms of Interaction
None known.

4.6 Pregnancy and lactation
Safety has not been established and animal toxicological studies are lacking, therefore the use of Nutrizym 22 capsules is not recommended.

4.7 Effects on ability to drive and use machines
Not known.

4.8 Undesirable effects
Hypersensitivity reactions may occur. As with any pancreatin extract, high doses may cause buccal and perianal irritation, in some cases resulting in inflammation.

Stricture of the ileo-caecum and large bowel, and colitis have been reported in children with cystic fibrosis taking Nutrizym 22. Abdominal symptoms (those not usually experienced by the patient) or changes in abdominal symptoms should be reviewed to exclude the possibility of colonic damage - especially if the patient is taking in excess of 10,000 units of lipase/kg/day.

4.9 Overdose
Inappropriately large doses could result in abdominal discomfort, nausea, vomiting and perianal irritation or inflammation.

5. PHARMACOLOGICAL PROPERTIES

5.1 Pharmacodynamic properties
The active ingredient is a preparation of porcine pancreas with lipase, amylase and protease activity. Lipase enzymes hydrolyse fats to glycerol and fatty acids. Amylase converts starch into dextrins and sugars and protease enzymes change proteins into proteoses and derived substances.

5.2 Pharmacokinetic properties
The active ingredient of Nutrizym 22 is pancreatin which is a substance involved in the digestive process. During the enzymatic degradation of food substances the enzymes themselves are degraded. Any breakdown products are those that would be expected to appear following normal digestion.

5.3 Preclinical safety data
Preclinical data are not available.

6. PHARMACEUTICAL PARTICULARS

6.1 List of excipients
Uncoated minitablets:

Castor Oil (hydrogenated)

Silicon dioxide, colloidal

Magnesium stearate

Sodium carboxymethylcellulose

Microcrystalline cellulose

Minitablet coating:

Simethicone emulsion

Methacrylic acid copolymer, type C (Eudragit L30D)

Talc

Triethyl citrate

Gelatin capsules:

Titanium dioxide

Iron oxide, red

Iron oxide, yellow

Gelatin

6.2 Incompatibilities
Not known.

6.3 Shelf life
Two years.

6.4 Special precautions for storage
Store below 25 degree C in tightly closed containers.

6.5 Nature and contents of container
Polyethylene or polypropylene containers with polyethylene tamper evident closures containing 50, 100, 200 or 500 capsules.

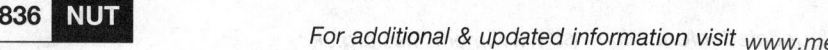

6.6 Instructions for use and handling
Not relevant.

7. MARKETING AUTHORISATION HOLDER
E Merck Ltd trading as

Merck Pharmaceuticals

(A Division of Merck Ltd)

Harrier House

High Street

West Drayton

Middlesex

UB7 7QG

8. MARKETING AUTHORISATION NUMBER(S)
PL 00493/0158

9. DATE OF FIRST AUTHORISATION/RENEWAL OF THE AUTHORISATION
17 August 1992 / 15 October 1997

10. DATE OF REVISION OF THE TEXT
13 August 2002

LEGAL CATEGORY
POM

NutropinAq 10mg/2ml

(Ipsen Ltd)

1. NAME OF THE MEDICINAL PRODUCT
NutropinAq 10 mg/2 ml solution for injection in a cartridge

2. QUALITATIVE AND QUANTITATIVE COMPOSITION
One cartridge contains 10 mg (30 IU) of somatropin, recombinant DNA origin, *Escherichia coli*. For excipients, see 6.1.

3. PHARMACEUTICAL FORM
Solution for injection in a cartridge.

4. CLINICAL PARTICULARS

4.1 Therapeutic indications
- Long-term treatment of children with growth failure due to inadequate endogenous growth hormone secretion,

- Long-term treatment of growth failure associated with Turner syndrome,

- Treatment of prepubertal children with growth failure associated with chronic renal insufficiency up to the time of renal transplantation,

- Replacement of endogenous growth hormone in adults with growth hormone deficiency of either childhood or adult-onset etiology. Growth hormone deficiency should be confirmed appropriately prior to treatment (see 4.4 Special warnings and special precautions for use).

4.2 Posology and method of administration
The diagnosis and management of somatropin therapy should be initiated and monitored by adequately experienced physicians.

The NutropinAq dosage and administration schedule should be individualised for each patient.

Dosage

Growth failure in children due to inadequate growth hormone secretion:

0.025 - 0.035 mg/kg bodyweight given as a daily subcutaneous injection.

Growth failure associated with Turner syndrome:

Up to 0.05 mg/kg bodyweight given as a daily subcutaneous injection.

Growth failure associated with chronic renal insufficiency:

Up to 0.05 mg/kg bodyweight given as a daily subcutaneous injection.

Somatropin therapy may be continued up to the time of renal transplantation.

Growth hormone deficiency in adults:

At the start of somatropin therapy, low initial doses of 0.15 - 0.3 mg are recommended, given as a daily subcutaneous injection. The dose should be adjusted stepwise, controlled by serum Insulin-Like Growth Factor-1 (IGF-1) values. The recommended final dose seldom exceeds 1.0 mg/day. In general, the lowest efficacious dose should be administered. In older or overweight patients, lower doses may be necessary.

Administration

The solution for injection should be administered subcutaneously each day. The site of injection should be changed.

4.3 Contraindications
Hypersensitivity to somatropin or to any of the excipients.

Somatropin should not be used for growth promotion in patients with closed epiphyses.

Growth hormone should not be used in patients with active neoplasm. NutropinAq therapy should be discontinued if evidence of tumour growth develops.

Growth hormone should not be initiated to treat patients with acute critical illness due to complications following open-heart or abdominal surgery, multiple accidental traumas or to treat patients having acute respiratory failure.

4.4 Special warnings and special precautions for use
In adults with growth hormone deficiency the diagnosis should be established depending on the etiology:

Adult-onset: The patient must have growth hormone deficiency as a result of hypothalamic or pituitary disease, and at least one other hormone deficiency diagnosed (except for prolactin). Test for growth hormone deficiency should not be performed until adequate replacement therapy for other hormone deficiencies have been instituted.

Childhood-onset: Patients who have had growth hormone deficiency as a child should be retested to confirm growth hormone deficiency in adulthood before replacement therapy with NutropinAq is started.

In patients with previous malignant disease, special attention should be given to signs and symptoms of relapse.

Patients with a history of an intracranial lesion should be examined frequently for progression or recurrence of the lesion.

NutropinAq is not indicated for the long term treatment of paediatric patients who have growth failure due to genetically confirmed Prader-Willi syndrome, unless they also have a diagnosis of growth hormone deficiency. There have been reports of sleep apnoea and sudden death after initiating therapy with growth hormone in paediatric patients with Prader-Willi syndrome who had one or more of the following risk factors: severe obesity, history of upper airway obstruction or sleep apnoea, or unidentified respiratory infection.

The effects of growth hormone on recovery were studied in two placebo-controlled clinical trials involving 522 adult patients who were critically ill due to complications following open-heart or abdominal surgery, multiple accidental traumas, or who were having acute respiratory failure. Mortality was higher (41.9 % vs. 19.3 %) among growth hormone treated patients (doses 5.3 - 8 mg/day) compared to those receiving placebo.

The safety of continuing somatropin treatment in patients with acute critical illness in intensive care units due to complications following open-heart or abdominal surgery, multiple accidental trauma or acute respiratory failure receiving replacement doses for approved indications has not been established. Therefore, the benefit-risk assessment for continuing treatment should be performed carefully.

Paediatric patients with endocrine disorders, including growth hormone deficiency, have a higher incidence of slipped capital femoral epiphyses. Any patient with the onset of a limp or complaint of hip or knee pain should be evaluated.

Because somatropin may reduce insulin sensitivity, patients should be monitored for evidence of glucose intolerance. For patients with diabetes mellitus, the insulin dose may require adjustment after NutropinAq therapy is instituted. Patients with diabetes or glucose intolerance should be monitored closely during somatropin therapy.

Intracranial hypertension with papilloedema, visual changes, headache, nausea and/or vomiting has been reported in a small number of patients treated with somatropin. Symptoms usually occur within the first eight weeks of the initiation of NutropinAq therapy. In all reported cases, intracranial hypertension-associated signs and symptoms resolved after reduction of the somatropin dose or termination of the therapy. Funduscopic examination is recommended at the initiation and periodically during the course of treatment.

Hypothyroidism may develop during treatment with somatropin, and untreated hypothyroidism may prevent optimal response to NutropinAq. Therefore, patients should have periodic thyroid function tests and should be treated with thyroid hormone when indicated. Patients with severe hypothyroidism should be treated accordingly prior to the start of NutropinAq therapy.

Since somatropin therapy following renal transplantation has not been adequately tested, NutropinAq treatment should be terminated after that surgery.

Concomitant treatment with glucocorticoids inhibits the growth-promoting effects of NutropinAq. Patients with ACTH deficiency should have their glucocorticoid replacement therapy carefully adjusted to avoid any inhibitory effect on growth. The use of NutropinAq in patients with chronic renal insufficiency receiving glucocorticoid therapy has not been evaluated.

4.5 Interaction with other medicinal products and other forms of Interaction

Limited published data indicate that growth hormone treatment increases cytochrome P450 mediated antipyrine clearance in man. Monitoring is advisable when NutropinAq is administered in combination with drugs known to be metabolised by CYP450 liver enzymes, such as corticosteroids, sex steroids, anticonvulsants, and cyclosporin.

4.6 Pregnancy and lactation

For NutropinAq, no clinical data on exposed pregnancies are available. Thus, the risk for humans is unknown. Although animal studies do not point to a potential risk during pregnancy, NutropinAq should be discontinued if pregnancy occurs.

It is not known whether somatropin is excreted in human milk, however, absorption of intact protein from the gastrointestinal tract of the infant is unlikely.

4.7 Effects on ability to drive and use machines

No studies on the effects of NutropinAq on the ability to drive and use machines have been performed.

Somatropin has no known effect on the ability to drive or to use machines.

4.8 Undesirable effects

Undesirable effects from a postmarketing surveillance program

Safety data from 9829 patients treated with Nutropin or NutropinAq - derived from a postmarketing surveillance program in the United States - demonstrate that approximately 2% of patients can be expected to experience drug-related adverse reactions.

Overall, 81 patients reported undesirable effects in the "Body as a Whole" body system. The number of subjects with adverse drugs reactions (ADRs) in other body systems was as follows: Cardiovascular: 5, Digestive: 9, Endocrine: 7, Haematological/Lymphatic: 2, Metabolic: 18, Musculoskeletal: 33, Nervous: 24, Skin: 11, Special Senses: 3, Urogenital: 13.

The most frequently reported ADR is injection site pain (0.5% of patients). Headache (0.16%) and bone disorder (0.33%) were reported with an uncommon frequency, and diabetes mellitus (0.05%), oedema/peripheral oedema/face oedema (0.08%), hyperglycaemia/glucose tolerance decreased (0.05%), intracranial hypertension (0.08%), CNS neoplasm (0.08%), urticaria (0.04%), naevi (0.04%) and gynaecomastia (0.07%) were reported with a rare frequency.

Rare ADRs which were reported in more than 1 patient were immune disorder (0.02%), cardiovascular disorder (0.02%), diarrhoea (0.02%), vomiting (0.02%), increased creatinine (0.02%), neuropathy (0.02%), abnormal kidney function (0.02%).

Patients with endocrinological disorders are more prone to develop an epiphysiolysis.

As with all drugs, a small percentage of patients may develop antibodies to the protein somatropin. The binding capacity of growth hormone antibodies was lower than 2 mg/l in NutropinAq subjects tested, which has not been associated with adversely affected growth rate.

Leukaemia has been reported in a small number of growth hormone deficient patients treated with growth hormone. A causal relationship to somatropin therapy is unlikely.

Children with chronic renal insufficiency receiving NutropinAq are more likely to develop intracranial hypertension, although children with GHD and Turner syndrome also have an increased incidence. The greatest risk is at the beginning of treatment. Peripheral oedema and carpal tunnel syndrome have been reported as side effects more frequently in adults than in children treated with somatropin.

Undesirable effects from clinical trials

The following table gives an overview of very common or common ADRs, which occurred in clinical trials performed in the United States in at least one of the four indications.

(see Table 1 on next page)

Uncommon ADRs are listed below. These events occurred in 1 out of all treated patients (0.15%) - unless otherwise indicated.

Body as a whole: injection site atrophy, injection site oedema, injection site haemorrhage, injection site hypersensitivity, injection site mass (0.5%), carcinoma, neoplasm, hypertrophy, abdominal pain.

Cardiovascular: vasodilatation (0.3%), hypertension, tachycardia.

Digestive: vomiting (0.6%), flatulence, nausea.

Haemic/Lymphatic: anaemia, lipodystrophy, hypoglycaemia, hyperphosphataemia.

Musculoskeletal: bone pain, muscle atrophy.

Nervous: somnolence, nystagmus, personality disorder, vertigo.

Skin/Appendages: skin atrophy, urticaria, exfoliative dermatitis, hirsutism, skin hypertrophy.

Special Senses: diplopia, papilloedema.

Urogenital: urinary incontinence, leukorrhoea, polyuria, urine frequency, urine abnormality, urine haemorrhage.

Compared to untreated Turner syndrome patients, no new or unexpected safety signals unique to Turner syndrome patients treated with somatropin were identified. The incidence of known complications of the underlying syndrome was not altered.

In patients with chronic renal insufficiency, there was no evidence that NutropinAq altered the rate of progression of renal failure or renal osteodystrophy.

4.9 Overdose

Acute overdose could lead to hyperglycaemia. Long-term overdose could result in signs and symptoms of gigantism and/or acromegaly consistent with the known effects of excess growth hormone.

5. PHARMACOLOGICAL PROPERTIES

5.1 Pharmacodynamic properties

Pharmacotherapeutic group: Somatropin and analogues

ATC Code: H01 AC 01

Somatropin stimulates growth rate and increases adult height in children who lack endogenous growth hormone. Treatment of growth hormone deficient adults with somatropin results in reduced fat mass, increased lean body mass and increased spine bone mineral density. Metabolic alterations in these patients include normalisation of IGF-1 serum levels.

In vitro and *in vivo* preclinical and clinical tests have demonstrated that somatropin is therapeutically equivalent to human growth hormone of pituitary origin.

Actions that have been demonstrated for human growth hormone include:

Tissue Growth

1. Skeletal growth: growth hormone and its mediator IGF-1 stimulate skeletal growth in growth hormone deficient children by an effect on the epiphyseal plates of long bones. This results in a measurable increase in body length until these growth plates fuse at the end of puberty.

2. Cell growth: Treatment with somatropin results in an increase in both the number and size of skeletal muscle cells.

3. Organ growth: Growth hormone increases the size of internal organs, including kidneys, and increases red blood cell mass.

Protein metabolism

Linear growth is facilitated in part by growth hormone-stimulated protein synthesis. This is reflected by nitrogen retention as demonstrated by a decline in urinary nitrogen excretion and blood urea nitrogen during growth hormone therapy.

Carbohydrate metabolism

Patients with inadequate growth hormone secretion sometimes experience fasting hypoglycaemia that is improved by treatment with somatropin. Growth hormone therapy may decrease insulin sensitivity and impair glucose tolerance.

Mineral metabolism

Somatropin induces retention of sodium, potassium and phosphorus. Serum concentration of inorganic phosphorus are increased in patients with growth hormone deficiency after NutropinAq therapy due to metabolic activity associated with bone growth and increased tubular reabsorption in the kidney. Serum calcium is not significantly altered by somatropin. Adults with growth hormone deficiency show low bone mineral density and in the childhood-onset patient, NutropinAq has been shown to increase spine bone mineral density in a dose-dependent manner.

Connective tissue metabolism

Somatropin stimulates the synthesis of chondroitin sulphate and collagen as well as the urinary excretion of hydroxyproline.

Body composition

Adult growth hormone deficient patients treated with somatropin at a mean dosage of 0.014 mg/kg bodyweight daily demonstrate a decrease in fat mass and increase in lean body mass. When these alterations are coupled with the increase in total body water and bone mass, the overall effect of somatropin therapy is to modify body composition, an effect that is maintained with continued treatment.

5.2 Pharmacokinetic properties

General characteristics

The pharmacokinetic properties of NutropinAq have only been investigated in healthy adult males.

Absorption: The absolute bioavailability of recombinant human growth hormone after subcutaneous administration is about 80%.

Distribution: Animal studies with somatropin showed that growth hormone localises to highly perfused organs, particularly the liver and kidney. The volume of distribution at steady state for somatropin in healthy adult males is about 50 ml/kg bodyweight, approximating the serum volume.

Metabolism: Both the liver and the kidney have been shown to be important protein catabolising organs for growth hormone. Animal studies suggest that the kidney is the dominant organ of clearance. Growth hormone is filtered at the glomerulus and reabsorbed in the proximal tubules. It is then cleaved within renal cells into its constituent amino acids, which return to the systemic circulation.

Elimination: After subcutaneous bolus administration, the mean terminal half-life $t_{1/2}$ of somatropin is about 2.3 hours. After intravenous bolus administration of somatropin, the mean terminal half-life $t_{1/2}\beta$ or $t_{1/2}\gamma$ is about 20 minutes and the mean clearance is reported to be in the range of 116 - 174 ml/h/kg.

Available literature data suggest that somatropin clearance is similar in adults and children.

Characteristics in patients

Clearance and mean terminal half-life $t_{1/2}$ of somatropin in adult and paediatric growth hormone deficient patients are similar to those observed in healthy subjects.

Children and adults with chronic renal failure and end-stage renal disease tend to have decreased clearance compared to normal subjects. Endogenous growth hormone production may also increase in some individuals with end-stage renal disease. However, no somatropin accumulation has been reported in children with chronic renal failure or end-stage renal disease dosed with current regimens.

Limited published data for exogenously-administered somatropin suggest absorption and elimination half-lives and time of maximum concentration t_{max} in Turner patients are similar to those observed in both normal and growth hormone deficient populations.

In patients with severe liver dysfunction a reduction in somatropin clearance has been noted. The clinical significance of this decrease is unknown.

5.3 Preclinical safety data

The toxicity of NutropinAq has been tested in rats and monkeys and no findings of toxicological relevance were revealed.

Due to its hormonal activity, somatropin may exert a promotional effect on tumour growth in tumour-bearing subjects. To date, this has not been confirmed in patients.

Local tolerance studies with NutropinAq showed no substantial adverse local reactions.

Studies in transgenic mice suggest a low antibody provoking potential of (aged) liquid Nutropin.

No common reproduction studies were performed. However, long-term treatment of monkeys during pregnancy and lactation and of newborn animals until adolescence, sexual maturity and reproduction did not indicate substantial disturbances of fertility, pregnancy, delivery, nursing or development of progeny.

6. PHARMACEUTICAL PARTICULARS

6.1 List of excipients

Sodium chloride,

Phenol,

Polysorbate 20,

Sodium citrate and citric acid anhydrous

Water for injections.

Table 1 Adverse Drug Reactions from Clinical Trials

	Growth failure due to inadequate growth hormone secretion	Growth failure associated with Turner syndrome	Growth failure associated with chronic renal insufficiency	Growth hormone deficiency in adults
Number of treated patients in clinical trials	236	108	171	127
Percentage of patients reporting adverse drug reactions (%)	16	10	29	59
Mean dosage of growth hormone (mg/kg/day)	0.043	0.054	0.050	0.014
Body as a Whole (n/%)				
Headache	7 (3%)	1 (1%)	7 (4%)	5 (4%)
Injection Site Haematoma	2 (1%)	1 (1%)	3 (2%)	(-)
Injection Site Inflammation	(-)	(-)	2 >1%)	(-)
Injection Site Pain	5 (2%)	(-)	2 >1%)	(-)
Injection Site Reaction	3 (1%)	1 (1%)	2 (1%)	(-)
Pain	6 (3%)	1 (1%)	8 (5%)	15 (12%)
Peritonitis	(-)	(-)	2 >1%)	(-)
Asthenia	(-)	(-)	1 (1%)	5 (4%)
Back Pain			(-)	2 (2%)
Lab Test Abnormal			(-)	2 (2%)
Endocrine (n/%)				
Hypothyroidism	1 (0%)	(-)	(-)	4 (3%)
Haemic/Lymphatic (n/%)				
Ecchymosis	3 (1%)	(-)	1 >1%)	(-)
Metabolic/Nutrition (n/%)				
Oedema	1 (0%)	(-)	(-)	31 (24%)
Peripheral Oedema	(-)	1 (0%)	(-)	30 (24%)
Glucose Tolerance Decreased	(-)	(-)	1 (1%)	4 (3%)
Hyperglycaemia	(-)	(-)	(-)	2 (2%)
Hyperlipaemia	(-)	(-)	(-)	3 (2%)
Creatinine Increased	(-)	(-)	2 >1%)	(-)
Tenosynovitis	(-)	(-)	(-)	7 (6%)
Bone Disorder	1 (0%)	(-)	4 (2%)	1 (1%)
Bone Necrosis	(-)	(-)	4 (2%)	(-)
Musculoskeletal (n/%)				
Arthralgia	3 (1%)	(-)	6 (4%)	23 (18%)
Joint Disorders	(-)	(-)	1 (1%)	13 (10%)
Arthrosis	(-)	(-)	(-)	3 (2%)
Myalgia	(-)	(-)	(-)	5 (4%)
Myasthenia	(-)	(-)	(-)	2 (2%)
Nervous (n/%)				
Paraesthesia	(-)	(-)	(-)	17 (13%)
Hypertonia	1 (0%)	(-)	(-)	2 (2%)
Insomnia	(-)	(-)	(-)	2 (2%)
CNS Neoplasm	3 >1%)	(-)	(-)	(-)
Skin Appendages (n/%)				
Rash	3 >1%)	(-)	1 (1%)	(-)
Urogenital (n/%)				
Menorrhagia	(-)	2 (2%)	(-)	(-)
Kidney Failure	(-)	(-)	3 (2%)	(-)
Breast Pain	(-)	(-)	(-)	4 (3%)
Gynaecomastia	(-)	(-)	(-)	2 (2%)

6.2 Incompatibilities
In the absence of compatibility studies, this medicinal productmust not be mixed with other medicinal products.

6.3 Shelf life
2 years

Chemical and physical in-use stability has been demonstrated for 28 days at 2°C - 8°C.

From a microbiological point of view, once opened, the product may be stored for a maximum of 28 days at 2°C - 8°C. The NutropinAq is designed to withstand a nominal (one hour maximum) period of time outside of the refrigerator on a daily basis. Do not remove the cartridge that is being used from the NutropinAq Pen between injections.

After first opening: the product may be stored for up to 28 days at 2°C - 8°C

6.4 Special precautions for storage
Store at 2°C - 8°C. Do not freeze.

Keep the container in the outer carton

A cartridge that is in the pen should not be removed during injections.

6.5 Nature and contents of container
2 ml of solution in a cartridge (Type I glass) closed with a stopper (butyl rubber) and a seal (rubber).

Pack sizes of 1, 3 and 6 cartridges.

Not all pack sizes may be marketed.

6.6 Instructions for use and handling
NutropinAq is supplied as a sterile solution with preservative for multiple use.

The solution should be clear immediately after removal from the refrigerator. If the solution is cloudy, the content must not be injected.

Gently swirl. Do not shake vigorously in order not to denature the protein.

NutropinAq is intended for use only with the NutropinAq Pen. Wipe the rubber seal of the NutropinAq with rubbing alcohol or an antiseptic solution to prevent contamination of the contents by microorganisms that may be introduced by repeated needle insertions. It is recommended that NutropinAq be administered using sterile, disposable needles.

The NutropinAq Pen allows for administration of a minimum dose of 0.1 mg to a maximum dose of 4.0 mg, in 0.1 mg increments.

7. MARKETING AUTHORISATION HOLDER
IPSEN Ltd.
190 Bath Road
Slough, Berkshire
SL1 3XE, United Kingdom

8. MARKETING AUTHORISATION NUMBER(S)
EU/1/00/164/003
EU/1/00/164/004
EU/1/00/164/005

9. DATE OF FIRST AUTHORISATION/RENEWAL OF THE AUTHORISATION
16 February 2001

10. DATE OF REVISION OF THE TEXT
6 December 2004

Nuvelle

(Schering Health Care Limited)

1. NAME OF THE MEDICINAL PRODUCT
Nuvelle™

2. QUALITATIVE AND QUANTITATIVE COMPOSITION
- Each white sugar-coated tablet contains:

Estradiol valerate 2.0mg

- Each pink sugar-coated tablet contains:

Estradiol valerate 2.0mg
Levonorgestrel 75 micrograms

3. PHARMACEUTICAL FORM
Sugar coated tablets for oral use.

4. CLINICAL PARTICULARS
4.1 Therapeutic indications
Hormone replacement therapy for the treatment of the climacteric syndrome.

Second line therapy for prevention of osteoporosis in postmenopausal women at high risk of future fractures who are intolerant of, or contraindicated for, other medicinal products approved for the prevention of osteoporosis.

For maximum prophylactic benefit treatment should commence as soon as possible after the menopause.

Bone mineral density measurements may help to confirm the presence of low bone mass.

Nuvelle is designed to provide hormone replacement therapy during and after the climacteric. The addition of a progestogen in the second half of each course helps to provide good control of the irregular cycles that are characteristic of the premenopausal phase and opposes the production of endometrial hyperplasia. Whilst ovarian hormone production is little affected, Nuvelle abolishes or improves the characteristic symptoms of the climacteric such as hot flushes, sweating attacks and sleep disorders.

Studies of bone mineral content have shown Nuvelle to be effective in the prevention of progressive bone loss following the menopause.

Nuvelle does not consistently inhibit ovulation and is therefore unsuitable for contraception.

4.2 Posology and method of administration
Adults, including the elderly:

If the patient is still menstruating, treatment should begin on the 5th day of menstruation. Patients whose periods are very infrequent or who are postmenopausal may start at any time, provided pregnancy has been excluded (see Section 4.4. Special warnings and special precautions for use).

One white tablet is taken daily for the first 16 days, followed by one pink tablet daily for 12 days. Thus, each pack contains 28 days treatment. Treatment is continuous, which means that the next pack follows immediately without a break. Bleeding usually occurs within the last few days of one pack and the first week of the next.

4.3 Contraindications
- Pregnancy (See Section 4.4. Special warnings and special precautions for use)
- severe disturbances of liver function
- previous or existing liver tumours
- jaundice or general pruritus during a previous pregnancy
- Dubin-Johnson syndrome
- Rotor syndrome
- active deep venous thrombosis, thromboembolic disorders, or a history of confirmed venous thromboembolism. (See also Special warnings and special precautions for use).
- sickle-cell anaemia
- suspected or existing hormone-dependent disorders or tumours of the uterus and breast
- undiagnosed irregular vaginal bleeding
- congenital disturbances of lipid metabolism
- a history of herpes gestationis
- otosclerosis with deterioration in previous pregnancies
- endometriosis
- severe diabetes with vascular changes
- mastopathy.

4.4 Special warnings and special precautions for use
Assessment of each woman prior to taking hormone replacement therapy (and at regular intervals thereafter) should include a personal and family medical history. Physical examination should be guided by this and by the contraindications (section 4.3) and warnings (section 4.4) for Nuvelle. During assessment of each individual woman clinical examination of the breasts and pelvic examination should be performed where clinically indicated rather than as a routine procedure. Women should be encouraged to participate in the national breast cancer screening programme (mammography) and the national cervical cancer screening programme (cervical cytology) as appropriate for their age. Breast awareness should also be encouraged and women advised to report any changes in their breasts to their doctor or nurse.

Before starting treatment, pregnancy must be excluded. If the expected bleeding fails to occur at about 28-day intervals, treatment should be stopped until pregnancy has been ruled out.

Persistent breakthrough bleeding during treatment is an indication for endometrial assessment which may include biopsy.

Epidemiological studies have suggested that hormone replacement therapy (HRT) is associated with an increased relative risk of developing venous thromboembolism (VTE) i.e. deep vein thrombosis or pulmonary embolism. The studies find a 2-3 fold increase for users compared with non-users which for healthy women amounts to a low risk of one extra case of VTE each year for every 5000 patients taking HRT.

Generally recognised risk factors for VTE include a personal or family history and severe obesity (Body Mass Index >30 kg/m^2). In women with these factors the benefits of treatment with HRT need to be carefully weighed against risks. There is no consensus about the possible role of varicose veins in VTE.

The risk of VTE may be temporarily increased with prolonged immobilisation, major trauma or major surgery. In women on HRT scrupulous attention should be given to prophylactic measures to prevent VTE following surgery. Where prolonged immobilisation is liable to follow elective surgery, particularly abdominal or orthopaedic surgery to the lower limbs, consideration should be given to temporarily stopping HRT 4 weeks earlier, if this is possible.

If venous thromboembolism develops after initiating HRT the drug should be discontinued.

Prolonged exposure to unopposed oestrogens increases the risk of development of endometrial carcinoma. The general consensus of opinion is that the addition of 12 days progestogen towards the end of the cycle, as in Nuvelle, diminishes the possibility of such a risk, and some investigators consider that it might be protective.

A reanalysis of original data from 51 epidemiological studies reported a small or moderate increase in the probability of having breast cancer *diagnosed* in women currently or recently using HRT. The findings may be due to biological effects of HRT, earlier diagnosis, or a combination of both. The relative risk increased with duration of treatment (by 2.3% per year of use) and returned to normal in the course of five years after cessation of HRT use. This increase in relative risk associated with duration of HRT use is comparable to the increase in relative risk when natural menopause is delayed in the absence of HRT (2.8% increase for each year older at menopause). Breast cancers diagnosed in current or recent users of HRT are more likely to be localised to the breast than those found in non-users. HRT use may not be associated with increased mortality from breast cancer.

Between the ages of 50 and 70, about 45 women in every 1000 not using HRT will have breast cancer diagnosed. It is estimated that among those who use HRT for 5 years starting at age 50, 2 extra cases of breast cancer will be detected by age 70 in every 1000 women. For those who use HRT for 10 years there will be 6 extra cases of breast cancer, and for 15 years use, 12 extra cases of breast cancer in every 1000 women during the 20 year period until age 70.

It is important that the increased risk of being diagnosed with breast cancer is discussed with the patient and weighed against the known benefits of HRT.

Treatment should be stopped at once if migrainous or frequent and unusually severe headaches occur for the first time, or if there are other symptoms that are possible prodromata of vascular occlusion.

Treatment should be stopped at once if jaundice or pregnancy occurs, if there is a significant rise in blood pressure, or an increase in epileptic seizures.

Some women are predisposed to cholestasis during steroid therapy. Diseases that are known to be subject to deterioration during pregnancy (e.g. multiple sclerosis, epilepsy, diabetes, benign breast disease, hypertension, cardiac or renal dysfunction, asthma, porphyria, tetany and otosclerosis) and women with a strong family history of breast cancer should be carefully observed during treatment.

Pre-existing fibroids may increase in size under the influence of oestrogens. If this is observed treatment should be discontinued.

In patients with mild chronic liver disease, liver function should be checked every 8 - 12 weeks.

In rare cases benign and, in even rarer cases, malignant liver tumours leading in isolated cases to life-threatening intra-abdominal haemorrhage have been observed after the use of hormonal substances such as those contained in Nuvelle. If severe upper abdominal complaints, enlarged liver, or signs of intra-abdominal haemorrhage occur, a liver tumour should be included in the differential diagnostic considerations.

4.5 Interaction with other medicinal products and other forms of Interaction
Hormonal contraception should be stopped when treatment with Nuvelle is started and the patient should be advised to take non-hormonal contraceptive precautions.

Drugs which induce hepatic microsomal enzyme systems e.g. barbiturates, phenytoin, rifampicin, accelerate the metabolism of oestrogen/progestogen combinations such as Nuvelle and may reduce their efficacy.

The requirement for oral antidiabetics or insulin can change.

4.6 Pregnancy and lactation
Contra-indicated.

4.7 Effects on ability to drive and use machines
None known.

4.8 Undesirable effects
During the first few months of treatment, breakthrough bleeding, spotting and breast tenderness or enlargement can occur. These are usually temporary and normally disappear after continued treatment. Other symptoms known to occur are: anxiety; increased appetite; bloating; palpitations; depressive symptoms; headache; migraine; dizziness; dyspepsia; leg pains; oedema; altered libido; nausea; rashes; vomiting; altered weight; chloasma.

4.9 Overdose
There have been no reports of ill-effects from overdosage, which it is, therefore, generally unnecessary to treat. There are no specific antidotes, and treatment should be symptomatic.

5. PHARMACOLOGICAL PROPERTIES

5.1 Pharmacodynamic properties
Nuvelle contains estradiol valerate (the valeric acid ester of the endogenous female oestrogen, estradiol) and the synthetic progestogen, levonorgestrel. Estradiol valerate provides hormone replacement during and after the climacteric. The addition of levonorgestrel in the second half of each course of tablets helps to provide good cycle control and opposes the development of endometrial hyperplasia.

Most studies show that oral administration of estradiol valerate to post-menopausal women increases serum high density lipoprotein cholesterol (HDL-C) and decreases low density lipoprotein cholesterol (LDL-C). Although epidemiological data are limited such alterations are recognised as potentially protective against the development of arterial disease. A possible attenuation of these effects may occur with the addition of a progestogen. However, at the doses used in Nuvelle, the 12 days of combined therapy with estradiol valerate and levonorgestrel have not been observed to be associated with any unwanted lipid effects.

5.2 Pharmacokinetic properties
1. Levonorgestrel (LNG)

Orally administered LNG is rapidly and completely absorbed. Following ingestion of one tablet of Nuvelle maximum drug serum levels of 1.9ng/ml were found at 1.3 hours. Thereafter, LNG serum levels decrease in two disposition phases. The first phase is described by a half-life of 0.5-1.5 hours and the terminal phase by a half-life of 20-27 hours. For LNG, a metabolic clearance rate from serum of about 1.5 ml/min/kg was determined. LNG is not excreted in unchanged form but as metabolites. LNG metabolites are excreted at about equal proportions with urine and faeces. The biotransformation follows the known pathways of steroid metabolism. No pharmacologically active metabolites are known.

LNG is bound to serum albumin and to SHBG. Only about 1.5% of the total serum drug levels are present as free steroid, but 65% are specifically bound to SHBG. The relative distribution (free, albumin-bound, SHBG-bound) depends on the SHBG concentrations in the serum. Following induction of the binding protein, the SHBG bound fraction increases while the unbound and the albumin-bound fraction decrease.

Following daily repeated administration, LNG concentrations in the serum increase by a factor of about 2. Steady-state conditions are reached within a few days. The pharmacokinetics of LNG is influenced by SHBG serum levels. Under treatment with Nuvelle SHBG levels will rise by about 40% during the oestrogen phase and remain constant or slightly decrease thereafter. The absolute bioavailability of LNG was determined to be almost 100% of the dose administered. The relative bioavailability was tested against an aqueous microcrystalline suspension and was found to be complete (108%).

About 0.1% of the maternal dose can be transferred via milk to the nursed infant.

2. Estradiol valerate (E_2 val)

E_2 val is completely absorbed from the Nuvelle tablet. During absorption and the first passage through the liver the steroid ester is cleaved into estradiol (E_2) and valeric acid. At the same time E_2 undergoes extensive further metabolism yielding E_2 conjugates, estrone (E_1) and E_1 conjugates. The pharmacologically most active metabolites of E_2 val are E_2 and E_1. Maximum serum levels of 25 pg E_2/ml and 180 pg E_1/ml are reached 5-7 hours after the administration of one Nuvelle tablet.

Mean E1 serum levels are 10-12 fold higher than mean E_2 serum concentrations. Serum levels of E_1 conjugates are about 25 fold higher than the E_1 serum levels.

E_2 is rapidly metabolised and the metabolic clearance rate has been determined to 30ml/min/kg. After oral intake of E_2 the half-life of the terminal disposition phase was about 13 hours for E_2. The respective half-life for E_1 serum level decline was about 20 hours. The daily use of Nuvelle will lead to an about 50% increase in E_2 serum levels and to twofold E_1 levels at steady state.

Estradiol is bound to about 97% to serum proteins, about 35% are specifically bound to SHBG. E_2 val is not excreted in unchanged form. The metabolites of estradiol are excreted via urine and bile with a half-life of about 1 day at a ratio of 9:1.

The absolute bioavailability of E_2 from E_2 val is about 3% of oral dose and thus in the same range like oral E_2 (5% of dose).

The relative bioavailability of E_2 val (reference: aqueous microcrystalline suspension) from Nuvelle tablets was complete (111-112%).

Estradiol and its metabolites are excreted into milk only to a minor extent.

5.3 Preclinical safety data
There are no preclinical data which could be of relevance to the prescriber and which are not already included in other relevant sections of the SPC.

6. PHARMACEUTICAL PARTICULARS

6.1 List of excipients
Nuvelle contains the following excipients: lactose, maize starch, povidone 25 000, povidone 700 000, talcum, magnesium stearate (E572), sucrose, macrogol 6000 (polyethylene glycol 6000), calcium carbonate (E170), glycerol (E422), montan glycol wax, yellow and red ferric oxide pigments (E172), titanium dioxide (E171).

6.2 Incompatibilities
Not applicable.

6.3 Shelf life
5 years.

6.4 Special precautions for storage
None.

6.5 Nature and contents of container
Packs containing aluminium foil and PVC blister strips.

Presentation:

Carton containing memo-packs of either 1 × 28 tablets or 3 × 28 tablets.

6.6 Instructions for use and handling
Not applicable.

7. MARKETING AUTHORISATION HOLDER
Schering Health Care Limited

The Brow

Burgess Hill

West Sussex RH15 9NE

8. MARKETING AUTHORISATION NUMBER(S)
PL/0053/0219

9. DATE OF FIRST AUTHORISATION/RENEWAL OF THE AUTHORISATION
7th October 1991/26th March 1997

10. DATE OF REVISION OF THE TEXT
4th December 2003

LEGAL CATEGORY
POM

Nuvelle Continuous

(Schering Health Care Limited)

1. NAME OF THE MEDICINAL PRODUCT
Nuvelle® Continuous

2. QUALITATIVE AND QUANTITATIVE COMPOSITION
Each tablet contains:

Estradiol (as hemihydrate) 2.0mg

Norethisterone acetate 1.0mg

3. PHARMACEUTICAL FORM
Film-coated tablets.

Each tablet is pink.

4. CLINICAL PARTICULARS

4.1 Therapeutic indications
Hormone replacement therapy for the treatment of menopausal symptoms such as night sweats and hot flushes in women who are at least 1 year past their menopause and who have an intact uterus. Prophylaxis and treatment of the postmenopausal sequelae of oestrogen withdrawal, including atrophic vaginitis and atrophic urethritis.

Second line therapy for prevention of osteoporosis in postmenopausal women at high risk of future fractures who are intolerant of, or contraindicated for, other medicinal products approved for the prevention of osteoporosis.

Although for maximum prophylactic benefit, hormone replacement therapy should commence as soon as possible, in the case of Nuvelle Continuous this should be at least one year past the menopause. If given in the earlier post-menopausal phase the incidence of bleeding is unacceptably high. Administration is continued without a break in therapy. The presence of continuous progestogen is designed to result in the absence of menstrual bleeding whilst also protecting against the development of endometrial hyperplasia.

Nuvelle Continuous does not consistently inhibit ovulation and is, therefore, unsuitable for contraception.

Combined preparations containing an oestrogen and progestogen are only necessary in patients with an intact uterus.

4.2 Posology and method of administration
Adults, including the elderly:

Nuvelle Continuous is only suitable for women who are at least one year past their menopause i.e. at least one year past their last natural menstrual bleed.

One pink tablet is taken daily without a break thus running one packet into the next. The treatment is designed to provide hormone replacement therapy without cyclical bleeding, but bleeding may occur in the first few cycles of use. It can be unpredictable but is unlikely to be excessive. Patients must be warned of this but reassured that this should diminish significantly and usually will cease. If significant bleeding continues, or if at any time bleeding or spotting becomes unacceptable, patients should consider discontinuing treatment or changing to sequential therapy. If all bleeding subsides within 3 weeks of stopping Nuvelle Continuous then further investigation may be unnecessary. Each case, however, should be assessed individually.

Prophylaxis of osteoporosis:

Hormone replacement therapy (HRT) has been found to be effective in the prevention of osteoporosis especially when started soon after the menopause and used for 5 years and probably up to 10 years or more. Treatment should ideally start as soon as possible after the onset of the menopause and certainly within 2 to 3 years, but benefit may also be obtained even if treatment is started at a later date. Protection appears to be effective for as long as treatment is continued. However, data beyond 10 years are limited. A careful re-appraisal of the risk-benefit ratio should be undertaken before treating for longer than 5 to 10 years.

Patients using hormone replacement therapy for the first time:

May begin Nuvelle Continuous at any time provided they are at least one year past the menopause and pregnancy has been excluded (see Special warnings and special precautions for use).

Patients changing from a sequential combined hormone replacement therapy:

In women transferred from sequential HRT, treatment should probably be started at the end of the scheduled bleed. Bleeding may occur in the first few cycles of use. If significant bleeding continues, or if at any time bleeding or spotting becomes unacceptable, patients should consider discontinuing Nuvelle Continuous treatment.

Children: Not recommended for children.

4.3 Contraindications

- known, suspected, or past history of cancer of the breast
- known or suspected oestrogen-dependent neoplasia. Vaginal bleeding of unknown aetiology
- known or suspected pregnancy
- active deep venous thrombosis, thromboembolic disorders, or a history of confirmed venous thromboembolism. (See also Special Warnings and Special Precautions for Use).
- acute or chronic liver disease or history of liver disease where the liver function tests have failed to return to normal
- Dubin-Johnson syndrome, Rotor syndrome.
- severe cardiac or severe renal disease
- hypersensitivity to any of the ingredients.

4.4 Special warnings and special precautions for use
Before starting treatment, pregnancy must be excluded.

If changing from a sequential combined preparation which generated regular bleeding a pregnancy test is not indicated. Absence of bleeding during Nuvelle Continuous therapy can be expected and is not a cause for anxiety.

Assessment of each woman prior to taking hormone replacement therapy (and at regular intervals thereafter) should include a personal and family medical history. Physical examination should be guided by this and by the contraindications (section 4.3) and warnings (section 4.4) for Nuvelle. During assessment of each individual woman clinical examination of the breasts and pelvic examination should be performed where clinically indicated rather than as a routine procedure. Women should be encouraged to participate in the national breast cancer screening programme (mammography) and the national cervical cancer screening programme (cervical cytology) as appropriate for their age. Breast awareness should also be encouraged and women advised to report any changes in their breasts to their doctor or nurse.

A reanalysis of original data from 51 epidemiological studies reported a small or moderate increase in the probability of having breast cancer *diagnosed* in women currently or recently using HRT. The findings may be due to biological effects of HRT, earlier diagnosis, or a combination of both. The relative risk increased with duration of treatment (by 2.3% per year of use) and returned to normal in the course of five years after cessation of HRT use. This increase in relative risk associated with duration of HRT use is comparable to the increase in relative risk when natural menopause is delayed in the absence of HRT (2.8% increase for each year older at menopause). Breast cancers diagnosed in current or recent users of HRT are more likely to be localised to the breast than those found in non-users. HRT use may not be associated with increased mortality from breast cancer.

Between the ages of 50 and 70, about 45 women in every 1000 not using HRT will have breast cancer diagnosed. It is estimated that among those who use HRT for 5 years starting at age 50, 2 extra cases of breast cancer will be detected by age 70 in every 1000 women. For those who use HRT for 10 years there will be 6 extra cases of breast cancer, and for 15 years use, 12 extra cases of breast cancer in every 1000 women during the 20 year period until age 70.

It is important that the increased risk of being diagnosed with breast cancer is discussed with the patient and weighed against the known benefits of HRT.

There is a need for caution when prescribing oestrogens in women who have a history of, or known breast nodules or fibrocystic disease.

Breakthrough bleeding may occasionally occur and can be the result of poor compliance or concurrent antibiotic use. It may however indicate endometrial pathology and therefore any doubt as to its cause is an indication for endometrial evaluation, including biopsy.

Treatment should be stopped at once if migrainous or frequent and unusually severe headaches occur for the first time or if there are any other symptoms that are possible prodromata of vascular occlusion e.g. sudden visual disturbances.

Treatment should be stopped at once if jaundice, cholestasis, hepatitis or pregnancy occurs, or if there is a significant rise in blood pressure, or an increase in epileptic seizures.

Epidemiological studies have suggested that hormone replacement therapy (HRT) is associated with an increased relative risk of developing venous thromboembolism (VTE) i.e. deep vein thrombosis or pulmonary embolism. The studies find a 2-3 fold increase for users compared with non-users which for healthy women amounts to a low risk of one extra case of VTE each year for every 5000 patients taking HRT.

Generally recognised risk factors for VTE include a personal or family history and severe obesity (Body Mass Index >30 kg/m^2). In women with these factors the benefits of treatment with HRT need to be carefully weighed against risks. There is no consensus about the possible role of varicose veins in VTE.

The risk of VTE may be temporarily increased with prolonged immobilisation, major trauma or major surgery. In women on HRT scrupulous attention should be given to prophylactic measures to prevent VTE following surgery. Where prolonged immobilisation is liable to follow elective surgery, particularly abdominal or orthopaedic surgery to the lower limbs, consideration should be given to temporarily stopping HRT 4 weeks earlier, if this is possible.

If venous thromboembolism develops after initiating therapy the drug should be discontinued.

There is an increased risk of gall bladder disease in women receiving postmenopausal oestrogens.

There is an increased risk of endometrial hyperplasia and carcinoma associated with unopposed oestrogen administered long term (for more than one year). However, the appropriate addition of a progestogen to the oestrogen regimen statistically lowers the risk.

Should endometriosis be reactivated under therapy with Nuvelle Continuous, therapy should be discontinued.

Diseases that are known to be subject to deterioration during pregnancy (e.g. multiple sclerosis, epilepsy, diabetes, benign breast disease, hypertension, cardiac or renal dysfunction, porphyria, asthma, migraine, tetany, systemic lupus erythematosus, and melanoma) and women with a strong family history of breast cancer should be carefully observed during treatment.

Because of the occurrence of herpes gestationis and the worsening of otosclerosis in pregnancy, it is thought that treatment with female hormones may have similar effects. Patients with these conditions should be carefully monitored. Similarly, patients with sickle-cell anaemia should be monitored because of the increased risk of thrombosis that accompanies this disease.

Patients with pre-existing fibroids should be closely monitored as fibroids may increase in size under the influence of oestrogens. If this is observed, treatment should be discontinued.

Oestrogens may cause fluid retention and therefore patients with renal or cardiac dysfunction should be carefully observed.

Most studies demonstrate that oestrogen replacement therapy has little effect on blood pressure. Some show that it may decrease blood pressure. In addition, studies on combined therapy show that the addition of a progestogen also has little effect on blood pressure. Rarely, idiosyncratic hypertension may occur. When oestrogens are administered to hypertensive women, supervision is necessary and blood pressure should be monitored at regular intervals.

In patients with mild chronic liver disease, liver function should be checked every 8-12 weeks. Results of liver function tests may be affected by HRT.

In rare cases benign and in even rarer cases malignant liver tumours leading in isolated cases to life-threatening intra-abdominal haemorrhage have been observed after the use of hormonal substances such as those contained in Nuvelle Continuous. If severe upper abdominal complaints, enlarged liver, or signs of intra-abdominal haemorrhage occur, a liver tumour should be considered in the differential diagnosis.

Diabetes should be carefully observed when initiating HRT as worsening of glucose tolerance may occur.

Nuvelle Continuous is not suitable for contraception, neither will it restore fertility. Therefore, where applicable, contraception should be practised with non-hormonal methods.

4.5 Interaction with other medicinal products and other forms of Interaction
Hormonal contraception should be stopped when treatment with Nuvelle Continuous is started and the patient should be advised to take non-hormonal contraceptive precautions if required.

Drugs which induce hepatic microsomal enzyme systems, e.g. barbiturates, carbamazepine, phenytoin, rifampicin, accelerate the metabolism of oestrogen/progestogen combinations such as Nuvelle Continuous and may reduce their efficacy.

The requirement for oral antidiabetics or insulin can change as a result of the effect on glucose tolerance.

There are some laboratory tests that can be influenced by oestrogens, such as tests for glucose tolerance, liver function or thyroid function.

4.6 Pregnancy and lactation
Contra-indicated.

4.7 Effects on ability to drive and use machines
None known.

4.8 Undesirable effects
During the first few months of treatment, breakthrough bleeding, spotting and breast tenderness or enlargement can occur. These are usually temporary and normally disappear after continued treatment. Other symptoms known to occur are: increased appetite; bloating; palpitations; anxiety/depressive symptoms; headache; migraine; dizziness; dyspepsia; leg pains; oedema; hypertension; altered libido; nausea; rashes; vomiting; altered weight; chloasma; melasma; increase in the size of uterine fibromyomata; reduced carbohydrate tolerance; dysmenorrhoea; premenstrual-like syndrome.

The following have also been reported with similar products, most of them rarely: vaginal candidiasis; change in cervical erosion; cystitis-like syndrome; breast secretion; abdominal cramps; erythema multiforme; erythema nodosum; haemorrhagic eruption; aggravated porphyria; loss of scalp hair; hirsutism; steepening of corneal curvature; intolerance to contact lenses; chorea.

Some women are predisposed to cholestasis during oestrogen therapy.

4.9 Overdose
Nausea and vomiting may occur with an overdose.

There are no specific antidotes and treatment should be symptomatic. Withdrawal bleeding may occur in females.

5. PHARMACOLOGICAL PROPERTIES

5.1 Pharmacodynamic properties
Nuvelle Continuous contains estradiol a naturally occurring oestrogen and the synthetic progestogen norethisterone acetate. Estradiol provides hormone replacement during and after the climacteric and the addition of norethisterone acetate opposes the development of endometrial hyperplasia.

Biochemical parameters of bone turnover are shown to fall significantly during long term use of 17β-estradiol in combination with norethisterone acetate, at the doses in this product. This reflects a decrease in the risk of developing osteoporosis or worsening of the condition as borne out by bone mineral density studies.

5.2 Pharmacokinetic properties
Natural oestrogens such as 17β-estradiol are readily and completely absorbed from the gastrointestinal tract. Estradiol is converted by the liver and other tissues to estrone, estriol and other metabolites. Estradiol is excreted into the bile and is then reabsorbed from the intestine. During this enterohepatic circulation degradation of the estradiol occurs. 90-95% of estradiol is excreted in the urine as biologically inactive glucuronides and sulphate conjugates.

Norethisterone acetate is rapidly absorbed from the gastrointestinal tract and transformed to norethisterone. It is then metabolised and excreted as glucuronides and sulphate conjugates which are eliminated with the urine and faeces. Approximately half the dose is recovered in the urine in the first 24 hours.

5.3 Preclinical safety data
There are no preclinical safety data which could be of relevance to the prescriber and which are not already included in other relevant sections of the SPC.

6. PHARMACEUTICAL PARTICULARS

6.1 List of excipients
Nuvelle Continuous contains the following excipients: lactose monohydrate, maize starch, povidone 25 000, talc, magnesium stearate (E572), methylhydroxypropyl cellulose, macrogol 6000, titanium dioxide (E171), ferric oxide pigment, red (E172).

6.2 Incompatibilities
None.

6.3 Shelf life
36 months.

6.4 Special precautions for storage
None.

6.5 Nature and contents of container
Container consists of 20 μm hard tempered aluminium foil and 250μm transparent PVC film blister strips packed in a cardboard carton.

Presentation: Carton containing memo-packs 3 × 28 tablets.

6.6 Instructions for use and handling
Not applicable.

7. MARKETING AUTHORISATION HOLDER
Schering Health Care Limited
The Brow
Burgess Hill
West Sussex RH15 9NE

8. MARKETING AUTHORISATION NUMBER(S)
PL 0053/0263

9. DATE OF FIRST AUTHORISATION/RENEWAL OF THE AUTHORISATION
12 January 1999

10. DATE OF REVISION OF THE TEXT
10 December 2004

LEGAL CATEGORY
POM

Nyogel 0.1% Eye Gel

(Novartis Pharmaceuticals UK Ltd)

1. NAME OF THE MEDICINAL PRODUCT
Nyogel® 0.1%, eye gel

2. QUALITATIVE AND QUANTITATIVE COMPOSITION
Timolol 1mg/g (as maleate)

1 g gel contains 1.37 mg timolol maleate, corresponding to 1 mg of timolol.

For excipients see section 6.1.

3. PHARMACEUTICAL FORM
Eye gel.

Practically colourless, opalescent, odourless gel, free of visible particulate matter.

4. CLINICAL PARTICULARS

4.1 Therapeutic indications
Timolol eye gel is used to reduce elevated intraocular pressure in the following conditions:

- ocular hypertension
- chronic open-angle glaucoma.

4.2 Posology and method of administration
Adults and children over the age of 12 years:

The recommended dosage is one drop of timolol eye gel in the affected eye(s) daily, preferably in the morning. Intraocular pressure should be reassessed 2 to 4 weeks after starting treatment, because response to treatment may take a few weeks to stabilise. If necessary, timolol eye gel can be used concomitantly with miotics, adrenaline and/or carbonic anhydrase inhibitors. To prevent the active substance from being washed out from the eye, an interval of at least 5 minutes between application of different drugs is required, and timolol eye gel should be the last one to be administered.

In case of transfer from other topical beta blocking agents: discontinue their use after a full day of therapy and start treatment with timolol eye gel the next day. Instill one drop in each affected eye once a day, preferably in the morning.

In case of transfer from a single antiglaucoma agent other than topical beta blocking agent:

Continue the agent and add one drop of timolol eye gel in each affected eye once a day. On the following day, discontinue the previous agent completely, and continue with timolol eye gel.

Elderly:

The above dosage can be used for the elderly.

Children under the age of 12 years:

Peadiatric use is not recommended.

Method of administration:

Timolol eye gel is to be instilled into the conjunctival cul-de-sac. It can be used also for long-term therapy.

For a correct dosing during application, the eye-drop bottle must be held vertically during administration.

The dispenser remains sterile until the original closure is broken. Patients should be instructed to avoid allowing the tip of the dispensing container to contact the eye or surrounding structures as this may contaminate the gel.

When using nasolacrimal occlusion or closing the eyelids for 3 minutes the systemic absorption may be reduced. This may result in a decrease in systemic side effects and an increase in local activity.

4.3 Contraindications
Timolol eye gel is contraindicated in patients with:

- bronchial asthma
- history of bronchial asthma or severe obstructive pulmonary disease
- sinus bradycardia
- second or third degree AV block
- overt cardiac failure
- cardiogenic shock
- severe peripheral circulatory disturbance (Raynaud's disease) and peripheral disorders
- Prinzmetal's angina
- untreated phaeochromocytoma
- hypotension
- corneal dystrophies
- hypersensitivity to timolol or to any of the excipients and/ or other beta-blocking agent
- severe allergic rhinitis and bronchial hyperreactivity.

Timolol eye gel is also contraindicated in case of association with:

- combination with fluctafenine

(see section 4.5. Interaction with other medicinal products and other forms of interaction)

- combination with sultopride

(see section 4.5. Interaction with other medicinal products and other forms of interaction).

4.4 Special warnings and special precautions for use
Like other topically applied ophthalmic drugs, timolol eye gel may be absorbed into the systemic circulation. This may cause similar undesirable side effects as seen with oral beta-blocking agents.

Therefore, it should be used with caution in patients with sick sinus syndrome, metabolic acidosis or low blood pressure.

Timolol eye gel should be administered with caution to patients having first degree atrioventricular block.

Cardiac failure should be ruled out before starting treatment. Patients with a history of severe cardiac disease should be monitored for early signs of possible cardiac failure. Beta-blocking agents may mask certain symptoms of hyperthyroidism, e.g. tachycardia. Patients suspected of developing thyrotoxicosis should be watched carefully to avoid abrupt withdrawal of beta-blocking agents, which might cause a thyroid storm.

Although the concentration of timolol in the plasma following application of timolol eye gel is lower than after administration of timolol eye drops, the product should generally not be used in combination with amiodarone, calcium antagonists, (bepridil, verapamil, diltiazem) or with beta blockers (see section 4.5 Interaction with other medicinal products and other forms of interaction).

Timolol eye gel has little or no effect on the pupil. When this eye gel is used to lower intraocular pressure in patients with angle-closure glaucoma, it should be given in combination with a miotic. In these patients, the immediate treatment objective is to open the angle by constriction of the pupil with a miotic agent.

Risk of anaphylactic reactions: Patients with a history of atopy or serious anaphylactic reactions to different allergens may be more sensitive to repeated exposure to allergens. The exposure may be accidental, diagnostic or therapeutic. When timolol eye gel is used in such patients, the normal epinephrine dose used to treat anaphylactic reactions may be insufficient.

Timolol eye gel contains benzalkonium chloride as a preservative. Benzalkonium chloride may precipitate in soft contact lenses.

Timolol eye gel has not been studied in patients using contact lenses, and therefore it should not be used with contact lenses.

Beta-blockers may increase the risk of rebound hypertension.

Caution should be exercised if timolol eye gel is used with systemic beta-blockers.

The use of timolol eye gel with an other topical beta-blocker is not recommended.

The concomitant administration of MAO inhibitors should be avoided.

As with any glaucoma treatment, regular examination of the intraocular pressure and cornea is recommended.

Diabetic patients should be advised to reinforce self-monitoring of their glycaemia at the beginning of treatment. Signs and symptoms of hypoglycaemia, especially tachycardia, palpitations and sweating may be masked.

4.5 Interaction with other medicinal products and other forms of Interaction
1. Other eye drops

If concomitant treatment with other eye drops is used, their administration should be separated by at least a 5 minute interval and the eye gel should be administered last.

Although timolol eye gel has little effect on the size of the pupil, mydriasis has occasionally been reported when timolol has been used with mydriatic agents such as epinephrine.

2. Other drugs

Despite the lower systemic exposure after instillation of the once daily timolol 0.1% eye gel compared to the twice daily timolol 0.5% eye drops, timolol may be absorbed systemically and interactions observed with oral beta-blockers may occur.

Combinations which are contraindicated

Floctafenine

In the event of shock or hypotension caused by floctafenine, beta-blockers attenuate compensatory cardiovascular mechanisms.

Sultopride

Increased risk of ventricular arrhythmia, particularly torsades de points.

Combinations which are not recommended

Amiodarone

Supression of compensatory sympathetic mechanisms may lead to conduction and myocardial contractility disorders.

Calcium antagonists

Bradyarrhythmias (excessive bradycardia, sinus arrest), sinoatrial or atrioventricular conduction disorders and cardiac failure via a synergistic effect.

The nature of any cardiovascular adverse effects tends to depend on the type of calcium-channel blocker used. Dihydropyridine derivatives, such as nifedipine, may lead to hypotension, whereas verapamil or diltiazem tend to cause AV conduction disturbances or left ventricular failure when used with beta-blocker.

Oral beta-blockers

When timolol eye gel is administered to patients receiving an oral beta-blocking agent, both the reduction in intraocular pressure and the effects of systemic beta-blockade may be intensified. The response of such patients should be closely observed.

Combinations requiring precautions for use

Catecholamine-depleting drugs (e.g. reserpine)

Close observation of the patient is also recommended when a beta-blocker is administered to patients receiving catecholamine-depleting drugs such as reserpine, because of possible additive effects and the production of hypotension and/or marked bradycardia which may produce vertigo, syncope, or postural hypotension.

Digitalis glycosides

The concomitant use of digitalis glycosides and beta-blockers may slow down atrioventricular conduction.

Class I anti-arrhythmic drugs

Class I anti-arrhythmic drugs (e.g. disopyramide, quinidine, lidocain i.v.) and amiodarone may have a potentiating effect on atrial conduction and thus induce a negative inotropic effect.

Volatile halogenated anaesthetic agents

Reductions in compensatory cardiovascular mechanisms by beta blockers (beta-adrenergic inhibition may be counteracted during surgery by beta-stimulants). As a general rule do not discontinue beta-blocker therapy and in any event, avoid a sudden discontinuation. The anaesthetist should be advised of this treatment.

Potentiation of the systemic beta-blocking effects of eye drops

and an increase in plasma levels of the beta-blocker have been reported when beta-blocker eye drops are combined with quinidine, probably due to inhibition of the beta-blocker metabolism by quinidine (described for timolol). In addition, cimetidine may increase the timolol concentration in the plasma.

Clonidine and other centrally acting antihypertensive agents (methyldopa, guanfacine, moxonidine, rilmenidine)

Close observation of the patient is recommended. To avoid rebound hypertension, abrupt withdrawal of the drugs should be avoided.

Insulin, oral hypoglycaemic agents

All beta blockers may mask certain symptoms of hypoglycaemia: palpitations and tachycardia.

Most of the non-cardioselective beta-blockers increase the frequency and severity of hypoglycaemia.

Warn the patient and particularly at the beginning of treatment, self-monitoring of glucose by the patient should be increased.

4.6 Pregnancy and lactation

Pregnancy

Clinically, to date, no teratogenic effect has been reported, and the results of controlled prospective studies performed with some beta-blockers have not shown any malformations at birth.

Experimental data did not show teratogenic effect.

Beta-blockers reduce placental perfusion, which may result in foetal death or premature delivery. In addition, undesirable effects, especially hypoglycaemia and bradycardia may also occur in fetuses.

In neonates born to treated mothers, beta-blocker activity persists for several days after birth and may cause bradycardia, respiratory distress and hypoglycaemia, but in general this is of no clinical consequence. However, as a result of depressed sympathetic compensatory mechanisms, cardiac failure, requiring intensive care, may occur. Administration of intravenous fluids should be avoided to reduce the risk of precipitating acute pulmonary oedema.

Therefore, timolol eye drops may be used during pregnancy, if necessary. If treatment is continued until delivery, close monitoring of the neonate (for heart rate and hypoglycaemia during the first 3 to 5 days after birth) is recommended.

Breast-feeding

An occurrence of hypoglycaemia and bradycardia with poorly protein-bound beta-blockers has been described in suckling infant. Therefore, breast-feeding is not recommended while using timolol eye drops.

4.7 Effects on ability to drive and use machines

No studies on the effect of this medicinal product on the ability to drive have been conducted. While driving vehicles or operating different machines, it should be taken into account that occasionally visual disturbances may occur including refractive changes, diplopia, ptosis, frequent episodes of mild and transient blurred vision and occasional episodes of dizziness or fatigue.

4.8 Undesirable effects

Like other topically applied ophthalmic drugs, timolol eye gel may be absorbed into the systemic circulation. This may cause similar undesirable effects as seen with oral beta-blocking agents.

Ocular reactions:

Symptoms of ocular irritation include:

- conjunctivitis
- blepharitis
- keratitis
- conjunctival hyperaemia
- decreased corneal sensitivity.

Blurred vision of short duration may occur in 30 to 50% of patients.

Other possible reactions are:

- visual disturbances, including refractive changes (due to withdrawal of miotic therapy in some cases)
- diplopia
- ptosis.

Dry eyes have been reported during beta-blocker therapy.

Cardiovascular reactions:

- bradycardia
- slowed atrioventricular conduction or increase in an existing atrioventricular block
- hypotension
- cardiac insufficiency
- heart block
- arrhythmia
- syncope
- cerebrovascular disturbances
- cerebral ischaemia
- palpitation
- Raynaud phenomenon
- cold hands and feet
- intermittent claudication
- cardiac arrest.

Respiratory reactions:

- bronchospasm (predominantly in patients with broncho-obstructive pulmonary disease)
- respiratory insufficiency
- dyspnoea
- cough.

Body as a whole:

- fatigue
- headache
- asthenia
- chest pain.

Skin reactions:

- hypersensitivity reactions
- local and generalised erythema including urticaria
- alopecia
- psoriatiform-like lesions or exacerbation of psoriasis.

The incidence of the symptoms is low, and in most cases the symptoms have cleared after discontinuation of treatment. The use of the medication should be discontinued if any such reaction is not otherwise explicable. Benzalkonium chloride is known to cause allergy.

Central nervous system/psychiatric reactions:

- dizziness
- depression
- insomnia
- nightmares
- memory loss
- paraesthesiae
- an increase in signs and symptoms of myasthenia gravis.

Gastrointestinal reactions:

- nausea
- vomiting
- diarrhoea
- dyspepsia
- gastralgia
- dry mouth.

Immunologics:

- systemic lupus erythematosus.

Metabolism and nutrition:

- hypoglycaemia.

Urogenital:

- sexual disfunction (such as decreased libido, impotence)
- syndrome of Peyronie.

Biologically:

rare cases of antinuclear antibodies have been observed, only exceptionally accompanied by clinical symptoms such as lupus syndrome, which regress at treatment discontinuation.

4.9 Overdose

No data specific to this preparation are available. The most common side effects caused by beta-blocker overdosage are symptomatic bradycardia, hypotension, bronchospasm, and acute cardiac insufficiency.

If overdosage occurs, the following measures should be considered:

1. Administration of activated charcoal, if the preparation has been taken orally. Studies have shown that timolol cannot be removed by haemodialysis.

2. Symptomatic bradycardia: Atropine sulphate, 0.25 to 2 mg intravenously, should be used to induce vagal blockade. If bradycardia persists, intravenous isoprenaline hydrochloride should be administered cautiously. In refractory cases, the use of a cardiac pacemaker should be considered.

3. Hypotension: A sympathomimetic agent such as dopamine, dobutamine or noradrenaline should be given. In refractory cases, the use of glucagon has been useful.

4. Bronchospasm: Isoprenaline hydrochloride should be given. Concomitant therapy with aminophylline may be considered.

5. Acute cardiac failure: Conventional therapy with digitalis, diuretics and oxygen should be instituted immediately. In refractory cases, the use of intravenous aminophylline is recommended.

This may be followed, if necessary, by glucagon, which has been found useful.

6. Heart blocks: Isoprenaline hydrochloride or a pacemaker should be used.

5. PHARMACOLOGICAL PROPERTIES

5.1 Pharmacodynamic properties

Pharmacotherapeutic group: Antiglaucoma preparations and miotics, beta blocking agents.

ATC code: S01ED01

Timolol is a non-selective beta-blocker that does not have any significant cardiac stimulating or direct cardiac depressant or local anaesthetic (membrane stabilizing) activity. When applied topically in the eye, it reduces both elevated and normal intraocular pressure. Although not all mechanisms of action of timolol are known yet, it is thought to primarily reduce the production of aqueous humour. It may also have a lesser effect on the outflow of aqueous humour. Unlike miotics, timolol reduces intraocular pressure with little effect on pupil size or visual acuity. Thus, impairment of vision or night blindness does not occur as with the use of miotics. In cataract patients, the impairment of vision, caused by lenticular opacities when the pupil is constricted, is avoided.

The onset of reduction in intraocular pressure following ocular administration of timolol can usually be detected within 30 minutes after eye drop administration. The maximum effect is achieved within about 2 hours from administration and significant lowering of intraocular pressure can be maintained for periods as long as 24 hours.

5.2 Pharmacokinetic properties

Timolol eye gel 0.1% is an eye-drop formulation in gel form, which due to the particular chemical characteristics, maximise the drug absorption in the eye and reduces its absorption into the systemic circulation.

The systemic absorption after topical administration of timolol eye gel 0.1% has been shown to be reduced by 90% as compared to timolol 0.5% eye drops. This is due to the 10 times lower daily timolol maleate dose. Timolol eye gel 0.1% had a significantly smaller effect on the peak heart rate in an exercise test as compared to timolol 0.5% solution.

Pharmacokinetic data from studies in healthy volunteers have shown that the mean value of the maximum plasma concentration is 0.18 ng/ml when timolol eye gel 1mg/g is given once daily, which is approximately 10 times lower than achieved after twice daily dosage of timolol eye drops 5mg/ml.

5.3 Preclinical safety data

No adverse local effects were observed in rabbits or dogs receiving timolol by ocular administration for 4 weeks.

Timolol was not mutagenic and did not affect fertility in rats.

Carcinogenicity studies produced an increased incidence of phaeochromocytomas in male rats, and mammary adenomas, pulmonary tumors and benign uterine polyps in mice, but only at high oral doses.

Repeated application of timolol eye gel did not produce any local or systemic intolerance in rabbits or dogs.

6. PHARMACEUTICAL PARTICULARS

6.1 List of excipients

Benzalkonium chloride

Sorbitol

Polyvinyl alcohol

Carbomer 974 P

Sodium acetate trihydrate

Lysine monohydrate

Water for injections

6.2 Incompatibilities

For information on use of the product with contact lenses see under 4.4.

6.3 Shelf life

18 months. The shelf-life after first opening is 4 weeks

6.4 Special precautions for storage

Keep the container in the outer carton in order to protect from light. Do not store above 25°C.

Store the dropper bottle upside down in the carton below 25°C after first opening.

Do not freeze.

6.5 Nature and contents of container

The eye-drop bottle contains 5g gel and it is made of low-density polyethylene (LDPE). The tip of the bottle is also of LDPE and the cap is of high-density polyethylene.

The following pack sizes are available: cartons containing 1 or 3 bottles of 5g. Not all pack sizes may be marketed.

6.6 Instructions for use and handling

No special requirements.

7. MARKETING AUTHORISATION HOLDER

Novartis Pharmaceuticals UK Ltd
Frimley Business Park
Frimley, Camberley
Surrey, GU16 7SR
UK.

8. MARKETING AUTHORISATION NUMBER(S)

PL 00101/0616

9. DATE OF FIRST AUTHORISATION/RENEWAL OF THE AUTHORISATION

20 January 2005

10. DATE OF REVISION OF THE TEXT

11 December, 2003

LEGAL CATEGORY

POM

Nystan Cream and Ointment

(E. R. Squibb & Sons Limited)

1. NAME OF THE MEDICINAL PRODUCT

NYSTAN CREAM AND OINTMENT

2. QUALITATIVE AND QUANTITATIVE COMPOSITION

Nystan Cream:	Pale buff, containing 100,000 units per gram nystatin in a vanishing-cream base.
Nystan Ointment:	Yellow to amber, containing 100,000 units per gram nystatin in a plastibase.

3. PHARMACEUTICAL FORM

Topical Cream and Ointment

4. CLINICAL PARTICULARS

4.1 Therapeutic indications

For the treatment of cutaneous and mucocutaneous mycoses, particularly those caused by *Candida Albicans*.

4.2 Posology and method of administration

Adults and children:

To be applied two to four times daily.

Elderly:

No specific dosage recommendations or precautions.

4.3 Contraindications

There are no known contra-indications or special precautions for topical application of nystatin.

4.4 Special warnings and special precautions for use

Children:

No specific precautions apply; systemic absorption is negligible.

4.5 Interaction with other medicinal products and other forms of Interaction

None known.

4.6 Pregnancy and lactation

No specific precautions apply; systemic absorption is negligible.

4.7 Effects on ability to drive and use machines

None known.

4.8 Undesirable effects

There have been no substantiated reports of sensitivity associated with topical nystatin.

4.9 Overdose

Since absorption of nystatin from the gastro-intestinal tract is negligible, accidental ingestion causes no systemic toxicity.

5. PHARMACOLOGICAL PROPERTIES

5.1 Pharmacodynamic properties

Actions:

Nystatin is a polyene, antifungal antibiotic active against a wide range of yeasts and yeast-like fungi, including *Candida albicans*.

5.2 Pharmacokinetic properties

Nystatin is formulated in oral and topical dosage forms and is not systemically absorbed from any of these preparations.

5.3 Preclinical safety data

No further relevant information.

6. PHARMACEUTICAL PARTICULARS

6.1 List of excipients

Nystan Cream:	Aluminium hydroxide, antifoam emulsion, benzyl alcohol, macrogol ether, perfume, propylene glycol, sorbitol, titanium dioxide, white soft paraffin, water.
Nystan Ointment:	Liquid paraffin and polyethylene resin.

6.2 Incompatibilities

None known.

6.3 Shelf life

Cream:	48 months.
Ointment	36 months

6.4 Special precautions for storage

Cream:	Do not store above 25°C. Avoid freezing.
Ointment	Do not store above 25°C.

6.5 Nature and contents of container

Aluminium tubes of 30g.

6.6 Instructions for use and handling

Not applicable.

7. MARKETING AUTHORISATION HOLDER

E. R. Squibb & Sons Limited
Uxbridge Business Park
Sanderson Road
Uxbridge
Middlesex UB8 1DH

8. MARKETING AUTHORISATION NUMBER(S)

Nystan Cream:	PL 0034/5058R
Nystan Ointment:	PL 0034/0161R

9. DATE OF FIRST AUTHORISATION/RENEWAL OF THE AUTHORISATION

Nystan Cream:	22 November 1990 / 22 January 2001
Nystan Ointment:	30 November 1990 / 19 January 2001

10. DATE OF REVISION OF THE TEXT

24 June 2005

Nystan Oral Suspension (Ready-Mixed) and Nystan Oral Tablets

(E. R. Squibb & Sons Limited)

1. NAME OF THE MEDICINAL PRODUCT

NYSTAN ORAL SUSPENSION (READY-MIXED) AND NYSTAN ORAL TABLETS.

2. QUALITATIVE AND QUANTITATIVE COMPOSITION

Ready mixed oral suspension containing 100,000 units nystatin per ml.

Tablets containing 500,000 units nystatin.

3. PHARMACEUTICAL FORM

Oral suspension and tablets

4. CLINICAL PARTICULARS

4.1 Therapeutic indications

Suspension:

The prevention and treatment of candidal infections of the oral cavity, oesophagus and intestinal tract. The suspension provides effective prophylaxis against oral candidosis in those born of mothers with vaginal candidosis.

Tablets:

Tablets for intestinal candidosis. Also for use in patients who may be susceptible to candidal overgrowth, e.g. patients with malignant disease especially if receiving cytotoxic drugs, and those patients receiving high doses or prolonged courses of antibiotics or corticosteroids.

4.2 Posology and method of administration

Adults:

Suspension:

For the treatment of denture sores, and oral infections in adults caused by *C.albicans*, 1ml of the suspension should be dropped into the mouth four times daily; it should be kept in contact with the affected areas as long as possible.

Tablets:

For the treatment of intestinal candidosis 1 tablet four times daily, but this dose may be doubled. For prophylaxis a total daily dosage of 1 million units has been found to suppress the overgrowth of *C.albicans* in patients receiving broad-spectrum antibiotic therapy.

Administration should be continued for 48 hours after clinical cure to prevent relapse.

Children:

Suspension:

In intestinal and oral candidosis (thrush) in infants and children, 1ml should be dropped into the mouth four times a day. The longer the suspension is kept in contact with the affected area in the mouth, before swallowing, the greater will be its effect.

For prophylaxis in the newborn the suggested dose is 1ml once daily.

Elderly:

No specific dosage recommendations or precautions.

4.3 Contraindications

Contra-indicated in patients with a history of hypersensitivity to any of the components.

4.4 Special warnings and special precautions for use

Nystan Oral Suspension contains sugar. Nystan oral preparations should not be used for treatment of systemic mycoses.

4.5 Interaction with other medicinal products and other forms of Interaction

None known.

4.6 Pregnancy and lactation

Animal reproductive studies have not been conducted with nystatin.

It is not known whether nystatin can cause foetal harm when administered to a pregnant women, however absorption of nystatin from the gastro-intestinal tract is negligible. Nystatin should be prescribed during pregnancy only if the potential benefits to be derived outweigh the possible risks involved.

Nursing Mothers:

Though gastro-intestinal absorption is insignificant, it is not known whether nystatin is excreted in human breast milk and caution should be exercised when nystatin is prescribed for nursing women.

4.7 Effects on ability to drive and use machines

None known.

4.8 Undesirable effects

Nystatin is generally well tolerated by all age groups, even during prolonged use. Rarely, oral irritation or sensitisation may occur. Nausea has been reported occasionally during therapy.

Large oral doses of Nystatin have occasionally produced diarrhoea, gastrointestinal distress, nausea and vomiting. Rash, including urticaria, has been reported rarely. Steven-Johnson Syndrome has been reported very rarely.

4.9 Overdose

Since the absorption of nystatin from the gastro-intestinal tract is negligible, overdosage or accidental ingestion causes no systemic toxicity.

5. PHARMACOLOGICAL PROPERTIES

5.1 Pharmacodynamic properties

Nystatin is an antifungal antibiotic active against a wide range of yeasts and yeast-like fungi, including *Candida albicans*.

5.2 Pharmacokinetic properties

Nystatin is formulated in oral and topical dosage forms and is not systemically absorbed from any of these preparations.

5.3 Preclinical safety data

No further relevant information.

6. PHARMACEUTICAL PARTICULARS

6.1 List of excipients

Oral Suspension:	Ethanol, flavours, glycerin, methyl parahydroxybenzoate, pH adjusters (hydrochloric acid, sodium hydroxide), propyl parahydroxybenzoate, sodium carboxymethylcellulose, sodium phosphate, sucrose, water.
Oral Tablets:	Carnauba wax, castor oil, chalk, iron oxide, lactose, magnesium stearate, maize starch, microcrystalline cellulose, polysorbate 20, povidone, shellac, sorbic acid, stearic acid, sucrose, talc, white beeswax.

6.2 Incompatibilities

None known.

6.3 Shelf life

Oral Suspension:	24 months
Oral Tablets:	36 months

6.4 Special precautions for storage

Do not store above 25°C

6.5 Nature and contents of container

Oral Suspension:	30ml amber glass bottle, packed in a cardboard carton with a graduated, polyethylene dropper.
Oral Tablets:	Amber glass bottle of 56 tablets, packed in a cardboard carton.

6.6 Instructions for use and handling

Oral Suspension:

Shake well before use.

Dilution is not recommended as this may reduce therapeutic efficacy.

7. MARKETING AUTHORISATION HOLDER

E.R. Squibb & Sons Limited
Uxbridge Business Park
Sanderson Road
Uxbridge
Middlesex UB8 1DH

8. MARKETING AUTHORISATION NUMBER(S)

Oral Suspension:	PL 0034/0130R
Oral Tablets:	PL 0034/5063R

9. DATE OF FIRST AUTHORISATION/RENEWAL OF THE AUTHORISATION

Oral Suspension:	28 November 1990 / 19 January 2001
Oral Tablets:	12 March 1996 / 13 March 2001

10. DATE OF REVISION OF THE TEXT

24 June 2005

Nystan Pastilles

(E. R. Squibb & Sons Limited)

1. NAME OF THE MEDICINAL PRODUCT

Nystan Pastilles

2. QUALITATIVE AND QUANTITATIVE COMPOSITION

Each pastille contains 100,000 I.U. of nystatin.

For excipients, see Section 6.1.

3. PHARMACEUTICAL FORM

Pastille

4. CLINICAL PARTICULARS

4.1 Therapeutic indications

For the prevention and treatment of oral candidosis.

4.2 Posology and method of administration

No food or drink should be taken for five minutes before or one hour after consumption of the pastille. The pastilles should be sucked slowly and retained in the mouth for as long as possible in accordance with the doctors instructions.

Adults:

One pastille to be sucked slowly, four times a day for 7-14 days.

Elderly:

No specific dosage recommendations or precautions.

Children:

One pastille to be sucked slowly, four times a day for 7-14 days.

4.3 Contraindications

Contraindicated in patients with a history of hypersensitivity to any of its components.

4.4 Special warnings and special precautions for use

Each Nystan pastille contains approximately 825mg of total glucose solids and 750mg of sucrose. As the pastilles contain sugar, they should be administered with caution to patients with disaccharide intolerance.

Nystan pastilles should not be used for treatment of systemic mycoses.

4.5 Interaction with other medicinal products and other forms of Interaction

None known.

4.6 Pregnancy and lactation

Animal reproductive studies have not been conducted with nystatin.

It is not known whether nystatin can cause foetal harm when administered to a pregnant women, however absorption of nystatin from the gastro intestinal tract is negligible. Nystatin should be prescribed during pregnancy only if the potential benefits to be derived outweigh the possible risks involved.

Though gastro intestinal absorption is insignificant, it is not known whether nystatin is excreted in human breast milk and caution should be exercised when nystatin is prescribed for nursing women.

4.7 Effects on ability to drive and use machines

None known.

4.8 Undesirable effects

Nystatin is generally well tolerated by all age groups, even during prolonged use. Rarely, oral irritation or sensitisation may occur. Nausea has been reported occasionally during therapy.

Large oral doses of Nystatin have occasionally produced diarrhoea, gastrointestinal distress, nausea and vomiting. Rash, including urticaria, has been reported rarely. Steven Johnson Syndrome has been reported very rarely.

4.9 Overdose

Since the absorption of nystatin from the gastro intestinal tract is negligible, overdosage causes no systemic toxicity.

5. PHARMACOLOGICAL PROPERTIES

5.1 Pharmacodynamic properties

Nystatin is an antifungal antibiotic active against a wide range of yeasts and yeast-like fungi, including *Candida albicans*.

5.2 Pharmacokinetic properties

Nystatin is formulated in oral and topical dosage forms and is not systemically absorbed from any of these presentations.

5.3 Preclinical safety data

No further relevant information.

6. PHARMACEUTICAL PARTICULARS

6.1 List of excipients

Aniseed oil, cinnamon oil, dextrose monohydrate, gelatin, liquid glucose, pH adjusters, silicone antifoam emulsion, sucrose and water.

6.2 Incompatibilities

None known.

6.3 Shelf life

24 months

6.4 Special precautions for storage

Do not store above 25°C.

6.5 Nature and contents of container

Pouch of paper/polyethylene/foil/polyethylene laminate (28 pastilles per pouch).

6.6 Instructions for use and handling

None stated.

7. MARKETING AUTHORISATION HOLDER

E.R. Squibb & Sons Limited
Uxbridge Business Park
Sanderson Road
Uxbridge
Middlesex UB8 1DH

8. MARKETING AUTHORISATION NUMBER(S)

PL 0034/0248

9. DATE OF FIRST AUTHORISATION/RENEWAL OF THE AUTHORISATION

09 May 1984 / 8 December 1995 / 23 January 2001

10. DATE OF REVISION OF THE TEXT

24 June 2005

Nystan Pessaries, Vaginal Cream

(E. R. Squibb & Sons Limited)

1. NAME OF THE MEDICINAL PRODUCT

Nystan Pessaries

Nystan Vaginal Cream

2. QUALITATIVE AND QUANTITATIVE COMPOSITION

Pessaries:	Each pessary contains 100,000 units nystatin
Cream:	Each 4g application contains 100,000 units nystatin

3. PHARMACEUTICAL FORM

Vaginal tablet

Vaginal cream

4. CLINICAL PARTICULARS

4.1 Therapeutic indications

The treatment of candidal vaginitis.

4.2 Posology and method of administration

Adults:

Pessaries: 1 or 2 pesssaries should be inserted high into the vagina for 14 consecutive nights, or longer, regardless of any intervening menstrual period.

Cream: Insert 1 or 2 applications (of 4g each) high into the vagina for 14 consecutive nights, or longer, regardless of any intervening menstrual period.

Children:

Cream: Vulvovaginal candidosis is rarely a problem in children. It is suggested that the vaginal cream is the most acceptable formulation for children.

Pessaries: Not recommended for children under 12 years.

Elderly:

No specific dosage recommendations or precautions.

4.3 Contraindications

There are no known contra-indications to the use of nystatin.

4.4 Special warnings and special precautions for use

Pessaries: No specific precautions apply.

Cream: Avoid contact between the cream and contraceptive diaphragms and condoms, since the rubber may be damaged by the preparation.

4.5 Interaction with other medicinal products and other forms of Interaction

None known.

4.6 Pregnancy and lactation

There is no evidence that nystatin is absorbed systemically from the vagina. However, as with all drugs, caution should be exercised in pregnancy. Care should be taken while using an applicator to prevent the possibility of mechanical trauma.

4.7 Effects on ability to drive and use machines

None known.

4.8 Undesirable effects

Nystan is well tolerated and no substantiated sensitivity reactions have been associated with its use. Some transient local discomfort may be experienced.

4.9 Overdose

Since the absorption of nystatin from the gastro-intestinal tract is negligible, overdosage or accidental ingestion causes no systemic toxicity.

5. PHARMACOLOGICAL PROPERTIES

5.1 Pharmacodynamic properties

Nystatin is an antifungal antibiotic active against a wide range of yeasts and yeast-like fungi, including *Candida albicans*.

5.2 Pharmacokinetic properties

Nystatin is formulated in oral and topical dosage forms and is not systemically absorbed from any of these preparations.

5.3 Preclinical safety data

No further relevant information.

6. PHARMACEUTICAL PARTICULARS

6.1 List of excipients

Pessaries:	Lactose, magnesium stearate, maize starch, microcrystalline cellulose.
Cream:	Aluminium hydroxide, antifoam emulsion, benzyl alcohol, macrogol ether, pH adjusters (hydrochloric acid, sodium hydroxide), propylene glycol, sorbitol, water, white soft paraffin.

6.2 Incompatibilities

None known.

6.3 Shelf life

Pessaries:	24 months
Cream:	24 months

6.4 Special precautions for storage

Pessaries:	Do not store above 25°C.
Cream:	Do not store above 25°C. Avoid freezing

6.5 Nature and contents of container

Pessaries:	Foil strip, packed in a carton with an applicator, in packs of 28 pessaries.
Cream:	60g aluminium tube, packed in a cardboard carton with a vaginal applicator.

6.6 Instructions for use and handling

Pessaries:	None stated.
Cream:	Dilution of the vaginal cream is not recommended as this may reduce therapeutic efficacy.

7. MARKETING AUTHORISATION HOLDER

E. R. Squibb & Sons Limited
Uxbridge Business Park
Sanderson Road
Uxbridge
Middlesex UB8 1DH

8. MARKETING AUTHORISATION NUMBER(S)

Pessaries:	PL 0034/5062R
Cream:	PL 0034/0137R

9. DATE OF FIRST AUTHORISATION/RENEWAL OF THE AUTHORISATION

Pessaries:	25th January 1991
Cream:	22nd November 1990/19 January 2001

10. DATE OF REVISION OF THE TEXT

24 June 2005

Occlusal

(Alliance Pharmaceuticals)

1. NAME OF THE MEDICINAL PRODUCT

Occlusal.

26% w/w cutaneous solution

2. QUALITATIVE AND QUANTITATIVE COMPOSITION

Salicylic Acid 26% w/w.

For excipients, see 6.1

3. PHARMACEUTICAL FORM

Cutaneous solution

A colourless to pale yellow solution with a characteristic smell of nail varnish

4. CLINICAL PARTICULARS

4.1 Therapeutic indications

Occlusal is indicated for the treatment and removal of common and plantar warts (verrucae).

4.2 Posology and method of administration

For topical application.

Prior to application soak wart in warm water for five minutes. Remove loose tissue with a brush, emery board, pumice or abrasive sponge, being careful to avoid causing pin-point bleeding or abrading the surrounding healthy skin. Dry thoroughly with a towel not used by others to avoid contagion. Carefully apply Occlusal twice to the wart using the brush applicator allowing the first application to dry before applying the second. Thereafter repeat treatment once daily or as directed by physician. Do not apply to surrounding healthy skin. Clinically visible improvement should occur in one to two weeks but maximum effect may be expected after four to six weeks.

There are no differences in dosage for children, adults or the elderly.

4.3 Contraindications

Occlusal should not be used by diabetics or patients with impaired blood circulation. Do not use on moles, birthmarks, unusual warts with hair growth, on facial warts, or in the anal or perineal region.

4.4 Special warnings and special precautions for use

Occlusal is for external use only. Do not permit contact with eyes or mucous membranes. If contact occurs flush with water for 15 minutes. Do not allow contact with normal skin around wart. Avoid using on areas of broken or damaged skin. Discontinue treatment if excessive irritation occurs.

4.5 Interaction with other medicinal products and other forms of Interaction

None known.

4.6 Pregnancy and lactation

The chronic use of this product during pregnancy and lactation, particularly when large areas of skin are involved, should be avoided.

4.7 Effects on ability to drive and use machines

None known.

4.8 Undesirable effects

A localised irritant reaction may occur if Occlusal is applied to normal skin surrounding the wart. This may normally be controlled by temporarily discontinuing the use of Occlusal and by being careful to apply the solution only to the wart itself when treatment is resumed.

4.9 Overdose

Salicylism can occur following large doses of salicylic acid or prolonged use of topical salicylic preparations, or in the unlikely event of accidental consumption.

5. PHARMACOLOGICAL PROPERTIES

5.1 Pharmacodynamic properties

Salicylic acid has bacteriostatic and fungicidal actions, but it is its keratolytic properties which are important for this medicinal product. When applied externally it produces slow and painless destruction of the epithelium. Salicylic acid is usually applied in the form of a paint in a collodian base (10 to 17%) or as a plaster (20 to 50%) to destroy warts or corns.

5.2 Pharmacokinetic properties

Not applicable.

5.3 Preclinical safety data

None presented.

6. PHARMACEUTICAL PARTICULARS

6.1 List of excipients

Polyvinyl butyral

Dibutyl phthalate

Isopropyl alcohol

Butyl acetate

Acrylates copolymer

6.2 Incompatibilities

Not applicable

6.3 Shelf life

2 years.

6.4 Special precautions for storage

Do not store above 25°C

6.5 Nature and contents of container

The product is presented in a 10ml amber glass bottle with cap brush assembly. The cap brush assembly comprises of a black cap and a white polythene wand nylon brush with stainless steel staple.

6.6 Instructions for use and handling

Occlusal is flammable and should be kept away from flame or fire. Keep the bottle tightly capped when not in use. Do not allow the solution to drip from the brush onto the bottle neck thread, otherwise subsequent opening of the bottle may be difficult.

7. MARKETING AUTHORISATION HOLDER

Alliance Pharmaceuticals Limited

Avonbridge House

2 Bath Road

Chippenham

Wiltshire, SN15 2BB

UK

8. MARKETING AUTHORISATION NUMBER(S)

PL 16853/0071

9. DATE OF FIRST AUTHORISATION/RENEWAL OF THE AUTHORISATION

7th September 1998/18th May 2005

10. DATE OF REVISION OF THE TEXT

May 2005

Octim Injection

(Ferring Pharmaceuticals Ltd)

1. NAME OF THE MEDICINAL PRODUCT

OCTIM® Injection

2. QUALITATIVE AND QUANTITATIVE COMPOSITION

Desmopressin acetate 15 micrograms per ml.

3. PHARMACEUTICAL FORM

Solution for injection.

4. CLINICAL PARTICULARS

4.1 Therapeutic indications

OCTIM Injection is indicated as follows:

1. To increase Factor VIII:C and Factor VIII:Ag in patients with mild to moderate haemophilia or von Willebrand's disease undergoing surgery or following trauma.

2. To test for fibrinolytic response.

4.2 Posology and method of administration

Mild to Moderate Haemophilia and von Willebrand's Disease:

By subcutaneous or intravenous administration.

The dose for adults, children and infants is 0.3 micrograms per kilogram body weight, administered by subcutaneous injection or intravenous infusion. Further doses may be administered at 12 hourly intervals so long as cover is required. As some patients have shown a diminishing response to successive doses, it is recommended that monitoring of Factor VIII levels should continue.

For intravenous infusion, the dose should be diluted in 50ml of 0.9% sodium chloride for injection and given over 20 minutes. This dose should be given immediately prior to surgery or following trauma. During administration of intravenous desmopressin, vasodilation may occur resulting in decreased blood pressure and tachycardia with facial flushing in some patients.

Increase of Factor VIII levels are dependent on basal levels and are normally between 2 and 5 times the pre-treatment levels. If results from a previous administration of desmopressin are not available then blood should be taken pre-dose and 20 minutes post-dose for assay of Factor VIII levels in order to monitor response.

Unless contraindicated, when surgery is undertaken tranexamic acid may be given orally at the recommended dose from 24 hours beforehand until healing is complete.

Fibrinolytic Response Testing:

By subcutaneous or intravenous administration.

The dose for adults and children is 0.3 micrograms per kilogram body weight, administered by subcutaneous injection or intravenous infusion.

For intravenous infusion, the dose should be diluted in 50ml of 0.9% sodium chloride for injection and given over 20 minutes.

A sample of venous blood should be taken 20 minutes after the administration. In patients with a normal response the sample should show fibrinolytic activity of euglobulin clot precipitate on fibrin plates of at least 240mm^2.

4.3 Contraindications

OCTIM Injection is contraindicated in cases of:

- habitual and psychogenic polydipsia
- unstable angina pectoris
- decompensated cardiac insufficiency
- von Willebrand's Disease Type IIB where the administration of desmopressin may result in pseudothrombocytopenia due to the release of abnormal clotting factors which cause platelet aggregation.

Fibrinolytic Response Testing should not be carried out in patients with hypertension, heart disease, cardiac insufficiency and other conditions requiring treatment with diuretic agents.

4.4 Special warnings and special precautions for use

Precautions to prevent fluid overload must be taken in:

- conditions characterised by fluid and/or electrolyte imbalance
- patients at risk for increased intracranial pressure.

Care should be taken with patients who have reduced renal function and/or cardiovascular disease.

When repeated doses are used to control bleeding in haemophilia or von Willebrand's disease, care should be taken to prevent fluid overload. Fluid should not be forced, orally or parenterally, and patients should only take as much fluid as they require to satisfy thirst. Intravenous infusions should not be left up as a routine after surgery. Fluid accumulation can be readily monitored by weighing the patient or by determining plasma sodium or osmolality.

Measures to prevent fluid overload must be taken in patients with conditions requiring treatment with diuretic agents.

Special attention must be paid to the risk of water retention. The fluid intake should be restricted to the least possible and the body weight should be checked regularly.

If there is a gradual increase of the body weight, decrease of serum sodium to below 130mmol/l or plasma osmolality to below 270mOsm/kg, the fluid intake must be reduced drastically and the administration of OCTIM Injection interrupted.

During administration of OCTIM Injection, it is recommended that the patient's blood pressure is monitored continuously.

OCTIM Injection does not reduce prolonged bleeding time in thrombocytopenia.

4.5 Interaction with other medicinal products and other forms of Interaction

Substances which are known to induce SIADH e.g. tricyclic antidepressants, selective serotonin re-uptake inhibitors, chlorpromazine and carbamazepine, may cause an additive antidiuretic effect leading to an increased risk of water retention and/or hyponatraemia.

NSAIDs may induce water retention and/or hyponatraemia.

4.6 Pregnancy and lactation

Pregnancy:

Data on a limited number (n=53) of exposed pregnancies in women with diabetes insipidus indicate rare cases of malformations in children treated during pregnancy. To date, no other relevant epidemiological data are available. Animal studies do not indicate direct or indirect harmful effects with respect to pregnancy, embryonal/fetal development, parturition or postnatal development.

Caution should be exercised when prescribing to pregnant women. Blood pressure monitoring is recommended due to the increased risk of pre-eclampsia.

Lactation:

Results from analyses of milk from nursing mothers receiving 300 micrograms desmopressin intranasally indicate that the amounts of desmopressin that may be transferred to the child are considerably less than the amounts required to influence diuresis or haemostasis.

4.7 Effects on ability to drive and use machines

None

4.8 Undesirable effects

Side-effects include headache, stomach pain and nausea. Isolated cases of allergic skin reactions and more severe general allergic reactions have been reported. Treatment with desmopressin without concomitant reduction of fluid intake may lead to water retention/hyponatraemia with accompanying symptoms of headache, nausea, vomiting, weight gain, decreased serum sodium and in serious cases, convulsions.

During intravenous infusion of OCTIM Injection, vasodilation may occur, resulting in decreased blood pressure and tachycardia with facial flushing. This side effect is normally avoided by infusing the product over 20 minutes.

4.9 Overdose

An overdose of OCTIM Injection leads to a prolonged duration of action with an increased risk of water retention and/or hyponatraemia.

Treatment:

Although the treatment of hyponatraemia should be individualised, the following general recommendations can be given. Hyponatraemia is treated by discontinuing the desmopressin treatment, fluid restriction and symptomatic treatment if needed.

5. PHARMACOLOGICAL PROPERTIES

5.1 Pharmacodynamic properties

Desmopressin is a structural analogue of vasopressin, with two chemical changes namely desamination of the N-terminal and replacement of the 8-L-Arginine by 8-D-Arginine. These changes have increased the antidiuretic activity and prolonged the duration of action. The pressor activity is reduced to less than 0.01% of the natural peptide as a result of which side-effects are rarely seen.

Like vasopressin, desmopressin also increases concentrations of Factor VIII:C, Factor VIII:Ag (vWF) and Plasminogen Activator (t-PA).

5.2 Pharmacokinetic properties

Following intravenous injection, plasma concentrations of desmopressin follow a biexponential curve. The initial fast phase of a few minutes duration and with a half life of less than 10 minutes is thought mainly to represent the diffusion of desmopressin from plasma to its volume of distribution. The second phase with a half life of 51-158 minutes represents the elimination rate of desmopressin from the body.

As a comparison, the half life of vasopressin is less than 10 minutes.

Subcutaneous administration of desmopressin results in a later T_{max} and lower C_{max} values but comparable bioavailability.

In vitro, in human liver microsome preparations, it has been shown that no significant amount of desmopressin is metabolised in the liver and thus human liver metabolism *in vivo* is not likely to occur.

It is unlikely that desmopressin will interact with drugs affecting hepatic metabolism, since desmopressin has been shown not to undergo significant liver metabolism in *in vitro* studies with human microsomes. However, formal *in vivo* interaction studies have not been performed.

5.3 Preclinical safety data

There are no pre-clinical data of relevance to the prescriber which are additional to those already included in other sections of the SPC.

6. PHARMACEUTICAL PARTICULARS

6.1 List of excipients

Sodium chloride Ph. Eur.

Hydrochloric acid Ph. Eur.

Water for injection Ph. Eur.

6.2 Incompatibilities

None

6.3 Shelf life

36 months.

6.4 Special precautions for storage

Store in a refrigerator at 2°C- 8°C and protect from light.

6.5 Nature and contents of container

Clear glass ampoules.

6.6 Instructions for use and handling

The injection is administered by subcutaneous injection or intravenous infusion.

For intravenous infusion, the dose should be diluted in 50ml of 0.9% sodium chloride for injection and given over 20 minutes.

7. MARKETING AUTHORISATION HOLDER

Ferring Pharmaceuticals Ltd.

The Courtyard

Waterside Drive

Langley

Berkshire SL3 6EZ.

8. MARKETING AUTHORISATION NUMBER(S)

PL 03194/0055

9. DATE OF FIRST AUTHORISATION/RENEWAL OF THE AUTHORISATION

11th February 2002

10. DATE OF REVISION OF THE TEXT

September 2002

11. LEGAL CATEGORY

POM

Octim Nasal Spray

(Ferring Pharmaceuticals Ltd)

1. NAME OF THE MEDICINAL PRODUCT

OCTIM® Nasal Spray

2. QUALITATIVE AND QUANTITATIVE COMPOSITION

Desmopressin acetate 150 micrograms per actuation

For excipients, see 6.1

3. PHARMACEUTICAL FORM

Nasal Spray, Solution

Clear, colourless solution

4. CLINICAL PARTICULARS

4.1 Therapeutic indications

OCTIM Nasal Spray is indicated as follows:

1) To increase Factor VIIIC and Factor VIII:Ag (vWf) in patients with mild to moderate haemophilia or von Willebrand's disease undergoing surgery, following trauma or with other bleeding episodes such as menorrhagia and epistaxis.

2) To test for fibrinolytic response.

4.2 Posology and method of administration

Mild to moderate haemophilia and von Willebrand's disease:

Adults (including the elderly) should take 300 micrograms (one spray into each nostril) half an hour before surgery or at bleeding.

Under direct medical supervision, further doses may be administered at 12 hourly intervals so long as cover is required. As some patients have shown a diminishing response to successive doses, Factor VIII levels should continue to be monitored.

Unless specifically directed by the doctor, when OCTIM Nasal Spray is self-administered by the patient, there should be an interval of at least three days between doses.

Increase of Factor VIII levels are dependent on basal levels and are normally between 2 and 5 times the pre-treatment levels. If results from a previous administration of desmopressin are not available then blood should be taken pre-dose and 60 minutes post-dose for assay of Factor VIII levels in order to monitor response.

Fibrinolytic response testing:

Adults (including the elderly) should take 300 micrograms (one spray in each nostril). A sample of venous blood should be taken 60 minutes later.

In patients with a normal response, the sample should show fibrinolytic activity of euglobulin clot precipitate on fibrin plates of at least 240mm^2.

4.3 Contraindications

OCTIM Nasal Spray is contraindicated in cases of:

- habitual and psychogenic polydipsia
- unstable angina pectoris
- decompensated cardiac insufficiency
- von Willebrand's Disease Type IIB where the administration of desmopressin may result in pseudothrombocytopenia due to the release of abnormal clotting factors which cause platelet aggregation.

Fibrinolytic response testing should not be carried out in patients with hypertension, heart disease, cardiac insufficiency and other conditions requiring treatment with diuretic agents.

4.4 Special warnings and special precautions for use

Precautions to prevent fluid overload must be taken in:

- conditions characterised by fluid and/or electrolyte imbalance
- patients at risk for increased intracranial pressure.

Care should be taken with patients who have reduced renal function and or cardiovascular disease or cystic fibrosis.

When repeated doses are used to control bleeding in haemophilia or von Willebrand's disease, care should be taken to prevent fluid overload. Patients should only take as much fluid as they require to satisfy thirst. Intravenous infusions should not be left up as a routine after surgery. Fluid accumulation can be readily monitored by weighing the patient or by determining plasma sodium or osmolality.

Measures to prevent fluid overload must be taken in patients with conditions requiring treatment with diuretic agents.

Special attention must be paid to the risk of water retention. The fluid intake should be restricted to the least possible and the body weight should be checked regularly.

If there is a gradual increase of the body weight, decrease of serum sodium to 130mmol/l or plasma osmolality to below 270mOsm/kg, the fluid intake must be reduced drastically and the administration of OCTIM Nasal Spray interrupted.

OCTIM Nasal Spray does not reduce prolonged bleeding time in thrombocytopenia.

4.5 Interaction with other medicinal products and other forms of Interaction

Indomethacin may augment the magnitude but not the duration of response to desmopressin.

Substances which are known to release antidiuretic hormone e.g. tricyclic antidepressants, chlorpromazine and carbamazepine, may cause an additive antidiuretic effect and increase the risk of water retention.

4.6 Pregnancy and lactation

Pregnancy:

OCTIM Nasal Spray should be given with caution to pregnant patients, although the oxytocic effect of desmopressin is very low.

Reproduction studies performed in rats and rabbits with doses of more than 100 times the human dose have revealed no evidence of a harmful action of desmopressin on the fetus. There have been rare reports of malformations in children born to mothers treated for diabetes insipidus during pregnancy. However, a review of available data suggests no increase in the rate of malformations in children exposed to desmopressin throughout pregnancy.

Lactation:

Results from analyses of milk from nursing mothers receiving 300 micrograms desmopressin intranasally indicate that the amounts of desmopressin that may be transferred to the child are considerably less than the amounts required to influence diuresis or haemostasis.

4.7 Effects on ability to drive and use machines

None

4.8 Undesirable effects

Side-effects include headache, stomach pain, nausea, nasal congestion, rhinitis and epistaxis. Isolated cases of allergic skin reactions and more severe general allergic reactions have been reported. Treatment with desmopressin without concomitant reduction of fluid intake may lead to water retention/hyponatraemia with accompanying symptoms of headache, nausea, vomiting, weight gain, decreased serum sodium and in serious cases, convulsions.

4.9 Overdose

Overdose of OCTIM Nasal Spray can lead to hyponatraemia and convulsions.

Treatment:

Overdosage increases the risk of fluid retention and hyponatraemia. If hyponatraemia occurs, desmopressin treatment should immediately be discontinued and fluid intake restricted until serum sodium is normalised.

5. PHARMACOLOGICAL PROPERTIES

5.1 Pharmacodynamic properties

Desmopressin is an analogue of the hormone vasopressin in which the antidiuretic activity has been enhanced by the order of 10, whilst the vasopressor effect has been reduced by the order of 1500. The duration of activity has also been extended.

Like vasopressin, desmopressin also increases concentrations of Factor VIII:C, Factor VIII:Ag (vWf) and plasminogen activator (t-PA)

5.2 Pharmacokinetic properties

ATC code H01B A02

Following intranasal administration, the bioavailability of desmopressin is of the order of 6-10%. Peak plasma levels are achieved in approximately 50 minutes and the mean plasma half-life is about three hours.

5.3 Preclinical safety data

There are no pre-clinical data of relevance to the prescriber which are additional to that already included in other sections of the SPC

6. PHARMACEUTICAL PARTICULARS

6.1 List of excipients

Sodium chloride

Citric acid monohydrate

Disodium phosphate dihydrate

Benzalkonium chloride soln 50%

Purified water

6.2 Incompatibilities

Not applicable

6.3 Shelf life

36 months

6.4 Special precautions for storage

Do not store above 25°C. Keep vial in the outer carton. Do not freeze.

6.5 Nature and contents of container

Multidose container, Type I glass vial with a pre-compression pump set comprising of a spray pump with a metering valve, nasal applicator and protection cap.

Pack size: 2.5ml (25 sprays)

6.6 Instructions for use and handling

None

7. MARKETING AUTHORISATION HOLDER

Ferring Pharmaceuticals Ltd.

The Courtyard

Waterside Drive

Langley

Berkshire SL3 6EZ

United Kingdom

8. MARKETING AUTHORISATION NUMBER(S)
PL 3194/0056

9. DATE OF FIRST AUTHORISATION/RENEWAL OF THE AUTHORISATION
25th October 2002

10. DATE OF REVISION OF THE TEXT
October 2004

11. LEGAL CATEGORY
POM

Ocufen

(Allergan Ltd)

1. NAME OF THE MEDICINAL PRODUCT
Ocufen

2. QUALITATIVE AND QUANTITATIVE COMPOSITION
Flurbiprofen sodium 0.03% w/v

3. PHARMACEUTICAL FORM
Eye drops.

4. CLINICAL PARTICULARS

4.1 Therapeutic indications
Ocufen is indicated for

1) the inhibition of intraoperative miosis. Ocufen does not have intrinsic mydriatic properties and does not replace mydriatic agents.

2) the management of post-operative and post-laser trabeculoplasty inflammation in the anterior segment of the eye in patients in whom steroid therapy is not recommended.

4.2 Posology and method of administration
Adult dosage: For the inhibition of intraoperative miosis, 1 drop is instilled every half hour starting 2 hours before surgery. The final drop should be given not less than 30 minutes before surgery.

To control post-operative and post-laser trabeculoplasty inflammation the dosing regimen above should be followed. Beginning twenty-four hours after surgery, one drop is administered four times daily for at least one week after laser trabeculoplasty or for two to three weeks after other surgery.

In accordance with standard practice, other topical medication should not be co-administered with Ocufen. When administering other topical medications, a minimum interval of 5 minutes between instillations is recommended.

Use in children: Safety and effectiveness in children have not been established.

Administration: Topical by instillation into the conjunctival sac.

4.3 Contraindications
Ocufen is contra-indicated in epithelial herpes simplex keratitis (dendritic keratitis) and in individuals hypersensitive to any component of the medication.

The potential exists for cross-sensitivity to acetylsalicylic acid and other non-steroidal anti-inflammatory drugs. Ocufen is contra-indicated in individuals who have previously exhibited sensitivities to these drugs.

Use of Ocufen is contra-indicated in patients with known haemostatic defects or who are receiving other medications which may prolong bleeding time. Ocufen is contra-indicated for intraocular use during surgical procedures.

4.4 Special warnings and special precautions for use
Wound healing may be delayed with the use of Ocufen.

There have been reports that Ocufen may cause an increased bleeding tendency of ocular tissues in conjunction with surgery.

Patients with a history of herpes simplex keratitis should be monitored closely.

4.5 Interaction with other medicinal products and other forms of Interaction
Although clinical studies with acetylcholine chloride and animal studies with acetylcholine chloride or carbachol revealed no interference, and there is no known pharmacological basis for an interaction, there have been reports that acetylcholine chloride and carbachol have been ineffective when used in some surgical patients treated with Ocufen.

4.6 Pregnancy and lactation
Use in pregnancy: Safety of use in pregnant women has not been established. Ocufen should be used during pregnancy only if the potential benefit justifies the potential risk to the foetus.

4.7 Effects on ability to drive and use machines
None known.

4.8 Undesirable effects
The most frequent adverse reactions reported with the use of Ocufen are transient burning and stinging on instillation, and other minor signs of ocular irritation.

4.9 Overdose
No adverse effects are likely to be experienced following overdosage.

5. PHARMACOLOGICAL PROPERTIES

5.1 Pharmacodynamic properties
Flurbiprofen sodium is a non steroidal anti inflammatory agent which inhibits prostaglandin synthesis by inhibition of the cyclo-oxygenase enzyme.

Ophthalmic surgery causes prostaglandin release, with the effect that prostaglandin-mediated miosis may occur.

Treatment with Ocufen prior to surgery has been shown to inhibit intra-operative miosis and it is believed that this is brought about by inhibition of ocular prostaglandin release.

The sympathetic nervous system is not affected by this mechanism and acetylcholine-induced miosis has not been found to be inhibited in clinical trials.

Prostaglandins have also been shown to be mediators of certain kinds of intraocular inflammatory processes. In studies performed on animal eyes, prostaglandins have been shown to produce disruption of the blood-aqueous humour barrier, vasodilation, increased vascular permeability, leukocytosis and increased intraocular pressure.

5.2 Pharmacokinetic properties
Flurbiprofen concentrations of 213 ng/ml in aqueous humour have been reported following half hourly treatment for two hours preceding surgery.

5.3 Preclinical safety data
There are no preclinical data of relevance to the prescriber which are additional to that already included in the Summary of Product Characteristics.

6. PHARMACEUTICAL PARTICULARS

6.1 List of excipients
Liquifilm (polyvinyl alcohol)
Potassium chloride
Sodium chloride
Sodium citrate dihydrate
Citric acid monohydrate
Sodium hydroxide or
Hydrochloric acid (to adjust pH)
Purified water

6.2 Incompatibilities
None known.

6.3 Shelf life
The shelf life is 24 months for the unopened vial. The vial should be discarded after a single dose.

6.4 Special precautions for storage
Store at or below 25°C.

6.5 Nature and contents of container
Clear, plastic unit dose vial, each containing 0.4 ml of solution.

6.6 Instructions for use and handling
Each vial of Ocufen should be used for a single dose and discarded after use.

7. MARKETING AUTHORISATION HOLDER
Allergan Limited
Coronation Road
High Wycombe
Bucks
HP12 3SH

8. MARKETING AUTHORISATION NUMBER(S)
PL 00426/0069

9. DATE OF FIRST AUTHORISATION/RENEWAL OF THE AUTHORISATION
28th June 1991/17th May 2005

10. DATE OF REVISION OF THE TEXT
17th May 2005

Oculotect

(Novartis Pharmaceuticals UK Ltd)

1. NAME OF THE MEDICINAL PRODUCT
Oculotect® 50 mg/ml, eye drops solution in single-dose containers

2. QUALITATIVE AND QUANTITATIVE COMPOSITION
One ml contains 50 mg povidone K 25
For excipients, see 6.1.

3. PHARMACEUTICAL FORM
Eye drops, solution in single-dose containers
Almost colourless, clear aqueous solution

4. CLINICAL PARTICULARS

4.1 Therapeutic indications
Symptomatic treatment of dry eyes

4.2 Posology and method of administration
One drop into the conjunctival sac of the eye 4 times daily, or as required, depending upon the severity of the disease. The contents of a single-dose container are sufficient for one administration into the left and right eye.

Single-dose containers must be discarded immediately after use. Unused contents must not be stored.

4.3 Contraindications
Hypersensitivity to the components of the product.

4.4 Special warnings and special precautions for use
None.

4.5 Interaction with other medicinal products and other forms of Interaction
If a patient instils other medication into the eyes (e.g. for glaucoma therapy), there must be an interval of at least 5 minutes between medications. Oculotect should always be instilled last.

4.6 Pregnancy and lactation
There is no experience relating to the safety of Oculotect eye drops during pregnancy and lactation. For this reason, use of the preparation during pregnancy and lactation is not recommended except for compelling reasons.

4.7 Effects on ability to drive and use machines
If vision is blurred patients must refrain from driving a car or operating machinery.

4.8 Undesirable effects
Occasionally, a mild, transient burning or sticky sensation may occur. Very rarely irritation or hypersensitivity reactions may occur.

4.9 Overdose
None Stated.

5. PHARMACOLOGICAL PROPERTIES

5.1 Pharmacodynamic properties
The product does not contain any active pharmacological compounds. Due to their physical properties, non-irritant water soluble polymers can be used for moistening and lubrication of the ocular surface.

5.2 Pharmacokinetic properties
Orally administered povidone with a molecular weight of 12600 is rapidly excreted in the urine, most in 11 hours.

Following intravenous administration, long-term accumulation of povidone can be avoided by reducing the proportion of povidone of molecular weight higher than 25000. Because of the relatively large size of the povidone molecule, penetration through the cornea is unlikely.

5.3 Preclinical safety data
After two years administration of 5 and 10 % PVP K25 (povidone) added to the feed of rats no toxic effects could be observed. No data on mutagenicity and teratogenicity are available.

6. PHARMACEUTICAL PARTICULARS

6.1 List of excipients
Boric acid
Calcium chloride
Potassium chloride
Magnesium chloride
Sodium chloride
Sodium hydroxide for pH adjustment
Sodium lactate
Water for injections
The product contains no preservative.

6.2 Incompatibilities
High salt concentrations, e.g. of sodium sulphate in cold and sodium chloride in warm conditions, can result in precipitation of povidone. Depending on the ionic strength of the solution methyl- and propylhydroxybenzoates easily form complexes with povidone.

6.3 Shelf life
Unopened single-dose container: 2 years

The contents of a single-dose container must be used immediately after first opening.

6.4 Special precautions for storage
Do not store above 25°C.

Keep container in the outer carton in order to protect from light.

6.5 Nature and contents of container
The container is a transparent 0.4 ml LDPE single-dose container. Carton boxes of 20, 60 and 120 single-dose containers. Not all pack sizes may be marketed.

6.6 Instructions for use and handling
The single-dose container itself is not sterile whereas the contents of single-dose containers remain sterile until the original closure is broken.

Oculotect eye drops in single-dose containers must be used immediately after a container has been opened. Single-dose containers must be discarded after the use. Unused contents must not be stored.

7. MARKETING AUTHORISATION HOLDER
Novartis Pharmaceuticals UK Ltd
Frimley Business Park
Frimley
Camberley
Surrey
GU16 7SR
United Kingdom

8. MARKETING AUTHORISATION NUMBER(S)
PL 00101/0611

9. DATE OF FIRST AUTHORISATION/RENEWAL OF THE AUTHORISATION
4 December 2001

10. DATE OF REVISION OF THE TEXT
17 December 2002

LEGAL CATEGORY
P

Oestrogel Pump Pack

(sanofi-aventis)

1. NAME OF THE MEDICINAL PRODUCT
Oestrogel™ Pump-Pack.

2. QUALITATIVE AND QUANTITATIVE COMPOSITION
Oestrogel contains oestradiol as active ingredient, 0.06% w/w.

3. PHARMACEUTICAL FORM
Transdermal gel.

4. CLINICAL PARTICULARS

4.1 Therapeutic indications
As oestrogen replacement therapy for the relief of symptoms due to natural or surgically induced menopause, such as vasomotor symptoms (hot flushes and sweating), atrophic vaginitis and atrophic urethritis.

Second line therapy for prevention of osteoporosis in post-menopausal women at high risk of future fractures who are intolerant of, or contraindicated for, other medicinal products approved for the prevention of osteoporosis.

4.2 Posology and method of administration
Adults and the Elderly
Menopausal symptoms:

Each measure from the dispenser is 1.25g of Oestrogel. Two measures (2.5g) of Oestrogel once daily (1.5mg 17β-oestradiol) is the usual starting dose, which in the majority of women will provide effective relief of symptoms. If after one month's treatment effective relief is not obtained, the dosage may be increased accordingly to a maximum of four measures (5g) of Oestrogel daily (3.0mg 17β-oestradiol).

Prevention of osteoporosis:

The minimum effective dose is 2.5g of Oestrogel once daily for most patients.

The lowest effective dose should be used for maintenance therapy. In women with an intact uterus the recommended dose of a progestogen should be administered for 12 days of each month, in accordance with the manufacturer's recommendations. Oestrogel should be administered daily on a continuous basis.

The correct dose of gel should be dispensed and applied to clean, dry, intact areas of skin e.g. on the arms and shoulders, or inner thighs. The area of application should be at least 750cm^2, twice the area of the template provided. One measure from the dispenser, or half the prescribed dose, should be applied to each arm/shoulder (or thigh). Oestrogel should NOT be applied on or near the breasts or on the vulval region.

Oestrogel should be allowed to dry for 5 minutes before covering the skin with clothing.

Children

Not recommended for children.

4.3 Contraindications
Pregnancy and lactation. Known or suspected cancer of the breast, genital tract or other oestrogen dependent neoplasia. Severe hepatic, renal or cardiac disease. Porphyria. Active deep vein thrombosis, thromboembolic disorders, or a confirmed history of these conditions. Endometrial hyperplasia, undiagnosed vaginal bleeding.

4.4 Special warnings and special precautions for use
Assessment of each women prior to taking hormone replacement therapy (and at regular intervals thereafter) should include a personal and family medical history. Physical examination should be guided by this and by the contra-indications (section 4.3) and warnings (section 4.4) for this product. During assessment of each individual woman, clinical examination of the breasts and pelvic examination should be performed where clinically indicated rather than as a routine procedure. Women should be encouraged to participate in the national breast cancer screening programme (mammography) and the national cervical cancer screening programme (cervical cytology) as appropriate for their age. Breast awareness should also be encouraged and women advised to report any changes in their breasts to their doctor or nurse.

Prolonged use of unopposed oestrogens may increase the risk of endometrial carcinoma. In women with an intact uterus the addition of a progestogen is therefore considered essential. Caution should be exercised in prescribing oestrogens for patients with mastopathy or a strong family history of breast cancer.

A reanalysis of original data from 51 epidemiological studies reported a small or moderate increase in the probability of having breast cancer diagnosed in women currently or recently using HRT. The findings may be due to biological effects of HRT, earlier diagnosis, or a combination of both. The relative risk increased with duration of treatment (by 2.3% per year of use) and returned to normal in the course of five years after cessation of HRT use. This is comparable to the increase in relative risk when natural menopause is delayed in the absence of HRT. Breast cancers diagnosed in current or recent users of HRT are more likely to be localised to the breast than those found in non-users. HRT use may not be associated with increased mortality from breast cancer.

Between the ages of 50 and 70, about 45 women in every 1000 not using HRT will have breast cancer diagnosed. It is estimated that among those who use HRT for 5 years starting at age 50, 2 cases of breast cancer will be detected by age 70 in every 1000 women. For those who use HRT for 10 years there will be 6 extra cases of breast cancer, and for 15 years use, 12 extra cases of breast cancer in every 1000 women during the 20 year period until age 70.

It is important that the increased risk of being diagnosed with breast cancer is discussed with the patient and weighed against the known benefits of HRT.

In patients with hypertension, or a history of it, blood pressure should be monitored at regular intervals. If hypertension develops in patients receiving oestrogens, treatment should be discontinued.

Epidemiological studies have suggested that hormone replacement therapy (HRT) is associated with an increased relative risk of developing venous thromboembolism (VTE) i.e. deep vein thrombosis or pulmonary embolism. The studies find a 2-3 fold increase for users compared with non-users which for healthy women amounts to a low risk of one extra case of VTE each year for every 5000 patients taking HRT.

Generally recognised risk factors for VTE include a personal or family history and severe obesity (Body Mass Index >30 kg/m^2). In women with these factors the benefits of treatment with HRT need to be carefully weighed against risks.

The risk of VTE may be temporarily increased with prolonged immobilisation, major trauma or major surgery. In women on HRT scrupulous attention should be given to prophylactic measures to prevent VTE following surgery. Where prolonged immobilisation is liable to follow elective surgery, particularly abdominal or orthopaedic surgery to the lower limbs, consideration should be given to temporarily stopping HRT 4 weeks earlier.

If venous thromboembolism develops after initiating therapy the drug should be discontinued.

Care should be taken with patients with cholelithiasis, a history of endometriosis, diabetes mellitus, migraine, otosclerosis or any other condition which is known to deteriorate during pregnancy.

The gel should be applied by the patient herself, not by anyone else, and skin contact, particularly with a male partner, should be avoided for one hour after application.

Washing the skin or contact with other skin products should be avoided until at least one hour after application of Oestrogel.

4.5 Interaction with other medicinal products and other forms of interaction
Treatment with surface active agents (e.g. sodium lauryl sulphate), or other drugs which alter barrier structure or function, could remove drug bound to the skin, altering transdermal flux. Therefore patients should avoid the use of strong skin cleansers and detergents (e.g. benzalkonium or benzothonium chloride products), skin care products of high alcoholic content (astringents, sunscreens) and keratolytics (e.g. salicylic acid, lactic acid).

The use of any concomitant skin medication which alters skin production (e.g. cytotoxic drugs) should be avoided.

4.6 Pregnancy and lactation
Use is contraindicated in pregnancy and during lactation.

4.7 Effects on ability to drive and use machines
None known.

4.8 Undesirable effects
Irritation, reddening of the skin or mild and transient erythema at the site of application have been occasionally reported. In this instance a different site of application should be used, but if the topical side-effects continue, consideration should be given to discontinuation of treatment.

Systemic side-effects with Oestrogel are rare but the following have been reported with oral oestrogen therapy:

Genito-urinary tract: increase in the size of uterine fibromyomata, excessive production of cervical mucus.

Breast: pain, enlargement and secretion.

Gastrointestinal tract: nausea

CNS: headache, migraine and mood changes.

4.9 Overdose
Pain in the breasts or excessive production of cervical mucus may be indicative of too high a dosage, but acute overdosage has not been reported and is unlikely to be a problem. Overdosages of oestrogen may cause nausea, and withdrawal bleeding may occur. There are no specific antidotes and treatment should be symptomatic.

5. PHARMACOLOGICAL PROPERTIES

5.1 Pharmacodynamic properties
As the major oestrogen secreted by the human ovary, oestradiol is crucial to the development and maintenance of the female reproductive system and secondary sex characteristics; it promotes growth and development of the vagina, uterus and fallopian tubes, and enlargement of the breasts. Indirectly it contributes to the shaping of the skeleton, maintenance of tone and elasticity of urogenital structures, changes in the epiphyses of the long bones that allow for pubertal growth spurt and its termination, growth of axillary and pubic hair and pigmentation of the nipples and genitals.

The onset of menopause results from a decline in the secretion of oestradiol and other oestrogens by the ovary resulting initially in the cessation of menstruation, followed by menopausal symptoms such as vasomotor symptoms (hot flushes and sweating), muscle cramps, myalgias, arthralgias, anxiety, atrophic vaginitis and kraurosis vulvae. Oestrogens are also an important factor in preventing bone loss and after the menopause women lose bone mineral content at an average rate of 15-20% in a ten year period.

5.2 Pharmacokinetic properties
Pharmacokinetic studies indicate that, when applied topically to a large area of skin in a volatile solvent, approximately 10% of the oestradiol is percutaneously absorbed into the vascular system, regardless of the age of the patient. Daily application of 2.5g or 5g Oestrogel over a surface area of 400-750cm^2 results in a gradual increase in oestrogen blood levels to steady state after approximately 3-5 days and provides circulating levels of both oestradiol and oestrone equivalent in absolute concentrations and in their respective ratio to those obtained during the early-mid follicular phase of the menstrual cycle.

Avoidance of first pass metabolism by the percutaneous route not only results in a physiologic ratio of oestradiol and oestrone, but also reduces the impact on hepatic biosynthesis of protein that has been demonstrated with orally administered oestrogens.

5.3 Preclinical safety data
No relevant information additional to that already contained in the SPC.

6. PHARMACEUTICAL PARTICULARS

6.1 List of excipients
Ethanol, carbomer, triethanolamine and purified water.

6.2 Incompatibilities
None known.

6.3 Shelf life
24 months.

6.4 Special precautions for storage
Do not store above 25°C.

6.5 Nature and contents of container
Rigid plastic container enclosing a LDPE bag fitted with a metering valve and closed with a polypropylene cap, containing 80g.

6.6 Instructions for use and handling
Not applicable.

7. MARKETING AUTHORISATION HOLDER
Hoechst Marion Roussel Limited

Broadwater Park

Denham

Uxbridge

Middlesex UB9 5HP

8. MARKETING AUTHORISATION NUMBER(S)
PL 13402/0020

9. DATE OF FIRST AUTHORISATION/RENEWAL OF THE AUTHORISATION
1 November 1997

10. DATE OF REVISION OF THE TEXT
December 2003

11. Legal Category
POM

Oilatum Cream

(Stiefel Laboratories (UK) Limited)

1. NAME OF THE MEDICINAL PRODUCT
Oilatum Cream

2. QUALITATIVE AND QUANTITATIVE COMPOSITION
Contains Light Liquid Paraffin 6.0% w/w and White Soft Paraffin 15.0% w/w in a cream base.

3. PHARMACEUTICAL FORM
Cream for topical application.

4. CLINICAL PARTICULARS

4.1 Therapeutic indications

Oilatum Cream is indicated in the treatment of contact dermatitis, atopic eczema, senile pruritus, ichthyosis and related dry skin conditions.

4.2 Posology and method of administration

Oilatum Cream may be used as often as required. Apply to the affected area and rub in well. It is especially effective after washing when the sebum content of the stratum corneum may be depleted resulting in excessive moisture loss.

Oilatum Cream is suitable for adults, children and the elderly.

4.3 Contraindications

Should not be used in patients with known hypersensitivity to any of the ingredients.

4.4 Special warnings and special precautions for use

None.

4.5 Interaction with other medicinal products and other forms of Interaction

None.

4.6 Pregnancy and lactation

There are no restrictions on the use of Oilatum Cream during pregnancy or lactation.

4.7 Effects on ability to drive and use machines

None.

4.8 Undesirable effects

May cause irritation in patients hypersensitive to any of the ingredients.

4.9 Overdose

Accidental ingestion may cause nausea and vomiting. Administer copious quantities of water as required. Excessive topical application should cause no untoward effects other than greasy skin.

5. PHARMACOLOGICAL PROPERTIES

5.1 Pharmacodynamic properties

Light Liquid Paraffin and White Soft Paraffin exert an emollient effect by forming an occlusive film which reduces trans-epidermal water loss, thus helping to maintain normal skin humidity levels. Polyvinyl pyrrolidone enhances the strength and longevity of the occlusive film formed by the oil on the skin.

5.2 Pharmacokinetic properties

Not applicable.

5.3 Preclinical safety data

White Soft Paraffin and Light Liquid Paraffin have been used in pharmaceutical and cosmetic preparations for many years. The formulation contains excipients that are commonly used in such preparations. The safety of these substances is well established by common use over long periods in man.

6. PHARMACEUTICAL PARTICULARS

6.1 List of excipients

PEG 1000 Monostearate

Cetostearyl alcohol

Glycerol

Potassium sorbate

Benzyl alcohol

Citric acid monohydrate

Povidone K29/32

Purified water

6.2 Incompatibilities

None.

6.3 Shelf life

Three years.

6.4 Special precautions for storage

None.

6.5 Nature and contents of container

Internally lacquered, membrane sealed aluminium tube fitted with a polypropylene screw cap and packed into a carton: pack size 40g.

High density polyethylene tube: pack size 150g.

6.6 Instructions for use and handling

None.

Administrative Data

7. MARKETING AUTHORISATION HOLDER

Stiefel Laboratories (UK) Ltd

Holtspur Lane

Wooburn Green

High Wycombe

Bucks HP10 0AU

8. MARKETING AUTHORISATION NUMBER(S)

PL 0174/0207

9. DATE OF FIRST AUTHORISATION/RENEWAL OF THE AUTHORISATION

24th January 2001

10. DATE OF REVISION OF THE TEXT

September 2005

Oilatum Emollient

(Stiefel Laboratories (UK) Limited)

1. NAME OF THE MEDICINAL PRODUCT

Oilatum Bath Formula

Oilatum Emollient

2. QUALITATIVE AND QUANTITATIVE COMPOSITION

Light Liquid Paraffin 63.4% w/w

3. PHARMACEUTICAL FORM

Liquid Bath Additive

4. CLINICAL PARTICULARS

4.1 Therapeutic indications

Oilatum Emollient is indicated in the treatment of contact dermatitis, atopic dermatitis, senile pruritus, ichthyosis and related dry skin conditions. Oilatum Emollient replaces oil and water and hydrates the keratin. Oilatum Emollient is particularly suitable for infant bathing. The preparation also overcomes the problem of cleansing the skin in conditions where the use of soaps, soap substitutes and colloid or oatmeal baths proves irritating.

4.2 Posology and method of administration

Oilatum Emollient should always be used with water, either added to the water or applied to wet skin.

Adult bath:

Add 1-3 capfuls to an 8-inch bath of water, soak for 10-20 minutes. Pat dry.

Infant bath:

Add ½-2 capfuls to a basin of water. Apply gently over entire body with a sponge. Pat dry.

Skin cleansing:

Rub a small amount of oil into wet skin. Rinse and pat dry. Where conditions permit, and particularly in cases of extensive areas of dry skin, Oilatum Emollient should be used as a bath oil, ensuring complete coverage by immersion. In addition to the therapeutic benefits, this method of use provides a means of sedating tense patients, particularly relevant in cases of acute pruritic dermatoses where relaxation of tension appears to relieve symptoms.

The product is suitable for use in adults, children and the elderly.

4.3 Contraindications

None

4.4 Special warnings and special precautions for use

The patient should be advised to use care to avoid slipping in the bath. If a rash or skin irritation occurs, stop using the product and consult your doctor.

4.5 Interaction with other medicinal products and other forms of Interaction

None known

4.6 Pregnancy and lactation

There is no, or inadequate, evidence of the safety of Oilatum Emollient in human pregnancy or lactation, but it has been in wide use for many years without ill consequence.

4.7 Effects on ability to drive and use machines

None

4.8 Undesirable effects

None

4.9 Overdose

Not applicable

5. PHARMACOLOGICAL PROPERTIES

5.1 Pharmacodynamic properties

Light liquid paraffin exerts an emollient effect by forming an occlusive oil film on the stratum corneum. This prevents excessive evaporation of water from the skin surface and aids in the prevention of dryness.

5.2 Pharmacokinetic properties

Not applicable

5.3 Preclinical safety data

Not applicable

6. PHARMACEUTICAL PARTICULARS

6.1 List of excipients

Acetylated Lanolin Alcohols

Isopropyl Palmitate

Polyethylene Glycol 400 dilaurate

Polyoxyethylene 40 sorbitol septaoleate

Floral Spice

6.2 Incompatibilities

None

6.3 Shelf life

5 years

6.4 Special precautions for storage

None

6.5 Nature and contents of container

High density polyethylene bottles with a screw cap. Capacity: 250ml and 500ml

6.6 Instructions for use and handling

There are no special instructions for use or handling

7. MARKETING AUTHORISATION HOLDER

Stiefel Laboratories (UK) Ltd

Holtspur Lane

Wooburn Green

High Wycombe

Bucks HP10 0AU

8. MARKETING AUTHORISATION NUMBER(S)

PL0174/5010R

9. DATE OF FIRST AUTHORISATION/RENEWAL OF THE AUTHORISATION

8 December 1989

10. DATE OF REVISION OF THE TEXT

April 1997

Oilatum Fragrance Free Junior

(Stiefel Laboratories (UK) Limited)

1. NAME OF THE MEDICINAL PRODUCT

Oilatum Fragrance Free Junior

2. QUALITATIVE AND QUANTITATIVE COMPOSITION

Light Liquid Paraffin 63.4% w/w

For excipients, see 6.1.

3. PHARMACEUTICAL FORM

Liquid bath additive.

4. CLINICAL PARTICULARS

4.1 Therapeutic indications

Oilatum Fragrance Free Junior is indicated in the treatment of contact dermatitis, atopic dermatitis, senile pruritus, ichthyosis and related dry skin conditions.

Route of administration:

Topical.

4.2 Posology and method of administration

Oilatum Fragrance Free Junior may be used as frequently as necessary.

Oilatum Fragrance Free Junior should always be used with water, either added to the water or applied to wet skin.

For adult add 1-3 capfuls to an 8 inch bath of water. Soak for 10-20 minutes. Pat dry.

For infants, add ½-2 capfuls to a basin of water. Apply gently over entire body with a sponge. Pat dry.

4.3 Contraindications

None.

4.4 Special warnings and special precautions for use

Patients should be advised to use care to avoid slipping in the bath. If a rash or skin irritation should occur, stop using the product and consult your doctor.

4.5 Interaction with other medicinal products and other forms of Interaction

None known.

4.6 Pregnancy and lactation

There is no or inadequate evidence of the safety of Oilatum Fragrance Free Junior in pregnancy and lactation, but it has been in wide use for many years without apparent ill consequence.

4.7 Effects on ability to drive and use machines

None.

4.8 Undesirable effects

None.

4.9 Overdose

Not applicable.

5. PHARMACOLOGICAL PROPERTIES

5.1 Pharmacodynamic properties

Light liquid paraffin exerts an emollient effect by forming an occlusive oil film in the stratum corneum. This prevents excessive evaporation of water from the skin surface and aids in the prevention of dryness.

5.2 Pharmacokinetic properties

Not applicable.

5.3 Preclinical safety data

None.

6. PHARMACEUTICAL PARTICULARS

6.1 List of excipients

Acetylated Lanolin Alcohols

Isopropyl Palmitate

Polyethylene Glycol 400 Dilaurate

Macrogol ester.

6.2 Incompatibilities

Not applicable.

6.3 Shelf life

For the product as packaged for sale: 5 years.

6.4 Special precautions for storage

None.

6.5 Nature and contents of container
High density polyethylene bottles with screw caps. Capacity 250ml, 500ml and 1000ml.

6.6 Instructions for use and handling
There are no special instructions for use or handling of Oilatum Fragrance Free Junior.

7. MARKETING AUTHORISATION HOLDER
Stiefel Laboratories (UK) Ltd
Holtspur Lane
Wooburn Green
High Wycombe
Bucks
HP10 0AU

8. MARKETING AUTHORISATION NUMBER(S)
PL: 0174/0182

9. DATE OF FIRST AUTHORISATION/RENEWAL OF THE AUTHORISATION
June 1993.

10. DATE OF REVISION OF THE TEXT
September 2005.

Oilatum Gel
(Stiefel Laboratories (UK) Limited)

1. NAME OF THE MEDICINAL PRODUCT
Oilatum Gel

2. QUALITATIVE AND QUANTITATIVE COMPOSITION
Light liquid paraffin 70% w/w

3. PHARMACEUTICAL FORM
Shower gel

4. CLINICAL PARTICULARS
4.1 Therapeutic indications
For the treatment of contact dermatitis, atopic dermatitis, senile pruritus, ichthyosis and related dry skin conditions.

4.2 Posology and method of administration
Topical

Adults, children and the elderly:
Oilatum Gel may be used as frequently as necessary. Oilatum Gel should always be applied to wet skin, normally as a shower gel.

Shower as usual. Apply Oilatum Gel liberally to wet skin and massage gently. Rinse briefly and lightly pat the skin dry.

4.3 Contraindications
None.

4.4 Special warnings and special precautions for use
Take care to avoid slipping in the shower.

Oilatum Gel should not be used on greasy skin.

4.5 Interaction with other medicinal products and other forms of Interaction
None.

4.6 Pregnancy and lactation
There is no or inadequate evidence of the safety of Oilatum Gel in human pregnancy and lactation. Topical preparations containing light liquid paraffin have been in wide use for many years without apparent ill consequence.

4.7 Effects on ability to drive and use machines
None.

4.8 Undesirable effects
None.

4.9 Overdose
Not applicable.

5. PHARMACOLOGICAL PROPERTIES
5.1 Pharmacodynamic properties
Light liquid paraffin exerts an emollient effect by forming an occlusive oil film on the stratum corneum. This prevents excessive evaporation of water from the skin surface and aids in the prevention of dryness.

5.2 Pharmacokinetic properties
Not applicable.

5.3 Preclinical safety data
There are no pre-clinical data of relevance to the prescriber which are additional to those already stated in other sections of the SPC.

6. PHARMACEUTICAL PARTICULARS
6.1 List of excipients
Polyethylene 617A
2-octadodecanol
Polyethylene glycol 400 dilaurate
Polyoxyethylene 40 sorbital septaoleate
Polyethylene glycol-2-myristyl ether propionate
Polyphenylmethyl siloxane copolymer
Floral spice

6.2 Incompatibilities
None.

6.3 Shelf life
a) For the product as packaged for sale
3 years

b) After first opening the container
Comply with expiry date

6.4 Special precautions for storage
Store below 25°C.

6.5 Nature and contents of container
High density polyethylene tube of 125g.

6.6 Instructions for use and handling
There are no special instructions for use or handling of Oilatum Gel.

Administrative Data
7. MARKETING AUTHORISATION HOLDER
Stiefel Laboratories (UK) Ltd
Holtspur Lane
Wooburn Green
High Wycombe
Bucks HP10 0AU

8. MARKETING AUTHORISATION NUMBER(S)
PL 0174/0072

9. DATE OF FIRST AUTHORISATION/RENEWAL OF THE AUTHORISATION
6th August 2004

10. DATE OF REVISION OF THE TEXT
5th September 2005

Oilatum Junior Bath Formula
(Stiefel Laboratories (UK) Limited)

1. NAME OF THE MEDICINAL PRODUCT
Oilatum Junior Bath Formula

2. QUALITATIVE AND QUANTITATIVE COMPOSITION
Light Liquid Paraffin 63.4% w/w

For excipients, see 6.1.

3. PHARMACEUTICAL FORM
Liquid bath additive.

4. CLINICAL PARTICULARS
4.1 Therapeutic indications
Oilatum Junior Bath Formula is indicated in the treatment of contact dermatitis, atopic dermatitis, senile pruritus, ichthyosis and related dry skin conditions.

Route of administration:
Topical.

4.2 Posology and method of administration
Oilatum Junior Bath Formula may be used as frequently as necessary.

Oilatum Junior Bath Formula should always be used with water, either added to the water or applied to wet skin.

For adult add 1-3 capfuls to an 8 inch bath of water. Soak for 10-20 minutes. Pat dry.

For infants, add ½-2 capfuls to a basin of water. Apply gently over entire body with a sponge. Pat dry.

4.3 Contraindications
None.

4.4 Special warnings and special precautions for use
Patients should be advised to use care to avoid slipping in the bath. If a rash or skin irritation should occur, stop using the product and consult your doctor.

4.5 Interaction with other medicinal products and other forms of Interaction
None known.

4.6 Pregnancy and lactation
There is no or inadequate evidence of the safety of Oilatum Junior Bath Formula in pregnancy and lactation, but it has been in wide use for many years without apparent ill consequence.

4.7 Effects on ability to drive and use machines
None.

4.8 Undesirable effects
None.

4.9 Overdose
Not applicable.

5. PHARMACOLOGICAL PROPERTIES
5.1 Pharmacodynamic properties
Light liquid paraffin exerts an emollient effect by forming an occlusive oil film in the stratum corneum. This prevents excessive evaporation of water from the skin surface and aids in the prevention of dryness.

5.2 Pharmacokinetic properties
Not applicable.

5.3 Preclinical safety data
None.

6. PHARMACEUTICAL PARTICULARS
6.1 List of excipients
Acetylated Lanolin Alcohols
Isopropyl Palmitate
Polyethylene Glycol 400 Dilaurate
Macrogol ester

6.2 Incompatibilities
Not applicable.

6.3 Shelf life
For the product as packaged for sale: 5 years.

6.4 Special precautions for storage
None.

6.5 Nature and contents of container
High density polyethylene bottles with screw caps. Capacity 150 and 300ml.

6.6 Instructions for use and handling
There are no special instructions for use or handling of Oilatum Junior Bath Formula.

7. MARKETING AUTHORISATION HOLDER
Stiefel Laboratories (UK) Ltd
Holtspur Lane
Wooburn Green
High Wycombe
Bucks
HP10 0AU

8. MARKETING AUTHORISATION NUMBER(S)
PL: 0174/0182

9. DATE OF FIRST AUTHORISATION/RENEWAL OF THE AUTHORISATION
June 1993.

10. DATE OF REVISION OF THE TEXT
September 2005.

Oilatum Plus
(Stiefel Laboratories (UK) Limited)

1. NAME OF THE MEDICINAL PRODUCT
Oilatum Plus
Oilatum Junior Flare-Up

2. QUALITATIVE AND QUANTITATIVE COMPOSITION
Light liquid paraffin 52.5% w/w, benzalkonium chloride solution 12.0% w/w, triclosan 2% w/w

3. PHARMACEUTICAL FORM
Solution

4. CLINICAL PARTICULARS
4.1 Therapeutic indications
Topical as a bath additive.

For the prophylactic treatment of eczemas at risk from infection.

4.2 Posology and method of administration
Oilatum Plus should always be diluted with water. It is an effective cleanser and should not be used with soap.

Adults and children: In an eight inch bath add 2 capfuls, in a four inch bath add 1 capful

Infants: Add 1 ml (just sufficient to cover the bottom of the cap) and mix well with water

Do not use for babies younger than 6 months

4.3 Contraindications
Patients with a known hypersensitivity to any of the ingredients should not use the product.

4.4 Special warnings and special precautions for use
Avoid contact of the undiluted product with the eyes. If the undiluted product comes into contact with the eye, reddening may occur. Eye irrigation should be performed for 15 minutes and then the eye examined under fluorescein stain. If there is persistent irritation or any uptake of fluorescein, the patient should be referred for ophthalmological opinion.

The product should not be used with soap.

4.5 Interaction with other medicinal products and other forms of Interaction
None known.

4.6 Pregnancy and lactation
No restrictions on the use of the product in pregnancy and lactation are proposed.

4.7 Effects on ability to drive and use machines
None known.

4.8 Undesirable effects
None known.

4.9 Overdose
The product is intended for topical use only. Accidental ingestion may cause gastro intestinal irritation with vomiting and diarrhoea. Vomiting may result in foam aspiration. In the case of accidental ingestion, give 1 to 2 glasses of milk or water to drink. If a large quantity of the product is

ingested, the patient should be observed in hospital and the use of activated charcoal may be considered.

5. PHARMACOLOGICAL PROPERTIES

5.1 Pharmacodynamic properties

Benzalkonium chloride and triclosan are anti-bacterial agents with proven efficacy against *Staphylococcus aureus*, the principal causative organism in infected eczemas.

Light liquid paraffin is an emollient widely used in the treatment of eczema.

5.2 Pharmacokinetic properties

Not Applicable.

5.3 Preclinical safety data

Not applicable.

6. PHARMACEUTICAL PARTICULARS

6.1 List of excipients

Acetylated lanolin alcohols

Isopropyl palmitate

Oleyl alcohol

Polyoxyethylene lauryl ether

6.2 Incompatibilities

None known.

6.3 Shelf life

a) For the product as packaged for sale

3 years

b) After first opening the container

Comply with expiry date

6.4 Special precautions for storage

None.

6.5 Nature and contents of container

White polyvinyl chloride or high density polyethylene bottles containing 500ml and 1000ml with white urea cap.

6.6 Instructions for use and handling

There are no special instructions for use or handling of Oilatum Plus/Oilatum Junior Flare-Up.

7. MARKETING AUTHORISATION HOLDER

Stiefel Laboratories (UK) Ltd.

Holtspur Lane,

Wooburn Green,

High Wycombe,

Bucks. HP10 0AU

8. MARKETING AUTHORISATION NUMBER(S)

PL 0174/0070

9. DATE OF FIRST AUTHORISATION/RENEWAL OF THE AUTHORISATION

16.2.90

10. DATE OF REVISION OF THE TEXT

08.07.98

Oily Phenol Injection BP

(UCB Pharma Limited)

1. NAME OF THE MEDICINAL PRODUCT

Oily Phenol Injection BP

2. QUALITATIVE AND QUANTITATIVE COMPOSITION

Phenol BP 5.00 % WV

3. PHARMACEUTICAL FORM

Sterile solution intended for parenteral use

4. CLINICAL PARTICULARS

4.1 Therapeutic indications

Scleropathy of haemorrhoids

4.2 Posology and method of administration

Injected into sub-mucosal layer at the base of the haemorrhoid

ADULTS

2-3 ml of oily phenol injection into the sub-mucosal layer at the base of the pile; Several injections may be given at different sites but not more than a total volume of 10 ml should be used at any one time.

CHILDREN

Use of this product is not advised

ELDERLY

No alternative dosage schedules have been suggested.

4.3 Contraindications

Hypersensitivity to any component of the preparation. Hypersensitivity to nuts.

4.4 Special warnings and special precautions for use

None stated

4.5 Interaction with other medicinal products and other forms of Interaction

None stated

4.6 Pregnancy and lactation

No adverse effects have been reported.

4.7 Effects on ability to drive and use machines

Effects of phenol oily injection are not likely to affect the patient's ability to drive and use machinery.

4.8 Undesirable effects

Side effects may include irritation and tissue necrosis.

4.9 Overdose

Not applicable

5. PHARMACOLOGICAL PROPERTIES

5.1 Pharmacodynamic properties

Oily phenol injection acts as an analgesic and thrombotic agent by numbimg the sensory nerve endings and precipitating proteins.

5.2 Pharmacokinetic properties

Phenol is absorbed from the gastro-intestinal tract and through skin and mucous membranes. It is metabolised to phenylglucoronide and phenylsulphate and small amounts are oxidised to catechol and quinol which are mainly conjugated. The metabolites are excreted in the urine; on oxidation to quinones they may tint the urine green.

5.3 Preclinical safety data

No data available

6. PHARMACEUTICAL PARTICULARS

6.1 List of excipients

Almond oil

6.2 Incompatibilities

Incompatible with alkaline salts, acetanilide, phenazone, piperazine, quinine salts, phenacetin and iron salts. Phenol coagulates albumin and gelatinises collodion.

6.3 Shelf life

3 years

6.4 Special precautions for storage

Store below 25 °C

6.5 Nature and contents of container

5 ml neutral glass (type 1) ampoules supplied in cartons of 10

6.6 Instructions for use and handling

None stated

7. MARKETING AUTHORISATION HOLDER

UCB Pharma Limited

208 Bath Road

Slough

Berkshire

SL1 3WE

UK

8. MARKETING AUTHORISATION NUMBER(S)

PL 0039/5690R

9. DATE OF FIRST AUTHORISATION/RENEWAL OF THE AUTHORISATION

20 March 1987 / 15 October 1997

10. DATE OF REVISION OF THE TEXT

June 2005

Olbetam Capsules 250

(Pharmacia Limited)

1. NAME OF THE MEDICINAL PRODUCT

Olbetam Capsules 250

2. QUALITATIVE AND QUANTITATIVE COMPOSITION

Acipimox INN 250.00 mg

3. PHARMACEUTICAL FORM

Red-brown/dark pink hard gelatin capsules, size no. 1, containing a white to cream powder.

4. CLINICAL PARTICULARS

4.1 Therapeutic indications

Olbetam is indicated for the treatment of lipid disorders characterised, according to Fredrickson, by elevated plasma levels of triglycerides (type IV hyperlipo-proteinaemia), or cholesterol (type IIA hyperlipoproteinaemia) and triglycerides and cholesterol (type IIB hyperlipoproteinaemia).

4.2 Posology and method of administration

To be given orally.

The daily dosage should be adjusted individually depending on plasma triglyceride and cholesterol levels.

The recommended dosage is one 250 mg capsule 2 or 3 times daily to be taken with or after meals. The lower dose is advised in type IV and the higher dose in types IIA and IIB hyperlipoproteinaemias.

Daily dosages of up to 1200 mg have been safely administered for long periods. Improvement in the plasma lipid's picture is usually seen within the first month of therapy.

In patients with slight renal impairment (creatinine clearance values > 60 ml/min) no dose reduction is required. For patients with moderate to severe renal impairment (creatinine clearance values between 60 and 30 ml/min) the dose needs to be reduced accordingly. Acipimox is eliminated entirely through the kidneys, therefore, accumulation can be expected and is related to the degree of renal impairment. It is advised that longer intervals are left between doses of the drug in patients with renal impairment.

4.3 Contraindications

Olbetam is contra-indicated in patients who are hypersensitive to the drug and those with peptic ulceration.

Olbetam should not be given to patients with severe renal impairment (creatinine clearance < 30 ml/min)

4.4 Special warnings and special precautions for use

Modification of hyperlipidaemia is recommended only for patients with hyperlipoproteinaemia of a degree and type considered appropriate for treatment.

Low cholesterol and low-fat diets, together with cessation of alcohol consumption, are preferable therapeutic approaches to be tried before starting treatment with Olbetam.

The absorption of Olbetam is not affected by the concomitant administration of cholestyramine.

Evidence of clinical efficacy in the prevention of heart disease has not been established.

The possible beneficial and adverse, long-term consequences of some drugs used in the hyperlipidaemias are still the subject of scientific discussion.

4.5 Interaction with other medicinal products and other forms of Interaction

No interaction has been shown with other lipid lowering agents. However, the combination with statins or fibrates should be used with caution due to reports of an increased risk of musculoskeletal events with nicotinic acid, as strict analog of acipimox, is used in combination with such lipid-lowering agents.

4.6 Pregnancy and lactation

There is no evidence from the animal studies that acipimox is teratogenic. However, a higher incidence of immature and underweight foetuses was seen in pregnant animals given higher doses of acipimox. This effect may be due to maternal toxicity.

There is only limited experience to date of administration of acipimox to humans therefore epidemiological data is not available. Taking into account the present experience of administration to humans of acipimox and that the safety of acipimox in human pregnancy has not yet been ascertained, it is recommended, therefore, that acipimox not be administered to women who are, or may be pregnant.

In the absence of animal data on the levels of acipimox excreted in milk, Olbetam should not be administered to women who are breast-feeding.

4.7 Effects on ability to drive and use machines

None stated.

4.8 Undesirable effects

The drug may induce skin vasodilatation giving rise to a sensation of heat, flushing or itching, especially at the beginning of therapy and also rash and erythema. These reactions usually disappear rapidly during the first day of treatment. Moderate gastric disturbances (heartburn, epigastric pain, nausea and diarrhoea) have been reported occasionally, as well as headache, malaise, eye symptoms (dry or gritty eye), myositis, myalgia, weakness, arthralgiaand urticaria. On rare occasions patients have developed angioedema and bronchospasm; and anaphylactoid reactions have also been reported.

4.9 Overdose

If toxic effects are observed, supportive care and symptomatic treatment should be administered.

5. PHARMACOLOGICAL PROPERTIES

5.1 Pharmacodynamic properties

Acipimox inhibits the release of fatty acids from adipose tissue and reduces the blood concentrations of very low density lipoproteins (VLDL or Pre-beta) and low density lipoproteins (LDL or beta) with a subsequent overall reduction in triglyceride and cholesterol levels.

Acipimox also has a favourable effect on high density lipoproteins (HDL or alpha) which increase during treatment.

5.2 Pharmacokinetic properties

Acipimox is rapidly and completely absorbed orally, reaching peak plasma levels within two hours. The half-life is about two hours. It does not bind to plasma proteins; it is not significantly metabolised and is eliminated almost completely intact by the urinary route.

5.3 Preclinical safety data

There is no evidence from the animal studies that acipimox is teratogenic. However, a higher incidence of immature and underweight foetuses was seen in pregnant animals given higher doses of acipimox. This effect may be due to maternal toxicity.

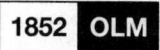

6. PHARMACEUTICAL PARTICULARS

6.1 List of excipients

Physically modified corn starch (STA-RX 1500)

Silica gel (Syloid 244) USP

Magnesium stearate Ph. Eur

Sodium lauryl sulphate Ph. Eur

Hard gelatin capsules shell:

Gelatin USP

Titanium dioxide (E171)

Iron oxide red (E172)

Iron oxide yellow (E172)

6.2 Incompatibilities

None stated.

6.3 Shelf life

48 months

6.4 Special precautions for storage

Store at a temperature below 30°C in a dry place.

6.5 Nature and contents of container

Packed in blisters of 10 capsules per strip, inside cartons. Each carton contains 90 capsules.

6.6 Instructions for use and handling

None given.

Administrative Data

7. MARKETING AUTHORISATION HOLDER

Pharmacia Limited

Davy Avenue

Milton Keynes

MK5 8PH

United Kingdom

8. MARKETING AUTHORISATION NUMBER(S)

PL 00032/0322

9. DATE OF FIRST AUTHORISATION/RENEWAL OF THE AUTHORISATION

2 May 2003

10. DATE OF REVISION OF THE TEXT

Legal Category

POM

OLMETEC film-coated tablets

(Sankyo Pharma UK Limited)

1. NAME OF THE MEDICINAL PRODUCT

Olmetec® 10 mg film-coated tablet

Olmetec® 20 mg film-coated tablet

Olmetec® 40 mg film-coated tablet

2. QUALITATIVE AND QUANTITATIVE COMPOSITION

Each tablet contains 10 mg of olmesartan medoxomil

Each tablet contains 20 mg of olmesartan medoxomil

Each tablet contains 40 mg of olmesartan medoxomil

For excipients, see 6.1

3. PHARMACEUTICAL FORM

Film-coated tablet.

Olmetec® 10and 20mg tablets: White, circular, film-coated tablets with C13 and C14 respectively embossed on one side.

Olmetec® 40mg tablets: White, oval, film-coated tablets with C15 embossed on one side.

4. CLINICAL PARTICULARS

4.1 Therapeutic indications

Treatment of essential hypertension.

4.2 Posology and method of administration

Adults

The recommended starting dose of olmesartan medoxomil is 10 mg once daily. In patients whose blood pressure is not adequately controlled at this dose, the dose of olmesartan medoxomil may be increased to 20 mg once daily as the optimal dose. If additional blood pressure reduction is required, olmesartan medoxomil dose may be increased to a maximum of 40 mg daily or hydrochlorothiazide therapy may be added.

The antihypertensive effect of olmesartan medoxomil is substantially present within 2 weeks of initiating therapy and is maximal by about 8 weeks after initiating therapy. This should be borne in mind when considering changing the dose regimen for any patient.

In order to assist compliance, it is recommended that Olmetec tablets be taken at about the same time each day, with or without food, for example at breakfast time.

Elderly

The maximum dose in elderly patients is 20 mg olmesartan medoxomil once daily, owing to limited experience of higher dosages in this patient group (see 5.2).

Renal impairment

The maximum dose in patients with mild to moderate renal impairment (creatinine clearance of 20 – 60 mL/min) is 20 mg olmesartan medoxomil once daily, owing to limited experience of higher dosages in this patient group. The use of olmesartan medoxomil in patients with severe renal impairment (creatinine clearance < 20 mL/min) is not recommended, since there is only limited experience in this patient group (see 5.2).

Hepatic impairment

The use of olmesartan medoxomil is not recommended in patients with hepatic impairment, since there is only limited experience in this patient group (see 4.4, 5.2).

Children and adolescents

The safety and efficacy of olmesartan medoxomil have not been established in children and adolescents up to 18 years of age.

4.3 Contraindications

Hypersensitivity to the active ingredient or any of the other excipients of Olmetec tablets (see 6.1).

Second and third trimesters of pregnancy (see 4.6).

Lactation (see 4.6).

Biliary obstruction (see 5.2).

4.4 Special warnings and special precautions for use

Intravascular volume depletion:

Symptomatic hypotension, especially after the first dose, may occur in patients who are volume and/or sodium depleted by vigorous diuretic therapy, dietary salt restriction, diarrhoea or vomiting. Such conditions should be corrected before the administration of olmesartan medoxomil.

Other conditions with stimulation of the renin-angiotensin-aldosterone system:

In patients whose vascular tone and renal function depend predominantly on the activity of the renin-angiotensin-aldosterone system (e.g. patients with severe congestive heart failure or underlying renal disease, including renal artery stenosis), treatment with other drugs that affect this system has been associated with acute hypotension, azotaemia, oliguria or, rarely, acute renal failure. The possibility of similar effects cannot be excluded with angiotensin II receptor antagonists.

Renovascular hypertension:

There is an increased risk of severe hypotension and renal insufficiency when patients with bilateral renal artery stenosis or stenosis of the artery to a single functioning kidney are treated with medicinal products that affect the renin-angiotensin-aldosterone system.

Renal impairment and kidney transplantation:

When olmesartan medoxomil is used in patients with impaired renal function, periodic monitoring of serum potassium and creatinine levels is recommended. Use of olmesartan medoxomil is not recommended in patients with severe renal impairment (creatinine clearance < 20 mL/min) (see 4.2, 5.2). There is no experience of the administration of olmesartan medoxomil in patients with a recent kidney transplant or in patients with end-stage renal impairment (i.e. creatinine clearance <12 mL/min).

Hepatic impairment:

There is currently limited experience in patients with mild to moderate hepatic impairment and no experience in patients with severe hepatic impairment, therefore use of olmesartan medoxomil in these patient groups is not recommended (see 4.2, 5.2).

Hyperkalaemia:

As with other angiotensin II antagonists and ACE inhibitors, hyperkalaemia may occur during treatment with olmesartan medoxomil, especially in the presence of renal impairment and/or heart failure (see 4.5). Close monitoring of serum potassium levels in at risk patients is recommended.

Lithium:

As with other angiotensin-II receptor antagonists, the combination of lithium and olmesartan medoxomil is not recommended (see 4.5).

Aortic or mitral valve stenosis; obstructive hypertrophic cardiomyopathy:

As with other vasodilators, special caution is indicated in patients suffering from aortic or mitral valve stenosis, or obstructive hypertrophic cardiomyopathy.

Primary aldosteronism:

Patients with primary aldosteronism generally will not respond to antihypertensive drugs acting through inhibition of the renin-angiotensin system. Therefore, the use of olmesartan medoxomil is not recommended in such patients.

Ethnic differences:

As with all other angiotensin II antagonists, the blood pressure lowering effect of olmesartan medoxomil is somewhat less in black patients than in non-black patients, possibly because of a higher prevalence of low-renin status in the black hypertensive population.

Other:

As with any antihypertensive agent, excessive blood pressure decrease in patients with ischaemic heart disease or ischaemic cerebrovascular disease could result in a myocardial infarction or stroke.

4.5 Interaction with other medicinal products and other forms of Interaction

Effects of other medicinal products on olmesartan medoxomil:

Potassium supplements and potassium sparing diuretics:

Based on experience with the use of other drugs that affect the renin-angiotensin system, concomitant use of potassium-sparing diuretics, potassium supplements, salt substitutes containing potassium or other drugs that may increase serum potassium levels (e.g. heparin) may lead to increases in serum potassium (see 4.4). Such concomitant use is therefore not recommended.

Other antihypertensive medications:

The blood pressure lowering effect of olmesartan medoxomil can be increased by concomitant use of other antihypertensive medications.

Non-steroidal anti-inflammatory drugs (NSAIDs):

NSAIDs (including acetylsalicylic acid at doses > 3g/day and also COX-2 inhibitors) and angiotensin-II receptor antagonists may act synergistically by decreasing glomerular filtration. The risk of the concomitant use of NSAIDs and angiotensin II antagonists is the occurrence of acute renal failure. Monitoring of renal function at the beginning of treatment should be recommended as well as regular hydration of the patient. Additionally, concomitant treatment can reduce the antihypertensive effect of angiotensin II receptor antagonists, leading to their partial loss of efficacy.

Other compounds:

After treatment with antacid (aluminium magnesium hydroxide), a modest reduction in bioavailability of olmesartan was observed. Coadministration of warfarin and digoxin had no effect on the pharmacokinetics of olmesartan.

Effects of olmesartan medoxomil on other medicinal products:

Lithium:

Reversible increases in serum lithium concentrations and toxicity have been reported during concomitant administration of lithium with angiotensin converting enzyme inhibitors and angiotensin II antagonists. Therefore use of olmesartan medoxomil and lithium in combination is not recommended (see 4.4). If use of the combination proves necessary, careful monitoring of serum lithium levels is recommended.

Other compounds:

Compounds which have been investigated in specific clinical studies in healthy volunteers include warfarin, digoxin, an antacid (magnesium aluminium hydroxide), hydrochlorothiazide and pravastatin. No clinically relevant interactions were observed and in particular olmesartan medoxomil had no significant effect on the pharmacokinetics or pharmacodynamics of warfarin or the pharmacokinetics of digoxin.

Olmesartan had no clinically relevant inhibitory effects on *in vitro* human cytochrome P450 enzymes 1A1/2, 2A6, 2C8/9, 2C19, 2D6, 2E1 and 3A4, and had no or minimal inducing effects on rat cytochrome P450 activities. Therefore *in vivo* interaction studies with known cytochrome P450 enzyme inhibitors and inducers were not conducted, and no clinically relevant interactions between olmesartan and drugs metabolised by the above cytochrome P450 enzymes are expected.

4.6 Pregnancy and lactation

Use in pregnancy (see 4.3):

There is no experience with the use of olmesartan medoxomil in pregnant women. However, drugs that act directly on the renin-angiotensin system administered during the second and third trimesters of pregnancy have been reported to cause foetal and neonatal injury (hypotension, renal dysfunction, oliguria and/or anuria, oligohydramnios, skull hypoplasia, intrauterine growth retardation, lung hypoplasia, facial abnormalities, limb contracture) and even death.

Thus, as for any drug in this class, olmesartan medoxomil is contraindicated during the second and third trimesters of pregnancy. In addition, olmesartan medoxomil must not be used during the first trimester. If pregnancy occurs during therapy, olmesartan medoxomil must be discontinued as soon as possible.

Use during lactation (see 4.3):

Olmesartan is excreted in the milk of lactating rats but it is not known whether olmesartan is excreted in human milk. Mothers must not breast-feed if they are taking olmesartan medoxomil.

4.7 Effects on ability to drive and use machines

The effect of Olmetec tablets on the ability to drive has not been specifically studied. With respect to driving vehicles or operating machines, it should be taken into account that occasionally dizziness or fatigue may occur in patients taking antihypertensive therapy.

4.8 Undesirable effects

Market experience

The following adverse reactions have been reported in post-marketing experience.

They are listed by System Organ Class and ranked under headings of frequency using the following convention: very common (⩾1/10); common (⩾1/100, <1/10);uncommon

(≥1/1,000, <1/100); rare (≥1/10,000, <1/1,000); very rare (<1/10,000) including isolated reports.

System Organ Class	*Very rare*
Blood and lymphatic system disorders	Thrombocytopenia
Nervous system disorders	Dizziness, headache
Respiratory, thoracic and mediastinal disorders	Cough
Gastrointestinal disorders	Abdominal pain, nausea, vomiting
Skin and subcutaneous tissue disorders	Pruritus, exanthem, rash Allergic conditions such as angioneurotic oedema, dermatitis allergic, face oedema and urticaria
Musculoskeletal and connective tissue disorders	Muscle cramp, myalgia
Renal and urinary disorders	Acute renal failure and renal insufficiency (See also under Investigations)
General disorders and administration site conditions	Asthenic conditions such as asthenia, fatigue, lethargy, malaise
Investigations	Abnormal renal function tests such as blood creatinine increased and blood urea increased Increased hepatic enzymes

Clinical trials

In double-blind, placebo-controlled monotherapy studies, the overall incidence of treatment-emergent adverse events was 42.4% on olmesartan medoxomil and 40.9% on placebo.

In placebo-controlled monotherapy studies, the only adverse drug reaction that was unequivocally related to treatment was dizziness (2.5% incidence on olmesartan medoxomil and 0.9% on placebo).

In long-term (2-year) treatment, the incidence of withdrawals due to adverse events on olmesartan medoxomil 10 - 20 mg once daily was 3.7%. The following adverse events have been reported across all clinical trials with olmesartan medoxomil (including trials with active as well as placebo control), irrespective of causality or incidence relative to placebo. They are listed by body system and ranked under headings of frequency using the conventions described above:

Central nervous system disorders:

Common: Dizziness

Uncommon: Vertigo

Cardiovascular disorders:

Rare: Hypotension

Uncommon: Angina pectoris

Respiratory system disorders:

Common: Bronchitis, cough, pharyngitis, rhinitis

Gastro-intestinal disorders:

Common: Abdominal pain, diarrhoea, dyspepsia, gastroenteritis, nausea

Skin and appendages disorders:

Uncommon: Rash

Musculoskeletal disorders:

Common: Arthritis, back pain, skeletal pain

Urinary system disorders:

Common: Haematuria, urinary tract infection

General disorders:

Common: Chest pain, fatigue, influenza-like symptoms, peripheral oedema, pain

Laboratory parameters

In placebo-controlled monotherapy studies, the incidence was somewhat higher on olmesartan medoxomil compared with placebo for hypertriglyceridaemia (2.0% versus 1.1%) and for raised creatine phosphokinase (1.3% versus 0.7%).

Laboratory adverse events reported across all clinical trials with olmesartan medoxomil (including trials without a placebo control), irrespective of causality or incidence relative to placebo, included:

Metabolic and nutritional disorders:

Common: Increased creatine phosphokinase, hypertriglyceridaemia, hyperuricaemia.

Rare: Hyperkalaemia

Liver and biliary disorders:

Common: Liver enzyme elevations.

4.9 Overdose

Only limited information is available regarding overdosage in humans. The most likely effect of overdosage is hypotension. In the event of overdosage, the patient should be carefully monitored and treatment should be symptomatic and supportive.

No information is available regarding the dialysability of olmesartan.

5. PHARMACOLOGICAL PROPERTIES

5.1 Pharmacodynamic properties

Pharmaco-therapeutic group:

Angiotensin II antagonists, ATC code CO9C A 08.

Olmesartan medoxomil is a potent, orally active, selective angiotensin II receptor (type AT_1) antagonist. It is expected to block all actions of angiotensin II mediated by the AT_1 receptor, regardless of the source or route of synthesis of angiotensin II. The selective antagonism of the angiotensin II (AT_1) receptors results in increases in plasma renin levels and angiotensin I and II concentrations, and some decrease in plasma aldosterone concentrations.

Angiotensin II is the primary vasoactive hormone of the renin-angiotensin-aldosterone system and plays a significant role in the pathophysiology of hypertension via the type 1 (AT_1) receptor.

In hypertension, olmesartan medoxomil causes a dose-dependent, long-lasting reduction in arterial blood pressure. There has been no evidence of first-dose hypotension, of tachyphylaxis during long-term treatment, or of rebound hypertension after cessation of therapy.

Once daily dosing with olmesartan medoxomil provides an effective and smooth reduction in blood pressure over the 24 hour dose interval. Once daily dosing produced similar decreases in blood pressure as twice daily dosing at the same total daily dose.

With continuous treatment, maximum reductions in blood pressure are achieved by 8 weeks after the initiation of therapy, although a substantial proportion of the blood pressure lowering effect is already observed after 2 weeks of treatment. When used together with hydrochlorothiazide, the reduction in blood pressure is additive and coadministration is well tolerated.

The effect of olmesartan on mortality and morbidity is not yet known.

5.2 Pharmacokinetic properties

Absorption and distribution

Olmesartan medoxomil is a prodrug. It is rapidly converted to the pharmacologically active metabolite, olmesartan, by esterases in the gut mucosa and in portal blood during absorption from the gastrointestinal tract.

No intact olmesartan medoxomil or intact side chain medoxomil moiety have been detected in plasma or excreta. The mean absolute bioavailability of olmesartan from a tablet formulation was 25.6%.

The mean peak plasma concentration (C_{max}) of olmesartan is reached within about 2 hours after oral dosing with olmesartan medoxomil, and olmesartan plasma concentrations increase approximately linearly with increasing single oral doses up to about 80 mg.

Food had minimal effect on the bioavailability of olmesartan and therefore olmesartan medoxomil may be administered with or without food.

No clinically relevant gender-related differences in the pharmacokinetics of olmesartan have been observed.

Olmesartan is highly bound to plasma protein (99.7%), but the potential for clinically significant protein binding displacement interactions between olmesartan and other highly bound coadministered drugs is low (as confirmed by the lack of a clinically significant interaction between olmesartan medoxomil and warfarin). The binding of olmesartan to blood cells is negligible. The mean volume of distribution after intravenous dosing is low (16 – 29 L).

Metabolism and elimination

Total plasma clearance was typically 1.3 L/h (CV, 19%) and was relatively slow compared to hepatic blood flow (ca 90 L/h). Following a single oral dose of ^{14}C-labelled olmesartan medoxomil, 10 - 16% of the administered radioactivity was excreted in the urine (the vast majority within 24 hours of dose administration) and the remainder of the recovered radioactivity was excreted in the faeces. Based on the systemic availability of 25.6%, it can be calculated that absorbed olmesartan is cleared by both renal excretion (ca 40%) and hepato-biliary excretion (ca 60%). All recovered radioactivity was identified as olmesartan. No other significant metabolite was detected. Enterohepatic recycling of olmesartan is minimal. Since a large proportion of olmesartan is excreted via the biliary route, use in patients with biliary obstruction is contraindicated (see 4.3).

The terminal elimination half life of olmesartan varied between 10 and 15 hours after multiple oral dosing. Steady state was reached after the first few doses and no further accumulation was evident after 14 days of repeated dosing. Renal clearance was approximately 0.5 – 0.7 L/h and was independent of dose.

Pharmacokinetics in special populations

Elderly:

In hypertensive patients, the AUC at steady state was increased by ca 35% in elderly patients (65 – 75 years old) and by ca 44% in very elderly patients (≥ 75 years old) compared with the younger age group (see 4.2).

Renal impairment:

In renally impaired patients, the AUC at steady state increased by 62%, 82% and 179% in patients with mild, moderate and severe renal impairment, respectively, compared to healthy controls (see 4.2, 4.4).

Hepatic impairment:

After single oral administration, olmesartan AUC values were 6% and 65% higher in mildly and moderately hepatically impaired patients, respectively, than in their corresponding matched healthy controls. The unbound fraction of olmesartan at 2 hours post-dose in healthy subjects, in patients with mild hepatic impairment and in patients with moderate hepatic impairment was 0.26%, 0.34% and 0.41%, respectively. Olmesartan medoxomil has not been evaluated in patients with severe hepatic impairment (see 4.2, 4.4).

5.3 Preclinical safety data

In chronic toxicity studies in rats and dogs, olmesartan medoxomil showed similar effects to other AT_1 receptor antagonists and ACE inhibitors: raised blood urea (BUN) and creatinine (through functional changes to the kidneys caused by blocking AT_1 receptors); reduction in heart weight; a reduction of red cell parameters (erythrocytes, haemoglobin, haematocrit); histological indications of renal damage (regenerative lesions of the renal epithelium, thickening of the basal membrane, dilatation of the tubules). These adverse effects caused by the pharmacological action of olmesartan medoxomil have also occurred in preclinical trials on other AT_1 receptor antagonists and ACE inhibitors and can be reduced by simultaneous oral administration of sodium chloride.

In both species, increased plasma renin activity and hypertrophy/hyperplasia of the juxtaglomerular cells of the kidney were observed. These changes, which are a typical effect of the class of ACE inhibitors and other AT_1 receptor antagonists, would appear to have no clinical relevance.

Like other AT_1 receptor antagonists olmesartan medoxomil was found to increase the incidence of chromosome breaks in cell cultures in vitro. No relevant effects were observed in several in vivo studies using olmesartan medoxomil at very high oral doses of up to 2000 mg/kg. The overall data of a comprehensive genotoxicity testing suggest that olmesartan is very unlikely to exert genotoxic effects under conditions of clinical use.

Olmesartan medoxomil was not carcinogenic, neither in rats in a 2 year study nor in mice when tested in two 6 month carcinogenicity studies using transgenic models.

In reproductive studies in rats, olmesartan medoxomil did not affect fertility and there was no evidence of a teratogenic effect. In common with other angiotensin II antagonists, survival of offspring was reduced following exposure to olmesartan medoxomil and pelvic dilatation of the kidney was seen after exposure of the dams in late pregnancy and lactation. In common with other antihypertensive agents, olmesartan medoxomil was shown to be more toxic to pregnant rabbits than to pregnant rats, however, there was no indication of a fetotoxic effect.

6. PHARMACEUTICAL PARTICULARS

6.1 List of excipients

Tablet core

Microcrystalline cellulose

Lactose monohydrate

Hydroxypropylcellulose

Magnesium stearate

Tablet coat

Titanium dioxide (E 171)

Talc

Hypromellose

6.2 Incompatibilities

Not applicable.

6.3 Shelf life

3 years.

6.4 Special precautions for storage

No special precautions for storage.

6.5 Nature and contents of container

Laminated polyamide/ aluminium/polyvinyl chloride/ aluminium blister pack.

Packs of 14, 28, 56 and 98 film-coated tablets.

Not all pack sizes may be marketed.

6.6 Instructions for use and handling

No special requirements.

7. MARKETING AUTHORISATION HOLDER
Sankyo Pharma UK Limited,
Sankyo House
Repton Place
White Lion Road
Amersham
Buckinghamshire HP7 9LP
United Kingdom

8. MARKETING AUTHORISATION NUMBER(S)
OLMETEC® 10mg: PL 08265/0015
OLMETEC® 20mg: PL 08265/0016
OLMETEC® 40mg: PL 08265/0017

9. DATE OF FIRST AUTHORISATION/RENEWAL OF THE AUTHORISATION
22nd May 2003

10. DATE OF REVISION OF THE TEXT
13th August 2004

11. LEGAL CATEGORY
POM

Omacor
(Solvay Healthcare Limited)

1. NAME OF THE MEDICINAL PRODUCT
Omacor, soft capsule

2. QUALITATIVE AND QUANTITATIVE COMPOSITION
Omega-3-acid ethyl esters 90 1000 mg
comprising 840 mg eicosapentaenoic acid (EPA) ethyl ester 46% and docosahexaenoic acid (DHA) ethyl ester 38%.
For one capsule
For excipients see 6.1

3. PHARMACEUTICAL FORM
Capsule, soft
Soft, oblong, transparent gelatin capsules containing pale yellow oil.

4. CLINICAL PARTICULARS
4.1 Therapeutic indications
Post Myocardial Infarction
Adjuvant treatment in secondary prevention after myocardial infarction, in addition to other standard therapy (e.g. statins, antiplatelet drugs, betablockers, ACE inhibitors).
Hypertriglyceridaemia
Endogenous hypertriglyceridaemia as a supplement to diet when dietary measures alone are insufficient to produce an adequate response:
- type IV in monotherapy,
- type IIb/III in combination with statins, when control of triglycerides is insufficient.

4.2 Posology and method of administration
Post Myocardial Infarction
One capsule daily.
Hypertriglyceridaemia
Initial treatment two capsules daily. If adequate response is not obtained, the dose may be increased to four capsules daily.
The capsules may be taken with food to avoid gastrointestinal disturbances.
There is no information regarding the use of Omacor in children, in elderly patients over 70 years of age, or in patients with hepatic impairment, and only limited information regarding the use in patients with renal impairment.

4.3 Contraindications
Hypersensitivity to any of the ingredients.

4.4 Special warnings and special precautions for use
Warnings
Because of the moderate increase in bleeding time (with the high dosage, i.e. 4 capsules), patients receiving anticoagulant therapy must be monitored and the dosage of anticoagulant adjusted if necessary (see section 4.5 Interaction with other Medicinal Products and other forms of Interaction). Use of this medication does not eliminate the need for the surveillance usually required for patients of this type.
Make allowance for the increased bleeding time in patients at high risk of haemorrhage (because of severe trauma, surgery, etc).
In the absence of efficacy and safety data, use of this medication in children is not recommended.
Omacor is not indicated in exogenous hypertriglyceridaemia (type 1 hyperchylomicronaemia). There is only limited experience in secondary endogenous hypertriglyceridaemia (especially uncontrolled diabetes).
There is no experience regarding hypertriglyceridaemia in combination with fibrates.

Special precaution
Regular monitoring of hepatic function (ASAT and ALAT) is required in patients with hepatic impairment (in particular with the high dosage, i.e. 4 capsules).

4.5 Interaction with other medicinal products and other forms of Interaction
Oral anticoagulants: See section 4.4 Special Warnings and Precautions for Use.
Omacor has been given in conjunction with warfarin without haemorrhagic complications. However, the prothrombin time must be checked when Omacor is combined with warfarin or when treatment with Omacor is stopped.

4.6 Pregnancy and lactation
Pregnancy
There are no adequate data from the use of Omacor in pregnant women.
Studies in animals have not shown reproductive toxicity. The potential risk for humans is unknown and therefore Omacor should not be used during pregnancy unless clearly necessary.
Lactation
There are no data on the excretion of Omacor in animal and human milk. Omacor should not be used during lactation.

4.7 Effects on ability to drive and use machines
Not applicable.

4.8 Undesirable effects
The frequencies of adverse events are ranked according to the following:
common (> 1/100, < 1/10); uncommon (>1/1000 < 1/100); rare (>1/10000, < 1/1000); very rare (< 1/10000), including isolated ADRs.
Gastrointestinal system disorders:
Common: dyspepsia, nausea
Uncommon: abdominal pain, gastrointestinal disorders, gastritis, abdominal pain upper
Rare: gastrointestinal pain
Very rare: lower gastrointestinal haemorrhage
Immune system disorders:
Uncommon: hypersensitivity
Infection:
Uncommon: gastroenteritis
Nervous system disorders:
Uncommon: dizziness, dysgeusia
Rare: headache
Metabolism system disorders:
Rare: hyperglycaemia
Hepatobiliary system disorders:
Rare: hepatic disorders
Vascular system disorders:
Very rare: hypotension
Respiratory system disorders:
Very rare: nasal dryness
Skin system disorders:
Rare: acne, rash pruritic
Very rare: urticaria
General disorders and administration site conditions:
Rare: Ill-defined disorders
Investigations:
Very rare: white blood count increased, blood lactate dehydrogenase increased
Moderate elevation of transaminases has been reported in patients with hypertriglyceridaemia.

4.9 Overdose
There are no special recommendations.
Administer symptomatic treatment.

5. PHARMACOLOGICAL PROPERTIES
5.1 Pharmacodynamic properties
SERUM LIPID-LOWERING AGENT / TRIGLYCERIDE REDUCER
(C: heart and circulation; serum lipid-lowering agents)
C10AX
The omega-3 series polyunsaturated fatty acids, eicosapentaenoic acid (EPA) and docosahexaenoic acid (DHA), are essential fatty acids.
Omacor is active on the plasma lipids by lowering triglyceride levels as a result of a fall in VLDL (very low density lipoprotein), and the substance is also active on haemostasis and blood pressure.
Omacor reduces the synthesis of triglycerides in the liver because EPA and DHA are poor substrates for the enzymes responsible for triglyceride synthesis and they inhibit esterification of other fatty acids.
The increase in peroxisomes of β-oxidation of fatty acids in the liver also contributes to the fall in triglycerides, by reducing the quantity of free fatty acids available for their synthesis. The inhibition of this synthesis lowers VLDL.
Omacor increases LDL-Cholesterol in some patients with hypertriglyceridaemia. A rise in HDL-Cholesterol is only small, significantly smaller than seen after administration of fibrates, and not consistent.
The long-term lipid-lowering effect (after more than one year) is not known. Otherwise there is no strong evidence that lowering triglycerides reduces the risk of ischaemic heart disease.
During treatment with Omacor, there is a fall in thromboxane A2 production and a slight increase in bleeding time. No significant effect has been observed on the other coagulation factors.
11324 patients, with recent MI (<3 months) and receiving a recommended preventative treatment associated with a Mediterranean diet, were randomised in the GISSI-Prevenzione study in order to receive Omacor (n=2836), vitamin E (n=2830), Omacor + vitamin E (n=2830) or no treatment (n=2828). GISSI-P was a multicentre, randomised, open-label study performed in Italy.
The results observed over 3.5 years, with Omacor 1g/day, have shown a significant reduction of a combined endpoint including all-cause death, non fatal MI and non fatal stroke (decrease in relative risk of 15% [2-26] p=0.0226 in patients taking Omacor alone compared to control, and of 10% [1-18] p=0.0482 in patients taking Omacor with or without vitamin E). A reduction of the second pre-specified endpoint criteria including cardiovascular deaths, non fatal MI and non-fatal stroke has been shown (decrease in relative risk of 20% [5-32] p=0.0082 in patients taking Omacor alone compared to control, decrease in relative risk of 11% [1-20] p= 0.0526 in patients taking Omacor with or without vitamin E). The secondary analysis for each component of the primary endpoints has shown a significant reduction of all cause deaths and cardiovascular deaths, but no reduction of non fatal cardiovascular events or fatal and non fatal strokes.

5.2 Pharmacokinetic properties
During and after absorption, there are three main pathways for the metabolism of the omega-3 fatty acids:
- the fatty acids are first transported to the liver where they are incorporated into various categories of lipoproteins and then channelled to the peripheral lipid stores;
- the cell membrane phospholipids are replaced by lipoprotein phospholipids and the fatty acids can then act as precursors for various eicosanoids;
- the majority is oxidised to meet energy requirements.
The concentration of omega-3 fatty acids, EPA and DHA, in the plasma phospholipids corresponds to the EPA and DHA incorporated into the cell membranes.
Animal pharmacokinetic studies have shown that there is a complete hydrolysis of the ethyl ester accompanied by satisfactory absorption and incorporation of EPA and DHA into the plasma phospholipids and cholesterol esters.

5.3 Preclinical safety data
No safety issues have been identified relevant to human use at the recommended daily intake.

6. PHARMACEUTICAL PARTICULARS
6.1 List of excipients
As antioxidant: Alpha-tocopherol
Capsule shell: Gelatin, glycerol, purified water

6.2 Incompatibilities
Not applicable

6.3 Shelf life
3 years

6.4 Special precautions for storage
Do not store above 25°C. Do not freeze.

6.5 Nature and contents of container
White high density polyethylene (HDPE) container.
- 28 capsules per container
- 100 capsules per container
- 10 × 28 capsules
Not all pack sizes may be marketed.

6.6 Instructions for use and handling
No special requirements.

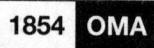

7. MARKETING AUTHORISATION HOLDER
Pronova Biocare a.s, 1327 Lysaker, Norway

8. MARKETING AUTHORISATION NUMBER(S)
PL 15905/0001

9. DATE OF FIRST AUTHORISATION/RENEWAL OF THE AUTHORISATION
9 July 1999

10. DATE OF REVISION OF THE TEXT
30 March 2004

One-Alpha Capsules
(Leo Laboratories Limited)

1. NAME OF THE MEDICINAL PRODUCT
One-Alpha® Capsules 1 microgram.
One-Alpha® Capsules 0.25 microgram.
One-Alpha® Capsules 0.5 microgram.

2. QUALITATIVE AND QUANTITATIVE COMPOSITION

One-Alpha Capsules 1 microgram: alfacalcidol (1-α hydroxyvitamin D3) 1 μg.

One-Alpha Capsules 0.25 microgram: alfacalcidol (1-α hydroxyvitamin D3) 0.25 μg.

One-Alpha Capsules 0.5 microgram: alfacalcidol 0.5 μg.

3. PHARMACEUTICAL FORM

One-Alpha Capsules 1 microgram: brown soft gelatin capsules.

One-Alpha Capsules 0.25 microgram: white soft gelatin capsules.

One-Alpha Capsules 0.5 microgram: red soft gelatin capsules.

4. CLINICAL PARTICULARS

4.1 Therapeutic indications

One-Alpha is indicated in all conditions where there is a disturbance of calcium metabolism due to impaired 1-α hydroxylation such as when there is reduced renal function. The main indications are:

a) Renal osteodystrophy

b) Hyperparathyroidism (with bone disease)

c) Hypoparathyroidism

d) Neonatal hypocalcaemia

e) Nutritional and malabsorptive rickets and osteomalacia

f) Pseudo-deficiency (D-dependent) rickets and osteomalacia

g) Hypophosphataemic vitamin D resistant rickets and osteomalacia

4.2 Posology and method of administration

Route of administration: oral

Initial dose for all indications:

Adults	1 microgram/day
Dosage in the elderly	0.5 microgram/day
Neonates and premature infants	0.05 - 0.1 microgram/kg/day
Children under 20 kg bodyweight	0.05 microgram/kg/day
Children over 20 kg bodyweight	1 microgram/day

The dose of One-Alpha should be adjusted thereafter to avoid hypercalcaemia according to the biochemical response. Indices of response include plasma levels of calcium (ideally corrected for protein binding), alkaline phosphatase, parathyroid hormone, as well as radiographic and histological investigations.

Plasma levels should initially be measured at weekly intervals. The daily dose of One-Alpha may be increased by increments of 0.25 - 0.5 microgram. When the dose is stabilised, measurements may be taken every 2 - 4 weeks.

Most adult patients respond to doses between 1 and 3 micrograms per day. When there is biochemical or radiographic evidence of bone healing, (and in hypoparathyroid patients when normal plasma calcium levels have been attained), the dose generally decreases. Maintenance doses are generally in the range of 0.25 to 1 microgram per day. If hypercalcaemia occurs, One-Alpha should be stopped until plasma calcium returns to normal (approximately 1 week) then restarted at half the previous dose.

(a) Renal bone disease:

Patients with relatively high initial plasma calcium levels may have autonomous hyperparathyroidism, often unresponsive to One-Alpha. Other therapeutic measures may be indicated.

Before and during treatment with One-Alpha, phosphate binding agents should be considered to prevent hyperphosphataemia. It is particularly important to make frequent plasma calcium measurements in patients with chronic renal failure because prolonged hypercalcaemia may aggravate the decline of renal function.

(b) Hyperparathyroidism:

In patients with primary or tertiary hyperparathyroidism about to undergo parathyroidectomy, pre-operative treatment with One-Alpha for 2-3 weeks alleviates bone pain and myopathy without aggravating pre-operative hypercalcaemia. In order to decrease post-operative hypocalcaemia, One-Alpha should be continued until plasma alkaline phosphatase levels fall to normal or hypercalcaemia occurs.

(c) Hypoparathyroidism:

In contrast to the response to parent vitamin D, low plasma calcium levels are restored to normal relatively quickly with One-Alpha. Severe hypocalcaemia is corrected more rapidly with higher doses of One-Alpha (e.g. 3-5 micrograms) together with calcium supplements.

(d) Neonatal hypocalcaemia:

Although the normal starting dose of One-Alpha is 0.05-0.1 microgram/kg/day (followed by careful titration) in severe cases doses of up to 2 microgram/kg/day may be required. Whilst ionised serum calcium levels may provide a guide to response, measurement of plasma alkaline phosphatase activity may be more useful. Levels of alkaline phosphatase approximately 7.5 times above the adult range indicates active disease.

A dose of 0.1 microgram/kg/day of One-Alpha has proven effective as prophylaxis against early neonatal hypocalcaemia in premature infants.

(e) Nutritional and malabsorptive rickets and osteomalacia:

Nutritional rickets and osteomalacia can be cured rapidly with One-Alpha. Malabsorptive osteomalacia (responding to large doses of IM or IV parent vitamin D) will respond to small doses of One-Alpha.

(f) Pseudo-deficiency (D-dependent) rickets and osteomalacia:

Although large doses of parent vitamin D would be required, effective doses of One-Alpha are similar to those required to heal nutritional vitamin D deficiency rickets and osteomalacia.

(g) Hypophosphataemic vitamin D-resistant rickets and osteomalacia:

Neither large doses of parent vitamin D nor phosphate supplements are entirely satisfactory. Treatment with One-Alpha at normal dosage rapidly relieves myopathy when present and increases calcium and phosphate retention. Phosphate supplements may also be required in some patients.

4.3 Contraindications

None known.

4.4 Special warnings and special precautions for use

None.

4.5 Interaction with other medicinal products and other forms of Interaction

Patients taking barbiturates or anticonvulsants may require larger doses of One-Alpha to produce the desired effect.

4.6 Pregnancy and lactation

There is inadequate evidence of safety of One-Alpha in human pregnancy but it has been in wide use for many years without apparent ill consequence. Animal studies have shown no hazard. If drug therapy is needed in pregnancy, One-Alpha can be used if there is no alternative.

Although it has not been established, it is likely that increased amounts of 1,25-dihydroxyvitamin D will be found in the milk of lactating mothers treated with One-Alpha. This may influence calcium metabolism in the infant.

4.7 Effects on ability to drive and use machines

Not applicable.

4.8 Undesirable effects

If hypercalcaemia occurs during treatment with One-Alpha, this can be rapidly corrected by stopping treatment until plasma calcium levels return to normal (about 1 week). One-Alpha may then be re-started at half the previous dose.

4.9 Overdose

Hypercalcaemia is treated by stopping One-Alpha. Severe hypercalcaemia may be additionally treated with a 'loop' diuretic and intravenous fluids, or with corticosteroids.

5. PHARMACOLOGICAL PROPERTIES

5.1 Pharmacodynamic properties

Alfacalcidol (One-Alpha) is converted rapidly in the liver to 1,25-dihydroxyvitamin D. This is the metabolite of vitamin D which acts as a regulator of calcium and phosphate metabolism. Since this conversion is rapid, the clinical effects of One-Alpha and 1,25-dihydroxyvitamin D are very similar.

Impaired 1-α hydroxylation by the kidneys reduces endogenous 1,25-dihydroxyvitamin D production. This contributes to the disturbances in mineral metabolism found in several disorders, including renal bone disease, hypoparathyroidism, neonatal hypocalcaemia and vitamin D dependent rickets. These disorders, which require high doses of parent vitamin D for their correction, will respond to small doses of One-Alpha.

The delay in response and high dosage required in treating these disorders with parent vitamin D makes dosage adjustment difficult. This can result in unpredictable hypercalcaemia which may take weeks or months to reverse. The major advantage of One-Alpha is the more rapid onset of response, which allows a more accurate titration of dosage. Should inadvertent hypercalcaemia occur it can be reversed within days of stopping treatment.

5.2 Pharmacokinetic properties

In patients with renal failure, 1-5 μg/day of 1α-hydroxyvitamin D (1α-OHD3) increased intestinal calcium and phosphorus absorption in a dose-related manner. This effect was observed within 3 days of starting the drug and conversely, it was reversed within 3 days of its discontinuation.

In patients with nutritional osteomalacia, increases in calcium absorption were noted within 6 hours of giving 1 μg 1α-OHD3 orally and usually peaked at 24 hours. 1α-OHD3 also produced increases in plasma inorganic phosphorus due to increased intestinal absorption and renal tubular reabsorption. This latter effect is a result of PTH suppression by 1α-OHD3. The effect of the drug on calcium was about double its effect on phosphorus absorption.

Patients with chronic renal failure have shown increased serum calcium levels within 5 days of receiving 1α-OHD3 in a dose of 0.5 - 1.0 μg/day. As serum calcium rose, PTH levels and alkaline phosphatase decreased toward normal.

5.3 Preclinical safety data

There are no pre-clinical data of relevance to the prescriber which are additional to that already included in other sections of the SPC.

6. PHARMACEUTICAL PARTICULARS

6.1 List of excipients

One-Alpha Capsules 1 microgram: sesame oil, dl-α-tocopherol, gelatin, glycerol, potassium sorbate, black iron oxide, red iron oxide.

One-Alpha Capsules 0.25 microgram: sesame oil, dl-α-tocopherol, gelatin, glycerol, potassium sorbate, titanium dioxide.

One-Alpha Capsules 0.5 microgram: sesame oil, dl-α-tocopherol, gelatin, glycerol, potassium sorbate, red iron oxide, titanium dioxide.

6.2 Incompatibilities

Not applicable.

6.3 Shelf life

3 years.

6.4 Special precautions for storage

Do not store above 25°C.

6.5 Nature and contents of container

PVC/AL blister of 30 (OP), with polyamide-coated aluminium cover.

6.6 Instructions for use and handling

None.

7. MARKETING AUTHORISATION HOLDER

Leo Laboratories Limited

Longwick Road

Princes Risborough

Bucks HP27 9RR

UK

8. MARKETING AUTHORISATION NUMBER(S)

One-Alpha Capsules 1 microgram: PL 0043/0050.

One-Alpha Capsules 0.25 microgram: PL 0043/0052.

One-Alpha Capsules 0.5 microgram: PL 0043/0206.

9. DATE OF FIRST AUTHORISATION/RENEWAL OF THE AUTHORISATION

One-Alpha Capsules 1 microgram: 26 January 1978/13 January 1994.

One-Alpha Capsules 0.25 microgram: 26 January 1978/31 March 1993.

One-Alpha Capsules 0.5 microgram: 22 September 1999.

10. DATE OF REVISION OF THE TEXT

One-Alpha Capsules 1 microgram: April 2000

One-Alpha Capsules 0.25 microgram: April 2000

One-Alpha Capsules 0.5 microgram: August 1999

LEGAL CATEGORY

POM

One-Alpha Drops

(Leo Laboratories Limited)

1. NAME OF THE MEDICINAL PRODUCT

One-Alpha Drops.

2. QUALITATIVE AND QUANTITATIVE COMPOSITION

Alfacalcidol 2 micrograms/ml

3. PHARMACEUTICAL FORM

Oral drops, solution.

4. CLINICAL PARTICULARS

4.1 Therapeutic indications

One-Alpha is indicated in all conditions where there is a disturbance of calcium metabolism due to impaired 1-α hydroxylation such as when there is reduced renal function. The main indications are:

a) Renal osteodystrophy

b) Hyperparathyroidism (with bone disease)

c) Hypoparathyroidism

d) Neonatal hypocalcaemia

e) Nutritional and malabsorptive rickets and osteomalacia

f) Pseudo-deficiency (D-dependent) rickets and osteomalacia

g) Hypophosphataemic vitamin D resistant rickets and osteomalacia

4.2 Posology and method of administration

One-Alpha Drops should be administered orally, using the integral dropper. One drop = 0.1 microgram.

Initial dose for all indications:

Adults	1 microgram/day
Dosage in the elderly	0.5 microgram/day
Neonates and premature infants	0.05 - 0.1 microgram/kg/day
Children under 20 kg bodyweight	0.05 microgram/kg/day
Children over 20 kg bodyweight	1 microgram/day

Half-drop doses should be rounded up to the next whole number of drops.

The dose of One-Alpha should be adjusted thereafter to avoid hypercalcaemia according to the biochemical response. Indices of response include plasma levels of calcium (ideally corrected for protein binding), alkaline phosphatase, parathyroid hormone, as well as radiographic and histological investigations.

Plasma levels should initially be measured at weekly intervals. The daily dose of One-Alpha may be increased by increments of 0.25 - 0.5 microgram. When the dose is stabilised, measurements may be taken every 2 - 4 weeks.

Most adult patients respond to doses between 1 and 3 micrograms per day. When there is biochemical or radiographic evidence of bone healing, (and in hypoparathyroid patients when normal plasma calcium levels have been attained), the dose generally decreases. Maintenance doses are generally in the range of 0.25 to 1 microgram per day. If hypercalcaemia occurs, One-Alpha should be stopped until plasma calcium returns to normal (approximately 1 week) then restarted at half the previous dose.

(a) Renal bone disease:
Patients with relatively high initial plasma calcium levels may have autonomous hyperparathyroidism, often unresponsive to One-Alpha. Other therapeutic measures may be indicated.

Before and during treatment with One-Alpha, phosphate binding agents should be considered to prevent hyperphosphataemia. It is particularly important to make frequent plasma calcium measurements in patients with chronic renal failure because prolonged hypercalcaemia may aggravate the decline of renal function.

(b) Hyperparathyroidism:
In patients with primary or tertiary hyperparathyroidism about to undergo parathyroidectomy, pre-operative treatment with One-Alpha for 2-3 weeks alleviates bone pain and myopathy without aggravating pre-operative hypercalcaemia. In order to decrease post-operative hypocalcaemia, One-Alpha should be continued until plasma alkaline phosphatase levels fall to normal or hypercalcaemia occurs.

(c) Hypoparathyroidism:
In contrast to the response to parent vitamin D, low plasma calcium levels are restored to normal relatively quickly with One-Alpha. Severe hypocalcaemia is corrected more rapidly with higher doses of One-Alpha (eg 3-5 micrograms) together with calcium supplements.

(d) Neonatal hypocalcaemia:
Although the normal starting dose of One-Alpha is 0.05-0.1 microgram/kg/day (followed by careful titration) in severe cases doses of up to 2 microgram/kg/day may be required. Whilst ionised serum calcium levels may provide a guide to response, measurement of plasma alkaline phosphatase activity may be more useful. Levels of alkaline phosphatase approximately 7.5 times above the adult range indicates active disease.

A dose of 0.1 microgram/kg/day of One-Alpha has proven effective as prophylaxis against early neonatal hypocalcaemia in premature infants.

(e) Nutritional and malabsorptive rickets and osteomalacia:
Nutritional rickets and osteomalacia can be cured rapidly with One-Alpha. Malabsorptive osteomalacia (responding to large doses of IM or IV parent vitamin D) will respond to small doses of One-Alpha.

(f) Pseudo-deficiency (D-dependent) rickets and osteomalacia:
Although large doses of parent vitamin D would be required, effective doses of One-Alpha are similar to those required to heal nutritional vitamin D deficiency rickets and osteomalacia.

(g) Hypophosphataemic vitamin D-resistant rickets and osteomalacia:
Neither large doses of parent vitamin D nor phosphate supplements are entirely satisfactory. Treatment with One-Alpha at normal dosage rapidly relieves myopathy when present and increases calcium and phosphate retention. Phosphate supplements may also be required in some patients.

4.3 Contraindications
None known.

4.4 Special warnings and special precautions for use
None.

4.5 Interaction with other medicinal products and other forms of Interaction
Patients taking barbiturates or anticonvulsants may require larger doses of One-Alpha to produce the desired effect.

4.6 Pregnancy and lactation
There is inadequate evidence of safety of One-Alpha in human pregnancy but it has been in wide use for many years without apparent ill consequence. Animal studies have shown no hazard. If drug therapy is needed in pregnancy, One-Alpha can be used if there is no alternative.

Although it has not been established, it is likely that increased amounts of 1,25-dihydroxyvitamin D will be found in the milk of lactating mothers treated with One-Alpha. This may influence calcium metabolism in the infant.

4.7 Effects on ability to drive and use machines
None known.

4.8 Undesirable effects
If hypercalcaemia occurs during treatment with One-Alpha, this can be rapidly corrected by stopping treatment until plasma calcium levels return to normal (about 1 week). One-Alpha may then be re-started at half the previous dose.

4.9 Overdose
Hypercalcaemia is treated by stopping One-Alpha. Severe hypercalcaemia may be additionally treated with a 'loop' diuretic and intravenous fluids, or with corticosteroids.

5. PHARMACOLOGICAL PROPERTIES

5.1 Pharmacodynamic properties
Alfacalcidol is converted rapidly in the liver to 1,25-dihydroxyvitamin D. This is the metabolite of vitamin D which acts as a regulator of calcium and phosphate metabolism. Since this conversion is rapid, the clinical effects of One-Alpha and 1,25-dihydroxyvitamin D are very similar.

Impaired 1-α hydroxylation by the kidneys reduces endogenous 1,25- dihydroxyvitamin D production. This contributes to the disturbances in mineral metabolism found in several disorders, including renal bone disease, hypoparathyroidism, neonatal hypocalcaemia and vitamin D dependent rickets. These disorders, which require high doses of parent vitamin D for their correction, will respond to small doses of One-Alpha.

The delay in response and high dosage required in treating these disorders with parent vitamin D makes dosage adjustment difficult. This can result in unpredictable hypercalcaemia which may take weeks or months to reverse. The major advantage of One-Alpha is the more rapid onset of response, which allows a more accurate titration of dosage. Should inadvertent hypercalcaemia occur it can be reversed within days of stopping treatment.

5.2 Pharmacokinetic properties
In patients with renal failure, 1-5 μg/day of 1α-hydroxyvitamin D (1α-OHD3) increased intestinal calcium and phosphorus absorption in a dose-related manner. This effect was observed within 3 days of starting the drug and, conversely, it was reversed within 3 days of its discontinuation.

In patients with nutritional osteomalacia, increases in calcium absorption were noted within 6 hours of giving 1 μg 1α-OHD3 orally and usually peaked at 24 hours. 1α-OHD3 also produced increases in plasma inorganic phosphorus due to increased intestinal absorption and renal tubular reabsorption. This latter effect is a result of PTH suppression by 1α-OHD3. The effect of the drug on calcium was about double its effect on phosphorus absorption.

Patients with chronic renal failure have shown increased serum calcium levels within 5 days of receiving 1α-OHD3 in a dose of 0.5 - 1.0 μg/day. As serum calcium rose, PTH levels and alkaline phosphatase decreased toward normal.

5.3 Preclinical safety data
There are no pre-clinical data of relevance to the prescriber which are additional to that already included in other sections of the SPC.

6. PHARMACEUTICAL PARTICULARS

6.1 List of excipients
Ethanol, polyoxyl 40 hydrogenated castor oil, methylparahydroxybenzoate, citric acid monohydrate, sodium citrate, sorbitol, dl-α-tocopherol and purified water.

6.2 Incompatibilities
None known.

6.3 Shelf life
3 years.

6.4 Special precautions for storage
Store at 2 - 8°C (in a refrigerator). Keep the container in the outer carton.

6.5 Nature and contents of container
Amber glass bottles of 10 ml with a polyethylene dropping device and a polypropylene screw cap.

6.6 Instructions for use and handling
None.

7. MARKETING AUTHORISATION HOLDER
Leo Laboratories Limited
Longwick Road
Princes Risborough
Bucks HP27 9RR
UK

8. MARKETING AUTHORISATION NUMBER(S)
PL 0043/0207

9. DATE OF FIRST AUTHORISATION/RENEWAL OF THE AUTHORISATION
3 March 2000.

10. DATE OF REVISION OF THE TEXT
November 1999

LEGAL CATEGORY
POM

One-Alpha Injection

(Leo Laboratories Limited)

1. NAME OF THE MEDICINAL PRODUCT
One-Alpha®Injection

2. QUALITATIVE AND QUANTITATIVE COMPOSITION
Alfacalcidol (1α-hydroxyvitamin D_3) 2 micrograms/ml.

3. PHARMACEUTICAL FORM
Injection

4. CLINICAL PARTICULARS

4.1 Therapeutic indications
One-Alpha is indicated in all conditions where there is a disturbance of calcium metabolism due to impaired 1 α-hydroxylation such as when there is reduced renal function.

The main indications are:

a) Renal osteodystrophy

b) Hyperparathyroidism (with bone disease)

c) Hypoparathyroidism

d) Neonatal hypocalcaemia

e) Nutritional and malabsorptive rickets and osteomalacia

f) Pseudo - deficiency (D - dependent) rickets and osteomalacia

g) Hypophosphataemic vitamin D resistant rickets and osteomalacia

4.2 Posology and method of administration
One-Alpha Injection should be administered intravenously as a bolus over approximately 30 seconds.

The dosage of One-Alpha Injection is the same as for One-Alpha in its oral presentations.

Initial dosage for all indications is:

Adults	1 microgram/day
Dosage in the elderly	0.5 microgram/day
Neonates and premature infants	0.05 - 0.1 microgram/kg/day
Children under 20 kg bodyweight	0.05 microgram/kg/day
Children over 20 kg bodyweight	1 microgram/day

The dose of One-Alpha should be adjusted thereafter to avoid hypercalcaemia according to the biochemical response.

Indices of response include plasma levels of calcium (ideally corrected for protein binding), alkaline phosphatase, parathyroid hormone, as well as radiographic and histological investigations.

Maintenance doses are generally in the range of 0.25 - 1 microgram per day.

When administered as intravenous injection to patients undergoing haemodialysis the initial dosage for adults is 1 microgram per dialysis. The maximum dose recommended is 6 micrograms per dialysis and not more than 12 micrograms per week. The injection should be administered into the return line from the haemodialysis machine at the end of each dialysis.

(a) Renal bone disease:
Patients with relatively high initial plasma calcium levels may have autonomous hyperparathyroidism, often unresponsive to One-Alpha. Other therapeutic measures may be indicated.

Before and during treatment with One-Alpha, phosphate binding agents should be considered to prevent hyperphosphataemia. It is particularly important to make frequent plasma calcium measurements in patients with chronic renal failure because prolonged hypercalcaemia may aggravate the decline of renal function.

(b) Hyperparathyroidism:
In patients with primary or tertiary hyperparathyroidism about to undergo parathyroidectomy, pre-operative treatment with One-Alpha for 2-3 weeks alleviates bone pain and myopathy without aggravating pre-operative hypercalcaemia. In order to decrease post-operative hypocalcaemia, One-Alpha should be continued until plasma alkaline phosphatase levels fall to normal or hypercalcaemia occurs.

(c) Hypoparathyroidism:
In contrast to the response to parent vitamin D, low plasma calcium levels are restored to normal relatively quickly with One-Alpha. Severe hypocalcaemia is corrected more rapidly with higher doses of One-Alpha (eg 3-5 micrograms) together with calcium supplements.

(d) Neonatal hypocalcaemia:
Although the normal starting dose of One-Alpha is 0.05-0.1 microgram/kg/day (followed by careful titration), in severe cases, doses of up to 2 microgram/kg/day may be required. Whilst ionised serum calcium levels may provide a guide to response, measurement of plasma alkaline phosphatase activity may be more useful. Levels of alkaline phosphatase approximately 7.5 times above the adult range indicates active disease.

(e) Nutritional and malabsorptive rickets and osteomalacia:
Nutritional rickets and osteomalacia can be cured rapidly with One-Alpha. Malabsorptive osteomalacia (responding to large doses of IM or IV parent vitamin D) will respond to small doses of One-Alpha.

(f) Pseudo-deficiency (D-dependent) rickets and osteomalacia:
Although large doses of parent vitamin D would be required, effective doses of One-Alpha are similar to those required to heal nutritional Vitamin D deficiency rickets and osteomalacia.

(g) Hypophosphataemic vitamin D-resistant rickets and osteomalacia:
Neither large doses of parent vitamin D nor phosphate supplements are entirely satisfactory. Treatment with One-Alpha at normal dosage rapidly relieves myopathy when present and increases calcium and phosphate retention. Phosphate supplements may also be required in some patients.

4.3 Contraindications
None known.

4.4 Special warnings and special precautions for use
During treatment with One-Alpha Injection serum calcium should be monitored regularly.

One-Alpha Injection should be avoided in patients with known sensitivity to injections containing propylene glycol and it should be used with caution in small premature infants.

4.5 Interaction with other medicinal products and other forms of Interaction
Patients taking barbiturates or anticonvulsants may require larger doses of One-Alpha to produce the desired effect.

4.6 Pregnancy and lactation
There is inadequate evidence of safety of One-Alpha in human pregnancy but it has been in wide use for many years without apparent ill consequence. Animal studies have shown no hazard. If drug therapy is needed in pregnancy, One-Alpha can be used if there is no alternative.

Although it has not been established, it is likely that increased amounts of 1,25 dihydroxyvitamin D will be found in the milk of lactating mothers treated with One-Alpha. This may influence calcium metabolism in the infant.

4.7 Effects on ability to drive and use machines
None known.

4.8 Undesirable effects
Rarely hypercalcaemia occurs during treatment with One-Alpha Injection. This can be rapidly corrected by stopping treatment until plasma calcium levels return to normal (about 1 week). One-Alpha may then be restarted at a reduced dose.

4.9 Overdose
Hypercalcaemia is treated by stopping One-Alpha. Severe hypercalcaemia may be additionally treated with a 'loop' diuretic and intravenous fluids, or with corticosteroids.

5. PHARMACOLOGICAL PROPERTIES

5.1 Pharmacodynamic properties
Alfacalcidol is converted rapidly in the liver to 1,25 dihydroxyvitamin D. This is the metabolite of vitamin D which acts as a regulator of calcium and phosphate metabolism. Since this conversion is rapid, the clinical effects of One-Alpha and 1,25 dihydroxyvitamin D are very similar.

Impaired 1 α-hydroxylation reduces 1,25 dihydroxyvitamin D production. This contributes to the disturbances in mineral metabolism found in several disorders, including renal bone disease, hypoparathyroidism, neonatal hypocalcaemia and vitamin D dependent rickets. These disorders, which require high doses of parent vitamin D for their correction, will respond to small doses of One-Alpha.

The delay in response and high dosage required in treating these disorders with parent vitamin D makes dosage adjustment difficult. This can result in unpredictable hypercalcaemia which may take weeks or months to reverse. The major advantage of One-Alpha is the more rapid onset of response, which allows a more accurate titration of dosage. Should inadvertent hypercalcaemia occur it can be reversed within days of stopping treatment.

5.2 Pharmacokinetic properties
In patients on regular haemodialysis administration of doses between 1 - 4 micrograms of intravenous 1 α-hydroxyvitamin D_3 resulted in increased levels of 1,25 dihydroxyvitamin D. Formation of 1,25 dihydroxyvitamin D_3 occurred within 1 hour after intravenous 1 α-hydroxyvitamin D_3 and peak concentrations were reached between 2 and 5 hours. Elimination half life of the formed 1,25 dihydroxyvitamin D was between 14 and 30 hours.

5.3 Preclinical safety data
There are no pre-clinical data of relevance to the prescriber which are additional to that already included in other sections of the SPC.

6. PHARMACEUTICAL PARTICULARS

6.1 List of excipients
Citric acid, ethanol, sodium citrate, propylene glycol and water for injection.

6.2 Incompatibilities
None known.

6.3 Shelf life
2 years.

6.4 Special precautions for storage
Store below 15°C.

6.5 Nature and contents of container
10 × 0.5ml amber glass ampoules.

10 × 1.0ml amber glass ampoules.

6.6 Instructions for use and handling
None.

7. MARKETING AUTHORISATION HOLDER
Leo Laboratories Limited

Longwick Road

Princes Risborough

Bucks

HP27 9RR

8. MARKETING AUTHORISATION NUMBER(S)
PL 0043/0183

9. DATE OF FIRST AUTHORISATION/RENEWAL OF THE AUTHORISATION
22 July 1991.

10. DATE OF REVISION OF THE TEXT
April 1996

LEGAL CATEGORY
POM

Opticrom Aqueous Eye Drops

(sanofi-aventis)

1. NAME OF THE MEDICINAL PRODUCT
Opticrom™ Aqueous Eye Drops

2. QUALITATIVE AND QUANTITATIVE COMPOSITION
Sodium cromoglicate 2.0% w/v.

3. PHARMACEUTICAL FORM
A clear colourless to pale yellow solution for administration to the eye.

4. CLINICAL PARTICULARS

4.1 Therapeutic indications
For the prophylaxis and symptomatic treatment of acute allergic conjunctivitis, chronic allergic conjunctivitis and vernal kerato conjunctivitis.

4.2 Posology and method of administration
Adults and children: one or two drops into each eye four times daily or as indicated by the doctor.

Elderly: no current evidence for alteration of the dose.

Route of administration: topical ophthalmic.

4.3 Contraindications
The product is contraindicated in patients who have shown hypersensitivity to Sodium cromoglicate, Benzalkonium chloride or Disodium edetate.

4.4 Special warnings and special precautions for use
Discard any remaining contents four weeks after opening the bottle.

As with other ophthalmic solutions containing Benzalkonium chloride, soft contact lenses should not be worn during treatment period.

4.5 Interaction with other medicinal products and other forms of Interaction
None known.

4.6 Pregnancy and lactation
As with all medication, caution should be exercised especially during the first trimester of pregnancy. Cumulative experience with Sodium cromoglicate suggests that it has no adverse effects on foetal development. It should be used in pregnancy only where there is a clear clinical need.

It is not known whether Sodium cromoglicate is excreted in human breast milk but, on the basis of its physicochemical properties, this is considered unlikely. There is no information to suggest the use of Sodium cromoglicate has any undesirable effects on the baby.

4.7 Effects on ability to drive and use machines
As with all eye drops, instillation of Opticrom may cause a transient blurring of vision.

4.8 Undesirable effects
Transient stinging and burning may occur after instillation. Other symptoms of local irritation have been reported rarely.

4.9 Overdose
No action other than medical observation should be necessary.

5. PHARMACOLOGICAL PROPERTIES

5.1 Pharmacodynamic properties
In vitro and *in vivo* animal studies have shown that Sodium cromoglicate inhibits the degranulation of sensitised mast cells which occurs after exposure to specific antigens. Sodium cromoglicate acts by inhibiting the release of histamine and various membrane derived mediators from the mast cell.

Sodium cromoglicate has demonstrated the activity *in vitro* to inhibit the degranulation of non-sensitised rat mast cells by phospholipase A and subsequent release of chemical mediators. Sodium cromoglicate did not inhibit the enzymatic activity of released phospholipase A on its specific substrate.

Sodium cromoglicate has no intrinsic vasoconstrictor or antihistamine activity.

5.2 Pharmacokinetic properties
Sodium cromoglicate is poorly absorbed. When multiple doses of Sodium cromoglicate ophthalmic solution are instilled into normal rabbit eyes, less than 0.07% of the administered dose of Sodium cromoglicate is absorbed into the systemic circulation (presumably by way of the eye, nasal passages, buccal cavity and gastrointestinal tract). Trace amounts (less than 0.01%) of the sodium cromoglicate does penetrate into the aqueous humour and clearance from this chamber is virtually complete within 24 hours after treatment is stopped.

In normal volunteers, analysis of drug excretion indicates that approximately 0.03% of Sodium cromoglicate is absorbed following administration to the eye.

5.3 Preclinical safety data
None stated.

6. PHARMACEUTICAL PARTICULARS

6.1 List of excipients
Benzalkonium chloride, Disodium edetate, Purified water.

6.2 Incompatibilities
None known.

6.3 Shelf life
3 years.

The eye drops should be used within 4 weeks of opening the container. Any remaining after this time should be discarded.

6.4 Special precautions for storage
Store below 30°C.

Protect from direct sunlight.

6.5 Nature and contents of container
Low density polyethylene bottle and plug with a polypropylene cap with a shrink type security seat containing 13.5 ml.

6.6 Instructions for use and handling
None.

7. MARKETING AUTHORISATION HOLDER
Aventis Pharma Ltd

50 Kings Hill Avenue

Kings Hill

West Malling

Kent

ME19 4AH

United Kingdom

8. MARKETING AUTHORISATION NUMBER(S)
PL 04425/0324

9. DATE OF FIRST AUTHORISATION/RENEWAL OF THE AUTHORISATION
28 February 2003

10. DATE OF REVISION OF THE TEXT
September 2004

11 LEGAL CLASSIFICATION
POM

Optimax

(Merck Pharmaceuticals)

1. NAME OF THE MEDICINAL PRODUCT
Optimax Tablets 500 mg

2. QUALITATIVE AND QUANTITATIVE COMPOSITION
Each tablet contains 500 mg L-tryptophan.

For excipients, see section 6.1.

3. PHARMACEUTICAL FORM
Tablet

White, capsule-shaped, engraved with 'Optimax' on one side, break line on the reverse

4. CLINICAL PARTICULARS

4.1 Therapeutic indications
In treatment-resistant depression after trials of standard antidepressant drug treatments, and as an adjunct to other anti-depressant medication.

Treatment with Optimax should only be initiated by hospital specialists. Patients may subsequently be prescribed Optimax in the community by their general practitioner.

4.2 Posology and method of administration
For oral use

Adults: The usual dose is two tablets, three times daily; for some patients, up to 6g L-tryptophan may be required.

Elderly: A lower dose may be appropriate, especially where there is evidence of renal or hepatic impairment.

Children: Not recommended. Safety has not been established.

4.3 Contraindications
Patients with a previous history of eosinophilia myalgia syndrome (EMS) following the use of L-tryptophan. This syndrome, which is a multisystem disorder, is characterised by raised eosinophils ($>1.0 \times 10^9$/L), and severe myalgia in the absence of either an infectious or neoplastic cause.

Patients with a known hypersensitivity to the active substance or any of the excipients.

4.4 Special warnings and special precautions for use
Eosinophilia Myalgia Syndrome (EMS) has been reported in association with the use of oral L-tryptophan-containing products. It is a multisystem disorder which is usually reversible but, rarely, fatal. Various investigations have not as yet identified the aetiological factors precisely.

The symptoms of EMS have been reported to include eosinophilia, arthralgia or myalgia, fever, dyspnoea, neuropathy, peripheral oedema and skin lesions which can include sclerosis or papular and urticarial lesions.

Caution should be exercised with patients who experience some but not all of the symptoms of EMS after taking L-tryptophan. Treatment should be withheld and the symptoms investigated until the possibility of EMS can be excluded.

The possible interaction between L-tryptophan and 5HT reuptake inhibitors could lead to the "serotonin syndrome" characterised by a combination of agitation, restlessness and gastro-intestinal symptoms including diarrhoea. Combinations with 5HT reuptake inhibitors should only be used with care (see Section 4.5).

4.5 Interaction with other medicinal products and other forms of Interaction
Where L-tryptophan is combined with an MAO Inhibitor the side effects of the latter may be enhanced. Use of L-tryptophan in combination with a 5HT reuptake inhibitor has the potential for increasing the severity of the adverse effects of the latter and could lead to serotonin syndrome (see Section 4.4).

In patients taking L-tryptophan in conjunction with phenothiazines or benzodiazepines there have been isolated reports of sexual disinhibition.

4.6 Pregnancy and lactation
Safety in pregnancy or lactation has not been established

4.7 Effects on ability to drive and use machines
L-tryptophan may produce drowsiness. Patients who drive and operate machinery should be warned of the possible hazard.

4.8 Undesirable effects
In some patients, L-tryptophan may cause a slight feeling of nausea which usually disappears within 2 or 3 days. Such nausea can be minimised by giving L-tryptophan after food. Other adverse reactions include headache and light-headedness.

4.9 Overdose
Drowsiness and vomiting may occur; supportive measures should be employed.

5. PHARMACOLOGICAL PROPERTIES

5.1 Pharmacodynamic properties
Pharmacotherapeutic group: Antidepressants

ATC Code: NO6A X 02

L-tryptophan is an essential dietary amino acid and, following hydroxylation and decarboxylation, is the major source of 5-hydroxytryptamine (5-HT). L-tryptophan, 5-HT and 5-HT metabolite levels are lower than normal in patients with depression. Administration of L-tryptophan re-establishes the inhibitory action of 5-HT on the amygdaloid nuclei, thereby reducing feelings of anxiety and depression.

5.2 Pharmacokinetic properties
L-tryptophan is readily absorbed after oral administration. The elimination half-life when administered orally or intravenously to healthy humans is in the range of 1-3 hours. L-tryptophan is bound to plasma proteins to a large extent and is eliminated primarily by metabolism.

5.3 Preclinical safety data
None reported

6. PHARMACEUTICAL PARTICULARS

6.1 List of excipients
Sta-RX Starch,

maize starch,

Explotab,

saccharin sodium,

magnesium stearate,

Aerosil

6.2 Incompatibilities
None known

6.3 Shelf life
3 years

6.4 Special precautions for storage
None

6.5 Nature and contents of container
Polypropylene bottle containing 84 tablets

6.6 Instructions for use and handling
Not applicable

7. MARKETING AUTHORISATION HOLDER
E Merck Ltd., t/a Merck Pharmaceuticals (A division of Merck Ltd), Harrier House, High Street, West Drayton, Middlesex, UB7 7QG, UK

8. MARKETING AUTHORISATION NUMBER(S)
PL 0493/5900

9. DATE OF FIRST AUTHORISATION/RENEWAL OF THE AUTHORISATION
11/01/82 / 08/07/02

10. DATE OF REVISION OF THE TEXT
November 2004

Oraldene

(Pfizer Consumer Healthcare)

1. NAME OF THE MEDICINAL PRODUCT
ORALDENE

2. QUALITATIVE AND QUANTITATIVE COMPOSITION
ORALDENE contains 0.1% w/v hexetidine.

3. PHARMACEUTICAL FORM
A clear red solution.

4. CLINICAL PARTICULARS

4.1 Therapeutic indications
ORALDENE is indicated for use in minor mouth infections including thrush, as an aid in the prevention and treatment of gingivitis, and in the management of sore throat and recurrent aphthous ulcers. ORALDENE is also of value in the alleviation of halitosis and pre- and post-dental surgery.

4.2 Posology and method of administration
Adults and children 12 years and over:

Topical administration to the buccal cavity.

Rinse the mouth, or gargle with at least 15 ml of undiluted solution, two or three times a day.

ORALDENE should not be swallowed in large quantities.

Children aged 6 to 11 years:

As recommended for adults.

Children under 6 years:

Not recommended.

The Elderly:

As recommended for adults.

4.3 Contraindications
None known.

4.4 Special warnings and special precautions for use
None known.

4.5 Interaction with other medicinal products and other forms of Interaction
No interactions are known.

4.6 Pregnancy and lactation
No formal studies have been conducted in man. However, on the basis of animal studies and, in theory, the negligible systemic absorption it is considered highly unlikely that the use of ORALDENE during pregnancy will present a risk to the foetus.

It is not known whether hexetidine is excreted in human breast milk, however, in view of the negligible amount of hexetidine which could be predicted to be systemically absorbed, it is unlikely that concentrations of hexetidine in the milk will present any risk to the neonate/infant.

4.7 Effects on ability to drive and use machines
ORALDENE is unlikely affect ability to drive or operate machinery.

4.8 Undesirable effects
ORALDENE is generally very well tolerated with a low potential for causing irritation, or sensitisation reactions. Prolonged use of ORALDENE is also well tolerated.

Patch testing with of hexetidine containing ointment was negative for irritation or sensitisation potential.

In a few individuals mild irritation (described as sore mouth, burning or itching) of the tongue and/or buccal tissues has been reported. Other side effects which are reported very rarely include transient anaesthesia and taste impairment.

4.9 Overdose
Signs and Symptoms of Overdose

There are no reports of alcohol intoxication from overdose with ORALDENE.

Hexetidine, at the strength present in ORALDENE, is non-toxic.

Acute alcoholic intoxication is extremely unlikely, however, it is theoretically possible that, if a massive dose were swallowed by a small child, alcoholic intoxication may occur due to the ethanol content.

There is no evidence to suggest that repeated, excessive administration of hexetidine would lead to hypersensitivity-type reactions.

Treatment of Overdose

Treatment of overdose is symptomatic, but rarely required. In the event of accidental ingestion of the contents of a bottle by a child, a doctor should be consulted immediately. Gastric lavage should be considered within two hours of ingestion and management should relate to treatment of alcoholic intoxication.

5. PHARMACOLOGICAL PROPERTIES

5.1 Pharmacodynamic properties
Hexetidine is a broad spectrum antimicrobial. It is active both in vivo and in vitro, against gram positive and negative bacterium, as well as yeasts (Candida albicans) and fungi.

5.2 Pharmacokinetic properties
Specific pharmacodynamic studies have not been carried out on ORALDENE in man.

The oral retention of hexetidine to mucous membranes and dental plaque has been observed. In studies using radiolabelled hexetidine it has been shown that retention on buccal tissues can extend to between 8 and 10 hours after a single oral rinse and in some cases hexetidine has been detected on oral tissues up to 65 hours post-treatment.

No absorption studies following the topical application of ORALDENE have been performed in man.

Pharmacokinetics in renal/hepatic impairment

There have been no specific studies of ORALDENE or hexetidine in renal/hepatic impairment.

Pharmacokinetics in elderly

There have been no specific studies of ORALDENE or hexetidine in the elderly.

5.3 Preclinical safety data
Pre-clinical safety data do not add anything of further significance to the prescriber.

6. PHARMACEUTICAL PARTICULARS

6.1 List of excipients
Polysorbate 60

Citric acid

Saccharin sodium

Peppermint flavour

Anise oil

Methyl salicylate

Levomenthol

Clove oil

Eucalyptus oil

Ethanol 96%

Azorubin (85%) (E122)

Purified water

6.2 Incompatibilities
None.

6.3 Shelf life
24 months.

6.4 Special precautions for storage
Do not store above 25°C. Keep container in outer carton.

6.5 Nature and contents of container
ORALDENE is presented in a clear 100 ml, 200 ml and 30 ml glass bottles, with white aluminium ROPP cap.

Each bottle is fitted with its own polypropylene measuring cup.

6.6 Instructions for use and handling
Shake well before use.

7. MARKETING AUTHORISATION HOLDER
Pfizer Consumer Healthcare

Alternative Trading Style:

Warner-Lambert Consumer Healthcare

Walton Oaks

Dorking Road

Walton-on-the-Hill

Surrey KT20 7NS

United Kingdom

8. MARKETING AUTHORISATION NUMBER(S)
PL 15513/0067

9. DATE OF FIRST AUTHORISATION/RENEWAL OF THE AUTHORISATION
29th April 1998

10. DATE OF REVISION OF THE TEXT
January 2004

Oraldene Icemint

(Pfizer Consumer Healthcare)

1. NAME OF THE MEDICINAL PRODUCT
ORALDENE ICEMINT

2. QUALITATIVE AND QUANTITATIVE COMPOSITION
ORALDENE ICEMINT contains 0.1% w/v hexetidine.

3. PHARMACEUTICAL FORM
Mouthwash.

A clear blue green mouthwash.

4. CLINICAL PARTICULARS
4.1 Therapeutic indications
ORALDENE ICEMINT is indicated for use in minor mouth infections including thrush, as an aid in the prevention and treatment of gingivitis, and in the management of sore throat and recurrent aphthous ulcers. ORALDENE ICEMINT is also of value in the alleviation of halitosis and pre- and post- dental surgery.

4.2 Posology and method of administration
Adults and children 12 years and over
Topical administration to the buccal cavity.

Rinse the mouth, or gargle with at least 15 ml of undiluted solution, two or three times a day.

ORALDENE ICEMINT should not be swallowed in large quantities.

Children aged 6 to 11 years
As recommended for adults.

Children under 6 years
Not recommended.

The Elderly
As recommended for adults.

4.3 Contraindications
None known.

4.4 Special warnings and special precautions for use
None known.

4.5 Interaction with other medicinal products and other forms of Interaction
No interactions are known.

4.6 Pregnancy and lactation
No formal studies have been conducted in man. However, on the basis of animal studies and, in theory, the negligible systemic absorption it is considered highly unlikely that the use of ORALDENE ICEMINT during pregnancy will present a risk to the foetus.

It is not known whether hexetidine is excreted in human breast milk, however, in view of the negligible amount of hexetidine which could be predicted to be systemically absorbed, it is unlikely that concentrations of hexetidine in the milk will present any risk to the neonate/infant.

4.7 Effects on ability to drive and use machines
ORALDENE ICEMINT is unlikely to affect ability to drive or operate machinery.

4.8 Undesirable effects
ORALDENE ICEMINT is generally very well-tolerated with a low potential for causing irritation, or sensitisation reactions. Prolonged use of ORALDENE ICEMINT is also well-tolerated.

Patch testing with of hexetidine containing ointment was negative for irritation or sensitisation potential.

In a few individuals mild irritation (described as sore mouth, burning or itching), of the tongue and/or buccal tissues has been reported. Other side effects which are reported very rarely include transient anaesthesia and taste impairment.

4.9 Overdose
Signs and Symptoms of Overdose
There are no reports of alcohol intoxication from overdose with ORALDENE ICEMINT.

Hexetidine, at the strength present in ORALDENE ICEMINT, is non-toxic.

Acute alcoholic intoxication is extremely unlikely, however, it is theoretically possible that, if a massive dose were swallowed by a small child, alcoholic intoxication may occur due to the ethanol content.

There is no evidence to suggest that repeated, excessive administration of hexetidine would lead to hypersensitivity-type reactions.

Treatment of Overdose
Treatment of overdose is symptomatic, but rarely required. In the event of accidental ingestion of the contents of a bottle by a child, a doctor should be consulted immediately. Gastric lavage should be considered within two hours of ingestion and management should relate to treatment of alcoholic intoxication.

5. PHARMACOLOGICAL PROPERTIES
5.1 Pharmacodynamic properties
Hexetidine is a broad spectrum antimicrobial. It is active both in vivo and in vitro, against gram positive and negative bacterium, as well as yeasts (Candida albicans) and fungi.

5.2 Pharmacokinetic properties
Specific pharmacodynamic studies have not been carried out on ORALDENE ICEMINT in man.

The oral retention of hexetidine to mucous membranes and dental plaque has been observed. In studies using radiolabelled hexetidine it has been shown that retention on buccal tissues can extend to between 8 and 10 hours after a single oral rinse and in some cases hexetidine has been detected on oral tissues up to 65 hours post-treatment.

No absorption studies following the topical application of ORALDENE ICEMINT have been performed in man.

Pharmacokinetics in renal/hepatic impairment
There have been no specific studies of ORALDENE ICEMINT or hexetidine in renal/hepatic impairment.

Pharmacokinetics in elderly
There have been no specific studies of ORALDENE ICEMINT or hexetidine in the elderly.

5.3 Preclinical safety data
Pre-clinical safety data does not add anything of further significance to the presciber.

6. PHARMACEUTICAL PARTICULARS
6.1 List of excipients
Polysorbate 60

Citric acid

Saccharin sodium

Ethanol 96%

Quinoline Yellow (70%) E104

Patent Blue V (85%) E131

Mint flavour

Purified water

6.2 Incompatibilities
None.

6.3 Shelf life
24 months

6.4 Special precautions for storage
Do not store above 25°C. Keep the container in the outer carton.

6.5 Nature and contents of container
ORALDENE ICEMINT is presented in a clear (Type 3) 200 ml glass bottles, with white aluminium ROPP cap fitted with PET wad or a 400ml PET bottle with aluminium ROPP cap fitted with PET wad.

Each bottle is fitted with its own polypropylene measuring cup.

6.6 Instructions for use and handling
Shake well before use.

7. MARKETING AUTHORISATION HOLDER
Pfizer Consumer Healthcare

Alternative Trading Style:

Warner-Lambert Consumer Healthcare

Walton Oaks

Dorking Road

Walton-on-the-Hill

Surrey KT20 7NS

United Kingdom

8. MARKETING AUTHORISATION NUMBER(S)
PL 15513/0107

9. DATE OF FIRST AUTHORISATION/RENEWAL OF THE AUTHORISATION
2 August 2001

10. DATE OF REVISION OF THE TEXT
January 2004

Oramorph Oral Solution

(Boehringer Ingelheim Limited)

1. NAME OF THE MEDICINAL PRODUCT
Oramorph Oral Solution 10 mg/5 ml

2. QUALITATIVE AND QUANTITATIVE COMPOSITION
Each 5 ml contains 10 mg of Morphine Sulphate BP.

3. PHARMACEUTICAL FORM
A clear, colourless solution for oral administration.

4. CLINICAL PARTICULARS
4.1 Therapeutic indications
For the relief of severe pain.

4.2 Posology and method of administration
Adults: Usual dose 10-20 mg (5-10 ml) every 4 hours.

Children 6-12 years: Maximum dose 5-10 mg (2.5-5 ml) every 4 hours.

Children 1-5 years: Maximum dose 5 mg (2.5 ml) every 4 hours.

Children under 1 year: Not recommended.

Dosage can be increased under medical supervision according to the severity of the pain and the patient's previous history of analgesic requirements. Reductions in dosage may be appropriate in the elderly.

Morphine Sulphate BP is readily absorbed from the gastrointestinal tract following oral administration. However, when Oramorph Oral Solution is used in place of parenteral morphine, a 50% to 100% increase in dosage is usually required in order to achieve the same level of analgesia.

4.3 Contraindications
Respiratory depression, obstructive airways disease, known morphine sensitivity, acute hepatic disease, acute alcoholism, head injuries, coma, convulsive disorders and where the intracranial pressure is raised. Concurrent administration of monoamine oxidase inhibitors or within two weeks of discontinuation of their use.

4.4 Special warnings and special precautions for use
Care should be exercised if morphine sulphate is given in the first 24 hours post-operatively, in hypothyroidism, and where there is reduced respiratory reserve, such as kyphoscoliosis, emphysema and severe obesity.

Morphine sulphate should not be given if paralytic ileus is likely to occur or where there is an obstructive bowel disorder. If constipation occurs, this may be treated with appropriate laxatives.

It is wise to reduce dosage in chronic hepatic and renal disease, myxoedema, adrenocortical insufficiency, prostatic hypertrophy or shock.

Tolerance and dependence may occur.

4.5 Interaction with other medicinal products and other forms of Interaction
Phenothiazine antiemetics may be given with morphine, but it should be noted that morphine potentiates the effects of tranquillisers, anaesthetics, hypnotics, sedatives and alcohol.

4.6 Pregnancy and lactation
Although morphine sulphate has been in general use for many years, there is inadequate evidence of safety in human pregnancy and lactation.

Morphine is known to cross the placenta, and is excreted in breast milk, and may thus cause respiratory depression in the newborn infant.

Medicines should not be used in pregnancy, especially the first trimester unless the expected benefit is thought to outweigh any possible risk to the foetus.

4.7 Effects on ability to drive and use machines
Morphine sulphate is likely to impair ability to drive and to use machinery.

4.8 Undesirable effects
Nausea, vomiting and confusion may be troublesome. If constipation occurs, this may be treated with appropriate laxatives. Morphine may cause dry mouth, sweating, facial flushing, vertigo, bradycardia, palpitations, orthostatic hypotension, hypothermia, restlessness, changes of mood and miosis. Micturition may be difficult and there may be ureteric or biliary spasm. There is also an antidiuretic effect. These effects are more common in ambulant patients than in those who are bedridden. Raised intracranial pressure occurs in some patients.

4.9 Overdose
Symptoms: Signs of morphine toxicity and overdosage are likely to consist of pin-point pupils, respiratory depression and hypotension. Circulatory failure and deepening coma may occur in more severe cases. Convulsions may occur in infants and children. Death may occur from respiratory failure.

Treatment of morphine overdose: Administer 400 microgram of naloxone intravenously. Repeat at 2-3 minute intervals as necessary, or by an infusion of 2mg in 500 ml of normal saline or 5 % dextrose (4 microgram/ml). Empty the stomach. A 0.02% aqueous solution of potassium permanganate may be used for lavage. Assist respiration if necessary. Maintain fluid and electrolyte levels.

5. PHARMACOLOGICAL PROPERTIES
5.1 Pharmacodynamic properties
Morphine binds to opiate receptors, which are located on the cell surfaces of the brain and nervous tissue. This action results in alteration of neurotransmitter release and calcium uptake. It has been postulated that this is the basis of the modulation of sensory input from afferent nerves sensitive to pain.

5.2 Pharmacokinetic properties
Morphine N-methyl ^{14}C sulphate administered orally to humans reaches a peak plasma level after around 15 minutes: levels of plasma-conjugated morphine peak at about 3 hours, and slowly decrease over the following 24 hours. After the first hour no significant differences in total plasma levels of radioactivity are seen whether administration is by intravenous, intramuscular, subcutaneous or oral route.

Morphine is a basic amine, and rapidly leaves the plasma and concentrates in the tissues. In animals it has been shown that a relatively small amount of free morphine crosses the blood-brain barrier. Morphine is metabolised in the liver and probably also in the mucosal cells of the small intestine. The metabolites recovered in the urine, in addition to free morphine, are morphine-3-glucuronide and morphine ethereal sulphate. These account for over 65 %

of administered radioactivity; further radioactivity can be recovered as exhaled $^{14}CO_2$.

5.3 Preclinical safety data
No further relevant preclinical data are available.

6. PHARMACEUTICAL PARTICULARS

6.1 List of excipients
Alcohol, corn syrup, sucrose, methyl hydroxybenzoate (E218), propyl hydroxybenzoate (E216) and purified water.

6.2 Incompatibilities
None stated.

6.3 Shelf life
3 years.

Discard Oramorph Oral Solution 90 days after first opening.

6.4 Special precautions for storage
Do not store above 25°C. Store in the original container.

6.5 Nature and contents of container
Registered Packs

Amber glass bottles with a tamper–evident, child resistant polypropylene closure with expanded PE liner are available in packs of 100 ml, 250 ml, 300 ml or 500 ml.

Marketed Packs

Oramorph Oral Solution is available in 100 ml, 300 ml, and 500 ml amber glass bottles with a tamper–evident, child resistant polypropylene closure an expanded PE liner.

6.6 Instructions for use and handling
None stated.

7. MARKETING AUTHORISATION HOLDER
Boehringer Ingelheim Limited

Ellesfield Avenue

Bracknell

Berkshire

RG12 8YS

United Kingdom

8. MARKETING AUTHORISATION NUMBER(S)
PL 0015/0122

9. DATE OF FIRST AUTHORISATION/RENEWAL OF THE AUTHORISATION
08.03.88 / 08.03.93

10. DATE OF REVISION OF THE TEXT
January 2005

11. Legal category
POM

02b/UK/SPC/5

Oramorph Unit Dose Vials

(Boehringer Ingelheim Limited)

1. NAME OF THE MEDICINAL PRODUCT
Oramorph Unit Dose Vials 10 mg/5 ml

Oramorph Unit Dose Vials 30 mg/5 ml

Oramorph Unit Dose Vials 100 mg/5 ml

2. QUALITATIVE AND QUANTITATIVE COMPOSITION
Oramorph Unit Dose Vials 10 mg/5 ml: each vial contains 10 mg Morphine Sulphate.

Oramorph Unit Dose Vials 30 mg/5 ml: each vial contains 30 mg Morphine Sulphate.

Oramorph Unit Dose Vials 100 mg/5 ml: each vial contains 100 mg Morphine Sulphate.

For excipients, see 6.1

3. PHARMACEUTICAL FORM
Oral solution.

Clear, colourless solution.

4. CLINICAL PARTICULARS

4.1 Therapeutic indications
For the relief of severe pain.

4.2 Posology and method of administration
Dosage and administration

Adults:	Usual starting dose 10-20 mg (5-10 ml) of 0.2 % Oramorph Unit Dose Vials every 4 hours
Children:	
Under 5 years:	Not recommended
6-12 years:	Maximum dose 10 mg (5 ml of Oramorph 0.2 % Unit Dose Vial) every 4 hours

The dosage can be increased under medical supervision according to the severity of the pain and the patient's previous history of analgesic requirements using Oramorph 0.6 % UDVs (30 mg morphine sulphate/5 ml) or Oramorph 2.0 % UDVs (100 mg morphine sulphate/5 ml).

Reductions in dosage may be appropriate in the elderly or where sedation is undesirable.

The required dose may be added to a soft drink immediately prior to administration.

4.3 Contraindications
Respiratory depression, obstructive airways disease, known morphine sensitivity, acute hepatic disease, acute alcoholism, head injuries, coma, convulsive disorders and where the intracranial pressure is raised. Concurrent administration of monoamine oxidase inhibitors or within two weeks of discontinuation of their use.

4.4 Special warnings and special precautions for use
Care should be exercised if morphine sulphate is given in the first 24 hours post operatively, in hypothyroidism, and where there is reduced respiratory reserve, such as kyphoscoliosis, emphysema and severe obesity.

Morphine sulphate should not be given if paralytic ileus is likely to occur or where there is an obstructive bowel disorder. If constipation occurs, this may be treated with appropriate laxatives. It is wise to reduce dosage in chronic hepatic and renal disease, myxoedema, adrenocortical insufficiency, prostatic hypertrophy or shock. Tolerance and dependence may occur.

4.5 Interaction with other medicinal products and other forms of Interaction
Phenothiazine anti-emetics may be given with morphine, but it should be noted that morphine potentiates the effect of tranquillisers, anaesthetics, hypnotics, sedatives and alcohol.

4.6 Pregnancy and lactation
Although morphine sulphate has been in general use for many years, there is inadequate evidence of safety in human pregnancy and lactation. Morphine is known to cross the placenta and is excreted in breast milk and may thus cause respiratory depression in the new born infant. Medicines should not be used in pregnancy, especially in the first trimester, unless the expected benefit outweighs any possible risk to the foetus.

4.7 Effects on ability to drive and use machines
Patients should be warned not to drive or operate dangerous machinery after taking Oramorph.

4.8 Undesirable effects
Side effects:

In routine clinical practice, the commonest side effects of morphine sulphate are nausea, vomiting, constipation, drowsiness and confusion. If constipation occurs, this may be treated with appropriate laxatives. Micturition may be difficult and there may be ureteric or biliary spasm. There is also an antidiuretic effect. Dry mouth, sweating, facial flushing, vertigo, bradycardia, palpitations, orthostatic hypotension, hypothermia, restlessness, changes of moods and miosis can also occur. These effects are more common in ambulant patients than in those who are bedridden. Raised intracranial pressure occurs in some patients. As a consequence of histamine release, urticaria and or pruritus may occur in some individuals.

4.9 Overdose
Signs of morphine toxicity and overdosage:

These are likely to consist of pin-point pupils, respiratory depression and hypotension. Circulatory failure and deepening coma may occur in more severe cases. Convulsions may occur in infants and children. Death may occur from respiratory failure.

Treatment of morphine overdosage:

Administer naloxone 0.4 mg intravenously. Repeat at 2-3 minute intervals as necessary, or by an infusion of 2 mg in 500 ml of normal saline or 5 % dextrose (4 micrograms/ml). Empty the stomach. A 0.02 % aqueous solution of potassium permanganate may be used for lavage. Assist respiration if necessary. Maintain fluid and electrolyte levels.

5. PHARMACOLOGICAL PROPERTIES

5.1 Pharmacodynamic properties
Morphine binds to opiate receptors located on the cell surfaces of the brain and nervous tissue. This action results in alteration of neurotransmitter release and calcium uptake. It has been postulated that this is the basis of the modulation of sensory input from afferent nerves sensitive to pain.

5.2 Pharmacokinetic properties
Morphine N-methyl ^{14}C sulphate administered orally to humans reaches a peak plasma level after around 15 minutes: levels of plasma-conjugated morphine peak at about 3 hours, and slowly decrease over the following 24 hours. After the first hour no significant differences in total plasma levels of radioactivity are seen whether administration is by intravenous, intramuscular, subcutaneous or oral route.

Morphine is a basic amine, and rapidly leaves the plasma and concentrates in the tissues. In animals it has been shown that a relatively small amount of free morphine crosses the blood-brain barrier. Morphine is metabolised in the liver and probably also in the mucosal cells of the small intestine. The metabolites recovered in the urine, in addition to free morphine, are morphine-3-glucuronide and morphine ethereal sulphate. These account for over 65 % of administered radioactivity; further radioactivity can be recovered as exhaled $^{14}CO_2$.

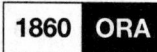

5.3 Preclinical safety data
No preclinical data are available which are additional to the experience gained in over many years.

6. PHARMACEUTICAL PARTICULARS

6.1 List of excipients
Disodium edetate, citric acid anhydrous, purified water.

6.2 Incompatibilities
None known

6.3 Shelf life
Two years.

Once opened, use immediately.

6.4 Special precautions for storage
Do not store above 25C.

Keep container in outer carton.

6.5 Nature and contents of container
Marketed packs:

5 ml low density polyethylene Unit Dose Vials packed into cartons containing 20 vials.

Non-marketed packs:

Cartons containing 6, 30, 50, 60, or 100 vials.

6.6 Instructions for use and handling
Discard any unused solution.

7. MARKETING AUTHORISATION HOLDER
Boehringer Ingelheim Limited

Ellesfield Avenue

Bracknell, Berkshire

RG12 8YS

United Kingdom

8. MARKETING AUTHORISATION NUMBER(S)

Oramorph UDVs 10 mg/5 ml	PL 00015/0157
Oramorph UDVs 30 mg/5 ml	PL 00015/0158
Oramorph UDVs 100 mg/5 ml	PL 00015/0159

9. DATE OF FIRST AUTHORISATION/RENEWAL OF THE AUTHORISATION
21 July 1992 / 21 July 1997

10. DATE OF REVISION OF THE TEXT
30th July 2002

11. Legal category

Oramorph UDVs 10 mg/5 ml	POM
Oramorph UDVs 30 mg/5 ml	POM CD
Oramorph UDVs 100 mg/5ml	POM CD

02e/UK/SPC/4 combined

Orap 4 mg tablets.

(Janssen-Cilag Ltd)

1. NAME OF THE MEDICINAL PRODUCT
Orap® 4 mg tablets.

2. QUALITATIVE AND QUANTITATIVE COMPOSITION
Each tablet contains pimozide 4 mg.

3. PHARMACEUTICAL FORM
Tablet

Green, circular, biconvex, normally arched tablets, cross-scored on one side and 'JANSSEN' on the other side.

4. CLINICAL PARTICULARS

4.1 Therapeutic indications
Orap is an antipsychotic of the diphenylbutyl-piperidine series and is indicated in:

• Chronic schizophrenia, for the treatment of symptoms and prevention of relapse.

• Other psychoses, especially paranoid and monosymptomatic hypochondriacal psychoses (eg delusional parasitosis).

4.2 Posology and method of administration
Orap is intended for once daily oral administration in adults and children over 12 years of age.

Since individual response to antipsychotic drugs is variable, dosage should be individually determined and is best initiated and titrated under close clinical supervision. In determining the initial dose, consideration should be given to the patient's age, severity of symptoms and previous response to other neuroleptic drugs. Dose increases should be made at weekly intervals or longer, and by increments of 2-4 mg in the daily dose.

The patient should be reviewed regularly to ensure the minimum effective dose is being used.

Chronic schizophrenia:

The dose ranges between 2 and 20 mg daily, with 2 mg as a starting dose. This may be increased according to response and tolerance to achieve an optimum response.

Other psychoses, paranoid states and monosymptomatic hypochondriacal psychoses (MHP):

An initial dose of 4 mg daily which may then be gradually increased, if necessary, according to response, to a maximum of 16 mg daily.

Use in elderly:

Elderly patients require half the normal starting dose of pimozide.

Method of Administration

Oral use.

4.3 Contraindications

In common with several other neuroleptics, pimozide has been reported to prolong the QT interval. It is, therefore, contra-indicated in patients with a pre-existing congenital prolongation of QT, or with a family history of this syndrome, and in patients with a history of cardiac arrhythmias. Orap should not be used in the case of acquired long QT interval, such as that associated with the concomitant use of drugs known to prolong the QT interval (see section 4.5 Interactions), known hypokalaemia or hypomagnesaemia, or clinically significant bradycardia.

Orap is also contra-indicated in patients with severe central nervous system depression and in patients with a known hypersensitivity to pimozide or other diphenylbutyl-piperidine derivatives. It should not be used in patients with depression or Parkinson's syndrome.

The concomitant use of orally or parenterally administered cytochrome P450 CYP 3A4 inhibiting drugs such as azole antimycotics, antiviral protease inhibitors, macrolide antibiotics and nefazodone is contra-indicated. The concomitant use of CYP 2D6 inhibiting drugs such as quinidine is also contra-indicated. The inhibition of either or both cytochrome P450 systems, may result in the elevation of pimozide blood concentration and increase the possibility of QT-prolongation.

4.4 Special warnings and special precautions for use

Please also refer to Drug Interactions section.

Caution is advised in patients with hepatic or renal dysfunction, phaeochromocytoma, thyrotoxicosis, epilepsy and conditions predisposing to epilepsy (eg alcohol withdrawal and brain damage).

It is recommended that a baseline ECG is undertaken in all patients prior to commencing treatment with pimozide in view of the cardiac contra-indications and in order to identify possible subsequent electrocardiographic changes.

It is further recommended that an ECG is repeated annually, or earlier if clinically indicated. Periodic assessment of cardiac function should be undertaken in those patients receiving pimozide in excess of 16 mg daily. If repolarisation changes (prolongation of QT interval, T-wave or U-wave changes) appear or arrhythmias develop, treatment should be reviewed and either gradually withdrawn or the dose reduced under close supervision.

Electrolyte disturbances should also be considered a risk factor (see also Contra-indications).

Drugs which may cause electrolyte disturbances are not recommended in patients receiving long-term pimozide (please also refer to the Drug Interactions section.)

As with other neuroleptics, cases of sudden unexpected death have been rarely reported with pimozide (generally in doses in excess of the current recommended maximum of 20 mg per day). Whilst the cause of death in these cases is not known with certainty, it is postulated that the QT prolongation seen with pimozide in some patients may have made the patients susceptible to some form of fatal arrhythmia (eg Torsades de Pointes). Whilst some of these patients were taking pimozide as a sole therapy, the remainder were also taking other drugs, including neuroleptics, implicated in the aetiology of arrhythmias.

In schizophrenia, the response to antipsychotic drug treatment may be delayed. If drugs are withdrawn, recurrence of symptoms may not become apparent for several weeks or months.

Acute withdrawal symptoms, including nausea, vomiting, sweating and insomnia, have been described after abrupt cessation of antipsychotic drugs. Recurrence of psychotic symptoms may also occur, and the emergence of involuntary movement disorders (such as akathisia, dystonia and dyskinesia) has been reported. Therefore, gradual withdrawal is advisable.

4.5 Interaction with other medicinal products and other forms of Interaction

Please also refer to the Precautions and Warnings and Contra-indications sections.

As with other neuroleptics, Orap may increase the central nervous system depression produced by other CNS depressant drugs, including alcohol, hypnotics, sedatives or strong analgesics.

Orap may impair the anti-Parkinson effect of levodopa. The dosage of anticonvulsants may need to be increased to take account of lowered seizure threshold.

Drugs known to prolong the QT interval are contra-indicated. Examples include certain antiarrhythmics, such as those of Class 1A (such as quinidine, disopyramide and procainamide) and Class III (such as amiodarone and sotalol), tricyclic antidepressants (such as amitriptyline), certain tetracyclic antidepressants (such as maprotiline), certain other antipsychotic medications (such as phenothiazines and sertindole), certain antihistamines (such as terfenadine), cisapride,, bretylium and certain antimalarials such as quinine and mefloquine. This list is not comprehensive.

There is an increased risk of extrapyramidal effects with anti-emetics such as metoclopramide.

Avoid concomitant use with sibutramine due to an increased risk of CNS toxicity.

Concomitant use with calcium channel blockers may result in an enhanced hypotensive effect.

Concurrent treatment with neuroleptics should be kept to a minimum as they may predispose to the cardiotoxic effects of pimozide. Particular care should be exercised in patients who are using depot neuroleptics. Low potency neuroleptics such as chlorpromazine and thioridazine should not be used concomitantly with pimozide.

Pimozide is metabolised mainly via the cytochrome P450 subtype 3A4 (CYP 3A4) enzyme system and, to a lesser extent, via the CYP 2D6 subtype.

In vitro data indicate that highly potent inhibitors of the CYP 3A4 enzyme system, such as azole antimycotics, antiviral protease inhibitors, macrolide antibiotics and nefazodone will inhibit the metabolism of pimozide, resulting in markedly elevated plasma levels of pimozide.

In vitro data also indicated that quinidine diminishes the CYP 2D6 dependent metabolism of pimozide.

Elevated pimozide levels may enhance the risk of QT-prolongation.

As grapefruit juice is known to inhibit the metabolism of CYP3A4 metabolised drugs, concomitant use of grapefruit juice with pimozide should be avoided. As CYP1A2 may also contribute to the metabolism of pimozide, prescribers should be aware of the theoretical potential for drug interactions with inhibitors of this enzymatic system.

Concurrent use of drugs causing electrolyte imbalance is not recommended. Diuretics should be avoided but, if necessary, potassium-sparing diuretics are preferred.

4.6 Pregnancy and lactation

The safety of Orap in human pregnancy has not been established. Studies in animals have not demonstrated teratogenic effects. As with other drugs, it is not advisable to administer Orap in pregnancy.

Orap may be excreted in breast milk. If the use of Orap is considered essential, breast feeding should be discontinued.

4.7 Effects on ability to drive and use machines

Orap may impair alertness, especially at the start of treatment. These effects may be potentiated by alcohol. Patients should be warned of the risks of sedation and advised not to drive or operate machinery during treatment until their susceptibility is known.

4.8 Undesirable effects

In common with all neuroleptics, extrapyramidal symptoms may occur. Anti-parkinson agents should not be prescribed routinely because of the possible risk of impairing pimozide's efficacy. They should only be given as required.

Tardive dyskinesia is common among patients treated with moderate to high doses of antipsychotic drugs for prolonged periods of time and may prove irreversible, particularly in patients over 50 years of age.

The potential seriousness and unpredictability of tardive dyskinesia, and the fact that it has occasionally been reported to occur when neuroleptic antipsychotic drugs have been prescribed for a relatively short period in low dosage, means that the prescribing of such agents requires especially careful assessment of risk versus benefit. Tardive dyskinesia can be precipitated or aggravated by anti-Parkinson drugs. Short-term dyskinesia may occur after abrupt drug withdrawal.

Epileptic fits have been reported even in low dosage. The elderly may be more liable to experience adverse effects.

Dose-related side effects, including drowsiness, insomnia, anxiety and gastro-intestinal symptoms, such as nausea, constipation or dyspepsia may occur. Dizziness, vertigo, weakness, excessive sweating, headache, dry mouth, loss of libido, impotence and hypotension have been reported, but autonomic symptoms are infrequent. QT-interval prolongation and/or ventricular arrhythmias have rarely been reported, and predominantly with high doses and in predisposed patients. Hypersensitivity reactions such as skin rash, itching, shortness of breath or swollen face have also rarely been reported.

Hormonal effects of antipsychotic neuroleptic drugs include hyperprolactinaemia, which may cause galactorrhoea, gynaecomastia and oligo- or amenorrhoea. Very rarely, cases have been reported of hyponatraemia, either due to polydipsia or to the syndrome of inappropriate secretion of anti-diuretic hormone. Neuroleptics may very rarely be associated with body temperature dysregulation.

Glycosuria has been reported.

In common with other antipsychotics, pimozide has been associated with rare cases of Neuroleptic Malignant Syndrome, an idiosyncratic response characterised by hyperthermia, muscle rigidity, autonomic instability, altered consciousness and coma. Signs of autonomic dysfunction such as tachycardia, labile arterial pressure and sweating may precede the onset of hyperthermia, acting as early warning signs. Recovery usually occurs within five to seven days of antipsychotic withdrawal. Affected patients should be carefully monitored. Dantrolene sodium, bromocriptine mesylate and ECT have all been reported as offering benefit in some patients with Neuroleptic Malignant Syndrome.

4.9 Overdose

In general, the signs and symptoms of overdose with Orap would be an exaggeration of known pharmacological effects, the most prominent of which would be severe extrapyramidal symptoms, hypotension or sedation. The risk of cardiac arrhythmias, possibly associated with QT-prolongation, should be considered. The patient may appear comatose with respiratory depression and hypotension which could be severe enough to produce a shock-like state.

Treatment:

There is no specific antidote to pimozide. Gastric lavage, establishment of a patent airway and, if necessary, mechanically assisted respiration are advised. Electrocardiographic monitoring should commence immediately and continue until the ECG returns to normal. Hypotension and circulatory collapse may be counteracted by the use of intravenous fluids, plasma or concentrated albumin, and vasopressor agents such as noradrenaline.

Adrenaline should not be used.

In cases of severe extrapyramidal symptoms, anti-Parkinson medication should be administered.

Because of the long half-life of pimozide, patients who have taken an overdose should be observed for at least 4 days.

5. PHARMACOLOGICAL PROPERTIES

5.1 Pharmacodynamic properties

Pimozide is an orally active neuroleptic drug which blocks central dopaminergic receptors. Pimozide antagonises many of the actions of amphetamine and apomorphine.

5.2 Pharmacokinetic properties

The mean serum elimination half-life in schizophrenic patients is approximately 55 hours. This is highly variable and may be as long as 150 hours in some individuals. There is a 13-fold interindividual difference in the area under the serum pimozide concentration-time curve and an equivalent degree of variation in peak serum levels among patients studied. The significance of this is unclear since there are few correlations between plasma levels and clinical findings.

5.3 Preclinical safety data

No relevant information additional to that contained elsewhere in the Summary of Product Characteristics.

6. PHARMACEUTICAL PARTICULARS

6.1 List of excipients

Calcium hydrogen phosphate dihydrate

Maize starch

Microcrystalline cellulose

Polyvidone K30

Talc

Cottonseed Oil Hydrogenated

Ferric oxide (E172)

Indigotindisulphonate (E132) - aluminium lake

Purified water*

* not in final product

6.2 Incompatibilities

None known.

6.3 Shelf life

5 years.

6.4 Special precautions for storage

Do not store above 25°C.

6.5 Nature and contents of container

PVC/aluminium foil blister packs, containing 100 tablets.

6.6 Instructions for use and handling

Not applicable.

7. MARKETING AUTHORISATION HOLDER

Janssen-Cilag Ltd

Saunderton

High Wycombe

Buckinghamshire

HP14 4HJ

UK

8. MARKETING AUTHORISATION NUMBER(S)

PL 0242/0038R

9. DATE OF FIRST AUTHORISATION/RENEWAL OF THE AUTHORISATION

Renewal of Authorisation: 17 October 1997

10. DATE OF REVISION OF THE TEXT

April 2002

11. Legal category

POM.

Orelox Paediatric Granules for Oral Suspension

(sanofi-aventis)

1. NAME OF THE MEDICINAL PRODUCT
Orelox™ Paediatric Granules for Oral Suspension.

2. QUALITATIVE AND QUANTITATIVE COMPOSITION
When reconstituted each 5ml volume contains 52mg of cefpodoxime proxetil (equivalent to 40mg cefpodoxime).

3. PHARMACEUTICAL FORM
Granules for the preparation of an oral suspension.

4. CLINICAL PARTICULARS
4.1 Therapeutic indications
Orelox is a bactericidal cephalosporin antibiotic active against a wide range of Gram-negative and Gram-positive organisms. It is indicated for the treatment of the following infections either before the infecting organism has been identified or when caused by bacteria of established sensitivity.

Indications include:

UPPER RESPIRATORY TRACT INFECTIONS caused by organisms sensitive to cefpodoxime, including acute otitis media, sinusitis, tonsillitis and pharyngitis.

Orelox should be reserved for recurrent or chronic infections, or for infections where the causative organism is known or suspected to be resistant to commonly used antibiotics.

LOWER RESPIRATORY TRACT INFECTIONS caused by organisms sensitive to cefpodoxime. Including pneumonia, acute bronchitis and when bacterial super-infection complicates bronchiolitis.

UPPER AND LOWER URINARY TRACT INFECTIONS caused by organisms sensitive to cefpodoxime including cystitis and acute pyelonephritis.

SKIN AND SOFT TISSUE INFECTIONS caused by organisms sensitive to cefpodoxime such as abscesses, cellulitis, infected wounds, furuncles, folliculitis, paronychia, carbuncles and ulcers.

4.2 Posology and method of administration
Route of administration: oral.

Adults and Elderly:

Not applicable for this product.

Children:

The recommended mean dosage for children is 8mg/kg/day administered in two divided doses at 12 hour intervals.

The following dosage regimen is proposed as a guide to prescribing:-

Below 6 months:	8mg/kg/day in 2 divided doses
6 months-2 years:	5.0 ml twice daily
3-8 years:	10.0 ml twice daily
Above 9 years:	12.5ml twice daily or 100mg tablet twice daily

Orelox should not be used in infants less than 15 days old, as no experience yet exists in this age group.

A measuring spoon (5ml) is provided with the bottle to aid correct dosing. One measuring spoon (5ml) contains the equivalent of 40 mg cefpodoxime.

The product should be taken during meals for optimal absorption.

Renal Impairment:

The dosage of Orelox does not require modification if creatinine clearance exceeds 40 $ml.min^{-1}/1.73m^2$.

Below this value, pharmacokinetic studies indicate an increase in plasma elimination half-life and the maximum plasma concentrations, and hence the dosage should be adjusted appropriately.

CREATININE CLEARANCE ML/MIN)	
39 – 10	Unit dose[1] administered as a single dose every 24 hours (i.e half of the usual adult dose).
< 10	Unit dose[1] administered as a single dose every 48 hours (i.e quarter of the usual adult dose).
Haemodialysis Patients	Unit dose[1] administered after each dialysis session.

NOTE:

[1]The unit dose is either 100mg or 200mg, depending on the type of infection.

Hepatic Impairment:

The dosage does not require modification in cases of hepatic impairment.

Instructions for Reconstitution:

Before preparing the suspension the silica gel desiccant contained in a capsule inside the cap must be removed and disposed of. The suspension is prepared by adding water to the bottle up to the calibrated mark and shaking thoroughly to obtain an evenly dispersed suspension.

4.3 Contraindications
Patients with hypersensitivity to cephalosporin antibiotics.

Patients with phenylketonuria since the product contains aspartame.

4.4 Special warnings and special precautions for use
Preliminary enquiry about allergy to penicillin is necessary before prescribing cephalosporins since cross allergy to penicillins occurs in 5-10% of cases.

Particular care will be needed in patients sensitive to penicillin: strict medical surveillance is necessary from the very first administration. Where there is doubt, medical assistance should be available at the initial administration, in order to treat any anaphylactic episode.

In patients who are allergic to other cephalosporins, the possibility of cross allergy to Orelox should be borne in mind. Orelox should not be given to those patients with a previous history of immediate type hypersensitivity to cephalosporins.

Hypersensitivity reactions (anaphylaxis) observed with beta-lactam antibiotics can be serious and occasionally fatal.

The onset of any manifestation of hypersensitivity indicates that treatment should be stopped.

Orelox is not the preferred antibiotic for the treatment of staphylococcal pneumonia and should not be used in the treatment of atypical pneumonia caused by organisms such as *Legionella*, *Mycoplasma* and *Chlamydia*.

In cases of severe renal insufficiency it may be necessary to reduce the dosage regimen dependent on the creatinine clearance.

Antibiotics should always be prescribed with caution in patients with a history of gastrointestinal disease, particularly colitis. Orelox may induce diarrhoea, antibiotic associated colitis and pseudomembranous colitis. These side-effects, which may occur more frequently in patients receiving higher doses for prolonged periods, should be considered as potentially serious. The presence of *C. difficile* should be investigated. In all potential cases of colitis, the treatment should be stopped immediately. The diagnosis should be confirmed by sigmoidoscopy and specific antibiotic therapy (vancomycin) substituted if considered clinically necessary. The administration of products which cause faecal stasis must be avoided. Although any antibiotic may cause pseudomembranous colitis, the risk may be higher with broad-spectrum drugs, such as the cephalosporins.

As with all beta-lactam antibiotics, neutropenia, and more rarely agranulocytosis may develop, particularly during extended treatment. For cases of treatment lasting longer than 10 days, blood count should therefore be monitored, and treatment discontinued if neutropenia is found.

Cephalosporins may be absorbed onto the surface of red cell membranes and react with antibiotics directed against the drug. This can produce a positive Coombs' test and very rarely, haemolytic anaemia. Cross-reactivity may occur with penicillin for this reaction.

The product should not be used in infants less than 15 days old as no clinical trial data in this age group yet exists.

Changes in renal function have been observed with antibiotics of the same class, particularly when given concurrently with potentially nephrotoxic drugs such as aminoglycosides and/or potent diuretics. In such cases, renal function should be monitored.

As with other antibiotics, the prolonged use of cefpodoxime proxetil may result in the overgrowth of non-susceptible organisms. With oral antibiotics the normal colonic flora may be altered, allowing overgrowth by clostridia with consequent pseudomembranous colitis. Repeated evaluation of the patient is essential and if superinfection occurs during therapy, appropriate measures should be taken.

4.5 Interaction with other medicinal products and other forms of Interaction
No clinically significant drug interactions have been reported during the course of clinical studies.

As with other cephalosporins, isolated cases showing development of a positive Coombs' test have been reported (see Precautions).

Studies have shown that bioavailability is decreased by approximately 30% when Orelox is administered with drugs which neutralise gastric pH or inhibit acid secretions. Therefore, such drugs as antacids of the mineral type and H_2 blockers such as ranitidine, which cause an increase in gastric pH, should be taken 2 or 3 hours after Orelox administration.

In contrast, drugs which decrease gastric pH such as pentagastrine will increase bioavailability. The clinical consequences remain to be established.

The bioavailability increases if the product is administered during meals.

A false positive reaction for glucose in the urine may occur with Benedict's or Fehling's solutions or with copper sulphate test tablets, but not with tests based on enzymatic glucose oxidase reactions.

4.6 Pregnancy and lactation
Not applicable.

4.7 Effects on ability to drive and use machines
Not applicable.

4.8 Undesirable effects
Possible side effects include gastrointestinal disorders such as diarrhoea, nausea, vomiting and abdominal pain and rash, urticaria and itching.

Occasional cases have been reported of headaches, dizziness, tinnitus, parethesia, asthenia and malaise. Rare cases of allergic reactions including hypersensitivity mucocutaneous reactions, skin rashes and pruritus. Occasional cases of bullous reactions including Stevens-Johnson syndrome, toxic epidermal necrolysis and erythema multiforme have also been received. Transient moderate elevations of ASAT, ALAT and alkaline phosphatases and/or bilirubin have been reported. These laboratory abnormalities which may also be explained by the infection, may rarely exceed twice the upper limit of the named range and elicit a pattern of liver injury, usually cholestatic and most often asymptomatic. Slight increases in blood urea and creatinine have also been reported. Exceptionally rare are the occurrence of liver damage and of haematological disorders such as reduction in haemoglobin, thrombocytosis, thrombocytopenia, leucopenia and eosinophilia. Haemolytic anaemia has extremely rarely been reported.

As with other cephalosporins there have been rare reports of anaphylactic reactions, bronchospasm, purpura and angiodema.

4.9 Overdose
In the event of overdosage with Orelox, supportive and symptomatic therapy is indicated.

In cases of overdosage, particularly in patients with renal insufficiency, encephalopathy may occur. The encephalopathy is usually reversible once cefpodoxime plasma levels have fallen.

5. PHARMACOLOGICAL PROPERTIES
5.1 Pharmacodynamic properties
Orelox (Cefpodoxime proxetil) is a beta-lactam antibiotic, a 3rd generation oral cephalosporin. It is the prodrug of cefpodoxime.

Following oral administration, Orelox is taken up by the gastro-intestinal wall where it is rapidly hydrolysed to cefpodoxime, a bactericidal antibiotic, which is then absorbed systemically.

BACTERIOLOGY:

The mechanism of action of cefpodoxime is based on inhibition of bacterial cell wall synthesis. It is stable to numerous beta-lactamases.

Cefpodoxime has been shown to possess *in vitro* bactericidal activity against numerous Gram-positive and Gram-negative bacteria.

ANTIBACTERIAL ACTIVITY:

It is highly active against the Gram-positive organisms:

- *Streptococcus pneumoniae*
- Streptococci of Groups A *(S. pyogenes)*, B *(S. agalactiae)*, C, F and G
- Other streptococci *(S. mitis, S. sanguis* and *S. salivarius)*
- *Propionibacterium acnes*
- *Corynebacterium diphtheriae*

It is highly active against the Gram-negative organisms:

- *Haemophilus influenzae* (beta-lactamase and non beta-lactamase producing strains)
- *Haemophilus para-influenzae* (beta-lactamase and non beta-lactamase producing strains)
- *Moraxella catarrhalis* (beta-lactamase and non beta-lactamase producing strains)
- *Escherichia coli*
- *Klebsiella* Spp. (*K. pneumoniae*)
- *Proteus mirabilis*

It is moderately active against:

- Methicillin-sensitive staphylococci, penicillinase and non-penicillinase producing strains *(S. aureus* and *S. epidermidis)*

In addition, as with many cephalosporins, the following are resistant to cefpodoxime.

- Enterococci
- Methicillin-resistant staphylococci (*S. aureus* and *S. coagulase* (negative))
- *Staphylococcus saprophyticus*
- *Pseudomonas aeruginosa* and *Pseudomonas* Spp.
- *Clostridium difficile*
- *Bacteroides fragilis* and related species

As with all antibiotics, whenever possible, sensitivity should be confirmed by *in vitro* testing.

5.2 Pharmacokinetic properties
Orelox is taken up in the intestine and is hydrolysed to the active metabolite cefpodoxime. When cefpodoxime proxetil is administered orally to fasting subjects as a tablet corresponding to 100mg of cefpodoxime, 51.5% is absorbed and absorption is increased by food intake. The volume of distribution is 32.3 l and peak levels of cefpodoxime occur 2 to 3 hrs after dosing. The maximum plasma concentration is 1.2mg/l and 2.5mg/l after doses of 100mg and 200mg respectively. Following administration of 100mg and 200mg twice daily over 14.5 days, the plasma pharmacokinetic parameters of cefpodoxime remain unchanged.

Serum protein binding of cefpodoxime, 40% principally to albumin. This binding is non saturable in type.

Concentrations of cefpodoxime in excess of the minimum inhibitory levels (MIC) for common pathogens can be achieved in lung parenchyma, bronchial mucosa, pleural fluid, tonsils, interstitial fluid and prostate tissue.

As the majority of cefpodoxime is eliminated in the urine, the concentration is high. (Concentrations in 0-4, 4-8, 8-12 hr fractions after a single dose exceed MIC_{90} of common urinary pathogens). Good diffusion of cefpodoxime is also seen into renal tissue, with concentrations above MIC_{90} of the common urinary pathogens, 3-12hrs after an administration of a single 200mg dose (1.6-3.1μG/G). Concentrations of cefpodoxime in the medullary and cortical tissues is similar.

Studies in healthy volunteers show median concentrations of cefpodoxime in the total ejaculate 6-12hrs following administration of a single 200mg dose to be above the MIC_{90} of *N. gonorrhoeae*.

The main route of excretion is renal, 80% is excreted unchanged in the urine, with an elimination half life of approx 2.4 hours.

CHILDREN

In children, studies have shown the maximum plasma concentration occurs approximately 2-4 hours after dosing. A single 5mg/kg dose in 4-12 year olds produced a maximum concentration similar to that in adults given a 200mg dose.

In patients below 2 years receiving repeated doses of 5mg/kg 12 hourly, the average plasma concentrations, 2hrs post dose, are between 2.7mg/l (1-6 months) and 2.0mg/l (7 months-2 years).

In patients between 1 month and 12 years receiving repeated doses of 5mg/kg 12 hourly, the residual plasma concentrations at steady state are between 0.2-0.3mg/l (1 month-2 years) and 0.1mg/l (2-12 years).

5.3 Preclinical safety data
Not applicable.

6. PHARMACEUTICAL PARTICULARS

6.1 List of excipients
The product contains anhydrous colloidal silica, aspartame, banana flavour, carboxymethylcellulose calcium, carboxymethylcellulose sodium, citric acid monohydrate, hydroxypropylcellulose, yellow iron oxide, lactose monohydrate, monosodium glutamate, potassium sorbate, sodium chloride, sorbitan trioleate, sucrose and talc.

6.2 Incompatibilities
None reported during clinical studies.

6.3 Shelf life
24 months.

Reconstituted suspension: can be stored for up to 10 days refrigerated (2-8°C).

6.4 Special precautions for storage
Bottles: unreconstituted product should be stored below 30°C.

6.5 Nature and contents of container
Amber glass bottle with a calibration marking. This is fitted with a polyethylene dehydrating capsule containing silica gel, closed by a cardboard disc make up part of closure. There is a polyethylene pilfer and childproof screw cap fitted with tight triseal joint.

Pack sizes of 100ml of suspension.

A 5ml plastic spoon is supplied with the pack.

6.6 Instructions for use and handling
Before preparing the suspension the silica gel desiccant contained in a capsule inside the cap must be removed and disposed of. The suspension is prepared by adding water to the bottle up to the calibrated mark and shaking thoroughly to obtain an evenly dispersed suspension.

7. MARKETING AUTHORISATION HOLDER
Aventis Pharma Ltd

50 Kings Hill Avenue

West Malling

Kent

ME19 4AH

United Kingdom

8. MARKETING AUTHORISATION NUMBER(S)
PL 04425/0251

9. DATE OF FIRST AUTHORISATION/RENEWAL OF THE AUTHORISATION
27 December 2002

10. DATE OF REVISION OF THE TEXT

11. Legal Category
POM

Orelox Tablets 100mg

(sanofi-aventis)

1. NAME OF THE MEDICINAL PRODUCT
Orelox™ Tablets 100mg.

2. QUALITATIVE AND QUANTITATIVE COMPOSITION
Each Orelox tablet contains 130mg of cefpodoxime proxetil (equivalent to 100mg cefpodoxime).

3. PHARMACEUTICAL FORM
Tablet for oral use.

4. CLINICAL PARTICULARS

4.1 Therapeutic indications
Orelox is a bactericidal cephalosporin antibiotic active against a wide range of Gram-negative and Gram-positive organisms. It is indicated for the treatment of the following infections either before the infecting organism has been identified or when caused by bacteria of established sensitivity.

UPPER RESPIRATORY TRACT INFECTIONS caused by organisms sensitive to cefpodoxime, including sinusitis.

In tonsillitis and pharyngitis, Orelox should be reserved for recurrent or chronic infections, or for infections where the causative organism is known or suspected to be resistant to commonly used antibiotics.

LOWER RESPIRATORY TRACT INFECTIONS caused by organisms sensitive to cefpodoxime, including acute bronchitis, relapses or exacerbations of chronic bronchitis and bacterial pneumonia.

UPPER AND LOWER URINARY TRACT INFECTIONS caused by organisms sensitive to cefpodoxime including cystitis and acute pyelonephritis.

SKIN AND SOFT TISSUE INFECTIONS caused by organisms sensitive to cefpodoxime such as abscesses, cellulitis, infected wounds, furuncles, folliculitis, paronychia, carbuncles and ulcers.

GONORRHOEA - uncomplicated gonococcal urethritis.

4.2 Posology and method of administration
Route of administration: oral.

ADULTS:

Adults with normal renal function:

UPPER RESPIRATORY TRACT INFECTIONS: For upper respiratory tract infections caused by organisms sensitive to cefpodoxime, including sinusitis. In tonsillitis and pharyngitis, Orelox should be reserved for recurrent or chronic infections, or for infections where the causative organism is known or suspected to be resistant to commonly used antibiotics. Sinusitis: 200mg twice daily. Other upper respiratory tract infections: 100mg twice daily.

LOWER RESPIRATORY TRACT INFECTIONS:For lower respiratory tract infections caused by organisms sensitive to cefpodoxime, including acute bronchitis, relapses or exacerbations of chronic bronchitis and bacterial pneumonia: 100-200 mg twice daily, dependent on the severity of the infection.

URINARY TRACT INFECTIONS:

Uncomplicated lower urinary tract infections: 100mg should be taken twice daily.

Uncomplicated upper urinary tract infections: 200mg should be taken twice daily.

Uncomplicated gonococcal urethritis: 200mg should be taken as a single dose.

SKIN AND SOFT TISSUE INFECTIONS: 200mg should be taken twice daily.

Tablets should be taken during meals for optimum absorption.

ELDERLY:

It is not necessary to modify the dose in elderly patients with normal renal function.

CHILDREN:

Orelox Paediatric is available to treat infants (over 15 days old) and children. Please refer to the separate Summary of Product Characteristics for details.

HEPATIC IMPAIRMENT:

The dosage does not require modification in cases of hepatic impairment.

RENAL IMPAIRMENT:

The dosage of Orelox does not require modification if creatinine clearance exceeds 40 ml/min.

Below this value, pharmacokinetic studies indicate an increase in plasma elimination half-life and the maximum plasma concentrations, and hence the dosage should be adjusted appropriately.

CREATININE CLEARANCE (ML/MIN)	
39 – 10	Unit dose[1] administered as a single dose every 24 hours (i.e half of the usual adult dose).
< 10	Unit dose[1] administered as a single dose every 48 hours (i.e quarter of the usual adult dose).
Haemodialysis Patients	Unit dose[1] administered after each dialysis session.

NOTE:

[1]The unit dose is either 100mg or 200mg, depending on the type of infection.

4.3 Contraindications
Hypersensitivity to cephalosporin antibiotics.

4.4 Special warnings and special precautions for use
Preliminary enquiry about allergy to penicillin is necessary before prescribing cephalosporins since cross allergy to penicillins occurs in 5-10% of cases.

Particular care will be needed in patients sensitive to penicillin: strict medical surveillance is necessary from the very first administration. Where there is doubt, medical assistance should be available at the initial administration, in order to treat any anaphylactic episode.

In patients who are allergic to other cephalosporins, the possibility of cross allergy to Orelox should be borne in mind. Orelox should not be given to those patients with a previous history of immediate type hypersensitivity to cephalosporins.

Hypersensitivity reactions (anaphylaxis) observed with beta-lactam antibiotics can be serious and occasionally fatal.

The onset of any manifestation of hypersensitivity indicates that treatment should be stopped.

Orelox is not the preferred antibiotic for the treatment of staphylococcal pneumonia and should not be used in the treatment of atypical pneumonia caused by organisms such as *Legionella*, *Mycoplasma* and *Chlamydia*.

In cases of severe renal insufficiency it may be necessary to reduce the dosage regimen dependent on the creatinine clearance.

Possible side effects include gastrointestinal disorders such as nausea, vomiting and abdominal pain. Antibiotics should always be prescribed with caution in patients with a history of gastrointestinal disease, particularly colitis. Orelox may induce diarrhoea, antibiotic associated colitis and pseudomembranous colitis. These side-effects, which may occur more frequently in patients receiving higher doses for prolonged periods, should be considered as potentially serious. The presence of *C. difficile* should be investigated. In all potential cases of colitis, the treatment should be stopped immediately. The diagnosis should be confirmed by sigmoidoscopy and specific antibiotic therapy (vancomycin) substituted if considered clinically necessary. The administration of products which cause faecal stasis must be avoided. Although any antibiotic may cause pseudomembranous colitis, the risk may be higher with broad-spectrum drugs, such as the cephalosporins.

As with all beta-lactam antibiotics, neutropenia, and more rarely agranulocytosis may develop, particularly during extended treatment. For cases of treatment lasting longer than 10 days, blood count should therefore be monitored, and treatment discontinued if neutropenia is found.

Cephalosporins may be absorbed onto the surface of red cell membranes and react with antibodies directed against the drug. This can produce a positive Coomb's test and very rarely, haemolytic anaemia. Cross-reactivity may occur with penicillin for this reaction.

Changes in renal function have been observed with antibiotics of the same class, particularly when given concurrently with potentially nephrotoxic drugs such as aminoglycosides and/or potent diuretics. In such cases, renal function should be monitored.

As with other antibiotics, the prolonged use of cefpodoxime proxetil may result in the overgrowth of non-susceptible organisms. With oral antibiotics the normal colonic flora may be altered, allowing overgrowth by clostridia with consequent pseudomembranous colitis. Repeated evaluation of the patient is essential and if superinfection occurs during therapy, appropriate measures should be taken.

4.5 Interaction with other medicinal products and other forms of Interaction
No clinically significant drug interactions have been reported during the course of clinical studies.

As with other cephalosporins, isolated cases showing development of a positive Coombs' test have been reported (see Precautions).

Studies have shown that bioavailability is decreased by approximately 30% when Orelox is administered with drugs which neutralise gastric pH or inhibit acid secretions. Therefore, such drugs as antacids of the mineral type and

H_2 blockers such as ranitidine, which cause an increase in gastric pH, should be taken 2 to 3 hours after Orelox administration.

The bioavailability increases if the product is administered during meals.

A false positive reaction for glucose in the urine may occur with Benedict's or Fehling's solutions or with copper sulphate test tablets, but not with tests based on enzymatic glucose oxidase reactions.

4.6 Pregnancy and lactation

Studies carried out in several animal species have not shown any teratogenic or foetotoxic effects. However, the safety of cefpodoxime proxetil in pregnancy has not been established and, as with all drugs, it should be administered with caution during the early months of pregnancy.

Cefpodoxime is excreted in human milk. Either breastfeeding or treatment of the mother should be stopped.

4.7 Effects on ability to drive and use machines

Attention should be drawn to the risk of dizzy sensations.

4.8 Undesirable effects

Possible side effects include gastrointestinal disorders such as diarrhoea, nausea, vomiting and abdominal pain.

Occasional cases have been reported of headaches, dizziness, tinnitus, parethesia, asthenia and malaise. Rare cases of allergic reactions include hypersensitivity mucocutaneous reactions, skin rashes and pruritus. Occasional cases of bullous reactions such as Stevens-Johnson syndrome, toxic epidermal necrolysis and erythema multiforme have also been received. Transient moderate elevations of ASAT, ALAT and alkaline phosphatases and/or bilirubin have been reported. These laboratory abnormalities which may be explained by the infection, may rarely exceed twice the upper limit of the named range and elicit a pattern of liver injury, usually cholestatic and most often asymptomatic. Slight increases in blood urea and creatinine have been reported. Exceptionally rare are the occurrence of liver damage and of haematological disorders such as reduction in haemoglobin, thrombocytosis, thrombocytopenia, leucopenia and eosinophilia. Haemolytic anaemia has been reported.

As with other cephalosporins there have been rare reports of anaphylactic reactions, bronchospasm, purpura and angiodema.

4.9 Overdose

In the event of overdosage with Orelox, supportive and symptomatic therapy is indicated.

In cases of overdosage, particularly in patients with renal insufficiency, encephalopathy may occur. The encephalopathy is usually reversible once cefpodoxime plasma levels have fallen.

5. PHARMACOLOGICAL PROPERTIES

5.1 Pharmacodynamic properties

Orelox (Cefpodoxime proxetil) is a beta-lactam antibiotic, a 3rd generation oral cephalosporin. It is the prodrug of cefpodoxime.

Following oral administration, Orelox is taken up by the gastro-intestinal wall where it is rapidly hydrolysed to cefpodoxime, a bactericidal antibiotic, which is then absorbed systemically.

BACTERIOLOGY:

The mechanism of action of cefpodoxime is based on inhibition of bacterial cell wall synthesis. It is stable to numerous beta-lactamases.

Cefpodoxime has been shown to possess *in vitro* bactericidal activity against numerous Gram-positive and Gram-negative bacteria.

It is highly active against the Gram-positive organisms:

- *Streptococcus pneumoniae*
- Streptococci of Groups A *(S. pyogenes)*, B *(S. agalactiae)*, C, F and G
- Other streptococci *(S. mitis, S. sanguis and S. salivarius)*
- *Corynebacterium diphtheriae*

It is highly active against the Gram-negative organisms:

- *Haemophilus influenzae* (beta-lactamase and non beta-lactamase producing strains)
- *Haemophilus para-influenzae* (beta-lactamase and non beta-lactamase producing strains)
- *Branhamella catarrhalis* (beta-lactamase and non beta-lactamase producing strains)
- *Neisseria meningitidis*
- *Neisseria gonorrhoeae*
- *Escherichia coli*
- *Klebsiella* Spp. *(K. pneumoniae, K. oxytoca)*
- *Proteus mirabilis*

It is moderately active against:

- Methicillin-sensitive staphylococci, penicillinase and non-penicillinase producing strains *(S. aureus* and *S. epidermidis)*

In addition, as with many cephalosporins, the following are resistant to cefpodoxime.

- Enterococci
- Methicillin-resistant staphylococci (*S. aureus* and *S. epidermidis)*
- *Staphylococcus saprophyticus*
- *Pseudomonas aeruginosa* and *Pseudomonas* Spp.
- *Clostridium difficile*
- *Bacteroides fragilis* and related species

As with all antibiotics, whenever possible, sensitivity should be confirmed by *in vitro* testing.

5.2 Pharmacokinetic properties

Orelox is taken up in the intestine and is hydrolysed to the active metabolite cefpodoxime. When cefpodoxime proxetil is administered orally to fasting subjects as a tablet corresponding to 100mg of cefpodoxime, 51.5% is absorbed and absorption is increased by food intake. The volume of distribution is 32.3 l and peak levels of cefpodoxime occur 2 to 3 hrs after dosing. The maximum plasma concentration is 1.2mg/l and 2.5mg/l after doses of 100mg and 200mg respectively. Following administration of 100mg and 200mg twice daily over 14.5 days, the plasma pharmacokinetic parameters of cefpodoxime remain unchanged.

Serum protein binding of cefpodoxime, 40% principally to albumin. This binding is non saturable in type.

Concentrations of cefpodoxime in excess of the minimum inhibitory levels (MIC) for common pathogens can be achieved in lung parenchyma, bronchial mucosa, pleural fluid, tonsils, interstitial fluid and prostate tissue.

As the majority of cefpodoxime is eliminated in the urine, the concentration is high. (Concentrations in 0-4, 4-8, 8-12 hr fractions after a single dose exceed MIC_{90} of common urinary pathogens). Good diffusion of cefpodoxime is also seen into renal tissue, with concentrations above MIC_{90} of the common urinary pathogens, 3-12hrs after an administration of a single 200mg dose (1.6-3.1μG/G). Concentrations of cefpodoxime in the medullary and cortical tissues is similar.

Studies in healthy volunteers show median concentrations of cefpodoxime in the total ejaculate 6-12hrs following administration of a single 200mg dose to be above the MIC_{90} of *N. gonorrhoeae.*

The main route of excretion is renal, 80% is excreted unchanged in the urine, with an elimination half life of approx 2.4 hours.

5.3 Preclinical safety data

Not applicable.

6. PHARMACEUTICAL PARTICULARS

6.1 List of excipients

The product contains magnesium stearate, carboxymethylcellulose calcium, hydroxypropylcellulose, sodium lauryl sulphate, lactose, ethyl alcohol and purified water. The coating contains titanium dioxide, talc and hydroxypropylmethylcellulose 6CP.

6.2 Incompatibilities

None reported during clinical studies.

6.3 Shelf life

36 months.

6.4 Special precautions for storage

Store below 25°C.

6.5 Nature and contents of container

Orelox tablets are supplied in blister packs of 10 tablets.

6.6 Instructions for use and handling

None.

7. MARKETING AUTHORISATION HOLDER

Aventis Pharma Ltd

50 Kings Hill Avenue

Kings Hill

West Malling

Kent

ME19 4AH

UK

8. MARKETING AUTHORISATION NUMBER(S)

PL 04425/0252

9. DATE OF FIRST AUTHORISATION/RENEWAL OF THE AUTHORISATION

22/4/02

10. DATE OF REVISION OF THE TEXT

11. Legal Category

POM

Orlept SF Liquid

(Wockhardt UK Ltd)

1. NAME OF THE MEDICINAL PRODUCT

Orlept (SF) liquid or Sodium Valproate Oral Solution BP

2. QUALITATIVE AND QUANTITATIVE COMPOSITION

Sodium Valproate 200mg in 5ml

For excipients, see 6.1

3. PHARMACEUTICAL FORM

Liquid for oral use

Clear, colourless viscous liquid.

4. CLINICAL PARTICULARS

4.1 Therapeutic indications

Sodium valproate is used in the treatment of all forms of epilepsy.

4.2 Posology and method of administration

Dosage requirements vary according to age and body weight and should be adjusted individually to achieve adequate seizure control. The liquid may be given in divided doses (twice daily).

Monotherapy: usual requirements are as follows:

Adults: Dosage should start at 600mg daily increasing by 200mg at three day intervals until control is achieved. This is generally within the dosage range 1000mg to 2000mg per day i.e. 20-30mg/kg body weight daily. Where adequate control is not achieved within this range the dose may be further increased to a maximum of 2500mg per day.

Children over 20kg: Initial dosage should be 400mg/day increasing until control is achieved. This is usually within the range 20-30mg/kg body weight per day.

Children under 20kg: 20mg/kg of body weight per day; in severe cases this may be increased up to 40mg/kg/day.

Use in the elderly: Care should be taken when adjusting dosage in the elderly since the pharmacokinetics of sodium valproate are modified. Dosage should be determined by seizure control.

Use in renal impairment:

Mild to moderate - Reduce dose

Severe - Alter dose according to free serum valproic acid concentration

Combined Therapy: In certain cases it may be necessary to raise the dose by 5 to 10mg/kg/day when used in combination with liver enzyme inducing drugs such as phenytoin, phenobarbitone and carbamazepine.

4.3 Contraindications

Liver disease or family history of severe hepatic dysfunction

Hypersensitivity to valproate

Porphyria

4.4 Special warnings and special precautions for use

Clinical symptoms are a more sensitive indicator in the early stages of hepatic failure than laboratory investigations. The onset of an acute illness, especially within the first six months, which may include symptoms of vomiting, lethargy or weakness, drowsiness, anorexia, jaundice or loss of seizure control is an indication for immediate withdrawal of the drug.

Patients should be instructed to report any such signs to the clinician should they occur.

Routine measurement of liver function should be undertaken in those at risk before and during the first six months of therapy including children under three years, especially those with severe seizure disorders associated with mental retardation, organic brain disease, metabolic or degenerative disorder.

The drug should be discontinued if signs of liver damage occur or if serum amylase levels are elevated.

Combination with other antiepileptics may increase the risk of liver damage and should therefore be avoided if possible (see Section 4.5 Interactions with Other Medicaments).

Consider dose adjustment in renal impairment (see Section 4.2 Posology and Method of Administration).

Severe pancreatitis, which may be fatal, has been reported. Medical evaluation (including measurement of serum amylase) should be undertaken in patients presenting with symptoms suggestive of pancreatitis (e.g. abdominal pain, nausea and vomiting) and valproate should be discontinued if pancreatitis is diagnosed. Patients should be advised to consult their doctor immediately if they develop symptoms suggestive of pancreatitis (See Section 4.8. Undesirable Effects).

Valproic acid inhibits the second stage of platelet aggregation. If spontaneous bruising or bleeding occurs or the prothrombin time is abnormally prolonged, medication should be withdrawn. Concomitant salicylates should be stopped if coagulation is affected. It is recommended that patients receiving sodium valproate are monitored for platelet function and clotting time before major surgery. Patients should be told how to recognise signs of blood disorders and advised to seek immediate medical advice.

Withdrawal of sodium valproate or transition to another antiepileptic should be made gradually to avoid precipitation of an increase in seizure frequency.

Sodium valproate may give false positives for ketone bodies in the urine testing of diabetics.

Sodium valproate very commonly causes weight gain, which may be marked and progressive. All patients should be warned of this risk at the initiation of therapy and appropriate strategies adopted to minimise weight gain.

Monitor body weight during sodium valproate therapy.

Pregnancy

Women of childbearing potential should not be started on sodium valproate without specialist neurological advice. Sodium valproate is the antiepileptic of choice in patients with certain types of epilepsy such as generalised epilepsy ± myoclonus/photosensitivity. For partial epilepsy, sodium valproate should be used only in those resistant to other treatment. Women who are likely to get pregnant should receive specialist advice because of the potential teratogenic risk to the foetus (see also section 4.6 Pregnancy and Lactation).

4.5 Interaction with other medicinal products and other forms of Interaction

Other antiepileptics:

Co-administration with other antiepileptics may be associated with enhanced effects, increased sedation, reduced plasma concentrations and enhanced toxicity (especially hepatic, see Section 4.4 Special Warnings and Precautions for Use), and can complicate monitoring of treatment.

Concomitant use of hepatic enzyme inducers (e.g. barbiturates, carbamazepine, phenytoin) may enhance metabolism of valproic acid. Valproic acid has been reported to have variable effects on blood levels of other hepatically metabolised or highly protein bound agents. Plasma levels of lamotrigine, primidone, phenobarbital, ethosuximide, and an active metabolite of carbamazepine may be increased. Plasma levels of phenytoin may be increased or reduced. Plasma levels of an active metabolite of oxcarbazepine are sometimes lowered.

Other drugs affecting clotting:

Caution is recommended when administering with other drugs affecting clotting (e.g. warfarin, aspirin). (See Section 4.4 Special Warnings and Precautions for Use).

Other hepatotoxic drugs:

Other hepatotoxic drugs should be avoided (including aspirin in children).

Antacids:

Absorption of sodium valproate may be increased when administered with aluminium and magnesium hydroxides.

Antidepressants and antipsychotics:

Antidepressants and antipsychotics may lower the threshold for convulsions and higher doses of sodium valproate may be needed.

Antimalarials:

Chloroquine and mefloquine antagonise the anticonvulsant effect of valproate.

Antiulcer drugs:

Cimetidine has been reported to decrease clearance.

Antivirals:

Plasma concentration of zidovudine possibly increased (risk of toxicity).

Lipid-lowering agents:

Cholestyramine may decrease valproate absorption; separate dosage by three hours.

4.6 Pregnancy and lactation

Pregnancy

From experience in treating mothers with epilepsy, the risk associated with the use of valproate during pregnancy has been described as follows:

Risk associated with epilepsy and antiepileptics

In offspring born to mothers with epilepsy receiving any anti-epileptic treatment, the overall rate of malformations has been demonstrated to be 2 to 3 times higher than the rate (approximately 3%) reported in the general population. Although an increased number of children with malformations has been reported in cases of multiple drug therapy, the respective role of treatments and disease in causing the malformations has not been formally established. Malformations most frequently encountered are cleft lip and cardiovascular malformations.

Epidemiological studies have suggested an association between in-utero exposure to sodium valproate and a risk of development delay. Many factors including maternal epilepsy may also contribute to this risk but it is difficult to quantify the relative contributions of these or of maternal anti-epileptic treatment. Notwithstanding those potential risks, no sudden discontinuation in the anti-epileptic therapy should be undertaken as this may lead to breakthrough seizures, which could have serious consequences for both the mother and the foetus.

Risk associated with valproate

In animals: teratogenic effects have been demonstrated in the mouse, rat and rabbit. There is animal experimental evidence that high plasma peak levels and the size of an individual dose are associated with neural tube defects.

In humans: an increased incidence of congenital abnormalities (including cases of facial dysmorphia, hypospadias and multiple malformations, particularly of the limbs) has been demonstrated in offspring born to mothers with epilepsy treated with valproate.

Valproate use is associated with neural tube defects such as myelomeningocele and spina bifida. The frequency of this effect is estimated to be 1 to 2%.

In view of the above data

When a woman is planning pregnancy, this provides as opportunity to review the need for anti-epileptic treatment.

Women of childbearing age should be informed of the risks and benefits of continuing anti-epileptic treatment throughout pregnancy.

Folate supplementation, **prior** to pregnancy, has been demonstrated to reduce the incidence of neural tube defects in the offspring of women at high risk. Although no direct evidence exists of such effects in women receiving anti-epileptic drugs, women should be advised to start taking folic acid supplementation (5mg) as soon as contraception is discontinued.

The available evidence suggests that anticonvulsant monotherapy is preferred. Dosage should be reviewed before conception and the lowest effective dose used, in divided doses, as abnormal pregnancy outcome tends to be associated with higher total daily dosage and with the size of an individual dose. The incidence of neural tube defects rises with increasing dosage, particularly above 1000 mg daily. The administration in several divided doses over the day and the use of a prolonged release formulation is preferable in order to avoid high peak plasma levels. During pregnancy, valproate anti-epileptic treatment should not be discontinued if it has been effective. Nevertheless, specialist prenatal monitoring should be instituted in order to detect the possible occurrence of a neural tube defect or any other malformation. Pregnancies should be carefully screened by ultrasound, and other techniques if appropriate (see Section 4.4 Special Warnings and Special Precautions for use).

Risk in the neonate

Very rare cases of haemorrhagic syndrome have been reported in neonates whose mothers have taken valproate during pregnancy. This haemorrhagic syndrome is related to hypofibrinogenaemia; afibrinogenaemia has also been reported and may be fatal. These are possibly associated with a decrease of coagulation factors. However, this syndrome has to be distinguished from the decrease of the vitamin-K factors induced by phenobarbitone and other anti-epileptic enzyme inducing drugs.

Therefore, platelet count, fibrinogen plasma level, coagulation tests and coagulation factors should be investigated in neonates.

Lactation

Excretion of valproate in breast milk is low, with a concentration between 1% to 10% of total maternal serum levels; up to now breast fed children that have been monitored during the neonatal period have not experienced clinical effects. There appears to be no contraindication to breast feeding by patients on valproate.

4.7 Effects on ability to drive and use machines

Sodium valproate in appropriate doses may not impair driving skills but driving should be restricted to patients whose seizures are adequately controlled. Administration of the drug may occasionally induce drowsiness.

4.8 Undesirable effects

Most frequently, gastrointestinal disturbances, particularly on initiation of therapy. Sodium valproate very commonly causes weight gain, which may be marked and progressive (see Section 4.4 Special Warnings and Special Precautions for Use). Less commonly, increased appetite.

Occasionally, neurological side effects (often with too high a dose or other antiepileptics), including tremor, drowsiness, ataxia, confusion, headache, lethargy, and, more rarely, encephalopathy, coma and reversible dementia associated with cerebral atrophy.

Increased alertness may occur, but occasionally aggression, hyperactivity and behavioural disturbances in children.

Inhibition of platelet aggregation, reduced fibrinogen, reversible prolongation of bleeding time, red cell hypoplasia, thrombocytopenia, leucopenia and bone marrow depression have been reported (see Section 4.4 Special Warnings and Precautions for Use).

Occasionally, rashes (risk increased with concomitant lamotrigine), including erythema multiforme, Stevens-Johnson syndrome and toxic epidermal necrolysis), transient alopecia with regrowth of curly hair, acne and hirsutism.

Transient elevation of liver enzyme levels is common and dose related. Liver dysplasia and hepatic failure (rarely fatal) occurs occasionally, usually in the first few months, necessitating withdrawal. Hyperammonaemia without liver failure (sometimes associated with neurological symptoms), and hyperglycinaemia have been reported.

Cases of life-threatening pancreatitis have been reported in both children and adults receiving valproate. Some of the cases have been described as haemorrhagic with a rapid progression from initial symptoms to death. Some cases have occurred shortly after initial use as well as after several years of use (see Section 4.4 Special Warnings and Precautions for Use).

Rarely, gynaecomastia, menstrual irregularity and amenorrhoea reversible defects in renal tubular function (Fanconi's syndrome), hearing loss.

Congenital malformations have been reported in women receiving anti-epileptic agents including sodium valproate during pregnancy.

4.9 Overdose

Treatment includes induced vomiting, gastric lavage, assisted ventilation and forced diuresis.

5. PHARMACOLOGICAL PROPERTIES

5.1 Pharmacodynamic properties

The mode of action of valproic acid in epilepsy is not fully understood but may involve an elevation of gamma-amino butyric acid levels in the brain.

5.2 Pharmacokinetic properties

Sodium valproate is rapidly and completely absorbed after oral administration; the rate of absorption is delayed by administration as enteric coated tablets.

Sodium valproate is extensively metabolised in the liver, it is excreted in the urine almost entirely in the form of its metabolites.

Sodium valproate is extensively bound to plasma protein. Peak plasma levels are attained 1-4 hours after oral dosing and the half-life is of the order of 8-22 hours.

Sodium valproate crosses the blood brain barrier and small amounts are excreted in milk. Data from animal studies indicate that sodium valproate crosses the placenta.

5.3 Preclinical safety data

There are no additional preclinical data of relevance to the prescriber that have not been included in the main body of the text.

6. PHARMACEUTICAL PARTICULARS

6.1 List of excipients

Maltitol Solution (Syrup)

Nipasept

Cherry flavour black NA D3923

3M Hydrochloride acid

3M Sodium hydroxide

Purified water

6.2 Incompatibilities

None known

6.3 Shelf life

24 months

6.4 Special precautions for storage

Do not store above 25°C

Store in the original package in order to protect from light

6.5 Nature and contents of container

100ml opaque HDPE bottles with polypropylene caps.

500ml and 2000ml amber glass bottles with black bakelite screw-on caps.

6.6 Instructions for use and handling

None.

Administrative Data

7. MARKETING AUTHORISATION HOLDER

CP Pharmaceuticals Ltd

Ash Road North

Wrexham

LL13 9UF

UK

8. MARKETING AUTHORISATION NUMBER(S)

4543/0323

9. DATE OF FIRST AUTHORISATION/RENEWAL OF THE AUTHORISATION

19/2/92

10. DATE OF REVISION OF THE TEXT

August 2003

Orlept Tablets 200mg

(Wockhardt UK Ltd)

1. NAME OF THE MEDICINAL PRODUCT

Orlept Tablets 200mg or Sodium Valproate Tablets BP 200mg.

2. QUALITATIVE AND QUANTITATIVE COMPOSITION

Sodium Valproate 200mg

For excipients, see 6.1

3. PHARMACEUTICAL FORM

Enteric coated tablets.

White to faintly yellowish round bevel edged tablets.

4. CLINICAL PARTICULARS

4.1 Therapeutic indications

Sodium valproate is used in the treatment of all forms of epilepsy.

4.2 Posology and method of administration

Dosage requirements vary according to age and body weight and should be adjusted individually to achieve adequate seizure control. The tablets may be given in divided doses.

Monotherapy: usual requirements are as follows:

Adults: Dosage should start at 600mg daily increasing by 200mg at three day intervals until control is achieved. This is generally within the dosage range 1000mg to 2000mg per day i.e. 20-30mg/kg body weight daily. Where adequate control is not achieved within this range the dose may be further increased to a maximum of 2500mg per day.

Children over 20kg: Initial dosage should be 400mg/day increasing until control is achieved. This is usually within the range 20-30mg/kg body weight per day.

Children under 20kg: 20mg/kg of body weight per day; in severe cases this may be increased up to 40mg/kg/day.

Use in the elderly: Care should be taken when adjusting dosage in the elderly since the pharmacokinetics of sodium valproate are modified. Dosage should be determined by seizure control.

Use in renal impairment:

Mild to moderate - Reduce dose

Severe - Alter dose according to free serum valproic acid concentration

Combined Therapy: In certain cases it may be necessary to raise the dose by 5 to 10mg/kg/day when used in combination with liver enzyme inducing drugs such as phenytoin, phenobarbitone and carbamazepine.

4.3 Contraindications

Liver disease or family history of severe hepatic dysfunction

Hypersensitivity to valproate

Porphyria

4.4 Special warnings and special precautions for use

Clinical symptoms are a more sensitive indicator in the early stages of hepatic failure than laboratory investigations. The onset of an acute illness, especially within the first six months, which may include symptoms of vomiting, lethargy or weakness, drowsiness, anorexia, jaundice or loss of seizure control is an indication for immediate withdrawal of the drug.

Patients should be instructed to report any such signs to the clinician should they occur.

Routine measurement of liver function should be undertaken in those at risk before and during the first six months of therapy including children under three years, especially those with severe seizure disorders associated withmental retardation, organic brain disease, metabolic or degenerativedisorder.

The drug should be discontinued if signs of liver damage occur or if serum amylase levels are elevated.

Combination with other antiepileptics may increase the risk of liver damage and should therefore be avoided if possible (see Section 4.5 Interactions with Other Medicaments).

Consider dose adjustment in renal impairment (see Section 4.2 Posology and Method of Administration).

Severe pancreatitis, which may be fatal, has been reported. Medical evaluation (including measurement of serum amylase) should be undertaken in patients presenting with symptoms suggestive of pancreatitis (e.g. abdominal pain, nausea and vomiting) and valproate should be discontinued if pancreatitis is diagnosed. Patients should be advised to consult their doctor immediately if they develop symptoms suggestive of pancreatitis (See Section 4.8. Undesirable Effects).

Valproic acid inhibits the second stage of platelet aggregation. If spontaneous bruising or bleeding occurs or the prothrombin time is abnormally prolonged, medication should be withdrawn. Concomitant salicylates should be stopped if coagulation is affected. It is recommended that patients receiving sodium valproate are monitored for platelet function and clotting time before major surgery. Patients should be told how to recognise signs of blood disorders and advised to seek immediate medical advice.

Withdrawal of sodium valproate or transition to another antiepileptic should be made gradually to avoid precipitation of an increase in seizure frequency.

Sodium valproate may give false positives for ketone bodies in the urine testing of diabetics.

Sodium valproate very commonly causes weight gain, which may be marked and progressive. All patients should be warned of this risk at the initiation of therapy and appropriate strategies adopted to minimise weight gain.

Monitor body weight during sodium valproate therapy.

Pregnancy

Women of childbearing potential should not be started on sodium valproate without specialist neurological advice. Sodium valproate is the antiepileptic of choice in patients with certain types of epilepsy such as generalised epilepsy ± myoclonus/photosensitivity. For partial epilepsy, sodium valproate should be used only in those resistant to other treatment. Women who are likely to get pregnant should receive specialist advice because of the potential teratogenic risk to the foetus (see also section 4.6 Pregnancy and Lactation).

4.5 Interaction with other medicinal products and other forms of Interaction

Other antiepileptics:

Co-administration with other antiepileptics may be associated with enhanced effects, increased sedation, reduced plasma concentrations and enhanced toxicity (especially hepatic, see Section 4.4 Special Warnings and Precautions for Use), and can complicate monitoring of treatment.

Concomitant use of hepatic enzyme inducers (e.g. barbiturates, carbamazepine, phenytoin) may enhance metabolism of valproic acid. Valproic acid has been reported to have variable effects on blood levels of other hepatically metabolised or highly protein bound agents. Plasma levels of lamotrigine, primidone, phenobarbital, ethosuximide, and an active metabolite of carbamazepine may be increased. Plasma levels of phenytoin may be increased or reduced. Plasma levels of an active metabolite of oxcarbazepine are sometimes lowered.

Other drugs affecting clotting:

Caution is recommended when administering with other drugs affecting clotting (e.g. warfarin, aspirin). (See Section 4.4 Special Warnings and Precautions for Use).

Other hepatotoxic drugs:

Other hepatotoxic drugs should be avoided (including aspirin in children).

Antacids:

Absorption of sodium valproate may be increased when administered with aluminium and magnesium hydroxides.

Antidepressants and antipsychotics:

Antidepressants and antipsychotics may lower the threshold for convulsions and higher doses of sodium valproate may be needed.

Antimalarials:

Chloroquine and mefloquine antagonise the anticonvulsant effect of valproate.

Antiulcer drugs:

Cimetidine has been reported to decrease clearance.

Antivirals:

Plasma concentration of zidovudine possibly increased (risk of toxicity).

Lipid-lowering agents:

Cholestyramine may decrease valproate absorption; separate dosage by three hours.

4.6 Pregnancy and lactation

Pregnancy

From experience in treating mothers with epilepsy, the risk associated with the use of valproate during pregnancy has been described as follows:

Risk associated with epilepsy and antiepileptics

In offspring born to mothers with epilepsy receiving any anti-epileptic treatment, the overall rate of malformations has been demonstrated to be 2 to 3 times higher than the rate (approximately 3%) reported in the general population. Although an increased number of children with malformations has been reported in cases of multiple drug therapy, the respective role of treatments and disease in causing the malformations has not been formally established. Malformations most frequently encountered are cleft lip and cardiovascular malformations.

Epidemiological studies have suggested an association between in-utero exposure to sodium valproate and a risk of development delay. Many factors including maternal epilepsy may also contribute to this risk but it is difficult to quantify the relative contributions of these or of maternal anti-epileptic treatment. Notwithstanding those potential risks, no sudden discontinuation in the anti-epileptic therapy should be undertaken as this may lead to breakthrough seizures, which could have serious consequences for both the mother and the foetus.

Risk associated with valproate

In animals: teratogenic effects have been demonstrated in the mouse, rat and rabbit. There is animal experimental evidence that high plasma peak levels and the size of an individual dose are associated with neural tube defects.

In humans: an increased incidence of congenital abnormalities (including cases of facial dysmorphia, hypospadias and multiple malformations, particularly of the limbs) has been demonstrated in offspring born to mothers with epilepsy treated with valproate.

Valproate use is associated with neural tube defects such as myelomeningocele and spina bifida. The frequency of this effect is estimated to be 1 to 2%.

In view of the above data

When a woman is planning pregnancy, this provides as opportunity to review the need for anti-epileptic treatment. Women of childbearing age should be informed of the risks and benefits of continuing anti-epileptic treatment throughout pregnancy.

Folate supplementation, **prior** to pregnancy, has been demonstrated to reduce the incidence of neural tube defects in the offspring of women at high risk. Although no direct evidence exists of such effects in women receiving anti-epileptic drugs, women should be advised to start taking folic acid supplementation (5mg) as soon as contraception is discontinued.

The available evidence suggests that anticonvulsant monotherapy is preferred. Dosage should be reviewed before conception and the lowest effective dose used, in divided doses, as abnormal pregnancy outcome tends to be associated with higher total daily dosage and with the size of an individual dose. The incidence of neural tube defects rises with increasing dosage, particularly above 1000 mg daily. The administration in several divided doses over the day and the use of a prolonged release formulation is preferable in order to avoid high peak plasma levels. During pregnancy, valproate anti-epileptic treatment should not be discontinued if it has been effective. Nevertheless, specialist prenatal monitoring should be instituted in order to detect the possible occurrence of a neural tube defect or any other malformation. Pregnancies should be carefully screened by ultrasound, and other techniques if appropriate (see Section 4.4 Special Warnings and Special Precautions for use).

Risk in the neonate

Very rare cases of haemorrhagic syndrome have been reported in neonates whose mothers have taken valproate during pregnancy. This haemorrhagic syndrome is related to hypofibrinogenaemia; afibrinogenaemia has also been reported and may be fatal. These are possibly associated with a decrease of coagulation factors. However, this syndrome has to be distinguished from the decrease of the vitamin-K factors induced by phenobarbitone and other anti-epileptic enzyme inducing drugs.

Therefore, platelet count, fibrinogen plasma level, coagulation tests and coagulation factors should be investigated in neonates.

Lactation

Excretion of valproate in breast milk is low, with a concentration between 1% to 10% of total maternal serum levels; up to now breast fed children that have been monitored during the neonatal period have not experienced clinical effects. There appears to be no contraindication to breast feeding by patients on valproate.

4.7 Effects on ability to drive and use machines

Sodium valproate in appropriate doses may not impair driving skills but driving should be restricted to patients whose seizures are adequately controlled. Administration of the drug may occasionally induce drowsiness.

4.8 Undesirable effects

Most frequently, gastrointestinal disturbances, particularly on initiation of therapy. Sodium valproate very commonly causes weight gain, which may be marked and progressive (see Section 4.4 Special Warnings and Special Precautions for Use). Less commonly, increased appetite.

Occasionally, neurological side effects (often with too high a dose or other antiepileptics), including tremor, drowsiness, ataxia, confusion, headache, lethargy, and, more rarely, encephalopathy, coma and reversible dementia associated with cerebral atrophy.

Increased alertness may occur, but occasionally aggression, hyperactivity and behavioural disturbances in children.

Inhibition of platelet aggregation, reduced fibrinogen, reversible prolongation of bleeding time, red cell hypoplasia, thrombocytopenia, leucopenia and bone marrow depression have been reported (see Section 4.4 Special Warnings and Precautions for Use).

Occasionally, rashes (risk increased with concomitant lamotrigine), including erythema multiforme, Stevens-Johnson syndrome and toxic epidermal necrolysis), transient alopecia with regrowth of curly hair, acne and hirsutism.

Transient elevation of liver enzyme levels is common and dose related. Liver dysplasia and hepatic failure (rarely fatal) occurs occasionally, usually in the first few months, necessitating withdrawal. Hyperammonaemia without liver failure (sometimesassociated with neurological symptoms), and hyperglycinaemia have been reported.

Cases of life-threatening pancreatitis have been reported in both children and adults receiving valproate. Some of the cases have been described as haemorrhagic with a rapid progression from initial symptoms to death. Some cases have occurred shortly after initial use as well as after several years of use (see Section 4.4 Special Warnings and Precautions for Use).

Rarely, gynaecomastia, menstrual irregularity and amenorrhoea, reversible defects in renal tubular function (Fanconi's syndrome), hearing loss.

Congenital malformations have been reported in women receiving anti-epileptic agents including sodium valproate during pregnancy.

4.9 Overdose

Treatment includes induced vomiting, gastric lavage, assisted ventilation and forced diuresis.

5. PHARMACOLOGICAL PROPERTIES

5.1 Pharmacodynamic properties

The mode of action of valproic acid in epilepsy is not fully understood but may involve an elevation of gamma-amino butyric acid levels in the brain.

5.2 Pharmacokinetic properties

Sodium valproate is rapidly and completely absorbed after oral administration; the rate of absorption is delayed by administration as enteric coated tablets.

Sodium valproate is extensively metabolised in the liver, it is excreted in the urine almost entirely in the form of its metabolites.

Sodium valproate is extensively bound to plasma protein. Peak plasma levels are attained 1-4 hours after oral dosing and the half-life is of the order of 8-22 hours.

Sodium valproate crosses the blood brain barrier and small amounts are excreted in milk. Data from animal studies indicate that sodium valproate crosses the placenta.

5.3 Preclinical safety data
There are no additional preclinical data of relevance to the prescriber that have not been included in the main body of the text.

6. PHARMACEUTICAL PARTICULARS

6.1 List of excipients
Microcrystalline cellulose anhydrous

Methylated colloidal anhydrous silica

Enzymatically hydrolysed gelatin

Calcium behenate

Talc

TabletCoating

Methacrylic acid copolymer

Talc

Triacetin

Titanium Dioxide

Polyethylene Glycol 6000

6.2 Incompatibilities
None known

6.3 Shelf life
24 months in polypropylene or polyethylene container or glass bottles.

24 months in blister strips of PVC/PVDC and aluminium foil.

6.4 Special precautions for storage
Do not store above 25°C.

Store in the original package in order to protect from moisture.

6.5 Nature and contents of container
Polypropylene or polyethylene containers or glass bottles containing 100 tablets.

Blister strips of rigid PVC/PVDC film and aluminium foil of 10 tablets used in multiples of 5, 6 or 10 giving pack sizes of 10, 50, 60 or 100 tablets.

6.6 Instructions for use and handling
None.

Administrative Data

7. MARKETING AUTHORISATION HOLDER
CP Pharmaceuticals Ltd

Ash Road North

Wrexham

LL13 9UF

UK

8. MARKETING AUTHORISATION NUMBER(S)
4543/0283

9. DATE OF FIRST AUTHORISATION/RENEWAL OF THE AUTHORISATION
14/05/91

10. DATE OF REVISION OF THE TEXT
August 2003

Orlept Tablets 500mg

(Wockhardt UK Ltd)

1. NAME OF THE MEDICINAL PRODUCT
Orlept Tablets 500mg or Sodium Valproate Tablets BP 500mg.

2. QUALITATIVE AND QUANTITATIVE COMPOSITION
Sodium Valproate 500mg

For excipients, see 6.1

3. PHARMACEUTICAL FORM
Enteric coated tablets.

White to faintly yellowish oval shaped tablets.

4. CLINICAL PARTICULARS

4.1 Therapeutic indications
Sodium valproate is used in the treatment of all forms of epilepsy.

4.2 Posology and method of administration
Dosage requirements vary according to age and body weight and should be adjusted individually to achieve adequate seizure control. The tablets may be given in divided doses.

Monotherapy: usual requirements are as follows:

Adults: Dosage should start at 600mg daily increasing by 200mg at three day intervals until control is achieved. This is generally within the dosage range 1000mg to 2000mg per day i.e. 20-30mg/kg body weight daily. Where adequate control is not achieved within this range the dose may be further increased to a maximum of 2500mg per day.

Children over 20kg: Initial dosage should be 400mg/day increasing until control is achieved. This is usually within the range 20-30mg/kg body weight per day.

Children under 20kg: 20mg/kg of body weight per day; in severe cases this may be increased up to 40mg/kg/day.

Use in the elderly: Care should be taken when adjusting dosage in the elderly since the pharmacokinetics of sodium valproate are modified. Dosage should be determined by seizure control.

Use in renal impairment:

Mild to moderate - Reduce dose

Severe - Alter dose according to free serum valproic acid concentration

Combined Therapy: In certain cases it may be necessary to raise the dose by 5 to 10mg/kg/day when used in combination with liver enzyme inducing drugs such as phenytoin, phenobarbitone and carbamazepine.

4.3 Contraindications
Liver disease or family history of severe hepatic dysfunction

Hypersensitivity to valproate

Porphyria

4.4 Special warnings and special precautions for use
Clinical symptoms are a more sensitive indicator in the early stages of hepatic failure than laboratory investigations. The onset of an acute illness, especially within the first six months, which may include symptoms of vomiting, lethargy or weakness, drowsiness, anorexia, jaundice or loss of seizure control is an indication for immediate withdrawal of the drug.

Patients should be instructed to report any such signs to the clinician should they occur.

Routine measurement of liver function should be undertaken in those at risk before and during the first six months of therapy including children under three years, especially those with severe seizure disorders associated with mental retardation, organic brain disease, metabolic or degenerative disorder.

The drug should be discontinued if signs of liver damage occur or if serum amylase levels are elevated.

Combination with other antiepileptics may increase the risk of liver damage and should therefore be avoided if possible (see Section 4.5 Interactions with Other Medicaments).

Consider dose adjustment in renal impairment (see Section 4.2 Posology and Method of Administration).

Severe pancreatitis, which may be fatal, has been reported. Medical evaluation (including measurement of serum amylase) should be undertaken in patients presenting with symptoms suggestive of pancreatitis (e.g. abdominal pain, nausea and vomiting) and valproate should be discontinued if pancreatitis is diagnosed. Patients should be advised to consult their doctor immediately if they develop symptoms suggestive of pancreatitis (See Section 4.8. Undesirable Effects).

Valproic acid inhibits the second stage of platelet aggregation. If spontaneous bruising or bleeding occurs or the prothrombin time is abnormally prolonged, medication should be withdrawn. Concomitant salicylates should be stopped if coagulation is affected. It is recommended that patients receiving sodium valproate are monitored for platelet function and clotting time before major surgery. Patients should be told how to recognise signs of blood disorders and advised to seek immediate medical advice.

Withdrawal of sodium valproate or transition to another antiepileptic should be made gradually to avoid precipitation of an increase in seizure frequency.

Sodium valproate may give false positives for ketone bodies in the urine testing of diabetics.

Sodium valproate very commonly causes weight gain, which may be marked and progressive. All patients should be warned of this risk at the initiation of therapy and appropriate strategies adopted to minimise weight gain.

Monitor body weight during sodium valproate therapy.

<u>*Pregnancy*</u>

Women of childbearing potential should not be started on sodium valproate without specialist neurological advice. Sodium valproate is the antiepileptic of choice in patients with certain types of epilepsy such as generalised epilepsy ± myoclonus/photosensitivity. For partial epilepsy, sodium valproate should be used only in those resistant to other treatment. Women who are likely to get pregnant should receive specialist advice because of the potential teratogenic risk to the foetus (see also section 4.6 Pregnancy and Lactation).

4.5 Interaction with other medicinal products and other forms of Interaction
Other antiepileptics:

Co-administration with other antiepileptics may be associated with enhanced effects, increased sedation, reduced plasma concentrations and enhanced toxicity (especially hepatic, see Section 4.4 Special Warnings and Precautions for Use), and can complicate monitoring of treatment.

Concomitant use of hepatic enzyme inducers (e.g. barbiturates, carbamazepine, phenytoin) may enhance metabolism of valproic acid. Valproic acid has been reported to have variable effects on blood levels of other hepatically metabolised or highly protein bound agents. Plasma levels of lamotrigine, primidone, phenobarbital, ethosuximide, and an active metabolite of carbamazepine may be increased. Plasma levels of phenytoin may be increased or reduced. Plasma levels of an active metabolite of oxcarbazepine are sometimes lowered.

Other drugs affecting clotting:

Caution is recommended when administering with other drugs affecting clotting (e.g. warfarin, aspirin). (See Section 4.4 Special Warnings and Precautions for Use).

Other hepatotoxic drugs:

Other hepatotoxic drugs should be avoided (including aspirin in children).

Antacids:

Absorption of sodium valproate may be increased when administered with aluminium and magnesium hydroxides.

Antidepressants and antipsychotics:

Antidepressants and antipsychotics may lower the threshold for convulsions and higher doses of sodium valproate may be needed.

Antimalarials:

Chloroquine and mefloquine antagonise the anticonvulsant effect of valproate.

Antiulcer drugs:

Cimetidine has been reported to decrease clearance.

Antivirals:

Plasma concentration of zidovudine possibly increased (risk of toxicity).

Lipid-lowering agents:

Cholestyramine may decrease valproate absorption; separate dosage by three hours.

4.6 Pregnancy and lactation

<u>*Pregnancy*</u>

From experience in treating mothers with epilepsy, the risk associated with the use of valproate during pregnancy has been described as follows:

Risk associated with epilepsy and antiepileptics

In offspring born to mothers with epilepsy receiving any anti-epileptic treatment, the overall rate of malformations has been demonstrated to be 2 to 3 times higher than the rate (approximately 3%) reported in the general population. Although an increased number of children with malformations has been reported in cases of multiple drug therapy, the respective role of treatments and disease in causing the malformations has not been formally established. Malformations most frequently encountered are cleft lip and cardiovascular malformations.

Epidemiological studies have suggested an association between in-utero exposure to sodium valproate and a risk of development delay. Many factors including maternal epilepsy may also contribute to this risk but it is difficult to quantify the relative contributions of these or of maternal anti-epileptic treatment. Notwithstanding those potential risks, no sudden discontinuation in the anti-epileptic therapy should be undertaken as this may lead to breakthrough seizures, which could have serious consequences for both the mother and the foetus.

Risk associated with valproate

In animals: teratogenic effects have been demonstrated in the mouse, rat and rabbit. There is animal experimental evidence that high plasma peak levels and the size of an individual dose are associated with neural tube defects.

In humans: an increased incidence of congenital abnormalities (including cases of facial dysmorphia, hypospadias and multiple malformations, particularly of the limbs) has been demonstrated in offspring born to mothers with epilepsy treated with valproate.

Valproate use is associated with neural tube defects such as myelomeningocele and spina bifida. The frequency of this effect is estimated to be 1 to 2%.

In view of the above data

When a woman is planning pregnancy, this provides as opportunity to review the need for anti-epileptic treatment. Women of childbearing age should be informed of the risks and benefits of continuing anti-epileptic treatment throughout pregnancy.

Folate supplementation, **prior** to pregnancy, has been demonstrated to reduce the incidence of neural tube defects in the offspring of women at high risk. Although no direct evidence exists of such effects in women receiving anti-epileptic drugs, women should be advised to start taking folic acid supplementation (5mg) as soon as contraception is discontinued.

The available evidence suggests that anticonvulsant monotherapy is preferred. Dosage should be reviewed before conception and the lowest effective dose used, in divided doses, as abnormal pregnancy outcome tends to be associated with higher total daily dosage and with the size of an individual dose. The incidence of neural tube defects rises with increasing dosage, particularly above 1000 mg daily. The administration in several divided doses over the day and the use of a prolonged release formulation is preferable in order to avoid high peak plasma levels. During pregnancy, valproate anti-epileptic treatment should not be discontinued if it has been effective. Nevertheless, specialist prenatal monitoring should be instituted in order to detect the possible occurrence of a neural tube defect or any other malformation. Pregnancies should be carefully screened by ultrasound, and other techniques if appropriate (see Section 4.4 Special Warnings and Special Precautions for use).

Risk in the neonate

Very rare cases of haemorrhagic syndrome have been reported in neonates whose mothers have taken valproate during pregnancy. This haemorrhagic syndrome is related to hypofibrinogenaemia; afibrinogenaemia has also been reported and may be fatal. These are possibly associated with a decrease of coagulation factors. However, this syndrome has to be distinguished from the decrease of the vitamin-K factors induced by phenobarbitone and other anti-epileptic enzyme inducing drugs.

Therefore, platelet count, fibrinogen plasma level, coagulation tests and coagulation factors should be investigated in neonates.

Lactation

Excretion of valproate in breast milk is low, with a concentration between 1% to 10% of total maternal serum levels; up to now breast fed children that have been monitored during the neonatal period have not experienced clinical effects. There appears to be no contraindication to breast feeding by patients on valproate.

4.7 Effects on ability to drive and use machines

Sodium valproate in appropriate doses may not impair driving skills but driving should be restricted to patients whose seizures are adequately controlled. Administration of the drug may occasionally induce drowsiness.

4.8 Undesirable effects

Most frequently, gastrointestinal disturbances, particularly on initiation of therapy. Sodium valproate very commonly causes weight gain, which may be marked and progressive (see Section 4.4 Special Warnings and Special Precautions for Use). Less commonly, increased appetite.

Occasionally, neurological side effects (often with too high a dose or other antiepileptics), including tremor, drowsiness, ataxia, confusion, headache, lethargy, and, more rarely, encephalopathy, coma and reversible dementia associated with cerebral atrophy.

Increased alertness may occur, but occasionally aggression, hyperactivity and behavioural disturbances in children.

Inhibition of platelet aggregation, reduced fibrinogen, reversible prolongation of bleeding time, red cell hypoplasia, thrombocytopenia, leucopenia and bone marrow depression have been reported (see Section 4.4 Special Warnings and Precautions for Use).

Occasionally, rashes (risk increased with concomitant lamotrigine), including erythema multiforme, Stevens-Johnson syndrome and toxic epidermal necrolysis), transient alopecia with regrowth of curly hair, acne and hirsutism.

Transient elevation of liver enzyme levels is common and dose related. Liver dysplasia and hepatic failure (rarely fatal) occurs occasionally, usually in the first few months, necessitating withdrawal. Hyperammonaemia without liver failure (sometimes associated with neurological symptoms), and hyperglycinaemia have been reported.

Cases of life-threatening pancreatitis have been reported in both children and adults receiving valproate. Some of the cases have been described as haemorrhagic with a rapid progression from initial symptoms to death. Some cases have occurred shortly after initial use as well as after several years of use (see Section 4.4 Special Warnings and Precautions for Use).

Rarely, gynaecomastia, menstrual irregularity and amenorrhoea, reversible defects in renal tubular function (Fanconi's syndrome), hearing loss.

Congenital malformations have been reported in women receiving anti-epileptic agents including sodium valproate during pregnancy.

4.9 Overdose

Treatment includes induced vomiting, gastric lavage, assisted ventilation and forced diuresis.

5. PHARMACOLOGICAL PROPERTIES

5.1 Pharmacodynamic properties

The mode of action of valproic acid in epilepsy is not fully understood but may involve an elevation of gamma-amino butyric acid levels in the brain.

5.2 Pharmacokinetic properties

Sodium valproate is rapidly and completely absorbed after oral administration; the rate of absorption is delayed by administration as enteric coated tablets.

Sodium valproate is extensively metabolised in the liver, it is excreted in the urine almost entirely in the form of its metabolites.

Sodium valproate is extensively bound to plasma protein. Peak plasma levels are attained 1-4 hours after oral dosing and the half-life is of the order of 8-22 hours.

Sodium valproate crosses the blood brain barrier and small amounts are excreted in milk. Data from animal studies indicate that sodium valproate crosses the placenta.

5.3 Preclinical safety data

There are no additional preclinical data of relevance to the prescriber that have not been included in the main body of the text.

6. PHARMACEUTICAL PARTICULARS

6.1 List of excipients

Microcrystalline cellulose anhydrous

Methylated colloidal anhydrous silica

Enzymatically hydrolysed gelatin

Calcium behenate

Talc

TabletCoating

Methacrylic acid copolymer

Talc

Triacetin

Titanium Dioxide

Polyethylene Glycol 6000

6.2 Incompatibilities

None known

6.3 Shelf life

24 months in polypropylene or polyethylene container or glass bottles.

24 months in blister strips of PVC/PVDC and aluminium foil.

6.4 Special precautions for storage

Do not store above 25°C.

Store in the original package in order to protect from moisture.

6.5 Nature and contents of container

Polypropylene or polyethylene containers or glass bottles containing 100 tablets.

Blister strips of rigid PVC/PVDC film and aluminium foil of 10 tablets used in multiples of 5, 6 or 10 giving pack sizes of 10, 50, 60 or 100 tablets.

6.6 Instructions for use and handling

None.

Administrative Data

7. MARKETING AUTHORISATION HOLDER

CP Pharmaceuticals Ltd

Ash Road North

Wrexham

LL13 9UF

UK

8. MARKETING AUTHORISATION NUMBER(S)

4543/0284

9. DATE OF FIRST AUTHORISATION/RENEWAL OF THE AUTHORISATION

14/12/89

10. DATE OF REVISION OF THE TEXT

August 2003

Ortho-Creme Contraceptive Cream

(Janssen-Cilag Ltd)

1. NAME OF THE MEDICINAL PRODUCT

ORTHO-CREME® Contraceptive Cream

2. QUALITATIVE AND QUANTITATIVE COMPOSITION

Contains 2.0% w/w of nonoxinol-9.

3. PHARMACEUTICAL FORM

Vaginal cream.

4. CLINICAL PARTICULARS

4.1 Therapeutic indications

For use as a spermicidal contraceptive in conjunction with barrier methods of contraception.

4.2 Posology and method of administration

For vaginal use.

For use by adult females only.

The cream should be spread over the surface of the diaphragm which will be in contact with the cervix and on the rim. The diaphragm must be allowed to remain *in situ* for at least six to eight hours after coitus. A fresh application of cream or other spermicides, eg ORTHO-FORMS® Contraceptive Pessaries, must be made prior to any subsequent act of coitus within this period of time, without removing the diaphragm. (A vaginal applicator should be used for inserting more cream.)

Douching is not recommended, but if it is desired it should be deferred for at least six hours after intercourse.

4.3 Contraindications

(i) Hypersensitivity to nonoxinol-9 or to any component of the preparation.

(ii) Patients with absent vaginal sensation, eg paraplegics and quadriplegics.

4.4 Special warnings and special precautions for use

(i) Spermicidal intravaginal preparations are intended for use in conjunction with barrier methods of contraception such as condoms, diaphragms and caps.

(ii) Where avoidance of pregnancy is important, the choice of contraceptive method should be made in consultation with a doctor or a family planning clinic.

(iii) This product does not protect against HIV (AIDS) or other sexually transmitted diseases (STDs). A latex condom should be used to protect against the spread of STDs. High frequency use of nonoxinol-9 has been reported to cause epithelial damage and increase the risk of HIV infection. Therefore women at risk of HIV/STD infection and who have multiple daily acts of intercourse should be advised to choose another method of contraception. Sexually active women should consider their individual HIV/STD infection risk when choosing a method of contraception.

(iv) If vaginal or penile irritation occurs, discontinue use. If symptoms worsen or continue for more than 48 hours medical advice should be sought.

4.5 Interaction with other medicinal products and other forms of Interaction

None known.

4.6 Pregnancy and lactation

There is no evidence from animal and human studies that nonoxinol-9 is teratogenic. Human epidemiological studies have not shown any firm evidence of adverse effects on the foetus. However some studies have shown that nonoxinol-9 may be embryotoxic in animals. This product should not be used if pregnancy is suspected or confirmed. Animal studies have detected nonoxinol-9 in milk after intravaginal administration. Use by lactating women has not been studied.

4.7 Effects on ability to drive and use machines

None known.

4.8 Undesirable effects

May cause irritation of the vagina or penis.

4.9 Overdose

If taken orally, the surfactant properties of this preparation may cause gastric irritation. General supportive therapy should be carried out. Hepatic and renal function should be monitored if medically indicated.

5. PHARMACOLOGICAL PROPERTIES

5.1 Pharmacodynamic properties

The standard *in vitro* test (Sander-Cramer) evaluating the effect of nonoxinol-9 on animal sperm motility has shown the compound to be a potent spermicide.

The site of action of nonoxinol-9 has been determined as the sperm cell membrane. The lipoprotein membrane is disrupted, increasing permeability, with subsequent loss of cell components and decreased motility. A similar effect on vaginal epithelial and bacterial cells is also found.

5.2 Pharmacokinetic properties

The intravaginal absorption and excretion of radiolabelled (^{14}C) nonoxinol-9 has been studied in non-pregnant rats and rabbits and in pregnant rats. No appreciable difference was found in the extent or rate of absorption in pregnant and non-pregnant animals. Plasma levels peaked at about one hour and recovery from urine as unchanged nonoxinol-9 accounted for approximately 15-25% and faeces approximately 70% of the administered dose as unchanged nonoxinol-9. Less than 0.3% was found in the milk of lactating rats. No metabolites were detected in any of the samples analysed.

5.3 Preclinical safety data

No relevant information additional to that contained elsewhere in the Summary of Product Characteristics.

6. PHARMACEUTICAL PARTICULARS

6.1 List of excipients

Benzoic acid (E 210)

Cetyl alcohol

Lavender compound 13091

Methyl hydroxybenzoate (E218)

Propyl hydroxybenzoate (E216)

Propylene glycol

Sodium carboxymethylcellulose

Sodium lauryl sulphate

Stearic acid

Triethanolmine

Acetic acid glacial

Castor oil

Potassium hydroxide

Sorbic acid (E200)

Purified water

6.2 Incompatibilities

Not applicable.

6.3 Shelf life

3 years.

6.4 Special precautions for storage

Do not store above 25°C.

6.5 Nature and contents of container

Epoxy-resin lined aluminium tubes of 70 g with polyethylene cap.

6.6 Instructions for use and handling

Not applicable.

Administrative Data

7. MARKETING AUTHORISATION HOLDER
Janssen-Cilag Ltd
Saunderton
High Wycombe
Bucks
HP14 4HJ
UK
www.janssen-cilag.co.uk

8. MARKETING AUTHORISATION NUMBER(S)
PL 0242/0248

9. DATE OF FIRST AUTHORISATION/RENEWAL OF THE AUTHORISATION
First Authorisation: 03/08/1995
Date of Renewal of Authorisation: 02/10/1996

10. DATE OF REVISION OF THE TEXT
23 October 2002

Legal Category GSL

Orthoforms Contraceptive Pessaries

(Janssen-Cilag Ltd)

1. NAME OF THE MEDICINAL PRODUCT
ORTHOFORMS Contraceptive Pessaries

2. QUALITATIVE AND QUANTITATIVE COMPOSITION
Nonoxinol-9, 5.0% w/w

3. PHARMACEUTICAL FORM
Pessary.

4. CLINICAL PARTICULARS

4.1 Therapeutic indications
For use as a spermicide contraceptive in conjunction with barrier methods of contraception.

4.2 Posology and method of administration
For vaginal use.

For use by adult females only.

The Orthoforms Contraceptive Pessary should be inserted as high as possible into the vagina approximately 10 minutes before intercourse to permit the pessary to melt.

Any subsequent acts of intercourse should not be undertaken before the insertion of an additional pessary.

4.3 Contraindications
Hypersensitivity to nonoxinol-9 or to any component of the preparation.

Patients with absent vaginal sensation, e.g. paraplegics and quadriplegics.

4.4 Special warnings and special precautions for use
Spermicidal intravaginal preparations are intended for use in conjunction with barrier methods of contraception such as condoms, diaphragms and caps.

Where avoidance of pregnancy is important the choice of contraceptive method should be made in consultation with a doctor or family planning clinic.

This product does not protect against HIV (AIDS) or other sexually transmitted diseases (STDs). A latex condom should be used to protect against the spread of STDs. High frequency use of nonoxinol-9 has been reported to cause epithelial damage and increase the risk of HIV infection. Therefore women at risk of HIV/STD infection and who have multiple daily acts of intercourse should be advised to choose another method of contraception. Sexually active women should consider their individual HIV/STD infection risk when choosing a method of contraception.

If vaginal or penile irritation occurs, discontinue use. If symptoms worsen or continue for more than 48 hours, medical advice should be sought.

4.5 Interaction with other medicinal products and other forms of Interaction
None known.

4.6 Pregnancy and lactation
There is no evidence from animal or human studies that nonoxinol-9 is teratogenic. Human epidemiological studies have not shown any firm evidence of adverse effects on the foetus. However, some studies have shown that nonoxinol-9 may be embryotoxic in animals. This product should not be used if pregnancy is suspected or confirmed.

Animal studies have detected nonoxinol-9 in milk after intravaginal administration. Use by lactating women has not been studied.

4.7 Effects on ability to drive and use machines
None known.

4.8 Undesirable effects
Orthoforms Contraceptive Pessaries may cause irritation of the vagina or penis.

4.9 Overdose
If taken orally, the surfactant properties of this preparation may cause gastric irritation. General supportive therapy should be carried out. Hepatic and renal function should be monitored if medically indicated.

5. PHARMACOLOGICAL PROPERTIES

5.1 Pharmacodynamic properties
The standard *in vitro* test (Sander-Cramer) evaluating the effect of nonoxinol-9 on animal sperm motility has shown the compound to be a potent spermicide.

The site of action of nonoxinol-9 has been determined as the sperm cell membrane. The lipoprotein membrane is disrupted, increasing permeability, with subsequent loss of cell components and decreased motility. A similar effect on vaginal epithelial and bacterial cells is also found.

5.2 Pharmacokinetic properties
The intravaginal absorption and excretion of radiolabelled (^{14}C) nonoxinol-9 has been studied in non-pregnant rats and rabbits and in pregnant rats. No appreciable difference was found in the extent or rate of absorption in pregnant and non-pregnant animals. Plasma levels peaked at about one hour and recovery from urine as unchanged nonoxinol-9 accounted for approximately 15-25% and faeces approximately 70% of the administered dose as unchanged nonoxinol-9. Less than 0.3% was found in the milk of lactating rats. No metabolites were detected in any of the samples analysed.

5.3 Preclinical safety data
See section 4.6 - 'Pregnancy and lactation'.

6. PHARMACEUTICAL PARTICULARS

6.1 List of excipients
Cetomacrogol 1000 BP

Citric acid monohydrate PhEur

Polyethylene glycol 1500

Polyethylene glycol 1000 BP

Purified water PhEur

6.2 Incompatibilities
None known.

6.3 Shelf life
36 months.

6.4 Special precautions for storage
Store in a cool place (8-15°C).

6.5 Nature and contents of container
Immediate container: polyvinylchloride/polyethylene laminate moulds.

Three strips of 5 pessaries are packed in an outer cardboard carton.

6.6 Instructions for use and handling
None stated.

7. MARKETING AUTHORISATION HOLDER
Janssen-Cilag Ltd
Saunderton
High Wycombe
Buckinghamshire
HP14 4HJ
UK

8. MARKETING AUTHORISATION NUMBER(S)
PL 0242/0247

9. DATE OF FIRST AUTHORISATION/RENEWAL OF THE AUTHORISATION
1 September 1995/02 October1996

10. DATE OF REVISION OF THE TEXT
23 October 2002

Legal status POM

Ortho-Gynest Cream

(Janssen-Cilag Ltd)

1. NAME OF THE MEDICINAL PRODUCT
Ortho-Gynest® Cream

2. QUALITATIVE AND QUANTITATIVE COMPOSITION
Estriol 0.01% w/w USP.

3. PHARMACEUTICAL FORM
Cream.

4. CLINICAL PARTICULARS

4.1 Therapeutic indications
Ortho-Gynest Cream is indicated for the treatment of atrophic vaginitis and kraurosis vulvae in post menopausal women, and for the treatment of pruritus vulvae and dyspareunia when associated with atrophic vaginal epithelium.

4.2 Posology and method of administration
For intravaginal use only.

The recommended initial daily dose is one applicatorful (0.5 mg estriol) inserted high into the vagina, preferably in the evening.

The lowest dose that will control symptoms should be chosen and medication should be discontinued as promptly as possible. Attempts to discontinue medication should be made at three to six month intervals following physical examination.

4.3 Contraindications
Although publications indicate that estriol may occupy a somewhat different position with respect to mammary and endometrial carcinomas than other oestrogens, contraindications for treatment with Ortho-Gynest Cream should be the same as for other oestrogen products.

Oestrogens should not be used in women with any of the following conditions:

- Known or suspected cancer of the breast
- Known or suspected oestrogen-dependent neoplasia
- Undiagnosed abnormal genital bleeding
- Active thrombophlebitis
- A past history of thrombophlebitis
- Active deep venous thrombosis, thrombo-embolic disorders, or a history of confirmed venous thrombo-embolism
- Markedly impaired liver function
- Congenital or existing disorder of lipid metabolism
- History during pregnancy of idiopathic jaundice
- Severe pruritus
- Herpes gestationis or otosclerosis
- Dubin-Johnson syndrome
- Rotor syndrome
- Pregnancy
- Hypersensitivity to arachis oil or peanuts

4.4 Special warnings and special precautions for use
Ortho-Gynest Cream contains arachis oil (peanut oil) and should not be applied by patients known to be allergic to peanuts (see Section 4.3). As there is a possible relationship between allergy to peanuts and allergy to soya, patients with soya allergy should also avoid Ortho-Gynest Cream.

Assessment of each woman prior to using hormone replacement therapy (and at regular intervals thereafter) should include a personal and family medical history. Physical examination should be guided by this and by the Contra-indications (Section 4.3) and Warnings (Section 4.4) for this product. During assessment of each individual woman clinical examination of the breasts and pelvic examination should be performed where clinically indicated rather than as a routine procedure. Women should be encouraged to participate in the national breast cancer screening programme (mammography) and the national cervical cancer screening programme (cervical cytology) as appropriate for their age. Breast awareness should also be encouraged and women advised to report any changes in their breasts to their doctor or nurse.

A pathologist should be advised of oestrogen therapy when relevant specimens are submitted.

If jaundice develops in any patient receiving oestrogen the medication should be discontinued while the cause is investigated.

Therapy should be discontinued immediately if pregnancy is suspected.

Oestrogen should be used with caution in patients with endometriosis.

Epidemiological studies have suggested that hormone replacement therapy (HRT) is associated with an increased relative risk of developing venous thrombo-embolism (VTE) ie deep vein thrombosis or pulmonary embolism. The studies found a 2-3 fold increase for users compared with non-users which for healthy women amounts to a low risk of one extra case of VTE each year for every 5000 patients taking HRT.

Generally recognised risk factors for VTE include a personal or family history and severe obesity (body mass index >30 kg/m^2). In women with these factors the benefits of treatment with HRT need to be carefully weighed against risks.

The risk of VTE may be temporarily increased with prolonged immobilisation, major trauma or major surgery. In women on HRT, scrupulous attention should be given to prophylactic measures to prevent VTE following surgery. Where prolonged immobilisation is liable to follow elective surgery, particularly abdominal or orthopaedic surgery to the lower limbs, consideration should be given to temporarily stopping HRT 4 weeks earlier, if this is possible.

If venous thrombo-embolism develops after initiating therapy the drug should be discontinued.

A re-analysis of original data from 51 epidemiological studies reported a small or moderate increase in the probability of having breast cancer *diagnosed* in women currently or recently using HRT. The findings may be due to biological effects of HRT, earlier diagnosis, or a combination of both. The relative risk increased with duration of treatment (by 2.3% per year of use) and returned to normal in the course of five years after cessation of HRT use. This is comparable to the increase in relative risk when natural menopause is delayed in the absence of HRT. Breast cancers diagnosed in current or recent users of HRT are more likely to be localised to the breast than those found in non-users. HRT use may not be associated with increased mortality from breast cancer.

Between the ages of 50 and 70, about 45 women in every 1,000 not using HRT will have breast cancer diagnosed. It is estimated that among those who use HRT for 5 years starting at age 50, 2 extra cases of breast cancer will be detected by age 70 in every 1,000 women. For those who use HRT for 10 years, there will be 6 extra cases of breast cancer, and for 15 years use, 12 extra cases of breast cancer in every 1,000 women during the 20 year period until age 70.

It is important that the increased risk of being diagnosed with breast cancer is discussed with the patient and weighed against the known benefits of HRT.

4.5 Interaction with other medicinal products and other forms of Interaction

Contact between contraceptive diaphragms or condoms and the cream must be avoided since the rubber may be damaged by this preparation.

4.6 Pregnancy and lactation

Ortho-Gynest Cream is contra-indicated in pregnancy.

4.7 Effects on ability to drive and use machines

None known.

4.8 Undesirable effects

– An increased risk of gall-bladder disease has been reported in women receiving post-menopausal oestrogens.

– Prolonged exposure to unopposed oestrogens may increase the risk of development of endometrial carcinoma.

– Benign hepatic adenomas appear to be associated with the use of oral contraceptives and although rare, these may rupture and cause death through intra-abdominal haemorrhage. Such lesions have not yet been reported in association with other oestrogen or progestogen preparations but should be considered in oestrogen users having abdominal pain and tenderness, abdominal mass or hypovolaemic shock.

– Elevated blood pressure may occur with the use of oestrogens in menopausal women.

– Oestrogens may aggravate cases of porphyria.

– Certain patients may develop undesirable manifestations of excessive oestrogenic stimulation such as abnormal or excessive uterine bleeding, mastodynia, etc. Pre-existing uterine fibroids may increase in size during oestrogen use.

– Patients with a past history of jaundice during pregnancy have an increased risk of recurrence of jaundice while receiving oestrogen therapy.

4.9 Overdose

Ortho-Gynest Cream is intended for intravaginal use. If accidental ingestion of large quantities of the product occurs, an appropriate method of gastric emptying may be used if considered desirable.

5. PHARMACOLOGICAL PROPERTIES

5.1 Pharmacodynamic properties

Estriol is a naturally occurring oestrogen which exerts specific effects on the vulva, vagina and cervix.

5.2 Pharmacokinetic properties

Estriol is rapidly absorbed from the vaginal mucosa. Peak plasma levels are reached within two hours and remain elevated for at least six hours.

5.3 Preclinical safety data

No relevant information additional to that contained elsewhere in the Summary of Product Characteristics.

6. PHARMACEUTICAL PARTICULARS

6.1 List of excipients

Benzoic acid

Arachis oil

Glyceryl monostearate

Glycerin

Glutamic acid

Purified water

6.2 Incompatibilities

None known.

6.3 Shelf life

2 years.

6.4 Special precautions for storage

Store at room temperature (not exceeding 25°C).

6.5 Nature and contents of container

Aluminium tube with screw cap containing 80 g [or 78]* cream supplied with a plastic vaginal applicator.

* not currently marketed.

6.6 Instructions for use and handling

The following instructions will appear in the Patient Information Leaflet.

How to apply the cream:

Ortho-Gynest Cream comes with a plastic applicator to be screwed onto the tube to help you put the right amount in your vagina.

1. Remove the cap from the tube and use the top of the cap to pierce the metal seal on the tube.

2. One end of the applicator has a plunger fitted. Screw the other end of the applicator onto the tube. Squeeze the tube so that the barrel of the applicator is completely filled with cream.

[Figure]

3. Unscrew the filled applicator and replace the cap on the tube.

4. Lie down, with knees bent and spread apart. Gently insert the open end of the applicator well into your vagina. Push the plunger firmly but gently as far as it will go to empty the cream into your vagina.

[Figure]

5. Keeping the plunger pressed firmly down, grip the applicator by the barrel and remove the empty applicator.

Keep the applicator clean

Clean it after each use with mild soap and warm (not boiling) water. Rinse it well. The plunger can be pulled free from the barrel to make cleaning easier. Simply pull the plunger out as far as possible and give it a sharp tug.

[Figure]

To put the applicator together again, insert the tip of the plunger into the barrel and push the plunger firmly.

If you lose or break the applicator you can get a new one from the pharmacist. Ask for the Ortho® Vaginal Applicator.

7. MARKETING AUTHORISATION HOLDER

Janssen-Cilag Limited

Saunderton

High Wycombe

Buckinghamshire

HP14 4HJ

UK

8. MARKETING AUTHORISATION NUMBER(S)

PL 00242/0249

9. DATE OF FIRST AUTHORISATION/RENEWAL OF THE AUTHORISATION

1 September 1995

10. DATE OF REVISION OF THE TEXT

December 2004

Legal category POM

Ortho-Gynest Pessaries

(Janssen-Cilag Ltd)

1. NAME OF THE MEDICINAL PRODUCT

ORTHO-GYNEST Pessaries.

2. QUALITATIVE AND QUANTITATIVE COMPOSITION

Estriol 0.5 mg.

3. PHARMACEUTICAL FORM

Pessary.

4. CLINICAL PARTICULARS

4.1 Therapeutic indications

1. Treatment of atrophic vaginitis and kraurosis vulvae in post-menopausal women.

2. Treatment of pruritus vulvae and dyspareunia associated with atrophic vaginal epithelium.

4.2 Posology and method of administration

For intravaginal administration.

The recommended initial dose is one pessary inserted daily high into the vagina, preferably in the evening. A maintenance dose of one pessary twice a week may be used after restoration of the vaginal mucosa has been achieved.

The lowest dose that will control symptoms should be chosen and medication should be discontinued as promptly as possible. Attempts to taper and discontinue medication should be made at three to six month intervals following physical examination.

4.3 Contraindications

Although publications indicate that estriol may occupy a somewhat different position with respect to mammary and endometrial carcinomas than other estrogens, contra-indications for treatment with Ortho-Gynest should be the same as for other estrogen products.

Estrogens should not be used in women with any of the following conditions: Known or suspected cancer of the breast, known or suspected estrogen-dependent neoplasia, undiagnosed abnormal genital bleeding, active thrombophlebitis or thrombo-embolic disorders, a past history of thrombophlebitis, active deep venous thrombosis, thrombo-embolic disorders, or a history of confirmed venous thromboembolism. Markedly impaired liver function. Congenital or existing disorders of lipid metabolism. History during pregnancy of idiopathic jaundice, severe pruritus, herpes gestationis or otosclerosis. Dubin-Johnson Syndrome. Rotor Syndrome. Pregnancy.

4.4 Special warnings and special precautions for use

Assessment of each woman prior to using hormone replacement therapy (and at regular intervals thereafter) should include a personal and family medical history. Physical examination should be guided by this and by the Contra-indications (Section 4.3) and Warnings (Section 4.4) for this product. During assessment of each individual woman clinical examination of the breasts and pelvic examination should be performed where clinically indicated rather than as a routine procedure. Women should be encouraged to participate in the national breast cancer screening programme (mammography) and the national cervical cancer screening programme (cervical cytology) as appropriate for their age. Breast awareness should also be encouraged and women advised to report any changes in their breasts to their doctor or nurse.

A pathologist should be advised of estrogen therapy when relevant specimens are submitted.

If jaundice develops in any patient receiving estrogen, the medication should be discontinued while the cause is investigated.

Therapy should be discontinued immediately if pregnancy is suspected.

Epidemiological studies have suggested that hormone replacement therapy (HRT) is associated with an increased relative risk of developing venous thrombo-embolism (VTE), ie deep vein thrombosis or pulmonary embolism. The studies find a 2-3 fold increase for users compared with non-users which for healthy women amounts to a low risk of one extra case of VTE each year for every 5,000 patients taking HRT.

Generally recognised risk factors for VTE include a personal or family history and severe obesity (body mass index >30 kg/m^2). In women with these factors the benefits of treatment with HRT need to be carefully weighed against risks.

The risk of VTE may be temporarily increased with prolonged immobilisation, major trauma or major surgery. In women on HRT scrupulous attention should be given to prophylactic measures to prevent VTE following surgery. Where prolonged immobilisation is liable to follow elective surgery, particularly abdominal or orthopaedic surgery to the lower limbs, consideration should be given to temporarily stopping HRT 4 weeks earlier, if this is possible.

If venous thrombo-embolism develops after initiating therapy the drug should be discontinued.

A re-analysis of original data from 51 epidemiological studies reported a small or moderate increase in the probability of having breast cancer *diagnosed* in women currently or recently using HRT. The findings may be due to biological effects of HRT, earlier diagnosis, or a combination of both. The relative risk increased with duration of treatment (by 2.3% per year of use) and returned to normal in the course of five years after cessation of HRT use. This is comparable to the increase in relative risk when natural menopause is delayed in the absence of HRT. Breast cancers diagnosed in current or recent users of HRT are more likely to be localised to the breast than those found in non-users. HRT use may not be associated with increased mortality from breast cancer.

Between the ages of 50 and 70, about 45 women in every 1,000 not using HRT will have breast cancer diagnosed. It is estimated that among those who use HRT for 5 years starting at age 50, 2 extra cases of breast cancer will be detected by age 70 in every 1,000 women. For those who use HRT for 10 years, there will be 6 extra cases of breast cancer, and for 15 years use, 12 extra cases of breast cancer in every 1,000 women during the 20 year period until age 70.

It is important that the increased risk of being diagnosed with breast cancer is discussed with the patient and weighed against the known benefits of HRT.

4.5 Interaction with other medicinal products and other forms of Interaction

None known.

4.6 Pregnancy and lactation

Ortho-Gynest Pessaries are contra-indicated in pregnancy.

4.7 Effects on ability to drive and use machines

None known.

4.8 Undesirable effects

An increased risk of gall bladder disease has been reported in women receiving post-menopausal estrogens.

Prolonged exposure to unopposed estrogens may increase the risk of development of endometrial carcinoma.

Benign hepatic adenomas appear to be associated with the use of oral contraceptives and, although rare, these may rupture and cause death through intra-abdominal haemorrhage. Such lesions have not yet been reported in association with other estrogen or progestogen preparations, but should be considered in estrogen users having abdominal pain and tenderness, abdominal mass or hypovolaemic shock.

Elevated blood pressure may occur with the use of estrogens in menopausal women.

Estrogens may aggravate cases of porphyria.

Certain patients may develop undesirable manifestations of excessive estrogenic stimulation such as abnormal or excessive uterine bleeding, mastodynia, etc. Pre-existing uterine fibroids may increase in size during estrogen use.

Patients with a past history of jaundice during pregnancy have an increased risk of recurrence of jaundice while receiving estrogen therapy.

4.9 Overdose
If accidental ingestion of large quantities of the product occurs, an appropriate method of gastric emptying may be used if considered desirable.

5. PHARMACOLOGICAL PROPERTIES

5.1 Pharmacodynamic properties
Estriol is a naturally occurring estrogen which exerts specific actions on the vulva, vagina and cervix.

5.2 Pharmacokinetic properties
Estriol is rapidly absorbed from the vaginal mucosa. Peak plasma estriol levels are achieved within 2 hours of therapy and remain elevated for at least 6 hours in the recumbent patient.

5.3 Preclinical safety data
There are no pre-clinical data of relevance to the prescriber which are additional to that already included in other sections of the Summary of Product Characteristics.

6. PHARMACEUTICAL PARTICULARS

6.1 List of excipients
Benzoic acid

Butylated hydroxytoluene

Polyethylene glycol 400

Polyethylene glycol 1000

Sorbitan monostearate

Witepsol S 55

6.2 Incompatibilities
None known.

6.3 Shelf life
Three years.

6.4 Special precautions for storage
Store at room temperature (maximum 25°C).

6.5 Nature and contents of container
PVC or PVC/PE moulds, containing 5 or 15 pessaries.

6.6 Instructions for use and handling
None.

7. MARKETING AUTHORISATION HOLDER
Janssen-Cilag Ltd

Saunderton

High Wycombe

Buckinghamshire

HP14 4HJ

UK

8. MARKETING AUTHORISATION NUMBER(S)
0242/0250

9. DATE OF FIRST AUTHORISATION/RENEWAL OF THE AUTHORISATION
Date of First Authorisation: 1 December 1995

10. DATE OF REVISION OF THE TEXT
December 2004

Legal category POM.

Orudis

(sanofi-aventis)

1. NAME OF THE MEDICINAL PRODUCT
Orudis

2. QUALITATIVE AND QUANTITATIVE COMPOSITION
In terms of the active ingredient

Capsules each containing 50mg Ketoprofen. Capsules each containing 100mg Ketoprofen.

3. PHARMACEUTICAL FORM
Capsules

4. CLINICAL PARTICULARS

4.1 Therapeutic indications
Recommended in the management of rheumatoid arthritis, osteoarthritis, ankylosing spondylitis, acute articular and periarticular disorders, (bursitis, capsulitis, synovitis, tendinitis), cervical spondylitis, low back pain (strain, lumbago, sciatica, fibrositis), painful musculoskeletal conditions, acute gout, dysmenorrhoea and control of pain and inflammation following orthopaedic surgery.

Orudis reduces joint pain and inflammation and facilitates increase in mobility and functional independence.

It does not cure the underlying disease.

4.2 Posology and method of administration
Oral dosage 50 - 100mg twice daily, morning and evening, depending on patient's weight and on the severity of symptoms.

Best results are obtained by titrating dosage to suit each patient: start with a low dosage in mild chronic disease and a high dosage in acute or severe disease. Some patients derive greater benefit by treatment with capsules only, some with a combined capsule/suppository regimen and others with a higher dosage at night time than at early morning. Where patients require a maximum oral dosage initially, an attempt should be made to reduce this dosage for maintenance since lower dosage might be better tolerated for purposes of long-term treatment.

Elderly: The elderly are at increased risk of the serious consequences of adverse reactions. If an NSAID is considered necessary, the lowest dose should be used and the patient should be monitored for GI bleeding for 4 weeks following initiation of NSAID therapy.

Paediatric dosage: Not established.

To limit occurrence of gastrointestinal disturbance, capsules should always be taken with food (milk, meals).

4.3 Contraindications
Active peptic ulceration, a history of recurrent peptic ulceration or chronic dyspepsia, severe renal dysfunction, disease in children (safety/dosage during long-term treatment has not been established).

Orudis should not be given to patients who have previously shown hypersensitivity reactions (e.g. asthma, rhinitis or urticaria) in response to ketoprofen, any of the other ingredients contained, or to aspirin, ibuprofen or other non-steroidal anti-inflammatory agents. As with other non-steroidal anti-inflammatory agents, severe bronchospasm might be precipitated in these subjects, and in patients suffering from or with a history of, bronchial asthma or allergic disease.

4.4 Special warnings and special precautions for use
Ketoprofen should be used with caution in patients with renal, hepatic or cardiac impairment. Inhibition of renal prostaglandin synthesis by non-steroidal anti-inflammatory agents may interfere with renal function especially in the presence of existing renal disease. The dose should be kept as low as possible and renal function should be monitored in these patients. NSAIDs should be given with care to patients with a history of heart failure or hypertension since oedema has been reported in association with ibuprofen administration.

Caution is required if NSAIDs are administered to patients suffering from, or with a previous history of, bronchial asthma, since ibuprofen has been reported to cause bronchospasm in such patients.

NSAIDs should only be given with care to patients with a history of gastrointestinal disease.

Orudis capsules should always be prescribed "to be taken with food" to minimise gastric intolerance.

Undesirable effects may be minimised by using the minimum effective dose for the shortest possible duration.

4.5 Interaction with other medicinal products and other forms of Interaction
Orudis is highly protein-bound. Concomitant use of other protein-binding drugs e.g. anticoagulants, sulphonamides, hydantoins, might necessitate modification of dosage in order to avoid increased levels of such drugs resulting from competition for plasma protein-binding sites.

Similar acting drugs such as aspirin or other NSAIDS should not be administered concomitantly with ketoprofen as the potential for adverse reactions is increased.

Serious interactions have been recorded after the use of high dose methotrexate with non-steroidal anti-inflammatory agents including ketoprofen. Decreased elimination of methotrexate has been reported.

NSAIDs should not be used for 8-12 days after mifepristone administration as NSAIDs can reduce the effect of mifepristone.

Care should be taken in patients treated with any of the following drugs, as interactions with NSAIDs have been reported in some patients:

Antihpertensives: Reduced antihypertensive effect.

Diuretics: Reduced diuretic effect. Diuretics can increase the risk of nephrotoxicity of NSAIDs.

Cardiac glycosides: NSAIDs may exacerbate cardiac failure, reduce GFR and increase plasma glycoside levels.

Lithium: Decreased elimination of lithium.

Cyclosporin: Increased risk of nephrotoxicity.

Corticosteroids: Increased risk of GI bleeding.

Quinolone antibiotics: Animal data indicate that NSAIDs can increase the risk of convulsions associated with quinolone antibiotics. Patients taking NSAIDs and quinolones may have an increased risk of developing convulsions.

4.6 Pregnancy and lactation
No embryopathic effects have been demonstrated in animals and there is epidemiological evidence of the safety of ketoprofen in human pregnancy. Nevertheless, it is recommended to avoid ketoprofen unless considered essential, in which case it should be discontinued within one week of expected confinement when NSAIDS might cause premature closure of the ductus arteriosus or persistent pulmonary hypertension in the neonate. They may also delay labour.

Trace amounts of ketoprofen are excreted in breast milk. Avoid use of ketoprofen unless considered essential.

4.7 Effects on ability to drive and use machines
CNS side effects have been observed in some patients (see section 4.8). If affected patients should not drive or operate machinery.

4.8 Undesirable effects
Adverse effects: minor adverse effects, frequently transient, consist for the most part of gastrointestinal effects such as indigestion, dyspepsia, nausea, vomiting, constipation, diarrhoea, heartburn and various types of abdominal discomfort. Other minor effects such as ulcerative stomatitis, headache, dizziness, mild confusion, vertigo, malaise, fatigue, drowsiness, paraesthesia, oedema, mood change and insomnia may occur less commonly.

Major gastrointestinal adverse effects such as melaena, haematemesis, peptic ulceration, gastrointestinal haemorrhage or perforation, may rarely occur.

Less commonly reported major adverse effects involving other organ systems include:

Hypersensitivity: Hypersensitivity reactions have been reported following treatment with NSAIDs. These may consist of non-specific allergic reactions and anaphylaxis; respiratory tract reactivity comprising asthma, aggravated asthma, bronchospasm or dyspnoea; or skin disorders, including rashes, pruritus, urticaria, purpura, angioedema and, less commonly, bullous dermatoses (including epidermal necrolysis and erythema multiforme).

Renal: Nephrotoxicity, including interstitial nephritis, nephrotic syndrome and renal failure.

Hepatic: Abnormal liver function, hepatitis and jaundice.

Neurological and special senses: Hallucinations, visual disturbances, optic neuritis, tinnitus.

Haematological: Thrombocytopenia, neutropenia, agranulocytosis, aplastic anaemia and haemolytic anaemia.

Dermatological: Photosensitivity, exfoliative dermatitis

As with other NSAIDs, rare cases of colitis, proctitis and ulcerative colitis have been reported. In such an event, all NSAID drugs, including ketoprofen, should be discontinued.

In all cases of major adverse effects Orudis should be withdrawn at once.

4.9 Overdose
Like other propionic acid derivatives, ketoprofen is of low toxicity in overdosage. Symptoms after acute ketoprofen intoxication are largely limited to drowsiness, abdominal pain and vomiting, but adverse effects seen after overdosage with propionic acid derivatives such as hypotension, bronchospasm and gastro-intestinal haemorrhage should be anticipated. Gastric lavage and correction of severe electrolyte abnormalities may need to be considered. Treatment is otherwise supportive and symptomatic.

5. PHARMACOLOGICAL PROPERTIES

5.1 Pharmacodynamic properties
Ketoprofen overall has the properties of a potent non-steroidal anti-inflammatory agent. It has the following pharmacological effects.

Anti-inflammatory

It inhibits the development of carageenan-induced abscesses in rats at 1mg/kg and

UV-radiation induced erythema in guinea pigs at 6mg/kg. It is also a potent inhibitor of PGE_2 and PGF_2 synthesis in guinea pigs and human chopped lung preparations.

Analgesic

Ketoprofen effectively reduced visceral pain in mice caused by phenyl benzoquinone or by bradykinin following P.O. administration at about 6mg/kg.

Antipyretic

Ketoprofen (2 and 6mg/kg) inhibited hyperthermia caused by s.c. injection of brewer's yeast in rats and, at 1mg/kg, hyperthermia caused by i.v. administration of antigonococcal vaccine to rabbits.

Ketoprofen at 10mg/kg i.v. did not affect the cardiovascular, respiratory, central nervous system or autonomic nervous systems.

5.2 Pharmacokinetic properties
Ketoprofen is completely absorbed from Orudis capsules and maximum plasma concentrations occur after ½ - 1 hour. It declines thereafter with a elimination half-life of about 2 - 3 hours. There is no accumulation on continued daily dosing.

5.3 Preclinical safety data
No additional data of relevance to the prescriber

6. PHARMACEUTICAL PARTICULARS

6.1 List of excipients

Lactose	BP
Magnesium Stearate	BP

Capsule shells (Elanco & Scherer)

Opaque purple cap

Brilliant Blue FCF (E133)

Erythrosine (E127)

Titanium Dioxide (E171)

Gelatin

Opaque green base

Brilliant Blue FCF (E133)

Yellow iron Oxide (E172)

Titanium Dioxide (E171)

Gelatin

Capsule shells (Capsulgel)

Opaque purple cap

Patent Blue V (E131)

Erythrosine (E127)

Titanium Dioxide (E171)

Gelatin

Opaque green base

Yellow iron Oxide (E172)

Patent Blue V (E131)

Titanium Dioxide (E171)

Gelatin

6.2 Incompatibilities
None stated

6.3 Shelf life
60 months

6.4 Special precautions for storage
Store in a dry place below 25C

Blister pack only - Store in a dry place below 25C. Protect from light.

6.5 Nature and contents of container
Securitainer or HDPE bottle containing 500 or 100 capsules

Cardboard carton containing blister packs of 56 or 112 capsules

6.6 Instructions for use and handling
None stated

7. MARKETING AUTHORISATION HOLDER
Hawgreen Ltd

4 Priory Hall

Stillorgan Road

Stillorgan

County Dublin

8. MARKETING AUTHORISATION NUMBER(S)
50mg capsules 17077 / 0015

100mg capsules 17077 / 0016

9. DATE OF FIRST AUTHORISATION/RENEWAL OF THE AUTHORISATION
01/09/98

10. DATE OF REVISION OF THE TEXT
January 2002

11. LEGAL CLASSIFICATION
POM

Orudis Suppositories 100mg

(sanofi-aventis)

1. NAME OF THE MEDICINAL PRODUCT
Orudis Suppositories 100mg

2. QUALITATIVE AND QUANTITATIVE COMPOSITION
In terms of the active ingredient

Ketoprofen BP 100 mg

3. PHARMACEUTICAL FORM
Suppository

4. CLINICAL PARTICULARS

4.1 Therapeutic indications
Orudis is a potent non steroidal anti-inflammatory analgesic agent and strong inhibitor of prostaglandin synthetase.

Orudis is recommended in the management of rheumatoid arthritis, osteoarthritis, ankylosing spondilitis, acute articular and peri-articular disorders (bursitis, capsulitis, synovitis, tendinitis), cervical spondylitis, low back pain (strain, lumbago, sciatica, fibrositis), painful musculo-skeletal conditions, acute gout and control of pain and inflammation following orthopaedic surgery.

Orudis reduces joint pain and inflammation and facilitates increase in mobility and functional independence. As with other non-steroidal anti-inflammatory agents, it does not cure the underlying disease.

4.2 Posology and method of administration
Rectal dosage is one suppository (100 mg) late at night supplemented as required with Orudis capsules during daytime.

Elderly: The elderly are at increased risk of the serious consequences of adverse reactions. If an NSAID is considered necessary, the lowest dose should be used and the patient should be monitored for GI bleeding for 4 weeks following initiation of NSAID therapy.

Paediatric dosage is not established.

Route of administration is rectal.

4.3 Contraindications
Active peptic ulceration, a history of recurrent peptic ulceration or chronic dyspepsia, severe renal dysfunction, disease in children (safety/dosage during long term treatment has not been established).

Orudis should not be given to patients who have previously shown hypersensitivity reactions (e.g. asthma, rhinitis or urticaria) in response to ketoprofen, any of the other ingredients contained, or to aspirin, ibuprofen or other non-steroidal anti-inflammatory agents. As with other non-steroidal anti-inflammatory agents, severe bronchospasm might be precipitated in these subjects, and in patients suffering from or with a history of, bronchial asthma or allergic disease.

Suppositories should not be used following recent proctitis or in association with haemorroids.

4.4 Special warnings and special precautions for use
Ketoprofen should be used with caution in patients with renal, hepatic or cardiac impairment. Inhibition of renal prostaglandin synthesis by non-steroidal anti-inflammatory agents may interfere with renal function especially in the presence of existing renal disease. The dose should be kept as low as possible and renal function should be monitored in these patients. NSAIDs should be given with care to patients with a history of heart failure or hypertension since oedema has been reported in association with NSAID administration.

Caution is required if NSAIDs are administered to patients suffering from, or with a previous history of, bronchial asthma, since NSAIDs have been reported to cause bronchospasm in such patients.

NSAIDs should only be given with care to patients with a history of gastrointestinal disease.

Undesirable effects may be minimised by using the minimum effective dose for the shortest possible duration.

4.5 Interaction with other medicinal products and other forms of Interaction
Ketoprofen is highly protein bound. Concomitant use of other protein-binding drugs e.g. anticoagulants, sulphonamides, hydantoins, might necessitate modification of dosage in order to avoid increased levels of such drugs resulting from competition for plasma protein-binding sites.

Similar acting drugs such as aspirin or other NSAIDs should not be administered concomitantly with ketoprofen as the potential for adverse reactions is increased.

Serious interactions have been recorded after the use of high dose methotrexate with non-steroidal anti-inflammatory agents, including ketoprofen. Decreased elimination of methotrexate has been reported.

NSAIDs should not be used for 8-12 days after mifepristone administration as NSAIDs can reduce the effect of mifepristone.

Care should be taken in patients treated with any of the following drugs, as interactions with NSAIDs have been reported in some patients:

Antihypertensives: Reduced anti-hypertensive effect.

Diuretics: Reduced diuretic effect. Diuretics can increase the risk of nephrotoxicity of NSAIDs.

Cardiac glycosides: NSAIDs may exacerbate cardiac failure, reduce GFR and increase plasma glycoside levels.

Lithium: Decreased elimination of lithium.

Cyclosporin: Increased risk of nephrotoxicity.

Corticosteroids: Increased risk of GI bleeding.

Anticoagulants: Enhanced anticoagulant effect.

Quinolone antibiotics: Animal data indicate that NSAIDs can increase the risk of convulsions associated with quinolone antibiotics. Patients taking NSAIDs and quinolones may have an increased risk of developing convulsions.

4.6 Pregnancy and lactation
No embryopathic effects have been demonstrated in animals and there is epidemiological evidence of the safety of ketoprofen in human pregnancy. Nevertheless, it is recommended to avoid ketoprofen unless considered essential in which case it should be discontinued within one week of expected confinement when NSAIDs might cause premature closure of the ductus arteriosus or persistent pulmonary hypertension in the neonate. They may also delay labour.

Trace amounts of ketoprofen are excreted in breast milk. Avoid use of ketoprofen unless it is considered essential.

4.7 Effects on ability to drive and use machines
CNS side effects have been observed in some patients (see section 4.8). If affected patients should not drive or operate machinery.

4.8 Undesirable effects
Adverse effects: minor adverse effects, frequently transient, consist for the most part of gastrointestinal effects such as indigestion, dyspepsia, nausea, vomiting, constipation, diarrhoea, heartburn and various types of abdominal discomfort. Other minor effects, such as, headache, dizziness, mild confusion, vertigo, drowsiness, oedema, mood change and insomnia may occur less commonly.

Major gastrointestinal adverse effects such as ulcerative stomatitis, melaena, haematemesis, peptic ulceration, gastrointestinal haemorrhage, or perforation, gastritis, duodenal ulcer, gastric ulcer may rarely occur.

Less commonly reported major adverse effects involving other organ systems include:

Hypersensitivity: Hypersensitivity reactions have been reported following treatment with NSAIDs. These may consist of non-specific allergic reactions and anaphylaxis; respiratory tract reactivity comprising asthma, aggravated asthma, bronchospasm or dyspnoea; or skin disorders, including rashes of various types, pruritus, urticaria, purpura, angioedema and, less commonly, bullous dermatoses (including epidermal necrolysis and erythema multiforme, and exfoliative dermatitis).

Renal: Nephrotoxicity in various forms, including interstitial nephritis, nephrotic syndrome and renal failure.

Hepatic: Abnormal liver function, hepatitis and jaundice.

Neurological and special senses: Hallucinations, visual disturbances, optic neuritis, tinnitus, paraesthesia, malaise, fatigue, depression

Haematological: Thrombocytopenia, neutropenia, agranulocytosis, aplastic anaemia and haemolytic anaemia.

Dermatological: Photosensitivity

As with other NSAIDs, rare cases of colitis, proctitis and ulcerative colitis have been reported. In such an event, all NSAID drugs, including ketoprofen, should be discontinued.

In all cases of major effects Orudis should be withdrawn at once.

4.9 Overdose
Like other propionic acid derivatives, ketoprofen is of low toxicity in overdosage. Symptoms after acute ketoprofen intoxication are largely limited to drowsiness, abdominal pain and vomiting, but adverse effects seen after overdosage with propionic acid derivatives such as hypotension, bronchospasm and gastro-intestinal haemorrhage should be anticipated. Gastric lavage and correction of severe electrolyte abnormalities may need to be considered. Treatment is otherwise supportive and symptomatic.

5. PHARMACOLOGICAL PROPERTIES

5.1 Pharmacodynamic properties
Ketoprofen overall has the properties of a potent non-steroidal anti-inflammatory agent. It has the following pharmacological effects:

Anti-inflammatory

It inhibits the development of carageenan-induced abscesses in rats at 1mg/kg and UV-radiation induced erythema in guinea pigs at 6mg/kg. It is also a potent inhibitor of PGE_2 and PGF_2 synthesis in guinea pig and human chopped lung preparations.

Analgesic

Ketoprofen effectively reduced visceral pain in mice caused by phenyl benzoquinone or by bradykinin following p.o. administration at about 6mg/kg.

Antipyretic

Ketoprofen (2 and 6mg/kg) inhibited hyperthermia caused by s.c injection of brewer's yeast in rats and, at 1mg/kg hyperthermia caused by i.v. administration of antigonococcal vaccine to rabbits.

Ketoprofen at 10mg/kg i.v. did not affect the cardiovascular, respiratory, central nervous system or autonomic nervous systems.

5.2 Pharmacokinetic properties
The bioavailability of ketoprofen from the suppository formulation (1 × 100 mg suppositories) has been compared with that from the capsule formulation (2 × 50 mg capsules). The results indicated that there was no significant difference between the bioavailability of the two dosage forms. It is for this reason that toxicological studies by the oral route are considered relevent to the present application for Orudis suppositories.

Ketoprofen is completely absorbed from Orudis capsules and maximum plasma concentrations occur after - 1 hour. It declines thereafter with an elimination half life of about 2-3 hours. There is no acculmulation on daily dosing.

5.3 Preclinical safety data
No additional pre-clinical data of relevance to the prescriber.

6. PHARMACEUTICAL PARTICULARS

6.1 List of excipients
Hydrophobic Silica

Hard Fat EP

6.2 Incompatibilities
None stated

6.3 Shelf life
36 months

6.4 Special precautions for storage
Store in a dry place below 25°C

6.5 Nature and contents of container
Cardboard carton containing sealed PVC/polyethylene laminate, 2 × 5 suppositories

6.6 Instructions for use and handling
None stated

7. MARKETING AUTHORISATION HOLDER
Hawgreen Ltd
4 Priory Hall
Stillorgan Road
Stillorgan
County Dublin

8. MARKETING AUTHORISATION NUMBER(S)
PL 17077/0017

9. DATE OF FIRST AUTHORISATION/RENEWAL OF THE AUTHORISATION
12 November 1991

10. DATE OF REVISION OF THE TEXT
January 2002

11. LEGAL CLASSIFICATION
POM

Oruvail

(sanofi-aventis)

1. NAME OF THE MEDICINAL PRODUCT
Oruvail

2. QUALITATIVE AND QUANTITATIVE COMPOSITION
Oruvail 100 contain in terms of the active ingredient Ketoprofen BP 100 mg

Oruvail 150 contain in terms of the active ingredient Ketoprofen BP 150 mg

Oruvail 200 contain in terms of the active ingredient Ketoprofen BP 200 mg

3. PHARMACEUTICAL FORM
Controlled release capsules

4. CLINICAL PARTICULARS

4.1 Therapeutic indications
Oruvail is recommended in the management of rheumatoid arthritis, osteoarthritis, ankylosing spondylitis, acute articular and peri-articular disorders, (bursitis, capsulitis, synovitis, tendinitis), cervical spondylitis, low back pain (strain, lumbago, sciatica, fibrositis), painful musculo-skeletal conditions, acute gout, dysmenorrhoea and control of pain and inflammation following orthopaedic surgery.

Oruvail reduces joint pain and inflammation and facilitates increase in mobility and functional independence. As with other non-steroidal anti-inflammatory agents, it does not cure the underlying disease.

4.2 Posology and method of administration
Adults: 100 - 200mg once daily, depending on patient weight and on severity of symptoms.

Elderly: The elderly are at increased risk of the serious consequences of adverse reactions. If an NSAID is considered necessary, the lowest dose should be used and the patient should be monitored for GI bleeding for 4 weeks following initiation of NSAID therapy.

Paediatric dosage not established.

Oruvail capsules are for oral administration. To be taken preferably with or after food.

4.3 Contraindications
Active peptic ulceration, a history of recurrent peptic ulceration or chronic dyspepsia, severe renal dysfunction.

Oruvail should not be given to patients who have previously shown hypersensitivity reactions (e.g. asthma, rhinitis or urticaria) in response to ketoprofen, any of the other ingredients contained, or to aspirin, ibuprofen or other non-steroidal anti-inflammatory agents. As with other non-steroidal anti-inflammatory agents, severe bronchospasm might be precipitated in these subjects, and in patients suffering from or with a history of, bronchial asthma or allergic disease.

4.4 Special warnings and special precautions for use
Ketoprofen should be used with caution in patients with renal, hepatic or cardiac impairment. Inhibition of renal prostaglandin synthesis by non-steroidal anti-inflammatory agents may interfere with renal function especially in the presence of existing renal disease. The dose should be kept as low as possible and renal function should be monitored in these patients. NSAIDs should be given with care to patients with a history of heart failure or hypertension since oedema has been reported in association with NSAID administration.

Caution is required if NSAIDs are administered to patients suffering from, or with a previous history of, bronchial asthma, since NSAIDs have been reported to cause bronchospasm in such patients.

NSAIDs should only be given with care to patients with a history of gastrointestinal disease. Oruvail capsules should always be prescribed, "to be taken with food" to minimise gastric intolerance

Undesirable effects may be minimised by using the minimum effective dose for the shortest possible duration.

4.5 Interaction with other medicinal products and other forms of Interaction
Ketoprofen is highly protein bound, concomitant use of other protein-binding drugs e.g. anticoagulants, sulphonamides, hydantoins, might necessitate modification of dosage in order to avoid increased levels of such drugs resulting from competition for plasma protein-binding sites.

Similar acting drugs such as aspirin or other NSAIDS should not be administered concomitantly with ketoprofen as the potential for adverse reactions is increased.

Serious interactions have been recorded after the use of high dose methotrexate with non-steroidal anti-inflammatory agents, including ketoprofen. Decreased elimination of methotrexate has been reported.

NSAIDs should not be used for 8-12 days after mifepristone administration as NSAIDs can reduce the effect of mifepristone.

Care should be taken in patients treated with any of the following drugs, as interactions with NSAIDs have been reported in some patients:

Antihpertensives: Reduced anti-hypertensive effect.

Diuretics: Reduced diuretic effect. Diuretics can increase the risk of nephrotoxicity of NSAIDs.

Cardiac glycosides: NSAIDs may exacerbate cardiac failure, reduce GFR and increase plasma glycoside levels.

Lithium: Decreased elimination of lithium.

Cyclosporin: Increased risk of nephrotoxicity.

Corticosteroids: Increased risk of GI bleeding.

Anticoagulants: Enhanced anticoagulant effect.

Quinolone antibiotics: Animal data indicate that NSAIDs can increase the risk of convulsions associated with quinolone antibiotics. Patients taking NSAIDs and quinolones may have an increased risk of developing convulsions.

4.6 Pregnancy and lactation
No embryopathic effects have been demonstrated in animals and there is epidemiological evidence of the safety of ketoprofen in human pregnancy. Nevertheless, it is recommended to avoid ketoprofen unless considered essential in which case it should be discontinued within one week of expected confinement when NSAIDS might cause premature closure of the ductus arteriosus or persistent pulmonary hypertension in the neonate. They may also delay labour.

Trace amounts of ketoprofen are excreted in breast milk. Avoid use of ketoprofen unless it is considered essential

4.7 Effects on ability to drive and use machines
CNS side effects have been observed in some patients (see section 4.8). If affected patients should not drive or operate machinery.

4.8 Undesirable effects
Adverse effects: minor adverse effects, frequently transient, consist for the most part of gastrointestinal effects such as indigestion, dyspepsia, nausea, vomiting, constipation, diarrhoea, heartburn and various types of abdominal discomfort. Other minor effects, such as, headache, dizziness, mild confusion, vertigo, drowsiness, oedema, mood change and insomnia may occur less commonly.

Major gastrointestinal adverse effects such as ulcerative stomatitis, melaena, haematemesis, peptic ulceration, gastrointestinal haemorrhage, or perforation, gastritis, duodenal ulcer, gastric ulcer may rarely occur.

Less commonly reported major adverse effects involving other organ systems include:

Hypersensitivity: Hypersensitivity reactions have been reported following treatment with NSAIDs. These may consist of non-specific allergic reactions and anaphylaxis; respiratory tract reactivity comprising asthma, aggravated asthma, bronchospasm or dyspnoea; or skin disorders, including rashes of various types, pruritus, urticaria, purpura, angioedema and, less commonly, bullous dermatoses (including epidermal necrolysis and erythema multiforme, and exfoliative dermatitis).

Renal: Nephrotoxicity in various forms, including interstitial nephritis, nephrotic syndrome and renal failure.

Hepatic: Abnormal liver function, hepatitis and jaundice.

Neurological and special senses: Hallucinations, visual disturbances, optic neuritis, tinnitus, paraesthesia, malaise, fatigue, depression

Haematological: Thrombocytopenia, neutropenia, agranulocytosis, aplastic anaemia and haemolytic anaemia.

Dermatological: Photosensitivity

As with other NSAIDs, rare cases of colitis, proctitis and ulcerative colitis have been reported. In such an event, all NSAID drugs, including ketoprofen, should be discontinued.

In all cases of major effects Oruvail should be withdrawn at once.

4.9 Overdose
Like other propionic acid derivatives, ketoprofen is of low toxicity in overdosage; symptoms after acute ketoprofen intoxication are largely limited to drowsiness, abdominal pain and vomiting, but adverse effects seen after overdosage with propionic acid derivatives such as hypotension, bronchospasm and gastro-intestinal haemorrhage should be anticipated.

Owing to the slow release characteristics of Oruvail, it should be expected that ketoprofen will continue to be absorbed for up to 16 hours after ingestion.

Gastric lavage, aimed at recovering pellets that may still be in the stomach should be performed if the patient is seen soon after ingestion. It should be possible to identify the pellets in the gastric contents. Correction of severe electrolyte abnormalities may need to be considered. Treatment is otherwise supportive and symptomatic.

Administration of activated charcoal in an attempt to reduce absorption of slowly-released ketoprofen should be considered

5. PHARMACOLOGICAL PROPERTIES

5.1 Pharmacodynamic properties
Ketoprofen overall has the properties of a potent non-steroidal anti- inflammatory agent. It has the following pharmacological effects:

Anti-inflammatory

It inhibits the development of carageenan-induced abscesses in rats at 1mg/kg, UV-radiation induced erythema in guinea pigs at 6mg/kg. It is also a potent inhibitor of PGE_2 and PFG_2 synthesis in guinea pig and human chopped lung preparations.

Analgesic

Ketoprofen effectively reduced visceral pain in mice caused by phenyl benzoquinone or by bradykinin following p.o. Administration at about 6mg/kg.

Antipyretic

Ketoprofen (2 and 6mg/kg) inhibited hyperthermia caused by s.c injection of brewer's yeast in rats and, at 1mg/kg hyperthermia caused by i.v. administration of anticoagulant vaccine to rabbits.

Ketoprofen at 10mg/kg i.v. did not affect the cardiovascular, respiratory, central nervous system or autonomic nervous systems.

5.2 Pharmacokinetic properties
Ketoprofen is slowly but completely absorbed from Oruvail capsules. Maximum plasma concentration occurs after 6 - 8 hours. It declines thereafter with a half-life of about 8 hours. There is no accumulation on continued daily dosing. Ketoprofen is very highly bound to plasma protein

5.3 Preclinical safety data
No additional data of relevance to the prescriber

6. PHARMACEUTICAL PARTICULARS

6.1 List of excipients

Pellets	
Sugar Spheres	NF
Colloidal Silicon Dioxide	EP
Shellac	NF
Ethyl Cellulose	NF
Talc	EP
Capsule shell - body	
Erythrocine (EEC 127)	
Gelatin	
Capsule shell - Cap	
Erythrocine (EEC 127)	
Patent Blue V (EEC 131)	
Titanium Dioxide (EEC 171)	
Gelatin	

6.2 Incompatibilities
None stated

6.3 Shelf life
36 months

6.4 Special precautions for storage
Securitainer / HDPE bottle: Store below 30°C in a dry place.

Blister pack: Store below 25°C in a dry place and protect from light.

6.5 Nature and contents of container
Securitainer or HDPE bottle containing 100 capsules.

UPVC/Aluminium foil blister or UPVC coated with PVDC aluminium foil blister containing either 28 or 4 capsules

6.6 Instructions for use and handling
None stated

7. MARKETING AUTHORISATION HOLDER
Hawgreen Limited

4 Priory Hall

Stillorgan Road

Stillorgan

County Dublin

Ireland

8. MARKETING AUTHORISATION NUMBER(S)
Oruvail 100 PL 17077/0020

Oruvail 150 PL 17077/0018

Oruvail 200 PL 17077/0019

9. DATE OF FIRST AUTHORISATION/RENEWAL OF THE AUTHORISATION
01/09/98

10. DATE OF REVISION OF THE TEXT
January 2002

11. LEGAL CLASSIFICATION:
POM

Oruvail Gel 2.5%

(sanofi-aventis)

1. NAME OF THE MEDICINAL PRODUCT
Oruvail™ Gel 2.5%.

2. QUALITATIVE AND QUANTITATIVE COMPOSITION
Ketoprofen BP 2.5% w/w.

3. PHARMACEUTICAL FORM
Gel.

4. CLINICAL PARTICULARS
4.1 Therapeutic indications
Ketoprofen is a non-steroidal anti-inflammatory drug. It has anti-inflammatory and analgesic actions.

Indications recommended for packs supplied within Pharmacy only legal status
Relief of backache, muscular pain and rheumatic pain, sprains and strains.

Relief of musculoskeletal pain and swelling caused by sports injuries.

Pain of non serious arthritis.

Indications recommended when prescribed by a physician as a Prescription Only Medicine
Relief of acute painful musculoskeletal conditions caused by trauma, such as sports injuries, sprains, strains and contusions.

Pain of non serious arthritis.

4.2 Posology and method of administration
Recommended dose and dosage schedule for packs supplied with Pharmacy only legal status
Adults: Apply a thin layer of gel to the affected area three times a day for up to 7 days. After the gel is applied it should be rubbed in well.

Elderly: As above.

Children: Not to be applied to children under 12 year of age.

Recommended dose and dosage schedule when prescribed by a physician as a Prescription Only Medicine
Adults: To be applied two to four times daily to the skin in the painful or inflamed region for up to 7 days. Apply gently but massage well to ensure gel penetration. The usual recommended dose is 15g per day (7.5 grams correspond to approximately 14cm of gel).

Elderly: There are no specific dosage recommendations for the elderly.

Children: Not recommended as safety in children has not been established.

4.3 Contraindications
Patients with a known hypersensitivity to ketoprofen or any of the excipients, aspirin or other non-steroidal anti-inflammatory agents; patients suffering from or with a history of bronchial asthma or allergic disease. Oruvail gel should be avoided in patients with exudative dermatoses, eczema, sores and infected skin lesions or broken skin. Oruvail gel should not be applied to mucous membranes, anal or genital areas, eyes or used with occlusive dressings.

4.4 Special warnings and special precautions for use
Although systemic effects are minimal, the gel should be used with caution in patients with severe renal impairment. Should a skin rash occur after gel application, treatment must be stopped. Do not apply Oruvail gel beneath occlusive dressings. Areas of skin treated with Oruvail gel should not be exposed directly to sunlight, or solarium ultraviolet light, either during treatment or for two weeks following treatment discontinuation. Keep the gel away from naked flames. Do not incinerate.

4.5 Interaction with other medicinal products and other forms of Interaction
Interactions are unlikely as serum concentrations following topical administration are low.

Serious interactions have been recorded after the use of high dose methotrexate with non-steroidal anti-inflammatory agents, including ketoprofen, when administered by the systemic route.

4.6 Pregnancy and lactation
No embryopathic effects have been demonstrated in animals and there is epidemiological evidence of the safety of ketoprofen in human pregnancy. Nevertheless, it is recommended that ketoprofen should be avoided during pregnancy. Non-steroidal anti-inflammatory drugs may also delay labour.

Trace amounts of ketoprofen are excreted in breast milk, therefore Oruvail Gel should not be used during breast feeding.

4.7 Effects on ability to drive and use machines
None known.

4.8 Undesirable effects
Adverse reactions: Skin reactions, including photosensitivity reactions, pruritus, localised erythema. These are usually mild and resolve after cessation of the gel. Cases of more severe reactions such as bullous or phylcytenar eczema which may spread or become generalised have occurred rarely.

4.9 Overdose
Overdose is unlikely by topical administration.

If accidentally ingested, the gel may cause systemic adverse effects depending on the amount ingested. However, if they occur, treatment should be supportive and symptomatic.

5. PHARMACOLOGICAL PROPERTIES
5.1 Pharmacodynamic properties
Ketoprofen is a non-steroidal anti-inflammatory drug. It has anti-inflammatory and analgesic actions.

5.2 Pharmacokinetic properties
Plasma and tissue levels of ketoprofen have been measured in 24 patients undergoing knee surgery. After repeated percutaneous administration of Oruvail gel the plasma levels were about 60 fold less (9 - 39 ng/g) than those obtained after a single oral dose of ketoprofen (490 - 3300 ng/g). Tissue levels at the area of application were within the same concentration range for the gel as for the oral treatment, although the gel was associated with a considerably higher inter-individual variability.

The bioavailability of ketoprofen after topical administration has been estimated to be approximately 5% of the level obtained after an orally administered dose, based on urinary excretion data.

The protein binding in plasma is approximately 99%. Ketoprofen is excreted through the kidneys mainly as glucuronide conjugate.

5.3 Preclinical safety data
No additional pre-clinical data of relevance to the prescriber.

6. PHARMACEUTICAL PARTICULARS
6.1 List of excipients
Carbopol, Triethanolamine, Lavender Oil, Ethanol and Purified water.

6.2 Incompatibilities
The gel should not be diluted.

6.3 Shelf life
36 months.

6.4 Special precautions for storage
Do not store above 25°C.

6.5 Nature and contents of container
Cardboard carton containing aluminium tube internally coated with polycondensed epoxyphenol varnish with the tip sealed with the same material containing either 30 or 100g of gel.

6.6 Instructions for use and handling
Wash your hands following application.

Keep gel away from naked flames.

Do not incinerate.

The tube should be closed after use.

7. MARKETING AUTHORISATION HOLDER
Rhone-Poulenc Rorer

RPR House

50 Kings Hill Avenue

Kings Hill

West Malling

Kent

ME19 4AH

8. MARKETING AUTHORISATION NUMBER(S)
PL 00012/0243

9. DATE OF FIRST AUTHORISATION/RENEWAL OF THE AUTHORISATION
28 July 1997

10. DATE OF REVISION OF THE TEXT
May 2003

11. Legal Category
POM for pack sizes larger than 30g.

P for pack sizes up to and including 30g.

Oruvail I.M. Injection

(sanofi-aventis)

1. NAME OF THE MEDICINAL PRODUCT
Oruvail IM Injection

2. QUALITATIVE AND QUANTITATIVE COMPOSITION
In terms of the active ingredient

Ketoprofen BP 100mg in 2 ml.

3. PHARMACEUTICAL FORM
Solution for IM injection

4. CLINICAL PARTICULARS
4.1 Therapeutic indications
Oruvail injection is recommended in the management of acute exacerbations of:

- Rheumatoid arthritis, osteoarthritis, ankylosing spondylitis.
- Periarticular conditions such as fibrositis, bursitis, capsulitis, tendinitis and tenosynovitis.
- Low back pain of musculoskeletal origin and sciatica.
- Other painful musculoskeletal conditions.
- Acute gout.
- Control of pain and inflammation following orthopaedic surgery.

4.2 Posology and method of administration
Adults: 50 to 100 mg every four hours, repeated up to a maximum of 200 mg in twenty-four hours. Following a satisfactory response, oral therapy should be instituted with Oruvail capsules. It is recommended that the injection should not normally be continued for longer than three days.

Elderly: As with other medications it is generally advisable in the elderly to begin ketoprofen therapy at the lower end of the dose range and to maintain such patients on the lowest effective dosage.

Paediatric dosage: not established.

Oruvail IM Injection is for intramuscular injection. It must not be given intravenously.

4.3 Contraindications
Active peptic ulceration, a history of recurrent peptic ulceration or chronic dyspepsia, severe renal dysfunction, sensitivity to aspirin or other non-steroidal anti-inflammatory agents.

4.4 Special warnings and special precautions for use
Inhibition of renal prostaglandin synthesis by non-steroidal anti-inflammatory agents may interfere with renal function especially in the presence of existing renal disease. Ketoprofen should therefore be used with caution in patients with renal impairment.

Severe bronchospasm might be precipitated in patients with a history of bronchial asthma or allergic disease.

Oruvail injection must not be given intravenously.

4.5 Interaction with other medicinal products and other forms of Interaction
Ketoprofen is highly protein bound. Concomitant use of other protein-binding drugs e.g. anticoagulants, sulphonamides, hydantoins, might necessitate modification of dosage in order to avoid increased levels of such drugs resulting from competition for plasma protein-binding sites.

Similar acting drugs such as aspirin or other NSAIDs should not be administered concomitantly with ketoprofen as the potential for adverse reactions is increased.

Serious interactions have been recorded after the use of high dose methotrexate with non-steroidal anti-inflammatory agents, including ketoprofen.

4.6 Pregnancy and lactation
No embryopathic effects have been demonstrated in animals and there is epidemiological evidence of the safety of ketoprofen in human pregnancy. Nevertheless, it is recommended to avoid ketoprofen unless considered essential in which case it should be discontinued within one week of expected confinement when NSAIDs might cause premature closure of the ductus arteriosus or persistent pulmonary hypertension in the neonate. They may also delay labour.

Trace amounts of ketoprofen are excreted in breast milk. Avoid use of ketoprofen unless it is considered essential.

4.7 Effects on ability to drive and use machines
CNS side effects have been observed in some patients (see section 4.8). If affected patients should not drive or operate machinery.

4.8 Undesirable effects
Adverse effects: minor adverse effects, frequently transient, consist for the most part of gastrointestinal effects such as indigestion, dyspepsia, nausea, constipation, diarrhoea, heartburn and various types of abdominal

discomfort. Other minor effects, such as headache, dizziness, mild confusion, vertigo, drowsiness, oedema, mood change and insomnia may occur less commonly.

Major gastrointestinal adverse effects such as peptic ulceration, haemorrhage, or perforation may rarely occur.

Major adverse effects involving other organ systems such as haematological reactions including thrombocytopenia, hepatic or renal damage, dermatological and photosensitivity reactions, bronchospasm and anaphylaxis are exceedingly rare.

Local reactions can occur and may include pain or a burning sensation. In all cases of major adverse effects Oruvail should be withdrawn at once.

4.9 Overdose

Like other propionic acid derivatives, ketoprofen is of low toxicity in overdosage. Symptoms after acute ketoprofen intoxication are largely limited to drowsiness, abdominal pain and vomiting, but adverse effects seen after overdosage with propionic acid derivatives such as hypotension, bronchospasm and gastro-intestinal haemorrhage should be anticipated. Treatment is otherwise supportive and symptomatic.

5. PHARMACOLOGICAL PROPERTIES

5.1 Pharmacodynamic properties

Ketoprofen is a pharmacopoeial non-steroidal anti-inflammatory drug (NSAID). It is a strong inhibitor of prostaglandin synthetase and potent analgesic agent. Studies in vitro and in vivo show that ketoprofen possesses powerful anti-inflammatory, antipyretic, antibradykinin and lysosomal membrane stabilising properties.

5.2 Pharmacokinetic properties

Peak concentrations of approximately 10 mg/L are reached at about 0.5-0.75 H after a 100 mg dose. The elimination half life is approximately 1.88 H. Apart from earlier Tmax values, there are no significant differences between the pharmacokinetics of Oruvail IM injection and conventional release capsules (Orudis).

5.3 Preclinical safety data

No additional data of relevance to the prescriber.

6. PHARMACEUTICAL PARTICULARS

6.1 List of excipients

Arginine	BP
Benzyl Alcohol	BP
Citric Acid anhydrous (E330)	BP
Water For Injections	BP

6.2 Incompatibilities

None stated

6.3 Shelf life

36 months

6.4 Special precautions for storage

Store below 30°C. Protect from light.

6.5 Nature and contents of container

Cartons containing 10 ampoules each having 2 ml. of injection.

6.6 Instructions for use and handling

None stated

7. MARKETING AUTHORISATION HOLDER

Hawgreen Limited
4 Priory Hall
Stillorgan Road
Stillorgan
County Dublin

8. MARKETING AUTHORISATION NUMBER(S)

PL 17077/0021

9. DATE OF FIRST AUTHORISATION/RENEWAL OF THE AUTHORISATION

1st September 1998

10. DATE OF REVISION OF THE TEXT

February 1997

Legal category: POM

Otosporin Ear Drops

(GlaxoSmithKline UK)

1. NAME OF THE MEDICINAL PRODUCT

Otosporin Ear Drops

2. QUALITATIVE AND QUANTITATIVE COMPOSITION

Polymyxin B Sulphate EP 10,000 units per ml
Neomycin Sulphate EP 3,400 units per ml
Hydrocortisone EP 1.0% w/v

3. PHARMACEUTICAL FORM

Liquid for topical application to humans

4. CLINICAL PARTICULARS

4.1 Therapeutic indications

Otosporin Ear Drops are indicated for the treatment of otitis externa due to, or complicated by, bacterial infection.

Route of Administration

Topical

In Vitro Activity

Otosporin Ear Drops are active against a wide range of bacterial pathogens. The range of activity includes:-

Gram-Positive Organisms:

Staphylococcus Epidermis and Staphylococcus Aureus:

Gram-Negative Organisms:

Enterobacter Spp.
Escherichia Spp.
Haemophilus Spp.
Klebsiella Spp.
Proteus Spp.
Pseudomonas Aeruginosa

Otosporin Ear Drops are not expected to be active against streptococci, including *Streptococcus Pyogenes*

Hydrocortisone possesses anti-inflammatory, anti-allergic and antipruritic activity.

4.2 Posology and method of administration

Adults

Following cleansing and drying of the external auditory meatus and canal as appropriate, three drops should be instilled into the affected ear three or four times daily. Alternatively, a gauze wick may be introduced into the external auditory canal and kept saturated with the solution; the wick may be left in place for 24 to 48 hours.

Treatment should not be continued for more than 7 days without medical supervision.

Soap should not be used for cleansing of the external auditory meatus and canal as it may inactivate the antibiotics.

Children

Otosporin Ear Drops are suitable for use in children (3 years and over) at the same dose as adults. A possibility of increased absorption exists in very young children, thus Otosporin Ear Drops are not recommended in neonates and infants (<3 years). (See 4.3 Contra-indications, 4.4 Special Warnings and Precautions for Use).

Use in the Elderly

As for adults. Caution should be exercised in cases where a decrease in renal function exists and significant systemic absorption of neomycin sulphate may occur (see 4.4 Special Warnings and Precautions for Use).

Use in Renal Impairment

Dosage should be reduced in patients with reduced renal function (see 4.4 Special Warnings and Precautions for Use).

4.3 Contraindications

The use of Otosporin Ear Drops is contra-indicated in patients in whom perforation of the tympanic membrane is known or suspected.

Due to the known ototoxic and nephrotoxic potential of neomycin sulphate, the use of Otosporin Ear Drops in large quantities or on large areas for prolonged periods of time is not recommended in circumstances where significant systemic absorption may occur.

The use of Otosporin Ear Drops is contra-indicated in patients who have demonstrated allergic hypersensitivity to any of the components of the preparation or to cross-sensitising substances such as framycetin, kanamycin, gentamicin and other related antibiotics.

The use of Otosporin Ear Drops is contra-indicated in the presence of untreated viral, fungal and tubercular infections.

A possibility of increased absorption exists in very young children, thus Otosporin Ear Drops are not recommended for use in neonates and infants (up to 3years). In neonates and infants, absorption by immature skin may be enhanced and renal function may be immature.

4.4 Special warnings and special precautions for use

Occasionally, delayed hypersensitivity to corticosteroids may occur. Treatment with topical steroid antibiotic combinations should not be continued for more than seven days in the absence of any clinical improvement, since prolonged use may lead to occult extension of infection due to the masking effect of the steroid. Prolonged use may also lead to skin sensitisation and the emergence of resistant organisms.

Following significant systemic absorption, aminoglycosides such as neomycin can cause irreversible ototoxicity; neomycin and polymyxin B sulphate have nephrotoxic potential and polymyxin B sulphate has neurotoxic potential.

All topically active corticosteroids possess the potential to suppress the pituitary-adrenal axis following systemic absorption. Development of adverse systemic effects due to the hydrocortisone component of Otosporin Ear Drops is considered to be unlikely, although the recommended dosage should not be exceeded, particularly in infants.

Prolonged, unsupervised, use should be avoided as it may lead to irreversible partial or total deafness, especially in the elderly and in patients with impaired renal function. In renal impairment the plasma clearance of neomycin is reduced (see Dosage in Renal Impairment).

Use in the immediate pre- and post- operative period is not advised as neomycin may rarely cause neuro-muscular block; because it potentiates skeletal muscle relaxant drugs, it may cause respiratory depression and arrest.

4.5 Interaction with other medicinal products and other forms of Interaction

Following significant systemic absorption, both neomycin sulphate and polymyxin b sulphate can intensify and prolong the respiratory depressant effects of neuromuscular blocking agents.

4.6 Pregnancy and lactation

There is little information to demonstrate the possible effect of topically applied neomycin in pregnancy and lactation. However, neomycin present in maternal blood can cross the placenta and may give rise to a theoretical risk of foetal toxicity thus use of Otosporin Ear Drops is not recommended in pregnancy or lactation.

4.7 Effects on ability to drive and use machines

None known.

4.8 Undesirable effects

The incidence of allergic hypersensitivity reactions to neomycin sulphate in the general population is low. There is, however, an increased incidence of hypersensitivity to neomycin in certain selected groups of patients in dermatological practice, particularly those with venous stasis eczema and ulceration, and chronic otitis externa.

Allergic hypersensitivity reactions following topical application of polymyxin B sulphate and hydrocortisone are rare.

Allergic hypersensitivity to neomycin following topical use may manifest itself as an eczematous exacerbation with reddening, scaling, swelling and itching or as a failure of the lesion to heal.

Stinging and burning have occasionally been reported when Otosporin Ear Drops gained access to the middle ear.

Otosporin Ear Drops should only be used in the ear and are not suitable for use in the eye.

4.9 Overdose

Symptoms and signs:-

Possible symptoms or signs associated with excessive use of Otosporin Ear Drops are those due to significant systemic absorption (see Special Warnings and Precautions for Use).

Management:-

Use of the product should be stopped and the patient's general status, hearing acuity, renal and neuromuscular functions should be monitored.

In overdose, blood concentrations of neomycin sulphate, and polymyxin B sulphate should be determined. Haemodialysis may reduce the serum level of neomycin sulphate.

5. PHARMACOLOGICAL PROPERTIES

5.1 Pharmacodynamic properties

Otosporin solution is a bactericidal preparation active against all the pathogens commonly found in bacterial infections of the ear. Polymyxin B is bactericidal against a wide range of gram negative bacilli including *Pseudomonas* Spp., *Escherichea coli*, *Enterobacter* Spp., *Klebsiella* Spp., and *Haemophilus influenzae*. It exerts a bactericidal effect by binding to acid phospholipids in the cell wall and membranes of the bacterium, thereby rendering ineffective the osmotic barrier normally provided by the cell membrane. This leads to escape of the cell contents and the death of the organism.

Neomycin sulphate is bactericidal against a wide range of gram positive and negative bacterial pathogens including *staphylococci, streptococci, Escherichia, Enterobacter, Klebsiella, Haemophilus, Proteus, Salmonella* and *Shigella* species. It is also active against some strains of the *pseudomonas aeruginosa* and against *mycobacterium tuberculosis* and *Neisseria gonorrhoea*. Neomycin exerts its bactericidal effect by interfering with the protein synthesis of susceptible organisms.

5.2 Pharmacokinetic properties

No data are available regarding the pharmacokinetics of this product. However since this is a topical preparation and significant systemic absorption is unlikely to occur, the data are irrelevant.

Systemically absorbed neomycin is predominantly excreted by the kidney and the total amount excreted in the urine varies between 30% and 50%. The pharmacokinetics of systemically absorbed polymyxin B has been described.

5.3 Preclinical safety data

None stated.

6. PHARMACEUTICAL PARTICULARS
6.1 List of excipients
Cetostearyl Alcohol EP
Sorbitan Laurate BP
Polysorbate 20 EP
Methyl Hydroxybenzoate EP
Dilute Sulphuric Acid BP
Purified Water EP

6.2 Incompatibilities
None known

6.3 Shelf life
36 months

6.4 Special precautions for storage
Protect from light
Store below 15°C

6.5 Nature and contents of container
Polypropylene bottles with integral nozzles and pilfer proof caps
5ml or 10ml pack sizes
Not all pack sizes may be marketed

6.6 Instructions for use and handling
None stated.

Administrative Data
7. MARKETING AUTHORISATION HOLDER
The Wellcome Foundation Ltd
Glaxo Wellcome House
Berkeley Avenue
Greenford
Middlesex
Trading as
GlaxoSmithKline UK
Stockley Park West
Uxbridge
Middlesex UB11 1BT

8. MARKETING AUTHORISATION NUMBER(S)
PL0003/5106R

9. DATE OF FIRST AUTHORISATION/RENEWAL OF THE AUTHORISATION
29/06/03

10. DATE OF REVISION OF THE TEXT
28/10/04

Otrivine
(Novartis Consumer Health)

1. NAME OF THE MEDICINAL PRODUCT
Otrivine Adult Nasal Drops
Otrivine Adult Nasal Spray
Otrivine Child Nasal Drops

2. QUALITATIVE AND QUANTITATIVE COMPOSITION
Otrivine Adult Nasal Drops/Otrivine Adult Nasal Spray (Xylometazoline Hydrochloride 0.1% w/v)
Otrivine Child Nasal Drops (Xylometazoline Hydrochloride 0.05% w/v)

3. PHARMACEUTICAL FORM
Otrivine Adult Nasal Drops/Otrivine Child Nasal Drops - Nasal drops, solution
Otrivine Adult Nasal Spray - Nasal spray, solution

4. CLINICAL PARTICULARS
4.1 Therapeutic indications
For the symptomatic relief of nasal congestion, perennial and allergic rhinitis (including hay fever), sinusitis.

4.2 Posology and method of administration
Otrivine Adult Nasal Drops - Adults, children over 12 years and the elderly: 2 or 3 drops in each nostril 2 or 3 times daily
Otrivine Adult Nasal Spray - Adults, children over 12 years and the elderly: One application in each nostril 2 or 3 times daily
Otrivine Child Nasal Drops - Children under 12 years: 1 or 2 drops in each nostril 1 or 2 times daily. Consult your doctor before use on infants under 2 years of age. Not to be used in infants less than 3 months of age.
Route of administration: Nasal use

4.3 Contraindications
Known hypersensitivity to Otrivine.
Patients with trans-sphenoidal hypophysectomy or surgery exposing the dura mater.

4.4 Special warnings and special precautions for use
Patients are advised not to take decongestants for more than seven consecutive days. Otrivine, like other preparations belonging to the same class of active substances, should be used only with caution in patients showing a strong reaction to sympathomimetic agents as evidenced by signs of insomnia, dizziness etc.

Otrivine Adult Nasal Drops/Otrivine Adult Nasal Spray/Otrivine Child Nasal Drops:
- Do not exceed the recommended dosage
- Decongestants should not be used for more than seven consecutive days. If symptoms persist consult your doctor
- Each Otrivine pack should be used by one person only to prevent any cross infection
- Some patients who have sensitive nasal passages may feel some local discomfort when applying nasal spray. Other side effects are very rare
- Keep medicines out of reach of children

Otrivine Adult Nasal Drops/Otrivine Adult Nasal Spray:
- If you are pregnant or taking other medicines or are under a doctor's care consult him before using Otrivine
- The adult drops or spray should not be used for infants or children under 12 years

Otrivine Child Nasal Drops:
- If your child is receiving medication or is under a doctor's care, consult him before giving Otrivine Child Nasal Drops
- Occasionally small children may show restlessness or sleep disturbance when Otrivine is used. If this occurs Otrivine should be stopped
- Expectant mothers should consult their doctors before using Otrivine for themselves

4.5 Interaction with other medicinal products and other forms of Interaction
None

4.6 Pregnancy and lactation
No foetal toxicity or fertility studies have been carried out in animals. In view of its potential systemic vasoconstrictor effect, it is advisable to take the precaution of not using Otrivine during pregnancy.
Otrivine Adult Nasal Drops/Otrivine Adult Nasal Spray – Label Warnings: If you are pregnant or taking any other medicines or are under a doctor's care, consult him before using Otrivine.
Otrivine Child Nasal Drops – Label Warnings: Expectant mothers should consult their doctor before using Otrivine for themselves.

4.7 Effects on ability to drive and use machines
None

4.8 Undesirable effects
The following side effects have occasionally been encountered: A burning sensation in the nose and throat, local irritation, nausea, headache, and dryness of the nasal mucosa.
Systemic cardiovascular effects have occurred, and this should be kept in mind when giving Otrivine to people with cardiovascular disease.

4.9 Overdose
No cases of overdosage in adults have yet been reported. In rare instances of accidental poisoning in children, the clinical picture has been marked chiefly by signs such as acceleration and irregularity of the pulse, elevated blood pressure, drowsiness, respiratory depression or irregularity. There is no specific treatment and appropriate supportive treatment should be initiated.

5. PHARMACOLOGICAL PROPERTIES
5.1 Pharmacodynamic properties
Otrivine is a sympathomimetic agent with marked alpha-adrenergic activity, and is intended for use in the nose. It constricts the nasal blood vessels, thereby decongesting the mucosa of the nose and neighbouring regions of the pharynx. This enables patients suffering from colds to breathe more easily through the nose. The effect of Otrivine begins within a few minutes and lasts for up to 10 hours. Otrivine is generally well tolerated and does not impair the function of ciliated epithelium.

5.2 Pharmacokinetic properties
Systemic absorption may occur following nasal application of xylometazoline hydrochloride solutions. It is not used systemically.

5.3 Preclinical safety data
There are no findings in the preclinical testing which are of relevance to the prescriber.

6. PHARMACEUTICAL PARTICULARS
6.1 List of excipients
Benzalkonium chloride, Sodium phosphate, Disodium edetate, Sodium acid phosphate, Sodium chloride, Sorbitol*, Hypromellose*, Water. *Not in Adult Spray

6.2 Incompatibilities
None

6.3 Shelf life
Unopened: 36 months (30 months for Menthol)
After the container is opened for the first time: 28 days

6.4 Special precautions for storage
Protect from heat

6.5 Nature and contents of container
Otrivine Adult and Otrivine Child Nasal Drops - Plastic bottle with pipette and bulb and protective cap in a cardboard carton.
Otrivine Adult Nasal Spray - Plastic bottle with spray plug and capillary in a cardboard carton.
Pack size: 10 ml

6.6 Instructions for use and handling
Keep all medicines out of the reach of children

7. MARKETING AUTHORISATION HOLDER
Novartis Consumer Health UK Limited
Wimblehurst Road
Horsham
West Sussex
RH12 5AB
Trading as: Novartis Consumer Health

8. MARKETING AUTHORISATION NUMBER(S)
Otrivine Adult Nasal Drops PL 00030/0115
Otrivine Adult Nasal Spray PL 00030/0116
Otrivine Child Nasal Drops PL 00030/0114

9. DATE OF FIRST AUTHORISATION/RENEWAL OF THE AUTHORISATION
Date of first authorisation: 1 October 1997

10. DATE OF REVISION OF THE TEXT
21 May 2001
Additional information
Legal category: GSL

Ovex Suspension
(Janssen-Cilag Ltd)

1. NAME OF THE MEDICINAL PRODUCT
OVEX SUSPENSION

2. QUALITATIVE AND QUANTITATIVE COMPOSITION
Each 5ml of suspension contains 100mg mebendazole.
For excipients, see section 6.1.

3. PHARMACEUTICAL FORM
Oral suspension
White homogeneous suspension

4. CLINICAL PARTICULARS
4.1 Therapeutic indications
For the treatment of gastrointestinal infestations of *Enterobius vermicularis* (threadworm).
There is no evidence that Ovex is effective in the treatment of cysticercosis.

4.2 Posology and method of administration
For oral administration.
Adults and children over 2 years: 1 × 5ml (1 dosing cup).
Care should be taken to avoid re-infection and it is strongly recommended that all members of the family are treated at the same time.
It is highly recommended that a second dose is taken after two weeks, if re-infection is suspected.

4.3 Contraindications
Ovex is contraindicated in pregnancy and in patients who have shown hypersensitivity to the product or any components.

4.4 Special warnings and special precautions for use
Ovex is not recommended in the treatment of children under 2 years. If symptoms do not disappear within a few days, consult your doctor.
A case-control studyof a single outbreak of Stevens-Johnson syndrome /toxic epidermal necrolysis (SJS/TEN) suggested a possible association with the concomitant use of metronidazole with mebendazole. Although there are no additional data on this potential interaction, concomitant use mebendazole and metronidazole should be avoided.

4.5 Interaction with other medicinal products and other forms of Interaction
Concomitant treatment with cimetidine may inhibit the metabolism of mebendazole in the liver, resulting in increased plasma concentrations of the drug.
Concomitant use of mebendazole and metronidazole should be avoided (see section 4.4).

4.6 Pregnancy and lactation
Use in pregnancy: Since Ovex is contra-indicated in pregnancy, patients who think they are or may be pregnant should not take this preparation.
Use in lactation: As it is not known whether mebendazole is excreted in human milk, it is not advisable to breast feed following administration of Ovex.

4.7 Effects on ability to drive and use machines
None known.

4.8 Undesirable effects
At the recommended dose, Ovex is generally well tolerated. However, patients with high parasitic burdens when treated with Ovex have manifested diarrhoea and abdominal pain.

Post-marketing experience

Within each system organ class, the adverse drug reactions are ranked under the headings of reporting frequency, using the following convention:

Very common >1/10) Common >1/100, < 1/10) Uncommon >1/1000, < 1/100) Rare >1/10000, < 1/1000) Very rare (< 1/10000) including isolated reports.

Immune system disorders

Very rare: hypersensitivity reactions such as anaphylactic and anaphylactoid reactions

Nervous system disorders

Very rare: convulsions in infants

Gastrointestinal disorders

Very rare: abdominal pain, diarrhoea (these symptoms can also be the result of the worm infestation itself)

Skin and subcutaneous tissue disorders

Very rare: toxic epidermal necrolysis, Stevens-Johnson syndrome (see also section 4.4), exanthema, angioedema, urticaria, rash

Adverse drug reactions reported with prolonged use at dosages substantially above those recommended

Liver function disturbances, hepatitis, glomerulonephritis and neutropenia.

4.9 Overdose

Symptoms

In the event of accidental overdosage, abdominal cramps, nausea, vomiting and diarrhoea may occur.

See also section 4.8. subheading 'Adverse drug reactions reported with prolonged use at dosages substantially above those recommended'.

Treatment

There is no specific antidote. Within the first hour after ingestion, gastric lavage may be performed. Activated charcoal may be given if considered appropriate.

5. PHARMACOLOGICAL PROPERTIES

5.1 Pharmacodynamic properties

Antinematodal agent: PO2C A01

In vitro and *in vivo* work suggests that mebendazole blocks the uptake of glucose by adult and larval forms of helminths, in a selective and irreversible manner. Inhibition of glucose uptake appears to lead to endogenous depletion of glycogen stores within the helminth. Lack of glycogen leads to decreased formation of ATP and ultrastructural changes in the cells.

There is no evidence that Ovex is effective in the treatment of cysticercosis.

5.2 Pharmacokinetic properties

Using a tracer dose of ^{3}H-mebendazole, the pharmacokinetics and bioavailability of a solution and iv drug have been examined. After oral administration the half-life was 0.93 hours. Absorption of this tracer dose was almost complete but low availability indicated a high first pass effect. At normal therapeutic doses it is very hard to measure levels in the plasma.

5.3 Preclinical safety data

Not applicable.

6. PHARMACEUTICAL PARTICULARS

6.1 List of excipients

Sucrose

Microcrystalline cellulose and sodium carboxymethyl cellulose

Methylcellulose 15 mPa.s

Methylparaben

Propylparaben

Sodium lauryl sulphate

Banana flavour 1

Citric acid, monohydrate

Purified water

6.2 Incompatibilities

Not applicable.

6.3 Shelf life

5 years.

6.4 Special precautions for storage

Keep out of the reach and sight of children.

6.5 Nature and contents of container

Amber glass flask containing 30 ml suspension, with either:

- Pilfer-proof screw cap. Cork insert in cap is coated on both sides with polyvinylchloride

or

- Child-resistant polypropylene screw cap, lined inside with a LDPE insert.

A 5ml natural polypropylene (food-grade) dosing cup is also provided, graduated for 2.5 ml and 5 ml.

6.6 Instructions for use and handling

Shake well before use.

7. MARKETING AUTHORISATION HOLDER

Janssen-Cilag Ltd
Saunderton
High Wycombe
Buckinghamshire
HP14 4HJ

8. MARKETING AUTHORISATION NUMBER(S)

PL 00242/0405

9. DATE OF FIRST AUTHORISATION/RENEWAL OF THE AUTHORISATION

24 November 2004

10. DATE OF REVISION OF THE TEXT

June 2005

Legal category P.

Ovex/Ovex Family Pack/Boots Threadworm Treatment.

(Janssen-Cilag Ltd)

1. NAME OF THE MEDICINAL PRODUCT

Ovex/Ovex Family Pack/Boots Threadworm Tablets.

2. QUALITATIVE AND QUANTITATIVE COMPOSITION

Mebendazole 100 mg.

3. PHARMACEUTICAL FORM

Tablet.

4. CLINICAL PARTICULARS

4.1 Therapeutic indications

For the treatment of gastrointestinal infestations of *Enterobius vermicularis* (threadworm).

There is no evidence that Ovex is effective in the treatment of cysticercosis.

4.2 Posology and method of administration

Ovex is for oral administration.

Adults and children over 2 years:

Take one tablet.

Tablets may be chewed or swallowed whole. Crush the tablet before giving it to a young child. Always supervise a child while they are taking this medicine. Care should be taken to avoid re-infection and it is strongly recommended that all members of the family are treated at the same time.

It is highly recommended that a second tablet is taken after two weeks, if re-infection is suspected.

4.3 Contraindications

Ovex is contra-indicated in pregnancy and in patients who have shown hypersensitivity to the product or any components.

4.4 Special warnings and special precautions for use

Ovex is not recommended in the treatment of children under 2 years.

If symptoms do not disappear within a few days, consult your doctor.

A case-control study of a single outbreak of Stevens-Johnson syndrome /toxic epidermal necrolysis (SJS/TEN) suggested a possible association with the concomitant use of metronidazole with mebendazole. Although there are no additional data on this potential interaction, concomitant use of mebendazole and metronidazole should be avoided.

4.5 Interaction with other medicinal products and other forms of Interaction

Concomitant treatment with cimetidine may inhibit the metabolism of mebendazole in the liver, resulting in increased plasma concentrations of the drug.

Concomitant use of mebendazole and metronidazole should be avoided (see section 4.4).

4.6 Pregnancy and lactation

Use in pregnancy

Since Ovex is contra-indicated in pregnancy patients who think they are or may be pregnant should not take this preparation.

Use in lactation

As it is not known whether mebendazole is excreted in human milk, it is not advisable to breast feed following administration of Ovex.

4.7 Effects on ability to drive and use machines

None known.

4.8 Undesirable effects

At the recommended dose, Ovex is generally well tolerated. However, patients with high parasitic burdens when treated with Ovex have manifested diarrhoea and abdominal pain.

Post-marketing experience

Within each system organ class, the adverse drug reactions are ranked under the headings of reporting frequency, using the following convention:

Very common >1/10) Common >1/100, < 1/10) Uncommon >1/1000, < 1/100) Rare >1/10000, < 1/1000) Very rare (< 1/10000) including isolated reports.

Immune system disorders

Very rare: hypersensitivity reactions such as anaphylactic and anaphylactoid reactions

Nervous system disorders

Very rare: convulsions in infants

Gastrointestinal disorders

Very rare: abdominal pain, diarrhoea (these symptoms can also be the result of the worm infestation itself)

Skin and subcutaneous tissue disorders

Very rare: toxic epidermal necrolysis, Stevens-Johnson syndrome (see also section 4.4), exanthema, angioedema, urticaria, rash

Adverse drug reactions reported with prolonged use at dosages substantially above those recommended

Liver function disturbances, hepatitis, glomerulonephritis and neutropenia.

4.9 Overdose

Symptoms

In the event of accidental overdosage, abdominal cramps, nausea, vomiting and diarrhoea may occur.

See also section 4.8. subheading 'Adverse drug reactions reported with prolonged use at dosages substantially above those recommended'.

Treatment

There is no specific antidote. Within the first hour after ingestion, gastric lavage may be performed. Activated charcoal may be given if considered appropriate.

5. PHARMACOLOGICAL PROPERTIES

5.1 Pharmacodynamic properties

In vitro and *in vivo* work suggests that mebendazole blocks the uptake of glucose by adult and larval forms of helminths, in a selective and irreversible manner. Inhibition of glucose uptake appears to lead to endogenous depletion of glycogen stores within the helminth. Lack of glycogen leads to decreased formation of ATP and ultrastructural changes in the cells.

There is no evidence that Ovex is effective in the treatment of cysticercosis.

5.2 Pharmacokinetic properties

Using a tracer dose of ^{3}H-mebendazole, the pharmacokinetics and bioavailability of a solution and iv drug have been examined. After oral administration the half-life was 0.93 hours. Absorption of this tracer dose was almost complete but low availability indicated a high first pass effect. At normal therapeutic doses it is very hard to measure levels in the plasma.

5.3 Preclinical safety data

Not applicable.

6. PHARMACEUTICAL PARTICULARS

6.1 List of excipients

Microcrystalline cellulose

Sodium starch glycollate

Talc

Maize starch

Sodium saccharin

Magnesium stearate

Cottonseed oil - hydrogenated

Orange flavour

Colloidal anhydrous silica

Sodium lauryl sulphate

Orange yellow S

Purified water*

2-propanol*

* not present in the final product

6.2 Incompatibilities

None known.

6.3 Shelf life

60 months.

6.4 Special precautions for storage

None.

6.5 Nature and contents of container

Blister pack: PVC genotherm glass clear and aluminium foil with heat seal lacquer.

Pack size: 1, 2, 4 and 8 tablets.

6.6 Instructions for use and handling

Not applicable.

7. MARKETING AUTHORISATION HOLDER

Janssen-Cilag Ltd
Saunderton
High Wycombe
Buckinghamshire
HP14 4HJ
UK

8. MARKETING AUTHORISATION NUMBER(S)

0242/0171

9. DATE OF FIRST AUTHORISATION/RENEWAL OF THE AUTHORISATION

23 August 1990/24 August 1995

10. DATE OF REVISION OF THE TEXT
June 2005

Legal category P.

Ovitrelle 250 micrograms

(Serono Ltd)

1. NAME OF THE MEDICINAL PRODUCT
Ovitrelle▼ 250 micrograms powder and solvent for solution for injection

2. QUALITATIVE AND QUANTITATIVE COMPOSITION
To ensure delivery of a 250 microgram dose, each vial contains 285 micrograms of choriogonadotropin alfa.

Choriogonadotropin alfa is produced by recombinant DNA technology in Chinese Hamster Ovary cells.

A dose of 250 micrograms is equivalent to approximately 6500 IU.

For excipients, see 6.1.

3. PHARMACEUTICAL FORM
Powder and solvent for solution for injection

4. CLINICAL PARTICULARS

4.1 Therapeutic indications
Ovitrelle is indicated in the treatment of

(i) Women undergoing superovulation prior to assisted reproductive techniques such as in vitro fertilisation (IVF): Ovitrelle is administered to trigger final follicular maturation and luteinisation after stimulation of follicular growth.

(ii) Anovulatory or oligo-ovulatory women: Ovitrelle is administered to trigger ovulation and luteinisation in anovulatory or oligo-ovulatory patients after stimulation of follicular growth

4.2 Posology and method of administration
Ovitrelle is intended for subcutaneous administration. The powder should be reconstituted immediately prior to use with the solvent provided.

Treatment with Ovitrelle should be performed under the supervision of a physician experienced in the treatment of fertility problems.

The following dosing regimen should be applied:

(i) Women undergoing superovulation prior to assisted reproductive techniques such as in vitro fertilisation (IVF):

One vial of Ovitrelle (250 micrograms) is administered 24 to 48 hours after the last administration of an FSH- or hMG preparation, i.e. when optimal stimulation of follicular growth is achieved.

(ii) Anovulatory or oligo-ovulatory women:

One vial of Ovitrelle (250 micrograms) is administered 24 to 48 hours after optimal stimulation of follicular growth is achieved. The patient is recommended to have coitus on the day of, and the day after, Ovitrelle injection.

4.3 Contraindications
Ovitrelle is contraindicated for safety reasons in case of:

- Tumours of the hypothalamus and pituitary gland
- Hypersensitivity to the active substance or to any of the excipients
- Ovarian enlargement or cyst due to reasons other than polycystic ovarian disease
- Gynaecological haemorrhages of unknown aetiology
- Ovarian, uterine or mammary carcinoma
- Extrauterine pregnancy in the previous 3 months
- Active thrombo-embolic disorders

Ovitrelle must not be used when an effective response cannot be obtained, for example:

- Primary ovarian failure
- Malformations of sexual organs incompatible with pregnancy
- Fibroid tumours of the uterus incompatible with pregnancy
- Postmenopausal women

4.4 Special warnings and special precautions for use
To date, there is no clinical experience with Ovitrelle in other indications commonly treated with urine derived human chorionic gonadotrophin.

Before starting treatment, the couple's infertility should be assessed as appropriate and putative contraindications for pregnancy evaluated. In particular, patients should be evaluated for hypothyroidism, adrenocortical deficiency, hyperprolactinemia and pituitary or hypothalamic tumours, and appropriate specific treatment given.

Special precautions should be taken before administering Ovitrelle to patients with clinically significant systemic disease where pregnancy could lead to a worsening of the condition.

Patients undergoing ovarian stimulation are at an increased risk of developing ovarian hyperstimulation syndrome (OHSS) due to multiple follicular development

Ovarian hyperstimulation syndrome may become a serious medical event characterised by large ovarian cysts which are prone to rupture and the presence of ascites within a clinical picture of circulatory dysfunction. Ovarian hyperstimulation syndrome due to excessive ovarian response can be avoided by withholding hCG administration. Patients should be advised to refrain from coitus or use barrier methods for at least 4 days.

Careful monitoring of estradiol levels and ovarian response, based on ultrasound is recommended prior to and during stimulation therapy, for all patients.

The risk of multiple pregnancy following assisted reproductive technologies is related to the number of embryos replaced. In patients undergoing induction of ovulation, the incidence of multiple pregnancies and births (mostly twins) is increased compared with natural conception.

To minimise the risk of OHSS and of multiple pregnancy, ultrasound scans as well as estradiol measurements are recommended. In anovulation, the risk of OHSS is increased by a serum estradiol level > 1500 pg/ml (5400 pmol/l) and more than 3 follicles of 14 mm or more in diameter. In assisted reproductive techniques, there is an increased risk of OHSS with a serum estradiol > 3000 pg/ml (11000 pmol/l) and 20 or more follicles of 12 mm or more in diameter. When the estradiol level is > 5500 pg/ml (20000 pmol/l) and when there are 40 or more follicles in total, it may be necessary to withhold hCG administration.

Adherence to recommended Ovitrelle dosage, regimen of administration and careful monitoring of therapy will minimise the incidence of ovarian hyperstimulation and multiple pregnancy.

The rate of miscarriage, in both anovulatory patients and women undergoing assisted reproductive techniques, is higher than that found in the normal population but comparable with the rates observed in women with other fertility problems.

Self-administration of Ovitrelle should only be performed by patients who are adequately trained and have access to expert advice.

4.5 Interaction with other medicinal products and other forms of Interaction
No clinically significant drug interactions have been reported during hCG therapy.

Following administration, Ovitrelle may interfere for up to ten days with the immunological determination of serum / urinary hCG, leading to a false positive pregnancy test.

During Ovitrelle therapy, a minor thyroid stimulation is possible, of which the clinical relevance is unknown.

4.6 Pregnancy and lactation
Considering the indication, Ovitrelle should not be used during pregnancy and lactation. For Ovitrelle no clinical data on exposed pregnancies are available. No reproduction studies with choriogonadotropin alfa in animals were performed (see 5.3). The potential risk for humans is unknown.

There are no data on the excretion of choriogonadotropin alfa in milk.

4.7 Effects on ability to drive and use machines
No studies on the effects on the ability to drive and use machines have been performed.

4.8 Undesirable effects
Ovitrelle is used to trigger final follicular maturation and early luteinisation after use of medicinal products for the stimulation of follicular growth. In this context, it is difficult to attribute undesirable effects to any one of the products used.

In comparative trials with different doses of Ovitrelle, the following undesirable effects were found to be associated with Ovitrelle in a dose-related fashion: ovarian hyperstimulation syndrome, and vomiting and nausea. Ovarian hyperstimulation syndrome was observed in approximately 4% of patients treated with Ovitrelle. Severe ovarian hyperstimulation syndrome was reported in less than 0.5% patients (section 4.4 Special warnings and special precautions for use).

In rare instances, thromboembolisms have been associated with menotrophin/hCG therapy. Although this adverse event was not observed, there is the possibility that this may also occur with Ovitrelle.

Ectopic pregnancy, ovarian torsion and other complications have been reported in patients after hCG administration. These are considered concomitant effects related to Assisted Reproductive Technologies (ART).

After best evidence assessment, the following undesirable effects may be observed after administration of Ovitrelle.

(i) Common >1/100, < 1/10)

Application site disorders: Local reaction/pain at injection site

General disorders: Headache, tiredness

Gastro-intestinal system disorders: Vomiting/nausea, abdominal pain

Reproductive disorders: Mild or moderate ovarian hyperstimulation syndrome

(ii) Uncommon >1/1000, <1/100)

Psychiatric disorders: Depression, irritability, restlessness

Gastro-intestinal system disorders: Diarrhoea

Reproductive disorders: Severe ovarian hyperstimulation syndrome, Breast pain

4.9 Overdose
No case of overdose has been reported.

Nevertheless, there is a possibility that ovarian hyperstimulation syndrome (OHSS) may result from an overdosage of Ovitrelle (see "4.4 Special warnings and special precautions for use").

5. PHARMACOLOGICAL PROPERTIES

5.1 Pharmacodynamic properties
Pharmacotherapeutic group: gonadotropins, ATC code: G03G A01

Ovitrelle is a medicinal product of chorionic gonadotropin produced by recombinant DNA techniques. It shares the amino acid sequence with urinary hCG. Chorionic gonadotropin binds on the ovarian theca (and granulosa) cells to a transmembrane receptor shared with the luteinising hormone, the LH/CG receptor.

The principal pharmacodynamic activity in women is oocyte meiosis resumption, follicular rupture (ovulation), corpus luteum formation and production of progesterone and estradiol by the corpus luteum.

In women, Chorionic gonadotropin acts as a surrogate LH-surge that triggers ovulation.

Ovitrelle is used to trigger final follicular maturation and early luteinisation after use of medicinal products for stimulation of follicular growth.

In comparative clinical trials, administration of a dose of 250 micrograms of Ovitrelle was as effective as 5000 IU and 10000 IU of urinary hCG in inducing final follicular maturation and early luteinisation in assisted reproductive techniques, and as effective as 5000 IU of urinary hCG in ovulation induction.

So far, there are no signs of antibody development in humans to Ovitrelle. Repeated exposure to Ovitrelle was investigated in male patients only. Clinical investigation in women for the indication of ART and anovulation was limited to one treatment cycle.

5.2 Pharmacokinetic properties
Following intravenous administration, choriogonadotropin alfa is distributed to the extracellular fluid space with a distribution half-life of around 4.5 hours. The steady-state volume of distribution and the total clearance are 6 l and 0.2 l/h, respectively. There are no indications that choriogonadotropin alfa is metabolised and excreted differently than endogenous hCG.

Following subcutaneous administration, choriogonadotropin alfa is eliminated from the body with a terminal half-life of about 30 hours, and the absolute bioavailability is about 40 %.

5.3 Preclinical safety data
Preclinical safety data reveal no intrinsic toxicity of choriogonadotropin alfa. Studies on carcinogenic potential were not performed. This is justified, given the proteinous nature of the active substance and the negative outcome of the genotoxicity testing.

Studies on reproduction were not performed in animals.

6. PHARMACEUTICAL PARTICULARS

6.1 List of excipients

Powder for solution for injection:

Sucrose

Phosphoric acid, concentrated

Sodium hydroxide

Solvent:

Water for injections

6.2 Incompatibilities
In the absence of compatibility studies, this medicinal product must not be mixed with other medicinal products.

6.3 Shelf life
2 years. For immediate and single use following first opening and reconstitution.

6.4 Special precautions for storage
Do not store above 25°C. Store in the original package.

6.5 Nature and contents of container
The powder container is a neutral colourless (type 1, Ph. Eur.) glass vial with a bromobutyl rubber stopper.

The solvent container is a neutral, colourless glass type 1 vial with a bromobutyl rubber stopper or a neutral, colourless glass type 1 ampoule.

The product is supplied in packs of 1, 2, 10 vials with the corresponding number of solvent containers.

6.6 Instructions for use and handling
Ovitrelle is for single use only. One vial of Ovitrelle can be reconstituted with 1 ml of the solvent before use. The reconstituted solution should not be administered if it contains particles or is not clear. Any unused product or waste material should be disposed of in accordance with local requirements.

7. MARKETING AUTHORISATION HOLDER
SERONO EUROPE LIMITED
56, Marsh Wall
London E14 9TP
United Kingdom

8. MARKETING AUTHORISATION NUMBER(S)

Authorisation number	Presentations
EU/1/00/165/001	Ovitrelle - 250 micrograms - powder and solvent for solution for injection – subcutaneous use – Powder: vial (glass), Solvent: ampoule (glass) – Powder: 250 micrograms, Solvent: 1 ml (250 micrograms/ml) – 1 vial + 1 ampoule
EU/1/00/165/002	Ovitrelle - 250 micrograms - powder and solvent for solution for injection – subcutaneous use – Powder: vial (glass), Solvent: ampoule (glass) – Powder: 250 micrograms, Solvent: 1 ml (250 micrograms/ml) – 2 vials + 2 ampoules
EU/1/00/165/003	Ovitrelle - 250 micrograms - powder and solvent for solution for injection – subcutaneous use – Powder: vial (glass), Solvent: ampoule (glass) – Powder: 250 micrograms, Solvent: 1 ml (250 micrograms/ml) – 10 vials + 10 ampoules
EU/1/00/165/004	Ovitrelle - 250 micrograms - powder and solvent for solution for injection – subcutaneous use – Powder: vial (glass), Solvent: vial (glass) – Powder: 250 micrograms, Solvent: 1 ml (250 micrograms/ml) – 1 vial + 1 vial
EU/1/00/165/005	Ovitrelle - 250 micrograms - powder and solvent for solution for injection – subcutaneous use – Powder: vial (glass), Solvent: vial (glass) – Powder: 250 micrograms, Solvent: 1 ml (250 micrograms/ml) – 2 vials + 2 vials
EU/1/00/165/006	Ovitrelle - 250 micrograms - powder and solvent for solution for injection – subcutaneous use – Powder: vial (glass), Solvent: vial (glass) – Powder: 250 micrograms, Solvent: 1 ml (250 micrograms/ml) – 10 vials + 10 vials

9. DATE OF FIRST AUTHORISATION/RENEWAL OF THE AUTHORISATION

2nd February 2001

10. DATE OF REVISION OF THE TEXT

20th July 2001

LEGAL STATUS

POM

NAME AND ADDRESS OF DISTRIBUTOR IN UK

Serono Pharmaceuticals Ltd

Bedfont Cross

Stanwell Road

Feltham

Middlesex

TW14 8NX

NAME AND ADDRESS OF DISTRIBUTOR IN IRELAND

Allphar Services Limited

Pharmaceutical Agents and Distributors

Belgard Road

Tallaght

Dublin 24

Ovitrelle 250 micrograms/0.5 ml prefilled syringe

(Serono Ltd)

1. NAME OF THE MEDICINAL PRODUCT

Ovitrelle® ▼ 250 micrograms/0.5ml, solution for injection in a pre-filled syringe

2. QUALITATIVE AND QUANTITATIVE COMPOSITION

Choriogonadotropin alfa*250 micrograms in 0.5ml. (equivalent to approximately 6500 IU)

* Produced by recombinant DNA technology in CHO

For excipients, see 6.1.

3. PHARMACEUTICAL FORM

Solution for injection

Clear colourless solution.

4. CLINICAL PARTICULARS

4.1 Therapeutic indications

Ovitrelle is indicated in the treatment of

(i) Women undergoing superovulation prior to assisted reproductive techniques such as in vitro fertilisation (IVF): Ovitrelle is administered to trigger final follicular maturation and luteinisation after stimulation of follicular growth.

(ii) Anovulatory or oligo-ovulatorywomen: Ovitrelle is administered to trigger ovulation and luteinisation in anovulatory or oligo-ovulatory patients after stimulation of follicular growth

4.2 Posology and method of administration

Ovitrelle is intended for subcutaneous administration.

Treatment with Ovitrelle should be performed under the supervision of a physician experienced in the treatment of fertility problems.

The following dosing regimen should be used:

Women undergoing superovulation prior to assisted reproductive techniques such as in vitro fertilisation (IVF):

One pre-filled syringe of Ovitrelle (250 micrograms) is administered 24 to 48 hours after the last administration of an FSH- or hMG preparation, i.e. when optimal stimulation of follicular growth is achieved.

Anovulatory or oligo-ovulatory women:

One pre-filled syringe of Ovitrelle (250 micrograms) is administered 24 to 48 hours after optimal stimulation of follicular growth is achieved. The patient is recommended to have coitus on the day of, and the day after, Ovitrelle injection.

4.3 Contraindications

Ovitrelle is contraindicated for safety reasons in case of:

- Tumours of the hypothalamus and pituitary gland
- Hypersensitivity to the active substance or to any of the excipients
- Ovarian enlargement or cyst due to reasons other than polycystic ovarian disease
- Gynaecological haemorrhages of unknown aetiology
- Ovarian, uterine or mammary carcinoma
- Extrauterine pregnancy in the previous 3 months
- Active thrombo-embolic disorders

Ovitrelle must not be used when an effective response cannot be obtained, for example:

- Primary ovarian failure
- Malformations of sexual organs incompatible with pregnancy
- Fibroid tumours of the uterus incompatible with pregnancy
- Postmenopausal women

4.4 Special warnings and special precautions for use

To date, there is no clinical experience with Ovitrelle in other indications commonly treated with urine derived human chorionic gonadotrophin.

Before starting treatment, the couple's infertility should be assessed as appropriate and putative contraindications for pregnancy evaluated. In particular, patients should be evaluated for hypothyroidism, adrenocortical deficiency, hyperprolactinemia and pituitary or hypothalamic tumours, and appropriate specific treatment given.

Special precautions should be taken before administering Ovitrelle to patients with clinically significant systemic disease where pregnancy could lead to a worsening of the condition.

Patients undergoing ovarian stimulation are at an increased risk of developing ovarian hyperstimulation syndrome (OHSS) due to multiple follicular development

Ovarian hyperstimulation syndrome may become a serious medical event characterised by large ovarian cysts which are prone to rupture and the presence of ascites within a clinical picture of circulatory dysfunction. Ovarian hyperstimulation syndrome due to excessive ovarian response can be avoided by withholding hCG administration. Patients should be advised to refrain from coitus or use barrier methods for at least 4 days.

Careful monitoring of estradiol levels and ovarian response, based on ultrasound is recommended prior to and during stimulation therapy, for all patients.

The risk of multiple pregnancy following assisted reproductive technologies is related to the number of embryos replaced. In patients undergoing induction of ovulation, the incidence of multiple pregnancies and births (mostly twins) is increased compared with natural conception.

To minimise the risk of OHSS and of multiple pregnancy, ultrasound scans as well as estradiol measurements are recommended. In anovulation, the risk of OHSS is increased by a serum estradiol level $>$ 1500 pg/ml (5400 pmol/l) and more than 3 follicles of 14 mm or more in diameter. In assisted reproductive techniques, there is an increased risk of OHSS with a serum estradiol $>$ 3000 pg/ml (11000 pmol/l) and 20 or more follicles of 12 mm or more in diameter. When the estradiol level is $>$ 5500 pg/ml (20000 pmol/l) and when there are 40 or more follicles in total, it may be necessary to withhold hCG administration.

Adherence to recommended Ovitrelle dosage, regimen of administration and careful monitoring of therapy will minimise the incidence of ovarian hyperstimulation and multiple pregnancy.

The rate of miscarriage, in both anovulatory patients and women undergoing assisted reproductive techniques, is higher than that found in the normal population but comparable with the rates observed in women with other fertility problems.

During Ovitrelle therapy, a minor thyroid stimulation is possible, of which the clinical relevance is unknown.

Self-administration of Ovitrelle should only be performed by patients who are adequately trained and have access to expert advice.

4.5 Interaction with other medicinal products and other forms of Interaction

No specific interaction studies with Ovitrelle and other medicines have been performed however no clinically significant drug interactions have been reported during hCG therapy. Following administration, Ovitrelle may interfere for up to ten days with the immunological determination of serum / urinary hCG, leading to a false positive pregnancy test.

4.6 Pregnancy and lactation

Considering the indication, Ovitrelle should not be used during pregnancy and lactation. For Ovitrelle no clinical data on exposed pregnancies are available. No reproduction studies with choriogonadotropin alfa in animals were performed (see 5.3). The potential risk for humans is unknown.

There are no data on the excretion of choriogonadotropin alfa in milk.

4.7 Effects on ability to drive and use machines

No studies on the effects on the ability to drive and use machines have been performed.

4.8 Undesirable effects

In comparative trials with different doses of Ovitrelle, the following undesirable effects were found to be associated with Ovitrelle in a dose-related fashion: ovarian hyperstimulation syndrome, and vomiting and nausea. Ovarian hyperstimulation syndrome was observed in approximately 4% of patients treated with Ovitrelle. Severe ovarian hyperstimulation syndrome was reported in less than 0.5% patients (section 4.4 Special warnings and special precautions for use).

In rare instances, thromboembolisms have been associated with menotrophin/hCG therapy. Although this adverse event was not observed, there is the possibility that this may also occur with Ovitrelle.

Ectopic pregnancy, ovarian torsion and other complications have been reported in patients after hCG administration. These are considered concomitant effects related to Assisted Reproductive Technologies (ART).

After best evidence assessment, the following undesirable effects may be observed after administration of Ovitrelle.

Common $>$1/100, $<$ 1/10)

Application site disorders: Local reaction/pain at injection site

General disorders: Headache, tiredness

Gastro-intestinal system disorders: Vomiting/nausea, abdominal pain

Reproductive disorders: Mild or moderate ovarian hyperstimulation syndrome

Uncommon $>$1/1000, $<$1/100)

Psychiatric disorders: Depression, irritability, restlessness

Gastro-intestinal system disorders: Diarrhoea

Reproductive disorders: Severe ovarian hyperstimulation syndrome, Breast pain

4.9 Overdose

No case of overdose has been reported.

Nevertheless, there is a possibility that ovarian hyperstimulation syndrome (OHSS) may result from an overdosage of Ovitrelle (see "4.4").

5. PHARMACOLOGICAL PROPERTIES

5.1 Pharmacodynamic properties

Pharmacotherapeutic group: gonadotropins, ATC code: G03G A08

Ovitrelle is a medicinal product of chorionic gonadotropin produced by recombinant DNA techniques. It shares the amino acid sequence with urinary hCG. Chorionic gonadotropin binds on the ovarian theca (and granulosa) cells to a transmembrane receptor shared with the luteinising hormone, the LH/CG receptor.

The principal pharmacodynamic activity in women is oocyte meiosis resumption, follicular rupture (ovulation), corpus luteum formation and production of progesterone and estradiol by the corpus luteum.

In women, Chorionic gonadotropin acts as a surrogate LH-surge that triggers ovulation.

Ovitrelle is used to trigger final follicular maturation and early luteinisation after use of medicinal products for stimulation of follicular growth.

In comparative clinical trials, administration of a dose of 250 micrograms of Ovitrelle was as effective as 5000 IU and 10000 IU of urinary hCG in inducing final follicular maturation and early luteinisation in assisted reproductive techniques, and as effective as 5000 IU of urinary hCG in ovulation induction.

So far, there are no signs of antibody development in humans to Ovitrelle. Repeated exposure to Ovitrelle was investigated in male patients only. Clinical investigation in women for the indication of ART and anovulation was limited to one treatment cycle.

5.2 Pharmacokinetic properties

Following intravenous administration, choriogonadotropin alfa is distributed to the extracellular fluid space with a distribution half-life of around 4.5 hours. The steady-state volume of distribution and the total clearance are 6 l and 0.2 l/h, respectively. There are no indications that choriogonadotropin alfa is metabolised and excreted differently than endogenous hCG.

Following subcutaneous administration, choriogonadotropin alfa is eliminated from the body with a terminal half-life of about 30 hours, and the absolute bioavailability is about 40 %.

A comparative study between the currently registered freeze-dried formulation and the liquid formulation showed bioequivalence between the two formulations.

5.3 Preclinical safety data

Preclinical safety data reveal no intrinsic toxicity of choriogonadotropin alfa. Studies on carcinogenic potential were not performed. This is justified, given the proteinous nature of the active substance and the negative outcome of the genotoxicity testing.

Studies on reproduction were not performed in animals.

6. PHARMACEUTICAL PARTICULARS

6.1 List of excipients

Mannitol

Methionine

Poloxamer 188

Diluted phosphoric acid

Sodium hydroxide

Water for injections

6.2 Incompatibilities

In the absence of compatibility studies, this medicinal product must not be mixed with other medicinal products.

6.3 Shelf life

18 months.

After opening, the product should be used immediately. However, the in-use stability has been demonstrated for 24 hours at +2° to 8°C.

6.4 Special precautions for storage

Store at 2°C – 8°C (in a refrigerator). Store in the original package. Within its shelf-life, the solution may be stored at or below 25°C for up to 30 days without being refrigerated again during this period. It must be discarded if not used after these 30 days.

6.5 Nature and contents of container

0.5ml of solution in a pre-filled syringe (type I glass) with a plunger stopper (halobutyl rubber) and plunger (plastic), and with a needle for injection (stainless) – pack of 1.

6.6 Instructions for use and handling

Only clear solution without particles should be used. Any unused product or waste material should be disposed of in accordance with local requirements.

For single use only.

7. MARKETING AUTHORISATION HOLDER

SERONO EUROPE LIMITED

56, Marsh Wall

London E14 9TP

United Kingdom

8. MARKETING AUTHORISATION NUMBER(S)

Authorisation number	Presentations
EU/1/00/165/007	Ovitrelle – 250 micrograms/0.5 ml – Solution for injection – 1 pre-filled syringe

9. DATE OF FIRST AUTHORISATION/RENEWAL OF THE AUTHORISATION

24th October 2003

10. DATE OF REVISION OF THE TEXT

NA

LEGAL STATUS

POM

NAME AND ADDRESS OF DISTRIBUTOR IN UK

Serono Ltd

Bedfont Cross

Stanwell Road

Feltham

Middlesex

TW14 8NX

NAME AND ADDRESS OF DISTRIBUTOR IN IRELAND

Allphar Services Limited

Pharmaceutical Agents and Distributors

Belgard Road

Tallaght

Dublin 24

Ovranette

(Wyeth Pharmaceuticals)

1. NAME OF THE MEDICINAL PRODUCT

Ovranette Tablets.

2. QUALITATIVE AND QUANTITATIVE COMPOSITION

Each tablet contains 0.15mg levonorgestrel and 0.03mg ethinylestradiol.

For excipients see 6.1

3. PHARMACEUTICAL FORM

Sugar-coated tablets.

4. CLINICAL PARTICULARS

4.1 Therapeutic indications

Oral contraception.

Treatment of endometriosis.

Treatment of spasmodic dysmenorrhoea and premenstrual tension.

Treatment of functional uterine bleeding (menorrhagia, metrorrhagia, metropathia haemorrhatica).

Emergency treatment of acute uterine bleeding.

4.2 Posology and method of administration

For oral administration

Dosage and Administration

First treatment cycle: 1 tablet daily for 21 days, starting with the tablet marked number 1, on the first day of the menstrual cycle. Additional contraception (barriers and spermicides) is not required.

Subsequent cycles: Each subsequent course is started when seven tablet-free days have followed the preceding course. A withdrawal bleed should occur during the 7 tablet-free days.

Changing from another 21 day combined oral contraceptive: The first tablet of Ovranette should be taken on the first day immediately after the end of the previous oral contraceptive course. Additional precautions are not required. A withdrawal bleed should not be expected until the end of the first pack.

Changing from an Every Day (ED) 28 day combined oral contraceptive: The first tablet of Ovranette should be taken on the day immediately after the day on which the last active pill in the ED pack has been taken. The remaining tablets in the ED pack should be discarded. Additional precautions are not required. A withdrawal bleed should not be expected until the end of the first pack.

Changing from a Progestogen-only-Pill (POP): The first tablet of Ovranette should be taken on the first day of menstruation even if the POP for that day has already been taken. The remaining tablets in the POP pack should be discarded. Additional precautions are not required.

Post-partum and post-abortum use: After pregnancy, combined oral contraception can be started in non-lactating women 21 days after a vaginal delivery, provided that the patient is fully ambulant and there are no puerperal complications. If the pill is started later than 21 days after delivery, then alternative contraception (barriers and spermicides) should be used until oral contraception is started and for the first 7 days of pill-taking. If unprotected intercourse has taken place after 21 days post partum, then oral contraception should not be started until the first menstrual bleed after childbirth. After miscarriage or abortion oral contraception may be started immediately.

Other indications:

Endometriosis: Continuous treatment with two tablets daily.

Spasmodic dysmenorrhoea, premenstrual tension: Dosage as for oral contraception.

Functional uterine bleeding: Two tablets are taken daily on a cyclic basis as for oral contraception. In the first one or two cycles it may be necessary to give four tablets, or in exceptional cases, five.

Emergency treatment of acute uterine bleeding: Four tablets are given initially and, if necessary, 4-8 tablets daily.

Elderly: Not applicable

Children: Not applicable

Special Circumstances Requiring Additional Contraception:

Missed Pills: If a tablet is delayed, it should be taken as soon as possible, and if it is taken within 12 hours of the correct time, additional contraception is not needed. Further tablets should then be taken at the usual time. If the delay exceeds 12 hours, the last missed pill should be taken when remembered, the earlier missed pills left in the pack and normal pill-taking resumed. If one or more tablets are omitted from the 21 days of pill-taking, addition contraception (barriers and spermicides) should be used for the next 7 days of pill-taking. In addition, if one or more pills are missed during the last 7 days of pill-taking, the subsequent pill-free interval should be disregarded and the next pack started the day after taking the last tablet from the previous pack. In this case, a period should not be expected until the end of the second pack. If the patient does not have a period at the end of the second pack, she must return to her doctor to exclude the possibility of pregnancy.

Gastro-intestinal upset: Vomiting or diarrhoea may reduce the efficacy by preventing full absorption. Additional contraception (barriers and spermicides) should be used during the stomach upset and for the 7 days following the upset. If these 7 days overrun the end of a pack, the next pack should be started without a break. In this case, a period should not be expected until the end of the second pack. If the patient does not have a period at the end of the second pack, she must return to her doctor to exclude the possibility of pregnancy.

Mild laxatives do not impair contraceptive action.

Interaction with other drugs:

Some drugs may reduce the efficacy of oral contraceptives (refer to "4.5. Interaction with other medicaments and other forms of interaction."). It is, therefore, advisable to use non-hormonal methods of contraception (barriers and spermicides) in addition to the oral contraceptive as long as an extremely high degree of protection is required during treatment with such drugs. The additional contraception should be used while the concurrent medication continues and for 7 days afterwards. If these extra precautions overrun the end of the pack, the next pack should be started without a break. In this case a withdrawal bleed should not be expected until the end of the second pack. If the patient does not have a withdrawal bleed at the end of the second pack, she must return to her doctor to exclude the possibility of pregnancy.

4.3 Contraindications

1. Suspected pregnancy

2. History of confirmed venous thromboembolism (VTE). Family history of idiopathic VTE. Other known risk factors for VTE

3. Arterial thrombotic disorders and a history of these conditions, disorders of lipid metabolism and other conditions in which, in individual cases, there is known or suspected to be a much increased risk of thrombosis

4. Sickle-cell anaemia

5. Acute or severe chronic liver diseases. Dubin-Johnson syndrome. Rotor syndrome. History, during pregnancy, of idiopathic jaundice or severe pruritus

6. History of herpes gestationis

7. Mammary or endometrial carcinoma, or a history of these conditions

8. Abnormal vaginal bleeding of unknown cause

9. Deterioration of otosclerosis during pregnancy

4.4 Special warnings and special precautions for use

Warnings:

1. Venous and Arterial Thrombosis and Thromboembolism

Use of COCs is associated with an increased risk of venous and arterial thrombotic and thromboembolic events.

Minimising exposure to oestrogens and progestogens is in keeping with good principles of therapeutics. For any particular oestrogen/progestogen combination, the dosage regimen prescribed should be one that contains the least amount of oestrogen and progestogen that is compatible with a low failure rate and the needs of the patient.

Unless clinically indicated otherwise, new users of COCs should be started on preparations containing less than 50μg of oestrogen.

Venous Thrombosis and Thromboembolism

Use of COCs increases the risk of venous thrombotic and thromboembolic events. Reported events include deep venous thrombosis and pulmonary embolism.

The use of any COC carries an increased risk of venous thrombotic and thromboembolic events compared with no use. The excess risk is highest during the first year a woman ever uses a combined oral contraceptive. This increased risk is less than the risk of venous thrombotic and thromboembolic events associated with pregnancy which is estimated as 60 cases per 100,000 woman-years. Venous thromboembolism is fatal in 1-2% of cases.

Some epidemiological studies have reported a greater risk of VTE for women using combined oral contraceptives containing desogestrel or gestodene (the so-called third generation pills) than for women using pills containing levonorgestrel (the so-called second generation pills).

The spontaneous incidence of VTE in healthy non-pregnant women (not taking any oral contraceptive) is about 5 cases per 100,000 women per year. The incidence in users of the second-generation pills (such as Ovranette) is about 15 per 100,000 women per year of use. The incidence in users of third generation pills is about 25 cases per 100,000 women per year of use; this excess incidence has not been satisfactorily explained by bias or confounding. The level of all these risks of VTE increases with age and is likely to be further increased in women with other known risk factors of VTE.

All this information should be taken into account when prescribing this COC. When counselling on the choice of contraceptive method(s) all of the above information should be considered.

The risk of venous thrombotic and thromboembolic events is further increased in women with conditions predisposing for venous thrombosis and thromboembolism. Caution must be exercised when prescribing COCs for such women.

Examples of predisposing conditions for venous thrombosis are:

- Certain inherited or acquired thrombophilias (the presence of an inherited thrombophilia may be indicated by a family history of venous thrombotic/thromboembolic events
- Obesity (body mass index of 30kg/m^2 or over)
- Surgery or trauma with increased risk of thrombosis (see reasons for discontinuation)
- Recent delivery or second-trimester abortion
- Prolonged immobilisation
- Increasing age
- Systemic Lupus Erythematosus (SLE)

The relative risk of post-operative thromboembolic complications has been reported to be increased two- or four-fold with the use of COCs (see reasons for discontinuation).

Since the immediate post-partum period is associated with an increased risk of thromboembolism, COCs should be started no earlier than day 28 after delivery or second-trimester abortion.

Arterial Thrombosis and Thromboembolism

The use of COCs increases the risk or arterial thrombotic and thromboembolic events. Reported events include myocardial infarction and cerebrovascular events (ischaemic and haemorrhagic stroke).

The risk of arterial thrombotic and thromboembolic events is further increased in women with underlying risk factors.

Caution must be exercised when prescribing COCs for women with risk factors for arterial thrombotic and thromboembolic events.

Examples of risk factors for arterial thrombotic and thromboembolic event are:

- Smoking, especially over the age of 35
- Certain inherited and acquired thrombophilias
- Hypertension
- Dyslipoproteinaemias
- Thrombogenic valvular heart disease, atrial fibillation
- Obesity (body mass index of 30kg/m^2)
- Increasing age
- Diabetes
- Systemic Lupus Erythematosus (SLE)

COC users with migraine (particularly migraine with aura) may be at increased risk of stroke.

There is no consensus about the possible role of varicose veins and superficial thrombophlebitis in venous thromboembolism

The suitability of a combined oral contraceptive should be judged according to the severity of such conditions in the individual case, and should be discussed with the patient before she decides to take it.

2. The risk of arterial thrombosis associated with combined oral contraceptives increases with age, and this risk is aggravated by cigarette smoking. The use of combined oral contraceptives by women in the older age group, especially those who are cigarette smokers, should therefore be discouraged and alternative methods used.

3. The possibility cannot be ruled out that certain chronic diseases may occasionally deteriorate during the use of combined oral contraceptives. (See 'Precautions').

4. Malignant liver tumours have been reported on rare occasions in long-term users of oral contraceptives. Benign hepatic tumours have also been associated with oral contraceptive usage. A hepatic tumour should be considered in the differential diagnosis when upper abdominal pain, enlarged liver or signs of intra-abdominal haemorrhage occur.

5. Numerous epidemiological studies have been reported on the risks of ovarian, endometrial, cervical and breast cancer in women using combined oral contraceptives. The evidence is clear that combined oral contraceptives offer substantial protection against both ovarian and endometrial cancer.

An increased risk of cervical cancer in long-term users of combined oral contraceptives has been reported in some studies, but there continues to be controversy about the extent to which this is attributable to the confounding effects of sexual behaviour and other factors.

A meta-analysis from 54 epidemiological studies reported that there is a slightly increased relative risk (RR = 1.24) of having breast cancer diagnosed in women who are currently using combined oral contraceptives (COCs). The observed pattern of increased risk may be due to an earlier diagnosis of breast cancer in COC users, the biological effects of COCs or a combination of both. The additional breast cancers diagnosed in current users of COCs or in women who have used COCs in the last ten years are more likely to be localised to the breast than those in women who never used COCs.

Breast cancer is rare among women under 40 years of age whether or not they take COCs. Whilst this background risk increases with age, the excess number of breast cancer

Figure 1

Estimated cumulative numbers of breast cancers per 10,000 women diagnosed in 5 years of use and up to 10 years after stopping COCs, compared with numbers of breast cancers diagnosed in 10,000 women who had never used COCs

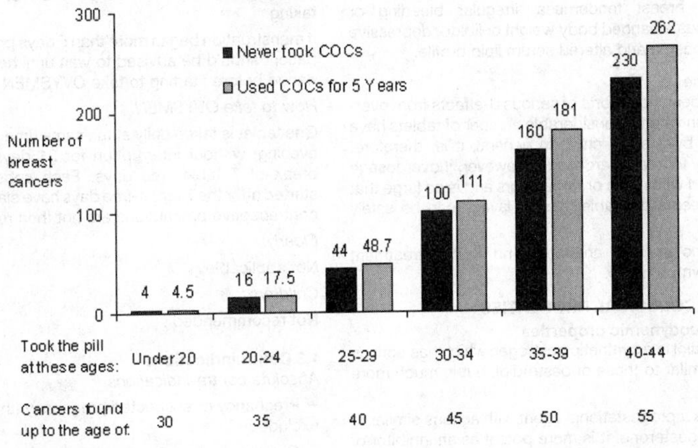

diagnoses in current and recent COC users is small in relation to the overall risk of breast cancer (see bar chart).

(see Figure 1 above)

The most important risk factor for breast cancer in COC users is the age women discontinue the COC; the older the age at stopping, the more breast cancers are diagnosed. Duration of use is less important and the excess risk gradually disappears during the course of the 10 years after stopping COC use such that by 10 years there appears to be no excess.

The possible increase in risk of breast cancer should be discussed with the user and weighed against the benefits of COCs taking into account the evidence that they offer substantial protection against the risk of developing certain other cancers (e.g. ovarian and endometrial cancer).

Reasons for stopping oral contraception immediately:

1. Occurrence of migraine in patients who have never previously suffered from it. Exacerbation of pre-existing migraine. Any unusually frequent or unusually severe headaches.

2. Any kind of acute disturbance of vision.

3. Suspicion of thrombosis or infarction including symptoms such as unusual pains in or swelling of the legs, stabbing pains on breathing, persistent cough or coughing blood, pain or tightness in the chest.

4. Six weeks before elective operations, or treatment of varicose veins by sclerotherapy and during immobilisation, e.g. after accidents, etc.

5. Significant rise in blood-pressure.

6. Jaundice.

7. Clear exacerbation of conditions known to be capable of deteriorating during oral contraception or pregnancy.

8. Pregnancy is a reason for stopping immediately because it has been suggested by some investigations that oral contraceptives taken in early pregnancy may slightly increase the risk of foetal malformations. Other investigations have failed to support these findings. The possibility therefore cannot be excluded, but it is certain that if a risk exists at all, it is very small.

If oral contraception is stopped for any reason and pregnancy is not desired, it is recommended that alternative non-hormonal methods of contraception (such as barriers or spermicides) are used to ensure contraceptive protection is maintained.

Precautions:

1. Assessment of women prior to starting oral contraceptives (and at regular intervals thereafter) should include a personal and family medical history of each woman. Physical examination should be guided by this and by the contraindications (section 4.3) and warnings (section 4.4) for this product. The frequency and nature of these assessments should be based upon relevant guidelines and should be adapted to the individual woman, but should include measurement of blood pressure and, if judged appropriate by the clinician, breast, abdominal and pelvic examination including cervical cytology.

2. Before starting treatment, pregnancy must be excluded.

3. The following conditions require careful observation during medication: a history of severe depressive states, varicose veins, diabetes, hypertension, epilepsy, otosclerosis, multiple sclerosis, porphyria, tetany, disturbed liver function, gall-stones, cardiovascular diseases, renal diseases, chloasma, uterine fibroids, asthma, the wearing of contact lenses, or any disease that is prone to worsen during pregnancy. The first appearance or deterioration of any of these conditions may indicate that the oral contraceptive should be stopped.

4. The risk of the deterioration of chloasma, which is often not fully reversible, is reduced by the avoidance of excessive exposure to sunlight.

Menstrual changes:

1. Reduction of menstrual flow: This is not abnormal and it is to be expected in some patients.

2. Missed menstruation: Occasionally withdrawal bleeding may not occur at all. If the tablets have been taken correctly, pregnancy is very unlikely but should be ruled out before a new course of tablets is started.

Intermenstrual bleeding:

Very light "spotting" or heavier "break through bleeding" may occur during tablet-taking, especially in the first few cycles. It appears to be generally of no significance, except where it indicates errors of tablet-taking, or where the possibility of interaction with other drugs exists. However, if irregular bleeding is persistent an organic cause should be considered.

4.5 Interaction with other medicinal products and other forms of Interaction

Some drugs accelerate the metabolism of oral contraceptives when taken concurrently and these include barbiturates, phenytoin, phenylbutazone and rifampicin. Other drugs suspected of having the capacity to reduce the efficacy of oral contraceptives include ampicillin and other antibiotics. It is therefore, advisable to use non-hormonal methods of contraception (barriers and spermicides). Please refer to "4.2 Posology and Method of Administration, Interaction with other drugs".

The response to metyrapone is less pronounced in women taking oral contraceptives.

ACTH function test remains unchanged. Reduction in corticosteroid excretion and elevation or plasma corticosteroids are due to increased cortisol binding capacity of plasma proteins.

Serum protein-bound iodine levels should not be used for evaluation of thyroid function as levels may rise due to increased thyroid hormone binding capacity of plasma proteins.

Erythrocyte sedimentation may be accelerated in absence of any disease due to change in proportion of plasma protein fractions. Increases in plasma copper, iron and alkaline phosphatase have been recorded.

The herbal remedy, St John's Wort (*Hypericum perforatum*) should not be taken concomitantly with this medicine as it could potentially lead to a loss of contraceptive effect.

4.6 Pregnancy and lactation

Pregnancy is a reason for stopping administration immediately because it have been suggested by some investigations that oral contraceptives taken in early pregnancy may slightly increase the risk of foetal malformations. Other investigations have failed to support these findings. The possibility therefore cannot be excluded, but it is certain that if a risk exists at all, it is very small. After pregnancy, combined oral contraception can be started in non-lactating women 21 days after vaginal delivery, provided that the patient is fully ambulant and there are no puerperal complications.

Please refer to recommended dosage schedule: Post-partum and post-abortum use.

Administration of oestrogens to lactating women may decrease the quantity or quality of the milk.

4.7 Effects on ability to drive and use machines

None known.

4.8 Undesirable effects

See 'Special Warnings and Special Precautions for Use'.

There is an increased risk of venous thromboembolism for all women using a combined oral contraceptive. For information on differences in risk between oral contraceptives, see Section 4.4.

Occasional side-effect may include nausea, vomiting, headaches, breast tenderness, irregular bleeding or missed bleeds, changed body weight or libido, depressive moods, chloasma and altered serum lipid profile.

4.9 Overdose

There have been no reports of serious ill-effects from overdosage, even when a considerable number of tablets have been taken by a small child. In general, it is, therefore, unnecessary to treat overdosage. However, if overdosage is discovered within two or three hours and is so large that treatment seems desirable, gastric lavage can be safely used.

There are no specific antidotes and further treatment should be symptomatic.

5. PHARMACOLOGICAL PROPERTIES

5.1 Pharmacodynamic properties

Ethinylestradiol is a synthetic oestrogen which has actions and uses similar to those of oestradiol, but is much more potent.

Norgestrel is a progestational agent with actions similar to those of progesterone. It is more potent as an inhibitor of ovulation than norethisterone and has androgenic activity.

5.2 Pharmacokinetic properties

Ethinylestradiol is absorbed by the gastro-intestinal tract. It is only slowly metabolised and excreted in the urine.

Norgestrel is absorbed from the gastrointestinal tract. Metabolites are excreted in the urine and faeces as glucuronide and sulphate conjugates.

5.3 Preclinical safety data

Nothing of relevance to the prescriber.

6. PHARMACEUTICAL PARTICULARS

6.1 List of excipients

Core: lactose, maize starch, povidone 25, magnesium stearate, talc, purified water.

Coating: sucrose, polyethylene glycol 6000, calcium carbonate, talc, povidone 90, glycerin, titanium dioxide, iron oxide yellow pigment E172, Wax E, purified water.

6.2 Incompatibilities

None known.

6.3 Shelf life

36 months.

6.4 Special precautions for storage

Store at or below room temperature.

6.5 Nature and contents of container

Aluminium foil and PVC blister packs of 21 tablets.

Cartons containing 1, 3 and 50 blisters.

6.6 Instructions for use and handling

Not applicable.

7. MARKETING AUTHORISATION HOLDER

John Wyeth & Brother Limited

t/a Wyeth Laboratories

Huntercombe Lane South

Taplow, Maidenhead

Berkshire SL6 0PH

8. MARKETING AUTHORISATION NUMBER(S)

PL 0011/0041

9. DATE OF FIRST AUTHORISATION/RENEWAL OF THE AUTHORISATION

26th February 1996

10. DATE OF REVISION OF THE TEXT

3rd March 2003

Ovysmen Oral Contraceptive Tablets

(Janssen-Cilag Ltd)

1. NAME OF THE MEDICINAL PRODUCT

OVYSMEN® Oral Contraceptive Tablets

2. QUALITATIVE AND QUANTITATIVE COMPOSITION

OVYSMEN are tablets for oral administration.

Each tablet contains norethisterone PhEur 0.5 mg and ethinylestradiol PhEur 0.035 mg.

3. PHARMACEUTICAL FORM

Tablet.

4. CLINICAL PARTICULARS

4.1 Therapeutic indications

Contraception and the recognised indications for such oestrogen/progestogen combinations.

4.2 Posology and method of administration

For Oral Administration

Adults

It is preferable that tablet intake from the first pack is started on the first day of menstruation in which case no extra contraceptive precautions are necessary.

If menstruation has already begun (that is 2, 3 or 4 days previously), tablet taking should commence on day 5 of the menstrual period. In this case, additional contraceptive precautions must be taken for the first 7 days of tablet taking.

If menstruation began more than 5 days previously then the patient should be advised to wait until her next menstrual period before starting to take OVYSMEN.

How to take OVYSMEN:

One tablet is taken daily at the same time (preferably in the evening) without interruption for 21 days, followed by a break of 7 tablet-free days. Each subsequent pack is started after the 7 tablet-free days have elapsed. Additional contraceptive precautions are not then required.

Elderly:

Not applicable

Children:

Not recommended

4.3 Contraindications

Absolute contra-indications

– Pregnancy or suspected pregnancy (that cannot yet be excluded).

– Circulatory disorders (cardiovascular or cerebrovascular) such as thrombophlebitis and thrombo-embolic processes, or a history of these conditions (including history of confirmed venous thrombo-embolism (VTE), family history of idiopathic VTE and other known risk factors for VTE), moderate to severe hypertension, hyperlipoproteinaemia. In addition the presence of more than one of the risk factors for arterial disease.

– Severe liver disease, cholestatic jaundice or hepatitis (viral or non-viral) or a history of these conditions if the results of liver function tests have failed to return to normal, and for 3 months after liver function tests have been found to be normal; a history of jaundice of pregnancy or jaundice due to the use of steroids, Rotor syndrome and Dubin-Johnson syndrome, hepatic cell tumours and porphyria.

– Cholelithiasis.

– Known or suspected oestrogen-dependent tumours; endometrial hyperplasia; undiagnosed vaginal bleeding.

– Systemic lupus erythematosus or a history of this condition.

– A history during pregnancy or previous use of steroids of:

- severe pruritus
- herpes gestationis
- a manifestation or deterioration of otosclerosis

Relative contra-indications:

If any relative contra-indication listed below is present, the benefits of oestrogen/progestogen-containing preparations must be weighed against the possible risk for each individual case and the patient kept under close supervision. In case of aggravation or appearance of any of these conditions whilst the patient is taking the pill, its use should be discontinued.

– Conditions implicating an increasing risk of developing venous thrombo-embolic complications, e.g. severe varicose veins or prolonged immobilisation or major surgery. Disorders of coagulation.

– Presence of any risk factor for arterial disease e.g. smoking, hyperlipidaemia or hypertension.

– Other conditions associated with an increased risk of circulatory disease such as latent or overt cardiac failure, renal dysfunction, or a history of these conditions.

– Epilepsy or a history of this condition.

– Migraine or a history of this condition.

– A history of cholelithiasis.

– Presence of any risk factor for oestrogen-dependent tumours; oestrogen-sensitive gynaecological disorders such as uterine fibromyomata and endometriosis.

– Diabetes mellitus.

– Severe depression or a history of this condition. If this is accompanied by a disturbance in tryptophan metabolism, administration of vitamin B6 might be of therapeutic value.

– Sickle cell haemoglobinopathy, since under certain circumstances, e.g. during infections or anoxia, oestrogen-containing preparations may induce thrombo-embolic process in patients with this condition.

– If the results of liver function tests become abnormal, use should be discontinued.

4.4 Special warnings and special precautions for use

Post partum administration

Following a vaginal delivery, oral contraceptive administration to non-breast-feeding mothers can be started 21 days post-partum provided the patient is fully ambulant and there are no puerperal complications. No additional contraceptive precautions are required. If post-partum administration begins more than 21 days after delivery, additional contraceptive precautions are required for the first 7 days of pill-taking.

If intercourse has taken place post-partum, oral contraceptive use should be delayed until the first day of the first menstrual period.

After miscarriage or abortion, administration should start immediately, in which case no additional contraceptive precautions are required.

Changing from a 21 day pill or 22 day pill to OVYSMEN

All tablets in the old pack should be finished. The first OVYSMEN tablet is taken the next day ie no gap is left between taking tablets nor does the patient need to wait for her period to begin. Tablets should be taken as instructed in 'How to take OVYSMEN' (see 4.2). Additional contraceptive precautions are not required. The patient will not have a period until the end of the first OVYSMEN pack, but this is not harmful, nor does it matter if she experiences some bleeding on tablet-taking days.

Changing from a combined every day pill (28 day tablets) to OVYSMEN

OVYSMEN should be started after taking the last active tablet from the 'Every day Pill' pack (ie after taking 21 or 22 tablets). The first OVYSMEN tablet is taken the next day ie no gap is left between taking tablets nor does the patient need to wait for her period to begin. Tablets should be taken as instructed in 'How to take OVYSMEN' (see 4.2). Additional contraceptive precautions are not required. Remaining tablets from the every day (ED) pack should be discarded.

The patient will not have a period until the end of the first OVYSMEN pack, but this is not harmful, nor does it matter if she experiences some bleeding on tablet-taking days.

Changing from a progestogen-only pill (POP or mini pill) to OVYSMEN

The first OVYSMEN tablet should be taken on the first day of the period, even if the patient has already taken a mini pill on that day. Tablets should be taken as instructed in 'How to take OVYSMEN' (see 4.2). Additional contraceptive precautions are not required. All the remaining progestogen-only pills in the mini pill pack should be discarded.

If the patient is taking a mini pill, then she may not always have a period, especially when she is breast-feeding. The first OVYSMEN tablet should be taken on the day after stopping the mini pill. All remaining pills in the mini pill packet must be discarded. Additional contraceptive precautions must be taken for the first 7 days.

To skip a period

To skip a period, a new pack of OVYSMEN should be started on the day after finishing the current pack (the patient skips the tablet-free days). Tablet-taking should be continued in the usual way.

During the use of the second pack she may experience slight spotting or break- through bleeding but contraceptive protection will not be diminished provided there are no tablet omissions.

The next pack of OVYSMEN is started after the usual 7 tablet-free days, regardless of whether the period has completely finished or not.

Reduced reliability

When OVYSMEN is taken according to the directions for use the occurrence of pregnancy is highly unlikely. However, the reliability of oral contraceptives may be reduced under the following circumstances:

(i) Forgotten tablets

If the patient forgets to take a tablet, she should take it as soon as she remembers and take the next one at the normal time. This may mean that two tablets are taken in one day. Provided she is less than 12 hours late in taking her tablet, OVYSMEN will still give contraceptive protection during this cycle and the rest of the pack should be taken as usual.

If she is more than 12 hours late in taking one or more tablets then she should take the last missed pill as soon as she remembers but leave the other missed pills in the pack. She should continue to take the rest of the pack as usual but must use extra precautions (eg sheath, diaphragm, plus spermicide) and follow the '7-day rule' (see Further Information for the '7-day rule').

If there are 7 or more pills left in the pack after the missed and delayed pills then the usual 7-day break can be left before starting the next pack. If there are less than 7 pills left in the pack after the missed and delayed pills then when the pack is finished the next pack should be started the next day. If withdrawal bleeding does not occur at the end of the second pack then a pregnancy test should be performed.

(ii) Vomiting or diarrhoea

If after tablet intake, vomiting or diarrhoea occurs, a tablet may not be absorbed properly by the body. If the symptoms disappear within 12 hours of tablet-taking, the patient should take an extra tablet from a spare pack and continue with the rest of the pack as usual.

However, if the symptoms continue beyond those 12 hours, additional contraceptive precautions are necessary for any sexual intercourse during the stomach or bowel upset and for the following 7 days (the patient must be advised to follow the '7-day rule').

(iii) Change in bleeding pattern

If after taking OVYSMEN for several months, there is a sudden occurrence of spotting or breakthrough bleeding (not observed in previous cycles) or the absence of withdrawal bleeding, contraceptive effectiveness may be reduced. If withdrawal bleeding fails to occur and none of the above mentioned events has taken place, pregnancy is highly unlikely and oral contraceptive use can be continued until the end of the next pack. (If withdrawal bleeding fails to occur at the end of the second cycle, tablet intake should be discontinued and pregnancy excluded before oral contraceptive use can be resumed.) However, if withdrawal bleeding is absent and any of the above mentioned events has occurred, tablet intake should be discontinued and pregnancy excluded before oral contraceptive use can be resumed.

Medical examination/consultation

Assessment of women prior to starting oral contraceptives (and at regular intervals thereafter) should include a personal and family medical history of each woman. Physical examination should be guided by this and by the contraindications (Section 4.3) and warnings (Section 4.4) for this product. The frequency and nature of these assessments should be based upon relevant guidelines and should be adapted to the individual woman, but should include measurement of blood pressure and, if judged appropriate by the clinician, breast, abdominal and pelvic examination including cervical cytology.

Caution should be observed when prescribing oral contraceptives to young women whose cycles are not yet stabilised.

Venous thrombo-embolic disease

An increased risk of venous thrombo-embolic disease (VTE) associated with the use of oral contraceptives is well established but is smaller than that associated with pregnancy, which has been estimated at 60 cases per 100,000 pregnancies. Some epidemiological studies have reported a greater risk of VTE for women using combined oral contraceptives containing desogestrel or gestodene (the so-called 'third generation' pills) than for women using pills containing levonorgestrel or norethisterone (the so-called 'second generation' pills).

The spontaneous incidence of VTE in healthy non-pregnant women (not taking any oral contraceptive) is about 5 cases per 100,000 per year. The incidence in users of second generation pills is about 15 per 100,000 women per year of use. The incidence in users of third generation pills is about 25 cases per 100,000 women per year of use; this excess incidence has not been satisfactorily explained by bias or confounding. The level of all of these risks of VTE increases with age and is likely to be further increased in women with other known risk factors for VTE such as obesity. The excess risk of VTE is highest during the first year a woman ever uses a combined oral contraceptive.

Surgery, varicose veins or immobilisation

In patients using oestrogen-containing preparations, the risk of deep vein thrombosis may be temporarily increased when undergoing a major operation (eg abdominal, orthopaedic), and surgery to the legs, medical treatment for varicose veins or prolonged immobilisation. Therefore, it is advisable to discontinue oral contraceptive use at least 4 to 6 weeks prior to these procedures if performed electively and to (re)start not less than 2 weeks after full ambulation. The latter is also valid with regard to immobilisation after an accident or emergency surgery. In case of emergency surgery, thrombotic prophylaxis is usually indicated e.g. with subcutaneous heparin.

Chloasma

Chloasma may occasionally occur, especially in women with a history of chloasma gravidarum. Women with a tendency to chloasma should avoid exposure to the sun or ultraviolet radiation whilst taking this preparation. Chloasma is often not fully reversible.

Laboratory tests

The use of steroids may influence the results of certain laboratory tests. In the literature, at least a hundred different parameters have been reported to possibly be influenced by oral contraceptive use, predominantly by the oestrogenic component. Among these are: biochemical parameters of the liver, thyroid, adrenal and renal function, plasma levels of (carrier) proteins and lipid/lipoprotein fractions and parameters of coagulation and fibrinolysis.

Further information

Additional contraceptive precautions

When additional contraceptive precautions are required, the patient should be advised either not to have sex, or to use a cap plus spermicide or for her partner to use a condom. Rhythm methods should not be advised as the pill disrupts the usual cyclical changes associated with the natural menstrual cycle e.g. changes in temperature and cervical mucus.

The 7-day rule

If any one tablet is forgotten for more than 12 hours.

If the patient has vomiting or diarrhoea for more than 12 hours.

Figure 1

Estimated number of breast cancers found in 10,000 women who took the Pill for 5 years then stopped, or who never took the Pill

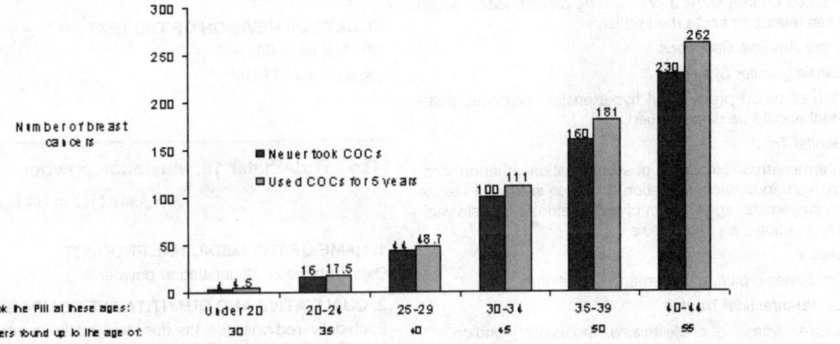

If the patient is taking any of the drugs listed under 'Interactions':

The patient should continue to take her tablets as usual and:

- Additional contraceptive precautions must be taken for the next 7 days.

But - if these 7 days run beyond the end of the current pack, the next pack must be started as soon as the current one is finished, i.e. no gap should be left between packs. (This prevents an extended break in tablet taking which may increase the risk of the ovaries releasing an egg and thus reducing contraceptive protection.) The patient will not have a period until the end of 2 packs but this is not harmful nor does it matter if she experiences some bleeding on tablet taking days.

4.5 Interaction with other medicinal products and other forms of Interaction

Irregular cycles and reduced reliability of oral contraceptives may occur when these preparations are used concomitantly with drugs such as anticonvulsants, barbiturates, antibiotics, (eg tetracyclines, ampicillin, rifampicin, etc.), griseofulvin, activated charcoal and certain laxatives. Special consideration should be given to patients being treated with antibiotics for acne. They should be advised to use a non-hormonal method of contraception, or to use an oral contraceptive containing a progestogen showing minimal androgenicity, which have been reported as helping to improve acne without using an antibiotic. Oral contraceptives may diminish glucose tolerance and increase the need for insulin or other antidiabetic drugs in diabetics.

The herbal remedy St John's Wort *(Hypericum perforatum)* should not be taken concomitantly with this medicine as this could potentially lead to a loss of contraceptive effect.

4.6 Pregnancy and lactation

OVYSMEN is contra-indicated for use during pregnancy or suspected pregnancy, since it has been suggested that combined oral contraceptives, in common with many other substances, might be capable of affecting the normal development of the child in the early stages of pregnancy. It can be definitely concluded, however, that, if a risk of abnormality exists at all, it must be very small.

Mothers who are breast-feeding should be advised not to use the combined pill since this may reduce the amount of breast-milk, but may be advised instead to use a progestogen-only pill (POP).

4.7 Effects on ability to drive and use machines

Not applicable.

4.8 Undesirable effects

Various adverse reactions have been associated with oral contraceptive use. The first appearance of symptoms indicative of any one of these reactions necessitates immediate cessation of oral contraceptive use while appropriate diagnostic and therapeutic measures are undertaken.

Serious Adverse Reactions

There is a general opinion, based on statistical evidence, that users of combined oral contraceptives experience more often than non-users various disorders of the coagulation. How often these disorders occur in users of modern low-oestrogen oral contraceptives is unknown, but there are reasons for suggesting that they may occur less often than with the older types of pill which contain more oestrogen.

Various reports have associated oral contraceptive use with the occurrence of deep venous thrombosis, pulmonary embolism and other embolisms. Other investigations of these oral contraceptives have suggested an increased risk of oestrogen and/or progestogen dose-dependent coronary and cerebrovascular accidents, predominantly in heavy smokers. Thrombosis has very rarely been reported to occur in other veins or arteries, e.g. hepatic, mesenteric, renal or retinal.

It should be noted that there is no consensus about often contradictory findings obtained in early studies. The physician should bear in mind the possibility of vascular accidents occurring and that there may not be full recovery from such disorders and they may be fatal. The physician should take into account the presence of risk factors for arterial disease and deep venous thrombosis when prescribing oral contraceptives. Risk factors for arterial disease include smoking, the presence of hyperlipidaemia, hypertension or diabetes.

Signs and symptoms of a thrombotic event may include: sudden severe pain in the chest, whether or not reaching to the left arm; sudden breathlessness; and unusual severe, prolonged headache, especially if it occurs for the first time or gets progressively worse, or is associated with any of the following symptoms: sudden partial or complete loss of vision or diplopia, aphasia, vertigo, a bad fainting attack or collapse with or without focal epilepsy, weakness or very marked numbness suddenly affecting one side or one part of the body, motor disturbances; severe pain in the calf of one leg; acute abdomen.

Cigarette smoking increases the risk of serious cardiovascular adverse reactions to oral contraceptive use. The risk increases with age and with heavy smoking and is more marked in women over 35 years of age. Women who use oral contraceptives should be strongly advised not to smoke.

The use of oestrogen-containing oral contraceptives may promote growth of existing sex steroid dependent tumours. For this reason, the use of these oral contraceptives in patients with such tumours is contra-indicated. Numerous epidemiological studies have been reported on the risk of ovarian, endometrial, cervical and breast cancer in women using combined oral contraceptives. The evidence is clear that combined oral contraceptives offer substantial protection against both ovarian and endometrial cancer. An increased risk of cervical cancer in long term users of combined oral contraceptives has been reported in some studies, but there continues to be controversy about the extent to which this is attributable to the confounding effects of sexual behaviour and other factors.

A meta-analysis from 54 epidemiological studies reported that there is a slightly increased relative risk (RR = 1.24) of having breast cancer diagnosed in women who are currently using combined oral contraceptives (COCs). The observed pattern of increased risk may be due to an earlier diagnosis of breast cancer in COC users, the biological effects of COCs or a combination of both. The additional breast cancers diagnosed in current users of COCs or in women who have used COCs in the last 10 years are more likely to be localised to the breast than those in women who never used COCs.

Breast cancer is rare among women under 40 years of age whether or not they take COCs. Whilst this background risk increases with age, the excess number of breast cancer diagnoses in current and recent COC users is small in relation to the overall risk of breast cancer (see bar chart).

The most important risk factor for breast cancer in COC users is the age women discontinue the COC; the older the age at stopping, the more breast cancers are diagnosed. Duration of use is less important and the excess risk gradually disappears during the course of the 10 years after stopping COC use such that by 10 years there appears to be no excess.

The possible increase in risk of breast cancer should be discussed with the user and weighed against the benefits of COCs taking into account the evidence that they offer substantial protection against the risk of developing certain other cancers (e.g. ovarian and endometrial cancer).

(see Figure 1 above)

Malignant hepatic tumours have been reported on rare occasions in long-term users of oral contraceptives. Benign hepatic tumours have also been associated with oral contraceptive usage. A hepatic tumour should be considered in the differential diagnosis when upper abdominal pain, enlarged liver or signs of intra-abdominal haemorrhage occur.

The use of oral contraceptives may sometimes lead to the development of cholestatic jaundice or cholelithiasis.

On rare occasions the use of oral contraceptives may trigger or reactivate systemic lupus erythematosus.

A further rare complication of oral contraceptive use is the occurrence of chorea which can be reversed by discontinuing the pill. The majority of cases of oral contraceptive-induced chorea show a pre-existing predisposition which often relates to acute rheumatism.

Other Adverse Reactions

Cardiovascular System

Rise of blood pressure. If hypertension develops, treatment should be discontinued.

Genital Tract

Intermenstrual bleeding, post-medication amenorrhoea, changes in cervical secretion, increase in size of uterine fibromyomata, aggravation of endometriosis, certain vaginal infections, eg candidiasis.

Breast

Tenderness, pain, enlargement, secretion.

Gastro-intestinal Tract

Nausea, vomiting, cholelithiasis, cholestatic jaundice.

Skin

Erythema nodosum, rash, chloasma, erythema multiforme, hirsutism, loss of scalp hair.

Eyes

Discomfort of the cornea if contact lenses are used.

CNS

Headache, migraine, mood changes, depression.

Metabolic

Fluid retention, change in body weight, reduced glucose tolerance.

Other

Changes in libido, leg cramps.

4.9 Overdose

There have been no reports of serious ill-health from overdosage even when a considerable number of tablets have been taken by a small child. In general, it is therefore unnecessary to treat overdosage. However, if overdosage is discovered within two or three hours and is large, then gastric lavage can be safely used. There are no antidotes and further treatment should be symptomatic.

5. PHARMACOLOGICAL PROPERTIES

5.1 Pharmacodynamic properties

OVYSMEN acts through the mechanism of gonadotrophin suppression by the oestrogenic and progestational actions of ethinylestradiol and norethisterone. The primary mechanism of action is inhibition of ovulation, but alterations to the cervical mucus and to the endometrium may also contribute to the efficacy of the product.

5.2 Pharmacokinetic properties

Norethisterone and ethinylestradiol are absorbed from the gastro-intestinal tract and metabolised in the liver. To obtain maximal contraceptive effectiveness the tablets should be taken as directed and at approximately the same time each day.

Because the active ingredients are metabolised in the liver, reduced contraceptive efficacy has been associated with concomitant use of oral contraceptives and rifampicin. A similar association has been suggested with oral contraceptives and barbiturates, phenytoin sodium, phenylbutazone, griseofulvin and ampicillin.

5.3 Preclinical safety data

The toxicology of norethisterone and ethinylestradiol has been extensively investigated in animal studies and through long term clinical experience with widespread use in contraceptives.

6. PHARMACEUTICAL PARTICULARS

6.1 List of excipients

Lactose (anhydrous)

Magnesium stearate

Pregelatinised starch

Methanol (does not appear in final product)

6.2 Incompatibilities

Not applicable.

6.3 Shelf life

Three years.

6.4 Special precautions for storage

Store at room temperature (below 25°C). Protect from light.

6.5 Nature and contents of container

Carton containing 3 PVC/foil blister strips of 21 tablets each.

6.6 Instructions for use and handling

Not applicable.

7. MARKETING AUTHORISATION HOLDER

Janssen-Cilag Limited
Saunderton
High Wycombe
Buckinghamshire
HP14 4HJ
UK

8. MARKETING AUTHORISATION NUMBER(S)

0242/0253

9. DATE OF FIRST AUTHORISATION/RENEWAL OF THE AUTHORISATION

1 September 1995

10. DATE OF REVISION OF THE TEXT

19th August 2004

Legal category POM

Oxis Turbohaler 12, inhalation powder

(AstraZeneca UK Limited)

1. NAME OF THE MEDICINAL PRODUCT

Oxis Turbohaler 12, inhalation powder.

2. QUALITATIVE AND QUANTITATIVE COMPOSITION

Each delivered dose (i.e. the dose leaving the mouthpiece) from Oxis Turbohaler 12 contains 9 micrograms formoterol fumarate dihydrate which is derived from a metered dose of 12 micrograms.

For excipients, see 6.1.

3. PHARMACEUTICAL FORM

Inhalation powder.

White powder.

4. CLINICAL PARTICULARS

4.1 Therapeutic indications

Oxis Turbohaler is indicated as add on therapy to maintenance treatment with inhaled corticosteroids, for the relief of broncho-obstructive symptoms and prevention of exercise-induced symptoms, in patients with asthma when adequate treatment with corticosteroids is not sufficient. Oxis Turbohaler is also indicated for the relief of broncho-obstructive symptoms in patients with chronic obstructive pulmonary disease (COPD).

4.2 Posology and method of administration

Use of doses above those normally required by the individual patient on more than 2 days per week, is a sign of suboptimal disease control and maintenance treatment should be reassessed.

Asthma:

In asthma, Oxis Turbohaler can be used once or twice daily ('regular dosage') and as 'relief medication' to relieve acute broncho-obstructive symptoms.

Adults aged > 18 years:

Relief medication: 1 inhalation for the relief of acute broncho-obstructive symptoms.

Regular dosage: 1 inhalation once or twice daily. Some patients may need 2 inhalations once or twice daily.

Prevention of exercise-induced bronchoconstriction: 1 inhalation before exercise.

The daily dose for regular use should not exceed 4 inhalations, however occasionally up to a maximum of 6 inhalations may be allowed within a 24-hour period.

No more than 3 inhalations should be taken on any single occasion.

Children and adolescents 6 years and older:

Relief medication: 1 inhalation for the relief of acute broncho-
obstructive symptoms.

Regular dosage: 1 inhalation once or twice daily.

Prevention of exercise-induced bronchoconstriction: 1 inhalation before exercise.

The regular daily dose should not exceed 2 inhalations, however, occasionally up to a maximum of 4 inhalations may be allowed within a 24-hour period. More than 1 inhalation should not be taken on any single occasion.

COPD:

Regular dosage: 1 inhalation once or twice daily.

The daily dose for regular use should not exceed 2 inhalations.

If required, additional inhalations above those prescribed for regular therapy may be used for relief of symptoms, up to a maximum total daily dose of 4 inhalations (regular plus as required). More than 2 inhalations should not be taken on any single occasion.

Special patient groups:

No adjustment of dose should be required in the elderly, or in patients with renal or hepatic impairment at the recommended normal doses. (See Special warnings and special precautions for use.)

NB! A lower strength is also available.

Oxis Turbohaler is inspiratory flow driven which means that, when the patient inhales through the mouthpiece, the substance will follow the inspired air into the airways.

Note! It is important to instruct the patient to breathe in forcefully and deeply through the mouthpiece to ensure that an optimal dose is obtained.

It is important to instruct the patient never to chew or bite on the mouthpiece and never to use the inhaler if it has been damaged or if the mouthpiece has become detached.

The patient may not taste or feel any medication when using Oxis Turbohaler due to the small amount of drug dispensed.

Detailed instructions for use are packed together with each inhaler.

4.3 Contraindications

Hypersensitivity to formoterol or to inhaled lactose.

4.4 Special warnings and special precautions for use

Asthmatic patients who require therapy with long acting β_2-agonists, should also receive optimal maintenance anti-inflammatory therapy with corticosteroids. Patients must be advised to continue taking their anti-inflammatory therapy after the introduction of Oxis Turbohaler even when symptoms decrease. Should symptoms persist, or treatment with β_2-agonists need to be increased, this indicates a worsening of the underlying condition and warrants a reassessment of the maintenance therapy. Oxis Turbohaler should not be initiated to treat a severe asthma exacerbation.

The maximum daily dose should not be exceeded. The long-term safety of regular treatment at higher doses than 36 micrograms per day in adults with asthma, 18 micrograms per day in children with asthma and 18 micrograms per day in patients with COPD, has not been established.

Frequent need of medication for the prevention of exercise-induced bronchoconstriction can be a sign of suboptimal asthma control, and warrants a reassessment of the asthma therapy and an evaluation of the compliance. If the patient needs prophylactic treatment for exercise-induced bronchoconstriction several times every week despite an adequate maintenance treatment (e.g. corticosteroids and long-acting β_2-agonists), the total asthma management should be reassessed by a specialist.

Caution should be observed when treating patients with thyrotoxicosis, phaeochromocytoma, hypertrophic obstructive cardiomyopathy, idiopathic subvalvular aortic stenosis, severe hypertension, aneurysm or other severe cardiovascular disorders, such as ischaemic heart disease, tachyarrhythmias or severe heart failure.

Formoterol may induce prolongation of the QTc-interval. Caution should be observed when treating patients with prolongation of the QTc-interval and in patients treated with drugs affecting the QTc-interval (see 4.5).

Due to the hyperglycaemic effects of β_2-agonists, additional blood glucose monitoring is recommended initially in diabetic patients.

Potentially serious hypokalaemia may result from β_2-agonist therapy. Particular caution is recommended in acute severe asthma as the associated risk may be augmented by hypoxia. The hypokalaemic effect may be potentiated by concomitant treatment with xanthine-derivatives, steroids and diuretics. The serum potassium levels should therefore be monitored.

As with other inhalation therapy, the potential for paradoxical bronchospasm should be considered.

Oxis Turbohaler contains lactose, 450 micrograms per delivered dose (corresponding to 600 micrograms per metered dose). This amount does not normally cause problems in lactose intolerant people.

Children up to the age of 6 years should not be treated with Oxis Turbohaler, as no sufficient experience is available for this group.

The effect of decreased liver or kidney function on the pharmacokinetics of formoterol and the pharmacokinetics in the elderly is not known. As formoterol is primarily eliminated via metabolism an increased exposure can be expected in patients with severe liver cirrhosis.

4.5 Interaction with other medicinal products and other forms of Interaction

No specific interaction studies have been carried out with Oxis Turbohaler.

Concomitant treatment with other sympathomimetic substances such as other β_2-agonists or ephedrine may potentiate the undesirable effects of Oxis Turbohaler and may require titration of the dose.

Concomitant treatment with xanthine derivatives, steroids or diuretics such as thiazides and loop diuretics may potentiate a rare hypokalaemic adverse effect of β_2-agonists. Hypokalaemia may increase the disposition towards arrhythmias in patients who are treated with digitalis glycosides.

There is a theoretical risk that concomitant treatment with other drugs known to prolong the QTc-interval may give rise to a pharmacodynamic interaction with fomoterol and increase the possible risk of ventricular arrhythmias. Examples of such drugs include certain antihistamines (e.g. terfenadine, astemizole, mizolastine), certain antiarrhythmics (e.g. quinidine, disopyramide, procainamide), erythromycin and tricyclic antidepressants.

There is an elevated risk of arrhythmias in patients receiving concomitant anaesthesia with halogenated hydrocarbons.

Beta-adrenergic blockers can weaken or inhibit the effect of Oxis Turbohaler. Oxis Turbohaler should therefore not be given together with beta-adrenergic blockers (including eye drops) unless there are compelling reasons.

4.6 Pregnancy and lactation

Clinical experience in pregnant women is limited. In animal studies formoterol has caused implantation losses as well as decreased early postnatal survival and birth weight. The effects appeared at considerably higher systemic exposures than those reached during clinical use of Oxis Turbohaler. Treatment with Oxis Turbohaler may be considered at all stages of pregnancy if needed to obtain asthma control and if the expected benefit to the mother is greater than any possible risk to the foetus.

It is not known whether formoterol passes into human breast milk. In rats, small amounts of formoterol have been detected in maternal milk. Administration of Oxis Turbohaler to women who are breastfeeding should only be considered if the expected benefit to the mother is greater than any possible risk to the child.

4.7 Effects on ability to drive and use machines

Oxis Turbohaler does not affect the ability to drive or use machines.

4.8 Undesirable effects

The most commonly reported adverse events of β_2-agonist therapy, such as tremor and palpitations, tend to be mild and disappear within days of treatment.

Common 1% to 10%	*Cardiac disorders:*	Palpitations
	Nervous system disorders:	Headache, tremor
Uncommon 0.1% to 1%	*Cardiac disorders:*	Tachycardia
	Musculoskeletal and connective tissue disorders:	Muscle cramps
	Psychiatric disorders:	Agitation, restlessness, sleep disturbance
Rare 0.01% to 0.1%	*Cardiac disorders:*	Cardiac arrhythmias, e.g. atrial fibrillation, supraventricular tachycardia, extrasystoles
	Gastrointestinal disorders:	Nausea
	Immune system disorders:	Hypersensitivity reactions, e.g. bronchospasm, exanthema, urticaria, pruritus
	Metabolism and nutrition disorders:	Hypokalaemia/hyperkalaemia
Very rare <0.01%	*Cardiac disorders:*	Angina pectoris
	Investigations:	Prolongation of the QTc-interval
	Metabolism and nutrition disorders:	Hyperglycaemia
	Nervous system disorders:	Taste disturbance, dizziness
	Vascular disorders:	Variations in blood pressure

As with all inhalation therapy, paradoxical bronchospasm may occur in very rare cases.

Treatment with β_2-agonists may result in an increase in blood levels of insulin, free fatty acids, glycerol and ketone bodies.

4.9 Overdose

There is limited clinical experience on the management of overdose. An overdose would likely lead to effects that are typical of β_2-agonists: tremor, headache, palpitations. Symptoms reported from isolated cases are tachycardia, hyperglycaemia, hypokalaemia, prolonged QTc-interval, arrhythmia, nausea and vomiting. Supportive and symptomatic treatment is indicated.

Use of cardioselective beta-blockers may be considered, but only subject to extreme caution since the use of β-adrenergic blocker medication may provoke bronchospasm. Serum potassium should be monitored.

5. PHARMACOLOGICAL PROPERTIES

5.1 Pharmacodynamic properties

Pharmacotherapeutic group: selective β_2-agonist, formoterol, ATC code: R03A C13.

Formoterol is a selective β_2-adrenoceptor agonist that produces relaxation of bronchial smooth muscle. Formoterol thus has a bronchodilating effect in patients with reversible airways obstruction. The bronchodilating effect sets in rapidly, within 1-3 minutes after inhalation and has a mean duration of 12 hours after a single dose.

5.2 Pharmacokinetic properties

Absorption

Inhaled formoterol is rapidly absorbed. Peak plasma concentration is reached about 10 minutes after inhalation.

In studies the mean lung deposition of formoterol after inhalation via Turbohaler ranged from 28-49% of the delivered dose (corresponding to 21-37% of the metered dose). The total systemic availability for the higher lung deposition was around 61% of the delivered dose (corresponding to 46% of the metered dose).

Distribution and metabolism

Plasma protein binding is approximately 50%.

Formoterol is metabolised via direct glucuronidation and O-demethylation. The enzyme responsible for O-demethylation has not been identified. Total plasma clearance and volume of distribution has not been determined.

Elimination

The major part of the dose of formoterol is eliminated via metabolism. After inhalation 8-13% of the delivered dose (corresponding to 6-10% of the metered dose) of formoterol is excreted unmetabolised in the urine. About 20% of an intravenous dose is excreted unchanged in the urine. The terminal half-life after inhalation is estimated to be 17 hours.

5.3 Preclinical safety data

The effects of formoterol seen in toxicity studies in rats and dogs were mainly on the cardiovascular system and consisted of hyperaemia, tachycardia, arrhythmias and myocardial lesions. These effects are known pharmacological manifestations seen after the administration of high doses of β_2-agonists.

A somewhat reduced fertility in male rats was observed at high systemic exposure to formoterol.

No genotoxic effects of formoterol have been observed in in-vitro or in vivo tests. In rats and mice a slight increase in the incidence of benign uterine leiomyomas has been observed. This effect is looked upon as a class-effect observed in rodents after long exposure to high doses of β_2-agonists.

6. PHARMACEUTICAL PARTICULARS

6.1 List of excipients

Lactose monohydrate.

6.2 Incompatibilities

Not applicable.

6.3 Shelf life

2 years.

6.4 Special precautions for storage

Do not store above 30°C. Should be stored with cover tightened.

6.5 Nature and contents of container

Oxis Turbohaler is a multidose, inspiratory flow driven, dry powder inhaler. The inhaler is made of plastic parts (PP, PC, HDPE, LDPE, LLDPE, PBT).

Each inhaler contains 60 doses.

Each pack contains either 60 doses (one inhaler),180 doses (three inhalers), 600 doses (10 Inhalers), 1080 doses (18 Inhalers), 1200 doses (20 inhalers).

Not all pack-sizes may be marketed.

6.6 Instructions for use and handling

No special requirements.

7. MARKETING AUTHORISATION HOLDER

AstraZeneca UK Ltd. 600 Capability Green

Luton

Bedfordshire

LU1 3LU

UK

8. MARKETING AUTHORISATION NUMBER(S)

PL17901/0153

9. DATE OF FIRST AUTHORISATION/RENEWAL OF THE AUTHORISATION

29th March 2003

10. DATE OF REVISION OF THE TEXT

15 October 2004

Oxis Turbohaler 6, inhalation powder

(AstraZeneca UK Limited)

1. NAME OF THE MEDICINAL PRODUCT

Oxis Turbohaler 6, inhalation powder.

2. QUALITATIVE AND QUANTITATIVE COMPOSITION

Each delivered dose (i.e. the dose leaving the mouthpiece) from Oxis Turbohaler 6 contains 4.5 micrograms formoterol fumarate dihydrate, which is derived from a metered dose of 6 micrograms.

For excipients, see 6.1.

3. PHARMACEUTICAL FORM

Inhalation powder.

White powder.

4. CLINICAL PARTICULARS

4.1 Therapeutic indications

Oxis Turbohaler is indicated as add on therapy to maintenance treatment with inhaled corticosteroids, for the relief of broncho-obstructive symptoms and prevention of exercise-induced symptoms, in patients with asthma when adequate treatment with corticosteroids is not sufficient. Oxis Turbohaler is also indicated for the relief of broncho-obstructive symptoms in patients with chronic obstructive pulmonary disease (COPD).

4.2 Posology and method of administration

Use of doses above those normally required by the individual patient on more than 2 days per week, is a sign of suboptimal disease control and maintenance treatment should be reassessed.

Asthma:

In asthma, Oxis turbohaler can be used once or twice daily ('regular dosage') and as 'relief medication' to relieve acute broncho-obstructive symptoms.

Adults aged > 18 years:

Relief medication: 1 or 2 inhalations for the relief of acute broncho-obstructive symptoms.

Regular dosage: 1 or 2 inhalations once or twice daily. Some patients may need 4 inhalations once or twice daily.

Prevention of exercise-induced bronchoconstriction: 2 inhalations before exercise.

The daily dose for regular use should not exceed 8 inhalations, however occasionally up to a maximum of 12 inhalations may be allowed within a 24-hour period.

No more than 6 inhalations should be taken on any single occasion.

Children and adolescents 6years and older:

Relief medication: 1 or 2 inhalations for the relief of acute broncho-

obstructive symptoms.

Regular dosage: 2 inhalations once or twice daily.

Prevention of exercise-induced bronchoconstriction: 1 or 2 inhalations before exercise.

The regular daily dose should not exceed 4 inhalations, however occasionally up to 8 inhalations may be allowed within a 24-hour period. No more than 2 inhalations should be taken on any single occasion.

COPD:

Regular dosage: 2 inhalations once or twice daily.

The daily dose for regular use should not exceed 4 inhalations.

If required, additional inhalations above those prescribed for regular therapy may be used for relief of symptoms, up to a maximum total daily dose of 8 inhalations (regular plus as required). More than 4 inhalations should not be taken on any single occasion.

Special patient groups:

No adjustment of dose should be required in the elderly, or in patients with renal or hepatic impairment at the recommended normal doses. (See Special warnings and special precautions for use.)

NB! A higher strength is available as an alternative for patients requiring 2 or more inhalations.

Oxis Turbohaler is inspiratory flow driven which means that, when the patient inhales through the mouthpiece, the substance will follow the inspired air into the airways.

Note! It is important to instruct the patient to breathe in forcefully and deeply through the mouthpiece to ensure that an optimal dose is obtained.

It is important to instruct the patient never to chew or bite on the mouthpiece and never to use the inhaler if it has been damaged or if the mouthpiece has become detached.

The patient may not taste or feel any medication when using Oxis Turbohaler due to the small amount of drug dispensed.

Detailed instructions for use are packed together with each inhaler.

4.3 Contraindications

Hypersensitivity to formoterol or to inhaled lactose.

4.4 Special warnings and special precautions for use

Asthmatic patients who require therapy with long acting β_2-agonists, should also receive optimal maintenance anti-inflammatory therapy with corticosteroids. Patients must be advised to continue taking their anti-inflammatory therapy after the introduction of Oxis Turbohaler even when symptoms decrease. Should symptoms persist, or treatment with β_2-agonists need to be increased, this indicates a worsening of the underlying condition and warrants a reassessment of the maintenance therapy. Oxis Turbohaler should not be initiated to treat a severe asthma exacerbation.

The maximum daily dose should not be exceeded. The long-term safety of regular treatment at higher doses than 36 micrograms per day in adults with asthma, 18 micrograms per day in children with asthma and 18 micrograms per day in patients with COPD, has not been established.

Frequent need of medication for the prevention of exercise-induced bronchconstriction can be a sign of suboptimal asthma control, and warrants a reassessment of the asthma therapy and an evaluation of the compliance. If the patient needs prophylactic treatment for exercise-induced bronchconstriction several times every week despite an adequate maintenance treatment (e.g. corticosteroids and long-acting β_2-agonists), the total asthma management should be reassessed by a specialist.

Caution should be observed when treating patients with thyrotoxicosis, phaeochromocytoma, hypertrophic obstructive cardiomyopathy, idiopathic subvalvular aortic stenosis, severe hypertension, aneurysm or other severe cardiovascular disorders, such as ischaemic heart disease, tachyarrhythmias or severe heart failure.

Formoterol may induce prolongation of the QTc-interval. Caution should be observed when treating patients with prolongation of the QTc-interval and in patients treated with drugs affecting the QTc-interval (see 4.5).

Due to the hyperglycaemic effects of β_2-agonists, additional blood glucose monitoring is recommended initially in diabetic patients.

Potentially serious hypokalaemia may result from β_2-agonist therapy. Particular caution is recommended in acute severe asthma as the associated risk may be augmented by hypoxia. The hypokalaemic effect may be potentiated by concomitant treatment with xanthine-derivatives, steroids and diuretics. The serum potassium levels should therefore be monitored.

As with other inhalation therapy, the potential for paradoxical bronchospasm should be considered.

Oxis Turbohaler contains lactose 450 micrograms per delivered dose (corresponding to 600 micrograms per metered dose). This amount does not normally cause problems in lactose intolerant people.

Children up to the age of 6 years should not be treated with Oxis Turbohaler, as no sufficient experience is available for this group.

The effect of decreased liver or kidney function on the pharmacokinetics of formoterol and the pharmacokinetics in the elderly is not known. As formoterol is primarily eliminated via metabolism an increased exposure can be expected in patients with severe liver cirrhosis.

4.5 Interaction with other medicinal products and other forms of Interaction

No specific interaction studies have been carried out with Oxis Turbohaler.

Concomitant treatment with other sympathomimetic substances such as other β_2-agonists or ephedrine may potentiate the undesirable effects of Oxis Turbohaler and may require titration of the dose.

Concomitant treatment with xanthine derivatives, steroids or diuretics such as thiazides and loop diuretics may potentiate a rare hypokalaemic adverse effect of β_2-agonists. Hypokalaemia may increase the disposition towards arrhythmias in patients who are treated with digitalis glycosides.

There is a theoretical risk that concomitant treatment with other drugs known to prolong the QTc-interval may give rise to a pharmacodynamic interaction with fomoterol and increase the possible risk of ventricular arrhythmias. Examples of such drugs include certain antihistamines (e.g. terfenadine, astemizole, mizolastine), certain antiarrhythmics (e.g. quinidine, disopyramide, procainamide), erythromycin and tricyclic antidepressants.

here is an elevated risk of arrhythmias in patients receiving concomitant anaesthesia with halogenated hydrocarbons.

Beta-adrenergic blockers can weaken or inhibit the effect of Oxis Turbohaler. Oxis Turbohaler should therefore not be given together with beta-adrenergic blockers (including eye drops) unless there are compelling reasons.

4.6 Pregnancy and lactation

Clinical experience in pregnant women is limited. In animal studies formoterol has caused implantation losses as well as decreased early postnatal survival and birth weight. The effects appeared at considerably higher systemic exposures than those reached during clinical use of Oxis Turbohaler. Treatment with Oxis Turbohaler may be considered at all stages of pregnancy if needed to obtain asthma control and if the expected benefit to the mother is greater than any possible risk to the foetus.

It is not known whether formoterol passes into human breast milk. In rats, small amounts of formoterol have been detected in maternal milk. Administration of Oxis Turbohaler to women who are breastfeeding should only be considered if the expected benefit to the mother is greater than any possible risk to the child.

4.7 Effects on ability to drive and use machines

Oxis Turbohaler does not affect the ability to drive or use machines.

4.8 Undesirable effects

The most commonly reported adverse events of β_2-agonist therapy, such as tremor and palpitations, tend to be mild and disappear within days of treatment.

Common 1% to 10%	*Cardiac disorders:* Palpitations *Nervous system disorders:* Headache, tremor
Uncommon 0.1% to 1%	*Cardiac disorders:* Tachycardia *Musculoskeletal and connective tissue disorders:* Muscle cramps *Psychiatric disorders:* Agitation, restlessness, sleep disturbance
Rare 0.01% to 0.1%	*Cardiac disorders:* Cardiac arrhythmias, e.g. atrial fibrillation, supraventricular tachycardia, extrasystoles *Gastrointestinal disorders:* Nausea *Immune system disorders:* Hypersensitivity reactions, e.g. bronchospasm, exanthema, urticaria, pruritus *Metabolism and nutrition disorders:* Hypokalaemia/hyperkalaemia
Very rare <0.01%	*Cardiac disorders:* Angina pectoris *Investigations:* Prolongation of the QTc-interval *Metabolism and nutrition disorders:* Hyperglycaemia *Nervous system disorders:* Taste disturbance, dizziness *Vascular disorders:* Variations in blood pressure

As with all inhalation therapy, paradoxical bronchospasm may occur in very rare cases.

reatment with β_2-agonists may result in an increase in blood levels of insulin, free fatty acids, glycerol and ketone bodies.

4.9 Overdose

There is limited clinical experience on the management of overdose. An overdose would likely lead to effects that are typical of β_2-agonists: tremor, headache, palpitations. Symptoms reported from isolated cases are tachycardia, hyperglycaemia, hypokalaemia, prolonged QTc-interval, arrhythmia, nausea and vomiting. Supportive and symptomatic treatment is indicated.

Use of cardioselective beta-blockers may be considered, but only subject to extreme caution since the use of β-adrenergic blocker medication may provoke bronchospasm. Serum potassium should be monitored.

5. PHARMACOLOGICAL PROPERTIES

5.1 Pharmacodynamic properties

Pharmacotherapeutic group: selective β_2-agonist, formoterol, ATC code: R03A C13.

Formoterol is a selective β_2-adrenoceptor agonist that produces relaxation of bronchial smooth muscle. Formoterol thus has a bronchodilating effect in patients with reversible airways obstruction. The bronchodilating effect sets in rapidly, within 1-3 minutes after inhalation and has a mean duration of 12 hours after a single dose.

5.2 Pharmacokinetic properties

Absorption

Inhaled formoterol is rapidly absorbed. Peak plasma concentration is reached about 10 minutes after inhalation.

In studies the mean lung deposition of formoterol after inhalation via Turbohaler ranged from 28-49% of the delivered dose (corresponding to 21-37% of the metered dose). The total systemic availability for the higher lung deposition was around 61% of the delivered dose (corresponding to 46% of the metered dose).

Distribution and metabolism

Plasma protein binding is approximately 50%.

Formoterol is metabolised via direct glucuronidation and O-demethylation. The enzyme responsible for O-demethylation has not been identified. Total plasma clearance and volume of distribution has not been determined.

Elimination

The major part of the dose of formoterol is eliminated via metabolism. After inhalation 8-13% of the delivered dose (corresponding to 6-10% of the metered dose) of formoterol is excreted unmetabolised in the urine. About 20% of an intravenous dose is excreted unchanged in the urine. The terminal half-life after inhalation is estimated to be 17 hours.

5.3 Preclinical safety data

The effects of formoterol seen in toxicity studies in rats and dogs were mainly on the cardiovascular system and consisted of hyperaemia, tachycardia, arrhythmias and myocardial lesions. These effects are known pharmacological manifestations seen after the administration of high doses of β_2-agonists.

A somewhat reduced fertility in male rats was observed at high systemic exposure to formoterol.

No genotoxic effects of formoterol have been observed in in-vitro or in vivo tests. In rats and mice a slight increase in the incidence of benign uterine leiomyomas has been observed. This effect is looked upon as a class-effect observed in rodents after long exposure to high doses of β_2-agonists.

6. PHARMACEUTICAL PARTICULARS

6.1 List of excipients

Lactose monohydrate.

6.2 Incompatibilities

Not applicable.

6.3 Shelf life

2 years.

6.4 Special precautions for storage

Do not store above 30°C. Should be stored with cover tightened.

6.5 Nature and contents of container

Oxis Turbohaler is a multidose, inspiratory flow driven, dry powder inhaler.

The inhaler is made of plastic parts (PP, PC, HDPE, LDPE, LLDPE, PBT).

Each inhaler contains 60 doses.

Each pack contains either 60 doses (one inhaler), 180 doses (three inhalers), 600 doses (10 Inhalers), 1080 doses (18 Inhalers), 1200 doses (20 inhalers).

Not all pack-sizes may be marketed.

6.6 Instructions for use and handling

No special requirements.

7. MARKETING AUTHORISATION HOLDER

AstraZeneca UK Ltd. 600 Capability Green

Luton

Bedfordshire

LU1 3LU

UK

8. MARKETING AUTHORISATION NUMBER(S)

PL 17901/0154

9. DATE OF FIRST AUTHORISATION/RENEWAL OF THE AUTHORISATION

29th March 2003

10. DATE OF REVISION OF THE TEXT

16 October 2004

OxyContin tablets

(Napp Pharmaceuticals Limited)

1. NAME OF THE MEDICINAL PRODUCT

OxyContin® 5 mg, 10 mg, 20 mg, 40 mg, 80 mg film-coated, prolonged release tablets ▼

2. QUALITATIVE AND QUANTITATIVE COMPOSITION

5 mg tablet contains 4.5 mg of oxycodone as 5 mg of oxycodone hydrochloride.

10 mg tablet contains 9.0 mg of oxycodone as 10 mg of oxycodone hydrochloride.

20 mg tablet contains 18.0 mg of oxycodone as 20 mg of oxycodone hydrochloride.

40 mg tablet contains 36.0 mg of oxycodone as 40 mg of oxycodone hydrochloride.

80 mg tablet contains 72.0 mg of oxycodone as 80 mg of oxycodone hydrochloride.

For excipients see section 6.1.

3. PHARMACEUTICAL FORM

Film coated, prolonged release, round, convex tablet.

The 5 mg tablets are light blue, marked OC on one side and 5 on the other.

The 10 mg tablets are white, marked OC on one side and 10 on the other.

The 20 mg tablets are pink, marked OC on one side and 20 on the other.

The 40 mg tablets are yellow, marked OC on one side and 40 on the other.

The 80 mg tablets are green, marked OC on one side and 80 on the other.

4. CLINICAL PARTICULARS

4.1 Therapeutic indications

For the treatment of moderate to severe pain in patients with cancer and post-operative pain.

For the treatment of severe pain requiring the use of a strong opioid.

4.2 Posology and method of administration

OxyContin tablets must be swallowed whole, and not chewed.

Elderly and adults over 18 years:

OxyContin tablets should be taken at 12-hourly intervals. The dosage is dependent on the severity of the pain, and the patient's previous history of analgesic requirements.

OxyContin is not intended for use as a prn analgesic.

Increasing severity of pain will require an increased dosage of ***OxyContin*** tablets using the 5 mg, 10 mg, 20 mg, 40 mg or 80 mg tablet strengths, either alone or in combination, to achieve pain relief. The correct dosage for any individual patient is that which controls the pain and is well tolerated for a full 12 hours. Patients should be titrated to pain relief unless unmanageable adverse drug reactions prevent this. If higher doses are necessary increases should be made, where possible, in 25% - 50% increments. The need for escape medication more than twice a day indicates that the dosage of ***OxyContin*** tablets should be increased.

The usual starting dose for opioid naïve patients or patients presenting with severe pain uncontrolled by weaker opioids is 10 mg, 12-hourly. Some patients may benefit from a starting dose of 5 mg to minimise the incidence of side effects. The dose should then be carefully titrated, as frequently as once a day if necessary, to achieve pain relief. For the majority of patients, the maximum dose is 200 mg 12-hourly. However, a few patients may require higher doses. Doses in excess of 1000 mg have been recorded.

Patients receiving oral morphine before ***OxyContin*** therapy should have their daily dose based on the following ratio: 10 mg of oral oxycodone is equivalent to 20 mg of oral morphine. It must be emphasised that this is a guide to the dose of ***OxyContin*** tablets required. Inter-patient variability requires that each patient is carefully titrated to the appropriate dose.

Controlled pharmacokinetic studies in elderly patients (aged over 65 years) have shown that, compared with younger adults, the clearance of oxycodone is only slightly reduced. No untoward adverse drug reactions were seen based on age, therefore adult doses and dosage intervals are appropriate.

Children under 18 years:

There were no studies in patients below 18 years of age, therefore ***OxyContin*** should not be used in patients under 18 years.

Adults with mild to moderate renal impairment and mild hepatic impairment:

The plasma concentration in this population may be increased. Therefore dose initiation should follow a conservative approach. Patients should be started on ***OxyContin*** 5 mg 12-hourly or ***OxyNorm*** liquid 2.5 mg 6-hourly and titrated to pain relief as described above.

Use in non-malignant pain:

Opioids are not first line therapy for chronic non-malignant pain, nor are they recommended as the only treatment. Types of chronic pain which have been shown to be alleviated by strong opioids include chronic osteoarthritic pain and intervertebral disc disease. The need for continued treatment in non-malignant pain should be assessed at regular intervals.

Cessation of therapy:

When a patient no longer requires therapy with oxycodone, it may be advisable to taper the dose gradually to prevent symptoms of withdrawal.

4.3 Contraindications

Hypersensitivity to any of the constituents, respiratory depression, head injury, paralytic ileus, acute abdomen, delayed gastric emptying, chronic obstructive airways disease, cor pulmonale, chronic bronchial asthma, hypercarbia, known oxycodone sensitivity or in any situation where opioids are contraindicated, moderate to severe hepatic impairment, severe renal impairment (creatinine clearance <10 ml/min), chronic constipation, concurrent administration of monoamine oxidase inhibitors or within 2 weeks of discontinuation of their use. Not recommended for pre-operative use or for the first 24 hours post-operatively. Patients with rare hereditary problems of galactose intolerance, the Lapp lactase deficiency or glucose-galactose malabsorption should not take this medicine. Pregnancy.

4.4 Special warnings and special precautions for use

The major risk of opioid excess is respiratory depression. As with all narcotics, a reduction in dosage may be advisable in hypothyroidism. Use with caution in patients with raised intracranial pressure, hypotension, hypovolaemia, toxic psychosis, diseases of the biliary tract, pancreatitis, inflammatory bowel disorders, prostatic hypertrophy, adrenocortical insufficiency, acute alcoholism, delirium tremens, chronic renal and hepatic disease or severe pulmonary disease, and debilitated, elderly and infirm patients. ***OxyContin*** tablets should not be used where there is a possibility of paralytic ileus occurring. Should paralytic ileus be suspected or occur during use, ***OxyContin*** tablets should be discontinued immediately. As with all opioid preparations, patients who are to undergo cordotomy or other pain relieving surgical procedures should not receive ***OxyContin*** tablets for 24 hours before surgery. If further treatment with ***OxyContin*** tablets is then indicated the dosage should be adjusted to the new post-operative requirement.

OxyContin 80 mg should not be used in patients not previously exposed to opioids. This tablet strength may cause fatal respiratory depression when administered to opioid naïve patients.

As with all opioid preparations, ***OxyContin*** tablets should be used with caution following abdominal surgery as opioids are known to impair intestinal motility and should not be used until the physician is assured of normal bowel function.

For appropriate patients who suffer with chronic non-malignant pain, opioids should be used as part of a comprehensive treatment programme involving other medications and treatment modalities. A crucial part of the assessment of a patient with chronic non-malignant pain is the patient's addiction and substance abuse history. ***OxyContin*** tablets should be used with particular care in patients with a history of alcohol and drug abuse.

If opioid treatment is considered appropriate for the patient, then the main aim of treatment is not to minimise the dose of opioid but rather to achieve a dose which provides adequate pain relief with a minimum of side effects. There must be frequent contact between physician and patient so that dosage adjustments can be made. It is strongly recommended that the physician defines treatment outcomes in accordance with pain management guidelines. The physician and patient can then agree to discontinue treatment if these objectives are not met.

OxyContin has an abuse liability similar to other strong opioids and should be used with caution in opioid dependent patients, or if the doctor or pharmacist is concerned about the risk of misuse. Oxycodone may be sought and abused by people with latent or manifest addiction disorders.

As with other opioids, infants who are born to dependent mothers may exhibit withdrawal symptoms and may have respiratory depression at birth.

OxyContin tablets must be swallowed whole, and not broken, chewed or crushed. The administration of broken, chewed or crushed ***OxyContin*** tablets leads to a rapid release and absorption of a potentially fatal dose of oxycodone (see Section 4.9). Abuse of the tablets by parenteral administration can be expected to result in other serious adverse events, such as local tissue necrosis, infection, pulmonary granulomas, increased risk of endocarditis, and valvular heart injury, which may be fatal.

4.5 Interaction with other medicinal products and other forms of Interaction

OxyContin, like other opioids, potentiates the effects of tranquillisers, anaesthetics, hypnotics, anti-depressants, sedatives, phenothiazines, neuroleptic drugs, alcohol, other opioids, muscle relaxants and antihypertensives. Monoamine oxidase inhibitors are known to interact with narcotic analgesics, producing CNS excitation or depression with hypertensive or hypotensive crisis. Concurrent administration of quinidine, an inhibitor of cytochrome P450-2D6, resulted in an increase in oxycodone C_{max} by 11%, AUC by 13%, and $t_{½}$ elim. by 14%. Also an increase in noroxycodone level was observed, (C_{max} by 50%; AUC by 85%, and $t_{½}$ elim. by 42%). The pharmacodynamic effects of oxycodone were not altered. This interaction may be observed for other potent inhibitors of cytochrome P450-2D6 enzyme. Cimetidine and inhibitors of cytochrome P450-3A such as ketoconazole and erythromycin may inhibit the metabolism of oxycodone.

4.6 Pregnancy and lactation

OxyContin tablets are not recommended for use in pregnancy nor during labour. Infants born to mothers who have received opioids during pregnancy should be monitored for respiratory depression.

Oxycodone may be secreted in breast milk and may cause respiratory depression in the newborn. ***OxyContin*** tablets should, therefore, not be used in breast-feeding mothers.

4.7 Effects on ability to drive and use machines

Oxycodone may modify patients' reactions to a varying extent depending on the dosage and individual susceptibility. Therefore patients should not drive or operate machinery if affected.

4.8 Undesirable effects

Adverse drug reactions are typical of full opioid agonists. Tolerance and dependence may occur (see *Tolerance and Dependence*, below). Constipation may be prevented with an appropriate laxative. If nausea and vomiting are troublesome, oxycodone may be combined with an anti-emetic.

Common (incidence of ≥1%) and uncommon (incidence of ≤1%) adverse drug reactions are listed in the table below.

Body System	Common	Uncommon
Gastrointestinal	Constipation	Biliary spasm
	Nausea	Dysphagia
	Vomiting	Eructation
	Dry mouth	Flatulence
	Anorexia	Gastrointestinal disorders
	Dyspepsia	Ileus
	Abdominal pain	Taste perversion
	Diarrhoea	Gastritis
		Hiccups
Central Nervous System	Headache	Vertigo
	Confusion	Hallucinations
	Asthenia	Hypertonia
	Faintness	Disorientation
	Dizziness	Mood changes
	Sedation	Restlessness
	Anxiety	Agitation
	Abnormal dreams	Depression
	Nervousness	Tremor
	Insomnia	Withdrawal syndrome
	Thought abnormalities	Amnesia
	Drowsiness	Hypoaesthesia
	Twitching	Hypotonia
		Malaise
		Paraesthesia
		Speech disorder
		Euphoria
		Dysphoria
		Seizure
		Vision abnormalities
Genitourinary		Urinary retention
		Ureteric spasm
		Impotence
		Amenorrhoea
		Decreased libido
Cardiovascular	Orthostatic hypotension	Palpitations
		Supraventricular tachycardia
		Hypotension
		Syncope
		Vasodilation
Metabolic and Nutritional		Dehydration
		Oedema
		Peripheral oedema
		Thirst
Respiratory	Bronchospasm	Overdose may produce respiratory depression
	Dyspnoea	
	Decreased cough reflex	
Dermatological	Rash	Dry skin
	Pruritus	Exfoliative dermatitis
		Urticaria
General	Sweating	Facial flushing
	Chills	Miosis
		Muscular rigidity
		Allergic reaction
		Fever
		Anaphylaxis

Tolerance and Dependence:

The patient may develop tolerance to the drug with chronic use and require progressively higher doses to maintain pain control. Prolonged use of ***OxyContin*** tablets may lead to physical dependence and a withdrawal syndrome may occur upon abrupt cessation of therapy. When a patient no longer requires therapy with oxycodone, it may be advisable to taper the dose gradually to prevent symptoms of withdrawal. The opioid abstinence or withdrawal syndrome is characterised by some or all of the following:

restlessness, lacrimation, rhinorrhea, yawning, perspiration, chills, myalgia and mydriasis. Other symptoms also may develop, including: irritability, anxiety, backache, joint pain, weakness, abdominal cramps, insomnia, nausea, anorexia, vomiting, diarrhoea, or increased blood pressure, respiratory rate or heart rate.

The development of psychological dependence (addiction) to opioid analgesics in properly managed patients with pain has been reported to be rare. However, data are not available to establish the true incidence of psychological dependence (addiction) in chronic pain patients.

OxyContin tablets should be used with particular care in patients with a history of alcohol and drug abuse.

4.9 Overdose

Signs of oxycodone toxicity and overdosage are pin-point pupils, respiratory depression and hypotension. Circulatory failure and somnolence progressing to stupor or deepening coma, skeletal muscle flaccidity, bradycardia and death may occur in more severe cases.

Treatment of oxycodone overdosage: Primary attention should be given to the establishment of a patent airway and institution of assisted or controlled ventilation.

In the case of massive overdosage, administer naloxone intravenously (0.4 to 2 mg for an adult and 0.01 mg/kg body weight for children), if the patient is in a coma or respiratory depression is present. Repeat the dose at 2 minute intervals if there is no response. If repeated doses are required then an infusion of 60% of the initial dose per hour is a useful starting point. A solution of 10 mg made up in 50 ml dextrose will produce 200 micrograms/ml for infusion using an IV pump (dose adjusted to the clinical response). Infusions are not a substitute for frequent review of the patient's clinical state. Intramuscular naloxone is an alternative in the event IV access is not possible. As the duration of action of naloxone is relatively short, the patient must be carefully monitored until spontaneous respiration is reliably re-established. Naloxone is a competitive antagonist and large doses (4 mg) may be required in seriously poisoned patients.

For less severe overdosage, administer naloxone 0.2 mg intravenously followed by increments of 0.1 mg every 2 minutes if required.

Naloxone should not be administered in the absence of clinically significant respiratory or circulatory depression secondary to oxycodone overdosage. Naloxone should be administered cautiously to persons who are known, or suspected, to be physically dependent on oxycodone. In such cases, an abrupt or complete reversal of opioid effects may precipitate pain and an acute withdrawal syndrome.

Additional/other considerations:

- Consider activated charcoal (50 g for adults, 10 -15 g for children), if a substantial amount has been ingested within 1 hour, provided the airway can be protected. It may be reasonable to assume that late administration of activated charcoal may be beneficial for prolonged release preparations; however there is no evidence to support this.
- **OxyContin** tablets will continue to release and add to the oxycodone load for up to 12 hours after administration and management of oxycodone overdosage should be modified accordingly. Gastric contents may need to be emptied as this can be useful in removing unabsorbed drug, particularly when a prolonged release formulation has been taken.

5. PHARMACOLOGICAL PROPERTIES

5.1 Pharmacodynamic properties

Pharmacotherapeutic group: Natural opium alkaloids

ATC code: NO2A AO5

Oxycodone is a full opioid agonist with no antagonist properties. It has an affinity for kappa, mu and delta opiate receptors in the brain and spinal cord. Oxycodone is similar to morphine in its action. The therapeutic effect is mainly analgesic, anxiolytic and sedative.

5.2 Pharmacokinetic properties

Compared with morphine, which has an absolute bioavailability of approximately 30%, oxycodone has a high absolute bioavailability of up to 87% following oral administration. Oxycodone has an elimination half-life of approximately 3 hours and is metabolised principally to noroxycodone and oxymorphone. Oxymorphone has some analgesic activity but is present in the plasma in low concentrations and is not considered to contribute to oxycodone's pharmacological effect.

The release of oxycodone from **OxyContin** tablets is biphasic with an initial relatively fast release providing an early onset of analgesia followed by a more controlled release which determines the 12 hour duration of action. The mean apparent elimination half-life of **OxyContin** is 4.5 hours which leads to steady-state being achieved in about one day.

Release of oxycodone from **OxyContin** tablets is independent of pH.

OxyContin tablets have an oral bioavailability comparable with conventional oral oxycodone, but the former achieve maximal plasma concentrations at about 3 hours rather than about 1 to 1.5 hours. Peak and trough concentrations of oxycodone from **OxyContin** tablets 10 mg administered 12-hourly are equivalent to those achieved from conventional oxycodone 5 mg administered 6-hourly.

OxyContin tablets 5 mg, 10 mg, 20 mg, 40 mg and 80 mg are bioequivalent in terms of both rate and extent of absorption. Ingestion of a standard high-fat meal does not alter the peak oxycodone concentration or the extent of oxycodone absorption from **OxyContin** tablets.

Elderly

The AUC in elderly subjects is 15% greater when compared with young subjects.

Gender

Female subjects have, on average, plasma oxycodone concentrations up to 25% higher than males on a body weight adjusted basis. The reason for this difference is unknown.

Patients with renal impairment

Preliminary data from a study of patients with mild to moderate renal dysfunction show peak plasma oxycodone and noroxycodone concentrations approximately 50% and 20% higher, respectively and AUC values for oxycodone, noroxycodone and oxymorphone approximately 60%, 60% and 40% higher than normal subjects, respectively. There was an increase in $t_{½}$ of elimination for oxycodone of only 1 hour.

Patients with mild to moderate hepatic impairment

Patients with mild to moderate hepatic dysfunction showed peak plasma oxycodone and noroxycodone concentrations approximately 50% and 20% higher, respectively, than normal subjects. AUC values were approximately 95% and 75% higher, respectively. Oxymorphone peak plasma concentrations and AUC values were lower by 15% to 50%. The $t_{½}$ elimination for oxycodone increased by 2.3 hours.

5.3 Preclinical safety data

Oxycodone was not mutagenic in the following assays: Ames Salmonella and E. Coli test with and without metabolic activation at doses of up to 5000 μg, chromosomal aberration test in human lymphocytes (in the absence of metabolic activation and with activation after 48 hours of exposure) at doses of up to 1500 μg/ml, and in the *in vivo* bone marrow micronucleus assay in mice (at plasma levels of up to 48 μg/ml). Mutagenic results occurred in the presence of metabolic activation in the human chromosomal aberration test (at greater than or equal to 1250 μg/ml) at 24 but not 48 hours of exposure and in the mouse lymphoma assay at doses of 50 μg/ml or greater with metabolic activation and at 400 μg/ml or greater without metabolic activation. The data from these tests indicate that the genotoxic risk to humans may be considered low.

Studies of oxycodone in animals to evaluate its carcinogenic potential have not been conducted owing to the length of clinical experience with the drug substance.

6. PHARMACEUTICAL PARTICULARS

6.1 List of excipients

Lactose monohydrate

Povidone

Ammoniomethacrylate co-polymer

Sorbic acid

Glyceryl triacetate

Stearyl alcohol

Talc

Magnesium stearate

Hypromellose (E464)

Titanium dioxide (E171)

Macrogol

In addition the tablets contain the following:

5 mg	Brilliant blue (E133)
10 mg	Hydroxypropylcellulose
20 mg and 40 mg	Polysorbate 80, iron oxide (E172).
80 mg	Hydroxypropylcellulose, iron oxide (E172), indigo carmine (E132)

6.2 Incompatibilities

Not applicable

6.3 Shelf life

Three years.

6.4 Special precautions for storage

Do not store above 25°C.

6.5 Nature and contents of container

PVC blister packs with aluminium foil backing containing 28 tablets (5 mg) or 56 tablets (10, 20, 40, 80 mg).

6.6 Instructions for use and handling

None.

7. MARKETING AUTHORISATION HOLDER

Napp Pharmaceuticals Ltd

Cambridge Science Park

Milton Road

Cambridge CB4 0GW

8. MARKETING AUTHORISATION NUMBER(S)

PL 16950/0097-0100, 0123

9. DATE OF FIRST AUTHORISATION/RENEWAL OF THE AUTHORISATION

10, 20, 40, 80 mg tablets: 5 March 1999/ 30 June 2005

5 mg tablets: 21 May 2002/ 30 June 2005

10. DATE OF REVISION OF THE TEXT

March 2005

11. Legal Category

CD (Sch 2) POM

® **OxyContin** and the Napp Device are Registered Trade Marks.

OxyNorm 10 mg/ml solution for injection or infusion

(Napp Pharmaceuticals Limited)

1. NAME OF THE MEDICINAL PRODUCT

OxyNorm® 10 mg/ml, solution for injection or infusion ▼

2. QUALITATIVE AND QUANTITATIVE COMPOSITION

Oxycodone hydrochloride 10 mg/ml

(equivalent to 9 mg/ml oxycodone)

For excipients, see section 6.1

3. PHARMACEUTICAL FORM

Solution for injection or infusion.

4. CLINICAL PARTICULARS

4.1 Therapeutic indications

For the treatment of moderate to severe pain in patients with cancer and post-operative pain.

For the treatment of severe pain requiring the use of a strong opioid

4.2 Posology and method of administration

Route of administration:

Subcutaneous injection or infusion

Intravenous injection or infusion.

Posology:

The dose should be adjusted according to the severity of pain, the total condition of the patient and previous or concurrent medication.

Adults over 18 years:

The following starting doses are recommended. A gradual increase in dose may be required if analgesia is inadequate or if pain severity increases.

i.v. (Bolus): Dilute to 1 mg/ml in 0.9% saline, 5% dextrose or water for injections. Administer a bolus dose of 1 to 10 mg slowly over 1-2 minutes.

Doses should not be administered more frequently than every 4 hours.

i.v. (Infusion): Dilute to 1 mg/ml in 0.9% saline, 5% dextrose or water for injections. A starting dose of 2 mg/hour is recommended.

i.v. (PCA): Dilute to 1 mg/ml in 0.9% saline, 5% dextrose or water for injections. Bolus doses of 0.03 mg/kg should be administered with a minimum lock-out time of 5 minutes.

s.c. (Bolus): Use as 10 mg/ml concentration. A starting dose of 5 mg is recommended, repeated at 4-hourly intervals as required.

s.c. (Infusion): Dilute in 0.9% saline, 5% dextrose or water for injections if required. A starting dose of 7.5 mg/day is recommended in opioid naïve patients, titrating gradually according to symptom control. Cancer patients transferring from oral oxycodone may require much higher doses (see below).

Transferring patients between oral and parenteral oxycodone:

The dose should be based on the following ratio: 2 mg of oral oxycodone is equivalent to 1 mg of parenteral oxycodone. It must be emphasised that this is a guide to the dose required. Inter-patient variability requires that each patient is carefully titrated to the appropriate dose.

Elderly:

Elderly patients should be treated with caution. The lowest dose should be administered with careful titration to pain control.

Patients with renal and hepatic impairment:

Patients with mild to moderate renal impairment and/or mild hepatic impairment should be treated with caution. The lowest dose should be given with careful titration to pain control.

Children under 18 years:

There are no data on the use of ***OxyNorm*** injection in patients under 18 years of age.

Use in non-malignant pain:

Opioids are not first line therapy for chronic non-malignant pain, nor are they recommended as the only treatment. Types of chronic pain which have been shown to be alleviated by strong opioids include chronic osteoarthritic pain and intervertebral disc disease. The need for continued treatment in non-malignant pain should be assessed at regular intervals.

Cessation of therapy:

When a patient no longer requires therapy with oxycodone, it may be advisable to taper the dose gradually to prevent symptoms of withdrawal.

4.3 Contraindications

OxyNorminjection is contraindicated in patients with known hypersensitivity to oxycodone or any of the other constituents; or in situation where opioids are contraindicated; respiratory depression; head injury; paralytic ileus; acute abdomen; chronic obstructive airways disease; cor pulmonale; chronic bronchial asthma; hypercarbia; moderate to severe hepatic impairment; severe renal impairment (creatinine clearance < 10 ml/min); chronic constipation; concurrent administration of monoamine oxidase inhibitors or within 2 weeks of discontinuation of their use; pregnancy.

4.4 Special warnings and special precautions for use

The major risk of opioid excess is respiratory depression. As with all opioids, a reduction in dosage may be advisable in hypothyroidism. Use with caution in patients with raised intracranial pressure, hypotension, hypovolaemia, toxic psychosis, diseases of the biliary tract, inflammatory bowel disorders, prostatic hypertrophy, adrenocortical insufficiency, acute alcoholism, delerium tremens, pancreatitis, chronic renal and hepatic disease or severe pulmonary disease and debilitated, elderly and infirm patients. ***OxyNorm*** injection should not be used where there is a possibility of paralytic ileus occurring. Should paralytic ileus be suspected or occur during use, ***OxyNorm*** injection should be discontinued immediately.

The patient may develop tolerance to oxycodone with chronic use and require progressively higher doses to maintain pain control. The patient may develop physical dependence in which case an abstinence syndrome may be seen following abrupt cessation.

For appropriate patients who suffer with chronic non-malignant pain, opioids should be used as part of a comprehensive treatment programme involving other medications and treatment modalities. A crucial part of the assessment of a patient with chronic non-malignant pain is the patient's addiction and substance abuse history. ***OxyNorm*** injection should be used with particular care in patients with a history of alcohol and drug abuse.

If opioid treatment is considered appropriate for the patient, then the main aim of treatment is not to minimise the dose of opioid but rather to achieve a dose which provides adequate pain relief with a minimum of side effects. There must be frequent contact between physician and patient so that dosage adjustments can be made. It is strongly recommended that the physician defines treatment outcomes in accordance with pain management guidelines. The physician and patient can then agree to discontinue treatment if these objectives are not met.

Oxycodone has an abuse liability similar to other strong opioids and should be used with caution in opioid dependent patients. Oxycodone may be sought and abused by people with latent or manifest addiction disorders.

4.5 Interaction with other medicinal products and other forms of Interaction

There is an enhanced CNS depressant effect with drugs such as tranquillisers, anaesthetics, hypnotics, antidepressants, sedatives, phenothiazines, neuroleptic drugs, alcohol, other opioids, muscle relaxants and antihypertensives. Monoamine oxidase inhibitors are known to interact with narcotic analgesics, producing CNS excitation or depression with hypertensive or hypotensive crisis.

Oxycodone is metabolised in part via the CYP2D6 and CYP3A4 pathways. While these pathways may be blocked by a variety of drugs, such blockade has not yet been shown to be of clinical significance with this agent.

4.6 Pregnancy and lactation

The effect of oxycodone in human reproduction has not been adequately studied. No studies on fertility or the post-natal effects of intrauterine exposure have been carried out. However, studies in rats and rabbits with oral doses of oxycodone equivalent to 3 and 47 times an adult dose of 160 mg/day respectively, did not reveal evidence of harm to the foetus due to oxycodone. ***OxyNorm*** injection is not recommended for use in pregnancy.

Oxycodone may be secreted in breast milk and may cause respiratory depression in the newborn. Oxycodone should therefore not be used in breast-feeding mothers.

4.7 Effects on ability to drive and use machines

Oxycodone may modify patients' reactions to a varying extent depending on the dosage and individual susceptibility. Therefore patients should not drive or operate machinery, if affected.

4.8 Undesirable effects

Adverse drug reactions are typical of full opioid agonists. Tolerance and dependence may occur (see *Tolerance and Dependence*, below). Constipation may be prevented with an appropriate laxative. If nausea or vomiting are troublesome, oxycodone may be combined with an antiemetic.

Common (incidence of ⩾ 1%) and uncommon (incidence of ⩽ 1%) adverse drug reactions to oxycodone are listed in the table below.

Body System	Common	Uncommon
Gastrointestinal	Constipation	Biliary spasm
	Nausea	Dysphagia
	Vomiting	Eructation
	Dry mouth	Flatulence
	Anorexia	Gastrointestinal disorders
	Dyspepsia	Ileus
	Abdominal pain	Taste perversion
	Diarrhoea	Gastritis
		Hiccups
Central Nervous System	Headache	Vertigo
	Confusion	Hallucinations
	Asthenia	Disorientation
	Faintness	Mood changes
	Dizziness	Restlessness
	Sedation	Agitation
	Anxiety	Depression
	Abnormal dreams	Tremor
	Nervousness	Withdrawal syndrome
	Insomnia	Amnesia
	Thought abnormalities	Hypoaesthesia
	Drowsiness	Hypertonia
	Twitching	Hypotonia
		Malaise
		Paraesthesia
		Speech disorder
		Euphoria
		Dysphoria
		Seizure
		Vision abnormalities
Genitourinary		Urinary retention
		Ureteric spasm
		Impotence
		Amenorrhoea
		Decreased libido
Cardiovascular	Orthostatic hypotension	Palpitations
		Supraventricular tachycardia
		Hypotension
		Syncope
		Vasodilation
Metabolic and Nutritional		Dehydration
		Oedema
		Peripheral oedema
		Thirst
Respiratory	Bronchospasm	Overdose may produce respiratory depression
	Dyspnoea	
	Decreased cough reflex	
Dermatological	Rash	Dry skin
	Pruritus	Exfoliative dermatitis
		Urticaria
General	Sweating	Facial flushing
	Chills	Miosis
		Allergic reaction
		Fever Anaphylaxis

Tolerance and Dependence:

The patient may develop tolerance to the drug with chronic use and require progressively higher doses to maintain pain control. Prolonged use of ***OxyNorm*** injection may lead to physical dependence and a withdrawal syndrome may occur upon abrupt cessation of therapy. When a patient no longer requires therapy with oxycodone, it may be advisable to taper the dose gradually to prevent symptoms of withdrawal. The opioid abstinence or withdrawal syndrome is characterised by some or all of the following: restlessness, lacrimation, rhinorrhoea, yawning, perspiration, chills, myalgia and mydriasis. Other symptoms also may develop, including: irritability, anxiety, backache, joint pain, weakness, abdominal cramps, insomnia, nausea, anorexia, vomiting, diarrhoea, or increased blood pressure, respiratory rate or heart rate.

The development of psychological dependence (addiction) to opioid analgesics in properly managed patients with pain has been reported to be rare. However, data are not available to establish the true incidence of psychological dependence (addiction) in chronic pain patients.

OxyNorm injection should be used with particular care in patients with a history of alcohol and drug abuse.

4.9 Overdose

Symptoms of overdosage

Signs of oxycodone toxicity and overdosage are pin-point pupils, respiratory depression and hypotension. Circulatory failure and somnolence progressing to stupor or coma, skeletal muscle flaccidity, bradycardia and death may occur in more severe cases.

Treatment of overdosage.

Primary attention should be given to the establishment of a patent airway and institution of assisted or controlled ventilation.

In the case of massive overdosage, administer naloxone 0.8 mg intravenously. Repeat at 2-3 minute intervals as necessary, or by an infusion of 2 mg in 500 ml of normal saline or 5% dextrose (0.004 mg/ml).

The infusion should be run at a rate related to the previous bolus doses administered and should be in accordance with the patient's response.

However, because the duration of action of naloxone is relatively short, the patient must be carefully monitored until spontaneous respiration is reliably re-established. Monitoring for a further 24-48 hours is then recommended in case of possible relapse.

For less severe overdosage, administer naloxone 0.2 mg intravenously followed by increments of 0.1 mg every 2 minutes if required.

Naloxone should not be administered in the absence of clinically significant respiratory or circulatory depression secondary to oxycodone overdosage. Naloxone should be administered cautiously to persons who are known, or suspected, to be physically dependent on oxycodone. In such cases, an abrupt or complete reversal of opioid effects may precipitate pain and an acute withdrawal syndrome.

5. PHARMACOLOGICAL PROPERTIES

5.1 Pharmacodynamic properties

N02A A05 Narcotic analgesic

Oxycodone is a full opioid agonist with no antagonist properties. It has an affinity for kappa, mu and delta opioid receptors in the brain and spinal cord. Oxycodone is similar to morphine in its action. The therapeutic effect is mainly analgesic, anxiolytic, antitussive and sedative.

5.2 Pharmacokinetic properties

Pharmacokinetic studies in healthy subjects demonstrated an equivalent availability of oxycodone from ***OxyNorm*** injection when administered by the intravenous and subcutaneous routes, as a single bolus dose or a continuous infusion over 8 hours.

Following absorption, oxycodone is distributed throughout the entire body. Approximately 45% is bound to plasma protein. It is metabolised in the liver to produce noroxycodone, oxymorphone and various conjugated glucuronides.

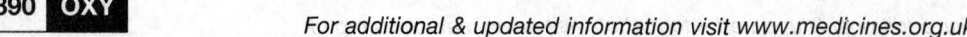

The analgesic effects of the metabolites are clinically insignificant.

The active drug and its metabolites are excreted in both urine and faeces.

The plasma concentrations of oxycodone are only minimally affected by age, being 15% greater in elderly as compared to young subjects.

Female subjects have, on average, plasma oxycodone concentrations up to 25% higher than males on a body weight adjusted basis.

The drug penetrates the placenta and can be found in breast milk.

When compared to normal subjects, patients with mild to severe hepatic dysfunction may have higher plasma concentrations of oxycodone and noroxycodone, and lower plasma concentrations of oxymorphone. There may be an increase in the elimination half-life of oxycodone and this may be accompanied by an increase in drug effects.

When compared to normal subjects, patients with mild to severe renal dysfunction may have higher plasma concentrations of oxycodone and its metabolites. There may be an increase in the elimination half-life of oxycodone and this may be accompanied by an increase in drug effects.

5.3 Preclinical safety data

Oxycodone was not mutagenic in the following assays: Ames Salmonella and E. Coli test with and without metabolic activation at doses of up to 5000 μg, chromosomal aberration test in human lymphocytes (in the absence of metabolic activation and with activation after 48 hours of exposure) at doses of up to 1500 μg/ml, and in the *in vivo* bone marrow micronucleus assay in mice (at plasma levels of up to 48 μg/ml). Mutagenic results occurred in the presence of metabolic activation in the human chromosomal aberration test (at greater than or equal to 1250 μg/ml) at 24 but not 48 hours of exposure and in the mouse lymphoma assay at doses of 50 μg/ml or greater with metabolic activation and at 400 μg/ml or greater without metabolic activation. The data from these tests indicate that the genotoxic risk to humans may be considered low.

Studies of oxycodone in animals to evaluate its carcinogenic potential have not been conducted owing to the length of clinical experience with the drug substance.

6. PHARMACEUTICAL PARTICULARS

6.1 List of excipients

Citric acid monohydrate

Sodium citrate

Sodium chloride

Hydrochloric acid, dilute

Sodium hydroxide

Water for injections

6.2 Incompatibilities

Cyclizine at concentrations of 3 mg/ml or less, when mixed with ***OxyNorm***injection, either undiluted or diluted with water for injections, shows no sign of precipitation over a period of 24 hours storage at room temperature. Precipitation has been shown to occur in mixtures with ***OxyNorm*** injection at cyclizine concentrations greater than 3 mg/ml or when diluted with 0.9% saline.

It is recommended that water for injections be used as a diluent when cyclizine and oxycodone hydrochloride are co-administered either intravenously or subcutaneously as an infusion.

Prochlorperazine is chemically incompatible with ***OxyNorm***injection.

6.3 Shelf life

3 years unopened.

After opening use immediately.

For further information see section 6.6.

6.4 Special precautions for storage

No special precautions for storage prior to opening.

For further information on use after opening see section 6.6.

6.5 Nature and contents of container

Clear glass ampoules: 1 ml and 2 ml.

Pack sizes: 5 ampoules.

6.6 Instructions for use and handling

The injection should be given immediately after opening the ampoule. Once opened any unused portion should be discarded. Chemical and physical in-use stability has been demonstrated for 24 hours at room temperature.

From a microbiological point of view, the product should be used immediately. If not used immediately, in-use storage times and conditions prior to use are the responsibility of the user and would normally not be longer than 24 hours at 2 to 8°C, unless reconstitution, dilution, etc has taken place in controlled and validated aseptic conditions.

OxyNorm injection, undiluted or diluted to 1 mg/ml with 0.9% w/v saline, 5% w/v dextrose or water for injections, is physically and chemically stable when in contact with representative brands of polypropylene or polycarbonate syringes, polyethylene or PVC tubing and PVC or EVA infusion bags, over a 24 hour period at room temperature.

The injection, whether undiluted or diluted to 1 mg/ml in the infusion fluids used in these studies and contained in the various assemblies, does not need to be protected from light.

Inappropriate handling of the undiluted solution after opening of the original ampoule, or of the diluted solutions may compromise the sterility of the product.

7. MARKETING AUTHORISATION HOLDER

Napp Pharmaceuticals Ltd

Cambridge Science Park

Milton Road

Cambridge CB4 0GW

8. MARKETING AUTHORISATION NUMBER(S)

PL 16950/0128

9. DATE OF FIRST AUTHORISATION/RENEWAL OF THE AUTHORISATION

14 April 2003

10. DATE OF REVISION OF THE TEXT

November 2003

11. Legal Category

CD (Sch 2) POM

® ***OxyNorm*** and the NAPP device are Registered Trade Marks.

OxyNorm 5, 10, 20 mg

(Napp Pharmaceuticals Limited)

1. NAME OF THE MEDICINAL PRODUCT

OxyNorm® 5, 10, 20 mg ▼

2. QUALITATIVE AND QUANTITATIVE COMPOSITION

Each capsule contains 4.5, 9, or 18 mg of oxycodone as 5, 10, or 20 mg of oxycodone hydrochloride.

For excipients, see section 6.1.

3. PHARMACEUTICAL FORM

Capsule, hard.

OxyNorm capsules 5 mg are orange/beige, printed ONR 5.

OxyNorm capsules 10 mg are white/beige, printed ONR 10.

OxyNorm capsules 20 mg are pink/beige, printed ONR 20.

4. CLINICAL PARTICULARS

4.1 Therapeutic indications

For the treatment of moderate to severe pain in patients with cancer and post-operative pain.

For the treatment of severe pain requiring the use of a strong opioid.

4.2 Posology and method of administration

Route of administration:

Oral

In common with other strong opioids, the need for continued treatment should be assessed at regular intervals.

Elderly and adults over 18 years:

OxyNorm capsules should be taken at 4-6 hourly intervals. The dosage is dependent on the severity of the pain, and the patient's previous history of analgesic requirements.

Increasing severity of pain will require an increased dosage of ***OxyNorm*** capsules. The correct dosage for any individual patient is that which controls the pain and is well tolerated throughout the dosing period. Patients should be titrated to pain relief unless unmanageable adverse drug reactions prevent this.

The usual starting dose for opioid naive patients or patients presenting with severe pain uncontrolled by weaker opioids is 5 mg, 4-6 hourly. The dose should then be carefully titrated, as frequently as once a day if necessary, to achieve pain relief. The majority of patients will not require a daily dose greater than 400 mg. However, a few patients may require higher doses.

Patients receiving oral morphine before oxycodone therapy should have their daily dose based on the following ratio: 10 mg of oral oxycodone is equivalent to 20 mg of oral morphine. It must be emphasised that this is a guide to the dose of ***OxyNorm*** capsules required. Inter-patient variability requires that each patient is carefully titrated to the appropriate dose.

Controlled pharmacokinetic studies in elderly patients (aged over 65 years) have shown that, compared with younger adults, the clearance of oxycodone is only slightly reduced. No untoward adverse drug reactions were seen based on age, therefore adult doses and dosage intervals are appropriate.

Adults with mild to moderate renal impairment and mild hepatic impairment. The plasma concentration in this patient population may be increased. Therefore, dose initiation should follow a conservative approach. The starting dose for opioid naive patients is 2.5 mg oxycodone 6-hourly, given as ***OxyNorm*** liquid.

Children under 18 years:

OxyNorm capsules should not be used in patients under 18 years.

Use in non-malignant pain:

Opioids are not first line therapy for chronic non-malignant pain, nor are they recommended as the only treatment. Types of chronic pain which have been shown to be alleviated by strong opioids include chronic osteoarthritic pain and intervertebral disc disease. The need for continued treatment in non-malignant pain should be assessed at regular intervals.

Cessation of Therapy:

When a patient no longer requires therapy with oxycodone, it may be advisable to taper the dose gradually to prevent symptoms of withdrawal.

4.3 Contraindications

Hypersensitivity to any of the constituents, respiratory depression, head injury, paralytic ileus, acute abdomen, delayed gastric emptying, chronic obstructive airways disease, cor pulmonale, chronic bronchial asthma, hypercarbia, known oxycodone sensitivity or in any situation where opioids are contraindicated, moderate to severe hepatic impairment, severe renal impairment (creatinine clearance < 10 ml/min), chronic constipation, concurrent administration of monoamine oxidase inhibitors or within 2 weeks of discontinuation of their use. Pregnancy.

4.4 Special warnings and special precautions for use

The major risk of opioid excess is respiratory depression. As with all narcotics, a reduction in dosage may be advisable in hypothyroidism. Use with caution in opioid dependent patients and in patients with raised intracranial pressure, hypotension, hypovolaemia, toxic psychosis, diseases of the biliary tract, pancreatitis, inflammatory bowel disorders, prostatic hypertrophy, adrenocortical insufficiency, acute alcoholism, delirium tremens, chronic renal and hepatic disease, or severe pulmonary disease and debilitated, elderly and infirm patients. ***OxyNorm*** capsules should not be used where there is a possibility of paralytic ileus occurring. Should paralytic ileus be suspected or occur during use, ***OxyNorm*** capsules should be discontinued immediately. As with all opioid preparations, patients who are to undergo cordotomy or other pain relieving surgical procedures should not receive ***OxyNorm*** capsules for 6 hours before surgery. If further treatment with oxycodone is then indicated the dosage should be adjusted to the new post-operative requirement.

Oxycodone should be used with caution following abdominal surgery as opioids are known to impair intestinal motility and should not be used until the physician is assured of normal bowel function.

For appropriate patients who suffer with chronic non-malignant pain, opioids should be used as part of a comprehensive treatment programme involving other medications and treatment modalities. A crucial part of the assessment of a patient with chronic non-malignant pain is the patient's addiction and substance abuse history. ***OxyNorm*** capsules should be used with particular care in patients with a history of alcohol and drug abuse.

If opioid treatment is considered appropriate for the patient, then the main aim of treatment is not to minimise the dose of opioid but rather to achieve a dose which provides adequate pain relief with a minimum of side effects. There must be frequent contact between physician and patient so that dosage adjustments can be made. It is strongly recommended that the physician defines treatment outcomes in accordance with pain management guidelines. The physician and patient can then agree to discontinue treatment if these objectives are not met.

Sunset yellow, a constituent of the 5 mg capsule, can cause allergic type reactions such as asthma. This is more common in people who are allergic to aspirin.

The capsules are printed with ink containing a small amount of benzoic acid. This is a mild irritant to the skin, eyes and mucous membranes.

Oxycodone has an abuse profile similar to other strong opioids. Oxycodone may be sought and abused by people with latent or manifest addiction disorders.

As with other opioids, infants who are born to dependent mothers may exhibit withdrawal symptoms and may have respiratory depression at birth.

The capsules should be swallowed whole, and not chewed or crushed. Abuse of oral dosage forms by parenteral administration can be expected to result in serious adverse events, which may be fatal.

4.5 Interaction with other medicinal products and other forms of Interaction

Oxycodone, like other opioids, potentiates the effects of tranquillisers, anaesthetics, hypnotics, anti-depressants, sedatives, phenothiazines, neuroleptic drugs, alcohol, muscle relaxants and antihypertensives. Monoamine oxidase inhibitors are known to interact with narcotic analgesics, producing CNS excitation or depression with hypertensive or hypotensive crisis. Concurrent administration of quinidine, an inhibitor of cytochrome P450-2D6, resulted in an increase in oxycodone C_{max} by 11%, AUC by 13%, and $t_{½}$ elim. by 14%. Also an increase in noroxycodone level was observed, (C_{max} by 50%, AUC by 85%, and $t_{½}$ elim. by 42%). The pharmacodynamic effects of oxycodone were not altered. This interaction may be observed for other potent inhibitors of cytochrome P450-2D6 enzyme. Cimetidine and inhibitors of cytochrome

P450-3A such as ketoconazole and erythromycin may inhibit the metabolism of oxycodone.

4.6 Pregnancy and lactation

OxyNorm capsules are not recommended for use in pregnancy nor during labour. Infants born to mothers who have received opioids during pregnancy should be monitored for respiratory depression.

Oxycodone may be secreted in breast milk and may cause respiratory depression in the newborn. ***OxyNorm*** capsules should, therefore, not be used in breast-feeding mothers.

4.7 Effects on ability to drive and use machines

Oxycodone may modify patients' reactions to a varying extent depending on the dosage and individual susceptibility. Therefore patients should not drive or operate machinery if affected.

4.8 Undesirable effects

Adverse drug reactions are typical of full opioid agonists. Tolerance and dependence may occur (see *Tolerance and Dependence*, below). Constipation may be prevented with an appropriate laxative. If nausea and vomiting are troublesome, oxycodone may be combined with an anti-emetic.

Common (incidence of ⩾ 1%) and uncommon (incidence of ⩽ 1%) adverse drug reactions are listed in the table below.

Body System	Common	Uncommon
Gastrointestinal	Constipation	Biliary spasm
	Nausea	Dysphagia
	Vomiting	Eructation
	Dry mouth	Flatulence
	Anorexia	Gastrointestinal disorders
	Dyspepsia	Ileus
	Abdominal pain	Taste perversion
	Diarrhoea	Gastritis
		Hiccups
Central Nervous System	Headache	Vertigo
	Confusion	Hallucinations
	Asthenia	Hypertonia
	Faintness	Disorientation
	Dizziness	Mood changes
	Sedation	Restlessness
	Anxiety	Agitation
	Abnormal dreams	Depression
	Nervousness	Tremor
	Insomnia	Withdrawal syndrome
	Thought abnormalities	Amnesia
	Drowsiness	Hypoaesthesia
	Twitching	Hypotonia
		Malaise
		Paraesthesia
		Speech disorder
		Euphoria
		Dysphoria
		Seizure
		Vision abnormalities
Genitourinary		Urinary retention
		Ureteric spasm
		Impotence
		Amenorrhoea
		Decreased libido
Cardiovascular	Orthostatic hypotension	Palpitations
		Supraventricular tachycardia
		Hypotension
		Syncope
		Vasodilation
Metabolic and Nutritional		Dehydration
		Oedema
		Peripheral oedema
		Thirst
Respiratory	Bronchospasm	Overdose may produce respiratory depression
		Dyspnoea
	Decreased cough reflex	
Dermatological	Rash	Dry skin
	Pruritus	Exfoliative dermatitis
		Urticaria
General	Sweating	Facial flushing
	Chills	Miosis
		Muscular rigidity
		Allergic reaction
		Fever Anaphylaxis

Tolerance and Dependence:

The patient may develop tolerance to the drug with chronic use and require progressively higher doses to maintain pain control. Prolonged use of ***OxyNorm*** capsules may lead to physical dependence and a withdrawal syndrome may occur upon abrupt cessation of therapy. When a patient no longer requires therapy with oxycodone, it may be advisable to taper the dose gradually to prevent symptoms of withdrawal. The opioid abstinence or withdrawal syndrome is characterised by some or all of the following: restlessness, lacrimation, rhinorrhoea, yawning, perspiration, chills, myalgia and mydriasis. Other symptoms also may develop, including: irritability, anxiety, backache, joint pain, weakness, abdominal cramps, insomnia, nausea, anorexia, vomiting, diarrhoea, or increased blood pressure, respiratory rate or heart rate.

The development of psychological dependence (addiction) to opioid analgesics in properly managed patients with pain has been reported to be rare. However, data are not available to establish the true incidence of psychological dependence (addiction) in chronic pain patients.

OxyNorm capsules should be used with particular care in patients with a history of alcohol and drug abuse.

4.9 Overdose

Signs of oxycodone toxicity and overdosage are pin-point pupils, respiratory depression and hypotension. Circulatory failure and somnolence progressing to stupor or deepening coma, skeletal muscle flaccidity, bradycardia and death may occur in more severe cases.

Treatment of oxycodone overdosage: Primary attention should be given to the establishment of a patent airway and institution of assisted or controlled ventilation.

In the case of massive overdosage, administer naloxone intravenously (0.4 to 2 mg for an adult and 0.01 mg/kg body weight for children), if the patient is in a coma or respiratory depression is present. Repeat the dose at 2 minute intervals if there is no response. If repeated doses are required then an infusion of 60% of the initial dose per hour is a useful starting point. A solution of 10 mg made up in 50 ml dextrose will produce 200 micrograms/ml for infusion using an IV pump (dose adjusted to the clinical response). Infusions are not a substitute for frequent review of the patient's clinical state. Intramuscular naloxone is an alternative in the event IV access is not possible. As the duration of action of naloxone is relatively short, the patient must be carefully monitored until spontaneous respiration is reliably established. Naloxone is a competitive antagonist and large doses (4 mg) may be required in seriously poisoned patients.

For less severe overdosage, administer naloxone 0.2 mg intravenously followed by increments of 0.1 mg every 2 minutes if required.

Naloxone should not be administered in the absence of clinically significant respiratory or circulatory depression secondary to oxycodone overdosage. Naloxone should be administered cautiously to persons who are known, or suspected, to be physically dependent on oxycodone. In such cases, an abrupt or complete reversal of opioid effects may precipitate pain and an acute withdrawal syndrome.

Additional/other considerations:

- Consider activated charcoal (50 g for adults, 10 -15 g for children), if a substantial amount has been ingested within 1 hour, provided the airway can be protected.
- Gastric contents may need to be emptied as this can be useful in removing unabsorbed drug.

5. PHARMACOLOGICAL PROPERTIES

5.1 Pharmacodynamic properties

Pharmacotherapeutic group: Natural opium alkaloids

ATC code: N02A A05

Oxycodone is a full opioid agonist with no antagonist properties. It has an affinity for kappa, mu and delta opiate receptors in the brain and spinal cord. The therapeutic effect is mainly analgesic, anxiolytic and sedative.

5.2 Pharmacokinetic properties

Compared with morphine, which has an absolute bioavailability of approximately 30%, oxycodone has a high absolute bioavailability of up to 87% following oral administration. Oxycodone has an elimination half-life of approximately 3 hours and is metabolised principally to noroxycodone via CYP450-3A and oxymorphone via CYP450-2D6. Oxymorphone has some analgesic activity but is present in the plasma in low concentrations and is not considered to contribute to oxycodone's pharmacological effect.

5.3 Preclinical safety data

Oxycodone was not mutagenic in the following assays: Ames Salmonella and E. Coli test with and without metabolic activation at doses of up to 5000 μg, chromosomal aberration test in human lymphocytes (in the absence of metabolic activation and with activation after 48 hours of exposure) at doses of up to 1500 μg/ml, and in the *in vivo* bone marrow micronucleus assay in mice (at plasma levels of up to 48 μg/ml). Mutagenic results occurred in the presence of metabolic activation in the human chromosomal aberration test (at greater than or equal to 1250 μg/ml) at 24 but not 48 hours of exposure and in the mouse lymphoma assay at doses of 50 μg/ml or greater with metabolic activation and at 400 μg/ml or greater without metabolic activation. The data from these tests indicate that the genotoxic risk to humans may be considered low. Studies of oxycodone in animals to evaluate its carcinogenic potential have not been conducted owing to the length of clinical experience with the drug substance.

6. PHARMACEUTICAL PARTICULARS

6.1 List of excipients

Cellulose, microcrystalline

Magnesium stearate

Titanium dioxide (E171)

Iron oxide (E172)

Indigo carmine (E132)

Sodium laurylsulphate

Gelatin

In addition, the 5 mg capsule contains Sunset Yellow (E110).

The capsules are printed with ink containing shellac, iron oxide (E172), industrial methylated spirits, n-butyl alcohol, soya lecithin, dimethyl siloxane, mono- and di-glycerides, methylcellulose, polyethylene glycol stearate, xanthan gum, benzoic acid, polyethylene glycol, sorbic acid.

6.2 Incompatibilities

Not applicable

6.3 Shelf life

Four years

6.4 Special precautions for storage

Do not store above 30°C.

6.5 Nature and contents of container

PVdC coated PVC blister packs with aluminium backing foil.

Pack size: 56 capsules.

6.6 Instructions for use and handling

None stated.

Administrative Data

7. MARKETING AUTHORISATION HOLDER

Napp Pharmaceuticals Ltd

Cambridge Science Park

Milton Road

Cambridge CB4 0GW

8. MARKETING AUTHORISATION NUMBER(S)

PL 16950/0106-0108

9. DATE OF FIRST AUTHORISATION/RENEWAL OF THE AUTHORISATION

26th October 1999/25 June 2005

10. DATE OF REVISION OF THE TEXT
March 2005

11. Legal Category
CD (Sch 2) POM

OxyNorm liquid and OxyNorm concentrate

(Napp Pharmaceuticals Limited)

1. NAME OF THE MEDICINAL PRODUCT
OxyNorm® liquid 5 mg/5 ml ▼

OxyNorm® concentrate 10 mg/ml ▼

2. QUALITATIVE AND QUANTITATIVE COMPOSITION
Each 5 ml ***OxyNorm*** liquid contains oxycodone base 4.5 mg as oxycodone hydrochloride 5 mg.

Each 1 ml ***OxyNorm*** concentrate contains oxycodone base 9 mg as oxycodone hydrochloride 10 mg.

For excipients, see section 6.1.

3. PHARMACEUTICAL FORM
OxyNorm liquid is a clear colourless/straw-coloured solution.

OxyNorm concentrate is a clear orange solution.

4. CLINICAL PARTICULARS
4.1 Therapeutic indications
For the treatment of moderate to severe pain in patients with cancer and post-operative pain.

For the treatment of severe pain requiring the use of a strong opioid.

4.2 Posology and method of administration
Route of administration:

Oral

Post-operative pain:

In common with other strong opioids, the need for continued treatment should be assessed at regular intervals.

Elderly and adults over 18 years:

OxyNorm liquids should be taken at 4-6 hourly intervals. The dosage is dependent on the severity of the pain, and the patient's previous history of analgesic requirements.

Increasing severity of pain will require an increased dosage of ***OxyNorm*** liquids. The correct dosage for any individual patient is that which controls the pain and is well tolerated throughout the dosing period. Patients should be titrated to pain relief unless unmanageable adverse drug reactions prevent this.

The usual starting dose for opioid naive patients or patients presenting with severe pain uncontrolled by weaker opioids is 5 mg, 4-6 hourly. The dose should then be carefully titrated, as frequently as once a day if necessary, to achieve pain relief. The majority of patients will not require a daily dose greater than 400 mg. However, a few patients may require higher doses.

Patients receiving oral morphine before oxycodone therapy should have their daily dose based on the following ratio: 10 mg of oral oxycodone is equivalent to 20 mg of oral morphine. It must be emphasised that this is a guide to the dose of ***OxyNorm*** liquids required. Inter-patient variability requires that each patient is carefully titrated to the appropriate dose.

Controlled pharmacokinetic studies in elderly patients (aged over 65 years) have shown that, compared with younger adults, the clearance of oxycodone is only slightly reduced. No untoward adverse drug reactions were seen based on age, therefore adult doses and dosage intervals are appropriate.

Adults with mild to moderate renal impairment and mild hepatic impairment: The plasma concentration in this patient population may be increased. Therefore, dose initiation should follow a conservative approach. The starting dose for opioid naive patients is 2.5 mg, 6-hourly.

Children under 18 years:

OxyNorm liquids should not be used in patients under 18 years.

Use in non-malignant pain:

Opioids are not first line therapy for chronic non-malignant pain, nor are they recommended as the only treatment. Types of chronic pain which have been shown to be alleviated by strong opioids include chronic osteoarthritic pain and intervertebral disc disease. The need for continued treatment in non-malignant pain should be assessed at regular intervals.

Cessation of therapy:

When a patient no longer requires therapy with oxycodone, it may be advisable to taper the dose gradually to prevent symptoms of withdrawal.

4.3 Contraindications
Respiratory depression, head injury, paralytic ileus, acute abdomen, delayed gastric emptying, chronic obstructive airways disease, cor pulmonale, chronic bronchial asthma, hypercarbia, known oxycodone sensitivity or in any situation where opioids are contraindicated, moderate to severe hepatic impairment, severe renal impairment (creatinine clearance < 10 ml/min), chronic constipation, concurrent administration of monoamine oxidase inhibitors or within 2 weeks of discontinuation of their use, pregnancy and lactation, hypersensitivity to any of the constituents of the product.

4.4 Special warnings and special precautions for use
The major risk of opioid excess is respiratory depression. As with all narcotics, a reduction in dosage may be advisable in hypothyroidism. Use with caution in opioid dependent patients and in patients with raised intracranial pressure, hypotension, hypovolaemia, toxic psychosis, diseases of the biliary tract, pancreatitis, inflammatory bowel disorders, prostatic hypertrophy, adrenocortical insufficiency, acute alcoholism, delirium tremens, chronic renal and hepatic disease, or severe pulmonary disease and debilitated, elderly and infirm patients. ***OxyNorm*** liquids should not be used where there is a possibility of paralytic ileus occurring. Should paralytic ileus be suspected or occur during use, ***OxyNorm*** liquids should be discontinued immediately. As with all opioid preparations, patients who are to undergo cordotomy or other pain relieving surgical procedures should not receive ***OxyNorm*** liquids for 6 hours before surgery. If further treatment with oxycodone is then indicated the dosage should be adjusted to the new post-operative requirement.

Oxycodone should be used with caution following abdominal surgery as opioids are known to impair intestinal motility and should not be used until the physician is assured of normal bowel function.

For appropriate patients who suffer with chronic non-malignant pain, opioids should be used as part of a comprehensive treatment programme involving other medications and treatment modalities. A crucial part of the assessment of a patient with chronic non-malignant pain is the patient's addiction and substance abuse history. ***OxyNorm*** liquids should be used with particular care in patients with a history of alcohol and drug abuse.

If opioid treatment is considered appropriate for the patient, then the main aim of treatment is not to minimise the dose of opioid but rather to achieve a dose which provides adequate pain relief with a minimum of side effects. There must be frequent contact between physician and patient so that dosage adjustments can be made. It is strongly recommended that the physician defines treatment outcomes in accordance with pain management guidelines. The physician and patient can then agree to discontinue treatment if these objectives are not met.

Sunset yellow, a constituent of ***OxyNorm*** concentrate, can cause allergic-type reactions such as asthma. This is more common in people who are allergic to aspirin.

Both ***OxyNorm*** liquid and ***OxyNorm*** concentrate contain the preservative sodium benzoate. This is a mild irritant to the skin, eyes and mucous membrane.

Oxycodone has an abuse profile similar to other strong opioids. Oxycodone may be sought and abused by people with latent or manifest addiction disorders.

As with other opioids, infants who are born to dependent mothers may exhibit withdrawal symptoms and may have respiratory depression at birth.

Abuse of oral dosage forms by parenteral administration can be expected to result in serious adverse events, which may be fatal.

4.5 Interaction with other medicinal products and other forms of Interaction
Oxycodone, like other opioids, potentiates the effects of tranquillisers, anaesthetics, hypnotics, anti-depressants, sedatives, phenothiazines, neuroleptic drugs, alcohol, other opioids, muscle relaxants and antihypertensives. Monoamine oxidase inhibitors are known to interact with narcotic analgesics, producing CNS excitation or depression with hypertensive or hypotensive crisis. Concurrent administration of quinidine, an inhibitor of cytochrome P450-2D6 with a modified release oxycodone tablet, resulted in an increase in oxycodone C_{max} by 11%, AUC by 13%, and $t_{1/2}$ elim. by 14%. Also an increase in noroxycodone level was observed, (C_{max} by 50%, AUC by 85%, and $t_{1/2}$ elim. by 42%). The pharmacodynamic effects of oxycodone were not altered. This interaction may be observed for other potent inhibitors of cytochrome P450-2D6 enzyme. Cimetidine and inhibitors of cytochrome P450-3A4 such as ketoconazole and erythromycin may inhibit the metabolism of oxycodone.

4.6 Pregnancy and lactation
OxyNorm liquids are not recommended for use in pregnancy nor during labour. Infants born to mothers who have received opioids during pregnancy should be monitored for respiratory depression.

Oxycodone may be secreted in breast milk and may cause respiratory depression in the newborn. ***OxyNorm*** liquids should, therefore, not be used in breast-feeding mothers.

4.7 Effects on ability to drive and use machines
Oxycodone may modify patients' reactions to a varying extent depending on the dosage and individual susceptibility. Therefore patients should not drive or operate machinery if affected.

4.8 Undesirable effects
Adverse drug reactions are typical of full opioid agonists. Tolerance and dependence may occur (see *Tolerance and Dependence*, below). Constipation may be prevented with an appropriate laxative. If nausea and vomiting are troublesome, oxycodone may be combined with an anti-emetic.

Common (incidence of ⩾ 1%) and uncommon (incidence of ⩽ 1%) adverse drug reactions are listed in the table below.

Body System	Common	Uncommon
Gastrointestinal	Constipation	Biliary spasm
	Nausea	Dysphagia
	Vomiting	Eructation
	Dry mouth	Flatulence
	Anorexia	Gastrointestinal disorders
	Dyspepsia	Ileus
	Abdominal pain	Taste perversion
	Diarrhoea	Gastritis
		Hiccups
Central Nervous System	Headache	Vertigo
	Confusion	Hallucinations
	Asthenia	Hypertonia
	Faintness	Disorientation
	Dizziness	Mood changes
	Sedation	Restlessness
	Anxiety	Agitation
	Abnormal dreams	Depression
	Nervousness	Tremor
	Insomnia	Withdrawal syndrome
	Thought abnormalities	Amnesia
	Drowsiness	Hypoaesthesia
	Twitching	Hypotonia
		Malaise
		Paraesthesia
		Speech disorder
		Euphoria
		Dysphoria
		Seizure
		Vision abnormalities
Genitourinary		Urinary retention
		Ureteric spasm
		Impotence
		Amenorrhoea
		Decreased libido
Cardiovascular	Orthostatic hypotension	Palpitations
		Supraventricular tachycardia
		Hypotension
		Syncope
		Vasodilation
Metabolic and Nutritional		Dehydration
		Oedema

		Peripheral oedema
		Thirst
Respiratory	Bronchospasm	Overdose may produce respiratory depression
	Dyspnoea	
	Decreased cough reflex	
Dermatological	Rash	Dry skin
	Pruritus	Exfoliative dermatitis
		Urticaria
General	Sweating	Facial flushing
	Chills	Miosis
		Muscular rigidity
		Allergic reaction
		Fever Anaphylaxis

Tolerance and Dependence:

The patient may develop tolerance to the drug with chronic use and require progressively higher doses to maintain pain control. Prolonged use of ***OxyNorm*** liquids may lead to physical dependence and a withdrawal syndrome may occur upon abrupt cessation of therapy. When a patient no longer requires therapy with oxycodone, it may be advisable to taper the dose gradually to prevent symptoms of withdrawal. The opioid abstinence or withdrawal syndrome is characterised by some or all of the following: restlessness, lacrimation, rhinorrhoea, yawning, perspiration, chills, myalgia and mydriasis. Other symptoms also may develop, including: irritability, anxiety, backache, joint pain, weakness, abdominal cramps, insomnia, nausea, anorexia, vomiting, diarrhoea, or increased blood pressure, respiratory rate or heart rate.

The development of psychological dependence (addiction) to opioid analgesics in properly managed patients with pain has been reported to be rare. However, data are not available to establish the true incidence of psychological dependence (addiction) in chronic pain patients.

OxyNorm liquids should be used with particular care in patients with a history of alcohol and drug abuse.

4.9 Overdose

Signs of oxycodone toxicity and overdosage are pin-point pupils, respiratory depression and hypotension. Circulatory failure and somnolence progressing to stupor or deepening coma, skeletal muscle flaccidity, bradycardia and death may occur in more severe cases.

Treatment of oxycodone overdosage: Primary attention should be given to the establishment of a patent airway and institution of assisted or controlled ventilation.

In the case of massive overdosage, administer naloxone intravenously (0.4 to 2 mg for an adult and 0.01 mg/kg body weight for children), if the patient is in a coma or respiratory depression is present. Repeat the dose at 2 minute intervals if there is no response. If repeated doses are required then an infusion of 60% of the initial dose per hour is a useful starting point. A solution of 10 mg made up in 50 ml dextrose will produce 200 micrograms/ml for infusion using an IV pump (dose adjusted to the clinical response). Infusions are not a substitute for frequent review of the patient's clinical state. Intramuscular naloxone is an alternative in the event IV access is not possible. As the duration of action of naloxone is relatively short, the patient must be carefully monitored until spontaneous respiration is reliably established. Naloxone is a competitive antagonist and large doses (4 mg) may be required in seriously poisoned patients.

For less severe overdosage, administer naloxone 0.2 mg intravenously followed by increments of 0.1 mg every 2 minutes if required.

Naloxone should not be administered in the absence of clinically significant respiratory or circulatory depression secondary to oxycodone overdosage. Naloxone should be administered cautiously to persons who are known, or suspected, to be physically dependent on oxycodone. In such cases, an abrupt or complete reversal of opioid effects may precipitate pain and an acute withdrawal syndrome.

Additional/other considerations:

- Consider activated charcoal (50 g for adults, 10 -15 g for children), if a substantial amount has been ingested within 1 hour, provided the airway can be protected.
- Gastric contents may need to be emptied as this can be useful in removing unabsorbed drug.

5. PHARMACOLOGICAL PROPERTIES

5.1 Pharmacodynamic properties

Pharmacotherapeutic group: Natural opium alkaloids

ATC code: N02A A05

Oxycodone is a full opioid agonist with no antagonist properties. It has an affinity for kappa, mu and delta opiate receptors in the brain and spinal cord. Oxycodone is similar to morphine in its action. The therapeutic effect is mainly analgesic, anxiolytic and sedative.

5.2 Pharmacokinetic properties

Compared with morphine, which has an absolute bioavailability of approximately 30%, oxycodone has a high absolute bioavailability of up to 87% following oral administration. Oxycodone has an elimination half life of approximately 3-4 hours and is metabolised principally to noroxycodone and oxymorphone. Oxymorphone has some analgesic activity but is present in the plasma at low concentrations and is not considered to contribute to oxycodone's pharmacological effect.

A pharmacokinetic study in healthy volunteers has demonstrated that, following administration of a single 10 mg dose, ***OxyNorm*** liquid 5 mg/5 ml and ***OxyNorm*** concentrate 10 mg/ml provided an equivalent rate and extent of absorption of oxycodone. Mean peak plasma concentrations of approximately 20 ng/ml were achieved within 1.5 hours of administration, median t_{max} values from both strengths of liquid being less than one hour.

Studies involving controlled release oxycodone have demonstrated that the oral bioavailability of oxycodone is only slightly increased (16%) in the elderly. In patients with renal and hepatic impairment, the bioavailability of oxycodone was increased by 60% and 90% respectively, and a reduced initial dose is recommended in these groups.

5.3 Preclinical safety data

Oxycodone was not mutagenic in the following assays: Ames Salmonella and E. Coli test with and without metabolic activation at doses of up to 5000 μg, chromosomal aberration test in human lymphocytes (in the absence of metabolic activation and with activation after 48 hours of exposure) at doses of up to 1500 μg/ml, and in the *in vivo* bone marrow micronucleus assay in mice (at plasma levels of up to 48 μg/ml). Mutagenic results occurred in the presence of metabolic activation in the human chromosomal aberration test (at greater than or equal to 1250 μg/ml) at 24 but not 48 hours of exposure and in the mouse lymphoma assay at doses of 50 μg/ml or greater with metabolic activation and at 400 μg/ml or greater without metabolic activation. The data from these tests indicate that the genotoxic risk to humans may be considered low. Studies of oxycodone in animals to evaluate its carcinogenic potential have not been conducted owing to the length of clinical experience with the drug substance.

6. PHARMACEUTICAL PARTICULARS

6.1 List of excipients

Saccharin sodium

Sodium benzoate

Citric acid monohydrate

Sodium citrate

Hydrochloric acid

Sodium hydroxide

Purified water

In addition, ***OxyNorm*** liquid contains hypromellose and ***OxyNorm*** concentrate contains Sunset Yellow (E110).

6.2 Incompatibilities

Not applicable.

6.3 Shelf life

Two years

6.4 Special precautions for storage

Do not store above 30°C

6.5 Nature and contents of container

OxyNorm liquid is supplied in 250 ml amber glass bottles with polyethylene/polypropylene screw caps. ***OxyNorm*** concentrate is supplied in 120 ml amber glass bottles with polyethylene/polypropylene caps. A graduated dropper or an oral syringe is also supplied with ***OxyNorm*** concentrate.

6.6 Instructions for use and handling

OxyNorm concentrate may be mixed with a soft drink for ease of administration and to improve palatability.

Administrative Data

7. MARKETING AUTHORISATION HOLDER

Napp Pharmaceuticals Ltd

Cambridge Science Park

Milton Road

Cambridge CB4 0GW

8. MARKETING AUTHORISATION NUMBER(S)

PL 16950/0003,4

9. DATE OF FIRST AUTHORISATION/RENEWAL OF THE AUTHORISATION

9th December 1999/ 25 June 2005

10. DATE OF REVISION OF THE TEXT

March 2005

11. Legal Category

CD (Sch 2) POM

® ***OxyNorm*** and the Napp Device are Registered Trade Marks

Pabrinex Intramuscular High Potency Injection

(Link Pharmaceuticals Ltd)

1. NAME OF THE MEDICINAL PRODUCT

Pabrinex Intramuscular High Potency

2. QUALITATIVE AND QUANTITATIVE COMPOSITION

Each No. 1 ampoule (5ml) contains:

Thiamine Hydrochloride BP	250mg
Riboflavin (as Phosphate Sodium BP)	4mg
Pyridoxine Hydrochloride BP	50mg

Each No. 2 ampoule (2ml) contains:

Ascorbic Acid BP	500mg
Nicotinamide BP	160mg

3. PHARMACEUTICAL FORM

Injection for intramuscular use: two (5ml, 2ml) amber glass ampoules containing sterile aqueous solutions which are to be mixed prior to administration.

4. CLINICAL PARTICULARS

4.1 Therapeutic indications

Rapid therapy of severe depletion or malabsorption of the water soluble vitamins B and C, particularly in alcoholism, after acute infections, post-operatively and in psychiatric states.

4.2 Posology and method of administration

Pabrinex is also available as an Intravenous High Potency Injection. Therefore before administration ensure that both the Summary of Product Characteristics and ampoule labels refer to the INTRAMUSCULAR injection.

The contents of one ampoule number 1 and one ampoule number 2 of Pabrinex Intramuscular High Potency (total 7ml) are drawn up into a syringe to mix them just before use, then injected slowly high into the gluteal muscle, 5cm below the iliac crest.

Adults: The contents of one pair of ampoules (7ml) twice daily for up to 7 days.

Elderly: As for adults.

Children: Pabrinex Intramuscular High Potency is rarely indicated for administration to children, however suitable doses are as follows:

Under 6 years	0.25 adult dose
6-10 years	0.33 adult dose
10-14 years	0.5 to 0.66 adult dose
14 years and over	adult dose

4.3 Contraindications

Known hypersensitivity to any of the active constituents.

4.4 Special warnings and special precautions for use

Repeated injections of preparations containing high concentrations of vitamin B_1 (thiamine) may give rise to anaphylactic shock. Mild allergic reactions such as sneezing or mild asthma are warning signs that further injections may give rise to anaphylactic shock. Facilities for treating anaphylactic reactions should be available whenever Pabrinex Intramuscular High Potency is administered.

Not for intravenous use.

4.5 Interaction with other medicinal products and other forms of Interaction

The content of pyridoxine may interfere with the effects of concurrent levodopa therapy.

4.6 Pregnancy and lactation

No adverse effects have been noted at recommended doses when used as clinically indicated.

4.7 Effects on ability to drive and use machines

None stated.

4.8 Undesirable effects

Occasionally, hypotension and mild paraesthesia from continued high doses of thiamine; occasionally mild ache at local site of injection.

4.9 Overdose

In the unlikely event of overdosage, treatment is symptomatic and supportive.

5. PHARMACOLOGICAL PROPERTIES

5.1 Pharmacodynamic properties

Pabrinex Intramuscular High Potency contains vitamins B_1, B_2, B_6, nicotinamide and vitamin C.

ATC code: A11EB

5.2 Pharmacokinetic properties

None supplied.

5.3 Preclinical safety data

There are no preclinical data of relevance to the prescriber which are additional to that already included in other sections of the Summary of Product Characteristics.

6. PHARMACEUTICAL PARTICULARS

6.1 List of excipients

Edetic acid, sodium hydroxide, benzyl alcohol, Water for Injections

6.2 Incompatibilities

None stated.

6.3 Shelf life

24 months.

6.4 Special precautions for storage

Store in a refrigerator at 2°C to 8°C. Do not freeze.

6.5 Nature and contents of container

Pabrinex Intramuscular High Potency is supplied in pairs of (5ml and 2ml) amber glass ampoules in packs of 10 pairs.

6.6 Instructions for use and handling

None stated.

7. MARKETING AUTHORISATION HOLDER

Link Pharmaceuticals Limited, Bishops Weald House, Albion Way, Horsham, West Sussex, RH12 1AH, United Kingdom

8. MARKETING AUTHORISATION NUMBER(S)

PL 12406/0004

9. DATE OF FIRST AUTHORISATION/RENEWAL OF THE AUTHORISATION

October 1998.

10. DATE OF REVISION OF THE TEXT

October 2002.

11. Legal Category

POM.

® Pabrinex is a registered trade mark

Pabrinex Intravenous High Potency Injection

(Link Pharmaceuticals Ltd)

1. NAME OF THE MEDICINAL PRODUCT

Pabrinex Intravenous High Potency

2. QUALITATIVE AND QUANTITATIVE COMPOSITION

(see Table 1 below)

(see Table 2 below)

3. PHARMACEUTICAL FORM

Injection for intravenous use: two 5ml or two 10ml amber glass ampoules containing sterile aqueous solutions which are to be mixed prior to administration.

4. CLINICAL PARTICULARS

4.1 Therapeutic indications

Rapid therapy of severe depletion or malabsorption of the water soluble vitamins B and C, particularly in alcoholism, after acute infections, post-operatively and in psychiatric states. Also used to maintain levels of vitamin B and C in patients on chronic intermittent haemodialysis.

Table 1

Each No. 1 ampoule contains:	5ml	or	10ml
Thiamine Hydrochloride BP	250mg		500mg
Riboflavin (as Phosphate Sodium BP)	4mg		8mg
Pyridoxine Hydrochloride BP	50mg		100mg

Table 2

Each No. 2 ampoule contains:	5ml	or	10ml
Ascorbic Acid BP	500mg		1000mg
Nicotinamide BP	160mg		320mg
Anhydrous Glucose BP	1000mg		2000mg

4.2 Posology and method of administration

Pabrinex is also available as an Intramuscular High Potency Injection. Therefore before administration ensure that both the Summary of Product Characteristics and ampoule labels refer to the INTRAVENOUS injection.

1) The preferred method of administration of Pabrinex Intravenous High Potency is by drip infusion. Equal volumes of the contents of ampoules number 1 and 2 should be added to 50ml to 100ml physiological saline or glucose 5% and infused over 15 to 30 minutes (see *"Special Precautions for Storage"* section).

2) For a combined injection volume of not more than 10ml (e.g. the contents of one 5ml ampoule number 1 and one 5ml ampoule number 2) the contents of the ampoules are drawn up into a syringe to mix them just before use, then injected slowly, over a period of 10 minutes, into a vein.

Adults:

Coma or delirium from alcohol, narcotics or barbiturates; collapse following continuous narcosis		
10ml Ampoule Number 1 OR **15ml Ampoule Number 1**	**PLUS** **PLUS**	**10ml Ampoule Number 2** OR **15ml Ampoule Number 2**
20ml to 30ml of the mixed ampoules diluted with 50ml to 100ml infusion solution (physiological saline or glucose 5%) administered over 15 to 30 minutes every 8 hours or at the discretion of the physician.		

Psychosis following narcosis or E.C.T; toxicity from acute infections		
5ml Ampoule Number 1	**PLUS**	**5ml Ampoule Number 2**
10ml of the mixed ampoules diluted with 50ml to 100ml infusion solution (physiological saline or glucose 5%) administered over 15 to 30 minutes twice daily for up to 7 days.		

Haemodialysis		
5ml Ampoule Number 1	**PLUS**	**5ml Ampoule Number 2**
10ml of the mixed ampoules diluted with 50ml to 100ml infusion solution (physiological saline or glucose 5%) administered over 15 to 30 minutes once every two weeks at the end of dialysis.		

Elderly: as for adults.

Children: Pabrinex Intravenous High Potency is rarely indicated for administration to children, however suitable doses are as follows:

Under 6 years	one quarter of the adult dose
6-10 years	one third of the adult dose
10-14 years	one half to two thirds of the adult dose
14 years and over	as for the adult dose

4.3 Contraindications
Known hypersensitivity to any of the active constituents.

4.4 Special warnings and special precautions for use
Repeated injections of preparations containing high concentrations of vitamin B_1 (thiamine) may give rise to anaphylactic shock. Mild allergic reactions such as sneezing or mild asthma are warning signs that further injections may give rise to anaphylactic shock. Facilities for treating anaphylactic reactions should be available whenever Pabrinex Intravenous High Potency is administered.

Not for intramuscular use.

4.5 Interaction with other medicinal products and other forms of Interaction
The content of pyridoxine may interfere with the effects of concurrent levodopa therapy.

4.6 Pregnancy and lactation
No adverse effects have been noted at recommended doses when used as clinically indicated.

4.7 Effects on ability to drive and use machines
None stated.

4.8 Undesirable effects
Occasionally, hypotension and mild paraesthesia from continued high doses of thiamine; occasionally mild ache at local site of injection.

4.9 Overdose
In the unlikely event of overdosage, treatment is symptomatic and supportive.

5. PHARMACOLOGICAL PROPERTIES

5.1 Pharmacodynamic properties
Pabrinex Intravenous High Potency contains vitamins B_1, B_2, B_6, nicotinamide, vitamin C and glucose.

ATC code: A11EB

5.2 Pharmacokinetic properties
Not supplied.

5.3 Preclinical safety data
There are no pre-clinical data of relevance to the prescriber which are additional to that already included in other sections of the Summary of Product Characteristics.

6. PHARMACEUTICAL PARTICULARS

6.1 List of excipients
Edetic acid, sodium hydroxide, Water for Injections

6.2 Incompatibilities
If it is necessary to administer Pabrinex Intravenous High Potency in infusion, it is recommended that Pabrinex IV HP is administered in physiological saline or glucose 5%.

6.3 Shelf life
24 months.

6.4 Special precautions for storage
Do not store above 25°C. Keep the container in the outer carton. Do not freeze.

Storage of diluted Pabrinex Intravenous High Potency

The stability of Pabrinex Intravenous High Potency in intravenous infusion fluids, at room temperature, is as follows:

Intravenous infusion fluid	In the light
Glucose 5%	7 hours
Physiological saline (sodium chloride 0.9%)	7 hours
Glucose 4.3% with sodium chloride 0.18%	4 hours
Glucose 5% with potassium chloride 0.3%	4 hours
Sodium lactate M/6	7 hours

Although no further specific data are available, the solutions are expected to be stable for longer periods when protected from light. Store diluted solutions at 2°C to 8°C if not used immediately. Do not freeze.

6.5 Nature and contents of container
Pabrinex Intravenous High Potency is supplied in pairs of amber glass ampoules of 5ml or 10ml. Pack sizes contain ten pairs of 5ml or five pairs of 10ml ampoules.

6.6 Instructions for use and handling
None stated.

7. MARKETING AUTHORISATION HOLDER
Link Pharmaceuticals Limited, Bishops Weald House, Albion Way, Horsham, West Sussex, RH12 1AH, United Kingdom

8. MARKETING AUTHORISATION NUMBER(S)
PL 12406/0003

9. DATE OF FIRST AUTHORISATION/RENEWAL OF THE AUTHORISATION
October 1998

10. DATE OF REVISION OF THE TEXT
June 2003

Palladone capsules

(Napp Pharmaceuticals Limited)

1. NAME OF THE MEDICINAL PRODUCT
PALLADONE® capsules 1.3 mg and 2.6 mg.

2. QUALITATIVE AND QUANTITATIVE COMPOSITION
PALLADONE capsules contain Hydromorphone Hydrochloride USP 1.3 mg or 2.6 mg.

3. PHARMACEUTICAL FORM
PALLADONE capsules 1.3 mg are orange/clear capsules marked HNR 1.3.

PALLADONE capsules 2.6 mg are red/clear capsules marked HNR 2.6.

4. CLINICAL PARTICULARS

4.1 Therapeutic indications
For the relief of severe pain in cancer.

4.2 Posology and method of administration
Route of administration

The capsules can be swallowed whole or opened and their contents sprinkled on to cold soft food.

Dosage and administration

Adults and children over 12 years

PALLADONE capsules should be used at 4-hourly intervals. The dosage is dependent upon the severity of the pain and the patient's previous history of analgesic requirements. 1.3 mg of hydromorphone has an efficacy approximately equivalent to 10 mg of morphine given orally. A patient presenting with severe pain should normally be started on a dosage of one PALLADONE capsule 4-hourly. Increasing severity of pain will require increased dosage of hydromorphone to achieve the desired relief.

Elderly and patients with renal impairment

The elderly and patients with renal impairment should be dose titrated with PALLADONE capsules in order to achieve adequate analgesia. It should be noted, however, that these patients may require a lower dosage to achieve adequate analgesia.

Patients with hepatic impairment

Contra-indicated.

Children under 12 years

Not recommended.

4.3 Contraindications
Respiratory depression, pregnancy, coma, acute abdomen, hepatic impairment, known hydromorphone sensitivity, concurrent administration of monoamine oxidase inhibitors or within 2 weeks of discontinuation of their use. Hydromorphone should be avoided in patients with raised intracranial pressure or head injury, and also in patients with convulsive disorders or acute alcoholism.

4.4 Special warnings and special precautions for use
As with all narcotics, a reduction in dosage may be advised in the elderly, in hypothyroidism, in chronic obstructive airways disease, in renal or adrenocortical insufficiency, prostatic hypertrophy, shock or reduced respiratory reserve. PALLADONE capsules are not recommended in the first 24 hours post-operatively. After this time they should be used with caution, particularly following abdominal surgery.

PALLADONE capsules should not be used where there is the possibility of paralytic ileus occurring. Should paralytic ileus be suspected or occur during use, PALLADONE capsules should be discontinued immediately.

Patients about to undergo cordotomy or other pain-relieving surgical procedures should not receive PALLADONE capsules for 4 hours prior to surgery. If further treatment with PALLADONE capsules is indicated, the dosage should be adjusted to the new post-operative requirement.

4.5 Interaction with other medicinal products and other forms of Interaction
Hydromorphone potentiates the effects of tranquillisers, anaesthetics, hypnotics and sedatives.

4.6 Pregnancy and lactation
PALLADONE capsules are not recommended in pregnancy or in the breast-feeding mother as there are insufficient animal or human data to justify such use.

4.7 Effects on ability to drive and use machines
Hydromorphone may cause drowsiness and patients should not drive or operate machinery if affected.

4.8 Undesirable effects
Hydromorphone may cause constipation, nausea and vomiting. Constipation may be treated with appropriate laxatives. When nausea and vomiting are troublesome, PALLADONE capsules can be readily combined with anti-emetics. Tolerance and dependence may occur.

4.9 Overdose
Signs of hydromorphone toxicity and overdosage are pinpoint pupils, respiratory depression and hypotension. Circulatory failure and deepening coma may occur in more severe cases.

Treatment of overdosage:

Primary attention should be given to the establishment of a patent airway and institution of assisted or controlled ventilation.

In the case of massive overdosage, administer naloxone 0.8 mg intravenously. Repeat at 2-3 minute intervals as necessary, or by an infusion of 2 mg in 500 ml of normal saline or 5% dextrose (0.004 mg/ml).

The infusion should be run at a rate related to the previous bolus doses administered and should be in accordance with the patient's response. However, because the duration of action of naloxone is relatively short, the patient must be carefully monitored until spontaneous respiration is reliably re-established.

For less severe overdosage, administer naloxone 0.2 mg intravenously followed by increments of 0.1 mg every 2 minutes if required.

Naloxone should not be administered in the absence of clinically significant respiratory or circulatory depression secondary to hydromorphone overdosage. Naloxone should be administered cautiously to persons who are known, or suspected, to be physically dependent on hydromorphone. In such cases, an abrupt or complete reversal of opioid effects may precipitate an acute withdrawal syndrome.

Gastric contents may need to be emptied as this can be useful in removing unabsorbed drug.

5. PHARMACOLOGICAL PROPERTIES

5.1 Pharmacodynamic properties
Like morphine, hydromorphone is an agonist of mu receptors. The pharmacological actions of hydromorphone and morphine do not differ significantly. The oral analgesic potency ratio of hydromorphone to morphine is approximately 5-10:1. Hydromorphone and related opioids produce their major effects on the central nervous system and bowel. The effects are diverse and include analgesia, drowsiness, changes in mood, respiratory depression, decreased gastrointestinal motility, nausea, vomiting, and alteration of the endocrine and autonomic nervous system.

5.2 Pharmacokinetic properties
Hydromorphone is absorbed from the gastrointestinal tract and undergoes pre-systemic elimination resulting in an oral bioavailability of about 50%. It is metabolised and excreted in the urine mainly as conjugated hydromorphone, dihydroisomorphine and dihydromorphine.

5.3 Preclinical safety data
There are no pre-clinical data of relevance to the prescriber which are additional to that already included in other sections of the SPC.

6. PHARMACEUTICAL PARTICULARS

6.1 List of excipients
Microcrystalline cellulose

Lactose (anhydrous)

Capsule shells

Gelatin

Erythrosine (E127)

Iron oxide (E172)

Titanium dioxide (E171)

Sodium dodecylsulphate

6.2 Incompatibilities
None known.

6.3 Shelf life
Two years.

6.4 Special precautions for storage
Store at or below 25°C. Protect from moisture.

6.5 Nature and contents of container
PVdC coated PVC blisters with aluminium backing foil containing 56 capsules.

6.6 Instructions for use and handling
None stated.

Administrative Data

7. MARKETING AUTHORISATION HOLDER
Napp Pharmaceuticals Limited

Cambridge Science Park

Milton Road

Cambridge

CB4 0GW

8. MARKETING AUTHORISATION NUMBER(S)
PL 16950/0049, 0050

9. DATE OF FIRST AUTHORISATION/RENEWAL OF THE AUTHORISATION
12 February 1997

10. DATE OF REVISION OF THE TEXT
June 2000

11. Legal Category
CD (Sch 2), POM

® Palladone and the Napp device are Registered Trade Marks.

Palladone SR capsules

(Napp Pharmaceuticals Limited)

1. NAME OF THE MEDICINAL PRODUCT
PALLADONE®SR capsules 2 mg, 4 mg, 8 mg, 16 mg, 24 mg.

2. QUALITATIVE AND QUANTITATIVE COMPOSITION
The capsules contain Hydromorphone Hydrochloride USP 2 mg, 4 mg, 8 mg, 16 mg, 24 mg.

3. PHARMACEUTICAL FORM
Hard gelatin capsule containing spherical controlled release pellets.

PALLADONE SR capsules 2 mg are yellow/white capsules marked HCR 2.

PALLADONE SR capsules 4 mg are pale blue/clear capsules marked HCR 4.

PALLADONE SR capsules 8 mg are pink/clear capsules marked HCR 8.

PALLADONE SR capsules 16 mg are brown/clear capsules marked HCR 16.

PALLADONE SR capsules 24 mg are dark blue/clear capsules marked HCR 24.

4. CLINICAL PARTICULARS

4.1 Therapeutic indications
For the relief of severe pain in cancer.

4.2 Posology and method of administration
Route of administration

The capsules can be swallowed whole or opened and their contents sprinkled on to cold soft food.

Dosage and administration

Adults and children over 12 years

PALLADONE SR capsules should be used at 12-hourly intervals. The dosage is dependent upon the severity of the pain and the patient's previous history of analgesic requirements. 4 mg of hydromorphone has an efficacy approximately equivalent to 30 mg of morphine sulphate given orally. A patient presenting with severe pain should normally be started on a dosage of 4 mg PALLADONE SR capsules 12-hourly. Increasing severity of pain will require increased dosage of hydromorphone to achieve the desired relief.

Elderly and patients with renal impairment

The elderly and patients with renal impairment should be dose titrated with PALLADONE SR capsules in order to achieve adequate analgesia. It should be noted, however, that these patients may require a lower dosage to achieve adequate analgesia.

Patients with hepatic impairment

Contra-indicated.

Children under 12 years

Not recommended.

4.3 Contraindications
Respiratory depression, pregnancy, coma, acute abdomen, hepatic impairment, known hydromorphone sensitivity, concurrent administration of monoamine oxidase inhibitors or within 2 weeks of discontinuation of their use. Use of PALLADONE SR capsules should be avoided in patients with raised intracranial pressure or head injury, and also in patients with convulsive disorders or acute alcoholism.

Pre-operative administration of PALLADONE SR capsules is not recommended and is not an approved indication.

4.4 Special warnings and special precautions for use
As with all narcotics, a reduction in dosage may be advised in the elderly, in hypothyroidism, in chronic obstructive airways disease, in renal or adrenocortical insufficiency, prostatic hypertrophy, shock or reduced respiratory reserve. PALLADONE SR capsules are not recommended in the first 24 hours post-operatively. After this time they should be used with caution, particularly following abdominal surgery.

PALLADONE SR capsules should not be used where there is the possibility of paralytic ileus occurring. Should paralytic ileus be suspected or occur during use, PALLADONE SR capsules should be discontinued.

Patients about to undergo cordotomy or other pain relieving surgical procedures should not receive PALLADONE SR capsules for 24 hours prior to surgery. If further treatment with PALLADONE SR capsules is indicated, then the dosage should be adjusted to the new post-operative requirement.

4.5 Interaction with other medicinal products and other forms of Interaction
Hydromorphone potentiates the effects of tranquillisers, anaesthetics, hypnotics and sedatives.

4.6 Pregnancy and lactation
PALLADONE SR capsules are not recommended in pregnancy or in the breast-feeding mother as there are insufficient animal or human data to justify such use.

4.7 Effects on ability to drive and use machines
Hydromorphone may cause drowsiness and patients should not drive or operate machinery if affected.

4.8 Undesirable effects
Hydromorphone may cause constipation, nausea and vomiting. Constipation may be treated with appropriate laxatives. When nausea and vomiting are troublesome, PALLADONE SR capsules can be readily combined with antiemetics. Tolerance and dependence may occur.

4.9 Overdose
Signs of hydromorphone toxicity and overdosage are pin-point pupils, respiratory depression and hypotension. Circulatory failure and deepening coma may occur in more severe cases.

Treatment of overdosage:

Primary attention should be given to the establishment of a patent airway and institution of assisted or controlled ventilation.

In the case of massive overdosage, administer naloxone 0.8 mg intravenously. Repeat at 2-3 minute intervals as necessary, or by an infusion of 2 mg in 500 ml of normal saline or 5% dextrose (0.004 mg/ml).

The infusion should be run at a rate related to the previous bolus doses administered and should be in accordance with the patient's response. However, because the duration of action of naloxone is relatively short, the patient must be carefully monitored until spontaneous respiration is reliably re-established. PALLADONE SR capsules will continue to release and add to the hydromorphone load for up to 12 hours after administration, and the management of the overdosage should be modified accordingly.

For less severe overdosage, administer naloxone 0.2 mg intravenously followed by increments of 0.1 mg every 2 minutes if required.

Naloxone should not be administered in the absence of clinically significant respiratory or circulatory depression secondary to hydromorphone overdosage. Naloxone should be administered cautiously to persons who are known, or suspected, to be physically dependent on hydromorphone. In such cases, an abrupt or complete reversal of opioid effects may precipitate an acute withdrawal syndrome.

Gastric contents may need to be emptied as this can be useful in removing unabsorbed drug, particularly when a modified release formulation has been taken.

5. PHARMACOLOGICAL PROPERTIES

5.1 Pharmacodynamic properties
Like morphine, hydromorphone is an agonist of mu receptors. The pharmacological actions of hydromorphone and morphine do not differ significantly. The oral analgesic potency ratio of hydromorphone to morphine is approximately 5-10:1. Hydromorphone and related opioids produce their major effects on the central nervous system and bowel. The effects are diverse and include analgesia, drowsiness, changes in mood, respiratory depression, decreased gastrointestinal motility, nausea, vomiting and alteration of the endocrine and autonomic nervous system.

5.2 Pharmacokinetic properties
Hydromorphone is absorbed from the gastrointestinal tract and undergoes pre-systemic elimination resulting in an oral bioavailability of about 50%. It is metabolised and excreted in the urine mainly as conjugated hydromorphone and with smaller amounts of unchanged hydromorphone, dihydroisomorphine and dihydromorphine. PALLADONE SR capsules have been formulated to produce therapeutic plasma levels following 12-hourly dosing.

5.3 Preclinical safety data
There are no pre-clinical data of relevance to the prescriber which are additional to that already included in other sections of the SPC.

6. PHARMACEUTICAL PARTICULARS

6.1 List of excipients
Microcrystalline cellulose

Hypromellose (15 cps)

Purified water

Ethylcellulose (N10)

Colloidal anhydrous silica

Dibutyl sebacate

Methanol

Dichloromethane

Capsule shells

Gelatin

Sodium Dodecylsulphate

The following colours are included in the capsule shells:

2 mg (E104, E171), 4 mg (E127, E132, E171), 8 mg (E127, E171), 16 mg (E171, E172), 24 mg (E132, E171).

6.2 Incompatibilities
None known.

6.3 Shelf life
Eighteen months.

6.4 Special precautions for storage
Do not store above 25°C. Store in the original package.

6.5 Nature and contents of container
PVdC/PVC blister packs with aluminium backing foil containing 56 capsules.

6.6 Instructions for use and handling
None stated.

Administrative Data

7. MARKETING AUTHORISATION HOLDER
Napp Pharmaceuticals Limited
Cambridge Science Park
Milton Road
Cambridge, CB4 0GW

8. MARKETING AUTHORISATION NUMBER(S)
PL 16950/0051-0055

9. DATE OF FIRST AUTHORISATION/RENEWAL OF THE AUTHORISATION
12 February 1997

10. DATE OF REVISION OF THE TEXT
June 2000

11. Legal category
CD (Sch 2), POM

® Palladone and the Napp device are Registered Trade Marks.

Paludrine Tablets

(AstraZeneca UK Limited)

1. NAME OF THE MEDICINAL PRODUCT
Paludrine Tablets

2. QUALITATIVE AND QUANTITATIVE COMPOSITION
Proguanil hydrochloride 100 mg

3. PHARMACEUTICAL FORM
Tablets for oral administration.

4. CLINICAL PARTICULARS

4.1 Therapeutic indications
Paludrine is an effective antimalarial agent. It is recommended for the prevention and suppression of malaria.

4.2 Posology and method of administration
Non-immune subjects entering a malarious area are advised to begin treatment with Paludrine 1 week before, or if this is not possible, then at least 2 days before entering the malarious area. The daily dose of Paludrine should be continued throughout exposure to risk and for 4 weeks after leaving the area.

Adults:	Two tablets (200 mg) daily.	
Children:	Under 1 year:	1/4 tablet (25 mg) daily
	1 to 4 years:	1/2 tablet (50 mg) daily
	5 to 8 years:	1 tablet (100 mg) daily
	9 to 14 years:	1 1/2 tablets (150 mg) daily
	Over 14 years:	Adult dose daily

The daily dose is best taken with water, after food, at the same time each day.

Provided the tablet fragment gives the minimum amount specified, precise accuracy in children's dosage is not essential since the drug possesses a wide safety margin.

For a young child, the dose may be administered crushed and mixed with milk, honey or jam. The treatment should be started at least two days before entering the malarious area and continued for the whole period of stay and 4 weeks after leaving the area.

Elderly patients: There are no special dosage recommendations for the elderly, but it may be advisable to monitor elderly patients so that optimum dosage can be individually determined.

Renal Impairment: Based on a theoretical model derived from a single dose pharmacokinetic study, the following guidance is given for adults with renal impairment. (See also Sections 4.3 and 4.4)

Creatinine clearance (ml/min/1.73 m²)	Dosage
⩾ 60	200 mg once daily (standard dose)
20 to 59	100 mg once daily
10 to 19	50 mg every second day
< 10	50 mg once weekly

The grade of renal impairment and/or the serum creatinine concentration may be approximately equated to creatinine clearance levels as indicated below.

Creatinine Clearance (ml/min/1.73 m²)	Approx* serum Creatinine (micromol/1)	Renal Impairment Grade (arbitrarily divided for dosage purposes)
⩾ 60	-	
20 to 59	150 to 300	Mild
10 to 19	300 to 700	Moderate
< 10	> 700	Severe

*Serum creatinine concentration is only an approximate guide to renal function unless corrected for age, weight and sex.

4.3 Contraindications
Paludrine should be used with caution in patients with severe renal impairment. (See also Sections 4.2 and 4.4)

4.4 Special warnings and special precautions for use
Paludrine should be used with caution in patients with severe renal impairment. (See also Section 4.2) There have been rare reports of haematological changes in such patients.

In any locality where drug-resistant malaria is known or suspected, it is essential to take local medical advice on what prophylactic regimen is appropriate. Prophylactic use of Paludrine alone may not be sufficient.

4.5 Interaction with other medicinal products and other forms of Interaction
Antacids may reduce the absorption of proguanil, so should be taken at least 2-3 hours apart.

Proguanil can potentiate the anticoagulant effect of warfarin and related anticoagulants through a possible interference with their metabolic pathways. Caution is advised when initiating or withdrawing malaria prophylaxis with Paludrine in patients on continuous treatment with anticoagulants.

4.6 Pregnancy and lactation
Pregnancy: Paludrine has been widely used for over 40 years and a causal connection between its use and any adverse effect on mother or foetus has not been established.

However, Paludrine should not be used during pregnancy unless, in the judgement of the physician, potential benefit outweighs the risk.

Malaria in pregnant women increases the risk of maternal death, miscarriage, still-birth and low birth weight with the associated risk of neonatal death. Although travel to malarious areas should be avoided during pregnancy, if this is unavoidable effective prophylaxis is therefore strongly advised in pregnant women.

Lactation: Although Paludrine is excreted in breast milk, the amount is insufficient to confer any benefit on the infant. Separate chemoprophylaxis for the infant is required.

4.7 Effects on ability to drive and use machines
There is no evidence to suggest that Paludrine causes sedation or is likely to affect concentration.

4.8 Undesirable effects
At normal dosage levels the side effect most commonly encountered is mild gastric intolerance, including diarrhoea and constipation. This usually subsides as treatment is continued.

Mouth ulceration and stomatitis have on occasion been reported. Isolated cases of skin reactions and reversible hair loss have been reported in association with the use of proguanil.

Rarely, allergic reactions, which manifest as urticaria or angioedema and very rarely vasculitis, have been reported.

Drug fever and cholestasis may very rarely occur in patients receiving Paludrine.

Haematological changes in patients with severe renal impairment have been reported.

4.9 Overdose
The following effects have been reported in cases of overdosage:

Haematuria, renal irritation, epigastric discomfort and vomiting. There is no specific antidote and symptoms should be treated as they arise.

5. PHARMACOLOGICAL PROPERTIES
5.1 Pharmacodynamic properties
Proguanil is an antimalarial drug and dihydrofolate reductase inhibitor. It acts like the other antifolate antimalarials by interfering with the folic-folinic acid systems and thus exerts its effect mainly at the time the nucleus is dividing. Since its activity is dependent on its metabolism, proguanil has a slow schizonticidal effect in the blood. It also has some schizonticidal activity in the tissues.

Proguanil is effective against the exoerythrocytic forms of some strains of plasmodium falciparum but it has little or no activity against the exoerythrocytic forms of p. Vivax. It has a marked sporonticidal effect against some strains of p falciparum; it does not kill the gametocytes, but renders them non-infective for the mosquito while the drug is present in the blood. Malaria parasites in the red blood cells are killed more rapidly by chloroquine or quinine than by proguanil, which is therefore not the best drug to use for the treatment of acute malaria.

Soon after proguanil was introduced, it was observed that the drug was inactive as an inhibitor of the in vitro growth of p. Gallinaceum and p. Cynomolgi, but that sera from dosed monkeys were active against p. Cynomolgi in vitro. These findings suggested that proguanil was activated in vivo.

Since that time it has been accepted by most investigators in this field that cycloguanil is the active metabolite of proguanil and that parent compound is inactive per se.

Cycloguanil acts by binding to the enzyme dihydrofolate reductase in the malaria parasite. The effect of this action is to prevent the completion of schizogony. This is seen in the asexual blood stages as an arrest of maturation of the developing schizonts and an accumulation of large, abnormal looking trophozoites.

Proguanil is highly active against the primary exoerythocytic forms of p. Falciparum and it has a fleeting inhibiting action on those of p. Vivax. Proguanil is therefore a valuable drug for causal prophylaxis in falciparum malaria.

5.2 Pharmacokinetic properties
Absorption: Rapid, reaching a peak at 3 to 4 hours. The active metabolite (cycloguanil) peaks somewhat later (4 to 9 hours).

Half-life: The half-life of proguanil is 14 to 20 hours, whilst cycloguanil has a half-life of the order of 20 hours. Accumulation during repeated dosing is therefore limited, steady-state being reached within approximately 3 days.

Metabolism: Transformation of proguanil into cycloguanil is associated with cytochrome P450, CYP 2C19, activity. A smaller part of the transformation of proguanil into cycloguanil is probably catalysed by CYP 3A4.

Elimination: Elimination occurs both in the faeces and, principally, in the urine.

In the event of a daily dose being missed, the blood levels fall rapidly but total disappearance of the drug only occurs 3 to 5 days after stopping treatment.

5.3 Preclinical safety data
Proguanil is a drug on which extensive clinical experience has been obtained. All relevant information for the prescriber is provided elsewhere in the Summary of Product Characteristics.

6. PHARMACEUTICAL PARTICULARS
6.1 List of excipients
Calcium carbonate

Gelatin

Magnesium stearate

Maize starch

6.2 Incompatibilities
None known.

6.3 Shelf life
5 years.

6.4 Special precautions for storage
Store below 30°C.

6.5 Nature and contents of container
HDPE bottles (100) and blister packs (98).

6.6 Instructions for use and handling
Use as directed by the prescriber.

7. MARKETING AUTHORISATION HOLDER
AstraZeneca UK Limited,

600 Capability Green,

Luton, LU1 3LU, UK.

8. MARKETING AUTHORISATION NUMBER(S)
PL 17901/0036

9. DATE OF FIRST AUTHORISATION/RENEWAL OF THE AUTHORISATION
18th June 2000

10. DATE OF REVISION OF THE TEXT
18th April 2005

Paludrine/Avloclor Anti-Malarial Travel Pack Chloroquine & Proguanil Anti-Malarial Tablets

(AstraZeneca UK Limited)

1. NAME OF THE MEDICINAL PRODUCT
Paludrine/Avloclor Anti-malarial Travel Pack.

Chloroquine and Proguanil Anti-malarial Tablets.

2. QUALITATIVE AND QUANTITATIVE COMPOSITION
Paludrine tablets containing 100 mg proguanil hydrochloride

Avloclor tablets containing 250 mg chloroquine phosphate, which is equivalent to 155 mg chloroquine base.

3. PHARMACEUTICAL FORM
Tablets.

4. CLINICAL PARTICULARS
4.1 Therapeutic indications
Prophylaxis and suppression of malaria.

4.2 Posology and method of administration
Non-immune subjects entering a malarious area are advised to begin daily treatment with Paludrine 1 week before, or if this is not possible, then at least 2 days before entering the malarious area. The daily dose of Paludrine should be continued throughout exposure to risk and for 4 weeks after leaving the area.

A single dose of Avloclor should be taken each week on the same day each week. Start one week before exposure to risk and continue until 4 weeks after leaving the malarious area.

Each dose should be taken with water after food.

Adults and children over 14 years: Take two Paludrine tablets daily as directed above. Take two Avloclor tablets once a week as directed above.

Children: Do not give to children under 1 year. The following single dose of Paludrine should be taken at the same time each day and the following single dose of Avloclor should be taken once a week on the same day each week.

	Paludrine (at the same time each day)	**Avloclor (on the same day each week)**
1 to 4 years	Half of a tablet	Half of a tablet
5 to 8 years	One tablet	One tablet
9 to 14 years	One and a half tablets	One and a half tablets

For a young child the dose may be administered crushed and mixed with milk, honey or jam.

Provided the Paludrine tablet fragment gives the minimum amount specified, precise accuracy in children's dosage is not essential since the drug possesses a wide safety margin.

The Avloclor dose given to children should be calculated on their body weight (5 mg chloroquine base/kg/week) and must not exceed the adult dose regardless of weight.

Elderly Patients: There are no special dosage recommendations for the elderly, but it may be advisable to monitor elderly patients so that optimum dosage can be individually determined.

Paludrine and Renal Impairment: Based on a theoretical model derived from a single dose pharmacokinetic study, the following guidance is given for adults with renal impairment. (See also Sections 4.3 and 4.4).

Creatinine clearance (ml/min/1.73 m²)	**Dosage**
⩾ 60	200 mg once daily (standard dose)
20 to 59	100 mg once daily
10 to 19	50 mg every second day
< 10	50 mg once weekly

The grade of renal impairment and/or the serum creatinine concentration may be approximately equated to creatinine clearance levels as indicated below.

Creatinine clearance (ml/min/1.73 m²)	**Approx* serum creatinine (micromol/1)**	**Renal Impairment Grade (arbitrarily divided for dosage purposes)**
⩾ 60	-	-
20 to 59	150 to 300	Mild
10 to 19	300 to 700	Moderate
< 10	> 700	Severe

*Serum creatinine concentration is only an approximate guide to renal function unless corrected for age, weight and sex.

Avloclor and Hepatic or Renally Impaired Patients: Caution is necessary when giving Avloclor to patients with renal disease or hepatic disease.

4.3 Contraindications
Known hypersensitivity to chloroquine or any other ingredients of the formulation.

4.4 Special warnings and special precautions for use
When used as malaria prophylaxis official guidelines and local information on prevalence of resistance to anti-malarial drugs should be taken into consideration.

Paludrine should be used with caution in patients with severe renal impairment. (See also Section 4.2). There have been rare reports of haematological changes in such patients. Caution is necessary when giving Avloclor to patients with renal disease.

Caution is necessary when giving Avloclor to patients with impaired hepatic function, particularly when associated with cirrhosis.

Caution is also necessary in patients with porphyria. Avloclor may precipitate severe constitutional symptoms and an increase in the amount of porphyrins excreted in the urine. This reaction is especially apparent in patients with high alcohol intake.

Avloclor should be used with care in patients with a history of epilepsy. Potential risks and benefits should be carefully evaluated before use in subjects taking anti-convulsant therapy or with a history of epilepsy as, rarely, cases of convulsions have been reported in association with chloroquine.

The use of Avloclor in patients with psoriasis may precipitate a severe attack.

Caution is advised in patients with glucose-6-phosphate dehydrogenase deficiency, as there may be a risk of haemolysis.

Prolonged or high dose Avloclor therapy:

Considerable caution is needed in the use of Avloclor for long-term high dosage therapy and such use should only be considered when no other drug is available.

Irreversible retinal damage and corneal changes may develop during long term therapy and after the drug has been discontinued. Ophthalmic examination prior to and at 3 – 6 monthly intervals during use is required if patients are receiving chloroquine

- At continuous high doses for longer than 12 months
- As weekly treatment for longer than 3 years
- When total consumption exceeds 1.6g/kg (cumulative dose 100g).

Full blood counts should be carried out regularly during extended treatment as bone marrow suppression may occur rarely.

4.5 Interaction with other medicinal products and other forms of Interaction

Antacids (aluminium, calcium and magnesium salts) may reduce the absorption of proguanil and chloroquine, so antacids should be taken well separated from Paludrine and Avloclor (at least two hours before or after).

If the patient is taking cyclosporin then chloroquine may cause an increase in cyclosporin levels.

Pre-exposure intradermal human diploid-cell rabies vaccine should not be administered to patients taking chloroquine as this may suppress antibody response. When vaccinated against rabies, that vaccine should precede the start of antimalarial dosing, otherwise the effectiveness of the vaccine might be reduced.

Chloroquine significantly reduces levels of praziquantel. Caution is therefore advised during co-administration. Prescribers may consider increasing the dose of praziquantel if the patient does not respond to the initial dose.

Amiodarone:	chloroquine and hydroxychloroquine increase the risk of cardiac arrhythmias including ventricular arrhythmias, bradycardias and cardiac conduction defect. Concurrent use is contra-indicated.
Anticoagulants:	proguanil can potentiate the anticoagulant effect of warfarin and related anticoagulants through a possible interference with their metabolic pathways. Caution is advised when initiating or withdrawing malaria prophylaxis with Paludrine in patients on continuous treatment with anticoagulants.
Other antimalarials:	increased risk of convulsion with mefloquine.
Cardiac glycosides:	hydroxychloroquine and possibly chloroquine increase plasma concentration of digoxin.
Parasympathomimetics:	chloroquine and hydroxychloroquine have potential to increase symptoms of myasthenia gravis and thus diminish effect of neostigmine and pyridostigmine.
Ulcer healing drugs:	cimetidine inhibits metabolism of chloroquine (increased plasma concentration).

4.6 Pregnancy and lactation

Pregnancy

Avloclor and Paludrine should not be used during pregnancy unless, in the judgement of the physician, potential benefit outweighs the risk.

Short-term malaria prophylaxis:

Malaria in pregnant women increases the risk of maternal death, miscarriage, still-birth and low birth weight with the associated risk of neonatal death. Travel to malarious areas should be avoided during pregnancy but, if this is not possible, women should receive effective prophylaxis.

Long-term high dose Avloclor therapy:

There is evidence to suggest that Avloclor given to women in high doses throughout pregnancy can give rise to foetal abnormalities including visual loss, ototoxicity and cochlear-vestibular dysfunction. Paludrine has been widely used for over 40 years and a causal connection between its use and any adverse effect on mother or foetus has not been established.

Lactation

Although both Paludrine and Avloclor are excreted in breast milk, the amount is too small to be harmful when used for malaria prophylaxis but as a consequence is insufficient to confer any benefit on the infant. Separate chemoprophylaxis for the infant is required. However, when long-term high doses of chloroquine are used for rheumatoid disease, breast feeding is not recommended.

4.7 Effects on ability to drive and use machines

Defects in visual accommodation may occur on first taking Avloclor and patients should be warned regarding driving or operating machinery.

There is no evidence to suggest that Paludrine causes sedation or is likely to affect concentration.

4.8 Undesirable effects

The adverse reactions which may occur at doses used in the prophylaxis of malaria are generally not of a serious nature. Where prolonged high dosage of chloroquine is required, i.e. in the treatment of rheumatoid arthritis, adverse reactions can be of a more serious nature.

Paludrine

At normal dosage levels the side effect most commonly encountered is mild gastric intolerance, including diarrhoea and constipation. This usually subsides as treatment is continued.

Mouth ulceration and stomatitis have on occasion been reported. Isolated cases of skin reactions and reversible hair loss have been reported in association with the use of proguanil.

Rarely, allergic reactions which manifest as urticaria or angioedema and very rarely vasculitis, have been reported.

Drug fever and cholestasis may very rarely occur in patients receiving Paludrine.

Haematological changes in patients with severe renal impairment have been reported.

Avloclor

Adverse reactions reported after Avloclor use are:

Cardiovascular:	hypotension and ECG changes (at high doses), cardiomyopathy.
Central nervous system:	convulsions and psychotic reactions including hallucinations (rare), anxiety, personality changes.
Eye disorders:	retinal degeneration, macular defects of colour vision, pigmentation, optic atrophy scotomas, field defects, blindness, corneal opacities and pigmented deposits, blurring of vision, difficulty in accommodation, diplopia.
Gastro-intestinal:	gastro-intestinal disturbances, nausea, vomiting, diarrhoea, abdominal cramps.
General:	headache.
Haematological:	bone marrow depression, aplastic anaemia, agranulocytosis, thrombocytopenia, neutropenia.
Hepatic:	changes in liver function, including hepatitis and abnormal liver function tests, have been reported rarely.
Hypersensitivity:	allergic and anaphylactic reactions, including urticaria, angioedema and vasculitis.
Hearing disorders:	tinnitus, reduced hearing, nerve deafness.
Muscular:	neuromyopathy and myopathy.
Skin:	macular, urticarial and purpuric skin eruptions, occasional depigmentation or loss of hair, erythema multiforme, Stevens-Johnson syndrome, toxic epidermal necrolysis, precipitation of psoriasis, pruritus, photosensitivity, lichen-planus type reaction, pigmentation of the skin and mucous membranes (long term use).

4.9 Overdose

Paludrine

The following effects have been reported in cases of overdosage:

Haematuria, renal irritation, epigastric discomfort and vomiting. There is no specific antidote and symptoms should be treated as they arise.

Avloclor

Chloroquine is highly toxic in overdose and children are particularly susceptible. The chief symptoms of overdosage include circulatory collapse due to a potent cardiotoxic effect, respiratory arrest and coma. Symptoms may progress rapidly after initial nausea and vomiting. Cardiac complications may occur without progressively deepening coma.

Death may result from circulatory or respiratory failure or cardiac arrhythmia. If there is no demonstrable cardiac output due to arrhythmias, asystole or electromechanical dissociation, external chest compression should be persisted with for as long as necessary, or until adrenaline and diazepam can be given (see below).

Gastric lavage should be carried out urgently, first protecting the airway and instituting artificial ventilation where necessary. There is a risk of cardiac arrest following aspiration of gastric contents in more serious cases. Activated charcoal left in the stomach may reduce absorption of any remaining chloroquine from the gut. Circulatory status (with central venous pressure measurement), respiration, plasma electrolytes and blood gases should be monitored, with correction of hypokalaemia and acidosis if indicated. Cardiac arrhythmias should not be treated unless life threatening; drugs with quinidine-like effects should be avoided. Intravenous sodium bicarbonate 1-2mmol/kg over 15 minutes may be effective in conduction disturbances, and DC shock is indicated for ventricular tachycardia and ventricular fibrillation.

Early administration of the following has been shown to improve survival in cases of serious poisoning:

1. Adrenaline infusion 0.25 micrograms/kg/min initially, with increments of 0.25 micrograms/kg/min until adequate systolic blood pressure (more than 100mm/Hg) is restored; adrenaline reduces the effects of chloroquine on the heart through its inotropic and vasoconstrictor effects.

2. Diazepam infusion (2mg/kg over 30 minutes as a loading dose, followed by 1-2mg/kg/day for up to 2-4 days). Diazepam may minimise cardiotoxicity.

Acidification of the urine, haemodialysis, peritoneal dialysis or exchange transfusion have not been shown to be of value in treating chloroquine poisoning. Chloroquine is excreted very slowly, therefore cases of overdosage require observation for several days.

5. PHARMACOLOGICAL PROPERTIES

5.1 Pharmacodynamic properties

Paludrine

Proguanil is an antimalarial drug and dihydrofolate reductase inhibitor. It acts like the other antifolate antimalarials by interfering with the folic-folinic acid systems and thus exerts its effect mainly at the time the nucleus is dividing. Since its activity is dependent on its metabolism, proguanil has a slow schizonticidal effect in the blood. It also has some schizonticidal activity in the tissues.

Proguanil is effective against the exoerythrocytic forms of some strains of *plasmodium falciparum* but it has little or no activity against the exoerythrocytic forms of *p. Vivax*. It has a marked sporonticidal effect against some strains of *p falciparum*; it does not kill the gametocytes, but renders them non-infective for the mosquito while the drug is present in the blood. Malaria parasites in the red blood cells are killed more rapidly by chloroquine or quinine than by proguanil, which is therefore not the best drug to use for the treatment of acute malaria.

Soon after proguanil was introduced, it was observed that the drug was inactive as an inhibitor of the in vitro growth of *p. Gallinaceum* and *p. Cynomolgi*, but that sera from dosed monkeys were active against *p. Cynomolgi* in vitro. These findings suggested that proguanil was activated in vivo.

Since that time it has been accepted by most investigators in this field that cycloguanil is the active metabolite of proguanil and that parent compound is inactive per se.

Cycloguanil acts by binding to the enzyme dihydrofolate reductase in the malaria parasite. The effect of this action is to prevent the completion of schizogony. This is seen in the asexual blood stages as an arrest of maturation of the developing schizonts and an accumulation of large, abnormal looking trophozoites.

Proguanil is highly active against the primary exoerythocytic forms of *p. Falciparum* and it has a fleeting inhibiting action on those of *p. Vivax*. Proguanil is therefore a valuable drug for causal prophylaxis in falciparum malaria.

Avloclor

The mode of action of chloroquine on plasmodia has not been fully elucidated. Chloroquine binds to and alters the properties of DNA. Chloroquine also binds to ferriprotoporphyrin IX and this leads to lysis of the plasmodial membrane.

In suppressive treatment, chloroquine inhibits the erythrocytic stage of development of plasmodia. In acute attacks of malaria, it interrupts erythrocytic schizogony of the parasite. Its ability to concentrate in parasitised erythrocytes may account for the selective toxicity against the erythrocytic stages of plasmodial infection.

5.2 Pharmacokinetic properties

Paludrine

Absorption: Rapid, reaching a peak at 3 to 4 hours. The active metabolite (cycloguanil) peaks somewhat later (4 to 9 hours).

Half-life: The half-life of proguanil is 14 to 20 hours, whilst cycloguanil has a half-life of the order of 20 hours. Accumulation during repeated dosing is therefore limited, steady-state being reached within approximately 3 days.

Metabolism: Transformation of proguanil into cycloguanil is associated with cytochrome P450, CYP 2C19, activity. A smaller part of the transformation of proguanil into cycloguanil is probably catalysed by CYP 3A4.

Elimination: Elimination occurs both in the faeces and, principally, in the urine.

In the event of a daily dose being missed, the blood levels fall rapidly but total disappearance of the drug only occurs 3 to 5 days after stopping treatment.

Avloclor

Studies in volunteers using single doses of chloroquine phosphate equivalent to 300mg base have found peak plasma levels to be achieved within one to six hours. These levels are in the region of 54-102 microgram/litre, the concentration in whole blood being some 4 to 10 times higher. Following a single dose, chloroquine may be detected in plasma for more than four weeks. Mean bioavailability from tablets of chloroquine phosphate is 89%. Chloroquine is widely distributed in body tissues such as the eyes, kidneys, liver, and lungs where retention is prolonged. The elimination of chloroquine is slow, with a multi exponential decline in plasma concentration. The initial distribution phase has a half-life of 2-6 days while the terminal elimination phase is 10-60 days. Approximately 50-70% of chloroquine in plasma is bound to the plasma proteins.

The principal metabolite is monodesethylchloroquine, which reaches a peak concentration of 10-20 microgram/litre within a few hours. Mean urinary recovery, within 3-13 weeks, is approximately 50% of the administered dose, most being unchanged drug and the remainder as metabolite. Chloroquine may be detected in urine for several months.

5.3 Preclinical safety data
Both Paludrine and Avloclor have been extensively used for many years in clinical practice. All relevant information for the prescriber is provided elsewhere in this document.

6. PHARMACEUTICAL PARTICULARS
6.1 List of excipients

Paludrine	**Avloclor**
Calcium carbonate	Magnesium stearate
Gelatin	Maize starch
Magnesium stearate	
Maize starch	

6.2 Incompatibilities
None known.

6.3 Shelf life
5 years.

6.4 Special precautions for storage
Do not store above 30°C. Store in the original package.

6.5 Nature and contents of container
PVC/PVDC Aluminium Foil Blister Pack of 112's containing 98 Paludrine and 14 Avloclor tablets.

6.6 Instructions for use and handling
No special instructions.

7. MARKETING AUTHORISATION HOLDER
AstraZeneca UK Limited,
600 Capability Green,
Luton, LU1 3LU, UK.

8. MARKETING AUTHORISATION NUMBER(S)
PL 17901/0037

9. DATE OF FIRST AUTHORISATION/RENEWAL OF THE AUTHORISATION
18th June 2000/5th November 2002

10. DATE OF REVISION OF THE TEXT
23rd June 2005

Pancrease Capsules

(Janssen-Cilag Ltd)

1. NAME OF THE MEDICINAL PRODUCT
Pancrease Capsules

2. QUALITATIVE AND QUANTITATIVE COMPOSITION
Each capsule contains no less than
Protease 330 BP units
Amylase 2900 BP units
Lipase 5000 BP units

3. PHARMACEUTICAL FORM
Capsule.

4. CLINICAL PARTICULARS
4.1 Therapeutic indications
Exocrine pancreatic enzyme deficiency as in cystic fibrosis, chronic pancreatitis, post pancreatectomy, post gastro-intestinal bypass surgery. (eg Billroth 11 gastroenterostomy), ductal obstruction from neoplasm (eg of the pancreas or common bile duct).

4.2 Posology and method of administration
For oral administration.
For adults and children

1 or 2 capsules during each meal and one capsule with snacks. Occasionally a third capsule with meals may be required depending upon individual requirements. Where swallowing of capsules is difficult, they may be opened and the beads taken with liquids or soft foods which do not require chewing. To protect the enteric coating, the beads should not be crushed or chewed.

4.3 Contraindications
Hypersensitivity to pork protein.

4.4 Special warnings and special precautions for use
Contact of the microspheres with food having a pH higher than 5.5.

4.5 Interaction with other medicinal products and other forms of Interaction
None known.

4.6 Pregnancy and lactation
The safety of Pancrease during pregnancy has not yet been established. Use of the product during pregnancy is therefore not recommended.

4.7 Effects on ability to drive and use machines
None known.

4.8 Undesirable effects
The most frequently reported adverse reactions are gastro-intestinal in nature. Less frequently, allergic type reactions have also been observed. Extremely high doses of exogenous pancreatic enzymes have been associated with hyperuricosuria and hyperuricaemia.

4.9 Overdose
No special warnings.

5. PHARMACOLOGICAL PROPERTIES
5.1 Pharmacodynamic properties
None stated.

5.2 Pharmacokinetic properties
None stated.

5.3 Preclinical safety data
Not applicable.

6. PHARMACEUTICAL PARTICULARS
6.1 List of excipients
Non pareil seeds
Povidone
Sodium starch glycollate
Cellulose acetate phthalate
Diethyl phthalate
Talc

6.2 Incompatibilities
None.

6.3 Shelf life
24 months.

6.4 Special precautions for storage
Keep bottle tightly closed.
Store at room temperature in a dry place.
Do not refrigerate.

6.5 Nature and contents of container
Securitainers or white polyethylene bottles and caps.
Pack size:100.

6.6 Instructions for use and handling
Not applicable.

7. MARKETING AUTHORISATION HOLDER
Janssen-Cilag Ltd
Saunderton
High Wycombe
Buckinghamshire
HP14 4HJ
UK

8. MARKETING AUTHORISATION NUMBER(S)
0242/0254

9. DATE OF FIRST AUTHORISATION/RENEWAL OF THE AUTHORISATION
1 July 1995/16 October 1998

10. DATE OF REVISION OF THE TEXT
September 1996

Pancrease HL Capsules

(Janssen-Cilag Ltd)

1. NAME OF THE MEDICINAL PRODUCT
Pancrease™ HL Capsules

2. QUALITATIVE AND QUANTITATIVE COMPOSITION
Each capsule contains pancreatin BP 387.45 mg, equivalent to not less than 25000 BP units of lipase, 22500 BP units of amylase and 1250 BP units of protease.

3. PHARMACEUTICAL FORM
Size 0, elongated hard gelatin capsule, with a white opaque body and a white opaque cap, each ringed with a red band and the letters HL in red, containing enterically coated minitablets.

4. CLINICAL PARTICULARS
4.1 Therapeutic indications
Exocrine pancreatic enzyme deficiency as in cystic fibrosis, chronic pancreatitis, post pancreatectomy, post gastro-intestinal bypass surgery (eg Billroth II gastroenterostomy), and ductal obstruction from neoplasm (eg of the pancreas or common bile duct).

4.2 Posology and method of administration
For oral administration.
Adults and children
One or two capsules during each meal and one capsule with snacks. The interindividual response to pancreatin supplements is variable and the number of capsules may need to be titrated to the individual based upon parameters of steatorrhoea and symptomatology. Further dose increases, if required, should be added slowly, with careful monitoring of response and symptomatology.

Where patients are already in receipt of lower unit dose enteric coated pancreatin supplements, then Pancrease HL Capsules may be substituted at one-third of the number of capsules of the previous preparation.

Where swallowing of capsules is difficult, then they may be opened and the minitablets taken with liquid or soft foods which do not require chewing. To protect the enteric coating, the minitablets should not be crushed or chewed.

It is important to ensure adequate hydration of patients at all times whilst dosing Pancrease HL Capsules.

Patients who are taking or have been given in excess of 10,000 units of lipase/kg/day are at risk of developing colon damage. The dose of Pancrease HL should usually not exceed this dose.

4.3 Contraindications
Hypersensitivity to pork protein or any excipient.
Children aged 15 or under with cystic fibrosis.

4.4 Special warnings and special precautions for use
Contact of the minitablets with food having a pH higher than 5.5 can dissolve the protective coating and will reduce the efficacy of the product.

4.5 Interaction with other medicinal products and other forms of Interaction
None stated.

4.6 Pregnancy and lactation
The safety of Pancrease HL during pregnancy has not yet been established. Consequently, use of the product in pregnancy is therefore not recommended.

4.7 Effects on ability to drive and use machines
None stated.

4.8 Undesirable effects
The most frequently reported adverse reactions are gastro-intestinal in nature such as abdominal discomfort, nausea and vomiting. Less frequently, allergic-type reactions of the skin have also been observed. Very high doses of exogenous pancreatic enzymes have been associated with hyperuricosuria and hyperuricaemia.

Stricture of the ileo-caecum and large bowel and colitis have been reported in children with cystic fibrosis taking Pancrease HL.

Abdominal symptoms (not usually experienced by the patient) or changes in abdominal symptoms should be reviewed to exclude the possibility of colonic damage, especially if the patient is taking in excess of 10,000 units of lipase/kg/day.

4.9 Overdose
Overdosage is unlikely and has not been experienced to date with Pancrease HL. Inappropriately large doses could result in symptoms such as abdominal discomfort, nausea, vomiting, perianal irritation or inflammation.

5. PHARMACOLOGICAL PROPERTIES
5.1 Pharmacodynamic properties
The enzymes catalyse the hydrolysis of fats into glycerol and fatty acids, protein into proteoses and derived substances, and starch into dextrins and sugars.

5.2 Pharmacokinetic properties
Pancreatin is not systemically absorbed from the gastro-intestinal tract.

5.3 Preclinical safety data
No relevant information additional to that contained elsewhere in the Summary of Product Characteristics.

6. PHARMACEUTICAL PARTICULARS
6.1 List of excipients
Caster oil, hydrogenated NF
Silicon dioxide, colloidal PhEur
Magnesium stearate PhEur
Sodium carboxymethylcellulose PhEur
Cellulose microcrystalline PhEur
<u>Coat composition</u>:
Simethicone emulsion USP
Methacryllic acid copolymer type C NF
Talc PhEur
Triethyl citrate NF
Purified water PhEur
<u>Capsule composition (body and cap)</u>:
Titanium dioxide PhEur
Gelatin PhEur
<u>Ink composition</u>:
Shellac
Industrial methylated spirits
Purified water PhEur
Soya lecithin (food grade)
2-ethoxyethanol
Dimethylpolysiloxane
Red iron oxide (E172)

6.2 Incompatibilities
None stated.

6.3 Shelf life
2 years.

6.4 Special precautions for storage
Keep bottle tightly closed. Store at room temperature (10°C - 25°C) in a dry place. Do not refrigerate.

6.5 Nature and contents of container
High density polyethylene bottles with a low density polyethylene snap top lid, containing 100 or 500 capsules.

6.6 Instructions for use and handling
Not applicable.

7. MARKETING AUTHORISATION HOLDER
Janssen-Cilag Ltd

Saunderton

High Wycombe

Buckinghamshire

HP14 4HJ

UK

8. MARKETING AUTHORISATION NUMBER(S)
0242/0255

9. DATE OF FIRST AUTHORISATION/RENEWAL OF THE AUTHORISATION
1 October 1995

10. DATE OF REVISION OF THE TEXT
May 1997

Legal category POM

Pancrex Granules

(Paines & Byrne Limited)

1. NAME OF THE MEDICINAL PRODUCT
Pancrex Granules.

2. QUALITATIVE AND QUANTITATIVE COMPOSITION
Pancreatin BP to provide enzymatic activity per gram not less than:

Free protease 300 BP units

Lipase 5000 BP units

Amylase 4000 BP units

3. PHARMACEUTICAL FORM
Granules.

4. CLINICAL PARTICULARS

4.1 Therapeutic indications
Pancrex is used to compensate for reduced intestinal enzyme activity in pancreatic deficiency states.

It is indicated for the treatment of fibrocystic disease of the pancreas (cystic fibrosis), chronic pancreatitis and pancreatic steatorrhoea following pancreatectomy. It may also be indicated following gastrectomy as an aid to digestion.

4.2 Posology and method of administration
Dosage should be adjusted according to the needs of the individual patient and the amount and type of food consumed.

The following dosage ranges provide a suitable basis for adjustment.

Adults, the Elderly, and Children

5 g - 10 g swallowed dry or mixed with a little water or milk just before meals

4.3 Contraindications
Hypersensitivity to the active ingredient (porcine pancreatin) or any of the excipients.

4.4 Special warnings and special precautions for use
Unsuitable for people with lactose insufficiency, galactosaemia or glucose/galactose malabsorption syndrome.

It is possible that some irritation of the skin of the mouth may occur if the granules are chewed or retained in the mouth. Irritation of the anus may also occur. A barrier cream may prevent this local irritation.

If the granules are mixed with liquids the resulting mixture should not be allowed to stand for more than one hour prior to use.

4.5 Interaction with other medicinal products and other forms of Interaction
None known.

4.6 Pregnancy and lactation
Safety in pregnancy has not been established. However, no teratogenic effects have been observed in clinical use.

4.7 Effects on ability to drive and use machines
None.

4.8 Undesirable effects
Rare cases of hyperuricosuria and hyperuricaemia have been reported when extremely high doses of pancreatin have been taken.

Strictures of the ileo-caecum and large bowel, and colitis, have been reported in children with cystic fibrosis taking high doses of pancreatic enzyme supplements. To date Pancrex and Pancrex V presentations have not been implicated in the development of colonic damage. However unusual abdominal symptoms or changes in abdominal symptoms should be reviewed to exclude the possibility of colonic damage especially if the patient is taking in excess of 10,000 units/kg/day of lipase.

4.9 Overdose
None stated.

5. PHARMACOLOGICAL PROPERTIES

5.1 Pharmacodynamic properties
Pancreatin is derived from porcine pancreas and contains the enzymes, amylase, protease and lipase. The enzymes have the same actions as pancreatic juice and when administered to patients with pancreatic insufficiency improve the ability to metabolise starches, proteins and fats.

5.2 Pharmacokinetic properties
Pancreatin hydrolyses fats to glycerol and fatty acids, changes proteins into proteases and derived substances, and converts starch into dextrins and sugars.

5.3 Preclinical safety data
No relevant pre-clinical safety data has been generated.

6. PHARMACEUTICAL PARTICULARS

6.1 List of excipients
Lactose, acacia, (E414) Opaseal P17-0200 containing IMS, polyvinyl acetate phthalate and stearic acid (E570).

This medicinal product contains approximately 70g of lactose per 100g. When taken according to the dosage recommendations each dose supplies up to 7g of lactose.

6.2 Incompatibilities
None known.

6.3 Shelf life
2 years.

6.4 Special precautions for storage
Store at a temperature not exceeding 15°C.

6.5 Nature and contents of container
Securitainer; 100, 300 and 500 g.

6.6 Instructions for use and handling
Not applicable.

Administrative Data

7. MARKETING AUTHORISATION HOLDER
Paines and Byrne Limited

Yamanouchi House

Pyrford Road

West Byfleet

Surrey

KT14 6RA

8. MARKETING AUTHORISATION NUMBER(S)
Product licence 0051/5003R

9. DATE OF FIRST AUTHORISATION/RENEWAL OF THE AUTHORISATION
First authorisation granted 1 May 1987 / October 2003

10. DATE OF REVISION OF THE TEXT
Date of partial revision = October 2003

11. Legal category
P

Pancrex V Capsules

(Paines & Byrne Limited)

1. NAME OF THE MEDICINAL PRODUCT
Pancrex V Capsules.

2. QUALITATIVE AND QUANTITATIVE COMPOSITION
Pancreatin BP to provide enzymatic activity per capsule not less than:

Free protease 430 BP units

Lipase 8000 BP units

Amylase 9000 BP units

3. PHARMACEUTICAL FORM
Capsule.

4. CLINICAL PARTICULARS

4.1 Therapeutic indications
Pancrex is used to compensate for reduced intestinal enzyme activity in pancreatic deficiency states.

It is indicated for the treatment of fibrocystic disease of the pancreas (cystic fibrosis), chronic pancreatitis and pancreatic steatorrhoea following pancreatectomy. It may also be indicated following gastrectomy as an aid to digestion.

4.2 Posology and method of administration
Dosage should be adjusted according to the needs of the individual patient and the amount and type of food consumed.

The following dosage ranges provide a suitable basis for adjustment.

Infants: the contents of 1 - 2 capsules mixed with feeds.

Older Children and Adults: the contents of 2 - 6 capsules with each snack or meal. The capsules may be swallowed.

The capsules may provide a suitable alternative to the enteric coated presentations in cases where the pH of the duodenum is not sufficiently alkaline to dissolve the enteric coat.

Capsules provide a simple and convenient method of dose measurement of pancreatin for administration to younger children requiring a low dose.

4.3 Contraindications
Hypersensitivity to the active ingredient (porcine pancreatin) or any of the excipients.

4.4 Special warnings and special precautions for use
It is possible that some irritation of the skin of the mouth may occur if capsules are chewed or the contents retained in the mouth. Irritation of the anus may also occur. A barrier cream may prevent this local irritation.

Allergic/asthmatic reactions have occasionally occurred on handling the capsule contents.

If the capsule contents are mixed with liquids or feeds the resulting mixture should not be allowed to stand for more than one hour prior to use.

4.5 Interaction with other medicinal products and other forms of Interaction
None known.

4.6 Pregnancy and lactation
Safety in pregnancy has not been established. However, no teratogenic effects have been observed in clinical use.

4.7 Effects on ability to drive and use machines
None.

4.8 Undesirable effects
Rare cases of hyperuricosuria and hyperuricaemia have been reported when extremely high doses of pancreatin have been taken.

Strictures of the ileo-caecum and large bowel, and colitis, have been reported in children with cystic fibrosis taking high doses of pancreatic enzyme supplements. To date Pancrex and Pancrex V presentations have not been implicated in the development of colonic damage. However unusual abdominal symptoms or changes in abdominal symptoms should be reviewed to exclude the possibility of colonic damage especially if the patient is taking in excess of 10,000 units/kg/day of lipase.

4.9 Overdose
None stated.

5. PHARMACOLOGICAL PROPERTIES

5.1 Pharmacodynamic properties
Pancreatin is derived from porcine pancreas and contains the enzymes, amylase, protease and lipase. The enzymes have the same actions as pancreatic juice and when administered to patients with pancreatic insufficiency improve the ability to metabolise starches, proteins and fats.

5.2 Pharmacokinetic properties
Pancreatin hydrolyses fats to glycerol and fatty acids, changes proteins into proteases and derived substances, and converts starch into dextrins and sugars.

5.3 Preclinical safety data
No relevant pre-clinical safety data has been generated.

6. PHARMACEUTICAL PARTICULARS

6.1 List of excipients
Aluminium oxide, magnesium stearate, microcrystalline cellulose gelatin, titanium dioxide, yellow iron oxide (E172), quinoline yellow (E104).

6.2 Incompatibilities
None known.

6.3 Shelf life
2 years.

6.4 Special precautions for storage
Store at a temperature not exceeding 15°C.

6.5 Nature and contents of container
Securitainer; 100, 300 and 500 capsules.

6.6 Instructions for use and handling
Not applicable.

Administrative Data

7. MARKETING AUTHORISATION HOLDER
Paines and Byrne Limited

Yamanouchi House

Pyrford Road

West Byfleet

Surrey

KT14 6RA

8. MARKETING AUTHORISATION NUMBER(S)
Product licence 0051/5043R

9. DATE OF FIRST AUTHORISATION/RENEWAL OF THE AUTHORISATION
First authorisation granted 13 November 1985

Renewal granted 31st May 2001.

10. DATE OF REVISION OF THE TEXT
Date of partial revision = October 2003.

11. Legal category
P

Pancrex V Capsules 125mg

(Paines & Byrne Limited)

1. NAME OF THE MEDICINAL PRODUCT
Pancrex V Capsules 125 mg.

2. QUALITATIVE AND QUANTITATIVE COMPOSITION
Pancreatin BP to provide enzymatic activity per capsule not less than:

Free protease 160 BP units

Lipase 2950 BP units

Amylase 3300 BP units

3. PHARMACEUTICAL FORM
Capsule.

4. CLINICAL PARTICULARS
4.1 Therapeutic indications
Pancrex is used to compensate for reduced intestinal enzyme activity in pancreatic deficiency states.

It is indicated for the treatment of fibrocystic disease of the pancreas (cystic fibrosis), chronic pancreatitis and pancreatic steatorrhoea following pancreatectomy. It may also be indicated following gastrectomy as an aid to digestion.

4.2 Posology and method of administration
These low dose capsules may be used when small amounts of Pancrex are required, for example for neonates.

Dosage should be adjusted according to the needs of the individual patient and the amount of food consumed.

The following dosage scale provides a suitable basis for adjustment.

Neonates: the contents of 1 - 2 capsules mixed with feeds.

4.3 Contraindications
Hypersensitivity to the active ingredient (porcine pancreatin) or any of the excipients.

4.4 Special warnings and special precautions for use
It is possible that some irritation of the skin of the mouth may occur if capsules 125 mg are chewed or the contents retained in the mouth. Irritation of the anus may also occur. A barrier cream may prevent this local irritation.

Allergic/asthmatic reactions have occasionally occurred on handling the capsule contents.

If the capsule contents are mixed with liquids or feeds the resulting mixture should not be allowed to stand for more than one hour prior to use.

4.5 Interaction with other medicinal products and other forms of Interaction
None known.

4.6 Pregnancy and lactation
Safety in pregnancy has not been established. However, no teratogenic effects have been observed in clinical use.

4.7 Effects on ability to drive and use machines
None.

4.8 Undesirable effects
Rare cases of hyperuricosuria and hyperuricaemia have been reported when extremely high doses of pancreatin have been taken.

Strictures of the ileo-caecum and large bowel, and colitis, have been reported in children with cystic fibrosis taking high doses of pancreatic enzyme supplements. To date Pancrex and Pancrex V presentations have not been implicated in the development of colonic damage. However unusual abdominal symptoms or changes in abdominal symptoms should be reviewed to exclude the possibility of colonic damage especially if the patient is taking in excess of 10,000 units/kg/day of lipase.

4.9 Overdose
None stated.

5. PHARMACOLOGICAL PROPERTIES
5.1 Pharmacodynamic properties
Pancreatin is derived from porcine pancreas and contains the enzymes, amylase, protease and lipase. The enzymes have the same actions as pancreatic juice and when administered to patients with pancreatic insufficiency improve the ability to metabolise starches, proteins and fats.

5.2 Pharmacokinetic properties
Pancreatin hydrolyses fats to glycerol and fatty acids, changes proteins into proteases and derived substances, and converts starch into dextrins and sugars.

5.3 Preclinical safety data
No relevant pre-clinical safety data has been generated.

6. PHARMACEUTICAL PARTICULARS
6.1 List of excipients
Aluminium oxide, magnesium stearate, microcrystalline cellulose.

6.2 Incompatibilities
None known.

6.3 Shelf life
2 years.

6.4 Special precautions for storage
Store at a temperature not exceeding 15°C.

6.5 Nature and contents of container
Securitainer; 300 and 500 capsules.

6.6 Instructions for use and handling
Not applicable.

Administrative Data
7. MARKETING AUTHORISATION HOLDER
Paines and Byrne Limited

Yamanouchi House

Pyrford Road

West Byfleet

Surrey

KT14 6RA

8. MARKETING AUTHORISATION NUMBER(S)
Product licence 0051/5104R

9. DATE OF FIRST AUTHORISATION/RENEWAL OF THE AUTHORISATION
First authorisation granted 13 November 1985

Renewal granted 4 November 2003

10. DATE OF REVISION OF THE TEXT
Date of partial revision = 4 November 2003

11. Legal category
P

Pancrex V Forte Tablets

(Paines & Byrne Limited)

1. NAME OF THE MEDICINAL PRODUCT
Pancrex V Forte Tablets

2. QUALITATIVE AND QUANTITATIVE COMPOSITION
Pancreatin BP to provide enzymatic activity per tablet not less than:

Free protease 330 BP units

Lipase 5600 BP units

Amylase 5000 BP units

3. PHARMACEUTICAL FORM
Tablet.

4. CLINICAL PARTICULARS
4.1 Therapeutic indications
Pancrex is used to compensate for reduced intestinal enzyme activity in pancreatic deficiency states.

It is indicated for the treatment of fibrocystic disease of the pancreas (cystic fibrosis), chronic pancreatitis and pancreatic steatorrhoea following pancreatectomy. It may also be indicated following gastrectomy as an aid to digestion.

4.2 Posology and method of administration
Dosage should be adjusted according to the needs of the individual patient and the amount and type of food consumed.

The following dosage ranges provide a suitable basis for adjustment.

Adults, the Elderly, and Children

6 - 10 tablets before each snack or meal, swallowed whole

4.3 Contraindications
Hypersensitivity to the active ingredient (porcine pancreatin) or any of the excipients.

4.4 Special warnings and special precautions for use
Unsuitable for people with lactase insufficiency, galactosaemia or glucose/galactose malabsorption syndrome.

Variations in response to treatment may be due to enteric coating. It is possible that some irritation of the skin of the mouth may occur if tablets are chewed or preparations retained in the mouth. Irritation of the anus may also occur. A barrier cream may prevent this local irritation.

4.5 Interaction with other medicinal products and other forms of Interaction
None known.

4.6 Pregnancy and lactation
Safety in pregnancy has not been established. However, no teratogenic effects have been observed in clinical use.

4.7 Effects on ability to drive and use machines
None.

4.8 Undesirable effects
Rare cases of hyperuricosuria and hyperuricaemia have been reported when extremely high doses of pancreatin have been taken.

Strictures of the ileo-caecum and large bowel, and colitis, have been reported in children with cystic fibrosis taking high doses of pancreatic enzyme supplements. To date Pancrex and Pancrex V presentations have not been implicated in the development of colonic damage. However unusual abdominal symptoms or changes in abdominal symptoms should be reviewed to exclude the possibility of colonic damage especially if the patient is taking in excess of 10,000 units/kg/day of lipase.

4.9 Overdose
None stated.

5. PHARMACOLOGICAL PROPERTIES
5.1 Pharmacodynamic properties
Pancreatin is derived from porcine pancreas and contains the enzymes, amylase, protease and lipase. The enzymes have the same actions as pancreatic juice and when administered to patients with pancreatic insufficiency improve the ability to metabolise starches, proteins and fats.

5.2 Pharmacokinetic properties
Pancreatin hydrolyses fats to glycerol and fatty acids, changes proteins into proteases and derived substances, and converts starch into dextrins and sugars.

5.3 Preclinical safety data
No relevant pre-clinical safety data has been generated.

6. PHARMACEUTICAL PARTICULARS
6.1 List of excipients
Lactose, povidone, stearic acid, Opaseal P17-28901 (containing IMS, titanium dioxide (E171), polyvinyl acetate phthalate, and stearic acid (E570)) talc, sucrose, acacia, calcium carbonate, titanium dioxide, Opalux AS 7000B (containing sucrose, sodium benzoate (E211), titanium dioxide (E171), and indigo carmine aluminium lake (E132)), syrup, Opagloss 6000P (containing ethanol, shellac (E904), white beeswax (E901), yellow carnuba wax (E903)).

This medicinal product contains approximately 0.13g of lactose. When taken according to the dosage recommendations each dose supplies up to 1.3g of lactose.

6.2 Incompatibilities
None known.

6.3 Shelf life
2 years.

6.4 Special precautions for storage
Store at a temperature not exceeding 15°C.

6.5 Nature and contents of container
Securitainer: 100, 250, 300 and 500 tablets.

6.6 Instructions for use and handling
Not applicable.

Administrative Data
7. MARKETING AUTHORISATION HOLDER
Paines and Byrne Limited

Yamanouchi House

Pyrford Road

West Byfleet

Surrey

KT14 6RA

United Kingdom

8. MARKETING AUTHORISATION NUMBER(S)
Product licence 0051/5000R

9. DATE OF FIRST AUTHORISATION/RENEWAL OF THE AUTHORISATION
First authorisation granted 22 November 1985 / October 2003

10. DATE OF REVISION OF THE TEXT
Date of partial revision = October 2003

11. Legal Category
P

Pancrex V Powder

(Paines & Byrne Limited)

1. NAME OF THE MEDICINAL PRODUCT
Pancrex V Powder

2. QUALITATIVE AND QUANTITATIVE COMPOSITION
Pancreatin BP to provide enzymatic activity per gram not less than:

Free protease 1400 BP units

Lipase 25000 BP units

Amylase 30000 BP units

3. PHARMACEUTICAL FORM
Powder.

4. CLINICAL PARTICULARS
4.1 Therapeutic indications
Pancrex is used to compensate for reduced intestinal enzyme activity in pancreatic deficiency states.

It is indicated for the treatment of fibrocystic disease of the pancreas (cystic fibrosis), chronic pancreatitis and pancreatic steatorrhoea following pancreatectomy. It may also be indicated following gastrectomy as an aid to digestion.

4.2 Posology and method of administration
Dosage should be adjusted according to the needs of the individual patient and the amount and type of food consumed.

The following dosage ranges provide a suitable basis for adjustment.

Adults, the Elderly, and Children

0.5 g - 2 g swallowed dry or mixed with a little water or milk before each snack or meal

New-born infants

0.25 g - 0.5 g with each feed

4.3 Contraindications
Hypersensitivity to the active ingredient (porcine pancreatin) or any of the excipients.

4.4 Special warnings and special precautions for use
It is possible that some irritation of the skin of the mouth may occur if the powder is retained in the mouth. Irritation of the anus may also occur. A barrier cream may prevent this local irritation.

Allergic/asthmatic reactions have occasionally occurred on handling the powder.

If the powder is mixed with liquids or feeds the resulting mixture should not be allowed to stand for more than one hour prior to use.

4.5 Interaction with other medicinal products and other forms of Interaction
None known.

4.6 Pregnancy and lactation
Safety in pregnancy has not been established. However, no teratogenic effects have been observed in clinical use.

4.7 Effects on ability to drive and use machines
None.

4.8 Undesirable effects
Rare cases of hyperuricosuria and hyperuricaemia have been reported when extremely high doses of pancreatin have been taken.

Strictures of the ileo-caecum and large bowel, and colitis, have been reported in children with cystic fibrosis taking high doses of pancreatic enzyme supplements. To date Pancrex and Pancrex V presentations have not been implicated in the development of colonic damage. However unusual abdominal symptoms or changes in abdominal symptoms should be reviewed to exclude the possibility of colonic damage especially if the patient is taking in excess of 10,000 units/kg/day of lipase.

4.9 Overdose
None stated.

5. PHARMACOLOGICAL PROPERTIES
5.1 Pharmacodynamic properties
Pancreatin is derived from porcine pancreas and contains the enzymes, amylase, protease and lipase. The enzymes have the same actions as pancreatic juice and when administered to patients with pancreatic insufficiency improve the ability to metabolise starches, proteins and fats.

5.2 Pharmacokinetic properties
Pancreatin hydrolyses fats to glycerol and fatty acids, changes proteins into proteases and derived substances, and converts starch into dextrins and sugars.

5.3 Preclinical safety data
No relevant pre-clinical safety data has been generated.

6. PHARMACEUTICAL PARTICULARS
6.1 List of excipients
None.

6.2 Incompatibilities
None known.

6.3 Shelf life
2 years.

6.4 Special precautions for storage
Store at a temperature not exceeding 15°C.

6.5 Nature and contents of container
Securitainer; 100 g, 250 g and 300 g.

6.6 Instructions for use and handling
Not applicable.

Administrative Data
7. MARKETING AUTHORISATION HOLDER
Paines and Byrne Limited

Yamanouchi House

Pyrford Road

West Byfleet

Surrey

KT14 6RA

8. MARKETING AUTHORISATION NUMBER(S)
Product licence 0051/5004R

9. DATE OF FIRST AUTHORISATION/RENEWAL OF THE AUTHORISATION
First authorisation granted 13 November 1985 / October 2003

10. DATE OF REVISION OF THE TEXT
Date of partial revision = October 2003

11. Legal Category
P

Pancrex V Tablets
(Paines & Byrne Limited)

1. NAME OF THE MEDICINAL PRODUCT
Pancrex V Tablets.

2. QUALITATIVE AND QUANTITATIVE COMPOSITION
Pancreatin BP to provide enzymatic activity per tablet not less than:

Free protease 110 BP units

Lipase 1900 BP units

Amylase 1700 BP units

3. PHARMACEUTICAL FORM
Tablet.

4. CLINICAL PARTICULARS
4.1 Therapeutic indications
Pancrex is used to compensate for reduced intestinal enzyme activity in pancreatic deficiency states.

It is indicated for the treatment of fibrocystic disease of the pancreas (cystic fibrosis), chronic pancreatitis and pancreatic steatorrhoea following pancreatectomy. It may also be indicated following gastrectomy as an aid to digestion.

4.2 Posology and method of administration
Dosage should be adjusted according to the needs of the individual patient and the amount and type of food consumed.

The following dosage ranges provide a suitable basis for adjustment.

Adults, the Elderly, and Children

5 - 15 tablets before each snack or meal, swallowed whole

4.3 Contraindications
Hypersensitivity to the active ingredient (porcine pancreatin) or any of the excipients.

4.4 Special warnings and special precautions for use
Unsuitable for people with lactase insufficiency, galactosaemia or glucose/galactose malabsorption syndrome.

Variations in response to treatment may be due to enteric coating. It is possible that some irritation of the skin of the mouth may occur if tablets are chewed or preparations retained in the mouth. Irritation of the anus may also occur. A barrier cream may prevent this local irritation.

4.5 Interaction with other medicinal products and other forms of Interaction
None known.

4.6 Pregnancy and lactation
Safety in pregnancy has not been established. However, no teratogenic effects have been observed in clinical use.

4.7 Effects on ability to drive and use machines
None.

4.8 Undesirable effects
Rare cases of hyperuricosuria and hyperuricaemia have been reported when extremely high doses of pancreatin have been taken.

Strictures of the ileo-caecum and large bowel, and colitis, have been reported in children with cystic fibrosis taking high doses of pancreatic enzyme supplements. To date Pancrex and Pancrex V presentations have not been implicated in the development of colonic damage. However unusual abdominal symptoms or changes in abdominal symptoms should be reviewed to exclude the possibility of colonic damage especially if the patient is taking in excess of 10,000 units/kg/day of lipase.

4.9 Overdose
None stated.

5. PHARMACOLOGICAL PROPERTIES
5.1 Pharmacodynamic properties
Pancreatin is derived from porcine pancreas and contains the enzymes, amylase, protease and lipase. The enzymes have the same actions as pancreatic juice and when administered to patients with pancreatic insufficiency improve the ability to metabolise starches, proteins and fats.

5.2 Pharmacokinetic properties
Pancreatin hydrolyses fats to glycerol and fatty acids, changes proteins into proteases and derived substances, and converts starch into dextrins and sugars.

5.3 Preclinical safety data
No relevant pre-clinical safety data has been generated.

6. PHARMACEUTICAL PARTICULARS
6.1 List of excipients
Lactose, povidone, stearic acid, Opaseal P17-28901 (containing IMS, titanium dioxide (E171), polyvinyl acetate phthalate, and stearic acid (E570)), talc, sucrose, acacia, calcium carbonate, titanium dioxide, Opalux AS 7000B (containing sucrose, sodium benzoate (E211), titanium dioxide (E171), and indigo carmine aluminium lake (E132)), syrup, Opagloss 6000P (containing ethanol, shellac (E904), white beeswax (E901), yellow carnuba wax (E903)).

This medicinal product contains approximately 0.055g of lactose. When taken according to the dosage recommendations each dose supplies up to 0.83g of lactose.

6.2 Incompatibilities
None known.

6.3 Shelf life
2 years.

6.4 Special precautions for storage
Store at a temperature not exceeding 15°C.

6.5 Nature and contents of container
Securitainer; 100, 300 and 500 tablets.

6.6 Instructions for use and handling
Not applicable.

Administrative Data
7. MARKETING AUTHORISATION HOLDER
Paines and Byrne Limited

Yamanouchi House

Pyrford Road

West Byfleet

Surrey

KT14 6RA

8. MARKETING AUTHORISATION NUMBER(S)
Product licence 0051/5002R

9. DATE OF FIRST AUTHORISATION/RENEWAL OF THE AUTHORISATION
First authorisation granted 30 October 1985 / October 2003

10. DATE OF REVISION OF THE TEXT
Date of partial revision = October 2003

11. LEGAL CATEGORY
P

PanOxyl 5 Cream
(Stiefel Laboratories (UK) Limited)

1. NAME OF THE MEDICINAL PRODUCT
PanOxyl 5 Cream.

2. QUALITATIVE AND QUANTITATIVE COMPOSITION
Benzoyl peroxide 5.0 % w/w.

For excipients, see 6.1.

3. PHARMACEUTICAL FORM
Cream for cutaneous use.

4. CLINICAL PARTICULARS
4.1 Therapeutic indications
PanOxyl 5 Cream is indicated for the treatment of acne vulgaris.

4.2 Posology and method of administration
Adults:

Apply to the whole of the affected area once daily. Washing with soap and water prior to application greatly enhances the efficacy of the preparation.

Elderly patients:

There are no specific recommendations. Acne vulgaris does not present in the elderly.

Paediatric use:

The product is not intended for use in pre-pubescent children since acne vulgaris rarely presents in this age group.

4.3 Contraindications
Patients with a known hypersensitivity to benzoyl peroxide should not use this product.

4.4 Special warnings and special precautions for use
Avoid contact with the eyes, mouth and other mucous membranes. Care should be taken when applying the product to the neck and other sensitive areas.

The product may bleach dyed fabrics.

4.5 Interaction with other medicinal products and other forms of Interaction
None.

4.6 Pregnancy and lactation
There are no restrictions on the use of the product during pregnancy or lactation.

4.7 Effects on ability to drive and use machines
None.

4.8 Undesirable effects
In normal use, a mild burning sensation will probably be felt on first application and a moderate reddening and peeling of the skin will occur within a few days. During the first few weeks of treatment a sudden increase in peeling will occur in most patients: this is not harmful and will normally subside in a day or two if treatment is temporarily discontinued.

4.9 Overdose
Not applicable.

5. PHARMACOLOGICAL PROPERTIES
5.1 Pharmacodynamic properties
Benzoyl peroxide has antibacterial activity against *Propionibacterium acnes*, the organism implicated in acne vulgaris. It has keratolytic activity and is sebostatic,

counteracting the hyperkeratinisation and excessive sebum production associated with acne.

5.2 Pharmacokinetic properties
Not applicable.

5.3 Preclinical safety data
Not applicable. Benzoyl peroxide has been in widespread use for many years.

6. PHARMACEUTICAL PARTICULARS

6.1 List of excipients
Macrogol 1000 monostearate
Stearic acid
Glyceryl monostearate
Isopropyl palmitate
Propylene glycol
Zinc stearate
Purified water

6.2 Incompatibilities
None.

6.3 Shelf life
For the product as packaged
3 years.
After first opening the container
Comply with expiry date.

6.4 Special precautions for storage
Store below 25°C.

6.5 Nature and contents of container
Internally lacquered aluminium tubes of 40g.

6.6 Instructions for use and handling
There are no special instructions for use or handling of PanOxyl 5 Cream.

7. MARKETING AUTHORISATION HOLDER
Stiefel Laboratories (UK) Ltd
Holtspur Lane
Wooburn Green
High Wycombe
Buckinghamshire
HP10 0AU

8. MARKETING AUTHORISATION NUMBER(S)
PL 00174/5007R.

9. DATE OF FIRST AUTHORISATION/RENEWAL OF THE AUTHORISATION
26.02.1990

10. DATE OF REVISION OF THE TEXT
September 2005.

Panoxyl Acne Gel 5, 10

(Stiefel Laboratories (UK) Limited)

1. NAME OF THE MEDICINAL PRODUCT
Panoxyl Acnegel 5
Panoxyl Acnegel 10

2. QUALITATIVE AND QUANTITATIVE COMPOSITION
Panoxyl Acnegel 5: Benzoyl peroxide B.P. 5.0% w/w
Panoxyl Acnegel 10: Benzoyl peroxide B.P. 10.0% w/w

3. PHARMACEUTICAL FORM
Gel for cutaneous use

4. CLINICAL PARTICULARS

4.1 Therapeutic indications
Indicated for the treatment of acne vulgaris

4.2 Posology and method of administration
Adults
Apply to the whole of the affected area once daily. Washing with soap and water prior to application greatly enhances the efficacy of the preparation.
Elderly Patients
There are no specific recommendations. Acne vulgaris does not present in the elderly.
Paediatric Use
The product is not intended for use in pre-pubescent children since acne vulgaris rarely presents in this age group.

4.3 Contraindications
Patients with a known hypersensitivity to any of the ingredients should not use the product.

4.4 Special warnings and special precautions for use
Avoid contact with the eyes, mouth and other mucous membranes. Care should be taken when applying the product to the neck and other sensitive areas.
The product may bleach dyed fabrics.

4.5 Interaction with other medicinal products and other forms of Interaction
None

4.6 Pregnancy and lactation
There are no restrictions on the use of the product during pregnancy or lactation.

4.7 Effects on ability to drive and use machines
None

4.8 Undesirable effects
In normal use, a mild burning sensation will probably be felt on first application and a moderate reddening and peeling of the skin will occur within a few days. During the first few weeks of treatment a sudden increase in peeling will occur in most patients; this is not harmful and will normally subside in a day or two if treatment is temporarily discontinued.

4.9 Overdose
Not applicable

5. PHARMACOLOGICAL PROPERTIES

5.1 Pharmacodynamic properties
Benzoyl peroxide has anti-bacterial activity against *Propionibacterium acnes*, the organism implicated in acne vulgaris. It has keratolytic activity and is sebostatic, counteracting the hyperkeratinisation and excessive sebum production associated with acne.

5.2 Pharmacokinetic properties
Not applicable

5.3 Preclinical safety data
Not applicable. Benzoyl peroxide has been in widespread use for many years.

6. PHARMACEUTICAL PARTICULARS

6.1 List of excipients
Colloidal Magnesium Aluminium Silicate
Hydroxypropylmethylcellulose
Polyoxyethylene lauryl ether
Denatured alcohol
Citric acid monohydrate
Alpine Essence 6565A
Purified water.

6.2 Incompatibilities
None

6.3 Shelf life
36 months

6.4 Special precautions for storage
Store in a cool place

6.5 Nature and contents of container
Internally lacquered aluminium tubes of 40g

6.6 Instructions for use and handling
There are no special instructions for use or handling the product.

7. MARKETING AUTHORISATION HOLDER
Stiefel Laboratories (UK) Ltd
Holtspur Lane
Wooburn Green
High Wycombe
Bucks HPIO OAU

8. MARKETING AUTHORISATION NUMBER(S)
Panoxyl Acnegel 5: PL0174/0019R
Panoxyl Acnegel 10: PL0174/0020R

9. DATE OF FIRST AUTHORISATION/RENEWAL OF THE AUTHORISATION
23.04.90

10. DATE OF REVISION OF THE TEXT
Panoxyl Acnegel 5: 08.08.94
Panoxyl Acnegel 10: 30.03.95

Panoxyl Aquagel 2.5, 5, 10

(Stiefel Laboratories (UK) Limited)

1. NAME OF THE MEDICINAL PRODUCT
PanOxyl Aquagel 2.5
PanOxyl Aquagel 5
PanOxyl Aquagel 10

2. QUALITATIVE AND QUANTITATIVE COMPOSITION
PanOxyl Aquagel 2.5: Benzoyl peroxide 2.5% w/w
PanOxyl Aquagel 5: Benzoyl peroxide 5% w/w
PanOxyl Aquagel 10: Benzoyl peroxide 10% w/w

3. PHARMACEUTICAL FORM
Gel

4. CLINICAL PARTICULARS

4.1 Therapeutic indications
The product is indicated for use in the topical treatment of acne vulgaris.

4.2 Posology and method of administration
Treatment should normally begin with PanOxyl Aquagel 2.5. Apply to the affected areas once daily. Washing prior to application enhances the efficacy of the preparation.

The reaction of the skin to benzoyl peroxide differs in individual patients. The higher concentration in PanOxyl Aquagel 5 or 10 may be required to produce a satisfactory response.

4.3 Contraindications
PanOxyl Aquagel should not be prescribed for patients with a known hypersensitivity to benzoyl peroxide.

4.4 Special warnings and special precautions for use
Avoid contact with the eyes, mouth and mucous membranes. Care should be taken when applying the product to the neck and other sensitive areas.
During the first few days of treatment a moderate reddening and peeling will occur. During the first few weeks of treatment a sudden increase in peeling will occur in most patients. This is not harmful and will normally subside within a day or two if treatment is discontinued. If excessive irritation, redness or peeling occurs, discontinue use.
The product may bleach dyed fabrics.

4.5 Interaction with other medicinal products and other forms of Interaction
None.

4.6 Pregnancy and lactation
There are no restriction on the use of PanOxyl Aquagel in pregnancy and lactation.

4.7 Effects on ability to drive and use machines
None.

4.8 Undesirable effects
None.

4.9 Overdose
Not applicable.

5. PHARMACOLOGICAL PROPERTIES

5.1 Pharmacodynamic properties
Benzoyl peroxide has sebostatic and keratolytic activity coupled with antibacterial activity against *Propionibacterium acnes*, the organism implicated in acne vulgaris. Its use in the treatment of acne is well established.

5.2 Pharmacokinetic properties
Not applicable.

5.3 Preclinical safety data
Not applicable. Benzoyl peroxide has been in widespread use for many years.

6. PHARMACEUTICAL PARTICULARS

6.1 List of excipients
Carbomer 940
Di-isopropanolamine
Propylene glycol
Polyoxyethylene lauryl ether
Sodium lauryl sulphate
Purified water

6.2 Incompatibilities
None.

6.3 Shelf life
2 years.

6.4 Special precautions for storage
Store below 25°C.

6.5 Nature and contents of container
Internally lacquered aluminium tubes with screw caps. Pack size: 40g

6.6 Instructions for use and handling
There are no special instructions for use or handling of PanOxyl Aquagel.

7. MARKETING AUTHORISATION HOLDER
Stiefel Laboratories (UK) Ltd
Holtspur Lane
Wooburn Green
High Wycombe
Bucks HP10 0AU

8. MARKETING AUTHORISATION NUMBER(S)
PanOxyl Aquagel 2.5: PL 0174/0049
PanOxyl Aquagel 5: PL 0174/0050
PanOxyl Aquagel 10: PL 0174/0051

9. DATE OF FIRST AUTHORISATION/RENEWAL OF THE AUTHORISATION
21.08.1984

10. DATE OF REVISION OF THE TEXT
30.06.1995

PanOxyl Wash 10%

(Stiefel Laboratories (UK) Limited)

1. NAME OF THE MEDICINAL PRODUCT
PanOxyl Wash 10%

2. QUALITATIVE AND QUANTITATIVE COMPOSITION
Benzoyl peroxide10.0% w/w

3. PHARMACEUTICAL FORM
Lotion for cutaneous use

4. CLINICAL PARTICULARS
4.1 Therapeutic indications
PanOxyl Wash 10% is indicated for the treatment of acne vulgaris.

4.2 Posology and method of administration
Adults
Wet the affected area with water and wash thoroughly with PanOxyl Wash. Rinse well with warm water, then rinse with cold water. Pat dry with a clean towel. Use once a day.

Elderly patients
There are no specific recommendations. Acne vulgaris does not present in the elderly.

Paediatric Use
The product is not intended for use in pre-pubescent children since acne vulgaris rarely presents in this age group.

4.3 Contraindications
Patients with a known hypersensitivity to any of the ingredients should not use the product.

4.4 Special warnings and special precautions for use
Avoid contact with the eyes, mouth and other mucous membranes. Care should be taken when applying the product to the neck and other sensitive areas.

The product may bleach dyed fabrics.

4.5 Interaction with other medicinal products and other forms of Interaction
None

4.6 Pregnancy and lactation
There are no restrictions on the use of the product during pregnancy or lactation.

4.7 Effects on ability to drive and use machines
None

4.8 Undesirable effects
In normal use, a mild burning sensation will probably be felt on first application and a moderate reddening and peeling of the skin will occur within a few days. During the first few weeks of treatment a sudden increase in peeling will occur in most patients; this is not harmful and will normally subside in a day or two if treatment is temporarily discontinued.

4.9 Overdose
Not applicable.

5. PHARMACOLOGICAL PROPERTIES
5.1 Pharmacodynamic properties
Benzoyl peroxide has antibacterial activity against *Propionibacterium acnes*, the organism implicated in acne vulgaris. It has keratolytic activity and is sebostatic, counteracting the hyperkeratinisation and excessive sebum production associated with acne.

5.2 Pharmacokinetic properties
Not applicable.

5.3 Preclinical safety data
Not applicable. Benzoyl peroxide has been in widespread use for many years.

6. PHARMACEUTICAL PARTICULARS
6.1 List of excipients
Magnesium aluminium silicate

Citric acid monohydrate

Sodium alkyl aryl polyether sulphonate

Sodium dihexyl sulphosuccinate

Sodium lauryl sulphoacetate

Hydroxypropylmethylcellulose

Polyoxyethylene lauryl ether

Imidurea

Purified water

6.2 Incompatibilities
None.

6.3 Shelf life
a) For the product as packaged for sale
2 years

b) After first opening the container
Comply with expiry date

6.4 Special precautions for storage
Store at room temperature

6.5 Nature and contents of container
Flip top polyethylene bottle containing 150 ml.

6.6 Instructions for use and handling
There are no special instructions for use or handling of PanOxyl Wash 10%.

7. MARKETING AUTHORISATION HOLDER
Stiefel Laboratories (UK) Ltd.

Holtspur Lane

Wooburn Green

High Wycombe

Bucks HP10 0AU

8. MARKETING AUTHORISATION NUMBER(S)
PL 0174/0048

9. DATE OF FIRST AUTHORISATION/RENEWAL OF THE AUTHORISATION
25.03.95

10. DATE OF REVISION OF THE TEXT
26.09.05

Paramax Tablets, Paramax Sachets
(sanofi-aventis)

1. NAME OF THE MEDICINAL PRODUCT
Paramax Tablets

Paramax Sachets

2. QUALITATIVE AND QUANTITATIVE COMPOSITION
2.1 Active ingredients:

Paracetamol BP

Metoclopramide Hydrochloride BP

2.2 Quantitative composition

500mg paracetamol BP with 5mg metoclopramide hydrochloride BP (calculated with reference to anhydrous substance).

3. PHARMACEUTICAL FORM
Tablets and sachets

4. CLINICAL PARTICULARS
4.1 Therapeutic indications
Paramax is indicated for the symptomatic treatment of migraine

4.2 Posology and method of administration
Paramax should be taken at the first warning of an attack. If symptoms persist, further doses may be taken at four-hourly intervals. Total dosage in any 24-hour period should not exceed the quantity stated.

The dosage recommendations given below should be strictly adhered to if side-effects of the dystonic type are to avoided. It should be noted that at total daily dosage of metoclopramide, especially for adolescents and young adults, should not normally exceed 0.5mg/kg body weight.

Usual Recommended Dosage (number of tablets or sachets)

	Initial dose at first warning of attack	Maximum dosage in any 24-hour period
Adults (including elderly patients)	2	6
Young adults (12-19 years)	1	3

Young adults and adolescents: Paramax should only be used after careful examination to avoid masking an underlying disorder, eg cerebral irritation. In the treatment of this group attention should be given primarily to bodyweight.

Children: A presentation of Paramax suitable for the treatment of children under 12 years of age is not available.

Paramax sachets are emptied into about $^1/_4$ of a glass of water and stirred before taking.

For oral administration only.

4.3 Contraindications
Hypersensitivity to paracetamol, metoclopramide or any other constituents.

Gastrointestinal haemorrhage, obstruction or perforation, since stimulation of gastrointestinal motility constitutes a risk in these situations.

History of neuroleptic or metoclopramide-induced tardive dyskinesia.

Confirmed epilepsy, since the frequency and severity of seizures may be increased.

Confirmed or suspected phaeochromocytoma, because of the risk of hypertensive crisis.

Combination with levodopa because of a mutual antagonism.

Metoclopramide should be not be used in the immediate post-operative period (up to 3-4 days) following pyloroplasty or gut anastomosis, as vigorous gastro-intestinal contractions may adversely affect healing.

4.4 Special warnings and special precautions for use
Patients should not take Paramax with any other paracetamol-containing products.

Care is advised in the administration of paracetamol to patients with severe renal or severe hepatic impairment. The hazards of overdose are greater in those with (non-cirrhotic) alcoholic liver disease.

Care should be exercised in the event of Paramax being prescribed concurrently with a phenothiazine since extra-pyramidal symptoms may occur with both products (see section 4.5).

Children, young patients and the elderly should be treated with care as they are at increased risk of extrapyramidal reactions (see section 4.8). Symptomatic treatment may be necessary (benzodiazepines in children and/or anticholinergic anti-parkinsonian drugs in adults).

If vomiting persists the patient should be re-assessed to exclude the possibility of an underlying disorder, e.g. cerebral irritation.

Care should be exercised in patients being treated with other centrally active drugs (see section 4.5).

Neuroleptic Malignant Syndrome (NMS), a potentially fatal symptom complex with hyperthermia, muscle rigidity, extrapyramidal symptoms, altered mental status and autonomic dysfunction, may occur. The management of NMS should include

1) immediate discontinuation of the product,

2) intensive symptomatic treatment and medical monitoring, and

3) treatment of any concomitant serious medical problems for which specific treatments are available.

Methemoglobinemia which could be related to NADH cytochrome b5 reductase deficiency has been reported. In such cases, metoclopramide should be immediately and permanently discontinued and appropriate measures initiated.

4.5 Interaction with other medicinal products and other forms of Interaction
Interactions with other medicinal products and other forms of interaction

Contraindicated combination:

<u>Levodopa</u>: Levodopa and metoclopramide have a mutual antagonism (see section 4.3)

Combination to be avoided:

<u>Alcohol</u>: Alcohol potentiates the sedative effect of metoclopramide.

Paracetamol may potentiate the effects of alcohol. Therefore, the risk of sedation and the effects of alcohol may be increased when Paramax is taken with alcohol.

Chloramphenicol: Paracetamol may increase the elimination half-life of chloramphenicol. <u>Oral contraceptives</u>: Oral contraceptives may increase the rate of paracetamol clearance.

Metoclopramide or domperidone: The speed of absorption of paracetamol may be increased by metoclopramide or domperidone.

Cholestyramine: The speed of absorption of paracetamol may be reduced by cholestyramine.

Warfarin and other coumarins: The anticoagulant effect of warfarin and other coumarins may be enhanced by prolonged regular use of paracetamol with increased risk of bleeding; occasional doses have no significant effect.

Combination to be taken into account:

Anticholinergics and morphine derivatives: Anticholinergics and morphine derivatives antagonise the effects of metoclopramide on the gastrointestinal motility.

<u>CNS depressants (morphine derivatives, hypnotics, anxiolytics, sedative H1 antihistamines, sedative antidepressants, barbiturates, clonidine and related):</u> Combination of CNS depressants with metoclopramide may result in potentiation of sedative effects.

Antipsychotics: Combination of antipsychotics with metoclopramide may result in potentiation of extrapyramidal effects.

Digoxin: Metoclopramide decreases the gastric absorption of digoxin. Therefore, dose adjustment may be required.

<u>Cyclosporine</u>: Metoclopramide increases cyclosporine bioavailability. Dose adjustment may be required. In one study, dosing requirements for cysclosporin were reduced by 20% when metoclopramide was administered concomitantly. To avoid toxicity, careful monitoring of cyclosporine plasma concentration in therefore required.

4.6 Pregnancy and lactation
Animal studies, carried out on the individual active components, have not demonstrated any teratogenic effect. These studies have not been carried out on the combination product. In the absence of a teratogenic effect in animals, a malformative effect in humans is not anticipated.

Exposure of pregnant women to the individual active components indicates no adverse effect on pregnancy or on the health of the foetus/new born child. To date, no epidemiological data are available for the combination product. Paramax should only be used during pregnancy when there are compelling reasons and it is not advised during the first trimester. Nevertheless, Paramax should only be used when there are compelling reasons and is not advised during the first trimester. Thereafter, patients should follow the advice of their doctor regarding its use.

During lactation, metoclopramide and paracetamol may be found in breast milk. In consequence, breast-feeding should be avoided.

4.7 Effects on ability to drive and use machines
Paramax may cause drowsiness. The ability to drive vehicles or operate machinery can be impaired, particularly if Paramax is administered with CNS depressants or alcohol.

4.8 Undesirable effects
Central nervous system and psychiatric disorders
The incidence of extrapyramidal symptoms in children and young adults may increase if the metoclopramide dosage

exceeds 0.5mg/kg body weight/day. Acute dystonia and dyskinesia, parkinsonian syndrome, akathisia (see section 4.4) may increase following administration of a single dose. Although, rarely, tardive dyskinesia may be irreversible.

- Reactions include spasm of the facial muscles, trismus, rhythmic protrusion of the tongue, a bulbar type of speech, spasm of extra-ocular muscles including oculogyric crises, unnatural positioning of the head and shoulders and opisthotonos. There may be a generalised increase in muscle tone. The majority of reactions occur within 36 hours of starting treatment and the effects usually disappear within 24 hours of withdrawal of the drug. Should treatment of a dystonic reaction be required, a benzodiazepine or an anticholinergic anti-Parkinsonian drug may be used.
- Tardive dyskinesia, particularly in elderly patients and following prolonged treatment.
- Drowsiness, restlessness, anxiety, confusion.
- Depressive tendency.
- Very rare (less than 0.01%) cases of seizures and neuroleptic malignant syndrome have been reported.

Gastro-intestinal disorders
- Diarrhoea

Haematological disorders
- Very rare (less than 0.01%) cases of methaemoglobinaemia which could be related to NADH cytochrome b5 reductase deficiency have been reported, particularly in neonates. (see section 4.4).
- Blood dyscrasias including thrombocytopenia and agranulocytosis,

Endocrine disorders
- Hyperprolactinaemia with (amenorrhea, galactorrhea, gynaecomastia).

Body as a whole
- Allergic reaction including anaphylaxis.
- Asthenia.
- Skin rash

Cardiovascular disorders
- Hypotension.
- Very rare (less than 0.01%) cases of bradycardia and heart block have been reported with metoclopramide, particularly the intravenous formulation.

Since extrapyramidal symptoms may occur with both metoclopramide and phenothiazines, care should be exercised in the event of both drugs being prescribed concurrently.

4.9 Overdose

Immediate treatment is essential in the management of paracetamol overdose. Despite a lack of significant early symptoms, patients should be referred to hospital urgently for immediate medical attention and any patient who had ingested around 7.5g or more of paracetamol in the proceeding 4 hours should undergo gastric lavage. Administration of oral methionine or intravenous N-acetylcysteine which may have a beneficial effect up to at least 48 hours after the overdose, may be required. General supportive measures must be available. Treatment for extrapyramidal disorders caused by metoclopramide overdose is symptomatic (benzodiazepines in children and/or anticholinergic anti-parkinsonian drugs in adults).

Symptoms of paracetamol overdosage in the first 24 hours are pallor, nausea, vomiting, anorexia, and abdominal pain. Liver damage may become apparent 12 to 48 hours after ingestion. Abnormalities of glucose metabolism and metabolic acidosis may occur. In severe poisoning, hepatic failure may progress to encephalopathy, coma and death. Acute renal failure with acute tubular necrosis may develop even in the absence of severe liver damage. Cardiac arrhythmias and pancreatitis have been reported.

Metoclopramide overdose may cause drowsiness, extrapyramidal disorders and convulsions.

Liver damage is possible in adults who have taken 10g or more of paracetamol.

5. PHARMACOLOGICAL PROPERTIES

5.1 Pharmacodynamic properties

The mechanism of action of metoclopramide in the gastrointestinal tract remains unclear and current hypotheses have been reviewed by Harrington et al (1983). It appears that metoclopramide has both central and local mechanisms of action; at the local level metoclopramide may have a direct effect on gastric muscle, stimulating contractility (Hay, 1975).

The addition of metoclopramide to paracetamol therapy for migraine has the additional benefit of combatting the nausea and vomiting which are often experienced by migraine sufferers. The antiemetic activity of metoclopramide is probably mediated, at least in part, by blockade of dopamine receptors in the chemoreceptor trigger zone for vomiting (Harrington et al 1983).

5.2 Pharmacokinetic properties

Published data concerning the pharmacokinetics of Paramax is limited. In a study involving four healthy volunteers in which plasma paracetamol concentrations were compared following administration of Paramax tablets (1g paracetamol + 10mg metoclopramide), Panadol tablets (1g paracetamol) and Solpadeine effervescent tablets (1g paracetamol + 16mg codeine phosphate + 16mg caffeine), absorption of paracetamol from Paramax tablets was found not to differ significantly from absorption from Panadol or Solpadeine (Dougall et al, 1983).

Oral paracetamol is largely absorbed from the small intestine, the rate of absorption depending on the rate of gastric emptying (Heading et al, 1973; Clements et al, 1978).

Gastric emptying is often severely delayed during migraine attacks (Kreel, 1969); absorption of oral paracetamol has been shown to be delayed and impaired in patients during a migraine attack compared to when the same patients are headache free (Tokala and Neuvonen, 1984). Metoclopramide stimulates gastric emptying and has been shown to accelerate absorption of paracetamol (Nimmo *et al.* 1973 and Crome *et al.* 1981).

5.3 Preclinical safety data

Paracetamol and metoclopramide hydrochloride are well established drug substances and results of preclinical testing are well documented.

6. PHARMACEUTICAL PARTICULARS

6.1 List of excipients

Paramax tablets:	Colloidal silica dioxide
	Magnesium stearate
	Microcrystalline cellulose
Paramax sachets:	Sodium carbonate
	Saccharin sodium
	Lemon flavour
	Sodium dihydrogen citrate, anhydrous
	Sodium bicarbonate

6.2 Incompatibilities

None stated

6.3 Shelf life

Shelf life allocation: 5 years

Do not use after expiry date given on the label

6.4 Special precautions for storage

Store in the original container. Do not store above 30°C.

6.5 Nature and contents of container

Paramax tablets: PVC aluminium blister packs of 42 tablets.

Paramax sachets: Packs of 42 sachets packed into cartons.

6.6 Instructions for use and handling

No special instructions for use

7. MARKETING AUTHORISATION HOLDER

Sanofi-Synthelabo
PO Box 597
Guildford
Surrey

8. MARKETING AUTHORISATION NUMBER(S)

PL 11723/0321

9. DATE OF FIRST AUTHORISATION/RENEWAL OF THE AUTHORISATION

12th December 2000

10. DATE OF REVISION OF THE TEXT

April 2003

Legal Category

POM

Paramol Soluble Tablets

(SSL International plc)

1. NAME OF THE MEDICINAL PRODUCT

Paramol Soluble Tablets.

2. QUALITATIVE AND QUANTITATIVE COMPOSITION

Paracetamol 500 mg

Dihydrocodeine tartrate 7.46 mg

3. PHARMACEUTICAL FORM

Effervescent tablet.

4. CLINICAL PARTICULARS

4.1 Therapeutic indications

For the treatment of mild to moderate pain; including headache, migraine, feverish conditions, period pain, toothache and other dental pain, back pain, muscular and joint pains, neuralgia, the aches and pains of cold and flu, and as an antipyretic.

4.2 Posology and method of administration

Oral.

Dosage and administration

Paramol Soluble Tablets should be taken during or after meals. The tablets should be dissolved in water.

Adults and children over 12 years

1 or 2 tablets every four to six hours. Do not exceed eight tablets in any 24-hour period.

Children under 12 years

Not recommended.

Elderly

Caution should be observed in increasing the dose in the elderly.

4.3 Contraindications

Known hypersensitivity to paracetamol, dihydrocodeine, other opioids or other constituents of the tablets.

Respiratory depression, obstructive airways disease, convulsive disorders.

Diarrhoea caused by poisoning until the toxic material has been eliminated, or diarrhoea associated with pseudomembranous colitis.

4.4 Special warnings and special precautions for use

Paramol Soluble Tablets should be used with caution in patients with:Hepatic function impairment (avoid if severe) and those with non-cirrhotic alcoholic liver disease. The hazards of overdose are greater in those with alcoholic liver disease. Prolonged use of Paramol Soluble Tablets may cause hepatic necrosis. Renal function impairment. Hypothyroidism (risk of depression and prolonged CNS depression is increased) Inflammatory bowel disease – risk of toxic megacolon Opioids should not be administered during an asthma attack Convulsions - may be induced or exacerbated Drug abuse, dependence (including alcoholism), enhanced instability, suicidal ideation or attempts – predisposed to drug abuse Head injuries or conditions where intracranial pressure is raised Gall bladder disease or gall stones - opioids may cause biliary contraction Gastro-intestinal surgery - use with caution after recent GI surgery as opioids may alter GI motility Prostatic hypertrophy or recent urinary tract surgery Adrenocortical insufficiency, e.g. Addison's Disease Hypotension and shock Myasthenia gravis Phaeochromocytoma - opioids may stimulate catecholamine release by inducing the release of endogenous histamine

The label will state:

Do not exceed the recommended dose.

Do not take with any other paracetamol-containing products. Immediate medical attention should be sought in the event of an overdose, even if you feel well.

May cause dizziness, if affected do not drive or operate machinery.

If symptoms persist, consult your doctor.

Keep out of the reach and sight of children.

The leaflet will state:

Immediate medical advice should be sought in the event of an overdose, even if you feel well, because of the risk of delayed, serious liver damage.

4.5 Interaction with other medicinal products and other forms of Interaction

The speed of absorption of paracetamol may be increased by metoclopramide or domperidone and absorption reduced by cholestyramine.

The anticoagulant effect of warfarin and other coumarins may be enhanced by prolonged regular daily use of paracetamol with increased risk of bleeding. Occasional doses have no significant effect.

The depressant effects of opioid analgesics are enhanced by other CNS depressants such as alcohol, anaesthetics, anxiolytics, hypnotics, tricyclic antidepressants and antipsychotics.

Dihydrocodeine tartrate may interact with monoamine oxidase inhibitors (MAOI's), such that opioids should not be used in patients taking MAOI's or within 14 days of stopping such treatment. If opioid analgesics are required they should be given with extreme caution.

The effects of dihydrocodeine tartrate in reducing gastrointestinal motility may interfere with the absorption of such as mexiletine, and may counteract the stimulatory effect of metoclopramide and domperidone.

Cimetidine inhibits the metabolism of some opioids

4.6 Pregnancy and lactation

Epidemiological studies in human pregnancy have shown no effects due to paracetamol used in the recommended dosage. However, paracetamol should be avoided in pregnancy unless considered essential by the physician.

Risk benefit must be considered because opioid analgesics cross the placenta. Studies in animals have shown opioids to cause delayed ossification in mice and increased resorption in rats.

Regular use during pregnancy may cause physical dependence in the fetus, leading to withdrawal symptoms in the neonate. During labour opioids enter the fetal circulation and may cause respiratory depression in the neonate.

Administration should be avoided during the late stages of labour and during the delivery of a premature infant.

Paracetamol is excreted in breast milk but not in a clinically significant amount.

Available published data do not contraindicate breast feeding; however some opioids are distributed in breast milk in small amounts and it is advisable to avoid administration of opioids in a breastfeeding woman.

4.7 Effects on ability to drive and use machines

Opioid analgesics can impair mental function and can cause blurred vision and dizziness. Patients should make sure they are not affected before driving or operating machinery.

4.8 Undesirable effects

Adverse effects of paracetamol are rare but hypersensitivity, including skin rash, may occur. There have been rare reports of blood dyscrasias including thrombocytopenia and agranulocytosis, but these were not necessarily causally related to paracetamol. Constipation if it occurs, is readily treated with a mild laxative. Nausea, headache, vertigo, dizziness and urinary retention may occur in a few patients.

4.9 Overdose

Paracetamol:

Symptoms: Pallor, nausea, vomiting, anorexia and abdominal pain in the first 24 hours. Liver damage may become apparent 12 to 48 hours after ingestion.

Abnormalities of glucose metabolism and metabolic acidosis may occur. In severe poisoning, hepatic failure may progress to encephalopathy, coma and death.

Acute renal failure with acute tubular necrosis may develop even in the absence of severe liver damage. Cardiac arrhythmias have been reported.

Liver damage is likely in adults who have taken 10g or more of paracetamol. It is considered that excess quantities of a toxic metabolite (usually adequately detoxified by glutathione when normal doses of paracetamol are ingested), become irreversibly bound to liver tissue.

Treatment: Immediate treatment is essential in the management of paracetamol overdose. Despite a lack of significant early symptoms, patients should be referred to hospital urgently for immediate medical attention and any patient who had ingested around 7.5g or more of paracetamol in the preceding 4 hours should undergo gastric lavage. Administration of oral methionine or intravenous N-acetylcysteine, which may have a beneficial effect up to at least 48 hours after the overdose, may be required.

General supportive measures must be available.

Opioids:

Symptoms: cold clammy skin, confusion, convulsions, severe drowsiness, tiredness, low blood pressure, pinpoint pupils of eyes, slow heart beat and respiratory rate coma.

Treatment: Treat respiratory depression or other life-threatening adverse effects first.

Empty the stomach via gastric lavage or induction of emesis.

The opioid antagonist naloxone (0.4-2mg subcutaneous) can be given and repeated at 2-3 minute intervals to a maximum of 10mg. Naloxone may also be given by intramuscular injection or intravenous infusion. The patient should be monitored as the duration of opioid analgesic may exceed that of the antagonist.

5. PHARMACOLOGICAL PROPERTIES

5.1 Pharmacodynamic properties

Paracetamol is an effective analgesic possessing a remarkably low level of side effects. Its broad clinical utility has been extensively reported, and it now largely replaces aspirin for routine use. Paracetamol is well tolerated, having a bland effect on gastric mucosa, unlike aspirin, it neither exacerbates symptoms of peptic ulcer nor precipitates bleeding. Dihydrocodeine tartrate has been widely used for a number of years as a powerful analgesic; 30 mg of dihydrocodeine has been reported to have analgesic potency equal to 60 or 120 mg codeine.

In addition the compound exhibits well-defined anti-tussive activity.

Fortifying paracetamol with 7.46 mg dihydrocodeine tartrate provides an effective combination of drugs for the treatment of severe pain.

5.2 Pharmacokinetic properties

Dihydrocodeine is well absorbed from the gastrointestinal tract. Like other phenanthrene derivatives, dihydrocodeine is mainly metabolised in the liver with the resultant metabolites being excreted mainly in the urine. Metabolism of dihydrocodeine includes o-demethylation, n-demethylation and 6-keto reduction.

Paracetamol is readily absorbed from the gastrointestinal tract with peak plasma concentrations occurring 30 minutes to 2 hours after ingestion. It is metabolised in the liver and excreted in the urine mainly as the glucuronide and sulphate conjugates.

5.3 Preclinical safety data

Not applicable.

6. PHARMACEUTICAL PARTICULARS

6.1 List of excipients

Citric acid (anhydrous, added as citric acid monohydrate)

Sodium hydrogen carbonate

Sodium carbonate (anhydrous)

Sodium benzoate

Saccharin sodium

Povidone

6.2 Incompatibilities

None known.

6.3 Shelf life

24 months.

6.4 Special precautions for storage

Store at or below 25°C.

6.5 Nature and contents of container

Blister packs: 43 μm soft tempered aluminium foil coated with 25 μm polyethylene on the inside.

Aluminium foil strip packs: 25 μm aluminium foil coated with 40g/m^2 paper and 12g/m^2 polyethylene on the outside and 18g/m^2 surlyn on the inside.

Pack sizes: 12, 24 tablets

6.6 Instructions for use and handling

None stated.

7. MARKETING AUTHORISATION HOLDER

Seton Products Ltd.

Tubiton House

Oldham

OL1 3HS

8. MARKETING AUTHORISATION NUMBER(S)

PL 11314/0058.

9. DATE OF FIRST AUTHORISATION/RENEWAL OF THE AUTHORISATION

20th December 1995.

10. DATE OF REVISION OF THE TEXT

December 2004

Paramol Tablets (New Capsule Shape)

(SSL International plc)

1. NAME OF THE MEDICINAL PRODUCT

Paramol Tablets.

2. QUALITATIVE AND QUANTITATIVE COMPOSITION

Paracetamol 500mg; Dihydrocodeine Tartrate 7.46mg.

3. PHARMACEUTICAL FORM

Tablets.

4. CLINICAL PARTICULARS

4.1 Therapeutic indications

For the treatment of mild to moderate pain and as anti-pyretic.

4.2 Posology and method of administration

Route of Administration: Oral. Recommended doses and dosage schedules: Paramol Tablets should, if possible, be taken during or after meals. Adults and children over 12 years: One or two tablets every four to six hours. Do not exceed 8 tablets in any 24 hour period. Children under 12 years: Not recommended. The Elderly: Caution should be exercised when increasing the dose in the elderly.

4.3 Contraindications

Hypersensitivity to paracetamol or any other constituents, respiratory depression, obstructive airways disease.

4.4 Special warnings and special precautions for use

Paramol Tablets should be given with caution to patients with allergic disorders and should not be given during an attack of asthma. Dosage should be reduced in the elderly, in hyperthyroidism and in chronic hepatic disease. An overdose can cause hepatic necrosis. Care is advised in the administration of paracetamol to patients with severe renal or severe hepatic impairment. The hazard of overdose is greater in those with non-cirrhotic alcoholic liver disease.

Do not exceed the recommended dose. Do not be take with any other paracetamol-containing products. Immediate medical attention should be sought in the event of an overdose, even if you feel well because of the risk of delayed, serious liver damage. If symptoms persist, consult your doctor. Keep out of reach of children.

4.5 Interaction with other medicinal products and other forms of Interaction

The speed of absorption of paracetamol may be increased by metoclopramide or domperidone and absorption reduced by cholyestyramine. The anticoagulant effect of warfarin and other coumarins may be enhanced by prolonged regular daily use of paracetamol with increased risk of bleeding; occasional doses have no significant effect. Additive central nervous system depression may occur with alcohol.

4.6 Pregnancy and lactation

Epidemiological studies in human pregnancy have shown no ill effects due to paracetamol used in the recommended dosage, but patients should follow the advice of their doctor regarding its use. Paracetamol is excreted in breast milk but not in a clinically significant amount. Available published data do not contraindicate breast-feeding.

4.7 Effects on ability to drive and use machines

None stated.

4.8 Undesirable effects

Adverse effects of paracetamol are rare but hypersensitivity, including skin rash, may occur. There have been rare reports of blood dyscrasias including thrombocytopenia and agranulocytosis, but these were not necessarily causally related to paracetamol. Constipation if it occurs, is readily treated with a mild laxative. Nausea, vertigo, headache and giddiness may occur in a few patients.

4.9 Overdose

Symptoms of paracetamol overdose in the first 24 hours are pallor, nausea, vomiting, anorexia and abdominal pain. Liver damage may become apparent 12 to 48 hours after ingestion. Abnormalities of glucose metabolism and metabolic acidosis may occur. In severe poisoning, hepatic failure may progress to encephalopathy, coma and death. Acute renal failure with acute tubular necrosis may develop even in the absence of severe liver damage. Cardiac arrhythmia's and pancreatitis have been reported. Liver damage is possible in adults who have taken 10g or more of paracetamol. It is considered that excess quantities of a toxic metabolite (usually adequately detoxified by glutathione when normal doses of paracetamol are ingested) become irreversibly bound to liver tissue. Treatment: Immediate treatment is essential in the management of paracetamol overdose. Despite a lack of significant early symptoms, patients should be referred to hospital urgently for immediate medical attention and any patient who has ingested around 7.5g or more of paracetamol in the preceding 4 hours should undergo gastric lavage. Administration of oral methionine or intravenous N-acetylcysteine, which may have a beneficial effect up to at least 48 hours after the overdose, may be required. General supportive measures must be available.

5. PHARMACOLOGICAL PROPERTIES

5.1 Pharmacodynamic properties

Paracetamol is an effective analgesic possessing a remarkably low level of side effects. It's broad clinical utility has been extensively reported and now largely replaces aspirin for routine use. Paracetamol is well tolerated, having a bland effect on the gastric mucosa, unlike aspirin, it neither exacerbates symptoms of peptic ulcer nor precipitates bleeding. Dihydrocodeine Tartrate has been widely used for a number of years as a powerful analgesic. 30mg of Dihydrocodeine has the analgesic potency of 60 to 120mg of codeine. In addition the product exhibits well defined anti-tussive activity. Fortifying paracetamol with dihydrocodeine tartrate provides an effective combination of drugs for the treatment of mild to moderate pain and acts as an anti-pyretic.

5.2 Pharmacokinetic properties

Dihydrocodeine is well absorbed from the gastrointestinal tract. Like other Phenanthrene derivatives, dihydrocodeine is largely metabolised in the liver with the resultant metabolites being excreted mainly in the urine. Metabolisom of dihyrocodeine includes O-Demethylation, N-Demthylation and 6-Ketoreduction. Paracetamol is readily absorbed from the gastro-intestinal tract with peak plasma concentrations occurring 30 minutes to 2 hours after ingestion. It is metabolised in the liver, and excreted in the urine mainly as glucuronide and sulphate conjugates.

5.3 Preclinical safety data

There are no pre-clinical tests performed on the product.

6. PHARMACEUTICAL PARTICULARS

6.1 List of excipients

Magnesium Stearate; Maize Starch; Povidone; Opadry White (Hypromellose, Titanium Dioxide and Macrogol 400)

6.2 Incompatibilities

None stated.

6.3 Shelf life

24 months.

6.4 Special precautions for storage

Do not store above 25°C.

6.5 Nature and contents of container

250μ PVC/PVDC blister packs with 25μ hard tempered aluminium backing foil containing 12, 24, or 32 tablets.

6.6 Instructions for use and handling

None stated.

7. MARKETING AUTHORISATION HOLDER

Seton Products Ltd., Tubiton House, Oldham OL1 3HS.

8. MARKETING AUTHORISATION NUMBER(S)

PL 11314/0128.

9. DATE OF FIRST AUTHORISATION/RENEWAL OF THE AUTHORISATION

17th September 1999.

10. DATE OF REVISION OF THE TEXT

November 2001.

Paraplatin 10 mg/ml Concentrate for Solution for Infusion

(Bristol-Myers Pharmaceuticals)

1. NAME OF THE MEDICINAL PRODUCT

Paraplatin 10mg/ml Concentrate for Solution for Infusion.

2. QUALITATIVE AND QUANTITATIVE COMPOSITION

Carboplatin 10mg/ml. The 5ml vial contains 50mg carboplatin, the 15ml vial contains 150mg carboplatin, the 45ml vial contains 450mg carboplatin and the 60ml vial contains 600mg carboplatin.

For excipients, see 6.1.

3. PHARMACEUTICAL FORM

Concentrate for solution for infusion.

A slightly yellow solution.

4. CLINICAL PARTICULARS

4.1 Therapeutic indications

Paraplatin is indicated for the treatment of:

1. advanced ovarian carcinoma of epithelial origin in:
   (a) first line therapy
   (b) second line therapy, after other treatments have failed.
2. small cell carcinoma of the lung.

4.2 Posology and method of administration

Dosage and Administration:

Paraplatin should be used by the intravenous route only. The recommended dosage of Paraplatin in previously untreated adult patients with normal kidney function is 400 mg/m^2 as a single i.v. dose administered by a 15 to 60 minutes infusion. Alternatively, see Calvert formula below:

Dose (mg) = target AUC (mg/ml × min) × [GFR ml/min + 25]

Target AUC	Planned Chemotherapy	Patient treatment status
5-7 mg/ml/min	single agent carboplatin	Previously untreated
4-6 mg/ml/min	single agent carboplatin	Previously treated
4-6 mg/ml/min	carboplatin plus cyclophosphamide	Previously untreated

Note: With the Calvert formula, the total dose of carboplatin is calculated in mg, not mg/m^2.

Therapy should not be repeated until four weeks after the previous Paraplatin course and/or until the neutrophil count is at least 2,000 cells/mm^3 and the platelet count is at least 100,000 cells/mm^3.

Reduction of the initial dosage by 20-25% is recommended for those patients who present with risk factors such as prior myelosuppressive treatment and low performance status (ECOG-Zubrod 2-4 or Karnofsky below 80).

Determination of the haematological nadir by weekly blood counts during the initial courses of treatment with Paraplatin is recommended for future dosage adjustment.

Impaired Renal Function:

The optimal use of Paraplatin in patients presenting with impaired renal function requires adequate dosage adjustments and frequent monitoring of both haematological nadirs and renal function.

Combination Therapy:

The optimal use of Paraplatin in combination with other myelosuppressive agents requires dosage adjustments according to the regimen and schedule to be adopted.

Paediatrics:

Sufficient usage of Paraplatin in paediatrics has not occurred to allow specific dosage recommendations to be made.

Elderly:

Dosage adjustment, initially or subsequently, may be necessary, dependent on the physical condition of the patient.

Dilution & Reconstitution:

The product must be diluted. See 6.6 Instructions for Use and Handling, (and disposal).

4.3 Contraindications

Paraplatin should not be used in patients with severe pre-existing renal impairment (creatinine clearance at or below 20ml/minute).

It should not be employed in severely myelosuppressed patients. It is also contra-indicated in patients with a history of severe allergic reactions to Paraplatin or other platinum containing compounds.

4.4 Special warnings and special precautions for use

Warnings:

Paraplatin should be administered by individuals experienced in the use of anti-neoplastic therapy.

Paraplatin myelosuppression is closely related to its renal clearance. Patients with abnormal kidney function or receiving concomitant therapy with other drugs with nephrotoxic potential are likely to experience more severe and prolonged myelotoxicity. Renal function parameters should therefore be carefully assessed before and during therapy. Paraplatin courses should not be repeated more frequently than monthly under normal circumstances. Thrombocytopenia, leukopenia and anaemia occur after administration of Paraplatin. Frequent monitoring of peripheral blood counts is recommended throughout and following therapy with Paraplatin. Paraplatin combination therapy with other myelosuppressive compounds must be planned very carefully with respect to dosages and timing in order to minimise additive effects. Supportive transfusional therapy may be required in patients who suffer severe myelosuppression.

Paraplatin can cause nausea and vomiting. Premedication with anti-emetics has been reported to be useful in reducing the incidence and intensity of these effects.

Renal and hepatic function impairment may be encountered with Paraplatin. Very high doses of Paraplatin (⩾5 times single agent recommended dose) have resulted in severe abnormalities in hepatic and renal function. Although no clinical evidence on compounding nephrotoxicity has been accumulated, it is recommended not to combine Paraplatin with aminoglycosides or other nephrotoxic compounds.

Infrequent allergic reactions to Paraplatin have been reported, e.g. erythematous rash, fever with no apparent cause or pruritus. Rarely anaphylaxis, angio-oedema and anaphylactoid reactions including bronchospasm, urticaria and facial oedema have occurred. These reactions are similar to those observed after administration of other platinum containing compounds and may occur within minutes. The incidence of allergic reactions may increase with previous exposure to platinum therapy; however, allergic reactions have been observed upon initial exposure to Paraplatin. Patients should be observed carefully for possible allergic reactions and managed with appropriate supportive therapy.

The carcinogenic potential of Paraplatin has not been studied but compounds with similar mechanisms of action and mutagenicity have been reported to be carcinogenic.

Precautions:

Peripheral blood counts and renal and hepatic function tests should be monitored closely. Blood counts at the beginning of the therapy and weekly to assess haematological nadir for subsequent dose adjustment are recommended. Neurological evaluations should also be performed on a regular basis.

4.5 Interaction with other medicinal products and other forms of Interaction

The use of Paraplatin with nephrotoxic compounds is not recommended.

4.6 Pregnancy and lactation

The safe use of Paraplatin during pregnancy has not been established: Paraplatin has been shown to be an embryotoxin and teratogen in rats. If Paraplatin is used during pregnancy the patient should be apprised of the potential hazard to the foetus. Women of child-bearing potential should be advised to avoid becoming pregnant.

Carboplatin has been shown to be mutagenic *in vivo* and *in vitro*.

Nursing Mothers:

It is not known whether Paraplatin is excreted in human milk.

4.7 Effects on ability to drive and use machines

None reported.

4.8 Undesirable effects

Incidences of adverse reactions reported hereunder are based on cumulative data obtained in a large group of patients with various pretreatment prognostic features.

Haematological toxicity:

Myelosuppression is the dose-limiting toxicity of Paraplatin. At maximum tolerated dosages of Paraplatin administered as a single agent, thrombocytopenia, with nadir platelet counts of less than 50 × 10^9/L, occurs in about a quarter of the patients.

The nadir usually occurs between days 14 and 21, with recovery within 35 days from the start of therapy. Leukopenia has also occurred in approximately 14% of patients but its recovery from the day of nadir (day 14-28) may be slower and usually occurs within 42 days from the start of therapy. Neutropenia with granulocyte counts below 1 × 10^9/L occurs in approximately one fifth of patients. Anaemia with haemoglobin values below 11g/dL has been observed in more than two-thirds of patients with normal base-line values.

Myelosuppression may be more severe and prolonged in patients with impaired renal function, extensive prior treatment, poor performance status and age above 65. Myelosuppression is also worsened by therapy combining Paraplatin with other compounds that are myelosuppressive.

Myelosuppression is usually reversible and not cumulative when Paraplatin is used as a single agent and at the recommended dosages and frequencies of administration.

Infectious complications have occasionally been reported. Haemorrhagic compli-cations, usually minor, have also been reported.

Nephrotoxicity:

Renal toxicity is usually not dose-limiting in patients receiving Paraplatin, nor does it require preventive measures such as high volume fluid hydration or forced diuresis. Nevertheless, increasing blood urea or serum creatinine levels can occur. Renal function impairment, as defined by a decrease in the creatinine clearance below 60 ml/min, may also be observed. The incidence and severity of nephrotoxicity may increase in patients who have impaired kidney function before Paraplatin treatment. It is not clear whether an appropriate hydration programme might overcome such an effect, but dosage reduction or discontinuation of therapy is required in the presence of severe alteration of renal function tests.

Decreases in serum electrolytes (sodium, magnesium, potassium and calcium) have been reported after treatment with Paraplatin but have not been reported to be severe enough to cause the appearance of clinical signs or symptoms.

Cases of hyponatraemia have been reported. Haemolytic uraemic syndrome has been reported rarely.

Gastrointestinal toxicity:

Nausea without vomiting occurs in about 15% of patients receiving Paraplatin; vomiting has been reported in over half of the patients and about one-fifth of these suffer severe emesis. Nausea and vomiting usually disappear within 24 hours after treatment and are usually responsive to (and may be prevented by) anti-emetic medication. A fifth of patients experience no nausea or vomiting.

Cases of anorexia have been reported.

Allergic reactions:

Infrequent allergic reactions to Paraplatin have been reported, e.g., erythematous rash, fever with no apparent cause orpruritus. Rarely, anaphylaxis, angio-oedema and anaphylactoid reactions, including bronchospasm, urticaria and facial oedema have occurred. (See Warnings.)

Ototoxicity:

Subclinical decrease in hearing acuity, consisting of high-frequency (4000-8000 Hz) hearing loss determined by audiogram, has been reported in 15% of the patients treated with Paraplatin. However, only 1% of patients present with clinical symptoms, manifested in the majority of cases by tinnitus. In patients who have been previously treated with cisplatin and have developed hearing loss related to such treatment, the hearing impairment may persist or worsen.

At higher than recommended doses in combination with other ototoxic agents, clinically significant hearing loss has been reported to occur in paediatric patients when Paraplatin Solution was administered.

Neurotoxicity:

The incidence of peripheral neuropathies after treatment with Paraplatin is 4%. In the majority of the patients neurotoxicity is limited to paraesthesia and decreased deep tendon reflexes. The frequency and intensity of this side effect increases in elderly patients and those previously treated with cisplatin.

Paraesthesia present before commencing Paraplatin therapy, particularly if related to prior cisplatin treatment, may persist or worsen during treatment with Paraplatin.

Ocular toxicity:

Transient visual disturbances, sometimes including transient sight loss, have been reported rarely with platinum therapy. This is usually associated with high dose therapy in renally impaired patients.

Injection site reactions:

Injection site reactions, including redness, swelling and pain, have been reported during post marketing surveillance. Necrosis associated with extravasation has also been reported.

Other:

Abnormalities of liver function tests (usually mild to moderate) have been reported with Paraplatin in about one-third of the patients with normal baseline values. The alkaline phosphatase level is increased more frequently than SGOT, SGPT or total bilirubin. The majority of these abnormalities regress spontaneously during the course of treatment.

Infrequent events consisting of taste alteration, asthenia, alopecia, fever and chills without evidence of infection have occurred.

4.9 Overdose

There is no known antidote for Paraplatin overdosage. The anticipated complications of overdosage would be related to myelosuppression as well as impairment of hepatic and renal function.

5. PHARMACOLOGICAL PROPERTIES

5.1 Pharmacodynamic properties

Carboplatin is an antineoplastic agent. Its activity has been demonstrated against several murine and human cell lines.

Carboplatin exhibited comparable activity to cisplatin against a wide range of tumours regardless of implant site.

Alkaline elution techniques and DNA binding studies have demonstrated the qualitatively similar modes of action of carboplatin and cisplatin. Carboplatin, like cisplatin, induces changes in the superhelical conformation of DNA which is consistent with a "DNA shortening effect".

5.2 Pharmacokinetic properties

Paraplatin has biochemical properties similar to that of cisplatin, thus producing predominantly interstrand and intrastrand DNA crosslinks. Following administration of Paraplatin in man, linear relationships exist between dose and plasma concentrations of total and free ultrafilterable platinum. The area under the plasma concentration versus time curve for total platinum also shows a linear relationship with the dose when creatinine clearance ⩾60ml/min.

Repeated dosing during four consecutive days did not produce an accumulation of platinum in plasma. Following the administration of Paraplatin reported values for the terminal elimination of half-lives of free ultrafilterable platinum and Paraplatin in man are approximately 6 hours and 1.5 hours respectively. During the initial phase, most of the free ultrafilterable platinum is present as Paraplatin. The terminal half-life for total plasma platinum is 24 hours. Approximately 87% of plasma platinum is protein bound within 24 hours following administration. Paraplatin is excreted primarily in the urine, with recovery of approximately 70% of the administered platinum within 24 hours. Most of the drug is excreted in the first 6 hours. Total body and renal clearances of free ultrafilterable platinum correlate with the rate of glomerular filtration but not tubular secretion.

5.3 Preclinical safety data

Paraplatin has been shown to be embryotoxic and teratogenic in rats. (See 4.6, Pregnancy and Lactation.) It is mutagenic *in vivo* and *in vitro* and although the carcinogenic potential of Paraplatin has not been studied, compounds with similar mechanisms of action and mutagenicity have been reported to be carcinogenic.

6. PHARMACEUTICAL PARTICULARS

6.1 List of excipients

Water for Injections.

6.2 Incompatibilities

Needles or intravenous sets containing aluminium parts that may come into contact with Paraplatin should not be used for preparation or administration of Paraplatin.

6.3 Shelf life

Unopened product:	18 months
After dilution:	8 hours at room temperature (15 - 25°C), or 24 hours under refrigeration (2 - 8°C)

6.4 Special precautions for storage

Do not store above 25°C. Protect from light.

When diluted as directed, it is recommended that any Paraplatin Solution should be discarded after 8 hours from dilution if stored at room temperature (15 - 25°C) or after 24 hours if stored refrigerated (2 - 8°C).

6.5 Nature and contents of container

Cardboard carton containing a Type I flint glass vial with a rubber or Daikyo compound Teflon coated stopper and aluminium closure with polypropylene top, containing either 50mg, 150mg, 450mg or 600mg carboplatin as a 10mg/ml solution.

6.6 Instructions for use and handling

This product is for single dose use only.

Reconstitution:

The product must be diluted before use. It may be diluted with 5% Glucose for Injection BP, or 0.9% Sodium Chloride for Injection BP, to concentrations as low as 0.5 mg/ml (500 micrograms/ml).

When diluted as directed, Paraplatin solutions are stable for eight hours stored at room temperature or 24 hours stored under refrigeration. Since no antibacterial preservatives are contained in the formulation, it is recommended that any Paraplatin solution be discarded after eight hours from dilution if stored at room temperature or after 24 hours if stored refrigerated. This product is for single dose use only.

Guidelines for the safe handling of anti-neoplastic agents:

1. Trained personnel should reconstitute the drug.
2. This should be performed in a designated area.
3. Adequate protective gloves should be worn.
4. Precautions should be taken to avoid the drug accidentally coming into contact with the eyes. In the event of contact with the eyes, wash with water and/or saline.
5. The cytotoxic preparation should not be handled by pregnant staff.
6. Adequate care and precautions should be taken in the disposal of items (syringes, needles, etc.) used to reconstitute cytotoxic drugs. Excess material and body waste may be disposed of by placing in double sealed polyethylene bags and incinerating at a temperature of 1,000 degrees C. Liquid waste may be flushed with copious amounts of water.
7. The work surface should be covered with disposable plastic-backed absorbent paper.
8. Use Luer-Lock fittings on all syringes and sets. Large bore needles are recommended to minimise pressure and the possible formation of aerosols. The latter may also be reduced by the use of a venting needle.

7. MARKETING AUTHORISATION HOLDER

Bristol-Myers Squibb Holdings Limited

(t/a Bristol-Myers Pharmaceuticals)

Uxbridge Business Park

Sanderson Road

Uxbridge

Middlesex UB8 1DH

8. MARKETING AUTHORISATION NUMBER(S)

PL 0125/0201

9. DATE OF FIRST AUTHORISATION/RENEWAL OF THE AUTHORISATION

27 February 1991 / 24 April 2002

10. DATE OF REVISION OF THE TEXT

22 July 2005

Pardelprin MR

(Alpharma Limited)

1. NAME OF THE MEDICINAL PRODUCT

PARDELPRIN MR CAPSULES 75mg

INDOMETACIN MODIFIED RELEASE CAPSULES

2. QUALITATIVE AND QUANTITATIVE COMPOSITION

Each capsule contains 75mg of Indometacin.

3. PHARMACEUTICAL FORM

Dark blue (head) and clear (body) hard gelatin Size 2 capsules printed "COX" and "IR" in grey.

4. CLINICAL PARTICULARS

4.1 Therapeutic indications

Non-steroidal analgesic and anti-inflammatory agent indicated in active rheumatoid arthritis, osteoarthritis, ankylosing spondylitis, degenerative joint disease of the hip, acute musculoskeletal disorders and low back pain. Also indicated in periarticular disorders such as bursitis, tendinitis, synovitis, tenosynovitis and capsulitis. Also indicated in inflammation, pain and oedema following orthopaedic procedures and the treatment of pain and associated symptoms of primary dysmenorrhoea.

4.2 Posology and method of administration

Posology

Pardelprin is for oral administration and should always be given with food or milk to reduce the chance of gastrointestinal disturbance. To minimise the evolution of unwanted reactions it is helpful in chronic conditions to start the therapy with a low dosage, increasing as required.

Adults: One capsule once or twice daily, depending on patient needs and response.

Dysmenorrhoea: One capsule a day, starting with onset of cramps or bleeding, and continuing for as long as symptoms usually last.

Elderly: Particular care should be taken with older patients who are more susceptible to side-effects from indometacin.

Children: Safety for use in children has not been established.

Method of Administration

Oral use.

4.3 Contraindications

Patients with angioneurotic oedema or who have, with aspirin or other non-steroidal anti-inflammatory drugs experienced acute asthmatic attacks, urticaria or rhinitis.

Active peptic ulcer, a history of recurrent gastro-intestinal lesions, sensitivity to indometacin or to aspirin.

Not to be used during pregnancy or during lactation as indometacin is secreted in breast milk.

Safety in children has not been established.

4.4 Special warnings and special precautions for use

In common with other anti-inflammatory analgesic antipyretic agents, indometacin may mask the signs and symptoms of infectious disease and this should be borne in mind in order to avoid delay in starting treatment for infections. Indometacin should be used with caution in patients with an existing, albeit controlled infection.

Particular care should be taken with older patients who are more susceptible to side-effects from indometacin.

It is reported that a few patients receiving non-steroidal anti-inflammatory drugs manifest borderline elevations in liver function test results; if these persist or worsen or symptoms of liver disease, a rash or eosinophilia develop, treatment with indometacin should be stopped. Periodic assessments to detect, at an early stage, unwanted effects on peripheral blood (anaemia) and liver function are advisable. The dexamethasone suppression test may give false negative results. An increase in plasma potassium concentration (including hyperkalaemia) has been reported even in the absence of renal impairment. Since indometacin is eliminated primarily by the kidney, patients with impaired renal function should be monitored closely and a lower daily dosage may be needed to avoid accumulation.

4.5 Interaction with other medicinal products and other forms of Interaction

Co-administration of diflunisal with indometacin increases the plasma level of indometacin by about a third with a concomitant decrease in renal clearance. Fatal gastro-intestinal haemorrhage has occurred. The combination should not be used.

Use of indometacin with aspirin or other salicylates is not recommended because there is no enhancement of therapeutic effect while the incidence of gastro-intestinal side-effects is increased. Moreover, co-administration of aspirin may decrease the blood concentration of indometacin.

Indometacin may decrease the tubular secretion of methotrexate thus potentiating toxicity; simultaneous use should be undertaken with caution.

Patients receiving anticoagulants should be observed carefully for alteration of prothrombin time even though clinical studies suggest no influence from indometacin or hypoprothrombinaemia induced by anticoagulants.

Indometacin can inhibit platelet aggregation - an effect which disappears within 24 hours of discontinuation; the bleeding time may be prolonged and this effect may be exaggerated in patients with an underlying haemostatic defect.

Indometacin and triamterene should not be administered together since reversible renal failure may be induced.

Co-administration of probenecid may increase plasma levels of indometacin.

Because indometacin may reduce the antihypertensive effect of beta-blockers, patients receiving dual therapy should have the antihypertensive effect of their therapy reassessed.

If the patient is receiving corticosteroids concomitantly, a reduction in dosage of these may be possible but should only be effected slowly under supervision.

Indometacin is an inhibitor of prostaglandin synthesis and therefore the following drug interactions may occur; indometacin may raise plasma lithium levels and reduce lithium clearance in subjects with steady state plasma lithium concentrations. At the onset of such combined therapy, plasma lithium concentration should be monitored more frequently.

Indometacin may reduce the diuretic and antihypertensive effect of thiazides and frusemide in some patients. Indometacin may cause blocking of the frusemide-induced increase in plasma renin activity.

4.6 Pregnancy and lactation

Not to be used during pregnancy or lactation as indometacin is secreted in breast milk.

4.7 Effects on ability to drive and use machines

Patients should be warned not to drive, or operate machinery, if they become dizzy.

4.8 Undesirable effects

The most common side effects are headache, dizziness and dyspepsia; patients should be warned that they may experience dizziness and should therefore avoid driving or undertaking other activities which require full alertness. If headache persists even after dosage reduction indometacin should be withdrawn.

Gastro-intestinal disorders which occur can be reduced by giving indometacin with food, milk or antacids. Ulceration of the oesophagus, stomach or duodenum may also occur, accompanied by haemorrhage and perforation (a few fatalities have been reported).

Intestinal ulceration has rarely been associated with stenosis and obstruction. Also, bleeding without obvious ulceration and perforation of pre-existing sigmoid lesions (such as diverticulum or carcinoma) have occurred; and increased abdominal pain in patients with ulcerative colitis (or the development of this condition) and regional ileitis have been rarely reported. If gastro-intestinal bleeding does occur treatment with indometacin should be discontinued.

Blood dyscrasias, particularly thrombocytopenia have been reported.

Oedema and increased blood pressure also sometimes occur, as does haematuria.

Hypersensitivity reactions include pruritus, urticaria, angiitis, erythema nodosum. Skin rash and hair loss may also occur.

Acute respiratory distress, including sudden dyspnoea and asthma, have been reported on rare occasions. Bronchospasm may be precipitated in patients suffering from, or with a previous history of, bronchial asthma or allergic disease.

Indometacin should be used with caution in patients with hepatic or renal dysfunction. Hepatitis and jaundice have been reported rarely.

Non-steroidal anti-inflammatory drugs may precipitate renal decompensation in those with renal or hepatic dysfunction, diabetes mellitus, advanced age, extracellular volume depletion, congestive cardiac failure, sepsis or concomitant use of other nephrotoxic drugs. Also, there have been reports of acute interstitial nephritis with haematuria, proteinuria and occasionally the nephrotic syndrome in long-term therapy with indometacin.

CNS: headache, dizziness or lightheadedness, depression, vertigo and fatigue are not uncommon; infrequently there may be confusion, anxiety or other psychiatric disturbances, drowsiness, convulsions, neuropathy or paraesthesia, involuntary movements, insomnia, aggravation of epilepsy or Parkinsonism. All are often transient and likely to abate or disappear with reduced or cessation of therapy.

Gastro-intestinal: nausea, anorexia, vomiting, epigastric discomfort or abdominal pain, constipation or diarrhoea all have been reported; more rarely, stomatitis, flatulence, ulceration at any point in the gastro-intestinal tract (even with resultant stenosis and obstruction), bleeding (even without obvious ulceration or from a diverticulum) and perforation of pre-existing sigmoid lesions have all been reported.

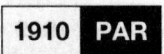

Hepatic: rarely hepatitis and jaundice (some fatalities have been reported).

Cardiovascular: oedema, increased blood pressure, hypotension, tachycardia, chest pain, arrhythmia, palpitations and congestive cardiac failure have been reported infrequently.

Renal: elevation of blood urea, haematuria, nephrotic syndrome, interstitial nephritis, renal insufficiency or failure have all been reported. In patients with renal, cardiac or hepatic impairment, caution is required since the use of non-steroidal anti-inflammatory drugs may result in deterioration of renal function. The dose should be kept as low as possible and renal function should be monitored.

Dermatological/hypersensitivity: itching, urticaria, angioneurotic oedema, angiitis, erythema nodosum, rash and exfoliative dermatitis all have been reported infrequently - as have Stevens Johnson syndrome, erythema multiforme, toxic epidermal necrolysis, hair loss, acute anaphylaxis (including sudden loss of blood pressure) and acute respiratory distress (including sudden dyspnoea, asthma and pulmonary oedema). There may be bronchospasm in patients with a history of bronchial asthma or other allergic disease.

Haematological: blood dyscrasias (thrombocytopenia, leucopenia, petechiae, ecchymosis, purpura, aplastic or haemolytic anaemia, agranulocytosis and bone marrow depression, disseminated intravascular coagulation) may occur infrequently.

Ocular: blurred vision and orbital and peri-orbital pain are seen infrequently. Corneal deposits and retinal disturbances have been reported in some patients with rheumatoid arthritis on prolonged therapy with indometacin, and ophthalmic examinations are desirable in patients given prolonged treatment.

Aural: tinnitus or hearing disturbances (rarely deafness) have been reported.

Genito-urinary: proteinuria, nephrotic syndrome, interstitial nephritis, renal insufficiency or failure all have been reported.

Other: hyperglycaemia, glycosuria, hyperkalemia, vaginal bleeding, epistaxis, breast changes (enlargement, tenderness, gynaecomastia), flushing, sweating and ulcerative stomatitis all have been reported rarely.

4.9 Overdose

Many of the unwanted symptoms associated with indometacin therapy may be seen. Treatment is symptomatic and supportive - emptying the stomach by induction of vomiting and/or lavage and use of activated charcoal. Antacid therapy may be useful. Close monitoring thereafter is required because intestinal ulceration may develop. It can be noted that indometacin has a biphasic plasma elimination with the terminal phase showing a half-life ranging between 2 and 12 hours.

5. PHARMACOLOGICAL PROPERTIES

5.1 Pharmacodynamic properties

Indometacin is a non-steroidal analgesic and anti-inflammatory agent.

5.2 Pharmacokinetic properties

The following pharmacokinetic particulars were obtained with Indometacin MR 75mg Capsules; (n=8)

$t_{1/2}\alpha$ 3.999 hours

$t_{1/2}\beta$ 3.853 hours

T_{max} 6.182 hours

C_{max} 2.192 μg/ml

AUC_{0-24} 31.190 μg/ml/hours

5.3 Preclinical safety data

None stated.

6. PHARMACEUTICAL PARTICULARS

6.1 List of excipients

Also contains: sucrose, corn starch, lactose, povidone, talc, magnesium stearate, polymers of methacrylic acid, acrylic acid esters and methacrylic acid esters. Capsule shell: titanium dioxide (E171), erythrosine (E127), indigotine (E132), yellow iron oxide (E172) and gelatin. Printing ink: shellac, soya lecithin (E322), dimethicone, titanium dioxide (E171), black iron oxide (E172).

6.2 Incompatibilities

See under interactions with other medicaments and other forms of interaction section.

6.3 Shelf life

Shelf-life

In the medicinal product as packaged for sale: 36 months.

Shelf-life after dilution/reconstitution

Not applicable.

Shelf-life after first opening

Not applicable.

6.4 Special precautions for storage

Store in a dry place below 25°C.

Protect from light.

6.5 Nature and contents of container

Capsule container: ie polypropylene securitainer with polyethylene closure.

Number of capsules per container: 28 or 100.

6.6 Instructions for use and handling

Not applicable.

Administrative Data

7. MARKETING AUTHORISATION HOLDER

Name or style and permanent address of registered place of business of the holder of the Marketing Authorisation:

Alpharma Limited

(Trading styles: Alpharma, Cox Pharmaceuticals)

Whiddon Valley

BARNSTAPLE

N Devon EX32 8NS

8. MARKETING AUTHORISATION NUMBER(S)

PL 0142/0436

9. DATE OF FIRST AUTHORISATION/RENEWAL OF THE AUTHORISATION

12.8.97

10. DATE OF REVISION OF THE TEXT

June 2005

Pariet 10mg & 20mg

(Eisai Ltd)

1. NAME OF THE MEDICINAL PRODUCT

PARIET® 10mg gastro-resistant tablet

PARIET® 20mg gastro-resistant tablet

2. QUALITATIVE AND QUANTITATIVE COMPOSITION

10mg rabeprazole sodium, equivalent to 9.42mg rabeprazole

20mg rabeprazole sodium, equivalent to 18.85mg rabeprazole

For excipients, see 6.1.

3. PHARMACEUTICAL FORM

Gastro-resistant tablet.

10mg: Pink, film coated biconvex tablet with 'E 241' printed on one side.

20mg: Yellow, film coated biconvex tablet with 'E 243' printed on one side.

4. CLINICAL PARTICULARS

4.1 Therapeutic indications

PARIET tablets are indicated for the treatment of:

- Active duodenal ulcer
- Active benign gastric ulcer
- Symptomatic erosive or ulcerative gastro-oesophageal reflux disease (GORD)
- Gastro-Oesophageal Reflux Disease Long-term Management (GORD Maintenance)
- Symptomatic treatment of moderate to very severe gastro-oesophageal reflux disease (symptomatic GORD)
- Zollinger-Ellison Syndrome
- In combination with appropriate antibacterial therapeutic regimens for the eradication of *Helicobacter pylori* in patients with peptic ulcer disease. See section 4.2

4.2 Posology and method of administration

Adults/elderly:

Active Duodenal Ulcer and Active Benign Gastric Ulcer: The recommended oral dose for both active duodenal ulcer and active benign gastric ulcer is 20mg to be taken once daily in the morning.

Most patients with active duodenal ulcer heal within four weeks. However a few patients may require an additional four weeks of therapy to achieve healing. Most patients with active benign gastric ulcer heal within six weeks. However again a few patients may require an additional six weeks of therapy to achieve healing.

Erosive or Ulcerative Gastro-Oesophageal Reflux Disease (GORD): The recommended oral dose for this condition is 20mg to be taken once daily for four to eight weeks.

Gastro-Oesophageal Reflux Disease Long-term Management (GORD Maintenance): For long-term management, a maintenance dose of PARIET 20 mg or 10 mg once daily can be used depending upon patient response.

Symptomatic treatment of moderate to very severe gastro-oesophageal reflux disease (symptomatic GORD): 10mg once daily in patients without oesophagitis. If symptom control has not been achieved during four weeks, the patient should be further investigated. Once symptoms have resolved, subsequent symptom control can be achieved using an on-demand regimen taking 10mg once daily when needed.

Zollinger-Ellison Syndrome: The recommended adult starting dose is 60 mg once a day. The dose may be titrated upwards to 120 mg/day based on individual patient needs. Single daily doses up to 100 mg/day may be given. 120 mg dose may require divided doses, 60 mg twice daily. Treatment should continue for as long as clinically indicated.

Eradication of H. pylori: Patients with *H. pylori* infection should be treated with eradication therapy. The following combination given for 7 days is recommended.

PARIET 20mg twice daily + clarithromycin 500mg twice daily and amoxicillin 1g twice daily.

For indications requiring once daily treatment PARIET tablets should be taken in the morning, before eating; and although neither the time of day nor food intake was shown to have any effect on rabeprazole sodium activity, this regimen will facilitate treatment compliance.

Patients should be cautioned that the PARIET tablets should not be chewed or crushed, but should be swallowed whole.

Renal and hepatic impairment: No dosage adjustment is necessary for patients with renal or hepatic impairment.

See section 4.4 Special Warnings and Precautions for Use of PARIET in the treatment of patients with severe hepatic impairment.

Children:

PARIET is not recommended for use in children, as there is no experience of its use in this group.

4.3 Contraindications

PARIET is contra-indicated in patients with known hypersensitivity to rabeprazole sodium, substituted benzimidazoles or to any excipient used in the formulation. PARIET is contra-indicated in pregnancy and during breast feeding.

4.4 Special warnings and special precautions for use

Symptomatic response to therapy with rabeprazole sodium does not preclude the presence of gastric or oesophageal malignancy, therefore the possibility of malignancy should be excluded prior to commencing treatment with PARIET.

Patients on long-term treatment (particularly those treated for more than a year) should be kept under regular surveillance.

Patients should be cautioned that PARIET tablets should not be chewed or crushed, but should be swallowed whole.

PARIET is not recommended for use in children, as there is no experience of its use in this group.

No evidence of significant drug related safety problems was seen in a study of patients with mild to moderate hepatic impairment versus normal age and sex matched controls. However because there are no clinical data on the use of PARIET in the treatment of patients with severe hepatic dysfunction the prescriber is advised to exercise caution when treatment with PARIET is first initiated in such patients.

4.5 Interaction with other medicinal products and other forms of Interaction

Rabeprazole sodium produces a profound and long lasting inhibition of gastric acid secretion. An interaction with compounds whose absorption is pH dependent may occur. Co-administration of rabeprazole sodium with ketoconazole or itraconazole may result in a significant decrease in antifungal plasma levels. Therefore individual patients may need to be monitored to determine if a dosage adjustment is necessary when ketoconazole or itraconazole are taken concomitantly with PARIET.

In clinical trials, antacids were used concomitantly with the administration of PARIET and, in a specific drug-drug interaction study, no interaction with liquid antacids was observed.

4.6 Pregnancy and lactation

Pregnancy:

There are no data on the safety of rabeprazole in human pregnancy. Reproduction studies performed in rats and rabbits have revealed no evidence of impaired fertility or harm to the foetus due to rabeprazole sodium, although low foeto-placental transfer occurs in rats. PARIET is contraindicated during pregnancy.

Lactation:

It is not known whether rabeprazole sodium is excreted in human breast milk. No studies in lactating women have been performed. Rabeprazole sodium is however excreted in rat mammary secretions. Therefore PARIET should not be used during breast feeding.

4.7 Effects on ability to drive and use machines

Based on the pharmacodynamic properties and the adverse events profile, it is unlikely that PARIET would cause an impairment of driving performance or compromise the ability to use machinery. If however, alertness is impaired due to somnolence, it is recommended that driving and operating complex machinery be avoided.

4.8 Undesirable effects

PARIET tablets were generally well tolerated during clinical trials. The observed undesirable effects have been generally mild/moderate and transient in nature. The most common adverse events are headache, diarrhoea and nausea. Adverse reactions reported as more than isolated cases are listed below, by system organ class and by frequency.

The following adverse events have been reported from clinical trial and post-marketed experience. However of those adverse reactions reported in Company sponsored clinical trials, only headache, diarrhoea, abdominal pain, asthenia, flatulence, rash and dry mouth were associated

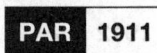

with the use of Pariet Tablets. Frequencies are defined as: common (> 1/100, < 1/10), uncommon (> 1/1,000, < 1/100), rare (>1/10,000, <1/1000) and very rare (<1/10,000).

(see Table 1 below)

4.9 Overdose

Experience to date with deliberate or accidental overdose is limited. The maximum established exposure has not exceeded 60mg twice daily, or 160mg once daily. Effects are generally minimal, representative of the known adverse event profile and reversible without further medical intervention. No specific antidote is known. Rabeprazole sodium is extensively protein bound and is, therefore, not dialysable. As in any case of overdose, treatment should be symptomatic and general supportive measures should be utilised.

5. PHARMACOLOGICAL PROPERTIES

5.1 Pharmacodynamic properties

ATC code: A02B C04

Mechanism of Action: Rabeprazole sodium belongs to the class of anti-secretory compounds, the substituted benzimidazoles, that do not exhibit anticholinergic or H_2 histamine antagonist properties, but suppress gastric acid secretion by the specific inhibition of the H^+/K^+-ATPase enzyme (the acid or proton pump). The effect is dose-related and leads to inhibition of both basal and stimulated acid secretion irrespective of the stimulus. Animal studies indicate that after administration, rabeprazole sodium rapidly disappears from both the plasma and gastric mucosa. As a weak base, rabeprazole is rapidly absorbed following all doses and is concentrated in the acid environment of the parietal cells. Rabeprazole is converted to the active sulphenamide form through protonation and it subsequently reacts with the available cysteines on the proton pump.

Anti-secretory Activity: After oral administration of a 20mg dose of rabeprazole sodium the onset of the anti-secretory effect occurs within one hour, with the maximum effect occurring within two to four hours. Inhibition of basal and food stimulated acid secretion 23 hours after the first dose of rabeprazole sodium are 69% and 82% respectively and the duration of inhibition lasts up to 48 hours. The inhibitory effect of rabeprazole sodium on acid secretion increases slightly with repeated once-daily dosing, achieving steady state inhibition after three days. When the drug is discontinued, secretory activity normalises over 2 to 3 days.

Serum Gastrin Effects: In clinical studies patients were treated once daily with 10 or 20mg rabeprazole sodium, for up to 43 months duration. Serum gastrin levels increased during the first 2 to 8 weeks reflecting the inhibitory effects on acid secretion and remained stable while treatment was continued. Gastrin values returned to pre-treatment levels, usually within 1 to 2 weeks after discontinuation of therapy.

Table 1

System Organ Class	Common	Uncommon	Rare	Very Rare
Infections and infestations	Infection			
Blood and the lymphatic system disorders			Neutropenia Leucopenia Thrombocytopenia Leucocytosis	
Immune system disorders			Acute systemic allergic reactions (for example facial swelling, hypotension and dyspnea)*	
Metabolism and nutrition disorders			Anorexia	
Psychiatric disorders	Insomnia	Nervousness Somnolence	Depression	
Nervous system disorders	Headache Dizziness			
Eye disorders			Visual disturbance	
Respiratory, thoracic and mediastinal disorders	Cough Pharyngitis Rhinitis	Bronchitis Sinusitis		
Gastrointestinal disorders	Diarrhoea Vomiting Nausea Abdominal pain Constipation Flatulence	Dyspepsia Dry mouth Eructation	Gastritis Stomatitis Taste disturbance	
Hepato-biliary disorders			Hepatitis Jaundice Hepatic encephalopathy**	
Skin and subcutaneous tissue disorders		Rash Erythema*	Pruritis Sweating Bullous reactions*	Erythema multiforme, toxic epidermal necrolysis (TEN), Stevens-Johnson syndrome (SJS)
Musculoskeletal, connective tissue and bone disorders	Non-specific pain/ back pain	Myalgia Leg cramps Arthralgia		
Renal and urinary disorders		Urinary tract infection	Interstitial nephritis	
General disorders and administration site conditions	Asthenia Flu-like syndrome	Chest pain Chills Fever		
Investigations		Increased hepatic enzymes**	Weight gain	

* Erythema, bullous reactions and acute systemic allergic reactions have usually resolved after discontinuation of therapy.

** Rare reports of hepatic encephalopathy have been received in patients with underlying cirrhosis. In treatment of patients with severe hepatic dysfunction the prescriber is advised to exercise caution when treatment with PARIET is first initiated in such patients (see section 4.4).

Human gastric biopsy specimens from the antrum and the fundus from over 500 patients receiving rabeprazole or comparator treatment for up to 8 weeks have not detected changes in ECL cell histology, degree of gastritis, incidence of atrophic gastritis, intestinal metaplasia or distribution of *H. pylori* infection. In over 250 patients followed for 36 months of continuous therapy, no significant change in findings present at baseline was observed.

Other Effects: Systemic effects of rabeprazole sodium in the CNS, cardiovascular and respiratory systems have not been found to date. Rabeprazole sodium, given in oral doses of 20mg for 2 weeks, had no effect on thyroid function, carbohydrate metabolism, or circulating levels of parathyroid hormone, cortisol, oestrogen, testosterone, prolactin, cholecystokinin, secretin, glucagon, follicle stimulating hormone (FSH), luteinising hormone (LH), renin, aldosterone or somatotrophic hormone.

Studies in healthy subjects have shown that rabeprazole sodium does not have clinically significant interactions with amoxicillin. Rabeprazole does not adversely influence plasma concentrations of amoxicillin or clarithromycin when co-administered for the purpose of eradicating upper gastrointestinal *H. pylori* infection.

5.2 Pharmacokinetic properties

Absorption: PARIET is an enteric-coated (gastro-resistant) tablet formulation of rabeprazole sodium. This presentation is necessary because rabeprazole is acid-labile. Absorption of rabeprazole therefore begins only after the tablet leaves the stomach. Absorption is rapid, with peak plasma levels of rabeprazole occurring approximately 3.5 hours after a 20mg dose. Peak plasma concentrations (C_{max}) of rabeprazole and AUC are linear over the dose range of 10mg to 40mg. Absolute bioavailability of an oral 20mg dose (compared to intravenous administration) is about 52% due in large part to pre-systemic metabolism. Additionally the bioavailability does not appear to increase with repeat administration. In healthy subjects the plasma half-life is approximately one hour (range 0.7 to 1.5 hours), and the total body clearance is estimated to be 283 ± 98 ml/min. There was no clinically relevant interaction with food. Neither food nor the time of day of administration of the treatment affect the absorption of rabeprazole sodium.

Distribution: Rabeprazole is approximately 97% bound to human plasma proteins.

Metabolism and excretion: Rabeprazole sodium, as is the case with other members of the proton pump inhibitor (PPI) class of compounds, is metabolised through the cytochrome P450 (CYP450) hepatic drug metabolising system. In vitro studies with human liver microsomes indicated that rabeprazole sodium is metabolised by isoenzymes of CYP450 (CYP2C19 and CYP3A4). In these studies, at expected human plasma concentrations rabeprazole neither induces nor inhibits CYP3A4; and although *in vitro* studies may not always be predictive of *in vivo* status these findings indicate that no interaction is expected between rabeprazole and cyclosporin. In humans the thioether (M1) and carboxylic acid (M6) are the main plasma metabolites with the sulphone (M2), desmethyl-thioether (M4) and mercapturic acid conjugate (M5) minor metabolites observed at lower levels. Only the desmethyl metabolite (M3) has a small amount of anti-secretory activity, but it is not present in plasma.

Following a single 20mg ^{14}C labelled oral dose of rabeprazole sodium, no unchanged drug was excreted in the urine. Approximately 90% of the dose was eliminated in urine mainly as the two metabolites: a mercapturic acid conjugate (M5) and a carboxylic acid (M6), plus two unknown metabolites. The remainder of the dose was recovered in faeces.

Gender: Adjusted for body mass and height, there are no significant gender differences in pharmacokinetic parameters following a single 20 mg dose of rabeprazole.

Renal dysfunction: In patients with stable, end-stage, renal failure requiring maintenance haemodialysis (creatinine clearance $\leqslant 5$ml/min/1.73m^2), the disposition of rabeprazole was very similar to that in healthy volunteers. The AUC and the C_{max} in these patients was about 35% lower than the corresponding parameters in healthy volunteers. The mean half-life of rabeprazole was 0.82 hours in healthy volunteers, 0.95 hours in patients during haemodialysis and 3.6 hours post dialysis. The clearance of the drug in patients with renal disease requiring maintenance haemodialysis was approximately twice that in healthy volunteers.

Hepatic dysfunction: Following a single 20 mg dose of rabeprazole to patients with chronic mild to moderate hepatic impairment the AUC doubled and there was a 2-3 fold increase in half-life of rabeprazole compared to the healthy volunteers. However, following a 20 mg dose daily for 7 days the AUC had increased to only 1.5-fold and the C_{max} to only 1.2-fold. The half-life of rabeprazole in patients with hepatic impairment was 12.3 hours compared to 2.1 hours in healthy volunteers. The pharmacodynamic response (gastric pH control) in the two groups was clinically comparable.

Elderly: Elimination of rabeprazole was somewhat decreased in the elderly. Following 7 days of daily dosing with 20mg of rabeprazole sodium, the AUC approximately doubled, the C_{max} increased by 60% and t½ increased by approximately 30% as compared to young healthy volunteers. However there was no evidence of rabeprazole accumulation.

CYP2C19 Polymorphism: Following a 20mg daily dose of rabeprazole for 7 days, CYP2C19 slow metabolisers, had AUC and t½ which were approximately 1.9 and 1.6 times the corresponding parameters in extensive metabolisers whilst Cmax had increased by only 40%.

5.3 Preclinical safety data

Pre-clinical effects were observed only at exposures sufficiently in excess of the maximum human exposure that make concerns for human safety negligible in respect of animal data.

Studies on mutagenicity gave equivocal results. Tests in mouse lymphoma cell line were positive, but *in vivo* micronucleus and *in vivo* and *in vitro* DNA repair tests were negative. Carcinogenicity studies revealed no special hazard for humans.

6. PHARMACEUTICAL PARTICULARS

6.1 List of excipients

Core tablet: Mannitol, magnesium oxide, low-substituted hyprolose, hyprolose, magnesium stearate

Undercoating: ethylcellulose, magnesium oxide

Enteric coating: hypromellose phthalate, diacetylated monoglycerides, talc, titanium dioxide (E171), red iron oxide (E172) – 10mg only, yellow iron oxide (E172) – 20mg only, carnauba wax

Printing ink – Pariet 10mg: pharmaceutical glaze black iron oxide (E172), propylene glycol, medicinal antifoam A.

Printing ink – Pariet 20mg: shellac food grade (E904), red iron oxide (E172), soya lecithin (E322), antifoam DC1510.

6.2 Incompatibilities

Not applicable.

6.3 Shelf life

2 years.

6.4 Special precautions for storage

Do not store above 25°C. Do not refrigerate

6.5 Nature and contents of container

Blister strips (aluminium/aluminium)

Pack sizes: 1, 7, 14, 15, 25, 28, 30, 50, 56, 75, 120 tablets

Not all pack sizes may be marketed.

6.6 Instructions for use and handling

No special requirements.

Administrative Data

7. MARKETING AUTHORISATION HOLDER

Eisai Ltd., Hammersmith International Centre,

3 Shortlands, London W6 8EE, United Kingdom.

8. MARKETING AUTHORISATION NUMBER(S)

Pariet 10mg: PL 10555/0010 (10mg tablets)

Pariet 20mg: PL10555/0008 (20mg tablets)

9. DATE OF FIRST AUTHORISATION/RENEWAL OF THE AUTHORISATION

8 May 1998/July 2003

10. DATE OF REVISION OF THE TEXT

September 2004

PARLODEL Capsules

(Novartis Pharmaceuticals UK Ltd)

1. NAME OF THE MEDICINAL PRODUCT

Parlodel® 5mg Capsules

Parlodel ® 10mg Capsules

2. QUALITATIVE AND QUANTITATIVE COMPOSITION

Parlodel 5mg Capsules

Active substance: Ergotaman-3', 6', 18-trione, 2-bromo-12'-hydroxy-2'-(1-methylethyl-5'-(2-methylpropyl)-, (5'alpha)-mono-methanesulphonate.

Blue opaque and white opaque oblong hard gelatine capsule coded in red "PS" containing 5.735mg of bromocriptine mesilate (equivalent to 5mg bromocriptine base).

For excipients, see 6.1

Parlodel 10mg Capsules

Active substance: Ergotaman-3', 6', 18-trione, 2-bromo-12'-hydroxy-2'-(1-methylethyl-5'-(2-methylpropyl)-, (5'alpha)-mono-methanesulphonate.

Each capsule contains 11.47mg of bromocriptine mesilate Ph Eur equivalent to 10mg of bromocriptine base.

For excipients, see 6.1

3. PHARMACEUTICAL FORM

Parlodel 5mg Capsules

Hard gelatin capsules

Parlodel 10mg Capsules

White, opaque hard shell capsule, size No 1, coded in red PARLODEL 10.

4. CLINICAL PARTICULARS

4.1 Therapeutic indications

Inhibition of lactation

The inhibition or suppression of puerperal lactation for medical reasons. Parlodel is not recommended for the routine suppression of lactation or for the relief of symptoms of post-partum pain and engorgement which can be adequately treated with simple analgesics and breast support.

Hyperprolactinaemia

The treatment of hyperprolactinaemia in men and women with hypogonadism and/or galactorrhoea.

Infertility

The treatment of hyperprolactinaemic infertility.

Parlodel has been used successfully in the treatment of a number of infertile women who do not have demonstrable hyperprolactinaemia.

Prolactinomas

In a number of specialised units, patients who have shown to have prolactin secreting adenomas have been treated successfully with Parlodel. In particular, Parlodel can be considered as a first choice of treatment in patients with macro-adenomas and as an alternative to the surgical procedure, transsphenoidal hypophysectomy, in patients with micro-adenomas.

Benign Breast Disease

The treatment of cyclical benign breast disease/cyclical pronounced mastalgia.

Menstrual Cycle Disorders/Premenstrual Symptoms

Cyclical menstrual disorders have also responded to Parlodel, particularly breast symptomatology, but in the premenstrual syndrome, there is also some evidence that other symptoms, such as headache, mood changes and bloatedness may be alleviated.

Acromegaly

Parlodel has been used in a number of specialised units, as an adjunct to surgery and/or radiotherapy to reduce circulating growth hormone in the management of acromegalic patients.

Parkinson's Disease

In the treatment of idiopathic Parkinson's Disease, Parlodel has been used both alone and in combination with Levodopa in the management of previously treated patients and those disabled by 'on-off' phenomena. Parlodel has been used with occasional benefit in patients who do not respond to or are unable to tolerate Levodopa and those whose response to Levodopa is declining.

4.2 Posology and method of administration

Parlodel should always be taken with food.

A number of disparate conditions are amenable to treatment with Parlodel and for this reason, the recommended dosage regimens are variable.

In most indications, irrespective of the final dose, the optimum response with the minimum of side effects is best achieved by gradual introduction of Parlodel. The following scheme is suggested: Initially, 1mg to 1.25mg at bed time, increasing after 2 to 3 days to 2mg to 2.5mg at bed time. Dosage may then be increased by 1mg to 2.5mg at 2 to 3 day intervals, until a dosage of 2.5mg twice daily is achieved. Further dosage increments, if necessary, should be added in a similar manner.

Prevention of Lactation

2.5mg on the day of delivery, followed by 2.5mg twice daily for 14 days. Treatment should be instituted within a few hours of parturition, once vital signs have been stabilised. Gradual introduction of Parlodel is not necessary in this indication.

Suppression of Lactation

2.5mg on first day, increasing after 2 to 3 days to 2.5mg twice daily for 14 days. Gradual introduction of Parlodel is not necessary in this indication.

Hypogonadism/Galactorrhea syndromes/Infertility

Introduce Parlodel gradually according to the suggested scheme. Most patients with hyperprolactinaemia have responded to 7.5mg daily, in divided doses, but doses of up to 30mg daily have been used. In infertile patients without demonstrably elevated serum prolactin levels, the usual dose is 2,5mg twice daily.

Prolactinomas

Introduce Parlodel gradually according to the suggested scheme. Dosage may then be increased by 2.5mg daily at 2 to 3 day intervals as follows: 2.5mg eight-hourly, 2.5mg six hourly, 5mg six-hourly. Patients have been responding to doses of up to 30mg daily.

Cyclical Benign Breast Disease/Cyclical Pronounced Mastalgia/Cyclical Menstrual Disorders

Introduce Parlodel gradually, according to the suggested scheme, until the recommended dosage of 2.5mg twice daily is reached.

For the treatment of premenstrual symptoms, treatment should begin on day 14 of the cycle, with 1.25mg daily, increasing the dose gradually up to 2.5mg twice daily until menstruation sets in.

Acromegaly

Introduce Parlodel gradually, according to the suggested scheme. Dosage may then be increased by 2.5mg daily at 2 to 3 day intervals as follows 2.5mg eight-hourly, 2.5mg six-hourly, 5mg six-hourly, 5mg six-hourly.

Parkinson's Disease

Introduce Parlodel gradually, as follows: Week 1: 1mg to 1.25mg at bed time. Week 2: 2mg to 2.5mg at bed time. Week 3: 2.5mg twice daily. Week 4: 2.5mg three times daily. Thereafter take three times a day increasing by 2.5mg every 3 to 14 days, depending on the patient's response. Continue until the optimum dose is reached. This will usually be between 10mg and 40mg daily. In patients already receiving Levodopa the dosage of this drug may gradually be decreased while the dosage daily of Parlodel is increased until the optimum balance is determined.

Use in Children

Administration of Parlodel is not appropriate for children less than 15 years old.

Use in Elderly

There is no clinical evidence that Parlodel poses a special risk to the elderly.

Use in Patients with Hepatic Impairment

In patients with impaired hepatic function, the speed of elimination may be retarded and plasma levels may increase, requiring dose adjustment.

4.3 Contraindications

Hypersensitivity to any of the components of Parlodel (see Qualitative and quantitative composition and 6.1 List of excipient or other ergot alkaloids.

Uncontrolled hypertension, hypertensive disorders of pregnancy (including eclampsia, pre-eclampsia or pregnancy-induced hypertension), hypertension post partum and in the puerperium. For use during pregnancy, see Section 4.6 – Pregnancy and Lactation.

Parlodel is contraindicated for use in the suppression of lactation or other non-life threatening indications in patients with a history of coronary artery disease or other severe cardiovascular conditions, or symptoms / history of severe psychiatric disorders.

Patients with severe cardiovascular disorders or psychiatric disorders taking Parlodel for the indication of macro-adenomas should only take it if the perceived benefits outweigh the potential risks. (see Section 4.4 Special Warnings and Precautions).

4.4 Special warnings and special precautions for use

Parlodel is contraindicated for use in the suppression of lactation or other non-life threatening indications in patients with severe coronary artery disease, or symptoms and/or a history of serious mental disorders (see Section 4.3 Contraindications).

In rare cases, serious adverse events, including hypertension, myocardial infarction, seizures, stroke or psychiatric disorders have been reported in postpartum women treated with Parlodel for inhibition of lactation. In some patients the development of seizures or stroke was preceded by severe headache and/or transient visual disturbances. (see Section 4.8 Undesirable Effects).

Patients with severe cardiovascular disorders or psychiatric disorders taking Parlodel for the indication of macro-adenomas should only take it if the perceived benefits outweigh the potential risks. (see Section 4.3 Contraindications).

Blood pressure should be carefully monitored, especially during the first days of therapy. Particular caution is required in patients who are on concomitant therapy with, or have recently been treated with drugs that can alter blood pressure. Although there is no conclusive evidence of an interaction between Parlodel and other ergot alkaloids, a concomitant course of these medications during the puerperium is not recommended. If hypertension, unremitting headache, or any signs of CNS toxicity develop, treatment should be discontinued immediately.

Hyperprolactinaemia may be idiopathic, drug-induced, or due to hypothalamic or pituitary disease. The possibility that hyperprolactinaemic patients may have a pituitary tumour should be recognised and complete investigation at specialized units to identify such patients is advisable. Parlodel will effectively lower prolactin levels in patients with pituitary tumours but does not obviate the necessity for radiotherapy or surgical intervention where appropriate in acromegaly.

Since patients with macro-adenomas of the pituitary might have accompanying hypopituitarism due to compression or destruction of pituitary tissue, one should make a complete evaluation of pituitary functions and institute appropriate substitution therapy prior to administration of Parlodel. In patients with secondary adrenal insufficiency, substitution with corticosteroids is essential.

The evolution of tumour size in patients with pituitary macro-adenomas should be carefully monitored and if evidence of tumour expansion develops, surgical procedures must be considered.

If in adenoma patients, pregnancy occurs after the administration of Parlodel, careful observation is mandatory. Prolactin-secreting adenomas may expand during pregnancy. In these patients, treatment with Parlodel often results in tumour shrinkage and rapid improvement of the visual fields defects. In severe cases, compression of the optic or other cranial nerves may necessitate emergency pituitary surgery.

Visual field impairment is a known complication of macroprolactinoma. Effective treatment with Parlodel leads to a reduction in hyperprolactinaemia and often to resolution of the visual impairment. In some patients, however, a secondary deterioration of visual fields may subsequently develop despite normalised prolactin levels and tumour shrinkage, which may result from traction on the optic chiasm which is pulled down into the now partially empty sella. In these cases the visual field defect may improve on reduction of bromocriptine dosage while there is some elevation of prolactin and some tumour re-expansion. Monitoring of visual fields in patients with macro-prolactinoma is therefore recommended for an early recognition of secondary field loss due to chiasmal herniation and adaptation of drug dosage.

Bromocriptine has been associated with somnolence and episodes of sudden sleep onset, particularly in patients with Parkinson's disease. Sudden onset of sleep during daily activities, in some cases without awareness or warning signs, has been reported very rarely. Patients must be informed of this and advised to exercise caution while driving or operating machines during treatment with bromocriptine. Patients who have experienced somnolence and/or an episode of sudden sleep onset must refrain from driving or operating machines. Furthermore, a reduction of dosage or termination of therapy may be considered.

In women suffering from prolactin-related fertility disorders, treatment with Parlodel results in ovulation. Patients who do not wish to conceive should be advised to practice a reliable method of contraception. Oral contraceptives have however, been reported to increase serum prolactin levels. When women of child-bearing age are treated with Parlodel for conditions not associated with hyperprolactinaemia the lowest effective dose should be used. This is in order to avoid suppression of prolactin to below normal levels, with consequent impairment of luteal function.

Gynaecological assessment, preferably including cervical and endometrial cytology, is recommended for women receiving Parlodel for extensive periods. Six monthly assessment is suggested for post-menopausal women and annual assessment for women with regular menstruation.

In patients to be treated for mastalgia and nodular and /or cystic breast alterations, malignancy must be excluded by appropriate diagnostic procedures.

A few cases of gastrointestinal bleeding and gastric ulcer have been reported. If this occurs,

Parlodel should be withdrawn. Patients with a history of evidence of peptic ulceration should be closely monitored when receiving the treatment.

Since, especially during the first few days of treatment, hypotensive reactions may occasionally occur and result in reduced alertness, particular care should be exercised when driving a vehicle or operating machinery.

Parlodel is an ergot derivative. Fibrotic and serosal inflammatory disorders such as pleuritis, pleural and pericardial effusion, pleural and, pulmonary fibrosis, constrictive pericarditis, and retroperitoneal fibrosis have occurred after prolonged usage of ergot derivatives. The factors predisposing patients to the risk of such disorders are not known, however, Parkinson's disease patients with a history of such disorders should not be treated with Parlodel, or any other ergot derivative, unless the potential benefit clearly outweighs the risk.

Attention should be paid to the signs and symptoms of

- pleuro-pulmonary disease such as dyspnoea, shortness of breath, persistent cough or chest pain
- renal insufficiency or ureteral/abdominal vascular obstruction that may occur with pain in the loin/flank and lower limb oedema as well as any possible abdominal masses or tenderness that may indicate retroperitoneal fibrosis
- cardiac failure as cases of pericardial fibrosis have often manifested as cardiac failure. Constrictive pericarditis should be excluded if such symptoms appear.

Appropriate investigations such as erythrocyte sedimentation rate, chest X-ray and serum creatinine measurements should be performed if necessary to support a diagnosis of a fibrotic disorder. It is also appropriate to perform baseline investigations of erythrocyte sedimentation rate or other inflammatory markers, lung function/chest X-ray and renal function prior to initiation of therapy.

These disorders can have an insidious onset and patients should be regularly and carefully monitored while taking Parlodel for manifestations of progressive fibrotic disorders. Parlodel should be withdrawn if fibrotic or serosal inflammatory changes are diagnosed or suspected.

4.5 Interaction with other medicinal products and other forms of Interaction

Tolerance to Parlodel may be reduced by alcohol.

Caution is required in patients who are on concomitant therapy with, or have recently been treated with drugs that can alter blood pressure.

No data suggests that therapeutic levels of bromocriptine inhibit CYP3A4 to a clinically significant level. However, bromocriptine has been shown to be an inhibitor of CYP3A4 in vitro and caution should be used when co-administering drug substances of this enzyme.

Although there is no conclusive evidence of an interaction between Parlodel and other ergot alkaloids, concomitant use of these medications during the puerperium is not recommended (See also Section 4.4 Special Warnings and Precautions)

The concomitant use of erythromycin, other macrolide antibiotics or octreotide may increase bromocriptine plasma levels.

Dopamine antagonists such as antipsychotics (phenothiazines, butyrophenones and thioxanthenes) may reduce the prolactin-lowering and antiparkinsonian effects of bromocriptine. Metoclopramide and domperidone may reduce the prolactin-lowering effect.

4.6 Pregnancy and lactation

If pregnancy occurs it is generally advisable to withdraw Parlodel after the first missed menstrual period.

Rapid expansion of pituitary tumours sometimes occurs during pregnancy and this may also occur in patients who have been able to conceive as a result of Parlodel therapy. As a precautionary measure, patients should be monitored to detect signs of pituitary enlargement so that Parlodel may be reintroduced if necessary. Based on the outcome of more than 2,000 pregnancies, the use of Parlodel to restore fertility has not been associated with an increased risk of abortion, premature delivery, multiple pregnancy or malformation in infants. Because this accumulated evidence suggests a lack of teratogenic or embryopathic effects in humans, maintenance of Parlodel treatment during pregnancy may be considered where there is a large tumour or evidence of expansion.

Lactation

Since Parlodel inhibits lactation, it should not be administered to mothers who elect to breast-feed.

4.7 Effects on ability to drive and use machines

Hypotensive reactions may be disturbing in some patients during the first few days of treatment and particular care should be exercised when driving vehicles or operating machinery.

Patients being treated with bromocriptine and presenting with somnolence and/or sudden sleep episodes must be advised not to drive or engage in activities where impaired alertness may put themselves or others at risk of serious injury or death (eg. Operating machines) until such recurrent episodes and somnolence have resolved (see also Section 4.4 Special Warnings and Precautions).

4.8 Undesirable effects

The occurrence of side-effects can be minimised by gradual introduction of the dose or a dose reduction followed by a more gradual titration. If necessary, initial nausea and/ or vomiting may be reduced by taking Parlodel during a meal and by the intake of a peripheral dopamine antagonist, such as domperidone, for a few days, at least one hour prior to the administration of Parlodel.

Adverse reactions are ranked under headings of frequency, using the following convention:- very common: ≥ 10 %; common: ≥ 1 % - < 10 %; uncommon: ≥ 0.1% - < 1 %; rare: ≥ 0.01% - < 0.1 %; very rare: < 0.01 %

Central Nervous System

Common: Headache, Drowsiness

Uncommon: Dizziness, Dyskinesia

Rare: Somnolence

Very Rare: Excess daytime somnolence and sudden sleep onset

Psychiatric

Uncommon: Confusion, Psychomotor agitation, Hallucinations

Gastrointestinal

Common: Nausea, Constipation

Uncommon: Vomiting

Very Rare: Gastrointestinal bleeding, Gastric ulcer

Cardiovascular System

Uncommon: Hypotension including orthostatic hypotension (which may in very rare instances lead to collapse)

Rare: Pericardial effusion, Constrictive pericarditis

Very Rare: Reversible pallor of fingers and toes induced by cold (especially in patients who have a history of Raynaud's phenomenon)

Respiratory System

Common: Nasal congestion

Uncommon: Dry mouth

Rare: Pleural effusion, pleural and pulmonary fibrosis, pleuritis

Musculoskeletal

Uncommon: Leg cramps

Skin and appendages

Uncommon: Allergic skin reactions, Hair loss

General conditions

Uncommon: Fatigue

Rare: Retroperitoneal fibrosis

Very Rarely: A syndrome resembling Neuroleptic Malignant Syndrome has been reported on withdrawal of Parlodel.

Post-partum women

In extremely rare cases (in postpartum women treated with Parlodel for the prevention of lactation) serious adverse events including hypertension, myocardial infarction, seizures, stroke or mental disorders have been reported, although the causal relationship is uncertain. In some patients the occurrence of seizures or stroke was preceded by severe headache and/or transient visual disturbances.

4.9 Overdose

Overdosage with Parlodel is likely to result in vomiting and other symptoms which could be due to over stimulation of dopaminergic receptors and might include confusion, hallucinations and hypotension. General supportive measures should be undertaken to remove any unabsorbed material and maintain blood pressure if necessary.

5. PHARMACOLOGICAL PROPERTIES

5.1 Pharmacodynamic properties

Pharmacotherapeutic group: dopamine agonist (ATC code N04B C01), prolactin inhibitor (ATC code G02C B01)

Parlodel, active ingredient bromocriptine, is an inhibitor of prolactin secretion and a stimulator of dopamine receptors. The areas of application of PARLODEL are divided into endocrinological and neurological indications. The pharmacological particulars will be discussed under each indication.

Endocrinological indications

Parlodel inhibits the secretion of the anterior pituitary hormone prolactin without affecting normal levels of other pituitary hormones. However, Parlodel is capable of reducing elevated levels of growth hormone (GH) in patients with acromegaly. These effects are due to stimulation of dopamine receptors.

In the puerperium prolactin is necessary for the initiation and maintenance of puerperal lactation. At other times increased prolactin secretion gives rise to pathological lactation (galactorrhoea) and/or disorders of ovulation and menstruation.

As a specific inhibitor of prolactin secretion, Parlodel can be used to prevent or suppress physiological lactation as well as to treat prolactin-induced pathological states. In amenorrhoea and/or anovulation (with or without galactorrhoea), Parlodel can be used to restore menstrual cycles and ovulation.

The customary measures taken during lactation suppression, such as the restriction of fluid intake are not necessary with Parlodel. In addition, Parlodel does not impair the puerperal involution of the uterus and does not increase the risk of thromboembolism.

Parlodel has been shown to arrest the growth or to reduce the size of prolactin-secreting pituitary adenomas (prolactinomas).

In acromegalic patients - apart from lowering the plasma levels of growth hormone and prolactin - Parlodel has a beneficial effect on clinical symptoms and on glucose tolerance.

Parlodel improves the clinical symptoms of the polycystic ovary syndrome by restoring a normal pattern of LH secretion.

In patients with benign breast disease, Parlodel reduces the size and number of cysts and/or nodules of the breast and alleviates the breast pain often associated with such conditions by normalising the underlying progesterone/ oestrogen imbalance. At the same time it reduces prolactin secretion in patients with elevated levels.

Neurological Indications

Because of its dopaminergic activity, Parlodel, in doses usually higher than those for endocrinological indications, is effective in the treatment of Parkinson's Disease, which is characterised by a specific nigrostriatal dopamine deficiency. The stimulation of dopamine receptors by Parlodel can in this condition restore the neurochemical balance within the striatum.

Clinically, Parlodel improves tremor, rigidity, bradykinesia and other Parkinsonian symptoms at all stages of the disease. Usually the therapeutic effect lasts over years (so far, good results have been reported in patients treated up to eight years). PARLODEL can be given either alone or - at early as well as advanced stages - combined with other anti-Parkinsonian drugs. Combination with Levodopa treatment results in enhanced anti-Parkinsonian effects, often making possible a reduction of the Levodopa dose. Parlodel offers particular benefit to patients on Levodopa treatment exhibiting a deteriorating therapeutic response or complications such as abnormal involuntary movements (choreatoid dykinesia and/or painful dystonia), end-of-dose failure, and 'on-off' phenomenon.

Parlodel improves the depressive symptomatology often observed in parkinsonian patients. This is due to its inherent antidepressant properties as substantiated by controlled studies in non-Parkinsonian patients with endogenous or psychogenic depression.

5.2 Pharmacokinetic properties

Following oral administration, Parlodel (bromocriptine) is rapidly and well absorbed. Peak plasma levels are reached within 1-3 hours. The prolactin-lowering effect occurs 1-2 hours after ingestion, reaches its maximum within about 5 hours and lasts for 8-12 hours.

Parlodel is extensively metabolised. In plasma the elimination half life is 3-4 hours for the parent drug and 50 hours for the inactive metabolites. The parent drug and its metabolites are also completely excreted via the liver with only 6%

being eliminated via the kidney. Parlodel is 96% bound to plasma proteins.

There is no evidence that the pharmacokinetic properties and tolerability of PARLODEL are directly affected by advanced age. However, in patients with impaired hepatic function, the speed of elimination may be retarded and plasma levels may increase, requiring dose adjustment.

5.3 Preclinical safety data

There are no other clinically relevant preclinical safety data in addition to those mentioned in other sections of the SmPC.

6. PHARMACEUTICAL PARTICULARS

6.1 List of excipients

Parlodel 5mg Capsules

Aerosil 200 (Standard), magnesium stearate, maleic acid, maize starch, lactose, indigo charmine (E132), titanium dioxide (E171), gelatin.

Parlodel 10mg Capsules

Aerosil 200 (Standard), magnesium stearate, maleic acid, lactose, maize starch, titanium dioxide (E171), gelatin.

6.2 Incompatibilities

None.

6.3 Shelf life

Parlodel 5mg Capsules

Opaque white PV/PVDC blister strip: 48 months.

Amber glass bottle: 60 months.

Parlodel 10mg Capsules

A shelf-life of 5 years (amber glass bottle) is applied to this product.

6.4 Special precautions for storage

Protect from light.

6.5 Nature and contents of container

Parlodel 5mg Capsules

Opaque white PV/PVDC blister strip containing 30 Parlodel 5mg capsules.

Amber glass bottle with a CRC closure containing 100 Parlodel 5mg capsules.

Parlodel 10mg Capsules

The capsules are packaged in amber glass bottles with a CRC closure containing 100 capsules.

6.6 Instructions for use and handling

None.

7. MARKETING AUTHORISATION HOLDER

Novartis Pharmaceuticals UK Limited

Trading as: Sandoz Pharmaceuticals

Frimley Business Park

Frimley

Camberley

Surrey

GU16 7SR

8. MARKETING AUTHORISATION NUMBER(S)

Parlodel 5mg Capsules 00101/0131.

Parlodel 10mg Capsules 00101/0108

9. DATE OF FIRST AUTHORISATION/RENEWAL OF THE AUTHORISATION

Parlodel 5mg Capsules 9 October 1981 / 27 October 1997

Parlodel 10mg Capsules 20 January 1977 / 15 May 1997

10. DATE OF REVISION OF THE TEXT

27 July 2004

Legal Category

POM

Parlodel Tablets

(Novartis Pharmaceuticals UK Ltd)

1. NAME OF THE MEDICINAL PRODUCT

Parlodel® 1mg Tablets

Parlodel® 2.5mg Tablets

2. QUALITATIVE AND QUANTITATIVE COMPOSITION

Active substance: Ergotaman-3', 6', 18-trione, 2-bromo-12'-hydroxy-2'-(1-methylethyl-5'-(2-methylpropyl)-, (5'alpha)-mono-methanesulphonate.

Parlodel 1mg Tablets

Bromocriptine mesilate Ph. Eur 1.147mg, equivalent to 1mg of bromocriptine base.

Parlodel 2.5mg Tablets

Bromocriptine mesilate Ph. Eur 2.87mg, equivalent to 2.5mg of bromocriptine base.

For excipients, see 6.1

3. PHARMACEUTICAL FORM

Parlodel 1mg Tablets

Each tablet is round, white, bevelled edged with a breakline on one side, marked with "PARLODEL 1" circumferentially on the reverse.

Parlodel 2.5mg Tablets

Each tablet is white, bevelled edged with a breakline on one side, marked with "PARLODEL 2.5" circumferentially on the reverse

4. CLINICAL PARTICULARS

4.1 Therapeutic indications

Inhibition of lactation

The inhibition or suppression of puerperal lactation for medical reasons. Parlodel is not recommended for the routine suppression of lactation or for the relief of symptoms of post-partum pain and engorgement which can be adequately treated with simple analgesics and breast support.

Hyperprolactinaemia

The treatment of hyperprolactinaemia in men and women with hypogonadism and/or galactorrhoea.

Infertility

The treatment of hyperprolactinaemic infertility.

Parlodel has been used successfully in the treatment of a number of infertile women who do not have demonstrable hyperprolactinaemia.

Prolactinomas

In a number of specialised units, patients who have shown to have prolactin secreting adenomas have been treated successfully with Parlodel. In particular, Parlodel can be considered as a first choice of treatment in patients with macro-adenomas and as an alternative to the surgical procedure, transsphenoidal hypophysectomy, in patients with micro-adenomas.

Benign Breast Disease

The treatment of cyclical benign breast disease/cyclical pronounced mastalgia.

Menstrual Cycle Disorders/Premenstrual Symptoms

Cyclical menstrual disorders have also responded to Parlodel, particularly breast symptomatology, but in the premenstrual syndrome, there is also some evidence that other symptoms, such as headache, mood changes and bloatedness may be alleviated.

Acromegaly

Parlodel has been used in a number of specialised units, as an adjunct to surgery and/or radiotherapy to reduce circulating growth hormone in the management of acromegalic patients.

Parkinson's Disease

In the treatment of idiopathic Parkinson's Disease, Parlodel has been used both alone and in combination with Levodopa in the management of previously untreated patients and those disabled by 'on-off' phenomena. Parlodel has been used with occasional benefit in patients who do not respond to or are unable to tolerate Levodopa and those whose response to Levodopa is declining.

4.2 Posology and method of administration

Parlodel should always be taken with food.

A number of disparate conditions are amenable to treatment with Parlodel and for this reason, the recommended dosage regimens are variable.

In most indications, irrespective of the final dose, the optimum response with the minimum of side effects is best achieved by gradual introduction of Parlodel. The following scheme is suggested: Initially, 1mg to 1.25mg at bed time, increasing after 2 to 3 days to 2mg to 2.5mg at bed time. Dosage may then be increased by 1mg at 2 to 3 day intervals, until a dosage of 2.5mg twice daily is achieved. Further dosage increments, if necessary, should be added in a similar manner.

Prevention of Lactation

2.5mg on the day of delivery, followed by 2.5mg twice daily for 14 days. Treatment should be instituted within a few hours of parturition once vital signs have been stabilised. Gradual introduction of Parlodel is not necessary in this indication.

Suppression of Lactation

2.5mg on first day, increasing after 2 to 3 days to 2.5mg twice daily for 14 days. Gradual introduction of Parlodel is not necessary in this indication.

Hypogonadism/Galactorrhea syndromes/Infertility

Introduce Parlodel gradually according to the suggested scheme.

Most patients with hyperprolactinaemia have responded to 7.5mg daily, in divided doses, but doses of up to 30mg daily have been used. In infertile patients without demonstrably elevated serum prolactin levels, the usual dose is 2.5mg twice daily.

Prolactinomas

Introduce Parlodel gradually according to the suggested scheme. Dosage may then be increased by 2.5mg daily at 2 to 3 day intervals, as follows:- 2.5mg eight hourly, 2.5mg six hourly, 5mg six hourly. Patients have responded to doses of up to 30mg daily.

Cyclical Benign Breast Disease/Cyclical Pronounced Mastalgia/Cyclical Menstrual Disorders

Introduce Parlodel gradually, according to the suggested scheme, until the recommended dosage of 2.5mg twice daily is reached.

For the treatment of premenstrual symptoms, treatment should begin on day 14 of the cycle, with 1.25mg daily, increasing the dose gradually up to 2.5mg twice daily until menstruation sets in.

Acromegaly

Introduce Parlodel gradually, according to the suggested scheme.

Dosage may then be increased by 2.5mg at 2 to 3 day intervals as follows: - 2.5mg eight-hourly, 2.5mg six-hourly, 5mg six-hourly.

Parkinson's Disease

Introduce Parlodel gradually, as follows: Week 1: 1mg to 1.25mg at bed time. Week 2: 2mg to 2.5mg at bed time. Week 3: 2.5mg twice daily. Week 4: 2.5mg three times daily. Thereafter take three times a day increasing by 2.5mg every 3 to 14 days, depending on the patient's response. Continue until the optimum dose is reached. This will usually be between 10mg and 40mg daily. In patients already receiving Levodopa the dosage of this drug may gradually be decreased, while the dosage of Parlodel is increased until the optimum balance is determined.

Use in Children

Administration of Parlodel is not appropriate for children less than 15 years old.

Use in Elderly

There is no clinical evidence that Parlodel poses a special risk to the elderly.

Use in Patients with Hepatic Impairment

In patients with impaired hepatic function, the speed of elimination may be retarded and plasma levels may increase, requiring dose adjustment.

4.3 Contraindications

Hypersensitivity to any of the components of Parlodel (see Qualitative and quantitative composition and 6.1 List of excipients) or other ergot alkaloids.

Uncontrolled hypertension, hypertensive disorders of pregnancy (including eclampsia, pre-eclampsia or pregnancy-induced hypertension), hypertension post partum and in the puerperium. For use during pregnancy, see Section 4.6 – Pregnancy and Lactation.

Parlodel is contraindicated for use in the suppression of lactation or other non-life threatening indications in patients with a history of coronary artery disease, or other severe cardiovascular conditions, or symptoms / history of severe psychiatric disorders.

Patients with these underlying conditions taking Parlodel for the indication of macro-adenomas should only take it if the perceived benefits outweigh the potential risks (see Section 4.4 Special Warnings and Precautions).

4.4 Special warnings and special precautions for use

Parlodel is contraindicated for use in the suppression of lactation or other non-life threatening indications in patients with severe coronary artery disease, or symptoms and/or a history of serious mental disorders (see Section 4.3 Contraindications).

In rare cases, serious adverse events, including hypertension, myocardial infarction, seizures, stroke or psychiatric disorders have been reported in postpartum women treated with Parlodel for inhibition of lactation. In some patients the development of seizures or stroke was preceded by severe headache and/or transient visual disturbances. (see Section 4.8, Undesirable Effects).

Patients with severe cardiovascular disorders or psychiatric disorders taking Parlodel for the indication of macro-adenomas should only take it if the perceived benefits outweigh the potential risks. (see Section 4.3 Contraindications).

Blood pressure should be carefully monitored, especially during the first days of therapy. Particular caution is required in patients who are on concomitant therapy with, or have recently been treated with drugs that can alter blood pressure. Although there is no conclusive evidence of an interaction between Parlodel and other ergot alkaloids, a concomitant course of these medications during the puerperium is not recommended. If hypertension, unremitting headache, or any signs of CNS toxicity develop, treatment should be discontinued immediately.

Hyperprolactinaemia may be idiopathic, drug-induced, or due to hypothalamic or pituitary disease. The possibility that hyperprolactinaemic patients may have a pituitary tumour should be recognised and complete investigation at specialised units to identify such patients is advisable. Parlodel will effectively lower prolactin levels in patients with pituitary tumours but does not obviate the necessity for radiotherapy or surgical intervention where appropriate in acromegaly.

Since patients with macro-adenomas of the pituitary might have accompanying hypopituitarism due to compression or destruction of pituitary tissue, one should make a complete evaluation of pituitary functions and institute appropriate substitution therapy prior to administration of Parlodel. In patients with secondary adrenal insufficiency, substitution with corticosteroids is essential.

The evolution of tumour size in patients with pituitary macro-adenomas should be carefully monitored and if evidence of tumour expansion develops, surgical procedures must be considered.

If in adenoma patients, pregnancy occurs after the administration of Parlodel, careful observation is mandatory. Prolactin-secreting adenomas may expand during pregnancy. In these patients, treatment with Parlodel often results in tumour shrinkage and rapid improvement of the visual fields defects. In severe cases, compression of the optic or other cranial nerves may necessitate emergency pituitary surgery.

Visual field impairment is a known complication of macroprolactinoma. Effective treatment with Parlodel leads to a reduction in hyperprolactinaemia and often to resolution of the visual impairment. In some patients, however, a secondary deterioration of visual fields may subsequently develop despite normalised prolactin levels and tumour shrinkage, which may result from traction on the optic chiasm which is pulled down into the now partially empty sella. In these cases the visual field defect may improve on reduction of bromocriptine dosage while there is some elevation of prolactin and some tumour re-expansion. Monitoring of visual fields in patients with macro-prolactinoma is therefore recommended for an early recognition of secondary field loss due to chiasmal herniation and adaptation of drug dosage.

Bromocriptine has been associated with somnolence and episodes of sudden sleep onset, particularly in patients with Parkinson's disease. Sudden onset of sleep during daily activities, in some cases without awareness or warning signs, has been reported very rarely. Patients must be informed of this and advised to exercise caution while driving or operating machines during treatment with bromocriptine. Patients who have experienced somnolence and/or an episode of sudden sleep onset must refrain from driving or operating machines. Furthermore, a reduction of dosage or termination of therapy may be considered.

In women suffering from prolactin-related fertility disorders, treatment with Parlodel results in ovulation. Patients who do not wish to conceive should be advised to practice a reliable method of contraception. Oral contraceptives have however, been reported to increase serum prolactin levels. When women of child-bearing age are treated with Parlodel for conditions not associated with hyperprolactinaemia the lowest effective dose should be used. This is in order to avoid suppression of prolactin to below normal levels, with consequent impairment of luteal function.

Gynaecological assessment, preferably including cervical and endometrial cytology, is recommended for women receiving Parlodel for extensive periods. Six monthly assessment is suggested for post-menopausal women and annual assessment for women with regular menstruation.

In patients to be treated for mastalgia and nodular and /or cystic breast alterations, malignancy must be excluded by appropriate diagnostic procedures.

A few cases of gastrointestinal bleeding and gastric ulcer have been reported. If this occurs, Parlodel should be withdrawn. Patients with a history of evidence of peptic ulceration should be closely monitored when receiving the treatment.

Since, especially during the first few days of treatment, hypotensive reactions may occasionally occur and result in reduced alertness, particular care should be exercised when driving a vehicle or operating machinery.

Parlodel is an ergot derivative. Fibrotic and serosal inflammatory disorders such as pleuritis, pleural and pericardial effusion, pleural and, pulmonary fibrosis, constrictive pericarditis, and retroperitoneal fibrosis have occurred after prolonged usage of ergot derivatives. The factors predisposing patients to the risk of such disorders are not known, however, Parkinson's disease patients with a history of such disorders should not be treated with Parlodel, or any other ergot derivative, unless the potential benefit clearly outweighs the risk.

Attention should be paid to the signs and symptoms of

- pleuro-pulmonary disease such as dyspnoea, shortness of breath, persistent cough or chest pain
- renal insufficiency or ureteral/abdominal vascular obstruction that may occur with pain in the loin/flank and lower limb oedema as well as any possible abdominal masses or tenderness that may indicate retroperitoneal fibrosis
- cardiac failure as cases of pericardial fibrosis have often manifested as cardiac failure. Constrictive pericarditis should be excluded if such symptoms appear.

Appropriate investigations such as erythrocyte sedimentation rate, chest X-ray and serum creatinine measurements should be performed if necessary to support a diagnosis of a fibrotic disorder. It is also appropriate to perform baseline investigations of erythrocyte sedimentation rate or other inflammatory markers, lung function/chest X-ray and renal function prior to initiation of therapy.

These disorders can have an insidious onset and patients should be regularly and carefully monitored while taking Parlodel for manifestations of progressive fibrotic disorders. Parlodel should be withdrawn if fibrotic or serosal inflammatory changes are diagnosed or suspected.

4.5 Interaction with other medicinal products and other forms of Interaction

Tolerance to Parlodel may be reduced by alcohol.

Caution is required in patients who are on concomitant therapy with, or have recently been treated with drugs that can alter blood pressure.

No data suggests that therapeutic levels of bromocriptine inhibit CYP3A4 to a clinically significant level. However, bromocriptine has been shown to be an inhibitor of CYP3A4 in vitro and caution should be used when co-administering drug substances of this enzyme.

Although there is no conclusive evidence of an interaction between Parlodel and other ergot alkaloids, concomitant use of these medications during the puerperium is not recommended (see also Section 4.4, Special Warnings and Precautions).

The concomitant use of erythromycin, other macrolide antibiotics or octreotide may increase bromocriptine plasma levels.

Dopamine antagonists such as antipsychotics (phenothiazines, butyrophenones and thioxanthenes) may reduce the prolactin-lowering and antiparkinsonian effects of bromocriptine. Metoclopramide and domperidone may reduce the prolactin-lowering effect.

4.6 Pregnancy and lactation

If pregnancy occurs it is generally advisable to withdraw Parlodel after the first missed menstrual period.

Rapid expansion of pituitary tumours sometimes occurs during pregnancy and this may also occur in patients who have been able to conceive as a result of Parlodel therapy. As a precautionary measure, patients should be monitored to detect signs of pituitary enlargement so that Parlodel may be reintroduced if necessary. Based on the outcome of more than 2,000 pregnancies, the use of Parlodel to restore fertility has not been associated with an increased risk of abortion, premature delivery, multiple pregnancy or malformation in infants. Because this accumulated evidence suggests a lack of teratogenic or embryopathic effects in humans, maintenance of Parlodel treatment during pregnancy may be considered where there is a large tumour or evidence of expansion.

Lactation

Since Parlodel inhibits lactation, it should not be administered to mothers who elect to breast-feed.

4.7 Effects on ability to drive and use machines

Hypotensive reactions may be disturbing in some patients during the first few days of treatment and particular care should be exercised when driving vehicles or operating machinery.

Patients being treated with bromocriptine and presenting with somnolence and/or sudden sleep episodes must be advised not to drive or engage in activities where impaired alertness may put themselves or others at risk of serious injury or death (eg. Operating machines) until such recurrent episodes and somnolence have resolved (see also Section 4.4 Special Warnings and Precautions).

4.8 Undesirable effects

The occurrence of side-effects can be minimised by gradual introduction of the dose or a dose reduction followed by a more gradual titration. If necessary, initial nausea and/or vomiting may be reduced by taking Parlodel during a meal and by the intake of a peripheral dopamine antagonist, such as domperidone, for a few days, at least one hour prior to the administration of Parlodel.

Adverse reactions are ranked under headings of frequency, using the following convention:- very common: $\geq 10\,\%$; common: $\geq 1\,\% - < 10\,\%$; uncommon: $\geq 0.1\,\% - < 1\,\%$; rare: $\geq 0.01\,\% - < 0.1\,\%$; very rare: $< 0.01\,\%$

Central Nervous System

Common: Headache, Drowsiness

Uncommon: Dizziness, Dyskinesia

Rare: Somnolence

Very Rare: Excess daytime somnolence and sudden sleep onset

Psychiatric

Uncommon: Confusion, Psychomotor agitation, Hallucinations

Gastrointestinal

Common: Nausea, Constipation

Uncommon: Vomiting

Very Rare: Gastrointestinal bleeding, Gastric ulcer

CardiovascularSystem

Uncommon: Hypotension including orthostatic hypotension (which may in very rare instances lead to collapse)

Rare: Pericardial effusion, Constrictive pericarditis

Very Rare: Reversible pallor of fingers and toes induced by cold (especially in patients who have a history of Raynaud's phenomenon)

RespiratorySystem

Common: Nasal congestion

Uncommon: Dry mouth

Rare: Pleural effusion, pleural and pulmonary fibrosis, pleuritis

Musculoskeletal

Uncommon: Leg cramps

Skin and appendages

Uncommon: Allergic skin reactions, Hair loss

General conditions

Uncommon: Fatigue

Rare: Retroperitoneal fibrosis

Very Rarely: A syndrome resembling Neuroleptic Malignant Syndrome has been reported on withdrawal of Parlodel.

Post-partum women

In extremely rare cases (in postpartum women treated with Parlodel for the prevention of lactation) serious adverse events including hypertension, myocardial infarction, seizures, stroke or mental disorders have been reported, although the causal relationship is uncertain. In some patients the occurrence of seizures or stroke was preceded by severe headache and/or transient visual disturbances.

4.9 Overdose

Overdosage with Parlodel is likely to result in vomiting and other symptoms which could be due to over stimulation of dopaminergic receptors and might include confusion, hallucinations and hypotension. General supportive measures should be undertaken to remove any unabsorbed material and maintain blood pressure if necessary.

Bromocriptine is associated with somnelence and has been associated very rarely with excessive daytime somnelence and sudden sleep onset episodes.

5. PHARMACOLOGICAL PROPERTIES

5.1 Pharmacodynamic properties

Pharmacotherapeutic group: Stimulator of dopamine agonist (ATC code N04B C01), prolactin inhibitor (ATC code G02C B01)

Parlodel, active ingredient bromocriptine, is an inhibitor of prolactin secretion and a stimulator of dopamine receptors. The areas of application of Parlodel are divided into endocrinological and neurological indications. The pharmacological particulars will be discussed under each indication.

Endocrinological indications

Parlodel inhibits the secretion of the anterior pituitary hormone prolactin without affecting normal levels of other pituitary hormones. However, Parlodel is capable of reducing elevated levels of growth hormone (GH) in patients with acromegaly. These effects are due to stimulation of dopamine receptors.

In the puerperium prolactin is necessary for the inhibition and maintenance of puerperal lactation. At other times increased prolactin secretion gives rise to pathological lactation (galactorrhoea) and/or disorders of ovulation and menstruation.

As a specific inhibitor of prolactin secretion, Parlodel can be used to prevent or suppress physiological lactation as well as to treat prolactin-induced pathological states. In amenorrhoea and/or anovulation (with or without galactorrhoea), Parlodel can be used to restore menstrual cycles and ovulation.

The customary measures taken during lactation suppression, such as the restriction of fluid intake are not necessary with Parlodel. In addition, Parlodel does not impair the puerperal involution of the uterus and does not increase the risk of thromboembolism.

Parlodel has been shown to arrest the growth or to reduce the size of prolactin-secreting pituitary adenomas (prolactinomas).

In acromegalic patients - apart from lowering the plasma levels of growth hormone and prolactin - Parlodel has a beneficial effect on clinical symptoms and on glucose tolerance.

Parlodel improves the clinical symptoms of the polycystic ovary syndrome by restoring a normal pattern of LH secretion.

In patients with benign breast disease, Parlodel reduces the size and number of cysts and/or nodules of the breast and alleviates the breast pain often associated with such conditions by normalising the underlying progesterone/oestrogen imbalance. At the same time it reduces prolactin secretion in patients with elevated levels.

Neurological Indications

Because of its dopaminergic activity, Parlodel, in doses usually higher than those for endocrinological indications, is effective in the treatment of Parkinson's Disease, which is characterised by a specific nigrostriatal dopamine deficiency. The stimulation of dopamine receptors by Parlodel can in this condition restore the neurochemical balance within the striatum.

Clinically, Parlodel improves tremor, rigidity, bradykinesia and other Parkinsonian symptoms at all stages of the disease. Usually the therapeutic effect lasts over years (so far, good results have been reported in patients treated up to eight years). Parlodel can be given either alone or - at early as well as advanced stages - combined with other anti-Parkinsonian drugs. Combination with Levodopa treatment results in enhanced anti-Parkinsonian effects, often making possible a reduction of the Levodopa dose. Parlodel offers particular benefit to patients on Levodopa treatment exhibiting a deteriorating therapeutic response or complications such as abnormal involuntary movements (choreoatoid dykinesia and/or painful dystonia), end-of-dose failure, and 'on-off' phenomenon.

Parlodel improves the depressive symptomatology often observed in Parkinsonian patients. This is due to its inherent antidepressant properties as substantiated by controlled studies in non-Parkinsonian patients with endogenous or psychogenic depression.

5.2 Pharmacokinetic properties

Following oral administration, Parlodel (bromocriptine) is rapidly and well absorbed. Peak plasma levels are reached within 1-3 hours. The prolactin-lowering effect occurs 1-2 hours after ingestion, reaches its maximum within about 5 hours and lasts for 8-12 hours.

The substance is extensively metabolised in the liver. The elimination of parent drug from plasma occurs biphasically, with a terminal half-life of about 15 hours. Parent drug and metabolites are almost completely excreted via the liver, with only 6% being eliminated via the kidney. Plasma protein-binding amounts to 96%.

There is no evidence that the pharmacokinetic properties and tolerability of Parlodel are directly affected by advanced age. However, in patients with impaired hepatic function, the speed of elimination may be retarded and plasma levels may increase, requiring dose adjustment.

5.3 Preclinical safety data

There are no other clinically relevant preclinical safety data in addition to those mentioned in other sections of the SmPC.

6. PHARMACEUTICAL PARTICULARS

6.1 List of excipients

Parlodel Tablets 1mg

Aerosil 200 (Standard) Ph. Eur., Disodium edetate BP, Magnesium stearate Ph. Eur., Maleic acid Ph.Eur., Maize starch Ph. Eur., Lactose Ph. Eur.

Parlodel Tablets 2.5mg

Aerosil 200 (Standard) Ph. Eur., Disodium edetate BP, Magnesium stearate Ph. Eur., Maleic acid Ph.Eur., Maize starch Ph. Eur., Lactose Ph. Eur.

6.2 Incompatibilities

None.

6.3 Shelf life

Parlodel Tablets 1mg

Opaque white PVC/PVDC blister strip: 24 months

Amber glass bottles: 24 months

Parlodel Tablets 2.5mg

Opaque white PVC/PVDC blister strip: 36 months

Amber glass bottles: 60 months

6.4 Special precautions for storage

Parlodel Tablets 1mg

Store below 25°C in a dry place. Protect from light.

Parlodel Tablets 2.5mg

Protect from direct light.

6.5 Nature and contents of container

Parlodel Tablets 1mg

Opaque white PVC/PVDC blister strip containing 100 Parlodel 1mg tablets.

Amber glass bottles with a CRC closure containing 30 and 100 Parlodel 1mg tablets.

Parlodel Tablets 2.5mg

Opaque white PVC/PVDC blister strip containing 30 Parlodel 2.5mg tablets.

Amber glass bottles with a CRC closure containing 100 and 500 Parlodel 2.5mg tablets.

6.6 Instructions for use and handling

None.

7. MARKETING AUTHORISATION HOLDER

Novartis Pharmaceuticals UK Limited

Trading as: Sandoz Pharmaceuticals

Frimley Business Park

Frimley

Camberley

Surrey

GU16 7SR

8. MARKETING AUTHORISATION NUMBER(S)

Parlodel Tablets 1mg 00101/0176

Parlodel Tablets 2.5mg 00101/0061

9. DATE OF FIRST AUTHORISATION/RENEWAL OF THE AUTHORISATION

Parlodel Tablets 1mg 11 June 1984 / 29 January 1999

Parlodel Tablets 2.5mg 14 January 1976 / 21 April 1998

10. DATE OF REVISION OF THE TEXT

27 July 2004

Legal Category

POM

Paroven Capsules

(Novartis Consumer Health)

1. NAME OF THE MEDICINAL PRODUCT

Paroven capsules 250 mg

2. QUALITATIVE AND QUANTITATIVE COMPOSITION

Active ingredient: Oxerutins 250 mg

3. PHARMACEUTICAL FORM

Capsules

4. CLINICAL PARTICULARS

4.1 Therapeutic indications

Relief of symptoms of oedema associated with chronic venous insufficiency.

4.2 Posology and method of administration

Adults and elderly: 2 capsules (500 mg) twice daily.

Children: not recommended for children under 12 years

4.3 Contraindications

Hypersensitivity to any of the ingredients.

4.4 Special warnings and special precautions for use

Treatment of leg oedema due to cardiac, renal or hepatic disease should be directed to the underlying cause; Paroven should not be used in these conditions. If leg pain and swelling do not improve, or get worse, the patient should consult their doctor.

4.5 Interaction with other medicinal products and other forms of Interaction

None reported. Oxerutins have been shown not to interact with warfarin anticoagulants.

4.6 Pregnancy and lactation

Clinical trials and animal studies have shown no increase in teratogenic (or other) hazard to the foetus if used in the recommended dosage during pregnancy. However, in keeping with current medical opinion, Paroven should not be used during the first trimester of pregnancy. In animal studies traces of oxerutins and/or their metabolites have been found in breast milk, but the levels are not considered to be of clinical relevance. The use of Paroven in lactating women is therefore at the physician's discretion.

4.7 Effects on ability to drive and use machines

None known.

4.8 Undesirable effects

Occasionally, mild adverse reactions (skin allergies, minor gastrointestinal disturbances, headaches and flushes) have been reported. They disappear rapidly on stopping treatment.

4.9 Overdose

No cases of overdosage with symptoms have been reported. No specific antidotes are known.

5. PHARMACOLOGICAL PROPERTIES

5.1 Pharmacodynamic properties

Oxerutins has uniquely useful therapeutic actions in the microcirculation and particularly in the post-capillary venous segment. Oxerutins reduces capillary leakage and hence oedema formation.

5.2 Pharmacokinetic properties

Not all conventional pharmacokinetic parameters are available due to technical difficulties. Oxerutins is absorbed from the gastrointestinal tract of mammals. Its metabolism is, in part, determined by the degree of hydroxyethylation of the aromatic ring systems of the constituent rutoside derivatives. Biliary excretion plays a major role in elimination in the animal species studied. It is, however, not clear if this route of elimination is equally important in man since quantitative data in humans are not available.

The same applies to entero-hepatic recycling.

5.3 Preclinical safety data

Not applicable.

6. PHARMACEUTICAL PARTICULARS

6.1 List of excipients

Polyethylene glycol

Gelatin

Titanium dioxide

Iron oxides

6.2 Incompatibilities

None.

6.3 Shelf life

60 months.

6.4 Special precautions for storage

Protect from moisture.

6.5 Nature and contents of container

Blister pack composed of PVC blisters sealed with aluminium foil.

Pack sizes: 120 capsules.

6.6 Instructions for use and handling

Medicines should be kept out of the reach of children.

7. MARKETING AUTHORISATION HOLDER

Novartis Consumer Health UK Ltd

Trading as Novartis Consumer Health

Wimblehurst Road

Horsham

West Sussex

RH12 5AB

UK

8. MARKETING AUTHORISATION NUMBER(S)

PL 0030/5002R

9. DATE OF FIRST AUTHORISATION/RENEWAL OF THE AUTHORISATION

19 July 1991

10. DATE OF REVISION OF THE TEXT

July 1997

Additional information

Legal category: P

Parvolex Injection

(UCB Pharma Limited)

1. NAME OF THE MEDICINAL PRODUCT

Parvolex Solution for Infusion.

2. QUALITATIVE AND QUANTITATIVE COMPOSITION

Acetylcysteine 200mg/ml.

For excipients, see 6.1.

3. PHARMACEUTICAL FORM

Solution for infusion.

4. CLINICAL PARTICULARS

4.1 Therapeutic indications

For the treatment of paracetamol overdosage.

4.2 Posology and method of administration

The injection is administered by intravenous infusion. The following infusion fluids may be used: 5% dextrose, 0.9% sodium chloride, 0.3% potassium chloride with 5% glucose, or 0.3% potassium chloride with 0.9% sodium chloride.

Adults:

An initial dose of 150mg/kg body weight of acetylcysteine is infused in 200ml of the recommended infusion fluid over 15 minutes, followed by 50mg/kg in 500ml infusion fluid over the next 4 hours, then 100mg/kg in 1 litre infusion fluid over the next 16 hours. (This gives a total dose of 300mg/kg in 20 hours.)

Children:

Children should be treated with the same doses and regimen as adults; however, the quantity of intravenous fluid used should be modified to take into account age and weight, as fluid overload is a potential danger. The National Poisons Centres in the UK have provided the following guidance:

Children weighing 20kg or more:

150mg/kg intravenous infusion in 100ml infusion fluid over 15 minutes; then 50mg/kg in 250ml infusion fluid over 4 hours; then 100mg/kg in 500ml infusion fluid over 16 hours.

Children under 20kg:

Volumes for infusion of the above doses are the responsibility of the prescriber and should be based on the daily maintenance requirements of the child by weight.

Critical times:

Acetylcysteine (Parvolex®) is very effective in preventing paracetamol-induced hepatotoxicity when administered during the first 8 hours after a paracetamol overdose. When administered after the first 8 hours, the protective effect diminishes progressively as the overdose-treatment interval increases. However, clinical experience indicates that acetylcysteine can still be of benefit when administered up to 24 hours after paracetamol overdose, without any change in its safety profile. It may also be administered after 24 hours in patients at risk of severe liver damage. In general, for patients presenting later than 24 hours after a paracetamol overdose, guidance should be sought from a National Poisons Centre.

Treatment 'nomogram':

Plasma paracetamol concentration in relation to time after the overdose is commonly used to determine whether a patient is at risk of hepatotoxicity and should, therefore, receive treatment with an antidote such as acetylcysteine.

For the majority of otherwise healthy patients, a line joining points of 200mg/l at 4 hours and 30mg/l at 15 hours on a semilogarithmic plot is used. (Treatment line A - see graph.) This line can be extended to 24 hours after overdose, based on a paracetamol half-life of 4 hours. It is recommended that patients whose plasma paracetamol concentrations fall on or above this line receive acetylcysteine. If there is doubt about the timing of the overdose, consideration should be given to treatment with acetylcysteine.

Patients with induced hepatic microsomal oxidase enzymes (such as chronic alcoholics and patients taking anticonvulsant drugs) are susceptible to paracetamol-induced hepatotoxicity at lower plasma paracetamol concentrations (see section 4.4 - Special Warnings and Precautions for Use) and should be assessed against treatment line B (see graph).

In patients who have taken staggered overdoses, blood levels are meaningless in relation to the treatment graph. These patients should all be considered for treatment with acetylcysteine.

NB: Blood samples taken less than 4 hours after a paracetamol overdose give unreliable estimates of the serum paracetamol concentration.

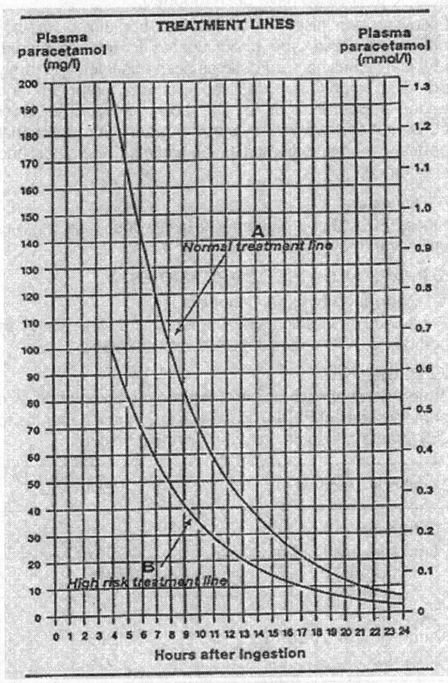

Plasma paracetamol concentrations in relation to time after overdosage as a guide to prognosis.

From guidelines agreed by National Poisons Centres - June 1995.

Parvolex is indicated in patients with values on or above the appropriate treatment line.

4.3 Contraindications

Hypersensitivity to any ingredient in the preparation.

4.4 Special warnings and special precautions for use

Precautions:

Administer with caution in patients with asthma or a history of bronchospasm.

Liver enzyme-inducing drugs; chronic alcohol abuse:

Patients taking drugs that induce liver enzymes, such as some anticonvulsant drugs (e.g. phenytoin, phenobarbitone, primidone and carbamazepam) and rifampicin, and patients who routinely consume alcohol above recommended levels are believed to be at risk of hepatotoxicity from paracetamol poisoning at lower plasma paracetamol concentrations than other patients. It is recommended that such patients whose plasma paracetamol concentrations fall on or above a treatment line joining 100mg/l at 4 hours after overdose and 15mg/l at 15 hours after overdose on a semilogarithmic plot (i.e. treatment line B - see graph), be given acetylcysteine.

Other patients predisposed to toxicity:

Patients suffering from malnutrition, for example, patients with anorexia or AIDS, may have depleted glutathione reserves. It has been recommended that paracetamol overdose in such patients be treated as for chronic alcohol consumers or patients taking anticonvulsant drugs (treatment line B - see graph).

4.5 Interaction with other medicinal products and other forms of Interaction

There are no known interactions.

4.6 Pregnancy and lactation

The safety of acetylcysteine in pregnancy has not been investigated in formal prospective clinical trials. However, clinical experience indicates that use of acetylcysteine in pregnancy for the treatment of paracetamol overdose is effective. Prior to use in pregnancy, the potential risks should be balanced against the potential benefits.

4.7 Effects on ability to drive and use machines

There are no known effects on ability to drive and use machines.

4.8 Undesirable effects

'Anaphylactoid' or 'hypersensitivity-like' reactions have been reported. They include nausea/vomiting, injection-site reactions, flushing, itching, rashes/urticaria, angioedema, bronchospasm/respiratory distress, hypotension, and rarely, tachycardia or hypertension. These have usually occurred between 15 and 60 minutes after the start of infusion. In many cases, symptoms have been relieved by stopping the infusion. Occasionally, an antihistamine drug may be necessary. Corticosteroids may occasionally be required. Once an anaphylactoid reaction is under control, the infusion can normally be restarted at the lowest infusion rate (100mg/kg in 1 litre over 16 hours).

In rare instances, the following side-effects have occurred: coughing, chest tightness or pain, puffy eyes, sweating, malaise, raised temperature, vasodilation, blurred vision, bradycardia, facial or eye pain, syncope, acidosis, thrombocytopenia, respiratory or cardiac arrest, stridor, anxiety, extravasation, arthropathy, arthralgia, deterioration of liver function, generalised seizure, cyanosis, lowered blood urea. Rare instances of fatality have also occurred.

Hypokalaemia and ECG changes have been noted in patients with paracetamol poisoning irrespective of the treatment given. Monitoring of plasma potassium concentration is, therefore, recommended.

If any side-effects to Parvolex® (acetylcysteine) develop, advice should be sought from a National Poisons Centre to ensure that the patients receives adequate treatment of the paracetamol overdose.

4.9 Overdose

There is a theoretical risk of hepatic encephalopathy. Overdosage of acetylcysteine has been reported to be associated with effects similar to the 'anaphylactoid' reactions noted in section 4.8 (Undesirable Effects), but they may be more severe. General supportive measures should be carried out. Such reactions are managed with antihistamines and steroids in the usual way. There is no specific antidote.

5. PHARMACOLOGICAL PROPERTIES

5.1 Pharmacodynamic properties

Acetylcysteine is considered to reduce the hepatic toxicity of NAPQI (n-acetyl-p-benzo-quinoneimine), the highly reactive intermediate metabolite following ingestion of a high dose of paracetamol, by at least two mechanisms. First, acetylcysteine acts as a precursor for the synthesis of glutathione and, therefore, maintains cellular glutathione at a level sufficient to inactivate NAPQI. This is thought to be the main mechanism by which acetylcysteine acts in the early stages of paracetamol toxicity.

Acetylcysteine has been shown to still be effective when infusion is started at up to 12 hours after paracetamol ingestion, when most of the analgesic will have been metabolised to its reactive metabolite. At this stage, acetylcysteine is thought to act by reducing oxidised thiol groups in key enzymes.

When acetylcysteine treatment is begun more than 8 to 10 hours after paracetamol overdose, its efficacy in preventing hepatotoxicity (based on serum indicators) declines progressively with further lengthening of the overdose-treatment interval (the time between paracetamol overdose and start of treatment). However, there is now evidence that it can still be beneficial when given up to 24 hours after overdose. At this late stage of paracetamol hepatotoxicity, acetylcysteine's beneficial effects may be due to its ability to improve systematic haemodynamics and oxygen transport, although the mechanism by which this may occur has yet to be determined.

5.2 Pharmacokinetic properties

Following intravenous administration of acetylcysteine using the standard 20-hour intravenous regimen, plasma levels of 300 to 900mg/l have been reported to occur shortly after the start of the infusion, falling to 11 to 90mg/l at the end of the infusion period. Elimination half-lives of 2 to 6 hours have been reported after intravenous dosing, with 20 to 30% of the administered dose being recovered unchanged in the urine.

Metabolism appears to be rapid and extensive. There is no information on whether acetylcysteine crosses the blood-brain barrier or the placenta, or whether it is excreted in breast milk.

5.3 Preclinical safety data

None stated.

6. PHARMACEUTICAL PARTICULARS

6.1 List of excipients

Disodium Edetate

Sodium Hydroxide

Water for Injections

6.2 Incompatibilities

Acetylcysteine is not compatible with rubber or metals, particularly iron, copper and nickel. Silicone rubber and plastic are satisfactory for use with Parvolex®.

A change in the colour of the solution to light purple has sometimes been noted and is not thought to indicate significant impairment of safety or efficacy.

6.3 Shelf life

3 years.

6.4 Special precautions for storage

Store below 25°C.

6.5 Nature and contents of container

Clear, Type I glass, 10ml snap ring ampoules. 10 × 10ml ampoules are packed in cartons.

6.6 Instructions for use and handling

Acetylcysteine to be diluted for intravenous infusion using either 5% dextrose, 0.9% sodium chloride, 0.3% potassium chloride with 5% glucose, or 0.3% potassium chloride with 0.9% sodium chloride. The volumes to be used are as directed in section 4.2.

7. MARKETING AUTHORISATION HOLDER

UCB Pharma Limited

208 Bath Road

Slough

Berkshire

SL1 3WE

UK

8. MARKETING AUTHORISATION NUMBER(S)

PL 00039/0410

9. DATE OF FIRST AUTHORISATION/RENEWAL OF THE AUTHORISATION

14 October 1992, 31 October 1997, June 2002

10. DATE OF REVISION OF THE TEXT

June 2005

11. Legal Category

POM

PEDIACEL

(Sanofi Pasteur MSD)

1. NAME OF THE MEDICINAL PRODUCT

PEDIACEL®▼

Suspension for Injection

Diphtheria, tetanus, five component acellular pertussis, inactivated poliomyelitis and *Haemophilus influenzae* type b conjugate vaccine (adsorbed).

2. QUALITATIVE AND QUANTITATIVE COMPOSITION

Each 0.5 millilitre dose contains:

Purified diphtheria toxoid	not less than 30 international units* (15 Lf)
Purified tetanus toxoid	not less than 40 international units* (5 Lf)
Purified pertussis toxoid (PT)	20 micrograms
Purified filamentous haemagglutinin (FHA)	20 micrograms
Purified fimbrial agglutinogens 2 and 3 (FIM)	5 micrograms
Purified pertactin (PRN)	3 micrograms
Inactivated type 1 poliovirus (Mahoney)	40 D antigen units**
Inactivated type 2 poliovirus (MEF-1)	8 D antigen units**
Inactivated type 3 poliovirus (Saukett)	32 D antigen units**
Haemophilus influenzae type b polysaccharide	
(polyribosylribitol phosphate)	10 micrograms
conjugated to tetanus toxoid (PRP-T)	20 micrograms

For excipients, see 6.1.

*As lower confidence limit (p=0.95) of activity measured according to the assay described in the European Pharmacopoeia

**or equivalent antigenic quantity determined by a suitable immunochemical method.

Active components of the vaccine are inactivated with either formaldehyde or glutaraldehyde.

Inactivated poliovirus components are produced using the Vero cell line.

3. PHARMACEUTICAL FORM

Suspension for injection in a vial.

4. CLINICAL PARTICULARS

4.1 Therapeutic indications

PEDIACEL® is indicated for use as a three dose regimen for the active immunisation of infants against diphtheria, tetanus, pertussis, poliomyelitis and invasive infections caused by *Haemophilus influenzae* type b.

PEDIACEL® may also be administered as a single dose in the second year of life to children who have previously completed a primary immunisation series with diphtheria, tetanus, pertussis, polio and Hib antigens (see sections 4.8 and 5.1) if this is in accordance with the national recommendations.

4.2 Posology and method of administration

Primary Immunisation Series in Infancy

The primary immunisation series in infancy, consisting of three doses of PEDIACEL®, may be commenced from two months of age according to national recommendations. A single 0.5 millilitre dose should be given on three separate occasions with at least one month between doses.

There are no data regarding the administration of PEDIACEL® for one or two doses and use of different vaccine(s) for other dose(s). Therefore, it is recommended that infants who receive PEDIACEL® for the first dose should also receive this vaccine for the second and third doses of the primary immunisation series.

Booster Dose

After completion of the primary series, a booster dose of Hib conjugate vaccine should be administered. The timing of this Hib conjugate booster dose should be in accordance with official recommendations.

A single 0.5 millilitre dose of PEDIACEL® may be used to provide the Hib booster dose if it is officially recommended to boost responses to all other antigens in the vaccine at the same time.

Based on safety and immunogenicity data from clinical studies, PEDIACEL® should preferably be given to children who received this same vaccine in infancy. However, if necessary, PEDIACEL® may be given at this age to children who received other vaccines in infancy.

PEDIACEL® should not be administered to children after reaching the fourth birthday.

Method of Administration

PEDIACEL® should be administered intramuscularly. The recommended injection sites are the anterolateral aspect of the thigh in infants and the deltoid region in older children.

4.3 Contraindications

PEDIACEL® should not be given to children who:

- Are known to be hypersensitive to any component of the vaccine (including neomycin, streptomycin and polymyxin B which may be present in trace amounts).

- Have had a previous severe local or general reaction to this vaccine or to any other vaccine that contains one or more of the antigenic components.

- Have experienced encephalopathy, not due to another identifiable cause, within 7 days of administration of a previous dose of any vaccine containing pertussis antigens (whole cell or acellular). Encephalopathy refers to a severe acute neurological illness with prolonged seizures and/or unconsciousness and/or focal neurological signs. In these circumstances the vaccination course should be continued with vaccines not containing a pertussis component.

- Have a fever or acute severe systemic illness. In this case vaccination should be postponed until the child has recovered. Minor infections without fever or systemic upset are not reasons to postpone vaccination.

4.4 Special warnings and special precautions for use

As with all vaccines, appropriate facilities and medication such as epinephrine (adrenaline) should be readily available for immediate use in case of anaphylaxis or hypersensitivity following injection.

If any of the following events are known to have occurred in temporal relation to a previous dose of a pertussis-containing vaccine, the decision to give further doses of pertussis-containing vaccines should be carefully considered:

- Temperature of ⩾40°C within 48 hours, not due to another identifiable cause.

- Hypotonic hyporesponsive episode (HHE): a syndrome characterised by acute diminution of sensory awareness or loss of consciousness, accompanied by pallor and muscle hypotonicity. The onset is usually 1-12 hours after vaccination and the episode may last from a few minutes up to 36 hours. Recovery is complete with no persistent sequelae.

- Persistent, inconsolable crying lasting more than 3 hours occurring within 48 hours of vaccination.

- Convulsions with or without fever occurring within 3 days of vaccination.

In children with a progressive, evolving or unstable neurological condition (including seizures), immunisation should be deferred until the condition is corrected or stable.

The immunogenicity of the vaccine may be reduced by immunosuppressive treatment or immunodeficiency. It is recommended to postpone vaccination until the end of such treatment or the resolution of disease. Nevertheless, vaccination of subjects with chronic immunodeficiency (such as those with HIV infection or on long-term immunosuppressive therapy) is recommended even though the immunological response may be impaired and the degree of protection may be limited.

Intramuscular injections should be given with care in patients with thrombocytopenia or bleeding disorders due to the risk of haemorrhage.

The vaccine should be given intramuscularly since subcutaneous administration increases the chances of an injection site reaction. Do not administer by intradermal or intravenous injection.

PEDIACEL® does not protect against infectious diseases caused by *Haemophilus influenzae* other than type b, or against meningitis caused by other organisms.

As with any vaccine, immunisation with PEDIACEL® may not protect all recipients from the infections that it is intended to prevent.

National recommendations for childhood immunisations should be consulted before administering this vaccine to children in or after the second year of life since this exact combination of antigens may not be considered appropriate and/or necessary after completion of the infant immunisation series.

4.5 Interaction with other medicinal products and other forms of Interaction

PEDIACEL® may be administered at the same time as, but as a separate injection to, meningococcal group C conjugate vaccines or hepatitis B vaccines. Injections should be made into separate sites and, preferably, into separate limbs.

Antibody responses to the Hib component of PEDIACEL® (PRP conjugated to tetanus toxoid; see section 2) were lower when a meningococcal group C CRM_{197} conjugate vaccine was co-administered as a separate injection than when a meningococcal group C tetanus toxoid conjugate vaccine was co-administered as a separate injection at 2, 3 and 4 months of age (see section 5.1). The clinical significance of these observations is unknown but the findings relating to meningococcal group C CRM_{197} conjugate vaccine may have implications for the timing of and need for a Hib conjugate booster dose.

The type of meningococcal conjugate vaccine that is co-administered may also affect responses to the diphtheria and tetanus components of PEDIACEL®. Anti-diphtheria responses were higher when a meningococcal group C CRM_{197} conjugate was co-administered with PEDIACEL® and anti-tetanus responses were higher when a meningococcal group C tetanus toxoid conjugate was co-administered. However, responses to both these antigens were satisfactory regardless of the type of meningococcal group C conjugate that was given (see section 5.1).

PEDIACEL® did not affect the proportions of infants with meningococcal group C serum bactericidal antibody (SBA) titres of at least 1:8 (measured with rabbit complement) when co-administered with either a CRM_{197} conjugate or a tetanus toxoid conjugate vaccine. However, the SBA geometric mean titres (GMTs) were numerically lower after co-administration with PEDIACEL® than were seen when these same meningococcal group C conjugate vaccines were co-administered with a whole cell pertussis (as DTwP) vaccine. Also, the SBA GMT when PEDIACEL® was co-administered with a meningococcal group C tetanus toxoid conjugate vaccine was significantly lower than that seen after co-administration with a CRM_{197} conjugate (see section 5.1). However, the clinical significance of the lower SBA GMTs is unknown.

There are no data on immune responses to hepatitis B vaccines when co-administered with PEDIACEL®. However, there are no safety concerns regarding co-administration.

Except for immunosuppressive therapy (see 4.4), no significant interaction with other treatments or biological products is anticipated.

4.6 Pregnancy and lactation

As PEDIACEL® is not intended for use in adults, or in children above the age of 4 years, information on the safety of the vaccine when used in pregnancy or lactation is not available.

4.7 Effects on ability to drive and use machines

Not applicable. This vaccine is intended for paediatric use.

4.8 Undesirable effects

In controlled clinical studies performed with PEDIACEL®, 71% of 451 infants immunised at 2, 4 and 6 months experienced a reaction (pain, erythema or oedema) at the injection site within the first 24 hours after vaccination. In 16% of infants the reaction was of moderate to severe intensity. Also, 64% of infants experienced a systemic reaction, which was of moderate to severe intensity in 16%.

There was a trend for an increased frequency of injection site reactions when a fourth dose of PEDIACEL® was given to 401 children in the second year of life. Pain was reported in 33%, erythema in 23% and oedema in 16% compared to rates of 18%, 11% and 11%, respectively, during the primary series. The frequency of systemic reactions was similar whether PEDIACEL® was administered in infancy or in the second year of life.

The reactions observed were as follows:

<u>Nervous system disorders</u>

Rare (0.01-0.1%):	Febrile convulsions.
	Hypotonic hyporesponsive episodes (HHE) (see section 4.4).

<u>Gastrointestinal disorders</u>

Common (1-10%):	Anorexia, diarrhoea and vomiting.

<u>General disorders and administration site conditions</u>

Very common (>10%):	Pain, erythema and oedema at the injection site.
	Irritability, malaise, increased crying and fever.
Very rare (<0.01%):	High fever (>40.5°C).
	Unusual high-pitched or inconsolable crying.
	Painless circumferential limb swelling following booster doses which resolve spontaneously.

In a controlled clinical study of PEDIACEL®, administered concomitantly with meningococcal group C conjugate vaccine, 71% of 121 infants immunised at 2, 3 and 4 months experienced a reaction (pain, erythema or oedema) at the PEDIACEL® injection site within the first seven days after vaccination. Also, 92% of infants experienced a systemic reaction within the first seven days after vaccination. The rates of moderate to severe reactions were similar to those described at 2, 4 and 6 months.

Acute allergic reactions have been reported after diphtheria, tetanus and/or pertussis vaccines. Manifestations include dyspnoea, cyanosis, urticaria, angioneurotic oedema, hypotension and, rarely, anaphylaxis.

A persistent nodule at the site of vaccination may occur with all adsorbed vaccines, particularly if administered into the superficial layers of the subcutaneous tissue. Rarely aseptic abscesses have been reported.

Following administration of vaccines containing *Haemophilus influenzae* type b conjugated to tetanus toxoid, atypical rashes have sometimes been observed and rarely urticarial eruptions, localised oedema, pruritus and oedematous reactions of the lower limbs. The latter consist of oedema with cyanosis or transient purpura that appears soon after immunisation and resolves rapidly and spontaneously.

4.9 Overdose

Since PEDIACEL® is presented in single dose vials, it is very unlikely that overdose might occur.

5. PHARMACOLOGICAL PROPERTIES

5.1 Pharmacodynamic properties

Therapeutic classification: Bacterial and viral vaccines combined, ATC codes J07CA02 and J07AG01.

<u>Immunogenicity</u>

Antibody responses at one month after completion of a primary series of PEDIACEL® given at 2, 4 and 6 months to 339 infants are summarised in the table below.

Antibody response	PEDIACEL®
Diphtheria	
Antitoxin ⩾0.01 IU/mL	100%
⩾0.1 IU/mL	79%
Tetanus	
Antitoxin ⩾0.01 EU/mL	100%
⩾0.1 EU/mL	99%
Pertussis†	
PT GMT (EU/mL)	87
FHA GMT (EU/mL)	155
Pertactin GMT (EU/mL)	55
Fimbriae GMT (EU/mL)	277
Poliomyelitis	
Type 1 antibody titre ⩾1:8	100%
Type 2 antibody titre ⩾1:8	100%
Type 3 antibody titre ⩾1:8	100%
Haemophilus influenzae type b‡	
Anti-PRP ⩾0.15 μg/mL	98%
Anti-PRP ⩾1.0 μg/mL	89%

†GMT Geometric mean titre; PT Pertussis toxoid; FHA Filamentous haemagglutinin

‡PRP Polyribosyl Ribitol Phosphate

Antibody responses were also assessed one month after completion of a primary series of PEDIACEL®, administered concomitantly with meningococcal group C conjugate vaccine, given at 2, 3 and 4 months to 121 infants. Serological responses were generally similar to those summarised above and to those seen in the comparator group who received diphtheria, tetanus, whole cell pertussis and PRP-T Hib combination vaccine and oral polio vaccine. These data are summarised in the table below.

(see Table 1 on next page)

Concomitant administration of meningococcal group C conjugate vaccine influenced the response to the PRP-T Hib component of PEDIACEL®, dependent upon the type of conjugate protein. The Hib response in infants who received PEDIACEL® and concomitant meningococcal group C tetanus conjugate vaccine was comparable to that observed in the whole cell pertussis comparator group. The mean anti-PRP antibody levels were 3.67 μg/mL and 4.01 μg/mL, respectively, with 98.1% and 100% achieving a level ⩾0.15 μg/mL. However, Hib antibody levels were lower in infants who received PEDIACEL® and a concomitant meningococcal group C CRM_{197} conjugate vaccine (mean anti-PRP antibody level of 1.26 μg/mL with 88.0% achieving a level ⩾0.15 μg/mL). Hib antibody levels were also lower in infants who received the whole cell pertussis comparator and concomitant meningococcal group C CRM_{197} conjugate vaccine (mean anti-PRP antibody level of 2.57 μg/mL) compared to those who received concomitant meningococcal group C tetanus conjugate vaccine (GMT 4.01 μg/mL).

The type of meningococcal conjugate vaccine also affected responses to the diphtheria and tetanus components of PEDIACEL®. Anti-diphtheria responses were higher when a meningococcal group C CRM_{197} conjugate was co-administered with PEDIACEL® and anti-tetanus responses were higher when a meningococcal group C tetanus toxoid conjugate was co-administered. However, responses to both these antigens were satisfactory regardless of the type of meningococcal group C conjugate that was given.

Table 1

Antibody response	PEDIACEL® + MCC-T†	PEDIACEL® + MCC-CRM$_{197}$‡	DTwP//Hib§ + OPV + MCC-T	DTwP//Hib + OPV + MCC-CRM$_{197}$
Diphtheria				
Antitoxin ⩾0.01 IU/mL	98%	100%	96%	98%
⩾0.1 IU/mL	13%	38%	19%	21%
Tetanus				
Antitoxin ⩾0.01 EU/mL	100%	100%	100%	100%
⩾0.1 EU/mL	100%	98%	100%	100%
Pertussis				
PT GMT (EU/mL)	75	83	104	94
FHA GMT (EU/mL)	53	51	28	24
Pertactin GMT (EU/mL)	32	33	81	59
Fimbriae GMT (EU/mL)	260	300	633	555
Poliomyelitis				
Type 1 ⩾1:8	100%	100%	100%	100%
Type 2 ⩾1:8	100%	100%	100%	100%
Type 3 ⩾1:8	98%	98%	98%	100%
***Haemophilus influenzae* type b**				
Anti-PRP ⩾0.15 μg/mL	98%	88%	100%	100%
Anti-PRP ⩾1.0 μg/mL	83%	62%	88%	77%
GMT (μg/mL)	3.67	1.26	4.01	2.57
Group C meningococcus				
SBA ⩾1:8	98%	100%	100%	100%
GMT	690	2165	3816	2674

† Meningococcal group C tetanus toxoid conjugate vaccine
‡ Meningococcal group C CRM$_{197}$ conjugate vaccine
§ Vaccine studied was Act-HIB® DTP

Concomitant administration of PEDIACEL® and meningococcal group C conjugate vaccine also influenced the meningococcal group C SBA GMTs, dependent upon the type of conjugate protein. However, the seroprotection rates were unaffected, remaining at 98-100%. The antibody levels in infants who received PEDIACEL® and concomitant meningococcal group C CRM$_{197}$ conjugate vaccine were comparable to those observed in the whole cell pertussis comparator group. Meningococcal group C antibody levels were lower in infants receiving PEDIACEL® and concomitant meningococcal group C tetanus conjugate vaccine compared to those receiving PEDIACEL® and concomitant meningococcal group C CRM$_{197}$ conjugate vaccine (SBA GMTs of 690 and 2165 respectively).

When PEDIACEL® was administered to children in the second year of life who had completed a primary immunisation series with all antigens, an anamnestic response was observed for all antigens. The interval between the completion of the primary series and the booster was not less than 10 months.

Efficacy

The efficacy of the acellular pertussis component of PEDIACEL® was assessed when given in combination with the diphtheria and tetanus toxoids to more than 18,000 Swedish infants at 3, 5 and 12 months. The relative risk for typical pertussis compared with a whole cell DTP vaccine was 0.85, and the relative risk for any pertussis was 1.4.

Immunogenicity data were obtained from 80 out of another 2,500 infants who were given the acellular pertussis component of PEDIACEL® at 2, 4 and 6 months in this study, and were compared with data from 58 infants immunised at 3, 5 and 12 months. The GMTs at one month after the third dose of each regimen were generally comparable for antibody to each of PT, FHA, pertactin and fimbrial agglutinogens.

GMTs seen in response to pertussis components in the same amounts as in PEDIACEL® were also found to be generally comparable with those recorded in a previous Swedish study, in which the same antigens (but with a lower dose of PT and FHA) were shown to be efficacious.

These data have also been compared with GMTs obtained after administration of three doses of PEDIACEL® to Canadian infants at 2, 4 and 6 months and found to be of the same order. Therefore, an extrapolation from the efficacy of the pertussis component in the Swedish trials appears to be supported.

5.2 Pharmacokinetic properties

Not applicable.

5.3 Preclinical safety data

Limited pre-clinical testing of PEDIACEL® and closely related products, mainly single dose rodent toxicity studies, revealed no special hazards for human health in addition to those identified in controlled clinical trials.

6. PHARMACEUTICAL PARTICULARS

6.1 List of excipients

Aluminium phosphate

2-phenoxyethanol

Polysorbate 80

Water for Injections

6.2 Incompatibilities

The vaccine should not be mixed with other vaccines or parenterally administered substances.

6.3 Shelf life

48 months.

6.4 Special precautions for storage

Store between +2°C and +8°C. Do not freeze; vaccine which has been frozen must not be used.

6.5 Nature and contents of container

PEDIACEL® is supplied in a Type I (Ph. Eur.) glass tubing vial with bromobutyl stopper (latex free).

Available in unit packs of one vial or packs of 10 vials.

Not all pack sizes may be marketed.

6.6 Instructions for use and handling

The vaccine should be used as supplied; no dilution or reconstitution is necessary.

Shake well immediately before use. The vaccine is a cloudy suspension.

Parenteral drug products should be inspected visually for extraneous particulate matter and discolouration prior to administration.

It is important to use a separate sterile syringe and needle for each individual to prevent transmission of infections from one person to another.

7. MARKETING AUTHORISATION HOLDER

Sanofi Pasteur MSD Limited

Mallards Reach

Bridge Avenue

Maidenhead

Berkshire

SL6 1QP

8. MARKETING AUTHORISATION NUMBER(S)

PL 06745/0120

9. DATE OF FIRST AUTHORISATION/RENEWAL OF THE AUTHORISATION

16 October 2002

10. DATE OF REVISION OF THE TEXT

May 2005

Pegasys 135 PFS

(Roche Products Limited)

1. NAME OF THE MEDICINAL PRODUCT

Pegasys®▼ 135 micrograms solution for injection in pre-filled syringe

2. QUALITATIVE AND QUANTITATIVE COMPOSITION

One pre-filled syringe contains

peginterferon alfa-2a*............................ 135 micrograms

in 0.5 ml of solution

* recombinant interferon alfa-2a produced by genetic engineering from *Escherichia coli* conjugated to bis-[monomethoxy polyethylene glycol] of a molecular mass, M_n, of 40 000.

For excipients, see section 6.1.

3. PHARMACEUTICAL FORM

Solution for injection in pre-filled syringe.

The solution is clear and colourless to light yellow.

4. CLINICAL PARTICULARS

4.1 Therapeutic indications

Chronic hepatitis B:

Pegasys is indicated for the treatment of HBeAg-positive or HBeAg-negative chronic hepatitis B in adult patients with compensated liver disease and evidence of viral replication, increased ALT and histologically verified liver inflammation and/or fibrosis (see 4.4 and 5.1).

Chronic hepatitis C:

Pegasys is indicated for the treatment of chronic hepatitis C in adult patients who are positive for serum HCV-RNA, including patients with compensated cirrhosis and/or co-infected with clinically stable HIV (see 4.4).

The optimal way to use Pegasys in patients with chronic hepatitis C is in combination with ribavirin. This combination is indicated in previously untreated patients as well as in patients who have previously responded to interferon alpha therapy and subsequently relapsed after treatment was stopped.

Monotherapy is indicated mainly in case of intolerance or contraindication to ribavirin.

4.2 Posology and method of administration

Treatment should be initiated only by a physician experienced in the treatment of patients with hepatitis B or C.

Please refer also to the ribavirin Summary of Product Characteristics (SPC) when Pegasys is to be used in combination with ribavirin.

Dose to be administered and duration of treatment

Chronic hepatitis B:

The recommended dosage and duration of Pegasys for both HBeAg-positive and HBeAg-negative chronic hepatitis B is 180 micrograms once weekly for 48 weeks by subcutaneous administration in the abdomen or thigh.

Chronic hepatitis C:

The recommended dose for Pegasys is 180 micrograms once weekly by subcutaneous administration in the abdomen or thigh given in combination with oral ribavirin or as monotherapy.

The dose of ribavirin to be used in combination with Pegasys is given in Table 1.

The ribavirin dose should be administered with food.

Duration of treatment

The duration of combination therapy with ribavirin for chronic hepatitis C depends on viral genotype. Patients infected with HCV genotype 1 regardless of viral load should receive 48 weeks of therapy.

Patients infected with HCV genotype 2/3 regardless of viral load should receive 24 weeks of therapy (see Table 1).

Table 1: Dosing Recommendations for Combination therapy for HCV Patients

(see Table 1 on next page)

In general, patients infected with genotype 4 are considered hard to treat and limited study data (N=66) are compatible with a posology as for genotype 1. When deciding on the duration of therapy, the presence of additional risk factors should also be considered. For patients infected with genotype 5 or 6, this posology should also be considered.

The recommended duration of Pegasys monotherapy is 48 weeks.

HIV-HCV Co-infection

The recommended dosage for Pegasys, alone or in combination with 800 milligrams of ribavirin, is 180 micrograms once weekly subcutaneously for 48 weeks, regardless of genotype. The safety and efficacy of combination therapy with ribavirin doses greater than 800 milligrams daily or a duration of therapy less than 48 weeks has not been studied.

Predictability of response and non-response

Early virological response by week 12, defined as a 2 log viral load decrease or undetectable levels of HCV RNA has been shown to be predictive for sustained response (see Tables 2 and 8).

Table 2: Predictive Value of Week 12 Virological Response at the Recommended Dosing Regimen while on Pegasys Combination Therapy

(see Table 2 on next page)

The negative predictive value for sustained response in patients treated with Pegasys in monotherapy was 98%.

A similar negative predictive value has been observed in HIV-HCV co-infected patients treated with Pegasys monotherapy or in combination with ribavirin (100% (130/130) or 98% (83/85), respectively). Positive predictive values of 45% (50/110) and 70% (59/84) were observed for genotype 1 and genotype 2/3 HIV-HCV co-infected patients receiving combination therapy.

Table 1 Dosing Recommendations for Combination therapy for HCV Patients

Genotype	Pegasys Dose	Ribavirin Dose	Duration
Genotype 1	180 micrograms	<75 kg = 1000 mg ≥75 kg = 1200 mg	48 weeks 48 weeks
Genotype 2/3	180 micrograms	800 mg	24 weeks

Table 2 Predictive Value of Week 12 Virological Response at the Recommended Dosing Regimen while on Pegasys Combination Therapy

Genotype	Negative			Positive		
	No response by week 12	No sustained response	Predictive Value	Response by week 12	Sustained response	Predictive Value
Genotype 1 (N=569)	102	97	**95%** (97/102)	467	271	**58%** (271/467)
Genotype 2 and 3 (N=96)	3	3	**100%** (3/3)	93	81	**87%** (81/93)

Table 3 Dose Adjustment for Adverse Reaction (For further guidance see also text above)

	Reduce Ribavirin to 600 mg	Withhold Ribavirin	Reduce Pegasys to 135/90/45 micrograms	Withhold Pegasys	Discontinue Combination
Absolute Neutrophil Count			< 750/mm^3	< 500/mm^3	
Platelet Count			< 50,000/mm^3 > 25,000/mm^3		< 25,000/mm^3
Haemoglobin - no cardiac disease	< 10 g/dl, and ≥ 8.5 g/dl	< 8.5 g/dl			
Haemoglobin - stable cardiac disease	decrease ≥ 2 g/dl during any 4 weeks	< 12 g/dl despite 4 weeks at reduced dose			

Dose adjustment for adverse reactions

General

Where dose adjustment is required for moderate to severe adverse reactions (clinical and/or laboratory) initial dose reduction to 135 micrograms is generally adequate. However, in some cases, dose reduction to 90 micrograms or 45 micrograms is necessary. Dose increases to or towards the original dose may be considered when the adverse reaction abates (see 4.4 and 4.8).

Haematological (see also Table3)

Dose reduction is recommended if the neutrophil count is < 750/mm^3. For patients with Absolute Neutrophil Count (ANC) < 500/mm^3 treatment should be suspended until ANC values return to > 1000/mm^3. Therapy should initially be re-instituted at 90 micrograms Pegasys and the neutrophil count monitored.

Dose reduction to 90 micrograms is recommended if the platelet count is < 50,000/mm^3. Cessation of therapy is recommended when platelet count decreases to levels < 25,000/mm^3.

Specific recommendations for management of treatment-emergent anaemia are as follows: ribavirin should be reduced to 600 milligrams/day (200 milligrams in the morning and 400 milligrams in the evening) if either of the following apply: (1) a patient without significant cardiovascular disease experiences a fall in haemoglobin to < 10 g/dl and ≥ 8.5 g/dl, or (2) a patient with stable cardiovascular disease experiences a fall in haemoglobin by ≥ 2 g/dl during any 4 weeks of treatment. A return to original dosing is not recommended. Ribavirin should be discontinued if either of the following apply: (1) A patient without significant cardiovascular disease experiences a fall in haemoglobin confirmed to < 8.5 g/dl; (2) A patient with stable cardiovascular disease maintains a haemoglobin value < 12 g/dl despite 4 weeks on a reduced dose. If the abnormality is reversed, ribavirin may be restarted at 600 milligrams daily, and further increased to 800 milligrams daily at the discretion of the treating physician. A return to original dosing is not recommended.

(see Table 3 above)

In case of intolerance to ribavirin, Pegasys monotherapy should be continued.

Liver function

Fluctuations in abnormalities of liver function tests are common in patients with chronic hepatitis C. As with other alpha interferons, increases in ALT levels above baseline (BL) have been observed in patients treated with Pegasys, including patients with a virological response.

In chronic hepatitis C clinical trials, isolated increases in ALT (≥ 10x ULN, or ≥ 2x BL for patients with a BL ALT ≥ 10x ULN) which resolved without dose-modification were observed in 8 of 451 patients treated with combination therapy. If ALT increase is progressive or persistent, the dose should be reduced initially to 135 micrograms. When increase in ALT levels is progressive despite dose reduction, or is accompanied by increased bilirubin or evidence of hepatic decompensation, therapy should be discontinued (see 4.4).

For chronic hepatitis B patients, transient flares of ALT levels sometimes exceeding 10 times the upper limit of normal are not uncommon, and may reflect immune clearance. Treatment should normally not be initiated if ALT is >10 times the upper limit of normal. Consideration should be given to continuing treatment with more frequent monitoring of liver function during ALT flares. If the Pegasys dose is reduced or withheld, therapy can be restored once the flare is subsiding (see 4.4).

Special populations

Elderly

Adjustments in the recommended dosage of 180 micrograms once weekly are not necessary when instituting Pegasys therapy in elderly patients (see 5.2).

Patients under the age of 18 years

The safety and efficacy of Pegasys have not been established in this population.

Patients with renal impairment

In patients with end stage renal disease, a starting dose of 135 micrograms should be used (see 5.2). Regardless of the starting dose or degree of renal impairment, patients should be monitored and appropriate dose reductions of Pegasys during the course of therapy should be made in the event of adverse reactions.

Patients with hepatic impairment

In patients with compensated cirrhosis (eg, Child-Pugh A), Pegasys has been shown to be effective and safe. Pegasys has not been evaluated in patients with decompensated cirrhosis (eg, Child-Pugh B or C or bleeding oesophageal varices) (see 4.3).

The Child-Pugh classification divides patients into groups A, B, and C, or "Mild", "Moderate" and "Severe" corresponding to scores of 5-6, 7-9 and 10-15, respectively.

Modified Assessment

Assessment	Degree of abnormality	Score
Encephalopathy	None Grade 1-2 Grade 3-4*	1 2 3
Ascites	Absent Slight Moderate	1 2 3
S-Bilirubin (mg/dl)	<2 2.0-3 >3	1 2 3
SI unit = μmol/l)	<34 34-51 >51	1 2 3
S-Albumin (g/dl)	>3.5 3.5-2.8 <2.8	1 2 3
INR	<1.7 1.7-2.3 >2.3	1 2 3

*Grading according to Trey, Burns and Saunders (1966)

4.3 Contraindications

- Hypersensitivity to the active substance, to alpha interferons, or to any of the excipients
- Autoimmune hepatitis
- Severe hepatic dysfunction or decompensated cirrhosis of the liver
- Neonates and young children up to 3 years old, because of the excipient benzyl alcohol
- A history of severe pre-existing cardiac disease, including unstable or uncontrolled cardiac disease in the previous six months (see 4.4)
- Pregnancy and lactation
- Initiation of Pegasys is contraindicated in HIV-HCV patients with cirrhosis and a Child-Pugh score ≥ 6

For contraindications to ribavirin, please refer also to the ribavirin Summary of Product Characteristics (SPC) when Pegasys is to be used in combination with ribavirin.

4.4 Special warnings and special precautions for use

Please refer also to the ribavirin Summary of Product Characteristics (SPC) when Pegasys is to be used in combination with ribavirin.

All patients in the chronic hepatitis C studies had a liver biopsy before inclusion, but in certain cases (ie, patients with genotype 2 or 3), treatment may be possible without histological confirmation. Current treatment guidelines should be consulted as to whether a liver biopsy is needed prior to commencing treatment.

In patients with normal ALT, progression of fibrosis occurs on average at a slower rate than in patients with elevated ALT. This should be considered in conjunction with other factors, such as HCV genotype, age, extrahepatic manifestations, risk of transmission, etc. which influence the decision to treat or not.

In patients co-infected with HIV-HCV, limited efficacy and safety data (N = 51) are available in subjects with CD4 counts less than 200 cells/uL. Caution is therefore warranted in the treatment of patients with low CD4 counts.

Laboratory tests prior to and during therapy

Prior to beginning Pegasys therapy, standard haematological and biochemical laboratory tests are recommended for all patients.

The following may be considered as baseline values for initiation of treatment:

- Platelet count ≥ 90,000/mm^3
- Absolute neutrophil counts ≥ 1500/mm^3
- Adequately controlled thyroid function (TSH and T4)

Haematological tests should be repeated after 2 and 4 weeks and biochemical tests should be performed at 4 weeks. Additional testing should be performed periodically during therapy.

In clinical trials, Pegasys treatment was associated with decreases in both total white blood cell (WBC) count and absolute neutrophil count (ANC), usually starting within the first 2 weeks of treatment (see 4.8). Progressive decreases after 8 weeks of therapy were infrequent. The decrease in ANC was reversible upon dose reduction or cessation of therapy (see 4.2).

Pegasys treatment has been associated with decreases in platelet count, which returned to pre-treatment levels during the post-treatment observation period (see 4.8). In some cases, dose modification may be necessary (see 4.2).

The occurrence of anaemia (haemoglobin <10 g/dl) has been observed in up to 15% of chronic hepatitis C patients in clinical trials on the combined treatment of Pegasys with ribavirin. The frequency depends on the treatment duration and the dose of ribavirin (see 4.8, Table 4). The risk of developing anaemia is higher in the female population.

As with other interferons, caution should be exercised when administering Pegasys in combination with other potentially myelosuppressive agents.

Endocrine System

Thyroid function abnormalities or worsening of pre-existing thyroid disorders have been reported with the use of alpha interferons, including Pegasys. Prior to initiation of

Pegasys therapy, TSH and T4 levels should be evaluated. Pegasys treatment may be initiated or continued if TSH levels can be maintained in the normal range by medication. TSH levels should be determined during the course of therapy if a patient develops clinical symptoms consistent with possible thyroid dysfunction (see 4.8). As with other interferons, hypoglycaemia, hyperglycaemia and diabetes mellitus have been observed with Pegasys (see 4.8).

Psychiatric and Central Nervous System (CNS)

If treatment with Pegasys is judged necessary in patients with existence or history of severe psychiatric conditions, this should only be initiated after having ensured appropriate individualised diagnostic and therapeutic management of the psychiatric condition.

Severe CNS effects, particularly depression, suicidal ideation and attempted suicide have been observed in some patients during interferon or peginterferon alfa therapy. Other CNS effects including aggressive behaviour, confusion and alterations of mental status have been observed with interferon or peginterferon alfa. If patients develop psychiatric or CNS problems when treated with Pegasys, including clinical depression, it is recommended that the patient be carefully monitored due to the potential seriousness of these undesirable effects. If symptoms persist or worsen, discontinue Pegasys therapy (see 4.8).

Cardiovascular system

Hypertension, supraventricular arrhythmias, congestive heart failure, chest pain and myocardial infarction have been associated with alpha interferon therapies, including Pegasys. It is recommended that patients who have pre-existing cardiac abnormalities have an electrocardiogram prior to initiation of Pegasys therapy. If there is any deterioration of cardiovascular status, therapy should be suspended or discontinued. In patients with cardiovascular disease, anaemia may necessitate dose reduction or discontinuation of ribavirin (see 4.2).

Liver function

In patients who develop evidence of hepatic decompensation during treatment, Pegasys should be discontinued. As with other alpha interferons, increases in ALT levels above baseline have been observed in patients treated with Pegasys, including patients with a viral response. When the increase in ALT levels is progressive and clinically significant, despite dose reduction, or is accompanied by increased direct bilirubin, therapy should be discontinued (see 4.2 and 4.8).

In chronic hepatitis B, unlike chronic hepatitis C, disease exacerbations during therapy are not uncommon and are characterised by transient and potentially significant increases in serum ALT. In clinical trials with Pegasys in HBV, marked transaminase flares have been accompanied by mild changes in other measures of hepatic function and without evidence of hepatic decompensation. In approximately half the case of flares exceeding 10 times the upper limit of normal, Pegasys dosing was reduced or withheld until the transaminase elevations subsided, while in the rest therapy was continued unchanged. More frequent monitoring of hepatic function was recommended in all instances.

Hypersensitivity

Serious, acute hypersensitivity reaction (eg, urticaria, angioedema, bronchoconstriction, anaphylaxis) have been rarely observed during alpha interferon therapy. If this occurs, therapy must be discontinued and appropriate medical therapy instituted immediately. Transient rashes do not necessitate interruption of treatment.

Autoimmune disease

The development of auto-antibodies and autoimmune disorders has been reported during treatment with alpha interferons. Patients predisposed to the development of autoimmune disorders may be at increased risk. Patients with signs or symptoms compatible with autoimmune disorders should be evaluated carefully, and the benefit-risk of continued interferon therapy should be reassessed (see also *Endocrine System* in 4.4 and 4.8).

Fever

While fever may be associated with the flu-like syndrome reported commonly during interferon therapy, other causes of persistent fever, particularly serious infections (bacterial, viral, fungal) must be ruled out, especially in patients with neutropenia.

Ocular changes

As with other interferons retinopathy including retinal haemorrhages, cotton wool spots, papilloedema, optic neuropathy and retinal artery or vein obstruction which may result in loss of vision have been reported in rare instances with Pegasys. All patients should have a baseline eye examination. Any patient complaining of decrease or loss of vision must have a prompt and complete eye examination. Patients with preexisting ophthalmologic disorders (eg, diabetic or hypertensive retinopathy) should receive periodic ophthalmologic exams during Pegasys therapy. Pegasys treatment should be discontinued in patients who develop new or worsening ophthalmologic disorders.

Pulmonary changes

As with other alpha interferons, pulmonary symptoms, including dyspnoea, pulmonary infiltrates, pneumonia, and pneumonitis have been reported during therapy with Pegasys. In case of persistent or unexplained pulmonary infiltrates or pulmonary function impairment, treatment should be discontinued.

Skin disorder

Use of alpha interferons has been rarely associated with exacerbation or provocation of psoriasis and sarcoidosis. Pegasys must be used with caution in patients with psoriasis, and in cases of onset or worsening of psoriatic lesions, discontinuation of therapy should be considered.

Transplantation

The safety and efficacy of Pegasys treatment have not been established in patients with liver transplantation.

HIV-HCV co-infected patients

Please refer to the respective Summary of Product Characteristics of the antiretroviral medicinal products that are to be taken concurrently with HCV therapy for awareness and management of toxicities specific for each product and the potential for overlapping toxicities with Pegasys with or without ribavirin. In study NR15961, patients concurrently treated with stavudine and interferon therapy with or without ribavirin, the incidence of pancreatitis and/or lactic acidosis was 3% (12/398).

Patients co-infected with HIV and receiving Highly Active Anti-Retroviral Therapy (HAART) may be at increased risk of developing lactic acidosis. Caution should therefore be exercised when adding Pegasys and ribavirin to HAART therapy (see ribavirin SPC).

Co-infected patients with advanced cirrhosis receiving HAART may also be at increased risk of hepatic decompensation and possibly death if treated with ribavirin in combination with interferons, including Pegasys. Baseline variables in co-infected cirrhotic patients that may be associated with hepatic decompensation include: increased serum bilirubin, decreased haemoglobin, increased alkaline phosphatase or decreased platelet count, and treatment with didanosine (ddI).

Co-infected patients should be closely monitored, assessing their Child-Pugh score during treatment, and should be immediately discontinued if they progress to a Child-Pugh score of 7 or greater.

4.5 Interaction with other medicinal products and other forms of Interaction

Administration of Pegasys 180 micrograms once weekly for 4 weeks in healthy male subjects did not show any effect on mephenytoin, dapsone, debrisoquine and tolbutamide pharmacokinetics profiles, suggesting that Pegasys has no effect on in vivo metabolic activity of cytochrome P450 3A4, 2C9, 2C19 and 2D6 isozymes.

In the same study, a 25% increase in the AUC of theophylline (marker of cytochrome P450 1A2 activity) was observed, demonstrating that Pegasys is an inhibitor of cytochrome P450 1A2 activity. Serum concentrations of theophylline should be monitored and appropriate dose adjustments of theophylline made for patients taking theophylline and Pegasys concomitantly. The interaction between theophylline and Pegasys is likely to be maximal after more than 4 weeks of Pegasys therapy.

Results from pharmacokinetic substudies of pivotal phase III trials demonstrated no pharmacokinetic interaction of lamivudine on Pegasys in HBV patients or between Pegasys and ribavirin in HCV patients.

HIV-HCV co-infected patients

No apparent evidence of drug interaction was observed in 47 HIV-HCV co-infected patients who completed a 12 week pharmacokinetic substudy to examine the effect of ribavirin on the intracellular phosphorylation of some nucleoside reverse transcriptase inhibitors (lamivudine and zidovudine or stavudine). However, due to high variability, the confidence intervals were quite wide. Plasma exposure of ribavirin did not appear to be affected by concomitant administration of nucleoside reverse transcriptase inhibitors (NRTIs).

Co-administration of ribavirin and didanosine is not recommended. Exposure to didanosine or its active metabolite (dideoxyadenosine 5'-triphosphate) is increased *in vitro* when didanosine is co-administered with ribavirin. Reports of fatal hepatic failure as well as peripheral neuropathy, pancreatitis, and symptomatic hyperlactatemia/lactic acidosis have been reported with use of ribavirin.

4.6 Pregnancy and lactation

There are no adequate data on the use of peginterferon alfa-2a in pregnant women. Studies in animals with interferon alfa-2a have shown reproductive toxicity (see 5.3) and the potential risk for humans is unknown. Pegasys should not be used during pregnancy.

Patients on treatment with Pegasys should take effective contraceptive measures.

It is not known whether peginterferon alfa-2a or any of the excipients of Pegasys are excreted in human milk. To avoid any potential for serious adverse reactions in nursing infants from Pegasys, a decision should be made whether to continue breast-feeding or to initiate Pegasys therapy, based on the importance of Pegasys therapy to the mother.

Use with ribavirin

Significant teratogenic and/or embryocidal effects have been demonstrated in all animal species exposed to ribavirin. Ribavirin therapy is contraindicated in women who are pregnant. Extreme care must be taken to avoid pregnancy in female patients or in partners of male patients taking ribavirin. Any birth control method can fail. Therefore, it is critically important that women of childbearing potential and their partners must use 2 forms of effective contraception simultaneously, during treatment and for 6 months after treatment has been concluded.

Please refer to the ribavirin Summary of Product Characteristics (SPC) when Pegasys is to be used in combination with ribavirin (especially see 4.3, 4.4 and 4.6 in the ribavirin SPC).

4.7 Effects on ability to drive and use machines

No studies on the effects on the ability to drive and use machines have been performed. Patients who develop dizziness, confusion, somnolence or fatigue should be cautioned to avoid driving or operating machinery.

4.8 Undesirable effects

Experience from clinical trials

The frequency and severity of the most commonly reported adverse reactions with Pegasys are similar to those reported with interferon alfa-2a. The most frequently reported adverse reactions with Pegasys 180 micrograms were mostly mild to moderate in severity and were manageable without the need for modification of doses or discontinuation of therapy.

Chronic Hepatitis B:

In clinical trials of 48 week treatment and 24 weeks follow-up, the safety profile for Pegasys in chronic hepatitis B was similar to that seen in chronic hepatitis C, although the frequency of reported adverse reactions was notably less in CHB (see Table 5). Eighty eight (88%) percent of Pegasys-treated patients experienced adverse reactions, as compared to 53% of patients in the lamivudine comparator group, while 6% of the Pegasys treated and 4% of the lamivudine treated patients experienced serious adverse events during the studies. Five percent of patients withdrew from Pegasys treatment due to adverse events or laboratory abnormalities, while less than 1% withdrew from lamivudine treatment for safety reasons. The withdrawal rates for patients with cirrhosis were similar to those of the overall population in each treatment group.

Chronic Hepatitis C:

HIV-HCV co-infected patients

In HIV-HCV co-infected patients, the clinical adverse event profiles reported for Pegasys, alone or in combination

Table 4 Safety Overview of Pegasys Treatment Regimens-Combination Therapy with Ribavirinfor HCV and HIV-HCV Patients

	HCV mono-infection Pegasys 180 mcg & **Ribavirin** 800 mg 24 weeks	**HCV mono-infection Pegasys** 180 mcg & **Ribavirin** 1000/1200 mg 48 weeks	**HIV-HCV co-infection Pegasys** 180 mcg & **Ribavirin** 800 mg 48 weeks
Serious adverse events	3%	11%	17%
Anaemia (haemoglobin < 10g/dl)	3%	15%	14%
Ribavirin dose modification	19%	39%	37%
Premature withdrawals due to adverse events	4%	10%	12%
Premature withdrawals due to laboratory abnormalities	1%	3%	3%

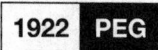

with ribavirin, were similar to those observed in HCV mono-infected patients (see Tables 4 and 5). Pegasys treatment was associated with decreases in absolute CD4+ cell counts within the first 4 weeks without a reduction in CD4+ cell percentage. The decrease in CD4+ cell counts was reversible upon dose reduction or cessation of therapy. The use of Pegasys had no observable negative impact on the control of HIV viremia during therapy or follow-up. Limited safety data (N= 31) are available in co-infected patients with CD4+ cell counts <200/μl.

Table 4 summarises the safety overview of different treatment regimens of Pegasys in combination with ribavirin for HCV and HIV-HCV patients.

Table 4: Safety Overview of Pegasys Treatment Regimens-Combination Therapy with Ribavirinfor HCV and HIV-HCV Patients

(see Table 4 on previous page)

(see Table 5)

Table 6: Undesirable Effects (<10% Incidence) Reported on Pegasys Monotherapy for HBV or HCV or In Combination with Ribavirin for HCV Patients

(see Table 6 on next page)

Very rarely, alpha interferons including Pegasys, used alone or in combination with ribavirin, may be associated with pancytopenia including aplastic anaemia.

For HIV-HCV patients receiving Pegasys and ribavirin combination therapy other undesirable effects have been reported in ⩾ 1% to ⩽ 2% of patients: hyperlactacidemia/lactic acidosis, influenza, pneumonia, affect lability, apathy, tinnitus, pharyngolaryngeal pain, cheilitis, acquired lipodystrophy and chromaturia.

Laboratory values

Pegasys treatment was associated with abnormal laboratory values: ALT increase, bilirubin increase, electrolyte disturbance (hypokalaemia, hypocalcaemia, hypophosphataemia), hyperglycaemia, hypoglycaemia and elevated triglycerides (see 4.4.). With both Pegasys monotherapy, and also the combined treatment with ribavirin, up to 2% of patients experienced increased ALT levels that led to dose modification or discontinuation of the treatment.

Treatment with Pegasys was associated with decreases in haematological values (leucopenia, neutropenia, lymphopenia, thrombocytopenia and haemoglobin), which generally improved with dose modification, and returned to pre-treatment levels within 4-8 weeks upon cessation of therapy (see 4.2 and 4.4).

Moderate (ANC: 0.749 - 0.5 × 10^9/l) and severe (ANC: < 0.5 × 10^9/l) neutropenia was observed respectively in 24% (216/887) and 5% (41/887) of patients receiving Pegasys 180 micrograms and ribavirin 1000/1200 milligrams for 48 weeks.

Anti-interferon antibodies

1-5% of patients treated with Pegasys developed neutralising anti-interferon antibodies. As with other interferons, a higher incidence of neutralising antibodies was seen in chronic hepatitis B. However in neither disease was this correlated with lack of therapeutic response.

Thyroid function

Pegasys treatment was associated with clinically significant abnormalities in thyroid laboratory values requiring clinical intervention (see 4.4). The frequencies observed (4.9%) in patients receiving Pegasys/ribavirin (NV15801) are similar to those observed with other interferons.

Laboratory values for HIV-HCV co-infected patients

Although haematological toxicities of neutropenia, thrombocytopenia and anaemia occurred more frequently in HIV-HCV patients, the majority could be managed by dose modification and the use of growth factors and infrequently required premature discontinuation of treatment. Decrease in ANC levels below 500 cells/mm^3 was observed in 13% and 11% of patients receiving Pegasys monotherapy and combination therapy, respectively. Decrease in platelets below 50,000/mm^3 was observed in 10% and 8% of patients receiving Pegasys monotherapy and combination therapy, respectively. Anaemia (haemoglobin < 10g/dL) was reported in 7% and 14% of patients treated with Pegasys monotherapy or in combination therapy, respectively.

4.9 Overdose

Overdoses involving between two injections on consecutive days (instead of weekly interval) up to daily injections for 1 week (ie, 1260 micrograms/week) have been reported. None of these patients experienced unusual, serious or treatment-limiting events. Weekly doses of up to 540 and 630 micrograms have been administered in renal cell carcinoma and chronic myelogenous leukaemia clinical trials, respectively. Dose limiting toxicities were fatigue, elevated liver enzymes, neutropenia and thrombocytopenia, consistent with interferon therapy.

5. PHARMACOLOGICAL PROPERTIES

5.1 Pharmacodynamic properties

Pharmacotherapeutic group: Immunostimulating Agent/Cytokine, ATC code: L03A B11

The conjugation of PEG reagent (bis-monomethoxypolyethylene glycol) to interferon alfa-2a forms a pegylated

Table 5 Undesirable Effects (⩾10% Incidence in Any Treatment Group) for HBV or HCV Patients

	HBV	HCV				
Body System	HCV	HCV	HCV	HCV	HIV-HCV	
	Pegasys	Pegasys	Pegasys	Pegasys	IFN alfa-2b	Pegasys
	180 mcg	180 mcg	180 mcg	180 mcg	3 MIU	180 mcg
			& Ribavirin	& Ribavirin	& Ribavirin	& Ribavirin
			800 mg	1000/ 1200 mg	1000/ 1200 mg	800 mg
	48 weeks	48 weeks	24 weeks	48 weeks	48 weeks	48 weeks
	N=448	N=827	N=207	N=887	N=443	N=288
	%		%	%	%	%
Metabolism & Nutrition						
Anorexia	13	16	20	27	26	23
Weight Decrease	4	5	2	7	10	16
Neuro/Psych Disorders						
Headache	23	52	48	47	49	35
Insomnia	6	20	30	32	37	19
Irritability	3	17	28	24	27	15
Depression	4	18	17	21	28	22
Dizziness	6	14	13	15	14	7
Concentration Impairment	2	9	8	10	13	2
Anxiety	3	6	8	8	12	8
Respiratory Disorder						
Dyspnoea	1	5	11	13	14	7
Cough	2	4	8	13	7	3
Gastrointestinal Disorders						
Nausea	6	24	29	28	28	24
Diarrhoea	6	16	15	14	10	16
Abdominal Pain	4	15	9	10	9	7
Skin						
Alopecia	17	22	25	24	33	10
Pruritus	6	12	25	21	18	5
Dermatitis	<1	9	15	16	13	1
Dry skin	1	5	13	12	13	4
Musculoskeletal						
Myalgia	25	37	42	38	49	32
Arthralgia	10	26	20	22	23	16
General						
Fatigue	21	49	45	49	53	40
Pyrexia	52	35	37	39	54	41
Rigors	6	30	30	25	34	16
Injection-Site Reaction	7	22	28	21	15	10
Asthenia	11	7	18	15	16	26
Pain	1	11	9	10	9	6

Table 6 Undesirable Effects (< 10% Incidence) Reported on Pegasys Monotherapy for HBV or HCV or In Combination with Ribavirin for HCV Patients

Body system	Common < 10% - 5%	Common < 5% -1%	Uncommon to Rare serious adverse events < 1% - < 0.1%
Infections and infestations		herpes simplex, upper respiratory infection, bronchitis, oral candidiasis	skin infection, pneumonia, otitis externa, endocarditis
Neoplasms benign and malignant			hepatic neoplasm
Blood and lymphatic system disorders		anaemia, lymphadenopathy, thrombocytopenia	
Immune system disorders			idiopathic or thrombotic thrombocytopenic purpura, thyroiditis, psoriasis, rheumatoid arthritis, systemic lupus erythematosus, sarcoidosis, anaphylaxis
Endocrine disorders		hypothyroidism, hyperthyroidism	diabetes
Psychiatric disorders	mood alteration, emotional disorders	nervousness, libido decreased, aggression,	suicidal ideation, suicide,
Nervous system disorders	memory impairment	taste disturbance, weakness, paraesthesia, hypoaesthesia, tremor, migraine, somnolence, hyperaesthesia, nightmares, syncope	peripheral neuropathy, coma
Eye disorders		vision blurred, eye inflammation, xerophthalmia, eye pain	corneal ulcer, retinopathy, retinal vascular disorder, retinal haemorrhage, papilledema, optic neuropathy, vision loss
Ear and labyrinth disorders		vertigo, earache	hearing loss
Cardiac disorders		palpitations, oedema peripheral, tachycardia	arrhythmia, supraventricular tachycardia, atrial fibrillation, congestive heart failure, angina, pericarditis, myocardial infarction
Vascular disorders		flushing	cerebral haemorrhage, hypertension
Respiratory, thoracic and mediastinal disorders		sore throat, dyspnoea exertional, epistaxis, nasopharyngitis, sinus congestion, rhinitis, nasal congestion	wheezing, interstitial pneumonitis with fatal outcome, pulmonary embolism
Gastrointestinal disorders	vomiting, dry mouth, dyspepsia	mouth ulceration, flatulence, gingival bleeding, stomatitis, dysphagia, glossitis	peptic ulcer, gastrointestinal bleeding, reversible pancreatic reaction (ie, amylase/lipase increase with or without abdominal pain)
Hepato-biliary disorders			hepatic failure, hepatic dysfunction, fatty liver, cholangitis
Skin and subcutaneous tissue disorders	rash, sweating increased	eczema, night sweats, psoriasis, photosensitivity reaction, urticaria, skin disorder	angioedema
Musculoskeletal, connective tissue and bone disorders	back pain	muscle cramps, neck pain, musculoskeletal pain, bone pain, arthritis, muscle weakness	myositis
Reproductive system and breast disorders		impotence	
General disorders and administration site conditions		malaise, lethargy, chest pain, hot flushes, thirst, influenza like illness	
Injury and poisoning			substance overdose

Table 7 Serological, Virological and Biochemical Responses in Chronic Hepatitis B

Response Parameter	HBeAg positive Study WV16240			HBeAg negative / anti-HBe positive Study WV16241		
	Pegasys 180 mcg & Placebo	Pegasys 180 mcg & Lamivudine 100 mg	Lamivudine 100 mg	Pegasys 180 mcg & Placebo	Pegasys 180 mcg & Lamivudine 100 mg	Lamivudine 100 mg
	(N=271)	(N=271)	(N=272)	(N=177)	(N=179)	(N=181)
HBeAg Sero-conversion	32% #	27%	19%	N/A	N/A	N/A
HBV DNA response *	32% #	34%	22%	43% #	44%	29%
ALT Normal-ization	41% #	39%	28%	59% #	60%	44%
HBsAg Sero-conversion	3% #	3%	0%	3%	2%	0%

*** For HBeAg-positive patients: HBV DNA < 10^5 copies/ml**
For HBeAg-negative / anti-HBe-positive patients: HBV DNA < 2×10^4 copies/ml
 # p-value (vs. lamivudine) ≤ 0.01 (stratified Cochran-Mantel-Haenszel test)

interferon alfa-2a (Pegasys). Pegasys possesses the *in vitro* antiviral and antiproliferative activities that are characteristic of interferon alfa-2a.

HCV RNA levels decline in a biphasic manner in responding patients with hepatitis C who have received treatment with 180 micrograms Pegasys. The first phase of decline occurs 24 to 36 hours after the first dose of Pegasys is followed by and the second phase of decline which continues over the next 4 to 16 weeks in patients who achieve a sustained response. Ribavirin had no significant effect on the initial viral kinetics over the first 4 to 6 weeks in patients treated with the combination of ribavirin and pegylated interferon alfa-2a or interferon alfa.

Chronic Hepatitis B:

Clinical trial results

All clinical trials recruited patients with chronic hepatitis B who had active viral replication measured by HBV DNA, elevated levels of ALT and a liver biopsy consistent with chronic hepatitis. Study WV16240 recruited patients who were positive for HBeAg, while study WV16241 recruited patients who were negative for HBeAg and positive for anti-HBe. In both studies the treatment duration was 48 weeks, with 24 weeks of treatment-free follow-up. Both studies compared Pegasys plus placebo vs Pegasys plus lamivudine vs lamivudine alone. No HBV-HIV co-infected patients were included in these clinical trials.

Response rates at the end of follow-up for the two studies are presented in Table 7. In study WV16240, the primary efficacy endpoints were HBeAg seroconversion and HBV-DNA below 10^5 copies/ml. In study WV16241, the primary efficacy endpoints were ALT normalisation and HBV-DNA below 2×10^4 copies/ml. HBV-DNA was measured by the COBAS AMPLICOR™ HBV MONITOR Assay (limit of detection 200 copies/ml).

A total of 283/1351 (21%) of patients had advanced fibrosis or cirrhosis, 85/1351 (6%) had cirrhosis. There was no difference in response rate between these patients and those without advanced fibrosis or cirrhosis.

Table 7: Serological, Virological and Biochemical Responses in Chronic Hepatitis B

(see Table 7)

Histological response was similar across the three treatment groups in each study; however, patients showing a sustained response 24 weeks after the end of treatment were significantly more likely to also show histological improvement.

All patients who completed the phase III studies were eligible for entry into a long-term follow-up study (WV16866). Among patients from study WV16240, who received Pegasys monotherapy and entered the long-term follow-up study, the rate of sustained HBeAg seroconversion 12 months after the end of therapy was 48% (73/153). In patients receiving Pegasys monotherapy in study WV16241, the rate of HBV DNA response and ALT normalization 12 months after end of treatment were 42% (41/97) and 59% (58/99), respectively.

Chronic Hepatitis C

Predictability of response

Please refer to section 4.2, in Table 2.

Dose-response in monotherapy

In a direct comparison with 90 micrograms, the 180 micrograms-dose was associated with superior sustained virological response in patients with cirrhosis, but in a study in non-cirrhotic patients very similar results were obtained with doses of 135 micrograms and 180 micrograms.

Confirmatory clinical trials

All clinical trials recruited interferon-naïve patients with chronic hepatitis C confirmed by detectable levels of serum HCV RNA, elevated levels of ALT (with the exception of study NR16071) and a liver biopsy consistent with chronic hepatitis. Study NV15495 specifically recruited patients with a histological diagnosis of cirrhosis (about 80%) or transition to cirrhosis (about 20%). Only HIV-HCV co-infected patients were included in the study NR15961 (see Table 10). These patients had stable HIV disease and mean CD4 T-cell count was about 500 cells/μl. Clinical trials in non-responders and in relapsers are in progress.

For HCV monoinfected patients and HIV-HCV co-infected patients, for treatment regimens, duration of therapy and study outcome see Tables 8, 9 and Table 10, respectively. Virological response was defined as undetectable HCV RNA as measured by the COBAS AMPLICOR™ HCV Test, version 2.0 (limit of detection 100 copies/ml equivalent to 50 International Units/ml) and sustained response as one negative sample approximately 6 months after end of therapy.

(see Table 8 on next page)

The virological responses of patients treated with Pegasys monotherapy and with Pegasys and ribavirin combination therapy in relation to genotype and viral load are summarised in Tables 9 and 10 for HCV monoinfected patients and HIV-HCV co-infected patients, respectively. The results of study NV15942 provide the rationale for recommending treatment regimens based on genotype (see Table 1).

The difference between treatment regimens was in general not influenced by viral load or presence/absence of cirrhosis; therefore treatment recommendations for genotype 1,2 or 3 are independent of these baseline characteristics.

Table 8 Virological Response in HCV Patients

	Pegasys Monotherapy				Pegasys Combination Therapy		
	non-cirrhotic and cirrhotic		cirrhotic		non-cirrhotic and cirrhotic		
	Study NV15496 + NV15497 + NV15801		Study NV15495		Study NV15942	Study NV15801	
	Pegasys	Interferon alfa-2a	Pegasys	Interferon alfa-2a	Pegasys	Pegasys	Interferon alfa-2a
	180 mcg	6 MIU/3 MIU	180 mcg	3 MIU	180 mcg	180 mcg	3 MIU
		&			&	&	&
		3 MIU			Ribavirin	Ribavirin	Ribavirin
					1000/1200	1000/1200	1000/1200
					mg	mg	mg
	(N=701)	(N=478)	(N=87)	(N=88)	(N=436)	(N=453)	(N=444)
	48 weeks	48 weeks	48 weeks	48 weeks	48 weeks	48 weeks	48 weeks
Response at End of Treatment	55 - 69%	22 - 28%	44%	14%	68%	69%	52%
Overall Sustained Response	28 - 39%	11 - 19%	30%*	8%*	63%	54%**	45%**

*** 95% CI for difference: 11% to 33% p-value (stratified Cochran-Mantel-Haenszel test) = 0.001**
**** 95% CI for difference: 3% to 16% p-value (stratified Cochran-Mantel-Haenszel test)=0.003**

Table 9: Sustained Virological Response Based on Genotype and Viral Load after Pegasys Combination Therapy with Ribavirin in HCV Patients

(see Table 9 below)

Superior efficacy of Pegasys compared to interferon alfa-2a was demonstrated also in terms of histological response, including patients with cirrhosis and/or HIV-HCV co-infection.

HIV-HCV co-infected patients

Table 10: Sustained Virological Response based on Genotype and Viral Load after Pegasys Combination Therapy with Ribavirin in HIV-HCV Co-infected Patients

(see Table 10 on next page)

HCV patients with normal ALT

In study NR16071, HCV patients with normal ALT values were randomized to receive Pegasys 180 micrograms/week and ribavirin 800 milligrams/day for either 24 or 48 weeks followed by a 24 week treatment free follow-up period or no treatment for 72 weeks. The SVRs reported in the treatment arms of this study were similar to the corresponding treatment arms from study NV15942.

5.2 Pharmacokinetic properties

Following a single subcutaneous injection of Pegasys 180 micrograms in healthy subjects, serum concentrations of peginterferon alfa-2a are measurable within 3 to 6 hours. Within 24 hours, about 80% of the peak serum concentration is reached. The absorption of Pegasys is sustained with peak serum concentrations reached 72 to 96 hours after dosing. The absolute bioavailability of Pegasys is 84% and is similar to that seen with interferon alfa-2a.

Peginterferon alfa-2a is found predominantly in the bloodstream and extracellular fluid as seen by the volume of distribution at steady-state (V_d) of 6 to 14 liters in humans after intravenous administration. From mass balance, tissue distribution and whole body autoradioluminography studies performed in rats, peginterferon alfa-2a is distributed to the liver, kidney and bone marrow in addition to being highly concentrated in the blood.

The metabolism of Pegasys is not fully characterised; however studies in rats indicate that the kidney is a major organ for excretion of radiolabelled material. In humans, the systemic clearance of peginterferon alfa-2a is about 100-fold lower than that of the native interferon alfa-2a. After intravenous administration, the terminal half-life of peginterferon alfa-2a is approximately 60 to 80 hours compared to values of 3-4 hours for standard interferon. The terminal half-life after subcutaneous administration is longer [50 to 130 hours]. The terminal half-life may not only reflect the elimination phase of the compound, but may also reflect the sustained absorption of Pegasys.

Dose-proportional increases in exposure of Pegasys are seen in healthy subjects and in patients with chronic hepatitis B or C after once-weekly dosing.

In chronic hepatitis B or C patients, peginterferon alfa-2a serum concentrations accumulate 2 to 3 fold after 6 to 8 weeks of once weekly dosing compared to single dose values. There is no further accumulation after 8 weeks of once weekly dosing. The peak to trough ratio after 48 weeks of treatment is about 1.5 to 2. Peginterferon alfa-2a serum concentrations are sustained throughout one full week (168 hours).

Patients with renal impairment

Renal impairment is associated with slightly decreased CL/F and prolonged half-life. In patients (n=3) with CL_{crea} between 20 and 40 ml/min, the average CL/F is reduced by 25% compared with patients with normal renal function. In patients with end stage renal disease undergoing haemodialysis, there is a 25% to 45% reduction in the clearance, and doses of 135 micrograms result in similar exposure as 180 micrograms doses in patients with normal renal function (see 4.2).

Gender

The pharmacokinetics of Pegasys after single subcutaneous injections were comparable between male and female healthy subjects.

Elderly

In subjects older than 62 years, the absorption of Pegasys after a single subcutaneous injection of 180 micrograms was delayed but still sustained compared to young healthy subjects (t_{max} of 115 hours vs. 82 hours, older than 62 years vs. younger, respectively). The AUC was slightly increased (1663 vs. 1295 ng·h/ml) but peak concentrations (9.1 vs. 10.3 ng/ml) were similar in subjects older than 62 years. Based on drug exposure, pharmacodynamic response and tolerability, a lower dose of Pegasys is not needed in the geriatric patient (see 4.2).

Hepatic impairment

The pharmacokinetics of Pegasys were similar between healthy subjects and patients with hepatitis B or C. Comparable exposure and pharmacokinetic profiles were seen in cirrhotic (Child-Pugh Grade A) and non-cirrhotic patients.

Site of administration

Subcutaneous administration of Pegasys should be limited to the abdomen and thigh, as the extent of absorption based on AUC was about 20% to 30% higher upon injection in the abdomen and thigh. Exposure to Pegasys was decreased in studies following administration of Pegasys in the arm compared to administration in the abdomen and thigh.

5.3 Preclinical safety data

The preclinical toxicity studies conducted with Pegasys were limited due to species specificity of interferons. Acute and chronic toxicity studies have been carried out in cynomolgus monkeys, and the findings observed in peginterferon dosed animals were similar in nature to those produced by interferon alfa-2a.

Reproductive toxicity studies have not been performed with Pegasys. As with other alpha interferons, prolongation of the menstrual cycle was observed following administration of peginterferon alfa-2a to female monkeys. Treatment with interferon alfa-2a resulted in a statistically significant increase in abortifacient activity in rhesus monkeys. Although no teratogenic effects were seen in the offspring delivered at term, adverse effects in humans cannot be excluded.

Pegasys plus ribavirin

When used in combination with ribavirin, Pegasys did not cause any effects in monkeys not previously seen with either active substance alone. The major treatment-related change was reversible mild to moderate anaemia, the severity of which was greater than that produced by either active substance alone.

Table 9 Sustained Virological Response Based on Genotype and Viral Load after Pegasys Combination Therapy with Ribavirin in HCV Patients

	Study NV15942				Study NV15801	
	Pegasys	Pegasys	Pegasys	Pegasys	Pegasys	Interferon alfa-2b
	180 mcg	180 mcg	180 mcg	180 mcg	180 mcg	3 MIU
	&	&	&	&	&	&
	Ribavirin	Ribavirin	Ribavirin	Ribavirin	Ribavirin	Ribavirin
	800 mg	1000/1200 mg	800 mg	1000/1200 mg	1000/1200 mg	1000/1200 mg
	24 weeks	24 weeks	48 weeks	48 weeks	48 weeks	48 weeks
Genotype 1 Low viral load High viral load	29% (29/101) 41% (21/51) 16% (8/50)	42% (49/118)* 52% (37/71) 26% (12/47)	41% (102/250)* 55% (33/60) 36% (69/190)	**52%** (142/271)* **65%** (55/85) **47%** (87/186)	45% (134/298) 53% (61/115) 40% (73/182)	36% (103/285) 44% (41/94) 33% (62/189)
Genotype 2/3 Low viral load High viral load	**84%** (81/96) **85%** (29/34) **84%** (52/62)	81% (117/144) 83% (39/47) 80% (78/97)	79% (78/99) 88% (29/33) 74% (49/66)	80% (123/153) 77% (37/48) 82% (86/105)	71% (100/140) 76% (28/37) 70% (72/103)	61% (88/145) 65% (34/52) 58% (54/93)
Genotype 4	(0/5)	(8/12)	(5/8)	(9/11)	(10/13)	(5/11)

* Pegasys 180 mcg ribavirin 1000/1200 mg, 48 w *vs.* Pegasys 180 mcg ribavirin 800 mg, 48 w: Odds Ratio (95% CI) = 1.52 (1.07 to 2.17) P-value (stratified Cochran-Mantel-Haenszel test) = 0.020
* Pegasys 180 mcg ribavirin 1000/1200 mg, 48 w *vs.* Pegasys 180 mcg ribavirin 1000/1200 mg, 24 w: Odds Ratio (95% CI) = 2.12 (1.30 to 3.46) P-value (stratified Cochran-Mantel-Haenszel test) = 0.002.

6. PHARMACEUTICAL PARTICULARS

6.1 List of excipients

sodium chloride
polysorbate 80
benzyl alcohol
sodium acetate
acetic acid
water for injections

6.2 Incompatibilities

In the absence of compatibility studies, Pegasys must not be mixed with other medicinal products.

6.3 Shelf life

3 years

6.4 Special precautions for storage

Store in a refrigerator (2°C-8°C). Do not freeze.

Store in the original package in order to protect from light.

6.5 Nature and contents of container

0.5 ml of solution for injection in pre-filled syringe (siliconised Type I glass) with a plunger stopper and tip cap (butyl rubber laminated on the product facing side with fluororesin) with a needle. Available in packs of 1, 4 or 12.

Table 10 Sustained Virological Response based on Genotype and Viral Load after Pegasys Combination Therapy with Ribavirin in HIV-HCV Co-infected Patients

Study NR15961			
	Interferon alfa-2a 3 MIU & **Ribavirin 800 mg** 48 weeks	**Pegasys** 180 mcg & **Placebo** 48 weeks	**Pegasys** 180 mcg & **Ribavirin 800 mg** 48 weeks
All patients	12% (33/285)*	20% (58/286)*	40% (116/289)*
Genotype 1	7% (12/171)	14% (24/175)	29% (51/176)
Low viral load	19% (8/42)	38% (17/45)	61% (28/46)
High viral load	3% (4/129)	5% (7/130)	18% (23/130)
Genotype 2-3	20% (18/89)	36% (32/90)	62% (59/95)
Low viral load	27% (8/30)	38% (9/24)	61% (17/28)
High viral load	17% (10/59)	35% (23/66)	63% (42/67)

* Pegasys 180 mcg ribavirin 800mg vs. Interferon alfa-2a 3MIU ribavirin 800mg: Odds Ratio (95% CI) = 5.40 (3.42 to 8.54), ...P-value (stratified Cochran-Mantel-Haenszel test) = < 0.0001

* Pegasys 180 mcg ribavirin 800mg vs. Pegasys 180μg: Odds Ratio (95% CI) = 2.89 (1.93 to 4.32), ...P-value (stratified Cochran-Mantel-Haenszel test) = < 0.0001

* Interferon alfa-2a 3MIU ribavirin 800mg vs. Pegasys 180mcg: Odds Ratio (95% CI) = 0.53 (0.33 to 0.85), ...P-value (stratified Cochran-Mantel-Haenszel test) = < 0.0084

6.6 Instructions for use and handling

The solution for injection is for single use only. It should be inspected visually for particulate matter and discoloration before administration.

Any unused product or waste material should be disposed of in accordance with local requirements.

7. MARKETING AUTHORISATION HOLDER

Roche Registration Limited
40 Broadwater Road
Welwyn Garden City
Hertfordshire, AL7 3AY
United Kingdom

8. MARKETING AUTHORISATION NUMBER(S)

EU/1/02/221/005
EU/1/02/221/006
EU/1/02/221/009

9. DATE OF FIRST AUTHORISATION/RENEWAL OF THE AUTHORISATION

20 June 2002

10. DATE OF REVISION OF THE TEXT

24 February 2005

Pegasys 180

(Roche Products Limited)

1. NAME OF THE MEDICINAL PRODUCT

Pegasys®▼ 180 micrograms solution for injection in pre-filled syringe

2. QUALITATIVE AND QUANTITATIVE COMPOSITION

One pre-filled syringe contains

peginterferon alfa-2a* .... 180 micrograms in 0.5 ml of solution

* recombinant interferon alfa-2a produced by genetic engineering from *Escherichia coli* conjugated to bis-[monomethoxy polyethylene glycol] of a molecular mass, M_n, of 40 000.

For excipients, see section 6.1.

3. PHARMACEUTICAL FORM

Solution for injection in pre-filled syringe.

The solution is clear and colourless to light yellow.

4. CLINICAL PARTICULARS

4.1 Therapeutic indications

Chronic hepatitis B:

Pegasys is indicated for the treatment of HBeAg-positive or HBeAg-negative chronic hepatitis B in adult patients with compensated liver disease and evidence of viral replication, increased ALT and histologically verified liver inflammation and/or fibrosis (see 4.4 and 5.1).

Chronic hepatitis C:

Pegasys is indicated for the treatment of chronic hepatitis C in adult patients who are positive for serum HCV-RNA, including patients with compensated cirrhosis and/or co-infected with clinically stable HIV (see 4.4).

The optimal way to use Pegasys in patients with chronic hepatitis C is in combination with ribavirin. This combination is indicated in previously untreated patients as well as in patients who have previously responded to interferon alpha therapy and subsequently relapsed after treatment was stopped.

Monotherapy is indicated mainly in case of intolerance or contraindication to ribavirin.

4.2 Posology and method of administration

Treatment should be initiated only by a physician experienced in the treatment of patients with hepatitis B or C.

Please refer also to the ribavirin Summary of Product Characteristics (SPC) when Pegasys is to be used in combination with ribavirin.

Dose to be administered and duration of treatment

Chronic hepatitis B:

The recommended dosage and duration of Pegasys for both HBeAg-positive and HBeAg-negative chronic hepatitis B is 180 micrograms once weekly for 48 weeks by subcutaneous administration in the abdomen or thigh.

Chronic hepatitis C:

The recommended dose for Pegasys is 180 micrograms once weekly by subcutaneous administration in the abdomen or thigh given in combination with oral ribavirin or as monotherapy.

The dose of ribavirin to be used in combination with Pegasys is given in Table 1.

The ribavirin dose should be administered with food.

Duration of treatment

The duration of combination therapy with ribavirin for chronic hepatitis C depends on viral genotype. Patients infected with HCV genotype 1 regardless of viral load should receive 48 weeks of therapy.

Patients infected with HCV genotype 2/3 regardless of viral load should receive 24 weeks of therapy (see Table1).

Table 1: Dosing Recommendations for Combination Therapy for HCV Patients

(see Table 1 below)

In general, patients infected with genotype 4 are considered hard to treat and limited study data (N=66) are compatible with a posology as for genotype 1. When deciding on the duration of therapy, the presence of additional risk factors should also be considered. For patients infected with genotype 5 or 6, this posology should also be considered.

The recommended duration of Pegasys monotherapy is 48 weeks.

HIV-HCV Co-infection

The recommended dosage for Pegasys, alone or in combination with 800 milligrams of ribavirin, is 180 micrograms once weekly subcutaneously for 48 weeks, regardless of genotype. The safety and efficacy of combination therapy with ribavirin doses greater than 800 milligrams daily or a duration of therapy less than 48 weeks has not been studied.

Predictability of response and non-response

Early virological response by week 12, defined as a 2 log viral load decrease or undetectable levels of HCV RNA has been shown to be predictive for sustained response (see Tables 2 and 8).

Table 2: Predictive Value of Week 12 Virological Response at the Recommended Dosing Regimen while on Pegasys Combination Therapy

(see Table 2 below)

The negative predictive value for sustained response in patients treated with Pegasys in monotherapy was 98%.

A similar negative predictive value has been observed in HIV-HCV co-infected patients treated with Pegasys monotherapy or in combination with ribavirin (100% (130/130) or 98% (83/85), respectively). Positive predictive values of 45% (50/110) and 70% (59/84) were observed for genotype 1 and genotype 2/3 HIV-HCV co-infected patients receiving combination therapy.

Dose adjustment for adverse reactions

General

Where dose adjustment is required for moderate to severe adverse reactions (clinical and/or laboratory) initial dose reduction to 135 micrograms is generally adequate. However, in some cases, dose reduction to 90 micrograms or 45 micrograms is necessary. Dose increases to or towards the original dose may be considered when the adverse reaction abates (see 4.4 and 4.8).

Haematological (see also Table 3)

Dose reduction is recommended if the neutrophil count is < 750/mm³. For patients with Absolute Neutrophil Count (ANC) < 500/mm³ treatment should be suspended until ANC values return to > 1000/mm³. Therapy should initially be re-instituted at 90 micrograms Pegasys and the neutrophil count monitored.

Dose reduction to 90 micrograms is recommended if the platelet count is < 50,000/mm³. Cessation of therapy is recommended when platelet count decreases to levels < 25,000/mm³.

Specific recommendations for management of treatment-emergent anaemia are as follows: ribavirin should be reduced to 600 milligrams /day (200 milligrams in the morning and 400 milligrams in the evening) if either of the following apply: (1) a patient without significant cardiovascular disease experiences a fall in haemoglobin to < 10 g/dl and ⩾ 8.5 g/dl, or (2) a patient with stable cardiovascular disease experiences a fall in haemoglobin by ⩾ 2 g/dl during any 4 weeks of treatment. A return to original dosing is not recommended. Ribavirin should be discontinued if either of the following apply: (1) A patient without significant cardiovascular disease experiences a fall in haemoglobin confirmed to < 8.5 g/dl; (2) A patient with stable cardiovascular disease maintains a haemoglobin value < 12 g/dl despite 4 weeks on a reduced dose. If the abnormality is reversed, ribavirin may be restarted at 600 milligrams daily, and further increased to 800 milligrams daily at the discretion of the treating physician. A return to original dosing is not recommended.

(see Table 3 on next page)

In case of intolerance to ribavirin, Pegasys monotherapy should be continued.

Liver function

Fluctuations in abnormalities of liver function tests are common in patients with chronic hepatitis C. As with other alpha interferons, increases in ALT levels above baseline

Table 1 Dosing Recommendations for Combination Therapy for HCV Patients

Genotype	Pegasys Dose	Ribavirin Dose	Duration
Genotype 1	180 micrograms	<75 kg = 1000 mg ⩾75 kg = 1200 mg	48 weeks 48 weeks
Genotype 2/3	180 micrograms	800 mg	24 weeks

Table 2 Predictive Value of Week 12 Virological Response at the Recommended Dosing Regimen while on Pegasys Combination Therapy

Genotype	Negative			Positive		
	No response by week 12	No sustained response	Predictive Value	Response by week 12	Sustained response	Predictive Value
Genotype 1 (N= 569)	102	97	**95%** (97/102)	467	271	**58%** (271/467)
Genotype 2 and 3 (N=96)	3	3	**100%** (3/3)	93	81	**87%** (81/93)

Table 3 Dose Adjustment for Adverse Reaction (For further guidance see also text above)

	Reduce Ribavirin to 600 mg	Withhold Ribavirin	Reduce Pegasys to 135/ 90/45 micrograms	Withhold Pegasys	Discontinue Combination
Absolute Neutrophil Count			< 750/mm^3	< 500/mm^3	
Platelet Count			< 50,000/mm^3 > 25,000/mm^3		< 25,000/mm^3
Haemoglobin - no cardiac disease	< 10 g/dl, and ⩾ 8.5 g/dl	< 8.5 g/dl			
Haemoglobin - stable cardiac disease	decrease ⩾ 2 g/dl during any 4 weeks	< 12 g/dl despite 4 weeks at reduced dose			

(BL) have been observed in patients treated with Pegasys, including patients with a virological response.

In chronic hepatitis C clinical trials, isolated increases in ALT (⩾ 10x ULN, or ⩾ 2x BL for patients with a BL ALT ⩾ 10x ULN) which resolved without dose-modification were observed in 8 of 451 patients treated with combination therapy. If ALT increase is progressive or persistent, the dose should be reduced initially to 135 micrograms. When increase in ALT levels is progressive despite dose reduction, or is accompanied by increased bilirubin or evidence of hepatic decompensation, therapy should be discontinued (see 4.4).

For chronic hepatitis B patients, transient flares of ALT levels sometimes exceeding 10 times the upper limit of normal are not uncommon, and may reflect immune clearance. Treatment should normally not be initiated if ALT is >10 times the upper limit of normal. Consideration should be given to continuing treatment with more frequent monitoring of liver function during ALT flares. If the Pegasys dose is reduced or withheld, therapy can be restored once the flare is subsiding (see 4.4).

<u>*Special populations*</u>

Elderly

Adjustments in the recommended dosage of 180 micrograms once weekly are not necessary when instituting Pegasys therapy in elderly patients (see 5.2).

Patients under the age of 18 years

The safety and efficacy of Pegasys have not been established in this population.

Patients with renal impairment

In patients with end stage renal disease, a starting dose of 135 micrograms should be used (see 5.2). Regardless of the starting dose or degree of renal impairment, patients should be monitored and appropriate dose reductions of Pegasys during the course of therapy should be made in the event of adverse reactions.

Patients with hepatic impairment

In patients with compensated cirrhosis (eg, Child-Pugh A), Pegasys has been shown to be effective and safe. Pegasys has not been evaluated in patients with decompensated cirrhosis (eg, Child-Pugh B or C or bleeding oesophageal varices) (see 4.3).

The Child-Pugh classification divides patients into groups A, B, and C, or "Mild", "Moderate" and "Severe" corresponding to scores of 5-6, 7-9 and 10-15, respectively.

Modified Assessment

Assessment	Degree of abnormality	Score
Encephalopathy	None Grade 1-2 Grade 3-4*	1 2 3
Ascites	Absent Slight Moderate	1 2 3
S-Bilirubin (mg/dl)	<2 2.0-3 >3	1 2 3
SI unit = μmol/l)	<34 34-51 >51	1 2 3
S-Albumin (g/dl)	>3.5 3.5-2.8 <2.8	1 2 3
INR	<1.7 1.7-2.3 >2.3	1 2 3

* Grading according to Trey, Burns and Saunders (1966)

4.3 Contraindications

• Hypersensitivity to the active substance, to alpha interferons, or to any of the excipients

• Autoimmune hepatitis

• Severe hepatic dysfunction or decompensated cirrhosis of the liver

• Neonates and young children up to 3 years old, because of the excipient benzyl alcohol

• A history of severe pre-existing cardiac disease, including unstable or uncontrolled cardiac disease in the previous six months (see 4.4)

• Pregnancy and lactation

• Initiation of Pegasys is contraindicated in HIV-HCV patients with cirrhosis and a Child-Pugh score ⩾ 6

For contraindications to ribavirin, please refer also to the ribavirin Summary of Product Characteristics (SPC) when Pegasys is to be used in combination with ribavirin.

4.4 Special warnings and special precautions for use

Please refer also to the ribavirin Summary of Product Characteristics (SPC) when Pegasys is to be used in combination with ribavirin.

All patients in the chronic hepatitis C studies had a liver biopsy before inclusion, but in certain cases (ie, patients with genotype 2 or 3), treatment may be possible without histological confirmation. Current treatment guidelines should be consulted as to whether a liver biopsy is needed prior to commencing treatment.

In patients with normal ALT, progression of fibrosis occurs on average at a slower rate than in patients with elevated ALT. This should be considered in conjunction with other factors, such as HCV genotype, age, extrahepatic manifestations, risk of transmission, etc. which influence the decision to treat or not.

In patients co-infected with HIV-HCV, limited efficacy and safety data (N = 51) are available in subjects with CD4 counts less than 200 cells/uL. Caution is therefore warranted in the treatment of patients with low CD4 counts.

Laboratory tests prior to and during therapy

Prior to beginning Pegasys therapy, standard haematological and biochemical laboratory tests are recommended for all patients.

The following may be considered as baseline values for initiation of treatment:

- Platelet count ⩾ 90,000/mm^3

- Absolute neutrophil counts ⩾ 1500/mm^3

- Adequately controlled thyroid function (TSH and T4).

Haematological tests should be repeated after 2 and 4 weeks and biochemical tests should be performed at 4 weeks. Additional testing should be performed periodically during therapy.

In clinical trials, Pegasys treatment was associated with decreases in both total white blood cell (WBC) count and absolute neutrophil count (ANC), usually starting within the first 2 weeks of treatment (see 4.8). Progressive decreases after 8 weeks of therapy were infrequent. The decrease in ANC was reversible upon dose reduction or cessation of therapy (see 4.2).

Pegasys treatment has been associated with decreases in platelet count, which returned to pre-treatment levels during the post-treatment observation period (see 4.8). In some cases, dose modification may be necessary (see 4.2).

The occurrence of anaemia (haemoglobin <10 g/dl) has been observed in up to 15% of chronic hepatitis C patients in clinical trials on the combined treatment of Pegasys with ribavirin. The frequency depends on the treatment duration and the dose of ribavirin (see 4.8, Table 4). The risk of developing anaemia is higher in the female population.

As with other interferons, caution should be exercised when administering Pegasys in combination with other potentially myelosuppressive agents.

Endocrine System

Thyroid function abnormalities or worsening of pre-existing thyroid disorders have been reported with the use of alpha interferons, including Pegasys. Prior to initiation of Pegasys therapy, TSH and T4 levels should be evaluated. Pegasys treatment may be initiated or continued if TSH levels can be maintained in the normal range by medication. TSH levels should be determined during the course of therapy if a patient develops clinical symptoms consistent with possible thyroid dysfunction (see 4.8). As with other interferons, hypoglycaemia, hyperglycaemia and diabetes mellitus have been observed with Pegasys (see 4.8).

Psychiatric and Central Nervous System (CNS)

If treatment with Pegasys is judged necessary in patients with existence or history of severe psychiatric conditions, this should only be initiated after having ensured appropriate individualised diagnostic and therapeutic management of the psychiatric condition.

Severe CNS effects, particularly depression, suicidal ideation and attempted suicide have been observed in some patients during interferon or peginterferon alfa therapy. Other CNS effects including aggressive behaviour, confusion and alterations of mental status have been observed with interferon or peginterferon alfa. If patients develop psychiatric or CNS problems when treated with Pegasys, including clinical depression, it is recommended that the patient be carefully monitored due to the potential seriousness of these undesirable effects. If symptoms persist or worsen, discontinue Pegasys therapy (see 4.8).

Cardiovascular system

Hypertension, supraventricular arrhythmias, congestive heart failure, chest pain and myocardial infarction have been associated with alpha interferon therapies, including Pegasys. It is recommended that patients who have preexisting cardiac abnormalities have an electrocardiogram prior to initiation of Pegasys therapy. If there is any deterioration of cardiovascular status, therapy should be suspended or discontinued. In patients with cardiovascular disease, anaemia may necessitate dose reduction or discontinuation of ribavirin (see 4.2).

Liver function

In patients who develop evidence of hepatic decompensation during treatment, Pegasys should be discontinued. As with other alpha interferons, increases in ALT levels above baseline have been observed in patients treated with Pegasys, including patients with a viral response. When the increase in ALT levels is progressive and clinically significant, despite dose reduction, or is accompanied by increased direct bilirubin, therapy should be discontinued (see 4.2 and 4.8).

In chronic hepatitis B, unlike chronic hepatitis C, disease exacerbations during therapy are not uncommon and are characterised by transient and potentially significant increases in serum ALT. In clinical trials with Pegasys in HBV, marked transaminase flares have been accompanied by mild changes in other measures of hepatic function and without evidence of hepatic decompensation. In approximately half the case of flares exceeding 10 times the upper limit of normal, Pegasys dosing was reduced or withheld until the transaminase elevations subsided, while in the rest therapy was continued unchanged. More frequent monitoring of hepatic function was recommended in all instances.

Hypersensitivity

Serious, acute hypersensitivity reaction (eg, urticaria, angioedema, bronchoconstriction, anaphylaxis) have been rarely observed during alpha interferon therapy. If this occurs, therapy must be discontinued and appropriate medical therapy instituted immediately. Transient rashes do not necessitate interruption of treatment.

Autoimmune disease

The development of auto-antibodies and autoimmune disorders has been reported during treatment with alpha interferons. Patients predisposed to the development of autoimmune disorders may be at increased risk. Patients with signs or symptoms compatible with autoimmune disorders should be evaluated carefully, and the benefit-risk of continued interferon therapy should be reassessed (see also *Endocrine System* in 4.4 and 4.8).

Fever

While fever may be associated with the flu-like syndrome reported commonly during interferon therapy, other causes of persistent fever, particularly serious infections (bacterial, viral, fungal) must be ruled out, especially in patients with neutropenia.

Ocular changes

As with other interferons retinopathy including retinal haemorrhages, cotton wool spots, papilloedema, optic neuropathy and retinal artery or vein obstruction which may result in loss of vision have been reported in rare instances with Pegasys. All patients should have a baseline eye examination. Any patient complaining of decrease or loss of vision must have a prompt and complete eye examination. Patients with preexisting ophthalmologic disorders (eg, diabetic or hypertensive retinopathy) should receive periodic ophthalmologic exams during Pegasys therapy. Pegasys treatment should be discontinued in patients who develop new or worsening ophthalmologic disorders.

Pulmonary changes

As with other alpha interferons, pulmonary symptoms, including dyspnoea, pulmonary infiltrates, pneumonia, and pneumonitis have been reported during therapy with Pegasys. In case of persistent or unexplained pulmonary infiltrates or pulmonary function impairment, treatment should be discontinued.

Skin disorder

Use of alpha interferons has been rarely associated with exacerbation or provocation of psoriasis and sarcoidosis. Pegasys must be used with caution in patients with psoriasis, and in cases of onset or worsening of psoriatic lesions, discontinuation of therapy should be considered.

Transplantation

The safety and efficacy of Pegasys treatment have not been established in patients with liver transplantation.

HIV/HCV co-infected patients

Please refer to the respective Summary of Product Characteristics of the antiretroviral medicinal products that are to be taken concurrently with HCV therapy for awareness and management of toxicities specific for each product and the potential for overlapping toxicities with Pegasys with or without ribavirin. In study NR15961, patients concurrently treated with stavudine and interferon therapy with or without ribavirin, the incidence of pancreatitis and/or lactic acidosis was 3% (12/398).

Patients co-infected with HIV and receiving Highly Active Anti-Retroviral Therapy (HAART) may be at increased risk of developing lactic acidosis. Caution should therefore be exercised when adding Pegasys and ribavirin to HAART therapy (see ribavirin SPC).

Co-infected patients with advanced cirrhosis receiving HAART may also be at increased risk of hepatic decompensation and possibly death if treated with ribavirin in combination with interferons, including Pegasys. Baseline variables in co-infected cirrhotic patients that may be associated with hepatic decompensation include: increased serum bilirubin, decreased haemoglobin, increased alkaline phosphatase or decreased platelet count, and treatment with didanosine (ddI).

Co-infected patients should be closely monitored, assessing their Child-Pugh score during treatment, and should be immediately discontinued if they progress to a Child-Pugh score of 7 or greater.

4.5 Interaction with other medicinal products and other forms of Interaction

Administration of Pegasys 180 micrograms once weekly for 4 weeks in healthy male subjects did not show any effect on mephenytoin, dapsone, debrisoquine and tolbutamide pharmacokinetics profiles, suggesting that Pegasys has no effect on in vivo metabolic activity of cytochrome P450 3A4, 2C9, 2C19 and 2D6 isozymes.

In the same study, a 25% increase in the AUC of theophylline (marker of cytochrome P450 1A2 activity) was observed, demonstrating that Pegasys is an inhibitor of cytochrome P450 1A2 activity. Serum concentrations of theophylline should be monitored and appropriate dose adjustments of theophylline made for patients taking theophylline and Pegasys concomitantly. The interaction between theophylline and Pegasys is likely to be maximal after more than 4 weeks of Pegasys therapy.

Results from pharmacokinetic substudies of pivotal phase III trials demonstrated no pharmacokinetic interaction of lamivudine on Pegasys in HBV patients or between Pegasys and ribavirin in HCV patients.

HIV-HCV co-infected patients

No apparent evidence of drug interaction was observed in 47 HIV-HCV co-infected patients who completed a 12 week pharmacokinetic substudy to examine the effect of ribavirin on the intracellular phosphorylation of some nucleoside reverse transcriptase inhibitors (lamivudine and zidovudine or stavudine). However, due to high variability, the confidence intervals were quite wide. Plasma exposure of ribavirin did not appear to be affected by concomitant administration of nucleoside reverse transcriptase inhibitors (NRTIs).

Co-administration of ribavirin and didanosine is not recommended. Exposure to didanosine or its active metabolite (dideoxyadenosine 5'-triphosphate) is increased *in vitro* when didanosine is co-administered with ribavirin. Reports of fatal hepatic failure as well as peripheral neuropathy, pancreatitis, and symptomatic hyperlactatemia/lactic acidosis have been reported with use of ribavirin.

4.6 Pregnancy and lactation

There are no adequate data on the use of peginterferon alfa-2a in pregnant women. Studies in animals with interferon alfa-2a have shown reproductive toxicity (see 5.3) and the potential risk for humans is unknown. Pegasys should not be used during pregnancy.

Patients on treatment with Pegasys should take effective contraceptive measures.

It is not known whether peginterferon alfa-2a or any of the excipients of Pegasys are excreted in human milk. To avoid any potential for serious adverse reactions in nursing infants from Pegasys, a decision should be made whether to continue breast-feeding or to initiate Pegasys therapy, based on the importance of Pegasys therapy to the mother.

Use with ribavirin

Significant teratogenic and/or embryocidal effects have been demonstrated in all animal species exposed to ribavirin. Ribavirin therapy is contraindicated in women who are pregnant. Extreme care must be taken to avoid pregnancy in female patients or in partners of male patients taking ribavirin. Any birth control method can fail. Therefore, it is critically important that women of childbearing potential and their partners must use 2 forms of effective contraception simultaneously, during treatment and for 6 months after treatment has been concluded.

Please refer to the ribavirin Summary of Product Characteristics (SPC) when Pegasys is to be used in combination with ribavirin (especially see 4.3, 4.4 and 4.6 in the ribavirin SPC).

4.7 Effects on ability to drive and use machines

No studies on the effects on the ability to drive and use machines have been performed. Patients who develop dizziness, confusion, somnolence or fatigue should be cautioned to avoid driving or operating machinery.

4.8 Undesirable effects

Experience from clinical trials

The frequency and severity of the most commonly reported adverse reactions with Pegasys are similar to those reported with interferon alfa-2a. The most frequently reported adverse reactions with Pegasys 180 micrograms were mostly mild to moderate in severity and were manageable without the need for modification of doses or discontinuation of therapy.

Chronic Hepatitis B:

In clinical trials of 48 week treatment and 24 weeks follow-up, the safety profile for Pegasys in chronic hepatitis B was similar to that seen in chronic hepatitis C, although the frequency of reported adverse reactions was notably less in CHB (see Table 5). Eighty eight (88%) percent of Pegasys-treated patients experienced adverse reactions, as compared to 53% of patients in the lamivudine comparator group, while 6% of the Pegasys treated and 4% of the lamivudine treated patients experienced serious adverse events during the studies. Five percent of patients withdrew from Pegasys treatment due to adverse events or laboratory abnormalities, while less than 1% withdrew from lamivudine treatment for safety reasons. The withdrawal rates for patients with cirrhosis were similar to those of the overall population in each treatment group.

Chronic Hepatitis C:

HIV-HCV co-infected patients

In HIV-HCV co-infected patients, the clinical adverse event profiles reported for Pegasys, alone or in combination with ribavirin, were similar to those observed in HCV mono-infected patients (see Tables 4 and 5). Pegasys treatment was associated with decreases in absolute CD4+ cell counts within the first 4 weeks without a reduction in CD4+ cell percentage. The decrease in CD4+ cell counts was reversible upon dose reduction or cessation of therapy. The use of Pegasys had no observable negative impact on the control of HIV viremia during therapy or follow-up. Limited safety data (N= 31) are available in co-infected patients with CD4+ cell counts $<200/\mu l$.

Table 4 summarises the safety overview of different treatment regimens of Pegasys in combination with ribavirin for HCV and HIV-HCV patients.

Table 4: Safety Overview of Pegasys Treatment Regimens-Combination Therapy with Ribavirin for HCV and HIV-HCV Patients

(see Table 4)

(see Table 5 on next page)

Table 6: Undesirable Effects (<10% Incidence) Reported on Pegasys Monotherapy for HBV or HCV or In Combination with Ribavirin for HCV Patients

(see Table 6 on page 1929)

Very rarely, alpha interferons including Pegasys, used alone or in combination with ribavirin, may be associated with pancytopenia including aplastic anaemia.

For HIV-HCV patients receiving Pegasys and ribavirin combination therapy other undesirable effects have been reported in ≥ 1% to ≤ 2% of patients: hyperlactacidemia/lactic acidosis, influenza, pneumonia, affect lability, apathy, tinnitus, pharyngolaryngeal pain, cheilitis, acquired lipodystrophy and chromaturia.

Laboratory values

Pegasys treatment was associated with abnormal laboratory values: ALT increase, bilirubin increase, electrolyte disturbance (hypokalaemia, hypocalcaemia, hypophosphataemia), hyperglycaemia, hypoglycaemia and elevated triglycerides (see 4.4.). With both Pegasys monotherapy, and also the combined treatment with ribavirin, up to 2% of patients experienced increased ALT levels that led to dose modification or discontinuation of the treatment.

Treatment with Pegasys was associated with decreases in haematological values (leucopenia, neutropenia, lymphopenia, thrombocytopenia and haemoglobin), which generally improved with dose modification, and returned to pre-treatment levels within 4-8 weeks upon cessation of therapy (see 4.2 and 4.4).

Moderate (ANC: $0.749 - 0.5 \times 10^9$/l) and severe (ANC: $< 0.5 \times 10^9$/l) neutropenia was observed respectively in 24% (216/887) and 5% (41/887) of patients receiving Pegasys 180 micrograms and ribavirin 1000/1200 milligrams for 48 weeks.

Anti-interferon antibodies

1-5% of patients treated with Pegasys developed neutralising anti-interferon antibodies. As with other interferons, a higher incidence of neutralising antibodies was seen in chronic hepatitis B. However in neither disease was this correlated with lack of therapeutic response.

Thyroid function

Pegasys treatment was associated with clinically significant abnormalities in thyroid laboratory values requiring clinical intervention (see 4.4). The frequencies observed (4.9%) in patients receiving Pegasys/ribavirin (NV15801) are similar to those observed with other interferons.

Laboratory values for HIV-HCV co-infected patients

Although haematological toxicities of neutropenia, thrombocytopenia and anaemia occurred more frequently in HIV-HCV patients, the majority could be managed by dose modification and the use of growth factors and infrequently required premature discontinuation of treatment. Decrease in ANC levels below 500 cells/mm3 was observed in 13% and 11% of patients receiving Pegasys monotherapy and combination therapy, respectively. Decrease in platelets below 50,000/mm3 was observed in 10% and 8% of patients receiving Pegasys monotherapy and combination therapy, respectively. Anaemia (haemoglobin < 10g/dL) was reported in 7% and 14% of patients treated with Pegasys monotherapy or in combination therapy, respectively.

4.9 Overdose

Overdoses involving between two injections on consecutive days (instead of weekly interval) up to daily injections for 1 week (ie, 1260 micrograms/week) have been reported. None of these patients experienced unusual, serious or treatment-limiting events. Weekly doses of up to 540 and 630 micrograms have been administered in renal cell carcinoma and chronic myelogenous leukaemia clinical trials, respectively. Dose limiting toxicities were fatigue, elevated liver enzymes, neutropenia and thrombocytopenia, consistent with interferon therapy.

5. PHARMACOLOGICAL PROPERTIES

5.1 Pharmacodynamic properties

Pharmacotherapeutic group: Immunostimulating Agent/Cytokine, ATC code: L03A B11

Table 4: Safety Overview of Pegasys Treatment Regimens-Combination Therapy with Ribavirin for HCV and HIV-HCV Patients

	HCV mono-infection Pegasys 180 mcg & **Ribavirin** 800 mg 24 weeks	**HCV mono-infection Pegasys** 180 mcg & **Ribavirin** 1000/1200 mg 48 weeks	**HIV-HCV co-infection Pegasys** 180 mcg & **Ribavirin** 800 mg 48 weeks
Serious adverse events	3%	11%	17%
Anaemia (haemoglobin < 10g/dl)	3%	15%	14%
Ribavirin dose modification	19%	39%	37%
Premature withdrawals due to adverse events	4%	10%	12%
Premature withdrawals due to laboratory abnormalities	1%	3%	3%

Table 5: Undesirable Effects (≥10% Incidence in Any Treatment Group) for HBV or HCV Patients

	HBV	HCV				
Body System		HCV	HCV	HCV	HCV	HIV-HCV
	Pegasys	Pegasys	Pegasys	Pegasys	IFN alfa-2b	Pegasys
	180 mcg	180 mcg	180 mcg	180 mcg	3 MIU	180 mcg
			& Ribavirin	& Ribavirin	& Ribavirin	& Ribavirin
			800 mg	1000/1200 mg	1000/1200 mg	800 mg
	48 weeks	48 weeks	24 weeks	48 weeks	48 weeks	48 weeks
	N=448	N=827	N=207	N=887	N=443	N=288
	%	%	%	%	%	%
Metabolism & Nutrition						
Anorexia	13	16	20	27	26	23
Weight Decrease	4	5	2	7	10	16
Neuro/Psych Disorders						
Headache	23	52	48	47	49	35
Insomnia	6	20	30	32	37	19
Irritability	3	17	28	24	27	15
Depression	4	18	17	21	28	22
Dizziness	6	14	13	15	14	7
Concentration Impairment	2	9	8	10	13	2
Anxiety	3	6	8	8	12	8
Respiratory Disorder						
Dyspnoea	1	5	11	13	14	7
Cough	2	4	8	13	7	3
Gastrointestinal Disorders						
Nausea	6	24	29	28	28	24
Diarrhoea	6	16	15	14	10	16
Abdominal Pain	4	15	9	10	9	7
Skin						
Alopecia	17	22	25	24	33	10
Pruritus	6	12	25	21	18	5
Dermatitis	<1	9	15	16	13	1
Dry skin	1	5	13	12	13	4
Musculoskeletal						
Myalgia	25	37	42	38	49	32
Arthralgia	10	26	20	22	23	16
General						
Fatigue	21	49	45	49	53	40
Pyrexia	52	35	37	39	54	41
Rigors	6	30	30	25	34	16
Injection-Site Reaction	7	22	28	21	15	10
Asthenia	11	7	18	15	16	26
Pain	1	11	9	10	9	6

The conjugation of PEG reagent (bis-monomethoxypolyethylene glycol) to interferon alfa-2a forms a pegylated interferon alfa-2a (Pegasys). Pegasys possesses the *in vitro* antiviral and antiproliferative activities that are characteristic of interferon alfa-2a.

HCV RNA levels decline in a biphasic manner in responding patients with hepatitis C who have received treatment with 180 micrograms Pegasys. The first phase of decline occurs 24 to 36 hours after the first dose of Pegasys and is followed by the second phase of decline which continues over the next 4 to 16 weeks in patients who achieve a sustained response. Ribavirin had no significant effect on the initial viral kinetics over the first 4 to 6 weeks in patients treated with the combination of ribavirin and pegylated interferon alfa-2a or interferon alfa.

Chronic Hepatitis B:

Clinical trial results

All clinical trials recruited patients with chronic hepatitis B who had active viral replication measured by HBV DNA, elevated levels of ALT and a liver biopsy consistent with chronic hepatitis. Study WV16240 recruited patients who were positive for HBeAg, while study WV16241 recruited patients who were negative for HBeAg and positive for anti-HBe. In both studies the treatment duration was 48 weeks, with 24 weeks of treatment-free follow-up. Both studies compared Pegasys plus placebo vs Pegasys plus lamivudine vs lamivudine alone. No HBV-HIV co-infected patients were included in these clinical trials.

Response rates at the end of follow-up for the two studies are presented in Table 7. In study WV16240, the primary efficacy endpoints were HBeAg seroconversion and HBV-DNA below 10^5 copies/ml. In study WV16241, the primary efficacy endpoints were ALT normalisation and HBV-DNA below 2×10^4 copies/ml. HBV-DNA was measured by the COBAS AMPLICOR® HBV MONITOR Assay (limit of detection 200 copies/ml).

A total of 283/1351 (21%) of patients had advanced fibrosis or cirrhosis, 85/1351 (6%) had cirrhosis. There was no difference in response rate between these patients and those without advanced fibrosis or cirrhosis.

Table 7: Serological, Virological and Biochemical Responses in Chronic Hepatitis B

(see Table 7 on next page)

Histological response was similar across the three treatment groups in each study; however, patients showing a sustained response 24 weeks after the end of treatment were significantly more likely to also show histological improvement.

All patients who completed the phase III studies were eligible for entry into a long-term follow-up study (WV16866). Among patients from study WV16240, who received Pegasys monotherapy and entered the long-term follow-up study, the rate of sustained HBeAg seroconversion 12 months after the end of therapy was 48% (73/153). In patients receiving Pegasys monotherapy in study WV16241, the rate of HBV DNA response and ALT normalization 12 months after end of treatment were 42% (41/97) and 59% (58/99), respectively.

Chronic Hepatitis C

Predictability of response

Please refer to section 4.2, in Table 2.

Dose-response in monotherapy

In a direct comparison with 90 micrograms, the 180 micrograms-dose was associated with superior sustained virological response in patients with cirrhosis, but in a study in non-cirrhotic patients very similar results were obtained with doses of 135 micrograms and 180 micrograms.

Confirmatory clinical trials

All clinical trials recruited interferon-naïve patients with chronic hepatitis C confirmed by detectable levels of serum HCV RNA, elevated levels of ALT (with the exception of study NR16071) and a liver biopsy consistent with chronic hepatitis. Study NV15495 specifically recruited patients with a histological diagnosis of cirrhosis (about 80%) or transition to cirrhosis (about 20%). Only HIV-HCV co-infected patients were included in the study NR15961 (see Table 10). These patients had stable HIV disease and mean CD4 T-cell count was about 500 cells/μl. Clinical trials in non-responders and in relapsers are in progress.

For HCV monoinfected patients and HIV-HCV co-infected patients, for treatment regimens, duration of therapy and study outcome see Tables 8, 9 and Table 10, respectively. Virological response was defined as undetectable HCV RNA as measured by the COBAS AMPLICOR® HCV Test, version 2.0 (limit of detection 100 copies/ml equivalent to 50 International Units/ml) and sustained response as one negative sample approximately 6 months after end of therapy.

(see Table 8 on page 1930)

The virological responses of patients treated with Pegasys monotherapy and with Pegasys and ribavirin combination therapy in relation to genotype and viral load are summarised in Tables 9 and 10 for HCV monoinfected patients and HIV-HCV co-infected patients, respectively. The results of study NV15942 provide the rationale for recommending treatment regimens based on genotype (see Table 1).

The difference between treatment regimens was in general not influenced by viral load or presence/absence of cirrhosis; therefore treatment recommendations for genotype 1,2 or 3 are independent of these baseline characteristics.

Table 9: Sustained Virological Response Based on Genotype and Viral Load after Pegasys Combination Therapy with Ribavirin in HCV Patients

(see Table 9 on page 1930)

Superior efficacy of Pegasys compared to interferon alfa-2a was demonstrated also in terms of histological response, including patients with cirrhosis and/or HIV-HCV co-infection.

HIV-HCV co-infected patients

Table 10: Sustained Virological Response based on Genotype and Viral Load after Pegasys Combination Therapy with Ribavirin in HIV-HCV Co-infected Patients

(see Table 10 on page 1930)

HCV patients with normal ALT

In study NR16071, HCV patients with normal ALT values were randomized to receive Pegasys 180 micrograms/week and ribavirin 800 milligrams/day for either 24 or 48 weeks followed by a 24 week treatment free follow-up period or no treatment for 72 weeks. The SVRs reported in the treatment arms of this study were similar to the corresponding treatment arms from study NV15942.

Table 6 Undesirable Effects (< 10% Incidence) Reported on Pegasys Monotherapy for HBV or HCV or In Combination with Ribavirin for HCV Patients

Body system	Common < 10% - 5%	Common < 5% -1%	Uncommon to Rare serious adverse events < 1% - < 0.1%
Infections and infestations		herpes simplex, upper respiratory infection, bronchitis, oral candidiasis	skin infection, pneumonia, otitis externa, endocarditis
Neoplasms benign and malignant			hepatic neoplasm
Blood and lymphatic system disorders		anaemia, lymphadenopathy, thrombocytopenia	
Immune system disorders			idiopathic or thrombotic thrombocytopenic purpura, thyroiditis, psoriasis, rheumatoid arthritis, systemic lupus erythematosus, sarcoidosis, anaphylaxis
Endocrine disorders		hypothyroidism, hyperthyroidism	diabetes
Psychiatric disorders	mood alteration, emotional disorders	nervousness, libido decreased, aggression,	suicidal ideation,suicide,
Nervous system disorders	memory impairment	taste disturbance, weakness, paraesthesia, hypoaesthesia, tremor, migraine, somnolence, hyperaesthesia, nightmares, syncope	peripheral neuropathy, coma
Eye disorders		vision blurred, eye inflammation, xerophthalmia, eye pain	corneal ulcer, retinopathy, retinal vascular disorder, retinal haemorrhage, papilledema, optic neuropathy, vision loss
Ear and labyrinth disorders		vertigo, earache	hearing loss
Cardiac disorders		palpitations, oedema peripheral, tachycardia	arrhythmia, supraventricular tachycardia, atrial fibrillation, congestive heart failure, angina, pericarditis, myocardial infarction
Vascular disorders		flushing	cerebral haemorrhage, hypertension
Respiratory, thoracic and mediastinal disorders		sore throat, dyspnoea exertional, epistaxis, nasopharyngitis, sinus congestion, rhinitis, nasal congestion	wheezing, interstitial pneumonitis with fatal outcome, pulmonary embolism
Gastrointestinal disorders	vomiting, dry mouth, dyspepsia	mouth ulceration, flatulence, gingival bleeding, stomatitis, dysphagia, glossitis	peptic ulcer, gastrointestinal bleeding, reversible pancreactic reaction (ie, amylase/lipase increase with or without abdominal pain)
Hepato-biliary disorders			hepatic failure, hepatic dysfunction, fatty liver, cholangitis
Skin and subcutaneous tissue disorders	rash, sweating increased	eczema, night sweats, psoriasis, photosensitivity reaction, urticaria, skin disorder	angioedema
Musculoskeletal, connective tissue and bone disorders	back pain	muscle cramps, neck pain, musculoskeletal pain, bone pain, arthritis, muscle weakness	myositis
Reproductive system and breast disorders		impotence	
General disorders and administration site conditions		malaise, lethargy, chest pain, hot flushes, thirst, influenza like illness	
Injury and poisoning			substance overdose

Table 7 Serological, Virological and Biochemical Responses in Chronic Hepatitis B

Response Parameter	HBeAg positive Study WV16240			HBeAg negative / anti-HBe positive Study WV16241		
	Pegasys 180 mcg & Placebo	Pegasys 180 mcg & Lamivudine 100 mg	Lamivudine 100 mg	Pegasys 180 mcg & Placebo	Pegasys 180 mcg & Lamivudine 100 mg	Lamivudine 100 mg
	(N=271)	(N=271)	(N=272)	(N=177)	(N=179)	(N=181)
HBeAg Sero-conversion	32% #	27%	19%	N/A	N/A	N/A
HBV DNA response *	32% #	34%	22%	43% #	44%	29%
ALT Normal-ization	41% #	39%	28%	59% #	60%	44%
HBsAg Sero-conversion	3% #	3%	0%	3%	2%	0%

* For HBeAg-positive patients: HBV DNA < 10^5 copies/ml

For HBeAg-negative / anti-HBe-positive patients: HBV DNA < 2 × 10^4 copies/ml

\# p-value (vs. lamivudine) ≤ 0.01 (stratified Cochran-Mantel-Haenszel test)

5.2 Pharmacokinetic properties

Following a single subcutaneous injection of Pegasys 180 micrograms in healthy subjects, serum concentrations of peginterferon alfa-2a are measurable within 3 to 6 hours. Within 24 hours, about 80% of the peak serum concentration is reached. The absorption of Pegasys is sustained with peak serum concentrations reached 72 to 96 hours after dosing. The absolute bioavailability of Pegasys is 84% and is similar to that seen with interferon alfa-2a.

Peginterferon alfa-2a is found predominantly in the bloodstream and extracellular fluid as seen by the volume of distribution at steady-state (V_d) of 6 to 14 liters in humans after intravenous administration. From mass balance, tissue distribution and whole body autoradioluminography studies performed in rats, peginterferon alfa-2a is distributed to the liver, kidney and bone marrow in addition to being highly concentrated in the blood.

The metabolism of Pegasys is not fully characterised; however studies in rats indicate that the kidney is a major organ for excretion of radiolabelled material. In humans, the systemic clearance of peginterferon alfa-2a is about 100-fold lower than that of the native interferon alfa-2a. After intravenous administration, the terminal half-life of peginterferon alfa-2a is approximately 60 to 80 hours compared to values of 3-4 hours for standard interferon. The terminal half-life after subcutaneous administration is longer [50 to 130 hours]. The terminal half-life may not only reflect the elimination phase of the compound, but may also reflect the sustained absorption of Pegasys.

Dose-proportional increases in exposure of Pegasys are seen in healthy subjects and in patients with chronic hepatitis B or C after once-weekly dosing.

In chronic hepatitis B or C patients, peginterferon alfa-2a serum concentrations accumulate 2 to 3 fold after 6 to 8 weeks of once weekly dosing compared to single dose values. There is no further accumulation after 8 weeks of once weekly dosing. The peak to trough ratio after 48 weeks of treatment is about 1.5 to 2. Peginterferon alfa-2a serum concentrations are sustained throughout one full week (168 hours).

Patients with renal impairment

Renal impairment is associated with slightly decreased CL/F and prolonged half-life. In patients (n=3) with CL_{crea} between 20 and 40 ml/min, the average CL/F is reduced by 25% compared with patients with normal renal function. In patients with end stage renal disease undergoing haemodialysis, there is a 25% to 45% reduction in the clearance, and doses of 135 micrograms result in similar exposure as 180 micrograms doses in patients with normal renal function (see 4.2).

Gender

The pharmacokinetics of Pegasys after single subcutaneous injections were comparable between male and female healthy subjects.

Elderly

In subjects older than 62 years, the absorption of Pegasys after a single subcutaneous injection of 180 micrograms was delayed but still sustained compared to young healthy subjects (t_{max} of 115 hours vs. 82 hours, older than 62 years vs. younger, respectively). The AUC was slightly increased (1663 vs. 1295 ng·h /ml) but peak concentrations (9.1 vs. 10.3 ng/ml) were similar in subjects older than 62 years. Based on drug exposure, pharmacodynamic response and tolerability, a lower dose of Pegasys is not needed in the geriatric patient (see 4.2).

Hepatic impairment

The pharmacokinetics of Pegasys were similar between healthy subjects and patients with hepatitis B or C. Comparable exposure and pharmacokinetic profiles were seen in cirrhotic (Child-Pugh Grade A) and non-cirrhotic patients.

Site of administration

Subcutaneous administration of Pegasys should be limited to the abdomen and thigh, as the extent of absorption based on AUC was about 20% to 30% higher upon injection in the abdomen and thigh. Exposure to Pegasys was decreased in studies following administration of Pegasys in the arm compared to administration in the abdomen and thigh.

5.3 Preclinical safety data

The preclinical toxicity studies conducted with Pegasys were limited due to species specificity of interferons. Acute and chronic toxicity studies have been carried out in cynomolgus monkeys, and the findings observed in peginterferon dosed animals were similar in nature to those produced by interferon alfa-2a.

Reproductive toxicity studies have not been performed with Pegasys. As with other alpha interferons, prolongation of the menstrual cycle was observed following administration of peginterferon alfa-2a to female monkeys. Treatment with interferon alfa-2a resulted in a statistically significant increase in abortifacient activity in rhesus monkeys. Although no teratogenic effects were seen in the offspring delivered at term, adverse effects in humans cannot be excluded.

Pegasys plus ribavirin

When used in combination with ribavirin, Pegasys did not cause any effects in monkeys not previously seen with

Table 8 Virological Response in HCV Patients

	Pegasys Monotherapy				Pegasys Combination Therapy		
	non-cirrhotic and cirrhotic		cirrhotic		non-cirrhotic and cirrhotic		
	Study NV15496 + NV15497 + NV15801		Study NV15495		Study NV15942	Study NV15801	
	Pegasys	Interferon alfa-2a	Pegasys	Interferon alfa-2a	Pegasys	Pegasys	Interferon alfa-2a
	180 mcg	6 MIU/3 MIU	180 mcg	3 MIU	180 mcg	180 mcg	3 MIU
		&			&	&	&
		3 MIU			Ribavirin	Ribavirin	Ribavirin
					1000/1200	1000/1200	1000/1200
					mg	mg	mg
	(N=701)	(N=478)	(N=87)	(N=88)	(N=436)	(N=453)	(N=444)
	48 weeks	48 weeks	48 weeks	48 weeks	48 weeks	48 weeks	48 weeks
Response at End of Treatment	55 - 69%	22 - 28%	44%	14%	68%	69%	52%
Overall Sustained Response	28 - 39%	11 - 19%	30%*	8%*	63%	54%**	45%**

*** 95% CI for difference: 11% to 33% p-value (stratified Cochran-Mantel-Haenszel test) = 0.001**
**** 95% CI for difference: 3% to 16% p-value (stratified Cochran-Mantel-Haenszel test)=0.003**

Table 9 Sustained Virological Response Based on Genotype and Viral Load after Pegasys Combination Therapy with Ribavirin in HCV Patients

	Study NV15942				Study NV15801	
	Pegasys	Pegasys	Pegasys	Pegasys	Pegasys	Interferon alfa-2b
	180 mcg	180 mcg	180 mcg	180 mcg	180 mcg	3 MIU
	&	&	&	&	&	&
	Ribavirin	Ribavirin	Ribavirin	Ribavirin	Ribavirin	Ribavirin
	800 mg	1000/1200 mg	800 mg	1000/1200 mg	1000/1200 mg	1000/1200 mg
	24 weeks	24 weeks	48 weeks	48 weeks	48 weeks	48 weeks
Genotype 1 Low viral load High viral load	29% (29/101) 41% (21/51) 16% (8/50)	42% (49/118)* 52% (37/71) 26% (12/47)	41% (102/250)* 55% (33/60) 36% (69/190)	**52%** (142/271)* **65%** (55/85) **47%** (87/186)	45% (134/298) 53% (61/115) 40% (73/182)	36% (103/285) 44% (41/94) 33% (62/189)
Genotype 2/3 Low viral load High viral load	**84%** (81/96) **85%** (29/34) **84%** (52/62)	81% (117/144) 83% (39/47) 80% (78/97)	79% (78/99) 88% (29/33) 74% (49/66)	80% (123/153) 77% (37/48) 82% (86/105)	71% (100/140) 76% (28/37) 70% (72/103)	61% (88/145) 65% (34/52) 58% (54/93)
Genotype 4	(0/5)	(8/12)	(5/8)	(9/11)	(10/13)	(5/11)

* Pegasys 180 mcg ribavirin 1000/1200 mg, 48 w *vs.* Pegasys 180 mcg ribavirin 800 mg, 48 w: Odds Ratio (95% CI) = 1.52 (1.07 to 2.17) P-value (stratified Cochran-Mantel-Haenszel test) = 0.020

* Pegasys 180 mcg ribavirin 1000/1200 mg, 48 w *vs.* Pegasys 180 mcg ribavirin 1000/1200 mg, 24 w: Odds Ratio (95% CI) = 2.12 (1.30 to 3.46) P-value (stratified Cochran-Mantel-Haenszel test) = 0.002.

Table 10 Sustained Virological Response based on Genotype and Viral Load after Pegasys Combination Therapy with Ribavirin in HIV-HCV Co-infected Patients

Study NR15961			
	Interferon alfa-2a **3 MIU** **&** **Ribavirin 800 mg** 48 weeks	**Pegasys** 180 mcg & **Placebo** 48 weeks	**Pegasys** 180 mcg & **Ribavirin 800 mg** 48 weeks
All patients	12% (33/285)*	20% (58/286)*	40% (116/289)*
Genotype 1	7% (12/171)	14% (24/175)	29% (51/176)
Low viral load	19% (8/42)	38% (17/45)	61% (28/46)
High viral load	3% (4/129)	5% (7/130)	18% (23/130)
Genotype 2-3	20% (18/89)	36% (32/90)	62% (59/95)
Low viral load	27% (8/30)	38% (9/24)	61% (17/28)
High viral load	17% (10/59)	35% (23/66)	63% (42/67)

* Pegasys 180 mcg ribavirin 800mg vs. Interferon alfa-2a 3MIU ribavirin 800mg: Odds Ratio (95% CI) = 5.40 (3.42 to 8.54), ...P-value (stratified Cochran-Mantel-Haenszel test) = < 0.0001

* Pegasys 180 mcg ribavirin 800mg vs. Pegasys 180μg: Odds Ratio (95% CI) = 2.89 (1.93 to 4.32), ...P-value (stratified Cochran-Mantel-Haenszel test) = < 0.0001

* Interferon alfa-2a 3MIU ribavirin 800mg vs. Pegasys 180mcg: Odds Ratio (95% CI) = 0.53 (0.33 to 0.85), ...P-value (stratified Cochran-Mantel-Haenszel test) = < 0.0084

either active substance alone. The major treatment-related change was reversible mild to moderate anaemia, the severity of which was greater than that produced by either active substance alone.

6. PHARMACEUTICAL PARTICULARS

6.1 List of excipients

sodium chloride

polysorbate 80

benzyl alcohol

sodium acetate

acetic acid

water for injections

6.2 Incompatibilities

In the absence of compatibility studies, Pegasys must not be mixed with other medicinal products.

6.3 Shelf life

3 years

6.4 Special precautions for storage

Store in a refrigerator (2°C-8°C). Do not freeze.

Store in the original package in order to protect from light.

6.5 Nature and contents of container

0.5 ml of solution for injection in pre-filled syringe (siliconised Type I glass) with a plunger stopper and tip cap (butyl rubber laminated on the product facing side with fluororesin) with a needle. Available in packs of 1, 4 or 12.

6.6 Instructions for use and handling

The solution for injection is for single use only. It should be inspected visually for particulate matter and discoloration before administration.

Any unused product or waste material should be disposed of in accordance with local requirements.

7. MARKETING AUTHORISATION HOLDER

Roche Registration Limited

40 Broadwater Road

Welwyn Garden City

Hertfordshire, AL7 3AY

United Kingdom

8. MARKETING AUTHORISATION NUMBER(S)

EU/1/02/221/007

EU/1/02/221/008

EU/1/02/221/010

9. DATE OF FIRST AUTHORISATION/RENEWAL OF THE AUTHORISATION

20 June 2002

10. DATE OF REVISION OF THE TEXT

24 February 2005

Pentacarinat 300mg

(sanofi-aventis)

1. NAME OF THE MEDICINAL PRODUCT

Pentacarinat 300mg

2. QUALITATIVE AND QUANTITATIVE COMPOSITION

in terms of the active ingredient

Pentamidine Isetionate BP 300 mg (Equivalent to 172.4 mg pentamidine base)

3. PHARMACEUTICAL FORM

Sterile powder for use after reconstitution

4. CLINICAL PARTICULARS

4.1 Therapeutic indications

Pentamidine is indicated in the treatment of:

Pneumonia due to Pneumocystis carinii (PCP)

Leishmaniasis including visceral and cutaneous

Early phase African sleeping sickness caused by Trypanosoma gambiense.

All indications can be treated by deep intramuscular injection or intravenous injection.

Pneumocystis carinii pneumonia can also be treated by the inhalation route.

Pentacarinat is also indicated in the prevention of Pneumocystis carinii pneumonia in patients infected by the human immunodeficiency virus (HIV) who have experienced a previous episode of PCP. Administration is by the inhalation route.

4.2 Posology and method of administration

Pentamidine powder is reconstituted before use with Water for Injections BP. For intravenous use the required dose of pentamidine isetionate is diluted further in 50-250ml of glucose intravenous infusion BP or 0.9% (normal) Sodium Chloride Injection BP.

The following dosage regimens are recommended for adults, children and infants.

Treatment:

Pneumocystis carinii pneumonia:

By slow iv infusion, 4 mg/kg bodyweight of pentamidine isetionate once daily for at least 14 days.

If administered by inhalation, two 300 mg vials are dissolved in 6 ml of water for injection and the resultant solution administered by a suitable nebuliser once daily for three weeks.

Leishmaniasis

Visceral: 3-4 mg/kg bodyweight of pentamidine isetionate on alternate days to a maximum of 10 injections, preferably by im injection. A repeat course may be necessary.

Cutaneous: 3-4 mg/kg bodyweight, once or twice weekly by im injection until the condition resolves.

Trypanosomiasis:

4mg/kg bodyweight of pentamidine isetionate once daily or on alternate days to a total of 7-10 injections. The im or iv infusion route may be used.

There are no specific dosage recommendations for the elderly.

In renal failure the following recommendations are made for a creatinine clearance of less than 10ml/min.:

P. carinii pneumonia: in life threatening cases, 4 mg/kg bodyweight once daily for 7 to 10 days, then 4 mg/kg bodyweight on alternate days, to complete the course of at least 14 doses. In less severe cases, 4 mg/kg bodyweight on alternate days, to complete the course of at least 14 doses.

No dosage reductions are necessary in renally impaired patients with leishmaniasis or trypanosomiasis.

Hepatic failure: no specific dosage recommendations.

Prevention

Dissolve the contents of one pentacarinat vial (300 mg pentamidine isetionate) in 4-6 ml water for injections BP.

In the prophylaxis of P. carinii pneumonia, the adult dosage is 300 mg every 4 weeks or 150mg every 2 weeks.

4.3 Contraindications

The drug should not be administered to patients with a known hypersensitivity to pentamidine.

4.4 Special warnings and special precautions for use

Pentamidine isetionate should be used with particular caution in patients with hepatic and/or renal dysfunction, hypertension or hypotension, hyperglycaemia or hypoglycaemia, leucopenia, thrombocytopenia or anaemia.

Fatalities due to severe hypotension, hypoglycaemia, acute pancreatitis and cardiac arrhythmias have been reported in patients treated with pentamidine isetionate, by both the intramuscular and intravenous routes. Baseline blood pressure should be established and patients should receive the drug lying down. Blood pressure should be closely monitored during administration and at regular intervals until treatment is concluded.

Therefore patients receiving pentamidine by inhalation should be closely monitored for the development of severe adverse reactions.

Pentamidine isetionate may prolong the QT interval. Cardiac arrhythmias indicative of QT prolongation, such as Torsades de Pointes, have been reported in isolated cases with administration of pentamidine isetionate. Therefore, pentamidine isetionate should be used with care in patients with coronary heart disease, a history of ventricular arrhythmias, uncorrected hypokalaemia and or hypomagnesaemia, bradycardia (< 50 bpm), or during concomitant administration of pentamidine isetionate with QT prolonging agents.

Particular caution is necessary if the QTc exceeds 500 msec whilst receiving pentamidine isetionate therapy, continuous cardiac monitoring should be considered in this case.

Should the QTc interval exceed 550 msec then an alternative regimen should be considered

Laboratory monitoring: The following tests should be carried out before, during and after therapy by the parenteral route:

I) Blood urea, nitrogen and serum creatinine daily during therapy.

II) Complete blood and platelet counts daily during therapy.

III) Fasting blood glucose measurements daily during therapy, and at regular intervals after completion of therapy. Hyperglycaemia and diabetes mellitus, with or without preceding hypoglycaemia have occurred up to several months after cessation of therapy.

IV) Liver function tests (LFTS) including bilirubin, alkaline phosphatase, aspartate aminotransferase (AST/GOT), and alkaline aminotransferase (ALT/GPT). If baseline measurements are normal and remain so during therapy, test weekly. When there is baseline elevation in LFTS and/or LFTS increase during therapy, continue monitoring weekly unless the patient is on other hepatotoxic agents, when monitoring every 3-5 days is appropriate.

V) Serum calcium, test weekly. Serum magnesium, test twice weekly.

VI) Electrocardiograms at regular intervals.

VII) Urine analysis and serum electrolytes daily during therapy.

The benefit of aerosolised pentamidine therapy in patients at high risk of a pneumothorax should be weighed against the clinical consequences of such a manifestation.

4.5 Interaction with other medicinal products and other forms of Interaction

Caution is advised when pentamidine isetionate is concomitantly used with drugs that are known to prolong the QT interval such as phenothiazines, tricyclic antidepressants, terfenadine and astemizole, IV erythromycin, halofantrine and quinolone antibiotics (see Warnings section).

4.6 Pregnancy and lactation

There is no evidence of the safety of pentamidine isetionate in human pregnancy. A miscarriage within the first trimester of pregnancy has been reported following aerosolised prophylactic administration. Pentamidine isetionate should not be administered to pregnant patients unless considered essential.

Lactation : The use of pentamidine isetionate is contra-indicated in breast feeding mothers unless considered essential by the physician.

4.7 Effects on ability to drive and use machines

Pentamidine has no known effect on the ability to drive and use machines.

4.8 Undesirable effects

Pentamidine isetionate may prolong the QT interval. Isolated cases of Torsades de Pointes have been reported with the administration of pentamidine isetionate.

Parenteral Route

Severe reactions which may be life threatening include hypotension, hypoglycaemia, pancreatitis, cardiac arrythmias, leucopenia, thrombocytopenia, acute renal failure, hypocalcaemia. A possible case of Stevens-Johnson syndrome has been reported.

Less severe reactions include azotemia, abnormal liver function tests, leucopenia, anaemia, thrombocytopenia, macroscopic haematuria, hypomagnesaemia, hyperkalaemia, nausea and vomiting, hypotension, dizziness, syncope, flushing, hypoglycaemia, hyperglycaemia, rash, taste disturbances.

Rhabdomyolysis has been rarely reported following intramuscular administration of pentamidine isetionate.

Local reactions can occur ranging in severity from discomfort and pain to induration, abscess formation and muscle necrosis.

Reversible renal side effects occur with the highest frequency (over 20% of patients) with a slightly lower frequency of local reactions.

Side effects including metabolic disturbances, hepatic, haematological, or hypotensive episodes occur much less frequently (5-10% patients).

Inhalation Route:

Bronchospasm has been reported to occur following use of the nebuliser. This has been particularly noted in patients who have a history of smoking or asthma. This can usually be controlled by prior use of bronchodilators.

The occurrence of cases of pneumothorax has been reported in patients presenting a history of PCP. Although the aetiology of the pneumothorax was not linked primarily to the aerosolised administration of pentamidine in the majority of cases, a causal relationship to pentamidine cannot be ruled out.

Local reactions involving the upper respiratory tract can occur ranging in severity from cough, shortness of breath and wheezing, bronchospasms to eosinophilic pneumonia.

Other side effects reported were hypotention, hypoglycaemia, acute pancreatitis, renal insufficiency rash, fever, decrease in appetite, taste disturbances, fatigue, lightheadedness and nausea.

4.9 Overdose

Treatment is symptomatic. Cardiac rhythm disorders, including Torsades de Pointes, have been reported following overdose of pentamidine isetionate.

5. PHARMACOLOGICAL PROPERTIES

5.1 Pharmacodynamic properties

Pentamidine isetionate is an aromatic diamine. It is an antiprotozoal agent which acts by interfering with DNA and folate transformation, and by the inhibition of RNA and protein synthesis.

5.2 Pharmacokinetic properties

After intravenous infusion, plasma levels of pentamidine fall rapidly during the first two hours to one twentieth of peak levels, followed by a much slower decline thereafter. After intramuscular administration, the apparent volume of distribution of pentamidine is significantly greater > 3 times) than that observed following intravenous administration.

Elimination of half-lives after parenteral administration were estimated to be about 6 hours after intravenous infusion in patients with a normal renal function. The elimination of half-life following intramuscular injection was found to be about 9 hours.

Following parenteral administration, pentamidine appears to be widely distributed in the body and probably accumulates in tissue, particularly the liver and kidney. Only a small amount is excreted unchanged in the urine.

When administered by the use of a nebuliser, human kinetic studies revealed significant differences when compared to parenteral administration. Aerosol administration resulted in a 10-fold increase in bronchial alveolar lavage (BAL) supernatant fluid and an 80-fold increase in BAL sediment concentrations in comparison with those seen with equivalent intravenous doses.

Limited data suggests that the half-life of pentamidine in BAL fluid is greater than 10 to 14 days. Peak plasma concentrations after inhalation therapy were found to be approximately 10% of those observed with equivalent intramuscular doses and less than 5% of those observed following intravenous administration. This suggests that systemic effects by the inhalation route are less likely.

Long term pulmonary parenchymal effects of aerosolised pentamidine are not known. Lung volume and alveolar capillary diffusion, however, have not been shown to be affected by high doses of pentamidine administered by inhalation to AIDS patients.

5.3 Preclinical safety data

No additional data of relevance to the prescriber

6. PHARMACEUTICAL PARTICULARS

6.1 List of excipients

Not applicable

6.2 Incompatibilities

Pentamidine isetionate solution should not be mixed with any injection solutions other than Water for Injections BP, Glucose Intravenous Infusion BP and 0.9% (normal) Sodium Chloride Injection BP.

6.3 Shelf life

60 months when unopened. After reconstitution 24 hours.

6.4 Special precautions for storage

Store the dry product below 30C.

Store the reconstituted product (for intravenous infusion) at 2-8C. Use within 24 hours.

6.5 Nature and contents of container

Cardboard carton containing 5 × 10 ml glass vials each with rubber bung and aluminium ring. Each vial contains 300 mg Pentamidine Isetionate BP.

6.6 Instructions for use and handling

This product should be reconstituted in a fume cupboard. Store the dry product below 30C. Store dilute reconstituted drug solutions between 2-8C, and discard all unused portions within 24 hours of preparation. Concentrated solutions for administration by the inhalation or intramuscular routes should be used immediately.

After reconstitution with Water for Injections BP, pentacarinat should not be mixed with any injection solutions other than Glucose Intravenous Infusion 5% BP and 0.9% (normal) Sodium Chloride Injection BP.

The optimal particle size for alveolar deposition is between 1 and 2 microns.

The freshly prepared solution should be administered by inhalation using a suitable nebuliser such as a Respirgard II (trade mark of Marquest Medical Products Inc.), Modified Acorn system 22 (trade mark of Medic-Aid) or an equivalent device with either a compressor or piped oxygen at a flow rate of 6 to 10 Litres/Minute.

The nebuliser should be used in a vacated, well ventilated room. Only staff wearing adequate protective clothing (mask, goggles, gloves) should be in the room when nebulisers are being used.

A suitable well fitted one-way system should be employed such that the nebuliser stores the aerosolised drug during exhalations and disperses exhaled pentamidine into a reservoir. A filter should be fitted to the exhaust line to reduce atmospheric pollution. It is advisable to use a suitable exhaust tube which vents directly through a window to the external atmosphere. Care should be taken to ensure that passers-by will not be exposed to the exhaust.

All bystanders including medical personnel, women of child bearing potential, pregnant women, children, and people with a history of asthma, should avoid exposure to atmospheric pentamidine resulting from nebuliser usage.

Dosage equivalence: 4 mG of pentamidine isetionate contains 2.3 mG pentamidine base; 1 mg of pentamidine base is equivalent to 1.74 mG pentamidine isetionate.

Displacement value: 300 mG of pentamidine isetionate displace approximately 0.15 ml of water.

7. MARKETING AUTHORISATION HOLDER

JHC Healthcare Ltd

5 Lower Merrion Street

Dublin 2

Eire

8. MARKETING AUTHORISATION NUMBER(S)

PL 16186/0001

9. DATE OF FIRST AUTHORISATION/RENEWAL OF THE AUTHORISATION

1 September 1997

10. DATE OF REVISION OF THE TEXT

January 2005

11. LEGAL CLASSIFICATION

POM

Pentacarinat Ready-to-Use Solution

(sanofi-aventis)

1. NAME OF THE MEDICINAL PRODUCT
Pentacarinat Ready-to-Use solution

2. QUALITATIVE AND QUANTITATIVE COMPOSITION
In terms of the active ingredient

Pentamidine Isetionate 300mg

(Equivalent to 172.4mg Pentamidine base)

3. PHARMACEUTICAL FORM
Nebuliser Solution

4. CLINICAL PARTICULARS

4.1 Therapeutic indications
Pentacarinat Ready-to-Use Solution is indicated in the treatment of Pneumocystis carinii pneumonia (PCP) in patients infected by the human immunodeficiency virus (HIV).

Pentacarinat Ready-to-Use Solution is also indicated for the prevention of Pneumocystis carinii pneumonia in patients infected by the human immunodeficiency virus who have experienced a previous episode of PCP.

4.2 Posology and method of administration
Adults

Treatment of Pneumocystis carinii pneumonia

600mg, (two bottles) given once daily for 3 weeks, administered by a suitable nebuliser.

Prevention of Pneumocystis cannii pneumonia

300mg given once a month or 150mg given every two weeks, administered using a suitable nebuliser.

There are no specific dosage recommendations for the elderly.

Hepatic failure

No information is available.

4.3 Contraindications
The drug should not be administered to patients with a known hypersensitivity to pentamidine.

4.4 Special warnings and special precautions for use
Fatalities due to severe hypotension, hypoglycaemia, acute pancreatitis and cardiac arrhythmias have been reported in patients treated with pentamidine isetionate, by both the intramusciar and intravenous routes. Therefore patients receiving pentamidine by inhalation should be closely monitored for the development of severe adverse reactions.

Pentamidine isetionate should be used with particular caution in patients with hepatic and/or renal dysfunction, hypertension, hyperglycaemia, hypoglycaemia, leucopenia, thrombocytopenia or anaemia. Bronchospasm has been reported to occur following the use of the nebuliser. This has been particularly noted in patients who have a history of smoking or asthma. This can be controlled by prior use of bronchodilators.

The benefit of aerosolised pentamidine therapy in patients at high risk of a pneumothorax should be weighed against the clinical consequences of such a manifestation.

Pentamidine isetionate may prolong the QT interval. Cardiac arrhythmias indicative of QT prolongation, such as Torsades de Pointes, have been reported in isolated cases with administration of pentamidine isetionate. Therefore, pentamidine isetionate should be used with care in patients with coronary heart disease, a history of ventricular arrhythmias, uncorrected hypokalaemia and or hypomagnesaemia, bradycardia (<50 bpm), or during concomitant administration of pentamidine isetionate with QT prolonging agents.

Particular caution is necessary if the QTc exceeds 500 msec whilst receiving pentamidine isetionate therapy, continuous cardiac monitoring should be considered in this case.

Should the QTc-interval exceed 550 msec then an alternative regimen should be considered.

4.5 Interaction with other medicinal products and other forms of Interaction
Caution is advised when pentamidine isetionate is concomitantly used with drugs that are known to prolong the QT interval such as phenothiazines, tricyclic antidepressants, terfenadine and astemizole, IV erythromycin, halofantrine, and quinolene antibiotics (see Warnings section).

4.6 Pregnancy and lactation
There is no evidence on the safety of aerosolised pentamidine in human pregnancy. A miscarriage within the first trimester of pregnancy has been reported following aerosolised prophylactic administration. Pentamidine isetionate should not be administered to pregnant patients unless considered essential. The use of pentamidine isetionate is contraindicated in breast feeding mothers unless considered essential by the physician.

4.7 Effects on ability to drive and use machines
Pentamidine has no known effect on the ability to drive and use machines.

4.8 Undesirable effects
Cases of pneumothorax have been reported in patients with a history of PCP. Although the aetiology of the pneumothorax was not linked primarily to the aerosolised administration of pentamidine in the majority of cases, a causal relationship cannot be ruled out. Local reactions involving the respiratory tract can occur, ranging in severity from cough, shortness of breath and wheezing, bronchospasms to eosinophilic pneumonia. Other adverse effects reported with the use of aerosolised pentamidine are rash, hypotension, hypoglycaemia, acute pancreatitis, renal insufficiency, fever, decrease in appetite, taste disturbances, fatigue, lightheadedness and nausea.

Pentamidine isetionate may prolong the QT interval. Isolated cases of Torsades de Pointes have been reported with the administration of pentamidine isetionate.

4.9 Overdose
Should overdosage occur, treatment is symptomatic.

Cardiac rhythm disorders, including Torsades de Pointes, have been reported following overdose of pentamidine isetionate.

5. PHARMACOLOGICAL PROPERTIES

5.1 Pharmacodynamic properties
Pentamidine isetionate is an aromatic diamine. It is an antiprotozoal agent which acts by interfering with DNA and folate transformation, and by the inhibition of RNA and protein synthesis.

5.2 Pharmacokinetic properties
When administered by the use of a nebuliser, human kinetic studies revealed significant differences when compared to parenteral administration. Aerosol administration resulted in a 10-fold increase in bronchial alveolar lavage (BAL) supematant fluid and an 80-fold increase in BAL sediment concentrations in comparison with those seen with equivalent parenteral doses.

Limited data suggests that the half life of pentamidine in BAL fluid is greater than 10-14 days.

Long term pulmonary parenchymal effects of aerosolised pentamidine are not known. Lung volume and alveolar capillary diffusion, however, have not been shown to be affected by high doses of pentamidine administered by inhalation to AIDS patients.

5.3 Preclinical safety data
No additional data of relevance to the prescriber.

6. PHARMACEUTICAL PARTICULARS

6.1 List of excipients

Glucose
Sodium acetate
Glacial acetic acid
Water for Injections

6.2 Incompatibilities
Pentamidine nebuliser solution should not be mixed with any other solution.

6.3 Shelf life
12 months.

6.4 Special precautions for storage
Store below 25°C. Do not refrigerate. See 6.6 (Instructions for Use/Handling)

6.5 Nature and contents of container
Low density polyethylene bottles and plug with yellow high density polyethylene tamper evident caps

6.6 Instructions for use and handling
Any solid material evident in the polyethylene bottle should be re-dissolved by gentle warming in the hand before use. The solution placed in the nebuliser reservoir should be visually inspected prior to use. Any solution containing particulate matter should be discarded and the nebuliser reservoir rinsed with sterile water prior to re-use.

The optimal particle size for alveolar deposition is between 1 and 2 microns.

The solution containing the required dosage should be administered by inhalation using a suitable nebuliser such as a Respirgard II (trade mark of Marquest Medical Products inc.), modified Acorn system 22 (trade mark of Medic-Aid) or an equivalent device with either a compressor or piped oxygen at a flow rate of 6 to 10 litres/minute.

The nebuliser should be used in a vacated well ventilated room. Only staff wearing adequate protective clothing (mask, goggles, gloves) should be in the room when nebulisers are being used.

A suitable well fitted one way system should be employed such that the nebuliser stores the aerosolised drug during exhalations and disperses exhaled pentamidine into a reservoir. A filter should be fitted to the exhaust line to reduce atmospheric pollution. It is advisable to use a suitable exhaust tube which vents directly through a window to the external atmosphere. Care should be taken to ensure that passers-by will not be exposed to the exhaust. All bystanders including medical personnel, women of child bearing potential, pregnant women, children and people with a history of asthma should avoid exposure to atmospheric pentamidine resulting from nebuliser usage.

Dosage equivalence: 4 mg pentamidine isethionate contain 2.3 mg pentamidine base. I mg pentamidine base is equivalent to 1.74 mg pentamidine isethionate.

7. MARKETING AUTHORISATION HOLDER
JHC Healthcare Ltd

5 Lower Merrion Street

Dublin 2

Eire

8. MARKETING AUTHORISATION NUMBER(S)
PL 16186/0002

9. DATE OF FIRST AUTHORISATION/RENEWAL OF THE AUTHORISATION
1st Seprember 1997

10. DATE OF REVISION OF THE TEXT
October 2004

Legal category: POM

Pentagastrin Injection BP

(Cambridge Laboratories)

1. NAME OF THE MEDICINAL PRODUCT
Pentagastrin Injection BP

2. QUALITATIVE AND QUANTITATIVE COMPOSITION
Pentagastrin BP 0.025% w/v

3. PHARMACEUTICAL FORM
Solution for Injection.

4. CLINICAL PARTICULARS

4.1 Therapeutic indications
Pentagastrin Injection BP is used for the diagnostic testing of gastric secretion.

4.2 Posology and method of administration
For administration either subcutaneously or by continuous intravenous infusion.

Adults (including the elderly) and Children

The following procedure is adopted for testing gastric secretion with Pentagastrin Injection BP:

The patient receives no medication (eg. antacids, etc.) that might affect the results of the test for 24 hours and no food for 12 hours before the test. On the morning of the test a radio-opaque tube (Leven no. 7 or Ryles's 12 – 16Fr.) is passed into the patients by the way of the nose. Radiological observation is used to ensure that the tube is correctly positioned in the lower part of the body of the stomach.

The tube is securely fastened to the patient's nose and forehead with adhesive tape to ensure that it is not displaced. The patient lies on his left side.

The gastric juices are then collected by applying continuous suction (at 30-50 mm Hg below atmospheric pressure) to this tube, supplemented by manual suction. The patient takes occasional deep breaths to improve collection. The basal secretion is obtained by collecting samples at 15 minute intervals over an hour.

Pentagastrin Injection BP is then given, either at a dose of:

(a) 6 micrograms/kg bodyweight subcutaneously, or

(b) 0.6 micrograms/kg/hour as a continuous intravenous infusion. A tuberculin syringe is used to give a dose correct to 0.01 ml.

If dilution is required normal saline may be used.

Specimens of the gastric juices are again collected over periods of 10 or 15 minutes. The volume of the sample is measured and it is immediately filtered through gauze into a bottle. The acidity of each sample is determined by titration.

4.3 Contraindications
When the patient has previously shown a severe idiosyncratic response to the drug, Pentagastrin Injection BP should not be administered.

4.4 Special warnings and special precautions for use
As pentagastrin stimulates gastric acid secretion it should be used with caution in patients with acute or bleeding peptic ulcer disease, though there is no clinical evidence to contraindicate use.

4.5 Interaction with other medicinal products and other forms of Interaction
None known.

4.6 Pregnancy and lactation
Pregnancy: Pentagastrin Injection BP should not be administered during pregnancy.

Lactation: no special precautions are required.

4.7 Effects on ability to drive and use machines
No precautions are required.

4.8 Undesirable effects
At the recommended dosage the incidence of side effects is extremely small, although very occasionally an individual may respond with hypotension and associated dizziness and faintness. Other unwanted effects reported are mild abdominal discomfort, abdominal cramps, nausea, vomiting, flushing, sweating, headaches, drowsiness or exhaustion, heaviness or weakness of the legs, allergic reactions,

bradycardia, tachycardia, anxiety and panic attacks. These effects disappear once administration of 'Pentagastrin Injection BP' has ceased.

4.9 Overdose
The form of presentation makes it unlikely that overdosage will occur, and no such occurrence has been reported. As maximal secretory response is produced by the normal dosage, increased dosage would be expected to have no sequel other than an accentuation of the known side effects.

5. PHARMACOLOGICAL PROPERTIES

5.1 Pharmacodynamic properties
Pentagastrin is a synthetic pentapeptide containing the carboxyl terminal tetrapeptide responsible for the actions of natural gastrins. The most prominent action of pentagastrin is to stimulate the secretion of gastric acid, pepsin and intrinsic factor. Additonally, it stimulates pancreatic secretion, inhibits absorption of water and electrolytes from the ileum, contracts the smooth muscle of the lower oesophageal sphincter and stomach (but delays gastric emptying time), relaxes the sphincter of Oddi and increases blood flow in the gastric mucosa.

5.2 Pharmacokinetic properties
Pentagastrin stimulates gastric acid secretion approximately ten minutes after subcutaneous injection, with peak response occurring in most cases twenty to thirty minutes after administration. Duration of activity is usually between sixty and eighty minutes.

Pentagastrin is rapidly absorbed after administration. Pentagastrin has a short half-live (10 minutes or less) in the circulation. It is metabolised primarily in the liver and excretion is mainly by the kidneys.

5.3 Preclinical safety data
Pentagastrin is a drug on which extensive clinical experience has been obtained. All relevant information for the prescriber is provided elsewhere in the Summary of Product Characteristics.

6. PHARMACEUTICAL PARTICULARS

6.1 List of excipients

List of Excipients Used in Manufacture

Sodium chloride Ph.Eur

Water for Injections Ph.Eur

Ammonium bicarbonate BP

N. Ammonia solution } pH Adjustment

N. Hydrochloric acid }

Final Excipient Composition in Solution

Sodium chloride

Ammonium chloride

Water

6.2 Incompatibilities
None known.

6.3 Shelf life
24 months

6.4 Special precautions for storage
Store away from light, below 4°C but above freezing.

6.5 Nature and contents of container
2 ml glass ampoules in boxes of 5.

6.6 Instructions for use and handling
If dilution is required Sodium Chloride Injection BP may be used. This solution should be prepared immediately before it is required for use.

7. MARKETING AUTHORISATION HOLDER
Cambridge Laboratories Limited

Deltic House

Kingfisher Way

Silverlink Business Park

Wallsend

Tyne & Wear

NE28 9NX

8. MARKETING AUTHORISATION NUMBER(S)
PL 12070/0020

9. DATE OF FIRST AUTHORISATION/RENEWAL OF THE AUTHORISATION
First authorisation 9/2/73

Renewed 15/10/95

10. DATE OF REVISION OF THE TEXT
June 2000

Pentasa Mesalazine Enema

(Ferring Pharmaceuticals Ltd)

1. NAME OF THE MEDICINAL PRODUCT
PENTASA® Mesalazine Enema.

2. QUALITATIVE AND QUANTITATIVE COMPOSITION
Each enema bottle contains mesalazine 1g in 100ml.

3. PHARMACEUTICAL FORM
Rectal suspension.

Each bottle contains 100ml of a colourless to faint yellow suspension containing 1g mesalazine

4. CLINICAL PARTICULARS

4.1 Therapeutic indications
PENTASA Mesalazine Enema is indicated for the treatment of ulcerative colitis affecting the distal colon and rectum.

4.2 Posology and method of administration
Adults: The recommended dosage is one enema at bedtime.

Children: Not recommended.

PENTASA Mesalazine Enemas are for rectal administration

4.3 Contraindications
PENTASA is contraindicated in:

- patients with known sensitivity to salicylates
- patients with severe liver and/or renal impairment
- patients allergic to any of the ingredients

4.4 Special warnings and special precautions for use
Serious blood dyscrasias have been reported rarely with mesalazine. Haematological investigations should be performed if the patient develops unexplained bleeding, bruising, purpura, anaemia, fever or sore throat. Treatment should be stopped if there is suspicion or evidence of blood dyscrasia.

Most patients who are intolerant or hypersensitive to sulphasalazine are able to use PENTASA without risk of similar reactions. However, caution is recommended when treating patients allergic to sulphasalazine (risk of allergy to salicylates). Caution is recommended in patients with impaired liver function.

It is recommended that mesalazine is used with extreme caution in patients with mild to moderate renal impairment (see section 4.3).

If a patient develops dehydration while on treatment with mesalazine, normal electrolyte levels and fluid balance should be restored as soon as possible.

Mesalazine induced cardiac hypersensitivity reactions (myocarditis and pericarditis) have been reported rarely. Treatment should be discontinued on suspicion or evidence of these reactions.

4.5 Interaction with other medicinal products and other forms of Interaction
The concurrent use of mesalazine with other known nephrotoxic agents, such as NSAIDs and azathioprine, may increase the risk of renal reactions (see section 4.4).

Concomitant treatment with mesalazine can increase the risk of blood dyscrasia in patients receiving azathioprine or 6-mercaptopurine.

4.6 Pregnancy and lactation
PENTASA should be used with caution during pregnancy and lactation and only if the potential benefit outweighs the possible hazards in the opinion of the physician.

Mesalazine is known to cross the placental barrier, but the limited data available on its use in pregnant women do not allow assessment of possible adverse effects. No teratogenic effects have been observed in animal studies.

Blood disorders (leucopenia, thrombocytopenia, anaemia) have been reported in new-borns of mothers being treated with PENTASA.

Mesalazine is excreted in breast milk. The mesalazine concentration in breast milk is lower than in maternal blood, whereas the metabolite, acetyl mesalazine appears in similar or increased concentrations. There is limited experience of the use of oral mesalazine in lactating women. No controlled studies with PENTASA during breast-feeding have been carried out. Hypersensitivity reactions like diarrhoea in the infant cannot be excluded.

4.7 Effects on ability to drive and use machines
No adverse effects.

4.8 Undesirable effects
Mesalazine may be associated with an exacerbation of the symptoms of colitis in those patients who have previously had such problems with sulphasalazine.

Undesirable effects are as follows:

Common (≥1% and <10%)	*Gastrointestinal disorders:* Nausea, vomiting, diarrhoea, abdominal pain
	Skin disorders: Rash (including urticaria and erythematous rash)
	General: Headache
Rare (≥0.01% and < 0.1%)	*Blood disorders:* Leucopenia (including granulocytopenia), neutropenia, agranulocytosis, aplastic anaemia, thrombocytopenia
	Nervous system disorders: Peripheral neuropathy
	Cardiac disorders: Myocarditis, pericarditis
	Respiratory disorders: Allergic lung reactions (including dyspnoea, coughing, allergic alveolitis, pulmonary eosinophilia, pulmonary infiltration, pneumonitis)
	Gastrointestinal disorders: Pancreatitis, increased amylase
	Liver: Abnormalities of hepatic function and hepatotoxicity (including, hepatitis, cirrhosis, hepatic failure)
	Urogenital: Abnormal renal function (including interstitial nephritis, nephrotic syndrome), urine discolouration (*see additional text)
	Collagen disorders: Lupus erythematosus-like reactions
Very rare (<0.01%)	*Blood disorders:* Anaemia, eosinophilia (as part of an allergic reaction) and pancytopenia
	Liver: Increased liver enzymes and bilirubin
	Skin disorders: Reversible alopecia, bullous skin reactions including erythema multiforme and Stevens-Johnson syndrome
	Musculo-skeletal disorders: Myalgia, arthralgia
	Allergic reactions: Hypersensitivity reactions, drug fever

*Renal failure has been reported. Mesalazine-induced nephrotoxicity should be suspected in patients developing renal dysfunction during treatment.

The mechanism of mesalazine induced myocarditis, pericarditis, pancreatitis, nephritis and hepatitis is unknown, but it might be of allergic origin.

Following rectal administration local reactions such as pruritus, rectal discomfort and urge may occur.

4.9 Overdose
Acute experience in animals:

Single oral doses of mesalazine of up to 5g/kg in pigs or a single intravenous dose of mesalazine at 920mg/kg in rats were not lethal.

Human experience:

No cases of overdose have been reported.

Management of overdose in man:

Symptomatic treatment at hospital. Close monitoring of renal function. Intravenous infusion of electrolytes may be used to promote diuresis.

5. PHARMACOLOGICAL PROPERTIES

5.1 Pharmacodynamic properties
Pharmacotherapeutic group: Intestinal anti-inflammatory agents.

Mechanism of action and pharmacodynamic effects:

Mesalazine is recognised as the active moiety of sulphasalazine in the treatment of ulcerative colitis. It is thought to act locally on the gut wall in inflammatory bowel disease, although its precise mechanism of action has not been fully elucidated.

Increased leucocyte migration, abnormal cytokine production, increased production of arachidonic acid metabolites, particularly leukotriene B4 and increased free radical formation in the inflamed intestinal tissue are all present in patients with inflammatory bowel disease. Mesalazine has in-vitro and in-vivo pharmacological effects that inhibit leucocyte chemotaxis, decrease cytokine and leukotriene production and scavenge for free radicals. It is currently unknown which, if any of these mechanisms play a predominant role in the clinical efficacy of mesalazine.

5.2 Pharmacokinetic properties
General characteristics of the active substance

Disposition and local availability:

PENTASA enemas are designed to provide the distal part of the intestinal tract with high concentrations of mesalazine and a low systemic absorption. The enemas have been shown to reach and cover the descending colon.

Biotransformation:

Mesalazine is metabolised both pre-systemically by the intestinal mucosa and systemically in the liver to N-acetyl mesalazine (acetyl mesalazine). The acetylation seems to be independent of the acetylator phenotype of the patient. Some acetylation also occurs through the action of colonic bacteria.

Acetyl mesalazine is thought to be clinically as well as toxicologically inactive, although this remains to be confirmed.

Absorption:

The absorption following rectal administration is low, but depends on the dose, the formulation and the extent of spread. Based on urine recoveries in healthy volunteers under steady-state conditions given a daily dose of 2g (1g × 2), about 15-20% of the dose is absorbed after administration of enemas.

Distribution:

Mesalazine and acetyl mesalazine do not cross the blood brain barrier. Protein binding of mesalazine is approximately 50% and of acetyl mesalazine about 80%.

Elimination:

The plasma half-life of pure mesalazine is approximately 40 minutes and for acetyl mesalazine approximately 70 minutes. Both substances are excreted in urine and faeces. The urinary excretion consists mainly of acetyl mesalazine.

Characteristics in patients:

The systematic absorption following administration of PENTASA enemas has been shown to be significantly decreased in patients with active ulcerative colitis compared to those in remission.

In patients with impaired liver and kidney functions, the resultant decrease in the rate of elimination and increased systemic concentration of mesalazine may constitute an increased risk of nephrotoxic adverse reactions.

5.3 Preclinical safety data

There are no pre-clinical data of relevance to the prescriber which are additional to that already included in other sections of the SPC.

6. PHARMACEUTICAL PARTICULARS

6.1 List of excipients

Disodium edetate

Sodium metabisulphite

Sodium acetate

Hydrochloric acid, concentrated

Purified water

6.2 Incompatibilities

None known.

6.3 Shelf life

24 months.

6.4 Special precautions for storage

Do not store above 25°C. Keep bottle in the outer carton.

6.5 Nature and contents of container

Polyethylene enema bottles fitted with a tip and valve for rectal application, supplied in nitrogen-filled aluminium-foil bags. Presented in cartons containing 7 × 100ml bottles individually foil-wrapped.

6.6 Instructions for use and handling

None.

7. MARKETING AUTHORISATION HOLDER

Ferring Pharmaceuticals Ltd.,

The Courtyard

Waterside Drive

Langley

Berkshire SL3 6EZ.

8. MARKETING AUTHORISATION NUMBER(S)

PL 3194/0027

9. DATE OF FIRST AUTHORISATION/RENEWAL OF THE AUTHORISATION

4th February 2004

10. DATE OF REVISION OF THE TEXT

February 2005

11. LEGAL CATEGORY

POM

Pentasa Sachet

(Ferring Pharmaceuticals Ltd)

1. NAME OF THE MEDICINAL PRODUCT

PENTASA® Sachet 1g prolonged release granules

2. QUALITATIVE AND QUANTITATIVE COMPOSITION

Mesalazine 1g

For excipients, see section 6.1

3. PHARMACEUTICAL FORM

Prolonged release granules

Whitish to pale brown granules

4. CLINICAL PARTICULARS

4.1 Therapeutic indications

Mild to moderate ulcerative colitis

4.2 Posology and method of administration

Ulcerative colitis

Active disease:

Individual dosage, up to 4g mesalazine daily divided into 2 - 4 doses.

Maintenance treatment:

Individual dosage, recommended dosage 2g mesalazine daily divided into 2 doses.

There is no dosage recommendation in children due to limited clinical data.

The granules must not be chewed.

The contents of the sachet should be emptied onto the tongue and washed down with some water or orange juice.

4.3 Contraindications

Hypersensitivity to mesalazine, any other component of the product, or salicylates.

Severe liver and/or renal impairment.

Children under 12 years of age.

4.4 Special warnings and special precautions for use

Caution is recommended when treating patients allergic to sulphasalazine (risk of allergy to salicylates).

Caution is recommended in patients with impaired liver or renal function and in patients with haemorrhagic diathesis. The drug is not recommended for use in patients with renal impairment. The renal function should be regularly monitored (e.g. serum creatinine), especially during the initial phase of treatment. Mesalazine induced nephrotoxicity should be suspected in patients developing renal dysfunction during treatment.

The concurrent use of other known nephrotoxic agents, such as NSAIDs and azathioprine, may increase the risk of renal reactions.

Caution is recommended in patients with active peptic ulcer.

Mesalazine-induced cardiac hypersensitivity reactions (myo-and pericarditis) have been reported rarely. Serious blood dyscrasias have been reported very rarely with mesalazine. Concomitant treatment with mesalazine can increase the risk of blood dyscrasia in patients receiving azathioprine or 6-mercaptopurine. Treatment should be discontinued on suspicion or evidence of these adverse reactions.

4.5 Interaction with other medicinal products and other forms of Interaction

No interactions between PENTASA Sachet and other drugs have been reported.

4.6 Pregnancy and lactation

PENTASA Sachet should not be used during pregnancy and lactation except when the potential benefits of the treatment outweigh the possible hazards in the opinion of the physician.

Pregnancy:

Mesalazine is known to cross the placental barrier. The limited data available on the use of this compound in pregnant women do not allow assessment of possible adverse effects. No teratogenic effects have been observed in animal studies and in a controlled human study.

Blood disorders (leucopenia, thrombocytopenia, anaemia) have been reported in new-borns of mothers being treated with PENTASA.

Lactation:

Mesalazine is excreted in breast milk. The mesalazine concentration in breast milk is lower than in maternal blood, whereas the metabolite - acetyl mesalazine- appears in similar or increased concentrations. No controlled studies with PENTASA during breast-feeding have been carried out. Only limited experience during lactation in women after oral application is available to date. Hypersensitivity reactions like diarrhoea can not be excluded.

4.7 Effects on ability to drive and use machines

None known.

4.8 Undesirable effects

The most frequent undesirable effects seen in clinical trials are diarrhoea (3%), nausea (3%), abdominal pain (3%), headache (3%), vomiting (1%) and rash (1%). Hypersensitivity reactions and drug fever may occasionally occur.

Frequency of adverse effects, based on clinical trials and reports from post-marketing surveillance

Common (≥ 1% and < 10%)	Nervous system disorders:	Headache
	Gastrointestinal disorders:	Diarrhoea, abdominal pain, nausea, vomiting
	Skin and subcutaneous tissue disorders	Rash incl. urticaria, exanthema
Rare (≥ 0.01% and < 0.1%)	Cardiac disorders:	myo*- and pericarditis*
	Gastrointestinal disorders:	Increased amylase, pancreatitis*
Very rare (< 0.01%)	Blood and the lymphatic system disorders:	Eosinophilia (as part of an allergic reaction), anaemia, aplastic anaemia, leucopenia (incl. granulocytopenia), thrombocytopenia, agranulocytosis, pancytopenia.
	Nervous system disorders:	Peripheral neuropathy
	Respiratory, thoracic and mediastinal disorders:	Allergic lung reactions (incl. pneumonitis)
	Hepato-biliary disorders:	Increased liver enzymes, hepatitis*
	Skin and subcutaneous tissue disorders:	Reversible alopecia
	Musculo-skeletal, connective tissue and bone disorders:	Myalgia, arthralgia, single cases of lupus erythematosus- like reactions
	Renal and urinary disorders:	Abnormal renal function (incl. interstitial nephritis*, nephrotic syndrome), urine discolouration

(*) The mechanism of mesalazine-induced myo- and pericarditis, pancreatitis, nephritis and hepatitis in unknown, but it might be of allergic origin.

It is important to note that several of these disorders can also be attributed to the inflammatory bowel disease itself.

Isolated reports of Quincke's oedema

Isolated reports on benign intracranial hypertension in adolescents.

4.9 Overdose

Experience in animals:

A single intravenous dose of mesalazine in rats of 920mg/kg and single oral doses of mesalazine in pigs up to 5g/kg were not lethal.

Human experience:

No experience

Management of overdose in man:

Symptomatic treatment at hospital. Close monitoring of renal function.

5. PHARMACOLOGICAL PROPERTIES

5.1 Pharmacodynamic properties

Pharmacotherapeutic group (ATC-Code): A07E C02

Mesalazine is the active component of sulphasalazine, which has been used for a long time in the treatment of ulcerative colitis and Crohn's disease.

The therapeutic value of mesalazine appears to be due to local effect on the inflamed intestinal tissue, rather than to systemic effect.

Increased leucocyte migration, abnormal cytokine production, increased production of arachidonic acid metabolites particularly leukotriene B4, and increased free radical formation in the inflamed intestinal tissue are all present in patients with inflammatory bowel disease. Mesalazine has in-vitro and in-vivo pharmacological effects that inhibit leucocyte chemotaxis, decrease cytokine and leukotriene production and scavenge for free radicals. The mechanism of action of mesalazine is, however, still not understood.

5.2 Pharmacokinetic properties

General Characteristics of the Active Substance

PENTASA Sachet prolonged release granules consist of ethylcellulose coated microgranules of mesalazine. Following administration mesalazine is continuously released from the individual microgranules throughout the gastrointestinal tract in any enteral pH conditions. The microgranules enter the duodenum within an hour of administration, independent of food co-administration. The average small intestinal transit time is approximately 3-4 hrs in healthy volunteers.

Biotransformation:

Mesalazine is metabolised into N-acetyl-mesalazine (acetyl mesalazine) both pre-systematically by the intestinal mucosa and systemically in the liver. Some acetylation also occurs through the action of colonic bacteria. The acetylation seems to be independent of the acetylator phenotype of the patient. Acetyl mesalazine is believed to be clinically as well as toxicologically inactive.

Absorption:

30-50% of an oral dose is absorbed, predominantly from the small intestine. Maximum plasma concentrations are seen 1-4 hours post-dose. The plasma concentration of mesalazine decreases gradually and is no longer detectable 12 hours post-dose. The plasma concentration curve for acetyl mesalazine follows the same pattern, but the concentration is generally higher and the elimination is slower.

The metabolic ratio of acetyl mesalazine to mesalazine in plasma after oral administration ranges from 3.5 to 1.3 after daily doses of 500mg × 3 and 2g × 3, respectively, implying a dose-dependent acetylation which may be subject to saturation.

Mean steady-state plasma concentrations of mesalazine are approximately 2 micromoles/l, 8 micromoles/l and 12 micromoles/l after 1.5g, 4g and 6g daily dosages, respectively. For acetyl mesalazine the corresponding concentrations are 6 micromoles/l, 13 micromoles/l and 16 micromoles/l.

unknown which, if any of these mechanisms play a predominant role in the clinical efficacy of mesalazine.

5.2 Pharmacokinetic properties

General characteristics of the active substance:

Disposition and local availability:

PENTASA suppositories are designed to provide the distal part of the intestinal tract with high concentrations of mesalazine and a low systemic absorption. They are used to treat the rectum.

Biotransformation:

Mesalazine is metabolised both pre-systemically by the intestinal mucosa and systemically in the liver to N-acetyl mesalazine (acetyl mesalazine). The acetylation seems to be independent of the acetylator phenotype of the patient. Some acetylation also occurs through the action of colonic bacteria.

Acetyl mesalazine is thought to be clinically as well as toxicologically inactive, although this remains to be confirmed.

Absorption:

The absorption following rectal administration is low, but depends on the dose, the formulation and the extent of spread. Based on urine recoveries in healthy volunteers under steady-state conditions given a daily dose of 2g (1g × 2), approximately 10% of the dose is absorbed after administration of suppositories.

Distribution:

Mesalazine and acetyl mesalazine do not cross the blood brain barrier. Protein binding of mesalazine is approximately 50% and of acetyl mesalazine about 80%.

Elimination:

The plasma half-life of pure mesalazine is approximately 40 minutes and for acetyl mesalazine approximately 70 minutes. Both substances are excreted in urine and faeces. The urinary excretion consists mainly of acetyl mesalazine.

Characteristics in patients:

In patients with impaired liver and kidney functions, the resultant decrease in the rate of elimination and increased systemic concentration of mesalazine may constitute an increased risk of nephrotoxic adverse reactions.

5.3 Preclinical safety data

There are no pre-clinical data of relevance to the prescriber which are additional to that already included in other sections of the SPC.

6. PHARMACEUTICAL PARTICULARS

6.1 List of excipients

Povidone Ph. Eur.

Macrogol 6000 Ph. Eur.

Magnesium stearate Ph. Eur.

Talc Ph. Eur.

6.2 Incompatibilities

None known

6.3 Shelf life

36 months

6.4 Special precautions for storage

Do not store above 25°C. Store in the original package.

6.5 Nature and contents of container

Double aluminium foil blister strips of 7 suppositories each.

Pack size: 28

6.6 Instructions for use and handling

None

7. MARKETING AUTHORISATION HOLDER

Ferring Pharmaceuticals Ltd.

The Courtyard

Waterside Drive

Langley

Berkshire SL3 6EZ

8. MARKETING AUTHORISATION NUMBER(S)

PL 3194/0045

9. DATE OF FIRST AUTHORISATION/RENEWAL OF THE AUTHORISATION

5th December 2002

10. DATE OF REVISION OF THE TEXT

February 2005

11. LEGAL CATEGORY

POM

Pentostam Injection

(GlaxoSmithKline UK)

1. NAME OF THE MEDICINAL PRODUCT

Pentostam Injection.

2. QUALITATIVE AND QUANTITATIVE COMPOSITION

Sodium Stibogluconate BP equivalent to 100 mg pentavalent antimony in each ml.

3. PHARMACEUTICAL FORM

Injection.

4. CLINICAL PARTICULARS

4.1 Therapeutic indications

Pentostam is indicated for the following diseases:

Visceral leishmaniasis (kala azar).

Cutaneous leishmaniasis.

South American mucocutaneous leishmaniasis.

Pentostam may also be of value in the treatment of leishmaniasis recidivans and diffuse cutaneous leishmaniasis in the New World.

Note: Cutaneous and diffuse cutaneous leishmaniasis caused by *Leishmania aethiopica*infections are unresponsive to treatment with pentavalent antimony compounds, including Pentostam, at conventional dosage, but may respond slowly at higher dosage.

4.2 Posology and method of administration

Route of administration

Except where otherwise stated, all doses should be given by the intravenous or intramuscular route.

All dosage recommendations are based on the findings of the WHO Expert Committee on leishmaniasis which met in 1984. There are no special recommendations for different age groups.

Visceral leishmaniasis: 10 to 20 mg Sb^{5+} (0.1 to 0.2 ml Pentostam)/kg bodyweight to a maximum of 850 mg (8.5 ml Pentostam) daily for a minimum period of 20 days. Patients should be examined for evidence of relapse after 2 and 6 months, and in Africa after 12 months.

Cutaneous leishmaniasis NOT caused by L. aethiopica: The dosage regimen outlined for visceral leishmaniasis is recommended. Alternatively, single, non-inflamed nodular lesions known not to be due to *L. braziliensis* may be treated with intralesional injections of 100 to 300 mg Sb^{5+} (1 to 3 ml Pentostam) repeated once or twice if necessary at intervals of 1 to 2 days. Infiltration must be thorough and produce complete blanching of the base of the lesion.

Individuals with cutaneous leishmaniasis due to *L. braziliensis* should be treated systematically for several days after the lesion is healed.

Note: After successful treatment of *L. braziliensis*, antileishmania antibody titres decline steadily over 4 to 24 months.

Muco-cutaneous leishmaniasis: Patients with parasitologically confirmed leishmaniasis should be treated with 20 mg Sb^{5+} (0.2 ml Pentostam)/kg bodyweight to a maximum of 850 mg (8.5 ml Pentostam) daily, continuing this dosage for several days longer than it takes to achieve parasitological and clinical cure.

In the event of relapse, a further course should be given for at least twice the previous duration.

Diffuse cutaneous leishmaniasis in the New World and leishmaniasis recidivans: Owing to the rarity of these conditions, precise data on dosage are not available. A dose of 10 to 20 mg Sb^{5+} (0.1 to 0.2 mg Pentostam)/kg bodyweight to a maximum of 850 mg (8.5 ml Pentostam) may be given daily for 2 to 3 weeks. If there is a response, then treatment should be maintained until several days after clinical cure of leishmaniasis recidivans and for several months after clinical and parasitological cure of diffuse cutaneous leishmaniasis.

Use in the elderly: There is little information on the effects of Pentostam on elderly individuals. If treatment of cutaneous leishmaniasis is necessary then local infiltration is preferred. The normal precautions should be strictly adhered to when treating older patients for visceral leishmaniasis.

4.3 Contraindications

Pentostam should not be given to any patient with significantly impaired renal function.

Pentostam should not be given to any patient who has experienced a serious adverse reaction to a previous dose.

4.4 Special warnings and special precautions for use

Intravenous injection should be administered very slowly over 5 minutes to reduce the risk of local thrombosis. In the unlikely event of coughing, vomiting or substernal pain occurring, administration should be discontinued immediately. In such cases, extreme care should be taken if Pentostam is re-administered by this route.

Successful treatment of mucocutaneous leishmaniasis may induce severe inflammation around the lesion. In cases of pharyngeal or tracheal involvement, this may be life-threatening. Under such circumstances, corticosteroids may be used.

Very rarely, anaphylactic shock may develop during treatment for which adrenaline injection and appropriate supportive measures should be given immediately.

Prolongation of the QTc interval has been observed in some patients taking sodium stibogluconate and appears to be dose-related. There have also been reports of fatal cardiac arrhythmias in patients receiving higher dose antimonial therapy for visceral leishmaniasis. Therefore, ECG monitoring is recommended before and during therapy with sodium stibogluconate. Where ECG monitoring is not available, the risks and benefits of sodium stibogluconate therapy should be assessed on an individual basis.

If clinically significant prolongation of QTc interval occurs, sodium stibogluconate should be discontinued. Electrocardiographic changes, notably alterations in T wave amplitude may be expected in the majority of patients given sodium stibogluconate, these appear to be reversible on cessation of therapy and are not of serious significance.

Sodium stibogluconate should be used with caution in patients with cardiovascular disease, a history of ventricular arrhythmias or other risk factors known to predispose towards QT prolongation: for example, those with congenital QTc prolongation or taking concomitant drugs known to significantly prolong the QT interval (e.g. class III antiarrhythmics such as sotalol and amiodarone).

As there appears to be a dose relationship in the development of ECG abnormalities, prior exposure to antimonial therapy should be considered when assessing a patient's suitability for initiating or continuing therapy with sodium stibogluconate.

Patients who have recently received other antimonial drugs should be monitored closely for signs of antimony intoxication such as bradycardia and cardiac arrhythmias during administration of sodium stibogluconate.

Intercurrent infections, such as pneumonia, should be sought and treated concomitantly.

High concentrations of antimony are found in the livers of animals after repeated dosage with pentavalent antimony. Pentostam should therefore be used with caution in patients with hepatic disease. However, some abnormalities of liver function may be expected in cases of visceral leishmaniasis. In such patients the benefit of pentavalent antimony treatment outweighs the risk. Pentostam may induce mild elevation of hepatic enzymes in serum which later return to normal.

The Pack for this product carries the following statements:

Keep out of the reach and sight of children

Do not store above 25°C. Do not freeze.

Protect from light

Poison

In addition the 100ml pack will have the following statement:

The contents should not be used more than 1 month after removing the first dose.

4.5 Interaction with other medicinal products and other forms of Interaction

No interactions with Pentostam have been reported.

4.6 Pregnancy and lactation

Although no effects on the foetus have been reported, Pentostam should be withheld during pregnancy unless the potential benefits to the patient outweigh the possible risk to the foetus.

Children should not be breast-fed by mothers receiving Pentostam.

4.7 Effects on ability to drive and use machines

None known.

4.8 Undesirable effects

Approximately 1 to 2% of patients complain of nausea, vomiting and/or diarrhoea and a slightly higher number of abdominal pain.

Other common side-effects include anorexia, malaise, myalgia, arthralgia headache and lethargy.

ECG changes, including reduction in T-wave amplitude, T-wave inversion and QT prolongation have been observed (see Section 4.4 Special Warnings and Precautions for Use).

Transient coughing immediately following injection was reported with varying frequency during several trials.

Intravenous injection of Pentostam may cause transient pain along the course of the vein and eventually thrombosis of that vein.

Transient rises in serum lipase and amylase usually occur during treatment with sodium stibogluconate. Symptomatic pancreatitis has also been reported.

During some early trials of sodium stibogluconate, pneumonia occurred in a small number of patients treated for visceral leishmaniasis and this occasionally proved fatal. Pneumonia is a feature of the visceral leishmaniasis disease process; however, it has been associated with the toxicity profile of trivalent antimony. It is, therefore, not possible to determine whether these cases were due to the disease or to Pentostam.

Other (rarely reported) side-effects include fever, rigor, sweating, vertigo, facial flushing, worsening of lesions on the cheek, bleeding from the nose or gum, substernal pain, jaundice and rash.

Transient reductions in platelets, white blood cells and haemoglobin.

4.9 Overdose

The main symptoms of antimony overdosage are gastrointestinal disturbances (nausea, vomiting and severe diarrhoea). Haemorrhagic nephritis and hepatitis may also occur.

There is only limited information on the use of chelating agents in the treatment of intoxication with antimony compounds. Dimercaprol has been reported to be effective: a dose of 200 mg by intramuscular injection, every six hours until recovery is complete, is suggested.

2,3-dimercaptosuccinic acid (DMSA) may also be effective treatment.

5. PHARMACOLOGICAL PROPERTIES

5.1 Pharmacodynamic properties

The mode of action of Pentostam is unknown. *In vitro* exposure of amastigotes to 500 mg Sb^{5+}/ml results in a greater than 50% decrease in parasite DNA, RNA protein and purine nucleoside triphosphate levels. It has been postulated that the reduction in ATP (adenosine triphosphate) and GTP (guanosine triphosphate) synthesis contributes to decreased macromolecular synthesis.

5.2 Pharmacokinetic properties

Following intravenous or intramuscular administration of sodium stibogluconate, antimony is excreted rapidly via the kidneys, the majority of the dose being detected in the first 12-hour urine collection. This rapid excretion is reflected by a marked fall in serum or whole blood antimony levels to approximately 1 to 4% of the peak level by 8 hours after an intravenous dose. During daily administration, there is a slow accumulation of sodium stibogluconate into the central compartment so that tissue concentrations reach a theoretical maximum level after at least 7 days.

5.3 Preclinical safety data

There are no preclinical data of relevance to the prescriber which are additional to that in other sections of the SPC.

6. PHARMACEUTICAL PARTICULARS

6.1 List of excipients

Chlorocresol BP

Glucono-delta-lactone HSE

Water for Injections EP

6.2 Incompatibilities

None known.

6.3 Shelf life

36 months.

6.4 Special precautions for storage

Do not store above 25°C. Do not freeze.

Protect from light.

6.5 Nature and contents of container

Amber glass vials sealed with synthetic butyl rubber closures and aluminium collars.

Pack sizes: 6 and 100ml.

6.6 Instructions for use and handling

No special instructions.

Administrative Data

7. MARKETING AUTHORISATION HOLDER

The Wellcome Foundation Ltd

Glaxo Wellcome House

Berkeley Avenue

Greenford

Middlesex

UB6 ONN

Trading as

GlaxoSmithKline UK

Stockley Park West

Uxbridge

Middlesex UB11 1BT

8. MARKETING AUTHORISATION NUMBER(S)

PL00003/5105R

9. DATE OF FIRST AUTHORISATION/RENEWAL OF THE AUTHORISATION

23 June 1998

10. DATE OF REVISION OF THE TEXT

18th April 2005

Pentrax Shampoo

(Alliance Pharmaceuticals)

1. NAME OF THE MEDICINAL PRODUCT

Pentrax Shampoo

2. QUALITATIVE AND QUANTITATIVE COMPOSITION

Fractar 5 HSE 7.71%

(equivalent to coal tar 4.3%)

3. PHARMACEUTICAL FORM

Shampoo

4. CLINICAL PARTICULARS

4.1 Therapeutic indications

For the relief of itching, irritation, redness, flaking and/or scaling due to dandruff, seborrhoeic dermatitis, or psoriasis of the scalp.

4.2 Posology and method of administration

For topical administration.

Adults:

Pentrax Shampoo should be massaged into wet hair and scalp to produce a lather. The hair should be rinsed and the procedure repeated applying a liberal amount of Pentrax and allowing the lather to remain on the hair for up to 10 minutes. Hair should be rinsed thoroughly.

Use at least twice weekly or as directed by a physician.

Children:

As for adults.

Elderly:

As for adults.

4.3 Contraindications

Pentrax Shampoo is contra-indicated in persons with a sensitivity to any of the ingredients.

4.4 Special warnings and special precautions for use

Avoid contact with the eyes. If shampoo gets into the eyes rinse thoroughly with water.

If the condition worsens or does not improve after regular use of the product as directed, consult a physician.

4.5 Interaction with other medicinal products and other forms of Interaction

None known.

4.6 Pregnancy and lactation

No limitations to the use of Pentrax shampoo during pregnancy or lactation are known.

4.7 Effects on ability to drive and use machines

None known.

4.8 Undesirable effects

There have been no reports of adverse effects following the use of Pentrax

Shampoo. However, coal tar may cause irritation to the skin. Erythema and hypersensitivity to coal tar has been reported. Although carcinogenicity of coal tar has been demonstrated in animal studies, no studies demonstration an increased risk to skin cancer with normal therapeutic use in humans has been reported. There is no unequivocal evidence to link the use of topically applied coal tar products, with skin cancer.

4.9 Overdose

There is no evidence of systemic absorption following the use of this shampoo.

There are no reports available of its ingestion.

5. PHARMACOLOGICAL PROPERTIES

5.1 Pharmacodynamic properties

Coal tar is an antipruritic, keratolytic and a weak antiseptic.

5.2 Pharmacokinetic properties

There is no evidence of systemic absorption following the use of Pentrax Shampoo.

5.3 Preclinical safety data

Tar preparations have been in wide use for many years. Although tar preparations containing polycyclic aromatic hydrocarbons (PAHs) have been demonstrated to be carcinogenic in the skin of experimental animals, present evidence, based on epidemiology studies and follow up trials, reveals no evidence of increased risk of skin or internal cancer, particularly when the product is used as directed.

6. PHARMACEUTICAL PARTICULARS

6.1 List of excipients

Dioctyl sodium sulphosuccinate

Laureth 23

Polyethylene glycol 8

Sodium lauryl sulphate

Cocamide DEA

Lauramine oxide

6.2 Incompatibilities

None known.

6.3 Shelf life

48 months.

6.4 Special precautions for storage

Store below 30°C.

6.5 Nature and contents of container

Pentrax Shampoo is supplied in a polyvinylchloride bottle with a polypropylene screw cap with triseal. Each bottle contains either 30ml, 120ml or 240ml of Pentrax Shampoo.

6.6 Instructions for use and handling

For external use only.

Keep out of reach of children.

7. MARKETING AUTHORISATION HOLDER

Alliance Pharmaceuticals Ltd

Avonbridge House

Bath Road

Chippenham

Wiltshire

SN15 2BB

8. MARKETING AUTHORISATION NUMBER(S)

PL 16853/0075

9. DATE OF FIRST AUTHORISATION/RENEWAL OF THE AUTHORISATION

1st July 1999

10. DATE OF REVISION OF THE TEXT

Aug 2004

Pepcid

(Merck Sharp & Dohme Limited)

1. NAME OF THE MEDICINAL PRODUCT

PEPCID® 20 mg Tablets

PEPCID® 40 mg Tablets

2. QUALITATIVE AND QUANTITATIVE COMPOSITION

'Pepcid' 20 mg, each tablet contains 20 mg of famotidine.

'Pepcid' 40 mg, each tablet contains 40 mg of famotidine.

3. PHARMACEUTICAL FORM

Film-coated tablets.

Beige, round-cornered square tablets, marked 'MSD 963' on one side and plain on the other.

Brown, round-cornered square tablets, marked 'MSD 964' on one side and plain on the other.

4. CLINICAL PARTICULARS

4.1 Therapeutic indications

Duodenal ulcer.

Prevention of relapses of duodenal ulceration.

Benign gastric ulcer.

Hypersecretory conditions such as Zollinger-Ellison syndrome.

Treatment of gastro-oesophageal reflux disease.

Prevention of relapse of symptoms and erosions or ulcerations associated with gastro-oesophageal reflux disease.

4.2 Posology and method of administration

In benign gastric and duodenal ulceration, the dose of 'Pepcid' is one 40 mg tablet at night.

Duodenal ulcer

The recommended initial dose is one 40 mg tablet of 'Pepcid' at night. Treatment should continue for four to eight weeks. In most patients, healing occurs on this regimen within four weeks. In those patients whose ulcers have not healed completely after four weeks, a further four-week period of treatment is recommended.

Maintenance therapy: For preventing the recurrence of duodenal ulceration, the reduced dose of 20 mg of 'Pepcid' at night is recommended.

Benign gastric ulcer

The recommended dose is one 40 mg tablet of 'Pepcid' at night. Treatment should continue for four to eight weeks unless endoscopy reveals earlier healing.

Zollinger-Ellison syndrome

Patients without prior antisecretory therapy should be started on 20 mg of 'Pepcid' every six hours. Dosage should then be adjusted to individual response: doses up to 800 mg daily have been used up to one year without the development of significant adverse effects or tachyphylaxis. Patients who have been receiving another H_2 antagonist may be switched directly to 'Pepcid' at a dose higher than that recommended for new cases. This starting dose will depend on the severity of the condition and the last dose of H_2 antagonist previously used.

Gastro-oesophageal reflux disease

The recommended dosage for the symptomatic relief of gastro-oesophageal reflux disease is 20 mg of famotidine twice daily, which may be given for six to twelve weeks. Most patients experience improvement after two weeks.

Where gastro-oesophageal reflux disease is associated with the presence of oesophageal erosion or ulceration, the recommended dosage is 40 mg of famotidine twice daily, which may be given for six to twelve weeks.

Maintenance therapy: For the prevention of recurrence of symptoms and erosions or ulcerations associated with gastro-oesophageal reflux disease, the recommended dosage is 20 mg of famotidine twice daily.

Use in the elderly: The recommended dosage in most elderly patients is the same as in younger patients for all indications (see above).

Use in impaired renal function: Since 'Pepcid' is excreted primarily by the kidney, caution should be observed in patients with severe renal impairment. The dose should be reduced to 20 mg *nocte* when creatinine clearance falls below 10 ml/min.

Paediatric use

The efficacy and safety of 'Pepcid' in children have not been established.

4.3 Contraindications

Hypersensitivity to any component of this product. Cross sensitivity in this class of compounds has been observed. Therefore 'Pepcid' should not be administered to patients with a history of hypersensitivity to other H_2-receptor antagonists.

4.4 Special warnings and special precautions for use

Gastric carcinoma

Gastric malignancy should be excluded prior to initiation of therapy of gastric ulcer with 'Pepcid'. Symptomatic response of gastric ulcer to therapy with 'Pepcid' does not preclude the presence of gastric malignancy.

Impaired renal function

Since 'Pepcid' is primarily excreted via the kidney, caution should be exercised when treating patients with impaired renal function. The dose should be reduced to 20 mg *nocte* when creatinine clearance falls below 10 ml/min.

4.5 Interaction with other medicinal products and other forms of Interaction

'Pepcid' does not inhibit the hepatic cytochrome P450 enzyme system. Furthermore, clinical studies have shown that famotidine does not potentiate the actions of warfarin, theophylline, phenytoin, diazepam, propranolol, aminopyrine and antipyrine, which are inactivated by this system.

4.6 Pregnancy and lactation

Pregnancy: 'Pepcid' is not recommended for use in pregnancy, and should be prescribed only if clearly needed. Before a decision is made to use 'Pepcid' during pregnancy, the physician should weigh the potential benefits from the drug against the possible risks involved.

Breast-feeding mothers: 'Pepcid' is secreted in human milk, therefore breast-feeding mothers should either stop breast-feeding or stop taking the drug.

4.7 Effects on ability to drive and use machines

None known.

4.8 Undesirable effects

Headache, dizziness, constipation, and diarrhoea have been reported rarely. Other side effects reported even less frequently included dry mouth, nausea and/or vomiting, abdominal discomfort or distension, anorexia, fatigue, rash, pruritus and urticaria, liver enzyme abnormalities, cholestatic jaundice, anaphylaxis, angioedema, arthralgia, muscle cramps, reversible psychic disturbances including depression, anxiety disorders, agitation, confusion and hallucinations. Toxic epidermal necrolysis has been reported very rarely with H_2-receptor antagonists. Pancytopenia, leucopenia, thrombocytopenia, agranulocytosis and isolated cases of worsening of existing hepatic disease have been reported; however, a causal relationship to therapy with 'Pepcid' has not been established. No clinically significant increase in endocrine or gonadal function has been reported. Gynaecomastia has been reported rarely. In most cases that were followed up, it was reversible on discontinuing treatment. As with other H_2-receptor antagonists, A-V block has been reported very rarely.

4.9 Overdose

There is no experience to date with overdosage. The usual measures to remove unabsorbed material from the gastrointestinal tract, clinical monitoring, and supportive therapy should be employed.

Patients with Zollinger-Ellison syndrome have tolerated doses up to 800 mg daily for more than a year without the development of significant adverse effects.

5. PHARMACOLOGICAL PROPERTIES

5.1 Pharmacodynamic properties

'Pepcid', in single oral doses of 5 mg to 40 mg, produced dose-related inhibition of basal and pentagastrin, betazole, or insulin-stimulated gastric secretion in healthy volunteers. The inhibition affected volume, acid, and pepsin content of the gastric juice. In patients with benign gastric or duodenal ulceration, similar inhibitory effects on gastric secretion were noted.

In volunteers given a second pentagastrin challenge 5-7 hours after the dose of 'Pepcid' the inhibition of gastric secretion persisted, in contrast to control subjects on cimetidine 300 mg or on placebo.

A single oral dose of 40 mg of 'Pepcid' given at 9 pm was effective for more than 12 hours after administration. The 40 mg dose also had some continuing effect through the breakfast meal. The 80 mg dose of 'Pepcid' administered at 9 pm had no longer duration of action than the 40 mg dose.

Basal serum gastrin levels were increased by 20 mg and 10 mg doses of 'Pepcid' in some studies but unchanged in others. Gastric emptying was not affected by 'Pepcid', nor were hepatic and portal blood flows altered. 'Pepcid' did not cause changes in endocrine function.

5.2 Pharmacokinetic properties

'Pepcid' obeys linear kinetics. 'Pepcid' is rapidly absorbed, with dose-related peak plasma concentrations reached in one to three hours. Bioavailability is not affected by the presence of food in the stomach. Repeated doses do not lead to accumulation of the drug.

Protein binding in the plasma is relatively low (15-20%). The plasma half-life after a single oral dose or multiple repeated doses (for 5 days) was approximately 3 hours.

Metabolism of the drug occurs in the liver, with formation of the inactive sulphoxide metabolite.

Approximately 25-60% of the oral dosage is excreted in the urine, mainly as unchanged drug. A small amount may be excreted as the sulphoxide.

5.3 Preclinical safety data

No relevant information.

6. PHARMACEUTICAL PARTICULARS

6.1 List of excipients

Magnesium Stearate (E572)

Microcrystalline Cellulose (E460)

Pregelatinised Starch

Talc

Hydroxypropyl Cellulose (E463)

Hypromellose (E464)

Red Iron Oxide (E172)

Titanium Dioxide (E171)

Yellow Iron Oxide (E172)

Carnauba Wax (E903)

6.2 Incompatibilities

None.

6.3 Shelf life

36 months.

6.4 Special precautions for storage

Do not store above 25°C.

6.5 Nature and contents of container

Opacified PVC-aluminium blister packs of 2 and 4 tablets and calendar packs of 28 tablets.

Amber glass, high density polyethylene or polypropylene bottles of 50 tablets.

6.6 Instructions for use and handling

None.

7. MARKETING AUTHORISATION HOLDER

Merck Sharp & Dohme Limited

Hertford Road, Hoddesdon, Hertfordshire EN11 9BU, UK.

8. MARKETING AUTHORISATION NUMBER(S)

20 mg tablet: PL 0025/0215

40 mg tablet: PL 0025/0216

9. DATE OF FIRST AUTHORISATION/RENEWAL OF THE AUTHORISATION

Date granted: 8 September 1987

Last Renewed: 13 July 1999

10. DATE OF REVISION OF THE TEXT

July 2003.

11. LEGAL CATEGORY

POM

® denotes registered trademark of Merck & Co., Inc., Whitehouse Station, NJ, USA

SPC.PCD.03.UK.0942

Percutol

(Pliva Pharma Ltd)

1. NAME OF THE MEDICINAL PRODUCT

Percutol Ointment

2. QUALITATIVE AND QUANTITATIVE COMPOSITION

The active ingredient of Percutol is glyceryl trinitrate 2 % w/w.

3. PHARMACEUTICAL FORM

A homogeneous cream coloured ointment.

4. CLINICAL PARTICULARS

4.1 Therapeutic indications

Prophylaxis of angina pectoris.

4.2 Posology and method of administration

Topical application.

Adults (including elderly):

The usual dose is 1 to 2 inches squeezed from the tube, although some patients may require more. This dose may be repeated every 3 to 4 hours as required.

The dose may be titrated to individual patients' needs by finding the dose that causes headache and then reducing this dose by half an inch. Half an inch of ointment should be applied on the first day, one inch on the second, etc. increasing by half an inch per day until headache occurs and then reducing by half an inch. If several applications per day are required the dose may need to be reduced.

The ointment may be conveniently measured and applied using the paper "Applirules" enclosed in the carton. After squeezing the required length of ointment onto the "Applirule" it should be pressed on to any convenient area of skin (e.g. chest, thigh, or arm) until the ointment is spread in a thin layer under the paper. The ointment should not be rubbed in. The "Applirule" may be secured in place with surgical tape.

Children:

The safety and efficacy of Percutol in children has not been established.

4.3 Contraindications

May be contra-indicated in patients with marked anaemia, or raised intra cranial pressure. Should not be employed in patients with known idiosyncrasies to nitrates.

Sildenafil has been shown to potentiate the hypotensive effects of nitrates, and its co-administration with nitrates or nitric oxide donors is therefore contra-indicated.

4.4 Special warnings and special precautions for use

In the elderly the development of postural hypotension may be more pronounced especially on sudden rising. Caution should be exercised in patients with cerebrovascular disease. As with other vasodilators chronic therapy should not be discontinued abruptly. The frequency of application and the dosage should gradually be reduced (over a period of 4 to 6 weeks).

4.5 Interaction with other medicinal products and other forms of Interaction

Some effects of glyceryl trinitrate are enhanced by alcohol.

The hypotensive effects of nitrates are potentiated by concurrent administration of sildenafil.

4.6 Pregnancy and lactation

The safety of Percutol in pregnancy is not established. The product should therefore be given during pregnancy, only if clearly needed. It is not known whether glyceryl trinitrate is excreted in human milk, therefore caution should be exercised when administered to a nursing mother.

4.7 Effects on ability to drive and use machines

Glyceryl trinitrate may cause dizziness. In consequence until the effect of treatment is known, patients should be warned not to take charge of vehicles or machinery.

4.8 Undesirable effects

Headache, flushing, dizziness or postural hypotension.

4.9 Overdose

A hypotensive headache is a sign of overdosage. High doses of glyceryl trinitrate may cause marked hypotension and collapse, however topical application reduces the likelihood of overdosage and the effect can be quickly terminated by washing the ointment off the skin.

5. PHARMACOLOGICAL PROPERTIES

5.1 Pharmacodynamic properties

The active ingredient relaxes smooth muscle and reduces blood pressure. Its use as a vasodilator in the prophylaxis and treatment of angina pectoris is well established.

5.2 Pharmacokinetic properties

In human volunteers the mean absorption of glyceryl trinitrate from 1 inch of ointment was 0.8mg/hour.

5.3 Preclinical safety data

There are no preclinical data of relevance to the prescriber which are additional to that already included in other sections of the SPC.

6. PHARMACEUTICAL PARTICULARS

6.1 List of excipients

Percutol also contains lanolin anhydrous USP, purified water USP, white petroleum USP, and lactose anhydrous USP.

6.2 Incompatibilities

None stated.

6.3 Shelf life

36 months.

6.4 Special precautions for storage

Store below 25°C.

6.5 Nature and contents of container

Collapsible aluminium tube containing 60g.

6.6 Instructions for use and handling

None stated.

7. MARKETING AUTHORISATION HOLDER

PLIVA Pharma Ltd.

Vision House

Bedford Road

Petersfield

Hampshire, GU32 3QB

8. MARKETING AUTHORISATION NUMBER(S)

PL 10622/0046

9. DATE OF FIRST AUTHORISATION/RENEWAL OF THE AUTHORISATION

1 July 1998

10. DATE OF REVISION OF THE TEXT

23 September 2002

11. Legal classification

Pharmacy

Perdix 15mg

(SCHWARZ PHARMA Limited)

1. NAME OF THE MEDICINAL PRODUCT

Perdix 15 mg

2. QUALITATIVE AND QUANTITATIVE COMPOSITION

Each Perdix 15 mg tablet contains moexipril hydrochloride 15 mg.

3. PHARMACEUTICAL FORM

Film-coated tablet.

4. CLINICAL PARTICULARS

4.1 Therapeutic indications

For the treatment of hypertension as monotherapy.

As second line therapy for the treatment of hypertension in combination with diuretics or calcium antagonists e.g. hydrochlorothiazide or nifedipine.

4.2 Posology and method of administration

Initial therapy:

In patients with uncomplicated essential hypertension not on diuretic therapy, the recommended initial dose is 7.5 mg once a day. Dosage should be adjusted according to blood pressure response. The maintenance dose is 7.5 mg to 15 mg moexipril daily, administered in a single dose. Some patients may benefit from a further increase to 30 mg per day.

Doses over 30 mg have been used, but do not appear to give a greater effect.

If blood pressure is not controlled with Perdix alone, a low dose of a diuretic may be added. Hydrochlorothiazide 12.5 mg has been shown to provide an additive effect.

With concomitant diuretic therapy, it may be possible to reduce the dose of Perdix.

Diuretic treated patients:

In hypertensive patients who are currently being treated with a diuretic, symptomatic hypotension may occur occasionally following the initial dose of Perdix. The diuretic should be discontinued, if possible, for two to three days before beginning therapy with Perdix to reduce the likelihood of hypotension (see "Warnings"). The dosage of Perdix should be adjusted according to blood pressure response. If the patient's blood pressure is not controlled with Perdix alone, diuretic therapy may be resumed as described above.

If the diuretic cannot be discontinued or the diuretic has recently been withdrawn, an initial dose of 3.75 mg (half 7.5 mg tablet) should be used under medical supervision for at least two hours and until blood pressure has stabilised for at least an additional hour (see "Warnings and Precautions").

Concomitant administration of Perdix with potassium supplements, potassium salt substitutes, or potassium-sparing diuretics may lead to increases of serum potassium (see "Precautions").

Nifedipine treated patients:

As add-on therapy, Perdix has been investigated in combination with nifedipine. If Perdix is used as add-on therapy to nifedipine, the starting dose of Perdix should be 3.75 mg (half 7.5 mg tablet).

Elderly patients:

In elderly patients, an initial dosage of 3.75 mg (half 7.5 mg tablet) once daily is recommended followed by titration to the optimal response.

Children:

Not recommended. Safety and efficacy in children has not been established.

Renal failure:

In patients with creatinine clearance ≤ 40 ml/min, an initial dose of 3.75 mg of moexipril (half 7.5 mg tablet) is recommended.

Hepatic cirrhosis:

In patients with hepatic cirrhosis, an initial dose of 3.75 mg of moexipril (half 7.5 mg tablet) is recommended.

Afro-Caribbean patients:

Where Perdix is used as a single agent in hypertension, Afro-Caribbean patients may show a reduced therapeutic response.

4.3 Contraindications

Perdix is contra-indicated in patients who are hypersensitive to this product and in patients with a history of angioedema related to previous treatment with an angiotensin converting enzyme inhibitor.

Perdix is contra-indicated in pregnancy since fetotoxicity has been observed for ACE inhibitors in animals. Although there is no experience with Perdix, other ACE inhibitors in human pregnancy have been associated with oligohydramnios and neonatal hypotension and/or anuria. It is not known whether moexipril passes into human breast milk, but since animal data indicate that moexipril and its metabolites are present in rat milk Perdix should not be given to nursing mothers.

4.4 Special warnings and special precautions for use

Warnings:

Angioedema:

Angioedema involving the extremities, face, lips, mucous membranes, tongue, glottis or larynx has been reported in patients treated with ACE inhibitors. If angioedema involves the tongue, glottis or larynx, airway obstruction may occur and be fatal. If laryngeal stridor or angioedema of the face, lips mucous membranes, tongue, glottis or extremities occur, treatment with Perdix should be discontinued and appropriate therapy instituted immediately. Where there is involvement of the tongue, glottis, or larynx, likely to cause airway obstruction, appropriate therapy, e.g. subcutaneous epinephrine solution 1:1000 (0.3 ml to 0.5 ml) should be promptly administered (see "Precautions").

Intestinal angioedema has been reported in patients treated with ACE inhibitors. These patients presented with abdominal pain (with or without nausea and vomiting); in some cases there was no prior history of facial angioedema and C1-esterase levels were normal. The angioedema was diagnosed by procedures including abdominal CT scan or ultrasound, or at surgery, and symptoms resolved after stopping the ACE inhibitor. Intestinal angioedema should be included in the differential diagnosis of patients on ACE inhibitors presenting with abdominal pain.

Cough:

During treatment with an ACE inhibitor a dry and non-productive cough may occur which disappears after discontinuation.

Hypotension:

Perdix can cause symptomatic hypotension. Like other ACE inhibitors, Perdix has been only rarely associated with hypotension in hypertensive patients receiving monotherapy. Symptomatic hypotension is most likely to occur in patients who have been volume – and/or salt – depleted as a result of prolonged diuretic therapy, dietary salt restriction, dialysis, diarrhoea, or vomiting. Volume and/or salt depletion should be corrected before initiating therapy with Perdix.

If hypotension occurs, the patient should be placed in a supine position and, if necessary, treated with intravenous infusion of physiological saline. Perdix treatment usually can be continued following restoration of blood pressure and volume.

Neutropenia/agranulocytosis:

ACE inhibitors have been shown to cause agranulocytosis and bone marrow depression, rarely in uncomplicated patients, but more frequently in patients with renal impairment, especially if they also have a collagen-vascular disease such as systemic lupus erythematosus or scleroderma. Available data from clinical trials of Perdix are insufficient to show that Perdix does not cause agranulocytosis at similar rates. Monitoring of white blood cell counts should be considered in patients with collagen-vascular disease, especially if the disease is associated with impaired renal function.

Proteinuria:

Proteinuria may occur, particularly in patients with existing renal function impairment or on higher doses of Perdix.

Dialysis:

Patients who are dialysed using high-flux polyacrylonitrile membranes and treated with ACE inhibitors may experience anaphylactoid reactions such as facial swelling, flushing, hypotension and dyspnoea within a few minutes of commencing haemodialysis. It is recommended that an alternative membrane or an alternative antihypertensive drug be used.

LDL apheresis/Desensibilisation:

During LDL (low-density lipoprotein) apheresis (in patients with severe hypercholesterinemia) life-threatening hypersensitivity reactions may occur in patients under ACE inhibitor therapy.

During desensibilisation therapy against insect poisons (e.g. bee or wasp stings) and concomitant treatment with an ACE inhibitor, life-threatening hypersensitivity reactions (e.g. blood pressure fall, dyspnoea, vomiting, allergic skin reactions) may occur.

If LDL apheresis or desensibilisation therapy against insect poisons is required, the ACE inhibitor should be substituted by a different antihypertensive drug temporarily.

Precautions:

Impaired renal function:

As a consequence of inhibiting the renin-angiotensin-aldosterone system, changes in renal function may be anticipated in susceptible individuals.

Oliguria and/or progressive azotemia and rarely acute renal failure and/or death have been reported in association with ACE inhibitors in patients with severe congestive heart failure whose renal function may depend on the activity of the renin-angiotensin-aldosterone system.

In hypertensive patients with renal artery stenosis in a solitary kidney or bilateral renal artery stenosis, increases in blood urea nitrogen and serum creatinine may occur. Experience with other angiotensin converting enzyme inhibitors suggests that these increases are usually reversible upon discontinuation of ACE inhibitor and/or diuretic therapy. In such patients, renal function should be monitored during the first few weeks of therapy.

Some hypertensive patients with no apparent pre-existing renal vascular disease have developed increases in blood urea nitrogen and serum creatinine, usually minor and transient, especially when Perdix has been given concomitantly with a diuretic. This is more likely to occur in patients with pre-existing renal impairment. Dosage reduction of Perdix and/or discontinuation of the diuretic may be required.

Evaluation of the hypertensive patient should always include assessment of renal function.

Impaired renal function decreases total clearance of moexiprilat and approximately doubles AUC.

Hyperkalaemia:

In clinical trials, hyperkalaemia (serum potassium greater than 10% above the upper limit of normal) has occurred in approximately 2.6% of hypertensive patients receiving Perdix. In most cases, these were isolated values, which resolved despite continued therapy. In clinical trials, 0.1% of patients (two patients) were discontinued from therapy due to an elevated serum potassium. Risk factors for the development of hyperkalaemia include renal insufficiency, diabetes mellitus and the concomitant use of potassium-sparing diuretics, potassium supplements and/or potassium-containing salt substitutes, which should be used cautiously, if at all, with Perdix (see "Precautions").

Hepatic cirrhosis:

Since Perdix is primarily metabolised by hepatic and gut wall esterases to its active moiety, moexiprilat, patients with impaired liver function could develop elevated plasma levels of unchanged Perdix. In a study in patients with alcoholic or biliary cirrhosis, the extent of hydrolysis was unaffected, although the rate was slowed. In these patients, the apparent total body clearance of moexiprilat was decreased and the plasma AUC approximately doubled.

Surgery/anaesthesia:

In patients undergoing surgery or during anaesthesia with agents that produce hypotension, Perdix will block the angiotensin II formation that could otherwise occur secondary to compensatory renin release. Hypotension that occurs as a result of this mechanism can be corrected by volume expansion.

Aortic stenosis/Hypertrophic cardiomyopathy:

Perdix should be used with caution in patients with an obstruction in the outflow tract of the left ventricle.

4.5 Interaction with other medicinal products and other forms of Interaction

Diuretics:

Excessive reductions in blood pressure, especially in patients in whom diuretic therapy was recently instituted, have been reported with ACE inhibitors. The possibility of hypotensive effects with Perdix can be minimised by discontinuing diuretic therapy or increasing salt intake for several days before initiation of treatment with Perdix. If this is not possible, the starting dose should be reduced (see also 4.2 and 4.4).

Nifedipine:

The co-administration of nifedipine with Perdix gives rise to an enhanced antihypertensive effect.

Potassium supplements and potassium-sparing diuretics:

Perdix can attenuate potassium loss caused by thiazide diuretics. Potassium-sparing diuretics (spironolactone, triamterene, amiloride, and others) or potassium supplements have been shown to increase the risk of hyperkalaemia when used concomitantly with ACE inhibitors. Therefore, if concomitant use of such agents is indicated, they should be given with caution and the patient's serum potassium should be monitored frequently.

Oral anticoagulants:

Interaction studies with warfarin failed to identify any clinically important effects on the serum concentrations of the anticoagulants or on their anticoagulant effects.

Lithium:

Increased serum lithium levels and symptoms of lithium toxicity have been reported in patients receiving ACE inhibitors during therapy with lithium. These drugs should be co-administered with caution, and frequent monitoring of serum lithium levels is recommended. If a diuretic is also used, the risk of lithium toxicity may be increased.

Anaesthetic drugs:

Perdix may enhance the hypotensive effects of certain anaesthetic drugs.

Narcotic drugs/Antipsychotics:

Postural hypotension may occur.

Allopurinol, cytostatic or immunosuppressive agents, systemic corticosteroids or procainamide:

Concomitant administration with Perdix may lead to an increased risk for leucopenia.

Non-Steroidal anti-inflammatory drugs:

The administration of NSAIDs may reduce the antihypertensive effect of Perdix. Furthermore, it has been reported that NSAIDs and ACE inhibitors exert an additive effect on increase in serum potassium, whereas renal function may decrease. These effects are in principle reversible, and occur especially in patients with compromised renal function.

Alcohol enhances the hypotensive effect of Perdix.

Other agents:

No clinically important pharmacokinetic interactions occurred when Perdix was administered concomitantly with hydrochlorothiazide, digoxin, cimetidine, or nifedipine in healthy volunteers. However, in hypertensive patients, the antihypertensive effect of Perdix was enhanced when given in combination with diuretics, or calcium antagonists.

4.6 Pregnancy and lactation

There is no experience in man. As it is known from other ACE inhibitors that they can adversely affect the foetus, especially during the second and third trimester, for safety reasons a change to a different antihypertensive drug should be made after pregnancy is confirmed in women who are receiving Perdix (see "Contra-indications") or in women planning to get pregnant.

It is not known whether Perdix is excreted in human milk. As animal data indicate that moexipril and its metabolites are present in rat milk, Perdix should not be administered to a nursing woman.

4.7 Effects on ability to drive and use machines

The intake of ACE inhibitors may – as any antihypertensive therapy – induce hypotension with subsequent impairment of reactivity. Alcohol intake may enhance this effect.

4.8 Undesirable effects

The most commonly reported undesirable effects (more than 1% of patients treated with Perdix in controlled trials) were cough (4.0%), headache (3.6%), dizziness (3.3%), fatigue (1.2%), flushing (1.2%), and rash (1.0%).

Other adverse experiences possibly or probably related, or of uncertain relationship to therapy, reported in controlled or uncontrolled clinical trials occurring in less than 1% of Perdix patients and less frequent clinically significant events which have been attributed to ACE inhibitors include the following:

Cardiovascular:

Symptomatic hypotension, postural hypotension, or syncope was seen in < 1% of patients; these reactions led to discontinuation of therapy in controlled trials in 2 patients (0.1%) who had received Perdix monotherapy and in 1 patient (0.05%) who had received Perdix with hydrochlorothiazide. Other reports included chest pain, angina/myocardial infarction, tachycardia, palpitations, rhythm disturbances, transient ischaemic attacks, cerebrovascular accident.

Renal:

Of hypertensive patients with no apparent pre-existing renal disease, 0.8% of patients receiving Perdix alone and 1.5% of patients receiving Perdix with hydrochlorothiazide have experienced increases in serum creatinine to at least 140% of their baseline values.

Acute renal failure has been reported for ACE inhibitors including Perdix (see section 4.4 Special Warnings and Precautions for use).

Gastrointestinal:

Abdominal pain, dyspepsia, constipation, nausea, vomiting, diarrhoea, appetite/weight change, dry mouth, pancreatitis, hepatitis.

Intestinal Angioedema:

Intestinal Angioedema has been reported in patients treated with ACE inhibitors (see section 4.4 Special Warnings and Precautions for use).

Respiratory:

Upper respiratory infection, pharyngitis, sinusitis/rhinitis, bronchospasm, dyspnoea.

Urogenital:

Renal insufficiency.

Dermatologic:

Occasionally allergic and hypersensitivity reactions can occur like rash, pruritus, urticaria, erythema multiforme, Stevens-Johnson syndrome, toxic epidermic necrolysis, psoriasis-like efflorescence, pemphigus and alopecia. This can be accompanied by fever, myalgia, arthralgia, eosinophilia and/or increased ANA-titres. ACE inhibitors have been associated with the onset of angioneurotic oedema in a small subset of patients involving the face and oropharyngeal tissues.

Neurological and psychiatric:

Headache or tiredness may occasionally occur; rarely there may be drowsiness, depression, sleep disturbances, impotence, tingling sensations, numbness or paraesthesia, disturbances of balance, confusion, tinnitus, blurred vision, and alterations of taste or a transient loss of taste.

Other

Sweating, flu syndrome, malaise.

Clinical Laboratory Test Findings:

Decreases in haemoglobin, haematocrit, platelets and white cell count and individual cases agranulocytosis or pancytopenia, as well as elevation of liver enzymes and serum bilirubin have been reported in a few patients. In patients with congenital deficiency concerning G-6-PDH individual cases of haemolytic anaemia have been reported.

In rare cases, especially in patients with impaired kidney function or collagen diseases, or those simultaneously receiving treatment will allopurinol, procainamide or certain drugs which suppress the defence reactions, there may be anaemia, thrombocytopenia, neutropenia, eosinophilia and in isolated cases, even agranulocytosis or pancytopenia.

Creatinine and blood urea nitrogen:

As with other ACE inhibitors, minor increases in blood urea nitrogen or serum creatinine, reversible upon discontinuation of therapy, were observed in approximately 1% of patients with essential hypertension who were treated with Perdix. Increases are more likely to occur in patients receiving concomitant diuretics or in patients with compromised renal function.

Potassium:

Since moexipril decreases aldosterone secretion, elevation of serum potassium can occur. Potassium supplements and potassium-sparing diuretics should be given with caution and the patient's serum potassium should be monitored frequently.

Other:

Clinically important changes in standard laboratory tests were rarely associated with Perdix administration. Elevations of liver enzymes and uric acid have been reported. In trials, less than 1% of moexipril-treated patients discontinued Perdix treatment because of laboratory abnormalities.

4.9 Overdose

Symptoms and treatment:

To date, no case of overdosage has been reported. Signs and symptoms expected in cases of overdosage would be related to hypotension and should be relieved by intravenous infusion of isotonic saline solution.

5. PHARMACOLOGICAL PROPERTIES

5.1 Pharmacodynamic properties

In animals as well as in humans, interactions between the renin-angiotensin-aldosterone system and the kallikrein-kinin system provide an important biochemical basis for blood pressure homeostasis. In hypertension the normal feedback mechanism formed by the renin-angiotensin system (RAS) may be dysfunctional, resulting in a self-perpetuating hypertensive condition.

Angiotensin converting enzyme (ACE) inhibitors were developed to interrupt this system and thereby to lower blood pressure. Perdix potently inhibits ACE and by this the formation of angiotensin II, the active agent of the RAS, thus blocking its vasoconstrictor and sodium-retaining effects with a consequent reduction in blood pressure.

Since ACE is identical is kininase II, an enzyme that degrades the potent vasodilator bradykinin, inhibition of ACE leads to an additional, non renin-mediated reduction in systemic blood pressure. The antihypertensive effects of ACE inhibitors are accompanied by a reduction in peripheral vascular resistance.

5.2 Pharmacokinetic properties

The prodrug moexipril is rapidly absorbed and de-esterified to the active metabolite moexiprilat. The pharmacokinetic parameters for moexipril and moexiprilat were similar after both single and multiple dose of moexipril and appear to be dose-proportional.

Moexipril and moexiprilat are moderately bound to plasma proteins, predominantly albumin. Therefore, concurrently administered drugs are unlikely to interfere with the binding of moexipril and moexiprilat in any clinically significant way. Metabolites of moexipril present in the diketopiperazine derivatives of moexipril and moexiprilat. Both, moexipril and moexiprilat are eliminated in the urine, and moexiprilat is eliminated in the faeces.

The pharmacokinetic profile of moexipril and moexiprilat should allow the same dosage recommendation in patients with mild to moderate renal dysfunction(Cl_{cr} > 40 ml/min) as in patients with normal renal function. With severe renal dysfunction, dosage reduction is recommended. In patients with liver cirrhosis, the pharmacokinetics of moexipril and moexiprilat were significantly altered as compared with normal subjects. In such patients, therapy with Perdix should be started with 3.75 mg (half 7.5 mg tablet).

There were no apparent pharmacokinetic drug interactions with HCTZ, digoxin, cimetidine, warfarin or nifedipine.

5.3 Preclinical safety data

Acute toxicity:

Findings of the acute toxicity studies in animals do not raise questions as to the safety of moexipril HCl as well as the main metabolite moexiprilat under the conditions of proposed clinical usage.

Subacute/chronic toxicity:

Subacute and chronic toxicity studies in rats and dogs with repeated oral administration of moexipril HCl up to 12 months, revealed mainly heart and kidney as target organs. The effects are completely comparable with those of other ACE inhibitors and can be interpreted as results of highly exaggerated pharmacological activity.

First unspecific drug-related side effects after long-term administration were seen at 75 mg/kg, i.e. a dose which corresponds 150 times the maximum recommended total daily dose in humans when compared on the basis of body weight.

Reproduction studies:

Studies in rats and rabbits including all segments of reproduction revealed no direct effects of moexipril HCl on fertility, reproduction and abnormalities in F_1 – or F_2 – pups.

Regarding precautions in women of child bearing potential and use during pregnancy and lactation see 4.3 and 4.6.

Mutagenicity:

As conclusion of different 'in vitro' and one 'in vivo' mutagenicity studies, the mutagenic potential of moexipril HCl for human beings should be extremely low.

Carcinogenicity:

Neither the long-term toxicity studies in rats and dogs nor special carcinogenicity studies in mice and rats over 78 and 104 weeks respectively, indicated neoplastigenic properties of moexipril HCl. Therefore, it can be concluded that the carcinogenic risk for human beings will be extremely low.

6. PHARMACEUTICAL PARTICULARS

6.1 List of excipients

Lactose monohydrate
Crospovidone
Light magnesium oxide
Gelatin
Magnesium stearate
Methylhydroxypropylcellulose
Hydroxypropylcellulose
Polyethyleneglycol 6000
Titanium dioxide
Ferric oxide
Purified water (not present in the finished product).

6.2 Incompatibilities

No incompatibilities have so far been demonstrated.

6.3 Shelf life

5 years

6.4 Special precautions for storage

Store in the original package.

6.5 Nature and contents of container

Calendar packs containing 28 tablets, 14 per Al/Al blister pack.

6.6 Instructions for use and handling

No special instruction necessary.

7. MARKETING AUTHORISATION HOLDER

SCHWARZ PHARMA Limited
Schwarz House
East Street
Chesham
Bucks HP5 1DG
England

8. MARKETING AUTHORISATION NUMBER(S)

PL 4438/0034

9. DATE OF FIRST AUTHORISATION/RENEWAL OF THE AUTHORISATION

03 November 2000

10. DATE OF REVISION OF THE TEXT

May 2005

Perdix 7.5mg

(SCHWARZ PHARMA Limited)

1. NAME OF THE MEDICINAL PRODUCT

Perdix 7.5 mg

2. QUALITATIVE AND QUANTITATIVE COMPOSITION

Each Perdix 7.5 mg tablet contains moexipril hydrochloride 7.5 mg.

3. PHARMACEUTICAL FORM

Film-coated tablet.

4. CLINICAL PARTICULARS

4.1 Therapeutic indications

For the treatment of hypertension as monotherapy.

As second line therapy for the treatment of hypertension in combination with diuretics or calcium antagonists e.g. hydrochlorothiazide or nifedipine.

4.2 Posology and method of administration

Initial therapy:

In patients with uncomplicated essential hypertension not on diuretic therapy, the recommended initial dose is 7.5 mg once a day. Dosage should be adjusted according to blood pressure response. The maintenance dose is 7.5 to 15 mg moexipril daily, administered in a single dose. Some patients may benefit from a further increase to 30 mg per day.

Doses over 30 mg have been used, but do not appear to give a greater effect.

If blood pressure is not controlled with Perdix alone, a low dose of a diuretic may be added. Hydrochlorothiazide 12.5 mg has been shown to provide an additive effect.

With concomitant diuretic therapy, it may be possible to reduce the dose of Perdix.

Diuretic treated patients:

In hypertensive patients who are currently being treated with a diuretic, symptomatic hypotension may occur occasionally following the initial dose of Perdix. The diuretic should be discontinued, if possible, for two to three days before beginning therapy with Perdix to reduce the likelihood of hypotension (see "Warnings"). The dosage of Perdix should be adjusted according to blood pressure response. If the patient's blood pressure is not controlled with Perdix alone, diuretic therapy may be resumed as described above.

If the diuretic cannot be discontinued or the diuretic has recently been withdrawn, an initial dose of 3.75 mg (half 7.5 mg tablet) should be used under medical supervision for at least two hours and until blood pressure has stabilized for at least an additional hour (see "Warnings and Precautions").

Concomitant administration of Perdix with potassium supplements, potassium salt substitutes, or potassium-sparing diuretics may lead to increases of serum potassium (see "Precautions").

Nifedipine treated patients:

As add-on therapy, Perdix has been investigated in combination with nifedipine. If Perdix is used as add-on therapy to nifedipine, the starting dose of Perdix should be 3.75 mg (half 7.5 mg tablet).

Elderly patients:

In elderly patients, an initial dosage of 3.75 mg (half 7.5 mg tablet) once daily is recommended followed by titration to the optimal response.

Children:

Not recommended. Safety and efficacy in children has not been established.

Renal failure:

In patients with creatinine clearance ⩽ 40 ml/min, an initial dose of 3.75 mg of moexipril (half 7.5 mg tablet) is recommended.

Hepatic cirrhosis:

In patients with hepatic cirrhosis, an initial dose of 3.75 mg of moexipril (half 7.5 mg tablet) is recommended.

Afro-Caribbean patients:

Where Perdix is used as a single agent in hypertension, Afro-Caribbean patients may show a reduced therapeutic response.

4.3 Contraindications

Perdix is contra-indicated in patients who are hypersensitive to this product and in patients with a history of angioedema related to previous treatment with an angiotensin converting enzyme inhibitor.

Perdix is contra-indicated in pregnancy since fetotoxicity has been observed for ACE inhibitors in animals. Although there is no experience with Perdix, other ACE inhibitors in human pregnancy have been associated with oligohydramnios and neonatal hypotension and/or anuria. It is not known whether moexipril passes into human breast milk, but since animal data indicate that moexipril and its metabolites are present in rat milk Perdix should not be given to nursing mothers.

4.4 Special warnings and special precautions for use

Warnings:

Angioedema:

Angioedema involving the extremities, face, lips, mucous membranes, tongue, glottis or larynx has been reported in patients treated with ACE inhibitors. If angioedema involves the tongue, glottis or larynx, airway obstruction may occur and be fatal. If laryngeal stridor or angioedema of the face, lips, mucous membranes, tongue, glottis or extremities occur, treatment with Perdix should be discontinued and appropriate therapy instituted immediately. Where there is involvement of the tongue, glottis, or larynx, likely to cause airway obstruction, appropriate therapy, e.g. subcutaneous epinephrine solution 1:1000 (0.3 ml to 0.5 ml) should be promptly administered (see "Precautions").

Intestinal angioedema has been reported in patients treated with ACE inhibitors. These patients presented with abdominal pain (with or without nausea and vomiting); in some cases there was no prior history of facial angioedema and C1-esterase levels were normal. The angioedema was diagnosed by procedures including abdominal CT scan or ultrasound, or at surgery, and symptoms resolved after stopping the ACE inhibitor. Intestinal angioedema should be included in the differential diagnosis of patients on ACE inhibitors presenting with abdominal pain.

Cough:

During treatment with an ACE inhibitor a dry and non-productive cough may occur which disappears after discontinuation.

Hypotension:

Perdix can cause symptomatic hypotension. Like other ACE inhibitors, Perdix has been only rarely associated with hypotension in hypertensive patients receiving monotherapy. Symptomatic hypotension is most likely to occur in patients who have been volume – and/or salt – depleted as a result of prolonged diuretic therapy, dietary salt restriction, dialysis, diarrhoea, or vomiting. Volume and/or salt depletion should be corrected before initiating therapy with Perdix.

If hypotension occurs, the patient should be placed in a supine position and, if necessary, treated with intravenous infusion of physiological saline. Perdix treatment usually can be continued following restoration of blood pressure and volume.

Neutropenia/agranulocytosis:

ACE inhibitors have been shown to cause agranulocytosis and bone marrow depression, rarely in uncomplicated patients, but more frequently in patients with renal impairment, especially if they also have a collagen-vascular disease such as systemic lupus erythematosus or scleroderma. Available data from clinical trials of Perdix are insufficient to show that Perdix does not cause agranulocytosis at similar rates. Monitoring of white blood cell counts should be considered in patients with collagen-vascular disease, especially if the disease is associated with impaired renal function.

Proteinuria:

Proteinuria may occur, particularly in patients with existing renal function impairment or on higher doses of Perdix.

Dialysis:

Patients who are dialysed using high-flux polyacrylonitrile membranes and treated with ACE inhibitors may experience anaphylactoid reactions such as facial swelling, flushing, hypotension and dyspnoea within a few minutes of commencing haemodialysis. It is recommended that an alternative membrane or an alternative antihypertensive drug be used.

LDL apheresis/Desensibilisation:

During LDL (low-density lipoprotein) apheresis (in patients with severe hypercholesterinemia) life-threatening hypersensitivity reactions may occur in patients under ACE inhibitor therapy.

During desensibilisation therapy against insect poisons (e.g. bee or wasp stings) and concomitant treatment with an ACE inhibitor, life-threatening hypersensitivity reactions (e.g. blood pressure fall, dyspnoea, vomiting, allergic skin reactions) may occur.

If LDL apheresis or desensibilisation therapy against insect poisons is required, the ACE inhibitor should be substituted by a different antihypertensive drug temporarily.

Precautions:

Impaired renal function:

As a consequence of inhibiting the renin-angiotensin-aldosterone system, changes in renal function may be anticipated in susceptible individuals.

Oliguria and/or progressive azotemia and rarely acute renal failure and/or death have been reported in association with ACE inhibitors in patients with severe congestive heart failure whose renal function may depend on the activity of the renin-angiotensin-aldosterone system.

In hypertensive patients with renal artery stenosis in a solitary kidney or bilateral renal artery stenosis, increases in blood urea nitrogen and serum creatinine may occur. Experience with other angiotensin converting enzyme inhibitors suggests that these increases are usually reversible upon discontinuation of ACE inhibitor and/or diuretic therapy. In such patients, renal function should be monitored during the first few weeks of therapy.

Some hypertensive patients with no apparent pre-existing renal vascular disease have developed increases in blood urea nitrogen and serum creatinine, usually minor and transient, especially when Perdix has been given concomitantly with a diuretic. This is more likely to occur in patients with pre-existing renal impairment. Dosage reduction of Perdix and/or discontinuation of the diuretic may be required.

Evaluation of the hypertensive patient should always include assessment of renal function.

Impaired renal function decreases total clearance of moexiprilat and approximately doubles AUC.

Hyperkalaemia:

In clinical trials, hyperkalaemia (serum potassium greater than 10% above the upper limit of normal) has occurred in approximately 2.6% of hypertensive patients receiving Perdix. In most cases, these were isolated values, which resolved despite continued therapy. In clinical trials, 0.1% of patients (two patients) were discontinued from therapy due to an elevated serum potassium. Risk factors for the development of hyperkalaemia include renal insufficiency, diabetes mellitus and the concomitant use of potassium-sparing diuretics, potassium supplements and/or potassium-containing salt substitutes, which should be used cautiously, if at all, with Perdix (see "Precautions").

Hepatic cirrhosis:

Since Perdix is primarily metabolised by hepatic and gut wall esterases to its active moiety, moexiprilat, patients with impaired liver function could develop elevated plasma levels of unchanged Perdix. In a study in patients with alcoholic or biliary cirrhosis, the extent of hydrolysis was unaffected, although the rate was slowed. In these patients, the apparent total body clearance of moexiprilat was decreased and the plasma AUC approximately doubled.

Surgery/anaesthesia:

In patients undergoing surgery or during anaesthesia with agents that produce hypotension, Perdix will block the angiotensin II formation that could otherwise occur secondary to compensatory renin release. Hypotension that occurs as a result of this mechanism can be corrected by volume expansion.

Aortic stenosis/hypertrophic cardiomyopathy:

Perdix should be used with caution in patients with an obstruction in the outflow tract of the left ventricle.

4.5 Interaction with other medicinal products and other forms of Interaction

Diuretics:

Excessive reductions in blood pressure, especially in patients in whom diuretic therapy was recently instituted, have been reported with ACE inhibitors. The possibility of hypotensive effects with Perdix can be minimised by discontinuing diuretic therapy or increasing salt intake for several days before initiation of treatment with Perdix. If this is not possible, the starting dose should be reduced (see also 4.2 and 4.4).

Nifedipine:

The co-administration of nifedipine with Perdix gives rise to an enhanced antihypertensive effect.

Potassium supplements and potassium-sparing diuretics:

Perdix can attenuate potassium loss caused by thiazide diuretics. Potassium-sparing diuretics (spironolactone, triamterene, amiloride, and others) or potassium supplements have been shown to increase the risk of hyperkalaemia when used concomitantly with ACE inhibitors. Therefore, if concomitant use of such agents is indicated, they should be given with caution and the patient's serum potassium should be monitored frequently.

Oral anticoagulants:

Interaction studies with warfarin failed to identify any clinically important effects on the serum concentrations of the anticoagulants or on their anticoagulant effects.

Lithium:

Increased serum lithium levels and symptoms of lithium toxicity have been reported in patients receiving ACE inhibitors during therapy with lithium. These drugs should be co-administered with caution, and frequent monitoring of serum lithium levels is recommended. If a diuretic is also used, the risk of lithium toxicity may be increased.

Anaesthetic drugs:

Perdix may enhance the hypotensive effects of certain anaesthetic drugs.

Narcotic drugs/Antipsychotics:

Postural hypotension may occur.

Allopurinol, cytostatic or immunosuppressive agents, systemic corticosteroids or procainamide:

Concomitant administration with Perdix may lead to an increased risk for leucopenia.

Non-Steroidal anti-inflammatory drugs:

The administration of NSAIDs may reduce the antihypertensive effect of Perdix. Furthermore, it has been reported that NSAIDs and ACE inhibitors exert an additive effect on increase in serum potassium, whereas renal function may decrease. These effects are in principle reversible, and occur especially in patients with compromised renal function.

Alcohol enhances the hypotensive effect of Perdix.

Other agents:

No clinically important pharmacokinetic interactions occurred when Perdix was administered concomitantly with hydrochlorothiazide, digoxin, cimetidine, or nifedipine in healthy volunteers. However, in hypertensive patients, the antihypertensive effect of Perdix was enhanced when given in combination with diuretics, or calcium antagonists.

4.6 Pregnancy and lactation

There is no experience in man. As it is known from other ACE inhibitors that they can adversely affect the foetus, especially during the second and third trimester, for safety reasons a change to a different antihypertensive drug should be made after pregnancy is confirmed in women who are receiving Perdix (see "Contra-indications") or in women planning to get pregnant.

It is not known whether Perdix is excreted in human milk. As animal data indicate that moexipril and its metabolites are present in rat milk, Perdix should not be administered to a nursing woman.

4.7 Effects on ability to drive and use machines

The intake of ACE inhibitors may – as any antihypertensive therapy – induce hypotension with subsequent impairment of reactivity. Alcohol intake may enhance this effect.

4.8 Undesirable effects

The most commonly reported undesirable effects (more than 1% of patients treated with Perdix in controlled trials) were cough (4.0%), headache (3.6%), dizziness (3.3%), fatigue (1.2%), flushing (1.2%), and rash (1.0%).

Other adverse experiences possibly or probably related, or of uncertain relationship to therapy, reported in controlled or uncontrolled clinical trials occurring in less than 1% of Perdix patients and less frequent clinically significant events which have been attributed to ACE inhibitors include the following:

Cardiovascular:

Symptomatic hypotension, postural hypotension, or syncope was seen in < 1% of patients; these reactions led to discontinuation of therapy in controlled trials in 2 patients (0.1%) who had received Perdix monotherapy and in 1 patient (0.05%) who had received Perdix with hydrochlorothiazide. Other reports included chest pain, angina/myocardial infarction, tachycardia, palpitations, rhythm disturbances, transient ischaemic attacks, cerebrovascular accident.

Renal:

Of hypertensive patients with no apparent pre-existing renal disease, 0.8% of patients receiving Perdix alone and 1.5% of patients receiving Perdix with hydrochlorothiazide have experienced increases in serum creatinine to at least 140% of their baseline values.

Acute renal failure has been reported for ACE inhibitors including Perdix (see section 4.4 Special Warnings and Precautions for use).

Gastrointestinal:

Abdominal pain, dyspepsia, constipation, nausea, vomiting, diarrhoea, appetite/weight change, dry mouth, pancreatitis, hepatitis.

Intestinal Angioedema:

Intestinal Angioedema has been reported in patients treated with ACE inhibitors (see section 4.4 Special Warnings and Precautions for use).

Respiratory:

Upper respiratory infection, pharyngitis, sinusitis/rhinitis, bronchospasm, dyspnoea.

Urogenital:

Renal insufficiency.

Dermatologic:

Occasionally allergic and hypersensitivity reactions can occur like rash, pruritus, urticaria, erythema multiforme, Stevens-Johnson syndrome, toxic epidermic necrolysis, psoriasis-like efflorescence, pemphigus and alopecia. This can be accompanied by fever, myalgia, arthralgia, eosinophilia and/or increased ANA-titres. ACE inhibitors have been associated with the onset of angioneurotic oedema in a small subset of patients involving the face and oropharyngeal tissues.

Neurological and psychiatric:

Headache or tiredness may occasionally occur; rarely there may be drowsiness, depression, sleep disturbances, impotence, tingling sensations, numbness or paraesthesia, disturbances of balance, confusion, tinnitus, blurred vision, and alterations of taste or a transient loss of taste.

Other:

Sweating, flu syndrome, malaise.

Clinical Laboratory Test Findings:

Decreases in haemoglobin, haematocrit, platelets and white cell count and individual cases of agranulocytosis or pancytopenia, as well as elevation of liver enzymes and serum bilirubin have been reported in a few patients. In patients with congenital deficiency concerning G-6-PDH individual cases of haemolytic anaemia have been reported.

In rare cases, especially in patients with impaired kidney function or collagen disease, or those simultaneously receiving treatment will allopurinol, procainamide or certain drugs which suppress the defence reactions, there may be anaemia, thrombocytopenia, neutropenia, eosinophilia and in isolated cases, even agranulocytosis or pancytopenia.

Creatinine and blood urea nitrogen:

As with other ACE inhibitors, minor increases in blood urea nitrogen or serum creatinine, reversible upon discontinuation of therapy, were observed in approximately 1% of patients with essential hypertension who were treated with Perdix. Increases are more likely to occur in patients receiving concomitant diuretics or in patients with compromised renal function.

Potassium:

Since moexipril decreases aldosterone secretion, elevation of serum potassium can occur. Potassium supplements and potassium-sparing diuretics should be given with caution and the patient's serum potassium should be monitored frequently.

Other:

Clinically important changes in standard laboratory tests were rarely associated with Perdix administration. Elevations of liver enzymes and uric acid have been reported. In trials, less than 1% of moexipril-treated patients discontinued Perdix treatment because of laboratory abnormalities.

4.9 Overdose

Symptoms and treatment:

To date, no case of overdosage has been reported. Signs and symptoms expected in cases of overdosage would be related to hypotension and should be relieved by intravenous infusion of isotonic saline solution.

5. PHARMACOLOGICAL PROPERTIES

5.1 Pharmacodynamic properties

In animals as well as in humans, interactions between the renin-angiotensin-aldosterone system and the kallikrein-kinin system provide an important biochemical basis for blood pressure homeostasis. In hypertension the normal feedback mechanism formed by the renin-angiotensin system (RAS) may be dysfunctional, resulting in a self-perpetuating hypertensive condition.

Angiotensin converting enzyme (ACE) inhibitors were developed to interrupt this system and thereby to lower blood pressure. Perdix potently inhibits ACE and by this the formation of angiotensin II, the active agent of the RAS, thus blocking its vasoconstrictor and sodium-retaining effects with a consequent reduction in blood pressure.

Since ACE is identical is kininase II, an enzyme that degrades the potent vasodilator bradykinin, inhibition of ACE leads to an additional, non renin-mediated reduction in systemic blood pressure. The antihypertensive effects of ACE inhibitors are accompanied by a reduction in peripheral vascular resistance.

5.2 Pharmacokinetic properties

The prodrug moexipril is rapidly absorbed and de-esterified to the active metabolite moexiprilat. The pharmacokinetic parameters for moexipril and moexiprilat were similar after both, single and multiple does of moexipril and appear to be dose-proportional.

Moexipril and moexiprilat are moderately bound to plasma proteins, predominately albumin. Therefore, concurrently administered drugs are unlikely to interfere with the binding of moexipril and moexiprilat in any clinically significant way. Metabolites of moexipril present in the diketopiperazine derivatives of moexipril and moexiprilat. Both, moexipril and moexiprilat are eliminated in the urine, and moexiprilat is eliminated in the faeces.

The pharmacokinetic profile of moexipril and moexiprilat should allow the same dosage recommendation in patients with mild to moderate renal dysfunction

(Cl_{cr} > 40 ml/min) as in patients with normal renal function. With severe renal dysfunction, dosage reduction is recommended. In patients with liver cirrhosis, the pharmacokinetics of moexipril and moexiprilat were significantly altered as compared with normal subjects. In such patients, therapy with Perdix should be started with 3.75 mg (half 7.5 mg tablet).

There were no apparent pharmacokinetic drug interactions with HCTZ, digoxin, cimetidine, warfarin or nifedipine.

5.3 Preclinical safety data

Acute toxicity:

Findings of the acute toxicity studies in animals do not raise questions as to the safety of moexipril HCl as well as the main metabolite moexiprilat under the conditions of proposed clinical usage.

Subacute/chronic toxicity:

Subacute and chronic toxicity studies in rats and dogs with repeated oral administration of moexipril HCl up to 12 months, revealed mainly heart and kidney as target organs. The effects are completely comparable with those of other ACE inhibitors and can be interpreted as results of highly exaggerated pharmacological activity.

First unspecific drug-related side-effects after long-term administration were seen at 75 mg/kg, i.e. a dose which corresponds 150 times the maximum recommended total daily dose in humans when compared on the basis of body weight.

Reproduction studies:

Studies in rats and rabbits including all segments of reproduction revealed no direct effects of moexipril HCl on fertility, reproduction and abnormalities in F_1 – or F_2 – pups.

Regarding precautions in women of child bearing potential and use during pregnancy and lactation see 4.3 and 4.6.

Mutagenicity:

As conclusion of different 'in vitro' and one 'in vivo' mutagenicity studies, the mutagenic potential of moexipril HCl for human beings should be extremely low.

Carcinogenicity:

Neither the long-term toxicity studies in rats and dogs nor special carcinogenicity studies in mice and rats over 78 and 104 weeks respectively, indicated neoplastigenic properties of moexipril HCl. Therefore, it can be concluded that the carcinogenic risk for human beings will be extremely low.

6. PHARMACEUTICAL PARTICULARS

6.1 List of excipients

Lactose monohydrate

Crospovidone

Light magnesium oxide

Gelatin

Magnesium stearate

Methylhydroxypropylcellulose

Hydroxypropylcellulose

Polyethyleneglycol 6000

Titanium dioxide

Ferric oxide

Purified water (not present in the finished product).

6.2 Incompatibilities

No incompatibilities have so far been demonstrated.

6.3 Shelf life

5 years

6.4 Special precautions for storage

Store in the original package.

6.5 Nature and contents of container

Calendar packs containing 28 tablets, 14 per Al/Al blister pack.

6.6 Instructions for use and handling

No special instruction necessary.

7. MARKETING AUTHORISATION HOLDER

SCHWARZ PHARMA Limited

Schwarz House

East Street

Chesham

Bucks HP5 1DG

England

8. MARKETING AUTHORISATION NUMBER(S)

PL 04438/0033

9. DATE OF FIRST AUTHORISATION/RENEWAL OF THE AUTHORISATION

03 November 2000

10. DATE OF REVISION OF THE TEXT

May 2005

Perfalgan 10 mg/ml Solution for Infusion

(Bristol-Myers Squibb Pharmaceuticals Ltd)

1. NAME OF THE MEDICINAL PRODUCT

PERFALGAN ▼ 10 mg/ml solution for infusion.

2. QUALITATIVE AND QUANTITATIVE COMPOSITION

1 ml contains 10 mg paracetamol

1 vial contains 50ml, equivalent to 500mg paracetamol.

1 vial contains 100 ml, equivalent to 1000 mg paracetamol.

For excipients, see section 6.1.

3. PHARMACEUTICAL FORM

Solution for infusion.

The solution is clear and slightly yellowish.

4. CLINICAL PARTICULARS

4.1 Therapeutic indications

PERFALGAN is indicated for the short-term treatment of moderate pain, especially following surgery, and for the short-term treatment of fever, when administration by intravenous route is clinically justified by an urgent need to treat pain or hyperthermia and/or when other routes of administration are not possible.

4.2 Posology and method of administration

Intravenous use.

The 100ml vial is restricted to adults, adolescents and children weighing more than 33 kg (approximately 11 years old).

The 50ml vial is restricted to children weighing from 10kg (approximately one year old) to 33kg.

Posology:

Adolescents and adults weighing more than 50 kg:

Paracetamol 1 g per administration, i.e. one 100 ml vial, up to four times a day.

The minimum interval between each administration must be 4 hours.

The maximum daily dose must not exceed 4 g.

Children weighing more than 33 kg (approximately 11 years old), adolescents and adults weighing less than 50 kg:

Paracetamol 15 mg/kg per administration, i.e. 1.5 ml solution per kg up to four times a day.

The minimum interval between each administration must be 4 hours.

The maximum daily dose must not exceed 60 mg/kg (without exceeding 3g).

Children weighing more than 10kg (approximately 1 year old) and weighing less than 33kg:

Paracetamol 15mg/kg per administration, i.e. 1.5ml solution per kg up to four times a day.

The minimum interval between each administration must be 4 hours.

The maximum daily dose must not exceed 60mg/kg (without exceeding 2g)

Severe renal insufficiency: it is recommended, when giving paracetamol to patients with severe renal impairment (creatinine clearance ⩽ 30 mL/min), that the minimum interval between each administration be increased to 6 hours (See section 5.2 Pharmacokinetic properties).

Method of administration:

The paracetamol solution is administered as a 15-minute intravenous infusion.

4.3 Contraindications

PERFALGAN is contraindicated:

- in patients with hypersensitivity to paracetamol or to propacetamol hydrochloride (prodrug of paracetamol) or to any of the excipients.

- in cases of severe hepatocellular insufficiency.

4.4 Special warnings and special precautions for use

Warnings

It is recommended that a suitable analgesic oral treatment be used as soon as this route of administration is possible.

In order to avoid the risk of overdose, check that no other medicines administered contain paracetamol.

Doses higher than those recommended entail the risk of very serious liver damage. Clinical signs and symptoms of liver damage are not usually seen until two days, and up to a maximum of 4-6 days, after administration. Treatment with antidote should be given as soon as possible (See section 4.9 Overdose).

Precautions for use

Paracetamol should be used with caution in cases of:

- hepatocellular insufficiency,
- severe renal insufficiency (creatinine clearance $\leqslant$ 30 mL/min) (see sections 4.2 Posology and method of administration and 5.2 Pharmacokinetic properties),
- chronic alcoholism,
- chronic malnutrition (low reserves of hepatic glutathione),
- dehydration.

4.5 Interaction with other medicinal products and other forms of Interaction

- Probenecid causes an almost 2-fold reduction in clearance of paracetamol by inhibiting its conjugation with glucuronic acid. A reduction in the paracetamol dose should be considered if it is to be used concomitantly with probenecid.
- Salicylamide may prolong the elimination t½ of paracetamol.
- Caution should be taken with the concomitant intake of enzyme-inducing substances (see section 4.9 Overdose).

4.6 Pregnancy and lactation

Pregnancy:

Clinical experience of the intravenous administration of paracetamol is limited. However, epidemiological data from the use of oral therapeutic doses of paracetamol indicate no undesirable effects in pregnancy or on the health of the foetus / newborn infant.

Prospective data on pregnancies exposed to overdoses did not show any increase in the risk of malformation.

No reproductive studies with the intravenous form of paracetamol have been performed in animals. However, studies with the oral route did not show any malformation or foetotoxic effects.

Nevertheless, PERFALGAN should only be used during pregnancy after a careful benefit-risk assessment. In this case, the recommended posology and duration must be strictly observed.

Lactation:

After oral administration, paracetamol is excreted into breast milk in small quantities. No undesirable effects on nursing infants have been reported. Consequently, PERFALGAN may be used in breast-feeding women.

4.7 Effects on ability to drive and use machines

Not relevant.

4.8 Undesirable effects

As with all paracetamol products, adverse drug reactions are rare >1/10000, <1/1000) or very rare (1<1/10000). They are described below:

(see Table 1)

Very rare cases of hypersensitivity reactions ranging from simple skin rash or urticaria to anaphylactic shock have been reported and require discontinuation of treatment.

Isolated reports of thrombocytopenia have been observed.

4.9 Overdose

There is a risk of poisoning, particularly in elderly subjects, in young children, in patients with liver disease, in cases of chronic alcoholism, in patients with chronic malnutrition and in patients receiving enzyme inducers. Overdosing may be fatal in these cases.

Symptoms generally appear within the first 24 hours and comprise: nausea, vomiting, anorexia, pallor and abdominal pain.

Overdose, 7.5 g or more of paracetamol in a single administration in adults or 140 mg/kg of body weight in a single administration in children, causes hepatic cytolysis likely to induce complete and irreversible necrosis, resulting in hepatocellular insufficiency, metabolic acidosis and encephalopathy which may lead to coma and death. Simultaneously, increased levels of hepatic transaminases (AST, ALT), lactate dehydrogenase and bilirubin are observed together with decreased prothrombin levels that may appear 12 to 48 hours after administration. Clinical symptoms of liver damage are usually evident initially after two days, and reach a maximum after 4 to 6 days.

Emergency measures

Immediate hospitalisation.

Before beginning treatment, take a blood sample for plasma paracetamol assay, as soon as possible after the overdose.

The treatment includes administration of the antidote, N-acetylcysteine (NAC) by the i.v. or oral route, if possible before the 10th hour. NAC can, however, give some degree of protection even after 10 hours, but in these cases prolonged treatment is given.

Symptomatic treatment.

Hepatic tests must be carried out at the beginning of treatment and repeated every 24 hours. In most cases hepatic transaminases return to normal in one to two weeks with full return of normal liver function. In very severe cases, however, liver transplantation may be necessary.

5. PHARMACOLOGICAL PROPERTIES

5.1 Pharmacodynamic properties

Pharmacotherapeutic group: OTHER ANALGESICS AND ANTIPYRETICS,

ATC Code: N02BE01

The precise mechanism of the analgesic and antipyretic properties of paracetamol has yet to be established; it may involve central and peripheral actions.

PERFALGAN provides onset of pain relief within 5 to 10 minutes after the start of administration. The peak analgesic effect is obtained in 1 hour and the duration of this effect is usually 4 to 6 hours.

PERFALGAN reduces fever within 30 minutes after the start of administration with a duration of the antipyretic effect of at least 6 hours.

5.2 Pharmacokinetic properties

Adults:

Absorption:

Paracetamol pharmacokinetics is linear up to 2 g after single administration and after repeated administration during 24 hours.

The bioavailability of paracetamol following infusion of 500mg and 1 g of PERFALGAN is similar to that observed following infusion of 1g and 2 g propacetamol (containing 500mg and 1 g paracetamol respectively). The maximal plasma concentration (Cmax) of paracetamol observed at the end of 15-minutes intravenous infusion of 500mg and 1 g of PERFALGAN is about 15μg/ml and 30 μg/ml respectively.

Distribution:

The volume of distribution of paracetamol is approximately 1 L/kg.

Paracetamol is not extensively bound to plasma proteins.

Following infusion of 1 g paracetamol, significant concentrations of paracetamol (about 1.5 μg/mL) were observed in the cerebrospinal fluid at and after the 20th minute following infusion.

Metabolism:

Paracetamol is metabolised mainly in the liver following two major hepatic pathways: glucuronic acid conjugation and sulphuric acid conjugation. The latter route is rapidly saturable at doses that exceed the therapeutic doses. A small fraction (less than 4%) is metabolised by cytochrome P450 to a reactive intermediate (N-acetyl benzoquinone imine) which, under normal conditions of use, is rapidly detoxified by reduced glutathione and eliminated in the urine after conjugation with cysteine and mercapturic acid. However, during massive overdosing, the quantity of this toxic metabolite is increased.

Elimination:

The metabolites of paracetamol are mainly excreted in the urine. 90% of the dose administered is excreted within 24 hours, mainly as glucuronide (60-80%) and sulphate (20-30%) conjugates. Less than 5% is eliminated unchanged. Plasma half-life is 2.7 hours and total body clearance is 18 L/h.

Table 1

Organ System	Rare >1/10000, <1/1000	Very rare <1/10000	Isolated Reports
General	Malaise	Hypersensitivity reaction	
Cardiovascular	Hypotension		
Liver	Increased levels of hepatic transaminases		
Platelet/blood			Thrombocytopenia Leucopenia, Neutropenia

Neonates, infants and children:

The pharmacokinetic parameters of paracetamol observed in infants and children are similar to those observed in adults, except for the plasma half-life that is slightly shorter (1.5 to 2 h) than in adults. In neonates, the plasma half-life is longer than in infants i.e. around 3.5 hours. Neonates, infants and children up to 10 years excrete significantly less glucuronide and more sulphate conjugates than adults. Total excretion of paracetamol and its metabolites is the same at all ages.

Special populations:

Renal insufficiency:

In cases of severe renal impairment (creatinine clearance 10-30 mL/min), the elimination of paracetamol is slightly delayed, the elimination half-life ranging from 2 to 5.3 hours. For the glucuronide and sulphate conjugates, the elimination rate is 3 times slower in subjects with severe renal impairment than in healthy subjects. Therefore when giving paracetamol to patients with severe renal impairment (creatinine clearance $\leqslant$ 30 mL/min), the minimum interval between each administration should be increased to 6 hours (see section 4.2. Posology and method of administration).

Elderly subjects:

The pharmacokinetics and the metabolism of paracetamol are not modified in elderly subjects. No dose adjustment is required in this population.

5.3 Preclinical safety data

Preclinical data reveal no special hazard for humans beyond the information included in other sections of the SmPC.

Studies on local tolerance of PERFALGAN in rats and rabbits showed good tolerability. Absence of delayed contact hypersensitivity has been tested in guinea pigs.

6. PHARMACEUTICAL PARTICULARS

6.1 List of excipients

Cysteine hydrochloride monohydrate

Disodium phosphate dihydrate

Hydrochloric acid

Mannitol

Sodium hydroxide

Water for Injections

6.2 Incompatibilities

PERFALGAN should not be mixed with other medicinal products.

6.3 Shelf life

2 years.

From a microbiological point of view, unless the method of opening precludes the risk of microbial contamination, the product should be used immediately. If not used immediately, in-use storage times and conditions are the responsibility of the user.

6.4 Special precautions for storage

Do not store above 30°C. Do not refrigerate or freeze.

6.5 Nature and contents of container

50ml and 100 ml Type II clear glass vial with bromobutyl stopper and an aluminium/plastic flip-off cap.

Pack size: pack of 12 vials.

6.6 Instructions for use and handling

Before administration, the product should be visually inspected for any particulate matter and discolouration. For single use only. Any unused solution should be discarded.

7. MARKETING AUTHORISATION HOLDER

Bristol-Myers Squibb Pharmaceuticals Ltd

141-149 Staines Road

Hounslow

Middlesex TW3 3JA

8. MARKETING AUTHORISATION NUMBER(S)

PL 11184/0094

9. DATE OF FIRST AUTHORISATION/RENEWAL OF THE AUTHORISATION

20 November 2002

10. DATE OF REVISION OF THE TEXT

July 2004

Periactin

(Merck Sharp & Dohme Limited)

1. NAME OF THE MEDICINAL PRODUCT

PERIACTIN® 4 mg Tablets

2. QUALITATIVE AND QUANTITATIVE COMPOSITION

Each 'Periactin' tablet contains cyproheptadine hydrochloride equivalent to 4 mg anhydrous cyproheptadine hydrochloride.

3. PHARMACEUTICAL FORM

White round bevelled edged tablet with a scoreline on one side and marked 'MSD 62' on the other.

4. CLINICAL PARTICULARS

4.1 Therapeutic indications

'Periactin' is a serotonin and histamine antagonist with anticholinergic and sedative properties.

In allergy and pruritus: 'Periactin' has a wide range of antiallergic and antipruritic activity, and can be used successfully in the treatment of acute and chronic allergic and pruritic conditions, such as dermatitis, including neurodermatitis and neurodermatitis circumscripta; eczema; eczematoid dermatitis; dermatographism; mild, local allergic reactions to insect bites; hay fever and other seasonal rhinitis; perennial allergic and vasomotor rhinitis; allergic conjunctivitis due to inhalant allergens and foods; urticaria; angioneurotic oedema; drug and serum reactions; anogenital pruritus; pruritus of chicken-pox.

'Periactin' is indicated as adjunctive therapy to adrenaline and other standard measures for the relief of anaphylactic reactions after the acute manifestations have been controlled.

In migraine and vascular headache: 'Periactin' has been reported to have beneficial effects in a significant number of patients having vascular types of headache. Many patients who have responded inadequately to all other agents have reported amelioration of symptoms with 'Periactin'. The characteristic headache and feeling of malaise may disappear within an hour or two of the first dose.

4.2 Posology and method of administration

Route of administration: oral.

There is no recommended dosage for children under 2 years old. 'Periactin' is not recommended for elderly, debilitated patients.

For the treatment of allergy and pruritus:

Dosage must be determined on an individual basis. The effect of a single dose usually lasts for four to six hours. For continuous effective relief, the daily requirement should be given in divided doses, usually three times a day, or as often as necessary, to provide continuous relief.

Adults: The therapeutic range is 4-20 mg (1 to 5 tablets) a day, most patients requiring 12-16 mg a day. It is recommended that dosage be initiated with 4 mg three times a day and then adjusted according to the weight and response of the patient up to a maximum of 32 mg a day.

Children aged 7-14 years: Usually 4 mg two or three times a day, according to the patient's weight and response. If an additional dose is required, it should be given at bedtime. Maximum 16 mg a day.

Children aged 2-6 years: Initially 2 mg two or three times a day, adjusted according to the patient's weight and response. If an additional dose is required, it should be given at bedtime. Maximum 12 mg a day.

For treatment of vascular headache and migraine

For both prophylactic and therapeutic use, an initial dose of 4 mg, repeated if necessary after half an hour. Patients who respond usually obtain relief with 8 mg, and this dose should not be exceeded within a 4- to 6-hour period.

Maintenance: 4 mg every four to six hours.

Use in the elderly: 'Periactin' should not be used in elderly, debilitated patients. Elderly patients are more likely to experience dizziness, sedation, and hypotension.

4.3 Contraindications

'Periactin' is contra-indicated in:

- patients undergoing therapy for an acute asthmatic attack;
- newborn or premature infants;
- breast-feeding mothers;
- patients with known sensitivity to cyproheptadine hydrochloride or drugs with similar chemical structure;
- concurrent use with monoamine oxidase inhibitors;
- glaucoma;
- patients with pyloroduodenal obstruction, stenosing peptic ulcer, symptomatic prostatic hypertrophy, predisposition to urinary retention or bladder neck obstruction;
- elderly, debilitated patients.

4.4 Special warnings and special precautions for use

Antihistamines should not be used to treat lower respiratory tract symptoms, including those of acute asthma.

The safety and efficacy of 'Periactin' is not established in children under 2 years old.

Antihistamines may diminish mental alertness; conversely, particularly in the young child, they may occasionally produce excitation.

Patients should be warned against engaging in activities requiring motor co-ordination and mental alertness, such as driving a car or operating machinery (see section 4.7 'Effects on ability to drive and use machines').

Rarely, prolonged therapy with antihistamines may cause blood dyscrasias.

Because 'Periactin' has an atropine-like action, it should be used cautiously in patients with a history of bronchial asthma, increased intra-ocular pressure, hyperthyroidism, cardiovascular disease, or hypertension.

4.5 Interaction with other medicinal products and other forms of Interaction

MAO inhibitors prolong and intensify the anticholinergic effects of antihistamines.

Antihistamines may have additive effects with alcohol and other CNS depressants, e.g. hypnotics, sedatives, tranquillisers and anti-anxiety agents.

Drugs with anti-serotonin activity, such as cyproheptadine, may interfere with serotonin-enhancing anti-depressants including selective serotonin re-uptake inhibitors (SSRI's). This may result in possible recurrence of depression and related symptoms.

Cyproheptadine may cause a false positive test result for tricyclic antidepressant drugs (TCA) when evaluating a urine drug screen. Because cyproheptadine and TCAs may produce similar overdose symptoms, physicians should carefully monitor patients for TCA toxicity in the event of combined overdose.

4.6 Pregnancy and lactation

The use of any drug in pregnancy or in women of child-bearing age requires that the potential benefit of the drug should be weighed against possible hazards to the embryo and foetus. It is not known whether 'Periactin' is excreted in human milk, and because of the potential for serious adverse reactions in breast-feeding infants from 'Periactin', a decision should be made whether to discontinue breast-feeding or to discontinue the drug, taking into account the importance of the drug to the mother (see section 4.3 'Contra-indications').

4.7 Effects on ability to drive and use machines

This product may cause drowsiness and somnolence. Patients receiving it should not drive or operate machinery unless it has been shown that their physical and mental capacity remains unaffected.

4.8 Undesirable effects

The side effects that appear frequently are drowsiness and somnolence. Many patients who initially complain of drowsiness may no longer do so after the first three to four days of continuous administration.

Side effects reported with antihistamines are:

Central nervous system: Sedation, sleepiness (often transient), dizziness, disturbed co-ordination, confusion, restlessness, excitation, nervousness, tremor, irritability, aggressive behaviour, insomnia, paraesthesiae, neuritis, convulsions, euphoria, hallucinations, hysteria, faintness.

Integumentary: Allergic manifestations of rash and oedema, excessive perspiration, urticaria, photosensitivity.

Special senses: Acute labyrinthitis, blurred vision, diplopia, vertigo, tinnitus.

Cardiovascular: Hypotension, palpitation, tachycardia, extrasystoles, anaphylactic shock.

Haematological: Haemolytic anaemia, leucopenia, agranulocytosis, thrombocytopenia.

Digestive system: Cholestasis, hepatic failure, hepatitis, hepatic function abnormality, dryness of mouth, epigastric distress, anorexia, nausea, vomiting, diarrhoea, constipation, jaundice.

Genito-urinary: Frequency and difficulty of micturition, urinary retention, early menses.

Respiratory: Dryness of the nose and throat, thickening of bronchial secretions, tightness of chest and wheezing, nasal stuffiness.

Miscellaneous: Fatigue, rigors, headache, increased appetite/weight gain.

4.9 Overdose

Antihistamine overdosage reactions may vary from CNS depression or stimulation to convulsions, respiratory and cardiac arrest and death, especially in infants and children. Atropine-like and gastro-intestinal symptoms may occur.

If vomiting has not occurred spontaneously, it should be induced in the conscious patient with syrup of ipecac. If the patient cannot vomit, gastric lavage with isotonic or half isotonic saline is indicated, followed by activated charcoal. Precautions against aspiration must be taken, especially in infants and children.

Life-threatening CNS signs and symptoms should be treated appropriately.

Saline cathartics usefully draw water into the bowel by osmosis to dilute bowel content rapidly.

Central stimulants must not be used, but vasopressors may be used to counteract hypotension.

5. PHARMACOLOGICAL PROPERTIES

5.1 Pharmacodynamic properties

Cyproheptadine hydrochloride is a serotonin and histamine antagonist with anticholinergic and sedative effects. Antiserotonin and antihistamine drugs appear to compete with serotonin and histamine, respectively, for receptor sites.

Cyproheptadine hydrochloride antagonises the following effects of serotonin, in laboratory animals:

Bronchoconstrictor (guinea-pig)

Vasopressor (dog)

Spasmogenic (isolated rat uterus)

Oedema (rat)

Lethal (haemophilus petussis-treated mouse)

In these effects it equals or surpasses the activity of many of the activities of specific serotonin antagonists, such as 1-Benzyl-2-methyl-5-methoxy-tryptame (BAS) and 1 Benzyl-2methyl-5-hydroxy-tryptamine (BMS), in contrast, specific antihistamines, even the most potent, show little or no serotonin antagonism.

Cyproheptadine hydrochloride antagonises or blocks the following effects of histamine in laboratory animals:

Bronchoconstrictor (guinea-pig)

Vasopressor (dog)

Spasmogenic (isolated rat uterus)

Anaphylactic shock, active and passive (guinea-pig and mouse)

Increased gastric secretion (Heidenhain pouch dog.)

It is unusual that cyproheptadine hydrochloride protects both the guinea-pig and mice against anaphylactic shock. In guinea-pigs, the pulmonary aspects of anaphylactic shock are attributable to the release of endogenous histamine and can be controlled by substances with specific antihistamine activity. In mice however, where histamine release seems to be less important and serotonin release may be involved, specific antihistamines are of little value in protecting against anaphylaxis. Thus the protective effect of cyproheptadine hydrochloride in mice may be an anti-serotonin effect.

The inhibitory effect of cyproheptadine in histamine-induced gastric secretion is also unusual as specific antihistamines do not influence this effect.

Cyproheptadine has appetite stimulation properties in laboratory animals.

5.2 Pharmacokinetic properties

After a single 4 mg oral dose of ^{14}C-labelled cyproheptadine hydrochloride in normal subjects given as tablets or syrup, 2 to 20% of the radioactivity was excreted in the stools. Only about 34% of the stool radioactivity was unchanged drug, corresponding to less than 5.7% of the dose. At least 40% of the administered radioactivity was excreted in the urine.

No significant difference in the mean urinary excretion exists between the tablet and syrup formulations. No detectable amounts of unchanged drug were present in the urine of patients on chronic 12-20 mg daily doses of 'Periactin' syrup. The principle metabolite found in human urine has been identified as a quaternary ammonium glucuronide conjugate of cyproheptadine. Elimination is diminished in renal insufficiency.

5.3 Preclinical safety data

No relevant information.

6. PHARMACEUTICAL PARTICULARS

6.1 List of excipients

'Periactin' tablets contain the following inactive ingredients: calcium hydrogen phosphate E341, lactose, magnesium stearate E572, potato starch and pregelatinised maize starch.

6.2 Incompatibilities

None known.

6.3 Shelf life

3 years.

6.4 Special precautions for storage

Do not store above 25°C. Store in the original package.

6.5 Nature and contents of container

30 tablets in opaque PVC blisters with hard-temper aluminium lidding.

6.6 Instructions for use and handling

None.

7. MARKETING AUTHORISATION HOLDER

Merck Sharp & Dohme Limited

Hertford Road, Hoddesdon, Hertfordshire EN11 9BU, UK.

8. MARKETING AUTHORISATION NUMBER(S)

Tablets PL 0025/5017R

9. DATE OF FIRST AUTHORISATION/RENEWAL OF THE AUTHORISATION

Licence granted: 3 October 1990

Last renewed: 7 May 1996

10. DATE OF REVISION OF THE TEXT

January 2004

LEGAL CATEGORY

P.

® denotes registered trademark of Merck & Co., Inc., Whitehouse Station, NJ, USA.

SPC-PCTT.02.UK.0765

FT 04.02.2004

Perinal Spray

(Dermal Laboratories Limited)

1. NAME OF THE MEDICINAL PRODUCT

PERINAL® SPRAY

2. QUALITATIVE AND QUANTITATIVE COMPOSITION

Hydrocortisone 0.2 % w/w; Lidocaine Hydrochloride 1.0% w/w.

3. PHARMACEUTICAL FORM

Colourless to pale yellow aqueous cutaneous spray solution.

4. CLINICAL PARTICULARS

4.1 Therapeutic indications

For the symptomatic relief of anal and perianal itch, irritation and pain, such as associated with haemorrhoids.

4.2 Posology and method of administration

The same dosage schedule applies to all age groups, although the spray is not normally recommended for children under 14 years unless on medical advice:-

Spray once over the affected area up to three times daily, depending on the severity of the condition.

4.3 Contraindications

Not to be used if sensitive to lidocaine or any of the other ingredients. Not to be used on broken or infected skin. Not to be used internally (inside the anus), or anywhere other than the anal area.

4.4 Special warnings and special precautions for use

Perinal Spray is intended for use for limited periods and so should not be used continuously for longer than 7 days without medical advice. Patients should be instructed to seek medical advice if they experience persistent pain or bleeding from the anus, especially where associated with a change in bowel habit, if the stomach is distended or if they are losing weight. Prompt medical treatment may be very important under such circumstances. Perinal Spray should be kept away from the eyes, nose and mouth.

The label will state:-

Perinal Spray should not be used during pregnancy, while breast feeding or by children under the age of 14 without medical advice. Keep spray away from the eyes, nose and mouth, and do not apply to broken or infected skin, or to any part of the body except the anal area. Prime pump before initial use by depressing its top once or twice. Wash hands, and replace cap after use. Consult your doctor if the condition does not improve, or if rectal bleeding occurs. Do not use continuously for more than 7 days, unless recommended by your doctor. Do not use if sensitive to any of the ingredients. For external use only.

4.5 Interaction with other medicinal products and other forms of Interaction

No known interactions. Medical supervision is required if used in conjunction with other medicines containing steroids, owing to possible additive effects.

4.6 Pregnancy and lactation

There is inadequate evidence of safety in human pregnancy. Topical administration of corticosteroids to pregnant animals can cause abnormalities of foetal development including cleft palate and intra-uterine growth retardation. There may therefore be a very small risk of such effects in the human foetus. The risk/benefit needs to be carefully assessed, therefore, before prescribing this medicine.

4.7 Effects on ability to drive and use machines

None known.

4.8 Undesirable effects

A temporary tingling sensation may be experienced locally after initial application. Hypersensitivity to lidocaine has rarely been reported.

4.9 Overdose

Under exceptional circumstances, if Perinal Spray is used excessively, particularly in young children, it is theoretically possible that adrenal suppression and skin thinning may occur. The symptoms are normally reversible on cessation of treatment.

5. PHARMACOLOGICAL PROPERTIES

5.1 Pharmacodynamic properties

The preparation combines the well-known local anti-inflammatory and anti-pruritic properties of hydrocortisone and the analgesic effect of lidocaine in an aqueous spray formulation. On application, finger contact with the affected area can be avoided which makes for improved hygiene, and lessens the risk of infection.

5.2 Pharmacokinetic properties

The active ingredients of the formulation are readily available for intimate contact with the skin and mucous membranes, as the preparation is sprayed in small droplets which dry after application to leave the active ingredients in close contact with the affected area.

Because the preparation is a clear solution, it is entirely homogeneous, and the availability of the active ingredient is optimal.

5.3 Preclinical safety data

No special information.

6. PHARMACEUTICAL PARTICULARS

6.1 List of excipients

Cetomacrogol 1000; Citric Acid Monohydrate; Sodium Citrate; Propyl Gallate; Phenoxyethanol; Purified Water.

6.2 Incompatibilities

None known.

6.3 Shelf life

30 months.

6.4 Special precautions for storage

Do not store above 25°C.

6.5 Nature and contents of container

30 ml collapsible laminate tube with metering-dose spray pump and cap, which is ozone-friendly.

The spray operates when held in any direction. It is *not* an aerosol and does *not* contain any potentially irritant propellants.

This is supplied as an original pack (OP).

6.6 Instructions for use and handling

Not applicable.

7. MARKETING AUTHORISATION HOLDER

Dermal Laboratories

Tatmore Place, Gosmore

Hitchin, Herts SG4 7QR, UK.

8. MARKETING AUTHORISATION NUMBER(S)

0173/0049.

9. DATE OF FIRST AUTHORISATION/RENEWAL OF THE AUTHORISATION

5 June 2002.

10. DATE OF REVISION OF THE TEXT

April 2004.

Periostat 20mg film-coated tablets

(Alliance Pharmaceuticals)

1. NAME OF THE MEDICINAL PRODUCT

PERIOSTAT® 20 mg film-coated tablets

2. QUALITATIVE AND QUANTITATIVE COMPOSITION

Each film-coated tablet contains 23.08 mg doxycycline hyclate equivalent to 20 mg doxycycline.

For excipients, see 6.1

3. PHARMACEUTICAL FORM

Film-coated tablet

White to off-white round tablets imprinted on one side with PS-20

4. CLINICAL PARTICULARS

4.1 Therapeutic indications

For patients with adult periodontitis. PERIOSTAT is indicated as an adjunct to supra-gingival and sub-gingival scaling and root planing, with oral hygiene instruction, carried out by a dental practitioner or hygienist as appropriate.

4.2 Posology and method of administration

Adults and the elderly:

PERIOSTAT 20 mg should be administered twice daily, at least one hour before meals or before bedtime. Tablets should be swallowed whole with adequate fluids (at least 100ml of water) and should be taken in an upright sitting or standing position (see 4.4: Special warnings and Precautions for Use).

PERIOSTAT is indicated for treatment periods of 3 months. PERIOSTAT should not be administered for more than 3 consecutive three month periods.

No dosage modification is necessary in elderly patients.

Renal Impairment:

No dosage adjustment is necessary in the presence of renal impairment.

Children:

For use in children, see 'Contraindications'.

4.3 Contraindications

In common with other drugs of the tetracycline class, PERIOSTAT is contra-indicated in infants and children up to 12 years of age.

Doxycycline should not be administered to patients who have shown hypersensitivity to doxycycline hyclate, other tetracyclines or to any of the excipients.

Patients known to have, or suspected to have, achlorhydria should not be prescribed doxycycline.

Use of doxycycline is contra-indicated during pregnancy and lactation (See 4.6 Pregnancy and lactation).

4.4 Special warnings and special precautions for use

Tablet forms of the tetracycline class of drugs may cause oesophageal irritation and ulceration. To avoid oesophageal irritation and ulceration, adequate fluids should be taken with this medication. PERIOSTAT should be swallowed whilst in an upright sitting or standing posture. Tablets taken in the evening should be taken well in advance of retiring (see 4.2: Posology and Method of Administration).

Whilst no overgrowth by opportunistic microorganisms such as yeast were noted during clinical studies, PERIOSTAT therapy may result in overgrowth of nonsusceptible microorganisms including fungi (with clinical symptoms of persistent bad breath, reddening of the gums, etc.). Periodic observation of the patient is essential. If overgrowth by resistant organisms appears, PERIOSTAT therapy should be discontinued and an appropriate treatment instituted.

PERIOSTAT should be used with caution in patients with a history of or predisposition to oral candidosis. The safety and effectiveness of PERIOSTAT has not been established for the treatment of periodontitis in patients with coexistent oral candidosis. Whilst not observed during clinical trials with PERIOSTAT, the use of tetracyclines may increase the incidence of vaginal candidosis.

The blood doxycycline levels in patients treated with PERIOSTAT are lower than in those treated with conventional antimicrobial formulations of doxycycline. As, however, there are no data to support safety in hepatic impairment at this lower dose, PERIOSTAT should be administered with caution to patients with hepatic impairment or to those receiving potentially hepatotoxic drugs.

Caution should be observed in the treatment of patients with myasthenia gravis who may be at risk of worsening of the condition.

All patients receiving doxycycline including PERIOSTAT should be advised to avoid excessive sunlight or artificial ultraviolet light while receiving doxycycline and to discontinue therapy if phototoxicity (e.g., skin eruption etc.) occurs. Sunscreen or sunblock should be considered. Treatment should cease at the first sign of skin erythema.

In common with the use of antimicrobial drugs in general, there is a risk of the development of pseudomembranous colitis with doxycycline treatment. In the event of the development of diarrhoea during treatment with PERIOSTAT, the possibility of pseudomembranous colitis should be considered and appropriate therapy instituted. This may include the discontinuation of doxycycline and the institution of specific antibiotic therapy (e.g vancomycin). Agents inhibiting peristalsis should not be employed in this situation.

In the event of a severe acute hypersensitivity reaction (e.g. anaphylaxis), treatment with PERIOSTAT must be stopped at once and the usual emergency measures taken (e.g. administration of antihistamines, corticosteroids, sympathomimetics and if necessary artificial respiration instituted).

4.5 Interaction with other medicinal products and other forms of Interaction

These recommendations regarding the potential interactions between doxycycline and other medications are based upon the larger doses generally used in antimicrobial formulations of doxycycline rather than with PERIOSTAT. However at the present time, insufficient data exist for reassurance that the interactions described with higher doses of doxycycline will not occur with PERIOSTAT.

The absorption of doxycycline from the gastro-intestinal tract may be inhibited by bi- or tri- valent ions such as aluminium, zinc, calcium (found for example in milk, dairy products and calcium-containing fruit juices), by magnesium (found for example in antacids) or by iron preparations, activated charcoal, cholestyramine, bismuth chelates and sucralfate. Therefore such medicines or foodstuffs should be taken after a period of 2 to 3 hours following ingestion of PERIOSTAT. Didanosine tablets may decrease the absorption of doxycycline due to the gastric pH increase as a consequence of the antacid content of the didanosine tablets. Didanosine should therefore be taken at least 2 hours after doxycycline. Quinapril may reduce the absorption of doxycycline due to the high magnesium content in quinapril tablets.

Doxycycline has been shown to potentiate the hypoglycaemic effect of sulfonylurea oral antidiabetic agents. If administered in combination with these drugs, blood sugar levels should be monitored and if necessary, the doses of the above drugs reduced.

Doxycycline has been shown to depress plasma prothrombin activity thereby potentiating the effect of anticoagulants of the dicoumarol type. If administered in combination with these agents, coagulation parameters, including INR, should be monitored and if necessary, the doses of the above drugs reduced. The possibility of an increased risk of bleeding events should be borne in mind.

When doxycycline is administered shortly before, during or after courses of isotretinoin, there is the possibility of potentiation between the drugs to cause reversible pressure increase in the intracranial cavity (pseudotumour cerebri). Concomitant administration should therefore be avoided.

Bacteriostatic drugs including doxycycline may interfere with the bacteriocidal action of penicillin and betalactam antibiotics. It is advisable that PERIOSTAT and betalactam antibiotics should not therefore be used in combination.

Rifampicin, barbiturates, carbamazepine, diphenylhydantoin, primidone, phenytoin, and chronic alcohol abuse, may accelerate the decomposition of doxycycline due to enzyme induction in the liver thereby decreasing its half-life. Sub-therapeutic doxycycline concentrations may result. Doxycycline used concurrently with cyclosporin has been reported to decrease the half-life of doxycycline.

Tetracyclines and methoxyflurane used in combination have been reported to result in fatal renal toxicity.

Tetracyclines used concurrently with oral contraceptives have in a few cases resulted in either breakthrough bleeding or pregnancy.

4.6 Pregnancy and lactation

Use in Pregnancy:

Studies in animals have not demonstrated a teratogenic effect. In humans, the use of tetracyclines during a limited number of pregnancies has not revealed any specific malformation to date. The administration of tetracyclines during the second and the third trimesters results in permanent discolouration of the deciduous teeth in the offspring.

As a consequence, PERIOSTAT is contraindicated during pregnancy (see 4.3: Contraindications).

Use in Lactation:

Tetracyclines are secreted into the milk of lactating women. PERIOSTAT should therefore not be used in breast-feeding mothers.

4.7 Effects on ability to drive and use machines

PEROISTAT has no or negligible influence on the ability to drive and use machines.

Nausea and dizziness have been reported during clinical studies with PERIOSTAT. Those affected should not drive or operate machinery.

4.8 Undesirable effects

The most commonly reported adverse reactions in Phase III trials were headache (26%) and common cold (22%). The following table lists those adverse reactions occurring in four Phase III trials conducted in 213 patients.

(see Table 1 below)

The following adverse reactions have been observed in patients receiving tetracyclines:-

Gastrointestinal: Anorexia, nausea, vomiting, diarrhoea, glossitis, dysphagia, enterocolitis and inflammatory lesions with monilial overgrowth in the anogenital region. Hepatotoxity has been reported rarely. These reactions have been caused by both the oral and parenteral administration of tetracyclines. Oesophagitis and oesophageal ulceration have been reported, most often in patients administered the hyclate salt in capsule form. Most of these patients took medication just prior to going to bed.

Skin: Maculo papular and erythematous rashes. Skin photosensitivity can occur. Exfoliative dermatitis has been reported but is uncommon.

Renal: An apparently dose related increase in blood urea has been reported with tetracyclines.

Blood: Thrombocytopenia, neutropenia, haemolytic anaemia and eosinophilia have been reported with tetracyclines.

Hypersensitivity reactions: Exacerbation of systemic lupus erythematosus, anaphylaxis, anaphylactoid purpura, pericarditis, urticaria, and angioneurotic oedema.

Other: Bulging fontanelles in infants and benign intracranial hypertension in adults has been reported with the use of tetracyclines. Treatment should cease if evidence of raised intracranial pressure develops. These conditions disappeared rapidly when the drug was discontinued. Brown-black microscopic discolouration of thyroid tissue has been reported with long-term use of tetracyclines. Thyroid function is normal.

Adverse reactions typical of the tetracycline class of drugs are less likely to occur during medication with PERIOSTAT, due to the reduced dosage and the relatively low serum levels involved. This assertion is supported by several clinical trials which suggest that no significant differences exist with regard to frequency of adverse events between active and placebo groupings. However, the clinician should always be aware of the possibility of adverse events occurring and should monitor patients accordingly.

4.9 Overdose

To date no significant acute toxicity has been described in the case of a single oral intake of a multiple of therapeutic doses of doxycycline. In case of overdosage there is, however, a risk of parenchymatous hepatic and renal damage and of pancreatitis.

The usual dose of PERIOSTAT is low when compared with the usual doses for doxycycline when used for antimicrobial therapy. Therefore clinicians should bear in mind that a significant proportion of overdoses are likely to produce blood concentrations of doxycycline within the therapeutic range of antimicrobial treatment, for which there is a large quantity of data supporting the safety of the drug. In these cases observation is recommended. In cases of significant overdosage, doxycycline therapy should be stopped immediately; and symptomatic measures undertaken as required. Intestinal absorption of unabsorbed doxycycline should be minimised by producing non-absorbable chelate complexes by the administration of magnesium or calcium salt containing antacids. Gastric lavage should be considered.

Dialysis does not alter serum half-life and thus would not be of benefit in treating cases of overdosage.

5. PHARMACOLOGICAL PROPERTIES

5.1 Pharmacodynamic properties

Pharmacotherapeutic group: Tetracyclines

ATC code: J01A A02

The active ingredient of PERIOSTAT, doxycycline, is synthetically derived from oxytetracycline, with a molecular formula of $C_{22}H_{24}N_2O_8 \bullet HCl \bullet ½\ C_2H_5OH \bullet ½\ H_2O$.

PERIOSTAT is an inhibitor of collagenase activity. Studies have shown that at the proposed 20 mg b.i.d. dose level, PERIOSTAT reduces the elevated collagenase activity in the gingival crevicular fluid of patients with chronic adult periodontitis, whilst not demonstrating any clinical evidence of anti-microbial activity.

Susceptibility

The dosage achieved with this product during administration is well below the concentration required to inhibit microorganisms commonly associated with adult periodontitis. Clinical studies with this product demonstrated no effect on total anaerobic and facultative bacteria in plaque samples from patients administered this dose regimen for 9 to 18 months. This product **SHOULD NOT** be used for reducing the numbers of, or eliminating, those microorganisms associated with periodontitis.

5.2 Pharmacokinetic properties

Absorption:

Doxycycline is almost completely absorbed after oral administration. Following ingestion of 20 mg doxycycline twice daily, mean maximum plasma concentrations were 0.79 μg/ml. Peak levels were generally achieved 2 hours after administration. Food intake reduced the extent of absorption by 10% and decreased and delayed the peak plasma levels.

Distribution:

Doxycycline is greater than 90% bound to plasma proteins and has an apparent volume of distribution of 50L.

Metabolism:

Major metabolic pathways of doxycycline have not been identified, however, enzyme inducers decrease the half-life of doxycycline.

Elimination:

Doxycycline is excreted in the urine and faeces as unchanged drug. Between 40% and 60% of an administered dose can be accounted for in the urine by 92 hours, and approximately 30% in the faeces. The terminal half-life after a single 20 mg doxycycline dose averaged 18h.

Special populations:

The half-life is not significantly altered in patients with severely impaired renal function. Doxycycline is not eliminated to any great extent during haemodialysis.

5.3 Preclinical safety data

The carcinogenic potential of doxycycline has been investigated and no changes indicative of a direct carcinogenic effect were seen. Increases in benign tumours of the mammary gland (fibroadenoma), uterus (polyp) and thyroid (C-cell adenoma), which are consistent with a hormonal effect, were observed in treated females. Doxycycline has shown no mutagenic activity and no convincing evidence of clastogenic activity.

Effects on fertility and reproductive performance and on pre- and post-natal toxicity have been assessed in rats over the dose range 50 to 500 mg/kg/day. At 50 mg/kg/day (88 times the human dose) there was a decrease in the straight-line velocity of sperm, but there was no apparent effect on male or female fertility or on sperm morphology. Maternal toxicity at 500 mg/kg/day was shown by noisy breathing, loose faeces, and transient reductions in both body weight gain and food consumption after parturition with a slight increase in the duration of gestation. No maternal toxicity was apparent at or below 100 mg/kg/day and there was no effect on the F1 generation at 50 mg/kg/day during parturition, lactation or post-weaning. Developmental toxicity studies have not been conducted, but doxycycline is known to cross the placenta.

Hyperpigmentation of the thyroid following administration of members of the tetracycline class has been observed in rats, minipigs, dogs and monkeys and thyroid hyperplasia has occurred in rats, dogs, chickens and mice.

The anticipated human dose for doxycycline, 20 mg b.i.d. is equivalent to ~0.5 mg/kg/day for a 70 kg man. At this dose plasma C_{max} and AUC_{0-24} were 780 ng/ml and 10954 ng*h/ml respectively.

Toxicity following repeated oral administration has been evaluated in rats and cynomolgus monkeys. Discolouration of the thyroid was a finding common to rats exposed at 25 mg/kg/day for 13 weeks or 20 mg/kg/day for 26 weeks, and to cynomolgus monkeys at 30 mg/kg/day for 1 year. C_{max} and AUC_{0-24} following a single oral dose of 25 mg/kg were 2.2 and 1.6 times respectively the values recorded in man. Dose-related increases in both the incidence and severity of tubular degeneration/regeneration in the kidney were seen following administration to cynomolgus monkeys for 28 days or 52 weeks. At 5 mg/kg/day, focal lesions were present after 28 days, but no lesions were present in monkeys treated for 52 weeks. Mean plasma C_{max} and AUC_{0-24} values at 28 days in monkeys receiving 5 mg/kg/day were 1235 ng/ml and 11600 ng*h/ml respectively and there was no evidence of accumulation.

In humans the use of tetracyclines during tooth development may cause permanent discolouration of the teeth (yellow-grey-brown). This reaction is more common during long-term use of the drug but has been observed following repeated short-term courses. Enamel hypoplasia has also been reported. As for other tetracyclines, doxycycline forms a stable calcium complex in any bone-forming tissue. A decrease in the fibula growth has been observed in premature infants given oral tetracycline in doses of 25 mg/kg every 6 hours. This reaction was shown to be reversible when the drug was discontinued.

6. PHARMACEUTICAL PARTICULARS

6.1 List of excipients

Tablet core:

Magnesium stearate

Microcrystalline cellulose

Film coating:

Lactose monohydrate

Hypromellose (E464)

Titanium dioxide (E171)

Triacetin

6.2 Incompatibilities

Not applicable.

6.3 Shelf life

Three years

6.4 Special precautions for storage

Do not store above 25°C.

6.5 Nature and contents of container

PVC Aclar/aluminium foil blisters containing 14 tablets. Carton pack sizes: 28 and 56 tablets.

A 120ml white high density polyethylene tablet container with child resistant polypropylene closure. Each HDPE container contains 60 tablets.

Not all pack sizes may be marketed.

6.6 Instructions for use and handling

No special requirements.

7. MARKETING AUTHORISATION HOLDER

Alliance Pharmaceuticals Limited

Avonbridge House

Bath Road

Chippenham

Wiltshire SN15 2BB

United Kingdom

8. MARKETING AUTHORISATION NUMBER(S)

PL 16853/0078

Table 1

Organ System	Undesirable Effect	Very Common >1/10)	Common >1/100), (<1/10)	Uncommon >1/1000), (<1/100)	Rare >1/10000), (<1/1000)
Infections & Infestations	Infection		4		
	Periodontal Abscess		8		
Respiratory	Common Cold	47			
	Flu Symptoms	24			
	Sinusitis		18		
	Coughing		9		
	Bronchitis		7		
Gastrointestinal	Dyspepsia		13		
	Diarrhoea		12		
	Acid Indigestion		8		
Skin Disorders	Rash		8		
Musculoskeletal	Toothache		14		
	Joint Pain		12		
	Back Pain		11		
	Pain		8		
	Muscle Pain			2	
	Gum Pain			1	
Reproductive	Menstrual Cramps		9		
General	Headache	55			
	Nausea		17		
	Tooth Disorder		13		
	Sore Throat		11		
	Sinus Headache		8		
Injury	Accidental Injury		11		

9. DATE OF FIRST AUTHORISATION/RENEWAL OF THE AUTHORISATION

4 March 2005

10. DATE OF REVISION OF THE TEXT

March 2005

LEGAL CATEGORY

POM

Persantin Ampoules

(Boehringer Ingelheim Limited)

1. NAME OF THE MEDICINAL PRODUCT

Persantin Ampoules 10 mg / 2 ml Solution for Infusion

2. QUALITATIVE AND QUANTITATIVE COMPOSITION

Dipyridamole 5 mg/ml. Each 2 ml ampoule contains 10 mg dipyridamole.

For excipients, see 6.1.

3. PHARMACEUTICAL FORM

Solution for infusion.

2ml glass ampoules containing a clear, yellow-coloured solution.

4. CLINICAL PARTICULARS

4.1 Therapeutic indications

Adults:

As an alternative to exercise stress in thallium-201 myocardial imaging, particularly in patients unable to exercise or in those for whom exercise may be contraindicated.

Children:

As an alternative to exercise stress in myocardial perfusion imaging, particularly in children unable to exercise or in those for whom exercise may be contraindicated. More specifically, this may include children with Kawasaki disease complicated by coronary artery involvement, or those with congenitally abnormal coronary circulations.

4.2 Posology and method of administration

The dose of intravenous PERSANTIN as an adjunct to thallium myocardial perfusion imaging should be adjusted according to the weight of the patient. The recommended dose is 0.142 mg/kg/minute (0.567 mg/kg total) infused over 4 minutes.

Thallium-201 should be injected within 3-5 minutes following the 4-minute infusion of PERSANTIN.

4.3 Contraindications

Hypersensitivity to any of the components of the product.

Patients with dysrhythmias, second- or third degree atrioventricular block or with sick sinus syndrome should not receive intravenous PERSANTIN (unless they have a functioning pacemaker). Patients with baseline hypotension (systolic blood pressure < 90 mmHg), recent unexplained syncope (within 4 weeks) or with recent transient ischaemic attacks are not suitable candidates for dipyridamole testing.

Patients with severe coronary artery disease, including unstable angina and recent myocardial infarction (within 4 weeks), left ventricular outflow obstruction or haemodynamic instability (e.g. decompensated heart failure).

Patients with bronchial asthma or a tendency to bronchospasm.

Patients with myasthenia gravis. (See Interactions.)

Pregnancy and lactation.

4.4 Special warnings and special precautions for use

The potential clinical information to be gained through use of intravenous PERSANTIN as an adjunct in myocardial imaging must be weighed against the risk to the patient. Comparable reactions to exercise-induced stress may occur. Therefore dipyridamole-thallium scanning should be performed with continuous ECG monitoring of the patient.

When myocardial imaging is performed with intravenous PERSANTIN, parenteral aminophylline should be readily available for relieving adverse effects such as bronchospasm or chest pain. Vital signs should be monitored during and for 10 - 15 minutes following the intravenous infusion of PERSANTIN and an electrocardiographic tracing should be obtained using at least one chest lead.

Sedation may be necessary in young children.

Use with caution in young infants with immature hepatic metabolism.

Should severe chest pain or bronchospasm occur, parenteral aminophylline may be administered by slow intravenous injection; for adults, doses ranging from 75 mg to 100 mg aminophylline, repeated if necessary, are appropriate; for children, doses of 3-5 mg/kg aminophylline have been used.

In the case of severe hypotension, the patient should be placed in a supine position with the head tilted down if necessary, before administration of parenteral aminophylline. If aminophylline does not relieve chest pain symptoms within a few minutes, sublingual nitroglycerin may be administered. If chest pain continues despite use of aminophylline and nitroglycerin, the possibility of myocardial infarction should be considered.

If the clinical condition of a patient with an adverse effect permits a one minute delay in the administration of parenteral aminophylline, thallium-201 may be injected and allowed to circulate for one minute before the injection of aminophylline. This will allow initial thallium perfusion imaging to be performed before reversal of the pharmacologic effects of PERSANTIN on the coronary circulation.

Patients being treated with regular oral doses of dipyridamole should not receive additional PERSANTIN Ampoules 10mg/2ml Solution for Infusion. Clinical experience suggests that patients being treated with oral dipyridamole who also require pharmacological stress testing with intravenous dipyridamole should discontinue drugs containing oral dipyridamole for twenty-four hours prior to stress testing.

Caution should be exercised in patients with known preexisting first-degree heart block.

4.5 Interaction with other medicinal products and other forms of Interaction

Xanthine derivatives (e.g. caffeine and theophylline) can potentially reduce the vasodilating effect of dipyridamole and should therefore be avoided 24 hours before myocardial imaging with PERSANTIN. For discontinuation of oral dipyridamole see section 4.4.

Dipyridamole increases plasma levels and cardiovascular effects of adenosine.

Dipyridamole may increase the hypotensive effect of drugs which reduce blood pressure.

Dipyridamole may counteract the anticholinesterase effect of cholinesterase inhibitors thereby potentially aggravating myasthenia gravis.

4.6 Pregnancy and lactation

Use of intravenous dipyridamole for cardiac stress testing in pregnancy and lactation is not recommended.

4.7 Effects on ability to drive and use machines

None stated.

4.8 Undesirable effects

Approximately 47% of patients given intravenous dipyridamole will experience an adverse event, of which 0.26% would be expected to be severe.

When using PERSANTIN as an adjunct to myocardial imaging, the following adverse events have been reported: cardiac death, cardiac arrest, myocardial infarction (rarely fatal), chest pain/angina pectoris, electrocardiographic changes (most commonly ST-T changes), arrhythmias (e.g.sinus node arrest, heart block, tachycardia, bradycardia, fibrillation), syncope and cerebrovascular events (e.g. stroke, TIA, seizures). PERSANTIN may cause severe hypotension and hot flushes.

Hypersensitivity reactions such as rash, urticaria, angiooedema, laryngospasm, severe bronchospasm, and very rarely anaphylactoid reactions have been reported.

Other adverse reactions reported include: abdominal pain, vomiting, diarrhoea, nausea, dizziness, headache, paraesthesia, myalgia, hypertension, blood pressure lability, fatigue and dyspepsia. A bitter taste has been experienced after i.v. injection.

4.9 Overdose

Symptoms:

Although there is no experience of overdose, the signs and symptoms that might be expected to occur include cardiac death, cardiac arrest, myocardial infarction, chest pain, angina pectoris, electrocardiographic changes, syncope, cerebrovascular events, hypotension, hot flushes, hypersensitivity reactions, anaphylactoid reactions, gastrointestinal symptoms, dizziness, headache, paraesthesia, myalgia, bitter taste and blood pressure lability.

Therapy:

Symptomatic therapy is recommended.

Should severe chest pain or brochospasm occur, parenteral aminophylline may be administered by slow intravenous injection; for adults, doses ranging from 75 to 100 mg aminophylline, repeated if necessary, are appropriate; for children, doses of 3-5 mg/kg aminophylline have been used. If aminophylline does not relieve chest pain symptoms within a few minutes, sublingual nitroglycerin may be administered. If chest pain continues despite use of aminophylline and nitroglycerin, the possibility of myocardial infarction should be considered.

Due to its wide distribution to tissues and its predominantly hepatic elimination, dipyridamole is not likely to be accessible to enhanced removal procedures.

5. PHARMACOLOGICAL PROPERTIES

5.1 Pharmacodynamic properties

Dipyridamole has two main actions:

1. Coronary vasodilator.

2. Inhibitor of platelet aggregation and adhesion.

5.2 Pharmacokinetic properties

Distribution:

Does not cross blood brain barrier; very small placental transfer; 1/17 of plasma concentration detectable in breast milk.

Protein binding:

97-99% Protein bound mainly to alpha 1-acid glycoprotein.

Metabolism:

Mainly in liver to a monoglucuronide.

Excretion:

95% of i.v. injection excreted via bile into faeces.

6. PHARMACEUTICAL PARTICULARS

6.1 List of excipients

Tartaric acid

Macrogol 600

Hydrochloric acid

Water for injections

6.2 Incompatibilities

None stated.

6.3 Shelf life

3 years.

6.4 Special precautions for storage

Keep container in the outer carton.

6.5 Nature and contents of container

Carton containing 5 × 2 ml clear Type I glass ampoules.

6.6 Instructions for use and handling

None stated.

7. MARKETING AUTHORISATION HOLDER

Boehringer Ingelheim Limited
Ellesfield Avenue
Bracknell
Berkshire
RG12 8YS
UK

8. MARKETING AUTHORISATION NUMBER(S)

PL 0015/0119

9. DATE OF FIRST AUTHORISATION/RENEWAL OF THE AUTHORISATION

23 April 1987 / 17 June 1997

10. DATE OF REVISION OF THE TEXT

July 2004

11. Legal Category

POM

P2a/UK/SPC/7

Persantin Retard 200mg

(Boehringer Ingelheim Limited)

1. NAME OF THE MEDICINAL PRODUCT

Persantin Retard 200 mg

2. QUALITATIVE AND QUANTITATIVE COMPOSITION

Each modified release capsule contains dipyridamole 200 mg.

For excipients, see 6.1

3. PHARMACEUTICAL FORM

Modified release capsules, hard.

Hard gelatin capsules consisting of a red cap and an orange body.

4. CLINICAL PARTICULARS

4.1 Therapeutic indications

- Secondary prevention of ischaemic stroke and transient ischaemic attacks either alone or in conjunction with aspirin.

- An adjunct to oral anti-coagulation for prophylaxis of thromboembolism associated with prosthetic heart valves.

4.2 Posology and method of administration

For oral administration.

Adults, including the elderly

The recommended dose is one capsule twice daily, usually one in the morning and one in the evening preferably with meals.

The capsules should be swallowed whole without chewing.

Children

PERSANTIN Retard 200 mg is not recommended for children.

4.3 Contraindications

Hypersensitivity to any component of the product.

4.4 Special warnings and special precautions for use

Among other properties, dipyridamole acts as a potent vasodilator. It should therefore be used with caution in patients with severe coronary artery disease including unstable angina and/or recent myocardial infarction, left ventricular outflow obstruction or haemodynamic instability (e.g. decompensated heart failure).

Patients being treated with regular oral doses of PERSANTIN Retard should not receive additional intravenous dipyridamole. Clinical experience suggests that patients being treated with oral dipyridamole who also require pharmacological stress testing with intravenous dipyridamole, should discontinue drugs containing oral dipyridamole for twenty-four hours prior to stress testing.

In patients with myasthenia gravis readjustment of therapy may be necessary after changes in dipyridamole dosage. (See Interactions).

PERSANTIN should be used with caution in patients with coagulation disorders.

4.5 Interaction with other medicinal products and other forms of Interaction

Dipyridamole increases the plasma levels and cardiovascular effects of adenosine. Adjustment of adenosine dosage should therefore be considered if use with dipyridamole is unavoidable.

There is evidence that the effects of acetylsalicylic acid and dipyridamole on platelet behaviour are additive.

When dipyridamole is used in combination with anticoagulants or acetylsalicylic acid, the statements on intolerance and risks for these preparations must be observed. Addition of dipyridamole to acetylsalicylic acid does not increase the incidence of bleeding events. When dipyridamole was administered concomitantly with warfarin, bleeding was no greater in frequency or severity than that observed when warfarin was administered alone.

Dipyridamole may increase the hypotensive effect of blood pressure lowering drugs and may counteract the anticholinesterase effect of cholinesterase inhibitors thereby potentially aggravating myasthenia gravis.

4.6 Pregnancy and lactation

There is inadequate evidence of safety in human pregnancy, but dipyridamole has been used for many years without apparent ill-consequence. Animal studies have shown no hazard. Nevertheless, medicines should not be used in pregnancy, especially the first trimester unless the expected benefit is thought to outweigh the possible risk to the foetus.

PERSANTIN Retard 200 mg should only be used during lactation if considered essential by the physician.

4.7 Effects on ability to drive and use machines

None stated.

4.8 Undesirable effects

Adverse reactions at therapeutic doses are usually mild. Vomiting, diarrhoea and symptoms such as dizziness, nausea, dyspepsia, headache and myalgia have been observed. These tend to occur early after initiating treatment and may disappear with continued treatment.

As a result of its vasodilating properties, PERSANTIN Retard 200 mg may cause hypotension, hot flushes and tachycardia. Worsening of the symptoms of coronary heart disease such as angina and arrhythmias.

Hypersensitivity reactions such as rash, urticaria, severe bronchospasm and angio-odema have been reported. In very rare cases, increased bleeding during or after surgery has been observed.

Isolated cases of thrombocytopenia have been reported in conjunction with treatment with PERSANTIN.

Dipyridamole has been shown to be incorporated into gallstones.

4.9 Overdose

Symptoms

Due to the low number of observations, experience with dipyridamole overdose is limited. Symptoms such as feeling warm, flushes, sweating, accelerated pulse, restlessness, feeling of weakness, dizziness, drop in blood pressure and anginal complaints can be expected.

Therapy

Symptomatic therapy is recommended. Administration of xanthine derivatives (e.g. aminophylline) may reverse the haemodynamic effects of dipyridamole overdose. ECG monitoring is advised in such a situation. Due to its wide distribution to tissues and its predominantly hepatic elimination, dipyridamole is not likely to be accessible to enhanced removal procedures.

5. PHARMACOLOGICAL PROPERTIES

5.1 Pharmacodynamic properties

The antithrombotic action of dipyridamole is based on its ability to modify various aspects of platelet function such as inhibition of platelet adhesion and aggregation, which have been shown to be factors associated with the initiation of thrombus formation, as well as lengthening shortened platelet survival time.

5.2 Pharmacokinetic properties

PERSANTIN Retard 200 mg given twice daily has been shown to be bioequivalent to the same total daily dose of PERSANTIN Tablets given in four divided doses.

Peak plasma concentrations are reached 2 - 3 hours after administration. Steady state conditions are reached within 3 days.

Metabolism of dipyridamole occurs in the liver predominantly by conjugation with glucuronic acid to form a monoglucuronide. In plasma about 70 - 80% of the total amount is present as parent compound and 20 - 30% as the monoglucuronide.

Renal excretion is very low (1 - 5%).

5.3 Preclinical safety data

Dipyridamole has been extensively investigated in animal models and no clinically significant findings have been observed at doses equivalent to therapeutic doses in humans.

6. PHARMACEUTICAL PARTICULARS

6.1 List of excipients

Tartaric acid

Povidone

Methacrylic acid - methyl methacrylate copolymer (1:2)

Talc

Acacia

Hypromellose

Hypromellose phthalate

Triacetin

Dimethicone 350

Stearic acid

and in the capsule shells

Gelatin

Titanium dioxide; E171

Red and yellow iron oxides; E172

6.2 Incompatibilities

Not applicable.

6.3 Shelf life

3 years.

Discard any capsules remaining 6 weeks after first opening.

6.4 Special precautions for storage

Do not store above 25°C.

6.5 Nature and contents of container

White polypropylene tubes with low-density polyethylene Air-sec stoppers filled with desiccating agent (90% white silicon gel/10% molecular sieves).

Packs contain 30, 60 or 100 capsules. Packs of 60 are marketed.

6.6 Instructions for use and handling

None.

7. MARKETING AUTHORISATION HOLDER

Boehringer Ingelheim Limited

Ellesfield Avenue

Bracknell

Berkshire

RG12 8YS

United Kingdom

8. MARKETING AUTHORISATION NUMBER(S)

PL 00015/0206

9. DATE OF FIRST AUTHORISATION/RENEWAL OF THE AUTHORISATION

3 February 1997

10. DATE OF REVISION OF THE TEXT

July 2004

11. Legal category

Prescription Only Medicine

P2b/UK/SPC/9

Pethidine Injection BP

(Wockhardt UK Ltd)

1. NAME OF THE MEDICINAL PRODUCT

Pethidine Injection BP

2. QUALITATIVE AND QUANTITATIVE COMPOSITION

Pethidine Hydrochloride 50mg/ml

3. PHARMACEUTICAL FORM

Solution for Injection

4. CLINICAL PARTICULARS

4.1 Therapeutic indications

Pethidine hydrochloride may be used in the management of severe pain, including pain associated with surgical procedures, as a pre-anaesthetic medication and in obstetric analgesia.

4.2 Posology and method of administration

Pethidine may be given by intramuscular, subcutaneous or slow intravenous injection. For intravenous administration the contents of the ampoule can be diluted to 10ml with water for injections giving a strength of 5mg/ml (1ml ampoule) or 10mg/ml (2ml ampoule).

Pre-anaesthetic medication

Administered about one hour before the operation.

Adults: 50mg-100mg by intramuscular injection

Elderly: 50mg-100mg by intramuscular injection

Elderly patients may be more sensitive to pethidine

Children: 1.0 to 2.0mg/kg by intramuscular injection

Obstetric analgesia

50-100mg may be given by intramuscular or subcutaneous injection as soon as contractions occur at regular intervals. The dose may be repeated after one to three hours if necessary up to a maximum of 400mg in 24 hours.

Management of severe pain, including post-operative pain

Adults: 25mg-100mg by intramuscular or subcutaneous injection every four hours

By slow intravenous injection 25mg-50mg repeated every four hours.

Elderly: 25mg-100mg by intramuscular or subcutaneous injection every four hours.

By slow intravenous injection 25mg-50mg repeated every four hours

Elderly patients may be more sensitive to pethidine. The total daily dose may need to be reduced in elderly patients receiving repeated doses. Initial doses should not exceed 25mg as this group of patients may be specially sensitive to the central depressant effect of the drug.

Children: 0.5mg - 2mg/kg by intramuscular injection every four hours

Renal or hepatic impairment

The dose should be reduced.

4.3 Contraindications

- Known hypersensitivity to pethidine.
- Severe renal impairment.
- Respiratory depression and obstructive airways disease.
- Concurrent use of monoamine oxidase inhibitors or within two weeks of their discontinuation.

4.4 Special warnings and special precautions for use

Repeated administration of pethidine may lead to dependence and tolerance developing. Abrupt withdrawal in patients who have developed tolerance may precipitate a withdrawal syndrome. Caution should be exercised in patients with a known tendency or history of drug abuse. Babies born to opioid dependent mothers may suffer withdrawal symptoms.

Use with caution or in reduced doses in patients with phaeochromocytoma, biliary tract disorders, hypothyroidism, adreno-cortical insufficiency, asthma, hypotension, shock, prostatic hypertrophy, inflammatory or obstructive bowel disorders, myasthenia gravis, supraventricular tachycardia, a history of convulsive disorders, acute alcoholism, raised intracranial pressure or head injury.

Pethidine neurotoxicity may be seen in patients with renal failure, cancer or sickle cell anaemia, during concomitant administration of anticholinergics or during prolonged administration of increasing pethidine doses.

Care should be exercised in treating infants, elderly or debilitated patients and those with hepatic or renal impairment.

Administration during labour may cause respiratory depression in the new born infant.

4.5 Interaction with other medicinal products and other forms of Interaction

The depressant effects of pethidine may be exaggerated and prolonged by central nervous system depressants including anaesthetics, phenobarbitone and phenytoin, phenothiazines, tricyclic antidepressants, sedatives, anxiolytics and hypnotics.

Concurrent use of pethidine with or within two weeks of taking MAOI antidepressants may cause severe CNS excitation and hypertension or CNS depression and hypotension.

Pethidine has an antagonistic effect on metoclopramide and domperidone and may delay absorption of mexiletine.

Cyclizine may counteract the haemodynamic benefits of opioids.

Alcohol can enhance the sedative and hypotensive effects of pethidine.

Cimetidine and disulfiram may inhibit the metabolism of opioid analgesics.

Hyperpyrexia and CNS toxicity have been reported when opioid analgesics are used with selegiline.

4.6 Pregnancy and lactation

As with all drugs used during pregnancy care should be taken in assessing the risk to benefit ratio.

There is inadequate evidence of safety in human pregnancy although pethidine has been used for many years without apparent ill consequence.

Pethidine is widely used for pain relief during labour and is known to cross the placenta and may cause respiratory depression in the new born infant.

Pethidine is excreted in breast milk and this should be taken into account when considering its use in patients during pregnancy or breast-feeding.

4.7 Effects on ability to drive and use machines

Pethidine causes drowsiness. Patients should not drive or use machines.

4.8 Undesirable effects

The most serious hazard of therapy is respiratory depression. The most common side-effects are sedation, nausea, constipation, confusion, vomiting and sweating. Other side-effects include dizziness, miosis, orthostatic hypotension, facial flushing, bradycardia, tachycardia, vertigo, mood changes, dry mouth, dependence, hypothermia, restlessness, hallucinations, urinary retention, urticaria, pruritus and raised intracranial pressure.

4.9 Overdose

a) Symptoms

Respiratory depression, cold, clammy skin and hypothermia, muscle flaccidity, bradycardia and hypotension, coma or stupor, convulsions; apnoea, circulatory collapse, cardiac arrest, respiratory arrest and death may occur in severe overdose following rapid intravenous administration.

b) Treatment

Respiration and circulation should be maintained. Naloxone is indicated if coma or bradypnoea are present - by intravenous injection 100-200 micrograms (1.5-3 micrograms/kg) initially, with increments of 100 micrograms every two minutes if the response is inadequate. The usual intravenous dose for children is 10 micrograms/kg, subsequent dose of 100 micrograms/kg if no response. In neonates, an intravenous dose of 10 micrograms/kg may be repeated every two to three minutes, if necessary.

A short acting muscle relaxant, intubation and controlled respiration may be needed to treat convulsions.

5. PHARMACOLOGICAL PROPERTIES

5.1 Pharmacodynamic properties

Pethidine hydrochloride is a synthetic opioid analgesic which acts primarily on the central nervous system. It has a shorter duration of action than morphine. The analgesic effect lasts approximately two to four hours.

5.2 Pharmacokinetic properties

Pethidine is rapidly absorbed after subcutaneous or intramuscular injection with a peak plasma concentration usually occurring after 45 minutes. Pethidine is metabolised in the liver by hydrolysis to pethidinic acid or demethylation to norpethidine and hydrolysis to norpethidinic acid followed by partial conjugation with glucuronic acid.

The majority of the drug is excreted via the kidney as unchanged pethidine and its metabolite norpethidine.

Pethidine is 30%-50% bound to plasma proteins. The plasma half- life in man is three to six hours. The metabolite norpethidine which is pharmacologically active, is eliminated more slowly with a half life of up to 20 hours.

5.3 Preclinical safety data

There are no additional pre-clinical data of relevance to the prescriber.

6. PHARMACEUTICAL PARTICULARS

6.1 List of excipients

Water for Injections

Hydrochloric acid) for pH

Sodium hydroxide) adjustment

6.2 Incompatibilities

Pethidine hydrochloride injection has been reported to be physically or chemically incompatible with solutions containing aminophylline, barbiturates (especially with thiopentone solution, which results in the formation of a pharmacologically inactive complex), heparin sodium, ephedrine sulphate, hydrocortisone sodium succinate, methicillin sodium, methyl prednisolone succinate, morphine sulphate, nitrofurantoin sodium, oxytetracycline hydrochloride, phenytoin sodium, sodium bicarbonate, sodium iodide, sulphadiazine sodium, sulphafurazole diethanolamine, tetracycline hydrochloride, thiamylal sodium.

Colour changes in solution have occurred when solutions of minocycline hydrochloride or tetracycline hydrochloride have been mixed with pethidine hydrochloride in 5% glucose injection. Precipitation has occurred on admixture with cefoperazone sodium or mezlocillin sodium. When mixed with nafcillin sodium an immediate cloudy appearance cleared on agitation.

Pethidine hydrochloride has also been reported to be incompatible with aciclovir sodium, imipenem, frusemide, idarubicin and solutions containing potassium iodide, aminosalicyclic acid and salicylamide. Specialised references should be consulted for specific compatibility information.

6.3 Shelf life

Two years from date of manufacture

6.4 Special precautions for storage

Keep ampoules in the outer carton

6.5 Nature and contents of container

Neutral glass ampoules containing 1ml or 2ml of solution in cartons of 5, 10 or 50 ampoules.

6.6 Instructions for use and handling

The injection is for single patient use.

The injection should be given immediately after opening the ampoule. Once opened any unused portion should be discarded. The injection should not be used if particles are present.

For slow intravenous administration the contents of the ampoule may be diluted to 10ml with water for injections. Chemical and physical in-use stability has been demonstrated for 24 hours at 25°C. From a microbiological point of view the product should be used immediately. If not used immediately, in-use storage times and conditions prior to use are the responsibility of the user and would normally not be longer than 24 hours at 2-8°C, unless dilution has taken place in controlled and validated aseptic conditions.

Administrative Data

7. MARKETING AUTHORISATION HOLDER

CP Pharmaceuticals Ltd

Ash Road North

Wrexham

LL13 9UF

8. MARKETING AUTHORISATION NUMBER(S)

4543/0408

9. DATE OF FIRST AUTHORISATION/RENEWAL OF THE AUTHORISATION

N/A

10. DATE OF REVISION OF THE TEXT

October 99

Pevaryl Topical Cream

(Janssen-Cilag Ltd)

1. NAME OF THE MEDICINAL PRODUCT

Pevaryl® Topical Cream.

2. QUALITATIVE AND QUANTITATIVE COMPOSITION

Econazole nitrate Ph.Eur. 1.0% w/w.

3. PHARMACEUTICAL FORM

Cream.

4. CLINICAL PARTICULARS

4.1 Therapeutic indications

For the treatment of fungal infections of the skin.

4.2 Posology and method of administration

Route of administration

For topical administration.

Dosage

The dosage regimen is the same for all patients.

Apply twice daily to the affected part and rub into the skin gently with the finger. Continue the application until all skin lesions are healed.

In the treatment of fungal infections of the nail, the cream should be applied once a day and covered with an occlusive dressing.

4.3 Contraindications

Care should be taken in the presence of eczematous dermatitis.

4.4 Special warnings and special precautions for use

Hypersensitivity has rarely been recorded, if it should occur, administration of the product should be discontinued.

4.5 Interaction with other medicinal products and other forms of Interaction

Econazole administered systemically is known to inhibit CYP3A4/2C9. Due to the limited systemic availability after topical application, clinically relevant interactions are rare. However, in patients on oral anticoagulants, such as warfarin, caution should be exercised and anticoagulant effect should be monitored.

4.6 Pregnancy and lactation

Only small amounts of the drug are absorbed through the skin and no teratogenic effects have been observed in animals. Hence the product may be used with caution during pregnancy.

4.7 Effects on ability to drive and use machines

None stated.

4.8 Undesirable effects

Rarely, transient local irritation may occur after immediate application. If this persists please contact your doctor for advice.

4.9 Overdose

This product is for topical application only.

If large amounts have been taken by mouth or swallowed, gastric emptying may be considered desirable.

5. PHARMACOLOGICAL PROPERTIES

5.1 Pharmacodynamic properties

Econazole nitrate is a broad spectrum antimycotic with activity against dermatophytes, yeasts and moulds. A clinically relevant action against Gram positive bacteria has also been found.

5.2 Pharmacokinetic properties

Econazole nitrate is only slightly absorbed from the skin. No active drug has been detected in the serum. Radio labelling shows that less than 0.1% of an oral dose is absorbed. Peak serum levels are achieved after 2 hours and 90% binds to plasma proteins. Metabolism is limited but occurs primarily in the liver with excretion of metabolites in the urine.

5.3 Preclinical safety data

No relevant information additional to that contained elsewhere in the Summary of Product Characteristics.

6. PHARMACEUTICAL PARTICULARS

6.1 List of excipients

Pegoxyl-7-stearate

Peglicol-5-oleate

Liquid paraffin

Butylated hydroxyanisole (E320)

Benzoic acid (E210)

Flower Perfume 4074

Purified water

6.2 Incompatibilities

None stated.

6.3 Shelf life

36 months.

6.4 Special precautions for storage

Do not store above 25°C.

6.5 Nature and contents of container

Resin lined, aluminium tubes containing 15 g or 30 g of cream.

6.6 Instructions for use and handling

Not applicable.

7. MARKETING AUTHORISATION HOLDER

Janssen-Cilag Limited

Saunderton

High Wycombe

Buckinghamshire

HP14 4HJ

UK

8. MARKETING AUTHORISATION NUMBER(S)

PL 00242/0259

9. DATE OF FIRST AUTHORISATION/RENEWAL OF THE AUTHORISATION

Date of first authorisation: 01/07/95

10. DATE OF REVISION OF THE TEXT

12/07/04.

Legal category P

Pharmaton Capsules

(Boehringer Ingelheim Limited Self-Medication Division)

1. NAME OF THE MEDICINAL PRODUCT

Pharmaton Capsules

2. QUALITATIVE AND QUANTITATIVE COMPOSITION

Each capsule contains:

Active Ingredients	Declaration per capsule
G115 Panax Ginseng extract [dry extract ethanolic 40%: 1.3 – 3:1]	40.0mg
Vitamin A Palmitate (Vit.A)	2667 IU
Colecalciferol (Vit.D3)	200 IU
D,L-α-Tocopherol acetate (Vit.E)	10mg
Thiamine mononitrate (Vit.B1)	1.4mg
Riboflavin (Vit.B2)	1.6mg
Pyridoxine hydrochloride (Vit.B6)	2.0mg
Cyanocobalamine (Vit.B12)	1.0mcg
Biotin	150.0mcg
Nicotinamide	18.0mg
Ascorbic acid	60.0mg
Folic acid	0.1mg
Copper(II) sulphate dried (Cu:2.0 mg)	5.6mg
Sodium selenite, dried (Se:50.0 mcg)	111.0mcg
Magnesium sulphate, dried (Mg:10.0 mg)	71.0mg
Iron(II) sulphate, dried (Fe:10.0 mg)	33.0mg
Zinc sulphate, monohydrate (Zn:1.0 mg)	2.75mg
Dibasic calcium phosphate, anhydrous (Ca:100.0 mg)	340.0mg
Lecithin (containing choline, inositol, linoleic acid, linolenic acid)	100.0mg

3. PHARMACEUTICAL FORM

Soft gelatin capsules for oral use.

4. CLINICAL PARTICULARS

4.1 Therapeutic indications

Pharmaton Capsules contain vitamins, minerals and standardised Ginseng Extract G115 in amounts which suit the body's daily requirements.

The capsules are indicated for relief of temporary periods of:

States of exhaustion (e.g. caused by stress), tiredness, feeling of weakness, vitality deficiency.

Prevention and treatment of symptoms caused by ill-balanced or deficient nutrition.

4.2 Posology and method of administration

For situations of short term tiredness and exhaustion, Pharmaton Capsules are recommended for 4 weeks. If symptoms have not shown any improvement after 4 weeks, consult a doctor. Pharmaton Capsules may be taken for periods of up to 12 weeks. For longer term use consult a doctor.

Adults: The recommended daily dosage is one to two capsules per day. The first capsule should preferably be taken with breakfast and the second with lunch.

Children: Not recommended for use in children

Elderly: There are no special dosage recommendations for the elderly.

4.3 Contraindications

Hypersensitivity to any of the ingredients. Hypercalcaemia and/or hypercalciuria, haemochromatosis, iron overload syndrome, hypervitaminosis A or D, concomitant retinoid (*eg* against acne) or vitamin D therapy, renal insufficiency, pregnancy.

4.4 Special warnings and special precautions for use

Patients with a family history of haemochromatosis should seek medical advice before taking Pharmaton Capsules.

An allowance should be made for vitamins or minerals obtained from other sources.

In states of exhaustion (eg caused by stress), clinical trials have shown that improvement starts usually within 4 weeks of treatment. If symptoms have not shown any improvement during that time, or you are concerned, please consult your doctor.

The label will state "Important warning: Contains iron. Keep out of the reach and sight of children, as overdose may be fatal". This will appear on the labelling within a rectangle in which there is no other information.

Pharmaton Capsules contain Arachis oil (peanut oil) and should not be taken by patients known to be allergic to peanut. As there is a possible relationship between allergy to peanut and allergy to Soya, patients with Soya allergy should also avoid Pharmaton Capsules.

4.5 Interaction with other medicinal products and other forms of Interaction

There is no evidence from clinical experience that Pharmaton Capsules interacts with other medications.

4.6 Pregnancy and lactation

Reproduction studies with animals using the standardized Panax ginseng extract G115 Pharmaton showed no adverse effects on fertility, nor any teratogenic effects. However, controlled studies with pregnant women are not available.

Controlled studies with women using multivitamin-mineral preparations at the usual dosage during the course of the first trimester resulted in no fetal risks. There are no signs indicating a risk if this type of preparation is taken during the second and third trimesters, and the probability of injuring the fetus appears to be very low.

Large doses of vitamin A (10,000 IU per day) have been found to be teratogenic if administered during the first trimester of pregnancy. Vitamin D given during the last trimester of pregnancy may cause hypercalcaemia in infants. As with many other medicines an assessment of benefits versus risks should be made before this product is administered during this period.

Pharmaton Capsules should not be taken during pregnancy or lactation.

4.7 Effects on ability to drive and use machines

None known

4.8 Undesirable effects

Gastrointestinal reactions (e.g. abdominal pain, nausea) have been reported rarely.

4.9 Overdose

Nervousness may occur following an overdose of the product.

The toxicity of the product in large overdoses is caused by the toxicity of the liposoluble vitamins A and D. A safe dose for both vitamins is considered to be 5-10 × RDA (each capsule contains the EU %RDA for vitamins A and D).

Prolonged supply of larger amounts (40-55 × RDA for Vitamin A; 10-25 × RDA for Vitamin D) can cause symptoms of chronic toxicity. Acute toxic symptoms are only seen at even higher doses.

Iron: Severe acute toxicity in man has been reported from doses of iron ranging from 12-1500 × RDA (each capsule contains the UK %RDA for iron). Most incidents of acute iron toxicity have resulted from accidental oral ingestion of iron pills by children. Longer-term doses of iron up to 6-7 × RDA have been reported to have no toxic effect.

Symptoms: Initial symptoms include nausea, vomiting, diarrhoea, abdominal pain, haematemesis, rectal bleeding, lethargy and circulatory collapse. Hyperglycaemia and metabolic acidosis may also occur.

Treatment: To minimise or prevent further absorption of the medication, as follows:

- Induce vomiting eg. by administration of an emetic
- Gastric lavage with desferrioxamine solution (2g/l). Then desferrioxamine (5 - 10g in 50-100ml water) should be introduced into the stomach to be retained.
- Severe poisoning: Shock and/or coma with high iron levels (serum iron >90mol/l in children, >142mol/l in adults); immediate supportive measures plus i.v. infusion of desferrioxamine should be instituted.
- Less severe poisoning: i.m. desferrioxamine is recommended (1g 4-6 hourly in children; 50mg/kg up to a maximum dose of 4g in adults).

5. PHARMACOLOGICAL PROPERTIES

5.1 Pharmacodynamic properties

Pharmaton Capsules exert a stimulant effect at physical and psychological levels through the combined action of various substances on the basic metabolic processes.

The standardised ginseng extract G115 raises the general level of cellular activity, which is expressed by a pronounced increase in the physical and mental capacity.

In animal experiments, it caused a reduction of lactic acid concentration in muscles during exercise. An increase in the dopamine and noradrenaline content and a reduction in the serotonin content in the brain stem could be observed.

Vitamins, minerals and trace elements correct and prevent impairment of the cell metabolism in situations with increased demands. Low supply of vitamins, minerals, and trace elements may cause disturbances, such as debility, tiredness, decrease in vitality, reduced force of resistance, and decelerated convalescence. The composition and dosages of the preparation were chosen according to the European RDA-requirements for food supplements.

Choline, inositol, linoleic acid and linolenic acid, in the form of lecithin, improve energy output and lipid metabolism.

5.2 Pharmacokinetic properties

Pharmacokinetic studies of Pharmaton Capsules have not been carried out, because of the complex composition of the product and the small quantities of the active ingredients contained. Moreover, these substances are well known.

Pharmacokinetic studies of the standardised ginseng extract G115 are not possible, because it is a complex extract. In the ginseng root more than 200 substances have been identified to date. Pharmacokinetic studies of individual purified ginsenosides have been carried out in various animal species:

Using radioactively labelled (^{14}C) Ginsenoside Rgl, originated from the standardized Panax ginseng extract G115 Pharmaton, a bioavailability of 30% was determined in mice.

With intraperitoneal application, depending on the tested animal species and the Ginsenoside type, a half-life of between 27 minutes and 14.5 hours was measured.

5.3 Preclinical safety data

Acute toxicity

The oral LD_{50} of the standardized Panax ginseng extract G115 Pharmaton is more than 5 g/kg of body weight in the mouse and the rat, and more than 2 g/kg in the mini-pig.

Reproduction toxicity

The effect of standardized Panax ginseng extract G115 Pharmaton on reproductive performance was studied in two generations of Sprague-Dawley rats. Animals of both sexes were fed either control diet or diet supplemented with the standardized Panax ginseng extract G115 Pharmaton at dose levels of 1.5, 5 or 15 mg/kg body weight/day. Parameters of reproduction and lactation in the treated groups were comparable to those of the controls for two generations of dams and pups. No treatment-related effects were seen in weekly body weights and food consumption, haematological and blood chemistry parameters, and ophthalmic, macroscopic and histopathological examinations.

Fetal toxicity

The standardized Panax ginseng extract G115 Pharmaton, administered to pregnant Wistar rats and pregnant New Zealand rabbits, caused no abnormality in the foetal development.

The rats were treated with 40 mg/kg/day from the 1st to the 15th day after mating.

The rabbits were treated with 20 mg/kg/day from the 7th to the 16th day after mating.

The fetuses were removed by caesarean section on the 21st day in the rats and on the 27th day in the rabbits.

6. PHARMACEUTICAL PARTICULARS

6.1 List of excipients

Capsule:

Rapeseed oil, refined

Hard fat

Ethyl vanillin

Arachis oil (peanut oil)

Triglycerides, medium chain

Gelatin

Lactose monohydrate

Silica, colloidal anhydrous

Capsule shell:

Gelatin

Glycerol 85%

Iron oxide red (E172)

Iron oxide black (E172)

6.2 Incompatibilities

None stated.

6.3 Shelf life

Glass bottle packs: 3 years

Blister packs: 2 years

6.4 Special precautions for storage

Do not store above 25°C

Keep the container tightly closed

6.5 Nature and contents of container

Registered Packs

Brown glass bottles (hydrolytical class III, Ph.Eur) with pilfer proof aluminium caps (with rubber inserts) containing either 30, 60, 90 or 100 capsules. Or Aluminium foil/polyvinylchloride/polyvinylidenchloride blister packs of 4, 30, 60, 90 and 100 capsules.

Current Marketed Packs

Brown glass bottles (hydrolytical class III, Ph.Eur) with pilfer proof aluminium caps (with rubber inserts) containing either 30, 60, or 100 capsules.

6.6 Instructions for use and handling

None stated.

7. MARKETING AUTHORISATION HOLDER

Boehringer Ingelheim Ltd., Trading as Pharmaton Natural Health Products

Self-Medication Division,

Ellesfield Avenue,

Bracknell,

Berkshire,

RG12 8YS.

8. MARKETING AUTHORISATION NUMBER(S)

PL 00015/0250

9. DATE OF FIRST AUTHORISATION/RENEWAL OF THE AUTHORISATION

1st January 1999

10. DATE OF REVISION OF THE TEXT

May 2004

P7a/UK/SPC/15

PHARMORUBICIN

(Pharmacia Limited)

1. NAME OF THE MEDICINAL PRODUCT

Pharmorubicin Rapid Dissolution 10 mg, 20 mg, 50 mg & 150 mg

Pharmorubicin Solution for Injection 2 mg/ml

2. QUALITATIVE AND QUANTITATIVE COMPOSITION

Pharmorubicin Rapid Dissolution 10 mg, 20 mg, 50 mg and 150 mg

After reconstitution, each vial contains 2 mg/ml epirubicin hydrochloride

5 ml vials contain 10 mg of epirubicin hydrochloride

10 ml vials contain 20 mg of epirubicin hydrochloride

25 ml vials contain 50 mg of epirubicin hydrochloride

75 ml vials contain 150 mg epirubicin hydrochloride.

Pharmorubicin Solution for Injection 2 mg/ml

Each vial contains 2 mg/ml epirubicin hydrochloride

5 ml vials contain 10 mg of epirubicin hydrochloride

10 ml vials contain 20 mg of epirubicin hydrochloride

25 ml vials contain 50 mg of epirubicin hydrochloride

100 ml vials contain 200 mg epirubicin hydrochloride.

For excipients, see section 6.1.

3. PHARMACEUTICAL FORM

Powder for solution for injection or infusion.

Solution for injection or infusion.

Red, freeze-dried, sterile, powder for injection containing 10 mg, 20 mg, 50 mg and 150 mg epirubicin hydrochloride.

Red, sterile, preservative-free, aqueous solution.

4. CLINICAL PARTICULARS

4.1 Therapeutic indications

Pharmorubicin has produced responses in a wide range of neoplastic conditions, including breast, ovarian, gastric, lung and colorectal carcinomas, malignant lymphomas, leukaemias and multiple myeloma.

Intravesical administration of Pharmorubicin has been found to be beneficial in the treatment of superficial bladder cancer, carcinoma-in-situ and in the prophylaxis of recurrences after transurethral resection.

4.2 Posology and method of administration

Intravenous administration: Pharmorubicin is not active when given orally and should not be injected intramuscularly or intrathecally.

It is advisable to give the drug via the tubing of a freely running IV saline infusion after checking that the needle is well placed in the vein. This method minimises the risk of drug extravasation and makes sure that the vein is flushed with saline after the administration of the drug. Extravasation of Pharmorubicin from the vein during injection may give rise to severe tissue lesions, even necrosis. Venous sclerosis may result from injection into small vessels or repeated injections into the same vein.

Conventional doses:

When Pharmorubicin is used as a single agent, the recommended dosage in adults is 60-90 mg/m^2 body area; the drug should be injected IV over 3-5 minutes and, depending on the patients' haematomedullary status, the dose should be repeated at 21 day intervals.

High doses:

Pharmorubicin as a single agent for the treatment of lung cancer at high doses should be administered according to the following regimens:

Lung cancer

Small cell lung cancer (previously untreated): 120 mg/m^2 day 1, every 3 weeks.

Non-small cell lung cancer (squamous, large cell, and adenocarcinoma previously untreated): 135 mg/m^2 day 1 or 45 mg/m^2 days 1, 2, 3, every 3 weeks.

Breast cancer

In the adjuvant treatment of early breast cancer patients with positive lymph nodes, intravenous doses of epirubicin ranging from 100 mg/m^2 (as a single dose on day 1) to 120 mg/m^2 (in two divided doses on days 1 and 8) every 3-4 weeks, in combination with intravenous cyclophosphamide and 5-fluorouracil and oral tamoxifen, are recommended.

The drug should be given as an I.V. bolus over 3-5 minutes or as an infusion up to 30 minutes. Lower doses (60-75 mg/m^2 for conventional treatment and 105-120 mg/ m^2 for high dose schedules) are recommended for patients whose bone marrow function has already been impaired by previous chemotherapy or radiotherapy, by age, or neoplastic bone-marrow infiltration. The total dose per cycle may be divided over 2-3 successive days.

When the drug is used in combination with other antitumour agents, the doses need to be adequately reduced. Since the major route of elimination of Pharmorubicin is the hepatobiliary system, the dosage should be reduced in patients with impaired liver function, in order to avoid an increase of overall toxicity. Moderate liver impairment (bilirubin: 1.4-3 mg/100ml) requires a 50% reduction of dose, while severe impairment (bilirubin > 3 mg/100 ml) necessitates a dose reduction of 75%.

Moderate renal impairment does not appear to require a dose reduction in view of the limited amount of Pharmorubicin excreted by this route.

Intravesical administration:

Pharmorubicin may be given by intravesical administration for the treatment of superficial bladder cancer and carcinoma-in-situ. It should not be used in this way for the treatment of invasive tumours which have penetrated the bladder wall where systemic therapy or surgery is more appropriate. Epirubicin has also been successfully used intravesically as a prophylactic agent after transurethral resection of superficial tumours in order to prevent recurrences.

While many regimens have been used, the following may be helpful as a guide: for therapy 8 × weekly instillations of 50 mg/50 ml (diluted with saline or distilled sterile water). In the case of local toxicity (chemical cystitis), a dose reduction to 30 mg per 50 ml is advised. For carcinoma-in-situ, depending on the individual tolerability of the patient, the dose may be increased up to 80 mg/50 ml. For prophylaxis, 4 × weekly administrations of 50 mg/ 50 ml followed by 11 × monthly instillations at the same dosage, is the schedule most commonly used

The solution should be retained intravesically for 1 hour. To avoid undue dilution with urine, the patient should be instructed not to drink any fluid in the 12 hours prior to instillation. During the instillation, the patient should be rotated occasionally and should be instructed to void at the end of the instillation time.

4.3 Contraindications

Pharmorubicin is contraindicated in patients with marked myelosuppression induced by previous treatment with other antitumour agents or by radiotherapy and in patients already treated with maximal cumulative doses of other anthracyclines such as Doxorubicin or Daunorubicin.

The drug is contraindicated in patients with current or previous history of cardiac impairment.

4.4 Special warnings and special precautions for use

Pharmorubicin should be administered only under the supervision of qualified physicians experienced in antiblastic and cytotoxic therapy. Treatment with high dose Pharmorubicin in particular requires the availability of facilities for the care of possible clinical complications due to myelosuppression.

Initial treatment calls for a careful baseline monitoring of various laboratory parameters and cardiac function.

During each cycle of treatment with Pharmorubicin, patients must be carefully and frequently monitored. Red and white blood cells, neutrophils and platelet counts should be carefully assessed both before and during each cycle of therapy. Leukopenia and neutropenia are usually transient with conventional and high-dose schedules, reaching a nadir between the 10th and 14th day and returning to normal values by the 21st day; they are more severe with high dose schedules. Very few patients, even receiving high doses, experience thrombocytopenia (< 100,000 platelets/mm^3).

Before starting therapy and if possible during treatment, liver function should be evaluated (SGOT, SGPT, alkaline phosphatase, bilirubin). A cumulative dose of 900-1000 mg/m^2 should only be exceeded with extreme caution with both conventional and high doses.

Above this level the risk of irreversible congestive cardiac failure increases greatly. There is objective evidence that the cardiac toxicity may occur rarely below this range. However, cardiac function must be carefully monitored during treatment to minimise the risk of cardiac failure of the type described for other anthracyclines.

Heart failure can appear even several weeks after discontinuing treatment, and may prove unresponsive to specific medical treatment. The potential risk of cardiotoxicity may increase in patients who have received concomitant, or prior, radiotherapy to the mediastinal pericardial area.

In establishing the maximal cumulative doses of Pharmorubicin, any concomitant therapy with potentially cardiotoxic drugs should be taken intoaccount.

It is recommended that an ECG before and after each treatment cycle should be carried out. Alterations in the ECG tracing, such as flattening or inversion of the T-wave, depression of the S-T segment, or the onset of arrhythmias, generally transient and reversible, need not necessarily be taken as indications to discontinue treatment.

Cardiomyopathy induced by anthracyclines, is associated with a persistent reduction of the QRS voltage, prolongation beyond normal limits of the systolic interval (PEP/ LVET) and a reduction of the ejection fraction. Cardiac monitoring of patients receiving Pharmorubicin treatment is highly important and it is advisable to assess cardiac function by non-invasive techniques such as ECG, echocardiography and, if necessary, measurement of ejection fraction by radionuclide angiography.

Like other cytotoxic agents, Pharmorubicin may induce hyperuricaemia as a result of rapid lysis of neoplastic cells. Blood uric acid levels should therefore be carefully checked so that this phenomenon may be controlled pharmacologically.

Pharmorubicin may impart a red colour to the urine for 1-2 days after administration.

4.5 Interaction with other medicinal products and other forms of Interaction

It is not recommended that Pharmorubicin be mixed with other drugs. But Pharmorubicin can be used in combination with other anticancer drugs.

Cimetidine increases the formation of the active metabolite of epirubicin and the exposure of the unchanged epirubicin by pharmacokinetic interaction.

4.6 Pregnancy and lactation

There is no conclusive information as to whether epirubicin may adversely affect human fertility or cause teratogenesis. Experimental data, however, suggest that epirubicin may harm the foetus. This product should not normally be administered to patients who are pregnant or to mothers who are breast-feeding. Like most other anti-cancer agents, epirubicin has shown mutagenic and carcinogenic properties in animals.

4.7 Effects on ability to drive and use machines

There have been no reports of particular adverse events relating to effects on ability to drive and to use machines.

4.8 Undesirable effects

Apart from myelosuppression and cardiotoxicity, the following adverse reactions have been described:

Alopecia, normally reversible, appears in 60-90% of treated cases; it is accompanied by lack of beard growth in males.

Mucositis may appear 5-10 days after the start of treatment, and usually involves stomatitis with areas of painful erosions, mainly along the side of the tongue and the sublingual mucosa.

Gastro-intestinal disturbances, such as nausea, vomiting and diarrhoea.

Hyperpyrexia.

Fever, chills and urticaria have been rarely reported; anaphylaxis may occur.

High doses of pharmorubicin have been safely administered in a large number of untreated patients having various solid tumours and has caused adverse events which are no different from those seen at conventional doses with the exception of reversible severe neutropenia (< 500 neutrophils/mm^3 for < 7 days) which occurred in the majority of patients. Only a few patients required hospitalisation and supportive therapy for severe infectious complications at high doses.

During intravesical administration, as drug absorption is minimal, systemic side effects are rare; more frequently chemical cystitis, sometimes haemorrhagic, has been observed.

Haematological

The occurrence of secondary acute myeloid leukaemia with or without a pre-leukaemic phase has been reported rarely in patients concurrently treated with epirubicin in association with DNA- damaging antineoplastic agents. Such cases could have a short (1-3 year) latency period.

4.9 Overdose

Very high single doses of epirubicin may be expected to cause acute myocardial degeneration within 24 hours and severe myelosuppression within 10-14 days. Treatment should aim to support the patient during this period and should utilise such measures as blood transfusion and reverse barrier nursing. Delayed cardiac failure has been seen with the anthracyclines up to 6 months after the overdose. Patients should be observed carefully and should, if signs of cardiac failure arise, be treated along conventional lines.

5. PHARMACOLOGICAL PROPERTIES

5.1 Pharmacodynamic properties

Pharmacotherapeutic group (ATC code) – L01D B

The mechanism of action of Pharmorubicin is related to its ability to bind to DNA. Cell culture studies have shown rapid cell penetration, localisation in the nucleus and inhibition of nucleic acid synthesis and mitosis. Pharmorubicin has proved to be active on a wide spectrum of experimental tumours including L1210 and P388 leukaemias, sarcomas SA180 (solid and ascitic forms), B16 melanoma, mammary carcinoma, Lewis lung carcinoma and colon carcinoma 38. It has also shown activity against human tumours transplanted into athymic nude mice (melanoma, mammary lung, prostatic and ovarian carcinomas).

5.2 Pharmacokinetic properties

In patients with normal hepatic and renal function, plasma levels after I.V. injection of 60-150mg/m^2 of the drug follow a tri-exponential decreasing pattern with a very fast first phase and a slow terminal phase with a mean half-life of about 40 hours. These doses are within the limits of pharmacokinetic linearity both in terms of plasma clearance values and metabolic pathway. The major metabolites that have been identified are epirubicinol (13-OH-epirubicin) and glucuronides of epirubicin and epirubicinol.

The 4'-O-glucuronidation distinguishes epirubicin from doxorubicin and may account for the faster elimination of epirubicin and its reduced toxicity. Plasma levels of the main metabolite, the 13-OH derivative (epirubicinol) are consistently lower and virtually parallel those of the unchanged drug.

Pharmorubicin is eliminated mainly through the liver; high plasma clearance values (0.9 l/min) indicate that this slow elimination is due to extensive tissue distribution.

Urinary excretion accounts for approximately 9-10% of the administered dose in 48 hours. Biliary excretion represents the major route of elimination, about 40% of the administered dose being recovered in the bile in 72 hours.

The drug does not cross the blood-brain-barrier. When Pharmorubicin is administered intravesically the systemic absorption is minimal.

5.3 Preclinical safety data

The main target organs in rat, rabbit and dog following repeated dosing were the haemolymphopoietic system, GI tract, kidney, liver and reproductive organs. Epirubicin was also cardiotoxic in the species tested.

It was genotoxic, and, like other anthracyclines, carcinogenic in rats.

Epirubicin was embryotoxic in rats. No malformations were seen in rats or rabbits, but like other anthracyclines and cytotoxic drugs, epirubicin must be considered potentially teratogenic.

A local tolerance study in rats and mice showed extravasation of epirubicin causes tissue necrosis.

6. PHARMACEUTICAL PARTICULARS

6.1 List of excipients

Pharmorubicin Rapid Dissolution 10 mg, 20 mg, 50 mg & 150 mg

Methyl hydroxybenzoate
Lactose monohydrate

Pharmorubicin Solution for Injection 2 mg/ml

Hydrochloric acid

Sodium chloride

Water for Injections

6.2 Incompatibilities

Prolonged contact with any solution of an alkaline pH should be avoided as it will result in hydrolysis of the drug. Pharmorubicin should not be mixed with heparin due to chemical incompatibility, which may lead to precipitation when the drugs are in certain proportions.

Pharmorubicin can be used in combination with other antitumour agents, but it is not recommended that it be mixed with other drugs.

6.3 Shelf life

a) Shelf life of the product as package for sale.

Pharmorubicin Rapid Dissolution 10 mg, 20 mg, 50 mg & 150 mg

Four years.

Pharmorubicin Solution for Injection 2 mg/ml

Glass vials: 3 years

Polypropylene Cytosafe TM vials: 3 years

b) Shelf life after first opening the container/reconstitution according to directions:

Pharmorubicin Solution for Injection does not contain a preservative or bacteriostatic agent. Vials are, therefore for single use only and any unused portion must be discarded after use.

From a microbiological point of view, the product should be used immediately after first penetration of the rubber stopper. If not used immediately, in use storage times and conditions are the responsibility of the user.

6.4 Special precautions for storage

Pharmorubicin Rapid Dissolution 10 mg, 20 mg, 50 mg & 150 mg

Keep the container in the outer carton

Pharmorubicin Solution for Injection 2 mg/ml

Store at 2°C - 8°C (in a refrigerator)

Keep the container in outer carton

6.5 Nature and contents of container

Pharmorubicin Rapid Dissolution 10 mg, 20 mg, 50 mg & 150 mg

5 ml, 10 ml, 50 ml and 75 ml colourless glass vial Type I with chlorobutyl rubber bung and aluminium snap cap.

Pharmorubicin Solution for Injection 2 mg/ml

Colourless glass 5ml, 10ml, 25ml, or 100ml vial (type I), with Teflon-faced chlorobutyl rubber bung and aluminium cap with inset grey polypropylene disk.

Colourless polypropylene 5ml, 10ml, 25ml or 100ml vial with Teflon-faced halobutyl rubber stopper and aluminium cap with plastic flip-off top:

6.6 Instructions for use and handling

Pharmorubicin Rapid Dissolution 10 mg, 20 mg, 50 mg & 150 mg only:

Preparation of the freeze-dried powder for intravenous administration. Dissolve in sodium chloride/water for injection. The vial contents will be under a negative pressure. To minimize aerosol formation during reconstitution, particular care should be taken when the needle is inserted. Inhalation of any aerosol produced during reconstitution must be avoided. After gentle agitation the reconstituted solution will be transparent and red in appearance.

The product should be dissolved in 0.9% sodium chloride or water for injection to get the final concentration of 2 mg/ml according to the following instructions:

Strength (mg)	Solvent volume (ml)
10	5
20	10
50	25
150	75

Pharmorubicin Rapid Dissolution 10 mg, 20 mg, 50 mg & 150 mg

Pharmorubicin Solution for Injection 2 mg/ml

Intravenous administration. Epirubicin should be administered into the tubing of a freely flowing intravenous infusion (0.9% sodium chloride). To minimize the risk of thrombosis or perivenous extravasation, the usual infusion times range between 3 and 20 minutes depending upon dosage and volume of the infusion solution. A direct push injection is not recommended due to the risk of extravasation, which may occur even in the presence of adequate blood return upon needle aspiration (see Warning and Precautions).

Discard any unused solution.

Intravesical administration. Epirubicin should be instilled using a catheter and retained intravesically for 1 hour. During instillation, the patient should be rotated to ensure that the vesical mucosa of the pelvis receives the most extensive contact with the solution. To avoid undue dilution with urine, the patient should be instructed not to drink any fluid in the 12 hours prior to instillation. The patient should be instructed to void at the end of the instillation.

Protective measures: The following protective recommendations are given due to the toxic nature of this substance:

Personnel should be trained in good technique for reconstitution and handling.

- Pregnant staff should be excluded from working with this drug.
- Personnel handling epirubicin should wear protective clothing: goggles, gowns and disposable gloves and masks.
- A designated area should be defined for reconstitution (preferably under a laminar flow system); the work surface should be protected by disposable, plastic-backed, absorbent paper.
- All items used for reconstitution, administration or cleaning, including gloves, should be placed in high-risk, waste disposal bags for high temperature incineration. Spillage or leakage should be treated with dilute sodium hypochlorite (1% available chlorine) solution, preferably by soaking, and then water.
- All cleaning materials should be disposed of as indicated previously.
- In case of skin contact thoroughly wash the affected area with soap and water or sodium bicarbonate solution. However, do not abrade the skin by using a scrub brush. In case of contact with the eye(s), hold back the eyelid of the affected eye(s), and flush with copious amounts of water for at least 15 minutes. Then seek medical evaluation by a physician.
- Always wash hands after removing gloves.

7. MARKETING AUTHORISATION HOLDER

Pharmacia Limited

Ramsgate Road

Sandwich

Kent

CT13 9NJ

United Kingdom

8. MARKETING AUTHORISATION NUMBER(S)

PL 00032/0275 (Pharmorubicin Solution for Injection 2 mg/ml)

PL 00032/0276 (Pharmorubicin Rapid Dissolution)

9. DATE OF FIRST AUTHORISATION/RENEWAL OF THE AUTHORISATION

14 May 2004

10. DATE OF REVISION OF THE TEXT

June 2005

Company Reference: PM 2_0

Phenergan 10mg Tablets

(sanofi-aventis)

1. NAME OF THE MEDICINAL PRODUCT

Phenergan™ 10 mg Tablets.

2. QUALITATIVE AND QUANTITATIVE COMPOSITION

Promethazine hydrochloride BP 10 mg.

3. PHARMACEUTICAL FORM

Pale blue film coated tablets marked PN 10 on one side.

4. CLINICAL PARTICULARS

4.1 Therapeutic indications

As symptomatic treatment for allergic conditions of the upper respiratory tract and skin including allergic rhinitis, urticaria and anaphylactic reactions to drugs and foreign proteins.

As an adjunct in preoperative sedation in surgery and obstetrics.

As an antiemetic.

For short term use:

Sedation and treatment of insomnia in adults.

As a paediatric sedative.

4.2 Posology and method of administration

Route of administration: Oral.

Not for use in children under the age of 2 years because the safety of such use has not been established.

As an antihistamine in allergy:

Children 2-5 years	The use of Phenergan Elixir is recommended for this age group.
Children 5-10 years	Either 10 or 20 mg as a single dose*. Or 10 mg bd. Maximum daily dose 20 mg.
Children over 10 years and adults (including elderly)	Initially 10 mg bd. Increasing to a maximum of 20 mg tds as required.

*Single doses are best taken at night.

As an antiemetic:

Children 2-5 years	The use of Phenergan Elixir is recommended for this age group.
Children 5-10 years	10 mg to be taken the night before the journey. To be repeated after 6–8 hours as required.
Children over 10 years and adults (including elderly)	20 mg to be taken the night before the journey. To be repeated after 6–8 hours as required.

Short term sedation:

Children 2-5 years	The use of Phenergan Elixir is recommended for this age group.
Children 5-10 years	20 mg as a single night time dose.
Children over 10 years and adults (including elderly)	20 to 50 mg as a single night time dose.

4.3 Contraindications

Phenergan should not be used in patients in coma or suffering from CNS depression of any cause. It must not be given to neonates, premature infants or patients hypersensitive to phenothiazines. Phenergan should be avoided in patients taking monoamine oxidase inhibitors up to 14 days previously.

4.4 Special warnings and special precautions for use

Phenergan may thicken or dry lung secretions and impair expectoration. It should therefore be used with caution in patients with asthma, bronchitis or bronchiectasis. Use with care in patients with severe coronary artery disease, narrow angle glaucoma, epilepsy or hepatic and renal insufficiency. Caution should be exercised in patients with bladder neck or pyloro-duodenal obstruction.

Promethazine may mask the warning signs of ototoxicity caused by ototoxic drugs e.g. salicylates. It may also delay the early diagnosis of intestinal obstruction or raised intracranial pressure through the suppression of vomiting.

Phenergan should not be used for longer than 7 days without seeking medical advice.

4.5 Interaction with other medicinal products and other forms of Interaction

Phenergan will enhance the action of any anticholinergic agent, tricyclic antidepressant, sedative or hypnotic. Alcohol should be avoided during treatment. Phenergan may interfere with immunological urine pregnancy tests to produce false-positive or false-negative results. Phenergan should be discontinued at least 72 hours before the start of skin tests as it may inhibit the cutaneous histamine response thus producing false-negative results.

4.6 Pregnancy and lactation

Phenergan should not be used in pregnancy unless the physician considers it essential. The use of Phenergan is not recommended in the 2 weeks prior to delivery in view of the risk of irritability and excitement in the neonate.

Available evidence suggests that the amount excreted in milk is insignificant. However, there are risks of neonatal irritability and excitement.

4.7 Effects on ability to drive and use machines

Because the duration of action may be up to 12 hours, patients should be advised that if they feel drowsy they should not drive or operate heavy machinery.

4.8 Undesirable effects

Side effects may be seen in a few patients: drowsiness, dizziness, restlessness, headaches, nightmares, tiredness, and disorientation. Anticholinergic side effects such as blurred vision, dry mouth and urinary retention occur occasionally. Infants are susceptible to the anticholinergic effects of promethazine, while other children may display paradoxical hyperexcitability. The elderly are particularly susceptible to the anticholinergic effects and confusion due to promethazine. Other side-effects include anorexia, gastric irritation, palpitations, hypotension, arrhythmias, extrapyramidal effects, muscle spasms and tic-like movements of the head and face. Anaphylaxis, jaundice and blood dyscrasias including haemolytic anaemia rarely occur. Photosensitive skin reactions have been reported. Strong sunlight should be avoided during treatment.

4.9 Overdose
Symptoms of severe overdosage are variable. They are characterised in children by various combinations of excitation, ataxia, incoordination, athetosis and hallucinations, while adults may become drowsy and lapse into coma. Convulsions may occur in both adults and children: coma or excitement may precede their occurrence. Cardiorespiratory depression is uncommon. If the patient is seen soon enough after ingestion, it should be possible to induce vomiting with ipecacuanha despite the antiemetic effect of promethazine; alternatively, gastric lavage may be used.

Treatment is otherwise supportive with attention to maintenance of adequate respiratory and circulatory status. Convulsions should be treated with diazepam or other suitable anticonvulsant.

5. PHARMACOLOGICAL PROPERTIES
5.1 Pharmacodynamic properties
Potent, long acting, antihistamine with additional anti-emetic central sedative and anti-cholinergic properties.

5.2 Pharmacokinetic properties
Promethazine is distributed widely in the body. It enters the brain and crosses the placenta. Promethazine is slowly excreted via urine and bile. Phenothiazines pass into the milk at low concentrations.

5.3 Preclinical safety data
No additional preclinical data of relevance to the prescriber.

6. PHARMACEUTICAL PARTICULARS
6.1 List of excipients
Lactose BP, Maize starch BP, Povidone K30 BP, Magnesium stearate BP, Polyethylene glycol 200, Opaspray M-1-4210A (contains E132 and E171), Pharmacoat 606.

6.2 Incompatibilities
None stated.

6.3 Shelf life
60 months.

6.4 Special precautions for storage
Protect from light. Store below 30°C.

6.5 Nature and contents of container
Opaque white 250μm uPVC coated with 40gsm PVdC, 20μm hard temper aluminium foil (coated with vinyl heat seal lacquer) backing, of 56 tablets.

6.6 Instructions for use and handling
None stated.

7. MARKETING AUTHORISATION HOLDER
Rhône-Poulenc Rorer
RPR House
50 Kings Hill Avenue
Kings Hill
West Malling
Kent ME19 4AH

8. MARKETING AUTHORISATION NUMBER(S)
PL 00012/5285R

9. DATE OF FIRST AUTHORISATION/RENEWAL OF THE AUTHORISATION
6 March 1998 / 26 Feb 2004

10. DATE OF REVISION OF THE TEXT
April 2005

Legal category: P

Phenergan 25mg and nightime tablets

(sanofi-aventis)

1. NAME OF THE MEDICINAL PRODUCT
Phenergan™ 25 mg Tablets.
Phenergan™ Nightime.

2. QUALITATIVE AND QUANTITATIVE COMPOSITION
Promethazine hydrochloride BP 25 mg.

3. PHARMACEUTICAL FORM
Pale blue film coated tablets marked PN 25 on one side.

4. CLINICAL PARTICULARS
4.1 Therapeutic indications
As symptomatic treatment for allergic conditions of the upper respiratory tract and skin including allergic rhinitis, urticaria and anaphylactic reactions to drugs and foreign proteins.

As an adjunct in preoperative sedation in surgery and obstetrics.

As an antiemetic.

For short term use:

Sedation and treatment of insomnia in adults.

As a paediatric sedative.

Phenergan Nightime:

For short term treatment of insomnia (sleeplessness) in adults.

4.2 Posology and method of administration
Route of administration: Oral.

Not for use in children under the age of 2 years because the safety of such use has not been established.

As an antihistamine in allergy:

Children 2-5 years	The use of Phenergan Elixir is recommended for this age group.
Children 5-10 years	25 mg as a single dose*. Maximum daily dose 25 mg.
Children over 10 years and adults (including elderly)	25 mg as a single dose*. Increasing to a maximum of 25 mg bd as required.

*Single doses are best taken at night.

As an antiemetic:

Children 2-5 years	The use of Phenergan Elixir is recommended for this age group.
Children 5-10 years	The use of Phenergan Elixir or Phenergan 10 mg Tablets is recommended.
Children over 10 years and adults (including elderly)	25 mg to be taken the night before the journey. To be repeated after 6–8 hours as required.

Short term sedation:

Children 2-5 years	The use of Phenergan Elixir is recommended for this age group.
Children 5-10 years	25 mg as a single night time dose.
Children over 10 years and adults (including elderly)	25 or 50 mg as a single night time dose.

Phenergan Nightime:

Adults (including elderly) only	25 or 50 mg as a single night time dose.

4.3 Contraindications
Phenergan should not be used in patients in coma or suffering from CNS depression of any cause. It must not be given to neonates, premature infants or patients hypersensitive to phenothiazines. Phenergan should be avoided in patients taking monoamine oxidase inhibitors up to 14 days previously.

4.4 Special warnings and special precautions for use
Phenergan may thicken or dry lung secretions and impair expectoration. It should therefore be used with caution in patients with asthma, bronchitis or bronchiectasis. Use with care in patients with severe coronary artery disease, narrow angle glaucoma, epilepsy or hepatic and renal insufficiency. Caution should be exercised in patients with bladder neck or pyloro-duodenal obstruction.

Promethazine may mask the warning signs of ototoxicity caused by ototoxic drugs e.g. salicylates. It may also delay the early diagnosis of intestinal obstruction or raised intracranial pressure through the suppression of vomiting.

Phenergan should not be used for longer than 7 days without seeking medical advice.

4.5 Interaction with other medicinal products and other forms of Interaction
Phenergan will enhance the action of any anticholinergic agent, tricyclic antidepressant, sedative or hypnotic. Alcohol should be avoided during treatment. Phenergan may interfere with immunological urine pregnancy tests to produce false-positive or false-negative results. Phenergan should be discontinued at least 72 hours before the start of skin tests as it may inhibit the cutaneous histamine response thus producing false-negative results.

4.6 Pregnancy and lactation
There is epidemiological evidence for the safety of promethazine in pregnancy and animal studies have shown no hazard. Nevertheless it should not be used in pregnancy unless the physician considers it essential. The use of Phenergan is not recommended in the 2 weeks prior to delivery in view of the risk of irritability and excitement in the neonate.

Available evidence suggests that the amount excreted in milk is insignificant. However, there are risks of neonatal irritability and excitement.

4.7 Effects on ability to drive and use machines
Because the duration of action may be up to 12 hours, patients should be advised that if they feel drowsy they should not drive or operate heavy machinery.

4.8 Undesirable effects
Side effects may be seen in a few patients: drowsiness, dizziness, restlessness, headaches, nightmares, tiredness, and disorientation. Anticholinergic side effects such as blurred vision, dry mouth and urinary retention occur occasionally. Infants are susceptible to the anticholinergic effects of promethazine, while other children may display paradoxical hyperexcitability. The elderly are particularly susceptible to the anticholinergic effects and confusion due to promethazine. Other side-effects include anorexia, gastric irritation, palpitations, hypotension, arrhythmias, extrapyramidal effects, muscle spasms and tic-like movements of the head and face. Anaphylaxis, jaundice and blood dyscrasias including haemolytic anaemia rarely occur. Photosensitive skin reactions have been reported. Strong sunlight should be avoided during treatment.

4.9 Overdose
Symptoms of severe overdosage are variable. They are characterised in children by various combinations of excitation, ataxia, incoordination, athetosis and hallucinations, while adults may become drowsy and lapse into coma. Convulsions may occur in both adults and children: coma or excitement may precede their occurrence. Cardiorespiratory depression is uncommon. If the patient is seen soon enough after ingestion, it should be possible to induce vomiting with ipecacuanha despite the antiemetic effect of promethazine; alternatively, gastric lavage may be used.

Treatment is otherwise supportive with attention to maintenance of adequate respiratory and circulatory status. Convulsions should be treated with diazepam or other suitable anticonvulsant.

5. PHARMACOLOGICAL PROPERTIES
5.1 Pharmacodynamic properties
Potent, long acting, antihistamine with additional anti-emetic central sedative and anti-cholinergic properties.

5.2 Pharmacokinetic properties
Promethazine is distributed widely in the body. It enters the brain and crosses the placenta. Promethazine is slowly excreted via urine and bile. Phenothiazines pass into the milk at low concentrations.

5.3 Preclinical safety data
No additional preclinical data of relevance to the prescriber.

6. PHARMACEUTICAL PARTICULARS
6.1 List of excipients
Lactose BP, Maize starch BP, Povidone K30 BP, Magnesium stearate BP, Polyethylene glycol 200, Opaspray M-1-4210A (contains E132 and E171), Pharmacoat 606.

6.2 Incompatibilities
None stated.

6.3 Shelf life
60 months.

6.4 Special precautions for storage
Protect from light. Store below 30°C.

6.5 Nature and contents of container
Opaque white 250μm uPVC coated with 40gsm PVdC. 20μm hard temper aluminium foil (coated with vinyl heat seal lacquer) backing of 14 (Phenergan Nightime) or 56 (Phenergan 25 mg) tablets.

6.6 Instructions for use and handling
None stated.

7. MARKETING AUTHORISATION HOLDER
Aventis Pharma Limited
50 Kings Hill Avenue
Kings Hill
West Malling
Kent ME19 4AH

8. MARKETING AUTHORISATION NUMBER(S)
PL 04425/0281

9. DATE OF FIRST AUTHORISATION/RENEWAL OF THE AUTHORISATION
23 January 2003

10. DATE OF REVISION OF THE TEXT
April 2005

11 LEGAL CLASSIFICATION
P

Phenergan Elixir

(sanofi-aventis)

1. NAME OF THE MEDICINAL PRODUCT
Phenergan Elixir.

2. QUALITATIVE AND QUANTITATIVE COMPOSITION
Promethazine hydrochloride EP 5 mg / 5 ml.

3. PHARMACEUTICAL FORM
Elixir.

4. CLINICAL PARTICULARS
4.1 Therapeutic indications
As symptomatic treatment for allergic conditions of the upper respiratory tract and skin including allergic rhinitis, urticaria and anaphylactic reactions to drugs and foreign proteins.

As an adjunct in preoperative sedation in surgery and obstetrics.

As an antiemetic.

For short term use:

Sedation and treatment of insomnia in adults.

As a paediatric sedative.

4.2 Posology and method of administration
Route of administration: Oral.

Not for use in children under the age of 2 years because the safety of such use has not been established.

As an antihistamine in allergy:

Children 2-5 years	Either 5–15 mg as a single dose. Or 5 mg bd. Maximum daily dose 15 mg.
Children 5-10 years	Either 10–25 mg as a single dose. Or 5-10 mg bd. Maximum daily dose 25 mg.
Children over 10 years and adults (including elderly)	Initially 10 mg bd. Increasing to a maximum of 20 mg tds as required.

As an antiemetic:

Children 2-5 years	5mg to be taken the night before the journey. To be repeated after 6–8 hours as required.
Children 5-10 years	10 mg to be taken the night before the journey. To be repeated after 6–8 hours as required.
Children over 10 years and adults (including elderly)	25 mg to be taken the night before the journey. To be repeated after 6–8 hours as required.

Short term sedation:

Children 2-5 years	15 or 20 mg as a single night time dose.
Children 5-10 years	20 or 25 mg as a single night time dose.
Children over 10 years and adults (including elderly)	25 or 50 mg as a single night time dose. The use of Phenergan tablets to provide these doses is recommended.

4.3 Contraindications
Phenergan should not be used in patients in coma or suffering from CNS depression of any cause. It must not be given to neonates, premature infants or patients hypersensitive to phenothiazines. Phenergan should be avoided in patients taking monoamine oxidase inhibitors up to 14 days previously.

The elixir contains hydrogenated glucose syrup and is not suitable for diabetics.

4.4 Special warnings and special precautions for use
Phenergan may thicken or dry lung secretions and impair expectoration. It should therefore be used with caution in patients with asthma, bronchitis or bronchiectasis. Use with care in patients with severe coronary artery disease, narrow angle glaucoma, epilepsy or hepatic and renal insufficiency. Caution should be exercised in patients with bladder neck or pyloro-duodenal obstruction.

Promethazine may mask the warning signs of ototoxicity caused by ototoxic drugs e.g. salicylates. It may also delay the early diagnosis of intestinal obstruction or raised intracranial pressure through the suppression of vomiting.

Phenergan Elixir should not be used for longer than 7 days without seeking medical advice.

4.5 Interaction with other medicinal products and other forms of Interaction
Phenergan will enhance the action of any anticholinergic agent, tricyclic antidepressant, sedative or hypnotic. Alcohol should be avoided during treatment. Phenergan may interfere with immunological urine pregnancy tests to produce false-positive or false-negative results. Phenergan should be discontinued at least 72 hours before the start of skin tests as it may inhibit the cutaneous histamine response thus producing false-negative results.

4.6 Pregnancy and lactation
Phenergan Elixir should not be used in pregnancy unless the physician considers it essential. The use of Phenergan is not recommended in the 2 weeks prior to delivery in view of the risk of irritability and excitement in the neonate.

Available evidence suggests that the amount excreted in milk is insignificant. However, there are risks of neonatal irritability and excitement.

4.7 Effects on ability to drive and use machines
Because the duration of action may be up to 12 hours, patients should be advised that if they feel drowsy they should not drive or operate heavy machinery.

4.8 Undesirable effects
Side effects may be seen in a few patients: drowsiness, dizziness, restlessness, headaches, nightmares, tiredness, and disorientation. Anticholinergic side effects such as blurred vision, dry mouth and urinary retention occur occasionally. Infants are susceptible to the anticholinergic effects of promethazine, while other children may display paradoxical hyperexcitability. The elderly are particularly susceptible to the anticholinergic effects and confusion due to promethazine. Other side effects include anorexia, gastric irritation, palpitations, hypotension, arrhythmias, extrapyramidal effects, muscle spasms and tic-like movements of the head and face. Anaphylaxis, jaundice and blood dyscrasias including haemolytic anaemia rarely occur. Photosensitive skin reactions have been reported. Strong sunlight should be avoided during treatment.

The preservatives used in Phenergan Elixir have been reported to cause hypersensitivity reactions, characterised by circulatory collapse with CNS depression in certain susceptible individuals with allergic tendencies.

4.9 Overdose
Symptoms of severe overdosage are variable. They are characterised in children by various combinations of excitation, ataxia, incoordination, athetosis and hallucinations, while adults may become drowsy and lapse into coma. Convulsions may occur in both adults and children: coma may precede their occurrence. Tachycardia may develop. Cardiorespiratory depression is not uncommon. If the patient is seen soon enough after ingestion, it should be possible to induce vomiting with ipecacuanha despite the antiemetic effect of promethazine; alternatively, gastric lavage may be used.

Treatment is otherwise supportive with attention to maintenance of adequate respiratory and circulatory status. Convulsions should be treated with diazepam or other suitable anticonvulsant.

5. PHARMACOLOGICAL PROPERTIES
5.1 Pharmacodynamic properties
Potent, long acting, antihistamine with additional anti-emetic central sedative and anti-cholinergic properties.

5.2 Pharmacokinetic properties
Promethazine is distributed widely in the body. It enters the brain and crosses the placenta. Promethazine is slowly excreted via urine and bile. Phenothiazines pass into the milk at low concentrations.

5.3 Preclinical safety data
No additional preclinical data of relevance to the prescriber.

6. PHARMACEUTICAL PARTICULARS
6.1 List of excipients
Hydrogenated glucose syrup, Citric acid anhydrous (E330) BP, Sodium citrate (E331) BP, Ascorbic acid (E300) BP, Sodium sulphite anhydrous (E221) BP, Sodium metabisulphite (E223) BP, Sodium benzoate (E211) BP, Orange juice flavour 510844E, Caramel HT (E150), Acesulphame potassium (E950), Demineralised water BP.

6.2 Incompatibilities
None stated.

6.3 Shelf life
24 months when unopened. 1 month when opened.

6.4 Special precautions for storage
Protect from light. Store below 25°C.

6.5 Nature and contents of container
Amber glass type III bottle containing 100 ml. Rolled on pilfer proof aluminium cap and PVDC emulsion coated wad, or HDPE/polypropylene child resistant cap with tamper evident band.

6.6 Instructions for use and handling
None stated.

7. MARKETING AUTHORISATION HOLDER
May and Baker Limited
trading as
May and Baker or Rhône-Poulenc Rorer or Rorer Pharmaceuticals or Pharmuka or
Theraplix or APS or Berk Pharmaceuticals
RPR House
50 Kings Hill Avenue
Kings Hill
West Malling
Kent ME19 4AH

8. MARKETING AUTHORISATION NUMBER(S)
PL 00012/5025R

9. DATE OF FIRST AUTHORISATION/RENEWAL OF THE AUTHORISATION
20 July 1988 / 11 June 2003

10. DATE OF REVISION OF THE TEXT
June 2003

Legal Category: P

Phenergan Injection

(sanofi-aventis)

1. NAME OF THE MEDICINAL PRODUCT
Phenergan Solution for Injection 2.5% w/v.

2. QUALITATIVE AND QUANTITATIVE COMPOSITION
Promethazine hydrochloride 2.5% w/v.

3. PHARMACEUTICAL FORM
Solution for injection.

4. CLINICAL PARTICULARS
4.1 Therapeutic indications
As symptomatic treatment for allergic conditions of the upper respiratory tract and skin including allergic rhinitis, urticaria and anaphylactic reactions to drugs and foreign proteins.

Sedation and treatment of insomnia in adults.

As an adjunct in preoperative sedation in surgery and obstetrics.

As a paediatric sedative.

Not for use in children under 2 years of age because the safety of such use has not been established.

Route of administration: Intramuscular or intravenous.

4.2 Posology and method of administration
The usual dose is 25 - 50 mg by deep intramuscular injection, or, in emergency, by slow intravenous injection after dilution of the 2.5% solution to 10 times its volume with water for injections immediately before use.

Maximum parenteral dose 100 mg.

Elderly: No specific dosage recommendations.

Children: 6.25 - 12.5 mg for children from 5 - 10 years by deep intramuscular injection.

4.3 Contraindications
Phenergan should not be used in patients in coma or suffering from CNS depression of any cause. It must not be given to neonates or premature infants. Phenergan should not be given to patients with a known hypersensitivity to promethazine or to any of the excipients. Phenergan should be avoided in patients taking monoamine oxidase inhibitors up to 14 days previously.

4.4 Special warnings and special precautions for use
Phenergan may thicken or dry lung secretions and impair expectoration. It should therefore be used with caution in patients with asthma, bronchitis or bronchiectasis. Use with care in patients with severe coronary artery disease, narrow angle glaucoma, epilepsy or hepatic and renal insufficiency. Caution should be exercised in patients with bladder neck or pyloro-duodenal obstruction. The use of promethazine should be avoided in children and adolescents with signs and symptoms suggestive of Reye's Syndrome.

Promethazine may mask the warning signs of ototoxicity caused by ototoxic drugs e.g. salicylates. It may also delay the early diagnosis of intestinal obstruction or raised intracranial pressure through the suppression of vomiting.

Intravenous injection should be performed with extreme care to avoid extravasation or inadvertent intra-arterial injection, which could lead to necrosis and peripheral gangrene. If a patient complains of pain during intravenous injection, stop the injection immediately, as this may be a sign of extravasation or inadvertent intra-arterial injection. Intramuscular injection must also be performed carefully to avoid inadvertent subcutaneous injection, which could lead to local necrosis.

4.5 Interaction with other medicinal products and other forms of Interaction
Phenergan will enhance the action of any anticholinergic agent, tricyclic antidepressant, sedative or hypnotic. Alcohol should be avoided during treatment. Phenergan may cause hypotension, and dosage adjustment of antihypertensive therapy may therefore be required. Phenergan may

lower the convulsive threshold, and dosage adjustment of anticonvulsant medication may therefore be required. Phenergan may interfere with immunological urine pregnancy tests to produce false-positive or false-negative results. Phenergan should be discontinued at least 72 hours before the start of skin tests as it may inhibit the cutaneous histamine response thus producing false-negative results. Phenergan injection may increase glucose tolerance.

4.6 Pregnancy and lactation

Phenergan Injection should not be used in pregnancy unless the physician considers it essential. The use of Phenergan is not recommended in the 2 weeks prior to delivery in view of the risk of irritability and excitement in the neonate.

Available evidence suggests that the amount excreted in milk is insignificant. However, there are risks of neonatal irritability and excitement.

4.7 Effects on ability to drive and use machines

Ambulant patients receiving Phenergan for the first time should not be in control of vehicles or machinery for the first few days until it is established that they are not hypersensitive to the central nervous effects of the drug and do not suffer from disorientation, confusion or dizziness.

4.8 Undesirable effects

Side effects may be seen in a few patients: drowsiness, dizziness, restlessness, headaches, nightmares, tiredness, and disorientation. Anticholinergic side effects such as blurred vision, dry mouth and urinary retention occur occasionally. Newborn and premature infants are susceptible to the anticholinergic effects of promethazine, while other children may display paradoxical hyperexcitability. The elderly are particularly susceptible to the anticholinergic effects and confusion due to promethazine. Other side-effects include anorexia, gastric irritation, palpitations, hypotension, arrhythmias, extrapyramidal effects, muscle spasms and tic-like movements of the head and face. Jaundice and blood dyscrasias including haemolytic anaemia rarely occur. Very rare cases of allergic reactions, including urticaria, rash, pruritus and anaphylaxis, have been reported. Photosensitive skin reactions have been reported; strong sunlight should be avoided during treatment.

The preservatives used in Phenergan Injection have been reported to cause hypersensitivity reactions, characterised by circulatory collapse with CNS depression in certain susceptible individuals with allergic tendencies.

4.9 Overdose

Symptoms of severe overdosage are variable. They are characterised in children by various combinations of excitation, ataxia, incoordination, athetosis and hallucinations, while adults may become drowsy and lapse into coma. Convulsions may occur in both adults and children: coma or excitement may precede their occurrence. Cardiorespiratory depression is uncommon. If the patient is seen soon enough after ingestion, it should be possible to induce vomiting with ipecacuanha despite the antiemetic effect of promethazine; alternatively, gastric lavage may be used.

Treatment is otherwise supportive with attention to maintenance of adequate respiratory and circulatory status. Convulsions should be treated with diazepam or other suitable anticonvulsant.

5. PHARMACOLOGICAL PROPERTIES

5.1 Pharmacodynamic properties

Potent, long acting, antihistamine with additional anti-emetic central sedative and anti-cholinergic properties.

5.2 Pharmacokinetic properties

Promethazine is slowly excreted via urine and bile. It is distributed widely in the body. It enters the brain and crosses the placenta. Phenothiazines pass into the milk at low concentrations.

5.3 Preclinical safety data

No additional data of relevance to the prescriber.

6. PHARMACEUTICAL PARTICULARS

6.1 List of excipients

Sodium sulphite anhydrous (E221), Sodium metabisulphite (E223), Water for injections.

6.2 Incompatibilities

None stated.

6.3 Shelf life

60 months.

6.4 Special precautions for storage

Protect from light. Keep container in the outer carton.

6.5 Nature and contents of container

Cardboard carton containing 10 × 1 ml ampoules.

6.6 Instructions for use and handling

Discoloured solutions should not be used.

7. MARKETING AUTHORISATION HOLDER

Aventis Pharma

RPR House

50 Kings Hill Avenue

Kings Hill

West Malling

Kent ME19 4AH

8. MARKETING AUTHORISATION NUMBER(S)

PL 00012/5054R

9. DATE OF FIRST AUTHORISATION/RENEWAL OF THE AUTHORISATION

30 October 1996 / 29 July 2002

10. DATE OF REVISION OF THE TEXT

June 2005

Legal category: POM

Phenylephrine Injection BP 10 mg/ml

(Sovereign Medical)

1. NAME OF THE MEDICINAL PRODUCT

Phenylephrine Injection BP 10 mg/ml

2. QUALITATIVE AND QUANTITATIVE COMPOSITION

Phenylephrine hydrochloride Ph Eur 1.0% w/v

3. PHARMACEUTICAL FORM

Sterile solution.

4. CLINICAL PARTICULARS

4.1 Therapeutic indications

For the treatment of hypotensive states, e.g. circulatory failure, during spinal anaesthesia or drug-induced hypotension.

4.2 Posology and method of administration

For subcutaneous, intramuscular, slow intravenous injection or intravenous infusion.

Adults

Phenylephrine Injection may be administered subcutaneously or intramuscularly in a dosage of 2 to 5 mg with further doses of 1 to 10 mg if necessary according to response, or in a dose of 100 to 500 micrograms by slow intravenous injection as a 0.1% solution, repeated as necessary after at least 15 minutes.

Alternatively, 10 mg in 500 ml of glucose 5% injection or sodium chloride 0.9% injection may be infused intravenously, initially at a rate of up to 180 micrograms per minute, reduced according to response to 30-60 micrograms per minute.

Children

100 microgram/kg bodyweight subcutaneously or intramuscularly.

Elderly

There is no need for dosage reduction in the elderly.

4.3 Contraindications

Patients taking monoamine oxidase inhibitors, or within 14 days of ceasing such treatment. Severe hypertension and hyperthyroidism.

4.4 Special warnings and special precautions for use

Great care should be exercised in administering Phenylephrine Injection to patients with pre-existing cardiovascular disease such as ischaemic heart disease, arrhythmias, occlusive vascular disease including arteriosclerosis, hypertension or aneurysms. Anginal pain may be precipitated in patients with angina pectoris.

Care is also required when given to patients with diabetes mellitus or closed-angle glaucoma.

Keep all medicines out of the reach of children.

4.5 Interaction with other medicinal products and other forms of Interaction

Phenylephrine may interact with cyclopropane and halothane and other halogenated inhalational anaesthetics, to induce ventricular fibrillation. An increased risk of arrhythmias may also occur if Phenylephrine Injection is given to patients receiving cardiac glycosides, quinidine or tricyclic antidepressants.

Phenylephrine may increase blood pressure and consequently reverse the action of many antihypertensive agents. Interactions of phenylephrine with alpha- and beta-receptor blocking drugs may be complex.

4.6 Pregnancy and lactation

The safety of phenylephrine during pregnancy and lactation has not been established. Administration of phenylephrine in late pregnancy or labour may cause foetal hypoxia and bradycardia. Excretion of phenylephrine in breast milk appears to be minimal.

4.7 Effects on ability to drive and use machines

No adverse effects known.

4.8 Undesirable effects

Extravasation of Phenylephrine Injection may cause tissue necrosis. Phenylephrine will cause a rise in blood pressure with headache and vomiting and this may produce cerebral haemorrhage and pulmonary oedema. There may also be a reflex bradycardia or tachycardia, other cardiac arrhythmias, anginal pain, palpitations and cardiac arrest, hypotension with dizziness, fainting and flushing may occur. Phenylephrine may induce difficulty in micturition and urinary retention, dyspnoea, altered metabolism including disturbances of glucose metabolism, sweating, hypersalivation, transient tingling and coolness of the skin and a temporary fullness of the head. Phenylephrine is without significant stimulating effects on the central nervous system at usual doses.

4.9 Overdose

Symptoms of overdosage include headache, vomiting, hypertension and reflex bradycardia and other cardiac arrhythmias.

Treatment should consist of symptomatic and supportive measures. The hypertensive effects may be treated with an alpha-adrenoceptor blocking drug, such as phentolamine, 5 to 60 mg i.v. over 10-30 minutes, repeated as necessary.

5. PHARMACOLOGICAL PROPERTIES

5.1 Pharmacodynamic properties

Phenylephrine hydrochloride is a sympathomimetic agent with mainly direct effects on adrenergic receptors. It has predominantly alpha-adrenergic activity and is without significant stimulating effects on the central nervous system at usual doses. After injection it produces peripheral vasoconstriction and increased arterial pressure; it also causes reflex bradycardia.

5.2 Pharmacokinetic properties

When injected subcutaneously or intramuscularly, phenylephrine takes 10 to 15 minutes to act. Subcutaneous and intramuscular injections are effective for up to about one and up to about two hours, respectively. Intravenous injections are effective for up to about 20 minutes. Phenylephrine is metabolised in the liver by monoamine oxidase. The metabolites, their route and rate of excretion have not been identified.

5.3 Preclinical safety data

Not applicable.

6. PHARMACEUTICAL PARTICULARS

6.1 List of excipients

N/1 sodium hydroxide for SP

N/1 hydrochloric acid for SP

Water for injections Ph Eur

Sterile N/1 sodium hydroxide for SP

Sterile N/1 hydrochloric acid for SP

6.2 Incompatibilities

Phenylephrine Injection has been stated to be incompatible with alkalis, ferric salts, phenytoin sodium and oxidising agents.

6.3 Shelf life

24 months.

6.4 Special precautions for storage

Store at 2-25°C. Protect from light.

6.5 Nature and contents of container

1 ml neutral glass ampoule with ceramic breakring.

Pack size: 10 ampoules.

6.6 Instructions for use and handling

Not applicable.

7. MARKETING AUTHORISATION HOLDER

Waymade Plc trading as Sovereign Medical

Sovereign House

Miles Gray Road

Basildon

Essex SS14 3FR

United Kingdom

8. MARKETING AUTHORISATION NUMBER(S)

PL 06464/0902

9. DATE OF FIRST AUTHORISATION/RENEWAL OF THE AUTHORISATION

17 November 1999

10. DATE OF REVISION OF THE TEXT

Phosphate Sandoz

(HK Pharma Limited)

1. NAME OF THE MEDICINAL PRODUCT

PHOSPHATE SANDOZ® Effervescent Tablets

2. QUALITATIVE AND QUANTITATIVE COMPOSITION

PHOSPHATE SANDOZ Effervescent Tablets containing 1.936g of sodium acid phosphate anhydrous.

3. PHARMACEUTICAL FORM

Effervescent Tablets

4. CLINICAL PARTICULARS

4.1 Therapeutic indications

Hypercalcaemia associated with such conditions as hyperparathyroidism, multiple myelomatosis and malignancy.

Hypophosphataemia associated with vitamin D resistant rickets and vitamin D resistant hypophosphataemic osteomalacia.

4.2 Posology and method of administration

PHOSPHATE SANDOZ Effervescent should be dissolved in 1/3 to 1/2 a tumblerful of water and taken orally.

Dosage should be adjusted to suit the requirements of individual patients. Excessive dosage has been reported to produce hypocalcaemia in isolated cases. Particular care should therefore be taken to ensure appropriate dosage in the elderly.

Adults

Hypercalcaemia: up to 6 tablets daily (adjustment being made according to requirements).

Vitamin D resistant hypophosphateaemic osteomalacia: 4-6 tablets daily.

Children under 5 years

Hypercalcaemia: up to 3 tablets daily (adjustment being made according to requirements).

Vitamin D resistant rickets: 2-3 tablets daily.

4.3 Contraindications
None.

4.4 Special warnings and special precautions for use
In cases of impaired renal function associated with hypercalcaemia and in cases where restricted sodium intake is required, eg. congestive cardiac failure, hypertension or pre-eclamptic toxaemia, the sodium (20.4mmol per tablet) and potassium (3.1mmol per tablet) content of PHOSPHATE SANDOZ should be taken into consideration. In cases of hypercalcaemia associated with impaired renal function and hyperphosphataemia, the main effect of oral phosphate is to bind calcium in the gut and thus reduce calcium absorption.

The effect of oral phosphate on serum phosphate is likely to be minimal, but close monitoring of serum levels is recommended.

Soft tissue calcification and nephrocalcinosis have been reported in isolated cases following intravenous therapy with phosphate.

This is thought to be a function of dosage and rapidity of phosphate administration. While such effects appear less likely to occur with oral phosphates, careful surveillance of patients is recommended, especially if on long term therapy.

4.5 Interaction with other medicinal products and other forms of Interaction
Concurrent administrations of antacids, containing agents such as aluminium hydroxide, may result in displacement of calcium from binding to oral phosphate, thus reducing efficacy.

4.6 Pregnancy and lactation
The safety of PHOSPHATE SANDOZ in human pregnancy has not been formally studied, but the drug has been widely used for many years without ill-consequence.

4.7 Effects on ability to drive and use machines
None.

4.8 Undesirable effects
Apart from gastro-intestinal upsets, nausea and diarrhoea, very few side effects have been reported.

4.9 Overdose
Excessive dosage has been reported to produce hypocalcaemia in isolated cases. This has proved reversible when dosage has been adjusted.

5. PHARMACOLOGICAL PROPERTIES

5.1 Pharmacodynamic properties
Oral administration of inorganic phosphates produces a fall in serum calcium in patients with hypercalcaemia. PHOSPHATE SANDOZ Effervescent Tablets also contain sodium ions which aid the correction of the dehydration and sodium depletion seen in hypercalcaemia.

5.2 Pharmacokinetic properties
Approximately two thirds of ingested phosphate is absorbed from the gastro-intestinal tract; most of the absorbed phosphate is then filtered by the glomeruli and subsequently undergoes reabsorption. Parathyroid hormone and vitamin D stimulate absorption of phosphate from the small intestine and its reabsorption from the proximal tubule. Virtually all absorbed phosphate is eventually excreted in the urine, the remainder being excreted in the faeces.

5.3 Preclinical safety data
PHOSPHATE SANDOZ Effervescent Tablets contain sodium acid phosphate, anhydrous, sodium bicarbonate and potassium bicarbonate (all of which are subject to pharmacopoeial monographs). The physiological, pharmacological and clinical toxicity of potassium salts are well documented and limited animal data are therefore available.

6. PHARMACEUTICAL PARTICULARS

6.1 List of excipients
Potassium bicarbonate, sodium bicarbonate, sodium saccharin, orange flavour 52.570 TP, polyethylene glycol 4000, sugar icing CP, citric acid anhydrous, water.

6.2 Incompatibilities
None.

6.3 Shelf life
36 months.

6.4 Special precautions for storage
Do not store above 25°C. Store in the original container. Keep the container tightly closed

6.5 Nature and contents of container
Polypropylene tubes of 20 effervescent tablets in boxes of 5 tubes (100 tablets).

6.6 Instructions for use and handling
None.

7. MARKETING AUTHORISATION HOLDER
HK Pharma Ltd
PO Box 105
HITCHIN
SG5 2GG

8. MARKETING AUTHORISATION NUMBER(S)
PL 16784/0001

9. DATE OF FIRST AUTHORISATION/RENEWAL OF THE AUTHORISATION
28th April 1998

10. DATE OF REVISION OF THE TEXT
October 2002

Phyllocontin Continus tablets 225mg, Phyllocontin Forte Continus tablets 350mg.

(Napp Pharmaceuticals Limited)

1. NAME OF THE MEDICINAL PRODUCT
PHYLLOCONTIN® CONTINUS® tablets 225 mg
PHYLLOCONTIN® Forte CONTINUS® tablets 350 mg

2. QUALITATIVE AND QUANTITATIVE COMPOSITION
Tablets containing 225 mg and 350 mg of Aminophylline Hydrate PhEur.

3. PHARMACEUTICAL FORM
Prolonged release tablets

PHYLLOCONTIN CONTINUS tablets 225 mg are pale yellow, film-coated tablets with the Napp logo on one side and SA on the other.

PHYLLOCONTIN Forte CONTINUS tablets 350 mg are pale yellow, film-coated tablets with the Napp logo on one side and SA 350 on the other.

4. CLINICAL PARTICULARS

4.1 Therapeutic indications
For the treatment and prophylaxis of bronchospasm associated with asthma, chronic obstructive pulmonary disease and chronic bronchitis. Also indicated in adults for the treatment of left ventricular and congestive cardiac failure.

4.2 Posology and method of administration
Route of Administration

Oral.

The tablets should be swallowed whole and not chewed.

Children: The maintenance dose (expressed as mg aminophylline) is 12 mg/kg twice daily adjusted to the nearest 100 mg. It is recommended that half the maintenance dose be given for the first week of therapy if the patient has not previously been receiving xanthine preparations.

Some children with chronic asthma require and tolerate much higher doses (13-20 mg/kg twice daily). Lower doses (based on the usual adult dose) may be required by adolescents. Not recommended for children under 3 years of age.

Adults: The usual dose is two PHYLLOCONTIN CONTINUS tablets 225 mg, or one or two PHYLLOCONTIN Forte CONTINUS tablets 350mg twice-daily following an initial week of therapy on one tablet twice-daily.

The Elderly: The dose should be adjusted following the response to the initial week of therapy on one tablet twice-daily.

Dose Titration: Patients vary in their response to xanthines and it may be necessary to titrate dosage individually. Steady state theophylline levels are generally attained 3-4 days after dose adjustment. If a satisfactory clinical response is not achieved, serum theophylline should be measured 4-6 hours after the last dose. Based on serum theophylline assay results dosage should be titrated using the following as a guide:

Peak serum theophylline level	Dosage adjustment to nearest 125 mg
< 10 micrograms/ml	Increase total daily dose by half
10-15 micrograms/ml	Increase total daily dose by one quarter if symptoms persist
16-20 micrograms/ml	No adjustment required
21-25 micrograms/ml	Decrease dose by one quarter
26-30 micrograms/ml	Miss next dose and decrease maintenance by one half

4.3 Contraindications
Should not be given concomitantly with ephedrine in children. Hypersensitivity to xanthines or any of the tablet constituents. Porphyria.

4.4 Special warnings and special precautions for use
The patient's response to therapy should be carefully monitored – worsening of asthma symptoms requires medical attention.

Use with caution in patients with cardiac arrhythmias, peptic ulcer, hyperthyroidism, severe hypertension, hepatic dysfunction, chronic alcoholism or acute febrile illness.

The half-life of theophylline may be prolonged in the elderly and in patients with heart failure, hepatic impairment or viral infections. Toxic accumulation may occur (see Section 4.9 overdose).

A reduction of dosage may be necessary in the elderly patient.

Avoid concomitant use with other xanthine-containing products.

The hypokalaemia resulting from beta agonist therapy, steroids, diuretics and hypoxia may be potentiated by xanthines. Particular care is advised in patients suffering from severe asthma who require hospitalisation. It is recommended that serum potassium levels are monitored in such situations.

Alternative treatment is advised for patients with a history of seizure activity.

4.5 Interaction with other medicinal products and other forms of Interaction
The following increase clearance and it may therefore be necessary to increase dosage to ensure a therapeutic effect: aminoglutethimide, carbamazepine, moracizine, phenytoin, rifampicin, sulphinpyrazone, barbiturates and Hypericum perforatum. Plasma concentrations of theophylline can be reduced by concomitant use of the herbal remedy St John's Wort (Hypericum perforatum). Smoking and alcohol consumption can also increase clearance of theophylline.

The following reduce clearance and a reduced dosage may therefore be necessary to avoid side-effects: allopurinol, carbimazole, cimetidine, ciprofloxacin, clarithromycin, diltiazem, disulfiram, erythromycin, fluconazole, interferon, isoniazid, isoprenaline, methotrexate, mexiletine, nizatidine, norfloxacin, oxpentifylline, propafenone, propranolol, ofloxacin, thiabendazole, verapamil, viloxazine hydrochloride and oral contraceptives. The concomitant use of theophylline and fluvoxamine should usually be avoided. Where this is not possible, patients should have their theophylline dose halved and plasma theophylline should be monitored closely.

Factors such as viral infections, liver disease and heart failure also reduce theophylline clearance. There are conflicting reports concerning the potentiation of theophylline by influenza vaccine and physicians should be aware that interaction may occur. A reduction of dosage may be necessary in elderly patients. Thyroid disease or associated treatment may alter theophylline plasma levels. There is also a pharmacological interaction with adenosine, benzodiazepines, halothane, lomustine and lithium and these drugs should be used with caution.

Theophylline may decrease steady state phenytoin levels.

4.6 Pregnancy and lactation
There are no adequate data from well controlled studies from the use of theophylline in pregnant women. Theophylline has been reported to give rise to teratogenic effects in mice, rats and rabbits (see section 5.3). The potential risk for humans is unknown. Theophylline should not be administered during pregnancy unless clearly necessary. Theophylline is secreted in breast milk, and may be associated with irritability in the infant, therefore it should only be given to breast feeding women when the anticipated benefits outweigh the risk to the child.

4.7 Effects on ability to drive and use machines
No known effects.

4.8 Undesirable effects
The side-effects usually associated with theophylline and xanthine derivatives such are nausea, gastric irritation, headache, CNS stimulation, tachycardia, palpitations, arrhythmias and convulsions.

4.9 Overdose
Over 3 g could be serious in an adult (40 mg/kg in a child). The fatal dose may be as little as 4.5 g in an adult (60 mg/kg in a child), but is generally higher.

Symptoms

Warning: Serious features may develop as long as 12 hours after overdosage with prolonged release formulations.

Alimentary features: Nausea, vomiting (which is often severe), epigastric pain and haematemesis. Consider pancreatitis if abdominal pain persists.

Neurological features: Restlessness, hypertonia, exaggerated limb reflexes and convulsions. Coma may develop in very severe cases.

Cardiovascular features: Sinus tachycardia is common. Ectopic beats and supraventricular and ventricular tachycardia may follow.

Metabolic features: Hypokalaemia due to shift of potassium from plasma into cells is common, can develop rapidly and may be severe. Hyperglycaemia, hypomagnesaemia and metabolic acidosis may also occur. Rhabdomyolysis may also occur.

Management

Activated charcoal or gastric lavage should be considered if a significant overdose has been ingested within 1-2 hours. Repeated doses of activated charcoal given by mouth can enhance theophylline elimination. Measure the plasma potassium concentration urgently, repeat frequently and correct hypokalaemia. BEWARE! If large amounts of potassium have been given, serious hyperkalaemia may develop during recovery. If plasma potassium is low, then the plasma magnesium concentration should be measured as soon as possible.

In the treatment of ventricular arrhythmias, proconvulsant antiarrhythmic agents such as lignocaine (lidocaine) should be avoided because of the risk of causing or exacerbating seizures.

Measure the plasma theophylline concentration regularly when severe poisoning is suspected, until concentrations are falling. Vomiting should be treated with an antiemetic such as metoclopramide or ondansetron.

Tachycardia with an adequate cardiac output is best left untreated. Beta-blockers may be given in extreme cases but not if the patient is asthmatic. Control isolated convulsions with intravenous diazepam. Exclude hypokalaemia as a cause.

5. PHARMACOLOGICAL PROPERTIES

5.1 Pharmacodynamic properties

Aminophylline (theophylline) is a bronchodilator. In addition it affects the function of a number of cells involved in the inflammatory processes associated with asthma and chronic obstructive airways disease. Of most importance may be enhanced suppressor T-lymphocyte activity and reduction of eosinophil and neutrophil function. These actions may contribute to an anti-inflammatory prophylactic activity in asthma and chronic obstructive airways disease. Theophylline stimulates the myocardium and produces a diminution of venous pressure in congestive heart failure leading to marked increase in cardiac output.

5.2 Pharmacokinetic properties

Aminophylline (theophylline) is well absorbed from PHYLLOCONTIN CONTINUS tablets and at least 60% may be bound to plasma proteins. The main urinary metabolites are 1,3 dimethyl uric acid and 3-methylxanthine. About 10% is excreted unchanged.

5.3 Preclinical safety data

In studies in which mice, rats and rabbits were dosed during the period of organogenesis, theophylline produced teratogenic effects.

6. PHARMACEUTICAL PARTICULARS

6.1 List of excipients

Hydroxyethylcellulose

Povidone [K25]

Cetostearyl alcohol

Purified talc

Magnesium stearate

Hypromellose (E464)

Macrogol 400

Industrial methylated spirit

Titanium dioxide (E171)

Iron oxide (E172)

6.2 Incompatibilities

Not applicable.

6.3 Shelf life

Three years

6.4 Special precautions for storage

Do not store above 25°C.

Store in the original package.

6.5 Nature and contents of container

PHYLLOCONTIN CONTINUS tablets 225 mg are available in PVC blister packs containing 56 tablets.

PHYLLOCONTIN Forte CONTINUS tablets are available in polypropylene containers containing 56 tablets.

6.6 Instructions for use and handling

None.

Administrative Data

7. MARKETING AUTHORISATION HOLDER

Napp Pharmaceuticals Ltd

Cambridge Science Park

Milton Road

Cambridge CB4 0GW

8. MARKETING AUTHORISATION NUMBER(S)

PL 16950/0057, 0058

9. DATE OF FIRST AUTHORISATION/RENEWAL OF THE AUTHORISATION

PHYLLOCONTIN CONTINUS tablets 225 mg - 7 July 1989/ 9 April 2002

PHYLLOCONTIN Forte CONTINUS tablets 350 mg - 17 August 1983/15 March 2001

10. DATE OF REVISION OF THE TEXT

July 2004

11. Legal Category

P

Physiotens Tablets 200,300 & 400 micrograms

(Solvay Healthcare Limited)

1. NAME OF THE MEDICINAL PRODUCT

Physiotens® Tablets 200/300/400 micrograms

2. QUALITATIVE AND QUANTITATIVE COMPOSITION

Each tablet contains 200, 300 or 400 micrograms moxonidine.

3. PHARMACEUTICAL FORM

Film coated tablets.

200 mcg: Light pink, round, biconvex, film-coated tablets imprinted '0.2' on one face.

300 mcg: Pale red, round, biconvex, film-coated tablets imprinted '0.3' on one face.

400 mcg: Dull red, round, biconvex, film-coated tablets imprinted '0.4' on one face.

4. CLINICAL PARTICULARS

4.1 Therapeutic indications

Mild to moderate essential or primary hypertension.

4.2 Posology and method of administration

Adults (including the elderly):

Treatment should be started with 200 micrograms of Physiotens in the morning. The dose may be titrated after three weeks to 400 micrograms, given as one dose or as divided doses (morning and evening) until a satisfactory response has been achieved. If the response is still unsatisfactory after a further three weeks' treatment, the dosage can be increased up to a maximum of 600 micrograms in divided doses (morning and evening).

A single dose of 400 micrograms of Physiotens and a daily dose of 600 micrograms in divided doses (morning and evening) should not be exceeded.

In patients with moderate renal dysfunction (GFR above 30 ml/min, but below 60 ml/min), the single dose should not exceed 200 micrograms and the daily dose should not exceed 400 micrograms of moxonidine.

The tablets should be taken with a little liquid. As the intake of food has no influence on the pharmacokinetic properties of moxonidine, the tablets may be taken before, during or after the meal.

Children (under 16 years):

Physiotens should not be given below the age of 16 years as insufficient therapeutic experience exists in this group.

4.3 Contraindications

Physiotens should not be used in cases of

- history of angioneurotic oedema
- hypersensitivity to any of the ingredients
- sick sinus syndrome or sino-atrial block
- 2nd or 3rd degree atrioventricular block
- bradycardia (below 50 beats/minute at rest)
- malignant arrhythmia
- severe heart failure (see Section 4.4)
- severe coronary artery disease or unstable angina
- severe liver disease
- severe renal dysfunction (GFR <30 ml/min, serum creatinine concentration >160 μmol/l).

Physiotens should not be used because of lack of therapeutic experience in cases of

- intermittent claudication
- Raynaud's disease
- Parkinson's disease
- epileptic disorders
- glaucoma
- depression
- pregnancy or lactation
- children below 16 years of age.

4.4 Special warnings and special precautions for use

If Physiotens is used in combination with a beta-blocker and the treatment has to be stopped, the beta-blocker should be stopped first and then Physiotens after a few days have elapsed.

In patients with moderate renal dysfunction (GFR above 30 but below 60 ml/min, serum creatinine above 105 but below 160 μmol), the hypotensive effect of Physiotens should be closely monitored, especially at the start of treatment.

Due to lack of therapeutic experience, the use of Physiotens concomitantly with alcohol or tricyclic antidepressants should be avoided.

Due to a lack of clinical data supporting the safety in patients with co-existing moderate heart failure, Physiotens must be used with caution in such patients.

Treatment with Physiotens should not be discontinued abruptly, but should be withdrawn gradually over a period of two weeks.

4.5 Interaction with other medicinal products and other forms of Interaction

Concurrent administration of other antihypertensive agents enhances the hypotensive effect of Physiotens.

The effect of sedatives and hypnotics may be intensified by Physiotens. The sedative effect of benzodiazepines can be enhanced by concurrent administration of Physiotens.

4.6 Pregnancy and lactation

As insufficient data are available, Physiotens should not be used during pregnancy.

Physiotens should not be used during lactation because it is excreted into breast milk.

4.7 Effects on ability to drive and use machines

No data are available to suggest that Physiotens adversely affects the ability to drive or operate machines. However, as somnolence and dizziness have been reported, patients should be cautioned about their ability to undertake potentially hazardous tasks such as driving and operating machinery if so affected.

4.8 Undesirable effects

At the start of treatment dry mouth is frequently observed, while headache, asthenia, dizziness, nausea, sleep disturbances and vasodilatation are observed occasionally. Sedation has been reported in less than 1% of patients. The frequency and intensity of these symptoms often decrease in the course of treatment.

Allergic skin reactions have been reported in very rare cases.

Isolated cases of angioedema have been reported.

4.9 Overdose

Oral dosages up to 2.0 mg/day have been tolerated without the occurrence of serious adverse events. The following case of accidental overdose with Physiotens by a 2 year old child has been reported:

The child ingested an unknown quantity of Physiotens. The maximum dosage possibly ingested was 14 mg. The child had the following symptoms: sedation, coma, hypotension, miosis and dyspnoea. Gastric lavage, glucose infusion, mechanically assisted ventilation and rest resulted in the complete disappearance of the symptoms in 11 hours.

Because of the pharmacodynamic properties of Physiotens, the following symptoms can be expected in adults: sedation, hypotension, orthostatic dysregulation, bradycardia, dry mouth. In rare cases emesis and paradoxical hypertension may occur.

No specific antidote is known. Phentolamine (Rogitine) may, depending on the dose, reverse part of the symptoms of moxonidine overdosage. Measures to support blood circulation are recommended.

5. PHARMACOLOGICAL PROPERTIES

5.1 Pharmacodynamic properties

In different animal models, Physiotens has been shown to be a potent antihypertensive agent. Available experimental data convincingly suggest that the site of the antihypertensive action of Physiotens is the central nervous system (CNS). Within the brainstem, Physiotens has been shown to selectively interact with I_1-imidazoline receptors. These imidazoline-sensitive receptors are concentrated in the rostral ventrolateral medulla, an area critical to the central control of the peripheral sympathetic nervous system. The net effect of this interaction with the I_1-imidazoline receptor appears to result in a reduced activity of sympathetic nerves (demonstrated for cardiac, splanchnic and renal sympathetic nerves).

Physiotens differs from other available centrally acting antihypertensives by exhibiting only low affinity to central α_2-adrenoceptors as compared to I_1-imidazoline receptors; α_2-adrenoceptors are considered the molecular target via which sedation and dry mouth, the most common undesired side effects of centrally acting antihypertensives, are mediated.

In humans, Physiotens leads to a reduction of systemic vascular resistance and consequently in arterial blood pressure.

5.2 Pharmacokinetic properties

Oral moxonidine treatment of rats and dogs resulted in rapid and almost complete absorption and peak plasma levels within <0.5 hours. Average plasma concentrations were comparable in both species after p.o. and i.v. administration. The elimination half-lives of radioactivity and unchanged compound were estimated to be 1-3 hours. Moxonidine and its two main metabolites (4,5-dehydromoxonidine and a guanidine derivative) was predominantly excreted in the urine. No indication of moxonidine cumulation was observed in either species during chronic toxicity studies after 52 weeks.

In humans, about 90% of an oral dose of moxonidine is absorbed; it is not subject to first-pass metabolism and its bio-availability is 88%. Food intake does not interfere with moxonidine pharmacokinetics. Moxonidine is 10-20% metabolised, mainly to 4,5-dehydromoxonidine and to a guanidine derivative by opening of the imidazoline ring. The hypotensive effect of 4,5-dehydromoxonidine is only 1/10, and that of the guanidine derivative is less than 1/100 of that of moxonidine. The maximum plasma levels of moxonidine are reached 30-180 minutes after the intake of a film-coated tablet.

Only about 7% of moxonidine is bound to plasma protein (Vd_{ss}=1.8 ± 0.4 l/kg). Moxonidine and its metabolites are eliminated almost entirely via the kidneys. More than 90% of the dose is eliminated via the kidneys in the first 24 hours after administration, while only about 1% is eliminated via the faeces. The cumulative renal excretion of unchanged moxonidine is about 50-75%.

The mean plasma elimination half-life of moxonidine is 2.2-2.3 hours, and the renal elimination half-life is 2.6-2.8 hours.

Pharmacokinetics in the elderly

Small differences between the pharmacokinetic properties of moxonidine in the healthy elderly and younger adults are unlikely to be clinically significant. As there is no accumulation of moxonidine, dosage adjustment is unnecessary provided renal function is normal.

Pharmacokinetics in children

No pharmacokinetic studies have been performed in children.

Pharmacokinetics in renal impairment

In moderately impaired renal function (GFR 30-60 ml/min), AUC increased by 85% and clearance decreased to 52%. In such patients the hypotensive effect of Physiotens should be closely monitored, especially at the start of treatment; additionally, single doses should not exceed 200 micrograms and the daily dose should not exceed 400 micrograms.

5.3 Preclinical safety data

Chronic oral treatment for 52 weeks of rats (with dosages of 0.12-4 mg/kg) and dogs (with dosages of 0.04-0.4 mg/kg) revealed significant effects of moxonidine only at the highest doses. Slight disturbances of electrolyte balance (decrease of blood sodium and increase of potassium, urea and creatinine) were found in the high dose rats and emesis and salivation only for the high dose dogs. In addition slight increases of liver weight were obvious for both high dose species.

Reproductive toxicology did not show moxonidine effects (at oral doses up to 6.4 mg/kg) on fertility of rats and development of the embryo and foetus. Neither was evidence seen of embryotoxic and teratogenic properties in the rat at oral doses up to 27 mg/kg and the rabbit up to 4.9 mg/kg, nor on peri- and post-natal development in the rat after oral dosage up to 9 mg/kg.

Five different studies also did not show any indication of mutagenic or genotoxic effects of moxonidine. In addition, carcinogenicity studies in rats and mice at oral doses of 0.1-7.0 mg/kg did not reveal any evidence of carcinogenic potential.

6. PHARMACEUTICAL PARTICULARS

6.1 List of excipients

Lactose, povidone, crospovidone, magnesium stearate, hypromellose, ethylcellulose, polyethylene glycol 6000, talc, red ferric oxide, titanium dioxide.

6.2 Incompatibilities

No incompatibilities are known.

6.3 Shelf life

2 years.

6.4 Special precautions for storage

Do not store above 25°C.

6.5 Nature and contents of container

The tablets are packed in blister strips of 14. The blister strips are made of PVC/PVdC or PVC film with covering Aluminium foil. Each carton contains 14, 28 or 84 tablets.

6.6 Instructions for use and handling

None.

7. MARKETING AUTHORISATION HOLDER

Solvay Healthcare Limited
Mansbridge Road
West End
Southampton
SO18 3JD

8. MARKETING AUTHORISATION NUMBER(S)

200 mcg: PL 00512/0152
300 mcg: PL 00512/0153
400 mcg: PL 00512/0154

9. DATE OF FIRST AUTHORISATION/RENEWAL OF THE AUTHORISATION

15 September 1997/ 5 April 2002

10. DATE OF REVISION OF THE TEXT

March 2002

Picolax

(Ferring Pharmaceuticals Ltd)

1. NAME OF THE MEDICINAL PRODUCT

PICOLAX®

2. QUALITATIVE AND QUANTITATIVE COMPOSITION

Each sachet contains the following active ingredients:

Sodium Picosulfate	10.0mg
Magnesium Oxide, Light	3.5g
Citric Acid, Anhydrous	12.0g

3. PHARMACEUTICAL FORM

Powder for oral solution

White crystalline powder.

4. CLINICAL PARTICULARS

4.1 Therapeutic indications

To clean the bowel prior to X-ray examination, endoscopy or surgery.

4.2 Posology and method of administration

Route of administration: Oral

A low residue diet is recommended on the day prior to the hospital procedure. To avoid dehydration during treatment with PICOLAX it is recommended to drink approximately 250ml per hour, of water or other clear fluid while the washout effect persists.

Directions for reconstitution:

Reconstitute the contents of one sachet in a cup of water (approximately 150ml). Stir for 2-3 minutes and drink the solution. If it becomes hot, wait until it cools sufficiently to drink.

Adults (including the elderly):

One sachet reconstituted in water as directed, taken before 8 am on the day before the procedure. Second sachet 6 to 8 hours later.

Children:

1 - 2 years; ¼ sachet morning, ¼ sachet afternoon

2 - 4 years; ½ sachet morning, ½ sachet afternoon

4 - 9 years; 1 sachet morning, ½ sachet afternoon

9 and above; adult dose

4.3 Contraindications

Hypersensitivity to any of the ingredients of the product, congestive cardiac failure, gastric retention, gastro-intestinal ulceration, toxic colitis, toxic megacolon, ileus, nausea and vomiting, acute surgical abdominal conditions such as acute appendicitis and known or suspected gastro-intestinal obstruction or perforation.

In patients with severely reduced renal function, accumulation of magnesium in plasma may occur. Another preparation should be used in such cases.

4.4 Special warnings and special precautions for use

Recent gastro-intestinal surgery. Care should also be taken in patients with renal impairment, heart disease or inflammatory bowel disease.

Use with caution in patients on drugs that might affect water and/or electrolyte balance e.g. diuretics, corticosteroids, lithium (see 4.5).

PICOLAX may modify the absorption of regularly prescribed oral medication and should be used with caution e.g. there have been isolated reports of seizures in patients on antiepileptics, with previously controlled epilepsy (see 4.5 and 4.8).

An inadequate oral intake of water and electrolytes could create clinically significant, deficiencies, particularly in less fit patients. In this regard, the elderly, debilitated individuals and patients at risk of hypokalaemia may need particular attention. Prompt corrective action should be taken to restore fluid/electrolyte balance in patients with signs or symptoms of hyponatraemia.

The period of bowel cleansing should not exceed 24 hours because longer preparation may increase the risk of water and electrolyte imbalance.

4.5 Interaction with other medicinal products and other forms of Interaction

As a purgative, PICOLAX increases the gastrointestinal transit rate. The absorption of other orally administered medicines (e.g. anti-epileptics, contraceptives, anti-diabetics, antibiotics) may therefore be modified during the treatment period (see 4.4).

The efficacy of PICOLAX is lowered by bulk-forming laxatives.

Care should be taken with patients already receiving drugs which may be associated with hypokalaemia (such as diuretics or corticosteroids, or drugs where hypokalaemia is a particular risk i.e. cardiac glycosides). Caution is also advised when PICOLAX is used in patients on NSAIDs or drugs known to induce SIADH e.g. tricyclic antidepressants, selective serotonin re-uptake inhibitors, antipsychotic drugs and carbamazepine as these drugs may increase the risk of water retention and/or electrolyte imbalance.

4.6 Pregnancy and lactation

Reproduction studies with sodium picosulfate performed in animals have revealed no evidence of a harmful action on the fetus. However, clinical experience of the use of PICOLAX during pregnancy is limited and caution should be observed, particularly during the first trimester.

Neither sodium picosulfate nor magnesium citrate have been shown to be excreted in breast milk.

4.7 Effects on ability to drive and use machines

Not applicable.

4.8 Undesirable effects

Adverse reactions to PICOLAX are very rare (<1 in10,000) and are presented below by System Organ Class and Preferred term.

Immune system disorders

Anaphylactoid reaction, hypersensitivity

Metabolism and nutrition disorders

Hyponatraemia

Nervous system disorders

Epilepsy, grand mal convulsion, convulsions, confusional state, headache

Gastrointestinal disorders

Vomiting, diarrhoea, abdominal pain, nausea, proctalgia

Skin and subcutaneous tissue disorders

Rash (including erythematous and maculo-papular rash), urticaria, pruritus, purpura

General disorders

Drug interaction

Hyponatraemia has been reported with or without associated convulsions (see 4.4). In epileptic patients, there have been isolated reports of seizure/grand mal convulsion without associated hyponatraemia (see 4.4 and 4.5). There have been isolated reports of anaphylactoid reaction (see 4.3).

4.9 Overdose

Overdosage would lead to profuse diarrhoea. Treatment is by general supportive measures and maintenance of fluid intake.

5. PHARMACOLOGICAL PROPERTIES

5.1 Pharmacodynamic properties

The active components of PICOLAX are sodium picosulfate, a stimulant cathartic, active locally in the colon, and magnesium citrate which acts as an osmotic laxative by retaining moisture in the colon. The action is of a powerful 'washing out' effect combined with peristaltic stimulation to clear the bowel prior to radiography, colonoscopy or surgery. The product is not intended for use as a routine laxative.

5.2 Pharmacokinetic properties

Both active components are locally active in the colon, and neither are absorbed in any detectable amounts.

5.3 Preclinical safety data

There are no pre-clinical data of relevance to the prescriber which are additional to that already included in other sections of the SPC.

6. PHARMACEUTICAL PARTICULARS

6.1 List of excipients

Potassium Bicarbonate, Granular

Saccharin Sodium

Natural, spray dried orange flavour which contains acacia gum, lactose, ascorbic acid, butylated hydroxyanisole.

6.2 Incompatibilities

None known

6.3 Shelf life

36 months

6.4 Special precautions for storage

Do not store above 25°C. Store in the original package.

6.5 Nature and contents of container

Sachet:

4 layers: paper-polyethylene-aluminium-surlyn

Each pack contains a pair of sachets that can be separated by tearing apart the perforated strip.

Weight of sachet contents: 16.1g

6.6 Instructions for use and handling

None

7. MARKETING AUTHORISATION HOLDER

Ferring Pharmaceuticals Limited, The Courtyard, Waterside Drive, Langley, Berkshire SL3 6EZ, United Kingdom

8. MARKETING AUTHORISATION NUMBER(S)

PL 3194/0014

9. DATE OF FIRST AUTHORISATION/RENEWAL OF THE AUTHORISATION

1st November 2001

10. DATE OF REVISION OF THE TEXT

December 2003

11. Legal Category

P

Piportil Depot Injection

(sanofi-aventis)

1. NAME OF THE MEDICINAL PRODUCT
Piportil Depot 5% w/v.

2. QUALITATIVE AND QUANTITATIVE COMPOSITION
in terms of the active ingredient

Pipotiazine palmitate 5.0% w/v

3. PHARMACEUTICAL FORM
Depot injection.

4. CLINICAL PARTICULARS

4.1 Therapeutic indications
For the maintenance treatment of schizophrenia and paranoid psychoses and prevention of relapse, especially where compliance with oral medication is a problem

4.2 Posology and method of administration
Patients should be stabilised on Piportil Depot under psychiatric supervision. Administration should be by deep intramuscular injection into the gluteal region. Wide variation of response can be expected. The following dosage recommendations are suitable for either indication.

Adults: Initially 25mg should be given to assess the response of the patient to the drug. Further doses should be administered at appropriate intervals, increasing by increments of 25 or 50mg until a satisfactory response is obtained. In clinical practice, Piportil Depot has been shown to have a long duration of action, allowing intervals of 4 weeks between injections for maintenance therapy.

Dosage should be adjusted under close supervision to suit each individual patient in order to obtain the best therapeutic response compatible with tolerance. The duration of action depends on the dose administered, allowing dosage intervals to be varied to suit individual circumstances.

Most patients respond favourably to a dose of 50-100mg every 4 weeks, the maximum recommended dose is 200mg every four weeks.

Elderly : Neuroleptics should be used cautiously in the elderly: A reduced starting dose is recommended, ie 5-10mg might be considered.

Children : Not recommended for use in children.

4.3 Contraindications
Piportil Depot should not be administered to patients in a comatose state or with marked cerebral atherosclerosis, phaeochromocytoma, renal or liver failure, severe cardiac insufficiency or hypersensitivity to other phenothiazine derivatives.

4.4 Special warnings and special precautions for use
Piportil Depot should be used with caution in patients suffering from or who have a history of, the following conditions: severe respiratory disease, epilepsy, alcohol withdrawal symptoms, brain damage, Parkinson's disease or marked extrapyramidal symptoms with previously used neuroleptics, personal or family history of narrow angle glaucoma, hypothyroidism, myasthenia gravis, prostatic hypertrophy, thyrotoxicosis. Care is required in very hot or very cold weather particularly in elderly frail patients.

Except in emergencies, it is recommended that the biochemical status and an ECG be performed as part of the initial evaluation in patients to be treated with a neuroleptic agent (see Section 4.8 Undesirable Effects).

Acute withdrawal symptoms, including nausea, vomiting, sweating, and insomnia have been described after abrupt cessation of antipsychotic drugs. Recurrence of psychotic symptoms may also occur, and the emergence of involuntary movement disorders (such as akathisia, dystonia and dyskinesia) has been reported. Therefore, gradual withdrawal is advisable.

4.5 Interaction with other medicinal products and other forms of Interaction
There is an increased risk of arrhythmias when antipsychotics are used with drugs which prolong the QT interval including certain antiarrhythmics, antidepressants and other antipsychotics.

The CNS depressant actions of neuroleptic agents may be intensified (additively) by alcohol, barbiturates and other sedatives. Respiratory depression may occur.

The hypotensive effect of most antihypertensive drugs especially alpha adrenoceptor blocking agents may be exaggerated by neuroleptics. This effect may also be observed with anaesthetics and opioid analgesics.

The mild anticholinergic effect of neuroleptics may be enhanced by other anticholinergic drugs possibly leading to constipation, heat stroke, etc.

The action of some drugs may be opposed by phenothiazine neuroleptics; these include amfetamine, levodopa, apomorphine, lisuride, pergolide, bromocriptine, cabergoline, clonidine, guanethidine, adrenaline.

Some drugs may possibly enhance the effects of phenothiazines including cimetidine.

Anticholinergic agents may reduce the antipsychotic effect of neuroleptics.

Some drugs interfere with absorption of neuroleptic agents: antacids, kaolin, anti-Parkinson drugs, lithium. Increases or decreases in the plasma concentrations of a number of drugs, e.g. propranolol, phenobarbitalhave been observed but were not of clinical significance. Concomitant use with ritonavir may possibly increase the plasma concentration of the antipsychotic.

High doses of neuroleptics reduce the response to hypoglycaemic agents, the dosage of which might have to be raised.

There is an increased risk of extrapyramidal effects with tetrabenazine and lithium, and an increased possibility of neurotoxicity with lithium. Sibutramine can lead to an increased risk of CNS toxicity.

Adrenaline must not be used in patients overdosed with phenothiazine neuroleptics. Most of the above interactions are of a theoretical nature and not dangerous. Simultaneous administration of desferrioxamine and prochlorperazine has been observed to induce a transient metabolic encephalopathy characterised by loss of consciousness for 48–72 hours.

It is possible that this may occur with Piportil since it shares many of the pharmacological properties of prochlorperazine.

Avoid concomitant use of clozapine with depot formulation as it cannot be withdrawn quickly if neutropenia occurs.

4.6 Pregnancy and lactation
There is inadequate evidence of safety of Piportil Depot in human pregnancy, although animal studies have shown no hazard. The drug should not be used during pregnancy or lactation unless the physician considers it essential.

4.7 Effects on ability to drive and use machines
Patients should be warned about drowsiness especially at the start of treatment and advised not to drive or operate machinery.

4.8 Undesirable effects
Minor side effects of neuroleptics are drowsiness, especially at the start of treatment, nasal stuffiness, dry mouth, insomnia, agitation and weight gain. Other possible adverse effects are listed below.

Liver function: jaundice, usually transient, occurs in a very small percentage of patients taking neuroleptics. A premonitory sign may be a sudden onset of fever after one to three weeks of treatment followed by the development of jaundice. Neuroleptic jaundice has the biochemical and other characteristics of obstructive jaundice and is associated with obstructions of the canaliculi by bile thrombi; the frequent presence of an accompanying eosinophilia indicates the allergic nature of this phenomenon. Treatment should be withheld on the development of jaundice.

Cardiorespiratory: Hypotension, usually postural, commonly occurs. Elderly or volume depleted subjects are particularly susceptible; it is more likely to occur after intramuscular administration.

Cardiac arrhythmias, including atrial arrhythmia, A-V block, ventricular tachycardia and fibrillation have been reported during neuroleptic therapy, possibly related to dosage. Pre-existing cardiac disease, old age, hypokalaemia and concurrent tricyclic antidepressants may predispose. ECG changes, usually benign, include very rare widened QT interval (as with other neuroleptics), ST depression, U-waves and T-wave changes.

Respiratory depression is possible in susceptible patients.

Blood picture: A mild leukopenia occurs in up to 30% of patients on prolonged high dosage of neuroleptics. Agranulocytosis may occur rarely; it is not dose-related. The occurrence of unexplained infections or fever requires immediate haematological investigation.

Extrapyramidal: Acute dystonias or dyskinesias, usually transitory, are commoner in children and young adults, and usually occur within the first 4 days of treatment or after dosage increases.

- Akathisia characteristically occurs after large initial doses.

- Parkinsonism is commoner in adults and the elderly. It usually develops after weeks or months of treatment. One or more of the following may be seen: tremor, rigidity, akinesia or other features of Parkinsonism. Commonly just tremor.

- Tardive dyskinesia: If this occurs it is usually, but not necessarily, after prolonged or high dosage. It can even occur after treatment has been stopped. Dosage should therefore be kept low whenever possible.

Skin and eyes: contact skin sensitisation is a serious but rare complication in those frequently handling preparations of phenothiazines; the greatest care must be taken to avoid contact of the drug with the skin. Skin rashes of various kinds may also be seen in patients treated with these drugs. Patients on high dosage should be warned that they may develop photosensitivity in sunny weather and should avoid exposure to direct sunlight.

Ocular changes and the development of a metallic greyish-mauve coloration of exposed skin have been noted in some individuals mainly females, who have received chlorpromazine continuously for long periods (four to eight years). Other neuroleptics have been implicated but less frequently.

Endocrine: hyperprolactinaemia which may result in galactorrhoea, gynaecomastia, amenorrhoea; impotence.

Neuroleptic malignant syndrome (hyperthermia, rigidity, autonomic dysfunction and altered consciousness) may occur with any neuroleptic.

4.9 Overdose
Symptoms of phenothiazine overdosage include drowsiness or loss of consciousness, hypotension, tachycardia, ECG changes, ventricular arrhythmias and hypothermia. Severe extrapyramidal dyskinesias may occur.

Generalised vasodilatation may result in circulatory collapse; raising the patient's legs may suffice, in severe cases, volume expansion by intravenous fluids may be needed; infusion fluids should be warmed before administration in order not to aggravate hypothermia.

Positive inotropic agents such as dopamine may be tried if fluid replacement is insufficient to correct the circulatory collapse. Peripheral vasoconstrictor agents are not generally recommended; avoid the use of adrenaline.

Ventricular or supraventricular tachy-arrhythmias usually respond to restoration of normal body temperature and correction of circulatory or metabolic disturbances. If they are persistent or life threatening, appropriate anti-arrhythmic therapy may be considered. Avoid lidocaine and, as far as possible, long acting anti-arrhythmic drugs.

Pronounced central nervous system depression requires airway maintenance or, in extreme circumstances, assisted respiration. Severe dystonic reactions usually respond to procyclidine (5-10mg) or orphenadrine (20-40mg) administered intramuscularly or intravenously. Convulsions should be treated with intravenous diazepam.

Neuroleptic malignant syndrome should be treated with cooling. Dantrolene sodium may be tried.

5. PHARMACOLOGICAL PROPERTIES

5.1 Pharmacodynamic properties
Slow release phenothiazine neuroleptic

5.2 Pharmacokinetic properties
There is little information about blood levels, distribution and excretion in humans. The rate of metabolism and excretion of phenothiazines decreases in old age

5.3 Preclinical safety data
There are no pre-clinical data of relevance to the prescriber which are additional to that already included in other sections of the SPC.

6. PHARMACEUTICAL PARTICULARS

6.1 List of excipients
Sesame oil (peroxide-free)

6.2 Incompatibilities
Piportil Depot injection should not be admixed with any other substance.

6.3 Shelf life
60 months

6.4 Special precautions for storage
Protect from light

6.5 Nature and contents of container
1 and 2ml clear glass ampoules- pack containing 10 ampoules.

6.6 Instructions for use and handling
None stated

7. MARKETING AUTHORISATION HOLDER
JHC Healthcare Ltd

5 Lower Merrion Street

Dublin 2

Eire

8. MARKETING AUTHORISATION NUMBER(S)
PL16186/0006

9. DATE OF FIRST AUTHORISATION/RENEWAL OF THE AUTHORISATION
1st September 1997

10. DATE OF REVISION OF THE TEXT
November 2004

Legal Classification: POM

Plaquenil Tablets

(sanofi-aventis)

1. NAME OF THE MEDICINAL PRODUCT
Plaquenil Tablets

2. QUALITATIVE AND QUANTITATIVE COMPOSITION
Hydroxychloroquine Sulphate BP 200mg

3. PHARMACEUTICAL FORM
Film coated tablet.

4. CLINICAL PARTICULARS

4.1 Therapeutic indications
Treatment of rheumatoid arthritis, juvenile chronic arthritis, discoid and systemic lupus erythematosus, and dermatological conditions caused or aggravated by sunlight.

4.2 Posology and method of administration

Adults (including the elderly)

The minimum effective dose should be employed. This dose should not exceed 6.5mg/kg/day (calculated from ideal body weight and not actual body weight) and will be either 200mg or 400mg per day.

In patients able to receive 400mg daily:

Initially 400mg daily in divided doses. The dose can be reduced to 200mg when no further improvement is evident. The maintenance dose should be increased to 400mg daily if the response lessens.

Children

The minimum effective dose should be employed and should not exceed 6.5mg/kg/day based on ideal body weight. The 200mg tablet is therefore not suitable for use in children with an ideal body weight of less than 31kg.

Each dose should be taken with a meal or glass of milk.

Hydroxychloroquine is cumulative in action and will require several weeks to exert its beneficial effects, whereas minor side effects may occur relatively early. For rheumatic disease treatment should be discontinued if there is no improvement by 6 months. In light-sensitive diseases, treatment should only be given during periods of maximum exposure to light.

The tablets are for oral administration.

4.3 Contraindications

- known hypersensitivity to 4-aminoquinoline compounds
- pre-existing maculopathy of the eye
- pregnancy (see section 4.6 Pregnancy and lactation).

4.4 Special warnings and special precautions for use

General

• The occurrence of retinopathy is very uncommon if the recommended daily dose is not exceeded. The administration of doses in excess of the recommended maximum is likely to increase the risk of retinopathy, and accelerate its onset.

• All patients should have an ophthalmological examination before initiating treatment with Plaquenil. Thereafter, ophthalmological examinations must be repeated at least every 12 months.

The examination should include testing visual acuity, careful ophthalmoscopy, fundoscopy and central visual field testing with a red target.

This examination should be more frequent and adapted to the patient in the following situations:

- daily dosage exceeds 6.5mg/kg lean body weight. Absolute body weight used as a guide to dosage could result in an overdosage in the obese.
- renal insufficiency
- visual acuity below 6/8
- age above 65 years
- cumulative dose more than 200 g.

Plaquenil should be discontinued immediately in any patient who develops a pigmentary abnormality, visual field defect, or any other abnormality not explainable by difficulty in accommodation or presence of corneal opacities. Patients should continue to be observed for possible progression of the changes.

Patients should be advised to stop taking the drug immediately and seek the advice of their prescribing doctor if any disturbances of vision are noted.

Plaquenil should be used with caution in patients taking medicines which may cause adverse ocular or skin reactions. Caution should also be applied when it is used in the following:

• patients with hepatic or renal disease, and in those taking drugs known to affect those organs. Estimation of plasma hydroxychloroquine levels should be undertaken in patients with severely compromised renal or hepatic function and dosage adjusted accordingly.

• patients with severe gastrointestinal, neurological or blood disorders.

Although the risk of bone marrow depression is low, periodic blood counts are advisable and Plaquenil should be discontinued if abnormalities develop.

Caution is also advised in patients with a sensitivity to quinine, those with glucose-6-phosphate dehydrogenase deficiency, those with porphyria cutanea tarda which can be exacerbated by hydroxychloroquine and in patients with psoriasis since it appears to increase the risk of skin reactions.

Patients with rare hereditary problems of galactose intolerance, the Lapp lactase deficiency or glucose-galactose malabsorption should not take this medicine.

Small children are particularly sensitive to the toxic effects of 4-aminoquinolines; therefore patients should be warned to keep Plaquenil out of the reach of children.

All patients on long-term therapy should undergo periodic examination of skeletal muscle function and tendon reflexes. If weakness occurs, the drug should be withdrawn.

4.5 Interaction with other medicinal products and other forms of Interaction

Hydroxychloroquine sulphate has been reported to increase plasma digoxin levels: serum digoxin levels should be closely monitored in patients receiving combined therapy.

Hydroxychloroquine sulphate may also be subject to several of the known interactions of chloroquine even though specific reports have not appeared. These include: potentiation of its direct blocking action at the neuromuscular junction by aminoglycoside antibiotics; inhibition of its metabolism by cimetidine which may increase plasma concentration of the antimalarial; antagonism of effect of neostigmine and pyridostigmine; reduction of the antibody response to primary immunisation with intradermal human diploid-cell rabies vaccine.

As with chloroquine, antacids may reduce absorption of hydroxychloroquine so it is advised that a 4 hour interval be observed between Plaquenil and antacid dosaging.

As hydroxychloroquine may enhance the effects of a hypoglycaemic treatment, a decrease in doses of insulin or antidiabetic drugs may be required.

4.6 Pregnancy and lactation

Pregnancy:

Hydroxychloroquine crosses the placenta. Data are limited regarding the use of hydroxychloroquine during pregnancy. It should be noted that 4-aminoquinolines in therapeutic doses have been associated with central nervous system damage, including ototoxicity (auditory and vestibular toxicity, congenital deafness), retinal hemorrhages and abnormal retinal pigmentation. Therefore Plaquenil should not be used in pregnancy.

Lactation:

Careful consideration should be given to using hydroxychloroquine during lactation, since it has been shown to be excreted in small amounts in human breast milk, and it is known that infants are extremely sensitive to the toxic effects of 4-aminoquinolines.

4.7 Effects on ability to drive and use machines

Impaired visual accommodation soon after the start of treatment has been reported and patients should be warned regarding driving or operating machinery. If the condition is not self-limiting, it will resolve on reducing the dose or stopping treatment.

4.8 Undesirable effects

• Ocular effects:

Retinopathy with changes in pigmentation and visual field defects can occur, but appears to be uncommon if the recommended daily dose is not exceeded. In its early form it appears reversible on discontinuation of Plaquenil. If allowed to develop, there may be a risk of progression even after treatment withdrawal.

Patients with retinal changes may be asymptomatic initially, or may have scotomatous vision with paracentral, pericentral ring types and temporal scotomas.

Corneal changes including oedema and opacities have been reported. They are either symptomless or may cause disturbances such as haloes, blurring of vision or photophobia. They may be transient and are reversible on stopping treatment.

Blurring of vision due to a disturbance of accommodation which is dose dependent and reversible may also occur.

• Dermatologic effects:

Skin rashes sometimes occur; pruritus, pigmentary changes in skin and mucous membranes, bleaching of hair and alopecia have also been reported. These usually resolve readily on stopping treatment.

Bullous eruptions including very rare cases of erythema multiforme and Stevens-Johnson syndrome, photosensitivity and isolated cases of exfoliative dermatitis have been reported. Very rare cases of acute generalised exanthematous pustulosis (AGEP) has to be distinguished from psoriasis, although hydroxychloroquine may precipitate attacks of psoriasis. It may be associated with fever and hyperleukocytosis. Outcome is usually favourable after drug withdrawal.

• Gastrointestinal effects:

Gastrointestinal disturbances such as nausea, diarrhoea, anorexia, abdominal pain and, rarely, vomiting may occur. These symptoms usually resolve immediately on reducing the dose or on stopping treatment.

• CNS effects:

Less frequently, dizziness, vertigo, tinnitus, hearing loss, headache, nervousness, emotional lability, toxic psychosis and convulsions have been reported.

• Neuromuscular effects:

Skeletal muscle myopathy or neuromyopathy leading to progressive weakness and atrophy of proximal muscle groups have been noted. Myopathy may be reversible after drug discontinuation, but recovery may take many months.

Associated mild sensory changes, depression of tendon reflexes and abnormal nerve conduction may be observed.

• Cardio-vascular effects:

Cardiomyopathy has been rarely reported.

Chronic toxicity should be suspected when conduction disorders (bundle branch block/atrioventricular heart block) as well as biventricular hypertrophy are found. Drug withdrawal may lead to recovery.

• Hematologic effects:

Rarely, there have been reports of bone-marrow depression.

Hydroxychloroquine may precipitate or exacerbate porphyria.

• Liver effects:

Isolated cases of abnormal liver function tests have been reported; rare cases of fulminant hepatic failure have also been reported.

4.9 Overdose

Overdosage with the 4-aminoquinolines is dangerous particularly in infants, as little as 1-2g having proved fatal.

The symptoms of overdosage may include headache, visual disturbances, cardiovascular collapse, convulsions, hypokalaemia, and rhythm and conduction disorders, followed by sudden and early respiratory and cardiac arrest. Since these effects may appear soon after taking a massive dose, treatment should be prompt and symptomatic. The stomach should be immediately evacuated, either by emesis or by gastric lavage. Activated charcoal in a dose at least five times of the overdose may inhibit further absorption if introduced into the stomach by tube following lavage and within 30 minutes of ingestion of the overdose.

Consideration should be given to administration of parenteral diazepam in cases of overdosage; it has been shown to be beneficial in reversing chloroquine cardiotoxicity.

Respiratory support and shock management should be instituted as necessary.

5. PHARMACOLOGICAL PROPERTIES

5.1 Pharmacodynamic properties

Antimalarial agents like chloroquine and hydroxychloroquine have several pharmacological actions which may be involved in their therapeutic effect in the treatment of rheumatic disease, but the role of each is not known. These include interaction with sulphydryl groups, interference with enzyme activity (including phospholipase, NADH - cytochrome C reductase, cholinesterase, proteases and hydrolases), DNA binding, stabilisation of lysosomal membranes, inhibition of prostaglandin formation, inhibition of polymorphonuclear cell chemotaxis and phagocytosis, possible interference with interleukin 1 production from monocytes and inhibition of neutrophil superoxide release.

5.2 Pharmacokinetic properties

Hydroxychloroquine has actions, pharmacokinetics and metabolism similar to those of chloroquine. Following oral administration, hydroxychloroquine is rapidly and almost completely absorbed. In one study, mean peak plasma hydroxychloroquine concentrations following a single dose of 400mg in healthy subjects ranged from 53-208ng/ml with a mean of 105ng/ml. The mean time to peak plasma concentration was 1.83 hours. The mean plasma elimination half-life varied, depending on the post-administration period, as follows: 5.9 hours at C_{max}-10 hours), 26.1 hours (at 10-48 hours) and 299 hours (at 48-504 hours). The parent compound and metabolites are widely distributed in the body and elimination is mainly via the urine, where 3% of the administered dose was recovered over 24 hours in one study

5.3 Preclinical safety data

There are no preclinical safety data of relevance to the prescriber, which are additional to that already included in other sections of the SPC.

6. PHARMACEUTICAL PARTICULARS

6.1 List of excipients

Lactose monohydrate, maize starch, magnesium stearate, polyvidone, Opadry OY-L-28900 (containing hypromellose, macrogol 4000, titanium dioxide (E171), lactose).

6.2 Incompatibilities

No incompatibilities are known.

6.3 Shelf life

36 months.

6.4 Special precautions for storage

Store below 25°C.

6.5 Nature and contents of container

200μm clear PVC/20μm aluminium foil blister pack containing 60 tablets.

6.6 Instructions for use and handling

None.

7. MARKETING AUTHORISATION HOLDER

Sanofi-Synthelabo
PO Box 597
Guildford
Surrey

8. MARKETING AUTHORISATION NUMBER(S)

PL 11723/0150

9. DATE OF FIRST AUTHORISATION/RENEWAL OF THE AUTHORISATION

27 August 1997

10. DATE OF REVISION OF THE TEXT

March 2003

Legal Category POM

Plavix (Sanofi Pharma Bristol-Myers Squibb SNC)

(Sanofi Pharma Bristol-Myers Squibb SNC)

1. NAME OF THE MEDICINAL PRODUCT
Plavix 75 mg film-coated tablets

2. QUALITATIVE AND QUANTITATIVE COMPOSITION
Clopidogrel hydrogen sulphate 97.875 mg (molar equivalent of 75 mg of clopidogrel base)

For excipients, see 6.1.

3. PHARMACEUTICAL FORM
Film-coated tablet.

Plavix 75 mg film-coated tablets are pink, round, biconvex, film-coated, and engraved with «75» on one side and «1171» on the other side.

4. CLINICAL PARTICULARS

4.1 Therapeutic indications
Clopidogrel is indicated for the prevention of atherothrombotic events in:

• Patients suffering from myocardial infarction (from a few days until less than 35 days), ischaemic stroke (from 7 days until less than 6 months) or established peripheral arterial disease.

• Patients suffering from non-ST segment elevation acute coronary syndrome (unstable angina or non-Q-wave myocardial infarction) in combination with acetylsalicylic acid (ASA).

For further information please refer to section 5.1.

4.2 Posology and method of administration
• Adults and elderly

Clopidogrel should be given as a single daily dose of 75 mg with or without food.

In patients with non-ST segment elevation acute coronary syndrome (unstable angina or non-Q-wave myocardial infarction), clopidogrel treatment should be initiated with a single 300 mg loading dose and then continued at 75 mg once a day (with ASA 75 mg-325 mg daily). Since higher doses of ASA were associated with higher bleeding risk it is recommended that the dose of ASA should not be higher than 100 mg. The optimal duration of treatment has not been formally established. Clinical trial data support use up to 12 months, and the maximum benefit was seen at 3 months(see section 5.1).

• Children and adolescents

Safety and efficacy in subjects below the age of 18 have not been established.

4.3 Contraindications
• Hypersensitivity to the active substance or to any of the excipients of the medicinal product.

• Severe liver impairment.

• Active pathological bleeding such as peptic ulcer or intracranial haemorrhage.

• Breast-feeding (see section 4.6).

4.4 Special warnings and special precautions for use
Due to the risk of bleeding and haematological undesirable effects, blood cell count determination and/or other appropriate testing should be promptly considered whenever clinical symptoms suggestive of bleeding arise during the course of treatment (see section 4.8). As with other antiplatelet agents, clopidogrel should be used with caution in patients who may be at risk of increased bleeding from trauma, surgery or other pathological conditions and in patients receiving treatment with ASA, non-steroidal anti-inflammatory drugs, heparin, glycoprotein IIb/IIIa inhibitors or thrombolytics. Patients should be followed carefully for any signs of bleeding including occult bleeding, especially during the first weeks of treatment and/or after invasive cardiac procedures or surgery. The concomitant administration of clopidogrel with warfarin is not recommended since it may increase the intensity of bleedings (see section 4.5).

If a patient is to undergo elective surgery and antiplatelet effect is not necessary, clopidogrel should be discontinued 7 days prior to surgery. Clopidogrel prolongs bleeding time and should be used with caution in patients who have lesions with a propensity to bleed (particularly gastrointestinal and intraocular).

Patients should be told that it might take longer than usual to stop bleeding when they take clopidogrel (alone or in combination with ASA), and that they should report any unusual bleeding (site or duration) to their physician. Patients should inform physicians and dentists that they are taking clopidogrel before any surgery is scheduled and before any new drug is taken.

Thrombotic Thrombocytopenic Purpura (TTP) has been reported very rarely following the use of clopidogrel, sometimes after a short exposure. It is characterised by thrombocytopenia and microangiopathic hemolytic anemia associated with either neurological findings, renal dysfunction or fever. TTP is a potentially fatal condition requiring prompt treatment including plasmapheresis.

In view of the lack of data, in patients with acute myocardial infarction with ST-segment elevation, clopidogrel therapy should not be initiated within the first few days following myocardial infarction.

In view of the lack of data, clopidogrel cannot be recommended in acute ischaemic stroke (less than 7 days).

Therapeutic experience with clopidogrel is limited in patients with renal impairment. Therefore clopidogrel should be used with caution in these patients.

Experience is limited in patients with moderate hepatic disease who may have bleeding diatheses. Clopidogrel should therefore be used with caution in this population.

4.5 Interaction with other medicinal products and other forms of Interaction
Warfarin: the concomitant administration of clopidogrel with warfarin is not recommended since it may increase the intensity of bleedings (see section 4.4).

Glycoprotein IIb/IIIa inhibitors: clopidogrel should be used with caution in patients who may be at risk of increased bleeding from trauma, surgery or other pathological conditions that receive concomitant glycoprotein IIb/IIIa inhibitors. (see section 4.4)

Acetylsalicylic acid (ASA): ASA did not modify the clopidogrel-mediated inhibition of ADP-induced platelet aggregation, but clopidogrel potentiated the effect of ASA on collagen-induced platelet aggregation. However, concomitant administration of 500 mg of ASA twice a day for one day did not significantly increase the prolongation of bleeding time induced by clopidogrel intake. A pharmacodynamic interaction between clopidogrel and acetylsalicylic acid is possible, leading to increased risk of bleeding. Therefore, concomitant use should be undertaken with caution (see section 4.4). However, clopidogrel and ASA have been administered together for up to one year (see section 5.1).

Heparin: in a clinical study conducted in healthy subjects, clopidogrel did not necessitate modification of the heparin dose or alter the effect of heparin on coagulation. Co-administration of heparin had no effect on the inhibition of platelet aggregation induced by clopidogrel. A pharmacodynamic interaction between clopidogrel and heparin is possible, leading to increased risk of bleeding. Therefore, concomitant use should be undertaken with caution (see section 4.4).

Thrombolytics: the safety of the concomitant administration of clopidogrel, rt-PA and heparin was assessed in patients with recent myocardial infarction. The incidence of clinically significant bleeding was similar to that observed when rt-PA and heparin are co-administered with ASA. The safety of the concomitant administration of clopidogrel with other thrombolytic agents has not been formally established and should be undertaken with caution (see section 4.4).

Non-Steroidal Anti-Inflammatory Drugs (NSAIDs): in a clinical study conducted in healthy volunteers, the concomitant administration of clopidogrel and naproxen increased occult gastrointestinal blood loss. However, due to the lack of interaction studies with other NSAIDs it is presently unclear whether there is an increased risk of gastrointestinal bleeding with all NSAIDs. Consequently, NSAIDs and clopidogrel should be co-administered with caution (see section 4.4).

Other concomitant therapy: a number of other clinical studies have been conducted with clopidogrel and other concomitant medications to investigate the potential for pharmacodynamic and pharmacokinetic interactions. No clinically significant pharmacodynamic interactions were observed when clopidogrel was co-administered with atenolol, nifedipine, or both atenolol and nifedipine. Furthermore, the pharmacodynamic activity of clopidogrel was not significantly influenced by the co-administration of phenobarbital, cimetidine, or oestrogen.

The pharmacokinetics of digoxin or theophylline were not modified by the co-administration of clopidogrel. Antacids did not modify the extent of clopidogrel absorption.

Data from studies with human liver microsomes indicated that the carboxylic acid metabolite of clopidogrel could inhibit the activity of Cytochrome P_{450} 2C9. This could potentially lead to increased plasma levels of drugs such as phenytoin and tolbutamide and the NSAIDs, which are metabolised by Cytochrome P_{450} 2C9. Data from the CAPRIE study indicate that phenytoin and tolbutamide can be safely co-administered with clopidogrel.

Apart from the specific drug interaction information described above, interaction studies with clopidogrel and some drugs commonly administered in patients with atherothrombotic disease have not been performed. However, patients entered into clinical trials with clopidogrel received a variety of concomitant medications including diuretics, beta blockers, ACEI, calcium antagonists, cholesterol lowering agents, coronary vasodilators, antidiabetic agents (including insulin), antiepileptic agents, hormone replacement therapy and GPIIb/IIIa antagonists without evidence of clinically significant adverse interactions.

4.6 Pregnancy and lactation
• Pregnancy

As no clinical data on exposed pregnancies are available, it is preferable not to use clopidogrel during pregnancy as a precautionary measure.

Animal studies do not indicate direct or indirect harmful effects with respect to pregnancy, embryonic/foetal development, parturition or postnatal development (see section 5.3).

• Lactation

Studies in rats have shown that clopidogrel and/or its metabolites are excreted in the milk. It is not known whether this medicinal product is excreted in human milk.

4.7 Effects on ability to drive and use machines
Clopidogrel has no or negligible influence on the ability to drive and use machines.

4.8 Undesirable effects
Clinical studies experience:

Clopidogrel has been evaluated for safety in more than 17,500 patients, including over 9,000 patients treated for 1 year or more. Clopidogrel 75 mg/day was well tolerated compared to ASA 325 mg/day in CAPRIE. The overall tolerability of clopidogrel in this study was similar to ASA, regardless of age, gender and race. The clinically relevant adverse effects observed in the CAPRIE and CURE studies are discussed below.

Haemorrhagic disorders:

In CAPRIE, in patients treated with either clopidogrel or ASA, the overall incidence of any bleeding was 9.3%. The incidence of severe cases was 1.4% for clopidogrel and 1.6% for ASA.

In patients that received clopidogrel, gastrointestinal bleeding occurred at a rate of 2.0%, and required hospitalisation in 0.7%. In patients that received ASA, the corresponding rates were 2.7% and 1.1%, respectively.

The incidence of other bleedings was higher in patients that received clopidogrel compared to ASA (7.3% vs. 6.5%). However, the incidence of severe events was similar in both treatment groups (0.6% vs. 0.4%). The most frequently reported events in both treatment groups were: purpura/bruising/haematoma, and epistaxis. Other less frequently reported events were haematoma, haematuria, and eye bleeding (mainly conjunctival).

The incidence of intracranial bleeding was 0.4% in patients that received clopidogrel and 0.5% for patients that received ASA.

In CURE, the administration of clopidogrel+ASA as compared to placebo+ASA was not associated with a statistically significant increase in life-threatening bleeds (event rates 2.2% vs. 1.8%) or fatal bleeds (0.2% vs. 0.2%), but the risk of major, minor and other bleedings was significantly higher with clopidogrel+ASA: non-life-threatening major bleeds (1.6% clopidogrel+ASA vs. 1.0% placebo+ASA), primarily gastrointestinal and at puncture sites, and minor bleeds (5.1% clopidogrel+ASA vs. 2.4% placebo+ASA). The incidence of intracranial bleeding was 0.1% in both groups.

The major bleeding event rate for clopidogrel+ASA was dose-dependent on ASA (<100mg: 2.6%; 100-200mg: 3.5%; >200mg: 4.9%) as was the major bleeding event rate for placebo+ASA (<100mg: 2.0%; 100-200mg: 2.3%; >200mg: 4.0%).

The risk of bleeding (life-threatening, major, minor, other) decreased during the course of the trial: 0-1 months [clopidogrel: 599/6259 (9.6%); placebo: 413/6303 (6.6%)], 1-3 months [clopidogrel: 276/6123 (4.5%); placebo: 144/6168 (2.3%)], 3-6 months [clopidogrel: 228/6037 (3.8%); placebo: 99/6048 (1.6%)], 6-9 months [clopidogrel: 162/5005 (3.2%); placebo: 74/4972 (1.5%)], 9-12 months [clopidogrel: 73/3841 (1.9%); placebo: 40/3844 (1.0%)].

There was no excess in major bleeds within 7 days after coronary bypass graft surgery in patients who stopped therapy more than five days prior to surgery (4.4% clopidogrel+ASA vs. 5.3% placebo+ASA). In patients who remained on therapy within five days of bypass graft surgery, the event rate was 9.6% for clopidogrel+ASA, and 6.3% for placebo+ASA.

Haematological disorders:

In CAPRIE, severe neutropenia ($<0.45 \times 10^9$/l) was observed in 4 patients (0.04%) that received clopidogrel and 2 patients (0.02%) that received ASA. Two of the 9599 patients who received clopidogrel and none of the 9586 patients who received ASA had neutrophil counts of zero. One case of aplastic anaemia occurred on clopidogrel treatment.

The incidence of severe thrombocytopenia ($<80 \times 10^9$/l) was 0.2% on clopidogrel and 0.1% on ASA.

In CURE, the numbers of patients with thrombocytopenia (19 clopidogrel+ASA vs. 24 placebo+ASA) or neutropenia (3 vs. 3) were similar in both groups.

Other clinically relevant adverse drug reactions pooled from CAPRIE and CURE studies with an incidence ≥ 0.1% as well as all serious and relevant ADR are listed below according to the World Health Organisation classification. Their frequency is defined using the following conventions: common > 1/100, <1/10); uncommon > 1/1,000, < 1/100); rare >1/10,000, <1/1,000).

- Central and peripheral nervous system disorders:

- Uncommon: Headache, Dizziness and Paraesthesia
- Rare: Vertigo

- Gastrointestinal system disorders

- Common: Dyspepsia, Abdominal pain and Diarrhoea
- Uncommon: Nausea, Gastritis, Flatulence, Constipation, Vomiting, Gastric ulcer and Duodenal ulcer

- Platelet, bleeding and clotting disorders

- Uncommon: Bleeding time increased and Platelets decreased

- Skin and appendages disorders:

- Uncommon: Rash and Pruritus

- White cell and RES disorders

- Uncommon: Leucopenia, Neutrophils decreased and Eosinophilia

Post-marketing experience:

Bleeding is the most common reaction reported in the post-marketing experience and was mostly reported during the first month of treatment.

Bleeding: some cases were reported with fatal outcome (especially intracranial, gastrointestinal and retroperitoneal haemorrhage); serious cases of skin bleeding (purpura), musculo-skeletal bleeding (haemarthrosis, haematoma), eye bleeding (conjunctival, ocular, retinal), epistaxis, respiratory tract bleeding (haemoptysis, pulmonary haemorrhage), haematuria and haemorrhage of operative wound have been reported; cases of serious haemorrhage have been reported in patients taking clopidogrel concomitantly with acetylsalicylic acid or clopidogrel with acetylsalicylic acid and heparin (see section 4.4).

In addition to clinical studies experience, the following adverse reactions have been spontaneously reported. Within each system organ class (MedDRA classification), they are ranked under heading of frequency. "Very rare" corresponds to < 1/10,000.

Blood and lymphatic system disorders:

- Very rare: Thrombotic Thrombocytopenic Purpura (TTP) (1/200,000 exposed patients) (see section 4.4), severe Thrombocytopenia (platelet count $\leqslant 30 \times 10^9$/l), Granulocytopenia, Agranulocytosis, Anaemia and Aplastic Anaemia/Pancytopenia.

Immune system disorders:

- Very rare: Anaphylactoid reactions, Serum sickness

Psychiatric disorders:

- Very rare: Confusion, Hallucinations

Nervous system disorders:

- Very rare: Taste disturbances

Vascular disorders:

- Very rare: Vasculitis, Hypotension

Respiratory, thoracic and mediastinal disorders:

- Very rare: Bronchospasm, Interstitial pneumonitis

Gastrointestinal disorders:

- Very rare: Colitis (including ulcerative or lymphocytic colitis), Pancreatitis, Stomatitis

Hepato-biliary disorders

- Very rare: Hepatitis, Acute liver failure

Skin and subcutaneous tissue disorders:

- Very rare: Angioedema, Bullous dermatitis (erythema multiforme, Stevens Johnson Syndrome..), rash erythematous, urticaria, eczema and lichen planus

Musculoskeletal, connective tissue and bone disorders:

- Very rare: Arthralgia, Arthritis, Myalgia

Renal and urinary disorders:

- Very rare: Glomerulonephritis

General disorders and administration site conditions

- Very rare: Fever

Investigations:

- Very rare: Abnormal liver function test, Blood creatinine increase

4.9 Overdose

Overdose following clopidogrel administration may lead to prolonged bleeding time and subsequent bleeding complications. Appropriate therapy should be considered if bleedings are observed.

No antidote to the pharmacological activity of clopidogrel has been found. If prompt correction of prolonged bleeding time is required, platelet transfusion may reverse the effects of clopidogrel.

5. PHARMACOLOGICAL PROPERTIES

5.1 Pharmacodynamic properties

Pharmacotherapeutical group: platelet aggregation inhibitors excl. Heparin, ATC Code: BO1AC/04.

Clopidogrel selectively inhibits the binding of adenosine diphosphate (ADP) to its platelet receptor, and the subsequent ADP-mediated activation of the GPIIb/IIIa complex, thereby inhibiting platelet aggregation. Biotransformation of clopidogrel is necessary to produce inhibition of platelet aggregation. Clopidogrel also inhibits platelet aggregation induced by other agonists by blocking the amplification of platelet activation by released ADP. Clopidogrel acts by irreversibly modifying the platelet ADP receptor. Consequently, platelets exposed to clopidogrel are affected for the remainder of their lifespan and recovery of normal platelet function occurs at a rate consistent with platelet turnover.

Repeated doses of 75 mg per day produced substantial inhibition of ADP-induced platelet aggregation from the first day; this increased progressively and reached steady state between Day 3 and Day 7. At steady state, the average inhibition level observed with a dose of 75 mg per day was between 40% and 60%. Platelet aggregation and bleeding time gradually returned to baseline values, generally within 5 days after treatment was discontinued.

The safety and efficacy of clopidogrel in preventing vascular ischaemic events have been evaluated in two double-blind studies: the CAPRIE study, a comparison of clopidogrel to ASA, and the CURE study, a comparison of clopidogrel in combination with ASA, to placebo with ASA.

The CAPRIE study included 19,185 patients with atherothrombosis as manifested by recent myocardial infarction (<35 days), recent ischaemic stroke (between 7 days and 6 months) or established peripheral arterial disease (PAD). Patients were randomised to clopidogrel 75 mg/day or ASA 325 mg/day, and were followed for 1 to 3 years. In the myocardial infarction subgroup, most of the patients received ASA for the first few days following the acute myocardial infarction.

Clopidogrel significantly reduced the incidence of new ischaemic events (combined end point of myocardial infarction, ischaemic stroke and vascular death) when compared to ASA. In the intention to treat analysis, 939 events were observed in the clopidogrel group and 1,020 events with ASA (relative risk reduction (RRR) 8.7%, [95% CI: 0.2 to 16.4]; p = 0.045), which corresponds, for every 1000 patients treated for 2 years, to 10 [CI: 0 to 20] additional patients being prevented from experiencing a new ischaemic event. Analysis of total mortality as a secondary endpoint did not show any significant difference between clopidogrel (5.8%) and ASA (6.0%).

In a subgroup analysis by qualifying condition (myocardial infarction, ischaemic stroke, and PAD) the benefit appeared to be strongest (achieving statistical significance at p = 0.003) in patients enrolled due to PAD (especially those who also had a history of myocardial infarction) (RRR = 23.7%; CI: 8.9 to 36.2) and weaker (not significantly different from ASA) in stroke patients (RRR = 7.3%; CI: -5.7 to 18.7). In patients who were enrolled in the trial on the sole basis of a recent myocardial infarction, clopidogrel was numerically inferior, but not statistically different from ASA (RRR = -4.0%; CI: -22.5 to 11.7). In addition, a subgroup analysis by age suggested that the benefit of clopidogrel in patients over 75 years was less than that observed in patients $\leqslant$75 years.

Since the CAPRIE trial was not powered to evaluate efficacy of individual subgroups, it is not clear whether the differences in relative risk reduction across qualifying conditions are real, or a result of chance.

The CURE study included 12,562 patients with non-ST segment elevation acute coronary syndrome (unstable angina or non-Q-wave myocardial infarction), and presenting within 24 hours of onset of the most recent episode of chest pain or symptoms consistent with ischaemia. Patients were required to have either ECG changes compatible with new ischaemia or elevated cardiac enzymes or troponin I or T to at least twice the upper limit of normal. Patients were randomised to clopidogrel (300 mg loading dose followed by 75 mg/day, N=6,259) or placebo (N=6,303), both given in combination with ASA (75-325 mg once daily) and other standard therapies. Patients were treated for up to one year. In CURE, 823 (6.6%) patients received concomitant GPIIb/IIIa receptor antagonist therapy. Heparins were administered in more than 90% of the patients and the relative rate of bleeding between clopidogrel and placebo was not significantly affected by the concomitant heparin therapy.

The number of patients experiencing the primary endpoint [cardiovascular (CV) death, myocardial infarction (MI), or stroke] was 582 (9.3%) in the clopidogrel-treated group and 719 (11.4%) in the placebo-treated group, a 20% relative risk reduction (95% CI of 10%-28%; p=0.00009) for the clopidogrel-treated group (17% relative risk reduction when patients were treated conservatively, 29% when they underwent PTCA with or without stent and 10% when they underwent CABG). New cardiovascular events (primary endpoint) were prevented, with relative risk reductions of 22% (CI: 8.6, 33.4), 32% (CI: 12.8, 46.4), 4% (CI: -26.9, 26.7), 6% (CI: -33.5, 34.3) and 14% (CI: -31.6, 44.2), during the 0-1, 1-3, 3-6, 6-9 and 9-12 month study intervals, respectively. Thus, beyond 3 months of treatment, the benefit observed in the clopidogrel + ASA group was not further increased, whereas the risk of haemorrhage persisted (see section 4.4).

The use of clopidogrel in CURE was associated with a decrease in the need of thrombolytic therapy (RRR = 43.3%; CI: 24.3%, 57.5%) and GPIIb/IIIa inhibitors (RRR = 18.2%; CI: 6.5%, 28.3%).

The number of patients experiencing the co-primary endpoint (CV death, MI, stroke or refractory ischaemia) was 1035 (16.5%) in the clopidogrel-treated group and 1187 (18.8%) in the placebo-treated group, a 14% relative risk reduction (95% CI of 6%-21%, p=0.0005) for the clopidogrel-treated group. This benefit was mostly driven by the statistically significant reduction in the incidence of MI [287 (4.6%) in the clopidogrel treated group and 363 (5.8%) in the placebo treated group]. There was no observed effect on the rate of rehospitalisation for unstable angina.

The results obtained populations with different characteristics (e.g. unstable angina or non-Q-wave MI, low to high risk levels, diabetes, need for revascularisation, age, gender, etc.) were consistent with the results of the primary analysis. The benefits observed with clopidogrel were independent of other acute and long-term cardiovascular therapies (such as heparin/LMWH, GPIIb/IIIa antagonists, lipid lowering drugs, beta blockers, and ACE-inhibitors). The efficacy of clopidogrel was observed independently of the dose of ASA (75-325 mg once daily).

5.2 Pharmacokinetic properties

After repeated oral doses of 75 mg per day, clopidogrel is rapidly absorbed. However, plasma concentrations of the parent compound are very low and below the quantification limit (0.00025 mg/l) beyond 2 hours. Absorption is at least 50%, based on urinary excretion of clopidogrel metabolites.

Clopidogrel is extensively metabolised by the liver and the main metabolite, which is inactive, is the carboxylic acid derivative, which represents about 85% of the circulating compound in plasma. Peak plasma levels of this metabolite (approx. 3mg/l after repeated 75 mg oral doses) occurred approximately 1 hour after dosing.

Clopidogrel is a prodrug. The active metabolite, a thiol derivative, is formed by oxidation of clopidogrel to 2-oxo-clopidogrel and subsequent hydrolysis. The oxidative step is regulated primarily by Cytochrome P_{450} isoenzymes 2B6 and 3A4 and to a lesser extent by 1A1, 1A2 and 2C19. The active thiol metabolite, which has been isolated *in vitro*, binds rapidly and irreversibly to platelet receptors, thus inhibiting platelet aggregation. This metabolite has not been detected in plasma.

The kinetics of the main circulating metabolite were linear (plasma concentrations increased in proportion to dose) in the dose range of 50 to 150 mg of clopidogrel.

Clopidogrel and the main circulating metabolite bind reversibly *in vitro* to human plasma proteins (98% and 94% respectively). The binding is non-saturable *in vitro* over a wide concentration range.

Following an oral dose of ^{14}C-labelled clopidogrel in man, approximately 50% was excreted in the urine and approximately 46% in the faeces in the 120-hour interval after dosing. The elimination half-life of the main circulating metabolite was 8 hours after single and repeated administration.

After repeated doses of 75 mg clopidogrel per day, plasma levels of the main circulating metabolite were lower in subjects with severe renal disease (creatinine clearance from 5 to 15 ml/min) compared to subjects with moderate renal disease (creatinine clearance from 30 to 60 ml/min) and to levels observed in other studies with healthy subjects. Although inhibition of ADP-induced platelet aggregation was lower (25%) than that observed in healthy subjects, the prolongation of bleeding was similar to that seen in healthy subjects receiving 75 mg of clopidogrel per day. In addition, clinical tolerance was good in all patients.

The pharmacokinetics and pharmacodynamics of clopidogrel were assessed in a single and multiple dose study in both healthy subjects and those with cirrhosis (Child-Pugh class A or B). Daily dosing for 10 days with clopidogrel 75 mg/day was safe and well tolerated. Clopidogrel C_{max} for both single dose and steady state for cirrhotics was many fold higher than in normal subjects. However, plasma levels of the main circulating metabolite together with the effect of clopidogrel on ADP-induced platelet aggregation and bleeding time were comparable between these groups.

5.3 Preclinical safety data

During preclinical studies in rat and baboon, the most frequently occurred effects were liver changes. These occurred at doses representing at least 25 times the exposure seen in humans receiving the clinical dose of 75 mg/day and were a consequence of an effect on hepatic metabolising enzymes. No effect on hepatic metabolising enzymes was observed in humans receiving clopidogrel at the therapeutic dose.

At very high doses, a poor gastric tolerability (gastritis, gastric erosions and/or vomiting) of clopidogrel was also reported in rat and baboon.

There was no evidence of carcinogenic effect when clopidogrel was administered for 78 weeks to mice and 104 weeks to rats when given at doses up to 77 mg/kg per day (representing at least 25 times the exposure seen in humans receiving the clinical dose of 75 mg/day).

Clopidogrel has been tested in a range of *in vitro* and *in vivo* genotoxicity studies, and showed no genotoxic activity.

Clopidogrel was found to have no effect on the fertility of male and female rats and was not teratogenic in either rats or rabbits. When given to lactating rats, clopidogrel caused a slight delay in the development of the offspring. Specific pharmacokinetic studies performed with radiolabelled clopidogrel have shown that the parent compound or its metabolites are excreted in the milk. Consequently, a direct effect (slight toxicity), or an indirect effect (low palatability) cannot be excluded.

6. PHARMACEUTICAL PARTICULARS

6.1 List of excipients

Core:

Mannitol (E421)

Macrogol 6000

Microcrystalline cellulose

Hydrogenated castor oil

Low substituted hydroxypropylcellulose

Coating:

Hypromellose (E464)

Lactose

Triacetin (E1518)

Titanium dioxide (E171)

Red iron oxide (E172)

Carnauba wax

6.2 Incompatibilities

Not applicable

6.3 Shelf life

3 years

6.4 Special precautions for storage

No special precautions for storage.

Store in the original package.

6.5 Nature and contents of container

28 film-coated tablets packed in PVC/PVDC/Aluminium blisters in cardboard cartons.

6.6 Instructions for use and handling

No special requirements

7. MARKETING AUTHORISATION HOLDER

Sanofi Pharma Bristol-Myers Squibb SNC

174 Avenue de France

F-75013 Paris - France

8. MARKETING AUTHORISATION NUMBER(S)

EU/1/98/069/001a - Cartons of 28 film-coated tablets in PVC/PVDC/Alu blisters

9. DATE OF FIRST AUTHORISATION/RENEWAL OF THE AUTHORISATION

8 October 2003

10. DATE OF REVISION OF THE TEXT

5 January 2005

Legal Category: POM

Plavix (Sanofi Synthelabo)

(sanofi-aventis)

1. NAME OF THE MEDICINAL PRODUCT

Plavix 75 mg film-coated tablets

2. QUALITATIVE AND QUANTITATIVE COMPOSITION

Clopidogrel hydrogen sulphate 97.875 mg (molar equivalent of 75 mg of clopidogrel base)

For excipients, see 6.1.

3. PHARMACEUTICAL FORM

Film-coated tablet.

Plavix 75 mg film-coated tablets are pink, round, biconvex, film-coated, and engraved with «75» on one side and «1171» on the other side.

4. CLINICAL PARTICULARS

4.1 Therapeutic indications

Clopidogrel is indicated for the prevention of atherothrombotic events in:

• Patients suffering from myocardial infarction (from a few days until less than 35 days), ischaemic stroke (from 7 days until less than 6 months) or established peripheral arterial disease.

• Patients suffering from non-ST segment elevation acute coronary syndrome (unstable angina or non-Q-wave myocardial infarction) in combination with acetylsalicylic acid (ASA).

For further information please refer to section 5.1.

4.2 Posology and method of administration

• Adults and elderly

Clopidogrel should be given as a single daily dose of 75 mg with or without food.

In patients with non-ST segment elevation acute coronary syndrome (unstable angina or non-Q-wave myocardial infarction), clopidogrel treatment should be initiated with a single 300 mg loading dose and then continued at 75 mg once a day (with ASA 75 mg-325 mg daily). Since higher doses of ASA were associated with higher bleeding risk it is recommended that the dose of ASA should not be higher than 100 mg. The optimal duration of treatment has not been formally established. Clinical trial data support use up to 12 months, and the maximum benefit was seen at 3 months(see section 5.1).

• Children and adolescents

Safety and efficacy in subjects below the age of 18 have not been established.

4.3 Contraindications

• Hypersensitivity to the active substance or to any of the excipients of the medicinal product.

• Severe liver impairment.

• Active pathological bleeding such as peptic ulcer or intracranial haemorrhage.

• Breast-feeding (see section 4.6).

4.4 Special warnings and special precautions for use

Due to the risk of bleeding and haematological undesirable effects, blood cell count determination and/or other appropriate testing should be promptly considered whenever clinical symptoms suggestive of bleeding arise during the course of treatment (see section 4.8). As with other antiplatelet agents, clopidogrel should be used with caution in patients who may be at risk of increased bleeding from trauma, surgery or other pathological conditions and in patients receiving treatment with ASA, non-steroidal anti-inflammatory drugs, heparin, glycoprotein IIb/IIIa inhibitors or thrombolytics. Patients should be followed carefully for any signs of bleeding including occult bleeding, especially during the first weeks of treatment and/or after invasive cardiac procedures or surgery. The concomitant administration of clopidogrel with warfarin is not recommended since it may increase the intensity of bleedings (see section 4.5).

If a patient is to undergo elective surgery and antiplatelet effect is not necessary, clopidogrel should be discontinued 7 days prior to surgery. Clopidogrel prolongs bleeding time and should be used with caution in patients who have lesions with a propensity to bleed (particularly gastrointestinal and intraocular).

Patients should be told that it might take longer than usual to stop bleeding when they take clopidogrel (alone or in combination with ASA), and that they should report any unusual bleeding (site or duration) to their physician. Patients should inform physicians and dentists that they are taking clopidogrel before any surgery is scheduled and before any new drug is taken.

Thrombotic Thrombocytopenic Purpura (TTP) has been reported very rarely following the use of clopidogrel, sometimes after a short exposure. It is characterised by thrombocytopenia and microangiopathic hemolytic anemia associated with either neurological findings, renal dysfunction or fever. TTP is a potentially fatal condition requiring prompt treatment including plasmapheresis.

In view of the lack of data, in patients with acute myocardial infarction with ST-segment elevation, clopidogrel therapy should not be initiated within the first few days following myocardial infarction.

In view of the lack of data, clopidogrel cannot be recommended in acute ischaemic stroke (less than 7 days).

Therapeutic experience with clopidogrel is limited in patients with renal impairment. Therefore clopidogrel should be used with caution in these patients.

Experience is limited in patients with moderate hepatic disease who may have bleeding diatheses. Clopidogrel should therefore be used with caution in this population.

4.5 Interaction with other medicinal products and other forms of Interaction

Warfarin: the concomitant administration of clopidogrel with warfarin is not recommended since it may increase the intensity of bleedings (see section 4.4).

Glycoprotein IIb/IIIa inhibitors: clopidogrel should be used with caution in patients who may be at risk of increased bleeding from trauma, surgery or other pathological conditions that receive concomitant glycoprotein IIb/IIIa inhibitors. (see section 4.4)

Acetylsalicylic acid (ASA): ASA did not modify the clopidogrel-mediated inhibition of ADP-induced platelet aggregation, but clopidogrel potentiated the effect of ASA on collagen-induced platelet aggregation. However, concomitant administration of 500 mg of ASA twice a day for one day did not significantly increase the prolongation of bleeding time induced by clopidogrel intake. A pharmacodynamic interaction between clopidogrel and acetylsalicylic acid is possible, leading to increased risk of bleeding. Therefore, concomitant use should be undertaken with caution (see section 4.4). However, clopidogrel and ASA have been administered together for up to one year (see section 5.1).

Heparin: in a clinical study conducted in healthy subjects, clopidogrel did not necessitate modification of the heparin dose or alter the effect of heparin on coagulation. Co-administration of heparin had no effect on the inhibition of platelet aggregation induced by clopidogrel. A pharmacodynamic interaction between clopidogrel and heparin is possible, leading to increased risk of bleeding. Therefore, concomitant use should be undertaken with caution (see section 4.4).

Thrombolytics: the safety of the concomitant administration of clopidogrel, rt-PA and heparin was assessed in patients with recent myocardial infarction. The incidence of clinically significant bleeding was similar to that observed when rt-PA and heparin are co-administered with ASA. The safety of the concomitant administration of clopidogrel with other thrombolytic agents has not been formally established and should be undertaken with caution (see section 4.4).

Non-Steroidal Anti-Inflammatory Drugs (NSAIDs): in a clinical study conducted in healthy volunteers, the concomitant administration of clopidogrel and naproxen increased occult gastrointestinal blood loss. However, due to the lack of interaction studies with other NSAIDs it is presently unclear whether there is an increased risk of gastrointestinal bleeding with all NSAIDs. Consequently, NSAIDs and clopidogrel should be co-administered with caution (see section 4.4).

Other concomitant therapy: a number of other clinical studies have been conducted with clopidogrel and other concomitant medications to investigate the potential for pharmacodynamic and pharmacokinetic interactions. No clinically significant pharmacodynamic interactions were observed when clopidogrel was co-administered with atenolol, nifedipine, or both atenolol and nifedipine. Furthermore, the pharmacodynamic activity of clopidogrel was not significantly influenced by the co-administration of phenobarbital, cimetidine, or oestrogen.

The pharmacokinetics of digoxin or theophylline were not modified by the co-administration of clopidogrel. Antacids did not modify the extent of clopidogrel absorption.

Data from studies with human liver microsomes indicated that the carboxylic acid metabolite of clopidogrel could inhibit the activity of Cytochrome P_{450} 2C9. This could potentially lead to increased plasma levels of drugs such as phenytoin and tolbutamide and the NSAIDs, which are metabolised by Cytochrome P_{450} 2C9. Data from the CAPRIE study indicate that phenytoin and tolbutamide can be safely co-administered with clopidogrel.

Apart from the specific drug interaction information described above, interaction studies with clopidogrel and some drugs commonly administered in patients with atherothrombotic disease have not been performed. However, patients entered into clinical trials with clopidogrel received a variety of concomitant medications including diuretics, beta blockers, ACEI, calcium antagonists, cholesterol lowering agents, coronary vasodilators, antidiabetic agents (including insulin), antiepileptic agents, hormone replacement therapy and GPIIb/IIIa antagonists without evidence of clinically significant adverse interactions.

4.6 Pregnancy and lactation

• Pregnancy

As no clinical data on exposed pregnancies are available, it is preferable not to use clopidogrel during pregnancy as a precautionary measure.

Animal studies do not indicate direct or indirect harmful effects with respect to pregnancy, embryonic/foetal development, parturition or postnatal development (see section 5.3).

• Lactation

Studies in rats have shown that clopidogrel and/or its metabolites are excreted in the milk. It is not known whether this medicinal product is excreted in human milk.

4.7 Effects on ability to drive and use machines

Clopidogrel has no or negligible influence on the ability to drive and use machines.

4.8 Undesirable effects

Clinical studies experience:

Clopidogrel has been evaluated for safety in more than 17,500 patients, including over 9,000 patients treated for 1 year or more. Clopidogrel 75 mg/day was well tolerated compared to ASA 325 mg/day in CAPRIE. The overall tolerability of clopidogrel in this study was similar to ASA, regardless of age, gender and race. The clinically relevant adverse effects observed in the CAPRIE and CURE studies are discussed below.

Haemorrhagic disorders:

In CAPRIE, in patients treated with either clopidogrel or ASA, the overall incidence of any bleeding was 9.3%. The incidence of severe cases was 1.4% for clopidogrel and 1.6% for ASA.

In patients that received clopidogrel, gastrointestinal bleeding occurred at a rate of 2.0%, and required hospitalisation in 0.7%. In patients that received ASA, the corresponding rates were 2.7% and 1.1%, respectively.

The incidence of other bleedings was higher in patients that received clopidogrel compared to ASA (7.3% vs. 6.5%). However, the incidence of severe events was similar in both treatment groups (0.6% vs. 0.4%). The most frequently reported events in both treatment groups were: purpura/bruising/haematoma, and epistaxis. Other less frequently reported events were haematoma, haematuria, and eye bleeding (mainly conjunctival).

The incidence of intracranial bleeding was 0.4% in patients that received clopidogrel and 0.5% for patients that received ASA.

In CURE, the administration of clopidogrel+ASA as compared to placebo+ASA was not associated with a statistically significant increase in life-threatening bleeds (event rates 2.2% vs. 1.8%) or fatal bleeds (0.2% vs. 0.2%), but the risk of major, minor and other bleedings was significantly higher with clopidogrel+ASA: non-life-threatening major bleeds (1.6% clopidogrel+ASA vs. 1.0% placebo+ASA), primarily gastrointestinal and at puncture sites, and minor bleeds (5.1% clopidogrel+ASA vs. 2.4% placebo+ASA). The incidence of intracranial bleeding was 0.1% in both groups.

The major bleeding event rate for clopidogrel+ASA was dose-dependent on ASA (<100mg: 2.6%; 100-200mg: 3.5%; >200mg: 4.9%) as was the major bleeding event rate for placebo+ASA (<100mg: 2.0%; 100-200mg: 2.3%; >200mg: 4.0%).

The risk of bleeding (life-threatening, major, minor, other) decreased during the course of the trial: 0-1 months [clopidogrel: 599/6259 (9.6%); placebo: 413/6303 (6.6%)], 1-3 months [clopidogrel: 276/6123 (4.5%); placebo: 144/6168 (2.3%)], 3-6 months [clopidogrel: 228/6037 (3.8%); placebo: 99/6048 (1.6%)], 6-9 months [clopidogrel: 162/5005 (3.2%); placebo: 74/4972 (1.5%)], 9-12 months [clopidogrel: 73/3841 (1.9%); placebo: 40/3844 (1.0%)].

There was no excess in major bleeds within 7 days after coronary bypass graft surgery in patients who stopped therapy more than five days prior to surgery (4.4% clopidogrel+ASA vs. 5.3% placebo+ASA). In patients who remained on therapy within five days of bypass graft surgery, the event rate was 9.6% for clopidogrel+ASA, and 6.3% for placebo+ASA.

Haematological disorders:

In CAPRIE, severe neutropenia (<0.45 × 10^9/l) was observed in 4 patients (0.04%) that received clopidogrel and 2 patients (0.02%) that received ASA. Two of the 9599 patients who received clopidogrel and none of the 9586 patients who received ASA had neutrophil counts of zero. One case of aplastic anaemia occurred on clopidogrel treatment.

The incidence of severe thrombocytopenia (<80 × 10^9/l) was 0.2% on clopidogrel and 0.1% on ASA.

In CURE, the numbers of patients with thrombocytopenia (19 clopidogrel+ASA vs. 24 placebo+ASA) or neutropenia (3 vs. 3) were similar in both groups.

Other clinically relevant adverse drug reactions pooled from CAPRIE and CURE studies with an incidence ≥ 0.1% as well as all serious and relevant ADR are listed below according to the World Health Organisation classification. Their frequency is defined using the following conventions: common > 1/100, <1/10); uncommon > 1/1,000, < 1/100); rare >1/10,000, <1/1,000).

- Central and peripheral nervous system disorders:

- Uncommon: Headache, Dizziness and Paraesthesia
- Rare: Vertigo

- Gastrointestinal system disorders

- Common: Dyspepsia, Abdominal pain and Diarrhoea
- Uncommon: Nausea, Gastritis, Flatulence, Constipation, Vomiting, Gastric ulcer and Duodenal ulcer

- Platelet, bleeding and clotting disorders

- Uncommon: Bleeding time increased and Platelets decreased

- Skin and appendages disorders:

- Uncommon: Rash and Pruritus

- White cell and RES disorders

- Uncommon: Leucopenia, Neutrophils decreased and Eosinophilia

Post-marketing experience:

Bleeding is the most common reaction reported in the post-marketing experience and was mostly reported during the first month of treatment.

Bleeding: some cases were reported with fatal outcome (especially intracranial, gastrointestinal and retroperitoneal haemorrhage); serious cases of skin bleeding (purpura), musculo-skeletal bleeding (haemarthrosis, haematoma), eye bleeding (conjunctival, ocular, retinal), epistaxis, respiratory tract bleeding (haemoptysis, pulmonary haemorrhage), haematuria and haemorrhage of operative wound have been reported; cases of serious haemorrhage have been reported in patients taking clopidogrel concomitantly with acetylsalicylic acid or clopidogrel with acetylsalicylic acid and heparin (see section 4.4).

In addition to clinical studies experience, the following adverse reactions have been spontaneously reported. Within each system organ class (MedDRA classification), they are ranked under heading of frequency. "Very rare" corresponds to <1/10,000.

Blood and lymphatic system disorders:

- Very rare: Thrombotic Thrombocytopenic Purpura (TTP) (1/200,000 exposed patients) (see section 4.4), severe Thrombocytopenia (platelet count ≤30 x10^9/l), Granulocytopenia, Agranulocytosis, Anaemia and Aplastic Anaemia/Pancytopenia.

Immune system disorders:

- Very rare: Anaphylactoid reactions, Serum sickness

Psychiatric disorders:

- Very rare: Confusion, Hallucinations

Nervous system disorders:

- Very rare: Taste disturbances

Vascular disorders:

- Very rare: Vasculitis, Hypotension

Respiratory, thoracic and mediastinal disorders:

- Very rare: Bronchospasm, Interstitial pneumonitis

Gastrointestinal disorders:

- Very rare: Colitis (including ulcerative or lymphocytic colitis), Pancreatitis, Stomatitis

Hepato-biliary disorders

- Very rare: Hepatitis, Acute liver failure

Skin and subcutaneous tissue disorders:

- Very rare: Angioedema, Bullous dermatitis (erythema multiforme, Stevens Johnson Syndrome..), rash erythematous, urticaria, eczema and lichen planus

Musculoskeletal, connective tissue and bone disorders:

- Very rare: Arthralgia, Arthritis, Myalgia

Renal and urinary disorders:

- Very rare: Glomerulonephritis

General disorders and administration site conditions

- Very rare: Fever

Investigations:

- Very rare: Abnormal liver function test, Blood creatinine increase

4.9 Overdose

Overdose following clopidogrel administration may lead to prolonged bleeding time and subsequent bleeding complications. Appropriate therapy should be considered if bleedings are observed.

No antidote to the pharmacological activity of clopidogrel has been found. If prompt correction of prolonged bleeding time is required, platelet transfusion may reverse the effects of clopidogrel.

5. PHARMACOLOGICAL PROPERTIES

5.1 Pharmacodynamic properties

Pharmacotherapeutical group: platelet aggregation inhibitors excl. Heparin, ATC Code: BO1AC/04.

Clopidogrel selectively inhibits the binding of adenosine diphosphate (ADP) to its platelet receptor, and the subsequent ADP-mediated activation of the GPIIb/IIIa complex, thereby inhibiting platelet aggregation. Biotransformation of clopidogrel is necessary to produce inhibition of platelet aggregation. Clopidogrel also inhibits platelet aggregation induced by other agonists by blocking the amplification of platelet activation by released ADP. Clopidogrel acts by irreversibly modifying the platelet ADP receptor. Consequently, platelets exposed to clopidogrel are affected for the remainder of their lifespan and recovery of normal platelet function occurs at a rate consistent with platelet turnover.

Repeated doses of 75 mg per day produced substantial inhibition of ADP-induced platelet aggregation from the first day; this increased progressively and reached steady state between Day 3 and Day 7. At steady state, the average inhibition level observed with a dose of 75 mg per day was between 40% and 60%. Platelet aggregation and bleeding time gradually returned to baseline values, generally within 5 days after treatment was discontinued.

The safety and efficacy of clopidogrel in preventing vascular ischaemic events have been evaluated in two double-blind studies: the CAPRIE study, a comparison of clopidogrel to ASA, and the CURE study, a comparison of clopidogrel in combination with ASA, to placebo with ASA.

The CAPRIE study included 19,185 patients with atherothrombosis as manifested by recent myocardial infarction (<35 days), recent ischaemic stroke (between 7 days and 6 months) or established peripheral arterial disease (PAD). Patients were randomised to clopidogrel 75 mg/day or ASA 325 mg/day, and were followed for 1 to 3 years. In the myocardial infarction subgroup, most of the patients received ASA for the first few days following the acute myocardial infarction.

Clopidogrel significantly reduced the incidence of new ischaemic events (combined end point of myocardial infarction, ischaemic stroke and vascular death) when compared to ASA. In the intention to treat analysis, 939 events were observed in the clopidogrel group and 1,020 events with ASA (relative risk reduction (RRR) 8.7%, [95% CI: 0.2 to 16.4]; p = 0.045), which corresponds, for every 1000 patients treated for 2 years, to 10 [CI: 0 to 20] additional patients being prevented from experiencing a new ischaemic event. Analysis of total mortality as a secondary endpoint did not show any significant difference between clopidogrel (5.8%) and ASA (6.0%).

In a subgroup analysis by qualifying condition (myocardial infarction, ischaemic stroke, and PAD) the benefit appeared to be strongest (achieving statistical significance at p = 0.003) in patients enrolled due to PAD (especially those who also had a history of myocardial infarction) (RRR = 23.7%; CI: 8.9 to 36.2) and weaker (not significantly different from ASA) in stroke patients (RRR = 7.3%; CI: -5.7 to 18.7). In patients who were enrolled in the trial on the sole basis of a recent myocardial infarction, clopidogrel was numerically inferior, but not statistically different from ASA (RRR = -4.0%; CI: -22.5 to 11.7). In addition, a subgroup analysis by age suggested that the benefit of clopidogrel in patients over 75 years was less than that observed in patients ≤75 years.

Since the CAPRIE trial was not powered to evaluate efficacy of individual subgroups, it is not clear whether the differences in relative risk reduction across qualifying conditions are real, or a result of chance.

The CURE study included 12,562 patients with non-ST segment elevation acute coronary syndrome (unstable angina or non-Q-wave myocardial infarction), and presenting within 24 hours of onset of the most recent episode of chest pain or symptoms consistent with ischaemia. Patients were required to have either ECG changes compatible with new ischaemia or elevated cardiac enzymes or troponin I or T to at least twice the upper limit of normal. Patients were randomised to clopidogrel (300 mg loading dose followed by 75 mg/day, N=6,259) or placebo (N=6,303), both given in combination with ASA (75-325 mg once daily) and other standard therapies. Patients were treated for up to one year. In CURE, 823 (6.6%) patients received concomitant GPIIb/IIIa receptor antagonist therapy. Heparins were administered in more than 90% of the patients and the relative rate of bleeding between clopidogrel and placebo was not significantly affected by the concomitant heparin therapy.

The number of patients experiencing the primary endpoint [cardiovascular (CV) death, myocardial infarction (MI), or stroke] was 582 (9.3%) in the clopidogrel-treated group and 719 (11.4%) in the placebo-treated group, a 20% relative risk reduction (95% CI of 10%-28%; p=0.00009) for the clopidogrel-treated group (17% relative risk reduction when patients were treated conservatively, 29% when they underwent PTCA with or without stent and 10% when they underwent CABG). New cardiovascular events (primary endpoint) were prevented, with relative risk reductions of 22% (CI: 8.6, 33.4), 32% (CI: 12.8, 46.4), 4% (CI: -26.9, 26.7), 6% (CI: -33.5, 34.3) and 14% (CI: -31.6, 44.2), during the 0-1, 1-3, 3-6, 6-9 and 9-12 month study intervals, respectively. Thus, beyond 3 months of treatment, the benefit observed in the clopidogrel + ASA group was not further increased, whereas the risk of haemorrhage persisted (see section 4.4).

The use of clopidogrel in CURE was associated with a decrease in the need of thrombolytic therapy (RRR = 43.3%; CI: 24.3%, 57.5%) and GPIIb/IIIa inhibitors (RRR = 18.2%; CI: 6.5%, 28.3%).

The number of patients experiencing the co-primary endpoint (CV death, MI, stroke or refractory ischaemia) was 1035 (16.5%) in the clopidogrel-treated group and 1187 (18.8%) in the placebo-treated group, a 14% relative risk reduction (95% CI of 6%-21%, p=0.0005) for the clopidogrel-treated group. This benefit was mostly driven by the statistically significant reduction in the incidence of MI [287 (4.6%) in the clopidogrel treated group and 363 (5.8%) in the placebo treated group]. There was no observed effect on the rate of rehospitalisation for unstable angina.

The results obtained populations with different characteristics (e.g. unstable angina or non-Q-wave MI, low to high risk levels, diabetes, need for revascularisation, age, gender, etc.) were consistent with the results of the primary analysis. The benefits observed with clopidogrel were independent of other acute and long-term cardiovascular therapies (such as heparin/LMWH, GPIIb/IIIa antagonists, lipid lowering drugs, beta blockers, and ACE-inhibitors). The efficacy of clopidogrel was observed independently of the dose of ASA (75-325 mg once daily).

5.2 Pharmacokinetic properties

After repeated oral doses of 75 mg per day, clopidogrel is rapidly absorbed. However, plasma concentrations of the parent compound are very low and below the quantification limit (0.00025 mg/l) beyond 2 hours. Absorption is at least 50%, based on urinary excretion of clopidogrel metabolites.

Clopidogrel is extensively metabolised by the liver and the main metabolite, which is inactive, is the carboxylic acid derivative, which represents about 85% of the circulating compound in plasma. Peak plasma levels of this metabolite (approx. 3mg/l after repeated 75 mg oral doses) occurred approximately 1 hour after dosing.

Clopidogrel is a prodrug. The active metabolite, a thiol derivative, is formed by oxidation of clopidogrel to 2-oxo-clopidogrel and subsequent hydrolysis. The oxidative step is regulated primarily by Cytochrome P_{450} isoenzymes 2B6 and 3A4 and to a lesser extent by 1A1, 1A2 and 2C19. The active thiol metabolite, which has been isolated *in vitro*, binds rapidly and irreversibly to platelet receptors, thus inhibiting platelet aggregation. This metabolite has not been detected in plasma.

The kinetics of the main circulating metabolite were linear (plasma concentrations increased in proportion to dose) in the dose range of 50 to 150 mg of clopidogrel.

Clopidogrel and the main circulating metabolite bind reversibly *in vitro* to human plasma proteins (98% and 94% respectively). The binding is non-saturable *in vitro* over a wide concentration range.

Following an oral dose of ^{14}C-labelled clopidogrel in man, approximately 50% was excreted in the urine and approximately 46% in the faeces in the 120-hour interval after dosing. The elimination half-life of the main circulating metabolite was 8 hours after single and repeated administration.

After repeated doses of 75 mg clopidogrel per day, plasma levels of the main circulating metabolite were lower in subjects with severe renal disease (creatinine clearance from 5 to 15 ml/min) compared to subjects with moderate renal disease (creatinine clearance from 30 to

60 ml/min) and to levels observed in other studies with healthy subjects. Although inhibition of ADP-induced platelet aggregation was lower (25%) than that observed in healthy subjects, the prolongation of bleeding was similar to that seen in healthy subjects receiving 75 mg of clopidogrel per day. In addition, clinical tolerance was good in all patients.

The pharmacokinetics and pharmacodynamics of clopidogrel were assessed in a single and multiple dose study in both healthy subjects and those with cirrhosis (Child-Pugh class A or B). Daily dosing for 10 days with clopidogrel 75 mg/day was safe and well tolerated. Clopidogrel C_{max} for both single dose and steady state for cirrhotics was many fold higher than in normal subjects. However, plasma levels of the main circulating metabolite together with the effect of clopidogrel on ADP-induced platelet aggregation and bleeding time were comparable between these groups.

5.3 Preclinical safety data

During preclinical studies in rat and baboon, the most frequently observed effects were liver changes. These occurred at doses representing at least 25 times the exposure seen in humans receiving the clinical dose of 75 mg/day and were a consequence of an effect on hepatic metabolising enzymes. No effect on hepatic metabolising enzymes was observed in humans receiving clopidogrel at the therapeutic dose.

At very high doses, a poor gastric tolerability (gastritis, gastric erosions and/or vomiting) of clopidogrel was also reported in rat and baboon.

There was no evidence of carcinogenic effect when clopidogrel was administered for 78 weeks to mice and 104 weeks to rats when given at doses up to 77 mg/kg per day (representing at least 25 times the exposure seen in humans receiving the clinical dose of 75 mg/day).

Clopidogrel has been tested in a range of in *vitro* and *in vivo* genotoxicity studies, and showed no genotoxic activity.

Clopidogrel was found to have no effect on the fertility of male and female rats and was not teratogenic in either rats or rabbits. When given to lactating rats, clopidogrel caused a slight delay in the development of the offspring. Specific pharmacokinetic studies performed with radiolabelled clopidogrel have shown that the parent compound or its metabolites are excreted in the milk. Consequently, a direct effect (slight toxicity), or an indirect effect (low palatability) cannot be excluded.

6. PHARMACEUTICAL PARTICULARS

6.1 List of excipients

Core:

Mannitol (E421)

Macrogol 6000

Microcrystalline cellulose

Hydrogenated castor oil

Low substituted hydroxypropylcellulose

Coating:

Hypromellose (E464)

Lactose

Triacetin (E1518)

Titanium dioxide (E171)

Red iron oxide (E172)

Carnauba wax

6.2 Incompatibilities

Not applicable

6.3 Shelf life

3 years

6.4 Special precautions for storage

No special precautions for storage.

Store in the original package.

6.5 Nature and contents of container

28 film-coated tablets packed in PVC/PVDC/Aluminium blisters in cardboard cartons.

6.6 Instructions for use and handling

No special requirements

7. MARKETING AUTHORISATION HOLDER

Sanofi Pharma Bristol-Myers Squibb SNC

174 Avenue de France

F-75013 Paris - France

8. MARKETING AUTHORISATION NUMBER(S)

EU/1/98/069/001a - Cartons of 28 film-coated tablets in PVC/PVDC/Alu blisters

9. DATE OF FIRST AUTHORISATION/RENEWAL OF THE AUTHORISATION

8 October 2003

10. DATE OF REVISION OF THE TEXT

5 January 2005

Legal Category: POM

Plavix 75mg Film-Coated Tablets(Bristol-Myers Squibb Pharmaceuticals Ltd)

(Bristol-Myers Squibb Pharmaceuticals Ltd)

1. NAME OF THE MEDICINAL PRODUCT

Plavix 75mg film-coated tablets.

2. QUALITATIVE AND QUANTITATIVE COMPOSITION

Clopidogrel hydrogen sulphate 97.875 mg (molar equivalent of 75 mg of clopidogrel base)

For excipients, see 6.1.

3. PHARMACEUTICAL FORM

Film-coated tablet.

Plavix 75 mg film-coated tablets are pink, round, biconvex, film-coated, and engraved with «75» on one side and «1171» on the other side.

4. CLINICAL PARTICULARS

4.1 Therapeutic indications

Clopidogrel is indicated for the prevention of atherothrombotic events in:

• Patients suffering from myocardial infarction (from a few days until less than 35 days), ischaemic stroke (from 7 days until less than 6 months) or established peripheral arterial disease.

• Patients suffering from non-ST segment elevation acute coronary syndrome (unstable angina or non-Q-wave myocardial infarction) in combination with acetylsalicylic acid (ASA).

For further information please refer to section 5.1.

4.2 Posology and method of administration

Adults and elderly:

Clopidogrel should be given as a single daily dose of 75 mg with or without food.

In patients with non-ST segment elevation acute coronary syndrome (unstable angina or non-Q-wave myocardial infarction), clopidogrel treatment should be initiated with a single 300 mg loading dose and then continued at 75 mg once a day (with ASA 75 mg - 325 mg daily). Since higher doses of ASA were associated with higher bleeding risk it is recommended that the dose of ASA should not be higher than 100 mg. The optimal duration of treatment has not been formally established. Clinical trial data support use up to 12 months, and the maximum benefit was seen at 3 months (see section 5.1).

Children and adolescents:

Safety and efficacy in subjects below the age of 18 have not been established.

4.3 Contraindications

• Hypersensitivity to the active substance or to any of the excipients of the medicinal product.

• Severe liver impairment.

• Active pathological bleeding such as peptic ulcer or intracranial haemorrhage.

• Breast-feeding (see section 4.6).

4.4 Special warnings and special precautions for use

Due to the risk of bleeding and haematological undesirable effects, blood cell count determination and/or other appropriate testing should be promptly considered whenever clinical symptoms suggestive of bleeding arise during the course of treatment (see section 4.8). As with other antiplatelet agents, clopidogrel should be used with caution in patients who may be at risk of increased bleeding from trauma, surgery or other pathological conditions and in patients receiving treatment with ASA, non-steroidal anti-inflammatory drugs, heparin, glycoprotein IIb/IIIa inhibitors or thrombolytics. Patients should be followed carefully for any signs of bleeding including occult bleeding, especially during the first weeks of treatment and/or after invasive cardiac procedures or surgery. The concomitant administration of clopidogrel with warfarin is not recommended since it may increase the intensity of bleedings (see section 4.5).

If a patient is to undergo elective surgery and an antiplatelet effect is not necessary, clopidogrel should be discontinued 7 days prior to surgery. Clopidogrel prolongs bleeding time and should be used with caution in patients who have lesions with a propensity to bleed (particularly gastrointestinal and intraocular).

Patients should be told that it may take longer than usual to stop bleeding when they take clopidogrel (alone or in combination with ASA), and that they should report any unusual bleeding (site or duration) to their physician. Patients should inform physicians and dentists that they are taking clopidogrel before any surgery is scheduled and before any new drug is taken.

Thrombotic Thrombocytopenic Purpura (TTP) has been reported very rarely following the use of clopidogrel, sometimes after a short exposure. It is characterised by thrombocytopenia and microangiopathic haemolytic anaemia associated with either neurological findings, renal dysfunction or fever. TTP is a potentially fatal condition requiring prompt treatment including plasmapheresis.

In view of the lack of data, in patients with acute myocardial infarction with ST-segment elevation, clopidogrel therapy should not be initiated within the first few days following myocardial infarction.

In view of the lack of data, clopidogrel cannot be recommended in acute ischaemic stroke (less than 7 days).

Therapeutic experience with clopidogrel is limited in patients with renal impairment. Therefore clopidogrel should be used with caution in these patients.

Experience is limited in patients with moderate hepatic disease who may have bleeding diatheses. Clopidogrel should therefore be used with caution in this population.

4.5 Interaction with other medicinal products and other forms of Interaction

Warfarin: the concomitant administration of clopidogrel with warfarin is not recommended since it may increase the intensity of bleedings (see section 4.4).

Glycoprotein IIb/IIIa inhibitors: Clopidogrel should be used with caution in patients who may be at risk of increased bleeding from trauma, surgery or other pathological conditions that receive concomitant glycoprotein IIb/IIIa inhibitors (see section 4.4).

Acetylsalicylic acid (ASA): ASA did not modify the clopidogrel-mediated inhibition of ADP-induced platelet aggregation but clopidogrel potentiated the effect of ASA on collagen-induced platelet aggregation. However, concomitant administration of 500 mg of ASA twice a day for one day did not significantly increase the prolongation of bleeding time induced by clopidogrel intake. A pharmacodynamic interaction between clopidogrel and acetylsalicylic acid is possible, leading to increased risk of bleeding. Therefore, concomitant use should be undertaken with caution (see section 4.4). However, clopidogrel and ASA have been administered together for up to one year (see section 5.1).

Heparin: In a clinical study conducted in healthy subjects, clopidogrel did not necessitate modification of the heparin dose or alter the effect of heparin on coagulation. Co-administration of heparin had no effect on the inhibition of platelet aggregation induced by clopidogrel. A pharmacodynamic interaction between clopidogrel and heparin is possible, leading to increased risk of bleeding. Therefore, concomitant use should be undertaken with caution (see section 4.4).

Thrombolytics: The safety of the concomitant administration of clopidogrel, rt-PA and heparin was assessed in patients with recent myocardial infarction. The incidence of clinically significant bleeding was similar to that observed when rt-PA and heparin are co-administered with ASA. The safety of the concomitant administration of clopidogrel with other thrombolytic agents has not been formally established and should be undertaken with caution (see section 4.4).

Non-Steroidal Anti-Inflammatory Drugs (NSAIDs): In a clinical study conducted in healthy volunteers, the concomitant administration of clopidogrel and naproxen increased occult gastrointestinal blood loss. However, due to the lack of interaction studies with other NSAIDs, it is presently unclear whether there is an increased risk of gastrointestinal bleeding with all NSAIDs. Consequently, NSAIDs and clopidogrel should be co-administered with caution (see section 4.4).

Other concomitant therapy: A number of other clinical studies have been conducted with clopidogrel and other concomitant medications to investigate the potential for pharmacodynamic and pharmacokinetic interactions. No clinically significant pharmacodynamic interactions were observed when clopidogrel was co-administered with atenolol, nifedipine, or both atenolol and nifedipine. Furthermore, the pharmacodynamic activity of clopidogrel was not significantly influenced by the co-administration of phenobarbital, cimetidine or oestrogen.

The pharmacokinetics of digoxin or theophylline were not modified by the co-administration of clopidogrel. Antacids did not modify the extent of clopidogrel absorption.

Data from studies with human liver microsomes indicated that the carboxylic acid metabolite of clopidogrel could inhibit the activity of Cytochrome P_{450} 2C9. This could potentially lead to increased plasma levels of drugs such as phenytoin and tolbutamide and the NSAIDs which are metabolised by Cytochrome P_{450} 2C9. Data from the CAPRIE study indicate that phenytoin and tolbutamide can be safely coadministered with clopidogrel.

Apart from the specific drug interaction information described above, interaction studies with clopidogrel and some drugs commonly administered in patients with atherothrombotic disease have not been performed. However, patients entered into clinical trials with clopidogrel received a variety of concomitant medications including diuretics, beta-blockers, ACEI, calcium antagonists, cholesterol lowering agents, coronary vasodilators, antidiabetic agents (including insulin), antiepileptic agents, hormone replacement therapy and GPIIb/IIIa antagonists without evidence of clinically significant adverse interactions.

4.6 Pregnancy and lactation

Pregnancy:

As no clinical data on exposed pregnancies are available, it is preferable not to use clopidogrel during pregnancy as a precautionary measure.

Animal studies do not indicate direct or indirect harmful effects with respect to pregnancy, embryonic/foetal development, parturition or postnatal development (see section 5.3).

Lactation:

Studies in rats have shown that clopidogrel and/or its metabolites are excreted in the milk. It is not known whether this medicinal product is excreted in human milk.

4.7 Effects on ability to drive and use machines

Clopidogrel has no or negligible influence on the ability to drive and use machines.

4.8 Undesirable effects

Clinical studies experience:

Clopidogrel has been evaluated for safety in more than 17,500 patients, including over 9,000 patients treated for 1 year or more. Clopidogrel 75 mg/day was well tolerated compared to ASA 325 mg/day in CAPRIE. The overall tolerability of clopidogrel in this study was similar to ASA, regardless of age, gender and race. The clinically relevant adverse effects observed in the CAPRIE and CURE studies are discussed below.

Haemorrhagic disorders:

In CAPRIE, in patients treated with either clopidogrel or ASA, the overall incidence of any bleeding was 9.3%. The incidence of severe cases was 1.4% for clopidogrel and 1.6% for ASA.

In patients that received clopidogrel, gastrointestinal bleeding occurred at a rate of 2.0%, and required hospitalisation in 0.7%. In patients that received ASA, the corresponding rates were 2.7% and 1.1%, respectively.

The incidence of other bleeding was higher in patients that received clopidogrel compared to ASA (7.3% vs. 6.5%). However, the incidence of severe events was similar in both treatment groups (0.6% vs. 0.4%). The most frequently reported events in both treatment groups were: purpura/bruising/haematoma and epistaxis. Other less frequently reported events were haematoma, haematuria and eye bleeding (mainly conjunctival).

The incidence of intracranial bleeding was 0.4% in patients that received clopidogrel and 0.5% for patients that received ASA.

In CURE, the administration of clopidogrel+ASA as compared to placebo+ASA was not associated with a statistically significant increase in life-threatening bleeds (event rates 2.2% vs. 1.8%) or fatal bleeds (0.2% vs. 0.2%), but the risk of major, minor and other bleedings was significantly higher with clopidogrel+ASA: non-life-threatening major bleeds (1.6% clopidogrel+ASA vs. 1.0% placebo+ASA), primarily gastrointestinal and at puncture sites, and minor bleeds (5.1% clopidogrel+ASA vs. 2.4% placebo+ASA). The incidence of intracranial bleeding was 0.1% in both groups.

The major bleeding event rate for clopidogrel+ASA was dose-dependent on ASA (<100mg: 2.6%; 100-200mg: 3.5%; >200mg: 4.9%) as was the major bleeding event rate for placebo+ASA (<100mg: 2.0%; 100-200mg: 2.3%; >200mg: 4.0%).

The risk of bleeding (life-threatening, major, minor, other) decreased during the course of the trial: 0-1 months [clopidogrel: 599/6259 (9.6%); placebo: 413/6303 (6.6%)], 1-3 months [clopidogrel: 276/6123 (4.5%); placebo: 144/6168 (2.3%)], 3-6 months [clopidogrel: 228/6037 (3.8%); placebo: 99/6048 (1.6%)], 6-9 months [clopidogrel: 162/5005 (3.2%); placebo: 74/4972 (1.5%)], 9-12 months [clopidogrel: 73/3841 (1.9%); placebo: 40/3844 (1.0%)].

There was no excess in major bleeds within 7 days after coronary bypass graft surgery in patients who stopped therapy more than five days prior to surgery (4.4% clopidogrel+ASA vs. 5.3% placebo+ASA). In patients who remained on therapy within five days of bypass graft surgery, the event rate was 9.6% for clopidogrel+ASA, and 6.3% for placebo+ASA.

Haematological disorders:

In CAPRIE, severe neutropenia ($<0.45 \times 10^9$/l) was observed in 4 patients (0.04%) that received clopidogrel and 2 patients (0.02%) that received ASA. Two of the 9599 patients who received clopidogrel and none of the 9586 patients who received ASA had neutrophil counts of zero. One case of aplastic anaemia occurred on clopidogrel treatment.

The incidence of severe thrombocytopenia ($<80 \times 10^9$/l) was 0.2% on clopidogrel and 0.1% on ASA.

In CURE, the numbers of patients with thrombocytopenia (19 clopidogrel+ASA vs. 24 placebo+ASA) or neutropenia (3 vs. 3) were similar in both groups.

Other clinically relevant adverse drug reactions pooled from CAPRIE and CURE studies with an incidence ≥ 0.1% as well as all serious and relevant ADR are listed below according to the World Health Organisation classification. Their frequency is defined using the following conventions: common (> 1/100, <1/10); uncommon (>1/1,000, <1/100); rare (>1/10,000, <1/1,000).

Central and peripheral nervous system disorders:

Uncommon: Headache, Dizziness and Paraesthesia

Rare: Vertigo

Gastrointestinal system disorders

Common: Dyspepsia, Abdominal pain and Diarrhoea

Uncommon: Nausea, Gastritis, Flatulence, Constipation, Vomiting, Gastric ulcer and Duodenal ulcer

Platelet, bleeding and clotting disorders:

Uncommon: Bleeding time increased and Platelets decreased

Skin and appendages disorders:

Uncommon: Rash and Pruritus

White cell and RES disorders:

Uncommon: Leucopenia, Neutrophils decreased and Eosinophilia

Post-marketing experience:

Bleeding is the most common reaction reported in the post-marketing experience and was mostly reported during the first month of treatment.

Bleeding: Some cases were reported with fatal outcome (especially intracranial, gastrointestinal and retroperitoneal haemorrhage); serious cases of skin bleeding (purpura), musculo-skeletal bleeding (haemarthrosis, haematoma), eye bleeding (conjunctival, ocular, retinal), epistaxis, respiratory tract bleeding (haemoptysis, pulmonary haemorrhage), haematuria and haemorrhage of operative wound have been reported; cases of serious haemorrhage have been reported in patients taking clopidogrel concomitantly with acetylsalicylic acid or clopidogrel with acetylsalicylic acid and heparin (see section 4.4).

In addition to clinical studies experience, the following adverse reactions have been spontaneously reported. Within each system organ class (MedDRA classification), they are ranked under heading of frequency. "very rare" corresponds to <1/10,000.

Blood and lymphatic system disorders:

Very rare: Thrombotic Thrombocytopenic Purpura (TTP) (1/200,000 exposed patients) (see section 4.4), severe Thrombocytopenia (platelet count $\leqslant 30 \times 10^9$/l), Granulocytopenia, Agranulocytosis, Anaemia and Aplastic Anaemia/Pancytopenia.

Immune system disorders:

Very rare: Anaphylactoid reactions, Serum Sickness.

Psychiatric disorders:

Very rare: Confusion, Hallucinations.

Nervous system disorders:

Very rare: Taste disturbances.

Vascular disorders:

Very rare: Vasculitis, Hypotension.

Respiratory, thoracic and mediastinal disorders:

Very rare: Bronchospasm, Interstitial Pneumonitis.

Gastrointestinal disorders:

Very rare: Colitis (including ulcerative or lymphocytic colitis), Pancreatitis, Stomatitis.

Hepato-biliary disorders:

Very rare: Hepatitis, Acute liver failure.

Skin and subcutaneous tissue disorders:

Very rare: Angioedema, Bullous dermatitis (erythema multiforme, Stevens-Johnson Syndrome..), rash erythematous, urticaria, eczema and lichen planus.

Musculoskeletal, connective tissue and bone disorders:

Very rare: Arthralgia, Arthritis, Myalgia.

Renal and urinary disorders

Very rare: Glomerulonephritis.

General disorders and administration site conditions:

Very rare: Fever.

Investigations:

Very rare: Abnormal liver function test, Blood creatinine increase.

4.9 Overdose

Overdose following clopidogrel administration may lead to prolonged bleeding time and subsequent bleeding complications. Appropriate therapy should be considered if bleedings are observed.

No antidote to the pharmacological activity of clopidogrel has been found. If prompt correction of prolonged bleeding time is required, platelet transfusion may reverse the effects of clopidogrel.

5. PHARMACOLOGICAL PROPERTIES

5.1 Pharmacodynamic properties

Pharmacotherapeutical group: platelet aggregation inhibitors excl. Heparin, ATC Code: BO1AC/04.

Clopidogrel selectively inhibits the binding of adenosine diphosphate (ADP) to its platelet receptor, and the subsequent ADP-mediated activation of the GPIIb/IIIa complex, thereby inhibiting platelet aggregation. Biotransformation of clopidogrel is necessary to produce inhibition of platelet aggregation. Clopidogrel also inhibits platelet aggregation induced by other agonists by blocking the amplification of platelet activation by released ADP. Clopidogrel acts by irreversibly modifying the platelet ADP receptor. Consequently, platelets exposed to clopidogrel are affected for the remainder of their lifespan and recovery of normal platelet function occurs at a rate consistent with platelet turnover.

Repeated doses of 75 mg per day produced substantial inhibition of ADP-induced platelet aggregation from the first day; this increased progressively and reached steady state between Day 3 and Day 7. At steady state, the average inhibition level observed with a dose of 75 mg per day was between 40% and 60%. Platelet aggregation and bleeding time gradually returned to baseline values, generally within 5 days after treatment was discontinued.

The safety and efficacy of clopidogrel in preventing vascular ischaemic events have been evaluated in two double-blind studies: the CAPRIE study, a comparison of clopidogrel to ASA, and the CURE study, a comparison of clopidogrel in combination with ASA, to placebo with ASA.

The CAPRIE study included 19,185 patients with atherothrombosis as manifested by recent myocardial infarction (<35 days), recent ischaemic stroke (between 7 days and 6 months) or established peripheral arterial disease (PAD). Patients were randomised to clopidogrel 75 mg/day or ASA 325 mg/day, and were followed for 1 to 3 years. In the myocardial infarction subgroup, most of the patients received ASA for the first few days following the acute myocardial infarction.

Clopidogrel significantly reduced the incidence of new ischaemic events (combined end point of myocardial infarction, ischaemic stroke and vascular death) when compared to ASA. In the intention to treat analysis, 939 events were observed in the clopidogrel group and 1,020 events with ASA (relative risk reduction (RRR) 8.7%, [95% CI: 0.2 to 16.4]; p = 0.045), which corresponds, for every 1000 patients treated for 2 years, to 10 [CI: 0 to 20] additional patients being prevented from experiencing a new ischaemic event. Analysis of total mortality as a secondary endpoint did not show any significant difference between clopidogrel (5.8%) and ASA (6.0%).

In a subgroup analysis by qualifying condition (myocardial infarction, ischaemic stroke and PAD) the benefit appeared to be strongest (achieving statistical significance at p = 0.003) in patients enrolled due to PAD (especially those who also had a history of myocardial infarction) (RRR = 23.7%; CI 8.9 to 36.2) and weaker (not significantly different from ASA) in stroke patients (RRR = 7.3%; CI: -5.7 to 18.7). In patients who were enrolled in the trial on the sole basis of a recent myocardial infarction, clopidogrel was numerically inferior, but not statistically different from ASA (RRR = -4.0%; CI: -22.5 to 11.7). In addition, a subgroup analysis by age suggested that the benefit of clopidogrel in patients over 75 years was less than that observed in patients ≤75 years.

Since the CAPRIE trial was not powered to evaluate efficacy of individual subgroups, it is not clear whether the differences in relative risk reduction across qualifying conditions are real, or a result of chance.

The CURE study included 12,562 patients with non-ST segment elevation acute coronary syndrome (unstable angina or non-Q-wave myocardial infarction), and presenting within 24 hours of onset of the most recent episode of chest pain or symptoms consistent with ischaemia. Patients were required to have either ECG changes compatible with new ischaemia or elevated cardiac enzymes or troponin I or T to at least twice the upper limit of normal. Patients were randomised to clopidogrel (300 mg loading dose followed by 75 mg/day, N=6,259) or placebo (N=6,303), both given in combination with ASA (75-325 mg once daily) and other standard therapies. Patients were treated for up to one year. In CURE, 823 (6.6%) patients received concomitant GPIIb/IIIa receptor antagonist therapy. Heparins were administered in more than 90% of the patients and the relative rate of bleeding between clopidogrel and placebo was not significantly affected by the concomitant heparin therapy.

The number of patients experiencing the primary endpoint [cardiovascular (CV) death, myocardial infarction (MI), or stroke] was 582 (9.3%) in the clopidogrel-treated group and 719 (11.4%) in the placebo-treated group, a 20% relative risk reduction (95% CI of 10%-28%; p = 0.00009) for the clopidogrel-treated group (17% relative risk reduction when patients were treated conservatively, 29% when they underwent PTCA with or without stent and 10% when they underwent CABG). New cardiovascular events (primary endpoint) were prevented, with relative risk reductions of 22% (CI: 8.6, 33.4), 32% (CI: 12.8, 46.4), 4% (CI: -26.9, 26.7), 6% (CI: -33.5, 34.3) and 14% (CI: -31.6, 44.2), during the 0-1, 1-3, 3-6, 6-9 and 9-12 month study intervals, respectively. Thus, beyond 3 months of treatment, the benefit observed in the clopidogrel + ASA group was not further increased, whereas the risk of haemorrhage persisted (see section 4.4).

The use of clopidogrel in CURE was associated with a decrease in the need of thrombolytic therapy (RRR = 43.3%; CI: 24.3%, 57.5%) and GPIIb/IIIa inhibitors (RRR = 18.2%; CI: 6.5%, 28.3%).

The number of patients experiencing the co-primary endpoint (CV death, MI, stroke or refractory ischaemia) was 1035 (16.5%) in the clopidogrel-treated group and 1187 (18.8%) in the placebo-treated group, a 14% relative risk reduction (95% CI of 6%-21%, p = 0.0005) for the clopidogrel-treated group. This benefit was mostly driven by the statistically significant reduction in the incidence of MI [287 (4.6%) in the clopidogrel treated group and 363 (5.8%) in the placebo treated group]. There was no observed effect on the rate of rehospitalisation for unstable angina.

The results obtained in populations with different characteristics (e.g. unstable angina or non-Q-wave MI, low to high risk levels, diabetes, need for revascularisation, age, gender, etc.) were consistent with the results of the primary analysis. The benefits observed with clopidogrel were independent of other acute and long-term cardiovascular therapies (such as heparin/LMWH, GPIIb/IIIa antagonists, lipid lowering drugs, beta blockers and ACE-inhibitors). The efficacy of clopidogrel was observed independently of the dose of ASA (75-325 mg once daily).

5.2 Pharmacokinetic properties

After repeated doses of 75 mg per day, clopidogrel is rapidly absorbed. However, plasma concentrations of the parent compound are very low and below the quantification limit (0.00025 mg/l) beyond 2 hours. Absorption is at least 50%, based on urinary excretion of clopidogrel metabolites.

Clopidogrel is extensively metabolised by the liver and the main metabolite, which is inactive, is the carboxylic acid derivative which represents about 85% of the circulating compound in plasma. Peak plasma levels of this metabolite (approx. 3 mg/l after repeated 75 mg oral doses) occurred approximately 1 hour after dosing.

Clopidogrel is a prodrug. The active metabolite, a thiol derivative, is formed by oxidation of clopidogrel to 2-oxo-clopidogrel and subsequent hydrolysis. The oxidative step is regulated primarily by Cytochrome P_{450} isoenzymes 2B6 and 3A4 and to a lesser extent by 1A1, 1A2 and 2C19. The active thiol metabolite, which has been isolated *in vitro*, binds rapidly and irreversibly to platelet receptors, thus inhibiting platelet aggregation. This metabolite has not been detected in plasma.

The kinetics of the main circulating metabolite were linear (plasma concentrations increased in proportion to dose) in the dose range of 50 to 150 mg of clopidogrel.

Clopidogrel and the main circulating metabolite bind reversibly *in vitro* to human plasma proteins (98% and 94% respectively). The binding is non-saturable *in vitro* over a wide concentration range.

Following an oral dose of ^{14}C-labelled clopidogrel in man, approximately 50% was excreted in the urine and approximately 46% in the faeces in the 120 hour interval after dosing. The elimination half-life of the main circulating metabolite was 8 hours after single and repeated administration.

After repeated doses of 75 mg clopidogrel per day, plasma levels of the main circulating metabolite were lower in subjects with severe renal disease (creatinine clearance from 5 to 15 ml/min) compared to subjects with moderate renal disease (creatinine clearance from 30 to 60 ml/min) and to levels observed in other studies with healthy subjects. Although inhibition of ADP-induced platelet aggregation was lower (25%) than that observed in healthy subjects, the prolongation of bleeding was similar to that seen in healthy subjects receiving 75 mg of clopidogrel per day. In addition, clinical tolerance was good in all patients.

The pharmacokinetics and pharmacodynamics of clopidogrel were assessed in a single and multiple dose study in both healthy subjects and those with cirrhosis (Child-Pugh Class A or B). Daily dosing for 10 days with clopidogrel 75 mg/day was safe and well tolerated. Clopidogrel C_{max} for both single dose and steady state for cirrhotics was many fold higher than in normal subjects. However, plasma levels of the main circulating metabolite together with the effect of clopidogrel on ADP-induced platelet aggregation and bleeding time were comparable between these groups.

5.3 Preclinical safety data

During preclinical studies in rat and baboon, the most frequently observed effects were liver changes. These occurred at doses representing at least 25 times the exposure seen in humans receiving the clinical dose of 75 mg/day and were a consequence of an effect on hepatic metabolising enzymes. No effect on hepatic metabolising enzymes were observed in humans receiving clopidogrel at the therapeutic dose.

At very high doses, a poor gastric tolerability (gastritis, gastric erosion and/or vomiting) of clopidogrel was also reported in rat and baboon.

There was no evidence of carcinogenic effect when clopidogrel was administered for 78 weeks to mice and 104 weeks to rats when given at doses up to 77 mg/kg per day (representing at least 25 times the exposure seen in humans receiving the clinical dose of 75 mg/day).

Clopidogrel has been tested in a range of *in vitro* and *in vivo* genotoxicity studies, and showed no genotoxic activity.

Clopidogrel was found to have no effect on the fertility of male and female rats and was not teratogenic in either rats or rabbits. When given to lactating rats, clopidogrel caused a slight delay in the development of the offspring. Specific pharmacokinetic studies performed with radiolabelled clopidogrel have shown that the parent compound or its metabolites are excreted in the milk. Consequently, a direct effect (slight toxicity) or an indirect effect (low palatability) cannot be excluded.

6. PHARMACEUTICAL PARTICULARS

6.1 List of excipients

Core:

Mannitol (E421)

Macrogol 6000,

Microcrystalline cellulose

Hydrogenated castor oil

Low substituted hydroxypropylcellulose.

Coating:

Hypromellose (E464)

Lactose

Triacetin (E1518)

Titanium dioxide (E171)

Red iron oxide (E172)

Carnauba wax.

6.2 Incompatibilities

Not applicable.

6.3 Shelf life

3 years.

6.4 Special precautions for storage

No special precautions for storage.

Store in the original package.

6.5 Nature and contents of container

28 film-coated tablets packed in PVC/PVDC/Aluminium blisters in cardboard cartons.

6.6 Instructions for use and handling

No special requirements.

7. MARKETING AUTHORISATION HOLDER

Sanofi Pharma Bristol-Myers Squibb SNC

174 Avenue de France

F-75013 Paris - France

8. MARKETING AUTHORISATION NUMBER(S)

EU/1/98/069/001a

9. DATE OF FIRST AUTHORISATION/RENEWAL OF THE AUTHORISATION

15 July 1998 / 08 October 2003

10. DATE OF REVISION OF THE TEXT

05 January 2005

Plendil 2.5mg, Plendil 5mg and Plendil 10mg.

(AstraZeneca UK Limited)

1. NAME OF THE MEDICINAL PRODUCT

Plendil 2.5mg, Plendil 5mg and Plendil 10mg.

2. QUALITATIVE AND QUANTITATIVE COMPOSITION

Plendil 2.5mg contains Felodipine Ph. Eur. 2.5mg

Plendil 5mg contains Felodipine Ph. Eur. 5mg

Plendil 10mg contains Felodipine Ph. Eur. 10mg

3. PHARMACEUTICAL FORM

Circular biconvex film coated extended-release tablets.

Plendil 2.5mg - yellow tablets coded A/FL and 2.5 on the reverse.

Plendil 5mg - pink tablets coded A/FM and 5 on the reverse.

Plendil 10mg - red-brown tablets coded A/FE and 10 on the reverse.

4. CLINICAL PARTICULARS

4.1 Therapeutic indications

In the management of hypertension and prophylaxis of chronic stable angina pectoris.

4.2 Posology and method of administration

For oral administration.

The tablets should be taken in the morning irrespective of food intake. Plendil tablets must not be chewed or crushed. They should be swallowed whole with half a glass of water.

Hypertension

Adults (including elderly) The dose should be adjusted to the individual requirements of the patient. The recommended starting dose is 5mg once daily. If necessary the dose may be further increased or another antihypertensive agent added. The usual maintenance dose is 5 - 10 mg once daily. Doses higher than 20mg daily are not usually needed. For dose titration purposes a 2.5mg tablet is available. In elderly patients an initial treatment with 2.5mg daily should be considered.

Angina pectoris

Adults The dose should be adjusted individually. Treatment should be started with 5mg once daily and if needed be increased to 10mg once daily.

Children The safety and efficacy of Plendil in children has not been established.

Plendil can be used in combination with β-blockers, ACE inhibitors or diuretics. The effects on blood pressure are likely to be additive and combination therapy will usually enhance the antihypertensive effect. Care should be taken to avoid hypotension.

In patients with severely impaired liver function the dose of felodipine should be low. The pharmacokinetics are not significantly affected in patients with impaired renal function.

4.3 Contraindications

Unstable angina pectoris.

Pregnancy.

Patient with a previous allergic reaction to Plendil or other dihydropyridines because of the theoretical risk of cross-reactivity.

Plendil should not be used in patients with clinically significant aortic stenosis, uncompensated heart failure, and during or within one month of a myocardial infarction.

As with other calcium channel blockers, Plendil should be discontinued in patients who develop cardiogenic shock.

4.4 Special warnings and special precautions for use

As with other vasodilators, Plendil may, in rare cases, precipitate significant hypotension with tachycardia which in susceptible individuals may result in myocardial ischaemia.

There is no evidence that Plendil is useful for secondary prevention of myocardial infarction.

The efficacy and safety of Plendil in the treatment of malignant hypertension has not been studied.

Plendil should be used with caution in patients with severe left ventricular dysfunction.

4.5 Interaction with other medicinal products and other forms of Interaction

Concomitant administration of substances which interfere with the cytochrome P4503A4enzyme system may affect plasma concentrations of felodipine. Enzyme inhibitors such as cimetidine, erythromycin, itraconazole and ketoconazole impair the elimination of felodipine, and Plendil dosage may need to be reduced when drugs are given concomitantly. Conversely, powerful enzyme inducing agents such as some anticonvulsants (phenytoin, carbamazepine, phenobarbitone) can increase felodipine elimination and higher than normal Plendil doses may be required in patients taking the drugs.

No dosage adjustment is required when Plendil is given concomitantly with digoxin.

Felodipine does not appear to affect the unbound fraction of other extensively plasma protein bound drugs such as warfarin.

Felodipine may increase the concentration of tacrolimus. When used together, the tacrolimus serum concentration should be followed and the tacrolimus dose may need to be adjusted.

Grapefruit juice results in increased peak plasma levels and bioavailability possibly due to an interaction with flavonoids in the fruit juice. This interaction has been seen with other dihydropyridine calcium antagonists and represents a class effect. Therefore grapefruit juice should not be taken together with Plendil tablets.

4.6 Pregnancy and lactation

Felodipine should not be given during pregnancy.

In a study on fertility and general reproductive performance in rats, a prolongation of parturition resulting in difficult labour, increased foetal deaths and early postnatal deaths were observed in the medium-and high-dose groups. Reproductive studies in rabbits have shown a dose-related reversible enlargement of the mammary glands of the parent animals and dose-related digital abnormalities in the foetuses when felodipine was administered during stages of early foetal development.

Felodipine has been detected in breast milk, but it is unknown whether it has harmful effects on the new-born.

4.7 Effects on ability to drive and use machines

None.

4.8 Undesirable effects

As with other calcium antagonists, flushing, headache, palpitations, dizziness and fatigue may occur. These reactions are usually transient and are most likely to occur at the start of treatment or after an increase in dosage.

As with other calcium antagonists ankle swelling, resulting from precapillary vasodilation, may occur. The degree of ankle swelling is dose related.

In patients with gingivitis/periodontitis, mild gingival enlargement has been reported with Plendil, as with other calcium antagonists. The enlargement can be avoided or reversed by careful dental hygiene.

As with other dihydropyridines, aggravation of angina has been reported in a small number of individuals especially after starting treatment. This is more likely to happen in patients with symptomatic ischaemic heart disease.

The following adverse events have been reported from clinical trials and from Post Marketing Surveillance. In the great majority of cases a causal relationship between these events and treatment with felodipine has not been established.

Skin: very rarely - leucocytoclastic vasculitis, rarely - rash and/or pruritus, and isolated cases of photosensitivity.

Musculoskeletal: in isolated cases arthralgia and myalgia.

Psychiatric: rarely impotence/sexual dysfunction.

Central and peripheral nervous system: headache, dizziness. In isolated cases paraesthesia.

Gastrointestinal: very rarely - gingivitis, in isolated cases abdominal pain, nausea, vomiting, gum hyperplasia.

Hepatic: in isolated cases increased liver enzymes.

Urinary system: very rarely urinary frequency.

Cardiovascular: rarely - tachycardia, palpitations and syncope.

Vascular (extracardiac): peripheral oedema, flush.

Other: very rarely - fever, rarely - fatigue, in isolated cases hypersensitivity reactions e.g. urticaria, angio-oedema.

4.9 Overdose

Symptoms: Overdosage may cause excessive peripheral vasodilatation with marked hypotension which may sometimes be accompanied by bradycardia.

Management: Activiated charcoal, induction of vomiting or gastric lavage, if appropriate or indicated. Severe hypotension should be treated symptomatically, with the patient placed supine and the legs elevated. Bradycardia, if present, should be treated with atropine 0.5-1mg i.v. If this is not sufficient, plasma volume should be increased by infusion of e.g. glucose, saline or dextran. Sympathomimetic drugs with predominant effect on the α_1-adrenoceptor may be given e.g. metaraminol or phenylephrine.

5. PHARMACOLOGICAL PROPERTIES

5.1 Pharmacodynamic properties

Felodipine is a vascular selective calcium antagonist, which lowers arterial blood pressure by decreasing peripheral vascular resistance. Due to the high degree of selectivity for smooth muscle in the arterioles, felodipine in therapeutic doses has no direct effect on cardiac contractility or conduction.

It can be used as monotherapy or in combination with other antihypertensive drugs, e.g. β-receptor blockers, diuretics or ACE-inhibitors, in order to achieve an increased antihypertensive effect. Felodipine reduces both systolic and diastolic blood pressure and can be used in isolated systolic hypertension. In a study of 12 patients, felodipine maintained its antihypertensive effect during concomitant therapy with indomethacin.

Because there is no effect on venous smooth muscle or adrenergic vasomotor control, felodipine is not associated with orthostatic hypotension.

Felodipine has anti-anginal and anti-ischaemic effects due to improved myocardial oxygen supply/demand balance. Coronary vascular resistance is decreased and coronary blood flow as well as myocardial oxygen supply are increased by felodipine due to dilation of both epicardial arteries and arterioles. Felodipine effectively counteracts coronary vasospasm. The reduction in systemic blood pressure caused by felodipine leads to decreased left ventricular afterload.

Felodipine improves exercise tolerance and reduces anginal attacks in patients with stable effort induced angina pectoris. Both symptomatic and silent myocardial ischaemia are reduced by felodipine in patients with vasospastic angina. Felodipine can be used as monotherapy or in combination with β-receptor blockers in patients with stable angina pectoris.

Felodipine possesses a mild natriuretic/diuretic effect and generalised fluid retention does not occur.

Felodipine is well tolerated in patients with concomitant disease such as congestive heart failure well-controlled on appropriate therapy, asthma and other obstructive pulmonary diseases, diabetes, gout, hyperlipidemia impaired renal function, renal transplant recipients and Raynaud's disease. Felodipine has no significant effect on blood glucose levels or lipid profiles.

Haemodynamic effects: The primary haemodynamic effect of felodipine is a reduction of total peripheral vascular resistance which leads to a decrease in blood pressure. These effects are dose-dependent. In patients with mild to moderate essential hypertension, a reduction in blood pressure usually occurs 2 hours after the first oral dose and lasts for at least 24 hours with a trough/peak ratio usually above 50%.

Plasma concentration of felodipine and decrease in total peripheral resistance and blood pressure are positively correlated.

Electrophysiological and other cardiac effects: Felodipine in therapeutic doses has no effect on cardiac contractility or atrioventricular conduction or refractoriness.

Renal effects: Felodipine has a natriuretic and diuretic effect. Studies have shown that the tubular reabsorption of filtered sodium is reduced. This counteracts the salt and water retention observed for other vasodilators. Felodipine dose not affect the daily potassium excretion. The renal vascular resistance is decreased by felodipine. Normal glomerular filtration rate is unchanged. In patients with impaired renal function glomerular filtration rate may increase.

Felodipine is well tolerated in renal transplant recipients.

Site and mechanism of action: The predominant pharmacodynamic feature of felodipine is its pronounced vascular versus myocardial selectivity. Myogenically active smooth muscles in arterial resistance vessels are particularly sensitive to felodipine.

Felodipine inhibits electrical and contractile activity of vascular smooth muscle cells via an effect on the calcium channels in the cell membrane.

5.2 Pharmacokinetic properties

Absorption and distribution: Felodipine is completely absorbed from the gastrointestinal tract after administration of felodipine extended release tablets.

The systemic availability of felodipine is approximately 15% in man and is independent of dose in the therapeutic dose range.

With the extended-release tablets the absorption phase is prolonged. This results in even felodipine plasma concentrations within the therapeutic range for 24 hours.

The plasma protein binding of felodipine is approximately 99%. It is bound predominantly to the albumin fraction.

Elimination and metabolism: The average half-life of felodipine in the terminal phase is 25 hours. There is no significant accumulation during long-term treatment. Felodipine is extensively metabolised by the liver and all identified metabolites are inactive. Elderly patients and patients with reduced liver function have an average higher plasma concentration of felodipine than younger patients.

About 70% of a given dose is excreted as metabolites in the urine; the remaining fraction is excreted in the faeces. Less than 0.5% of a dose is recovered unchanged in the urine.

The kinetics of felodipine are not changed in patients with renal impairment.

5.3 Preclinical safety data

Felodipine is a calcium antagonist and lowers arterial blood pressure by decreasing vascular resistance. In general a reduction in blood pressure is evident 2 hours after the first oral dose and at steady state lasts for at least 24 hours after dose.

Felodipine exhibits a high degree of selectivity for smooth muscles in the arterioles and in therapeutic doses has no direct effect on cardiac contractility. Felodipine does not affect venous smooth muscle and adrenergic vasomotor control.

Electrophysiological studies have shown that felodipine has no direct effect on conduction in the specialised conducting system of the heart and no effect on the AV nodal refractories.

Plendil possesses a mild natriuretic/diuretic effect and does not produce general fluid retention, nor affect daily potassium excretion. Plendil is well tolerated in patients with congestive heart failure.

6. PHARMACEUTICAL PARTICULARS

6.1 List of excipients

Polyoxyl 40 hydrogenated castor oil, Hydroxypropyl cellulose, Propyl gallate, Hydroxypropyl methylcellulose, Sodium aluminium silicate, Microcrystalline cellulose, Lactose anhydrous, Sodium stearyl fumarate, Macrogol, Colour Titanium dioxide (E171), Colour Iron oxide yellow (E172) and Carnauba wax.

6.2 Incompatibilities

None stated.

6.3 Shelf life

Plendil 2.5mg – 30 months

Plendil 5mg – 3 years

Plendil 10mg – 3 years

6.4 Special precautions for storage

Do not store above 25°C.

6.5 Nature and contents of container

1. HDPE Bottles - White, high density polyethylene (PE) bottles with PE screw caps. A break-off ring guarantees the integrity of the unopened package. Each bottle contains 100 tablets.

2. Aclar® Blisters - Press through blister package of aluminium form foil with an aluminium foil as enclosure web. Each blister strip contains 7 tablets. A single pack may contain 7, 14, 28, 56 or 112 tablets as multiples of blisters of 7.

3. Tristar® Blisters - Press through packages of thermoformed PVC/PVDC with an aluminium foil as enclosure web. Each blister strip contains 7 tablets. A single pack may contain 7, 14, 28, 56 or 112 tablets as multiples of blisters of 7.

4. PVC/PVDC Blisters - Press through blister package of PVC/PVDC form foil with an aluminium foil as enclosure web. Each blister strip contains 7 tablets. A single pack may contain 7, 14, 28, 56 or 112 tablets as multiples of blisters of 7.

6.6 Instructions for use and handling

None Stated

7. MARKETING AUTHORISATION HOLDER

AstraZeneca UK Ltd.,
600 Capability Green,
Luton, LU1 3LU, UK.

8. MARKETING AUTHORISATION NUMBER(S)

Plendil 2.5mg PL 17901/0156

Plendil 5mg PL 17901/0157

Plendil 10mg PL 17901/0155

9. DATE OF FIRST AUTHORISATION/RENEWAL OF THE AUTHORISATION

Plendil 2.5mg Date MA granted: 03-02-02

Plendil 5mg Date MA granted: 03-02-02

Plendil 10mg Date MA granted: 03-02-02

10. DATE OF REVISION OF THE TEXT

5th September 2003

Pletal

(Otsuka Pharmaceuticals (UK) Ltd)

1. NAME OF THE MEDICINAL PRODUCT

PLETAL® ▼ 100 mg Tablet

2. QUALITATIVE AND QUANTITATIVE COMPOSITION

Each PLETAL® ▼ 100 mg Tablet contains 100 mg of cilostazol.

3. PHARMACEUTICAL FORM

Tablet

White, round, flat faced tablets embossed with "OG30" on one side.

4. CLINICAL PARTICULARS

4.1 Therapeutic indications

Pletal is indicated for the improvement of the maximal and pain-free walking distances in patients with intermittent claudication, who do not have rest pain and who do not have evidence of peripheral tissue necrosis.

4.2 Posology and method of administration

The recommended dosage of cilostazol is 100 mg twice a day. Cilostazol should be taken 30 minutes before or two hours after breakfast and the evening meal. Taking cilostazol with food has been shown to increase the maximum plasma concentrations (C_{max}) of cilostazol, which may be associated with an increased incidence of adverse effects.

Treatment for 16-24 weeks can result in a significant improvement in walking distance. Some benefit may be observed following treatment for 4-12 weeks.

The elderly

There are no special dosage requirements for the elderly.

Children

Safety and efficacy in children have not been established.

Renal Impairment

No dose adjustment is necessary in patients with a creatinine clearance of >25 ml/min. Cilostazol is contraindicated in patients with a creatinine clearance of ≤25 ml/min.

Hepatic Impairment

No dosage adjustment is necessary in patients with mild hepatic disease. There are no data in patients with moderate or severe hepatic impairment. Since cilostazol is extensively metabolised by hepatic enzymes, it is contraindicated in patients with moderate or severe hepatic impairment.

4.3 Contraindications

– Known hypersensitivity to cilostazol or any of the inactive ingredients

– Severe renal impairment: creatinine clearance of ≤ 25 ml/min

– Moderate or severe hepatic impairment

– Congestive heart failure

– Pregnancy and lactation

– Patients with any known predisposition to bleeding (e.g. active peptic ulceration, recent (within six months) haemorrhagic stroke, surgery within the previous three months, proliferative diabetic retinopathy, poorly controlled hypertension)

– Patients taking inhibitors of CYP3A4 or of CYP2C19 (e.g. cimetidine, diltiazem, erythromycin, ketoconazole, lansoprazole, omeprazole and inhibitors of HIV-1 proteases). Further detailed information can be found in Section 4.4 *Special Warnings and Special Precautions for Use* and Section 4.5 *Interactions*

– Patients with any history of ventricular tachycardia, ventricular fibrillation or multifocal ventricular ectopics, whether or not adequately treated, and in patients with prolongation of the QTc interval

4.4 Special warnings and special precautions for use

Patients should be warned to report any episode of bleeding or easy bruising whilst on therapy. In case of retinal bleeding administration of cilostazol should be stopped. Refer to Sections 4.3 *Contraindications* and 4.5 *Interactions with Other Medicaments and Other Forms of Interaction* for further advice on bleeding.

It is recommended that caution be exercised during co-administration with substrates of CYP3A4 or CYP2C19 (e.g. cisapride, midazolam, nifedipine and verapamil). Cilostazol is contraindicated in patients taking inhibitors of CYP3A4 or CYP2C19. See Section 4.3 *Contraindications* and Section 4.5 *Interactions* for further information.

Cilostazol is relatively highly protein bound and thus there is a theoretical potential that antiplatelet activity could be enhanced as a result of displacement by other highly bound drugs.

Caution should be exercised when prescribing cilostazol for patients with atrial or ventricular ectopy and patients with atrial fibrillation or flutter.

Caution is needed when co-administering cilostazol with any other agent which has the potential to reduce blood pressure due to the possibility that there may be an additive hypotensive effect with a reflex tachycardia. Refer also to Section 4.8 *Undesirable Effects*.

4.5 Interaction with other medicinal products and other forms of Interaction

Inhibitors of platelet aggregation

Cilostazol is a PDE III inhibitor with anti-platelet activity. In a clinical study in healthy subjects, cilostazol 150mg b.i.d. for five days did not result in prolongation of bleeding time.

Aspirin

Short term (⩽4 days) co-administration of aspirin with cilostazol suggested a 23-25% increase in inhibition of ADP-induced *ex vivo* platelet aggregation when compared to aspirin alone. There was no additive or synergistic effect on arachidonic acid induced platelet aggregation when compared to aspirin alone. There were no apparent trends toward a greater incidence of haemorrhagic adverse effects in patients taking cilostazol and aspirin compared to patients taking placebo and equivalent doses of aspirin. It is recommended that the daily dose of aspirin should not exceed 80 mg.

Clopidogrel

Concomitant administration of cilostazol 150 mg b.i.d. and clopidogrel 75 mg daily for five days did not have a notable effect on the pharmacokinetics of cilostazol, with an increase in AUC of only 9%. However, the AUC of the dehydro metabolite, which has 3-4 times the potency of cilostazol in inhibiting platelet aggregation, increased by 24%. Concomitant administration did not have any effect on platelet count, prothrombin time (PT) or activated partial thromboplastin time (aPTT). All subjects in the study had a prolongation of bleeding time on clopidogrel alone and it was not possible to determine whether there was an additive effect on bleeding times during concomitant administration with cilostazol. Caution is advised when co-administering cilostazol with any drug that inhibits platelet aggregation. Consideration should be given to monitoring the bleeding time at intervals.

Anticoagulants

In a single-dose clinical study, no inhibition of the metabolism of warfarin or an effect on the

Coagulation parameters (PT, aPTT, bleeding time) was observed. However, caution is advised in patients receiving both cilostazol and any anticoagulant agent, and frequent monitoring is required to reduce the possibility of bleeding.

Cytochrome P-450 (CYP) Enzyme Inhibitors

Cilostazol is extensively metabolised by CYP enzymes, particularly CYP3A4 and to a lesser extent CYP2C19 although other enzymes are involved. Some of the metabolites, particularly the dehydro metabolite, possess cilostazol-like activity. The effects of co-administration with CYP enzyme inhibitors are complex and cilostazol is contraindicated in patients taking inhibitors of CYP3A4 or CYP2C19. Examples of the many drugs which are known to inhibit either of these isoenzymes are given in Section 4.3.

Administration of 100 mg cilostazol on the seventh day of erythromycin (a moderate inhibitor of CYP3A4) 500 mg t.i.d. resulted in an increase in AUC cilostazol by 74%, accompanied by a 24% decrease in AUC of the dehydro metabolite but with notable increases in AUC of the 4'-trans-hydroxy metabolite.

Co-administration of single doses of ketoconazole (a strong inhibitor of CYP3A4 and an inhibitor of 2C19) 400 mg and cilostazol 100 mg resulted in a > 2-fold increase in AUC of cilostazol and increased systemic exposure to 4'-trans-hydroxymetabolite.

In healthy subjects dosed with cilostazol 100 mg b.i.d., mean AUC cilostazol increased by 44% on co-administration with diltiazem (an inhibitor of CYP3A4) at 180 mg once daily. Co-administration did not affect exposure to the dehydro metabolite but there were increases in AUC of the 4'-trans-hydroxy metabolite. In patients in clinical trials, concomitant use with diltiazem was shown to increase the AUC of cilostazol by 53%.

Administration of a single dose of 100 mg cilostazol with 240 ml grapefruit juice did not have a notable effect on the pharmacokinetics of cilostazol.

Administration of a single dose of 100 mg cilostazol on day 7 of dosing with omeprazole (inhibits CYP2C19) 40 mg once daily increased Cmax and AUC cilostazol by 18% and 26%, respectively. Cmax and AUC of the dehydro metabolite increased by 29% and 69% while exposure to the 4'-trans-hydroxy metabolite decreased by 31%.

Cytochrome P-450 Enzyme Substrates

Cilostazol was shown to inhibit CYP3A4, CYP2C19 and CYP2C9 *in vitro*, but only at concentrations several times higher than the maximal circulating level at therapeutic dosages. An interaction study with warfarin did not demonstrate significant effects on the pharmacokinetics of R-warfarin (substrate of CYP3A4) or S-warfarin (substrate of CYP2C9). However, the AUCs for lovastatin (substrate for CYP3A4) and its β-hydroxy acid were increased by more than 70% when given with cilostazol.

Caution is advised when cilostazol is administered along with drugs which are substrates of CYP2C19 or CYP3A4 especially those with a narrow therapeutic index. Examples of the many drugs which are the substrates of either of these isoenzymes are given in Section 4.4.

4.6 Pregnancy and lactation

Pregnancy

Studies in animals have shown reproductive toxicity (see section 5.3). There is no experience of the use of cilostazol in human pregnancy. Therefore cilostazol should not be used during pregnancy.

Lactation

The transfer of cilostazol to breast milk has been reported in animal studies. Therefore cilostazol should not be used in nursing mothers.

4.7 Effects on ability to drive and use machines

Cilostazol may cause dizziness and patients should be warned to exercise caution before they drive or operate machinery.

4.8 Undesirable effects

Clinical trials

The most commonly reported adverse reactions in clinical trials were headache (in > 30%), diarrhoea and abnormal stools (in >15% each). These reactions were usually of mild to moderate intensity and were sometimes alleviated by reducing the dose.

Adverse reactions reported as being at least possibly drug-related and occurring more commonly with Pletal 100 mg b.i.d. than in the placebo groups in clinical trials are listed below.

The frequencies correspond with: Very common: >1/10

Common >1/100, ⩽ 1/10

Uncommon >1/1,000, ⩽ 1/100

Rare >1/10,000, ⩽ 1/1000

Very rare ⩽1/10,000

Blood and the lymphatic system disorders

Common: Ecchymosis,

Uncommon Anaemia

Rare Bleeding time increased, thrombocythemia

Haemorrhagic disorders

Uncommon: Haemorrhages (eye, nose, gastrointestinal, cardiovascular)

Endocrine disorders

Uncommon Diabetes mellitus *Metabolism and nutrition disorders*

Common Oedema (peripheral, face).

Uncommon Hyperglycaemia

Nervous system disorders

Common Dizziness

Uncommon Insomnia, anxiety, abnormal dreams

Cardiac disorders

Common Palpitation, tachycardia, angina pectoris, arrhythmia, ventricular extrasystoles

Uncommon Myocardial infarction, atrial fibrillation, congestive heart failure, supraventricular tachycardia, ventricular tachycardia, syncope, postural hypotension

Respiratory, thoracic and mediastinal disorders

Common Rhinitis

Uncommon Dyspnoea, pneumonia, cough

Gastrointestinal disorders

Very Common Diarrhoea, abnormal stools.

Common Nausea and vomiting, dyspepsia, flatulence.

Uncommon Gastritis

Skin and subcutaneous tissue disorders

Common Rash, pruritus

Musculoskeletal, connective tissue and bone disorders

Uncommon Myalgia.

Renal and urinary disorders

Rare Kidney failure, kidney function abnormal

General disorders and administration site conditions

Very Common Headache

Common Chest pain, abdominal pain, asthenia

Uncommon Chills, allergic reaction

An increase in the incidence of palpitation and peripheral oedema was observed when cilostazol was combined with other vasodilators that cause reflex tachycardia e.g. dihydropyridine calcium channel blockers.

The only adverse event resulting in discontinuation of therapy in ⩾3% of patients treated with cilostazol was headache. Other frequent causes of discontinuation included palpitation and diarrhoea (both 1.1%).

Cilostazol *per se* may carry an increased risk of bleeding and this risk may be potentiated by co-administration with any other agent with such potential.

The risk of intraocular bleeding may be higher in patients with diabetes.

Post-marketing experience

Additional reactions not reported during clinical trials but reported rarely or very rarely in the post-marketing period are listed below.

Infections and infestations: Interstitial pneumonia

Blood and the lymphatic system disorders: Bleeding tendency, thrombocytopenia, granulocytopenia, agranulocytosis, leucopenia

Haemorrhagic disorders: Haemorrhages (cerebral, respiratory tract, pulmonary, muscle)

Metabolism and nutrition disorders: Anorexia

Nervous system disorders: Paresis, hypaesthesia

Eye disorders: Conjunctivitis

Ear and labyrinth disorders: Tinnitus

Vascular disorders: Hot flushes, hypertension, hypotension

Hepato-biliary disorders: Hepatitis, hepatic function abnormal, jaundice

Skin and subcutaneous tissue disorders: Subcutaneous haemorrhage, eczema, skin eruptions including Stevens-Johnson syndrome or toxic epidermal necrolysis, urticaria

Renal and urinary disorder: Haematuria, increased urinary frequency

General disorders and administration site conditions: Pyrexia, malaise, pain

Investigations: Uric acid level increased, BUN increased, blood creatinine increased

4.9 Overdose

Information on acute overdose in humans is limited. The signs and symptoms can be anticipated to be severe headache, diarrhoea, tachycardia and possibly cardiac arrhythmias.

Patients should be observed and given supportive treatment. The stomach should be emptied by induced vomiting or gastric lavage, as appropriate.

5. PHARMACOLOGICAL PROPERTIES

5.1 Pharmacodynamic properties

Pharmacotherapeutic group: Antithrombotic agents, platelet aggregation inhibitor excl. heparin.

ATC code: B01A C

From data generated in eight placebo-controlled studies (where 1,374 patients were exposed to the drug), it has been demonstrated that cilostazol improves exercise capacity as judged by changes in Absolute Claudication Distance (ACD, or maximal walking distance) and Initial Claudication Distance (ICD, or pain-free walking distance) upon treadmill testing. Following 24 weeks treatment, increases in ACD ranged from 76.2-142.6 metres, whilst ICD increases ranged from 44.0-102.5 metres.

A pooled analysis across the eight studies indicated that there was a significant overall post-baseline improvement in maximal walking distance (ACD) for cilostazol relative to placebo of about 20%. This effect appeared lower in diabetics (15%) than in non-diabetics (24%).

Animal studies have shown cilostazol to have vasodilator effects and this has been demonstrated in small studies in man where ankle blood flow was measured by strain gauge plethysmography. Cilostazol also inhibits smooth muscle cell proliferation in rat and human smooth muscle cells *in vitro*, and inhibits the platelet release reaction of platelet-derived growth factor and PF-4 in human platelets.

Studies in animals and in man (*in vivo* and *ex vivo*) have shown that cilostazol causes reversible inhibition of platelet aggregation. The inhibition is effective against a range of aggregants (including shear stress, arachidonic acid, collagen, ADP and adrenaline); in man the inhibition lasts for up to 12 hours, and on cessation of administration of cilostazol recovery of aggregation occurred within 48-96 hours, without rebound hyperaggregability.

A 12-week study of cilostazol at 100 mg b.i.d. compared to placebo produced a statistically significant increase in HDL cholesterol of about 10% (0.10 mmol/L), and a statistically significant decrease in triglycerides of about 15% (0.33 mmol/L).

5.2 Pharmacokinetic properties

Following multiple doses of cilostazol 100 mg twice daily in patients with peripheral vascular disease, steady state is achieved within 4 days.

The C_{max} of cilostazol and its primary circulating metabolites increase less than proportionally with increasing doses. However, the AUC for cilostazol and its metabolites increase approximately proportionally with dose.

The apparent elimination half-life of cilostazol is 10.5 hours. There are two major metabolites, a dehydro-cilostazol and a 4'-trans-hydroxy cilostazol, both of which have similar apparent half-lives. The dehydro metabolite is 4-7 times as active a platelet anti-aggregant as the parent compound and the 4'-trans-hydroxy metabolite is one fifth as active.

Cilostazol is eliminated predominantly by metabolism and subsequent urinary excretion of metabolites. The primary isoenzymes involved in its metabolism are cytochrome P-450 CYP3A4, to a lesser extent, CYP2C19, and to an even lesser extent CYP1A2.

The primary route of elimination is urinary (74%) with the remainder excreted in the faeces. No measurable amount of unchanged cilostazol is excreted in the urine, and less than 2% of the dose is excreted as the dehydro-cilostazol metabolite. Approximately 30% of the dose is excreted in the urine as the 4'-trans-hydroxy metabolite. The remainder is excreted as metabolites, none of which exceed 5% of the total excreted.

Cilostazol is 95-98% protein bound, predominantly to albumin. The dehydro metabolite and 4'-trans-hydroxy metabolite are 97.4% and 66% protein bound respectively.

There is no evidence that cilostazol induces hepatic microsomal enzymes.

The pharmacokinetics of cilostazol and its metabolites were not significantly affected by age or gender in healthy subjects aged between 50-80 years.

In subjects with severe renal impairment, the free fraction of cilostazol was 27% higher and both C_{max} and AUC were 29% and 39% lower respectively than in subjects with normal renal function. The C_{max} and AUC of the dehydro metabolite were 41% and 47% lower respectively in the severely renally impaired subjects compared to subjects with normal renal function. The C_{max} and AUC of 4'-trans-hydroxy cilostazol were 173% and 209% greater in subjects with severe renal impairment. The drug should not be administered to patients with a creatinine clearance <25ml/min (see Section 4.3 *Contraindications*).

There are no data in patients with moderate to severe hepatic impairment and since cilostazol is extensively metabolised by hepatic enzymes, the drug should not be used in such patients (see Section 4.3 *Contraindications*).

5.3 Preclinical safety data

Toxicodynamic effects were consistent with those expected for compounds of this class. Most of these responses were exaggerated physiological or pharmacological effects.

There were functional disturbances in the gastrointestinal tract at high dose levels, particularly in non-rodents. Changes in the cardiovascular system, especially in dogs, probably due to exaggerated pharmacological effects, were observed.

There were no unusual findings suggestive of any unexpected target organ toxicity due to repeated administration of cilostazol to laboratory animals.

Cilostazol is not a genotoxic mutagen. Two-year carcinogenicity studies have been conducted by the oral (dietary) route of administration in rats at doses up to 500 mg/kg/day, and in mice at doses up to 1000 mg/kg/day. No unusual neoplastic outcomes were observed in these studies.

In rats dosed during pregnancy, foetal weights were decreased. In addition, an increase in foetuses with external, visceral and skeletal abnormalities was noted at high dose levels. At lower dose levels, retardations of ossification were observed. Exposure in late pregnancy resulted in an increased incidence of stillbirths and lower offspring weights. An increased incidence of retardation of ossification of the sternum was observed in rabbits.

6. PHARMACEUTICAL PARTICULARS

6.1 List of excipients

Maize starch, microcrystalline cellulose, carmellose calcium, hypromellose and magnesium stearate.

6.2 Incompatibilities

Not applicable.

6.3 Shelf life

3 years.

6.4 Special precautions for storage

No special precautions for storage.

6.5 Nature and contents of container

Cartons containing 20, 28, 30, 50, 56, 100, 112 and 168 tablets packed in PVC/Aluminium blisters.

6.6 Instructions for use and handling

No special requirements.

7. MARKETING AUTHORISATION HOLDER

Otsuka Pharmaceutical Europe Ltd
9th Floor, Commonwealth House
2 Chalkhill Road
Hammersmith
London W6 8DW
UK

8. MARKETING AUTHORISATION NUMBER(S)

PL 11515/0001

9. DATE OF FIRST AUTHORISATION/RENEWAL OF THE AUTHORISATION

21 March 2000

10. DATE OF REVISION OF THE TEXT

25 October 2002

Pneumovax II

(Sanofi Pasteur MSD)

1. NAME OF THE MEDICINAL PRODUCT

PNEUMOVAX® II Vial

Pneumococcal Polysaccharide Vaccine

2. QUALITATIVE AND QUANTITATIVE COMPOSITION

The 0.5 mL dose of vaccine contains 25 micrograms of each of the following 23 pneumococcal serotypes: 1, 2, 3, 4, 5, 6B, 7F, 8, 9N, 9V, 10A, 11A, 12F, 14, 15B, 17F, 18C, 19F, 19A, 20, 22F, 23F, 33F.

For excipients, see 6.1.

3. PHARMACEUTICAL FORM

Solution for injection in a vial

4. CLINICAL PARTICULARS

4.1 Therapeutic indications

PNEUMOVAX® II is recommended for active immunisation against disease caused by the pneumococcal serotypes included in the vaccine. The vaccine is recommended for individuals 2 years of age or older in whom there is an increased risk of morbidity and mortality from pneumococcal disease. The specific at risk categories of persons to be immunised are to be determined on the basis of official recommendations.

The safety and efficacy of the vaccine have not been established in children under 2 years of age, in whom the antibody response may be poor.

The vaccine is not effective for the prevention of acute otitis media, sinusitis and other common upper respiratory tract infections.

4.2 Posology and method of administration

Primary vaccination: one single dose of 0.5 millilitre by intramuscular or subcutaneous injection.

Special dosing:

It is recommended that pneumococcal vaccine should preferably be given at least two weeks before elective splenectomy or the initiation of chemotherapy or other immunosuppressive treatment. Vaccination during chemotherapy or radiation therapy should be avoided.

Following completion of chemotherapy and/or radiation therapy for neoplastic disease, immune responses to vaccination may remain diminished, and the vaccine may not be protective. Full recovery of the immune response to vaccination may take two years or more depending upon the degree of immunosuppression that accompanies the illness and its treatment. (See 4.4 Special warnings and precautions for use.) Accordingly, the vaccine should not be administered any sooner than three months after completion of such therapy. A longer delay may be appropriate for patients who have received intensive or prolonged treatment.

Persons with asymptomatic or symptomatic HIV infection should be vaccinated as soon as possible after their diagnosis is confirmed.

Revaccination

One single dose of 0.5 millilitre by intramuscular or subcutaneous injection.

The specific timing of, and need for, revaccination should be determined on the basis of official recommendations.

Revaccination at an interval of less than three years is not recommended because of an increased risk of adverse reactions. However, revaccination is generally well tolerated with intervals of three years or longer between doses. A modestly increased rate of self-limited local reactions has been observed compared with primary vaccination.

There are limited clinical data regarding administration of more than two doses of PNEUMOVAX® II.

Healthy adults and children should not be revaccinated routinely.

Adults

Revaccination is recommended for persons at increased risk of serious pneumococcal infection who were given pneumococcal vaccine more than five years earlier or for those known to have a rapid decline in pneumococcal antibody levels.

For selected populations (e.g., asplenics) who are known to be at high risk of fatal pneumococcal infections, revaccination at three years should be considered.

Children

Revaccination after three years should be considered for children 10 years old or younger at highest risk for pneumococcal infection (e.g., those with nephrotic syndrome, asplenia or sickle cell disease).

4.3 Contraindications

Hypersensitivity to any component of the vaccine.

4.4 Special warnings and special precautions for use

Delay the use of the vaccine in any significant febrile illness, other active infection or when a systemic reaction would pose a significant risk except when this delay may involve even greater risk.

PNEUMOVAX® II should never be injected intravascularly, and precautions should be taken to make sure the needle does not enter a blood vessel. Also, the vaccine should not be injected intradermally, as injection by that route is associated with increased local reactions.

If the vaccine is administered to patients who are immunosuppressed due to either an underlying condition or medical treatment (e.g., immunosuppressive therapy such as cancer chemotherapy or radiation therapy), the expected serum antibody response may not be obtained after a first or second dose. Accordingly, such patients may not be as well protected against pneumococcal disease as immunocompetent individuals.

For patients receiving immunosuppressive therapy, the time to recovery of the immune response varies with the illness and the therapy. Significant improvement in antibody response has been observed for some patients during the two years following the completion of chemotherapy or other immunosuppressive therapy (with or without radiation), particularly as the interval between the end of treatment and pneumococcal vaccination increased. (See 4.2 Posology and method of administration, Special Dosing.)

As with any vaccine, adequate treatment provisions including epinephrine (adrenaline) should be available for immediate use should an acute anaphylactic reaction occur.

Required prophylactic antibiotic therapy against pneumococcal infection should not be stopped after pneumococcal vaccination.

Patients at especially increased risk of serious pneumococcal infection (e.g., asplenics and those who have received immunosuppressive therapy for any reason), should be advised regarding the possible need for early antimicrobial treatment in the event of severe, sudden febrile illness.

Pneumococcal vaccine may not be effective in preventing infection resulting from basilar skull fracture or from external communication with cerebrospinal fluid.

There are limited clinical data regarding administration of more than two doses of PNEUMOVAX® II. (See 4.2 Posology and method of administration, Revaccination.)

4.5 Interaction with other medicinal products and other forms of Interaction

Pneumococcal vaccine can be administered simultaneously with influenza vaccine as long as different needles and injection sites are used.

4.6 Pregnancy and lactation

Use during pregnancy

It is not known whether the vaccine can cause fetal harm or affect reproduction capacity when administered to a pregnant woman; the vaccine can be given to pregnant women only if clearly needed (potential benefit must justify any potential risk to the fetus).

In animals, no reproductive data are available.

Use during lactation

It is not known whether this vaccine is excreted in human milk. Caution should be exercised when PNEUMOVAX® II is administered to a nursing mother.

4.7 Effects on ability to drive and use machines

There is no information to suggest that PNEUMOVAX® II affects the ability to drive or operate machinery.

4.8 Undesirable effects

The following adverse experiences have been reported with PNEUMOVAX® II in clinical trials and/or post-marketing experience:

The most common adverse experiences (> 1/10) reported in clinical trials were:

Fever (≤38.8°C) and injection site reactions, consisting of soreness, erythema, warmth, swelling and local induration.

Very rarely, injection site cellulitis with short onset time from vaccine administration has also been reported during post-marketing experience.

Other adverse experiences reported in clinical trials and/or in post-marketing experience include:

Body as a whole

Asthenia

Fever (>38.8° C)

Malaise

Digestive System

Nausea

Vomiting

Hematological/Lymphatic System

Lymphadenitis

Thrombocytopenia in patients with stabilized idiopathic thrombocytopenic purpura

Hemolytic anaemia in patients who have had other hematologic disorders

Hypersensitivity

Anaphylactoid reactions

Serum sickness

Musculoskeletal System
Arthralgia
Arthritis
Myalgia
Nervous System
Headache
Paresthesia
Radiculoneuropathy
Guillain-Barré Syndrome
Skin
Rash
Urticaria.

4.9 Overdose
No specific information is available on the treatment of overdose with PNEUMOVAX® II.

5. PHARMACOLOGICAL PROPERTIES
5.1 Pharmacodynamic properties
Pharmacotherapeutic group: pneumococcal vaccines, ATC code: J07 AL

The vaccine is prepared from purified pneumococcal capsular polysaccharide antigens derived from the 23 serotypes that account for approximately 90% of invasive pneumococcal disease types.

The presence of type-specific humoral antibodies is generally thought to be effective in preventing pneumococcal disease. When postvaccination antibody levels have been compared to prevaccination levels or negative control sera, the vaccine has been demonstrated to be immunogenic for each of the 23 capsular types contained in the vaccine. As measured by either radioimmunoassay or enzyme immunoassay, most persons (85 to 95%) respond by making antibody to most or all of the 23 antigens. Protective type- specific capsular polysaccharide antibody levels usually appear by the third week following vaccination.

Although the duration of the protective effect of the vaccine is unknown, previous studies with other pneumococcal vaccines suggest that induced antibodies to some serotypes may decline as soon as 3 to 5 years after vaccination, dependent on the serotype and the population. A more rapid decline in antibody levels may occur in some groups (e.g., children). Limited published data suggest that antibody levels may also decline more rapidly in the elderly.

The results from one epidemiologic study suggest that vaccination may provide protection for at least 9 years after receipt of the initial dose of vaccine. Decreasing estimates of effectiveness have been reported with increasing interval after vaccination, particularly among the very elderly (persons aged ⩾ 85 years).

The protective level of anticapsular polysaccharide antibody has not been established for pneumococcal infection caused by any specific capsular type. However, ⩾ 2-fold increase in antibody level following vaccination was associated with efficacy in clinical trials of polyvalent pneumococcal polysaccharide vaccines.

The efficacy of polyvalent pneumococcal polysaccharide vaccine was established for pneumococcal pneumonia and bacteremia in randomized controlled trials that were conducted among novice gold miners in South Africa. Protective efficacy for pneumococcal pneumonia, the primary endpoint in these studies, with a 6-valent vaccine was 76.1%; and with a 12-valent preparation was 91.7%.

Subsequently, several trials have assessed the effectiveness of the vaccine in preventing invasive pneumococcal disease in target populations. These studies have generally found vaccine effectiveness to be 50 to 70% among persons for whom the vaccine is recommended (see Section 4.1 Therapeutic indications). Effectiveness has been demonstrated in persons with diabetes mellitus, chronic cardiac or pulmonary disease, and anatomic asplenia. Vaccination effectiveness in persons with other high risk conditions has not been shown, because the numbers of patients available for study are generally too small.

One study found that vaccination was significantly protective against invasive pneumococcal disease caused by several individual serotypes (e.g., 1, 3, 4, 8, 9V, and 14). For other serotypes, the numbers of cases detected in this study were too small, and thus evidence on effectiveness was inconclusive.

5.2 Pharmacokinetic properties
Since PNEUMOVAX® II is a vaccine, pharmacokinetic studies were not performed.

5.3 Preclinical safety data
No preclinical safety testing was performed using PNEUMOVAX® II.

6. PHARMACEUTICAL PARTICULARS
6.1 List of excipients
Phenol
Sodium chloride
Water for injections

6.2 Incompatibilities
Do not mix with other vaccines/drugs.

6.3 Shelf life
30 months.

6.4 Special precautions for storage
Store at +2 to +8°C.
DO NOT FREEZE.
If frozen, the vaccine should not be used.

6.5 Nature and contents of container
0.5 mL of solution in vial (type I glass) with stopper (rubber) with a flip off cap (plastic), pack of 1, 10 or 20.

6.6 Instructions for use and handling
The vaccine should be used directly as supplied; no dilution or reconstitution is necessary. The vaccine is a clear, colourless solution.

Administrative Data
7. MARKETING AUTHORISATION HOLDER
Sanofi Pasteur MSD Limited
Mallards Reach
Bridge Avenue
Maidenhead
Berkshire
SL6 1QP

8. MARKETING AUTHORISATION NUMBER(S)
PL 6745/0103

9. DATE OF FIRST AUTHORISATION/RENEWAL OF THE AUTHORISATION
3 May 2000

10. DATE OF REVISION OF THE TEXT
April 2005

Poliomyelitis Vaccine Live (Oral) PhEur (Monodose)

(GlaxoSmithKline UK)

1. NAME OF THE MEDICINAL PRODUCT
Poliomyelitis Vaccine, Live (Oral) Ph. Eur. (Monodose®)

2. QUALITATIVE AND QUANTITATIVE COMPOSITION
1 dose (Three drops; 0.135 ml) contains:
Live attenuated poliovirus (oral)
type 1 (strain LSc, 2ab) not less than 10^6 $TCID_{50}$
type 2 (strain P712 Ch,2ab) not less than 10^5 $TCID_{50}$
type 3 (strain Leon 12a, 1b) not less than $10^{5.5}$ $TCID_{50}$
There is an overage of $10^{0.5}$.5TCID50/dose for each polio virus type
Produced in human diploid (MRC-5) cells
For excipients, see section 6.1

3. PHARMACEUTICAL FORM
Oral drops, solution.

4. CLINICAL PARTICULARS
4.1 Therapeutic indications
Active immunisation against poliomyelitis.

4.2 Posology and method of administration
For oral use only. Not for injection.

Dosage
Adults and Children:
Three drops of vaccine from the monodose tube constitute one dose, which may be given with syrup or on a lump of sugar to mask the bitter salty taste of the magnesium chloride. Do not administer on foods, which contain preservatives.

For a complete schedule, three doses of the vaccine should be given at intervals of at least four weeks.

Other unvaccinated members of the same household (including adults) should be advised vaccination at the same time as the vaccinee.

4.3 Contraindications
The vaccine should not be used in the presence of acute febrile illness or intercurrent infection, persistent diarrhoea, or vomiting or other gastrointestinal disturbance (a minor infection is not a contraindication). The vaccine should also not be given in the presence of impaired immune response including leukaemia, lymphoma, generalised malignancy or treatment with corticosteroids, cytotoxic drugs or irradiation.

The vaccine should not be administered to subjects with known systemic hypersensitivity to any of the constituents of the vaccine, or to subjects having shown signs of hypersensitivity after previous administration of the vaccine.

4.4 Special warnings and special precautions for use
The vaccine may contain trace amounts of polymyxin B and neomycin which should not contra-indicate its use except in those with a history of severe anaphylaxis due to these antibiotics.

Contacts of recent vaccinees should be advised of the need for strict personal hygiene as vaccine strain polio virus may persist in faeces for up to six weeks after vaccination.

In immunocompetent recipients previous vaccination with inactivated poliomyelitis vaccine is not a contra-indication.

HIV-positive asymptomatic individuals may receive live polio vaccine but excretion of the vaccine virus in the faeces may continue for longer than in normal individuals. Household contacts should be warned of this and for the need for strict personal hygiene, including hand washing after nappy changes for an HIV-positive infant.

For HIV-positive symptomatic individuals, IPV may be used instead of OPV at the discretion of the clinician.

Diarrhoea or vomiting (including gastrointestinal infections) may interfere with replication ('take' rate).

4.5 Interaction with other medicinal products and other forms of Interaction
At least three weeks should normally intervene between the administration of any two live vaccines. Poliomyelitis vaccine can, however, be given simultaneously with measles mumps and rubella vaccines and with DTP vaccine. In this case the injectable vaccines should be given at different sites.

No data has been generated on the simultaneous administration of oral poliomyelitis vaccine with oral typhoid vaccine therefore the theoretical possibility of an interaction between the two products cannot be ruled out.

Poliomyelitis vaccine has been given at the same time as BCG or hepatitis b vaccines.

In some populations and groups of vaccinees lower seroconversion rates have been observed. Due to various non-specific factors all three vaccine viruses may not replicate optimally in the gut of susceptible subjects, even after three doses.

4.6 Pregnancy and lactation
Pregnant women should not be given oral poliomyelitis vaccine unless they are at definite risk from poliomyelitis.

The effect on breastfed infants of the administration of oral poliomyelitis vaccine to their mothers has not been evaluated in clinical studies.

4.7 Effects on ability to drive and use machines
Not applicable.

4.8 Undesirable effects
Non-specific signs and symptoms such as fever, malaise, headache, vomiting and diarrhoea have been described after immunisation.

Paralysis temporally associated with vaccination has been reported very rarely in recipients or contacts.

Anaphylaxis has been reported extremely rarely. As polio vaccine is mostly given concomitantly with other vaccines, causal relationship to polio vaccine is usually very difficult to establish.

4.9 Overdose
Occasional reports of overdosage have been received. Overdosage has not resulted in ill effects.

5. PHARMACOLOGICAL PROPERTIES
5.1 Pharmacodynamic properties
Active immunisation against poliomyelitis.

5.2 Pharmacokinetic properties
Not applicable.

5.3 Preclinical safety data
Preclinical safety data conforms with WHO recommendations.

6. PHARMACEUTICAL PARTICULARS
6.1 List of excipients
Magnesium chloride
Arginine
Polysorbate 80
Purified Water

6.2 Incompatibilities
None

6.3 Shelf life
12 months.

6.4 Special precautions for storage
Store in the original container to protect from light and store between 2°C and 8°C in a refrigerator.

6.5 Nature and contents of container
Polyethylene tube fitted with a nozzle and a cap containing 1 dose of vaccine. When inverted the cap may be twisted to break off the nozzle and expel the contents.

6.6 Instructions for use and handling
Before administration the contents of the tube should be inspected for particulate matter, in line with good vaccination practice. In the event that the nozzle falls into the tube, dispose of it as described in point 5. This is a precaution, however, as it is unlikely that the nozzle could be expelled

from the tube. **Do not administer directly into the vaccinee's mouth as the tube may slip and cause choking.**

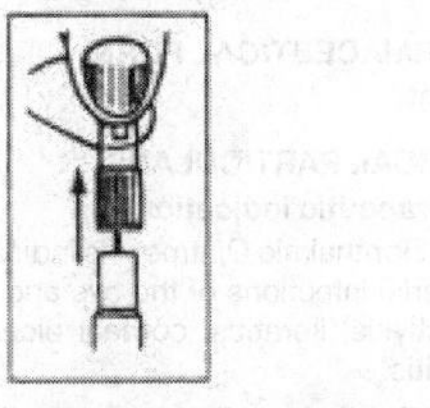

1. Pull off the protective cap from the top of the tube.

2. Turn the cap upside-down, replace the cap vertically over the nozzle as shown.

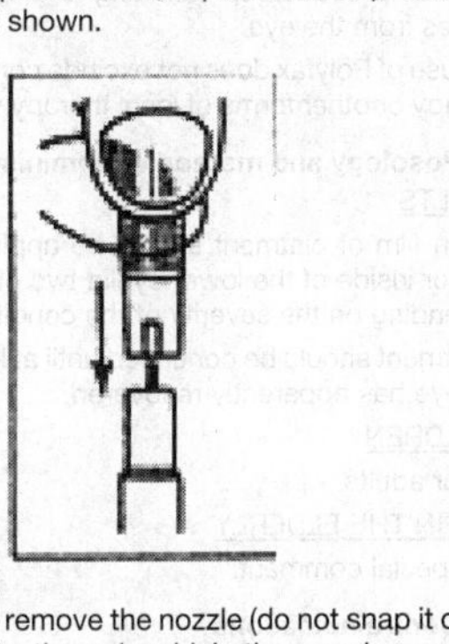

3. Twist the cap to remove the nozzle (do not snap it off) to leave a clean hole through which the vaccine can be expelled.

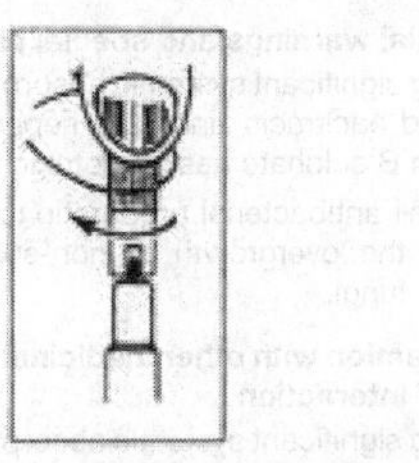

4. Invert the tube and expel three drops (one dose) onto a spoon or sugar cube for administration. Do not administer directly into the vaccinee's mouth as the tube may slip and cause choking.

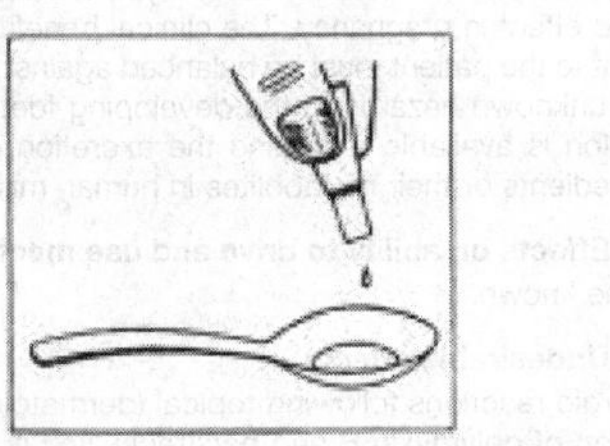

5. Since the vaccine contains live attenuated polio virus, care should be taken to avoid transfer or spillage. Tube, cap and also spoons should be disposed of safely, preferably by heat inactivation or incineration, according to locally agreed procedures.

Administrative Data

7. MARKETING AUTHORISATION HOLDER

SmithKline Beecham PLC

Great West Road,

Brentford, Middlesex TW8 9GS

Trading as:

GlaxoSmithKline UK,

Stockley Park West,

Uxbridge,

Middlesex UB11 1BT

8. MARKETING AUTHORISATION NUMBER(S)

PL 10592/0039

9. DATE OF FIRST AUTHORISATION/RENEWAL OF THE AUTHORISATION

19 November 1999

10. DATE OF REVISION OF THE TEXT

2 August 2004

11. Legal Status

POM

Poliomyelitis Vaccine (Inactivated)

(Sanofi Pasteur MSD)

1. NAME OF THE MEDICINAL PRODUCT

Poliomyelitis Vaccine (Inactivated) ▼

Suspension for injection in a pre-filled syringe

2. QUALITATIVE AND QUANTITATIVE COMPOSITION

Each dose (0.5 ml) contains:

Inactivated type 1 polio virus (Mahoney)[1] 40 D-antigen[2] units[3]

Inactivated type 2 polio virus (MEF-1)[1] 8 D-antigen[2] units[3]

Inactivated type 3 polio virus (Saukett)[1] 32 D-antigen[2] units[3]

[1]Cultivated on Vero cells

[2]Quantity of antigen in the Final Bulk Product, according to WHO (TRS 673, 1982)

[3]Or equivalent nominal amount of poliovirus of each type expressed in European Pharmacopoeia Units of D-antigen (parallel line method)

For excipients, see 6.1.

3. PHARMACEUTICAL FORM

Suspension for injection in a pre-filled syringe.

The vaccine is a clear and colourless suspension.

4. CLINICAL PARTICULARS

4.1 Therapeutic indications

Poliomyelitis Vaccine (Inactivated) is indicated for active immunisation against poliomyelitis as follows:

Primary immunisation from 2 months of age (see section 5.1)

Revaccination (boosting) in children, adolescents and adults in accordance with official recommendations (see section 4.2) and taking into account the pharmacodynamic properties of the vaccine (see section 5.1).

4.2 Posology and method of administration

Posology

Primary vaccination:

The primary immunisation schedule consists of three doses of 0.5 ml administered from two months of age according to official recommendations. There should be an interval of at least 1 month between doses.

Revaccination (boosting):

After completion of a primary immunisation series, booster doses should be given to maintain immunity. The need for and the timing of booster doses should be assessed in accordance with official recommendations.

Poliomyelitis Vaccine (Inactivated) may be used as a booster in individuals who have received one or more doses of an oral poliomyelitis vaccine previously.

Method of Administration

Poliomyelitis Vaccine (Inactivated) should be administered by intramuscular injection. In infants and small children the preferred site is the anterolateral upper thigh. In older subjects, the deltoid muscle is the preferred site. Poliomyelitis Vaccine (Inactivated) may also be administered subcutaneously in certain circumstances (see section 4.4).

The vaccine must not be administered by intravascular injection.

4.3 Contraindications

Hypersensitivity to any component of Poliomyelitis Vaccine (Inactivated).

Hypersensitivity to streptomycin, neomycin or polymixin B, which may be present in the vaccine as trace residues of manufacture.

Vaccination should be deferred in the presence of any acute febrile illness.

4.4 Special warnings and special precautions for use

As with all vaccines, appropriate facilities and medication for resuscitation should be readily available for immediate use in case of anaphylaxis or other severe hypersensitivity reaction following injection.

As with any injectable vaccine, Poliomyelitis Vaccine (Inactivated) must be administered with caution to subjects with thrombocytopenia or a bleeding disorder since bleeding may occur following intramuscular administrations. The vaccine may be administered by subcutaneous injection in such cases.

The immune response to the vaccine may be reduced by immunosuppressive treatment or immunodeficiency states. If possible, vaccination should be postponed until after immune recovery. Vaccination of HIV-infected subjects or subjects with chronic immunodeficiency, such as AIDS, is recommended even if the antibody response might be limited. In these cases, the immune response should be measured in order to assess the degree of protection and possible need for additional doses.

4.5 Interaction with other medicinal products and other forms of Interaction

As for other inactivated viral vaccines, concomitant administration with other vaccine(s) given at different injection sites is unlikely to interfere with immune responses to any of the antigens.

Poliomyelitis Vaccine (Inactivated) must not be mixed with other vaccines or vaccine components in the same syringe. Other vaccines that are to be given at the same time should be administered at different anatomical sites with different syringes and needles.

Administration of the vaccine to persons deficient in producing antibodies, whether due to disease or immunosuppressive therapy, may not elicit a protective immune response (see also section 4.4).

4.6 Pregnancy and lactation

Preclinical data are insufficient with respect to effects on pregnancy and embryo-foetal development, parturition and postnatal development. There are not enough data on the use of this vaccine in pregnant women to assess the potential risk. Therefore, Poliomyelitis Vaccine (Inactivated) should be given to pregnant women only if clearly needed.

Breast-feeding is not a contraindication for vaccination.

4.7 Effects on ability to drive and use machines

No studies on the effects on the ability to drive or use machines have been performed.

However, some of the adverse events mentioned under "Undesirable effects" may affect the ability to drive or operate machinery (see section 4.8).

4.8 Undesirable effects

The adverse events are ranked under headings of frequency using the following convention:

Very common: $\geqslant$ 10%

Common: $\geqslant$ 1% and < 10%

Uncommon: $\geqslant$ 0.1% and < 1%

Rare: $\geqslant$ 0.01% and < 0.1%

Very rare: < 0.01%, including isolated reports

Data from clinical studies

A total of 5,841 vaccinees from different age groups (infants, toddlers, children, adolescents and adults) have received combined vaccines containing IPV and/or IPV associated with other vaccines (i.e. containing tetanus and low dose diphtheria toxoids or containing diphtheria, tetanus and acellular pertussis components) during clinical studies.

In these studies, local reactions including redness, pain, mass and swelling at the injection site were uncommonly to very commonly reported.

The most common ($\geqslant$1%) systemic events observed were:

Ear and labyrinth disorders

Vertigo

Gastro-intestinal disorders

Vomiting, nausea, diarrhoea

General Disorders and Administration Site Conditions

Fever

Musculo-skeletal and connective tissue disorders

Myalgia, arthralgia

Nervous system disorders

Headache, drowsiness, dizziness

Psychiatric disorders

Irritability, inconsolable crying, insomnia

Data from Post-marketing surveillance

Based on spontaneous reporting, the following additional adverse events have been reported during the commercial use of IPV.

These events have been very rarely reported, however exact incidence rates cannot precisely be calculated.

Blood and lymphatic system disorders

Lymphadenopathy

- General Disorders and Administration Site Conditions

- Injection site reactions such as injection site oedema or rash within 48 hours following the vaccination and lasting one or two days.

- Influenza-like symptoms, mostly the same day as the vaccination.

Immune system disorders

Type I hypersensitivity reaction to any component of the vaccine such as allergic reaction, anaphylactic reaction or anaphylactic shock

- Nervous system disorders

- Short-lasting convulsions, fever convulsions, within a few days following vaccination,

- Transient and mild paraesthesia (mainly of limbs) within two weeks after vaccination.

Psychiatric disorders

Within the first hours or days following vaccination and shortly resolving:

agitation, somnolence

Skin and subcutaneous disorders

Rash, urticaria

4.9 Overdose

No case of overdose has been reported.

5. PHARMACOLOGICAL PROPERTIES

5.1 Pharmacodynamic properties

J07B (Viral vaccines) F (Poliomyelitis vaccines) 03 (Poliomyelitis, trivalent, inactivated, whole virus).

Three doses administered to infants have elicited almost 100% immune responses at the 1:8 cut-off in recent studies with combination vaccines. IPV alone or in combinations has produced almost 100% responses at this level when used to boost subjects in a variety of age groups and previous vaccination histories.

There are no clinical trial data on use for primary immunisation beyond infancy. However, referring to the World

Health Organization's recommendations, IPV can be given to children, adolescents and adults.

5.2 Pharmacokinetic properties

Evaluation of pharmacokinetic properties is not required for vaccines.

5.3 Preclinical safety data

Preclinical data including single dose, repeated dose and local tolerance studies revealed no unexpected findings and no target organ toxicity.

6. PHARMACEUTICAL PARTICULARS

6.1 List of excipients

2-phenoxyethanol, ethanol, formaldehyde, medium 199 without phenol red (complex mixture of amino acids (including phenylalanine), mineral salts, vitamins and other components (including glucose), supplemented with polysorbate 80 and diluted in water for injections).

6.2 Incompatibilities

In the absence of compatibility studies, the vaccine must not be mixed with other medicinal products.

6.3 Shelf life

3 years

6.4 Special precautions for storage

Store in a refrigerator between +2°C and +8°C.

Do not freeze. Discard the vaccine if it has been frozen.

Keep container in outer carton.

6.5 Nature and contents of container

0.5 ml of suspension in pre-filled syringe (type I glass) with a plunger stopper (bromobutyl/chlorobutyl elastomer), with or without needles.

Packs of 1, 10 and 20.

Not all pack sizes may be marketed.

6.6 Instructions for use and handling

The vaccine should be visually inspected for any foreign particulate matter and for any change in physical appearance (see Section 3) before administration.

It should not be used if it is cloudy or contains particles.

The vaccine should reach room temperature before administration.

Any unused vaccine or waste material should be disposed of in accordance with local requirements.

7. MARKETING AUTHORISATION HOLDER

Sanofi Pasteur MSD Limited
Mallards Reach
Bridge Avenue
Maidenhead, Berkshire
SL6 1QP

8. MARKETING AUTHORISATION NUMBER(S)

PL 06745/0126

9. DATE OF FIRST AUTHORISATION/RENEWAL OF THE AUTHORISATION

14th April 2004

10. DATE OF REVISION OF THE TEXT

May 2005

Polyfax Ointment

(Pliva Pharma Ltd)

1. NAME OF THE MEDICINAL PRODUCT

Polyfax Ointment

2. QUALITATIVE AND QUANTITATIVE COMPOSITION

Polymyxin B Sulphate 10,000 IU

Bacitracin zinc 500 IU

3. PHARMACEUTICAL FORM

Ointment

4. CLINICAL PARTICULARS

4.1 Therapeutic indications

Topical antibacterial agent. Polyfax Ointment is indicated for the treatment of infected wounds, burns, skin grafts, ulcers, pyoderma, sycosis barbae, impetigo, and in secondarily infected skin lesions of scabies, pediculosis, tinea pedis and contact and allergic dermatitis.

4.2 Posology and method of administration

ADULTS

Polyfax Ointment should be applied thinly over the affected area, which is best left exposed. Two or more applications a day may be necessary, depending on the severity of the condition.

CHILDREN

As for adults.

USE IN THE ELDERLY

No specific studies have been carried out in the elderly, however, it may be advisable to monitor renal function in these patients and if there is any impairment then caution should be exercised.

4.3 Contraindications

Hypersensitivity to bacitracin, Polymyxins or cross-sensitising substances.

4.4 Special warnings and special precautions for use

The following statements take into account the possibility that the constituent drugs of Polyfax Ointment may be absorbed to a significant degree after topical application. However, the normal use of Polyfax is unlikely to present any risk of systemic toxicity unless the application were excessive e.g. more than 200 g per day in adults or proportionately less in children and in patients with compromised renal function.

Following significant systemic absorption polymyxin B sulphate and bacitracin zinc have nephrotoxic potential and polymixin B sulphate has neurotoxic potential.

As with all antibacterial preparations prolonged use may result in the overgrowth of non-susceptible organisms including fungi.

4.5 Interaction with other medicinal products and other forms of Interaction

Following significant systemic absorption, polymyxin B can intensify and prolong the respiratory depressant effects of neuromuscular blocking agents.

4.6 Pregnancy and lactation

Due to lack of detailed information, the use of Polyfax Ointment during pregnancy and lactation cannot be recommended in circumstances where significant systemic absorption of the active ingredients may occur.

No information is available regarding the excretion of the active ingredients of their metabolites in human milk.

4.7 Effects on ability to drive and use machines

None known.

4.8 Undesirable effects

Allergic reactions following topical application of polymyxin B and bacitracin zinc have rarely been reported.

Anaphylactic reactions have been reported, as rare events, following topical application of zinc bacitracin.

4.9 Overdose

In the unlikely event of significant systemic absorption of the active ingredients of Polyfax Ointment occurring, signs of neurotoxicity and nephrotoxicity may be noted. In such an event, the patient's general status and renal function should be monitored and blood levels of polymyxin B and zinc bacitracin determined.

5. PHARMACOLOGICAL PROPERTIES

5.1 Pharmacodynamic properties

Polymyxin and Bacitracin zinc are both bactericidal antibiotics. The former exerts its action by binding with the cellular membrane and the latter by inhibiting bacterial cell wall development.

5.2 Pharmacokinetic properties

Not applicable.

5.3 Preclinical safety data

There are no preclinical data of relevance to the prescriber which are additional to that in other sections of the SmPC.

6. PHARMACEUTICAL PARTICULARS

6.1 List of excipients

White soft paraffin, B.P.

6.2 Incompatibilities

None known.

6.3 Shelf life

5 years.

6.4 Special precautions for storage

Store below 25C.

6.5 Nature and contents of container

Lacquered aluminium tubes with polyolefin screw caps.

Pack sizes: 4g, 20g, 90g

6.6 Instructions for use and handling

No special instructions.

Administrative Data

7. MARKETING AUTHORISATION HOLDER

PLIVA Pharma Limited
Vision House
Bedford Road
Petersfield
Hampshire
GU32 3QB

8. MARKETING AUTHORISATION NUMBER(S)

PL 10622/0155

9. DATE OF FIRST AUTHORISATION/RENEWAL OF THE AUTHORISATION

22 April 2003

10. DATE OF REVISION OF THE TEXT

April 2005

Polyfax Ophthalmic Ointment

(Pliva Pharma Ltd)

1. NAME OF THE MEDICINAL PRODUCT

Polyfax Ophthalmic Ointment

2. QUALITATIVE AND QUANTITATIVE COMPOSITION

10,000 IU Polymyxin B Sulphate EP per gram of ointment

500 IU Bacitracin Zinc EP per gram of ointment

3. PHARMACEUTICAL FORM

Ointment

4. CLINICAL PARTICULARS

4.1 Therapeutic indications

Polyfax Ophthalmic Ointment is indicated for the treatment of bacterial infections of the eye and its adnexa, including conjunctivitis, keratitis, corneal ulceration and ulcerative blepharitis.

Polyfax Ophthalmic Ointment may be applied both pre- and post-operatively to prevent ocular infection following surgical procedures, including the removal of foreign bodies from the eye.

The use of Polyfax does not exclude concomitant systemic therapy or other forms of local therapy where appropriate.

4.2 Posology and method of administration

ADULTS

A thin film of ointment should be applied to the affected part or inside of the lower eyelid two or more times a day depending on the severity of the condition.

Treatment should be continued until at least two days after the eye has apparently recovered.

CHILDREN

As for adults.

USE IN THE ELDERLY

No special comment.

4.3 Contraindications

Hypersensitivity to bacitracin, Polymixin B Sulphate or cross-sensitising substances.

4.4 Special warnings and special precautions for use

Following significant systemic absorption polymyxin B sulphate and bacitracin zinc have nephrotoxic potential and polymixin B sulphate has neurotoxic potential.

As with all antibacterial preparations prolonged use may result in the overgrowth of non-susceptible organisms including fungi.

4.5 Interaction with other medicinal products and other forms of Interaction

Following significant systemic absorption, polymixin B sulphate can intensify and prolong the respiratory depressant effects of neuromuscular blocking agents.

4.6 Pregnancy and lactation

Polyfax has been used for several years without any untoward effect in pregnancy. The clinical benefit of the treatment to the patient must be balanced against any possible but unknown hazards to the developing foetus. No information is available regarding the excretion of the active ingredients or their metabolites in human milk.

4.7 Effects on ability to drive and use machines

None known.

4.8 Undesirable effects

Allergic reactions following topical (dermatological) application of polymyxin B and bacitracin zinc is rare but has been reported.

As with other antibacterial preparations, prolonged use may result in the overgrowth of non-susceptible organisms, including fungi.

4.9 Overdose

Not applicable

5. PHARMACOLOGICAL PROPERTIES

5.1 Pharmacodynamic properties

Polymyxin B sulphate and bacitracin zinc are both bactericidal antibiotics. The former exerts its action by binding with the cellular membrane and the latter by inhibiting bacterial cell wall development.

It has been shown in animal studies that both Polymyxin B Sulphate and Bacitracin Zinc may be absorbed into the aqueous humour following topical application to the eye, especially in circumstances where the cornea is either abraded or inflamed.

In vitro activity: Gram positive: Species of staphylococcus; streptococcus, including *S. Pyogenes* (B haemolytic streptococcus) and *S. Pneumoniae* (Pneumococcus); and corynebacterium.

Gram negative: Species of pseudomonas (including *P. Aeruginosa*), haemophilus, klebsiella. enterobacter, escherichia and neisseria.

5.2 Pharmacokinetic properties

Not applicable.

5.3 Preclinical safety data

There are no preclinical data of relevance to the prescriber which are additional to that in other sections of the SmPC.

6. PHARMACEUTICAL PARTICULARS

6.1 List of excipients

White Petrolatum USP.

6.2 Incompatibilities

None known.

6.3 Shelf life
5 years.

6.4 Special precautions for storage
Store below 25°C.

6.5 Nature and contents of container
Pack size 4g

Lacquered ophthalmic ointment tubes with polyolefin screw caps.

6.6 Instructions for use and handling
No special instructions.

7. MARKETING AUTHORISATION HOLDER
PLIVA Pharma Limited

Vision House

Bedford Road

Petersfield

Hampshire

GU32 3QB

8. MARKETING AUTHORISATION NUMBER(S)
PL 10622/0156

9. DATE OF FIRST AUTHORISATION/RENEWAL OF THE AUTHORISATION
22 April 2003

10. DATE OF REVISION OF THE TEXT
22 March 2005

Polytar AF

(Stiefel Laboratories (UK) Limited)

1. NAME OF THE MEDICINAL PRODUCT
Polytar AF

2. QUALITATIVE AND QUANTITATIVE COMPOSITION
Tar Blend 1% w/w, Zinc Pyrithione 1% w/w in a shampoo base

Tar Blend comprises:

Pine tar, Cade oil, Coal Tar Solution, Arachis Oil extract of Coal Tar.

3. PHARMACEUTICAL FORM
Medicated Shampoo

4. CLINICAL PARTICULARS

4.1 Therapeutic indications
Polytar AF is indicated in the topical treatment of scalp disorders such as dandruff, seborrhoeic dermatitis and psoriasis.

4.2 Posology and method of administration
Shake the bottle before use. Wet the hair and massage Polytar AF into the hair, scalp and surrounding skin. Leave for 2-3 minutes, then rinse thoroughly.

Polytar AF should be used two or three times weekly for at least 3 weeks or until the condition clears.

4.3 Contraindications
Polytar AF should not be used by patients with known hypersensitivity to any of the ingredients.

4.4 Special warnings and special precautions for use
Avoid contact with the eyes. Tar products may cause skin irritation, rashes and, rarely, photosensitivity. Zinc pyrithione may cause dermatitis, should this occur, Polytar AF should be discontinued.

4.5 Interaction with other medicinal products and other forms of Interaction
None known.

4.6 Pregnancy and lactation
The safety of Polytar AF in human pregnancy and lactation has not been established.

4.7 Effects on ability to drive and use machines
None.

4.8 Undesirable effects
None.

4.9 Overdose
Not applicable.

5. PHARMACOLOGICAL PROPERTIES

5.1 Pharmacodynamic properties
Tar blend:

Tars suppress DNA synthesis in hyperplastic skin, this inhibits mitotic activity and protein synthesis. By decreasing proliferation and dermal infiltration, they promote a return to normal keratinisation. Tars also have vasoconstricting astringent and antipruritic properties.

Zinc Pyrithione:

Zinc Pyrithione has antibacterial and antifungal properties. It is fungicidal against the pathogenic yeasts of the pityrosporum genus which are implicated in dandruff and seborrhoeic dermatitis.

5.2 Pharmacokinetic properties
Not Applicable.

5.3 Preclinical safety data
Not Applicable.

6. PHARMACEUTICAL PARTICULARS

6.1 List of excipients
Coconut diethanolamide

Triethanolamine Lauryl Sulphate

Carbomer

Sodium Hydroxide

Hypromellose

Octoxinol

Glycerol

Imidurea

Purified Water

6.2 Incompatibilities
None

6.3 Shelf life
24 months

6.4 Special precautions for storage
Store below 25° C.

6.5 Nature and contents of container
High density polyethylene bottles of 150ml & 250ml

6.6 Instructions for use and handling
There are no special instructions for use or handling of Polytar AF.

7. MARKETING AUTHORISATION HOLDER
Stiefel Laboratories (UK) Ltd

Holtspur Lane

Wooburn Green

High Wycombe

Bucks HP10 0AU

8. MARKETING AUTHORISATION NUMBER(S)
PL 0174/0071

9. DATE OF FIRST AUTHORISATION/RENEWAL OF THE AUTHORISATION
16th March 1992.

10. DATE OF REVISION OF THE TEXT
March 1997.

Polytar Emollient

(Stiefel Laboratories (UK) Limited)

1. NAME OF THE MEDICINAL PRODUCT
Polytar Emollient

2. QUALITATIVE AND QUANTITATIVE COMPOSITION
Tar Blend 25.00% w/w, Light Liquid Paraffin 35.00% w/w.

Tar Blend comprises:

Pine tar BP 30% w/w, Cade oil BPC 30% w/w, Coal Tar Solution BP 10% w/w, Arachis Oil extract of Coal Tar BP 30% w/w.

3. PHARMACEUTICAL FORM
Liquid bath additive.

4. CLINICAL PARTICULARS

4.1 Therapeutic indications
Topical.

Polytar Emollient is indicated in the treatment of psoriasis, eczema, atopic and pruritic dermatoses. The use of Polytar Emollient may be combined with ultraviolet radiation and other adjunctive therapy. Polytar Emollient is also of value in removing loose psoriatic scales and paste following dithranol treatment.

4.2 Posology and method of administration
Adults, children and the elderly:

Two to four capfuls of Polytar Emollient should be added to an 8 inch bath and the patient instructed to soak for 20 minutes.

4.3 Contraindications
None.

4.4 Special warnings and special precautions for use
Patients should be instructed to guard against slipping when entering or leaving the bath. If skin irritation occurs and persists, discontinue use and consult your doctor. Tar products may stain baths and fabrics.

4.5 Interaction with other medicinal products and other forms of Interaction
None known.

4.6 Pregnancy and lactation
There is no, or inadequate evidence of the safety of Polytar Emollient in human pregnancy and lactation but it has been in wide use for many years without apparent ill consequence.

4.7 Effects on ability to drive and use machines
None.

4.8 Undesirable effects
Tar products may cause skin irritation, rashes and rarely, photosensitivity. In the event of such a reaction, discontinue use and consult your doctor.

4.9 Overdose
Not applicable.

5. PHARMACOLOGICAL PROPERTIES

5.1 Pharmacodynamic properties
Tar preparations have keratoplastic and antipruritic activity and are widely used as topical therapy for a range of dermatoses. The use of emollient bath oils in the management of widespread dry and itching skin is well established. Mineral oil exerts its emollient effect by skin absorption. The combination of tar blend with an emollient therefore provides a pharmacological active product with emollient properties.

5.2 Pharmacokinetic properties
Not applicable.

6. PHARMACEUTICAL PARTICULARS

6.1 List of excipients
Octylphenoxypolythoxy Ethanol

Sorbitan Monooleate

Polyethylene Glycol 400 Dilaurate

Isopropyl Palmitate

6.2 Incompatibilities
None.

6.3 Shelf life
36 months

6.4 Special precautions for storage
None.

6.5 Nature and contents of container
Polyvinyl chloride bottles fitted with a screw cap containing 500ml.

6.6 Instructions for use and handling
There are no special instructions for use or handling of Polytar Emollient.

7. MARKETING AUTHORISATION HOLDER
Stiefel Laboratories (UK) Ltd

Holtspur Lane

Wooburn Green

High Wycombe

Bucks

UP10 0AU

8. MARKETING AUTHORISATION NUMBER(S)
PL 00174/5011R

9. DATE OF FIRST AUTHORISATION/RENEWAL OF THE AUTHORISATION
30th November 1994

10. DATE OF REVISION OF THE TEXT
September 2005

Polytar Liquid

(Stiefel Laboratories (UK) Limited)

1. NAME OF THE MEDICINAL PRODUCT
Polytar Liquid

2. QUALITATIVE AND QUANTITATIVE COMPOSITION
Tar Blend 1% w/w

Tar Blend comprises:

Pine tar, cade oil, coal tar solution, arachis oil extract of coal tar.

3. PHARMACEUTICAL FORM
Medicated Shampoo

4. CLINICAL PARTICULARS

4.1 Therapeutic indications
Polytar Liquid is indicated in the treatment of scalp disorders including psoriasis, dandruff, seborrhoea, eczema and pruritus. Polytar Liquid is also of value in the removal of ointments and pastes used in the treatment of psoriasis.

4.2 Posology and method of administration
The hair should be wetted and sufficient Polytar Liquid applied to produce an abundant lather. The scalp and adjacent areas should be vigorously massaged with the fingertips. The hair should then be thoroughly rinsed and the procedure repeated.

Polytar Liquid should be used once or twice weekly.

4.3 Contraindications
Patients with a known hypersensitivity to any of the ingredients should not use the product.

4.4 Special warnings and special precautions for use
There are no special warnings or precautions.

4.5 Interaction with other medicinal products and other forms of Interaction
There are no known interactions with other medicaments or other forms of interaction.

4.6 Pregnancy and lactation
There is no, or inadequate evidence of the safety of Polytar Liquid in human pregnancy and lactation, but it has been in wide use for many years without apparent ill consequence.

4.7 Effects on ability to drive and use machines
The use of this product will not affect the ability to drive and to use machines.

4.8 Undesirable effects
Tar products may cause skin irritation, rashes and rarely, photosensitivity. If irritation occurs and persists, treatment should be discontinued.

4.9 Overdose
The product is intended for external use only. It is applied to the scalp and rinsed off. Use of an excessive quantity is not a cause for concern.

5. PHARMACOLOGICAL PROPERTIES

5.1 Pharmacodynamic properties
Tars suppress DNA synthesis in hyperplastic skin, inhibiting mitotic activity and protein synthesis. They decrease epidermal proliferation and dermal infiltration and thus promote a return to normal keratinisation.

Tars also have vasoconstrictor, antipruritic and antiseptic properties.

5.2 Pharmacokinetic properties
The product is applied topically and acts at the site of application. The potential for systemic absorption from a wash off shampoo is extremely low.

5.3 Preclinical safety data
Tar preparations have been in widespread use for many years and their safety in humans has been established.

6. PHARMACEUTICAL PARTICULARS

6.1 List of excipients
Oleyl alcohol
Coconut diethanolamide
Hexylene glycol
Polysorbate 80
Triethanolamide lauryl sulphate
Sodium chloride
Citric acid
Octylphenoxypolyethoxy ethanol
Imidurea
Fragrance 5412
Purified Water

6.2 Incompatibilities
There are no known incompatibilities.

6.3 Shelf life
a) For the product as packaged for sale
3 years
b) After first opening the container
Comply with expiry date

6.4 Special precautions for storage
There are no special precautions for storage.

6.5 Nature and contents of container
High density polyethylene bottles of 150ml, 250ml and 500ml.

6.6 Instructions for use and handling
There are no special instructions for use or handling of Polytar Liquid.

Administrative Data

7. MARKETING AUTHORISATION HOLDER
Stiefel Laboratories (UK) Ltd
Holtspur Lane
Wooburn Green
High Wycombe
Bucks HP10 0AU

8. MARKETING AUTHORISATION NUMBER(S)
PL 0174/5016R

9. DATE OF FIRST AUTHORISATION/RENEWAL OF THE AUTHORISATION
12 May 2000

10. DATE OF REVISION OF THE TEXT
September 2005

Polytar Plus
(Stiefel Laboratories (UK) Limited)

1. NAME OF THE MEDICINAL PRODUCT
Polytar Plus

2. QUALITATIVE AND QUANTITATIVE COMPOSITION
Tar Blend 1% w/w

3. PHARMACEUTICAL FORM
Medicated shampoo for topical use.

4. CLINICAL PARTICULARS

4.1 Therapeutic indications
Polytar Plus is indicated as an aid in the treatment of scalp disorders such as psoriasis, seborrhoea, pruritus, and dandruff. Polytar Plus is also of value in the removal of ointments and pastes used in the treatment of psoriasis.

4.2 Posology and method of administration
The following dosages and schedules are applicable for adults, children and the elderly.

The hair should be wetted and sufficient Polytar Plus applied to produce an abundant lather. The scalp and adjacent areas should be vigorously massaged with the fingertips. The hair should then be thoroughly rinsed and the procedure repeated.

Polytar Plus should be used once or twice weekly.

4.3 Contraindications
None stated.

4.4 Special warnings and special precautions for use
None stated.

4.5 Interaction with other medicinal products and other forms of Interaction
None stated.

4.6 Pregnancy and lactation
There are no restrictions on the use of Polytar Plus during pregnancy or lactation.

4.7 Effects on ability to drive and use machines
None stated.

4.8 Undesirable effects
None stated.

4.9 Overdose
None stated.

5. PHARMACOLOGICAL PROPERTIES

5.1 Pharmacodynamic properties
While the mode of action of tars are not fully established, their therapeutic effect has been observed over many years. It has been postulated that tars work by exerting a cytostatic action following an initial cytoproliferative effect. This slowing of the keratinisation process in the epidermal layer and reduction in the rate of epidermal turnover promoting a return to normal keratinisation.

5.2 Pharmacokinetic properties
Not applicable. The product acts at the site of application.

5.3 Preclinical safety data
Not applicable.

6. PHARMACEUTICAL PARTICULARS

6.1 List of excipients
Coconut diethanolamide, Hexylene glycol, Volpo N10, Oleyl alcohol, Polysorbate 80, Triton X100, Fragrance 5412, Polypeptide SF, Imadozolidinyl Urea, Triethanolamine Lauryl Sulphate, Citric acid, Purified water

6.2 Incompatibilities
None stated.

6.3 Shelf life
a) For the product as packaged for sale
3 years
b) After first opening the container
Comply with expiry date

6.4 Special precautions for storage
None

6.5 Nature and contents of container
Polyethylene screw top bottles of 500ml

6.6 Instructions for use and handling
There are no special instructions for use or handling of Polytar Plus.

7. MARKETING AUTHORISATION HOLDER
Stiefel Laboratories (UK) Ltd
Holtspur Lane,
Wooburn Green,
High Wycombe,
Bucks HP10 0AU

8. MARKETING AUTHORISATION NUMBER(S)
PL 0174/0037

9. DATE OF FIRST AUTHORISATION/RENEWAL OF THE AUTHORISATION
02 December 1977.

10. DATE OF REVISION OF THE TEXT
December 1997.

Ponstan Capsules 250mg
(Chemidex Pharma Ltd.)

1. NAME OF THE MEDICINAL PRODUCT
Ponstan® Capsules 250mg

2. QUALITATIVE AND QUANTITATIVE COMPOSITION
Mefenamic acid BP 250mg

3. PHARMACEUTICAL FORM
A practically white to greyish or creamy-white powder in a No 1 hard gelatin capsule having an ivory opaque body and powder blue opaque cap imprinted "PONSTAN 250".

4. CLINICAL PARTICULARS

4.1 Therapeutic indications
Mefenamic acid is a non-steroidal anti-inflammatory agent with analgesic properties, and a demonstrable antipyretic effect. It has been shown to inhibit prostaglandin activity.

Indications

1. As an anti-inflammatory analgesic for the symptomatic relief of rheumatoid arthritis (including Still's Disease), osteoarthritis, and pain including muscular, traumatic and dental pain, headaches of most aetiology, post-operative and post-partum pain; pyrexia in children.
2. Primary dysmenorrhoea.
3. Menorrhagia due to dysfunctional causes and presence of an IUD when other pelvic pathology has been ruled out.

4.2 Posology and method of administration
Adults

2 capsules (500mg) three times daily.

In menorrhagia to be administered on the first day of excessive bleeding and continued according to the judgment of the physician.

In dysmenorrhoea to be administered at the onset of menstrual pain and continued according to the judgment of the physician.

Elderly (Over 65 Years)

As for adults.

Whilst no pharmacokinetic or clinical studies specific to the elderly have been undertaken with Ponstan, it has been used at normal dosage in trials which included many elderly patients.

Ponstan should be used with caution in elderly patients suffering from dehydration and renal disease.

Non-oliguric renal failure and proctocolitis have been reported mainly in elderly patients who have not discontinued Ponstan after the development of diarrhoea.

Children

It is recommended that children under 12 years of age should be given Ponstan Paediatric Suspension (50mg / 5ml).

Do not exceed the stated dose.

4.3 Contraindications
Precaution should be taken in patients hypersensitive to mefenamic acid.

Mefenamic acid is contra-indicated in inflammatory bowel disease and in patients suffering from peptic and / or intestinal ulceration, and in patients with renal or hepatic impairment.

Because the potential exists for cross-sensitivity to aspirin or other non-steroidal anti-inflammatory drugs, mefenamic acid should not be given to patients in whom these drugs induce symptoms of bronchospasm, allergic rhinitis, or urticaria.

4.4 Special warnings and special precautions for use
Precaution should be taken in patients suffering from dehydration and renal disease, particularly the elderly.

In dysmenorrhoea and menorrhagia lack of response should alert the physician to investigate other causes.

Caution should be exercised when treating patients suffering from epilepsy.

4.5 Interaction with other medicinal products and other forms of Interaction
Concurrent therapy with other plasma protein binding drugs may necessitate a modification in dosage. In the case of anticoagulants the dose of the anticoagulant may need to be reduced. Concurrent administration of mefenamic acid with oral anticoagulant drugs requires careful prothrombin time monitoring.

The following interactions have been reported with NSAIDs but have not necessarily been associated with Ponstan Capsules:

Antihypertensives and diuretics: a reduction in antihypertensive and diuretic effect has been observed.

Cardiac glycosides: NSAIDs may exacerbate cardiac failure and increases in plasma cardiac glycoside levels may occur when renal function is affected.

Lithium and methotrexate: Elimination of these drugs can be reduced.

Cyclosporin: The risk of nephrotoxicity of cyclosporin may be increased with NSAIDs.

Mifepristone: NSAIDs should not be taken for 8-12 days after mifepristone administration, NSAIDs can reduce the effects of mifepristone.

Corticosteroids: Concomitant use may increase the risk of gastrointestinal bleeding.

Quinolone antibiotics: Animal data indicates that NSAIDs can increase the risk of convulsions associated with quinolone antibiotics. Patients taking NSAIDs and quinolones may have an increased risk of developing convulsions.

Other analgesics: Concomitant use of two or more NSAIDs should be avoided.

4.6 Pregnancy and lactation
Safety in pregnancy has not been established and because of the effects of drugs in this class on the foetal cardiovascular system, the use of mefenamic acid in pregnant women is not recommended.

Trace amounts of mefenamic acid may be present in breast milk and transmitted to the nursing infant. Therefore, mefenamic acid should not be taken by nursing mothers.

4.7 Effects on ability to drive and use machines
Drowsiness and dizziness have rarely been reported.

4.8 Undesirable effects
Diarrhoea occasionally occurs following the use of mefenamic acid. Although this may occur soon after starting treatment, it may also occur after several months of continuous use. The diarrhoea has been investigated in some patients who have continued this drug in spite of its continued presence. These patients were found to have associated proctocolitis. If diarrhoea does develop the drug should be withdrawn immediately and this patient should not receive mefenamic acid again.

Skin rashes have been observed following the administration of mefenamic acid and the occurrence of a rash is a definite indication to withdraw medication. There have been rare reports of Stevens-Johnson syndrome, Lyell's syndrome (toxic epidermal necrolysis) and erythema multiforme.

Serious gastrointestinal toxicity such as bleeding, ulceration, and perforation can occur at any time with or without warning symptoms, in patients treated chronically with NSAID therapy. GI bleeding has been associated with a previous history of peptic ulcer, smoking and alcohol use.

Elderly or debilitated patients seem to tolerate ulceration or bleeding less well than other individuals and most spontaneous reports of fatal GI events are in this population.

As with other prostaglandin inhibitors allergic glomerulonephritis had occurred occasionally. There have also been reports of acute interstitial nephritis with haematuria and proteinuria and occasionally nephrotic syndrome. Non-oliguric renal failure has been reported on a few occasions in elderly patients with dehydration usually from diarrhoea. Toxicity has been seen in patients with pre-renal conditions leading to a reduction in renal blood flow or blood volume.

Patients at greatest risk of this reaction are those with impaired renal function, heart failure, liver dysfunction, those taking diuretics and the elderly. The drug should not be administered to patients with significantly impaired renal function. It has been suggested that the recovery is more rapid and complete than with other forms of analgesic induced renal impairment, with discontinuation of NSAID therapy being typically followed by recovery to the pre-treatment state.

Thrombocytopenic purpura has been reported with mefenamic acid. In some cases reversible haemolytic anemia has occurred. Temporary lowering of the white blood cell count which may have been due to mefenamic acid has been reported. Rarely eosinophilia, agranulocytosis, pancytopenia and aplastic anaemia have been reported. Blood studies should therefore be carried out during long term administration and the appearance of any dyscrasia is an indication to discontinue therapy.

Bronchospasm and/or urticaria may be precipitated in patients suffering from, or with a previous history of, bronchial asthma or allergic disease.

Borderline elevations of one or more liver function tests may occur in some patients receiving mefenamic acid therapy. A patient with symptoms and/or signs suggesting liver dysfunction, or in whom an abnormal liver test has occurred, should have their therapy discontinued. Patients on prolonged therapy should be kept under surveillance with particular attention to liver dysfunction. Pancreatitis and cholestatic jaundice have also been reported.

Other adverse reactions: Nausea, vomiting, abdominal pain, headache, facial oedema, laryngeal oedema and anaphylaxis. Drowsiness, dizziness, abnormal vision, palpitations, glucose intolerance in diabetic patients and hypotension have rarely been reported.

Note: A positive reaction in certain tests for bile in the urine of patients receiving mefenamic acid has been demonstrated to be due to the presence of the drug and its metabolites and not to the presence of bile.

4.9 Overdose
Gastric lavage in the conscious patient and intensive supportive therapy where necessary. Vital functions should be monitored and supported. Activated charcoal has been shown to be a powerful adsorbent for mefenamic acid and its metabolites. Studies in experimental animals and human volunteers have shown that a 5 to 1 ratio of charcoal to mefenamic acid results in considerable suppression of absorption of the drug. Haemodialysis is of little value since mefenamic acid and its metabolites are firmly bound to plasma proteins. Overdose has led to fatalities.

Mefenamic acid has a tendency to induce tonic-clonic (grand mal) convulsions in overdose. Acute renal failure and coma have been reported with mefenamic acid overdose. It is important that the recommended dose is not exceeded and the regime adhered to since some reports have involved daily dosages under 3g.

5. PHARMACOLOGICAL PROPERTIES

5.1 Pharmacodynamic properties
ANIMAL MODELS

Mefenamic acid is a non-steroidal anti-inflammatory drug (NSAID) with anti- inflammatory, analgesic and antipyretic properties.

Its anti-inflammatory effect was first established in the UV erythema model of inflammation. Further studies included inhibition of granulation tissue growth into subcutaneous cotton pellets in rats and carrageenin induced rat paw oedema tests.

Antipyretic activity was demonstrated in yeast-induced pyresis in rats. In this model its antipyretic activity was roughly equal to that of phenylbutazone and flufenamic acid, but less than that of indomethacin.

Analgesic activity was demonstrated in tests involving pain sensitivity of rats paws inflamed by brewers yeast. Mefenamic acid was less potent than flufenamic acid in this model.

Prostaglandins are implicated in a number of disease processes including:

inflammation, modulation of the pain response, dysmenorrhoea, menorrhagia and pyrexia.

In common with most NSAID's mefenamic acid inhibits the action of prostaglandin synthetase (cyclo oxygenase). This results in a reduction in the rate of prostaglandin synthesis and reduced prostaglandin levels.

The anti-inflammatory activity of NSAID's in the rat paw oedema test has been correlated with their ability to inhibit prostaglandin synthetase. When mefenamic acid is ranked in both these tests it falls between indomethacin and phenylbutazone and it is probable that inhibition of prostaglandin synthesis contributes to the pharmacological activity and clinical efficacy of mefenamic acid.

There is also considerable evidence that the fenamates inhibit the action of prostaglandins after they have been formed. They therefore both inhibit the synthesis and response to prostaglandins. This double blockade may well be important in their mode of action.

5.2 Pharmacokinetic properties
Absorption and Distribution
Mefenamic acid is absorbed from the gastro intestinal tract. Peak levels of 10mg/l occur two hours after the administration of a 1g oral dose to adults.

Metabolism
Mefenamic acid is extensively metabolised, first to A3 hydroxymethyl derivative (metabolite I) and then A3 carboxyl derivative (metabolite II). Both metabolites undergo secondary conjugation to form glucuronides.

Elimination
Fifty two percent of a dose is recovered from the urine, 6% as mefenamic acid, 25% as metabolite I and 21% as metabolite II. Assay of stools over a 3 day period accounted for 10-20% of the dose chiefly as unconjugated metabolite II.

The plasma levels of unconjugated mefenamic acid decline with a half life of approximately two hours.

5.3 Preclinical safety data
Pre-clinical safety data does not add anything of further significance to the prescriber.

6. PHARMACEUTICAL PARTICULARS

6.1 List of excipients
Lactose, gelatin, sodium lauryl sulphate, potable water*, titanium dioxide (E171), patent blue (E131), quinoline yellow (E104), erythrosine (E127).

*not detectable

6.2 Incompatibilities
None known.

6.3 Shelf life
36 months

6.4 Special precautions for storage
Store at a temperature not exceeding 30 °C.

6.5 Nature and contents of container
a) Securitainer (polypropylene body and polyethylene cap). Pack size: 500.

b) High density polyethylene (HDPE) bottle fitted with a white low density polyethylene (LDPE) tamper evident 'J' cap. Pack size: 100 and 500.

c) Polyvinylchloride/aluminium foil blister pack. Pack size: 6,10,12,20,30,50,100 and 168.

6.6 Instructions for use and handling
Not applicable.

ADMINSTRATIVE DATA

7. MARKETING AUTHORISATION HOLDER
Chemidex Pharma Limited
Chemidex House
Egham Business Village
Crabtree Road
Egham
Surrey TW20 8RB
United Kingdom

8. MARKETING AUTHORISATION NUMBER(S)
PL 17736/0006

9. DATE OF FIRST AUTHORISATION/RENEWAL OF THE AUTHORISATION
31st December 2001

10. DATE OF REVISION OF THE TEXT

Ponstan Forte Tablets 500mg

(Chemidex Pharma Ltd.)

1. NAME OF THE MEDICINAL PRODUCT
Ponstan® Forte Tablets 500mg

2. QUALITATIVE AND QUANTITATIVE COMPOSITION
Mefenamic acid BP 500mg

3. PHARMACEUTICAL FORM
Yellow film coated tablet, inscribed 'Ponstan' on one side

4. CLINICAL PARTICULARS

4.1 Therapeutic indications
Mefenamic acid is a non-steroidal anti-inflammatory agent with analgesic properties, and a demonstrable antipyretic effect. It has been shown to inhibit prostaglandin activity.

Indications

1. As an anti-inflammatory analgesic for the symptomatic relief of rheumatoid arthritis (including Still's Disease), osteoarthritis, and pain including muscular, traumatic and dental pain, headaches of most aetiology, post-operative and post-partum pain.

2. Primary dysmenorrhoea.

3. Menorrhagia due to dysfunctional causes and presence of an IUD when other pelvic pathology has been ruled out.

4.2 Posology and method of administration
Adults

1 tablet (500mg) three times daily.

In menorrhagia to be administered on the first day of excessive bleeding and continued according to the judgement of the physician

In dysmenorrhoea to be administered at the onset of menstrual pain and continued according to the judgement of the physician.

Elderly (over 65 Years)

As for adults.

Whilst no pharmacokinetic or clinical studies specific to the elderly have been undertaken with Ponstan, it has been used at normal dosage in trials which included many elderly patients.

Ponstan should be used with caution in elderly patients suffering from dehydration and renal disease. Non-oliguric renal failure and proctocolitis have been reported mainly in elderly patients who have not discontinued Mefenamic Acid after the development of diarrhoea.

Children

It is recommended that children under 12 years of age should be given Ponstan Paediatric Suspension (50mg/5ml).

Do not exceed the stated dose.

4.3 Contraindications
Patients hypersensitive to mefenamic acid. Mefenamic acid is contra-indicated in inflammatory bowel disease and in patients suffering from peptic and/or intestinal ulceration, and in patients with renal or hepatic impairment.

Because the potential exists for cross-sensitivity to aspirin or other non-steroidal anti-inflammatory drugs, mefenamic acid should not be given to patients in whom these drugs induce symptoms of bronchopsasm, allergic rhinitis, or urticaria.

4.4 Special warnings and special precautions for use
Precaution should be taken in patients suffering from dehydration and renal disease, particularly the elderly.

In dysmenorrhoea and menorrhagia lack of response should alert the physician to investigate other causes.

Caution should be exercised when treating patients suffering from epilepsy.

4.5 Interaction with other medicinal products and other forms of Interaction
Concurrent therapy with other plasma protein binding drugs may necessitate a modification in dosage. In the case of anticoagulants the dose of the anticoagulant may need to be reduced. Concurrent administration of mefenamic acid with oral anticoagulant drugs requires careful prothrombin time monitoring.

The following interactions have been reported with NSAIDS but have not necessarily been associated with Ponstan Tablets:

Antihypertensives and diuretics: a reduction in antihypertensive and diuretic effect has been observed.

Cardiac glycosides: NSAIDs may exacerbate cardiac failure and increases in plasma cardiac glycoside levels may occur when renal function is affected.

Lithium and methotrexate: Elimination of these drugs can be reduced.

Cyclosporin: The risk of nephrotoxicity of cyclosporin may be increased with NSAIDs.

Mifepristone: NSAIDs should not be taken for 8-12 days after mifepristone administration, NSAIDs can reduce the effects of mifepristone.

Corticosteroids: Concomitant use may increase the risk of gastrointestinal bleeding.

Quinolone antibiotics: Animal data indicates that NSAIDs can increase the risk of convulsions associated with quinolone antibiotics. Patients taking NSAIDs and quinolones may have an increased risk of developing convulsions.

Other analgesics: Concomitant use of two or more NSAIDs should be avoided.

4.6 Pregnancy and lactation
Safety in pregnancy has not been established and because of the effects of drugs in this class on the foetal cardiovascular system, the use of mefenamic acid in pregnant women is not recommended.

Trace amounts of mefenamic acid may be present in breast milk and transmitted to the nursing infant. Therefore, mefenamic acid should not be taken by nursing mothers.

4.7 Effects on ability to drive and use machines
Drowsiness and dizziness have rarely been reported.

4.8 Undesirable effects
Diarrhoea occasionally occurs following the use of mefenamic acid. Although this may occur soon after starting treatment, it may also occur after several months of continuous use. The diarrhoea has been investigated in some patients who have continued this drug in spite of its continued presence. These patients were found to have associated proctocolitis. If diarrhoea does develop the drug should be withdrawn immediately and this patient should not receive mefenamic acid again.

Skin rashes have been observed following the administration of mefenamic acid and the occurrence of a rash is a definite indication to withdraw medication. There have been rare reports of Steven-Johnson syndrome, Lyell's syndrome (toxic epidermal necrolysis) and erythema multiforme.

Serious gastrointestinal toxicity such as bleeding, ulceration, and perforation can occur at any time with or without warning symptoms, in patients treated chronically with NSAID therapy. GI bleeding has been associated with a previous history of peptic ulcer, smoking and alcohol use.

Elderly or debilitated patients seem to tolerate ulceration or bleeding less well than other individuals and most spontaneous reports of fatal GI events are in this population.

As with other prostaglandin inhibitors allergic glomerulonephritis has occurred occasionally. There have also been reports of acute interstitial nephritis with haematuria and proteinuria and occasionally nephrotic syndrome. Non-oliguric renal failure has been reported on a few occasions in elderly patients with dehydration usually from diarrhoea. Toxicity has been seen in patients with pre-renal conditions leading to a reduction in renal blood flow or blood volume. Patients at greatest risk of this reaction are those with impaired renal function, heart failure, liver dysfunction, those taking diuretics and the elderly. The drug should not be administered to patients with significantly impaired renal function. It has been suggested that the recovery is more rapid and complete than with other forms of analgesic induced renal impairment, with discontinuation of NSAID therapy being typically followed by recovery to the pre-treatment state.

Thrombocytopenic purpura has been reported with mefenamic acid. In some cases reversible haemolytic anaemia has occurred. Temporary lowering of the white blood cell count which may have been due to mefenamic acid has been reported. Rarely eosinophilia, agranulocytosis, pancytopenia and aplastic anaemia have been reported. Blood studies should therefore be carried out during long term administration and the appearance of any dyscrasia is an indication to discontinue therapy.

Bronchospasm and/or urticaria may be precipitated in patients suffering from, or with a previous history of, bronchial asthma or allergic disease.

Borderline elevations of one or more liver function tests may occur in some patients receiving mefenamic acid therapy. A patient with symptoms and/or signs suggesting liver dysfunction, or in whom an abnormal liver test has occurred, should have their therapy discontinued. Patients on prolonged therapy should be kept under surveillance with particular attention to liver dysfunction. Pancreatitis and cholestatic jaundice have also been reported.

Other adverse reactions: Nausea, vomiting, abdominal pain, headache, facial oedema, laryngeal oedema and anaphylaxis. Drowsiness, dizziness, abnormal vision, palpitations, glucose intolerance in diabetic patients and hypotension have rarely been reported.

NOTE: A positive reaction in certain tests for bile in the urine of patients receiving mefenamic acid has been demonstrated to be due to the presence of the drug and its metabolites and not to the presence of bile.

4.9 Overdose
Gastric lavage in the conscious patient and intensive supportive therapy where necessary. Vital functions should be monitored and supported. Activated charcoal has been shown to be a powerful adsorbent for mefenamic acid and its metabolites. Studies in experimental animals and human volunteers have shown that a 5 to 1 ratio of charcoal to mefenamic acid results in considerable suppression of absorption of the drug. Haemodialysis is of little value since mefenamic acid and its metabolites are firmly bound to plasma proteins. Overdose has led to fatalities.

Mefenamic acid has a tendency to induce tonic-clonic (grand mal) convulsions in overdose. Acute renal failure and coma have been reported with mefenamic acid overdose. It is important that the recommended dose is not exceeded and the regime adhered to since some reports have involved daily dosages under 3g.

5. PHARMACOLOGICAL PROPERTIES
5.1 Pharmacodynamic properties
ANIMAL MODELS

Mefenamic acid is non-steroidal anti-inflammatory drug (NSAID) with anti-inflammatory, analgesic and antipyretic properties.

Its anti-inflammatory effect was first established in the UV erythema model of inflammation. Further studies included inhibition of granulation tissue growth into subcutaneous cotton pellets in rats and carrageenin induced rat paw oedema tests.

Antipyretic activity was demonstrated in yeast-induced pyresis in rats. In this model its antipyretic activity was roughly equal to that of phenylbutazone and flufenamic acid, but less than that of indomethacin.

Analgesic activity was demonstrated in tests involving pain sensitivity of rats paws inflamed by brewers yeast. Mefenamic acid was less potent than flufenamic acid in this model.

Prostaglandins are implicated in a number of disease processes including inflammation, modulation of the pain response, dysmenorrhoea, menorrhagia and pyrexia.

In common with most NSAIDs mefenamic acid inhibits the action of prostaglandin synthetase (cyclo oxygenase). This results in a reduction in the rate of prostaglandin synthesis and reduced prostaglandin levels.

The anti-inflammatory activity of NSAIDs in the rat paw oedema test has been correlated with their ability to inhibit prostaglandin synthetase. When mefenamic acid is ranked in both these tests it falls between indomethacin and phenylbutazone and it is probable that inhibition of prostaglandin synthesis contributes to the pharmacological activity and clinical efficacy of mefenamic acid.

There is also considerable evidence that the fenamates inhibit the action of prostaglandins after they have been formed. They therefore both inhibit the synthesis and response to prostaglandins. This double blockade may well be important in their mode of action.

5.2 Pharmacokinetic properties
Absorption and Distribution
Mefenamic acid is absorbed from the gastro intestinal tract. Peak levels of 10mg/l occur two hours after the administration of a 1g oral dose to adults.

Metabolism
Mefenamic acid is extensively metabolised, first to A3 hydroxymethyl derivative (metabolite I) and then A3 carboxyl derivative (metabolite II). Both metabolites undergo secondary conjugation to form glucuronides.

Elimination
Fifty two percent of a dose is recovered from the urine, 6% as mefenamic acid, 25% as metabolite I and 21% as metabolite II. Assay of stools over a 3 day period accounted for 10-20% of the dose chiefly as unconjugated metabolite II.

The plasma levels of unconjugated mefenamic acid decline with a half life of approximately two hours.

5.3 Preclinical safety data
Preclinical safety data does not add anything of further significance to the prescriber.

6. PHARMACEUTICAL PARTICULARS
6.1 List of excipients
Lactose, pregelatinised starch, maize starch, polyvidone, silicon dioxide, talc, magnesium stearate, croscarmellose sodium type A, sodium lauryl sulphate, purified water*, Opadry OY-LS-22808 (H.P.M.C.2910 15cps, lactose, polyethylene glycol 4000, vanillin, E104, E110, E171), Opaglos AG7350 (purified water, beeswax white, carnauba wax yellow, polysorbate 20, sorbic acid).

*not detectable

6.2 Incompatibilities
None Known

6.3 Shelf life
36 months for amber polystyrene bottle

48 months for blister and HDPE DUMA and polypropylene container

6.4 Special precautions for storage
Store below 30°C.

6.5 Nature and contents of container
a) Aluminium foil/pvc blister pack in cardboard carton. Pack sizes: 100

b) HDPE DUMA and polypropylene container. Pack sizes: 100 and 500

c) Amber polystyrene bottle with a high density polyethene anti-arthritic closure. Pack sizes: 6, 12, 84, 100 and 500.

6.6 Instructions for use and handling
Not applicable

7. MARKETING AUTHORISATION HOLDER
Chemidex Pharma Limited

Chemidex House

Egham Business Village

Crabtree Road

Egham

Surrey TW20 8RB

United Kingdom

8. MARKETING AUTHORISATION NUMBER(S)
PL 17736/0007

9. DATE OF FIRST AUTHORISATION/RENEWAL OF THE AUTHORISATION
31st December 2001

10. DATE OF REVISION OF THE TEXT

Pork Actrapid

(Novo Nordisk Limited)

1. NAME OF THE MEDICINAL PRODUCT
Pork Actrapid®

2. QUALITATIVE AND QUANTITATIVE COMPOSITION
Insulin Injection

Active ingredient: Porcine insulin 100 iu/ml

3. PHARMACEUTICAL FORM
Sterile solution for injection.

4. CLINICAL PARTICULARS
4.1 Therapeutic indications
Treatment of diabetes mellitus.

4.2 Posology and method of administration
Adults and children:

The dosage is determined by the physician according to the needs of the patient.

Pork Actrapid is usually administered subcutaneously, but may also be given by intramuscular or intravenous injection. When injected subcutaneously, injection into the abdominal wall ensures a faster absorption than from other regions of the body; injection into a lifted skin fold minimises the risk of intramuscular injection.

When used alone Pork Actrapid is usually given three or four times daily; it is most commonly used in regimens where an intermediate or long-acting insulin is given in addition. Pork Actrapid may be mixed in the syringe with insulin suspensions to intensify their initial effect. The Pork Actrapid should be drawn into the syringe first and the injection given immediately after mixing.

Pork Actrapid does not contain a buffer; for this reason it should not be used in ambulatory insulin infusion pumps because of the risk of needle or catheter blockage.

Use in the elderly:

There are no precautions concerning the use of insulin which are specific to the elderly diabetic. However, injection procedures may be difficult for the infirm or the confused patient and the simplest regimen consistent with keeping the patient symptom-free should be considered.

4.3 Contraindications
Insulin is contra-indicated in hypoglycaemia.

Hypersensitivity to porcine insulin or any of the excipients.

4.4 Special warnings and special precautions for use
Injection of Pork Actrapid should be followed by a meal within approximately 30 minutes of administration.

The use of dosages which are inadequate, or discontinuation of treatment, especially in insulin-dependent diabetics, may lead to hyperglycaemia and diabetic ketoacidosis; conditions which are potentially lethal.

Transfer of patients to this highly purified porcine insulin may lead to changes in glycaemic control; adjustments in therapy should be made under the guidance of a physician. The following general guidelines apply:

For patients currently controlled on highly purified porcine insulin no dosage change is expected other than routine adjustments made in order to maintain stable diabetic control. Patients currently controlled on mixed species or bovine insulin may require a dosage adjustment dependent upon dosage, purity, species and formulation of the insulin preparation(s) currently administered.

Patients whose blood glucose control is greatly improved, e.g. by intensified insulin therapy, may experience a change in their usual warning symptoms of hypoglycaemia and possibly lose some or all of the symptoms and should be advised accordingly.

4.5 Interaction with other medicinal products and other forms of Interaction
Concomitant use of other drugs may influence insulin requirements. The following substances may enhance the hypoglycaemic effect of insulin: alcohol, non-selective beta adrenergic blocking agents, monoamine oxidase inhibitors (MAOI), ACE inhibitors, salicylate, anabolic steroids.

Other drugs may increase insulin requirements: oral contraceptives, thyroid hormones, corticosteroids, thiazides and sympathomimetics. Beta adrenergic blocking agents may blur the symptoms of hypoglycaemia. Alcohol may intensify and prolong the hypoglycaemic effect of insulin.

Diabetic patients treated with drugs other than insulin should discuss possible interactions with the prescribing physician.

4.6 Pregnancy and lactation
Intensified control in the treatment of pregnant insulin-dependent diabetics is recommended. Insulin requirements usually fall in the first trimester and increase during the second and third trimester. Insulin does not pass the placental barrier. Breast feeding is not contra-indicated.

4.7 Effects on ability to drive and use machines
The patient's ability to concentrate and react may be impaired as a result of hypoglycaemia. This may constitute a risk in situations where these abilities are of special importance (e.g. driving a car or operating machinery).

Patients should be advised to take precautions to avoid hypoglycaemia whilst driving, this is particularly important in those who have reduced or absent awareness of the warning signs of hypoglycaemia or have frequent episodes of hypoglycaemia. The advisability of driving should be considered in these circumstances.

4.8 Undesirable effects
At initiation of insulin therapy, oedema and refraction anomalies may occur; these are usually transitory. The same applies to local hyper-sensitivity reactions (swelling and itching at the injection site) which usually disappear during continued treatment.

Persistent allergies to this insulin are very rare. Lipodystrophy at injection sites is also rare and should be prevented by constantly changing injection sites.

4.9 Overdose
Overdosage causes hypoglycaemia; symptoms are variable but may include confusion, palpitations, sweating, malaise and loss of consciousness.

In the event of an overdose, glucose should be given if the patient is conscious. Where the patient is unconscious an intramuscular, subcutaneous or intravenous injection of glucagon should be given and oral carbohydrate administered when the patient responds. Alternatively intravenous glucose may be administered; it must be given if there is no response to glucagon.

If severe hypoglycaemia is not treated it can cause temporary or permanent brain damage and death.

5. PHARMACOLOGICAL PROPERTIES
5.1 Pharmacodynamic properties
Porcine insulin is a hypoglycaemic agent in man; promotes uptake of glucose into liver, muscle and adipose tissue, inhibits gluconeogenesis and promotes lipogenesis.

5.2 Pharmacokinetic properties
Pork Actrapid is a neutral solution of porcine insulin. When injected subcutaneously it has a duration of action of some ½ to 8 hours and its maximum effect is exerted between 1 and 3 hours after injection.

5.3 Preclinical safety data
Not applicable.

6. PHARMACEUTICAL PARTICULARS
6.1 List of excipients
Glycerol (E422)

m-Cresol

Zinc Oxide

Sodium hydroxide

Hydrochloric acid

Water for Injections

6.2 Incompatibilities
Due to the high risk of precipitation in some pump catheters, Pork Actrapid is not recommended for use in ambulatory insulin infusion pumps.

6.3 Shelf life
30 months.

The vial in use may be kept at room temperature (maximum 25°C) for up to 6 weeks.

6.4 Special precautions for storage
Store between 2°C and 8°C. Avoid freezing.

6.5 Nature and contents of container
10ml glass vial, closed with rubber disc and aluminium cap. The rubber disc/aluminium cap is covered with a plastic, tamper-evident cap which must be removed before use of the vial. The plastic cap cannot be replaced once removed from the vial.

6.6 Instructions for use and handling
Each carton contains a patient information leaflet with instructions for use.

7. MARKETING AUTHORISATION HOLDER
Novo Nordisk Limited

Broadfield Park, Brighton Road

Crawley, West Sussex RH11 9RT

8. MARKETING AUTHORISATION NUMBER(S)
PL 3132/0121

9. DATE OF FIRST AUTHORISATION/RENEWAL OF THE AUTHORISATION
Date of first grant: 10.7.98

10. DATE OF REVISION OF THE TEXT
March 1997, April 2002

11 LEGAL CATEGORY
POM (Prescription Only Medicine).

Pork Insulatard

(Novo Nordisk Limited)

1. NAME OF THE MEDICINAL PRODUCT
Pork Insulatard®

2. QUALITATIVE AND QUANTITATIVE COMPOSITION
Isophane Insulin Injection.

Active ingredient: Porcine insulin 100 iu/ml

3. PHARMACEUTICAL FORM
Sterile suspension for injection.

4. CLINICAL PARTICULARS
4.1 Therapeutic indications
The treatment of insulin-requiring diabetics.

4.2 Posology and method of administration
Adults and children:

The dosage is determined by the physician according to the needs of the patient.

Pork Insulatard is usually administered subcutaneously, but may also be given intramuscularly. The thigh is the recommended site for subcutaneous injection; injection into a lifted skin fold minimises the risk of intramuscular injection.

Use in the elderly:

Clearance rates may be reduced in the elderly due to declining renal function. Insulin may, therefore have a more prolonged action. Dose requirements should be regularly reviewed.

4.3 Contraindications
Insulin is contra-indicated in hypoglycaemia.

4.4 Special warnings and special precautions for use
Care must be taken to avoid hypoglycaemia.

The use of dosages which are inadequate, or discontinuation of treatment, especially in insulin-dependent diabetics, may lead to hyperglycaemia and diabetic ketoacidosis; conditions which are potentially lethal.

Patients whose blood glucose control is greatly improved, e.g. by intensified insulin therapy, may experience a change in their usual warning symptoms of hypoglycaemia and possibly lose some or all of the symptoms and should be advised accordingly.

4.5 Interaction with other medicinal products and other forms of Interaction
Concomitant use of other drugs may influence insulin requirements. The following substances may enhance the hypoglycaemic effect of insulin: alcohol, non-selective beta adrenergic blocking agents, monoamine oxidase inhibitors (MAOI), ACE inhibitors, salicylate, anabolic steroids.

Other drugs may increase insulin requirements: oral contraceptives, thyroid hormones, corticosteroids, thiazides and sympathomimetics. Beta adrenergic blocking agents may blur the symptoms of hypoglycaemia. Alcohol may intensify and prolong the hypoglycaemic effect of insulin.

Diabetic patients treated with drugs other than insulin should discuss possible interactions with the prescribing physician.

4.6 Pregnancy and lactation
Intensified control in the treatment of pregnant insulin-dependent diabetics is recommended. Insulin requirements usually fall in the first trimester and increase during the second and third trimester.

Breast feeding is not contra-indicated.

4.7 Effects on ability to drive and use machines
The patient's ability to concentrate and react may be impaired as a result of hypoglycaemia. This may constitute a risk in situations where these abilities are of special importance (e.g. driving a car or operating machinery).

Patients should be advised to take precautions to avoid hypoglycaemia whilst driving, this is particularly important in those who have reduced or absent awareness of the warning signs of hypoglycaemia or have frequent episodes of hypoglycaemia. The advisability of driving should be considered in these circumstances.

4.8 Undesirable effects
At initiation of insulin therapy, oedema and refraction anomalies may occur; these are usually transitory. The same applies to local hyper-sensitivity reactions (swelling and itching at the injection site) which usually disappear during continued treatment.

Persistent allergies to purified insulin are rare. Lipodystrophy at injection sites is also rare and should be prevented by constantly changing injection sites.

4.9 Overdose
Overdose causes hypoglycaemia; symptoms are variable but may include confusion, palpitations, sweating, malaise and loss of consciousness.

In the event of an overdose, glucose should be given if the patient is conscious. Where the patient is unconscious an intramuscular, subcutaneous or intravenous injection of glucagon should be given and oral carbohydrate administered when the patient responds. Alternatively intravenous glucose may be administered; it must be given if there is no response to glucagon.

If severe hypoglycaemia is not treated it can cause temporary or permanent brain damage and death.

5. PHARMACOLOGICAL PROPERTIES
5.1 Pharmacodynamic properties
Insulin has a blood glucose lowering effect.

5.2 Pharmacokinetic properties
Pork Insulatard is an isophane porcine insulin preparation. When injected subcutaneously it has a duration of action of some 1½ to 24 hours and its maximum effect is exerted between 4 and 12 hours after injection.

When injected intramuscularly, the onset of action is more rapid, while the overall duration of action is shorter, provided the injection site is well perfused muscle.

5.3 Preclinical safety data
None stated.

6. PHARMACEUTICAL PARTICULARS
6.1 List of excipients
Glycerol (E422)

m-Cresol

Phenol

Disodium phosphate dihydrate

Sodium hydroxide

Hydrochloric acid

Zinc Oxide

Protamine Sulphate

Water for Injections

6.2 Incompatibilities
None stated.

6.3 Shelf life
30 months.

6.4 Special precautions for storage
Store between 2°C and 8°C. Avoid freezing and direct sunlight.

6.5 Nature and contents of container
10ml glass vial, closed with rubber disc and aluminium cap. The rubber disc/aluminium cap is covered with a plastic, tamper-evident cap which must be removed before use of the vial. The plastic cap cannot be replaced once removed from the vial.

6.6 Instructions for use and handling
Each carton contains a patient information leaflet with instructions for use.

7. MARKETING AUTHORISATION HOLDER
Novo Nordisk Limited

Broadfield Park, Brighton Road

Crawley, West Sussex RH11 9RT

8. MARKETING AUTHORISATION NUMBER(S)
PL 3132/0018

9. DATE OF FIRST AUTHORISATION/RENEWAL OF THE AUTHORISATION
Date of first grant: 8 February 1982

Date of last renewal: 20 May 1997

10. DATE OF REVISION OF THE TEXT
June 2002

11 LEGAL CATEGORY
POM

Pork Mixtard 30

(Novo Nordisk Limited)

1. NAME OF THE MEDICINAL PRODUCT
Pork Mixtard® 30

2. QUALITATIVE AND QUANTITATIVE COMPOSITION
Biphasic Isophane Insulin Injection 30/70.

Active ingredient: Porcine insulin 100 iu/ml

3. PHARMACEUTICAL FORM
Sterile suspension for injection.

4. CLINICAL PARTICULARS
4.1 Therapeutic indications
The treatment of insulin-requiring diabetics.

4.2 Posology and method of administration
Adults and children:

The dosage is determined by the physician according to the needs of the patient.

Pork Mixtard 30 is usually administered subcutaneously, but may also be given intramuscularly. The abdominal wall or thigh are recommended sites for subcutaneous injection; injection into a lifted skin fold minimises the risk of intramuscular injection.

Use in the elderly:

Clearance rates may be reduced in the elderly due to declining renal function. Insulin may, therefore have a more prolonged action. Dose requirements should be regularly reviewed.

4.3 Contraindications
Insulin is contra-indicated in hypoglycaemia.

4.4 Special warnings and special precautions for use
Injection of Pork Mixtard 30 should be followed by a meal within approximately 30 minutes of administration.

The use of dosages which are inadequate, or discontinuation of treatment, especially in insulin-dependent diabetics, may lead to hyperglycaemia and diabetic ketoacidosis; conditions which are potentially lethal.

Patients whose blood glucose control is greatly improved, e.g. by intensified insulin therapy, may experience a change in their usual warning symptoms of hypoglycaemia and possibly lose some or all of the symptoms and should be advised accordingly.

4.5 Interaction with other medicinal products and other forms of Interaction
Concomitant use of other drugs may influence insulin requirements. The following substances may enhance the hypoglycaemic effect of insulin: alcohol, non-selective beta adrenergic blocking agents, monoamine oxidase inhibitors (MAOI), ACE inhibitors, salicylate, anabolic steroids.

Other drugs may increase insulin requirements: oral contraceptives, thyroid hormones, corticosteroids, thiazides and sympathomimetics. Beta adrenergic blocking agents may blur the symptoms of hypoglycaemia. Alcohol may intensify and prolong the hypoglycaemic effect of insulin.

Diabetic patients treated with drugs other than insulin should discuss possible interactions with the prescribing physician.

4.6 Pregnancy and lactation
Intensified control in the treatment of pregnant insulin-dependent diabetics is recommended. Insulin requirements usually fall in the first trimester and increase during the second and third trimester.

Breast feeding is not contra-indicated.

4.7 Effects on ability to drive and use machines
The patient's ability to concentrate and react may be impaired as a result of hypoglycaemia. This may constitute a risk in situations where these abilities are of special importance (e.g. driving a car or operating machinery).

Patients should be advised to take precautions to avoid hypoglycaemia whilst driving, this is particularly important in those who have reduced or absent awareness of the warning signs of hypoglycaemia or have frequent episodes of hypoglycaemia. The advisability of driving should be considered in these circumstances.

4.8 Undesirable effects
At initiation of insulin therapy, oedema and refraction anomalies may occur; these are usually transitory. The same applies to local hyper-sensitivity reactions (swelling and itching at the injection site) which usually disappear during continued treatment.

Persistent allergies to purified insulin are rare. Lipodystrophy at injection sites is also rare and should be prevented by constantly changing injection sites.

4.9 Overdose
Overdose causes hypoglycaemia; symptoms are variable but may include confusion, palpitations, sweating, malaise and loss of consciousness.

In the event of an overdose, glucose should be given if the patient is conscious. Where the patient is unconscious an intramuscular, subcutaneous or intravenous injection of glucagon should be given and oral carbohydate administered when the patient responds. Alternatively intravenous glucose may be administered; it must be given if there is no response to glucagon.

If severe hypoglycaemia is not treated it can cause temporary or permanent brain damage and death.

5. PHARMACOLOGICAL PROPERTIES
5.1 Pharmacodynamic properties
Insulin has a blood glucose lowering effect.

5.2 Pharmacokinetic properties
Pork Mixtard 30 consists of soluble and isophane porcine insulin in the ratio 3:7. When injected subcutaneously it has a duration of action of some ½ up to 24 hours and its maximum effect is exerted between 4 and about 8 hours after injection.

When injected intramuscularly, the onset of action is more rapid, while the overall duration of action is shorter, provided the injection site is well perfused muscle.

5.3 Preclinical safety data
None stated

6. PHARMACEUTICAL PARTICULARS
6.1 List of excipients
Glycerol (E422)

m-Cresol

Phenol

Disodium phosphate dihydrate

Sodium hydroxide

Hydrochloric acid

Zinc Oxide

Protamine Sulphate

Water for Injections

6.2 Incompatibilities
None stated.

6.3 Shelf life
30 months.

6.4 Special precautions for storage
Store between 2°C and 8°C. Avoid freezing and direct sunlight.

6.5 Nature and contents of container
10ml glass vial, closed with rubber disc and aluminium cap. The rubber disc/aluminium cap is covered with a plastic, tamper-evident cap which must be removed before use of the vial. The plastic cap cannot be replaced once removed from the vial.

6.6 Instructions for use and handling
Each carton contains a patient information leaflet with instructions for use.

7. MARKETING AUTHORISATION HOLDER
Novo Nordisk Limited

Broadfield Park, Brighton Road

Crawley, West Sussex RH11 9RT

8. MARKETING AUTHORISATION NUMBER(S)
PL 3132/0021

9. DATE OF FIRST AUTHORISATION/RENEWAL OF THE AUTHORISATION
Date of first grant: 8 February 1982

Date of last renewal: 19 May 1997

10. DATE OF REVISION OF THE TEXT
June 2003

11 LEGAL CATEGORY
POM

Posalfilin Ointment

(Norgine Limited)

1. NAME OF THE MEDICINAL PRODUCT
POSALFILIN Ointment.

2. QUALITATIVE AND QUANTITATIVE COMPOSITION
Each 10g tube of POSALFILIN Ointment contains 20% w/w Podophyllum Resin BP and 25% w/w Salicylic Acid BP.

3. PHARMACEUTICAL FORM
Dark brown ointment.

4. CLINICAL PARTICULARS
4.1 Therapeutic indications
For the treatment of plantar warts.

4.2 Posology and method of administration
Adults (including the elderly) and Children: A corn ring should be placed around the wart, cutting the ring to fit if necessary. A minimal amount of ointment should be applied to the exposed wart, taking care to avoid normal skin. The wart and corn ring should be covered with a plaster and the treatment repeated daily. When the wart appears soft and spongy, it should be left exposed and allowed to drop off. If the wart remains, the procedure should be repeated.

4.3 Contraindications
Use in pregnancy, breastfeeding mothers, bleeding or friable warts. Patients with peripheral neuropathy, diabetes mellitus or peripheral vascular insufficiency. Should not be used on the skin of the face, armpits or ano-genital region.

4.4 Special warnings and special precautions for use
The patient should be warned that POSALFILIN Ointment is caustic to healthy skin, if such inflammation occurs, treatment should be suspended.

4.5 Interaction with other medicinal products and other forms of Interaction
None known.

4.6 Pregnancy and lactation
Contraindicated in pregnancy and breastfeeding mothers.

4.7 Effects on ability to drive and use machines
There is no effect on the ability to drive and use machines.

4.8 Undesirable effects
Misapplication of POSALFILIN to healthy skin may cause inflammation, desquamation or necrosis. If applied to delicate areas of skin such as the ano-genital area, the skin may be seriously damaged, to an extent dependent on the amount applied.

4.9 Overdose
Over-application can cause cutaneous necrosis and should be treated as a caustic burn.

5. PHARMACOLOGICAL PROPERTIES
5.1 Pharmacodynamic properties
The salicylic acid macerates the horny layer covering the wart and allows the podophyllum to penetrate the wart where it has a specific cytotoxic effect on the nuclei of the hyperplastic cells.

5.2 Pharmacokinetic properties
Not applicable, as POSALFILIN Ointment applied topically directly to the wart.

5.3 Preclinical safety data
There are no preclinical data of relevance to the prescriber, which are additional to that already included in other sections of the SPC.

6. PHARMACEUTICAL PARTICULARS
6.1 List of excipients
Yellow Soft Paraffin BP

Liquid Paraffin BP

6.2 Incompatibilities
None known.

6.3 Shelf life
The shelf life is 4 years.

6.4 Special precautions for storage
Do not store above 25°C.

6.5 Nature and contents of container
Aluminium tube containing 10g of ointment.

6.6 Instructions for use and handling
None.

7. MARKETING AUTHORISATION HOLDER
Norgine Limited

Chaplin House

Widewater Place

Moorhall Road

Harefield

UXBRIDGE

Middlesex' UB9 6NS

United Kingdom

8. MARKETING AUTHORISATION NUMBER(S)
PL 00322/5901R

9. DATE OF FIRST AUTHORISATION/RENEWAL OF THE AUTHORISATION
28th October 1996

10. DATE OF REVISION OF THE TEXT
16 August 2004

Legal Category: **P**

Potaba Capsules

(Glenwood Laboratories Ltd)

1. NAME OF THE MEDICINAL PRODUCT
Potaba®(Potassium para-aminobenzoate)

2. QUALITATIVE AND QUANTITATIVE COMPOSITION
Capsules: white/white gelatin capsule shell containing the active ingredient 500mg of potassium para-aminobenzoate powder.

3. PHARMACEUTICAL FORM
Capsules: White/white size zero gelatin capsules containing 500mg potassium para-aminobenzoate with Potaba 51 on the shell.

4. CLINICAL PARTICULARS
4.1 Therapeutic indications
Peyronie's Disease

Scleroderma

4.2 Posology and method of administration
Potaba capsules should be taken orally; six capsules four times daily with food.

Children: not recommended.

4.3 Contraindications
Potaba should not be given to patients taking sulphonamides as it will inactivate this medication.

4.4 Special warnings and special precautions for use
Treatment with Potaba should be interrupted during periods of low food intake (egg, during fasting, anorexia, nausea). This is to avoid the possible development of hypoglycaemia.

Potaba treatment should be given cautiously to patients with renal impairment and treatment discontinued if a hypersensitivity reaction occurs.

Potaba should not be taken by patients on sulphonamides; Potaba may cause inactivation of this medication.

4.5 Interaction with other medicinal products and other forms of Interaction
With the exception of sulphonamides, no interactions with other medicaments have been established.

4.6 Pregnancy and lactation
No information is available on this, therefore it is not recommended.

4.7 Effects on ability to drive and use machines
There is no evidence that Potaba has any effect on ability to drive or use machines.

4.8 Undesirable effects
Treatment with Potaba should be interrupted during periods of low food intake, (e.g. during fasting, anorexia, nausea). This is to avoid the possible development of hypoglycaemia.

No serious adverse effects have been reported in patients treated with Potaba.

4.9 Overdose
No particular problems are expected following overdosage with Potaba. Symptomatic and supportive therapy should be given as appropriate.

5. PHARMACOLOGICAL PROPERTIES

5.1 Pharmacodynamic properties
P. Aminobenzoate is considered a member of the Vitamin B complex. Small amounts are found in cereal, eggs, milk and meats. Detectable amounts are normally present in human blood, spinal fluid, urine and sweat. The pharmacological action of this chemical has not been clearly established, but it has been suggested that the antifibrosis activity of Potaba is brought about by the drug increasing oxygen uptake at the tissue level. Fibrosis is believed to occur from either too much serotonin or too little monoamine oxidase activity over a period of time. The activity of monoamine oxidase is dependant on an adequate oxygen supply. By increasing oxygen supply at tissue level Potaba enhances monoamine oxidase activity thereby preventing or bringing about regression of fibrosis.

5.2 Pharmacokinetic properties
Potaba is rapidly absorbed and metabolised as food. Excretion is through renal function.

5.3 Preclinical safety data
N/A

6. PHARMACEUTICAL PARTICULARS

6.1 List of excipients
None

6.2 Incompatibilities
Sulphonamides.

6.3 Shelf life
Capsules: three years from date of manufacture.

6.4 Special precautions for storage
Store below 25°C.

6.5 Nature and contents of container
:
White polypropylene tube with tamper-evident polyethylene cap. A filla may be inserted to reduce ullage.

Containers of 240 × 500mg capsules.

6.6 Instructions for use and handling

7. MARKETING AUTHORISATION HOLDER
Glenwood Laboratories Ltd.,

Jenkins Dale,

Chatham

Kent ME4 5RD

8. MARKETING AUTHORISATION NUMBER(S)
Potaba Capsules: 00245/5001R

9. DATE OF FIRST AUTHORISATION/RENEWAL OF THE AUTHORISATION
March 1998

10. DATE OF REVISION OF THE TEXT
June 2002

Potaba Sachets

(Glenwood Laboratories Ltd)

1. NAME OF THE MEDICINAL PRODUCT
Potaba®(Potassium para-aminobenzoate)

2. QUALITATIVE AND QUANTITATIVE COMPOSITION
Envules: foil laminate sachets containing 3g of potassium para-aminobenzoate.

3. PHARMACEUTICAL FORM
Envule; contains 3g potassium para-aminobenzoate; white/off-white powder.

4. CLINICAL PARTICULARS

4.1 Therapeutic indications
Peyronie's Disease
Scleroderma

4.2 Posology and method of administration
Potaba envules should be taken orally; four times daily with food; dissolve the powder in fruit juice.

Children: not recommended.

4.3 Contraindications
Potaba should not be given to patient taking sulphonamides as it will inactivate this medication.

4.4 Special warnings and special precautions for use
Treatment with Potaba should be interrupted during periods of low food intake (eg, during fasting, anorexia, nausea). This is to avoid the possible development of hypoglycaemia.

Potaba treatment should be given cautiously to patients with renal impairment and treatment discontinued if a hypersensitivity reaction occurs.

Potaba should not be taken by patients on sulphonamides; Potaba may cause inactivation of this medication.

4.5 Interaction with other medicinal products and other forms of Interaction
With the exception of sulphonamides, no interactions with other medicaments have been established.

4.6 Pregnancy and lactation
No information is available on this, therefore it is not recommended.

4.7 Effects on ability to drive and use machines
There is no evidence that Potaba has any effect on ability to drive or use machines.

4.8 Undesirable effects
Treatment with Potaba should be interrupted during periods of low food intake, (eg during fasting, anorexia, nausea.) This is to avoid the possible development of hypoglycaemia.

No serious adverse effects have been reported in patients treated with Potaba.

4.9 Overdose
No particular problems are expected following overdosage with Potaba. Symptomatic and supportive therapy should be given as appropriate.

5. PHARMACOLOGICAL PROPERTIES

5.1 Pharmacodynamic properties
P. Aminobenzoate is considered a member of the Vitamin B complex. Small amounts are found in cereal, eggs, milk and meats. Detectable amounts are normally present in human blood, spinal fluid, urine and sweat. The pharmacological action of this chemical has not been clearly established, but it has been suggested that the antifibrosis activity of Potaba is brought about by the drug increasing oxygen uptake at the tissue level. Fibrosis is believed to occur from either too much serotonin or too little monoamine oxidase activity over a period of time. The activity of monoamine oxidase is dependant on an adequate oxygen supply. By increasing oxygen supply at tissue level Potaba enhances monoamine oxidase activity thereby preventing or bringing about regression of fibrosis.

5.2 Pharmacokinetic properties
Potaba is rapidly absorbed and metabolised as food. Excretion is through renal function.

5.3 Preclinical safety data
N/A

6. PHARMACEUTICAL PARTICULARS

6.1 List of excipients
None in this presentation.

6.2 Incompatibilities
Sulphonamides.

6.3 Shelf life
Envules: five years from date of manufacture.

6.4 Special precautions for storage
Store below 25°C.

6.5 Nature and contents of container
Cardboard outer containing 40 × 3g foil laminate sachets.

6.6 Instructions for use and handling
Not applicable

7. MARKETING AUTHORISATION HOLDER
Glenwood Laboratories Ltd.,

Jenkins Dale,

Chatham

Kent ME4 5RD

8. MARKETING AUTHORISATION NUMBER(S)
Potaba Envules: 00245/5000R

9. DATE OF FIRST AUTHORISATION/RENEWAL OF THE AUTHORISATION
March 1998

10. DATE OF REVISION OF THE TEXT
April 02

Potaba Tablets

(Glenwood Laboratories Ltd)

1. NAME OF THE MEDICINAL PRODUCT
Potaba®(Potassium para-aminobenzoate)

2. QUALITATIVE AND QUANTITATIVE COMPOSITION
Tablets; white/off white tablet containing 500mg of potassium para-aminobenzoate and excipients as under section 6.1 "excipients".

3. PHARMACEUTICAL FORM
Tablet: contains 500mg potassium para-aminobenzoate; white/off-white plain biconvex 11.00mm in diameter.

4. CLINICAL PARTICULARS

4.1 Therapeutic indications
Peyronie's Disease
Scleroderma

4.2 Posology and method of administration
Potaba tablets should be taken orally; six tablets, crushed in juice, four times daily with food.

Children: not recommended.

4.3 Contraindications
Potaba should not be given to patient taking sulphonamides as it will inactivate this medication.

4.4 Special warnings and special precautions for use
Treatment with Potaba should be interrupted during periods of low food intake (eg, during fasting, anorexia, nausea). This is to avoid the possible development of hypoglycaemia.

Potaba treatment should be given cautiously to patients with renal impairment and treatment discontinued if a hypersensitivity reaction occurs.

Potaba should not be taken by patients on sulphonamides; Potaba may cause inactivation of this medication.

4.5 Interaction with other medicinal products and other forms of Interaction
With the exception of sulphonamides, no interactions with other medicaments have been established.

4.6 Pregnancy and lactation
No information is available on this, therefore it is not recommended.

4.7 Effects on ability to drive and use machines
There is no evidence that Potaba has any effect on ability to drive or use machines.

4.8 Undesirable effects
Treatment with Potaba should be interrupted during periods of low food intake, (eg during fasting, anorexia, nausea.) This is to avoid the possible development of hypoglycaemia.

No serious adverse effects have been reported in patients treated with Potaba.

4.9 Overdose
No particular problems are expected following overdosage with Potaba. Symptomatic and supportive therapy should be given as appropriate.

5. PHARMACOLOGICAL PROPERTIES

5.1 Pharmacodynamic properties
P. Aminobenzoate is considered a member of the Vitamin B complex. Small amounts are found in cereal, eggs, milk and meats. Detectable amounts are normally present in human blood, spinal fluid, urine and sweat. The pharmacological action of this chemical has not been clearly established, but it has been suggested that the antifibrosis activity of Potaba is brought about by the drug increasing oxygen uptake at the tissue level. Fibrosis is believed to occur from either too much serotonin or too little monoamine oxidase activity over a period of time. The activity of monoamine oxidase is dependant on an adequate oxygen supply. By increasing oxygen supply at tissue level Potaba enhances monoamine oxidase activity thereby preventing or bringing about regression of fibrosis.

5.2 Pharmacokinetic properties
Potaba is rapidly absorbed and metabolised as food. Excretion is through renal function.

5.3 Preclinical safety data
N/A

6. PHARMACEUTICAL PARTICULARS

6.1 List of excipients
Sucrose BP;

Acacia BP;

Ethylcellulose.;

Industrial Methylated Spirit (11 litres/100,000 tablets);

Magnesium stearate BP;

Stearic acid BPC;

Maize starch BP.

6.2 Incompatibilities
Sulphonamides.

6.3 Shelf life
Tablets: three years from date of manufacture.

6.4 Special precautions for storage
Store below 25°C.

6.5 Nature and contents of container
White polypropylene tube with tamper-evident polyethylene cap. A filla may be inserted to reduce ullage.

Containers of 120 × 500mg tablets and also 1,000 × 500mg tablets.

6.6 Instructions for use and handling

7. MARKETING AUTHORISATION HOLDER
Glenwood Laboratories Ltd.,

Jenkins Dale,

Chatham

Kent ME4 5RD

8. MARKETING AUTHORISATION NUMBER(S)
Potaba Tablets: 00245/5002R

9. DATE OF FIRST AUTHORISATION/RENEWAL OF THE AUTHORISATION
March 1998

10. DATE OF REVISION OF THE TEXT
January 02, November 1998; December 1997, November 1996, June 1996 (revised from December 1995)

Potassium Iodate Tablets 85mg

(Cambridge Laboratories)

1. NAME OF THE MEDICINAL PRODUCT
Potassium Iodate 85mg Tablets

2. QUALITATIVE AND QUANTITATIVE COMPOSITION
Each tablet contains 85mg Potassium Iodate.

For excipients see Section 6.1.

3. PHARMACEUTICAL FORM
Tablet.

Off white, round tablet with star shaped double break line, engraved 2202.

4. CLINICAL PARTICULARS

4.1 Therapeutic indications
Potassium Iodate is indicated as a thyroid blocking agent to prevent the uptake of radioactive iodine, which is a potential hazard arising from the application of nuclear energy.

4.2 Posology and method of administration
For oral administration.

Administration should take place within 3 hours of any accident, or up to 10 hours after an accident, however, this is less effective.

A single daily dose should be administered. Repeated daily administration is necessary in situations involving prolonged exposure. However, pregnant and lactating women should ordinarily receive not more than two doses and neonates not more than one dose.

Tablets	Iodine equivalent
Adults 2 tablets	100 mg
Children aged 3-12 years 1 tablet	50 mg
Children aged 1 month – 3 years ½ tablet	25 mg

For children half of one tablet may be crushed and mixed with milk or water before administration.

Neonates (birth – 1 month)

12.5 mg iodine equivalent should be given as a standard solution preparation where possible. Under emergency conditions, ½ tablet (25 mg iodine equivalent) may be given; careful hormonal follow-up is advised in such cases.

Elderly

The recommended adult dose is appropriate.

4.3 Contraindications
Potassium Iodate is contra-indicated in patients with known iodine sensitivity, renal failure, hypocomplementaemic vasculitis or dermatitis herpetiformis.

4.4 Special warnings and special precautions for use
Patients with thyrotoxicosis treated medically, or patients with a past history of thyrotoxicosis treated medically who are now off treatment and apparently in remission, may be at risk.

Iodine induced hyperthyroidism may be precipitated in patients with asymptomatic nodular goitre or latent Graves' disease, who are not under medical care.

Potassium salts should be given cautiously to patients with renal or adrenal insufficiency, acute dehydration or heat cramp.

Care should be exercised if potassium salts are given concomitantly with potassium-sparing diuretics, as hyperkalaemia may result.

4.5 Interaction with other medicinal products and other forms of Interaction
Several drugs, such as captopril, enalopril and the thiazide diuretics can induce hyperkalaemia and this effect may be enhanced if Potassium Iodate is also administered.

The effect of quinidine on the heart is increased by increased plasma concentrations of potassium.

Hyperkalaemia results from the interaction between potassium salts and amiloride, triamterene or aldosterone antagonists.

4.6 Pregnancy and lactation
Teratogenic effects such as congenital goitre and hypothyroidism have been reported when iodides, and therefore presumably iodate, are administered to pregnant women.

However, in the event of a nuclear accident, the proper use of Potassium Iodate in low doses, over a short period of time, as a thyroid blocking agent is not contra-indicated. Prophylactic administration of iodate to the pregnant mother should also be effective for the foetus.

4.7 Effects on ability to drive and use machines
No effect.

4.8 Undesirable effects
Since experience with Potassium Iodate is limited, presumably the following side effects which can occur with potassium iodide can also be associated with Potassium Iodate.

Hypersensitivity reactions such as skin rashes, swollen salivary glands; headache, bronchospasm and gastrointestinal disturbances can be mild or severe and may be dose dependent.

An overactive thyroid gland, thyroiditis, and an enlarged thyroid gland with or without development or myxoedema have also been reported.

Continued administration may lead to mental depression, nervousness, sexual impotence and insomnia.

4.9 Overdose
In overdose, symptoms or iodism, such as headache, pain and swelling of the salivary glands, fever or laryngitis may occur.

In acute iodine poisoning large quantities of milk and starch mucilage should be given.

Aspiration and lavage with starch mucilage or lavage with activated charcoal should be considered.

Electrolyte and water losses should be replaced and the circulation should be maintained. Pethidine (100 mg) or morphine sulphate (10 mg) may be given for pain. A tracheostomy may become necessary.

Haemodialysis may reduce excessively elevated serum iodine concentrations.

5. PHARMACOLOGICAL PROPERTIES

5.1 Pharmacodynamic properties
The iodine released from iodide and iodate on absorption from the gut is taken up rapidly and preferentially by the cells of the thyroid gland. Once in the thyroid, it is rapidly incorporated into organic molecules that are synthesised into thyroid hormones and ultimately released into the general circulation.

If excessive amounts of stable iodate are administered to normal adults, the iodine uptake mechanism of the thyroid is saturated and little or no further iodine is taken up. This effectively blocks the uptake of radioactive iodine in the event of accidental exposure to radioiodines.

5.2 Pharmacokinetic properties
Iodine absorbed from the gut is taken up rapidly and preferentially by the cells of the thyroid gland. Renal clearance of iodide/iodate is usually in the range of 30 to 50 ml of serum/minute, is closely related to glomerular filtration, and is little affected by the iodate load. Most radioiodine not taken up by the thyroid gland after a single oral bolus of iodate is excreted in the urine over the subsequent 48-hour period.

5.3 Preclinical safety data
Preclinical information has not been included because the safety profile of Potassium Iodate has been established after many years of clinical use.

6. PHARMACEUTICAL PARTICULARS

6.1 List of excipients
The tablet contains Calcium Hydrogen Phosphate, Croscarmellose Sodium, Microcrystalline Cellulose and Magnesium Stearate.

6.2 Incompatibilities
None known.

6.3 Shelf life
Containers - 24 months

Blisters - 24 months

6.4 Special precautions for storage
Do not store above 25°C.

Store in original container.

6.5 Nature and contents of container
In polypropylene containers with caps or child resistant closures in packs of 50, 100, 500 or 1000 tablets.

Blister strips in multiples of 10 or 100 tablets.

6.6 Instructions for use and handling
Not applicable.

7. MARKETING AUTHORISATION HOLDER
Cambridge Laboratories Ltd, Deltic House, Kingfisher Way, Silverlink Business Park, Wallsend, Tyne and Wear NE28 9NX

8. MARKETING AUTHORISATION NUMBER(S)
PL 12070/0025

9. DATE OF FIRST AUTHORISATION/RENEWAL OF THE AUTHORISATION
19 October 2001

10. DATE OF REVISION OF THE TEXT
22 October 2001

23 October 2001

Powergel

(A. Menarini Pharma U.K. S.R.L.)

1. NAME OF THE MEDICINAL PRODUCT
Powergel.

2. QUALITATIVE AND QUANTITATIVE COMPOSITION
Powergel contains ketoprofen BP 2.5g/100g.

3. PHARMACEUTICAL FORM
A colourless, non-greasy, non-staining gel with an aromatic fragrance for topical application.

4. CLINICAL PARTICULARS

4.1 Therapeutic indications
For local relief of pain and inflammation associated with soft tissue injuries and acute strains and sprains.

4.2 Posology and method of administration
Powergel should be applied topically to the affected area two or three times daily. Maximum duration of use should not exceed 7 days if supplied by a pharmacist or 10 days if supplied on prescription. Powergel should be applied with gentle massage only.

Adults and elderly: Apply 5 to 10cm of gel (100-200mg ketoprofen) with each application.

Children under 12 years of age: Not recommended as experience in children is limited.

4.3 Contraindications
Hypersensitivity to ketoprofen or aspirin or other non-steroidal anti-inflammatory drugs. Severe bronchospasm might be precipitated in these patients and in those suffering from, or with a history of, bronchial asthma or allergic disease. Hence Powergel should not be administered to patients in whom aspirin or other NSAIDs have caused asthma, rhinitis or urticaria.

4.4 Special warnings and special precautions for use
Powergel should not be applied to open wounds or lesions of the skin, or near the eyes. Powergel should be used with caution in patients with renal impairment. Keep out of the reach of children.

Discontinue use if rash develops.

Hands should be washed immediately after use.

Not for use with occlusive dressing.

Topical application of large amounts may result in systemic effects, including hypersensitivity and asthma.

The treated areas should not be exposed to direct sunlight, including solarium during treatment or for the following two weeks.

"P" warning: If symptoms persist after 7 days, consult your doctor.

4.5 Interaction with other medicinal products and other forms of Interaction
No interactions of Powergel with other drugs have been reported. It is, however, advisable to monitor patients under treatment with coumarinic substances.

4.6 Pregnancy and lactation
No embryopathic effects have been demonstrated in animals and there is no epidemiological evidence of the safety of ketoprofen in human pregnancy. Therefore, it is recommended to avoid ketoprofen unless considered essential in which case it should be discontinued within one week of expected confinement when NSAIDs might cause premature closure of the ductus arteriosus or persistent pulmonary hypertension in the neonate. They may also delay labour. Trace amounts of ketoprofen are excreted in breast milk after systemic administration.

4.7 Effects on ability to drive and use machines
None known.

4.8 Undesirable effects
The prolonged use of products for topical administration may cause hypersensitivity phenomena. In such cases the treatment should be discontinued and a suitable alternative therapy instituted. Skin photosensitivity has been reported in isolated cases. Although not known for topical use of ketoprofen, the following adverse events are reported for systemic use: Minor adverse events, frequently transient, consist of gastrointestinal effects such as indigestion, dyspepsia, nausea, constipation, diarrhoea, heartburn and various types of abdominal discomfort. Other minor effects such as headache, dizziness, mild confusion, vertigo, drowsiness, oedema, mood change and insomnia may occur less frequently. Major gastrointestinal adverse events such as peptic ulceration, haemorrhage or perforation may rarely occur. Haematological reactions including thrombocytopenia, hepatic or renal

damage, dermatological reactions, bronchospasm and anaphylaxis are exceedingly rare.

4.9 Overdose
Considering the low blood levels of ketoprofen by the percutaneous route, no overdosage phenomena have been described yet.

5. PHARMACOLOGICAL PROPERTIES

5.1 Pharmacodynamic properties
Ketoprofen is an inhibitor of both the cyclo-oxygenase and lipoxygenase pathways. Inhibition of prostaglandin synthesis provides for potent anti-inflammatory, analgesic and antipyretic effects. Lipoxygenase inhibitors appear to attenuate cell-mediated inflammation and thus retard the progression of tissue destruction in inflamed joints. In addition, Ketoprofen is a powerful inhibitor of bradykinin (a chemical mediator of pain and inflammation), it stabilises lysosomal membranes against osmotic damage and prevents the release of lysosomal enzymes that mediate tissue destruction in inflammatory reactions.

5.2 Pharmacokinetic properties
Powergel allows the site specific topical delivery of ketoprofen with very low plasma concentrations of drug. Therapeutic levels in the affected tissues provide relief from pain and inflammation, yet will satisfactorily overcome the problem of significant systemic unwanted effects.

5.3 Preclinical safety data
There are no preclinical data of relevance to the prescriber which are additional to that already included in other parts of the SPC.

6. PHARMACEUTICAL PARTICULARS

6.1 List of excipients
Powergel contains the following excipients: carbomer 940, ethanol, neroli essence, lavender essence, triethanolamine, purified water.

6.2 Incompatibilities
Not applicable.

6.3 Shelf life
5 years.

6.4 Special precautions for storage
Store below 25°C.

6.5 Nature and contents of container
Soft aluminium tube, treated inside with non-toxic epoxy resin. The tubes are packed in cardboard together with a package insert. The following pack sizes are approved:

P: 30g pack

POM: 30g sample pack, 50g pack, 2x50g twin pack, 100g pack

6.6 Instructions for use and handling
Not applicable.

7. MARKETING AUTHORISATION HOLDER
A Menarini Industrie Farmaceutiche Ruinite srl

Via Sette Santi, 3

50131 Florence

Italy

8. MARKETING AUTHORISATION NUMBER(S)
PL 10649/0001.

9. DATE OF FIRST AUTHORISATION/RENEWAL OF THE AUTHORISATION
28th January 1993/13th January 2004

10. DATE OF REVISION OF THE TEXT
November 2003

Legal Category
P (30g pack, maximum duration of use 7 days).

POM (30g sample pack, 50g pack, 2x50g twinpack, 100g pack).

Pragmatar Cream

(Alliance Pharmaceuticals)

1. NAME OF THE MEDICINAL PRODUCT
Pragmatar Cream

2. QUALITATIVE AND QUANTITATIVE COMPOSITION
4% w/w cetyl alcohol-coal tar distillate, 3% w/w precipitated sulphur PhEur and 3% w/w salicylic acid PhEur

3. PHARMACEUTICAL FORM
A smooth textured, buff coloured cream with a slightly perfumed tarry odour.

4. CLINICAL PARTICULARS

4.1 Therapeutic indications
Treatment of dandruff, other seborrhoeic conditions, and common scaly skin disorders.

4.2 Posology and method of administration
For topical application to the skin.

Adults and children:

For mild dandruff, apply the cream once a week when the hair is washed. For more severe cases, treat the entire scalp daily at bedtime, applying lightly but thoroughly with the fingertips. The cream can be washed out the next morning or left as a pleasant hair dressing. For other indicated subacute or chronic skin disorders, apply daily in small quantities to affected areas only.

Infants:

The cream may be diluted by mixing with a few drops of water in the palm of the hand.

4.3 Contraindications
Do not use in patients who are sensitive to sulphur, or in the presence of acute local infection.

4.4 Special warnings and special precautions for use
Use with care near the eyes, mucous membranes or on acutely inflamed areas. If any cream should accidentally enter the eye, flush with normal saline solution. Avoid use on genital or rectal areas.

4.5 Interaction with other medicinal products and other forms of Interaction
None known.

4.6 Pregnancy and lactation
If used according to the directions, no hazards are expected.

4.7 Effects on ability to drive and use machines
None known.

4.8 Undesirable effects
No side-effects are to be expected if the cream is used according to directions. Excessive use, however, may cause erythema and irritation. Very rarely, coal tar preparations may cause photosensitivity.

4.9 Overdose
If ingestion occurs, gastro-intestinal disturbances may follow. Treatment consists of rinsing out the mouth together with symptomatic measures if necessary. Even with massive ingestion, salicylate poisoning seems unlikely.

5. PHARMACOLOGICAL PROPERTIES

5.1 Pharmacodynamic properties
Pragmatar has mild antipruritic, antiseptic and keratolytic properties.

5.2 Pharmacokinetic properties
Coal tar is a complex intricate compound with a variable composition. As a result, it is not possible to perform normal pharmacokinetic analysis as for other medications. Consequently, there are no reliable data on the rate of absorption, blood levels or excretion of coal tar. However, the conspicuous absence of systemic toxicity over many years of use has led most clinicians to conclude that there is little or no systemic absorption of coal tar.

Salicylic acid is absorbed through skin when applied in ointments, and systemic poisoning has occurred from excessive application to large areas of skin. After absorption, salicylic acid is distributed throughout most body tissues and transcellular fluids, primarily by a pH-dependent passive process. It is mainly metabolised by the liver and excreted via the kidneys, and has a half-life of 2 to 3 hours in low doses.

5.3 Preclinical safety data
No formal preclinical studies have been undertaken with Pragmatar, as its active ingredients are all well established pharmaceuticals.

6. PHARMACEUTICAL PARTICULARS

6.1 List of excipients
Sodium carboxymethylcellulose, glycerol, sodium lauryl sulphate, cetyl alcohol, liquid paraffin, perfume bouquet, water.

6.2 Incompatibilities
None known.

6.3 Shelf life
3 years.

6.4 Special precautions for storage
Store below 30°C. Replace cap tightly after use.

6.5 Nature and contents of container
Printed aluminium internally lacquered tubes of 25g or 100g with screw-on cap of urea formaldehyde high density polythene or polypropylene.

6.6 Instructions for use and handling
No special instructions.

Administrative Data

7. MARKETING AUTHORISATION HOLDER
Alliance Pharmaceuticals Ltd

Avonbridge House

Bath Road

Chippenham

Wiltshire

SN15 2BB

8. MARKETING AUTHORISATION NUMBER(S)
PL16853/0025

9. DATE OF FIRST AUTHORISATION/RENEWAL OF THE AUTHORISATION
30 June 1999

10. DATE OF REVISION OF THE TEXT
May 2001

11. Legal Status
P

Alliance, Alliance Pharmaceuticals and associated devices are registered Trademarks of Alliance Pharmaceuticals Ltd.

Praxilene

(Merck Pharmaceuticals)

1. NAME OF THE MEDICINAL PRODUCT
Praxilene 100mg Capsules

2. QUALITATIVE AND QUANTITATIVE COMPOSITION
100mg naftidrofuryl oxalate equivalent to 81.0 mg naftidrofuryl and 19.0 mg oxalate.

3. PHARMACEUTICAL FORM
Capsule

4. CLINICAL PARTICULARS

4.1 Therapeutic indications
Peripheral vascular disorders - intermittent claudication, night cramps, rest pain, incipient gangrene, trophic ulcers, Raynaud's Syndrome, diabetic arteriopathy and acrocyanosis.

Cerebral vascular disorders - cerebral insufficiency and cerebral atherosclerosis, particularly where these manifest themselves as mental deterioration and confusion in the elderly.

4.2 Posology and method of administration
Peripheral vascular disorders - one or two capsules three times daily for a minimum of three months, or at the discretion of the physician.

Cerebral vascular disorders - one 100mg capsule three times daily for a minimum of three months, or at the discretion of the physician.

There is no recommended use for children.

Administration:

For oral administration. The capsules should be swallowed whole during meals with a sufficient amount of water (minimum) of one glass.

4.3 Contraindications
Hypersensitivity to the drug. Patients with a history of hyperoxaluria or recurrent calcium-containing stones.

4.4 Special warnings and special precautions for use
A sufficient amount of liquid should be taken during treatment to maintain an adequate level of diuresis.

4.5 Interaction with other medicinal products and other forms of Interaction
None known.

4.6 Pregnancy and lactation
Pregnancy: There is no, or inadequate, evidence of the safety of naftidrofuryl oxalate in human pregnancy, but it has been in wide use for many years without apparent ill consequence, animal studies having shown no hazard. If drug therapy is needed in pregnancy, this drug can be used if there is no safer alternative.

Lactation: No information is available.

4.7 Effects on ability to drive and use machines
None known.

4.8 Undesirable effects
Naftidrofuryl oxalate is normally well tolerated in the dosage recommended. Occasionally nausea, epigastric pain and rashes have been noted.

Rarely, hepatitis has been reported. Very rarely, calcium oxalate kidney stones have been reported.

4.9 Overdose
Signs and symptoms: Depression of cardiac conduction and convulsions may occur.

Treatment: The stomach should be emptied by gastric lavage and emesis. Activated charcoal may be employed if necessary. Cardiovascular function and respiration should be monitored and, in severe cases, electrical pacemaking or the use of isoprenaline should be considered. Convulsions may be managed by diazepam.

5. PHARMACOLOGICAL PROPERTIES

5.1 Pharmacodynamic properties
Naftidrofuryl oxalate has been shown to exert a direct effect on intracellular metabolism. Thus it has been shown in man and animals that it produces an increase of ATP levels and a decrease of lactic acid levels in ischaemic conditions, evidence for an enhancement of cellular oxidative capacity. Furthermore, naftidrofuryl oxalate is a powerful spasmolytic agent.

5.2 Pharmacokinetic properties
Naftidrofuryl oxalate is well absorbed when given orally. Peak plasma levels occur about 30 minutes after dosing and the half life is about an hour, although inter subject variation is relatively high. Accumulation does not occur at a dose level of 200mg three times daily.

The drug becomes extensively bound to plasma proteins and is excreted principally via the urine, all in the form of metabolites.

5.3 Preclinical safety data
No toxic effects were seen in animal studies which provide additional information to that obtained in man. In repeated dose studies the no effect level was 25mg/kg/day or greater. There was no evidence of effects on reproduction below doses which caused maternal toxicity.

6. PHARMACEUTICAL PARTICULARS

6.1 List of excipients
Talc
Magnesium Stearate
Purified Water*
Denatured Ethanol*
Capsule Shells:
Erythrosine (E127)
Titanium Dioxide (E171)
Gelatine
Printing ink:
Black iron oxide (E172)
*Not present in final product

6.2 Incompatibilities
None known.

6.3 Shelf life
36 months.

6.4 Special precautions for storage
Store below 20 degree C in a dry place away from light.

6.5 Nature and contents of container
Pack size 10 (medical sample), 21 and 84 capsules:-
Cardboard carton containing blister strips comprising heat-sealable PVC (250μm) and aluminium foil (30μm).
Pack size 100 and 500:
Polyethylene securitainers with tamper evident closures.

6.6 Instructions for use and handling
None.

7. MARKETING AUTHORISATION HOLDER
Merck Ltd
t/a Merck Pharmaceuticals (a division of Merck Ltd)
Harrier House
High Street
West Drayton
Middlesex
UB7 7QG

8. MARKETING AUTHORISATION NUMBER(S)
PL 11648/0064

9. DATE OF FIRST AUTHORISATION/RENEWAL OF THE AUTHORISATION
28 July 2004

10. DATE OF REVISION OF THE TEXT

LEGAL CATEGORY
POM

Pred Forte
(Allergan Ltd)

1. NAME OF THE MEDICINAL PRODUCT
Pred Forte

2. QUALITATIVE AND QUANTITATIVE COMPOSITION
1% w/v prednisolone acetate

3. PHARMACEUTICAL FORM
Eye Drops

4. CLINICAL PARTICULARS

4.1 Therapeutic indications
For short-term treatment of steroid-responsive inflammatory conditions of the eye, after excluding the presence of viral, fungal and bacterial pathogens.

4.2 Posology and method of administration
Route of administration is by ocular instillation.

Adults: One to two drops instilled into the conjunctival sac two to four times daily. During the initial 24 to 48 hours the dosing frequency may be safely increased to 2 drops every hour. Care should be taken not to discontinue therapy prematurely.

Children and elderly patients: Pred Forte has not specifically been studied in these patient groups. No adjustment in the adult dosage regimen is recommended.

4.3 Contraindications
Acute untreated purulent ocular infections. Acute superficial herpes simplex (dendritic keratitis); vaccinia, varicella and most other viral diseases of the cornea and conjunctiva. Fungal diseases of the eye. Ocular tuberculosis. Sensitivity to any component of the formulation.

4.4 Special warnings and special precautions for use
Acute purulent infections of the eye may be masked or enhanced by the use of topical steroids. Pred Forte contains no antimicrobial agent. If infection is present, appropriate measures must be taken to counteract the infective organisms.

Fungal infections of the cornea have been reported coincidentally with long-term steroid application and fungal invasion may be suspected in any persistent corneal ulceration where a steroid has been used, or is in use.

Various ocular diseases and long-term use of topical corticosteroids have been known to cause corneal or scleral thinning. Use of topical corticosteroids in the presence of thin corneal or scleral tissue may lead to perforation.

Pred Forte contains benzalkonium chloride as a preservative and should not be used in patients continuing to wear soft (hydrophilic) contact lenses.

Patients with a history of herpes simplex keratitis should be treated with caution. Use of steroid medication in the presence of stromal herpes simplex requires caution and should be followed by frequent, mandatory, slit-lamp microscopy.

Use of topical corticosteroids may cause an increase in intraocular pressure in certain individuals. This may result in damage to the optic nerve with resultant defects in visual fields. It is advisable that intraocular pressure be checked frequently during treatment with Pred Forte.

4.5 Interaction with other medicinal products and other forms of Interaction
None known

4.6 Pregnancy and lactation
There is inadequate evidence of safety in human pregnancy. Administration of corticosteroids to pregnant animals can cause abnormalities of foetal development including cleft palate and intra-uterine growth retardation. There may therefore be a very small risk of such defects in the human foetus.

4.7 Effects on ability to drive and use machines
Pred Forte may cause short-lasting blurring of vision upon instillation. If affected, the patient should not use machinery/electric tools or drive until vision has returned to normal.

4.8 Undesirable effects
Ocular: irritation, burning or stinging sensations, allergic reaction, blurred vision; increased intraocular pressure; secondary ocular infections from fungi or viruses liberated from ocular tissues; perforation of the globe when used in conditions where there is a thinning of the cornea or sclera. Posterior subcapsular cataract formation has been reported after heavy or protracted use of topical ophthalmic corticosteroids.

Systemic: extensive topical use of corticosteroids may lead to systemic side effects.

4.9 Overdose
There is no clinical experience of overdosage. Acute overdosage is unlikely to occur via the ophthalmic route.

5. PHARMACOLOGICAL PROPERTIES

5.1 Pharmacodynamic properties
Prednisolone acetate is a synthetic adrenocorticoid with the general properties of prednisolone. Adrenocorticoids diffuse across cell membranes to complex with cytoplasmic receptors and subsequently stimulate synthesis of enzymes with anti-inflammatory effects. Glucocorticoids inhibit the oedema, fibrin deposition, capillary dilation and phagocytic migration of the acute inflammatory response as well as capillary proliferation, deposition of collagen and scar formation.

Prednisolone acetate has, on a weight to weight basis, a potency three to five times that of hydrocortisone.

5.2 Pharmacokinetic properties
Prednisolone acetate has been shown to penetrate rapidly the cornea after topical application of a suspension preparation. Aqueous humour T_{max} occurs between 30 and 45 minutes after installation. The half life of prednisolone acetate in human aqueous humour is approximately 30 minutes.

5.3 Preclinical safety data
Not applicable

6. PHARMACEUTICAL PARTICULARS

6.1 List of excipients
Benzalkonium chloride
Hydroxypropylmethylcellulose
Polysorbate 80
Boric acid
Sodium citrate
Sodium chloride
Disodium edetate
Purified water

6.2 Incompatibilities
None known

6.3 Shelf life
24 months unopened.
28 days after first opening.

6.4 Special precautions for storage
Do not store above 25°C. Do not freeze.

6.5 Nature and contents of container
5 ml and 10 ml bottles and dropper tips composed of low density polyethylene. Screw caps are medium impact polystyrene.

6.6 Instructions for use and handling
Shake the bottle well before use.

7. MARKETING AUTHORISATION HOLDER
Allergan Limited
Coronation Road
High Wycombe
Buckinghamshire HP12 3SH

8. MARKETING AUTHORISATION NUMBER(S)
PL 00426/0051

9. DATE OF FIRST AUTHORISATION/RENEWAL OF THE AUTHORISATION
18th March 2003

10. DATE OF REVISION OF THE TEXT
29th November 2003

Predfoam
(Forest Laboratories UK Limited)

1. NAME OF THE MEDICINAL PRODUCT
PREDFOAM

2. QUALITATIVE AND QUANTITATIVE COMPOSITION
Each metered dose contains 31.4mg of the active ingredient prednisolone sodium metasulphobenzoate, equivalent to prednisolone 20.0mg.

3. PHARMACEUTICAL FORM
Aerosol foam for rectal administration

4. CLINICAL PARTICULARS

4.1 Therapeutic indications
Treatment of proctitis and ulcerative colitis.

4.2 Posology and method of administration
For adults and elderly patients:

One metered dose rectally once or twice daily for 2 weeks, extending treatment for a further 2 weeks when a good response is obtained. Use should be discontinued at the discretion of the physician once the disease is stable and under control.

For children:

Not recommended.

4.3 Contraindications
Corticosteroids are contra-indicated in local conditions where infection might be masked or healing impaired, e.g. peritonitis fistulae, intestinal obstruction, perforation of the bowel.

4.4 Special warnings and special precautions for use
This product should be used with extreme caution in the presence of severe ulcerative colitis. The possibility of masking local or systemic infection should be borne in mind when using this product.

For rectal use only

4.5 Interaction with other medicinal products and other forms of Interaction
None stated

4.6 Pregnancy and lactation
There is inadequate evidence of safety in human pregnancy. Topical administration of corticosteroids to pregnant animals can cause abnormalities in foetal development including cleft palate and intrauterine growth retardation. There may therefore be a very small risk of such effects in the human foetus.

4.7 Effects on ability to drive and use machines
None stated

4.8 Undesirable effects
The consequences of systemic absorption should be considered if Predfoam is used extensively over prolonged periods. As with all rectal corticosteroids, prolonged continuous use is undesirable.

4.9 Overdose
Overdosage by this route is unlikely.

5. PHARMACOLOGICAL PROPERTIES

5.1 Pharmacodynamic properties
Prednisolone sodium metasulphobenzoate is a synthetic glucocorticoid with anti-inflammatory action. The product is given rectally to enable local treatment and to reduce side-effects associated with systemic administration of steroids.

5.2 Pharmacokinetic properties
None stated

5.3 Preclinical safety data
There are no preclinical data of relevance to the prescriber which are additional to that already included in other sections of the SPC.

6. PHARMACEUTICAL PARTICULARS

6.1 List of excipients

Non-ionic Emulsifying Wax

Cetostearyl Alcohol

Oleyl Alcohol

Technical White Oils

Phenoxyethanol

Sorbic Acid

Polysorbate 20

Disodium Edetate

Sodium Hydroxide

Purified Water

Butane 48

6.2 Incompatibilities

None stated

6.3 Shelf life

4 years

6.4 Special precautions for storage

Pressurised container containing a flammable propellant. Do not store above 25°C. Protect from sunlight and do not expose to temperatures exceeding 50°C. Do not pierce or burn even after use. Do not spray on naked flame or any incandescent material.

Do not refrigerate

6.5 Nature and contents of container

Each pack contains an aluminium aerosol can fitted with a metering valve containing sufficient for 14 doses plus 14 disposable applicators.

6.6 Instructions for use and handling

Shake canister before use. When using for the first time remove and discard the small plastic safety tag from under the button. An applicator nozzle is then pushed on to the side arm of the canister. The semi-circular cut-out on the cap is lined up with the nozzle.

The easiest way to administer Predfoam is to stand with one foot raised on a chair and gently insert the nozzle tip into the rectum. Smearing the nozzle with lubricating jelly may help insertion. Holding the canister with the dose button pointing down, press the button on the canister firmly and release. Only press the button once so as not to exceed the recommended dose.

7. MARKETING AUTHORISATION HOLDER

Forest Laboratories UK Limited

Bourne Road

Bexley

Kent DA5 1NX

8. MARKETING AUTHORISATION NUMBER(S)

PL 0108/0101

9. DATE OF FIRST AUTHORISATION/RENEWAL OF THE AUTHORISATION

9 September 1986 / 7 October 1998

10. DATE OF REVISION OF THE TEXT

September 1998

11. Legal Category

POM

Prednisolone 25mg

(sanofi-aventis)

1. NAME OF THE MEDICINAL PRODUCT

Prednisolone 25mg Tablets

2. QUALITATIVE AND QUANTITATIVE COMPOSITION

Prednisolone EP 25.0mg

3. PHARMACEUTICAL FORM

Tablets

4. CLINICAL PARTICULARS

4.1 Therapeutic indications

Collagen Diseases:-

Systemic Lupus Erythematous, Acute Rheumatic Fever

Haematological Disorders:-

Acute granulocytic Leukaemia, Acute Monocytic Leukaemia, Chronic Lymphocytic Leukaemia, Thromcytopenia, Haemolytic Anaemia.

Miscellaneous:-

Ulcerative Colitis

Pemphigus

Nephrosis

4.2 Posology and method of administration

Route of Administration: Oral

In the initial treatment of acute illnesses such as described under 'Therapeutic Indications', daily doses of 75mg or more may be needed. The daily dose should be taken in the morning after breakfast.

In alternate day therapy, the average daily dose is doubled and given every other day in the morning after breakfast.

For further information with reference to dosage see 'Special Warnings and Special Precautions for Use'.

4.3 Contraindications

Systemic fungal and viral infections: acute bacterial infections unless specific anti-infective therapy is given.

Hypersensitivity to any ingredient.

4.4 Special warnings and special precautions for use

1. A patient information leaflet should be supplied with this product.

2. Adrenal cortical atrophy develops during prolonged therapy and may persist for years after stopping treatment. Withdrawal of corticosteroids after prolonged therapy must therefore always be gradual to avoid acute adrenal insufficiency, being tapered off over weeks or months according to the dose and duration of treatment. During prolonged therapy any intercurrent illness, trauma or surgical procedure will require temporary increase in dosage; if corticosteroids have been stopped following prolonged therapy they may need to be temporarily re-introduced.

3. Undesirable effects may be minimised by using the lowest effective dose for the minimum period and by administering the daily requirement as a single morning dose or whenever possible as a single morning dose on alternative days. Frequent patient review is required to appropriately titrate the dose against disease activity.

4. Care and frequent patient monitoring is necessary in patients with the following complaints: diabetes mellitus (or a family history of diabetes), osteoporosis (post-menopausal women are particularly at risk), hypertension, congestive heart failure, patients with a history of severe or pre-existing affective disorders (especially a history of steroid psychosis), glaucoma or a family history of glaucoma, previous corticosteroid induces myopathy, epilepsy, liver failure, renal insufficiency or peptic ulceration.

5. Suppression of the inflammatory response and immune function increases the susceptibility to infections and their severity. The clinical presentation may often be atypical and serious infections such as septicaemia and tuberculosis may be masked and may reach an advanced stage before being recognised.

6. Chicken pox is of particular concern since this normally minor illness may be fatal in immunosuppressed patients. Patients (or parents of children) without a definite history of chicken pox should be advised to avoid close personal contact with chickenpox or herpes zoster and if exposed they should seek urgent medical attention. Passive immunisation with varicella/zoster immunoglobulin (vzig) is needed by exposed non-immune patients who are receiving systemic corticosteroids or who have used them within the previous 3 months, this should be given within 10 days of exposure to chickenpox. If a diagnosis of chickenpox is confirmed, the illness warrants specialist care and urgent treatment. Corticosteroids should not be stopped and the dose may need to be increased.

7. Corticosteroids should be given with care in patients with a history of tuberculosis or the characteristic appearance of tuberculosis disease on X-Ray. The emergence of tuberculosis can however, be prevented by the prophylactic use of anti-tuberculosis therapy.

8. Live virus vaccines should not be administered to patients with impaired immune-responsiveness. If inactivated vaccines are administered to such individuals, the expected serum antibody response may not be obtained.

9. Patients should carry 'steroid treatment' cards which give a clear guidance on the precautions to be taken to minimise risk and which provide details of prescriber, drug, dosage and the duration of treatment.

10. Withdrawal symptoms and signs: too rapid a reduction of corticosteroid dosage following prolonged treatment can lead to acute adrenal insufficiency, hypotension and death. A 'withdrawal syndrome' may also occur including fever, myalgia, arthralgia, rhinitis, conjunctivitis, painful itchy skin nodules and loss of weight.

11. Use in children: corticosteroids cause dose-related growth retardation in infancy, childhood and adolescence which may be irreversible

12. Use in elderly: the common adverse effects of systemic corticosteroids may be associated with more serious consequences in old age, especially osteoporosis, hypertension, hypokalaemia, diabetes, susceptibility to infection and thinning of the skin. Close clinical supervision is required to avoid life threatening reactions.

In patients who have received more than physiological doses of systemic corticosteroids (approximately 7.5mg prednisolone or equivalent) for greater than 3 weeks, withdrawal should not be abrupt. How dose reduction should be carried out depends largely on whether the disease is likely to relapse on withdrawal of systemic corticosteroids but there is uncertainty about HPA suppression, the dose of systemic corticosteroid may be reduced rapidly to physiological doses. Once a daily dose equivalent to 7.5mg of prednisolone is reached, dose reduction should be slower to allow HPA-axis to recover.

Abrupt withdrawal of systemic corticosteroid treatment, which has continued up to 3 weeks is appropriate if it is considered that the disease is unlikely to relapse. Abrupt withdrawal of doses of up to 40mg daily prednisolone, or equivalent for 3 weeks is unlikely to lead to clinically relevant HPA-axis suppression, in the majority of patients. In the following patients groups, gradual withdrawal of systemic corticosteroid therapy should be considered even after courses lasting 3 weeks or less:

• Patients who have had repeated courses of systemic corticosteroids, particularly if taken for greater than 3 weeks.

• When a short course has been prescribed within one year of cessation of long term therapy.

• Patients who may have reasons for adrenocortical insufficiency other than exogenous corticosteroid therapy.

• Patients receiving doses of systemic corticosteroid greater than 40mg daily of prednisolone or equivalent

• Patients repeatedly taking doses in the evening.

4.5 Interaction with other medicinal products and other forms of Interaction

Rifampicin, rifabutin, carbamazepine, phenobarbitone and other barbiturates, phenytoin, phenyl butazone, primidone and aminoglutethimide enhance the metabolism of corticosteroids and its therapeutic effects may be reduced.

The desired effects of hypoglycaemic agents (including insulin), anti-hypertensives and diuretics are antagonised by the corticosteroids and the hypokalaemic effects of acetazolamide, loop diuretics, thiazide diuretics and carbenoxolone are enhanced.

The efficacy of coumarin anticoagulants may be enhanced by concurrent corticosteroid therapy and close monitoring of the INR or prothrombin time is required to avoid spontaneous bleeding.

The renal clearance of salicylates increased by corticosteroids and steroid withdrawal may result in salicylate intoxication.

In patients treated with systemic corticosteroids, use of non-depolarizing muscle relaxants can result in prolonged relaxation and acute myopathy. Risk factors for this include prolonged and high dose corticosteroids treatment and prolonged duration of muscle paralysis. This interaction is more likely to occur following prolonged ventililation (such as in an ITU setting).

Corticosteroid requirements may be reduced in patients taking estrogens (e.g. contraceptive products)

4.6 Pregnancy and lactation

Pregnancy: The ability of corticosteroids to cross the placenta varies between individual drugs, however, 88% of prednisolone is inactivated as it crosses the placenta. Administration of corticosteroids to pregnant animals can cause abnormalities of foetal development including cleft palate, intra-uterine growth retardation and affects on brain growth and development. There is no evidence that corticosteroids cause an increased incidence of congenital abnormalities, such as cleft palate/lip in man. However, when administered for prolonged periods or repeatedly during pregnancy, corticosteroids may increase the risk of intrauterine growth retardation. Hypoadrenalism may occur in the neonate following prenatal exposure to corticosteroids but usually resolves spontaneously after birth and is rarely clinically important. As with all other drugs, corticosteroids should only be prescribed when the benefits to the mother and child outweigh the risks. When corticosteroids are essential however, patients with abnormal pregnancies may be treated as though they were in a non-gravid state.

Lactation: Corticosteroids are excreted in small amounts in breast milk, however, doses of up to 40mg daily of prednisolone are unlikely to cause systemic effects in the infant. Infants of mothers taking higher doses than this may have a degree of adrenal suppression but the benefits of breast feeding are likely to outweigh any theoretic risk.

4.7 Effects on ability to drive and use machines

Not applicable.

4.8 Undesirable effects

The incidence of predictable undesirable effects including hypothalamic-pituitary-adrenal suppression correlates with the relative potency of the drug, dosage, timing of administration and duration of treatment. (see 'Special Warnings and Precautions for Use'.)

1. Endocrine and metabolic: suspension of growth in infancy, childhood and adolescence, menstrual irregularities, amenorrhoea, cushingoid facies, hirsutism and weight gain, decreased carbohydrate tolerance with development of classical symptoms of diabetes mellitus, increased need for insulin or oral hypoglycaemic agents in diabetes, negative nitrogen balance due to protein catabolism and negative calcium balance.

2. Suppression of the inflammatory response and immune function increases the susceptibility to infections and their severity. The clinical presentation may often be atypical and serious infections such as septicaemia and tuberculous may be masked and may reach an advanced stage before being recognised.

3. Gastro-intestinal: peptic ulceration with perforation and haemorrhage. Fatalities have been reported: perforation of the small and large bowel, particularly in patients with inflammatory bowel disease; other gastro-intestinal side effects include dyspepsia, abdominal distension, oesophageal ulceration and candidiasis, acute pancreatitis.

4. Musculo-skeletal: muscle weakness, proximal myopathy, wasting and loss of muscle mass, osteoporosis, vertebral compression fractures, avascular necrosis of bone, pathological fractures of long bones and rupture of tendons. Acute myopathy may be precipitated in patients administered non-depolarising muscle relaxants (See section 4.5).

5. Fluid and electrolyte disturbance: sodium and water retention leading to congestive heart failure in susceptible subjects, hypertension, potassium loss and hypokalaemic alkalosis.

6. Dermatological: impaired wound healing, skin atrophy, petechial haemorrhage and ecchymoses, erythema, telangiectasia, skin striae and acne.

7. Neuropsychiatric: euphoria may be marked and may lead to dependence. Insomnia, hypomania and depression have all been reported. Schizophrenia may be aggravated. There is increased risk of raised intracranial pressure and papilloedema in children (pseudotumour cerebri) usually after treatment withdrawal. Aggravation of epilepsy. Psychological dependence may be marked.

8. Opthalmic: increased intra-ocular pressure with development of glaucoma, papilloedema, posterior subcapsular cataracts, corneal and scleral thinning or perforation after prolonged use. Viral or fungal ophthalmic disease may be reignited or spread.

9. Miscellaneous: opportunistic infections occur more frequently in corticosteroid recipients; hypersensitivity including anaphylaxis, thromboembolism and increased appetite have also been reported. Clinical reactivation of previously dormant tuberculosis, leukcytosis (sometimes an almost leukaemoid-like reaction) may occur.

4.9 Overdose
In the event of an overdose, supportive and symptomatic therapy is indicated.

5. PHARMACOLOGICAL PROPERTIES

5.1 Pharmacodynamic properties
Prednisolone is a well absorbed glucocorticoid that exists in a metabolically active form.

5.2 Pharmacokinetic properties
Prednisolone is readily absorbed from gastro-intestinal tract. Peak plasma concentration is obtained 1-2 hours after oral administration and it had a plasma half-life of 2-3 hours.

It is excreted in the urine as free and conjugated metabolites together with an appreciable proportion of unchanged prednisolone.

5.3 Preclinical safety data
None stated

6. PHARMACEUTICAL PARTICULARS

6.1 List of excipients
Lactose, Potato Starch, Pregelatinised Maize Starch, Magnesium Stearate, Talc (purified).

6.2 Incompatibilities
None known

6.3 Shelf life
Blister Pack: 36 months

6.4 Special precautions for storage
Blister Pack: Protect from light. Store below 25°C in a dry place.

6.5 Nature and contents of container
Blister packs of 56 tablets

(Opaque PVC blisters / aluminium foil)

6.6 Instructions for use and handling
None Stated.

7. MARKETING AUTHORISATION HOLDER
Aventis Pharma Limited
50 Kings Hill Avenue
Kings Hill
West Malling
Kent
ME19 4AH
United Kingdom

8. MARKETING AUTHORISATION NUMBER(S)
PL 04425/0333

9. DATE OF FIRST AUTHORISATION/RENEWAL OF THE AUTHORISATION
8th March 2002

10. DATE OF REVISION OF THE TEXT
April 2003

Legal category: POM

Prednisolone Tablets BP

(Wockhardt UK Ltd)

1. NAME OF THE MEDICINAL PRODUCT
Prednisolone Tablets BP 1mg
Prednisolone Tablets BP 5mg

2. QUALITATIVE AND QUANTITATIVE COMPOSITION
Prednisolone BP 1.0mg
Prednisolone BP 5.0mg

3. PHARMACEUTICAL FORM
Tablet for oral use

4. CLINICAL PARTICULARS

4.1 Therapeutic indications
Suppression of inflammatory and allergic disorders

4.2 Posology and method of administration
Route of administration - Oral

Adults including the elderly

The lowest effective dose should be used for the minimum period in order to minimise side effects (see 'other special warnings and precautions')

Initially:

5mg to 60mg daily in divided doses, as a single dose in the morning after breakfast, or as a double dose on alternative days. They should be taken with or after food. The dose can often be reduced within a few days but may need to be continued for several weeks or months.

Maintenance:

2.5 to 15mg daily, but higher doses may be needed. Cushingoid side-effects more likely above 7.5mg daily.

Children

Prednisolone should be used only when specifically indicated, in a minimal dosage and for the shortest possible time (see other special warnings and precautions)

4.3 Contraindications
Systemic infection unless specific anti-infective therapy is employed. Hypersensitivity to any ingredient.

4.4 Special warnings and special precautions for use
A patient information leaflet should be supplied with this product

Undesirable effects may be minimised by using the lowest effective dose for the minimum period, and by administering the daily requirement as a single morning dose or whenever possible as a single morning dose on alternate days. Frequent patient review is required to appropriately titrate the dose against disease activity (see dosage section)

Adrenal suppression. Adrenal cortical atrophy develops during prolonged therapy and may persist for years after stopping treatment. Withdrawal of corticosteroids after prolonged therapy must therefore always be gradual to avoid acute adrenal insufficiency, being tapered off over weeks or months according to the dose and duration of treatment.

In patients who have received more than physiological doses of systemic corticosteroids (approximately 7.5mg prednisolone or equivalent) for longer than three weeks, withdrawal should not be abrupt. How dose reduction should be carried out depends largely on whether the disease is likely to relapse as the dose of systemic corticosteroids is reduced. Recommendations for initial reduction have varied from as little as steps of 1mg monthly to 2.5mg to 5mg every three to seven days. Adrenal function should be monitored throughout. Clinical assessment of disease activity may be needed during withdrawal. If the disease is unlikely to relapse on withdrawal of systemic corticosteroids but there is uncertainty about hypothalamic-pituitary-adrenal (HPA) suppression, the dose of systemic corticosteroid may be reduced rapidly to physiological doses. Once a daily dose equivalent to 7.5mg of prednisolone is reached, dose reduction should be slower to allow the HPA-axis to recover.

Abrupt withdrawal of systemic corticosteroid treatment which has continued up to three weeks is appropriate if it is considered that the disease is unlikely to relapse. Abrupt withdrawal of doses of up to 40mg daily of prednisolone, or equivalent, for three weeks, is unlikely to lead to clinically relevant HPA-axis suppression, in the majority of patients. In the following patient groups, gradual withdrawal of systemic corticosteroid therapy should be considerdeven after courses lasting three weeks or less:

- Patients who have had repeated courses of systemic corticosteroids, particularly if taken for longer than three weeks.
- When a short course has been prescribed within one year of cessation of long term therapy (months or years).
- Patients who may have reasons for adrenocortical insufficiency other than exogenous corticosteroid therapy.
- Patients receiving doses of systemic corticosteroid greater than 40mg daily of prednisolone (or equivalent),
- Patients repeatedly taking doses in the evening.

Patients should carry 'steroid treatment' cards which give clear guidance on the precautions to be taken to minimise risk and which provide details of prescriber, drug, dosage and the duration of treatment.

Anti-inflammatory/ immunosuppressive effects and infection. Suppression of the inflammatory response and immune function increases the susceptibility to infections and their severity. The clinical presentation may often be atypical and serious infections such as septicaemia and tuberculosis may be masked and may reach an advanced stage before being recognised. During prolonged therapy any intercurrent illness, trauma or surgical procedures will require a temporary increase in dosage, if corticosteroids have been stopped following prolonged therapy they may need to be temporarily re-introduced.

Chickenpox is of particular concern since this normally minor illness may be fatal in immunosuppressed patients. Patients (or parents of children) without a definite history of chickenpox should be advised to avoid close personal contact with chickenpox or herpes zoster and if exposed they should seek urgent medical attention. Passive immunisation with varicella zoster immunoglobulin (vzig) is needed by exposed non-immune patients who are receiving systemic corticosteroids or who have used them within the previous 3 months; this should be given within 10 days of exposure to chickenpox. **If a diagnosis of chickenpox is confirmed, the illness warrants specialist care and urgent treatment. Corticosteroids should not be stopped and the dose may need to be increased.**

Live vaccines should not be given to individuals with impaired immune responsiveness. The antibody response to other vaccines may be diminished.

Particular care is required when considering the use of systemic corticosteroids in patients with the following conditions and frequent patient monitoring is necessary.

a) osteoporosis (post menopausal females are particularly at risk)

b) hypertension or congestive heart failure

c) existing or previous history of severe affective disorders (especially previous steroid psychosis)

d) diabetes mellitus (or a family history of diabetes)

e) history of, or active tuberculosis

f) glaucoma (or a family history of glaucoma)

g) previous corticosteroid-induced myopathy

h) liver failure

i) renal insufficiency

j) epilepsy

k) peptic ulceration

Use in children - corticosteroids cause dose-related growth retardation in infancy, childhood and adolescence, which may be irreversible.

Use in the elderly - the common adverse effects of systemic corticosteroids may be associated with more serious consequences in old age, especially osteoporosis, hypertension, hypokalaemia, diabetes, susceptibility to infection and thinning of the skin. Close clinical supervision is required to avoid life-threatening reactions.

4.5 Interaction with other medicinal products and other forms of Interaction
Rifampicin, rifabutin, carbamazepine, phenobarbitone, phenytoin, primidone and aminoglutethimide enhance the metabolism of prednisolone and its therapeutic effects may be reduced.

The desired effects of hypoglycaemic agents (including insulin), antihypertensives and diuretics are antagonised by corticosteroids and the hypokalaemic effects of acetazolamide loop diuretics, thiazide diuretics and carbenoxolone are enhanced. The efficacy of coumarin anticoagulants may be enhanced by current corticosteroid therapy and close monitoring of the INR or prothrombin time is required to avoid spontaneous bleeding. The renal clearance of salicylates is increased by corticosteroids and steroid withdrawal may result in salicylate intoxication.

4.6 Pregnancy and lactation
Pregnancy

The ability of corticosteroids to cross the placenta varies between individual drugs, however, 88% of prednisolone is inactivated as it crosses the placenta.

Administration of corticosteroids to pregnant animals can cause abnormalities of foetal development including cleft palate, intra-uterine growth retardation and effects on brain growth and development. There is no evidence that corticosteroids result in an increased incidence of congenital abnormalities, such as cleft palate/lip in man. However, when administered for prolonged periods or repeatedly during pregnancy, corticosteroids may increase the risk of intra-uterine growth retardation. Hypoadrenalism may, in theory, occur in the neonate following prenatal exposure to corticosteroids but usually resolves spontaneously following birth and is rarely clinically important. As with all drugs, corticosteroids should only be prescribed when the benefits to the mother and child outweigh the risks. When corticosteroids are essential however, patients with normal pregnancies may be treated as though they were in the non-gravid state. Patients with pre-eclampsia or fluid retention require dose monitoring

Lactation

Corticosteroids are excreted in small amounts in breast milk. However, doses of up to 40mg daily of prednisolone are unlikely to cause systemic effects in the infant. Infants of mothers taking higher doses than this may have a degree of adrenal suppression but the benefits of breastfeeding are likely to outweigh any theoretical risk.

4.7 Effects on ability to drive and use machines
None

4.8 Undesirable effects

The incidence of predictable undesirable effects, including hypothalamic-pituitary-adrenal suppression correlates with the relative potency of the drug, dosage, timing of administration and the duration of treatment (see other special warnings and precautions)

Endocrine/metabolic - suppression of the hypothalamic-pituitary-adrenal axis, growth suppression in infancy, childhood and adolescence, menstrual irregularity and amenorrhoea. Cushingoid facies, hirsutism, weight gain, impaired carbohydrate tolerance with increased requirement for anti-diabetic therapy. Negative protein and calcium balance. Increased appetite.

Anti-inflammatory and immunosuppressive effects - increased susceptibility and severity of infections with suppression of clinical symptoms and signs, opportunistic infections, recurrence of dormant tuberculosis (see other special warnings and precautions).

Musculoskeletal - osteoporosis, vertebral and long bone fractures, avascular osteonecrosis, tendon rupture. Proximal myopathy, muscular weakness.

Fluid and electrolyte disturbance - sodium and water retention, hypertension, potassium loss, hypokalaemic alkalosis, oedema.

Neuropsychiatric - euphoria, psychological dependence, depression, insomnia and aggravation of schizophrenia. Increased intra-cranial pressure with papilloedema in children (pseudotumour cerebri), usually after treatment withdrawal. Aggravation of epilepsy.

Ophthalmic - increased intra-ocular pressure, glaucoma, papilloedema, posterior subcapsular cataracts, corneal or scleral thinning, exacerbation of ophthalmic viral of fungal diseases.

Gastrointestinal - dyspepsia, peptic ulceration with perforation and haemorrhage, acute pancreatitis, candidiasis.

Dermatological - impaired healing, skin atrophy, bruising, telangiectasia, striae, acne.

General - hypersensitivity including anaphylaxis, has been reported. Leucocytosis. Thromboembolism.

Withdrawal symptoms and signs - too rapid a reduction of corticosteroid dosage following prolonged treatment can lead to acute adrenal insufficiency, hypotension and death (see Special Warnings and Precautions for Use). A 'withdrawal syndrome' may also occur including, fever, myalgia, arthralgia, rhinitis, conjunctivitis, painful itchy skin nodules, loss of weight, mental changes, vomiting, hypotension and dehydration.

4.9 Overdose

Treatment is unlikely to be needed; serum electrolytes should be monitored.

5. PHARMACOLOGICAL PROPERTIES

5.1 Pharmacodynamic properties

The major therapeutic use of prednisolone is based on the anti-inflammatory and immunosuppressive activities of glucocorticoids. The suppression of inflammatory response is independent of the initiating stimulus and the action is mainly local. Some important components of the mechanism underlying the anti-inflammatory effects of corticosteroids are:

(i) inhibition of the adherence of neutrophils and monocyte-macrophages to the capillary endothelial cells of the inflamed area,

(ii) blocking of the effect of macrophage migration inhibitory factor,

(iii) decreased activation of plasminogen to plasmin, and

(iv) inhibition of phospholipase A_2 activity thereby lowering the formation of prostaglandins, leukotrienes and related compounds.

This suppression of inflammatory response by corticoids may also be a key feature of the way they counteract complications that arise from cell-mediated immune reactions. An acute effect of such steroids is sequestration of lymphocytes from blood although lysis of tissues also occurs, e.g. in lymphatic malignancies. At therapeutic dose levels corticoids do not seem to have any significant effect on circulating antibodies or on the metabolism of complement.

The two major targets of glucocorticoids, such as prednisolone, would be the liver (induction of enzymes, e.g. those involved in gluconeogenesis and amino acid degradation) and the lymphatic system (growth inhibitory actions which ultimately may result in cell death). The central feature of these hormonal actions is the combination of the steroid with an intracellular receptor, producing conformational changes that expose the DNA-binding domain on the receptor. The binding of the steroid receptor complex to specific sequences, known as hormone response elements, brings about transcriptional activation or repression of specific genes.

5.2 Pharmacokinetic properties

Prednisolone is readily absorbed from the gastrointestinal tract and already exists in a metabolically active form.

Peak plasma concentrations of prednisolone are obtained one or two hours after administration by mouth, and it has a usual plasma half-life of two to four hours. Its initial absorption, but not its overall bioavailability, is affected by food.

Prednisolone is extensively bound to plasma proteins, although less so than hydrocortisone (cortisol).

Prednisolone is excreted in the urine as free and conjugated metabolites, together with an appreciable proportion of unchanged prednisolone. Prednisolone crosses the placenta and small amounts are excreted in breast milk.

Prednisolone has a biological half-life lasting several hours, intermediate between those of hydrocortisone (cortisol) and the longer acting glucocorticoids, such as dexamethasone. It is this intermediate duration of action that makes it suitable for the alternate day administration regimens that have been found to reduce the risk of adrenocortical insufficiency, yet provide adequate corticosteroid coverage in some disorders.

5.3 Preclinical safety data

Teratogenic effects of glucocorticoids have not been demonstrated in the human. Although malignancies are known to arise in patients undergoing immunosuppression with corticosteroids, any role of these compounds in the induction of tumours remain uncertain. The classic toxic effects of prednisolone like drugs are given under adverse reactions.

6. PHARMACEUTICAL PARTICULARS

6.1 List of excipients

Lactose

Maize starch

Stearic acid

Purified talc

Magnesium Stearate

6.2 Incompatibilities

None

6.3 Shelf life

Three years

6.4 Special precautions for storage

Store below 25°C

6.5 Nature and contents of container

50 tablets in amber glass bottles or 100, 500 and 1000 tablets in polypropylene or polyethylene containers.

28 or 56 tablets in blister pack strips of 250 micron white rigid PVC and 20 micron hard tempered aluminium foil coated with PVC compatible heat seal lacquer on the reverse side.

28 or 56 tablets in polypropylene or polyethylene containers in cartons.

6.6 Instructions for use and handling

Not applicable

Administrative Data

7. MARKETING AUTHORISATION HOLDER

CP Pharmaceuticals Ltd, Ash Road North, Wrexham, LL13 9UF

8. MARKETING AUTHORISATION NUMBER(S)

Prednisolone Tablets BP 1mg 4543/5987

Prednisolone Tablets BP 5mg 4543/5988

9. DATE OF FIRST AUTHORISATION/RENEWAL OF THE AUTHORISATION

Renewed 11 December 1995

10. DATE OF REVISION OF THE TEXT

August 1998

DATE OF REVISION AUGUST 1998

Predsol Drops Eye & Ear

(UCB Pharma Limited)

1. NAME OF THE MEDICINAL PRODUCT

Predsol Drops for Eye and Ear

2. QUALITATIVE AND QUANTITATIVE COMPOSITION

Prednisolone Sodium Phosphate EP 0.5% w/v

3. PHARMACEUTICAL FORM

Sterilised clear and colourless aqueous solution

4. CLINICAL PARTICULARS

4.1 Therapeutic indications

Short term treatment of steroid responsive inflammatory conditions of the eye after clinical exclusion of bacterial, viral and fungal infections. Non-infected inflammatory conditions of the ear.

4.2 Posology and method of administration

Eyes

1 or 2 drops instilled into the eyes every one or two hours until control is achieved, when the frequency may be reduced.

Ears

2 or 3 drops instilled into the ear every two or three hours until control is achieved, when the frequency can be reduced.

Frequency of dosing depends on clinical response. If there is no clinical response within 7 days treatment, the drops should be discontinued. Treatment should be the lowest effective dose for the shortest possible time. After more prolonged treatment (over 6-8 weeks), the drops should be withdrawn slowly to avoid relapse.

4.3 Contraindications

Bacterial, viral, fungal tuberculous or purulent conditions of the eye. Use is contraindicated if glaucoma is present or where herpetic keratitis (e.g. dendritic ulcer) is considered a possibility. Inadvertent use of topical steroids in the latter condition can lead to the extension of the ulcer and marked visual deterioration. Hypersensitivity to the preparation.

In the ear, topical corticosteroids are contraindicated in patients with fungal diseases of the auricular structure, and in those with a perforated tympanic membrane.

4.4 Special warnings and special precautions for use

Topical corticosteroids should never be given for an undiagnosed red eye as inappropriate use is potentially blinding.

Prolonged use may lead to the risk of adrenal suppression in infants.

Ophthalmological treatment with corticosteroid preparations should not be repeated or prolonged without regular review to exclude raised intraocular pressure, cataract formation or unsuspected infections.

The use of corticosteroids may reduce resistance to or mask the signs of infection. Appropriate anti-infective agents should be used if infection is present.

4.5 Interaction with other medicinal products and other forms of Interaction

Predsol Drops contain benzalkonium chloride as a preservative and, therefore, should not be given to treat patients who wear soft contact lenses.

4.6 Pregnancy and lactation

Safety for use in pregnancy and lactation has not been established. There is inadequate evidence of safety in human pregnancy. Topical administration of corticosteroids to pregnant animals can cause abnormalities of foetal development including cleft palate and intrauterine growth retardation. There may be a very small risk of such effects in the human foetus.

4.7 Effects on ability to drive and use machines

May cause transient blurring of vision on instillation. Warn patients not to drive or operate hazardous machinery unless vision is clear.

4.8 Undesirable effects

Hypersensitivity reactions usually of the delayed type may occur leading to irritation, burning, stinging, itching and dermatitis.

Topical corticosteroid use may result in increased intraocular pressure leading to optic nerve damage, reduced visual acuity and visual field defects. Other side effects include mydriasis, ptosis, epithelial punctate keratitis and possible corneal or scleral malacia. Within a few days after discontinuing topical ophthalmic corticosteroid therapy and occasionally during therapy, acute anterior uveitis has occurred in patients (mainly blacks) without pre-existing ocular inflammation or infection.

Intensive or prolonged use of topical corticosteroids may lead to formation of posterior subcapsular cataracts.

In those diseases causing thinning of the cornea or sclera, corticosteroid therapy may result in thinning of the globe leading to perforation.

4.9 Overdose

Long term intensive topical use may lead to systemic effects. Oral ingestion of the contents of one bottle (up to 10ml) is unlikely to lead to any serious adverse effects.

5. PHARMACOLOGICAL PROPERTIES

5.1 Pharmacodynamic properties

Not available.

5.2 Pharmacokinetic properties

Not applicable.

5.3 Preclinical safety data

Not available.

6. PHARMACEUTICAL PARTICULARS

6.1 List of excipients

Benzalkonium chloride solution EP

Sodium chloride EP

Sodium acid phosphate EP

Disodium edetate EP

Sodium hydroxide EP

Phosphoric acid EP

Purified water EP

6.2 Incompatibilities

Not known.

6.3 Shelf life

18 months unopened.

4 weeks after first opening.

6.4 Special precautions for storage

Store at a temperature not exceeding 25°C. Avoid freezing. Always replace bottle in carton to protect contents from light. Sterility of the drops is assured until cap seal is broken.

6.5 Nature and contents of container

Single 5ml or 10ml bottle with nozzle insert moulded in natural low density polyethylene closed with a tamper evident high density polyethylene cap.

6.6 Instructions for use and handling

Store below 25°C. Protect from light.

7. MARKETING AUTHORISATION HOLDER

UCB Pharma Limited

208 Bath Road

Slough

Berkshire

SL1 3WE

UK

8. MARKETING AUTHORISATION NUMBER(S)

PL 00039/0393

9. DATE OF FIRST AUTHORISATION/RENEWAL OF THE AUTHORISATION

4 December 1992

10. DATE OF REVISION OF THE TEXT

June 2005

Predsol Retention Enema

(UCB Pharma Limited)

1. NAME OF THE MEDICINAL PRODUCT

Predsol Retention Enema

2. QUALITATIVE AND QUANTITATIVE COMPOSITION

20mg prednisolone as the sodium phosphate ester.

For excipients, see 6.1

3. PHARMACEUTICAL FORM

Rectal Solution

100ml disposable plastic bottles, each containing 20mg prednisolone as the sodium phosphate ester in a buffered solution. The product complies with the specification for Prednisolone Enema BP.

4. CLINICAL PARTICULARS

4.1 Therapeutic indications

Predsol Retention Enema provides local corticosteroid treatment for rectal and rectosigmoidal disease in ulcerative colitis and Crohn's disease.

4.2 Posology and method of administration

Adults

1 enema used nightly, for 2 to 4 weeks. Treatment may be continued in patients showing progressive improvement, but it should not be persisted with if the response has been inadequate. Some patients may relapse after an interval but are likely to respond equally well to a repeated course of treatment.

The enema is used each night on retiring. It may be warmed before administration by placing the bottle in a vessel of warm water for a few minutes. Before use lie in bed on the left side with knees drawn up. Hold the bottle upwards. Place hand in the protective plastic cover and remove the cap from the bottle. Attach the nozzle and lubricate with petroleum jelly. Gently insert about half the length of the nozzle into the rectum. The bottle should then be squeezed gently until it is emptied, taking a minute or two to do so. The nozzle should then be removed from the rectum. Invert the plastic protective cover around the bottle and discard the whole unit. The patient should then roll over to lie face down for 3 to 5 minutes but may sleep in any comfortable position.

Although predsol enema is applied locally, it should be born in mind that there is likely to be substantial systemic absorption, especially when the bowel is inflamed.

The volume of the enema is considered to be the optimum to ensure maximum coverage of the affected area. However, undesirable effects may be minimised by using for the minimum period. Frequent patient review is required to monitor therapeutic effect against disease activity.

Children

Predsol retention enema as packed is not suitable for use in children.

Route of Administration:

Rectal

4.3 Contraindications

Systemic or local infection unless specific anti-infective therapy is employed. Hypersensitivity to any ingredient.

4.4 Special warnings and special precautions for use

Although Predsol Enema is applied locally, it should be borne in mind that there is likely to be substantial systemic absorption, especially when the bowel is inflamed.

The volume of the enema is considered to be the optimum to ensure maximum coverage of the affected area, however, undesirable effects may be minimised by using for the minimum period. Frequent patient review is required to monitor therapeutic effect against disease activity (see 'Posology and Method of Administration').

Suppression of the inflammatory response and immune system increases the susceptibility to infections and their severity. The clinical presentation may often be atypical and serious infections such as septicaemia and tuberculosis may be masked and may reach an advanced stage before being recognised.

Chickenpox is of particular concern since this normally minor illness may be fatal in immunosuppressed patients. Patients without a definite history of chickenpox should be advised to avoid close contact with chickenpox or herpes zoster and if exposed they should seek medical attention. Passive immunisation with varicella zoster immunoglobulin (VZIG) is needed by exposed non-immune patients who are receiving systemic corticosteroids or who have used them within the previous 3 months; this should be given within 10 days of exposure to chickenpox. If a diagnosis of chickenpox is confirmed, the illness warrants special care and urgent treatment. Corticosteroids should not be stopped and the dose may need to be increased.

Patients should be advised to take particular care to avoid exposure to measles and to seek immediate medical advice if exposure occurs. Prophylaxis with intramuscular normal immunoglobulin may be needed.

Live vaccines should not be given to individuals with impaired immune responsiveness. The antibody response to other vaccines may be diminished.

Corticosteroid treatment may reduce the response of the pituitary adrenal axis to stress, and relative insufficiency can persist for up to a year after withdrawal of prolonged therapy. Withdrawal of corticosteroids after prolonged therapy must therefore always be gradual to avoid acute adrenal insufficiency, being tapered off over weeks or months according to the dose and the duration of treatment. During prolonged therapy any intercurrent illness, trauma or surgical procedure will require a temporary increase in dosage; if corticosteroids have been stopped following prolonged therapy they may need to be temporarily re-introduced.

Special precautions

Particular care is required when considering the use of systemic corticosteroids in patients with the following conditions and frequent patient monitoring is necessary.

A. Osteoporosis (post-menopausal females are particularly at risk).

B. Hypertension or congestive heart failure.

C. Existing or previous history of severe affective disorders (especially previous steroid psychosis).

D. Diabetes mellitus (or a family history of diabetes).

E. History of tuberculosis.

F. Glaucoma (or a family history of glaucoma).

G. Previous corticosteroid-induced myopathy.

H. Liver failure - blood levels of corticosteroid may be increased, as with other drugs which are metabolised in the liver.

I. Renal insufficiency.

J. Epilepsy.

K. Peptic ulceration.

L. Hypothroidism

M. Recent myocardial infarction.

Patients should carry "Steroid treatment" cards which give clear guidance on the precautions to be taken to minimise risk and which provide details of the prescriber, drug, dosage and the duration of treatment.

Use in the Elderly

The common adverse effects of systemic corticosteroids may be associated with more serious consequences in old age, especially osteoporosis, hypertension, hypokalaemia, diabetes, susceptibility to infection and thinning of the skin. Close clinical supervision is required to avoid life-threatening reactions.

4.5 Interaction with other medicinal products and other forms of Interaction

Systemic absorption of prednisolone should be borne in mind, especially when there is local inflammation. Thus the following interactions are possible:

Analgesics:

Increased risk of gastro-intestinal bleeding and ulceration with aspirin and NSAIDs; the renal clearance of salicylates is increased by corticosteroids and steroid withdrawal may result in salicylate intoxication.

Antibacterials:

Rifamycins accelerate metabolism of corticosteroids (reduced effect); erythromycin inhibits metabolism of methylprednisolone and possibly other corticosteroids.

Anticoagulants:

The efficacy of coumarin anticoagulants may be enhanced by concurrent corticosteroid therapy and close monitoring of the INR or prothrombin time is required to avoid spontaneous bleeding.

Antidiabetics:

Antagonism of hypoglycaemic effect.

Antiepileptics:

Carbamazepine, phenobarbital, phenytoin and primidone accelerate metabolism of corticosteroids (reduced effect).

Antifungals:

Increased risk of hypokalaemia with amphotericin (avoid concomitant use unless corticosteroids are required to control reactions); ketoconazole inhibits metabolism of methylprednisolone and possibly other corticosteroids.

Antihypertensives:

Antagonism of hypotensive effect.

Antivirals:

Ritonavir possibly increases plasma concentration of prednisolone.

Cardiac Glycosides:

Increased toxicity if hypokalaemia occurs with corticosteroids.

Ciclosporin:

Increased plasma concentrations of prednisolone.

Cytotoxics:

Increased risk of haematological toxicity with methotrexate.

Diuretics:

Antagonism of diuretic effect; acetazolamide, loop diuretics, and thiazides increased risk of hypokalaemia.

Hormone antagonists:

Aminoglutethimide accelerates metabolism of corticosteroids (reduced effect).

Mifepristone:

Effects of corticosteroids may be reduced for 3-4 days after mifepristone.

Oral Contraceptives:

Alteration in the plasma protein binding and metabolism of prednisolone caused by oestrogens, with or without progesterone, can result in exposure of women to increased levels of unbound prednisolone for prolonged periods of time.

Somatropin:

The growth promoting effect of somatropin may be inhibited.

Sympathomimetics:

Increased risk of hypokalaemia if high doses of corticosteroids given with high doses of bambuterol, fenoterol, formoterol, ritodrine, salbutamol, salmeterol, and terbutaline.

Theophylline:

Increased risk of hypokalaemia.

Ulcer-healing drugs:

Carbenoxolone increases the risk of hypokalaemia.

Vaccines:

Live vaccines should not be given to individuals with impaired immune response as a result of treatment with large doses of corticosteroids.

4.6 Pregnancy and lactation

Topical administration of corticosteroids to pregnant animals can cause abnormalities of foetal development including cleft palate and intrauterine growth retardation. There may therefore be a very small risk of such effects in the human foetus. Also, hypoadrenalism may occur in the neonate. When corticosteroids are essential however, patients with normal pregnancies may be treated as though they were in the non-gravid state. Patients with pre-eclampsia or fluid retention require close monitoring.

Corticosteroids are excreted in small amounts in breast milk and infants of mothers taking pharmacological doses of steroids should be monitored carefully for signs of adrenal suppression.

4.7 Effects on ability to drive and use machines

None known.

4.8 Undesirable effects

The incidence of predictable undesirable effects, including hypothalamic - pituitary - adrenal suppression correlates with the relative systemic potency of the drug, dosage, timing of administration and the duration of treatment (see 'Special Warnings and Precautions for Use').

Endocrine/metabolic

Suppression of the hypothalamic - pituitary - adrenal axis, growth suppression in infancy, childhood and adolescence, menstrual irregularity and amenorrhoea. Cushingoid Facies, hirsutism, weight gain, impaired carbohydrate tolerance with increased requirement for antidiabetic therapy. Negative protein and calcium balance. Increased appetite.

Anti-inflammatory and immunosuppressive effects

Increased susceptibility and severity of infections with suppression of clinical symptoms and signs. Opportunistic infections, recurrence of dormant tuberculosis (see 'Special Warnings and Precautions for Use').

Musculoskeletal

Osteoporosis, vertebral and long bone fractures, avascular osteonecrosis, tendon rupture, proximal myopathy.

Fluid and electrolyte disturbance

Sodium and water retention, hypertension, potassium loss, hypokalaemic alkalosis.

Neuropsychiatric

Euphoria, psychological dependence, depression, insomnia, and aggravation of schizophrenia. Increased intracranial pressure with papilloedema in children (pseudotumour cerebri), usually after treatment withdrawal. Aggravation of epilepsy.

Ophthalmic

Increased intra-ocular pressure, glaucoma, papilloedema, posterior subcapsular cataracts, corneal or scleral thinning, exacerbation of ophthalmic viral or fungal diseases.

Cardiac

Myocardial rupture following recent myocardial infarction.

Gastrointestinal

Nausea, hiccups, dyspepsia, peptic ulceration with perforation and haemorrhage, acute pancreatitis, candidiasis.

Dermatological

Impaired healing, skin atrophy, bruising, telangiectasia, striae, acne.

General

Hypersensitivity including anaphylaxis, has been reported. Leucocytosis. Thrombo-embolism.

Withdrawal symptoms and signs

Too rapid a reduction of corticosteroid dosage following prolonged treatment can lead to acute adrenal insufficiency, hypotension and in severe cases this could be fatal.

A 'withdrawal syndrome' may also occur including fever, myalgia, arthralgia, rhinitis, conjunctivitis, painful itchy skin nodules and loss of weight.

4.9 Overdose

Treatment is unlikely to be needed in cases of acute overdosage.

5. PHARMACOLOGICAL PROPERTIES

5.1 Pharmacodynamic properties

ATC Code: A07E A01

Not applicable

5.2 Pharmacokinetic properties

Not applicable.

5.3 Preclinical safety data

None stated.

6. PHARMACEUTICAL PARTICULARS

6.1 List of excipients

Nipastat GL 75

Disodium edetate

Sodium acid phosphate

Disodium hydrogen phosphate anhydrous AR

Sodium hydroxide

Purified water

6.2 Incompatibilities

None known.

6.3 Shelf life

24 months.

6.4 Special precautions for storage

Do not store above 25°C. Keep the container in the outer carton.

6.5 Nature and contents of container

Each 100ml single dose is supplied in a low density polythene bottle with a low density polythene cap, with a separate PVC nozzle. Seven bottles, plastic protective covers and instructions for use are supplied in each box.

6.6 Instructions for use and handling

None stated.

7. MARKETING AUTHORISATION HOLDER

UCB Pharma Limited
208 Bath Road
Slough
Berkshire
SL1 3WE
UK

8. MARKETING AUTHORISATION NUMBER(S)

PL 00039/0396

9. DATE OF FIRST AUTHORISATION/RENEWAL OF THE AUTHORISATION

14 October 1992

10. DATE OF REVISION OF THE TEXT

June 2005

Predsol Suppositories

(UCB Pharma Limited)

1. NAME OF THE MEDICINAL PRODUCT

Predsol Suppositories.

2. QUALITATIVE AND QUANTITATIVE COMPOSITION

5mg prednisolone as the sodium phosphate ester.

For excipients, see 6.1

3. PHARMACEUTICAL FORM

Suppository

4. CLINICAL PARTICULARS

4.1 Therapeutic indications

Prednisolone is a glucocorticosteroid which is about four times as potent as hydrocortisone on a weight for weight basis.

Predsol Suppositories are indicated for the treatment of haemorrhagic and granular proctitis and the anal complications of Crohn's disease.

4.2 Posology and method of administration

Rectal administration in adults and children:

One suppository inserted at night and one in the morning after defaecation. When the response is good, treatment is usually continued for some months. If symptoms recur later, treatment should be resumed.

4.3 Contraindications

Systemic or local infection unless specific anti-infective therapy is employed.

Hypersensitivity to any ingredient.

4.4 Special warnings and special precautions for use

Although Predsol Suppositories are applied locally, it should be borne in mind that there is likely to be substantial systemic absorption, especially when the bowel is inflamed.

Undesirable effects may be minimised by using for a minimum period. Frequent patient review is required to monitor therapeutic effect against disease activity.

Suppression of the inflammatory response and immune function increases the susceptibility to infections and their severity. The clinical presentation may often be atypical and serious infections such as septicaemia and tuberculosis may be masked and may reach an advanced stage before being recognised.

Chickenpox is of particular concern since this normally minor illness may be fatal in immunosuppressed patients. Patients without a definite history of chickenpox should be advised to avoid close personal contact with chickenpox or herpes zoster and if exposed they should seek urgent medical attention. Passive immunisation with varicella zoster immunoglobulin (VZIG) is needed by exposed non-immune patients who are receiving systemic corticosteroids or who have used them within the previous 3 months; this should be given within 10 days of exposure to chickenpox. If a diagnosis of chickenpox is confirmed, the illness warrants specialist care and urgent treatment. Corticosteroids should not be stopped and the dose may need to be increased.

Patients should be advised to take particular care to avoid exposure to measles and to seek immediate medical advice if exposure occurs. Prophylaxis with intramuscular normal immunoglobulin may be needed.

Live vaccines should not be given to individuals with impaired immune responsiveness. The antibody response to other vaccines may be diminished.

Corticosteroid treatment may reduce the response of the pituitary adrenal axis to stress, and relative insufficiency can persist for up to a year after withdrawal of prolonged therapy. Withdrawal of corticosteroids after prolonged therapy must therefore always be gradual to avoid acute adrenal insufficiency, being tapered off over weeks or months according to the dose and duration of treatment. During prolonged therapy any intercurrent illness, trauma or surgical procedure will require a temporary increase in dosage. If corticosteroids have been stopped following prolonged therapy they may need to be temporarily re-introduced.

Special precautions:

Particular care is required when considering the use of systemic corticosteroids in patients with the following conditions and frequent patient monitoring is necessary.

A. Osteoporosis (post-menopausal females are particularly at risk).

B. Hypertension or congestive heart failure.

C. Existing or previous history of severe affective disorders (especially previous steroid psychosis).

D. Diabetes mellitus (or a family history of diabetes).

E. History of tuberculosis.

F. Glaucoma (or a family history of glaucoma).

G. Previous corticosteroid-induced myopathy.

H. Liver failure - blood levels of corticosteroid may be increased, (as with other drugs which are metabolised in the liver).

I. Renal insufficiency.

J. Epilepsy.

K. Peptic ulceration.

L. Hypothyroidism.

M. Recent myocardial infarction.

Patients should carry 'steroid treatment' cards which give clear guidance on the precautions to be taken to minimise risk and which provide details of prescriber, drug, dosage and the duration of treatment.

Use in the elderly:

The common adverse effects of systemic corticosteroids may be associated with more serious consequences in old age, especially osteoporosis, hypertension, hypokalaemia, diabetes, susceptibility to infection and thinning of the skin. Close clinical supervision is required to avoid life-threatening reactions.

4.5 Interaction with other medicinal products and other forms of Interaction

Systemic absorption of prednisolone should be borne in mind, especially when there is local inflammation. Thus the following interactions are possible:

Analgesics:

Increased risk of gastro-intestinal bleeding and ulceration with aspirin and NSAIDs; the renal clearance of salicylates is increased by corticosteroids and steroid withdrawal may result in salicylate intoxication.

Antibacterials:

Rifamycins accelerate metabolism of corticosteroids (reduced effect); erythromycin inhibits metabolism of methylprednisolone and possibly other corticosteroids.

Anticoagulants:

The efficacy of coumarin anticoagulants may be enhanced by concurrent corticosteroid therapy and close monitoring of the INR or prothrombin time is required to avoid spontaneous bleeding.

Antidiabetics:

Antagonism of hypoglycaemic effect.

Antiepileptics:

Carbamazepine, phenobarbital, phenytoin and primidone accelerate metabolism of corticosteroids (reduced effect).

Antifungals:

Increased risk of hypokalaemia with amphotericin (avoid concomitant use unless corticosteroids are required to control reactions); ketoconazole inhibits metabolism of methylprednisolone and possibly other corticosteroids.

Antihypertensives:

Antagonism of hypotensive effect.

Antivirals:

Ritonavir possibly increases plasma concentration of prednisolone.

Cardiac Glycosides:

Increased toxicity if hypokalaemia occurs with corticosteroids.

Ciclosporin:

Increased plasma concentrations of prednisolone.

Cytotoxics:

Increased risk of haematological toxicity with methotrexate.

Diuretics:

Antagonism of diuretic effect; acetazolamide, loop diuretics, and thiazides increased risk of hypokalaemia.

Hormone antagonists:

Aminoglutethimide accelerates metabolism of corticosteroids (reduced effect).

Mifepristone:

Effects of corticosteroids may be reduced for 3-4 days after mifepristone.

Oral Contraceptives:

Alteration in the plasma protein binding and metabolism of prednisolone caused by oestrogens, with or without progesterone, can result in exposure of women to increased levels of unbound prednisolone for prolonged periods of time.

Somatropin:

The growth promoting effect of somatropin may be inhibited.

Sympathomimetics:

Increased risk of hypokalaemia if high doses of corticosteroids given with high doses of bambuterol, fenoterol, formoterol, ritodrine, salbutamol, salmeterol, and terbutaline.

Theophylline:

increased risk of hypokalaemia.

Ulcer-healing drugs:

Carbenoxolone increases the risk of hypokalaemia.

Vaccines:

Live vaccines should not be given to individuals with impaired immune response as a result of treatment with large doses of corticosteroids.

4.6 Pregnancy and lactation

There is inadequate evidence of safety in human pregnancy. Topical administration of corticosteroids to pregnant animals can cause abnormalities of foetal development including cleft palate and intrauterine growth retardation. There may therefore be a very small risk of such effects in the human foetus. Also, hypoadrenalism may occur in the neonate. When corticosteroids are essential however, patients with normal pregnancies may be treated as though they were in the non-gravid state. Patients with pre-eclampsia or fluid retention require close monitoring.

Corticosteroids are excreted in small amounts in breast milk and infants of mothers taking pharmacological doses of steroids should be monitored carefully for signs of adrenal suppression.

4.7 Effects on ability to drive and use machines
None known.

4.8 Undesirable effects
The incidence of predictable undesirable effects, including hypothalamic-pituitary-adrenal (HPA) axis suppression correlates with the relative systemic potency of the drug, dosage, timing of administration and the duration of treatment (see Other Special Warnings and Precautions).

Endocrine/metabolic:
Suppression of the hypothalamic-pituitary-adrenal axis, growth suppression in infancy, childhood and adolescence, menstrual irregularity and amenorrhoea. Cushingoid facies, hirsutism, weight gain, impaired carbohydrate tolerance with increased requirement for antidiabetic therapy. Negative protein and calcium balance. Increased appetite.

Anti-inflammatory and immunosuppressive effects:
Increased susceptibility and severity of infections with suppression of clinical symptoms and signs, opportunistic infections, recurrence of dormant tuberculosis (see Other Special Warnings and Precautions).

Musculoskeletal:
Osteoporosis, vertebral and long bone fractures, avascular osteonecrosis, tendon rupture, proximal myopathy.

Fluid and electrolyte disturbance:
Sodium and water retention, hypertension, potassium loss, hypokalaemic alkalosis.

Neuropsychiatric:
Euphoria, psychological dependence, depression, insomnia, and aggravation of schizophrenia. Increased intracranial pressure with papilloedema in children (pseudotumour cerebri), usually after treatment withdrawal. Aggravation of epilepsy.

Ophthalmic:
Increased intra-ocular pressure, glaucoma, papilloedema, posterior subcapsular cataracts, corneal or scleral thinning, exacerbation of ophthalmic viral or fungal diseases.

Cardiac
Myocardial rupture following recent myocardial infarction.

Gastrointestinal:
Nausea, hiccups, dyspepsia, peptic ulceration with perforation and haemorrhage, acute pancreatitis, candidiasis.

Dermatological:
Impaired healing, skin atrophy, bruising, telangiectasia, striae, acne.

General:
Hypersensitivity including anaphylaxis, has been reported. Leucocytosis. Thrombo-embolism.

Withdrawal symptoms and signs:
Too rapid a reduction of corticosteroid dosage following prolonged treatment can lead to acute adrenal insufficiency, hypotension and in severe cases this could be fatal.

A 'withdrawal syndrome' may also occur including; fever, myalgia, arthralgia, rhinitis, conjunctivitis, painful itchy skin nodules and loss of weight.

4.9 Overdose
Treatment is unlikely to be needed in cases of acute overdosage.

5. PHARMACOLOGICAL PROPERTIES

5.1 Pharmacodynamic properties
ATC: A07E A01

Prednisolone sodium phosphate is an active corticosteroid with topical anti-inflammatory activity.

5.2 Pharmacokinetic properties
Corticosteroids are metabolised mainly in the liver but also in the kidney and are excreted in the urine.

Synthetic corticosteroids such as prednisolone have increased potency when compared with the natural corticosteroids, due to their slower metabolism and lower protein-binding affinity.

5.3 Preclinical safety data
None stated.

6. PHARMACEUTICAL PARTICULARS

6.1 List of excipients
Witepsol H15.

6.2 Incompatibilities
None known.

6.3 Shelf life
2 years.

6.4 Special precautions for storage
Store below 25°C.

6.5 Nature and contents of container
Fin sealed plastic cavities moulded from 100 micron non-toxic PVC. Each cartoned plastic mould contains 10 suppositories (2 strips of 5 suppositories).

6.6 Instructions for use and handling

7. MARKETING AUTHORISATION HOLDER
UCB Pharma Limited
208 Bath Road
Slough
Berkshire
SL1 3WE
UK

8. MARKETING AUTHORISATION NUMBER(S)
PL 00039/0395

9. DATE OF FIRST AUTHORISATION/RENEWAL OF THE AUTHORISATION
23 February 1993.

10. DATE OF REVISION OF THE TEXT
June 2005

Predsol-N Drops for Eye & Ear

(UCB Pharma Limited)

1. NAME OF THE MEDICINAL PRODUCT
Predsol-N Drops for Eye and Ear

2. QUALITATIVE AND QUANTITATIVE COMPOSITION
Prednisolone Sodium Phosphate EP 0.5% w/v

Neomycin Sulphate EP 0.5% w/v

3. PHARMACEUTICAL FORM
Solution

4. CLINICAL PARTICULARS

4.1 Therapeutic indications
Eye:

For the short-term treatment of steroid responsive conditions of the eye when prophylactic antibiotic treatment is also required, after excluding the presence of fungal and viral disease.

Ear:

Otitis externa or other steroid responsive conditions where prophylactic antibiotic treatment is also required.

4.2 Posology and method of administration
Adults (and the elderly) and children:

Frequency of dosing depends on clinical response. If there is no clinical response within 7 days treatment, the drops should be discontinued.

Treatment should be the lowest effective dose for the shortest possible time. Normally, do not give for more than 7 days, unless under expert supervision. After more prolonged treatment (over 6-8 weeks), the drops should be withdrawn slowly to avoid relapse.

Eye:

1 or 2 drops applied to each affected eye up to six times daily depending upon clinical response.

Ear:

2 or 3 drops instilled into each ear three or four times daily.

4.3 Contraindications
Viral, fungal, tuberculous or purulent conditions of the eye. Use is contraindicated if glaucoma is present or herpetic keratitis (e.g. dendritic ulcer) is considered a possibility. Use of topical steroids in the latter condition can lead to extension of the ulcer and marked visual deterioration. Otitis externa should not be treated when the eardrum is perforated because of the risk of ototoxicity. Hypersensitivity to the preparation.

4.4 Special warnings and special precautions for use
Topical corticosteroids should never to given for an undiagnosed red eye as inappropriate use is potentially blinding.

Treatment with corticosteroid/antibiotic combinations should not be continued for more than 7 days in the absence of any clinical improvement, since prolonged use may lead to occult extension of infection due to the masking effect of the steroid. Prolonged use may also lead to skin sensitisation and the emergence of resistant organisms.

Prolonged use may lead to the risk of adrenal suppression in infants.

Ophthalmological treatment with corticosteroid preparations should not be repeated or prolonged without regular review to exclude raised intraocular pressure, cataract formation or unsuspected infections.

Aminoglycoside antibiotics may cause irreversible, partial or total deafness when given systemically or when applied topically to open wounds or damaged skin. This effect is dose related and is enhanced by renal or hepatic impairment. Although this effect has not been reported following topical ocular use, the possibility should be considered when high dose topical treatment is given to small children or infants.

4.5 Interaction with other medicinal products and other forms of Interaction
Predsol-N Drops contain benzalkonium chloride as a preservative and, therefore, should not be used to treat patients who wear soft contact lenses.

4.6 Pregnancy and lactation
Safety for use in pregnancy and lactation has not been established. There is inadequate evidence of safety in human pregnancy. Topical administration of corticosteroids to pregnant animals can cause abnormalities of foetal development including cleft palate and intrauterine growth retardation. There may, therefore, be a very small risk of such effects in the human foetus. There is a risk of foetal ototoxicity if aminoglycoside antibiotic preparations are administered during pregnancy.

4.7 Effects on ability to drive and use machines
May cause transient blurring of vision on instillation. Warn patients not to drive or operate hazardous machinery unless vision is clear.

4.8 Undesirable effects
Hypersensitivity reactions, usually of the delayed type, may occur leading to irritation, burning, stinging, itching, dermatitis, contact conjunctivitis and erythema.

Topical corticosteroid use may result in increased intraocular pressure leading to optic nerve damage, reduced visual acuity and visual field defects.

Intensive or prolonged use of topical corticosteroids may lead to formation of posterior subcapsular cataracts.

In those diseases causing thinning of the cornea or sclera, corticosteroid therapy may result in thinning of the globe leading to perforation.

Other side effects include mydriasis, ptosis, epithelial punctate keratitis and possible corneal or scleral malacia. Within a few days after discontinuing topical ophthalmic corticosteroid therapy and occasionally during therapy, acute anterior uveitis has occurred in patients (mainly blacks) without pre-existing ocular inflammation or infection.

4.9 Overdose
Long term intensive topical use may lead to systemic effects. Oral ingestion of the contents of one bottle (up to 10ml) is unlikely to lead to any serious adverse effects.

5. PHARMACOLOGICAL PROPERTIES

5.1 Pharmacodynamic properties
Prednisolone has topical corticosteroid activity. The presence of neomycin should prevent the development of bacterial infection.

5.2 Pharmacokinetic properties
Not applicable as the drops are applied topically.

5.3 Preclinical safety data
Not available.

6. PHARMACEUTICAL PARTICULARS

6.1 List of excipients
Benzalkonium Chloride EP
Disodium Edetate EP
Polyethylene Glycol 300 EP
Sodium Formate EP
Anhydrous Sodium Sulphate EP
Disodium Hydrogen Phosphate Anhydrous HSE
Sodium Acid Phosphate EP
Sodium Hydroxide EP
Phosphoric Acid EP
Purified Water EP

6.2 Incompatibilities
None known.

6.3 Shelf life
18 months unopened.

4 weeks after first opening.

6.4 Special precautions for storage
Store below 25°C.

Avoid freezing.

Always replace bottle in carton to protect contents from light.

Sterility of the drops is assured until cap seal is broken.

6.5 Nature and contents of container
Single 5ml or 10ml bottle with nozzle insert moulded in natural, low density polyethylene closed with a tamper evident high density polyethylene cap.

6.6 Instructions for use and handling
None

7. MARKETING AUTHORISATION HOLDER
UCB Pharma Limited
208 Bath Road
Slough
Berkshire
SL1 3WE
UK

8. MARKETING AUTHORISATION NUMBER(S)
PL 00039/0394

9. DATE OF FIRST AUTHORISATION/RENEWAL OF THE AUTHORISATION
2 December 1992

10. DATE OF REVISION OF THE TEXT
June 2005

Pregaday Tablets

(UCB Pharma Limited)

1. NAME OF THE MEDICINAL PRODUCT
Pregaday Tablets

2. QUALITATIVE AND QUANTITATIVE COMPOSITION
Each tablets contains Ferrous Fumarate EP 322.00 mg and Folic Acid EP 0.35 mg.

3. PHARMACEUTICAL FORM
Film-coated tablet

4. CLINICAL PARTICULARS

4.1 Therapeutic indications
There is evidence that a daily intake of 100mg of elemental iron in the ferrous form is adequate to prevent development of iron deficiency in expectant mothers. If a mild iron deficiency is present when Pregaday administration is started, this will be corrected by increased absorption of iron.

The daily folate requirement rises steeply during the final trimester of pregnancy, and evidence of maternal depletion may be found. To ensure normal tissue folate levels in the mother after delivery a daily supplement of about 300 micrograms is required during the second and third trimester of pregnancy. This does not obscure the blood picture of addisonian pernicious anaemia.

Pregaday Tablets are indicated during the second and third trimester of pregnancy for prophylaxis against iron deficiency and megaloblastic anaemia of pregnancy. Pregaday Tablets are not intended as a treatment for established megaloblastic anaemia.

4.2 Posology and method of administration
Adults:

It is usual to begin therapy with Pregaday Tablets about the thirteenth week of pregnancy (see precautions) either as routine prophylaxis or selectively if the haemoglobin concentration is less than 11g/100 ml (less than 75% normal).

One tablet should be taken daily by mouth.

Children: Not applicable

4.3 Contraindications
Known hypersensitivity to the product, Vitamin B_{12} deficiency, paroxysmal nocturnal haemoglobinuria, haemosiderosis, haemochromatosis, active peptic ulcer, repeated blood transfusion, regional enteritis and ulcerative colitis.

Pregaday must not be used in the treatment of anaemias other than those due to iron deficiency.

4.4 Special warnings and special precautions for use
The label will state

"Important warning: Contains Iron. Keep out of reach and sight of children, as overdose may be fatal".

This will appear on the front of the pack within a rectangle in which there is no other information.

Some post-gastrectomy patients show poor absorption of iron. Care is needed when treating iron deficiency anaemia in patients with treated or controlled peptic ulceration. Caution should be exercised when administering folic acid to patients who may have folate dependent tumours.

Since anaemia due to combined iron and vitamin B_{12} or folate deficiencies may be microcytic in type, patients with microcytic anaemia resistant to therapy with iron alone should be screened for vitamin B_{12} or folate deficiency.

Pregaday tablets should be kept out of the reach of children.

4.5 Interaction with other medicinal products and other forms of Interaction
Iron reduces the absorption of penicillamine. Iron compounds impair the bioavailability of fluoroquinolones, levodopa, carbidopa, thyroxine and bisphosphonates.

Absorption of both iron and antibiotic may be reduced if Pregaday is given with tetracycline.

Absorption of both iron and zinc are reduced if taken concomitantly.

Concurrent administration of antacids may reduce absorption of iron. Co-trimoxazole, chloramphenicol, sulphasalazine, aminopterin, methotrexate, pyrimethamine or sulphonamides may interfere with folate metabolism.

Serum levels of anticonvulsant drugs may be reduced by administration of folate.

Oral chloramphenicol delays plasma iron clearance, incorporation of iron into red blood cells and interferes with erythropoiesis.

Some inhibition of iron absorption may occur if it is taken with cholestyramine, trientine, tea, eggs or milk.

Administration of oral iron may increase blood pressure in patients receiving methyldopa.

Coffee may be a factor in reducing iron bioavailability.

Neomycin may alter the absorption of iron.

4.6 Pregnancy and lactation
Administration of Pregaday Tablets during the first trimester of pregnancy may be undesirable.

A minority of pregnant women are not protected by physiological doses of folic acid. The development of anaemia despite prophylaxis with Pregaday Tablets calls for investigation.

4.7 Effects on ability to drive and use machines
None

4.8 Undesirable effects
Gastro-intestinal disorders have been reported including gastro-intestinal discomfort, anorexia, nausea, vomiting, constipation, diarrhoea. Darkening of the stools may occur.

Rarely allergic reactions may occur.

4.9 Overdose
Acute overdose of oral iron requires emergency treatment. In young children

200-250 mg/kg ferrous fumarate is considered to be extremely dangerous.

Symptoms and signs of abdominal pain, vomiting and diarrhoea appear within 60 minutes. Cardiovascular collapse with coma may follow. Some improvement may occur after this phase which, in some patients, is followed by recovery. In others, after about 16 hours, deterioration may occur involving diffuse vascular congestion, pulmonary oedema, convulsions, anuria, hypothermia, severe shock, metabolic acidosis, coagulation abnormalities and hypoglycaemia.

Vomiting should be induced immediately, followed as soon as possible by parenteral injection of desferrioxamine mesylate, and then gastric lavage. In the meantime, it is helpful to give milk and/or 5% sodium bicarbonate solution by mouth.

Dissolve 2 g desferrioxamine mesylate in 2 to 3 ml of water for injections and give intramuscularly. A solution of 5 g desferrioxamine in 50 to 100 ml of fluid may be left in the stomach. If desferrioxamine is not available, leave 300 ml of 1 % to 5 % sodium bicarbonate in the stomach. Fluid replacement is essential.

Recovery may be complicated by long-term sequelae such as hepatic necrosis, pyloric stenosis or acute toxic encephalitis which may lead to CNS damage.

5. PHARMACOLOGICAL PROPERTIES

5.1 Pharmacodynamic properties
There is evidence that a daily dose of 100mg of elemental iron in the ferrous form is adequate to prevent development of iron deficiency in expectant mothers. If a mild iron deficiency is present when Pregaday administration is started, this will be corrected by increased absorption of iron. The daily folate requirement rises steeply during the final trimester of pregnancy, and evidence of maternal depletion may be found. To ensure normal tissue folate levels in the mother after delivery a daily supplement of about 300 micrograms is required during the second and third trimester of pregnancy. This does not obscure the blood picture of addisonian pernicious anaemia.

5.2 Pharmacokinetic properties
Iron is absorbed chiefly in the duodenum and jejunum, absorption being aided by the acid secretion of the stomach and being more readily effected when the iron is in the ferrous state.

Folic acid is absorbed mainly from the proximal part of the small intestine. Folate polyglutamates are considered to be de-conjugated to monoglutamates during absorption. Folic acid rapidly appears in the blood, where it is extensively bound to plasma proteins. The amounts of folic acid absorbed from normal diets are rapidly distributed in body tissues and about 4 to 5 micrograms is excreted in the urine daily. When larger amounts are absorbed, a high proportion is metabolised in the liver to other active forms of folate and a proportion is stored as reduced and methylated folate. Larger amounts of folate are rapidly excreted in the urine.

5.3 Preclinical safety data
Not stated

6. PHARMACEUTICAL PARTICULARS

6.1 List of excipients
The tablet cores also contain maize starch EP, sodium lauryl sulphate EP, gelatin EP and liquid paraffin EP. The film coat contains **either** hydroxypropylmethyl cellulose EP (E464), acetylated monoglyceride and Opaspray pink **or** hydroxypropylmethyl cellulose EP (E464), propylene glycol EP and Opaspray pink.

Opaspray pink contains hydroxypropyl cellulose (E463), red iron oxide(E172) and titanium dioxide (E171).

6.2 Incompatibilities
None

6.3 Shelf life
36 months

6.4 Special precautions for storage
Protect from light, store below 25°C

6.5 Nature and contents of container
Cartons containing two calendar blister packs of 14 tablets prepared from PVdC coated opaque 250 micron PVC film and 20 micron tempered aluminium foil.

6.6 Instructions for use and handling
Not applicable

7. MARKETING AUTHORISATION HOLDER
UCB Pharma Limited
208 Bath Road
Slough
Berkshire
SL1 3WE
UK

8. MARKETING AUTHORISATION NUMBER(S)
PL 00039/0398

9. DATE OF FIRST AUTHORISATION/RENEWAL OF THE AUTHORISATION
23 February 1993

10. DATE OF REVISION OF THE TEXT
June 2005

Premarin Tablets

(Wyeth Pharmaceuticals)

1. NAME OF THE MEDICINAL PRODUCT
Premarin 0.625mg.

Premarin 1.25mg.

2. QUALITATIVE AND QUANTITATIVE COMPOSITION
Tablets containing 0.625mg or 1.25mg Conjugated Estrogens USP.

3. PHARMACEUTICAL FORM
Premarin 0.625mg tablets are maroon oval sugar-coated tablets.

Premarin 1.25mg tablets are yellow oval sugar-coated tablets.

4. CLINICAL PARTICULARS

4.1 Therapeutic indications
– Hormone replacement therapy for estrogen deficiency symptoms in postmenopausal women.

– Second line therapy for prevention of osteoporosis in postmenopausal women at high risk of future fractures who are intolerant of, or contraindicated for, other medicinal products approved for the prevention of osteoporosis.

4.2 Posology and method of administration
__Adults:__

Premarin is an estrogen only HRT.

Premarin 0.625-1.25mg daily is the usual starting dose for women without a uterus. Continuous administration is recommended.

For treatment of postmenopausal symptoms the lowest effective dose should be used. HRT should only be continued as long as the benefit in alleviation of severe symptoms outweighs the risk.

__Prophylaxis of osteoporosis__:

The minimum effective dose is 0.625mg daily for most patients. (See section 5.1 Pharmacodynamic Properties).

__Concomitant progestogen use for women with a uterus__

In women with a uterus, where the addition of a progestogen is necessary it should be added for at least 12-14 days every 28 day cycle to reduce the risk to the endometrium.

The benefits of the lower risk of endometrial hyperplasia and endometrial cancer due to adding progestogen should be weighed against the increased risk of breast cancer (see sections 4.4 Special Warnings and Precautions for Use and 4.8 Undesirable effects).

In women who are not taking hormone replacement therapy or women who switch from a continuous combined hormone replacement therapy product, treatment may be started on any convenient day. In women transferring from a sequential hormone replacement therapy regimen, treatment should begin the day following completion of the prior regimen.

Unless there is a previous diagnosis of endometriosis, it is not recommended to add a progestogen in hysterectomised women.

__Forgotten tablet:__ If a tablet is forgotten, it should be taken as soon as the patient remembers, therapy should then be continued as before. If more than one tablet has been forgotten only the most recent tablet should be taken, the patient should not take double the usual dose to make up for missed tablets.

Missed pills may cause breakthrough bleeding in women with a uterus.

__Elderly__

There are no special dosage requirements for elderly patients, but as with all medicines, the lowest effective dose should be used.

__Children__

Not recommended

4.3 Contraindications

1. Known, past or suspected breast cancer

2. Known or suspected estrogen-dependent malignant tumours (e.g. endometrial cancer)

3. Undiagnosed abnormal genital bleeding

4. Untreated endometrial hyperplasia

5. Active or past history of venous thromboembolism (e.g. deep vein thrombosis, pulmonary embolism)

6. Active or recent arterial thromboembolic disease (e.g. angina, myocardial infarction)

7. Acute liver disease or history of liver disease where the liver function tests have failed to return to normal

8. Known hypersensitivity to the active substances or to any of the excipients of Premarin tablets

9. Porphyria

4.4 Special warnings and special precautions for use

1. Medical examination/Follow up

Before initiating or reinstituting HRT, a complete personal and family medical history should be taken. Physical (including pelvic and breast) examination should be guided by the contraindications and warnings for use. During treatment, periodic check-ups are recommended of a frequency and nature adapted to the individual women. Women should be advised what changes in their breasts should be reported to their doctor or nurse. Investigations, including mammography, should be carried out in accordance with currently accepted screening practices, modified to the clinical needs of the individual. A careful appraisal of the risks and benefits should be undertaken at least annually in women treated with hormone replacement therapy.

In women with an intact uterus, the benefits of the lower risk of endometrial hyperplasia and endometrial cancer due to adding progestogen should be weighed against the increased risk of breast cancer (see below and Section 4.8 Undesirable effects).

2. Conditions that need supervision

If any of the following conditions are present, have occurred previously, and/or have been aggravated during pregnancy or previous hormone treatment, the patient should be closely supervised. It should be taken into account that these conditions may recur or be aggravated during treatment with Premarin, in particular:

– Leiomyoma (uterine fibroids) or endometriosis

– A family history of, or other risk factors for, thromboembolic disorders (see below)

– Risk factors for estrogen dependent tumours (e.g. first degree heredity for breast cancer)

– Hypertension

– Liver disorders (e.g. liver adenoma)

– Diabetes mellitus with or without vascular involvement

– Cholelithiasis

– Migraine or (severe) headaches

– Systemic lupus erythematosus (SLE)

– A history of endometrial hyperplasia (see below)

– Epilepsy

– Asthma

– Otosclerosis

3. Reasons for immediate withdrawal of therapy

Therapy should be discontinued if a contra-indication is discovered and in the following situations:

– Jaundice or deterioration in liver function

– Significant increase in blood pressure

– New onset of migraine-type headache

– Pregnancy

4. Endometrial Hyperplasia

The risk of endometrial hyperplasia and carcinoma is increased when estrogens are administered alone for prolonged periods. The addition of a progestogen for at least 12 days of the cycle in non-hysterectomised women reduces, but may not eliminate, this risk (see section 4.8 Undesirable Effects).

The reduction in risk to the endometrium should be weighed against the increase in the risk of breast cancer of added progestogen (see 'Breast Cancer' below and section 4.8 Undesirable Effects).

Break-through bleeding and spotting may occur during the first months of treatment. If break-through bleeding or spotting appears after some time on therapy, or continues after treatment has been discontinued, the reason should be investigated, which may include endometrial biopsy to exclude endometrial malignancy.

Unopposed estrogen stimulation may lead to pre-malignant or malignant transformation in the residual foci of endometriosis. Therefore, the addition of progestogens to estrogen replacement therapy should be considered in women who have undergone hysterectomy because of endometriosis, especially if they are known to have residual endometriosis (but see above).

5. Breast Cancer

Randomised controlled trials and epidemiological studies have reported an increased risk of breast cancer in women taking estrogen or estrogen-progestogen combinations for HRT for several years (see Section 4.8 Undesirable Effects). An observational study of almost 829,000 women has shown that, compared to never-users, use of estrogen-progestogen combined HRT is associated with a higher risk of breast cancer (RR = 2.00, 95%CI: 1.88 - 2.12) than use of estrogens alone (RR = 1.30, 95%CI: 1.21 – 1.40). In this study the magnitude of the increase in breast cancer risk was similar for all estrogen-only preparations, irrespective of the type, dose or route of administration of the estrogen (oral, transdermal and implanted). Likewise the magnitude of the increased risk was similar for all estrogen plus progestogen preparations, irrespective of the type of progestogen or the number of days of addition per cycle. For all HRT, an excess risk becomes apparent within 1-2 years of starting treatment and increases with the duration of use of HRT but begins to decline when HRT is stopped and by 5 years reaches the same level as in women who have never taken HRT.

The increase in risk applies to all women studied, although the relative risk was significantly higher in those with a lean or normal body build (body mass index or BMI of $<25kg/m^2$) compared to those with a BMI of $\geqslant 25kg/m^2$.

At present the effect of HRT on the diagnosis of breast tumours remains unclear – all women should be encouraged to report any changes in their breasts to their doctor or nurse.

6. Venous thromboembolism

Hormone replacement therapy (HRT) is associated with a higher relative risk of developing venous thromboembolism (VTE) i.e. deep vein thrombosis or pulmonary embolism. One randomised controlled trial and epidemiological studies found a two to threefold higher risk for users compared with non-users. For non- users it is estimated that the number of cases of VTE that will occur over a 5-year period is about 3 per 1000 women aged 50-59 years and 8 per 1000 women aged between 60-69 years. It is estimated that in healthy women who use HRT for 5 years, the number of additional cases of VTE over a 5-year period will be between 2 and 6 (best estimate = 4) per 1000 women aged 50-59 years and between 5 and 15 (best estimate = 9) per 1000 women aged 60-69 years. The occurrence of such an event is more likely in the first year of HRT than later.

Generally recognised risk factors for VTE include a personal or family history and severe obesity (Body Mass Index $>30kg/m^2$) and systemic lupus erythematosus (SLE). There is no consensus about the possible role of varicose veins in VTE.

Patients with a history of VTE or known thrombophilic states have an increased risk of VTE. HRT may add to this risk. Personal or strong family history of thromboembolism or recurrent spontaneous abortion should be investigated in order to exclude a thrombophilic predisposition. Until a thorough evaluation of thrombophilic factors has been made or anticoagulant treatment initiated, use of HRT in such patients should be viewed as contraindicated. Those women already on anticoagulant treatment require careful consideration of the benefit-risk of use of HRT.

The risk of VTE may be temporarily increased with prolonged immobilisation, major trauma or major surgery. As in all postoperative patients scrupulous attention should be given to prophylactic measures to prevent VTE following surgery. Where prolonged immobilisation is liable to follow elective surgery, particularly abdominal or orthopaedic surgery to the lower limbs, consideration should be given to temporarily stopping HRT 4-6 weeks earlier, if this is possible. Treatment should not be restarted until the woman is completely mobilised.

If VTE develops after initiating therapy, the drug should be discontinued. Patients should be told to contact their doctors immediately when they are aware of potential thromboembolic symptoms (e.g. painful swelling of a leg, sudden pain in the chest, dyspnoea).

7. Coronary Artery Disease (CAD)

There is no evidence from randomised controlled trials of cardiovascular benefit with continuous combined conjugated estrogens and MPA. Large clinical trials showed a possible increased risk of cardiovascular morbidity in the first year of use and no benefit thereafter. For other HRT products, there are as yet no randomised controlled trials examining benefit in cardiovascular morbidity or mortality. Therefore, it is uncertain whether these findings also extend to other HRT products.

8. Stroke

One large randomised clinical trial (WHI-trial) found, as a secondary outcome, an increased risk of stroke in healthy women during treatment with continuous combined conjugated estrogens and MPA. For women who do not use HRT, it is estimated that the number of cases of stroke that will occur over a 5 year period is about 3 per 1000 women aged 50-59 years and 11 per 1000 women aged 60-69 years. It is estimated that for women who use conjugated estrogens and MPA for 5 years, the number of additional cases will be between 0 and 3 (best estimate =1) per 1000 users aged 50-59 years and between 1 and 9 (best estimate = 4) per 1000 users aged 60-69 years. It is unknown whether the increased risk also extends to other HRT products.

9. Ovarian Cancer

Long-term (at least 5-10 years) use of estrogen-only HRT products in hysterectomised women has been associated with an increased risk of ovarian cancer in some epidemiological studies. It is uncertain whether long-term use of combined HRT confers different risk than estrogen-only products.

Other Conditions

10. Estrogens may cause fluid retention and therefore patients with cardiac or renal dysfunction should be carefully observed. Patients with terminal renal insufficiency should be closely observed, since it is expected that the level of circulating active ingredients in Premarin is increased.

11. The use of estrogen may influence the laboratory results of certain endocrine tests and liver enzymes.

Estrogens increase thyroid binding globulin (TBG), leading to increased circulating total thyroid hormone, as measured by protein-bound iodine (PBI), T4 levels (by column or by radio-immunoassay) or T3 levels (by radio-immunoassay). T3 resin uptake is decreased, reflecting the elevated TBG. Free T4 and free T3 concentrations are unaltered.

Other binding proteins may be elevated in serum, i.e. corticoid binding globulin (CBG), sex-hormone-binding globulin (SHBG) leading to increased circulating corticosteroids and sex steroids, respectively. Free or biologically active hormone concentrations are unchanged. Other plasma proteins may be increased (angiotensinogen/renin substrate, alpha-I-antitrypsin, ceruloplasmin).

Some patients dependent on thyroid hormone replacement therapy may require increased doses in order to maintain their free thyroid hormone levels in an acceptable range. Therefore, patients should have their thyroid function monitored more frequently when commencing concurrent treatment in order to maintain their free thyroid hormone levels in an acceptable range.

12. A worsening of glucose tolerance may occur in patients taking estrogens and therefore diabetic patients should be carefully observed while receiving hormone replacement therapy.

13. There is an increase in the risk of gallbladder disease in women receiving HRT (see conditions that need supervision)

14. Women with pre-existing hypertriglyceridemia should be followed closely during estrogen replacement or hormone replacement therapy, since rare cases of large increases of plasma triglycerides leading to pancreatitis have been reported with estrogen therapy in this condition.

15. Estrogens should be used with caution in individuals with severe hypocalcaemia

16. At present there is no established screening programme for determining women at risk of developing osteoporotic fracture. Epidemiological studies suggest a number of individual risk factors which contribute to the development of postmenopausal osteoporosis. These include: early menopause; family history of osteoporosis; thin, small frame; cigarette use; recent prolonged systemic corticosteroid use.

If several risk factors are present in a patient consideration should be give to treatment.

4.5 Interaction with other medicinal products and other forms of Interaction

The metabolism of estrogens may be increased by concomitant use of substances known to induce drug-metabolising enzymes, specifically cytochrome P450 enzymes, such as anticonvulsants (e.g. phenobarbital, phenytoin, carbamazepine) and anti-infectives (e.g. rifampicin, rifabutin, nevirapine, efavirenz).

Ritonavir and nelfinavir, although known as strong inhibitors, by contrast exhibit inducing properties when used concomitantly with steroid hormones.

Herbal preparations containing St John's wort *(Hypericum perforatum)* may induce the metabolism of estrogens.

Clinically, an increased metabolism of estrogens and progestogens may lead to decreased effect and changes in the uterine bleeding profile.

The response to metyrapone may be reduced.

4.6 Pregnancy and lactation

Premarin is not indicated during pregnancy.

For women with a uterus

If pregnancy occurs during medication with Premarin treatment should be withdrawn immediately. The results of most epidemiological studies to date relevant to inadvertent foetal exposure to estrogens indicate no teratogenic or foetotoxic effects.

Lactation:

Premarin is not indicated during lactation.

4.7 Effects on ability to drive and use machines

None known.

4.8 Undesirable effects

See also 4.4 Special Warnings and Special Precautions for Use.

Adverse drug reactions (ADRs)

The adverse reactions listed in the table are based on post-marketing spontaneous (reporting rate), clinical trials and class-effects.

System Organ Class	Adverse Reaction
Reproductive system & breast disorders	Breakthrough bleeding/ spotting; Breast pain, tenderness, enlargement, discharge; Change in menstrual flow; Change in cervical ectropion and secretion; Dysmenorrhoea; Galactorrhoea; Increased size of uterine leiomyomata
Gastrointestinal disorders	Nausea; Bloating; Abdominal pain; Vomiting; Pancreatitis
Nervous	Dizziness; Headache; Migraine; Nervousness; Stroke; Exacerbation of epilepsy
Musculoskeletal, connective tissue and bone disorders	Arthralgias; Leg cramps
Psychiatric disorders	Changes in libido; Mood disturbances; Depression; Irritability
Vascular disorders	Pulmonary embolism; Superficial thrombophlebitis and deep venous thrombophlebitis
Cardiac Disorders	Myocardial Infarction
General disorders and administration site disorders	Oedema
Skin and subcutaneous tissue disorders	Alopecia; Chloasma/melasma; Hirsutism; Pruritus; Rash
Infections and infestations	Vaginitis, including vaginal candidiasis
Immune system disorders	Urticaria: Angioedoema: Anaphylactic/anaphylactoid reactions
Metabolism and nutrition disorders	Glucose intolerance
Eye disorders	Intolerance to contact lenses
Respiratory, thoracic and mediastinal disorders	Exacerbation of asthma
Hepatobiliary	Gallbladder disease
Neoplasms benign and malignant	Breast cancer*; Fibrocystic breast changes; Ovarian cancer; Endometrial Cancer
Investigations	Changes in weight (increase or decrease); Increased triglycerides

Breast Cancer

The risk of breast cancer increases with the number of years of HRT usage. According to data from a recent epidemiological study in about 829,000 postmenopausal women, the best estimate of the risk is that for women not using HRT, in total 32 in every 1000 are expected to have breast cancer diagnosed between the ages of 50 and 65 years. Among those with current or recent use of estrogen-only replacement therapy, it is estimated that the total number of additional cases during the corresponding period will be between 0 and 3 (best estimate = 1.5) per 1000 for 5 years' use and between 3 and 7 (best estimate = 5) per 1000 for 10 years' use (see table). Among those with current or recent use of estrogen plus progestogen combined HRT, it is estimated that the total number of additional cases will be between 5 and 7 (best estimate = 6) per 1000 for 5 years' use and between 18 and 20 (best estimate = 19) per 1000 for 10 years' use (See section 4.4 Special Warnings and Precautions for Use). The number of additional cases of breast cancer is broadly similar for women who start HRT irrespective of age at start of HRT use (between the ages of 45-65).

	No of additional cases of breast cancer diagnosed per 1000 women (95% confidence intervals)	
Type of HRT	5 years of use	10 years of use
Estrogen-only	1.5 (0-3)	5 (3-7)
Combined	6 (5-7)	19 (18-20)

Endometrial Cancer

In women with an intact uterus, the risk of endometrial hyperplasia and endometrial cancer increases with the increasing duration of use of unopposed estrogens and is substantially reduced by the addition of a progestogen (see section 4.4 Special Warnings and Precautions for Use). According to data from epidemiological studies the best estimate of the risk of endometrial cancer is that for women not using HRT, about 5 in every 1000 are expected to have endometrial cancer diagnosed between the ages of 50 and 65. It is estimated that, among those who use estrogen-only replacement therapy, there will be 4 additional cases per 100 after 5 years' use and 10 additional cases per 1000 after 10 years' use. Adding a progestogen to estrogen-only therapy substantially reduces, but may not eliminate, the increased risk.

Other adverse reactions reported in association with estrogen/progestogen treatment including Premarin:

- Estrogen-dependent neoplasms benign and malignant, e.g. endometrial hyperplasia, endometrial cancer
- Venous thromboembolism, i.e. deep leg or pelvic venous thrombosis and pulmonary embolism, is more frequent among hormone replacement therapy users than among non-users. For further information, see section 4.3 Contra-indications and 4.4 Special Warnings and Precautions for Use.
- Retinal vascular thrombosis
- Myocardial infarction
- Increases in blood pressure
- Cholestatic jaundice
- Enlargement of hepatic haemangiomas
- Skin and subcutaneous disorders: erythema multiforme, erythema nodosum, vascular purpura
- Exacerbation of chorea
- Exacerbation of porphyria,
- Exacerbation of hypocalcaemia
- Exacerbation of otosclerosis

4.9 Overdose

Numerous reports of ingestion of large doses of estrogen-containing oral contraceptives by young children indicate that acute serious ill effects do not occur. Overdosage of estrogen may cause nausea and vomiting, and withdrawal bleeding may occur in females. There is no specific antidote and further treatment should be symptomatic.

5. PHARMACOLOGICAL PROPERTIES

5.1 Pharmacodynamic properties

ATC Code: G03C A57

Conjugated Estrogens

The active ingredients are primarily the sulphate esters of estrone, equilin sulphates, 17α-estradiol and 17β-estradiol. These substitute for the loss of estrogen production in menopausal women, and alleviate menopausal symptoms. Estrogens prevent bone loss following menopause or ovariectomy.

Relief of estrogen-deficiency symptoms

In a 1-year clinical trial (n=2,808), vasomotor symptoms were assessed for efficacy during the first 12 weeks of treatment in a subset of symptomatic women (n=241) who had at least 7 moderate or severe hot flushes daily or 50 moderate to severe hot flushes during the week before randomisation. Premarin 0.625mg was shown to be statistically better than placebo at weeks 4, 8 and 12 for relief of both frequency and severity of moderate to severe vasomotor symptoms.

Prevention of osteoporosis

Estrogen deficiency at menopause is associated with an increasing bone turnover and decline in bone mass. Therefore, if possible, treatment for prevention of osteoporosis should start as soon as possible after the onset of menopause in women with increased risk for future osteoporotic fractures. The effect of estrogens on the bone mineral density is dose-dependent. Protection appears to be effective for as long as treatment is continued.

After 3 years of treatment with Premarin 0.625mg, the increase in lumbar spine bone mineral density (BMD) was 3.46% ± 0.68. The percentage of women who maintained (less than 1% BMD loss per year) or gained BMD in lumbar zone during treatment was 92%.

Premarin 0.625mg also had an effect on hip BMD. The increase after 3 years was 1.31% ± 0.55 at total hip. The percentage of women who maintained (less than 1% BMD loss per year) or gained BMD in hip zone during treatment was 88%.

5.2 Pharmacokinetic properties

Absorption

Conjugated estrogens are soluble in water and are well absorbed from the gastrointestinal tract after release from the drug formulation. The Premarin tablets release conjugated estrogens slowly over several hours. The pharmacodynamic profile of unconjugated and conjugated estrogens following a dose of 2 × 0.625mg is provided in Table 1.

Distribution

The distribution of exogenous estrogen is similar to that of endogenous estrogens. Estrogens are widely distributed in the body and are generally found in higher concentrations in the sex hormone target organs. Estrogens circulate in the blood largely bound to sex hormone binding globulin (SHBG) and albumin.

Metabolism

Exogenous estrogens are metabolised in the same manner as endogenous estrogens. Circulating estrogens exist in dynamic equilibrium of metabolic interconversions. These transformations take place mainly in the liver. Estradiol is converted reversibly to estrone, and both can be converted to estriol, which is the major urinary metabolite. Estrogens also undergo enterohepatic recirculation via sulphate and glucuronide conjugation in the liver, biliary secretion of conjugates into the intestine, and hydrolysis in the gut following reabsorption. In post-menopausal women a significant proportion of the circulating estrogens exists as sulphate conjugates, especially estrone sulphate, which serves as a circulating reservoir for the formation of more active estrogens.

Excretion

Estriol, estrone and estradiol are excreted in the urine along with glucuronide and sulphate conjugates.

Table 1 – Pharmacokinetic parameters for Premarin

Pharmacokinetic profile for unconjugated estrogens following a dose of 2 × 0.625mg

(see Table 1 below)

Pharmacokinetic profile for conjugated estrogens following a dose of 2 × 0.625mg

(see Table 2 below)

5.3 Preclinical safety data

Long-term continuous administration of natural and synthetic estrogens in certain animal species increases the frequency of carcinomas of the breast, cervix, vagina and liver.

Table 1 – Pharmacokinetic parameters for Premarin

Drug PK Parameter Arithmetic Mean (%CV)	C_{max} (pg/mL)	t_{max} (h)	$t_{1/2}$ (h)	AUC (pg.h/mL)*
Estrone	139 (37)	8.8 (20)	28.0 (13)	5016 (34)
baseline-adjusted estrone	120 (42)	8.8 (20)	17.4 (37)	2956 (39)
Equilin	66 (42)	7.9 (19)	13.6 (52)	1210 (37)

* $t_{1/2}$ = terminal-phase disposition half-life (0.693/γ)

Table 2

Drug PK Parameter Arithmetic Mean (%CV)	C_{max} (ng/mL)	t_{max} (h)	$t_{1/2}$ (h)	AUC (pg.h/mL)*
total estrone	7.3 (41)	7.3 (51)	15.0 (25)	134 (42)
baseline-adjusted total estrone	7.1 (41)	7.3 (25)	13.6 (27)	122 (39)
total equilin	5.0 (42)	6.2 (26)	10.1 (27)	65 (45)

* $t_{1/2}$ = terminal-phase disposition half-life (0.693/γ)

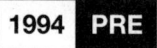

6. PHARMACEUTICAL PARTICULARS

6.1 List of excipients

Premarin 0.625mg: Calcium sulphate, carnauba wax, microcrystalline cellulose, glyceryl mono-oleate, lactose, magnesium stearate, methylcellulose, macrogol, shellac solution (pharmaceutical glaze), sucrose, titanium dioxide (E171), and opalux maroon colour AS-3910†.

† Opalux maroon colour contains sucrose, purified water, erythrosine (E127), titanium dioxide (E171), sunset yellow (E110), indigo carmine (E132), polyvinylpyrrolidone and sodium benzoate.

Premarin 1.25mg: Calcium sulphate, carnauba wax, microcrystalline cellulose, glyceryl mono-oleate, lactose, magnesium stearate, methylcellulose, macrogol, shellac solution (pharmaceutical glaze), sucrose, titanium dioxide (E171), colours E110, E104.

6.2 Incompatibilities
Not applicable.

6.3 Shelf life
Three years.

6.4 Special precautions for storage
Do not store above 25°C.

6.5 Nature and contents of container
Polyvinylchloride (PVC)/Aluminium foil blisters containing 28 tablets. One carton pack contains 3 blisters.

Securitainers containing 100 tablets

PVC/Aluminium foil blisters containing 21 tablets

6.6 Instructions for use and handling
Not applicable.

7. MARKETING AUTHORISATION HOLDER
John Wyeth and Brother Limited
Trading as: Wyeth Pharmaceuticals
Huntercombe Lane South
Taplow, Maidenhead,
Berkshire, SL6 0PH

8. MARKETING AUTHORISATION NUMBER(S)
Premarin tablets 0.625mg: PL 0011/0165.
Premarin tablets 1.25mg: PL 0011/0166.

9. DATE OF FIRST AUTHORISATION/RENEWAL OF THE AUTHORISATION
1972.

10. DATE OF REVISION OF THE TEXT
Approved 11th February 2005

Premarin Vaginal Cream

(Wyeth Pharmaceuticals)

1. NAME OF THE MEDICINAL PRODUCT
Premarin® Vaginal Cream.

2. QUALITATIVE AND QUANTITATIVE COMPOSITION
Each 1 gram of the cream contains 0.625mg conjugated estrogens USP.

3. PHARMACEUTICAL FORM
Cream for intravaginal or topical administration.

4. CLINICAL PARTICULARS

4.1 Therapeutic indications
Short-term treatment of atrophic vaginitis and post-menopausal atrophic urethritis, kraurosis vulvae.

4.2 Posology and method of administration

Dosage and Administration

Adults: The usual recommended dose is 1 to 2g daily administered intravaginally or topically to the vaginal area, depending on the severity of the condition. Administration should be cyclic (e.g. three weeks on and one week off). It should start on the fifth day of bleeding in the patient who is menstruating and arbitrarily if not.

For treatment of postmenopausal symptoms the lowest effective dose should be used. HRT should only be continued as long as the benefit in alleviation of severe symptoms outweighs the risk.

The addition of a progestogen is not needed during treatment with Premarin Vaginal Cream (see Section 4.4 Special Warnings and Precautions for Use)

Missed dose: If the patient forgets to apply a dose, it should be applied as soon as possible. The patient should not use doubled their usual dose to make up for missed applications.

Elderly: There are no special dosage requirements for elderly patients, but as with all medicines, the lowest effective dose should be used.

Children: Not recommended.

4.3 Contraindications

1. Known past or suspected cancer of the breast.

2. Known or suspected estrogen-dependent malignant tumours (e.g. endometrial cancer)

3. Undiagnosed abnormal genital bleeding.

4. Untreated endometrial hyperplasia

5. Active or past history of venous thromboembolism (e.g. deep vein thrombosis, pulmonary embolism)

6. Active or recent arterial thromboembolic disease (e.g. angina, myocardial infarction)

7. Acute liver disease or history of liver disease where the liver function tests have failed to return to normal.

8. Known hypersensitivity to the active substance or to any of the excipients of Premarin Vaginal Cream.

9. Porphyria

4.4 Special warnings and special precautions for use
Due to estrogen absorption following the application of Premarin Vaginal Cream, prolonged administration might result in systemic effects. Therefore, the following warnings and precautions should be considered.

1. Medical Examination/Follow up

Before initiating or reinstituting HRT, a complete personal and family medical history should be taken. Physical (including pelvic and breast) examination should be guided by the contraindications and warnings for use. During treatment, periodic check-ups are recommended of a frequency and nature adapted to the individual women. Women should be advised what changes in their breasts should be reported to their doctor or nurse. Investigations, including mammography, should be carried out in accordance with currently accepted screening practices, modified to the clinical needs of the individual. A careful appraisal of the risks and benefits should be undertaken at least annually in women treated with hormone replacement therapy.

2. Conditions that need supervision

If any of the following conditions are present, have occurred previously, and/or have been aggravated during pregnancy or previous hormone treatment, the patient should be closely supervised. It should be taken into account that these conditions may recur or be aggravated during treatment with Premarin, in particular:

– Leiomyoma (uterine fibroids) or endometriosis

– A family history of, or other risk factors for, thromboembolic disorders (see below)

– Risk factors for estrogen dependent tumours (e.g. first degree heredity for breast cancer)

– Hypertension

– Liver disorders (e.g. liver adenoma)

– Diabetes mellitus with or without vascular involvement

– Cholelithiasis

– Migraine or (severe) headaches

– Systemic lupus erythematosus (SLE)

– A history of endometrial hyperplasia (see below)

– Epilepsy

– Asthma

– Otosclerosis

3. Reasons for immediate withdrawal of therapy

Therapy should be discontinued if a contra-indication is discovered and in the following situations:

– Jaundice or deterioration in liver function

– Significant increase in blood pressure

– New onset of migraine-type headache

– Pregnancy

4. Endometrial Hyperplasia

The risk of endometrial hyperplasia and carcinoma is increased when systemic estrogens are administered alone for prolonged periods of time. The endometrial safety of long-term or repeated use of topical vaginal estrogens is uncertain. Therefore, if repeated, treatment should be reviewed at least annually, with special consideration given to any symptoms of endometrial hyperplasia or carcinoma.

If break-through bleeding or spotting appears at any time on therapy, the reason should be investigated, which may include endometrial biopsy to exclude endometrial malignancy.

5. Breast Cancer

Randomised controlled trials and epidemiological studies have reported an increased risk of breast cancer in women taking estrogen or estrogen-progestogen combinations for HRT for several years (see Section 4.8 Undesirable Effects). An observational study of almost 829,000 women has shown that, compared to never-users, use of estrogen-progestogen combined HRT is associated with a higher risk of breast cancer (RR = 2.00, 95%CI: 1.88 - 2.12) than use of estrogens alone (RR = 1.30, 95%CI: 1.21 – 1.40). In this study the magnitude of the increase in breast cancer risk was similar for all estrogen-only preparations, irrespective of the type, dose or route of administration of the estrogen (oral, transdermal and implanted). Likewise the magnitude of the increased risk was similar for all estrogen plus progestogen preparations, irrespective of the type of progestogen or the number of days of addition per cycle. For all HRT, an excess risk becomes apparent within 1-2 years of starting treatment and increase with the duration of use of HRT but begins to decline when HRT is stopped and by 5 years reaches the same level as in women who have never taken HRT.

The increase in risk applies to all women studied, although the relative risk was significantly higher in those with a lean or normal body build (body mass index or BMI of <25kg/m^2) compared to those with a BMI of ≥25kg/m^2.

At present the effect of HRT on the diagnosis of breast tumours remains unclear - all women should be encouraged to report any changes in their breasts to their doctor or nurse.

6. Venous Thromboembolism

Hormone replacement therapy (HRT) is associated with a higher relative risk of developing venous thromboembolism (VTE) i.e. deep vein thrombosis or pulmonary embolism. One randomised controlled trial and epidemiological studies found a two to threefold higher risk for users compared with non-users. For non- users it is estimated that the number of cases of VTE that will occur over a 5-year period is about 3 per 1000 women aged 50-59 years and 8 per 1000 women aged between 60-69 years. It is estimated that in healthy women who use HRT for 5 years, the number of additional cases of VTE over a 5-year period will be between 2 and 6 (best estimate = 4) per 1000 women aged 50-59 years and between 5 and 15 (best estimate = 9) per 1000 women aged 60-69 years. The occurrence of such an event is more likely in the first year of HRT than later.

Generally recognised risk factors for VTE include a personal or family history and severe obesity (Body Mass Index >30kg/m^2) and systemic lupus erythematosus (SLE). There is no consensus about the possible role of varicose veins in VTE.

Patients with a history of VTE or known thrombophilic states have an increased risk of VTE. HRT may add to this risk. Personal or strong family history of thromboembolism or recurrent spontaneous abortion should be investigated in order to exclude a thrombophilic predisposition. Until a thorough evaluation of thrombophilic factors has been made or anticoagulant treatment initiated, use of HRT in such patients should be viewed as contraindicated. Those women already on anticoagulant treatment require careful consideration of the benefit-risk of use of HRT.

The risk of VTE may be temporarily increased with prolonged immobilisation, major trauma or major surgery. As in all postoperative patients scrupulous attention should be given to prophylactic measures to prevent VTE following surgery. Where prolonged immobilisation is liable to follow elective surgery, particularly abdominal or orthopaedic surgery to the lower limbs, consideration should be given to temporarily stopping HRT 4 weeks earlier, if this is possible. Treatment should not be restarted until the woman is completely mobilised.

If venous thromboembolism develops after initiating therapy the drug should be discontinued. Patients should be told to contact their doctors immediately when they are aware of potential thromboembolic symptoms (e.g. painful swelling of leg, sudden pain in the chest, dyspnoea).

7. Coronary Artery Disease (CAD)

There is no evidence from randomised controlled trials of cardiovascular benefit with continuous combined conjugated estrogens and MPA. Large clinical trials showed a possible increased risk of cardiovascular morbidity in the first year of use and no benefit thereafter. For other HRT products, there are as yet no randomised controlled trials examining benefit in cardiovascular morbidity or mortality. Therefore, it is uncertain whether these findings also extend to other HRT products.

8. Stroke

One large randomised clinical trial (WHI-trial) found, as a secondary outcome, an increased risk of stroke in healthy women during treatment with continuous combined conjugated estrogens and MPA. For women who do not use HRT, it is estimated that the number of cases of stroke that will occur over a 5 year period is about 3 per 1000 women aged 50-59 years and 11 per 1000 women aged 60-69 years. It is estimated that for women who use conjugated estrogens and MPA for 5 years, the number of additional cases will be between 0 and 3 (best estimate =1) per 1000 users aged 50-59 years and between 1 and 9 (best estimate = 4) per 1000 users aged 60-69 years. It is unknown whether the increased risk also extends to other HRT products.

9. Ovarian Cancer

Long term (at least 5 –10 years) use of estrogen-only HRT products in hysterectomised women has been associated with an increased risk of ovarian cancer in some epidemiological studies. It is uncertain whether long-term use of combined HRT confers different risk than estrogen-only products.

Other Conditions

10. Estrogens may cause fluid retention and therefore patients with cardiac or renal dysfunction should be carefully observed. Patients with terminal renal insufficiency should be closely observed, since it is expected that the level of circulating active ingredients in Premarin is increased.

11. Women with an intact uterus of child-bearing potential should be advised to adhere to non-hormonal contraceptive methods.

Premarin Vaginal Cream has been shown to weaken latex condoms. The potential for Premarin Vaginal Cream to weaken and contribute to the failure of condoms, diaphragms or cervical caps made of latex or rubber should be considered. If there is still a possibility that a patient could become pregnant, they should be advised to use an alternative form of non-hormonal contraceptive.

12. The use of estrogen may influence the laboratory results of certain endocrine tests and liver enzymes.

Estrogens increase thyroid binding globulin (TBG), leading to increased circulating total thyroid hormone, as measured by protein-bound iodine (PBI), T4 levels (by column or by radio-immunoassay) or T3 levels (by radio-immunoassay). T3 resin uptake is decreased, reflecting the elevated TBG. Free T4 and free T3 concentrations are unaltered.

Other binding proteins may be elevated in serum, i.e. corticoid binding globulin (CBG), sex-hormone-binding globulin (SHBG) leading to increased circulating corticosteroids and sex steroids, respectively. Free or biologically active hormone concentrations are unchanged. Other plasma proteins may be increased (angiotensinogen/renin substrate, alpha-I-antitrypsin, ceruloplasmin).

Some patients dependent on thyroid hormone replacement therapy may require increased doses in order to maintain their free thyroid hormone levels in an acceptable range. Therefore, patients should have their thyroid function monitored more frequently when commencing concurrent treatment in order to maintain their free thyroid hormone levels in an acceptable range.

13. There is an increase in the risk of gallbladder disease in women receiving HRT (see conditions that need supervision)

14. A worsening of glucose tolerance may occur in patients taking estrogens and therefore diabetic patients should be carefully observed while receiving hormone replacement therapy.

15. Women with pre-existing hypertriglyceridemia should be followed closely during estrogen replacement or hormone replacement therapy, since rare cases of large increases of plasma triglycerides leading to pancreatitis have been reported with estrogen therapy in this condition.

16. Estrogens should be used with caution in individuals with severe hypocalcaemia

4.5 Interaction with other medicinal products and other forms of Interaction

The metabolism of estrogens may be increased by concomitant use of substances known to induce drug-metabolising enzymes, specifically cytochrome P450 enzymes, such as anticonvulsants (e.g. phenobarbital, phenytoin, carbamazepine) and anti-infectives (e.g. rifampicin, rifabutin, nevirapine, efavirenz).

Ritonavir and nelfinavir, although known as strong inhibitors, by contrast exhibit inducing properties when used concomitantly with steroid hormones.

Herbal preparations containing St John's wort *(Hypericum perforatum)* may induce the metabolism of estrogens.

Clinically, an increased metabolism of estrogens and progestogens may lead to decreased effect and changes in the uterine bleeding profile.

The response to metyrapone may be reduced.

4.6 Pregnancy and lactation

Premarin is not indicated during pregnancy.

For women with a uterus:

If pregnancy occurs during medication with Premarin, treatment should be withdrawn immediately. The results of most epidemiological studies to date relevant to inadvertent foetal exposure to estrogens indicate no teratogenic or foetotoxic effects.

Lactation:

Premarin is not indicated during lactation.

4.7 Effects on ability to drive and use machines

Not applicable.

4.8 Undesirable effects

See also 4.4 Special Warnings and Special Precautions for Use.

Adverse drug reactions (ADRs)

The following adverse reactions have been reported with Premarin Vaginal Cream or are undesirable effects associated with estrogens.

System Organ Class	Adverse Reaction
Reproductive system	Breakthrough bleeding/ spotting Application site reactions of vulvovaginal discomfort including burning, irritation, and genital pruritus Vaginal discharge Increased size of uterine leiomyomata Endometrial hyperplasia
Breast disorders	Breast pain, tenderness, enlargement, discharge
Gastrointestinal disorders	Nausea, vomiting bloating, abdominal pain Pancreatitis
Nervous system disorders	Dizziness, headache, migraine, nervousness, stroke
Musculoskeletal, connective tissue and bone disorders	Arthralgias, leg cramps
Psychiatric disorders	Changes in libido, mood disturbances, irritability, depression
Vascular disorders	Pulmonary embolism. Venous thromboembolism
Cardiac disorders	Myocardial Infarction
General disorders and administration site conditions	Oedema Exacerbation of otosclerosis
Skin and subcutaneous tissue disorders	Alopecia Chloasma, hirsutism, pruritus, rash Erythema multiforme, erythema nodosum
Hepatobiliary disorder	Gallbladder disease Cholestatic jaundice
Infections and Infestations	Vaginitis, including vaginal candidiasis Cystitis
Neoplasms benign and malignant (including cysts and polyps)	Breast cancer*, Fibrocystic breast changes Endometrial cancer, Enlargement of hepatic haemangiomas
Immune system disorders	Urticaria, Angioedema, Anaphylactic/anaphylactoid reactions, Hypersensitivity
Metabolism and nutrition disorders	Glucose intolerance
Eye Disorders	Intolerance to contact lenses
Investigations	Changes in weight (increase or decrease) Increased triglycerides Increases in blood pressure

Breast Cancer

The risk of breast cancer increases with the number of years of HRT usage. According to data from a recent epidemiological study in about 829,000 postmenopausal women, the best estimate of the risk is that for women not using HRT, in total 32 in every 1000 are expected to have breast cancer diagnosed between the ages of 50 and 65 years. Among those with current or recent use of estrogen-only replacement therapy, it is estimated that the total number of additional cases during the corresponding period will be between 0 and 3 (best estimate = 1.5) per 1000 for 5 years' use and between 3 and 7 (best estimate = 5) per 1000 for 10 years' use (see table). Among those with current or recent use of estrogen plus progestogen combined HRT, it is estimated that the total number of additional cases will be between 5 and 7 (best estimate = 6) per 1000 for 5 years' use and between 18 and 20 (best estimate = 19) per 1000 for 10 years' use (See section 4.4 Special Warnings and Precautions for Use). The number of additional cases of breast cancer is broadly similar for women who start HRT irrespective of age at start of HRT use (between the ages of 45-65).

	No of additional cases of breast cancer diagnosed per 1000 women (95% confidence intervals)	
Type of HRT	5 years of use	10 years of use
Estrogen-only	1.5 (0-3)	5 (3-7)
Combined	6 (5-7)	19 (18-20)

Other adverse reactions reported in association with estrogen/progestogen treatment including Premarin Vaginal Cream:

- Estrogen-dependent neoplasms benign and malignant, e.g. endometrial hyperplasia, endometrial cancer
- Venous thromboembolism, i.e. deep leg or pelvic venous thrombosis and pulmonary embolism, is more frequent among hormone replacement therapy users than among non-users. For further information, see section 4.3 Contraindications and 4.4 Special Warnings and Precautions for Use.
- Retinal vascular thrombosis
- Myocardial infarction
- Increases in blood pressure
- Cholestatic jaundice
- Enlargement of hepatic haemangiomas
- Skin and subcutaneous disorders: erythema multiforme, erythema nodosum, vascular purpura
- Exacerbation of chorea
- Exacerbation of porphyria,
- Exacerbation of hypocalcaemia
- Exacerbation of otosclerosis

4.9 Overdose

Numerous reports of ingestion of large doses of estrogen-containing oral contraceptives by young children indicate that acute serious ill effects do not occur. Overdosage of estrogen may cause nausea and vomiting, and withdrawal bleeding may occur in females. There is no specific antidote and further treatment should be symptomatic.

5. PHARMACOLOGICAL PROPERTIES

5.1 Pharmacodynamic properties

ATC Code: G03C A57

Conjugated Estrogens

Conjugated estrogen cream has identical pharmacological actions to endogenous estrogens. The active ingredients are primarily the sulphate esters of estrone, equilin sulphates, 17α-estradiol and 17β-estradiol. These substitute for the loss of estrogen production in menopausal women, and alleviate menopausal symptoms.

5.2 Pharmacokinetic properties

Absorption

The estrogens in Premarin Vaginal Cream are absorbed systemically.

Distribution

The distribution of exogenous estrogen is similar to that of endogenous estrogens. Estrogens are widely distributed in the body and are generally found in higher concentrations in the sex hormone target organs. Estrogens circulate in the blood largely bound to sex hormone binding globulin (SHBG) and albumin.

Metabolism

Exogenous estrogens are metabolised in the same manner as endogenous estrogens. Circulating estrogens exist in dynamic equilibrium of metabolic interconversions. These transformations take place mainly in the liver. Estradiol is converted reversibly to estrone, and both can be converted to stroll, which is the major urinary metabolite. Estrogens also undergo enterohepatic recirculation via sulphate and glucuronide conjugation in the liver, biliary secretion of conjugates into the intestine, and hydrolysis in the gut following reabsorption. In post-menopausal women a significant proportion of the circulating estrogens exists as sulphate conjugates, especially estrone sulphate, which serves as a circulating reservoir for the formation of more active estrogens.

Excretion

Estriol, estrone and estradiol are excreted in the urine along with glucuronide and sulphate conjugates.

5.3 Preclinical safety data

There are no preclinical data of relevance to the prescriber which are additional to that already included in other sections of the SPC.

6. PHARMACEUTICAL PARTICULARS

6.1 List of excipients

Liquid paraffin, glyceryl monostearate, cetyl alcohol, cetyl esters wax, white wax, methyl stearate, sodium lauryl sulphate, phenylethyl alcohol, glycerin, propylene glycol monostearate, purified water.

6.2 Incompatibilities

Not applicable.

6.3 Shelf life

2 years.

6.4 Special precautions for storage

Do not store above 25°C.

6.5 Nature and contents of container

Primary container: Aluminium tube with a white screw-on cap, containing 42.5g of cream.

Secondary container: Cardboard carton.

6.6 Instructions for use and handling

Not applicable.

7. MARKETING AUTHORISATION HOLDER

John Wyeth and Brother Limited

Trading as Wyeth Pharmaceuticals

Huntercombe Lane South

Taplow, Maidenhead

Berkshire, SL6 0PH

8. MARKETING AUTHORISATION NUMBER(S)

PL 0011/0163.

9. DATE OF FIRST AUTHORISATION/RENEWAL OF THE AUTHORISATION

22 November 1990 / 12 December 1995

10. DATE OF REVISION OF THE TEXT

Approved 11th February 2005

* Trade marks

Premique

(Wyeth Pharmaceuticals)

1. NAME OF THE MEDICINAL PRODUCT

Premique*.

2. QUALITATIVE AND QUANTITATIVE COMPOSITION

Premique is a tablet for oral administration containing conjugated estrogens† 0.625mg and medroxyprogesterone acetate (MPA) 5.0mg.

†Conjugated estrogens contain sodium estrone sulphate, sodium equilin sulphate, 17α-dihydroequilin, 17α-estradiol, equilenin, 17α-dihydroequilenin, 17β-dihydroequilin, 17β-dihydroequilenin, 17β-estradiol and 8,9-dehydro-estrone.

For excipients see 6.1.

3. PHARMACEUTICAL FORM

Coated tablet.

Light blue oval biconvex sugar coated tablet.

4. CLINICAL PARTICULARS

4.1 Therapeutic indications

Hormone replacement therapy for estrogen deficiency symptoms in postmenopausal women with an intact uterus.

Second line therapy for prevention of osteoporosis in postmenopausal women at high risk of future fractures who are intolerant of, or contraindicated for, other medicinal products approved for the prevention of osteoporosis.

4.2 Posology and method of administration

Premique is taken orally in a continuous combined 28-day regimen of one tablet daily with no break between packs.

In women who are not taking hormone replacement therapy or women who switch from another continuous combined hormone replacement therapy product, treatment may be started on any convenient day. In women transferring from a sequential hormone replacement therapy regimen, treatment should begin the day following completion of the prior regimen.

For treatment of postmenopausal symptoms: The usual starting dose is one tablet 0.625mg/5.0mg per day.

For prevention and management of osteoporosis associated with estrogen deficiency: The usual starting dose is one tablet 0.625mg/5.0mg per day. (see section 5.1 Pharmacodynamic Properties).

Maintenance/Continuation/Extended treatment

For treatment of postmenopausal symptoms, the lowest effective dose should be used. HRT should only be continued as long as the benefit in alleviation of severe symptoms outweighs the risk.

The benefits of the lower risk of endometrial hyperplasia and endometrial cancer due to adding a progestogen should be weighed against the increased risk of breast cancer (see sections 4.4 Special Warnings and Precautions for Use and 4.8 Undesirable Effects).

Forgotten tablet: If a tablet is forgotten, it should be taken as soon as the patient remembers, therapy should then be continued as before. If more than one tablet has been forgotten only the most recent tablet should be taken, the patient should not take double the usual dose to make up for missed tablets.

Missed pills may cause breakthrough bleeding.

Elderly:

There are no special dosage requirements for elderly patients, but, as with all medicines, the lowest effective dose should be used.

Children:

Not recommended

4.3 Contraindications

1. Known, past or suspected breast cancer.

2. Known or suspected estrogen-dependent malignant tumours (e.g. endometrial cancer)

3. Undiagnosed abnormal genital bleeding.

4. Untreated endometrial hyperplasia

5. Active or past history of venous thromboembolism (e.g. deep vein thrombosis, pulmonary embolism)

6. Active or recent arterial thromboembolic disease (e.g. angina, myocardial infarction)

7. Acute liver disease or history of liver disease where the liver function tests have failed to return to normal.

8. Known hypersensitivity to the active substances or to any of the excipients of Premique tablets.

9. Porphyria

4.4 Special warnings and special precautions for use

1. Medical examination/Follow up

Before initiating or reinstituting HRT, a complete personal and family medical history should be taken. Physical (including pelvic and breast) examination should be guided by the contraindications and warnings for use. During treatment, periodic check-ups are recommended of a frequency and nature adapted to the individual women. Women should be advised what changes in their breasts should be reported to their doctor or nurse. Investigations, including mammography, should be carried out in accordance with currently accepted screening practices, modified to the clinical needs of the individual. A careful appraisal of the risks and benefits should be undertaken at least annually in women treated with hormone replacement therapy.

In women with an intact uterus, the benefits of the lower risk of endometrial hyperplasia and endometrial cancer due to adding progestogen should be weighed against the increased risk of breast cancer (see below and Section 4.8 Undesirable Effects).

2. Conditions that need supervision

If any of the following conditions are present, have occurred previously, and/or have been aggravated during pregnancy or previous hormone treatment, the patient should be closely supervised. It should be taken into account that these conditions may recur or be aggravated during treatment with Premique, in particular:

– Leiomyoma (uterine fibroids) or endometriosis

– A family history of, or other risk factors for, thromboembolic disorders (see below)

– Risk factors for estrogen dependent tumours (e.g. 1st degree heredity for breast cancer)

– Hypertension

– Liver disorders (e.g. liver adenoma)

– Diabetes mellitus with or without vascular involvement

– Cholelithiasis

– Migraine or (severe) headaches

– Systemic lupus erythematosus (SLE)

– A history of endometrial hyperplasia (see below)

– Epilepsy

– Asthma

– Otosclerosis

3. Reasons for immediate withdrawal of therapy

Therapy should be discontinued if a contra-indication is discovered and in the following situations:

– Jaundice or deterioration in liver function

– Significant increase in blood pressure

– New onset of migraine-type headache

– Pregnancy

4. Endometrial Hyperplasia

The risk of endometrial hyperplasia and carcinoma is increased when estrogens are administered alone for prolonged periods. The addition of a progestogen for at least 12 days of the cycle in non-hysterectomised women reduces, but may not eliminate, this risk (see section 4.8 Undesirable Effects). Unless there is a previous diagnosis of endometriosis it is not recommended to add a progestogen in hysterectomised women (see 4.4 – Special Warnings and Precautions for Use).

The reduction in risk to the endometrium should be weighed against the increase in the risk of breast cancer of added progestogen (see 'Breast cancer' below and Section 4.8 Undesirable Effects).

Break-through bleeding and spotting may occur during the first months of treatment. If break-through bleeding or spotting appears after some time on therapy, or continues after treatment has been discontinued, the reason should be investigated, which may include endometrial biopsy to exclude endometrial malignancy.

5. Breast Cancer

Randomised controlled trials and epidemiological studies have reported an increased risk of breast cancer in women taking estrogen or estrogen-progestogen combinations for HRT for several years (see Section 4.8 Undesirable Effects). An observational study of almost 829,000 women has shown that, compared to never-users, use of estrogen-progestogen combined HRT is associated with a higher risk of breast cancer (RR = 2.00, 95%CI: 1.88 - 2.12) than use of estrogens alone (RR = 1.30, 95%CI: 1.21 – 1.40). In this study the magnitude of the increase in breast cancer risk was similar for all estrogen-only preparations, irrespective of the type, dose or route of administration of the estrogen (oral, transdermal and implanted). Likewise the magnitude of the increased risk was similar for all estrogen plus progestogen preparations, irrespective of the type of progestogen or the number of days of addition per cycle. For all HRT, an excess risk becomes apparent within 1-2 years of starting treatment and increases with the duration of use of HRT but begins to decline when HRT is stopped and by 5 years reaches the same level as in women who have never taken HRT.

The increase in risk applies to all women studied, although the relative risk was significantly higher in those with a lean or normal body build (body mass index or BMI of $<25kg/m^2$) compared to those with a BMI of $\geqslant 25kg/m^2$.

At present the effect of HRT on the diagnosis of breast tumours remains unclear – all women should be encouraged to report any changes in their breasts to their doctor or nurse.

6. Venous thromboembolism

Hormone replacement therapy (HRT) is associated with a higher relative risk of developing venous thromboembolism (VTE) i.e. deep vein thrombosis or pulmonary embolism. One randomised controlled trial and epidemiological studies found a two to threefold higher risk for users compared with non-users. For non- users it is estimated that the number of cases of VTE that will occur over a 5-year period is about 3 per 1000 women aged 50-59 years and 8 per 1000 women aged between 60-69 years. It is estimated that in healthy women who use HRT for 5 years, the number of additional cases of VTE over a 5-year period will be between 2 and 6 (best estimate 4) per 1000 women aged 50-59 years and between 5 and 15 (best estimate = 9) per 1000 women aged 60-69 years. The occurrence of such an event is more likely in the first year of HRT than later.

Generally recognised risk factors for VTE include a personal or family history and severe obesity (Body Mass Index $>30kg/m^2$) and systemic lupus erythematosus (SLE). There is no consensus about the possible role of varicose veins in VTE.

Patients with a history of VTE or known thrombophilic states have an increased risk of VTE. HRT may add to this risk. Personal or strong family history of thromboembolism or recurrent spontaneous abortion should be investigated in order to exclude a thrombophilic predisposition. Until a thorough evaluation of thrombophilic factors has been made or anticoagulant treatment initiated, use of HRT in such patients should be viewed as contraindicated. Those women already on anticoagulant treatment require careful consideration of the benefit-risk of use of HRT.

The risk of VTE may be temporarily increased with prolonged immobilisation, major trauma or major surgery. As in all postoperative patients scrupulous attention should be given to prophylactic measures to prevent VTE following surgery. Where prolonged immobilisation is liable to follow elective surgery, particularly abdominal or orthopaedic surgery to the lower limbs, consideration should be given to temporarily stopping HRT 4-6 weeks earlier, if this is possible. Treatment should not be restarted until the woman is completely mobilised.

If venous thromboembolism develops after initiating therapy the drug should be discontinued. Patients should be told to contact their doctors immediately when they are aware of potential thromboembolic symptoms (e.g. painful swelling of a leg, sudden pain in the chest, dyspnoea).

7. Coronary Artery Disease (CAD)

There is no evidence from randomised controlled trials of cardiovascular benefit with continuous combined conjugated estrogens and MPA. Large clinical trials showed a possible increased risk of cardiovascular morbidity in the first year of use and no benefit thereafter. For other HRT products, there are as yet no randomised controlled trials examining benefit in cardiovascular morbidity or mortality. Therefore, it is uncertain whether these findings also extend to other HRT products.

8. Stroke

One large randomised clinical trial (WHI-trial) found, as a secondary outcome, an increased risk of stroke in healthy women during treatment with continuous combined conjugated estrogens and MPA. For women who do not use HRT, it is estimated that the number of cases of stroke that will occur over a 5 year period is about 3 per 1000 women aged 50-59 years and 11 per 1000 women aged 60-69 years. It is estimated that for women who use conjugated estrogens and MPA for 5 years, the number of additional cases will be between 0 and 3 (best estimate =1) per 1000 users aged 50-59 years and between 1 and 9 (best estimate = 4) per 1000 users aged 60-69 years. It is unknown whether the increased risk also extends to other HRT products.

9. Ovarian Cancer

Long term (at least 5 –10 years) use of estrogen-only HRT products in hysterectomised women has been associated with an increased risk of ovarian cancer in some epidemiological studies. It is uncertain whether long-term use of combined HRT confers different risk than estrogen-only products.

Other Conditions

10. Estrogens/progestogens may cause fluid retention and therefore patients with cardiac or renal dysfunction should be carefully observed. Patients with terminal renal insufficiency should be closely observed, since it is expected that the level of circulating active ingredients in Premique is increased.

11. The use of estrogen may influence the laboratory results of certain endocrine tests and liver enzymes.

Estrogens increase thyroid binding globulin (TBG), leading to increased circulating total thyroid hormone, as measured by protein-bound iodine (PBI), T4 levels (by column or by radio-immunoassay) or T3 levels (by radio-immunoassay). T3 resin uptake is decreased, reflecting the elevated TBG. Free T4 and free T3 concentrations are usually unaltered.

Other binding proteins may be elevated in serum, i.e. corticoid binding globulin (CBG), sex-hormone-binding globulin (SHBG) leading to increased circulating corticosteroids and sex steroids, respectively. Free or biologically active hormone concentrations are usually unchanged. Other plasma proteins may be increased (angiotensinogen/renin substrate, alpha-I-antitrypsin, ceruloplasmin).

Some patients dependent on thyroid hormone replacement therapy may require increased doses in order to maintain their free thyroid hormone levels in an acceptable range. Therefore, patients should have their thyroid function monitored more frequently when commencing concurrent treatment in order to maintain their free thyroid hormone levels in an acceptable range.

12. There is an increase in the risk of gallbladder disease in women receiving HRT (see conditions that need supervision)

13. A worsening of glucose tolerance may occur in some patients on estrogen/progestogen therapy and therefore diabetic patients should be carefully observed while receiving hormone replacement therapy.

14. Women with pre-existing hypertriglyceridemia should be followed closely during estrogen replacement or hormone replacement therapy, since rare cases of large increases of plasma triglycerides leading to pancreatitis have been reported with estrogen therapy in this condition.

15. Estrogens should be used with caution in individuals with severe hypocalcaemia

16. Epidemiological studies suggest a number of individual risk factors which contribute to the development of postmenopausal osteoporosis. These include: early menopause; family history of osteoporosis; thin, small frame; cigarette use; recent prolonged systemic corticosteroid use. If several of these risk factors are present in a patient, consideration should be given to treatment.

4.5 Interaction with other medicinal products and other forms of Interaction

The metabolism of estrogens and progestogens may be increased by concomitant use of substances known to induce drug-metabolising enzymes, specifically cytochrome P450 enzymes, such as anticonvulsants (e.g. phenobarbital, phenytoin, carbamazepine) and anti-infectives (e.g. rifampicin, rifabutin, nevirapine, efavirenz).

Ritonavir and nelfinavir, although known as strong inhibitors, by contrast exhibit inducing properties when used concomitantly with steroid hormones.

Herbal preparations containing St John's wort *(Hypericum perforatum)* may induce the metabolism of estrogens and progestogens.

Clinically, an increased metabolism of estrogens and progestogens may lead to decreased effect and changes in the uterine bleeding profile.

The response to metyrapone may be reduced.

Aminogluthimide administered concomitantly with MPA may significantly depress the bioavailiablity of MPA.

4.6 Pregnancy and lactation

Pregnancy:

Premique is not indicated during pregnancy. If pregnancy occurs during medication with Premique treatment should be withdrawn immediately.

Clinically, data on a limited number of exposed pregnancies indicate no adverse effects of MPA on the foetus.

The results of most epidemiological studies to date relevant to inadvertent foetal exposure to combinations of estrogens and progestogens indicate no teratogenic or foetotoxic effect.

Lactation:

Premique is not indicated during lactation.

4.7 Effects on ability to drive and use machines

Premique should not affect the ability to drive or use machinery.

4.8 Undesirable effects

See also Section 4.4 Special Warnings and Special Precautions for Use.

Adverse drug reactions (ADRs)

The adverse reactions listed in the table are based on post-marketing spontaneous (reporting rate), clinical trials and class-effects. Breast pain is a very common adverse event reported in ⩾ 10% of patients.

System Organ Class	Adverse Reaction
Reproductive system & breast disorders	Breakthrough bleeding/ dysmenorrhoea, spotting; Breast pain, tenderness, enlargement, discharge Change in menstrual flow; Change in cervical ectropion and secretion Galactorrhoea; Increased size of uterine leiomyomata
Gastrointestinal disorders	Nausea; Bloating; Abdominal pain; Vomiting; Pancreatitis
Nervous	Anxiety; Dizziness; Headache (including migraine); Exacerbation of epilepsy; Stroke
Musculoskeletal, connective tissue and bone disorders	Arthralgias; Leg cramps
Psychiatric	Depression; Changes in libido; Mood disturbances; Irritability
Vascular	Pulmonary embolism; Deep Venous thrombophlebitis, Superficial thrombophlebitis,
Cardiac disorders	Myocardial Infarction
General disorders and administration site disorders	Oedema
Skin and subcutaneous tissue disorders	Alopecia; Acne; Pruritus; Chloasma/melasma; Hirsutism; Rash
Infections and infestations	Vaginitis, including vaginal candidiasis
Immune system disorders	Urticaria; Angioedeoma; Anaphylactic/anaphylactoid reactions
Metabolism and nutrition disorders	Glucose intolerance
Eye disorders	Intolerance to contact lenses
Respiratory, thoracic and mediastinal disorders	Exacerbation of asthma
Hepatobiliary	Gallbladder disease
Neoplasms benign and malignant	Breast cancer*; Fibrocystic breast changes; Ovarian Cancer
Investigations	Changes in weight (increase or decrease)

Breast cancer

** The risk of breast cancer increases with the number of years of HRT usage. According to data from a recent epidemiological study in about 829,000 postmenopausal women, the best estimate of the risk is that for women not using HRT, in total 32 in every 1000 are expected to have breast cancer diagnosed between the ages of 50 and 65 years. Among those with current or recent use of estrogen-only replacement therapy, it is estimated that the total number of additional cases during the corresponding period will be between 0 and 3 (best estimate = 1.5) per 1000 for 5 years' use and between 3 and 7 (best estimate = 5) per 1000 for 10 years' use (see table). Among those with current or recent use of estrogen plus progestogen combined HRT, it is estimated that the total number of additional cases will be between 5 and 7 (best estimate = 6) per 1000 for 5 years' use and between 18 and 20 (best estimate = 19) per 1000 for 10 years' use (See section 4.4 Special Warnings and Precautions for Use). The number of additional cases of breast cancer is broadly similar for women who start HRT irrespective of age at start of HRT use (between the ages of 45-65).*

	No of additional cases of breast cancer diagnosed per 1000 women (95% confidence intervals)	
Type of HRT	*5 years of use*	*10 years of use*
Estrogen-only	*1.5 (0-3)*	*5 (3-7)*
Combined	*6 (5-7)*	*19 (18-20)*

Endometrial Cancer

In women with an intact uterus, the risk of endometrial hyperplasia and endometrial cancer increases with the increasing duration of use of unopposed estrogens and is substantially reduced by the addition of a progestogen (see section 4.4 Special Warnings and Precautions for Use). According to data from epidemiological studies the best estimate of the risk of endometrial cancer is that for women not using HRT, about 5 in every 1000 are expected to have endometrial cancer diagnosed between the ages of 50 and 65. It is estimated that, among those who use estrogen-only replacement therapy, there will be 4 additional cases per 100 after 5 years' use and 10 additional cases per 1000 after 10 years' use. Adding a progestogen to estrogen-only therapy substantially reduces, but may not eliminate, the increased risk.

Other adverse reactions reported in association with estrogen/progestogen treatment including Premique:

- Estrogen-dependent neoplasms benign and malignant, e.g. endometrial hyperplasia, endometrial cancer
- Venous thromboembolism, i.e. deep leg or pelvic venous thrombosis and pulmonary embolism, is more frequent among hormone replacement therapy users than among non-users. For further information, see section 4.3 Contra-indications and 4.4 Special Warnings and Precautions for Use.
- Retinal vascular thrombosis
- Myocardial infarction
- Stroke
- Increases in blood pressure
- Cholestatic jaundice
- Enlargement of hepatic haemangiomas
- Skin and subcutaneous disorders: erythema multiforme, erythema nodosum, vascular purpura
- Exacerbation of chorea
- Exacerbation of porphyria
- Exacerbation of hypocalcaemia
- Exacerbation of otosclerosis

4.9 Overdose

Numerous reports of ingestion of large doses of estrogen/progestogen-containing oral contraceptives by young children indicate that acute serious ill effects do not occur. Overdosage of estrogens may cause nausea and vomiting, and withdrawal bleeding may occur in females. There is no specific antidote and further treatment should be symptomatic.

5. PHARMACOLOGICAL PROPERTIES

5.1 Pharmacodynamic properties

ATC Code: GO3F A12

Conjugated Estrogens

The active ingredients are primarily the sulphate esters of estrone, equilin sulphates, 17α-estradiol and 17β-estradiol. These substitute for the loss of estrogen production in menopausal women, and alleviate menopausal symptoms. Estrogens prevent bone loss following menopause or ovariectomy.

Progestogen:

As estrogens promote the growth of the endometrium, unopposed estrogens increase the risk of endometrial hyperplasia and cancer. The addition of a progestogen reduces but does not eliminate the estrogen-induced risk of endometrial hyperplasia in non-hysterectomised women.

Relief of estrogen-deficiency symptoms

In a 1-year clinical trial (n=2,808), vasomotor symptoms were assessed for efficacy during the first 12 weeks of treatment in a subset of symptomatic women (n=241) who had at least 7 moderate or severe hot flushes daily or 50 moderate to severe hot flushes during the week before randomisation. Premique 0.625mg/2.5mg (conjugated estrogens/medroxyprogesterone acetate) was shown to be statistically better than placebo at weeks 4, 8 and 12 for relief of both frequency and severity of moderate to severe vasomotor symptoms.

In two clinical trials, the incidence of amenorrhoea (no bleeding or spotting) increased over time in women treated with Premique 0.625mg/2.5mg. Amenorrhoea was seen in 68% of women at cycle 6 and 77% of women at cycle 12. Breakthrough bleeding and/or spotting appeared in 48% during the first 3 months, and in 24% of women during months 10-12 of treatment.

Prevention of osteoporosis

Estrogen deficiency at menopause is associated with an increasing bone turnover and decline in bone mass. Therefore, if possible, treatment for prevention of osteoporosis should start as soon as possible after the onset of menopause in women with increased risk for future osteoporotic fractures. The effect of estrogens on the bone mineral density is dose-dependent. Protection appears to be effective for as long as treatment is continued.

After 3 years of treatment with Premique 0.625mg/2.5mg, the increase in lumbar spine bone mineral density (BMD) was 4.87% ± 0.66. The percentage of women who maintained (less than 1% BMD loss per year) or gained BMD in lumbar zone during treatment was 92%.

Premique 0.625mg/2.5mg also had an effect on hip BMD. The increase after 3 years was 1.94% ± 0.44 at total hip. The percentage of women who maintained (less than 1% BMD loss per year) or gained BMD in hip zone during treatment was 88%.

5.2 Pharmacokinetic properties

Absorption

Conjugated estrogens are soluble in water and are well absorbed from the gastrointestinal tract after release from the drug formulation. However Premique contains a formulation of medroxyprogesterone acetate (MPA) that is immediately released and conjugated estrogens that are slowly released over several hours. MPA is well absorbed from the gastrointestinal tract. Table 1 summarises the mean pharmacokinetic parameters for unconjugated and conjugated estrogens, and medroxyprogesterone acetate following administration of 2 Premique 0.625/2.5mg and 2 Premique 0.625/5mg tablets to healthy postmenopausal women.

Table 1 – Pharmacokinetic parameters for Premique

Pharmacokinetic parameters for unconjugated and conjugated estrogens (CE) and medroxyprogesterone acetate (MPA)

(see Table 1 below)

Distribution

The distribution of exogenous estrogens is similar to that of endogenous estrogens. Estrogens are widely distributed in the body and are generally found in higher concentrations in the sex hormone target organs. Estrogens circulate in the blood largely bound to sex hormone biding globulin (SHBG) and albumin. MPA is approximately 90% bound to plasma proteins but does not bind to SHBG.

Metabolism

Exogenous estrogens are metabolised in the same manner as endogenous estrogens. Circulating estrogens exist in a dynamic equilibrium of metabolic interconversions. These transformations take place mainly in the liver. Oestradiol is converted reversibly to estrone, and both can be converted to oestriol, which is the major urinary metabolite. Estrogens also undergo enterohepatic recirculation via sulphate and glucuronide conjugation in the liver, biliary secretion of conjugates into the intestine, and hydrolysis in the gut followed by reabsorption. In postmenopausal women a significant proportion of the circulating estrogens exists as sulphate conjugates, especially estrone sulphate, which serves as a circulating reservoir for the formation of more active estrogens. Metabolism and elimination of MPA occur primarily in the liver via hydroxylation, with subsequent conjugation and elimination in the urine.

Excretion

Estradiol, estrone and estriol are excreted in the urine along with glucuronide and sulphate conjugates. Most metabolites of MPA are extracted as glucuronide conjugates with only minor amounts secreted as sulphates.

5.3 Preclinical safety data

Long-term continuous administration of natural and synthetic estrogens in certain animal species increases the frequency of carcinomas of the breast, cervix, vagina and liver.

In a two-year oral study in which female rats were exposed to MPA dosages of up to 5000μg/kg/day in their diets (50 times higher - based on AUC values - than the level observed in women taking 10mg of MPA), a dose-related increase in pancreatic islet cell tumours (adenomas and carcinomas) occurred. Pancreatic tumour incidence was increased at 1000 and 5000μg/kg/day, but not at 200μg/kg/day.

The cortisol activity of MPA at these high doses is thought to increase serum glucose in rats which reactively stimulates the beta cells of the pancreatic islets to produce insulin. This repeated stimulation is thought to cause the tumours in rats. Similar lesions are not likely to occur in humans since the endocrine system of rats is more sensitive to hormones than that of women. When MPA is combined with estrogen, MPA binds to fewer glucocorticosteriod receptors and thus has less effect on plasma glucose. In humans, the diabetogenic response to MPA at therapeutic doses is slight. Moreover, an extensive literature search revealed no evidence that MPA causes pancreatic tumours in humans.

6. PHARMACEUTICAL PARTICULARS

6.1 List of excipients

Tablet core:

Lactose monohydrate

Methylcellulose

Magnesium stearate

Calcium phosphate tribasic

Tablet coating:

Calcium sulphate anhydrous

Polyethylene glycol

Glyceryl mono-oleate

Shellac

Microcrystalline cellulose

Sucrose

Titanium dioxide

Povidone

Carnauba wax

Colour (E132)

6.2 Incompatibilities

None known.

6.3 Shelf life

Three years.

6.4 Special precautions for storage

Do not store above 25°C.

6.5 Nature and contents of container

Polyvinylchloride (PVC)/Aluminium foil blister pack of 14 tablets. Cartons of 2 blisters (28 tablets) or 6 blisters (84 tablets).

6.6 Instructions for use and handling

No special instructions.

Table 1 – Pharmacokinetic parameters for Premique

Drug	2 × 0.625mg CE/2.5mg MPA Combination Tablets (n=54)				2 × 0.625mg CE/5mg MPA Combination Tablets (n=51)			
PK Parameter Arithmetic Mean (%CV)	C_{max} (pg/mL)	t_{max} (h)	$t_{1/2}$- (h)	AUC (pg.h/mL)	C_{max} (pg/mL)	t_{max} (h)	$t_{1/2}$- (h)	AUC (pg.h/mL)
Unconjugated Estrogens								
Estrone	175(23)	7.6(24)	31.6(23)	5358(34)	124(43)	10(35)	62.2(137)	6303(40)
BA*-Estrone	159(26)	7.6(24)	16.9(34)	3313(40)	104(49)	10(35)	26.0(100)	3136(51)
Equilin	71(31)	5.8(34)	9.9(35)	951(43)	54(43)	8.9(34)	15.5(53)	1179(56)
PK Parameter Arithmetic Mean (%CV)	C_{max} (pg/mL)	t_{max} (h)	$t_{1/2}$- (h)	AUC (pg.h/mL)	C_{max} (pg/mL)	t_{max} (h)	$t_{1/2}$- (h)	AUC (pg.h/mL)
Conjugated Estrogens								
Total Estrone	6.6(38)	6.1(28)	20.7(34)	116(59)	6.3(48)	9.1(29)	23.6(36)	151(42)
BA* - Total Estrone	6.4(39)	6.1(28)	15.4(34)	100(57)	6.2(48)	9.1(29)	20.6(35)	139(40)
Total Equilin	5.1(45)	4.6(35)	11.4(25)	50(70)	4.2(52)	7.0(36)	17.2(131)	72(50)
PK Parameter Arithmetic Mean (%CV)	C_{max} (pg/mL)	t_{max} (h)	$t_{1/2}$- (h)	AUC (pg.h/mL)	C_{max} (pg/mL)	t_{max} (h)	$t_{1/2}$- (h)	AUC (pg.h/mL)
Medroxyprogesterone acetate								
MPA	1.5(40)	2.8(54)	37.6(30)	37(30)	4.8(31)	2.4(50)	46.3(39)	102(28)

BA* = Baseline adjusted

$T_{1/2}$ = apparent terminal phase disposition half life (0.693/λ_z)

7. MARKETING AUTHORISATION HOLDER

John Wyeth and Brother Limited

Trading as: Wyeth Pharmaceuticals

Huntercombe Lane South

Taplow, Maidenhead

Berkshire SL6 0PH

8. MARKETING AUTHORISATION NUMBER(S)

PL 00011/0212.

9. DATE OF FIRST AUTHORISATION/RENEWAL OF THE AUTHORISATION

27th September 1995

10. DATE OF REVISION OF THE TEXT

Approved 11 February 2005

* Trade Mark

Premique Cycle

(Wyeth Pharmaceuticals)

1. NAME OF THE MEDICINAL PRODUCT

Premique Cycle.

2. QUALITATIVE AND QUANTITATIVE COMPOSITION

Premique Cycle is a combination of conjugated estrogens* USP and medroxyprogesterone acetate (MPA) Ph.Eur.

Premique Cycle is composed of 14 tablets containing 0.625mg conjugated estrogens and 14 combination tablets containing 0.625mg conjugated estrogens and 10mg MPA.

*Conjugated estrogens contain sodium estrone sulphate, sodium equilin sulphate, 17α-dihydroequilin, 17α-estradiol, equilenin, 17α-dihydroequilenin, 17β-dihydroequilin, 17β-dihydroequilenin, 17β-estradiol and 8,9-dehydro-estrone.

3. PHARMACEUTICAL FORM

Premique Cycle is available for oral administration as conjugated estrogens 0.625mg tablets and conjugated estrogens/MPA (0.625mg/10mg) combination tablets. Conjugated estrogens 0.625mg tablets are white, oval, biconvex sugar-coated tablets marked "0.625". Conjugated estrogens/MPA (0.625mg/10mg) combination tablets are green, oval, biconvex sugar-coated tablets marked "0.625/10".

4. CLINICAL PARTICULARS

4.1 Therapeutic indications

• Hormone replacement therapy for estrogen deficiency symptoms in menopausal and postmenopausal women

• Second line therapy for prevention of osteoporosis in postmenopausal women at high risk of future fractures who are intolerant of, or contraindicated for, other medicinal products approved for the prevention of osteoporosis.

4.2 Posology and method of administration

Adults:

Premique Cycle is available for oral use in a sequential regimen for treatment of women with a uterus. That is, for the first 14 days of each cycle (days 1-14), one white tablet containing conjugated estrogens 0.625mg is taken daily, and for the last 14 days (days 15-28), one green tablet containing conjugated estrogens 0.625mg and MPA 10mg is taken daily. There should be no break between packs.

For most post-menopausal women, therapy may be commenced at any convenient time, although if the patient is still menstruating, commencement on the first day of bleeding is recommended. In women transferring from another sequential hormone replacement therapy regimen, treatment should begin the day following completion of the prior regimen.

Patients should be advised that a regular withdrawal bleed will usually occur at the end of one cycle of Premique Cycle and the beginning of the next.

For treatment of postmenopausal symptoms: Conjugated estrogens 0.625mg daily for the first 14 days of each cycle, followed by conjugated estrogens/MPA (0.625mg/10mg) combination tablet daily on days 15 to 28.

For prevention and treatment of osteoporosis associated with estrogen deficiency: Conjugated estrogens 0.625mg daily for the first 14 days and conjugated estrogens/MPA (0.625mg/10mg) combination tablet taken daily on days 15 to 28. (See section 5.1 Pharmacological Properties)

Maintenance/Continuation/Extended Treatment:

For treatment of postmenopausal symptoms, the lowest effective dose should be used. HRT should only be continued as long as the benefit in alleviation of severe symptoms outweighs the risk.

The benefits of the lower risk of endometrial hyperplasia and endometrial cancer due to adding a progestogen should be weighed against the increased risk of breast cancer (see sections 4.4 Special Warnings and Precautions for Use and 4.8 Undesirable Effects).

Forgotten tablet: If a tablet is forgotten, it should be taken as soon as the patient remembers, therapy should then be continued as before. If more than one tablet has been forgotten only the most recent tablet should be taken.

The patient should not take double the usual dose to make up for the missed tablet.

Missed pills may cause breakthrough bleeding.

Elderly:

There are no special dosage requirements for elderly patients, but, as with all medicines, the lowest effective dose should be used.

Children:

Not recommended.

4.3 Contraindications

1. Known, past or suspected cancer of the breast.

2. Known or suspected estrogen-dependent malignant tumours (e.g. endometrial cancer)

3. Undiagnosed abnormal genital bleeding.

4. Untreated endometrial hyperplasia

5. Active or past history of venous thromboembolism (e.g. deep vein thrombosis, pulmonary embolism)

6. Active or recent arterial thromboembolic disease (e.g. angina, myocardial infarction)

7. Acute liver disease or history of liver disease where the liver function tests have failed to return to normal.

8. Known hypersensitivity to the active substances or to any of the excipients of Premique Cycle tablets.

9. Porphyria

4.4 Special warnings and special precautions for use

1. Medical examination/Follow up

Before initiating or reinstituting HRT, a complete personal and family medical history should be taken. Physical (including pelvic and breast) examination should be guided by the contraindications and warnings for use. During treatment, periodic check-ups are recommended of a frequency and nature adapted to the individual women. Women should be advised what changes in their breasts should be reported to their doctor or nurse. Investigations, including mammography, should be carried out in accordance with currently accepted screening practices, modified to the clinical needs of the individual. A careful appraisal of the risks and benefits should be undertaken at least annually in women treated with hormone replacement therapy.

In women with an intact uterus, the benefits of the lower risk of endometrial hyperplasia and endometrial cancer due to adding progestogen should be weighed against the increased risk of breast cancer (see below and Section 4.8 Undesirable Effects).

2. Conditions that need supervision

If any of the following conditions are present, have occurred previously, and/or have been aggravated during pregnancy or previous hormone treatment, the patient should be closely supervised. It should be taken into account that these conditions may recur or be aggravated during treatment with Premique Cycle, in particular:

- Leiomyoma (uterine fibroids) or endometriosis
- A family history of, or other risk factors for, thromboembolic disorders (see below)
- Risk factors for estrogen dependent tumours (e.g. 1st degree heredity for breast cancer)
- Hypertension
- Liver disorders (e.g. liver adenoma)
- Diabetes mellitus with or without vascular involvement
- Cholelithiasis
- Migraine or (severe) headaches
- Systemic lupus erythematosus (SLE)
- A history of endometrial hyperplasia (see below)
- Epilepsy
- Asthma
- Otosclerosis

3. Reasons for immediate withdrawal of therapy

Therapy should be discontinued if a contra-indication is discovered and in the following situations:

- Jaundice or deterioration in liver function
- Significant increase in blood pressure
- New onset of migraine-type headache
- Pregnancy

4. Endometrial Hyperplasia

The risk of endometrial hyperplasia and carcinoma is increased when estrogens are administered alone for prolonged periods. The addition of a progestogen for at least 12 days of the cycle in non-hysterectomised women reduces, but may not eliminate, this risk (see section 4.8 Undesirable Effects). Unless there is a previous diagnosis of endometriosis it is not recommended to add a progestogen in hysterectomised women (see 4.4 – Special Warnings and Precautions for Use).

The reduction in risk to the endometrium should be weighed against the increase in the risk of breast cancer of added progestogen (see 'Breast cancer' below and Section 4.8 Undesirable Effects).

Break-through bleeding and spotting may occur during the first months of treatment. If break-through bleeding or spotting appears after some time on therapy, or continues after treatment has been discontinued, the reason should be investigated, which may include endometrial biopsy to exclude endometrial malignancy.

5. Breast Cancer

Randomised controlled trials and epidemiological studies have reported an increased risk of breast cancer in women taking estrogen or estrogen-progestogen combinations for HRT for several years (see Section 4.8 Undesirable Effects). An observational study of almost 829,000 women has shown that, compared to never-users, use of estrogen-progestogen combined HRT is associated with a higher risk of breast cancer (RR = 2.00, 95%CI: 1.88 - 2.12) than use of estrogens alone (RR = 1.30, 95%CI: 1.21 – 1.40). In this study the magnitude of the increase in breast cancer risk was similar for all estrogen-only preparations, irrespective of the type, dose or route of administration of the estrogen (oral, transdermal and implanted). Likewise the magnitude of the increased risk was similar for all estrogen plus progestogen preparations, irrespective of the type of progestogen or the number of days of addition per cycle. For all HRT, an excess risk becomes apparent within 1-2 years of starting treatment and increases with the duration of use of HRT but begins to decline when HRT is stopped and by 5 years reaches the same level as in women who have never taken HRT.

The increase in risk applies to all women studied, although the relative risk was significantly higher in those with a lean or normal body build (body mass index or BMI of $<25kg/m^2$) compared to those with a BMI of $\geqslant 25kg/m^2$.

At present the effect of HRT on the diagnosis of breast tumours remains unclear – all women should be encouraged to report any changes in their breasts to their doctor or nurse.

6. Venous thromboembolism

Hormone replacement therapy (HRT) is associated with a higher relative risk of developing venous thromboembolism (VTE) i.e. deep vein thrombosis or pulmonary embolism. One randomised controlled trial and epidemiological studies found a two to threefold higher risk for users compared with non-users. For non- users it is estimated that the number of cases of VTE that will occur over a 5-year period is about 3 per 1000 women aged 50-59 years and 8 per 1000 women aged between 60-69 years. It is estimated that in healthy women who use HRT for 5 years, the number of additional cases of VTE over a 5-year period will be between 2 and 6 (best estimate 4) per 1000 women aged 50-59 years and between 5 and 15 (best estimate = 9) per 1000 women aged 60-69 years. The occurrence of such an event is more likely in the first year of HRT than later.

Generally recognised risk factors for VTE include a personal or family history and severe obesity (Body Mass Index $>30kg/m^2$) and systemic lupus erythematosus (SLE). There is no consensus about the possible role of varicose veins in VTE.

Patients with a history of VTE or known thrombophilic states have an increased risk of VTE. HRT may add to this risk. Personal or strong family history of thromboembolism or recurrent spontaneous abortion should be investigated in order to exclude a thrombophilic predisposition. Until a thorough evaluation of thrombophilic factors has been made or anticoagulant treatment initiated, use of HRT in such patients should be viewed as contraindicated. Those women already on anticoagulant treatment require careful consideration of the benefit-risk of use of HRT.

The risk of VTE may be temporarily increased with prolonged immobilisation, major trauma or major surgery. As in all postoperative patients, scrupulous attention should be given to prophylactic measures to prevent VTE following surgery. Where prolonged immobilisation is liable to follow elective surgery, particularly abdominal or orthopaedic surgery to the lower limbs, consideration should be given to temporarily stopping HRT 4-6 weeks earlier, if this is possible. Treatment should not be restarted until the woman is completely mobilised.

If venous thromboembolism develops after initiating therapy, the drug should be discontinued. Patients should be told to contact their doctors immediately when they are aware of potential thromboembolic symptoms (e.g. painful swelling of a leg, sudden pain in the chest, dyspnoea).

7. Coronary Artery Disease (CAD)

There is no evidence from randomised controlled trials of cardiovascular benefit with continuous combined conjugated estrogens and MPA. Large clinical trials showed a possible increased risk of cardiovascular morbidity in the first year of use and no benefit thereafter. For other HRT products, there are as yet no randomised controlled trials examining benefit in cardiovascular morbidity or mortality. Therefore, it is uncertain whether these findings also extend to other HRT products.

8. Stroke

One large randomised clinical trial (WHI-trial) found, as a secondary outcome, an increased risk of stroke in healthy women during treatment with continuous combined conjugated estrogens and MPA. For women who do not use HRT, it is estimated that the number of cases of stroke that will occur over a 5 year period is about 3 per 1000 women aged 50-59 years and 11 per 1000 women aged 60-69 years. It is estimated that for women who use conjugated estrogens and MPA for 5 years, the number of additional cases will be between 0 and 3 (best estimate =1) per 1000 users aged 50-59 years and between 1 and 9 (best estimate = 4) per 1000 users aged 60-69 years. It is unknown whether the increased risk also extends to other HRT products.

9. Ovarian Cancer

Long term (at least 5-10 years) use of estrogen-only HRT products in hysterectomised women has been associated with an increased risk of ovarian cancer in some epidemiological studies. It is uncertain whether long-term use of combined HRT confers different risk than estrogen-only products.

Other Conditions

10. Estrogens/progestogens may cause fluid retention and therefore patients with cardiac or renal dysfunction should be carefully observed. Patients with terminal renal insufficiency should be closely observed, since it is expected that the level of circulating active ingredients in Premique Cycle is increased.

11. The use of estrogen may influence the laboratory results of certain endocrine tests and liver enzymes.

Estrogens increase thyroid binding globulin (TBG), leading to increased circulating total thyroid hormone, as measured by protein-bound iodine (PBI), T4 levels (by column or by radio-immunoassay) or T3 levels (by radio-immunoassay). T3 resin uptake is decreased, reflecting the elevated TBG. Free T4 and free T3 concentrations are unaltered.

Other binding proteins may be elevated in serum, i.e. corticoid binding globulin (CBG), sex-hormone-binding globulin (SHBG) leading to increased circulating corticosteroids and sex steroids, respectively. Free or biologically active hormone concentrations are unchanged. Other plasma proteins may be increased (angiotensinogen/renin substrate, alpha-I-antitrypsin, ceruloplasmin).

Some patients dependent on thyroid hormone replacement therapy may require increased doses in order to maintain their free thyroid hormone levels in an acceptable range. Therefore, patients should have their thyroid function monitored more frequently when commencing concurrent treatment in order to maintain their free thyroid hormone levels in an acceptable range.

12. There is an increase in the risk of gallbladder disease in women receiving HRT (see conditions that need supervision)

13. A worsening of glucose tolerance may occur in some patients on estrogen/progestogen therapy and therefore diabetic patients should be carefully observed while receiving hormone replacement therapy.

14. Women with pre-existing hypertriglyceridemia should be followed closely during estrogen replacement or hormone replacement therapy, since rare cases of large increases of plasma triglycerides leading to pancreatitis have been reported with estrogen therapy in this condition.

15. Estrogens should be used with caution in individuals with severe hypocalcaemia

16. Epidemiological studies suggest a number of individual risk factors which contribute to the development of postmenopausal osteoporosis. These include: early menopause; family history of osteoporosis; thin, small frame; cigarette use; recent prolonged systemic corticosteroid use. If several of these risk factors are present in a patient, consideration should be given to estrogen replacement therapy.

4.5 Interaction with other medicinal products and other forms of Interaction

The metabolism of estrogens and progestogens may be increased by concomitant use of substances known to induce drug-metabolising enzymes, specifically cytochrome P450 enzymes, such as anticonvulsants (e.g. phenobarbital, phenytoin, carbamazepine) and anti-infectives (e.g. rifampicin, rifabutin, nevirapine, efavirenz).

Ritonavir and nelfinavir, although known as strong inhibitors, by contrast exhibit inducing properties when used concomitantly with steroid hormones.

Herbal preparations containing St John's wort *(Hypericum perforatum)* may induce the metabolism of estrogens and progestogens.

Clinically, an increased metabolism of estrogens and progestogens may lead to decreased effect and changes in the uterine bleeding profile.

The response to metyrapone may be reduced.

Aminogluthimide administered concomitantly with MPA may significantly depress the bioavailablity of MPA.

4.6 Pregnancy and lactation

Pregnancy:

Premique Cycle is not indicated during pregnancy. If pregnancy occurs during medication with Premique treatment should be withdrawn immediately.

Clinically, data on a limited number of exposed pregnancies indicate no adverse effects of MPA on the foetus.

The results of most epidemiological studies to date relevant to inadvertent foetal exposure to combinations of estrogens and progestogens indicate no teratogenic or foetotoxic effect.

Lactation:

Premique Cycle is not indicated during lactation.

4.7 Effects on ability to drive and use machines

Premique Cycle should not affect the ability to drive or use machines.

4.8 Undesirable effects

See also 4.4 Special Warnings and Special Precautions for Use.

Adverse drug reactions (ADRs)

The adverse reactions listed in the table are based on post-marketing spontaneous (reporting rate), clinical trials and class-effects. Breast pain is a very common adverse event reported in ⩾ 10% of patients.

System Organ Class	Adverse Reaction
Reproductive system & breast disorders	Breakthrough bleeding/ dysmenorrhoea, spotting; Breast pain, tenderness, enlargement, discharge Change in menstrual flow; Change in cervical ectropion and secretion Galactorrhoea; Increased size of uterine leiomyomata
Gastrointestinal disorders	Nausea; Bloating; Abdominal pain; Vomiting; Pancreatitis
Nervous	Anxiety; Dizziness; Headache (including migraine); Exacerbation of epilepsy;
Musculoskeletal, connective tissue and bone disorders	Arthralgias; Leg cramps
Psychiatric	Depression; Changes in libido; Mood disturbances; Irritability
Vascular	Pulmonary embolism; Deep Venous thrombophlebitis, Superficial thrombophlebitis
Cardiac disorders	Myocardial Infarction
General disorders and administration site disorders	Oedema
Skin and subcutaneous tissue disorders	Alopecia; Acne; Pruritus; Chloasma/melasma; Hirsutism; Rash
Infections and infestations	Vaginitis, including vaginal candidiasis
Immune system disorders	Urticaria; Angioedeoma; Anaphylactic/anaphylactoid reactions
Metabolism and nutrition disorders	Glucose intolerance
Eye disorders	Intolerance to contact lenses
Respiratory, thoracic and mediastinal disorders	Exacerbation of asthma
Hepatobiliary	Gallbladder disease
Neoplasms benign and malignant	Breast cancer*; Fibrocystic breast changes; Ovarian Cancer
Investigations	Changes in weight (increase or decrease)

Breast cancer

* The risk of breast cancer increases with the number of years of HRT usage. According to data from a recent epidemiological study in about 829,000 postmenopausal women, the best estimate of the risk is that for women not using HRT, in total 32 in every 1000 are expected to have breast cancer diagnosed between the ages of 50 and 65 years. Among those with current or recent use of estrogen-only replacement therapy, it is estimated that the total number of additional cases during the corresponding period will be between 0 and 3 (best estimate = 1.5) per 1000 for 5 years' use and between 3 and 7 (best estimate = 5) per 1000 for 10 years' use (see table). Among those with current or recent use of estrogen plus progestogen combined HRT, it is estimated that the total number of additional cases will be between 5 and 7 (best estimate = 6) per 1000 for 5 years' use and between 18 and 20 (best estimate = 19) per 1000 for 10 years' use (See section 4.4 Special Warnings and Precautions for Use). The number of additional cases of breast cancer is broadly similar for women who start HRT irrespective of age at start of HRT use (between the ages of 45-65).

	No of additional cases of breast cancer diagnosed per 1000 women (95% confidence intervals)	
Type of HRT	5 years of use	10 years of use
Estrogen-only	1.5 (0-3)	5 (3-7)
Combined	6 (5-7)	19 (18-20)

Endometrial Cancer

In women with an intact uterus, the risk of endometrial hyperplasia and endometrial cancer increases with the increasing duration of use of unopposed estrogens and is substantially reduced by the addition of a progestogen (see section 4.4 Special Warnings and Precautions for Use). According to data from epidemiological studies the best estimate of the risk of endometrial cancer is that for women not using HRT, about 5 in every 1000 are expected to have endometrial cancer diagnosed between the ages of 50 and 65. It is estimated that, among those who use estrogen-only replacement therapy, there will be 4 additional cases per 100 after 5 years' use and 10 additional cases per 1000 after 10 years' use. Adding a progestogen to estrogen-only therapy substantially reduces, but may not eliminate, the increased risk.

Other adverse reactions reported in association with estrogen/progestogen treatment including Premique Cycle:

- Estrogen-dependent neoplasms benign and malignant, e.g. endometrial hyperplasia, endometrial cancer
- Venous thromboembolism, i.e. deep leg or pelvic venous thrombosis and pulmonary embolism, is more frequent among hormone replacement therapy users than among non-users. For further information, see section 4.3 Contra-indications and 4.4 Special Warnings and Precautions for Use.
- Retinal vascular thrombosis
- Myocardial infarction
- Stroke
- Increases in blood pressure
- Cholestatic jaundice
- Enlargement of hepatic haemangiomas
- Skin and subcutaneous disorders: erythema multiforme, erythema nodosum, vascular purpura
- Exacerbation of chorea
- Exacerbation of porphyria
- Exacerbation of hypocalcaemia
- Exacerbation of otosclerosis

4.9 Overdose

Numerous reports of ingestion of large doses of estrogen/ progestogen-containing oral contraceptives by young children indicate that acute serious ill effects do not occur. Overdosage of estrogens may cause nausea and vomiting and withdrawal bleeding may occur in females. There is no specific antidote and further treatment should be symptomatic.

5. PHARMACOLOGICAL PROPERTIES

5.1 Pharmacodynamic properties

ATC Code: GO3F A12

Conjugated Estrogens

The active ingredients are primarily the sulphate esters of estrone, equilin sulphates, 17α-estradiol and 17β-estradiol. These substitute for the loss of estrogen production in menopausal women, and alleviate menopausal symptoms. Estrogens prevent bone loss following menopause or ovariectomy.

Progestogen:

As estrogens promote the growth of the endometrium, unopposed estrogens increase the risk of endometrial hyperplasia and cancer. The addition of a progestogen reduces but does not eliminate the estrogen-induced risk of endometrial hyperplasia in non-hysterectomised women.

Relief of estrogen-deficiency symptoms

In a 1-year clinical trial (n=2,808), vasomotor symptoms were assessed for efficacy during the first 12 weeks of treatment in a subset of symptomatic women (n=241) who had at least 7 moderate or severe hot flushes daily or 50 moderate to severe hot flushes during the week before randomisation. Premique 0.625mg/2.5mg (conjugated estrogens/medroxyprogesterone acetate) was shown to be statistically better than placebo at weeks 4, 8 and 12 for relief of both frequency and severity of moderate to severe vasomotor symptoms.

In two clinical trials, the incidence of amenorrhoea (no bleeding or spotting) increased over time in women treated with Premique 0.625mg/2.5mg. Amenorrhoea was seen in 68% of women at cycle 6 and 77% of women at cycle 12. Breakthrough bleeding and/or spotting appeared in 48% during the first 3 months, and in 24% of women during months 10-12 of treatment.

Prevention of osteoporosis

Estrogen deficiency at menopause is associated with an increasing bone turnover and decline in bone mass. Therefore, if possible, treatment for prevention of osteoporosis should start as soon as possible after the onset of menopause in women with increased risk for future osteoporotic fractures. The effect of estrogens on the bone mineral density is dose-dependent. Protection appears to be effective for as long as treatment is continued.

After 3 years of treatment with Premique 0.625mg/2.5mg, the increase in lumbar spine bone mineral density (BMD) was 4.87% ± 0.66. The percentage of women who maintained (less than 1% BMD loss per year) or gained BMD in lumbar zone during treatment was 92%.

Premique 0.625mg/2.5mg also had an effect on hip BMD. The increase after 3 years was 1.94% ± 0.44 at total hip. The percentage of women who maintained (less than 1% BMD loss per year) or gained BMD in hip zone during treatment was 88%.

5.2 Pharmacokinetic properties

Absorption

Conjugated estrogens are soluble in water and are well absorbed from the gastrointestinal tract after release from the drug formulation. However Premique contains a formulation of medroxyprogesterone acetate (MPA) that is immediately released and conjugated estrogens that are slowly released over several hours. MPA is well absorbed from the gastrointestinal tract. Table 1 summarises the mean pharmacokinetic parameters for unconjugated and conjugated estrogens, and medroxyprogesterone acetate following administration of 2 Premique 0.625/2.5mg and 2 Premique 0.625/5mg tablets to healthy postmenopausal women.

Distribution

The distribution of exogenous estrogens is similar to that of endogenous estrogens. Estrogens are widely distributed in the body and are generally found in higher concentrations in the sex hormone target organs. Estrogens circulate in the blood largely bound to sex hormone binding globulin (SHBG) and albumin. MPA is approximately 90% bound to plasma proteins but does not bind to SHBG.

Metabolism

Exogenous estrogens are metabolised in the same manner as endogenous estrogens. Circulating estrogens exist in a dynamic equilibrium of metabolic interconversions. These transformations take place mainly in the liver. Estradiol is converted reversibly to estrone, and both can be converted to estriol, which is the major urinary metabolite. Estrogens also undergo enterohepatic recirculation via sulphate and glucuronide conjugation in the liver, biliary secretion of conjugates into the intestine, and hydrolysis in the gut followed by reabsorption. In postmenopausal women a significant proportion of the circulating estrogens exists as sulphate conjugates, especially estrone sulphate, which serves as a circulating reservoir for the formation of more active estrogens. Metabolism and elimination of MPA occur primarily in the liver via hydroxylation, with subsequent conjugation and elimination in the urine.

Excretion

Estradiol, estrone and estriol are excreted in the urine along with glucuronide and sulphate conjugates. Most metabolites of MPA are extracted as glucuronide conjugates with only minor amounts secreted as sulphates.

Table 1 – Pharmacokinetic parameters for Premique

Pharmacokinetic parameters for unconjugated and conjugated estrogens (CE) and medroxyprogesterone acetate (MPA)

(see Table 1 on next page)

5.3 Preclinical safety data

Long-term continuous administration of natural and synthetic estrogens in certain animal species increases the frequency of carcinomas of the breast, cervix, vagina and liver.

In a two-year oral study in which female rats were exposed to MPA dosages of up to 5000μg/kg/day in their diets (50 times higher – based on AUC values – than the level observed in women taking 10mg of MPA), a dose-related increase in pancreatic islet cell tumours (adenomas and carcinomas) occurred. Pancreatic tumour incidence was increased at 1000 and 5000μg/kg/day, but not at 200μg/kg/day.

The cortisol activity of MPA at these high doses is thought to increase serum glucose in rats which reactively stimulates the beta cells of the pancreatic islets to produce insulin. This repeated stimulation is thought to cause the tumours in rats. Similar lesions are not likely to occur in humans, since the endocrine system of rats is more sensitive to hormones than that of women. When MPA is combined with estrogen, MPA binds to fewer glucocorticosteroid receptors and thus has less effect on plasma glucose. In humans, the diabetogenic response to MPA at therapeutic doses is slight. Moreover, an extensive literature search revealed no evidence that MPA causes pancreatic tumours in humans.

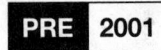

Table 1 – Pharmacokinetic parameters for Premique

Drug	2 × 0.625mg CE/2.5mg MPA Combination Tablets (n=54)				2 × 0.625mg CE/5mg MPA Combination Tablets (n=51)			
PK Parameter Arithmetic Mean (%CV)	C_{max} (pg/mL)	t_{max} (h)	$t_{1/2-}$ (h)	AUC (pg.h/mL)	C_{max} (pg/mL)	t_{max} (h)	$t_{1/2-}$ (h)	AUC (pg.h/mL)
Unconjugated Estrogens								
Estrone	175(23)	7.6(24)	31.6(23)	5358(34)	124(43)	10(35)	62.2(137)	6303(40)
BA*-Estrone	159(26)	7.6(24)	16.9(34)	3313(40)	104(49)	10(35)	26.0(100)	3136(51)
Equilin	71(31)	5.8(34)	9.9(35)	951(43)	54(43)	8.9(34)	15.5(53)	1179(56)
PK Parameter Arithmetic Mean (%CV)	C_{max} (pg/mL)	t_{max} (h)	$t_{1/2-}$ (h)	AUC (pg.h/mL)	C_{max} (pg/mL)	t_{max} (h)	$t_{1/2-}$ (h)	AUC (pg.h/mL)
Conjugated Estrogens								
Total Estrone	6.6(38)	6.1(28)	20.7(34)	116(59)	6.3(48)	9.1(29)	23.6(36)	151(42)
BA* - Total Estrone	6.4(39)	6.1(28)	15.4(34)	100(57)	6.2(48)	9.1(29)	20.6(35)	139(40)
Total Equilin	5.1(45)	4.6(35)	11.4(25)	50(70)	4.2(52)	7.0(36)	17.2(131)	72(50)
PK Parameter Arithmetic Mean (%CV)	C_{max} (pg/mL)	t_{max} (h)	$t_{1/2-}$ (h)	AUC (pg.h/mL)	C_{max} (pg/mL)	t_{max} (h)	$t_{1/2-}$ (h)	AUC (pg.h/mL)
Medroxyprogesterone acetate								
MPA	1.5(40)	2.8(54)	37.6(30)	37(30)	4.8(31)	2.4(50)	46.3(39)	102(28)

BA* = Baseline adjusted

$T_{1/2}$ = apparent terminal phase disposition half life ($0.693/\lambda_z$)

6. PHARMACEUTICAL PARTICULARS

6.1 List of excipients

White (conjugated estrogens) tablets: calcium phosphate tribasic, calcium sulphate, carnauba wax, microcrystalline cellulose, glyceryl mono-oleate, lactose, magnesium stearate, methylcellulose, macrogol, shellac, sucrose, titanium dioxide (E171) and edible printing ink†.

Green (conjugated estrogens/MPA) combination tablets: calcium phosphate tribasic, calcium sulphate, carnauba wax, microcrystalline cellulose, glyceryl mono-oleate, lactose, magnesium stearate, methylcellulose, methyl hydroxybenzoate, macrogol, povidone, propyl hydroxybenzoate, shellac, sodium benzoate, sucrose, indigo carmine (E132), titanium dioxide (E171), iron oxide yellow (E172) and edible printing ink†.

† contains iron oxide black (E172), shellac, propylene glycol, ethanol, ethyl acetate, N-Butyl alcohol.

6.2 Incompatibilities

None known.

6.3 Shelf life

Two years.

6.4 Special precautions for storage

Store in the original package. Do not store above 25°C.

6.5 Nature and contents of container

Primary container

Polyvinylchloride (PVC)/Aluminium foil blister pack.

Secondary container

Cardboard carton.

Presentation

Cartons containing 3 blisters. Each blister contains 14 conjugated estrogen tablets 0.625mg and 14 conjugated estrogen 0.625mg/MPA 10mg tablets.

6.6 Instructions for use and handling

No special instructions.

7. MARKETING AUTHORISATION HOLDER

John Wyeth and Brother Limited

Trading as: Wyeth Pharmaceuticals

Taplow, Maidenhead,

Berkshire SL6 0PH,

England, UK.

8. MARKETING AUTHORISATION NUMBER(S)

PL 0011/0239

9. DATE OF FIRST AUTHORISATION/RENEWAL OF THE AUTHORISATION

30 April 1999.

10. DATE OF REVISION OF THE TEXT

Approved 11th February 2005

Premique Low Dose 0.3mg/1.5mg Coated Tablets

(Wyeth Pharmaceuticals)

1. NAME OF THE MEDICINAL PRODUCT

Premique Low Dose 0.3 mg/1.5 mg coated tablets.

2. QUALITATIVE AND QUANTITATIVE COMPOSITION

Premique Low Dose 0.3 mg/1.5 mg coated tablets are for oral administration containing conjugated estrogens† 0.3 mg and medroxyprogesterone acetate (MPA) 1.5 mg.

†Conjugated estrogens contain the sodium sulphate conjugates of estrone, equilin, 17α-dihydroequilin, 17α-estradiol, 17β-dihydroequilin, 17α-dihydroequilenin, 17β-dihydroequilenin, equilenin, 17β-estradiol and Δ8,9-dehydro-estrone.

For excipients, see section 6.1.

3. PHARMACEUTICAL FORM

Coated tablet.

Cream oval biconvex sugar coated tablet marked 'W 0.3/1.5' in black ink.

4. CLINICAL PARTICULARS

4.1 Therapeutic indications

Hormone replacement therapy for estrogen deficiency symptoms in postmenopausal women with an intact uterus.

4.2 Posology and method of administration

Premique Low Dose is taken orally in a continuous combined 28-day regimen of one tablet daily with no break between packs.

In women who are not taking hormone replacement therapy or women who switch from another continuous combined hormone replacement therapy product, treatment may be started on any convenient day. In women transferring from a sequential hormone replacement therapy regimen, treatment should begin the day following completion of the prior regimen.

For treatment of postmenopausal symptoms: Take one tablet per day.

Breakthrough bleeding and spotting may occur in the early stages of Premique Low Dose therapy. If breakthrough bleeding persists and endometrial abnormality has been ruled out, a higher dose of treatment or cyclic therapy should be considered as an alternative.

The lowest dose and regimen that will control symptoms should be chosen.

Maintenance/Continuation/Extended treatment

For treatment of postmenopausal symptoms, the lowest effective dose should be used. HRT should only be continued as long as the benefit in alleviation of severe symptoms outweighs the risk.

The benefits of the lower risk of endometrial hyperplasia and endometrial cancer due to adding a progestogen should be weighed against the increased risk of breast cancer (see section 4.4 Special warnings and special precautions for use and section 4.8 Undesirable effects)

Forgotten tablet: If a tablet is forgotten, it should be taken as soon as the patient remembers, therapy should then be continued as before. If more than one tablet has been forgotten only the most recent tablet should be taken, the patient should not take double the usual dose to make up for missed tablets.

Missed pills may cause breakthrough bleeding.

Elderly:

There are no special dosage requirements for elderly patients, but, as with all medicines, the lowest effective dose should be used.

Children:

Not recommended

4.3 Contraindications

1. Known, past or suspected breast cancer.
2. Known or suspected estrogen-dependent malignant tumours (e.g. endometrial cancer)
3. Undiagnosed abnormal genital bleeding.
4. Untreated endometrial hyperplasia
5. Active or past history of venous thromboembolism (e.g. deep vein thrombosis, pulmonary embolism)
6. Active or recent arterial thromboembolic disease (e.g. angina, myocardial infarction)
7. Acute liver disease or history of liver disease where the liver function tests have failed to return to normal.
8. Known hypersensitivity to the active substances or to any of the excipients of Premique Low Dose tablets.
9. Porphyria

4.4 Special warnings and special precautions for use

Medical examination/Follow up

Before initiating or reinstituting HRT, a complete personal and family medical history should be taken. Physical (including pelvic and breast) examination should be guided by the contraindications and warnings for use. During treatment, periodic check-ups are recommended of a frequency and nature adapted to the individual woman. Women should be advised what changes in their breasts should be reported to their doctor or nurse. Investigations, including mammography, should be carried out in accordance with currently accepted screening practices, modified to the clinical needs of the individual. A careful appraisal of the risks and benefits should be undertaken at least annually in women treated with hormone replacement therapy.

In women with an intact uterus, the benefits of the lower risk of endometrial hyperplasia and endometrial cancer due to adding progestogen should be weighed against the increased risk of breast cancer (see below and section 4.8 Undesirable effects).

Conditions that need supervision

If any of the following conditions are present, have occurred previously, and/or have been aggravated during pregnancy or previous hormone treatment, the patient should be closely supervised. It should be taken into account that these conditions may recur or be aggravated during treatment with Premique Low Dose, in particular:

– Leiomyoma (uterine fibroids) or endometriosis
– A family history of, or other risk factors for, thromboembolic disorders (see below)
– Risk factors for estrogen dependent tumours (e.g. 1st degree heredity for breast cancer)
– Hypertension
– Liver disorders (e.g. liver adenoma)
– Diabetes mellitus with or without vascular involvement
– Cholelithiasis
– Migraine or (severe) headaches
– Systemic lupus erythematosus (SLE)
– A history of endometrial hyperplasia (see below)
– Epilepsy
– Asthma
– Otosclerosis

Reasons for immediate withdrawal of therapy

Therapy should be discontinued if a contra-indication is discovered and in the following situations:

– Jaundice or deterioration in liver function
– Significant increase in blood pressure
– New onset of migraine-type headache
– Pregnancy

Endometrial Hyperplasia

The risk of endometrial hyperplasia and carcinoma is increased when estrogens are administered alone for prolonged periods. The addition of a progestogen for at least 12 days of the cycle in non-hysterectomised women reduces, but may not eliminate, this risk (see section 4.8 Undesirable effects). Unless there is a previous diagnosis of endometriosis it is not recommended to add a progestogen in hysterectomised women.

The reduction in risk to the endometrium should be weighed against the increase in the risk of breast cancer of added progestogen (see 'Breast Cancer' below and section 4.8 Undesirable effects).

Break-through bleeding and spotting may occur during the first months of treatment. If break-through bleeding or spotting appears after some time on therapy, or continues after treatment has been discontinued, the reason should be investigated, which may include endometrial biopsy to exclude endometrial malignancy.

Breast Cancer

Randomised controlled trials and epidemiological studies have reported an increased risk of breast cancer in women taking estrogens or estrogen-progestogen combinations for HRT for several years (see Section 4.8 Undesirable effects). An observational study of almost 829,000 women has shown that, compared to never-users, use of estrogen-progestogen combined HRT is associated with a higher risk of breast cancer (RR = 2.00, 95%CI: 1.88 - 2.12) than use of estrogens alone (RR = 1.30, 95%CI: 1.21 – 1.40). In this study the magnitude of the increase in breast cancer risk was similar for all estrogen-only preparations, irrespective of the type, dose or route of administration of the estrogen (oral, transdermal and implanted). Likewise the magnitude of the increased risk was similar for all estrogen plus progestogen preparations, irrespective of the type of progestogen or the number of days of addition per cycle. For all HRT, an excess risk becomes apparent within 1-2 years of starting treatment and increase with the duration of use of HRT but begins to decline when HRT is stopped and by 5 years reaches the same level as in women who have never taken HRT.

The increase in risk applies to all women studied, although the relative risk was significantly higher in those with a lean or normal body build (body mass index or BMI of <25kg/m^2) compared to those with a BMI of ⩾25kg/m^2.

At present the effect of HRT on the diagnosis of breast tumours remains unclear – all women should be encouraged to report any changes in their breasts to their doctor or nurse.

Venous thromboembolism

Hormone replacement therapy (HRT) is associated with a higher relative risk of developing venous thromboembolism (VTE) i.e. deep vein thrombosis or pulmonary embolism. One randomised controlled trial and epidemiological studies found a two to threefold higher risk for users compared with non-users. For non- users it is estimated that the number of cases of VTE that will occur over a 5-year period is about 3 per 1000 women aged 50-59 years and 8 per 1000 women aged between 60-69 years. It is estimated that in healthy women who use HRT for 5 years, the number of additional cases of VTE over a 5-year period will be between 2 and 6 (best estimate 4) per 1000 women aged 50-59 years and between 5 and 15 (best estimate = 9) per 1000 women aged 60-69 years. The occurrence of such an event is more likely in the first year of HRT than later.

Generally recognised risk factors for VTE include a personal or family history and severe obesity (Body Mass Index >30 kg/m^2) and systemic lupus erythematosus (SLE). There is no consensus about the possible role of varicose veins in VTE.

Patients with a history of VTE or known thrombophilic states have an increased risk of VTE. HRT may add to this risk. Personal or strong family history of thromboembolism or recurrent spontaneous abortion should be investigated in order to exclude a thrombophilic predisposition. Until a thorough evaluation of thrombophilic factors has been made or anticoagulant treatment initiated, use of HRT in such patients should be viewed as contraindicated. Those women already on anticoagulant treatment require careful consideration of the benefit-risk of use of HRT.

The risk of VTE may be temporarily increased with prolonged immobilisation, major trauma or major surgery. As in all postoperative patients scrupulous attention should be given to prophylactic measures to prevent VTE following surgery. Where prolonged immobilisation is liable to follow elective surgery, particularly abdominal or orthopaedic surgery to the lower limbs, consideration should be given to temporarily stopping HRT 4-6 weeks earlier, if this is possible. Treatment should not be restarted until the woman is completely mobilised.

If venous thromboembolism develops after initiating therapy the drug should be discontinued. Patients should be told to contact their doctors immediately when they are aware of potential thromboembolic symptoms (e.g. painful swelling of a leg, sudden pain in the chest, dyspnoea).

Coronary Artery Disease (CAD)

There is no evidence from randomised controlled trials of cardiovascular benefit with continuous combined conjugated estrogens and MPA. Large clinical trials showed a possible increased risk of cardiovascular morbidity in the first year of use and no benefit thereafter. For other HRT products, there are as yet no randomised controlled trials examining benefit in cardiovascular morbidity or mortality. Therefore, it is uncertain whether these findings also extend to other HRT products.

Stroke

One large randomised clinical trial (WHI-trial) found, as a secondary outcome, an increased risk of stroke in healthy women during treatment with continuous combined conjugated estrogens and MPA. For women who do not use HRT, it is estimated that the number of cases of stroke that will occur over a 5 year period is about 3 per 1000 women aged 50-59 years and 11 per 1000 women aged 60-69 years. It is estimated that for women who use conjugated estrogens and MPA for 5 years, the number of additional cases will be between 0 and 3 (best estimate =1) per 1000 users aged 50-59 years and between 1 and 9 (best estimate = 4) per 1000 users aged 60-69 years. It is unknown whether the increased risk also extends to other HRT products.

Ovarian Cancer

Long term (at least 5 –10 years) use of estrogen-only HRT products in hysterectomised women has been associated with an increased risk of ovarian cancer in some epidemiological studies. It is uncertain whether long-term use of combined HRT confers different risk than estrogen-only products.

Other Conditions

• Estrogens/progestogens may cause fluid retention and therefore patients with cardiac or renal dysfunction should be carefully observed. Patients with terminal renal insufficiency should be closely observed, since it is expected that the level of circulating active ingredients in Premique Low Dose is increased.

• The use of estrogen may influence the laboratory results of certain endocrine tests and liver enzymes.

Estrogens increase thyroid binding globulin (TBG), leading to increased circulating total thyroid hormone, as measured by protein-bound iodine (PBI), T4 levels (by column or by radio-immunoassay) or T3 levels (by radio-immunoassay). T3 resin uptake is decreased, reflecting the elevated TBG. Free T4 and free T3 concentrations are usually unaltered.

Other binding proteins may be elevated in serum, i.e. corticoid binding globulin (CBG), sex-hormone-binding globulin (SHBG) leading to increased circulating corticosteroids and sex steroids, respectively. Free or biologically active hormone concentrations are usually unchanged. Other plasma proteins may be increased (angiotensinogen/renin substrate, alpha-I-antitrypsin, ceruloplasmin).

Some patients dependent on thyroid hormone replacement therapy may require increased doses in order to maintain their free thyroid hormone levels in an acceptable range. Therefore, patients should have their thyroid function monitored more frequently when commencing concurrent treatment in order to maintain their free thyroid hormone levels in an acceptable range.

• There is an increase in the risk of gallbladder disease in women receiving HRT (see conditions that need supervision)

• A worsening of glucose tolerance may occur in some patients on estrogen/progestogen therapy and therefore diabetic patients should be carefully observed while receiving hormone replacement therapy.

• Women with pre-existing hypertriglyceridemia should be followed closely during estrogen replacement or hormone replacement therapy, since rare cases of large increases of plasma triglycerides leading to pancreatitis have been reported with estrogen therapy in this condition.

• Estrogens should be used with caution in individuals with severe hypocalcaemia

• Epidemiological studies suggest a number of individual risk factors which contribute to the development of postmenopausal osteoporosis. These include: early menopause; family history of osteoporosis; thin, small frame; cigarette use; recent prolonged systemic corticosteroid use. If several of these risk factors are present in a patient, consideration should be given to treatment.

• Patients with rare hereditary problems of fructose intolerance, galactose intolerance, the Lapp lactase deficiency, glucose-galactose malabsorption or sucrase-isomaltase insufficiency should not take this medicine.

4.5 Interaction with other medicinal products and other forms of Interaction

The metabolism of estrogens and progestogens may be increased by concomitant use of substances known to induce drug-metabolising enzymes, specifically cytochrome P450 enzymes, such as anticonvulsants (e.g. phenobarbital, phenytoin, carbamazepine) and anti-infectives (e.g. rifampicin, rifabutin, nevirapine, efavirenz).

Ritonavir and nelfinavir, although known as strong inhibitors, by contrast exhibit inducing properties when used concomitantly with steroid hormones.

Herbal preparations containing St John's wort (Hypericum perforatum) may induce the metabolism of estrogens and progestogens.

Clinically, an increased metabolism of estrogens and progestogens may lead to decreased effect and changes in the uterine bleeding profile.

The response to metyrapone may be reduced.

Aminoglutethimide administered concomitantly with MPA may significantly depress the bioavailiablity of MPA.

4.6 Pregnancy and lactation

Pregnancy:

Premique Low Dose is not indicated during pregnancy. If pregnancy occurs during medication with Premique Low Dose treatment should be withdrawn immediately.

Clinically, data on a limited number of exposed pregnancies indicate no adverse effects of MPA on the foetus.

The results of most epidemiological studies to date relevant to inadvertent foetal exposure to combinations of estrogens and progestogens indicate no teratogenic or foetotoxic effect.

Lactation:

Premique Low Dose is not indicated during lactation.

4.7 Effects on ability to drive and use machines

Premique Low Dose should not affect the ability to drive or use machinery.

4.8 Undesirable effects

See also Section 4.4 Special warnings and special precautions for use.

Adverse drug reactions (ADRs)

The adverse reactions listed in the table are based on post-marketing spontaneous (reporting rate), clinical trials and class-effects. Breast pain is a very common adverse event reported in ⩾ 10% of patients.

(see Table 1 on next page)

Breast Cancer

The risk of breast cancer increases with the number of years of HRT usage. According to data from a recent epidemiological study in about 829,000 postmenopausal women, the best estimate of the risk is that for women not using HRT, in total 32 in every 1000 are expected to have breast cancer diagnosed between the ages of 50 and 65 years. Among those with current or recent use of estrogen-only replacement therapy, it is estimated that the total number of additional cases during the corresponding period will be between 0 and 3 (best estimate = 1.5) per 1000 for 5 years' use and between 3 and 7 (best estimate = 5) per 1000 for 10 years' use (see table). Among those with current or recent use of estrogen plus progestogen combined HRT, it is estimated that the total number of additional cases will be between 5 and 7 (best estimate = 6) per 1000 for 5 years' use and between 18 and 20 (best estimate = 19) per 1000 for 10 years' use (See section 4.4 Special warnings and special precautions for use). The number of additional cases of breast cancer is broadly similar for women who start HRT irrespective of age at start of HRT use (between the ages of 45-65).

Type of HRT	No of additional cases of breast cancer diagnosed per 1000 women (95% confidence intervals)	
	5 years of use	10 years of use
Estrogen-only	1.5 (0-3)	5 (3-7)
Combined	6 (5-7)	19 (18-20)

Endometrial Cancer

In women with an intact uterus, the risk of endometrial hyperplasia and endometrial cancer increases with increasing duration of use of unopposed estrogens and is substantially reduced by the addition of a progestogen (see section 4.4 Special warnings and special precautions for use). According to data from epidemiological studies, the best estimate of the risk of endometrial cancer is that for women not using HRT, about 5 in every 1000 are expected to have endometrial cancer diagnosed between the ages of 50 and 65. It is estimated that among those who use estrogen-only replacement therapy, there will be 4 additional cases per 1000 after 5 year's use and 10 additional cases per 1000 after 10 years' use. Adding a progestogen to estrogen-only therapy substantially reduces, but may not eliminate, this increased risk.

Other adverse reactions reported in association with estrogen/progestogen treatment including conjugated estrogens/MPA:

• Estrogen-dependent neoplasms benign and malignant, e.g. endometrial hyperplasia, endometrial cancer

• Venous thromboembolism, i.e. deep leg or pelvic venous thrombosis and pulmonary embolism, is more frequent among hormone replacement therapy users than among non-users. For further information, see section 4.3 Contraindications and 4.4 Special warnings and special precautions for use.

• Retinal vascular thrombosis

• Myocardial infarction

• Stroke

• Increases in blood pressure

• Cholestatic jaundice

• Enlargement of hepatic haemangiomas

• Skin and subcutaneous disorders: erythema multiforme, erythema nodosum, vascular purpura

• Exacerbation of chorea

• Exacerbation of porphyria

• Exacerbation of hypocalcaemia

• Exacerbation of otosclerosis

4.9 Overdose

Numerous reports of ingestion of large doses of estrogen/progestogen-containing oral contraceptives by young

Table 1

System Organ Class	Common ADRs (> 1/100, < 1/10)	Uncommon ADRs (> 1/1000, < 1/100)	Rare ADRs (> 1/10000, < 1/1000)
Reproductive system & breast disorders	Breakthrough bleeding/spotting; Breast pain, tenderness, enlargement, discharge	Change in menstrual flow; Change in cervical ectropion and secretion	Galactorrhoea; Increased size of uterine leiomyomata
Gastrointestinal disorders	None	Nausea; Bloating; Abdominal pain	Vomiting; Pancreatitis
Nervous system disorders	None	Dizziness; Headache; Migraine; Anxiety	Stroke/cerebrovascular accidents; Exacerbation of epilepsy
Musculoskeletal, connective tissue and bone disorders	Arthralgias; Leg cramps	None	None
Psychiatric disorders	Depression	Changes in libido; Mood disturbances	Irritability
Vascular disorders	None	Venous thrombosis	Pulmonary embolism; Superficial thrombophlebitis
General disorders and administration site conditions	None	Oedema	None
Skin and subcutaneous tissue disorders	None	Alopecia; Acne; Pruritus	Chloasma/melasma; Hirsutism; Rash
Infections and infestations	Vaginitis	Vaginal candidiasis	None
Immune system disorders	None	None	Anaphylactic/ anaphylactoid reactions, including urticaria and angioedema
Metabolism and nutrition disorders	None	None	Glucose intolerance
Eye disorders	None	Intolerance to contact lenses	None
Respiratory, thoracic and mediastinal disorders	None	None	Exacerbation of asthma
Hepatobiliary disorders	None	Gallbladder disease	None
Neoplasms, benign and malignant (including cysts & polyps)	None	None	Breast cancer; Fibrocystic breast changes, Ovarian Cancer
Investigations	Changes in weight (increase or decrease)	None	None

children indicate that acute serious ill effects have not been observed. Overdosage of estrogens may cause nausea, and withdrawal bleeding may occur in females.

Should large overdosages occur and medical concerns arise, the standard practices of gastric evacuation, activated charcoal administration, and general supportive therapy may be applicable.

5. PHARMACOLOGICAL PROPERTIES

5.1 Pharmacodynamic properties

ATC Code: GO3F A12 (Medroxyprogesterone & estrogen)

Conjugated Estrogens

The active ingredients are primarily the sulphate esters of estrone, equilin sulphates, 17α-estradiol and 17β-estradiol. These substitute for the loss of estrogen production in menopausal women, and alleviate menopausal symptoms.

Progestogen:

As estrogens promote the growth of the endometrium, unopposed estrogens increase the risk of endometrial hyperplasia and cancer. The addition of a progestogen reduces but does not eliminate the estrogen-induced risk of endometrial hyperplasia in non-hysterectomised women.

Relief of estrogen-deficiency symptoms

In a 1-year clinical trial (n=2,808), vasomotor symptoms were assessed for efficacy during the first 12 weeks of treatment in a subset of symptomatic women (n=241) who had at least 7 moderate or severe hot flushes daily or 50 moderate to severe hot flushes during the week before randomisation. Premique 0.625mg/2.5mg (conjugated estrogens/medroxyprogesterone acetate) was shown to be statistically better than placebo at weeks 4, 8 and 12 for relief of both frequency and severity of moderate to severe vasomotor symptoms.

In two clinical trials, the incidence of amenorrhoea (no bleeding or spotting) increased over time in women treated with Premique 0.625 mg/2.5 mg. Amenorrhoea was seen in 68% of women at cycle 6 and 77% of women at cycle 12. Breakthrough bleeding and/or spotting appeared in 48% during the first 3 months, and in 24% of women during months 10-12 of treatment.

5.2 Pharmacokinetic properties

Absorption

Conjugated estrogens are soluble in water and are well absorbed from the gastrointestinal tract after release from the drug formulation. However Premique Low Dose contains a formulation of medroxyprogesterone acetate (MPA) that is immediately released and conjugated estrogens that are slowly released over several hours. MPA is well absorbed from the gastrointestinal tract. Table 2 summarises the mean pharmacokinetic parameters for unconjugated and conjugated estrogens, and medroxyprogesterone acetate following administration of 2 Premique Low Dose 0.3 /1.5 mg and 2 Premique Low Dose 0.45/1.5 mg tablets to healthy postmenopausal women.

Distribution

The distribution of exogenous estrogens is similar to that of endogenous estrogens. Estrogens are widely distributed in the body and are generally found in higher concentrations in the sex hormone target organs. Estrogens circulate in the blood largely bound to sex hormone binding globulin (SHBG) and albumin. MPA is approximately 90% bound to plasma proteins but does not bind to SHBG.

Metabolism

Exogenous estrogens are metabolised in the same manner as endogenous estrogens. Circulating estrogens exist in a dynamic equilibrium of metabolic interconversions. These transformations take place mainly in the liver. Estradiol is converted reversibly to estrone, and both can be converted to estriol, which is the major urinary metabolite. Estrogens also undergo enterohepatic recirculation via sulphate and glucuronide conjugation in the liver, biliary secretion of conjugates into the intestine, and hydrolysis in the gut followed by reabsorption. In postmenopausal women a significant proportion of the circulating estrogens exists as sulphate conjugates, especially estrone sulphate, which serves as a circulating reservoir for the formation of more active estrogens. Metabolism and elimination of MPA occur primarily in the liver via hydroxylation, with subsequent conjugation and elimination in the urine.

Excretion

Estradiol, estrone and estriol are excreted in the urine along with glucuronide and sulphate conjugates. Most metabolites of MPA are extracted as glucuronide conjugates with only minor amounts secreted as sulphates.

Table 2 – Pharmacokinetic parameters for Premique Low Dose

(see Table 2 on next page)

5.3 Preclinical safety data

Long-term continuous administration of natural and synthetic estrogens in certain animal species increases the frequency of carcinomas of the breast, cervix, vagina and liver.

In a two-year oral study in which female rats were exposed to MPA dosages of up to 5000μg/kg/day in their diets (50 times higher - based on AUC values - than the level observed in women taking 10mg of MPA), a dose-related increase in pancreatic islet cell tumours (adenomas and carcinomas) occurred. Pancreatic tumour incidence was increased at 1000 and 5000μg/kg/day, but not at 200μg/kg/day.

The cortisol activity of MPA at these high doses is thought to increase serum glucose in rats which reactively stimulates the beta cells of the pancreatic islets to produce insulin. This repeated stimulation is thought to cause the tumours in rats. Similar lesions are not likely to occur in humans since the endocrine system of rats is more sensitive to hormones than that of women. When MPA is combined with estrogen, MPA binds to fewer glucocorticosteriod receptors and thus has less effect on plasma glucose. In humans, the diabetogenic response to MPA at therapeutic doses is slight. Moreover, an extensive literature search revealed no evidence that MPA causes pancreatic tumours in humans.

6. PHARMACEUTICAL PARTICULARS

6.1 List of excipients

Tablet core:

Lactose monohydrate
Methylcellulose
Magnesium stearate
Calcium phosphate

Tablet coating:

Macrogol
Glyceryl mono-oleate
Shellac
Calcium sulphate
Microcrystalline cellulose
Sucrose
Titanium dioxide (E171)
Povidone
Carnauba wax
Yellow Ferric Oxide (E172)

Printing on tablet:

Black Tek Print SW-9008 (shellac, propylene glycol, black iron oxide (E172) and potassium hydroxide).

6.2 Incompatibilities

Not applicable.

6.3 Shelf life

24 months.

6.4 Special precautions for storage

Do not store above 25°C.

6.5 Nature and contents of container

Polyvinylchloride (PVC)/Aluminium foil blister pack of 28 tablets. Each carton contains 1 or 3 blister packs.

6.6 Instructions for use and handling

Not applicable.

Table 2 – Pharmacokinetic parameters for Premique Low Dose

Drug	2 × 0.3 mg CE/1.5 mg MPA Combination (n=30)				2 × 0.45 mg CE/1.5 mg MPA Combination (n=61)			
PK Parameter Arithmetic Mean (%CV)	C_{max} (pg/mL)	t_{max} (h)	$t_{1/2}$ (h)	*AUC* (pg.h/mL)	C_{max} (pg/mL)	t_{max} (h)	$t_{1/2}$ (h)	*AUC* (pg.h/mL)
Unconjugated Estrogens								
Estrone	79 (35)	9.4 (86)	51.3 (30)	5029 (45)	91 (30)	9.8 (47)	48.9 (28)	5786 (42)
BA*-Estrone	56 (46)	9.4 (86)	19.8 (39)	1429 (49)	67 (37)	9.8 (47)	21.5 (49)	2042 (52)
Equilin	30 (43)	7.9 (42)	14.0 (75)	590 (42)	35 (40)	8.5 (34)	16.4 (49)	825 (44)
PK Parameter Arithmetic Mean (%CV)	C_{max} (pg/mL)	t_{max} (h)	$t_{1/2}$ (h)	*AUC* (ng.h/mL)	C_{max} (ng/mL)	t_{max} (h)	$t_{1/2}$ (h)	*AUC* (ng.h/mL)
Conjugated Estrogens								
Total Estrone	2.4 (38)	7.1 (27)	26.5 (33)	62 (48)	3.0 (37)	8.2 (39)	25.9 (23)	78 (40)
BA* - Total Estrone	2.2 (36)	7.1 (27)	16.3 (32)	41 (44)	2.8 (36)	8.2 (39)	16.9 (36)	56 (39)
Total Equilin	1.5 (47)	5.5 (29)	11.5 (24)	22 (41)	1.9 (42)	7.2 (33)	12.2 (25)	31 (52)
PK Parameter Arithmetic Mean (%CV)	C_{max} (ng/mL)	t_{max} (h)	$t_{1/2}$ (h)	*AUC* (ng.h/mL)	C_{max} (ng/mL)	t_{max} (h)	$t_{1/2}$ (h)	*AUC* (ng.h/mL)
Medroxyprogesterone acetate								
MPA	1.2 (42)	2.8 (61)	42.3 (34)	29.4 (30)	1.2 (42)	2.7 (52)	47.2 (41)	32.0 (36)

BA* = Baseline adjusted

C_{max} = peak plasma concentration

t_{max} = time peak concentration occurs

$t_{1/2}$ = apparent terminal-phase disposition half life (0.693/λ_z)

AUC = total area under the concentration-time curve

7. MARKETING AUTHORISATION HOLDER

John Wyeth & Brother Limited
Trading as: Wyeth Pharmaceuticals
Huntercombe Lane South
Taplow
Maidenhead
Berkshire SL6 0PH

8. MARKETING AUTHORISATION NUMBER(S)

PL 00011/0256

9. DATE OF FIRST AUTHORISATION/RENEWAL OF THE AUTHORISATION

08 March 2004

10. DATE OF REVISION OF THE TEXT

8th March 2004

Prempak-C

(Wyeth Pharmaceuticals)

1. NAME OF THE MEDICINAL PRODUCT

Prempak-C

2. QUALITATIVE AND QUANTITATIVE COMPOSITION

Prempak-C 0.625mg consists of 28 tablets containing 0.625mg conjugated estrogens USP, and 12 tablets containing 0.15mg norgestrel.

Prempak-C 1.25mg consists of 28 tablets containing 1.25mg conjugated estrogens USP, and 12 tablets containing 0.15mg norgestrel.

3. PHARMACEUTICAL FORM

Prempak-C 0.625mg: Oval maroon sugar coated tablets each containing conjugated estrogens USP 0.625mg. Round light brown sugar coated tablets containing norgestrel 0.15mg.

Prempak-C 1.25mg: Oval yellow sugar coated tablets each containing conjugated estrogens USP 1.25mg. Round light brown sugar coated tablets containing norgestrel 0.15mg.

4. CLINICAL PARTICULARS

4.1 Therapeutic indications

• Hormone replacement therapy for estrogen deficiency symptoms in menopausal and postmenopausal women

• Second line therapy for prevention of osteoporosis in postmenopausal women at high risk of future fractures who are intolerant of, or contraindicated for, other medicinal products approved for the prevention of osteoporosis.

4.2 Posology and method of administration

__Adults__:

Prempak-C is available for oral use in a sequential regimen for treatment of women with a uterus. The recommended starting dose is 0.625mg-1.25mg conjugated estrogens daily. One norgestrel tablet should be taken daily from day 17 to day 28 of estrogen therapy. Continuous estrogen administration is recommended. For maintenance, the lowest effective dose should be used.

__For treatment of postmenopausal symptoms__:

0.625-1.25mg conjugated estrogens daily depending on the response of the individual. One norgestrel tablet should be taken daily from day 17 to day 28 of estrogen therapy.

__Prophylaxis of osteoporosis__:

The minimum effective dose is 0.625mg daily for most patients. One norgestrel tablet should be taken daily from day 17 to day 28 of estrogen therapy. (See section 5.1 Pharmacological Properties)

For most postmenopausal women therapy may be commenced at any convenient time although if the patient is still menstruating, commencement on first day of bleeding is recommended. In women transferring from another sequential hormone replacement therapy regimen, treatment should begin the day following completion of the prior regimen. Withdrawal bleeding usually occurs within three to seven days after the last norgestrel tablet.

For treatment of postmenopausal symptoms, the lowest effective dose should be used. HRT should only be continued as long as the benefit in alleviation of severe symptoms outweighs the risk.

The benefits of the lower risk of endometrial hyperplasia and endometrial cancer due to adding a progestogen should be weighed against the increased risk of breast cancer (see sections 4.4 Special Warnings and Precautions for Use and 4.8 Undesirable Effects).

__Forgotten tablet__: If a tablet is forgotten, it should be taken as soon as the patient remembers, therapy should then be continued as before. If more than one tablet has been forgotten only the most recent tablet should be taken. The patient should not take double the usual dose to make up for the missed tablet.

Missed pills may cause breakthrough bleeding.

__Elderly__:

There are no special dosage requirements for elderly patients, but as with all medicines, the lowest effective dose should be used.

__Children__:

Not recommended.

4.3 Contraindications

1. Known, past or suspected cancer of the breast
2. Known or suspected estrogen-dependent malignant tumours (e.g. endometrial cancer)
3. Undiagnosed abnormal genital bleeding
4. Untreated endometrial hyperplasia
5. Active or past history of venous thromboembolism (e.g. deep vein thrombosis, pulmonary embolism)
6. Active or recent arterial thromboembolic disease (e.g. angina, myocardial infarction)
7. Acute liver disease or history of liver disease where the liver function tests have failed to return to normal
8. Known hypersensitivity to the active substances or to any of the excipients of Prempak-C tablets
9. Porphyria

4.4 Special warnings and special precautions for use

__1. Medical examination/Follow up__

Before initiating or reinstituting HRT, a complete personal and family medical history should be taken. Physical (including pelvic and breast) examination should be guided by the contraindications and warnings for use. During treatment, periodic check-ups are recommended of a frequency and nature adapted to the individual women. Women should be advised what changes in their breasts should be reported to their doctor or nurse. Investigations, including mammography, should be carried out in accordance with currently accepted screening practices, modified to the clinical needs of the individual. A careful appraisal of the risks and benefits should be undertaken at least annually in women treated with hormone replacement therapy.

In women with an intact uterus, the benefits of the lower risk of endometrial hyperplasia and endometrial cancer due to adding progestogen should be weighed against the increased risk of breast cancer (see below and Section 4.8 Undesirable Effects).

__2. Conditions that need supervision__

If any of the following conditions are present, have occurred previously, and/or have been aggravated during pregnancy or previous hormone treatment, the patient should be closely supervised. It should be taken into account that these conditions may recur or be aggravated during treatment with Prempak-C, in particular:

– Leiomyoma (uterine fibroids) or endometriosis
– A family history of, or other risk factors for, thromboembolic disorders (see below)
– Risk factors for estrogen dependent tumours (e.g. 1st degree heredity for breast cancer)
– Hypertension
– Liver disorders (e.g. liver adenoma)
– Diabetes mellitus with or without vascular involvement
– Cholelithiasis
– Migraine or (severe) headaches
– Systemic lupus erythematosus (SLE)
– A history of endometrial hyperplasia (see below)
– Epilepsy
– Asthma
– Otosclerosis

__3. Reasons for immediate withdrawal of therapy__

Therapy should be discontinued if a contra-indication is discovered and in the following situations:

– Jaundice or deterioration in liver function
– Significant increase in blood pressure
– New onset of migraine-type headache
– Pregnancy

__4. Endometrial Hyperplasia__

The risk of endometrial hyperplasia and carcinoma is increased when estrogens are administered alone for prolonged periods. The addition of a progestogen for at least 12 days of the cycle in non-hysterectomised women reduces, but may not eliminate, this risk (see section 4.8 Undesirable Effects). Unless there is a previous diagnosis of endometriosis it is not recommended to add a progestogen in hysterectomised women (see 4.4 – Special Warnings and Precautions for Use).

The reduction in risk to the endometrium should be weighed against the increase in the risk of breast cancer of added progestogen (see 'Breast cancer' below and Section 4.8 Undesirable Effects).

Break-through bleeding and spotting may occur during the first months of treatment. If break-through bleeding or spotting appears after some time on therapy, or continues after treatment has been discontinued, the reason should be investigated, which may include endometrial biopsy to exclude endometrial malignancy.

5. Breast Cancer

Randomised controlled trials and epidemiological studies have reported an increased risk of breast cancer in women taking estrogen or estrogen-progestogen combinations for HRT for several years (see Section 4.8 Undesirable Effects). An observational study of almost 829,000 women has shown that, compared to never-users, use of estrogen-progestogen combined HRT is associated with a higher risk of breast cancer (RR = 2.00, 95%CI: 1.88 - 2.12) than use of estrogens alone (RR = 1.30, 95%CI: 1.21 – 1.40). In this study the magnitude of the increase in breast cancer risk was similar for all estrogen-only preparations, irrespective of the type, dose or route of administration of the estrogen (oral, transdermal and implanted). Likewise the magnitude of the increased risk was similar for all estrogen plus progestogen preparations, irrespective of the type of progestogen or the number of days of addition per cycle. For all HRT, an excess risk becomes apparent within 1-2 years of starting treatment and increase with the duration of use of HRT but begins to decline when HRT is stopped and by 5 years reaches the same level as in women who have never taken HRT.

The increase in risk applies to all women studied, although the relative risk was significantly higher in those with a lean or normal body build (body mass index or BMI of <25kg/m^2) compared to those with a BMI of ⩾25kg/m^2.

At present the effect of HRT on the diagnosis of breast tumours remains unclear – all women should be encouraged to report any changes in their breasts to their doctor or nurse.

6. Venous thromboembolism

Hormone replacement therapy (HRT) is associated with a higher relative risk of developing venous thromboembolism (VTE) i.e. deep vein thrombosis or pulmonary embolism. One randomised controlled trial and epidemiological studies found a two to threefold higher risk for users compared with non-users. For non- users it is estimated that the number of cases of VTE that will occur over a 5-year period is about 3 per 1000 women aged 50-59 years and 8 per 1000 women aged between 60-69 years. It is estimated that in healthy women who use HRT for 5 years, the number of additional cases of VTE over a 5-year period will be between 2 and 6 (best estimate = 4) per 1000 women aged 50-59 years and between 5 and 15 (best estimate = 9) per 1000 women aged 60-69 years. The occurrence of such an event is more likely in the first year of HRT than later.

Generally recognised risk factors for VTE include a personal or family history and severe obesity (Body Mass Index >30kg/m^2) and systemic lupus erythematosus (SLE). There is no consensus about the possible role of varicose veins in VTE.

Patients with a history of VTE or known thrombophilic states have an increased risk of VTE. HRT may add to this risk. Personal or strong family history of thromboembolism or recurrent spontaneous abortion should be investigated in order to exclude a thrombophilic predisposition. Until a thorough evaluation of thrombophilic factors has been made or anticoagulant treatment initiated, use of HRT in such patients should be viewed as contraindicated. Those women already on anticoagulant treatment require careful consideration of the benefit-risk of use of HRT.

The risk of VTE may be temporarily increased with prolonged immobilisation, major trauma or major surgery. As in all post-operative patients, scrupulous attention should be given to prophylactic measures to prevent VTE following surgery. Where prolonged immobilisation is liable to follow elective surgery, particularly abdominal or orthopaedic surgery to the lower limbs, consideration should be given to temporarily stopping HRT 4-6 weeks earlier, if this is possible. Treatment should not be restarted until the woman is completely mobilised.

If venous thromboembolism develops after initiating therapy the drug should be discontinued. Patients should be told to contact their doctors immediately when they are aware of potential thromboembolic symptoms (e.g. painful swelling of a leg, sudden pain in the chest, dyspnoea).

7. Coronary Artery Disease (CAD)

There is no evidence from randomised controlled trials of cardiovascular benefit with continuous combined conjugated estrogens and MPA. Large clinical trials showed a possible increased risk of cardiovascular morbidity in the first year of use and no benefit thereafter. For other HRT products, there are as yet no randomised controlled trials examining benefit in cardiovascular morbidity or mortality. Therefore, it is uncertain whether these findings also extend to other HRT products.

8. Stroke

One large randomised clinical trial (WHI-trial) found, as a secondary outcome, an increased risk of stroke in healthy women during treatment with continuous combined conjugated estrogens and MPA. For women who do not use HRT, it is estimated that the number of cases of stroke that will occur over a 5 year period is about 3 per 1000 women aged 50-59 years and 11 per 1000 women aged 60-69 years. It is estimated that for women who use conjugated estrogens and MPA for 5 years, the number of additional cases will be between 0 and 3 (best estimate =1) per 1000 users aged 50-59 years and between 1 and 9 (best estimate = 4) per 1000 users aged 60-69 years. It is unknown whether the increased risk also extends to other HRT products.

9. Ovarian Cancer

Long term (at least 5-10 years) use of estrogen-only HRT products in hysterectomised women has been associated with an increased risk of ovarian cancer in some epidemiological studies. It is uncertain whether long-term use of combined HRT confers different risk than estrogen-only products.

Other Conditions

10. Estrogens/progestogens may cause fluid retention and therefore patients with cardiac or renal dysfunction should be carefully observed. Patients with terminal renal insufficiency should be closely observed, since it is expected that the level of circulating active ingredients in Prempak-C is increased.

11. The use of estrogen may influence the laboratory results of certain endocrine tests and liver enzymes.

Estrogens increase thyroid binding globulin (TBG), leading to increased circulating total thyroid hormone, as measured by protein-bound iodine (PBI), T4 levels (by column or by radio-immunoassay) or T3 levels (by radio-immunoassay). T3 resin uptake is decreased, reflecting the elevated TBG. Free T4 and free T3 concentrations are unaltered however, some patients dependent on thyroid hormone replacement therapy may require increased doses in order to maintain their free thyroid hormone levels in an acceptable range.

Other binding proteins may be elevated in serum, i.e. corticoid binding globulin (CBG), sex-hormone-binding globulin (SHBG) leading to increased circulating corticosteroids and sex steroids, respectively. Free or biologically active hormone concentrations are unchanged. Other plasma proteins may be increased (angiotensinogen/renin substrate, alpha-I-antitrypsin, ceruloplasmin).

Some patients dependent on thyroid hormone replacement therapy may require increased doses in order to maintain their free thyroid hormone levels in an acceptable range. Therefore, patients should have their thyroid function monitored more frequently when commencing concurrent treatment in order to maintain their free thyroid hormone levels in an acceptable range.

12. Changed estrogen levels may affect certain endocrine and liver function tests.

13. There is an increase in the risk of gallbladder disease in women receiving HRT (see conditions that need supervision).

14. A worsening of glucose tolerance may occur in patients taking estrogens and therefore diabetic patients should be carefully observed while receiving hormone replacement therapy.

15. Women with pre-existing hypertriglyceridemia should be followed closely during estrogen replacement or hormone replacement therapy, since rare cases of large increases of plasma triglycerides leading to pancreatitis have been reported with estrogen therapy in this condition.

16. Estrogens should be used with caution in individuals with severe hypocalcaemia

17. Epidemiological studies suggest a number of individual risk factors which contribute to the development of postmenopausal osteoporosis. These include: early menopause; family history of osteoporosis; thin, small frame; cigarette use; recent prolonged systemic corticosteroid use. If several of these risk factors are present in a patient, consideration should be given to estrogen replacement therapy.

4.5 Interaction with other medicinal products and other forms of Interaction

The metabolism of estrogens and progestogens may be increased by concomitant use of substances known to induce drug-metabolising enzymes, specifically cytochrome P450 enzymes, such as anticonvulsants (e.g. phenobarbital, phenytoin, carbamazepine) and anti-infectives (e.g. rifampicin, rifabutin, nevirapine, efavirenz).

Ritonavir and nelfinavir, although known as strong inhibitors, by contrast exhibit inducing properties when used concomitantly with steroid hormones.

Herbal preparations containing St John's wort *(Hypericum perforatum)* may induce the metabolism of estrogens and progestogens.

Clinically, an increased metabolism of estrogens and progestogens may lead to decreased effect and changes in the uterine bleeding profile.

The response to metyrapone may be reduced.

4.6 Pregnancy and lactation

Pregnancy:

Prempak-C is not indicated during pregnancy. If pregnancy occurs during medication with Prempak-C treatment should be withdrawn immediately.

Clinically, data on a limited number of exposed pregnancies indicate no adverse effects of MPA on the foetus.

The results of most epidemiological studies to date relevant to inadvertent foetal exposure to combinations of estrogens and progestogens indicate no teratogenic or foetotoxic effect.

Lactation:

Prempak-C is not indicated during lactation.

4.7 Effects on ability to drive and use machines

None known.

4.8 Undesirable effects

See also 4.4 Special Warnings and Special Precautions for Use.

Adverse drug reactions (ADRs)

The adverse reactions listed in the table are based on post-marketing spontaneous (reporting rate), clinical trials and class-effects.

System Organ Class	Adverse Reaction
Reproductive system & breast disorders	Breakthrough bleeding/ spotting; Dysmenorrhoea; Change in menstrual flow; Change in cervical ectropion and secretion; Increased size of uterine leiomyomata (fibroids) Breast pain, tenderness, enlargement, discharge; galactorrhoea;
Gastrointestinal disorders	Nausea; Bloating; Abdominal pain; Vomiting; Pancreatitis
Nervous system disorders	Anxiety; Dizziness; Headache (including migraine); Exacerbation of epilepsy; Stroke
Musculoskeletal, connective tissue and bone disorders	Arthralgias; Leg cramps
Psychiatric disorders	Depression; Changes in libido; Mood disturbances; Irritability
Vascular disorders	Pulmonary embolism; Deep Venous thrombophlebitis, Superficial thrombophlebitis
Cardiac disorders	Myocardial Infarction
General disorders and administration site disorders	Oedema
Skin and subcutaneous tissue disorders	Alopecia; Acne; Pruritus; Chloasma/ melasma; Hirsutism; Rash
Infections and infestations	Vaginitis, including vaginal candidiasis
Immune system disorders	Urticaria; Angioedeoma; Anaphylactic/ anaphylactoid reactions
Metabolism and nutrition disorders	Glucose intolerance
Eye disorders	Intolerance to contact lenses
Respiratory, thoracic and mediastinal disorders	Exacerbation of asthma
Hepatobiliary	Gallbladder disease
Neoplasms benign and malignant	Breast cancer*; Fibrocystic breast changes; Ovarian Cancer
Investigations	Changes in weight (increase or decrease)

Breast cancer

* The risk of breast cancer increases with the number of years of HRT usage. According to data from a recent epidemiological study in about 829,000 postmenopausal women, the best estimate of the risk is that for women not using HRT, in total 32 in every 1000 are expected to have breast cancer diagnosed between the ages of 50 and 65 years. Among those with current or recent use of estrogen-only replacement therapy, it is estimated that the total number of additional cases during the corresponding

period will be between 0 and 3 (best estimate = 1.5) per 1000 for 5 years' use and between 3 and 7 (best estimate = 5) per 1000 for 10 years' use (see table). Among those with current or recent use of estrogen plus progestogen combined HRT, it is estimated that the total number of additional cases will be between 5 and 7 (best estimate = 6) per 1000 for 5 years' use and between 18 and 20 (best estimate = 19) per 1000 for 10 years' use (See section 4.4 Special Warnings and Precautions for Use). The number of additional cases of breast cancer is broadly similar for women who start HRT irrespective of age at start of HRT use (between the ages of 45-65).

	No of additional cases of breast cancer diagnosed per 1000 women (95% confidence intervals)	
Type of HRT	5 years of use	10 years of use
Estrogen-only	1.5 (0-3)	5 (3-7)
Combined	6 (5-7)	19 (18-20)

Endometrial Cancer

In women with an intact uterus, the risk of endometrial hyperplasia and endometrial cancer increases with the increasing duration of use of unopposed estrogens and is substantially reduced by the addition of a progestogen (see section 4.4 Special Warnings and Precautions for Use). According to data from epidemiological studies the best estimate of the risk of endometrial cancer is that for women not using HRT, about 5 in every 1000 are expected to have endometrial cancer diagnosed between the ages of 50 and 65. It is estimated that, among those who use estrogen-only replacement therapy, there will be 4 additional cases per 100 after 5 years' use and 10 additional cases per 1000 after 10 years' use. Adding a progestogen to estrogen-only therapy substantially reduces, but may not eliminate, the increased risk.

Other adverse reactions reported in association with estrogen/progestogen treatment including Prempak-C:

- Estrogen-dependent neoplasms benign and malignant, e.g. endometrial hyperplasia, endometrial cancer
- Venous thromboembolism, i.e. deep leg or pelvic venous thrombosis and pulmonary embolism, is more frequent among hormone replacement therapy users than among non-users. For further information, see section 4.3 Contra-indications and 4.4 Special Warnings and Precautions for Use.
- Retinal vascular thrombosis
- Myocardial infarction
- Stroke
- Increases in blood pressure
- Cholestatic jaundice
- Enlargement of hepatic haemangiomas
- Skin and subcutaneous disorders: erythema multiforme, erythema nodosum, vascular purpura
- Exacerbation of chorea
- Exacerbation of porphyria
- Exacerbation of hypocalcaemia
- Exacerbation of otosclerosis

4.9 Overdose

Numerous reports of ingestion of large doses of estrogen-containing oral contraceptives by young children indicate that acute serious ill effects do not occur. Overdosage of estrogen may cause nausea and vomiting, and withdrawal bleeding may occur in females. There is no specific antidote, and further treatment should be symptomatic.

5. PHARMACOLOGICAL PROPERTIES

5.1 Pharmacodynamic properties

ATC Code: G03F A10

Conjugated Estrogens

The active ingredients are primarily the sulphate esters of estrone, equilin sulphates, 17α-estradiol and 17β-estradiol. These substitute for the loss of estrogen production in menopausal women, and alleviate menopausal symptoms. Estrogens prevent bone loss following menopause or ovariectomy.

Progestogen:

As estrogens promote the growth of the endometrium, unopposed estrogens increase the risk of endometrial hyperplasia and cancer. The addition of a progestogen reduces but does not eliminate the estrogen-induced risk of endometrial hyperplasia in non-hysterectomised women.

The following data are from studies done with a different progestogen to that in Prempak-C. However, since the effect is due to the conjugated estrogens, these results can be extrapolated to other conjugated estrogen plus progestogen combination products.

Relief of estrogen-deficiency symptoms

In a 1-year clinical trial (n=2,808), vasomotor symptoms were assessed for efficacy during the first 12 weeks of treatment in a subset of symptomatic women (n=241) who had at least 7 moderate or severe hot flushes daily or 50 moderate to severe hot flushes during the week before randomisation. Premique 0.625 mg/2.5 mg(conjugated estrogens/medroxyprogesterone acetate) was shown to be statistically better than placebo at weeks 4, 8 and 12 for relief of both frequency and severity of moderate to severe vasomotor symptoms.

Prevention of osteoporosis

Estrogen deficiency at menopause is associated with an increasing bone turnover and decline in bone mass. Therefore, if possible, treatment for prevention of osteoporosis should start as soon as possible after the onset of menopause in women with increased risk for future osteoporotic fractures. The effect of estrogens on the bone mineral density is dose-dependent. Protection appears to be effective for as long as treatment is continued.

After 3 years of treatment with Premique 0.625 mg/2.5 mg, the increase in lumbar spine bone mineral density (BMD) was 4.87% ± 0.66. The percentage of women who maintained (less than 1% BMD loss per year) or gained BMD in lumbar zone during treatment was 92%.

Premique 0.625 mg/2.5 mg also had an effect on hip BMD. The increase after 3 years was 1.94% ± 0.44 at total hip. The percentage of women who maintained (less than 1% BMD loss per year) or gained BMD in hip zone during treatment was 88%.

5.2 Pharmacokinetic properties

Conjugated Estrogens

Absorption

Conjugated estrogens are soluble in water and are well absorbed from the gastrointestinal tract after release from the drug formulation. Premarin tablets (conjugated estrogens only) release conjugated estrogens slowly over several hours. The pharmacodynamic profile of unconjugated and conjugated estrogens following a dose of 2 × 0.625mg is provided in Table 1.

Distribution

The distribution of exogenous estrogen is similar to that of endogenous estrogens. Estrogens are widely distributed in the body and are generally found in higher concentrations in the sex hormone target organs. Estrogens circulate in the blood largely bound to sex hormone binding globulin (SHBG) and albumin.

Metabolism

Exogenous estrogens are metabolised in the same manner as endogenous estrogens. Circulating estrogens exist in dynamic equilibrium of metabolic interconversions. These transformations take place mainly in the liver. Estradiol is converted reversibly to estrone, and both can be converted to estriol, which is the major urinary metabolite. Estrogens also undergo enterohepatic recirculation via sulphate and glucuronide conjugation in the liver, biliary secretion of conjugates into the intestine, and hydrolysis in the gut following reabsorption. In post-menopausal women a significant proportion of the circulating estrogens exists as sulphate conjugates, especially estrone sulphate, which serves as a circulating reservoir for the formation of more active estrogens.

Excretion

Estriol, estrone and estradiol are excreted in the urine along with glucuronide and sulphate conjugates.

Table 1 – Pharmacokinetic parameters for Premarin

Pharmacokinetic profile for unconjugated estrogens following a dose of 2 × 0.625mg

(see Table 1)

Pharmacokinetic profile for conjugated estrogens following a dose of 2 × 0.625mg

(see Table 2)

Norgestrel

Norgestrel is a racemic mixture consisting of a levo-rotatory isomer, which is biologically inactive, and the biologically active dextro-rotatory isomer, commonly known as levonorgestrel.

The biologically active isomer, levonorgestrel, is rapidly and almost completely absorbed after administration by mouth, and undergoes little first pass hepatic metabolism. It is highly bound to plasma proteins; 42 to 68% to sex hormone binding globulin and 30 to 56% to albumin. Levonorgestrel and norgestrel are metabolised in the liver to sulphate and glucuronide conjugates, which are excreted in the urine and to a lesser extent in the faeces.

The pharmacokinetic profile of levonorgestrel following an oral dose of 150 micrograms and repeat dosing performed until a steady state was achieved is provided in Table 3.

The proportion of levonorgestrel bound to sex hormone binding globulin is higher when it is given with an estrogen. This indicates that the pharmacokinetic parameters for each active substance will differ when used in combination.

Table 3 – Pharmacokinetic parameters for Levonorgestrel following a dose of 150 microgram and repeat dosing until steady state achieved

(see Table 3)

5.3 Preclinical safety data

Long-term continuous administration of natural and synthetic estrogens in certain animal species increases the frequency of carcinoma of the breast, cervix, vagina and liver.

6. PHARMACEUTICAL PARTICULARS

6.1 List of excipients

0.625 mg Conjugated estrogen tablets:

Calcium sulphate, carnauba wax, microcrystalline cellulose, glyceryl mono-oleate, lactose, magnesium stearate,

Table 1 – Pharmacokinetic parameters for Premarin

Drug PK Parameter Arithmetic Mean (%CV)	C_{max} (pg/mL)	t_{max} (h)	$t_{1/2}$ (h)	AUC (pg.h/mL)*
estrone	139 (37)	8.8 (20)	28.0 (13)	5016 (34)
baseline-adjusted estrone	120 (42)	8.8 (20)	17.4 (37)	2956 (39)
equilin	66 (42)	7.9 (19)	13.6 (52)	1210 (37)

* $t_{1/2}$ = terminal-phase disposition half-life (0.693/γ)

Table 2

Drug PK Parameter Arithmetic Mean (%CV)	C_{max} (ng/mL)	t_{max} (h)	$t_{1/2}$ (h)	AUC (pg.h/mL)*
total estrone	7.3 (41)	7.3 (51)	15.0 (25)	134 (42)
baseline-adjusted total estrone	7.1 (41)	7.3 (25)	13.6 (27)	122 (39)
total equilin	5.0 (42)	6.2 (26)	10.1 (27)	65 (45)

* $t_{1/2}$ = terminal-phase disposition half-life (0.693/γ)

Table 3 – Pharmacokinetic parameters for Levonorgestrel following a dose of 150 microgram and repeat dosing until steady state achieved

PK Parameter Mean value (SD provided in square brackets)	**C_{max} (μg/L)**	**t_{max} (h)**	**$t_{1/2DIST}$ (h)**	**$t_{1/2\beta}$ (h)**	**Vd (L)**	**CL (ml/min/kg)**	**AUC (μg/L·h)**
Single Dose (150μg)	4.3 [1.3]	1.2 [0.5]	0.6 [0.2]	13.9 [3.2]	108 [37]	1.5 [0.6]	30.9 [11.9]
Repeat dose (to steady state)	2.7 [0.3]	1.0 [0.3]	0.5 [0.2]	17.4 [3.6]	226 [61]	2.5 [0.4]	25.0 [5.9]

methylcellulose, macrogol, shellac solution, sucrose, titanium dioxide (E171), and opalux maroon colour AS-3910†.

† Opalux maroon colour contains sucrose, purified water, erythrosine (E127), titanium dioxide (E171), sunset yellow (E110), indigo carmine (E132), polyvinylpyrrolidone and sodium benzoate.

1.25 mg Conjugated estrogen tablets:

Calcium sulphate, carnauba wax, microcrystalline cellulose, glyceryl mono-oleate, lactose, magnesium stearate, methylcellulose, syrup, macrogol, shellac solution, sucrose, titanium dioxide (E171), colours E110, E104.

Norgestrel tablets:

Bleached wax, calcium carbonate, carnauba wax, lactose, magnesium stearate, macrogol, polyvinyl pyrrolidone, starch, sucrose, talc, titanium dioxide (E171), colour E172.

6.2 Incompatibilities
Not applicable.

6.3 Shelf life
Three years.

6.4 Special precautions for storage
Do not store above 25°C.

6.5 Nature and contents of container
Polyvinylchloride (PVC)/Aluminium foil blisters containing 28 conjugated estrogen and 12 norgestrel tablets. One carton pack contains 3 blisters.

6.6 Instructions for use and handling
Not applicable.

7. MARKETING AUTHORISATION HOLDER
John Wyeth and Brother Limited
Trading as: Wyeth Pharmaceuticals
Huntercombe Lane South
Taplow, Maidenhead
Berkshire, SL6 0PH

8. MARKETING AUTHORISATION NUMBER(S)
Prempak-C tablets 0.625mg PL 0011/0161
Prempak-C tablets 1.25mg PL 0011/0162

9. DATE OF FIRST AUTHORISATION/RENEWAL OF THE AUTHORISATION
1982.

10. DATE OF REVISION OF THE TEXT
11th February 2005

Preparation H Clear Gel

(Wyeth Consumer Healthcare)

1. NAME OF THE MEDICINAL PRODUCT
Preparation H Clear Gel

2. QUALITATIVE AND QUANTITATIVE COMPOSITION
Active Ingredients:
Hamamelis Water 50.0%w/w

3. PHARMACEUTICAL FORM
Gel for topical application

4. CLINICAL PARTICULARS

4.1 Therapeutic indications
Relief of the symptoms of Haemorrhoids i.e. pain, irritation and itching. Helps to shrink the tissues swollen by inflammation. Lubricant for easing painful bowel movements when the skin is dry and sore.

4.2 Posology and method of administration
Adults: For topical administration to the anal region. Apply freely night and morning and after each bowel movement. The applicator may be screwed onto the neck of the tube to assist in application of the product. The nozzle should only be inserted into the anal canal so as to avoid application to the rectum.

Elderly: As for adults.

Children: Not to be used except on the advice of a doctor.

4.3 Contraindications
History of sensitivity to any of the constituents.

4.4 Special warnings and special precautions for use
Persons who suffer from haemorrhoids are advised to consult a doctor.

Keep all medicines out of the reach of children.

4.5 Interaction with other medicinal products and other forms of Interaction
None known.

4.6 Pregnancy and lactation
There are no known problems with the use of witch-hazel in pregnancy and lactation.

4.7 Effects on ability to drive and use machines
None.

4.8 Undesirable effects
Occasionally stinging at the time of application may occur. Very rarely eczematous dermatitis has been reported.

4.9 Overdose
Preparation H Gel is not to be swallowed. Medical intervention is not required following ingestion. However, ingestion of witch-hazel is not recommended.

5. PHARMACOLOGICAL PROPERTIES

5.1 Pharmacodynamic properties
Hamamelis has astringent, anti-haemorrhagic and anti-inflammatory properties and is cooling on application.

5.2 Pharmacokinetic properties
Preparation H Clear Gel is for topical application and has a localised effect.

5.3 Preclinical safety data
None Stated

6. PHARMACEUTICAL PARTICULARS

6.1 List of excipients
Purified Water PhEur
Hydroxyethylcellulose PhEur
Propylene Glycol PhEur
Sodium Citrate PhEur
Methyl Hydroxybenzoate PhEur
Disodium Edetate PhEur
Propyl Hydroxybenzoate PhEur
Citric Acid Monohydrate PhEur

6.2 Incompatibilities
None known.

6.3 Shelf life
3 years.

6.4 Special precautions for storage
Do not store above 25 °C

6.5 Nature and contents of container
10g/25g/50g lacquered aluminium tube or 10g/25g/50g aluminium polyethylene laminate tube packed in a cardboard carton.

6.6 Instructions for use and handling
Lubricate applicator before each application and clean thoroughly after use.

7. MARKETING AUTHORISATION HOLDER
Whitehall Laboratories Limited
Huntercombe Lane South
Taplow
Maidenhead
Berkshire
SL6 0PH

8. MARKETING AUTHORISATION NUMBER(S)
PL 00165/0129.

9. DATE OF FIRST AUTHORISATION/RENEWAL OF THE AUTHORISATION
8 October 1998

10. DATE OF REVISION OF THE TEXT
October 2001

Preparation H Ointment

(Wyeth Consumer Healthcare)

1. NAME OF THE MEDICINAL PRODUCT
Preparation H ointment

2. QUALITATIVE AND QUANTITATIVE COMPOSITION
Active Ingredients
Yeast Cell Extract 1.0%w/w
Shark Liver Oil 3.0%w/w

3. PHARMACEUTICAL FORM
Ointment

4. CLINICAL PARTICULARS

4.1 Therapeutic indications
Relief of symptoms of haemorrhoids i.e. pain, irritation and itching. Helps to shrink the tissue swollen by inflammation. Lubricant in easing painful bowel movements when skin is dry and sore.

4.2 Posology and method of administration
For topical administration

Adults: Apply freely night and morning, and after each bowel movement.

Elderly: As for adults

Children: Not to be used except on the advice of a doctor.

4.3 Contraindications
Known history of sensitivity to any of the ingredients.

4.4 Special warnings and special precautions for use
Persons suffering from haemorrhoids are advised to consult a doctor.

4.5 Interaction with other medicinal products and other forms of Interaction
None Known.

4.6 Pregnancy and lactation
Preparation H has been used satisfactorily by a large number of pregnant women for many years without adverse or harmful effects being reported on the health of either the unborn or the new-born child.

4.7 Effects on ability to drive and use machines
None.

4.8 Undesirable effects
None Known.

4.9 Overdose
Preparation H is not to be swallowed: If you accidentally swallow any, seek medical advice.

5. PHARMACOLOGICAL PROPERTIES

5.1 Pharmacodynamic properties
Not applicable.

5.2 Pharmacokinetic properties
Not applicable.

5.3 Preclinical safety data
Not applicable.

6. PHARMACEUTICAL PARTICULARS

6.1 List of excipients
White Soft Paraffin
Liquid Paraffin
Light Liquid Paraffin
Wool Fat
Wool Alcohols
Thyme Oil Red
Methyl parahyroxybenzoate
Propyl parahyroxybenzoate
Glycerin

6.2 Incompatibilities
None known.

6.3 Shelf life
36 months

6.4 Special precautions for storage
Do not store above 25°C

6.5 Nature and contents of container
Collapsible aluminium tube with latex crimp seal and polypropylene tube nozzle and cap. Pack sizes 5g, 10g, 25g and 50g. Also available is a 25g tube as described above, packaged together with a re-sealable pouch containing 15 non-medicated moistened rayon tissues.

6.6 Instructions for use and handling
Not applicable.

7. MARKETING AUTHORISATION HOLDER
Whitehall Laboratories Limited *trading as* Wyeth Consumer Healthcare
Huntercombe Lane South
Taplow
Maidenhead
Berkshire SL6 OPH

8. MARKETING AUTHORISATION NUMBER(S)
PL0165/5014R

9. DATE OF FIRST AUTHORISATION/RENEWAL OF THE AUTHORISATION
23 January 1991

10. DATE OF REVISION OF THE TEXT
December 2004

Preparation H Suppositories

(Wyeth Consumer Healthcare)

1. NAME OF THE MEDICINAL PRODUCT
Preparation H suppositories

2. QUALITATIVE AND QUANTITATIVE COMPOSITION
Yeast Cell Extract 1.0%w/w
Shark Liver Oil 3.0%w/w

3. PHARMACEUTICAL FORM
Suppositories

4. CLINICAL PARTICULARS

4.1 Therapeutic indications
Relief of symptoms of haemorrhoids i.e. pain, irritation and itching. Helps to shrink the tissue swollen by inflammation. Lubricant in easing painful bowel movements.

4.2 Posology and method of administration
For rectal administration

Adults: Insert one suppository, rounded end first, into the rectum, morning and night, and after each bowel movement.

Elderly: As for adults

Children: Not to be used except on the advice of a doctor.

4.3 Contraindications
Known history of sensitivity to any of the ingredients.

4.4 Special warnings and special precautions for use
Persons suffering from haemorrhoids are advised to consult a doctor.

4.5 Interaction with other medicinal products and other forms of Interaction
None Known.

4.6 Pregnancy and lactation
Preparation H has been used satisfactorily by a large number of pregnant women for many years without adverse or harmful effects being reported on the health of either the unborn or the new-born child.

4.7 Effects on ability to drive and use machines
None.

4.8 Undesirable effects
None Known.

4.9 Overdose
Not applicable.

5. PHARMACOLOGICAL PROPERTIES

5.1 Pharmacodynamic properties
Not applicable.

5.2 Pharmacokinetic properties
Not applicable.

5.3 Preclinical safety data
Not applicable.

6. PHARMACEUTICAL PARTICULARS

6.1 List of excipients
Hard Fat

Hydrocarbon Wax

Polyethylene Glycol 600 Dilaurate

Cocoa Butter

Glycerin

6.2 Incompatibilities
None known.

6.3 Shelf life
24 months

6.4 Special precautions for storage
Do not store above 25°C

6.5 Nature and contents of container
PVC/Polyethylene strips for injection moulding, in a carton. Cartons contain 6, 12, 24 or 48 suppositories.

6.6 Instructions for use and handling
Not applicable.

7. MARKETING AUTHORISATION HOLDER
Whitehall Laboratories Limited *trading as* Wyeth Consumer Healthcare

Huntercombe Lane South

Taplow

Maidenhead

Berkshire SL6 0PH

8. MARKETING AUTHORISATION NUMBER(S)
PL0165/5015R

9. DATE OF FIRST AUTHORISATION/RENEWAL OF THE AUTHORISATION
18 January 1991

10. DATE OF REVISION OF THE TEXT
December 2004

Prescal

(Novartis Pharmaceuticals UK Ltd)

1. NAME OF THE MEDICINAL PRODUCT
PRESCAL® Tablets 2.5mg

2. QUALITATIVE AND QUANTITATIVE COMPOSITION
One tablet contains 2.5mg isradipine INN

3. PHARMACEUTICAL FORM
Yellow circular flat bevelled edge, angle scored tablets, 6mm in diameter, marked NM on one side and CIBA on the other

4. CLINICAL PARTICULARS

4.1 Therapeutic indications
PRESCAL is recommended for the treatment of essential hypertension

4.2 Posology and method of administration
Route of administration: oral

PRESCAL can be administered with or without food.

The recommended dosage is 2.5 mg twice a day (i.e. about every 12 hours). Treatment for 3-4 weeks is required for the maximum effect to develop. If blood pressure is not adequately controlled after this period patients may require a dosage of 5 mg twice a day, or if more appropriate, the addition of a low dose of another anti-hypertensive agent i.e. thiazide diuretic or beta-blocker. Exceptionally some patients may require up to 10mg twice a day. PRESCAL can also be added to an ongoing regimen of other anti-hypertensive agents.

Use in the elderly and patients with impaired or renal function

In elderly patients, or where hepatic or renal function is impaired, a more suitable starting dose is 1.25 mg twice a day for hypertension. However, the dosage may be increased according to the requirements of the individual patient. Once daily maintenance treatment with 2.5 mg or 5 mg may be sufficient in some hypertensive patients.

Use in children

The efficacy and safety of PRESCAL has not been established in children and is therefore not recommended in these patients.

4.3 Contraindications
Patients with a previous allergic reaction to isradipine and other dihydropyridines because of the theoretical risk of cross-reactivity.

Dihydropyridines, including PRESCAL Tablets, should be discontinued in patients who develop cardiogenic shock. They should also not be used in patients with symptomatic or tight aortic stenosis, and during or within one month of myocardial infarction.

Dihydropyridines including PRESCAL Tablets should not be used for the prevention of secondary myocardial infarctions and they have not been approved for the treatment of hypertensive crisis.

Dihydropyridines, including PRESCAL Tablets, should not be used in patients with unstable angina.

4.4 Special warnings and special precautions for use
As for other calcium antagonists PRESCAL does not give protection against the danger of abrupt beta-blocker withdrawal. Beta-blockers should therefore be withdrawn gradually, preferably over 8-10 days.

Caution should be taken when treating patients with documented or strongly suspected sick sinus syndrome who are not fitted with a pacemaker.

PRESCAL should be used with caution in patients with poor cardiac reserve.

Care is recommended when treating patients with a low systolic blood pressure.

There is no evidence that PRESCAL interferes with glucose metabolism, however, diabetic patients should be initially monitored in accordance with good clinical practice.

4.5 Interaction with other medicinal products and other forms of Interaction
The bioavailability of isradipine is not affected by co-administration of food. However, the lag time to absorption and time to peak plasma concentration may be delayed by about one hour.

The pharmacokinetics of isradipine are not modified by the concomitant administration of digoxin, propranolol, or hydrochlorothiazide. Nor are the kinetics of digoxin or hydrochlorothiazide altered by the concomitant administration of PRESCAL. However, PRESCAL increases the bioavailability of propranolol, but this does not appear to be of any clinical significance. Isradipine is non-specifically bound to proteins. Enzyme inducing anti-convulsants may be associated with reduced levels of isradipine.

As with other dihypropyridines, PRESCAL should not be taken with grapefruit juice because bioavailability may be increased.

Concurrent administration of cimetidine, an inhibitor of the cytochrome P_{450} system, results in an increase of about 50% in the bioavailability of PRESCAL whereas concomitant administration of rifampicin, an inducer of the cytochrome P_{450} system, greatly reduces the plasma concentrations of PRESCAL. Therefore, when PRESCAL is administered together with other drugs which alter the activity of the cytochrome P_{450} system, patients should be monitored carefully and doses of these drugs altered accordingly.

4.6 Pregnancy and lactation
Although some dihydropyridine compounds have been found to be teratogenic in animals, animal data in the rat and rabbit on isradipine provide no evidence for a teratogenic or embryotoxic effect. There is insufficient experience of the drug in pregnant women to justify its use during pregnancy, unless the potential benefit to the mother is expected to outweigh any potential risk to the offspring. Pre-natal observations in animals suggest that high doses of isradipine may cause prolongation of labour.

Animal data indicate that small quantities of isradipine may be excreted in the breast milk. Therefore breast-feeding should not be undertaken by mothers treated with PRESCAL.

4.7 Effects on ability to drive and use machines
None.

4.8 Undesirable effects
Clinical studies indicate that PRESCAL is well tolerated with an overall incidence of adverse events similar to that of placebo when used in doses up to 2.5 mg twice a day. Generally side effects are mild, dose dependent and tend to disappear or decrease in intensity as treatment is continued. Discontinuation of therapy is generally not required. Those side effects mentioned most often are related to the vasodilating properties of PRESCAL: headache, flushing, dizziness, tachycardia and palpitation, and localised peripheral oedema of non-cardiac origin; hypotension is uncommon and there have been no reports of orthostatic hypotension.

Non-specific side effects are rare and include: weight gain, fatigue, abdominal discomfort, and skin rash.

Elevations of serum transaminases have been observed on very rare occasions; these changes were reversible both spontaneously and on following PRESCAL withdrawal.

As with other dihydropyridines, aggravation of underlying angina has been reported in a small number of individuals especially after starting treatment. This is more likely to happen in patients with symptomatic ischaemic heart disease. PRESCAL should be discontinued under medical supervision in patients who develop unstable angina.

4.9 Overdose

Symptoms

Available data on calcium antagonists suggest that overdosage would result in marked and prolonged systemic hypotension requiring cardiovascular support, with monitoring of cardiac and respiratory functions and attention to possible cerebral ischaemia (elevation of the lower extremities) and to circulating blood volume (intravenous fluid or plasma volume expanders).

Management

In cases of severe hypotension, vasoconstrictors could be beneficial provided there is no contra-indication to their use. Intravenous calcium may help to reverse the effect of calcium entry blockade. Animal data suggest the risk for cardio-depression with PRESCAL should be minimal, but depression of the sinus node may occur in which case temporary pacemaker treatment may be useful.

Since isradipine is bound to plasma proteins to a very large extent, dialysis cannot be expected to be of benefit.

5. PHARMACOLOGICAL PROPERTIES

5.1 Pharmacodynamic properties
Isradipine is a dihydropyridine calcium antagonist with a higher affinity for calcium channels in arterial smooth muscle than for those in the myocardium. Thus it produces vasodilation of peripheral coronary and cerebral arteries without notably depressing cardiac function. As a result of the vasodilation of peripheral arteries, the arterial blood pressure is lowered; the attending after-load reduction improves myocardial contractility and increases cardiac output, while myocardial oxygen consumption decreases. In animal studies isradipine has been observed to exert a cardioprotective effect against ischaemic injury without cardiodepression.

5.2 Pharmacokinetic properties
Following oral administration of PRESCAL, isradipine is completely absorbed (90-95%) from the gastro-intestinal tract and undergoes extensive first pass metabolism resulting in a bioavailability of 15-24%. Single oral doses are detectable in the plasma within 20 minutes and peak plasma concentrations are reached approximately 2 hours after intake. Isradipine is approximately 95% bound to plasma proteins.

No clear correlation between renal function and pharmacokinetic parameters has been found; both an increase and a decrease in bioavailability has been observed in patients with impaired renal function. The bioavailability of isradipine was increased in elderly patients with impaired renal function.

5.3 Preclinical safety data
None available

6. PHARMACEUTICAL PARTICULARS

6.1 List of excipients
Sodium lauryl sulphate, magnesium stearate, polyvinylpyrrolidone, maize starch, lactose, purified water

6.2 Incompatibilities
None

6.3 Shelf life
60 months

6.4 Special precautions for storage
Protect from light

6.5 Nature and contents of container
56 tablets in White opaque PVC/PVdC blister pack in outer box cardboard container; PVC 250 micron, PVdC 60 GSM, Aluminium foil 20 micron

56 tablets in Red transparent PVC/PVdC blister pack in outer box cardboard container; PVC 200 micron, PVdC 60 GSM, Aluminium foil 20 micron

6.6 Instructions for use and handling
None

7. MARKETING AUTHORISATION HOLDER
Novartis Pharmaceuticals UK Ltd

Trading as Ciba Laboratories

Frimley Business Park

Frimley

Camberley

Surrey

GU16 7SR

8. MARKETING AUTHORISATION NUMBER(S)
00101/0537

9. DATE OF FIRST AUTHORISATION/RENEWAL OF THE AUTHORISATION
17 November 1997 / 08 February 1999

10. DATE OF REVISION OF THE TEXT
08 February 2002

LEGAL CATEGORY
POM

PRESERVEX film-coated tablets 100 mg

(UCB Pharma Limited)

1. NAME OF THE MEDICINAL PRODUCT
PRESERVEX® film-coated tablets 100 mg

2. QUALITATIVE AND QUANTITATIVE COMPOSITION
Aceclofenac. 100 mg

3. PHARMACEUTICAL FORM
Preservex film-coated tablets 100 mg are presented as white round film-coated tablets, 8 mm in diameter, with an "A" embossed on one side.

4. CLINICAL PARTICULARS

4.1 Therapeutic indications
Preservex is indicated for the relief of pain and inflammation in osteoarthritis, rheumatoid arthritis and ankylosing spondylitis.

4.2 Posology and method of administration
Preservex film-coated tablets are supplied for oral administration and should be swallowed whole with a sufficient quantity of liquid. When Preservex was administered to fasting and fed healthy volunteers only the rate and not the extent of aceclofenac absorption was affected and as such Preservex should be taken preferably with or after food.

Adults

The recommended dose is 200 mg daily, taken as two separate 100 mg doses, one tablet in the morning and one in the evening.

Children

There are no clinical data on the use of Preservex in children and therefore it is not recommended for use in children.

Elderly

The pharmacokinetics of Preservex are not altered in elderly patients, therefore it is not considered necessary to modify the dose or dose frequency.

As with other non-steroidal anti-inflammatory drugs (NSAIDs), caution should be exercised in the treatment of elderly patients, who are generally more prone to adverse reactions, and who are more likely to be suffering from impaired renal, cardiovascular or hepatic function and receiving concomitant medication. The elderly should be monitored for GI bleeding for 4 weeks following initiation of NSAID therapy.

Renal insufficiency

There is no evidence that the dosage of Preservex needs to be modified in patients with mild renal impairment, but as with other NSAIDs caution should be exercised (see also Precautions).

Hepatic insufficiency

There is some evidence that the dose of Preservex should be reduced in patients with hepatic impairment and it is suggested that an initial daily dose of 100 mg be used.

4.3 Contraindications
NSAIDs should not be administered to patients with a history of or active or suspected peptic ulcer or gastro-intestinal bleeding.

Preservex should not be given to patients with moderate to severe renal impairment.

Preservex should not be prescribed during pregnancy, unless there are compelling reasons for doing so. The lowest effective dosage should be used.

Preservex should not be administered to patients previously sensitive to aceclofenac or in whom aspirin or NSAIDs precipitate attacks of asthma, acute rhinitis or urticaria or who are hypersensitive to these drugs. Preservex is contraindicated in cases where there is hypersensitivity to any of its constituents.

4.4 Special warnings and special precautions for use
Warnings:

Gastro-intestinal: Close medical surveillance is imperative in patients with symptoms indicative of gastro-intestinal disorders, with a history suggestive of gastro-intestinal ulceration, with ulcerative colitis or with Crohn's disease, bleeding diathesis or haematological abnormalities.

Gastro-intestinal bleeding or ulcerative perforation, haematemesis and melaena have in general more serious consequences in the elderly. They can occur at any time during treatment, with or without warning symptoms or a previous history. In the rare instances where gastro-intestinal bleeding or ulceration occurs in patients receiving Preservex, the drug should be withdrawn.

Hepatic: Close medical surveillance is also imperative in patients suffering from severe impairment of hepatic function.

Hypersensitivity reactions: As with other NSAIDs, allergic reactions, including anaphylactic/anaphylactoid reactions, can also occur without earlier exposure to the drug.

Precautions:

Renal: Patients with mild renal or cardiac impairment and the elderly should be kept under surveillance, since the use of NSAIDs may result in deterioration of renal function. The lowest effective dose should be used and renal function monitored regularly.

The importance of prostaglandins in maintaining renal blood flow should be taken into account in patients with impaired cardiac or renal function, those being treated with diuretics or recovering from major surgery. Effects on renal function are usually reversible on withdrawal of Preservex.

Hepatic: If abnormal liver function tests persist or worsen, clinical signs or symptoms consistent with liver disease develop or if other manifestations occur (eosinophilia, rash), Preservex should be discontinued. Hepatitis may occur without prodromal symptoms.

Use of Preservex in patients with hepatic porphyria may trigger an attack.

Haematological: Preservex may reversibly inhibit platelet aggregation (see anticoagulants under 'Interactions').

Cardiovascular: NSAIDs should be given with care to patients with a history of heart failure or hypertension since oedema has been reported in association with NSAID administration.

Long-term treatment: All patients who are receiving NSAIDs should be monitored as a precautionary measure e.g. renal failure hepatic function (elevation of liver enzymes may occur) and blood counts.

Fertility: NSAIDs may impair fertility and is not recommended in women trying to conceive. The temporary discontinuation of aceclofenac should be considered in women having difficulties to conceive or undergoing investigations for infertility

Use with caution in patients suffering from or with a history of bronchial asthma since NSAIDs have been known to cause bronchospasm in such patients.

4.5 Interaction with other medicinal products and other forms of Interaction
Lithium: Preservex, like many NSAIDs, may increase plasma concentrations of lithium

Cardiac Glycosides: Through their renal effects, NSAIDs may increase plasma glycoside (including digoxin) levels, exacerbate cardiac failure and reduce the glomerular filtration rate in patients receiving glycosides.

Diuretics: Preservex, like other NSAIDs, may inhibit the activity of diuretics. Although it was not shown to affect blood pressure control when co-administered with bendrofluazide, interactions with other diuretics cannot be ruled out. When concomitant administration with potassium-sparing diuretics is employed, serum potassium should be monitored. Diuretics can increase the risk of nephrotoxicity of NSAIDs.

Anticoagulants: Like other NSAIDs, Preservex may enhance the activity of anticoagulants. Close monitoring of patients on combined anticoagulant and Preservex therapy should be undertaken.

Antidiabetic agents: Clinical studies have shown that diclofenac can be given together with oral antidiabetic agents with influencing their clinical effect. However, there have been isolated reports of hypoglycaemic and hyperglycaemic effects. Thus with Preservex, consideration should be given to adjustment of the dosage of hypoglycaemic agents.

Methotrexate: Caution should be exercised if NSAIDs and methotrexate are administered within 24 hours of each other, since NSAIDs may increase plasma levels, resulting in increased toxicity.

Mifepristone: NSAIDs should not be used for 8-12 days after mifepristone administration as NSAIDs can reduce the effect of mifepristone.

Other NSAIDs and steroids: Concomitant therapy with aspirin, other NSAIDs and steroids may increase the frequency of adverse reactions, including the risk of GI bleeding.

Cyclosporin: Cyclosporin nephrotoxicity may be increased by the effect of NSAIDs on renal prostaglandins.

Quinolone antimicrobials: Convulsions may occur due to an interaction between quinolones and NSAIDs. This may occur in patients with or without a previous history of epilepsy or convulsions. Therefore, caution should be exercised when considering the use of a quinolone in patients who are already receiving a NSAID.

4.6 Pregnancy and lactation
Pregnancy: There is no information on the use of Preservex during pregnancy. The regular use of NSAIDs during the last trimester of pregnancy may decrease uterine tone and contraction. NSAID use may also result in premature closure of the foetal ductus arteriosus *in utero* and possibly persistent pulmonary hypertension of the new born, delay onset and increase duration of labour.

Animal studies indicate that there was no evidence of teratogenesis in rats although the systemic exposure was low and in rabbits, treatment with aceclofenac (10 mg/kg/day) resulted in a series of morphological changes in some foetuses.

Lactation: There is no information on the secretion of Preservex to breast milk; there was however no notable transfer of radio-labelled (14C) aceclofenac to the milk of lactating rats.

The use of Preservex should therefore be avoided in pregnancy and lactation unless the potential benefits to the other outweigh the possible risks to the foetus.

Fertility: see precautions.

4.7 Effects on ability to drive and use machines
Patients suffering from dizziness, vertigo, or other central nervous system disorders whilst taking NSAIDs should refrain from driving or handling dangerous machinery.

4.8 Undesirable effects
The majority of adverse reactions reported have been reversible and of a minor nature. The most frequent are gastro-intestinal disorders, in particular dyspepsia, abdominal pain, nausea and diarrhoea, and occasional occurrence of dizziness. Dermatological complaints including pruritus and rash and abnormal hepatic enzyme and serum creatinine levels have also been reported with the frequencies indicated in the following table.

If serious adverse reactions occur, Preservex should be withdrawn.

The following is a table of adverse reactions reported during clinical studies and after authorisation, grouped by System-Organ Class and estimated frequencies.

(see Table 1 on next page)

Other rare or very rare class-effects reported with NSAIDs in general are:

Blood and lymphatic disorders – Aplastic anaemia

Psychiatric Disorders – Hallucination, Confusional state

Nervous System Disorders – Optic neuritis, somnolence

Ear and labyrinth disorders – Tinnitus

Respiratory, thoracic and mediastinal disorders – Aggravated asthma

Gastrointestinal System – Duodenal ulcer, Gastrointestinal perforation

Skin and Subcutaneous tissue disorders – Toxic epidermal necrolysis, Erythema multiforme, Exfoliative dermatitis, photosensitivity reaction

Renal and Urinary Disorders– Interstitial nephritis

General disorders and administration site conditions: Malaise

4.9 Overdose
Management of acute poisoning with NSAIDs essentially consists of supportive and symptomatic measures.

There are no human data available on the consequences of Preservex overdosage. The therapeutic measures to be taken are: absorption should be prevented as soon as possible after overdosage by means of gastric lavage and treatment with activated charcoal; supportive and symptomatic treatment should be given for complications such as hypotension, renal failure, convulsions, gastro-intestinal irritation, and respiratory depression; specific therapies such as forced diuresis, dialysis or haemoperfusion are probably of no help in eliminating NSAIDs due to their high rate of protein binding and extensive metabolism.

5. PHARMACOLOGICAL PROPERTIES

5.1 Pharmacodynamic properties
Aceclofenac is a non-steroidal agent with marked anti-inflammatory and analgesic properties.

The mode of action of aceclofenac is largely based on the inhibition to prostaglandin synthesis. Aceclofenac is a potent inhibitor of the enzyme cyclo-oxygenase, which is involved in the production of prostaglandins.

5.2 Pharmacokinetic properties
After oral administration, aceclofenac is rapidly and completely absorbed as unchanged drug. Peak plasma concentrations are reached approximately 1.25 to 3.00 hours following ingestion. Aceclofenac penetrates into the synovial fluid, where the concentrations reach approximately 57% of those in plasma. The volume of distribution is approximately 25 L.

The mean plasma elimination half-life is around 4 hours. Aceclofenac is highly protein-bound (>99%). Aceclofenac circulates mainly as unchanged drug. 4'-Hydroxyaceclofenac is the main metabolite detected in plasma. Approximately two-thirds of the administered dose is excreted via the urine, mainly as hydroxymetabolites.

No changes in the pharmacokinetics of aceclofenac have been detected in the elderly.

5.3 Preclinical safety data
The results from preclinical studies conducted with aceclofenac are consistent with those expected for NSAIDs. The principal target organ was the gastro-intestinal tract. No unexpected findings were recorded.

Aceclofenac was not considered to have any mutagenic activity in three *in vitro* studies and an *in vivo* study in the mouse.

Table 1

MedDRa SOC	Common < 10% - > 1%	Uncommon < 1% - > 0.1%	Rare < 0.1%- > 0.01%	Very rare/ isolated reports < 0.01%
Blood and lymphatic system disorders			Anaemia	Granulocytopenia Thrombocytopenia Neutropenia Haemolytic anaemia
Immune system disorders			Anaphylactic reaction (including shock) Hypersensitivity	
Metabolism and nutrition disorders				Hyperkalemia
Psychiatric disorders				Depression Abnormal dreams Insomnia
Nervous system disorders	Dizziness			Paraesthesia Tremor Somnolence Headache Dysgeusia (abnormal taste)
Eye disorders			Visual disturbance	
Ear and labyrinth disorders				Vertigo
Cardiac disorders				Palpitations
Vascular disorders				Flushing Hot flush
Respiratory, thoracic and mediastinal disorders			Dyspnoea	Bronchospasm Stridor
Gastrointestinal disorders	Dyspepsia Abdominal pain Nausea Diarrhoea	Flatulence Gastritis Constipation Vomiting Mouth ulceration	Melaena	Stomatitis Haematemesis Gastrointestinal haemorrhage Gastric ulcer Pancreatitis
Hepatobiliary disorders				Hepatitis Jaundice
Skin and subcutaneous tissue disorders		Pruritus Rash Dermatitis Urticaria	Face oedema	Purpura Dermatitis bullous
Renal and urinary disorders				Renal insufficiency Nephrotic syndrome
General disorders and administration site conditions				Oedema Fatigue Cramps in legs
Investigations	Hepatic enzyme increased	Blood urea increased Blood creatinine increased		Blood alkaline phosphatase increased Weight increase

Aceclofenac was not found to be carcinogenic in either the mouse or rat.

6. PHARMACEUTICAL PARTICULARS

6.1 List of excipients

The excipients used in Preservex film-coated tablets 100 mg are those commonly recommended for use in pharmaceutical preparations. These are microcrystalline cellulose, sodium croscarmellose, povidone, glyceryl palmitostearate and the film coat, containing partially substituted hydroxypropyl methylcellulose, microcrystalline cellulose, polyoxyethylene 40 stearate and titanium dioxide.

6.2 Incompatibilities

None known.

6.3 Shelf life

The shelf-life for this product shall not exceed three years from the date of manufacture.

6.4 Special precautions for storage

Do not store above 30°C.

6.5 Nature and contents of container

The immediate container for Preservex film-coated tablets 100 mg is a laminated aluminium/aluminium foil pack. Each foil strip contains either 10 or 14 tablets. One, two, four or six foil strips will be provided with a patient information leaflet inside a carton.

6.6 Instructions for use and handling

None stated.

7. MARKETING AUTHORISATION HOLDER

Almirall Prodesfarma SA

General Mitre 151

08022 Barcelona

Spain

8. MARKETING AUTHORISATION NUMBER(S)

PL 16973 / 0001

9. DATE OF FIRST AUTHORISATION/RENEWAL OF THE AUTHORISATION

22 May 2000

10. DATE OF REVISION OF THE TEXT

May 2005

Prestim Tablets

(Valeant Pharmaceuticals Ltd)

1. NAME OF THE MEDICINAL PRODUCT

Prestim Tablets

2. QUALITATIVE AND QUANTITATIVE COMPOSITION

Each tablet contains timolol maleate 10mg and bendroflumethiazide 2.5mg.

3. PHARMACEUTICAL FORM

Tablet.

4. CLINICAL PARTICULARS

4.1 Therapeutic indications

Prestim tablets are indicated for the treatment of mild to moderate hypertension.

4.2 Posology and method of administration

Prestim tablets are for oral administration.

The recommended dosage range is 1 to 4 tablets daily. The dosage can be taken in the morning or in two divided doses, morning and evening.

If blood pressure control is not achieved on 4 tablets daily, consideration should be given to titrating timolol and bendroflumethiazide separately or adding another agent with hypotensive activity.

__Dosage in the elderly__

Initiate treatment with 1 tablet daily and thereafter adjust according to response.

4.3 Contraindications

Anuria. Prestim should not be used in patients with renal failure or with a history of hypersensitivity to the thiazides.

Uncontrolled heart failure, bradycardia, cardiogenic shock, history of bronchospasm, bronchial asthma, chronic obstructive pulmonary disease, patients receiving adrenergic augmenting drugs (monoamine oxidase inhibitors and tricyclic antidepressants), sick sinus syndrome (including sino-atrial block), Prinzmetals angina, untreated phaeochromocytoma, hypersensitivity to any of the constituents, second to 3rd degree heart block, metabolic acidosis, hypotension, and severe peripheral circulatory disturbances.

Anaesthesia with agents that produce myocardial depression, such as chloroform and ether.

Prestim is contraindicated in pregnancy.

4.4 Special warnings and special precautions for use

__Cardiovascular__

The continued depression of sympathetic drive through beta-blockade may lead to cardiac failure. All patients should be observed for evidence of cardiac failure, and if it occurs, digitalisation should be considered.

Beta-blockers should not be used in patients with untreated congestive heart failure. This condition should first be stabilised

In patients with ischaemic heart disease, treatment should not be discontinued suddenly. The dosage should gradually be reduced, i.e. over 1-2 weeks. If necessary, replacement therapy should be initiated at the same time, to prevent exacerbation of angina pectoris.

Beta-blockers may induce bradycardia. If the pulse rate decreases to less than 50-55 beats per minute at rest and the patient experiences symptoms related to the bradycardia, the dosage should be reduced.

In patients with peripheral circulatory disorders (Raynaud's disease or syndrome, intermittent claudication), beta-blockers should be used with great caution as aggravation of these disorders may occur.

Metabolic/endocrine

Caution should be exercised in patients with diabetes mellitus, spontaneous hypoglycaemia, impaired renal or hepatic function

Beta-blockers may mask the symptoms of thyrotoxicosis or hypoglycaemia.

__Other warnings__:

Patients with a history of psoriasis should take beta-blockers only after careful consideration.

Beta-blockers may increase sensitivity to allergens and the seriousness of anaphylactic reactions.

The following statement will appear on the label of this product: 'Do not take this medicine if you have a history of wheezing or asthma'.

There have been reports of skin rashes and/or dry eyes associated with the use of beta-adrenergic blocking drugs. The reported incidence is small and in most cases the symptoms have cleared when treatment was withdrawn. Discontinuance of the drug should be considered if any such reaction is not otherwise explicable, cessation of therapy with the beta-blocker should be gradual.

4.5 Interaction with other medicinal products and other forms of Interaction

As with other diuretics, Prestim should not be administered concurrently with lithium salts. Diuretics can reduce lithium clearance resulting in high serum levels of lithium.

The depressant effect of beta-blocking drugs on myocardial contractility and on intracardiac conduction may be increased by concomitant use with other drugs having similar effects. Serious effects have been reported with verapamil, disopyramide, lignocaine and tocainide and may be anticipated with diltiazem, quinidine, amiodarone and any of the class 1 antiarrhythmic agents. Special care is necessary when any of these agents are given intravenously in patients who are receiving beta-blockers.

Concurrent administration of digitalis glycosides may increase the atrio-ventricular conduction time.

Beta-blockers increase the risk of 'rebound hypertension' when taken with clonidine. When clonidine is used in conjunction with non-selective beta-blockers such as timolol, treatment with clonidine should be continued for some time after treatment with the beta-blocker has been discontinued.

Concomitant administration of tricyclic antidepressants, barbiturates and phenothiazines, dihydropyridine derivatives such as nifedipine or antihypertensive agents may increase the blood pressure lowering effect.

Beta-blockers may intensify the blood sugar lowering effect of insulin and oral antidiabetic drugs.

Anaesthesia

The anaesthesiologist should be informed when the patient is receiving a beta-blocking agent. Concomitant use of beta blockers and anaesthetics may attenuate reflex tachycardia and increase the risk of hypotension.

The withdrawal of beta blocking drugs prior to surgery is not necessary in the majority of patients. If beta-blockade is interrupted in preparation for surgery, therapy should be discontinued at least 24 hours beforehand.

Continuation of beta-blockade reduces the risk of arrhythmias during induction and intubation, however the risk of hypertension may be increased. Anaesthetic agents such as ether, cyclopropane and trichloroethylene should not be used whereas halothane, isoflurane, nitrous oxide, intravenous induction agents, muscle relaxants, narcotic analgesics and local anaesthetic agents are all compatible with beta-adrenergic blockade. Local anaesthetics with added vasoconstrictors, e.g. adrenaline, should be avoided. The patient may be protected against vagal reactions by intravenous administration of atropine.

The bioavailability of beta-blockers will be increased by co-administration with cimetidine or hydralazine and reduced with rifampicin.

Alcohol induces increased plasma levels of hepatically metabolised beta-blockers such as timolol.

Some prostaglandin synthetase inhibiting drugs have been shown to impair the antihypertensive effect of beta-blocking drugs.

The effect of sympathomimetic agents, e.g. isoprenaline, salbutamol, will be reduced by concomitant use of beta blockers. In addition, sympathomimetics may counteract the effect of beta-blocking agents.

Caution is recommended when administering to patients on catecholamine depleting drugs such as reserpine or guanethidine.

4.6 Pregnancy and lactation

Prestim is contraindicated in pregnancy. Both constituents cross the placenta and appear in breast milk therefore breastfeeding is not recommended.

Beta-blockers reduce placental perfusion, which may result in intrauterine foetal death, immature and premature deliveries. In addition, adverse effects (especially hypoglycaemia and bradycardia) may occur in foetus and neonate. There is an increased risk of cardiac and pulmonary complications in the neonate in the postnatal period.

4.7 Effects on ability to drive and use machines

None known. When driving vehicles or operating machines it should be taken into account that occasionally dizziness or fatigue may occur.

4.8 Undesirable effects

Side effects associated with beta blockade e.g. gastrointestinal symptoms, dizziness, insomnia, sedation, depression, weakness, dyspnoea, bradycardia, heart block, bronchospasm and heart failure. Thiazide diuretics may cause excessive depletion of fluid and electrolytes during prolonged or intense use. Symptoms are muscle pain or fatigue, thirst and oliguria. With thiazide diuretics hypokalaemia is more severe in patients already depleted of potassium, as in renal or hepatic insufficiency. Coma may be precipitated in hepatic cirrhosis. The thiazides may induce hyperglycaemia and glycosuria in diabetic and other susceptible patients. The thiazides increase blood urea, which is most pronounced in patients with renal disease and pre-existing retention of nitrogen. Hyperuricaemia sometimes can occur. Reports of other adverse reactions to the thiazides include skin rashes with associated photosensitivity, necrotising vasculitis, acute pancreatitis, blood dyscrasias and aggravation of pre-existing myopia.

4.9 Overdose

The most common signs of overdosage are bradycardia, hypotension, bronchospasm and acute cardiac failure. Suggested treatments are as follows:

Severe bradycardia: IV atropine sulphate 0.25 - 2 mg

If bradycardia persists, IV isoprenaline 25 micrograms may be given.

Severe hypotension: IV noradrenaline or adrenaline

Bronchospasm: isoprenaline hydrochloride, orciprenaline or salbutamol.

Acute cardiac failure: digitalis, diuretics and oxygen. In refractory cases, IV aminophylline and IV glucagon 0.5 - 1mg have been reported useful.

General measures should be taken to restore blood volume, maintain blood pressure and correct electrolyte imbalance.

5. PHARMACOLOGICAL PROPERTIES

5.1 Pharmacodynamic properties

Timolol maleate is a non-selective Beta-adrenoceptor antagonist with marked hypotensive activity.

Bendroflumethiazide is a thiazide diuretic, which has a moderate duration of activity.

It has been shown that beta-blocking agents used in combination with a thiazide diuretic potentiates the effects of this diuretic giving an enhanced antihypertensive effect. This may be due to the inhibition of renin release or concomitant regional haemodynamic changes. This means that a relatively lower dose of the beta-blocker is required.

5.2 Pharmacokinetic properties

Timolol maleate is well absorbed, extensively metabolised in the liver and eliminated through the kidney with a half-life of 2.5 to 5 hours (the biological half-life is somewhat longer). The beta-blocking effect of timolol is apparent within 30 minutes of administration and has been shown to last for up to 24 hours. It has low to moderate lipid solubility. Protein binding is reported to be low. It crosses the placenta and appears in breast milk.

Bendroflumethiazide has been reported to be completely absorbed from the gastro-intestinal tract and to have a plasma half-life of about 3 or 4 hours. It is highly bound to plasma protein. There is evidence that bendroflumethiazide is fairly extensively metabolised; about 30% is excreted unchanged in the urine. The diuretic effect of bendroflumethiazide is usually complete in 12-18 hours.

5.3 Preclinical safety data

There are no pre-clinical data of relevance to the prescriber, which are additional to that already included in other sections of the SPC.

6. PHARMACEUTICAL PARTICULARS

6.1 List of excipients

Microcrystalline cellulose, starch, magnesium stearate.

6.2 Incompatibilities

None known.

6.3 Shelf life

The shelf life of Prestim tablets is three years.

6.4 Special precautions for storage

Store below 25°C.

6.5 Nature and contents of container

Glass bottles of 30 tablets, 100 and 500 tablets.

Glass bottle of 14 tablets (sample pack).

6.6 Instructions for use and handling

None.

Administrative Data

7. MARKETING AUTHORISATION HOLDER

Valeant Pharmaceuticals Ltd

Cedarwood

Chineham Business Park

Crockford Lane

Basingstoke

Hampshire

RG24 8WD

United Kingdom

8. MARKETING AUTHORISATION NUMBER(S)

PL 15142/0025

9. DATE OF FIRST AUTHORISATION/RENEWAL OF THE AUTHORISATION

31 December 2000

10. DATE OF REVISION OF THE TEXT

May 2004

Prevenar

(Wyeth Pharmaceuticals)

1. NAME OF THE MEDICINAL PRODUCT

Prevenar▼ suspension for injection

Pneumococcal saccharide conjugated vaccine, adsorbed

Prevenar▼ suspension for injection in pre-filled syringe

Pneumococcal saccharide conjugated vaccine, adsorbed

2. QUALITATIVE AND QUANTITATIVE COMPOSITION

Each 0.5 ml dose contains:

Pneumococcal polysaccharide serotype 4* 2 micrograms

Pneumococcal polysaccharide serotype 6B* 4 micrograms

Pneumococcal polysaccharide serotype 9V* 2 micrograms

Pneumococcal polysaccharide serotype 14* 2 micrograms

Pneumococcal oligosaccharide serotype 18C* 2 micrograms

Pneumococcal polysaccharide serotype 19F* 2 micrograms

Pneumococcal polysaccharide serotype 23F* 2 micrograms

* Conjugated to the CRM_{197} carrier protein and adsorbed on aluminium phosphate (0.5 mg)

For excipients, see 6.1.

3. PHARMACEUTICAL FORM

Suspension for injection.

Suspension for injection in pre-filled syringe

4. CLINICAL PARTICULARS

4.1 Therapeutic indications

Active immunisation against invasive disease (including sepsis, meningitis, bacteraemic pneumonia, bacteraemia) caused by *Streptococcus pneumoniae* serotypes 4, 6B, 9V, 14, 18C, 19F and 23F in:

- infants and young children from 2 months of age to 2 years of age

- previously unvaccinated children aged 2 years to 5 years (for high-risk subjects, see section 4.4).

For the number of doses to be administered in the different age groups, see section 4.2.

The use of Prevenar should be determined on the basis of official recommendations taking into consideration variability of serotype epidemiology in different geographical area as well as the impact of invasive disease in different age groups (see sections 4.4, 4.8 and 5.1).

4.2 Posology and method of administration

The vaccine should be given by intramuscular injection. The preferred sites are anterolateral aspect of the thigh (vastus lateralis muscle) in infants or the deltoid muscle of the upper arm in young children.

Infants aged 2 - 6 months: three doses, each of 0.5 ml, the first dose usually given at 2 months of age and with an interval of at least 1 month between doses.

A fourth dose is recommended in the second year of life.

Previously unvaccinated older infants and children:

Infants aged 7 - 11 months: two doses, each of 0.5 ml, with an interval of at least 1 month between doses. A third dose is recommended in the second year of life.

Children aged 12 - 23 months: two doses, each of 0.5 ml, with an interval of at least 2 months between doses.

Children aged 24 months – 5years: one single dose.

The need for a booster dose after these immunisation schedules has not been established.

Immunisation schedules:

The immunisation schedules for Prevenar should be based on official recommendations.

4.3 Contraindications

Hypersensitivity to the active substances or to any of the excipients, or to diphtheria toxoid.

4.4 Special warnings and special precautions for use

As with other vaccines, the administration of Prevenar should be postponed in subjects suffering from acute moderate or severe febrile illness.

As with all injectable vaccines, appropriate medical treatment and supervision should always be readily available in case of a rare anaphylactic event following the administration of the vaccine.

Prevenar will not protect against other *Streptococcus pneumoniae* serotypes than those included in the vaccine nor other micro-organisms that cause invasive disease or otitis media.

This vaccine should not be given to infants or children with thrombocytopenia or any coagulation disorder that would contraindicate intramuscular injection unless the potential benefit clearly outweighs the risk of administration.

Although some antibody response to diphtheria toxoid may occur, immunisation with this vaccine does not substitute for routine diphtheria immunisation.

For children from 2 years through 5 years of age, a single dose immunisation schedule was used. A higher rate of local reactions has been observed in children older than 24 months of age compared with infants (see section 4.8).

Children with impaired immune responsiveness, whether due to the use of immunosuppressive therapy, a genetic defect, HIV infection, or other causes, may have reduced antibody response to active immunisation.

Safety and immunogenicity data are limited in children with sickle cell disease and not yet available for children in other specific high-risk groups for invasive pneumococcal disease (e.g. children with congenital and acquired splenic dysfunction, HIV-infected, malignancy, nephrotic syndrome). Vaccination in high-risk groups should be considered on an individual basis.

Children below 2 years old (including those at high risk) should receive the appropriate-for-age Prevenar vaccination series (see section 4.2). The use of pneumococcal conjugate vaccine does not replace the use of 23-valent pneumococcal polysaccharide vaccines in children ⩾ 24 months of age with conditions (such as sickle cell disease, asplenia, HIV infection, chronic illness or who are immunocompromised) placing them at higher risk for invasive disease due to *Streptococcus pneumoniae*. Children ⩾ 24 months of age at high risk, previously immunised with Prevenar should receive 23-valent pneumococcal polysaccharide vaccine whenever recommended. Based on limited data, the interval between the pneumococcal conjugate vaccine (Prevenar) and the 23-valent pneumococcal polysaccharide vaccine should not be less than 8 weeks. Only limited data are available to inform the use of mixed schedules of pneumococcal conjugate vaccine and 23-valent pneumococcal polysaccharide vaccine in previously unimmunised high-risk children 2-5 years of age. Use of schedules may be considered on an individual basis taking into account current national recommendation.

When Prevenar is co-administered with hexavalent vaccines (DTaP/Hib(PRP-T)/IPV/HepB), the physician should be aware that data from clinical studies indicate that the rate of febrile reactions was higher compared to that occurring following the administration of hexavalent vaccines alone. These reactions were mostly moderate (less than or equal to 39 °C) and transient (see section 4.8).

Antipyretic treatment should be initiated according to local treatment guidelines.

Prophylactic antipyretic medication is recommended:

- for all children receiving Prevenar simultaneously with vaccines containing whole cell pertussis because of higher rate of febrile reactions (see section 4.8).

- for children with seizure disorders or with a prior history of febrile seizures.

Do not administer Prevenar intravenously.

4.5 Interaction with other medicinal products and other forms of Interaction

Prevenar can be administered simultaneously with other paediatric vaccines in accordance with the recommended immunisation schedules. Different injectable vaccines should always be given at different injection sites.

The immune response to routine paediatric vaccines co-administered with Prevenar at different injection sites was assessed in 7 controlled clinical studies. The antibody response to Hib tetanus protein conjugate (PRP-T), tetanus and Hepatitis B (HepB) vaccines was similar to controls. For CRM-based Hib conjugate vaccine, enhancement of antibody responses to Hib and diphtheria in the infant series was observed. At the booster, some suppression of Hib antibody level was observed but all children had protective levels. Inconsistent reduction in response to pertussis antigens as well as to inactivated polio vaccine (IPV) were observed. The clinical relevance of these interactions is unknown. Limited results from open label studies showed an acceptable response to MMR and varicella.

Data on concomitant administration of Prevenar with Infanrix hexa (DTaP/Hib(PRP-T)/IPV/HepB vaccine) have shown no clinically relevant interference in the antibody response to each of the individual antigens when given as a 3-dose primary vaccination.

Sufficient data regarding interference on the concomitant administration of other hexavalent vaccines with Prevenar are currently not available.

Data on concomitant administration with meningococcal C conjugate vaccines are not available, but data on an investigational combination vaccine containing the same 7 pneumococcal serotypes conjugated antigens of Prevenar and serogroup C meningococcal conjugated antigen of Meningitec has shown no clinically relevant interference in the antibody response to each of the individual antigens, suggesting that concomitant administration of Prevenar and CRM conjugate meningococcal C vaccines would not result in any immunologic interference when given as a 3-dose primary vaccination in the 1st year of life.

4.6 Pregnancy and lactation

Prevenar is not intended for use in adults. Information on the safety of the vaccine when used during pregnancy and lactation is not available.

4.7 Effects on ability to drive and use machines

Not relevant

4.8 Undesirable effects

The safety of the vaccine was assessed in different controlled clinical studies in which more than 18,000 healthy infants (6 weeks to 18 months) were included. The majority of the safety experience comes from the efficacy trial in which 17,066 infants received 55,352 doses of Prevenar. Also safety in previously unvaccinated older children has been assessed.

In all studies, Prevenar was administered concurrently with the recommended childhood vaccines.

Amongst the most commonly reported adverse reactions were injection site reactions and fever.

No consistent increased local or systemic reactions within repeated doses were seen throughout the primary series or with the booster dose, the exceptions being a higher rate of transient tenderness (36.5 %) and tenderness that interfered with limb movement (18.5 %) were seen with the booster dose.

In older children receiving a single dose of vaccine, a higher rate of local reactions has been observed than that previously described in infancy. These reactions were primarily transient in nature. In a post- licensure study involving 115 children between 2-5 years of age, tenderness was reported in up to 39.1 % of children; in 15.7 % of children the tenderness interfered with limb movement. Redness was reported in 40.0 % of children, and induration was reported in 32.2 % of subjects. Redness or induration ≥2cm in diameter was reported in 22.6 % and 13.9 % of children respectively.

When Prevenar is co-administered with hexavalent vaccines (DTaP/Hib(PRP-T)/IPV/HepB), fever ⩾ 38 °C per dose was reported in 28.3 % to 48.3 % of infants in the group receiving Prevenar and the hexavalent vaccine at the same time as compared to 15.6 % to 23.4 % in the group receiving the hexavalent vaccine alone. Fever of greater than 39.5 °C per dose was observed in 0.6 to 2.8 % of infants receiving Prevenar and hexavalent vaccines (see section 4.4).

Reactogenicity was higher in children receiving whole cell pertussis vaccines concurrently. In a study, including 1,662 children, fever of ⩾ 38 °C was reported in 41.2 % of children who received Prevenar simultaneously with DTP as compared to 27.9 % in the control group. Fever of > 39 °C was reported in 3.3 % of children compared to 1.2 % in the control group.

Undesirable effects reported in clinical trials or from the post-marketing experience are listed in the following table per body system and per frequency and this is for all age groups. The frequency is defined as follows: very common: ⩾ 10 %, common: ⩾ 1 % and < 10 %, uncommon: ⩾ 0.1 % and < 1 %, rare: ⩾ 0.01 % and < 0.1 %, very rare: < 0.01 %.

Blood and lymphatic system disorders:

Very rare: Lymphadenopathy localised to the region of the injection site.

Nervous system disorders:

Rare: Seizures, including febrile seizures.

Gastrointestinal disorders:

Very common: Decreased appetite, vomiting, diarrhoea.

Skin and subcutaneous tissue disorders:

Uncommon: Rash/urticaria.

Very rare: Erythema multiforme.

General disorders and administration site conditions:

Very common: Injection site reactions (e.g. erythema, induration/swelling, pain/tenderness); fever ⩾ 38 °C, irritability, drowsiness, restless sleep.

Common: Injection site swelling/induration and erythema >2.4 cm, tenderness interfering with movement, fever > 39 °C.

Rare: Hypotonic hyporesponsive episode, injection site hypersensitivity reactions (e.g. dermatitis, pruritus, urticaria).

Immune system disorders:

Rare: Hypersensitivity reaction including face oedema, angioneurotic oedema, dyspnoea, bronchospasm, anaphylactic/anaphylactoid reaction including shock.

4.9 Overdose

There have been reports of overdose with Prevenar, including cases of administration of a higher than recommended dose and cases of subsequent doses administered closer than recommended to the previous dose. No undesirable effects were reported in the majority of individuals. In general, adverse events reported with overdose have also been reported with recommended single doses of Prevenar.

5. PHARMACOLOGICAL PROPERTIES

5.1 Pharmacodynamic properties

Pharmacotherapeutic group: pneumococcal vaccines, ATC code: J07AL

Estimates of efficacy against invasive disease were obtained in the US population where vaccine serogroup coverage ranged from 89 - 93 %. Epidemiological data between 1998 and 2003 indicated that in Europe coverage is lower and varies from country to country. The coverage established for children less than 2 years of age is lower in the Northern part and higher in the Southern part of Europe. Consequently, Prevenar will cover between 71 % and 86 % of isolates from invasive pneumococcal disease (IPD) in European children less than 2 years of age. More than 80 % of the antimicrobial resistant strains are covered by the serotypes included in the vaccine. The vaccine serotype coverage in the paediatric population decreases with increasing age. In European children between 2 to 5 years of age, Prevenar should cover about 50 % to 75 % of the clinical isolates responsible for invasive pneumococcal disease. The decrease in the incidence of IPD seen in older children may be partly due to naturally acquired immunity.

Efficacy against invasive disease

Efficacy against invasive disease was assessed in a large-scale randomised double-blind clinical trial in a multiethnic population in Northern California (Kaiser Permanente trial). More than 37,816 infants were immunised with either Prevenar or a control vaccine (meningococcal conjugate group C vaccine), at 2, 4, 6 and 12-15 months of age. At the time of the study, the serotypes included in the vaccine accounted for 89 % of IPD.

A total of 52 cases of invasive disease caused by vaccine serotype had accumulated in a blinded follow-up period through April 20, 1999. The estimate of vaccine serotype-specific efficacy was 94 % (81, 99 - 95 % CI) in the intent-to-treat population and 97 % (85, 100 - 95 % CI) in the per protocol (fully immunised) population (40 cases). The corresponding estimates for vaccine serogroups are 92 % (79, 98 - 95 % CI) for the intent-to-treat population and 97 % (85, 100 - 95 % CI) for the fully immunised population.

In Europe, the estimates of effectiveness range from 65 % to 79 % when considering vaccine coverage of serogroups causing invasive disease.

In the Kaiser trial, efficacy was 87 % (7, 99 - 95 % CI) against bacteraemic pneumonia due to vaccine serotypes of *S. pneumoniae.*

Effectiveness (no microbiological confirmation of diagnosis was performed) against pneumonia was also assessed. The estimated risk reduction for clinical pneumonia with abnormal X-ray was 33 % (6, 52 - 95 % CI) and for clinical pneumonia with consolidation was 73 % (36, 90 - 95 % CI) in the intent-to-treat analysis.

Additional clinical data

Results from clinical trials support efficacy of Prevenar against otitis media due to vaccine serotypes, but the effectiveness was lower than in invasive disease.

Efficacy of Prevenar against acute otitis media (AOM) was assessed as a primary endpoint in a randomised double-blind clinical trial of 1,662 Finnish infants and as a secondary endpoint in the Northern California trial. The estimate for vaccine efficacy against vaccine-serotype AOM in the Finnish trial was 57 % (44, 67 - 95 % CI). In the intent-to-treat analysis the vaccine efficacy was 54 % (41, 64 - 95 % CI). A 34 % increase in AOM due to non-vaccine serogroups was observed in immunised subjects. However, the overall benefit was a statistically significant reduction (34 %) in the incidence of all pneumococcal AOM.

For recurrent otitis media (⩾ 3 episodes in 6 months or 4 in 12 months), the impact of the vaccine was a statistically non-significant 16 % reduction (-6, 35 - 95 % CI) in the Finnish trial. In the Northern California trial, the impact of the vaccine was a statistically significant 9.5 % reduction (3, 15 - 95 % CI). In Northern California, there was also a 20 % (2, 35 - 95 % CI) reduction in the placement of ear tubes in vaccine recipients.

In the Finnish trial, the impact of the vaccine on total number of episodes of otitis media regardless of etiology was a statistically non-significant 6 % reduction (-4, 16 - 95% CI) while in the Northern California trial the impact of the vaccine was a statistically significant 7 % reduction (4, 10 - 95% CI).

Immunogenicity

Vaccine-induced antibody to capsular polysaccharide-specific of each serotype are considered protective against invasive disease. The minimum protective antibody concentration against invasive disease has not been determined for any serotype.

A significant antibody response was seen following three and four doses to all vaccine serotypes in infants that received Prevenar, although geometric mean concentrations varied among serotypes. For all serotypes, peak primary series responses were seen after 3 doses, with boosting following the 4th dose. Prevenar induces functional antibodies to all vaccine serotypes, as measured by opsonophagocytosis following the primary series. Long-term persistence of antibodies after completion of immunisation has not been investigated in infants and older children (catch-up immunisation).

A plain polysaccharide challenge at 13 months following the primary series with Prevenar elicited an anamnestic antibody response for the 7 serotypes included in the vaccine which is indicative for priming.

A significant antibody response to all vaccine serotypes was seen after one dose of Prevenar in children aged 2 to 5 years. The vaccination with one dose of Prevenar in children aged 2 to 5 years resulted in similar immune responses to that seen following the primary series in infants and toddlers who were less than 2 years of age, in whom clinical effectiveness (protection) was demonstrated. Efficacy trials in the 2-to 5-year-old population have not been conducted.

Data on the immunogenicity of Prevenar administered at 3 and 5 months with a booster dose at 12 months of age are available from an open-label, uncontrolled clinical study conducted in Sweden in 83 infants. At the age of 13 months, one month after dose 3, geometric mean concentration (GMC) of serotype-specific antibody concentrations were substantially increased, ranging from 4.59 microgram/ml (serotype 23F) to 11.67 microgram/ml (serotype 14) and were comparable for all serotypes to those achieved following a fourth dose in European or U.S. infants immunised with a 4-dose series. However, at the age of 6 months, after 2 doses, GMC values for the seven vaccine serotypes were not all comparable to those seen in infants after 3 doses. For five serotypes, the GMC values ranged from 2.47 microgram/ml (serotype 18C) to 5.03 microgram/ml (serotype 19F), but for serotype 6B the GMC was 0.3 microgram/ml and for 23F the GMC was 0.88 microgram/ml.

Lower antibody levels after two priming doses at 3 and 5 months of age to two serotypes (6B and 23F) as compared to a 3-dose priming schedule were observed at the 6 months time point. Responses to the third (booster) dose indicated adequate priming and resulted in comparable antibody levels to all serotypes as after the booster dose in the 3-dose priming schedule. The clinical relevance of these observations remains unknown.

5.2 Pharmacokinetic properties

Evaluation of pharmacokinetic properties is not available for vaccines.

5.3 Preclinical safety data

A repeated dose toxicity study of pneumococcal conjugate vaccine in rabbits revealed no evidence of any significant local or systemic toxic effects.

6. PHARMACEUTICAL PARTICULARS

6.1 List of excipients

Sodium chloride

Water for injections

6.2 Incompatibilities

In the absence of compatibility studies, this medicinal product must not be mixed with other medicinal products.

6.3 Shelf life

Suspension for injection and Suspension for injection in pre-filled syringe:

3 years

6.4 Special precautions for storage

Suspension for injection and Suspension for injection in pre-filled syringe:

Store at 2 °C – 8 °C (in a refrigerator).

Do not freeze.

6.5 Nature and contents of container

0.5 ml suspension for injection in vial (Type I glass) with a grey butyl rubberstopper - pack size of 1 and 10 vials without syringe/needles. Pack size of 1 vial with syringe and 2 needles (1 for withdrawal, 1 for injection).

0.5 ml suspension for injection in pre-filled syringe (Type I glass) with a plunger rod (polypropylene). Pack size of 1 and 10 with or without needle.

Not all pack sizes may be marketed.

6.6 Instructions for use and handling

Upon storage, a white deposit and clear supernatant can be observed.

The vaccine should be well shaken to obtain a homogeneous white suspension and be inspected visually for any particulate matter and/or variation of physical aspect prior to administration. Do not use if the content appears otherwise.

7. MARKETING AUTHORISATION HOLDER

Wyeth Lederle Vaccines S.A.

Rue du Bosquet, 15

B-1348 Louvain-la-Neuve

Belgium

8. MARKETING AUTHORISATION NUMBER(S)

EU/1/00/167/001 – 1 × glass vial EU/1/00/167/002 – 10 × glass vial

EU/1/00/167/003 – 1 × pre-filled syringe

EU/1/00/167/004 – 10 × pre-filled syringe

EU/1/00/167/005 – 1 × glass vial with 1 syringe and 2 needles

EU/1/00/167/006 – 1 × pre-filled syringe with separate needle

EU/1/00/167/007 – 10 × pre-filled syringe with separate needles

9. DATE OF FIRST AUTHORISATION/RENEWAL OF THE AUTHORISATION

EU/1/00/167/001 – 02/02/2001

EU/1/00/167/002 – 02/02/2001

EU/1/00/167/003 – 02/02/2001

EU/1/00/167/004 – 02/02/2001

EU/1/00/167/005 – 02/02/2001

EU/1/00/167/006 – 02/02/2001

EU/1/00/167/007 – 02/02/2001

10. DATE OF REVISION OF THE TEXT

26 January 2005

Priadel Liquid

(sanofi-aventis)

1. NAME OF THE MEDICINAL PRODUCT

Priadel Liquid.

2. QUALITATIVE AND QUANTITATIVE COMPOSITION

A clear, colourless, pineapple flavoured, sugar free syrup containing 520mg lithium citrate equivalent to 200mg lithium carbonate per 5ml.

3. PHARMACEUTICAL FORM

Syrup.

4. CLINICAL PARTICULARS

4.1 Therapeutic indications

1. Treatment of mania and hypomania.

2. Lithium may also be tried in the treatment of some patients with recurrent bipolar depression, where treatment with other antidepressants has been unsuccessful.

3. Prophylactic treatment of recurrent affective disorders.

4. Control of aggressive or self-mutilating behaviour.

4.2 Posology and method of administration

A simple treatment schedule has been evolved which except for some minor variations should be followed whether using Priadel Liquid therapeutically or prophylactically. The minor variations to this schedule depend on the elements of the illness being treated and these are described later.

1. In patients of average weight (70kg) an initial daily dose of 10-30ml Priadel Liquid (equivalent to 400-1200mg lithium carbonate) should be given in divided doses, ideally twice a day. When changing between lithium preparations serum lithium levels should first be checked, then Priadel Liquid therapy commenced at a daily dose as close as possible to the dose of the other form of lithium. As bioavailability varies from product to product (particularly with regard to slow release preparations) a change of product should be regarded as initiation of new treatment.

2. Four to five days after starting treatment (and never longer than one week) a blood sample should be taken for the estimation of serum lithium level.

3. The objective is to adjust the Priadel Liquid dose so as to maintain the serum lithium level permanently within the diurnal range of 0.5-1.5mmol/l. In practice, the blood sample should be taken 12 hours after the previous dose of Priadel Liquid. "Target" serum lithium concentrations at 12 hours should be 0.5-0.8mmol/l.

Priadel Liquid is supplied with a 2.5/5ml double ended spoon to provide dosage adjustments equivalent to 100mg and 200mg lithium carbonate respectively. Serum lithium levels should be monitored weekly until stabilisation is achieved.

4. Lithium therapy should not be initiated unless adequate facilities for routine monitoring of serum concentrations are available. Following stabilisation of serum lithium levels, the period between subsequent estimations can be increased gradually but should not normally exceed three months. Additional measurements should be made following alteration of dosage, on development of intercurrent disease, signs of manic or depressive relapse, following significant change in sodium or fluid intake, or if signs of lithium toxicity occur.

5. Whilst a high proportion of acutely ill patients may respond within three to seven days of the commencement of therapy with Priadel Liquid it should be continued through any recurrence of the affective disturbance. This is important as the full prophylactic effect may not occur for 6 to 12 months after the initiation of therapy.

6. In patients who show a positive response with Priadel Liquid, treatment is likely to be long term. Careful clinical appraisal of the patient should be exercised throughout medication (see Precautions).

Prophylactic treatment of recurrent affective disorders: It is recommended that the described treatment schedule is followed.

Treatment of acute mania, hypomania and recurrent bipolar depression: It is likely that a higher than normal Priadel Liquid intake may be necessary during an acute phase. As soon as control of mania or depression is achieved, the serum lithium level should be determined and it may be necessary, dependent on the results, to lower the dose of Priadel Liquid and re-stabilise serum lithium levels. In all other details the described treatment schedule is recommended.

Elderly:

Elderly patients or those below 50kg in weight, often require lower lithium dosage to achieve therapeutic serum levels. Starting doses of 200mg to 400mg are recommended taken twice daily. Dosage increments of 200 to 400mg every 3 to 5 days are usual. Total daily doses of 800 to 1800mg may be necessary to achieve effective blood lithium levels of 0.8 to 1.0 mmol/L. For prophylaxis, the dosage necessary to reach a blood lithium level of 0.4 to 0.8 mmol/L is generally in the range of 600 to 1200 mg/day.

Children and adolescents:

Not recommended.

4.3 Contraindications

- Hypersensitivity to lithium or to any of the excipients.
- Cardiac disease.
- Clinically significant renal impairment.
- Untreated hypothyroidism.
- Breast-feeding.
- Patients with low body sodium levels, including for example dehydrated patients or those on low sodium diets.
- Addison's disease.

4.4 Special warnings and special precautions for use

- When considering Priadel therapy, it is necessary to ascertain whether patients are receiving lithium in any other form. If so, check serum levels before proceeding.
- Before beginning a lithium treatment:

– it is important to ensure that renal function is normal.

– cardiac function should be assessed.

– thyroid function should be evaluated. Patients should be euthyroid before initiation of lithium therapy.

- Renal, cardiac and thyroid functions should be reassessed periodically.
- The possibility of hypothyroidism and renal dysfunction arising during prolonged treatment should be borne in mind and periodic assessments made.
- Patients receiving long term lithium therapy should be warned by the physician and be given clear instructions regarding the symptoms of impending intoxication (see 4.9 Overdosage). They should be warned of the urgency of immediate action should these symptoms appear, and also of the need to maintain a constant and adequate salt and water intake. Treatment should be discontinued immediately on the first signs of toxicity (see 4.9 Overdosage).
- Patients should be warned to report if polyuria or polydipsia develop. Episodes of nausea, vomiting, diarrhoea, fluid deprivation (e.g. excessive sweating), and/or other conditions leading to salt/water depletion <u>should</u> also be reported. Drugs likely to upset electrolyte balance such as diuretics (including severe dieting) <u>should</u> also be reported. In these cases, lithium dosage should be closely monitored and reduction of dosage may be necessary.
- Caution should be exercised to ensure that diet and fluid intake are normal in order to maintain a stable electrolyte balance. This may be of special importance in very hot weather or work environment. Infectious diseases including colds, influenza, gastro-enteritis and urinary infections may alter fluid balance and thus affect serum lithium levels. Treatment should be discontinued during any intercurrent infection and should only be reinstituted after the patient's physical health has returned to normal.
- Elderly patients are particularly liable to lithium toxicity. Use with care as lithium excretion may also be reduced. They may exhibit adverse reactions at serum levels ordinarily tolerated by younger patients.

4.5 Interaction with other medicinal products and other forms of Interaction

<u>Interactions which increase lithium concentrations:</u>

If one of the following drugs is initiated, lithium dosage should either be adjusted or concomitant treatment stopped, as appropriate:

- Metronidazole.
- Non-steroidal anti-inflammatory drugs (monitor serum lithium concentrations more frequently if NSAID therapy is initiated or discontinued).
- ACE inhibitors.
- Diuretics (thiazides show a paradoxical antidiuretics effect resulting in possible water retention and lithium intoxication). If a thiazide diuretic has to be prescribed for a lithium-treated patient, lithium dosage should first be reduced and the patient re-stabilised with frequent monitoring. Similar precautions should be exercised on diuretic withdrawal.
- Other drugs affecting electrolyte balance, e.g. steroids, may alter lithium excretion and should therefore be avoided.
- Tetracyclines.

<u>Interactions which decrease serum lithium concentrations:</u>

- Xanthines (theophylline, caffeine).
- Sodium bicarbonate containing products.
- Diuretics (osmotic and carbonic anhydrase inhibitors).
- Urea.

<u>Interactions causing neurotoxicity:</u>

- Neuroleptics (particularly haloperidol at higher dosages), flupentixol, diazepam, thioridazine, fluphenazine, chlorpromazine and clozapine may lead in rare cases to neurotoxicity in the form of confusion, disorientation, lethargy, tremor, extra-pyramidal symptoms and myoclonus.
- Methyldopa.
- Selective Serotonin Re-uptake Inhibitors (e.g. fluvoxamine and fluxetine) as this combinationmay precipitate a serotoninergic syndrome, which justifies immediate discontinuation of treatment.
- Calcium channel blockers may lead to a risk of neurotoxicity in the form of ataxia, confusion and somnolence, reversible after discontinuation of the drug. Lithium concentrations may be increased.
- Carbamazepine may lead to dizziness, somnolence, confusion and cerebellar symptoms.

Lithium may prolong the effects of neuromuscular blocking agents. There have been reports of interaction between lithium and phenytoin, indomethacin and other prostaglandin-synthetase inhibitors.

4.6 Pregnancy and lactation

4.6.1

Pregnancy

Lithium therapy should not be used during pregnancy, especially during the first trimester, unless considered essential. There is epidemiological evidence that it may be harmful to the foetus in human pregnancy. Lithium crosses the placental barrier. In animal studies lithium has been reported to interfere with fertility, gestation and foetal development. An increase in cardiac and other abnormalities, especially Ebstein anomaly, are reported. Therefore, a pre-natal diagnosis such as ultrasound and electrocardiogramexamination is strongly recommended. In certain cases where a severe risk to the patient could exist if treatment were stopped, lithium has been continued during pregnancy.

If it is considered essential to maintain lithium treatment during pregnancy, serum lithium levels should be closely monitored and measured frequently since renal function changes gradually during pregnancy and suddenly at parturition. Dosage adjustments are required. It is recommended that lithium be discontinued shortly before delivery and reinitiated a few days *post-partum*.

Neonates may show signs of lithium toxicity necessitating fluid therapy in the neonatal period. Neonates born with low serum lithium concentrations may have a flaccid appearance that returns to normal without any treatment.

4.6.2 Women of child-bearing potential

It is advisable that women treated with lithium should adopt adequate contraceptive methods. In case of a planned pregnancy, it is strongly recommended to discontinue lithium therapy.

4.6.3 Lactation

Since adequate human data on use during lactation, adequate animal reproduction studies are not available and as lithium is secreted in breast milk, bottle-feeding is recommended (see section 4.3 Contraindications).

4.7 Effects on ability to drive and use machines

As lithium may cause disturbances of the CNS, patients should be warned of the possible hazards when driving or operating machinery.

4.8 Undesirable effects

Side effects are usually related to serum lithium concentration and are less common in patients with plasma lithium concentrations below 1.0 mmol/l.

Initial therapy: fine tremor of the hands, polyuria and thirst may occur.

Body as a whole: muscle weakness, peripheral oedema.

Cardiovascular: cardiac arrhythmia (NOS), mainly bradycardia, sinus node dysfunction, peripheral circulatory collapse, hypotension, oedema, ECG changes such as reversible flattening or inversion of T-waves and QT prolongation, cardiomyopathy.

CNS: ataxia, hyperactive deep tendon reflexes, extrapyramidal symptoms, seizures, slurred speech, dizziness, nystagmus, stupor, coma, pseudotumor cerebi, myasthenia gravis, vertigo, giddiness, dazed feeling, memory impairment.

Dermatology: alopecia, acne, folliculitis, pruritis, aggravation or occurrence of psoriasis, allergic rashes, acneiform eruptions, papular skin disorders, cutaneous ulcers.

Endocrine: euthyroid goitre, hypothyroidism, hyperthyroidism and thyrotoxicosis. Lithium-induced hypothyroidism may be managed successfully with concurrent thyroxine. Hypercalcaemia, hypermagnesaemia, hyperparathyroidism have been reported.

Gastrointestinal: anorexia, nausea, vomiting, diarrhoea, excessive salivation, dry mouth, abdominal discomfort, taste disorder, gastritis

Haematological: leucocytosis.

Metabolic and Nutrional: weight gain, hyperglycemia,

Renal: polydipsia and/or polyuria, symptoms of nephrogenic diabetes insipidus, histological renal changes with inerstitial fibrosis after long term treatment.

High serum concentrations of lithium including episodes of acute lithium toxicity may aggravate these changes. The minimum clinically effective dose of lithium should always be used. In patients who develop polyuria and/or polydipsia, renal function should be monitored, e.g. with measurement of blood urea, serum creatinine and urinary protein levels in addition to the routine serum lithium assessment.

Reproductive: sexual dysfunction.

Senses: dysgeusia, blurred vision, scotomata.

Rare cases of nephrotic syndrome, speech disorder, confusion, impaired consciousness, myoclony and abnormal reflex have been reported.

If any of the above symptoms appear, treatment should be stopped immediately and arrangements made for serum lithium measurement.

4.9 Overdose

The toxic effects which are indicative of impending lithium intoxication fall into three groups:

• Gastrointestinal: increasing anorexia, diarrhoea and vomiting.

• Central nervous system: muscle weakness, lack of co-ordination, drowsiness or lethargy progressing to giddiness with ataxia, nystagmus, tinnitus, blurred vision, dysarthria and myoclonia. Lack of co-ordination and/or coarse tremor of the extremities and lower jaw may occur, especially with serum levels above the therapeutic range. Muscle weakness and muscle hyperirritability, choreoathetoid movements and toxic psychosis have also been described.

• Other: ECG changes (flat or inverted T waves, QT prolongation), dehydration and electrolyte disturbances.

• Acute renal failure has been reported rarely with lithium toxicity.

At blood levels above 2-3 mmol/L, there may be a large output of dilute urine and renal insufficiency, with increasing confusion, seizures, coma and death. There is no specific antidote to lithium poisoning. In the event of accumulation, lithium should be stopped and serum assessment should be carried out every six hours.

Treatment consists of the induction of vomiting and/or gastric lavage together with supportive and symptomatic measures. Particular attention should be paid to maintenance of fluid and electrolyte balance and adequate renal function. Where convulsions are present, diazepam may be used.

Osmotic diuresis (mannitol or urea infusion) or alkalinisation of the urine (sodium lactate or sodium bicarbonate) should be initiated.

Peritoneal or haemodialysis should be instituted promptly:

- if the serum lithium level is over 4.0 mmol/L,

- if there is a deterioration in the patient's condition,

- or if the serum lithium concentration is not falling at a rate corresponding to a half-life of under 30 hours.

This should be continued until there is no lithium in the serum or dialysis fluid. Serum lithium levels should be monitored for at least a further week to take account of any possible rebound in serum lithium levels as a result of delayed diffusion from body tissues.

5. PHARMACOLOGICAL PROPERTIES

5.1 Pharmacodynamic properties

The mode of action of lithium is still not fully understood. However, lithium modifies the production and turnover of certain neurotransmitters, particularly serotonin, and it may also block dopamine receptors.

It modifies concentrations of some electrolytes, particularly calcium and magnesium, and it may reduce thyroid activity.

5.2 Pharmacokinetic properties

Lithium has a half-life of about 24 hours although this increases to about 36 hours in the elderly due to a progressive decrease in renal lithium clearance with age. Lithium is 95% eliminated in the urine. Time to peak serum level for an immediate release product, such as Priadel Liquid, is about 1.5 hours and complete bioavailability would be expected.

6. PHARMACEUTICAL PARTICULARS

6.1 List of excipients

Other ingredients include:

Ethanol, xantural 180, saccharin sodium, sorbic acid, citric acid, pineapple flavour, purified water.

6.2 Incompatibilities

None known.

6.3 Shelf life

Two years.

6.4 Special precautions for storage

Store at or below 25°C. Protect from direct sunlight.

6.5 Nature and contents of container

Priadel Liquid is supplied in an amber glass bottle fitted with a one-piece polypropylene screw cap. Packs are available in 150ml and 300ml volumes.

6.6 Instructions for use and handling

Dilution of Priadel Liquid is not recommended. There are no special precautions for handling.

7. MARKETING AUTHORISATION HOLDER

Sanofi-Synthelabo

PO Box 597

Guildford

Surrey

8. MARKETING AUTHORISATION NUMBER(S)

11723/0333

9. DATE OF FIRST AUTHORISATION/RENEWAL OF THE AUTHORISATION

12 December 2000

10. DATE OF REVISION OF THE TEXT

June 2004

Legal category: POM

Priadel, Priadel 200

(sanofi-aventis)

1. NAME OF THE MEDICINAL PRODUCT

Priadel.

Priadel 200.

2. QUALITATIVE AND QUANTITATIVE COMPOSITION

Priadel tablets contain 400mg lithium carbonate.

Priadel 200 tablets contain 200mg lithium carbonate.

3. PHARMACEUTICAL FORM

Priadel: White, circular, bi-convex tablets engraved PRIADEL on one side, scored on the other side, in a controlled release formulation.

Priadel 200: White, scored, capsule-shaped tablets engraved P200 on one side, in a controlled release formulation.

4. CLINICAL PARTICULARS

4.1 Therapeutic indications

1. In the management of acute manic or hypomanic episodes.

2. In the management of episodes of recurrent depressive disorders where treatment with other antidepressants has been unsuccessful.

3. In the prophylaxis against bipolar affective disorders.

4. Control of aggressive behaviour or intentional self harm.

4.2 Posology and method of administration

A simple treatment schedule has been evolved which except for some minor variations should be followed whether using Priadel therapeutically or prophylactically. The minor variations to this schedule depend on the elements of the illness being treated and these are described later.

1. In patients of average weight (70kg) an initial dose of 400-1,200mg of Priadel may be given as a single daily dose in the morning or on retiring. Alternatively, the dose may be divided and given morning and evening. The tablets should not be crushed or chewed. When changing between lithium preparations serum lithium levels should first be checked, then Priadel therapy commenced at a daily dose as close as possible to the dose of the other form of lithium. As bioavailability varies from product to product (particularly with regard to retard or slow release preparations) a change of product should be regarded as initiation of new treatment.

2. Four to five days after starting treatment (and never longer than one week) a blood sample should be taken for the estimation of serum lithium level.

3. The objective is to adjust the Priadel dose so as to maintain the serum lithium level permanently within the diurnal range of 0.5-1.5mmol/l. In practice, the blood sample should be taken between 12 and 24 hours after the previous dose of Priadel. "Target" serum lithium concentrations at 12 and 24 hours are shown in the table below.

"Target" serum lithium concentration (mmol/L)

	At 12 hours	At 24 hours
Once daily dosage	0.7 – 1.0	0.5 – 0.8
Twice daily dosage	0.5 – 0.8	

Both strengths have break lines, therefore they can be divided accurately to provide dosage requirements as small as 100mg. Serum lithium levels should be monitored weekly until stabilisation is achieved.

4. Lithium therapy should not be initiated unless adequate facilities for routine monitoring of serum concentrations are available. Following stabilisation of serum lithium levels, the period between subsequent estimations can be increased gradually but should not normally exceed three months. Additional measurements should be made following alteration of dosage, on development of intercurrent disease, signs of manic or depressive relapse, following significant change in sodium or fluid intake, or if signs of lithium toxicity occur.

5. Whilst a high proportion of acutely ill patients may respond within three to seven days of the commencement of Priadel therapy, Priadel should be continued through any recurrence of the affective disturbance. This is important as the full prophylactic effect may not occur for 6 to 12 months after the initiation of therapy.

6. In patients who show a positive response to Priadel therapy, treatment is likely to be long term. Careful clinical appraisal of the patient should be exercised throughout medication (see precautions).

Prophylactic treatment of bipolar affective disorders and control of aggressive behaviour or intentional self harm: It is recommended that the described treatment schedule is followed.

Treatment of acute manic or hypomanic episodes and recurrent depressive disorders: it is likely that a higher than normal Priadel intake may be necessary during an acute phase and divided doses would be required here. Therefore as soon as control of mania or depression is achieved, the serum lithium level should be determined and it may be necessary, dependent on the results, to lower the dose of Priadel and re-stabilise serum lithium levels. In all other details the described treatment schedule is recommended.

Elderly:

Elderly patients or those below 50kg in weight, often require lower lithium dosage to achieve therapeutic serum levels. Starting doses of 200mg to 400mg are recommended. Dosage increments of 200 to 400mg every 3 to 5 days are usual. Total daily doses of 800 to 1800mg may be necessary to achieve effective blood lithium levels of 0.8 to 1.0 mmol/L. For prophylaxis, the dosage necessary to reach a blood lithium level of 0.4 to 0.8 mmol/L is generally in the range of 600 to 1200 mg/day.

Children and adolescents:

Not recommended.

4.3 Contraindications

• Hypersensitivity to lithium or to any of the excipients.

• Cardiac disease.

• Clinically significant renal impairment.

• Untreated hypothyroidism.

- Breast-feeding.
- Patients with low body sodium levels, including for example dehydrated patients or those on low sodium diets.
- Addison's disease.

4.4 Special warnings and special precautions for use

- When considering Priadel therapy, it is necessary to ascertain whether patients are receiving lithium in any other form. If so, check serum levels before proceeding.
- Before beginning a lithium treatment:

– it is important to ensure that renal function is normal.

– cardiac function should be assessed.

– thyroid function should be evaluated. Patients should be euthyroid before initiation of lithium therapy.

- Renal, cardiac and thyroid functions should be re-assessed periodically.
- The possibility of hypothyroidism and renal dysfunction arising during prolonged treatment should be borne in mind and periodic assessments made.
- Patients receiving long term lithium therapy should be warned by the physician and be given clear instructions regarding the symptoms of impending intoxication (see 4.9 Overdosage). They should be warned of the urgency of immediate action should these symptoms appear, and also of the need to maintain a constant and adequate salt and water intake. Treatment should be discontinued immediately on the first signs of toxicity (see 4.9 Overdosage).
- Patients should be warned to report if polyuria or polydipsia develop. Episodes of nausea, vomiting, diarrhoea, fluid deprivation (e.g. excessive sweating), and/or other conditions leading to salt/water depletion should also be reported. Drugs likely to upset electrolyte balance such as diuretics (including severe dieting) should also be reported. In these cases, lithium dosage should be closely monitored and reduction of dosage may be necessary.
- Caution should be exercised to ensure that diet and fluid intake are normal in order to maintain a stable electrolyte balance. This may be of special importance in very hot weather or work environment. Infectious diseases including colds, influenza, gastro-enteritis and urinary infections may alter fluid balance and thus affect serum lithium levels. Treatment should be discontinued during any intercurrent infection and should only be reinstituted after the patient's physical health has returned to normal.
- Elderly patients are particularly liable to lithium toxicity. Use with care as lithium excretion may also be reduced. They may exhibit adverse reactions at serum levels ordinarily tolerated by younger patients.

4.5 Interaction with other medicinal products and other forms of Interaction

Interactions which increase lithium concentrations:

If one of the following drugs is initiated, lithium dosage should either be adjusted or concomitant treatment stopped, as appropriate:

- Metronidazole.
- Non-steroidal anti-inflammatory drugs (monitor serum lithium concentrations more frequently if NSAID therapy is initiated or discontinued).
- ACE inhibitors.
- Diuretics (thiazides show a paradoxical antidiuretics effect resulting in possible water retention and lithium intoxication). If a thiazide diuretic has to be prescribed for a lithium-treated patient, lithium dosage should first be reduced and the patient re-stabilised with frequent monitoring. Similar precautions should be exercised on diuretic withdrawal.
- Other drugs affecting electrolyte balance, e.g. steroids, may alter lithium excretion and should therefore be avoided.
- Tetracyclines.

Interactions which decrease serum lithium concentrations:

- Xanthines (theophylline, caffeine).
- Sodium bicarbonate containing products.
- Diuretics (osmotic and carbonic anhydrase inhibitors).
- Urea.

Interactions causing neurotoxicity:

- Neuroleptics (particularly haloperidol at higher dosages), flupentixol, diazepam, thioridazine, fluphenazine, chlorpromazine and clozapine may lead in rare cases to neurotoxicity in the form of confusion, disorientation, lethargy, tremor, extra-pyramidal symptoms and myoclonus.
- Methyldopa.
- Selective Serotonin Re-uptake Inhibitors (e.g. fluvoxamine and fluxetine) as this combinationmay precipitate a serotoninergic syndrome, which justifies immediate discontinuation of treatment.
- Calcium channel blockers may lead to a risk of neurotoxicity in the form of ataxia, confusion and somnolence, reversible after discontinuation of the drug. Lithium concentrations may be increased.
- Carbamazepine may lead to dizziness, somnolence, confusion and cerebellar symptoms

Lithium may prolong the effects of neuromuscular blocking agents. There have been reports of interaction between lithium and phenytoin, indomethacin and other prostaglandin-synthetase inhibitors.

4.6 Pregnancy and lactation

4.6.1 Pregnancy

Lithium therapy should not be used during pregnancy, especially during the first trimester, unless considered essential. There is epidemiological evidence that it may be harmful to the foetus in human pregnancy. Lithium crosses the placental barrier. In animal studies lithium has been reported to interfere with fertility, gestation and foetal development. An increase in cardiac and other abnormalities, especially Ebstein anomaly, are reported. Therefore, a pre-natal diagnosis such as ultrasound and electrocardiogramexamination is strongly recommended. In certain cases where a severe risk to the patient could exist if treatment were stopped, lithium has been continued during pregnancy.

If it is considered essential to maintain lithium treatment during pregnancy, serum lithium levels should be closely monitored and measured frequently since renal function changes gradually during pregnancy and suddenly at parturition. Dosage adjustments are required. It is recommended that lithium be discontinued shortly before delivery and reinitiated a few days *post-partum.*

Neonates may show signs of lithium toxicity necessitating fluid therapy in the neonatal period. Neonates born with low serum lithium concentrations may have a flaccid appearance that returns to normal without any treatment.

4.6.2 Women of child-bearing potential

It is advisable that women treated with lithium should adopt adequate contraceptive methods. In case of a planned pregnancy, it is strongly recommended to discontinue lithium therapy.

4.6.3 Lactation

Since adequate human data on use during lactation, adequate animal reproduction studies are not available and as lithium is secreted in breast milk, bottle-feeding is recommended (see section 4.3 Contraindications).

4.7 Effects on ability to drive and use machines

As lithium may cause disturbances of the CNS, patients should be warned of the possible hazards when driving or operating machinery.

4.8 Undesirable effects

Side effects are usually related to serum lithium concentration and are less common in patients with plasma lithium concentrations below 1.0 mmol/l.

Initial therapy: fine tremor of the hands, polyuria and thirst may occur.

Body as a whole: muscle weakness, peripheral oedema.

Cardiovascular: cardiac arrhythmia (NOS), mainly bradycardia, sinus node dysfunction, peripheral circulatory collapse, hypotension, oedema, ECG changes such as reversible flattening or inversion of T-waves and QT prolongation, cardiomyopathy.

CNS: ataxia, hyperactive deep tendon reflexes, extrapyramidal symptoms, seizures, slurred speech, dizziness, nystagmus, stupor, coma, pseudotumor cerebi, myasthenia gravis, vertigo, giddiness, dazed feeling, memory impairment.

Dermatology: alopecia, acne, folliculitis, pruritis, aggravation or occurrence of psoriasis, allergic rashes, acneiform eruptions, papular skin disorders, cutaneous ulcers.

Endocrine: euthyroid goitre, hypothyroidism, hyperthyroidism and thyrotoxicosis. Lithium-induced hypothyroidism may be managed successfully with concurrent thyroxine. Hypercalcaemia, hypermagnesaemia, hyperparathyroidism have been reported.

Gastrointestinal: anorexia, nausea, vomiting, diarrhoea, excessive salivation, dry mouth, abdominal discomfort, taste disorder, gastritis.

Haematological: leucocytosis.

Metabolic and Nutrional: weight gain, hyperglycemia.

Renal: polydipsia and/or polyuria, symptoms of nephrogenic diabetes insipidus, histological renal changes with interstitial fibrosis after long term treatment.

High serum concentrations of lithium including episodes of acute lithium toxicity may aggravate these changes. The minimum clinically effective dose of lithium should always be used. In patients who develop polyuria and/or polydipsia, renal function should be monitored, e.g. with measurement of blood urea, serum creatinine and urinary protein levels in addition to the routine serum lithium assessment.

Reproductive: sexual dysfunction.

Senses: dysgeusia, blurred vision, scotomata.

Rare cases of nephrotic syndrome, speech disorder, confusion, impaired consciousness, myoclony and abnormal reflex have been reported.

If any of the above symptoms appear, treatment should be stopped immediately and arrangements made for serum lithium measurement.

4.9 Overdose

The toxic effects which are indicative of impending lithium intoxication fall into three groups:

- Gastrointestinal: increasing anorexia, diarrhea and vomiting.
- Central nervous system: muscle weakness, lack of co-ordination, drowsiness or lethargy progressing to giddiness with ataxia, nystagmus, tinnitus, blurred vision, dysarthria and myoclonia. Lack of co-ordination and/or coarse tremor of the extremities and lower jaw may occur, especially with serum levels above the therapeutic range. Muscle weakness and muscle hyperirritability, choreoathetoid movements and toxic psychosis have also been described.
- Other: ECG changes (flat or inverted T waves, QT prolongation), dehydration and electrolyte disturbances.
- Acute renal failure has been reported rarely with lithium toxicity.

At blood levels above 2-3 mmol/L, there may be a large output of dilute urine and renal insufficiency, with increasing confusion, seizures, coma and death. There is no specific antidote to lithium poisoning. In the event of accumulation, lithium should be stopped and serum assessment should be carried out every six hours.

Treatment consists of the induction of vomiting and/or gastric lavage together with supportive and symptomatic measures. Particular attention should be paid to maintenance of fluid and electrolyte balance and adequate renal function. Where convulsions are present, diazepam may be used.

Osmotic diuresis (mannitol or urea infusion) or alkalinisation of the urine (sodium lactate or sodium bicarbonate) should be initiated.

Peritoneal or haemodialysis should be instituted promptly:

- if the serum lithium level is over 4.0 mmol/L,

- if there is a deterioration in the patient's condition,

- or if the serum lithium concentration is not falling at a rate corresponding to a half-life of under 30 hours.

This should be continued until there is no lithium in the serum or dialysis fluid. Serum lithium levels should be monitored for at least a further week to take account of any possible rebound in serum lithium levels as a result of delayed diffusion from body tissues.

5. PHARMACOLOGICAL PROPERTIES

5.1 Pharmacodynamic properties

The mode of action of lithium is still not fully understood. However, lithium modifies the production and turnover of certain neurotransmitters, particularly serotonin, and it may also block dopamine receptors.

It modifies concentrations of some electrolytes, particularly calcium and magnesium, and it may reduce thyroid activity.

5.2 Pharmacokinetic properties

Lithium has a half life of about 24-hours although this increases to about 36-hours in the elderly due to a progressive decrease in renal lithium clearance with age. Lithium is 95% eliminated in the urine. Time to peak serum level for controlled release Priadel tablets is about 2 hours and approximately 90% bioavailability would be expected.

5.3 Preclinical safety data

Nothing of therapeutic relevance.

6. PHARMACEUTICAL PARTICULARS

6.1 List of excipients

Priadel contains Glycerol monostearate, glycerol distearate, mannitol, acacia spray dried, sodium laurilsulfate, magnesium stearate, maize starch and sodium starch glycolate (Type A).

Priadel 200 contains precirol, precireol/imwitor blend, mannitol, acacia powder, sodium laurilsulfate, magnesium stearate, maize starch and sodium starch glycolate (Type A).

6.2 Incompatibilities

None stated

6.3 Shelf life

Three years

6.4 Special precautions for storage

Store in a cool, dry place.

6.5 Nature and contents of container

Pack sizes: Blister packs 100

6.6 Instructions for use and handling

Not applicable

7. MARKETING AUTHORISATION HOLDER

Sanofi-Synthelabo

PO Box 597

Guildford

Surrey

8. MARKETING AUTHORISATION NUMBER(S)

Priadel: 11723/0331

Priadel 200: 11723/0332

9. DATE OF FIRST AUTHORISATION/RENEWAL OF THE AUTHORISATION

Priadel: 12 December 2000

Priadel 200: 10 November 2000

10. DATE OF REVISION OF THE TEXT
Priadel: October 2004

Priadel 200: September 2004

Legal category: POM

Primacor Injection

(sanofi-aventis)

1. NAME OF THE MEDICINAL PRODUCT
Primacor Injection

2. QUALITATIVE AND QUANTITATIVE COMPOSITION
Milrinone 1mg/ml.

3. PHARMACEUTICAL FORM
Solution for Injection.

Clear, colourless to pale yellow liquid.

4. CLINICAL PARTICULARS

4.1 Therapeutic indications
Primacor Injection is indicated for the short-term treatment of severe congestive heart failure unresponsive to conventional maintenance therapy, and for the treatment of patients with acute heart failure, including low output states following cardiac surgery.

4.2 Posology and method of administration
For intravenous administration.

Adults: Primacor Injection should be given as a loading dose of 50mcg/kg administered over a period of 10 minutes usually followed by a continuous infusion at a dosage titrated between 0.375mcg/kg/min and 0.75mcg/kg/min according to haemodynamic and clinical response, but should not exceed 1.13mg/kg/day total dose.

The following provides a guide to maintenance infusion delivery rate based upon a solution containing milrinone 200mcg/ml prepared by adding 40ml diluent per 10ml ampoule (400ml diluent per 100ml Primacor Injection). 0.45% saline, 0.9% saline or 5% dextrose may be used as diluents.

Primacor Injection Dose (mcg/kg/min)	Infusion Delivery Rate (ml/kg/hr)
0.375	0.11
0.400	0.12
0.500	0.15
0.600	0.18
0.700	0.21
0.750	0.22

Solutions of different concentrations may be used according to patient fluid requirements. The duration of therapy should depend upon the patient's response. In congestive cardiac failure, patients have been maintained on the infusion for up to 5 days, although the usual period is 48 to 72 hours. In acute states following cardiac surgery, it is unlikely that treatment need be maintained for more than 12 hours.

Use in patients with impaired renal function: Data obtained from patients with severe renal impairment but without heart failure have demonstrated that the presence of renal impairment significantly increases the terminal elimination half-life of milrinone. For patients with clinical evidence of renal impairment, the following maintenance infusion rates are recommended using the infusion solution described above.

Creatinine Clearance (ml/min/1.73m^2)	Primacor Injection Dose (mcg/kg/min)	Maintenance Infusion Delivery Rate (ml/kg/hr)
5	0.20	0.06
10	0.23	0.07
20	0.28	0.08
30	0.33	0.10
40	0.38	0.11
50	0.43	0.13

The infusion rate should be adjusted according to haemodynamic response.

Use in elderly patients: Experience so far suggests that no special dosage recommendations are necessary.

Use in children: Safety and effectiveness in children and adolescents under 18 years of age have not been established. Primacor Injection should only be used when the potential benefits outweigh the potential risks.

4.3 Contraindications
Hypersensitivity to milrinone or other ingredients of the preparation.

4.4 Special warnings and special precautions for use
The use of inotropic agents such as milrinone during the acute phase of a myocardial infarction may lead to an undesirable increase in myocardial oxygen consumption (MVO_2). Primacor Injection is not recommended immediately following acute myocardial infarction until safety and efficacy have been established in this situation.

Careful monitoring should be maintained during Primacor Injection therapy including blood pressure, heart rate, clinical state, electro-cardiogram, fluid balance, electrolytes and renal function (i.e. serum creatinine).

In patients with severe obstructive aortic or pulmonary valvular disease or hypertrophic subaortic stenosis, Primacor Injection should not be used in place of surgical relief of the obstruction. In these conditions it is possible that a drug with inotropic / vasodilator properties might aggravate outflow obstruction.

Supraventricular and ventricular arrhythmias have been observed in the high risk population treated with Primacor Injection. In some patients an increase in ventricular ectopy including non-sustained ventricular tachycardia has been observed which did not affect patient safety or outcome.

As Primacor Injection produces a slight enhancement in A-V node conduction, there is a possibility of an increased ventricular response rate in patients with uncontrolled atrial flutter / fibrillation. Consideration should therefore be given to digitalisation or treatment with other agents to prolong A-V node conduction time prior to starting Primacor Injection therapy, and to discontinuing the therapy if arrhythmias occur.

The potential for arrhythmia, present in heart failure itself, may be increased by many drugs or a combination of drugs. Patients receiving Primacor Injection should be closely monitored during infusion and the infusion should be stopped if arrhythmias develop.

Milrinone may induce hypotension as a consequence of its vasodilatory activity, therefore caution should be exercised when Primacor Injection is administered to patients who are hypotensive prior to treatment. The rate of infusion should be slowed or stopped in patients showing excessive decreases in blood pressure.

If prior vigorous diuretic therapy is suspected of having caused significant decreases in cardiac filling pressure Primacor Injection should be cautiously administered while monitoring blood pressure, heart rate and clinical symptomatology.

Improvement in cardiac output with resultant diuresis may necessitate a reduction in the dose of diuretic. Potassium loss due to excessive diuresis may necessitate a reduction in the dose of diuretic. Potassium loss due to excessive diuresis may predispose digitalised patients to arrhythmias. Therefore, hypokalaemia should be corrected by potassium supplementation in advance of, or during, the use of Primacor Injection.

4.5 Interaction with other medicinal products and other forms of Interaction
None have been observed during Primacor Injection therapy (*but see Section 6.2, Incompatibilities*).

Whilst there is a theoretical potential interaction with calcium channel blockers, there has been no evidence of a clinically significant interaction to date.

Milrinone has a favourable inotropic effect in fully digitalised patients without causing signs of glycoside toxicity.

4.6 Pregnancy and lactation
Although animal studies have not revealed evidence of drug-induced foetal damage or other deleterious effects on reproductive function, the safety of milrinone in human pregnancy has not yet been established. It should be used during pregnancy only if the potential benefit justifies the potential risk to the foetus.

Caution should be exercised when Primacor Injection is administered to nursing women, since it is not known whether milrinone is excreted in human milk.

4.7 Effects on ability to drive and use machines
Not applicable.

4.8 Undesirable effects
Adverse reactions have been ranked under heading of system-organ class and frequency using the following convention: very commonly >= 1/10); commonly >= 1/100, <1/10); uncommonly >= 1/1,000, <1/100); rarely >= 1/10,000, <1/1,000); very rarely (<1/10,000).

Cardiovascular disorders:

- Commonly:
- Ventricular ectopic activity
- Non sustained or sustained ventricular tachycardia
- Supraventricular arrhythmias
- Hypotension
- Uncommonly:
- Ventricular fibrillation
- Angina/chest pain
- Very rarely: Torsades de pointes

The incidence of arrhythmias has not been related to dose or plasma levels of milrinone. These arrhythmias are rarely life threatening. If present, they are often associated with certain underlying factors such as pre-existing arrhythmias, metabolic abnormalities (e.g. hypokalaemia) abnormal digoxin levels and catheter insertion.

Haematological disorders:

- Uncommonly: Thrombocytopenia

General disorders:

- Very rarely: Anaphylactic shock

Respiratory disorders:

- Very rarely: Bronchospasm

Liver disorders:

- Uncommonly: liver function tests abnormality

Nervous System disorders:

- Commonly: Headaches, usually mild to moderate in severity
- Uncommonly: Tremor

Skin disorders:

- Very rarely: skin reactions such as rash, including at injection site.

Metabolic disorders:

- Uncommonly: Hypokalaemia

4.9 Overdose
Overdose of intravenous Primacor may produce hypotension (because of its vasodilatory effect) and cardiac arrhythmia. If this occurs, Primacor Injection administration should be reduced or temporarily discontinued until the patient's condition stabilises. No specific antidote is known, but general measures for circulatory support should be taken.

5. PHARMACOLOGICAL PROPERTIES

5.1 Pharmacodynamic properties
Milrinone is a positive inotrope and vasodilator, with little chronotropic activity. It also improves left ventricular diastolic relaxation. It differs in structure and mode of action from the digitalis glycosides, catecholamines or angiotensin converting enzyme inhibitors. It is a selective inhibitor of peak III phosphodiesterase isoenzyme in cardiac and vascular muscle. It produces slight enhancement of A-V node conduction, but no other significant electro-physiological effects.

In clinical studies Primacor Injection has been shown to produce prompt improvements in the haemodynamic indices of congestive heart failure, including cardiac output, pulmonary capillary wedge pressure and vascular resistance, without clinically significant effect on heart rate or myocardial oxygen consumption. Haemodynamic improvement during intravenous Primacor therapy is accompanied by clinical symptomatic improvement in congestive cardiac failure, as measured by change in New York Heart Association classification.

5.2 Pharmacokinetic properties
Following intravenous injections of 12.5 to 125mcg/kg to congestive heart failure patients, Primacor Injection had a volume of distribution of 0.38 l/kg/hr, a mean terminal elimination half-life of 2.3 hours, and a clearance of 0.13 l/kg/hr. Following intravenous infusions of 0.2 to 0.7mcg/kg/min to congestive heart failure patients, the drug had a volume of distribution of about 0.45 l/kg, a mean terminal elimination half-life of 2.4 hours, and a clearance of 0.14 l/kg/hr. These pharmacokinetic parameters were not dose-dependent, and the area under the plasma concentration versus time curve following injection was significantly dose-dependent.

The primary route of excretion of milrinone in man is via the urine. Elimination in normal subjects via the urine is rapid, with approximately 60% recovered within the first two hours following dosing, and approximately 90% recovered within the first eight hours following dosing. The mean renal clearance of milrinone is approximately 0.3 l/min, indicative of active secretion.

5.3 Preclinical safety data
There are no preclinical data of relevance to the prescriber which are additional to that already in other sections of the SPC.

6. PHARMACEUTICAL PARTICULARS

6.1 List of excipients
Lactic Acid, Dextrose Anhydrous, Water for Injection, Sodium Hydroxide.

6.2 Incompatibilities
Frusemide or bumetanide should not be administered in intravenous lines containing Primacor Injection since precipitation occurs on admixture. Sodium Bicarbonate Intravenous infusion should not be used for dilution.

Other drugs should not be mixed with Primacor Injection until further compatibility data are available.

6.3 Shelf life
48 months when unopened. A diluted solution of Primacor Injection should be used within 24 hours.

6.4 Special precautions for storage
Do not store above 25°C. Do not freeze.

6.5 Nature and contents of container
Type 1 10ml or 20ml flint glass ampoules packed in lots of 10.

6.6 Instructions for use and handling
Infusion solutions diluted as recommended with 0.45% saline, 0.9% saline or 5% dextrose should be freshly prepared before use. Parenteral drug products should be examined visually and should not be used if particulate matter or discolouration are present.

7. MARKETING AUTHORISATION HOLDER

Sanofi-Synthelabo Limited (*trading as Sanofi Winthrop*)
One Onslow Street
Guildford
Surrey GU1 4YS
or trading as:
Sanofi-Synthelabo
PO Box 597
Guildford
Surrey

8. MARKETING AUTHORISATION NUMBER(S)

PL 11723/0064

9. DATE OF FIRST AUTHORISATION/RENEWAL OF THE AUTHORISATION

1st June 2003

10. DATE OF REVISION OF THE TEXT

February 2004

Legal Category: POM

Primaxin IM Injection

(Merck Sharp & Dohme Limited)

1. NAME OF THE MEDICINAL PRODUCT

'Primaxin' IM 500 mg Injection

2. QUALITATIVE AND QUANTITATIVE COMPOSITION

'Primaxin' IM 500 mg Injection contains 500 mg imipenem (as the monohydrate) with 500 mg cilastatin (as the sodium salt).

3. PHARMACEUTICAL FORM

Powder for suspension for injection.

'Primaxin' IM is available as vials containing sterile white to light yellow powder.

4. CLINICAL PARTICULARS

4.1 Therapeutic indications

Broad-spectrum beta-lactam antibiotic.

'Primaxin' contains:

imipenem, a member of a class of beta-lactam antibiotics - the thienamycins cilastatin sodium, a specific enzyme inhibitor, that blocks the metabolism of imipenem in the kidney and substantially increases the concentration of unchanged imipenem in the urinary tract.

'Primaxin' is bactericidal against an unusually wide spectrum of Gram-positive, Gram-negative, aerobic and anaerobic pathogens. 'Primaxin' is useful for treating single and polymicrobic infections, and initiating therapy prior to identification of the causative organisms.

'Primaxin' is indicated for the treatment of the following infections due to susceptible organisms:

'Primaxin' IM

Lower respiratory tract infections (except those caused by *Pseudomonas aeruginosa*)

Intra-abdominal infections

Genito-urinary infections

Gynaecological infections

Bone and joint infections

(There is limited experience in patients with these infections.)

Skin and soft tissue infections

Note: 'Primaxin' is not indicated against central nervous system infections.

'Primaxin' is indicated against mixed infections caused by susceptible aerobic and anaerobic bacteria. The majority of these infections are associated with contamination by faecal flora, or flora originating from the vagina, skin, and mouth. In these mixed infections, 'Primaxin' is usually effective against *Bacteroides fragilis* sp., the most commonly encountered anaerobic pathogen, which is usually resistant to the aminoglycosides, cephalosporins and penicillins.

Consideration should be given to official local guidance (e.g. national recommendations) on the appropriate use of bacterial agents.

Susceptibility of the causative organism to the treatment should be tested (if possible), although therapy may be initiated before the results are available.

4.2 Posology and method of administration

The total daily dosage and route of administration of 'Primaxin' should be based on the type or severity of infection, consideration of degree of susceptibility of the pathogen(s), renal function and bodyweight. Doses cited are based on a bodyweight of ⩾70 kg. The total daily requirement should be given in equally divided doses.

The dosage recommendations that follow specify the amounts of imipenem to be given. An equivalent amount of cilastatin is provided with this. 'Primaxin' IM 500 mg provides the equivalents of 500 mg anhydrous imipenem and 500 mg cilastatin.

Use in the elderly

Age does not usually affect the tolerability and efficacy of 'Primaxin'. The dosage should be determined by the severity of the infection, the susceptibility of the causative organism(s), the patient's clinical condition, and renal function.

Intramuscular administration

This formulation is for intramuscular use only and should not be administered intravenously.

Note: All recommended doses refer to the imipenem fraction of 'Primaxin'.

Adults

A single 500 mg dose of the intramuscular formulation may be used for the treatment of urethritis or cervicitis due to non-penicillinase-producing *Neisseria gonorrhoea.*

The intramuscular formulation may be used as an alternative to the intravenous formulation in the treatment of mild and moderate infections. For severe or life-threatening conditions the intravenous formulation route is recommended.

'Primaxin' IM should be given by deep intramuscular injection into a large muscle mass (such as the gluteal muscle or lateral part of the thigh).

Usual adult intramuscular dose

(see Table 1 below)

In infants and children

The safety and efficacy of the intramuscular formulation have not been studied in the paediatric group.

In patients with renal insufficiency

The safety and efficacy of the intramuscular formulation have not been studied in patients with renal insufficiency.

4.3 Contraindications

Hypersensitivity to this product.

As lidocaine HCl (lignocaine) is used as a diluent with 'Primaxin' IM, 'Primaxin' IM is contra-indicated in patients with known or suspected hypersensitivity to local anaesthetics of the amide type. 'Primaxin' IM with lidocaine (lignocaine) is also contra-indicated in patients with severe shock or heart block.

4.4 Special warnings and special precautions for use

Warning

There is some clinical and laboratory evidence of partial cross-allergenicity between 'Primaxin' and the other beta-lactam antibiotics, penicillins and cephalosporins. Severe reactions (including anaphylaxis) have been reported with most beta-lactam antibiotics.

Before initiating therapy with 'Primaxin', careful inquiry should be made concerning previous hypersensitivity reactions to beta-lactam antibiotics. If an allergic reaction to 'Primaxin' occurs, the drug should be discontinued.

Pseudomembranous colitis, reported with virtually all antibiotics, can range from mild to life-threatening in severity. 'Primaxin' should be prescribed with caution in patients with a history of gastro-intestinal disease, particularly colitis. Treatment-related diarrhoea should always be considered as a pointer to this diagnosis. While studies indicate that a toxin of *Clostridium difficile* is one of the primary causes of antibiotic-associated colitis, other causes should be considered.

Paediatric use

'Primaxin' IM: Tolerability and efficacy of 'Primaxin' IM have not yet been studied in the paediatric group; therefore, at present, 'Primaxin' IM is not recommended for use in this group.

Central nervous system: Patients with CNS disorders and/or compromised renal function (accumulation of 'Primaxin' may occur) have shown CNS side effects, especially when recommended dosages based on bodyweight and renal function were exceeded. Hence it is recommended that the dosage schedules of 'Primaxin' should be strictly adhered to, and established anticonvulsant therapy continued.

If focal tremors, myoclonus or convulsions occur, the patient should be evaluated neurologically and placed on anticonvulsant therapy if not already instituted. If these symptoms continue, the dosage should be reduced, or 'Primaxin' withdrawn completely.

Use in patients with renal insufficiency

'Primaxin' IM: Safety and efficacy of 'Primaxin' IM have not yet been studied in patients with renal insufficiency; therefore, at present, 'Primaxin' IM is not recommended for use in this group.

4.5 Interaction with other medicinal products and other forms of Interaction

There are no data on adverse drug interactions. However, concomitant probenecid has been shown to double the plasma level and half-life of cilastatin, but with no effect on its urinary recovery.

Concomitant probenecid showed only minimal increases in plasma level and half-life of imipenem, with urinary recovery of active imipenem decreased to approximately 60% of the administered dose.

4.6 Pregnancy and lactation

Pregnant monkeys showed evidence of maternal and foetal toxicity with bolus injections at doses equivalent to twice the human dose.

The use of 'Primaxin' in pregnant women has not been studied and 'Primaxin' should therefore not be given in pregnancy unless the anticipated benefit to the mother outweighs the possible risk to the foetus.

'Primaxin' has been detected in human milk. If the use of 'Primaxin' is deemed essential, the mother should stop breast-feeding.

4.7 Effects on ability to drive and use machines

There are no specific data; however, some of the CNS side effects, such as dizziness, psychic disturbances, confusion and seizures, may affect the ability to drive or operate machinery.

4.8 Undesirable effects

Side effects

'Primaxin' is generally well tolerated. Side effects rarely require cessation of therapy and are generally mild and transient; serious side effects are rare.

Local reactions: erythema, local pain and induration, thrombophlebitis.

Allergic reactions/skin: rash, pruritus, urticaria, erythema multiforme, Stevens-Johnson Syndrome, angioedema, toxic epidermal necrolysis (rarely), exfoliative dermatitis (rarely), candidiasis, fever including drug fever, anaphylactic reactions.

Gastro-intestinal: nausea, vomiting, diarrhoea, staining of teeth and/or tongue. Pseudomembranous colitis has been reported.

Blood: eosinophilia, leucopenia, neutropenia including agranulocytosis, thrombocytopenia, thrombocytosis, decreased haemoglobin, and prolonged prothrombin time. A positive direct Coombs test may develop.

Liver function: increases in serum transaminases, bilirubin and/or serum alkaline phosphatase, hepatitis (rarely) have been reported.

Renal function: oliguria/anuria, polyuria, acute renal failure (rarely). The role of 'Primaxin' in changes in renal function is difficult to assess, since factors predisposing to pre-renal uraemia or to impaired renal function usually have been present. Elevated serum creatinine and blood urea have been seen. A harmless urine discoloration, not to be confused with haematuria, has been seen.

Nervous system/psychiatric: myoclonic activity, psychic disturbances including hallucinations, paraesthesia, confusional states or convulsions have been reported.

Special senses: hearing loss, taste perversion.

Other reported reactions with an unknown causal relationship

Gastro-intestinal: haemorrhagic colitis, gastro-enteritis, abdominal pain, glossitis, tongue papillar hypertrophy, heartburn, pharyngeal pain, increased salivation.

Central nervous system: dizziness, somnolence, encephalopathy, vertigo, headache.

Special senses: tinnitus.

Respiratory: chest discomfort, dyspnoea, hyperventilation, thoracic spine pain.

Cardiovascular: hypotension, palpitations, tachycardia.

Skin: flushing, cyanosis, hyperhidrosis, skin texture changes, pruritus vulvae.

Body as a whole: polyarthralgia, asthenia/weakness.

Blood: Haemolytic anaemia, pancytopenia, bone marrow depression.

4.9 Overdose

No specific information is available on the treatment of overdosage with 'Primaxin'. Imipenem-cilastatin sodium is haemodialysable; however, usefulness of this procedure in the overdosage setting is unknown.

5. PHARMACOLOGICAL PROPERTIES

Pharmacotherapeutic group: Antibacterials for systemic use

ATC code: J01D H51

5.1 Pharmacodynamic properties

Mechanism of Action:

Imipenem is a potent inhibitor of bacterial cell wall synthesis and is highly reactive towards penicillin-binding protein. Imipenem is more potent in its bactericidal effect than other antibiotics studied. Imipenem also provides excellent stability to degradative bacterial beta-lactamases. Imipenem

Table 1 Usual adult intramuscular dose

IM administration

Type or severity of infection	Dose of imipenem	Dosage interval	Total daily dose
Gonococcal urethritis/cervicitis	500 mg	single dose	0.5 g
Mild infections	500 mg	12 hours	1.0 g
Moderate infections	750 mg	12 hours	1.5 g

is therefore active against a high percentage of organisms resistant to other beta-lactam antibiotics.

Cilastatin sodium is a competitive, reversible, and specific inhibitor of dehydropeptidase-I, the renal enzyme which metabolises and inactivates imipenem. Cilastatin sodium is devoid of intrinsic antibacterial activity itself and does not affect the antibacterial activity of imipenem.

Bacteriology

'Primaxin' has a unique anti-bacterial spectrum. Against Gram-negative species, 'Primaxin' shares the spectrum of the newer cephalosporins and penicillins; against Gram-positive species 'Primaxin' exerts the high bacterial potency previously associated only with narrow-spectrum beta-lactam antibiotics and the first-generation cephalosporins.

The antibiotic spectrum of 'Primaxin' is broader than that of other antibiotics studied and includes virtually all clinically significant pathogenic genera.

In-vitro tests show that imipenem acts synergistically with aminoglycoside antibiotics against some isolates of *Pseudomonas aeruginosa*.

Breakpoints (NCCLS)

The general MIC susceptibility test breakpoints to separate sensitive (S) pathogens from resistant (R) pathogens are: S $\leqslant$4 mcg/mL, R $\geqslant$ 16 mcg/mL.

For *Haemophilus spp.* S $\leqslant$ 4 mcg/mL, R MIC breakpoint not defined.

For *Neisseria gonorrhoeae* MIC breakpoints not defined.

For *Streptococcus pneumoniae* S $\leqslant$ 0.12 mcg/mL, R $\geqslant$ 1 mcg/mL

For streptococci other than *S. pneumoniae* MIC breakpoints not defined.

<u>Susceptibility</u>

The prevalence of resistance may vary geographically and with time for selected species and local information on resistance is desirable, particularly when treating severe infections. The information below gives only approximate guidance on the probability as to whether the microorganism will be susceptible to 'Primaxin' or not.

Organism	Prevalence of Resistance (Range) [European Union]
SUSCEPTIBLE	
Gram-positive aerobes:	
Bacillus spp	
Enterococcus faecalis	0 to 7%
Erysipelothrix rhusiopathiae	
Listeria monocytogenes	
Nocardia spp	
Pediococcus spp	
Staphylococcus aureus (methicillin susceptible, including penicillinase-producing strains	0%
Staphylococcus epidermidis (methicillin susceptible, including penicillinase-producing strains)	0 to 7%
Staphylococcus saprophyticus	0%
*Streptococcus agalactiae**	
Streptococcus Group C	
Streptococcus Group G	
Streptococcus pneumoniae	0%
Streptococcus pneumoniae, PRSP	0 to 83%
*Streptococcus pyogenes**	
*Viridans group streptococci** (including alpha and gamma hemolytic strains)	
Gram-negative aerobes:	
Achromobacter spp.	
Acinetobacter baumannii	0 to 67%
Aeromonas hydrophila	0 to 50%
Alcaligenes spp	
Bordetella bronchicanis	
Bordetella bronchiseptica	
Bordetella pertussis	
Brucella melitensis	
Burkholderia pseudomallei (formerly *Pseudomonas pseudomallei)*	
Burkholderia stutzeri (formerly *Pseudomonas stutzeri)*	
Campylobacter spp.	
Capnocytophaga spp.	
Citrobacter freundii	0%
Citrobacter koseri (formerly *Citrobacter diversus*	0%
Eikenella corrodens	
Enterobacter aerogenes	0%
Enterobacter agglomerans	
Enterobacter cloacae	0 to 13%
Escherichia coli	0%
Gardnerella vaginalis	
Haemophilus ducreyi	
Haemophilus influenzae (including beta-lactamase-producing strains)*	
*Haemophilus parainfluenzae**	
Hafnia alvei	0%
Klebsiella oxytoca	0%
Klebsiella ozaenae	
Klebsiella pneumoniae	0%
Moraxella catarrhalis	0%
Morganella morgani (formerly *Proteus morganii)*	0 to 7%
Neisseria gonorrhoeae (including penicillinase-producing strains)*	
Neisseria meningitidis	
Pasteurella spp	0%
Pasteurella multocida	
Plesiomonas shigelloides	
Proteus mirabilis	0%
Proteus vulgaris	0 to 8%
Providencia alcalifaciens	
Providencia rettgeri (formerly *Proteus rettgeri)*	0 to 20%
Providencia stuartii	0%
Pseudomonas aeruginosa	0 to 20%
Pseudomonas fluorescens	
Pseudomonas putida	
Salmonella spp	0%
Salmonella typhi	
Serratia spp	
Serratia proteamaculans (formerly *Serratia liquefaciens)*	
Serratia marcescens	0%
Shigella spp.	0%
Yersinia spp (formerly *Pasteurella)*	
Yersinia enterocolitica	
Yersinia pseudotuberculosis	
Gram-positive Anaerobes:	
Actinomyces spp	
Bifidobacterium spp.	
Clostridium spp	0%
Clostridium pefringens	
Eubacterium spp.	
Lactobacillus spp.	
Mobiluncus spp.	
Microaerophilic streptococci	
Peptococcus spp.	
Peptostreptococcus spp.	0%
Propionibacterium spp (including *P. acnes)*	
Gram-negative Anaerobes:	
Bacteroides spp.	6%
Bacteroides distasonis	
Bacteroides fragilis	0 to 7%
Bacteroides ovatus	
Bacteroides thetaitaomicron	0%
Bacteroides uniformis	
Bacteroides vulgatus	
Bilophila wadsworthia	
Fusobacterium spp.	
Fusobacterium necrophorum	
Fusobacterium nucleatum	
Porphyromonas asaccharolytica (formerly *Bacteroides asaccharolytica bivius)*	
Prevotella bivia (formerly *Bacteroides bivius)*	
Prevotella disiens (formerly *Bacteroides disiens)*	
Prevotella intermedia (formerly *Bacteroides intermedius)*	
Prevotella melaninogenica (formerly *Bacteroides melaninogenicus)*	
Veillonella spp	
Others:	
Mycobacterium fortuitum	
Myobacterium smegmatis	
RESISTANT	
Gram-positive Aerobes:	
Enterococcus faecium	
methicillin-resistant staphylococci	
Gram-negative Aerobes:	
Stenotrophomonas maltophilia (formerly Xanthomonas maltophilia, formerly Pseudomonas maltophilia)	
(Some strains of *Burkholderia cepacia* (formerly *Pseudomonas cepacia)*	

*Resistant breakpoint not defined.

Mechanism/s of Resistance

For species considered susceptible to imipenem, resistance was uncommon in surveillance studies in Europe. In resistant isolates, resistance to other antibacterial agents of the carbapenem class was seen in some, but not all isolates. Imipenem is effectively stable to hydrolysis by most classes of beta-lactamases, including penicillinases, cephalosporinases and extended spectrum beta-lactamases, but not metallo-beta-lactamases. Although effectively stable to beta-lactamase activity, resistance, when seen, is generally due to a combination of decreased permeability and low-level beta-lactamase hydrolysis.

The mechanism of action of imipenem differs from that of other classes of antibiotics, such as quinolones, aminoglycosides, macrolides and tetracyclines. There is no target-based cross-resistance between imipenem and these substances. However, micro-organisms may exhibit resistance to more than one class of antibacterial agents when the mechanism is, or includes, impermeability to some compounds.

5.2 Pharmacokinetic properties

'Primaxin' IM

Bioavailability of imipenem and cilastatin sodium after 500 mg IM is 85% and 94% respectively. Plasma concentrations of imipenem for 500 mg IM exceed 1.5 mcg/ml at 8 hours, which is better than after intravenous dosing with 'Primaxin'. Plasma and urine levels support the use of intramuscular 'Primaxin' in the treatment of mild to moderate infections with organisms susceptible to imipenem.

5.3 Preclinical safety data

No relevant data.

6. PHARMACEUTICAL PARTICULARS

6.1 List of excipients

'Primaxin' IM contains no inactive ingredients.

6.2 Incompatibilities

None.

6.3 Shelf life

'Primaxin' IM is 36 months.

6.4 Special precautions for storage

Vials of dry 'Primaxin' should be stored in a dry place below 25°C. The container should be kept in the outer carton until immediately before use.

'Primaxin' IM must be used immediately after reconstitution.

6.5 Nature and contents of container

'Primaxin' IM 500 mg strength is available in nominal 13 ml Type I clear glass vials, siliconised with grey butyl rubber stoppers (West Formula 1888, plain or Teflon coated, 1816) and aluminium collar seals with plastic flip-off tops.

6.6 Instructions for use and handling

Preparation of intramuscular suspension

The following table is provided for convenience in reconstituting 'Primaxin' IM with 1% lidocaine (lignocaine) solution for intramuscular use.

Strength	Volume of 1% lidocaine solution to be added (ml)	Final volume (ml)
'Primaxin' IM 500 mg	2	2.8

Shake to prepare a white to light-tan-coloured suspension. Variation of colour within this range does not affect potency. Use immediately after making up. Lidocaine (lignocaine) with 'Primaxin' IM should not be used if patients are known or suspected to be hypersensitive to local anaesthetics of the amide type. Lidocaine (lignocaine) should also not be used with 'Primaxin' IM in patients with severe shock or heart block.

7. MARKETING AUTHORISATION HOLDER

Merck Sharp & Dohme Limited

Hertford Road, Hoddesdon, Hertfordshire EN11 9BU

8. MARKETING AUTHORISATION NUMBER(S)

'Primaxin' IM 500/500 mg: PL 0025/0230

9. DATE OF FIRST AUTHORISATION/RENEWAL OF THE AUTHORISATION

'Primaxin' IM 500/500 mg: Licence first granted 23 March 1991

10. DATE OF REVISION OF THE TEXT

October 2003.

LEGAL CATEGORY:

P.O.M.

SPC.TENIM.02.UK.0848

Primaxin IV Injection

(Merck Sharp & Dohme Limited)

1. NAME OF THE MEDICINAL PRODUCT

'Primaxin' IV 500 mg Injection

2. QUALITATIVE AND QUANTITATIVE COMPOSITION

'Primaxin' IV 500 mg Injection contains 500 mg imipenem (as the monohydrate) with 500 mg cilastatin (as the sodium salt).

3. PHARMACEUTICAL FORM

Powder for solution for infusion.

'Primaxin' IV is available as vials containing sterile white to light yellow powder.

'Primaxin' IV 500 mg Injection is also available in a monovial which has a built-in transfer needle to allow constitution of the product directly into an infusion bag.

4. CLINICAL PARTICULARS

4.1 Therapeutic indications

Broad-spectrum beta-lactam antibiotic.

'Primaxin' contains:

imipenem, a member of a class of beta-lactam antibiotics - the thienamycins cilastatin sodium, a specific enzyme inhibitor, that blocks the metabolism of imipenem in the kidney and substantially increases the concentration of unchanged imipenem in the urinary tract.

'Primaxin' is bactericidal against an unusually wide spectrum of Gram-positive, Gram-negative, aerobic and anaerobic pathogens. 'Primaxin' is useful for treating single and polymicrobic infections, and initiating therapy prior to identification of the causative organisms.

'Primaxin' is indicated for the treatment of the following infections due to susceptible organisms:

'Primaxin' IV

Lower respiratory tract infections

Intra-abdominal infections

Genito-urinary infections

Gynaecological infections

Septicaemia

Bone and joint infections

Skin and soft tissue infections

Note: 'Primaxin' is not indicated against central nervous system infections.

'Primaxin' is indicated against mixed infections caused by susceptible aerobic and anaerobic bacteria. The majority of these infections are associated with contamination by faecal flora, or flora originating from the vagina, skin, and mouth. In these mixed infections, 'Primaxin' is usually effective against *Bacteroides fragilis* sp., the most commonly encountered anaerobic pathogen, which is usually resistant to the aminoglycosides, cephalosporins and penicillins.

Consideration should be given to official local guidance (e.g. national recommendations) on the appropriate use of bacterial agents.

Susceptibility of the causative organism to the treatment should be tested (if possible), although therapy may be initiated before the results are available.

Prophylaxis: 'Primaxin' IV is also indicated for the prevention of certain post-operative infections in patients undergoing contaminated or potentially contaminated surgical procedures or where the occurrence of post-operative infection could be especially serious.

4.2 Posology and method of administration

The total daily dosage and route of administration of 'Primaxin' should be based on the type or severity of infection, consideration of degree of susceptibility of the pathogen(s), renal function and bodyweight. Doses cited are based on a bodyweight of ≥70 kg. The total daily requirement should be given in equally divided doses.

The dosage recommendations that follow specify the amounts of imipenem to be given. An equivalent amount of cilastatin is provided with this. One vial of 'Primaxin' IV 500 mg provides the equivalent of 500 mg anhydrous imipenem and 500 mg cilastatin.

Use in the elderly

Age does not usually affect the tolerability and efficacy of 'Primaxin'. The dosage should be determined by the severity of the infection, the susceptibility of the causative organism(s), the patient's clinical condition, and renal function.

INTRAVENOUS ADMINISTRATION

This formulation should not be used intramuscularly. The dosage of 'Primaxin' IV should be determined by the severity of the infection, the antibiotic susceptibility of the causative organism(s) and the condition of the patient.

Note: All recommended doses refer to the imipenem fraction of 'Primaxin'.

Adults (based on 70 kg bodyweight): The usual adult daily dosage is 1-2 g administered in 3-4 equally divided doses (see chart below). In infections due to less sensitive organisms, the daily dose may be increased to a maximum dose of 50 mg/kg/day (not exceeding 4 g daily).

Usual adult intravenous dosage

Each dose of 250 mg or 500 mg should be given by intravenous infusion over 20-30 minutes. Each dose of 1000 mg should be infused over 40-60 minutes. In patients who develop nausea during infusion, the infusion rate may be slowed.

(see Table 1 below)

Primaxin' has been used successfully as monotherapy in immunocompromised cancer patients for confirmed or suspected infections such as sepsis.

Prophylactic use

For prophylaxis against post-surgical infections in adults, 1 g 'Primaxin' IV should be given intravenously on induction of anaesthesia and 1 g three hours later. For high-risk (i.e. colorectal) surgery, two additional 0.5 g doses can be given at 8 and 16 hours after induction.

In patients with renal insufficiency

As in patients with normal renal function, dosing is based on the severity of the infection. The maximum dosage for patients with various degrees of renal functional impairment is shown in the following table. Doses cited are based on a bodyweight of 70 kg. Proportionate reduction in dose administered should be made for patients with lower bodyweight.

Maximum dosage in relation to renal function

(see Table 2 below)

Patients with a creatinine clearance of ≤5 ml/min should not receive 'Primaxin' IV unless haemodialysis is started within 48 hours.

'Primaxin' is cleared by haemodialysis. The patient should receive 'Primaxin' IV immediately after haemodialysis and at 12-hourly intervals thereafter. Dialysis patients, especially those with background CNS disease, should be carefully monitored; patients on haemodialysis should receive 'Primaxin' IV only when the benefit outweighs the potential risk of convulsions (see 4.4 'Special warnings and special precautions for use').

There are currently inadequate data to recommend the use of 'Primaxin' IV for patients on peritoneal dialysis.

Paediatric dosage

(see Table 3 on next page)

The maximum daily dose should not exceed 2 g.

Children over 40 kg bodyweight should receive adult doses.

Table 1

IV administration

Severity of infection	Dose	Dosage interval	Total daily dose
Mild	250 mg	6 hours	1.0 g
Moderate	500 mg	8 hours	1.5 g
Severe – fully susceptible	500 mg	6 hours	2.0 g
Severe and/or life-threatening infections due to less sensitive organisms (primarily some strains of *P.aeruginosa*)	1000 mg 1000 mg	8 hours 6 hours	3.0 g 4.0 g

Table 2 Maximum dosage in relation to renal function

Renal function	Creatinine clearance (ml/min)	Dose (mg)	Dosage interval (hrs)	Maximum total daily dose* (g)
Mild impairment	31-70	500	6 - 8	1.5 - 2
Moderate impairment	21-30	500	8 - 12	1 - 1.5
Severe** impairment	0-20	250-500	12	0.5 - 1.0

* The higher dose should be reserved for infections caused by less susceptible organisms.

** Patients with creatinine clearance of 6-20 ml/min should be treated with 250 mg (or 3.5 mg/kg, whichever is lower) every 12 hours for most pathogens. When the 500 mg dose is used in these patients there may be an increased risk of convulsions.

Table 3 Paediatric dosage

Age	Dose	Dosage interval	Total daily dose
3 months of age and older (less than 40 kg bodyweight)	15 mg/kg	6 hours	60 mg/kg

Clinical data are insufficient to recommend an optimal dose for children under 3 months of age or infants and children with impaired renal function.

'Primaxin' IV is not recommended for the therapy of meningitis. If meningitis is suspected an appropriate antibiotic should be used.

'Primaxin' IV may be used in children with sepsis as long as they are not suspected of having meningitis.

4.3 Contraindications

Hypersensitivity to this product.

4.4 Special warnings and special precautions for use

Warning

There is some clinical and laboratory evidence of partial cross-allergenicity between 'Primaxin' and the other beta-lactam antibiotics, penicillins and cephalosporins. Severe reactions (including anaphylaxis) have been reported with most beta-lactam antibiotics.

Before initiating therapy with 'Primaxin', careful inquiry should be made concerning previous hypersensitivity reactions to beta-lactam antibiotics. If an allergic reaction to 'Primaxin' occurs, the drug should be discontinued and appropriate measures undertaken.

Pseudomembranous colitis, reported with virtually all antibiotics, can range from mild to life-threatening in severity. 'Primaxin' should be prescribed with caution in patients with a history of gastro-intestinal disease, particularly colitis. Treatment-related diarrhoea should always be considered as a pointer to this diagnosis. While studies indicate that a toxin of *Clostridium difficile* is one of the primary causes of antibiotic-associated colitis, other causes should be considered.

Paediatric use

'Primaxin' IV: Efficacy and tolerability in infants under 3 months of age have yet to be established; therefore, 'Primaxin' IV is not recommended for use below this age.

Central nervous system: Patients with CNS disorders and/or compromised renal function (accumulation of 'Primaxin' may occur) have shown CNS side effects, especially when recommended dosages based on bodyweight and renal function were exceeded. Hence it is recommended that the dosage schedules of 'Primaxin' should be strictly adhered to, and established anticonvulsant therapy continued.

If focal tremors, myoclonus or convulsions occur, the patient should be evaluated neurologically and placed on anticonvulsant therapy if not already instituted. If these symptoms continue, the dosage should be reduced, or 'Primaxin' withdrawn completely.

Use in patients with renal insufficiency

Patients with creatinine clearances of $\leq$5 ml/min should not receive 'Primaxin' IV unless haemodialysis is instituted within 48 hours. For patients on haemodialysis, 'Primaxin' IV is recommended only when the benefit outweighs the potential risk of convulsions.

4.5 Interaction with other medicinal products and other forms of Interaction

General seizures have been reported in patients who received ganciclovir and 'Primaxin' IV. These drugs should not be used concomitantly unless the potential benefit outweighs the risk.

Concomitant probenecid has been shown to double the plasma level and half-life of cilastatin, but with no effect on its urinary recovery.

Concomitant probenecid showed only minimal increases in plasma level and half-life of imipenem, with urinary recovery of active imipenem decreased to approximately 60% of the administered dose.

4.6 Pregnancy and lactation

Pregnant monkeys showed evidence of maternal and foetal toxicity with bolus injections at doses equivalent to twice the human dose.

The use of 'Primaxin' in pregnant women has not been studied and 'Primaxin' should therefore not be given in pregnancy unless the anticipated benefit to the mother outweighs the possible risk to the foetus.

'Primaxin' has been detected in human milk. If the use of 'Primaxin' is deemed essential, the mother should stop breast-feeding.

4.7 Effects on ability to drive and use machines

There are no specific data; however, some of the CNS side-effects, such as dizziness, psychic disturbances, confusion and seizures, may affect the ability to drive or operate machinery.

4.8 Undesirable effects

Side effects

'Primaxin' is generally well tolerated. Side effects rarely require cessation of therapy and are generally mild and transient; serious side effects are rare.

Local reactions: erythema, local pain and induration, thrombophlebitis.

Allergic: rash, pruritus, urticaria, erythema multiforme, Stevens-Johnson syndrome, angioedema, toxic epidermal necrolysis (rarely), exfoliative dermatitis, (rarely) candidiasis, fever including drug fever, anaphylactic reactions.

Gastro-intestinal: nausea, vomiting, diarrhoea, staining of teeth and/or tongue. Pseudomembranous colitis has been reported.

Blood: eosinophilia, leucopenia, neutropenia including agranulocytosis, thrombocytopenia, thrombocytosis, decreased haemoglobin and prolonged prothrombin time. A positive direct Coombs test may develop.

Liver function: mild increases in serum transaminases, bilirubin and/or serum alkaline phosphatase, hepatitis rarely have been reported.

Renal function: oliguria/anuria, polyuria, acute renal failure (rarely). The role of 'Primaxin' in changes in renal function is difficult to assess, since factors predisposing to pre-renal uraemia or to impaired renal function usually have been present. Elevated serum creatinine and blood urea have been seen. A harmless urine discoloration, not to be confused with haematuria, has been seen in children.

Central nervous system: myoclonic activity, psychic disturbances including hallucinations, paraesthesia, confusional states or convulsions have been reported.

Granulocytopenic patients: drug-related nausea and/or vomiting appear to occur more frequently in granulocytopenic patients than in non-granulocytopenic patients treated with 'Primaxin'.

Special senses: hearing loss, taste perversion.

Other reported reactions with an unknown causal relationship

Gastro-intestinal: haemorrhagic colitis, gastro-enteritis, abdominal pain, glossitis, tongue papillar hypertrophy, heartburn, pharyngeal pain, increased salivation.

Central nervous system: dizziness, somnolence, encephalopathy, vertigo, headache.

Special senses: tinnitus.

Respiratory: chest discomfort, dyspnoea, hyperventilation, thoracic spine pain.

Cardiovascular: hypotension, palpitations, tachycardia.

Skin: flushing, cyanosis, hyperhidrosis, skin texture changes, pruritus vulvae.

Body as a whole: polyarthralgia, asthenia/weakness.

Blood: haemolytic anaemia, pancytopenia, bone marrow depression.

4.9 Overdose

No specific information is available on the treatment of overdosage with 'Primaxin'.

Imipenem-cilastatin sodium is haemodialysable. However, usefulness of this procedure in the overdosage setting is unknown.

5. PHARMACOLOGICAL PROPERTIES

Pharmacotherapeutic group: Antibacterials for systemic use.

ATC code: J01D H51

5.1 Pharmacodynamic properties

Mechanism of Action

Imipenem is a potent inhibitor of bacterial cell wall synthesis and is highly reactive towards penicillin-binding protein. Imipenem is more potent in its bactericidal effect than other antibiotics studied. Imipenem also provides excellent stability to degradative bacterial beta-lactamases. Imipenem is therefore active against a high percentage of organisms resistant to other beta-lactam antibiotics.

Cilastatin sodium is a competitive, reversible, and specific inhibitor of dehydropeptidase-I, the renal enzyme which metabolises and inactivates imipenem. Cilastatin sodium is devoid of intrinsic antibacterial activity itself and does not affect the antibacterial activity of imipenem.

Bacteriology

'Primaxin' has a unique anti-bacterial spectrum. Against Gram-negative species, 'Primaxin' shares the spectrum of the newer cephalosporins and penicillins; against Gram-positive species 'Primaxin' exerts the high bacterial potency previously associated only with narrow-spectrum beta-lactam antibiotics and the first-generation cephalosporins.

The antibiotic spectrum of 'Primaxin' is broader than that of other antibiotics studied and includes virtually all clinically significant pathogenic genera.

In vitro tests show that imipenem acts synergistically with aminoglycoside antibiotics against some isolates of *pseudomonas aeruginosa*.

Breakpoints (NCCLS)

The general MIC susceptibility test breakpoints to separate sensitive (S) pathogens from resistant (R) pathogens are: S $\leqslant$4 mcg/mL, R $\geqslant$ 16 mcg/mL.

For *Haemophilus spp.* S $\leqslant$ 4 mcg/mL, R MIC breakpoint not defined.

For *Neisseria gonorrhoeae* MIC breakpoints not defined.

For *Streptococcus pneumoniae* S $\leqslant$ 0.12 mcg/mL, R $\geqslant$ 1 mcg/mL

For streptococci other than *S. pneumoniae* MIC breakpoints not defined.

Susceptibility

The prevalence of resistance may vary geographically and with time for selected species and local information on resistance is desirable, particularly when treating severe infections. The information below gives only approximate guidance on the probability as to whether the microorganism will be susceptible to 'Primaxin' or not.

Organism	Prevalence of Resistance (Range) [European Union]
SUSCEPTIBLE	
Gram-positive aerobes:	
Bacillus spp	
Enterococcus faecalis	0 to 7%
Erysipelothrix rhusiopathiae	
Listeria monocytogenes	
Nocardia spp	
Pediococcus spp	
Staphylococcus aureus (methicillin susceptible, including penicillinase-producing strains	0%
Staphylococcus epidermidis (methicillin susceptible, including penicillinase-producing strains)	0 to 7%
Staphylococcus saprophyticus	0%
*Streptococcus agalactiae**	
Streptococcus Group C	
Streptococcus Group G	
Streptococcus pneumoniae	0%
Streptococcus pneumoniae, PRSP	0 to 83%
*Streptococcus pyogenes**	
*Viridans group streptococci** (including alpha and gamma hemolytic strains)	
Gram-negative aerobes:	
Achromobacter spp.	
Acinetobacter baumannii	0 to 67%
Aeromonas hydrophila	0 to 50%
Alcaligenes spp	
Bordetella bronchicanis	
Bordetella bronchiseptica	
Bordetella pertussis	
Brucella melitensis	
Burkholderia pseudomallei (formerly *pseudomonas pseudomallei)*	
Burkholderia stutzeri (formerly *pseudomonas stutzeri)*	
Campylobacter spp.	
Capnocytophaga spp.	
Citrobacter freundii	0%
Citrobacter koseri (formerly *Citrobacter diversus*	0%
Eikenella corrodens	
Enterobacter aerogenes	0%

Enterobacter agglomerans	
Enterobacter cloacae	0 to 13%
Eschericia coli	0%
Gardnerella vaginalis	
Haemophilus ducreyi	
Haemophilus influenzae (including beta-lactamase-producing strains)*	
*Haemophilus parainfluenzae**	
Hafnia alvei	0%
Klebsiella oxytoca	0%
Klebsiella ozaenae	
Klebsiella pneumoniae	0%
Moraxella catarrhalis	0%
Morganella morganii (formerly *Proteus morganii*)	0 to 7%
Neisseria gonorrhoeae (including penicillinase-producing strains)*	
Neisseria meningitidis	
Pasteurella spp	0%
Pasteurella multocida	
Plesiomonas shigelloides	
Proteus mirabilis	0%
Proteus vulgaris	0 to 8%
Providencia alcalifaciens	
Providencia rettgeri (formerly *Proteus rettgeri*)	0 to 20%
Providencia stuartii	0%
Pseudomonas aeruginosa	0 to 20%
Pseudomonas fluorescens	
Pseudomonas putida	
Salmonella spp	0%
Salmonella typhi	
Serratia spp	
Serratia proteamaculans (formerly *Serratia liquefaciens*)	
Serratia marcescens	0%
Shigella spp.	0%
Yersinia spp (formerly Pasteurella)	
Yersinia enterocolitica	
Yersinia pseudotuberculosis	
Gram-positive Anaerobes:	
Actinomyces spp	
Bifidobacterium spp.	
Clostridium spp	0%
Clostridium pefringens	
Eubacterium spp.	
Lactobacillus spp.	
Mobiluncus spp.	
Microaerophilic streptococci	
Peptococcus spp.	
Peptostreptococcus spp.	0%
Propionibacterium spp (including *P. acnes*)	
Gram-negative Anaerobes:	
Bacteroides spp.	6%
Bacteroides distasonis	
Bacteroides fragilis	0 to 7%
Bacteroides ovatus	
Bacteroides thetaitaomicron	0%
Bacteroides uniformis	
Bacteroides vulgatus	
Bilophila wadsworthia	
Fusobacterium spp.	
Fusobacterium necrophorum	
Fusobacterium nucleatum	
Porphyromonas asaccharolytica (formerly *Bacteroides asaccharolytica bivius*)	
Prevotella bivia (formerly *Bacteroides bivius*)	
Prevotella disiens (formerly *Bacteroides disiens*)	
Prevotella intermedia (formerly *Bacteroides intermedius*)	
Prevotella melaninogenica (formerly *Bacteroides melaninogenicus*)	
Veillonella spp	
Others:	
Mycobacterium fortuitum	
Myobacterium smegmatis	
RESISTANT	
Gram-positive Aerobes:	
Enterococcus faecium	
methicillin-resistant staphylococci	
Gram-negative Aerobes:	
Stenotrophomonas maltophilia (formerly *Xanthomonas maltophilia*, formerly *Pseudomonas maltophilia*)	
(Some strains of *Burkholderia cepacia* (formerly *Pseudomonas cepacia*)	

*Resistant breakpoint not defined.

Mechanism/s of Resistance

For species considered susceptible to imipenem, resistance was uncommon in surveillance studies in Europe. In resistant isolates, resistance to other antibacterial agents of the carbapenem class was seen in some, but not all isolates. Imipenem is effectively stable to hydrolysis by most classes of beta-lactamases, including penicillinases, cephalosporinases and extended spectrum beta-lactamases, but not metallo-beta-lactamases. Although effectively stable to beta-lactamase activity, resistance, when seen, is generally due to a combination of decreased permeability and low-level beta-lactamase hydrolysis.

The mechanism of action of imipenem differs from that of other classes of antibiotics, such as quinolones, aminoglycosides, macrolides and tetracyclines. There is no target-based cross-resistance between imipenem and these substances. However, micro-organisms may exhibit resistance to more than one class of antibacterial agents when the mechanism is, or includes, impermeability to some compounds.

5.2 Pharmacokinetic properties
'Primaxin' IV

The product is administered intravenously, therefore bioavailability data are not relevant.

Imipenem: Peak plasma levels of 36.4 mcg/ml after 500 mg, half-life 62.0 (±3.9) mins; plasma clearance 225.5 (±15.9) ml/min.

Co-administration of cilastatin sodium increases plasma concentrations of imipenem and increases the AUC by about 20%. There is also a decrease in plasma clearance (194.9 ml/min) and an increase in renal clearance, urinary recovery and urinary concentration.

5.3 Preclinical safety data
No relevant data.

6. PHARMACEUTICAL PARTICULARS

6.1 List of excipients
The only inactive ingredient in 'Primaxin' IV is sodium bicarbonate.

6.2 Incompatibilities
'Primaxin' is chemically incompatible with lactate and should not be reconstituted with diluents containing lactate. 'Primaxin' IV can, however, be administered into an IV tubing through which a lactate solution is being infused. 'Primaxin' should not be mixed or physically added to other antibiotics.

6.3 Shelf life
24 months.

6.4 Special precautions for storage
Vials of dry 'Primaxin' should be stored below 25°C. The container should be kept in the outer carton until immediately before use.

After reconstitution 'Primaxin' IV can be kept at room temperature (below 25°C) for up to three hours or under refrigeration (below 4°C) for up to 24 hours.

6.5 Nature and contents of container
'Primaxin' IV 500 mg strength is available in Type III or Type I clear glass vials with grey butyl rubber stoppers (West Formula 1816 or 1888 or Kashima Teflon coated) and aluminium collar seals with plastic flip-off tops. The vial size for 'Primaxin' IV 500 mg strength is 100 ml.

'Primaxin' IV 500 mg strength is available in nominal 20 ml vials and stoppers of the same materials with 'monovial' transfer system closures.

6.6 Instructions for use and handling
Preparation of intravenous solution

The following table is provided for convenience in reconstituting 'Primaxin' IV for intravenous infusion.

Strength	Volume of diluent added (ml)	Approximate concentration of imipenem (mg/ml)
'Primaxin' IV 500 mg	100	5

Compatibility and stability

In keeping with good clinical and pharmaceutical practice, 'Primaxin' IV should be administered as a freshly prepared solution. On the few occasions where changing circumstances make this impracticable, reconstituted 'Primaxin' IV retains satisfactory potency for three hours at room temperature (up to 25°C) or 24 hours in a refrigerator (below 4°C) when prepared in any of the following diluents: 0.9% Sodium Chloride Injection; 5% Dextrose and 0.9% Sodium Chloride; 5% Dextrose and 0.225% Sodium Chloride; 5% Mannitol.

'Primaxin' IV is chemically incompatible with lactate and should not be reconstituted with diluents containing lactate. 'Primaxin' IV can, however, be administered into an IV tubing through which a lactate solution is being infused.

'Primaxin' should not be mixed with, or physically added to, other antibiotics.

Addition of 'Primaxin' IV Injection in a Monovial to an infusion solution

(see Table 4 on next page)

7. MARKETING AUTHORISATION HOLDER
Merck Sharp & Dohme Limited

Hertford Road, Hoddesdon, Hertfordshire EN11 9BU

8. MARKETING AUTHORISATION NUMBER(S)
PL 0025/0229

9. DATE OF FIRST AUTHORISATION/RENEWAL OF THE AUTHORISATION
Licence first granted 30 June 1988

Licence last renewed 4 August 1994

10. DATE OF REVISION OF THE TEXT
October 2003

LEGAL CATEGORY
POM

SPC.TEN-IV.02.UK.0849

Table 4 Addition of 'Primaxin' IV Injection in a Monovial to an infusion solution

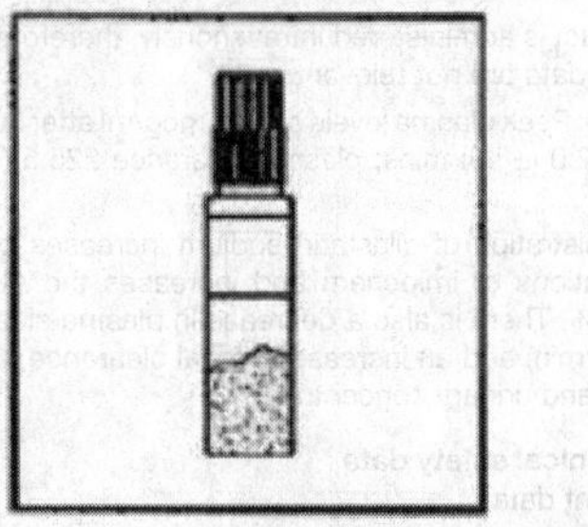

Step 1
EXAMINE
Examine the vial for any foreign material in the powder and make sure the tamper-evident seal between the cap and the vial is intact.

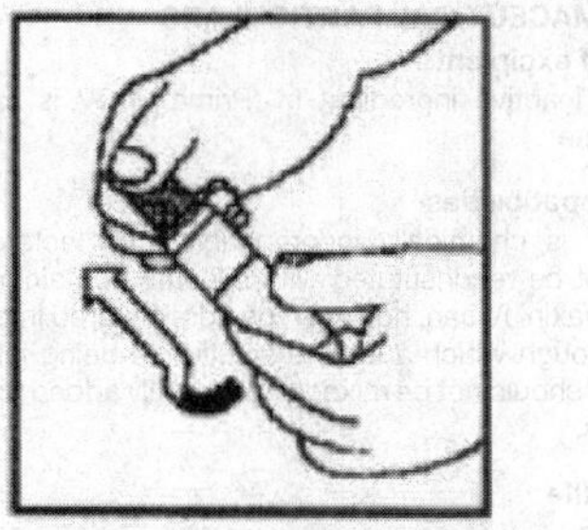

Step 2
REMOVE CAP
Remove the cap by first twisting it and pulling it up to break the tamper-evident seal.

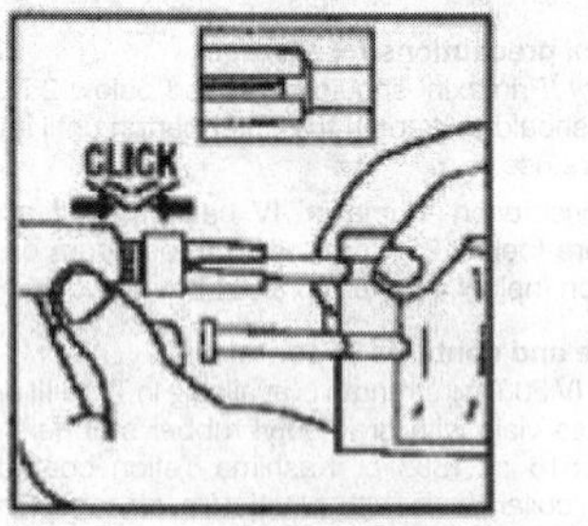

Step 3
CONNECT
Insert
the needle into the infusion-bag connector. *Push*
the needle-holder and vial together until they click into place.

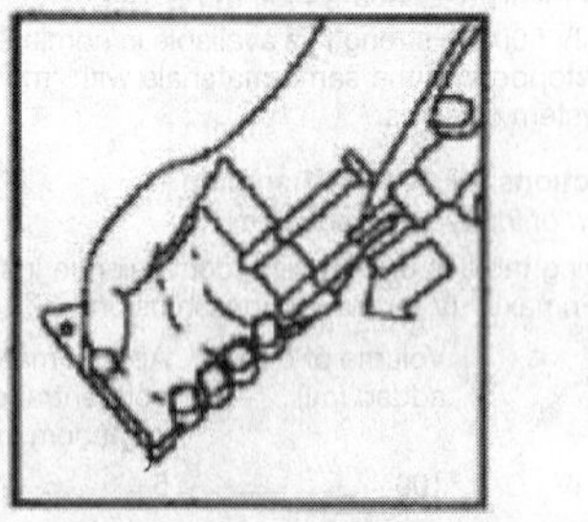

Step 4
MIX
Hold the vial in an upright position. *Squeeze*
the infusion bag several times to transfer the diluent into the vial. Shake the vial to reconstitute the substance.

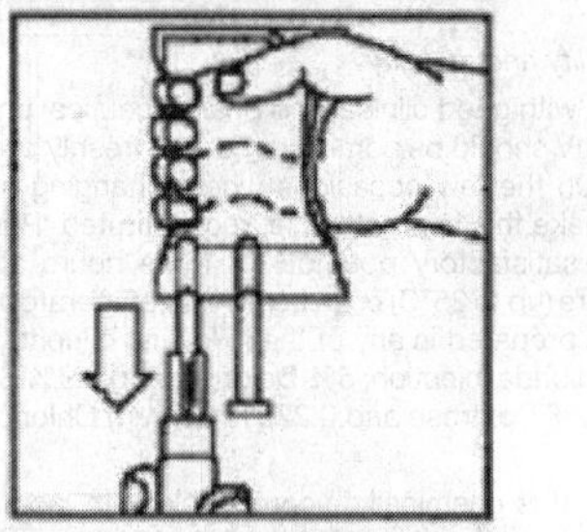

Step 5
TRANSFER
Now reverse the connected IV assembly, holding the vial upside down. Squeeze the infusion bag several times. This will create an over-pressure in the vial, allowing the contents of the vial to be transferred back into the infusion bag. Repeat steps 4 and 5 until the vial is completely empty

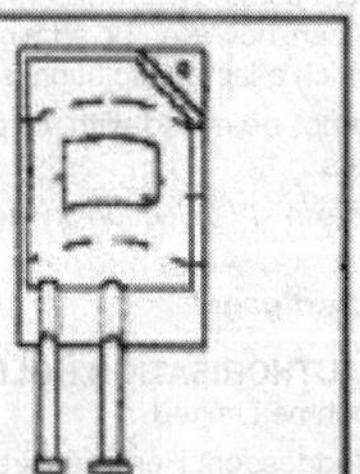

Step 6
IDENTIFY
Fill out the peel-off label on the vial and *affix*
it to the infusion bag for proper identification.

Primolut N

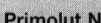

(Schering Health Care Limited)

1. NAME OF THE MEDICINAL PRODUCT
Primolut N®

2. QUALITATIVE AND QUANTITATIVE COMPOSITION
Each tablet contains 5 milligrams of norethisterone BP.

3. PHARMACEUTICAL FORM
Tablet.

White, uncoated tablets impressed with 'AN' in a regular hexagon on one side.

4. CLINICAL PARTICULARS

4.1 Therapeutic indications

Metropathia haemorrhagica. Premenstrual syndrome. Postponement of menstruation. Endometriosis. Menorrhagia. Dysmenorrhoea.

4.2 Posology and method of administration

Oral administration.

Not intended for use in children.

Metropathia haemorrhagica (dysfunctional uterine bleeding): 1 tablet 3 times daily for 10 days. Bleeding is arrested usually within 1-3 days. A withdrawal bleeding resembling normal menstruation occurs within 2-4 days after discontinuing treatment.

Prophylaxis against recurrence of dysfunctional bleeding: If there are no signs of resumption of normal ovarian function (no rise in the second half of the cycle of the morning temperature, which should be measured daily) recurrence must be anticipated. Cyclical bleeding can be established with 1 tablet twice daily from the 19th to the 26th day of the cycle.

Premenstrual syndrome (including premenstrual mastalgia): Premenstrual symptoms such as headache, migraine, breast discomfort, water retention, tachycardia, and psychological disturbances may be relieved by the administration of 2-3 tablets daily from the 19th to the 26th day of the cycle. Treatment should be repeated for several cycles. When treatment is stopped, the patient may remain symptom-free for a number of months.

Postponement of menstruation: In cases of too frequent menstrual bleeding, and in special circumstances (e.g. operations, travel, sports) the postponement of menstruation is possible. 1 tablet of Primolut N three times daily, starting 3 days before the expected onset of menstruation. A normal period should occur 2-3 days after the patient has stopped taking tablets.

Endometriosis (pseudo-pregnancy therapy): Long-term treatment is commenced on the 5th day of the cycle with 2 tablets of Primolut N daily for the first few weeks. In the event of spotting, the dosage is increased to 4, and, if necessary, 5 tablets daily. After bleeding has ceased, the initial dose is usually sufficient. Duration of treatment: 4-6 months continuously, or longer if necessary.

Menorrhagia (hypermenorrhoea): 1 tablet 2-3 times a day from the 19th to the 26th day of the cycle (counting the first day of menstruation as day 1).

Dysmenorrhoea: Functional or primary dysmenorrhoea is almost invariably relieved by the suppression of ovulation. 1 tablet three times daily for 20 days, starting on the fifth day of the cycle (the first day of menstruation counting as day 1). Treatment should be maintained for three to four cycles followed by treatment-free cycles. A further course of therapy may be employed if symptoms return.

4.3 Contraindications

1. Pregnancy.
2. Severe disturbances of liver function.
3. Dubin-Johnson syndrome.
4. Rotor syndrome.
5. Previous or existing liver tumours.
6. History during pregnancy of idiopathic jaundice, severe pruritus or herpes gestationis.
7. Current thromboembolic processes.
8. Hypersensitivity to the active substances or to any of the excipients.

4.4 Special warnings and special precautions for use

There is a general opinion, based on statistical evidence, that users of combined oral contraceptives experience, more often than non-users, venous thromboembolism, arterial thrombosis, including cerebral and myocardial infarction, and subarachnoid haemorrhage. Full recovery from such disorders does not always occur, and it should be realised that in a few cases they are fatal. Although Primolut N does not contain oestrogen, one should keep the possibility of an increased thromboembolic risk in mind, particularly where there is a history of thromboembolic disease or in the presence of severe diabetes with vascular changes or sickle-cell anaemia.

In rare cases benign, and in even rarer cases, malignant liver tumours leading in isolated cases to life-threatening intra-abdominal haemorrhage have been observed after the use of hormonal substances such as the one contained in Primolut N. If severe upper abdominal complaints, liver enlargement or signs of intra-abdominal haemorrhage occur, a liver tumour should be included in the differential diagnosis and, if necessary, the preparation should be withdrawn.

Primolut N can influence carbohydrate metabolism. Parameters of carbohydrate metabolism should be examined carefully in all diabetics before and regularly during treatment.

Reasons for stopping Primolut N immediately

1. Occurrence for the first time of migrainous headaches or more frequent occurrence of unusually severe headaches
2. Sudden perceptual disorders (e.g. disturbances of vision or hearing)
3. First signs of thrombophlebitis or thromboembolic symptoms, feeling of pain and tightness in the chest
4. Pending operations (six weeks beforehand), immobilisation (e.g. after accidents)
5. Onset of jaundice, hepatitis, general pruritus
6. Significant rise in blood pressure
7. Pregnancy.

4.5 Interaction with other medicinal products and other forms of Interaction

None known.

4.6 Pregnancy and lactation

The administration of Primolut N during pregnancy is contraindicated.

4.7 Effects on ability to drive and use machines
None known.

4.8 Undesirable effects
Side-effects rarely occur in doses of 15mg daily. Amongst those recorded are slight nausea, exacerbation of epilepsy, migraine and various skin disorders. With extremely high doses there may be cholestatic liver changes.

4.9 Overdose
There have been no reports of ill-effects from overdosage and treatment is generally unnecessary. There are no special antidotes, and treatment should be symptomatic.

5. PHARMACOLOGICAL PROPERTIES

5.1 Pharmacodynamic properties
Norethisterone has progestational actions similar to those of progesterone, but is a more potent inhibitor of ovulation and has weak oestrogenic and androgenic properties. It is used to treat a number of disorders of the menstrual cycle.

5.2 Pharmacokinetic properties
Norethisterone is absorbed from the gastro-intestinal tract and its effects last for at least 24 hours. It is excreted in the urine.

5.3 Preclinical safety data
There are no preclinical safety data which could be of relevance to the prescriber and which are not already included in other relevant sections of the SPC.

6. PHARMACEUTICAL PARTICULARS

6.1 List of excipients
lactose

maize starch

magnesium stearate

6.2 Incompatibilities
Not known.

6.3 Shelf life
5 years.

6.4 Special precautions for storage
Not applicable.

6.5 Nature and contents of container
Cardboard carton containing 3 blisters of 10 tablets.

6.6 Instructions for use and handling
Keep out of the reach of children.

7. MARKETING AUTHORISATION HOLDER
Schering Health Care Limited

The Brow

Burgess Hill

West Sussex

RH15 9NE

8. MARKETING AUTHORISATION NUMBER(S)
0053/5033R

9. DATE OF FIRST AUTHORISATION/RENEWAL OF THE AUTHORISATION
7/9/99

10. DATE OF REVISION OF THE TEXT
16th February, 2002

LEGAL CATEGORY
POM

Prioderm Cream Shampoo

(SSL International plc)

1. NAME OF THE MEDICINAL PRODUCT
Prioderm Cream Shampoo.

2. QUALITATIVE AND QUANTITATIVE COMPOSITION
Malathion USP 1.0% w/w.

3. PHARMACEUTICAL FORM
Cream shampoo.

4. CLINICAL PARTICULARS

4.1 Therapeutic indications
The source of infestation should be sought and treated. For the treatment of head louse and pubic louse infection.

4.2 Posology and method of administration
For topical external use only. As this product does not contain alcohol, it may be more suitable for those with asthma or eczema. Adults, the elderly and children aged 6 months and over: *For head lice:* Wet the hair thoroughly with warm water and apply sufficient shampoo to work up a rich lather and ensure that no part of the scalp is uncovered. Pay special attention to the back of the neck and the area behind the ears. Take care to avoid the eyes. Leave for at least five minutes. Rinse thoroughly with clean warm water and repeat procedure. While the hair is still wet, comb with an ordinary comb. The fine-toothed louse comb can then be used to remove the dead lice and eggs. This treatment should be carried out a total of three times at three day intervals, and should not be repeated within a 3 week period. *For pubic lice:* Application and dosage are as for the head. Apply the lotion to the pubic hair and the hair between the legs and anus. Children aged 6 months and under: On medical advice only.

4.3 Contraindications
None stated.

4.4 Special warnings and special precautions for use
As with all shampoos, avoid contact with the eyes. Children under 6 months should only be treated under medical supervision. When Prioderm Cream Shampoo is used by a school nurse or other health officer in the mass treatment of large numbers of children, it is advisable that protective plastic or rubber gloves be worn. Continued prolonged treatment with this product should be avoided. It should not be used for more than three times at three day intervals, and then not repeated within a three week period. Keep out of the reach of children.

4.5 Interaction with other medicinal products and other forms of Interaction
None stated.

4.6 Pregnancy and lactation
Prioderm Cream Shampoo is not known to have any effect on fertility, pregnancy and lactation. Its use in pregnant or lactating women is not recommended unless there is an overdue need.

4.7 Effects on ability to drive and use machines
None stated.

4.8 Undesirable effects
None stated.

4.9 Overdose
In the event of deliberate or accidental ingestion, empty stomach contents by gastric lavage and keep patient warm. In the event of massive ingestion, atropine or pralidoxime may be required to counteract cholinesterase inhibition.

5. PHARMACOLOGICAL PROPERTIES

5.1 Pharmacodynamic properties
Prioderm Cream Shampoo contains malathion, a widely used organophosphorus insecticide which is active by cholinesterase inhibition. It is effective against a wide range of insects, but is one of the least toxic organophosphorus insecticides since it is rapidly detoxified by plasma carboxylesterases.

5.2 Pharmacokinetic properties
Prioderm Cream Shampoo is applied topically to the affected area.

5.3 Preclinical safety data
None stated.

6. PHARMACEUTICAL PARTICULARS

6.1 List of excipients
Sodium Lauryl Sulphate paste; Cetostearyl Alcohol; Lauric Diethanolamide; Ethoxylated Lanolin (50%); Methyl Hydroxybenzoate; Propyl Hydroxybenzoate; Hydrochloric Acid; Citric Acid (anhydrous); Dibasic Sodium Phosphate; Colour Yellow (E110); Sodium Edetate; Perfume M&B 1658; Purified Water.

6.2 Incompatibilities
None stated.

6.3 Shelf life
18 months unopened.

6.4 Special precautions for storage
Store at or below 20°C.

6.5 Nature and contents of container
Cartoned, internally lacquered aluminium tube with polyethylene caps containing 40 g of product.

6.6 Instructions for use and handling
Not applicable.

7. MARKETING AUTHORISATION HOLDER
Seton Products Limited, Tubiton House, Oldham, OL1 3HS.

8. MARKETING AUTHORISATION NUMBER(S)
PL 11314/0051.

9. DATE OF FIRST AUTHORISATION/RENEWAL OF THE AUTHORISATION
6th October 1995 / 8th September 2000.

10. DATE OF REVISION OF THE TEXT
September 2000.

Prioderm Lotion

(SSL International plc)

1. NAME OF THE MEDICINAL PRODUCT
Prioderm Lotion.

2. QUALITATIVE AND QUANTITATIVE COMPOSITION
Malathion 0.5% w/v.

3. PHARMACEUTICAL FORM
Cutaneous solution.

4. CLINICAL PARTICULARS

4.1 Therapeutic indications
For the eradication of head lice infestation.

4.2 Posology and method of administration
Adults, the elderly and children aged 6 months and over: For topical external use only. For head lice: Rub the lotion gently into the scalp until all the hair and scalp is thoroughly moistened. Allow to dry naturally in a well ventilated room. Do not use a hairdryer or other artificial heat. Live lice will be eradicated after a minimum treatment period of two hours. However, the lotion should be left on the head for a further period of 8-10 hours to ensure that all lice eggs are totally eradicated. Shampoo in the normal manner. Rinse and comb the hair whilst wet to remove the dead lice. In the event of early reinfestation, Prioderm Lotion may be applied again provided 7 days have elapsed since the first application. Residual protective effect is variable of short duration and should not be relied upon. Not to be used on children under the age of 6 months, except on medical advice.

4.3 Contraindications
Not to be used on infants less than 6 months old except under medical supervision. Known sensitivity to malathion.

4.4 Special warnings and special precautions for use
Avoid contact with the eyes. Protect the eyes at all times by covering the eye area with a towel. In the event of contact with the eyes, rinse thoroughly with water. If there is persistent irritation, seek medical advice immediately. Do not cover the head until the hair has dried completely. It is advisable that nursing staff involved in repeated applications should wear gloves when carrying out treatment. Prioderm Lotion is for external use only and should be kept out of the reach of children. Keep away from exposed flames or lighted objects (e.g. cigarettes, gas and electric fires) during application and while hair is wet. Continued prolonged treatment with Prioderm Lotion should be avoided. It should not be used more than once a week and for not more than three consecutive weeks. Alcohol based products may cause a stinging sensation on patients with sensitive skin or wheezing in asthmatic people. In such cases, it may be more appropriate to use a liquid that does not contain isopropyl alcohol.

4.5 Interaction with other medicinal products and other forms of Interaction
None stated.

4.6 Pregnancy and lactation
No known effects in human pregnancy and lactation. However, as with all medicines, use with caution.

4.7 Effects on ability to drive and use machines
None stated.

4.8 Undesirable effects
Very rarely skin irritation has been reported with malathion products.

4.9 Overdose
In the event of deliberate or accidental ingestion, empty stomach by gastric lavage. Treatment: Atropine and pralidoxime may be required to counteract cholinesterase inhibition.

5. PHARMACOLOGICAL PROPERTIES

5.1 Pharmacodynamic properties
Prioderm Lotion contains malathion, a widely used organophosphorus insecticide which is active by cholinesterase inhibition. It is effective against a wide range of insects, but is one of the least toxic organophosphorus insecticides since it is rapidly detoxified by plasma carboxylesterases. Malathion kills insects by inhibiting their nervous system.

5.2 Pharmacokinetic properties
Prioderm Lotion is applied topically to the affected area.

5.3 Preclinical safety data
There are no preclinical data of relevance to the prescriber, which are additional to that included in other sections of the Summary of Product Characteristics.

6. PHARMACEUTICAL PARTICULARS

6.1 List of excipients
Isopropyl Alcohol; D-Limonene 17449; Terpineol 18689; Perfume Loxol P6160; Citric Acid; Shellsol T

6.2 Incompatibilities
None stated.

6.3 Shelf life
24 months.

6.4 Special precautions for storage
Do not store above 25°C. Keep container in the outer carton.

6.5 Nature and contents of container
Cartoned, clear or amber glass bottles with low density polyethylene caps and high density polypropylene sprinkler inserts containing either 50 or 200 ml of product.

6.6 Instructions for use and handling
Not applicable.

7. MARKETING AUTHORISATION HOLDER
Seton Products Limited, Tubiton House, Oldham, OL1 3HS.

8. MARKETING AUTHORISATION NUMBER(S)
PL 11314/0123.

9. DATE OF FIRST AUTHORISATION/RENEWAL OF THE AUTHORISATION
11th June 1999/ 24th December 2004

10. DATE OF REVISION OF THE TEXT
December 2004

Priorix

(GlaxoSmithKline UK)

1. NAME OF THE MEDICINAL PRODUCT
Priorix®

2. QUALITATIVE AND QUANTITATIVE COMPOSITION
Each 0.5 ml dose of the reconstituted vaccine contains:
- not less than $10^{3.0}$ $CCID_{50}$* of the Schwarz measles
- not less than $10^{3.7}$ $CCID_{50}$ of the RIT 4385 mumps, and
- - not less than $10^{3.0}$ $CCID_{50}$ of the Wistar RA 27/3 rubella virus strains.

*$CCID_{50}$ – Cell Culture Infective Dose 50

3. PHARMACEUTICAL FORM
Lyophilised vaccine for reconstitution with the sterile diluent provided.

4. CLINICAL PARTICULARS
4.1 Therapeutic indications
Priorix is indicated for active immunisation against measles, mumps and rubella.

4.2 Posology and method of administration
Posology
0.5 ml of the reconstituted vaccine constitutes one dose.

Priorix may be used for both primary immunisation and revaccination of children over 12 months of age, adolescents and adults. The vaccine should be given according to the recommended schedule.

Priorix may be given to subjects who have previously been vaccinated with other measles, mumps and rubella vaccines.

Children who suffered idiopathic thrombocytopenic purpura (ITP) within 6 weeks of the first dose of MMR (or its component vaccines) should have their serological status evaluated at the time the second dose is due. If serology testing suggests that a child is not fully immune against measles, mumps and rubella then a second dose of MMR is recommended.

Method of Administration
Priorix is for subcutaneous injection.

It may also be given by intramuscular injection. A limited number of subjects received Priorix intramuscularly in clinical trials in which an adequate immune response was obtained for all three components.

PRIORIX SHOULD UNDER NO CIRCUMSTANCES BE ADMINISTERED INTRAVASCULARLY.

Alcohol and other disinfecting agents must be allowed to evaporate from the skin before injection of the vaccine since they can inactivate the attenuated viruses in the vaccine.

4.3 Contraindications
Priorix is contra-indicated in subjects with known systemic hypersensitivity to any component of the vaccine or to neomycin (see also Section 4.4.) A history of contact dermatitis to neomycin is not a contra-indication.

Priorix must not be administered to pregnant women. Furthermore, pregnancy must be avoided for one month after vaccination (see Section 4.6).

Priorix should not be given to subjects with impaired immune responses. These include patients with primary or secondary immunodeficiencies.

However, measles, mumps, rubella-combined vaccines can be given to asymptomatic HIV-infected persons without adverse consequences to their illness and may be considered for those who are symptomatic.

As with other vaccines, the administration of Priorix should be postponed in subjects suffering from acute severe febrile illness. The presence of a minor infection, however, is not a contra-indication for vaccination.

4.4 Special warnings and special precautions for use
As with all injectable vaccines, appropriate medical treatment and supervision should always be readily available in case of a rare anaphylactic event following the administration of the vaccine.

Vaccines produced in chick embryo tissue cultures have been shown not to contain egg proteins in sufficient amounts to elicit hypersensitivity reactions. Persons having egg allergies, that are not anaphylactic in nature, can be considered for vaccination.

Priorix should be given with caution to persons with a history or family history of allergic diseases or those with a history or family history of convulsions.

Limited protection against measles may be obtained by vaccination up to 72 hours after exposure to natural measles.

Infants below 12 months of age may not respond sufficiently to the measles component of the vaccine, due to the possible persistence of maternal measles antibodies. This should not preclude the use of the vaccine in younger infants (<12 months) since vaccination may be indicated in some situations such as high-risk areas. In these circumstances revaccination at or after 12 months of age should be considered.

Children who suffered idiopathic thrombocytopenic purpura (ITP) within 6 weeks of the first dose of MMR (or its component vaccines) should have their serological status evaluated at the time the second dose is due. If serology testing suggests that a child is not fully immune against measles, mumps and rubella then a second dose of MMR is recommended.

Transmission of measles virus from vaccinees to susceptible contacts has never been documented. Pharyngeal excretion of the rubella virus is known to occur about 7 to 28 days after vaccination with peak excretion around the 11th day. However there is no evidence of transmission of this excreted vaccine virus to susceptible contacts. Studies have shown that recipients of the Jeryl Lynn strain of mumps virus vaccine do not spread this virus to susceptible contacts and that the virus cannot be isolated from blood, urine or saliva.

As with any vaccine, vaccination with Priorix may not result in complete protection of all vaccinees against the infections it is intended to prevent.

4.5 Interaction with other medicinal products and other forms of Interaction
Although data on the concomitant administration of Priorix and other vaccines are not available, it is generally accepted that measles, mumps and rubella-combined vaccine may be given at the same time as the oral polio vaccine (OPV) or inactivated polio vaccine (IPV), the injectable trivalent diphtheria, tetanus and pertussis vaccines (DTPw/DTPa) and *Haemophilus influenzae* type b (Hib). Concomitant vaccines should be given by separate injections into different body sites.

If Priorix cannot be given at the same time as other live attenuated vaccines, an interval of at least three weeks should be left between vaccinations.

In subjects who have received human gammaglobulins or a blood transfusion, vaccination should be delayed for at least three months because of the likelihood of vaccine failure due to passively acquired mumps, measles and rubella antibodies. However, if Priorix is being given primarily to achieve protection against rubella, the vaccine may be given within three months of the administration of an immunoglobulin preparation or a blood transfusion. In such instances, serological testing should be performed approximately 8-12 weeks later in order to assess the need for re-immunisation.

If tuberculin testing has to be done it should be carried out before, or simultaneously with, vaccination since it has been reported that live measles (and possibly mumps) vaccine may cause a temporary depression of tuberculin skin sensitivity. This anergy may last for four to six weeks and tuberculin testing should not be performed within that period after vaccination to avoid false negative results.

4.6 Pregnancy and lactation
Pregnancy
Priorix is contra-indicated in pregnant women. Furthermore, pregnancy should be avoided for one month after vaccination.

Lactation
There are little human data regarding use in breast-feeding women. Persons can be vaccinated where the benefit outweighs the risk.

4.7 Effects on ability to drive and use machines
The vaccine is unlikely to produce an effect on the ability to drive and use machines.

4.8 Undesirable effects
In controlled clinical studies in children aged from 9 months to 2 years, signs and symptoms were actively monitored on more than 5400 vaccinees during a 42-day follow-up period. The vaccinees were also requested to report any clinical events during the study period. The following adverse reactions were considered to have at least a suspected causal relationship with vaccination.

Frequencies are reported as:
Very common: ≥ 10%
Common: ≥ 1% and < 10%
Uncommon: ≥ 0.1% and < 1%
Rare: ≥ 0.01% and < 0.1%
Very rare: < 0.01%

Injection site:
common: local redness, pain and swelling

Body as a whole:
common: fever > 38.5°C when measured orally or by the axillary route

Central and peripheral nervous system:
uncommon: febrile convulsions
very rare: peripheral neuritis

Endocrine:
uncommon: parotid swelling

Gastro-intestinal system:
uncommon: diarrhoea, vomiting

Psychiatric:
uncommon: nervousness

Resistance mechanism:
uncommon: viral infection, otitis media

Respiratory system:
uncommon: pharyngitis, upper respiratory tract infection, rhinitis, bronchitis, coughing

Skin and appendages:
Common: rash

White cell and reticuloendothelial system:
Uncommon: lymphadenopathy

During post-marketing surveillance, the following reactions have been reported in temporal association with Priorix vaccination:

Body as a whole:
very rare:, allergic reactions (including anaphylactic reactions)

Central and peripheral nervous system:
very rare: meningitis

Platelet, bleeding and clotting:
very rare: thrombocytopenia, thrombocytopenic purpura

Skin and appendages:
very rare: erythema multiforme

As in natural rubella infection, arthralgia, or in isolated cases, chronic arthritis as well as myalgia, exanthema and swollen lymph nodes may occur two to four weeks after administration of live rubella vaccines. The incidence of joint reactions increases with the age of the vaccinee. Cases of exudative arthritis are extremely rare.

In comparative studies with other measles, mumps and rubella vaccines, the incidences of local pain, redness and swelling reported with Priorix were low, while the incidences of other adverse reactions were similar.

4.9 Overdose
Not applicable.

5. PHARMACOLOGICAL PROPERTIES
5.1 Pharmacodynamic properties
The safety and immunogenicity of Priorix in adolescents and adults has not been specifically studied in clinical trials.

In clinical studies in children aged from 12 months to 2 years Priorix has been demonstrated to be highly immunogenic. Following primary vaccination with a single dose of Priorix in the second year of life antibodies against measles were detected in 98.0%, against mumps in 96.1% and against rubella in 99.3% of previously seronegative vaccinees.

One hundred and fifty five children aged 10 – 22 months at immunisation were followed up for 12 months post vaccination. All remained seropositive for anti-measles and anti-rubella antibodies. 88.4% were still seropositive at month 12 for anti-mumps antibody. This percentage is in line with what was observed for other measles, mumps and rubella-combined vaccines (87%).

5.2 Pharmacokinetic properties
Not applicable.

5.3 Preclinical safety data
Not applicable.

6. PHARMACEUTICAL PARTICULARS
6.1 List of excipients
Vaccine: The vaccine contains the following amino acids: L-alanine,

L-arginine, glycine, L-histidine, L-isoleucine, L-leucine, L-lysine HC1,

L-methionine, L-phenylalanine, L-proline, L-serine, L-threonine,

L-tryptophan, L-tyrosine, L-valine, L-aspartic acid, L-cysteine, L-cystine,

L-hydroxproline, and, lactose, mannitol, sorbitol. The vaccine may also contain residual amounts of neomycin 25 micrograms maximum.

Diluent: Water for injections.

6.2 Incompatibilities
Priorix should not be mixed with other vaccines in the same syringe.

6.3 Shelf life
The shelf-life of Priorix is two years when the vaccine is stored according to recommendations (see Section 6.4.) The shelf lives of the vaccine and diluent are not identical, therefore their expiry dates are different. The outer carton bears the earlier of the two expiry dates and this date must be respected. The carton and ALL its contents should be discarded on reaching the outer carton expiry date.

6.4 Special precautions for storage
Priorix should be stored in a refrigerator between 2°C and 8°C and protected from light. Do not freeze.

During transport, recommended conditions of storage should be respected, particularly in hot climates.

6.5 Nature and contents of container
Priorix is presented as a whitish to slightly pink pellet in a glass vial. The sterile diluent is clear and colourless and presented in a glass prefilled syringe or ampoule. Due to minor variation of its pH, the reconstituted vaccine may vary in colour from light orange to light red without deterioration of the vaccine's potency.

Vials, prefilled syringes and ampoules are made of neutral glass type I, which conforms to European Pharmacopoeia requirements.

6.6 Instructions for use and handling
The diluent and reconstituted vaccine should be inspected visually for any foreign particulate matter and/or variation of physical aspects prior to administration. In the event of either being observed, discard the diluent or reconstituted vaccine.

The vaccine must be reconstituted by adding **the entire contents** of the supplied container of diluent to the vial containing the pellet. After the addition of the diluent to the pellet, the mixture should be well shaken until the pellet is completely dissolved in the diluent.

Inject the **entire contents** of the vial.

It is normal practice to administer the vaccine immediately after reconstitution with the diluent provided. However, the vaccine may still be used up to 3 hours after reconstitution or to the end of the vaccination session whichever is sooner.

Administrative Data

7. MARKETING AUTHORISATION HOLDER
SmithKline Beecham plc

Great West Road, Brentford, Middlesex TW8 9GS

Trading as

GlaxoSmithKline UK

Stockley Park West

Uxbridge

Middlesex

UB11 1BT

8. MARKETING AUTHORISATION NUMBER(S)
10592/0110

9. DATE OF FIRST AUTHORISATION/RENEWAL OF THE AUTHORISATION
4 December 1997

10. DATE OF REVISION OF THE TEXT
3 September 2004

11. Legal Category
POM

Procarbazine Capsules 50mg

(Cambridge Laboratories)

1. NAME OF THE MEDICINAL PRODUCT
Procarbazine Capsules 50mg

2. QUALITATIVE AND QUANTITATIVE COMPOSITION
Each capsule contains 58.3mg Procarbazine hydrochloride (equivalent to 50mg of Procarbazine).

3. PHARMACEUTICAL FORM
Capsules with opaque ivory cap and body.

4. CLINICAL PARTICULARS

4.1 Therapeutic indications
The main indication is Hodgkin's disease (lymphadenoma).

Procarbazine may also be useful in other advanced lymphomata and a variety of solid tumours which have proved resistant to other forms of therapy.

4.2 Posology and method of administration
In combination chemotherapeutic regimens:

Procarbazine is usually administered concomitantly with other appropriate cytostatic drugs in repeated four- to six-weekly cycles. In most such combination chemotherapy regimens currently in use (eg. the so-called MOPP schedule with mustine, Vincristine and Prednisone) Procarbazine is given daily on the first 10 - 14 days of each cycle in a dosage of 100mg per sq. metre of body surface (to nearest 50mg).

As sole therapeutic agent: Adults:

Treatment should begin with small doses which are increased gradually up to a maximum daily dose of 250 or 300mg divided as evenly as possible throughout the day.

Initial dosage scheme

(see Table 1 below)

Further procedure:

Treatment should be continued with 250 or 300mg daily until the greatest possible remission has been obtained, after which a maintenance dose is given.

Maintenance dose:

50 - 150mg daily. Treatment should be continued until a total dose of at least 6g has been given. Otherwise, a negative result is not significant.

Elderly:

Procarbazine should be used with caution in the elderly. Patients in this group should be observed very closely for signs of early failure or intolerance of treatment.

Children:

If, on the recommendation of a physician, a children's dosage is required, 50mg daily should be given for the first week. Daily dosage should then be maintained at 100mg per sq. metre of body surface (to nearest 50mg) until leucopenia or thrombocytopenia occurs or maximum response is obtained.

Procarbazine capsules are for oral administration.

4.3 Contraindications
Pre-existing severe leucopenia or thrombocytopenia from any cause; severe hepatic or renal damage.

Procarbazine should not be used in the management of non-malignant disease.

4.4 Special warnings and special precautions for use
Procarbazine should be given only under the supervision of a physician who is experienced in cancer chemotherapy and having facilities for regular monitoring of clinical and haematological effects during and after administration.

Introduction of therapy should only be effected under hospital conditions.

Caution is advisable in patients with hepatic or renal dysfunction, cardiovascular or cerebrovascular disease, phaeochromocytoma, or epilepsy.

Regular blood counts are of great importance. If during the initial treatment the total white cell count falls to 3,000 per mm^3 or the platelet count to 80,000 per mm^3, treatment should be suspended temporarily until the leucocyte and/or platelet levels recover, when therapy with the maintenance dose may be resumed.

Treatment should be interrupted on the appearance of allergic skin reactions.

Procarbazine has been shown to be carcinogenic in animals. The increased risk of carcinogenicity in man should be borne in mind when long-term management of patients is proposed.

4.5 Interaction with other medicinal products and other forms of Interaction
Procarbazine is a weak MAO inhibitor and therefore interactions with certain foodstuffs and drugs, although very rare, must be borne in mind. Thus, owing to possible potentiation of the effect of barbiturates, narcotic analgesics (especially Pethidine), drugs with anticholinergic effects (including phenothiazine derivatives and tricyclic antidepressants), other central nervous system depressants (including anaesthetic agents) and anti-hypertensive agents, these drugs should be given concurrently with caution and in low doses. Intolerance to alcohol (Disulfiram-like reaction) may occur.

4.6 Pregnancy and lactation
Procarbazine is teratogenic in animals. Isolated human foetal malformations have been reported following MOPP combination therapy. Therefore Procarbazine should not be administered to patients who are pregnant unless considered absolutely essential by the physician. Procarbazine should not be given to breast feeding mothers.

4.7 Effects on ability to drive and use machines
None known.

4.8 Undesirable effects
Loss of appetite and nausea occur in most cases, sometimes with vomiting. These symptoms are usually confined to the first few days of treatment and then tend to disappear.

Procarbazine causes leucopenia and thrombocytopenia. These haematological changes are almost always reversible and seldom require complete cessation of therapy.

4.9 Overdose
Signs of overdosage include severe nausea and vomiting, dizziness, hallucinations, depression and convulsions; hypotension or tachycardia may occur.

Gastric lavage and general supportive treatment should be performed, with prophylactic treatment against possible infection, and frequent blood counts.

Table 1 Initial dosage scheme

1st day:	50mg	4th day:	200mg
2nd day:	100mg	5th day:	250mg
3rd day:	150mg	6th day et seq:	250-300mg

5. PHARMACOLOGICAL PROPERTIES

5.1 Pharmacodynamic properties
Procarbazine, a methylhydrazine derivative, is a cytostatic agent with weak MAO inhibitor properties. Its exact mode of action on tumour cells is unknown. It may be effective in patients who have become resistant to radiation therapy and other cytostatic agents.

5.2 Pharmacokinetic properties
Procarbazine is readily absorbed from the gastrointestinal tract. It is rapidly metabolised, the primary circulating metabolite is the azo derivative while the major urinary metabolite has been shown to be N-isopropyl-terephthalamic acid.

5.3 Preclinical safety data
There are no pre-clinical data of relevance to the prescriber which are additional to that already included in other sections of the SPC.

6. PHARMACEUTICAL PARTICULARS

6.1 List of excipients
Mannitol

Maize starch

Talc

Magnesium stearate

Capsule shell components:

Gelatin

Yellow iron oxide E172

Titanium dioxide E171

6.2 Incompatibilities
None known.

6.3 Shelf life
Three years.

6.4 Special precautions for storage
Procarbazine capsules should be stored in a dry place; the recommended maximum storage temperature is 25°C

6.5 Nature and contents of container
Blister packs of 50 capsules.

6.6 Instructions for use and handling
Handling guidelines:

Undamaged capsules present minimal risk of contamination, but in accordance with good hygiene requirements, direct handling should be avoided. As with all cytotoxics, precautions should be taken to avoid exposing staff during pregnancy.

Waste material may be disposed of by incineration.

7. MARKETING AUTHORISATION HOLDER
Cambridge Laboratories Limited

Deltic House

Kingfisher Way

Silverlink Business Park

Wallsend

Tyne & Wear

NE28 9NX

8. MARKETING AUTHORISATION NUMBER(S)
PL 12070/0004

9. DATE OF FIRST AUTHORISATION/RENEWAL OF THE AUTHORISATION
10 November 1992

10. DATE OF REVISION OF THE TEXT
March 2000

Proctofoam

(Meda Pharmaceuticals)

1. NAME OF THE MEDICINAL PRODUCT
Proctofoam

2. QUALITATIVE AND QUANTITATIVE COMPOSITION
Hydrocortisone Acetate 1.0% w/w

Pramoxine Hydrochloride 1.0% w/w

3. PHARMACEUTICAL FORM
Rectal foam

4. CLINICAL PARTICULARS

4.1 Therapeutic indications
For the short term (not more than 5 - 7 days) relief of the symptoms of itching, irritation, discomfort or pain associated with local, non infective anal or perianal conditions.

4.2 Posology and method of administration
One applicator full per rectum two or three times daily and after each bowel evacuation (up to a maximum of four times daily). For perianal administration, apply a small quantity on two fingers.

Not recommended for use in children.

4.3 Contraindications
Hypersensitivity to pramoxine hydrochloride or to any component of the preparation.

Bacterial, viral or fungal infection.

4.4 Special warnings and special precautions for use
Not for prolonged use. Contact sensitisation to local anaesthetics is common following prolonged application.

Seek medical advice if symptoms worsen, or do not improve within 7 days or if bleeding occurs.

Shake vigorously before use, use at room temperature, keep out of the reach of children. For external use only.

Rectal examination must be performed to exclude serious pathology before initiating treatment with Proctofoam.

4.5 Interaction with other medicinal products and other forms of Interaction
None known.

4.6 Pregnancy and lactation
Safety for use in pregnancy and lactation has not been established.

There is inadequate evidence of safety in human pregnancy. Topical administration of corticosteroids to pregnant animals can cause abnormalities to foetal development including cleft palate and intrauterine growth retardation. There may be a very small risk of such effects in the human foetus. No data is available on the use of topical corticosteroids and local anaesthetic agents in nursing mothers. However, the product has been used by nursing mothers for many years without apparent ill consequence.

4.7 Effects on ability to drive and use machines
None known.

4.8 Undesirable effects
Although uncommon at this dosage; local burning, irritation, allergic dermatitis, secondary infection and skin atrophy may occur. Systemic absorption of topical corticosteroids has produced reversible suppression of the hypothalamic - pituitary - adrenal axis and manifestations of Cushing's syndrome.

4.9 Overdose
Excess use of topical corticosteroids may produce systemic adverse effects.

5. PHARMACOLOGICAL PROPERTIES

5.1 Pharmacodynamic properties
Pramoxine Hydrochloride is a surface anaesthetic and thus relieves the pain of anal and perianal conditions.

The use of steroids in inflammatory conditions is well known.

5.2 Pharmacokinetic properties
Not applicable.

5.3 Preclinical safety data
None stated.

6. PHARMACEUTICAL PARTICULARS

6.1 List of excipients
Cetyl Alcohol
Emulsifying Wax
Methyl Parahydroxybenzoate
Polyoxyethylene (10), Stearyl Ether
Propylene Glycol
Propyl Parahydroxybenzoate
Triethanolamine
Purified Water
Propellant HP-70 Consisting of:
- Isobutane
- Propane

6.2 Incompatibilities
Compatibility with barrier methods of contraception has not been demonstrated.

6.3 Shelf life
30 months.

6.4 Special precautions for storage
Pressurised container containing flammable propellant. Protect from sunlight. Do not expose to temperatures above 50°C. Do not spray on a naked flame or any incandescent material. Keep away from sources of ignition - no smoking. Do not pierce or burn, even after use.

Do not refrigerate.

6.5 Nature and contents of container
Aerosol canister containing 20 g of product plus 1.2 g of inert propellant. A 10% overage of product and propellant is included to ensure the required number of doses can be achieved.

6.6 Instructions for use and handling
1. Shake the canister vigorously for 30 seconds before each use.

2. Withdraw the plunger slowly until it stops at the catch line.

3. Holding upright, insert the canister top into the applicator tip. Make sure you hold the plunger and applicator body firmly with your fingers.

4. Press down a number of times on the canister top with your fingers. Each press releases a small amount of foam. When the applicator is half full of foam, stop for a few seconds until the foam stops expanding.

5. Press down again to complete filling to the fill line.

6. For internal use
Stand with one leg raised on a chair, or lie down on your left side. Insert gently into the back passage and push the plunger fully into the applicator.

7. For external use
Expel a small quantity of foam onto a tissue, pad or two fingers and apply the foam to the affected area.

These instructions are provided on the leaflet with illustrations to assist understanding.

7. MARKETING AUTHORISATION HOLDER
Meda Pharmaceuticals Ltd
Sherwood House
7 Gregory Boulevard
Nottingham
NG7 6LB
UK
Trading as:
Meda Pharmaceuticals
Regus House
Herald Way
Pegasus Business Park
Castle Donington
Derbyshire
DE74 2TZ
UK

8. MARKETING AUTHORISATION NUMBER(S)
PL 19477/0010

9. DATE OF FIRST AUTHORISATION/RENEWAL OF THE AUTHORISATION
First authorisation: December 1972
Last renewal: 29 July 1997

10. DATE OF REVISION OF THE TEXT
11 Nov 2003

Proctosedyl Ointment
(sanofi-aventis)

1. NAME OF THE MEDICINAL PRODUCT
Proctosedyl Ointment

2. QUALITATIVE AND QUANTITATIVE COMPOSITION
Cichocaine Hydrochloride (Micro) BP 0.5 %ww, Hydrocortisone (Micro) EP 0.5 %ww

3. PHARMACEUTICAL FORM
Yellowish-white translucent greasy ointment.

4. CLINICAL PARTICULARS

4.1 Therapeutic indications
The local anaesthetic cinchocaine relieves pain and relaxes sphincteric spasm. Pruritis and inflammation are relieved by hydrocortisone, which also decreases serious discharge.

Proctosedyl is, therefore, useful for the short term relief (not more than 7 days) of pain, irritation and pruritis associated with haemorrhoids and pruritis ani.

4.2 Posology and method of administration
Apply the ointment in small quantities with the finger, on the painful or pruritic area, morning and evening and after each stool. For deep application attach cannula to tube, insert to full extent and squeeze tube gently from lower end whilst withdrawing.

The ointment may be used separately or concurrently with the suppositories.

4.3 Contraindications
Known hypersensitivity to any of the ingredients.

Not for use in the presence of infections.

4.4 Special warnings and special precautions for use
Apply only to the region of the rectum and anus and surrounding skin. Hydrocortisone can cause thinning and damage to the skin especially of the face.

As with all preparations containing topical steroids, the possibility of systemic absorption should be considered. In particular, long-term continuous therapy should be avoided in infants. Adrenal suppression can occur even without occlusion.

4.5 Interaction with other medicinal products and other forms of Interaction
None known.

4.6 Pregnancy and lactation
In pregnant animals, administration of corticosteroids can cause abnormalities of foetal development. The relevance of this finding to human beings has not been established. However, topical steroids should not be used extensively in pregnancy, i.e. in large amounts or for long periods.

4.7 Effects on ability to drive and use machines
None.

4.8 Undesirable effects
In persons sensitive to any of the ingredients, skin rash may occur. Although less likely to cause adrenal suppression when applied topically, Hydrocortisone, applied to a large enough area, especially of damaged skin for long enough, or if under occlusive dressing, may have this adverse effect.

4.9 Overdose
Not applicable.

5. PHARMACOLOGICAL PROPERTIES

5.1 Pharmacodynamic properties
Cinchocaine is a local anaesthetic of the amide type.

Hydrocortisone is a glucocorticoid with anti-inflammatory and other properties.

5.2 Pharmacokinetic properties
The literature states that absorption of hydrocortisone does occur through the skin, particularly denuded skin. However, this absorption is not of a clinical significance as hydrocortisone topically, has only rarely been associated with side effects resulting from pituitary adrenal suppression.

Cinchocaine is little absorbed through the intact skin, but absorbed through mucous membranes. Like other local anaesthetics of the amide type, cinchocaine is metabolised in the liver.

5.3 Preclinical safety data
None stated.

6. PHARMACEUTICAL PARTICULARS

6.1 List of excipients
Wool fat, liquid paraffin, white soft paraffin.

6.2 Incompatibilities
None stated.

6.3 Shelf life
36 months

6.4 Special precautions for storage
Store below 25°C.

6.5 Nature and contents of container
Aluminium tube with plastic cannula (30g tubes).

6.6 Instructions for use and handling
None stated.

7. MARKETING AUTHORISATION HOLDER
Aventis Pharma Limited
50 Kings Hill Avenue
Kings Hill
West Malling
Kent ME19 4AH
UK

8. MARKETING AUTHORISATION NUMBER(S)
PL 04425/0207

9. DATE OF FIRST AUTHORISATION/RENEWAL OF THE AUTHORISATION
21 July 2005

10. DATE OF REVISION OF THE TEXT
July 2005

Legal category: POM

Proctosedyl Suppositories
(sanofi-aventis)

1. NAME OF THE MEDICINAL PRODUCT
Proctosedyl Suppositories

2. QUALITATIVE AND QUANTITATIVE COMPOSITION
Cinchocaine Hydrochloride (micro) BP 5mg

Hydrocortisone (micro) EP 5mg

3. PHARMACEUTICAL FORM
Smooth off-white suppositories.

4. CLINICAL PARTICULARS

4.1 Therapeutic indications
The local anaesthetic Cinchocaine relieves pain and relaxes sphincteric spasm. Pruritis and inflammation are relieved by Hydrocortisone which also decreases serous discharge. Proctosedyl is, therefore, useful for the short term relief (not more than 7 days) of pain, irritation and pruritis associated with haemorrhoids, pruritis ani.

4.2 Posology and method of administration
Adults (including the elderly) and children:

A suppository is inserted morning and evening, and after each stool. The ointment may be used concurrently with the suppositories.

4.3 Contraindications
Known hypersensitivity to any of the ingredients. Not for use in the presence of infections.

4.4 Special warnings and special precautions for use
As with all preparations containing topical steroids, the possibility of systemic absorption should be considered. In particular, long-term continuous therapy should be avoided in infants. Adrenal suppression can occur even without occlusion.

4.5 Interaction with other medicinal products and other forms of Interaction
None known.

4.6 Pregnancy and lactation
In pregnant animals, administration of corticosteroids can cause abnormalities of foetal development. The relevance of this finding to human beings has not been established. However, topical steroids should not be used extensively in pregnancy, i.e. in large amounts or for long periods.

4.7 Effects on ability to drive and use machines
None.

4.8 Undesirable effects
In persons sensitive to any of the ingredients, anal irritation may occur.

4.9 Overdose
Not applicable.

5. PHARMACOLOGICAL PROPERTIES

5.1 Pharmacodynamic properties
Cinchocaine is a local anaesthetic of the amide type.

Hydrocortisone is a glucocorticoid with anti-inflammatory and other properties.

5.2 Pharmacokinetic properties
The literature states that absorption of Hydrocortisone does occur through the skin, particularly denuded skin. However, this absorption is not of a clinical significance as Hydrocortisone topically has only rarely been associated with side effects resulting from pituitary adrenal suppression.

Cinchocaine is little absorbed through the intact skin, but absorbed through mucous membranes. Like other local anaesthetics of the amide type, Cinchocaine is metabolised in the liver.

5.3 Preclinical safety data
None stated.

6. PHARMACEUTICAL PARTICULARS

6.1 List of excipients
Suppocire AM

6.2 Incompatibilities
Not applicable.

6.3 Shelf life
18 months.

6.4 Special precautions for storage
Store at 2°C - 8°C

6.5 Nature and contents of container
Each suppository is contained in a pocket formed from white PVC/PE laminate in packs of 12.

6.6 Instructions for use and handling
None stated.

7. MARKETING AUTHORISATION HOLDER
Aventis Pharma Limited
50 Kings Hill Avenue
Kings Hill
West Malling
Kent ME19 4AH
UK

8. MARKETING AUTHORISATION NUMBER(S)
PL 04425/0208

9. DATE OF FIRST AUTHORISATION/RENEWAL OF THE AUTHORISATION
21 July 2005

10. DATE OF REVISION OF THE TEXT
July 2005

Legal category: POM

Pro-Epanutin Concentrate for infusion / Solution for injection

(Pfizer Limited)

1. NAME OF THE MEDICINAL PRODUCT
Pro-Epanutin Concentrate for infusion / Solution for injection

2. QUALITATIVE AND QUANTITATIVE COMPOSITION
One ml of Pro-Epanutin contains 75mg of fosphenytoin sodium (equivalent to 50mg of phenytoin sodium) and referred to as 50mg PE (see Section 4.2).

Each 10ml vial contains 750mg of fosphenytoin sodium (equivalent to 500mg of phenytoin sodium) and referred to as 500mg PE.

For excipients, see Section 6.1.

3. PHARMACEUTICAL FORM
Concentrate for infusion / Solution for injection.

Pro-Epanutin is a clear, colourless to pale yellow, sterile solution.

4. CLINICAL PARTICULARS

4.1 Therapeutic indications
Pro-Epanutin is indicated:

- for the control of status epilepticus of the tonic-clonic (grand mal) type **(see Section 4.2 Posology and Method of Administration)**.
- for prevention and treatment of seizures occurring in connection with neurosurgery and/or head trauma.
- as substitute for oral phenytoin if oral administration is not possible and/or contra-indicated.

4.2 Posology and method of administration
IMPORTANT NOTE: Throughout all Pro-Epanutin product labelling, the amount and concentration of fosphenytoin is always expressed in terms of phenytoin sodium equivalents (PE) to avoid the need to perform molecular weight-based adjustments when converting between fosphenytoin and phenytoin sodium doses. Pro-Epanutin should always be prescribed and dispensed in phenytoin sodium equivalent units (PE). Note, however, that fosphenytoin has important differences in administration from parenteral phenytoin sodium (see Section 4.4 Special Warnings and Precautions for Use).

Phenytoin sodium equivalents (PE):
1.5mg of fosphenytoin is equivalent to 1mg PE (phenytoin sodium equivalent)

Administration:
Pro-Epanutin may be administered by IV infusion or by IM injection. The intramuscular route should be considered when there is not an urgent need to control seizures. Pro-Epanutin should not be administered by IM route in emergency situations such as status epilepticus.

Products with particulate matter or discoloration should not be used.

Intravenous infusion:
For IV infusion, Pro-Epanutin should be diluted in 5% glucose or 0.9% sodium chloride solution. The concentration should range from 1.5 to 25mg PE/ml.

Because of the risk of hypotension, the recommended rate of administration by IV infusion in routine clinical settings is 50-100mg PE/minute. Even in an emergency, **it should not exceed 150mg PE/minute**. The use of a device controlling the rate of infusion is recommended.

Please refer to tables 1 to 10 for examples of dosing, dilution and infusion time calculations.

Continuous monitoring of electrocardiogram, blood pressure and respiratory function for the duration of the infusion is essential. The patient should also be observed throughout the period where maximal plasma phenytoin concentrations occur. This is approximately 30 minutes after the end of the Pro-Epanutin infusions.

Cardiac resuscitative equipment should be available **(see Section 4.4 Special Warnings and Precautions for Use)**.

DOSAGE IN ADULTS

Status Epilepticus

Loading dose:

In order to obtain rapid seizure control in patients with continuous seizure activity, IV diazepam or lorazepam should be administered prior to administration of Pro-Epanutin.

The loading dose of Pro-Epanutin is 15mg PE/kg administered as a single dose by IV infusion

Recommended IV infusion rate: 100 to 150mg PE/min. **(should not exceed 150mg PE/minute even for emergency use).**

Examples of infusion times are presented in Table 1.

Intramuscular administration of Pro-Epanutin is contra-indicated in the treatment of status epilepticus. If administration of Pro-Epanutin does not terminate seizures, the use of alternative anticonvulsants should be considered.

Table 1:

Status Epilepticus: Examples of IV loading doses of 15mg PE/kg, and recommendations for dilution (to 25mg PE/ml) and IV infusion times (at maximum rate of 150mg PE/min by body weight)

(see Table 1 below)

Maintenance dose:

The recommended maintenance dose of Pro-Epanutin of 4 to 5mg PE/kg/day may be given by IV infusion or by IM injection. The total daily dose may be given in one or two divided doses.

Recommended IV infusion rate for maintenance dose: 50 to 100mg PE/minute.

Examples of infusion times are provided in Table 2.

Maintenance doses should be adjusted according to patient response and trough plasma phenytoin concentrations **(see Therapeutic Drug Monitoring)**.

Transfer to maintenance therapy with oral phenytoin should be made when appropriate.

Table 2:

Status Epilepticus: Examples for maximum IV maintenance doses of 5mg PE/kg, recommendations for dilution* (to 25mg PE/ml or to 1.5mg PE/ml), and IV infusion times (at maximum rate of 100mg PE/minute) by body weight

(see Table 2 on next page)

Treatment or Prophylaxis of Seizures

Loading dose:

The loading dose of Pro-Epanutin is 10 to 15mg PE/kg given as a single dose by IV infusion or by IM injection.

Recommended IV infusion rate for treatment or prophylaxis of seizures: 50 to 100mg PE/minute **(should not exceed 150mg PE/minute).**

Examples of infusion times are presented in Table 3.

Table 3:

Treatment or Prophylaxis of seizures: Examples for IV loading doses of 10mg PE/kg[a], and recommendations for dilution* (to 25mg PE/ml or to 1.5mg PE/ml) and IV infusion times (at maximum rate of 100mg PE/minute) by body weight

(see Table 3 on next page)

Maintenance dose:

The recommended maintenance dose of Pro-Epanutin of 4 to 5mg PE/kg/day may be given by IV infusion or by IM injection. The total daily dose may be given in one or two divided doses.

Recommended IV infusion rate for maintenance dose: 50 to 100mg PE/minute.

Examples of infusion times are presented in Table 4.

Maintenance doses should be adjusted according to patient response and trough plasma phenytoin concentrations **(see Therapeutic Drug Monitoring)**.

Transfer to maintenance therapy with oral phenytoin should be made when appropriate.

Table 1

Weight (kg)	Dose (mg PE)	Volume of Pro-Epanutin (50mg PE/ml)		Volume (ml) of diluent (5% glucose or 0.9% sodium chloride) for final concentration of 25mg PE/ml	Minimum Infusion Time (mins) to achieve the maximum recommended infusion rate of 150mg PE / minute
		No. of 10ml vials to open	Volume (ml) to draw up		
100	1500	3	30	30	10
95	1425	3	28.5	28.5	9.5
90	1350	3	27	27	9
85	1275	3	25.5	25.5	8.5
80	1200	3	24	24	8
75	1125	3	22.5	22.5	7.5
70	1050	3	21	21	7
65	975	2	19.5	19.5	6.5
60	900	2	18	18	6
55	825	2	16.5	16.5	5.5
50	750	2	15	15	5
45	675	2	13.5	13.5	4.5

Table 4:

Treatment or Prophylaxis of seizures: Examples for maximum IV maintenance doses of 5mg PE/kg, recommendations for dilution* (to 25mg PE/ml or to 1.5mg PE/ml), and IV infusion times (at maximum infusion rate of 100mg PE/minute) by body weight

(see Table 4)

Temporary substitution of oral phenytoin therapy with Pro-Epanutin.

The same dose and dosing frequency as for oral phenytoin therapy should be used and can be administered by IV infusion or by IM injection.

Recommended IV infusion rate for temporary substitution dosing: 50 to 100mg PE/minute.

Examples of infusion times are presented in Table 5.

Therapeutic drug monitoring may be useful whenever switching between products and/or routes of administration. Doses should be adjusted according to patient response and trough plasma phenytoin concentrations (see **Therapeutic Drug Monitoring**).

Fosphenytoin has not been evaluated systemically for more than 5 days.

Table 5:

Temporary substitution of oral phenytoin therapy: Examples of equivalent doses and recommendations for dilution* (to 25mg PE/ml or to 1.5mg PE/ml), and IV infusion times (at maximum rate of 100mg PE/minute)

(see Table 5)

DOSAGE IN CHILDREN

Pro-Epanutin may be administered to children (ages 5 and above) by IV infusion only, at the same mg PE/kg dose used for adults. The doses of Pro-Epanutin for children have been predicted from the known pharmacokinetics of Pro-Epanutin in adults and children aged 5 to 10 years and of parenteral phenytoin in adults and children.

Status Epilepticus

Loading dose

In order to obtain rapid seizure control in patients with continuous seizure activity IV diazepam or lorazepam should be administered prior to administration of Pro-Epanutin.

The loading dose of Pro-Epanutin is 15mg PE/kg administered as a single dose by IV infusion

Recommended IV infusion rate: 2 to 3mg PE/kg/min. **(should not exceed 3mg PE/kg/minute or 150mg PE/minute).**

The recommended infusion rate is presented in Table 6.

If administration of Pro-Epanutin does not terminate seizures, the use of alternative anticonvulsants should be considered.

Table 6:

Status Epilepticus: Examples of IV loading doses of 15mg PE/kg and recommendations for dilution (to 25mg PE/ml) and IV infusion times (at 3mg PE/kg/minute) by body weight

(see Table 6 on next page)

Maintenance dose:

The recommended maintenance dose of Pro-Epanutin of 4 to 5mg PE/kg/day may be given by IV infusion. The total daily dose may be given in one to four divided doses.

Recommended IV infusion rate for maintenance dosing: 1 to 2mg PE/kg/minute **(should not exceed 100mg PE/minute).**

The recommended infusion time is presented in Table 7.

Maintenance doses should be adjusted according to patient response and trough plasma phenytoin concentrations **(see Therapeutic Drug Monitoring).**

Transfer to maintenance therapy with oral phenytoin should be made when appropriate.

Table 7:

Status Epilepticus: Examples for maximum IV maintenance doses of 5mg PE/kg, recommendations for dilution* (to 25mg PE/ml or to 1.5mg PE/ml) and IV infusion times (at maximum rate of 2mg PE/kg/minute) by body weight

(see Table 7 on next page)

Treatment or Prophylaxis of Seizures

Loading dose:

The loading dose of Pro-Epanutin is 10 to 15mg PE/kg given as a single dose by IV infusion.

Recommended IV infusion rate fortreatment or prophylaxis of seizures: 1 to 2mg PE/kg/minute **(should not exceed 3mg PE/kg/minute or 150mg PE/minute).**

The recommended infusion time is presented in Table 8.

Table 8:

Treatment or Prophylaxis of seizures: Examples for IV loading doses of 10mg PE/kg[a], and recommendations for dilution* (to 25mg PE/ml or to 1.5mg PE/ml) and IV infusion times (at maximum rate of 2mg PE/kg/minute) by body weight

(see Table 8 on next page)

Maintenance dose:

The recommended maintenance dose of Pro-Epanutin of 4 to 5mg PE/kg/day may be given by IV infusion. The total daily dose may be given in one to four divided doses.

Table 2

Weight (kg)	Dose (mg PE)	Volume of Pro-Epanutin (50mg PE/ml)		Volume (ml) of diluent* (5% glucose or 0.9% sodium chloride)		Minimum Infusion Time (mins) to achieve the maximum recommended infusion rate of 100mg PE / minute
		No. of 10ml vials to open	Volume (ml) to draw up	for final concentration of 25mg PE/ml	for final concentration of 1.5mg PE/ml	
100	500	1	10	10	323	5
90	450	1	9	9	291	4.5
80	400	1	8	8	259	4
70	350	1	7	7	226	3.5
60	300	1	6	6	194	3
50	250	1	5	5	162	2.5

***For IV infusion the final concentration should range between 1.5 and 25mg PE/ml**

Table 3

Weight (kg)	Dose (mg PE)	Volume of Pro-Epanutin (50mg PE/ml)		Volume (ml) of diluent* (5% glucose or 0.9% sodium chloride)		Minimum Infusion Time (mins) to achieve the maximum recommended infusion rate of 100mg PE / minute
		No. of 10ml vials to open	Volume (ml) to draw up	for final concentration of 25mg PE/ml	for final concentration of 1.5mg PE/ml	
100	1000	2	20	20	647	10
90	900	2	18	18	582	9
80	800	2	16	16	517	8
70	700	2	14	14	453	7
60	600	2	12	12	388	6
50	500	1	10	10	323	5

***For IV infusion the final concentration should range between 1.5 and 25mg PE/ml**

[a] Please refer to Table 1 for examples of calculations for loading doses of 15mg PE/kg

Table 4

Weight (kg)	Dose (mg PE)	Volume of Pro-Epanutin (50mg PE/ml)		Volume (ml) of diluent* (5% glucose or 0.9% sodium chloride)		Minimum Infusion Time (mins) to achieve the maximum recommended infusion rate of 100mg PE / minute
		No. of 10ml vials to open	Volume (ml) to draw up	for final concentration of 25mg PE/ml	for final concentration of 1.5mg PE/ml	
100	500	1	10	10	323	5
90	450	1	9	9	291	4.5
80	400	1	8	8	259	4
70	350	1	7	7	226	3.5
60	300	1	6	6	194	3
50	250	1	5	5	162	2.5

***For IV infusion the final concentration should range between 1.5 to 25mg PE/ml**

Table 5

Dose (mg phenytoin sodium)	Dose (mg PE)	Volume of Pro-Epanutin (50mg PE/ml)		Volume (ml) of diluent* (5% glucose or 0.9% sodium chloride)		Minimum Infusion Time (mins) to achieve the maximum recommended infusion rate of 100mg PE / minute
		No. of 10ml vials to open	Volume (ml) to draw up	for final concentration of 25mg PE/ml	for final concentration of 1.5mg PE/ml	
500	500	1	10	10	323	5
450	450	1	9	9	291	4.5
400	400	1	8	8	259	4
350	350	1	7	7	226	3.5
300	300	1	6	6	194	3
250	250	1	5	5	162	2.5

***For IV infusion the final concentration should range between 1.5 to 25mg PE/ml**

Table 6

Weight (kg)	Dose (mg PE)	Volume of Pro-Epanutin (50mg PE/ml)		Volume (ml) of diluent (5% glucose or 0.9% sodium chloride) for final concentration of 25mg PE/ml	Minimum Infusion Time (mins) to achieve the maximum recommended infusion rate of 3mg PE /kg/ minute
		No. of 10ml vials to open	Volume (ml) to draw up		
35	525	2	10.5	10.5	5
32.5	487.5	1	9.75	9.75	5
30	450	1	9	9	5
27.5	412.5	1	8.25	8.25	5
25	375	1	7.5	7.5	5
22.5	337.5	1	6.75	6.75	5
20	300	1	6	6	5
17.5	262.5	1	5.25	5.25	5

Table 7

Weight (kg)	Dose (mg PE)	Volume of Pro-Epanutin (50mg PE/ml)		Volume (ml) of diluent* (5% glucose or 0.9% sodium chloride)		Minimum Infusion Time (mins) to achieve the maximum recommended infusion rate of 2mg PE /kg/ minute
		No. of 10ml vials to open	Volume (ml) to draw up	for final concentration of 25mg PE/ml	for final concentration of 1.5mg PE/ml	
35	175	1	3.5	3.5	113	2.5
32.5	162.5	1	3.25	3.25	105	2.5
30	150	1	3	3	97	2.5
27.5	137.5	1	2.75	2.75	89	2.5
25	125	1	2.5	2.5	81	2.5
22.5	112.5	1	2.25	2.25	73	2.5
20	100	1	2	2	65	2.5
17.5	87.5	1	1.75	1.75	57	2.5

***For IV infusion the final concentration should range between 1.5 and 25mg PE/ml**

Table 8

Weight (kg)	Dose (mg PE)	Volume of Pro-Epanutin (50mg PE/ml)		Volume (ml) of diluent* (5% glucose or 0.9% sodium chloride)		Minimum Infusion Time (mins) to achieve the maximum recommended infusion rate of 2mg PE /kg/ minute
		No. of 10ml vials to open	Volume (ml) to draw up	for final concentration of 25mg PE/ml	for final concentration of 1.5mg PE/ml	
35	350	1	7	7	226	5
32.5	325	1	6.5	6.5	210	5
30	300	1	6	6	194	5
27.5	275	1	5.5	5.5	178	5
25	250	1	5	5	161	5
22.5	225	1	4.5	4.5	145	5
20	200	1	4	4	129	5
17.5	175	1	3.5	3.5	113	5

***For IV infusion the final concentration should range between 1.5 to 25mg PE/ml [a]**
Please refer to Table 1 for examples of calculations for loading doses of 15mg PE/kg

Recommended IV infusion rate for maintenance dosing: 1 to 2mg PE/kg/minute **(should not exceed 100mg PE/minute).**

The recommended infusion time is presented in Table 9.

Maintenance doses should be adjusted according to patient response and trough plasma phenytoin concentrations **(see Therapeutic Drug Monitoring).**

Transfer to maintenance therapy with oral phenytoin should be made when appropriate.

Table 9:

Treatment or Prophylaxis of seizures: Examples for maximum IV maintenance doses of 5mg PE/kg, recommendations for dilution* (to 25mg PE/ml or to 1.5mg PE/kg), and IV infusion times (at a maximum rate of 2mg PE/kg/minute) by body weight

(see Table 9 on next page)

Temporary substitution of oral phenytoin therapy with Pro-Epanutin.

The same dose and dosing frequency as for oral phenytoin therapy should be administered by IV infusion.

Recommended IV infusion rate for temporary substitution dosing: 1 to 2 mg PE/kg/minute **(should not exceed 50 to 100 mg PE/minute.)**

The recommended infusion time is presented in Table 10.

Therapeutic drug monitoring may be useful whenever switching between products and/or routes of administration. Doses should be adjusted according to patient response and trough plasma phenytoin concentrations **(see Therapeutic Drug Monitoring).**

Fosphenytoin has not been evaluated systemically for more than 5 days.

Table 10:

Temporary substitution of oral phenytoin therapy: Examples of equivalent doses and recommendations for dilution* (to 25mg PE/ml or to 1.5mg PE/ml), and IV infusion times (at maximum rate of 2mg PE/kg/minute)

(see Table 10 on next page)

ELDERLY PATIENTS

A lower loading dose and/or infusion rate, and lower or less frequent maintenance dosing of Pro-Epanutin may be required. Phenytoin metabolism is slightly decreased in elderly patients. A 10% to 25% reduction in dose or rate may be considered and careful clinical monitoring is required.

PATIENTS WITH RENAL OR HEPATIC DISEASE

Except in the treatment of status epilepticus, a lower loading dose and/or infusion rate, and lower or less frequent maintenance dosing may be required in patients with renal and/or hepatic disease or in those with hypoalbuminaemia. A 10% to 25% reduction in dose or rate may be considered and careful clinical monitoring is required.

The rate of conversion of IV Pro-Epanutin to phenytoin but not the clearance of phenytoin may be increased in these patients. Plasma unbound phenytoin concentrations may also be elevated. It may therefore, be more appropriate to measure plasma unbound phenytoin concentrations rather than plasma total phenytoin concentrations in these patients.

Therapeutic drug monitoring:

Prior to complete conversion, immunoanalytical techniques may significantly overestimate plasma phenytoin concentrations due to cross-reactivity with fosphenytoin. Chromatographic assay methods (e.g. HPLC) accurately quantitate phenytoin concentrations in biological fluids in the presence of fosphenytoin. It is advised that blood samples to assess phenytoin concentration ***should not*** be obtained for at least 2 hours after IV Pro-Epanutin infusion or 4 hours after IM Pro-Epanutin injection.

Optimal seizure control without clinical signs of toxicity occurs most often with plasma total phenytoin concentrations of between 10 and 20mg/l (40 and 80micromoles/l) or plasma unbound phenytoin concentrations of between 1 and 2mg/l (4 and 8micromoles/l).

Plasma phenytoin concentrations sustained above the optimal range may produce signs of acute toxicity **(see Section 4.4 Special Warnings and Precautions for Use).**

Phenytoin capsules are approximately 90% bioavailable by the oral route. Phenytoin, supplied as Pro-Epanutin, is 100% bioavailable by both the IM and IV routes. For this reason, plasma phenytoin concentrations may increase when IM or IV Pro-Epanutin is substituted for oral phenytoin sodium therapy. However, it is not necessary to adjust the initial doses when substituting oral phenytoin with Pro-Epanutin or vice versa.

Therapeutic drug monitoring may be useful whenever switching between products and/or routes of administration.

4.3 Contraindications

Hypersensitivity to fosphenytoin sodium or the excipients of Pro-Epanutin, or to phenytoin or other hydantoins.

Parenteral phenytoin affects ventricular automaticity. Pro-Epanutin is therefore, contra-indicated in patients with sinus bradycardia, sino-atrial block, second and third degree A-V block and Adams-Stokes syndrome.

Acute intermittent porphyria.

4.4 Special warnings and special precautions for use

Doses of Pro-Epanutin are always expressed as their phenytoin sodium equivalents (PE = phenytoin sodium equivalent). Therefore, when Pro-Epanutin is dosed as PE do not make any adjustment in the recommended doses when substituting Pro-Epanutin for phenytoin sodium or vice versa.

Note, however, that Pro-Epanutin has important differences in administration from parenteral phenytoin sodium. Pro-Epanutin should not be administered intravenously at a rate greater than 150mg PE/min while the maximum intravenous infusion rate for phenytoin is 50mg/min (see Section 4.2 Posology and Method of Administration).

Phenytoin is not effective in absence seizures. If tonic-clonic seizures are present simultaneously with absence seizures, combined drug therapy is recommended.

Cardiovascular disease:

Pro-Epanutin should be used with caution in patients with hypotension and severe myocardial insufficiency. Severe cardiovascular reactions including atrial and ventricular conduction depression and ventricular fibrillation, and sometimes, fatalities have been reported following phenytoin and fosphenytoin administration. Hypotension may also occur following IV administration of high doses and/or high infusion rates of Pro-Epanutin and even within

Table 9

Weight (kg)	Dose (mg PE)	Volume of Pro-Epanutin (50mg PE/ml)		Volume (ml) of diluent* (5% glucose or 0.9% sodium chloride)		Minimum Infusion Time (mins) to achieve the maximum recommended infusion rate of 2mg PE /kg/ minute
		No. of 10ml vials to open	Volume (ml) to draw up	for final concentration of 25mg PE/ml	for final concentration of 1.5mg PE/ml	
35	175	1	3.5	3.5	113	2.5
32.5	162.5	1	3.25	3.25	105	2.5
30	150	1	3	3	97	2.5
27.5	137.5	1	2.75	2.75	89	2.5
25	125	1	2.5	2.5	81	2.5
22.5	112.5	1	2.25	2.25	73	2.5
20	100	1	2	2	65	2.5
17.5	87.5	1	1.75	1.75	57	2.5

***For IV infusion the final concentration should range between 1.5 and 25mg PE/ml**

Table 10

Dose (mg phenytoin sodium) 5mg/kg	Dose (mg PE)	Volume of Pro-Epanutin (50mg PE/ml)		Volume (ml) of diluent* (5% glucose or 0.9% sodium chloride)		Minimum Infusion Time (mins) to achieve the maximum recommended infusion rate of 2mg PE /kg/ minute
		No. of 10ml vials to open	Volume (ml) to draw up	for final concentration of 25mg PE/ml	for final concentration of 1.5mg PE/ml	
175	175	1	3.5	3.5	113	2.5
150	150	1	3	3	97	2.5
125	125	1	2.5	2.5	81	2.5
100	100	1	2	2	65	2.5
75	75	1	1.5	1.5	49	2.5
50	50	1	1	1	32	2.5

***For IV infusion the final concentration should range between 1.5 to 25mg PE/ml**

recommended doses and rates. A reduction in the rate of administration or discontinuation of dosing may be necessary **(see Section 4.2 Posology and Method of Administration).**

Patients with an acute cerebrovascular event may be at increased risk of hypotension and require particularly close monitoring.

Withdrawal Precipitated Seizure/Status Epilepticus:

Abrupt withdrawal of antiepileptic drugs may increase seizure frequency and may lead to status epilepticus.

Rash:

Pro-Epanutin should be discontinued if a skin rash or signs of an allergic or hypersensitivity reaction or syndrome appear. Rapid substitution with an alternative antiepileptic drug not belonging to the hydantoin chemical class may be necessary.

Hypersensitivity Syndrome and Hepatoxicity:

A hypersensitivity reaction or syndrome has been associated with phenytoin administration. Fever, skin eruptions and lymphadenopathy may occur within the first two months of treatment. Hepatotoxicity is often associated with this hypersensitivity syndrome. Acute hepatotoxicities, including acute hepatic failure, jaundice, hepatomegaly and elevated serum transaminase levels have also been reported. Recovery from acute hepatotoxicity may be prompt, however fatal outcomes have also occurred.

Pro-Epanutin should be discontinued immediately following signs of acute hepatotoxicity and not readministered. Leucocytosis, eosinophilia and arthralgias may also occur. Although still rare, there may be an increased incidence of hypersensitivity reactions in black patients.

Lymphadenopathy:

Lymphadenopathy (local or generalised) including benign lymph node hyperplasia, pseudolymphoma, lymphoma and Hodgkin's Disease have been associated with administration of phenytoin, although a cause and effect relationship has not been established. It is therefore, important to eliminate other types of lymph node pathology before discontinuing therapy with Pro-Epanutin. Lymph node involvement may occur with or without symptoms and signs resembling serum sickness, e.g. fever, rash and liver involvement, as part of the hypersensitivity syndrome described above. In all cases of lymphadenopathy, long term follow-up observations are indicated and every effort should be made to achieve seizure control using alternative antiepileptic drugs.

Acute toxicity:

Confusional states referred to as "delirium", "psychosis" or "encephalopathy" or rarely irreversible cerebellar dysfunction may occur if plasma phenytoin concentrations are sustained above the optimal therapeutic range. Plasma phenytoin concentrations should be determined at the first sign of acute toxicity **(see Section 4.2 Posology and Method of Administration: Therapeutic Drug Monitoring).** If plasma phenytoin concentrations are excessive, the dose of Pro-Epanutin should be reduced. If symptoms persist, administration of Pro-Epanutin should be discontinued.

Renal or Hepatic Disease:

Pro-Epanutin should be used with caution in patients with renal and/or hepatic disease, or in those with hypoalbuminaemia. Alterations in dosing may be necessary in patients with impaired kidney or liver function, elderly patients or those who are gravely ill **(see Section 4.2 Posology and Method of Administration).** These patients may show early signs of phenytoin toxicity or an increase in the severity of adverse events due to alterations in Pro-Epanutin and phenytoin pharmacokinetics.

The phosphate load provided by Pro-Epanutin is 0.0037mmol phosphate/mg fosphenytoin sodium. Caution is advised when administering Pro-Epanutin in patients requiring phosphate restriction, such as those with severe renal impairment.

Sensory Disturbances:

Overall these occur in 13% of the patients exposed to Pro-Epanutin. Transient itching, burning, warmth or tingling in the groin during and shortly after intravenous infusion of Pro-Epanutin may occur. The sensations are not consistent with the signs of an allergic reaction and may be avoided or minimised by using a slower rate of IV infusion or by temporarily stopping the infusion.

Diabetes:

Phenytoin may raise blood glucose in diabetic patients.

Alcohol Use:

Acute alcohol intake may increase plasma phenytoin concentrations while chronic alcohol use may decrease plasma phenytoin concentrations.

4.5 Interaction with other medicinal products and other forms of Interaction

Drug interactions which may occur following the administration of Pro-Epanutin are those that are expected to occur with drugs known to interact with phenytoin. Phenytoin metabolism is saturable and other drugs that utilise the same metabolic pathways may alter plasma phenytoin concentrations. There are many drugs which may increase or decrease plasma phenytoin concentrations. Equally phenytoin may affect the metabolism of a number of other drugs because of its potent enzyme-inducing potential. Determination of plasma phenytoin concentrations is especially helpful when possible drug interactions are suspected **(see Section 4.2 Posology and Method of Administration: Therapeutic Drug Monitoring).**

No drugs are known to interfere with the conversion of fosphenytoin to phenytoin.

Phenytoin is extensively bound to plasma proteins and is prone to competitive displacement. Drugs highly bound to albumin could also increase the fosphenytoin unbound fraction with the potential to increase the rate of conversion of fosphenytoin to phenytoin. Phenytoin is metabolised by hepatic cytochrome P450 enzymes. Inhibition of phenytoin metabolism may produce significant increases in plasma phenytoin concentrations and increase the risk of phenytoin toxicity. Phenytoin is also a potent inducer of hepatic drug-metabolising enzymes.

The following drug interactions are the most commonly occurring drug interactions with phenytoin:

Drugs that may ***increase*** plasma phenytoin concentrations include: acute alcohol intake, amiodarone, chloramphenicol, chlordiazepoxide, diazepam, dicoumarol, disulfiram, oestrogens, fluoxetine, H_2-antagonists (e.g. cimetidine), halothane, isoniazid, methylphenidate, phenothiazines, phenylbutazone, salicylates, succinimides (e.g. ethosuximide), sulphonamides, tolbutamide, trazodone, viloxazine, antifungal agents (e.g. amphotericin B, fluconazole, ketoconazole, miconazole and itraconazole) and omeprazole.

Drugs that may ***decrease*** plasma phenytoin concentrations include carbamazepine, chronic alcohol abuse, reserpine, folic acid, sucralfate and vigabatrin.

Drugs that may either ***increase*** or ***decrease*** plasma phenytoin concentrations include: phenobarbitone, valproic acid, sodium valproate, antineoplastic agents, ciprofloxacin and certain antacids. Similarly, the effects of phenytoin on plasma phenobarbitone, valproic acid and sodium valproate concentrations are unpredictable.

Although not a true pharmacokinetic interaction, tricyclic antidepressants and phenothiazines may precipitate seizures in susceptible patients and Pro-Epanutin dosage may need to be adjusted.

Drugs whose efficacy is impaired by phenytoin include: anticoagulants, corticosteroids, dicoumarol, digitoxin, doxycycline, oestrogens, furosemide, oral contraceptives, rifampicin, quinidine, theophylline, vitamin D, antifungal agents, antineoplastic agents and clozapine.

Drugs whose effect is enhanced by phenytoin include: warfarin.

Drug/Laboratory Test Interactions:

Phenytoin may decrease serum concentrations of T_4. It may also produce low results in dexamethasone or metyrapone tests. This may be an artifact. Phenytoin may cause increased blood glucose or serum concentrations of alkaline phosphatase and gamma glutamyl transpeptidase (GGT). Phenytoin may affect blood calcium and blood sugar metabolism tests.

Phenytoin has the potential to lower serum folate levels.

4.6 Pregnancy and lactation

An increase in seizure frequency may occur during pregnancy because of altered phenytoin pharmacokinetics. Periodic measurement of plasma phenytoin concentrations may be valuable in the management of pregnant women as a guide to appropriate adjustment of dosage **(see Section 4.2 Posology and Method of Administration: Therapeutic Drug Monitoring).** However, postpartum restoration of the original dosage will probably be indicated.

If this drug is used during pregnancy, or if the patient becomes pregnant while taking the drug, the patient should be informed of the potential harm to the foetus.

Prenatal exposure to phenytoin may increase the risks for congenital malformations and other adverse developmental outcomes. Increased frequencies of major malformations (such as orofacial clefts and cardiac defects), minor anomalies (dysmorphic facial features, nail and digit hypoplasia), growth abnormalities (including microcephaly) and mental deficiency have been reported among children born to epileptic women who took phenytoin alone or in combination with other antiepileptic drugs during pregnancy. There have also been several reported cases of malignancies, including neuroblastoma, in children whose mothers received phenytoin during pregnancy. The overall incidence of malformations for children of epileptic women treated with antiepileptic drugs (phenytoin and/or others) during pregnancy is about 10% or two-to-three-fold that in the general population. However, the relative contribution of antiepileptic drugs and other factors associated with epilepsy to this increased risk are uncertain and in most cases it has not been possible to attribute specific developmental abnormalities to particular antiepileptic drugs.

It might be necessary to give vitamin K to the mother during the last gestational month. Neonates of the mother receiving Pro-Epanutin should be monitored for haemorrhagic diathesis and if necessary additional vitamin K should be administered.

Foetal toxicity, developmental toxicity and teratogenicity were observed in offspring of rats given fosphenytoin during pregnancy, similar to those reported with phenytoin. No developmental effects were observed in offspring of pregnant rabbits given fosphenytoin; malformations have been reported in offspring of pregnant rabbits with phenytoin at ⩾75mg/kg.

It is not known whether Pro-Epanutin is excreted in human milk. Following administration of oral phenytoin, phenytoin appears to be excreted in low concentrations in human milk. Therefore, breast-feeding is not recommended for women receiving Pro-Epanutin.

4.7 Effects on ability to drive and use machines

Caution is recommended in patients performing skilled tasks (e.g. driving or operating machinery) as treatment with fosphenytoin may cause central nervous system adverse effects such as dizziness and drowsiness **(see Section 4.8 Undesirable Effects)**.

4.8 Undesirable effects

The following adverse events have been reported in clinical trials in adults receiving Pro-Epanutin. The list also includes adverse effects that have been reported following both the acute and chronic use of phenytoin.

Central Nervous System:

Central nervous system effects are the most common side effects seen following administration of Pro-Epanutin or phenytoin and are usually dose-related. Nystagmus, dizziness, paraesthesia, ataxia, tremor, incoordination, stupor, vertigo, euphoria, drowsiness, motor twitching, transient nervousness, slurred speech, mental confusion and insomnia.

There have also been rare reports of phenytoin-induced dyskinesias, including chorea, dystonia and asterixis, similar to those induced by phenothiazines or other neuroleptic drugs. A predominantly sensory peripheral polyneuropathy has been observed in patients receiving long-term phenytoin therapy. Tonic seizures have also been reported. The incidence and severity of adverse events related to the CNS and sensory disturbances were greater at higher doses and rates.

Cardiovascular and Respiratory systems:

Hypotension, vasodilation, severe cardiotoxic reactions with atrial and ventricular conduction depression (including bradycardia and all degrees of heart block), asystole ventricular fibrillation and cardiovascular collapse. Some of these reactions have been fatal. **(see Section 4.4 Special Warnings and Precautions for Use)**.

Alterations in respiratory function (including respiratory arrest), pneumonitis.

Haemopoietic system:

Ecchymosis, thrombocytopenia, leucopenia, granulocytopenia, agranulocytosis, pancytopenia with or without bone marrow suppression and aplastic anaemia have been occasionally reported with phenytoin administration. Some of these reports have been fatal.

Liver or Kidney:

Toxic hepatitis, liver damage, interstitial nephritis.

Gastrointestinal System:

Nausea, vomiting, dry mouth, taste perversion, constipation.

Skin and Connective Tissue:

Pruritus, rash **(see Section 4.4 Special Warnings and Precautions for Use)**, coarsening of the facial features, enlargement of the lips, gingival hyperplasia, hirsutism, hypertrichosis, Peyronie's disease and Dupuytren's contracture may occur rarely.

Special Senses:

Tinnitus, ear disorder, taste perversion, abnormal vision.

Immune System:

Hypersensitivity syndrome **(see Section 4.4 Special Warnings and Precautions for Use)**, systemic lupus erythematosus, periarteritis nodosa, immunoglobulin abnormalities.

Body as a whole:

Headache, pain, asthenia, chills, injection site reaction, injection site pain, polyarthropathy, hyperglycaemia.

No trends in laboratory changes were observed in Pro-Epanutin treated patients.

4.9 Overdose

Nausea, vomiting, lethargy, tachycardia, bradycardia, asystole, cardiac arrest, hypotension, syncope, hypocalcaemia, metabolic acidosis and death have been reported in cases of overdosage with Pro-Epanutin.

Initial symptoms of Pro-Epanutin toxicity are those associated with acute phenytoin toxicity. These are nystagmus, ataxia and dysarthria. Other signs include tremor, hyperreflexia, lethargy, slurred speech, nausea, vomiting, coma and hypotension. There is a risk of potentially fatal respiratory or circulatory depression. There are marked variations among individuals with respect to plasma phenytoin concentrations where toxicity occurs. Lateral gaze nystagmus usually appears at 20mg/l, ataxia at 30mg/l and dysarthria and lethargy appear when the plasma concentration is over 40mg/l. However, phenytoin concentrations as high as 50mg/l have been reported without evidence of toxicity. As much as 25 times the therapeutic phenytoin dose has been taken, resulting in plasma phenytoin concentrations over 100mg/l, with complete recovery.

Treatment is non-specific since there is no known antidote to Pro-Epanutin or phenytoin overdosage. The adequacy of the respiratory and circulatory systems should be carefully observed and appropriate supportive measures employed. Haemodialysis can be considered since phenytoin is not completely bound to plasma proteins. Total exchange transfusion has been used in the treatment of severe intoxication in children. In acute overdosage the possibility of the use of other CNS depressants, including alcohol, should be borne in mind.

Formate and phosphate are metabolites of fosphenytoin and therefore, may contribute to signs of toxicity following overdosage. Signs of formate toxicity are similar to those of methanol toxicity and are associated with severe anion-gap metabolic acidosis. Large amounts of phosphate, delivered rapidly, could potentially cause hypocalcaemia with paraesthesia, muscle spasms and seizures. Ionised free calcium levels can be measured and, if low, used to guide treatment.

5. PHARMACOLOGICAL PROPERTIES

5.1 Pharmacodynamic properties

ATC-Code: N03AB

Pro-Epanutin is a prodrug of phenytoin and accordingly, its anticonvulsant effects are attributable to phenytoin.

The pharmacological and toxicological effects of fosphenytoin sodium include those of phenytoin.

The cellular mechanisms of phenytoin thought to be responsible for its anticonvulsant actions include modulation of voltage-dependent sodium channels of neurones, inhibition of calcium flux across neuronal membranes, modulation of voltage-dependent calcium channels of neurones and enhancement of the sodium-potassium ATPase activity of neurones and glial cells. The modulation of sodium channels may be a primary anticonvulsant mechanism because this property is shared with several other anticonvulsants in addition to phenytoin.

5.2 Pharmacokinetic properties

Fosphenytoin is a pro-drug of phenytoin and it is rapidly converted into phenytoin mole for mole.

Fosphenytoin Pharmacokinetics

Absorption/Bioavailability:

When Pro-Epanutin is administered by IV infusion, maximum plasma fosphenytoin concentrations are achieved at the end of the infusion. Fosphenytoin is completely bioavailable following IM administration of Pro-Epanutin. Peak concentrations occur at approximately 30 minutes post-dose. Plasma fosphenytoin concentrations following IM administration are lower but more sustained than those following IV administration due to the time required for absorption of fosphenytoin from the injection site.

Distribution:

Fosphenytoin is extensively bound (95% to 99%) to human plasma proteins, primarily albumin. Binding to plasma proteins is saturable with the result that the fraction unbound increases as total fosphenytoin concentrations increase. Fosphenytoin displaces phenytoin from protein binding sites. The volume of distribution of fosphenytoin increases with fosphenytoin sodium dose and rate and ranges from 4.3 to 10.8L.

Metabolism and Excretion:

The hydrolysis of fosphenytoin to phenytoin yields 2 metabolites, phosphate and formaldehyde. Formaldehyde is subsequently converted to formate, which is in turn metabolised via a folate dependent mechanism. Although phosphate and formaldehyde (formate) have potentially important biological effects, these effects typically occur at concentrations considerably in excess of those obtained when Pro-Epanutin is administered under conditions of use recommended in this labelling.

The conversion half-life of fosphenytoin to phenytoin is approximately 15 minutes. The mechanism of fosphenytoin conversion has not been determined but phosphatases probably play a major role. Each mmol of fosphenytoin is metabolised to 1mmol of phenytoin, phosphate and formate.

Fosphenytoin is not excreted in urine.

Phenytoin Pharmacokinetics (after Pro-Epanutin administration):

The pharmacokinetics of phenytoin following IV administration of Pro-Epanutin, are complex and when used in an emergency setting (e.g. status epilepticus), differences in rate of availability of phenytoin could be critical. Studies have, therefore, empirically determined an infusion rate for Pro-Epanutin that gives a rate and extent of phenytoin systemic availability similar to that of a 50mg/min phenytoin sodium infusion. Because Pro-Epanutin is completely absorbed and converted to phenytoin following IM administration, systemic phenytoin concentrations are generated that are similar enough to oral phenytoin to allow essentially interchangeable use and to allow reliable IM loading dose administration.

The following table displays pharmacokinetic parameters of fosphenytoin and phenytoin following IV and IM Pro-Epanutin administration.

Mean Pharmacokinetic Parameter Values by Route of Pro-Epanutin Administration.

(see Table 11 below)

Absorption/Bioavailability:

Fosphenytoin sodium is rapidly and completely converted to phenytoin following IV or IM Pro-Epanutin administration. Therefore, the bioavailability of phenytoin following administration of Pro-Epanutin is the same as that following parenteral administration of phenytoin.

Distribution:

Phenytoin is highly bound to plasma proteins, primarily albumin, although to a lesser extent than fosphenytoin. In the absence of fosphenytoin, approximately 12% of total plasma phenytoin is unbound over the clinically relevant concentration range. However, fosphenytoin displaces phenytoin from plasma protein binding sites. This increases the fraction of phenytoin unbound (up to 30% unbound) during the period required for conversion of fosphenytoin to phenytoin (approximately 0.5 to 1 hour postinfusion).

The volume of distribution for phenytoin ranges from 24.9 to 36.8L.

Metabolism and Excretion:

Phenytoin derived from administration of Pro-Epanutin is extensively metabolised in the liver and excreted in urine primarily as 5-(p-hydroxy-phenyl)-5-phenylhydantoin and its glucuronide; little unchanged phenytoin (1%-5% of the Pro-Epanutin dose) is recovered in urine. Phenytoin hepatic metabolism is saturable and, following administration of single IV Pro-Epanutin doses of 400 to 1200mg PE, total and unbound phenytoin AUC values increase disproportionately with dose. Mean total phenytoin half-life values (12.0 to 28.9 hr) following Pro-Epanutin administration at these doses are similar to those after equal doses of parenteral phenytoin and tend to be longer at higher plasma phenytoin concentrations.

Characteristics in Patients

Patients with Renal or Hepatic Disease:

Fosphenytoin conversion to phenytoin is more rapid in patients with renal or hepatic disease than with other patients because of decreased plasma protein binding, secondary to hypoalbuminaemia, occurring in these disease states. The extent of conversion to phenytoin is not affected. Phenytoin metabolism may be reduced in patients with hepatic impairment resulting in increased plasma phenytoin concentrations **(see Section 4.2 Posology and Method of Administration)**.

Elderly Patients:

Patient age had no significant impact on fosphenytoin pharmacokinetics. Phenytoin clearance tends to decrease with increasing age (20% less in patients over 70 years of

Table 11 Mean Pharmacokinetic Parameter Values by Route of Pro-Epanutin Administration

				Fosphenytoin			Total Phenytoin		Free (Unbound) Phenytoin	
Route	Dose (mg PE)	Dose (mg PE/kg)	Infusion Rate (mg PE/min)	Cmax (μg/ml)	tmax (hr)	t½ (min)	Cmax (μg/ml)	tmax (hr)	Cmax (μg/ml)	tmax (hr)
Intramuscular	855	12.4	–	18.5	0.61	41.2	14.3	3.23	2.02	4.16
Intravenous	1200	15.6	100	139	0.19	18.9	26.9	1.18	2.78	0.52
Intravenous	1200	15.6	150	156	0.13	20.5	28.2	0.98	3.18	0.58

Dose = Fosphenytoin dose (phenytoin sodium equivalents [mgPE] or phenytoin sodium equivalents/kg [mg PE/kg]).
Infusion Rate = Fosphenytoin infusion rate (mg phenytoin sodium equivalents/min [mg PE/min]).
Cmax = Maximum plasma analyte concentration (μg/ml).
tmax = Time of Cmax (hr).
t½ = Terminal elimination half-life (min).

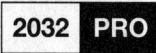

age relative to that in patients 20-30 years of age) **(see Section 4.2 Posology and Method of Administration).**

Gender:

Gender had no significant impact on fosphenytoin or phenytoin pharmacokinetics.

Children:

Limited studies in children (age 5 to 10) receiving Pro-Epanutin have shown similar concentration-time profiles of fosphenytoin and phenytoin to those observed in adult patients receiving comparable mg PE/kg doses.

5.3 Preclinical safety data

The systemic toxicity of fosphenytoin is qualitatively and quantitatively similar to that of phenytoin at comparable exposures.

Carcinogenicity studies with fosphenytoin are not available. Since fosphenytoin is a prodrug of phenytoin, the carcinogenicity results with phenytoin can be extrapolated. An increased incidence of hepatocellular tumors was observed after administration of phenytoin in 1 of 3 studies in rats and 2 of 3 studies in mice. Lymphomas were also observed in susceptible strains of mice. These rodent tumors are of uncertain clinical significance.

Genetic toxicity studies showed that fosphenytoin was not mutagenic in bacteria or in mammalian cells *in vitro*. It was clastogenic in cultured V79 Chinese hamster lung cells in the presence of metabolic activation, but not in an *in vivo* mouse bone marrow micronucleus test. Phenytoin is not genotoxic *in vivo*.

Local irritation following IV or IM dosing or inadvertent perivenous administration was less severe with fosphenytoin than with phenytoin and was generally comparable to that observed with vehicle injections. The potential of fosphenytoin to induce intra-arterial irritation was not assessed.

6. PHARMACEUTICAL PARTICULARS

6.1 List of excipients

Water for injection, trometamol buffer adjusted to pH 8.6 to 9.0 with hydrochloric acid.

6.2 Incompatibilities

This medicinal product must not be mixed with other medicinal products except those mentioned in Section 6.6.

6.3 Shelf life

2 years.

6.4 Special precautions for storage

Store at 2°C to 8°C (under refrigeration). The undiluted product may be stored at room temperature (8°C to 25°C) for up to 24 hours.

6.5 Nature and contents of container

10ml sulphur treated Type I glass vials (10ml solution) with a Teflon coated stopper, an aluminium seal and flip-off cap.

Boxes of 10 vials with 10ml solution for injection.

6.6 Instructions for use and handling

Pro-Epanutin must be diluted to a concentration ranging from 1.5 to 25mg PE/ml prior to infusion, with 5% glucose or 0.9% saline solution for injection. See Section 4.2 for dilution information. After dilution Pro-Epanutin is suitable only for immediate use.

For single use only. After opening, unused product should be discarded.

Vials that develop particulate matter should not be used.

7. MARKETING AUTHORISATION HOLDER

Pfizer Limited,

Sandwich,

Kent,

CT13 9NJ

8. MARKETING AUTHORISATION NUMBER(S)

PL 00057/0551

9. DATE OF FIRST AUTHORISATION/RENEWAL OF THE AUTHORISATION

28th July 2004

10. DATE OF REVISION OF THE TEXT

May 2005

Prograf Capsules, Concentrate for Infusion

(Astellas Pharma Limited)

1. NAME OF THE MEDICINAL PRODUCT

Prograf® 0.5 mg Capsules

Prograf® 1 mg Capsules

Prograf® 5 mg Capsules

Prograf® 5 mg/mL Concentrate for Infusion

2. QUALITATIVE AND QUANTITATIVE COMPOSITION

Capsules containing 0.5 mg, 1 mg and 5 mg tacrolimus (INN), respectively.

Concentrate for intravenous infusion containing tacrolimus (INN) 5 mg per 1 mL.

For excipients see 6.1.

3. PHARMACEUTICAL FORM

Hard gelatin capsules.

Concentrate for intravenous infusion.

4. CLINICAL PARTICULARS

4.1 Therapeutic indications

Primary immunosuppression in liver and kidney allograft recipients and liver and kidney allograft rejection resistant to conventional immunosuppressive regimens.

4.2 Posology and method of administration

General Considerations

The recommended initial dosages presented below are intended to act solely as a guideline. Prograf dosing should always be adjusted according to individual patient requirements aided by blood level monitoring.

Prograf is routinely administered in conjunction with other immunosuppressive agents in the initial post-operative period. The Prograf dose may vary depending upon the immunosuppressive regimen chosen.

Route of Administration

Prograf can be administered intravenously or orally. In general, dosing may commence orally; if necessary, by administering the capsule contents suspended in water, via nasogastric tubing.

Mode of Intake

Prograf 0.5 mg Capsules / Prograf 1 mg Capsules / Prograf 5 mg Capsules

It is recommended that the oral daily dose should be taken in two divided doses (e.g. morning and evening). The capsules should be swallowed with fluid, preferably water.

Based on pharmacokinetic considerations, the capsules should be taken on an empty stomach or at least 1 hour before or 2 – 3 hours after a meal, to achieve maximal absorption (see Section 5.2). However, no discernible food effect was observed in kidney transplant patients.

Prograf 5 mg/mL Concentrate for Infusion

NB: Prograf 5mg/mL Concentrate for Infusion must not be injected undiluted.

The concentrate for infusion should be diluted in 5% dextrose solution or in physiological saline solution in polyethylene or glass bottles. The concentration of a solution for final infusion produced in this way should be in the range of 0.004-0.1 mg/mL. The total volume of infusion during 24 hours should be in the range of 20-250 mL. The solution should not be given as a bolus.

The content of the concentrate for infusion is not compatible with PVC.

The solution for final use should be used up within 24 hours.

Maximum Whole Blood Concentration Levels

Clinical studies analysis suggests that the majority of patients can be successfully managed if the blood concentrations of tacrolimus are maintained below 20 ng/mL.

It is necessary to consider the clinical condition of the patient when interpreting whole blood level concentrations. If the blood levels are below the limit of quantification of the assay and the patient's clinical condition is satisfactory, then the dose should not be adjusted.

In clinical practice, 12-hour trough whole blood levels are generally 5-20 ng/mL early post transplant.

Duration of Dosing

To suppress graft rejection, immunosuppression must be maintained; consequently, no limit to the duration of oral therapy can be given.

Patients should be converted from intravenous to oral medication as soon as individual circumstances permit. Intravenous therapy should not be continued for more than seven days.

Administration with Other Therapies

Prograf is normally administered together with other immunosuppressive agents. The dose used may vary depending upon the other immunosuppressive regimen used. Prograf should not be given together with cyclosporin.

If allograft rejection or adverse events occur, alteration to the immunosuppressive regimen should be considered.

Dosage recommendations

Liver transplantation

Primary immunosuppression – adults

Oral Prograf therapy should commence at 0.10 - 0.20 mg/kg per day administered as two divided doses (e.g. morning and evening). Administration should commence approximately 6 hours after the completion of surgery.

If the dose cannot be administered orally as a result of the clinical condition of the patient, intravenous therapy of 0.01 - 0.05 mg/kg per day should be initiated as a continuous 24-hour infusion.

Primary immunosuppression - children

Experience with initial oral administration in paediatric patients is limited.

An initial oral dose of 0.30 mg/kg per day should be administered in two divided doses (e.g. morning and evening). If the clinical condition of the patient prevents oral dosing, an initial intravenous dose of 0.05 mg/kg per day should be administered as a continuous 24-hour infusion.

Maintenance therapy – adults and children

Prograf concentrate for infusion 5 mg/mL is administered for initial treatment only. In general, Prograf Concentrate for Infusion 5 mg/mL should not be used for maintenance therapy. For maintenance of the graft, patients are treated with Prograf Capsules.

Prograf doses are usually reduced during maintenance therapy. When Prograf is administered in combination with corticosteroids, these may often be reduced and in rare cases the treatment has continued as monotherapy. Post transplant improvement in the condition of the patient may alter the pharmacokinetics of tacrolimus and may necessitate dose adjustment.

Dosing should be based primarily on clinical assessments of rejection and tolerability in each patient individually. If clinical signs of rejection are apparent, alteration of the immunosuppressive regimen should be considered.

In general, paediatric patients require doses 1½ - 2 times higher than the adult doses to achieve similar blood levels.

Rejection therapy – adults and children

Increased Prograf doses, supplemental corticosteroid therapy and introduction of short courses of mono-/polyclonal antibodies have all been used to manage rejection episodes. If signs of toxicity are noted (e.g. pronounced adverse event - see section 4.8) the dose of Prograf may need to be reduced.

For information on conversion from cyclosporin to Prograf, refer to guidelines in "Dose Adjustments in Specific Patient Populations" at the end of this dosing section.

Kidney transplantation

Primary immunosuppression - adults

Prograf therapy should commence at a daily dose of 0.15 - 0.30 mg/kg per day administered as two divided doses (e.g. morning and evening). Administration should commence within 24 hours after the completion of surgery.

If the dose cannot be administered orally as a result of the clinical condition of the patient, intravenous therapy of 0.05 - 0.10 mg/kg per day should be initiated as a continuous 24-hour infusion.

Primary immunosuppression – children

Experience with initial oral administration in paediatric patients is limited.

An initial daily dose of 0.30 mg/kg should be administered in two divided doses. If the clinical condition of the patient prevents oral dosing, an initial intravenous dose of 0.1 mg/kg per day should be administered as a continuous 24-hour infusion.

Maintenance therapy – adults and children

Prograf concentrate for infusion 5 mg/mL is administered for initial treatment only. In general, Prograf Concentrate for Infusion 5 mg/mL should not be used for maintenance therapy. For maintenance of the graft, patients are treated with Prograf Capsules.

Prograf doses are usually reduced during maintenance therapy. When Prograf is administered in combination with corticosteroids, these may often be reduced and in rare cases the treatment has continued as monotherapy. Post transplant improvement in the condition of the patient may alter the pharmacokinetics of tacrolimus and may necessitate dose adjustment.

Dosing should be based primarily on clinical assessments of rejection and tolerability in each patient individually. If clinical signs of rejection are apparent, alteration of the immunosuppressive regimen should be considered.

In general, paediatric patients require doses 1½ - 2 times higher than the adult doses to achieve similar blood levels.

Rejection therapy – adults and children

Increased Prograf doses, supplemental corticosteroid therapy and introduction of short courses of mono-/polyclonal antibodies have all been used to manage rejection episodes. If signs of toxicity are noted (e.g. pronounced adverse event - see section 4.8) the dose of Prograf may need to be reduced.

For information on conversion from cyclosporin to Prograf, refer to guidelines in "Dose Adjustments in Specific Patient Populations" at the end of this dosing section.

Dosage adjustments in specific patient populations – all indications

Patients with liver impairment: Dose reduction may be necessary in patients with severe liver impairment in order to maintain the trough blood levels within the recommended target range.

Patients with kidney impairment: As the pharmacokinetics of tacrolimus are unaffected by renal function, no dose adjustment should be required. However, owing to the nephrotoxic potential of tacrolimus careful monitoring of renal function is recommended (including serial serum creatinine concentrations, calculation of creatinine clearance and monitoring of urine output). The blood concentration of tacrolimus is not reduced by dialysis.

Elderly patients: There is no evidence currently available to indicate that dosing should be adjusted in elderly patients.

Conversion from cyclosporin: Co-administration of cyclosporin and Prograf may increase the half-life of cyclosporin and exacerbate any toxic effects. Care should therefore be taken when converting patients from cyclosporin- to

Prograf-based therapy. Prograf therapy should be initiated after considering cyclosporin blood concentrations and the clinical condition of the patient. Dosing should be delayed in the presence of elevated cyclosporin blood levels. In practice, Prograf therapy has been initiated 12 - 24 hours after discontinuation of cyclosporin. Treatment should begin with the initial oral dose recommended for primary immunosuppression in that particular allograft (in both adult and paediatric patients).

Monitoring of cyclosporin blood levels should be continued following conversion as the clearance of cyclosporin might be affected.

Monitoring of Whole Blood Concentrations

Various assays have been used to measure blood or plasma levels. Comparison of the levels in published literature with those found in clinical practice should be made with knowledge of the assay methods employed. In current clinical practice, blood levels are monitored using immunoassay methods.

Drug level monitoring is recommended during the early post transplantation period, following dose adjustment of Prograf therapy after switching from another immunosuppressive regimen or following co-administration of drugs which are likely to lead to a drug to drug interaction. Blood trough levels of Prograf should also be monitored periodically during maintenance therapy.

The frequency of blood level monitoring should be based on clinical need. As tacrolimus has a long half-life, it can take several days for adjustments in Prograf dosing to be reflected in changes in blood levels.

4.3 Contraindications

Pregnancy.

Known hypersensitivity to tacrolimus or other macrolides.

Prograf 0.5 mg Capsules / Prograf 1 mg Capsules / Prograf 5 mg Capsules

Known hypersensitivity to other ingredients of the capsules.

Prograf 5 mg/mL Concentrate for Infusion

Known hypersensitivity to polyoxyethylated castor oil (HCO-60) or structurally related compounds.

4.4 Special warnings and special precautions for use

Prograf therapy requires careful monitoring by adequately qualified and equipped personnel. The drug should only be prescribed, and changes in immunosuppressive therapy should only be initiated, by physicians experienced in immunosuppressive therapy and the management of transplant patients. The physician responsible for maintenance therapy should have complete information requisite for the follow-up patient.

Dose and/or blood level adjustment should only be undertaken by the transplant centre responsible for the transplant patient.

Patients should be thoroughly controlled. In particular during the first months post transplant, close monitoring of the patient is required.

Regular monitoring of the following parameters should be undertaken on a routine basis: blood pressure, ECG, visual status, blood glucose levels, blood levels of potassium and other electrolytes, creatinine, BUN, haematology parameters, coagulation values and liver function tests. If clinically relevant alterations of these parameters are seen, the dose of tacrolimus should be reviewed.

Renal function tests should be performed at frequent intervals. In particular during the first days post transplant, monitoring of urinary output should be performed. If necessary the dose should be adjusted.

Several types of neurological and CNS disorders have been reported in association with Prograf therapy. For this reason, patients exhibiting such adverse events should be controlled very carefully. Occurrence of severe CNS symptoms should prompt immediate dose review. It has been reported that in some cases severe tremor and/or motoric (expressive) aphasia may be indicators for severe CNS disorders.

Ventricular hypertrophy or hypertrophy of the septum and rare cases of cardiomyopathy have been reported in association with administration of Prograf. Most of these have been reversible following dose reduction or drug discontinuation, occurring primarily in children having tacrolimus blood trough levels much higher than the recommended maximum levels. Factors which may increase the risk of this condition are pre-existing cardiac disease, corticosteroid usage, hypertension, renal or hepatic dysfunction, infections and fluid overload and oedema. Monitoring of cardiovascular function using such procedures as echocardiography with or without ECG pre- and post transplant (e.g. within the first three months and then at nine months to one year) is advised for high-risk patients. If abnormalities develop, dose reduction of Prograf therapy or discontinuation and change to alternative immunosuppressive therapy should be considered.

As with other potent immunosuppressive compounds, patients treated with Prograf have been reported to develop EBV-associated lymphoproliferative disorders. In patients switched to Prograf, this may be attributable to over-immunosuppression before commencing therapy with this agent. Patients switched to Prograf rescue therapy should not receive concomitantly anti-lymphocyte treatment. Very young (< 2 years), EBV-sero-negative children have been reported to have an increased risk of developing a lymphoproliferative disorder. Therefore, in this patient group, EBV serology should be ascertained before starting treatment with Prograf. During treatment, careful monitoring is recommended.

In view of the potential risk of malignancies, patients who spend extended periods in the sun, or are otherwise exposed to UV light, should apply a high protection suncream.

If accidentally administered arterially or perivasally, Prograf Concentrate for Infusion 5 mg/mL may cause irritation at the injection site.

Prograf should not be administered together with cyclosporin.

Prograf Concentrate for Infusion contains polyoxyethylated castor oil which has been reported to cause anaphylactoid reactions. These reactions consist of flushing of the face and upper thorax, acute respiratory distress with dyspnoea and wheezing, blood pressure changes and tachycardia. Caution is therefore necessary in patients who have previously received, by intravenous injection or infusion, preparations containing polyoxyethylated castor oil (such as HCO-60) and patients with an allergenic predisposition. Animal studies have shown that the risk of anaphylaxis may be reduced by slow infusion of polyoxyethylated castor oil containing drugs or by the prior administration of an antihistamine.

4.5 Interaction with other medicinal products and other forms of Interaction

Potential interactions

Pharmacokinetic interactions

Tacrolimus is extensively metabolised via the hepatic microsomal cytochrome P-450 3A4 isoenzyme (CYP3A4). Concomitant use of drugs or herbal remedies (for example St. John's Wort) known to inhibit or induce CYP3A4 may affect the metabolism of tacrolimus and thereby increase or decrease the blood level of tacrolimus.

Tacrolimus also shows a broad and powerful inhibitory effect on CYP3A4 dependent metabolism; thus concomitant use of tacrolimus with drugs known to be metabolised by CYP3A4 dependent pathways may affect the metabolism of such drugs (e.g. cortisone, testosterone).

Tacrolimus is extensively bound to plasma proteins. Possible interactions with other drugs known to have high affinity for plasma proteins should be considered (e.g., NSAIDs, oral anticoagulants, or oral antidiabetics).

Pharmacodynamic interactions (synergistic effects)

Concurrent use of tacrolimus with drugs known to have nephrotoxic or neurotoxic effects may increase the level of toxicity (e.g., aminoglycosides, gyrase inhibitors, vancomycin, trimethoprim-sulphamethoxazole, cotrimoxazole, NSAIDs, ganciclovir or aciclovir).

As tacrolimus treatment may be associated with hyperkalaemia, or may increase pre-existing hyperkalaemia, the following should be avoided:

- high potassium intake, or
- potassium-sparing diuretics (e.g., amiloride, triamterene, or spironolactone).

Other interactions

During treatment with tacrolimus, vaccinations may be less effective and the use of live attenuated vaccines should be avoided.

Clinically relevant interactions

The following interactions of tacrolimus with co-administered drugs were observed clinically. The underlying mechanism of interaction is known. Drugs marked with an asterisk * will require dose adjustment of tacrolimus in nearly all patients. Other drugs listed below may require dose adjustment in individual cases.

The following drugs inhibit CYP3A4 and have been shown to increase the blood levels of tacrolimus:

- ketoconazole*, fluconazole*, itraconazole*, clotrimazole
- nifedipine, nicardipine
- erythromycin*, clarithromycin, josamycin
- HIV protease inhibitors
- danazol, ethinyl oestradiol
- calcium antagonists such as diltiazem
- omeprazole
- nefazodone

The following drugs induce CYP3A4 and have been shown to decrease the blood levels of tacrolimus:

- rifampicin* (rifampin)
- phenytoin*
- phenobarbitone

Tacrolimus has been shown to increase the blood level of phenytoin.

Methylprednisolone has been reported both to increase and to decrease tacrolimus plasma levels.

Enhanced nephrotoxicity has been observed, following the administration of either of the following drugs in conjunction with tacrolimus:

- amphotericin B
- ibuprofen

The half-life of cyclosporin has been shown to increase when tacrolimus is given simultaneously. In addition, synergistic/additive nephrotoxic effects can occur. For these reasons, the combined administration of cyclosporin and tacrolimus is not recommended and care should be taken when administering tacrolimus to patients who have previously received cyclosporin.

Food interactions

Grapefruit juice has been reported to increase the blood level of tacrolimus by inhibiting the activity of CYP3A4.

Interactions observed in animals

In rats, tacrolimus decreased the clearance and increased the half-life of pentabarbitone and antipyrine.

Potential interactions

Substances inhibiting the cytochrome P-450 3A system

Based on studies in vitro, the following substances may be regarded as potential inhibitors of metabolism: bromocriptine, cortisone, dapsone, ergotamine, gestodene, lidocaine, mephenytoin, miconazole, midazolam, nilvadipine, norethindrone, quinidine, tamoxifen, (triacetyl)oleandomycin and verapamil.

Substances inducing the cytochrome P-450 3A system

Carbamazepine, metamizole and isoniazide induce cytochrome P-450 3A.

Tacrolimus inhibition of cytochrome P-450 3A system-mediated metabolism of other substances

As tacrolimus may alter the metabolism of steroid-based contraceptive agents, particular care should be exercised when deciding upon contraceptive measures.

4.6 Pregnancy and lactation

Prograf is contraindicated in pregnancy.

In animal studies (rats and rabbits) Prograf has been shown to be teratogenic at doses which also demonstrated maternal toxicity. Preclinical and human data show that the drug is able to cross the placenta. The possibility of pregnancy should therefore be excluded before initiating Prograf therapy.

As Prograf may alter the metabolism of oral contraceptives, other forms of contraception should be used.

Preclinical data in rats suggest that tacrolimus is excreted into breast milk. Human data on effects of the drug during the lactation period is limited. As detrimental effects on the newborn cannot be excluded, women should not breastfeed whilst receiving tacrolimus.

4.7 Effects on ability to drive and use machines

Tacrolimus is associated with visual and neurological disturbances. Individuals who are affected by such disorders should not drive a car or operate dangerous machinery. This effect may be enhanced when tacrolimus is given together with alcohol.

4.8 Undesirable effects

The adverse drug reaction (ADR) profile associated with immunosuppressive agents is often difficult to establish owing to the underlying disease and the concurrent use of multiple medications.

Many of the ADRs stated below are reversible and/or respond to dose reduction. Oral administration appears to be associated with a lower incidence of adverse events compared with intravenous use.

The ADRs are listed below in descending order by frequency of occurrence: very common (>10%), common (>1/100, <1/10), uncommon (> 1/1,000, < 1/100), rare (> 1/10,000, <1/1,000) or very rare (< 1/10,000 including isolated reports).

Haematological and lymphatic system

common:	anaemia
	leukopenia
	thrombocytopenia
	haemorrhage
	leukocytosis
	coagulation disorders
uncommon:	impairment of the hematopoietic system, including pancytopenia
	thrombotic microangiopathy

Metabolism and electrolytes

very common:	hyperglycaemia
	hyperkalaemia
	diabetes mellitus
common:	hypomagnesaemia
	hyperlipidaemia
	hypophosphataemia
	hypokalaemia
	hyperuricaemia
	hypocalcaemia
	acidosis
	hyponatraemia
	hypervolaemia
	other electrolyte abnormalities
	dehydration

uncommon:	hypoproteinaemia
	hyperphosphataemia
	increased amylase
	hypoglycaemia

Nervous system / Sensory system

very common:	tremor
	headache
	insomnia
common:	sensation disorders (e.g. paraesthesia)
	vision abnormalities
	confusion
	depression
	dizziness
	agitation
	neuropathy
	convulsion
	incoordination
	psychosis
	anxiety
	nervousness
	abnormal dreams
	impaired consciousness
	emotional lability
	hallucinations
	otological disturbances
	thinking abnormalities
	encephalopathy
uncommon:	hypertonia
	eye disorders
	amnesia
	cataract
	speech disorders
	paralysis
	coma
	deafness
very rare:	blindness

Cardiovascular system

very common:	hypertension
common:	hypotension
	tachycardia
	cardiac arrhythmias and conduction abnormalities
	thromboembolic and ischemic events
	angina pectoris
	vascular diseases
uncommon:	ECG abnormalities
	infarction
	heart failure
	shock
	myocardial hypertrophy
	cardiac arrest

Respiratory system

common:	impairment of the respiratory function (e.g. dyspnoea)
	pleural effusion
uncommon:	atelectasis
	asthma

Digestive system / Liver

very common:	diarrhoea
	nausea and/or vomiting
common:	dysfunction of the digestive system (e.g. dyspepsia)
	abnormal liver function tests
	abdominal pain
	constipation
	weight and appetite changes
	inflammatory and ulcerative disorders of the digestive system
	jaundice
	bile duct and gall bladder abnormalities
uncommon:	Ascites
	ileus
	lesion of liver tissue (e.g. cirrhosis, necrosis)
	pancreatitis
rare:	liver failure

Skin

common:	pruritus
	alopecia
	rash
	sweating
	acne
	photosensitivity
uncommon:	hirsutism
rare:	Lyell's syndrome
very rare:	Stevens-Johnson's syndrome

Musculoskeletal system

common:	cramps
uncommon:	joint disorders
	myasthenia

Kidney

very common:	abnormal kidney function (e.g. increase in serum creatinine)
common:	lesion of kidney tissue (e.g. tubular necrosis)
	kidney failure
uncommon:	proteinuria

Miscellaneous

very common:	localised pain (e.g. arthralgia)
common:	fever
	peripheral oedema
	asthenia
	dysfunction of urination
uncommon:	organ oedema
	disorders of female genitals

Malignancies

Patients receiving immunosuppressive therapy are at increased risk of developing malignancies. Benign and malignant neoplasms including EBV-associated lymphoproliferative disorders and skin malignancies have been reported in association with tacrolimus treatment.

Hypersensitivity Reactions

Allergic and anaphylactoid reactions have been observed in patients receiving tacrolimus.

Infections

As is well-known for other potent immunosuppressive agents, patients receiving tacrolimus are frequently at risk for infections (viral, bacterial, fungal or protozoal). The course of pre-existing infections may be aggravated. Both generalised and localised infections can occur.

4.9 Overdose

Experience of overdosage is limited.

Early clinical experience (when initial induction doses were two or three times greater than those currently recommended) suggested that symptoms of overdosage may include renal, neurological and cardiac disturbances, effects on glucose intolerance, hypertension and electrolyte disorders (eg hyperkalaemia). Over-immunosuppression may increase the risk of severe infections.

Isolated reports on overdose of tacrolimus indicate that nausea, vomiting, tremor, increased liver enzyme values, headache, lethargy, urticaria, and nephrotoxicity and infections may occur.

Liver function clearly influences all pre- and post operative pharmacokinetic variables. Patients with failing liver grafts or those switched from other immunosuppressive therapy to tacrolimus should be monitored carefully to avoid overdosage.

No specific antidote to Prograf therapy is available. If overdosage occurs, general supportive measures and symptomatic treatment should be conducted.

Based on its high molecular weight, poor aqueous solubility and extensive erythrocyte and plasma protein binding, it is anticipated that tacrolimus will not be dialysable. In isolated patients with very high plasma concentrations of tacrolimus, haemofiltration and haemodiafiltration have been reported to considerably decrease the tacrolimus levels. In cases of oral intoxication, gastric lavage and/or the use of adsorbents (such as activated charcoal) may be helpful.

5. PHARMACOLOGICAL PROPERTIES

5.1 Pharmacodynamic properties

Pharmacotherapeutic Group

Macrolide immunosuppressant

Mechanism of action and pharmacodynamic effects

At the molecular level, the effects of tacrolimus appear to be mediated by binding to a cytosolic protein (FKBP12) which is responsible for the intracellular accumulation of the compound. The FKBP12-tacrolimus complex specifically and competitively binds to and inhibits calcineurin, leading to a calcium-dependent inhibition of T-cell signal transduction pathways, thereby preventing transcription of a discrete set of lymphokine genes.

Tacrolimus is a highly potent immunosuppressive agent and has proven activity in experiments both in vitro and in vivo.

In particular, tacrolimus inhibits the formation of cytotoxic lymphocytes, which are mainly responsible for graft rejection. The drug suppresses T-cell activation and T-helper-cell dependent B-cell proliferation, as well as the formation of lymphokines (such as interleukins-2, -3 and γ-interferon) and the expression of the interleukin-2 receptor.

In studies in vivo, Prograf has been shown to be efficacious in transplantation of the liver and kidney.

5.2 Pharmacokinetic properties

Absorption

In animal models, tacrolimus has been shown to be absorbed throughout the gastrointestinal tract; the major site of absorption being identified as the upper gastrointestinal tract.

In man absorption of tacrolimus from the gastrointestinal tract after oral administration is variable. Peak concentrations (C_{max}) of tacrolimus in blood are achieved in approximately 1 – 3 hours. In some patients, the drug appears to be continuously absorbed over a prolonged period yielding a relatively flat absorption profile. Mean (± sd) absorption parameters are listed in the following table:

(see Table 1 below)

After oral administration (0.30 mg/kg per day) to liver transplant patients, steady state concentrations of tacrolimus were achieved within three days in the majority of patients.

In stable liver transplant patients, the oral bioavailability of Prograf was reduced when it was administered after a meal of moderate fat content. Decreases in AUC (27%) and C_{max} (50%) and an increase in t_{max} (173%) in whole blood were evident. Both the rate and extent of absorption of tacrolimus were reduced when Prograf was administered with food.

Bile does not influence the absorption of tacrolimus and therefore treatment may commence orally.

A strong correlation exists between the AUC and the whole blood trough levels at steady state. Monitoring of whole blood trough levels therefore provides a good estimate of systemic exposure.

Distribution and elimination

In man the disposition of tacrolimus after intravenous infusion may be described as biphasic.

In the systemic circulation, tacrolimus binds strongly to erythrocytes resulting in an approximate 20:1 distribution ratio of whole blood/plasma concentrations. In plasma, the drug is highly bound (>98.8%) to plasma proteins, mainly to serum albumin and α-1-acid glycoprotein.

Tacrolimus is extensively distributed in the body. The steady-state volume of distribution based on plasma concentrations is approximately 1300 L (healthy subjects). Corresponding data based on whole blood averaged 47.6 L.

Tacrolimus is a low-clearance drug. In healthy subjects, the average total body clearance (TBC) estimated from whole blood concentrations was 2.25 L/h. In adult liver and kidney transplant patients, values of 4.1 L/h and 6.7 L/h, respectively, have been observed. Paediatric liver transplant recipients have a TBC approximately twice that of adult liver transplant patients.

There is evidence that the pharmacokinetics of tacrolimus change with improving clinical condition of the patients. In liver transplant patients, the mean oral dose was decreased by 28% from Day 7 to Month 6 after transplantation, to maintain similar mean trough level of tacrolimus.

Table 1

Population	Daily Dose (mg/kg)	C_{max} (ng/mL)	t_{max} (hours)	Bioavailability (%)
Adult liver transplant (Steady state)	0.30	74.1	3.0	21.8 (± 6.3)
Paediatric liver transplant (Steady state)	0.30	37.0 (± 26.5)	2.1 (± 1.3)	25 (± 20)
Adult kidney transplant (Steady state)	0.30	44.3 (± 21.9)	1.5	20.1 (± 11.0)
Healthy subjects (Single dose)	1 × 5 mg 5 × 1 mg	28.6 (± 8.6) 36.2 (± 13.8)	1.4 (± 0.6) 1.3 (± 0.4)	14.4 (± 6.0) 17.4 (± 7.0)

Changes in clearance and/or bioavailability were suggested as probable causes for this effect.

The half-life of tacrolimus is long and variable. In healthy subjects, the mean half-life in whole blood is approximately 43 hours. In adult and paediatric liver transplant patients, it averaged 11.7 hours and 12.4 hours, respectively, compared with 15.6 hours in adult kidney transplant recipients.

Metabolism and biotransformation

Eight metabolites have so far been characterised using models in vitro; of these, only one metabolite showed significant immunosuppressive activity.

Excretion

Following intravenous and oral administration of [^{14}C]-labelled tacrolimus, most of the radioactivity was eliminated in the faeces. Approximately 2% of the radioactivity was eliminated in the urine. Less than 1% of unchanged tacrolimus was detected in the urine and faeces, indicating that tacrolimus is almost completely metabolised prior to elimination: bile being the principal route of elimination.

5.3 Preclinical safety data

Mutagenicity

Relevant tests *in vitro* and *in vivo* showed no signs of a mutagenic potential of tacrolimus.

Carcinogenicity

In chronic, one year toxicity studies (rats and baboons) and in long-term carcinogenicity studies (mouse 18 months and rat 24 months at maximum tolerable daily dose of 2.5-5 mg/kg) no signs of a direct tumorigenic potential of tacrolimus were seen.

Reproduction toxicity

In rats, fertility, embryonic and foetal development, birth and peri- and post-natal development were only impaired when receiving clearly toxic dosages (3.2 mg/kg per day). The only exception was a reversible reduction of the foetal birth weights at a dose of 0.1 mg/kg per day. Furthermore in rabbits, toxic effects on the embryos and on the foetus were observed. Again, these were limited to doses of 1.0 mg/kg per day which showed significant toxicity in maternal animals. Based on these observations, Prograf should not be administered to pregnant women.

6. PHARMACEUTICAL PARTICULARS

6.1 List of excipients

Prograf 0.5 mg Capsules / Prograf 1 mg Capsules / Prograf 5 mg Capsules

Hypromellose, croscarmellose sodium, lactose, magnesium stearate and titanium dioxide (E 171). In addition, Prograf 0.5 mg Capsules contain yellow iron oxide (E 172) and Prograf 5 mg Capsules contain red iron oxide (E 172).

Prograf 0.5 mg Capsules

The printing ink contains shellac, soya lecithin and dimethyl polysiloxane, and red iron oxide (E 172).

Prograf 5 mg/mL Concentrate for Infusion

Polyoxyethylene hydrogenated castor oil, dehydrated alcohol.

6.2 Incompatibilities

Prograf is not compatible with PVC plastics.

Mixed infusions between a solution prepared with Prograf 5 mg/mL Concentrate for Infusion and other drugs should be avoided. In particular mixed infusions with drugs exhibiting a marked alkaline reaction in solution (e.g. aciclovir, ganciclovir) must not be administered because tacrolimus can degrade in this condition.

6.3 Shelf life

Prograf 0.5 mg Capsules

Aluminium-wrapped blisters: 24 months.

After opening of the aluminium wrapper the capsules are stable for 12 months.

Prograf 1 mg Capsules / Prograf 5 mg Capsules

Aluminium-wrapped blisters: 36 months.

After opening of the aluminium wrapper the capsules are stable for 12 months.

Prograf 5 mg/mL Concentrate for Infusion

24 months when protected from light and stored at temperatures up to 25°C.

To be used within 24 hours when reconstituted with 5% dextrose solution or physiological saline in polyethylene or glass containers.

6.4 Special precautions for storage

Prograf 0.5 mg Capsules

Aluminium-wrapped blisters: store in the original package.

Unwrapped aluminium blisters: do not store above 25°C, store in the original package. The patients should be instructed accordingly.

Prograf 1 mg Capsules / Prograf 5 mg Capsules

Once the aluminium wrapper is opened the capsules in the blister strips are stable for 12 months. The individual blister strips should be kept in a dry place. The patients should be instructed accordingly.

Prograf 5 mg/mL Concentrate for Infusion

Store below 25°C.

Protect from light.

6.5 Nature and contents of container

Prograf 0.5 mg Capsules / Prograf 1 mg Capsules / Prograf 5 mg Capsules

The blister sheet consists of PVC/PVdC/Aluminium. There are ten capsules per blister sheet.

Prograf 0.5 mg Capsules: Five or ten blisters are packaged with one desiccant sachet in an aluminium wrapper inside a cardboard outer carton.

Prograf 1 mg Capsules: Three, five or ten blisters are packaged with one desiccant sachet in an aluminium wrapper inside a cardboard outer carton.

Prograf 5 mg Capsules: Three, or five blisters are packaged with one desiccant sachet in an aluminium wrapper inside a cardboard outer carton.

Prograf 5 mg/mL Concentrate for Infusion

Concentrate for infusion (solution) in transparent glass ampoules. Pack size of 10.

6.6 Instructions for use and handling

Prograf 0.5 mg Capsules / Prograf 1 mg Capsules / Prograf 5 mg Capsules

Capsules should be taken immediately following removal from the blister. In addition, patients should be cautioned not to swallow the desiccant sachet contained within the aluminium wrapper.

Prograf 5 mg/mL Concentrate for Infusion

Prograf 5mg/mL Concentrate for infusion must not be injected undiluted. The solution should not be given as a bolus.

Prograf Concentrate for infusion should be diluted with 5% dextrose solution or physiological saline in polyethylene, polypropylene or glass containers.

Tubing, syringes and any other equipment used to administer Prograf should not contain PVC.

The concentration of a solution for infusion should be within the range 0.004 - 0.100 mg/mL. The total volume of infusion during a 24-hour period should be in the range 20 - 500 mL.

After constitution, infusion solutions should be used within 24 hours.

Unused concentrate for infusion in an opened ampoule or unused reconstituted solution, should be disposed of immediately to avoid contamination.

7. MARKETING AUTHORISATION HOLDER

Fujisawa Ltd
62 London Road
Staines
Middlesex
TW18 4HN
United Kingdom

8. MARKETING AUTHORISATION NUMBER(S)

Prograf 0.5 mg Capsules	PL 13424/0004
Prograf 1 mg Capsules	PL 13424/0001
Prograf 5 mg Capsules	PL 13424/0002
Prograf 5 mg/mL Concentrate for Infusion	PL 13424/0003

9. DATE OF FIRST AUTHORISATION/RENEWAL OF THE AUTHORISATION

Prograf 0.5 mg Capsules

September 1999

Prograf 1 mg Capsules / Prograf 5 mg Capsules

July 1999

Prograf 5 mg/mL Concentrate for Infusion

July 1999

10. DATE OF REVISION OF THE TEXT

June 2002

Progynova 1mg

(Schering Health Care Limited)

1. NAME OF THE MEDICINAL PRODUCT

Progynova® 1mg

2. QUALITATIVE AND QUANTITATIVE COMPOSITION

Each memo pack contains 28 tablets each containing estradiol valerate 1.0 mg.

3. PHARMACEUTICAL FORM

Sugar coated tablet for oral administration.

4. CLINICAL PARTICULARS

4.1 Therapeutic indications

Hormone replacement therapy for the treatment of the climacteric syndrome in menopausal women. In women with a uterus, a progestogen should be added to Progynova for 12 days each month.

4.2 Posology and method of administration

Adults: One tablet of Progynova 1mg to be taken daily. For maintenance the lowest effective dose should be used.

Treatment is continuous, which means that the next pack follows immediately without a break.

Children: not recommended.

4.3 Contraindications

1. Pregnancy and lactation

2. Severe disturbances of liver function (including porphyria), previous or existing liver tumours, jaundice or general pruritus during a previous pregnancy, Dubin-Johnson syndrome, Rotor syndrome

3. Severe cardiac or severe renal disease.

4. Active deep venous thrombosis, thromboembolic disorders, or a history of confirmed venous thromboembolism. (See also Special Warnings and Special Precautions for Use).

5. Suspected or existing hormone-dependent disorders or tumours.

6. Tumours of the uterus or breast

7. Congenital disturbances of lipid metabolism

8. Severe diabetes with vascular changes

9. Hypersensitivity to any of the ingredients.

4.4 Special warnings and special precautions for use

Before starting treatment pregnancy must be excluded.

Assessment of each woman prior to taking hormone replacement therapy (and at regular intervals thereafter) should include a personal and family medical history. Physical examination should be guided by this and by the contraindications (section 4.3) and warnings (section 4.4) for Progynova. During assessment of each individual woman clinical examination of the breasts and pelvic examination should be performed where clinically indicated rather than as a routine procedure. Women should be encouraged to participate in the national breast cancer screening programme (mammography) and the national cervical cancer screening programme (cervical cytology) as appropriate for their age. Breast awareness should also be encouraged and women advised to report any changes in their breasts to their doctor or nurse.

A reanalysis of original data from 51 epidemiological studies reported a small or moderate increase in the probability of having breast cancer *diagnosed* in women currently or recently using HRT. The findings may be due to biological effects of HRT, earlier diagnosis, or a combination of both. The relative risk increased with duration of treatment (by 2.3% per year of use) and returned to normal in the course of five years after cessation of HRT use. This increase in relative risk associated with duration of HRT use is comparable to the increase in relative risk when natural menopause is delayed in the absence of HRT (2.8% increase for each year older at menopause). Breast cancers diagnosed in current or recent users of HRT are more likely to be localised to the breast than those found in non-users. HRT use may not be associated with increased mortality from breast cancer.

Between the ages of 50 and 70, about 45 women in every 1000 not using HRT will have breast cancer diagnosed. It is estimated that among those who use HRT for 5 years starting at age 50, 2 extra cases of breast cancer will be detected by age 70 in every 1000 women. For those who use HRT for 10 years there will be 6 extra cases of breast cancer, and for 15 years use, 12 extra cases of breast cancer in every 1000 women during the 20 year period until age 70.

It is important that the increased risk of being diagnosed with breast cancer is discussed with the patient and weighed against the known benefits of HRT.

There is a need for caution when prescribing oestrogens in women who have a history of, or known, breast nodules or fibrocystic disease.

Treatment should be stopped at once if migrainous or frequent and unusually severe headaches occur for the first time, or if there are any other symptoms that are possible prodromata of vascular occlusion e.g. sudden visual disturbances.

Treatment should be stopped at once if jaundice, cholestasis, hepatitis, or pregnancy occurs or if there is a significant rise in blood-pressure or an increase in epileptic seizures.

Epidemiological studies have suggested that hormone replacement therapy (HRT) is associated with an increased relative risk of developing venous thromboembolism (VTE) i.e. deep vein thrombosis or pulmonary embolism. The studies find a 2-3 fold increase for users compared with non-users which for healthy women amounts to a low risk of one extra case of VTE each year for every 5000 patients taking HRT.

Generally recognised risk factors for VTE include a personal or family history and severe obesity (Body Mass Index >30 kg/m^2). In women with these factors the benefits of treatment with HRT need to be carefully weighed against risks. There is no consensus about the possible role of varicose veins in VTE.

The risk of VTE may be temporarily increased with prolonged immobilisation, major trauma or major surgery. In women on HRT scrupulous attention should be given to prophylactic measures to prevent VTE following surgery. Where prolonged immobilisation is liable to follow elective surgery, particularly abdominal or orthopaedic surgery to the lower limbs, consideration should be given to temporarily stopping HRT 4 weeks earlier, if this is possible.

If venous thromboembolism develops after initiating therapy the drug should be discontinued.

There is an increased risk of gall bladder disease in women receiving post menopausal oestrogens.

In women with an intact uterus, there is an increased risk of endometrial hyperplasia and carcinoma associated with unopposed oestrogen administered long term (for more than one year). However, the appropriate addition of a progestogen to the oestrogen regimen statistically lowers the risk.

Should endometriosis be reactivated under therapy with Progynova, therapy should be discontinued.

Diseases that are known to be subject to deterioration during pregnancy (e.g. multiple sclerosis, epilepsy, diabetes, benign breast disease, hypertension, cardiac or renal dysfunction, asthma, migraine, tetany, systemic lupus erythematosus and melanoma) and women with a strong family history of breast cancer should be carefully observed during treatment.

Because of the occurrence of herpes gestationis and the worsening of otosclerosis in pregnancy, it is thought that treatment with female hormones may have similar effects. Patients with these conditions should be carefully monitored. Similarly, patients with sickle-cell anaemia should be monitored because of the increased risk of thrombosis that accompanies this disease.

Patients with pre-existing fibroids should be closely monitored as fibroids may increase in size under the influence of oestrogens. If this is observed, treatment should be discontinued.

Oestrogens may cause fluid retention and therefore patients with renal or cardiac dysfunction should be carefully observed.

Most studies demonstrate that oestrogen replacement therapy has little effect on blood pressure. Some show that it may decrease blood pressure. In addition, studies on combined therapy show that the addition of a progestogen also has little effect on blood pressure. Rarely, idiosyncratic hypertension may occur. When oestrogens are administered to hypersensitive women, supervision is necessary and blood pressure should be monitored at regular intervals.

In patients with mild chronic liver disease, liver function should be checked every 8-12 weeks. Results of liver function tests may be affected by HRT.

In rare cases benign and in even rarer cases malignant liver tumours leading in isolated cases to life-threatening intra-abdominal haemorrhage have been observed after the use of hormonal substances such as the one contained in Progynova. A hepatic tumour should be considered in the differential diagnosis if upper abdominal pain, enlarged liver or signs of intra-abdominal haemorrhage occur.

Diabetes should be carefully observed when initiating HRT as worsening of the glucose tolerance may occur.

In women with a uterus, contraception should be practised with non-hormonal methods.

4.5 Interaction with other medicinal products and other forms of Interaction
Drugs which induce hepatic microsomal enzyme systems e.g. barbiturates, carbamazepine, phenytoin, rifampicin accelerate the metabolism of oestrogen products such as Progynova and may reduce their efficacy.

The requirement for oral antidiabetics or insulin can change as a result of the effect on glucose tolerance.

There are some laboratory tests that can be influenced by oestrogens, such as tests for glucose tolerance, liver function or thyroid function.

4.6 Pregnancy and lactation
Contra-indicated

4.7 Effects on ability to drive and use machines
None known.

4.8 Undesirable effects
During the first few months of treatment, breast tenderness or enlargement can occur. These are usually temporary and normally disappear after continued treatment. Other symptoms known to occur are dyspepsia, flatulence, nausea, vomiting, leg pains, anxiety, depressive symptoms, increased appetite, abdominal pain and bloating, altered weight, oedema, palpitations, altered libido, headache, dizziness, epistaxis, hypertension, rashes, thrombophlebitis, mucous vaginal discharge, general pruritus. Some women are predisposed to cholestasis during steroid therapy.

4.9 Overdose
Nausea and vomiting may occur with an overdose. There are no specific antidotes, and treatment should be symptomatic. Withdrawal bleeding may occur in females with a uterus.

5. PHARMACOLOGICAL PROPERTIES
5.1 Pharmacodynamic properties
Progynova contains estradiol valerate, (the valeric-acid ester of the endogenous female oestrogen, estradiol). Estradiol valerate provides hormone replacement during the climacteric.

Most studies show that oral administration of estradiol valerate to post-menopausal women increases serum high density lipoprotein cholesterol (HDL-C) and decreases low density lipoprotein cholesterol (LDL-C). Although epidemiological data are limited such alterations are recognised as potentially protective against the development of arterial disease.

5.2 Pharmacokinetic properties
After oral administration estradiol valerate is quickly and completely absorbed.

Already after 0.5 - 3 hours peak plasma levels of estradiol, the active drug substance, are measured. As a rule, after 6 - 8 hours a second maximum appears, possibly indicating an entero-hepatic circulation of estradiol.

Esterases in plasma and the liver quickly decompose estradiol valerate into estradiol and valerianic acid. Further decomposition of valerianic acid through β-oxidation leads to C_2-units and results in CO_2 and water as end products. Estradiol itself undergoes several hydroxylating steps. Its metabolites as well as the unchanged substance are finally conjugated. Intermediate products of metabolism are oestrone and oestriol, which exhibit a weak oestrogenic activity of their own, although this activity is not so pronounced as with estradiol. The plasma concentration of conjugated oestrone is about 25 to 30 fold higher than the concentration of unconjugated oestrone. In a study using radioactive labelled estradiol valerate about 20% of radioactive substances in the plasma could be characterised as unconjugated steroids, 17% as glucuronized steroids and 33% as steroid sulphates. About 30% of all substances could not be extracted from the aqueous phase and, therefore, represent probably metabolites of high polarity.

Estradiol and its metabolites are mainly excreted by the kidneys (relation of urine:faeces = 9:1). Within 5 days about 78 - 96% of the administered dose are excreted with an excretion half-life of about 27 hours.

In plasma, estradiol is mainly found in its protein-bound form. About 37% are bound to SHBG and 61% to albumin. Cumulation of estradiol after daily repetitive intake of Progynova does not need to be expected.

The absolute bioavailability of estradiol amounts to 3 - 5% of the oral dose of estradiol valerate.

5.3 Preclinical safety data
There are no preclinical safety data which could be of relevance to the prescriber and which are not already included in other relevant sections of the SPC.

6. PHARMACEUTICAL PARTICULARS
6.1 List of excipients
Lactose monohydrate

Maize Starch

Povidone 25,000

Talc

Magnesium Stearate [E572]

Sucrose

Povidone 700,000

Macrogol 6,000

Calcium Carbonate [E170]

Titanium Dioxide [E171]

Glycerol 85% [E422]

Montan Glycol Wax

Ferric oxide pigment

Purified water

6.2 Incompatibilities
None known.

6.3 Shelf life
5 years.

6.4 Special precautions for storage
None.

6.5 Nature and contents of container
Container consists of aluminium foil and PVC blister strips packed in a cardboard carton.

Presentation:

Carton containing memo-packs of either 1 × 28 tablets or 3 × 28 tablets.

6.6 Instructions for use and handling
None.

7. MARKETING AUTHORISATION HOLDER
Schering Health Care Limited

The Brow

Burgess Hill

West Sussex

RH15 9NE

8. MARKETING AUTHORISATION NUMBER(S)
0053/0057.

9. DATE OF FIRST AUTHORISATION/RENEWAL OF THE AUTHORISATION
14th April 1972/24th May 1993.

10. DATE OF REVISION OF THE TEXT
20th March 2001

LEGAL CATEGORY
POM

Progynova 2mg

(Schering Health Care Limited)

1. NAME OF THE MEDICINAL PRODUCT
Progynova® 2mg.

2. QUALITATIVE AND QUANTITATIVE COMPOSITION
Each memo pack contains 28 tablets each containing estradiol valerate 2.0 mg.

3. PHARMACEUTICAL FORM
Sugar coated tablet for oral administration.

4. CLINICAL PARTICULARS
4.1 Therapeutic indications
In menopausal women:

1. Hormone replacement therapy for the treatment of the climacteric syndrome.

2. Second line therapy for prevention of osteoporosis in postmenopausal women at high risk of future fractures who are intolerant of, or contraindicated for, other medicinal products approved for the prevention of osteoporosis.

In women with a uterus, a progestogen should be added to Progynova for 12 days each month.

4.2 Posology and method of administration
Adults:

Climacteric syndrome: One tablet to be taken daily. For maintenance the lowest effective dose should be used.

Prophylaxis of osteoporosis: One tablet to be taken daily.

For maximum prophylactic benefit, treatment should commence as soon as possible after onset of the menopause.

Bone mineral density measurements may help to confirm the presence of low bone mass.

Treatment is continuous, which means that the next pack follows immediately without a break.

Children: not recommended

4.3 Contraindications
1. Pregnancy and lactation.

2. Severe disturbances of liver function (including porphyria), previous or existing liver tumours, jaundice or general pruritus during a previous pregnancy, Dubin-Johnson syndrome, Rotor syndrome.

3. Severe cardiac or severe renal disease.

4. Active deep venous thrombosis, thromboembolic disorders, or a history of confirmed venous thromboembolism. (See also Special Warnings and Special Precautions for use).

5. Suspected or existing hormone-dependent disorders or tumours.

6. Tumours of the uterus or breast

7. Congenital disturbances of lipid metabolism.

8. Severe diabetes with vascular changes.

9. Hypersensitivity to any of the ingredients

4.4 Special warnings and special precautions for use
Before starting treatment pregnancy must be excluded

Assessment of each woman prior to taking hormone replacement therapy (and at regular intervals thereafter) should include a personal and family medical history. Physical examination should be guided by this and by the contra-indications (section 4.3) and warnings (section 4.4) for Progynova. During assessment of each individual woman clinical examination of the breasts and pelvic examination should be performed where clinically indicated rather than as a routine procedure. Women should be encouraged to participate in the national breast cancer screening programme (mammography) and the national cervical cancer screening programme (cervical cytology) as appropriate for their age. Breast awareness should also be encouraged and women advised to report any changes in their breasts to their doctor or nurse.

A reanalysis of original data from 51 epidemiological studies reported a small or moderate increase in the probability of having breast cancer *diagnosed* in women currently or recently using HRT. The findings may be due to biological effects of HRT, earlier diagnosis, or a combination of both. The relative risk increased with duration of treatment (by 2.3% per year of use) and returned to normal in the course of five years after cessation of HRT use. This increase in relative risk associated with duration of HRT use is comparable to the increase in relative risk when natural menopause is delayed in the absence of HRT (2.8% increase for each year older at menopause). Breast cancers diagnosed in current or recent users of HRT are more likely to be localised to the breast than those found in non-users. HRT use may not be associated with increased mortality from breast cancer.

Between the ages of 50 and 70, about 45 women in every 1000 not using HRT will have breast cancer diagnosed. It is estimated that among those who use HRT for 5 years starting at age 50, 2 extra cases of breast cancer will be detected by age 70 in every 1000 women. For those who use HRT for 10 years there will be 6 extra cases of breast cancer, and for 15 years use, 12 extra cases of breast cancer in every 1000 women during the 20 year period until age 70.

It is important that the increased risk of being diagnosed with breast cancer is discussed with the patient and weighed against the known benefits of HRT.

There is a need for caution when prescribing oestrogens in women who have a history of, or known, breast nodules or fibrocystic disease.

Treatment should be stopped at once if migrainous or frequent and unusually severe headaches occur for the first time, or if there are any other symptoms that are possible prodromata of vascular occlusion e.g. sudden visual disturbances.

Treatment should be stopped at once if jaundice, cholestasis, hepatitis, or pregnancy occurs or if there is a significant rise in blood-pressure or an increase in epileptic seizures.

Epidemiological studies have suggested that hormone replacement therapy (HRT) is associated with an increased relative risk of developing venous thromboembolism (VTE) i.e. deep vein thrombosis or pulmonary embolism. The studies find a 2-3 fold increase for users compared with non-users which for healthy women amounts to a low risk of one extra case of VTE each year for every 5000 patients taking HRT.

Generally recognised risk factors for VTE include a personal or family history and severe obesity (Body Mass Index >30 kg/m^2). In women with these factors the benefits of treatment with HRT need to be carefully weighed against risks. There is no consensus about the possible role of varicose veins in VTE.

The risk of VTE may be temporarily increased with prolonged immobilisation, major trauma or major surgery. In women on HRT scrupulous attention should be given to prophylactic measures to prevent VTE following surgery. Where prolonged immobilisation is liable to follow elective surgery, particularly abdominal or orthopaedic surgery to the lower limbs, consideration should be given to temporarily stopping HRT 4 weeks earlier, if this is possible.

If venous thromboembolism develops after initiating therapy the drug should be discontinued.

There is an increased risk of gall bladder disease in women receiving post menopausal oestrogens.

In women with an intact uterus, there is an increased risk of endometrial hyperplasia and carcinoma associated with unopposed oestrogen administered long term (for more than one year). However, the appropriate addition of a progestogen to the oestrogen regimen statistically lowers the risk.

Should endometriosis be reactivated under therapy with Progynova, therapy shoud be discontinued.

Diseases that are known to be subject to deterioration during pregnancy (e.g. multiple sclerosis, epilepsy, diabetes, benign breast disease, hypertension, cardiac or renal dysfunction, asthma, migraine, tetany, systemic lupus erythematosus and melanoma) and women with a strong family history of breast cancer should be carefully observed during treatment.

Because of the occurrence of herpes gestationis and the worsening of otosclerosis in pregnancy, it is thought that treatment with female hormones may have similar effects. Patients with these conditions should be carefully monitored. Similarly, patients with sickle-cell anaemia should be monitored because of the increased risk of thrombosis that accompanies this disease.

Patients with pre-existing fibroids should be closely monitored as fibroids may increase in size under the influence of oestrogens. If this is observed, treatment should be discontinued.

Oestrogens may cause fluid retention and therefore patients with renal or cardiac dysfunction should be carefully observed.

Most studies demonstrate that oestrogen therapy has little effect on blood pressure. Some show that it may decrease blood pressure. In addition, studies on combined therapy show that the addition of a progestogen also has little effect on blood pressure. Rarely, idiosyncratic hypertension may occur. When oestrogens are administered to hypertensive women, supervision is necessary and blood pressure should be monitored at regular intervals.

In patients with mild chronic liver disease, liver function should be checked every 8-12 weeks. Results of liver function tests may be affected by HRT.

In rare cases benign and in even rarer cases malignant liver tumours leading in isolated cases to life-threatening intra-abdominal haemorrhage have been observed after the use of hormonal substances such as the one contained in Progynova. A hepatic tumour should be considered in the differential diagnosis if upper abdominal pain, enlarged liver or signs of intra-abdominal haemorrhage occur.

Diabetes should be carefully observed when initiating HRT as worsening of the glucose tolerance may occur.

In women with a uterus, contraception should be practised with non-hormonal methods.

4.5 Interaction with other medicinal products and other forms of Interaction

Drugs which induce hepatic microsomal enzyme systems e.g. barbiturates, carbamazepine, phenytoin, rifampicin accelerate the metabolism of oestrogen products such as Progynova and may reduce their efficacy.

The requirement for oral antidiabetics or insulin can change as a result of the effect on glucose tolerance.

There are some laboratory tests that can be influenced by oestrogens, such as tests for glucose tolerance, liver function or thyroid function.

4.6 Pregnancy and lactation

Contra-indicated

4.7 Effects on ability to drive and use machines

None known

4.8 Undesirable effects

During the first few months of treatment, breast tenderness or enlargement can occur. These are usually temporary and normally disappear after continued treatment. Other symptoms known to occur are dyspepsia, flatulence, nausea, vomiting, leg pains, anxiety, depressive symptoms, increased appetite, abdominal pain and bloating, altered weight, oedema, palpitations, altered libido, headache, dizziness, epistaxis, hypertension, rashes, thrombophlebitis, mucous vaginal discharge, general pruritus. Some women are predisposed to cholestasis during steroid therapy.

4.9 Overdose

Nausea and vomiting may occur with an overdose. There are no specific antidotes, and treatment should be symptomatic. Withdrawal bleeding may occur in females with a uterus.

5. PHARMACOLOGICAL PROPERTIES

5.1 Pharmacodynamic properties

Progynova contains estradiol valerate, (the valeric-acid ester of the endogenous female oestrogen, estradiol).

Estradiol valerate provides hormone replacement during the climacteric.

Most studies show that oral administration of estradiol valerate to post-menopausal women increases serum high density lipoprotein cholesterol (HDL-C) and decreases low density lipoprotein cholesterol (LDL-C). Although epidemiological data are limited such alterations are recognised as potentially protective against the development of arterial disease.

5.2 Pharmacokinetic properties

After oral administration estradiol valerate is quickly and completely absorbed.

Already after 0.5 - 3 hours peak plasma levels of estradiol, the active drug substance, are measured. As a rule, after 6 - 8 hours a second maximum appears, possibly indicating an entero-hepatic circulation of estradiol.

Esterases in plasma and the liver quickly decompose estradiol valerate into estradiol and valerianic acid. Further decomposition of valerianic acid through β-oxidation leads to C2-units and results in CO2 and water as end products. Estradiol itself undergoes several hydroxylating steps. Its metabolites as well as the unchanged substance are finally conjugated. Intermediate products of metabolism are oestrone and oestriol, which exhibit a weak oestrogenic activity of their own, although this activity is not so pronounced as with estradiol. The plasma concentration of conjugated oestrone is about 25 to 30 fold higher than the concentration of unconjugated oestrone. In a study using radioactive labelled estradiol valerate about 20% of radioactive substances in the plasma could be characterised as unconjugated steroids, 17% as glucuronized steroids and 33% as steroid sulphates. About 30% of all substances could not be extracted from the aqueous phase and, therefore, represent probably metabolites of high polarity.

Estradiol and its metabolites are mainly excreted by the kidneys (relation of urine:faeces = 9:1). Within 5 days about 78 - 96% of the administered dose are excreted with an excretion half-life of about 27 hours.

In plasma, estradiol is mainly found in its protein-bound form. About 37% are bound to SHBG and 61% to albumin. Cumulation of estradiol after daily repetitive intake of Progynova does not need to be expected.

The absolute bioavailability of estradiol amounts to 3 - 5% of the oral dose of estradiol valerate.

5.3 Preclinical safety data

There are no preclinical safety data which could be of relevance to the prescriber and which are not already included in other relevant sections of the SPC.

6. PHARMACEUTICAL PARTICULARS

6.1 List of excipients

Lactose monohydrate

Maize Starch

Povidone 25000

Talc

Magnesium Stearate [E572]

Sucrose

Povidone 700,000

Macrogol 6000

Calcium Carbonate [E170]

Titanium Dioxide [E171]

Glycerol 85% [E422]

Montan Glycol Wax

Indigo Carmine [E132]

Purified Water

6.2 Incompatibilities

None known.

6.3 Shelf life

5 years.

6.4 Special precautions for storage

None.

6.5 Nature and contents of container

Container consists of aluminium foil and PVC blister strips packed in a cardboard carton

Presentation: Carton containing memo-packs of either 1 × 28 tablets or 3 × 28 tablets.

6.6 Instructions for use and handling

None.

7. MARKETING AUTHORISATION HOLDER

Schering Health Care Limited

The Brow

Burgess Hill

West Sussex

RH15 9NE

8. MARKETING AUTHORISATION NUMBER(S)

0053/0058

9. DATE OF FIRST AUTHORISATION/RENEWAL OF THE AUTHORISATION

14 April 1972/24th May 1993.

10. DATE OF REVISION OF THE TEXT

4th December 2003

LEGAL CATEGORY

POM

Progynova TS 50, Progynova TS 100

(Schering Health Care Limited)

1. NAME OF THE MEDICINAL PRODUCT

Progynova® TS 50, Progynova® TS 100

2. QUALITATIVE AND QUANTITATIVE COMPOSITION

Estradiol transdermal system:

Progynova TS 50: 12.5 cm^2 patch contains 3.8 mg of estradiol (formed from 3.9mg of estradiol hemihydrate)

Progynova TS 100: 25 cm^2 patch contains 7.6 mg of estradiol (formed from 7.8 mg of estradiol hemihydrate)

Nominal average absorption rates of 50μg/day and 100μg/day were calculated for Progynova TS 50 and Progynova TS 100 respectively.

3. PHARMACEUTICAL FORM

Transdermal patch

Transdermal delivery system comprising a patch containing estradiol in an acrylate adhesive matrix. The transdermal delivery from a patch is maintained over 7 days. The active component of the system is estradiol. The remaining components of the system are pharmacologically inactive.

4. CLINICAL PARTICULARS

4.1 Therapeutic indications

• Hormone replacement therapy for oestrogen deficiency symptoms in postmenopausal women more than 1 year postmenopause.

• Prevention of osteoporosis in postmenopausal women at high risk of future fractures who are intolerant of, or contra-indicated for, other medicinal products approved for the prevention of osteoporosis.

(See also Section 4.4)

4.2 Posology and method of administration

• Posology

Progynova TS patches are oestrogen-only patches applied to the skin once weekly.

For initiation and continuation of treatment of postmenopausal symptoms, the lowest effective dose for the shortest duration (see also Section 4.4) should be used. Treatment to control menopausal symptoms should be initiated with the lowest Progynova TS patch dose. If considered necessary, a higher dosed patch should be used. Once treatment is established the lowest effective dose patch necessary for relief of symptoms should be used.

For prevention of postmenopausal osteoporosis Progynova TS 50 is recommended. Women receiving Progynova TS 100 for postmenopausal symptoms can continue at this dose.

In women with an intact uterus, a progestogen should be added to Progynova TS patches for at least 12-14 days each month. Unless there is a previous diagnosis of endometriosis, it is not recommended to add a progestogen in hysterectomised women.

For continuous use: The patches should be applied once weekly on a continuous basis, each used patch being removed after 7 days and a fresh patch applied to a different site.

For cyclical use: The patches may also be prescribed on a cyclical basis. Where this is the preferred option, the patches should be applied weekly for 3 consecutive weeks followed by a 7-day interval, without a patch being applied, before the next course.

• How to start Progynova TS patches

Women who do not take oestrogens or women who change from a continuous combined HRT product may start treatment at any time.

Patients changing from a continuous sequential HRT regimen, should begin the day following completion of the prior regimen.

Patients changing from a cyclic HRT regimen should begin the day after the treatment-free period.

• Missed or lost patch

In the event that a patch falls off before 7 days are up, it may be reapplied. If necessary, a new patch should be applied for the remainder of the 7-day dosing interval.

If the patient forgets to replace a patch, this should be done as soon as possible after she remembers it. The next patch has to be used after the normal 7-day interval.

After several days without replacement of a new patch there is an increased likelihood of breakthrough bleeding and spotting.

• Mode of application

Following removal of the protective liner the adhesive side of Progynova TS patches should be placed on a clean, dry area of the skin of the trunk or buttocks. Progynova TS patches should not be applied to the breasts. The sites of application should be rotated, with an interval of at least one week between applications to a particular site. The area selected should not be oily, damaged, or irritated. The waistline should be avoided since tight clothing may rub the patch off. The patch should be applied immediately after opening the pouch and removing the protective liner. The patch should be pressed firmly in place with the palm of the hand for about 10 seconds, making sure there is good contact, especially around the edges.

The patch should be changed once weekly.

If the patch is applied correctly, the patient can bath or shower as usual. The patch might, however, become detached from the skin in very hot bath water or in the sauna.

Children

Not recommended for children

4.3 Contraindications

• Known, past or suspected breast cancer

• Known or suspected oestrogen dependent malignant tumours, e.g. endometrial cancer

• Undiagnosed genital bleeding

• Untreated endometrial hyperplasia

• Previous idiopathic or current venous thromboembolism (deep venous thrombosis, pulmonary embolism)

• Active or recent arterial thromboembolic disease (e.g. angina, myocardial infarction)

• Acute liver disease, or history of liver disease as long as liver function tests have failed to return to normal

• Porphyria

• Known hypersensitivity to the active substance or any of the excipients

4.4 Special warnings and special precautions for use

For the treatment of postmenopausal symptoms, HRT should only be initiated for symptoms that adversely affect quality of life. In all cases, a careful appraisal of the risks and benefits should be undertaken al least annually and HRT should only be continued as long as the benefit outweighs the risk.

Medical examination/follow up:

• Before initiating or reinstituting HRT, a complete personal and family medical history should be taken. Physical (including pelvic and breasts) examination should be guided by this and by the contraindications and warnings for use. During treatment, periodic check-ups are recommended of a frequency and nature adapted to the individual woman. Women should be advised what changes in their breasts should be reported to their doctor or nurse. Investigations, including mammography, should be carried out in accordance with currently accepted screening practices, modified to the clinical needs of the individual.

Conditions which need supervision

• If any of the following conditions are present, have occurred previously, and/or have been aggravated during pregnancy or previous hormone treatment, the patient should be closely supervised. It should be taken into account that these conditions may recur or be aggravated during treatment with Progynova TS patches, in particular:

- Leiomyoma (uterine fibroids) or endometriosis
- A history of, or risk factors for, thromboembolic disorders (see below)
- Risk factors for oestrogen dependent tumours, e.g. 1 st degree heredity for breast cancer
- Hypertension
- Liver disorders (e.g. liver adenoma)
- Diabetes mellitus with or without vascular involvement
- Cholelithiasis
- Migraine or (severe) headache
- Systemic lupus erythematosus.
- A history of endometrial hyperplasia (see below)
- Epilepsy
- Asthma
- Otosclerosis

Reasons for immediate withdrawal of therapy:

Therapy should be discontinued in case a contra-indication is discovered and in the following situations:

- Jaundice or deterioration in liver function
- Significant increase in blood pressure
- New onset of migraine-type headache
- Pregnancy

Endometrial hyperplasia

• The risk of endometrial hyperplasia and carcinoma is increased when oestrogens are administered alone for prolonged periods (see section 4.8). The addition of a progestogen for at least 12 days per cycle in non-hysterectomised women greatly reduces this risk.

• For Progynova TS 100 (100 μg/day) the endometrial safety of added progestogens has not been studied.

• Break-through bleeding and spotting may occur during the first months of treatment. If break-through bleeding or spotting appears after some time on therapy, or continues after treatment has been discontinued, the reason should be investigated, which may include endometrial biopsy to exclude endometrial malignancy.

• Unopposed oestrogen stimulation may lead to premalignant or malignant transformation in the residual foci of endometriosis. Therefore, the addition of progestogens to oestrogen replacement therapy should be considered in women who have undergone hysterectomy because of endometriosis, if they are known to have residual endometriosis.

Breast cancer

• A randomised placebo-controlled trial, the Women's Health Initiative study (WHI), and epidemiological studies, including the Million Women Study (MWS), have reported an increased risk of breast cancer in women taking oestrogens, oestrogen-progestogen combinations or tibolone for HRT for several years (see Section 4.8).

• For all HRT, an excess risk becomes apparent within a few years of use and increases with duration of intake but returns to baseline within a few (at most five) years after stopping treatment.

• In the MWS, the relative risk of breast cancer with conjugated equine oestrogens (CEE) or estradiol (E2) was greater when a progestogen was added, either sequentially or continuously, and regardless of type of progestogen. There was no evidence of a difference in risk between the different routes of administration.

• In the WHI study, the continuous combined conjugated equine oestrogen and medroxyprogesterone acetate (CEE + MPA) product used was associated with breast cancers that were slightly larger in size and more frequently had local lymph node metastases compared to placebo.

• HRT, especially oestrogen-progestogen combined treatment, increases the density of mammographic images which may adversely affect the radiological detection of breast cancer.

Venous thromboembolism

• HRT is associated with a higher relative risk of developing venous thromboembolism (VTE), i.e. deep vein thrombosis or pulmonary embolism. One randomised controlled trial and epidemiological studies found a two- to threefold higher risk for users compared with non-users. For non-users, it is estimated that the number of cases of VTE that occur over a 5 year period is about 3 per 1000 women aged 50-59 years and 8 per 1000 women aged between 60-69 years. It is estimated that in healthy women who use HRT for 5 years, the number of additional cases of VTE over a 5 year period will be between 2 and 6 (best estimate = 4) per 1000 women aged 50-59 years and between 5 and 15 (best estimate = 9) per 1000 women aged 60-69 years. The occurrence of such an event is more likely in the first year of HRT than later.

• Generally recognised risk factors for VTE include a personal history or family history, severe obesity (BMI > 30 kg/m ^{2}) and systemic lupus erythematosus (SLE). There is no consensus about the possible role of varicose veins in VTE.

• Patients with a history of VTE or known thrombophilic states have an increased risk of VTE. HRT may add to this risk. Personal or strong family history of thromboembolism or recurrent spontaneous abortion should be investigated in order to exclude a thrombophilic predisposition. Until a thorough evaluation of thrombophilic factors has been made or anticoagulant treatment initiated, use of HRT in such patients should be viewed as contraindicated. Those women already on anticoagulant treatment require careful consideration of the benefit-risk of use of HRT.

• The risk of VTE may be temporarily increased with prolonged immobilisation, major trauma or major surgery. As in all postoperative patients, scrupulous attention should be given to prophylactic measures to prevent VTE following surgery. Where prolonged immobilisation is liable to follow elective surgery, particularly abdominal or orthopaedic surgery to the lower limbs, consideration should be given to temporarily stopping HRT 4 to 6 weeks earlier, if possible. Treatment should not be restarted until the woman is completely mobilised.

• If VTE develops after initiating therapy, the drug should be discontinued. Patients should be told to contact their doctors immediately when they are aware of a potential thromboembolic symptom (e.g. painful swelling of a leg, sudden pain in the chest, dyspnoea).

Coronary artery disease (CAD)

• There is no evidence from randomised controlled trials of cardiovascular benefit with continuous combined conjugated oestrogens and medroxyprogesterone acetate (MPA). Two large clinical trials (WHI and HERS, i.e. Heart and Estrogen/progestin Replacement Study) showed a possible increased risk of cardiovascular morbidity in the first year of use and no overall benefit. For other HRT products there are only limited data from randomised controlled trials examining effects in cardiovascular morbidity and mortality. Therefore, it is uncertain whether these findings also extend to other HRT products.

Stroke

• One large randomised clinical trial (WHI-trial) found, as a secondary outcome, an increased risk of ischaemic stroke in healthy women during treatment with continuous combined conjugated oestrogens and MPA. For women who do not use HRT, it is estimated that the number of cases of stroke that will occur over a 5 year period is about 3 per 1000 women aged 50-59 years and 11 women per 1000 women aged 60-69 years. It is estimated that for women who use conjugated oestrogens and MPA for 5 years, the number of additional cases will be between 0 and 3 (best estimate = 1) per 1000 users aged 50-59 years and between 1 and 9 (best estimate = 4) per 1000 users aged 60-69 years. It is unknown whether the increased risk also extends to other HRT products.

Ovarian cancer

• Long-term (at least 5-10 years) use of oestrogen only HRT products in hysterectomised women has been associated with an increased risk of ovarian cancer in some epidemiological studies. It is uncertain whether long-term use of combined HRT confers a different risk than oestrogen-only products.

Other conditions

• Oestrogens may cause fluid retention, and therefore patients with cardiac or renal dysfunction should be carefully observed. Patients with terminal renal insufficiency should be closely observed, since it is expected that the level of circulating active ingredients in Progynova TS is increased.

• Women with pre-existing hypertriglyceridemia should be followed closely during oestrogen replacement or hormone replacement therapy, since rare cases of large increases of plasma triglycerides leading to pancreatitis have been reported with oestrogen therapy in this condition.

• Oestrogens increase thyroid binding globulin (TBG), leading to increased circulating total thyroid hormone, as measured by protein-bound iodine (PBI), T4 levels (by column or by radio-immunoassay) or T3 levels (by radio-immunoassay). T3 resin uptake is decreased, reflecting the elevated TBG. Free T4 and free T3 concentrations are unaltered. Other binding proteins may be elevated in serum, i.e. corticoid binding globulin (CBG), sex-hormone-binding globulin (SHBG) leading to increased circulating corticosteroids and sex steroids, respectively. Free or biological active hormone concentrations are unchanged. Other plasma proteins may be increased (angiotensinogen/renin substrate, alpha-I-antitrypsin, ceruloplasmin).

• Chloasma may occasionally occur, especially in women with a history of chloasma gravidarum. Women with a tendency to chloasma should minimise exposure to the sun or ultraviolet radiation whilst taking HRT.

• There is no conclusive evidence for improvement of cognitive function. There is some evidence from the WHI trial of increased risk of probable dementia in women who start using continuous combined CEE and MPA after the age of 65. It is unknown whether the findings apply to younger postmenopausal women or other HRT products.

4.5 Interaction with other medicinal products and other forms of Interaction

The metabolism of oestrogens may be increased by concomitant use of substances known to induce drug-metabolising enzymes, specifically cytochrome P450 enzymes, such as anticonvulsants (e.g. phenobarbital, phenytoin, carbamezapin) and anti- infectives (e.g. rifampicin, rifabutin, nevirapine, efavirenz).

Ritonavir and nelfinavir, although known as strong inhibitors, by contrast exhibit inducing properties when used concomitantly with steroid hormones. Herbal preparations containing St. John's wort (Hypericum perforatum) may induce the metabolism of oestrogens.

At transdermal administration, the first-pass effect in the liver is avoided and, thus, transdermally applied oestrogens might be less affected than oral hormones by enzyme inducers.

Clinically, an increased metabolism of oestrogens and progestogens may lead to decreased effect and changes in the uterine bleeding profile.

4.6 Pregnancy and lactation

• **Pregnancy**

Progynova TS is not indicated during pregnancy. If pregnancy occurs during medication with Progynova TS treatment should be withdrawn immediately.

The results of most epidemiological studies to date relevant to inadvertent foetal exposure to oestrogens indicate no teratogenic or foetotoxic effects.

• **Lactation**

Progynova TS is not indicated during lactation.

4.7 Effects on ability to drive and use machines

None known.

4.8 Undesirable effects

During the first few months of treatment, breakthrough bleeding, spotting and breast tenderness or enlargement can occur. These are usually temporary and normally disappear after continued treatment. The table below lists adverse drug reactions recorded in clinical studies as well as adverse drug reactions reported post-marketing. Adverse drug reactions were recorded in 3 phase III clinical studies (n = 611 women at risk) and were included in the table when considered at least possibly related to treatment with 50 μg/day estradiol or 100 μg/day estradiol, respectively, following transdermal application.

The experience of adverse drug reactions is overall expected in 76% of the patients. Adverse drug reactions appearing in > 10% of patients in clinical trials were application site reactions and breast pain.

(see Table 1)

Table 1

Organ system	Adverse events reported in clinical trials		Adverse events reported post marketing
	Common (⩾ 1/100, < 1/10)	Uncommon (⩾ 1/1000, < 1/100)	
BODY AS A WHOLE	Pain.	Fatigue, abnormal laboratory test[1], asthenia[1], fever[1], flu syndrome[1], malaise[1].	
CARDIOVASCULAR SYSTEM	-	Migraine, palpitations, superficial phlebitis[1], hypertension[1].	
DIGESTIVE SYSTEM	Flatulence, nausea.	Increased appetite, constipation, dyspepsia[1], diarrhoea[1], rectal disorder[1].	Abdominal pain, bloating (abdominal distension), cholestatic jaundice
METABOLIC and NUTRITIONAL DISORDER	Oedema, weight gain.	Hypercholesteremia[1].	
HAEMATOLOGICAL and LYMPHATIC SYSTEM	-	Purpura[1].	
MUSCULOSKELETAL SYSTEM	-	Joint disorder, muscle cramps.	
RESPIRATORY SYSTEM	-	Dyspnoea[1], rhinitis[1].	
NERVOUS SYSTEM	Depression, dizziness, nervousness, lethargy, headache, increased sweating, hot flushes.	Anxiety, insomnia, apathy, emotional lability, impaired concentration, paraesthesia, libido changed, euphoria[1], tremor[1], agitation[1].	
SKIN and APPENDAGES	Application site pruritus, rash.	Acne, alopecia, dry skin, benign breast neoplasm, breast enlargement, breast tenderness, nail disorder[1], skin nodule[1], hirsutism[1]	Contact dermatitis, eczema, breast pain
UROGENITAL SYSTEM	Menstrual disorder, vaginal discharge, disorder of vulva/vagina.	Increased urinary frequency/urgency, benign endometrial neoplasm, endometrial hyperplasia, urinary incontinence[1], cystitis[1], urine discoloration[1], haematuria[1], uterine disorder[1].	Uterine fibroids
SPECIAL SENSES		Abnormal vision[1], dry eye[1]	

[1] have been reported in single cases. Given the small study population (n=611) it cannot be determined based on these results if the events are uncommon or rare.

Breast cancer

According to evidence from a large number of epidemiological studies and one randomised placebo-controlled trial, the Women's Health Initiative (WHI), the overall risk of breast cancer increases with increasing duration of HRT use in current or recent HRT users.

For *oestrogen-only* HRT, estimates of relative risk (RR) from a reanalysis of original data from 51 epidemiological studies (in which >80% of HRT use was oestrogen-only HRT) and from the epidemiological Million Women Study (MWS) are similar at 1.35 (95% CI 1.21-1.49) and 1.30 (95% CI 1.21-1.40), respectively.

For *oestrogen plus progestogen* combined HRT, several epidemiological studies have reported an overall higher risk for breast cancer than with oestrogens alone.

The MWS reported that, compared to never users, the use of various types of oestrogen-progestogen combined HRT was associated with a higher risk of breast cancer (RR = 2.00, 95% CI: 1.88-2.12) than use of oestrogens alone (RR = 1.30, 95% CI: 1.21-1.40) or use of tibolone (RR = 1.45, 95% CI 1.25-1.68).

The WHI trial reported a risk estimate of 1.24 (95% CI 1.01-1.54) after 5.6 years of use of oestrogen-progestogen combined HRT (CEE + MPA) in all users compared with placebo.

The absolute risks calculated from the MWS and the WHI trial are presented below:

The MWS has estimated, from the known average incidence of breast cancer in developed countries, that:

Ø For women not using HRT, about 32 in every 1000 are expected to have breast cancer diagnosed between the ages of 50 and 64 years.

Ø For 1000 current or recent users of HRT, the number of *additional* cases during the corresponding period will be

Ø For users of *oestrogen-only* replacement therapy

• between 0 and 3 (best estimate = 1.5) for 5 years' use

• between 3 and 7 (best estimate = 5) for 10 years' use.

Ø For users of *oestrogen plus progestogen* combined HRT,

• between 5 and 7 (best estimate = 6) for 5 years' use

• between 18 and 20 (best estimate = 19) for 10 years' use.

The WHI trial estimated that after 5.6 years of follow-up of women between the ages of 50 and 79 years, an *additional* 8 cases of invasive breast cancer would be due to *oestrogen-progestogen combined* HRT (CEE + MPA) per 10,000 women years. According to calculations from the trial data, it is estimated that:

Ø For 1000 women in the placebo group,

• about 16 cases of invasive breast cancer would be diagnosed in 5 years.

Ø For 1000 women who used *oestrogen + progestogen combined* HRT (CEE + MPA), the number of *additional* cases would be

• between 0 and 9 (best estimate = 4) for 5 years' use.

The number of additional cases of breast cancer in women who use HRT is broadly similar for women who start HRT irrespective of age at start of use (between the ages of 45-65) see section 4.4).

Endometrial cancer

In women with an intact uterus, the risk of endometrial hyperplasia and endometrial cancer increases with increasing duration of use of unopposed oestrogens. According to data from epidemiological studies, the best estimate of the risk is that for women not using HRT, about 5 in every 1000 are expected to have endometrial cancer diagnosed between the ages of 50 and 65. Depending on the duration of treatment and oestrogen dose, the reported increase in endometrial cancer risk among unopposed oestrogen users varies from 2- to 12-fold greater compared with non-users. Adding a progestogen to oestrogen-only therapy greatly reduces this increased risk.

Other adverse reactions have been reported in association with oestrogen/progestogen treatment:

- Oestrogen-dependent neoplasms benign and malignant, e.g. endometrial cancer.

- Venous thromboembolism, i.e. deep leg or pelvic venous thrombosis and pulmonary embolism, is more frequent among hormone replacement therapy users than among non-users. For further information, see section 4.3 Contra-indications and 4.4 Special warnings and precautions for use.

- Myocardial infarction and stroke (see also section 4.4).

- Gall bladder disease.

- Skin and subcutaneous disorders: chloasma, erythema multiforme, erythema nodosum, vascular purpura.

- Probable dementia (see section 4.4).

4.9 Overdose

Overdosage is unlikely with this type of application. Nausea, vomiting and withdrawal bleeding may occur in some women. There is no specific antidote and treatment should be symptomatic. The patch(es) should be removed.

5. PHARMACOLOGICAL PROPERTIES

5.1 Pharmacodynamic properties

Progynova TS contains synthetic 17β-estradiol, which is chemically and biologically identical to endogenous human estradiol. It substitutes for the loss of oestrogen production in menopausal women, and alleviates menopausal symptoms. Oestrogens prevent bone loss following menopause or ovariectomy.

• Relief of oestrogen-deficiency symptoms

- Relief of menopausal symptoms was achieved during the first few weeks of treatment.

• Prevention of osteoporosis

- Oestrogen deficiency at menopause is associated with an increasing bone turnover and decline in bone mass. The effect of oestrogens on the bone mineral density is dose-dependent. However, in clinical trials, the efficacy of Progynova TS 100 was not significantly better than the efficacy of Progynova TS 50 for the prevention of postmenopausal osteoporosis. Protection appears to be effective for as long as treatment is continued. After discontinuation of HRT, bone mass is lost at a rate similar to that in untreated women.

- Evidence from the WHI trial and meta-analysed trials shows that current use of HRT alone or in combination with a progestogen – given to predominantly healthy women – reduces the risk of hip, vertebral, and other osteoporotic fractures. HRT may also prevent fractures in women with low bone density and/or established osteoporosis, but the evidence for that is limited.

5.2 Pharmacokinetic properties

Absorption

After dermal application of Progynova TS, estradiol is continuously released and transported across intact skin leading to sustained circulating levels of estradiol during 7-day treatment period as shown in figure 1. The systemic availability of estradiol after transdermal administration is about 20 times higher than that after oral admin istration. This difference is due to the absence of first pass metabolism when estradiol is given by the transdermal route. The major pharmacokinetic parameters of estradiol are summarised in the following table:

(see Table 2 below)

Figure 1: Mean baseline uncorrected serum 17 β-estradiol concentrations vs. time profile following application of Progynova TS 50 and Progynova TS 100

(see Figure 1 below)

Distribution

The distribution of exogenous oestrogens is similar to that of endogenous oestrogens. The apparent volume of distribution of estradiol after single intravenous administration is about 1 l/kg. Oestrogens circulate in the blood largely bound to serum proteins. About 61 % of estradiol is bound non-specifically to serum albumin and about 37 % specifically to sex hormone binding globulin (SHBG).

Metabolism

After transdermal administration, the biotransformation of estradiol leads to concentrations of estrone and of the respective conjugates within the range as seen during the early follicular phase in the reproductive life period, indicated by an estradiol/estrone serum level ratio of approximately 1. Unphysiologically high estrone levels as a result of the intensive "first pass" metabolism during oral estradiol hormone replacement therapy, reflected in estradiol/estrone ratios as low as 0.1, are avoided.

The biotransformation of the transdermally administered estradiol is the same as that of the endogenous hormone: Estradiol is mainly metabolized in the liver but also extrahepatically e.g. in gut, kidney, skeletal muscles and target organs. These processes involve the formation of estrone, estriol, catecholoestrogens and sulfate and glucuronide conjugates of these compounds, which are less oestrogenic or even nonoestrogenic.

Excretion

The total serum clearance of estradiol following single intravenous administration, shows high variability in the range of 10-30 ml/min/kgEstradiol and its metabolites are excreted in the bile and undergo a so-called enterohepatic circulation. Ultimately estradiol its metabolites are mainly excreted as sulfates and glucuronides with the urine.

Steady-state conditions

Accumulation of estradiol and estrone was not observed following multiple 1-week patch applications. Accordingly, steady-state serum levels of estradiol and estrone correspond to those observed after a single application.

5.3 Preclinical safety data

In primary dermal irritation studies, application of Progynova TS patches resulted in mild irritation related to mechanical trauma at removal. Progynova TS patches had no dermal sensitising potential.

The components of the adhesive matrix of Progynova TS patches (monomer and polymer) have been studied extensively and, at many multiples of the projected human exposure, present a low risk. Additional excipients used in the adhesive matrix are either generally regarded as safe for use in food components or considered acceptable as an inactive ingredient for prescription and topical transdermal products.

The adhesive backing and release liner of Progynova TS patches were tested in biological test methods and were considered to be compatible with biologic systems.

6. PHARMACEUTICAL PARTICULARS

6.1 List of excipients

Isooctyl acrylate/acrylamide/vinyl acetate copolymer, ethyl oleate, isopropyl myristate, glycerol monolaurate mounted on a polyester release liner and protected with a polyethylene backing film.

6.2 Incompatibilities

None so far known.

6.3 Shelf life

3 years.

6.4 Special precautions for storage

Do not store unpouched. Apply immediately upon removal from the protective pouch.

6.5 Nature and contents of container

Protective pouch containing a patch with a surface area of 12.5 cm^2 or 25 cm^2. The patches comprise two layers. From the visible surface to the surface attached to the skin these are: a translucent polyethylene film; a drug reservoir of estradiol in an acrylate adhesive matrix; a protective liner of release-coated polyester film which is attached to the adhesive surface and must be removed prior to use.

Each patch is sealed in a multilaminate pouch containing a desiccant. The pouch consists of polyester film/aluminium foil/Barex 210 film.

Packs containing 4 patches.

Packs containing 12 patches.

6.6 Instructions for use and handling

The patch should be used according to the instructions under "Posology and method of administration" (Section 4.2).

Store all drugs properly and keep them out of reach of children.

Table 2

Transdermal Delivery System	Daily Delivery Rate, mg/day	Application Site	AUC(0-tlast) ngxh/mL / nmolxh/L	Cmax pg/mL / pmol/L	Cavg pg/mL / pmol/L	tmax h	Cmin pg/mL / pmol/L
Progynova TS 50	0.050	Abdomen	5.44 / 20	55 / 202	35 / 129	26	30 / 110
Progynova TS 100	0.100	Abdomen	11.5 / 42	110 / 404	70 / 257	31	56 / 206

Figure 1: Mean baseline uncorrected serum 17 β-estradiol concentrations vs. time profile following application of Progynova TS 50 and Progynova TS 100

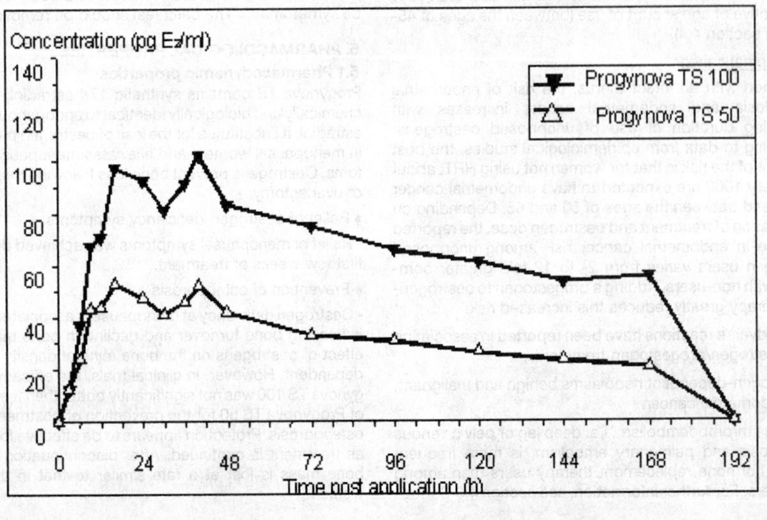

7. MARKETING AUTHORISATION HOLDER

Schering Health Care Limited
The Brow
Burgess Hill
West Sussex, RH15 9NE

8. MARKETING AUTHORISATION NUMBER(S)

Progynova TS 50: 0053/0241

Progynova TS 100: 0053/0242

9. DATE OF FIRST AUTHORISATION/RENEWAL OF THE AUTHORISATION

11th July 2000

10. DATE OF REVISION OF THE TEXT

8th March 2004

Legal category

POM

Proleukin powder for solution for infusion

(Chiron Corporation Limted)

1. NAME OF THE MEDICINAL PRODUCT

PROLEUKIN 18 × 10^6 IU

Powder for solution for infusion

2. QUALITATIVE AND QUANTITATIVE COMPOSITION

After reconstitution with 1.2 ml water for injection, according to the instructions (see section 6.6), each 1 ml solution contains 18 × 10^6 IU (1.1 mg) aldesleukin.

Each vial of Proleukin powder for solution for infusion contains 22 × 10^6 IU aldesleukin. Aldesleukin is produced by recombinant DNA technology using an *Escherichia coli* strain which contains a genetically engineered modification of the human Interleukin-2 (IL-2) gene.

For excipients, see section 6.1.

3. PHARMACEUTICAL FORM

Powder for solution for infusion.

The powder is sterile, white and lyophilized.

4. CLINICAL PARTICULARS

4.1 Therapeutic indications

Treatment of metastatic renal cell carcinoma.

Risk factors associated with decreased response rates and median survival are:

- A performance status of ECOG* 1 or greater
- More than one organ with metastatic disease sites
- A period of < 24 months between initial diagnosis of primary tumour and the date the patient is evaluated for Proleukin treatment.

*) ECOG (Eastern Cooperative Oncology Group) 0 = normal activity, 1 = symptoms but ambulatory; 2 = in bed less than 50% of time; 3 = in bed more than 50% of time.

Response rates and median survival decrease with the number of risk factors present. Patients positive for all three risk factors should not be treated with Proleukin.

4.2 Posology and method of administration

Proleukin should be administered intravenously by continuous infusion. The following dosage regimen is recommended to treat adult patients with metastatic renal cell carcinoma.

18 × 10^6 IU per m^2 per 24-hours as a continuous infusion for 5 days, followed by 2-6 days without active substance, an additional 5 days of intravenous Proleukin as a continuous infusion and 3 weeks without active substance. This constitutes one induction cycle. After the 3-week rest period of the first cycle, a second induction cycle should be given.

Up to four maintenance cycles (18 × 10^6 IU per m^2 as continuous infusion for 5 days) may be given with 4-week intervals to patients who respond or have disease stabilization.

If a patient cannot tolerate the recommended dosage regimen, the dose should be reduced or the administration interrupted until the toxicity has moderated. It is not known to what extent dose reduction affects response rates and median survival.

Elderly: Elderly patients may be more susceptible to the side effects of Proleukin and caution is recommended in the treatment of such patients.

Children: Safety and efficacy of Proleukin in children have not yet been established.

4.3 Contraindications

Proleukin therapy is contraindicated in the following patients:

1. Patients with hypersensitivity to the active substance or to any of the excipients.

2. Patients with a performance status of ECOG ⩾ 2*.

3. Patients with a simultaneous presence of a performance status of ECOG 1 or greater*) and more than one organ with metastatic disease sites and a period of < 24 months between initial diagnosis of primary tumour and the date the patient is evaluated for Proleukin treatment.

4. Patients with a significant history or current evidence of severe cardiac disease. In questionable cases a stress test should be performed.

5. Patients with evidence of active infection requiring antibiotic therapy.

6. Patients with a Pa O_2 < 60 mm Hg during rest.

7. Patients with pre-existing severe major organ dysfunction.

8. Patients with Central Nervous System (CNS) metastases or seizure disorders, with the exception of patients with successfully treated brain metastases (negative computerized tomography (CT); neurologically stable).

In addition, it is recommended to exclude the following patients:

1. Patients with White Blood Count (WBC) < 4.000/mm^3; platelets < 100.000/mm^3; hematocrit (HCT) < 30%.

2. Patients with serum bilirubin and creatinine outside normal range.

3. Patients with organ allografts.

4. Patients who are likely to require corticosteroids.

5. Patients with pre-existing auto-immune disease.

*) ECOG: see section 4.1.

4.4 Special warnings and special precautions for use

Patient screening

See also section 4.3.

Clinical studies have shown that patients with metastatic renal cell carcinoma can be divided into 4 distinct risk groups, predictive for survival and to some extent response, following Proleukin therapy. The 4 risk groups are defined by the number of risk factors present at treatment start: the very low risk group has no risk factor, the low risk group one risk factor, the median group any combination of 2 risk factors, and the high risk group has the simultaneous presence of all 3 risk factors. Response rates and median survival decrease with the number of risk factors present. Patients positive for all three risk factors should not be treated with Proleukin.

Risk factors associated with decreased response rates and median survival are:

- A performance status of ECOG 1 or greater
- More than one organ with metastatic disease sites
- A period of < 24 months between initial diagnosis of primary tumour and the date the patient is evaluated for Proleukin treatment.

Warnings

It is recommended to exclude the following patients from treatment with Proleukin:

1. Patients with White Blood Count (WBC) < 4,000/mm^3; platelets < 100,000/mm^3; hematocrit (HCT) < 30%.

2. Patients with serum bilirubin and creatinine outside normal range.

3. Patients who are likely to require corticosteroids.

4. Patients with pre-existing auto-immune disease.

Proleukin administration has been associated with capillary leak syndrome (CLS), which is characterized by a loss of vascular tone and extravasation of plasma proteins and fluid into the extravascular space. CLS results in hypotension and reduced organ perfusion. Severe CLS resulting in death has been reported. Capillary leak syndrome usually begins within hours after initiation of Proleukin treatment. The frequency and severity are lower after subcutaneous administration than with continuous intravenous infusion. In some patients hypotension resolves without therapy. In others, treatment is required with cautious use of intravenous fluids, albumin or, in more refractory cases, low-dose dopamine. If these measures are not successful, the Proleukin therapy should be interrupted.

If intravenous fluids are administered, care must be taken to weigh potential benefits of the expansion of intravascular volume against the risk of pulmonary oedema secondary to capillary leakage.

Proleukin may exacerbate pre-existing autoimmune disease, resulting in life threatening complications. Because not all patients who develop interleukin-2-associated autoimmune phenomena have a pre-existing history of autoimmune disease, awareness and close monitoring for thyroid abnormalities or other potentially autoimmune phenomena is warranted. A few patients with quiescent Crohn's disease had activation of their disease following treatment with Proleukin, requiring surgical intervention.

Proleukin administration should be discontinued in patients developing severe lethargy or somnolence; continued administration may result in coma.

Pulmonary function should be monitored closely in patients who develop rales or increased respiratory rate, or who complain of dyspnoea. Some patients may require intubation for management of transient respiratory failure. Intubation has only been reported for patients treated with intravenous Proleukin.

Patients may experience mental status changes including irritability, confusion, or depression while receiving Proleukin. Although generally reversible when administration of medicinal product is discontinued, these mental status changes may persist for several days. Proleukin may alter patient response to psychotropic medicinal products (see section 4.5).

Since Proleukin administration results in reversible elevation of hepatic transaminases, serum bilirubin, serum urea and serum creatinine, patients with pre-existing renal or hepatic dysfunction should be closely monitored. Renal or hepatic metabolism or excretion of concomitantly administered medicinal products may be altered by the administration of Proleukin. Other medicinal products with known nephrotoxic or hepatotoxic potential should be used with caution (see section 4.5).

There is a possibility of disturbances in the glucose metabolism in diabetes patients when Proleukin is administered subcutaneously.

Precautions for use

Proleukin should only be used under the supervision of a qualified physician, experienced in the use of cancer chemotherapeutic agents. It is recommended that patients are admitted to a specialized unit having the facilities of an intensive care unit for monitoring the patient's relevant clinical and laboratory parameters.

Should serious adverse events occur, dosage should be modified according to section 4.2. It is important to note that adverse reactions, although sometimes serious or in rare cases life-threatening, are manageable and usually, although not invariably, resolve within 1 or 2 days of cessation of Proleukin therapy. The decision to resume therapy should be based on the severity and spectrum of the clinical toxicity.

Proleukin may exacerbate disease symptoms in patients with clinically unrecognized or untreated CNS metastases. All patients should have adequate evaluation and treatment of CNS metastases prior to receiving Proleukin therapy.

Proleukin may exacerbate effusions from serosal surfaces. Consideration should be given to treating these prior to initiation of Proleukin therapy, particularly when effusions are located in anatomic sites where worsening may lead to impairment of major organ function (e.g. pericardial effusions).

Baseline electrocardiogram (ECG) (+ stress test if indicated), performance status, vital signs, objective evaluation for coronary vascular disease and, in patients with a history of smoking or respiratory disease, pulmonary function tests with arterial blood gases are recommended as adjuncts to history and physical examination in the pretreatment evaluation of patients.

Pre-existing bacterial infections should be treated prior to initiation of Proleukin therapy. Toxicities associated with Proleukin administration may be exacerbated by concurrent bacterial infection.

Administration of Proleukin may be associated with an increased incidence and/or severity of bacterial infection, including septicaemia, bacterial endocarditis, septic thrombophlebitis, peritonitis and pneumonia. This has mainly been reported after intravenous administration. Except for several cases due to *Escherichia coli*, causative organisms have been *Staphylococcus aureus* or *Staphylococcus epidermidis*. During continuous intravenous infusion of Proleukin an increased incidence and/or severity of local catheter site infection has been reported. Patients with central lines in place should be treated prophylactically with antibiotics.

Proleukin administration results in fever and gastrointestinal adverse reactions in most patients treated at the recommended dose. Concomitant therapy with paracetamol can be instituted at the time of Proleukin administration to reduce fever. Pethidine may be added to control the rigours associated with fever. Anti-emetics and antidiarrhoeals may be used as needed to treat other gastrointestinal adverse reactions. Some patients with pruritic rash benefit from concomitant administration of antihistamines.

Laboratory and clinical tests: In addition to those tests normally required for monitoring patients with metastatic renal cell carcinoma, the following tests are recommended for all patients on Proleukin therapy, prior to beginning treatment and then periodically thereafter:

- *Standard haematologic tests* – including WBC (with differential and platelet counts). Proleukin administration may cause anaemia and thrombocytopenia.

- *Blood chemistry* - including fluid and electrolyte balance, renal and hepatic function tests. Proleukin may cause renal dysfunction with oliguria, and reversible elevation of hepatic transaminases, serum bilirubin, serum urea and serum creatinine.

- *Chest x-rays.*

4.5 Interaction with other medicinal products and other forms of Interaction

Fatal Tumour Lysis Syndrome has been reported in combination with treatment with cis-platinum, vinblastine and dacarbazine. Concomitant use of the mentioned active substances is therefore not recommended.

Severe rhabdomyolysis and myocardial injury, including myocardial infarction, myocarditis and ventricular hypokinesia appear to be increased in patients receiving Proleukin (intravenously) and interferon-alpha concurrently.

There has also been exacerbation or the initial presentation of a number of autoimmune and inflammatory disorders observed following concurrent use of interferon-alpha and Proleukin, including crescentic immunoglobulin A (IgA) glomerulonephritis, oculo-bulbar myasthenia gravis, inflammatory arthritis, thyroiditis, bullous pemphigoid, and Stevens-Johnson syndrome.

Concomitantly administered glucocorticoids may decrease the activity of Proleukin. However, patients who develop life-threatening signs or symptoms may be treated with dexamethasone until toxicity resolves to an acceptable level.

Concurrent administration of medicinal products with hepatotoxic, nephrotoxic, myelotoxic, or cardiotoxic effects may increase the toxicity of Proleukin in these systems.

Antihypertensive agents, such as beta-blockers, may potentiate the hypotension seen with Proleukin.

Renal or hepatic metabolism or excretion of concomitantly administered medicinal products may be altered by the administration of Proleukin. Other medicinal products with known nephrotoxic or hepatotoxic potential should be used with caution (see section 4.4).

Proleukin may affect central nervous function. Therefore, interactions could occur following concomitant administration of centrally acting medicinal products. Proleukin may alter patient response to psychotropic medicinal products (see section 4.4).

Use of contrast media after Proleukin administration may result in a recall of the toxicity observed during Proleukin administration. Most events were reported to occur within 2 weeks after the last dose of Proleukin, but some occurred months later.

Hypersensitivity reactions have been reported in patients receiving combination regimens containing sequential high dose Proleukin and antineoplastic agents, specifically, dacarbazine, cis-platinum, tamoxifen and interferon-alpha. These reactions consisted of erythema, pruritus, and hypotension and occurred within hours of administration of chemotherapy. These events required medical intervention in some patients.

4.6 Pregnancy and lactation

Both sexually active men and women should use effective methods of contraception during treatment.

There are no adequate data on the use of aldesleukin in pregnant women.

Experimental animal studies are insufficient to assess the safety with respect to reproduction, development of the embryo or foetus, the course of gestation and peri- and postnatal development. Proleukin has been shown to have embryolethal and maternal toxic effects in rats. (see also section 5.3). The potential risk for humans is unknown.

Proleukin should not be used during pregnancy unless the potential benefit to the patient justifies the potential risk to the foetus.

It is not known whether this drug is excreted in human milk. Because the potential for serious adverse reactions in nursing infants is unknown, mothers should not breast feed their infants during treatment.

4.7 Effects on ability to drive and use machines

Proleukin causes adverse events that affect the ability to drive and operate machines.

Patients should not drive or operate machines until they have recovered from the undesirable effects.

4.8 Undesirable effects

Frequency and severity of adverse reactions to Proleukin have generally been shown to be dependent on dose and schedule. For information on the toxicity of subcutaneous use review the Summary of Product Characteristics (SPC) of Proleukin powder for solution for injection.

Most adverse reactions are self-limited and might reverse within 1 to 2 days of discontinuation of therapy. A small number of patients (3%) died of treatment related adverse reactions.

Explanatory table of frequency of undesirable effects

Very common	> 1/10
Common	> 1/100 but < 1/10
Uncommon	> 1/1,000 but < 1/100
Rare	> 1/10,000 but < 1/1,000
Very rare	< 1/10,000

(see Table 1 on next page)

Additional information

Cardiac arrhythmias (supraventricular and ventricular), angina pectoris, myocardial infarction, respiratory insufficiency requiring intubation, gastrointestinal bleeding or infarction, renal insufficiency, oedema and mental status changes may be associated with capillary leak syndrome (see section 4.4). The frequency and severity of capillary leak syndrome are lower after subcutaneous administration than with continuous intravenous infusion.

Cerebral vasculitis, both isolated and in combination with other manifestations, has been reported. Cutaneous and

Table 1

System	Very common	Common	Uncommon	Rare
Cardiovascular	mild to severe hypotension, mild to severe tachycardia	mild to severe arrhythmia, hypertension, phlebitis	angina pectoris, thrombosis, palpitations, transient ECG changes, cardiovascular disorders including myocardial infarction, myocarditis, cardiomyopathy	ventricular hypokinesia, pulmonary embolism
Kidneys	mild to severe oliguria with elevated serum urea and serum creatinine	haematuria	renal failure	
Respiratory tract	mild to severe dyspnoea, cough	mild to severe pulmonary oedema, mild to severe cyanosis, hypoxia, respiratory tract infection, mild to severe pleural effusions	haemoptysis	adult respiratory distress syndrome
Liver		mild to severe hyperbilirubinemia, mild to severe elevation of hepatic transaminases and alkaline phosphatase		
Gastrointestinal tract	mild to severe nausea with or without vomiting, mild to moderate diarrhoea, mild to severe anorexia	dysphagia, dyspepsia, constipation, gastrointestinal bleeding (including rectal hemorrhage), haematemesis		gastritis, cholecystitis, activation of quiescent Crohn's disease
Blood*	mild to severe anaemia, mild to severe thrombocytopenia	mild to moderate leucopenia, moderate coagulation disorders	epistaxis, haemorrhage	
Nervous system	moderate to severe anxiety, mild to severe confusion, mild to severe dizziness, mild to severe somnolence	mental status changes including irritability, moderate to severe agitation, paraesthesia, syncope, depression, hallucinations, speech disorders	mild to severe central or peripheral motor neurological disorders, paralysis	convulsions, lethargy, coma, cortical lesions
Abnormal laboratory findings		hyperglycaemia, hypocalcaemia, hyperkalaemia	hypo- or hyperthyroidism	
Skin and mucous membranes	mild to severe erythema/rash, mild to severe pruritus, mild to severe skin exfoliation	mild to moderate conjunctivitis, mild to moderate mucositis, alopecia, nasal congestion	mild to severe vitiligo	
Other adverse reactions	mild to moderate weight gain with oedema, mild to severe fever with or without chills, mild to severe malaise and fatigue, mild to severe headache	moderate to severe pain, moderate to severe arthralgia, myalgia, ascitis		hypersensitivity reactions, anaphylaxis, diabetes mellitus

* Note: During treatment most patients experience lymphocytopenia and eosinophilia, with a rebound lymphocytosis within 24-48 hours following treatment. These are not considered adverse reactions and may be related to the mechanism of antitumour activity of Proleukin.

leukocytoplastic hypersensitivity vasculitis has been reported. Some of these cases are responsive to corticosteroids.

The following undesirable effects have been reported rarely in association with concurrent interferon alpha treatment: crescentic IgA glomerulonephritis, oculo-bulbar myasthenia gravis, inflammatory arthritis, thyroiditis, bullous pemphigoid, rhabdomyolysis and Stevens-Johnson syndrome. Severe rhabdomyolysis and myocardial injury, including myocardial infarction, myocarditis and ventricular hypokinesia appear to be increased in patients receiving Proleukin (intravenously) and interferon-alpha concurrently (see section 4.5).

Bacterial infection or exacerbation of bacterial infection, including septicaemia, bacterial endocarditis, septic thrombophlebitis, peritonitis, pneumonia, and local catheter site infection has been reported (see section 4.4).

Liver failure with fatal outcome, haemolytic anaemia, agranulocytosis, aplastic anaemia, serious coagulation disorders (including Disseminated Intravascular Coagulation), optic neuropathy, Stevens-Johnson syndrome have been reported rarely after subcutaneous administration.

4.9 Overdose

Adverse reactions following the use of Proleukin are dose-related.

Therefore patients can be expected to experience these events in an exaggerated fashion when the recommended dose is exceeded.

Adverse reactions generally will reverse when the medicinal product is stopped. Any continuing symptoms should be treated supportively.

5. PHARMACOLOGICAL PROPERTIES

5.1 Pharmacodynamic properties

ATC classification system: immunostimulants, cytokines and immunomodulators, interleukins, aldesleukin

ATC code: L03A C01

Proleukin acts as a regulator of the immune response. The biological activities of aldesleukin and native human IL-2, a naturally occurring lymphokine, are comparable.

The administration of aldesleukin in murine tumour models has been shown to reduce both tumour growth and spread. The exact mechanism by which aldesleukin-mediated immunostimulation leads to antitumour activity is not yet known.

5.2 Pharmacokinetic properties

Absorption

The serum half-life curves of aldesleukin in humans following short intravenous (bolus) administration can be described as bi-exponential. The half-life in the α phase is 13 minutes and the half-life in the β phase is 85 minutes. The α phase accounts for clearance of 87% of a bolus injection. Observed serum levels are proportional to the dose of aldesleukin.

The subcutaneous kinetics can be described by a one-compartment model. The IL-2 absorption half-life is 45 minutes, while the elimination half-life is 5.3 hours. The longer half-life estimate, compared with the intravenous result is probably due to continued absorption of IL-2 from the subcutaneous injection site during the plasma elimination phase. Absolute bioavailability ranges between 35-47%.

Elimination

The kidney is the major clearance route of recombinant IL-2 (rIL-2) in animals, and most of the injected dose is metabolized in the kidney with no biologically active aldesleukin appearing in the urine. A secondary elimination pathway is receptor- mediated uptake. This active process is induced after chronic dosing. After an aldesleukin-free period between dosing cycles, the clearance of IL-2 is restored to its original value.

The observed clearance rates in humans after short intravenous infusion (15 minutes) and after 24-hour continuous intravenous infusion approximate renal glomerular filtration clearance and range from 140-300 ml/min.

5.3 Preclinical safety data

Animal studies are insufficient with respect to effects on fertility, embryo/foetal development and peri- and post-natal development. In a study with intravenous application of Proleukin in rats maternal toxicity and an increased embryolethality was seen in all tested dose-groups (0.5-2mg/kg/day).

6. PHARMACEUTICAL PARTICULARS

6.1 List of excipients

Mannitol (E421)

Sodium dodecyl sulphate

Sodium dihydrogen phosphate (pH adjuster)

Disodium hydrogen phosphate (pH adjuster)

6.2 Incompatibilities

Reconstitution and dilution procedures other than those recommended may result in incomplete delivery of bioactivity and/or formation of biologically inactive protein.

Use of Bacteriostatic Water for Injection or Sodium Chloride Injection 0.9% should be avoided because of increased aggregation.

Proleukin must not be mixed with other medicinal products except those mentioned in section 6.6.

It is recommended that devices or administration sets containing in-line filters are not used for delivery of Proleukin. Bioassays have shown significant loss of aldesleukin when filters are used.

6.3 Shelf life

2 years

After reconstitution: 24 hours

Diluted Proleukin should be used within 48 hours after reconstitution, which includes the time taken for infusion.

6.4 Special precautions for storage

Store at 2 to 8 °C (in a refrigerator). Do not freeze.

When reconstituted and diluted according to the directions, chemical and physical in-use stability has been demonstrated for up to 48 hours when stored at refrigerated and room temperatures (2 to 30 °C).

From a microbiological point of view, the reconstituted product should be used immediately. If not used immediately, in-use storage times and conditions prior to use are the responsibility of the user and would normally not be longer than 24 hours at 2 to 8 °C, unless reconstitution / dilution has taken place in controlled and validated aseptic conditions.

6.5 Nature and contents of container

Proleukin is supplied in 5 ml single-use clear Type I glass vials with a stopper of synthetic rubber. The product is supplied in carton boxes of 1 or 10 vials.

Not all pack sizes may be marketed.

6.6 Instructions for use and handling

Reconstitution of Proleukin powder for solution for infusion:

Vials must be reconstituted with 1.2 ml of Water for Injections. After reconstitution the obtained solution contains 18 million IU aldesleukin per millilitre. The reconstituted solution has a pH of 7.5 (range 7.2 – 7.8).

Using sterilised injection syringe and injection needle, inject 1.2 ml Water for Injections into the vial of Proleukin. Direct the diluent against the side of the vial to avoid excessive foaming. Swirl gently to facilitate complete dissolution of the powder. Do not shake. The appropriate dose can then be withdrawn with a sterile injection syringe and diluted for administration.

As for all parenteral medicinal products, inspect the reconstituted solution visually for particulate matter and discoloration prior to administration.

The solution may be slightly yellow.

The product should be brought to room temperature prior to administration.

Dilution directions:

The total daily dose of reconstituted aldesleukin should be diluted as necessary to up to 500 ml with glucose 50 mg/ml (5%) solution for infusion containing 1 mg/ml (0.1%) human albumin, and infused over a 24-hour period.

Order of addition: human albumin should be added and mixed with the glucose solution prior to the addition of the reconstituted aldesleukin. Human albumin is added to protect against loss of bioactivity.

For single use only. Any unused solution, the vial, and the syringe used for the reconstituted solution should be adequately disposed of, in accordance with local requirements for the handling of biohazardous waste.

7. MARKETING AUTHORISATION HOLDER

Chiron B.V.

Paasheuvelweg 30

1105 BJ Amsterdam

The Netherlands

8. MARKETING AUTHORISATION NUMBER(S)

PL 08800/0002

9. DATE OF FIRST AUTHORISATION/RENEWAL OF THE AUTHORISATION

January 29, 1992/ December 1, 1999

10. DATE OF REVISION OF THE TEXT

November 2004

Proleukin powder for solution for injection

(Chiron Corporation Limted)

1. NAME OF THE MEDICINAL PRODUCT

PROLEUKIN 18 × 10^6 IU

Powder for solution for injection

2. QUALITATIVE AND QUANTITATIVE COMPOSITION

After reconstitution with 1.2 ml water for injection, according to the instructions (see section 6.6), each 1 ml solution contains 18 × 10^6 IU (1.1 mg) aldesleukin.

Each vial of Proleukin powder for solution for injection contains 22 × 10^6 IU aldesleukin. Aldesleukin is produced by recombinant DNA technology using an *Escherichia coli* strain which contains a genetically engineered modification of the human Interleukin-2 (IL-2) gene.

For excipients, see section 6.1.

3. PHARMACEUTICAL FORM

Powder for solution for injection

The powder is sterile, white and lyophilized.

4. CLINICAL PARTICULARS

4.1 Therapeutic indications

Treatment of metastatic renal cell carcinoma.

Risk factors associated with decreased response rates and median survival are:

- A performance status of ECOG* 1 or greater
- More than one organ with metastatic disease sites
- A period of < 24 months between initial diagnosis of primary tumour and the date the patient is evaluated for Proleukin treatment.

*) ECOG (Eastern Cooperative Oncology Group) 0 = normal activity, 1 = symptoms but ambulatory; 2 = in bed less than 50% of time; 3 = in bed more than 50% of time.

Response rates and median survival decrease with the number of risk factors present. Patients positive for all three risk factors should not be treated with Proleukin.

4.2 Posology and method of administration

Proleukin will be administered by subcutaneous injection (s.c.). The following dosage regimen is recommended to treat adult patients with metastatic renal cell carcinoma.

18 × 10^6 IU as subcutaneous (s.c.) injection every day for 5 days, followed by 2 days rest. For the following 3 weeks 18 × 10^6 IU s.c. on days 1 and 2 of each week followed by 9 × 10^6 IU on days 3-5. On days 6 and 7 no treatment is administered. After 1 week rest this 4-week cycle should be repeated.

Maintenance cycles as described above may be given to patients who respond or have disease stabilisation.

If a patient cannot tolerate the recommended dosage regimen, the dose should be reduced or the administration interrupted until the toxicity has moderated. It is not known to what extent dose reduction affects response rates and median survival.

Elderly: Elderly patients may be more susceptible to the side effects of Proleukin and caution is recommended in the treatment of such patients.

Children: Safety and efficacy of Proleukin in children have not yet been established.

4.3 Contraindications

Proleukin therapy is contraindicated in the following patients:

1. Patients with hypersensitivity to the active substance or to any of the excipients.

2. Patients with a performance status of ECOG ⩾ 2*.

3. Patients with a simultaneous presence of a performance status of ECOG 1 or greater* <u>and</u> more than one organ with metastatic disease sites <u>and</u> a period of < 24 months between initial diagnosis of primary tumour and the date the patient is evaluated for Proleukin treatment.

4. Patients with a significant history or current evidence of severe cardiac disease. In questionable cases a stress test should be performed.

5. Patients with evidence of active infection requiring antibiotic therapy.

6. Patients with a Pa O_2 < 60 mm Hg during rest.

7. Patients with pre-existing severe major organ dysfunction.

8. Patients with Central Nervous System (CNS) metastases or seizure disorders, with the

9. exception of patients with successfully treated brain metastases (negative computerized tomography (CT); neurologically stable).

In addition, it is recommended to exclude the following patients:

1. Patients with White Blood Count (WBC) < 4.000/mm^3; platelets < 100.000/mm^3; hematocrit (HCT) < 30%.

2. Patients with serum bilirubin and creatinine outside normal range.

3. Patients with organ allografts.

4. Patients who are likely to require corticosteroids.

5. Patients with pre-existing auto-immune disease.

*) ECOG: see section 4.1.

4.4 Special warnings and special precautions for use

<u>Patient screening</u>

See also section 4.3.

Clinical studies have shown that patients with metastatic renal cell carcinoma can be divided into 4 distinct risk groups, predictive for survival and to some extent response, following Proleukin therapy. The 4 risk groups are defined by the number of risk factors present at treatment start: the very low risk group has no risk factor, the low risk group one risk factor, the median group any combination of 2 risk factors, and the high risk group has the simultaneous presence of all 3 risk factors. Response rates and median survival decrease with the number of risk factors present. Patients positive for all three risk factors should not be treated with Proleukin.

Risk factors associated with decreased response rates and median survival are:

- A performance status of ECOG 1 or greater
- More than one organ with metastatic disease sites
- A period of < 24 months between initial diagnosis of primary tumour and the date the patient is evaluated for Proleukin treatment.

<u>Warnings</u>

It is recommended to exclude the following patients from treatment with Proleukin:

1. Patients with White Blood Count (WBC) < 4,000/mm^3; platelets < 100,000/mm^3; haematocrit (HCT) < 30%.

2. Patients with serum bilirubin and creatinine outside normal range.

3. Patients who are likely to require corticosteroids.

4. Patients with pre-existing auto-immune disease.

Proleukin administration has been associated with capillary leak syndrome (CLS), which is characterized by a loss of vascular tone and extravasation of plasma proteins and fluid into the extravascular space. CLS results in hypotension and reduced organ perfusion. Severe CLS resulting in death has been reported. Capillary leak syndrome usually begins within hours after initiation of Proleukin treatment. The frequency and severity are lower after subcutaneous administration than with continuous intravenous infusion. In some patients hypotension resolves without therapy. In others, treatment is required with cautious use of intravenous fluids, albumin or, in more refractory cases, low-dose dopamine. If these measures are not successful, the Proleukin therapy should be interrupted.

If intravenous fluids are administered, care must be taken to weigh potential benefits of the expansion of intravascular volume against the risk of pulmonary oedema secondary to capillary leakage.

Proleukin may exacerbate pre-existing autoimmune disease, resulting in life threatening complications. Because not all patients who develop interleukin-2-associated autoimmune phenomena have a pre-existing history of autoimmune disease, awareness and close monitoring for thyroid abnormalities or other potentially autoimmune phenomena is warranted. A few patients with quiescent Crohn's disease had activation of their disease following treatment with Proleukin, requiring surgical intervention.

Proleukin administration should be discontinued in patients developing severe lethargy or somnolence; continued administration may result in coma.

Pulmonary function should be monitored closely in patients who develop rales or increased respiratory rate, or who complain of dyspnoea. Some patients may require intubation for management of transient respiratory failure. Intubation has only been reported for patients treated with intravenous Proleukin.

Patients may experience mental status changes including irritability, confusion, or depression while receiving Proleukin. Although generally reversible when administration of medicinal product is discontinued, these mental status changes may persist for several days. Proleukin may alter patient response to psychotropic medicinal products (see section 4.5).

Since Proleukin administration results in reversible elevation of hepatic transaminases, serum bilirubin, serum urea and serum creatinine, patients with pre-existing renal or hepatic dysfunction should be closely monitored. Renal or hepatic metabolism or excretion of concomitantly administered medicinal products may be altered by the administration of Proleukin. Other medicinal products with known nephrotoxic or hepatotoxic potential should be used with caution (see section 4.5).

There is a possibility of disturbances in the glucose metabolism in diabetes patients when Proleukin is administered subcutaneously.

<u>Precautions for use</u>

Proleukin should only be used under the supervision of a qualified physician, experienced in the use of cancer chemotherapeutic agents. Subcutaneous treatment can be administered in an outpatient setting by qualified health care professionals.

Should serious adverse events occur, dosage should be modified according to 4.2. It is important to note that adverse reactions, although sometimes serious or in rare cases life-threatening, are manageable and usually, although not invariably, resolve within 1 or 2 days of cessation of Proleukin therapy. The decision to resume therapy should be based on the severity and spectrum of the clinical toxicity.

Proleukin may exacerbate disease symptoms in patients with clinically unrecognized or untreated CNS metastases. All patients should have adequate evaluation and treatment of CNS metastases prior to receiving Proleukin therapy.

Proleukin may exacerbate effusions from serosal surfaces. Consideration should be given to treating these prior to initiation of Proleukin therapy, particularly when effusions are located in anatomic sites where worsening may lead to impairment of major organ function (e.g. pericardial effusions).

Baseline electrocardiogram (ECG) (+ stress test if indicated), performance status, vital signs, objective evaluation for coronary vascular disease and, in patients with a history of smoking or respiratory disease, pulmonary function tests with arterial blood gases are recommended as adjuncts to history and physical examination in the pretreatment evaluation of patients.

Pre-existing bacterial infections should be treated prior to initiation of Proleukin therapy. Toxicities associated with Proleukin administration may be exacerbated by concurrent bacterial infection.

Administration of Proleukin may be associated with an increased incidence and/or severity of bacterial infection, including septicaemia, bacterial endocarditis, septic thrombophlebitis, peritonitis and pneumonia. This has mainly been reported after intravenous administration. Except for several cases due to *Escherichia coli*, causative organisms have been *Staphylococcus aureus* or *Staphylococcus epidermidis*. In patients on subcutaneous treatment injection site reactions are common, sometimes with necrosis. The effects can be reduced by changing the injection site over the body.

Proleukin administration results in fever and gastrointestinal adverse reactions in most patients treated at the recommended dose. Concomitant therapy with paracetamol can be instituted at the time of Proleukin administration to reduce fever. Pethidine may be added to control the rigours associated with fever. Anti-emetics and antidiarrhoeals may be used as needed to treat other gastrointestinal adverse reactions. Some patients with pruritic rash benefit from concomitant administration of antihistamines.

<u>*Laboratory and clinical tests:*</u> In addition to those tests normally required for monitoring patients with metastatic renal cell carcinoma, the following tests are recommended for all patients on Proleukin therapy, prior to beginning treatment and then periodically thereafter:

- *Standard haematologic tests* – including WBC (with differential and platelet counts). Proleukin administration may cause anaemia and thrombocytopenia.
- *Blood chemistry* - including fluid and electrolyte balance, renal and hepatic function tests. Proleukin may cause renal dysfunction with oliguria, and reversible elevation of hepatic transaminases, serum bilirubin, serum urea and serum creatinine.
- *Chest x-rays.*

4.5 Interaction with other medicinal products and other forms of Interaction

Fatal Tumour Lysis Syndrome has been reported in combination with treatment with cis-platinum, vinblastine and dacarbazine. Concomitant use of the mentioned active substances is therefore not recommended.

Severe rhabdomyolysis and myocardial injury, including myocardial infarction, myocarditis and ventricular hypokinesia appear to be increased in patients receiving Proleukin (intravenously) and interferon-alpha concurrently.

There has also been exacerbation or the initial presentation of a number of autoimmune and inflammatory disorders observed following concurrent use of interferon-alpha and Proleukin, including crescentic immunoglobulin A (IgA) glomerulonephritis, oculo-bulbar myasthenia gravis, inflammatory arthritis, thyroiditis, bullous pemphigoid, and Stevens-Johnson syndrome.

Concomitantly administered glucocorticoids may decrease the activity of Proleukin. However, patients who develop life-threatening signs or symptoms may be treated with dexamethasone until toxicity resolves to an acceptable level.

Concurrent administration of medicinal products with hepatotoxic, nephrotoxic, myelotoxic, or cardiotoxic effects may increase the toxicity of Proleukin in these systems.

Antihypertensive agents, such as beta-blockers, may potentiate the hypotension seen with Proleukin.

Renal or hepatic metabolism or excretion of concomitantly administered medicinal products may be altered by the administration of Proleukin. Other medicinal products with known nephrotoxic or hepatotoxic potential should be used with caution (see section 4.4).

Proleukin may affect central nervous function. Therefore, interactions could occur following concomitant administration of centrally acting medicinal products. Proleukin may alter patient response to psychotropic medicinal products (see section 4.4).

Use of contrast media after Proleukin administration may result in a recall of the toxicity observed during Proleukin administration. Most events were reported to occur within 2 weeks after the last dose of Proleukin, but some occurred months later.

Hypersensitivity reactions have been reported in patients receiving combination regimens containing sequential high dose Proleukin and antineoplastic agents, specifically, dacarbazine, cis-platinum, tamoxifen and interferon-alpha. These reactions consisted of erythema, pruritus, and hypotension and occurred within hours of administration of chemotherapy. These events required medical intervention in some patients.

4.6 Pregnancy and lactation

Both sexually active men and women should use effective methods of contraception during treatment.

There are no adequate data from the use of aldesleukin in pregnant women.

Experimental animal studies are insufficient to assess the safety with respect to reproduction, development of the embryo or foetus, the course of gestation and peri- and postnatal development. Proleukin has been shown to have embryolethal and maternal toxic effects in rats. (see also section 5.3).

The potential risk for humans is unknown.

Proleukin should not be used during pregnancy unless the potential benefit to the patient justifies the potential risk to the foetus.

It is not known whether this drug is excreted in human milk. Because the potential for serious adverse reactions in nursing infants is unknown, mothers should not breast feed their infants during treatment.

4.7 Effects on ability to drive and use machines

Proleukin causes adverse events that affect the ability to drive and operate machines. Patients should not drive or operate machines until they have recovered from the undesirable effects.

4.8 Undesirable effects

Frequency and severity of adverse reactions to Proleukin have generally been shown to be dependent on dose and schedule. For information on the toxicity of intravenous use review the Summary of Product Characteristics (SPC) of Proleukin powder for solution for infusion.

Most adverse reactions are self-limited and might reverse within 1 to 2 days of discontinuation of therapy. A small number of patients (less than 1%) died of treatment related adverse reactions.

Explanatory table of frequency of undesirable effects

Very common	> 1/10
Common	> 1/100 but < 1/10
Uncommon	> 1/1,000 but < 1/100
Rare	> 1/10,000 but < 1/1,000
Very rare	< 1/10,000

(see Table 1)

Table 1

System	Very common	Common	Uncommon	Rare
Cardiovascular	hypotension, chest pain including angina pectoris	hypertension, tachycardia	arrhythmia, cardiovascular disorder, myocardial ischaemia, myocardial infarct	cardiovascular disorders including heart failure, (thrombo-) phlebitis, pulmonary embolism
Kidneys		elevated serum urea and serum creatinine, oliguria	haematuria, renal failure	
Respiratory tract	dyspnoea, cough		respiratory tract infection	pulmonary oedema, pleural effusions
Liver		elevation of hepatic transaminases, alkaline phosphatase and lactic dehydrogenase	hyperbilirubinaemia	liver failure with fatal outcome
Gastrointestinal tract	nausea with or without vomiting, diarrhoea, anorexia, stomatitis	constipation, gastrointestinal bleeding	cheilitis, gastritis	pancreatitis, intestinal obstruction
Blood*		anaemia, thrombocytopenia, leucopenia	haemorrhage	haemolytic anaemia, agranulocytosis, aplastic anaemia, serious coagulation disorders (including Disseminated Intravascular Coagulation)
Nervous system	dizziness	mental status changes including irritability, anxiety, confusion, somnolence, central or peripheral neural disorders (including paraesthesia and neuropathy), depression, insomnia	agitation, convulsions, hallucinations	
Eye Disorder				optic neuropathy
Abnormal laboratory findings		hyperglycaemia	hypo- or hyperthyroidism hypo- and hypercalcaemia, hyperkalaemia	hypoglycaemia
Skin and mucous membranes	injection site reaction, erythema/rash, injection site pain, injection site inflammation	injection site nodules, skin exfoliation, pruritus, sweating	alopecia, mucositis	injection site necrosis, conjunctivitis, vesiculobullous rash, Stevens-Johnson syndrome
Other adverse reactions	fever with or without chills, malaise, headache, pain, weight loss	arthralgia, weight gain, oedema, dehydration, myalgia, hypothermia	Myasthenia, hypersentivity reactions (including Quincke's oedema), taste loss	anaphylaxis,

* Note: During treatment most patients experience lymphocytopenia and eosinophilia, with a rebound lymphocytosis within 24-48 hours following treatment. These are not considered adverse reactions and may be related to the mechanism of antitumour activity of Proleukin.

Additional information

Cardiac arrhythmias (supraventricular and ventricular), angina pectoris, myocardial infarction, respiratory insufficiency requiring intubation, gastrointestinal bleeding or infarction, renal insufficiency, oedema and mental status changes may be associated with capillary leak syndrome (see section 4.4). The frequency and severity of capillary leak syndrome are lower after subcutaneous administration than with continuous intravenous infusion.

Cerebral vasculitis, both isolated and in combination with other manifestations, has been reported. Cutaneous and leukocytoplastic hypersensitivity vasculitis has been reported. Some of these cases are responsive to corticosteroids.

The following undesirable effects have been reported rarely in association with concurrent interferon alpha treatment: crescentic IgA glomerulonephritis, oculo-bulbar myasthenia gravis, inflammatory arthritis, thyroiditis, bullous pemphigoid, rhabdomyolysis and Stevens-Johnson syndrome. Severe rhabdomyolysis and myocardial injury, including myocardial infarction, myocarditis and ventricular hypokinesia appear to be increased in patients receiving Proleukin (intravenously) and interferon-alpha concurrently (see section 4.5).

Bacterial infection or exacerbation of bacterial infection, including septicaemia, bacterial endocarditis, septic thrombophlebitis, peritonitis, and pneumonia has been reported, mainly after intravenous administration.

4.9 Overdose

Adverse reactions following the use of Proleukin are dose-related. Therefore patients can be expected to experience these events in an exaggerated fashion when the recommended dose is exceeded. Adverse reactions generally will reverse when the medicinal product is stopped. Any continuing symptoms should be treated supportively.

5. PHARMACOLOGICAL PROPERTIES

5.1 Pharmacodynamic properties

ATC classification system: immunostimulants, cytokines and immunomodulators, interleukins, aldesleukin

ATC code: L03A C01

Proleukin acts as a regulator of the immune response. The biological activities of aldesleukin and native human IL-2, a naturally occurring lymphokine, are comparable.

The administration of aldesleukin in murine tumour models has been shown to reduce both tumour growth and spread. The exact mechanism by which aldesleukin-mediated immunostimulation leads to antitumour activity is not yet known.

5.2 Pharmacokinetic properties

Absorption

The serum half-life curves of aldesleukin in humans following short intravenous (bolus) administration can be described as bi-exponential. The half-life in the α phase is 13 minutes and the half-life in the β phase is 85 minutes. The α phase accounts for clearance of 87% of a bolus injection. Observed serum levels are proportional to the dose of aldesleukin.

The subcutaneous kinetics can be described by a one-compartment model. The IL-2 absorption half life is 45 minutes, while the elimination half life is 5.3 hours. The longer half-life estimate, compared with the intravenous result is probably due to continued absorption of IL-2 from the subcutaneous injection site during the plasma elimination phase. Absolute bioavailability ranges between 35-47%.

Elimination

The kidney is the major clearance route of recombinant IL-2 (rIL-2) in animals, and most of the injected dose is metabolized in the kidney with no biologically active aldesleukin appearing in the urine. A secondary elimination pathway is receptor- mediated uptake. This active process is induced after chronic dosing. After an aldesleukin-free period between dosing cycles, the clearance of IL-2 is restored to its original value.

The observed clearance rates in humans after short intravenous infusion (15 minutes) and after 24-hour continuous intravenous infusion approximate renal glomerular filtration clearance and range from 140-300 ml/min.

5.3 Preclinical safety data

Animal studies are insufficient with respect to effects on fertility, embryo/foetal development and peri- and postnatal development. In a study with intravenous application of Proleukin in rats maternal toxicity and an increased embryolethality was seen in all tested dose-groups (0.5- 2mg/kg/day).

6. PHARMACEUTICAL PARTICULARS

6.1 List of excipients

Mannitol (E421)

Sodium dodecyl sulphate

Sodium dihydrogen phosphate (pH adjuster)

Disodium hydrogen phosphate (pH adjuster)

6.2 Incompatibilities

Reconstitution procedures other than those recommended may result in incomplete delivery of bioactivity and/or formation of biologically inactive protein.

Use of Bacteriostatic Water for Injection or Sodium Chloride Injection 0.9% should be avoided because of increased aggregation.

Proleukin must not be mixed with other medicinal products except those mentioned in section 6.6.

It is recommended that devices or administration sets containing in-line filters are not used for delivery of Proleukin. Bioassays have shown significant loss of aldesleukin when filters are used.

6.3 Shelf life

2 years

After reconstitution: 24 hours

6.4 Special precautions for storage

Store at 2 to 8 °C (in a refrigerator). Do not freeze.

When reconstituted according to the directions, chemical and physical in-use stability has been demonstrated for up to 48 hours when stored at refrigerated and room temperatures (2 to 30 °C).

From a microbiological point of view, the reconstituted product should be used immediately. If not used immediately, in-use storage times and conditions prior to use are the responsibility of the user and would normally not be longer than 24 hours at 2 to 8 °C, unless reconstitution has taken place in controlled and validated aseptic conditions.

6.5 Nature and contents of container

Proleukin is supplied in 5 ml single-use clear Type I glass vials with a stopper of synthetic rubber. The product is supplied in carton boxes of 1 or 10 vials.

Not all pack sizes may be marketed.

6.6 Instructions for use and handling

Reconstitution of Proleukin powder for solution for injection:

Vials must be reconstituted with 1.2 ml of Water for Injections. After reconstitution the obtained solution contains 18 million IU aldesleukin per millilitre. The reconstituted solution has a pH of 7.5 (range 7.2 – 7.8).

Using sterilised injection syringe and injection needle, inject 1.2 ml Water for Injections into the vial of Proleukin. Direct the diluent against the side of the vial to avoid excessive foaming. Swirl gently to facilitate complete dissolution of the powder. Do not shake. The appropriate dose can then be withdrawn with a sterile injection syringe and injected.

As for all parenteral medicinal products, inspect the reconstituted solution visually for particulate matter and discoloration prior to administration. The solution may be slightly yellow.

The product should be brought to room temperature prior to administration.

For single use only. Any unused solution, the vial, and the syringe used for the reconstituted solution should be adequately disposed of, in accordance with local requirements for the handling of biohazardous waste.

7. MARKETING AUTHORISATION HOLDER

Chiron B.V.

Paasheuvelweg 30

1105 BJ Amsterdam

The Netherlands

8. MARKETING AUTHORISATION NUMBER(S)

PL 08800/0019

9. DATE OF FIRST AUTHORISATION/RENEWAL OF THE AUTHORISATION

22 December 1998/ 1 April 2003

10. DATE OF REVISION OF THE TEXT

November 2004

Promixin 1 MIU Powder for Nebuliser Solution

(Profile Pharma Limited)

1. NAME OF THE MEDICINAL PRODUCT

Promixin, 1 MIU, Powder for Nebuliser Solution

2. QUALITATIVE AND QUANTITATIVE COMPOSITION

Each vial contains 1 million International Units (1 MIU) which is approximately equivalent to 80 mg of colistimethate sodium.

3. PHARMACEUTICAL FORM

Powder for nebuliser solution

4. CLINICAL PARTICULARS

4.1 Therapeutic indications

Promixin is indicated for the treatment by nebulisation of colonisation and infections of the lung due to susceptible *Pseudomonas aeruginosa* in patients with cystic fibrosis.

Consideration should be given to official guidance on the appropriate use of antibacterial agents.

4.2 Posology and method of administration

Sputum cultures should be obtained to confirm colonisation with *Pseudomonas aeruginosa* sensitive to colistimethate sodium prior to initiating treatment with Promixin.

The following information provides guidance on recommended doses and the dose should be adjusted according to clinical response.

Recommended doses are:

Children >2 years and adults: 1-2 MIU two or three times daily

The dosage is determined by the severity and type of infection, and renal function of the patient.

The dose may be varied across this range depending on the condition being treated.

Initial colonisation with *Pseudomonas aeruginosa* sensitive to colistimethate sodium may be treated with a 3 week course of 2 MIU twice daily in conjunction with other parenteral or oral antibiotics.

For frequent, recurrent infections (Less than three positive cultures of *Pseudomonas aeruginosa* sensitive to colistimethate sodium in a six month period) the dose may be increased up to a maximum of 2 MIU three times daily for up to 3 months, in conjunction with other parenteral or oral antibiotics.

Chronic colonisation (Three or more positive cultures of *Pseudomonas aeruginosa* sensitive to colistimethate sodium in a 6 month period) may require long term therapy with 1 to 2 MIU twice daily. Additional parenteral or oral antibiotics may need to be administered to treat acute exacerbations of pulmonary infection.

Nebulised Promixin should be administered after physiotherapy and other inhaled treatments, where used. Other inhaled therapies may include agents to reduce the viscoelasticity of sputum and bronchodilators (see Section 4.4).

Colistimethate sodium is renally excreted and is nephrotoxic if high serum concentrations are achieved. Whilst this is unlikely during inhalation therapy, serum concentration estimations are recommended especially in patients with renal impairment.

Where there is renal impairment, excretion may be delayed and the daily dosage (magnitude of dose and dose interval) must be adjusted in relation to renal function to prevent accumulation of colistimethate sodium as indicated in the table.

Suggested modification of dosage of Promixin for patients with impaired renal function

(see Table 1)

Promixin can be administered by nebulisation using a suitable nebuliser (see Section 6.6 Instructions for Use/ Handling).

4.3 Contraindications

Promixin is contraindicated in patients with known hypersensitivity to colistimethate sodium.

Colistimethate sodium is known to reduce the amount of acetylcholine released from the pre-synaptic neuromuscular junction and therefore should not be used in patients with myasthenia gravis.

4.4 Special warnings and special precautions for use

Nebulisation of colistimethate sodium may induce coughing or bronchospasm. It is advisable to administer the first dose under medical supervision. Pre-dosing with a bronchodilator is recommended and should be routine, especially if this is part of the patient's current therapeutic regimen. FEV_1 should be evaluated pre and post dosing. If there is evidence of colistimethate sodium induced bronchial hyperreactivity in a patient not receiving pre-treatment bronchodilators the test should be repeated on a separate occasion using a bronchodilator. Evidence of bronchial hyperreactivity in the presence of a bronchodilator may indicate an allergic response and Promixin should be discontinued. Bronchospasm that occurs should be treated as medically indicated.

Bronchial hyperreactivity in response to colistimethate sodium may develop with continued use over time and it is recommended that pre and post treatment FEV_1s are evaluated at regular clinic visits.

Use with caution in renal impairment as colistimethate sodium is renally excreted.

Nephrotoxicity or neurotoxicity may rarely occur especially if the recommended dose is exceeded (see also section 4.5).

Use with extreme caution in patients with porphyria.

4.5 Interaction with other medicinal products and other forms of Interaction

Due to the effects of colistimethate sodium on the release of acetylcholine, non-depolarising muscle relaxants should be used with extreme caution in patients receiving Promixin as their effects could be prolonged.

Concomitant use of inhaled colistimethate sodium with other medications that are nephrotoxic or neurotoxic (e.g. cephalothin sodium, aminoglycosides, non-depolarising muscle relaxants) including those which are administered by the i.v. or i.m. routes should only be undertaken with the greatest caution.

4.6 Pregnancy and lactation

Safety in human pregnancy has not been established. There is evidence that colistimethate sodium crosses the

Table 1 Suggested modification of dosage of Promixin for patients with impaired renal function

	Degree of Renal Impairment			
	Normal	**Mild**	**Moderate**	**Severe**
Creatinine (μmol/L)	60 – 105	106 - 129	130 - 214	215 – 340
Creatinine Clearance (% of normal)	76 to 100	40 to 75	25 to 40	Less than 25
Dose				
Unit dose (MIU)	1.3 to 2	1 to 1.5	1	1 to 1.5
Frequency (Times per day)	3	2	1 or 2	Every 36 hours
Total Daily Dose (MIU)	4 to 6	2 to 3	1 to 2	0.6 to 1

placenta and consequently there is potential for foetal toxicity if administered during pregnancy. Animal studies are insufficient with respect to effects on reproduction Promixin should only be given during pregnancy if the benefits outweigh any potential risk.

Colistimethate sodium is excreted in breast milk, breast feeding is not recommended during therapy.

4.7 Effects on ability to drive and use machines

Neurotoxicity, characterised by dizziness, confusion or visual disturbances have been reported following parenteral administration of colistimethate sodium. If these effects occur patients should be warned against driving or operating machinery.

4.8 Undesirable effects

The commonest undesirable effects following nebulisation of colistimethate sodium are coughing and bronchospasm (indicated by chest tightness which may be detected by a decrease in FEV_1) in approximately 10% of patients.

Cases of sore throat or sore mouth have been reported. This may be due to hypersensitivity or superinfection with *Candida* species.

Hypersensitivity reactions such as skin rash have been known to occur. In the event that such reactions occur, treatment with colistimethate sodium should be withdrawn.

Impairment of renal function has been reported, usually following use of higher than recommended i.v. or i.m. doses in patients with normal renal function, or failure to reduce the i.v. or i.m dosage in patients with renal impairment or when used concomitantly with other nephrotoxic antibiotics. The effect is usually reversible on discontinuation of therapy.

High serum concentrations of colistimethate sodium, which may be associated with overdosage or failure to reduce the dosage in patients with renal impairment, have been known to lead to neurotoxicity. Concomitant use with either curariform agents or antibiotics with similar neurotoxic effects can also lead to neurotoxicity. Dose reduction of colistimethate sodium may relieve symptoms. Neurotoxic effects that have been reported include: vertigo, transient facial paraesthesia, slurred speech, vasomotor instability, visual disturbances, confusion, psychosis and apnoea.

4.9 Overdose

Overdosage may cause apnoea, muscle weakness and renal insufficiency. No antidote is available.

Management of overdose is by means of supportive treatment and measures designed to increase clearance of colistimethate sodium such as inducing an osmotic diuresis with mannitol, peritoneal dialysis or prolonged haemodialysis.

5. PHARMACOLOGICAL PROPERTIES

5.1 Pharmacodynamic properties

Pharmacotherapeutic group: other antibacterials, Polymyxins.

ATC code: J01XB01

General properties

Colistimethate sodium is a polymyxin antibiotic and is derived from *Bacillus polymyxa var. colistinus.* It is a polypeptide and is active against a number of aerobic, Gram-negative bacteria.

The polymyxin antibiotics are surface active agents and act by binding to and changing the permeability of the bacterial cell membrane causing bacterial cell death. Polymyxins are bactericidal against Gram-negative bacteria with a hydrophobic outer membrane.

Breakpoints

Susceptible (S) $\leqslant$ 4 mg/L Resistant (R) $\geqslant$ 8 mg/L

Susceptibility

The table below lists bacterial species which are regarded as susceptible to colistimethate sodium. Bacterial resistance may vary according to region and information on resistant species in a specific area is desirable, particularly when treating severe infections. Only bacteria likely to be relevant to the clinical indication are listed.

SUSCEPTIBLE BACTERIA	RESISTANT BACTERIA
Acinetobacter species *Haemophilus influenzae* *Klebsiella* species *Pseudomonas aeruginosa*	*Brucella* species *Burkholderia cepacia* and related species *Serratia* species *Proteus mirabilis*

Resistance

Colistimethate sodium acquired resistance in mucoid *Pseudomonas aeruginosa* has been reported to be approximately 3%. Susceptibility testing should be performed on patients who are treated on a long term basis.

Cross resistance

Polymyxins including colistimethate sodium differ in their mechanism of action compared with other antibiotics and there is evidence to show that Gram-negative bacteria resistant to other antibiotics may be susceptible to colistimethate sodium. The resistance to polymyxins is not crossed with other antibiotic families.

5.2 Pharmacokinetic properties

Absorption

Gastrointestinal absorption is negligible hence the swallowing of colistimethate sodium deposited in the nasopharynx is unlikely to add to the systemic exposure. Absorption following lung administration appears to be variable and clinical work has shown that resultant serum concentrations may range from undetectable to rarely exceeding 4 mg/L (50,000 IU/L) compared to serum concentrations of 10–20 mg/L (approx. 125,000-250,000 IU/L) following intravenous use. Absorption following lung administration is influenced by the nebuliser system, aerosol droplet size and disease state of the lungs. A study in cystic fibrosis patients showed that colistimethate sodium was undetectable in the urine after 1 MIU were inhaled twice daily for 3 months. This is despite the fact that excretion is known to be primarily via the urine.

Distribution

Colistimethate sodium shows a low level of protein binding. Polymyxin antibiotics are known to persist in muscle tissue, liver, kidney, heart and brain.

Pharmacokinetics

Serum concentrations and pharmacokinetics in 5 patients receiving inhaled colistimethate sodium

Parameter	160 mg (Approximately 2 MIU) Nebulised Colistimethate Sodium
$AUC_{0\text{-}4}$ (h/mg/L)	165.9 ± 76.5
C_{max} (mg/L)	0.051 ± 0.0244
T_{max} (h)	1.9 ± 1.2
Ka (h^{-1})	3.0 ± 1.8
$t_{½}$ (h)	10.4 ± 3.6
Cl/F	0.27 ± 0.15

Volume of distribution has been calculated to be 0.09 L/Kg in a single study in patients with cystic fibrosis (CF).

Biotransformation

Colistimethate sodium undergoes conversion to its base *in vivo*. Approximately 80% of the parenteral dose is recoverable unchanged in the urine. There is no biliary excretion.

Elimination

There is no information on the elimination of colistimethate sodium following nebulisation.

Following i.v. administration excretion is primarily renal with 40% of a parenteral dose recovered in the urine within 8 hours and around 80% in 24 hours. It follows that dose should be reduced in the renally impaired in order to prevent accumulation. Refer to Section 4.2.

The elimination half-life is approximately 1.5 hours following i.v. administration to healthy adults. This compares with an elimination half-life of 3.4 ± 1.4 hours when CF patients were given a single 30 minute i.v. infusion.

Colistimethate sodium kinetics appear to be similar in all patient groups provided renal function is normal.

5.3 Preclinical safety data

Animal studies are insufficient with respect to effects on reproduction.

Data on potential genotoxicity are limited and carcinogenicity data for colistimethate sodium are lacking. Colistimethate sodium has been shown to induce chromosomal aberrations in human lymphocytes, *in vitro*. This effect may be related to a reduction in mitotic index, which was also observed.

6. PHARMACEUTICAL PARTICULARS

6.1 List of excipients

None

6.2 Incompatibilities

The addition of other antibiotics to solutions of Promixin may lead to precipitation.

6.3 Shelf life

2 years

Use immediately after reconstitution.

6.4 Special precautions for storage

No special precautions for storage

6.5 Nature and contents of container

The product is supplied in clear type I clear glass vials sealed with a siliconised chlorobutyl type I rubber stopper and protected by a 20 mm aluminium tear-off cap incorporating a red flip-up central plastic top. The product is supplied in packs of 30 vials. Each pack also contains a Prodose Disc™ to enable use with a Prodose AAD® system.

6.6 Instructions for use and handling

Promixin may be reconstituted with Water for Injections (WFI) or a mixture of 50:50 WFI:0.9% saline to produce an hypotonic or isotonic solution. When reconstituted, Promixin may be used with any conventional nebuliser suitable for delivery of antibiotic solutions.

Promixin is supplied with a Prodose Disc for use with the Prodose AAD System.

For instructions on the use of Promixin with a Prodose AAD System please refer to detailed instructions provided with the device.

Any unused solution remaining in the nebuliser must be discarded following treatment.

Conventional nebulisers operate on a continuous flow basis and it is likely that some nebulised drug will be released into the local environment. When used with a conventional nebuliser, Promixin should be administered in a well-ventilated room, particularly in hospitals where several patients may be using nebulisers at the same time. Tubing or filters may be used to prevent waste aerosol from entering the environment.

7. MARKETING AUTHORISATION HOLDER

Profile Pharma Limited

Heath Place

Bognor Regis

West Sussex

PO22 9SL

United Kingdom

8. MARKETING AUTHORISATION NUMBER(S)

PL 19419/0001

9. DATE OF FIRST AUTHORISATION/RENEWAL OF THE AUTHORISATION

20 February 2003

10. DATE OF REVISION OF THE TEXT

February 2004

11. Legal category

POM

Propaderm Cream

(GlaxoSmithKline UK)

1. NAME OF THE MEDICINAL PRODUCT

Propaderm Cream

2. QUALITATIVE AND QUANTITATIVE COMPOSITION

Beclometasone Dipropionate BP 0.025% w/w

3. PHARMACEUTICAL FORM

Cream

4. CLINICAL PARTICULARS

4.1 Therapeutic indications

Propaderm Cream is indicated for the treatment of the various forms of eczema in children and adults including atopic and discoid eczemas; primary irritant and allergic dermatitis; psoriasis (excluding widespread plaque psoriasis); neurodermatoses including lichen simplex; intertrigo; discoid lupus erythematosus.

Propaderm Cream is often appropriate for moist or weeping surfaces and Propaderm Ointment for dry, lichenfield or scaly lesions but this is not invariably so.

4.2 Posology and method of administration

Route of Administration: Topical

Dosage and Administration

Propaderm preparations should be applied thinly over the whole of the affected area and gently rubbed in. Initially, application should be made twice daily, but when improvement is seen, the intervals between applications may be extended and treatment eventually stopped. If no improvement is seen within two to four weeks, reassessment of the diagnosis, or referral may be necessary. After cessation of treatment, should the condition recur, twice daily treatment should be re-instituted. However, when improvement is seen again, the intervals between application may be gradually extended until maintenance dosing of application every third or fourth day is achieved. This is likely to avoid subsequent reappearance of the condition.

The beneficial effects may be enhanced by preliminary use of hot soaks, or by intermittent applications or occlusive dressings.

4.3 Contraindications

Propaderm should not be applied to the eyes. Rosacea, acne vulgaris; peri-oral dermatitis. Primary cutaneous viral infections (e.g. herpes simplex, chickenpox). Hypersensitivity to the preparation. Varicose ulcers or any other statis ulcers.

Use of Propaderm preparations is not indicated in the treatment of primarily infected skin lesions caused by infection with fungi (e.g. candidiasis, tinea) or bacteria (e.g. impetigo); primary or secondary infections due to yeasts; perianal and genital pruritus; dermatoses in children under 1 year of age, including dermatitis and napkin eruptions.

4.4 Special warnings and special precautions for use

Long-term continuous therapy should be avoided where possible, particularly in infants and children, as adrenal suppression can occur even without occlusion.

The face, more than the other areas of the body, may exhibit atrophic changes after prolonged treatment with potent topical corticosteroids. This must be borne in mind when treating such conditions as psoriasis, discoid lupus erythematosus and severe eczema. If applied to the eyelids, care is needed to ensure that the preparation does not enter the eye, as glaucoma might result.

If used in childhood, or on the face, courses should be limited if possible to five days and occlusion should not be used.

Topical corticosteroids may be hazardous in psoriasis for a number of reasons including rebound relapses, development of tolerance, risk of generalised pustular psoriasis and development of local or systemic toxicity due to impaired barrier function of the skin. If used in psoriasis careful patient supervision is important.

Appropriate antimicrobial therapy should be used whenever treating inflammatory lesions which have become infected. Any spread of infection requires withdrawal of topical corticosteroid therapy and systemic administration of antimicrobial agents.

Bacterial infection is encouraged by the warm, moist conditions induced by occlusive dressings, and so the skin should be cleansed before a fresh dressing is applied.

4.5 Interaction with other medicinal products and other forms of Interaction
None stated.

4.6 Pregnancy and lactation
There is inadequate evidence of safety in human pregnancy. Topical administration of corticosteroids to pregnant animals can cause abnormalities of fetal development including cleft palate and intrauterine growth retardation. There may therefore be a very small risk of such effects in the human fetus.

4.7 Effects on ability to drive and use machines
None stated.

4.8 Undesirable effects
Prolonged and intensive treatment with highly active corticosteroid preparations may cause local atrophic changes in the skin such as thinning, striae, and dilatation of the superficial blood vessels, particularly when occlusive dressings are used or when skin folds are involved.

As with other topical corticosteroids, prolonged use of large amounts, or treatment of extensive areas, can result in sufficient systemic absorption to produce the features of hypercorticism. The effect is more likely to occur in infants and children, and if occlusive dressings are used. In infants, the napkin may act as an occlusive dressing.

Should systemic corticosteroid effects arise from application of Propaderm preparations topical treatment should be discontinued. If adrenal function is impaired the patient will need to be protected from any harmful effects of stress with oral corticosteroid preparations until normal adrenal function is established.

There are reports of pigmentation changes and hypertrichosis with topical steroids.

In rare instances, treatment of psoriasis with corticosteroids (or its withdrawal) is thought to have provoked the pustular form of the disease (see precautions).

Propaderm Cream is usually well tolerated, but if signs of hypersensitivity appear, application should stop immediately. Exacerbation of symptoms may occur.

4.9 Overdose
Should systemic corticosteroid effects arise from application of Propaderm preparations, topical treatment should be discontinued. If adrenal function is impaired the patient will need to be protected from any harmful effects of stress with oral corticosteroids preparations until normal adrenal function is established.

5. PHARMACOLOGICAL PROPERTIES

5.1 Pharmacodynamic properties
Beclometasone dipropionate is an active corticosteroid with topical anti-inflammatory activity.

5.2 Pharmacokinetic properties
The extent of percutaneous absorption of topical corticosteroid is determined by many factors including the vehicle, the integrity of the epidermal barrier, and the use of occlusive dressings.

Topical corticosteroids can be absorbed from normal intact skin. Inflammation and/or other disease processes in the skin increase percutaneous absorption. Occlusive dressings substantially increase the percutaneous absorption of topical corticosteroids.

Once absorbed through the skin, topical corticosteroids are handled through pharmacokinetic pathways similar to systemically administered corticosteroids. Corticosteroids are bound to plasma proteins in varying degrees. Corticosteroids are metabolised primarily by the liver and are then excreted by the kidneys.

5.3 Preclinical safety data
There are no preclinical data of relevance to the prescriber which are additional to that in other sections of the SmPC.

6. PHARMACEUTICAL PARTICULARS

6.1 List of excipients
Chlorocresol
Cetomacrogol 1000
Cetostearyl Alcohol
White Soft Paraffin
Liquid Paraffin
Sodium Acid Phosphate
Phosphoric Acid
Sodium Hydroxide
Purified Water

6.2 Incompatibilities
None stated.

6.3 Shelf life
36 months

6.4 Special precautions for storage
Store below 25°C and protect from light.

6.5 Nature and contents of container
Collapsible aluminium tubes internally coated with an epoxy resin based lacquer, and closed with a wadless polypropylene cap.

Pack size: 15g, 30g, 50g.

Not all pack sizes may be marketed.

6.6 Instructions for use and handling
No special instructions.

Administrative Data

7. MARKETING AUTHORISATION HOLDER
Glaxo Wellcome UK Ltd
Trading as GlaxoSmithKline UK
Stockley Park West
Uxbridge
Middlesex UB11 1BT

8. MARKETING AUTHORISATION NUMBER(S)
PL10949/0038

9. DATE OF FIRST AUTHORISATION/RENEWAL OF THE AUTHORISATION
28 June 1999

10. DATE OF REVISION OF THE TEXT
13th December 2004

Propaderm Ointment

(GlaxoSmithKline UK)

1. NAME OF THE MEDICINAL PRODUCT
Propaderm Ointment

2. QUALITATIVE AND QUANTITATIVE COMPOSITION
Beclometasone Dipropionate BP 0.025% w/w

3. PHARMACEUTICAL FORM
Ointment

4. CLINICAL PARTICULARS

4.1 Therapeutic indications
Propaderm Ointment is indicated for the treatment of the various forms of eczema in children and adults including atopic and discoid eczemas; primary irritant and allergic dermatitis; psoriasis (excluding widespread plaque psoriasis); neurodermatoses including lichen simplex; intertrigo; discoid lupus erythematosus.

Propaderm Cream is often appropriate for moist or weeping surfaces and Propaderm Ointment for dry, lichenified or scaly lesions but this is not invariably so.

4.2 Posology and method of administration
Propaderm preparations should be applied thinly over the whole of the affected area and gently rubbed in. Initially, application should be made twice daily, but when improvement is seen, the intervals between applications may be extended and treatment eventually stopped. If no improvement is seen within two to four weeks, reassessment of the diagnosis, or referral may be necessary. After cessation of treatment, should the condition recur, twice daily treatment should be re-instituted. However, when improvement is seen again, the intervals between application may be gradually extended until maintenance dosing of application every third or fourth day is achieved. This is likely to avoid subsequent reappearance of the condition.

The beneficial effects may be enhanced by preliminary use of hot soaks, or by intermittent applications or occlusive dressings.

For topical administration.

4.3 Contraindications
Propaderm should not be applied to the eyes. Rosacea, acne vulgaris; peri-oral dermatitis. Primary cutaneous viral infections (e.g. herpes simplex, chickenpox). Hypersensitivity to the preparation. Varicose ulcers or any other statis ulcers.

Use of Propaderm preparations is not indicated in the treatment of primarily infected skin lesions caused by infection with fungi (e.g. candidiasis, tinea) or bacteria (e.g. impetigo); primary or secondary infections due to yeasts; perianal and genital pruritus; dermatoses in children under 1 year of age, including dermatitis and napkin eruptions.

4.4 Special warnings and special precautions for use
Long-term continuous therapy should be avoided where possible, particularly in infants and children, as adrenal suppression can occur even without occlusion.

The face, more than the other areas of the body, may exhibit atrophic changes after prolonged treatment with potent topical corticosteroids. This must be borne in mind when treating such conditions as psoriasis, discoid lupus erythematosus and severe eczema. If applied to the eyelids, care is needed to ensure that the preparation does not enter the eye, as glaucoma might result.

If used in childhood, or on the face, courses should be limited if possible to five days and occlusion should not be used.

Topical corticosteroids may be hazardous in psoriasis for a number of reasons including rebound relapses, development of tolerance, risk of generalised pustular psoriasis and development of local or systemic toxicity due to impaired barrier function of the skin. If used in psoriasis careful patient supervision is important.

Appropriate antimicrobial therapy should be used whenever treating inflammatory lesions, which have become infected. Any spread of infection requires withdrawal of topical corticosteroid therapy and systemic administration of antimicrobial agents.

Bacterial infection is encouraged by the warm, moist conditions induced by occlusive dressings, and so the skin should be cleansed before a fresh dressing is applied.

4.5 Interaction with other medicinal products and other forms of Interaction
None stated.

4.6 Pregnancy and lactation
There is inadequate evidence of safety in human pregnancy. Topical administration of corticosteroids to pregnant animals can cause abnormalities of foetal development including cleft palate and intrauterine growth retardation. There may therefore be a very small risk of such effects in the human foetus.

4.7 Effects on ability to drive and use machines
None stated.

4.8 Undesirable effects
Prolonged and intensive treatment with highly active corticosteroid preparations may cause local atrophic changes in the skin such as thinning, striae, and dilatation of the superficial blood vessels, particularly when occlusive dressings are used or when skin folds are involved.

As with other topical corticosteroids, prolonged use of large amounts, or treatment of extensive areas, can result in sufficient systemic absorption to produce the features of hypercorticism. The effect is more likely to occur in infants and children, and if occlusive dressings are used. In infants, the napkin may act as an occlusive dressing.

Should systemic corticosteroid effects arise from application of Propaderm preparations, topical treatment should be discontinued. If adrenal function is impaired the patient will need to be protected from any harmful effects of stress with oral corticosteroid preparations until normal adrenal function is established.

There are reports of pigmentation changes and hypertrichosis with topical steroids.

In rare instances, treatment of psoriasis with corticosteroids (or its withdrawal) is thought to have provoked the pustular form of the disease (see Precautions).

Propaderm Ointment is usually well tolerated, but if signs of hypersensitivity appear, application should stop immediately. Exacerbation of symptoms may occur.

4.9 Overdose
Should systemic corticosteroid effects arise from application of Propaderm preparations, topical treatment should be discontinued. If adrenal function is impaired the patient will need to be protected from any harmful effects of stress with oral corticosteroids preparations until normal adrenal function is established.

5. PHARMACOLOGICAL PROPERTIES

5.1 Pharmacodynamic properties
Beclometasone dipropionate is an active corticosteroid with topical anti-inflammatory activity.

5.2 Pharmacokinetic properties
The extent of percutaneous absorption of topical corticosteroid is determined by many factors including the vehicle, the integrity of the epidermal barrier, and the use of occlusive dressings.

Topical corticosteroids can be absorbed from normal intact skin. Inflammation and/or other disease processes in the skin increase percutaneous absorption. Occlusive dressings substantially increase the percutaneous absorption of topical corticosteroids.

Once absorbed through the skin, topical corticosteroids are handled through pharmacokinetic pathways similar to systemically administered corticosteroids. Corticosteroids are bound to plasma proteins in varying degrees. Corticosteroids are metabolised primarily by the liver and are then excreted by the kidneys.

5.3 Preclinical safety data
There are no preclinical data of relevance to the prescriber, which are additional to that in other sections of the SmPC.

6. PHARMACEUTICAL PARTICULARS

6.1 List of excipients
Propylene Glycol EP
White Soft Paraffin BP

6.2 Incompatibilities
None stated.

6.3 Shelf life
36 months

6.4 Special precautions for storage
Store below 25°C and protect from light.

6.5 Nature and contents of container
Collapsible aluminium tube internally either uncoated or coated with an epoxy resin based lacquer, and closed with a wadless polypropylene cap.

Pack size: 15g, 30g, 50g.

Not all pack sizes may be marketed.

6.6 Instructions for use and handling
No special instructions.

Administrative Data

7. MARKETING AUTHORISATION HOLDER
Glaxo Wellcome UK Ltd

trading as GlaxoSmithKline UK

Stockley Park West

Uxbridge

Middlesex

UB11 1BT

8. MARKETING AUTHORISATION NUMBER(S)
PL 10949/0039

9. DATE OF FIRST AUTHORISATION/RENEWAL OF THE AUTHORISATION
4 March 1999

10. DATE OF REVISION OF THE TEXT
13th December 2004

Propecia 1mg tablets

(Merck Sharp & Dohme Limited)

1. NAME OF THE MEDICINAL PRODUCT
PROPECIA® 1 mg Tablets

2. QUALITATIVE AND QUANTITATIVE COMPOSITION
Each tablet of 'Propecia' contains 1 mg of finasteride as the active ingredient.

3. PHARMACEUTICAL FORM
Film-coated tablet. Tan octagonal, film-coated, convex tablets, marked with a 'P' logo on one side and 'PROPECIA' on the other.

4. CLINICAL PARTICULARS

4.1 Therapeutic indications
'Propecia' is indicated for the treatment of men with male pattern hair loss (androgenetic alopecia) to increase hair growth and prevent further hair loss.

'Propecia' is **not** indicated for use in women or children and adolescents.

4.2 Posology and method of administration
The recommended dosage is one 1 mg tablet daily. 'Propecia' may be taken with or without food.

There is no evidence that an increase in dosage will result in increased efficacy.

Efficacy and duration of treatment should continuously be assessed by the treating physician. Generally, three to six months of once daily treatment are required before evidence of stabilisation of hair loss can be expected. Continuous use is recommended to sustain benefit. If treatment is stopped, the beneficial effects begin to reverse by six months and return to baseline by 9 to 12 months.

No dosage adjustment is required in patients with renal insufficiency.

No data are available on the concomitant use of 'Propecia' and topical minoxidil in male pattern hair loss.

4.3 Contraindications
'Propecia' is contraindicated for use in women due to the risk in pregnancy (see 4.6 'Pregnancy and lactation') and in patients with hypersensitivity to any component of this product.

'Propecia' is not indicated for use in women or children and adolescents.

'Propecia' should not be taken by men who are taking 'Proscar' (finasteride 5 mg) or any other 5α-reductase inhibitor for benign prostatic hyperplasia or any other condition.

4.4 Special warnings and special precautions for use
In clinical studies with 'Propecia' in men 18-41 years of age, the mean value of serum prostate-specific antigen (PSA) decreased from 0.7 ng/ml at baseline to 0.5 ng/ml at month 12. This decrease in serum PSA concentrations needs to be considered, if during treatment with 'Propecia', a patient requires a PSA assay. In this case the PSA value should be doubled before making a comparison with the results from untreated men.

4.5 Interaction with other medicinal products and other forms of Interaction
No drug interactions of clinical importance have been identified. Finasteride does not appear to affect the cytochrome P450-linked drug metabolising enzyme system. Compounds which have been tested in man have included antipyrine, digoxin, glibenclamide, propranolol, theophylline and warfarin and no interactions were found.

Although specific interaction studies were not performed, in clinical studies finasteride doses of 1 mg or more were used concomitantly with ACE inhibitors, paracetamol, alpha blockers, benzodiazepines, beta blockers, calcium-channel blockers, cardiac nitrates, diuretics, H_2 antagonists, HMG-CoA reductase inhibitors, prostaglandin synthetase inhibitors (NSAIDs), and quinolones, without evidence of clinically significant adverse interactions.

4.6 Pregnancy and lactation
Use during pregnancy

'Propecia' is contra-indicated for use in women due to the risk in pregnancy.

Because of the ability of type II 5α-reductase inhibitors to inhibit conversion of testosterone to dihydrotestosterone (DHT) in some tissues, these drugs, including finasteride, may cause abnormalities of the external genitalia of a male foetus when administered to a pregnant woman.

Exposure to finasteride: risk to male foetus

A small amount of finasteride, less than 0.001% of the 1 mg dose per ejaculation, has been detected in the seminal fluid of men taking 'Propecia'. Studies in Rhesus monkeys have indicated that this amount is unlikely to constitute a risk to the developing male foetus (see Section 5.3).

During continual collection of adverse experiences, post-marketing reports of exposure to finasteride during pregnancy via semen of men taking 1 mg or higher doses have been received for eight live male births, and one retrospectively-reported case concerned an infant with simple hypospadias. Causality cannot be assessed on the basis of this single retrospective report and hypospadias is a relatively common congenital anomaly with an incidence ranging from 0.8 to 8 per 1000 live male births. In addition, a further nine live male births occurred during clinical trials following exposure to finasteride via semen, during pregnancy, and no congenital anomalies have been reported.

Crushed or broken tablets of 'Propecia' should not be handled by women when they are or may potentially be pregnant because of the possibility of absorption of finasteride and the subsequent potential risk to a male foetus. 'Propecia' tablets are coated to prevent contact with the active ingredient during normal handling, provided that the tablets are not broken or crushed.

Use during lactation

'Propecia' is contraindicated for use in lactation.

4.7 Effects on ability to drive and use machines
There are no data to suggest that 'Propecia' affects the ability to drive or use machines.

4.8 Undesirable effects
Side effects, which usually have been mild, generally have not required discontinuation of therapy.

Finasteride for male pattern hair loss has been evaluated for safety in clinical studies involving more than 3,200 men. In three 12-month, placebo-controlled, double-blind, multicentre studies of comparable design, the overall safety profiles of 'Propecia' and placebo were similar. Discontinuation of therapy due to any clinical adverse experience occurred in 1.7% of 945 men treated with 'Propecia' and 2.1% of 934 men treated with placebo.

In these studies, the following drug-related adverse experiences were reported in ≥1% of men treated with 'Propecia': decreased libido ('Propecia', 1.8% vs. placebo, 1.3%) and erectile dysfunction (1.3%, 0.7%). In addition, decreased volume of ejaculate was reported in 0.8% of men treated with 'Propecia' and 0.4% of men treated with placebo. Resolution of these side effects occurred in men who discontinued therapy with 'Propecia' and in many who continued therapy. The effect of 'Propecia' on ejaculate volume was measured in a separate study and was not different from that seen with placebo.

By the fifth year of treatment with 'Propecia', the proportion of patients reporting each of the above side effects decreased to ≤0.3%.

Finasteride has also been studied for prostate cancer risk reduction at 5 times the dosage recommended for male pattern hair loss. In a 7-year placebo-controlled trial that enrolled 18,882 healthy men, of whom 9060 had prostate needle biopsy data available for analysis, prostate cancer was detected in 803 (18.4%) men receiving finasteride 5 mg and 1147 (24.4%) men receiving placebo. In the finasteride 5 mg group, 280 (6.4%) men had prostate cancer with Gleason scores of 7-10 detected on needle biopsy vs. 237 (5.1%) men in placebo group. Of the total cases of prostate cancer diagnosed in this study, approximately 98% were classified as intracapsular (stage T1 or T2). The relationship between long-term use of finasteride 5 mg and tunours with Gleason scores of 7-10 is unknown.

The following undesirable effects have been reported in post-marketing use: ejaculation disorder; breast tenderness and enlargement; hypersensitivity reactions including rash, pruritus, urticaria and swelling of the lips and face; and testicular pain.

4.9 Overdose
In clinical studies, single doses of finasteride up to 400 mg and multiple doses of finasteride up to 80 mg/day for three months did not result in side effects.

No specific treatment of overdosage with 'Propecia' is recommended.

5. PHARMACOLOGICAL PROPERTIES

5.1 Pharmacodynamic properties
Finasteride is a competitive and specific inhibitor of type II 5α-reductase. Finasteride has no affinity for the androgen receptor and has no androgenic, anti-androgenic, oestrogenic, anti-oestrogenic, or progestational effects. Inhibition of this enzyme blocks the peripheral conversion of testosterone to the androgen DHT, resulting in significant decreases in serum and tissue DHT concentrations. Finasteride produces a rapid reduction in serum DHT concentration, reaching significant suppression within 24 hours of dosing.

Hair follicles contain type II 5α-reductase. In men with male pattern hair loss, the balding scalp contains miniaturised hair follicles and increased amounts of DHT. Administration of finasteride decreases scalp and serum DHT concentrations in these men. Men with a genetic deficiency of type II 5α-reductase do not suffer from male pattern hair loss. Finasteride inhibits a process responsible for miniaturisation of the scalp hair follicles, which can lead to reversal of the balding process.

Studies in men

Clinical studies were conducted in 1879 men aged 18 to 41 with mild to moderate, but not complete, vertex hair loss and/or frontal/mid-area hair loss. In the two studies in men with vertex hair loss (n=1553), 290 men completed 5 years of treatment with Propecia vs. 16 patients on placebo. In these two studies, efficacy was assessed by the following methods: (i) hair count in a representative 5.1cm² area of scalp, (ii) patient self assessment questionnaire, (iii) investigator assessment using a seven point scale, and (iv) photographic assessment of standardised paired photographs by a blinded expert panel of dermatologists using a seven point scale.

In these 5- year studies men treated with 'Propecia' improved compared to both baseline and placebo beginning as early as 3 months, as determined by both the patient and investigator assessments of efficacy. With regard to hair count, the primary endpoint in these studies, increases compared to baseline were demonstrated starting at 6 months (the earliest time point assessed) through to the end of the study. In men treated with 'Propecia' these increases were greatest at 2 years and gradually declined thereafter to the end of 5 years; whereas hair loss in the placebo group progressively worsened compared to baseline over the entire 5 year period. In 'Propecia' treated patients, a mean increase from baseline of 88 hairs *[p <0.01; 95% CI (77.9, 97.80; n=433]* in the representative 5.1 cm² area was observed at 2 years and an increase from baseline of 38 hairs *[p <0.01; 95% CI (20.8, 55.6); n=219]* was observed at 5 years, compared with a decrease from baseline of 50 hairs *[p <0.01; 95% CI (-80.5, -20.6);n=47]* at 2 years and a decrease from baseline of 239 hairs *[p <0.01; 95% CI (-304.4, -173.4); n=15]* at 5 years in patients who received placebo. Standardised photographic assessment of efficacy demonstrated that 48% of men treated with finasteride for 5 years were rated as improved, and an additional 42% were rated as unchanged. This is in comparison to 25% of men treated with placebo for 5 years who were rated as improved or unchanged. These data demonstrate that treatment with 'Propecia' for 5 years resulted in a stabilisation of the hair loss that occurred in men treated with placebo.

An additional 48-week, placebo-controlled study designed to assess the effect of 'Propecia' on the phases of the hair-growth cycle (growing phase [anagen] and resting phase [telogen]) in vertex baldness enrolled 212 men with androgenetic alopecia. At baseline and 48 weeks, total, anagen and telogen hair counts were obtained in a 1-cm² target area of the scalp. Treatment with 'Propecia' led to improvements in anagen hair counts, while men in the placebo group lost anagen hair. At 48 weeks, men treated with 'Propecia' showed net increases in total and anagen hair counts of 17 hairs and 27 hairs, respectively, compared to placebo. This increase in anagen hair count, compared to total hair count, led to a net improvement in the anagen-to-telogen ratio of 47% at 48 weeks for men treated with 'Propecia', compared to placebo. These data provide direct evidence that treatment with 'Propecia' promotes the conversion of hair follicles into the actively growing phase.

Studies in women

Lack of efficacy was demonstrated in post-menopausal women with androgenetic alopecia who were treated with 'Propecia' in a 12 month, placebo-controlled study (n=137). These women did not show any improvement in hair count, patient self-assessment, investigator assessment, or ratings based on standardised photographs, compared with the placebo group.

5.2 Pharmacokinetic properties
Absorption

Relative to an intravenous reference dose, the oral bioavailability of finasteride is approximately 80%. The bioavailability is not affected by food. Maximum finasteride plasma concentrations are reached approximately two hours after dosing and the absorption is complete after six to eight hours.

Distribution

Protein binding is approximately 93%. The volume of distribution of finasteride is approximately 76 litres.

At steady state following dosing with 1 mg/day, maximum finasteride plasma concentration averaged 9.2 ng/ml and was reached 1 to 2 hours postdose; AUC $_{(0\text{-}24\ hr)}$ was 53 ng•hr/ml.

Finasteride has been recovered in the cerebrospinal fluid (CSF), but the drug does not appear to concentrate preferentially to the CSF. A small amount of finasteride has also been detected in the seminal fluid of subjects receiving the drug.

Biotransformation

Finasteride is metabolised primarily via the cytochrome P450 3A4 enzyme subfamily. Following an oral dose of ^{14}C-finasteride in man, two metabolites of the drug were identified that possess only a small fraction of the 5α-reductase inhibitory activity of finasteride.

Elimination

Following an oral dose of ^{14}C-finasteride in man, 39% of the dose was excreted in the urine in the form of metabolites (virtually no unchanged drug was excreted in the urine) and 57% of total dose was excreted in the faeces.

Plasma clearance is approximately 165 ml/min.

The elimination rate of finasteride decreases somewhat with age. Mean terminal half-life is approximately 5-6 hours in men 18-60 years of age and 8 hours in men more than 70 years of age. These findings are of no clinical significance and hence, a reduction in dosage in the elderly is not warranted.

Characteristics in patients

No adjustment in dosage is necessary in non-dialysed patients with renal impairment.

5.3 Preclinical safety data

In general, the findings in laboratory animal studies with oral finasteride were related to the pharmacological effects of 5α-reductase inhibition.

Intravenous administration of finasteride to pregnant rhesus monkeys at doses as high as 800 ng/day during the entire period of embryonic and foetal development resulted in no abnormalities in male foetuses. This represents at least 750 times the highest estimated exposure of pregnant women to finasteride from semen. In confirmation of the relevance of the Rhesus model for human foetal development, oral administration of finasteride 2 mg/kg/day (100 times the recommended human dose or approximately 12 million times the highest estimated exposure to finasteride from semen) to pregnant monkeys resulted in external genital abnormalities in male foetuses. No other abnormalities were observed in male foetuses and no finasteride-related abnormalities were observed in female foetuses at any dose.

6. PHARMACEUTICAL PARTICULARS

6.1 List of excipients

Lactose, microcrystalline cellulose E460, pregelatinised maize starch, sodium starch glycollate, docusate sodium, magnesium stearate E572, hypromellose E464, hydroxypropyl cellulose E463, titanium dioxide, talc, yellow iron oxide E172, red iron oxide E172.

6.2 Incompatibilities

Not applicable.

6.3 Shelf life

36 months.

6.4 Special precautions for storage

Do not store above 30°C. Store in original package.

6.5 Nature and contents of container

Aluminium blisters lidded with aluminium foil, containing 28 tablets.

6.6 Instructions for use and handling

Crushed or broken tablets of 'Propecia' should not be handled by women when they are or may potentially be pregnant (see 4.6 'Pregnancy and lactation').

7. MARKETING AUTHORISATION HOLDER

Merck Sharp & Dohme Limited

Hertford Road, Hoddesdon, Hertfordshire EN11 9BU, UK.

8. MARKETING AUTHORISATION NUMBER(S)

PL 0025/0351

9. DATE OF FIRST AUTHORISATION/RENEWAL OF THE AUTHORISATION

20 September 1999/ 21 July 2005

10. DATE OF REVISION OF THE TEXT

August 2005

LEGAL CATEGORY

POM

® denotes registered trademark of Merck & Co., Inc., Whitehouse Station, NJ, USA.

SPC.PPC.05.UK.2216 F.T. 18 08 05

Propine

(Allergan Ltd)

1. NAME OF THE MEDICINAL PRODUCT

PROPINE®

2. QUALITATIVE AND QUANTITATIVE COMPOSITION

Dipivefrin hydrochloride 0.1% w/v.

3. PHARMACEUTICAL FORM

Eye drops.

4. CLINICAL PARTICULARS

4.1 Therapeutic indications

To control intraocular pressure in patients with chronic open angle glaucoma or ocular hypertensive patients with anterior chamber open angles.

4.2 Posology and method of administration

The usual dosage is one drop in the affected eye(s) every 12 hours.

4.3 Contraindications

a) Patients suffering from closed angle glaucoma

b) Hypersensitivity to any component of the formulation

4.4 Special warnings and special precautions for use

Dipivefrin should be used with caution in patients with narrow angles since dilation of the pupil may trigger an attack of angle closure glaucoma.

Macular oedema is a rare occurrence with adrenaline use in aphakic patients. Prompt reversal generally follows discontinuance of the drug. Macular oedema with dipivefrin does present as a possibility in the aphakic patient.

PROPINE® should be used in caution with patients who have hypertension, heart disease or hyperthyroidism.

This product contains benzalkonium chloride and should not be used by patients continuing to wear soft (hydrophilic) contact lenses.

4.5 Interaction with other medicinal products and other forms of Interaction

Systemic absorption is a possibility for PROPINE® and consequently there is potential for the following interactions to occur:

Mono-amine oxidase inhibitors: There is an elevated risk of adrenergic reactions with concomitant use of MAOIs. These interactions may occur up to 14 days after ceasing the concomitant MAOI therapy.

Tricyclic antidepressants: The pressor response to adrenergic agents and the risk of cardiac arrhythmia may be exacerbated in those patients receiving concomitant tricyclic antidepressants. Upon their cessation the pressor response may persist for up to several days.

Halogenated anaesthetics: PROPINE® should not be administered during general anaesthesia with those anaesthetic agents which sensitise the myocardium to sympathomimetics since under these circumstances there is an elevated risk of ventricular fibrillation.

4.6 Pregnancy and lactation

The safety of intensive or protracted use of dipivefrin during pregnancy has not been substantiated. Caution should be exercised when PROPINE® is administered to a nursing mother.

4.7 Effects on ability to drive and use machines

Mydriasis may occur in some patients. Do not drive or operate machinery if affected.

4.8 Undesirable effects

a) Cardiovascular: tachycardia, arrhythmias and hypertension have been reported with ocular administration of adrenaline, and may occur rarely with dipivefrin therapy.

b) Ocular: the most frequently reported side effects are conjunctival hyperaemia, and burning and stinging on instillation.

Rebound vasodilation, mydriasis and allergic reactions, including blepharoconjunctivitis have been reported occasionally.

Adrenochrome deposits in the conjunctiva and cornea have been associated rarely with the use of dipivefrin.

Follicular conjunctivitis has been reported during long term therapy with dipivefrin. The condition is reversible upon discontinuation of the drug.

c) Body as a Whole: headache may occur rarely with dipivefrin (and is occasionally associated with hypertension and tachycardia).

4.9 Overdose

There are no data available on overdosage with PROPINE®, which is unlikely to occur via the ocular route.

5. PHARMACOLOGICAL PROPERTIES

5.1 Pharmacodynamic properties

Dipivefrin is a prodrug that is converted inside the eye to adrenaline. Conversion takes place by enzyme hydrolysis.

Adrenaline, an adrenergic agonist, appears to exert its action by decreasing aqueous production and enhancing aqueous outflow facility.

5.2 Pharmacokinetic properties

Onset of action after instillation is about 30 minutes. Time to peak effect is about 1 hour.

5.3 Preclinical safety data

-

6. PHARMACEUTICAL PARTICULARS

6.1 List of excipients

Benzalkonium chloride

Disodium edetate

Sodium chloride

Hydrochloric acid (to adjust pH)

Purified water

6.2 Incompatibilities

None known

6.3 Shelf life

The shelf life of the unopened bottle is 18 months. Once opened, the shelf life is 28 days.

6.4 Special precautions for storage

Store at 25°C or less.

6.5 Nature and contents of container

White, low density polyethylene 5 ml and 10 ml fill dropper bottle and tip in single or triple packs; white, medium impact polystyrene (MIPS) screw cap or compliance screw cap (C-cap®).

6.6 Instructions for use and handling

No special instructions required.

7. MARKETING AUTHORISATION HOLDER

Allergan Ltd

Coronation Road

High Wycombe

Bucks

HP12 3SH

8. MARKETING AUTHORISATION NUMBER(S)

PL 00426/0040

9. DATE OF FIRST AUTHORISATION/RENEWAL OF THE AUTHORISATION

27th May 2002

10. DATE OF REVISION OF THE TEXT

22nd February 2002

Propylthiouracil Tablets BP 50mg

(Celltech Manufacturing Services Limited)

1. NAME OF THE MEDICINAL PRODUCT

Propylthiouracil Tablets BP 50mg

2. QUALITATIVE AND QUANTITATIVE COMPOSITION

Propylthiouracil BP 50mg

3. PHARMACEUTICAL FORM

White biconvex uncoated tablets engraved Evans 184 on one face and plain on the other.

4. CLINICAL PARTICULARS

4.1 Therapeutic indications

1. Management of hyperthyroidism, including the treatment of Graves' disease and thyrotoxicosis.

2. Amelioration of hyperthyroidism in preparation for surgical treatment.

3. An adjunct to radioactive iodine therapy.

4. In juvenile hyperthyroidism to delay ablative therapy.

5. To manage thyrotoxic crisis.

4.2 Posology and method of administration

Propylthiouracil is administered by the oral route.

Adults:

Management of Hyperthyroidism

The initial dose of propylthiouracil is between 300mg and 600mg given as a single daily dose. This dose should be maintained until the patient becomes euthyroid. The dose should then be reduced gradually to a maintenance dose of between 50mg and 150mg, taken as a single daily dose.

Daily doses can be divided if preferred.

Preparation for Surgery

As for management of hyperthyroidism, until the patient becomes euthyroid.

Adjunct to Radioactive Iodine Therapy

As for management of hyperthyroidism, for several weeks prior to radio-iodine treatment. Withdraw propylthiouracil 2 to 4 days before irradiation. The dosage of radio-iodine may need to be adjusted because propylthiouracil may have a radioprotective effect.

Management of Thyrotoxic Crisis

200mg every 4 to 6 hours for the first 24 hours, decrease the dose as the crisis subsides.

Elderly

The adult dose should apply, but caution is advised in the presence of renal or hepatic impairment, where a dosage reduction may be justified.

Children:

Juvenile Hyperthyroidism

Children aged 6 - 10 years: Initial dose of 50-150mg daily

Children over 10 years: Initial dose of 150-300mg (or 150mg/m^2) daily

Maintenance dose is determined by the patient's response.

Treatment of Hyperthyroidism in Neonates:

5-10mg/kg daily.

No other specific children's doses are known.

4.3 Contraindications
A known hypersensitivity to propylthiouracil.

4.4 Special warnings and special precautions for use
Patients should be made aware that the development of certain adverse effects (fever, mouth ulcers, rashes, sore throat) may be an indication of agranulocytosis, a serious reaction to the drug, and they should contact their doctor immediately as treatment should be stopped. A full blood count should be performed if there is clinical evidence of infection. Likewise propylthiouracil should be used with extreme caution in patients receiving other drugs known to cause agranulocytosis. Use propylthiouracil with caution in patients more than 40 years old.

Decrease the dose of propylthiouracil in renal failure. If the glomerular filtration rate is 10-50ml/min, decrease dose by 25%. If the GFR is <10ml/min decrease dose by 50%.

Propylthiouracil may cause hypothrombinaemia and bleeding so prothrombin time should be monitored during therapy, especially prior to surgery.

Discontinue propylthiouracil if clinically important evidence of abnormal liver function occurs.

Prolonged therapy and/or excessive doses of propylthiouracil may cause hypothyroidism so thyroid function should be monitored regularly.

4.5 Interaction with other medicinal products and other forms of Interaction
The response of the thyroid gland to propylthiouracil may be impaired by a concurrent high iodine intake.

Drug induced changes in thyroid status may affect the dosage requirements for theophylline and digitalis. The doses of digitalis and theophylline may need to be reduced as thyroid function returns to normal.

4.6 Pregnancy and lactation
Propylthiouracil crosses the placenta and can induce fetal goitre and hypothyroidism. The lowest dose possible should be used after carefully weighing the mother's needs against the risk to the fetus.

Propylthiouracil is present in breast milk in small amounts and neonatal development should be closely monitored in any nursing mother treated with this drug.

4.7 Effects on ability to drive and use machines
Propylthiouracil has no documented effects on the ability to drive or use machines.

4.8 Undesirable effects
Minor adverse effects of propylthiouracil include: rash, urticaria, pruritus, abnormal hair loss, skin pigmentation, oedema, nausea, vomiting, epigastric distress, loss of taste, arthralgia, myalgia, paresthesia and headache.

Leucopenia is a common adverse effect, but it is usually mild and reversible.

Agranulocytosis is the most serious adverse effect of propylthiouracil, but the incidence is very low. It tends to occur within the first two months of therapy and patients over the age of 40 years and receiving larger doses are at greater risk.

Other severe, but infrequent adverse events include: aplastic anaemia; drug fever; lupus-like syndrome; severe hepatic reactions (including encephalopathy, fulminant hepatic necrosis and death); periarteritis; hypoprothrombinaemia; thrombocytopenia and bleeding.

Nephritis, interstitial pneumonitis, cutaneous vasculitis and polymyositis have also been reported.

Propylthiouracil-induced hepatoxicity is rare and usually manifests as hepatocellular hepatitis with or without jaundice. Cholestatic jaundice has also occurred. Adverse liver effects are generally reversible on cessation of propylthiouracil.

4.9 Overdose
Symptoms of propylthiouracil overdose include: nausea, vomiting, epigastric distress, headache, fever, arthralgia, pruritus, oedema and pancytopenia, exfoliative dermatitis and hepatitis have occurred. Agranulocytosis is the most severe potential adverse effect due to acute propylthiouracil toxicity.

The treatment of propylthiouracil overdose should aim to minimise the amount of drug absorbed into the circulation. Following acute toxicity the stomach should be emptied by gastric lavage or emesis. Activated charcoal may also be employed. General symptomatic and supportive measures should then be instituted. A full blood analysis should be considered because of the slight risk of haematological complications and appropriate therapy given if bone marrow depression develops.

There is no specific antidote for propylthiouracil.

5. PHARMACOLOGICAL PROPERTIES

5.1 Pharmacodynamic properties
Propylthiouracil blocks the production of thyroid hormones by inhibiting the enzyme thyroid peroxidase. This prevents the incorporation of iodine into tyrosyl residues of thyroglobulin and inhibits the coupling of the iodotyrosyl residues to form iodothyronine. It also interferes with the oxidation of iodide ion and iodotyrosyl groups.

Propylthiouracil does not inhibit the action or release of already formed thyroid hormone nor does it interfere with the effectiveness of circulating or exogenously administered thyroid hormone. It does, however, inhibit the peripheral de-iodination of thyroxine to tri-iodothyronine. Propylthiouracil also causes a gradual reduction in the level of circulating thyroid stimulating immunoglobulins in Grave's disease.

5.2 Pharmacokinetic properties
Absorption

Propylthiouracil is rapidly absorbed from the gastro-intestinal tract and has a bioavailability of 50-75%.

Half-Life

The elimination half-life of propylthiouracil is estimated to be 1-2 hours. The elimination half-life may be increased in hepatic and renal impairment and a dosage reduction may be warranted. Despite its short half-life, propylthiouracil is retained in the thyroid gland for at least 24 hours.

Distribution

Propylthiouracil appears to be concentrated in the thyroid gland. It readily crosses the placenta and is distributed into breast milk. About 80% of propylthiouracil is protein bound.

Metabolism

Propylthiouracil undergoes rapid first-pass metabolism in the liver where it is metabolised to its glucuronic acid conjugate.

Excretion

Propylthiouracil is mainly excreted in the urine as the glucuronic acid conjugate. Very little unchanged drug is excreted in the urine and negligible amounts are excreted in the faeces.

5.3 Preclinical safety data
None stated.

6. PHARMACEUTICAL PARTICULARS

6.1 List of excipients
Alginic acid PH EUR

Maize starch PH EUR

Lactose 170 mesh PH EUR

Magnesium stearate PH EUR

Povidone 30 PH EUR

6.2 Incompatibilities
None known.

6.3 Shelf life
36 months.

6.4 Special precautions for storage
Store below 25°C.

6.5 Nature and contents of container
Pigmented polypropylene containers fitted with a tamper evident closure containing 7, 14, 21, 28, 30, 50, 56, 60, 84, 90, 100, 112, 120 or 500 tablets.

6.6 Instructions for use and handling
No special precautions are required.

Administrative Data

7. MARKETING AUTHORISATION HOLDER
Celltech Manufacturing Services Limited

Vale of Bardsley

Ashton-under-Lyne

Lancashire

OL7 9RR, UK

8. MARKETING AUTHORISATION NUMBER(S)
PL 18816/0014

9. DATE OF FIRST AUTHORISATION/RENEWAL OF THE AUTHORISATION
18 July 2001

10. DATE OF REVISION OF THE TEXT

Proscar

(Merck Sharp & Dohme Limited)

1. NAME OF THE MEDICINAL PRODUCT
PROSCAR®

(finasteride)

2. QUALITATIVE AND QUANTITATIVE COMPOSITION
Each tablet contains 5 mg of finasteride.

3. PHARMACEUTICAL FORM
Blue-coloured, apple-shaped, film-coated tablets marked 'Proscar' on one side and 'MSD 72' on the other.

4. CLINICAL PARTICULARS

4.1 Therapeutic indications
'Proscar' is indicated for the treatment and control of benign prostatic hyperplasia (BPH) in patients with an enlarged prostate to:

– cause regression of the enlarged prostate, improve urinary flow and improve the symptoms associated with BPH

– reduce the incidence of acute urinary retention and the need for surgery including transurethral resection of the prostate (TURP) and prostatectomy.

4.2 Posology and method of administration
The recommended adult dose is one 5 mg tablet daily, with or without food.

'Proscar' can be administered alone or in combination with the alpha-blocker doxazosin (see section 5.1 'Pharmacodynamic properties').

Although early improvement in symptoms may be seen, treatment for at least six months may be necessary to assess whether a beneficial response has been achieved. Thereafter, treatment should be continued long term.

No dosage adjustment is required in the elderly or in patients with varying degrees of renal insufficiency (creatinine clearances as low as 9 ml/min).

There are no data available in patients with hepatic insufficiency.

'Proscar' is contra-indicated in children.

4.3 Contraindications
Hypersensitivity to any component of this product; women who are or may potentially be pregnant; children.

4.4 Special warnings and special precautions for use
General

Patients with large residual urine volume and/or severely diminished urinary flow should be carefully monitored for obstructive uropathy.

Effects on prostate-specific antigen (PSA) and prostate cancer detection

No clinical benefit has yet been demonstrated in patients with prostate cancer treated with 'Proscar'.

Digital rectal examination, as well as other evaluations for prostate cancer, should be carried out on patients with BPH prior to initiating therapy with 'Proscar' and periodically thereafter. Generally, when PSA assays are performed a baseline PSA>10 ng/ml (Hybritech) prompts further evaluation and consideration of biopsy; for PSA levels between 4 and 10 ng/ml, further evaluation is advisable. There is considerable overlap in PSA levels among men with and without prostate cancer. Therefore, in men with BPH, PSA values within the normal reference range do not rule out prostate cancer regardless of treatment with 'Proscar'. A baseline PSA <4 ng/ml does not exclude prostate cancer.

'Proscar' causes a decrease in serum PSA concentrations by approximately 50% in patients with BPH even in the presence of prostate cancer. This decrease in serum PSA levels in patients with BPH treated with 'Proscar' should be considered when evaluating PSA data and does not rule out concomitant prostate cancer. This decrease is predictable over the entire range of PSA values, although it may vary in individual patients. In patients treated with 'Proscar' for six months or more, PSA values should be doubled for comparison with normal ranges in untreated men. This adjustment preserves the sensitivity and specificity of the PSA assay and maintains its ability to detect prostate cancer.

Any sustained increase in PSA levels of patients treated with finasteride should be carefully evaluated, including consideration of non-compliance to therapy with 'Proscar'.

Percent free PSA (free to total PSA ratio) is not significantly decreased by 'Proscar' and remains constant even under the influence of 'Proscar'. When percent free PSA is used as an aid in the detection of prostate cancer, no adjustment is necessary.

4.5 Interaction with other medicinal products and other forms of Interaction
No clinically important drug interactions have been identified. 'Proscar' does not appear to significantly affect the cytochrome P450-linked drug metabolising enzyme system. Compounds which have been tested in man include propranolol, digoxin, glibenclamide, warfarin, theophylline, and antipyrine and no clinically meaningful interactions were found.

Other concomitant therapy: Although specific interaction studies were not performed in clinical studies, 'Proscar' was used concomitantly with ACE inhibitors, alpha-blockers, beta-blockers, calcium channel blockers, cardiac nitrates, diuretics, H_2 antagonists, HMG-CoA reductase inhibitors, non-steroidal anti-inflammatory drugs (NSAIDs) including aspirin and paracetamol, quinolones and benzodiazepines without evidence of clinically significant adverse interactions.

4.6 Pregnancy and lactation
Pregnancy: 'Proscar' is contra-indicated in women who are or may potentially be pregnant.

Because of the ability of Type II 5 α-reductase inhibitors to inhibit conversion of testosterone to dihydrotestosterone, these drugs, including finasteride, may cause abnormalities of the external genitalia of a male foetus when administered to a pregnant woman.

In animal developmental studies, dose-dependent development of hypospadias were observed in the male offspring of pregnant rats given finasteride at doses ranging from 100 μg/kg/day to 100 mg/kg/day, at an incidence of 3.6% to 100%. Additionally, pregnant rats produced male offspring with decreased prostatic and seminal vesicular weights, delayed preputial separation, transient nipple development and decreased anogenital distance, when given finasteride at doses below the recommended human dose. The critical period during which these effects can be induced has been defined in rats as days 16-17 of gestation.

The changes described above are expected pharmacological effects of Type II 5 α-reductase inhibitors. Many of the changes, such as hypospadias, observed in male rats exposed *in utero* to finasteride are similar to those reported in male infants with a genetic deficiency of Type II 5 α-reductase. It is for these reasons that 'Proscar' is contra-indicated in women who are or may potentially be pregnant.

No effects were seen in female offspring exposed *in utero* to any dose of finasteride.

Exposure to finasteride - risk to male foetus

Women should not handle crushed or broken tablets of 'Proscar' when they are or may potentially be pregnant because of the possibility of absorption of finasteride and the subsequent potential risk to a male foetus (see 'Pregnancy'). 'Proscar' tablets are coated and will prevent contact with the active ingredient during normal handling, provided that the tablets have not been broken or crushed.

Small amounts of finasteride have been recovered from the semen in subjects receiving 'Proscar' 5 mg/day. It is not known whether a male foetus may be adversely affected if his mother is exposed to the semen of a patient being treated with finasteride. Therefore, when the patient's sexual partner is or may potentially be pregnant, the patient should either avoid exposure of his partner to semen (e.g. by use of a condom) or discontinue 'Proscar'.

Lactation: 'Proscar' is not indicated for use in women. It is not known whether finasteride is excreted in human milk.

4.7 Effects on ability to drive and use machines

None reported.

4.8 Undesirable effects

'Proscar' is well tolerated. In controlled clinical studies where patients received 5 mg of finasteride over periods of up to four years, the following adverse reactions were considered possibly, probably or definitely drug-related and occurred with a frequency greater than placebo and greater than or equal to 1%: impotence, decreased libido, ejaculation disorder, decreased volume of ejaculate; breast enlargement, breast tenderness and rash. There was no evidence of increased adverse experiences with increased duration of treatment with 'Proscar' and the incidence of new drug-related sexual adverse experiences decreased with duration of treatment.

Medical therapy of prostatic symptoms (MTOPS)

The MTOPS study compared finasteride 5 mg/day (n=768), doxazosin 4 or 8 mg/day (n=756), combination therapy of finasteride 5 mg/day and doxazosin 4 or 8 mg/day (n=786), and placebo (n=737). In this study, the safety and tolerability profile of the combination therapy was generally consistent with the profiles of the individual components. The incidence of ejaculation disorder events without regard to drug relationship were: finasteride 8.3%, doxazosin 5.3%, combination 15.0%, placebo 3.9%.

Other long-term data

In a 7 year placebo-controlled trial that enrolled 18,882 healthy men, of 9060 had prostate needle biopsy data available for analysis, prostate cancer was detected in 803 (18.4%) men receiving 'Proscar' and 1147 (24.4%) men receiving placebo. In the 'Proscar' group, 280 (6.4%) of men had prostate cancer with Gleason scores of 7-10 detected on needle biopsy vs 237 (5.1%). Of the total cases of prostate cancer diagnosed in this study, approximately 98% were classified as intracapsular (stage T1 or T2). The relationship between long-term use of 'Proscar' and tumours with Gleason scores of 7-10 is unknown.

Post Marketing Experience

The following additional adverse experiences have been reported in post-marketing experience:

– hypersensitivity reactions, including pruritus, urticaria and swelling of the lips and face

– testicular pain.

Laboratory test findings

Serum PSA concentration is correlated with patient age and prostatic volume, and prostatic volume is correlated with patient age. When PSA laboratory determinations are evaluated, consideration should be given to the fact that PSA levels generally decrease in patients treated with 'Proscar'. In most patients, a rapid decrease in PSA is seen within the first months of therapy, after which time PSA levels stabilise to a new baseline. The post-treatment baseline approximates half of the pre-treatment value. Therefore, in typical patients treated with 'Proscar' for six months or more, PSA values should be doubled for comparison to normal ranges in untreated men.

For clinical interpretation see 'Special warnings and precautions for use', *Effects on prostate-specific antigen (PSA) and prostate cancer detection.*

No other difference was observed in patients treated with placebo or 'Proscar' in standard laboratory tests.

4.9 Overdose

No specific treatment of overdosage with 'Proscar' is recommended. Patients have received single doses of 'Proscar' up to 400 mg and multiple doses of 'Proscar' up to 80 mg/day for up to three months without any adverse effects.

5. PHARMACOLOGICAL PROPERTIES

5.1 Pharmacodynamic properties

Finasteride is a competitive inhibitor of human 5 α-reductase, an intracellular enzyme which metabolises testosterone into the more potent androgen, dihydrotestosterone (DHT). In benign prostatic hyperplasia (BPH), enlargement of the prostate gland is dependent upon the conversion of testosterone to DHT within the prostate. 'Proscar' is highly effective in reducing circulating and intraprostatic DHT. Finasteride has no affinity for the androgen receptor.

In clinical studies of patients with moderate to severe symptoms of BPH, an enlarged prostate on digital rectal examination and low residual urinary volumes, 'Proscar' reduced the incidence of acute retention of urine from 7/100 to 3/100 over four years and the need for surgery (TURP or prostatectomy) from 10/100 to 5/100. These reductions were associated with a 2-point improvement in QUASI-AUA symptom score (range 0-34), a sustained regression in prostate volume of approximately 20% and a sustained increase in urinary flow rate.

Medical therapy of prostatic symptoms

The Medical Therapy of Prostatic Symptoms (MTOPS) Trial was a 4- to 6-year study in 3047 men with symptomatic BPH who were randomised to receive finasteride 5 mg/day, doxazosin 4 or 8 mg/day*, the combination of finasteride 5 mg/day and doxazosin 4 or 8 mg/day*, or placebo. The primary endpoint was time to clinical progression of BPH, defined as a $\geqslant$4 point confirmed increase from baseline in symptom score, acute urinary retention, BPH-related renal insufficiency, recurrent urinary tract infections or urosepsis, or incontinence. Compared to placebo, treatment with finasteride, doxazosin, or combination therapy resulted in a significant reduction in the risk of clinical progression of BPH by 34(p=0.002), 39 (p<0.001), and 67% (p<0.001), respectively. The majority of the events (274 out of 351) that constituted BPH progression were confirmed $\geqslant$4 point increases in symptom score; the risk of symptom score progression was reduced by 30 (95% CI 6 to 48%), 46 (95% CI 25 to 60%), and 64% (95% CI 48 to 75%) in the finasteride, doxazosin, and combination groups, respectively, compared to placebo. Acute urinary retention accounted for 41 of the 351 events of BPH progression; the risk of developing acute urinary retention was reduced by 67(p=0.011), 31 (p=0.296), and 79% (p=0.001) in the finasteride, doxazosin, and combination groups, respectively, compared to placebo. Only the finasteride and combination therapy groups were significantly different from placebo.

*Titrated from 1 mg to 4 or 8 mg as tolerated over a 3-week period

5.2 Pharmacokinetic properties

After an oral dose of ^{14}C-finasteride in man, 39% of the dose was excreted in the urine in the form of metabolites (virtually no unchanged drug was excreted in the urine), and 57% of total dose was excreted in the faeces. Two metabolites have been identified which possess only a small fraction of the Type II 5 α-reductase activity of finasteride.

The oral bioavailability of finasteride is approximately 80%, relative to an intravenous reference dose, and is unaffected by food. Maximum plasma concentrations are reached approximately two hours after dosing and the absorption is complete within 6-8 hours. Protein binding is approximately 93%. Plasma clearance and the volume of distribution are approximately 165 ml/min and 76 l, respectively.

In the elderly, the elimination rate of finasteride is somewhat decreased. Half-life is prolonged from a mean half-life of approximately six hours in men aged 18-60 years to eight hours in men aged more than 70 years. This is of no clinical significance and does not warrant a reduction in dosage.

In patients with chronic renal impairment, whose creatinine clearance ranged from 9-55 ml/min, the disposition of a single dose of ^{14}C-finasteride was not different from that in healthy volunteers. Protein binding also did not differ in patients with renal impairment. A portion of the metabolites which normally is excreted renally was excreted in the faeces. It therefore appears that faecal excretion increases commensurate to the decrease in urinary excretion of metabolites. Dosage adjustment in non-dialysed patients with renal impairment is not necessary.

There are no data available in patients with hepatic insufficiency.

Finasteride has been found to cross the blood-brain barrier. Small amounts of finasteride have been recovered in the seminal fluid of treated patients.

5.3 Preclinical safety data

No further information provided.

6. PHARMACEUTICAL PARTICULARS

6.1 List of excipients

Cellulose, Microcrystalline (E460)

Docusate sodium

Lactose monohydrate

Magnesium stearate (E572)

Pregelatinised maize starch

Sodium starch glycollate Type A

Yellow iron oxide (E172)

Hydroxypropylcellulose (E463)

Indigo carmine aluminium lake (E132)

Hypromellose (E464)

Talc

Titanium dioxide (E171)

6.2 Incompatibilities

None reported.

6.3 Shelf life

Three years.

6.4 Special precautions for storage

Do not store above 30°C. Store in the original package.

6.5 Nature and contents of container

Opaque PVC/PE/PVDC blisters lidded with aluminium foil; packs of 28 tablets.

6.6 Instructions for use and handling

Women should not handle crushed or broken 'Proscar' Tablets when they are or may potentially be pregnant (see 'Contra-indications, 'Pregnancy and lactation', *Exposure to finasteride - risk to male foetus).*

7. MARKETING AUTHORISATION HOLDER

Merck Sharp & Dohme Limited

Hertford Road, Hoddesdon, Hertfordshire EN11 9BU, UK.

8. MARKETING AUTHORISATION NUMBER(S)

PL 0025/0279.

9. DATE OF FIRST AUTHORISATION/RENEWAL OF THE AUTHORISATION

July 1997.

10. DATE OF REVISION OF THE TEXT

Date of approval: February 2004.

LEGAL CATEGORY

POM

® denotes registered trademark of Merck & Co., Inc., Whitehouse Station, NJ, USA.

SPC.PSC.03.UK.1025

Prostap 3 Leuprorelin Acetate Depot Injection 11.25mg

(Wyeth Pharmaceuticals)

1. NAME OF THE MEDICINAL PRODUCT

PROSTAP 3 Leuprorelin Acetate Depot Injection 11.25mg.

2. QUALITATIVE AND QUANTITATIVE COMPOSITION

PROSTAP 3 Powder: 11.25mg contains leuprorelin acetate (equivalent to 10.72mg base).

Sterile Vehicle: Each ml contains sodium carboxymethyl cellulose 5mg, mannitol 50mg, polysorbate 80 1mg in water for injections.

3. PHARMACEUTICAL FORM

Prolonged release powder for suspension for injection by subcutaneous (advanced prostate cancer) or intramuscular (endometriosis) administration after reconstitution with the Sterile Vehicle.

4. CLINICAL PARTICULARS

4.1 Therapeutic indications

(i) Treatment of advanced prostatic cancer.

(ii) Management of endometriosis, including pain relief and reduction of endometriotic lesions.

4.2 Posology and method of administration

Dosage

Advanced Prostatic Cancer: The usual recommended dose is 11.25mg presented as a three month depot injection and administered as a single subcutaneous injection at intervals of three months. The majority of patients will respond to this dosage. PROSTAP 3 therapy should not be discontinued when remission or improvement occurs. As with other drugs administered regularly by injection, the injection site should be varied periodically.

Response to PROSTAP 3 therapy should be monitored by clinical parameters and by measuring prostate-specific antigen (PSA) serum levels. Clinical studies have shown that testosterone levels increased during the first 4 days of treatment in the majority of non-orchidectomised patients. They then decreased and reached castrate levels by 2-4 weeks. Once attained, castrate levels were maintained as long as drug therapy continued. If a patient's response appears to be sub-optimal, then it would be advisable to confirm that serum testosterone levels have reached or are remaining at castrate levels. Transient increases in acid phosphatase levels sometimes occur early in the treatment period but usually return to normal or near normal values by the 4th week of treatment.

Endometriosis: The recommended dose is 11.25mg administered as a single intramuscular injection every 3 months for a period of 6 months only. Treatment should be initiated during the first 5 days of the menstrual cycle.

In women receiving GnRH analogues for the treatment of endometriosis, the addition of hormone replacement therapy (HRT – an oestrogen and progestogen) has been shown to reduce bone mineral density loss and vasomotor symptoms. Therefore if appropriate, HRT should be co-administered with PROSTAP 3 taking into account the risks and benefits of each treatment.

Elderly: As for adults

Children (under 18 years): Prostap 3 is not recommended in children as the safety and efficacy have not been established.

Administration

The vial of PROSTAP 3 microsphere powder should be reconstituted immediately prior to administration by subcutaneous or intramuscular injection.

Remove flip-cap from vial of PROSTAP 3 Powder and cap from pre-filled syringe containing 2ml Sterile Vehicle. Ensure a 23 gauge needle is fixed securely by screwing needle hub onto the syringe and inject whole contents of syringe into vial of PROSTAP 3 Powder using an aseptic technique. Remove the syringe/needle and keep aseptic. Shake the vial gently for 15-20 seconds to produce a uniform cloudy suspension of PROSTAP 3.

Immediately draw up suspension into syringe taking care to exclude air bubbles. Change the needle on syringe using a 23 gauge needle if the suspension is to be administered subcutaneously or alternatively a 21 gauge needle for intramuscular administration. Having cleaned an appropriate injection site and ensured that the needle is fixed securely, administer the suspension by subcutaneous or intramuscular injection as appropriate taking care not to enter a blood vessel. Apply sterile dressing to injection site if required.

The injection should be given as soon as possible after mixing. If any settling of suspension occurs in vial or syringe, re-suspend by gentle shaking and administer immediately.

No other fluid can be used for reconstitution of PROSTAP 3 Powder.

4.3 Contraindications

Hypersensitivity to any of the ingredients or to synthetic Gn-RH or Gn-RH derivatives.

Women: PROSTAP is contra-indicated in women who are or may become pregnant while receiving the drug. PROSTAP should not be used in women who are breastfeeding or have undiagnosed abnormal vaginal bleeding.

Men:There are no known contra-indications to the use of PROSTAP in men.

4.4 Special warnings and special precautions for use

Development or aggravation of diabetes may occur, therefore diabetic patients may require more frequent monitoring of blood glucose during treatment with PROSTAP.

Hepatic dysfunction and jaundice with elevated liver enzyme levels have been reported. Therefore, close observation should be made and appropriate measures taken if necessary.

Spinal fracture, paralysis, hypotension and worsening of depression have been reported.

Men: In the initial stages of therapy, a transient rise in levels of testosterone, dihydro-testosterone and acid phosphatase may occur. In some cases, this may be associated with a "flare" or exacerbation of the tumour growth resulting in temporary deterioration of the patient's condition. These symptoms usually subside on continuation of therapy. "Flare" may manifest itself as systemic or neurological symptoms in some cases.

In order to reduce the risk of flare, an anti-androgen may be administered beginning 3 days prior to leuprorelin therapy and continuing for the first two to three weeks of treatment. This has been reported to prevent the sequelae of an initial rise in serum testosterone.

Patients at risk of ureteric obstruction or spinal cord compression should be considered carefully and closely supervised in the first few weeks of treatment. These patients should be considered for prophylactic treatment with anti-androgens. Should urological/neurological complications occur, these should be treated by appropriate specific measures.

If an anti-androgen is used over a prolonged period, due attention should be paid to the contra-indications and precautions associated with its extended use.

Whilst the development of pituitary adenomas has been noted in chronic toxicity studies at high doses in some animal species, this has not been observed in long term clinical studies with leuprorelin acetate.

Women: During the early phase of endometriosis therapy, sex steroids temporarily rise above baseline because of the physiological effect of the drug. Therefore, a worsening of clinical signs and symptoms may be observed during the initial days of therapy, but these will dissipate with continued therapy.

When receiving GnRH analogues for the treatment of endometriosis, the addition of HRT (an oestrogen and progestogen) has been shown to reduce bone mineral density loss and vasomotor symptoms (see 'Posology and Method of Administration' section 4.2 for further information).

The induced hypo-oestrogenic state results in a small loss in bone density over the course of treatment, some of which may not be reversible. The extent of bone demineralisation due to hypo-oestrogenaemia is proportional to time and, consequently, is the adverse event responsible for limiting the duration of therapy to 6 months. The generally accepted level of bone loss with LHRH analogues such as PROSTAP is 5%. In clinical studies with PROSTAP the levels varied between 2.3% and 15.7% depending on the method of measurement. During one six-month treatment period, this bone loss should not be important. In patients with major risk factors for decreased bone mineral content such as chronic alcohol and/or tobacco use, strong family history of osteoporosis, or chronic use of drugs that can reduce bone mass such as anticonvulsants or corticosteroids, PROSTAP therapy may pose an additional risk. In these patients, the risks and benefits must be weighed carefully before therapy with PROSTAP is instituted.

In women with submucous fibroids there have been reports of severe bleeding following administration of PROSTAP as a consequence of the acute degeneration of the fibroids. Patients should be warned of the possibility of abnormal bleeding or pain in case earlier surgical intervention is required.

PROSTAP may cause an increase in uterine cervical resistance, which may result in difficulty in dilating the cervix for intrauterine surgical procedures.

Precautions

Men: Patients with urinary obstruction and patients with metastatic vertebral lesions should begin PROSTAP therapy under close supervision for the first few weeks of treatment.

Women: Since menstruation should stop with effective doses of PROSTAP, the patient should notify her physician if regular menstruation persists.

4.5 Interaction with other medicinal products and other forms of Interaction

None have been reported.

4.6 Pregnancy and lactation

Safe use of leuprorelin acetate in pregnancy has not been established clinically. Studies in animals have shown reproductive toxicity (see section 5.3). Before starting treatment with PROSTAP, pregnancy must be excluded. There have been reports of foetal malformation when PROSTAP has been given during pregnancy.

PROSTAP should not be used in women who are breastfeeding.

When used 3-monthly at the recommended dose, PROSTAP usually inhibits ovulation and stops menstruation. Contraception is not ensured, however, by taking PROSTAP and therefore patients should use non-hormonal methods of contraception during treatment.

Patients should be advised that if they miss successive doses of PROSTAP, breakthrough bleeding or ovulation may occur with the potential for conception. Patients should be advised to see their physician if they believe they may be pregnant. If a patient becomes pregnant during treatment, the drug must be discontinued. The patient must be appraised of this evidence and the potential for an unknown risk to the foetus.

4.7 Effects on ability to drive and use machines

The ability to drive and use machines may be impaired due to visual disturbances and dizziness.

4.8 Undesirable effects

Side effects seen with PROSTAP are due mainly to the specific pharmacological action, namely increases and decreases in certain hormone levels.

Adverse events which have been reported infrequently include peripheral oedema, pulmonary embolism, hypertension, palpitations, fatigue, muscle weakness, diarrhoea, nausea, vomiting, anorexia, fever/chills, headache (occasionally severe), hot flushes, arthralgia, myalgia, dizziness, insomnia, depression, paraesthesia, visual disturbances, weight changes, jaundice, increases in liver function test values and irritation at the injection site. Changes in blood lipids and alteration of glucose tolerance have also been reported which may affect diabetic control. Thrombocytopenia and leucopenia have been reported rarely. Hypersensitivity reactions including rash, pruritis, urticaria and, rarely, wheezing or interstitial pneumonitis have also been reported. Anaphylactic reactions are rare.

Spinal fracture, paralysis, hypotension and worsening of depression have been reported (see 'Special Warnings and Precautions for Use' section 4.4).

A reduction in bone mass may occur with the use of GnRH agonists.

Infarction of pre-existing pituitary adenoma has also been reported rarely after administration of both short- and long-acting GnRH agonists.

Men:In cases where a "tumour flare" occurs after PROSTAP therapy, an exacerbation may occur in any symptoms or signs due to disease, for example, bone pain, urinary obstruction etc. These symptoms subside on continuation of therapy.

Impotence and decreased libido will be expected with PROSTAP therapy.

The administration of PROSTAP is often associated with hot flushes and sometimes sweating.

Gynaecomastia has been reported occasionally.

Women: Those adverse events occurring most frequently with PROSTAP are associated with hypo-oestrogenism; the most frequently reported are hot flushes, mood swings including depression (occasionally severe), and vaginal dryness. Oestrogen levels return to normal after treatment is discontinued.

The induced hypo-oestrogenic state results in a small loss in bone density over the course of treatment, some of which may not be reversible (see 'Special Warnings and Precautions for Use' section 4.4).

Breast tenderness or change in breast size may occur occasionally. Hair loss has also been reported occasionally.

Vaginal haemorrhage may occur during therapy due to acute degeneration of submucous fibroids (see 'Special Warnings and Precautions for Use' section 4.4).

4.9 Overdose

There is no clinical experience with the effects of an acute overdose of leuprorelin acetate. In animal studies, doses of up to 500 times the recommended human dose resulted in dyspnoea, decreased activity and local irritation at the injection site. In cases of overdosage, the patients should be monitored closely and management should be symptomatic and supportive.

5. PHARMACOLOGICAL PROPERTIES

5.1 Pharmacodynamic properties

PROSTAP 3 contains leuprorelin acetate, a synthetic non-apeptide analogue of naturally occurring gonadotrophin releasing hormone (GnRH), which possesses greater potency than the natural hormone. Leuprorelin acetate is a peptide and therefore unrelated to the steroids. Chronic administration results in an inhibition of gonadotrophin production and subsequent suppression of ovarian and testicular steroid secretion. This effect is reversible on discontinuation of therapy.

Administration of leuprorelin acetate results in an initial increase in circulating levels of gonadotrophins, which leads to a transient increase in gonadal steroid levels in both men and women. Continued administration of leuprorelin acetate results in a decrease of gonadotrophin and sex steroid levels. In men serum testosterone levels, initially raised in response to early luteinising hormone (LH) release, fall to castrate levels in about 2-4 weeks.

PROSTAP 3 is inactive when given orally.

5.2 Pharmacokinetic properties

Leuprorelin acetate is well absorbed after subcutaneous and intramuscular injections. It binds to the luteinising hormone releasing hormone (LHRH) receptors and is rapidly degraded. An initially high plasma level of leuprorelin peaks at around 3 hours after a PROSTAP 3 subcutaneous injection, followed by a decrease to maintenance levels in 7 to 14 days. PROSTAP 3 provides continuous plasma levels for up to 117 days resulting in suppression of testosterone to below castration level within 4 weeks of the first injection in the majority of patients.

The metabolism, distribution and excretion of leuprorelin acetate in humans have not been fully determined.

5.3 Preclinical safety data

Animal studies have shown that leuprorelin acetate has a high acute safety factor. No major overt toxicological problems have been seen during repeated administration. Whilst the development of pituitary adenomas has been noted in chronic toxicity studies at high doses in some animal species, this has not been observed in long-term clinical studies. No evidence of mutagenicity or teratogenicity has been shown. Animal reproductive studies showed increased foetal mortality and decreased foetal weights reflecting the pharmacological effects of this LHRH antagonist.

6. PHARMACEUTICAL PARTICULARS

6.1 List of excipients

Poly (D-L lactic acid), Mannitol.

6.2 Incompatibilities

No other fluid other than the Sterile Vehicle provided for PROSTAP 3 can be used for the reconstitution of PROSTAP 3 Powder.

6.3 Shelf life

36 months unopened.

Once reconstituted with sterile vehicle, the suspension should be administered immediately.

6.4 Special precautions for storage
Store at or below room temperature (25°C), in the original container. Protect from light.

6.5 Nature and contents of container
Vials containing 11.25mg leuprorelin acetate as microsphere powder. Prefilled syringes containing 2ml of Sterile Vehicle.

6.6 Instructions for use and handling
See 6.2 above.

7. MARKETING AUTHORISATION HOLDER
John Wyeth and Brother Limited. Trading as:

Wyeth Pharmaceuticals, Huntercombe Lane South,

Taplow, Maidenhead,

Berkshire SL6 0PH, UK.

8. MARKETING AUTHORISATION NUMBER(S)
PROSTAP 3: PL 00011/0295

Sterile Vehicle: PL 00011/0272

9. DATE OF FIRST AUTHORISATION/RENEWAL OF THE AUTHORISATION
16 December 2004.

10. DATE OF REVISION OF THE TEXT
16 December 2004

*Registered Trademark of Takeda.

Wyeth [logo]

Further Information may be obtained from:

Wyeth Pharmaceuticals, Huntercombe Lane South,

Taplow, Maidenhead, Berkshire SL6 0PH, United Kingdom

Telephone: 01628 415330

Takeda [logo]

Under licence agreement with Takeda Chemical Industries, Ltd., Japan.

Prostap SR

(Wyeth Pharmaceuticals)

1. NAME OF THE MEDICINAL PRODUCT
PROSTAP* SR Leuprorelin Acetate Depot Injection 3.75mg.

2. QUALITATIVE AND QUANTITATIVE COMPOSITION
Each dose of PROSTAP SR Powder 3.75mg contains leuprorelin acetate equivalent to 3.57mg base.

3. PHARMACEUTICAL FORM
Prolonged release powder for suspension for injection by subcutaneous or intramuscular administration after reconstitution with the Sterile Vehicle.

4. CLINICAL PARTICULARS

4.1 Therapeutic indications
(i) Treatment of advanced prostatic cancer.

(ii) Management of endometriosis, including pain relief and reduction of endometriotic lesions.

(iii) Endometrial preparation prior to intrauterine surgical procedures including endometrial ablation or resection.

(iv) Preoperative management of uterine fibroids to reduce their size and associated bleeding.

4.2 Posology and method of administration

Dosage

Advanced Prostatic Cancer: The usual recommended dose is 3.75mg administered as a single subcutaneous or intramuscular injection every month. The majority of patients will respond to a 3.75mg dose. PROSTAP therapy should not be discontinued when remission or improvement occurs. As with other drugs administered chronically by injection, the injection site should be varied periodically.

Response to PROSTAP therapy may be monitored by clinical parameters and by measuring serum levels of testosterone and acid phosphatase. Clinical studies have shown that testosterone levels increased during the first 4 days of treatment in the majority of non-orchidectomised patients. They then decreased and reached castrate levels by 2-4 weeks. Once attained, castrate levels were maintained as long as drug therapy continued. Transient increases in acid phosphatase levels sometimes occur early in the treatment period but usually return to normal or near normal values by the 4th week of treatment.

Endometriosis: The recommended dose is 3.75mg administered as a single subcutaneous or intramuscular injection every month for a period of 6 months only. Treatment should be initiated during the first 5 days of the menstrual cycle.

In women receiving GnRH analogues for the treatment of endometriosis, the addition of hormone replacement therapy (HRT - an oestrogen and progestogen) has been shown to reduce bone mineral density loss and vasomotor symptoms. Therefore if appropriate, HRT should be co-administered with PROSTAP taking into account the risks and benefits of each treatment.

Endometrial preparation prior to intrauterine surgery: A single 3.75mg subcutaneous or intramuscular injection 5-6 weeks prior to surgery. Therapy should be initiated during days 3 to 5 of the menstrual cycle.

Preoperative management of uterine fibroids: The recommended dose is 3.75mg administered as a single subcutaneous or intramuscular injection every month, usually for 3-4 months but for a maximum of six months.

Elderly: As for adults.

Children: Safety and efficacy in children have not been established.

Administration

The vial of PROSTAP SR microcapsule powder should be reconstituted immediately prior to administration by subcutaneous or intramuscular injection. Remove flip-cap from vial of PROSTAP SR Powder and cap from prefilled syringe containing 1ml of Sterile Vehicle. Ensure 23 gauge needle is fixed securely to the syringe and inject whole contents of syringe into vial of PROSTAP SR Powder using an aseptic technique. Remove the syringe/needle and keep aseptic. Shake vial gently for 15-20 seconds to produce a uniform cloudy suspension of PROSTAP.

Immediately draw up suspension into syringe taking care to exclude air bubbles. Change the needle on syringe using a 23 gauge needle if the suspension is to be administered subcutaneously or alternatively a 21 gauge needle for intramuscular administration. Having cleaned an appropriate injection site and ensured that the needle is fixed securely, administer the suspension by subcutaneous or intramuscular injection as appropriate taking care not to enter a blood vessel. Apply sterile dressing to injection site if required.

The injection should be given as soon as possible after mixing. If any settling of suspension occurs in vial or syringe, re-suspend by gentle shaking and administer immediately.

No other fluid can be used for reconstitution of PROSTAP SR Powder.

4.3 Contraindications
Hypersensitivity to any of the ingredients or to synthetic Gn-RH or Gn-RH derivatives.

Women: PROSTAP is contra-indicated in women who are or may become pregnant while receiving the drug. PROSTAP should not be used in women who are breastfeeding or have undiagnosed abnormal vaginal bleeding.

Men: There are no known contra-indications to the use of PROSTAP in men.

4.4 Special warnings and special precautions for use
Diabetic patients may require more frequent monitoring of blood glucose during treatment with PROSTAP.

Spinal fracture, paralysis, hypotension and worsening of depression have been reported.

Men: In the initial stages of therapy, a transient rise in levels of testosterone, dihydrotestosterone and acid phosphatase may occur. In some cases, this may be associated with a "flare" or exacerbation of the tumour growth resulting in temporary deterioration of the patient's condition. These symptoms usually subside on continuation of therapy. "Flare" may manifest itself as systemic or neurological symptoms in some cases.

In order to reduce the risk of "flare", an anti-androgen may be administered beginning 3 days prior to leuprorelin therapy and continuing for the first two to three weeks of treatment. This has been reported to prevent the sequelae of an initial rise in serum testosterone.

Patients at risk of ureteric obstruction or spinal cord compression should be considered carefully and closely supervised in the first few weeks of treatment. These patients should be considered for prophylactic treatment with anti-androgens. Should urological/neurological complications occur, these should be treated by appropriate specific measures.

If an anti-androgen is used over a prolonged period, due attention should be paid to the contra-indications and precautions associated with its extended use.

Whilst the development of pituitary adenomas has been noted in chronic toxicity studies at high doses in some animal species, this has not been observed in long term clinical studies with PROSTAP.

Women: When considering the preoperative treatment of fibroids it is mandatory to confirm the diagnosis of fibroids and exclude an ovarian mass, either visually by laparoscopy or by ultrasonography or other investigative technique, as appropriate, before PROSTAP therapy is instituted.

During the early phase of therapy, sex steroids temporarily rise above baseline because of the physiological effect of the drug. Therefore, an increase in clinical signs and symptoms may be observed during the initial days of therapy, but these will dissipate with continued therapy.

The induced hypo-oestrogenic state results in a small loss in bone density over the course of treatment, some of which may not be reversible. The extent of bone demineralisation due to hypo-oestrogenaemia is proportional to time and, consequently, is the adverse event responsible for limiting the duration of therapy to 6 months. The generally accepted level of bone loss with LHRH analogues such as PROSTAP is 5%. In clinical studies with PROSTAP the levels varied between 2.3% and 15.7% depending on the method of measurement. During one six-month treatment period, this bone loss should not be important. In patients with major risk factors for decreased bone mineral content such as chronic alcohol and/or tobacco use, strong family history of osteoporosis, or chronic use of drugs that can reduce bone mass such as anticonvulsants or corticosteroids, PROSTAP therapy may pose an additional risk. In these patients, the risks and benefits must be weighed carefully before therapy with PROSTAP is instituted. This is particularly important in women with uterine fibroids where age related bone loss may have already begun to occur.

Therefore, before using PROSTAP for the preoperative treatment of uterine fibroids, patients with major risk factors for decreased bone mineral content (see above) should have their bone density measured and where results are below the normal (5th percentile by DEXA scan) range, PROSTAP therapy should not be started.

In women with submucous fibroids there have been reports of severe bleeding following the administration of PROSTAP as a consequence of the acute degeneration of the fibroids. Patients should be warned of the possibility of abnormal bleeding or pain in case earlier surgical intervention is required.

PROSTAP may cause an increase in uterine cervical resistance, which may result in difficulty in dilating the cervix for intrauterine surgical procedures.

In women receiving GnRH analogues for the treatment of endometriosis, the addition of HRT (an oestrogen and progestogen) has been shown to reduce bone mineral density loss and vasomotor symptoms.

Precautions

Men: Patients with urinary obstruction and patients with metastatic vertebral lesions should begin PROSTAP therapy under close supervision for the first few weeks of treatment.

Women: Since menstruation should stop with effective doses of PROSTAP, the patient should notify her physician if regular menstruation persists.

4.5 Interaction with other medicinal products and other forms of Interaction
None have been reported.

4.6 Pregnancy and lactation
Safe use of leuprorelin acetate in pregnancy has not been established clinically.

Studies in animals have shown reproductive toxicity (see section 5.3). Before starting treatment with PROSTAP, pregnancy must be excluded. There have been reports of foetal malformation when Prostap has been given during pregnancy.

PROSTAP should not be used in women who are breastfeeding.

When used monthly at the recommended dose, PROSTAP usually inhibits ovulation and stops menstruation. Contraception is not ensured, however, by taking PROSTAP and therefore patients should use non-hormonal methods of contraception during treatment.

Patients should be advised that if they miss successive doses of PROSTAP, breakthrough bleeding or ovulation may occur with the potential for conception. Patients should be advised to see their physician if they believe they may be pregnant. If a patient becomes pregnant during treatment, the drug must be discontinued. The patient must be appraised of this evidence and the potential for an unknown risk to the foetus.

4.7 Effects on ability to drive and use machines
The ability to drive and use machines may be impaired due to visual disturbances and dizziness.

4.8 Undesirable effects
Side effects seen with PROSTAP are due mainly to the specific pharmacological action, namely increases and decreases in certain hormone levels. Adverse events which have been reported infrequently include peripheral oedema, pulmonary embolism, hypertension, palpitations, fatigue, muscle weakness, diarrhoea, nausea, vomiting, anorexia, fever/chills, headache (occasionally severe), hot flushes, arthralgia, myalgia, dizziness, insomnia, paraesthesia, visual disturbances, weight changes, increases in liver function test values and irritation at the injection site. Changes in blood lipids and alteration of glucose tolerance have also been reported which may affect diabetic control. Thrombocytopenia and leucopenia have been reported rarely. Hypersensitivity reactions including rash, pruritus, urticaria, and rarely, wheezing or interstitial pneumonitis have also been reported. Anaphylactic reactions are rare.

Spinal fracture, paralysis, hypotension and worsening of depression have been reported (see 'Special Warnings and Precautions for Use' section 4.4).

Infarction of pre-existing pituitary adenoma has been reported rarely after administration of both short- and long-acting GnRH agonists.

Men: In cases where a "tumour flare" occurs after PROSTAP therapy, an exacerbation may occur in any symptoms or signs due to disease, for example, bone pain, urinary obstruction etc. These symptoms subside on continuation of therapy.

Impotence and decreased libido will be expected with PROSTAP therapy.

The administration of PROSTAP is often associated with hot flushes and sometimes sweating.

Gynaecomastia has been reported occasionally.

Women: Those adverse events occurring most frequently with PROSTAP are associated with hypo-oestrogenism; the most frequently reported are hot flushes, mood swings including depression (occasionally severe), and vaginal dryness. Oestrogen levels return to normal after treatment is discontinued.

The induced hypo-oestrogenic state results in a small loss in bone density over the course of treatment, some of which may not be reversible (see 'Special Warnings and Precautions for Use' section 4.4).

Breast tenderness or change in breast size may occur occasionally. Hair loss has also been reported occasionally.

Vaginal haemorrhage may occur during therapy due to acute degeneration of submucous fibroids (see 'Special Warnings and Precautions for Use' section 4.4).

4.9 Overdose

There is no clinical experience with the effects of an acute overdose of PROSTAP. In animal studies, doses of up to 500 times the recommended human dose resulted in dyspnoea, decreased activity and local irritation at the injection site. In cases of overdose, the patients should be monitored closely and management should be symptomatic and supportive.

5. PHARMACOLOGICAL PROPERTIES

5.1 Pharmacodynamic properties

PROSTAP is a synthetic nonapeptide analogue of naturally occurring gonadotrophin releasing hormone (GnRH) which possesses greater potency than the natural hormone. PROSTAP is a peptide and therefore unrelated to the steroids. Chronic administration results in an inhibition of gonadotrophin production and subsequent suppression of ovarian and testicular steroid secretion. This effect is reversible on discontinuation of therapy.

Administration of leuprorelin acetate results in an initial increase in circulating levels of gonadotrophins which leads to a transient increase in gonadal steroid levels in both men and women. Continued administration of leuprorelin acetate results in a decrease of gonadotrophin and sex steroid levels. In men serum testosterone levels, initially raised in response to early luteinising hormone (LH) release, fall to castrate levels in about 2-4 weeks. Oestradiol levels will decrease to postmenopausal levels in premenopausal women within one month of initiating treatment.

The drug is well absorbed from the subcutaneous or intramuscular route, binds to luteinising hormone releasing hormone (LHRH) receptors and is rapidly degraded. In this dose form, an initial high level of leuprorelin in the plasma is achieved within 3 hours followed by a drop over 24-48 hours to maintenance levels of 0.3-0.8ng/ml and a slow decline thereafter. Effective levels persist for 30-40 days after a single dose. PROSTAP is inactive when given orally.

5.2 Pharmacokinetic properties

Studies submitted show that single intramuscular or subcutaneous doses of leuprorelin acetate over the dose range 3.75 to 15mg results in detectable levels of leuprorelin for more than 28 days, good bioavailability, a consistent and predictable pharmacokinetic profile, and biological efficacy at plasma levels of less than 0.5ng/ml. The pharmacokinetic profile is similar to that seen in animal studies using the compound, with an initial high level of drug released from the microcapsules during reconstitution and injection followed by a plateau over a 2-3 week period before levels gradually become undetectable. There appears to be no significant difference between the routes of administration (im vs sc) in biological effectiveness or pharmacokinetics.

The metabolism, distribution and excretion of leuprorelin acetate in humans have not been fully determined.

5.3 Preclinical safety data

A teratogenic effect has been observed in rabbits but not in rats.

6. PHARMACEUTICAL PARTICULARS

6.1 List of excipients

PROSTAP SR Powder:

Gelatin, copoly (DL-lactic acid/glycolic acid) 75:25 mol%, mannitol.

Sterile Vehicle:

Each ml contains sodium carboxymethyl cellulose 5mg, mannitol 50mg and polysorbate 80 1mg in water for injections.

6.2 Incompatibilities

None reported.

6.3 Shelf life

36 months unopened.

Chemical and Physical in-use stability has been demonstrated for 24 hours at 25°C.

From a microbiological point of view, once reconstituted with Sterile Vehicle, the product should be used immediately. If not used immediately, in-use storage times and conditions prior to use are the responsibility of the user and would normally not be longer than 24 hours at 2 to 8°C, unless reconstitution has taken place in controlled and validated aseptic conditions.

6.4 Special precautions for storage

Do not store above 25°C. Store in the original container and protect from light.

6.5 Nature and contents of container

Vials containing 3.75mg leuprorelin acetate as microcapsule powder.

Prefilled syringes containing 1ml of Sterile Vehicle.

6.6 Instructions for use and handling

PROSTAP SR Powder 3.75mg: A sterile, lyophilised, white odourless PLGA microcapsule powder for subcutaneous or intramuscular injection after reconstitution with the Sterile Vehicle (4 week depot injection).

PLGA = copoly (DL-lactic acid/glycolic acid) 75:25mol%.

Sterile Vehicle: Prefilled syringes containing 1ml of clear, colourless, slightly viscous, Sterile Vehicle for reconstitution of the microcapsules.

7. MARKETING AUTHORISATION HOLDER

John Wyeth & Brother Limited Trading as:

Wyeth Pharmaceuticals

Huntercombe Lane South, Taplow, Maidenhead, Berks SL6 0PH, UK.

8. MARKETING AUTHORISATION NUMBER(S)

PL 00011/0271 PROSTAP SR.

PL 00011/0272 Sterile Vehicle.

9. DATE OF FIRST AUTHORISATION/RENEWAL OF THE AUTHORISATION

16 December 2004

10. DATE OF REVISION OF THE TEXT

16 December 2004

[Wyeth] logo

Distributed by Wyeth Pharmaceuticals,

Huntercombe Lane South, Taplow, Maidenhead,

Berks., UK, SL6 0PH.

Telephone (01628) 415330

[Takeda] logo

Under Licence Agreement with Takeda Chemical Industries

Ltd, Japan

* Registered Trademark of Takeda Chemical Industries.

Prostin E2 Sterile Solution 10 mg/ml Intravenous

(Pharmacia Limited)

1. NAME OF THE MEDICINAL PRODUCT

Prostin E2 Sterile Solution 10 mg/ml

2. QUALITATIVE AND QUANTITATIVE COMPOSITION

Each ml contains 10 mg dinoprostone.

3. PHARMACEUTICAL FORM

Colourless, sterile solution, which after appropriate dilution is intended for intravenous administration to human beings

4. CLINICAL PARTICULARS

4.1 Therapeutic indications

Oxytocic agent. Therapeutic termination of pregnancy, missed abortion and hydatidiform mole by the intravenous route.

4.2 Posology and method of administration

Adults: Ampoule contents must be diluted before use and full instructions on method of dilution and dosage are given on the package insert which should be consulted prior to initiation of therapy. The following is a guide to dosage:

Dilute with normal saline or 5% dextrose according to the package insert to produce a 5 micrograms/ml solution. The 5 micrograms/ml solution is infused at 2.5 micrograms/minute for 30 minutes and then maintained or increased to 5 micrograms/minute. The rate should be maintained for at least 4 hours before increasing further.

Elderly: Not applicable

Children: Not applicable

4.3 Contraindications

Prostin E2 Sterile Solution should not be used where the patient is sensitive to prostaglandins.

Prostin E2 Sterile Solution 10 mg/ml is not recommended in the following circumstances:

1. For patients in whom oxytocic drugs are generally contra-indicated or where prolonged contractions of the uterus are considered inappropriate such as:

Cases with a history of Caesarean section or major uterine surgery.

Cases where there is evidence of a potential for obstructed labour.

2. In patients with a past history of, or existing, pelvic inflammatory disease, unless adequate prior treatment has been instituted.

3. Patients with active cardiac, pulmonary, renal or hepatic disease.

4.4 Special warnings and special precautions for use

This product is only available to hospitals and clinics with specialised obstetric units and should only be used where 24-hour resident medical cover is provided

Use caution in handling this product to prevent contact with skin. Wash hands thoroughly with soap and water after administration.

It is advised that Prostin E2 Sterile Solution should not be administered by the intramyometrial route since there have been reports of a possible association between this route of administration and cardiac arrest in severely ill patients.

Caution should be exercised in the administration of Prostin E2 Sterile Solution in patients with:

(i) Asthma or a history of asthma.

(ii) Epilepsy or a history of epilepsy.

(iii) Glaucoma or raised intra-ocular pressure.

(iv) Compromised cardiovascular, hepatic, or renal function.

(v) Hypertension.

As with any oxytocic agent, Prostin E2 Sterile Solution should be used with caution in patients with compromised (scarred) uteri.

Animal studies lasting several weeks at high doses have shown that prostaglandins of the E and F series can induce proliferation of bone. Such effects have also been noted in newborn infants who received prostaglandin E_1 during prolonged treatment. There is no evidence that short-term administration of prostaglandin E_2 can cause similar bone effects.

4.5 Interaction with other medicinal products and other forms of Interaction

Since it has been found that prostaglandins potentiate the effect of oxytocin, it is not recommended that these drugs are used together. If used in sequence, the patient's uterine activity should be carefully monitored.

4.6 Pregnancy and lactation

Prostin E2 Sterile Solution 10 mg/ml is only used during pregnancy for therapeutic termination of pregnancy, missed abortion and hydatidiform mole. There has been some evidence in animals of a low order of teratogenic activity, therefore, if abortion does not occur or is suspected to be incomplete as a result of prostaglandin therapy, (as in spontaneous abortion, where the process is sometimes incomplete), the appropriate treatment for complete evacuation of the pregnant uterus should be instituted in all instances.

Prostaglandins are excreted in breast milk. This is not expected to be a hazard given the circumstances in which the product is used.

4.7 Effects on ability to drive and use machines

Not applicable

4.8 Undesirable effects

The most commonly reported events are vomiting, nausea and diarrhoea. Certain rare events that should be especially noted are: hypersensitivity to the drug; uterine rupture; and cardiac arrest. Other adverse events, in decreasing order of severity, reported with use of dinoprostone are:

Pulmonary/amniotic fluid embolism; Uterine hypercontractility or hypertonus; Hypertension - systemic (maternal); Bronchospasm/asthma; Rapid cervical dilation; Fever; Back ache; Rash.

In addition, with intravenous use, transient vasovagal symptoms, including flushing, shivering, headache and dizziness, have been recorded. Local tissue irritation and erythema have occurred. No evidence of thrombophlebitis has been recorded and local tissue erythema at the infusion site has disappeared within two to five hours after infusion. A temporary pyrexia and elevated WBC are not unusual, but both have reverted after termination of infusion.

4.9 Overdose

Uterine hypertonus or unduly severe uterine contractions have rarely been encountered, but might be anticipated to result from overdosage. Treatment of overdosage must be, at this time, symptomatic, as clinical studies with prostaglandin antagonists have not progressed to the point where recommendations may be made. If evidence of excessive uterine activity or side-effects appears, the rate of infusion should be decreased or discontinued. In cases of massive overdosage resulting in extreme uterine hypertonus, appropriate obstetric procedures are indicated.

5. PHARMACOLOGICAL PROPERTIES

5.1 Pharmacodynamic properties

Dinoprostone is a prostaglandin of the E series with actions on smooth muscle. It induces contraction of uterine muscle at any stage of pregnancy.

5.2 Pharmacokinetic properties

5.2 a General characteristics of active substance

Dinoprostone is rapidly metabolised in the body. Intravenous administration results in very rapid distribution and metabolism, with only 3% of unchanged drug remaining in the blood after 15 minutes. At least nine prostaglandin E_2 metabolites have been identified in human blood and urine.

5.2 b Characteristics in patients

No special characteristics. See "Special warnings and special precautions for use" for further information.

5.3 Preclinical safety data

There are no pre-clinical data of relevance to the prescriber which are additional to that already included in other sections of the SPC.

6. PHARMACEUTICAL PARTICULARS

6.1 List of excipients

Dehydrated alcohol.

6.2 Incompatibilities

None known

6.3 Shelf life

24 months.

6.4 Special precautions for storage

Special precautions for product and admixture storage

Store in a refrigerator at 4°C. Once diluted, the diluted solution should be stored in a refrigerator at 4°C and used within 24 hours.

6.5 Nature and contents of container

Ph. Eur. Type I glass ampoule, containing 0.5 ml sterile solution, packed in a carton.

6.6 Instructions for use and handling

Use caution in handling this product to prevent contact with skin. Wash hands thoroughly with soap and water after administration.

7. MARKETING AUTHORISATION HOLDER

Pharmacia Limited

Davy Avenue

Milton Keynes

MK5 8PH

UK

8. MARKETING AUTHORISATION NUMBER(S)

PL 0032/0021R

9. DATE OF FIRST AUTHORISATION/RENEWAL OF THE AUTHORISATION

27 June 1986/17 November 1998

10. DATE OF REVISION OF THE TEXT

April 2001

Legal Category

POM.

Prostin E2 Sterile Solution 10mg/ml Extra-Amniotic

(Pharmacia Limited)

1. NAME OF THE MEDICINAL PRODUCT

Prostin E2 Sterile Solution 10 mg/ml.

2. QUALITATIVE AND QUANTITATIVE COMPOSITION

Each ml contains 10 mg dinoprostone.

3. PHARMACEUTICAL FORM

Colourless, sterile solution, which after appropriate dilution is intended for extra-amniotic administration to human beings.

4. CLINICAL PARTICULARS

4.1 Therapeutic indications

Oxytocic agent. The therapeutic termination of pregnancy, by the extra-amniotic route.

4.2 Posology and method of administration

Adults: Ampoule contents must be diluted before use and full instructions on method of dilution and dosage are given on the package insert which should be consulted prior to initiation of therapy. The following is a guide to dosage:

Dilute with the 50ml of diluent provided according to the package insert to produce a 100 micrograms/ml solution. The 100 micrograms/ml solution is instilled via a 12-14 French gauge Foley catheter. Initial instillation is 1ml, then dependent on uterine response, 1 or 2 ml usually at two hour intervals.

Elderly: Not applicable

Children: Not applicable

4.3 Contraindications

Prostin E2 Sterile Solution should not be used where the patient is sensitive to prostaglandins.

Prostin E2 Sterile Solution 10 mg/ml is not recommended in the following circumstances:

1. For patients in whom oxytocic drugs are generally contra-indicated or where prolonged contractions of the uterus are considered inappropriate such as:
   Cases with a history of Caesarean section or major uterine surgery;
   Cases where there is evidence of a potential for obstructed labour;
2. In patients with a past history of; or existing, pelvic inflammatory disease, unless adequate prior treatment has been instituted.
3. In patients with cervicitis or vaginal infections.
4. Patients with active cardiac, pulmonary, renal or hepatic disease.

4.4 Special warnings and special precautions for use

This product is only available to hospitals and clinics with specialised obstetric units and should only be used where 24-hour resident medical cover is provided

Use caution in handling this product to prevent contact with skin. Wash hands thoroughly with soap and water after administration.

It is advised that Prostin E2 Sterile Solution should not be administered by the intramyometrial route since there have been reports of a possible association between this route of administration and cardiac arrest in severely ill patients.

Caution should be exercised in the administration of Prostin E2 Sterile Solution to patients with:

(i) asthma or a history of asthma;

(ii) epilepsy or a history of epilepsy;

(iii) glaucoma or raised intra-ocular pressure;

(iv) compromised cardiovascular, hepatic, or renal function.

(v) hypertension

As with any oxytocic agent, Prostin E2 Sterile Solution should be used with caution in patients with compromised (scarred) uteri.

Animal studies lasting several weeks at high doses have shown that prostaglandins of the E and F series can induce proliferation of bone. Such effects have also been noted in newborn infants who received prostaglandin E_1 during prolonged treatment. There is no evidence that short-term administration of prostaglandin E_2 can cause similar bone effects.

4.5 Interaction with other medicinal products and other forms of Interaction

Since it has been found that prostaglandins potentiate the effect of oxytocin, it is not recommended that these drugs are used together. If used in sequence, the patient's uterine activity should be carefully monitored.

4.6 Pregnancy and lactation

Pregnancy Code D

Prostin E2 Sterile Solution 10 mg/ml is only used during pregnancy for therapeutic termination of pregnancy. There has been some evidence in animals of a low order of teratogenic activity, therefore, if abortion does not occur or is suspected to be incomplete as a result of prostaglandin therapy, (as in spontaneous abortion, where the process is sometimes incomplete), the appropriate treatment for complete evacuation of the pregnant uterus should be instituted in all instances.

Prostaglandins are excreted in breast milk. This is not expected to be a hazard given the circumstances in which the product is used.

4.7 Effects on ability to drive and use machines

Not applicable

4.8 Undesirable effects

The most commonly reported events are vomiting, nausea and diarrhoea. Certain rare events that should be especially noted are: hypersensitivity to the drug; uterine rupture; and cardiac arrest. Other adverse effects, in decreasing order of severity reported with use of dinoprostone are:

Pulmonary/amniotic fluid embolism;

Uterine hypercontractility or hypertonus;

Hypertension - systemic (maternal);

Bronchospasm/asthma;

Rapid cervical dilation;

Fever;

Back ache;

Rash.

A temporary pyrexia and elevated WBC are not unusual, but both have reverted after termination of therapy. In extra-amniotic therapy, the possibility of local infection must be considered and appropriate therapy initiated if necessary.

4.9 Overdose

Uterine hypertonus or unduly severe uterine contractions have rarely been encountered, but might be anticipated to result from overdosage. Treatment of overdosage must be, at this time, symptomatic, as clinical studies with prostaglandin antagonists have not progressed to the point where recommendations may be made. If evidence of excessive uterine activity or side-effects appears, the rate of infusion should be decreased or discontinued. In cases of massive overdosage resulting in extreme uterine hypertonus, appropriate obstetric procedures are indicated.

5. PHARMACOLOGICAL PROPERTIES

5.1 Pharmacodynamic properties

Dinoprostone is a prostaglandin of the E series with actions on smooth muscle. It induces contraction of uterine muscle at any stage of pregnancy.

5.2 Pharmacokinetic properties

General characteristics of active substance

Dinoprostone is rapidly metabolised in the body. Intravenous administration results in very rapid distribution and metabolism, with only 3% of unchanged drug remaining in the blood after 15 minutes. At least nine prostaglandin E_2 metabolites have been identified in human blood and urine.

Characteristics in Patients

No special characteristics. See "Special Warnings and Precautions for use" for further information.

5.3 Preclinical safety data

In mice and rats, the oral LD_{50} values were >500mg/kg and 141-513 mg/kg respectively.

Three month oral administration to rats resulted in significantly heavier stomach weights for treated compared with untreated rats, which effect was reversible on treatment cessation. Treated rats had a dose related acanthotic squamous glandular junction and thickened glandular gastric mucosal epithelium. No significant alterations were recognized in routine evaluation of the stemebrae and the femur.

A fourteen day oral toxicity study in dogs showed a maximum tolerated dose of 6-20 mg/kg/day. All treated dogs had microscopic evidence of increased fundic and pyloric mucus. The fundic and pyloric mucosa were thickened, having a cobblestone appearance and had an increased gastric mucus in both 20 mg/kg/day treated dogs and the 60 mg/kg/day male dog. These were the only gross and microscopic drug related changes observed.

Satisfactory results were obtained in intravenous and intramuscular tolerability tests performed in dog and monkey.

Teratogenic effects were observed in rats injected subcutaneously with 0.5 mg/animal. No teratogenic effects were seen in the rabbit at dosage levels of up to 1.5 mg/kg day.

No evidence of mutagenicity was obtained using the Ames Assay, the DNA Damage/Alkaline Elution Assay and the micronucleus test.

6. PHARMACEUTICAL PARTICULARS

6.1 List of excipients

Dehydrated alcohol BP

6.2 Incompatibilities

None known

6.3 Shelf life

24 months.

6.4 Special precautions for storage

Store in a refrigerator at 4°C. The product after dilution should be stored in a refrigerator at 4°C and should not be kept for more than 48 hours.

6.5 Nature and contents of container

Ph. Eur. Type I glass ampoule, containing 0.5 ml sterile solution, packed in a carton, together with a vial containing diluent.

6.6 Instructions for use and handling

Use caution in handling this product to prevent contact with skin. Wash hands thoroughly with soap and water after administration.

7. MARKETING AUTHORISATION HOLDER

Pharmacia Limited

Davy Avenue

Milton Keynes

MK5 8PH

8. MARKETING AUTHORISATION NUMBER(S)

PL 0032/0026R

9. DATE OF FIRST AUTHORISATION/RENEWAL OF THE AUTHORISATION

1 July 1986 / 18 March 1997

10. DATE OF REVISION OF THE TEXT

May 2001

Legal Category

POM.

Prostin E2 Sterile Solution 1mg/ml Intravenous

(Pharmacia Limited)

1. NAME OF THE MEDICINAL PRODUCT

Prostin E2 Sterile Solution 1 mg/ml.

2. QUALITATIVE AND QUANTITATIVE COMPOSITION
Each ml contains 1 mg dinoprostone.

3. PHARMACEUTICAL FORM
Colourless, sterile solution, which after appropriate dilution is intended for intravenous administration to human beings.

4. CLINICAL PARTICULARS
4.1 Therapeutic indications
The induction of labour by the intravenous route.

4.2 Posology and method of administration
Adults

Ampoule contents must be diluted before use and full instructions on method of dilution and dosage are given on the package insert which should be consulted prior to initiation of therapy. The following is a guide to dosage:

Dilute with normal saline or 5% dextrose according to the package insert to produce a 1.5 micrograms/ml solution. The 1.5 micrograms/ml solution is infused at 0.25 micrograms/minute for 30 minutes and then maintained or increased. Cases of fetal death *in utero* may require higher doses. An initial rate of 0.5 micrograms/minute may be used with stepwise increases, at intervals of not less than one hour.

Elderly

Not applicable

Children

Not applicable

4.3 Contraindications
Prostin E2 Sterile Solution should not be used where the patient is sensitive to prostaglandins.

Prostin E2 Sterile Solution 1 mg/ml is not recommended in the following circumstances:

1. For patients in whom oxytocic drugs are generally contra-indicated or where prolonged contractions of the uterus are considered inappropriate such as:

Cases with a history of Caesarean section or major uterine surgery;

Cases where there is cephalopelvic disproportion;

Cases in which fetal malpresentation is present;

Cases where there is clinical suspicion or definite evidence of pre-existing fetal distress;

Cases in which there is a history of difficult labour and/or traumatic delivery;

Grand multiparae with over five previous term pregnancies.

2. In patients with a past history of, or existing, pelvic inflammatory disease, unless adequate prior treatment has been instituted.

3. In patients where there is clinical suspicion or definite evidence of placenta praevia or unexplained vaginal bleeding during this pregnancy.

4. Patients with active cardiac, pulmonary, renal or hepatic disease.

4.4 Special warnings and special precautions for use

This product is only available to hospitals and clinics with specialised obstetric units and should only be used where 24-hour resident medical cover is provided

Use caution in handling this product to prevent contact with skin. Wash hands thoroughly with soap and water after administration.

It is advised that Prostin E2 Sterile Solution should not be administered by the intramyometrial route since there have been reports of a possible association between this route of administration and cardiac arrest in severely ill patients.

Caution should be exercised in the administration of Prostin E2 Sterile Solution 1 mg/ml for the induction of labour in patients with:

(i) asthma or a history of asthma.

(ii) epilepsy or a history of epilepsy.

(iii) glaucoma or raised intra-ocular pressure.

(iv) compromised cardiovascular, hepatic, or renal function.

(v) hypertension.

As with any oxytocic agent, Prostin E2 Sterile Solution should be used with caution in patients with compromised (scarred) uteri.

In labour induction, cephalopelvic relationships should be carefully evaluated before use of Prostin E2 Sterile Solution. During use, uterine activity, fetal status and the progression of cervical dilation should be carefully monitored to detect possible evidence of undesired responses, e.g. hypertonus, sustained uterine contractions, or fetal distress. In cases where there is a known history of hypertonic uterine contractility or tetanic uterine contractions, it is recommended that uterine activity and the state of the fetus (where applicable) should be continuously monitored throughout labour. The possibility of uterine rupture should be borne in mind where high-tone uterine contractions are sustained.

Animal studies lasting several weeks at high doses have shown that prostaglandins of the E and F series can induce proliferation of bone. Such effects have also been noted in newborn infants who received prostaglandin E_1 during prolonged treatment. There is no evidence that short-term administration of prostaglandin E_2 can cause similar bone effects.

4.5 Interaction with other medicinal products and other forms of Interaction
Since it has been found that prostaglandins potentiate the effect of oxytocin, it is not recommended that these drugs are used together. If used in sequence, the patient's uterine activity should be carefully monitored.

4.6 Pregnancy and lactation
Pregnancy Code A

Prostin E2 Sterile Solution 1 mg/ml is only used during pregnancy, to induce labour.

Prostaglandins are excreted in breast milk. This is not expected to be a hazard given the circumstances in which the product is used.

4.7 Effects on ability to drive and use machines
Not applicable

4.8 Undesirable effects
The most commonly reported events are vomiting, nausea and diarrhoea. Certain rare events that should be especially noted are: hypersensitivity to the drug; uterine rupture; and cardiac arrest. Other adverse effects, reported in decreasing order of severity are:

Pulmonary/amniotic fluid embolism

Abruptio placenta

Stillbirth, neonatal death

Uterine hypercontractility or hypertonus

Fetal distress

Hypertension - systemic (maternal)

Bronchospasm/asthma

Rapid cervical dilation

Fever

Back ache

Rash

Transient vasovagal symptoms, including flushing, shivering, headache and dizziness, have been recorded with intravenous use of prostaglandin E_2. Local tissue irritation and erythema have occurred. No evidence of thrombophlebitis has been recorded and local tissue erythema at the infusion site has disappeared within two to five hours after infusion. A temporary pyrexia and elevated WBC are not unusual, but both have reverted after termination of infusion.

In addition, other adverse reactions that have been seen with the use of Prostin E2 for term labour induction have included: uterine hypercontractility with fetal bradycardia; uterine hypercontractility without fetal bradycardia; and low Apgar scores in the newborn.

4.9 Overdose
Uterine hypertonus or unduly severe uterine contractions have rarely been encountered, but might be anticipated to result from overdosage. In the rare instance where temporary discontinuation of therapy is not effective in reversing fetal distress or uterine hypertonus, then prompt delivery is indicated. Treatment of overdosage must be, at this time, symptomatic, since clinical studies with prostaglandin antagonists have not progressed to the point where recommendations may be made.

5. PHARMACOLOGICAL PROPERTIES
5.1 Pharmacodynamic properties
Dinoprostone is a prostaglandin of the E series with actions on smooth muscle. It induces contraction of uterine muscle at any stage of pregnancy.

5.2 Pharmacokinetic properties
5.2 a General Characteristics of Active Substance

Dinoprostone is rapidly metabolised in the body. Intravenous administration results in very rapid distribution and metabolism, with only 3% of unchanged drug remaining in the blood after 15 minutes. At least nine prostaglandin E_2 metabolites have been identified in human blood and urine.

5.2 b Characteristics in Patients

No special characteristics. See "Special warnings and special precautions for use" for further information.

5.3 Preclinical safety data
There are no pre-clinical data of relevance which are additional to that already included in other sections of the SPC.

6. PHARMACEUTICAL PARTICULARS
6.1 List of excipients
Dehydrated alcohol

6.2 Incompatibilities
None known

6.3 Shelf life
24 months.

6.4 Special precautions for storage
Store in a refrigerator at 4°C. The product after dilution should be stored in a refrigerator at 4°C and should not be kept for more than 24 hours.

6.5 Nature and contents of container
Ph. Eur. Type I glass ampoule, containing 0.75 ml sterile solution, packed in a carton.

6.6 Instructions for use and handling
Use caution in handling this product to prevent contact with skin. Wash hands thoroughly with soap and water after administration.

7. MARKETING AUTHORISATION HOLDER
Pharmacia Limited

Davy Avenue

Milton Keynes

MK5 8PH

UK

8. MARKETING AUTHORISATION NUMBER(S)
PL 0032/0020R

9. DATE OF FIRST AUTHORISATION/RENEWAL OF THE AUTHORISATION
27 June 1986/17 November 1998

10. DATE OF REVISION OF THE TEXT
April 2001

Legal Category
POM.

Prostin E2 Vaginal Gel 1mg, 2mg

(Pharmacia Limited)

1. NAME OF THE MEDICINAL PRODUCT
Prostin E2 Vaginal Gel 1 mg and 2 mg.

2. QUALITATIVE AND QUANTITATIVE COMPOSITION
Each 3 g gel (2.5 ml) contains 1 mg or 2 mg dinoprostone.

3. PHARMACEUTICAL FORM
Translucent, thixotropic gel.

4. CLINICAL PARTICULARS
4.1 Therapeutic indications
Oxytocic. Prostin E2 Vaginal Gel is indicated for the induction of labour, when there are no fetal or maternal contra-indications.

4.2 Posology and method of administration
Adults: In primigravida patients with unfavourable induction features (Bishop score of 4 or less), an initial dose of 2 mg should be administered vaginally. In other patients an initial dose of 1 mg should be administered vaginally.

In both groups of patients, a second dose of 1 mg or 2 mg may be administered after 6 hours as follows:

1 mg should be used where uterine activity is insufficient for satisfactory progress of labour.

2 mg may be used where response to the initial dose has been minimal.

Maximum dose 4 mg in unfavourable primigravida patients or 3 mg in other patients (see "Precautions").

The gel should be inserted high into the posterior fornix avoiding administration into the cervical canal. The patient should be instructed to remain recumbent for at least 30 minutes.

Elderly

Not applicable

Children

Not applicable

4.3 Contraindications
Prostin E2 Vaginal Gel should not be used where the patient is sensitive to prostaglandins or other constituents of the gel.

Prostin E2 Vaginal Gel is not recommended in the following circumstances:

1. For patients in whom oxytocic drugs are generally contra-indicated or where prolonged contractions of the uterus are considered inappropriate such as:

Cases with a history of Caesarean section or major uterine surgery;

Cases where there is cephalopelvic disproportion;

Cases in which fetal malpresentation is present;

Cases where there is clinical suspicion or definite evidence of pre-existing fetal distress;

Cases in which there is a history of difficult labour and/or traumatic delivery;

Grand multiparae with over five previous term pregnancies.

2. Patients with ruptured membranes.

3. In patients with a past history of, or existing, pelvic inflammatory disease, unless adequate prior treatment has been instituted.

4. In patients where there is clinical suspicion or definite evidence of placenta praevia or unexplained vaginal bleeding during this pregnancy.

5. Patients with active cardiac, pulmonary, renal or hepatic disease.

4.4 Special warnings and special precautions for use

This product is only available to hospitals and clinics with specialised obstetric units and should only be used where 24-hour resident medical cover is provided.

Use the total contents of the syringe for one patient only. Discard after use. Use caution in handling the product to prevent contact with skin. Wash hands thoroughly with soap and water after administration.

Prostin E2 Vaginal Gel and Prostin E2 Vaginal Tablets are not bioequivalent.

Caution should be exercised in the administration of Prostin E2 Vaginal Gel for the induction of labour in patients with:

(i) asthma or a history of asthma;

(ii) epilepsy or a history of epilepsy;

(iii) glaucoma or raised intra-ocular pressure;

(iv) compromised cardiovascular, hepatic, or renal function;

(v) hypertension

As with any oxytocic agent, Prostin E2 Vaginal Gel should be used with caution in patients with compromised (scarred) uteri.

In labour induction, cephalopelvic relationships should be carefully evaluated before use of Prostin E2 Vaginal Gel. During use, uterine activity, fetal status and the progression of cervical dilation should be carefully monitored to detect possible evidence of undesired responses, e.g. hypertonus, sustained uterine contractions, or fetal distress.

In cases where there is a known history of hypertonic uterine contractility or tetanic uterine contractions, it is recommended that uterine activity and the state of the fetus (where applicable) should be continuously monitored throughout labour. The possibility of uterine rupture should be borne in mind where high-tone uterine contractions are sustained.

Animal studies lasting several weeks at high doses have shown that prostaglandins of the E and F series can induce proliferation of bone. Such effects have also been noted in newborn infants who received prostaglandin E_1 during prolonged treatment. There is no evidence that short-term administration of prostaglandin E_2 can cause similar bone effects.

4.5 Interaction with other medicinal products and other forms of Interaction

Since it has been found that prostaglandins potentiate the effect of oxytocin, it is not recommended that these drugs are used together. If used in sequence, the patient's uterine activity should be carefully monitored.

4.6 Pregnancy and lactation

Pregnancy Code A

Prostin E2 Vaginal Gel is only used during pregnancy, to induce labour.

Prostaglandins are excreted in breast milk. This is not expected to be a hazard given the circumstances in which the product is used.

4.7 Effects on ability to drive and use machines

Not applicable

4.8 Undesirable effects

The most commonly reported events are vomiting, nausea and diarrhoea. Certain rare events that should be especially noted are: hypersensitivity to the drug; uterine rupture; and cardiac arrest. Other adverse events, in decreasing order of severity, reported with use of dinoprostone are:

Pulmonary/amniotic fluid embolism;

Abruptio placenta;

Stillbirth, neonatal death;

Uterine hypercontractility or hypertonus;

Fetal distress;

Hypertension - systemic (maternal);

Bronchospasm/asthma;

Rapid cervical dilation;

Fever;

Backache;

Rash;

Vaginal symptoms - warmth, irritation, pain.

In addition, other adverse reactions that have been seen with the use of prostaglandin E_2 for term labour induction have included: uterine hypercontractility with fetal bradycardia; uterine hypercontractility without fetal bradycardia; and low Apgar scores in the newborn.

4.9 Overdose

Uterine hypertonus or unduly severe uterine contractions have rarely been encountered, but might be anticipated to result from overdosage. Where there is evidence of fetal distress or uterine hypertonus, then prompt delivery is indicated. Treatment of overdosage must be, at this time, symptomatic, since clinical studies with prostaglandin antagonists have not progressed to the point where recommendations may be made.

5. PHARMACOLOGICAL PROPERTIES

5.1 Pharmacodynamic properties

Dinoprostone is a prostaglandin of the E series which induces myometrial contractions and promotes cervical ripening.

5.2 Pharmacokinetic properties

General characteristics of active substance

When given vaginally, PGE_2 is rapidly absorbed. Plasma levels of 15-keto PGE_2 equivalents peak at 1.5 hours after administration of a 5 mg dose. *In vitro* work indicates that PGE_2 is 73% bound to human plasma albumin. It is rapidly metabolised in the lungs, kidneys, spleen and liver, with a single pass of the circulatory system converting 90% of an injected PGE_2 dose to metabolites.

Characteristics in patients

No special characteristics. See "Special warnings and special precautions for use" for further information.

5.3 Preclinical safety data

There are no pre-clinical data of relevance which are additional to those already included in other sections of the SPC.

6. PHARMACEUTICAL PARTICULARS

6.1 List of excipients

Triacetin and colloidal silicon dioxide

6.2 Incompatibilities

None known

6.3 Shelf life

Prostin E2 Vaginal Gel has a shelf-life of 24 months when stored in a refrigerator at 2-8°C.

6.4 Special precautions for storage

Store in a refrigerator at 2-8°C.

6.5 Nature and contents of container

Polyethylene syringe containing 3 g or 2.5 ml of gel.

6.6 Instructions for use and handling

Use the total contents of the syringe for one patient only. Discard after use. Use caution in handling this product to prevent contact with skin. Wash hands thoroughly with soap and water after administration.

7. MARKETING AUTHORISATION HOLDER

Pharmacia Limited

Davy Avenue

Milton Keynes

MK5 8PH

UK

8. MARKETING AUTHORISATION NUMBER(S)

Prostin E2 Vaginal Gel 1 mg: PL 0032/0123

Prostin E2 Vaginal Gel 2 mg: PL 0032/0124

9. DATE OF FIRST AUTHORISATION/RENEWAL OF THE AUTHORISATION

30 April 1986/17 November 1998

10. DATE OF REVISION OF THE TEXT

April 2001

Legal Category

POM

Prostin E2 Vaginal Tablets

(Pharmacia Limited)

1. NAME OF THE MEDICINAL PRODUCT

Prostin E2 Vaginal Tablets 3mg

2. QUALITATIVE AND QUANTITATIVE COMPOSITION

Dinoprostone HSE 3 mg

3. PHARMACEUTICAL FORM

Tablet for vaginal administration

4. CLINICAL PARTICULARS

4.1 Therapeutic indications

Oxytocic. Prostin E2 Vaginal Tablets 3mg are indicated for the induction of labour, especially in patients with favourable induction features, when there are no fetal or maternal contra-indications.

4.2 Posology and method of administration

Method of administration: Vaginal tablets are administered by insertion high into the posterior fornix.

One tablet to be inserted high into the posterior fornix. A second tablet may be inserted after six to eight hours if labour is not established. Maximum dose 6 mg.

Children: Not applicable

Elderly: Not applicable

4.3 Contraindications

Prostin E2 Vaginal Tablets should not be used where the patient is sensitive to prostaglandins or other constituents of the tablet.

Prostin E2 Vaginal Tablets are not recommended in the following circumstances:

1. For patients in whom oxytocic drugs are generally contra-indicated or where prolonged contractions of the uterus are considered inappropriate such as:

- Cases with a history of Caesarean section or major uterine surgery;
- Cases where there is cephalopelvic disproportion;
- Cases in which fetal malpresentation is present;
- Cases where there is clinical suspicion or definite evidence of pre-existing fetal distress;
- Cases in which there is a history of difficult labour and/or traumatic delivery;
- Grand multiparae with over five previous term pregnancies.

2. Patients with ruptured membranes.

3. In patients with a past history of, or existing, pelvic inflammatory disease, unless adequate prior treatment has been instituted.

4. In patients where there is clinical suspicion or definite evidence of placenta praevia or unexplained vaginal bleeding during this pregnancy.

5. Patients with active cardiac, pulmonary, renal or hepatic disease.

4.4 Special warnings and special precautions for use

This product is only available to hospitals and clinics with specialised obstetric units and should only be used where 24-hour resident medical cover is provided

Use caution in handling this product to prevent contact with skin. Wash hands thoroughly with soap and water after administration.

Caution should be exercised in the administration of Prostin E2 Vaginal Tablets for the induction of labour in patients with:

(i) asthma or a history of asthma;

(ii) epilepsy or a history of epilepsy;

(iii) glaucoma or raised intra-ocular pressure;

(iv) compromised cardiovascular, hepatic, or renal function;

(v) hypertension

As with any oxytocic agent, Prostin E2 Vaginal Tablets should be used with caution in patients with compromised (scarred) uteri.

In labour induction, cephalopelvic relationships should be carefully evaluated before use of Prostin E2 Vaginal Tablets. During use, uterine activity, fetal status and the progression of cervical dilation should be carefully monitored to detect possible evidence of undesired responses, e.g. hypertonus, sustained uterine contractions, or fetal distress.

In cases where there is a known history of hypertonic uterine contractility or tetanic uterine contractions, it is recommended that uterine activity and the state of the fetus (where applicable) should be continuously monitored throughout labour. The possibility of uterine rupture should be borne in mind where high-tone uterine contractions are sustained.

4.5 Interaction with other medicinal products and other forms of Interaction

Since it has been found that prostaglandins potentiate the effect of oxytocin, it is not recommended that these drugs are used together. If used in sequence, the patient's uterine activity should be carefully monitored.

4.6 Pregnancy and lactation

Prostin E2 Vaginal Tablets are only used during pregnancy, to induce labour.

Prostaglandins are excreted in breast milk. This is not expected to be a hazard given the circumstances in which the product is used.

4.7 Effects on ability to drive and use machines

Not applicable

4.8 Undesirable effects

The most commonly reported events are vomiting, nausea and diarrhoea. Certain rare events that should be especially noted are: hypersensitivity to the drug; uterine rupture; and cardiac arrest. Other adverse events, in decreasing order of severity, reported with use of dinoprostone are:

Pulmonary/amniotic fluid embolism;

Abruptio placenta;

Stillbirth, neonatal death;

Uterine hypercontractility or hypertonus;

Fetal distress;

Hypertension - systemic (maternal);

Bronchospasm/asthma;

Rapid cervical dilation;

Fever;

Backache;

Rash;

Vaginal symptoms - warmth, irritation, pain.

In addition, other adverse reactions that have been seen with the use of prostaglandin E_2 for term labour induction have included: altered fetal heart rate patterns; uterine hypercontractility with fetal bradycardia; uterine hypercontractility without fetal bradycardia; and low Apgar scores in the newborn.

4.9 Overdose

Uterine hypertonus or unduly severe uterine contractions have rarely been encountered, but might be anticipated to result from overdosage. Where there is evidence of fetal distress or uterine hypertonus, then prompt delivery is indicated. Treatment of overdosage must be, at this time, symptomatic, since clinical studies with prostaglandin antagonists have not progressed to the point where recommendations may be made. It is currently believed that vomiting produced by overdosage may act as a self-limiting factor in protecting the patient.

5. PHARMACOLOGICAL PROPERTIES

5.1 Pharmacodynamic properties

Dinoprostone is a prostaglandin of the E series with actions on smooth muscle; the endogenous substance is termed prostaglandin E2 (PGE_2). It induces contraction of uterine muscle at any stage of pregnancy and is reported to act predominantly as a vasodilator on blood vessels and as a bronchodilator on bronchial muscle. It is postulated that vaginal absorption of PGE_2 stimulates endogenous PGE_2 and $PGF_{2\alpha}$ production, similar to that which is seen in spontaneous labour.

5.2 Pharmacokinetic properties

Following insertion of the tablet, PGE_2 absorption (as measured by the presence of PGE_2 metabolites) increases to reach a peak at about 40 minutes. PGE_2 is rapidly metabolised to 13, 14-dihydro, 15-keto PGE_2 which is converted to 13, 14-dihydro, 15-keto PGA_2 which binds covalently to albumen.

There has been found to be inter-patient variability regarding systemic absorption of PGE_2. This can be attributed to different conditions of the vaginal mucosa between patients.

5.3 Preclinical safety data

Animal studies lasting several weeks at high doses have shown that prostaglandins of the E and F series can induce proliferation of bone. Such effects have also been noted in newborn infants who received prostaglandin E_1 during prolonged treatment. There is no evidence that short-term administration of prostaglandin E_2 can cause similar bone effects.

6. PHARMACEUTICAL PARTICULARS

6.1 List of excipients

Lactose

Microcrystalline Cellulose

Colloidal Silicon Dioxide

Maize Starch

Magnesium Stearate

6.2 Incompatibilities

None known

6.3 Shelf life

24 months.

6.4 Special precautions for storage

Store in a refrigerator.

Where the tablets are pack in a bottle, the tablets should be used within one month of opening the bottle.

6.5 Nature and contents of container

Amber glass bottle with screw cap and tac seal. Each bottle contains a desiccant capsule and 4 tablets.

Aluminium foil strip of 4 tablets, each box containing 4 or 8 tablets.

6.6 Instructions for use and handling

Wash hands thoroughly with soap and water after administration.

7. MARKETING AUTHORISATION HOLDER

Pharmacia Limited

Davy Avenue

Milton Keynes

MK5 8PH

UK

8. MARKETING AUTHORISATION NUMBER(S)

PL 0032/0074

9. DATE OF FIRST AUTHORISATION/RENEWAL OF THE AUTHORISATION

15 March 1982/15 March 1998

10. DATE OF REVISION OF THE TEXT

June 2003

Legal category: POM

Prostin VR Sterile Solution

(Pharmacia Limited)

1. NAME OF THE MEDICINAL PRODUCT

Prostin™ VR Sterile Solution

2. QUALITATIVE AND QUANTITATIVE COMPOSITION

Each 1 ml contains 500 micrograms (0.5 mg) alprostadil.

3. PHARMACEUTICAL FORM

Sterile solution for injection.

4. CLINICAL PARTICULARS

4.1 Therapeutic indications

Prostin VR is indicated to temporarily maintain the patency of the ductus arteriosus until corrective or palliative surgery can be performed in infants who have congenital defects and who depend upon the patent ductus for survival. Such congenital heart defects include pulmonary atresia, pulmonary stenosis, tricuspid atresia, tetralogy of Fallot, interruption of the aortic arch, co-arctation of the aorta, aortic stenosis, aortic atresia, mitral atresia, or transposition of the great vessels with or without other defects.

4.2 Posology and method of administration

For administration by intravenous drip or constant rate infusion pump.

In infants with lesions restricting pulmonary blood flow (blood is flowing through the ductus arteriosus from the aorta to the pulmonary artery), Prostin VR may be administered by continuous infusion through an umbilical artery catheter placed at or just above the junction of the descending aorta and the ductus arteriosus, or intravenously. Adverse effects have occurred with both routes of administration, but the types of reactions are different. A higher incidence of flushing has been associated with intra-arterial than with intravenous administration.

The infusion is generally initiated at a rate of 0.05 to 0.1 micrograms alprostadil per kilogram of body weight per minute. The most experience has been with 0.1 micrograms/kg/min. After a therapeutic response (an increase in pO_2 in neonates with restricted pulmonary blood flow or an increase in systemic blood pressure and blood pH in neonates with restricted systemic blood flow) has been obtained, the infusion rate should be reduced to the lowest possible dosage that will maintain the desired response.

Dilution instructions:

To prepare infusion solutions, dilute 1 ml of Prostin VR Sterile Solution with sterile 0.9% Sodium Chloride Intravenous Infusion or sterile 5% Dextrose Intravenous Infusion. If undiluted Prostin VR Sterile Solution comes in direct contact with a plastic container, plasticisers are leached from the sidewalls. The solution may turn hazy and the appearance of the container may change. Should this occur, the solution should be discarded and the plastic container should be replaced. This appears to be a concentration-dependent phenomenon. To minimise the possibility of haze formation, Prostin VR Sterile Solution should be added directly to the intravenous infusion solution, avoiding contact with the walls of plastic containers. Dilute to volumes appropriate for the delivery system available. Prepare fresh infusion solutions every 24 hours. Discard any solution more than 24 hours old.

PARTICULAR CARE SHOULD BE TAKEN IN CALCULATING AND PREPARING DILUTIONS OF PROSTIN VR

4.3 Contraindications

None.

4.4 Special warnings and special precautions for use

Warnings: Only the recommended Prostin VR dosages should be administered and only by medically trained personnel in hospitals or other facilities with immediately available intensive care.

Approximately 10-12% of neonates with congenital heart defects treated with Prostin VR Sterile Solution experienced apnoea. Apnoea is most often seen in neonates weighing less than 2 kg at birth and usually appears during the first hour of drug infusion. Therefore, Prostin VR Sterile Solution should be used where ventilatory assistance is immediately available.

Precautions: Prostin VR Sterile Solution (alprostadil) should be infused for the shortest time and at the lowest dose which will produce the desired effects. The risk of long-term infusion of Prostin VR should be weighed against the possible benefits that critically ill infants may derive from its administration.

Cortical proliferation of the long bones has followed long-term infusions of alprostadil in infants and dogs. The proliferation in infants regressed after withdrawal of the drug.

Use Prostin VR Sterile Solution cautiously in neonates with histories of bleeding tendencies.

Care should be taken to avoid the use of Prostin VR Sterile Solution in neonates with respiratory distress syndrome (hyaline membrane disease), which sometimes can be confused with cyanotic heart disease. If full diagnostic facilities are not immediately available, cyanosis (pO_2 less than 40 mm Hg) and restricted pulmonary blood flow apparent on an X-ray are good indicators of congenital heart defects.

In all infants, commencing when infusion starts, intermittently monitor arterial pressure by umbilical artery catheter, auscultation, or with a Doppler transducer. Should arterial pressure fall significantly, decrease the rate of infusion immediately.

A weakening of the wall of the ductus arteriosus and pulmonary artery has been reported, particularly during prolonged administration.

The administration of alprostadil to neonates may result in gastric outlet obstruction secondary to antral hyperplasia. This effect appears to be related to duration of therapy and cumulative dose of the drug. Neonates receiving alprostadil at recommended doses for more than 120 hours should be closely monitored for evidence of antral hyperplasia and gastric outlet obstruction.

Long-term carcinogenicity and fertility studies have not been done. The Ames and Alkaline Elution assays reveal no potential for mutagenesis.

4.5 Interaction with other medicinal products and other forms of Interaction

No drug interactions have been reported to occur between Prostin VR and the standard therapy employed in neonates with congenital heart defects. Standard therapy includes antibiotics, such as penicillin or gentamicin; vasopressors, such as dopamine or isoproterenol; cardiac glycosides; and diuretics, such as frusemide.

4.6 Pregnancy and lactation

This product is for use in children only.

4.7 Effects on ability to drive and use machines

Not applicable

4.8 Undesirable effects

The most frequent adverse reactions observed with Prostin VR infusion in neonates with ductal-dependent congenital heart defects are related to the drug's known pharmacological effects. These include, in decreasing frequency, transient pyrexia, apnoea, bradycardia, seizures, hypotension, tachycardia, and diarrhoea. The relationship of the following adverse events, in decreasing frequency, to the drug is unknown: sepsis, cardiac arrest, disseminated intravascular coagulation, hypokalaemia, and oedema. Cutaneous vasodilation (flushing) is the only event related to the route of administration, occurring more frequently during intra-arterial administration.

4.9 Overdose

Apnoea, bradycardia, pyrexia, hypotension and flushing may be signs of drug overdose. If apnoea or bradycardia occur, the infusion should be discontinued and the appropriate medical treatment initiated. Caution should be used if the infusion is restarted. If pyrexia or hypotension occur, the infusion rate should be reduced until these symptoms subside. Flushing is usually attributed to incorrect intra-arterial catheter placement and is usually alleviated by repositioning the tip of the catheter.

5. PHARMACOLOGICAL PROPERTIES

5.1 Pharmacodynamic properties

Prostaglandins are potent vasoactive derivatives of arachadonic acid that exert vasomotor, metabolic and cellular effects on the pulmonary and coronary circulation. The E series of prostaglandins produces vasodilation of the systemic and coronary circulation in most species: these prostaglandins have been used for maintaining the patency of the ductus arteriosus in children.

5.2 Pharmacokinetic properties

Based on studies in several animal species, intravenous or arterially administered prostaglandin E_1 is very rapidly metabolised and distributed throughout the entire body, with the exception of the CNS, where distribution, though detectable, is markedly reduced. The primary organisms for metabolism and inactivation of prostaglandin E_1 are probably the lung, liver and kidney which remove and metabolise 40-95% of the prostaglandin E_1 in a single pass through the organ. A number of other tissues possess lesser, but significant, capacity to metabolise prostaglandin E_1. The predominant metabolites found in plasma, 15-oxo-prostaglandin E_1 and 13,14-dihydro-15 oxo-prostaglandin E_1 are extensively metabolised by β and ω-oxidation prior to excretion, primarily by the kidney. Few urinary metabolites of prostaglandin E_1 have been characterised, but are widely believed to be analogous to those reported in detail for prostaglandin E_2 and prostaglandin $F_{2\alpha}$. Excretion is essentially complete within 24 hours after dosing, with no intact prostaglandin E_1 being found in urine and no evidence of tissue retention of prostaglandin E_1 or metabolites. In three species, rat, rabbit and lamb, the prostaglandin metabolising activity of lung from near-term fetal animals has been shown to be at least as effective as that of adults.

5.3 Preclinical safety data

See section "Undesirable effects".

6. PHARMACEUTICAL PARTICULARS

6.1 List of excipients

Dehydrated ethanol

6.2 Incompatibilities

Diluted solutions of Prostin VR should be infused from glass or hard plastic containers, or PVC infusion bags. If undiluted Prostin VR Sterile Solution comes in direct contact with a plastic container, plasticisers are leached from the sidewalls. This appears to be a concentration-dependent phenomenon.

6.3 Shelf life

Three years.

6.4 Special precautions for storage

Store in a refrigerator.

6.5 Nature and contents of container
Glass ampoule, containing 1 ml solution.

6.6 Instructions for use and handling
Diluted solutions should be used within 24 hours.

7. MARKETING AUTHORISATION HOLDER
Pharmacia Limited
Davy Avenue
Milton Keynes
MK5 8PH

8. MARKETING AUTHORISATION NUMBER(S)
0032/0083

9. DATE OF FIRST AUTHORISATION/RENEWAL OF THE AUTHORISATION
Date of Grant: 23 July 1981
Date of Renewal: 17 April 1997

10. DATE OF REVISION OF THE TEXT
April 2001

Legal Category
POM.

Prosulf

(Wockhardt UK Ltd)

1. NAME OF THE MEDICINAL PRODUCT
Prosulf
Protamine Sulphate Injection BP

2. QUALITATIVE AND QUANTITATIVE COMPOSITION
Protamine Sulphate 10mg/ml

3. PHARMACEUTICAL FORM
Solution for injection
A clear, colourless solution.

4. CLINICAL PARTICULARS
4.1 Therapeutic indications
Protamine sulphate is used to counteract the anticoagulant effect of heparin: before surgery; after renal dialysis; after open-heart surgery; if excessive bleeding occurs and when an overdose has inadvertently been given.

4.2 Posology and method of administration
Adults:
Prosulf should be administered by slow intravenous injection over a period of about 10 minutes. No more than 50mg of protamine sulphate should be given in any one dose.

The dose is dependent on the amount and type of heparin to be neutralised, its route of administration and the time elapsed since it was last given, since heparin is continuously being excreted. Ideally, the dose required to neutralise the action of heparin should be guided by blood coagulation studies or calculated from a protamine neutralisation test.

Patients should be carefully monitored using either the activated partial thromboplastin time or the activated coagulation time, carried out 5-15 minutes after protamine sulphate administration. Further doses may be needed because protamine is cleared from the blood more rapidly than heparin, especially low molecular weight heparin.

In gross excess, protamine itself acts as an anticoagulant.

Neutralisation of unfractionated (UF) heparins:

1mg of protamine sulphate will usually neutralise at least 100 international units of mucous heparin or 80 units of lung heparin. The dose of protamine sulphate should be reduced if more than 15 minutes have elapsed since intravenous injection.

For example, if 30-60 minutes have elapsed since heparin was injected intravenously, 0.5-0.75mg protamine sulphate per 100 units of mucous heparin is recommended. If two hours or more have elapsed, 0.25-0.375mg per 100 units of mucous heparin should be administered.

If the patient is receiving an intravenous infusion of heparin, the infusion should be stopped and 25-50mg of protamine sulphate given by slow intravenous injection.

If heparin was administered subcutaneously, 1mg protamine sulphate should be given per 100 units of mucous heparin - 25-50mg by slow intravenous injection and the balance by intravenous infusion over 8-16 hours.

In the reversal of UF heparin following cardiopulmonary bypass, either a standard dose of protamine may be given, as above, or the dose may be titrated according to the activated clotting time.

Neutralisation of low molecular weight (LMW) heparins:

A dose of 1mg per 100 units is usually recommended but the manufacturer's own guidelines should be consulted.

The anti-Xa activity of LMW heparins may not be completely reversible with protamine sulphate and may persist for up to 24 hours after administration.

The longer half-life of LMW heparins (approximately twice that of UF heparin) should also be borne in mind when estimating the dose of protamine sulphate required in relation to the time which has elapsed since the last heparin dose.

Theoretically, the dose of protamine sulphate should be halved when one half-life has elapsed since the last LMW heparin dose. Intermittent injections or continuous infusion of protamine sulphate have been recommended for the neutralisation of LMW heparin following subcutaneous administration, as there may be continuing absorption from the subcutaneous depot.

Elderly:
There is no current evidence for alteration of the recommended dose.

Children:
Safety and efficacy in children have not been established. Not recommended.

4.3 Contraindications
None known.

4.4 Special warnings and special precautions for use
Too rapid administration of protamine sulphate may cause severe hypotension and anaphylactoid reactions. Facilities for resuscitation and treatment of shock should be available.

Protamine sulphate is not suitable for reversing the effects of oral anticoagulants. Caution should be observed when administering protamine sulphate to patients who may be at increased risk of allergic reaction to protamine. These patients include those who have previously undergone procedures such as coronary angioplasty or cardio-pulmonary by-pass which may include use of protamine, diabetics who have been treated with protamine insulin, patients allergic to fish and men who have had a vasectomy or are infertile and may have antibodies to protamine.

Patients undergoing prolonged procedures involving repeated doses of protamine should be subject to careful monitoring of clotting parameters. A rebound bleeding effect may occur up to 18 hours post-operatively which responds to further doses of protamine.

4.5 Interaction with other medicinal products and other forms of Interaction
None known.

4.6 Pregnancy and lactation
As with most drugs, to be used only if clearly indicated in pregnancy and with caution during lactation.

4.7 Effects on ability to drive and use machines
None.

4.8 Undesirable effects
When used at doses in excess of that required to neutralise the anticoagulant effect of heparin, protamine sulphate exerts its own anticoagulant effect. Following injection of protamine sulphate the following effects have been observed; a sudden fall in blood pressure, bradycardia, pulmonary and systemic hypertension, dyspnoea, transitory flushing and a feeling of warmth, back pain, nausea and vomiting, lassitude. Hypersensitivity reactions, including angioedema and fatal anaphylaxis, have been reported. There have been rare instances of noncardiogenic pulmonary oedema with prolonged hypotension, with significant morbidity and mortality.

4.9 Overdose
Symptoms:- Overdosage may cause hypotension, bradycardia and dyspnoea with a sensation of warmth, nausea, vomiting, lassitude and transitory flushing.

Treatment:- Includes monitoring of coagulation tests, respiratory ventilation and symptomatic treatment. If bleeding is a problem, fresh frozen plasma or fresh whole blood should be given.

5. PHARMACOLOGICAL PROPERTIES
5.1 Pharmacodynamic properties
Although protamine is a potent antidote for heparin, its precise mechanism of action is unknown. However, when the strongly basic protamine combines with the strongly acid heparin, a stable salt is formed lacking in anticoagulant activity. 1mg of protamine sulphate neutralises between 80 and 120 units of heparin. However, methods of standardisation and the use of heparin from different sources (mucosal, lung) may produce different responses to protamine.

5.2 Pharmacokinetic properties
The onset of action of protamine occurs within five minutes following intravenous administration. The fate of the protamine-heparin complex is unknown, but it may be partially degraded, thus freeing heparin.

5.3 Preclinical safety data
No data are available.

6. PHARMACEUTICAL PARTICULARS
6.1 List of excipients
Sodium Chloride
Hydrochloric Acid 3M
Sodium Hydroxide 3M
Water for Injections

6.2 Incompatibilities
Protamine sulphate is incompatible with certain antibiotics, including several cephalosporins and penicillin.

6.3 Shelf life
48 months

6.4 Special precautions for storage
Store between 15°C and 25°C.

6.5 Nature and contents of container
5ml and 10ml neutral type 1 hydrolytic glass ampoules in pack sizes of 10 ampoules in cartons.

6.6 Instructions for use and handling
Not applicable.

Administrative Data
7. MARKETING AUTHORISATION HOLDER
CP Pharmaceuticals Ltd
Ash Road North
Wrexham
LL13 9UF

8. MARKETING AUTHORISATION NUMBER(S)
4543/0234

9. DATE OF FIRST AUTHORISATION/RENEWAL OF THE AUTHORISATION
17 May 1991

10. DATE OF REVISION OF THE TEXT
September 2000

Protamine Sulphate Injection BP

(UCB Pharma Limited)

1. NAME OF THE MEDICINAL PRODUCT
Protamine Sulphate Injection BP

2. QUALITATIVE AND QUANTITATIVE COMPOSITION
Protamine Sulphate Salmine 10mg/ml

3. PHARMACEUTICAL FORM
Sterile Solution

4. CLINICAL PARTICULARS
4.1 Therapeutic indications
Neutralisation of the anticoagulant effect of heparin therapy and the treatment of heparin overdose.

4.2 Posology and method of administration
Adults: Protamine Sulphate Injection should be administered by slow intravenous injection (max rate 5 mg/min) over a period of 10 minutes. The dose is dependent on the amount of heparin to be neutralised. One mg of Protamine Sulphate will usually neutralise at least 100 IU of mucous heparin or 80 IU of lung heparin if given within 15 minutes of heparin administration. If more than 15 minutes has elapsed since heparin administration then less Protamine is required due to the rapid excretion of heparin.

Not more than 50 milligrams of Protamine Sulphate should be administered in a ten minute period.

The requirement for protamine may be monitored by APTT (Activated Partial Thromboplastin Time) or other appropriate test of clotting ability.

To antagonise heparin bolus:

Time Elapsed	Protamine dose needed/100 IU Heparin
30 min	1.00 -1.5 mg
30-60 min	0.50- 0.7 mg
2 hours	0.25- 0.375 mg

To antagonise heparin infusion:
25-50mg after stopping infusion

To antagonise heparin subcutaneous injection:
1-1.5 mg/ 100 IU heparin. 25-50 mg can be given by slow IV injection and the remainder by slow IV infusion over 8-16 hours (or the expected duration of absorption of heparin), or 2 hourly divided doses.

To antagonise heparin during extracorporeal circulation:
1.5 mg per 100 IU heparin. Sequential APTTs may be needed to calculate correct dosage.

Children and Elderly: There are no reports to suggest that the recommended adult dose should not also be used in children and the elderly.

4.3 Contraindications
Previous life threatening reaction to protamine.

4.4 Special warnings and special precautions for use
Not more than 50 milligrams of Protamine Sulphate (5 ml Protamine Sulphate Injection BP) should be administered in a 10 minute period.

Protamine Sulphate only partially reverses the effects of low molecular weight heparins. Consult the relevant manufacturer's product information for anti-Xa neutralisation, as the extent and time of neutralisation are dependent on the individual low molecular weight heparin.

Hypersensitivity reactions can occur: patients at risk include those who have received protamine-insulin preparations (Isophane insulin) and those with allergy to residual fish antigens that remain after purification and those who have had protamine before. There are reports of vasectomised or infertile men who have anti-protamine antibodies making them potential reactors to protamine.

When insufficient protamine is administered a heparin rebound occurs within 5 hours of neutralisation, which may be associated with clinical bleeding. This phenomenon has been described mainly in patients undergoing extra-corporeal circulation in arterial and cardiac surgery or in dialysis procedures.

It responds to further doses of protamine

Protamine sulphate is not suitable for reversing the effect of oral anti-coagulants.

4.5 Interaction with other medicinal products and other forms of Interaction

Protamine interferes with fluorescence methods of estimating plasma catecholamines.

4.6 Pregnancy and lactation

There is insufficient information as to whether this drug may affect fertility in humans or have a teratogenic potential or other adverse affects on the foetus. Reproduction studies have not been performed in animals. It is not known whether protamine sulphate is distributed into breast milk.

4.7 Effects on ability to drive and use machines

Not applicable.

4.8 Undesirable effects

Intravenous injections of Protamine Sulphate, particularly if administered rapidly, may cause a sensation of warmth, flushing of the skin, hypotension, bradycardia and dyspnoea. Nausea, vomiting and lassitude may also occur.

Urticaria and other hypersensitivity reactions including severe cardiovascular collapse, bronchospasm and death may occur rarely. Therefore this drug should only be given when resuscitation techniques and measures for the treatment of anaphylactic shock are readily available. Catastrophic pulmonary vasoconstriction and oedema may be associated with protamine use following cardiac surgery.

4.9 Overdose

Overdose of protamine sulphate may cause bleeding. Protamine has a weak anticoagulant effect due to an interaction with platelets and with many proteins including fibrinogen.

5. PHARMACOLOGICAL PROPERTIES

5.1 Pharmacodynamic properties

When administered alone, protamine sulphate has a weak anticoagulant effect. However, when given in the presence of heparin (which is strongly acidic), a stable salt is formed which results in the loss of anticoagulant activity of both drugs.

5.2 Pharmacokinetic properties

When used with heparin, protamine sulphate's effects are almost immediate and persist for approximately 2 hours.

5.3 Preclinical safety data

None available

6. PHARMACEUTICAL PARTICULARS

6.1 List of excipients

Water for Injections BP, Sulphuric Acid BP and Sodium Hydroxide BP

6.2 Incompatibilities

Protamine Sulphate is incompatible with certain antibiotics, including several of the cephalosporins and penicillins.

6.3 Shelf life

36 months

6.4 Special precautions for storage

Store below 25°C

6.5 Nature and contents of container

5 ml neutral glass ampoules

6.6 Instructions for use and handling

No special requirements

7. MARKETING AUTHORISATION HOLDER

UCB Pharma Limited
208 Bath Road
Slough
Berkshire
SL1 3WE
UK

8. MARKETING AUTHORISATION NUMBER(S)

PL 00039/5697R

9. DATE OF FIRST AUTHORISATION/RENEWAL OF THE AUTHORISATION

24 January 1991

10. DATE OF REVISION OF THE TEXT

June 2005

POM

Protamine Sulphate Injection BP 1%

(Sovereign Medical)

1. NAME OF THE MEDICINAL PRODUCT

Protamine Sulphate Injection BP 1%

2. QUALITATIVE AND QUANTITATIVE COMPOSITION

Protamine Sulphate Injection BP 1% contains protamine sulphate 10 mg/ml in sodium chloride 0.9% w/v.

3. PHARMACEUTICAL FORM

Sterile solution for injection.

4. CLINICAL PARTICULARS

4.1 Therapeutic indications

Protamine sulphate neutralises the anticoagulant action of heparin. It is given by intravenous injection to restore the original coagulation time of the blood in patients receiving heparin, and in the treatment of haemorrhage due to heparin overdosage.

4.2 Posology and method of administration

For intravenous injection.

The dose is calculated from the results of determinations of the amount required to produce an acceptable blood clotting time in the patient.

Protamine sulphate is given by slow intravenous injection, being administered at the rate of 5 ml of the 1% solution over a period of ten minutes. 1 ml of Protamine Sulphate Injection BP 1% is required to neutralise the anticoagulant activity of approximately 850 Units of heparin (lung) or 1100 Units of heparin (mucous) that has been injected within the previous fifteen minutes.

As more time elapses after the heparin injection, so proportionately less protamine sulphate is required. Ideally, the dosage of protamine sulphate should be controlled by serial measurements of the patient's coagulation time. This helps to avoid an excess of protamine sulphate which, having some anticoagulant effect itself, can prolong coagulation time.

The anticoagulant effect of Heparin Retard injection can be counteracted by the intravenous injection of up to 5 ml of Protamine Sulphate Injection BP 1% over ten minutes. Because of the prolonged action of Heparin Retard, the dosage of protamine sulphate is best controlled by measurements of coagulation time.

4.3 Contraindications

Protamine Sulphate Injection is contra-indicated in patients who are known to be hypersensitive to protamine.

4.4 Special warnings and special precautions for use

Protamine sulphate should be used with caution in patients with a known hypersensitivity to fish, in vasectomised or infertile males, and in patients who have received protamine-containing insulin or previous protamine sulphate therapy.

Not more than 50 mg of protamine sulphate, i.e. 5 ml of Protamine Sulphate Injection BP 1%, should usually be given at any one time. Protamine sulphate is a specific antidote to heparin and is not suitable for reversing the action of indirect anticoagulants such as coumarin and indanedione derivatives.

4.5 Interaction with other medicinal products and other forms of Interaction

Protamine sulphate may increase the magnitude and/or duration of action of non-depolarising neuromuscular blocking agents.

4.6 Pregnancy and lactation

The safety of protamine sulphate during pregnancy and lactation has not been established.

Neither animal nor human reproduction studies have been conducted, and therefore the drug should only be used during pregnancy when clearly needed. It is not known whether protamine sulphate is distributed into breast milk and the drug should be used with caution during lactation.

4.7 Effects on ability to drive and use machines

No adverse effects known.

4.8 Undesirable effects

Intravenous injections of protamine sulphate, particularly if given rapidly, may cause hypotension, bradycardia and dyspnoea. A sensation of warmth, transitory flushing, nausea, vomiting and lassitude may also occur. Occasionally, hypersensitivity reactions including urticaria, angioedema, pulmonary oedema, anaphylaxis and anaphylactoid reactions have been reported.

4.9 Overdose

Protamine sulphate is a weak anticoagulant and overdosage may theoretically result in bleeding. Usually, no specific therapy is required.

5. PHARMACOLOGICAL PROPERTIES

5.1 Pharmacodynamic properties

Protamine sulphate is strongly basic and acts as a heparin antagonist by complexing with the strongly acidic heparin sodium or heparin calcium to form a stable complex.

5.2 Pharmacokinetic properties

Protamine sulphate has a rapid onset of action. Following intravenous administration, neutralisation of heparin occurs within 5 minutes. Although the metabolic fate of the protamine-heparin complex is not known, it appears that the complex is partially degraded, thus freeing heparin.

5.3 Preclinical safety data

Not applicable.

6. PHARMACEUTICAL PARTICULARS

6.1 List of excipients

Water for injections, sodium chloride for injections, sodium hydroxide and/or hydrochloric acid as pH adjusters.

6.2 Incompatibilities

Protamine sulphate is incompatible with certain antibiotics, including several penicillins and cephalosporins.

6.3 Shelf life

36 months

6.4 Special precautions for storage

Store at 15 to 25°C. Do not refrigerate.

6.5 Nature and contents of container

One point cut ampoule.

Pack sizes: 6 × 10 ml ampoules
5 × 10 ml ampoules

6.6 Instructions for use and handling

None.

Administrative Data

7. MARKETING AUTHORISATION HOLDER

Waymade PLC
Trading as Sovereign Medical
Sovereign House
Miles Gray Road
Basildon
Essex, SS14 3FR
United Kingdom

8. MARKETING AUTHORISATION NUMBER(S)

PL 06464/0903

9. DATE OF FIRST AUTHORISATION/RENEWAL OF THE AUTHORISATION

17 November 1999

10. DATE OF REVISION OF THE TEXT

19/05/2000

Legal Category

POM

Protelos

(Servier Laboratories Limited)

1. NAME OF THE MEDICINAL PRODUCT

▼PROTELOS 2 g granules for oral suspension

2. QUALITATIVE AND QUANTITATIVE COMPOSITION

Each sachet contains 2 g of strontium ranelate.

For excipients, see section 6.1.

3. PHARMACEUTICAL FORM

Granules for oral suspension

Yellow granules

4. CLINICAL PARTICULARS

4.1 Therapeutic indications

Treatment of postmenopausal osteoporosis to reduce the risk of vertebral and hip fractures (see section 5.1).

4.2 Posology and method of administration

The recommended daily dose is one 2 g sachet once daily by oral administration.

Due to the nature of the treated disease, strontium ranelate is intended for long-term use.

The absorption of strontium ranelate is reduced by food, milk and derivative products and therefore, PROTELOS should be administered in-between meals. Given the slow absorption, PROTELOS should be taken at bedtime, preferably at least two hours after eating (see sections 4.5 and 5.2).

The granules in the sachets must be taken as a suspension in a glass of water. Although in-use studies have demonstrated that strontium ranelate is stable in suspension for 24 hours after preparation, the suspension should be drunk immediately after being prepared.

Patients treated with strontium ranelate should receive vitamin D and calcium supplements if dietary intake is inadequate.

Use in the elderly

The efficacy and safety of strontium ranelate have been established in a broad age range (up to 100 years at inclusion) of postmenopausal women with osteoporosis. No dosage adjustment is required in relation to age.

Use in renal impairment

No dosage adjustment is required in patients with mild-to-moderate renal impairment (30-70 ml/min creatinine clearance) (see section 5.2). Strontium ranelate is not recommended for patients with severe renal impairment (creatinine clearance below 30 ml/min) (see sections 4.4 and 5.2).

Use in hepatic impairment

As strontium ranelate is not metabolised, no dosage adjustment is required in patients with hepatic impairment.

Use in children and adolescents

The efficacy and safety of strontium ranelate have not been established in children and adolescents and use in these age groups is not recommended.

4.3 Contraindications

Hypersensitivity to the active substance or to any of the excipients.

4.4 Special warnings and special precautions for use

In the absence of bone safety data in patients with severe renal impairment treated with strontium ranelate, PROTELOS is not recommended in patients with a creatinine clearance below 30 ml/min (see section 5.2). In accordance with good medical practice, periodic assessment of renal function is recommended in patients with chronic renal impairment. Continuation of treatment with PROTELOS in patients developing severe renal impairment should be considered on an individual basis.

In phase III placebo-controlled studies, strontium ranelate treatment was associated with an increase in the annual incidence of venous thromboembolism (VTE), including pulmonary embolism (see section 4.8). The cause of this finding is unknown. Protelos should be used with caution in patients at increased risk of VTE, including patients with a past history of VTE. When treating patients at risk, or developing risk of VTE, particular attention should be given to possible signs and symptoms of VTE and adequate preventive measures taken.

Strontium interferes with colorimetric methods for the determination of blood and urinary calcium concentrations. Therefore, in medical practice, inductively coupled plasma atomic emission spectrometry or atomic absorption spectrometry methods should be used to ensure an accurate assessment of blood and urinary calcium concentrations.

PROTELOS contains a source of phenylalanine, which may be harmful for people with phenylketonuria.

4.5 Interaction with other medicinal products and other forms of Interaction

Food, milk and derivative products, and medicinal products containing calcium may reduce the bioavailability of strontium ranelate by approximately 60-70%. Therefore, administration of PROTELOS and such products should be separated by at least two hours (see section 5.2).

An *in vivo* clinical interaction study showed that the administration of aluminium and magnesium hydroxides either two hours before or together with strontium ranelate caused a slight decrease in the absorption of strontium ranelate (20-25% AUC decrease), while absorption was almost unaffected when the antacid was given two hours after strontium ranelate. It is therefore preferable to take antacids at least two hours after PROTELOS. However, when this dosing regimen is impractical due to the recommended administration of PROTELOS at bedtime, concomitant intake remains acceptable.

As divalent cations can form complexes with oral tetracycline and quinolone antibiotics at the gastro-intestinal level and thereby reduce their absorption, simultaneous administration of strontium ranelate with these medicinal products is not recommended. As a precautionary measure, PROTELOS treatment should be suspended during treatment with oral tetracycline or quinolone antibiotics.

No interaction was observed with oral supplementation of vitamin D.

No evidence of clinical interactions or relevant increase of blood strontium levels with medicinal products expected to be commonly prescribed concomitantly with PROTELOS in the target population were found during clinical trials. These included: nonsteroidal anti-inflammatory agents (including acetylsalicylic acid), anilides (such as paracetamol), H_2 blockers and proton pump inhibitors, diuretics, digoxin and cardiac glycosides, organic nitrates and other vasodilators for cardiac diseases, calcium channel blockers, beta blockers, ACE inhibitors, angiotensin II antagonists, selective beta-2 adrenoceptor agonists, oral anticoagulants, platelet aggregation inhibitors, statins, fibrates and benzodiazepine derivatives.

4.6 Pregnancy and lactation

PROTELOS is only intended for use in postmenopausal women.

No clinical data on exposed pregnancies are available for strontium ranelate. At high doses, animal studies have shown reversible bone effects in the offspring of rats and rabbits treated during pregnancy (see section 5.3). If PROTELOS is used inadvertently during pregnancy, treatment must be stopped.

Strontium is excreted in milk. Strontium ranelate should not be given to nursing women.

4.7 Effects on ability to drive and use machines

Strontium ranelate has no or negligible influence on the ability to drive and use machines.

4.8 Undesirable effects

PROTELOS has been studied in clinical trials involving nearly 8,000 participants. Long-term safety has been evaluated in postmenopausal women with osteoporosis treated for up to 56 months with strontium ranelate 2 g/day (n=3,352) or placebo (n=3,317) in phase III studies. Mean age was 75 years at inclusion and 23% of the patients enrolled were 80 to 100 years of age.

Overall incidence rates for adverse events with strontium ranelate did not differ from placebo and adverse events were usually mild and transient. The most common adverse events consisted of nausea and diarrhoea, which were generally reported at the beginning of treatment with no noticeable difference between groups afterwards. Discontinuation of therapy was mainly due to nausea (1.3% and 2.2% in the placebo and strontium ranelate groups respectively).

Adverse reactions, defined as adverse events considered at least possibly attributable to strontium ranelate treatment in phase III studies are listed below using the following convention (frequencies *versus* placebo): very common (>1/10); common (>1/100, <1/10); uncommon (>1/1,000, <1/100); rare (>1/10,000, <1/1,000); very rare (<1/10,000).

Nervous system disorders

Common: headache (3.0% vs. 2.4%)

Gastrointestinal disorders

Common: nausea (6.6% vs. 4.3%), diarrhoea (6.5% vs. 4.6%), loose stools (1.1% vs. 0.2%)

Skin and subcutaneous tissue disorders

Common: dermatitis (2.1% vs. 1.6%), eczema (1.5% vs. 1.2%)

There were no differences in the nature of adverse events between treatment groups regardless of whether patients were aged below or above 80 at inclusion.

In phase III studies, the annual incidence of venous thromboembolism (VTE) observed over 4 years was approximately 0.7%, with a relative risk of 1.42 (CI 1.02; 1.98, p=0.036) in strontium ranelate treated patients as compared to placebo (see section 4.4).

In phase III studies, over 4 years, nervous system disorders were reported with higher frequency in patients treated with strontium ranelate, compared with placebo: disturbances in consciousness (2.5% vs. 2.0%), memory loss (2.4% vs. 1.9 %) and seizures (0.3% vs. 0.1%).

Laboratory test findings

Transient emergent increases (> 3 times the upper limit of the normal range) in creatine kinase (CK) activity (musculo-skeletal fraction) were reported in 1.0% and 0.4% of the strontium ranelate and placebo groups respectively. In most cases, these values spontaneously reverted to normal without change in treatment.

4.9 Overdose

Good tolerance was shown in a clinical study investigating the repeated administration of 4 g strontium ranelate per day over 25 days in healthy postmenopausal women. Single administration of doses up to 11 g in healthy young male volunteers did not cause any particular symptoms.

Following episodes of overdoses during clinical trials (up to 4 g/day for a maximal duration of 147 days), no clinically relevant events were observed.

Administration of milk or antacids may be helpful to reduce the absorption of the active substance. In the event of substantial overdose, vomiting may be considered to remove unabsorbed active substance.

5. PHARMACOLOGICAL PROPERTIES

5.1 Pharmacodynamic properties

Pharmacotherapeutic group: Drugs for the treatment of bone diseases - Other drugs affecting bone structure and mineralisation

ATC code: M05BX03

In vitro, strontium ranelate:

- increases bone formation in bone tissue culture as well as osteoblast precursor replication and collagen synthesis in bone cell culture;

- reduces bone resorption by decreasing osteoclast differentiation and resorbing activity.

This results in a rebalance of bone turnover in favour of bone formation.

The activity of strontium ranelate was studied in various non-clinical models. In particular, in intact rats, strontium ranelate increases trabecular bone mass, trabeculae number and thickness; this results in an improvement of bone strength.

In bone tissue of treated animals and humans, strontium is mainly adsorbed onto the crystal surface and only slightly substitutes for calcium in the apatite crystal of newly formed bone. Strontium ranelate does not modify the bone crystal characteristics. In iliac crest bone biopsies obtained after up to 60 months of treatment with strontium ranelate 2 g/day in phase III trials, no deleterious effects on bone quality or mineralisation were observed.

The combined effects of strontium distribution in bone (see section 5.2) and increased X-ray absorption of strontium as compared to calcium, leads to an amplification of bone mineral density (BMD) measurement by dual-photon X-ray absorptiometry (DXA). Available data indicate that these factors account for approximately 50% of the measured change in BMD over 3 years of treatment with PROTELOS 2 g/day. This should be taken into account when interpreting BMD changes during treatment with PROTELOS. In phase III studies, which demonstrated the anti-fracture efficacy of PROTELOS treatment, measured mean BMD increased from baseline with PROTELOS by approximately 4% per year at the lumbar spine and 2% per year at the femoral neck, reaching 13% to 15% and 5% to 6% respectively after 3 years, depending on the study.

In phase III studies, as compared to placebo, biochemical markers of bone formation (bone-specific alkaline phosphatase and C-terminal propeptide of type I procollagen) increased and those of bone resorption (serum C-telopeptide and urinary N-telopeptide cross links) decreased from the third month of treatment up to 3 years.

Secondary to the pharmacological effects of strontium ranelate, slight decreases in calcium and parathyroid hormone (PTH) serum concentrations, increases in blood phosphorus concentrations and in total alkaline phosphatase activity were observed, with no observed clinical consequences.

Clinical efficacy

Osteoporosis is defined as BMD of the spine or hip 2.5 SD or more below the mean value of a normal young population. A number of risk factors are associated with postmenopausal osteoporosis including low bone mass, low bone mineral density, early menopause, a history of smoking and a family history of osteoporosis. The clinical consequence of osteoporosis is fractures. The risk of fractures is increased with the number of risk factors.

Treatment of postmenopausal osteoporosis:

The anti-fracture studies program of PROTELOS was made up of two placebo-controlled phase III studies: SOTI study and TROPOS study. SOTI involved 1,649 postmenopausal women with established osteoporosis (low lumbar BMD and prevalent vertebral fracture) and a mean age of 70 years. TROPOS involved 5,091 postmenopausal women with osteoporosis (low femoral neck BMD and prevalent fracture in more than half of them) and a mean age of 77 years. Together, SOTI and TROPOS enrolled 1,556 patients over 80 years at inclusion (23.1% of the study population). In addition to their treatment (2 g/day strontium ranelate or placebo), the patients received adapted calcium and vitamin D supplements throughout both studies.

PROTELOS reduced the relative risk of new vertebral fracture by 41% over 3 years in the SOTI study (table 1). The effect was significant from the first year. Similar benefits were demonstrated in women with multiple fractures at baseline. With respect to clinical vertebral fractures (defined as fractures associated with back pain and/or a body height loss of at least 1 cm), the relative risk was reduced by 38%. PROTELOS also decreased the number of patients with a body height loss of at least 1 cm as compared to placebo. Quality of life assessment on the QUALIOST specific scale as well as the General Health perception score of the SF-36 general scale indicated benefit of PROTELOS, compared with placebo.

Efficacy of PROTELOS to reduce the risk of new vertebral fracture was confirmed in the TROPOS study, including for osteoporotic patients without fragility fracture at baseline.

(see Table 1 on next page)

In patients over 80 years of age at inclusion, a pooled analysis of SOTI and TROPOS studies showed that PROTELOS reduced the relative risk of experiencing new vertebral fractures by 32% over 3 years (incidence of 19.1% with strontium ranelate vs. 26.5% with placebo).

In an *a-posteriori* analysis of patients from the pooled SOTI and TROPOS studies with baseline lumbar spine and / or femoral neck BMD in the osteopenic range and without prevalent fracture but with at least one additional risk factor for fracture (N=176), PROTELOS reduced the risk of a first vertebral fracture by 72% over 3 years (incidence of vertebral fracture3.6% with strontium ranelate vs. 12.0% with placebo).

An *a-posteriori* analysis was performed on a subgroup of patients from the TROPOS study of particular medical interest and at high-risk of fracture [defined by a femoral neck BMD T-score ⩽ -3 SD (manufacturer's range corresponding to -2.4 SD using NHANES III) and an age ⩾ 74 years (n=1,977, i.e. 40% of the TROPOS study population)]. In this group, over 3 years of treatment, PROTELOS reduced the risk of hip fracture by 36% relative to the placebo group (table 2).

(see Table 2 on next page)

5.2 Pharmacokinetic properties

Strontium ranelate is made up of 2 atoms of stable strontium and 1 molecule of ranelic acid, the organic part permitting the best compromise in terms of molecular weight, pharmacokinetics and acceptability of the medicinal product. The pharmacokinetics of strontium and ranelic acid have been assessed in healthy young men and healthy postmenopausal women, as well as during long-term exposure in postmenopausal osteoporotic women including elderly women.

Due to its high polarity, the absorption, distribution and binding to plasma proteins of ranelic acid are low. There is

Table 1 Incidence of patients with vertebral fracture and relative risk reduction

	Placebo	PROTELOS	Relative Risk Reduction vs. placebo (95%CI), p value
SOTI	N=723	N=719	
New vertebral fracture over 3 years	32.8%	20.9%	41% (27-52), p<0.001
New vertebral fracture over the 1st year	11.8%	6.1%	49% (26-64), p<0.001
New clinical vertebral fracture over 3 years	17.4%	11.3%	38% (17-53), p<0.001
TROPOS	N=1823	N=1817	
New vertebral fracture over 3 years	20.0%	12.5%	39% (27-49), p<0.001

Table 2 Incidence of patients with hip fracture and relative risk reduction in patients with BMD ≤ -2.4 SD (NHANES III) and age ≥ 74 years

	Placebo	PROTELOS	Relative Risk Reduction vs. placebo (95%CI), p value
TROPOS	N=995	N=982	
Hip fracture over 3 years	6.4%	4.3%	36% (0-59), p=0.046

no accumulation of ranelic acid and no evidence of metabolism in animals and humans. Absorbed ranelic acid is rapidly eliminated unchanged via the kidneys.

Absorption

The absolute bioavailability of strontium is about 25% (range 19-27%) after an oral dose of 2 g strontium ranelate. Maximum plasma concentrations are reached 3-5 hours after a single dose of 2 g. Steady state is reached after 2 weeks of treatment. Intake of strontium ranelate with calcium or food reduces the bioavailability of strontium by approximately 60-70%, compared with administration 3 hours after a meal. Due to the relatively slow absorption of strontium, food and calcium intake should be avoided both before and after administration of PROTELOS. Oral supplementation with vitamin D has no effect on strontium exposure.

Distribution

Strontium has a volume of distribution of about 1 l/kg. The binding of strontium to human plasma proteins is low (25%) and strontium has a high affinity for bone tissue. Measurement of strontium concentration in iliac crest bone biopsies from patients treated for up to 60 months with strontium ranelate 2 g/day indicate that bone strontium concentrations may reach a plateau after about 3 years of treatment. There are no data in patients to demonstrate elimination kinetics of strontium from bone off-therapy.

Biotransformation

As a divalent cation, strontium is not metabolised. Strontium ranelate does not inhibit cytochrome P450 enzymes.

Elimination

The elimination of strontium is time and dose independent. The effective half-life of strontium is about 60 hours. Strontium excretion occurs via the kidneys and the gastrointestinal tract. Its plasma clearance is about 12 ml/min (CV 22%) and its renal clearance about 7 ml/min (CV 28%).

Pharmacokinetics in special clinical situations

Elderly

Population pharmacokinetic data showed no relationship between age and apparent clearance of strontium in the target population.

Patients with renal impairment

In patients with mild-to-moderate renal impairment (30-70 ml/min creatinine clearance), strontium clearance decreases as creatinine clearance decreases (approximately 30% decrease over the creatinine clearance range 30 to 70 ml/min) and thereby induces an increase in strontium plasma levels. In phase III studies, 85% of the patients had a creatinine clearance between 30 and 70 ml/min and 6% below 30 ml/min at inclusion, and the mean creatinine clearance was about 50 ml/min. No dosage adjustment is therefore required in patients with mild-to-moderate renal impairment.

There is no pharmacokinetic data in patients with severe renal impairment (creatinine clearance below 30 ml/min).

Patients with hepatic impairment

There is no pharmacokinetic data in patients with hepatic impairment. Due to the pharmacokinetic properties of strontium, no effect is expected.

5.3 Preclinical safety data

Preclinical data revealed no special hazard for humans based on conventional studies of safety pharmacology, genotoxicity and carcinogenic potential.

Chronic oral administration of strontium ranelate at high doses in rodents induced bone and tooth abnormalities, mainly consisting of spontaneous fractures and delayed mineralisation. These effects were reported at bone strontium levels 2-3 times higher than long-term clinical bone strontium levels and were reversible after cessation of treatment.

Developmental toxicity studies in rats and rabbits resulted in bone and tooth abnormalities (e.g. bent long bones and wavy ribs) in the offspring. In rats, these effects were reversible 8 weeks after cessation of treatment.

6. PHARMACEUTICAL PARTICULARS

6.1 List of excipients

Aspartame (E951)

Maltodextrin

Mannitol (E421)

6.2 Incompatibilities

Not applicable.

6.3 Shelf life

3 years.

6.4 Special precautions for storage

This medicinal product does not require any special storage conditions.

6.5 Nature and contents of container

Paper/polyethylene/aluminium/polyethylene sachets.

Pack sizes

Boxes containing 7, 14, 28, 56, 84 or 100 sachets.

Not all pack sizes may be marketed.

6.6 Instructions for use and handling

No special requirements.

7. MARKETING AUTHORISATION HOLDER

LES LABORATOIRES SERVIER

22, rue Garnier

92200 Neuilly-sur-Seine

France

8. MARKETING AUTHORISATION NUMBER(S)

EU/1/04/288/003

9. DATE OF FIRST AUTHORISATION/RENEWAL OF THE AUTHORISATION

21st September 2004

10. DATE OF REVISION OF THE TEXT

September 2004

Prothiaden Capsules 25mg

(Abbott Laboratories Limited)

1. NAME OF THE MEDICINAL PRODUCT

Prothiaden Capsules 25 mg

Dosulepin Capsules BP 25 mg

2. QUALITATIVE AND QUANTITATIVE COMPOSITION

Each Prothiaden/ Dosulepin Capsule contains 25 mg Dosulepin Hydrochloride BP.

3. PHARMACEUTICAL FORM

Red/brown, hard gelatin capsules bearing the overprint 'P25' in white.

Generic version is unmarked.

4. CLINICAL PARTICULARS

4.1 Therapeutic indications

Prothiaden is indicated in the treatment of symptoms of depressive illness, especially where an anti-anxiety effect is required.

4.2 Posology and method of administration

For oral administration

Adults: Initially 75 mg/day in divided doses or as a single dose at night, increasing to 150 mg/day. In certain circumstances, *e.g.* in hospital use, dosages up to 225 mg daily have been used.

Suggested regimens: 25 or 50 mg three times daily or, alternatively, 75 or 150 mg as a single dose at night. Should the regimen of 150 mg as a single night-time dose be adopted, it is better to give a smaller dose for the first few days.

Elderly: 50 to 75 mg daily initially. As with any antidepressant, the initial dose should be increased with caution under close supervision. Half the normal adult dose may be sufficient to produce a satisfactory clinical response.

Children: Not recommended.

4.3 Contraindications

Prothiaden is contra-indicated following recent myocardial infarction, and in patients with any degree of heart block or other cardiac arrhythmias. It is also contra-indicated in mania and severe liver disease.

4.4 Special warnings and special precautions for use

It may be two to four weeks from the start of treatment before there is an improvement in the patient's depression; the subject should be monitored closely during this period. The anxiolytic effect may be observed within a few days of commencing treatment.

The elderly are particularly liable to experience adverse effects with antidepressants, especially agitation, confusion and postural hypotension. Patients posing a high risk of suicide require close supervision.

Prothiaden should be avoided in patients with a history of epilepsy and in patients with narrow-angle glaucoma or symptoms suggestive of prostatic hypertrophy. Use with caution in patients with cardiovascular disorders.

Tricyclic antidepressants potentiate the central nervous depressant action of alcohol. Anaesthetics given during tri/tetracyclic antidepressant therapy may increase the risk of arrhythmias and hypotension. If surgery is necessary, the anaesthetist should be informed that a patient is being so treated.

On stopping treatment, it is recommended that antidepressants should be withdrawn gradually, wherever possible.

4.5 Interaction with other medicinal products and other forms of Interaction

Prothiaden should not be given concurrently with a monoamine oxidase inhibitor, nor within fourteen days of ceasing such treatment. The concomitant administration of Prothiaden and SSRIs should be avoided since increases in plasma tricyclic antidepressant levels have been reported following the co-administration of some SSRIs.

Prothiaden may alter the pharmacological effect of some concurrently administered drugs including CNS depressants such as alcohol and narcotic analgesics; the effect of these will be potentiated as will be the effects of adrenaline and noradrenaline (some local anaesthetics contain these sympathomimetics). Anaesthetics given during tri/tetracyclic antidepressant therapy may increase the risk of arrhythmias and hypotension.

Prothiaden has quinidine-like actions on the heart. For this reason, its concomitant use with other drugs which may affect cardiac conduction (*e.g.* sotalol, terfenadine, astemizole, halofantrine) should be avoided.

The hypotensive activity of certain antihypertensive agents (*e.g.* bethanidine, debrisoquine, guanethidine) may be reduced by Prothiaden. It is advisable to review all antihypertensive therapy during treatment with tricyclic antidepressants.

Barbiturates may decrease and methylphenidate may increase the serum concentration of dothiepin and thus affect its antidepressant action.

There is no evidence that dothiepin interferes with standard laboratory tests.

4.6 Pregnancy and lactation

Treatment with Prothiaden should be avoided during pregnancy, unless there are compelling reasons. There is inadequate evidence of safety of the drug during human pregnancy.

There is evidence that dosulepin is secreted in breast milk but this is at levels which are unlikely to cause problems.

4.7 Effects on ability to drive and use machines

Initially, Prothiaden may impair alertness; patients likely to drive vehicles or operate machinery should be warned of this possibility.

4.8 Undesirable effects

The following adverse effects, although not necessarily all reported with dothiepin, have occurred with other tricyclic antidepressants:

Atropine-like side effects including dry mouth, disturbances of accommodation, tachycardia, constipation and hesitancy of micturition are common early in treatment, but usually lessen.

Other adverse effects include drowsiness, sweating, postural hypotension, tremor and skin rashes. Interference with sexual function may occur.

Potentially serious adverse effects are rare. These include depression of the bone marrow, agranulocytosis, hepatitis (including altered liver function), cholestatic jaundice, convulsions and inappropriate ADH secretion.

Psychotic manifestations, including mania and paranoid delusions, may be exacerbated during treatment with tricyclic antidepressants.

Withdrawal symptoms may occur on abrupt cessation of tricyclic therapy and include insomnia, irritability and excessive perspiration. Similar symptoms in neonates whose mothers received tricyclic antidepressants during the third trimester have also been reported.

Cardiac arrhythmias and severe hypotension are likely to occur with high dosage or in deliberate overdosage. They may also occur in patients with pre-existing heart disease taking normal dosage.

4.9 Overdose

Symptoms of overdosage may include dryness of the mouth, excitement, ataxia, drowsiness, loss of consciousness, muscle twitching, convulsions, widely dilated pupils, hyperreflexia, sinus tachycardia, cardiac arrhythmias, hypotension, hypothermia, depression of respiration, visual hallucinations, delirium, urinary retention, paralytic ileus, and respiratory or metabolic alkalosis.

Treatment should consist of gastric lavage. When the patient is unconscious or the cough reflex depressed, the lungs should be protected by a cuffed endotracheal tube. Repeated gastric/intestinal aspiration or repeated administration of activated charcoal may remove drug and metabolites excreted into the gut via the bile. Continuous ECG monitoring is advisable. Abnormalities of cardiac rhythm and epileptic convulsions may occur and should be treated accordingly. Forced diuresis is not recommended. Bed rest is advisable, even after recovery.

5. PHARMACOLOGICAL PROPERTIES

5.1 Pharmacodynamic properties

Dosulepin is a tricyclic antidepressant which acts by increasing transmitter levels at central synapses, so producing a clinical antidepressant effect.

Dosulepin, in common with other tricyclics, inhibits the reuptake of noradrenaline and 5-hydroxytryptamine, with a significantly greater action on the reuptake of noradrenaline. In addition, dosulepin inhibits the neuronal uptake of dopamine.

As a consequence of its effects on monoamine levels, dosulepin appears to produce adaptive changes in the brain by reducing or down-regulating both noradrenaline receptor numbers and noradrenaline-induced cyclic-AMP formation.

5.2 Pharmacokinetic properties

Dosulepin is readily absorbed from the gastrointestinal tract and extensively metabolised in the liver. Metabolites include northiaden, dosulepin-S-oxide and northiaden-S-oxide. dosulepin is excreted in the urine, mainly in the form of metabolites; appreciable amounts are also excreted in the faeces. A half-life of about 50 hours has been reported for dosulepin and its metabolites.

5.3 Preclinical safety data

Not applicable.

6. PHARMACEUTICAL PARTICULARS

6.1 List of excipients

Maize starch, magnesium stearate, lactose, gelatin, red iron oxide, yellow iron oxide, yellow iron oxide, erythrocin, titanium dioxide, shellac, polymethylsiloxane, soya lecithin.

The generic version does not contain shellac, soya lecithin or polydimethylsiloxane.

6.2 Incompatibilities

None stated

6.3 Shelf life

Unopened shelf-life is 36 months for all pack sizes.

6.4 Special precautions for storage

None stated.

6.5 Nature and contents of container

A 280 ml rectangular amber glass bottle, fitted with a white tinplate cap having a waxed aluminium faced pulpboard liner.

Pack size 600.

A 50 ml rectangular amber glass bottle, fitted with a tinplate cap having a waxed aluminium faced pulpboard liner, or a child resistant polypropylene cap fitted with a lectraseal liner.

Pack size 100

A high density polyethylene bottle with a cap and aluminium-faced pulpboard liner. The caps for packs which contain 100 units or less will be a clic-loc cap, for those containing more than 100 units per pack the cap will be a standard polypropylene cap.

Pack size: 100 and 600.

6.6 Instructions for use and handling

None stated.

7. MARKETING AUTHORISATION HOLDER

Abbott Laboratories Limited, Queenborough, Kent, ME11 5EL, United Kingdom

8. MARKETING AUTHORISATION NUMBER(S)

PL 00037/0363

9. DATE OF FIRST AUTHORISATION/RENEWAL OF THE AUTHORISATION

28 February 2002

10. DATE OF REVISION OF THE TEXT

November 2004

Prothiaden Tablets 75 mg

(Abbott Laboratories Limited)

1. NAME OF THE MEDICINAL PRODUCT

Prothiaden Tablets 75 mg

Dosulepin Tablets 75 mg

2. QUALITATIVE AND QUANTITATIVE COMPOSITION

Each Prothiaden/Dosulepin Tablet contains 75 mg Dosulepin Hydrochloride BP.

3. PHARMACEUTICAL FORM

Red, sugar-coated tablets, bearing the overprint 'P75' in white.

Generic version is unmarked.

4. CLINICAL PARTICULARS

4.1 Therapeutic indications

Prothiaden is indicated in the treatment of symptoms of depressive illness, especially where an anti-anxiety effect is required.

4.2 Posology and method of administration

For oral administration.

Adults: Initially 75 mg/day in divided doses or as a single dose at night, increasing to 150 mg/day. In certain circumstances, *e.g.* in hospital use, dosages up to 225 mg daily have been used.

Suggested regimens: 25 or 50 mg three times daily or, alternatively, 75 or 150 mg as a single dose at night. Should the regimen of 150 mg as a single night-time dose be adopted, it is better to give a smaller dose for the first few days.

Elderly: 50 to 75 mg daily initially. As with any antidepressant, the initial dose should be increased with caution under close supervision. Half the normal adult dose may be sufficient to produce a satisfactory clinical response.

Children: Not recommended.

4.3 Contraindications

Prothiaden is contra-indicated following recent myocardial infarction, and in patients with any degree of heart block or other cardiac arrhythmias. It is also contra-indicated in mania and severe liver disease.

4.4 Special warnings and special precautions for use

It may be two to four weeks from the start of treatment before there is an improvement in the patient's depression; the subject should be monitored closely during this period. The anxiolytic effect may be observed within a few days of commencing treatment.

The elderly are particularly liable to experience adverse effects with antidepressants, especially agitation, confusion and postural hypotension. Patients posing a high risk of suicide require close supervision.

Prothiaden should be avoided in patients with a history of epilepsy and in patients with narrow-angle glaucoma or symptoms suggestive of prostatic hypertrophy. Use with caution in patients with cardiovascular disorders.

Tricyclic antidepressants potentiate the central nervous depressant action of alcohol. Anaesthetics given during tri/tetracyclic antidepressant therapy may increase the risk of arrhythmias and hypotension. If surgery is necessary, the anaesthetist should be informed that a patient is being so treated.

On stopping treatment, it is recommended that antidepressants should be withdrawn gradually, wherever possible.

4.5 Interaction with other medicinal products and other forms of Interaction

Prothiaden should not be given concurrently with a monoamine oxidase inhibitor, nor within fourteen days of ceasing such treatment. The concomitant administration of Prothiaden and SSRIs should be avoided since increases in plasma tricyclic antidepressant levels have been reported following the co-administration of some SSRIs.

Prothiaden may alter the pharmacological effect of some concurrently administered drugs including CNS depressants such as alcohol and narcotic analgesics; the effect of these will be potentiated as will be the effects of adrenaline and noradrenaline (some local anaesthetics contain these sympathomimetics). Anaesthetics given during tri/tetracyclic antidepressant therapy may increase the risk of arrhythmias and hypotension.

Prothiaden has quinidine-like actions on the heart. For this reason, its concomitant use with other drugs which may affect cardiac conduction (*e.g.* sotalol, terfenadine, astemizole, halofantrine) should be avoided.

The hypotensive activity of certain antihypertensive agents (*e.g.* bethanidine, debrisoquine, guanethidine) may be reduced by Prothiaden. It is advisable to review all antihypertensive therapy during treatment with tricyclic antidepressants.

Barbiturates may decrease and methylphenidate may increase the serum concentration of dosulepin and thus affect its antidepressant action.

There is no evidence that dosulepin interferes with standard laboratory tests.

4.6 Pregnancy and lactation

Treatment with Prothiaden should be avoided during pregnancy, unless there are compelling reasons. There is inadequate evidence of safety of the drug during human pregnancy.

There is evidence that dosulepin is secreted in breast milk but this is at levels which are unlikely to cause problems.

4.7 Effects on ability to drive and use machines

Initially, Prothiaden may impair alertness; patients likely to drive vehicles or operate machinery should be warned of this possibility.

4.8 Undesirable effects

The following adverse effects, although not necessarily all reported with dosulepin, have occurred with other tricyclic antidepressants:

Atropine-like side effects including dry mouth, disturbances of accommodation, tachycardia, constipation and hesitancy of micturition are common early in treatment, but usually lessen.

Other adverse effects include drowsiness, sweating, postural hypotension, tremor and skin rashes. Interference with sexual function may occur.

Potentially serious adverse effects are rare. These include depression of the bone marrow, agranulocytosis, hepatitis (including altered liver function), cholestatic jaundice, convulsions and inappropriate ADH secretion.

Psychotic manifestations, including mania and paranoid delusions, may be exacerbated during treatment with tricyclic antidepressants.

Withdrawal symptoms may occur on abrupt cessation of tricyclic therapy and include insomnia, irritability and excessive perspiration. Similar symptoms in neonates whose mothers received tricyclic antidepressants during the third trimester have also been reported.

Cardiac arrhythmias and severe hypotension are likely to occur with high dosage or in deliberate overdosage. They may also occur in patients with pre-existing heart disease taking normal dosage.

4.9 Overdose

Symptoms of overdosage may include dryness of the mouth, excitement, ataxia, drowsiness, loss of consciousness, muscle twitching, convulsions, widely dilated pupils, hyperreflexia, sinus tachycardia, cardiac arrhythmias, hypotension, hypothermia, depression of respiration, visual hallucinations, delirium, urinary retention, paralytic ileus, and respiratory or metabolic alkalosis.

Treatment should consist of gastric lavage. When the patient is unconscious or the cough reflex depressed, the lungs should be protected by a cuffed endotracheal tube. Repeated gastric/intestinal aspiration or repeated administration of activated charcoal may remove drug and metabolites excreted into the gut via the bile. Continuous ECG monitoring is advisable. Abnormalities of cardiac rhythm and epileptic convulsions may occur and should be treated accordingly. Forced diuresis is not recommended. Bed rest is advisable, even after recovery.

5. PHARMACOLOGICAL PROPERTIES

5.1 Pharmacodynamic properties

dosulepin is a tricyclic antidepressant which acts by increasing transmitter levels at central synapses, so producing a clinical antidepressant effect.

dosulepin, in common with other tricyclics, inhibits the reuptake of noradrenaline and 5-hydroxytryptamine, with a significantly greater action on the reuptake of noradrenaline. In addition, dosulepin inhibits the neuronal uptake of dopamine.

As a consequence of its effects on monoamine levels, dosulepin appears to produce adaptive changes in the brain by reducing or down-regulating both noradrenaline receptor numbers and noradrenaline-induced cyclic-AMP formation.

5.2 Pharmacokinetic properties

dosulepin is readily absorbed from the gastrointestinal tract and extensively metabolised in the liver. Metabolites include northiaden, dosulepin-S-oxide and northiaden-S-oxide. dosulepin is excreted in the urine, mainly in the form of metabolites; appreciable amounts are also excreted in the faeces. A half-life of about 50 hours has been reported for dosulepin and its metabolites.

5.3 Preclinical safety data

Not applicable.

6. PHARMACEUTICAL PARTICULARS

6.1 List of excipients

Refined sugar, tricalcium phosphate, maize starch, talc, povidone, liquid glucose, magnesium stearate, sandarac or sandarac tablet varnish, ponceau 4R, sunset yellow, titanium dioxide, shellac, white beeswax, sodium benzoate, polydimethylsiloxane, soya lecithin.

The generic version does not contain shellac, polydimethylsiloxane or soya lecithin.

6.2 Incompatibilities
Not applicable.

6.3 Shelf life
36 months.

6.4 Special precautions for storage
None.

6.5 Nature and contents of container
Blister pack containing 28 tablets.

6.6 Instructions for use and handling
None.

7. MARKETING AUTHORISATION HOLDER
Abbott Laboratories Limited
Queenborough
Kent
ME11 5EL
United Kingdom

8. MARKETING AUTHORISATION NUMBER(S)
PL 00037/0376

9. DATE OF FIRST AUTHORISATION/RENEWAL OF THE AUTHORISATION
28 February 2002

10. DATE OF REVISION OF THE TEXT
November 2004

Protirelin Ampoules

(Cambridge Laboratories)

1. NAME OF THE MEDICINAL PRODUCT
Protirelin Ampoules

2. QUALITATIVE AND QUANTITATIVE COMPOSITION
Each ampoule contains 200micrograms of Protirelin (Thyrotrophin-releasing hormone, TRH) in 2ml of solution.

3. PHARMACEUTICAL FORM
Solution for Injection

4. CLINICAL PARTICULARS

4.1 Therapeutic indications
The administration of Protirelin provides a means of assessing thyroid function and the reserve of TSH in the pituitary gland and is recommended as a test procedure where such assessment is indicated.

It is particularly useful as a diagnostic test for:

1. Mild hyperthyroidism
2. Ophthalmic Graves' disease
3. Mild or preclinical hypothyroidism
4. Hypopituitarism
5. Hypothalamic disease

It may also be used in place of the T_3 suppression test.

4.2 Posology and method of administration
Protirelin ampoules are for intravenous injection.

Intravenous injection

Tests employing intravenous Protirelin are based on the serum TSH response to a standard dose. They provide a means of both quantitative and qualitative assessment of thyroid function. It is essential for each laboratory to establish its own normal range of values for serum TSH before attempting quantitative assessment of Protirelin responses by this means.

Intravenous Protirelin test

a) Blood sample taken for control TSH assay.

b) Protirelin 200μg given as a single bolus injection.

c) Blood sample taken 20 minutes after injection for peak TSH assay.

d) If necessary, a further blood sample may be taken 60 minutes after injection to detect a delayed TSH response.

The ampoule solution should not be diluted.

The elderly

The use of Protirelin in the elderly has been well documented. Dosage requirements and the side-effects are similar to those of younger adults. The response may be decreased in elderly subjects, but this does not interfere with the interpretation of the test results.

Children up to the age of 12

The procedures for administering Protirelin to children are identical to those outlined above. An intravenous dose of 1μg/kg bodyweight may be used.

Interpretation of results

Interpretation of the responses to Protirelin is based on the increase in TSH and/or PBI, T_3 or T_4 levels from the basal values. In normal subjects, there is a prompt rise in serum levels of TSH. The changes observed in various conditions are briefly outlined below:

1. Hyperthyroidism - no rise in serum TSH or thyroid hormone levels.
2. Ophthalmic Graves' disease - often no rise in serum TSH or thyroid hormone levels.
3. Primary hypothyroidism - exaggerated and prolonged rise in serum TSH but no change in thyroid hormone levels.
4. Hypopituitarism - absent or impaired TSH or thyroid hormone response implies diminished TSH reserve.
5. Hypothalamic disease - a rise in serum TSH or thyroid hormone levels can occur in the presence of hypothyroidism; delayed responses are common.

The Protirelin test provides, in most instances, information similar to that obtained from a T_3 suppression test in that an absent or impaired response usually correlates with an absent or impaired response to T_3 suppression.

4.3 Contraindications
There are no absolute contra-indications to Protirelin.

4.4 Special warnings and special precautions for use
In view of the postulated effect of bolus injections of Protirelin on smooth muscle, patients with bronchial asthma or other types of obstructive airways disease should be closely monitored. Caution should always be observed in patients with myocardial ischaemia and severe hypopituitarism.

4.5 Interaction with other medicinal products and other forms of Interaction
The secretion of thyrotrophin appears to be modulated by dopaminergic and noradrenergic pathways. The TSH response to Protirelin may be reduced by thyroid hormones, levodopa, phenothiazines, salicylates, bromocriptine, carbamazepine, lithium and by pharmacological doses of corticosteroids.

An increased response may be seen in subjects taking metoclopramide, amiodarone or theophyllines and in men taking oestrogens. Over-treatment with antithyroid drugs may also cause an enhanced response.

4.6 Pregnancy and lactation
Animal studies and clinical experience have shown no evidence of hazard in human pregnancy at the recommended dosage. Nevertheless, the established medical principle of not administering drugs during early pregnancy should be observed.

Breast enlargement and leaking of milk have been reported following the administration of protirelin to lactating women.

4.7 Effects on ability to drive and use machines
None known.

4.8 Undesirable effects
Protirelin is well tolerated. Following rapid intravenous injection, side-effects of a mild and transient nature may be experienced. These comprise nausea, a desire to micturate, a feeling of flushing, slight dizziness and a peculiar taste, and have been attributed to a local action of the bolus of Protirelin on the muscle of the gastro-intestinal and genito-urinary tracts. A transient increase in pulse rate and blood pressure may also be noted.

4.9 Overdose
No symptoms of overdosage have been noted in patients receiving up to 1mg i.v.

5. PHARMACOLOGICAL PROPERTIES

5.1 Pharmacodynamic properties
Pharmacotherapeutic group: V04CJ.

Protirelin stimulates the secretion of thyroid stimulating hormone (TSH). Intravenous injection results in a prompt rise in serum TSH levels in normal subjects, peak levels being observed about twenty minutes after administration. There is a concomitant rise in serum levels of prolactin.

5.2 Pharmacokinetic properties
TSH rapidly disappears from the plasma after intravenous injection. Over 90% is removed within 20 minutes with a half life of about 5.3 minutes. About 5.5% of the dose is excreted in the urine, mostly within 30 minutes.

5.3 Preclinical safety data
There are no pre-clinical data of relevance to the prescriber which are additional to that already included in other sections of the SPC.

6. PHARMACEUTICAL PARTICULARS

6.1 List of excipients
Mannitol Ph.Eur

Glacial acetic acid Ph.Eur

Water for Injections Ph.Eur

6.2 Incompatibilities
None known.

6.3 Shelf life
Three years.

6.4 Special precautions for storage
The recommended maximum storage temperature is 30°C.

6.5 Nature and contents of container
Clear glass ampoules coded with orange and black colour rings each containing 2ml of solution, in packs of 10 ampoules.

6.6 Instructions for use and handling
None.

Administrative Data

7. MARKETING AUTHORISATION HOLDER
Cambridge Laboratories Limited
Deltic House
Kingfisher Way
Silverlink Business Park
Wallsend
Tyne & Wear
NE28 9NX

8. MARKETING AUTHORISATION NUMBER(S)
PL 12070/0009

9. DATE OF FIRST AUTHORISATION/RENEWAL OF THE AUTHORISATION
October 2002

10. DATE OF REVISION OF THE TEXT
July 2003

Protium 20 mg tablet

(ALTANA Pharma Limited)

1. NAME OF THE MEDICINAL PRODUCT
Protium® 20 mg gastro-resistant tablets.

2. QUALITATIVE AND QUANTITATIVE COMPOSITION
One gastro-resistant tablet contains

20 mg Pantoprazole (as pantoprazole sodium sesquihydrate 22.6 mg).

For excipients see 6.1.

3. PHARMACEUTICAL FORM
Gastro-resistant tablet.

A yellow, oral biconvex film coated tablet imprinted with "P20" in brown ink on one side.

4. CLINICAL PARTICULARS

4.1 Therapeutic indications
For the treatment of mild reflux disease and associated symptoms (e.g. heartburn, acid regurgitation, pain on swallowing).

For long-term management and prevention of relapse in reflux oesophagitis.

Prevention of gastroduodenal ulcers induced by non-selective non-steroidal anti-inflammatory drugs (NSAIDs) in patients at risk with a need for continuous NSAID treatment (see section 4.4).

4.2 Posology and method of administration - recommended dosage:

Mild reflux disease and associated symptoms (e.g. heartburn, acid regurgitation, pain on swallowing)

The recommended oral dosage is one gastro-resistant tablet Protium® 20 mg per day. Symptom relief is generally accomplished within 2-4 weeks, and a 4-week treatment period is usually required for healing of associated oesophagitis. If this is not sufficient, healing will normally be achieved within a further 4 weeks. When symptom relief has been achieved, reoccurring symptoms can be controlled using an on-demand regimen of 20 mg once daily, when required. A switch to continuous therapy may be considered in case satisfactory symptom control cannot be maintained with on-demand treatment.

Long-term management and prevention of relapse in reflux oesophagitis

For long-term management, a maintenance dose of one gastro-resistant tablet Protium® 20 mg per day is recommended, increasing to 40 mg pantoprazole per day if a relapse occurs. Protium® 40 mg is available for this case. After healing of the relapse the dosage can be reduced again to 20 mg pantoprazole.

Prevention of gastroduodenal ulcers induced by non-selective non-steroidal anti-inflammatory drugs (NSAIDs) in patients at risk with a need for continuous NSAID treatment

The recommended oral dosage is one gastro-resistant tablet Protium® 20 mg per day.

Note:

A daily dose of 20 mg pantoprazole should not be exceeded in patients with severe liver impairment.

No dose adjustment is necessary in elderly patients or in those with impaired renal function.

General instructions:

Protium® 20 mg gastro-resistant tablets should not be chewed or crushed, and should be swallowed whole with liquid before a meal.

4.3 Contraindications
Protium® 20 mg should not be used in cases of known hypersensitivity to the active ingredient or/and any of the other constituents of Protium® 20 mg.

4.4 Special warnings and special precautions for use

Special warnings

None.

Table 1

Frequency Organ system	common (≥1% - <10%)	uncommon (≥0.1% - <1%)	Very rare (<0.01%)
Gastrointestinal Disorders	Upper abdominal pain; Diarrhoea; Constipation; Flatulence	Nausea	
General disorders and administration site conditions			Peripheral edema subsiding after termination of therapy
Hepatobiliary disorders			Severe hepatocellular damage leading to jaundice with or without hepatic failure
Immune system disorders			Anaphylactic reactions including anaphylactic shock
Investigations			Increased liver enzymes (transaminases, γ-GT); Elevated triglycerides; Increased body temperature subsiding after termination of therapy
Musculoskeletal, connective tissue disorders			Myalgia subsiding after termination of therapy
Nervous system disorders	Headache	Dizziness; Disturbances in vision (blurred vision)	
Psychiatric disorders			Mental depression subsiding after termination of therapy
Renal and urinary disorders			Interstitial nephritis
Skin and sub-cutaneous tissue disorders		Allergic reactions such as pruritus and skin rash	Urticaria; Angioedema; Severe skin reactions such as Stevens Johnson Syndrome, Erythema Multi-forme, Lyell-Syndrome; Photosensitivity

Special precautions for use

In patients with severe liver impairment the liver enzymes should be monitored regularly during treatment with pantoprazole, particularly on long-term use. In the case of a rise of the liver enzymes Protium® 20 mg should be discontinued.

The use of Protium® 20 mg as a preventive of gastroduodenal ulcers induced by non-selective non-steroidal anti-inflammatory drugs (NSAIDs) should be restricted to patients who require continued NSAID treatment and have an increased risk to develop gastrointestinal complications.

The increased risk should be assessed according to individual risk factors, e.g. high age >65 years), history of gastric or duodenal ulcer or upper gastrointestinal bleeding.

Pantoprazole, as all acid-blocking medicines, may reduce the absorption of vitamin B12 (cyanocobalamin) due to hypo- or achlorhydria. This should be considered in patients with reduced body stores or risk factors for reduced vitamin B12 absorption on long-term therapy.

In long term treatment, especially when exceeding a treatment period of 1 year, patients should be kept under regular surveillance.

Note:

Prior to treatment a malignant disease of the oesophagus or stomach should be excluded as the treatment with pantoprazole may alleviate the symptoms of malignant diseases and can thus delay diagnosis.

Patients who do not respond after 4 weeks should be investigated.

To date there has been no experience with treatment in children.

4.5 Interaction with other medicinal products and other forms of Interaction

Protium® 20 mg may reduce or increase the absorption of drugs whose bioavailability is pH-dependent (e.g. ketoconazole).

Pantoprazole is metabolized in the liver via the cytochrome P450 enzyme system. An interaction of pantoprazole with other drugs or compounds which are metabolized using the same enzyme system cannot be excluded. However, no clinically significant interactions were observed in specific tests with a number of such drugs or compounds, namely carbamazepine, caffeine, diazepam, diclofenac, digoxin, ethanol, glibenclamide, metoprolol, naproxen, nifedipine, phenprocoumon, phenytoin, piroxicam, theophylline, warfarin and an oral contraceptive.

There were also no interactions with concomitantly administered antacids.

4.6 Pregnancy and lactation

Clinical experience in pregnant women is limited. In animal reproduction studies, signs of slight fetotoxicity were observed at doses above 5 mg/kg. There is no information on the excretion of pantoprazole into human breast milk. Pantoprazole tablets should only be used when the benefit to the mother is considered greater than the potential risk to the foetus/baby.

4.7 Effects on ability to drive and use machines

There are no known effects on the ability to drive and use machines.

4.8 Undesirable effects

(see Table 1 above)

4.9 Overdose

There are no known symptoms of over-dosage in man. Doses up to 240 mg i.v. were administered over 2 minutes and were well tolerated.

In the case of over-dosage with clinical signs of intoxication, the usual rules of intoxication therapy apply.

5. PHARMACOLOGICAL PROPERTIES

5.1 Pharmacodynamic properties

Proton pump inhibitors

ATC Code: AO2BC02

Pantoprazole is a substituted benzimidazole which inhibits the secretion of hydrochloric acid in the stomach by specific action on the proton pumps of the parietal cells.

Pantoprazole is converted to its active form in the acidic canaliculi of the parietal cells where it inhibits the H^+, K^+-ATPase enzyme, i. e. the final stage in the production of hydrochloric acid in the stomach. The inhibition is dose-dependent and affects both basal and stimulated acid secretion. In most patients, freedom from symptoms is achieved in 2 weeks. As with other proton pump inhibitors and H_2 receptor inhibitors, treatment with pantoprazole causes a reduced acidity in the stomach and thereby an increase in gastrin in proportion to the reduction in acidity. The increase in gastrin is reversible. Since pantoprazole binds to the enzyme distal to the cell receptor level, the substance can affect hydrochloric acid secretion independently of stimulation by other substances (acetylcholine, histamine, gastrin). The effect is the same whether the product is given orally or intravenously.

The fasting gastrin values increase under pantoprazole. On short-term use, in most cases they do not exceed the normal upper limit. During long-term treatment, gastrin levels double in most cases. An excessive increase, however, occurs only in isolated cases. As a result, a mild to moderate increase in the number of specific endocrine (ECL) cells in the stomach is observed in a minority of cases during long-term treatment (simple to adenomatoid hyperplasia). However, according to the studies conducted so far, the formation of carcinoid precursors (atypical hyperplasia) or gastric carcinoids as were found in animal experiments (see Section 5.3) can be ruled out for humans for a 1-year treatment period.

An influence of a long term treatment with pantoprazole exceeding one year cannot be completely ruled out on endocrine parameters of the thyroid and liver enzymes according to results in animal studies.

5.2 Pharmacokinetic properties

- General pharmacokinetics

Pantoprazole is rapidly absorbed and the maximal plasma concentration is achieved even after one single 20 mg oral dose. On average at about 2.0 h - 2.5 h p.a. the maximum serum concentrations of about 1-1.5 μg/ml are achieved, and these values remain constant after multiple administration. Volume of distribution is about 0.15 l/kg and clearance is about 0.1 l/h/kg.

Terminal half-life is about 1 h. There were a few cases of subjects with delayed elimination. Because of the specific binding of pantoprazole to the proton pumps of the parietal cell the elimination half-life does not correlate with the much longer duration of action (inhibition of acid secretion).

Pharmacokinetics do not vary after single or repeated administration. In the dose range of 10 to 80 mg, the plasma kinetics of pantoprazole are linear after both oral and intravenous administration.

Pantoprazole's serum protein binding is about 98%. The substance is almost exclusively metabolized in the liver. Renal elimination represents the major route of excretion (about 80%) for the metabolites of pantoprazole, the rest is excreted with the faeces. The main metabolite in both the serum and urine is desmethylpantoprazole which is conjugated with sulphate. The half-life of the main metabolite (about 1.5 h) is not much longer than that of pantoprazole.

- Bioavailability

Pantoprazole is completely absorbed after oral administration. The absolute bioavailability from the tablet was found to be about 77%. Concomitant intake of food had no influence on AUC, maximum serum concentration and thus bioavailability. Only the variability of the lag-time will be increased by concomitant food intake.

- Characteristics in patients/special groups of subjects

No dose reduction is requested when pantoprazole is administered to patients with restricted kidney function (incl. dialysis patients). As with healthy subjects, pantoprazole's half-life is short. Only very small amounts of pantoprazole can be dialyzed. Although the main metabolite has a moderately delayed half-life (2 - 3h), excretion is still rapid and thus accumulation does not occur.

Although for patients with liver cirrhosis (classes A and B according to *Child*) the half-life values increased to between 3 and 6 h and the AUC values increased by a factor of 3 - 5, the maximum serum concentration only increased slightly by a factor of 1.3 compared with healthy subjects.

A slight increase in AUC and Cmax in elderly volunteers compared with younger counterparts is also not clinically relevant.

5.3 Preclinical safety data

Preclinical data reveal no special hazard to humans based on conventional studies of safety pharmacology, repeated dose toxicity and genotoxicity.

In the 2-year carcinogenicity studies (corresponding to lifetime treatment) in rats, neuroendocrine neoplasms were found. In addition, squamous cell papillomas were found in the forestomach of rats in one study. The mechanism leading to the formation of gastric carcinoids by substituted benzimidazoles has been carefully investigated and allows the conclusion that it is a secondary reaction to the massively elevated serum gastrin levels occurring in the rat during chronic high-dose treatment.

In the two-year rodent studies an increased number of liver tumors was observed in rats (in one rat study only) and in female mice and was interpreted as being due to pantoprazole's high metabolic rate in the liver.

A slight increase of neoplastic changes of the thyroid was observed in the group of rats receiving the highest dose (200 mg/kg) in one 2 year study. The occurrence of these neoplasms is associated with the pantoprazole-induced changes in the breakdown of thyroxine in the rat liver. As the therapeutic dose in man is low, no side effects on the thyroid glands are expected.

From mutagenicity studies, cell transformation tests and a DNA binding study it is concluded that pantoprazole has no genotoxic potential.

Investigations revealed no evidence of impaired fertility or teratogenic effects.

Penetration of the placenta was investigated in the rat and was found to increase with advanced gestation. As a result, concentration of pantoprazole in the foetus is increased shortly before birth.

6. PHARMACEUTICAL PARTICULARS

6.1 List of excipients

Sodium carbonate

Mannitol

Crospovidone

Povidone K90

Calcium stearate

Hypromellose

Povidone K25

Propylene glycol

Methacrylic acid-ethylacrylate-copolymer (1:1)

Polysorbate 80

Sodium laurilsulphate

Triethyl citrate

Titanium dioxide E 171

Yellow ferric oxide E 172

Printing ink (shellac, red, black and yellow ferric oxide E172, soya lecithin, titanium dioxide E171, antifoam DC 1510)

6.2 Incompatibilities

Not applicable.

6.3 Shelf life

3 years.

6.4 Special precautions for storage

No special precautions for storage.

6.5 Nature and contents of container

Packs: bottles (HDPE container with LDPE closure) and ALU/ALU blisters with:

7 gastro-resistant tablets

14 and 15* gastro-resistant tablets

28 and 30* gastro-resistant tablets

56 and 60* gastro-resistant tablets

84 gastro-resistant tablets

100* gastro-resistant tablets

112 gastro-resistant tablets

Hospital packs: bottles (HDPE container with LDPE closure) and ALU/ALU blisters with:

50 gastro-resistant tablets

84 gastro-resistant tablets

90 gastro-resistant tablets

112 gastro-resistant tablets

140* gastro-resistant tablets

140 (10x14*) (5x28*) gastro-resistant tablets

700 (5x140*) gastro-resistant tablets

280 (20x14*), (10x28*) gastro-resistant tablets

500 gastro-resistant tablets

*authorised in the Reference Member State

Note: Not all pack sizes may be marketed.

6.6 Instructions for use and handling

No special requirements.

7. MARKETING AUTHORISATION HOLDER

ALTANA Pharma AG

Byk-Gulden-Str. 2

D-78467 Konstanz

Germany

8. MARKETING AUTHORISATION NUMBER(S)

PL 20141/0001

9. DATE OF FIRST AUTHORISATION/RENEWAL OF THE AUTHORISATION

7 January 1999/18 March 2004

10. DATE OF REVISION OF THE TEXT

1st July 2005

11. LEGAL STATUS

POM

Protium® is a registered trademark of ALTANA Pharma AG, Germany

Protium 40 mg i.v.

(ALTANA Pharma Limited)

1. NAME OF THE MEDICINAL PRODUCT

Protium® i.v. powder for solution for injection.

2. QUALITATIVE AND QUANTITATIVE COMPOSITION

One vial contains:

40mg pantoprazole (as pantoprazole sodium).

For excipients see 6.1.

3. PHARMACEUTICAL FORM

Powder for solution for injection. A white to almost white dry substance.

4. CLINICAL PARTICULARS

4.1 Therapeutic indications

For symptomatic improvement and healing of gastrointestinal diseases which require a reduction in acid secretion:

- duodenal ulcer
- gastric ulcer
- moderate and severe reflux oesophagitis
- Zollinger-Ellison Syndrome and other pathological hypersecretory conditions

Note: Prior to treatment of gastric ulcer, the possibility of malignancy should be excluded as treatment with Protium® i.v. may alleviate the symptoms of malignant ulcers and can thus delay diagnosis.

4.2 Posology and method of administration

Protium® i.v. is for intravenous administration ONLY and must NOT be given by any other route. Protium® i.v. is recommended only if oral application is not appropriate.

Duodenal ulcer, gastric ulcer, moderate and severe reflux oesophagitis

The recommended intravenous dosage is one vial (40 mg pantoprazole) of Protium® i.v. per day.

Long-term management of Zollinger-Ellison Syndrome and other pathological hypersecretory conditions

Patients should start their treatment with a daily dose of 80 mg Protium® i.v. Thereafter, the dosage can be titrated up or down as needed using measurements of gastric acid secretion to guide. With doses above 80 mg daily, the dose should be divided and given twice daily. A temporary increase of the dosage above 160 mg pantoprazole is possible but should not be applied longer than required for adequate acid control.

In case a rapid acid control is required, a starting dose of 2×80 mg Protium® i.v. is sufficient to manage a decrease of acid output into the target range (<10 mEq/h) within one hour in the majority of patients. Transition from Protium® i.v. to the oral formulation of Protium® should be performed as soon as it is clinically justified.

A ready-to-use intravenous solution is prepared by injecting 10 ml of 0.9% sodium chloride injection into the vial containing the lyophilised powder.

This freshly prepared solution should be administered intravenously over 2 to 15 minutes, either as a slow injection or it may be further diluted with 100 ml of 0.9% sodium chloride injection, or 5% glucose injection, and administered as a short-term infusion.

Protium® i.v. should not be reconstituted with diluents other than those stated.

After preparation, the solution must be used within 12 hours.

With an exception of the treatment of patients with Zollinger-Ellison-Syndrome and other pathological hypersecretory conditions, the duration of treatment with the active ingredient pantoprazole should not exceed 8 weeks.

In most patients, freedom from symptoms is achieved rapidly.

As soon as oral therapy is possible, treatment with Protium® i.v. should be discontinued.

Data are available on i.v. use for up to 7 days. Thereafter, oral Protium® treatment should be administered in compliance with the approved dosage regimen.

Duodenal ulcer:

Duodenal ulcers generally heal within 2 weeks. If a 2-week period of treatment is not sufficient, healing will be achieved in almost all cases within a further 2 weeks.

Gastric ulcer:

A 4-week period is usually required for the treatment of gastric ulcers. If this is not sufficient, healing will usually be achieved within a further 4 weeks.

Gastro-Oesophageal Reflux:

A 4-week period is usually required for the treatment of gastro-oesophageal reflux. If this is not sufficient, healing will usually be achieved within a further 4 weeks.

Elderly:

No dose adjustment is necessary in the elderly.

Patients with impaired renal function:

No dose adjustment is necessary in patients with renal impairment.

Patients with severe liver impairment:

In patients with severe liver impairment, the daily dose should be reduced to 20 mg pantoprazole. Furthermore, in these patients the liver enzymes should be monitored during Protium® i.v. therapy. In case of a rise in the liver enzymes, Protium® i.v. should be discontinued.

Children:

There is no information on the use of pantoprazole in children. Therefore Protium® i.v. should not be used in children.

4.3 Contraindications

Protium® i.v. should not be used in cases of known hypersensitivity to pantoprazole.

4.4 Special warnings and special precautions for use

Protium® i.v. is for intravenous administration ONLY and must NOT be given by any other route.

Protium® i.v. is recommended only if oral application is not appropriate.

4.5 Interaction with other medicinal products and other forms of Interaction

As with other acid secretion inhibitors, changes in absorption may be observed when drugs whose absorption is pH-dependent, e.g. ketoconazole, are taken concomitantly.

Pantoprazole is metabolised in the liver via the cytochrome P450 enzyme system. Although studies have shown that pantoprazole has no significant effect on cytochrome P450, an interaction of pantoprazole with other drugs or compounds which are metabolised using the same enzyme system cannot be excluded.

However, no clinically significant interactions were observed in specific tests with a number of such drugs/compounds, namely antipyrine, caffeine, carbamazepine, diazepam, diclofenac, digoxin, ethanol, glibenclamide, metoprolol, naproxen, nifedipine, phenprocoumon, phenytoin, piroxicam, theophylline, warfarin and an oral contraceptive. There were also no interactions with concomitantly administered antacids.

4.6 Pregnancy and lactation

Use during pregnancy:

There is no information about the safety of pantoprazole during pregnancy in humans. Animal experiments have revealed no signs of foetal damage, but reproduction studies have revealed reduced litter weight and delayed development of the skeleton at doses above 15 mg/kg.

During pregnancy, Protium® i.v. should not be used unless the benefit exceeds the potential risk.

Use during lactation:

There is no information about the safety of pantoprazole during breast-feeding in humans. In the rat, not more than 0.02% of the administered dose is excreted via the breast milk.

During breast-feeding, Protium® i.v. should not be used unless the benefit exceeds the potential risk.

4.7 Effects on ability to drive and use machines

Pantoprazole does not affect the ability to drive and use machines.

4.8 Undesirable effects

(see Table 1 on next page)

4.9 Overdose

There are no known symptoms of overdosage in man. However, pantoprazole is very specific in action and no particular problems are anticipated. Doses up to 240 mg i.v. were administered without obvious adverse effects.

As pantoprazole is extensively protein bound, it is not readily dialysable. Apart from symptomatic and supportive treatment, no specific therapeutic recommendations can be made.

5. PHARMACOLOGICAL PROPERTIES

5.1 Pharmacodynamic properties

Proton pump inhibitors

ATC code: A02BC02

Pantoprazole is a proton pump inhibitor, i.e. it inhibits specifically and dose-proportionally the gastric H^+/K^+-ATPase enzyme which is responsible for acid secretion in the parietal cells of the stomach.

The substance is a substituted benzimidazole which accumulates in the acidic environment of the parietal cells after absorption. There it is converted into the active form, a cyclic sulphenamide, which binds to the H^+/K^+-ATPase, thus inhibiting the proton pump and causing potent and long-lasting suppression of basal and stimulated gastric acid secretion. As pantoprazole acts distally to the receptor level, it can inhibit gastric acid secretion irrespective of the nature of the stimulus (acetylcholine, histamine, gastrin).

Pantoprazole's selectivity is due to the fact that it can only exert its full effect in a strongly acidic environment (pH<3), remaining mostly inactive at higher pH values. As a result, its complete pharmacological and thus therapeutic effect can only be achieved in the acid-secretory parietal cells. By means of a feedback mechanism, this effect is diminished at the same rate as acid secretion is inhibited.

Pantoprazole has the same effect whether administered orally or intravenously.

Following intravenous or oral administration, pantoprazole inhibits the pentagastrin-stimulated gastric acid secretion. In volunteers, acid secretion was inhibited by 56% following the first i.v. administration of 30 mg and by 99% after 5 days. With an oral dose of 40 mg, inhibition was 51% on day 1 and 85% on day 7. Basal 24 hour acidity was reduced by 37% and 98%, respectively.

The fasting gastrin values increased under pantoprazole but in most cases they did not exceed the normal upper limit. Following completion of a course of oral treatment, the median gastrin levels clearly declined again.

5.2 Pharmacokinetic properties

General Pharmacokinetics

Terminal half-life is about 1 hour. Volume of distribution is about 0.15 L/kg, clearance is about 0.1 L/h/kg and Cmax is approximately 5.53 mg/l.

Table 1

Frequency Organ System	common (≥1% - <10%)	uncommon (≥0.1% - <1%)	Very rare (<0.01%)
Gastrointestinal disorders	Upper abdominal pain; Diarrhoea; Constipation; Flatulence	Nausea	
General disorders and administration site conditions			Injection site thrombophlebitis; Peripheral edema subsiding after termination of therapy
Hepatobiliary disorders			Severe hepatocellular damage leading to jaundice with or without hepatic failure
Immune system disorders			Anaphylactic reactions including anaphylactic shock
Investigations			Increased liver enzymes (transaminases, γ-GT); Elevated triglycerides; Increased body temperature subsiding after termination of therapy
Musculoskeletal, connective tissue disorders			Myalgia subsiding after termination of therapy
Nervous system disorders	Headache	Dizziness; Disturbances in vision (blurred vision)	
Psychiatric disorders			Mental depression subsiding after termination of therapy
Renal and urinary disorders			Interstitial nephritis
Skin and sub-cutaneous tissue disorders		Allergic reactions such as pruritus and skin rash	Urticaria; Angioedema; Severe skin reactions such as Stevens Johnson Syndrome; Erythema Multi-forme; Lyell-Syndrome; Photosensitivity

Pharmacokinetics do not vary after single or repeated administration. The plasma kinetics of pantoprazole are linear after both oral and intravenous administration.

Studies with pantoprazole in humans reveal no interaction with the cytochrome P450-system of the liver. There was no induction of the P450-system seen as tested after chronic administration with antipyrine as a marker. Also, no inhibition of metabolism was observed after concomitant administration of pantoprazole with either antipyrine, caffeine, carbamazepine, diazepam, diclofenac, digoxin, ethanol, glibenclamide, metropolol, naproxen, nifedipine, phenprocoumon, phenytoin, piroxicam, theophylline, or oral contraceptives. Concomitant administration of pantoprazole with warfarin has no influence on warfarin's effect on the coagulation factors.

Pantoprazole's plasma protein binding is about 98%. The substance is almost exclusively metabolised in the liver. Renal elimination represents the major route of excretion (about 80%) for the metabolites of pantoprazole; the rest are excreted in the faeces. The main metabolite in both the plasma and urine is desmethylpantoprazole which is conjugated with sulphate. The half-life of the main metabolites (about 1.5 hours) is not much longer than that of pantoprazole.

Characteristics in patients/special groups of subjects:

Although for patients with hepatic cirrhosis (classes A and B according to Child) the half-time values increased to between 7 and 9 hours and the AUC values increased by a factor of 5 to 7, the maximum plasma concentration only increased slightly by a factor of 1.5 compared with healthy subjects. As pantoprazole has a good safety profile and is well tolerated it can be given to patients with mild to moderate liver impairment.

No dose reduction is required when pantoprazole is administered to patients with impaired kidney function (including dialysis patients). As with healthy subjects, pantoprazole's half-life is short. Only very small amounts of pantoprazole are dialysed. Although the main metabolite has a moderately delayed half-life (2-3 hours), excretion is still rapid and thus accumulation does not occur.

A slight increase in AUC and Cmax in elderly volunteers compared with younger counterparts is also not clinically relevant.

5.3 Preclinical safety data

Acute toxicity

In acute toxicity studies in mice, the LD_{50} values were found to be 370 mg/kg bodyweight for i.v. administration and around 700 mg/kg bodyweight for oral administration.

In the rat, the corresponding values were around 240 mg/kg for i.v. administration and 900 mg/kg for oral administration.

Chronic toxicity

Hypergastrinaemia and morphologic changes of the mucosa were observed in studies investigating repeated administration for up to 12 months in the rat and dog. Most of the effects were reversible and attributable solely to the drug action, i.e. suppression of acid secretion.

In long-term studies in the rat and dog, there was an increase in stomach and liver weights, the increase being reversible after the substance was discontinued. The increase in liver weight following highly toxic doses was seen as a result of the induction of drug-metabolising enzymes.

Thyroid activation in two rat experiments is due to the rapid metabolism of thyroid hormones in the liver and has also been described in a similar form for other drugs. Changes in the thyroid and associated reduced degradation of cholesterol have been observed in one-year studies in the rat and dog. Hypertrophy of the thyroid and increases in cholesterol levels are reversible.

In studies in the dog, a species-species specific pulmonary oedema was observed. The animal-specific metabolite which was responsible for the oedema could not be identified in man.

Carcinogenicity

In a 2-year carcinogenicity study in rats - which corresponds to lifetime treatment for rats - ECL cell carcinoids were found. The mechanism leading to the formation of gastric carcinoids by substituted benzimidazoles has been carefully investigated and allows the conclusion that it is a secondary reaction to the massively elevated serum gastrin levels occurring in the rat during treatment. In addition, rats have more ECL cells in the mucosa of the glandular stomach than man, so that a larger number of responder cells for the increased gastrin values can become active.

ECL cell neoplasms were not observed in either the study in mice (24 months) or in long-term studies in the dog. In clinical studies (40 - 80 mg for 1 year), ECL cell density slightly increased.

In the two year studies, an increased number of neoplastic changes of the liver was observed in rats and female mice and was interpreted as being due to pantoprazole's high rate of metabolism in the liver.

A slight increase of neoplastic changes of the thyroid was observed in the group of rats receiving the highest dose. The occurrence of these neoplasms is associated with the pantoprazole-induced changes in the breakdown of thyroxine in the rat liver. In man, no changes in the thyroid hormones T3, T4 and TSH were observed. This high dose phenomenon in the rat is therefore not relevant for man.

Mutagenicity

In mutagenicity studies, there were no indications of a mutagenic action in vivo or in vitro.

Reproduction toxicology

Investigations revealed no evidence of impaired fertility or teratogenic effects. Penetration of the placenta was investigated in the rat and was found to increase with advanced gestation. As a result, the concentration of pantoprazole in the foetus is increased shortly before birth, regardless of the route of administration.

In humans, there is no experience of the use of the drug during pregnancy.

6. PHARMACEUTICAL PARTICULARS

6.1 List of excipients

Edetate disodium dehydrate, sodium hydroxide.

6.2 Incompatibilities

Protium® i.v. is not compatible with acidic solutions.

6.3 Shelf life

3 years.

The reconstituted solution must be used within 12 hours after preparation.

Any unused portion should be discarded.

6.4 Special precautions for storage

Do not store above 25°C. Keep container in outer carton.

6.5 Nature and contents of container

10 ml glass vial (type 1 acc. to Ph.Eur.), with an aluminium cap and rubber stopper.

Dose units: 1, 5 and 20 vials.

6.6 Instructions for use and handling

A ready-to-use intravenous solution is prepared by injecting 10 ml of physiological sodium chloride solution into the vial containing the lyophilised powder.

This freshly prepared solution should be administered intravenously over 2 to 15 minutes, either as a slow injection or it may be further diluted with 100 ml of 0.9% sodium chloride injection, or 5% glucose injection, and administered as a short-term infusion.

Protium® i.v. should not be reconstituted with diluents other than those stated. The reconstituted solution has a pH of 9 - 10.

Once reconstituted, from a microbiological point of view, the product should be used immediately. If not used immediately, in-use storage times and conditions prior to use are the responsibility of the user and would normally not be longer than 12 hours at not more than 25°C.

Any product that has remained in the container or the visual appearance of which has changed (e.g. if cloudiness or precipitation is observed) has to be discarded. The content of the vial is for single use only.

7. MARKETING AUTHORISATION HOLDER

ALTANA Pharma AG

Byk-Gulden Strae 2

D-78467 Konstanz, Germany

8. MARKETING AUTHORISATION NUMBER(S)

PL 20141/0003

9. DATE OF FIRST AUTHORISATION/RENEWAL OF THE AUTHORISATION

1 April 2003

10. DATE OF REVISION OF THE TEXT

May 2005

11. LEGAL STATUS

POM

Protium® is a registered trademark of ALTANA Pharma AG, Germany

Protium 40 mg tablet

(ALTANA Pharma Limited)

1. NAME OF THE MEDICINAL PRODUCT

Protium® (or Panselect) 40 mg gastro resistant tablets.

2. QUALITATIVE AND QUANTITATIVE COMPOSITION

One gastro resistant tablet contains:

40 mg Pantoprazole (as pantoprazole sodium sesquihydrate).

For excipients see 6.1.

3. PHARMACEUTICAL FORM

Gastro-resistant coated tablet for oral use.

A yellow, oval, biconvex, film-coated tablet imprinted with "P 40" in brown ink on one side.

4. CLINICAL PARTICULARS

4.1 Therapeutic indications

For symptomatic improvement and healing of gastrointestinal diseases which require a reduction in acid secretion:

- Duodenal ulcer
- Gastric ulcer
- Moderate and severe reflux oesophagitis

- Zollinger-Ellison-Syndrome and other pathological hypersecretory conditions

- Eradication of *Helicobacter pylori*, in combination with two antibiotics in patients with duodenal ulcer or gastritis.

In the case of combination therapy for the eradication of *Helicobacter pylori*, the Summaries of Product Characteristics of the respective drugs should be observed.

4.2 Posology and method of administration

The recommended dosage in duodenal ulcer, gastric ulcer and gastro-oesophageal reflux is one enteric-coated tablet per day. Protium® should not be chewed or crushed, and should be swallowed whole with water either before or during breakfast.

In combination therapy for the eradication of *Helicobacter pylori*, the recommended dose is one tablet taken twice daily. The second Protium® tablet should be taken before the evening meal. Combination therapy should be implemented for 7 days. At the end of the 7 days' combination period, pantoprazole may be continued to ensure the healing of the ulcer. For duodenal ulcers, this may require an additional 1 to 3 weeks.

The safety of longer-term use is generally well established. Long-term administration of pantoprazole has a safety profile similar to that observed with short-term treatment, and is well tolerated. Except for patients with Zollinger-Ellison-Syndrome and other pathological hypersecretory conditions, the treatment with Protium® 40mg should not exceed 8 weeks, as experience with long-term administration in man is insufficient.

In most patients, freedom from symptoms is achieved rapidly. Except for patients with pathological hypersecretory conditions including Zollinger-Ellison syndrome, the treatment with Protium® should not exceed 8 weeks, as experience in man is insufficient. In a few instances, there may be benefit in extending treatment beyond 8 weeks to ensure healing.

Duodenal ulcer:

Duodenal ulcers generally heal within 2 weeks. If a 2-week period of treatment is not sufficient, healing will be achieved in almost all cases within a further 2 weeks.

Gastric ulcer:

A 4-week period is usually required for the treatment of gastric ulcers. If this is not sufficient, healing will usually be achieved within a further 4 weeks.

Gastro-Oesophageal Reflux:

A 4-week period is usually required for the treatment of gastro-oesophageal reflux. If this is not sufficient, healing will usually be achieved within a further 4 weeks.

Long-term management of Zollinger-Ellison-Syndrome and other pathological hypersecretory conditions:

For the long-term management of Zollinger-Ellison-Syndrome and other pathological hypersecretory conditions patients should start their treatment with a daily dose of 80 mg (2 tablets of Protium® 40 mg). Thereafter, the dosage can be titrated up or down as needed using measurements of gastric acid secretion to guide. With doses above 80 mg daily, the dose should be divided and given twice daily. A temporary increase of the dosage above 160 mg pantoprazole is possible but should not be applied longer than required for adequate acid control.

Treatment duration in Zollinger-Ellison-Syndrome and other pathological hypersecretory conditions is not limited and should be adapted according to clinical needs.

Eradication of *Helicobacter pylori* (*H. pylori*):

The use of Protium® in combination with two antibiotics (triple therapy) is recommended. The following combinations have been shown to be effective:

(a) Protium® 40 mg twice daily,

plus 1000 mg amoxycillin twice daily

and 500 mg clarithromycin twice daily

(b) Protium® 40 mg twice daily,

plus 400 mg metronidazole twice daily

and 250 mg clarithromycin twice daily

The second Protium® tablet should be taken before the evening meal. Combination therapy should be implemented for 7 days.

Elderly:

No dose adjustment is necessary in the elderly. However, the daily dose of 40 mg pantoprazole should not be exceeded. An exception is combination therapy for eradication of *H. pylori*, where elderly patients should receive the usual pantoprazole dose (2 × 40 mg/day) during 1 week treatment.

Patients with impaired renal function:

No dose adjustment is necessary in patients with impaired renal function. However, the daily dose of 40mg pantoprazole should not be exceeded. For this reason, *H. pylori* triple therapy is not appropriate in these patients.

Patients with hepatic cirrhosis:

Due to an increased AUC and a modified metabolism of pantoprazole in patients with hepatic cirrhosis, the dose regimen should be reduced to one tablet every other day. For this reason, *H. pylori* triple therapy is not appropriate in these patients.

Children:

There is no information on the use of pantoprazole in children. Therefore pantoprazole tablets should not be used in children.

4.3 Contraindications

Protium® may not be used in cases of known hypersensitivity to any of its constituents.

4.4 Special warnings and special precautions for use

In patients with severe liver impairment, particularly those on long-term use, liver enzymes should be monitored regularly during treatment with pantoprazole. In the case of a rise in liver enzymes, Protium® should be discontinued.

To date, there has been no experience with treatment in children.

Note:

Prior to treatment of gastric ulcer, the possibility of malignancy should be excluded as treatment with Protium® may alleviate the symptoms of malignant ulcers and can thus delay diagnosis.

Decreased gastric acidity due to any means – including proton pump inhibitors – increases gastric counts of bacteria normally present in the gastrointestinal tract. Treatment with acid-reducing drugs may lead to a slightly increased risk of gastrointestinal infections, such as *Salmonella* and *Campylobacter*.

In patients with Zollinger-Ellison-Syndrome and other pathological hypersecretory conditions requiring long-term treatment, pantoprazole, as all acid-blocking medicines, may reduce the absorption of vitamin B12 (cyanocobalamin) due to hypo- or achlorhydria. This should be considered if respective clinical symptoms are observed.

4.5 Interaction with other medicinal products and other forms of Interaction

As with other acid secretion inhibitors, changes in absorption may be observed when drugs whose absorption is pH-dependent, e.g. ketoconazole, are taken concomitantly.

Pantoprazole is metabolised in the liver via the cytochrome P450 enzyme system. Although studies have shown that pantoprazole has no significant effect on cytochrome P450, an interaction of pantoprazole with other drugs or compounds, which are metabolised using the same enzyme system, cannot be excluded.

However, no clinically significant interactions were observed in specific tests with a number of such drugs/compounds, namely antipyrine, carbamazepine, caffeine, diazepam, diclofenac, digoxin, ethanol, glibenclamide, metoprolol, naproxen, nifedipine, phenprocoumon, phenytoin, piroxicam, theophylline, warfarin and an oral contraceptive. There were also no interactions with concomitantly administered antacids.

4.6 Pregnancy and lactation

Clinical experience in pregnant women is limited. In animal reproduction studies, signs of slight fetotoxicity were observed at doses above 5 mg/kg. There is no information on the excretion of pantoprazole into human breast milk.

During pregnancy and breast feeding, Protium® should only be used when the benefit exceeds the potential risk.

4.7 Effects on ability to drive and use machines

Pantoprazole does not affect the ability to drive and use machines.

4.8 Undesirable effects

(see Table 1 below)

4.9 Overdose

There are no known symptoms of over dosage in man. However, pantoprazole is very specific in action and no particular problems are anticipated. Doses up to 240 mg i.v. were administered without obvious adverse effects. As pantoprazole is extensively protein bound, it is not readily dialysable.

Apart from symptomatic and supportive treatment, no specific therapeutic recommendations can be made.

5. PHARMACOLOGICAL PROPERTIES

5.1 Pharmacodynamic properties

Proton Pump Inhibitors.

ATC code: A02BC02.

Pantoprazole is a proton pump inhibitor, i.e. it inhibits specifically and dose-proportionally the gastric H^+/K^+-ATPase enzyme, which is responsible for acid secretion in the parietal cells of the stomach.

The substance is a substituted benzimidazole, which accumulates, in the acidic environment of the parietal cells after absorption. There it is converted into the active form, a cyclic sulphenamide, which binds to the H^+/K^+-ATPase, thus inhibiting the proton pump and causing potent and long-lasting suppression of basal and stimulated gastric acid secretion. As pantoprazole acts distally to the receptor level, it can inhibit gastric acid secretion irrespective of the nature of the stimulus (acetylcholine, histamine, gastrin).

Pantoprazole's selectivity is due to the fact that it can only exert its full effect in a strongly acidic environment ($pH < 3$), remaining mostly inactive at higher pH values. As a result, its complete pharmacological and thus therapeutic effect can only be achieved in the acid-secretory parietal cells. By means of a feedback mechanism, this effect is diminished at the same rate as acid secretion is inhibited.

Pantoprazole has the same effect whether administered orally or intravenously.

Table 1

Frequency Organ system	common (≥1% - <10%)	uncommon (≥0.1% - <1%)	Very rare (<0.01%)
Gastrointestinal Disorders	Upper abdominal pain; Diarrhoea; Constipation; Flatulence	Nausea	
General disorders and administration site conditions			Peripheral edema subsiding after termination of therapy
Hepatobiliary disorders			Severe hepatocellular damage leading to jaundice with or without hepatic failure
Immune system disorders			Anaphylactic reactions including anaphylactic shock
Investigations			Increased liver enzymes (transaminases, γ-GT); Elevated triglycerides; Increased body temperature subsiding after termination of therapy
Musculoskeletal, connective tissue disorders			Arthralgia, myalgia subsiding after termination of therapy
Nervous system disorders	Headache	Dizziness; Disturbances in vision (blurred vision)	
Psychiatric disorders			Mental depression subsiding after termination of therapy
Renal and urinary disorders			Interstitial nephritis
Skin and sub-cutaneous tissue disorders		Allergic reactions such as pruritus and skin rash	Urticaria; Angioedema; Severe skin reactions such as Stevens Johnson Syndrome, Erythema Multi-forme, Lyell-Syndrome; Photosensitivity

Following intravenous or oral administration, pantoprazole inhibits the pentagastrin-stimulated gastric acid secretion. In volunteers, acid secretion was inhibited by 56% following the first i.v. administration of 30 mg and by 99% after 5 days. With an oral dose of 40 mg, inhibition was 51% on day 1 and 85% on day 7. Basal 24-hour acidity was reduced by 37% and 98%, respectively.

The fasting gastrin values increased under pantoprazole but in most cases they did not exceed the normal upper limit. Following completion of a course of oral treatment, the median gastrin levels clearly declined again.

5.2 Pharmacokinetic properties

General Pharmacokinetics

Pantoprazole is rapidly absorbed and the maximal plasma concentration is achieved even after one single 40 mg oral dose. On average, the maximum serum concentrations are approximately 2-3 μg/ml about 2.5 hours post-administration and these values remain constant after multiple administration. Terminal half-life is about 1 hour. Volume of distribution is about 0.15 l/kg and clearance is about 0.1 l/h/kg. There were a few cases of subjects with delayed elimination. Because of the specific activation within the parietal cell, the elimination half-life does not correlate with the much longer duration of action (inhibition of acid secretion).

Pharmacokinetics does not vary after single or repeated administration. The plasma kinetics of pantoprazole are linear after both oral and intravenous administration.

Studies with pantoprazole in humans reveal no interaction with the cytochrome P450-system of the liver. There was no induction of the P450-system seen as tested after chronic administration with antipyrine as a marker. Also, no inhibition of metabolism was observed after concomitant administration of pantoprazole with either antipyrine, caffeine, carbamazepine, diazepam, diclofenac, digoxin, ethanol, glibenclamide, metoprolol, naproxen, nifedipine, phenprocoumon, phenytoin, piroxicam, theophylline and oral contraceptives. Concomitant administration of pantoprazole with warfarin has no influence on warfarin's effect on the coagulation factors.

The absolute bioavailability of the tablet is about 77%. Concomitant intake of food or antacids had no influence on AUC, maximum serum concentrations and thus bioavailability.

Pantoprazole's plasma protein binding is about 98%. The substance is almost exclusively metabolised in the liver. Renal elimination represents the major route of excretion (about 80%) for the metabolites of pantoprazole; the rest are excreted in the faeces. The main metabolite in both the plasma and urine is desmethylpantoprazole, which is conjugated with sulphate. The half-life of the main metabolites (about 1.5 hours) is not much longer than that of pantoprazole.

Characteristics in patients/special groups of subjects

Although for patients with hepatic cirrhosis (classes A and B according to *Child*) the half-time values increased to between 7 and 9 hours and the AUC values increased by a factor of 5 to 7, the maximum plasma concentration only increased slightly by a factor of 1.5 compared with healthy subjects. Therefore the dose regimen in patients with hepatic cirrhosis should be reduced to one tablet every other day.

No dose reduction is required when pantoprazole is administered to patients with impaired kidney function (including dialysis patients). As with healthy subjects, pantoprazole's half-life is short. Only very small amounts of pantoprazole are dialysed. Although the main metabolite has a moderately delayed half-life (2-3 hours), excretion is still rapid and thus accumulation does not occur.

A slight increase in AUC and Cmax in elderly volunteers compared with younger counterparts is also not clinically relevant.

5.3 Preclinical safety data

Acute toxicity

In acute toxicity studies in mice, the LD_{50} values were found to be 370 mg/kg bodyweight for i.v. administration and around 700 mg/kg bodyweight for oral administration.

In the rat, the corresponding values were around 240 mg/kg for i.v. administration and 900 mg/kg for oral administration.

Chronic toxicity

Hypergastrinaemia and morphologic changes of the mucosa were observed in studies investigating repeated administration for up to 12 months in the rat and dog. Most of the effects were reversible and attributable solely to the drug action, i.e. suppression of acid secretion.

In long-term studies in the rat and dog, there was an increase in stomach and liver weights; the increase being reversible after the substance was discontinued. The increase in liver weight following highly toxic doses was seen as a result of the induction of drug-metabolising enzymes.

Thyroid activation in two rat experiments is due to the rapid metabolism of thyroid hormones in the liver and has also been described in a similar form for other drugs. Changes in the thyroid and associated reduced degradation of cholesterol have been observed in one-year studies in the rat and dog. Hypertrophy of the thyroid and increases in cholesterol levels are reversible.

In studies in the dog, a species-species specific pulmonary oedema was observed. The animal-specific metabolite, which was responsible for the oedema, could not be identified in man.

Carcinogenicity

In a 2-year carcinogenicity study in rats - which corresponds to lifetime treatment for rats - ECL cell carcinoids were found. The mechanism leading to the formation of gastric carcinoids by substituted benzimidazoles has been carefully investigated and allows the conclusion that it is a secondary reaction to the massively elevated serum gastrin levels occurring in the rat during treatment. In addition, rats have more ECL cells in the mucosa of the glandular stomach than man, so that a larger number of responder cells for the increased gastrin values can become active.

ECL cell neoplasms were not observed in either the study in mice (24 months) or in long-term studies in the dog. In clinical studies (40 - 80 mg for 1 year), ECL cell density slightly increased.

In the two-year studies, an increased number of neoplastic changes of the liver was observed in rats and female mice and was interpreted as being due to pantoprazole's high rate of metabolism in the liver.

A slight increase of neoplastic changes of the thyroid was observed in the group of rats receiving the highest dose. The occurrence of these neoplasms is associated with the pantoprazole-induced changes in the breakdown of thyroxine in the rat liver. In man, no changes in the thyroid hormones T3, T4 and TSH were observed. This high dose phenomenon in the rat is therefore not relevant for man.

Mutagenicity

In mutagenicity studies, there were no indications of a mutagenic action *in vivo* or *in vitro.*

Reproduction toxicology

Investigations revealed no evidence of impaired fertility or teratogenic effects. Penetration of the placenta was investigated in the rat and was found to increase with advanced gestation. As a result, the concentration of pantoprazole in the foetus is increased shortly before birth, regardless of the route of administration.

In humans, there is no experience of the use of the drug during pregnancy.

6. PHARMACEUTICAL PARTICULARS

6.1 List of excipients

Crospovidone

Mannitol (=0.0036 BU)

Hypromellose

Methylacrylic acid-ethyl acrylate copolymer (1:1)

Sodium carbonate

Propylene glycol

Povidone K90

Calcium stearate

Triethyl citrate

Povidone K25

Titanium dioxide (E 171)

Polysorbate 80

Sodium lauril sulphate

Yellow iron oxide (E 172)

Printing ink

6.2 Incompatibilities

Not applicable.

6.3 Shelf life

Pantoprazole tablets are stable over a period of 3 years.

6.4 Special precautions for storage

Blister packaging: Do not store above 25°C

PE-bottle: Do not store above 30°C

6.5 Nature and contents of container

Protium® is distributed in PE-bottles or Alu/Alu blisters, packed in carton boxes.

Dose units: 7, 14, 28 gastro-resistant coated tablets

2 tablet starter pack

6.6 Instructions for use and handling

No special requirements.

7. MARKETING AUTHORISATION HOLDER

ALTANA Pharma AG

Byk Gulden Straße 2

D-78467 Konstanz

Germany

8. MARKETING AUTHORISATION NUMBER(S)

PL 20141/0002

9. DATE OF FIRST AUTHORISATION/RENEWAL OF THE AUTHORISATION

13 August 2003

10. DATE OF REVISION OF THE TEXT

November 2004

11. LEGAL STATUS

POM

Protium® is a registered trademark of ALTANA Pharma AG, Germany

Protopic 0.03% ointment

(Astellas Pharma Limited)

1. NAME OF THE MEDICINAL PRODUCT

Protopic®▼0.03% ointment

2. QUALITATIVE AND QUANTITATIVE COMPOSITION

1 g of Protopic 0.03% ointment contains 0.3 mg of tacrolimus as tacrolimus monohydrate (0.03%).

For excipients, see 6.1.

3. PHARMACEUTICAL FORM

Ointment

A white to slightly yellowish ointment.

4. CLINICAL PARTICULARS

4.1 Therapeutic indications

Treatment of moderate to severe atopic dermatitis in adults who are not adequately responsive to or are intolerant of conventional therapies. Treatment of moderate to severe atopic dermatitis in children (2 years of age and above) who failed to respond adequately to conventional therapies.

4.2 Posology and method of administration

Protopic should be prescribed by physicians with experience in the treatment of atopic dermatitis.

Protopic ointment should be applied as a thin layer to affected areas of the skin. Protopic ointment may be used on any part of the body, including face, neck and flexure areas, except on mucous membranes. Protopic ointment should not be applied under occlusion (see 4.4).

Each affected region of the skin should be treated with Protopic until clearance occurs and then treatment should be discontinued. Generally, improvement is seen within one week of starting treatment. If no signs of improvement are seen after two weeks of treatment, further treatment options should be considered. Protopic can be used for short term and intermittent long term treatment.

Use in children (2 years of age and above)

Treatment should be started twice a day for up to three weeks. Afterwards the frequency of application should be reduced to once a day until clearance of the lesion (see 4.4).

Use in adults (16 years of age and above)

Protopic is available in two strengths, Protopic 0.03% and Protopic 0.1% ointment. Treatment should be started with Protopic 0.1% twice a day and treatment should be continued until clearance of the lesion. If symptoms recur, twice daily treatment with Protopic 0.1% should be restarted. An attempt should be made to reduce the frequency of application or to use the lower strength Protopic 0.03% ointment if the clinical condition allows.

Use in elderly (65 years of age and above)

Specific studies have not been conducted in elderly patients. However, the clinical experience available in this patient population has not shown the necessity for any dosage adjustment.

As clinical efficacy studies were performed with abrupt cessation of treatment, no information is available on whether tapering of the dosage would reduce recurrence rate.

4.3 Contraindications

Hypersensitivity to macrolides in general, to tacrolimus or to any of the excipients.

4.4 Special warnings and special precautions for use

The effect of treatment with Protopic ointment on the developing immune system of children, especially the young, has not yet been established and this should be taken into account when prescribing to this age group (see 4.1).

The use of Protopic ointment has not been evaluated in children below the age of 2 years.

Exposure of the skin to sunlight should be minimised and the use of ultraviolet (UV) light from a solarium, therapy with UVB or UVA in combination with psoralens (PUVA) should be avoided during use of Protopic ointment (see 5.3). Physicians should advise patients on appropriate sun protection methods, such as minimisation of the time in the sun, use of a sunscreen product and covering of the skin with appropriate clothing.

Emollients should not be applied to the same area within 2 hours of applying Protopic ointment. Concomitant use of other topical preparations has not been assessed. There is no experience with concomitant use of systemic steroids or immunosuppressive agents.

Protopic ointment has not been evaluated for its efficacy and safety in the treatment of clinically infected atopic dermatitis. Before commencing treatment with Protopic ointment, clinical infections at treatment sites should be cleared. Patients with atopic dermatitis are predisposed to superficial skin infections. Treatment with Protopic may be associated with an increased risk of herpes viral infections (herpes simplex dermatitis [eczema herpeticum], herpes simplex [cold sores], Kaposi's varicelliform eruption). In the presence of these infections, the balance of risks and benefits associated with Protopic use should be evaluated.

Beyond 4 years of treatment, the potential for local immunosuppression (possibly resulting in infections or cutaneous malignancies) is unknown (see 5.1).

Lymphadenopathy was uncommonly (0.8%) reported in clinical trials. The majority of these cases related to infections (skin, respiratory tract, tooth) and resolved with appropriate antibiotic therapy. Transplant patients receiving immunosuppressive regimens (e.g. systemic tacrolimus) are at increased risk for developing lymphoma; therefore patients who receive Protopic and who develop lymphadenopathy should be monitored to ensure that the lymphadenopathy resolves. In case of persistent lymphadenopathy, the aetiology of the lymphadenopathy should be investigated. In the absence of a clear aetiology for the lymphadenopathy or in the presence of acute infectious mononucleosis, discontinuation of Protopic should be considered.

Care should be taken to avoid contact with eyes and mucous membranes. If accidentally applied to these areas, the ointment should be thoroughly wiped off and/or rinsed off with water.

The use of Protopic ointment under occlusion has not been studied in patients. Occlusive dressings are not recommended.

As with any topical medicinal product, patients should wash their hands after application if the hands are not intended for treatment.

Tacrolimus is extensively metabolised in the liver and although blood concentrations are low following topical therapy, the ointment should be used with caution in patients with hepatic failure (see 5.2).

The use of Protopic ointment in patients with genetic epidermal barrier defects such as Netherton's syndrome is not recommended due to the potential for permanently increased systemic absorption of tacrolimus. The safety of Protopic ointment has not been established in patients with generalised erythroderma.

4.5 Interaction with other medicinal products and other forms of Interaction

Formal topical drug interaction studies with tacrolimus ointment have not been conducted.

Tacrolimus is not metabolised in human skin, indicating that there is no potential for percutaneous interactions that could affect the metabolism of tacrolimus.

Systemically available tacrolimus is metabolised via the hepatic Cytochrome P450 3A4 (CYP3A4). Systemic exposure from topical application of tacrolimus ointment is low (< 1.0 ng/ml) and is unlikely to be affected by concomitant use of substances known to be inhibitors of CYP3A4. However, the possibility of interactions cannot be ruled out and the concomitant systemic administration of known CYP3A4 inhibitors (e.g. erythromycin, itraconazole, ketoconazole and diltiazem) in patients with widespread and/or erythrodermic disease should be done with caution.

A potential interaction between vaccination and application of Protopic ointment has not been investigated. Because of the potential risk of vaccination failure, vaccination should be administered prior to commencement of treatment, or during a treatment-free interval with a period of 14 days between the last application of Protopic and the vaccination. In case of live attenuated vaccination, this period should be extended to 28 days or the use of alternative vaccines should be considered.

4.6 Pregnancy and lactation

The use of tacrolimus ointment has not been studied in pregnant women. Studies in animals have shown reproductive toxicity following systemic administration (see 5.3).

Protopic ointment should not be used during pregnancy.

Human data demonstrate that, after systemic administration, tacrolimus is excreted into breast milk. Although clinical data have shown that systemic exposure from application of tacrolimus ointment is low, breast-feeding during treatment with Protopic ointment is not recommended.

4.7 Effects on ability to drive and use machines

No studies on the effects on the ability to drive or use machines have been performed. Protopic ointment is administered topically and is unlikely to have an effect on the ability to drive or use machines.

4.8 Undesirable effects

In clinical studies approximately 50% of patients experienced some type of skin irritation adverse reaction at the site of application. Burning sensation and pruritus were very common, usually mild to moderate in severity and tended to resolve within one week of starting treatment. Erythema was a common skin irritation adverse reaction. Sensation of warmth, pain, paraesthesia and rash at the site of application were also commonly observed. Alcohol intolerance (facial flushing or skin irritation after consumption of an alcoholic beverage) was common.

Patients may be at an increased risk of folliculitis, acne and herpes viral infections.

Adverse reactions with suspected relationship to treatment are listed below by system organ class. Frequencies are defined as very common (> 1/10), common (> 1/100, < 1/10) and uncommon (> 1/1,000, < 1/100).

General disorders and administration site conditions

Very common:	Application site burning, application site pruritus
Common:	Application site warmth, application site erythema, application site pain, application site irritation, application site paraesthesia, application site rash

Infections and infestations

Common:	Herpes viral infections (herpes simplex dermatitis [eczema herpeticum], herpes simplex [cold sores], Kaposi's varicelliform eruption)

Skin and subcutaneous tissue disorders

Common:	Folliculitits, pruritus
Uncommon:	Acne

Nervous system disorders

Common:	Paraesthesias and dysaesthesias (hyperaesthesia, burning sensation)

Metabolism and nutrition disorders

Common:	Alcohol intolerance (facial flushing or skin irritation after consumption of an alcoholic beverage)

The following adverse reactions have been reported during post-marketing experience:

Skin and subcutaneous tissue disorders: Rosacea

4.9 Overdose

Overdosage following topical administration is unlikely.

If ingested, general supportive measures may be appropriate. These may include monitoring of vital signs and observation of clinical status. Due to the nature of the ointment vehicle, induction of vomiting or gastric lavage is not recommended.

5. PHARMACOLOGICAL PROPERTIES

5.1 Pharmacodynamic properties

Pharmacotherapeutic group: Other dermatologicals, ATC code: D11AX14

Mechanism of action and pharmacodynamic effects

The mechanism of action of tacrolimus in atopic dermatitis is not fully understood. While the following have been observed, the clinical significance of these observations in atopic dermatitis is not known.

Via its binding to a specific cytoplasmic immunophilin (FKBP12), tacrolimus inhibits calcium-dependent signal transduction pathways in T cells, thereby preventing the transcription and synthesis of IL-2, IL-3, IL-4, IL-5 and other cytokines such as GM-CSF, TNF-α and IFN-γ.

In vitro, in Langerhans cells isolated from normal human skin, tacrolimus reduced the stimulatory activity towards T cells. Tacrolimus has also been shown to inhibit the release of inflammatory mediators from skin mast cells, basophils and eosinophils.

In animals, tacrolimus ointment suppressed inflammatory reactions in experimental and spontaneous dermatitis models that resemble human atopic dermatitis. Tacrolimus ointment did not reduce skin thickness and did not cause skin atrophy in animals.

In patients with atopic dermatitis, improvement of skin lesions during treatment with tacrolimus ointment was associated with reduced Fc receptor expression on Langerhans cells and a reduction of their hyperstimulatory activity towards T cells. Tacrolimus ointment does not affect collagen synthesis in humans.

Results from clinical studies in patients

The efficacy and safety of Protopic was assessed in more than 13,500 patients treated with tacrolimus ointment in Phase I to Phase III clinical trials. Data from four major trials are presented here.

In a six-month multicentre double-blind randomised trial, 0.1% tacrolimus ointment was administered twice-a-day to adults with moderate to severe atopic dermatitis and compared to a topical corticosteroid based regimen (0.1% hydrocortisone butyrate on trunk and extremities, 1% hydrocortisone acetate on face and neck). The primary endpoint was the response rate at month 3 defined as the proportion of patients with at least 60% improvement in the mEASI (modified Eczema Area and Severity Index) between baseline and month 3. The response rate in the 0.1% tacrolimus group (71.6%) was significantly higher than that in the topical corticosteroid based treatment group (50.8%; p<0.001; Table 1). The response rates at month 6 were comparable to the 3-month results.

Table 1 Efficacy at month 3

	Topical corticosteroid regimen§ (N=485)	Tacrolimus 0.1% (N=487)
Response rate of ⩾ 60% improvement in mEASI (Primary Endpoint)§§	50.8%	71.6%
Improvement ⩾ 90% in Physician's Global Evaluation	28.5%	47.7%

§ Topical corticosteroid regimen = 0.1% hydrocortisone butyrate on trunk and extremities, 1% hydrocortisone acetate on face and neck

§§ higher values = greater improvement

The incidence and nature of most adverse events were similar in the two treatment groups. Skin burning, herpes simplex, alcohol intolerance (facial flushing or skin sensitivity after alcohol intake), skin tingling, hyperaesthesia, acne and fungal dermatitis occurred more often in the tacrolimus treatment group. There were no clinically relevant changes in the laboratory values or vital signs in either treatment group throughout the study.

In the second trial, children aged from 2 to 15 years with moderate to severe atopic dermatitis received twice daily treatment for three weeks of 0.03% tacrolimus ointment, 0.1% tacrolimus ointment or 1% hydrocortisone acetate ointment. The primary endpoint was the area-under-the-curve (AUC) of the mEASI as a percentage of baseline averaged over the treatment period. The results of this multicentre, double-blind, randomised trial showed that tacrolimus ointment, 0.03% and 0.1%, is significantly more effective (p<0.001 for both) than 1% hydrocortisone acetate ointment (Table 2).

Table 2 Efficacy at week 3

(see Table 2 below)

The incidence of local skin burning was higher in the tacrolimus treatment groups than in the hydrocortisone group. Pruritus decreased over time in the tacrolimus groups but not in the hydrocortisone group. There were no clinically relevant changes in the laboratory values or vital signs in either treatment group throughout the clinical trial.

The purpose ofthe third multicentre, double-blind, randomised studywas the assessment of efficacy and safety of 0.03% tacrolimus ointment applied once or twice a day relative to twice daily administration of 1% hydrocortisone acetate ointment in children with moderate to severe atopic dermatitis. Treatment duration was for up to three weeks.

Table 3 Efficacy at week 3

(see Table 3 on next page)

The primary endpoint was defined as the percentage decrease in mEASI from the baseline to end of treatment. A statistically significant better improvement was shown for once daily and twice daily 0.03% tacrolimus ointment compared to twice daily hydrocortisone acetate ointment (p<0.001 for both). Twice daily treatment with 0.03% tacrolimus ointment was more effective than once daily administration (Table 3). The incidence of local skin burning was higher in the tacrolimus treatment groups than in the hydrocortisone group. There were no clinically relevant changes in the laboratory values or vital signs in either treatment group throughout the study.

In the fourth trial, approximately 800 patients (aged ⩾ 2 years) received 0.1% tacrolimus ointment intermittently or continuously in an open-label, long-term safety study for

Table 2 Efficacy at week 3

	Hydrocortisone acetate 1% (N=185)	Tacrolimus 0.03% (N=189)	Tacrolimus 0.1% (N=186)
Median mEASI as Percentage of Baseline mean AUC (Primary Endpoint)§	64.0%	44.8%	39.8%
Improvement ⩾90% in Physician's Global Evaluation	15.7%	38.5%	48.4%

§ lower values = greater improvement

Table 3 Efficacy at week 3

	Hydrocortisone acetate 1% Twice daily (N=207)	Tacrolimus 0.03% Once daily (N=207)	Tacrolimus 0.03% Twice daily (N=210)
Median mEASI Percentage Decrease (Primary Endpoint)§	47.2%	70.0%	78.7%
Improvement ⩾ 90% in Physician's Global Evaluation	13.6%	27.8%	36.7%

§ higher values = greater improvement

up to four years, with 300 patients receiving treatment for at least three years and 79 patients receiving treatment for a minimum of 42 months. Based on changes from baseline in EASI score and body surface area affected, patients regardless of age had improvement in their atopic dermatitis at all subsequent time points. In addition, there was no evidence of loss of efficacy throughout the duration of the clinical trial. The overall incidence of adverse events tended to decrease as the study progressed for all patients independent of age. The three most common adverse events reported were flu-like symptoms (cold, common cold, influenza, upper respiratory infection, etc.), pruritus and skin burning. No adverse events previously unreported in shorter duration and/or previous studies were observed in this long-term study.

5.2 Pharmacokinetic properties

Clinical data have shown that tacrolimus concentrations in systemic circulation after topical administration are low and, when measurable, transient.

Absorption

Data from healthy human subjects indicate that there is little or no systemic exposure to tacrolimus following single or repeated topical application of tacrolimus ointment.

Most atopic dermatitis patients (adults and children) treated with single or repeated application of tacrolimus ointment (0.03 - 0.3%) had blood concentrations < 1.0 ng/ml. When observed, blood concentrations exceeding 1.0 ng/ml were transient. Systemic exposure increases with increasing treatment areas. However, both the extent and the rate of topical absorption of tacrolimus decrease as the skin heals. In both adults and children with an average of 50% body surface area treated, systemic exposure (i.e. AUC) of tacrolimus from Protopic is approximately 30-fold less than that seen with oral immunosuppressive doses in kidney and liver transplant patients. The lowest tacrolimus blood concentration at which systemic effects can be observed is not known.

There was no evidence of systemic accumulation of tacrolimus in patients (adults and children) treated for prolonged periods (up to one year) with tacrolimus ointment.

Distribution

As systemic exposure is low with tacrolimus ointment, the high binding of tacrolimus (>98.8%) to plasma proteins is considered not to be clinically relevant.

Following topical application of tacrolimus ointment, tacrolimus is selectively delivered to the skin with minimal diffusion into the systemic circulation.

Metabolism

Metabolism of tacrolimus by human skin was not detectable. Systemically available tacrolimus is extensively metabolised in the liver via CYP3A4.

Elimination

When administered intravenously, tacrolimus has been shown to have a low clearance rate. The average total body clearance is approximately 2.25 l/h. The hepatic clearance of systemically available tacrolimus could be reduced in subjects with severe hepatic impairment, or in subjects who are co-treated with drugs that are potent inhibitors of CYP3A4.

Following repeated topical application of the ointment the average half-life of tacrolimus was estimated to be 75 hours for adults and 65 hours for children.

5.3 Preclinical safety data

Repeated dose toxicity and local tolerance

Repeated topical administration of tacrolimus ointment or the ointment vehicle to rats, rabbits and micropigs was associated with slight dermal changes such as erythema, oedema and papules.

Long-term topical treatment of rats with tacrolimus led to systemic toxicity including alterations of kidneys, pancreas, eyes and nervous system. The changes were caused by high systemic exposure of rodents resulting from high transdermal absorption of tacrolimus. Slightly lower body weight gain in females was the only systemic change observed in micropigs at high ointment concentrations (3%).

Rabbits were shown to be especially sensitive to intravenous administration of tacrolimus, reversible cardiotoxic effects being observed.

Mutagenicity

In vitro and *in vivo* tests did not indicate a genotoxic potential of tacrolimus.

Carcinogenicity

Systemic carcinogenicity studies in mice (18 months) and rats (24 months) revealed no carcinogenic potential of tacrolimus.

In a 24-month dermal carcinogenicity study performed in mice with 0.1% ointment, no skin tumours were observed. In the same study an increased incidence of lymphoma was detected in association with high systemic exposure.

In a photocarcinogenicity study, albino hairless mice were chronically treated with tacrolimus ointment and UV radiation. Animals treated with tacrolimus ointment showed a statistically significant reduction in time to skin tumour (squamous cell carcinoma) development and an increase in the number of tumours. It is unclear whether the effect of tacrolimus is due to systemic immunosuppression or a local effect. The relevance of these findings for man is unknown.

Reproduction toxicity

Embryo/foetal toxicity was observed in rats and rabbits, but only at doses that caused significant toxicity in maternal animals. Reduced sperm function was noted in male rats at high oral doses.

6. PHARMACEUTICAL PARTICULARS

6.1 List of excipients

White soft paraffin

Liquid paraffin

Propylene carbonate

White beeswax

Hard paraffin

6.2 Incompatibilities

Not applicable.

6.3 Shelf life

3 years

6.4 Special precautions for storage

Do not store above 25°C.

6.5 Nature and contents of container

Laminate tube with an inner lining of low-density-polyethylene fitted with a white polypropylene screw cap.

Package sizes: 10 g, 30 g and 60 g. Not all pack sizes may be marketed.

6.6 Instructions for use and handling

No special requirements.

7. MARKETING AUTHORISATION HOLDER

Astellas Pharma GmbH

Neumarkter Str. 61

D-81673 München

Germany

8. MARKETING AUTHORISATION NUMBER(S)

EU/1/02/201/001

EU/1/02/201/002

EU/1/02/201/005

9. DATE OF FIRST AUTHORISATION/RENEWAL OF THE AUTHORISATION

28.02.2002

10. DATE OF REVISION OF THE TEXT

09.09.2005

Protopic 0.1% ointment

(Astellas Pharma Limited)

1. NAME OF THE MEDICINAL PRODUCT

Protopic® ▼ 0.1% ointment

2. QUALITATIVE AND QUANTITATIVE COMPOSITION

1 g of Protopic 0.1% ointment contains 1.0 mg of tacrolimus as tacrolimus monohydrate (0.1%).

For excipients, see 6.1.

3. PHARMACEUTICAL FORM

Ointment

A white to slightly yellowish ointment.

4. CLINICAL PARTICULARS

4.1 Therapeutic indications

Treatment of moderate to severe atopic dermatitis in adults who are not adequately responsive to or are intolerant of conventional therapies.

4.2 Posology and method of administration

Protopic should be prescribed by physicians with experience in the treatment of atopic dermatitis.

Protopic ointment should be applied as a thin layer to affected areas of the skin. Protopic ointment may be used on any part of the body, including face, neck and flexure areas, except on mucous membranes. Protopic ointment should not be applied under occlusion (see 4.4).

Each affected region of the skin should be treated with Protopic until clearance occurs and then treatment should be discontinued. Generally, improvement is seen within one week of starting treatment. If no signs of improvement are seen after two weeks of treatment, further treatment options should be considered. Protopic can be used for short term and intermittent long term treatment.

Use in adults (16 years of age and above)

Protopic is available in two strengths, Protopic 0.03% and Protopic 0.1% ointment. Treatment should be started with Protopic 0.1% twice a day and treatment should be continued until clearance of the lesion. If symptoms recur, twice daily treatment with Protopic 0.1% should be restarted. An attempt should be made to reduce the frequency of application or to use the lower strength Protopic 0.03% ointment if the clinical condition allows.

Use in elderly (65 years of age and above)

Specific studies have not been conducted in elderly patients. However, the clinical experience available in this patient population has not shown the necessity for any dosage adjustment.

As clinical efficacy studies were performed with abrupt cessation of treatment, no information is available on whether tapering of the dosage would reduce recurrence rate.

4.3 Contraindications

Hypersensitivity to macrolides in general, to tacrolimus or to any of the excipients.

4.4 Special warnings and special precautions for use

The use of Protopic ointment has not been evaluated in children below the age of 2 years.

Exposure of the skin to sunlight should be minimised and the use of ultraviolet (UV) light from a solarium, therapy with UVB or UVA in combination with psoralens (PUVA) should be avoided during use of Protopic ointment (see 5.3). Physicians should advise patients on appropriate sun protection methods, such as minimisation of the time in the sun, use of a sunscreen product and covering of the skin with appropriate clothing.

Emollients should not be applied to the same area within 2 hours of applying Protopic ointment. Concomitant use of other topical preparations has not been assessed. There is no experience with concomitant use of systemic steroids or immunosuppressive agents.

Protopic ointment has not been evaluated for its efficacy and safety in the treatment of clinically infected atopic dermatitis. Before commencing treatment with Protopic ointment, clinical infections at treatment sites should be cleared. Patients with atopic dermatitis are predisposed to superficial skin infections. Treatment with Protopic may be associated with an increased risk of herpes viral infections (herpes simplex dermatitis [eczema herpeticum], herpes simplex [cold sores], Kaposi's varicelliform eruption). In the presence of these infections, the balance of risks and benefits associated with Protopic use should be evaluated.

Beyond 4 years of treatment, the potential for local immunosuppression (possibly resulting in infections or cutaneous malignancies) is unknown (see 5.1).

Lymphadenopathy was uncommonly (0.8%) reported in clinical trials. The majority of these cases related to infections (skin, respiratory tract, tooth) and resolved with appropriate antibiotic therapy. Transplant patients receiving immunosuppressive regimens (e.g. systemic tacrolimus) are at increased risk for developing lymphoma; therefore patients who receive Protopic and who develop lymphadenopathy should be monitored to ensure that the lymphadenopathy resolves. In case of persistent lymphadenopathy, the aetiology of the lymphadenopathy should be investigated. In the absence of a clear aetiology for the lymphadenopathy or in the presence of acute infectious mononucleosis, discontinuation of Protopic should be considered.

Care should be taken to avoid contact with eyes and mucous membranes. If accidentally applied to these areas, the ointment should be thoroughly wiped off and/or rinsed off with water.

The use of Protopic ointment under occlusion has not been studied in patients. Occlusive dressings are not recommended.

As with any topical medicinal product, patients should wash their hands after application if the hands are not intended for treatment.

Tacrolimus is extensively metabolised in the liver and although blood concentrations are low following topical therapy, the ointment should be used with caution in patients with hepatic failure (see 5.2).

The use of Protopic ointment in patients with genetic epidermal barrier defects such as Netherton's syndrome is not recommended due to the potential for permanently increased systemic absorption of tacrolimus. The safety of

Protopic ointment has not been established in patients with generalised erythroderma.

4.5 Interaction with other medicinal products and other forms of Interaction
Formal topical drug interaction studies with tacrolimus ointment have not been conducted.

Tacrolimus is not metabolised in human skin, indicating that there is no potential for percutaneous interactions that could affect the metabolism of tacrolimus.

Systemically available tacrolimus is metabolised via the hepatic Cytochrome P450 3A4 (CYP3A4). Systemic exposure from topical application of tacrolimus ointment is low (< 1.0 ng/ml) and is unlikely to be affected by concomitant use of substances known to be inhibitors of CYP3A4. However, the possibility of interactions cannot be ruled out and the concomitant systemic administration of known CYP3A4 inhibitors (e.g. erythromycin, itraconazole, ketoconazole and diltiazem) in patients with widespread and/or erythrodermic disease should be done with caution.

A potential interaction between vaccination and application of Protopic ointment has not been investigated. Because of the potential risk of vaccination failure, vaccination should be administered prior to commencement of treatment, or during a treatment-free interval with a period of 14 days between the last application of Protopic and the vaccination. In case of live attenuated vaccination, this period should be extended to 28 days or the use of alternative vaccines should be considered.

4.6 Pregnancy and lactation
The use of tacrolimus ointment has not been studied in pregnant women. Studies in animals have shown reproductive toxicity following systemic administration (see 5.3).

Protopic ointment should not be used during pregnancy.

Human data demonstrate that, after systemic administration, tacrolimus is excreted into breast milk. Although clinical data have shown that systemic exposure from application of tacrolimus ointment is low, breast-feeding during treatment with Protopic ointment is not recommended.

4.7 Effects on ability to drive and use machines
No studies on the effects on the ability to drive or use machines have been performed. Protopic ointment is administered topically and is unlikely to have an effect on the ability to drive or use machines.

4.8 Undesirable effects
In clinical studies approximately 50% of patients experienced some type of skin irritation adverse reaction at the site of application. Burning sensation and pruritus were very common, usually mild to moderate in severity and tended to resolve within one week of starting treatment. Erythema was a common skin irritation adverse reaction. Sensation of warmth, pain, paraesthesia and rash at the site of application were also commonly observed. Alcohol intolerance (facial flushing or skin irritation after consumption of an alcoholic beverage) was common.

Patients may be at an increased risk of folliculitis, acne and herpes viral infections.

Adverse reactions with suspected relationship to treatment are listed below by system organ class. Frequencies are defined as very common (>1/10), common (>1/100, <1/10) and uncommon (>1/1,000, <1/100).

General disorders and administration site conditions

Very common: Application site burning, application site pruritus

Common: Application site warmth, application site erythema, application site pain, application site irritation, application site paraesthesia, application site rash

Infections and infestations

Common: Herpes viral infections (herpes simplex dermatitis [eczema herpeticum], herpes simplex [cold sores], Kaposi's varicelliform eruption)

Skin and subcutaneous tissue disorders

Common: Folliculitis, pruritus

Uncommon: Acne

Nervous system disorders

Common: Paraesthesias and dysaesthesias (hyperaesthesia, burning sensation)

Metabolism and nutrition disorders

Common: Alcohol intolerance (facial flushing or skin irritation after consumption of an alcoholic beverage)

The following adverse reactions have been reported during post-marketing experience:

Skin and subcutaneous tissue disorders: Rosacea

4.9 Overdose
Overdosage following topical administration is unlikely.

If ingested, general supportive measures may be appropriate. These may include monitoring of vital signs and observation of clinical status. Due to the nature of the ointment vehicle, induction of vomiting or gastric lavage is not recommended.

5. PHARMACOLOGICAL PROPERTIES

5.1 Pharmacodynamic properties
Pharmacotherapeutic group: Other dermatologicals, ATC code: D11AX14

Mechanism of action and pharmacodynamic effects

The mechanism of action of tacrolimus in atopic dermatitis is not fully understood. While the following have been observed, the clinical significance of these observations in atopic dermatitis is not known.

Via its binding to a specific cytoplasmic immunophilin (FKBP12), tacrolimus inhibits calcium-dependent signal transduction pathways in T cells, thereby preventing the transcription and synthesis of IL-2, IL-3, IL-4, IL-5 and other cytokines such as GM-CSF, TNF-α and IFN-γ.

In vitro, in Langerhans cells isolated from normal human skin, tacrolimus reduced the stimulatory activity towards T cells. Tacrolimus has also been shown to inhibit the release of inflammatory mediators from skin mast cells, basophils and eosinophils.

In animals, tacrolimus ointment suppressed inflammatory reactions in experimental and spontaneous dermatitis models that resemble human atopic dermatitis. Tacrolimus ointment did not reduce skin thickness and did not cause skin atrophy in animals.

In patients with atopic dermatitis, improvement of skin lesions during treatment with tacrolimus ointment was associated with reduced Fc receptor expression on Langerhans cells and a reduction of their hyperstimulatory activity towards T cells. Tacrolimus ointment does not affect collagen synthesis in humans.

Results from clinical studies in patients

The efficacy and safety of Protopic was assessed in more than 13,500 patients treated with tacrolimus ointment in Phase I to Phase III clinical trials. Data from four major trials are presented here.

In a six-month multicentre double-blind randomised trial, 0.1% tacrolimus ointment was administered twice-a-day to adults with moderate to severe atopic dermatitis and compared to a topical corticosteroid based regimen (0.1% hydrocortisone butyrate on trunk and extremities, 1% hydrocortisone acetate on face and neck). The primary endpoint was the response rate at month 3 defined as the proportion of patients with at least 60% improvement in the mEASI (modified Eczema Area and Severity Index) between baseline and month 3. The response rate in the 0.1% tacrolimus group (71.6%) was significantly higher than that in the topical corticosteroid based treatment group (50.8%; p<0.001; Table 1). The response rates at month 6 were comparable to the 3-month results.

Table 1 Efficacy at month 3

	Topical corticosteroid regimen§ (N=485)	Tacrolimus 0.1% (N=487)
Response rate of ⩾ 60% improvement in mEASI (Primary Endpoint)§§	50.8%	71.6%
Improvement ⩾ 90% in Physician's Global Evaluation	28.5%	47.7%

§ Topical corticosteroid regimen = 0.1% hydrocortisone butyrate on trunk and extremities, 1% hydrocortisone acetate on face and neck

§§ higher values = greater improvement

The incidence and nature of most adverse events were similar in the two treatment groups. Skin burning, herpes simplex, alcohol intolerance (facial flushing or skin sensitivity after alcohol intake), skin tingling, hyperaesthesia, acne and fungal dermatitis occurred more often in the tacrolimus treatment group. There were no clinically relevant changes in the laboratory values or vital signs in either treatment group throughout the study.

In the second trial, children aged from 2 to 15 years with moderate to severe atopic dermatitis received twice daily treatment for three weeks of 0.03% tacrolimus ointment, 0.1% tacrolimus ointment or 1% hydrocortisone acetate ointment. The primary endpoint was the area-under-the-curve (AUC) of the mEASI as a percentage of baseline averaged over the treatment period. The results of this multicentre, double-blind, randomised trial showed that tacrolimus ointment, 0.03% and 0.1%, is significantly more effective (p<0.001 for both) than 1% hydrocortisone acetate ointment (Table 2).

Table 2 Efficacy at week 3

(see Table 2 below)

The incidence of local skin burning was higher in the tacrolimus treatment groups than in the hydrocortisone group. Pruritus decreased over time in the tacrolimus groups but not in the hydrocortisone group. There were no clinically relevant changes in the laboratory values or vital signs in either treatment group throughout the clinical trial.

The purpose of the third multicentre, double-blind, randomised study was the assessment of efficacy and safety of 0.03% tacrolimus ointment applied once or twice a day relative to twice daily administration of 1% hydrocortisone acetate ointment in children with moderate to severe atopic dermatitis. Treatment duration was for up to three weeks.

Table 3 Efficacy at week 3

(see Table 3 below)

The primary endpoint was defined as the percentage decrease in mEASI from the baseline to end of treatment. A statistically significant better improvement was shown for once daily and twice daily 0.03% tacrolimus ointment compared to with twice daily hydrocortisone acetate ointment (p<0.001 for both). Twice daily treatment with 0.03% tacrolimus ointment was more effective than once daily administration (Table 3). The incidence of local skin burning was higher in the tacrolimus treatment groups than in the hydrocortisone group. There were no clinically relevant changes in the laboratory values or vital signs in either treatment group throughout the study.

In the fourth trial, approximately 800 patients (aged ⩾ 2 years) received 0.1% tacrolimus ointment intermittently or continuously in an open-label, long-term safety study for up to four years, with 300 patients receiving treatment for at least three years and 79 patients receiving treatment for a minimum of 42 months. Based on changes from baseline in EASI score and body surface area affected, patients regardless of age had improvement in their atopic dermatitis at all subsequent time points. In addition, there was no evidence of loss of efficacy throughout the duration of the clinical trial. The overall incidence of adverse events tended to decrease as the study progressed for all patients independent of age. The three most common adverse events reported were flu-like symptoms (cold, common cold, influenza, upper respiratory infection, etc.), pruritus and skin burning. No adverse events previously unreported in shorter duration and/or previous studies were observed in this long-term study.

5.2 Pharmacokinetic properties
Clinical data have shown that tacrolimus concentrations in systemic circulation after topical administration are low and, when measurable, transient.

Table 2 Efficacy at week 3

	Hydrocortisone acetate 1% (N=185)	Tacrolimus 0.03% (N=189)	Tacrolimus 0.1% (N=186)
Median mEASI as Percentage of baseline mean AUC (Primary Endpoint)§	64.0%	44.8%	39.8%
Improvement ⩾ 90% in Physician's Global Evaluation	15.7%	38.5%	48.4%

§ lower values = greater improvement

Table 3 Efficacy at week 3

	Hydrocortisone acetate 1% Twice daily (N=207)	Tacrolimus 0.03% Once daily (N=207)	Tacrolimus 0.03% Twice daily (N=210)
Median mEASI Percentage Decrease (Primary Endpoint)§	47.2%	70.0%	78.7%
Improvement ⩾ 90% in Physician's Global Evaluation	13.6%	27.8%	36.7%

§ higher values = greater improvement

Absorption

Data from healthy human subjects indicate that there is little or no systemic exposure to tacrolimus following single or repeated topical application of tacrolimus ointment.

Most atopic dermatitis patients (adults and children) treated with single or repeated application of tacrolimus ointment (0.03 - 0.3%) had blood concentrations < 1.0 ng/ml. When observed, blood concentrations exceeding 1.0 ng/ml were transient. Systemic exposure increases with increasing treatment areas. However, both the extent and the rate of topical absorption of tacrolimus decrease as the skin heals. In both adults and children with an average of 50% body surface area treated, systemic exposure (i.e. AUC) of tacrolimus from Protopic is approximately 30-fold less than that seen with oral immunosuppressive doses in kidney and liver transplant patients. The lowest tacrolimus blood concentration at which systemic effects can be observed is not known.

There was no evidence of systemic accumulation of tacrolimus in patients (adults and children) treated for prolonged periods (up to one year) with tacrolimus ointment.

Distribution

As systemic exposure is low with tacrolimus ointment, the high binding of tacrolimus (>98.8%) to plasma proteins is considered not to be clinically relevant.

Following topical application of tacrolimus ointment, tacrolimus is selectively delivered to the skin with minimal diffusion into the systemic circulation.

Metabolism

Metabolism of tacrolimus by human skin was not detectable. Systemically available tacrolimus is extensively metabolised in the liver via CYP3A4.

Elimination

When administered intravenously, tacrolimus has been shown to have a low clearance rate. The average total body clearance is approximately 2.25 l/h. The hepatic clearance of systemically available tacrolimus could be reduced in subjects with severe hepatic impairment, or in subjects who are co-treated with drugs that are potent inhibitors of CYP3A4.

Following repeated topical application of the ointment the average half-life of tacrolimus was estimated to be 75 hours for adults and 65 hours for children.

5.3 Preclinical safety data

Repeated dose toxicity and local tolerance

Repeated topical administration of tacrolimus ointment or the ointment vehicle to rats, rabbits and micropigs was associated with slight dermal changes such as erythema, oedema and papules.

Long-term topical treatment of rats with tacrolimus led to systemic toxicity including alterations of kidneys, pancreas, eyes and nervous system. The changes were caused by high systemic exposure of rodents resulting from high transdermal absorption of tacrolimus. Slightly lower body weight gain in females was the only systemic change observed in micropigs at high ointment concentrations (3%).

Rabbits were shown to be especially sensitive to intravenous administration of tacrolimus, reversible cardiotoxic effects being observed.

Mutagenicity

In vitro and *in vivo* tests did not indicate a genotoxic potential of tacrolimus.

Carcinogenicity

Systemic carcinogenicity studies in mice (18 months) and rats (24 months) revealed no carcinogenic potential of tacrolimus.

In a 24-month dermal carcinogenicity study performed in mice with 0.1% ointment, no skin tumours were observed. In the same study an increased incidence of lymphoma was detected in association with high systemic exposure.

In a photocarcinogenicity study, albino hairless mice were chronically treated with tacrolimus ointment and UV radiation. Animals treated with tacrolimus ointment showed a statistically significant reduction in time to skin tumour (squamous cell carcinoma) development and an increase in the number of tumours. It is unclear whether the effect of tacrolimus is due to systemic immunosuppression or a local effect. The relevance of these findings for man is unknown.

Reproduction toxicity

Embryo/foetal toxicity was observed in rats and rabbits, but only at doses that caused significant toxicity in maternal animals. Reduced sperm function was noted in male rats at high oral doses.

6. PHARMACEUTICAL PARTICULARS

6.1 List of excipients

White soft paraffin

Liquid paraffin

Propylene carbonate

White beeswax

Hard paraffin

6.2 Incompatibilities

Not applicable.

6.3 Shelf life

3 years

6.4 Special precautions for storage

Do not store above 25°C.

6.5 Nature and contents of container

Laminate tube with an inner lining of low-density-polyethylene fitted with a white polypropylene screw cap.

Package sizes: 10 g, 30 g and 60 g. Not all pack sizes may be marketed.

6.6 Instructions for use and handling

No special requirements.

7. MARKETING AUTHORISATION HOLDER

Astellas Pharma GmbH

Neumarkter Str. 61

D-81673 München

Germany

8. MARKETING AUTHORISATION NUMBER(S)

EU/1/02/201/003

EU/1/02/201/004

EU/1/02/201/006

9. DATE OF FIRST AUTHORISATION/RENEWAL OF THE AUTHORISATION

28.02.2002

10. DATE OF REVISION OF THE TEXT

09.09.2005

Provera Tablets 10 mg

(Pharmacia Limited)

1. NAME OF THE MEDICINAL PRODUCT

Provera Tablets 10 mg

2. QUALITATIVE AND QUANTITATIVE COMPOSITION

Each tablet contains 10 mg medroxyprogesterone acetate Ph. Eur.

3. PHARMACEUTICAL FORM

Tablets for oral use

4. CLINICAL PARTICULARS

4.1 Therapeutic indications

Progestogen. Indicated for dysfunctional (anovulatory) uterine bleeding, secondary amenorrhoea and for mild to moderate endometriosis.

4.2 Posology and method of administration

Oral.

Adults:

Dysfunctional (anovulatory) uterine bleeding: 2.5-10 mg daily for 5-10 days commencing on the assumed or calculated 16th-21st day of the cycle. Treatment should be given for two consecutive cycles. When bleeding occurs from a poorly developed proliferative endometrium, conventional oestrogen therapy may be employed in conjunction with medroxyprogesterone acetate in doses of 5-10 mg for 10 days.

Secondary amenorrhoea: 2.5-10 mg daily for 5-10 days beginning on the assumed or calculated 16th to 21st day of the cycle. Repeat the treatment for three consecutive cycles. In amenorrhoea associated with a poorly developed proliferative endometrium, conventional oestrogen therapy may be employed in conjunction with medroxyprogesterone acetate in doses of 5-10 mg for 10 days.

Mild to moderate endometriosis: Beginning on the first day of the menstrual cycle, 10 mg three times a day for 90 consecutive days. Breakthrough bleeding, which is self-limiting, may occur. No additional hormonal therapy is recommended for the management of this bleeding.

Elderly: Not applicable

Children: not applicable

4.3 Contraindications

Use in patients with a known sensitivity to medroxyprogesterone acetate.

Use in patients with impaired liver function or with active liver disease.

Before using Provera, the general medical condition of the patient should be carefully evaluated. This evaluation should exclude the presence of genital or breast neoplasia before considering the use of Provera.

4.4 Special warnings and special precautions for use

Whether administered alone or in conjunction with oestrogens, Provera should not be employed in patients with abnormal uterine bleeding until a definite diagnosis has been established and the possibility of genital malignancy eliminated.

Rare cases of thrombo-embolism have been reported with use of Provera, especially at higher doses. Causality has not been established.

Doses of up to 30 mg a day may not suppress ovulation and patients should be advised to take adequate contraceptive measures, where appropriate.

Provera, especially in high doses, may cause weight gain and fluid retention. With this in mind, caution should be exercised in treating any patient with a pre-existing medical condition, such as epilepsy, migraine, asthma, cardiac or renal dysfunction, that might be adversely affected by weight gain or fluid retention.

Some patients receiving Provera may exhibit a decreased glucose tolerance. The mechanism for this is not known. This fact should be borne in mind when treating all patients and especially known diabetics.

Patients with a history of treatment for mental depression should be carefully monitored while receiving Provera therapy. Some patients may complain of premenstrual like depression while on Provera therapy.

4.5 Interaction with other medicinal products and other forms of Interaction

Aminoglutethimide administered concurrently with Provera may significantly depress the bioavailability of Provera.

Interactions with other medicinal treatments (including oral anti-coagulants) have rarely been reported, but causality has not been determined. The possibility of interaction should be borne in mind in patients receiving concurrent treatment with other drugs.

4.6 Pregnancy and lactation

A negative pregnancy test should be demonstrated before starting therapy. Medroxyprogesterone acetate and its metabolites are secreted in breast milk, but there is no evidence to suggest that this presents any hazard to the child.

4.7 Effects on ability to drive and use machines

No adverse effect has been reported.

4.8 Undesirable effects

The following medical events, listed in order of seriousness rather than frequency of occurrence, have been occasionally to rarely associated with the use of progestogens:

Rare anaphylactoid-like reactions.

Psychic: nervousness, insomnia, somnolence, fatigue, depression, dizziness and headache.

Skin and mucous membranes: urticaria, pruritus, rash, acne, hirsutism and alopecia.

Gastro-intestinal: nausea.

Breast: tenderness and galactorrhoea.

Miscellaneous: change in weight.

4.9 Overdose

In animals Provera has been shown to be capable of exerting an adreno-corticoid effect, but this has not been reported in the human, following usual dosages. The oral administration of Provera at a rate of 100 mg per day has been shown to have no effect on adrenal function.

5. PHARMACOLOGICAL PROPERTIES

5.1 Pharmacodynamic properties

Medroxyprogesterone acetate has actions and uses similar to those of progesterone.

MPA has minimal androgenic activity compared to progesterone and virtually no oestrogenic activity.

Progestogens are used in the treatment of dysfunctional uterine bleeding, secondary amenorrhoea and endometriosis.

5.2 Pharmacokinetic properties

MPA is rapidly absorbed from the G-I tract with a single oral dose of 10-250 mg. The time taken to reach the peak serum concentration (T_{max}) was 2-6 hours and the average peak serum concentration (C_{max}) was 13-46.89 mg/ml.

Unmetabolised MPA is highly plasma protein bound. MPA is metabolised in the liver.

6. PHARMACEUTICAL PARTICULARS

6.1 List of excipients

Lactose

Sucrose

Maize Starch

Liquid Paraffin

Talc

Calcium Stearate

6.2 Incompatibilities

None known.

6.3 Shelf life

Five years.

6.4 Special precautions for storage

Glass bottles: None.

Blister packs: Store below 25°C

6.5 Nature and contents of container

HDPE tamper-evident bottles with LDPE push-fit tamper evident caps, containing 50 tablets.

Aluminium foil/PVC blisters, containing 10, 20, 30, 50, 90 or 100 tablets.

6.6 Instructions for use and handling

None.

7. MARKETING AUTHORISATION HOLDER
Pharmacia Limited
Davy Avenue
Milton Keynes
MK5 8PH
UK

8. MARKETING AUTHORISATION NUMBER(S)
PL 0032/0151

9. DATE OF FIRST AUTHORISATION/RENEWAL OF THE AUTHORISATION
8 January 1996

10. DATE OF REVISION OF THE TEXT
March 2000
August 2001

Legal Category
POM.

Provera Tablets 100 mg

(Pharmacia Limited)

1. NAME OF THE MEDICINAL PRODUCT
Provera Tablets 100 mg or Medroxyprogesterone Acetate Tablets 100 mg.

2. QUALITATIVE AND QUANTITATIVE COMPOSITION
1 tablet contains 100 mg medroxyprogesterone acetate.

For excipients, see 6.1.

3. PHARMACEUTICAL FORM
Tablet

4. CLINICAL PARTICULARS

4.1 Therapeutic indications
Progestogen indicated for the treatment of certain hormone dependent neoplasms, such as:

1. Endometrial carcinoma
2. Renal cell carcinoma
3. Carcinoma of the breast in post menopausal women.

4.2 Posology and method of administration
Route of administration: Oral

Adults

Endometrial and renal cell carcinoma 200-600 mg daily.

Breast carcinoma 400-1500 mg per day.

The incidence of minor side-effects, such as indigestion and weight gain, increase with increase in dose.

Response to hormonal therapy may not be evident until after at least 8-10 weeks of therapy.

Elderly patients

This product has been used primarily in the older age group for the treatment of malignancies. There is no evidence to suggest that the older age group is any less prepared to handle the drug metabolically than is the younger patient. Therefore the same dosage, contra-indications, and precautions would apply to either age group.

Children

The product is not anticipated for paediatric use in the indications recommended.

4.3 Contraindications
Medroxyprogesterone acetate is contraindicated in the following conditions:

- thrombophlebitis, thrombo-embolic disorders, and where there is a high risk of developing such manifestations [presence or history of atrial fibrillation, valvular disorders, endocarditis, heart failure, pulmonary embolism; thrombo-embolic ischaemic attack (TIA), cerebral infarction; atherosclerosis; immediate post surgery period]
- hypercalcaemia in patients with osseous metastases
- known sensitivity to medroxyprogesterone acetate or any component of the drug.
- impaired liver function, or with active liver disease.
- missed abortion, metrorrhagia, known or suspected pregnancy.
- undiagnosed vaginal bleeding.
- previous idiopathic or current venous thromboembolism (deep vein thrombosis, pulmonary embolism).
- active or recent arterial thromboembolic disease (e.g. angina, myocardial infarction).
- suspected or early breast carcinoma

Progestogens are known to be porphyrogenic. Patients with a history of attacks or aged under 30 are at greatest risk of an acute attack while on progesterone treatment. A careful assessment of potential benefit should be made where this risk is present.

4.4 Special warnings and special precautions for use
Warnings

In the treatment of carcinoma of breast occasional cases of hypercalcaemia have been reported.

Unexpected vaginal bleeding during therapy with medroxyprogesterone acetate should be investigated.

Medication should not be readministered pending examination if there is sudden partial or complete loss of vision or if there is a sudden onset of proptosis, diplopia or migraine. If examination reveals papilloedema or retinal vascular lesions, medication should not be readministered.

Medroxyprogesterone acetate may produce Cushingoid symptoms.

Some patients receiving medroxyprogesterone acetate may exhibit suppressed adrenal function. Medroxyprogesterone acetate may decrease ACTH and hydrocortisone blood levels.

Treatment with medroxyprogesterone acetate should be discontinued in the event of:

- jaundice or deterioration in liver function
- significant increase in blood pressure
- new onset of migraine-type headache

Precautions

Before using Provera the general medical condition of the patient should be carefully evaluated.

This product should be used under the supervision of a specialist and the patients kept under regular surveillance.

Animal studies have shown that Provera possesses adrenocorticoid activity. This has also been reported in man, therefore patients receiving large doses continuously and for long periods should be observed closely for signs normally associated with adrenocorticoid therapy, such as hypertension, sodium retention, oedema, etc. Care is needed in treating patients with diabetes and/or arterial hypertension.

Patients with the following conditions should be carefully monitored while taking progestogens:

- Conditions which may be influenced by potential fluid retention
  - o Epilepsy
  - o Migraine
  - o Asthma
  - o Cardiac dysfunction
  - o Renal dysfunction
- History of mental depression
- Diabetes (a decrease in glucose tolerance has been observed in some patients)
- Hyperlipidaemia.

The pathologist (laboratory) should be informed of the patient's use of medroxyprogesterone acetate if endometrial or endocervical tissue is submitted for examination.

The physician/laboratory should be informed that medroxyprogesterone acetate may decrease the levels of the following endocrine biomarkers:

- Plasma/urinary steroids (e.g., cortisol, oestrogen, pregnanediol, progesterone, testosterone)
- Plasma/urinary gonadotrophins (e.g., LH and FSH)
- Sex-hormone-binding-globulin

The use of medroxyprogesterone acetate in oncology indications may also cause partial adrenal insufficiency (decrease in pituitary-adrenal axis response) during Metyrapone testing. Thus the ability of adrenal cortex to respond to ACTH should be demonstrated before metyrapone is administered.

Although medroxyprogesterone acetate has not been causally associated with the induction of thromboembolic disorders, any patient with a history or who develops this kind of event while undergoing therapy with medroxyprogesterone acetate should have her status and need for treatment carefully assessed before continuing therapy.

Risk of venous thromboembolism (VTE)
The risk of VTE has not been assessed for progesterone alone. However, VTE is a known risk factor of oestrogen-only and combined hormone replacement therapy. When prescribing medroxyprogesterone acetate for oncology indications the following precautions and risk factors should be considered in the light of the patient's condition, the dose of medroxyprogesterone acetate and the duration of therapy:

- Generally recognised risk factors for VTE include a personal or family history of VTE or known thromboembolic states, severe obesity (BMI> 30 kg/m^2) and systemic lupus erythematosus
- The risk of VTE may be temporarily increased with prolonged immobilisation, major trauma or major surgery.
- If VTE develops after initiating therapy, medroxyprogesterone acetate should be discontinued. Patients should be told to contact their doctor immediately if they become aware of a symptom suggestive of potential thromboembolism (e.g. painful swelling of a leg, sudden pain in the chest, dyspnoea)

4.5 Interaction with other medicinal products and other forms of Interaction
Interaction with other medicaments

The metabolism of progestogens may be increased by concomitant administration of compounds known to induce drug-metabolising enzymes, specifically cytochrome P450 enzymes. These compounds include anticonvulsants (e.g., phenobarbital, phenytoin, carbamezapine) and anti-infectives (e.g., rifampicin, rifabutin, nevirapine, efavirenz,).

Ritonavir and nelfinavir, although known as strong inhibitors, by contrast exhibit inducing properties when used concomitantly with steroid hormones. Herbal preparations containing St John's Wort (Hypericum Perforatum) may induce the metabolism of progestogens. Progestogen levels may therefore be reduced.

Aminoglutethimide has been reported to decrease plasma levels of some progestogens.

Concurrent administration of cyclosporin and MPA has been reported to lead to increased plasma cyclosporin levels and/or decreased plasma MPA levels.

Interactions with oral anti-coagulants have been reported rarely, but causality has not been established.

When used in combination with cytotoxic drugs, it is possible that progestogens may reduce the haematological toxicity of chemotherapy.

Special care should be taken when progestogens are administered with other drugs which also cause fluid retention, such as NSAIDs and vasodilators.

Other forms of interaction

Progestogens can influence certain laboratory tests (e.g., tests for hepatic function, thyroid function and coagulation).

4.6 Pregnancy and lactation
Pregnancy
Medroxyprogesterone acetate is contraindicated in women who are pregnant. If medroxyprogesterone acetate is used during pregnancy, or if the patient becomes pregnant while using this drug, the patient should be apprised of the potential hazard to the foetus.

Some reports suggest an association between intrauterine exposure to progestational drugs in the first trimester of pregnancy and genital abnormalities in male and female foetuses.

Infants from unintentional pregnancies that occur 1 to 2 months after injection of medroxyprogesterone acetate injectable suspension may be at an increased risk of low birth weight, which, in turn, is associated with an increased risk of neonatal death. The attributable risk is low because pregnancies while on medroxyprogesterone acetate are uncommon.

Lactation
Medroxyprogesterone acetate and/or its metabolites are secreted in breast milk. Therefore, the use of Provera whilst breast-feeding is not recommended.

4.7 Effects on ability to drive and use machines
No adverse effect has been reported.

4.8 Undesirable effects
Reactions occasionally associated with the use of progestogens, particularly in high doses, are:

Breast: Tenderness, mastodynia or galactorrhoea.

Genitourinary: Abnormal uterine bleeding (irregular, increase, decrease), amenorrhoea, alterations of cervical secretions, cervical erosions, prolonged anovulation.

Central nervous system: Confusion, euphoria, loss of concentration, nervousness, insomnia, somnolence, fatigue, dizziness, depression, vision disorders and headache.

Skin and mucous membranes: sensitivity reactions ranging from pruritus, urticaria, angioneurotic oedema to generalised rash and anaphylaxis have been occasionally reported. Acne and alopecia or hirsutism have been reported in a few cases.

Allergy: Hypersensitivity reactions (e.g., anaphylaxis or anaphylactoid reactions, angioedema).

Gastro-intestinal/hepatobiliary: Constipation, diarrhoea, dry mouth, disturbed liver function, jaundice, vomiting, nausea and indigestion.

Metabolic and nutritional: Adrenergic-like effects (e.g., fine hand tremors, sweating, tremors, cramps in calves at night), corticoid-like effects (e.g., Cushingoid Syndrome), decreased glucose tolerance, diabetic cataract, exacerbation of diabetes mellitus, glycosuria.

Cardiovascular: cerebral and myocardial infarction, congestive heart failure, increased blood pressure, palpitations, pulmonary embolism, retinal thrombosis, tachycardia, thromboembolic disorders, thrombophlebitis,

Haematological: elevation of white blood cells and platelet count.

Miscellaneous: Change in appetite, changes in libido, oedema/fluid retention, hypercalcaemia, malaise, hyperpyrexia, weight gain, moon facies.

4.9 Overdose
No action required other than cessation of therapy.

5. PHARMACOLOGICAL PROPERTIES

5.1 Pharmacodynamic properties
Pharmacotherapeutic group: Progestogens. ATC Code: L02A B.

Medroxyprogesterone acetate has the pharmacological action of a progestogen.

5.2 Pharmacokinetic properties
Medroxyprogesterone acetate is absorbed from the gastro intestinal tract with a single oral dose of 10-250 mg. The

time taken to reach the peak serum concentration (T_{max}) was 2-6 hours and the average peak serum concentration (C_{max}) was 13-46.89 mg/ml.

Unmetabolised medroxyprogesterone acetate is highly plasma protein bound. Medroxyprogesterone acetate is metabolised in the liver.

Medroxyprogesterone acetate is primarily metabolised by faecal excretion as glucuronide conjugated metabolite.

Metabolised medroxyprogesterone acetate is excreted more rapidly and in a greater percentage following oral doses than after aqueous intramuscular injection

5.3 Preclinical safety data
No further preclinical safety data are available.

6. PHARMACEUTICAL PARTICULARS
6.1 List of excipients
Microcrystalline cellulose

Maize starch

Gelatin (Byco C)

Macrogol 400

Sodium starch glycollate

Docusate sodium

Sodium benzoate

Magnesium stearate

Isopropyl alcohol

Purified water

6.2 Incompatibilities
Not applicable.

6.3 Shelf life
36 months if stored in glass/HDPE bottles, or 24 month in blister packs.

6.4 Special precautions for storage
Store below 25°C.

Bottle packs only: keep in a well closed container.

6.5 Nature and contents of container
Amber glass bottle with screw cap containing 100 tablets.

HDPE bottle with tamper evident cap containing 100 tablets.

PVC/aluminium strip containing 30, 60 or 100 tablets.

6.6 Instructions for use and handling
None.

7. MARKETING AUTHORISATION HOLDER
Pharmacia Limited

Davy Avenue

Milton Keynes

MK5 8PH

UK

8. MARKETING AUTHORISATION NUMBER(S)
PL 0032/0111

9. DATE OF FIRST AUTHORISATION/RENEWAL OF THE AUTHORISATION
7 November 1983/30 January 1996

10. DATE OF REVISION OF THE TEXT
June 2004

Company Ref: PV 1_0

Provera Tablets 2.5 mg

(Pharmacia Limited)

1. NAME OF THE MEDICINAL PRODUCT
Provera Tablets 2.5 mg

2. QUALITATIVE AND QUANTITATIVE COMPOSITION
Each tablet contains 2.5 mg medroxyprogesterone acetate Ph. Eur.

3. PHARMACEUTICAL FORM
Tablets for oral use

4. CLINICAL PARTICULARS
4.1 Therapeutic indications
Progestogen. Indicated for dysfunctional (anovulatory) uterine bleeding, secondary amenorrhoea and for mild to moderate endometriosis.

4.2 Posology and method of administration
Oral.

Adults:

Dysfunctional (anovulatory) uterine bleeding: 2.5-10 mg daily for 5-10 days commencing on the assumed or calculated 16th-21st day of the cycle. Treatment should be given for two consecutive cycles. When bleeding occurs from a poorly developed proliferative endometrium, conventional oestrogen therapy may be employed in conjunction with medroxyprogesterone acetate in doses of 5-10 mg for 10 days.

Secondary amenorrhoea: 2.5-10 mg daily for 5-10 days beginning on the assumed or calculated 16th to 21st day of the cycle. Repeat the treatment for three consecutive cycles. In amenorrhoea associated with a poorly developed proliferative endometrium, conventional oestrogen therapy may be employed in conjunction with medroxyprogesterone acetate in doses of 5-10 mg for 10 days.

Mild to moderate endometriosis: Beginning on the first day of the menstrual cycle, 10 mg three times a day for 90 consecutive days.

Elderly: Not applicable

Children: Not applicable

4.3 Contraindications
Use in patients with a known sensitivity to medroxyprogesterone acetate.

Use in patients with impaired liver function or with active liver disease.

Before using Provera, the general medical condition of the patient should be carefully evaluated. This evaluation should exclude the presence of genital or breast neoplasia before considering the use of Provera.

4.4 Special warnings and special precautions for use
Whether administered alone or in conjunction with oestrogens, Provera should not be employed in patients with abnormal uterine bleeding until a definite diagnosis has been established and the possibility of genital malignancy eliminated.

Rare cases of thrombo-embolism have been reported with use of Provera, especially at higher doses. Causality has not been established.

Doses of up to 30 mg a day may not suppress ovulation and patients should be advised to take adequate contraceptive measures, where appropriate.

Provera, especially in high doses, may cause weight gain and fluid retention. With this in mind, caution should be exercised in treating any patient with a pre-existing medical condition, such as epilepsy, migraine, asthma, cardiac or renal dysfunction, that might be adversely affected by weight gain or fluid retention.

Some patients receiving Provera may exhibit a decreased glucose tolerance. The mechanism for this is not known. This fact should be borne in mind when treating all patients and especially known diabetics.

Patients with a history of treatment for mental depression should be carefully monitored while receiving Provera therapy. Some patients may complain of premenstrual like depression while on Provera therapy.

4.5 Interaction with other medicinal products and other forms of Interaction
Aminoglutethimide administered concurrently with Provera may significantly depress the bioavailability of Provera.

Interactions with other medicinal treatments (including oral anti-coagulants) have rarely been reported, but causality has not been determined. The possibility of interaction should be borne in mind in patients receiving concurrent treatment with other drugs.

4.6 Pregnancy and lactation
A negative pregnancy test should be demonstrated before starting therapy. Medroxyprogesterone acetate and its metabolites are secreted in breast milk, but there is no evidence to suggest that this presents any hazard to the child.

4.7 Effects on ability to drive and use machines
No adverse effect has been reported.

4.8 Undesirable effects
The following medical events, listed in order of seriousness rather than frequency of occurrence, have been occasionally to rarely associated with the use of progestogens:

Rare anaphylactoid-like reactions.

Psychic: nervousness, insomnia, somnolence, fatigue, depression, dizziness and headache.

Skin and mucous membranes: urticaria, pruritus, rash, acne, hirsutism and alopecia.

Gastro-intestinal: nausea.

Breast: tenderness and galactorrhoea.

Miscellaneous: change in weight.

4.9 Overdose
In animals Provera has been shown to be capable of exerting an adreno-corticoid effect, but this has not been reported in the human, following usual dosages. The oral administration of Provera at a rate of 100 mg per day has been shown to have no effect on adrenal function.

5. PHARMACOLOGICAL PROPERTIES
5.1 Pharmacodynamic properties
Medroxyprogesterone acetate has actions and uses similar to those of progesterone.

MPA has minimal androgenic activity compared to progesterone and virtually no oestrogenic activity.

Progestogens are used in the treatment of dysfunctional uterine bleeding, secondary amenorrhoea and endometriosis.

5.2 Pharmacokinetic properties
MPA is rapidly absorbed from the G-I tract with a single oral dose of 10-250 mg. The time taken to reach the peak serum concentration (T_{max}) was 2-6 hours and the average peak serum concentration (C_{max}) was 13-46.89 mg/ml.

Unmetabolised MPA is highly plasma protein bound. MPA is metabolised in the liver.

MPA is primarily metabolised by faecal excretion as glucuronide conjugated metabolite.

Metabolised MPA is excreted more rapidly and in a greater percentage following oral doses than after aqueous intramuscular injection

5.3 Preclinical safety data
None stated

6. PHARMACEUTICAL PARTICULARS
6.1 List of excipients

Lactose	Ph Eur.
Sucrose	Ph Eur.
Maize Starch	Ph Eur.
Liquid Paraffin	Ph Eur.
Talc	Ph Eur.
Calcium Stearate	NF
E110	
Purified Water	Ph Eur.

6.2 Incompatibilities
None known.

6.3 Shelf life
36 months

6.4 Special precautions for storage
Store bottle pack at controlled room temperature (15-30°C)

Store blister pack below 25°C

6.5 Nature and contents of container
HDPE tamper-evident bottles with LDPE push-fit tamper evident caps, containing 100 tablets.

Aluminium foil/PVC blisters, containing 10, 30, 50 or 100 tablets.

6.6 Instructions for use and handling
None.

7. MARKETING AUTHORISATION HOLDER
Pharmacia Limited

Davy Avenue

Milton Keynes

MK5 8PH

UK

8. MARKETING AUTHORISATION NUMBER(S)
PL 0032/0168

9. DATE OF FIRST AUTHORISATION/RENEWAL OF THE AUTHORISATION
Date of first authorisation: 28/5/92

Renewal of authorisation: 28/5/97

10. DATE OF REVISION OF THE TEXT
March 2000

January 2002

Legal Category
POM.

Provera Tablets 200 mg

(Pharmacia Limited)

1. NAME OF THE MEDICINAL PRODUCT
Provera® Tablets 200 mg

2. QUALITATIVE AND QUANTITATIVE COMPOSITION
Medroxyprogesterone acetate Ph. Eur. 200 mg per tablet

3. PHARMACEUTICAL FORM
Tablet

4. CLINICAL PARTICULARS
4.1 Therapeutic indications
Progestogen indicated for the treatment of certain hormone dependent neoplasms, such as:

1. Endometrial carcinoma
2. Renal cell carcinoma
3. Carcinoma of the breast in post menopausal women.

4.2 Posology and method of administration
Adults

Endometrial and renal cell carcinoma 200-400 mg daily.

Breast carcinoma 400-800 mg per day. Doses of 1000 mg daily have been given although the incidence of minor side-effects, such as indigestion and weight gain, increase with increase in dose.

Response to hormonal therapy may not be evident until after at least 8-10 weeks of therapy.

Elderly patients

This product has been used primarily in the older age group for the treatment of malignancies. There is no evidence to suggest that the older age group is any less prepared to handle the drug metabolically than is the younger patient. Therefore the same dosage, contra-indications, and precautions would apply to either age group.

Children

The product is not anticipated for paediatric use in the indications recommended.

4.3 Contraindications

Use in patients with a known sensitivity to medroxyprogesterone acetate.

Use in patients with impaired liver function, or with active liver disease.

4.4 Special warnings and special precautions for use

Warnings

In the treatment of carcinoma of breast occasional cases of hypercalcaemia have been reported.

Any patient who develops an acute impairment of vision, proptosis, diplopia or migraine headache should be carefully evaluated opthalmologically to exclude the presence of papilloedema or retinal vascular regions before continuing medication.

Precautions

Animal studies have shown that Provera possesses adrenocorticoid activity. This has also been reported in man, therefore patients receiving large doses continuously and for long periods should be observed closely. Because progestogens may cause some degree of fluid retention, conditions that might be influenced by this factor, such as epilepsy, migraine, asthma, cardiac or renal dysfunction, require careful observation.

Patients who have a history of mental depression should be carefully observed and the drug discontinued if the depression recurs to a serious degree. A decrease in glucose tolerance has been observed in some patients on progestogens. The mechanism of this decrease is obscure. For this reason diabetic patients should be carefully observed while receiving progestogen therapy.

Before using Provera the general medical condition of the patient should be carefully evaluated.

This product should be used under the supervision of a specialist and the patients kept under regular surveillance.

Rare cases of thrombo-embolism have been reported with use of Provera but causality has not been established.

4.5 Interaction with other medicinal products and other forms of Interaction

Aminoglutethimide administered concurrently with Provera may significantly depress the bioavailability of Provera.

Interactions with other medicinal treatments (including oral anti-coagulants) have rarely been reported, but causality has not been determined. The possibility of interaction should be born in mind in patients receiving concurrent treatment with other drugs.

4.6 Pregnancy and lactation

The administration of large doses to pregnant women has resulted in the observation of some instances of female foetal masculinisation. Doctors should therefore check that patients are not pregnant before commencing treatment.

Medroxyprogesterone acetate and/or its metabolites are secreted in breast milk but there is no evidence to suggest that this presents any hazard to the child.

4.7 Effects on ability to drive and use machines

No adverse effect has been reported.

4.8 Undesirable effects

Reactions occasionally associated with the use of progestogens, particularly in high doses, are:

Breast: Tenderness or galactorrhoea.

Psychic: nervousness, insomnia, somnolence, fatigue, dizziness, depression and headache.

Skin and mucous membranes: sensitivity reactions, ranging from pruritus, urticaria, angioneurotic oedema, to generalised rash and anaphylaxis have been occasionally reported. Acne and alopecia or hirsutism have been reported in a few cases.

Gastro-intestinal: nausea and indigestion have been noted particularly with the higher doses.

Miscellaneous: hyperpyrexia, weight gain, moon facies, increased blood pressure.

4.9 Overdose

No action required other than cessation of therapy.

5. PHARMACOLOGICAL PROPERTIES

5.1 Pharmacodynamic properties

Pharmotherapeutic group (ATC code) L02A B

Medroxyprogesterone acetate has the pharmacological action of a progestogen.

5.2 Pharmacokinetic properties

Medroxyprogesterone acetate is absorbed from the gastro intestinal tract with a single oral dose of 10-250 mg. The time taken to reach the peak serum concentration (Tmax) was 2-6 hours and the average peak serum concentration (Cmax) was 13-46.89 mg/ml.

Unmetabolised MPA is highly plasma protein bound. MPA is metabolised in the liver.

MPA is primarily metabolised by faecal excretion as glucuronide conjugated metabolite.

Metabolised MPA is excreted more rapidly and in a greater percentage following oral doses than after aqueous intramuscular injection

5.3 Preclinical safety data

No further preclinical safety data are available.

6. PHARMACEUTICAL PARTICULARS

6.1 List of excipients

Microcrystalline cellulose Ph. Eur.

Maize starch Ph. Eur.

Byco C

Polyethylene glycol 400 USP

Sodium starch glycollate BP

Docusate sodium with sodium benzoate

Magnesium stearate Ph. Eur.

Isopropyl alcohol BP

Purified water Ph. Eur.

6.2 Incompatibilities

Not applicable.

6.3 Shelf life

36 months if stored in glass/HDPE bottles or 24 month in blister packs.

6.4 Special precautions for storage

Store below 25°C.

Bottle packs only: keep in a well closed container.

6.5 Nature and contents of container

Amber glass bottle with screw cap containing 100 tablets.

HDPE bottle with tamper evident cap containing 100 tablets.

PVC/aluminium strip containing 30, 60 or 100 tablets.

6.6 Instructions for use and handling

None.

7. MARKETING AUTHORISATION HOLDER

Pharmacia Limited

Davy Avenue

Milton Keynes

MK5 8PH

UK

8. MARKETING AUTHORISATION NUMBER(S)

PL 0032/0112

9. DATE OF FIRST AUTHORISATION/RENEWAL OF THE AUTHORISATION

7 November 1983/30 January 1996

10. DATE OF REVISION OF THE TEXT

April 2001

Legal Category

POM.

Provera Tablets 400 mg

(Pharmacia Limited)

1. NAME OF THE MEDICINAL PRODUCT

Provera® Tablets 400 mg

2. QUALITATIVE AND QUANTITATIVE COMPOSITION

Medroxyprogesterone acetate BP, 400 mg.

3. PHARMACEUTICAL FORM

Tablets for oral use

4. CLINICAL PARTICULARS

4.1 Therapeutic indications

Oral progestogen for the treatment of certain hormone dependant neoplasms, such as:

1. Endometrial carcinoma.
2. Renal cell carcinoma.
3. Carcinoma of breast in post menopausal women.

4.2 Posology and method of administration

Adults

Endometrial and renal cell carcinoma 200-400 mg daily.

Breast carcinoma 400-800 mg daily. Doses of 1000 mg daily have been given although the incidence of minor side-effects, such as indigestion and weight gain, increase with the increase in dose.

Response to hormonal therapy may not be evident until after at least 8-10 weeks of therapy.

Elderly patients

Normal adult dose appropriate.

Children

The product is not anticipated for paediatric use in the indications recommended.

4.3 Contraindications

Use in patients with a known sensitivity to medroxyprogesterone acetate.

Use in patients with impaired liver function or active liver disease.

4.4 Special warnings and special precautions for use

Warnings

In the treatment of carcinoma of breast occasional cases of hypercalcaemia have been reported.

Any patient who develops an acute impairment of vision, proptosis, diplopia or migraine headache should be carefully evaluated ophthalmologically to exclude the presence of papilloedema or retinal vascular lesions before continuing medication.

Precautions

Animal studies show that Provera possesses adrenocorticoid activity. This has also been reported in man, therefore patients receiving large doses continuously and for long periods should be observed closely. Because progestogen may cause some degree of fluid retention, conditions which might be influenced by this factor, such as epilepsy, migraine, asthma, cardiac or renal dysfunction, require careful observation.

Patients who have a history of mental depression should be carefully observed and the drug discontinued if the depression recurs to a serious degree. A decrease in glucose tolerance has been observed in some patients on progestogens. The mechanism of this decrease is obscure. For this reason diabetic patients should be carefully observed while receiving progestogen therapy. Before using Provera the general medical condition of the patient should be carefully evaluated.

This product should be used under the supervision of a specialist and the patient kept under regular surveillance.

Rare cases of thrombo-embolism have been reported with use of Provera, but causality has not been established.

4.5 Interaction with other medicinal products and other forms of Interaction

Aminoglutethimide administered concurrently with Provera may significantly depress the bioavailability of Provera.

Interactions with other medicinal treatments (including oral anti-coagulants) have rarely been reported, but causality has not been determined. The possibility of interaction should be born in mind in patients receiving concurrent treatment with other drugs.

4.6 Pregnancy and lactation

The administration of large doses to pregnant women has resulted in the observation of some instances of female foetal masculinisation. Doctors should therefore check that patients are not pregnant before commencing treatment. Medroxyprogesterone acetate and/or its metabolites are secreted in breast milk but there is no evidence to suggest that this presents any hazard to the child.

4.7 Effects on ability to drive and use machines

No adverse effect has been reported.

4.8 Undesirable effects

Reactions occasionally associated with the use of progestogens, particularly in high doses, are:

Breast: Tenderness or galactorrhoea.

Psychic: Nervousness, insomnia, somnolence, fatigue, dizziness, depression and headache.

Skin and mucous membranes: Sensitivity reactions ranging from pruritus, urticaria, angioneurotic oedema, to generalised rash and anaphylaxis have occasionally been reported. Acne, alopecia or hirsutism have been reported in a few cases.

Gastro-intestinal: Nausea and indigestion have been noted particularly with the higher doses.

Miscellaneous: Hyperpyrexia, weight gain, moon facies, increased blood pressure.

4.9 Overdose

No action required other than cessation of therapy.

5. PHARMACOLOGICAL PROPERTIES

5.1 Pharmacodynamic properties

Medroxyprogesterone acetate has the pharmacological action of a progestogen.

5.2 Pharmacokinetic properties

The comparative bioavailability of medroxyprogesterone acetate (MPA) in sixteen healthy male volunteers was determined following the oral ingestion of 400 mg MPA as two Provera 200 mg tablets or as one Provera 400mg tablet. It is concluded that the bioavailability appeared to be equivalent in this group of volunteers.

5.3 Preclinical safety data

No further preclinical safety data available.

6. PHARMACEUTICAL PARTICULARS

6.1 List of excipients

Microcrystalline cellulose

Corn Starch

Byco C

Polyethylene glycol 400

Sodium starch glycollate

Docusate sodium

Sodium benzoate

Magnesium stearate

Isopropyl alcohol

Purified water

6.2 Incompatibilities

Not applicable.

6.3 Shelf life

The shelf life for Provera Tablets 400 mg is 36 months

6.4 Special precautions for storage
Store at controlled room temperature (15-30°C)

6.5 Nature and contents of container
Glass/HDPE bottles of 60 tablets

PVC aluminium blisters of 30 tablets

6.6 Instructions for use and handling
None stated.

7. MARKETING AUTHORISATION HOLDER
Pharmacia Limited
Davy Avenue
Milton Keynes
MK5 8PH
UK

8. MARKETING AUTHORISATION NUMBER(S)
PL 0032/0131

9. DATE OF FIRST AUTHORISATION/RENEWAL OF THE AUTHORISATION
Date of first authorisation: 29 April 1986

Date of renewal of authorisation: 21 May 1998

10. DATE OF REVISION OF THE TEXT
April 2001

Legal Category
POM.

Provera Tablets 5 mg

(Pharmacia Limited)

1. NAME OF THE MEDICINAL PRODUCT
Provera Tablets 5 mg

2. QUALITATIVE AND QUANTITATIVE COMPOSITION
Medroxyprogesterone Acetate Ph. Eur. 5 mg.

3. PHARMACEUTICAL FORM
Tablets.

4. CLINICAL PARTICULARS
4.1 Therapeutic indications
Progestogen.

Indicated for dysfunctional (anovulatory) uterine bleeding, secondary amenorrhoea and for mild to moderate endometriosis.

4.2 Posology and method of administration
Tablets for oral administration.

Adults

Dysfunctional (anovulatory) uterine bleeding: 2.5-10 mg daily for 5-10 days commencing on the assumed or calculated 16th-21st day of the cycle. Treatment should be given for two consecutive cycles. When bleeding occurs from a poorly developed proliferative endometrium, conventional oestrogen therapy may be employed in conjunction with medroxyprogesterone acetate in doses of 5-10 mg for 10 days.

Secondary amenorrhoea: 2.5-10 mg daily for 5-10 days beginning on the assumed or calculated 16th-21st day of the cycle. Repeat the treatment for three consecutive cycles. In amenorrhoea associated with a poorly developed proliferative endometrium, conventional oestrogen therapy may be employed in conjunction with medroxyprogesterone acetate in doses of 5-10 mg for 10 days.

Mild to moderate endometriosis: beginning on the first day of the menstrual cycle, 10 mg three times a day for 90 consecutive days. Breakthrough bleeding, which is self-limiting, may occur. No additional hormonal therapy is recommended for the management of this bleeding.

Elderly
Not applicable.

Children
Not applicable.

4.3 Contraindications
Use in patients with known hypersensitivity to medroxyprogesterone acetate.

Use in patients with impaired liver function, or with active liver disease.

Before using Provera, the general medical condition of the patient should be carefully evaluated. This evaluation should exclude the presence of genital or breast neoplasia before considering the use of Provera.

4.4 Special warnings and special precautions for use
Precautions:

Whether administered alone or in conjunction with oestrogens, Provera should not be employed in patients with abnormal uterine bleeding until a definite diagnosis has been established and the possibility of genital malignancy eliminated.

Provera, especially in high doses, may cause weight gain and fluid retention. With this in mind, caution should be exercised in treating any patient with a pre-existing medical condition, such as epilepsy, migraine, asthma, cardiac or renal dysfunction, that might be adversely affected by weight gain or fluid retention.

Rare cases of thrombo-embolism have been reported with use of Provera, especially at higher doses. Causality has not been established.

Some patients receiving Provera may exhibit a decreased glucose tolerance. The mechanism for this is not known. This fact should be borne in mind when treating all patients and especially known diabetics.

Patients with a history of treatment for mental depression should be carefully monitored while receiving Provera therapy. Some patients may complain of premenstrual like depression while on Provera therapy.

Warning:

Doses of up to 30 mg a day may not suppress ovulation and patients should be advised to take adequate contraceptive measures, where appropriate.

4.5 Interaction with other medicinal products and other forms of Interaction
Aminoglutethimide administered concurrently with Provera may significantly depress the bioavailability of Provera.

Interactions with other medicinal treatments (including oral anti-coagulants) have rarely been reported, but causality has not been determined. The possibility of interaction should be borne in mind in patients receiving concurrent treatment with other drugs.

4.6 Pregnancy and lactation
A negative pregnancy test should be demonstrated before starting therapy. Medroxyprogesterone acetate and/or its metabolites are secreted in breast milk but there is no evidence to suggest that this presents any hazard to the child.

4.7 Effects on ability to drive and use machines
No adverse effect has been reported.

4.8 Undesirable effects
The following medical events, listed in order of seriousness rather than frequency of occurrence, have been occasionally to rarely associated with the use of progestogens:

Rare anaphylactoid-like reactions.

Psychic: nervousness, insomnia, somnolence, fatigue, depression, dizziness and headache.

Skin and mucous membranes: urticaria, pruritus, rash, acne, hirsutism and alopecia.

Gastro-intestinal: nausea.

Breast: tenderness and galactorrhoea.

Miscellaneous: change in weight.

4.9 Overdose
In animals Provera has been shown to be capable of exerting an adreno-corticoid effect but this has not been reported in the human, following usual dosages. The oral administration of Provera at a rate of 100 mg per day has been shown to have no effect on adrenal function.

5. PHARMACOLOGICAL PROPERTIES
5.1 Pharmacodynamic properties
Medroxyprogesterone acetate (MPA) has actions and uses similar to those of progesterone.

MPA has minimal androgenic activity compared to progesterone and virtually no oestrogenic activity.

Progestogen are used in the treatment of dysfunctional uterine bleeding, secondary amenorrhoea and endometriosis.

5.2 Pharmacokinetic properties
MPA is rapidly absorbed from the G.I. tract with a single oral dose of 10-250 mg. The time taken to reach the peak serum concentration (T_{max}) was 2-6 hours and the average peak serum concentration (C_{max}) was from 13-46.89 mg/ml.

Unmetabolised MPA is highly plasma protein bound. MPA is metabolised in the liver.

MPA is primarily eliminated by faecal excretion as a glucoronide conjugated metabolite.

Metabolised MPA is excreted more rapidly and in a greater percentage following oral doses than after aqueous IM injection.

5.3 Preclinical safety data
No further pre-clinical safety data are available.

6. PHARMACEUTICAL PARTICULARS
6.1 List of excipients

Lactose	Ph Eur.
Starch	Ph Eur.
Sucrose	Ph Eur.
Liquid Paraffin	Ph Eur.
Calcium Stearate	NF
Talc	Ph Eur.
FD & C Blue No. 2 Aluminium Lake	HSE
Purified Water	Ph Eur.

6.2 Incompatibilities
None.

6.3 Shelf life
24 months if stored in blister strips

60 months if stored in either amber glass bottles with screw caps or HDPE bottles with tamper evident caps.

6.4 Special precautions for storage
Blister packs: Store below 25°C.

Bottle packs: Store at room temperature.

6.5 Nature and contents of container
Blister strips of 250 micron opaque PVC/20 micron aluminium foil containing 10, 20 or 100 tablets or amber glass bottles with screw caps or HDPE bottles with tamper evident caps containing 100 tablets.

6.6 Instructions for use and handling
None given.

7. MARKETING AUTHORISATION HOLDER
Pharmacia Limited
Davy Avenue
Milton Keynes
MK5 8PH
UK

8. MARKETING AUTHORISATION NUMBER(S)
PL 0032/5035R

9. DATE OF FIRST AUTHORISATION/RENEWAL OF THE AUTHORISATION
Date of First Authorisation: 8 January 1988

Date of Renewal of Authorisation: 13 March 2000

10. DATE OF REVISION OF THE TEXT
March 2000

August 2001

Legal Category
POM.

Provigil 100 mg Tablets, Provigil 200 mg Tablets

(Cephalon UK Limited)

1. NAME OF THE MEDICINAL PRODUCT
PROVIGIL®▼ 100 mg tablets

PROVIGIL®▼ 200 mg tablets

2. QUALITATIVE AND QUANTITATIVE COMPOSITION
Modafinil 100 mg per tablet.

Modafinil 200 mg per tablet.

For excipients, see 6.1.

3. PHARMACEUTICAL FORM
Tablet

White to off-white, capsule-shaped tablets, debossed with "PROVIGIL" on one side and "100 MG" on the other.

White to off-white, scored, capsule-shaped tablets, debossed with "PROVIGIL" on one side and "200 MG" on the other.

4. CLINICAL PARTICULARS
4.1 Therapeutic indications
PROVIGIL is indicated for the treatment of excessive sleepiness associated with chronic pathological conditions, including narcolepsy, obstructive sleep apnoea/hypopnoea syndrome and moderate to severe chronic shift work sleep disorder.

4.2 Posology and method of administration
Adults
Narcolepsy and Obstructive Sleep Apnoea / Hypopnoea Syndrome

The recommended daily dose is 200-400 mg, commencing at 200 mg and titrated according to clinical response. PROVIGIL may be taken as two divided doses in the morning and at noon, or as a single dose in the morning, according to physician assessment of the patient and the patient's response. Tablets should be swallowed whole.

For patients with obstructive sleep apnoea / hypopnoea syndrome, PROVIGIL treats the symptoms of excessive daytime sleepiness associated with the condition. In addition to this symptomatic treatment, disease-modifying interventions (e.g., Continuous Positive Airway Pressure) should be commenced or continued.

Moderate to Severe Chronic Shift Work Sleep Disorder

The recommended daily dose is 200 mg. PROVIGIL should be taken as a single dose approximately 1 hour prior to the start of the work shift. Tablets should be swallowed whole.

Elderly
There are limited data available on the use of PROVIGIL in elderly patients. In view of the generally lower hepatic and renal clearance expected in an elderly population, it is recommended that patients over 65 years of age should commence therapy at 100 mg daily. The maximum dose of 400 mg per day should only be used in the absence of renal or hepatic impairment.

Hepatic and renal failure
The dose in patients with severe hepatic or renal failure should be reduced by half (100-200 mg per day).

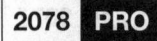

Children
Because safety and effectiveness in controlled studies in children have not been established the use of PROVIGIL is not recommended in children.

4.3 Contraindications
PROVIGIL is contra-indicated for use during pregnancy and lactation, or in patients with uncontrolled moderate to severe hypertension, or arrhythmia. PROVIGIL is also contra-indicated in patients with known hypersensitivity to PROVIGIL or any component of the preparation.

4.4 Special warnings and special precautions for use
Patients with major anxiety should only receive treatment with PROVIGIL in a specialist unit.

Sexually active women of child-bearing potential should be established on a contraceptive programme before taking PROVIGIL (also see 4.5 with respect to potential interaction with oral contraceptives).

Blood pressure and heart rate should be monitored in hypertensive patients.

In patients with obstructive sleep apnoea / hypopnoea syndrome, the underlying condition and any associated cardiovascular pathology should be monitored.

Patients should be advised that PROVIGIL is not a replacement for sleep and good sleep hygiene should be maintained.

It is recommended that PROVIGIL tablets not be used in patients with a history of left ventricular hypertrophy or cor pulmonale. PROVIGIL should not be used in patients with mitral valve prolapse who have experienced the mitral valve prolapse syndrome when previously receiving CNS stimulants. This syndrome may present with ischaemic ECG changes, chest pain or arrhythmia.

Whilst studies with modafinil have demonstrated a low potential for dependence, the possibility of dependence with long-term use cannot be entirely excluded.

PROVIGIL tablets contain lactose and therefore should not be used in patients with rare hereditary problems of galactose intolerance, the Lapp lactase deficiency, or glucose-galactose malabsorption.

4.5 Interaction with other medicinal products and other forms of Interaction
Modafinil may increase its own metabolism via induction of CYP3A4/5 activity but the effect is modest and unlikely to have significant clinical consequences.

Anticonvulsants: Co-administration of potent inducers of CYP activity, such as carbamazepine and phenobarbital, could reduce the plasma levels of modafinil.

Due to a possible inhibition of CYP2C19 by modafinil and suppression of CYP2C9 the clearance of phenytoin may be decreased when PROVIGIL is administered concomitantly. Patients should be monitored for signs of phenytoin toxicity, and repeated measurements of phenytoin plasma levels may be appropriate upon initiation or discontinuation of treatment with PROVIGIL.

Oral contraceptives: The effectiveness of oral contraceptives may be impaired due to induction of CYP3A4/5 by modafinil. When oral contraceptives are used, a product containing 50 micrograms or more of ethinylestradiol should be taken or alternative/ concomitant methods of contraception should be considered. Adequate contraception will require continuation of these methods for two cycles after stopping PROVIGIL.

Antidepressants: A number of tricyclic antidepressants and selective serotonin reuptake inhibitors are largely metabolised by CYP2D6. In patients deficient in CYP2D6 (approximately 10% of a Caucasian population) a normally ancillary metabolic pathway involving CYP2C19 becomes more important. As modafinil may inhibit CYP2C19, lower doses of antidepressants may be required in such patients.

Anticoagulants: Due to possible suppression of CYP2C9 by modafinil the clearance of warfarin may be decreased when PROVIGIL is administered concomitantly. Prothrombin times should be monitored regularly during the first 2 months of PROVIGIL use and after changes in PROVIGIL dosage.

Other drugs: Drugs that are largely eliminated via CYP2C19 metabolism, such as diazepam, propranolol and omeprazole may have reduced clearance upon co-administration of PROVIGIL and may thus require dosage reduction. In addition, *in vitro* induction of CYP1A2, CYP2B6 and CYP3A4/5 activities has been observed in human hepatocytes, which were it to occur *in vivo*, could decrease the blood levels of drugs metabolised by these enzymes, thereby possibly decreasing their therapeutic effectiveness. Results from clinical interaction studies suggest that the largest effects may be on substrates of CYP3A4/5 that undergo significant presystemic elimination, particularly via CYP3A enzymes in the gastrointestinal tract. Examples include ciclosporin, HIV-protease inhibitors, buspirone, triazolam, midazolam and most of the calcium channel blockers and statins. In a case report, a 50% reduction in ciclosporin concentration was observed in a patient receiving ciclosporin in whom concurrent treatment with modafinil was initiated.

4.6 Pregnancy and lactation
There are no adequate data from the use of modafinil in pregnant women.

Modafinil was non-teratogenic in rats and rabbits at doses greater than the maximum clinical dose. However, plasma levels in preclinical studies, due to metabolic auto-induction, were less than or similar to that expected in patients.

Modafinil and its acid and sulphone metabolites pass into milk of lactating rats (see 5.3). It is not known whether modafinil passes into human milk.

Modafinil use during pregnancy and lactation is contra-indicated.

4.7 Effects on ability to drive and use machines
There is no information available concerning the effects of PROVIGIL on vehicle driving and/or the ability to use machinery. Undesirable effects such as blurred vision or dizziness might affect ability to drive (see 4.8 Undesirable Effects).

4.8 Undesirable effects
The adverse events considered to be at least possibly related to treatment, from clinical trials involving 1561 patients taking PROVIGIL were as follows (very common $>10\%$, common $>1\%$ - 10%, uncommon $>0.1\%$ - 1%).

The most commonly reported adverse drug reaction is headache, affecting approximately 21% of patients. This is usually mild or moderate, dose-dependent and disappears within a few days.

Body as a whole
Very common: headache

Common: abdominal pain, asthenia, chest pain

Uncommon: back pain, minor allergic reaction (e.g., hayfever symptoms), neck pain

Cardiovascular
Common: tachycardia, palpitation, vasodilatation

Uncommon: hypertension, abnormal ECG, extrasystoles, arrhythmia, bradycardia, hypotension

Digestive
Common: nausea, dry mouth, diarrhoea, decreased appetite, dyspepsia, constipation

Uncommon: flatulence, reflux, vomiting, increased appetite, thirst, dysphagia, glossitis, mouth ulcers

Endocrine
Uncommon: diabetes mellitus

Haemic and lymphatic
Uncommon: eosinophilia, leucopenia

Metabolic and nutritional
Common: abnormal liver function tests

Dose related increases in alkaline phosphatase and gamma glutamyl transferase have been observed.

Uncommon: peripheral oedema, weight increase, weight decrease, hypercholesterolaemia, hyperglycaemia

Musculoskeletal
Uncommon: myalgia, myasthenia, leg cramps, arthralgia, twitch

Nervous system
Common: nervousness, insomnia, anxiety, dizziness, somnolence, depression, abnormal thinking, confusion, paraesthesia

Uncommon: sleep disorder, dyskinesia, hypertonia, hyperkinesia, agitation, amnesia, abnormal dreams, emotional lability, migraine, tremor, vertigo, decreased libido, hostility, CNS stimulation, depersonalisation, hypoaesthesia, incoordination, movement disorder, personality disorder, speech disorder

Respiratory system
Uncommon: pharyngitis, dyspnoea, rhinitis, increased cough, asthma, epistaxis, sinusitis

Skin and appendages
Uncommon: sweating, rash, acne, pruritis

Special senses
Common: blurred vision

Uncommon: taste perversion, abnormal vision, dry eye

Urogenital system
Uncommon: abnormal urine, urinary frequency, menstrual disorder

4.9 Overdose
Symptoms most often accompanying modafinil overdose, alone or in combination with other drugs have included: insomnia; central nervous system symptoms such as restlessness, disorientation, confusion, excitation and hallucination; digestive changes such as nausea and diarrhoea; and cardiovascular changes such as tachycardia, bradycardia, hypertension and chest pain.

Management:
Induced emesis or gastric lavage should be considered. Hospitalisation and surveillance of psychomotor status; cardiovascular monitoring or surveillance until the patient's symptoms have resolved are recommended.

5. PHARMACOLOGICAL PROPERTIES

5.1 Pharmacodynamic properties
Therapeutic class: centrally acting sympathomimetic (ATC Code: N06BA07).

Modafinil promotes wakefulness in a variety of species, including man. The precise mechanism(s) through which modafinil promotes wakefulness is unknown.

In pre-clinical models, modafinil does not appear to be a direct or indirect acting alpha$_1$-adrenoceptor or dopamine receptor agonist. The wakefulness induced by amphetamine, but not by modafinil, is antagonised by the dopamine receptor antagonist haloperidol. Equal wakefulness-promoting doses of methylphenidate and amphetamine increase neuronal activation throughout the brain, but modafinil selectively and prominently increases neuronal activation in more discrete regions of the brain, especially in the hypothalamus.

In man, modafinil restores and/or improves the level and duration of wakefulness and daytime alertness in a dose-related manner. Administration of modafinil results in electrophysiological changes indicative of increased alertness and improvements in objective measures of ability to sustain wakefulness. Modafinil opposes the impairment of cognitive, psychomotor and neurosensorial performance induced by sleep deprivation. These changes are produced without any adverse changes in behaviour and appetite.

In patients with narcolepsy, morning administration of 400 mg modafinil or administration of 200 mg modafinil in the morning and at noon does not adversely affect nocturnal sleep.

5.2 Pharmacokinetic properties
Modafinil is a racemic compound, whose enantiomers have different pharmacokinetics. The half-life of *l*-modafinil is approximately three times that of the *d* enantiomer, as is the total systemic exposure (AUC) to *l*-modafinil. Apparent steady state is reached after 2-4 days of dosing.

Absorption
Modafinil is readily absorbed, with peak plasma concentrations occurring at 2-4 hours. Food has no effect on overall modafinil bioavailability but t_{max} may be delayed by approximately one hour if PROVIGIL is taken with food.

Distribution
Modafinil is well distributed in body tissue with an apparent volume of distribution larger than the volume of total body water. In human plasma, *in vitro*, modafinil is moderately bound to plasma protein (approximately 60%, mainly to albumin). This degree of protein binding is such that the risk of interaction with strongly bound drugs is unlikely.

Biotransformation
Modafinil is metabolised in the liver to two major metabolites, modafinil acid and modafinil sulphone, by esterase enzymes and CYP3A4/5, respectively. In preclinical models, the metabolites did not appear to contribute to the arousal effects of modafinil. *In vitro* studies using human hepatocytes have demonstrated that modafinil slightly induces the following in a concentration-dependent manner: CYP1A2, CYP2B6 and CYP3A4. In addition, the activity of CYP2C9 was suppressed in the hepatocytes. In human liver microsomes, modafinil and modafinil sulphone produced partial competitive, reversible inhibition of CYP2C19 at concentrations expected during clinical use (see 4.5).

Elimination
The excretion of modafinil and its metabolites is chiefly renal, with a small proportion being eliminated unchanged ($<10\%$). The elimination half-life of modafinil after multiple doses is 15 hours and enables a treatment regimen based upon 1 or 2 doses per day.

Linearity/non-linearity
The pharmacokinetics of modafinil are linear and independent of the dose administered in the dose range of 200 to 600 mg once daily. Systemic exposure increases in proportion to doses administered.

Renal failure/hepatic impairment
In severe chronic renal failure the pharmacokinetics of modafinil were unaltered but exposure to modafinil acid was increased 9 fold (see 4.2). There is minimal information available regarding the safety of such levels of this metabolite. In patients with severe hepatic impairment, oral clearance of modafinil was decreased by about 60% and the steady state concentration of modafinil was doubled. The dose of PROVIGIL should be reduced by half in patients with severe hepatic or renal impairment (see 4.2).

Elderly
Elderly patients may have diminished renal and/or hepatic function and dosage reductions should be considered (see 4.2).

5.3 Preclinical safety data
Toxicology studies by single and repeated dosing have revealed no particular toxic action in animals.

Reproduction function studies have revealed no effect on fertility, nor any teratogenic effect, nor any effect on viability, growth or development of the offspring.

Modafinil is not considered to be mutagenic or carcinogenic.

Animal exposure to modafinil, based on actual plasma levels in the general toxicology, reproductive and carcinogenicity studies, was less than or similar to that expected in humans. This circumstance is the result of metabolic auto-induction noted in the pre-clinical studies. However, animal exposure on a mg/kg dose basis to modafinil in the general toxicology, reproductive and carcinogenicity studies was greater than the expected exposure, calculated on a similar basis, in humans.

In the rat peri-post-natal study, modafinil concentration in milk was about 11.5 times higher than in plasma.

6. PHARMACEUTICAL PARTICULARS

6.1 List of excipients

Provigil 100 mg tablets

Lactose monohydrate

Maize starch

Magnesium silicate

Croscarmellose sodium

Povidone K90

Talc

Magnesium stearate

Provigil 200 mg tablets

Lactose monohydrate

Pregelatinised starch

Microcrystalline cellulose

Croscarmellose sodium

Povidone K29/32

Magnesium stearate

6.2 Incompatibilities

Not applicable

6.3 Shelf life

Three years.

6.4 Special precautions for storage

No special precautions for storage.

6.5 Nature and contents of container

Provigil 100 mg tablets

PVC/PE/Aclar/Aluminium blisters containing 10 tablets

Provigil 200 mg tablets

Opaque PVC/PVDC/Aluminium blisters containing 10 tablets

Packs containing 30, 60 or 90 tablets.

Not all pack sizes may be marketed.

6.6 Instructions for use and handling

Not applicable

7. MARKETING AUTHORISATION HOLDER

Cephalon UK Limited

11/13 Frederick Sanger Road

Surrey Research Park

Guildford

Surrey GU2 7YD

United Kingdom

8. MARKETING AUTHORISATION NUMBER(S)

Provigil 100 mg tablets - PL 16260/0001

Provigil 200 mg tablets - PL 16260/0002

9. DATE OF FIRST AUTHORISATION/RENEWAL OF THE AUTHORISATION

PL 16260/0001 - 14 October 1997 / 14 October 2002

PL 16260/0002 – 2 December 2002

10. DATE OF REVISION OF THE TEXT

PL 16260/0001 - December 2003

PL 16260/0002 – September 2004

Provigil and Cephalon are registered trademarks.

Pro-Viron

(Schering Health Care Limited)

1. NAME OF THE MEDICINAL PRODUCT

Pro-viron®

2. QUALITATIVE AND QUANTITATIVE COMPOSITION

Each tablet contains 25mg mesterolone.

3. PHARMACEUTICAL FORM

Tablets.

4. CLINICAL PARTICULARS

4.1 Therapeutic indications

Androgen deficiency or male infertility when associated with primary or secondary male hypogonadism.

4.2 Posology and method of administration

The following dosages are recommended:

Adults:

Initially: 3 or 4 tablets daily for several months, followed by maintenance therapy of 2-3 tablets (50-75mg) daily.

Children:

Not recommended in children

4.3 Contraindications

Pro-viron is contraindicated in the presence of prostatic carcinoma since androgens can stimulate the growth of an existing carcinoma. Previous or existing liver tumours. Hypersensitivity to the active substances or to any of the excipients.

4.4 Special warnings and special precautions for use

Androgens are not suitable for enhancing muscular development in healthy individuals or for increasing physical ability. Regular examination of the prostate during treatment is advised, in order to exclude prostatic carcinoma.

In rare cases benign, and in even rarer cases, malignant liver tumours leading in isolated cases to life-threatening intra-abdominal haemorrhage have been observed after the use of hormonal substances such as the one contained in Pro - viron. If severe upper abdominal complaints, liver enlargement or signs of intra- abdominal haemorrhage occur, the possibility of a liver tumour should be included in the differential diagnosis.

Frequent or persistent erections of the penis may occur (see section 4.8 "Undesirable effects").

4.5 Interaction with other medicinal products and other forms of Interaction

None known.

4.6 Pregnancy and lactation

Not applicable.

4.7 Effects on ability to drive and use machines

None known.

4.8 Undesirable effects

If, in individual cases, frequent or persistent erections occur, the dose should be discontinued in order to avoid injury to the penis.

4.9 Overdose

There have been no reports of ill-effects from overdosage and treatment is generally unncessary. If overdosage is discovered within two to three hours and is so large that treatment seems desirable, gastric lavage can safely be used.

5. PHARMACOLOGICAL PROPERTIES

5.1 Pharmacodynamic properties

Pro-viron is an orally active androgen. The presence of a methyl group at C-1 confers special properties on this steroid which, unlike testosterone and all its derivatives that are used for androgen therapy, is not metabolised to oestrogen.

This difference almost certainly accounts for the observation that, in its usual therapeutic dosage in normal men, Pro-viron does not significantly depress the release of gonadotrophins from the pituitary. Hence (1) spermatogenesis is unimpaired (2) unlike other androgens, which suppress and therefore replace endogenous androgens, Pro-viron supplements endogenous androgens.

In contrast to other orally active androgens, liver tolerance is excellent (a fact probably related to the absence of 17-alkyl substitution of the steroid nucleus).

5.2 Pharmacokinetic properties

Following oral ingestion mesterolone is rapidly and almost completely absorbed in a wide dose range of 25 - 100 mg. The intake of Pro-viron generates maximum serum drug levels of 3.1 ± 1.1 ng/ml after 1.6 ± 0.6 hours. Thereafter, drug levels in serum decrease with a terminal half-life of 12 - 13 hours. Mesterolone is 98% bound to serum proteins., 40% to albumin and 58% to SHBG (sex hormone binding globulin).

Mesterolone is rapidly inactivated by metabolism. The metabolic clearance rate from serum accounts for 4.4 ± 1.6 $ml \cdot min^{-1} \cdot kg^{-1}$. There is no renal excretion of unchanged drug. The main metabolite has been identified as 1α-methyl-androsterone, which - in conjugated form - accounts for 55 - 70 % of renally excreted metabolites. The ratio of the main metabolite glucuronide to sulphate is about 12:1. A further metabolite 1α-methyl-5α-androstane-3α,17β-diol has been recognized, which accounted for about 3 % of renally eliminated metabolites. No metabolic conversion into oestrogens or corticoids has been observed. 77% of the mesterolone metabolites are excreted via the urine and 13% with the faeces. 50% of the dose is excreted in the urine within 24 hours and 90% within 7 days via the faeces and urine.

The absolute bioavailability of mesterolone is about 3 % of the oral dose.

5.3 Preclinical safety data

There are no preclinical data which could be of relevance to the prescriber and which are not already included in other relevant sections of the SPC.

6. PHARMACEUTICAL PARTICULARS

6.1 List of excipients

Lactose

maize starch

povidone 25 000 (E1201)

methyl parahydroxybenzoate (E218)

propyl parahydroxybenzoate (E216)

magnesium stearate (E572)

6.2 Incompatibilities

None known.

6.3 Shelf life

5 years.

6.4 Special precautions for storage

None

6.5 Nature and contents of container

3 blister packs of 10 tablets contained in a cardboard outer pack.

6.6 Instructions for use and handling

Store all drugs properly and keep them out of reach of children.

7. MARKETING AUTHORISATION HOLDER

Schering Health Care Limited

The Brow

Burgess Hill

West Sussex RH15 9NE

8. MARKETING AUTHORISATION NUMBER(S)

0053/0030

9. DATE OF FIRST AUTHORISATION/RENEWAL OF THE AUTHORISATION

24th July 2002

10. DATE OF REVISION OF THE TEXT

24th July 2002

LEGAL CATEGORY

POM

Prozac 20mg and 60mg hard capsules, and 20mg per 5ml oral liquid

(Eli Lilly and Company Limited)

1. NAME OF THE MEDICINAL PRODUCT

Prozac* 20mg hard capsules.

Prozac 60mg hard capsules.

Prozac 20mg per 5ml oral liquid.

2. QUALITATIVE AND QUANTITATIVE COMPOSITION

Each 20mg capsule contains fluoxetine hydrochloride equivalent to 20mg of fluoxetine.

Each 60mg capsule contains fluoxetine hydrochloride equivalent to 60mg of fluoxetine.

Each 5ml of oral liquid contains fluoxetine hydrochloride equivalent to 20mg of fluoxetine.

For excipients, see section 6.1.

3. PHARMACEUTICAL FORM

Hard capsules.

The 20mg capsules are green and yellow, printed 'Prozac 20mg'.

The 60mg capsules are yellow, printed '3109'.

Oral liquid (clear, colourless, mint odoured).

4. CLINICAL PARTICULARS

4.1 Therapeutic indications

Major depressive episodes.

Obsessive-compulsive disorder.

Bulimia nervosa: Prozac is indicated as a complement of psychotherapy for the reduction of binge-eating and purging activity.

4.2 Posology and method of administration

For oral administration to adults only.

Major depressive episodes: Adults and the elderly: 20mg/day to 60mg/day. A dose of 20mg/day is recommended as the initial dose. Although there may be an increased potential for undesirable effects at higher doses, a dose increase may be considered after three weeks if there is no response.

In agreement with the consensus statement of the WHO, antidepressant medication should be continued for at least 6 months.

Obsessive-compulsive disorder: Adults and the elderly: 20mg/day to 60mg/day. A dose of 20mg/day is recommended as the initial dose. Although there may be an increased potential for side-effects at higher doses, a dose increase may be considered after two weeks if there is no response. If no improvement is observed within 10 weeks, treatment with fluoxetine should be reconsidered. If a good therapeutic response has been obtained, treatment can be continued at a dosage adjusted on an individual basis. While there are no systematic studies to answer the question of how long to continue fluoxetine treatment, OCD is a chronic condition and it is reasonable to consider continuation beyond 10 weeks in responding patients. Dosage adjustments should be made carefully, on an individual patient basis, to maintain the patient at the lowest effective dose. The need for treatment should be reassessed periodically. Some clinicians advocate concomitant behavioural psychotherapy for patients who have done well on pharmacotherapy.

Long-term efficacy (more than 24 weeks) has not been demonstrated in OCD.

Bulimia nervosa: Adults and the elderly: A dose of 60mg/day is recommended. Long-term efficacy (more than 3 months) has not been demonstrated in bulimia nervosa.

All indications: The recommended dose may be increased or decreased. Doses above 80mg/day have not been systematically evaluated.

Fluoxetine may be administered as a single or divided dose, during or between meals.

When dosing is stopped, active drug substances will persist in the body for weeks. This should be borne in mind when starting or stopping treatment. Dosage tapering is unnecessary in most patients.

The capsule and liquid dosage forms are bioequivalent.

Children: The use of fluoxetine in children and adolescents (under the age of 18) is not recommended, as safety and efficacy have not been established.

Elderly: Caution is recommended when increasing the dose, and the daily dose should generally not exceed 40mg. Maximum recommended dose is 60mg/day.

A lower or less frequent dose (eg, 20mg every second day) should be considered in patients with hepatic impairment (see section 5.2), or in patients where concomitant medication has the potential for interaction with Prozac (see section 4.5).

4.3 Contraindications

Hypersensitivity to fluoxetine or to any of its excipients.

Monoamine oxidase inhibitors: Cases of serious and sometimes fatal reactions have been reported in patients receiving an SSRI in combination with a monoamine oxidase inhibitor (MAOI), and in patients who have recently discontinued an SSRI and have been started on a MAOI. Treatment of fluoxetine should only be started 2 weeks after discontinuation of an irreversible MAOI and the following day after discontinuation of a reversible MAOI-A.

Some cases presented with features resembling serotonin syndrome (which may resemble, and be diagnosed as, neuroleptic malignant syndrome). Cyproheptadine or dantrolene may benefit patients experiencing such reactions. Symptoms of a drug interaction with a MAOI include: hyperthermia, rigidity, myoclonus, autonomic instability with possible rapid fluctuations of vital signs, mental status changes that include confusion, irritability, and extreme agitation, progressing to delirium and coma.

Therefore, fluoxetine is contra-indicated in combination with a non-selective MAOI. Similarly, at least 5 weeks should elapse after discontinuing fluoxetine treatment before starting a MAOI. If fluoxetine has been prescribed chronically and/or at a high dose, a longer interval should be considered.

The combination of fluoxetine with a reversible MAOI (eg, moclobemide) is not recommended. Treatment with fluoxetine can be initiated the following day after discontinuation of a reversible MAOI.

4.4 Special warnings and special precautions for use

Warnings

Rash and allergic reactions: Rash, anaphylactoid events, and progressive systemic events, sometimes serious (involving skin, kidney, liver, or lung), have been reported. Upon the appearance of rash or of other allergic phenomena for which an alternative aetiology cannot be identified, fluoxetine should be discontinued.

Precautions

Seizures: Seizures are a potential risk with antidepressant drugs. Therefore, as with other antidepressants, fluoxetine should be introduced cautiously in patients who have a history of seizures. Treatment should be discontinued in any patient who develops seizures or where there is an increase in seizure frequency. Fluoxetine should be avoided in patients with unstable seizure disorders/epilepsy, and patients with controlled epilepsy should be carefully monitored.

Mania: Antidepressants should be used with caution in patients with a history of mania/hypomania. As with all antidepressants, fluoxetine should be discontinued in any patient entering a manic phase.

Hepatic/renal function: Fluoxetine is extensively metabolised by the liver and excreted by the kidneys. A lower dose, eg, alternate day dosing, is recommended in patients with significant hepatic dysfunction. When given fluoxetine 20mg/day for 2 months, patients with severe renal failure (GFR < 10ml/min) requiring dialysis showed no difference in plasma levels of fluoxetine or norfluoxetine compared to controls with normal renal function.

Cardiac disease: No conduction abnormalities that resulted in heart block were observed in the ECG of 312 patients who received fluoxetine in double-blind clinical trials. However, clinical experience in acute cardiac disease is limited, therefore caution is advisable.

Weight loss: Weight loss may occur in patients taking fluoxetine but it is usually proportional to baseline body weight.

Diabetes: In patients with diabetes, treatment with an SSRI may alter glycaemic control. Hypoglycaemia has occurred during therapy with fluoxetine, and hyperglycaemia has developed following discontinuation. Insulin and/or oral hypoglycaemic dosage may need to be adjusted.

Suicide: As improvement may not occur during the first few weeks of treatment, in common with all antidepressants, patients should be closely monitored during this period. The possibility of a suicide attempt is inherent in depression and may persist until significant remission occurs. It is general clinical experience with all therapies for depression that the risk of suicide may increase in the early stages of recovery.

Haemorrhage: There have been reports of cutaneous bleeding abnormalities, such as ecchymosis and purpura, with SSRIs. Ecchymosis has been reported as an infrequent event during treatment with fluoxetine. Other haemorrhagic manifestations (eg, gynaecological haemorrhages, gastro-intestinal bleedings, and other cutaneous or mucous bleedings) have been reported rarely. Caution is advised in patients taking SSRIs, particularly in concomitant use with oral anticoagulants, drugs known to affect platelet function (eg, atypical antipsychotics, such as clozapine, phenothiazines, most TCAs, aspirin, NSAIDs), or other drugs that may increase risk of bleeding, as well as in patients with a history of bleeding disorders.

Electroconvulsive therapy (ECT): There have been rare reports of prolonged seizures in patients on fluoxetine receiving ECT treatment, therefore caution is advisable.

St John's Wort: An increase in serotonergic effects, such as serotonin syndrome, may occur when selective serotonin reuptake inhibitors and herbal preparations containing St John's Wort (*Hypericum perforatum*) are used together.

On rare occasions, development of a serotonin syndrome or neuroleptic malignant syndrome-like events have been reported in association with treatment of fluoxetine, particularly when given in combination with other serotonergic (among others, L-tryptophan) and/or neuroleptic drugs. As these syndromes may result in potentially life-threatening conditions, treatment with fluoxetine should be discontinued if such events (characterised by clusters of symptoms, such as hyperthermia, rigidity, myoclonus, autonomic instability with possible rapid fluctuations of vital signs, mental status changes, including confusion, irritability, extreme agitation, progressing to delirium and coma) occur, and supportive symptomatic treatment should be initiated.

4.5 Interaction with other medicinal products and other forms of Interaction

Half-life: The long elimination half-lives of both fluoxetine and norfluoxetine should be borne in mind (see section 5.2) when considering pharmacodynamic or pharmacokinetic drug interactions (eg, when switching from fluoxetine to other antidepressants).

Monoamine oxidase inhibitors: See section 4.3.

Not recommended combinations: MAOI-A (see section 4.3).

Combinations requiring precautions for use: MAOI-B (selegeline): risk of serotonin syndrome. Clinical monitoring is recommended.

Phenytoin: Changes in blood levels have been observed when combined with fluoxetine. In some cases manifestations of toxicity have occurred. Consideration should be given to using conservative titration schedules of the concomitant drug and to monitoring clinical status.

Serotonergic drugs: Co-administration with serotonergic drugs (eg, tramadol, triptans) may increase the risk of serotonin syndrome. Use with triptans carries the additional risk of coronary vasoconstriction and hypertension.

Lithium and tryptophan: There have been reports of serotonin syndrome when SSRIs have been given with lithium or tryptophan and, therefore, the concomitant use of fluoxetine with these drugs should be undertaken with caution. When fluoxetine is used in combination with lithium, closer and more frequent clinical monitoring is required.

CYP2D6 isoenzyme: Because fluoxetine's metabolism (like tricyclic antidepressants and other selective serotonin antidepressants) involves the hepatic cytochrome CYP2D6 isoenzyme system, concomitant therapy with drugs also metabolised by this enzyme system may lead to drug interactions. Concomitant therapy with drugs predominantly metabolised by this isoenzyme, and which have a narrow therapeutic index (such as flecainide, encainide, carbamazepine, and tricyclic antidepressants), should be initiated at or adjusted to the low end of their dose range. This will also apply if fluoxetine has been taken in the previous 5 weeks.

Oral anticoagulants: Altered anticoagulant effects (laboratory values and/or clinical signs and symptoms), with no consistent pattern, but including increased bleeding, have been reported uncommonly when fluoxetine is co-administered with oral anticoagulants. Patients receiving warfarin therapy should receive careful coagulation monitoring when fluoxetine is initiated or stopped (see section 4.4).

Electroconvulsive therapy (ECT): There have been rare reports of prolonged seizures in patients on fluoxetine receiving ECT treatment, therefore caution is advisable.

Alcohol: In formal testing, fluoxetine did not raise blood alcohol levels or enhance the effects of alcohol. However, the combination of SSRI treatment and alcohol is not advisable.

St John's Wort: In common with other SSRIs, pharmacodynamic interactions between fluoxetine and the herbal remedy St John's Wort (*Hypericum perforatum*) may occur, which may result in an increase of undesirable effects.

4.6 Pregnancy and lactation

Pregnancy: Data on a large number of exposed pregnancies do not indicate a teratogenic effect of fluoxetine. Fluoxetine can be used during pregnancy, but caution should be exercised, especially during late pregnancy or just prior to the onset of labour, since the following effects have been reported in neonates: irritability, tremor, hypotonia, persistent crying, difficulty in sucking or in sleeping. These symptoms may indicate either serotonergic effects or a withdrawal syndrome. The time to occur and the duration of these symptoms may be related to the long half-life of fluoxetine (4-6 days) and its active metabolite, norfluoxetine (4-16 days).

Lactation: Fluoxetine and its metabolite, norfluoxetine, are known to be excreted in human breast milk. Adverse events have been reported in breast-feeding infants. If treatment with fluoxetine is considered necessary, discontinuation of breast-feeding should be considered; however, if breast-feeding is continued, the lowest effective dose of fluoxetine should be prescribed.

4.7 Effects on ability to drive and use machines

Although fluoxetine has been shown not to affect psychomotor performance in healthy volunteers, any psychoactive drug may impair judgement or skills. Patients should be advised to avoid driving a car or operating hazardous machinery until they are reasonably certain that their performance is not affected.

4.8 Undesirable effects

Undesirable effects may decrease in intensity and frequency with continued treatment and do not generally lead to cessation of therapy.

In common with other SSRIs, the following undesirable effects have been seen:

Body as a whole: Hypersensitivity (eg, pruritus, rash, urticaria, anaphylactoid reaction, vasculitis, serum sickness-like reaction, angioedema) (see sections 4.3 and 4.4), chills, serotonin syndrome, photosensitivity, and, very rarely, toxic epidermal necrolysis (Lyell syndrome).

Digestive system: Gastro-intestinal disorders (eg, diarrhoea, nausea, vomiting, dyspepsia, dysphagia, taste perversion), dry mouth. Abnormal liver function tests have been reported rarely. Very rare cases of idiosyncratic hepatitis.

Nervous system: Headache, sleep abnormalities (eg, abnormal dreams, insomnia), dizziness, anorexia, fatigue (eg, somnolence, drowsiness), euphoria, transient abnormal movement (eg, twitching, ataxia, tremor, myoclonus), seizures, and psychomotor restlessness. Hallucinations, manic reaction, confusion, agitation, anxiety and associated symptoms (eg, nervousness), impaired concentration and thought process (eg, depersonalisation), panic attacks (these symptoms may be due to the underlying disease), and, very rarely, serotonin syndrome.

Urogenital system: Urinary retention, urinary frequency.

Reproductive disorders: Sexual dysfunction (delayed or absent ejaculation, anorgasmia), priapism, galactorrhoea.

Miscellaneous: Alopecia, yawn, abnormal vision (eg, blurred vision, mydriasis), sweating, vasodilatation, arthralgia, myalgia, postural hypotension, ecchymosis. Other haemorrhagic manifestations (eg, gynaecological haemorrhages, gastro-intestinal bleedings, and other cutaneous or mucous bleedings) have been reported rarely (see section 4.4).

Hyponatraemia: Hyponatraemia (including serum sodium below 110mmol/l) has been rarely reported and appeared to be reversible when fluoxetine was discontinued. Some cases were possibly due to the syndrome of inappropriate antidiuretic hormone secretion. The majority of reports were associated with older patients, and patients taking diuretics or otherwise volume depleted.

Respiratory system: Pharyngitis, dyspnoea. Pulmonary events (including inflammatory processes of varying histopathology and/or fibrosis) have been reported rarely. Dyspnoea may be the only preceding symptom.

When stopping treatment, withdrawal symptoms have been reported in association with SSRIs, although the available evidence does not suggest this is due to dependence. Common symptoms include dizziness, paraesthesia, headache, anxiety, and nausea, the majority of which are mild and self-limiting. Fluoxetine has been only rarely associated with such symptoms. Plasma fluoxetine and norfluoxetine concentrations decrease gradually at the conclusion of therapy, which makes dosage tapering unnecessary in most patients.

4.9 Overdose

Cases of overdose of fluoxetine alone usually have a mild course. Symptoms of overdose have included nausea, vomiting, seizures, cardiovascular dysfunction ranging from asymptomatic arrhythmias to cardiac arrest, pulmonary dysfunction, and signs of altered CNS status ranging from excitation to coma. Fatality attributed to overdose of fluoxetine alone has been extremely rare. Cardiac and vital signs monitoring are recommended, along with general symptomatic and supportive measures. No specific antidote is known.

Forced diuresis, dialysis, haemoperfusion, and exchange transfusion are unlikely to be of benefit. Activated charcoal, which may be used with sorbitol, may be as or more effective than emesis or lavage. In managing overdosage, consider the possibility of multiple drug involvement. An extended time for close medical observation may be needed in patients who have taken excessive quantities of a tricyclic antidepressant if they are also taking, or have recently taken, fluoxetine.

5. PHARMACOLOGICAL PROPERTIES

5.1 Pharmacodynamic properties

Fluoxetine is a selective inhibitor of serotonin reuptake, and this probably accounts for the mechanism of action. Fluoxetine has practically no affinity to other receptors such as α_1-, α_2-, and β-adrenergic; serotonergic; dopaminergic; histaminergic$_1$; muscarinic; and GABA receptors.

Major depressive episodes: Clinical trials in patients with major depressive episodes have been conducted versus placebo and active controls. Prozac has been shown to be significantly more effective than placebo, as measured by the Hamilton Depression Rating Scale (HAM-D). In these studies, Prozac produced a significantly higher rate of response (defined by a 50% decrease in the HAM-D score) and remission, compared to placebo.

Obsessive-compulsive disorder: In short-term trials (under 24 weeks), fluoxetine was shown to be significantly more effective than placebo. There was a therapeutic effect at 20mg/day, but higher doses (40 or 60mg/day) showed a higher response rate. In long-term studies (three short-term studies extension phase and a relapse prevention study) efficacy has not been shown.

Bulimia nervosa: In short-term trials (under 16 weeks), in out-patients fulfilling DSM-III-R-criteria for bulimia nervosa, fluoxetine 60mg/day was shown to be significantly more effective than placebo for the reduction of bingeing and purging activities. However, for long-term efficacy no conclusion can be drawn.

Two placebo-controlled studies were conducted in patients meeting Pre-Menstrual Dysphoric Disorder (PMDD) diagnostic criteria according to DSM-IV. Patients were included if they had symptoms of sufficient severity to impair social and occupational function and relationships with others. Patients using oral contraceptives were excluded. In the first study of continuous 20mg daily dosing for 6 cycles, improvement was observed in the primary efficacy parameter (irritability, anxiety, and dysphoria). In the second study, with intermittent luteal phase dosing (20mg daily for 14 days) for 3 cycles, improvement was observed in the primary efficacy parameter (Daily Record of Severity of Problems score). However, definitive conclusions on efficacy and duration of treatment cannot be drawn from these studies.

5.2 Pharmacokinetic properties

Absorption: Fluoxetine is well absorbed from the gastro-intestinal tract after oral administration. The bioavailability is not affected by food intake.

Distribution: Fluoxetine is extensively bound to plasma proteins (about 95%) and it is widely distributed (volume of distribution: 20-40 l/kg). Steady-state plasma concentrations are achieved after dosing for several weeks. Steady-state concentrations after prolonged dosing are similar to concentrations seen at 4 to 5 weeks.

Metabolism: Fluoxetine has a non-linear pharmacokinetic profile with first pass liver effect. Maximum plasma concentration is generally achieved 6 to 8 hours after administration. Fluoxetine is extensively metabolised by the polymorphic enzyme CYP2D6. Fluoxetine is primarily metabolised by the liver to the active metabolite norfluoxetine (desmethylfluoxetine), by desmethylation.

Elimination: The elimination half-life of fluoxetine is 4 to 6 days and for norfluoxetine 4 to 16 days. These long half-lives are responsible for persistence of the drug for 5-6 weeks after discontinuation. Excretion is mainly (about 60%) via the kidney. Fluoxetine is secreted into breast milk.

At-Risk Populations

Elderly: Kinetic parameters are not altered in healthy elderly when compared to younger subjects.

Hepatic insufficiency: In case of hepatic insufficiency (alcoholic cirrhosis), fluoxetine and norfluoxetine half-lives are increased to 7 and 12 days, respectively. A lower or less frequent dose should be considered.

Renal insufficiency: After single-dose administration of fluoxetine in patients with mild, moderate, or complete (anuria) renal insufficiency, kinetic parameters have not been altered when compared to healthy volunteers. However, after repeated administration, an increase in steady-state plateau of plasma concentrations may be observed.

5.3 Preclinical safety data

There is no evidence of carcinogenicity, mutagenicity, or impairment of fertility from *in vitro* or animal studies.

6. PHARMACEUTICAL PARTICULARS

6.1 List of excipients

The liquid contains:

Benzoic acid

Sucrose

Glycerin

Mint flavour (containing 0.23% alcohol)

Purified water

The capsules contain:

Starch flowable

Dimeticone

Capsule components:

Patent blue V (E131) (20mg capsules only)

Yellow iron oxide (E172)

Titanium dioxide (E171)

Gelatin

Pharmaceutical grade edible printing ink components:

Formulation 1:

Shellac

Propylene glycol

Ammonium hydroxide

Black iron oxide (E172)

Formulation 2:

Shellac

Soya lecithin

Antifoam DC 1510

Black iron oxide (E172)

6.2 Incompatibilities

Not applicable.

6.3 Shelf life

20 mg capsules:

Three years.

60 mg capsules and liquid:

Two years.

6.4 Special precautions for storage

Do not store above 25°C.

6.5 Nature and contents of container

20 mg capsules:

PVC/aluminium blister packs of 2, 28, 30, and 98 capsules.

60 mg capsules:

PVC/aluminium blister packs of 7, 14, 28, 30, 56, 60, and 98 capsules.

Liquid: Glass bottles containing 70ml oral liquid. The pack may include a measuring cup or syringe.

Not all pack sizes may be marketed.

6.6 Instructions for use and handling

Not applicable.

7. MARKETING AUTHORISATION HOLDER

Eli Lilly and Company Limited
Kingsclere Road
Basingstoke
Hampshire
RG21 6XA
England

8. MARKETING AUTHORISATION NUMBER(S)

20mg capsules:	PL 0006/0195
60mg capsules:	PL 0006/0198
Liquid:	PL 0006/0272

9. DATE OF FIRST AUTHORISATION/RENEWAL OF THE AUTHORISATION

Capsules:

Date of first authorisation:	25 November 1988
Date of last renewal of the authorisation:	15 March 2005

Liquid:

Date of first authorisation:	28 October 1992
Date of last renewal of the authorisation:	15 March 2005

10. DATE OF REVISION OF THE TEXT

September 2004

LEGAL CATEGORY

POM

*PROZAC (fluoxetine hydrochloride) is a trademark of Eli Lilly and Company.

PZ39M

Psoriderm Bath Emulsion

(Dermal Laboratories Limited)

1. NAME OF THE MEDICINAL PRODUCT

PSORIDERM™ BATH EMULSION

2. QUALITATIVE AND QUANTITATIVE COMPOSITION

Distilled Coal Tar 40.0% w/v.

3. PHARMACEUTICAL FORM

Bath additive. Buff coloured liquid emulsion.

4. CLINICAL PARTICULARS

4.1 Therapeutic indications

For use topically as an aid in the treatment of sub-acute and chronic psoriasis.

4.2 Posology and method of administration

For adults, children and the elderly. Add 30 ml of the emulsion to a standard bath of warm water. Soak for 5 minutes, pat dry.

4.3 Contraindications

Not to be used in cases of sensitivity to any of the ingredients.

4.4 Special warnings and special precautions for use

Do not use product undiluted. Keep away from the eyes and broken or inflamed skin. Replace cap after use. Avoid spillage. For external use only.

4.5 Interaction with other medicinal products and other forms of Interaction

None known.

4.6 Pregnancy and lactation

No special precautions.

4.7 Effects on ability to drive and use machines

None known.

4.8 Undesirable effects

Local side-effects do not normally occur. In rare cases of skin irritation, discontinue treatment.

4.9 Overdose

There are no known toxic effects resulting from excessive use of Psoriderm Bath Emulsion. If accidentally swallowed, patients should contact a doctor or hospital immediately.

5. PHARMACOLOGICAL PROPERTIES

5.1 Pharmacodynamic properties

Coal tar has been used dermatologically for hundreds of years and has been shown to be safe and effective in the treatment of scaly skin conditions such as psoriasis. The British Pharmacopoeia contains monographs on coal tar and coal tar solution, and many formulations of coal tar are used in hospitals throughout the country. The coal tar used in Psoriderm Bath Emulsion has been specially distilled and is based on a neutral fraction which has been shown to be effective in the treatment of psoriasis.

The precise mechanism of action of coal tar is not understood, largely as a result of it comprising up to 10,000 components. There is evidence that topical application of coal tar improves psoriasis by reducing the excessive rate of mitotic epidermal cell division.

5.2 Pharmacokinetic properties

Dry scales, which are a common feature of psoriasis, generally reduce the effectiveness of topically applied treatments by reducing absorption of the active ingredient. An established means of overcoming this problem is to add a mild softening agent such as lecithin. In the case of Psoriderm Bath Emulsion, however, no such softening agent is included because the dosage and administration regime involves prolonged soaking (5 minutes) in a warm water emulsion which achieves a similar effect.

5.3 Preclinical safety data

None.

6. PHARMACEUTICAL PARTICULARS

6.1 List of excipients

Polysorbate 20; Triethanolamine; Phenoxyethanol; Water.

6.2 Incompatibilities

None known.

6.3 Shelf life

36 months.

6.4 Special precautions for storage

Do not store above 25°C.

6.5 Nature and contents of container

Amber glass bottle containing 200 ml. This is supplied as an original pack (OP).

6.6 Instructions for use and handling

Not applicable.

7. MARKETING AUTHORISATION HOLDER

Dermal Laboratories
Tatmore Place, Gosmore
Hitchin, Herts SG4 7QR, UK.

8. MARKETING AUTHORISATION NUMBER(S)

0173/5003R.

9. DATE OF FIRST AUTHORISATION/RENEWAL OF THE AUTHORISATION

26 May 2000.

10. DATE OF REVISION OF THE TEXT

May 2000.

Psoriderm Cream

(Dermal Laboratories Limited)

1. NAME OF THE MEDICINAL PRODUCT

PSORIDERM™ CREAM

2. QUALITATIVE AND QUANTITATIVE COMPOSITION

Distilled Coal Tar 6.0% w/w; Lecithin 0.4% w/w.

3. PHARMACEUTICAL FORM

Buff coloured cream.

4. CLINICAL PARTICULARS

4.1 Therapeutic indications

For the topical treatment of sub-acute and chronic psoriasis, including psoriasis of the scalp and flexures.

4.2 Posology and method of administration
For adults, children and the elderly. Apply to the affected area once or twice daily, or as recommended by the physician. Wash hands after use.

4.3 Contraindications
Not to be used for acute, sore or pustular psoriasis or in the presence of infection. Not to be used in cases of sensitivity to any of the ingredients.

4.4 Special warnings and special precautions for use
Keep away from the eyes and mucous membranes, genital or rectal areas. Avoid cuts and grazes or infected skin. Replace cap after use. Avoid spillage. For external use only.

4.5 Interaction with other medicinal products and other forms of Interaction
None known.

4.6 Pregnancy and lactation
No special precautions.

4.7 Effects on ability to drive and use machines
None known.

4.8 Undesirable effects
Local side-effects do not normally occur. In rare cases of skin irritation, acne-like eruptions or photosensitivity, discontinue treatment. Rarely, Psoriderm Cream may stain skin, hair or fabric.

4.9 Overdose
There are no known toxic effects resulting from excessive use of Psoriderm Cream.

5. PHARMACOLOGICAL PROPERTIES

5.1 Pharmacodynamic properties
Coal tar has been used dermatologically for hundreds of years and has been shown to be safe and effective in the treatment of scaly skin conditions such as psoriasis. The British Pharmacopoeia contains monographs on coal tar and coal tar solution, and many formulations of coal tar are used in hospitals throughout the country. The coal tar used in Psoriderm Cream has been specially distilled and is based on a neutral fraction which has been shown to be effective in the treatment of psoriasis.

The precise mechanism of action of coal tar is not understood, largely as a result of it comprising up to 10,000 components. There is evidence that topical application of coal tar improves psoriasis by reducing the excessive rate of mitotic epidermal cell division.

Lecithin is a well known phospholipid which is present in foodstuffs. It is added to Psoriderm Cream to soften psoriasis scales and thereby enhance the absorption of the coal tar.

5.2 Pharmacokinetic properties
Not applicable.

5.3 Preclinical safety data
No relevant information additional to that contained elsewhere in the SPC.

6. PHARMACEUTICAL PARTICULARS

6.1 List of excipients
Stearic Acid; Isopropyl Palmitate; Propylene Glycol; Triethanolamine; Phenoxyethanol; Purified Water.

6.2 Incompatibilities
None known.

6.3 Shelf life
36 months.

6.4 Special precautions for storage
Do not store above 25°C.

6.5 Nature and contents of container
Amber glass jar containing 225 ml. This is supplied as an original pack (OP).

6.6 Instructions for use and handling
Not applicable.

7. MARKETING AUTHORISATION HOLDER
Dermal Laboratories

Tatmore Place, Gosmore

Hitchin, Herts SG4 7QR, UK.

8. MARKETING AUTHORISATION NUMBER(S)
0173/5000R.

9. DATE OF FIRST AUTHORISATION/RENEWAL OF THE AUTHORISATION
18 September 2000.

10. DATE OF REVISION OF THE TEXT
February 2001.

Psoriderm Scalp Lotion

(Dermal Laboratories Limited)

1. NAME OF THE MEDICINAL PRODUCT
PSORIDERM® SCALP LOTION

2. QUALITATIVE AND QUANTITATIVE COMPOSITION
Distilled Coal Tar 2.5% w/v; Lecithin 0.3% w/v.

3. PHARMACEUTICAL FORM
Golden brown coloured foaming therapeutic shampoo.

4. CLINICAL PARTICULARS

4.1 Therapeutic indications
For the topical treatment of psoriasis of the scalp.

4.2 Posology and method of administration
For adults, children and the elderly. Wet the hair thoroughly. Apply a small amount of the shampoo to the scalp, and massage gently until a rich lather has been generated. Retain on the scalp for a few minutes. Remove excess lather with the hands before rinsing with warm water. Repeat the above procedure.

4.3 Contraindications
Not to be used for acute psoriasis. Not to be used in cases of sensitivity to any of the ingredients.

4.4 Special warnings and special precautions for use
Keep away from the eyes and mucous membranes. Replace cap after use. Avoid spillage. For external use only.

4.5 Interaction with other medicinal products and other forms of Interaction
None known.

4.6 Pregnancy and lactation
No special precautions.

4.7 Effects on ability to drive and use machines
None known.

4.8 Undesirable effects
Local side-effects do not normally occur. In rare cases of skin irritation, discontinue treatment.

4.9 Overdose
There are no known toxic effects resulting from excessive use of Psoriderm Scalp Lotion.

5. PHARMACOLOGICAL PROPERTIES

5.1 Pharmacodynamic properties
Coal tar has been used dermatologically for hundreds of years and has been shown to be safe and effective in the treatment of scaly scalp conditions such as psoriasis. The British Pharmacopoeia contains monographs on coal tar and coal tar solution, and many formulations of coal tar are used in hospitals throughout the country. The coal tar used in Psoriderm Scalp Lotion has been specially distilled and is based on a neutral fraction which has been shown to be effective in the treatment of psoriasis.

The precise mechanism of action of coal tar is not understood, largely as a result of it comprising up to 10,000 components. There is evidence that topical application of coal tar improves psoriasis by reducing the excessive rate of mitotic epidermal cell division.

Lecithin is a well known phospholipid which is present in foodstuffs. It is added to Psoriderm Scalp Lotion to soften psoriasis scales and thereby enhance the absorption of the coal tar.

5.2 Pharmacokinetic properties
Not applicable.

5.3 Preclinical safety data
Not applicable.

6. PHARMACEUTICAL PARTICULARS

6.1 List of excipients
Triethanolamine Lauryl Sulphate; Lauric Acid Diethanolamide; Disodium Edetate; Sodium Chloride; Phenoxyethanol; Purified Water.

6.2 Incompatibilities
None known.

6.3 Shelf life
36 months.

6.4 Special precautions for storage
Do not store above 25°C.

6.5 Nature and contents of container
White plastic bottle containing 250 ml. This is supplied as an original pack (OP).

6.6 Instructions for use and handling
Not applicable.

7. MARKETING AUTHORISATION HOLDER
Dermal Laboratories

Tatmore Place, Gosmore

Hitchin, Herts SG4 7QR, UK.

8. MARKETING AUTHORISATION NUMBER(S)
0173/5001R.

9. DATE OF FIRST AUTHORISATION/RENEWAL OF THE AUTHORISATION
18 September 2000.

10. DATE OF REVISION OF THE TEXT
September 2000.

Pulmicort Inhaler

(AstraZeneca UK Limited)

1. NAME OF THE MEDICINAL PRODUCT
Pulmicort® Inhaler

200 micrograms per actuation, pressurised inhalation suspension

2. QUALITATIVE AND QUANTITATIVE COMPOSITION
Pulmicort Inhaler contains budesonide 200 micrograms per actuation (puff).

For excipients, see 6.1.

3. PHARMACEUTICAL FORM
Pulmicort Inhaler is a pressurised inhalation suspension. The suspension is delivered via a pressurised metered dose inhaler (pMDI).

Pulmicort Inhaler may also be administered via Nebuhaler® and Nebuchamber®.

4. CLINICAL PARTICULARS

4.1 Therapeutic indications
Bronchial asthma.

4.2 Posology and method of administration
For oral inhalation.

Adults, including the elderly: 200 micrograms twice daily, in the morning and in the evening. During periods of severe asthma, the daily dosage can be increased up to 1600 micrograms.

In patients whose asthma is well controlled, the daily dose may be reduced below 400 micrograms, but should not go below 200 micrograms.

The dose should be reduced to the minimum needed to maintain good asthma control.

Children:50 to 400 micrograms, to be given twice daily. During periods of severe asthma, the daily dose can be increased up to 800 micrograms.

The dose should be reduced to the minimum needed to maintain good asthma control.

Patients maintained on oral glucocorticosteroids

Pulmicort Inhaler may permit replacement or significant reduction in the dosage of oral glucocorticosteroids while maintaining asthma control. For further information on the withdrawal of oral corticosteroids, see section 4.4.

Pulmicort Inhaler with NebuChamber ®:

Pulmicort Inhaler with NebuChamber consists of a Pulmicort Inhaler attached to a 250ml, non-electrostatic metal spacer, with uni-directional inspiratory and expiratory valves.

The use of Pulmicort Inhaler with NebuChamber {*CE mark*} is recommended to enable patients with difficulty in co-ordinating inhalation with actuation, such as infants, young children, the poorly co-operative or the elderly, to derive greater therapeutic benefit. The use of the NebuChamber spacer device obviates the need to co-ordinate breathing and actuation, whilst also reducing oropharyngeal absorption of budesonide. NebuChamber has been designed to maximise the deposition from a pressurised metered dose inhaler in these patient groups.

Use of Pulmicort Inhaler with Nebuhaler ®:

Nebuhaler is a spacer device available separately that is compatible for use with Pulmicort. Nebuhaler is a Medical Device. Nebuhaler is a 750ml plastic cone with a one-way valve. The use of the Nebuhaler spacer device is recommended to enable patients with difficulty co-ordinating conventional aerosols to derive greater delivery and subsequent therapeutic benefits.

Method of Administration

Instructions for the correct use of Pulmicort Inhaler:

Note: It is important to instruct the patient

- To carefully read the instructions for use in the patient information leaflet, which is packed with each inhaler.
- To shake the inhaler thoroughly before each actuation, in order to mix the contents of the inhaler properly.
- To breathe in slowly and deeply through the mouthpiece and to release the dose whilst continuing to breathe in.

On actuation of Pulmicort Inhaler, a suspension of the substance is pumped out of the canister at a high velocity. When the patient inhales through the mouthpiece at the same time as releasing a dose, the substance will follow the inspired air into the airways.

Instructions for the correct use of Pulmicort Inhaler with NebuChamber:

Note: It is important to instruct the patient:

- To carefully read the instructions for use in the patient information leaflet, which is packed with each inhaler.
- To shake the inhaler thoroughly, in order to mix the contents of the inhaler properly.

On actuation of the aerosol, the dose is released into the inhalation chamber. The inhalation chamber is then emptied by two slow deep breaths. Young children may need to breathe 5 - 10 times through the mouthpiece. For further doses, the procedure is repeated. For young children who are unable to breathe through the mouthpiece, a face mask can be used. Compatible face masks are available separately and care should be taken to ensure a good fit is achieved.

4.3 Contraindications
History of hypersensitivity to budesonide or any of the excipients. No other specific contraindications are known, but special care is needed in patients with lung tuberculosis, fungal and viral infections in the airways.

4.4 Special warnings and special precautions for use
Patients not dependent on steroids: Treatment with the recommended doses of Pulmicort usually gives a therapeutic benefit within 7 days. However, certain patients may have an excessive collection of mucus secretion in the bronchi. In these cases, a short course of oral corticosteroids (usually 1 to 2 weeks) should be given in addition to the aerosol. After the course of the oral drug, the inhaler alone should be sufficient therapy. Exacerbations of asthma caused by bacterial infections are usually controlled by appropriate antibiotic treatment and possibly increasing the Pulmicort dosage or, if necessary, by giving systemic steroids.

Steroid-dependent patients: Transfer of patients on oral steroids to treatment with Pulmicort demands special care, mainly due to the slow restitution of the disturbed hypothalamic-pituitary function, caused by extended treatment with oral corticosteroids. When the Pulmicort treatment is initiated, the patient should be in a relatively stable phase. Pulmicort is then given, in combination with the previously used oral steroid dose, for about 10 days.

After this period of time, the reduction of oral steroid dose can be started, with a dose reduction corresponding to about 1 mg prednisolone per day, every week. The oral dose is thus reduced to the lowest level which, in combination with Pulmicort, gives a stable respiratory capacity.

In many cases, it may eventually be possible to completely substitute the oral steroid with Pulmicort treatment, but other cases may have to be maintained on a low oral steroid dosage.

Some patients may experience uneasiness during the withdrawal period due to a decreased steroid effect. The physician may have to explain the reason for the Pulmicort treatment in order to encourage the patient to continue. The length of time needed for the body to regain its natural production of corticosteroid in sufficient amounts is often extensive. Prolonged treatment with high doses of inhaled corticosteroids, particularly higher than the recommended doses, may result in clinically significant adrenal suppression. Additional systemic corticosteroid cover should be considered during periods of stress or elective surgery.

During transfer from oral therapy to Pulmicort, a generally lower systemic steroid action will be experienced which may result in the appearance of allergic or arthritic symptoms such as rhinitis, eczema and muscle and joint pain. Specific treatment should be initiated for these conditions. A general insufficient glucocorticosteroid effect should be suspected if, in rare cases, symptoms such as tiredness, headache, nausea and vomiting should occur. In these cases a temporary increase in the dose of oral glucocorticosteroids is sometimes necessary.

As with other inhalation therapy, paradoxical bronchospasm may occur, with an immediate increase in wheezing after dosing. If a severe reaction occurs, treatment should be reassessed and an alternative therapy instituted if necessary.

Systemic effects of inhaled corticosteroids may occur, particularly at high doses prescribed for prolonged periods. These effects are much less likely to occur than with oral corticosteroids. Possible systemic effects include adrenal suppression, growth retardation in children and adolescents, decrease in bone mineral density, cataract and glaucoma.

It is important, therefore, that the dose of inhaled corticosteroid is titrated to the lowest dose at which effective control of asthma is maintained.

It is recommended that the height of children receiving prolonged treatment with inhaled corticosteroids is regularly monitored. If growth is slowed, therapy should be reviewed with the aim of reducing the dose of inhaled corticosteroid, if possible, to the lowest dose at which effective control of asthma is maintained. In addition, consideration should be given to referring the patient to a paediatric respiratory specialist.

If patients find short-acting bronchodilator treatment ineffective, or they need more inhalations than usual, medical attention must be sought. In this situation consideration should be given to the need for or an increase in their regular therapy, e.g., higher doses of inhaled budesonide, the addition of a long-acting beta agonist or a course of oral glucocorticosteroid.

Reduced liver function may affect the elimination of glucocorticosteroids. The plasma clearance following an intravenous dose of budesonide however was similar in cirrhotic patients and in healthy subjects. After oral ingestion systemic availability of budesonide was increased by compromised liver function due to decreased first pass metabolism. The clinical relevance of this to treatment with Pulmicort is unknown as no data exist for inhaled budesonide, but increases in plasma levels and hence an increased risk of systemic adverse effects could be expected.

In vivo studies have shown that oral administration of ketoconazole and itraconazole (known inhibitors of CYP3A4 activity in the liver and in the intestinal mucosa) causes an increase in the systemic exposure to budesonide. Concomitant treatment with ketoconazole and itraconazole or other potent CYP3A4 inhibitors should be avoided (see section 4.5 Interactions). If this is not possible, the time interval between administration of the interacting drugs should be as long as possible. A reduction in the dose of budesonide should also be considered.

4.5 Interaction with other medicinal products and other forms of Interaction
The metabolism of budesonide is primarily mediated by CYP3A4, one of the cytochrome p450 enzymes. Inhibitors of this enzyme, e.g. ketoconazole and itraconazole, can therefore increase systemic exposure to budesonide, (see Section 4.4 Special Warnings and Special Precautions for Use and Section 5.2 Pharmacokinetic Properties). Other potent inhibitors of CYP3A4 are also likely to markedly increase plasma levels of budesonide.

4.6 Pregnancy and lactation
Data on approximately 2000 exposed pregnancies indicate no increased teratogenic risk associated with the use of inhaled budesonide. In animal studies, glucocorticosteroids have been shown to induce malformations (see Section 5.3). This is not likely to be relevant for humans given recommended doses, but therapy with inhaled budesonide should be regularly reviewed and maintained at the lowest effective dose.

The administration of budesonide during pregnancy requires that the benefits for the mother be weighed against the risk for the foetus. Inhaled glucocorticosteroids should be considered in preference to oral glucocorticosteroids because of the lower systemic effects at the doses required to achieve similar pulmonary responses. There is no information regarding the passage of budesonide into breast milk.

4.7 Effects on ability to drive and use machines
Pulmicort Inhaler does not affect the ability to drive or operate machinery.

4.8 Undesirable effects
Clinical trials, literature reports and post-marketing experience suggest that the following adverse drug reactions may occur:

Common (>1/100, <1/10)	• Mild irritation in the throat • Candida infection in the oropharynx • Hoarseness • Coughing
Rare (>1/10 000, <1/1 000)	• Nervousness, restlessness, depression, behavioural disturbances • Immediate and delayed hypersensitivity reactions including rash, contact dermatitis, urticaria, angioedema and bronchospasm • Skin bruising

The candida infection in the oropharynx is due to drug deposition. Advising the patient to rinse the mouth out with water after each dosing will minimise the risk. The incidence should be less with the NebuChamber® and Nebuhaler®, as these reduce oral deposition.

As with other inhalation therapy, paradoxical bronchospasm may occur in very rare cases (see Section 4.4).

Systemic effects of inhaled corticosteroids may occur, particularly at high doses prescribed for prolonged periods. These effects are much less likely to occur than with oral corticosteroids. Possible systemic effects include adrenal suppression, growth retardation in children and adolescents, decrease in bone mineral density, cataract and glaucoma. The effect is probably dependent on dose, exposure time, concomitant and previous steroid exposure, and individual sensitivity.

4.9 Overdose
The only harmful effect that follows inhalation of large amounts of the drug over a short period is suppression of hypothalamic-pituitary-adrenal (HPA) axis function. No special emergency action needs to be taken. Treatment with Pulmicort Inhaler should be continued at the recommended dose to control the asthma.

5. PHARMACOLOGICAL PROPERTIES

5.1 Pharmacodynamic properties
Budesonide is a glucocorticosteroid which possesses a high local anti-inflammatory action, with a lower incidence and severity of adverse effects than those seen with oral corticosteroids.

Pharmacotherapeutic group: Other drugs for obstructive airway diseases, inhalants, glucocorticoids. ATC Code: RO3B A02.

Topical anti-inflammatory effect
The exact mechanism of action of glucocorticosteroids in the treatment of asthma is not fully understood. Anti-inflammatory actions, such as inhibition of inflammatory mediator release and inhibition of cytokine-mediated immune response are probably important.

A clinical study in asthmatics comparing inhaled and oral budesonide at doses calculated to achieve similar systemic bioavailability demonstrated statistically significant evidence of efficacy with inhaled but not oral budesonide compared with placebo. Thus, the therapeutic effect of conventional doses of inhaled budesonide may be largely explained by its direct action on the respiratory tract.

In a provocation study pre-treatment with budesonide for four weeks has shown decreased bronchial constriction in immediate as well as late asthmatic reactions.

Onset of effect
After a single dose of orally inhaled budesonide, delivered via dry powder inhaler, improvement of the lung function is achieved within a few hours. After therapeutic use of orally inhaled budesonide delivered via dry powder inhaler, improvement in lung function has been shown to occur within 2 days of initiation of treatment, although maximum benefit may not be achieved for up to 4 weeks.

Airway reactivity
Budesonide has also been shown to decrease airway reactivity to histamine and methacholine in hyper-reactive patients.

Exercise-induced asthma
Therapy with inhaled budesonide has effectively been used for prevention of exercise-induced asthma.

Growth
Limited data from long term studies suggest that most children and adolescents treated with inhaled budesonide ultimately achieve their adult target height. However, an initial small but transient reduction in growth (approximately 1 cm) has been observed. This generally occurs within the first year of treatment (see section 4.4).

HPA axis function
Studies in healthy volunteers with inhaled budesonide (administered as a dry powder via Turbohaler) have shown dose-related effects on plasma and urinary cortisol. At recommended doses, Pulmicort Turbohaler, causes less effect on the adrenal function than prednisolone 10mg, as shown by ACTH tests.

5.2 Pharmacokinetic properties
In healthy volunteers, inhalation of tritium radiolabelled budesonide quickly gives a high plasma concentration and shows good lung deposition and minimal lung biotransformation, thus prolonging duration of action. Systemic availability after inhalation is approximately 70%.

Plasma concentration decreases exponentially with a plasma half-life of 2 ± 0.2 hours.

The metabolism of budesonide is primarily mediated by CYP3A4, one of the cytochrome p450 enzymes. Rapid systemic biotransformation, with relatively inactive metabolites, thereby minimises the risk of systemic effects.

In a study, 100 mg ketoconazole taken twice daily, increased plasma levels of concomitantly administered oral budesonide (single dose of 10 mg) on average, by 7.8-fold. Information about this interaction is lacking for inhaled budesonide, but marked increases in plasma levels could be expected.

5.3 Preclinical safety data
The acute toxicity of budesonide is low and of the same order of magnitude and type as that of the reference glucocorticoids studied (beclomethasone dipropionate, fluocinolone acetonide).

Results from subacute and chronic toxicity studies show that the systemic effects of budesonide are less severe than, or similar to, those observed after administration of the other glucocorticosteroids, e.g. decreased body weight gain and atrophy of lymphoid tissues and adrenal cortex.

An increased incidence of brain gliomas in male rats, in a carcinogenicity study, could not be verified in a repeat study in which the incidence of gliomas did not differ between any of the groups on active treatment (budesonide, prednisolone, triamcinolone acetonide) and the control groups.

Liver changes (primary hepatocellular neoplasms) found in male rats in the original carcinogenicity study were noted again in the repeat study with budesonide, as well as with the reference glucocorticosteroids. These effects are most probably related to a receptor effect and thus represent a class effect.

Available clinical experience shows no indication that budesonide, or other glucocorticosteroids, induce brain gliomas or primary heptocellular neoplasms in man.

In animal reproduction studies, corticosteroids such as budesonide have been shown to induce malformations (cleft palate, skeletal malformations). However, these animal experimental results do not appear to be relevant in humans at the recommended doses.

Animal studies have also identified an involvement of excess prenatal glucocorticosteroids, in increased risk for intrauterine growth retardation, adult cardiovascular disease and permanent changes in glucocorticoid receptor density, neurotransmitter turnover and behaviour at exposures below the teratogenic dose range.

6. PHARMACEUTICAL PARTICULARS

6.1 List of excipients

Sorbitan trioleate, trichlorodifluoromethane (CFC 12), dichlorotetrafluoroethane (CFC 114) and trichlorofluoromethane (CFC 11).

6.2 Incompatibilities

None known.

6.3 Shelf life

2 years.

6.4 Special precautions for storage

Do not store above 30°C.

Do not puncture or expose the canister to high temperatures (40°C) or direct sunlight, even when empty.

6.5 Nature and contents of container

Pulmicort Inhaler is a pressurised metered dose inhaler delivering 200 micrograms budesonide in each actuation.

Pulmicort Inhaler consists of an aluminium vial with a metering valve which is fitted into a plastic device through which the dose is released.

100 and 200 actuation packs are available.

Pulmicort Inhaler is also available with NebuChamber. NebuChamber is a medical device. NebuChamber is a non-electrostatic metal spacer consisting of a 250ml inhalation chamber with unidirectional inspiratory and expiratory valves.

NebuChamber is constructed of stainless steel, it is entirely free of electrostatic forces. Drug delivery will not be affected by any electrostatic forces in the NebuChamber.

6.6 Instructions for use and handling

See *Section 4.2 Posology and Method of Administration*.

Pulmicort Inhaler may also be used in conjunction with a Nebuhaler spacer device. Nebuhaler is a Medical Device supplied separately with full instructions for use.

7. MARKETING AUTHORISATION HOLDER

AstraZeneca UK Ltd.,

600 Capability Green

Luton

LU1 3LU, UK.

8. MARKETING AUTHORISATION NUMBER(S)

PL 17901/0158

9. DATE OF FIRST AUTHORISATION/RENEWAL OF THE AUTHORISATION

12th August 2002

10. DATE OF REVISION OF THE TEXT

4th April 2005

Pulmicort LS Inhaler

(AstraZeneca UK Limited)

1. NAME OF THE MEDICINAL PRODUCT

Pulmicort® LS Inhaler, 50 micrograms per actuation, pressurised inhalation suspension.

2. QUALITATIVE AND QUANTITATIVE COMPOSITION

Pulmicort LS Inhaler contains budesonide, 50 micrograms per actuation (puff).

For excipients see 6.1.

3. PHARMACEUTICAL FORM

Pulmicort LS Inhaler is a pressurised inhalation suspension. The suspension is delivered via a pressurised metered dose inhaler (pMDI).

Pulmicort LS inhaler may also be administered via the Nebuhaler®.

4. CLINICAL PARTICULARS

4.1 Therapeutic indications

Pulmicort LS Inhaler is recommended in patients with bronchial asthma.

4.2 Posology and method of administration

Adults: 200 micrograms twice daily, in the morning and in the evening. During periods of severe asthma, the daily dosage can be increased up to 1600 micrograms.

In patients whose asthma is well controlled, the daily dose may be reduced below 400 micrograms, but should not go below 200 micrograms.

The dose should be reduced to the minimum needed to maintain good asthma control.

Children: 50 to 400 micrograms to be given twice daily. During periods of severe asthma, the daily dose can be increased up to 800 micrograms.

The dose should be reduced to the minimum needed to maintain good asthma control.

Elderly: Dosage as for adults.

Patients maintained on oral glucocorticosteroids

Pulmicort Inhaler may permit replacement or significant reduction in the dosage of oral glucocorticosteroids while maintaining asthma control. For further information on the withdrawal of oral corticosteroids, see section 4.4

Instructions for the correct use of Pulmicort LS Inhaler:

Note: It is important to instruct the patient

- To carefully read the instructions for use in the patient information leaflet, which is packed with each inhaler.
- To shake the inhaler thoroughly before each actuation, in order to mix the contents of the inhaler properly.
- To breathe in slowly and deeply through the mouthpiece and to release the dose whilst continuing to breathe in.

On actuation of Pulmicort LS Inhaler, a suspension of the substance is pumped out of the canister at a high velocity. When the patient inhales through the mouthpiece at the same time as releasing a dose, the substance will follow the inspired air into the airways.

4.3 Contraindications

History of hypersensitivity to budesonide or any of the excipients. No other specific contraindications are known, but special care is needed in patients with lung tuberculosis, fungal and viral infections in the airways.

4.4 Special warnings and special precautions for use

Patients not dependent on steroids: Treatment with the recommended doses of Pulmicort LS Inhaler usually gives a therapeutic benefit within 7 days. However, certain patients may have an excessive collection of mucous secretion in the bronchi, which reduces penetration of the active substance into the airways. In these cases, a short course of oral corticosteroids (usually 1 to 2 weeks) should be given in addition to the aerosol. After the course of the oral drug, the inhaler alone should be sufficient therapy. Exacerbations of asthma caused by bacterial infections are usually controlled by appropriate antibiotic treatment and possibly increasing the Pulmicort LS Inhaler dosage or, if necessary, by giving systemic steroids.

Steroid-dependent patients: Transfer of patients dependent upon oral steroids to treatment with Pulmicort LS Inhaler demands special care, mainly due to the slow restitution of the disturbed hypothalamic-pituitary function, caused by extended treatment with oral corticosteroids. When the Pulmicort LS Inhaler treatment is initiated, the patient should be in a relatively stable phase. Pulmicort LS Inhaler is then given in combination with the previously used oral steroid dose, for about 10 days.

After this period of time, the reduction of the oral corticosteroid dose can be started, with a dose reduction corresponding to about 1 mg prednisolone per day, every week. The oral dose is thus reduced to the lowest level which, in combination with Pulmicort LS Inhaler, gives a stable respiratory capacity.

In many cases, it may eventually be possible to completely substitute the oral steroid with Pulmicort LS Inhaler, but other cases may have to be maintained on a low steroid dosage.

Some patients may experience unease during the withdrawal period due to a decreased steroid effect. The physician may have to explain the reason for the Pulmicort LS Inhaler treatment in order to encourage the patient to continue. The length of time needed for the body to regain its natural production of corticosteroid in sufficient amounts is often extensive. Prolonged treatment with high doses of inhaled corticosteroids, particularly higher than the recommended doses, may result in clinically significant adrenal suppression. Additional systemic corticosteroid cover should be considered during periods of stress or elective surgery.

During transfer from oral therapy to Pulmicort LS Inhaler, a generally lower systemic steroid action will be experienced which may result in the appearance of allergic or arthritic symptoms such as rhinitis, eczema, and muscle and joint pain. Specific treatment should be initiated for these conditions. A general insufficient glucocorticosteroid effect should be suspected if, in rare cases, symptoms such as tiredness, headache, nausea and vomiting should occur. In these cases a temporary increase in the dose of oral glucocorticosteroids is sometimes necessary.

As with other inhalation therapy, paradoxical bronchospasm may occur, with an immediate increase in wheezing after dosing. If a severe reaction occurs, treatment should be reassessed and an alternative therapy instituted if necessary.

Systemic effects of inhaled corticosteroids may occur, particularly at high doses prescribed for prolonged periods. These effects are much less likely to occur than with oral corticosteroids. Possible systemic effects include adrenal suppression, growth retardation in children and adolescents, decrease in bone mineral density, cataract and glaucoma.

It is important, therefore, that the dose of inhaled corticosteroid is titrated to the lowest dose at which effective control of asthma is maintained.

It is recommended that the height of children receiving prolonged treatment with inhaled corticosteroids is regularly monitored. If growth is slowed, therapy should be reviewed with the aim of reducing the dose of inhaled corticosteroid, if possible, to the lowest dose at which effective control of asthma is maintained. In addition, consideration should be given to referring the patient to a paediatric respiratory specialist.

If patients find short-acting bronchodilator treatment ineffective, or they need more inhalations than usual, medical attention must be sought. In this situation consideration should be given to the need for or an increase in their regulartherapy, e.g., higher doses of inhaled budesonide, the addition of a long-acting beta agonist or a course of oral glucocorticosteroid.

Reduced liver function may affect the elimination of glucocorticosteroids. The plasma clearance following an intravenous dose of budesonide however was similar in cirrhotic patients and in healthy subjects. After oral ingestion systemic availability of budesonide was increased by compromised liver function due to decreased first pass metabolism. The clinical relevance of this to treatment with Pulmicort is unknown as no data exist for inhaled budesonide, but increases in plasma levels and hence an increased risk of systemic adverse effects could be expected.

In vivo studies have shown that oral administration of ketoconazole and itraconazole (known inhibitors of CYP3A4 activity in the liver and in the intestinal mucosa) causes an increase in the systemic exposure to budesonide. Concomitant treatment with ketoconazole and itraconazole or other potent CYP3A4 inhibitors should be avoided (see section 4.5 Interactions). If this is not possible, the time interval between administration of the interacting drugs should be as long as possible. A reduction in the dose of budesonide should also be considered.

4.5 Interaction with other medicinal products and other forms of Interaction

The metabolism of budesonide is primarily mediated by CYP3A4, one of the cytochrome p450 enzymes. Inhibitors of this enzyme, e.g. ketoconazole and itraconazole, can therefore increase systemic exposure to budesonide, (see Section 4.4 Special Warnings and Special Precautions for Use and Section 5.2 Pharmacokinetic Properties). Other potent inhibitors of CYP3A4 are also likely to markedly increase plasma levels of budesonide.

4.6 Pregnancy and lactation

Data on approximately 2000 exposed pregnancies indicate no increased teratogenic risk associated with the use of inhaled budesonide. In animal studies, glucocorticosteroids have been shown to induce malformations (see Section 5.3). This is not likely to be relevant for humans given recommended doses, but therapy with inhaled budesonide should be regularly reviewed and maintained at the lowest effective dose.

The administration of budesonide during pregnancy requires that the benefits for the mother be weighed against the risk for the foetus. Inhaled glucocorticosteroids should be considered in preference to oral glucocorticosteroids because of the lower systemic effects at the doses required to achieve similar pulmonary responses. There is no information regarding the passage of budesonide into breast milk.

4.7 Effects on ability to drive and use machines

Pulmicort LS Inhaler does not affect ability to drive or use machines.

4.8 Undesirable effects

Clinical trials, literature reports and post-marketing experience suggest that the following adverse drug reactions may occur:

Common (>1/100, <1/10)	• Mild irritation in the throat • Candida infection in the oropharynx • Hoarseness • Coughing
Rare (>1/10 000, <1/1 000)	• Nervousness, restlessness, depression, behavioural disturbances • Immediate and delayed hypersensitivity reactions including rash, contact dermatitis, urticaria, angioedema and bronchospasm • Skin bruising

The candida infection in the oropharynx is due to drug deposition. Advising the patient to rinse the mouth out with water after each dosing will minimise the risk. The incidence should be less with the Nebuhaler®, as this reduces oral deposition.

As with other inhalation therapy, paradoxical bronchospasm may occur in very rare cases (see Section 4.4).

Systemic effects of inhaled corticosteroids may occur, particularly at high doses prescribed for prolonged periods. These effects are much less likely to occur than with oral corticosteroids. Possible systemic effects include adrenal suppression, growth retardation in children and adolescents, decrease in bone mineral density, cataract and glaucoma. The effect is probably dependent on dose, exposure time, concomitant and previous steroid exposure, and individual sensitivity.

4.9 Overdose

The only harmful effect that follows inhalation of large amounts of the drug over a short period is suppression of hypothalamic-pituitary-adrenal (HPA) function. No special emergency action needs to be taken. Treatment with

Pulmicort LS Inhaler should be continued at the recommended dose to control the asthma.

5. PHARMACOLOGICAL PROPERTIES

5.1 Pharmacodynamic properties

Budesonide is a glucocorticosteroid which possesses a high local anti-inflammatory action, with a lower incidence and severity of adverse effects than those seen with oral corticosteroids

Pharmacotherapeutic group: Other drugs for obstructive airway diseases, inhalants, glucocorticoids. ATC Code: RO3B A02.

Topical anti-inflammatory effect

The exact mechanism of action of glucocorticosteroids in the treatment of asthma is not fully understood. Anti-inflammatory actions, such as inhibition of inflammatory mediator release and inhibition of cytokine-mediated immune response are probably important.

A clinical study in asthmatics comparing inhaled and oral budesonide at doses calculated to achieve similar systemic bioavailability demonstrated statistically significant evidence of efficacy with inhaled but not oral budesonide compared with placebo. Thus, the therapeutic effect of conventional doses of inhaled budesonide may be largely explained by its direct action on the respiratory tract.

In a provocation study pre-treatment with budesonide for four weeks has shown decreased bronchial constriction in immediate as well as late asthmatic reactions.

Onset of effect

After a single dose of orally inhaled budesonide, delivered via dry powder inhaler, improvement of the lung function is achieved within a few hours. After therapeutic use of orally inhaled budesonide delivered via dry powder inhaler, improvement in lung function has been shown to occur within 2 days of initiation of treatment, although maximum benefit may not be achieved for up to 4 weeks.

Airway reactivity

Budesonide has also been shown to decrease airway reactivity to histamine and methacholine in hyper-reactive patients.

Exercise-induced asthma

Therapy with inhaled budesonide has effectively been used for prevention of exercise-induced asthma.

Growth

Limited data from long term studies suggest that most children and adolescents treated with inhaled budesonide ultimately achieve their adult target height. However, an initial small but transient reduction in growth (approximately 1 cm) has been observed. This generally occurs within the first year of treatment (see section 4.4).

HPA axis function

Studies in healthy volunteers with inhaled budesonide (administered as a dry powder via Turbohaler) have shown dose-related effects on plasma and urinary cortisol. At recommended doses, Pulmicort Turbohaler, causes less effect on the adrenal function than prednisolone 10mg, as shown by ACTH tests.

5.2 Pharmacokinetic properties

Budesonide is a glucocorticosteroid with high local anti-inflammatory effect.

Budesonide undergoes extensive biotransformation in the liver, to metabolites of low glucocorticosteroid activity. The glucocorticosteroid activity of the major metabolites 6β-hydroxybudesonide and 16α-hydroxyprednisolone, is less than 1% of that of budesonide. The metabolism of budesonide is primarily mediated by CYP3A4, one of the cytochrome p450 enzymes.

In a study, 100 mg ketoconazole taken twice daily, increased plasma levels of concomitantly administered oral budesonide (single dose of 10 mg) on average, by 7.8-fold. Information about this interaction is lacking for inhaled budesonide, but marked increases in plasma levels could be expected.

About 10% of the dose is deposited in the lungs. Of the fraction of budesonide which is swallowed, approximately 90% is inactivated at first passage through the liver. The maximal plasma concentration after inhalation of 1 mg budesonide is about 2.1 nmol/L and is reached after about 10 minutes.

5.3 Preclinical safety data

The acute toxicity of budesonide is low and of the same order of magnitude and type as that of the reference glucocorticosteroids studied (beclomethasone dipropionate, fluocinolone acetonide).

Results from subacute and chronic toxicity studies show that the systemic effects of budesonide are less severe than, or similar to, those observed after administration of the other glucocorticosteroids, e.g. decreased body-weight gain and atrophy of lymphoid tissues and adrenal cortex.

An increased incidence of brain gliomas in male rats, in a carcinogenicity study, could not be verified in a repeat study in which the incidence of gliomas did not differ between any of the groups on active treatment (budesonide, prednisolone, triamcinolone acetonide) and the control groups.

Liver changes (primary hepatocellular neoplasms) found in male rats in the original carcinogenicity study were noted again in the repeat study with budesonide, as well as with the reference glucocorticosteroids. These effects are most probably related to a receptor effect and thus represent a class effect.

Available clinical experience shows no indication that budesonide, or other glucocorticosteroids, induce brain gliomas or primary hepatocellular neoplasms in man.

In animal reproduction studies, corticosteroids such as budesonide have been shown to induce malformations (cleft palate, skeletal malformations). However, these animal experimental results do not appear to be relevant in humans at the recommended doses.

Animal studies have also identified an involvement of excess prenatal glucocorticosteroids, in increased risk for intrauterine growth retardation, adult cardiovascular disease and permanent changes in glucocorticoid receptor density, neurotransmitter turnover and behaviour at exposures below the teratogenic dose range.

6. PHARMACEUTICAL PARTICULARS

6.1 List of excipients

Sorbitan trioleate, trichlorofluoromethane, dichlorotetrafluoroethane, dichlorodifluoromethane.

6.2 Incompatibilities

None known.

6.3 Shelf life

24 months

6.4 Special precautions for storage

Do not store above 30°C.

Do not puncture or expose the canister to high temperatures (40°C) or direct sunlight, even when empty.

6.5 Nature and contents of container

Aluminium canister containing 200 metered doses of budesonide, fitted with a valve to deliver 50 micrograms budesonide per actuation. The canister fits into a plastic adaptor made of polypropylene, with a removable cover made of polypropylene or polyethylene.

6.6 Instructions for use and handling

See Section 4.2 Posology and Method of Administration.

7. MARKETING AUTHORISATION HOLDER

AstraZeneca UK Ltd.,
600 Capability Green,
Luton, LU1 3LU, UK.

8. MARKETING AUTHORISATION NUMBER(S)

PL 17901/0159

9. DATE OF FIRST AUTHORISATION/RENEWAL OF THE AUTHORISATION

28th June 2002

10. DATE OF REVISION OF THE TEXT

4th April 2004

Pulmicort Respules 0.5mg & 1mg Nebuliser Suspension

(AstraZeneca UK Limited)

1. NAME OF THE MEDICINAL PRODUCT

Pulmicort® Respules® 0.5 mg, nebuliser suspension.

Pulmicort® Respules® 1 mg, nebuliser suspension.

2. QUALITATIVE AND QUANTITATIVE COMPOSITION

Pulmicort® Respules® 0.5 mg, nebuliser suspension:

Budesonide 0.25 mg/ml. Each 2 ml Respule contains 0.5 mg budesonide.

Pulmicort® Respules® 1 mg, nebuliser suspension:

Budesonide 0.5 mg/ml. Each 2 ml Respule contains 1 mg budesonide.

For excipients, see 6.1.

3. PHARMACEUTICAL FORM

A white to off-white nebuliser suspension.

4. CLINICAL PARTICULARS

4.1 Therapeutic indications

Pulmicort Respules contain the potent, non-halogenated, corticosteroid, budesonide, for use in bronchial asthma, in patients where use of a pressurised inhaler or dry powder formulation is unsatisfactory or inappropriate.

Pulmicort Respules are also recommended for use in infants and children with acute laryngotracheobronchitis - croup.

4.2 Posology and method of administration

Dosage schedules: Pulmicort Respules should be administered from suitable nebulisers. The dose delivered to the patient varies depending on the nebulising equipment used. The nebulisation time and the dose delivered is dependent on flow rate, volume of nebuliser chamber and fill volume. An air-flow rate of 6 - 8 litres per minute through the device should be employed. A suitable fill volume for most nebulisers is 2 - 4 ml. The dosage of Pulmicort Respules should be adjusted to the need of the individual. The dose should be reduced to the minimum needed to maintain good asthma control.

Bronchial asthma

Initiation of therapy

When treatment is started, during periods of severe asthma and while reducing or discontinuing oral glucocorticosteroids, the recommended dose of Pulmicort Respules is:

Adults (including elderly): Usually 1 – 2 mg twice daily. In very severe cases the dosage may be further increased.

Children 12 years and older: Dosage as for adults.

Children 3 months to 12 years: 0.5 – 1 mg twice daily.

Maintenance

The maintenance dose should be individualised and bethe lowest dose which keeps the patient symptom-free.

Adults (including elderly and children 12 years and older): 0.5 - 1 mg twice daily.

Children 3 months to 12 years: 0.25 - 0.5 mg twice daily.

Patients maintained on oral glucocorticosteroids

Pulmicort Respules may permit replacement or significant reduction in dosage of oral glucocorticosteroids while maintaining asthma control. For further information on the withdrawal of oral corticosteroids, see section 4.4.

Dose division and miscibility

Pulmicort Respules can be mixed with 0.9% saline and with solutions for nebulisation of terbutaline, salbutamol, fenoterol, acetylcysteine, sodium cromoglycate or ipratropium bromide.

Recommended Dosage Table

Dose (mg)	Pulmicort Respules 0.5 mg nebuliser solution (0.25 mg/ml) Volume (ml)	Pulmicort Respules 1 mg nebuliser solution (0.5 mg/ml) Volume (ml)
0.25	1	-
0.5	2	1
0.75	3	-
1.0	4	2
1.5	6	3
2.0	8	4

Where an increased therapeutic effect is desired, especially in those patients without major mucus secretion in the airways, an increased dose of Pulmicort is recommended, rather than combined treatment with oral corticosteroids, because of the lower risk of systemic effects.

Acute laryngotracheobronchitis – croup

In infants and children with croup, the usual dose is 2 mg of nebulised budesonide. This dose is given as a single administration, or as two 1 mg doses separated by 30 minutes.

Instruction for correct use of Pulmicort Respules

The Respule should be detached from the strip, shaken gently and opened by twisting off the wing tab. The contents of the Respule should be gently squeezed into the nebuliser cup. The empty Respule should be thrown away and the top of the nebuliser cup replaced.

Pulmicort Respules should be administered via a jet nebuliser equipped with a mouthpiece or suitable face mask. The nebuliser should be connected to an air compressor with an adequate air flow (6-8 L/min), and the fill volume should be 2-4ml.

Note: It is important to instruct the patient

- to carefully read the instructions for use in the patient information leaflet which are packed together with each nebuliser.
- that Ultrasonic nebulisers are not suitable for the administration of Pulmicort Respules and therefore are not recommended.
- Pulmicort Respules can be mixed with 0.9% saline and with solutions for nebulisation of terbutaline, salbutamol, fenoterol, acetylcysteine, sodium cromoglycate and ipratropium bromide.
- to rinse the mouth out with water after inhaling the prescribed dose to minimise the risk of oropharyngeal thrush.
- to wash the facial skin with water after using the face mask to prevent irritation.
- to adequately clean and maintain the nebuliser according to the manufacturer's instructions.

The dosage of Pulmicort Respules should be adjusted to the need of the individual.

4.3 Contraindications

History of hypersensitivity to budesonide or any of the excipients.

4.4 Special warnings and special precautions for use

Special care is needed in patients with pulmonary tuberculosis and viral infections of the airways.

Non steroid-dependent patients: A therapeutic effect is usually reached within 10 days. In patients with excessive mucus secretion in the bronchi, a short (about 2 weeks) additional oral corticosteroid regimen can be given initially. After the course of the oral drug, Pulmicort Respules alone should be sufficient therapy.

Steroid-dependent patients: When transfer from oral corticosteroid to treatment with Pulmicort is initiated, the patient should be in a relatively stable phase. Pulmicort is then given, in combination with the previously used oral steroid dose, for about 10 days.

After that, the oral steroid dose should be gradually reduced (by, for example, 2.5 mg prednisolone or the equivalent each month), to the lowest possible level. In many cases, it is possible to completely substitute Pulmicort for the oral corticosteroid.

During transfer from oral therapy to Pulmicort, a generally lower systemic corticosteroid action will be experienced, which may result in the appearance of allergic or arthritic symptoms such as rhinitis, eczema and muscle and joint pain. Specific treatment should be initiated for these conditions. A general insufficient glucocorticosteroid effect should be suspected if, in rare cases, symptoms such as tiredness, headache, nausea and vomiting should occur. In these cases a temporary increase in the dose of oral glucocorticosteroids is sometimes necessary.

As with other inhalation therapy, paradoxical bronchospasm may occur, with an immediate increase in wheezing after dosing. If a severe reaction occurs, treatment should be reassessed and an alternative therapy instituted if necessary.

Prolonged treatment with high doses of inhaled corticosteroids, particularly higher than the recommended doses, may result in clinically significant adrenal suppression. Additional systemic corticosteroid cover should be considered during periods of stress or elective surgery.

Systemic effects of inhaled corticosteroids may occur, particularly at high doses prescribed for prolonged periods. These effects are much less likely to occur than with oral corticosteroids. Possible systemic effects include adrenal suppression, growth retardation in children and adolescents, decrease in bone mineral density, cataract and glaucoma.

It is important, therefore, that the dose of inhaled corticosteroid is titrated to the lowest dose at which effective control of asthma is maintained.

It is recommended that the height of children receiving prolonged treatment with inhaled corticosteroids is regularly monitored. If growth is slowed, therapy should be reviewed, with the aim of reducing the dose of inhaled corticosteroid, if possible, to the lowest dose at which effective control of asthma is maintained. In addition, consideration should be given to referring the patient to a paediatric respiratory specialist.

Pulmicort Respules is not intended for rapid relief of acute episodes of asthma where an inhaled short-acting bronchodilator is required. If patients find short-acting bronchodilator treatment ineffective, or they need more inhalations than usual, medical attention must be sought. In this situation consideration should be given to the need for or an increase in their regular therapy, e.g., higher doses of inhaled budesonide or the addition of a long-acting beta agonist, or for a course of oral glucocorticosteroid.

Reduced liver function may affect the elimination of glucocorticosteroids. The plasma clearance following an intravenous dose of budesonide however was similar in cirrhotic patients and in healthy subjects. After oral ingestion systemic availability of budesonide was increased by compromised liver function due to decreased first pass metabolism. The clinical relevance of this to treatment with Pulmicort is unknown as no data exist for inhaled budesonide, but increases in plasma levels and hence an increased risk of systemic adverse effects could be expected.

In vivo studies have shown that oral administration of ketoconazole and itraconazole (known inhibitors of CYP3A4 activity in the liver and in the intestinal mucosa causes an increase in the systemic exposure to budesonide. Concomitant treatment with ketoconazole and itraconazole or other potent CYP3A4 inhibitors should be avoided (see section 4.5 Interactions). If this is not possible, the time interval between administration of the interacting drugs should be as long as possible. A reduction in the dose of budesonide should also be considered.

The nebuliser chamber should be cleaned after every administration. Wash the nebuliser chamber and mouthpiece or face-mask in hot water using a mild detergent. Rinse well and dry, by connecting the nebuliser chamber to the compressor or air inlet.

4.5 Interaction with other medicinal products and other forms of Interaction

The metabolism of budesonide is primarily mediated by CYP3A4, one of the cytochrome p450 enzymes. Inhibitors of this enzyme, e.g. ketoconazole and itraconazole, can therefore increase systemic exposure to budesonide, (see Section 4.4 Special Warnings and Special Precautions for Use and Section 5.2 Pharmacokinetic Properties). Other potent inhibitors of CYP3A4 are also likely to markedly increase plasma levels of budesonide.

4.6 Pregnancy and lactation

Data on approximately 2000 exposed pregnancies indicate no increased teratogenic risk associated with the use of inhaled budesonide. In animal studies, glucocorticosteroids have been shown to induce malformations (see Section 5.3). This is not likely to be relevant for humans given recommended doses, but therapy with inhaled budesonide should be regularly reviewed and maintained at the lowest effective dose.

The administration of budesonide during pregnancy requires that the benefits for the mother be weighed against the risk for the foetus. Inhaled glucocorticosteroids should be considered in preference to oral glucocorticosteroids because of the lower systemic effects at the doses required to achieve similar pulmonary responses. There is no information regarding the passage of budesonide into breast milk.

4.7 Effects on ability to drive and use machines

Pulmicort does not affect the ability to drive or use machinery.

4.8 Undesirable effects

Clinical trials, literature reports and post-marketing experience suggest that the following adverse drug reactions may occur:

Common (>1/100, <1/10)	• Mild irritation in the throat • Candida infection in the oropharynx • Hoarseness • Coughing
Rare (>1/10 000, <1/1 000)	• Nervousness, restlessness, depression, behavioural disturbances • Immediate and delayed hypersensitivity reactions including rash, contact dermatitis, urticaria, angioedema and bronchospasm • Skin bruising

The candida infection in the oropharynx is due to drug deposition. Advising the patient to rinse the mouth out with water after each dosing will minimise the risk.

As with other inhalation therapy, paradoxical bronchospasm may occur in very rare cases (see Section 4.4).

Systemic effects of inhaled corticosteroids may occur, particularly at high doses prescribed for prolonged periods. These effects are much less likely to occur than with oral corticosteroids. Possible systemic effects include adrenal suppression, growth retardation in children and adolescents, decrease in bone mineral density, cataract and glaucoma. The effect is probably dependent on dose, exposure time, concomitant and previous steroid exposure, and individual sensitivity.

Facial skin irritation has occurred in some cases when a nebuliser with a face mask has been used. To prevent irritation, the facial skin should be washed with water after use of the face mask.

4.9 Overdose

Pulmicort Respules contains 0.1 mg/ml disodium edetate which has been shown to cause bronchoconstriction at levels above 1.2 mg/ml. Acute overdose with Pulmicort should not present a clinical problem.

5. PHARMACOLOGICAL PROPERTIES

5.1 Pharmacodynamic properties

Budesonide is a glucocorticosteroid which possesses a high local anti-inflammatory action, with a lower incidence and severity of adverse effects than those seen with oral corticosteroids.

Pharmacotherapeutic group: Other drugs for obstructive airway diseases, inhalants, glucocorticoids. ATC Code: RO3B A02.

Topical anti-inflammatory effect

The exact mechanism of action of glucocorticosteroids in the treatment of asthma is not fully understood. Anti-inflammatory actions, such as inhibition of inflammatory mediator release and inhibition of cytokine-mediated immune response are probably important.

A clinical study in asthmatics comparing inhaled and oral budesonide at doses calculated to achieve similar systemic bioavailability demonstrated statistically significant evidence of efficacy with inhaled but not oral budesonide compared with placebo. Thus, the therapeutic effect of conventional doses of inhaled budesonide may be largely explained by its direct action on the respiratory tract.

In a provocation study pre-treatment with budesonide for four weeks has shown decreased bronchial constriction in immediate as well as late asthmatic reactions.

Onset of effect

After a single dose of orally inhaled budesonide, delivered via dry powder inhaler, improvement of the lung function is achieved within a few hours. After therapeutic use of orally inhaled budesonide delivered via dry powder inhaler, improvement in lung function has been shown to occur within 2 days of initiation of treatment although maximum benefit may not be achieved for up to 4 weeks.

Airway reactivity

Budesonide has also been shown to decrease airway reactivity to histamine and methacholine in hyperreactive patients.

Exercise-induced asthma

Therapy with inhaled budesonide has effectively been used for prevention of exercise-induced asthma.

Growth

Limited data from long-term studies suggest that most children and adolescents treated with inhaled budesonide ultimately achieve their adult target height. However, an initial small but transient reduction in growth (approximately 1 cm) has been observed. This generally occurs within the first year of treatment (see section 4.4).

5.2 Pharmacokinetic properties

Budesonide undergoes an extensive biotransformation in the liver, to metabolites of low glucocorticosteroid activity. The glucocorticosteroid activity of the major metabolites, 6β-hydroxybudesonide and 16α-hydroxyprednisolone, is less than 1% of that of budesonide. The metabolism of budesonide is primarily mediated by CYP3A4, one of the cytochrome p450 enzymes.

In a study, 100 mg ketoconazole taken twice daily, increased plasma levels of concomitantly administered oral budesonide (single dose of 10 mg) on average, by 7.8-fold. Information about this interaction is lacking for inhaled budesonide, but marked increases in plasma levels could be expected.

Of the fraction of budesonide which is swallowed, approximately 90% is inactivated at first passage through the liver. The maximal plasma concentration after inhalation of 1 mg budesonide, delivered via dry powder inhaler, is about 3.5 nmol/L and is reached after about 20 minutes.

5.3 Preclinical safety data

The acute toxicity of budesonide is low and of the same order of magnitude and type as that of the reference glucocorticosteroids studied (beclomethasone dipropionate, fluocinolone acetonide).

Results from subacute and chronic toxicity studies show that the systemic effects of budesonide are less severe than, or similar to, those observed after administration of other glucocorticosteroids, e.g. decreased body-weight gain and atrophy of lymphoid tissues and adrenal cortex.

An increased incidence of brain gliomas in male rats, in a carcinogenicity study, could not be verified in a repeat study in which the incidence of gliomas did not differ between any of the groups on active treatment (budesonide, prednisolone, triamcinolone acetonide) and the control groups.

Liver changes (primary hepatocellular neoplasms) found in male rats in the original carcinogenicity study were noted again in the repeat study with budesonide, as well as with the reference glucocorticosteroids. These effects are most probably related to a receptor effect and thus represent a class effect.

Available clinical experience shows that there are no indications that budesonide, or other glucocorticosteroids, induce brain gliomas or primary hepatocellular neoplasms in man.

In animal reproduction studies, corticosteroids such as budesonide have been shown to induce malformations (cleft palate, skeletal malformations). However, these animal experimental results do not appear to be relevant in humans at the recommended doses.

Animal studies have also identified an involvement of excess prenatal glucocorticosteroids, in increased risk for intrauterine growth retardation, adult cardiovascular disease and permanent changes in glucocorticoid receptor density, neurotransmitter turnover and behaviour at exposures below the teratogenic dose range.

6. PHARMACEUTICAL PARTICULARS

6.1 List of excipients

Disodium edetate, sodium chloride, polysorbate 80, citric acid anhydrous, sodium citrate, water purified.

6.2 Incompatibilities

None known.

6.3 Shelf life

24 months

Use within 3 months of opening the foil envelope.

Use Respule within 12 hours of opening.

6.4 Special precautions for storage

Do not store above 30°C. Store the Respules in the foil envelope to protect them from light.

6.5 Nature and contents of container

Single dose unit made of LD-polyethylene. Each single dose unit contains 2 ml of suspension. Sheets of 5 units are packed in a heat sealed envelope of foil laminate. 4 heat sealed envelopes are packed into a carton.

6.6 Instructions for use and handling

See section 4.2.

7. MARKETING AUTHORISATION HOLDER
AstraZeneca UK Ltd,
600 Capability Green,
Luton, LU1 3LU, UK.

8. MARKETING AUTHORISATION NUMBER(S)
Pulmicort® Respules® 0.5 mg, nebuliser suspension: PL 17901/0160.

Pulmicort® Respules® 1 mg, nebuliser suspension: PL 17901/0161.

9. DATE OF FIRST AUTHORISATION/RENEWAL OF THE AUTHORISATION
11th June 2002 / 15th Oct 2003

10. DATE OF REVISION OF THE TEXT
4th April 2005

Pulmicort Turbohaler 100

(AstraZeneca UK Limited)

1. NAME OF THE MEDICINAL PRODUCT
Pulmicort® Turbohaler® 100.

2. QUALITATIVE AND QUANTITATIVE COMPOSITION
Budesonide 100 micrograms/actuation.

There are no inactive ingredients.

3. PHARMACEUTICAL FORM
Breath-actuated metered dose powder inhaler.

4. CLINICAL PARTICULARS

4.1 Therapeutic indications
Pulmicort is recommended in patients with bronchial asthma.

4.2 Posology and method of administration
Pulmicort Turbohaler is for oral inhalation

When transferring patients to Turbohaler from other devices, treatment should be individualised, whether once or twice daily dosing is being used. The drug and method of delivery should be considered.

Divided doses (twice daily):

The dosage should be individualised.

The dose should always be reduced to the minimum needed to maintain good asthma control.

Adults (including elderly) and children over 12 years of age: When starting treatment, during periods of severe asthma and while reducing or discontinuing oral glucocorticosteroids, the dosage in adults should be 200 - 1600 micrograms daily, in divided doses.

In less severe cases and children over 12 years of age, 200 - 800 micrograms daily, in divided doses, may be used. During periods of severe asthma, the daily dosage can be increased to up to 1600 micrograms, in divided doses.

Children 12 years of age and under: 200 - 800 micrograms daily, in divided doses. During periods of severe asthma, the daily dose can be increased to up to 800 micrograms.

Once daily dosage:

The dosage should be individualised.

The dose should always be reduced to the minimum needed to maintain good asthma control.

Adults (including elderly) and children over 12 years of age: 200 micrograms to 400 micrograms may be used in patients with mild to moderate asthma who have not previously received inhaled glucocorticosteroids.

Up to 800 micrograms may be used by patients with mild to moderate asthma already controlled on inhaled steroids (e.g. budesonide or beclomethasone dipropionate), administered twice daily.

Children 12 years of age and under: 200 micrograms to 400 micrograms may be used in children with mild to moderate asthma who have not previously received inhaled glucocorticosteroids, or who are already controlled on inhaled steroids (e.g. budesonide or beclomethasone dipropionate), administered twice daily.

The patient should be transferred to once daily dosing at the same equivalent total daily dose; the drug and method of delivery should be considered. The dose should subsequently be reduced to the minimum needed to maintain good asthma control.

Patients should be instructed to take the once daily dose in the evening. It is important that the dose is taken consistently and at a similar time each evening.

There are insufficient data to make recommendations for the transfer of patients from newer inhaled steroids to once daily Pulmicort Turbohaler.

Patients, in particular those receiving once daily treatment, should be advised that if their asthma deteriorates (e.g. increased frequency of bronchodilator use or persistent respiratory symptoms) they should double their steroid dose, by administering it twice daily, and should contact their doctor as soon as possible.

In patients where an increased therapeutic effect is desired, an increased dose of Pulmicort is recommended because of the lower risk of systemic effects as compared with a combined treatment with oral glucocorticosteroids.

Patients maintained on oral glucocorticosteroids

Pulmicort Turbohaler may permit replacement or significant reduction in dosage of oral glucocorticosteroids while maintaining asthma control. For further information on the withdrawal of oral corticosteroids, see section 4.4.

Patients should be reminded of the importance of taking prophylactic therapy regularly, even when they are asymptomatic. A short-acting inhaled bronchodilator should be made available for the relief of acute asthma symptoms.

Instructions for the correct use of Pulmicort Turbohaler

Turbohaler is inspiratory flow-driven which means that, when the patient inhales through the mouthpiece, the substance will follow the inspired air into the airways.

Note: It is important to instruct the patient:

- To carefully read the instructions for use in the patient information leaflet, which is packed with each Turbohaler
- To breathe in forcefully and deeply through the mouthpiece to ensure that an optimal dose is delivered to the lungs
- Never to breathe out through the mouthpiece
- To rinse the mouth out with water and spit it out, or to brush the teeth after inhaling the prescribed dose, to minimise the risk of oropharyngeal thrush

The patient may not taste or feel any medication when using Turbohaler due to the small amount of drug dispensed.

4.3 Contraindications
Active pulmonary tuberculosis.

Hypersensitivity to budesonide.

4.4 Special warnings and special precautions for use
Special care is needed in patients with quiescent lung tuberculosis, fungal and viral infections in the airways.

Non steroid-dependent patients: A therapeutic effect is usually reached within 10 days. In patients with excessive mucus secretion in the bronchi, a short (about 2 weeks) additional oral corticosteroid regimen can be given initially.

Steroid-dependent patients: When transferral from oral steroids to Pulmicort Turbohaler is started, the patient should be in a relatively stable phase. A high dose of Pulmicort Turbohaler is then given in combination with the previously used oral steroid dose for about 10 days.

After that, the oral steroid dose should be gradually reduced (by for example 2.5 milligrams prednisolone or the equivalent each month) to the lowest possible level. In many cases, it is possible to completely substitute Pulmicort for the oral steroid.

During transfer from oral therapy to Pulmicort, a generally lower systemic steroid action will be experienced which may result in the appearance of allergic or arthritic symptoms such as rhinitis, eczema and muscle and joint pain. Specific treatment should be initiated for these conditions. During the withdrawal of oral steroids, patients may feel unwell in a non-specific way, even though respiratory function is maintained or improved. Patients should be encouraged to continue with Pulmicort therapy whilst withdrawing the oral steroid, unless there are clinical signs to indicate the contrary. A general insufficient glucocorticosteroid effect should be suspected if, in rare cases, symptoms such as tiredness, headache, nausea and vomiting should occur. In these cases a temporary increase in the dose of oral glucocorticosteroids is sometimes necessary.

As with other inhalation therapy, paradoxical bronchospasm may occur, with an immediate increase in wheezing after dosing. If a severe reaction occurs, treatment should be reassessed and an alternative therapy instituted if necessary.

Patients who have previously been dependent on oral steroids may, as a result of prolonged systemic steroid therapy, experience the effects of impaired adrenal function. Recovery may take a considerable amount of time after cessation of oral steroid therapy, hence oral steroid-dependent patients transferred to budesonide may remain at risk from impaired adrenal function for some considerable time. In such circumstances, HPA axis functions should be monitored regularly.

Acute exacerbations of asthma may need an increase in the dose of Pulmicort or additional treatment with a short course of oral corticosteroid and/or an antibiotic, if there is an infection. The patient should be advised to use a short-acting inhaled bronchodilator as rescue medication to relieve acute asthma symptoms.

If patients find short-acting bronchodilator treatment ineffective or they need more inhalations than usual, medical attention must be sought. In this situation consideration should be given to the need for or an increase in their regular therapy, e.g., higher doses of inhaled budesonide or the addition of a long-acting beta agonist, or for a course of oral glucocorticosteroid.

Prolonged treatment with high doses of inhaled corticosteroids, particularly higher than the recommended doses, may result in clinically significant adrenal suppression. Additional systemic corticosteroid cover should be considered during periods of stress or elective surgery. These patientsshould be instructed to carry a steroid warning card indicating their needs. Treatment with supplementary systemic steroids or Pulmicort should not be stopped abruptly.

Systemic effects of inhaled corticosteroids may occur, particularly at high doses prescribed for prolonged periods. These effects are much less likely to occur than with oral corticosteroids. Possible systemic effects include adrenal suppression, growth retardation in children and adolescents, decrease in bone mineral density, cataract and glaucoma.

It is important, therefore, that the dose of inhaled corticosteroid is titrated to the lowest dose at which effective control of asthma is maintained.

It is recommended that the height of children receiving prolonged treatment with inhaled corticosteroids is regularly monitored. If growth is slowed, therapy should be reviewed with the aim of reducing the dose of inhaled corticosteroid, if possible, to the lowest dose at which effective control of asthma is maintained. In addition, consideration should be given to referring the patient to a paediatric respiratory specialist.

Reduced liver function may affect the elimination of glucocorticosteroids. The plasma clearance following an intravenous dose of budesonide however was similar in cirrhotic patients and in healthy subjects. After oral ingestion systemic availability of budesonide was increased by compromised liver function due to decreased first pass metabolism. The clinical relevance of this to treatment with Pulmicort is unknown as no data exist for inhaled budesonide, but increases in plasma levels and hence an increased risk of systemic adverse effects could be expected.

In vivo studies have shown that oral administration of ketoconazole and itraconazole (known inhibitors of CYP3A4 activity in the liver and in the intestinal mucosa causes an increase in the systemic exposure to budesonide. Concomitant treatment with ketoconazole and itraconazole or other potent CYP3A4 inhibitors should be avoided (see section 4.5 Interactions). If this is not possible, the time interval between administration of the interacting drugs should be as long as possible. A reduction in the dose of budesonide should also be considered.

4.5 Interaction with other medicinal products and other forms of Interaction
The metabolism of budesonide is primarily mediated by CYP3A4, one of the cytochrome p450 enzymes. Inhibitors of this enzyme, e.g. ketoconazole and itraconazole, can therefore increase systemic exposure to budesonide, (see Section 4.4 Special Warnings and Special Precautions for Use and Section 5.2 Pharmacokinetic Properties). Other potent inhibitors of CYP3A4 are also likely to markedly increase plasma levels of budesonide.

4.6 Pregnancy and lactation
Data on approximately 2000 exposed pregnancies indicate no increased teratogenic risk associated with the use of inhaled budesonide. In animal studies, glucocorticosteroids have been shown to induce malformations (see Section 5.3). This is not likely to be relevant for humans given recommended doses, but therapy with inhaled budesonide should be regularly reviewed and maintained at the lowest effective dose.

The administration of budesonide during pregnancy requires that the benefits for the mother be weighed against the risk for the foetus. Inhaled glucocorticosteroids should be considered in preference to oral glucocorticosteroids because of the lower systemic effects at the doses required to achieve similar pulmonary responses.

There is no information regarding the passage of budesonide into breast milk.

4.7 Effects on ability to drive and use machines
Pulmicort Turbohaler does not affect the ability to drive or to use machines.

4.8 Undesirable effects
Clinical trials, literature reports and post-marketing experience suggest that the following adverse drug reactions may occur:

Common (>1/100, <1/10)	• Mild irritation in the throat • Candida infection in the oropharynx • Hoarseness • Coughing
Rare (>1/10 000, <1/1 000)	• Nervousness, restlessness, depression, behavioural disturbances • Immediate and delayed hypersensitivity reactions including rash, contact dermatitis, urticaria, angioedema and bronchospasm • Skin bruising

The candida infection in the oropharynx is due to drug deposition. Advising the patient to rinse the mouth out with water after each dosing will minimise the risk.

As with other inhalation therapy, paradoxical bronchospasm may occur in very rare cases (see Section 4.4).

Systemic effects of inhaled corticosteroids may occur, particularly at high doses prescribed for prolonged periods. These effects are much less likely to occur than with oral corticosteroids. Possible systemic effects include adrenal suppression, growth retardation in children and adolescents, decrease in bone mineral density, cataract and glaucoma. The effect is probably dependent on dose, exposure time, concomitant and previous steroid exposure, and individual sensitivity.

4.9 Overdose

The only harmful effect that follows inhalation of large amounts of the drug over a short period is suppression of hypothalamic-pituitary-adrenal (HPA) function. No special emergency action needs to be taken. Treatment with Pulmicort Turbohaler should be continued at the recommended dose to control the asthma.

5. PHARMACOLOGICAL PROPERTIES

5.1 Pharmacodynamic properties

Budesonide is a glucocorticosteroid which possesses a high local anti-inflammatory action, with a lower incidence and severity of adverse effects than those seen with oral corticosteroids.

Pharmacotherapeutic group: Other drugs for obstructive airway diseases, inhalants, glucocorticoids. ATC Code: RO3B A02.

Topical anti-inflammatory effect

The exact mechanism of action of glucocorticosteroids in the treatment of asthma is not fully understood. Anti-inflammatory actions, such as inhibition of inflammatory mediator release and inhibition of cytokine-mediated immune response are probably important.

A clinical study in asthmatics comparing inhaled and oral budesonide at doses calculated to achieve similar systemic bioavailability demonstrated statistically significant evidence of efficacy with inhaled but not oral budesonide compared with placebo. Thus, the therapeutic effect of conventional doses of inhaled budesonide may be largely explained by its direct action on the respiratory tract.

In a provocation study pre-treatment with budesonide for four weeks has shown decreased bronchial constriction in immediate as well as late asthmatic reactions.

Onset of effect

After a single dose of orally inhaled budesonide, delivered via dry powder inhaler, improvement of the lung function is achieved within a few hours. After therapeutic use of orally inhaled budesonide delivered via dry powder inhaler, improvement in lung function has been shown to occur within 2 days of initiation of treatment, although maximum benefit may not be achieved for up to 4 weeks.

Airway reactivity

Budesonide has also been shown to decrease airway reactivity to histamine and methacholine in hyper-reactive patients.

Exercise-induced asthma

Therapy with inhaled budesonide has effectively been used for prevention of exercise-induced asthma.

Growth

Limited data from long term studies suggest that most children and adolescents treated with inhaled budesonide ultimately achieve their adult target height. However, an initial small but transient reduction in growth (approximately 1 cm) has been observed. This generally occurs within the first year of treatment (see section 4.4).

HPA axis function

Studies in healthy volunteers with Pulmicort Turbohaler have shown dose-related effects on plasma and urinary cortisol. At recommended doses, Pulmicort Turbohaler, causes less effect on the adrenal function than prednisolone 10mg, as shown by ACTH tests.

5.2 Pharmacokinetic properties

After inhalation via Turbohaler, about 25 - 30% of the metered dose is deposited in the lungs.

Of the fraction which is swallowed, approximately 90% is inactivated by first pass metabolism in the liver.

The maximal plasma concentration after inhalation of 1 milligram budesonide is about 3.5 nmol/L and is reached after about 20 minutes.

Budesonide undergoes an extensive degree (approximately 90%) of biotransformation in the liver, to metabolites of low glucocorticosteroid activity. The glucocorticosteroid activity of the major metabolites, 6β-hydroxybudesonide and 16α-hydroxyprednisolone, is less than 1% of that of budesonide. The metabolism of budesonide is primarily mediated by CYP3A4, one of the cytochrome p450 enzymes.

In a study, 100 mg ketoconazole taken twice daily, increased plasma levels of concomitantly administered oral budesonide (single dose of 10 mg) on average, by 7.8-fold. Information about this interaction is lacking for inhaled budesonide, but marked increases in plasma levels could be expected.

5.3 Preclinical safety data

The acute toxicity of budesonide is low and of the same order of magnitude and type as that of the reference glucocorticosteroids studied (beclomethasone dipropionate, fluocinolone acetonide).

Results from subacute and chronic toxicity studies show that the systemic effects of budesonide are less severe than, or similar to, those observed after administration of the other glucocorticosteroids, e.g. decreased body-weight gain and atrophy of lymphoid tissues and adrenal cortex.

An increased incidence of brain gliomas in male rats, in a carcinogenicity study, could not be verified in a repeat study in which the incidence of gliomas did not differ between any of the groups on active treatment (budesonide, prednisolone, triamcinolone acetonide) and the control groups.

Liver changes (primary hepatocellular neoplasms) found in male rats in the original carcinogenicity study were noted again in the repeat study with budesonide, as well as with the reference glucocorticosteroids. These effects are most probably related to a receptor effect and thus represent a class effect.

Available clinical experience shows no indication that budesonide, or other glucocorticosteroids, induce brain gliomas or primary hepatocellular neoplasms in man.

In animal reproduction studies, corticosteroids such as budesonide have been shown to induce malformations (cleft palate, skeletal malformations). However, these animal experimental results do not appear to be relevant in humans at the recommended doses.

Animal studies have also identified an involvement of excess prenatal glucocorticosteroids, in increased risk for intrauterine growth retardation, adult cardiovascular disease and permanent changes in glucocorticoid receptor density, neurotransmitter turnover and behaviour at exposures below the teratogenic dose range.

6. PHARMACEUTICAL PARTICULARS

6.1 List of excipients

Pulmicort Turbohaler contains only active drug, budesonide. There are no propellants, lubricants, preservatives, carrier substances or other additives.

6.2 Incompatibilities

None known.

6.3 Shelf life

24 months.

6.4 Special precautions for storage

Do not store above 30°C.

6.5 Nature and contents of container

Polyethylene container consisting of a cover screwed onto a bottom plate. Inside this is the inhaler with its main parts: a mouthpiece, a dosing mechanism and a substance store.

The device also contains a desiccant.

100 micrograms/actuation. 200 actuations.

6.6 Instructions for use and handling

See section 4.2

7. MARKETING AUTHORISATION HOLDER

AstraZeneca UK Ltd

600 Capability Green,

Luton, LU1 3LU, UK.

8. MARKETING AUTHORISATION NUMBER(S)

PL 17901/0162

9. DATE OF FIRST AUTHORISATION/RENEWAL OF THE AUTHORISATION

18th June 2002

10. DATE OF REVISION OF THE TEXT

4th April 2005

Pulmicort Turbohaler 200

(AstraZeneca UK Limited)

1. NAME OF THE MEDICINAL PRODUCT

Pulmicort® Turbohaler® 200.

2. QUALITATIVE AND QUANTITATIVE COMPOSITION

Budesonide 200 micrograms/actuation.

There are no inactive ingredients.

3. PHARMACEUTICAL FORM

Breath-actuated metered dose powder inhaler.

4. CLINICAL PARTICULARS

4.1 Therapeutic indications

Pulmicort is recommended in patients with bronchial asthma.

4.2 Posology and method of administration

Pulmicort Turbohaler is for oral inhalation.

When transferring patients to Turbohaler from other devices, treatment should be individualised, whether once or twice daily dosing is being used. The drug and method of delivery should be considered.

Divided doses (twice daily):

The dosage should be individualised.

The dose should always be reduced to the minimum needed to maintain good asthma control.

Adults (including elderly) and children over 12 years of age: When starting treatment, during periods of severe asthma and while reducing or discontinuing oral glucocorticosteroids, the dosage in adults should be 200 - 1600 micrograms daily, in divided doses.

In less severe cases and children over 12 years of age, 200 - 800 micrograms daily, in divided doses, may be used. During periods of severe asthma, the daily dosage can be increased to up to 1600 micrograms, in divided doses.

Children 12 years of age and under: 200 - 800 micrograms daily, in divided doses. During periods of severe asthma, the daily dose can be increased up to 800 micrograms.

Once daily dosage:

The dosage should be individualised.

The dose should always be reduced to the minimum needed to maintain good asthma control.

Adults (including elderly) and children over 12 years of age: 200 micrograms to 400 micrograms may be used in patients with mild to moderate asthma who have not previously received inhaled glucocorticosteroids.

Up to 800 micrograms may be used by patients with mild to moderate asthma already controlled on inhaled steroids (e.g. budesonide or beclomethasone dipropionate), administered twice daily.

Children 12 years of age and under: 200 micrograms to 400 micrograms may be used in children with mild to moderate asthma who have not previously received inhaled glucocorticosteroids, or who are already controlled on inhaled steroids (e.g. budesonide or beclomethasone dipropionate), administered twice daily.

The patient should be transferred to once daily dosing at the same equivalent total daily dose; the drug and method of delivery should be considered. The dose should subsequently be reduced to the minimum needed to maintain good asthma control.

Patients should be instructed to take the once daily dose in the evening. It is important that the dose is taken consistently and at a similar time each evening.

There are insufficient data to make recommendations for the transfer of patients from newer inhaled steroids to once daily Pulmicort Turbohaler.

Patients, in particular those receiving once daily treatment, should be advised that if their asthma deteriorates (e.g. increased frequency of bronchodilator use or persistent respiratory symptoms) they should double their steroid dose, by administering it twice daily, and should contact their doctor as soon as possible.

In patients where an increased therapeutic effect is desired, an increased dose of Pulmicort is recommended because of the lower risk of systemic effects as compared with a combined treatment with oral glucocorticosteroids.

Patients maintained on oral glucocorticosteroids

Pulmicort Turbohaler may permit replacement or significant reduction in dosage of oral glucocorticosteroids while maintaining asthma control. For further information on the withdrawal of oral corticosteroids, see section 4.4.

Patients should be reminded of the importance of taking prophylactic therapy regularly, even when they are asymptomatic. A short-acting inhaled bronchodilator should be made available for the relief of acute asthma symptoms.

Instructions for the correct use of Pulmicort Turbohaler

Turbohaler is inspiratory flow-driven which means that, when the patient inhales through the mouthpiece, the substance will follow the inspired air into the airways.

Note: It is important to instruct the patient:

- To carefully read the instructions for use in the patient information leaflet, which is packed with each Turbohaler
- To breathe in forcefully and deeply through the mouthpiece to ensure that an optimal dose is delivered to the lungs
- Never to breathe out through the mouthpiece
- To rinse the mouth out with water and spit it out, or to brush the teeth after inhaling the prescribed dose, to minimise the risk of oropharyngeal thrush

The patient may not taste or feel any medication when using Turbohaler due to the small amount of drug dispensed.

4.3 Contraindications

Active pulmonary tuberculosis.

Hypersensitivity to budesonide.

4.4 Special warnings and special precautions for use

Special care is needed in patients with quiescent lung tuberculosis, fungal and viral infections in the airways.

Non steroid-dependent patients: A therapeutic effect is usually reached within 10 days. In patients with excessive mucus secretion in the bronchi, a short (about 2 weeks) additional oral corticosteroid regimen can be given initially.

Steroid-dependent patients: When transferral from oral steroids to Pulmicort Turbohaler is started, the patient should be in a relatively stable phase. A high dose of Pulmicort Turbohaler is then given in combination with the previously used oral steroid dose for about 10 days.

After that, the oral steroid dose should be gradually reduced (by for example 2.5 milligrams prednisolone or the equivalent each month) to the lowest possible level. In many cases, it is possible to completely substitute Pulmicort for the oral steroid.

During transfer from oral therapy to Pulmicort, a generally lower systemic steroid action will be experienced which may result in the appearance of allergic or arthritic symptoms such as rhinitis, eczema and muscle and joint pain. Specific treatment should be initiated for these conditions. During the withdrawal of oral steroids, patients may feel unwell in a non-specific way, even though respiratory function is maintained or improved. Patients should be encouraged to continue with Pulmicort therapy whilst withdrawing the oral steroid, unless there are clinical signs to indicate the contrary. A general insufficient glucocorticosteroid effect should be suspected if, in rare cases, symptoms such as tiredness, headache, nausea and vomiting should occur. In these cases a temporary increase in the dose of oral glucocorticosteroids is sometimes necessary.

As with other inhalation therapy, paradoxical bronchospasm may occur, with an immediate increase in wheezing after dosing. If a severe reaction occurs, treatment should be reassessed and an alternative therapy instituted if necessary.

Patients who have previously been dependent on oral steroids may, as a result of prolonged systemic steroid therapy, experience the effects of impaired adrenal function. Recovery may take a considerable amount of time after cessation of oral steroid therapy, hence oral steroid-dependent patients transferred to budesonide may remain at risk from impaired adrenal function for some considerable time. In such circumstances, HPA axis functions should be monitored regularly.

Acute exacerbations of asthma may need an increase in the dose of Pulmicort or additional treatment with a short course of oral corticosteroid and/or an antibiotic, if there is an infection. The patient should be advised to use a short-acting inhaled bronchodilator as rescue medication to relieve acute asthma symptoms.

If patients find short-acting bronchodilator treatment ineffective or they need more inhalations than usual, medical attention must be sought. In this situation consideration should be given to the need for or an increase in their regular therapy, e.g., higher doses of inhaled budesonide or the addition of a long-acting beta agonist, or for a course of oral glucocorticosteroid.

Prolonged treatment with high doses of inhaled corticosteroids, particularly higher than the recommended doses, may result in clinically significant adrenal suppression. Additional systemic corticosteroid cover should be considered during periods of stress or elective surgery. These patientsshould be instructed to carry a steroid warning card indicating their needs. Treatment with supplementary systemic steroids or Pulmicort should not be stopped abruptly.

Systemic effects of inhaled corticosteroids may occur, particularly at high doses prescribed for prolonged periods. These effects are much less likely to occur than with oral corticosteroids. Possible systemic effects include adrenal suppression, growth retardation in children and adolescents, decrease in bone mineral density, cataract and glaucoma.

It is important, therefore, that the dose of inhaled corticosteroid is titrated to the lowest dose at which effective control of asthma is maintained.

It is recommended that the height of children receiving prolonged treatment with inhaled corticosteroids is regularly monitored. If growth is slowed, therapy should be reviewed with the aim of reducing the dose of inhaled corticosteroid, if possible, to the lowest dose at which effective control of asthma is maintained. In addition, consideration should be given to referring the patient to a paediatric respiratory specialist.

Reduced liver function may affect the elimination of glucocorticosteroids. The plasma clearance following an intravenous dose of budesonide however was similar in cirrhotic patients and in healthy subjects. After oral ingestion systemic availability of budesonide was increased by compromised liver function due to decreased first pass metabolism. The clinical relevance of this to treatment with Pulmicort is unknown as no data exist for inhaled budesonide, but increases in plasma levels and hence an increased risk of systemic adverse effects could be expected.

In vivo studies have shown that oral administration of ketoconazole and itraconazole (known inhibitors of CYP3A4 activity in the liver and in the intestinal mucosa causes an increase in the systemic exposure to budesonide. Concomitant treatment with ketoconazole and itraconazole or other potent CYP3A4 inhibitors should be avoided (see section 4.5 Interactions). If this is not possible, the time interval between administration of the interacting drugs should be as long as possible. A reduction in the dose of budesonide should also be considered.

4.5 Interaction with other medicinal products and other forms of Interaction

The metabolism of budesonide is primarily mediated by CYP3A4, one of the cytochrome p450 enzymes. Inhibitors of this enzyme, e.g. ketoconazole and itraconazole, can therefore increase systemic exposure to budesonide, (see Section 4.4 Special Warnings and Special Precautions for Use and Section 5.2 Pharmacokinetic Properties). Other potent inhibitors of CYP3A4 are also likely to markedly increase plasma levels of budesonide.

4.6 Pregnancy and lactation

Data on approximately 2000 exposed pregnancies indicate no increased teratogenic risk associated with the use of inhaled budesonide. In animal studies, glucocorticosteroids have been shown to induce malformations (see Section 5.3). This is not likely to be relevant for humans given recommended doses, but therapy with inhaled budesonide should be regularly reviewed and maintained at the lowest effective dose.

The administration of budesonide during pregnancy requires that the benefits for the mother be weighed against the risk for the foetus. Inhaled glucocorticosteroids should be considered in preference to oral glucocorticosteroids because of the lower systemic effects at the doses required to achieve similar pulmonary responses.

There is no information regarding the passage of budesonide into breast milk.

4.7 Effects on ability to drive and use machines

Pulmicort Turbohaler does not affect the ability to drive or to use machines.

4.8 Undesirable effects

Clinical trials, literature reports and post-marketing experience suggest that the following adverse drug reactions may occur:

Common (>1/100, <1/10)	• Mild irritation in the throat • Candida infection in the oropharynx • Hoarseness • Coughing
Rare (>1/10 000, <1/1 000)	• Nervousness, restlessness, depression, behavioural disturbances • Immediate and delayed hypersensitivity reactions including rash, contact dermatitis, urticaria, angioedema and bronchospasm • Skin bruising

The candida infection in the oropharynx is due to drug deposition. Advising the patient to rinse the mouth out with water after each dosing will minimise the risk.

As with other inhalation therapy, paradoxical bronchospasm may occur in very rare cases (see Section 4.4).

Systemic effects of inhaled corticosteroids may occur, particularly at high doses prescribed for prolonged periods. These effects are much less likely to occur than with oral corticosteroids. Possible systemic effects include adrenal suppression, growth retardation in children and adolescents, decrease in bone mineral density, cataract and glaucoma. The effect is probably dependent on dose, exposure time, concomitant and previous steroid exposure, and individual sensitivity.

4.9 Overdose

The only harmful effect that follows inhalation of large amounts of the drug over a short period is suppression of hypothalamic-pituitary-adrenal (HPA) function. No special emergency action needs to be taken. Treatment with Pulmicort Turbohaler should be continued at the recommended dose to control the asthma.

5. PHARMACOLOGICAL PROPERTIES

5.1 Pharmacodynamic properties

Budesonide is a glucocorticosteroid which possesses a high local anti-inflammatory action, with a lower incidence and severity of adverse effects than those seen with oral corticosteroids.

Pharmacotherapeutic group: Other drugs for obstructive airway diseases, inhalants, glucocorticoids. ATC Code: RO3B A02.

Topical anti-inflammatory effect

The exact mechanism of action of glucocorticosteroids in the treatment of asthma is not fully understood. Anti-inflammatory actions, such as inhibition of inflammatory mediator release and inhibition of cytokine-mediated immune response are probably important.

A clinical study in asthmatics comparing inhaled and oral budesonide at doses calculated to achieve similar systemic bioavailability demonstrated statistically significant evidence of efficacy with inhaled but not oral budesonide compared with placebo. Thus, the therapeutic effect of conventional doses of inhaled budesonide may be largely explained by its direct action on the respiratory tract.

In a provocation study pre-treatment with budesonide for four weeks has shown decreased bronchial constriction in immediate as well as late asthmatic reactions.

Onset of effect

After a single dose of orally inhaled budesonide, delivered via dry powder inhaler, improvement of the lung function is achieved within a few hours. After therapeutic use of orally inhaled budesonide delivered via dry powder inhaler, improvement in lung function has been shown to occur within 2 days of initiation of treatment, although maximum benefit may not be achieved for up to 4 weeks.

Airway reactivity

Budesonide has also been shown to decrease airway reactivity to histamine and methacholine in hyper-reactive patients.

Exercise-induced asthma

Therapy with inhaled budesonide has effectively been used for prevention of exercise-induced asthma.

Growth

Limited data from long term studies suggest that most children and adolescents treated with inhaled budesonide ultimately achieve their adult target height. However, an initial small but transient reduction in growth (approximately 1 cm) has been observed. This generally occurs within the first year of treatment (see section 4.4).

HPA axis function

Studies in healthy volunteers with Pulmicort Turbohaler have shown dose-related effects on plasma and urinary cortisol. At recommended doses, Pulmicort Turbohaler, causes less effect on the adrenal function than prednisolone 10mg, as shown by ACTH tests.

5.2 Pharmacokinetic properties

After inhalation via Turbohaler, about 25 - 30% of the metered dose is deposited in the lungs.

Of the fraction which is swallowed, approximately 90% is inactivated by first pass metabolism in the liver.

The maximal plasma concentration after inhalation of 1 milligram budesonide is about 3.5 nmol/L and is reached after about 20 minutes.

Budesonide undergoes an extensive degree (approximately 90%) of biotransformation in the liver, to metabolites of low glucocorticosteroid activity. The glucocorticosteroid activity of the major metabolites, 6β-hydroxybudesonide and 16α-hydroxyprednisolone, is less than 1% of that of budesonide. The metabolism of budesonide is primarily mediated by CYP3A4, one of the cytochrome p450 enzymes.

In a study, 100 mg ketoconazole taken twice daily, increased plasma levels of concomitantly administered oral budesonide (single dose of 10 mg) on average, by 7.8-fold. Information about this interaction is lacking for inhaled budesonide, but marked increases in plasma levels could be expected.

5.3 Preclinical safety data

The acute toxicity of budesonide is low and of the same order of magnitude and type as that of the reference glucocorticosteroids studied (beclomethasone dipropionate, fluocinolone acetonide).

Results from subacute and chronic toxicity studies show that the systemic effects of budesonide are less severe than, or similar to, those observed after administration of the other glucocorticosteroids, e.g. decreased body-weight gain and atrophy of lymphoid tissues and adrenal cortex.

An increased incidence of brain gliomas in male rats, in a carcinogenicity study, could not be verified in a repeat study in which the incidence of gliomas did not differ between any of the groups on active treatment (budesonide, prednisolone, triamcinolone acetonide) and the control groups.

Liver changes (primary hepatocellular neoplasms) found in male rats in the original carcinogenicity study were noted again in the repeat study with budesonide, as well as with the reference glucocorticosteroids. These effects are most probably related to a receptor effect and thus represent a class effect.

Available clinical experience shows no indication that budesonide, or other glucocorticosteroids, induce brain gliomas or primary hepatocellular neoplasms in man.

In animal reproduction studies, corticosteroids such as budesonide have been shown to induce malformations (cleft palate, skeletal malformations). However, these animal experimental results do not appear to be relevant in humans at the recommended doses.

Animal studies have also identified an involvement of excess prenatal glucocorticosteroids, in increased risk for intrauterine growth retardation, adult cardiovascular disease and permanent changes in glucocorticoid receptor density, neurotransmitter turnover and behaviour at exposures below the teratogenic dose range.

6. PHARMACEUTICAL PARTICULARS

6.1 List of excipients

Pulmicort Turbohaler contains only active drug, budesonide. There are no propellants, lubricants, preservatives, carrier substances or other additives.

6.2 Incompatibilities

None known.

6.3 Shelf life

24 months.

6.4 Special precautions for storage

Do not store above 30°C.

6.5 Nature and contents of container
Polyethylene container consisting of a cover screwed onto a bottom plate. Inside this is the inhaler with its main parts: a mouthpiece, a dosing mechanism and a substance store. The device also contains a desiccant.

200 micrograms/actuation, 100 actuations.

6.6 Instructions for use and handling
See section 4.2

7. MARKETING AUTHORISATION HOLDER
AstraZeneca UK Ltd.

600 Capability Green,

Luton, LU1 3LU, UK.

8. MARKETING AUTHORISATION NUMBER(S)
PL 17901/0163

9. DATE OF FIRST AUTHORISATION/RENEWAL OF THE AUTHORISATION
18th June 2002

10. DATE OF REVISION OF THE TEXT
4th April 2005

Pulmicort Turbohaler 400

(AstraZeneca UK Limited)

1. NAME OF THE MEDICINAL PRODUCT
Pulmicort® Turbohaler® 400.

2. QUALITATIVE AND QUANTITATIVE COMPOSITION
Budesonide 400 micrograms/actuation.

There are no inactive ingredients.

3. PHARMACEUTICAL FORM
Breath-actuated metered dose powder inhaler.

4. CLINICAL PARTICULARS

4.1 Therapeutic indications
Pulmicort is recommended in patients with bronchial asthma.

4.2 Posology and method of administration
Pulmicort Turbohaler is for oral inhalation.

When transferring patients to Turbohaler from other devices, treatment should be individualised, whether once or twice daily dosing is being used. The drug and method of delivery should be considered.

Divided doses (twice daily):

The dosage should be individualised.

The dose should always be reduced to the minimum needed to maintain good asthma control.

Adults (including elderly) and children over 12 years of age: When starting treatment, during periods of severe asthma and while reducing or discontinuing oral glucocorticosteroids, the dosage in adults should be 200 - 1600 micrograms daily, in divided doses.

In less severe cases and children over 12 years of age, 200 - 800 micrograms daily, in divided doses, may be used. During periods of severe asthma, the daily dosage can be increased to up to 1600 micrograms, in divided doses.

Children 12 years of age and under: 200 - 800 micrograms daily, in divided doses. During periods of severe asthma, the daily dose can be increased up to 800 micrograms.

Once daily dosage:

The dosage should be individualised.

The dose should always be reduced to the minimum needed to maintain good asthma control.

Adults (including elderly) and children over 12 years of age: 200 micrograms to 400 micrograms may be used in patients with mild to moderate asthma who have not previously received inhaled glucocorticosteroids.

Up to 800 micrograms may be used by patients with mild to moderate asthma already controlled on inhaled steroids (e.g. budesonide or beclomethasone dipropionate), administered twice daily.

Children 12 years of age and under: 200 micrograms to 400 micrograms may be used in children with mild to moderate asthma who have not previously received inhaled glucocorticosteroids, or who are already controlled on inhaled steroids (e.g. budesonide or beclomethasone dipropionate), administered twice daily.

The patient should be transferred to once daily dosing at the same equivalent total daily dose; the drug and method of delivery should be considered. The dose should subsequently be reduced to the minimum needed to maintain good asthma control.

Patients should be instructed to take the once daily dose in the evening. It is important that the dose is taken consistently and at a similar time each evening.

There are insufficient data to make recommendations for the transfer of patients from newer inhaled steroids to once daily Pulmicort Turbohaler.

Patients, in particular those receiving once daily treatment, should be advised that if their asthma deteriorates (e.g. increased frequency of bronchodilator use or persistent respiratory symptoms) they should double their steroid dose, by administering it twice daily, and should contact their doctor as soon as possible.

In patients where an increased therapeutic effect is desired, an increased dose of Pulmicort is recommended because of the lower risk of systemic effects as compared with a combined treatment with oral glucocorticosteroids.

Patients maintained on oral glucocorticosteroids

Pulmicort Turbohaler may permit replacement or significant reduction in dosage of oral glucocorticosteroids while maintaining asthma control. For further information on the withdrawal of oral corticosteroids, see section 4.4.

Patients should be reminded of the importance of taking prophylactic therapy regularly, even when they are asymptomatic. A short-acting inhaled bronchodilator should be made available for the relief of acute asthma symptoms.

Instructions for the correct use of Pulmicort Turbohaler

Turbohaler is inspiratory flow-driven which means that, when the patient inhales through the mouthpiece, the substance will follow the inspired air into the airways.

Note: It is important to instruct the patient:

- To carefully read the instructions for use in the patient information leaflet, which is packed with each Turbohaler
- To breathe in forcefully and deeply through the mouthpiece to ensure that an optimal dose is delivered to the lungs
- Never to breathe out through the mouthpiece
- To rinse the mouth out with water and spit it out, or to brush the teeth after inhaling the prescribed dose, to minimise the risk of oropharyngeal thrush

The patient may not taste or feel any medication when using Turbohaler due to the small amount of drug dispensed.

4.3 Contraindications
Active pulmonary tuberculosis.

Hypersensitivity to budesonide.

4.4 Special warnings and special precautions for use
Special care is needed in patients with quiescent lung tuberculosis, fungal and viral infections in the airways.

Non steroid-dependent patients: A therapeutic effect is usually reached within 10 days. In patients with excessive mucus secretion in the bronchi, a short (about 2 weeks) additional oral corticosteroid regimen can be given initially.

Steroid-dependent patients: When transferral from oral steroids to Pulmicort Turbohaler is started, the patient should be in a relatively stable phase. A high dose of Pulmicort Turbohaler is then given in combination with the previously used oral steroid dose for about 10 days.

After that, the oral steroid dose should be gradually reduced (by for example 2.5 milligrams prednisolone or the equivalent each month) to the lowest possible level. In many cases, it is possible to completely substitute Pulmicort for the oral steroid.

During transfer from oral therapy to Pulmicort, a generally lower systemic steroid action will be experienced which may result in the appearance of allergic or arthritic symptoms such as rhinitis, eczema and muscle and joint pain. Specific treatment should be initiated for these conditions. During the withdrawal of oral steroids, patients may feel unwell in a non-specific way, even though respiratory function is maintained or improved. Patients should be encouraged to continue with Pulmicort therapy whilst withdrawing the oral steroid, unless there are clinical signs to indicate the contrary. A general insufficient glucocorticosteroid effect should be suspected if, in rare cases, symptoms such as tiredness, headache, nausea and vomiting should occur. In these cases a temporary increase in the dose of oral glucocorticosteroids is sometimes necessary.

As with other inhalation therapy, paradoxical bronchospasm may occur, with an immediate increase in wheezing after dosing. If a severe reaction occurs, treatment should be reassessed and an alternative therapy instituted if necessary.

Patients who have previously been dependent on oral steroids may, as a result of prolonged systemic steroid therapy, experience the effects of impaired adrenal function. Recovery may take a considerable amount of time after cessation of oral steroid therapy, hence oral steroid-dependent patients transferred to budesonide may remain at risk from impaired adrenal function for some considerable time. In such circumstances, HPA axis functions should be monitored regularly.

Acute exacerbations of asthma may need an increase in the dose of Pulmicort or additional treatment with a short course of oral corticosteroid and/or an antibiotic, if there is an infection. The patient should be advised to use a short-acting inhaled bronchodilator as rescue medication to relieve acute asthma symptoms.

If patients find short-acting bronchodilator treatment ineffective or they need more inhalations than usual, medical attention must be sought. In this situation consideration should be given to the need for or an increase in their regular therapy, e.g., higher doses of inhaled budesonide or the addition of a long-acting beta agonist, or for a course of oral glucocorticosteroid.

Prolonged treatment with high doses of inhaled corticosteroids, particularly higher than the recommended doses, may result in clinically significant adrenal suppression. Additional systemic corticosteroid cover should be considered during periods of stress or elective surgery. These patientsshould be instructed to carry a steroid warning card indicating their needs. Treatment with supplementary systemic steroids or Pulmicort should not be stopped abruptly.

Systemic effects of inhaled corticosteroids may occur, particularly at high doses prescribed for prolonged periods. These effects are much less likely to occur than with oral corticosteroids. Possible systemic effects include adrenal suppression, growth retardation in children and adolescents, decrease in bone mineral density, cataract and glaucoma.

It is important, therefore, that the dose of inhaled corticosteroid is titrated to the lowest dose at which effective control of asthma is maintained.

It is recommended that the height of children receiving prolonged treatment with inhaled corticosteroids is regularly monitored. If growth is slowed, therapy should be reviewed with the aim of reducing the dose of inhaled corticosteroid, if possible, to the lowest dose at which effective control of asthma is maintained. In addition, consideration should be given to referring the patient to a paediatric respiratory specialist.

Reduced liver function may affect the elimination of glucocorticosteroids. The plasma clearance following an intravenous dose of budesonide however was similar in cirrhotic patients and in healthy subjects. After oral ingestion systemic availability of budesonide was increased by compromised liver function due to decreased first pass metabolism. The clinical relevance of this to treatment with Pulmicort is unknown as no data exist for inhaled budesonide, but increases in plasma levels and hence an increased risk of systemic adverse effects could be expected.

In vivo studies have shown that oral administration of ketoconazole and itraconazole (known inhibitors of CYP3A4 activity in the liver and in the intestinal mucosa causes an increase in the systemic exposure to budesonide. Concomitant treatment with ketoconazole and itraconazole or other potent CYP3A4 inhibitors should be avoided (see section 4.5 Interactions). If this is not possible, the time interval between administration of the interacting drugs should be as long as possible. A reduction in the dose of budesonide should also be considered.

4.5 Interaction with other medicinal products and other forms of Interaction
The metabolism of budesonide is primarily mediated by CYP3A4, one of the cytochrome p450 enzymes. Inhibitors of this enzyme, e.g. ketoconazole and itraconazole, can therefore increase systemic exposure to budesonide, (see Section 4.4 Special Warnings and Special Precautions for Use and Section 5.2 Pharmacokinetic Properties). Other potent inhibitors of CYP3A4 are also likely to markedly increase plasma levels of budesonide.

4.6 Pregnancy and lactation
Data on approximately 2000 exposed pregnancies indicate no increased teratogenic risk associated with the use of inhaled budesonide. In animal studies, glucocorticosteroids have been shown to induce malformations (see Section 5.3). This is not likely to be relevant for humans given recommended doses, but therapy with inhaled budesonide should be regularly reviewed and maintained at the lowest effective dose.

The administration of budesonide during pregnancy requires that the benefits for the mother be weighed against the risk for the foetus. Inhaled glucocorticosteroids should be considered in preference to oral glucocorticosteroids because of the lower systemic effects at the doses required to achieve similar pulmonary responses.

There is no information regarding the passage of budesonide into breast milk.

4.7 Effects on ability to drive and use machines
Pulmicort Turbohaler does not affect the ability to drive or to use machines.

4.8 Undesirable effects
Clinical trials, literature reports and post-marketing experience suggest that the following adverse drug reactions may occur:

Common (>1/100, <1/10)	• Mild irritation in the throat • Candida infection in the oropharynx • Hoarseness • Coughing
Rare (>1/10 000, <1/1 000)	• Nervousness, restlessness, depression, behavioural disturbances • Immediate and delayed hypersensitivity reactions including rash, contact dermatitis, urticaria, angioedema and bronchospasm • Skin bruising

The candida infection in the oropharynx is due to drug deposition. Advising the patient to rinse the mouth out with water after each dosing will minimise the risk.

As with other inhalation therapy, paradoxical bronchospasm may occur in very rare cases (see Section 4.4).

Systemic effects of inhaled corticosteroids may occur, particularly at high doses prescribed for prolonged periods. These effects are much less likely to occur than with oral corticosteroids. Possible systemic effects include adrenal suppression, growth retardation in children and adolescents, decrease in bone mineral density, cataract and glaucoma. The effect is probably dependent on dose, exposure time, concomitant and previous steroid exposure, and individual sensitivity.

4.9 Overdose

The only harmful effect that follows inhalation of large amounts of the drug over a short period is suppression of hypothalamic-pituitary-adrenal (HPA) function. No special emergency action needs to be taken. Treatment with Pulmicort Turbohaler should be continued at the recommended dose to control the asthma.

5. PHARMACOLOGICAL PROPERTIES

5.1 Pharmacodynamic properties

Budesonide is a glucocorticosteroid which possesses a high local anti-inflammatory action, with a lower incidence and severity of adverse effects than those seen with oral corticosteroids.

Pharmacotherapeutic group: Other drugs for obstructive airway diseases, inhalants, glucocorticoids. ATC Code: RO3B A02.

Topical anti-inflammatory effect

The exact mechanism of action of glucocorticosteroids in the treatment of asthma is not fully understood. Anti-inflammatory actions, such as inhibition of inflammatory mediator release and inhibition of cytokine-mediated immune response are probably important.

A clinical study in asthmatics comparing inhaled and oral budesonide at doses calculated to achieve similar systemic bioavailability demonstrated statistically significant evidence of efficacy with inhaled but not oral budesonide compared with placebo. Thus, the therapeutic effect of conventional doses of inhaled budesonide may be largely explained by its direct action on the respiratory tract.

In a provocation study pre-treatment with budesonide for four weeks has shown decreased bronchial constriction in immediate as well as late asthmatic reactions.

Onset of effect

After a single dose of orally inhaled budesonide, delivered via dry powder inhaler, improvement of the lung function is achieved within a few hours. After therapeutic use of orally inhaled budesonide delivered via dry powder inhaler, improvement in lung function has been shown to occur within 2 days of initiation of treatment, although maximum benefit may not be achieved for up to 4 weeks.

Airway reactivity

Budesonide has also been shown to decrease airway reactivity to histamine and methacholine in hyper-reactive patients.

Exercise-induced asthma

Therapy with inhaled budesonide has effectively been used for prevention of exercise-induced asthma.

Growth

Limited data from long term studies suggest that most children and adolescents treated with inhaled budesonide ultimately achieve their adult target height. However, an initial small but transient reduction in growth (approximately 1 cm) has been observed. This generally occurs within the first year of treatment (see section 4.4).

HPA axis function

Studies in healthy volunteers with Pulmicort Turbohaler have shown dose-related effects on plasma and urinary cortisol. At recommended doses, Pulmicort Turbohaler, causes less effect on the adrenal function than prednisolone 10mg, as shown by ACTH tests.

5.2 Pharmacokinetic properties

After inhalation via Turbohaler, about 25 - 30% of the metered dose is deposited in the lungs.

Of the fraction which is swallowed, approximately 90% is inactivated by first pass metabolism in the liver.

The maximal plasma concentration after inhalation of 1 milligram budesonide is about 3.5 nmol/L and is reached after about 20 minutes.

Budesonide undergoes an extensive degree (approximately 90%) of biotransformation in the liver, to metabolites of low glucocorticosteroid activity. The glucocorticosteroid activity of the major metabolites, 6β-hydroxybudesonide and 16α-hydroxyprednisolone, is less than 1% of that of budesonide. The metabolism of budesonide is primarily mediated by CYP3A4, one of the cytochrome p450 enzymes.

In a study, 100 mg ketoconazole taken twice daily, increased plasma levels of concomitantly administered oral budesonide (single dose of 10 mg) on average, by 7.8-fold. Information about this interaction is lacking for inhaled budesonide, but marked increases in plasma levels could be expected.

5.3 Preclinical safety data

The acute toxicity of budesonide is low and of the same order of magnitude and type as that of the reference glucocorticosteroids studied (beclomethasone dipropionate, fluocinolone acetonide).

Results from subacute and chronic toxicity studies show that the systemic effects of budesonide are less severe than, or similar to, those observed after administration of the other glucocorticosteroids, e.g. decreased body-weight gain and atrophy of lymphoid tissues and adrenal cortex.

An increased incidence of brain gliomas in male rats, in a carcinogenicity study, could not be verified in a repeat study in which the incidence of gliomas did not differ between any of the groups on active treatment (budesonide, prednisolone, triamcinolone acetonide) and the control groups.

Liver changes (primary hepatocellular neoplasms) found in male rats in the original carcinogenicity study were noted again in the repeat study with budesonide, as well as with the reference glucocorticosteroids. These effects are most probably related to a receptor effect and thus represent a class effect.

Available clinical experience shows no indication that budesonide, or other glucocorticosteroids, induce brain gliomas or primary hepatocellular neoplasms in man.

In animal reproduction studies, corticosteroids such as budesonide have been shown to induce malformations (cleft palate, skeletal malformations). However, these animal experimental results do not appear to be relevant in humans at the recommended doses.

Animal studies have also identified an involvement of excess prenatal glucocorticosteroids, in increased risk for intrauterine growth retardation, adult cardiovascular disease and permanent changes in glucocorticoid receptor density, neurotransmitter turnover and behaviour at exposures below the teratogenic dose range.

6. PHARMACEUTICAL PARTICULARS

6.1 List of excipients

Pulmicort Turbohaler contains only active drug, budesonide. There are no propellants, lubricants, preservatives, carrier substances or other additives.

6.2 Incompatibilities

None known.

6.3 Shelf life

24 months.

6.4 Special precautions for storage

Do not store above 30°C.

6.5 Nature and contents of container

Polyethylene container consisting of a cover screwed onto a bottom plate. Inside this is the inhaler with its main parts: a mouthpiece, a dosing mechanism and a substance store.

The device also contains a desiccant.

400 micrograms/actuation, 50 actuations.

6.6 Instructions for use and handling

See section 4.2

7. MARKETING AUTHORISATION HOLDER

AstraZeneca UK Ltd

600 Capability Green,

Luton, LU1 3LU, UK.

8. MARKETING AUTHORISATION NUMBER(S)

PL 17901/0164

9. DATE OF FIRST AUTHORISATION/RENEWAL OF THE AUTHORISATION

18th June 2002

10. DATE OF REVISION OF THE TEXT

4th April 2005

Pulmozyme

(Roche Products Limited)

1. NAME OF THE MEDICINAL PRODUCT

Pulmozyme 2500 U/ 2.5ml, nebuliser solution

2. QUALITATIVE AND QUANTITATIVE COMPOSITION

Each ampoule contains 2500 U (corresponding to 2.5mg) of dornase alfa* per 2.5ml corresponding to 1000 U/ml or 1mg/ml**.

*phosphorylated glycosylated protein human deoxyribonuclease 1 produced in Chinese Hamster Ovary Cell Line CHO A14.16-1 MSB #757 by recombinant DNA technology

**1 Genentech unit/ml = 1μg/ml

For excipients, see section *6.1*.

3. PHARMACEUTICAL FORM

Nebuliser solution

Clear, colourless solution.

4. CLINICAL PARTICULARS

4.1 Therapeutic indications

Management of cystic fibrosis patients with a forced vital capacity (FVC) of greater than 40% of predicted and over 5 years of age to improve pulmonary function.

4.2 Posology and method of administration

2.5mg (corresponding to 2,500 U) deoxyribonuclease I by inhalation once daily. Inhale the contents of one ampoule (2.5ml of solution) undiluted using a recommended jet nebuliser/compressor system (see section *6.6 Instructions for use/handling*).

Some patients over the age of 21 years may benefit from twice daily dosage.

Most patients gain optimal benefit from regular daily use of Pulmozyme. In studies in which Pulmozyme was given in an intermittent regimen, improvement in pulmonary function was lost on cessation of therapy. Patients should therefore be advised to take their medication every day without a break.

Patients should continue their regular medical care, including their standard regimen of chest physiotherapy.

Administration can be safely continued in patients who experience exacerbation of respiratory tract infection.

Safety and efficacy have not yet been demonstrated in patients under the age of 5 years, or in patients with forced vital capacity less than 40% of predicted.

4.3 Contraindications

Hypersensitivity to the active ingredient or its excipients.

4.4 Special warnings and special precautions for use

None.

4.5 Interaction with other medicinal products and other forms of Interaction

Pulmozyme can be effectively and safely used in conjunction with standard cystic fibrosis therapies such as antibiotics, bronchodilators, pancreatic enzymes, vitamins, inhaled and systemic corticosteroids, and analgesics.

4.6 Pregnancy and lactation

Pregnancy

The safety of dornase alfa has not been established in pregnant women. Animal studies do not indicate direct or indirect harmful effects with respect to pregnancy, or embryofoetal development (see section *5.3 Preclinical safety data*). Caution should be exercised when prescribing dornase alfa to pregnant women.

Lactation

As it is not known whether dornase alfa is excreted in human milk, caution should be exercised when dornase alfa is administered to a breast-feeding woman (see section *5.3 Preclinical safety data).*

4.7 Effects on ability to drive and use machines

No effects on the patient's ability to drive and use machines have been reported.

4.8 Undesirable effects

The adverse event data reflect the clinical trial and post-marketing experience of using Pulmozyme at the recommended dose regimen.

Adverse reactions attributed to Pulmozyme are rare (< 1/1000). In most cases, the adverse reactions are mild and transient in nature and do not require alterations in Pulmozyme dosing.

Body as a whole: Chest pain (pleuritic / non-cardiac), fever

Special senses: Conjunctivitis

Gastrointestinal system: Dyspepsia

Respiratory system: Voice alteration (hoarseness), pharyngitis (inflammation of the throat), dyspnoea, laryngitis, rhinitis, decreased lung function

Skin and Appendages: Rash, urticaria

Patients who experience adverse events common to cystic fibrosis can, in general, safely continue administration of Pulmozyme as evidenced by the high percentage of patients completing clinical trials with Pulmozyme.

In clinical trials, few patients experienced adverse events resulting in permanent discontinuation from dornase alfa, and the discontinuation rate was observed to be similar between placebo (2%) and dornase alfa (3%).

Upon initiation of dornase alfa therapy, as with any aerosol, pulmonary function may decline and expectoration of sputum may increase.

Less than 5% of patients treated with dornase alfa have developed antibodies to dornase alpha and none of these patients have developed IgE antibodies to dornase alfa. Improvement in pulmonary function tests has still occurred even after the development of antibodies to dornase alfa.

4.9 Overdose

Pulmozyme overdosage has not been established. Single-dose inhalation studies in rats and monkeys at doses up to 180-fold higher than doses routinely used in clinical studies are well tolerated. Oral administration of dornase alfa in doses up to 200mg/kg are also well tolerated by rats.

In clinical studies, CF patients have received up to 20mg dornase alfa BID for up to six days and 10mg BID intermittently (2 weeks on/2 weeks off drug) for 168 days. Both dose regimens were shown to be well tolerated.

5. PHARMACOLOGICAL PROPERTIES

5.1 Pharmacodynamic properties

Pharmacotherapeutic group: respiratory system, ATC code: R 05 C B13.

Recombinant human DNase is a genetically engineered version of a naturally occurring human enzyme which cleaves extracellular DNA.

Retention of viscous purulent secretions in the airways contributes both to reduced pulmonary function and to exacerbations of infection. Purulent secretions contain very high concentrations of extracellular DNA, a viscous polyanion released by degenerating leukocytes, which accumulate in response to infection. *In vitro*, dornase alfa hydrolyses DNA in sputum and greatly reduces the viscoelasticity of cystic fibrosis sputum.

5.2 Pharmacokinetic properties

Absorption

Inhalation studies conducted in rats and non-human primates show a low percentage of dornase alfa systemic absorption, < 15% for rats and < 2% for monkeys. Consistent with the results of these animal studies, dornase alfa administered to patients as an inhaled aerosol shows low systemic exposure.

Absorption of dornase alfa from the gastrointestinal tract following oral administration to rats is negligible.

DNase is normally present in human serum. Inhalation of up to 40mg of dornase alfa for up to 6 days did not result in a significant elevation of serum DNase concentration above normal endogenous levels. No increase in serum DNase concentration greater than 10ng/ml was observed. Following administration of 2,500 U (2.5mg) of dornase alfa twice daily for 24 weeks, mean serum DNase concentrations were no different from the mean pre-treatment baseline value of 3.5 ± 0.1ng/ml; suggesting low systemic absorption or accumulation.

Distribution

Studies in rats and monkeys have shown that, following intravenous administration, dornase alfa was cleared rapidly from the serum. The initial volume of distribution was similar to serum volume in these studies.

Inhalation of 2,500 U (2.5mg) dornase alfa results in a mean sputum concentration of dornase alfa of approximately 3μg/ml within 15 minutes in CF patients. Concentrations of dornase alfa in sputum rapidly decline following inhalation.

Elimination

Studies in rats indicate that, following aerosol administration the disappearance half-life of dornase alfa from the lungs is 11 hours.

No pharmacokinetic data are available in very young or geriatric animals.

5.3 Preclinical safety data

Studies of dornase alfa in rabbits and rodents show no evidence of impaired fertility, teratogenicity, or effects on development.

In a study performed in lactating cynomolgus monkeys, receiving high doses of dornase alfa by the intravenous route, low concentrations (< 0.1% of the concentrations seen in the serum of pregnant cynomolgus monkeys), were detectable in the maternal milk. When administered to humans according to the dosage recommendation, there is minimal systemic absorption of dornase alfa; therefore no measurable concentrations of dornase alfa would be expected in human milk.

6. PHARMACEUTICAL PARTICULARS

6.1 List of excipients

Sodium Chloride

Calcium Chloride Dihydrate

Water for Injections

6.2 Incompatibilities

Pulmozyme is an unbuffered aqueous solution and should not be diluted or mixed with other drugs or solutions in the nebuliser bowl. Mixing of this solution could lead to adverse structural and/or functional changes in Pulmozyme or the admixed compound.

6.3 Shelf life

2 years.

6.4 Special precautions for storage

Store in a refrigerator (2°C - 8°C).

Keep the ampoule in the outer carton in order to protect from light.

A single brief exposure to elevated temperatures (less than or equal to 24 hours at up to 30°C) does not affect product stability.

6.5 Nature and contents of container

2.5 ml of nebuliser solution in an ampoule (low density polyethylene plastic).

Pack sizes of 6 and 30.

6.6 Instructions for use and handling

The contents of one 2.5mg (2,500 U) single-use ampoule of Pulmozyme sterile solution for inhalation should be inhaled once a day using a recommended jet nebuliser.

- Pulmozyme should not be mixed with other drugs or solutions in the nebuliser (see section *6.2 Incompatibilities*).
- The complete contents of a single ampoule should be placed in the bowl of a jet nebuliser/compressor system, such as the Hudson T Up-draft II/Pulmo-Aide, Airlife Misty/Pulmo-Aide, customised Respirgard/Pulmo-Aide, or Acorn II/Pulmo-Aide.
- Pulmozyme may also be used in conjunction with a reusable jet nebuliser/compressor system, such as the Pari LL/Inhalierboy, Pari LC/Inhalierboy or Master, Aiolos/2 Aiolos, Side Stream/CR50 or MobilAire or Porta-Neb.
- Ultrasonic nebulisers may be unsuitable for delivery of Pulmozyme because they may inactivate Pulmozyme or have unacceptable aerosol delivery characteristics.
- The manufacturers' instructions on the use and maintenance of the nebuliser and compressor should be followed.
- Containment of the aerosol is not necessary.
- Pulmozyme ampoules are for single administration only.

7. MARKETING AUTHORISATION HOLDER

Roche Products Limited

40 Broadwater Road

Welwyn Garden City

Hertfordshire, AL7 3AY

United Kingdom

8. MARKETING AUTHORISATION NUMBER(S)

PL 0031/0335

9. DATE OF FIRST AUTHORISATION/RENEWAL OF THE AUTHORISATION

Date of last renewal: January 2005

10. DATE OF REVISION OF THE TEXT

April 2004

Pulmozyme is a registered trade mark

Puri-Nethol Tablets

(GlaxoSmithKline UK)

1. NAME OF THE MEDICINAL PRODUCT

Puri-Nethol 50 mg tablets

2. QUALITATIVE AND QUANTITATIVE COMPOSITION

	mg/tab
Mercaptopurine	50.0

3. PHARMACEUTICAL FORM

Tablets

4. CLINICAL PARTICULARS

4.1 Therapeutic indications

Cytotoxic agent.

Puri-Nethol is indicated for the treatment of acute leukaemia. It may be utilised in remission induction and it is particularly indicated for maintenance therapy in: acute lymphoblastic leukaemia; acute myelogenous leukaemia. Puri-Nethol may be used in the treatment of chronic granulocytic leukaemia.

4.2 Posology and method of administration

For oral administration

Dosage in adults and children:

For adults and children the usual starting dose is 2.5 mg/kg bodyweight per day, or 50-75 mg/m^2 body surface area per day, but the dose and duration of administration depend on the nature and dosage of other cytotoxic agents given in conjunction with Puri-Nethol.

The dosage should be carefully adjusted to suit the individual patient.

Puri-Nethol has been used in various combination therapy schedules for acute leukaemia and the literature should be consulted for details.

Dosage in the elderly:

No specific studies have been carried out in the elderly. However, it is advisable to monitor renal and hepatic function in these patients, and if there is any impairment, consideration should be given to reducing the Puri-Nethol dosage.

Dosage in renal impairment:

Consideration should be given to reducing the dosage in patients with impaired renal function.

Dosage in hepatic function:

Consideration should be given to reducing the dosage in patients with impaired hepatic function.

In general:

When Zyloric (allopurinol) and 6-mercaptopurine are administered concomitantly it is essential that only a quarter of the usual dose of 6-mercaptopurine is given since Zyloric (allopurinol) decreases the rate of catabolism of 6-mercaptopurine.

4.3 Contraindications

Hypersensitivity to any component of the preparation.

In view of the seriousness of the indications there are no other absolute contra-indications.

4.4 Special warnings and special precautions for use

Puri-Nethol is an active cytotoxic agent for use only under the direction of physicians experienced in the administration of such agents.

Safe handling of Puri-Nethol Tablets:

See section 6.6 Instructions for Use/Handling

Monitoring:

Treatment with Puri-Nethol causes bone marrow suppression leading to leucopenia and thrombocytopenia and, less frequently, to anaemia. Full blood counts must be taken daily during remission induction and careful monitoring of haematological parameters should be conducted during maintenance therapy.

The leucocyte and platelet counts continue to fall after treatment is stopped, so at the first sign of an abnormally large fall in the counts, treatment should be interrupted immediately.

Bone marrow suppression is reversible if Puri-Nethol is withdrawn early enough.

During remission induction in acute myelogenous leukaemia the patient may frequently have to survive a period of relative bone marrow aplasia and it is important that adequate supportive facilities are available.

There are individuals with an inherited deficiency of the enzyme thiopurine methyltransferase (TPMT) who may be unusually sensitive to the myelosuppresive effect of 6-mercaptopurine and prone to developing rapid bone marrow depression following the initiation of treatment with Puri-Nethol. This problem could be exacerbated by coadministration with drugs that inhibit TPMT, such as olsalazine, mesalazine or sulphasalazine. Some laboratories offer testing for TPMT deficiency, although these tests have not been shown to identify all patients at risk of severe toxicity. Therefore close monitoring of blood counts is still necessary.

Puri-Nethol is hepatotoxic and liver function tests should be monitored weekly during treatment. More frequent monitoring may be advisable in those with pre-existing liver disease or receiving other potentially hepatotoxic therapy. The patient should be instructed to discontinue Puri-Nethol immediately if jaundice becomes apparent.

During remission induction when rapid cell lysis is occurring, uric acid levels in blood and urine should be monitored as hyperuricaemia and/or hyperuricosuria may develop, with the risk of uric acid nephropathy.

Cross resistance usually exists between 6-mercaptopurine and 6-thioguanine.

The dosage of 6-mercaptopurine may need to be reduced when this agent is combined with other drugs whose primary or secondary toxicity is myelosuppression.

Mutagenicity and carcinogenicity:

Increases in chromosomal aberrations were observed in the peripheral lymphocytes of leukaemic patients, in a hypernephroma patient who received an unstated dose of 6-mercaptopurine and in patients with chronic renal disease treated at doses of 0.4 – 1.0 mg/kg/day.

In view of its action on cellular deoxyribonucleic acid (DNA) 6-mercaptopurine is potentially carcinogenic and consideration should be given to the theoretical risk of carcinogenisis with this treatment.

Two cases have been documented of the occurrence of acute nonlymphatic leukaemia in patients who received 6-mercaptopurine, in combination with other drugs, for non-neoplastic disorders. A single case has been reported where a patient was treated for pyoderma gangrenosum with 6-mercaptopurine and later developed acute nonlymphatic leukaemia, but it is not clear whether this was part of the natural history of the disease or if the 6-mercaptopurine played a causative role.

A patient with Hodgkins Disease treated with 6-mercaptopurine and multiple additional cytotoxic agents developed acute myelogenous leukaemia.

Twelve and a half years after 6-mercaptopurine treatment for myasthenia gravis a female patient developed chronic myeloid leukaemia.

4.5 Interaction with other medicinal products and other forms of Interaction

When Zyloric (allopurinol) and Puri-Nethol are administered concomitantly it is essential that only a quarter of the usual dose of Puri-Nethol is given since Zyloric decreases the rate of catabolism of Puri-Nethol.

Inhibition of the anticoagulant effect of warfarin, when given with Puri-Nethol, has been reported.

As there is *in vitro* evidence that aminosalicylate derivatives (eg. olsalazine, mesalazine or sulphasalazine) inhibit the TPMT enzyme, they should be administered with caution to patients receiving concurrent Puri-Nethol therapy (see Special Warnings and Precautions for Use).

4.6 Pregnancy and lactation

Teratogenicity:

Puri-Nethol has been shown to be embryotoxic in rats at doses that are not toxic to the mother. It has also proven to be embryolethal when administered at higher doses in the first half of the gestation period.

Normal offspring have been born after Puri-Nethol therapy administered during human pregnancy, but abortion, prematurity and malformation have been reported. A leukaemia patient treated with 6-mercaptopurine 100 mg/day (plus splenic irradiation) throughout pregnancy gave birth to a normal, premature baby. A second baby, born to the same mother who was treated as before, together with busulphan 4 mg/day, had multiple severe abnormalities, including corneal opacities, microphthalmia, cleft palate and hypoplasia of the thyroid and ovaries.

Effects on fertility:

The effect of Puri-Nethol therapy on human fertility is largely unknown but there are reports of successful fatherhood/motherhood after receiving treatment during childhood or adolescence. Transient profound oligospermia was observed in a young man who received 6-mercaptopurine 150 mg/day plus prednisone 80 mg/day for acute leukaemia. Two years after cessation of the chemotherapy, he had a normal sperm count and he fathered a normal child.

Pregnancy:

The use of Puri-Nethol should be avoided whenever possible during pregnancy, particularly during the first trimester. In any individual case the potential hazard to the foetus must be balanced against the expected benefit to the mother.

As with all cytotoxic chemotherapy, adequate contraceptive precautions should be advised if either partner is receiving Puri-Nethol tablets.

Lactation:

6-Mercaptopurine has been detected in the breast milk of renal transplant patients receiving immunosuppressive therapy with azathioprine, a pro-drug of 6-mercaptopurine and thus mothers receiving Puri-Nethol should not breastfeed.

4.7 Effects on ability to drive and use machines

There are no data on the effect of 6-mercaptopurine on driving performance or the ability to operate machinery. A detrimental effect on these activities cannot be predicted from the pharmacology of the drug.

4.8 Undesirable effects

The main side effect of treatment with Puri-Nethol is bone marrow suppression leading to leucopenia and thrombocytopenia. Puri-Nethol is hepatotoxic in animals and man. The histological findings in man have shown hepatic necrosis and biliary stasis. The incidence of hepatotoxicity varies considerably and can occur with any dose but more frequently when the recommended dose of 2.5 mg/kg bodyweight daily or 75 mg/m^2 body surface area per day is exceeded.

Monitoring of liver function tests may allow early detection of liver toxicity. This is usually reversible if Puri-Nethol therapy is stopped soon enough, but fatal liver damage has occurred.

Anorexia, nausea and vomiting have occasionally been noted.

Oral ulceration has been reported during Puri-Nethol therapy and rarely intestinal ulceration has occurred.

Rare complications are drug fever and skin rash.

Pancreatitis has been reported in association with the unlicensed use of 6-mercaptopurine in the treatment of inflammatory bowel disease.

Alopecia has been reported.

4.9 Overdose

Symptoms and signs:

Gastrointestinal effects, including nausea, vomiting and diarrhoea and anorexia may be early symptoms of overdosage having occurred. The principal toxic effect is on the bone marrow, resulting in myelosuppression. Haematological toxicity is likely to be more profound with chronic overdosage than with a single ingestion of Puri-Nethol. Liver dysfunction and gastroenteritis may also occur.

The risk of overdosage is also increased when Zyloric is being given concomitantly with Puri-Nethol (see Interaction with other Medicaments and other forms of Interaction).

Management:

As there is no known antidote the blood picture should be closely monitored and general supportive measures, together with appropriate blood transfusion, instituted if necessary. Active measures (such as the use of activated charcoal or gastric lavage) may not be effective in the event of 6-mercaptopurine overdose unless the procedure can be undertaken within 60 minutes of ingestion.

5. PHARMACOLOGICAL PROPERTIES

5.1 Pharmacodynamic properties

Pharmacotherapeutic group:

6-Mercaptopurine is sulphydryl analogue of the purine base hypoxanthine and acts as a cytotoxic antimetabolite.

Mode of Action:

6-Mercaptopurine is an inactive pro-drug which acts as a purine antagonist but requires cellular uptake and intracellular anabolism to thioguanine nucleotides for cytotoxicity. The 6-mercaptopurine metabolites inhibit *de novo* purine synthesis and purine nucleotide interconversions. The thioguanine nucleotides are also incorporated into nucleic acids and this contributes to the cytotoxic effects of the drug.

5.2 Pharmacokinetic properties

The bioavailability of oral 6-mercaptopurine shows considerable inter-individual variability, which probably results from its first-pass metabolism (when administered orally at a dosage of 75 mg/m^2 to 7 paediatric patients, the bioavailability averaged 16% of the administered dose, with a range of 5 to 37%).

The elimination half-life of 6-mercaptopurine is 90 ± 30 minutes, but the active metabolites have a longer half-life (approximately 5 hours) than the parent drug. The apparent body clearance is 4832 ± 2562 ml/min/m^2. There is low entry of 6-mercaptopurine into the cerebrospinal fluid.

The main method of elimination for 6-mercaptopurine is by metabolic alteration. The kidneys eliminate approximately 7% of 6-mercaptopurine unaltered within 12 hours of the drug being administered. Xanthine oxidase is the main catabolic enzyme of 6-mercaptopurine and it converts the drug into the inactive metabolite, 6-thiouric acid. This is excreted in the urine.

5.3 Preclinical safety data

Puri-Nethol in common with other antimetabolites is potentially mutagenic in man and chromosome damage has been reported in mice, rats and man.

6. PHARMACEUTICAL PARTICULARS

6.1 List of excipients

Lactose

Maize Starch

Hydrolysed Starch

Stearic Acid

Magnesium Stearate

Purified Water

6.2 Incompatibilities

None known

6.3 Shelf life

60 months

6.4 Special precautions for storage

Store below 25°C. Keep the bottle tightly closed.

6.5 Nature and contents of container

Amber glass bottles with child resistant high density polyethylene closures with induction heat seal liners.

Pack size: 25 tablets

6.6 Instructions for use and handling

Safe handling:

It is recommended that the handling of Puri-Nethol tablets follows the "Guidelines for the Handling of Cytotoxic Drugs", according to prevailing local recommendations and/or regulations.

It is advisable that care be taken when handling or halving these tablets not to contaminate hands or inspire drug.

Disposal:

Puri-Nethol tablets surplus to requirements should be destroyed in a manner appropriate to the prevailing local regulations for the destruction of dangerous substances.

Administrative Data

7. MARKETING AUTHORISATION HOLDER

The Wellcome Foundation Ltd	trading as	GlaxoSmithKline
Glaxo Wellcome House		UK Stockley Park
Berkeley Avenue		West Uxbridge
Greenford		Middlesex UB11 1BT
Middlesex UB6 0NN		

8. MARKETING AUTHORISATION NUMBER(S)

PL 00003/5227R

9. DATE OF FIRST AUTHORISATION/RENEWAL OF THE AUTHORISATION

27 April 1998

10. DATE OF REVISION OF THE TEXT

31 July 2005

11. Legal Status

POM

Pylorid Tablets

(GlaxoSmithKline UK)

1. NAME OF THE MEDICINAL PRODUCT

Pylorid tablets.

2. QUALITATIVE AND QUANTITATIVE COMPOSITION

Each tablet contains 400 mg of ranitidine bismuth citrate (INN).

3. PHARMACEUTICAL FORM

Film coated tablets.

These tablets are light blue, octagonal capsule-shaped identified by a logo on one face.

4. CLINICAL PARTICULARS

4.1 Therapeutic indications

Eradication of *Helicobacter pylori* and prevention of relapse of peptic ulcer disease when administered in co-prescription with appropriate antibiotic(s).

Treatment of duodenal ulcer and benign gastric ulcer.

4.2 Posology and method of administration

Pylorid should be taken twice daily (morning and evening), preferably with food.

Eradication of *Helicobacter pylori* and prevention of relapse of peptic ulcer disease:-

The following dosage regimens have been shown to be clinically effective. Selection of the appropriate regimen should be based on patient tolerability and local prescribing habits/availability of the antibiotic(s).

7 -day triple therapy regimens:-

The recommended dose of Pylorid is 400 mg twice daily taken orally with antibiotics as detailed below:-

clarithromycin 500 mg twice daily with either	metronidazole 400 mg or 500 mg twice daily
or	amoxycillin 1 g twice daily
clarithromycin 250 mg twice daily with	metronidazole 400 mg or 500 mg twice daily

Alternatively, 14-day dual therapy regimens may be given as follows:

Pylorid 400 mg twice daily with either	clarithromycin 500 mg two or three times daily
or	in cases where clarithromycin cannot be given, amoxycillin 500 mg four times daily, although the latter resulted in lower eradication rates.

If symptoms recur and the patient is *H. pylori* positive, a further course of Pylorid together with an alternative antibiotic regimen may be considered.

To facilitate ulcer healing, therapy with Pylorid 400 mg twice daily may be continued to 28 days.

Treatment of Peptic Ulcer Disease:-

Duodenal Ulcer: Pylorid 400 mg twice daily for 4 weeks. Treatment may be extended for a further 4 weeks.

Benign Gastric Ulcer: Pylorid 400 mg twice daily for 8 weeks.

Pylorid is not indicated for long-term (maintenance) therapy; more than two 8-week courses in any one year should be avoided because of the possibility of accumulation of bismuth. If 4-week courses of therapy are given, up to a maximum of 16 weeks of treatment may be given in any one year.

Elderly patients:- Ranitidine and bismuth exposure is increased in elderly patients as a result of decreased renal clearance. (See renal impairment (below) and Section 4.3 Contra-indications).

Children: There are no data available on the use of Pylorid tablets in children. Therefore, they are not recommended for use in children.

Renal Impairment: Ranitidine and bismuth exposure is increased in patients with renal impairment as a result of decreased clearance. As with other bismuth-containing drugs, Pylorid should not be used in patients with moderate to severe renal impairment ie, creatinine clearance typically < 25 mL/min. (See Section 4.3 Contra-indications).

Hepatic Impairment: There is no information regarding the use of Pylorid tablets in patients with hepatic impairment. However, as ranitidine and bismuth in the systemic circulation are eliminated mainly by renal clearance, no dosage adjustment is necessary in hepatically impaired patients.

4.3 Contraindications

Pylorid tablets are contra-indicated in patients known to have hypersensitivity to any of the ingredients.

Pylorid is contra-indicated for long-term (maintenance) therapy.

As with other bismuth-containing drugs, Pylorid should not be used in patients with moderate to severe renal impairment (i.e., creatinine clearance typically <25 mL/min).

4.4 Special warnings and special precautions for use

The possibility of malignancy should be excluded before commencement of therapy in patients with gastric ulcer, as treatment with Pylorid tablets may mask symptoms of gastric carcinoma.

Pylorid tablets should be avoided in patients with a history of acute porphyria.

When co-prescription with antibiotic(s) is clinically indicated, the relevant prescribing information should be consulted prior to initiation of therapy.

4.5 Interaction with other medicinal products and other forms of Interaction

An increase in median trough plasma bismuth concentrations has been observed when Pylorid is co-administered with clarithromycin, however, this has not been associated with any adverse clinical sequelae in clinical trials. This increase was not observed in clinical studies in patients receiving 7-day triple therapy with Pylorid, clarithromycin and either metronidazole or amoxycillin. Clarithromycin levels are unaffected by the administration of ranitidine bismuth citrate, although systemic exposure to the active metabolite of clarithromycin is increased. The ranitidine absorption from Pylorid tablets is increased when co-administered with clarithromycin. This enhanced ranitidine exposure is of no clinical concern due to the wide therapeutic index of ranitidine.

Food causes a decrease in bismuth absorption which is not of any clinical relevance. Limited data suggest increased ulcer healing when Pylorid tablets are administered with food. (See Section 4.2 Posology).

The co-administration of antacids with Pylorid tablets does not result in any clinically relevant effect.

4.6 Pregnancy and lactation

The safety of ranitidine bismuth citrate in human pregnancy has not been established. As animal reproductive studies are not always predictive of human response, Pylorid tablets should not be used in pregnancy.

It has been demonstrated in animal reproductive studies that during repeat dosing, low levels of ranitidine and bismuth cross the placenta. There was no evidence that ranitidine bismuth citrate induced any major malformations in either foetal rats or rabbits after maternal administration at high dose levels. Embryo/foetal lethality in rabbits, as a consequence of the maternal susceptibility to antimicrobial agents, together with minor effects of skeletal development in both rats and rabbits, were a result of dose levels considerably in excess of clinical exposure and were related to maternal toxicity.

It has been demonstrated that during repeat dosing of ranitidine bismuth citrate in the lactating rat, low levels of ranitidine and bismuth are secreted in the milk with consequent exposure of the pups. The passage of ranitidine bismuth citrate into human breast milk has not been evaluated.

Consequently, Pylorid tablets should not be used by women who are breast feeding.

4.7 Effects on ability to drive and use machines

None reported.

4.8 Undesirable effects

The following convention has been utilised for the classification of undesirable effects: very common ($<1/10$), common $>1/100$, $<1/10$), uncommon $>1/1000$, $<1/100$), rare $>1/10,000$, $<1/1000$), very rare ($<1/10,000$). Adverse event frequencies have been estimated from spontaneous reports from post-marketing data.

Blood and Lymphatic System Disorders:-

Uncommon: Anaemia

Immune System Disorders:-

Rare: Hypersensitivity reactions.

Very rare: Anaphylaxis.

Nervous System Disorders:-

Very rare: Headache

Gastrointestinal Disorders:-

Common: Black stools, black tongue. Blackening of the stools is frequently reported with bismuth-containing drugs. As with other medicines containing bismuth, ranitidine bismuth citrate may cause blackening of the tongue.

Uncommon: Gastric pain

Very rare: Diarrhoea, abdominal discomfort

Hepato-biliary Disorders:-

Uncommon: Abnormal liver function tests. Treatment with Pylorid tablets may cause transient changes in the liver enzymes SGPT (ALT) and SGOT (AST).

Skin and Subcutaneous Tissue Disorders:-

Rare: Skin rash

Very rare: Pruritus

The following have been reported as adverse events in patients treated with ranitidine hydrochloride. Because ranitidine hydrochloride. is used for longer treatment periods, the relevance of some of the events to the clinical use of Pylorid tablets is unknown.

Blood and Lymphatic System Disorders:-

Very rare: Blood count changes (leucopenia, thrombocytopenia). These are usually reversible. Agranulocytosis or pancytopenia, sometimes with marrow hypoplasia or marrow aplasia.

Immune System Disorders:-

Rare: Hypersensitivity reactions (urticaria, angioneurotic oedema, fever, bronchospasm, hypotension and chest pain).

Very rare: Anaphylactic shock.

These events have been reported after a single dose.

Psychiatric Disorders:-

Very rare: Reversible mental confusion, depression and hallucinations.

These have been reported predominantly in severely ill and elderly patients.

Nervous System Disorders:-

Very rare: Headache (sometimes severe), dizziness and reversible involuntary movement disorders.

Eye Disorders:-

Very rare: Reversible blurred vision. There have been reports of blurred vision, which is suggestive in a change in accommodation.

Cardiac Disorders:-

Very rare: As with other H2 receptor antagonists bradycardia, A-V block and asystole (injection only).

Vascular Disorders:-

Very rare: Vasculitis.

Gastrointestinal Disorders:-

Very rare: Acute pancreatitis, diarrhoea.

Hepatobiliary Disorders:-

Rare: Transient and reversible changes in liver function tests.

Very rare: Hepatitis (hepatocellular, hepatocanalicular or mixed) with or without jaundice, these are usually reversible.

Skin and Subcutaneous Tissue Disorders:-

Rare: Skin rash

Very rare: Erythema multiforme, alopecia.

Musculoskeletal and Connective Tissue Disorders:-

Very rare: Musculoskeletal symptoms such as arthralgia and myalgia

Renal and Urinary Disorders:-

Very rare: Acute interstitial nephritis

Reproductive System and Breast Disorders:-

Very rare: Reversible impotence, breast symptoms in men.

4.9 Overdose

Administration of ranitidine bismuth citrate in acute animal studies at very high dosages has been associated with nephrotoxicity. In cases of overdose, gastric lavage and appropriate supportive therapy would be indicated.

5. PHARMACOLOGICAL PROPERTIES

5.1 Pharmacodynamic properties

Pharmaco-therapeutic group:

Pylorid tablets are histamine H_2-receptor antagonists, with anti-*Helicobacter pylori*, and mucosal protective activity.

Mechanism of action:

Ranitidine bismuth citrate inhibits basal and stimulated secretion of gastric acid, reducing both the volume and the acid and pepsin content of the secretion, is bactericidal to *Helicobacter pylori, in vitro*, and has gastric mucosal-protective actions.

These pharmacodynamic properties depend on the dissociation of ranitidine bismuth citrate into ranitidine and bismuth components. The biological and anti-*H. pylori* activity of the latter is related to the solubility of dissociated bismuth from ranitidine bismuth citrate. As the absorption of bismuth from ranitidine bismuth citrate is minimal (see Section 5.2 Pharmacokinetic Properties) the *H. pylori* activity is a local effect. Even in acidic conditions, which lead to precipitation of bismuth, sufficient bismuth from ranitidine bismuth citrate remains soluble to inhibit the growth of *H. pylori*.

5.2 Pharmacokinetic properties

Bismuth absorption from Pylorid tablets is less than 1% of the bismuth dose administered, and is similar in healthy volunteers, male and female subjects, patients with peptic ulcer disease and gastritis patients. The rate of absorption of ranitidine and bismuth is rapid, the time to peak plasma levels typically being 1-3 hr and 15-60 min, respectively. The absorption of bismuth from Pylorid tablets is dependent on intragastric pH and increases if the intragastric pH is raised to ≥ 6 prior to dosing. However the co-administration of antacids has no clinically relevant effect (see Section 4.5 Interactions).

Ranitidine is cleared primarily by renal clearance (approximately 500 mL/min). This accounts for approximately 70% of the total clearance, which is approximately 700 mL/min. Ranitidine is rapidly eliminated from the body, with a half-life of about 3 hours after oral dosing; and does not accumulate in the plasma with twice daily dosing.

Bismuth in the systemic circulation is cleared from the body mainly by renal clearance (approximately 50 mL/min). Multiple half-lives describe the distribution and elimination of bismuth. The mean terminal plasma half-life of bismuth is 20.7 days and the mean terminal half-life of bismuth urinary excretion is 45.1 days. Bismuth accumulates in plasma upon twice daily Dosing with Pylorid tablets. Within 3 months of completing a 4- or 8-week course of treatment with Pylorid, plasma concentrations and urinary excretion of bismuth have returned to pre-treatment levels in most patients.

Ranitidine and bismuth exposure is increased in patients with renal impairment and the elderly as a result of decreased renal clearance.

Patients with moderate to severe renal impairment (creatinine clearance typically < 25 mL/min) should not be given Pylorid tablets (see Section 4.2 Posology and Section 4.3 Contraindications).

5.3 Preclinical safety data

In acute animal studies at high dosages, nephrotoxicity was observed in all species studied.

In local tolerance studies ranitidine bismuth citrate was slightly irritating to abraded guinea pig skin. It was also a weak skin contact sensitiser in the guinea pig "split adjuvant" test.

No mutagenic activity was seen in standard genotoxicity tests with ranitidine bismuth citrate. A weak clastogenic effect was seen *in vitro*. This can be accounted for as an effect of a bismuth containing compound as it also occurred with bismuth citrate, at bismuth equivalent concentrations of 33 μg/mL for ranitidine bismuth citrate compared to 26 μg/mL for bismuth citrate. As no genotoxic activity was demonstrated *in vivo* these findings are not considered to be of any clinical significance.

Evidence of bismuth accumulation in tissues to steady state was observed following long-term repeat dosing in animal studies. To avoid the possibility of bismuth accumulation, ranitidine bismuth citrate is not indicated for maintenance therapy in man.

6. PHARMACEUTICAL PARTICULARS

6.1 List of excipients

Tablet core:-

Sodium carbonate (anhydrous) USNF.

Microcrystalline cellulose PhEur.

Polyvidone K30 PhEur.

Magnesium stearate PhEur.

Tablet film coat:-

Hydroxypropylmethyl cellulose PhEur (E464).

Titanium dioxide PhEur (E171).

Triacetin USP.

Indigo carmine aluminium lake (E132).

6.2 Incompatibilities

None reported.

6.3 Shelf life

3 years.

6.4 Special precautions for storage

Do not store Pylorid tablets above 30°C.

6.5 Nature and contents of container

Cartons containing 14, 28, or 56 tablets in a double foil blister pack.

6.6 Instructions for use and handling

None.

Administrative Data

7. MARKETING AUTHORISATION HOLDER

Glaxo Group Limited
Greenford Road
Greenford
Middlesex
UB6 0NN
United Kingdom.

8. MARKETING AUTHORISATION NUMBER(S)

14213/0001

9. DATE OF FIRST AUTHORISATION/RENEWAL OF THE AUTHORISATION

28 July 2000

10. DATE OF REVISION OF THE TEXT

24th June 2005

11. Legal Status

POM

Pyralvex

(Norgine Limited)

1. NAME OF THE MEDICINAL PRODUCT

PYRALVEX.

2. QUALITATIVE AND QUANTITATIVE COMPOSITION

PYRALVEX contains the following active ingredients in each 1ml of solution:

Rhubarb Extract	50 mg (equivalent to 5 mg anthraquinone glycosides)
Salicylic Acid	10 mg

3. PHARMACEUTICAL FORM

Oromucosal solution.

4. CLINICAL PARTICULARS

4.1 Therapeutic indications

For the symptomatic relief of pain associated with recurrent mouth ulcers and denture irritation.

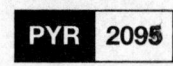

4.2 Posology and method of administration

Adults (including the elderly): To be applied to the inflamed oral mucosa (after removing any dentures) three or four times daily using the brush provided.

Children: Not recommended below the age of 12 years.

4.3 Contraindications

None known.

4.4 Special warnings and special precautions for use

Each bottle of PYRALVEX should be used by only one person.

4.5 Interaction with other medicinal products and other forms of Interaction

None known.

4.6 Pregnancy and lactation

There is no evidence to suggest that PYRALVEX should not be used during pregnancy or lactation.

4.7 Effects on ability to drive and use machines

None.

4.8 Undesirable effects

None known.

4.9 Overdose

Not applicable.

5. PHARMACOLOGICAL PROPERTIES

5.1 Pharmacodynamic properties

Pharmacological studies have shown that the active ingredients of PYRALVEX display anti-inflammatory, analgesic and anti-microbial properties, which are the basis of its clinical efficacy.

5.2 Pharmacokinetic properties

Systemic availability of PYRALVEX is unlikely to be significant, owing to the low levels of ingredients administered.

5.3 Preclinical safety data

Preclinical studies indicate that at clinically effective doses, the ingredients in PYRALVEX are unlikely to have any potential for toxic effects.

6. PHARMACEUTICAL PARTICULARS

6.1 List of excipients

Ethanol

Water

6.2 Incompatibilities

None known.

6.3 Shelf life

The shelf life is 3 years.

6.4 Special precautions for storage

Store below 25°C.

6.5 Nature and contents of container

An amber glass bottle with brush applicator containing 10ml of solution.

6.6 Instructions for use and handling

Avoid rinsing of the mouth or eating for 15 minutes after application. Any discolouration which may occur will disappear during normal cleaning of the teeth.

7. MARKETING AUTHORISATION HOLDER

Norgine Limited

Chaplin House

Widewater Place

Moorhall Road

Harefield

UXBRIDGE

Middlesex, UB9 6NS

United Kingdom

8. MARKETING AUTHORISATION NUMBER(S)

PL 00322/5013

9. DATE OF FIRST AUTHORISATION/RENEWAL OF THE AUTHORISATION

May 1972.

10. DATE OF REVISION OF THE TEXT

October 1996.

Legal Category: **P**

Questran & Questran Light

(Bristol-Myers Pharmaceuticals)

1. NAME OF THE MEDICINAL PRODUCT

QUESTRAN

QUESTRAN LIGHT

2. QUALITATIVE AND QUANTITATIVE COMPOSITION

Each sachet contains 4g anhydrous colestyramine (a basic anion-exchange resin).

3. PHARMACEUTICAL FORM

Powder for oral administration.

4. CLINICAL PARTICULARS

4.1 Therapeutic indications

Questran is used for:

1. Primary prevention of coronary heart disease in men between 35 and 59 years of age and with primary hypercholesterolaemia who have not responded to diet and other appropriate measures.
2. Reduction of plasma cholesterol in hypercholesterolaemia, particularly in those patients who have been diagnosed as Fredrickson's Type II (high plasma cholesterol with normal or slightly elevated triglycerides).
3. Relief of pruritus associated with partial biliary obstruction and primary biliary cirrhosis.
4. Relief of diarrhoea associated with ileal resection, Crohn's disease, vagotomy and diabetic vagal neuropathy.
5. Management of radiation-induced diarrhoea.

4.2 Posology and method of administration

Adults:

As a precautionary measure, where concurrent drug therapy exists then such drugs should be administered at least one hour before or 4-6 hours after Questran.

Questran should not be taken in its dry form.

Questran should be administered mixed with water or a suitable liquid, such as fruit juice, and stirred to a uniform consistency.

Questran may also be mixed with skimmed milk, thin soups, pulpy fruits with high moisture content, e.g. apple sauce, etc.

1. For primary prevention of coronary heart disease and to reduce cholesterol: After initial introduction over a three to four week period, 3 to 6 Questran sachets per day, administered either as a single daily dose or in divided doses up to four times daily, according to dosage requirements and patient acceptability. Dosage may be modified according to response and can be increased to 9 sachets per day if necessary. Occasional slight gastro-intestinal upsets, e.g. constipation, may occur when starting Questran. These usually pass with continued usage of Questran and are minimised by starting therapy gradually.

(see Table 1 below)

2. To relieve pruritus: One or two sachets daily are usually sufficient.
3. To relieve diarrhoea: As for reduction of cholesterol but it may be possible to reduce this dosage. In all patients presenting with diarrhoea induced by bile acid malabsorption, if a response is not seen within 3 days, then alternative therapy should be initiated.

Children:

Children 6 - 12 years: The initial dose is determined by the following formula:

$$\frac{\text{Child's Weight in Kg x Adult Dose}}{70}$$

Subsequent dosage adjustment may be necessary where clinically indicated.

Children under 6 years: The dose has not been established in infants and children under 6 years.

Elderly:

No dosage adjustment is necessary.

4.3 Contraindications

Questran is contra-indicated in patients who have shown hypersensitivity to any of the product ingredients.

In patients with complete biliary obstruction, since Questran cannot be effective where bile is not secreted into the intestine.

4.4 Special warnings and special precautions for use

Reduction of serum folate concentrations has been reported in children with familial hypercholesterolaemia. Supplementation with folic acid should be considered in these cases.

Questran: Diabetic patients should be warned that each sachet of Questran contains 3.79 g sucrose.

Questran Light contains aspartame, a source of phenylalanine.

4.5 Interaction with other medicinal products and other forms of Interaction

Questran may delay or reduce the absorption of certain drugs (such as digitalis, tetracycline, chlorothiazide, warfarin and thyroxine). The response to concomitant medication should be closely monitored and appropriate adjustments made if necessary.

Questran may interfere with the pharmacokinetics of drugs that undergo enterohepatic recirculation.

Patients should take other drugs at least one hour before or 4-6 hours after Questran to minimise possible interference with their absorption.

4.6 Pregnancy and lactation

The safety of colestyramine in pregnancy and lactation has not been established and the possibility of interference with absorption of fat soluble vitamins should be considered.

4.7 Effects on ability to drive and use machines

None.

4.8 Undesirable effects

Since Questran may interfere with the absorption of fat soluble vitamins, the diet may require supplementation with Vitamins A, D and K during prolonged high dose administration.

Chronic use of Questran may be associated with increased bleeding tendency due to hypoprothrombinaemia associated with Vitamin K deficiency. This will usually respond promptly to parenteral Vitamin K administration; recurrences can be prevented by oral administration of Vitamin K.

Hyperchloraemic acidosis has occasionally been reported following the prolonged use of anion exchange resins.

Gastro-intestinal side effects are those most frequently reported. The principal complaint is constipation which may be controlled with the usual remedies, and frequently disappears on continued usage of Questran. Large doses of Questran can cause diarrhoea.

Taste disturbance and skin irritation have been reported rarely but causal relationship to colestyramine remains undetermined. Rare reports of intestinal obstruction have been received.

4.9 Overdose

One case of medication error experienced heartburn and nausea after taking colestyramine 27g t.i.d. for a week. The potential problem in overdosage would be obstruction of the gastrointestinal tract.

5. PHARMACOLOGICAL PROPERTIES

5.1 Pharmacodynamic properties

Cholesterol is a major, if not the sole precursor of bile acids. During normal digestion, bile acids are secreted via the bile from the liver and gall bladder into the small intestine. Bile acids emulsify the fat and lipid materials present in foods, thus facilitating absorption. A major portion of the bile acids secreted are reabsorbed from the ileum and returned via the portal vein to the liver, thus completing the enterohepatic cycle. Only very small amounts of bile acids are found in normal serum.

Colestyramine resin absorbs and combines with the bile acids in the intestine to form an insoluble complex which is excreted in the faeces. This results in a continuous, though partial, removal of bile acids from the enterohepatic circulation by preventing their reabsorption. The increased faecal loss of bile acids leads to an increased oxidation of cholesterol to bile acids and a decrease in serum cholesterol levels and low density lipoprotein serum levels. Colestyramine is hydrophilic but it is not soluble in water, nor is it hydrolysed by digestive enzymes.

In patients with partial biliary obstruction, the reduction of serum bile acid levels reduces excess bile acids deposited in the dermal tissue with resultant decrease in pruritus.

5.2 Pharmacokinetic properties

Colestyramine is not absorbed from the digestive tract.

5.3 Preclinical safety data

No further significant information.

6. PHARMACEUTICAL PARTICULARS

6.1 List of excipients

Questran:	Acacia, citric acid anhydrous, orange juice flavour, polysorbate 80, propylene glycol alginate, sucrose.
Questran Light:	Aspartame, citric acid anhydrous, colloidal anhydrous silica, orange juice flavour, propylene glycol alginate, xanthan gum.

6.2 Incompatibilities

None known.

6.3 Shelf life

Questran:	48 months
Questran Light:	36 months

6.4 Special precautions for storage

Do not store above 30°C. Store in a dry place.

6.5 Nature and contents of container

Original packs containing 50 laminate sachets composed of paper, polyethylene and aluminium.

6.6 Instructions for use and handling

No special instructions.

7. MARKETING AUTHORISATION HOLDER

Bristol-Myers Squibb Holdings Limited

t/a Bristol-Myers Pharmaceuticals

Uxbridge Business Park

Sanderson Road

Uxbridge

Middlesex UB8 1DH

8. MARKETING AUTHORISATION NUMBER(S)

Questran:	PL 0125/5009R
Questran Light:	PL 0125/0192

9. DATE OF FIRST AUTHORISATION/RENEWAL OF THE AUTHORISATION

Questran:	22 January 1987 / 23 April 2002
Questran Light:	25 July 1988 / 18 September 1998

10. DATE OF REVISION OF THE TEXT

July 2005

Table 1

Final dose required	Week1	Week 2	Week 3	Week 4
	Sachets per day			
3	1	2	3	3
4	1	2	3	4
6	1	2	3	6

Rabies Vaccine BP

(Sanofi Pasteur MSD)

1. NAME OF THE MEDICINAL PRODUCT

Mérieux Inactivated Rabies Vaccine (MIRV)

Rabies Vaccine BP Pasteur Mérieux.

2. QUALITATIVE AND QUANTITATIVE COMPOSITION

Active Ingredient:

Inactivated Rabies Virus ... not less than 2.5 International Units per dose

Strain PM/WI 38 1503-3M

3. PHARMACEUTICAL FORM

Single dose vial of lyophilised vaccine and single dose syringe of diluent.

4. CLINICAL PARTICULARS

4.1 Therapeutic indications

For prophylactic immunisation against rabies. Treatment of patients following suspected rabies contact.

4.2 Posology and method of administration

Administer by intramuscular or deep subcutaneous injection. The vaccine should be administered into the deltoid region.

Adults, Elderly and Children

Prophylaxis:

Three injections each of 1 millilitre given on days 0, 7 and 28. A single reinforcing dose should be given at two or three year intervals to those at continued risk.

If, for whatever reason, it has not been possible to give a full course of three injections, it is probable that, in the majority of subjects, two doses may be adequate to confer protection, provided these were given four weeks apart. Subjects receiving only two injections who remain at continued risk should receive a reinforcing dose 6-12 months later, with further reinforcing doses given at two to three year intervals.

Treatment

(i) In persons known to have adequate prophylaxis:

In the event of contact with a suspected rabid animal, two further boosters should be given on day 0 and on day 3 to 7.

(ii) *In persons with no, or possibly inadequate, prophylaxis:*

The first injection of rabies vaccine should be given as soon as possible after the suspected contact (day 0) and followed by five further doses on days 3, 7, 14, 30 and 90. The use of Human Rabies Immunoglobulin on day 0 should be considered, but only in persons with no adequate prophylaxis. The treatment schedule may be stopped if the animal concerned is found conclusively to be free of rabies.

4.3 Contraindications

There are no absolute contra-indications to Rabies Vaccine BP, although if there were evidence of hypersensitivity, subsequent doses should not be given except for treatment.

4.4 Special warnings and special precautions for use

In subjects with a history of allergy there may be an increased risk of side-effects and this possibility should be taken into account.

As with all vaccines, appropriate facilities and medication such as epinephrine (adrenaline) should be readily available for immediate use in case of anaphylaxis or hypersensitivity following injection.

4.5 Interaction with other medicinal products and other forms of Interaction

None known.

4.6 Pregnancy and lactation

Because of the potential consequences of inadequately treated rabies exposure and because there is no indication that foetal abnormalities have been associated with rabies vaccination, pregnancy is not considered a contra-indication to post-exposure prophylaxis. If there is substantial risk of exposure to rabies, pre-exposure prophylaxis may also be indicated during pregnancy.

4.7 Effects on ability to drive and use machines

No adverse effects reported.

4.8 Undesirable effects

Minor local reactions:

pain, erythema, oedema, itching and induration at the injection site.

General reactions:

moderate fever, shivering, malaise, asthenia, headaches, dizziness, paraesthesia, arthralgia, myalgia, gastro-intestinal disorders (nausea, abdominal pains), allergic skin reactions (urticaria, rash, itching, oedema) have been reported with use of the vaccine. Exceptional cases of neuropathy have been reported.

In rarer cases:

anaphylactic reactions, serum sickness type reactions (following booster dose). Remedial facilities such as adrenaline should always therefore be available during vaccination. The vaccine contains traces of neomycin.

In subjects with a history of allergic reactions to previous doses of human diploid cell rabies vaccine, there may be an increased risk of side-effects and this should be taken into account.

4.9 Overdose

Not applicable.

5. PHARMACOLOGICAL PROPERTIES

5.1 Pharmacodynamic properties

The vaccine is a lyophilised, stabilised suspension of inactivated Wistar rabies virus strain PM/WI 38-1503-3M, cultured in human diploid cells (MRC_5) and inactivated by beta-propiolactone.

5.2 Pharmacokinetic properties

Not applicable.

5.3 Preclinical safety data

None stated.

6. PHARMACEUTICAL PARTICULARS

6.1 List of excipients

Human albumin.

Trace quantities of neomycin.

Diluent: Water for Injections (1 millilitre).

6.2 Incompatibilities

None known.

6.3 Shelf life

3 years

6.4 Special precautions for storage

Store between +2°C and +8°C. Do not freeze.

6.5 Nature and contents of container

Lyophilised vaccine - Single dose type 1 glass (Ph Eur) vial with elastomeric stopper and aluminium overcap.

Diluent - 1 millilitre disposable syringe type 1 glass (Ph Eur) with elastomeric cap.

6.6 Instructions for use and handling

Use immediately after reconstitution.

Shake well immediately before use.

Discard any unused vaccine one hour after reconstitution.

The lyophilised vaccine is coloured off white, but after reconstitution with the diluent supplied, it turns a pinkish colour due to the presence of phenol red.

7. MARKETING AUTHORISATION HOLDER

Sanofi Pasteur MSD Limited

Mallards Reach

Bridge Avenue

Maidenhead

Berkshire

SL6 1QP

8. MARKETING AUTHORISATION NUMBER(S)

PL 6745/0053

9. DATE OF FIRST AUTHORISATION/RENEWAL OF THE AUTHORISATION

7 November 1994

10. DATE OF REVISION OF THE TEXT

May 2005

11. LEGAL CATEGORY

POM

Rabipur (Masta Ltd)

(MASTA Ltd)

1. NAME OF THE MEDICINAL PRODUCT

Rabipur $\geqslant$ 2.5 IU/ml, powder and solvent for solution for injection

Rabies vaccine for human use prepared in cell cultures

2. QUALITATIVE AND QUANTITATIVE COMPOSITION

After reconstitution, 1 dose (1 ml) contains:

Rabies virus* (Inactivated, strain Flury LEP) .... $\geqslant$ 2.5 IU

* produced on purified chick embryo cells

For excipients, see Section 6.1.

3. PHARMACEUTICAL FORM

Powder and solvent for solution for injection.

A clear colourless solution results after reconstitution of the white freeze-dried powder with the clear and colourless solvent.

4. CLINICAL PARTICULARS

4.1 Therapeutic indications

a) Pre-exposure prophylaxis (before possible risk of exposure to rabies)

b) Post-exposure treatment (after known or possible exposure to rabies)

Consideration should be given to national and/or WHO guidance regarding the prevention of rabies.

4.2 Posology and method of administration

Posology

The recommended single intramuscular dose is 1 ml in all age groups.

Whenever possible according to vaccine availablility, it is recommended that one type of cell culture vaccine should be used throughout the course of pre- or post-exposure immunisation. However, adherence to the recommended schedules is of critical importance for post-exposure treatment, even if another type of cell culture vaccine has to be used.

PRE-EXPOSURE PROPHYLAXIS

Primary immunisation

In previously unvaccinated persons, an initial course of pre-exposure prophylaxis consists of three doses (each of 1 ml) administered on days 0, 7 and 21 or 28.

Booster doses

The need of intermittent serological testing for the presence of antibody $\geqslant$ 0.5 IU/ml (as assessed by the Rapid Focus-Fluorescent inhibition Test) and the administration of booster doses should be assessed in accordance with official recommendations.

The following provides general guidance:

- Testing for neutralising antibodies at 6-month intervals is usually recommended if the risk of exposure is high (e. g. Laboratory staff working with rabies virus).
- In persons who are considered to be at continuing risk of exposure to rabies (e. g. veterinarians and their assistants, wildlife workers, hunters), a serological test should usually be performed at least every 2 years, with shorter intervals if appropriate to the perceived degree of risk.
- In above mentioned cases, a booster dose should be given should the antibody titre fall below 0.5 IU/ml.
- Alternatively, booster doses may be given at official recommended intervals without prior serological testing, according to the perceived risk. Experience shows that reinforcing doses are generally required every 2-5 years.

Rabipur may be used for booster vaccination after prior immunisation with human diploid cell rabies vaccine.

POST-EXPOSURE TREATMENT

Post-exposure immunisation should begin as soon as possible after exposure and should be accompanied by local measures to the site of inoculation so as to reduce the risk of infection. Official guidance should be sought regarding the appropriate concomitant measures that should be taken to prevent establishment of infection (see also section 4.4).

Previously fully immunised individuals:

For WHO exposure categories II and III, and in category I cases where there is uncertainty regarding the correct classification of exposure (see Table 1 below), two doses (each of 1 ml) should be administered, one each on days 0 and 3. On a case by case basis, schedule A (see Table 2 below) may be applied if the last dose of vaccine was given more than two years previously.

Table 1: Immunisation schedules appropriate to different types of exposure (WHO 2002)

Exposure Category	Type of contact with suspect or confirmed rabid domestic or wild animal, or animal unavailable for observation[(a)]	Recommended treatment
I	Touching or feeding of animals	None, if reliable case history is available.
	Licks on intact skin	In case of unreliable case history, treat according to schedule A (see Table 2).
	Touching of inoculated animal lure with intact skin	

II	Nibbling of uncovered skin Minor scratches or abrasions without bleeding Licks on broken skin Touching of inoculated animal lure with skin damaged	Administer vaccine immediately [(b)] as in schedule A (see Table 2). In case of uncertainty and/or exposure in a high-risk area, administer active and passive treatment as in schedule B (see Table 2). (See also footnote [c)])
III	Single or multiple transdermal bites or scratches Contamination of mucous membrane with saliva (i. e. licks) Touching of inoculated animal lure with mucous membrane or fresh skin wound	Administer rabies immunoglobulin and vaccine immediately [(b)] as in schedule B (see Table 2). (See also footnote [c)])

[a)] Exposure to rodents, rabbits and hares seldom, if ever, requires specific anti-rabies treatment.

[b)] If an apparently healthy dog or cat in or from a low-risk area is placed under observation, it may be justified to delay specific treatment.

[c)] Stop treatment if animal is a cat or dog and remains healthy throughout an observation period of 10 days or if animal is euthanised and found to be negative for rabies by appropriate laboratory techniques. Except in the case of threatened or endangered species, other domestic and wild animals suspected as rabid should be euthanised and their tissues examined using appropriate laboratory techniques.

Individuals unimmunised or with uncertain immune status

Depending on the WHO category as in Table 1, treatment according to schedules A or B (see Table 2 below) may be required for previously unimmunised persons and for those who have received fewer than 3 doses of vaccine or who have received a vaccine of doubtful potency.

Table 2: Post-exposure treatment of subjects with no or uncertain immune status

Schedule A Active immunisation after exposure is required	Schedule B Active and passive immunisation after exposure are required
One injection of Rabipur i.m. on days: 0, 3, 7, 14, 28 (5-doses schedule) Or One dose of Rabipur is given into the right deltoid muscle and one dose into the left deltoid muscle on day 0, and one dose is applied into the deltoid muscle on days 7 and 21 (2-1-1 regimen). In small children the vaccine is to be given into the thighs.	Give Rabipur as in schedule A + 1 × 20 IU/kg body weight human rabies immunoglobulin* concomitantly with the first dose of Rabipur. If HRIG is not available at the time of the first vaccination it must be administered not later than 7 days after the first vaccination.

* Observe manufacturer's instructions regarding administration

Immunocompromised patients and patients with a particularly high risk of contracting rabies

For immunocompromised patients, those with multiple wounds and/or wounds on the head or other highly innervated areas, and those for whom there is a delay before initiation of treatment, it is recommended that:

- The days 0, 3, 7, 14 and 28 immunisation regimen should be used for these cases

- Two doses of vaccine may be given on day 0. That is, a single dose of 1 ml vaccine should be injected into the right deltoid and another single dose into the left deltoid muscle. In small children, one dose should be given into the anterolateral region of each thigh.

Severely immunosuppressed patients may not develop an immunologic response after rabies vaccination. Therefore, prompt and appropriate wound care after an exposure is an essential step in preventing death. In addition, rabies immune globulin should be administered in all immunosuppressed patients experiencing Category II and Category III wounds.

In immunocompromised patients, the neutralising antibody titre should be measured 14 days after the first injection. Patients with a titre that is less than 0.5 IU/ml should be given another two doses of vaccine simultaneously and as soon as possible. Further checks on the antibody titre should be made and further doses of vaccine should be administered as necessary.

In all cases, the immunisation schedule must be followed exactly as recommended, even if the patient does not present for treatment until a considerable time has elapsed since exposure.

Method of Administration

The vaccine should be given by intramuscular injection into the deltoid muscle, or into the anterolateral region of the thigh in small children.

It must not be given by intra-gluteal injection.

Do not administer by intravascular injection (see Section 4.4).

4.3 Contraindications

Post-exposure treatment

There are no contraindications to vaccination when post-exposure treatment is indicated. However, subjects considered to be at risk of a severe hypersensitivity reaction should receive an alternative rabies vaccine if a suitable product is available (see also section 4.4 regarding previous hypersensitivity reactions).

Pre-exposure prophylaxis

Rabipur should not be administered to subjects with a history of a severe hypersensitivity reaction to any of the ingredients in the vaccine. Note that the vaccine may contain polygeline, traces of neomycin, chlortetracycline, amphotericin B and chick proteins (see also section 4.4).

Vaccination should be delayed in subjects suffering from an acute febrile illness. Minor infections are not a contra-indication to vaccination.

4.4 Special warnings and special precautions for use

As with all vaccines, appropriate medical treatment should be immediately available for use in the rare event of an anaphylactic reaction to the vaccine.

A history of allergy to eggs or a positive skin test to ovalbumin does not necessarily indicate that a subject will be allergic to Rabipur. However, subjects who have a history of a severe hypersensitivity reaction to eggs or egg products should not receive the vaccine for pre-exposure prophylaxis. Such subjects should not receive the vaccine for post-exposure treatment unless a suitable alternative vaccine is not available, in which case all injections should be administered with close monitoring and with facilities for emergency treatment.

Similarly, subjects with a history of a severe hypersensitivity reaction to any of the other ingredients in Rabipur such as polygeline (stabilizer), or to amphotericin B, chlortetracycline or neomycin (which may be present as trace residues) should not receive the vaccine for pre-exposure prophylaxis. The vaccine should not be given to such persons for post-exposure treatment unless a suitable alternative vaccine is not available, in which case precautions should be taken as above.

Do not administer by intravascular injection.

If the vaccine is inadvertently administered into a blood vessel there is a risk of severe adverse reactions, including shock

After contact with animals which are suspected carriers of rabies, it is essential to observe the following procedures (according to WHO 1997):

Immediate wound treatment

In order to remove rabies virus, immediately cleanse wound with soap and flush thoroughly with water. Then treat with alcohol (70%) or iodine solution. Where possible, bite injuries should not be closed with a suture, or only sutured to secure apposition.

Tetanus vaccination and rabies immunoglobulin administration

Prophylaxis against tetanus should be implemented when necessary.

In cases of indicated passive immunisation, as much of the recommended dose of human rabies immunoglobulin (HRIG) as anatomically feasible should be applied as deeply as possible in and around the wound. Any remaining HRIG should be injected intramuscularly at a site distant from the vaccination site, preferably intragluteally. For detailed information plesase refer to the SmPC and/or package insert of HRIG.

4.5 Interaction with other medicinal products and other forms of Interaction

Patients who are immunocompromised, including those receiving immunosuppressive therapy, may not mount an adequate response to rabies vaccine. Therefore, it is recommended that serological responses should be monitored in such patients and additional doses given as necessary (see section 4.2 for details).

Administration of rabies immunoglobulin may be necessary for management but may attenuate the effects of concomitantly administered rabies vaccine. Therefore, it is important that rabies immunoglobulin should be administered once only for treating each at-risk exposure and with adherence to the recommended dose.

Other essential inactivated vaccines may be given at the same time as Rabipur. Different injectable inactivated vaccines should be administered into separate injection sites.

4.6 Pregnancy and lactation

No cases of harm attributable to use of Rabipur during pregnancy have been observed. While it is not known whether Rabipur enters breast milk, no risk to the breast-feeding infant has been identified. Rabipur may be administered to pregnant and breastfeeding women when post-exposure treatment is required.

The vaccine may also be used for pre-exposure prophylaxis during pregnancy and in breastfeeding women if it is considered that the potential benefit outweighs any possible risk to the fetus/infant.

4.7 Effects on ability to drive and use machines

The vaccine is unlikely to produce an effect on ability to drive and use machines.

4.8 Undesirable effects

In clinical studies the most commonly reported solicited adverse reactions were injection site pain (30 –85 %, mainly pain due to injection) or injection site induration (15 - 35 %). Most injection site reactions were not severe and resolved within 24 to 48 hours after injection. Furthermore, the following undesirable effects were observed in clinical trials and/or during the post-marketing period:

(see Table 3 on next page)

4.9 Overdose

No symptoms of overdose are known.

5. PHARMACOLOGICAL PROPERTIES

5.1 Pharmacodynamic properties

ATC-Code: J07B G01

Pre-exposure Prophylaxis

In clinical trials with previously unimmunised subjects, almost all subjects achieve a protective antibody titre (⩾ 0.5 IU/ml) by day 28 of a primary series of three injections of Rabipur when given according to the recommended schedule by the intramuscular route.

As antibody titres slowly decrease, booster doses are required to maintain antibody levels above 0.5 IU/ml. However, persistence of protective antibody titres for 2 years after immunisation with Rabipur without additional booster has been found to be 100 % in clinical trials.

In clinical trials, a booster dose of Rabipur elicited a 10-fold or higher increase in Geometric Mean Titres (GMTs) by day 30. It has also been demonstrated that individuals who had previously been immunised with Human Diploid Cell Vaccine (HDCV) developed a rapid anamnestic response when boosted with Rabipur.

Persistence of antibody titres has been shown for 14 years in a limited number (n = 28) of subjects tested.

Nevertheless, the need for and timing of boosting should be assessed on a case by case basis, taking into account official guidance (see also section 4.2).

Post-exposure Treatment

In clinical studies, Rabipur elicited neutralising antibodies (⩾ 0.5 IU/ml) in 98% of patients within 14 days and in 99-100% of patients by day 28 – 38, when administered according to the WHO-recommended schedule of five intramuscular injections of 1 ml, one each on days 0, 3, 7, 14 and 28.

Concomitant administration of either Human Rabies Immunoglobulin (HRIG) or Equine Rabies Immunoglobulin (ERIG) with the first dose of rabies vaccine caused a slight decrease in GMTs. However, this was not considered to be clinically relevant.

5.2 Pharmacokinetic properties

Not applicable.

5.3 Preclinical safety data

Preclinical data including single-dose, repeated dose and local tolerance studies revealed no unexpected findings and no target organ toxicity. No genotoxicity and reproductive toxicity studies have been performed.

6. PHARMACEUTICAL PARTICULARS

6.1 List of excipients

Powder:

TRIS-(hydroxymethyl)-aminomethane

Sodium chloride

Disodium edetate (Titriplex III)

Potassium-L-glutamate

Polygeline

Sucrose

Solvent:

Water for injections

6.2 Incompatibilities

This vaccine should not be mixed with other medicinal products.

6.3 Shelf life

4 years

6.4 Special precautions for storage

Store at +2 to +8° C (in a refrigerator).

Table 3

Standard system organ class	Frequency	Adverse reactions
General disorders and administration site condition	Very common > 1/10	Injection site pain, injection site reaction, injection site induration
	Common > 1/100, < 1/10	Asthenia, malaise, fever, fatigue, influenza like illness, injection site erythema
Cardiac disorders	Rare > 1/10.000, <1/1.000	Circulatory reactions (such as palpitations or hot flush)
Blood and lymphatic system disorders	Common > 1/100, < 1/10	Lymphadenopathy
Ear and labyrinth disorders	Very rare < 1/10.000	Vertigo
Eye disorders	Rare > 1/10.000, < 1/1.000	Visual disturbance
Nervous system disorders*	Common > 1/100, < 1/10	Headache
	Rare > 1/10.000, < 1/1.000	Paraesthesia
	Very rare < 1/10.000	Nervous system disorders (such as paresis or Guillain-Barré-Syndrome)
Skin disorders	Common > 1/100, < 1/10	Rash
Immune system disorders	Rare > 1/10.000, < 1/1.000	Allergic reactions (such as anaphylaxis, bronchospasm, oedema, urticaria or pruritus)
Musculosceletal and connective tissue disorders	Common > 1/100, < 1/10	Myalgia, arthralgia
Gastrointestinal disorders	Common > 1/100, < 1/10	Gastrointestinal disorder (such as nausea or abdominal pain)

* Statistically there is no indication of increasing frequencies of primary manifestations or triggered attacks of autoimmune diseases (e.g. multiple sclerosis) after vaccination. However, in individual cases it cannot be absolutely excluded that a vaccination may trigger an episode in patients with corresponding genetic disposition. According to the current state of scientific knowledge vaccinations are not the cause of autoimmune diseases.

6.5 Nature and contents of container

Pack containing

Powder in a vial (type I glass) with stopper (chlorobutyl)

1 ml solvent for solution in an ampoule (type I glass)

with or without disposable syringe (polypropylene with natural rubber plunger stopper)

Not all pack sizes may be marketed.

6.6 Instructions for use and handling

The vaccine should be visually inspected both before and after reconstitution for any foreign particulate matter and or change in physical appearance. The vaccine must not be used if any change in the appearance of the vaccine has taken place. For appearance see Section 3.

The powder for solution should be reconstituted using the solvent for solution supplied and carefully agitated prior to injection. The reconstituted vaccine should be used immediately.

Any unused vaccine or waste material should be disposed of in accordance with local requirements.

7. MARKETING AUTHORISATION HOLDER

Chiron Behring GmbH & Co KG

P.O. Box 16 30

D-35006 Marburg

Germany

8. MARKETING AUTHORISATION NUMBER(S)

PL 16033/0008

9. DATE OF FIRST AUTHORISATION/RENEWAL OF THE AUTHORISATION

24 September 2003

10. DATE OF REVISION OF THE TEXT

June 2004

Rapamune

(Wyeth Pharmaceuticals)

1. NAME OF THE MEDICINAL PRODUCT

Rapamune ▼ 1 mg coated tablets

Rapamune ▼ 2 mg coated tablets

Rapamune ▼ 1mg/ml oral solution in 60ml bottle.

2. QUALITATIVE AND QUANTITATIVE COMPOSITION

Each 1mg tablet contains 1 mg sirolimus.

Each 2mg tablet contains 2 mg sirolimus.

Each ml contains 1 mg sirolimus

For excipients, see section 6.1

3. PHARMACEUTICAL FORM

Coated tablet.

1mg: White coloured, triangular-shaped coated tablet marked "RAPAMUNE 1 mg" on one side.

2mg: Yellow to beige coloured, triangular-shaped coated tablet marked "RAPAMUNE 2 mg" on one side.

or

Oral solution.

4. CLINICAL PARTICULARS

4.1 Therapeutic indications

Rapamune is indicated for the prophylaxis of organ rejection in adult patients at low to moderate immunological risk receiving a renal transplant. It is recommended that Rapamune be used initially in combination with ciclosporin microemulsion and corticosteroids for 2 to 3 months. Rapamune may be continued as maintenance therapy with corticosteroids only if ciclosporin microemulsion can be progressively discontinued (see sections 4.2 and 5.1).

4.2 Posology and method of administration

Rapamune is for oral use only.

Treatment should be initiated by and remain under the guidance of an appropriately qualified specialist in transplantation.

Use in adults

Initial therapy (2 to 3 months post-transplantation): The usual dosage regimen for Rapamune is a 6 mg oral loading dose, administered as soon as possible after transplantation, followed by 2 mg once daily. The Rapamune dose should then be individualised, to obtain whole blood trough levels of 4 to 12 ng/ml (chromatographic assay; see *Therapeutic drug monitoring*). Rapamune therapy should be optimised with a tapering regimen of steroids and ciclosporin microemulsion. Suggested ciclosporin trough concentration ranges for the first 2 to 3 months after transplantation are 150 to 400 ng/ml (monoclonal assay or equivalent technique).

Maintenance Therapy: Ciclosporin should be progressively discontinued over 4 to 8 weeks and the Rapamune dose should be adjusted to obtain whole blood trough levels of 12 to 20 ng/ml (chromatographic assay; see *Therapeutic drug monitoring*). Rapamune should be given with corticosteroids. In patients for whom ciclosporin withdrawal is either unsuccessful or cannot be attempted, the combination of ciclosporin and Rapamune should not be maintained for more than 3 months post-transplantation. In such patients, when clinically appropriate, Rapamune should be discontinued and an alternative immunosuppressive regimen instituted.

Use in black recipients: There is limited information indicating that black renal transplant recipients (predominantly African-American) require higher doses and trough levels of sirolimus to achieve the same efficacy as observed in non-black patients. Currently, the efficacy and safety data are too limited to allow specific recommendations for use of sirolimus in black recipients.

Use in children and adolescents (< 18 years): There is insufficient experience to recommend the use of sirolimus in children and adolescents. Limited pharmacokinetic information is available in children (see section 5.2).

Use in elderly patients (> 65 years): Clinical studies with Rapamune oral solution did not include a sufficient number of patients > 65 years of age to determine whether they will respond differently than younger patients. Sirolimus trough concentration data in 35 renal transplant patients > 65 years of age were similar to those in the adult population (n = 822) from 18 to 65 years of age. Rapamune tablets administered to 12 renal transplant patients > 65 years of age also gave similar results to adult patients (n = 167) 18 to 65 years of age.

Use in patients with renal impairment: No dosage adjustment is required (see section 5.2).

Use in patients with mild or moderate hepatic impairment: It is recommended that sirolimus whole blood trough levels be closely monitored in patients with impaired hepatic function. It is not necessary to modify the Rapamune loading dose (see section 5.2).

Use in patients with severe hepatic impairment: Sirolimus pharmacokinetics have not been evaluated in patients with severe hepatic impairment.

Therapeutic drug monitoring: Most patients who received 2 mg of Rapamune 4 hours after ciclosporin had whole blood trough concentrations of sirolimus within the 4 to 12 ng/ml target range. Optimal therapy requires therapeutic drug concentration monitoring in all patients. Whole blood sirolimus levels should be closely monitored in the following populations: (1) in patients with hepatic impairment; (2) when inducers or inhibitors of CYP3A4 are concurrently administered and after their discontinuation (see section 4.5); and/or (3) if ciclosporin dosing is markedly reduced or discontinued, as these populations are most likely to have special dosing requirements.

To minimise variability, Rapamune should be taken at the same time in relation to ciclosporin, 4 hours after the ciclosporin dose, and consistently either with or without food (see section 5.2). Optimally, adjustments in Rapamune dosage should be based on more than a single trough level obtained > 5 days after a previous dosing change. Patients can be switched from the solution to the tablet formulation on a mg per mg basis. It is recommended that a trough concentration be taken 1 or 2 weeks after switching formulations or tablet strength to confirm that the trough concentration is within the recommended target range.

Following the discontinuation of ciclosporin therapy, a target trough range of 12 to 20 ng/ml (chromatographic assay) is recommended. Ciclosporin inhibits the metabolism of sirolimus, and consequently, sirolimus levels will decrease when ciclosporin is discontinued unless the sirolimus dose is increased. On average, the sirolimus dose will need to be 4-fold higher to account for both the absence of the pharmacokinetic interaction (2-fold increase) and the augmented immunosuppressive requirement in the absence of ciclosporin (2-fold increase). The rate at which the dose of sirolimus is increased should correspond to the rate of ciclosporin elimination.

The recommended ranges for sirolimus are based on chromatographic methods. On average, chromatographic methods, with either ultraviolet or mass spectrometric detection, yield results that are approximately 20% lower than the immunoassay whole blood concentration determinations. Adjustments to the targeted range should be made according to the assay utilised to determine sirolimus trough concentrations. Therefore, comparison between concentrations in the published literature and an individual patient concentration using current assays must be made with detailed knowledge of the assay methods employed.

Therapeutic drug monitoring should not be the sole basis for adjusting sirolimus therapy. Careful attention should be made to clinical signs/symptoms, tissue biopsies, and laboratory parameters.

Other considerations for use: Ciclosporin (microemulsion) and other medicinal or non-medicinal products may interact with sirolimus (see section 4.5).

4.3 Contraindications

Hypersensitivity to sirolimus or any of the excipients.

4.4 Special warnings and special precautions for use

Rapamune has not been adequately studied in patients at high immunological risk (see section 5.1)

Concomitant use with other immunosuppressive agents

Sirolimus has been administered concurrently with the following agents in clinical studies: ciclosporin, azathioprine, mycophenolate mofetil, corticosteroids and cytotoxic antibodies. Sirolimus in combination with other immunosuppressive agents has not been extensively investigated.

Immunosuppressants may affect response to vaccination. During treatment with immunosuppressants, including Rapamune, vaccination may be less effective. The use of live vaccines should be avoided during treatment with Rapamune.

The pharmacokinetics of Rapamune have not been studied in patients with severe hepatic impairment. It is recommended that sirolimus whole blood trough levels be closely monitored in hepatically impaired patients.

Co-administration of sirolimus with strong inhibitors of CYP3A4 (such as ketoconazole, voriconazole, itraconazole, telithromycin or clarithromycin) or inducers of CYP3A4 (such as rifampin, rifabutin) is not recommended (see section 4.5).

Increased susceptibility to infection and the possible development of lymphoma and other malignancies, particularly of the skin, may result from immunosuppression (see section 4.8). Oversuppression of the immune system can also increase susceptibility to infection including opportunistic infections, fatal infections, and sepsis.

The safety and efficacy of Rapamune as immunosuppressive therapy have not been established in liver or lung transplant patients, and therefore, such use is not recommended.

In two clinical studies in *de novo* liver transplant patients the use of sirolimus plus ciclosporin or tacrolimus was associated with an increase in hepatic artery thrombosis, mostly leading to graft loss or death.

Cases of bronchial anastomotic dehiscence, most fatal, have been reported in *de novo* lung transplant patients when sirolimus has been used as part of an immunosuppressive regimen.

Hypersensitivity reactions, including anaphylactic/anaphylactoid reactions, have been associated with the administration of sirolimus (see section 4.8).

As usual for patients with increased risk for skin cancer, exposure to sunlight and UV light should be limited by wearing protective clothing and using a sunscreen with a high protection factor.

Cases of *Pneumocystis carinii* pneumonia have been reported in patients not receiving antimicrobial prophylaxis. Therefore, antimicrobial prophylaxis for *Pneumocystis carinii* pneumonia should be administered for the first 12 months following transplantation.

Cytomegalovirus (CMV) prophylaxis is recommended for 3 months after transplantation, particularly for patients at increased risk for CMV disease.

The use of Rapamune in renal transplant patients was associated with increased serum cholesterol and triglycerides that may require treatment. Patients administered Rapamune, should be monitored for hyperlipidemia using laboratory tests and if hyperlipidemia is detected, subsequent interventions such as diet, exercise, and lipid-lowering agents should be initiated. The risk/benefit should be considered in patients with established hyperlipidemia before initiating an immunosuppressive regimen including Rapamune. Similarly the risk/benefit of continued Rapamune therapy should be re-evaluated in patients with severe refractory hyperlipidemia.

In clinical trials, the concomitant administration of Rapamune and HMG-CoA reductase inhibitors and/or fibrates was well tolerated. During Rapamune therapy, patients administered an HMG-CoA reductase inhibitor and/or fibrate, should be monitored for the possible development of rhabdomyolysis and other adverse effects as described in the respective Summary of Product Characteristics of these agents.

Renal function should be monitored during concomitant administration of Rapamune and ciclosporin. Appropriate adjustment of the immunosuppression regimen should be considered in patients with elevated serum creatinine levels. Caution should be exercised when co-administering other agents that are known to have a deleterious effect on renal function.

Patients treated with ciclosporin and Rapamune beyond 3 months had higher serum creatinine levels and lower calculated glomerular filtration rates compared to patients treated with ciclosporin and placebo or azathioprine controls. Patients who were successfully withdrawn from ciclosporin had lower serum creatinine levels and higher calculated glomerular filtration rates compared to patients remaining on ciclosporin. Until further clinical data are available, the continued co-administration of ciclosporin and Rapamune as maintenance therapy cannot be recommended. Sirolimus tablets contain sucrose and lactose. In those patients with a history of sucrase insufficiency, isomaltase insufficiency, fructose intolerance, glucose malabsorption, galactose malabsorption, galactose intolerance (e.g., galactosemia), or Lapp lactase deficiency, a careful risk/benefit assessment should be performed prior to prescribing sirolimus tablets.

4.5 Interaction with other medicinal products and other forms of Interaction

Sirolimus is extensively metabolised by the CYP3A4 isozyme in the intestinal wall and liver. Sirolimus is also a substrate for the multidrug efflux pump, P-glycoprotein (P-gp) located in the small intestine. Therefore, absorption and the subsequent elimination of sirolimus may be influenced by substances that affect these proteins. Inhibitors of CYP3A4 (such as ketoconazole, voriconazole, itraconazole, telithromycin, or clarithromycin) decrease the metabolism of sirolimus and increase sirolimus levels. Inducers of CYP3A4 (such as rifampin or rifabutin) increase the metabolism of sirolimus and decrease the sirolimus levels. Co-administration of sirolimus with strong inhibitors of CYP3A4 or inducers of CYP3A4 is not recommended (see section 4.4).

Ciclosporin (CYP3A4 substrate): The rate and extent of sirolimus absorption from Rapamune tablets and solution were significantly increased by ciclosporin A (CsA). Sirolimus administered concomitantly (5 mg), and at 2h (5 mg) and 4h (10 mg) after CsA (300 mg) resulted in increased sirolimus AUC by approximately 183%, 141%, and 80% respectively. The effect of CsA was also reflected by increases in sirolimus C_{max} and t_{max}. When given 2 hours before CsA administration, sirolimus C_{max} and AUC were not affected. Single-dose sirolimus did not affect the pharmacokinetics of ciclosporin (microemulsion) in healthy volunteers when administered simultaneously or 4 hours apart. It is recommended that Rapamune be administered 4 hours after ciclosporin (microemulsion).

Rifampicin (CYP3A4 inducer): Administration of multiple doses of rifampicin decreased sirolimus whole blood concentrations following a single 10 mg dose of Rapamune oral solution. Rifampicin increased the clearance of sirolimus by approximately 5.5-fold and decreased AUC and C_{max} by approximately 82% and 71%, respectively. Co-administration of sirolimus and rifampicin is not recommended (see section 4.4).

Ketoconazole (CYP3A4 inhibitor): Multiple-dose ketoconazole administration significantly affected the rate and extent of absorption and sirolimus exposure from Rapamune oral solution as reflected by increases in sirolimus C_{max}, t_{max}, and AUC of 4.3-fold, 1.4-fold, and 10.9-fold, respectively. Co-administration of sirolimus and ketoconazole is not recommended (see section 4.4).

Voriconazole (CYP3A4 inhibitor): Co-administration of sirolimus (2 mg single dose) with multiple-dose administration of oral voriconazole (400 mg every 12 hours for 1 day, then 100 mg every 12 hours for 8 days) in healthy subjects has been reported to increase sirolimus C_{max} and AUC by an average of 7-fold and 11-fold respectively. Co-administration of sirolimus and voriconazole is not recommended (see section 4.4).

Diltiazem (CYP3A4 inhibitor): The simultaneous oral administration of 10 mg of Rapamune oral solution and 120 mg of diltiazem significantly affected the bioavailability of sirolimus. Sirolimus C_{max}, t_{max}, and AUC were increased 1.4-fold, 1.3-fold, and 1.6-fold, respectively. Sirolimus did not affect the pharmacokinetics of either diltiazem or its metabolites, desacetyldiltiazem and desmethyldiltiazem. If diltiazem is administered, sirolimus blood levels should be monitored and a dose adjustment may be necessary.

Verapamil (CYP3A4 inhibitor): Multiple-dose administration of verapamil and sirolimus oral solution significantly affected the rate and extent of absorption of both drugs. Whole blood sirolimus C_{max}, t_{max}, and AUC were increased 2.3-fold, 1.1-fold, and 2.2 fold, respectively. Plasma S-(-) verapamil C_{max} and AUC were both increased 1.5-fold, and t_{max} was decreased 24%. Sirolimus levels should be monitored and appropriate dose reductions of both medications should be considered.

Erythromycin (CYP3A4 inhibitor): Multiple-dose administration of erythromycin and sirolimus oral solution significantly increased the rate and extent of absorption of both drugs. Whole blood sirolimus C_{max}, t_{max}, and AUC were increased 4.4-fold, 1.4-fold, and 4.2-fold, respectively. The C_{max}, t_{max}, and AUC of plasma erythromycin base were increased 1.6-fold, 1.3-fold, and 1.7-fold, respectively. Sirolimus levels should be monitored and appropriate dose reductions of both medications should be considered.

Oral contraceptives: No clinically significant pharmacokinetic interaction was observed between Rapamune oral solution and 0.3 mg norgestrel/0.03 mg ethinyl estradiol. Although the results of a single dose-drug interaction study with an oral contraceptive suggest the lack of a pharmacokinetic interaction, the results cannot exclude the possibility of changes in the pharmacokinetics that might affect the efficacy of the oral contraceptive during long-term treatment with Rapamune.

Other possible interactions: Moderate and weak inhibitors of CYP3A4 may decrease the metabolism of sirolimus and increase sirolimus blood levels (e.g. **calcium channel blockers:** nicardipine; **antifungal agents**: clotrimazole, fluconazole; **antibiotics:** troleandomycin; **other substances:** bromocriptine, cimetidine, danazol, **protease inhibitors**).

Inducers of CYP3A4 may increase the metabolism of sirolimus and decrease sirolimus blood levels (e.g. St. John's Wort, (*Hypericum perforatum*); **anticonvulsants:** carbamazepine, phenobarbital, phenytoin).

Although sirolimus inhibits human liver microsomal cytochrome P_{450} CYP2C9, CYP2C19, CYP2D6, and CYP3A4/5 *in vitro*, the active substance is not expected to inhibit the activity of these isozymes *in vivo* since the sirolimus concentrations necessary to produce inhibition are much higher than those observed in patients receiving therapeutic doses of Rapamune. Inhibitors of P-gp may decrease the efflux of sirolimus from intestinal cells and increase sirolimus levels.

Grapefruit juice affects CYP3A4 mediated metabolism and should therefore be avoided.

Pharmacokinetic interactions may be observed with gastrointestinal prokinetic agents such as cisapride and metoclopramide.

No clinically significant pharmacokinetic interaction was observed between sirolimus and any of the following substances: acyclovir, atorvastatin, digoxin, glibenclamide, methylprednisolone, nifedipine, prednisolone, and trimethoprim/sulphamethoxazole.

4.6 Pregnancy and lactation

There are no adequate data from the use of Rapamune in pregnant women. Studies in animals have shown reproductive toxicity (see section 5.3). The potential risk for humans is unknown. Rapamune should not be used during pregnancy unless clearly necessary. Effective contraception must be used during Rapamune therapy and for 12 weeks after Rapamune has been stopped.

Following administration of radiolabelled sirolimus, radioactivity is excreted in the milk of lactating rats. It is not known whether sirolimus is excreted in human milk. Because of the potential for adverse reactions in nursing infants from sirolimus, nursing should be discontinued during therapy.

4.7 Effects on ability to drive and use machines

No studies on the effects on the ability to drive and use machines have been performed.

4.8 Undesirable effects

The list below contains adverse reactions seen in clinical trials and post-marketing reports. Only events for which there is at least reasonable suspicion of a causal relationship to Rapamune treatment are listed.

The majority of patients in clinical trials were treated with ciclosporin and corticosteroids; thus the frequency of adverse reactions listed includes Rapamune administration combined with ciclosporin and corticosteroids.

The incidence of adverse events may increase as the trough sirolimus level increases.

The frequency of the adverse reactions taken from clinical trial data listed below was determined in 5 clinical trials in renal transplantation. These included 2 randomised, double-blind, multicentre controlled trials in which 499 renal transplant patients received Rapamune oral solution 2 mg/day and 477 received Rapamune oral solution 5 mg/day together with ciclosporin and corticosteroids. One randomised, open-label study enrolling 477 patients compared the tablet (238 patients) and the solution (239 patients). Additionally, 2 open-label studies enrolled 771 patients who initially received Rapamune (246 patients received oral solution and 525 received tablets) and ciclosporin. These patients were randomised to continue ciclosporin therapy or to have ciclosporin withdrawn after 2 to 3 months post-transplant. Overall, the safety profile of Rapamune tablets did not differ from that of the oral solution formulation in clinical trials.

Adverse reactions are listed according to the following categories:

Very common:	>1/10
Common:	>1/100, <1/10
Uncommon:	>1/1000, <1/100
Rare:	>1/10,000, <1/1000

Body as a whole:

Very common: Lymphocele, peripheral oedema

Common: Abnormal healing; fever; oedema; fungal, viral, and bacterial infections (such as mycobacterial infections, Epstein-Barr virus, CMV, and Herpes zoster); Herpes simplex; sepsis

Cardiac disorders:

Common: Tachycardia

Vascular disorders:

Common: Venous thromboembolism

Gastrointestinal disorders:

Very common: Abdominal pain, diarrhoea

Common: Stomatitis

Uncommon: Pancreatitis

Blood and the lymphatic system disorders:

Very common: Anaemia; thrombocytopenia

Common: Leucopenia; neutropenia; thrombotic thrombocytopenic purpura/haemolytic uremia syndrome

Uncommon: Lymphoma/post transplant lymphoproliferative disorder; pancytopenia

Immune system disorders:

Rare: Hypersensitivity reactions, including anaphylactic/anaphylactoid reactions (see section 4.4)

Metabolism and nutrition disorders:

Very common: Hypercholesterolemia, hypertriglyceridemia (hyperlipemia); hypokalaemia; increased lactic dehydrogenase (LDH)

Common: Liver function tests abnormal; increased SGOT, increased SGPT

Musculoskeletal, connective tissue and bone disorders:

Very common: Arthralgia

Common: Bone necrosis

Respiratory, thoracic and mediastinal disorders:

Common: Epistaxis; pneumonia; pneumonitis

Skin and subcutaneous tissue disorders:

Very common: Acne

Common: Rash

Renal and urinary disorders:

Very common: Urinary tract infection

Common: Pyelonephritis

Immunosuppression increases the susceptibility to the development of lymphoma and other malignancies, particularly of the skin (see section 4.4).

Cases of interstitial lung disease (including pneumonitis and infrequently bronchiolitis obliterans organising pneumonia (BOOP) and pulmonary fibrosis), some fatal, with no identified infectious etiology have occurred in patients receiving immunosuppressive regimens including Rapamune. In some cases, the interstitial lung disease has resolved upon discontinuation or dose reduction of Rapamune. The risk may be increased as the trough sirolimus level increases.

Hepatotoxicity has been reported, the risk may increase as the trough sirolimus level increases. Rare reports of fatal hepatic necrosis have been reported with elevated trough sirolimus levels.

Abnormal healing following transplant surgery has been reported, including fascial dehiscence and anastomotic disruption (e.g. wound, vascular, airway, ureteral, biliary).

In an ongoing study evaluating the safety and efficacy of conversion from calcineurin inhibitors to sirolimus (target levels of 12 - 20 ng/mL) in maintenance renal transplant patients, enrollment was stopped in the subset of patients (n=90) with a baseline glomerular filtration rate of less than 40 mL/min. There was a higher rate of serious adverse events including pneumonia, acute rejection, graft loss and death in this sirolimus treatment arm (n=60, median time post-transplant 36 months).

4.9 Overdose

At present, there is minimal experience with overdose. One patient experienced an episode of atrial fibrillation after ingestion of 150 mg of Rapamune. In general, the adverse effects of overdose are consistent with those listed in Section 4.8. General supportive measures should be initiated in all cases of overdose. Based on the poor aqueous solubility and high erythrocyte and plasma protein binding of Rapamune, it is anticipated that Rapamune will not be dialysable to any significant extent.

5. PHARMACOLOGICAL PROPERTIES

5.1 Pharmacodynamic properties

Pharmacotherapeutic group: selective immunosuppressant agents. ATC code: L04A A10.

Sirolimus inhibits T cell activation induced by most stimuli, by blocking calcium dependent and calcium independent intracellular signal transduction. Studies demonstrated that its effects are mediated by a mechanism that is different from that of ciclosporin, tacrolimus, and other immunosuppressive agents. Experimental evidence suggests that sirolimus binds to the specific cytosolic protein FKPB-12 and that the FKPB 12-sirolimus complex inhibits the activation of the mammalian Target Of Rapamycin (mTOR), a critical kinase for cell cycle progression. The inhibition of mTOR results in blockage of several specific signal transduction pathways. The net result is the inhibition of lymphocyte activation, which results in immunosuppression.

In animals, sirolimus has a direct effect on T and B cell activation suppressing immune mediated reactions such as allograft rejection.

Patients at low to moderate immunological risk were studied in the ciclosporin elimination-sirolimus maintenance trials which included patients receiving a renal allograft from a cadaveric or living donor. In addition, re- transplant recipients whose previous grafts survived for at least 6 months after transplantation were included. Ciclosporin was not withdrawn in patients experiencing Banff Grade 3 acute rejection episodes, who were dialysis-dependent, who had a serum creatinine > 400 μmol/l, or who had inadequate renal function to support ciclosporin withdrawal. Patients at high immunological risk of graft loss were not studied in sufficient number in the ciclosporin elimination-sirolimus maintenance trials and are not recommended for this treatment regimen.

5.2 Pharmacokinetic properties

Much of the general pharmacokinetic information was obtained using the oral solution, which is summarised first. Information directly related to the tablet formulation is summarised specifically in the *Oral Tablet* section.

Oral solution

Following administration of the oral solution, sirolimus is rapidly absorbed, with a time to peak concentration of 1 hour in healthy subjects receiving single doses and 2 hours in patients with stable renal allografts receiving multiple doses. The systemic availability of sirolimus in combination with simultaneously administered ciclosporin (Sandimune) is approximately 14%. Upon repeated administration, the average blood concentration of sirolimus is increased approximately 3-fold. The terminal half-life in stable renal transplant patients after multiple oral doses was 62 ± 16 h. The effective half-life, however, is shorter and mean steady-state concentrations were achieved after 5 to 7 days. The blood to plasma ratio (B/P) of 36 indicates that sirolimus is extensively partitioned into formed blood elements.

Pharmacokinetic parameters for sirolimus obtained from 19 renal transplant patients receiving microemulsion ciclosporin (4 hours prior to Rapamune) and corticosteroids, following daily doses of 2 mg Rapamune solution in a Phase III clinical trial, were; $C_{max,ss}$ 12.2 ± 6.2 ng/ml, $t_{max,ss}$ 3.01 ± 2.40 h, AUC $_{\tau,ss}$ 158 ± 70 ng•h/ml, CL/F/W 182 ± 72 ml/h/kg (parameters calculated from LC-MS/MS assay results). There was no significant difference in any of these parameters over time up to 6 months after transplantation. Mean sirolimus whole blood trough levels from the same Phase III trial were 9 ng/ml (5 to 14 ng/ml, immunoassay; n=226) for the 2 mg per day dose and 17 ng/ml (10 to 28 ng/ml, immunoassay; n=219) for the 5 mg per day dose.

Sirolimus is a substrate for both cytochrome P450 IIIA4 (CYP3A4) and P-glycoprotein. Sirolimus is extensively metabolised by O-demethylation and/or hydroxylation. Seven major metabolites, including hydroxyl, demethyl, and hydroxydemethyl, are identifiable in whole blood. Sirolimus is the major component in human whole blood and contributes to greater than 90% of the immunosuppressive activity. After a single dose of [^{14}C] sirolimus in healthy volunteers, the majority (91.1%) of radioactivity was recovered from the faeces, and only a minor amount (2.2%) was excreted in urine.

Clinical studies of Rapamune did not include a sufficient number of patients > 65 years of age to determine whether they will respond differently than younger patients. Sirolimus trough concentration data in 35 renal transplant patients > 65 years of age were similar to those in the adult population (n = 822) from 18 to 65 years of age.

In healthy volunteers, a high fat meal altered the bioavailability characteristics of oral liquid sirolimus. There was a 34% decrease in the peak blood sirolimus concentration (C_{max}), a 3.5-fold increase in the time to peak concentration (t_{max}), and a 35% increase in total exposure (AUC). It is recommended that Rapamune be taken consistently either with or without food. The use of orange juice and water to dilute Rapamune were equivalent with respect to C_{max}, and AUC. Grapefruit juice affects CYP3A4 mediated metabolism and must therefore be avoided.

In paediatric patients on dialysis (30% to 50% reduction in glomerular filtration rate) within age ranges of 5 to 11 years and 12 to 18 years, the mean weight-normalised CL/F was larger for younger paediatric patients (580 ml/h/kg) than for older paediatric patients (450 ml/h/kg) as compared with adults (287 ml/h/kg). There was a large variability for individuals within the age groups.

In mild and moderate hepatically impaired patients (Child-Pugh classification of A or B), mean values for sirolimus AUC and $t_{1/2}$ were increased 61% and 43%, respectively, and CL/F was decreased 33% compared with normal healthy subjects. Sirolimus pharmacokinetics were not evaluated in patients with severe hepatic impairment.

The pharmacokinetics of sirolimus were similar in various populations with renal function ranging from normal to absent (dialysis patients).

Oral Tablet

In healthy subjects, the mean extent of bioavailability of sirolimus after single-dose administration of the tablet formulation is about 27% higher relative to the oral solution. The mean C_{max} was decreased by 35% and mean t_{max} increased by 82%. The difference in bioavailability was less marked upon steady-state administration to renal transplant recipients, and therapeutic equivalence has been demonstrated in a randomised study of 477 patients. When switching patients between oral solution and tablet formulations, it is recommended to give the same dose and to verify the sirolimus trough concentration 1 to 2 weeks later to assure that it remains within recommended target ranges. Also when switching between different tablet strengths, verification of trough concentrations is recommended.

In 24 healthy volunteers receiving Rapamune tablets with a high-fat meal, C_{max}, t_{max} and AUC showed increases of 65%, 32%, and 23%, respectively. To minimise variability, Rapamune tablets should be taken consistently with or without food. Grapefruit juice affects CYP3A4-mediated metabolism and must, therefore, be avoided.

Sirolimus concentrations, following the administration of Rapamune tablets (5 mg) to healthy subjects as single doses are dose-proportional between 5 and 40 mg.

Initial Therapy (2 to 3 months post-transplant): In most patients receiving Rapamune tablets with a loading dose of 6 mg followed by an initial maintenance dose of 2 mg, whole blood sirolimus trough concentrations rapidly achieved steady-state concentrations within the recommended target range (4 to 12 ng/ml, chromatographic assay). Sirolimus pharmacokinetic parameters following daily doses of 2 mg Rapamune tablets administered in combination with ciclosporin microemulsion (4 hours prior to Rapamune tablets) and corticosteroids in 13 renal transplant patients, based on data collected at months 1 and 3 after transplantation, were: $C_{min,ss}$, 7.39 ± 2.18 ng/ml; $C_{max,ss}$, 15.0 ± 4.9 ng/ml; $t_{max,ss}$, 3.46 ± 2.40 h; AUC $_{\tau,ss}$, 230 ± 67 ng•h/ml; CL/F/WT, 139 ± 63 ml/h/kg (parameters calculated from LC-MS/MS assay results). The corresponding results for the oral solution in the same clinical trial were $C_{min,ss}$ 5.40 ± 2.50 ng/ml, $C_{max,ss}$ 14.4 ± 5.3 ng/ml, $t_{max,ss}$ 2.12 ± 0.84 h, AUC $_{\tau,ss}$ 194 ± 78 ng•h/ml, CL/F/W 173 ± 50 ml/h/kg. Whole blood trough sirolimus concentrations, as measured by LC/MS/MS, were significantly correlated (r^2 = 0.85) with AUC $_{\tau,ss}$.

Based on monitoring in all patients during the period of concomitant therapy with ciclosporin, mean (10th, 90th percentiles) troughs (by immunoassay) and daily doses were 10.8 ± 3.8 ng/ml (6.3 to 15.8 ng/ml) and 2.1 ± 0.70 mg (1.5 to 2.7 mg), respectively.

Maintenance therapy: From month 3 to month 12, following discontinuation of ciclosporin, mean (10th, 90th percentiles) troughs (by immunoassay) and daily doses were 23.3 ± 5.1 ng/ml (16.9 to 29.6 ng/ml) and 8.2 ± 4.2 mg (3.6 to 13.6 mg), respectively. Therefore, the sirolimus dose was approximately 4-fold higher to account for both the absence of the pharmacokinetic interaction with ciclosporin (2-fold increase) and the augmented immunosuppressive requirement in the absence of ciclosporin (2-fold increase).

5.3 Preclinical safety data

Adverse reactions not observed in clinical studies, but seen in animals at exposure levels similar to clinical exposure levels and with possible relevance to clinical use were as follows: pancreatic islet cell vacuolation, testicular tubular degeneration, gastrointestinal ulceration, bone fractures and calluses, hepatic haematopoiesis, and pulmonary phospholipidosis.

Sirolimus was not mutagenic in the *in vitro* bacterial reverse mutation assays, the Chinese Hamster Ovary cell chromosomal aberration assay, the mouse lymphoma cell forward mutation assay, or the *in vivo* mouse micronucleus assay.

Carcinogenicity studies conducted in mouse and rat showed increased incidences of lymphomas (male and female mouse), hepatocellular adenoma and carcinoma (male mouse) and granulocytic leukaemia (female mouse). It is known that malignancies (lymphoma) secondary to the chronic use of immunosuppressive agents can occur and have been reported in patients in rare instances. In mouse, chronic ulcerative skin lesions were increased. The changes may be related to chronic immunosuppression. In rat, testicular interstitial cell adenomas were likely indicative of a species dependent response to luteinising hormone levels and are usually considered of limited clinical relevance.

In reproduction toxicity studies decreased fertility in male rats was observed. Partly reversible reductions in sperm counts were reported in a 13-week rat study. Reductions in testicular weights and/or histological lesions (e.g. tubular atrophy and tubular giant cells) were observed in rats and in a monkey study. In rats, sirolimus caused embryo/foetotoxicity that was manifested as mortality and reduced foetal weights (with associated delays in skeletal ossification). (See section 4.6).

6. PHARMACEUTICAL PARTICULARS

6.1 List of excipients

Tablet core:

Lactose monohydrate

Macrogol

Magnesium stearate

Talc

1 mg Tablet coating:

Macrogol

Glyceryl monooleate

Pharmaceutical glaze

Anhydrous calcium sulphate

Microcrystalline cellulose

Sucrose

Titanium dioxide

Poloxamer 188

Povidone

Carnauba wax:

Red opacode S-1-15038 (shellac glaze ~45% in SD-45 alcohol, red iron oxide (E172), isopropyl alcohol, propylene glycol, ammonium hydroxide, simethicone emulsion 30%).

2 mg Tablet coating:

Macrogol

Glyceryl monooleate

Pharmaceutical glaze

Anhydrous calcium sulphate

Microcrystalline cellulose

Sucrose

Titanium dioxide

Brown iron oxide (E172)

Yellow iron oxide (E172)

Poloxamer 188

Povidone

Carnauba wax:

Red opacode S-1-15038 (shellac glaze ~45% in SD-45 alcohol, red iron oxide (E172), isopropyl alcohol, propylene glycol, ammonium hydroxide, simethicone emulsion 30%).

Solution: Polysorbate 80

Phosal 50 PG (phosphatidylcholine, propylene glycol, mono-, di-glycerides, ethanol (1.5% to 2.5%), soya fatty acids, and ascorbyl palmitate).

6.2 Incompatibilities

Rapamune tablets: Not applicable

Rapamune solution must not be diluted in grapefruit juice or any other liquid other than water or orange juice. See Instructions for use and handling, section 6.6.

6.3 Shelf life

1 mg/ml oral solution

18 months

1mg tablet

2 years

2mg tablet

23 months

Bottle

30 days for opened bottle.

24 hours in the dosing syringe (at room temperature, but not to exceed 25°C).

After dilution, (see Instructions for use and handling, section 6.6) the preparation should be used immediately.

6.4 Special precautions for storage

1 mg tablet

Keep the blister in the outer carton in order to protect from light.

2 mg tablet

Keep the blister in the outer carton in order to protect from light. Do not store above 25°C

Bottle

Store at 2°C to 8°C (in a refrigerator). Store in the original container in order to protect from light.

If necessary, the patient may store the bottles at room temperatures up to 25°C for a short period of time (24 hours).

6.5 Nature and contents of container

Tablet

Clear polyvinyl chloride (PVC)/polyethylene (PE)/polychlorotrifluoroethylene (Aclar) aluminium blister packages of 30 and 100 tablets. Not all pack sizes may be marketed.

Bottles

60 ml type III amber glass bottles with syringe adapter and 30 amber, plastic dosing syringes.

6.6 Instructions for use and handling

Tablets

No special requirements.

Bottles

The dosing syringe should be used to withdraw the prescribed amount of Rapamune from the bottle. Empty the correct amount of Rapamune from the syringe into only a glass or plastic container with at least 60 ml of water or orange juice. No other liquids, including grapefruit juice, should be used for dilution. Stir vigorously and drink at once. Refill the container with an additional volume (minimum of 120 ml) of water or orange juice, stir vigorously, and drink at once.

7. MARKETING AUTHORISATION HOLDER

Wyeth Europa Ltd.

Huntercombe Lane South

Taplow, Maidenhead

Berkshire, SL6 0PH

United Kingdom

8. MARKETING AUTHORISATION NUMBER(S)

EU/1/01/171/001 – 60 ml bottle

EU/1/01/171/007 – 1 mg Tablet (pack of 30)

EU/1/01/171/009 – 2mg Tablet (pack of 30)

9. DATE OF FIRST AUTHORISATION/RENEWAL OF THE AUTHORISATION

EU/1/01/171/001 – 13/03/2001

EU/1/01/171/007 – 12/04/2002

EU/1/01/171/009 – 10/01/2003

10. DATE OF REVISION OF THE TEXT

28 April 2005

Rapifen

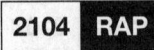

(Janssen-Cilag Ltd)

1. NAME OF THE MEDICINAL PRODUCT

Rapifen™

2. QUALITATIVE AND QUANTITATIVE COMPOSITION

Each ml of Rapifen contains alfentanil hydrochloride 544 micrograms, equivalent to 500 micrograms alfentanil base.

3. PHARMACEUTICAL FORM

Aqueous injection.

4. CLINICAL PARTICULARS

4.1 Therapeutic indications

As an analgesic supplement for use before and during anaesthesia.

It is indicated for:

1. Short procedures and outpatient surgery.

2. Procedures of medium and long duration when given as a bolus followed by supplemental doses or by continuous infusion.

At very high doses, Rapifen may be used as an anaesthetic induction agent in ventilated patients.

4.2 Posology and method of administration

For intravenous administration.

Rapifen by the intravenous route can be administered to both adults and children. The dosage of Rapifen should be individualised according to age, bodyweight, physical status, underlying pathological condition, use of other drugs and type of surgery and anaesthesia. The usual recommended dosage regimen is as follows:

Adults	Initial	*Supplemental*
Spontaneous respiration	500 μg (1 ml)	250 μg (0.5 ml)
Assisted ventilation	30-50 $\mu g/kg$	15 $\mu g/kg$
Children	Initial	*Supplemental*
Assisted ventilation	30-50 $\mu g/kg$	15 $\mu g/kg$

If desired, Rapifen can be mixed with sodium chloride injection BP, dextrose injection BP or compound sodium lactate injection BP (Hartmann's solution). Such dilutions are compatible with plastic bags and giving sets. These dilutions should be used within 24 hours of preparation.

Children may require higher or more frequent dosing owing to a shorter half-life of Rapifen in this age group. The elderly and debilitated may require lower or less frequent dosing owing to a longer half-life of Rapifen in this age group (dilution may be helpful).

In spontaneously breathing patients, the initial bolus dose should be given slowly over about 30 seconds (dilution may be helpful).

After intravenous administration in unpremedicated adult patients, 1 ml Rapifen may be expected to have a peak effect in 90 seconds and to provide analgesia for 5-10 minutes. Periods of more painful stimuli may be overcome by the use of small increments of Rapifen. For procedures of longer duration, additional increments will be required.

In ventilated patients, the last dose of alfentanil should not be given later than about 10 minutes before the end of surgery to avoid the continuation of respiratory depression after surgery is complete.

In ventilated patients undergoing longer procedures, Rapifen may be infused at a rate of 0.5-1 microgram/kg/minute. Adequate plasma concentrations of alfentanil will only be achieved rapidly if this infusion is preceded by a loading dose of 50-100 microgram/kg given as a bolus or fast infusion over 10 minutes.

Lower doses may be adequate, for example, in geriatric patients or where anaesthesia is being supplemented by other agents.

The infusion should be discontinued up to 30 minutes before the anticipated end of surgery.

Increasing the infusion rate may prolong recovery. Supplementation of the anaesthetic, if required, for periods of painful stimuli, is best managed by extra bolus doses of Rapifen (1-2 ml) or low concentrations of a volatile agent for brief periods.

Patients with severe burns presenting for dressing, etc, have received a loading dose of 18-28 $\mu g/kg/min$ for up to 30 minutes without requiring mechanical ventilation. In heart surgery, when used as a sole anaesthetic, doses in the range of 12-50 mg/hour have been used.

4.3 Contraindications

Obstructive airways disease or respiratory depression if not ventilating.

Concurrent administration with monoamine oxidase inhibitors or within 2 weeks of their discontinuation.

Administration in labour or before clamping of the cord during caesarean section due to the possibility of respiratory depression in the newborn infant.

Patients with a known intolerance to alfentanil and other morphinomimetics.

4.4 Special warnings and special precautions for use

Warnings: Following administration of Rapifen, a fall in blood pressure may occur. The magnitude of this effect may be exaggerated in the hypovolaemic patient or in the presence of concomitant sedative medication. Appropriate measures to maintain a stable arterial pressure should be taken.

Significant respiratory depression will occur following administration of Rapifen in doses in excess of 1 mg and is dose-related. This and the other pharmacological effects of Rapifen are usually of short duration and can be reversed by the specific opioid antagonists (eg naloxone). Additional doses of the antagonists may be necessary because the respiratory depression may last longer than the duration of action of the opioid antagonist.

Like other opioids, alfentanil may cause bradycardia, an effect that may be marked and rapid in onset but which can be antagonised by atropine. Particular care must be taken following treatment with drugs which may depress the heart or increase vagal tone, such as anaesthetic agents or beta-blockers, since they may predispose to bradycardia or hypotension. Heart rate and blood pressure should therefore be monitored carefully. If hypotension or bradycardia occur, appropriate measures should be instituted.

Asystole following bradycardia has been reported on very rare occasions in non-atropinised patients. Therefore it is advisable to be prepared to administer an anticholinergic drug.

Precautions: It is wise to reduce the dosage in the elderly and debilitated patients. In hypothyroidism, pulmonary disease, decreased respiratory reserve, alcoholism and liver or renal impairment the dosage should be titrated with care and prolonged monitoring may be required.

Patients on chronic opioid therapy or with a history of opioid abuse may require higher doses.

Rapifen may induce muscle rigidity during induction. Rigidity, which may also involve the thoracic muscles, can be avoided by the following measures:

- Slow iv injection (usually sufficient for lower doses);
- Premedication with a benzodiazepine;
- Administration of a muscle relaxant just prior to administration of Rapifen.

Non-epileptic (myo)clonic movements can occur.

As with all potent opioids, profound analgesia is accompanied by marked respiratory depression, which may persist into or recur in the early postoperative period. Care should be taken after infusions or large doses of alfentanil to ensure that adequate spontaneous breathing has been established and maintained in the absence of stimulation before discharging the patient from the recovery area. Resuscitation equipment and narcotic antagonists should be readily available. Hyperventilation during anaesthesia may alter the patient's response to CO_2, thus affecting respiration postoperatively.

The use of rapid bolus injections of opioids should be avoided in patients with compromised intracerebral compliance; in such patients a transient decrease in the mean arterial pressure has occasionally been accompanied by a transient reduction of the cerebral perfusion pressure.

4.5 Interaction with other medicinal products and other forms of Interaction

Alfentanil is metabolised mainly via the human cytochrome P450 3A4 enzyme. Available human pharmacokinetic data indicate that the metabolism of alfentanil may be inhibited by fluconazole, erythromycin, diltiazem and cimetidine (known cytochrome P450 3A4 enzyme inhibitors). *In vitro* data suggest that other potent cytochrome P450 3A4 enzyme inhibitors (eg ketoconazole, itraconazole, ritonavir) may also inhibit the metabolism of alfentanil. This could increase the risk of prolonged or delayed respiratory depression. The concomitant use of such drugs requires special patient care and observation; in particular, it may be necessary to lower the dose of Rapifen.

Treatment with drugs which may depress the heart or increase vagal tone, such as beta-blockers and anaesthetic agents, may predispose to bradycardia or hypotension. Bradycardia and possibly asystole can occur when Rapifen is combined with non-vagolytic muscle relaxants.

The use of opioid premedication, barbiturates, benzodiazepines, neuroleptics, halogenic gases and other non-selective CNS depressants may enhance or prolong the respiratory depressant effects of alfentanil.

If other narcotic or CNS depressant drugs are used concurrently with alfentanil, the effects of the drugs can be expected to be additive. When patients have received such drugs the dose of alfentanil required will be less than usual. Likewise, following the administration of alfentanil, the dose of other CNS-depressant drugs should be reduced.

4.6 Pregnancy and lactation

Although no teratogenic or acute embryotoxic effects have been observed in animal experiments, insufficient data are available to evaluate any harmful effects in man.

Consequently, it is necessary to consider possible risks and potential advantages before administering this drug to pregnant patients.

I.V. administrationduring childbirth (including Caesarian section) is not recommended, because alfentanil crosses the placenta and because the foetal respiratory centre is particularly sensitive to opiates. If, however, Rapifen is administered, an antidote should always be at hand for the child.

Alfentanil may appear in breast milk. It is therefore recommended that breast feeding is not initiated within 24 hours of treatment.

4.7 Effects on ability to drive and use machines

Where early discharge is envisaged, patients should be advised not to drive or operate machinery for the 24 hours following administration.

4.8 Undesirable effects

Adverse events reported in association with Rapifen use in clinical trials are listed below by decreasing frequency within each body system.

Frequency estimate: Very common >10%; Common >1% to <10%; Uncommon >0.1% to <1%.

Application Site Disorders

Uncommon: Injection site pain

Body As a Whole – General Disorders

Uncommon: Shivering, Allergic reactions (such as anaphylaxis, bronchospasm, urticaria)

Cardiovascular Disorders, General

Common: Hypotension, Hypertension

Central & Peripheral Nervous System Disorders

Common: Muscle rigidity (which may also involve the thoracic muscles), Myoclonic movements, Dizziness

Uncommon: Headache

Gastro-Intestinal System Disorders

Very Common: Nausea, Vomiting

Heart Rate and Rhythm Disorders

Common: Bradycardia, Tachycardia

Uncommon: Arrhythmia

Isolated reports: Asystole

Psychiatric Disorders

Common: Somnolence

Uncommon: Disorientation, Agitation, Euphoria

Respiratory System Disorders

Common: Apnoea, Respiratory depression

Uncommon: Cough, Recurrence of respiratory depression, Laryngospasm, Hiccup

Skin and Appendages Disorders

Uncommon: Pruritus, Sweating

Vision Disorders

Uncommon: Blurred/double vision

4.9 Overdose

The manifestations of alfentanil overdose are generally an extension of its pharmacological action, which include the following:

	Action
Bradycardia	Anticholinergics such as atropine or glycopyrrolate.
Hypoventilation or apnoea	O_2 administration, assisted or controlled respiration and an opioid antagonist may be required.
Muscle rigidity	Intravenous neuromuscular blocking agent may be given.

If hypotension is severe or persists, the possibility of hypovolaemia should be considered and controlled with appropriate parenteral fluid administration.

The suggested treatments given above do not preclude the use of other clinically indicated counter measures.

Body temperature and adequate fluid intake should be maintained and the patient observed for 24 hours. A specific opioid antagonist (eg naloxone) should be available to treat respiratory depression.

5. PHARMACOLOGICAL PROPERTIES

5.1 Pharmacodynamic properties

The analgesic potency of Rapifen is one quarter that of fentanyl. The duration of action of Rapifen is one third that on an equianalgesic dose of fentanyl and is clearly dose-related. Its depressant effects on respiratory rate and alveolar ventilation are also of shorter duration than those of fentanyl.

The onset of action of Rapifen is four times more rapid than that of an equianalgesic dose of fentanyl. The peak analgesic and respiratory depressant effects occur within 90 seconds.

In man, alfentanil at therapeutic doses had no detrimental effects of myocardial performance. The cardiovascular stability is remarkable both in healthy and poor-risk patients. The only changes seen in blood pressure and heart rate are transient, slight decreases occurring immediately after induction. The incidence and degree of respiratory depression is less and of shorter duration after alfentanil than with fentanyl. Like other narcotic analgesics, alfentanil increases the amplitude of the EEG and reduces its frequency. Alfentanil reduces intraocular pressure by about 45%. It blocks increases in plasma cortisol and in plasma antidiuretic and growth hormones throughout surgery and prevents increases in plasma catecholamines up to but not during or after cardiopulmonary bypass in patients undergoing open heart surgery.

5.2 Pharmacokinetic properties

After bolus injections ranging from 2.4 to 125 μg/kg, plasma levels in man decay triexponentially with a terminal half life of approximately 90 minutes. Total distribution volume varies from 0.4 to 1.0 L/kg, indicating a limited distribution of alfentanil to the tissues. Plasma clearance, varying from 3.3 to 8.3 ml/kg/min represents approximately one third of liver plasma flow indicating that elimination of alfentanil is not flow dependent. Since only 0.4% of the dose is excreted with the urine as unchanged drug, elimination of alfentanil occurs mainly by metabolism.

These main parameters in patients undergoing surgery are similar to those in healthy volunteers. Only when the drug was given as the sole anaesthetic in a continuous high infusion over about 5 hours was the clearance of alfentanil reduced resulting in a plasma half-life of about 200 minutes, the distribution volume not being markedly changed.

Plasma protein binding of alfentanil is 92%, mainly due to a strong binding to the 'acute phase' α_1 acid-glycoprotein. It is not bound to the blood cells. Pharmacokinetics were comparable in rats, dogs and man. In children, Rapifen has been shown to have a much shorter half-life than adults, whereas the elderly show a longer half-life for Rapifen.

5.3 Preclinical safety data

Preclinical effects observed were only at exposures considered sufficiently in excess of the maximum human exposure indicating little relevance to clinical use.

6. PHARMACEUTICAL PARTICULARS

6.1 List of excipients

Sodium chloride

Water for injection

0.1N Sodium hydroxide*

0.1N Hydrochloric acid*

* for occasional pH adjustment only

6.2 Incompatibilities

See 'Dosage and dosage schedules'.

6.3 Shelf life

5 years.

6.4 Special precautions for storage

Store in a controlled drug store, at or below 25°C.

6.5 Nature and contents of container

Colourless glass one-point-cut ampoules (PhEur, Type I).

Pack size: packs of 10 × 2 ml ampoules; packs of 5 and 10 × 10 ml ampoules.

6.6 Instructions for use and handling

None stated.

7. MARKETING AUTHORISATION HOLDER

Janssen-Cilag Limited

Saunderton

High Wycombe

Buckinghamshire

HP14 4HJ

UK

8. MARKETING AUTHORISATION NUMBER(S)

PL 0242/0091

9. DATE OF FIRST AUTHORISATION/RENEWAL OF THE AUTHORISATION

27 July 1983/30 March 1999

10. DATE OF REVISION OF THE TEXT

17 November 2004

Legal category POM

Rapifen Intensive Care

(Janssen-Cilag Ltd)

1. NAME OF THE MEDICINAL PRODUCT

Rapifen® Intensive Care

2. QUALITATIVE AND QUANTITATIVE COMPOSITION

Alfentanil hydrochloride 5.44 mg equivalent to 5 mg alfentanil base per ml.

3. PHARMACEUTICAL FORM

Solution for injection.

4. CLINICAL PARTICULARS

4.1 Therapeutic indications

Rapifen Intensive Care is a potent opioid analgesic with a very rapid onset of action. It is indicated for analgesia and suppression of respiratory activity in mechanically ventilated patients on intensive care and to provide analgesic cover for painful manoeuvres. It will aid compliance with mechanical ventilation, and tolerance of the endotracheal tube. Intravenous bolus doses of Rapifen (0.5 mg/ml) may be used to provide additional pain relief during brief painful procedures such as physiotherapy, endotracheal suction, etc. Despite being mechanically ventilated, patients may be awake in the presence of adequate analgesia.

At the proposed doses, Rapifen Intensive Care has no sedative activity. Therefore supplementation with an appropriate hypnotic or sedative agent is recommended. Admixture is not advisable due to the need to individually titrate both agents.

Alfentanil given by infusion should only be given in areas where facilities are available to deal with respiratory depression and where continuous monitoring is performed. Alfentanil should only be prescribed by physicians familiar with the use of potent opioids when given by continuous IV infusion.

4.2 Posology and method of administration

Method of Administration

For intravenous infusions.

Dosage

Rapifen Intensive Care should be diluted with sodium chloride intravenous infusion BP, glucose intravenous infusion BP, or compound sodium lactate intravenous infusion BP (Hartmann's solution). Such dilutions are compatible with plastic bags and giving sets. These dilutions should be used within 24 hours of preparation.

Once the patient has been intubated, mechanical ventilation can be initiated using the following dosage regimen:

The recommended initial infusion rate for mechanically ventilated adult patients is 2 mg per hour (equivalent to 0.4 ml per hour of undiluted Rapifen Intensive Care). For a 70 kg patient, this corresponds to approximately 30 micrograms per kilogram per hour.

More rapid control may initially be gained by using a loading dose. For example, a dose of 5 mg may be given in divided doses over a period of 10 minutes, during which time careful monitoring of blood pressure and heart rate should be performed. If hypotension or bradycardia occurs, the rate of administration should be reduced accordingly and other appropriate measures instituted.

The dose to produce the desired effects should then be individually determined and reassessed regularly to ensure that the optimum dose is being used.

In clinical trials, patient requirements have generally been met with doses of 0.5 to 10 mg alfentanil per hour.

Additional bolus doses of 0.5-1.0 mg alfentanil may be given to provide analgesia during short painful procedures.

The elderly and those patients with liver impairment and hypothyroidism will require lower doses. Obese patients may require a dose based on their lean body mass.

Adolescents and young adults will require higher than average doses. There is little experience of use of alfentanil to treat children in intensive care.

The maximum recommended duration of treatment with alfentanil infusions is 4 days.

Present data suggest that clearance of alfentanil is unaltered in renal failure. However there is an increased free fraction and hence dosage requirements may be less than in the patient with normal renal function.

4.3 Contraindications

Known intolerance of alfentanil or other morphinomimetics.

4.4 Special warnings and special precautions for use

Warnings:

Following administration of Rapifen Intensive Care, a fall in blood pressure may occur. The magnitude of this effect may be exaggerated in the hypovolaemic patient or in the presence of concomitant sedative medication. Appropriate measures to maintain a stable arterial pressure should be taken.

Like other opioids, alfentanil may cause bradycardia, an effect which may be marked and rapid in onset but which can be antagonised by atropine.

Particular care must be taken following treatment with drugs which may depress the heart or increase vagal tone, such as anaesthetic agents or beta-blockers since they may predispose to bradycardia or hypotension. Heart rate and blood pressure should therefore be monitored carefully. If hypotension or bradycardia occurs, the rate of administration of alfentanil should be reduced and other appropriate measures instituted. Asystole following bradycardia has been reported on very rare occasions in non-atropinised patients. Therefore it is advisable to be prepared to administer an anticholinergic drug.

Care must be taken if the patient has received monoamine oxidase inhibitors within the previous 2 weeks.

Significant respiratory depression will occur following administration of alfentanil in doses in excess of 1 mg and is dose-related. If necessary for assessment purposes, naloxone or other specific antagonists may be administered to reverse the opioid respiratory depression and other pharmacological effects of alfentanil. More than one dose of naloxone may be required in view of its short half life.

Muscle rigidity (morphine-like effect) may occur, in which case neuromuscular blocking drugs may be helpful.

Precautions:

It is wise to reduce the dosage in the elderly and debilitated patient. In hypothyroidism, pulmonary disease, decreased respiratory reserve, alcoholism and liver or renal impairment the dosage should be titrated with care and prolonged monitoring may be required.

Patients on chronic opioid therapy or with a history of opioid abuse may require higher doses.

Non-epileptic (myo)clonic movements can occur.

As with all potent opioids, profound analgesia is accompanied by marked respiratory depression, which may persist into or recur in the early post infusion period. Care should therefore be taken throughout the weaning period and adequate spontaneous respiration should be established and maintained in the absence of stimulation or ventilatory support. Following cessation of the infusion, the patient should be closely observed for at least 6 hours. Prior use of opioid medication may enhance or prolong the respiratory depressant effects of alfentanil.

The use of rapid bolus injections of opioids should be avoided in patients with compromised intracerebral compliance; in such patients a transient decrease in the mean arterial pressure has occasionally been accompanied by a transient reduction of the cerebral perfusion pressure.

4.5 Interaction with other medicinal products and other forms of Interaction

Alfentanil is metabolised mainly via the human cytochrome P450 3A4 enzyme. Available human pharmacokinetic data indicate that the metabolism of alfentanil may be inhibited by fluconazole, erythromycin, diltiazem and cimetidine (known cytochrome P450 3A4 enzyme inhibitors). *In vitro* data suggest that other potent cytochrome P450 3A4 enzyme inhibitors (e.g. ketoconazole, itraconazole, ritonavir) may also inhibit the metabolism of alfentanil. This could increase the risk of prolonged or delayed respiratory depression. The concomitant use of such drugs requires special patient care and observation; in particular, it may be necessary to lower the dose of Rapifen.

Treatment with drugs which may depress the heart or increase vagal tone, such as beta-blockers and anaesthetic agents, may predispose to bradycardia or hypotension. Bradycardia and possibly asystole can occur when Rapifen Intensive Care is combined with non-vagolytic muscle relaxants.

Prior use of opioid premedication, barbiturates, benzodiazepines, neuroleptics, halogenic gases and other non-selective CNS depressants may enhance or prolong the respiratory depressant effects of alfentanil.

If other narcotic or CNS depressant drugs are used concurrently with alfentanil, the effects of the drugs can be expected to be additive. When patients have received such drugs, the dose of alfentanil required will be less than usual. Likewise, following the administration of alfentanil, the dose of other CNS-depressant drugs should be reduced.

4.6 Pregnancy and lactation

Although no teratogenic or acute embryotoxic effects have been observed in animal experiments, insufficient data are available to evaluate any harmful effects in man.

Consequently, it is necessary to consider possible risks and potential advantages before administering this drug to pregnant patients.

I.V. administrationduring childbirth (including Caesarian section) is not recommended, because alfentanil crosses the placenta and because the foetal respiratory centre is particularly sensitive to opiates. If, however, Rapifen is administered, an antidote should always be at hand for the child.

Alfentanil may appear in breast milk. It is therefore recommended that breast feeding is not initiated within 24 hours of treatment.

4.7 Effects on ability to drive and use machines

Where early discharge is envisaged, patients should be advised not to drive or operate machinery for the 24 hours following administration.

4.8 Undesirable effects

Adverse events reported in association with Rapifen use in clinical trials are listed below by decreasing frequency within each body system.

Frequency estimate: Very common >10%; Common >1% to <10%; Uncommon >0.1% to <1%.

Application Site Disorders

Uncommon: Injection site pain

Body As a Whole – General Disorders

Uncommon: Shivering, Allergic reactions (such as anaphylaxis, bronchospasm, urticaria)

Cardiovascular Disorders, General

Common: Hypotension, Hypertension

Central & Peripheral Nervous System Disorders

Common: Muscle rigidity (which may also involve the thoracic muscles), Myoclonic movements, Dizziness

Uncommon: Headache

Gastro-Intestinal System Disorders

Very Common: Nausea, Vomiting

Heart Rate and Rhythm Disorders

Common: Bradycardia, Tachycardia

Uncommon: Arrhythmia

Isolated reports: Asystole

Psychiatric Disorders

Common: Somnolence

Uncommon: Disorientation, Agitation, Euphoria

Respiratory System Disorders

Common: Apnoea, Respiratory depression

Uncommon: Cough, Recurrence of respiratory depression, Laryngospasm, Hiccup

Skin and Appendages Disorders

Uncommon: Pruritus, Sweating

Vision Disorders

Uncommon: Blurred/double vision

4.9 Overdose

The manifestations of alfentanil overdose are generally an extension of its pharmacological action, which include the following:-

	Action:
Bradycardia:	Anticholinergics such as atropine or glycopyrrolate;
Hypoventilation or apnoea:	O_2 administration, assisted or controlled respiration and an opioid antagonist may be required;
Muscle rigidity:	Intravenous neuromuscular blocking agent may be given.

The suggested treatments given above do not preclude the use of other clinically indicated counter measures.

Body temperature and adequate fluid intake should be maintained and the patient observed for 24 hours.

A specific narcotic antagonist (eg naloxone) should be available to treat respiratory depression.

5. PHARMACOLOGICAL PROPERTIES

5.1 Pharmacodynamic properties

In man, alfentanil at therapeutic doses has no detrimental effects on myocardial performance. The cardiovascular stability is remarkable both in healthy and poor-risk patients. The only changes seen in blood pressure and heart rate were transient, slight decreases occurring immediately after induction. The incidence and degree of respiratory depression is less and of shorter duration after alfentanil than with fentanyl. Like other narcotic analgesics, alfentanil increases the amplitude of the EEG and reduces its frequency. Alfentanil reduces intraocular pressure by about 45%. It blocks increases in plasma cortisol and in plasma antidiuretic and growth hormones throughout surgery, and prevents increases in plasma catecholamines up to, but not during or after, cardiopulmonary bypass in patients undergoing open heart surgery.

5.2 Pharmacokinetic properties

After bolus injections ranging from 2.4 to 125 μg/kg, plasma levels in man decay triexponentially with a terminal half life of approx. 90 minutes. Total distribution volume varies from 0.4 to 1.0 l/kg, indicating a limited distribution of alfentanil to the tissues. Plasma clearance, varying from 3.3 to 8.3 ml/kg/min represents approximately one third of liver plasma flow indicating that elimination of alfentanil is not flow dependent. Since only 0.4% of the dose is excreted with the urine as unchanged drug, elimination of alfentanil occurs mainly by metabolism.

These main parameters in patients undergoing surgery are similar to those in healthy volunteers. Only when the drug was given as the sole anaesthetic in a continuous high infusion over about 5 hours was the clearance of alfentanil reduced resulting in a plasma half-life of about 200 minutes, the distribution volume not being markedly changed.

Plasma protein binding of alfentanil is 92%, mainly due to a strong binding to the 'acute phase' α_1-acid-glycoprotein. It is not bound to the blood cells. Pharmacokinetics were comparable in rats, dogs and man. In children, alfentanil has been shown to have a much shorter half-life than adults, whereas the elderly show a longer half-life for alfentanil, after IV bolus doses.

5.3 Preclinical safety data

Preclinical effects observed were only at exposures considered sufficiently in excess of the maximum human exposure indicating little relevance to clinical use.

6. PHARMACEUTICAL PARTICULARS

6.1 List of excipients

Sodium chloride

Water for injections

Sodium hydroxide 0.1 N

Hydrochloric acid 0.1 N

6.2 Incompatibilities

See Section 4.2 Posology and Method of administration.

6.3 Shelf life

60 months.

6.4 Special precautions for storage

Store in the controlled drug store, at or below 25°C.

6.5 Nature and contents of container

Type I USP clear glass ampoules containing 1 ml, packed in 5s or 10s.

6.6 Instructions for use and handling

None.

7. MARKETING AUTHORISATION HOLDER

Janssen-Cilag Limited
Saunderton
High Wycombe
Buckinghamshire
HP14 4HJ
UK

8. MARKETING AUTHORISATION NUMBER(S)

PL 0242/0137

9. DATE OF FIRST AUTHORISATION/RENEWAL OF THE AUTHORISATION

Date of first Authorisation: 31/07/89

Date of Renewal: 23/06/00

10. DATE OF REVISION OF THE TEXT

17 November 2004

Rapilysin 10 U

(Roche Products Limited)

1. NAME OF THE MEDICINAL PRODUCT

Rapilysin 10 U powder and solvent for solution for injection.

2. QUALITATIVE AND QUANTITATIVE COMPOSITION

1 vial contains 0.56 g powder for solution for injection with 10 U reteplase (INN)

1 prefilled syringe contains 10 ml water for injections.

The reconstituted solution contains 1 U reteplase per ml.

Potency of reteplase is expressed in units (U) by using a reference standard which is specific for reteplase and is not comparable with units used for other thrombolytic agents.

For excipients see 6.1.

3. PHARMACEUTICAL FORM

Powder and solvent for solution for injection.

Appearance: white powder (lyophilisate) and clear colourless liquid.

4. CLINICAL PARTICULARS

4.1 Therapeutic indications

Rapilysin is indicated for the thrombolytic treatment of suspected myocardial infarction with persistent ST elevation or recent left Bundle Branch Block within 12 hours after the onset of AMI symptoms.

4.2 Posology and method of administration

Treatment with reteplase should be initiated as soon as possible after the onset of AMI symptoms.

Reteplase is supplied as a freeze-dried substance in vials. The lyophilisate is reconstituted with the contents of the accompanying syringe (see chapter 6.6 Instructions for use and handling).

The reconstituted solution must be used immediately. Visual inspection of the solution is necessary after reconstitution. Only clear, colourless solutions should be injected. If the solution is not clear and colourless it should be discarded.

Heparin and Rapilysin are incompatible when*combined in solution*. Other incompatibilities may also exist. No other medication should be added to the injection solution (see below and 6.2. Incompatibilities). Rapilysin should be injected preferably through an intravenous line whose sole purpose is the injection of Rapilysin. No other medication should be injected through the line reserved for Rapilysin, neither at the same time, nor prior to, nor following Rapilysin injection. This applies to all products including heparin, and acetylsalicylic acid, which should be administered before and following the administration of reteplase to reduce the risk of re-thrombosis.

In those patients where the same line has to be used, this line (including Y-line) must be flushed thoroughly with 0.9% sodium chloride or 5% dextrose solution prior to and following the Rapilysin injection.

Dosage of Rapilysin

Rapilysin is administered as a 10 U bolus dose followed by a second 10 U bolus dose 30 minutes later (double bolus).

Each bolus is administered as a slow intravenous injection within 2 minutes. Ensure that the injection is not mistakenly given paravenously.

Heparin and acetylsalicylic acid should be administered before and following the administration of Rapilysin to reduce the risk of rethrombosis.

Dosage of Heparin

The recommended dose of heparin is 5000 I.U. given as a bolus injection prior to reteplase therapy followed by an infusion of 1000 I.U. per hour starting after the second reteplase bolus. Heparin should be administered for at least 24 hours, preferably for 48 – 72 hours, aiming to keep aPTT values 1.5 to 2 times normal.

Dosage of Acetylsalicylic Acid

The initial dose of acetylsalicylic acid prior to thrombolysis should be at least 250 mg (250 – 350 mg) followed by 75 – 150 mg/day at least until discharge.

4.3 Contraindications

Rapilysin is contraindicated in patients with known hypersensitivity to the active substance (reteplase), polysorbate 80 or any of the other ingredients.

Because thrombolytic therapy increases the risk of bleeding, reteplase is contra-indicated in the following situations:

- known haemorrhagic diathesis

- patients with current concomitant therapy with oral anticoagulants (e.g. warfarin sodium)

- intracranial neoplasm, arteriovenous malformation or aneurysm
- neoplasm with increased bleeding risk
- history of cerebrovascular accident
- recent (< 10 days) prolonged and vigorous external heart massage
- severe uncontrolled hypertension
- active peptic ulceration
- portal hypertension (oesophageal varices)
- severe liver or renal dysfunction
- acute pancreatitis, pericarditis, bacterial endocarditis
- within 3 months of severe bleeding, major trauma or major surgery (e.g. coronary artery bypass graft, intracranial or intraspinal surgery or trauma), obstetrical delivery, organ biopsy, previous puncture of noncompressible vessels.

4.4 Special warnings and special precautions for use

Reteplase should be used by physicians experienced in the use of thrombolytic treatment and with the facilities to monitor that use.

Each patient being considered for therapy with reteplase should be carefully evaluated.

For information on product incompatibilities see section 4.2.

Bleeding

The most common complication encountered during reteplase therapy is bleeding. In the following conditions the risks of reteplase therapy may be increased and should be weighed against the anticipated benefits:

- cerebrovascular disease
- systolic blood pressure at entry >160 mmHg
- recent gastrointestinal or genitourinary bleeding (within 10 days)
- high likelihood of left heart thrombus, e.g. mitral stenosis with atrial fibrillation
- septic thrombophlebitis or occluded arteriovenous cannula at seriously infected site
- age over 75 years
- any other condition in which bleeding constitutes a significant hazard or would be particularly difficult because of its location.

The concomitant use of heparin anticoagulation may contribute to bleeding. As fibrin is lysed during reteplase therapy, bleeding from recent puncture sites may occur. Therefore, thrombolytic therapy requires careful attention to all possible bleeding sites (including catheter insertion sites, arterial and venous puncture sites, cutdown sites and needle puncture sites). The use of rigid catheter as well as intramuscular injections and nonessential handling of the patient should be avoided during treatment with reteplase.

Caution should be employed when used with other drugs affecting haemostasis such as heparin, low-molecular-weight heparins, heparinoids, oral anticoagulants and antiplatelet agents other than acetylsalicylic acid, such as dipyridamole, ticlopidine, clopidogrel or glycoprotein IIb/IIIa receptor antagonists.

Should serious bleeding, in particular cerebral haemorrhage, occur any concomitant heparin should be terminated immediately. In addition, the second bolus of reteplase should not be given if the serious bleeding occurs before it is administered. In general, however, it is not necessary to replace the coagulation factors because of the relatively short half-life of reteplase. Most patients who have bleeding can be managed by interruption of thrombolytic and anticoagulant therapy, volume replacement and manual pressure applied to an incompetent vessel. Protamine should be considered if heparin has been administered within 4 hours of the onset of bleeding. In the patients who fail to respond to these conservative measures, judicious use of transfusion products may be indicated. Transfusions of cryoprecipitate, fibrinogen, fresh frozen plasma and platelets should be considered with clinical and laboratory reassessment after each administration. A target fibrinogen level of 1 g/l is desirable with cryoprecipitate or fibrinogen infusion.

At present, insufficient data in patients with a diastolic blood pressure >100 mmHg prior to thrombolytic therapy are available for reteplase.

Arrhythmias

Coronary thrombolysis may result in arrhythmias associated with reperfusion. It is strongly recommended that antiarrhythmic therapy for bradycardia and/or ventricular tachyarrhythmias (e.g. ventricular tachycardia or fibrillation) be available when reteplase is administered.

Readministration

Since at present there is no experience with readministration of reteplase, the readministration is not recommended. However, no antibody formation to the reteplase molecule has been observed.

If an anaphylactoid reaction occurs, the injection should be discontinued immediately and appropriate therapy should be initiated.

Use in children

Safety and effectiveness of reteplase in children have not been established. Treatment of children is not recommended.

4.5 Interaction with other medicinal products and other forms of Interaction

No formal interaction studies with reteplase and drugs commonly administered in patients with AMI have been performed. Retrospective analyses of clinical studies did not reveal any clinically relevant interactions with drugs used concomitantly with reteplase in patients with acute myocardial infarction. Heparin, vitamin K antagonists and drugs that alter platelet function (such as acetylsalicylic acid, dipyridamole and abciximab) may increase the risk of bleeding if administered prior to, during or after reteplase therapy.

Attention should be paid to this effect especially during periods of low plasma fibrinogen (up to about 2 days after fibrinolytic therapy of AMI).

For information on product incompatibilities see section 4.2.

4.6 Pregnancy and lactation

There are no adequate data on the use of reteplase in pregnant women. The only relevant available animal data refer to studies performed in rabbits, which showed vaginal bleedings associated with abortions (see 5.3) The potential risk for humans is unknown.

Except in life-threatening situations, Rapilysin 10 U should not be used in pregnant women.

It is not known whether reteplase is excreted into breast milk. Breast milk should be discarded within the first 24 hours after thrombolytic therapy.

4.7 Effects on ability to drive and use machines

Not applicable.

4.8 Undesirable effects

The frequency of the adverse drug reactions is described using the following convention:

Very common	> 1/10
Common	> 1/100, <1/10
Uncommon	> 1/1,000, <1/100
Rare	> 1/10,000, <1/1,000
Very rare	< 1/10,000, (including isolated reports)

Haemorrhage

The most frequent adverse drug reaction associated with reteplase treatment is haemorrhage.

- very commonly: bleeding at the injection site (e.g. haematoma)
- commonly: as gastrointestinal (haematemesis, melena), gingival or genitourinary bleeding
- uncommonly: haemopericardium, retroperitoneal bleeding, cerebral haemorrhage, epistaxis, haemoptysis, eye haemorrhage and ecchymosis were observed.

Reports of intracranial bleeding, many of which are fatal, are of particular concern.

Systolic blood pressure over 160 mmHg before thrombolysis with reteplase was associated with greater risk for cerebral bleeding. The risk of intracranial bleeding and fatal intracranial bleeding increases with increasing age. Blood transfusions were rarely required. Death and permanent disability are not uncommonly reported in patients who have experienced stroke (including intracranial bleeding) and other serious bleeding episodes.

Cardiovascular disorders

As with other thrombolytic agents, the following events have been reported as sequelae of myocardial infarction and / or thrombolytic administration.

- *very commonly*: recurrent ischaemia / angina, hypotension and heart failure / pulmonary oedema
- *commonly*: arrhythmias (e.g. AV block, atrial fibrillation / flutter, ventricular tachycardia / fibrillation, electromechanical dissociation (EMD)), cardiac arrest, cardiogenic shock and reinfarction
- *uncommonly*: mitral regurgitation, pulmonary embolism, other systemic embolism / cerebral embolism and ventricular septal defect.

These cardiovascular events can be life-threatening and may lead to death.

- Nervous system disorders

- *uncommonly:* cerebral haemorrhage was observed.
- *isolated reports:* events related to the nervous system (e.g. epileptic seizure, convulsion, aphasia, speech disorder, delirium, acute brain syndrome, agitation, confusion, depression, psychosis).

Ischaemic or haemorrhagic cerebrovascular events may be contributing or underlying conditions.

- General disorders and administration site conditions

- *very commonly*: haemorrhage at the injection site (e.g. haematoma); a local reaction at injection site for example a burning sensation can occur.

- Immune system disorders

- *uncommonly*: hypersensitivity reactions (e.g. allergic reactions)
- *isolated reports*: serious anaphylaxis/ anaphylactoid reactions.

Available evidence on reteplase does not indicate an antibody-mediated origin of these hypersensitivity reactions.

4.9 Overdose

In the event of overdosage one might expect depletion of fibrinogen and other blood coagulation components (e.g. coagulation factor V) with a consequent risk of bleeding.

For further information see 4.4 Special warnings and special precautions for use, section *Bleeding*.

5. PHARMACOLOGICAL PROPERTIES

5.1 Pharmacodynamic properties

Pharmaco-therapeutic group: antithrombotic agent, ATC Code: **B 01 A D**

Reteplase is a recombinant plasminogen activator that catalyzes the cleavage of endogenous plasminogen to generate plasmin. This plasminogenolysis occurs preferentially in the presence of fibrin. Plasmin in turn degrades fibrin, which is the main component of the matrix of thrombi, thereby exerting its thrombolytic action.

Reteplase (10+10 U) dose-dependently reduces plasma fibrinogen levels by about 60 to 80%. The fibrinogen level normalises within 2 days. As with other plasminogen activators a rebound phenomenon then occurs during which fibrinogen levels reach a maximum within 9 days and remain elevated for up to 18 days.

Reductions of plasma levels of plasminogen and α2-antiplasmin normalise within 1 to 3 days. Coagulation factor V, clotting factor VIII, α2-macroglobulin, and C1-esterase inhibitor are only slightly reduced and normalise within 1 to 2 days. Plasminogen activator inhibitor 1 (PAI-1) activity can be reduced to around zero, but rapidly normalises within two hours showing a rebound phenomenon. Prothrombin activation fragment 1 levels and thrombin-antithrombin III-complexes increase during thrombolysis indicating thrombin production of which the clinical relevance is unknown.

A large comparative mortality trial (INJECT) in approx. 6000 patients showed that reteplase reduced the incidence of heart failure (secondary efficacy criterion) in a significant manner and was at least equally effective in terms of reducing mortality (primary efficacy criterion) when compared to streptokinase. In two clinical trials aiming primarily at coronary artery patency (RAPID I and II) reteplase was associated with higher early patency rates (primary efficacy criterion), as well as with a lower incidence of heart failure (secondary efficacy criterion) than alteplase (3 hour and "accelerated" dosage regimens). A clinical trial in approximately 15 000 patients comparing reteplase with the accelerated dose regimen of alteplase (GUSTO III) (2:1 randomisation reteplase: alteplase) did not show statistically different results for the primary endpoint of 30-day mortality (reteplase: 7.47%, alteplase 7.23%, p = 0.61) or for the combined endpoint of 30-day mortality and non-fatal disabling stroke (reteplase: 7.89%, alteplase 7.88%, p = 0.99). Overall stroke rates were 1.64% in the reteplase and 1.79% in the alteplase group. In the reteplase group, 49.4% of these strokes were fatal and 27.1% were disabling. In the alteplase group 33.0% were fatal and 39.8% were disabling.

5.2 Pharmacokinetic properties

Following intravenous bolus injection of 10 + 10 U in patients with acute myocardial infarction reteplase antigen is distributed in plasma with a dominant half-life ($t1/2\alpha$) of 18±5 min and eliminated with a terminal half-life ($t1/2\beta$) of 5.5 hours±12.5 min at a clearance rate of 121±25 ml/min. Reteplase activity is cleared from the plasma at a rate of 283±101 ml/min, resulting in a dominant half-life ($t1/2\alpha$) of 14.6±6.7 min and a terminal half-life ($t1/2\beta$) of 1.6 hours±39 min. Only minor amounts of reteplase were immunologically detected in the urine. Exact data on the main elimination routes for reteplase in humans are not available and the consequences of hepatic or renal insufficiency are not known. Experiments in rats indicate that the liver and the kidneys are the main organs of active uptake and lysosomal degradation.

Additional studies in human plasma samples *in vitro* suggest that complexation with C1-inactivator, α2-antiplasmin and α2-antitrypsin contributes to the inactivation of reteplase in plasma. The relative contribution of the inhibitors to inactivation of reteplase decreases as follows: C1-inactivator > α2-antiplasmin > α2-antitrypsin.

The half-life of reteplase was increased in patients with AMI as compared to healthy volunteers. An additional increase of half-life of activity in patients with myocardial infarction and severely impaired liver and renal function cannot be excluded, but no clinical data of pharmacokinetics of reteplase in these patients are available. Animal data show that in case of severely impaired renal function with a pronounced increase in serum creatinine and serum urea an increase in half-life of reteplase has to be expected. Mild impairment of renal function did not significantly affect the pharmacokinetic properties of reteplase.

5.3 Preclinical safety data

Acute toxicity studies were performed in rats, rabbits and monkeys. Subacute toxicity studies were performed in rats, dogs and monkeys. The predominant acute symptom after single high doses of reteplase in rats and rabbits was transient apathy shortly after injection. In cynomolgus monkeys, the sedative effect ranged from slight apathy to unconsciousness, caused by a reversible dose-related drop in blood pressure. There was increased local haemorrhage at the injection site.

Subacute toxicity studies did not reveal any unexpected adverse events. In dogs repeated dosing of the human peptide reteplase led to immunologic-allergic reactions. Genotoxicity of reteplase was excluded by a complete battery of tests at different genetic end points in vitro and in vivo.

Reproductive toxicity studies were performed in rats (fertility and embryo-foetotoxicity study including a littering phase) and in rabbits (embryo-foetotoxicity study, dose-range finding only). In rats, a species insensitive to the pharmacological effects of reteplase, there were no adverse effects on fertility, embryo-foetal development and offspring. In rabbits, vaginal bleedings and abortions possibly associated to prolonged haemostasis, but no foetal abnormalities were noted. A pre- and postnatal toxicity study was not performed with reteplase.

6. PHARMACEUTICAL PARTICULARS

6.1 List of excipients

Tranexamic acid, di-potassium-hydrogen phosphate, phosphoric acid, sucrose, polysorbate 80.

6.2 Incompatibilities

Heparin and Rapilysin are incompatible when combined in solution. Other incompatibilities may also exist. No other medication should be added to the injection solution.

No other medication should be injected through the line reserved for Rapilysin either at the same time, or prior to, or following Rapilysin injection. This applies to all products including heparin and acetylsalicylic acid, which should be administered before and following the administration of reteplase to reduce the risk of re-thrombosis.

In those patients where the same line has to be used, this line (including Y-line) must be flushed thoroughly with a 0.9% sodium chloride or 5% dextrose solution prior to and following the Rapilysin injection (see 4.2 Posology and method of administration).

6.3 Shelf life

Rapilysin 10 U vials have a shelf-life of 3 years.

When reconstituted as directed, the solution must be used immediately.

6.4 Special precautions for storage

Do not store Rapilysin 10 U above 25°C.

Keep the container in the outer carton in order to protect from light.

6.5 Nature and contents of container

Each pack contains:

2 vials with powder for solution for injection

2 syringes with solvent

2 reconstitution devices and 2 needles 19 G 1

6.6 Instructions for use and handling

Use aseptic technique throughout.

1. Remove the protective flip-cap from the vial of Rapilysin 10 U and clean the rubber closure with an alcohol wipe.

2. Open the package containing the reconstitution spike, remove both protective caps from the reconstitution spike.

3. Insert the spike through the rubber closure into the vial of Rapilysin 10 U.

4. Take the 10 ml syringe out of the package. Remove the tip cap from the syringe. Connect the syringe to the reconstitution spike and transfer the 10 ml of solvent into the vial of Rapilysin 10 U.

5. With the reconstitution spike and syringe still attached to the vial, swirl the vial gently to dissolve the Rapilysin 10 U powder. DO NOT SHAKE.

6. The reconstituted preparation results in a clear, colourless solution. If the solution is not clear and colourless it should be discarded.

7. Heparin and Rapilysin are incompatible when combined in solution. Other incompatibilities may also exist. No other medication should be added to the injection solution.

8. Withdraw 10 ml of Rapilysin 10 U solution back into the syringe. A small amount of solution may remain in the vial due to overfill.

9. Disconnect the syringe from the reconstitution spike and attach the sterile needle provided. The dose is now ready for intravenous administration.

7. MARKETING AUTHORISATION HOLDER

Roche Registration Limited

40 Broadwater Road

Welwyn Garden City

Hertfordshire AL7 3 AY

United Kingdom

8. MARKETING AUTHORISATION NUMBER(S)

EU/1/96/018/001

9. DATE OF FIRST AUTHORISATION/RENEWAL OF THE AUTHORISATION

9 November 2001

10. DATE OF REVISION OF THE TEXT

August 2003

Rapitil Eye Drops

(sanofi-aventis)

1. NAME OF THE MEDICINAL PRODUCT

Rapitil™ Eye Drops

2. QUALITATIVE AND QUANTITATIVE COMPOSITION

Nedocromil sodium 2.0% w/v.

3. PHARMACEUTICAL FORM

Presented as a 5 ml sterile, preserved, aqueous solution containing 2% nedocromil sodium in a dropper bottle for administration to the eye.

4. CLINICAL PARTICULARS

4.1 Therapeutic indications

For the prevention, relief and treatment of allergic conjunctivitis, including seasonal allergic conjunctivitis, allergic conjunctivitis and vernal kerato-conjunctivitis.

4.2 Posology and method of administration

Adults (including the elderly) and children aged 6 years and over:

In seasonal allergic conjunctivitis: one drop into each eye twice daily, increasing when necessary to four times daily. In seasonal allergic conjunctivitis therapy should be restricted to 12 weeks.

In vernal kerato-conjunctivitis: one drop into each eye four times daily.

Adults (including the elderly):

In perennial allergic conjunctivitis: one drop into each eye twice daily, increasing when necessary to four times daily.

Rapitil should be used regularly to ensure optimum control of symptoms.

There is only limited clinical trial evidence with Rapitil in children aged below 6 years, therefore use in this age range cannot be recommended.

4.3 Contraindications

Contraindicated in patients with known hypersensitivity to any constituent of the formulation.

4.4 Special warnings and special precautions for use

Patients who use soft contact lenses should be advised not to wear them during the treatment period. In patients who continue to use hard or gas-permeable contact lenses during treatment with the eye drops, the lenses should be taken out of the eye prior to instillation and not inserted again for at least 10 minutes.

4.5 Interaction with other medicinal products and other forms of Interaction

None has been reported.

4.6 Pregnancy and lactation

Studies in pregnant and lactating animals have failed to reveal a hazard with nedocromil sodium. However, as with all medications caution should be exercised during pregnancy (especially during the first trimester) and whilst breast feeding.

On the basis of animal studies and its physicochemical properties it is considered that only negligible amounts of nedocromil sodium may pass into human breast milk. There is no information to suggest that the use of nedocromil sodium by nursing mothers has any undesirable effects upon the baby.

4.7 Effects on ability to drive and use machines

No sedative effects have been reported.

4.8 Undesirable effects

Transient stinging and burning may occur after instillation. Other symptoms of local irritation have been reported rarely. Some patients have reported a distinctive taste.

4.9 Overdose

Animal studies have not shown evidence of toxic effects of nedocromil sodium even at high dosage, nor have extended human studies revealed any safety hazard with the drug. Overdosage is unlikely, therefore, to cause problems. However, if suspected, treatment should be supportive and directed to the control of the relevant symptoms.

5. PHARMACOLOGICAL PROPERTIES

5.1 Pharmacodynamic properties

Rapitil, the ophthalmic preparation of nedocromil sodium, displays specific anti-allergic and anti-inflammatory properties. Nedocromil sodium has been shown to prevent the release of inflammatory mediators from a range of inflammatory cell types.

5.2 Pharmacokinetic properties

Following topical ophthalmic administration, less than 4% of the dose is absorbed following multiple dosing. Absorption occurs primarily through the nasal mucosa as approximately 80% of the ophthalmic dose drains into the nose via the naso-lachrymal duct, although 1-2% of the dose may be absorbed orally.

Nedocromil sodium is reversibly bound to plasma proteins and is not metabolised, but is excreted unchanged in bile and urine. The drug is rapidly cleared from the plasma (plasma clearance 10.2 ± 1.3 ml/min/kg - elimination half-life 5.3 ± 0.9 min) and accumulation does not occur.

5.3 Preclinical safety data

Animal studies have failed to reveal toxic effects with nedocromil sodium even at high doses.

6. PHARMACEUTICAL PARTICULARS

6.1 List of excipients

Benzalkonium chloride, Sodium chloride, Disodium edetate.

6.2 Incompatibilities

None known.

6.3 Shelf life

36 months.

6.4 Special precautions for storage

Store below 25°C, away from direct sunlight. Discard any remaining contents four weeks after opening the bottle.

6.5 Nature and contents of container

A plastic dropper bottle containing 5ml of sterile, aqueous solution for administration to the eye.

6.6 Instructions for use and handling

Please refer to enclosed package insert.

7. MARKETING AUTHORISATION HOLDER

Aventis Pharma Ltd

50 Kings Hill Avenue

West Malling

Kent ME19 4AH

United Kingdom

8. MARKETING AUTHORISATION NUMBER(S)

PL 04425/0285

9. DATE OF FIRST AUTHORISATION/RENEWAL OF THE AUTHORISATION

26 February 2004

10. DATE OF REVISION OF THE TEXT

11 LEGAL CLASSIFICATION

POM

Rapolyte

(Provalis Healthcare)

1. NAME OF THE MEDICINAL PRODUCT

RAPOLYTE®

2. QUALITATIVE AND QUANTITATIVE COMPOSITION

Sodium chloride 0.35 g

Potassium chloride 0.3 g

Sodium citrate 0.6 g

Anhydrous dextrose 4 g

3. PHARMACEUTICAL FORM

Crystalline Powder

4. CLINICAL PARTICULARS

4.1 Therapeutic indications

For the treatment of fluid and electrolyte loss associated with diarrhoea.

4.2 Posology and method of administration

For oral administration

Dosage:

The actual volume of reconstituted Rapolyte® taken should be determined by the physician, depending on the patient's weight and the stage and severity of the condition (see 6.6 Instructions for Use/Handling). Daily intake may be based on a volume of 150 ml/kg bodyweight for infants and 20-40 ml/kg bodyweight for adults and children. A reasonable approximation is:

Infants:

One to one and a half times the usual feed volume.

Children:

One sachet after every loose motion.

Adults:

One sachet after every loose motion.

In the initial stages (24 hours) of treatment of diarrhoea, all foods, including cows and artificial milk, should be stopped. After 24-48 hours, when symptoms have subsided, the normal diet should be resumed, but this should be gradual to avoid worsening or prolonging the diarrhoea. A suggested regimen for the treatment of infantile diarrhoea is given below:

(see Table 1 at top of next page)

In breast fed infants, it is suggested that the infant is given the appropriate volume of Rapolyte® and then put to the breast until satisfied. Where vomiting is present with the diarrhoea, it is advisable that small amounts of Rapolyte® be taken frequently. However, it is important that the whole of the required volume of Rapolyte® is taken. With normal renal function it is difficult to over-rehydrate by mouth, and where there is doubt about the exact dosage, more rather than less should be taken.

4.3 Contraindications

None known. However, there may be a number of conditions where treatment with Rapolyte® will be inappropriate, e.g. intestinal obstruction requiring surgical intervention.

Table 1

Day	Volume of Rapolyte® solution (ml)	Volume of artificial milk feed (ml)	Total volume in 24 hours (ml)
1	150 × wt*	0 × wt	150 × wt
2	120 × wt	30 × wt	150 × wt
3	90 × wt	60 × wt	150 × wt
4	60 × wt	90 × wt	150 × wt
5	30 × wt	120 × wt	150 × wt
6	0 × wt	150 × wt	150 × wt

*weight in kilograms

4.4 Special warnings and special precautions for use
Cow's milk and artificial milk feeds in infants should be stopped for 24 hours and gradually reintroduced when the diarrhoea has lessened. However, breast feeding should be continued.

For oral administration only
Rapolyte® should not be reconstituted in diluents other than water. Each sachet should always be dissolved in 200 ml of water. A weaker solution than recommended will not contain the optimum glucose and electrolyte concentration, and a stronger solution than recommended may give rise to electrolyte imbalance. If the diarrhoea does not improve promptly, the patient should be reassessed. The sachet should be stored in a cool, dry place.

4.5 Interaction with other medicinal products and other forms of Interaction
None known.

4.6 Pregnancy and lactation
Not contra-indicated when used as directed for the conditions specified.

4.7 Effects on ability to drive and use machines
None known.

4.8 Undesirable effects
None known.

4.9 Overdose
Not applicable.

5. PHARMACOLOGICAL PROPERTIES

5.1 Pharmacodynamic properties
Sodium chloride:
Maintains the osmotic tension of the blood and tissues; changes in osmotic tension influence the movement of fluids and diffusion of salts in cellular tissues.

Potassium chloride:
Potassium is important in the ionic exchange of cellular metabolism and a sufficient concentration of potassium is necessary for the efficient working of cardiac muscle and nervous tissue.

Sodium Citrate:
Corrects metabolic acidosis.

Dextrose:
Readily absorbed carbohydrate, which enhances the absorption of water and electrolytes from the bowel.

5.2 Pharmacokinetic properties
Sodium chloride:
Readily absorbed from the gastro-intestinal tract: present in all body fluids, but mainly found in extra cellular fluids; osmotic equilibrium maintained by excretion of surplus in urine.

Potassium chloride:
Readily absorbed from the gastro-intestinal tract; potassium excretion mainly in urine.

Sodium citrate:
After absorption it increases the alkali reserve of the plasma with an increased excretion of urine, which is rendered less acid.

Dextrose:
Absorbed from gastro-intestinal tract and oxidised or stored in the liver as glycogen.

5.3 Preclinical safety data
Not applicable.

6. PHARMACEUTICAL PARTICULARS

6.1 List of excipients
Available in four flavours, each contain the following excipients:

Rapolyte® - Raspberry flavour.

Rapolyte® - Blackcurrant flavour.

Rapolyte® - Tutti Frutti flavour.

Rapolyte® - Natural: No excipients.

6.2 Incompatibilities
None known.

6.3 Shelf life
36 months.

6.4 Special precautions for storage
Store in a cool, dry place.

6.5 Nature and contents of container
Sachets consisting of paper, aluminium foil and polyethylene, in packs of 4, 5, 6, 12, 18, 20 and 25.

6.6 Instructions for use and handling
Reconstitution:

The contents of each sachet should be dissolved in 200ml (approximately 7 fluid ounces) or drinking water. Use fresh drinking water for adults and children. For infants, and where drinking water is unavailable, the water should be freshly boiled and cooled. The solution should be made up immediately before use. If refrigerated, the solution may be stored for up to 24 hours; otherwise any solution remaining an hour after reconstitution should be discarded. The solution must not be boiled.

Administrative Data

7. MARKETING AUTHORISATION HOLDER
Helsinn Birex Pharmaceuticals Ltd.

Damastown

Mulhaddart

Dublin 15

Ireland

8. MARKETING AUTHORISATION NUMBER(S)
PL 12333/0001 – Raspberry Flavour

PL 12333/0002 – Blackcurrant Flavour

PL 12333/0003 – Tutti Frutti Flavour

PL 12333/0004 – Natural Flavour

9. DATE OF FIRST AUTHORISATION/RENEWAL OF THE AUTHORISATION
30 June 1999.

10. DATE OF REVISION OF THE TEXT
May 2001

11. LEGAL CATEGORY
GSL

Raptiva 100 mg/ml

(Serono Ltd)

1. NAME OF THE MEDICINAL PRODUCT
Raptiva®▼ 100 mg/ml powder and solvent for solution for injection

2. QUALITATIVE AND QUANTITATIVE COMPOSITION
Each vial contains a retrievable amount of 125 mg of efalizumab.

Reconstitution with the solvent yields a solution containing efalizumab at 100 mg/ml.

Efalizumab is a recombinant humanized monoclonal antibody produced in genetically engineered Chinese Hamster Ovary (CHO) cells. Efalizumab is an IgG1 kappa immunoglobulin, containing human constant region sequences and murine light- and heavy-chain complementary determining region sequences.

For excipients, see section 6.1.

3. PHARMACEUTICAL FORM
Powder and solvent for solution for injection.

The powder is a white to off white cake.

The solvent is a clear, colourless liquid.

4. CLINICAL PARTICULARS

4.1 Therapeutic indications
Treatment of adult patients with moderate to severe chronic plaque psoriasis who have failed to respond to, or who have a contraindication to, or are intolerant to other systemic therapies including cyclosporine, methotrexate and PUVA (see section 5.1 – Clinical Efficacy).

4.2 Posology and method of administration
Treatment with Raptiva should be initiated by a physician specialised in dermatology.

An initial single dose of 0.7 mg/kg body weight is given followed by weekly injections of 1.0 mg/kg body weight (maximum single dose should not exceed a total of 200 mg). The volume to be injected should be calculated as follows:

Dose	Volume to be injected per 10 kg body weight
Single initial dose: 0.7 mg/kg	0.07 ml
Subsequent doses: 1 mg/kg	0.1 ml

The duration of therapy is 12 weeks. Therapy may be continued only in patients who responded to treatment (PGA good or better). For discontinuation guidance see section 4.4.

Children and adolescents (< 18 years)

The safety and efficacy of Raptiva in this age group (< 18 years old) have not been studied. Raptiva should not be used in this age group.

Use in the elderly (≥ 65 years)

The dosage and administration schedule in the elderly should be the same as for adults (see also section 4.4).

Patients with renal or hepatic impairment

No studies have been conducted in patients with renal or hepatic impairment. Raptiva should be used with caution in this patient population.

Method of administration

Raptiva is for subcutaneous injection. Injection sites should be rotated.

For instructions for use see section 6.6.

After proper training in the reconstitution and injection technique, patients may self-inject with Raptiva, if their physician determines that this is appropriate.

4.3 Contraindications
Hypersensitivity to efalizumab or to any of the excipients.

Patients with history of malignancies.

Patients with active tuberculosis and other severe infections.

Patients with specific forms of psoriasis like guttate, erythrodermic or pustular psoriasis as sole or predominant form of psoriasis.

Patients with immunodeficiencies.

4.4 Special warnings and special precautions for use
Effects on the immune system

a) Infections

Raptiva, may affect host defenses against infections. The impact of treatment with Raptiva on the development and course of active and/or chronic infections is not fully understood. Patients developing an infection during treatment with Raptiva should be monitored and according to severity Raptiva should be discontinued. In a patient with history of clinically significant recurring infections, Raptiva should be used with caution.

b) Vaccinations

No data are available on the effects of vaccination or on the secondary transmission of infection by live vaccines in patients receiving Raptiva. Patients should not receive acellular, live and live-attenuated vaccines during Raptiva treatment. Before vaccination, treatment with Raptiva should be withheld for 8 weeks and can resume 2 weeks after vaccination.

c) Malignancies and lymphoproliferative disorders

It is not known whether Raptiva can increase the risk of malignancies and lymphoproliferative disorders. Raptiva should be discontinued if a malignancy develops while the patient is on treatment (see sections 4.3 and 4.8).

Raptiva has not been studied in combination with immunosuppressive systemic antipsoriasis medicinal products. Therefore, combination therapies with these products are not recommended (see section 4.5).

Thrombocytopenia

Thrombocytopenia may occur during Raptiva treatment and may be associated with clinical signs such as echymoses, spontaneous bruising or bleeding from muco-cutaneous tissues. If these manifestations occur, efalizumab should be stopped immediately, a platelet count should be performed and appropriate symptomatic treatment should be instituted immediately (see section 4.8).

Platelet counts are recommended upon initiating and periodically while receiving Raptiva treatment. It is recommended that assessments be more frequent when initiating therapy (e.g., monthly) and may decrease in frequency with continued treatment (e.g., every 3 months).

Hypersensitivity and allergic reactions

As with any recombinant product, Raptiva is potentially immunogenic. Consequently, if any serious hypersensitivity or allergic reaction occurs, Raptiva should be discontinued immediately and appropriate therapy initiated (see sections 4.3 and 4.8).

Arthritis

Cases of arthritis have been observed during treatment with Raptiva. In such circumstances it is recommended to discontinue Raptiva treatment.

Psoriasis

During treatment with Raptiva, cases of exacerbation of psoriasis, including pustular, erythrodermic, and guttate subtypes, have been observed (see section 4.8). In such cases, it is recommended to discontinue treatment with Raptiva.

Abrupt discontinuation of treatment may cause a recurrence or exacerbation of plaque psoriasis including erythrodermic and pustular psoriasis.

Discontinuation

Management of patients discontinuing Raptiva includes close observation. In case of recurrence or exacerbation of disease, the treating physician should institute the most appropriate psoriasis treatment as necessary.

In case re-treatment with Raptiva is indicated the same guidance should be followed as under Posology and method of administration. Re-treatment may be associated with lower or inadequate response to Raptiva than in the earlier treatment periods. Therapy may be continued only in those patients who respond adequately to treatment.

Special patient populations

No differences in safety or efficacy were observed between elderly (⩾ 65 years) patients and younger patients. As there is a higher incidence of infections in the elderly population in general, caution should be used in treating the elderly.

Raptiva has not been studied in patients with renal or hepatic impairment and should therefore be used with caution in such patients. See section 4.8 regarding the effects on the hepatic function.

4.5 Interaction with other medicinal products and other forms of Interaction

There have been no formal drug interaction studies performed with Raptiva.

No data are available on the effects of vaccination or on the secondary transmission of infection by live vaccines in patients receiving Raptiva. Patients should not receive acellular, live and live-attenuated vaccines during Raptiva treatment. See section 4.4.

Given the mechanism of action of efalizumab, its effects on the immune system may be potentiated by systemic immunosuppressives commonly used for the treatment of psoriasis (see section 4.4).

Raptiva has been used in combination with topical corticosteroids in psoriasis patients without any untoward effects nor with any observable significant beneficial effect of the combination therapy above monotherapy with efalizumab.

4.6 Pregnancy and lactation

Pregnancy

In general, immunoglobulins are known to cross the placental barrier. There is only incidental clinical experience with efalizumab in pregnant women. Animal studies indicate an impairment of the immune function of the offspring (see section 5.3). Pregnant women should not be treated with Raptiva.

Women of childbearing potential should be advised to use appropriate contraception.

Lactation

Excretion of efalizumab in human milk has not been investigated, however immunoglobulins are expected to be excreted in human milk. Moreover, an antibody analogue of efalizumab was shown to be excreted in milk of mice. Women should not breastfeed during treatment with Raptiva.

4.7 Effects on ability to drive and use machines

No studies on the effects on the ability to drive and use machines have been performed. Based on the pharmacological mechanism of action of efalizumab, the use of Raptiva is not expected to affect patient's ability to drive and use machines.

4.8 Undesirable effects

The most frequent symptomatic adverse drug reactions (ADRs) observed during Raptiva therapy were mild to moderate dose-related acute flu-like symptoms including headache, fever, chills, nausea and myalgia. In large placebo-controlled clinical studies, these reactions were observed in approximately 41% of Raptiva-treated patients and 24% in placebo-treated patients over 12 weeks of treatment. After initiation of therapy, these reactions were generally less frequent and occurred at similar rates to that seen in the placebo group from the third and subsequent weekly injections.

Antibodies to efalizumab were detected in only 6% of patients. In this small number of patients no differences were observed in pharmacokinetics, pharmacodynamics, clinically noteworthy adverse events or clinical efficacy.

Adverse events (Preferred Terms) in the overall population studied clinically with Raptiva are listed below by frequency of occurrence and by MedDRA System Organ Class.

(see Table 1)

Table 1

System Organ Class	Very common (>1/10)	Common (>1/100, <1/10)	Uncommon (>1/1,000, <1/100)	Rare (>1/10,000, <1/1,000)	Very rare (<1/10,000)
Blood and the lymphatic system disorders	Leukocytosis and lymphocytosis		Thrombocytopenia		
Skin and subcutaneous tissue disorders		Psoriasis	Urticaria		
Musculoskeletal and connective disorders		Arthralgia Psoriatic arthritis (exacerbation/ flare)			
General disorders and administration site conditions	Flu-like symptoms including, fever, headaches, chills, nausea and myalgia	Hypersensitivity reactions, back pain, asthenia	Injection site reactions		
Investigations		Elevation of alkaline Phosphatase Elevation of ALT			

The safety profile in the target population as defined in section 4.1 is similar to the safety profile in the overall population treated during clinical development of Raptiva as presented above.

Analysis following long-term use in a cohort of 158 patients with moderate to severe psoriasis receiving Raptiva 1 mg/kg/week for 108 weeks did not show any noteworthy differences in frequency of adverse events as compared to 12 weeks of exposure to Raptiva. Safety data beyond 12 weeks in the target population are not yet available.

Additional Information

Leucocytosis and lymphocytosis: in large placebo-controlled clinical studies, between 40 and 50% of patients developed sustained asymptomatic lymphocytosis during Raptiva therapy. All values were between 2.5 fold and 3.5 fold the ULN (Upper Limit of Normal). Lymphocyte count returned to baseline after therapy discontinuation. Slight elevation in absolute neutrophil count and eosinophil count were observed but in a smaller proportion of patients.

Thrombocytopenia: in the combined safety database of 3291 Raptiva-treated patients, there were nine occurrences (0.3%) of thrombocytopenia with less than 52,000 cells per μl reported. Four of these patients had clinical signs of thrombocytopenia. Based on available platelet count measurements, the onset of platelet decline was between 8 and 12 weeks after the first dose of Raptiva in 5 patients, but occurred later in the other patients. In one patient, thrombocytopenia occurred 3 weeks after treatment discontinuation. The platelet count nadirs occurred between 12 and 72 weeks after the first dose of Raptiva. (See section 4.4)

Psoriasis: in the first 12 weeks of placebo-controlled studies, the rate of psoriasis adverse events was 3.2% in the Raptiva-treated patients and 1.4% in the placebo-treated patients. Among 3291 patients in the combined safety database, 39 patients presented an erythrodermic or pustular psoriasis (1.2%). Seventeen of these events occurred after discontinuation of Raptiva, while 22 occurred during treatment. In the cases occurring during treatment, most of these events (16/22) occurred in patients presenting no response to Raptiva. Cases occurring after discontinuation were observed both in patients responding or not responding to Raptiva treatment.

Psoriatic arthritis: in the first 12 weeks of placebo-controlled studies, psoriatic arthritis and exacerbation or flare of psoriatic arthritis were observed in 1.8% of Raptiva-treated patients and placebo-treated patients. In these studies, the incidence of other types of arthritis-related adverse events were similar between the Raptiva and placebo groups.

Flu-like symptoms: in large placebo-controlled clinical studies, approximately 20% of patients in excess of placebo reported flu-like symptoms including headaches, chills, fever, nausea and myalgia. The percentage of patients reporting flu-like symptoms was greatest with the first injection and decreased by more than 50% with the second injection. These symptoms diminished thereafter to a percentage comparable to that of patients treated with placebo. Headache was the most frequent of the flu-like symptoms. None of those events was serious and less than 5% were considered severe. Overall less than 1% of patients discontinued therapy because of acute flu-like symptoms.

Hypersensitivity and allergic disorders: in large placebo-controlled clinical studies, the percentage of patients experiencing an adverse event suggestive of hypersensitivity, including urticaria, rash and allergic reactions was slightly higher in the Raptiva group (8%) than in the placebo group (7%). No case of anaphylaxis has been reported with the use of Raptiva. (See section 4.4)

Elevation of alkaline phosphatase: in large placebo-controlled clinical studies approximately 4.5% of patients developed sustained elevation of alkaline phosphatase throughout Raptiva therapy compared to 1% in placebo patients. All values were between 1.5 fold and 3 fold the ULN, and returned to baseline levels after therapy discontinuation.

Elevation of ALT: about 5.7% of patients developed elevation in ALT during Raptiva therapy compared to 3.5% in placebo. All occurrences were asymptomatic and values above 2.5 fold ULN were not more frequent in the Raptiva group than in the placebo group. All values returned to baseline levels upon therapy discontinuation.

Infections: other therapies that alter T-lymphocyte function have been associated with increased risk of developing serious infections. In placebo controlled clinical trials, infection rates in Raptiva-treated patients was approximately 27.3% versus 24.0% in placebo-treated patients. In the target population studied in study IMP24011, the infection rate in Raptiva-treated patients was approximately 25.7% versus 22.3% in placebo-treated patients. In both controlled and uncontrolled studies, the overall incidence of hospitalization for infections was 1.6 per 100 patient-years for Raptiva-treated patients compared with 1.2 per 100 patient-years for placebo- treated patients. The most frequent serious infections were pneumonia, cellulitis, infections not otherwise specified and sepsis. (See section 4.4)

Class adverse reactions

Neoplasms benign and malignant: a higher rate of malignancies has been associated with therapies affecting the immune system. In placebo controlled clinical trials, the overall incidences of malignancy (the majority of which were non-melanoma skin cancers) were similar in Raptiva-treated patients and in placebo-treated patients. In addition, the incidences of specific tumours in Raptiva patients were in line with those observed in control psoriasis populations. Among psoriasis patients who received Raptiva at any dose, the overall incidence of malignancies of any kind was 1.7 per 100 patient-years for Raptiva-treated patients compared with 1.6 per 100 patient-years for placebo-treated patients. Experience with Raptiva has not shown evidence of risk of developing malignancy exceeding that expected in the psoriasis population. (See section 4.4)

4.9 Overdose

In a clinical study, where subjects were exposed to higher doses of efalizumab (up to 10 mg/kg intravenous), one subject receiving 3 mg/kg intravenous dose experienced hypertension, chills, and fever on the day of study drug dosing, which required hospitalization. Another subject who received 10 mg/kg intravenous experienced severe vomiting following administration of efalizumab, which also required hospitalization. Both occurrences fully resolved without any sequelae. Doses up to 4 mg/kg/week subcutaneously for 10 weeks have been administered without any toxic effect.

There is no known antidote to Raptiva or any specific treatment for Raptiva overdose other than withholding treatment and patient observation. In case of overdose, it is recommended that the patient be monitored under close medical care and appropriate symptomatic treatment instituted immediately.

5. PHARMACOLOGICAL PROPERTIES

5.1 Pharmacodynamic properties

Pharmacotherapeutic group: selective immunosuppressive agents, ATC code: L04AA21

Mechanism of action

Efalizumab is a recombinant humanized monoclonal antibody that binds specifically to the CD11a subunit of LFA-1 (lymphocyte function-associated antigen-1), a leukocyte cell surface protein.

By this mechanism, efalizumab inhibits the binding of LFA-1 to ICAM-1, which interferes with T lymphocytes adhesion to other cell types. LFA-1 is present on activated T lymphocytes, and ICAM-1 is up-regulated on endothelial cells and keratinocytes in psoriasis plaques. By preventing LFA-1/ICAM binding, efalizumab may alleviate signs and symptoms of psoriasis by inhibiting several stages in the immunologic cascade.

Pharmacodynamic effects

In studies using an initial dose of 0.7 mg/kg followed by 11 weekly doses of 1.0 mg/kg, efalizumab maximally reduced expression of CD11a on circulating T lymphocytes to approximately 15-30% of pre-dose baseline values and saturated CD11a to <5% of baseline available CD11a binding sites. The full effect was seen 24 to 48 hours after the first dose, and was maintained between weekly doses. Within 5 to 8 weeks following the 12th and final dose of efalizumab administered at 1.0 mg/kg/wk, CD11a levels returned to within a range of ±25% of baseline values.

Another pharmacodynamic marker, consistent with the mechanism of action of efalizumab, was the increase in the absolute counts of circulating leukocytes observed during efalizumab treatment. Increased absolute counts were apparent within 24 hours of the first dose, remained elevated with weekly dosing, and returned to baseline after treatment cessation. The largest increase occurred in the absolute count of circulating lymphocytes. In clinical trials, mean lymphocyte counts approximately doubled relative to baseline in subjects receiving 1.0 mg/kg/wk of Raptiva. The increase included CD4 T-lymphocytes, CD8 T-lymphocytes, B-lymphocytes, and natural killer (NK) cells, although NK cells and CD4 cells increased less relative to other cell types. At a dose of 1.0 mg/kg/wk subcutaneous efalizumab, lymphocyte levels returned to within 10% of baseline by 8 weeks post last dose.

Clinical efficacy

The efficacy of Raptiva versus other systemic therapies in patients with moderate to severe psoriasis has not been evaluated in studies directly comparing Raptiva with other systemic therapies. The present results of Raptiva versus placebo in these patients indicate a modest efficacy of Raptiva (in terms of PASI 75 response rate) (see Table 3). Based on the clinical development data generated (see Table 2) and limited long-term experience, Raptiva is recommended for use in patients as defined in section 4.1.

Failure on prior systemic therapies is defined as insufficient response (PASI < 50 or PGA less than good), or worsening of disease in patients while on treatment, and who were adequately dosed for a sufficiently long duration to assess response with at least each of the 3 major systemic therapies as available.

The safety and efficacy of Raptiva in moderate to severe plaque psoriasis patients has been demonstrated in five randomized, double-blind, placebo-controlled trials at the recommended dose (n=1742). There are no comparative data with Raptiva versus other systemic psoriasis therapies. The largest study IMP24011 (n=793) included patients (n=526) who were not controlled by, contraindicated to, or intolerant to two or more systemic therapies as judged from the patients' histories of psoriasis treatment. In all studies, the primary endpoint was the proportion of patients with a ⩾ 75% improvement in the Psoriasis Area and Severity Index score (a PASI 75 response) relative to baseline when assessed one week after a 12-week treatment course. Secondary endpoints included the proportion of subjects who achieved a rating of Minimal or Clear on a static global assessment by the physician, the Overall Lesion Severity (OLS), the proportion of patients with a ⩾ 50% improvement in PASI score (a PASI 50 response) relative to baseline after 12 weeks of treatment, the time-course of mean PASI percentage improvement from baseline, improvement in the Dermatology Life Quality Index (DLQI), Psoriasis Symptom Assessment (PSA), the Physician's Global Assessment (PGA) of change, change in the PASI thickness component, and change in the body surface area affected.

In all five studies, patients randomized to the Raptiva group achieved statistically significantly better responses than placebo on the primary endpoint. The same results were confirmed in patients that were unsuitable for other systemic therapies (study IMP24011) (see Table 2 below).

(see Table 2)

Table 2 Primary Endpoint: Proportion of Subjects with ⩾75% improvement in PASI after 12 weeks of Treatment (PASI 75)

Patient population IMP24011	Placebo	Efalizumab [a] 1.0 mg/kg/wk	Treatment Effect [95% CI]
All patients	4% (n=264)	31% (n=529) [b]	27% [22%, 32%]
Patients who are not controlled by, contraindicated to, or intolerant to two or more systemic therapies *	3% (n=184)	30% (n=342) [b]	27% [21%, 32%]

[a] p-values compared efalizumab with placebo using logistic regression including baseline PASI score, prior treatment for psoriasis and geographical region as covariates.

[b] $p<0.001$.

* As judged from the patients' histories of psoriasis treatments

In all five studies, patients randomized to the Raptiva dose group achieved statistically significantly better responses than placebo on the primary endpoint (PASI 75 response) (see Table 3 below) and on all the secondary efficacy endpoints.

(see Table 3)

Table 3 Primary Endpoint: Proportion of Subjects with ⩾75% improvement in PASI after 12 weeks of Treatment (PASI 75)

Study	Placebo	Efalizumab [a] 1.0 mg/kg/wk	Treatment Effect [95% CI]
ACD2390g *	4% (n=187)	27% (n=369) [b]	22% [16%, 29%]
ACD2058g	2% (n=170)	39% (n=162) [b]	37% [28%, 46%]
ACD2059g *	5% (n=122)	22% (n=232) [b]	17% [9%, 27%]
ACD2600g *	3% (n=236)	24% (n=450) [b]	21% [15%, 27%]
IMP24011 *	4% (n=264)	31% (n=529) [b]	27% [22%, 32%]

[a] IMP24011: p-values compared efalizumab with placebo using logistic regression including baseline PASI score, prior treatment for psoriasis and geographical region as covariates.

Other studies: p-values compared each efalizumab group with placebo using Fisher's exact test within each study.

[b] $p<0.001$.

* The efalizumab used in the study is the Genentech manufactured product

Time to relapse (⩾50% loss of improvement) was evaluated in Study ACD2058g for patients who were classified as responders (⩾75% improvement on PASI) after 12 weeks of treatment. The median time to relapse among PASI responders ranged from 59 to 74 days following the last Raptiva dose in the initial treatment period.

(see Table 4)

Table 4 Summary of Overall Patient Exposure from Clinical Trials

Treatment duration completed	24 weeks	48 weeks	96 weeks	108 weeks
Number of Patients	1053	221	171	158

Long term data up to 108 weeks have been obtained in an uncontrolled study in 158 patients with moderate to severe psoriasis (ACD2243g) (See Table 4 above). About 72% of the patients (122 of 170) in the cohort were PASI 75 responders. When all the drop outs of the maintenance cohort were considered as non responders, the PASI 75 responder rate was 42% (122 of 290 patients).

5.2 Pharmacokinetic properties

Absorption:

After subcutaneous administration of efalizumab peak plasma concentrations are reached after 1-2 days. Comparison with intravenous data indicated an average bioavailability of about 50% at the recommended dose level of 1.0 mg/kg/wk subcutaneous.

Distribution:

Steady state was achieved at week 4. At the 1 mg/kg/wk dose level (with an initial dose of 0.7 mg/kg the first week), mean efalizumab plasma trough values were 11.1±7.9 μg/ml. Measurements of volume of distribution of the central compartment after single intravenous doses were 110 ml/kg at dose 0.03 mg/kg and 58 ml/kg at dose 10 mg/kg.

Biotransformation:

The metabolism of efalizumab is through internalisation followed by intracellular degradation as a consequence of either binding to cell surface CD11a or through endocytosis. The expected degradation products are small peptides and individual amino acids which are eliminated by glomerular filtration. Cytochrome P450 enzymes as well as conjugation reactions are not involved in the metabolism of efalizumab.

Elimination:

Efalizumab is cleared by nonlinear saturable elimination (dose dependent). Mean steady state clearance is 24 ml/kg/day (range 5-76 ml/kg/day) at 1 mg/kg/day subcutaneous.

The elimination half-life was about 5.5-10.5 days at 1 mg/kg/day subcutaneous. T_{end} at steady state is 25 days (range 13-35 days). Weight is the most significant covariate affecting efalizumab clearance.

Non-linearity:

Efalizumab shows dose-dependent nonlinear pharmacokinetics which can be explained by its saturable specific binding to cell surface receptors CD11a. It appeared that the receptor mediated clearance of efalizumab was saturated when plasma efalizumab concentrations were above 1 μg/ml.

Through population pharmacokinetic analysis, weight was found to affect efalizumab clearance. Covariates as baseline PASI, baseline lymphocyte count and age had modest effects on clearance; gender and ethnic origin had no effect. The pharmacokinetics of efalizumab in paediatric patients have not been studied. The effect of renal or hepatic impairment on the pharmacokinetics of efalizumab has not been studied.

Antibodies to efalizumab were detected in only 6% of patients evaluated. In this small number of patients no differences were observed in either pharmacodynamic or pharmacokinetic parameters.

5.3 Preclinical safety data

Efalizumab does not cross-react with CD11a from species other than humans and chimpanzees. Therefore, conventional non-clinical safety data with the medicinal product are limited and do not allow for a comprehensive safety assessment. Inhibitory effects were observed on the humoral and T-cell dependent immune responses. In pups of mice treated with an antibody analogue of efalizumab, a decrease in T-cell dependent immunity was observed up to at least 11 weeks of age. Only at 25 weeks of age was this decrease no longer significant.

Otherwise, the effects observed in non-clinical studies could be related to the pharmacology of efalizumab.

No lymphomas were observed following 6 months treatment with an antibody analogue of efalizumab in a 6 months study with p53 +/+ wild type mice.

No teratogenic effects were seen in mice during organogenesis.

6. PHARMACEUTICAL PARTICULARS

6.1 List of excipients

Powder for solution for injection:

Polysorbate 20

Histidine

Histidine hydrochloride monohydrate

Sucrose

Solvent:

Water for injections

6.2 Incompatibilities

In the absence of compatibility studies, this medicinal product must not be mixed with other medicinal products.

6.3 Shelf life

2 years.

After reconstitution, an immediate use is recommended (see also section 6.4).

6.4 Special precautions for storage

Store in a refrigerator (2°C – 8°C). Do not freeze.

Store in the original package to protect from light.

From a microbiological point of view, the product should be used immediately after first opening and reconstitution. If not used immediately, in-use storage times and conditions prior to use are the responsibility of the user and would normally not be longer than 24 hours at 2°C to 8°C, unless reconstitution has taken place in controlled and validated aseptic conditions. Physico-chemical stability of the reconstituted product has been shown for 24 hours at 2°C to 8°C.

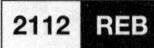

6.5 Nature and contents of container

Powder:

Colourless type I glass vial with a butyl rubber stopper, and aluminum seal fitted with a flip-off plastic cap.

Solvent:

Type I glass pre-filled syringe.

Raptiva is available in:

Packs of 1 vial of powder, 1 pre-filled syringe of solvent, 1 needle for reconstitution and 1 needle for injection.

Packs of 4 vials of powder, 4 pre-filled syringes of solvent, 4 needles for reconstitution and 4 needles for injection.

Not all pack sizes may be marketed.

6.6 Instructions for use and handling

Raptiva is for single use only.

One vial of Raptiva should be reconstituted with the solvent before use. Reconstitution of the single-use vial with 1.3 ml of the supplied water for injections yields approximately 1.5 ml of solution to deliver 100 mg per 1 ml of Raptiva. The maximum retrievable dose is 125 mg per 1.25 ml of Raptiva.

The solution should reconstitute in not more than 5 minutes. The reconstituted solution is a clear to slightly opalescent, colourless to pale yellow solution, and should not be administered if it contains particles or is not clear.

Detailed instructions for use are provided in the package leaflet.

Any unused product or waste material should be disposed of in accordance with local requirements.

7. MARKETING AUTHORISATION HOLDER

Serono Europe Ltd.

56 Marsh Wall

London E14 9TP

United Kingdom

8. MARKETING AUTHORISATION NUMBER(S)

Raptiva – 1 vial EU/1/04/291/001

Raptiva – 4 vials EU/1/04/291/002

9. DATE OF FIRST AUTHORISATION/RENEWAL OF THE AUTHORISATION

20 September 2004

10. DATE OF REVISION OF THE TEXT

LEGAL STATUS

POM

NAME AND ADDRESS OF DISTRIBUTOR IN UK

Serono Ltd

Bedfont Cross

Stanwell Road

Feltham

Middlesex

TW14 8NX

Tel. 020 8818 7200

NAME AND ADDRESS OF DISTRIBUTOR IN IRELAND

Allphar Services Limited

Pharmaceutical Agents and Distributors

Belgard Road

Tallaght

Dublin 24

Tel. (01) 404 1600

Rebetol 200mg hard capsules

(Schering-Plough Ltd)

1. NAME OF THE MEDICINAL PRODUCT

Rebetol 200 mg hard capsules

2. QUALITATIVE AND QUANTITATIVE COMPOSITION

Each Rebetol capsule contains 200 mg of ribavirin.

For excipients, see section 6.1.

3. PHARMACEUTICAL FORM

Hard capsule

The hard capsules are white, opaque and imprinted with blue ink.

4. CLINICAL PARTICULARS

4.1 Therapeutic indications

Rebetol is indicated for the treatment of chronic hepatitis C and must only be used as part of a combination regimen with peginterferon alfa-2b (adults) or interferon alfa-2b (adults, children (3-years of age or older), and adolescents). Rebetol monotherapy must not be used.

There is no safety or efficacy information on the use of Rebetol with other forms of interferon (i.e., not alfa-2b), or on the use of Rebetol with peginterferon alfa-2b in children or adolescents.

Please refer also to the peginterferon alfa-2b or interferon alfa-2b Summary of Product Characteristics (SPC) for prescribing information particular to that product.

__Naïve patients__

Adult patients: Rebetol is indicated, in combination with peginterferon alfa-2b or interferon alfa-2b, for the treatment of adult patients with chronic hepatitis C, not previously treated, without liver decompensation, with elevated ALT, who are positive for serum HCV-RNA (see section **4.4**).

Children and adolescents: Rebetol is intended for use, in a combination regimen with interferon alfa-2b, for the treatment of children and adolescents 3 years of age and older, who have chronic hepatitis C, not previously treated, without liver decompensation, and who are positive for serum HCV-RNA.

The decision to treat should be made on a case by case basis, taking into account any evidence of disease progression such as hepatic inflammation and fibrosis, as well as prognostic factors for response, HCV genotype and viral load. The expected benefit of treatment should be weighed against the safety findings observed for paediatric subjects in the clinical trials (see sections **4.4, 4.8** and **5.1**).

__Relapse patients__

Adult patients: Rebetol is indicated, in combination with peginterferon alfa-2b or interferon alfa-2b, for the treatment of adult patients with chronic hepatitis C who have previously responded (with normalisation of ALT at the end of treatment) to interferon alpha monotherapy but who have subsequently relapsed.

4.2 Posology and method of administration

Treatment should be initiated, and monitored, by a physician experienced in the management of chronic hepatitis C.

__Dose to be administered__

The dose of Rebetol is based on patient body weight (**Table 1**). Rebetol capsules are to be administered orally each day in two divided doses (morning and evening) with food.

Adult patients: Rebetol must be used in combination with either peginterferon alfa-2b (1.5 micrograms/kg/week) or interferon alfa-2b (3 million international units [MIU] three times a week). The choice of combination regimen is based on the characteristics of the patient. The regimen administered should be selected based on the anticipated efficacy and safety of the combination treatment for an individual patient (see section **5.1**).

Table 1 Rebetol dose based on body weight

Patient weight (kg)	Daily Rebetol dose	Number of 200 mg capsules
< 65	800 mg	4 [a]
65 – 85	1,000 mg	5 [b]
> 85	1,200 mg	6 [c]

a: 2 morning, 2 evening

b: 2 morning, 3 evening

c: 3 morning, 3 evening

Rebetol Capsules in combination with pegylated interferon alfa-2b:

Duration of treatment

Predictability of sustained virological response: Patients infected with virus genotype 1who fail to achieve virological response at Week 12 are highly unlikely to become sustained virological responders (see also section **5.1**).

• **Genotype 1**: For patients who exhibit virological response at week 12, treatment should be continued for another nine month period (i.e., a total of 48 weeks).

In the subset of patients with genotype 1 infection and low viral load (< 600,000 IU/ml) who become HCV RNA negative at treatment week 4 and remain HCV RNA negative at week 24, the treatment could either be stopped after this 24 week treatment course or pursued for an additional 24 weeks (i.e. overall 48 weeks treatment duration). However, an overall 24 weeks treatment duration may be associated with a higher risk of relapse than a 48 weeks treatment duration (see section **5.1**).

• **Genotypes 2 or 3**: It is recommended that all patients be treated for 24 weeks.

• **Genotype 4**: In general, patients infected with genotype 4 are considered harder to treat and limited study data (n=66) indicate they are compatible with a posology for genotype 1.

Rebetol Capsules in combination with interferon alfa-2b:

Duration of treatment: Based on the results of clinical trials, it is recommended that patients be treated for at least six months. During those clinical trials in which patients were treated for one year, patients who failed to show a virological response after six months of treatment (HCV-RNA below lower limit of detection) were unlikely to become sustained virological responders (HCV-RNA below lower limit of detection six months after withdrawal of treatment).

• **Genotype 1**: Treatment should be continued for another six month period (i.e., a total of one year) in patients who exhibit negative HCV-RNA after six months of treatment.

• **Genotypes Non-1:** The decision to extend therapy to one year in patients with negative HCV-RNA after six months of treatment should be based on other prognostic factors (e.g., age > 40 years, male gender, bridging fibrosis).

Children aged three years and older, and adolescents: (for patients who weigh < 47 kg, or are unable to swallow capsules, please refer to the SPC for ribavirin 40 mg/ml oral solution).

In clinical studies performed in this population ribavirin and interferon alfa-2b were used in doses of 15 mg/kg/day and 3 MIU/m² three times a week respectively (**Table 2**).

Rebetol capsules are to be administered orally each day in two divided doses with food (morning and evening).

Table 2 Rebetol paediatric dose based on body weight

Patient weight (kg)	Daily Rebetol dose	Number of 200 mg capsules
47 - 49	600 mg	3 capsules [a]
50 - 65	800 mg	4 capsules [b]
> 65	Refer to adult dosing table (Table 1)	

a 1 morning, 2 evening

b 2 morning, 2 evening

Duration of treatment in children and adolescents

__Genotype 1:__ The recommended duration of treatment is 1 year. Patients who fail to achieve virological response at 12 weeks are highly unlikely to become sustained virological responders (negative predictive value 96 %). Virological response is defined as absence of detectable HCV-RNA at Week 12 of treatment. Treatment should be discontinued in these patients.

__Genotype 2 or 3:__ The recommended duration of treatment is 24 weeks.

Virological responses after 1 year of treatment and 6 months of follow-up were 36 % for genotype 1 and 81 % for genotype 2/3/4.

Dose modification for all patients

If severe adverse reactions or laboratory abnormalities develop during therapy with Rebetol and peginterferon alfa-2b or interferon alfa-2b, modify the dosages of each product if appropriate, until the adverse reactions abate. Guidelines were developed in clinical trials for dose modification (see Dosage modification guidelines, **Table 3**).

(see Table 3 on next page)

Special populations

Use in renal impairment: The pharmacokinetics of ribavirin are altered in patients with renal dysfunction due to reduction of apparent clearance in these patients (see section **5.2**). Therefore, it is recommended that renal function be evaluated in all patients prior to initiation of Rebetol. Patients with creatinine clearance < 50 ml/minute must not be treated with Rebetol (see section **4.3**). If serum creatinine rises to > 2 mg/dl (**Table 3**), Rebetol and peginterferon alfa-2b/interferon alfa-2b must be discontinued.

Use in hepatic impairment: No pharmacokinetic interaction appears between ribavirin and hepatic function (see section **5.2**). Therefore, no dose adjustment of Rebetol is required in patients with hepatic impairment.

Use in the elderly (⩾ 65 years of age): There does not appear to be a significant age-related effect on the pharmacokinetics of ribavirin. However, as in younger patients, renal function must be determined prior to administration of Rebetol (see section **5.2**).

Use in patients under the age of 18 years: Rebetol as capsules or oral solution may be used in combination with interferon alfa-2b in children (3 years of age and older) and adolescents. The selection of formulation is based on individual characteristics of the patient (see section **4.1**). Safety and effectiveness of Rebetol with pegylated or other forms of interferon (i.e. not alfa-2b) in these patients have not been evaluated.

Patients co-infected with HCV/HIV: Patients taking NRTI treatment in association with ribavirin and interferon alfa-2b or peginterferon alfa-2b may be at increased risk of mitochondrial toxicity, lactic acidosis and hepatic decompensation (see section **4.4**). Please refer also to the relevant product information for antiretroviral medicinal products.

4.3 Contraindications

- Hypersensitivity to the active substance or to any of the excipients.

- Pregnant women (see sections **4.4, 4.6** and **5.3**). Rebetol must not be initiated until a report of a negative pregnancy test has been obtained immediately prior to initiation of therapy.

- Women who are breast-feeding.

- A history of severe pre-existing cardiac disease, including unstable or uncontrolled cardiac disease, in the previous six months (see section **4.4**).

Table 3 Dosage modification guidelines

Laboratory Values	Reduce only Rebetol daily dose adult to 600 mg/day*, paediatric to 7.5 mg/kg, if:	Reduce only peginterferon alfa-2b (adult) or interferon alfa-2b dose (adult and paediatric) to one-half dose, if:	Discontinue combination therapy if:
Haemoglobin	< 10 g/dl	-	< 8.5 g/dl
Adult: Haemoglobin in: patients with history of stable cardiac disease Paediatric: not applicable (see section **4.4**)	≥ 2 g/dl decrease in haemoglobin during any 4 week period during treatment (permanent dose reduction)		< 12 g/dl after 4 weeks of dose reduction
White blood cells	-	$< 1.5 \times 10^9$/l	$< 1.0 \times 10^9$/l
Neutrophils	-	$< 0.75 \times 10^9$/l	$< 0.5 \times 10^9$/l
Platelets	-	Adult $< 50 \times 10^9$/l Paediatric $< 80 \times 10^9$/l	Adult $< 25 \times 10^9$/l Paediatric $< 50 \times 10^9$/l
Bilirubin – Direct	-	-	2.5 × ULN**
Bilirubin – Indirect	> 5 mg/dl	-	Adult > 4 mg/dl Paediatric > 5 mg/dl (for > 4 weeks)
Creatinine	-	-	> 2.0 mg/dl
ALT/AST	-	-	2 × baseline and > 10 × ULN**

* Administered in two divided doses, in the morning and in the evening.

** Upper limit of normal

- Severe, debilitating medical conditions, including patients with chronic renal failure, patients with creatinine clearance < 50 ml/minute and/or on haemodialysis.

- Severe hepatic dysfunction or decompensated cirrhosis of the liver.

- Haemoglobinopathies (e.g., thalassemia, sickle-cell anaemia).

Children and adolescents:

- Existence of, or history of severe psychiatric condition, particularly severe depression, suicidal ideation, or suicide attempt.

Because of co-administration with peginterferon alfa-2b or interferon alfa-2b:

- Autoimmune hepatitis; or history of autoimmune disease.

4.4 Special warnings and special precautions for use

Based on results of clinical trials, the use of ribavirin as monotherapy is not effective and Rebetol must not be used alone. The safety and efficacy of this combination have been established only using ribavirin capsules together with peginterferon alfa-2b or interferon alfa-2b solution for injection.

There is no experience with Rebetol in combination with peginterferon alfa-2b in patients who have relapsed after Rebetol + interferon alfa-2b therapy.

All patients in the chronic hepatitis C studies had a liver biopsy before inclusion, but in certain cases (i.e. patients with genotype 2 and 3), treatment may be possible without histological confirmation. Current treatment guidelines should be consulted as to whether a liver biopsy is needed prior to commencing treatment.

Teratogenic risk:

Female patients: Rebetol must not be used by women who are pregnant (see section **4.3**). Extreme care must be taken to avoid pregnancy in female patients (see sections **4.6** and **5.3**).

Male patients and their female partners: Extreme care must be taken to avoid pregnancy in partners of male patients taking Rebetol (see sections **4.6** and **5.3**).

Haemolysis: A decrease in haemoglobin levels to < 10 g/dl was observed in up to 14 % of adult patients and 7 % of children and adolescents treated with Rebetol in combination with peginterferon alfa-2b (adults only) or interferon alfa-2b (adults and children or adolescents) in clinical trials. Although ribavirin has no direct cardiovascular effects, anaemia associated with Rebetol may result in deterioration of cardiac function, or exacerbation of the symptoms of coronary disease, or both. Thus, Rebetol must be administered with caution to patients with pre-existing cardiac disease (see section **4.3**). Cardiac status must be assessed before start of therapy and monitored clinically during therapy; if any deterioration occurs, therapy must be stopped (see section **4.2**).

Cardiovascular: Adult patients with a history of congestive heart failure, myocardial infarction and/or previous or current arrhythmic disorders must be closely monitored. It is recommended that those patients who have pre-existing cardiac abnormalities have electrocardiograms taken prior to and during the course of treatment. Cardiac arrhythmias (primarily supraventricular) usually respond to conventional therapy but may require discontinuation of therapy. There are no data in children or adolescents with a history of cardiac disease.

Acute hypersensitivity: If an acute hypersensitivity reaction (e.g., urticaria, angioedema, bronchoconstriction, anaphylaxis) develops, Rebetol must be discontinued immediately and appropriate medical therapy instituted. Transient rashes do not necessitate interruption of treatment.

Liver function: Any patient developing significant liver function abnormalities during treatment must be monitored closely. Discontinue treatment in patients who develop prolongation of coagulation markers which might indicate liver decompensation.

Psychiatric and Central Nervous System (CNS): Severe CNS effects, particularly depression, suicidal ideation and attempted suicide have been observed in some patients during Rebetol combination therapy with peginterferon alfa-2b or interferon alfa-2b. Among children and adolescents, suicidal ideation or attempts were reported more frequently compared to adult patients (2.4 % versus 1 %) during treatment and during the 6-month follow-up after treatment. As in adult patients, children and adolescents experienced other psychiatric adverse events (e.g., depression, emotional lability, and somnolence). Other CNS effects including aggressive behaviour, confusion and alterations of mental status have been observed with alpha interferon. If patients develop psychiatric or CNS problems, including clinical depression, it is recommended that patients be carefully monitored by the prescribing physician during treatment and in the follow-up period. If such symptoms appear, the potential seriousness of these undesirable effects must be borne in mind by the prescribing physician. If psychiatric symptoms persist or worsen, or suicidal ideation is identified, it is recommended that treatment with Rebetol and peginterferon alfa-2b or interferon alfa-2b be discontinued, and the patient followed, with psychiatric intervention as appropriate.

Patients with existence of or history of severe psychiatric conditions: If treatment with ribavirin is judged necessary in adult patients with existence or history of severe psychiatric conditions, this should only be initiated after having ensured appropriate individualised diagnostic and therapeutic management of the psychiatric condition. The use of ribavirin in children and adolescents with existence of or history of severe psychiatric conditions is contraindicated (see section **4.3**).

Supplemental monitoring specific for children and adolescents

Growth and Development: During a 1-year course of therapy there was a decrease in the rate of linear growth (mean percentile decrease of 9 %) and a decrease in the rate of weight gain (mean percentile decrease of 13 %). A general reversal of these trends was noted during the 6 months follow-up post treatment. However, based on interim data from a long-term follow-up study, 12 (14 %) of 84 children had a > 15 percentile decrease in rate of linear growth, of whom 5 (6 %) children had a > 30 percentile decrease despite being off treatment for more than 1 year. There are no data on long term effects on growth and development and on sexual maturation.

Thyroid Monitoring: Approximately 12 % of children treated with Rebetol and interferon alfa-2b developed increase in TSH. Another 4 % had a transient decrease below the lower limit of normal. Prior to initiation of interferon alfa-2b therapy, TSH levels must be evaluated and any thyroid abnormality detected at that time must be treated with conventional therapy. Interferon alfa-2b therapy may be initiated if TSH levels can be maintained in the normal range by medication. Thyroid dysfunction during treatment with Rebetol and interferon alfa-2b has been observed. If thyroid abnormalities are detected, the patient's thyroid status should be evaluated and treated as clinically appropriate. Children and adolescents should be monitored every 3 months for evidence of thyroid dysfunction (e.g. TSH).

HCV/HIV Coinfection: Caution should be taken in HIV-positive subjects co-infected with HCV who receive nucleoside reverse transcriptase inhibitor (NRTI) treatment and associated interferon alfa-2b/ribavirin treatment. In the HIV-positive population receiving an NRTI regimen, physicians should carefully monitor markers of mitochondrial toxicity and lactic acidosis when ribavirin is associated.

Co-infected patients with advanced cirrhosis receiving HAART may be at increased risk of hepatic decompensation and death. Adding treatment with alfa interferons alone or in combination with ribavirin may increase the risk in this patient subset.

Laboratory tests: Standard haematologic tests and blood chemistries (complete blood count [CBC] and differential, platelet count, electrolytes, serum creatinine, liver function tests, uric acid) must be conducted in all patients prior to initiating therapy. Acceptable baseline values that may be considered as a guideline prior to initiation of Rebetol therapy:

- Haemoglobin — Adult: ≥ 12 g/dl (females); ≥ 13 g/dl (males); Paediatric: ≥ 11 g/dl (females); ≥ 12 g/dl (males)
- Platelets — ≥ 100,000/mm^3
- Neutrophil Count — ≥ 1,500/mm^3

Laboratory evaluations are to be conducted at weeks 2 and 4 of therapy, and periodically thereafter as clinically appropriate.

For females of childbearing potential: Female patients must have a routine pregnancy test performed monthly during treatment and for four months thereafter. Female partners of male patients must have a routine pregnancy test performed monthly during treatment and for seven months thereafter (see section **4.6**).

Uric acid may increase with Rebetol due to haemolysis; therefore, the potential for development of gout must be carefully monitored in pre-disposed patients.

Use in patients with rare hereditary disorders: Each Rebetol capsule contains 40 mg of lactose.

Patients with rare hereditary problems of galactose intolerance, the Lapp lactase deficiency or glucose-galactose malabsorption should not take this medicine.

4.5 Interaction with other medicinal products and other forms of Interaction

Results of *in vitro* studies using both human and rat liver microsome preparations indicated no cytochrome P450 enzyme mediated metabolism of ribavirin. Ribavirin does not inhibit cytochrome P450 enzymes. There is no evidence from toxicity studies that ribavirin induces liver enzymes. Therefore, there is a minimal potential for P450 enzyme-based interactions.

No interaction studies have been conducted with Rebetol and other medicinal products, except for peginterferon alfa-2b, interferon alfa-2b and antacids.

Interferon alfa-2b: No pharmacokinetic interactions were noted between Rebetol and peginterferon alfa-2b or interferon alfa-2b in a multiple-dose pharmacokinetic study.

Antacid: The bioavailability of ribavirin 600 mg was decreased by co-administration with an antacid containing magnesium aluminium and simethicone; AUC_{tf} decreased 14 %. It is possible that the decreased bioavailability in this study was due to delayed transit of ribavirin or modified pH. This interaction is not considered to be clinically relevant.

Nucleoside analogs: Ribavirin was shown *in vitro* to inhibit phosphorylation of zidovudine and stavudine. The clinical significance of these findings is unknown. However, these *in vitro* findings raise the possibility that concurrent use of Rebetol with either zidovudine or stavudine might lead to increased HIV plasma viraemia. Therefore, it is recommended that plasma HIV RNA levels be closely monitored in patients treated with Rebetol concurrently with either of these two agents. If HIV RNA levels increase, the use of Rebetol concomitantly with reverse transcriptase inhibitors must be reviewed.

Use of nucleoside analogs, alone or in combination with other nucleosides, has resulted in lactic acidosis. Pharmacologically, ribavirin increases phosphorylated metabolites of purine nucleosides in vitro. This activity could potentiate the risk of lactic acidosis induced by purine nucleoside analogs (e.g. didanosine or abacavir).

Any potential for interactions may persist for up to two months (five half-lives for ribavirin) after cessation of Rebetol therapy due to the long half-life (see section **5.2**).

There is no evidence that ribavirin interacts with non-nucleoside reverse transcriptase inhibitors or protease inhibitors.

4.6 Pregnancy and lactation

The use of Rebetol is contraindicated during pregnancy.

Preclinical data:

- Fertility: In animal studies, ribavirin produced reversible effects on spermatogenesis (see section **5.3**).

- Teratogenicity: Significant teratogenic and/or embryocidal potential have been demonstrated for ribavirin in all animal species in which adequate studies have been conducted, occurring at doses as low as one twentieth of the recommended human dose (see section **5.3**).

- Genotoxicity: Ribavirin induces genotoxicity (see section **5.3**).

Female patients: Rebetol must not be used by females who are pregnant (see sections **4.3, 4.4** and **5.3**). Extreme care must be taken to avoid pregnancy in female patients. Rebetol therapy must not be initiated until a report of a negative pregnancy test has been obtained immediately prior to initiation of therapy. Females of childbearing potential and their partners must each use an effective contraceptive during treatment and for four months after treatment has been concluded; routine monthly pregnancy tests must be performed during this time (see section **4.4**). If pregnancy does occur during treatment or within four months from stopping treatment, the patient must be advised of the significant teratogenic risk of ribavirin to the foetus.

Male patients and their female partners: Extreme care must be taken to avoid pregnancy in partners of male patients taking Rebetol (see sections **4.3, 4.4** and **5.3**). Ribavirin accumulates intracellularly and is cleared from the body very slowly. It is unknown whether the ribavirin that is contained in sperm will exert its potential teratogenic or genotoxic effects on the human embryo/foetus. Although data on approximately 300 prospectively followed pregnancies with paternal exposure to ribavirin have not shown an increased risk of malformation compared to the general population, nor any specific pattern of malformation, male patients and their female partners of childbearing age must be counselled to each use an effective contraceptive during treatment with Rebetol and for seven months after treatment Men whose partners are pregnant must be instructed to use a condom to minimise delivery of ribavirin to the partner.

Lactation: It is not known whether ribavirin is excreted in human milk. Because of the potential for adverse reactions in nursing infants, nursing must be discontinued prior to initiation of treatment.

4.7 Effects on ability to drive and use machines

Rebetol has no or negligible influence on the ability to drive or use machines; however, peginterferon alfa-2b or interferon alfa-2b used in combination may have an effect. Thus, patients who develop fatigue, somnolence, or confusion during treatment must be cautioned to avoid driving or operating machinery.

4.8 Undesirable effects

Adult patients:

The safety of Rebetol capsules is evaluated from data from three clinical trials in patients with no previous exposure to interferon (interferon-naïve patients): two trials studied Rebetol in combination with interferon alfa-2b, one trial studied Rebetol in combination with peginterferon alfa-2b.

Patients who are treated with interferon alfa-2b and ribavirin after previous relapse from interferon therapy or who are treated for a shorter period are likely to have an improved safety profile than that described below.

Table 4 describes the regimens and patient exposure from the trial experience for one year of treatment in interferon-naïve patients. Undesirable effects reported for these patients are presented in **Table 5**.

Table 4 Regimens and patient exposure

Treatment	Regimen	Number of patients treated for one year
Rebetol + peginterferon alfa-2b	Rebetol (> 10.6 mg/kg/day) + peginterferon alfa-2b (1.5 micrograms/kg/week)	188
Rebetol + interferon alfa-2b	Rebetol (1,000/1,200 mg/day) + interferon alfa-2b (3 MIU three times a week)	505

(see Table 5)

Table 5 Undesirable effects reported (1 % - ⩾ 10 % incidence) in adult patients taking Rebetol capsules with pegylated interferon alfa-2b or interferon alfa-2b injection

Body system	**⩾ 10 %**	**5 % - < 10 %**	**1 % - < 5 %**
Application site disorder	Injection site inflammation, injection site reaction		Injection site pain
Autonomic nervous system	Dry mouth	Sweating increased	Flushing, lacrimal gland disorder
Blood and lymphatic system	Anaemia, neutropenia		Lymphopenia, lymphadenopathy
Body as a whole	Headache, fatigue, fever, rigors, flu-like symptoms, asthenia, weight decrease	Chest pain, right upper quadrant pain	Malaise, neoplasm unspecified, peripheral oedema
Cardio-vascular		Tachycardia	Hypotension, hypertension, palpitation, syncope, cardiac murmur
Central and peripheral nervous	Dizziness	Paresthaesia	Confusion, decreased libido, hyperaesthesia, hypoaesthesia, tremor, migraine, hypertonia, ataxia, abnormal crying, dysphonia
Endocrine		Hypothyroidism	Hyperthyroidism
Gastro-intestinal	Nausea, anorexia, diarrhoea, abdominal pain, vomiting	Constipation, dyspepsia, taste perversion	Flatulence, gingival bleeding, glossitis, loose stools, stomatitis, ulcerative stomatitis, gingivitis, colitis, taste loss
Hearing and vestibular			Vertigo, hearing impairment/loss, tinnitus, earache
Liver and biliary			Hepatomegaly, jaundice
Metabolic and nutritional			Hyperglycaemia, hyperuricaemia, hypocalcaemia, thirst, dehydration
Musculoskeletal	Myalgia, arthralgia, musculoskeletal pain		Arthritis
Platelet, bleeding and clotting			Thrombocytopenia, bruise
Psychiatric	Depression, irritability, insomnia, anxiety, concentration impaired, emotional lability	Agitation, nervousness	Aggressive behaviour, somnolence, apathy, increased appetite, abnormal dreaming, psychosis, sleep disorder, suicidal ideation
Reproductive disorder,		Female: menorrhagia, menstrual disorder	Female: Amenorrhea, dysmenorrhea, breast pain, ovarian disorder, vaginal disorder. Male: impotence
Resistance disorder	Viral infection		Herpes simplex, fungal infection, otitis media
Respiratory system	Cough, dyspnoea, pharyngitis	Nonproductive cough, rhinitis	Bronchitis, nasal congestion, respiratory disorder, rhinorrhea, sinusitis, epistaxis
Skin and appendages	Alopecia, pruritus, skin dry, rash		Eczema, abnormal hair texture, photosensitivity reaction, erythema, erythematous rash, maculopapular rash, acne, dermatitis, psoriasis, aggravated psoriasis, skin disorder
Urinary/renal system			Micturition frequency, urinary tract infection, urine abnormal, prostatitis, polyuria
Visual Disorder		Blurred vision	Conjunctivitis, abnormal vision, eye pain

A reduction in haemoglobin concentrations by > 4 g/dl was observed in 30 % of patients treated with Rebetol and peginterferon alfa-2b and 37 % of patients treated with Rebetol + interferon alfa-2b. Haemoglobin levels dropped below 10 g/dl in up to 14 % of adult patients and 7 % of children and adolescents treated with Rebetol in combination with either peginterferon alfa-2b (adults only) or interferon alfa-2b.

Most cases of anaemia, neutropaenia, and thrombocytopaenia were mild (WHO grades 1 or 2). There were some cases of more severe neutropenia in patients treated with Rebetol in combination with peginterferon alfa-2b (WHO grade 3: 39 of 186 [21 %]; and WHO grade 4: 13 of 186 [7 %]); WHO grade 3 leukopenia was also reported in 7 % of this treatment group.

In a clinical trial, life-threatening psychiatric events reported in patients treated with Rebetol in combination with peginterferon alfa-2b or interferon alfa-2b included suicidal ideation (1 %) and attempted suicide (0.4 %). Following marketing, psychosis and hallucination have been reported rarely.

An increase in uric acid and indirect bilirubin values associated with haemolysis was observed in some patients treated with Rebetol used in combination with peginterferon alfa-2b or interferon alfa-2b in clinical trials, but values returned to baseline levels by four weeks after the end of therapy. Among those patients with elevated uric acid levels, very few patients treated with the combination developed clinical gout, none of which required treatment modification or discontinuation from the clinical trials.

Following the marketing of Rebetol in combination with peginterferon alfa-2b or interferon alfa-2b, the following events have been reported very rarely:

Blood and the lymphatic system disorders

Aplastic anaemia

Metabolism and nutrition disorders

Mitochondrial toxicity and lactic acidosis have been reported in HIV-positive patients receiving NRTI regimen and associated-ribavirin for co-HCV infection.

Hepatobiliary disorders

Pancreatitis

Skin and Subcutaneous tissue disorders

Erythema multiforme, Stevens Johnson syndrome, toxic epidermal necrolysis.

Children and adolescents

In clinical trials of 118 children or adolescents 3 to 16 years of age, 6 % discontinued therapy due to adverse events. In general, the adverse event profile in the limited paediatric population studied was similar to that observed in adults, although there is a paediatric-specific concern regarding growth inhibition, as decrease in height (mean percentile decrease of growth velocity of 9 %) and weight (mean percentile decrease of 13 %) percentile were observed during treatment (see section **4.4**). Furthermore, suicidal ideation or attempts were reported more frequently compared to adult patients (2.4 % vs 1 %) during treatment and during the 6 month follow-up after treatment. As in adult patients, children and adolescents also experienced other psychiatric adverse events (e.g., depression, emotional lability, and somnolence) (see section **4.4**). In addition, injection site disorders, fever, anorexia, vomiting, and emotional lability occurred more frequently in children and adolescents compared to adult patients. Dose modifications were required in 30 % of patients, most commonly for anaemia and neutropaenia.

Undesirable effects reported in paediatric clinical trials, and not previously reported at an incidence ⩾ 1 % in adults, are shown in **Table 5a**. All effects reported at a ⩾ 10 % incidence in paediatric trials were previously reported in adults (**Table 5**) and are not repeated in the paediatric table.

(see Table 5a)

Table 5a Undesirable effects in paediatric clinical trials (⩾ 1% of patients treated with Rebetol + interferon alfa-2b injection)

Body system	**⩾ 10%**	**5 % - < 10%**	**1 % - < 5%**
Application site disorder	Injection site reaction, injection site inflammation	Injection site pain	
Autonomic nervous system			Flushing, lacrimal gland disorder, sweating increased
Body as a whole	Fatigue, fever, headache, influenza-like symptoms, malaise, rigors, growth rate decrease (height and/or weight decrease for age)		Asthenia, chest pain, erythema, neoplasm (unspecified), oedema, right upper quadrant pain
Central and peripheral nervous	Dizziness	Tremor	Confusion, dysphonia, hyperkinesia, hyperaesthesia, hypoaesthesia, paresthaesia, urinary incontinence
Endocrine	Hypothyroidism		Hyperthyroidism, virilism
Gastrointestinal	Abdominal pain, anorexia, diarrhoea, nausea, vomiting		Constipation, dyspepsia, gastroenteritis, gastroesophogeal reflux, gastrointestinal disorder, glossitis, loose stools, mouth ulceration, rectal disorder, stomatitis, stomatitis ulcerative, toothache, tooth disorder
Infection and infestations			Tooth abscess
Liver and biliary			Hepatic function abnormal
Metabolic and nutritional			Hypertriglyceridemia, hyperuricemia
Musculoskeletal	Arthralgia, musculoskeletal pain, myalgia		
Platelet, bleeding and clotting			Bruise, thrombocytopaenia
Psychiatric	Depression, emotional lability, insomnia, irritability	Agitation, somnolence	Aggressive reaction, anxiety, apathy, increased appetite, behavior disorder, concentration impaired, abnormal dreaming, nervousness, sleep disorder, somnambulism, suicidal ideation
Red blood cell	Anaemia		
Renal and urinary			Enuresis, micturition disorder, urinary tract infection
Reproductive disorder, female and male			Female: amenorrhea, menorrhagia, menstrual disorder, vaginal disorder, vaginitis Male: testicular pain
Resistance mechanism disorder	Viral infection		Bacterial infection, fungal infection, herpes simplex, otitis media
Respiratory system	Pharyngitis	Epistaxis	Coughing, dyspnoea, nasal congestion, nasal irritation, pulmonary infection, rhinorrhea, sneezing, tachypnea
Skin and appendages	Alopecia, rash	Pruritus	Acne, eczema, skin laceration, nail disorder, dry skin, photosensitivity reaction, maculopapular rash, skin discolouration, skin disorder
Vascular (extracardiac)		Pallor	Raynaud's disease
Vision			Conjunctivitis, eye pain, abnormal vision
White cell and resistance	Neutropenia		Lymphadenopathy

4.9 Overdose

In clinical trials with Rebetol used in combination with peginterferon alfa-2b or interferon alfa-2b, the maximum overdose reported was a total dose of 10 g of Rebetol (50 × 200 mg capsules) and 39 MIU of interferon alfa-2b (13 subcutaneous injections of 3 MIU each) taken in one day by a patient in an attempt at suicide. The patient was observed for two days in the emergency room, during which time no adverse event from the overdose was noted.

5. PHARMACOLOGICAL PROPERTIES

5.1 Pharmacodynamic properties

Pharmacotherapeutic group: Direct acting antivirals, nucleosides and nucleotides (excl. reverse transcriptase inhibitors), ATC code: J05A B04.

Ribavirin (Rebetol) is a synthetic nucleoside analogue which has shown *in vitro* activity against some RNA and DNA viruses. The mechanism by which Rebetol in combination with peginterferon alfa-2b or interferon alfa-2b exerts its effects against HCV is unknown. Oral formulations of Rebetol monotherapy have been investigated as therapy for chronic hepatitis C in several clinical trials. Results of these investigations showed that Rebetol monotherapy had no effect on eliminating hepatitis virus (HCV-RNA) or improving hepatic histology after six to 12 months of therapy and six months of follow-up.

Rebetol clinical trials in adults

The use of Rebetol in combination treatment with peginterferon alfa-2b or interferon alfa-2b was evaluated in five clinical trials. Eligible patients for these trials had chronic hepatitis C confirmed by a positive HCV-RNA polymerase chain reaction assay (PCR) (> 30 IU/ml), a liver biopsy consistent with a histological diagnosis of chronic hepatitis with no other cause for the chronic hepatitis, and abnormal serum ALT.

Relapse patients

Two trials examined the use of Rebetol + interferon alfa-2b combination treatment in relapse patients (C95-144 and I95-145); 345 chronic hepatitis patients who had relapsed after previous interferon treatment were treated for six months with a six month follow-up. Combination therapy with Rebetol + interferon alfa-2b resulted in a sustained virological response that was ten-fold higher than that with interferon alfa-2b alone (49 % vs 5 %, $p < 0.0001$). This benefit was maintained irrespective of standard predictors of response to interferon alfa-2b such as virus level, HCV genotype and histological staging.

Naïve patients

Three trials examined the use of interferon in naïve patients, two with Rebetol + interferon alfa-2b (C95-132 and I95-143) and one with Rebetol + peginterferon alfa-2b (C/I98-580). In all cases the treatment was for one year with a follow-up of six months. The sustained response at the end of follow-up was significantly increased by the addition of Rebetol to interferon alfa-2b (41 % vs 16 %, $p < 0.001$).

In clinical trials C95-132 and I95-143, Rebetol + interferon alfa-2b combination therapy proved to be significantly more effective than interferon alfa-2b monotherapy (a doubling in sustained response). Combination therapy also decreased the relapse rate. This was true for all HCV genotypes, particularly Genotype 1, in which the relapse rate was reduced by 30 % compared with interferon alfa-2b monotherapy.

In clinical trial C/I98-580, 1,530 naïve patients were treated for one year with one of the following combination regimens:

- Rebetol (800 mg/day) + peginterferon alfa-2b (1.5 micrograms/kg/week) (n = 511).
- Rebetol (1,000/1,200 mg/day) + peginterferon alfa-2b (1.5 micrograms/kg/week for one month followed by 0.5 microgram/kg/week for 11 months) (n = 514).
- Rebetol (1,000/1,200 mg/day) + interferon alfa-2b (3 MIU three times as week) (n = 505).

In this trial, the combination of Rebetol and peginterferon alfa-2b (1.5 micrograms/kg/week) was significantly more effective than the combination of Rebetol and interferon alfa-2b, particularly in patients infected with Genotype 1. Sustained response was assessed by the response rate six months after the cessation of treatment.

HCV genotype and baseline virus load are prognostic factors which are known to affect response rates. However, response rates in this trial were shown to be dependent also on the dose of Rebetol administered in combination with peginterferon alfa-2b or interferon alfa-2b. In those patients that received > 10.6 mg/kg Rebetol (800 mg dose in typical 75 kg patient), regardless of genotype or viral load, response rates were significantly higher than in those patients that received ⩽ 10.6 mg/kg Rebetol (**Table 5b**), while response rates in patients that received > 13.2 mg/kg Rebetol were even higher.

(see Table 5b on next page)

In a separate trial, 224 patients with genotype 2 or 3 received peginterferon alfa-2b, 1.5 microgram/kg subcutaneously, once weekly, in combination with ribavirin 800 mg –1,400 mg p.o. for 6 months (based on body weight, only three patients weighing > 105 kg, received the1,400 mg dose, which has not yet been validated) (**Table 6**). Twenty-four % had bridging fibrosis or cirrhosis (Knodell 3/4).

Table 6. Virologic Response at End of Treatment, Sustained Virologic Response and Relapse by HCV Genotype and Viral Load*

(see Table 6)

The 6 month treatment duration in this trial was better tolerated than one year of treatment in the pivotal combination trial; for discontinuation 5 % vs. 14 %, for dose modification 18 % vs. 49 %.

In a non-comparative trial, 235 patients with genotype 1 and low viral load (< 600,000 IU/ml) received peginterferon alfa-2b, 1.5 microgram/kg subcutaneously, once weekly, in combination with weight adjusted Rebetol. The overall sustained response rate after a 24-week treatment duration was 50 %. Forty-one percent of subjects (97/235) had nondetectable plasma HCV-RNA levels at Week 4 and Week 24 of therapy. In this subgroup, there was a 92 % (89/97) sustained virological response rate. The high sustained response rate in this subgroup of patients was identified in an interim analysis (n=49) and prospectively confirmed (n=48).

Limited historical data indicate that treatment for 48 weeks might be associated with a higher sustained response rate (11/11) and with a lower risk of relapse (0/11 as compared to 7/96 following 24 weeks of treatment).

Predictability of sustained virological response

Virological response by week 12, defined as a 2-log viral load decrease or undetectable levels of HCV RNA has been shown to be predictive for sustained response (**Table 7**).

(see Table 7)

Rebetol clinical trials in children and adolescents:

Children and adolescents 3 to 16 years of age with compensated chronic hepatitis C and detectable HCV-RNA (assessed by a central laboratory using a research-based RT-PCR assay) were enrolled in two multicentre trials and received Rebetol 15 mg/kg per day plus interferon alfa-2b 3 MIU/m^2 3 times a week for 1 year followed by 6 months follow-up after treatment. A total of 118 patients were enrolled: 57 % male, 80 % Caucasian, and 78 % genotype 1, 64 % ⩽ 12 years of age. The population enrolled mainly consisted in children with mild to moderate hepatitis C. Sustained virological response rates in children and adolescents were similar to those in adults. Due to the lack of data in children with severe progression of the disease, and the potential for undesirable effects, the benefit/risk of the combination of ribavirin and interferon alfa-2b needs to be carefully considered in this population (see sections **4.1**, **4.4** and **4.8**).

Study results are summarized in **Table 8**.

Table 8. Virological response in previously untreated children and adolescents

	Rebetol 15 mg/kg/day + interferon alfa-2b 3 MIU/m^2 3 times a week
Overall Response[1] (n=118)	54 (46 %)*
Genotype 1 (n=92)	33 (36 %)*
Genotype 2/3/4 (n=26)	21 (81 %)*

* Number (%) of patients

1. Defined as HCV-RNA below limit of detection using a research based RT-PCR assay at end of treatment and during follow-up period

Table 5b Sustained response rates with Rebetol + peginterferon alfa-2b (by Rebetol dose [mg/kg], genotype and viral load)

HCV Genotype	Rebetol dose (mg/kg)	P 1.5/R	P 0.5/R	I/R
All Genotypes	**All**	**54 %**	**47 %**	**47 %**
	⩽ 10.6	50 %	41 %	27 %
	> 10.6	61 %	48 %	47 %
Genotype 1	**All**	**42 %**	**34 %**	**33 %**
	⩽ 10.6	38 %	25 %	20 %
	> 10.6	48 %	34 %	34 %
Genotype 1 ⩽ 600,000 IU/ml	All	73 %	51 %	45 %
	⩽ 10.6	74 %	25 %	33 %
	> 10.6	71 %	52 %	45 %
Genotype 1 > 600,000 IU/ml	All	30 %	27 %	29 %
	⩽ 10.6	27 %	25 %	17 %
	> 10.6	37 %	27 %	29 %
Genotype 2/3	**All**	**82 %**	**80 %**	**79 %**
	⩽ 10.6	79 %	73 %	50 %
	> 10.6	88 %	80 %	80 %

P1.5/R Rebetol (800 mg) + peginterferon alfa-2b (1.5 micrograms/kg)

P0.5/R Rebetol (1,000/1,200 mg) + peginterferon alfa-2b (1.5 to 0.5 microgram/kg)

I/R Rebetol (1,000/1,200 mg) + interferon alfa-2b (3 MIU)

Table 6. Virologic Response at End of Treatment, Sustained Virologic Response and Relapse by HCV Genotype and Viral Load*

	Rebetol 800-1,400 mg/day Plus peginterferon alfa-2b 1.5 μg/kg Once Weekly		
	End of Treatment Response	Sustained Virologic Response	Relapse
All Subjects	**94 % (211/224)**	**81 % (182/224)**	**12 % (27/224)**
HCV 2	**100 % (42/42)**	**93 % (39/42)**	**7 % (3/42)**
⩽ 600,000 IU/ml	**100 % (20/20)**	**95 % (19/20)**	**5 % (1/20)**
> 600,000 IU/mL	**100 % (22/22)**	**91 % (20/22)**	**9 % (2/22)**
HCV 3	**93 % (169/182)**	**79 % (143/182)**	**14 % (24/166)**
⩽ 600,000 IU/ml	**93 % (92/99)**	**86 % (85/99)**	**8 % (7/91)**
> 600,000 IU/ml	**93 % (77/83)**	**70 % (58/83)**	**23 % (17/75)**

* Any subject with an undetectable HCV-RNA level at the Follow-Up Week 12 visit and missing data at the Follow-Up Week 24 visit was considered a sustained responder. Any subject with missing data in and after the Follow-Up Week 12 window was considered to be a non-responder at Week 24 of follow-up.

Table 7 Predictability of sustained response by viral response at week 12 and genotype*

Treatment	Genotype	Viral response at week 12	Sustained response	Negative predictive value
Rebetol (>10.6mg/kg) +peginterferon alfa-2b 1.5 48-week treatment	1	Yes 75 % (82/110)	71 % (58/82)	
		No 25 % (28/110)	0 % (0/28)	100 %
Rebetol 800-1400 mg +peginterferon alfa-2b 1.5 24-week treatment	2 and 3	Yes 99 % (213/215)	83 % (177/213)	—
		No 1 % (2/215)	50 % (1/2)	50 %

*reflects patients with 12 week data available

5.2 Pharmacokinetic properties

Ribavirin is absorbed rapidly following oral administration of a single dose (mean T_{max}= 1.5 hours), followed by rapid distribution and prolonged elimination phases (single dose half-lives of absorption, distribution and elimination are 0.05, 3.73 and 79 hours, respectively). Absorption is extensive with approximately 10 % of a radiolabelled dose excreted in the faeces. However, absolute bioavailability is approximately 45 %-65 %, which appears to be due to first pass metabolism. There is a linear relationship between dose and AUC_{tf} following single doses of 200-1,200 mg ribavirin. Volume of distribution is approximately 5,000 l. Ribavirin does not bind to plasma proteins.

Ribavirin has been shown to produce high inter- and intra-subject pharmacokinetic variability following single oral doses (intrasubject variability of approximately 30 % for both AUC and C_{max}), which may be due to extensive first pass metabolism and transfer within and beyond the blood compartment.

Ribavirin transport in non-plasma compartments has been most extensively studied in red cells, and has been identified to be primarily via an e_s-type equilibrative nucleoside transporter. This type of transporter is present on virtually all cell types and may account for the high volume of distribution of ribavirin. The ratio of whole blood:plasma ribavirin concentrations is approximately 60:1; the excess of ribavirin in whole blood exists as ribavirin nucleotides sequestered in erythrocytes.

Ribavirin has two pathways of metabolism: 1) a reversible phosphorylation pathway; 2) a degradative pathway involving deribosylation and amide hydrolysis to yield a triazole carboxyacid metabolite. Both ribavirin and its triazole carboxamide and triazole carboxylic acid metabolites are also excreted renally.

Upon multiple dosing, ribavirin accumulates extensively in plasma with a six-fold ratio of multiple-dose to single-dose AUC_{12hr}. Following oral dosing with 600 mg BID, steady-state was reached by approximately four weeks, with mean steady state plasma concentrations approximately 2,200 ng/ml. Upon discontinuation of dosing the half-life was approximately 298 hours, which probably reflects slow elimination from non-plasma compartments.

Food effect: The bioavailability of a single oral dose of ribavirin was increased by co-administration of a high fat meal (AUC_{tf} and C_{max} both increased by 70 %). It is possible that the increased bioavailability in this study was due to delayed transit of ribavirin or modified pH. The clinical relevance of results from this single dose study is unknown. In the pivotal clinical efficacy trial, patients were instructed to take ribavirin with food to achieve the maximal plasma concentration of ribavirin.

Renal function: Single-dose ribavirin pharmacokinetics were altered (increased AUC_{tf} and C_{max}) in patients with renal dysfunction compared with control subjects (creatinine clearance > 90 ml/minute). This appears to be due to reduction of apparent clearance in these patients. Ribavirin concentrations are essentially unchanged by haemodialysis.

Hepatic function: Single-dose pharmacokinetics of ribavirin in patients with mild, moderate or severe hepatic dysfunction (Child-Pugh Classification A, B or C) are similar to those of normal controls.

Elderly patients (⩾ 65 years of age): Specific pharmacokinetic evaluations for elderly subjects have not been performed. However, in a population pharmacokinetic study, age was not a key factor in the kinetics of ribavirin; renal function is the determining factor.

Population pharmacokinetic analysis was performed using sparsely sampled serum concentration values from four controlled clinical trials. The clearance model developed showed that body weight, gender, age, and serum creatinine were the main covariates. For males, clearance was approximately 20 % higher than for females. Clearance increased as a function of body weight and was reduced at ages greater than 40 years. Effects of these covariates on ribavirin clearance appear to be of limited clinical significance due to the substantial residual variability not accounted for by the model.

Children and adolescents: Multiple-dose pharmacokinetic properties for Rebetol capsules and interferon alfa-2b in children and adolescents with chronic hepatitis C between 5 and 16 years of age are summarized in **Table 9**. The pharmacokinetics of Rebetol and interferon alfa-2b (dose-normalized) are similar in adults and children or adolescents.

Table 9. Mean (% CV) multiple-dose pharmacokinetic parameters for interferon alfa-2b and Rebetol capsules when administered to children or adolescents with chronic hepatitis C

Parameter	Rebetol 15 mg/kg/day as 2 divided doses (n = 17)	Interferon alfa-2b 3 MIU/m^2 3 times a week (n = 54)
T_{max} (hr)	1.9 (83)	5.9 (36)
C_{max} (ng/ml)	3,275 (25)	51 (48)
AUC*	29,774 (26)	622 (48)
Apparent clearance l/hr/kg	0.27 (27)	Not done

*AUC_{12} (ng.hr/ml) for Rebetol; AUC_{0-24} (IU.hr/ml) for interferon alfa-2b

5.3 Preclinical safety data

Ribavirin: Ribavirin is embryotoxic or teratogenic, or both, at doses well below the recommended human dose in all animal species in which studies have been conducted. Malformations of the skull, palate, eye, jaw, limbs, skeleton and gastrointestinal tract were noted. The incidence and severity of teratogenic effects increased with escalation of the dose. Survival of foetuses and offspring was reduced.

Erythrocytes are a primary target of toxicity for ribavirin in animal studies. Anaemia occurs shortly after initiation of dosing, but is rapidly reversible upon cessation of treatment.

In 3- and 6-month studies in mice to investigate ribavirin-induced testicular and sperm effects, abnormalities in sperm, occurred at doses of 15 mg/kg and above. These doses in animals produce systemic exposures well below those achieved in humans at therapeutic doses. Upon cessation of treatment, essentially total recovery from ribavirin-induced testicular toxicity occurred within one or two spermatogenic cycles (see section **4.6**).

Genotoxicity studies have demonstrated that ribavirin does exert some genotoxic activity. Ribavirin was active in the Balb/3T3 *in vitro* Transformation Assay. Genotoxic activity was observed in the mouse lymphoma assay, and at doses of 20-200 mg/kg in a mouse micronucleus assay. A dominant lethal assay in rats was negative, indicating that if mutations occurred in rats they were not transmitted through male gametes.

Conventional carcinogenicity rodent studies with low exposures compared to human exposure under therapeutic conditions (factor 0.1 in rats and 1 in mice) did not reveal tumorigenicity of ribavirin. In addition, in a 26 week carcinogenicity study using the heterozygous p53(+/-) mouse model, ribavirin did not produce tumours at the maximally tolerated dose of 300 mg/kg (plasma exposure factor approximately 2.5 compared to human exposure). These studies suggest that a carcinogenic potential of ribavirin in humans is unlikely.

Ribavirin plus interferon alfa-2b: When used in combination with peginterferon alfa-2b or interferon alfa-2b, ribavirin did not cause any effects not previously seen with either active substance alone. The major treatment-related change was a reversible mild to moderate anaemia, the severity of which was greater than that produced by either active substance alone.

No studies have been conducted in juvenile animals to examine the effects of treatment on growth, development, sexual maturation, and behaviour.

6. PHARMACEUTICAL PARTICULARS

6.1 List of excipients

Capsule contents:

Microcrystalline cellulose,

Lactose monohydrate,

Croscarmellose sodium,

Magnesium stearate.

Capsule shell:

Gelatine,

Titanium dioxide.

Capsule imprint:

Shellac,

Propylene glycol,

Ammonium hydroxide,

Colouring agent (E 132).

6.2 Incompatibilities

Not applicable

6.3 Shelf life

2 years

6.4 Special precautions for storage

Do not store above 30°C.

6.5 Nature and contents of container

Ribavirin capsules are packaged in blisters consisting of polyvinyl chloride (PVC)/polyethylene (PE)/polyvinylidene chloride (PVdC).

Ribavirin capsules are supplied as:

- 7 foil blisters of 12 capsules (for a total of 84 capsules)
- 14 foil blisters of 10 capsules (for a total of 140 capsules)
- 14 foil blisters of 12 capsules (for a total of 168 capsules)

Not all pack sizes may be marketed.

6.6 Instructions for use and handling

No special requirements

7. MARKETING AUTHORISATION HOLDER

SP Europe

73, rue de Stalle

B-1180 Bruxelles

Belgium

8. MARKETING AUTHORISATION NUMBER(S)

EU/1/99/107/001 84 hard capsules

EU/1/99/107/002 140 hard capsules

EU/1/99/107/003 168 hard capsules

9. DATE OF FIRST AUTHORISATION/RENEWAL OF THE AUTHORISATION

Date of first authorisation: 7 May 1999

Date of last renewal: 02 September 2004

10. DATE OF REVISION OF THE TEXT

31 August 2005

Legal Category

Prescription Only Medicine

Rebetol/EU/09-05/9

Rebif 22 micrograms or 44 micrograms - solution for injection

(Serono Ltd)

1. NAME OF THE MEDICINAL PRODUCT

Rebif® 22 micrograms or 44 micrograms - solution for injection

2. QUALITATIVE AND QUANTITATIVE COMPOSITION

Rebif 22 micrograms (Interferon beta-1a) contains 22 micrograms (6 million IU*) of Interferon beta-1a per pre-filled syringe.

Rebif 44 micrograms (Interferon beta-1a) contains 44 micrograms (12 million IU*) of Interferon beta-1a per pre-filled syringe.

.*: measured by cytopathic effect (CPE) bioassay against the in-house IFN beta-1a standard which is calibrated against the current international NIH standard (GB-23-902-531).

For excipients, see section 6.1.

3. PHARMACEUTICAL FORM

Solution for injection

4. CLINICAL PARTICULARS

4.1 Therapeutic indications

Rebif is indicated for the treatment of patients with multiple sclerosis and with 2 or more relapses within the last two years. Efficacy has not been demonstrated in patients with secondary progressive multiple sclerosis without ongoing relapse activity. See section 5.1.

4.2 Posology and method of administration

Rebif is available in two strengths: 22 micrograms and 44 micrograms.

The recommended posology of Rebif is 44 micrograms given three times per week by subcutaneous injection. Rebif 22 micrograms, also given three times per week by subcutaneous injection, is recommended for patients who cannot tolerate the higher dose in view of the treating specialist. Treatment should be initiated under supervision of a physician experienced in the treatment of the disease.

When first starting treatment with Rebif, in order to allow tachyphylaxis to develop thus reducing adverse events, it is recommended that 8.8 micrograms (0.1 ml of the 44 micrograms strength or 0.2 ml of the 22 micrograms strength) be administered during the initial 2 weeks of therapy, 22 micrograms (0.25 ml of the 44 micrograms strength or the total of the 22 micrograms strength) be administered in weeks 3 and 4, and the total of the 44 micrograms strength be administered from the fifth week onwards.

There is no experience with Rebif in children under 16 years of age with multiple sclerosis and therefore Rebif should not be used in this population.

At the present time, it is not known for how long patients should be treated. Safety and efficacy with Rebif have not been demonstrated beyond 4 years of treatment. It is recommended that patients should be evaluated at least every second year in the 4 year period after initiation of treatment with Rebif and a decision for longer-term treatment should then be made on an individual basis by the treating physician.

4.3 Contraindications

Interferon beta-1a is contraindicated in patients with a known hypersensitivity to natural or recombinant interferon beta, human serum albumin, or any other component of the formulation.

Interferon beta-1a is contraindicated in pregnant patients (also see section 4.6), patients with severe depressive disorders and/or suicidal ideation, and in epileptic patients with a history of seizures not adequately controlled by treatment

(see section 4.4 and section 4.8).

4.4 Special warnings and special precautions for use

Patients should be informed of the most common adverse events associated with interferon beta administration, including symptoms of the flu-like syndrome (see section 4.8). These symptoms tend to be most prominent at the initiation of therapy and decrease in frequency and severity with continued treatment.

Interferons should be used with caution in patients with depression. Depression and suicidal ideation are known to occur in increased frequency in the multiple sclerosis population and in association with interferon use. Patients treated with Interferon beta-1a should be advised to immediately report any symptoms of depression and/or suicidal ideation to their prescribing physician. Patients exhibiting depression should be monitored closely during therapy with Interferon beta-1a and treated appropriately. Cessation of therapy with Interferon beta-1a should be considered (see also section 4.3 and section 4.8).

Caution should be exercised when administering Interferon beta-1a to patients with pre-existing seizure disorders. For patients without a pre-existing seizure disorder who develop seizures during therapy with Interferon beta-1a, an aetiological basis should be established and appropriate anti-convulsant therapy instituted prior to resuming Interferon beta-1a treatment (see also section 4.3 and section 4.8).

Patients with cardiac disease, such as angina, congestive heart failure or arrhythmia, should be closely monitored for worsening of their clinical condition during initiation of therapy with Interferon beta-1a. Symptoms of the flu-like syndrome associated with Interferon beta-1a therapy may prove stressful to patients with cardiac conditions.

Injection site necrosis (ISN) has been reported in patients using Rebif (see section 4.8). To minimise the risk of injection site necrosis patients should be advised to:

- use an aseptic injection technique
- rotate the injection sites with each dose.

The procedure for the self-administration by the patient should be reviewed periodically especially if injection site reactions have occurred.

If the patient experiences any break in the skin, which may be associated with swelling or drainage of fluid from the injection site, the patient should be advised to consult with their physician before continuing injections with Rebif. If the patient has multiple lesions, Rebif should be discontinued until healing has occurred. Patients with single lesions may continue provided that the necrosis is not too extensive.

Patients should be advised about the abortifacient potential of interferon beta (see section 4.6 and section 5.3).

In clinical trials with Rebif, asymptomatic elevations of hepatic transaminases (particularly ALT) were common and 1-3 % of patients developed elevations of hepatic transaminases above 5 times the upper limit of normal (ULN). Dose reduction of Rebif should be considered if ALT rises above 5 times the ULN, and gradually re-escalated when enzyme levels have normalised. Rebif should be initiated with caution in patients with a history of significant liver disease, clinical evidence of active liver disease, alcohol abuse or increased serum ALT >2.5 times ULN). Serum ALT levels should be monitored prior to the start of therapy, at months 1, 3 and 6 on therapy and periodically thereafter in the absence of clinical symptoms. Treatment with Rebif should be stopped if icterus or other clinical symptoms of liver dysfunction appear (see section 4.8).

Rebif, like other interferons beta, has a potential for causing severe liver injury (see section 4.8) including acute hepatic failure. The mechanism for the rare symptomatic hepatic dysfunction is not known. No specific risk factors have been identified.

Laboratory abnormalities are associated with the use of interferons. The overall incidence of these is slightly higher with Rebif 44 than Rebif 22 mcg. Therefore, in addition to those laboratory tests, normally required for monitoring patients with multiple sclerosis, and in addition to liver enzyme monitoring, complete and differential blood cell counts, and platelet counts are also recommended during Interferon beta-1a therapy. These should be more frequent when initiating Rebif 44 micrograms.

Patients being treated with Rebif may occasionally develop new or worsening thyroid abnormalities. Thyroid function testing is recommended at baseline and if abnormal, every 6-12 months following initiation of therapy. If tests are normal at baseline, routine testing is not needed but should be performed if clinical findings of thyroid dysfunction appear (see section 4.8).

Caution should be used, and close monitoring considered when administering Interferon beta-1a to patients with severe renal and hepatic failure and to patients with severe myelosuppression.

Serum neutralising antibodies against Interferon beta-1a may develop. The precise incidence of antibodies is as yet uncertain. Clinical data suggest that after 24 to 48 months of treatment with Rebif 22 micrograms, approximately 24% of patients develop persistent serum antibodies to Interferon beta-1a. After 24 to 48 months of treatment with Rebif 44 micrograms, approximately 13 to 14% of patients develop persistent serum antibodies to Interferon beta-1a. The presence of antibodies has been shown to attenuate the pharmacodynamic response to Interferon beta-1a (Beta-2 microglobulin and neopterin). Although the clinical significance of the induction of antibodies has not been fully elucidated, the development of neutralising antibodies is associated with reduced efficacy on clinical and MRI variables. If a patient responds poorly to therapy with Rebif, and has neutralising antibodies, the treating physician should reassess the benefit/risk ratio of continued Rebif therapy.

The use of various assays to detect serum antibodies and differing definitions of antibody positivity limits the ability to compare antigenicity among different products.

Only sparse safety and efficacy data are available from non-ambulatory patients with multiple sclerosis.

4.5 Interaction with other medicinal products and other forms of Interaction

No formal drug interaction studies have been conducted with Rebif (Interferon beta-1a) in humans.

Interferons have been reported to reduce the activity of hepatic cytochrome P450-dependent enzymes in humans and animals. Caution should be exercised when administering Rebif in combination with medicinal products that have a narrow therapeutic index and are largely dependent on the hepatic cytochrome P450 system for clearance, e.g. antiepileptics and some classes of antidepressants.

The interaction of Rebif with corticosteroids or ACTH has not been studied systematically. Clinical studies indicate that multiple sclerosis patients can receive Rebif and corticosteroids or ACTH during relapses.

4.6 Pregnancy and lactation

Because of potential hazards to the foetus, Rebif is contra-indicated in pregnancy.

There are no studies of interferon beta-1a in pregnant women. At high doses, in monkeys, abortifacient effects were observed with other interferons (see section 5.3). It cannot be excluded that such effects will be observed in humans.

Fertile women receiving Rebif should take appropriate contraceptive measures. Patients planning for pregnancy and those becoming pregnant should be informed of the potential hazards of interferons to the foetus and Rebif should be discontinued.

It is not known whether Rebif is excreted in human milk. Because of the potential for serious adverse reactions in nursing infants, a decision should be made either to discontinue nursing or to discontinue Rebif therapy.

4.7 Effects on ability to drive and use machines

Less commonly reported central nervous system-related adverse events associated with the use of interferon beta might influence the patient's ability to drive or use machines (see section 4.8).

4.8 Undesirable effects

a) General description

Approximately 40% of patients treated with Rebif can expect to experience the typical interferon flu-like syndrome within the first six months after starting treatment. Most patients will also experience reactions at the injection site, predominantly mild inflammation or erythema. Asymptomatic increases in laboratory parameters of hepatic function and decreases in WBC are also common.

The majority of adverse reactions observed with IFN-beta-1a are usually mild and reversible, and respond well to dose reductions. In case of severe or persistent undesirable effects, the dose of Rebif may be temporarily lowered or interrupted, at the discretion of the physician.

b) Adverse reactions by frequency

The adverse reactions reported below are classified according to frequency of occurrence as follows:

Very Common	> 1/10
Common	1/100 - 1/10
Uncommon	1/1000 - 1/100
Rare	1/10 000 - 1/ 1000
Very Rare	< 1/10000

Adverse reactions identified in clinical studies: the data presented is obtained from pooled clinical studies in multiple sclerosis (placebo=824 patients; Rebif 22 mcg TIW= 398 patients; Rebif 44 mcg TIW= 727 patients) and shows the frequency of adverse reactions observed at six-month (excess over placebo).

Application site disorders:

Very Common: Injection site inflammation, injection site reaction.

Common: Injection site pain.

Uncommon: Injection site necrosis, injection site abscess, injection site mass

Body as a whole - General disorders

Very Common: Influenza-like symptoms, headache

Common: Myalgia, arthralgia, fatigue, rigors, fever

Liver and biliary system disorders

Very Common: Asymptomatic transaminase increase

Skin and appendages disorders

Common: pruritus, rash, erythematous rash, maculo-papular rash.

Red blood cell and white cell disorders

Common: Neutropenia, lymphopenia, leucopenia, thrombocytopenia, anemia.

Endocrine Disorders

Uncommon: Thyroid dysfunction (elevated T3, T4, reduced TSH)

Gastrointestinal disorders

Common: diarrhoea, vomiting, nausea

Psychiatric disorders

Common: depression, insomnia

Adverse reactions identified during post-marketing surveillance.

Body as a whole:

Very rare: Anaphylactic reaction

Skin and appendages disorders

Very rare: angioedema, urticaria, erythema multiforme, erythema multiforme-like skin reactions, hair loss

Liver and biliary system disorders

Rare: Hepatitis with or without icterus.

Central and peripheral nervous system disorders

Very rare: seizures

Vascular (extra-cardiac) disorders

Very rare: thromboembolic events

Psychiatric disorders

Very rare: suicide attempt

c) Information characterising individual serious and/or frequently-occurring adverse reactions

Rebif, like other interferons beta, has a potential for causing severe liver injury. The mechanism for the rare symptomatic hepatic dysfunction is not known. The majority of the cases of severe liver injury occurred within the first six months of treatment. No specific risk factors have been identified. Treatment with Rebif should be stopped if icterus or other clinical symptoms of liver dysfunction appear (see Section 4.4).

d) Adverse reactions that apply to the pharmacological class.

The administration of interferons has been associated with anorexia, dizziness, anxiety, arrhythmias, vasodilation, palpitation, menorrhagia and metrorrhagia.

An increased formation of autoantibodies may occur during treatment with interferon beta.

4.9 Overdose

No case of overdose has been reported. However, in case of overdosage, patients should be hospitalised for observation and appropriate supportive treatment should be given.

5. PHARMACOLOGICAL PROPERTIES

5.1 Pharmacodynamic properties

Pharmacotherapeutic group: cytokines, ATC code: L03 AB.

Interferons (IFNs) are a group of endogenous glycoproteins endowed with immunomodulatory, antiviral and antiproliferative properties.

Rebif (Interferon beta-1a) is composed of the native amino acid sequence of natural human interferon beta. It is produced in mammalian cells (Chinese Hamster Ovary) and is therefore glycosylated like the natural protein.

The precise mechanism of action of Rebif in multiple sclerosis is still under investigation.

The safety and efficacy of Rebif has been evaluated in patients with relapsing-remitting multiple sclerosis at doses ranging from 11 to 44 micrograms (3-12 million IU), administered subcutaneously three times per week. At licensed posology, Rebif has been demonstrated to decrease the incidence (approximately 30% over 2 years) and severity of clinical relapses. The proportion of patients with disability progression, as defined by at least one point increase in EDSS confirmed three months later, was reduced from 39% (placebo) to 30% (Rebif 22 micrograms), or to 27% (Rebif 44 micrograms). Over 4 years the reduction in the mean exacerbation rate was 22% in patients treated with Rebif 22 micrograms, and 29% in patients treated with Rebif 44 micrograms group compared with a group of patients treated with placebo for 2 years and then either Rebif 22 or Rebif 44 micrograms for 2 years.

In a 3-year study in patients with secondary progressive multiple sclerosis, Rebif had no significant effect on progression of disability, but relapse rate was reduced by approximately 30%. If the patient population was divided into 2 subgroups (those with and those without relapses in the 2-year period prior to study entry), there was no effect on disability in patients without relapses, but in patients with relapses, the proportion with progression in disability at the end of the study was reduced from 70% (placebo) to 57% (Rebif 22 microgram and 44 microgram combined). These results obtained in a subgroup of patients a posteriori should be interpreted cautiously.

Rebif has not yet been investigated in patients with primary progressive multiple sclerosis, and should not be used in such patients.

5.2 Pharmacokinetic properties

In healthy volunteers after intravenous administration, interferon beta-1a exhibits a sharp multi-exponential decline, with serum levels proportional to the dose. The initial half-life is in the order of minutes and the terminal half-life is several hours, with the possible presence of a deep compartment. When administered by the subcutaneous or intramuscular routes, serum levels of interferon beta remain low, but are still measurable up to 12 to 24 hours post-dose. Subcutaneous and intramuscular administrations of Rebif produce equivalent exposure to interferon beta. Following a single 60 microgram dose, the maximum peak concentration, as measured by immunoassay, is around 6 to 10 IU/ml, occurring on average around 3 hours after the dose. After subcutaneous administration at the same dose repeated every 48 hours for 4 doses, a moderate accumulation occurs (about 2.5 × for AUC).

Regardless of the route of dosing, pronounced pharmacodynamic changes are associated with the administration of Rebif. After a single dose, intracellular and serum activity of 2-5A synthetase and serum concentrations of beta$_2$-microglobulin and neopterin increase within 24 hours, and start to decline within 2 days. Intramuscular and subcutaneous administrations produce fully superimposable responses. After repeated subcutaneous administration every 48 hours for 4 doses, these biological responses remain elevated, with no signs of tolerance development.

Interferon beta-1a is mainly metabolised and excreted by the liver and the kidneys.

5.3 Preclinical safety data

Rebif was tested in toxicology studies of up to 6 months in duration in monkeys and 3 months in rats and caused no overt signs of toxicity.

Rebif has been shown to be neither mutagenic nor clastogenic. Rebif has not been investigated for carcinogenicity.

A study on embryo/foetal toxicity in monkeys showed no evidence of reproductive disturbances. Based on observations with other alpha and beta interferons, an increased risk of abortions cannot be excluded. No information is available on the effects of the interferon beta-1a on male fertility.

6. PHARMACEUTICAL PARTICULARS

6.1 List of excipients

Mannitol, human serum albumin, sodium acetate, acetic acid, sodium hydroxide, water for injections.

6.2 Incompatibilities

Not applicable.

6.3 Shelf life

2 years at 2-8 °C (in a refrigerator).

At the user, 30 days below 25 °C

6.4 Special precautions for storage
Store in a refrigerator (2°C -8°C). Do not freeze. Store in the original package in order to protect from light. Should refrigeration be temporarily unavailable, Rebif can, at the user, be stored below 25°C for up to 30 days, then put back in the refrigerator and used before the expiry date.

6.5 Nature and contents of container
Rebif 22 micrograms and 44 micrograms (Interferon beta-1a) is available as a package of 3 or 12 individual doses of Rebif solution for injection (0.5 ml) filled in a 1 ml glass syringe with a stainless steel needle.

6.6 Instructions for use and handling
The solution for injection in a pre-filled syringe is ready for use. It may also be administered with a suitable auto-injector.

Any unused product or waste material should be disposed of in accordance with local requirements.

7. MARKETING AUTHORISATION HOLDER
Serono Europe Limited
56 Marsh Wall
London E14 9TP
United Kingdom

8. MARKETING AUTHORISATION NUMBER(S)
EU/1/98/063/003- Rebif 22 micrograms 12 pre-filled syringes
EU/1/98/063/006- Rebif 44 micrograms 12 pre-filled syringes

9. DATE OF FIRST AUTHORISATION/RENEWAL OF THE AUTHORISATION

Rebif 22 micrograms:	Rebif 44 micrograms:
Date of first authorisation:	Date of first authorisation:
4th May 1998	29th March 1999
Date of last renewal:	Date of last renewal:
4th June 2003	4th June 2003

10. DATE OF REVISION OF THE TEXT
22 July 2004

LEGAL STATUS
POM

NAME AND ADDRESS OF DISTRIBUTOR IN UK
Serono Ltd
Bedfont Cross
Stanwell Road
Feltham
Middlesex
TW14 8NX
Tel. 020 8818 7200

NAME AND ADDRESS OF DISTRIBUTOR IN IRELAND
Allphar Services Limited
Pharmaceutical Agents and Distributors
Belgard Road
Tallaght
Dublin 24

Prepared: 17-09-04

Rectogesic 0.4% Rectal Ointment

(Strakan Pharmaceuticals Ltd)

1. NAME OF THE MEDICINAL PRODUCT
▼Rectogesic® 0.4% Rectal Ointment.

2. QUALITATIVE AND QUANTITATIVE COMPOSITION
Glyceryl trinitrate (GTN): 0.4% w/w (4 mg/g).

For excipients, see 6.1.

3. PHARMACEUTICAL FORM
Rectal ointment. Rectogesic® 0.4% Rectal Ointment is an off-white smooth opaque ointment formulation.

4. CLINICAL PARTICULARS

4.1 Therapeutic indications
Rectogesic® 0.4% Rectal Ointment is indicated for relief of pain associated with chronic anal fissure.

4.2 Posology and method of administration
Adults and elderly:

Rectogesic® Rectal Ointment is supplied in 30g tubes with a 2.5 cm dosing line on the outside carton. A finger covering, such as cling film or a finger cot, may be placed on the finger to be used to apply the ointment. (Finger cots to be obtained separately from local pharmacy or surgical supplies retailer or cling film from local store.) The finger is placed along side the line and a strip of ointment the length of the line is expressed onto the end of the finger by gently squeezing the tube. The amount of ointment expressed is approximately 375 mg (1.5 mg GTN). The covered finger is then gently inserted into the anal canal to the first interphalangeal joint (knuckle) and applied circumferentially to the anal canal.

The dose delivered from the 0.4% ointment is 1.5 mg glyceryl trinitrate. The dose is to be applied intra-anally every twelve hours. Treatment may be continued until the pain abates, up to a maximum of 8 weeks.

Children: Rectogesic® 0.4% Rectal Ointment should not be used in children as safety andeffectiveness in children-under the age of 18 years have not been established.

4.3 Contraindications
Rectogesic® 0.4% Rectal Ointment is contraindicated in those patients who are known to be hypersensitive to glyceryl trinitrate or to any of the excipients in the ointment or have a known idiosyncratic reaction to organic nitrates.

Rectogesic® 0.4% Rectal Ointment is contraindicated for concomitant treatment with sildenafil citrate (Viagra®), tadalafil (Cialis®), vardenafil (Levitra®) and with nitric oxide (NO) donors, such as isosorbide dinitrate and amyl or butyl-nitrite.

Rectogesic® 0.4% Rectal Ointment is contraindicated in patients with postural hypotension, hypotension or uncorrected hypovolaemia as the use of glyceryl trinitrate in such states could produce severe hypotension or shock, increased intracranial pressure (e.g. head trauma or cerebral haemorrhage) or inadequate cerebral circulation; in patients with migraine or recurrent headache, in patients with aortic or mitral stenosis, hypertrophic obstructive cardiomyopathy, constrictive pericarditis or pericardial tamponade; marked anaemia or closed-angle glaucoma.

4.4 Special warnings and special precautions for use
Rectogesic® 0.4% Rectal Ointment should be used with caution in patients who have severe hepatic or renal disease.

Excessive hypotension, especially for prolonged periods of time, must be avoided because of possible deleterious effects on the brain, heart, liver and kidney from poor perfusion and the attendant risk of ischaemia, thrombosis and altered function of these organs. Patients should be advised to change position slowly when changing from lying or sitting to upright to minimize postural hypotension. Paradoxical bradycardia and increased angina pectoris may accompany glyceryl trinitrate-induced hypotension.

Alcohol may enhance the hypotensive effects of glyceryl trinitrate.

If the physician elects to use glyceryl trinitrate ointment for patients with acute myocardial infarction or congestive heart failure, careful clinical and haemodynamic monitoring must be used to avoid the potential hazards of hypotension and tachycardia.

4.5 Interaction with other medicinal products and other forms of Interaction
Concomitant treatment with other vasodilators, calcium antagonists, ACE inhibitors, beta blockers, diuretics, anti-hypertensives, tricyclic anti-depressants and major tranquillisers, as well as the consumption of alcohol, may potentiate the blood pressure lowering effects of Rectogesic®.

Co-administration of Rectogesic® with dihydroergotamine may increase the bioavailability of dihydroergotamine and lead to coronary vasoconstriction. The possibility that the ingestion of acetylsalicylic acid and non-steroidal anti-inflammatory drugs might diminish the therapeutic response to Rectogesic® cannot be excluded.

4.6 Pregnancy and lactation
Pregnancy: As with all drugs, Rectogesic® 0.4% Rectal Ointment should not be prescribed during pregnancy, particularly during the first trimester, unless there are compelling reasons for doing so.

Lactation: It is not known whether glyceryl trinitrate is excreted in human milk. Because many drugs are excreted in human milk, caution should be exercised when Rectogesic® 0.4% Rectal Ointment is administered to nursing mothers.

4.7 Effects on ability to drive and use machines
Rectogesic® 0.4% Rectal Ointment may cause dizziness, light-headedness, blurred vision, headache or tiredness in some patients, especially on first use. Patients should be cautioned about driving or operating machinery while using Rectogesic® 0.4% Rectal Ointment.

4.8 Undesirable effects
In patients treated with Rectogesic® 0.4% Rectal Ointment, the most common adverse event was dose-related headache which occurred with an incidence of 50%. Other less common adverse events noted in clinical trials include pain, nausea, vomiting, rectal bleeding, rectal disorder, anal burning and itching, dizziness, reflex tachycardia.

Adverse reactions to glyceryl trinitrate 2% ointment (used in the prophylaxis of angina pectoris) are generally dose-related and almost all of these reactions are the result of vasodilator activity. Headache, which may be severe, is the most commonly reported side effect. Headache may be recurrent with each daily dose, especially at higher doses. Transient episodes of light-headedness, occasionally related to blood pressure changes, also may occur. Hypotension occurs infrequently, but in some patients may be severe enough to warrant discontinuation of therapy. Syncope, crescendo angina and rebound hypertension have been reported but are uncommon. Allergic reactions to glyceryl trinitrate are uncommon, and the great majority of those reported have been cases of contact dermatitis or fixed drug eruptions occurring in patients receiving glyceryl trinitrate in ointments or patches. There have been a few reports of genuine anaphylactoid reactions and these reactions can probably occur in patients receiving glyceryl trinitrate by any route. Extremely rarely, ordinary doses of organic nitrates have caused methaemoglobinaemia in normal–seeming patients.

4.9 Overdose
Accidental overdose of Rectogesic® 0.4% Rectal Ointment may result in hypotension and reflex tachycardia. No specific antagonist of the vasodilator effects of nitroglycerin is known, and no intervention has been subjected to controlled study as a therapy for nitroglycerin overdose. Because the hypotension associated with nitroglycerin overdose is the result of venodilation and arterial hypovolaemia, prudent therapy in this situation should be directed toward increasing central fluid volume. Passive elevation of the patient's legs may be sufficient, but intravenous infusion of normal saline or similar fluid may also be necessary.

5. PHARMACOLOGICAL PROPERTIES

5.1 Pharmacodynamic properties
The principal pharmacologic action of glyceryl trinitrate is mediated via the release of nitric oxide. When glyceryl trinitrate ointment is applied by the intra-anal route, the internal anal sphincter becomes relaxed.

Hypertonicity of the internal but not the external anal sphincter is a predisposing factor in the formation of anal fissures. The blood vessels to the anoderm course through the internal anal sphincter (IAS). Therefore hypertonicity of the IAS may thereby decrease blood flow and cause ischaemia to this region.

Distension of the rectum results in the anorector inhibitory reflex and relaxation of the internal anal sphincter. The nerves mediating this reflex lie in the wall of the gut. Release of the neurotransmitter NO from nerves of this type play a significant role in the physiology of the internal anal sphincter. Specifically, NO mediates the anorector inhibitory reflex in man, relaxing the IAS.

The link between IAS hypertonicity and spasm and the presence of an anal fissure has been established. Patients with chronic anal fissure have a significantly higher mean maximum resting anal pressure than controls and anodermal blood flow in chronic anal fissure patients was significantly lower than in controls. In patients whose fissures healed following a sphincterotomy, a reduction in anal pressure and improvement in anodermal blood flow was demonstrated, providing further evidence for the ischaemic nature of anal fissure. Topical application of a NO donor (glyceryl trinitrate) relaxes the anal sphincter, resulting in a reduction of anal pressure and an improvement in anoderm blood flow.

5.2 Pharmacokinetic properties
The volume of distribution of glyceryl trinitrate is about 3 L/kg and is cleared from this volume at extremely rapid rates, with a resulting serum half-life of about 3 minutes. The observed clearance rates (close to 1 L/kg/min) greatly exceed hepatic blood flow. The known sites of extrahepatic metabolism include red blood cells and vascular walls. The initial products in the metabolism of glyceryl trinitrate are inorganic nitrate and the 1,2 and 1,3-dinitroglycerols. The dinitrates are less effective vasodilators than glyceryl trinitrate, but they are longer lived in the serum. Their contribution to the relaxation of the internal anal sphincter is unknown. The dinitrates are further metabolised to non-vasoactive mononitrates and ultimately to glycerol and carbon dioxide. In six healthy subjects, the average bioavailability of glyceryl trinitrate applied to the anal canal as a 0.2% ointment was approximately 50% of the 0.75 mg dose.

5.3 Preclinical safety data
No systemic toxicity studies have been conducted with Rectogesic® 0.4% Rectal Ointment. Repeated oral dosing with glyceryl trinitrate in the rat and dog produced methaemoglobinaemia. In rats, testicular atrophy and aspermatogenesis, and hepatocellular carcinoma developed depending upon the dose (markedly in excess of those used in man) and duration of dosing.

6. PHARMACEUTICAL PARTICULARS

6.1 List of excipients
Propylene glycol
Lanolin
Sorbitan sesquioleate
Hard paraffin
White soft paraffin

6.2 Incompatibilities
None known.

6.3 Shelf life
36 months

6.4 Special precautions for storage
Do not store above 25°C. Do not freeze.

6.5 Nature and contents of container
30g open-ended, unlined printed aluminium tubes with end sealant and white low-density polyethylene non-piercing caps.

6.6 Instructions for use and handling
None stated.

7. MARKETING AUTHORISATION HOLDER

CELLEGY UK LIMITED

Ruskin House

40/41 Museum Street

London

WC1A 1LT

UK

8. MARKETING AUTHORISATION NUMBER(S)

PL 19075/0003

9. DATE OF FIRST AUTHORISATION/RENEWAL OF THE AUTHORISATION

24 August 2004

10. DATE OF REVISION OF THE TEXT

February 2005

Reductil 10mg & 15mg

(Abbott Laboratories Limited)

1. NAME OF THE MEDICINAL PRODUCT

Reductil 10 mg capsules, hard

Reductil 15 mg capsules, hard

2. QUALITATIVE AND QUANTITATIVE COMPOSITION

One capsule of Reductil 10 mg contains 10 mg of sibutramine hydrochloride monohydrate (equivalent to 8.37 mg of sibutramine).

One capsule of Reductil 15 mg contains 15 mg of sibutramine hydrochloride monohydrate (equivalent to 12.55 mg of sibutramine).

For excipients, see 6.1

3. PHARMACEUTICAL FORM

10 mg Hard capsule with a blue cap and yellow body

15 mg Hard capsule with a blue cap and white body

4. CLINICAL PARTICULARS

4.1 Therapeutic indications

Reductil 10 mg / 15 mg is indicated as adjunctive therapy within a weight management programme for:

- Patients with nutritional obesity and a body mass index (BMI) of 30 kg/m^2 or higher

- Patients with nutritional excess weight and a BMI of 27 kg/m^2 or higher, if other obesity-related risk factors such as type 2 diabetes or dyslipidaemia are present.

Note:

Reductil may only be prescribed to patients who have not adequately responded to an appropriate weight-reducing regimen alone, ie patients who have difficulty achieving or maintaining >5% weight loss within 3 months.

Treatment with Reductil 10 mg / 15 mg should only be given as part of a long-term integrated therapeutic approach for weight reduction under the care of a physician experienced in the treatment of obesity. An appropriate approach to obesity management should include dietary and behavioural modification as well as increased physical activity. This integrated approach is essential for a lasting change in eating habits and behaviour which is fundamental to the long-term maintenance of the reduced weight level once Reductil is stopped. Patients should change their lifestyle while on Reductil so that they are able to maintain their weight once drug treatment has ceased. They should be informed that, if they fail to do so, they may regain weight. Even after cessation of Reductil continued monitoring of the patient by the physician should be encouraged.

4.2 Posology and method of administration

Adults: The initial dose is one (1) capsule of Reductil 10 mg swallowed whole, once daily, in the morning, with liquid (eg a glass of water). The capsule can be taken with or without food.

In those patients with an inadequate response to Reductil 10 mg (defined as less than 2 kg weight loss after four (4) weeks treatment), the dose may be increased to one (1) capsule of Reductil 15 mg once daily, provided that Reductil 10 mg was well tolerated.

Treatment must be discontinued in patients who have responded inadequately to Reductil 15 mg (defined as less than 2 kg weight loss after four (4) weeks treatment). Non-responders are at a higher risk of undesirable effects (see section 4.8 "Undesirable Effects").

Duration of treatment:

Treatment must be discontinued in patients who have not responded adequately, ie whose weight loss stabilises at less than 5% of their initial bodyweight or whose weight loss within three (3) months after starting therapy has been less than 5% of their initial bodyweight. Treatment should not be continued in patients who regain 3 kg or more after previously achieved weight loss.

In patients with associated co-morbid conditions, it is recommended that treatment with Reductil 10 mg / 15 mg should only be continued if it can be shown that the weight loss induced is associated with other clinical benefits, such as improvements in lipid profile in patients with dyslipidaemia or glycaemic control of type 2 diabetes.

Reductil 10 mg / 15 mg should only be given for periods up to one year. Data on use over one year is limited.

4.3 Contraindications

- Known hypersensitivity to sibutramine hydrochloride monohydrate or to any of the excipients

- Organic causes of obesity

- History of major eating disorders

- Psychiatric illness. Sibutramine has shown potential antidepressant activity in animal studies and, therefore it cannot be excluded that sibutramine could induce a manic episode in bipolar patients.

- Gilles de la Tourette's syndrome

- Concomitant use, or use during the past two weeks, of monoamine oxidase inhibitors or of other centrally-acting drugs for the treatment of psychiatric disorders (such as antidepressants, antipsychotics) or for weight reduction, or tryptophan for sleep disturbances.

- History of coronary artery disease, congestive heart failure, tachycardia, peripheral arterial occlusive disease, arrhythmia or cerebrovascular disease (stroke or TIA)

- Inadequately controlled hypertension >145/90 mmHg; see section 4.4 "Special warnings and special precautions")

- Hyperthyroidism

- Severe hepatic impairment

- Severe renal impairment

- Benign prostatic hyperplasia with urinary retention

- Phaeochromocytoma

- Narrow angle glaucoma

- History of drug, medication or alcohol abuse

- Pregnancy and lactation (see section 4.6 "Pregnancy and lactation")

- Children and young adults up to the age of 18 years, owing to insufficient data

- Patients above 65 years of age, owing to insufficient data.

4.4 Special warnings and special precautions for use

Warnings:

Blood pressure and pulse rate should be monitored in all patients on Reductil 10 mg / 15mg, as sibutramine has caused clinically relevant increases in blood pressure in some patients. In the first three months of treatment, these parameters should be checked every 2 weeks; between month 4 and 6 these parameters should be checked once monthly and regularly thereafter, at maximum intervals of three months. Treatment should be discontinued in patients who have an increase, at two consecutive visits, in resting heart rate of $\geq$10 bpm or systolic/diastolic blood pressure of $\geq$ 10 mmHg. In previously well-controlled hypertensive patients, if blood pressure exceeds 145/90 mmHg at two consecutive readings, treatment should be discontinued (see section 4.8 "Undesirable effects, cardiovascular system"). In patients with sleep apnoea syndrome particular care should be taken in monitoring blood pressure.

- For use of sibutramine concomitantly with sympathomimetics, please refer to section 4.5.

- Although sibutramine has not been associated with primary pulmonary hypertension, it is important, in view of general concerns with anti-obesity drugs, to be on the look out for symptoms such as progressive dyspnoea, chest pain and ankle oedema in the course of routine check-ups. The patient should be advised to consult a doctor immediately if these symptoms occur.

- Reductil 10 mg / 15 mg should be given with caution to patients with epilepsy.

- Increased plasma levels have been observed in the assessment of sibutramine in patients with mild to moderate hepatic impairment. Although no adverse effects have been reported, Reductil 10 mg / 15 mg should be used with caution in these patients.

- Although only inactive metabolites are excreted by the renal route, Reductil 10 mg / 15 mg should be used with caution in patients with mild to moderate renal impairment.

- Reductil 10 mg / 15 mg should be given with caution to patients who have a family history of motor or verbal tics.

- Women of child-bearing potential should employ adequate contraception whilst taking Reductil 10 mg / 15 mg.

- There is the possibility of drug abuse with CNS-active drugs. However, available clinical data have shown no evidence of drug abuse with sibutramine.

- There are general concerns that certain anti-obesity drugs are associated with an increased risk of cardiac valvulopathy. However, clinical data show no evidence of an increased incidence with sibutramine.

- Patients with a history of major eating disorders, such as anorexia nervosa and bulimia nervosa, are contraindicated. No data are available for sibutramine in the treatment of patients with binge (compulsive) eating disorder.

- Sibutramine should be given with caution to patients with open angle glaucoma and those who are at risk of raised intraocular pressure, e.g. family history.

- In common with other agents that inhibit serotonin reuptake, there is a potential for an increased risk of bleeding in patients taking sibutramine. Sibutramine should, therefore, be used with caution in patients predisposed to bleeding events and those taking concomitant medications known to affect haemostasis or platelet function.

- Cases of depression, suicidal ideation and suicide have been reported rarely in patients on sibutramine treatment. Special attention is therefore required in patients with a history of depression. If signs or symptoms of depression occur during the treatment with sibutramine, the discontinuation of sibutramine and commencement of an appropriate treatment should be considered.

- Reductil 10 mg / 15 mg contains lactose and therefore should not be used in patients with rare hereditary problems of galactose intolerance, Lapp lactase deficiency or glucose-galactose malabsorption.

4.5 Interaction with other medicinal products and other forms of Interaction

Sibutramine and its active metabolites are eliminated by hepatic metabolism; the main enzyme involved is CYP3A4, and CYP2C9 and CYP1A2 can also contribute. Caution should be exercised on concomitant administration of Reductil 10 mg / 15 mg with drugs which affect CYP3A4 enzyme activity (see section 5.2 "Pharmacokinetic properties"). CYP3A4 inhibitors include ketoconazole, itraconazole, erythromycin, clarithromycin, troleandomycin and cyclosporin. Co-administration of ketoconazole or erythromycin with sibutramine increased plasma concentrations (AUC) of sibutramine active metabolites (23% or 10% respectively) in an interaction study. Mean heart rate increased by up to 2.5 beats per minute more than on sibutramine alone.

Rifampicin, phenytoin, carbamazepine, phenobarbital and dexamethasone are CYP3A4 enzyme inducers and may accelerate sibutramine metabolism, although this has not been studied experimentally.

The simultaneous use of several drugs, each of which increases levels of serotonin in the brain, may give rise to serious interactions. This phenomenon is called serotonin syndrome and may occur in rare cases in connection with the simultaneous use of a selective serotonin reuptake inhibitor [SSRI] together with certain antimigraine drugs (such as sumatriptan, dihydroergotamine), or along with certain opioids (such as pentazocine, pethidine, fentanyl, dextromethorphan), or in the case of simultaneous use of two SSRIs.

As sibutramine inhibits serotonin reuptake (among other effects), Reductil 10 mg / 15mg should not be used concomitantly with other drugs which also raise serotonin levels in the brain.

Concomitant use of Reductil 10 mg / 15 mg with other drugs which may raise the blood pressure or heart rate (e.g. sympathomimetics) has not been systematically evaluated. Drugs of this type include certain cough, cold and allergy medications (eg ephedrine, pseudoephedrine), and certain decongestants (eg xylometazoline). Caution should be used when prescribing Reductil 10 mg / 15 mg to patients who use these medicines.

Reductil 10 mg / 15 mg does not impair the efficacy of oral contraceptives.

At single doses, there was no additional impairment of cognitive or psychomotor performance when sibutramine was administered concomitantly with alcohol. However, the consumption of alcohol is not compatible with the recommended dietary measures as a general rule.

No data on the concomitant use of Reductil 10 mg / 15 mg with orlistat are available.

Two weeks should elapse between stopping sibutramine and starting monoamine oxidase inhibitors.

4.6 Pregnancy and lactation

Use in pregnancy: Sibutramine should not be used during pregnancy. It is generally considered inappropriate for weight-reducing drugs to be used during pregnancy, so women of childbearing potential should employ an adequate method of contraception while taking sibutramine and notify their physician if they become pregnant or intend to become pregnant during therapy. No controlled studies with Reductil have been conducted in pregnant women. Studies in pregnant rabbits have shown effects on reproduction at maternally toxic doses (see section 5.3 "Preclinical safety data"). The relevance of these findings to humans is unknown.

Use in lactation: It is not known whether sibutramine is excreted in human breast milk and therefore administration of Reductil 10 mg / 15 mg is contraindicated during lactation.

4.7 Effects on ability to drive and use machines

Although sibutramine did not affect psychomotor or cognitive performance in healthy volunteers, any centrally-acting drug may impair judgement, thinking or motor skills. Therefore, patients should be cautioned that their ability to drive a vehicle, operate machinery or work in a hazardous environment may be impaired when taking Reductil 10 mg / 15 mg.

4.8 Undesirable effects

Most side effects reported with sibutramine occurred at the start of treatment (during the first 4 weeks). Their severity and frequency diminished over time. They were generally not serious, did not entail discontinuation of treatment, and were reversible.

The side effects observed in phase II/III clinical trials are listed below by body system (very common > 1/10, common $\leq$1/10 and > 1/100):

Body system	Frequency	Undesirable effects
Cardiovascular system (see detailed information below)	Common	Tachycardia Palpitations Raised blood pressure/ hypertension Vasodilation (hot flush)
Gastrointestinal system	Very common	Constipation
	Common	Nausea Haemorrhoid aggravation
Central nervous system	Very common	Dry mouth Insomnia
	Commom	Light-headedness Paraesthesia Headache Anxiety
Skin	Common	Sweating
Sensory functions	Common	Taste perversion

Cardiovascular system

A mean increase in resting systolic and diastolic blood pressure of 2-3 mmHg, and a mean increase in heart rate of 3-7 beats per minute have been observed. Higher increases in blood pressure and heart rate cannot be excluded in isolated cases.

Any clinically significant increase in blood pressure and pulse rate tends to occur early on in treatment (first 4-12 weeks). Therapy should be discontinued in such cases (see Section 4.4 "Special warnings and special precautions.").

For use of Reductil 10 mg / 15 mg in patients with hypertension, see section 4.3 "Contraindications" and 4.4 "Special warnings and special precautions".

Clinically significant adverse events seen in clinical studies and during postmarketing surveillance are listed below by body system:

Blood and lymphatic system disorders:

Thrombocytopenia, Henoch-Schonlein purpura

Cardiovascular disorders:

Atrial fibrillation, paroxysmal supraventricular tachycardia

Immune system disorders:

Allergic hypersensitivity reactions ranging from mild skin eruptions and urticaria to angioedema and anaphylaxis have been reported

Psychiatric disorders:

Agitation

Depression in patients both with and without a prior history of depression (see section 4.4).

Nervous system disorders:

SeizuresSerotonin syndrome in combination with other agents affecting serotonin release (section 4.5).

Transient short-term memory disturbance

Eye disorders:

Blurred vision

Gastrointestinal disorders:

Diarrhoea, vomiting

Skin and subcutaneous tissue disorders:

Alopecia, rash, urticaria

Renal and urinary disorders:

Acute interstitial nephritis, mesangiocapillary glomerulonephritis, urinary retention

Reproductive system and breast disorders:

Abnormal ejaculation/orgasm, impotence, menstrual cycle disorders, metrorrhagia

Investigations:

Reversible increases in liver enzymes

Other:

Withdrawal symptoms such as headache and increased appetite have rarely been reported

4.9 Overdose

There is limited experience of overdosing with sibutramine. No specific therapeutic measures are recommended and there is no specific antidote. Treatment should consist of the general measures employed in the management of overdosing, such as keeping airways unobstructed, monitoring of cardiovascular functions and general symptomatic and supportive measures. Early administration of activated charcoal may delay the absorption of sibutramine. Gastric lavage may also be of benefit. Cautious use of beta-blockers may be indicated in patients with elevated blood pressure or tachycardia.

There are a number of reports of overdose in humans (including accidental ingestion by children as young as 18 months) where doses of up to 500 mg sibutramine hydrochloride monohydrate were ingested. A heart rate of 160 beats per minute was observed in one patient who took 500 mg sibutramine hydrochloride monohydrate. Except in one case of multiple drug intoxication with alcohol (where the patient died, possibly due to inhalation of vomit), there were no complications and the individuals made a full recovery.

5. PHARMACOLOGICAL PROPERTIES

5.1 Pharmacodynamic properties

Pharmacotherapeutic group: anti-obesity drug, ATC code A08A A10.

Sibutramine produces its therapeutic effects predominantly via its active secondary and primary amine metabolites (metabolite 1 and metabolite 2) which are inhibitors of noradrenaline, serotonin (5-hydroxytryptamine; 5-HT) and dopamine reuptake. In human brain tissue, metabolite 1 and metabolite 2 are ~3-fold more potent as in vitro inhibitors of noradrenaline and serotonin reuptake than of dopamine reuptake. Plasma samples taken from sibutramine-treated volunteers caused significant inhibition of both noradrenaline reuptake (73%) and serotonin reuptake (54%) with no significant inhibition of dopamine reuptake (16%). Sibutramine and its metabolites are neither monoamine-releasing agents nor are they monoamine oxidase inhibitors. They have no affinity with a large number of neurotransmitter receptors, including serotonergic (5-HT_1, 5-HT_{1A}, 5-HT_{1B}, 5-HT_{2A}, 5-HT_{2C}), adrenergic (β_1, β_2, β_3, α_1, α_2), dopaminergic (D_1-like, D_2-like), muscarinic, histaminergic (H_1), benzodiazepine and NMDA receptors.

In animal models using lean growing and obese rats, sibutramine produces a reduction in bodyweight gain. This is believed to result from its impact on food intake, ie by enhancing satiety, but enhanced thermogenesis also contributes to weight loss. These effects have been shown to be mediated by the inhibition of serotonin and noradrenaline re-uptake.

In clinical trials in man, Reductil was shown to effect weight loss by enhancing satiety. Data are also available which demonstrate a thermogenic effect of Reductil by attenuating the adaptive decline in resting metabolic rate during weight loss. Weight loss induced by Reductil is accompanied by beneficial changes in serum lipids and glycaemic control in patients with dyslipidaemia and type 2 diabetes, respectively.

In obese patients with type 2 diabetes mellitus weight loss with sibutramine was associated with mean reductions of 0.6% (unit) in HbA_{1c}. Similarly, in obese patients with dyslipidaemia, weight loss was associated with increases in HDL cholesterol of 12-22% and reductions in triglycerides of 9-21%.

5.2 Pharmacokinetic properties

Sibutramine is well absorbed and undergoes extensive first-pass metabolism. Peak plasma levels (C_{max}) were achieved 1.2 hours after a single oral dose of 20 mg of sibutramine hydrochloride monohydrate. The half-life of the parent compound is 1.1 hours. The pharmacologically active metabolites 1 and 2 reach C_{max} in three hours with elimination half-lives of 14 and 16 hours, respectively. Linear kinetics have been demonstrated over the dose range of 10 to 30 mg, with no dose-related change in the elimination half-lives but a dose-proportionate increase in plasma concentrations. On repeated dosing, steady-state concentrations of metabolites 1 and 2 are achieved within 4 days, with an approximately 2-fold accumulation. The pharmacokinetics of sibutramine and its metabolites in obese subjects are similar to those in normal weight subjects. The relatively limited data available so far provide no evidence of a clinically relevant difference in the pharmacokinetics of males and females. The pharmacokinetic profile observed in elderly healthy subjects (mean age 70 years) was similar to that seen in young healthy subjects. In subjects with moderate hepatic impairment, bioavailability of the active metabolites was 24% higher after a single dose of sibutramine. Plasma protein binding of sibutramine and its metabolites 1 and 2 amounts to approximately 97%, 94% and 94%, respectively. Hepatic metabolism is the major route of elimination of sibutramine and its active metabolites 1 and 2. Other (inactive) metabolites are excreted primarily via the urine, at a urine: faeces ratio of 10: 1.

In vitro hepatic microsome studies indicated that CYP3A4 is the major cytochrome P450 isoenzyme responsible for sibutramine metabolism. In vitro, there was no indication of an affinity with CYP2D6, a low capacity enzyme involved in pharmacokinetic interactions with various drugs. Further in vitro studies have revealed that sibutramine has no significant effect on the activity of the major P450 isoenzymes, including CYP3A4. The CYP450s involved in the further metabolism of metabolite 2 were shown (in vitro) to be CYP3A4 and CYP2C9. Although there are no data at present, it is likely that CYP3A4 is also involved in further metabolism of metabolite 1.

5.3 Preclinical safety data

The toxicity of sibutramine seen after single doses in experimental animals has generally been a result of exaggerated pharmacodynamic effects. Longer-term treatment was associated with only mild pathological changes and secondary or species-related findings. It follows that they are unlikely to present concerns during the proper clinical use of sibutramine. Reproduction studies were conducted in rats and rabbits. In rabbits, one study showed a slightly higher incidence of fetal cardiovascular anomalies in the treatment groups than in the control group, while another study showed a lower incidence than in controls. In addition, in the latter study but not in the former, the treatment group had slightly more fetuses with two minor anomalies (a tiny thread-like ossified connection between the maxilla and jugal bones, and very slight differences in the spacing of the roots of some small arteries from the aortic arch). The relevance of these findings to humans is unknown. Sibutramine's use in human pregnancy has not been investigated. Extensive genetic toxicity tests disclosed no evidence of sibutramine-induced mutagenicity. Studies in rodents have shown that sibutramine has no carcinogenic potential relevant to man.

6. PHARMACEUTICAL PARTICULARS

6.1 List of excipients

Capsule content: lactose monohydrate, magnesium stearate, microcrystalline cellulose, colloidal anhydrous silica.

Capsule shell (10 mg): indigo carmine (E 132), titanium dioxide (E 171), gelatin, sodium lauryl sulphate, quinoline yellow (E 104).

Capsule shell (15 mg): indigo carmine (E 132), titanium dioxide (E 171), gelatin, sodium lauryl sulphate.

Printing ink: dimethicone, iron oxides and hydroxides (E 172), shellac, soybean lecithin (E 322), titanium dioxide (E 171).

6.2 Incompatibilities

Not applicable

6.3 Shelf life

3 years

6.4 Special precautions for storage

Do not store above 25°C. Store in the original package.

6.5 Nature and contents of container

Reductil 10 mg / 15 mg, capsules in a PVC/PVDC blister strip pack.

Calendar pack containing 28 capsules (4 weeks)

6.6 Instructions for use and handling

No special requirements

7. MARKETING AUTHORISATION HOLDER

Abbott Laboratories Limited

Queenborough

Kent

ME11 5EL

United Kingdom

8. MARKETING AUTHORISATION NUMBER(S)

Reductil 10 mg: PL 0037/0326

Reductil 15 mg: PL 0037/0327

9. DATE OF FIRST AUTHORISATION/RENEWAL OF THE AUTHORISATION

14 January 2004

10. DATE OF REVISION OF THE TEXT

February 2005

Refacto

(Wyeth Pharmaceuticals)

1. NAME OF THE MEDICINAL PRODUCT

ReFacto 250 IU, ReFacto 500 IU, ReFacto 1000 IU, ReFacto 2000 IU powder and solvent for solution for injection.

2. QUALITATIVE AND QUANTITATIVE COMPOSITION

ReFacto is presented as a lyophilised powder for solution for injection containing nominally 250 IU, 500 IU, 1000 IU or 2000 IU moroctocog alfa (recombinant coagulation factor VIII) per vial.

The product contains approximately 62.5 IU/ml, 125 IU/ml, 250 IU/ml or 500 IU/ml recombinant coagulation factor VIII when reconstituted with 4 ml of 0.9% w/v sodium chloride solution for injection.

The potency (IU) is determined using the European Pharmacopoeia chromogenic assay. The specific activity of ReFacto is approximately 11000 IU/mg protein.

ReFacto contains recombinant coagulation factor VIII (INN=moroctocog alfa). Moroctocog alfa is a purified protein that has 1438 amino acids. It has an amino acid sequence that is comparable to the 90 + 80 kDa form of factor VIII (i.e. B-domain deleted), and post-translational modifications that are similar to those of the plasma-derived molecule. Recombinant coagulation factor VIII is a glycoprotein that is secreted by genetically engineered mammalian cells derived from a Chinese hamster ovary (CHO) cell line.

For excipients, see 6.1.

3. PHARMACEUTICAL FORM

Powder and solvent for solution for injection.

4. CLINICAL PARTICULARS

4.1 Therapeutic indications

Treatment and prophylaxis of bleeding in patients with haemophilia A (congenital factor VIII deficiency).

ReFacto does not contain von Willebrand factor and hence is not indicated in von Willebrand's disease.

4.2 Posology and method of administration

Treatment should be initiated under the supervision of a physician experienced in the treatment of haemophilia A.

Posology

ReFacto is appropriate for use in adults and children of all ages, including new-borns. Safety and efficacy studies have been performed both in previously treated children and adolescents (n=31, ages 8-18 years) and in previously untreated neonates, infants and children (n=101, ages <1-52 months). The labelled potency of ReFacto is based on the European Pharmacopoeial chromogenic substrate assay. With ReFacto, the chromogenic assay yields results which are higher than the results obtained with the one-stage clotting assay.

When monitoring patients' factor VIII activity levels during treatment, it is strongly recommended that the European Pharmacopoeial chromogenic substrate assay be used.

The dosage and duration of the substitution therapy depend on the severity of the factor VIII deficiency, on the location and extent of bleeding, and on the patient's clinical condition. Doses administered should be titrated to the patient's clinical response. In the presence of an inhibitor, higher doses or appropriate specific treatment may be required. Dosage adjustment for patients with renal or hepatic impairment has not been studied in clinical trials.

The number of units of factor VIII administered is expressed in International Units (IU), which are related to the current WHO standard for factor VIII products. Factor VIII activity in plasma is expressed either as a percentage (relative to normal human plasma) or in International Units (relative to an International Standard for factor VIII in plasma). One International Unit (IU) of factor VIII activity is equivalent to the quantity of factor VIII in one ml of normal human plasma. The calculation of the required dosage of factor VIII is based upon the empirical finding that 1 International Unit (IU) of factor VIII per kg body weight raises the plasma factor VIII activity by 2 IU/dl per IU/kg administered. The required dosage is determined using the following formula:

Required units = body weight (kg) × desired factor VIII rise (% or IU/dl) × 0.5 (IU/kg per IU/dl)

The amount to be administered and the frequency of administration should always be oriented to the clinical effectiveness in the individual case.

In the case of the following haemorrhagic events, the factor VIII activity should not fall below the given plasma levels (in % of normal or in IU/dl) in the corresponding period. The following table can be used to guide dosing in bleeding episodes and surgery:

Degree of haemorrhage/ Type of surgical procedure	Factor VIII level required (% or IU/dl)	Frequency of doses (hours)/ Duration of therapy (days)
Haemorrhage		
Early haemarthrosis, muscle bleeding or oral bleeding	20-40	Repeat every 12 to 24 hours. At least 1 day, until the bleeding episode as indicated by pain is resolved or healing is achieved.
More extensive haemarthrosis, muscle bleeding or haematoma	30-60	Repeat infusion every 12-24 hours for 3-4 days or more until pain and acute disability are resolved.
Life threatening haemorrhages	60-100	Repeat infusion every 8 to 24 hours until threat is resolved
Surgery		
Minor including tooth extraction	30-60	Every 24 hours, at least 1 day, until healing is achieved.
Major	80-100 (pre- and post-operative)	Repeat infusion every 8-24 hours until adequate wound healing, then therapy for at least another 7 days to maintain a factor VIII activity of 30% to 60% (IU/dl)

During the course of treatment, appropriate determination of factor VIII levels is advised to guide the dose to be administered and the frequency of repeated infusions. In the case of major surgical interventions in particular, precise monitoring of the substitution therapy by means of coagulation analysis (plasma factor VIII activity) is indispensable. Individual patients may vary in their response to factor VIII, achieving different levels of *in vivo* recovery and demonstrating different half-lives.

For long-term prophylaxis against bleeding in patients with severe haemophilia A, the usual doses are 20 to 40 IU of factor VIII per kg body weight at intervals of 2 to 3 days. In some cases, especially in younger patients, shorter dosage intervals or higher doses may be necessary.

In a clinical trial setting the mean dose per infusion of ReFacto for bleeding episodes in children less than 6 years of age was higher than the mean dose administered to older children and adults (51.3 IU/kg and 29.3 IU/kg, respectively).

Children less than 6 years of age on a prophylaxis regimen during the clinical trials used an average dose of 50 IU/kg of ReFacto and experienced an average of 6.1 bleeding episodes per year. Older children and adults on a prophylaxis regimen used an average dose of 27 IU/kg and experienced an average of 10 bleeding episodes per year.

Patients using ReFacto should be monitored for the development of factor VIII inhibitors. If expected factor VIII activity plasma levels are not attained, or if bleeding is not controlled with an appropriate dose, an assay should be performed to determine if a factor VIII inhibitor is present. If the inhibitor is present at levels less than 10 Bethesda Units (BU), administration of additional antihaemophilic factor may neutralize the inhibitor. In patients with high levels of inhibitor, (eg. above 10 BU), factor VIII therapy may not be effective and other therapeutic options should be considered. Management of such patients should be directed by physicians with experience in the care of patients with haemophilia. See also 4.4.

Method of administration

ReFacto is administered by intravenous (IV) injection after reconstitution of the lyophilised powder for injection with 0.9% w/v sodium chloride solution for injection (provided). The reconstituted solution should be used within 3 hours.

ReFacto should be injected intravenously over several minutes. The rate of administration should be determined by the patient's comfort level.

4.3 Contraindications

Hypersensitivity to the active substance or to any of the excipients. Known allergic reaction to mouse or hamster proteins.

4.4 Special warnings and special precautions for use

As with any intravenous protein product, allergic type hypersensitivity reactions are possible. The product contains traces of mouse and hamster proteins. Patients should be informed of the early signs of hypersensitivity reactions including hives, generalised urticaria, tightness of the chest, wheezing, hypotension, and anaphylaxis. If allergic or anaphylactic reactions occur, administration of ReFacto should be discontinued immediately, and an appropriate treatment must be initiated. In case of shock, the current medical standards for shock-treatment should be observed. Patients should be advised to discontinue use of the product and contact their physician/ or seek immediate emergency care, depending on the type/severity of the reaction, is any of these symptoms occur.

The formation of neutralising antibodies (inhibitors) to factor VIII is a known complication in the management of individuals with haemophilia A. These inhibitors are usually IgG immunoglobulins directed against the factor VIII procoagulant activity, which are quantified in Bethesda Units (BU) per ml of plasma using the modified assay. The risk of developing inhibitors is correlated to the exposure to antihaemophilic factor VIII, this risk being highest within the first 20 exposure days. In the post-marketing setting, high and low titre inhibitors have been observed in previously treated patients. Patients treated with recombinant coagulation factor VIII should be carefully monitored for the development of inhibitors by appropriate clinical observations and laboratory tests. See also 4.8. Undesirable effects.

Reports of lack of effect, mainly in prophylaxis patients, have been received in the clinical trials and in the post-marketing setting. The reported lack of effect has been described as bleeding into target joints, bleeding into new joints or a subjective feeling by the patient of new onset bleeding. When switching to ReFacto it is important to individually titrate and monitor each patient's dose in order to ensure an adequate therapeutic response.

In the interest of patients, it is recommended that, whenever possible, every time that ReFacto is administered to them, the name and batch number of the product is recorded.

4.5 Interaction with other medicinal products and other forms of Interaction

No interactions of recombinant factor VIII products with other medicinal products are known.

4.6 Pregnancy and lactation

Animal reproduction studies have not been conducted with factor VIII. Based on the rare occurrence of haemophilia A in women, experience regarding the use of factor VIII during pregnancy and breast-feeding is not available. Therefore, factor VIII should be used during pregnancy and lactation only if clearly indicated.

4.7 Effects on ability to drive and use machines

There are no indications that ReFacto may impair the ability to drive or operate machines.

4.8 Undesirable effects

Hypersensitivity or allergic reactions (which may include angioedema, burning and stinging at the infusion site, chills, flushing, generalized urticaria, headache, hives, hypotension, lethargy, nausea, restlessness, tachycardia, tightness of the chest, tingling, vomiting, wheezing) have been observed infrequently, and may in some cases progress to severe anaphylaxis (including shock).

On rare occasions, fever has been observed.

The following adverse events have also been reported: dyspnoea, venous access catheter complications, paraesthesia, transaminase elevation, dizziness, somnolence, fatigue, perspiration, blurred vision, coughing, acne, altered taste, anorexia, gastritis, gastroenteritis, pain, pruritis, rash, increased bilirubin and slight creatine phosphokinase muscle brain isotype (CK MB) elevation.

The occurrence of neutralising antibodies (inhibitors) is well known in the treatment of patients with haemophilia A.

In a clinical trial, 32 out of 101 (32%) previously untreated patients treated with ReFacto developed inhibitors: 16 out of 101 (16%) with a titre > 5 BU and 16 out of 101 (16%) with a titre ⩽ 5 BU. The median number of exposure days up to inhibitor development in these patients was 12 days (range 3 - 49 days). Of the 16 patients with high titres, 15 received immune tolerance (IT) treatment. Of the 16 patients with low titres IT treatment was started in 10. IT had an efficacy of 73% for patients with high titres and 90% for those with low titres.

For all 101 treated PUPs, regardless of inhibitor development, the median number of exposure days is 197 days (range 1-1299 days).

In a clinical trial of ReFacto, one of 113 (0.9%) previously treated patients developed an inhibitor. Inhibitor development occurred in the same time frame as the development of monoclonal gammopathy of uncertain significance. The development of this inhibitor was associated with a bleeding episode that failed to respond to ReFacto treatment. Also there have been spontaneous postmarketing reports of high titre inhibitors involving previously treated patients.

Twenty of 113 (18%) previously treated patients (PTPs) had an increase in anti-CHO antibody titre, without any apparent clinical effect. Six of 113 PTPs (5.3%) had an increase in anti-mouse IgG antibody titre, without any apparent clinical effect.

Very rarely development of antibodies to hamster protein has been measured, but there were no clinical sequelae.

If any reaction takes place that is thought to be related to the administration of ReFacto, the rate of infusion should be decreased or the infusion stopped, as dictated by the response of the patient.

4.9 Overdose

No symptoms of overdose have been reported with recombinant coagulation factor VIII products.

5. PHARMACOLOGICAL PROPERTIES

5.1 Pharmacodynamic properties

Pharmacotherapeutic group: antihaemorrhagics blood coagulation factor VIII;

ATC code: B02BD02.

ReFacto, recombinant coagulation factor VIII is a glycoprotein with an approximate molecular mass of 170,000 Da consisting of 1438 amino acids. ReFacto is a recombinant DNA-based substance which has functional characteristics comparable to those of endogenous factor VIII. Factor VIII activity is greatly reduced in patients with haemophilia A and therefore replacement therapy is necessary.

When infused into a haemophiliac patient, factor VIII binds to von Willebrand factor in the patient's circulation.

Activated factor VIII acts as a cofactor for activated factor IX accelerating the conversion of factor X to activated factor X. Activated factor X converts prothrombin into thrombin. Thrombin then converts fibrinogen into fibrin and a clot is formed. Haemophilia A is a sex-linked hereditary disorder of blood coagulation due to decreased levels of factor VIII:C and results in profuse bleeding into joints, muscles or internal organs, either spontaneously or as a result of accidental or surgical trauma. By replacement therapy the plasma levels of factor VIII are increased, thereby enabling a temporary correction of the factor deficiency and correction of the bleeding tendencies.

Pharmacodynamic data on ReFacto in the form of incremental recovery (k-value, IU/dl per IU/kg) are available at baseline for 45 children less than 6 years of age (age range 1 – 44 months). On average in this population, the incremental recovery was 1.7 ± 0.4 IU/dl per IU/kg (range 0.2 - 2.8) as compared with average incremental recovery of 2.4 ± 0.4 IU/dl per IU/kg (range 1.1 – 3.8) in 85 older children and adults.

5.2 Pharmacokinetic properties

The pharmacokinetic parameters derived from a crossover study of ReFacto in 18 previously treated patients are listed in the table below.

PK parameter	Mean	SD	Median
AUC_{0-t} (IU-h/ml)	19.9	4.9	19.9
$t_{1/2}$ (h)	14.8	5.6	12.7
CL (ml/h/kg)	2.4	0.75	2.3
MRT (h)	20.2	7.4	18.0
K-value (IU/dl increase in FVIII:C per IU/kg FVIII given)	2.4	0.38	2.5

Results obtained from this pharmacokinetic study, using a central laboratory for the analysis of plasma samples, showed that the one-stage assay gave results which were approximately 50% of the values obtained with the chromogenic assay (see 4.2).

In additional clinical studies, pharmacokinetic parameters measured using the chromogenic assay were determined for previously treated patients (PTPs) and previously untreated patients (PUPs). In PTPs (n=101), ReFacto had a recovery at Week 0 of 2.4 ± 0.4 IU/dl per IU/kg (range 1.1 to 3.8 IU/dl per IU/kg). In measurements over 4 years of use, the mean incremental recovery was reproducible and ranged from 2.3 to 2.5 IU/dl per IU/kg. A subset of 37 study subjects had evaluable pharmacokinetic profiles at both baseline and Month 12 that were stable. In PUPs (n=59), ReFacto had a mean recovery at Week 0 of 1.5 ± 0.6IU/dl per IU/kg (range 0.2 to 2.8 IU/dl per IU/kg). Recovery for PUPs was stable over time (5 visits during a 2 year period) and ranged from 1.5 to 1.8 IU/dl per IU/kg of ReFacto.

5.3 Preclinical safety data

In preclinical studies ReFacto was used to safely and effectively restore haemostasis. ReFacto and plasma-derived factor VIII demonstrated similar toxicological profiles when tested in repeated dose toxicology studies in animals.

ReFacto shows no genotoxic properties in the mouse micronucleus assay. No other mutagenicity studies and no investigations on carcinogenesis, impairment of fertility or foetal development have been conducted.

6. PHARMACEUTICAL PARTICULARS

6.1 List of excipients

Powder

Sucrose

Calcium chloride

L-histidine

Polysorbate 80

Sodium chloride

Solvent

Sodium chloride

6.2 Incompatibilities

This medicinal product must not be mixed with other medicinal products, including other infusion solutions.

Only the provided infusion set should be used. Treatment failure can occur as a consequence of human coagulation factor VIII adsorption to the internal surfaces of some infusion equipment.

6.3 Shelf life

2 years.

The reconstituted solution should be used immediately or within 3 hours.

6.4 Special precautions for storage

Store at 2°C - 8°C. Do not freeze.

For the purpose of ambulatory use, the product may be removed from the refrigerator for one single period of maximum 3 months at room temperature (do not store above 25°C).

The product may not be returned to refrigerated storage after storage at room temperature. During storage, avoid prolonged exposure of the ReFacto vial to light.

6.5 Nature and contents of container

The container-closure system for ReFacto consists of an injection vial, 10 ml, glass type I, stoppered with a bromobutyl rubber stopper and sealed with a flip off seal.

Each vial of ReFacto is provided with one prefilled syringe containing 4 ml of 0.9% w/v sodium chloride solution for injection, and accessories required for reconstitution and administration (vial adapter, alcohol swabs, sterile infusion set, plaster and gauze).

6.6 Instructions for use and handling

Do not use after the expiry date given on the label.

Reconstitute lyophilised ReFacto powder for injection with the supplied diluent (0.9% w/v sodium chloride solution) from the prefilled syringe provided. Gently rotate the vial until all powder is dissolved.

ReFacto, when reconstituted, contains polysorbate-80, which is known to increase the rate of di-(2-ethylhexyl)phthalate (DEHP) extraction from polyvinyl chloride (PVC). This should be considered during the preparation and administration of ReFacto, including storage time elapsed in a PVC container following reconstitution. It is important that the recommendations in 4.2 POSOLOGY AND METHOD OF ADMINISTRATION be followed closely.

After reconstitution, the solution is drawn back into the syringe. The solution should be clear and colourless. The solution should be discarded if visible particulate matter or discolouration is observed.

After reconstitution, the medicinal product should be used immediately or within 3 hours.

Any unused product or waste material should be disposed of in accordance with local requirements.

7. MARKETING AUTHORISATION HOLDER

Wyeth Europa Ltd

Huntercombe Lane South

Taplow, Maidenhead

Berkshire, SL6 0PH

United Kingdom

8. MARKETING AUTHORISATION NUMBER(S)

ReFacto 250 IU powder and solvent for solution for injection: EU/1/99/103/001

ReFacto 500 IU powder and solvent for solution for injection: EU/1/99/103/002

ReFacto 1000 IU powder and solvent for solution for injection: EU/1/99/103/003

ReFacto 2000 IU powder and solvent for solution for injection: EU/1/99/103/004

9. DATE OF FIRST AUTHORISATION/RENEWAL OF THE AUTHORISATION

19 December 2002

10. DATE OF REVISION OF THE TEXT

Approved 28 July 2005

Refolinon Injection 2 ml / 10 ml

(Pharmacia Limited)

1. NAME OF THE MEDICINAL PRODUCT

Refolinon Injection

2. QUALITATIVE AND QUANTITATIVE COMPOSITION

Clear pale yellow liquid for injection containing leucovorin 3 mg/ml in ampoules of 2 ml and 10 ml, as the calcium salt

3. PHARMACEUTICAL FORM

Solution for injection

4. CLINICAL PARTICULARS

4.1 Therapeutic indications

Leucovorin (Folinic Acid) is the formyl derivative of tetrahydrofolic acid and is an intermediate product of the metabolism of folic acid. Leucovorin is used in cytotoxic therapy as an antidote to folic acid antagonists such as methotrexate. Leucovorin is effective in the treatment of megaloblastic anaemia due to folate deficiency.

Warning: Leucovorin should not be given simultaneously with a folic acid antagonist, for the purpose of reducing or preventing clinical toxicity, as the therapeutic effect of the antagonist may be nullified.

4.2 Posology and method of administration

Adults and Children:

Leucovorin rescue: depending upon the dose of methotrexate administered.

Dosage regimens of Leucovorin Calcium vary. Up to 120 mg Leucovorin Calcium are generally given, usually in divided doses over 12-24 hours by intramuscular injection, bolus intravenous injection or intravenous infusion in normal saline. This is followed by 12-15 mg intramuscularly or 15 mg orally every 6 hours for 48 hours. Rescue therapy is usually started 24 hours after the commencement of methotrexate administration. If overdosage of methotrexate is suspected, the dose of Leucovorin Calcium should be equal to or greater than the dose of methotrexate and should be administered within one hour of the methotrexate administration.

4.3 Contraindications

None stated.

4.4 Special warnings and special precautions for use

High dose methotrexate therapy together with Leucovorin rescue should only be carried out under the direction of physicians experienced in antitumour chemotherapy.

Calcium Folinate should not be used for the treatment of pernicious anaemia or other megaloblastic anaemia where vitamin B12 is deficient.

4.5 Interaction with other medicinal products and other forms of Interaction

Leucovorin should not be given simultaneously with a folic acid antagonist, for the purpose of reducing or preventing clinical toxicity, as the therapeutic effect of the antagonist may be nullified.

4.6 Pregnancy and lactation

None stated.

4.7 Effects on ability to drive and use machines

None stated.

4.8 Undesirable effects

Adverse reactions to Leucovorin Calcium are rare, but following parenteral administration occasional pyrexial reactions have been reported.

4.9 Overdose

None stated.

5. PHARMACOLOGICAL PROPERTIES

5.1 Pharmacodynamic properties

Methotrexate Rescue:

Leucovorin (5-Formyltetrahydrofolate) acts partly by providing a fresh supply of tetrahydrofolate and also by competitively displacing methotrexate from dihydrofolate reductase so that its excretion is accelerated (methotrexate binds to the enzyme dihydrofolate reductase which is responsible for reducing dietary folic acid to dihydrofolate and tetrahydrofolate thus inhibiting its action).

Megaloblastic Anaemia:

Leucovorin is an active folic acid derivative and it can therefore relieve pathological conditions associated with folic acid deficiency, e.g. megaloblastic anaemia.

5.2 Pharmacokinetic properties

The bioavailability of Leucovorin following administration of both tablet and parenteral formulations is comparable. After 30 minutes approximately 90% of the total reduced folates were assayed as 5-methyltetrahydrofolate following oral administration compared with only 72% following I.M. administration. The half-life of Leucovorin after reaching peak plasma levels was 35-45 minutes by both routes. Peak serum tetrahydrofolate levels were reached 2 hours after oral administration and approximately 40 minutes after I.M. adminstration.

5.3 Preclinical safety data

None stated.

6. PHARMACEUTICAL PARTICULARS

6.1 List of excipients

Sodium Chloride

Sodium Hydroxide

Hydrochloric Acid

Water for injections

6.2 Incompatibilities

None stated.

6.3 Shelf life

24 Months

6.4 Special precautions for storage

Store at 2°C – 8°C and protect from light.

6.5 Nature and contents of container

Type 1 colourless glass ampoules containing 2 or 10 ml. Packs of 5 or 10 ampoules.

6.6 Instructions for use and handling

Protect from light.

7. MARKETING AUTHORISATION HOLDER

Pharmacia Limited

Davy Avenue

Milton Keynes

MK5 8PH

United Kingdom

8. MARKETING AUTHORISATION NUMBER(S)

PL 00032/0346

9. DATE OF FIRST AUTHORISATION/RENEWAL OF THE AUTHORISATION

17th July 2002

10. DATE OF REVISION OF THE TEXT

16th December 2004

Refolinon Tablets

(Pharmacia Limited)

1. NAME OF THE MEDICINAL PRODUCT

Refolinon Tablets

2. QUALITATIVE AND QUANTITATIVE COMPOSITION

Leucovorin calcium equivalent to

leucovorin (folinic acid) 15.0 mg

3. PHARMACEUTICAL FORM

Uncoated tablet for oral use

4. CLINICAL PARTICULARS

4.1 Therapeutic indications

Leucovorin (folinic acid) is the formyl derivative of tetrahydrofolic acid and is an intermediate product of the metabolism of folic acid. Leucovorin is used in cytotoxic therapy as an antidote to folic acid antagonists such as methotrexate. Leucovorin is effective in the treatment of megaloblastic anaemia.

4.2 Posology and method of administration
To be given orally.

Adults and children:

Leucovorin rescue: Depending upon the dose of methotrexate administered, dosage regimens of leucovorin calcium vary. Up to 120 mg leucovorin calcium are generally given, usually in divided doses over 12-24 hours by intramuscular injection, bolus intravenous injection or intravenous infusion in normal saline. This is followed by 12-15 mg intramuscularly or 15 mg orally every 6 hours for 48 hours. Rescue therapy is usually started 24 hours after the commencement of methotrexate administration.

If overdosage of methotrexate is suspected, the dose of leucovorin calcium should be equal to or greater than the dose of methotrexate and should be administered within one hour of the methotrexate administration.

Megaloblastic anaemia (folate deficiency): 15 mg (one tablet) leucovorin per day.

4.3 Contraindications
None stated.

4.4 Special warnings and special precautions for use
High dose methotrexate therapy together with leucovorin rescue should only be carried out under the direction of physicians experienced in antitumour chemotherapy.

Calcium folinate should not be used for the treatment of pernicious anaemia where vitamin B_{12} is deficient.

4.5 Interaction with other medicinal products and other forms of Interaction
Leucovorin should not be given simultaneously with a folic acid antagonist, for the purpose of reducing or preventing clinical toxicity, as the therapeutic effect of the antagonist may be nullified.

4.6 Pregnancy and lactation
None stated.

4.7 Effects on ability to drive and use machines
None known.

4.8 Undesirable effects
Adverse reactions to leucovorin calcium are rare, but following parenteral administration occasional pyrexial reactions have been reported.

4.9 Overdose
There are no special instructions.

5. PHARMACOLOGICAL PROPERTIES

5.1 Pharmacodynamic properties
Methotrexate rescue: Leucovorin (5-formyltetrahydrofolinate) acts partly by providing a fresh supply of tetrahydrofolate and also by competitively displacing methotrexate from dihydrofolate reductase so that its excretion is accelerated (methotrexate binds to the enzyme dihydrofolate reductase which is responsible for reducing dietary folic acid to dihydrofolate and tetrahydrofolate thus inhibiting its action.

Megaloblastic anaemia: Leucovorin is an active folic acid derivative and it can therefore relieve pathological conditions associated with folic acid deficiency e.g. megaloblastic anaemia.

5.2 Pharmacokinetic properties
The bioavailability of leucovorin following administration of both tablet and parenteral formulations is comparable. After 30 minutes approximately 90% of the total reduced folates were assayed as 5-methyltetrahydrofolate following oral administration compared with only 72% following i.m. administration. The half-life of leucovorin after reaching peak plasma levels was 35-45 minutes by both routes. Peak serum tetrahydrofolate levels were reached 2 hours after oral administration and approximately 40 minutes after i.m administration.

5.3 Preclinical safety data
None stated.

6. PHARMACEUTICAL PARTICULARS

6.1 List of excipients
Avicel PH101 NF

Magnesium stearate Ph. Eur

Lactose Ph. Eur

6.2 Incompatibilities
None known.

6.3 Shelf life
60 months.

6.4 Special precautions for storage
None stated.

6.5 Nature and contents of container
The tablets are contained in white high density polyethylene containers with polyethylene screw closures. The bottles contain 30 or 100 tablets.

6.6 Instructions for use and handling
The tablets are contained in white high density polyethylene containers with polyethylene screw closures. The bottles contain 30 or 100 tablets.

7. MARKETING AUTHORISATION HOLDER
Pharmacia Ltd

Davy Avenue

Milton Keynes

MK5 8PH

United Kingdom

8. MARKETING AUTHORISATION NUMBER(S)
PL 00032/0347

9. DATE OF FIRST AUTHORISATION/RENEWAL OF THE AUTHORISATION
15 December 2003

10. DATE OF REVISION OF THE TEXT
03 February 2004

Regaine for Men Extra Strength

(Pfizer Consumer Healthcare)

1. NAME OF THE MEDICINAL PRODUCT
Regaine for Men Extra Strength

2. QUALITATIVE AND QUANTITATIVE COMPOSITION
Minoxidil 50 mg/ml (5%w/v).

3. PHARMACEUTICAL FORM
Cutaneous Solution

4. CLINICAL PARTICULARS

4.1 Therapeutic indications
Regaine for Men Extra Strength is indicated for the treatment of alopecia androgenetica in men.

Onset and degree of hair regrowth may be variable among users. Although trends in the data suggest that those users who are younger, who have been balding for a shorter period of time or who have a smaller area of baldness on the vertex are more likely to respond to Regaine for Men Extra Strength, individual responses cannot be predicted.

4.2 Posology and method of administration
Men aged 18-65:

Hair and scalp should be thoroughly dry prior to topical application of Regaine for Men Extra Strength. A dose of 1 ml Regaine for Men Extra Strength cutaneous solution should be applied to the total affected areas of the scalp twice daily. The total dosage should not exceed 2 ml. If fingertips are used to facilitate drug application, hands should be washed afterwards.

It may take twice daily applications for 2 months or more before evidence of hair growth can be expected.

If hair regrowth occurs, twice daily applications of Regaine for Men Extra Strength are necessary for continued hair growth. Anecdotal reports indicate that regrown hair may disappear three to four months after stopping Regaine for Men Extra Strength application and the balding process will continue.

Users should discontinue treatment if there is no improvement after one year.

The method of application varies according to the disposable applicator used:

Pump spray applicator: this is useful for large areas. Aim the pump at the centre of the bald area, press once and spread with fingertips over the entire bald area. Repeat for a total of 6 times to apply a dose of 1 ml. Avoid breathing spray mist.

Extended spray-tip applicator: this is useful for small areas, or under hair. The pump spray applicator must be in place in order to use this additional applicator. Use in the same way as the pump spray.

Rub-on applicator: squeeze the upright bottle once to fill the 1 ml chamber to the black line. Invert bottle, dab on scalp, and spread Regaine for Men Extra Strength over the entire bald area until chamber is empty.

Children and the Elderly

Not recommended. The safety and effectiveness of Regaine for Men Extra Strength in users aged under 18 or over 65 has not been established.

4.3 Contraindications
Regaine for Men Extra Strength is contraindicated:

– in women

– in users with a history of sensitivity to minoxidil, ethanol, or propylene glycol

– in users with treated or untreated hypertension

– in users with any scalp abnormality (including psoriasis and sunburn)

– in users with a shaved scalp

– if occlusive dressings or other topical medical preparations are being used.

4.4 Special warnings and special precautions for use
Before using Regaine for Men Extra Strength, the user should determine that the scalp is normal and healthy.

The patient should stop using Regaine for Men Extra Strength and see a doctor if hypotension is detected or if the patient is experiencing chest pain, rapid heart beat, faintness or dizziness, sudden unexplained weight gain, swollen hands or feet or persistent redness.

Patients with known cardiovascular disease or cardiac arrhythmia should contact a physician before using Regaine for Men Extra Strength.

Regaine for Men Extra Strength is for external use only. Do not apply to areas of the body other than the scalp

Hands should be washed thoroughly after applying the solution. Inhalation of the spray mist should be avoided.

Regaine for Men Extra Strength cutaneous solution contains alcohol, which will cause burning and irritation of the eye. In the event of accidental contact with sensitive surfaces (eye, abraded skin and mucous membranes) the area should be bathed with large amounts of cool tap water.

Regaine for Men Extra Strength contains propylene glycol, which may cause skin irritation.

Some patients have experienced changes in hair colour and/or texture with Regaine for Men Extra Strength use.

Users should be aware that, whilst extensive use of Regaine for Men Extra Strength has not revealed evidence that sufficient minoxidil is absorbed to have systemic effects, greater absorption because of misuse, individual variability, unusual sensitivity or decreased integrity of the epidermal barrier caused by inflammation or disease processes in the skin (eg. excoriations of the scalp, or scalp psoriasis) could lead, at least theoretically, to systemic effects.

4.5 Interaction with other medicinal products and other forms of Interaction
Topical drugs, such as tretinoin or dithranol, which alter the stratum corneum barrier, could result in increased absorption of minoxidil if applied concurrently. Although it has not been demonstrated clinically, there exists the theoretical possibility of absorbed minoxidil potentiating orthostatic hypotension caused by peripheral vasodilators.

4.6 Pregnancy and lactation
There is no evidence as to drug safety in human pregnancy nor is there evidence from animal work that it is free from hazard. Regaine for Men Extra Strength should not be used during pregnancy or lactation.

4.7 Effects on ability to drive and use machines
Based on the pharmacodynamic and overall safety profile of minoxidil, it is not expected that Regaine for Men Extra Strength would interfere with the ability to drive or operate machinery.

4.8 Undesirable effects
Several thousand patients have used topical minoxidil in clinical trials where a comparison with an inactive solution was made. Dermatological reactions (e.g. irritation, itching) occurred in patients using both solutions. This has been explained by the presence of propylene glycol in both the active and inactive solution.

Reactions reported in commercial marketing experience include: hypertrichosis (unwanted non-scalp hair including facial hair growth in women), local erythema, itching, dry skin/scalp flaking, and exacerbation of hair loss.

Some consumers reported increased hair shedding upon initiation of therapy with Regaine for Men Extra Strength. This is most likely due to minoxidil's action of shifting hairs from the resting telogen phase to the growing anagen phase (old hairs fall out as new hairs grow in their place). This temporary increase in hair shedding generally occurs two to six weeks after beginning treatment and subsides within a couple of weeks. If shedding persists >2 weeks), users should stop using Regaine for Men Extra Strength and consult their doctor.

Particular attention was paid to body systems, such as cardiovascular and metabolic, which might have some relevance based on the pharmacology of minoxidil. There was no increased risk to users due to drug related medical reactions in these, or other, body system categories.

Users should stop using Regaine for Men Extra Strength if they experience chest-pain, tachycardia, faintness, dizziness, sudden unexplained weight gain, swollen hands or feet or persistent redness or irritation of the scalp. Rare cases of hypotension have been reported.

4.9 Overdose
Increased systemic absorption of minoxidil may potentially occur if higher-than-recommended doses of Regaine for Men Extra Strength are applied to larger surface areas of the body or areas other than the scalp. There are no known cases of minoxidil overdosage resulting from topical administration of Regaine for Men Extra Strength.

Because of the concentration of minoxidil in Regaine for Men Extra Strength, accidental ingestion has the potential of producing systemic effects related to the pharmacological action of the drug (2 ml of Regaine for Men Extra Strength contains 100 mg minoxidil; the maximum recommended adult dose for oral minoxidil administration in the treatment of hypertension). Signs and symptoms of minoxidil overdosage would primarily be cardiovascular effects associated with sodium and water retention, and tachycardia. Fluid retention can be managed with appropriate diuretic therapy. Clinically significant tachycardia can be controlled by administration of a beta-adrenergic blocking agent.

5. PHARMACOLOGICAL PROPERTIES

5.1 Pharmacodynamic properties

The effect of Regaine for Men Extra Strength has been assessed in a phase III clinical trial conducted over a 48 week treatment period.

In this study Regaine for Men Extra Strength (5% minoxidil cutaneous solution) was compared to the product vehicle without the minoxidil active ingredient and also to 2% minoxidil cutaneous solution.

The primary efficacy criterion was non-vellus hair count in a $1.0cm^2$ reference area of affected scalp. The mean changes observed in this parameter in these studies were significantly in favour of active treatment. A significant dose effect was also demonstrated. The results are summarized in the following table:

Mean change in non-vellus hair count in reference $1cm^2$ area of scalp compared with baseline

(see Table 1)

Table 1 Mean change in non-vellus hair count in reference $1cm^2$ area of scalp compared with baseline

	Regaine for Men Extra Strength (n=139) Minoxidil 5%	(n=142) Minoxidil 2%	(n=71) Vehicle	Pairwise comparison
Baseline	151.1	143.6	152.4	
	Mean change from baseline	Mean change from baseline	Mean change from baseline	
8 weeks	+29.7	+24.9	+14.3	5>2>vehicle
16 weeks	+35.3	+29.8	+15.3	5>2>vehicle
32 weeks	+29.0	+22.2	+7.7	5>2>vehicle
48 weeks	+18.6	+12.7	+3.9	5>2>vehicle

Efficacy was further assessed by comparing photographs taken at various timepoints with baseline.

Assessment was undertaken by patients using a 100mm visual analogue scale and assessing scalp coverage where point 0 represented much less scalp coverage, 50mm no difference and 100mm much more scalp coverage. In addition, an assessment was undertaken by 2 blinded reviewers who compared photographs taken at baseline and after 48 weeks. Differences were assessed using a 7 point categorical scale viz:

Dense growth
Moderate growth
Minimal growth
No change
Minimal loss
Moderate loss
Dense loss

The results of these analyses were as follows:

Patient evaluation of change in scalp coverage

(see Table 2)

Table 2 Patient evaluation of change in scalp coverage

	Regaine for Men Extra Strength (n=139) Minoxidil 5%	(n=142) Minoxidil 2%	(n=71) Vehicle	Pairwise comparison
	mm	mm	mm	
16 weeks	63.5	58.2	51.4	5>2>vehicle
32 weeks	63.4	58.0	52.0	5>2>vehicle
48 weeks	62	56.9	51.0	5>2>vehicle

Photographic Evaluation of Clinical Response (Reviewer 1)

(see Table 3)

Table 3 Photographic Evaluation of Clinical Response (Reviewer 1)

	Dense Growth %	Moderate Growth %	Minimal Growth %	No change %	Hair Loss %	Unable to rate
Minoxidil 5%	2.2	37.4	22.3	31.7	5.0	1.4
Minoxidil 2%	2.8	19.7	21.1	50.0	2.8	3.5
Vehicle	0	7.0	22.5	60.0	9.9	0

Photographic Evaluation of Clinical Response (Reviewer 2)

(see Table 4)

Table 4 Photographic Evaluation of Clinical Response (Reviewer 2)

	Dense Growth %	Moderate Growth %	Minimal Growth %	No change %	Hair Loss %	Unable to rate
Minoxidil 5%	10.1	20.1	23.7	28.8	6.5	10.8
Minoxidil 2%	3.5	12.0	22.5	47.2	1.4	13.4
Vehicle	0	7.0	9.9	60.6	14.1	8.5

Based upon these photographic data, around 60% of the patients experienced an increased scalp coverage after 48 weeks treatment with Regaine for Men Extra Strength as defined by re-growth of hair; compared with around 23% at an average for those who received vehicle alone. Of these, around 35% treated with Regaine for Men Extra Strength experienced dense or moderate regrowth compared with around 7% who received vehicle alone. In addition 30% of patients who received Regaine for Men Extra Strength were adjudged to have no change between the photographic assessments of hair growth compared with 60% who received vehicle alone. Stabilisation of hair loss (expressed both as regrowth of hair and no continuation of hair loss) can therefore be expected in about 4 out of 5 of patients using Regaine for Men Extra Strength compared with 3 out of 4 patients using vehicle alone.

Regaine for Men Extra Strength may therefore be considered by men who wish to achieve a faster onset and greater degree of hair regrowth than would be expected through the use of Regaine Regular Strength.

The mechanism by which minoxidil stimulates hair growth is not fully understood, but minoxidil can reverse the hair loss process of androgenetic alopecia by the following means:

- increasing the diameter of the hair shaft
- stimulating anagen growth
- prolonging the anagen phase
- stimulating anagen recovery from the telegon phase

As a peripheral vasodilator minoxidil enhances microcirculation to hair follicles. The Vascular Endothelial Growth Factor (VEGF) is stimulated by minoxidil and VEGF is presumably responsible of the increased capillary fenestration, indicative of a high metabolic activity, observed during the anagen phase.

5.2 Pharmacokinetic properties

The failure to detect evidence of systemic effects during treatment with Regaine for Men Extra Strength reflects the poor absorption of topical minoxidil, which averages about 1.7% (range 0.3-4.5%) of the total applied dose from normal intact skin.

Absorption is about 2% when applied topically to shaved scalps of hypertensive users. Increasing the amount of drug applied or increasing the frequency of application of Regaine for Men Extra Strength also results in increased absorption.

The use of Regaine for Men Extra Strength in conjunction with occlusion (plastic dressings), application to sunburn areas, and increasing the surface area of application has minimal to no effect on the absorption of topical minoxidil.

Results of extensive pharmacokinetic studies indicate that the three major factors by which topical minoxidil absorption is increased are: increasing the dose applied, increasing the frequency of dosing and decreasing the barrier function of the stratum corneum.

Serum minoxidil levels and systemic effects resulting from administration of Regaine for Men Extra Strength are governed by the drug's absorption rate through the skin. Following cessation of topical dosing of Regaine for Men Extra Strength, approximately 95% of the systemically absorbed drug is eliminated within 4 days. Minoxidil and its metabolites are excreted principally in the urine.

5.3 Preclinical safety data

6. PHARMACEUTICAL PARTICULARS

6.1 List of excipients

Propylene glycol

Ethanol

Water

6.2 Incompatibilities

None known.

6.3 Shelf life

24 months

6.4 Special precautions for storage

Regaine for Men Extra Strength is flammable. Store below 25°C.

6.5 Nature and contents of container

HDPE bottle with spray-pump/dabbing applicator containing 60 ml of solution. Packs contain either one or three bottles.

6.6 Instructions for use and handling

The solution is flammable and exposure of the container and contents to naked flames should be avoided during use, storage and disposal.

Administrative Data

7. MARKETING AUTHORISATION HOLDER

Pfizer Consumer Healthcare
Walton Oaks
Dorking Road
Walton-on-the-Hill
Surrey
KT20 7NS
United Kingdom

8. MARKETING AUTHORISATION NUMBER(S)

PL 15513/0148

9. DATE OF FIRST AUTHORISATION/RENEWAL OF THE AUTHORISATION

28 June 2005

10. DATE OF REVISION OF THE TEXT

Regaine for Men Regular Strength

(Pfizer Consumer Healthcare)

1. NAME OF THE MEDICINAL PRODUCT

Regaine for Men Regular Strength

2. QUALITATIVE AND QUANTITATIVE COMPOSITION

Minoxidil 20 mg/ml (2%w/v).

For excipients see section 6.1.

3. PHARMACEUTICAL FORM

Cutaneous Solution (to be applied to the scalp)

4. CLINICAL PARTICULARS

4.1 Therapeutic indications

Regainefor MenRegular Strength is indicated for the treatment of alopecia androgenetica in men aged between 18 and 65.

Onset and degree of hair regrowth may be variable among users. Although trends in the data suggest that those users who are younger, who have been balding for a shorter period of time or who have a smaller area of baldness on the vertex are more likely to respond to Regaine for Men Regular Strength, individual responses cannot be predicted.

4.2 Posology and method of administration

Menaged 18-65:

Hair and scalp should be thoroughly dry prior to topical application of Regaine for Men Regular Strength. A dose of 1 ml Regaine for Men Regular Strength cutaneous solution should be applied to the total affected areas of the scalp twice daily. The total dosage should not exceed 2 ml. If fingertips are used to facilitate drug application, hands should be washed afterwards.

It may take twice daily applications for four months or more before evidence of hair growth can be expected.

If hair regrowth occurs, twice daily applications of Regaine for Men Regular Strength are necessary for continued hair growth. Anecdotal reports indicate that regrown hair may disappear three to four months after stopping Regaine for Men Regular Strength application and the balding process will continue.

Users should discontinue treatment if there is no improvement after one year.

The method of application varies according to the disposable applicator used:

Pump spray applicator: this is useful for large areas. Aim the pump at the centre of the bald area, press once and spread with fingertips over the entire bald area. Repeat for a total of 6 times to apply a dose of 1 ml. Avoid breathing spray mist.

Extended spray-tip applicator: this is useful for small areas, or under hair. The pump spray applicator must be in place in order to use this additional applicator. Use in the same way as the pump spray.

Rub-on applicator: squeeze the upright bottle once to fill the 1 ml chamber to the black line. Invert bottle, dab on scalp, and spread Regaine for Men Regular Strength over the entire bald area until chamber is empty.

Children and the Elderly

Not recommended. The safety and effectiveness of Regaine for Men Regular Strength in users aged under 18 or over 65 has not been established.

4.3 Contraindications

Regaine for Men Regular Strength is contra-indicated:

– in users with a history of sensitivity to minoxidil, ethanol, or propylene glycol

– in users with treated or untreated hypertension

– in users with any scalp abnormality (including psoriasis and sunburn)

– in users with a shaved scalp

– if occlusive dressings or other topical medical preparations are being used.

4.4 Special warnings and special precautions for use

Before using Regaine for Men Regular Strength, the user should determine that the scalp is normal and healthy.

The patient should stop using Regaine for MenRegular Strength and see a doctor if hypotension is detected or if the patient is experiencing chest pain, rapid heart beat, faintness or dizziness, sudden unexplained weight gain, swollen hands or feet or persistent redness.

Patients with known cardiovascular disease or cardiac arrhythmia should contact a physician before using Regaine for Men Regular Strength.

Regaine for Men Regular Strength is for external use only. Do not apply to areas of the body other than the scalp.

Hands should be washed thoroughly after applying the solution. Inhalation of the spray mist should be avoided.

Regaine for Men Regular Strength contains alcohol, which will cause burning and irritation of the eye. In the event of accidental contact with sensitive surfaces (eye, abraded skin and mucous membranes) the area should be bathed with large amounts of cool tap water.

Regaine for Men Regular Strength contains propylene glycol, which may cause skin irritation.

Some patients have experienced changes in hair colour and/or texture with use of Regaine for MenRegular Strength.

Patients should be advised to consult their doctor or pharmacist if they are concerned at any time during treatment with Regaine for Men Regular Strength.

Users should be aware that, whilst extensive use of Regaine for Men Regular Strength has not revealed evidence that sufficient minoxidil is absorbed to have systemic effects, greater absorption because of misuse, individual variability, unusual sensitivity or decreased integrity of the epidermal barrier caused by inflammation or disease processes in the skin (e.g. excoriations of the scalp, or scalp psoriasis) could lead, at least theoretically, to systemic effects.

4.5 Interaction with other medicinal products and other forms of Interaction

Topical drugs, such as corticosteroids, tretinoin, dithranol or petrolatum which alter the stratum corneum barrier, could result in increased absorption of minoxidil if applied concurrently. Although it has not been demonstrated clinically, there exists the theoretical possibility of absorbed minoxidil potentiating orthostatic hypotension caused by peripheral vasodilators.

4.6 Pregnancy and lactation

There are no adequate data from the use of minoxidil in pregnant women. Studies in animals have shown reproductive toxicity (see Section 5.3). The potential risk for humans is unknown. Regaine should not be used during pregnancy.

In pregnant rats administered a single subcutaneous dose of 0.9 mg/kg minoxidil, the concentrations in foetuses were 19% to 28% of the maternal plasma concentration.

It is recommended that breast-feeding should be discontinued during treatment with Regaine.

4.7 Effects on ability to drive and use machines

Based on the pharmacodynamic and overall safety profile of minoxidil, it is not expected that Regaine for Men Regular Strength would interfere with the ability to drive or operate machinery.

4.8 Undesirable effects

In placebo controlled trials, the overall frequency of medical events in females in all body system categories was approximately five times that of males.

Several thousand patients have used topical minoxidil in clinical trials where a comparison with an inactive solution was made. Dermatological reactions (e.g. irritation, itching) occurred in patients using both solutions. This has been explained by the presence of propylene glycol in both the active and inactive solution.

Reactions reported in commercial marketing experience include: hypertrichosis (unwanted non-scalp hair including facial hair growth in women), local erythema, itching, dry skin/scalp flaking, and exacerbation of hair loss. Users should stop using Regaine for MenRegular Strength if they experience persistent redness or irritation of the scalp.

Some consumers reported increased hair shedding upon initiation of therapy with Regaine for MenRegular Strength. This is most likely due to minoxidil's action of shifting hairs from the resting telogen phase to the growing anagen phase (old hairs fall out as new hairs grow in their place). This temporary increase in hair shedding generally occurs two to six weeks after beginning treatment and subsides within a couple of weeks. If shedding persists >2 weeks), users should stop using Regaine for MenRegular Strength and consult their doctor.

Particular attention has been paid to body systems, such as cardiovascular and metabolic, which might have some relevance based on the pharmacology of minoxidil. There was no increased risk to users due to drug related medical reactions in these, or other, body system categories.

Users should stop using Regaine for MenRegular Strength if they experience chest-pain, tachycardia, faintness, dizziness, sudden unexplained weight gain, or swollen hands or feet. Rare cases of hypotension have been reported.

4.9 Overdose

Increased systemic absorption of minoxidil may potentially occur if higher-than-recommended doses of Regaine for Men Regular Strength are applied to larger surface areas of the body or areas other than the scalp. There are no known cases of minoxidil overdosage resulting from topical administration of Regaine for Men Regular Strength.

Because of the concentration of minoxidil in Regaine for Men Regular Strength, accidental ingestion has the potential of producing systemic effects related to the pharmacological action of the drug (5ml of Regaine for Men Regular Strength contains 100mg minoxidil; the maximum recommended adult dose for oral minoxidil administration in the treatment of hypertension). Signs and symptoms of minoxidil overdosage would primarily be cardiovascular effects associated with sodium and water retention, and tachycardia. Fluid retention can be managed with appropriate diuretic therapy. Clinically significant tachycardia can be controlled by administration of a beta-adrenergic blocking agent.

5. PHARMACOLOGICAL PROPERTIES

5.1 Pharmacodynamic properties

Individual responses to Regaine for Men Regular Strength are variable and unpredictable.

The effect of Regaine for Men Regular Strength has been assessed in phase III clinical trials in men conducted over a 48 week treatment period. In these studies Regaine for Men Regular Strength was compared to the product vehicle without the minoxidil active ingredient. The primary efficacy criterion was non-vellus hair count in a 1.0cm^2 reference area of affected scalp. The mean changes observed in this parameter in these studies were significantly in favour of Regaine for MenRegular Strength and were as follows:

Mean change in non-vellus hair count in reference 1cm^2 area of scalp compared with baseline

(see Table 1)

In addition, efficacy was further assessed by comparing photographs taken at various timepoints with baseline. Assessment was undertaken by patients using a 100mm visual analogue scale where point 0 represented much less scalp coverage, 50mm no difference and 100mm much more scalp coverage. The results were as follows.

Patient evaluation of change in scalp coverage

(see Table 2)

Assessment was also undertaken by 2 blinded reviewers who compared photographs taken at baseline and after 48 weeks. Differences were assessed using a 7 point categorical scale viz:

Dense growth

Moderate growth

Minimal Growth

No change

Minimal loss

Moderate loss

Dense loss

The results were as follows:

Photographic Evaluation of Clinical Response (Reviewer 1)

(see Table 3 on next page)

Photographic Evaluation of Clinical Response (Reviewer 2)

(see Table 4 on next page)

Based upon the photographic data around 40% of the patients experienced an increased scalp coverage after 48 weeks treatment with Regaine for Men Regular Strength as defined by regrowth of hair compared with 23% at an average for those who received vehicle alone. Around 19% treated with Regaine for Men Regular Strength experienced dense or moderate regrowth compared with around 7% who received vehicle alone. In addition 49% of patients who received Regaine for Men Regular Strength were adjudged to have no change between the photographic

Table 1 Mean change in non-vellus hair count in reference 1cm^2 area of scalp compared with baseline

	Regaine for Men Regular Strength (minoxidil 2%)	Vehicle	Pairwise comparison
Baseline	143.6	152.4	
	Mean change from baseline	Mean change from baseline	
16 weeks	+29.8	+15.3	**2>vehicle**
32 weeks	+22.2	+7.7	**2>vehicle**
48 weeks	+12.7	+3.9	**2>vehicle**

Table 2 Patient evaluation of change in scalp coverage

	Regaine for Men Regular Strength	Vehicle	Pairwise comparison
	mm	**mm**	
16 weeks	58.2	51.4	**2>vehicle**
32 weeks	58.0	52.0	**2>vehicle**
48 weeks	56.9	51.0	**2>vehicle**

Table 3 Photographic Evaluation of Clinical Response (Reviewer 1)

	Dense Growth %	Moderate Growth %	Minimal Growth %	No change %	Hair Loss %	Unable to rate
Regaine for Men Regular Strength	2.8	19.7	21.1	50.0	2.8	3.5
Placebo	0	7.0	22.5	60.6	9.9	0

Table 4 Photographic Evaluation of Clinical Response (Reviewer 2)

	Dense Growth %	Moderate Growth %	Minimal Growth %	No change %	Hair Loss %	Unable to rate
Regaine for Men Regular Strength	3.5	12.0	22.5	47.2	1.4	13.4
Placebo	0	7.0	9.9	60.6	14.1	8.5

assessments of hair growth compared with 60% who received vehicle alone. Stabilisation of hair loss (i.e. regrowth or no loss) can therefore be expected in about 4 out of 5 patients using Regaine for Men Regular Strength compared with 3 out of 4 patients using vehicle alone.

The mechanism by which minoxidil stimulates hair growth is not fully understood, but minoxidil can reverse the hair loss process of androgenetic alopecia by the following means:

- increase the diameter of the hair shaft
- stimulate anagen growth
- prolong the anagen phase
- stimulate anagen recovery from the telogen phase

As a peripheral vasodilator minoxidil enhances microcirculation to hair follicles. The Vascular Endothelial Growth Factor (VEGF) is stimulated by minoxidil and VEGF is presumably responsible of the increased capillary fenestration, indicative of a high metabolic activity, observed during the anagen phase.

5.2 Pharmacokinetic properties

The failure to detect evidence of systemic effects during treatment with Regaine for Men Regular Strength reflects the poor absorption of topical minoxidil, which averages about 1.4% (range 0.3-4.5%) of the total applied dose from normal intact skin. Absorption is about 2% when applied topically to shaved scalps of hypertensive users. Increasing the amount of drug applied or increasing the frequency of application of Regaine for Men Regular Strength also results in increased absorption.

Results of extensive pharmacokinetic studies indicate that the three major factors by which topical minoxidil absorption is increased are: increasing the dose applied, increasing the frequency of dosing and decreasing the barrier function of the stratum corneum.

Serum minoxidil levels and systemic effects resulting from administration of Regaine for Men Regular Strength are governed by the drug's absorption rate through the skin. Following cessation of topical dosing of Regaine for Men Regular Strength, approximately 95% of the systemically absorbed drug is eliminated within 4 days. Minoxidil and its metabolites are excreted principally in the urine.

5.3 Preclinical safety data

Preclinical data reveal no special hazards for humans based on conventional studies of safety pharmacology, repeated dose toxicity, genotoxicity or carcinogenic potential.

Cardiac effects of minoxidil in dogs are species-specific in terms of the low doses that cause profound haemodynamic effects and associated changes in the heart. Available data indicate that similar cardiac effects do not occur in humans treated topically or orally with minoxidil.

In rat fertility studies, minoxidil at dose levels between 3 and 80 mg/kg exhibited adverse effects on fertility. Animal reproduction toxicity studies have shown a risk to the foetus at exposure levels that in comparison to levels obtained in humans are very high (doses that ranged from 569- to 1139-fold anticipated human exposures) and showing signs for maternal toxicity.

6. PHARMACEUTICAL PARTICULARS

6.1 List of excipients

Propylene glycol

Ethanol

Water

6.2 Incompatibilities

None known.

6.3 Shelf life

48 months

6.4 Special precautions for storage

Regaine for Men Regular Strength is flammable. Do not store above 25°C.

6.5 Nature and contents of container

HDPE bottle with spray-pump/dabbing applicator containing 60 ml of solution.

Pack size: 1 × 60 ml.

6.6 Instructions for use and handling

The solution is flammable. Do not use while smoking, or near any naked flame or strong heat source. Avoid exposure of the container and contents to naked flames during use, storage and disposal.

Administrative Data

7. MARKETING AUTHORISATION HOLDER

Pfizer Consumer Healthcare

Walton Oaks

Dorking Road

Walton-on-the-Hill

Surrey

KT20 7NS

8. MARKETING AUTHORISATION NUMBER(S)

PL 15513/0150

9. DATE OF FIRST AUTHORISATION/RENEWAL OF THE AUTHORISATION

9 June 2005

10. DATE OF REVISION OF THE TEXT

9 June 2005

Regaine for Women Regular Strength

(Pfizer Consumer Healthcare)

1. NAME OF THE MEDICINAL PRODUCT

Regaine for Women Regular Strength

2. QUALITATIVE AND QUANTITATIVE COMPOSITION

Minoxidil 20 mg/ml (2% w/v).

For excipients see section 6.1.

3. PHARMACEUTICAL FORM

Cutaneous Solution (to be applied to the scalp)

4. CLINICAL PARTICULARS

4.1 Therapeutic indications

Regainefor WomenRegular Strength is indicated for the treatment of alopecia androgenetica in women aged between 18 and 65.

Onset and degree of hair regrowth may be variable among users. Although trends in the data suggest that those users who are younger, whose hair has been thinning for a shorter period of time or who have a smaller area of thinning on the vertex are more likely to respond to Regaine for Women Regular Strength, individual responses cannot be predicted.

4.2 Posology and method of administration

Womenaged 18-65:

Hair and scalp should be thoroughly dry prior to topical application of Regaine for Women Regular Strength. A dose of 1 ml Regaine for Women Regular Strength cutaneous solution should be applied to the total affected areas of the scalp twice daily. The total dosage should not exceed 2 ml. If fingertips are used to facilitate drug application, hands should be washed afterwards.

It may take twice daily applications for four months or more before evidence of hair growth can be expected.

If hair regrowth occurs, twice daily applications of Regaine for Women Regular Strength are necessary for continued hair growth. Anecdotal reports indicate that regrown hair may disappear three to four months after stopping Regaine for Women Regular Strength application and the balding process will continue.

Users should discontinue treatment if there is no improvement after one year.

The method of application varies according to the disposable applicator used:

Pump spray applicator: this is useful for large areas. Aim the pump at the centre of the bald area, press once and spread with fingertips over the entire bald area. Repeat for a total of 6 times to apply a dose of 1 ml. Avoid breathing spray mist.

Extended spray-tip applicator: this is useful for small areas, or under hair. The pump spray applicator must be in place in order to use this additional applicator. Use in the same way as the pump spray.

Rub-on applicator: squeeze the upright bottle once to fill the 1 ml chamber to the black line. Invert bottle, dab on scalp, and spread Regaine for Women Regular Strength over the entire bald area until chamber is empty.

Children and the Elderly

Not recommended. The safety and effectiveness of Regaine for Women Regular Strength in users aged under 18 or over 65 has not been established.

4.3 Contraindications

Regaine for Women Regular Strength is contra-indicated:

– in users with a history of sensitivity to minoxidil, ethanol, or propylene glycol

– in users with treated or untreated hypertension

– in users with any scalp abnormality (including psoriasis and sunburn)

– in users with a shaved scalp

– if occlusive dressings or other topical medical preparations are being used.

4.4 Special warnings and special precautions for use

Before using Regaine for Women Regular Strength, the user should determine that the scalp is normal and healthy.

The patient should stop using Regaine for Women Regular Strength and see a doctor if hypotension is detected or if the patient is experiencing chest pain, rapid heart beat, faintness or dizziness, sudden unexplained weight gain, swollen hands or feet or persistent redness.

Patients with known cardiovascular disease or cardiac arrhythmia should contact a physician before using Regaine for Women Regular Strength.

Regaine for Women Regular Strength is for external use only. Do not apply to areas of the body other than the scalp. Hands should be washed thoroughly after applying the solution. Inhalation of the spray mist should be avoided.

Regaine for Women Regular Strength contains alcohol, which will cause burning and irritation of the eye. In the event of accidental contact with sensitive surfaces (eye, abraded skin and mucous membranes) the area should be bathed with large amounts of cool tap water.

Regaine for Women Regular Strength contains propylene glycol, which may cause skin irritation.

Some patients have experienced changes in hair colour and/or texture with use of Regaine for Women Regular Strength.

Patients should be advised to consult their doctor or pharmacist if they are concerned at any time during treatment with Regaine for Women Regular Strength.

Users should be aware that, whilst extensive use of Regaine for Women Regular Strength has not revealed evidence that sufficient minoxidil is absorbed to have systemic effects, greater absorption because of misuse, individual variability, unusual sensitivity or decreased integrity of the epidermal barrier caused by inflammation or disease processes in the skin (e.g. excoriations of the scalp, or scalp psoriasis) could lead, at least theoretically, to systemic effects.

4.5 Interaction with other medicinal products and other forms of Interaction

Topical drugs, such as corticosteroids, tretinoin, dithranol or petrolatum which alter the stratum corneum barrier, could result in increased absorption of minoxidil if applied concurrently. Although it has not been demonstrated clinically, there exists the theoretical possibility of absorbed minoxidil potentiating orthostatic hypotension caused by peripheral vasodilators.

4.6 Pregnancy and lactation

There are no adequate data from the use of minoxidil in pregnant women. Studies in animals have shown reproductive toxicity (see Section 5.3). The potential risk for humans is unknown. Regaine should not be used during pregnancy.

In pregnant rats administered a single subcutaneous dose of 0.9 mg/kg minoxidil, the concentrations in foetuses were 19% to 28% of the maternal plasma concentration.

It is recommended that breast-feeding should be discontinued during treatment with Regaine.

4.7 Effects on ability to drive and use machines

Based on the pharmacodynamic and overall safety profile of minoxidil, it is not expected that Regaine for Women Regular Strength would interfere with the ability to drive or operate machinery.

4.8 Undesirable effects

In placebo controlled trials, the overall frequency of medical events in females in all body system categories was approximately five times that of males.

Several thousand patients have used topical minoxidil in clinical trials where a comparison with an inactive solution was made. Dermatological reactions (e.g. irritation, itching) occurred in patients using both solutions. This has been explained by the presence of propylene glycol in both the active and inactive solution.

Reactions reported in commercial marketing experience include: hypertrichosis (unwanted non-scalp hair including facial hair growth in women), local erythema, itching, dry skin/scalp flaking, and exacerbation of hair loss. Users should stop using Regaine if they experience persistent redness or irritation of the scalp.

Some consumers reported increased hair shedding upon initiation of therapy with Regaine. This is most likely due to minoxidil's action of shifting hairs from the resting telogen phase to the growing anagen phase (old hairs fall out as new hairs grow in their place). This temporary increase in hair shedding generally occurs two to six weeks after beginning treatment and subsides within a couple of weeks. If shedding persists >2 weeks), users should stop using Regaine and consult their doctor.

Particular attention has been paid to body systems, such as cardiovascular and metabolic, which might have some relevance based on the pharmacology of minoxidil. There was no increased risk to users due to drug related medical reactions in these, or other, body system categories.

Users should stop using Regaine if they experience chest-pain, tachycardia, faintness, dizziness, sudden unexplained weight gain, or swollen hands or feet. Rare cases of hypotension have been reported.

4.9 Overdose

Increased systemic absorption of minoxidil may potentially occur if higher-than-recommended doses of Regaine for Women Regular Strength are applied to larger surface areas of the body or areas other than the scalp. There are no known cases of minoxidil overdosage resulting from topical administration of Regaine for Women Regular Strength.

Because of the concentration of minoxidil in Regaine for Women Regular Strength, accidental ingestion has the potential of producing systemic effects related to the pharmacological action of the drug (5ml of Regaine for Women Regular Strength contains 100mg minoxidil; the maximum recommended adult dose for oral minoxidil administration in the treatment of hypertension). Signs and symptoms of minoxidil overdosage would primarily be cardiovascular effects associated with sodium and water retention, and tachycardia. Fluid retention can be managed with appropriate diuretic therapy. Clinically significant tachycardia can be controlled by administration of a beta-adrenergic blocking agent.

5. PHARMACOLOGICAL PROPERTIES

5.1 Pharmacodynamic properties

Individual responses to Regaine for Women Regular Strength are variable and unpredictable.

The effect of Regaine for Women Regular Strength has been assessed in phase III clinical trials in women conducted over a 48 week treatment period. In these studies Regaine for Women Regular Strength was compared to the product vehicle without the minoxidil active ingredient. The primary efficacy criterion was non-vellus hair count in a 1.0 cm^2 reference area of affected scalp. The mean changes observed in this parameter in these studies were significantly in favour of Regaine and were as follows:

Mean change in non-vellus hair count in reference 1 cm^2 area of scalp compared with baseline

(see Table 1 below)

Using non-vellus hair count as an efficacy criteria, Regaine for Women Regular Strength has also been shown to stabilise hair loss (defined as regrowth or no loss) in 88% of patients compared with 69% of patients who received vehicle in one trial following 48 weeks treatment and in 87% of patients compared with 73% of patients who received vehicle in a further trial following 32 weeks treatment.

Female patients' own evaluations in clinical studies have shown that hair growth was reported by approximately 60% of females after 8 months of Regaine for Women Regular Strength usage.

Patient evaluation of visible hair growth

	% of Females reporting regrowth after 8 months Regaine for Women Regular Strength usage	% of Females reporting regrowth after 4 months Product vehicle usage
Minimal re-growth	30-40	29-33
Moderate to dense re-growth	20-25	7-12
Total	55-59	40-41

In addition, Regaine for Women Regular Strength has also been shown to stabilise hair loss (shown as regrowth or no loss) in 4 out of 5 females as calculated from two clinical studies that showed stabilisation with 88 and 87% respectively while corresponding figures for vehicle were 69 and 74%.

The mechanism by which minoxidil stimulates hair growth is not fully understood, but minoxidil can reverse the hair loss process of androgenetic alopecia by the following means:

- increase the diameter of the hair shaft
- stimulate anagen growth
- prolong the anagen phase
- stimulate anagen recovery from the telogen phase

As a peripheral vasodilator minoxidil enhances microcirculation to hair follicles. The Vascular Endothelial Growth Factor (VEGF) is stimulated by minoxidil and VEGF is presumably responsible for the increased capillary fenestration, indicative of a high metabolic activity, observed during the anagen phase.

5.2 Pharmacokinetic properties

The failure to detect evidence of systemic effects during treatment with Regaine for Women Regular Strength reflects the poor absorption of topical minoxidil, which averages about 1.4% (range 0.3-4.5%) of the total applied dose from normal intact skin. Absorption is about 2% when applied topically to shaved scalps of hypertensive users. Increasing the amount of drug applied or increasing the frequency of application of Regaine for Women Regular Strength also results in increased absorption.

Results of extensive pharmacokinetic studies indicate that the three major factors by which topical minoxidil absorption is increased are: increasing the dose applied, increasing the frequency of dosing and decreasing the barrier function of the stratum corneum.

Serum minoxidil levels and systemic effects resulting from administration of Regaine for Women Regular Strength are governed by the drug's absorption rate through the skin. Following cessation of topical dosing of Regaine for Women Regular Strength, approximately 95% of the systemically absorbed drug is eliminated within 4 days. Minoxidil and its metabolites are excreted principally in the urine.

5.3 Preclinical safety data

Preclinical data reveal no special hazards for humans based on conventional studies of safety pharmacology, repeated dose toxicity, genotoxicity or carcinogenic potential.

Cardiac effects of minoxidil in dogs are species-specific in terms of the low doses that cause profound haemodynamic effects and associated changes in the heart. Available data indicate that similar cardiac effects do not occur in humans treated topically or orally with minoxidil.

In rat fertility studies, minoxidil at dose levels between 3 and 80 mg/kg exhibited adverse effects on fertility. Animal reproduction toxicity studies have shown a risk to the foetus at exposure levels that in comparison to levels obtained in humans are very high (doses that ranged from 569- to 1139-fold anticipated human exposures) and showing signs for maternal toxicity.

Table 1 Mean change in non-vellus hair count in reference 1 cm^2 area of scalp compared with baseline

	Regaine for Women Regular Strength (minoxidil 2%)	Vehicle	Pairwise comparison
Baseline	150.4	138.4	
	Mean change from baseline	Mean change from baseline	
16 weeks	+35.9	+20.0	2>vehicle
32 weeks	+26.7	+15.2	2>vehicle
48 weeks	+20.7	+9.4	2>vehicle

6. PHARMACEUTICAL PARTICULARS

6.1 List of excipients

Propylene glycol
Ethanol
Water

6.2 Incompatibilities

None known.

6.3 Shelf life

48 months

6.4 Special precautions for storage

Regaine for Women Regular Strength is flammable. Do not store above 25°C.

6.5 Nature and contents of container

HDPE bottle with spray-pump/dabbing applicator containing 60 ml of solution.

Pack size: 1 × 60 ml.

6.6 Instructions for use and handling

The solution is flammable. Do not use while smoking, or near any naked flame or strong heat source. Avoid exposure of the container and contents to naked flames during use, storage and disposal.

Administrative Data

7. MARKETING AUTHORISATION HOLDER

Pfizer Consumer Healthcare
Walton Oaks
Dorking Road
Walton-on-the-Hill
Surrey
KT20 7NS
United Kingdom

8. MARKETING AUTHORISATION NUMBER(S)

PL 15513/0149

9. DATE OF FIRST AUTHORISATION/RENEWAL OF THE AUTHORISATION

7th March 2005

10. DATE OF REVISION OF THE TEXT

7th March 2005

Regranex 0.01% gel

(Janssen-Cilag Ltd)

1. NAME OF THE MEDICINAL PRODUCT

REGRANEX 0.01% gel

2. QUALITATIVE AND QUANTITATIVE COMPOSITION

REGRANEX contains 100 μg of becaplermin per gram of gel. Becaplermin is a recombinant human Platelet Derived Growth Factor-BB (rhPDGF-BB). It is produced by insertion of the gene for the B chain of human platelet derived growth factor into the yeast, *Saccharomyces cerevisiae*. rhPDGF-BB is a dimeric protein with a molecular weight of approximately 24,500 daltons.

For excipients, see 6.1.

3. PHARMACEUTICAL FORM

Gel

REGRANEX is a clear colourless to straw-coloured preserved gel.

4. CLINICAL PARTICULARS

4.1 Therapeutic indications

REGRANEX is indicated, in association with other good wound care measures, to promote granulation and thereby the healing of full-thickness, neuropathic, chronic, diabetic ulcers less than or equal to 5 cm^2.

4.2 Posology and method of administration

Treatment with REGRANEX should be initiated and monitored by physicians (specialists or non-specialists) who are experienced in the management of diabetic wounds.

REGRANEX should always be used in conjunction with good wound care consisting of initial debridement (to remove all the necrotic and/or infected tissue), additional debridement as necessary and a non-weight-bearing regimen to alleviate pressure on the ulcer. Wound-related infection should be identified and treated with appropriate antimicrobial therapy prior to the use of REGRANEX. Prior to the use of REGRANEX, related underlying conditions such as osteomyelitis and peripheral arteriopathy should be excluded or treated if present. Osteomyelitis should be assessed by X-ray examination. Peripheral arteriopathy should be excluded by assessment of the pedal pulses or other techniques. Ulcers with a suspicious appearance should be biopsied to exclude malignancy.

REGRANEX should be applied as a continuous thin layer to the entire ulcerated area(s) once daily using a clean application aid. The site(s) of application should then be covered by a moist saline gauze dressing that maintains a moist wound-healing environment. REGRANEX should not be used in conjunction with occlusive dressings.

REGRANEX should not be used for more than 20 weeks in any individual patient.

If during treatment with REGRANEX no meaningful healing progress is evident after the first ten weeks of continuous therapy, treatment should be re-evaluated, and factors known to compromise healing (such as osteomyelitis, ischaemia, infection) should be re-assessed. Therapy should be continued to the maximum of 20 weeks as long as healing progress is seen on periodic evaluations.

REGRANEX is not intended for repeated use.

REGRANEX has not been studied in children.

4.3 Contraindications

- Known hypersensitivity to the active substance or to any of the excipients of this product
- Known neoplasm(s) at or near the site(s) of application.

4.4 Special warnings and special precautions for use

Safety and effectiveness in children and adolescents below the age of 18 years have not been established.

In view of the lack of data, REGRANEX should be used with caution in patients with known malignancies.

REGRANEX should not be used in patients with ulcers that are not of primarily neuropathic origin, such as those due to arteriopathy or other factors.

REGRANEX should not be used in clinically infected ulcers. Infection should be treated prior to the use of REGRANEX. Should a wound become infected during REGRANEX therapy, the product should be discontinued until the infective process is controlled.

REGRANEX should not be used in ulcers of baseline surface area > 5 cm^2, or for more than 20 weeks in any individual. There are insufficient data to support safe use of the product for more than 20 weeks (see 5.1 Pharmacodynamic properties). Efficacy has not been demonstrated for ulcers of baseline surface area > 5 cm^2.

4.5 Interaction with other medicinal products and other forms of Interaction

It is not known whether REGRANEX interacts with other topical medications applied to the ulcer site. Consequently, it is recommended that REGRANEX should not be applied to the ulcer site in conjunction with other topical medications.

4.6 Pregnancy and lactation

Pregnancy

No studies in pregnant women have been conducted. Therefore, REGRANEX should not be used in pregnant women.

Nursing mothers

It is not known whether becaplermin is excreted in human milk. Therefore, REGRANEX should not be used in nursing mothers.

4.7 Effects on ability to drive and use machines

Not relevant.

4.8 Undesirable effects

The following adverse events, which are not clearly related to REGRANEX therapy, were reported in the randomised clinical trials: Infection, skin ulceration, skin disorder, including erythema and pain. Bullous eruption and oedema were reported rarely.

Rare cases (frequency $\geqslant$1/10000, <1/1000) of hypertrophic granulation have been reported in post marketing experience.

4.9 Overdose

Since absorption is insignificant from the site of topical application, no untoward systemic events are expected.

5. PHARMACOLOGICAL PROPERTIES

5.1 Pharmacodynamic properties

Pharmacotherapeutic group: Preparation for treatment of wounds and ulcers, ATC code: D 03 AX06

REGRANEX contains becaplermin, a recombinant human Platelet Derived Growth Factor-BB (rhPDGF-BB). Becaplermin is produced by insertion of the gene for the B chain of human platelet derived growth factor into the yeast, *Saccharomyces cerevisiae*. The biological activity of becaplermin includes promoting the chemotactic recruitment and proliferation of cells involved in wound repair. Thus it helps the growth of normal tissue for healing. In animal wound models, the predominant effect of becaplermin is to enhance the formation of granulation tissue. From data combined from 4 clinical trials conducted over a 20 week treatment phase for ulcers of baseline surface area less than or equal to 5 cm^2, 47% of ulcers treated with becaplermin 100 μg/g gel completely healed, compared to 35% which were treated with placebo gel alone. Subjects recruited into these studies were diabetic adults aged 19 years or over who were suffering from at least one stage III or IV diabetic ulcer of at least 8 weeks duration.

Since becaplermin is a growth factor, which stimulates the proliferation of cells, it must be cautiously used in patients with malignancies.

5.2 Pharmacokinetic properties

Absorption

Clinical absorption studies were conducted in patients with a mean diabetic ulcer area of 10.5 cm^2 (range 2.3 - 43.5 cm^2). Following 14 consecutive daily topical applications of REGRANEX, only insignificant systemic absorption of becaplermin occurred.

5.3 Preclinical safety data

Becaplermin was not mutagenic in a battery of *in vitro* and *in vivo* tests. Since absorption is insignificant from the site of topical application, carcinogenesis and reproductive toxicity studies have not been conducted with REGRANEX. In the process of healing the wound, becaplermin induces cell proliferation. However, skin tumours have not been reported in the clinical trials at the site of application or in close proximity.

In a preclinical study designed to determine the effects of PDGF on exposed bone, rats injected at the metatarsals with 3 or 10 μg/site (concentration of 30 or 100 μg/ml/site) of becaplermin every other day for 13 days displayed histological changes indicative of accelerated bone remodelling consisting of periosteal hyperplasia and subperiosteal bone resorption and exostosis. The soft tissue adjacent to the injection site had fibroplasia with accompanying mononuclear cell infiltration reflective of the ability of PDGF to stimulate connective tissue growth.

Preclinical absorption studies through full-thickness wounds were conducted in rats with a wound area of 1.4 - 1.6 cm^2. Systemic absorption of a single dose and multiple applications for 5 consecutive days of becaplermin to those wounds was insignificant.

6. PHARMACEUTICAL PARTICULARS

6.1 List of excipients

carmellose sodium (E466)

sodium chloride

sodium acetate

glacial acetic acid (E260)

methyl parahydroxybenzoate (methylparaben) (E218)

propyl parahydroxybenzoate (propylparaben) (E216)

m-cresol

lysine hydrochloride

water for injections

6.2 Incompatibilities

There are no known incompatibilities.

6.3 Shelf life

1 year.

Use within 6 weeks after first opening.

6.4 Special precautions for storage

Store in a refrigerator (2°C - 8°C). Do not freeze.

6.5 Nature and contents of container

REGRANEX is supplied in 15 g laminated polyethylene-lined multidose tubes.

6.6 Instructions for use and handling

(See section 4.2).

- A tube of REGRANEX should be used on a single patient only.
- Care should be taken during use to avoid microbial contamination and spoilage.
- Hands should be washed thoroughly before applying REGRANEX.
- The tip of the tube should not come into contact with the wound or any other surface.
- The use of a clean application aid is recommended and contact with other parts of the body should be avoided.
- Before each application, the ulcer should be gently rinsed with saline or water to remove residual gel.
- The tube should be closed tightly after each use.
- After treatment is completed, any unused gel should be discarded.

7. MARKETING AUTHORISATION HOLDER

JANSSEN-CILAG INTERNATIONAL NV

Turnhoutseweg, 30

B-2340 Beerse

Belgium

8. MARKETING AUTHORISATION NUMBER(S)

EU/1/99/101/001

9. DATE OF FIRST AUTHORISATION/RENEWAL OF THE AUTHORISATION

March 29, 1999/March 31 2004

10. DATE OF REVISION OF THE TEXT

31 March 2004

Regulan Lemon/Lime Flavour.

(Procter & Gamble Pharmaceuticals UK Limited)

1. NAME OF THE MEDICINAL PRODUCT

Lemon/Lime Flavour Regulan.

2. QUALITATIVE AND QUANTITATIVE COMPOSITION

Lemon/Lime Flavour Regulan contains 3.4g of Ispaghula Husk, BP.

3. PHARMACEUTICAL FORM

Premeasured, single-dose sachets containing a lemon/lime flavoured beige, fine ground powder, which when reconstituted with water is intended for administration as an oral solution.

4. CLINICAL PARTICULARS

4.1 Therapeutic indications

For the relief of constipation and for patients who need to increase their daily fibre intake.

4.2 Posology and method of administration

The measured dosage should be poured into a glass and 150ml (¼ pint) of cool water, milk, fruit juice or other liquid added, stirred, and taken immediately. Additional liquid may be taken if required. Adequate fluid intake should be maintained.

Adults and children over 12 years

Usual dosage is the entire contents of one sachet taken one to three times daily.

Elderly

No alteration in dosage necessary.

Children 6-12 years

A reduced dosage based upon age of the child should be given. ½ - 1 level teaspoonful one to three times daily.

4.3 Contraindications

Not to be given to patients with intestinal obstruction, faecal impaction, colonic atony or hypersensitivity to ispaghula.

4.4 Special warnings and special precautions for use

Lemon/Lime Flavour Regulan should always be taken as a liquid suspension and should be drunk immediately after mixing. The last dose should not be taken immediately before going to bed since impaired or reduced gastric motility may impair the intestinal passage and then cause sub-obstruction. The drug may cause allergic reactions in people sensitive to inhaled or ingested ispaghula powder.

It may be advisable to supervise treatment in the elderly or debilitated and patients with intestinal narrowing or decreased motility, as rare instances of gastrointestinal obstruction have been reported with mucilloid preparations when taken, contrary to the administration instructions, with insufficient liquid.

Each sachet contains 26mg of phenylalanine and this should be considered in phenylketonuric patients.

The colouring agent, Sunset Yellow, can cause allergic type reactions including asthma. Allergy is more common in those people who are allergic to aspirin.

4.5 Interaction with other medicinal products and other forms of Interaction

None known.

4.6 Pregnancy and lactation

Controlled studies in pregnant and lactating women are not available, but the product has been in wide use for many years without apparent ill consequence and animal studies have shown no hazard. Ispaghula is not thought to be absorbed nor is it thought to enter breast milk. Nevertheless the benefits of therapy should be weighed against the possible risks if used during pregnancy and lactation.

4.7 Effects on ability to drive and use machines

None known.

4.8 Undesirable effects

Allergy and gastrointestinal obstruction or impaction have been reported with hydrophilic mucilloid preparations.

4.9 Overdose

No instances of true overdosage have been reported. If overdosage should occur there is no specific treatment and symptomatic measures should be employed.

5. PHARMACOLOGICAL PROPERTIES

5.1 Pharmacodynamic properties

The active constituent, ispaghula husk, is the epidermis and collapsed adjacent layers removed from the dried ripe seeds of plantago ovata, containing mucilage and hemicelluloses.

The ispaghula husk is not absorbed and produces its effect as a bulking agent by physical means alone.

5.2 Pharmacokinetic properties

Not applicable.

5.3 Preclinical safety data

None stated.

6. PHARMACEUTICAL PARTICULARS

6.1 List of excipients

Contains maltodextrin, citric acid, citrus flavour, aspartame (E951), and Sunset Yellow FCF (E110). Lemon/Lime flavour Regulan is sugar free and gluten free. Each sachet contains 0.23 mmol of sodium.

6.2 Incompatibilities

None known.

6.3 Shelf life

Three years.

6.4 Special precautions for storage

Store in a dry place not above 25°C.

6.5 Nature and contents of container

Paper / aluminium foil / polyethylene sachets. The product is available in packs of 30 sachets.

6.6 Instructions for use and handling

A patient leaflet is provided with details of use and handling of the product.

7. MARKETING AUTHORISATION HOLDER
Procter & Gamble (Health & Beauty Care) Limited
The Heights, Brooklands,
Weybridge,
Surrey, KT13 0XP
UK

8. MARKETING AUTHORISATION NUMBER(S)
PL 0129/0113
PA 441/34/1

9. DATE OF FIRST AUTHORISATION/RENEWAL OF THE AUTHORISATION
15 September 1992

10. DATE OF REVISION OF THE TEXT
April 2000

Regulan Orange Flavour.

(Procter & Gamble Pharmaceuticals UK Limited)

1. NAME OF THE MEDICINAL PRODUCT
Orange Flavour Regulan.

2. QUALITATIVE AND QUANTITATIVE COMPOSITION
Orange Flavour Regulan contains 3.4g of Ispaghula Husk, BP.

3. PHARMACEUTICAL FORM
Premeasured, single-dose sachets containing an orange flavoured beige, fine ground powder, which when reconstituted with water is intended for administration as an oral solution.

4. CLINICAL PARTICULARS
4.1 Therapeutic indications
For the relief of constipation and for patients who need to increase their daily fibre intake.

4.2 Posology and method of administration
The measured dosage should be poured into a glass and 150ml (¼ pint) of cool water, milk, fruit juice or other liquid added, stirred, and taken immediately. Additional liquid may be taken if required. Adequate fluid intake should be maintained.

Adults and children over 12 years

Usual dosage is the entire contents of one sachet taken one to three times daily.

Elderly

No alteration in dosage necessary.

Children 6-12 years

A reduced dosage based upon age of the child should be given. ½ - 1 level teaspoonful one to three times daily.

4.3 Contraindications
Not to be given to patients with intestinal obstruction, faecal impaction, colonic atony or hypersensitivity to ispaghula.

4.4 Special warnings and special precautions for use
Orange Flavour Regulan should always be taken as a liquid suspension and should be drunk immediately after mixing. The last dose should not be taken immediately before going to bed since impaired or reduced gastric motility may impair the intestinal passage and then cause subobstruction. The drug may cause allergic reactions in people sensitive to inhaled or ingested ispaghula powder.

It may be advisable to supervise treatment in the elderly or debilitated and patients with intestinal narrowing or decreased motility, as rare instances of gastrointestinal obstruction have been reported with mucilloid preparations when taken, contrary to the administration instructions, with insufficient liquid.

Each sachet contains 26mg of phenylalanine and this should be considered in phenylketonuric patients.

The colouring agent, Sunset Yellow, can cause allergic type reactions including asthma. Allergy is more common in those people who are allergic to aspirin.

4.5 Interaction with other medicinal products and other forms of Interaction
None known.

4.6 Pregnancy and lactation
Controlled studies in pregnant and lactating women are not available, but the product has been in wide use for many years without apparent ill consequence and animal studies have shown no hazard. Ispaghula is not thought to be absorbed nor is it thought to enter breast milk. Nevertheless the benefits of therapy should be weighed against the possible risks if used during pregnancy and lactation.

4.7 Effects on ability to drive and use machines
None known.

4.8 Undesirable effects
Allergy and gastrointestinal obstruction or impaction have been reported with hydrophilic mucilloid preparations.

4.9 Overdose
No instances of true overdosage have been reported. If overdosage should occur there is no specific treatment and symptomatic measures should be employed.

5. PHARMACOLOGICAL PROPERTIES
5.1 Pharmacodynamic properties
The active constituent, ispaghula husk, is the epidermis and collapsed adjacent layers removed from the dried ripe seeds of plantago ovata, containing mucilage and hemicelluloses.

The ispaghula husk is not absorbed and produces its effect as a bulking agent by physical means alone.

5.2 Pharmacokinetic properties
Not applicable.

5.3 Preclinical safety data
None stated.

6. PHARMACEUTICAL PARTICULARS
6.1 List of excipients
Contains maltodextrin, citric acid, orange flavour, aspartame (E951), and Sunset Yellow FCF (E110). Orange flavour Regulan is sugar free and gluten free. Each sachet contains 0.23 mmol of sodium.

6.2 Incompatibilities
None known.

6.3 Shelf life
Three years.

6.4 Special precautions for storage
Store in a dry place not above 25°C.

6.5 Nature and contents of container
Paper / aluminium foil / polyethylene sachets. The product is available in packs of 30 sachets.

6.6 Instructions for use and handling
A patient leaflet is provided with details of use and handling of the product.

7. MARKETING AUTHORISATION HOLDER
Procter & Gamble (Health & Beauty Care) Limited
The Heights, Brooklands,
Weybridge,
Surrey, KT13 0XP
UK

8. MARKETING AUTHORISATION NUMBER(S)
PL 0129/0114
PA 441/34/2

9. DATE OF FIRST AUTHORISATION/RENEWAL OF THE AUTHORISATION
15 September 1992

10. DATE OF REVISION OF THE TEXT
April 2000

Regurin 20mg Tablets

(Galen Limited)

1. NAME OF THE MEDICINAL PRODUCT
Regurin 20mg Tablets.

2. QUALITATIVE AND QUANTITATIVE COMPOSITION
The active ingredient is trospium chloride. Each coated tablet contains 20mg trospium chloride.

For excipients, see 6.1.

3. PHARMACEUTICAL FORM
Coated tablet.

Brownish-yellow, glossy coated, biconvex tablets.

4. CLINICAL PARTICULARS
4.1 Therapeutic indications
Symptomatic treatment of urge incontinence and/or increased urinary frequency and urgency as may occur in patients with overactive bladder (e.g. idiopathic or neurologic detrusor overactivity).

4.2 Posology and method of administration
One coated tablet twice daily (equivalent to 40mg of trospium chloride per day).

In patients with severe renal impairment (creatinine clearance between 10 and 30ml/min/1.73 m^2) the recommended dosage is: One coated tablet per day or every second day (equivalent to 20mg of trospium chloride per day or every second day).

The coated tablet should be swallowed whole with a glass of water before meals on an empty stomach.

The need for continued treatment should be reassessed at regular intervals of 3-6 months.

Since no data are available, use in children under 12 years of age is contra-indicated.

4.3 Contraindications
Trospium chloride is contra-indicated in patients with urinary retention, severe gastro-intestinal condition (including toxic megacolon), myasthenia gravis, narrow-angle glaucoma and tachyarrhythmia.

Trospium chloride is also contra-indicated in patients who have demonstrated hypersensitivity to the active substance or to any of the excipients.

4.4 Special warnings and special precautions for use
Trospium chloride should be used with caution by patients:

- with obstructive conditions of the gastro-intestinal tract such as pyloric stenosis
- with obstruction of the urinary flow with the risk of formation of urinary retention
- with autonomic neuropathy
- with hiatus hernia associated with reflux oesophagitis
- in whom fast heart rates are undesirable e.g. those with hyperthyroidism, coronary artery disease and congestive heart failure.

As there are no data in patients with severe hepatic impairment, treatment of these patients with trospium chloride is not recommended. In patients with mild to moderate liver impairment caution should be exercised.

Trospium chloride is mainly eliminated by renal excretion. Marked elevations in the plasma levels have been observed in patients with severe renal impairment. Therefore in this population but also in patients with mild to moderate renal impairment caution should be exercised (see 4.2).

Before commencing therapy organic causes of urinary frequency, urgency, and urge incontinence, such as heart diseases, diseases of the kidneys, polydipsia, or infections, or tumours of urinary organs should be excluded.

Regurin contains lactose monohydrate, sucrose and wheat starch. Patients with rare hereditary problems of galactose intolerance, the Lapp lactase deficiency or glucose-galactose malabsorption should not take this medicine. Patients with rare hereditary problems of fructose intolerance or sucrase-isomaltase insufficiency should not take this medicine.

Patients with wheat allergy (different from coeliac disease) should not take this medicine. Apart from that, trospium chloride is suitable for people with coeliac disease.

4.5 Interaction with other medicinal products and other forms of Interaction
Pharmacodynamic interactions:

The following potential pharmacodynamic interactions may occur: Potentiation of the effect of drugs with anticholinergic action (such as amantadine, tricyclic antidepressants), enhancement of the tachycardic action of β-sympathomimetics; decrease in efficacy of pro-kinetic agents (e.g. metoclopramide).

Since trospium chloride may influence gastro-intestinal motility and secretion, the possibility cannot be excluded that the absorption of other concurrently administered drugs may be altered.

Pharmacokinetic interactions:

An inhibition of the absorption of trospium chloride with drugs like guar, cholestyramine and colestipol cannot be excluded. Therefore the simultaneous administration of these drugs with trospium chloride is not recommended.

Metabolic interactions of trospium chloride have been investigated in vitro on cytochrome P450 enzymes involved in drug metabolism (P450 1A2, 2A6, 2C9, 2C19, 2D6, 2E1, 3A4). No influence on their metabolic activities were observed. Since trospium chloride is metabolised only to a low extent and since ester hydrolysis is the only relevant metabolic pathway, no metabolic interactions are expected.

4.6 Pregnancy and lactation
Animal studies do not indicate direct or indirect harmful effects with respect to pregnancy, embryonal/foetal development, parturition or postnatal development (see section 5.3). In rats, placental transfer and passage into the maternal milk of trospium chloride occurs.

For Regurin 20mg no clinical data on exposed pregnancies are available.

Caution should be exercised when prescribing to pregnant or breast-feeding women.

4.7 Effects on ability to drive and use machines
Principally, disorders of accommodation can lower the ability to actively participate in road traffic and to use machines.

However, examinations of parameters characterising the ability to participate in road traffic (visual orientation, general ability to react, reaction under stress, concentration and motor coordination) have not revealed any effects of trospium chloride.

4.8 Undesirable effects
Anticholinergic effects such as dry mouth, dyspepsia and constipation may occur during treatment with trospium chloride.

Very common (>10%):	gastro-intestinal system: dry mouth
Common (> 1%):	gastro-intestinal system: dyspepsia, constipation, abdominal pain, nausea
Uncommon (>1%):	gastro-intestinal system: flatulence

Rare (< 0.1%):	urinary system: micturition disorders (e.g. formation of residual urine) cardiovascular system: tachycardiavision disorders: disorders of accommodation (this applies in particular to patients who are hypermetropic and whose vision has not been adequately corrected) gastro-intestinal system: diarrhoearespiratory system: dyspnoeaskin: rashbody as a whole: asthenia, chest pain
Very rare (< 0.01%):	urinary system: urinary retention cardiovascular system: tachyarrhythmia musculoskeletal system: myalgia, arthralgia skin: angio-oedema liver and biliary system: mild to moderate increase in serum transaminase levels body as a whole: anaphylaxiscentral nervous system: headache, dizziness.

4.9 Overdose

After the administration of a maximum single dose of 360mg trospium chloride to healthy volunteers, dryness of the mouth, tachycardia and disorders of micturition were observed to an increased extent. No manifestations of severe overdosage or intoxication in humans have been reported to date. Increased anticholinergic symptoms are to be expected as signs of intoxication.

In the case of intoxication the following measures should be taken:

- gastric lavage and reduction of absorption (e.g. activated charcoal)
- local administration of pilocarpine to glaucoma patients
- catheterisation in patients with urinary retention
- treatment with a parasympathomimetic agent (e.g. neostigmine) in the case of severe symptoms
- administration of beta blockers in the case of insufficient response, pronounced tachycardia and/or circulatory instability (e.g. initially 1mg propranolol intravenously along with monitoring of ECG and blood pressure).

5. PHARMACOLOGICAL PROPERTIES

5.1 Pharmacodynamic properties

Pharmacotherapeutic group: Urinary Antispasmodic, ATC code G04BD15.

Trospium chloride is a quaternary derivative of nortropane and therefore belongs to the class of parasympatholytic or anticholinergic drugs, as it competes concentration-dependently with acetylcholine, the body's endogenous transmitter at postsynaptic, parasympathic binding sites.

Trospium chloride binds with high affinity to muscarinic receptors of the so called M_1-, M_2- and M_3- subtypes and demonstrates negligible affinity to nicotinic receptors.

Consequently, the anticholinergic effect of trospium chloride exerts a relaxing action on smooth muscle tissue and organ functions mediated by muscarinic receptors. Both in preclinical as well as in clinical experiments, trospium chloride diminishes the contractile tone of smooth muscle in the gastro-intestinal and genito-urinary tract.

Furthermore, it can inhibit the secretion of bronchial mucus, saliva, sweat and the occular accommodation. No effects on the central nervous system have so far been observed.

In two specific safety studies in healthy volunteers trospium chloride has been proven not to affect cardiac repolarisation, but has been shown to have a consistent and dose dependent heart rate accelerating effect.

A long term clinical trial with trospium chloride 20mg bid found an increase of QT> 60 ms in 1.5% (3/197) of included patients. The clinical relevance of these findings has not been established. Routine safety monitoring in two other placebo-controlled clinical trials of three months duration do not support such an influence of trospium chloride: In the first study an increase of QTcF>=60 msec was seen in 4/258 (1.6%) in trospium-treated patients versus 9/256 (3.5%) in placebo-treated patients. Corresponding figures in the second trial were 8/326 (2.5%) in trospium-treated patients versus 8/325 (2.5%) in placebo-treated patients.

5.2 Pharmacokinetic properties

After oral administration of trospium chloride maximum plasma levels are reached at 4-6 hours. Following a single dose of 20mg the maximum plasma level is about 4ng/ml. Within the tested interval, 20 to 60mg as a single dose, the plasma levels are proportional to the administered dose. The absolute bioavailability of a single oral dose of 20mg of trospium chloride (1 coated tablet Regurin 20mg) is 9.6 ± 4.5% (mean value ± standard deviation). At steady state the intraindividual variability is 16%, the interindividual variability is 36%.

Simultaneous intake of food, especially high fat diets, reduces the bioavailability of trospium chloride. After a high-fat meal mean C_{max} and AUC are reduced to 15-20% of the values in the fasted state.

Trospium chloride exhibits diurnal variability in exposure with a decrease of both C_{max} and AUC for evening relative to morning doses.

Most of the systemically available trospium chloride is excreted unchanged by the kidneys, though a small portion (10% of the renal excretion) appears in the urine as the spiroalcohol, a metabolite formed by ester hydrolysis. The terminal elimination half-life is in the range of 10-20 hours. No accumulation occurs. The plasma protein binding is 50-80%.

Pharmacokinetic data in elderly patients suggests no major differences. There are also no gender differences.

In a study in patients with severe renal impairment (creatinine clearance 8-32ml/min) mean AUC was 4-fold higher, C_{max} was 2-fold higher and the mean half-life was prolonged 2-fold compared with healthy subjects.

Pharmacokinetic results of a study with mildly and moderately hepatically impaired patients do not suggest a need for dose adjustment in patients with hepatic impairment, and are consistent with the limited role of hepatic metabolism in the elimination of trospium chloride.

5.3 Preclinical safety data

Preclinical data reveal no special hazard to humans based on conventional studies of safety pharmacology, repeated dose toxicity, genotoxicity, carcinogenicity, and toxicity to reproduction.

Placental transfer and passage of trospium chloride into the maternal milk occurs in rats.

6. PHARMACEUTICAL PARTICULARS

6.1 List of excipients

Tablet core:

Wheat starch

Microcrystalline cellulose

Lactose monohydrate

Povidone

Croscarmellose sodium

Stearic acid

Silica colloidal anhydrous

Talc

Tablet coat:

Sucrose

Carmellose sodium

Talc

Silica colloidal anhydrous

Calcium carbonate E170

Macrogol 8000

Titanium dioxide (E171)

Iron oxide hydrate yellow (E172)

Beeswax white

Carnauba wax

Note for diabetics: 1 coated tablet corresponds to 0.06g carbohydrate (equivalent to 0.005 bread units).

6.2 Incompatibilities

Not applicable.

6.3 Shelf life

5 years.

6.4 Special precautions for storage

This medicinal product does not require any special storage conditions.

6.5 Nature and contents of container

PVC foiled aluminium blister.

Packs sizes approved: 2, 20, 28, 30, 40, 50, 56, 60, 90, 100, 120, 150, 200, 500, 600, 1000, 1200, 2000.

Not all pack sizes may be marketed.

6.6 Instructions for use and handling

No special requirements.

7. MARKETING AUTHORISATION HOLDER

Madaus AG

51101 Cologne

Germany.

8. MARKETING AUTHORISATION NUMBER(S)

PL 4638/0013.

9. DATE OF FIRST AUTHORISATION/RENEWAL OF THE AUTHORISATION

14 September 2000/17 August 2004.

10. DATE OF REVISION OF THE TEXT

16 December 2004

Relcofen (ibuprofen) tablet 200mg

(Alpharma Limited)

1. NAME OF THE MEDICINAL PRODUCT

IBUPROFEN TABLETS BP 200mg

2. QUALITATIVE AND QUANTITATIVE COMPOSITION

Each tablet contains 200mg Ibuprofen PhEur.

3. PHARMACEUTICAL FORM

Pink sugar-coated tablets.

4. CLINICAL PARTICULARS

4.1 Therapeutic indications

POM product:

Ibuprofen is a non-steroidal anti-inflammatory agent with analgesic and antipyretic activity. It is indicated for:

1) The treatment of rheumatoid arthritis, osteoarthritis, ankylosing spondylitis and other non-rheumatoid (seronegative) arthropathies.

2) The treatment of non-articular rheumatic conditions and soft-tissue injuries including capsulitis, tenosynovitis, bursitis, low-back pain, strains and sprains.

P product (Relcofen):

For the relief of rheumatic and muscular pain, backache, migraine, headache, period pain, neuralgia, dental pain, feverishness, symptoms of colds and influenza.

4.2 Posology and method of administration

Posology

POM product:

Adults and children over 12 years: The recommended dosage is 1200-1800mg daily in divided doses. In acute or severe conditions the dosage may be increased until the acute phase has been brought under control, providing the dosage does not exceed 2400mg in any 24 hour period. The 600mg tablet offers a convenient dosage form where higher dosages are required. Some patients may be maintained on 600-1200mg daily.

Elderly: The elderly are at increased risk of the serious consequences of adverse reactions. If an NSAID is considered necessary, the lowest dose should be used and the patient should be monitored for GI bleeding for 4 weeks following the initiation of NSAID therapy.

Children under 12 years: Not recommended.

P product (Relcofen):

Dosage: Adults, the elderly and children over 12 years: 1-2 tablets three times a day swallowed whole with water. The dose should not be repeated more frequently than every four hours and no more than 6 tablets in any 24 hour period. To be taken preferably with or after food.

Not suitable for children under 12 years.

Method of Adminstration

For oral use.

4.3 Contraindications

A known hypersensitivity to ibuprofen or any other ingredients in the product; patients with a known history of, or active, peptic ulceration. Ibuprofen should not be given to patients in whom aspirin or other NSAIDs induce the symptoms of asthma, rhinitis, angioedema or urticaria.

4.4 Special warnings and special precautions for use

Bronchospasm may be precipitated in patients suffering from, or with a previous history of, bronchial asthma; therefore ibuprofen should be used with extreme caution in these patients. Fluid retention and oedema have been reported in association with ibuprofen; therefore the drug should be used with caution in patients with a history of cardiac decompensation or hypertension.

Undesirable effects may be minimised by using the minimum effective dose for the shortest possible duration.

The elderly are at increased risk of the serious consequences of adverse reactions.

Ibuprofen should be given under close supervision to patients with a history of upper gastrointestinal tract disease.

As with other NSAIDs, long-term administration of ibuprofen to animals has resulted in renal papillary necrosis and other abnormal renal pathology. In humans, there have been reports of acute interstitial nephritis with haematuria, proteinuria, and occasionally nephrotic syndrome.

A second form of renal toxicity has been seen in patients with prerenal conditions leading to a reduction in renal blood flow or blood volume, where the renal prostaglandins have a supportive role in the maintenance of renal perfusion. In these patients, administration of a NSAID may cause a dose dependent reduction in prostaglandin formation and may precipitate overt renal decompensation. Patients at greatest risk of this reaction are those with impaired renal function, heart failure, liver dysfunction, those taking diuretics and the elderly. Cessation of NSAID therapy is typically followed by recovery to the pre-treatment state.

In patients with renal, cardiac or hepatic impairment, caution is required since the use of NSAIDs may result in deterioration of renal function. The dose should be kept as low as possible and renal function should be monitored.

OTC & POM Label Warning

The label will state: Do not use if you have ever had a stomach ulcer or are allergic to ibuprofen or aspirin. If you are allergic to are taking any other painkiller, pregnant, or suffer from asthma speak to your doctor before taking ibuprofen. Do not exceed the stated dose. Keep out of the reach of children. If symptoms persist, consult your doctor.

4.5 Interaction with other medicinal products and other forms of Interaction

In therapeutic doses, no evidence of significant interactions with other commonly used drugs have yet been observed. In common with other NSAIDs, however, ibuprofen should be used with caution in patients receiving oral anticoagulants and diuretics, including frusemide and thiazides. NSAIDs may diminish the effect of anti-hypertensives.

Ibuprofen has been shown to produce a clinically relevant elevation of plasma lithium levels and a reduction in renal lithium clearance in a volunteer study. This effect has been attributed to inhibition of renal prostaglandin synthesis. Therefore, when ibuprofen and lithium are concurrently administered, patients should be carefully observed for signs of lithium toxicity.

Cardiac glycosides: NSAIDs may exacerbate cardiac failure, reduce GFR and increase plasma cardiac glycoside levels.

Methotrexate: Decreases elimination of methotrexate.

Cyclosporin: increased risk of nephrotoxicity with NSAIDs.

Mifepristone: NSAIDs should not be used for 8-12 days after mifepristone administration as NSAIDs can reduce the effects of mifepristone.

Other analgesics: Avoid concomitant use of two or more NSAIDs.

Corticosteroids: Increased risk of GI bleeding.

Quinolone antibiotics: Animal data indicate that NSAIDs can increase the risk of convulsions associated with quinolone antibiotics. Patients taking NSAIDs and quinolones may have an increased risk of developing convulsions.

4.6 Pregnancy and lactation

Ibuprofen does not appear to be teratogenic in animals; however, the use of ibuprofen in pregnancy should, if possible, be avoided. Congenital abnormalities have been reported in association with ibuprofen administration in man; however, these are low in frequency and do not appear to follow any discernible pattern. Due to the known effects of NSAIDs on the foetal cardiovascular system (closure of the ductus arteriosus), use during late pregnancy should be avoided. As with other drugs known to inhibit prostaglandin synthesis, an increased incidence of dystocia and delayed parturition occurred in rats. The onset of labour may be delayed and duration of labour increased. Ibuprofen appears in breast-milk in very low concentration and is unlikely to adversely affect the breast-fed infant.

4.7 Effects on ability to drive and use machines

None known.

4.8 Undesirable effects

Gastrointestinal: abdominal pain, nausea and dyspepsia, occasionally peptic ulcer and gastrointestinal haemorrhage, vomiting, diarrhoea, melaena, haematemesis, ulcerative stomatitis have been reported following administration. Less frequently, gastritis, duodenal ulcer, gastric ulcer and gastrointestinal perforation have been observed.

Hypersensitivity: hypersensitivity reactions have been reported following treatment with NSAIDs. These may consist of (a) non-specific allergic reactions and anaphylaxis, (b) respiratory tract reactivity comprising asthma, aggravated asthma, bronchospasm or dyspnoea, or (c) assorted skin disorders, including rashes of various types, pruritis, urticaria, purpura, angiodema and, less commonly, bullous dermatoses (including epidermal necrolysis and erythema multiforme).

Cardiovascular: oedema has been reported in association with NSAID treatment.

Other: other adverse effects reported less commonly include:

Renal: nephrotoxicity in various forms, including interstitial nephritis, nephrotic syndrome and renal failure.

Hepatic: abnormal liver function, hepatitis and jaundice.

Neurological and special senses: visual disturbances, optic neuritis, headaches, paraesthesia, depression, confusion, hallucinations, tinnitus, vertigo, dizziness, malaise, fatigue and drowsiness.

Haematological: thrombocytopenia, neutropenia, agranulocytosis, aplastic anaemia and haemolytic anaemia.

Dermatological: photosensitivity.

Other effects: lupus erythematosus syndrome with aseptic meningitis.

4.9 Overdose

Symptoms of headache, vomiting, drowsiness and hypotension.

There is no specific antidote to ibuprofen. Gastric lavage may be carried out and, if necessary, correction of serum electrolytes.

5. PHARMACOLOGICAL PROPERTIES

5.1 Pharmacodynamic properties

Ibuprofen has analgesic, antipyretic and anti-inflammatory properties. Ibuprofen inhibits prostaglandin synthesis.

Ibuprofen has prominent anti-inflammatory effect in addition to having analgesic and antipyretic actions. The analgesic effects of ibuprofen are due to both a peripheral and a central effect, and are distinct from its property as an anti-inflammatory drug. Ibuprofen is a potent inhibitor of the enzyme cyclo-oxygenase which thus results in a marked reduction in prostaglandin synthesis.

Ibuprofen also inhibits the synthesis of some lipoxygenase products, especially 11 and 15-monohydroxyeicosatetranoic acid (HETE) but it has no effect on the generation of 5-HETE and leukotriene B4.

Ibuprofen also inhibits the migration of polymorphonuclear leucocytes but the role of this in its anti-inflammatory action is not clear.

Inhibition of prostaglandin biosynthesis prevents their hyperalgesic effect upon sensory nerves. Inhibition of vasodilator prostanoid formation (PGE) diminishes the vascularity and transudation of fluid which are two of the principal manifestations of inflammation.

5.2 Pharmacokinetic properties

Ibuprofen is rapidly absorbed following administration and is rapidly distributed throughout the whole body. The excretion is rapid and complete via the kidneys.

Maximum plasma concentrations are reached 45 minutes after ingestion if taken on an empty stomach. When taken with food peak levels are observed at 1 to 2 hours. These times may vary with different dosage forms.

The half-life of ibuprofen is about 2 hours.

In limited studies, ibuprofen appears in the breast milk in very low concentrations.

About 1% is excreted in urine as unchanged ibuprofen and about 14% as conjugated ibuprofen.

5.3 Preclinical safety data

Not applicable.

6. PHARMACEUTICAL PARTICULARS

6.1 List of excipients

Also contains: beeswax, carmellose sodium, colloidal silica, dimethicone, gelatin, hydrochloric acid, kaolin, shellac, sodium lauryl sulphate, sucrose, E127, E170, E171, E172, E211, E322, E414, E460, E463, E553.

6.2 Incompatibilities

None known.

6.3 Shelf life

Shelf-life

Three years from the date of manufacture.

Shelf-life after dilution/reconstitution

Not applicable.

Shelf-life after first opening

Not applicable.

6.4 Special precautions for storage

Store below 25°C in a dry place.

6.5 Nature and contents of container

The product containers are rigid injection moulded polypropylene or injection blow-moulded polyethylene containers with polyfoam wad or polyethylene ullage filler and snap-on polyethylene caps or child-resistant closures; in case any supply difficulties should arise the alternative is amber glass containers with screw caps. An alternative closure for polyethylene containers is a polypropylene, twist on, push down and twist off child-resistant, tamper-evident lid.

OTC packs include a child-resistant closure.

The product may also be supplied in blister packs in cartons:

a) Carton: Printed carton manufactured from white folding box board.

b) Blister pack: (i) 250μm white rigid PVC. (ii) Surface printed 20μm hard temper aluminium foil with 5-7g/M^2 PVC and PVdC compatible heat seal lacquer on the reverse side.

Pack sizes: 28s, 56s, 60s, 84s, 100s, 112s, 168s, 250s, 500s, 1000s.

OTC pack sizes: 12s, 20s, 24s, 48s, 96s.

Product may also be supplied in bulk packs, for reassembly purposes only, in polybags contained in tins, skillets or polybuckets filled with suitable cushioning material. Bulk packs are included for *temporary* storage of the finished product before final packaging into the proposed marketing containers.

Maximum size of bulk packs: 28,000.

6.6 Instructions for use and handling

Not applicable.

Administrative Data

7. MARKETING AUTHORISATION HOLDER

Alpharma Limited (Trading style: Alpharma, Cox Pharmaceuticals)

Whiddon Valley

BARNSTAPLE

N Devon EX32 8NS

8. MARKETING AUTHORISATION NUMBER(S)

PL 0142/0304

9. DATE OF FIRST AUTHORISATION/RENEWAL OF THE AUTHORISATION

26.10.90 (Renewed 1/00)

10. DATE OF REVISION OF THE TEXT

October 2002

Relcofen (ibuprofen) tablet 400mg

(Alpharma Limited)

1. NAME OF THE MEDICINAL PRODUCT

IBUPROFEN TABLETS BP 400mg

2. QUALITATIVE AND QUANTITATIVE COMPOSITION

Each tablet contains 400mg Ibuprofen PhEur.

3. PHARMACEUTICAL FORM

Pink sugar-coated tablets.

4. CLINICAL PARTICULARS

4.1 Therapeutic indications

POM product:

Ibuprofen is a non-steroidal anti-inflammatory agent with analgesic and antipyretic activity. It is indicated for:

1) The treatment of rheumatoid arthritis, osteoarthritis, ankylosing spondylitis and other non-rheumatoid (seronegative) arthropathies.

2) The treatment of non-articular rheumatic conditions and soft-tissue injuries including capsulitis, tenosynovitis, bursitis, low-back pain, strains and sprains.

P product (Relcofen):

For the relief of rheumatic and muscular pain, backache, migraine, headache, period pain, neuralgia, dental pain, feverishness, symptoms of colds and influenza.

4.2 Posology and method of administration

Posology

POM product:

Adults and children over 12 years: The recommended dosage is 1200-1800mg daily in divided doses. In acute or severe conditions the dosage may be increased until the acute phase has been brought under control, providing the dosage does not exceed 2400mg in any 24 hour period. The 600mg tablet offers a convenient dosage form where higher dosages are required. Some patients may be maintained on 600-1200mg daily.

Elderly: The elderly are at increased risk of the serious consequences of adverse reactions. If an NSAID is considered necessary, the lowest dose should be used and the patient should be monitored for GI bleeding for 4 weeks following initiation of NSAID therapy.

Children under 12 years: Not recommended.

P product (Relcofen):

Dosage: Adults, the elderly and children over 12 years: 1 tablet three times a day swallowed whole with water. The dose should not be repeated more frequently than every four hours and no more than 3 tablets in any 24 hour period. To be taken preferably with or after food.

Not suitable for children under 12 years.

Method of Adminstration

For oral use.

4.3 Contraindications

A known hypersensitivity to ibuprofen or any other ingredients in the product; patients with a known history of, or active, peptic ulceration. Ibuprofen should not be given to patients in whom aspirin or other NSAIDs induce the symptoms of asthma, rhinitis, angioedema or urticaria.

4.4 Special warnings and special precautions for use

Bronchospasm may be precipitated in patients suffering from, or with a previous history of, bronchial asthma; therefore ibuprofen should be used with extreme caution in these patients. Fluid retention and oedema have been reported in association with ibuprofen; therefore the drug should be used with caution in patients with a history of cardiac decompensation or hypertension.

Undesirable effects may be minimised by using the minimum effective dose for the shortest possible duration.

The elderly are at increased risk of the serious consequences of adverse reactions.

Ibuprofen should be given under close supervision to patients with a history of upper gastrointestinal tract disease.

As with other NSAIDs, long-term administration of ibuprofen to animals has resulted in renal papillary necrosis and other abnormal renal pathology. In humans, there have been reports of acute interstitial nephritis with haematuria, proteinuria, and occasionally nephrotic syndrome.

A second form of renal toxicity has been seen in patients with prerenal conditions leading to a reduction in renal blood flow or blood volume, where the renal prostaglandins have a supportive role in the maintenance of renal perfusion. In these patients, administration of a NSAID may cause a dose dependent reduction in prostaglandin formation and may precipitate overt renal decompensation. Patients at greatest risk of this reaction are those with impaired renal function, heart failure, liver dysfunction, those taking diuretics and the elderly. Cessation of NSAID therapy is typically followed by recovery to the pre-treatment state.

In patients with renal, cardiac or hepatic impairment, caution is required since the use of NSAIDs may result in deterioration of renal function. The dose should be kept as low as possible and renal function should be monitored.

OTC & POM Label Warning

The label will state: Do not use if you have ever had a stomach ulcer or are allergic to ibuprofen or aspirin. If you are allergic to are taking any other painkiller, pregnant, or suffer from asthma speak to your doctor before taking ibuprofen. Do not exceed the stated dose. Keep out of the reach of children. If symptoms persist, consult your doctor.

4.5 Interaction with other medicinal products and other forms of Interaction

In therapeutic doses, no evidence of significant interactions with other commonly used drugs have yet been observed. In common with other NSAIDs, however, ibuprofen should be used with caution in patients receiving oral anticoagulants and diuretics, including frusemide and thiazides. NSAIDs may diminish the effect of anti-hypertensives.

Ibuprofen has been shown to produce a clinically relevant elevation of plasma lithium levels and a reduction in renal lithium clearance in a volunteer study. This effect has been attributed to inhibition of renal prostaglandin synthesis. Therefore, when ibuprofen and lithium are concurrently administered, patients should be carefully observed for signs of lithium toxicity.

Cardiac glycosides: NSAIDs may exacerbate cardiac failure, reduce GFR and increase plasma cardiac glycoside levels.

Methotrexate: Decreases elimination of methotrexate.

Cyclosporin: increased risk of nephrotoxicity with NSAIDs.

Mifepristone: NSAIDs should not be used for 8-12 days after mifepristone administration as NSAIDs can reduce the effects of mifepristone.

Other analgesics: Avoid concomitant use of two or more NSAIDs.

Corticosteroids: Increased risk of GI bleeding.

Quinolone antibiotics: Animal data indicate that NSAIDs can increase the risk of convulsions associated with quinolone antibiotics. Patients taking NSAIDs and quinolones may have an increased risk of developing convulsions.

4.6 Pregnancy and lactation

Ibuprofen does not appear to be teratogenic in animals; however, the use of ibuprofen in pregnancy should, if possible, be avoided. Congenital abnormalities have been reported in association with ibuprofen administration in man; however, these are low in frequency and do not appear to follow any discernible pattern. Due to the known effects of NSAIDs on the foetal cardiovascular system (closure of the ductus arteriosus), use during late pregnancy should be avoided. As with other drugs known to inhibit prostaglandin synthesis, an increased incidence of dystocia and delayed parturition occurred in rats. The onset of labour may be delayed and duration of labour increased. Ibuprofen appears in breast-milk in very low concentration and is unlikely to adversely affect the breast-fed infant.

4.7 Effects on ability to drive and use machines

None known.

4.8 Undesirable effects

Gastrointestinal: abdominal pain, nausea and dyspepsia, occasionally peptic ulcer and gastrointestinal haemorrhage, vomiting, diarrhoea, melaena, haematemesis, ulcerative stomatitis have been reported following administration. Less frequently, gastritis, duodenal ulcer, gastric ulcer and gastrointestinal perforation have been observed.

Hypersensitivity: hypersensitivity reactions have been reported following treatment with NSAIDs. These may consist of (a) non-specific allergic reactions and anaphylaxis, (b) respiratory tract reactivity comprising asthma, aggravated asthma, bronchospasm or dyspnoea, or (c) assorted skin disorders, including rashes of various types, pruritis, urticaria, purpura, angiodema and, less commonly, bullous dermatoses (including epidermal necrolysis and erythema multiforme).

Cardiovascular: oedema has been reported in association with NSAID treatment.

Other: other adverse effects reported less commonly include:

Renal: nephrotoxicity in various forms, including interstitial nephritis, nephrotic syndrome and renal failure.

Hepatic: abnormal liver function, hepatitis and jaundice.

Neurological and special senses: visual disturbances, optic neuritis, headaches, paraesthesia, depression, confusion, hallucinations, tinnitus, vertigo, dizziness, malaise, fatigue and drowsiness.

Haematological: thrombocytopenia, neutropenia, agranulocytosis, aplastic anaemia and haemolytic anaemia.

Dermatological: photosensitivity.

Other effects: lupus erythematosus syndrome with aseptic meningitis.

4.9 Overdose

Symptoms of headache, vomiting, drowsiness and hypotension.

There is no specific antidote to ibuprofen. Gastric lavage may be carried out and, if necessary, correction of serum electrolytes.

5. PHARMACOLOGICAL PROPERTIES

5.1 Pharmacodynamic properties

Ibuprofen has analgesic, antipyretic and anti-inflammatory properties. Ibuprofen inhibits prostaglandin synthesis.

Ibuprofen has prominent anti-inflammatory effect in addition to having analgesic and antipyretic actions. The analgesic effects of ibuprofen are due to both a peripheral and a central effect, and are distinct from its property as an anti-inflammatory drug. Ibuprofen is a potent inhibitor of the enzyme cyclo-oxygenase which thus results in a marked reduction in prostaglandin synthesis.

Ibuprofen also inhibits the synthesis of some lipoxygenase products, especially 11 and 15-monohydroxyeicosatetranoic acid (HETE) but it has no effect on the generation of 5-HETE and leukotriene B4.

Ibuprofen also inhibits the migration of polymorphonuclear leucocytes but the role of this in its anti-inflammatory action is not clear.

Inhibition of prostaglandin biosynthesis prevents their hyperalgesic effect upon sensory nerves. Inhibition of vasodilator prostanoid formation (PGE) diminishes the vascularity and transudation of fluid which are two of the principal manifestations of inflammation.

5.2 Pharmacokinetic properties

Ibuprofen is rapidly absorbed following administration and is rapidly distributed throughout the whole body. The excretion is rapid and complete via the kidneys.

Maximum plasma concentrations are reached 45 minutes after ingestion if taken on an empty stomach. When taken with food peak levels are observed at 1 to 2 hours. These times may vary with different dosage forms.

The half-life of ibuprofen is about 2 hours.

In limited studies, ibuprofen appears in the breast milk in very low concentrations.

About 1% is excreted in urine as unchanged ibuprofen and about 14% as conjugated ibuprofen.

5.3 Preclinical safety data

Not applicable.

6. PHARMACEUTICAL PARTICULARS

6.1 List of excipients

Also contains: beeswax, carmellose sodium, colloidal silica, dimethicone, gelatin, hydrochloric acid, kaolin, shellac, sodium lauryl sulphate, sucrose, E127, E170, E171, E172, E211, E322, E414, E460, E463, E553.

6.2 Incompatibilities

None known.

6.3 Shelf life

Shelf-life

Three years from the date of manufacture.

Shelf-life after dilution/reconstitution

Not applicable.

Shelf-life after first opening

Not applicable.

6.4 Special precautions for storage

Store below 25°C in a dry place.

6.5 Nature and contents of container

The product containers are rigid injection moulded polypropylene or injection blow-moulded polyethylene containers with polyethylene wad or polyethylene ullage filler and snap-on polyethylene caps or child-resistant closures; in case any supply difficulties should arise the alternative is amber glass containers with screw caps. An alternative closure for polyethylene containers is a polypropylene, twist on, push down and twist off child-resistant, tamper-evident lid.

OTC packs include a child-resistant closure.

The product may also be supplied in blister packs in cartons:

a) Carton: Printed carton manufactured from white folding box board.

b) Blister pack: (i) 250μm white rigid PVC. (ii) Surface printed 20μm hard temper aluminium foil with 5-7g/M^2 PVC and PVdC compatible heat seal lacquer on the reverse side.

Pack sizes: 28s, 56s, 60s, 84s, 100s, 112s, 168s, 250s, 500s, 1000s.

OTC pack sizes: 12s, 20s, 24s, 48s, 96s.

Product may also be supplied in bulk packs, for reassembly purposes only, in polybags contained in tins, skillets or polybuckets filled with suitable cushioning material. Bulk packs are included for *temporary* storage of the finished product before final packaging into the proposed marketing containers.

Maximum size of bulk packs: 16,000.

6.6 Instructions for use and handling

Not applicable.

Administrative Data

7. MARKETING AUTHORISATION HOLDER

Alpharma Limited (Trading style: Alpharma, Cox Pharmaceuticals)

Whiddon Valley

BARNSTAPLE

N Devon EX32 8NS

8. MARKETING AUTHORISATION NUMBER(S)

PL 0142/0305

9. DATE OF FIRST AUTHORISATION/RENEWAL OF THE AUTHORISATION

26.10.90 (Renewed 1/00)

10. DATE OF REVISION OF THE TEXT

October 2002

Relenza 5mg/dose inhalation powder.

(GlaxoSmithKline UK)

1. NAME OF THE MEDICINAL PRODUCT

Relenza 5mg/dose, inhalation powder, pre-dispensed.

2. QUALITATIVE AND QUANTITATIVE COMPOSITION

Each pre-dispensed quantity of inhalation powder (one blister) contains 5 mg zanamivir. Each delivered inhalation (the amount that leaves the mouthpiece of the Diskhaler) contains 3.6 mg zanamivir.

For excipients, see section 6.1.

3. PHARMACEUTICAL FORM

Inhalation powder, pre-dispensed.

4. CLINICAL PARTICULARS

4.1 Therapeutic indications

Relenza is indicated for treatment of both influenza A and B in adults and adolescents ($\geqslant$ 12 years) who present with symptoms typical of influenza when influenza is circulating in the community.

4.2 Posology and method of administration

Treatment should begin as soon as possible, within 48 hours after onset of symptoms.

Relenza is for administration to the respiratory tract by oral inhalation only, using the Diskhaler device provided. One blister should be utilised for each inhalation.

The recommended dose of Relenza is two inhalations (2 × 5 mg) twice daily for five days, providing a total daily inhaled dose of 20 mg.

Inhaled drugs, e.g. asthma medication, should be administered prior to administration of Relenza (see section 4.4).

Impaired Renal or Hepatic Function: No dose modification is required. (See section 5.2).

Elderly patients: No dose modification is required. (See section 5.2).

4.3 Contraindications

Hypersensitivity to any ingredient of the preparation (see Pharmaceutical Particulars, 6.1 List of excipients).

4.4 Special warnings and special precautions for use

Due to the limited number of patients with severe asthma or with other chronic respiratory disease, patients with unstable chronic illnesses or immunocompromised patients (see Section 5.1) who have been treated, it has not been possible to demonstrate the efficacy and safety of Relenza in these groups. Efficacy of zanamivir in elderly patients $\geqslant$ 65 years has not been established (see section 5.1).

There have been very rare reports of patients being treated with Relenza who have experienced bronchospasm and/or decline in respiratory function which may be acute and/or serious. Some of these patients did not have any previous history of respiratory disease. Any patients experiencing such reactions should discontinue Relenza and seek medical evaluation immediately.

Due to the limited experience, patients with severe asthma require a careful consideration of the risk in relation to the expected benefit, and Relenza should not be administered unless close medical monitoring and appropriate clinical facilities are available in case of bronchoconstriction. In patients with persistent asthma or severe COPD, management of the underlying disease should be optimised during therapy with Relenza.

Should zanamivir be considered appropriate for patients with asthma or chronic obstructive pulmonary disease, the patient should be informed of the potential risk of bronchospasm with Relenza and should have a fast acting bronchodilator available. Patients on maintenance inhaled bronchodilating therapy should be advised to use their bronchodilators before taking Relenza (see section 4.2).

4.5 Interaction with other medicinal products and other forms of Interaction

Zanamivir is not protein bound and not hepatically metabolised or modified. Clinically significant drug interactions are unlikely. Zanamivir, when given for 28 days, did not impair the immune response to influenza vaccine.

4.6 Pregnancy and lactation

Pregnancy: The safe use of Relenza during pregnancy has not been established.

In rats and rabbits zanamivir has been shown to cross the placenta. High doses of zanamivir were not associated with malformations in rats or rabbits and only minor alterations were reported. The potential risk for humans is unknown. Relenza should not be used in pregnancy unless the expected benefit to the mother is thought to outweigh any possible risk to the foetus.

Lactation: In rats zanamivir has been shown to be secreted into milk. There is no information on secretion into breast milk in humans.

The use of zanamivir is not recommended in mothers who are breast feeding.

4.7 Effects on ability to drive and use machines

None known

4.8 Undesirable effects

There have been rare reports of patients with previous history of respiratory disease (asthma, COPD) and very rare reports of patients without previous history of respiratory disease, who have experienced acute bronchospasm and/or serious decline in respiratory function after use of Relenza (see section 4.4).

The adverse events considered at least possibly related to the treatment are listed below by body system, organ class and absolute frequency. Frequencies are defined as very common $>1/10$), common $>1/100$, $<1/10$), uncommon $>1/1000$, $<1/100$), rare $>1/10,000$, $<1/1000$), very rare ($<1/10,000$).

Immune system disorders

Very rare: allergic-type reaction including facial and oropharyngeal oedema

Respiratory, thoracic and mediastinal disorders:

Very rare: bronchospasm, dyspnea, throat tightness or constriction

Skin and subcutaneous tissue disorders:

Very rare: rash, urticaria

4.9 Overdose

Accidental overdose is unlikely due to the physical limitations of the presentation, the route of administration and the poor oral bioavailability (2 to 3%) of zanamivir. Doses of zanamivir up to 64 mg/day (approximately 3 times the maximum daily recommended dose) have been administered by oral inhalation (by nebuliser) without adverse effects. Additionally, systemic exposure by intravenous administration of up to 1200 mg/day for five days showed no adverse effect.

5. PHARMACOLOGICAL PROPERTIES

5.1 Pharmacodynamic properties

ATC code J05AH01

Mechanism of action

Zanamivir is a selective inhibitor of neuraminidase, the influenza virus surface enzyme. Neuraminidase inhibition occurred in vitro at very low zanamivir concentrations (50% inhibition at 0.64nM – 7.9nM against influenza A and B strains). Viral neuraminidase aids the release of newly formed virus particles from infected cells, and may facilitate access of virus through mucus to epithelial cell surfaces, to allow viral infection of other cells. The inhibition of this enzyme is reflected in both *in vitro* and *in vivo* activity against influenza A and B virus replication, and encompasses all of the known neuraminidase subtypes of influenza A viruses.

The activity of zanamivir is extracellular. It reduces the propagation of both influenza A and B viruses by inhibiting the release of infectious influenza virions from the epithelial cells of the respiratory tract. Influenza viral replication occurs in the superficial epithelium of the respiratory tract. The efficacy of topical administration of zanamivir to this site has been confirmed in clinical studies. To date, virus with reduced susceptibility to zanamivir has not been detected in samples obtained pre and post treatment from patients in clinicalstudies.

Clinical experience

Relenza alleviates the symptoms of influenza and reduces their median duration by 1.5 days (range 0.25 – 2.5 days) as detailed in the table below. The efficacy of Relenza has been demonstrated in otherwise healthy subjects when treatment is initiated within 48 hours after the onset of symptoms. No treatment benefit has been documented for patients with afebrile disease ($<37.8°C$).

Five Phase III randomised, placebo-controlled, parallel-group, multicentre treatment studies (NAIB3001, NAIA3002, NAIB3002, NAI30008 and NAI30012) have been conducted with zanamivir for the treatment of naturally acquired influenza A and B. Study NAI30008 recruited only patients with asthma (n=399), COPD (n=87), or asthma and COPD (n=32) and study NAI30012 recruited only elderly (≥65 years) patients (n=358). The Intent to Treat population of these five studies comprised 2471 patients of which 1266 received 10 mg zanamivir b.i.d by oral inhalation. The primary endpoint was identical for all five Phase III studies, i.e. time to alleviation of clinically significant signs and symptoms of influenza. Alleviation was defined as no fever, i.e. temperature $<37.8°C$ and feverishness score of 'none'('same as normal/none' in NAI30012), and headache, myalgia, cough and sore throat recorded as 'none' ('same as normal/none' in NAI30012) or 'mild' and maintained for 24 hours.

Comparison of Median Time (Days) to Alleviation of Influenza Symptoms: Influenza Positive Population

(see Table 1)

The median time to alleviation of influenza symptoms in elderly subjects (≥ 65 years) was not significantly reduced.

In the Intent to Treat (ITT) population the difference in time to alleviation of symptoms was 1.0 day (95% CI: 0.5 to 1.5) in the combined analysis of NAIB3001, NAIA3002 and NAIB3002, 1.0 day (95% CI: 0 to 2) in study NAI30008, and 1.0 day (95% CI −1.0 to 3.0) in study NAI30012.

In a combined analysis of patients with influenza B (n=163), including 79 treated with zanamivir, a 2.0 day treatment benefit was observed (95%CI: 0.50 to 3.50).

In the pooled analysis of 3 phase III studies in influenza positive, predominantly healthy adults, the incidence of complications was 152/558 (27%) in placebo recipients and 119/609 (20%) in zanamivir recipients (relative risk 0.73; 95% CI 0.59 to 0.90, p=0.004). In study NAI30008 enrolling patients with asthma and COPD the incidence of complications was 56/153 (37%) in influenza-positive placebo recipients and 52/160 (33%) in influenza positive zanamivir recipients (relative risk 0.89; 95% CI: 0.65 to 1.21, p=0.520). In study NAI30012 enrolling elderly patients the incidence of complications was 46/114 (40%) in influenza positive placebo recipients and 39/120 (33%) in influenza positive zanamivir recipients (relative risk 0.80, 95% CI: 0.57 to 1.13, p=0.256).

In a placebo controlled study in patients with predominantly mild/moderate asthma and/or Chronic Obstructive Pulmonary Disease (COPD) there was no clinically significant difference between zanamivir and placebo in forced expiratory volume in one second (FEV_1) or peak expiratory flow rate (PEFR) measured during treatment or after the end of treatment.

Table 1 Comparison of Median Time (Days) to Alleviation of Influenza Symptoms: Influenza Positive Population

Study	Placebo	Zanamivir 10mg inhaled twice daily	Difference in Days	(95% CI) p-value
NAIB3001	n=160 6.0	n=161 4.5	1.5	(0.5, 2.5) 0.004
NAIA3002	n=257 6.0	n=312 5.0	1.0	(0.0, 1.5) 0.078
NAIB3002	n=141 7.5	n=136 5.0	2.5	(1.0, 4.0) <0.001
Combined analysis of NAIB3001, NAIA3002, and NAIB3002	n=558 6.5	n=609 5.0	1.5	(1.0, 2.0) <0.001
Asthma/COPD study				
NAI30008	n=153 7.0	n=160 5.5	1.5	(0.5, 3.25) 0.009
Elderly study				
NAI30012	n=114 7.5	n=120 7.25	0.25	(-2.0 to 3.25) 0.609

5.2 Pharmacokinetic properties

Absorption: Pharmacokinetic studies in humans have shown that the absolute oral bioavailability of the drug is low (mean (min, max) is 2%(1%, 5%)). Similar studies of orally inhaled zanamivir indicate that approximately 10-20% of the dose is systemically absorbed, with serum concentrations generally peaking within 1-2 hours. The poor absorption of the drug results in low systemic concentrations and therefore there is no significant systemic exposure to zanamivir after oral inhalation. There is no evidence of modification in the kinetics after repeated dosing with oral inhaled administration.

Distribution: After oral inhalation, zanamivir is widely deposited at high concentrations throughout the respiratory tract, thus delivering the drug to the site of influenza infection. Following a single 10mg dose the concentrations of zanamivir were measured in induced sputum. Zanamivir concentrations of 337 (range 58-1593) and 52 (range 17-286) fold above the median viral neuraminidase IC_{50} were measured at 12h and 24h respectively. The high concentrations of zanamivir in the respiratory tract will result in the rapid onset of inhibition of the viral neuraminidase. The major immediate site of deposition is the oropharynx (mean 78%) from where zanamivir was rapidly eliminated to the GI-tract. The early deposition in total lungs ranged between 8 and 21%.

Metabolism: Zanamivir has been shown to be renally excreted as unchanged drug, and does not undergo metabolism. *In vitro* studies demonstrated that zanamivir did not affect the activity of a range of probe substrates for cytochrome P450 isoenzymes (CYP1A/2, A6, 2C9, 2C18, 2D6, 2E1, 3A4) in human hepatic microsomes, nor did it induce cytochrome P450 expression in rats, suggesting that metabolic interactions between zanamivir and other drugs are unlikely *in vivo*.

Elimination: The serum half-life of zanamivir following administration by oral inhalation ranges from 2.6 to 5.05 hours. It is entirely excreted unchanged in the urine. Total clearance ranges from 2.5 to 10.9 L/h as approximated by urinary clearance. Renal elimination is completed within 24 hours.

Patients with renal impairment: Inhaled zanamivir results in approximately 10%-20% of the inhaled dose being absorbed. In the severe renal impairment group from the single IV zanamivir dose trial subjects were sampled after a dose of 2 mg or twice to four times the expected exposure from inhalation. Using the normal dosing regimen (10mg bid), the predicted exposure at Day 5 is 40 fold lower than what was tolerated in healthy subjects after repeated iv administration. Given the importance of local concentrations, the low systemic exposure, and the previous tolerance of much higher exposures no dose adjustment is advised.

Patients with hepatic impairment: Zanamivir is not metabolised, therefore dose adjustment in patients with hepatic impairment is not required.

Elderly patients: At the therapeutic daily dose of 20mg, bioavailabilty is low (10-20%), and as a result there is no significant systemic exposure of patients to zanamivir. Any alteration of pharmacokinetics that may occur with age is unlikely to be of clinical consequence and no dose modification is recommended.

5.3 Preclinical safety data

General toxicity studies did not indicate any significant toxicity of zanamivir. Zanamivir was not genotoxic and no clinically relevant findings were observed in long term carcinogenicity studies in rats and mice.

6. PHARMACEUTICAL PARTICULARS

6.1 List of excipients

Lactose monohydrate (which contains milk protein).

6.2 Incompatibilities

Not applicable

6.3 Shelf life

3 years

6.4 Special precautions for storage

Do not store above 30°C.

6.5 Nature and contents of container

Relenza inhalation powder is packed in a circular aluminium foil disk (a Rotadisk) with four regularly distributed blisters. An inspiration driven inhaler made of plastic (a Diskhaler) is used for administration of doses (the contents of 2 blisters constitute a dose) from these foil disks, and is provided in the pack.

The pack contains 1 or 5 foil disks and a Diskhaler.

6.6 Instructions for use and handling

The inhaler (Diskhaler) is loaded with a disk containing inhalation powder packed in individual blisters. These blisters are pierced when the inhaler is used, and with a deep inhalation the powder can then be inhaled through the mouthpiece down into the respiratory tract. Detailed instructions for use are enclosed in the pack.

Administrative Date

7. MARKETING AUTHORISATION HOLDER

GlaxoSmithKline AB

Box 263

431 23 Mölndal

8. MARKETING AUTHORISATION NUMBER(S)
14997

9. DATE OF FIRST AUTHORISATION/RENEWAL OF THE AUTHORISATION
1999-02-09 / 2004-02-09

10. DATE OF REVISION OF THE TEXT
2004-11-27

Relestat
(Allergan Ltd)

1. NAME OF THE MEDICINAL PRODUCT
Relestat▼, 0.5 mg/ml, eye drops, solution.

2. QUALITATIVE AND QUANTITATIVE COMPOSITION
One ml of eye drops, solution, contains 0.5 mg of epinastine hydrochloride.

(equivalent to 0.436 mg epinastine)

For excipients, see 6.1.

3. PHARMACEUTICAL FORM
Eye drops, solution.

A clear colourless solution.

4. CLINICAL PARTICULARS
4.1 Therapeutic indications
Treatment of the symptoms of seasonal allergic conjunctivitis.

4.2 Posology and method of administration
The recommended dose for adults is one drop instilled in each affected eye twice daily, during the symptomatic period.

There is no experience with the use of Relestat for more than 8 weeks.

The contents of the bottle remain sterile until the original closure is broken by twisting the cap to pierce the dropper tip. To avoid contamination do not touch any surface with the dropper tip.

If more than one topical ophthalmic medicinal product is being used, the medicinal products should be administered at least 10 minutes apart.

Elderly patients

Relestat has not been studied in elderly patients. Post-marketing safety data from the tablet formulation of epinastine hydrochloride (up to 20 mg once daily) indicates that there are no particular safety issues for elderly patients compared with adult patients. As such, no dosage adjustment is considered to be necessary.

Children and Adolescents

Relestat may be used in adolescents (12 years of age and older) at the same dosage as in adults.

Hepatic impairment

Relestat has not been studied in patients with hepatic impairment. Post-marketing safety data from the tablet formulation of epinastine hydrochloride (up to 20 mg once daily) indicates that the incidence of adverse reactions was higher in this group compared with adult patients without hepatic impairment. The daily dose of a 10 mg epinastine hydrochloride tablet is more than 100-fold higher than the daily dose following Relestat. In addition, the metabolism of epinastine in humans is minimal (<10%). Therefore, no dosage adjustment is considered to be necessary.

Renal impairment

Relestat has not been studied in patients with renal impairment. Post-marketing safety data from the tablet formulation of epinastine hydrochloride (up to 20 mg once daily) indicate that there are no particular safety issues for patients with renal impairment. As such, no dosage adjustment is considered to be necessary.

4.3 Contraindications
Hypersensitivity to epinastine or to any excipient.

4.4 Special warnings and special precautions for use
Benzalkonium chloride is commonly used as a preservative in ophthalmic products and has been reported rarely to cause punctate keratopathy and/or toxic ulcerative keratopathy.

Benzalkonium chloride may be absorbed by and discolour soft contact lenses and therefore patients should be instructed to wait until 10-15 minutes after instillation of Relestat before inserting contact lenses. Relestat should not be administered while wearing contact lenses.

4.5 Interaction with other medicinal products and other forms of Interaction
No drug-drug interactions are anticipated in humans since systemic concentrations of epinastine are extremely low following ocular dosing. In addition, epinastine is mainly excreted unchanged in humans indicating a low level of metabolism. Specific interaction studies with other medicinal products have not been performed with Relestat.

4.6 Pregnancy and lactation
Pregnancy

Data on a limited number (11) of exposed pregnancies indicate no adverse effects of epinastine on pregnancy or on the health of the foetus/newborn child. To date, no other relevant epidemiological data are available. Animal studies do not indicate direct or indirect harmful effects with respect to pregnancy, embryonic/foetal development, parturition or postnatal development (see section 5.3).

Caution should be exercised when prescribing to pregnant women.

Lactation

Epinastine is excreted in the breast milk of rats, but it is not known if epinastine is excreted in human milk. Due to the lack of experience, caution should be exercised when prescribing to breast-feeding women.

4.7 Effects on ability to drive and use machines
Based on the pharmacodynamic profile, reported adverse reactions and specific psychometric studies, epinastine has no or negligible influence on the ability to drive and use machines.

If transient blurred vision occurs at instillation, the patient should wait until the vision clears before driving or using machinery.

4.8 Undesirable effects
In clinical studies, the overall incidence of adverse drug reactions following Relestat was less than 10%. No serious adverse reactions occurred. Most were ocular and mild. The most common adverse reaction was burning sensation in eye (mostly mild); all other adverse reactions were uncommon.

The following adverse drug reactions were reported during clinical trials with Relestat:

Eye disorders

Common (>1/100, <1/10): burning sensation

Uncommon (>1/1000, <1/100): allergic conjunctivitis, blepharoptosis, conjunctival oedema, conjunctival hyperaemia, eye discharge, eye dryness, irritation, itching, increased sensitivity, photophobia, visual disturbance

Nervous system disorders

Uncommon (>1/1000, <1/100): headache

Respiratory, thoracic and mediastinal disorders

Uncommon (>1/1000, <1/100): asthma, nasal irritation, rhinitis

Gastrointestinal disorders

Uncommon (>1/1000, <1/100): oral dryness, taste alteration

Skin and subcutaneous tissue disorders

Uncommon (>1/1000, <1/100): pruritus

4.9 Overdose
After instillation of 0.3% epinastine hydrochloride eye drops 3 times daily (corresponds to 9 times the recommended daily dose) reversible miosis, without influence on visual acuity or other ocular parameters, was observed.

The 5 ml bottle of Relestat contains 2.5 mg of epinastine hydrochloride. A tablet formulation is marketed at a once daily dose of up to 20 mg epinastine hydrochloride, as such, intoxication after oral ingestion of the ophthalmic formulation is not expected even if the whole content of the bottle is swallowed.

No case of overdose with Relestat has been reported.

5. PHARMACOLOGICAL PROPERTIES
5.1 Pharmacodynamic properties
Pharmacotherapeutic group: Ophthalmologicals; Decongestants and Antiallergics; Other antiallergics

ATC code: S01G X 10

Epinastine is a topically active, direct H_1-receptor antagonist. Epinastine has a high binding affinity for the histamine H_1-receptor and a 400 times lower affinity for the histamine H_2-receptor. Epinastine also possesses affinity for the α_1-, α_2-, and the 5-HT_2 –receptor. It has low affinity for cholinergic, dopaminergic and a variety of other receptor sites. Epinastine does not penetrate the blood/brain barrier and, therefore, does not induce side effects of the central nervous system, i.e., it is non-sedative.

Following topical eye application in animals, epinastine showed evidence for antihistaminic activity, a modulating effect on the accumulation of inflammatory cells, and mast cell stabilising activity.

In provocation studies with allergens in humans, epinastine was able to ameliorate ocular symptoms following ocular antigen challenge. The duration of the effect was at least 8 hours.

5.2 Pharmacokinetic properties
Following administration of one drop of Relestat in each eye twice daily, an average maximum plasma concentration of 0.042 ng/ml is reached after about two hours. Epinastine has a volume of distribution of 417 litres and is 64% bound to plasma proteins. The clearance is 928 ml/min and the terminal plasma elimination half-life is about 8 hours. Less than 10% is metabolised. Epinastine is mainly excreted renally unchanged. The renal elimination is mainly via active tubular secretion.

Preclinical studies *in vitro* and *in vivo* show that epinastine binds to melanin and accumulates in the pigmented ocular tissues of rabbits and monkeys. *In vitro* data indicate that the binding to melanin is moderate and reversible.

5.3 Preclinical safety data
Preclinical data revealed no special hazard for humans based on conventional studies of safety pharmacology, repeated dose toxicity, genotoxicity, carcinogenic potential and toxicity to reproduction.

6. PHARMACEUTICAL PARTICULARS
6.1 List of excipients
Benzalkonium chloride, disodium edetate, sodium chloride, sodium dihydrogen phosphate dihydrate, sodium hydroxide/hydrochloric acid, purified water.

6.2 Incompatibilities
Not applicable.

6.3 Shelf life
2 years.

After first opening: 4 weeks.

6.4 Special precautions for storage
Keep the bottle in the outer carton in order to protect from light.

Do not store above 25°C.

6.5 Nature and contents of container
5 ml polyethylene bottle with a white polystyrene screw cap with spike device for opening the bottle.

6.6 Instructions for use and handling
No special requirements

7. MARKETING AUTHORISATION HOLDER
Allergan Pharmaceuticals Ireland

Castlebar Road

Westport

Co. Mayo

Ireland

8. MARKETING AUTHORISATION NUMBER(S)
PL 05179/0004

9. DATE OF FIRST AUTHORISATION/RENEWAL OF THE AUTHORISATION
5th August 2003

10. DATE OF REVISION OF THE TEXT
1st February 2005

Relifex Dispersible Tablets
(Meda Pharmaceuticals)

1. NAME OF THE MEDICINAL PRODUCT
Relifex Dispersible Tablets.

2. QUALITATIVE AND QUANTITATIVE COMPOSITION
Each tablet contains 500 mg nabumetone.

3. PHARMACEUTICAL FORM
Off-white, round, flat, bevelled, dispersible tablets.

4. CLINICAL PARTICULARS
4.1 Therapeutic indications
Nabumetone is a non-acidic non-steroidal anti-inflammatory agent which is a relatively weak inhibitor of prostaglandin synthesis. However, following absorption from the gastrointestinal tract it is rapidly metabolised in the liver to the principal active metabolite, 6-methoxy-2-naphthylacetic acid (6-MNA), a potent inhibitor of prostaglandin synthesis.

It is indicated for the treatment of osteoarthritis and rheumatoid arthritis requiring anti-inflammatory and analgesic treatment.

4.2 Posology and method of administration
Adults

The recommended daily dose is 1 g taken as a single dose at bedtime.

For severe or persistent symptoms, or during acute exacerbations, an additional 500 mg-1 g may be given as a morning dose.

Elderly

In common with many drugs, blood levels may be higher in elderly patients. The recommended daily dose of 1 g should not be exceeded in this age group and in some cases 500 mg may give satisfactory relief.

The elderly are at increased risk of the serious consequences of adverse reactions. If an NSAID is considered necessary, the lowest dose should be used and patients should be monitored for gastrointestinal bleeding for 4 weeks following initiation of NSAID therapy.

Children

There are no clinical data to recommend use of Relifex in children.

Administration

Oral.

The tablets should be stirred into a glass of water before taking and drunk immediately.

4.3 Contraindications
Active peptic ulceration or a history of peptic ulceration. Severe hepatic impairment (e.g. cirrhosis). Patients in

whom aspirin or other NSAIDs precipitate asthmatic attacks, urticaria or acute rhinitis. Hypersensitivity to the drug.

4.4 Special warnings and special precautions for use
Caution is required if administered to patients suffering from, or with a previous history of, bronchial asthma since ibuprofen has been reported to cause bronchospasm in such patients.

NSAIDs should only be given with care to patients with a history of gastrointestinal disease.

Peripheral oedema has been observed in some patients. Relifex should therefore be used with caution in patients with fluid retention, hypertension or heart failure.

Use in patients with impaired renal function: Urine is the major excretion route for the metabolites of Relifex. In patients with impaired renal function (creatinine clearance less than 30 ml/minute), dosage reduction should be considered. It is consistent with good clinical practice that patients with known renal impairment should be monitored regularly during therapy.

Liver function: Fluctuations in some parameters of liver function, particularly alkaline phosphatase, are frequently observed in patients with chronic inflammatory disorders; there is no evidence that Relifex accentuates these changes. However patients with abnormal liver function should be monitored closely.

Undesirable effects may be minimised by using the minimum effective dose for the shortest possible duration.

4.5 Interaction with other medicinal products and other forms of Interaction
Other analgesics: avoid the concomitant use of two or more NSAIDs (including aspirin).

Corticosteroids: increased risk of GI bleeding.

As the major circulating metabolite of Relifex is highly protein bound, patients receiving concurrent treatment with oral anti-coagulants, hydantoin anticonvulsants or sulphonylurea hypoglycaemics should be monitored for signs of overdosage of these drugs. Dosages should be adjusted if necessary.

Some NSAIDs are known to increase plasma concentrations of cardiac glycosides, lithium and methotrexate and may decrease the therapeutic efficacy of diuretics and antihypertensives. Such drugs may also induce hyperkalaemia when administered with potassium-sparing diuretics. Interaction studies between Relifex and these other drugs have not been performed; caution in co-administration is therefore recommended.

NSAIDs should not be used 8-12 days after mifepristone administration, as they could affect the efficacy of mifepristone treatment.

Aluminium hydroxide gel, paracetamol and aspirin have not affected the bioavailability of Relifex in volunteer subjects.

Animal data indicate that some NSAIDs can increase the risk of convulsions associated with quinoline antibiotics. Patients taking NSAIDs and quinolines may have an increased risk of developing convulsions. However, to date there have been no reports of such interactions with Relifex.

4.6 Pregnancy and lactation
Studies in experimental animals have shown no teratogenic potential. As is common with other compounds administered to animals at doses high enough to be maternally toxic, indications of embryotoxicity were noted (studies in the rabbit 300 mg/kg dose). High doses in rats (320 mg/kg) delayed parturition; this effect is considered to be due to inhibition of prostaglandin synthesis. The active metabolite of nabumetone has been found in the milk of lactating animals.

Safety in human pregnancy has not been established. Relifex is not recommended during human pregnancy or in mothers who are breast feeding.

4.7 Effects on ability to drive and use machines
Dizziness, drowsiness, visual disturbances or headaches are possible undesirable effects after taking NSAIDs, if affected, patients should not drive or operate machinery.

4.8 Undesirable effects
Reported gastrointestinal side effects include dry mouth, faecal occult blood, diarrhoea, dyspepsia, nausea, constipation, abdominal pain, vomiting, haematemesis, ulcerative stomatis, gastritis, flatulence, gastrointestinal bleeding, ulceration and perforation. Headache, dizziness, fatigue, confusion, sedation, depression, insomnia, tinnitus, abnormal vision, oedema, menorrhagia, paraesthesia, hallucinations, vertigo, malaise, anaphylaxis and anaphylactoid reaction have also been reported. Skin reactions including rash, pruritus, urticaria, alopecia and photosensitivity reactions may occur. The following hypersensitivity reactions may occur: non-specific allergic reactions, respiratory reactivity comprising asthma, aggravated asthma, bronchospasm, dyspnoea and angioedema. The following hepatic side effects have been reported very rarely: elevated liver function tests, jaundice and hepatic failure.

As with other NSAIDs, severe skin eruptions, e.g. Stevens Johnson syndrome and toxic epidermal necrolysis have been reported very rarely. Blood dyscrasias including leucopenia and thrombocytopenia have also been reported very rarely.

As with other NSAIDs, there have been rare reports of renal adverse effects, including nephrotic syndrome and renal failure.

In clinical trials, increases in doses above 1 g did not lead to an increase in the incidence of side effects. However, the lowest effective dose should always be used.

4.9 Overdose
There is no specific antidote. Treatment is with gastric lavage followed by activated charcoal using up to 60 g orally in divided doses with appropriate supportive therapy.

5. PHARMACOLOGICAL PROPERTIES

5.1 Pharmacodynamic properties
Nabumetone is a non-acidic non-steroidal anti-inflammatory agent which is a relatively weak inhibitor of prostaglandin synthesis. A notable feature of the animal pharmacology is the lack of effect on the gastric mucosa. Following absorption from the gastrointestinal tract nabumetone is rapidly metabolised in the liver to the principal active metabolite, 6-methoxy-2-naphthylacetic acid (6-MNA) a potent inhibitor of prostaglandin synthesis.

5.2 Pharmacokinetic properties
Although nabumetone is absorbed essentially intact through the small intestine, extensive metabolism occurs during the first pass through the liver. As a result, concentrations in plasma of nabumetone are barely detectable after oral dosage. Intravenous studies in rats with nabumetone indicate it to be rapidly distributed throughout the body, in keeping with its highly lipophilic character. The active metabolite, 6-MNA, binds strongly to plasma proteins; it is distributed into inflamed tissue and crosses the placenta into foetal tissue. It is found in the milk of lactating females. 6-MNA is eliminated by metabolism, principally conjugation with glucuronic acid, and o-demethylation followed by conjugation, the main route of excretion being the urine. The plasma elimination half-life is about 1 day in man.

5.3 Preclinical safety data
Not applicable.

6. PHARMACEUTICAL PARTICULARS

6.1 List of excipients
Croscarmellose sodium

Povidone

Sodium lauryl sulphate

Saccharin sodium

Peppermint dry flavour

Vanilla flavour

Magnesium stearate

Microcrystalline cellulose

6.2 Incompatibilities
Not applicable.

6.3 Shelf life
36 months.

6.4 Special precautions for storage
None.

6.5 Nature and contents of container
500 mg: Blister packs containing 10 or 60 tablets.

6.6 Instructions for use and handling
None.

Administrative Data

7. MARKETING AUTHORISATION HOLDER
Meda Phamaceuticals Ltd.

Sherwood House

7 Gregory Boulevard

Nottingham

NG7 6LB

UK

Trading as:

Meda Pharmaceuticals

Regus House

Herald Way

Pegasus Business Park

Castle Donington

Derbyshire

DE74 2TZ

UK

8. MARKETING AUTHORISATION NUMBER(S)
PL 19477/0002.

9. DATE OF FIRST AUTHORISATION/RENEWAL OF THE AUTHORISATION
15 May 2002.

10. DATE OF REVISION OF THE TEXT
20 September 2002.

11. Legal Status
POM.

Relifex Suspension

(Meda Pharmaceuticals)

1. NAME OF THE MEDICINAL PRODUCT
'Relifex' Suspension

2. QUALITATIVE AND QUANTITATIVE COMPOSITION
Each 5 ml contains 500 mg nabumetone.

3. PHARMACEUTICAL FORM
A white to off-white suspension.

4. CLINICAL PARTICULARS

4.1 Therapeutic indications
Nabumetone is a non-acidic non-steroidal anti-inflammatory agent which is a relatively weak inhibitor of prostaglandin synthesis. However, following absorption from the gastrointestinal tract it is rapidly metabolised in the liver to the principal active metabolite, 6-methoxy-2-naphthylacetic acid (6-MNA), a potent inhibitor of prostaglandin synthesis.

It is indicated for the treatment of osteoarthritis and rheumatoid arthritis requiring anti-inflammatory and analgesic treatment.

4.2 Posology and method of administration

Adults

The recommended daily dose is 10 ml suspension (1 g) taken as a single dose at bedtime.

For severe or persistent symptoms, or during acute exacerbations, an additional 5 or 10 ml suspension (500 mg-1 g) may be given as a morning dose.

Elderly

In common with many drugs, blood levels may be higher in elderly patients. The recommended daily dose of 1 g should not be exceeded in this age group and in some cases 500 mg may give satisfactory relief.

The elderly are at increased risk of the serious consequences of adverse reactions. If an NSAID is considered necessary, the lowest dose should be used and the patients should be monitored for gastrointestinal bleeding for 4 weeks following initiation of NSAID therapy.

Children

There are no clinical data to recommend use of 'Relifex' in children.

Administration

Oral.

4.3 Contraindications
Active peptic ulceration or a history of peptic ulceration. Severe hepatic impairment (e.g. cirrhosis). Patients in whom aspirin or other NSAIDs precipitate asthmatic attacks, urticaria or acute rhinitis. Hypersensitivity to the drug.

4.4 Special warnings and special precautions for use

Caution is required if administered to patients suffering from, or with a previous history of, bronchial asthma since ibuprofen has been reported to cause bronchospasm in such patients.

NSAIDs should only be given with care to patients with a history of gastrointestinal disease.

Peripheral oedema has been observed in some patients. 'Relifex' should therefore be used with caution in patients with fluid retention, hypertension or heart failure.

Use in patients with impaired renal function: Urine is the major excretion route for the metabolites of 'Relifex'. In patients with impaired renal function (creatinine clearance less than 30 ml/minute), dosage reduction should be considered. It is consistent with good clinical practice that patients with known renal impairment should be monitored regularly during therapy.

Liver function: Fluctuations in some parameters of liver function, particularly alkaline phosphatase, are frequently observed in patients with chronic inflammatory disorders; there is no evidence that 'Relifex' accentuates these changes. However patients with abnormal liver function should be monitored closely.

Undesirable effects may be minimised by using the minimum effective dose for the shortest possible duration.

4.5 Interaction with other medicinal products and other forms of Interaction
Other analgesics: avoid the concomitant use of two or more NSAIDs (including aspirin).

Corticosteroids: increased risk of GI bleeding.

As the major circulating metabolite of 'Relifex' is highly protein bound, patients receiving concurrent treatment with oral anti-coagulants, hydantoin anticonvulsants or sulphonylurea hypoglycaemics should be monitored for signs of overdosage of these drugs. Dosages should be adjusted if necessary.

Some NSAIDs are known to increase plasma concentrations of cardiac glycosides, lithium and methotrexate and may decrease the therapeutic efficacy of diuretics and antihypertensives. Such drugs may also induce hyperkalaemia when administered with potassium-sparing diuretics. Interaction studies between 'Relifex' and these other drugs have not been performed; caution in co-administration is therefore recommended.

NSAIDs should not be used 8-12 days after mifepristone administration, as they could affect the efficacy of mifepristone treatment.

Aluminium hydroxide gel, paracetamol and aspirin have not affected the bioavailability of 'Relifex' in volunteer subjects.

Animal data indicate that some NSAIDs can increase the risk of convulsions associated with quinoline antibiotics. Patients taking NSAIDs and quinolines may have an increased risk of developing convulsions. However, to date there have been no reports of such interactions with 'Relifex'.

4.6 Pregnancy and lactation

Studies in experimental animals have shown no teratogenic potential. As is common with other compounds administered to animals at doses high enough to be maternally toxic, indications of embryotoxicity were noted (studies in the rabbit 300 mg/kg dose). High doses in rats (320 mg/kg) delayed parturition; this effect is considered to be due to inhibition of prostaglandin synthesis. The active metabolite of nabumetone has been found in the milk of lactating animals.

Safety in human pregnancy has not been established. 'Relifex' is not recommended during human pregnancy or in mothers who are breast feeding.

4.7 Effects on ability to drive and use machines

Dizziness, drowsiness, visual disturbances or headaches are possible undesirable effects after taking NSAIDs, if affected, patients should not drive or operate machinery.

4.8 Undesirable effects

Reported gastrointestinal side effects include dry mouth, faecal occult blood, diarrhoea, dyspepsia, nausea, constipation, abdominal pain, vomiting, haematemesis, ulcerative stomatis, gastritis, flatulence, gastrointestinal bleeding, ulceration and perforation. Headache, dizziness, fatigue, confusion, sedation, depression, insomnia, tinnitus, abnormal vision, oedema, menorrhagia, paraesthesia, hallucinations, vertigo, malaise, anaphylaxis and anaphylactoid reaction have also been reported. Skin reactions including rash, pruritus, urticaria, alopecia and photosensitivity reactions may occur. The following hypersensitivity reactions may occur: non-specific allergic reactions, respiratory reactivity comprising asthma, aggravated asthma, bronchospasm, dyspnoea and angioedema. The following hepatic side effects have been reported very rarely: elevated liver function tests, jaundice and hepatic failure.

As with other NSAIDs, severe skin eruptions, e.g. Stevens Johnson syndrome and toxic epidermal necrolysis have been reported very rarely. Blood dyscrasias including leucopenia and thrombocytopenia have also been reported very rarely.

As with other NSAIDs, there have been rare reports of renal adverse effects, including nephrotic syndrome and renal failure.

In clinical trials, increases in doses above 1 g did not lead to an increase in the incidence of side effects. However, the lowest effective dose should always be used.

4.9 Overdose

There is no specific antidote. Treatment is with gastric lavage followed by activated charcoal using up to 60 g orally in divided doses with appropriate supportive therapy.

5. PHARMACOLOGICAL PROPERTIES

5.1 Pharmacodynamic properties

Nabumetone is a non-acidic non-steroidal anti-inflammatory agent which is a relatively weak inhibitor of prostaglandin synthesis. A notable feature of the animal pharmacology is the lack of effect on the gastric mucosa. Following absorption from the gastrointestinal tract nabumetone is rapidly metabolised in the liver to the principal active metabolite, 6-methoxy-2-naphthylacetic acid (6-MNA) a potent inhibitor of prostaglandin synthesis.

5.2 Pharmacokinetic properties

Although nabumetone is absorbed essentially intact through the small intestine, extensive metabolism occurs during the first pass through the liver. As a result, concentrations in plasma of nabumetone are barely detectable after oral dosage. Intravenous studies in rats with nabumetone indicate it to be rapidly distributed throughout the body, in keeping with its highly lipophilic character. The active metabolite, 6-MNA, binds strongly to plasma proteins; it is distributed into inflamed tissue and crosses the placenta into foetal tissue. It is found in the milk of lactating females. 6-MNA is eliminated by metabolism, principally conjugation with glucuronic acid, and o-demethylation followed by conjugation, the main route of excretion being the urine. The plasma elimination half-life is about 1 day in man.

5.3 Preclinical safety data

Not applicable.

6. PHARMACEUTICAL PARTICULARS

6.1 List of excipients

Methylcellulose

Xanthan gum

Sorbitol

Sodium benzoate

Liquid vanilla flavour

Liquid buttermint flavour

Monoammonium glycyrrhizinate

Glycerin

Dilute Hydrochloric Acid

Purified Water

6.2 Incompatibilities

Not applicable.

6.3 Shelf life

36 months.

6.4 Special precautions for storage

None.

6.5 Nature and contents of container

HDPE bottles each containing 300 ml

6.6 Instructions for use and handling

None.

Administrative Data

7. MARKETING AUTHORISATION HOLDER

Meda Pharmaceuticals Ltd.

Sherwood House

7 Gregory Boulevard

Nottingham

NG7 6LB

UK

Trading as:

Meda Pharmaceuticals

Regus House

Herald Way

Pegasus Business Park

Castle Donington

Derbyshire

DE74 2TZ

UK

8. MARKETING AUTHORISATION NUMBER(S)

PL 19477/0004

9. DATE OF FIRST AUTHORISATION/RENEWAL OF THE AUTHORISATION

09 May 2002

10. DATE OF REVISION OF THE TEXT

Legal Status

POM

Relifex Tablets

(Meda Pharmaceuticals)

1. NAME OF THE MEDICINAL PRODUCT

Relifex Tablets

2. QUALITATIVE AND QUANTITATIVE COMPOSITION

Each tablet contains 500 mg nabumetone.

3. PHARMACEUTICAL FORM

Dark red, film-coated tablets marked 'Relifex' on one side and "500" on the other.

4. CLINICAL PARTICULARS

4.1 Therapeutic indications

Nabumetone is a non-acidic non-steroidal anti-inflammatory agent which is a relatively weak inhibitor of prostaglandin synthesis. However, following absorption from the gastrointestinal tract it is rapidly metabolised in the liver to the principal active metabolite, 6-methoxy-2-naphthylacetic acid (6-MNA), a potent inhibitor of prostaglandin synthesis.

It is indicated for the treatment of osteoarthritis and rheumatoid arthritis requiring anti-inflammatory and analgesic treatment.

4.2 Posology and method of administration

Relifex 500mg tablets should be taken preferably with or after food.

Adults

The recommended daily dose is two tablets (1 g) taken as a single dose at bedtime.

For severe or persistent symptoms, or during acute exacerbations, an additional one or two tablets (500 mg-1 g) may be given as a morning dose.

Elderly

In common with many drugs, blood levels may be higher in elderly patients. The recommended daily dose of 1 g should not be exceeded in this age group and in some cases 500 mg may give satisfactory relief.

The elderly are at increased risk of the serious consequences of adverse reactions. If an NSAID is considered necessary, the lowest dose should be used and the patients should be monitored for gastrointestinal bleeding for 4 weeks following initiation of NSAID therapy.

Children

There are no clinical data to recommend use of 'Relifex' in children.

Administration

Oral.

4.3 Contraindications

Active peptic ulceration or a history of peptic ulceration. Severe hepatic impairment (e.g. cirrhosis). Patients in whom aspirin or other NSAIDs precipitate asthmatic attacks, urticaria or acute rhinitis. Hypersensitivity to the drug.

4.4 Special warnings and special precautions for use

Caution is required if administered to patients suffering from, or with a previous history of, bronchial asthma since ibuprofen has been reported to cause bronchospasm in such patients.

NSAIDs should only be given with care to patients with a history of gastrointestinal disease.

Peripheral oedema has been observed in some patients. 'Relifex' should therefore be used with caution in patients with fluid retention, hypertension or heart failure.

Use in patients with impaired renal function: Urine is the major excretion route for the metabolites of 'Relifex'. In patients with impaired renal function (creatinine clearance less than 30 ml/minute), dosage reduction should be considered. It is consistent with good clinical practice that patients with known renal impairment should be monitored regularly during therapy.

Liver function: Fluctuations in some parameters of liver function, particularly alkaline phosphatase, are frequently observed in patients with chronic inflammatory disorders; there is no evidence that 'Relifex' accentuates these changes. However patients with abnormal liver function should be monitored closely.

Undesirable effects may be minimised by using the minimum effective dose for the shortest possible duration.

4.5 Interaction with other medicinal products and other forms of Interaction

Other analgesics: avoid the concomitant use of two or more NSAIDs (including aspirin)

Corticosteroids: Increased risk of GI bleeding.

As the major circulating metabolite of 'Relifex' is highly protein bound, patients receiving concurrent treatment with oral anti-coagulants, hydantoin anticonvulsants or sulphonylurea hypoglycaemic drugs should be monitored for signs of overdosage of these drugs. Dosages should be adjusted if necessary.

Some NSAIDs are known to increase plasma concentrations of cardiac glycosides, lithium and methotrexate and may decrease the therapeutic efficacy of diuretics and antihypertensives. Such drugs may also induce hyperkalaemia when administered with potassium-sparing diuretics. Interaction studies between 'Relifex' and these other drugs have not been performed; caution in co-administration is therefore recommended.

NSAIDs should not be used 8-12 days after mifepristone administration, as they could affect the efficacy of mifepristone treatment.

Aluminium hydroxide gel, paracetamol and aspirin have not affected the bioavailability of 'Relifex' in volunteer subjects.

Animal data indicate that some NSAIDs can increase the risk of convulsions associated with quinoline antibiotics. Patients taking NSAIDs and quinolines may have an increased risk of developing convulsions. However, to date there have been no reports of such interactions with 'Relifex'.

4.6 Pregnancy and lactation

Studies in experimental animals have shown no teratogenic potential. As is common with other compounds administered to animals at doses high enough to be maternally toxic, indications of embryotoxicity were noted (studies in the rabbit 300 mg/kg dose). High doses in rats (320 mg/kg) delayed parturition; this effect is considered to be due to inhibition of prostaglandin synthesis. The active metabolite of nabumetone has been found in the milk of lactating animals.

Safety in human pregnancy has not been established. 'Relifex' is not recommended during human pregnancy or in mothers who are breast feeding.

4.7 Effects on ability to drive and use machines

Dizziness, drowsiness, visual disturbances or headaches are possible undesirable effects after taking NSAIDs, if affected, patients should not drive or operate machinery.

4.8 Undesirable effects

Reported gastrointestinal side effects include dry mouth, faecal occult blood, diarrhoea, dyspepsia, nausea, constipation, abdominal pain, vomiting, haematemesis, ulcerative stomatis, gastritis, flatulence, gastrointestinal bleeding, ulceration and perforation. Headache, dizziness, fatigue, confusion, sedation, depression, insomnia, tinnitus, abnormal vision, oedema, menorrhagia, paraesthesia, hallucinations, vertigo, malaise, anaphylaxis and anaphylactoid reaction have also been reported. Skin reactions including rash, pruritus, urticaria, alopecia and photosensitivity reactions may occur. The following hypersensitivity reactions may occur: non-specific allergic reactions, respiratory reactivity comprising asthma, aggravated asthma, bronchospasm, dyspnoea and angioedema. The following hepatic side effects have been reported very rarely: elevated liver function tests, jaundice and hepatic failure.

As with other NSAIDs, severe skin eruptions, e.g. Stevens Johnson syndrome and toxic epidermal necrolysis have been reported very rarely. Blood dyscrasias including leucopenia and thrombocytopenia have also been reported very rarely.

As with other NSAIDs, there have been rare reports of renal adverse effects, including nephrotic syndrome and renal failure.

In clinical trials, increases in doses above 1 g did not lead to an increase in the incidence of side effects. However, the lowest effective dose should always be used.

4.9 Overdose
There is no specific antidote. Treatment is with gastric lavage followed by activated charcoal using up to 60 g orally in divided doses with appropriate supportive therapy.

5. PHARMACOLOGICAL PROPERTIES
5.1 Pharmacodynamic properties
Nabumetone is a non-acidic non-steroidal anti-inflammatory agent which is a relatively weak inhibitor of prostaglandin synthesis. A notable feature of the animal pharmacology is the lack of effect on the gastric mucosa. Following absorption from the gastrointestinal tract nabumetone is rapidly metabolised in the liver to the principal active metabolite, 6-methoxy-2-naphthylacetic acid (6-MNA) a potent inhibitor of prostaglandin synthesis.

5.2 Pharmacokinetic properties
Although nabumetone is absorbed essentially intact through the small intestine, extensive metabolism occurs during the first pass through the liver. As a result, concentrations in plasma of nabumetone are barely detectable after oral dosage. Intravenous studies in rats with nabumetone indicate it to be rapidly distributed throughout the body, in keeping with its highly lipophilic character. The active metabolite, 6-MNA, binds strongly to plasma proteins; it is distributed into inflamed tissue and crosses the placenta into foetal tissue. It is found in the milk of lactating females. 6-MNA is eliminated by metabolism, principally conjugation with glucuronic acid, and o-demethylation followed by conjugation, the main route of excretion being the urine. The plasma elimination half-life is about 1 day in man.

5.3 Preclinical safety data
Not applicable.

6. PHARMACEUTICAL PARTICULARS
6.1 List of excipients
Sodium starch glycollate
Sodium lauryl sulphate
Hydroxypropylmethylcellulose
Magnesium stearate
Microcrystalline cellulose
Red carmine
Yellow iron oxide
Titanium dioxide
Talc
Polyethylene glycol
Saccharin sodium
Liquid caramel flavour
Purified water
Carnuba wax

6.2 Incompatibilities
Not applicable.

6.3 Shelf life
36 months.

6.4 Special precautions for storage
The tablets should be protected from light.

6.5 Nature and contents of container
HDPE bottles each containing 56 tablets.

6.6 Instructions for use and handling
None.

Administrative Data
7. MARKETING AUTHORISATION HOLDER
Meda Phamaceuticals Ltd.
Sherwood House
7 Gregory Boulevard
Nottingham
NG7 6LB
UK

Trading as:
Meda Pharmaceuticals
Regus House
Herald Way
Pegasus Business Park
Castle Donington
Derbyshire
DE74 2TZ
UK

8. MARKETING AUTHORISATION NUMBER(S)
PL 19477/0001

9. DATE OF FIRST AUTHORISATION/RENEWAL OF THE AUTHORISATION
09 May 02

10. DATE OF REVISION OF THE TEXT

11. Legal Status
POM

Relpax - 20 mg and 40 mg
(Pfizer Limited)

1. NAME OF THE MEDICINAL PRODUCT
RELPAX ® ▼20mg and 40mg Film-Coated Tablets.

2. QUALITATIVE AND QUANTITATIVE COMPOSITION
Each film-coated tablet contains 20mg, and 40mg eletriptan (as hydrobromide).

For excipients, see section 6.1.

3. PHARMACEUTICAL FORM
Film-coated tablet.

Round, convex orange tablets debossed with 'REP 20' and 'REP 40' on one side and 'Pfizer' on the other.

4. CLINICAL PARTICULARS
4.1 Therapeutic indications
Acute treatment of the headache phase of migraine attacks, with or without aura.

4.2 Posology and method of administration
RELPAX tablets should be taken as early as possible after the onset of migraine headache but they are also effective if taken at a later stage during a migraine attack.

RELPAX, if taken during the aura phase, has not been demonstrated to prevent migraine headache and therefore RELPAX should only be taken during the headache phase of migraine.

RELPAX tablets should not be used prophylactically.

The tablets should be swallowed whole with water.

Adults (18-65 years of age):

The recommended initial dose is 40mg.

If headache returns within 24 hours: If the migraine headache recurs within 24 hours of an initial response, a second dose of the same strength of RELPAX has been shown to be effective in treating the recurrence. If a second dose is required, it should not be taken within 2 hours of the initial dose.

If no response is obtained: If a patient does not achieve a headache response to the first dose of RELPAX within 2 hours, a second dose should not be taken for the same attack as clinical trials have not adequately established efficacy with the second dose. Clinical trials show that patients who do not respond to the treatment of an attack are still likely to respond to the treatment of a subsequent attack.

Patients who do not obtain satisfactory efficacy after an appropriate trial of 40mg, (e.g. good tolerability and failure to respond in 2 out of 3 attacks), may be effectively treated with 80mg (2 × 40mg) in subsequent migraine attacks (see section 5.1 Pharmacodynamic Properties – Further information on Clinical Trials). A second dose of 80mg should not be taken within 24 hours.

The maximum daily dose should not exceed 80mg (see section 4.8 Undesirable effects).

Elderly (over 65 years of age)
The safety and effectiveness of eletriptan in patients over 65 years of age have not been systematically evaluated due to the small number of such patients in clinical trials. Use of RELPAX in the elderly is therefore not recommended.

Adolescents (12-17 years of age)
The efficacy of RELPAX has not been established in this population and its use is therefore not recommended in this age group.

Children (6-11 years of age)
The safety and efficacy of RELPAX in children have not been evaluated. Therefore the use of RELPAX is not recommended in this age group (see 5.2 Pharmacokinetic Properties).

Hepatic Impairment
No dose adjustment is required in patients with mild or moderate hepatic impairment. As RELPAX has not been studied in patients with severe hepatic impairment, it is contra-indicated in these patients.

Renal Impairment
As the blood pressure effects of RELPAX are amplified in renal impairment (see 4.4 Special Warnings and Precautions for Use), a 20mg initial dose, is recommended in patients with mild or moderate renal impairment. The maximum daily dose should not exceed 40mg. RELPAX is contra-indicated, in patients with severe renal impairment.

4.3 Contraindications
Hypersensitivity to eletriptan hydrobromide or to any of the excipients.

Patients with severe hepatic or severe renal impairment.

Moderately severe or severe hypertension, or untreated mild hypertension.

Patients with confirmed coronary heart disease, including ischaemic heart disease (angina pectoris, previous myocardial infarction or confirmed silent ischaemia), objective or subjective symptoms of ischaemic heart disease or Prinzmetal's angina.

Patients with significant arrhythmias or heart failure.

Patients with peripheral vascular disease.

Patients with a history of cerebrovascular accident (CVA) or transient ischaemic attack (TIA).

Administration of ergotamine, or derivatives of ergotamine (including methysergide), within 24hr before or after treatment with eletriptan (see 4.5 Interactions with other medicinal products and other forms of interaction). Concomitant administration of other 5-HT_1 receptor agonists with eletriptan.

4.4 Special warnings and special precautions for use
RELPAX should not be used together with potent CYP3A4 inhibitors eg. ketoconazole, itraconazole, erythromycin, clarithromycin, josamycin and protease inhibitors (ritonavir, indinavir and nelfinavir).

RELPAX should only be used where a clear diagnosis of migraine has been established. RELPAX is not indicated for the management of hemiplegic, ophthalmoplegic, or basilar migraine.

RELPAX should not be given for the treatment of 'atypical' headaches, i.e. headaches, which may be related to a possibly serious condition (stroke, aneurysm rupture) where cerebrovascular vasoconstriction may be harmful.

Eletriptan can be associated with transient symptoms including chest pain and tightness, which may be intense and involve the throat (see 4.8 Undesirable effects). Where such symptoms are thought to indicate ischaemic heart disease, no further dose should be taken and appropriate evaluation should be carried out.

RELPAX should not be given without prior evaluation, to patients in whom unrecognised cardiac disease is likely, or to patients at risk of coronary artery disease (CAD) [e.g. patients with hypertension, diabetes, smokers or users of nicotine substitution therapy, men over 40 years of age, post-menopausal women and those with a strong family history of CAD]. Cardiac evaluations may not identify every patient who has cardiac disease and, in very rare cases, serious cardiac events have occurred, in patients without underlying cardiovascular disease when 5-HT_1 agonists have been administered. Patients in whom CAD is established, should not be given RELPAX (see 4.3 Contra-indications).

5-HT_1 receptor agonists have been associated with coronary vasospasm. In rare cases, myocardial ischaemia or infarction, have been reported with 5-HT_1 receptor agonists.

Undesirable effects may be more common during concomitant use of triptans and herbal preparations containing St. John's wort (Hypericum perforatum)

Within the clinical dose range, slight and transient increases in blood pressure have been seen with eletriptan doses of 60mg or greater. However, these increases have not been associated with clinical sequelae in the clinical trial programme. The effect was much more pronounced in renally impaired and elderly subjects. In renally impaired subjects, the range of mean maximum increases in systolic blood pressure was 14 -17mmHg (normal 3mmHg) and for diastolic blood pressure was 14 -21mmHg (normal 4mmHg). In elderly subjects, the mean maximum increase in systolic blood pressure was 23mmHg compared with 13mmHg in young adults (placebo 8mmHg).

Excessive use of any anti-migraine medicinal product can lead to daily chronic headaches requiring a therapeutic window.

4.5 Interaction with other medicinal products and other forms of Interaction
Effect of other medicinal products on eletriptan

In the pivotal clinical trials of eletriptan no evidence of interaction with beta-blockers, tricyclic antidepressants, selective serotonin re-uptake inhibitors and flunarizine was reported but data from formal clinical interaction studies with these medicinal products are not available (other than propranolol, see below).

Population pharmacokinetic analysis of clinical studies has suggested that the following medicinal products (beta-blockers, tricyclic antidepressants, selective serotonin re-uptake inhibitors, oestrogen based hormone replacement therapy, oestrogen containing oral contraceptives and calcium channel blockers) are unlikely to have an effect on the pharmacokinetic properties of eletriptan.

Eletriptan is not a substrate for MAO. Therefore there is no expectation of an interaction between eletriptan and MAO inhibitors. Therefore no formal interaction study has been undertaken.

In clinical studies with propranolol (160mg), verapamil (480mg) and fluconazole (100mg) the C_{max} of eletriptan was increased 1.1 fold, 2.2 fold and 1.4 fold respectively. The increase in eletriptan's AUC being 1.3 fold, 2.7 fold and 2.0 fold respectively. These effects are not considered clinically significant as there were no associated increases in blood pressure or adverse events compared to administering eletriptan alone.

In clinical studies with erythromycin (1000mg) and ketoconazole (400mg), specific and potent inhibitors of CYP3A4, significant increases in eletriptan C_{max} (2 and 2.7- fold) and AUC (3.6 and 5.9- fold) respectively, were observed. This increased exposure was associated with an increase in eletriptan $t_{1/2}$ from 4.6 to 7.1 hours for erythromycin and from 4.8 to 8.3 hours for ketoconazole (see 5.2 Pharmacokinetic Properties). Therefore, RELPAX should not be used together with potent CYP3A4 inhibitors eg. ketoconazole, itraconazole, erythromycin, clarithromycin, josamycin and protease inhibitors (ritonavir, indinavir and nelfinavir).

In clinical studies with oral (caffeine/ergotamine) administered 1 and 2 hours after eletriptan, minor though additive increases in blood pressure were observed which are predictable based on the pharmacology of the two drugs. Therefore it is recommended that either ergotamine-containing or ergot-type medications (e.g. dihydroergotamine) should not be taken within 24 hours of eletriptan dosing. Conversely, at least 24 hours should elapse after the administration of an ergotamine-containing preparation before eletriptan is given.

Effect of eletriptan on other medicinal products

There is no *in vitro* or *in vivo* evidence that clinical doses (and associated concentrations) of eletriptan will inhibit or induce cytochrome P450 enzymes including CYP3A4 drug metabolising enzymes and therefore it is considered that eletriptan is unlikely to cause clinically important drug interactions mediated by these enzymes.

4.6 Pregnancy and lactation

Pregnancy: For RELPAX no clinical data on exposed pregnancies are available. Animal studies do not indicate direct or indirect harmful effects with respect to pregnancy, embryonal/fetal development, parturition or postnatal development. RELPAX should be used during pregnancy only if clearly needed.

Lactation: Eletriptan is excreted in human breast milk. In one study of 8 women given a single dose of 80mg, the mean total amount of eletriptan in breast milk over 24 hours in this group was 0.02% of the dose. Nevertheless, caution should be exercised when considering the administration of RELPAX to women who are breast-feeding. Infant exposure can be minimised by avoiding breast-feeding for 24 hours after treatment.

4.7 Effects on ability to drive and use machines

Migraine or treatment with RELPAX may cause drowsiness or dizziness in some patients. Patients should be advised to evaluate their ability to perform complex tasks such as driving during migraine attacks and following administration of RELPAX.

4.8 Undesirable effects

RELPAX has been administered in clinical trials to over 5000 subjects, taking one or two doses of RELPAX 20, 40 or 80mg. The most common adverse reactions noted were asthenia, somnolence, nausea and dizziness. In randomised clinical studies using doses of 20, 40 and 80mg, a trend for a dose-dependency of the incidence of adverse events has been shown. The table below contains all adverse events seen on RELPAX that are considered treatment related and treatment emergent which occur at an incidence greater than placebo.

(see Table 1)

Table 1

Organ system	Very common > 1/10)	Common > 1/100, < 1/10)	Uncommon > 1/1000, < 1/100)	Rare > 1/10000, < 1/1000)
General Disorders and Administration Site Conditions		Asthenia, Chest symptoms (pain, tightness, pressure) and Chills	Malaise, Face oedema	Shock
Cardiac Disorders		Palpitation, Tachycardia,	Peripheral vascular disorder	Bradycardia
Vascular Disorders		Sensation of warmth or flushing.		
Gastrointestinal Disorders		Abdominal pain Nausea, Dry mouth, Dyspepsia	Diarrhoea, Anorexia, and Glossitis	Constipation, Oesophagitis, Tongue oedema and Eructation
Ear and Labyrinth Disorders		Vertigo		
Hemic and Lymphatic				Lymphadenopathy
Metabolic and nutritional			Thirst, Oedema and Peripheral oedema	Bilirubinaemia and Increased AST
Musculoskeletal, Connective Tissue and Bone Disorders:		Back pain, Myalgia	Arthralgia, Arthrosis and Bone pain	Arthritis and Myopathy
Nervous System Disorders		Somolence, Headache, Dizziness, Tingling or abnormal sensation, Hypertonia, Hypoaesthesia, Myasthenia	Tremor, Hyperaesthesia, Thinking abnormal, Agitation, Insomnia, Confusion, Ataxia, Depersonalisation, Euphoria, Hypokinesia, Speech disorder, Depression and Stupor	Emotional lability and Twitching
Respiratory, Thoracic and Mediastinal Disorders		Pharyngitis Throat tightness	Dyspnea, Rhinitis, Respiratory disorder and Yawn	Asthma Respiratory tract infection and Voice alteration
Skin and Subcutaneous Tissue Disorder		Sweating	Rash and Pruritis	Skin disorder and Urticaria
Special senses			Abnormal vision, Ear pain, Eye pain, Photophobia, Taste perversion, Tinnitus and Lacrimation disorder	Conjunctivitis
Urogenital			Urinary frequency, Urinary tract disorder and Polyuria	Breast pain and Menorrhagia

In post-marketing experience, the following undesirable effects have been reported:

Immune System Disorders: Allergic reactions, some of which may be serious.

Some of the symptoms reported as adverse events may be associated symptoms of the migraine attack. The common adverse events seen with RELPAX are typical of adverse events reported with $5\text{-}HT_1$ agonists as a class.

4.9 Overdose

Subjects have received single doses of 120mg without significant adverse effects. However, based on the pharmacology of this class, hypertension or other more serious cardiovascular symptoms could occur on overdose.

In cases of overdose, standard supportive measures should be adopted as required. The elimination half-life of eletriptan is about 4 hours, and therefore monitoring of patients and provision of general supportive therapy after overdose with eletriptan should continue for at least 20 hours or while signs and symptoms persist.

It is unknown what effect haemodialysis or peritoneal dialysis has on the serum concentrations of eletriptan.

5. PHARMACOLOGICAL PROPERTIES

5.1 Pharmacodynamic properties

Pharmacotherapeutic group: Selective Serotonin ($5HT_1$) receptor agonists ATC code: NO2C C

Mode of action/pharmacology: Eletriptan is a selective agonist at the vascular $5\text{-}HT_{1B}$ and neuronal $5\text{-}HT_{1D}$ receptors. Eletriptan also exhibits high affinity for the $5\text{-}HT_{1F}$ receptor which may contribute to its anti-migraine mechanism of action. Eletriptan has modest affinity for the human recombinant $5\text{-}HT_{1A}$, $5\text{-}HT_{2B}$, $5\text{-}HT_{1E}$ and $5\text{-}HT_7$ receptors.

Further Information on Clinical Trials

The efficacy of RELPAX in the acute treatment of migraine has been evaluated in 10 placebo-controlled trials that included about 4000 patients who received RELPAX at doses of 20 to 80mg. Headache relief occurred as early as 30 minutes following oral dosing. Response rates (i.e. reduction of moderate or severe headache pain to no or mild pain) 2 hours after dosing were 59-77% for the 80mg dose, 54-65% for the 40mg dose, 47-54% for the 20mg dose, and 19-40% following placebo. RELPAX was also effective in the treatment of associated symptoms of migraine such as vomiting, nausea, photophobia and phonophobia.

The recommendation for dose titration to 80mg, is derived from open label long term studies and from a short term double blind study, where only a trend towards statistical significance was observed.

RELPAX remains effective in menstrually associated migraine. RELPAX, if taken during the aura phase, has not been demonstrated to prevent migraine headache and therefore RELPAX should only be taken during the headache phase of migraine.

In a non placebo controlled pharmacokinetic study of patients with renal impairment, larger elevations in blood pressure were recorded after an 80mg dose of RELPAX than with normal volunteers (see Section 4.4). This cannot be explained by any pharmacokinetic changes and so may represent a specific pharmacodynamic response to eletriptan in patients with renal impairment.

5.2 Pharmacokinetic properties

Absorption:

Eletriptan is rapidly and well absorbed across the gastrointestinal tract (at least 81%) after oral administration. Absolute oral bioavailability across males and females is approximately 50%. The median T_{max} is 1.5 hours after oral dosing. Linear pharmacokinetics were demonstrated over the clinical dose range (20-80mg).

The AUC and C_{max} of eletriptan were increased by approximately 20-30% following oral administration with a high fat meal. Following oral administration during a migraine attack, there was a reduction of approximately 30% in AUC and T_{max} was increased to 2.8 hours.

Following repeated doses (20mg tid) for 5-7 days, the pharmacokinetics of eletriptan remained linear and accumulation was predictable. On multiple dosing of larger doses (40mg tid and 80mg bid), the accumulation of eletriptan over 7 days was greater than predicted (approximately 40%).

Distribution:

The volume of distribution of eletriptan following IV administration is 138L indicating distribution into the tissues. Eletriptan is only moderately protein bound (approximately 85%).

Metabolism:

In vitro studies indicate that eletriptan is primarily metabolised by hepatic cytochrome P-450 enzyme CYP3A4. This finding is substantiated by increased plasma concentrations of eletriptan following co-administration with erythromycin and ketoconazole, known selective and potent CYP3A4 inhibitors. *In vitro* studies also indicate a small involvement of CYP2D6 although clinical studies do not indicate any evidence of polymorphism with this enzyme.

There are two major circulating metabolites identified that significantly contribute to plasma radioactivity following administration of C^{14}-labelled eletriptan. The metabolite formed by N-oxidation, has demonstrated no activity in animal *in vitro* models. The metabolite formed by N-demethylation, has been demonstrated to have similar activity to eletriptan in animal *in vitro* models. A third area of radioactivity in plasma has not been formally identified, but is most likely to be a mixture of hydroxylated metabolites which have also been observed excreted in urine and faeces.

The plasma concentrations of the N-demethylated active metabolite are only 10-20% of those of parent and so would not be expected to significantly contribute to the therapeutic action of eletriptan.

Elimination:

Mean total plasma clearance of eletriptan following IV administration is 36 L/h with a resultant plasma half-life of approximately 4 hours. The mean renal clearance following oral administration is approximately 3.9 L/h. Non-renal clearance accounts for approximately 90% of the total clearance indicating that eletriptan is eliminated primarily by metabolism.

Pharmacokinetics in Special Patient Groups

Gender

A meta analysis across clinical pharmacology studies and a population pharmacokinetic analysis of clinical trial data indicate that gender does not have any clinically significant influence on plasma concentrations of eletriptan.

Elderly (over 65 years of age)

Though not statistically significant, there is a small reduction (16%) in clearance associated with a statistically significant increased half-life (from approximately 4.4 hours to 5.7 hours) between elderly (65-93 years) and younger adult subjects.

Adolescents (12-17 years of age)

The pharmacokinetics of eletriptan (40mg and 80mg) in adolescent migraine patients dosed between attacks, were similar to those seen in healthy adults.

Children (6-11 years of age)

The clearance of eletriptan is unchanged in children relative to adolescents. However the volume of distribution is lower in children resulting in higher plasma levels than would be predicted following the same dose in adults.

Hepatic Impairment

Subjects with hepatic impairment (Child-Pugh A and B) demonstrated a statistically significant increase in both AUC (34%) and half-life. There was a small increase in C_{max} (18%). This small change in exposure is not considered clinically relevant.

Renal Impairment

Subjects with mild (creatinine clearance 61-89ml/min), moderate (creatinine clearance 31-60ml/min) or severe (creatinine clearance <30ml/min) renal impairment did not have any statistically significant alterations in their eletriptan pharmacokinetics or plasma protein binding. Blood pressure elevations were observed in this group.

5.3 Preclinical safety data

Preclinical data, revealed no special hazard for humans based on conventional studies of safety pharmacology, repeated dose toxicity, genotoxicity, carcinogenicity and toxicity to reproduction.

6. PHARMACEUTICAL PARTICULARS

6.1 List of excipients

Core Tablet: Microcrystalline cellulose, lactose monohydrate, croscarmellose sodium and magnesium stearate.

Film Coat: titanium dioxide (E171), hypromellose, lactose monohydrate, glycerol triacetate and Sunset Yellow Aluminium Lake (E110).

6.2 Incompatibilities

Not Applicable.

6.3 Shelf life

3 years

6.4 Special precautions for storage

This medicinal product does not require any special storage conditions.

HDPE bottles: Keep the container tightly closed.

6.5 Nature and contents of container

Opaque PVC/Aclar/Aluminium blister packs containing 2, 3, 4, 6, 10, 18, 30 and 100 tablets (20, 40mg).

HDPE bottles with child-resistant HDPE/PP closures containing 30 and 100 tablets (20, 40mg).

Not all pack sizes may be marketed.

6.6 Instructions for use and handling

No special requirements.

7. MARKETING AUTHORISATION HOLDER

Pfizer Limited
Sandwich
Kent, CT13 9NJ
United Kingdom

8. MARKETING AUTHORISATION NUMBER(S)

PL 00057/0452

PL 00057/0453

9. DATE OF FIRST AUTHORISATION/RENEWAL OF THE AUTHORISATION

12 February 2001

10. DATE OF REVISION OF THE TEXT

17 December 2003

11. LEGAL CATEGORY

POM

Company reference: RP4_0

Remedeine and Remedeine forte tablets

(Napp Pharmaceuticals Limited)

1. NAME OF THE MEDICINAL PRODUCT

REMEDEINE® and REMEDEINE FORTE® tablets

2. QUALITATIVE AND QUANTITATIVE COMPOSITION

REMEDEINE tablets contain Paracetamol 500 mg and Dihydrocodeine Tartrate BP 20 mg.

REMEDEINE FORTE tablets contain Paracetamol 500 mg and Dihydrocodeine Tartrate BP 30 mg.

3. PHARMACEUTICAL FORM

White to off-white, circular, flat faced tablets with a bevelled edge.

REMEDEINE tablets are engraved PD/20 on one side.

REMEDEINE FORTE tablets are engraved PD/30 on one side.

4. CLINICAL PARTICULARS

4.1 Therapeutic indications

For the treatment of severe pain.

4.2 Posology and method of administration

Route of Administration

Oral.

REMEDEINE\REMEDEINE FORTE tablets should, if possible, be taken during or after meals.

Adults and children over 12 years

1 or 2 tablets every four to six hours.

Do not exceed eight tablets in any 24-hour period.

Children under 12 years

Not recommended.

Elderly

One tablet every 4 - 6 hours increasing to two tablets every 4 - 6 hours if required and tolerated. Caution should be exercised when increasing the dose in the elderly.

4.3 Contraindications

Respiratory depression, obstructive airways disease, hypersensitivity to paracetamol, dihydrocodeine or other tablet constituents.

4.4 Special warnings and special precautions for use

REMEDEINE\REMEDEINE FORTE tablets should be given with caution in patients with allergic disorders and should not be given during an attack of asthma. Caution should also be observed if there is marked impairment of liver function, advanced kidney disease and in chronic alcoholics.

Do not exceed the recommended dose.

Patients should be advised not to take other paracetamol-containing products concurrently.

Dosage should be reduced in the elderly, in hypothyroidism and in chronic hepatic disease. An overdose can cause hepatic necrosis.

Dihydrocodeine should be used with caution in patients taking monoamine oxidase inhibitors and should be avoided in those patients with raised intracranial pressure or head injury.

Use with caution in patients with prostatic hypertrophy since dihydrocodeine may cause urinary retention.

In patients already habituated to a drug such as pethidine, the substitution of dihydrocodeine in equi-analgesic doses has led to the appearance of abstinence symptoms. This suggests that dihydrocodeine, despite its effectiveness as an analgesic, has a low addiction potential. Nevertheless, when dihydrocodeine is prescribed for chronic use the physician should take care to avoid any unnecessary increase in dosage especially when there is a previous history of drug dependence or abuse.

4.5 Interaction with other medicinal products and other forms of Interaction

Additive CNS depression may occur with alcohol, and other CNS depressants such as anxiolytics, anti-depressants, hypnotics and anti-psychotics. The rate of absorption of paracetamol may be increased by metoclopramide or domperidone and absorption of paracetamol may be reduced by cholestyramine.

The anti-coagulant effect of warfarin and other coumarins may be enhanced by prolonged regular use of paracetamol with increased risk of bleeding.

4.6 Pregnancy and lactation

Epidemiological studies in human pregnancy have shown no effects due to paracetamol or dihydrocodeine. However, both drugs should be avoided during pregnancy unless considered essential by the physician.

Paracetamol is excreted in breast milk but not in a clinically significant amount. Available published data do not contra-indicate breast feeding.

4.7 Effects on ability to drive and use machines

Dihydrocodeine may cause drowsiness and, if affected, patients should not drive or operate machinery.

4.8 Undesirable effects

Constipation, if it occurs, is readily treated with a mild laxative.

Other side-effects of dihydrocodeine which may occur in a few patients, are nausea, vomiting, headache, vertigo, giddiness, urinary retention, pruritus, sedation, dysphoria, hallucinations and allergic reactions including skin rashes.

Adverse effects of paracetamol are rare but hypersensitivity reactions including skin rash, blood dyscrasias, acute pancreatitis have been reported.

4.9 Overdose

Symptoms of paracetamol overdosage in the first 24 hours are pallor, nausea, vomiting, anorexia and abdominal pain. Liver damage may become apparent 12 to 48 hours after ingestion. Abnormalities of glucose metabolism and metabolic acidosis may occur. In severe poisoning, hepatic failure may progress to encephalopathy, coma and death. Acute renal failure with acute tubular necrosis may develop even in the absence of severe liver damage. Cardiac arrhythmias have been reported.

Liver damage is likely in adults who have taken 10 g or more of paracetamol. It is considered that excess quantities of a toxic metabolite (usually adequately detoxified by glutathione when normal doses of paracetamol are ingested), become irreversibly bound to liver tissue.

Immediate treatment is essential in the management of paracetamol overdose. Despite a lack of significant early symptoms, patients should be referred to hospital urgently for immediate medical attention and any patient who has ingested around 7.5 g or more of paracetamol in the preceding 4 hours should undergo gastric lavage. Administration of oral methionine or intravenous N-acetylcysteine which may have a beneficial effect up to at least 48 hours after the overdose, may be required. General supportive measures must be available.

Severe respiratory depression due to dihydrocodeine can be treated with naloxone hydrochloride 0.8 to 2 mg intravenously, repeated as required at 2 or 3 minute intervals.

5. PHARMACOLOGICAL PROPERTIES

5.1 Pharmacodynamic properties

Paracetamol is an effective analgesic possessing a remarkably low level of side effects. Its broad clinical utility has been extensively reported, and it now largely replaces aspirin for routine use. Paracetamol is well tolerated; having a bland effect on gastric mucosa, unlike aspirin, it neither exacerbates symptoms of peptic ulcer nor precipitates bleeding. Dihydrocodeine tartrate has been widely used for a number of years as a powerful analgesic.

In addition the compound exhibits well-defined anti-tussive activity.

Fortifying paracetamol with dihydrocodeine tartrate provides an effective combination of drugs for the treatment of severe pain.

5.2 Pharmacokinetic properties

Dihydrocodeine is well absorbed from the gastrointestinal tract. Like other phenanthrene derivatives, dihydrocodeine is mainly metabolised in the liver with the resultant metabolites being excreted mainly in the urine.

Metabolism of dihydrocodeine includes 0-demethylation, N-demethylation and 6-keto reduction.

Paracetamol is readily absorbed from the gastrointestinal tract with peak plasma concentrations occurring 30 minutes to 2 hours after ingestion. It is metabolised in the liver and excreted in the urine as the glucuronide and sulphate conjugates.

5.3 Preclinical safety data

There are no pre-clinical data of relevance to the prescriber which are additional to that already included in other sections of the SPC.

6. PHARMACEUTICAL PARTICULARS

6.1 List of excipients

Magnesium Stearate

Starch Maize Special

6.2 Incompatibilities

None known.

6.3 Shelf life

Three years.

6.4 Special precautions for storage
Store at or below 30°C protected from moisture.

6.5 Nature and contents of container
REMEDEINE tablets are available in polypropylene containers with polyethylene lids containing 56 or 112 tablets.

REMEDEINE FORTE tablets are available in polypropylene containers with polyethylene lids containing 56 tablets.

6.6 Instructions for use and handling
None

Administrative Data

7. MARKETING AUTHORISATION HOLDER
Napp Pharmaceuticals Ltd
Cambridge Science Park
Milton Road
Cambridge CB4 0GW
Tel: 01223 424444

8. MARKETING AUTHORISATION NUMBER(S)
PL 16950/0059, 0060

9. DATE OF FIRST AUTHORISATION/RENEWAL OF THE AUTHORISATION
20 November 1991/14 January 1998

10. DATE OF REVISION OF THE TEXT
February 2004

11. Legal Category
POM

® The Napp device, REMEDEINE and REMEDEINE FORTE are Registered Trade Marks.

Remicade 100mg powder for concentrate for solution for infusion

(Schering-Plough Ltd)

1. NAME OF THE MEDICINAL PRODUCT
Remicade 100 mg powder for concentrate for solution for infusion.

2. QUALITATIVE AND QUANTITATIVE COMPOSITION
Each vial of Remicade contains 100 mg of infliximab, a chimeric IgG1 monoclonal antibody manufactured from a recombinant cell line cultured by continuous perfusion. After reconstitution each ml contains 10 mg of infliximab.

For excipients, see section 6.1.

3. PHARMACEUTICAL FORM
Powder for concentrate for solution for infusion.

4. CLINICAL PARTICULARS

4.1 Therapeutic indications

Rheumatoid arthritis:

Remicade, in combination with methotrexate, is indicated for:

the reduction of signs and symptoms as well as the improvement in physical function in:

- patients with active disease when the response to disease-modifying drugs, including methotrexate, has been inadequate.
- patients with severe, active and progressive disease not previously treated with methotrexate or other DMARDs.

In these patient populations, a reduction in the rate of the progression of joint damage, as measured by x-ray, has been demonstrated (see section 5.1).

Crohn's disease

Remicade is indicated for:

- treatment of severe, active Crohn's disease, in patients who have not responded despite a full and adequate course of therapy with a corticosteroid and an immunosuppressant; or who are intolerant to or have medical contraindications for such therapies.
- treatment of fistulising, active Crohn's disease, in patients who have not responded despite a full and adequate course of therapy with conventional treatment (including antibiotics, drainage and immunosuppressive therapy).

Ankylosing spondylitis

Remicade is indicated for:

Treatment of ankylosing spondylitis, in patients who have severe axial symptoms, elevated serological markers of inflammatory activity and who have responded inadequately to conventional therapy.

Psoriatic arthritis:

Remicade, in combination with methotrexate, is indicated for:

Treatment of active and progressive psoriatic arthritis in patients who have responded inadequately to disease-modifying anti-rheumatic drugs.

4.2 Posology and method of administration
Remicade is for intravenous use in adults and has not been studied in children (0-17 years).

Remicade treatment is to be administered under the supervision and monitoring of specialised physicians experienced in the diagnosis and treatment of rheumatoid arthritis, inflammatory bowel diseases, or ankylosing spondylitis. Patients treated with Remicade should be given the package leaflet and the special Alert card.

The recommended infusion time is 2 hours. All patients administered Remicade are to be observed for at least 1-2 hours post infusion for acute infusion-related reactions. Emergency equipment, such as adrenaline, antihistamines, corticosteroids and an artificial airway must be available. Patients may be pretreated with e.g., an antihistamine, hydrocortisone and/or paracetamol and infusion rate may be slowed in order to decrease the risk of infusion related reactions especially if infusion-related reactions have occurred previously (see section 4.4).

During Remicade treatment, other concomitant therapies, e.g., corticosteroids and immunosuppressants should be optimised.

Rheumatoid arthritis

3 mg/kg given as an intravenous infusion over a 2-hour period followed by additional 3 mg/kg infusion doses at 2 and 6 weeks after the first infusion, then every 8 weeks thereafter.

Remicade must be given concomitantly with methotrexate.

Available data suggest that the clinical response is usually achieved within 12 weeks of treatment. Continued therapy should be carefully reconsidered in patients who show no evidence of therapeutic benefit within this time period.

Severe, active Crohn's disease

5 mg/kg given as an intravenous infusion over a 2-hour period. Available data do not support further infliximab treatment, in patients not responding within 2 weeks to the initial infusion. In responding patients, the alternative strategies for continued treatment are:

- Maintenance: Additional infusions of 5 mg/kg at 2 and 6 weeks after the initial dose, followed by infusions every 8 weeks or
- Readministration: Infusion of 5 mg/kg if signs and symptoms of the disease recur (see 'Readministration' below and section 4.4).

Fistulising, active Crohn's disease

An initial 5 mg/kg infusion given over a 2-hour period is to be followed with additional 5 mg/kg infusion doses at 2 and 6 weeks after the first infusion. If a patient does not respond after these 3 doses, no additional treatment with infliximab should be given.

In responding patients, the strategies for continued treatment are:

- Additional infusions of 5 mg/kg every 8 weeks or
- Readministration if signs and symptoms of the disease recur followed by infusions of 5 mg/kg every 8 weeks (see 'Readministration' below and section 4.4).

In Crohn's disease, experience with readministration if signs and symptoms of disease recur is limited and comparative data on the benefit / risk of the alternative strategies for continued treatment are lacking.

Ankylosing spondylitis

5 mg/kg given as an intravenous infusion over a 2-hour period followed by additional 5 mg/kg infusion doses at 2 and 6 weeks after the first infusion, then every 6 to 8 weeks. If a patient does not respond by 6 weeks (i.e. after 2 doses), no additional treatment with infliximab should be given.

Psoriatic arthritis

5 mg/kg given as an intravenous infusion over a 2-hour period followed by additional 5 mg/kg infusion doses at 2 and 6 weeks after the first infusion, then every 8 weeks thereafter. Efficacy and safety have been demonstrated in combination with methotrexate.

Readministration for Crohn's disease and rheumatoid arthritis

If the signs and symptoms of disease recur, Remicade can be readministered within 16 weeks following the last infusion. In clinical studies, delayed hypersensitivity reactions have been uncommon and have occurred after drug free intervals of less than 1 year (see section 4.4 and 4.8: delayed hypersensitivity). The safety and efficacy of readministration after a drug free interval of more than 16 weeks has not been established. This applies to both Crohn's disease patients and rheumatoid arthritis patients.

Readministration for ankylosing spondylitis

The safety and efficacy of readministration, other than every 6 to 8 weeks, has not been established.

Readministration for psoriatic arthritis

The safety and efficacy of readministration, other than every 8 weeks, has not been established.

For preparation and administration instructions, see section 6.6.

4.3 Contraindications
Patients with tuberculosis or other severe infections such as sepsis, abscesses, and opportunistic infections (see section 4.4).

Patients with moderate or severe heart failure (NYHA class III/IV) (see sections 4.4 and 4.8).

Remicade must not be given to patients with a history of hypersensitivity to infliximab (see section 4.8), to other murine proteins, or to any of the excipients.

4.4 Special warnings and special precautions for use

Infusion reactions and hypersensitivity

Infliximab has been associated with acute infusion-related reactions, including anaphylactic shock, and delayed hypersensitivity reactions (see section 4.8: "Undesirable effects").

Acute infusion reactions including anaphylactic reactions may develop during (within seconds) or within a few hours following infusion. If acute infusion reactions occur, the infusion must be interrupted immediately. Emergency equipment, such as adrenaline, antihistamines, corticosteroids and an artificial airway must be available. Patients may be pretreated with e.g., an antihistamine, hydrocortisone and/or paracetamol to prevent mild and transient effects.

Antibodies to infliximab may develop and have been associated with an increased frequency of infusion reactions. A low proportion of the infusion reactions was serious allergic reactions. In Crohn's disease patients, an association between development of antibodies to infliximab and reduced duration of response has also been observed. Concomitant administration of immunomodulators has been associated with lower incidence of antibodies to infliximab and a reduction in the frequency of infusion reactions. The effect of concomitant immunomodulator therapy was more profound in episodically treated patients than in patients given maintenance therapy. Patients who discontinue immunosuppressants prior to or during Remicade treatment are at greater risk of developing these antibodies. Antibodies to infliximab can not always be detected in serum samples. If serious reactions occur, symptomatic treatment must be given and further Remicade infusions must not be administered (see section 4.8: "Immunogenicity").

In clinical trials, delayed hypersensitivity reactions have been reported. Available data suggest an increased risk for delayed hypersensitivity with increasing drug free interval. Advise patients to seek immediate medical advice if they experience any delayed adverse event (see section 4.8: "Delayed hypersensitivity"). If patients are retreated after a prolonged period, they must be closely monitored for signs and symptoms of delayed hypersensitivity.

Infections

Patients must be monitored closely for infections including tuberculosis before, during and after treatment with Remicade. Because the elimination of infliximab may take up to six months, monitoring should be continued throughout this period. Further treatment with Remicade must not be given if a patient develops a serious infection or sepsis.

Tumour necrosis factor alpha (TNFα) mediates inflammation and modulates cellular immune responses. Experimental data show that TNFα is essential for the clearing of intracellular infections. Clinical experience shows that host defence against infection is compromised in some patients treated with infliximab. It should be noted that suppression of TNFα may also mask symptoms of infection such as fever.

Opportunistic infections and other infections including sepsis and pneumonia have been observed in patients treated with infliximab, some of these infections have been fatal.

Cases of active tuberculosis including miliary tuberculosis and tuberculosis with extrapulmonary location have been reported in patients treated with Remicade. Some of these cases had a fatal outcome.

Before starting treatment with Remicade, all patients must be evaluated for both active and inactive ('latent') tuberculosis. This evaluation should include a detailed medical history with personal history of tuberculosis or possible previous contact with tuberculosis and previous and/or current immunosuppressive therapy. Appropriate screening tests, i.e. tuberculin skin test and chest x-ray, should be performed in all patients (local recommendations may apply). It is recommended that the conduct of these tests should be recorded in the patient's alert card. Prescribers are reminded of the risk of false negative tuberculin skin test results especially in patients who are severely ill or immunocompromised.

If active tuberculosis is diagnosed, Remicade therapy must not be initiated (see section 4.3)

If inactive ('latent') tuberculosis is diagnosed, prophylactic anti-tuberculosis therapy must be started before the initiation of Remicade, and in accordance with local recommendations. In this situation, the benefit/ risk balance of Remicade therapy should be very carefully considered.

Patients with fistulising Crohn's disease with acute suppurative fistulas must not initiate Remicade therapy until a source for possible infection, specifically abscess, has been excluded (see section 4.3).

All patients should be informed to seek medical advice if signs/symptoms suggestive of tuberculosis (e.g. persistent cough, wasting/weight loss, low-grade fever) appear during or after Remicade treatment.

Reactivation of hepatitis B occurred in patients receiving Remicade who are chronic carriers of this virus (i.e. surface antigen positive). Chronic carriers of hepatitis B should be appropriately evaluated and monitored prior to the initiation of and during treatment with Remicade.

Hepatobiliary events

Very rare cases of jaundice and non-infectious hepatitis, some with features of autoimmune hepatitis, have been observed in the post-marketing experience of Remicade. Isolated cases of liver failure resulting in liver transplantation or death have occurred. Patients with symptoms or signs of liver dysfunction should be evaluated for evidence or liver injury. If jaundice and/or ALT elevations $\geqslant$ 5 times the upper limit of normal develop(s), Remicade should be discontinued, and a thorough investigation of the abnormality should be undertaken.

Concurrent administration of TNF-alpha inhibitor and anakinra

Serious infections were seen in clinical studies with concurrent use of anakinra and another TNFα-blocking agent, etanercept, with no added clinical benefit compared to etanercept alone. Because of the nature of the adverse events seen with combination of etanercept and anakinra therapy, similar toxicities may also result from the combination of anakinra and other TNFα-blocking agents. Therefore, the combination of Remicade and anakinra is not recommended.

Vaccinations

No data are available on the response to vaccination with live vaccines or on the secondary transmission of infection by live vaccines in patients receiving anti-TNF therapy. It is recommended that live vaccines not be given concurrently.

Autoimmune processes

The relative deficiency of TNFα caused by anti-TNF therapy may result in the initiation of an autoimmune process. If a patient develops symptoms suggestive of a lupus-like syndrome following treatment with Remicade and is positive for antibodies against double-stranded DNA, further treatment with Remicade must not be given (see section 4.8: "Anti-nuclear antibodies (ANA)/Double-stranded DNA (dsDNA) antibodies").

Neurological events

Infliximab and other agents that inhibit TNFα have been associated in rare cases with optic neuritis, seizure and new onset of exacerbation of clinical symptoms and/or radiographic evidence of demyelinating disorders, including multiple sclerosis. In patients with pre-existing or recent onset of central nervous system demyelinating disorders, the benefits and risks of Remicade treatment should be carefully considered before initiation of Remicade therapy.

Malignancies and lymphoproliferative disorders:

In the controlled portions of clinical trials of TNF-blocking agents, more cases of lymphoma have been observed among patients receiving a TNF blocker compared with control patients. However, the occurrence was rare, and the follow up period of placebo in patients was shorter than for patients receiving TNF-blocking therapy. Furthermore, there is an increased background lymphoma risk in rheumatoid arthritis patients with longstanding, highly active, inflammatory disease, which complicates the risk estimation. With the current knowledge, a possible risk for the development of lymphomas or other malignancies in patients treated with a TNF-blocking agent cannot be excluded.

No studies have been conducted that include patients with a history of malignancy or that continue treatment in patients who develop malignancy while receiving Remicade. Thus additional caution should be exercised in considering Remicade treatment of these patients (see section 4.8).

Heart failure

Remicade should be used with caution in patients with mild heart failure (NYHA class I/II). Patients should be closely monitored and Remicade must not be continued in patients who develop new or worsening symptoms of heart failure (see sections 4.3 and 4.8).

Others

Treatment with Remicade has not been studied in children 0-17 years with rheumatoid arthritis or Crohn's disease. Until safety and efficacy data in children are available, such treatment is to be avoided.

The pharmacokinetics of infliximab in elderly patients has not been studied. Studies have not been performed in patients with liver or renal disease (see section 5.2).

There are insufficient preclinical data to draw conclusions on the effects of infliximab on fertility and general reproductive function (see section 5.3).

There is limited safety experience of surgical procedures in Remicade treated patients. The long half life of Remicade should be taken into consideration if a surgical procedure is planned. A patient who requires surgery while on Remicade should be closely monitored for infections, and appropriate actions should be taken.

There is limited safety experience of Remicade treatment in patients who have undergone arthroplasty.

Treatment of patients with intestinal strictures due to Crohn's disease is not recommended since the risk/benefit relationship in this patient population has not been established.

4.5 Interaction with other medicinal products and other forms of Interaction

In rheumatoid arthritis and Crohn's disease patients, there are indications that concomitant use of methotrexate and other immunomodulators reduces the formation of antibodies against infliximab and increases the plasma concentrations of infliximab. However, the results are uncertain due to limitations in the methods used for serum analyses of infliximab and antibodies against infliximab. Corticosteroids do not appear to affect the pharmacokinetics of infliximab to a clinically relevant extent. The combination of Remicade and anakinra is not recommended (see section 4.4). Nothing is known regarding possible interactions between infliximab and other active substances.

4.6 Pregnancy and lactation

Pregnancy

Post-marketing reports from approximately 300 pregnancies exposed to infliximab do not indicate unexpected effects on pregnancy outcome. Due to its inhibition of TNFα, infliximab administered during pregnancy could affect normal immune responses in the newborn. In a developmental toxicity study conducted in mice using an analogous antibody that selectively inhibits the functional activity of mouse TNFα, there was no indication of maternal toxicity, embryotoxicity or teratogenicity (see section 5.3).

The available clinical experience is too limited to exclude a risk, and administration of infliximab is therefore not recommended during pregnancy.

Women of childbearing potential

Women of childbearing potential must use adequate contraception to prevent pregnancy and continue its use for at least 6 months after the last Remicade treatment.

Lactation

It is not known whether infliximab is excreted in human milk or absorbed systemically after ingestion. Because human immunoglobulins are excreted in milk, women must not breast feed for at least 6 months after Remicade treatment.

4.7 Effects on ability to drive and use machines

No studies on the effects on the ability to drive and use machines have been performed.

4.8 Undesirable effects

In clinical studies with infliximab, adverse drug reactions (ADRs) were observed in approximately 60% of infliximab-treated patients and 40% of placebo-treated patients. The adverse reactions listed in table 1 are based on experience from clinical trials. Within the organ system classes, adverse reactions are listed under headings of frequency using the following categories: common (> 1/100, < 1/10); uncommon (> 1/1000, < 1/100); rare (> 1/10,000, < 1/1,000). Infusion-related reactions were the most common ADRs reported. Infusion-related reactions (dyspnoea, urticaria and headache) were the most common cause for discontinuation.

Table 1

Undesirable Effects in Clinical Studies

Infections and infestations Common:	Viral infection (e.g. influenza, herpes infections)
Uncommon:	Abscess, cellulitis, moniliasis, sepsis, bacterial infection, tuberculosis, fungal infection, hordeolum
Blood and lymphatic disorders Uncommon:	Anaemia, leukopoenia, lymphadenopathy, lymphocytosis, lymphopenia, neutropenia, thrombocytopenia
Immune System disorders Common:	Serum sickness-like reactions
Uncommon:	Lupus-like syndrome, respiratory tract allergic reactions, anaphylactic reactions
Psychiatric disorders Uncommon:	Depression, confusion, agitation, amnesia, apathy, nervousness, somnolence, insomnia
Nervous system disorders Common:	Headache, vertigo/dizziness
Uncommon:	Exacerbation of demyelinating disease suggestive of multiple sclerosis
Rare:	Meningitis
Eye disorders Uncommon:	Conjunctivitis, endophthalmitis, keratoconjunctivitis, periorbital oedema,
Cardiac disorders Uncommon:	Syncope, bradycardia, palpitations, cyonosis, arrhythmia, worsening heart failure.
Rare:	Tachycardia
Vascular disorders Common:	Flushing
Uncommon:	Ecchymosis/haematoma, hot flushes, hypertension, hypotension, petechia, thrombophleblitis, vasospasm, peripheral ischaemia,
Rare:	Circulatory failure,
Respiratory, thoracic and mediastinal disorders	
Common:	Upper respiratory tract infection, lower respiratory tract infection (e.g. bronchitis, pneumonia), dyspnoea, sinusitis
Uncommon:	Epistaxis, bronchospasm, pleurisy, pulmonary oedema
Rare:	Pleural effusion
Gastrointestinal disorders Common:	Nausea, diarrhoea, abdominal pain, dyspepsia
Uncommon:	Constipation, gastroesophageal reflux, cheilitis, diverticulitis
Rare:	Intestinal perforation, intestinal stenosis, gastrointestinal hemorrhage.
Hepatobiliary disorders Uncommon:	Abnormal hepatic function, cholecystitis
Rare:	Hepatitis
Skin and subcutaneous tissue disorders	
Common:	Rash, pruritus, urticaria, increased sweating, dry skin
Uncommon:	Fungal dermatitis/ onychomycosis, eczema/ seborrhoea, bullous eruption, furunculosis, hyperkeratosis, rosacea, verruca, abnormal skin pigmentation/colouration, alopoecia
Musculoskeletal and connective tissue disorders	
Uncommon:	Myalgia, arthralgia, back pain
Renal and urinary disorders Uncommon:	Urinary tract infection, pyelonephritis
Reproductive System and breast disorders	
Uncommon:	Vaginitis
General disorders and administration site conditions	
Common:	Fatigue, chest pain, infusion-related reactions, fever

Uncommon:	Injection site reactions, oedema, pain, chills/rigors, impaired healing.
Rare:	Granulomatous lesion
Investigations Common:	Elevated hepatic transaminases
Uncommon:	Autoantibodies, complement factor abnormality

Table 2
Undesirable effects in Post-marketing reports

(common > 1/100, < 1/10; uncommon > 1/1000, < 1/100; rare > 1/10,000, < 1/1000; very rare < 1/10,000, including isolated reports).

Infections and infestations	
Rare:	Opportunistic infections (such as tuberculosis, atypical mycobacteria, pneumocystosis, histoplasmosis, coccidioidomycosis, cryptococcosis, aspergillosis, listeriosis and candidiasis)
Very Rare:	Salmonellosis, reactivation of hepatitis B
Blood and lymphatic system disorders	
Rare:	Pancytopenia
Very Rare:	Haemolytic anaemia, idiopathic thrombocytopenic purpura, thrombotic thrombocytopenic purpura, agranulocytosis
Immune system disorders	
Uncommon:	Anaphylactic reactions
Rare:	Anaphylactic shock, serum sickness, vasculitis
Nervous system disorders	
Rare:	Demyelinating disorders (such as multiple sclerosis and optic neuritis), Guillain-Barré syndrome, neuropathies, numbness, tingling, seizure
Very Rare:	Transverse myelitis
Cardiac disorders	
Rare:	Worsening heart failure, new onset heart failure
Very rare:	Pericardial effusion
Respiratory, thoracic and mediastinal disorders	
Rare:	Interstitial pneumonitis/fibrosis
Gastrointestinal disorders	
Rare:	Pancreatitis
Hepatobiliary disorders	
Rare:	Hepatitis
Very rare:	Hepatocellular damage, jaundice, liver failure, autoimmune hepatitis
Skin and subcutaneous tissue disorders	
Rare:	Vasculitis (primarily cutaneous)
General disorders and administration site conditions	
Common:	Infusion-related reactions

Infusion-related reactions: An infusion-related reaction was defined in clinical studies as any adverse event occurring during an infusion or within 1 to 2 hours after an infusion. In clinical studies, approximately 20% of infliximab-treated patients compared with approximately 10% of placebo-treated patients experienced an infusion-related effect. Approximately 3% of patients discontinued treatment due to infusion reactions and all patients recovered with or without medical therapy.

In post-marketing experience, cases of anaphylactic-like reactions, including laryngeal/pharyngeal oedema and severe bronchospasm, and seizure have been associated with Remicade administration.

Delayed hypersensitivity: In clinical studies delayed hypersensitivity reactions have been uncommon and have occurred after drug free intervals of less than 1 year. Signs and symptoms included myalgia and/or arthralgia with fever and/or rash with some patients also experiencing pruritus, facial, hand or lip edema, dysphagia, urticaria, sore throat and headache.

There are insufficient data on the incidence of delayed hypersensitivity reactions after drug free intervals of more than 1 year but limited data from clinical trials suggest an increased risk for delayed hypersensitivity with increasing drug free interval.

In a 1-year trial with repeated infusions in patients with Crohn's disease (ACCENT I study), the incidence of serum sickness-like reactions was 2.4%.

Immunogenicity: Patients who developed antibodies to infliximab were more likely (approximately 2-3 fold) to develop infusion-related reactions. Use of concomitant immunosuppressant agents appeared to reduce the frequency of infusion-related reactions.

In clinical studies using single and multiple infliximab doses ranging from 1 to 20 mg/kg, antibodies to infliximab were detected in 140 of 980 (14%) patients with any immunosuppressant therapy, and in 92 of 383 (24%) patients without immunosuppressant therapy. In rheumatoid arthritis patients who received the recommended repeated treatment dose regimens with methotrexate, 6 of 77 (8%) patients developed antibodies to infliximab. Of Crohn's disease patients who received maintenance treatment, approximately 6-13% developed antibodies to infliximab. The antibody incidence was 2-3 fold higher for patients treated episodically. Due to methodological limitations, a negative assay did not exclude the presence of antibodies to infliximab. Some patients who developed high titres of antibodies to infliximab had evidence of reduced efficacy (see section 4.4: "Infusion reactions and hypersensitivity").

Infections: In clinical studies 36% of infliximab-treated patients were treated for infections compared with 25% of placebo-treated patients.

In RA trials, the incidence of serious infections including pneumonia was higher in infliximab plus MTX treated patients compared with methotrexate alone especially at doses of 6 mg/kg or greater (see section 4.4).

In postmarketing spontaneous reporting, infections are the most common serious adverse event. Some of the cases have resulted in fatal outcome. Nearly 50% of reported deaths have been associated with infection. Cases of tuberculosis, sometimes fatal, including miliary tuberculosis and tuberculosis with extrapulmonary location have been reported (see section 4.4).

Malignancies and lymphoproliferative disorders: In clinical studies with infliximab and during long-term follow-up of 4 years, representing 8800 patient years, 8 cases of lymphomas and 43 other malignancies were detected as compared with 9 malignancies and 0 lymphoma in placebo-treated patients observed during 1274 patient years. The overall rate of malignancies in these patients was similar to that expected for an age-, gender- and race-matched general population. From August 1998 to August 2004, 1367 cases of suspected malignancies have been reported from post-marketing, clinical trials and registries (229 in Crohn's disease patients, 942 in rheumatoid arthritis patients and 196 in patients with other or unknown indications). Among those there were 242 lymphoma cases. During this period, the estimated exposure is 1,350,000 patient years (see section 4.4: Special Warnings and Special Precautions for Use – "Malignancies".

Heart failure: In a phase II study aimed at evaluating Remicade in congestive heart failure (CHF), higher incidence of mortality due to worsening of heart failure were seen in patients treated with Remicade, especially those treated with the higher dose of 10 mg/kg (i.e. twice the maximum approved dose). In this study 150 patients with NYHA Class III-IV CHF (left ventricular ejection fraction ≤35%) were treated with 3 infusions of Remicade 5 mg/kg, 10 mg/kg, or placebo over 6 weeks. At 38 weeks, 9 of 101 patients treated with Remicade (2 at 5 mg/kg and 7 at 10 mg/kg) died compared to one death among the 49 patients on placebo.

There have been post-marketing reports of worsening heart failure, with and without identifiable precipitating factors, in patients taking Remicade. There have also been rare post-marketing reports of new onset heart failure, including heart failure in patients without known pre-existing cardiovascular disease. Some of these patients have been under 50 years of age.

Hepatobiliary events: In clinical trials, mild or moderate elevations of ALT and AST have been observed in patients receiving Remicade without progression to severe hepatic injury. Elevations of aminotransferases were observed (ALT more common than AST) in a greater proportion of patients receiving Remicade than in controls, both when Remicade was given as monotherapy and when it was used in combination with other immunosuppressive agents. Most aminotransferase abnormalities were transient; however, a small number of patients experienced more prolonged elevations. In general, patients who developed ALT and AST elevations were asymptomatic, and the abnormalities decreased or resolved with either continuation or discontinuation of Remicade, or modification of concomitant medications. ALT elevations ≥ 5 times the upper limit of normal were observed in 1% of patients receiving Remicade. In post-marketing surveillance, very rare cases of jaundice and hepatitis, some with features of autoimmune hepatitis, have been reported in patients receiving Remicade (see section 4.4).

Antinuclear antibodies (ANA)/Anti-double-stranded DNA (dsDNA) antibodies: Approximately half of infliximab-treated patients in clinical studies who were ANA negative at baseline developed a positive ANA during the study compared with approximately one-fifth of placebo-treated patients. Anti-dsDNA antibodies were newly detected in approximately 17% of infliximab-treated patients compared with 0% of placebo-treated patients. At the last evaluation, 57% infliximab-treated patients remained anti-dsDNA positive. Reports of lupus and lupus-like syndromes, remain uncommon.

4.9 Overdose

Single doses up to 20 mg/kg have been administered without toxic effects. There is no clinical experience of overdose.

5. PHARMACOLOGICAL PROPERTIES

5.1 Pharmacodynamic properties

Pharmacotherapeutic group: Selective immunosuppressive agents, ATC code: LO4AA12.

Pharmacodynamic properties: Infliximab is a chimeric human-murine monoclonal antibody that binds with high affinity to both soluble and transmembrane forms of TNFα but not to lymphotoxin α (TNFβ). Infliximab inhibits the functional activity of TNFα in a wide variety of *in vitro* bioassays. Infliximab prevented disease in transgenic mice that develop polyarthritis as a result of constitutive expression of human TNFα and when administered after disease onset, it allowed eroded joints to heal. *In vivo*, infliximab rapidly forms stable complexes with human TNFα, a process that parallels the loss of TNFα bioactivity.

Elevated concentrations of TNFα have been found in the joints of rheumatoid arthritis patients and correlate with elevated disease activity. In rheumatoid arthritis, treatment with infliximab reduced infiltration of inflammatory cells into inflamed areas of the joint as well as expression of molecules mediating cellular adhesion, chemoattraction and tissue degradation. After infliximab treatment, patients exhibited decreased levels of serum interleukin 6 (IL-6) and C-reactive protein (CRP) compared with baseline. Peripheral blood lymphocytes further showed no significant decrease in number or in proliferative responses to *in vitro* mitogenic stimulation when compared with untreated patients' cells.

Histological evaluation of colonic biopsies, obtained before and 4 weeks after administration of infliximab, revealed a substantial reduction in detectable TNFα. Infliximab treatment of Crohn's disease patients was also associated with a substantial reduction of the commonly elevated serum inflammatory marker, CRP. Total peripheral white blood cell counts were minimally affected in infliximab-treated patients, although changes in lymphocytes, monocytes and neutrophils reflected shifts towards normal ranges. Peripheral blood mononuclear cells (PBMC) from infliximab-treated patients showed undiminished proliferative responsiveness to stimuli compared with untreated patients, and no substantial changes in cytokine production by stimulated PBMC were observed following treatment with infliximab. Analysis of lamina propria mononuclear cells obtained by biopsy of the intestinal mucosa showed that infliximab treatment caused a reduction in the number of cells capable of expressing TNFα and interferonγ. Additional histological studies provided evidence that treatment with infliximab reduces the infiltration of inflammatory cells into affected areas of the intestine and the presence of inflammation markers at these sites.

Clinical Efficacy

Rheumatoid arthritis

The efficacy of infliximab was assessed in two multicentre, randomised, double-blind, pivotal trials: ATTRACT and ASPIRE. In both studies concurrent use of stable doses of folic acid, oral corticosteroids (≤ 10 mg/day) and/or non-steroidal anti-inflammatory drugs was permitted.

The primary endpoints were the reduction of signs and symptoms as assessed by the American College of Rheumatology criteria (ACR20 for ATTRACT, landmark ACR-N for ASPIRE), the prevention of structural joint damage, and the improvement in physical function. A reduction in signs and symptoms was defined to be at least a 20% improvement (ACR20) in both tender and swollen joint counts, and in 3 of the following 5 criteria: (1) evaluator's global assessment, (2) patient's global assessment, (3) functional/disability measure, (4) visual analogue pain scale and (5) erythrocyte sedimentation rate or C-reactive protein. ACR-N uses the same criteria as the ACR20, calculated by taking the lowest percent improvement in swollen joint count, tender joint count, and the median of the remaining 5 components of the ACR response. Structural joint damage (erosions and joint space narrowing) in both hands and feet was measured by the change from baseline in the total van der Heijde-modified Sharp score (0-440). The Health Assessment Questionnaire (HAQ; scale 0-3) was used to measure patients' average change from baseline scores over time, in physical function.

The ATTRACT trial evaluated responses at 30, 54 and 102 weeks in a placebo-controlled study of 428 patients with active rheumatoid arthritis despite treatment with methotrexate. Approximately 50% of patients were in functional Class III. Patients received placebo, 3 mg/kg or 10 mg/kg infliximab at weeks 0, 2 and 6, and then every 4 or 8 weeks thereafter. All patients were on stable methotrexate doses (median 15 mg/wk) for 6 months prior to enrolment and were to remain on stable doses throughout the study.

Results from week 54 (ACR20, total van der Heijde-modified Sharp score and HAQ) are shown in Table 3. Higher degrees of clinical response (ACR50 and ACR70) were observed in all infliximab groups at 30 and 54 weeks compared with methotrexate alone.

A reduction in the rate of the progression of structural joint damage (erosions and joint space narrowing) was observed in all infliximab groups at 54 weeks (Table 3).

The effects observed at 54 weeks were maintained through 102 weeks. Due to a number of treatment withdrawals, the magnitude of the effect difference between infliximab and the methotrexate alone group can not be defined.

Table 3

Effects on ACR20, Structural Joint Damage and Physical Function at week 54, ATTRACT

(see Table 3)

Table 3 Effects on ACR20, Structural Joint Damage and Physical Function at week 54, ATTRACT

		infliximab[b]				
	Control[a]	3 mg/kg q 8 wks	3 mg/kg q 4 wks	10 mg/ kg q 8 wks	10 mg/kg q 4 wks	All infliximab[b]
Patients with ACR20 response/ patients evaluated (%)[c]	15/88 (17%)	36/86 (42%)	41/86 (48%)	51/87 (59%)	48/81 (59%)	176/340 (52%)
Total score[d] (van der Heijde-modified Sharp score)						
Change from baseline (Mean ± SD[c])	7.0 ± 10.3	1.3 ± 6.0	1.6 ± 8.5	0.2 ± 3.6	-0.7 ± 3.8	0.6 ± 5.9
Median[c] (Interquartile range)	4.0 (0.5,9.7)	0.5 (-1.5,3.0)	0.1 (-2.5,3.0)	0.5 (-1.5,2.0)	-0.5 (-3.0,1.5)	0.0 (-1.8,2.0)
Patients with no deterioration/ patients evaluated (%)[c]	13/64 (20%)	34/71 (48%)	35/71 (49%)	37/77 (48%)	44/66 (67%)	150/285 (53%)
HAQ change from baseline over time[e] (patients evaluated)	87	86	85	87	81	339
Mean ± SD[c]	0.2 ± 0.3	0.4 ± 0.3	0.5 ± 0.4	0.5 ± 0.5	0.4 ± 0.4	0.4 ± 0.4

a: control = All patients had active RA despite treatment with stable methotrexate doses for 6 months prior to enrolment and were to remain on stable doses throughout the study. Concurrent use of stable doses of oral corticosteroids (⩽ 10 mg/day) and/or non-steroidal anti-inflammatory drugs was permitted, and folate supplementation was given.

b: all infliximab doses given in combination with methotrexate and folate with some on corticosteroids and/or non-steroidal anti-inflammatory drugs

c: $p < 0.001$, for each infliximab treatment group vs. control

d: greater values indicate more joint damage.

e: HAQ = Health Assessment Questionnaire; greater values indicate less disability.

The ASPIRE trial evaluated responses at 54 weeks in 1004 methotrexate naïve patients with early (⩽ 3 years disease duration, median 0.6 years) active rheumatoid arthritis (median swollen and tender joint count of 19 and 31, respectively). All patients received methotrexate (optimised to 20 mg/wk by week 8) and either placebo, 3 mg/kg or 6 mg/kg infliximab at weeks 0, 2 and 6 and every 8 week thereafter. Results from week 54 are shown in Table 4.

Aftr 54 weeks of treatment, both doses of infliximab + methotrexate resulted in statistically significantly greater improvement in signs and symptoms compared to methotrexate alone as measured by the proportion of patients achieving ACR20, 50 and 70 responses.

In ASPIRE, more than 90% of patients had at least two evaluable x-rays. Reduction in the rate of progression of structural damage was observed at weeks 30 and 54 in the infliximab + methotrexate groups compared to methotrexate alone.

Table 4

Effects on ACRn, Structural Joint Damage and Physical Function at week 54, ASPIRE

(see Table 4)

Table 4 Effects on ACRn, Structural Joint Damage and Physical Function at week 54, ASPIRE

		infliximab + MTX		
	Placebo + MTX	3 mg/kg	6 mg/kg	Combined
Subjects randomised	282	359	363	722
Percentage ACR improvement Mean ± SD[a]	24.8 ± 59.7	37.3 ± 52.8	42.0 ± 47.3	39.6 ± 50.1
Change from baseline in total van der Heijde modified Sharp score[b].				
Mean ± SD[a] Median	3.70 ± 9.61 0.43	0.42 ± 5.82 0.00	0.51 ± 5.55 0.00	0.46 ± 5.68 0.00
Improvement from baseline in HAQ averaged over time from week 30 to week 54[c] Mean ± SD[d]	0.68 ± 0.63	0.80 ± 0.65	0.88 ± 0.65	0.84 ± 0.65

a: $p < 0.001$, for each infliximab treatment group vs. control

b: greater values indicate more joint damage.

c: HAQ = Health Assessment Questionnaire; greater values indicate less disability.

d: $p = 0.030$ and < 0.001 for the 3mg/kg and 6mg/kg treatment groups respectively vs. placebo + MTX.

<u>Crohn's disease</u>

Induction treatment in severe active Crohn's disease

The efficacy of a single dose treatment with infliximab was assessed in 108 patients with active Crohn's disease (Crohn's Disease Activity Index (CDAI) ⩾ 220 ⩽ 400) in a randomised, double-blinded, placebo-controlled, dose-response study. Of these 108 patients, 27 were treated with the recommended dosage of infliximab 5 mg/kg. All patients had experienced an inadequate response to prior conventional therapies. Concurrent use of stable doses of conventional therapies was permitted, and 92% of patients continued to receive these medications.

The primary endpoint was the proportion of patients who experienced a clinical response, defined as a decrease in CDAI by ⩾ 70 points from baseline at the 4-week evaluation and without an increase in Crohn's disease medications or surgery for Crohn's disease. Patients who responded at week 4 were followed to week 12. Secondary endpoints included the proportion of patients in clinical remission at week 4 (CDAI < 150) and clinical response over time.

At week 4, following a single dose of study medication, 22/27 (81%) of infliximab-treated patients receiving a 5 mg/kg dose achieved a clinical response vs. 4/25 (16%) of the placebo-treated patients ($p < 0.001$). Also at week 4, 13/27 (48%) of infliximab-treated patients achieved a clinical remission (CDAI < 150) vs. 1/25 (4%) of placebo-treated patients. A response was observed within 2 weeks, with a maximum response at 4 weeks. At the last observation at 12 weeks, 13/27 (48%) of infliximab-treated patients were still responding.

Maintenance treatment in severe active Crohn's disease

The efficacy of repeated infusions with infliximab was studied in a 1-year clinical study.

A total of 573 patients with active Crohn's disease (CDAI ⩾ 220 ⩽ 400) received a single infusion of 5 mg/kg at week 0. Sixty-eight of these patients (12%) belonged to the population defined in the indication (see section 4.1). Three hundred and thirty-five patients (58%) responding to the 5 mg/kg infusion at week 2 were randomised to one of three treatment groups; a placebo maintenance group, 5 mg/kg maintenance group and 10 mg/kg maintenance group, receiving repeated infusions at week 2, 6 and every eight weeks.

At week 30, a significantly greater proportion of patients in the combined infliximab maintenance treatment group (42%) achieved clinical remission, compared with patients in the placebo maintenance group (21%). Median time to loss of response was 46 weeks in the combined infliximab maintenance treatment group vs. 19 weeks in the placebo maintenance group ($p<0.001$). Similar results were obtained in the subgroup analyses of the population defined in the indication (see section 4.1).

Improvements in quality of life measures were seen for both the IBDQ and SF-36 scores in the infliximab maintenance groups compared with the placebo maintenance group at week 30 ($p<0.001$).

Induction treatment in fistulising active Crohn's disease

The efficacy was assessed in a randomised, double-blinded, placebo-controlled study in 94 patients with fistulising Crohn's disease who had fistulae that were of at least 3 months' duration. Thirty-one of these patients were treated with infliximab 5 mg/kg. Approximately 93% of the patients had previously received antibiotic or immunosuppressive therapy.

Concurrent use of stable doses of conventional therapies was permitted, and 83% of patients continued to receive at least one of these medications. Patients received three doses of either placebo or infliximab at weeks 0, 2 and 6. Patients were followed up to 26 weeks. The primary endpoint was the proportion of patients who experienced a clinical response, defined as ⩾ 50% reduction from baseline in the number of fistulae draining upon gentle compression on at least two consecutive visits (4 weeks apart), without an increase in medication or surgery for Crohn's disease.

Sixty-eight percent (21/31) of infliximab-treated patients receiving a 5 mg/kg dose regimen achieved a clinical response vs. 26% (8/31) placebo-treated patients ($p = 0.002$). The median time to onset of response in the infliximab-treated group was 2 weeks. The median duration of response was 12 weeks. Additionally, closure of all fistulae was achieved in 55% of infliximab-treated patients compared with 13% of placebo-treated patients ($p = 0.001$).

Maintenance treatment in fistulising active Crohn's disease

The efficacy of repeated infusions with infliximab in patients with fistulising Crohn's disease was studied in a 1-year clinical study. A total of 306 patients received 3 doses of infliximab 5 mg/kg at week 0,2 and 6. At baseline, 87% of the patients had perianal fistulae, 14% had abdominal fistulae, 9% had rectovaginal fistulae. The median CDAI score was 180. One-hundred and ninety-five patients responding to the 3 doses (for definition of response see description of primary endpoint for the study above) were randomised at week 14 to receive either placebo or 5 mg/kg infliximab every 8 weeks through week 46. A significantly longer time to loss of response was seen in the infliximab maintenance group compared to the placebo maintenance group ($p<0.001$). Median time to loss of response was >40 weeks in the infliximab group compared with 14 weeks in the placebo group.

Most patients had a loss of response due to increase in medication for Crohn's disease and not because of a <50% reduction in number of draining fistulas. At week 54, the infliximab group showed greater improvement in CDAI score from baseline compared with placebo ($p=0.04$). There was no significant difference between placebo and infliximab for the proportion of patients with sustained closure of all fistulas through week 54, for symptoms such as proctalgia, abscesses and urinary tract infection or for number of newly developed fistulas during treatment.

Ankylosing spondylitis

Efficacy and safety were studied in a double-blind, placebo-controlled investigator initiated, multicenter study evaluating infliximab in 70 patients with active ankylosing spondylitis (disease activity [Bath Ankylosing Spondylitis Disease Activity Index (BASDAI) score > 4] and pain [NRS score >4]). During the 3 month double-blind phase, patients received either 5 mg/kg infliximab or placebo at weeks 0, 2, 6 (35 patients in each group). Starting at week 12, placebo patients were switched to infliximab and all patients subsequently received 5 mg/kg infliximab every 6 weeks up to week 54.

Treatment with infliximab resulted in improvement in signs and symptoms, as assessed by the BASDAI, with 57% of infliximab treated patients achieving at least 50% reduction from baseline in BASDAI score (mean baseline score was 6.5 in the infliximab group and 6.3 in the placebo group), compared with 9% of placebo patients ($p<0.01$). Improvement was observed at week 2 and was maintained through week 54. Physical function and quality of life (SF36) were improved similarly. In the trial, efficacy was not shown in HLA-B27 negative patients (n=7).

Psoriatic Arthritis

Efficacy and safety were studied in a double-blind, placebo-controlled, multicenter study evaluating infliximab in 104 patients with active polyarticular psoriatic arthritis. In total 74 subjects were on at least one concomitant DMARD, and among those 58 patients were treated with methotrexate. During the 16-week double-blind phase, patients received either 5 mg/kg infliximab or placebo at weeks 0, 2, 6, and 14 (52 patients in each group). Starting at week 16, placebo patients were switched to infliximab and all patients subsequently received 5 mg/kg infliximab every 8 weeks up to week 46.

Treatment with infliximab resulted in improvement in signs and symptoms, as assessed by the ACR criteria, with 65% of infliximab-treated patients achieving ACR 20 at week 16, compared with 10% of placebo-treated patients ($p<0.01$). Improvement (ACR 20 and 50) was observed as early as week 2 and was maintained through week 50 (ACR 20, 50, and 70). Decreases in parameters of peripheral activity characteristic of psoriatic arthritis (such as number of swollen joints, number of painful/tender joints, dactylitis and presence of enthesopathy) were seen in the infliximab-treated patients.

Infliximab-treated patients also demonstrated improvement in physical function as assessed by HAQ (mean change from baseline to week 16 of 0.6 vs. 0 for placebo-treated patients).

5.2 Pharmacokinetic properties

Single intravenous infusions of 1, 3, 5, 10 or 20 mg/kg of infliximab yielded dose proportional increases in the maximum serum concentration (C_{max}) and area under the concentration-time curve (AUC). The volume of distribution at steady state (median V_d of 3.0 to 4.1 litres) was not dependent on the administered dose and indicated that infliximab is predominantly distributed within the vascular compartment. No time-dependency of the pharmacokinetics was observed. The elimination pathways for infliximab have not been characterised. Unchanged infliximab was not detected in urine. No major age- or weight-related differences in clearance or volume of distribution were observed in rheumatoid arthritis patients. The pharmacokinetics of infliximab in elderly patients has not been studied. Studies have not been performed in patients with liver or renal disease.

At single doses of 3, 5, or 10 mg/kg, the median C_{max} values were 77, 118 and 277 micrograms/ml, respectively. The median terminal half-life at these doses ranged from 8 to 9.5 days. In most patients, infliximab could be detected in the serum for at least 8 weeks after the recommended single dose of 5 mg/kg for Crohn's disease and the rheumatoid arthritis maintenance dose of 3 mg/kg every 8 weeks.

Repeated administration of infliximab (5 mg/kg at 0, 2 and 6 weeks in fistulising Crohn's disease, 3 or 10 mg/kg every 4 or 8 weeks in rheumatoid arthritis) resulted in a slight accumulation of infliximab in serum after the second dose. No further clinically relevant accumulation was observed. In most fistulising Crohn's disease patients, infliximab was detected in serum for 12 weeks (range 4-28 weeks) after administration of the regimen.

5.3 Preclinical safety data

Infliximab does not cross react with TNFα from species other than human and chimpanzees. Therefore, conventional preclinical safety data with infliximab are limited. In a developmental toxicity study conducted in mice using an analogous antibody that selectively inhibits the functional activity of mouse TNFα, there was no indication of maternal toxicity, embryotoxicity or teratogenicity. In a fertility and general reproductive function study, the number of pregnant mice was reduced following administration of the same analogous antibody. It is not known whether this finding was due to effects on the males and/or the females. In a 6-month repeated dose toxicity study in mice, using the same analogous antibody against mouse TNFα, crystalline deposits were observed on the lens capsule of some of the treated male mice. No specific ophthalmologic examinations have been performed in patients to investigate the relevance of this finding for humans. Long-term studies have not been performed to evaluate the carcinogenic potential of infliximab. Studies in mice deficient in TNFα demonstrated no increase in tumours when challenged with known tumour initiators and/or promoters.

6. PHARMACEUTICAL PARTICULARS

6.1 List of excipients

Sucrose, polysorbate 80, monobasic sodium phosphate, dibasic sodium phosphate.

6.2 Incompatibilities

In the absence of incompatibility studies, this medicinal product must not be mixed with other medicinal products.

6.3 Shelf life

3 years.

Chemical and physical stability of the reconstituted solution has been demonstrated for 24 hours at room temperature (25°C). From a microbiological point of view, the product should be used as soon as possible but within 3 hours of reconstitution and dilution. If not used immediately, in use storage times and conditions prior to use are the responsibility of the user and should not be longer than 24 hours at 2 to 8°C.

6.4 Special precautions for storage

Store in a refrigerator (2°C - 8°C). Do not freeze.

6.5 Nature and contents of container

Remicade is supplied as a lyophilised powder in single-use glass (Type 1) vials with rubber stoppers and aluminium crimps protected by plastic caps. Remicade is available in packs of 1, 2 or 3 vials. Not all pack sizes may be marketed.

6.6 Instructions for use and handling

1. Calculate the dose and the number of Remicade vials needed. Each Remicade vial contains 100 mg infliximab. Calculate the total volume of reconstituted Remicade solution required.

2. Under aseptic conditions, reconstitute each Remicade vial with 10 ml of water for injections, using a syringe equipped with a 21-gauge (0.8 mm) or smaller needle. Remove flip-top from the vial and wipe the top with a 70% alcohol swab. Insert the syringe needle into the vial through the centre of the rubber stopper and direct the stream of water for injections to the glass wall of the vial. Do not use the vial if the vacuum is not present. Gently swirl the solution by rotating the vial to dissolve the lyophilised powder. Avoid prolonged or vigorous agitation. DO NOT SHAKE. Foaming of the solution on reconstitution is not unusual. Allow the reconstituted solution to stand for 5 minutes. Check that the solution is colourless to light yellow and opalescent. The solution may develop a few fine translucent particles, as infliximab is a protein. Do not use if opaque particles, discoloration, or other foreign particles are present.

3. Dilute the total volume of the reconstituted Remicade solution dose to 250 ml with sodium chloride 9mg/ml (0.9%) solution for infusion. This can be accomplished by withdrawing a volume of the sodium chloride 9mg/ml (0.9%) solution for infusion from the 250-ml glass bottle or infusion bag equal to the volume of reconstituted Remicade. Slowly add the total volume of reconstituted Remicade solution to the 250-ml infusion bottle or bag. Gently mix.

4. Administer the infusion solution over a period of not less than 2 hours (at not more than 2 ml/min). Use only an infusion set with an in-line, sterile, non-pyrogenic, low protein-binding filter (pore size 1.2 micrometer or less). Since no preservative is present, it is recommended that the administration of the solution for infusion is to be started as soon as possible and within 3 hours of reconstitution and dilution. When reconstitution and dilution are performed under aseptic conditions, Remicade infusion solution can be used within 24 hours if stored at 2°C to 8°C. Do not store any unused portion of the infusion solution for reuse.

5. No physical biochemical compatibility studies have been conducted to evaluate the co-administration of Remicade with other agents. Do not infuse Remicade concomitantly in the same intravenous line with other agents.

6. Visually inspect parenteral medicinal products for particulate matter or discolouration prior to administration. Do not use if visibly opaque particles, discolouration or foreign particulates are observed.

7. Discard any unused portion of the solution.

7. MARKETING AUTHORISATION HOLDER

Centocor B.V.

Einsteinweg 101

2333 CB Leiden

The Netherlands

8. MARKETING AUTHORISATION NUMBER(S)

EU/1/99/116/001

EU/1/99/116/002

EU/1/99/116/003

9. DATE OF FIRST AUTHORISATION/RENEWAL OF THE AUTHORISATION

Date of first authorisation: 13th August 1999

Date of last renewal: 13th August 2004

10. DATE OF REVISION OF THE TEXT

1st August 2005

LEGAL CATEGORY

Prescription Only Medicine

Remicade/EU/8-05/18

Reminyl Oral Solution

(Shire Pharmaceuticals Limited)

1. NAME OF THE MEDICINAL PRODUCT

Reminyl® 4 mg/ml Oral Solution

2. QUALITATIVE AND QUANTITATIVE COMPOSITION

1 ml Reminyl oral solution contains 4 mg galantamine (as hydrobromide).

For excipients, see 6.1.

3. PHARMACEUTICAL FORM

Oral solution. Reminyl oral solution is clear and colourless.

4. CLINICAL PARTICULARS

4.1 Therapeutic indications

Galantamine is indicated for the symptomatic treatment of mild to moderately severe dementia of the Alzheimer type.

4.2 Posology and method of administration

Adults/elderly

Administration

Galantamine should be administered twice a day, preferably with morning and evening meals. Ensure adequate fluid intake during treatment (See section 4.8).

Starting dose

The recommended starting dose is 8 mg/day (4 mg twice a day) for four weeks.

Maintenance dose

- The initial maintenance dose is 16 mg/day (8 mg twice a day) and patients should be maintained on 16 mg/day for at least 4 weeks.
- An increase to the maintenance dose of 24 mg/day (12 mg twice a day) should be considered on an individual basis after appropriate assessment including evaluation of clinical benefit and tolerability.
- In individual patients not showing an increased response or not tolerating 24 mg/day, a dose reduction to 16 mg/day should be considered.
- Maintenance treatment can be continued for as long as therapeutic benefit for the patient exists. Therefore, the clinical benefit of galantamine should be reassessed on a regular basis. Discontinuation should be considered when evidence of a therapeutic effect is no longer present.
- There is no rebound effect after abrupt discontinuation of treatment (e.g. in preparation for surgery).

Children

Galantamine is not recommended for use in children.

Hepatic and renal impairment

Galantamine plasma levels may be increased in patients with moderate to severe hepatic or renal impairment. In patients with moderately impaired hepatic function, based on pharmacokinetic modelling, it is recommended that dosing should begin with 4 mg once daily, preferably taken in the morning, for at least one week. Thereafter, patients should proceed with 4 mg b.i.d. for at least 4 weeks. In these patients, daily doses should not exceed 8 mg b.i.d. In patients with severe hepatic impairment (Child-Pugh score greater than 9), the use of galantamine is contraindicated (see section 4.3). No dosage adjustment is required for patients with mild hepatic impairment.

For patients with a creatinine clearance greater than 9 ml/min no dosage adjustment is required. In patients with severe renal impairment (creatinine clearance less than 9 ml/min), the use of galantamine is contraindicated (see section 4.3).

Concomitant treatment

In patients treated with potent CYP2D6 or CYP3A4 inhibitors (e.g. ketoconazole) dose reductions can be considered (see section 4.5).

4.3 Contraindications

- Galantamine should not be administered to patients with a known hypersensitivity to galantamine hydrobromide or to any excipients used in the formulations.
- Since no data are available on the use of galantamine in patients with severe hepatic (Child-Pugh score greater than 9) and severe renal (creatinine clearance less than 9 ml/min) impairment, galantamine is contraindicated in these populations. Galantamine is contra-indicated in patients who have both significant renal and hepatic dysfunction.

4.4 Special warnings and special precautions for use

A diagnosis of Alzheimer's dementia should be made according to current guidelines by an experienced physician. Therapy with galantamine should occur under the supervision of a physician and should only be initiated if a caregiver is available who will regularly monitor drug intake by the patient.

Patients with Alzheimer's disease lose weight. Treatment with cholinesterase inhibitors, including galantamine, has been associated with weight loss in these patients. During therapy, patient's weight should be monitored.

As with other cholinomimetics, galantamine should be given with caution in the following conditions:

Cardiovascular conditions: because of their pharmacological action, cholinomimetics may have vagotonic effects on heart rate (e.g. bradycardia). The potential for this action may be particularly important to patients with 'sick sinus syndrome' or other supraventricular cardiac conduction disturbances or who use drugs that significantly reduce heart rate concomitantly, such as digoxin and beta blockers.

Gastrointestinal conditions: patients at increased risk of developing peptic ulcers, e.g. those with a history of ulcer disease or those predisposed to these conditions, should be monitored for symptoms. The use of galantamine is not recommended in patients with gastro-intestinal obstruction or recovering from gastro-intestinal surgery.

Neurological Conditions: cholinomimetics are believed to have some potential to cause generalised convulsions. However, seizure activity may also be a manifestation of Alzheimer's disease. In clinical trials there was no increase in incidence of convulsions with galantamine compared with placebo. In rare cases an increase in cholinergic tone may worsen Parkinsonian symptoms.

Pulmonary Conditions: cholinomimetics should be prescribed with care for patients with a history of severe asthma or obstructive pulmonary disease.

Genitourinary: the use of galantamine is not recommended in patients with urinary outflow obstruction or recovering from bladder surgery.

Anaesthesia: galantamine, as a cholinomimetic is likely to exaggerate succinylcholinetype muscle relaxation during anaesthesia.

Methyl parahydroxybenzoate and propyl parahydroxybenzoate may cause allergic reactions (possibly delayed).

4.5 Interaction with other medicinal products and other forms of Interaction

Pharmacodynamic interactions

Because of its mechanism of action, galantamine should not be given concomitantly with other cholinomimetics. Galantamine antagonises the effect of anticholinergic medication. As expected with cholinomimetics, a pharmacodynamic interaction is possible with drugs that significantly reduce the heart rate (e.g. digoxin and beta blockers). Galantamine, as a cholinomimetic, is likely to exaggerate succinylcholine-type muscle relaxation during anaesthesia.

Pharmacokinetic interactions

Multiple metabolic pathways and renal excretion are involved in the elimination of galantamine.

Concomitant administration with food slows the absorption rate of galantamine but does not affect the extent of absorption. It is recommended that galantamine be taken with food in order to minimise cholinergic side effects.

Other drugs affecting the metabolism of galantamine

Formal drug interaction studies showed an increase in galantamine bioavailability of about 40% during co-administration of paroxetine (a potent CYP2D6 inhibitor) and of 30% and 12% during co-treatment with ketoconazole and erythromycin (both CYP3A4 inhibitors). Therefore, during initiation of treatment with potent inhibitors of CYP2D6 (e.g. quinidine, paroxetine, fluoxetine or fluvoxamine) or CYP3A4 (e.g. ketoconazole, ritonavir) patients may experience an increased incidence of cholinergic side effects, predominantly nausea and vomiting. Under these circumstances, based on tolerability, a reduction of the galantamine maintenance dose can be considered (see section 4.2).

Effect of galantamine on the metabolism of other drugs

Therapeutic doses of galantamine (12 mg b.i.d.) had no effect on the kinetics of digoxin and warfarin (see also pharmacodynamic interactions).

4.6 Pregnancy and lactation

Pregnancy

For galantamine no clinical data on exposed pregnancies are available. Animal studies indicate a slightly delayed development in foetuses and neonates (see section 5.3). Caution should be exercised when prescribing to pregnant women.

Lactation

It is not known whether galantamine is excreted in human breast milk and there are no studies in lactating women. Therefore, women on galantamine should not breast-feed.

4.7 Effects on ability to drive and use machines

Galantamine may cause dizziness and somnolence, which could affect the ability to drive or use machines, especially during the first weeks after initiation of treatment.

4.8 Undesirable effects

The most common adverse events observed in clinical trials (incidence $\geqslant$ 5% and twice the frequency of placebo) were nausea, vomiting, diarrhoea, abdominal pain, dyspepsia, anorexia, fatigue, dizziness, headache, somnolence and weight decrease. Nausea, vomiting and anorexia were more commonly observed in women.

Other common adverse events observed in clinical trials (incidence $\geqslant$ 5% and $\geqslant$ placebo) were confusion, fall, injury, insomnia, rhinitis and urinary tract infection.

The majority of these adverse events occurred during the titration period. Nausea and vomiting, the most frequent adverse events, lasted less than a week in most cases and the majority of patients had only one episode.

Prescription of anti-emetics and ensuring adequate fluid intake may be useful in these instances.

Adverse reactions observed during clinical trials and post marketing experience.

(see Table 1)

Frequencies are defined as: very common (> 1/10), common (> 1/100, < 1/10), uncommon (> 1/1,000, < 1/100), rare (> 1/10,000, < 1/1,000) and very rare (< 1/10,000)

Some of these adverse events may be attributable to cholinomimetic properties of galantamine or in some cases may represent manifestations or exacerbations of the underlying disease processes common in the elderly population.

4.9 Overdose

Symptoms

Signs and symptoms of significant overdosing of galantamine are predicted to be similar to those of overdosing of other cholinomimetics. These effects generally involve the central nervous system, the parasympathetic nervous system, and the neuromuscular junction. In addition to muscle weakness or fasciculations, some or all of the signs of a cholinergic crisis may develop: severe nausea, vomiting, gastro-intestinal cramping, salivation, lacrimation, urination, defecation, sweating, bradycardia, hypotension, collapse and convulsions. Increasing muscle weakness together with tracheal hypersecretions and bronchospasm, may lead to vital airway compromise.

In a post-marketing report, bradycardia, QT prolongation, ventricular tachycardia and torsades de pointes accompanied by a brief loss of consciousness were reported in association with an inadvertent ingestion of eight 4 mg tablets (32 mg total) on a single day.

Treatment

As in any case of overdose, general supportive measures should be used. In severe cases, anticholinergics such as atropine can be used as a general antidote for cholinomimetics. An initial dose of 0.5 to 1.0 mg i.v. is recommended, with subsequent doses based on the clinical response.

Because strategies for the management of overdose are continually evolving, it is advisable to contact a poison control centre to determine the latest recommendations for the management of an overdose.

5. PHARMACOLOGICAL PROPERTIES

5.1 Pharmacodynamic properties

Pharmacotherapeutic group: Antidementia drugs; ATC-code: N06DA04.

Galantamine, a tertiary alkaloid is a selective, competitive and reversible inhibitor of acetylcholinesterase. In addition, galantamine enhances the intrinsic action of acetylcholine on nicotinic receptors, probably through binding to an allosteric site of the receptor. As a consequence, an increased activity in the cholinergic system associated with improved cognitive function can be achieved in patients with dementia of the Alzheimer type.

Clinical studies

The dosages of galantamine effective in placebo-controlled clinical trials with a duration of 5 to 6 months were 16, 24 and 32 mg/day. Of these doses 16 and 24 mg/day were judged to have the best benefit/risk and were retained as recommended maintenance doses. Galantamine's efficacy has been shown using outcome measures which evaluate the three major symptom complexes of the disease and a global scale: the ADAS-Cog (a performance based measure of cognition), DAD and ADCS-ADL-Inventory (measurements of basic and instrumental Activities of Daily Living), the Neuropsychiatric Inventory (a scale that measures behavioural disturbances) and the CIBIC-plus (a global assessment by an independent physician based on a clinical interview with the patient and caregiver).

Composite responder analysis based on at least 4 points improvement in ADAS-Cog/11 compared to baseline and CIBIC-plus unchanged + improved (1-4), and DAD/ADL score unchanged + improved.

(see Table 2 on next page)

The results of a 26-week double-blind placebo-controlled trial, in which patients with vascular dementia and patients with Alzheimer's disease and concomitant cerebrovascular disease ("mixed dementia") were included, indicate that the symptomatic effect of galantamine is maintained in patients with Alzheimer's disease and concomitant cerebrovascular disease. In a post-hoc subgroup analysis, no statistically significant effect was observed in the subgroup of patients with vascular dementia alone.

In a second 26-week placebo-controlled trial in patients with probable vascular dementia, no clinical benefit of galantamine treatment was demonstrated.

5.2 Pharmacokinetic properties

Galantamine is an alkalinic compound with one ionisation constant (pKa 8.2). It is slightly lipophilic and has a partition coefficient (Log P) between n-octanol/buffer solution (pH 12) of 1.09. The solubility in water (pH 6) is 31 mg/ml. Galantamine has three chiral centres, the S, R, S-form is the naturally occurring form. Galantamine is partially metabolised by various cytochromes, mainly CYP2D6 and CYP3A4. Some of the metabolites formed during the

Table 1 Adverse reactions observed during clinical trials and post marketing experience

System Organ Class	Very Common	Common	Uncommon	Rare	Very Rare
Infections and infestations		Rhinitis			
Blood disorders				Hypokalaemia	
Metabolism and nutrition disorders		Anorexia			
Psychiatric disorders		Insomnia Confusion		Hallucinations Agitation Aggression	
Nervous system disorders		Dizziness Somnolence		Syncope Convulsions	Tremor Worsening of Parkinsonism
Cardiac disorders				Severe Bradycardia	Hypotension AV block
Gastrointestinal disorders	Vomiting Nausea	Diarrhoea Abdominal pain Dyspepsia			Gastrointestinal bleeding Dysphagia
Skin and subcutaneous tissue disorders				Rash	Increased sweating
Renal and urinary disorders		Urinary tract infections			Dehydration
General disorders and administration site conditions		Headache Fatigue			
Investigations		Weight decrease			
Injury and poisoning		Fall Injury			

degradation of galantamine have been shown to be active *in vitro* but are of no importance *in vivo*.

GENERAL CHARACTERISTICS OF GALANTAMINE

Absorption

The absorption is rapid, with a t_{max} of about 1 hour after both tablets and oral solution. The absolute bioavailability of galantamine is high, 88.5 ± 5.4%. The presence of food delays the rate of absorption and reduces C_{max} by about 25%, without affecting the extent of absorption (AUC).

Distribution

The mean volume of distribution is 175 L. Plasma protein binding is low, 18%.

Metabolism

Up to 75% of galantamine dosed is eliminated via metabolism. *In vitro* studies indicate that CYP2D6 is involved in the formation of O-desmethylgalantamine and CYP3A4 is involved in the formation of N-oxide-galantamine. The levels of excretion of total radioactivity in urine and faeces were not different between poor and extensive CYP2D6 metabolisers. In plasma from poor and extensive metabolisers, unchanged galantamine and its glucuronide accounted for most of the sample radioactivity. None of the active metabolites of galantamine (norgalantamine, O-desmethylgalantamine and O-desmethyl-norgalantamine) could be detected in their unconjugated form in plasma from poor and extensive metabolisers after single dosing. Norgalantamine was detectable in plasma from patients after multiple dosing, but did not represent more than 10% of the galantamine levels. *In vitro* studies indicated that the inhibition potential of galantamine with respect to the major forms of human cytochrome P450 is very low.

Elimination

Galantamine plasma concentration declines bi-exponentially, with a terminal half-life in the order of 7-8 h in healthy subjects. Typical oral clearance in the target population is about 200 mL/min with intersubject variability of 30% as derived from the population analysis. Seven days after a single oral dose of 4 mg ^{3}H-galantamine, 90-97% of the radioactivity is recovered in urine and 2.2 - 6.3% in faeces. After i.v. infusion and oral administration, 18-22% of the dose was excreted as unchanged galantamine in the urine in 24 hours, with a renal clearance of 68.4 ± 22.0 ml/min, which represents 20-25% of the total plasma clearance.

Dose-linearity

After repeated oral dosing of 12 and 16 mg galantamine b.i.d., mean trough and peak plasma concentrations fluctuated between 29 - 97 ng/ml and 42 - 137 ng/ml. The pharmacokinetics of galantamine are linear in the dose range of 4 - 16 mg b.i.d. In patients taking 12 or 16 mg b.i.d., no accumulation of galantamine was observed between months 2 and 6.

CHARACTERISTICS IN PATIENTS

Data from clinical trials in patients indicate that the plasma concentrations of galantamine in patients with Alzheimer's disease are 30-40% higher than in healthy young subjects. Based upon the population pharmacokinetic analysis, clearance in female subjects is 20% lower as compared to males. No major effects of age per se or race are found on the galantamine clearance. The galantamine clearance in poor metabolisers of CYP2D6 is about 25% lower than in extensive metabolisers, but no bimodality in the population is observed. Therefore, the metabolic status of the patient is not considered to be of clinical relevance in the overall population.

The pharmacokinetics of galantamine in subjects with mild hepatic impairment (Child-Pugh score of 5-6) were comparable to those in healthy subjects. In patients with moderate hepatic impairment (Child-Pugh score of 7-9), AUC and half-life of galantamine were increased by about 30% (see section 4.2).

Elimination of galantamine decreases with decreasing creatinine clearance as observed in a study with renally impaired subjects. Compared to Alzheimer patients, peak and trough plasma concentrations are not increased in patients with a creatinine clearance of ⩾ 9 ml/min. Therefore, no increase in adverse events is expected and no dosage adjustments are needed (see section 4.2).

PHARMACOKINETIC/PHARMACODYNAMIC RELATIONSHIP

No apparent correlation between average plasma concentrations and efficacy parameters (i.e. Change in ADAS-Cog11 and CIBIC-plus at Month 6) were observed in the large Phase III trials with a dose-regimen of 12 and 16 mg b.i.d. These results indicate that maximal effects may be obtained at the studied doses.

Plasma concentrations in patients experiencing syncope were within the same range as in the other patients at the same dose.

The occurrence of nausea is shown to correlate with higher peak plasma concentrations (see section 4.5).

5.3 Preclinical safety data

Preclinical data reveal no special hazard for humans other than those expected from the pharmacodynamic effect of galantamine. This assumption is based on conventional studies of safety pharmacology, repeated dose toxicity, genotoxicity and carcinogenic potential.

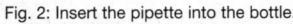

Table 2 Composite responder analysis based on at least 4 points improvement in ADAS-Cog/11 compared to baseline and CIBIC-plus unchanged + improved (1-4), and DAD/ADL score unchanged + improved

Treatment	At least 4 points improvement from baseline in ADAS-Cog/11 and CIBIC-plus Unchanged+Improved							
	Change in DAD ⩾ 0 GAL-USA-1 and GAL-INT-1 (Month 6)				Change in ADCS/ADL-Inventory ⩾ 0 GAL-USA-10 (Month 5)			
	n	n (%) of responder	Comparison with placebo		n	n (%) of responder	Comparison with placebo	
			Diff (95%CI)	p-value†			Diff (95%CI)	p-value†
Classical ITT								
Placebo	422	21 (5.0)	-	-	273	18 (6.6)	-	-
Gal 16 mg/day	-	-	-	-	266	39 (14.7)	8.1 (3, 13)	0.003
Gal 24 mg/day	424	60 (14.2)	9.2 (5, 13)	<0.001	262	40 (15.3)	8.7 (3, 14)	0.002
*Trad. LOCF**								
Placebo	412	23 (5.6)	-	-	261	17 (6.5)	-	-
Gal 16 mg/day	-	-	-	-	253	36 (14.2)	7.7 (2, 13)	0.005
Gal 24 mg/day	399	58 (14.5)	8.9 (5, 13)	<0.001	253	40 (15.8)	9.3 (4, 15)	0.001

† CMH test of difference from placebo.

* LOCF: Last Observation Carried Forward.

Table 3

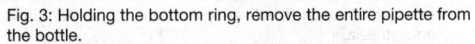

To open the bottle and use the pipette:

Fig. 1: The bottle comes with a child-proof cap, and should be opened as follows:

- Push the plastic screw cap down while turning it counter clockwise.

- Remove the unscrewed cap.

Fig. 1

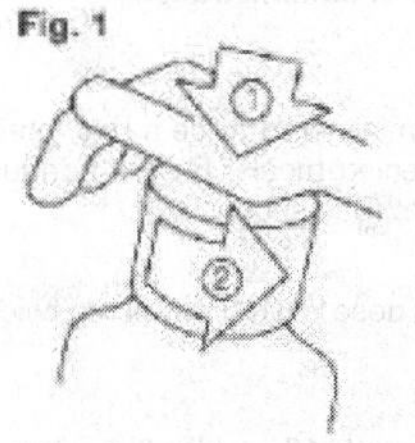

Fig. 2

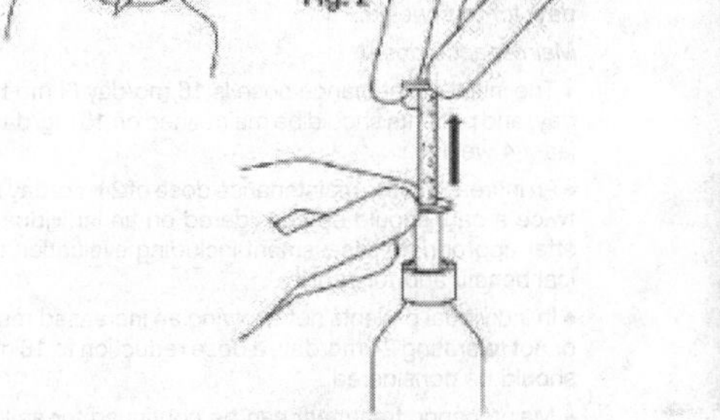

Fig. 2: Insert the pipette into the bottle.

While holding the bottom ring, pull the top ring up to the mark corresponding to the number of millilitres you need to give.

Fig. 3

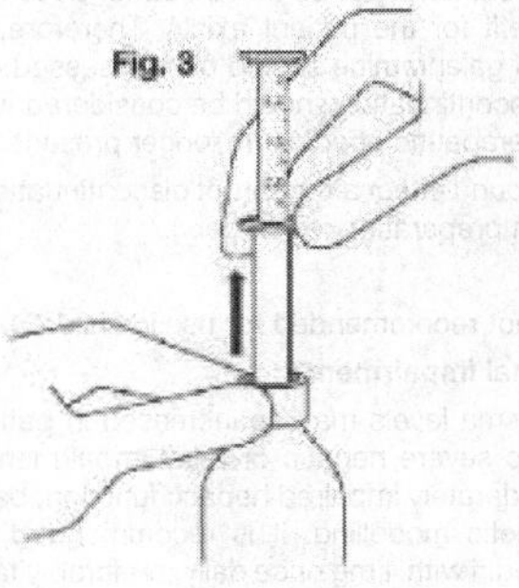

Fig. 3: Holding the bottom ring, remove the entire pipette from the bottle.

Empty the pipette into any non-alcoholic drink by sliding the upper ring down and drink it immediately.

Close the bottle.

Rinse the pipette with some water.

Reproduction toxicity studies showed a slight delay in development in rats and rabbits, at doses which are below the threshold of toxicity in the pregnant females.

6. PHARMACEUTICAL PARTICULARS

6.1 List of excipients

Methyl parahydroxybenzoate, propyl parahydroxybenzoate, sodium saccharin, sodium hydroxide and purified water.

6.2 Incompatibilities

Not applicable.

6.3 Shelf life

2 years. After first opening: 3 months.

6.4 Special precautions for storage

Do not freeze.

6.5 Nature and contents of container

The oral solution is packaged in a 100 ml amber glass bottle with a LDPE insert, a PP/LDPE child resistant closure and a HDPE/LDPE/PS pipette of 6 ml, calibrated in millilitres. The pipette has a minimum volume of 0.5 ml and a maximum volume of 4 ml.

6.6 Instructions for use and handling

(see Table 3 above)

7. MARKETING AUTHORISATION HOLDER

Shire Pharmaceuticals Limited

Hampshire International Business Park

Chineham

Basingstoke

Hampshire RG24 8EP

United Kingdom.

8. MARKETING AUTHORISATION NUMBER(S)

PL 08557/0042

9. DATE OF FIRST AUTHORISATION/RENEWAL OF THE AUTHORISATION

14 September 2000

10. DATE OF REVISION OF THE TEXT

November 2004

LEGAL CATEGORY

POM

Reminyl Tablets

(Shire Pharmaceuticals Limited)

1. NAME OF THE MEDICINAL PRODUCT

Reminyl® 4 mg Tablets

Reminyl 8 mg Tablets

Reminyl 12 mg Tablets

2. QUALITATIVE AND QUANTITATIVE COMPOSITION

Each Reminyl 4 mg tablet contains 4 mg galantamine (as hydrobromide).

Each Reminyl 8 mg tablet contains 8 mg galantamine (as hydrobromide).

Each Reminyl 12 mg tablet contains 12 mg galantamine (as hydrobromide).

For excipients, see 6.1.

3. PHARMACEUTICAL FORM

Film-coated tablet.

Reminyl 4 mg tablet: 4 mg galantamine as off-white, circular, biconvex tablets with the inscription "JANSSEN" on one side and "G4" on the other side

Reminyl 8 mg tablet: 8 mg galantamine as pink, circular, biconvex tablets with the inscription "JANSSEN" on one side and "G8" on the other side

Reminyl 12 mg tablet: 12 mg galantamine as orange-brown, circular, biconvex tablets with the inscription "JANSSEN" on one side and "G12" on the other side

4. CLINICAL PARTICULARS

4.1 Therapeutic indications

Galantamine is indicated for the symptomatic treatment of mild to moderately severe dementia of the Alzheimer type.

4.2 Posology and method of administration

Adults/Elderly

Administration

Galantamine should be administered twice a day, preferably with morning and evening meals. Ensure adequate fluid intake during treatment (See section 4.8).

Starting dose

The recommended starting dose is 8 mg/day (4 mg twice a day) for four weeks.

Maintenance dose

• The initial maintenance dose is 16 mg/day (8 mg twice a day) and patients should be maintained on 16 mg/day for at least 4 weeks.

• An increase to the maintenance dose of 24 mg/day (12 mg twice a day) should be considered on an individual basis after appropriate assessment including evaluation of clinical benefit and tolerability.

• In individual patients not showing an increased response or not tolerating 24 mg/day, a dose reduction to 16 mg/day should be considered.

• Maintenance treatment can be continued for as long as therapeutic benefit for the patient exists. Therefore, the clinical benefit of galantamine should be reassessed on a regular basis. Discontinuation should be considered when evidence of a therapeutic effect is no longer present.

• There is no rebound effect after abrupt discontinuation of treatment (e.g. in preparation for surgery).

Children

Galantamine is not recommended for use in children.

Hepatic and renal impairment

Galantamine plasma levels may be increased in patients with moderate to severe hepatic or renal impairment. In patients with moderately impaired hepatic function, based on pharmacokinetic modelling, it is recommended that dosing should begin with 4 mg once daily, preferably taken in the morning, for at least one week. Thereafter, patients should proceed with 4 mg b.i.d. for at least 4 weeks. In these patients, daily doses should not exceed 8 mg b.i.d. In patients with severe hepatic impairment (Child-Pugh score greater than 9), the use of galantamine is contraindicated (see section 4.3). No dosage adjustment is required for patients with mild hepatic impairment.

For patients with a creatinine clearance greater than 9 ml/min no dosage adjustment is required. In patients with severe renal impairment (creatinine clearance less than 9 ml/min), the use of galantamine is contraindicated (see section 4.3)

Concomitant treatment

In patients treated with potent CYP2D6 or CYP3A4 inhibitors (e.g. ketoconazole) dose reductions can be considered (see section 4.5).

4.3 Contraindications

• Galantamine should not be administered to patients with a known hypersensitivity to galantamine hydrobromide or to any excipients used in the formulations.

• Since no data are available on the use of galantamine in patients with severe hepatic (Child-Pugh score greater than 9) and severe renal (creatinine clearance less than 9 ml/min) impairment, galantamine is contraindicated in these populations. Galantamine is contra-indicated in patients who have both significant renal and hepatic dysfunction.

4.4 Special warnings and special precautions for use

A diagnosis of Alzheimer's dementia should be made according to current guidelines by an experienced physician. Therapy with galantamine should occur under the supervision of a physician and should only be initiated if a caregiver is available who will regularly monitor drug intake by the patient.

Patients with Alzheimer's disease lose weight. Treatment with cholinesterase inhibitors, including galantamine, has been associated with weight loss in these patients. During therapy, patient's weight should be monitored.

As with other cholinomimetics, galantamine should be given with caution in the following conditions:

Cardiovascular conditions: because of their pharmacological action, cholinomimetics may have vagotonic effects on heart rate (e.g. bradycardia). The potential for this action may be particularly important to patients with 'sick sinus syndrome' or other supraventricular cardiac conduction disturbances or who use drugs that significantly reduce heart rate concomitantly, such as digoxin and beta blockers.

Gastrointestinal conditions: patients at increased risk of developing peptic ulcers, e.g. those with a history of ulcer disease or those predisposed to these conditions, should be monitored for symptoms. The use of galantamine is not recommended in patients with gastro-intestinal obstruction or recovering from gastro-intestinal surgery.

Neurological Conditions: cholinomimetics are believed to have some potential to cause generalised convulsions. However, seizure activity may also be a manifestation of Alzheimer's disease. In clinical trials there was no increase in incidence of convulsions with galantamine compared with placebo. In rare cases an increase in cholinergic tone may worsen Parkinsonian symptoms.

Pulmonary Conditions: cholinomimetics should be prescribed with care for patients with a history of severe asthma or obstructive pulmonary disease.

Genitourinary: the use of galantamine is not recommended in patients with urinary outflow obstruction or recovering from bladder surgery.

Anaesthesia: galantamine, as a cholinomimetic is likely to exaggerate succinylcholinetype muscle relaxation during anaesthesia.

Orange yellow S aluminium lake (E110), present in the 12 mg tablet, may cause allergic reactions.

Patients with rare hereditary problems of galactose intolerance, the Lapp lactase deficiency or glucose-galactose malabsorption should not take this medicine.

4.5 Interaction with other medicinal products and other forms of Interaction

Pharmacodynamic interactions

Because of its mechanism of action, galantamine should not be given concomitantly with other cholinomimetics. Galantamine antagonises the effect of anticholinergic medication. As expected with cholinomimetics, a pharmacodynamic interaction is possible with drugs that significantly reduce the heart rate (e.g. digoxin and beta blockers). Galantamine, as a cholinomimetic, is likely to exaggerate succinylcholine-type muscle relaxation during anaesthesia.

Pharmacokinetic interactions

Multiple metabolic pathways and renal excretion are involved in the elimination of galantamine.

Concomitant administration with food slows the absorption rate of galantamine but does not affect the extent of absorption. It is recommended that galantamine be taken with food in order to minimise cholinergic side effects.

Other drugs affecting the metabolism of galantamine

Formal drug interaction studies showed an increase in galantamine bioavailability of about 40% during co-administration of paroxetine (a potent CYP2D6 inhibitor) and of 30% and 12% during co-treatment with ketoconazole and erythromycin (both CYP3A4 inhibitors). Therefore, during initiation of treatment with potent inhibitors of CYP2D6 (e.g. quinidine, paroxetine, fluoxetine or fluvoxamine) or CYP3A4 (e.g. ketoconazole, ritonavir) patients may experience an increased incidence of cholinergic side effects, predominantly nausea and vomiting. Under these circumstances, based on tolerability, a reduction of the galantamine maintenance dose can be considered (see section 4.2).

Effect of galantamine on the metabolism of other drugs

Therapeutic doses of galantamine (12 mg b.i.d.) had no effect on the kinetics of digoxin and warfarin (see also pharmacodynamic interactions).

4.6 Pregnancy and lactation

Pregnancy

For galantamine no clinical data on exposed pregnancies are available. Animal studies indicate a slightly delayed development in foetuses and neonates (see section 5.3). Caution should be exercised when prescribing to pregnant women.

Lactation

It is not known whether galantamine is excreted in human breast milk and there are no studies in lactating women. Therefore, women on galantamine should not breast-feed.

4.7 Effects on ability to drive and use machines

Galantamine may cause dizziness and somnolence, which could affect the ability to drive or use machines, especially during the first weeks after initiation of treatment.

4.8 Undesirable effects

The most common adverse events observed in clinical trials (incidence ⩾ 5% and twice the frequency of placebo) were nausea, vomiting, diarrhoea, abdominal pain, dyspepsia, anorexia, fatigue, dizziness, headache, somnolence and weight decrease. Nausea, vomiting and anorexia were more commonly observed in women.

Other common adverse events observed in clinical trials (incidence ⩾ 5% and ⩾ placebo) were confusion, fall, injury, insomnia, rhinitis and urinary tract infection.

The majority of these adverse events occurred during the titration period. Nausea and vomiting, the most frequent adverse events, lasted less than a week in most cases and the majority of patients had only one episode. Prescription of anti-emetics and ensuring adequate fluid intake may be useful in these instances.

Adverse reactions observed during clinical trials and post marketing experience.

(see Table 1 on next page)

Frequencies are defined as: very common (>1/10), common (> 1/100, < 1/10), uncommon (> 1/1,000, < 1/100), rare (>1/10,000, <1/1,000) and very rare (<1/10,000).

Some of these adverse events may be attributable to cholinomimetic properties of galantamine or in some cases may represent manifestations or exacerbations of the underlying disease processes common in the elderly population.

4.9 Overdose

Symptoms

Signs and symptoms of significant overdosing of galantamine are predicted to be similar to those of overdosing of other cholinomimetics. These effects generally involve the central nervous system, the parasympathetic nervous system, and the neuromuscular junction. In addition to muscle weakness or fasciculations, some or all of the signs of a cholinergic crisis may develop: severe nausea, vomiting, gastro-intestinal cramping, salivation, lacrimation, urination, defecation, sweating, bradycardia, hypotension, collapse and convulsions. Increasing muscle weakness together with tracheal hypersecretions and bronchospasm, may lead to vital airway compromise.

In a post-marketing report, bradycardia, QT prolongation, ventricular tachycardia and torsades de pointes accompanied by a brief loss of consciousness were reported in association with an inadvertent ingestion of eight 4 mg tablets (32 mg total) on a single day.

Treatment

As in any case of overdose, general supportive measures should be used. In severe cases, anticholinergics such as atropine can be used as a general antidote for cholinomimetics. An initial dose of 0.5 to 1.0 mg i.v. is recommended, with subsequent doses based on the clinical response.

Because strategies for the management of overdose are continually evolving, it is advisable to contact a poison control centre to determine the latest recommendations for the management of an overdose.

5. PHARMACOLOGICAL PROPERTIES

5.1 Pharmacodynamic properties

Pharmacotherapeutic group: Antidementia drugs; ATC-code: N06DA04.

Galantamine, a tertiary alkaloid is a selective, competitive and reversible inhibitor of acetylcholinesterase. In addition, galantamine enhances the intrinsic action of acetylcholine on nicotinic receptors, probably through binding to an allosteric site of the receptor. As a consequence, an increased activity in the cholinergic system associated with improved cognitive function can be achieved in patients with dementia of the Alzheimer type.

Clinical studies

The dosages of galantamine effective in placebo-controlled clinical trials with a duration of 5 to 6 months were 16, 24 and 32 mg/day. Of these doses 16 and 24 mg/day were judged to have the best benefit/risk and were retained as recommended maintenance doses. Galantamine's efficacy has been shown using outcome measures which evaluate the three major symptom complexes of the disease and a global scale: the ADAS-Cog (a performance based measure of cognition), DAD and ADCS-ADL-Inventory (measurements of basic and instrumental Activities of Daily Living), the Neuropsychiatric Inventory (a scale that measures behavioural disturbances) and the CIBIC-plus (a global assessment by an independent physician based on a clinical interview with the patient and caregiver).

Composite responder analysis based on at least 4 points improvement in ADAS-Cog/11 compared to baseline and CIBIC-plus unchanged + improved (1-4), and DAD/ADL score unchanged + improved.

(see Table 2 on next page)

The results of a 26-week double-blind placebo-controlled trial, in which patients with vascular dementia and patients with Alzheimer's disease and concomitant cerebrovascular disease ("mixed dementia") were included, indicate that the symptomatic effect of galantamine is maintained

Table 1 Adverse reactions observed during clinical trials and post marketing experience

System Organ Class	Very Common	Common	Uncommon	Rare	Very Rare
Infections and infestations		Rhinitis			
Blood disorders				Hypokalaemia	
Metabolism and nutrition disorders		Anorexia			
Psychiatric disorders		Insomnia Confusion		Hallucinations Agitation Aggression	
Nervous system disorders		Dizziness Somnolence		Syncope Convulsions	Tremor Worsening of Parkinsonism
Cardiac disorders				Severe Bradycardia	Hypotension AV block
Gastrointestinal disorders	Vomiting Nausea	Diarrhoea Abdominal pain Dyspepsia			Gastrointestinal bleeding Dysphagia
Skin and subcutaneous tissue disorders				Rash	Increased sweating
Renal and urinary disorders		Urinary tract infections			Dehydration
General disorders and administration site conditions		Headache Fatigue			
Investigations		Weight decrease			
Injury and poisoning		Fall Injury			

Table 2 Composite responder analysis based on at least 4 points improvement in ADAS-Cog/11 compared to baseline and CIBIC-plus unchanged + improved (1-4), and DAD/ADL score unchanged + improved

	At least 4 points improvement from baseline in ADAS-Cog/11 and CIBIC-plus Unchanged+Improved							
	Change in DAD ⩾ 0 GAL-USA-1 and GAL-INT-1 (Month 6)				Change in ADCS/ADL-Inventory ⩾ 0 GAL-USA-10 (Month 5)			
Treatment	n	n (%) of responder	Comparison with placebo		n	n (%) of responder	Comparison with placebo	
			Diff (95%CI)	p-value†			Diff (95%CI)	p-value†
Classical ITT								
Placebo	422	21 (5.0)	-	-	273	18 (6.6)	-	-
Gal 16 mg/day	-	-	-	-	266	39 (14.7)	8.1 (3, 13)	0.003
Gal 24 mg/day	424	60 (14.2)	9.2 (5, 13)	<0.001	262	40 (15.3)	8.7 (3, 14)	0.002
Trad. LOCF*								
Placebo	412	23 (5.6)	-	-	261	17 (6.5)	-	-
Gal 16 mg/day	-	-	-	-	253	36 (14.2)	7.7 (2, 13)	0.005
Gal 24 mg/day	399	58 (14.5)	8.9 (5, 13)	<0.001	253	40 (15.8)	9.3 (4, 15)	0.001

† CMH test of difference from placebo.

* LOCF: Last Observation Carried Forward.

in patients with Alzheimer's disease and concomitant cerebrovascular disease. In a post-hoc subgroup analysis, no statistically significant effect was observed in the subgroup of patients with vascular dementia alone.

In a second 26-week placebo-controlled trial in patients with probable vascular dementia, no clinical benefit of galantamine treatment was demonstrated.

5.2 Pharmacokinetic properties

Galantamine is an alkalinic compound with one ionisation constant (pKa 8.2). It is slightly lipophilic and has a partition coefficient (Log P) between n-octanol/buffer solution (pH 12) of 1.09. The solubility in water (pH 6) is 31 mg/ml. Galantamine has three chiral centres, the S, R, S-form is the naturally occurring form. Galantamine is partially metabolised by various cytochromes, mainly CYP2D6 and CYP3A4. Some of the metabolites formed during the degradation of galantamine have been shown to be active *in vitro* but are of no importance *in vivo*.

GENERAL CHARACTERISTICS OF GALANTAMINE

Absorption

The absorption is rapid, with a t_{max} of about 1 hour after both tablets and oral solution. The absolute bioavailability of galantamine is high, 88.5 ± 5.4%. The presence of food delays the rate of absorption and reduces C_{max} by about 25%, without affecting the extent of absorption (AUC).

Distribution

The mean volume of distribution is 175 L. Plasma protein binding is low, 18%.

Metabolism

Up to 75% of galantamine dosed is eliminated via metabolism. *In vitro* studies indicate that CYP2D6 is involved in the formation of O-desmethylgalantamine and CYP3A4 is involved in the formation of N-oxide-galantamine. The levels of excretion of total radioactivity in urine and faeces were not different between poor and extensive CYP2D6 metabolisers. In plasma from poor and extensive metabolisers, unchanged galantamine and its glucuronide accounted for most of the sample radioactivity. None of the active metabolites of galantamine (norgalantamine, O-desmethylgalantamine and O-desmethyl-norgalantamine) could be detected in their unconjugated form in plasma from poor and extensive metabolisers after single dosing. Norgalantamine was detectable in plasma from patients after multiple dosing, but did not represent more than 10% of the galantamine levels. *In vitro* studies indicated that the inhibition potential of galantamine with respect to the major forms of human cytochrome P450 is very low.

Elimination

Galantamine plasma concentration declines bi-exponentially, with a terminal half-life in the order of 7-8 h in healthy subjects. Typical oral clearance in the target population is about 200 mL/min with intersubject variability of 30% as derived from the population analysis. Seven days after a single oral dose of 4 mg ^{3}H-galantamine, 90-97% of the radioactivity is recovered in urine and 2.2 – 6.3% in faeces. After i.v. infusion and oral administration, 18-22% of the dose was excreted as unchanged galantamine in the urine in 24 hours, with a renal clearance of 68.4 ± 22.0 ml/min, which represents 20-25% of the total plasma clearance.

Dose-linearity

After repeated oral dosing of 12 and 16 mg galantamine b.i.d., mean trough and peak plasma concentrations fluctuated between 29 – 97 ng/ml and 42 – 137 ng/ml. The pharmacokinetics of galantamine are linear in the dose range of 4 - 16 mg b.i.d. In patients taking 12 or 16 mg b.i.d., no accumulation of galantamine was observed between months 2 and 6.

CHARACTERISTICS IN PATIENTS

Data from clinical trials in patients indicate that the plasma concentrations of galantamine in patients with Alzheimer's disease are 30-40% higher than in healthy young subjects. Based upon the population pharmacokinetic analysis, clearance in female subjects is 20% lower as compared to males. No major effects of age per se or race are found on the galantamine clearance. The galantamine clearance in poor metabolisers of CYP2D6 is about 25% lower than in extensive metabolisers, but no bimodality in the population is observed. Therefore, the metabolic status of the patient is not considered to be of clinical relevance in the overall population.

The pharmacokinetics of galantamine in subjects with mild hepatic impairment (Child-Pugh score of 5-6) were comparable to those in healthy subjects. In patients with moderate hepatic impairment (Child-Pugh score of 7-9), AUC and half-life of galantamine were increased by about 30% (see section 4.2).

Elimination of galantamine decreases with decreasing creatinine clearance as observed in a study with renally impaired subjects. Compared to Alzheimer patients, peak and trough plasma concentrations are not increased in patients with a creatinine clearance of ⩾ 9 ml/min. Therefore, no increase in adverse events is expected and no dosage adjustments are needed (see section 4.2).

PHARMACOKINETIC/PHARMACODYNAMIC RELATIONSHIP

No apparent correlation between average plasma concentrations and efficacy parameters (i.e. Change in ADAS-Cog11 and CIBIC-plus at Month 6) were observed in the large Phase III trials with a dose-regimen of 12 and 16 mg b.i.d. These results indicate that maximal effects may be obtained at the studied doses.

Plasma concentrations in patients experiencing syncope were within the same range as in the other patients at the same dose.

The occurrence of nausea is shown to correlate with higher peak plasma concentrations (see section 4.5).

5.3 Preclinical safety data

Preclinical data reveal no special hazard for humans other than those expected from the pharmacodynamic effect of galantamine. This assumption is based on conventional studies of safety pharmacology, repeated dose toxicity, genotoxicity and carcinogenic potential.

Reproduction toxicity studies showed a slight delay in development in rats and rabbits, at doses, which are below the threshold of toxicity in the pregnant females.

6. PHARMACEUTICAL PARTICULARS

6.1 List of excipients

Tablet core:

Colloidal anhydrous silica, crospovidone, lactose monohydrate, magnesium stearate and microcrystalline cellulose.

Film-coating:

Hypromellose, propylene glycol, talc and titanium dioxide (E171).

The 4 mg tablets also contain yellow ferric oxide (E172).

The 8 mg tablets contain red ferric oxide (E172).

The 12 mg tablets contain red ferric oxide and orange yellow S aluminium lake (E110).

6.2 Incompatibilities

Not applicable.

6.3 Shelf life

2 years.

6.4 Special precautions for storage

No special precautions for storage.

6.5 Nature and contents of container

The tablets are packaged in a PVC-PE-PVDC/Alu blister that hold 14 tablets.

Available pack sizes: 4 mg, 8 mg, 12 mg: 56 tablets.

6.6 Instructions for use and handling
No special requirements.

7. MARKETING AUTHORISATION HOLDER
Shire Pharmaceuticals Limited
Hampshire International Business Park
Chineham
Basingstoke
Hampshire RG24 8EP
United Kingdom

8. MARKETING AUTHORISATION NUMBER(S)
4 mg tablets: PL 08557/0039
8 mg tablets: PL 08557/0040
12 mg tablets: PL 08557/0041

9. DATE OF FIRST AUTHORISATION/RENEWAL OF THE AUTHORISATION
14 September 2000

10. DATE OF REVISION OF THE TEXT
November 2004

LEGAL CATEGORY
POM

Reminyl XL 8mg, 16mg and 24mg prolonged release capsules

(Shire Pharmaceuticals Limited)

1. NAME OF THE MEDICINAL PRODUCT
Reminyl XL 8 mg prolonged release capsules
Reminyl XL 16 mg prolonged release capsules
Reminyl XL 24 mg prolonged release capsules

2. QUALITATIVE AND QUANTITATIVE COMPOSITION
Each Reminyl XL 8 mg prolonged release capsule, hard contains galantamine hydrobromide, equivalent to 8 mg galantamine.

Each Reminyl XL 16 mg prolonged release capsule, hard contains galantamine hydrobromide, equivalent to 16 mg galantamine.

Each Reminyl XL 24 mg prolonged release capsule, hard contains galantamine hydrobromide, equivalent to 24 mg galantamine.

For excipients, see section 6.1.

3. PHARMACEUTICAL FORM
Prolonged release capsule, hard

8mg: White opaque, size 4 hard capsules with the inscription "G8", containing white to off-white pellets.

16mg: Pink opaque, size 2 hard capsules with the inscription "G16", containing white to off-white pellets.

24mg: Caramel opaque, size 1 hard capsules with the inscription "G24", containing white to off-white pellets.

4. CLINICAL PARTICULARS
4.1 Therapeutic indications
Reminyl XL is indicated for the symptomatic treatment of mild to moderately severe dementia of the Alzheimer type.

4.2 Posology and method of administration
Adults/elderly
Administration

Reminyl XL prolonged release capsules should be administered once-daily in the morning, preferably with food. The capsules should be swallowed whole together with some liquid. The capsules must not be chewed or crushed.

Ensure adequate fluid intake during treatment (see section 4.8).

Starting dose

The recommended starting dose is 8 mg/day for 4 weeks.

Maintenance dose

• The initial maintenance dose is 16 mg/day and patients should be maintained on 16 mg/day for at least 4 weeks.

• An increase to the maintenance dose of 24 mg/day should be considered on an individual basis after appropriate assessment including evaluation of clinical benefit and tolerability.

• In individual patients not showing an increased response or not tolerating 24 mg/day, a dose reduction to 16 mg/day should be considered.

• Maintenance treatment can be continued for as long as therapeutic benefit for the patient exists. Therefore, the clinical benefit of Reminyl XL should be reassessed on a regular basis. Discontinuation should be considered when evidence of a therapeutic effect is no longer present.

• There is no rebound effect after abrupt discontinuation of treatment (e.g. in preparation for surgery).

Children
Reminyl XL is not recommended for use in children.

Hepatic and renal impairment
Galantamine plasma levels may be increased in patients with moderate to severe hepatic or renal impairment. In patients with moderately impaired hepatic function, based on pharmacokinetic modelling, it is recommended that dosing should begin with 8 mg prolonged release capsule once every other day, preferably taken in the morning, for one week. Thereafter, patients should proceed with 8 mg once-daily for four weeks. In these patients, daily doses should not exceed 16 mg. In patients with severe hepatic impairment (Child-Pugh score greater than 9), the use of Reminyl XL is contraindicated (see section 4.3). No dosage adjustment is required for patients with mild hepatic impairment.

For patients with a creatinine clearance greater than 9 ml/min no dosage adjustment is required. In patients with severe renal impairment (creatinine clearance less than 9 ml/min), the use of Reminyl XL is contraindicated (see section 4.3).

Concomitant treatment
In patients treated with potent CYP2D6 or CYP3A4 inhibitors, dose reductions can be considered (see section 4.5).

4.3 Contraindications
Reminyl XL should not be administered to patients with a known hypersensitivity to galantamine hydrobromide or to any of the excipients.

Since no data are available on the use of Reminyl XL in patients with severe hepatic (Child-Pugh score greater than 9) and severe renal (creatinine clearance less than 9 ml/min) impairment, Reminyl XL is contraindicated in these populations. Reminyl XL is contraindicated in patients who have both significant renal and hepatic dysfunction.

4.4 Special warnings and special precautions for use
A diagnosis of Alzheimer's dementia should be made according to current guidelines by an experienced physician. Therapy with Reminyl XL should occur under the supervision of a physician and should only be initiated if a caregiver is available who will regularly monitor medicinal product intake by the patient.

Patients with Alzheimer's disease lose weight. Treatment with cholinomimetics, including Reminyl XL, has been associated with weight loss in these patients. During therapy, patient's weight should be monitored.

The use of Reminyl XL in patients with other types of dementia or other type of memory impairment has not been investigated.

As with other cholinomimetics, Reminyl XL should be given with caution in the following conditions:

Cardiovascular conditions

Because of their pharmacological action, cholinomimetics may have vagotonic effects on heart rate (e.g. bradycardia). The potential for this action may be particularly important to patients with "sick sinus syndrome" or other supraventricular cardiac conduction disturbances or in those who use medicinal products that significantly reduce heart rate concomitantly, such as digoxin and beta-blockers.

Gastrointestinal conditions

Patients at increased risk of developing peptic ulcers, e.g. those with a history of ulcer disease or those predisposed to these conditions, should be monitored for symptoms. The use of Reminyl XL is not recommended in patients with gastrointestinal obstruction or recovering from gastrointestinal surgery.

Neurological conditions

Cholinomimetics are believed to have some potential to cause generalised convulsions. However, seizure activity may also be a manifestation of Alzheimer's disease. In clinical trials there was no increase in incidence of convulsions with Reminyl XL compared with placebo. In rare cases an increase in cholinergic tone may worsen Parkinsonian symptoms.

Pulmonary conditions

Cholinomimetics should be prescribed with care for patients with a history of severe asthma or obstructive pulmonary disease.

Genitourinary

The use of Reminyl XL is not recommended in patients with urinary outflow obstruction or recovering from bladder surgery.

Anaesthesia

Reminyl XL, as a cholinomimetic is likely to exaggerate succinylcholine-type muscle relaxation during anaesthesia, especially in cases of pseudocholinesterase deficiency.

Other

Patients with rare hereditary problems of fructose intolerance, glucose-galactose malabsorption or sucrase-isomaltase insufficiency should not take this medicine.

4.5 Interaction with other medicinal products and other forms of Interaction
Pharmacodynamic interactions
Because of its mechanism of action, galantamine should not be given concomitantly with other cholinomimetics (such as ambenonium, donepezil, neostigmine, pyridostigmine, rivastigmine or systemically administered pilocarpine). Galantamine has the potential to antagonise the effect of anticholinergic medication. Should anticholinergic medication such as atropine be abruptly stopped there is a potential risk that galantamine's effect could be exacerbated. As expected with cholinomimetics, a pharmacodynamic interaction is possible with medicinal products that significantly reduce the heart rate such as digoxin, beta-blockers, certain calcium-channel blocking agents and amiodarone. Caution should be taken with medicinal products that have potential to cause *torsades de pointes*. In such cases an ECG should be considered.

Galantamine, as a cholinomimetic, is likely to exaggerate succinylcholine-type muscle relaxation during anaesthesia, especially in cases of pseudocholinesterase deficiency.

Pharmacokinetic interactions
Multiple metabolic pathways and renal excretion are involved in the elimination of galantamine. The possibility of clinically relevant interactions is low. However, the occurrence of significant interactions may be clinically relevant in individual cases.

Concomitant administration with food slows the absorption rate of galantamine but does not affect the extent of absorption. It is recommended that Reminyl XL be taken with food in order to minimise cholinergic side effects.

Other medicinal products affecting the metabolism of galantamine

Formal drug interaction studies showed an increase in galantamine bioavailability of about 40% during co-administration of paroxetine (a potent CYP2D6 inhibitor) and of 30% and 12% during co-treatment with ketoconazole and erythromycin (both CYP3A4 inhibitors). Therefore, during initiation of treatment with potent inhibitors of CYP2D6 (e.g. quinidine, paroxetine or fluoxetine) or CYP3A4 (e.g. ketoconazole or ritonavir) patients may experience an increased incidence of cholinergic adverse reactions, predominantly nausea and vomiting. Under these circumstances, based on tolerability, a reduction of the Reminyl XL maintenance dose can be considered (see section 4.2).

Effect of galantamine on the metabolism of other medicinal products

Therapeutic doses of Reminyl XL 24 mg/day had no effect on the kinetics of digoxin, although pharmacodynamic interactions may occur (see also pharmacodynamic interactions).

Therapeutic doses of Reminyl XL 24 mg/day had no effect on the kinetics and prothrombin time of warfarin.

4.6 Pregnancy and lactation
Pregnancy
For Reminyl XL no clinical data on exposed pregnancies are available. Animal studies indicate a slightly delayed development in foetuses and neonates (see section 5.3). Caution should be exercised when prescribing to pregnant women.

Lactation
It is not known whether galantamine is excreted in human breast milk and there are no studies in lactating women. Therefore, women on Reminyl XL should not breast-feed.

4.7 Effects on ability to drive and use machines
Reminyl XL may cause dizziness and somnolence, which could affect the ability to drive or use machines, especially during the first weeks after initiation of treatment.

4.8 Undesirable effects
The most common adverse events observed in clinical trials (incidence ⩾ 5% and twice the frequency of placebo) were nausea, vomiting, diarrhoea, abdominal pain, dyspepsia, anorexia, fatigue, dizziness, headache, somnolence and weight decrease. Nausea, vomiting and anorexia were more commonly observed in women.

Other common adverse events observed in clinical trials (incidence ⩾ 5% and ⩾ placebo) were confusion, depression, fall, injury, insomnia, rhinitis and urinary tract infection.

In a randomised, double-blind, placebo controlled, clinical trial, adverse events that occurred with once-daily treatment with Reminyl XL prolonged release capsules were similar in frequency and nature to those seen with Reminyl tablets.

The majority of these adverse events occurred during the titration period. Nausea and vomiting, the most frequent adverse events, lasted less than a week in most cases and the majority of patients had only one episode. Prescription of anti-emetics and ensuring adequate fluid intake may be useful in these instances.

Adverse Events Observed During Clinical Trials and Post Marketing Experience.

(see Table 1 on next page)

Frequencies are defined as: very common (>1/10), common (> 1/100, < 1/10), uncommon (> 1/1,000, < 1/100), rare (>1/10,000, <1/1,000) and very rare (<1/10,000).

Some of these adverse events may be attributable to cholinomimetic properties of galantamine or in some cases may represent manifestations or exacerbations of the underlying disease processes common in the elderly population.

4.9 Overdose
Symptoms
Signs and symptoms of significant overdosing of Reminyl XL are predicted to be similar to those of overdosing of other cholinomimetics. These effects generally involve the central nervous system, the parasympathetic nervous system, and the neuromuscular junction. In addition to muscle weakness or fasciculations, some or all of the signs of a cholinergic crisis may develop: severe nausea, vomiting, gastrointestinal cramping, salivation, lacrimation, urination, defecation, sweating, bradycardia, hypotension,

collapse and convulsions. Increasing muscle weakness together with tracheal hypersecretions and bronchospasm, may lead to vital airway compromise.

In a post-marketing report, bradycardia, QT prolongation, ventricular tachycardia and *torsade de pointes* accompanied by a brief loss of consciousness were reported in association with an inadvertent ingestion of eight 4 mg tablets (32 mg total) on a single day.

Treatment

As in any case of overdose, general supportive measures should be used. In severe cases, anticholinergics such as atropine can be used as a general antidote for cholinomimetics. An initial dose of 0.5 to 1.0 mg i.v. is recommended, with subsequent doses based on the clinical response.

Because strategies for the management of overdose are continually evolving, it is advisable to contact a poison control centre to determine the latest recommendations for the management of an overdose.

5. PHARMACOLOGICAL PROPERTIES

5.1 Pharmacodynamic properties

Pharmacotherapeutic group: Antidementia drugs; ATC-code: N06DA04.

Galantamine, a tertiary alkaloid is a selective, competitive and reversible inhibitor of acetylcholinesterase. In addition, galantamine enhances the intrinsic action of acetylcholine on nicotinic receptors, probably through binding to an allosteric site of the receptor. As a consequence, an increased activity in the cholinergic system associated with improved cognitive function can be achieved in patients with dementia of the Alzheimer type.

Clinical studies

Reminyl XL was originally developed in the form of immediate release tablets (Reminyl) for twice-daily administration. The dosages of Reminyl effective in these placebo-controlled clinical trials with a duration of 5 to 6 months were 16, 24 and 32 mg/day. Of these doses 16 and 24 mg/day were judged to have the best benefit/risk and were retained as recommended maintenance doses. Reminyl's efficacy has been shown using outcome measures which evaluate the three major symptom complexes of the disease and a global scale: the ADAS-cog/11 (a performance based measure of cognition), DAD and ADCS-ADL-Inventory (measurements of basic and instrumental Activities of Daily Living), the Neuropsychiatric Inventory (a scale that measures behavioural disturbances) and the CIBIC-plus (a global assessment by an independent physician based on a clinical interview with the patient and caregiver).

Composite Responder Analysis Based on at Least 4 Points Improvement in ADAS-cog/11 Compared to Baseline and CIBIC-plus Unchanged + Improved (1-4), and DAD/ADL Score Unchanged + Improved. See Table Below.

(see Table 2)

The efficacy of Reminyl XL prolonged release capsules was studied in a randomised, double-blind, placebo-controlled trial, GAL-INT-10, using a 4-week dose escalation, flexible dosing regimen of 16 or 24 mg/day for a treatment duration of 6 months. Reminyl immediate release tablets (Gal-IR) were added as a positive control arm. Efficacy was evaluated using the ADAS-cog/11 and the CIBIC-plus scores as co-primary efficacy criteria, and ADCS-ADL and NPI scores as secondary end-points. Reminyl XL prolonged release capsules (Gal-PR) demonstrated statistically significant improvements in the ADAS-cog/11 score compared to placebo, but were not statistically different in the CIBIC-plus score compared to placebo. The results of the ADCS-ADL score were statistically significantly better compared to placebo at week 26.

Composite Responder Analysis at Week 26 Based on at Least 4 Points Improvement from Baseline in ADAS-cog/11, Total ADL Score Unchanged + Improved (⩾0) and No Worsening in CIBIC-plus Score (1-4). See Table Below.

(see Table 3)

5.2 Pharmacokinetic properties

Galantamine is an alkalinic compound with one ionisation constant (pKa 8.2). It is slightly lipophilic and has a partition coefficient (Log P) between n-octanol/buffer solution (pH 12) of 1.09. The solubility in water (pH 6) is 31 mg/ml. Galantamine has three chiral centres. The S, R, S-form is the naturally occurring form. Galantamine is partially metabolised by various cytochromes, mainly CYP2D6 and CYP3A4. Some of the metabolites formed during the degradation of galantamine have been shown to be active *in vitro*but are of no importance *in vivo*.

General characteristics of galantamine

Absorption

The absolute bioavailability of galantamine is high, 88.5 ± 5.4%. Reminyl XL prolonged release capsules are bioequivalent to the twice-daily immediate release tablets with respect to AUC_{24h} and C_{min}. The C_{max} value is reached after 4.4 hours and is about 24% lower than that of the tablet. Food has no significant effect on AUC of the prolonged release capsules. C_{max} was increased by about 12% and T_{max} increased by about 30 minutes when the capsule was given after food. However, these changes are unlikely to be clinically significant.

Table 1 Adverse Events Observed During Clinical Trials and Post Marketing Experience

System Organ Class	Very Common	Common	Uncommon	Rare	Very Rare
Infections and infestations		Rhinitis			
Blood disorders				Hypokalaemia	
Metabolism and nutrition disorders		Anorexia			
Psychiatric disorders		Insomnia Confusion Depression		Hallucinations Agitation Aggression	
Nervous system disorders		Dizziness Somnolence		Syncope Convulsions	Tremor Worsening of Parkinsonism
Cardiac disorders				Severe bradycardia	Hypotension AV block
Gastrointestinal disorders	Vomiting Nausea	Diarrhoea Abdominal pain Dyspepsia			Gastrointestinal bleeding Dysphagia
Skin and subcutaneous tissue disorders				Rash	Increased sweating
Renal and urinary disorders		Urinary tract infections			Dehydration
General disorders and administration site conditions		Headache Fatigue			
Investigations		Weight decrease			
Injury and poisoning		Fall Injury			

Table 2 Composite Responder Analysis Based on at Least 4 Points Improvement in ADAS-cog/11 Compared to Baseline and CIBIC-plus Unchanged + Improved (1-4), and DAD/ADL Score Unchanged + Improved

At least 4 points improvement from baseline in ADAS-cog/11 and CIBIC-plus Unchanged + Improved								
Treatment	Change in DAD ⩾ 0 GAL-USA-1 and GAL-INT-1 (Month 6)				Change in ADCS/ADL-Inventory ⩾ 0 GAL-USA-10 (Month 5)			
	N	n (%) of responder	Comparison with placebo		n	n (%) of responder	Comparison with placebo	
			Diff (95%CI)	p-value†			Diff (95%CI)	p-value†
Classical ITT								
Placebo	422	21 (5.0)	-	-	273	18 (6.6)	-	-
Gal 16 mg/day	-	-	-	-	266	39 (14.7)	8.1 (3, 13)	0.003
Gal 24 mg/day	424	60 (14.2)	9.2 (5, 13)	<0.001	262	40 (15.3)	8.7 (3, 14)	0.002
*Trad. LOCF**								
Placebo	412	23 (5.6)	-	-	261	17 (6.5)	-	-
Gal 16 mg/day	-	-	-	-	253	36 (14.2)	7.7 (2, 13)	0.005
Gal 24 mg/day	399	58 (14.5)	8.9 (5, 13)	<0.001	253	40 (15.8)	9.3 (4, 15)	0.001

† CMH test of difference from placebo.

* LOCF: Last Observation Carried Forward.

Table 3 Composite Responder Analysis at Week 26 Based on at Least 4 Points Improvement from Baseline in ADAS-cog/11, Total ADL Score Unchanged + Improved (⩾0) and No Worsening in CIBIC-plus Score (1-4)

GAL-INT-10	Placebo	Gal-IR†	Gal-PR*	p-value (Gal-PR* vs. Placebo)
	(n = 245)	(n = 225)	(n = 238)	
Composite Response: n (%)	20 (8.2)	43 (19.1)	38 (16.0)	0.008

† Immediate release tablets

* Prolonged release capsules

Distribution

The mean volume of distribution is 175 l. Plasma protein binding is low, 18%.

Metabolism

Up to 75% of galantamine dosed is eliminated via metabolism. *In vitro* studies indicate that CYP2D6 is involved in the formation of O-desmethylgalantamine and CYP3A4 is involved in the formation of N-oxide-galantamine. The levels of excretion of total radioactivity in urine and faeces were not different between poor and extensive CYP2D6 metabolisers. In plasma from poor and extensive metabolisers, unchanged galantamine and its glucuronide accounted for most of the sample radioactivity. None of the active metabolites of galantamine (norgalantamine, O-desmethylgalantamine and O-desmethyl-norgalantamine) could be detected in their unconjugated form in plasma from poor and extensive metabolisers after single dosing. Norgalantamine was detectable in plasma from patients after multiple dosing, but did not represent more than 10%

of the galantamine levels. *In vitro* studies indicated that the inhibition potential of galantamine with respect to the major forms of human cytochrome P450 is very low.

Elimination

Galantamine plasma concentration declines bi-exponentially, with a terminal half-life around 8-10 hours in healthy subjects. Typical oral clearance in the target population is about 200 ml/min with intersubject variability of 30% as derived from the population analysis of immediate release tablets. Seven days after a single oral dose of 4 mg ^{3}H-galantamine, 90-97% of the radioactivity is recovered in urine and 2.2-6.3% in faeces. After i.v. infusion and oral administration, 18-22% of the dose was excreted as unchanged galantamine in the urine in 24 hours, with a renal clearance of 68.4 ±22.0 ml/min, which represents 20-25% of the total plasma clearance.

Dose-linearity

Galantamine pharmacokinetics of Reminyl XL prolonged release capsules are dose proportional within the studied dose range of 8 mg to 24 mg in elderly and young age groups.

Characteristics in patients

Data from clinical trials in patients indicate that the plasma concentrations of galantamine in patients with Alzheimer's disease are 30% to 40% higher than in healthy young subjects primarily due to the advanced age and reduced kidney function. Based upon the population pharmacokinetic analysis, clearance in female subjects is 20% lower as compared to males. The galantamine clearance in poor metabolisers of CYP2D6 is about 25% lower than in extensive metabolisers, but no bimodality in the population is observed. Therefore, the metabolic status of the patient is not considered to be of clinical relevance in the overall population.

The pharmacokinetics of galantamine in subjects with mild hepatic impairment (Child-Pugh score of 5 to 6) were comparable to those in healthy subjects. In patients with moderate hepatic impairment (Child-Pugh score of 7 to 9), AUC and half-life of galantamine were increased by about 30% (see section 4.2).

Elimination of galantamine decreases with decreasing creatinine clearance as observed in a study with renally impaired subjects. Compared to Alzheimer patients, peak and trough plasma concentrations are not increased in patients with a creatinine clearance of $\geq$ 9 ml/min. Therefore, no increase in adverse events is expected and no dosage adjustments are needed (see section 4.2).

Pharmacokinetic/pharmacodynamic relationship

No apparent correlation between average plasma concentrations and efficacy parameters (i.e. change in ADAS-cog/11 and CIBIC-plus at month 6) were observed in the large Phase III trials with a dose-regimen of 12 and 16 mg twice-daily.

Plasma concentrations in patients experiencing syncope were within the same range as in the other patients at the same dose.

The occurrence of nausea is shown to correlate with higher peak plasma concentrations (see section 4.5).

5.3 Preclinical safety data

Preclinical data reveal no special hazard for humans other than those expected from the pharmacodynamic effect of galantamine. This assumption is based on conventional studies of safety pharmacology, repeated dose toxicity, genotoxicity and carcinogenic potential.

Reproduction toxicity studies showed a slight delay in development in rats and rabbits, at doses that are below the threshold of toxicity in the pregnant females.

6. PHARMACEUTICAL PARTICULARS

6.1 List of excipients

Prolonged release pellets

Diethyl phthalate

Ethylcellulose

Hypromellose

Macrogol

Maize starch

Sucrose

Capsules

Gelatin

Titanium dioxide (E171)

The 16 mg capsule also contains red ferric oxide (E172).

The 24 mg capsule also contains red ferric oxide (E172) and yellow ferric oxide (E172).

Imprinting ink

Benzoic acid (E210)

Black ferric oxide (E172)

Dimethyl siloxanes

Glycerides

Lecithin (soya) (E322)

Methylcellulose

Polyethylene glycol

Polyethylene glycol stearate

Shellac

Sorbic acid

Xanthum gum

6.2 Incompatibilities

Not applicable.

6.3 Shelf life

2 years.

6.4 Special precautions for storage

Do not store above 30°C.

6.5 Nature and contents of container

Available pack sizes:

8 mg

28 prolonged release capsules, hard (PVC-PE-PVDC/Aluminium blister)

16 mg

28 prolonged release capsules, hard (PVC-PE-PVDC/Aluminium blister)

24 mg

28 prolonged release capsules, hard (PVC-PE-PVDC/Aluminium blister)

6.6 Instructions for use and handling

No special requirements.

7. MARKETING AUTHORISATION HOLDER

Shire Pharmaceuticals Limited

Hampshire International Business Park

Chineham

Basingstoke

Hampshire RG24 8EP

United Kingdom

8. MARKETING AUTHORISATION NUMBER(S)

8mg : PL 08557/0052

16mg : PL 08557/0053

24mg : PL 08557/0054

9. DATE OF FIRST AUTHORISATION/RENEWAL OF THE AUTHORISATION

06 January 2005

10. DATE OF REVISION OF THE TEXT

LEGAL CATEGORY

POM

Reopro 2mg/ml solution for injection or infusion.

(Eli Lilly and Company Limited)

1. NAME OF THE MEDICINAL PRODUCT

ReoPro* 2mg/ml solution for injection or infusion.

2. QUALITATIVE AND QUANTITATIVE COMPOSITION

Abciximab 2mg/ml (10mg/5ml vial).

For excipients, see section 6.1.

3. PHARMACEUTICAL FORM

Solution for injection or infusion.

4. CLINICAL PARTICULARS

4.1 Therapeutic indications

ReoPro is indicated as an adjunct to heparin and aspirin for:

1. Percutaneous Coronary Intervention

The prevention of ischaemic cardiac complications in patients undergoing percutaneous coronary intervention (balloon angioplasty, atherectomy, and stent). (See section 5.1.)

2. Unstable Angina

The short-term (1-month) reduction of the risk of myocardial infarction, in patients with unstable angina, not responding to full conventional therapy who have been scheduled for percutaneous coronary intervention.

4.2 Posology and method of administration

ReoPro is for intravenous (IV) administration in adults.

Adults:

The recommended dose of ReoPro is a 0.25mg/kg intravenous bolus immediately followed by a 0.125 microgram/kg/min (to a maximum of 10 microgram/min) continuous intravenous infusion.

For the stabilisation of unstable angina patients, the bolus dose followed by the infusion should be started up to 24 hours prior to the possible intervention and concluded 12 hours after the intervention.

For the prevention of ischaemic cardiac complications in patients undergoing percutaneous coronary intervention, and who are not currently receiving a ReoPro infusion, the bolus should be administered 10 to 60 minutes prior to the intervention followed by the infusion for 12 hours.

Administration Instructions:

1. Parenteral drug products should be inspected visually for particulate matter prior to administration. Preparations of ReoPro containing visibly opaque particles should NOT be used.

2. Hypersensitivity reactions should be anticipated whenever protein solutions such as ReoPro are administered. Adrenaline, dopamine, theophylline, antihistamines, and corticosteroids should be available for immediate use. If symptoms of an allergic reaction or anaphylaxis appear, the infusion should be stopped immediately. Subcutaneous administration of 0.3 to 0.5ml of aqueous adrenaline (1:1000 dilution), and use of corticosteroids, respiratory assistance, and other resuscitative measures are essential.

3. As with all parenteral drug products, aseptic procedures should be used during the administration of ReoPro.

4. Withdraw the necessary amount of ReoPro for the bolus injection into a syringe. Filter the bolus injection using a sterile, non-pyrogenic, low protein-binding 0.2/0.22μm or 5.0μm syringe filter. The bolus should be administered over one (1) minute.

5. Withdraw the necessary amount of ReoPro for the continuous infusion into a syringe. Inject into an appropriate container of sterile 0.9% saline or 5% dextrose and infuse at the calculated rate via a continuous infusion pump. The continuous infusion should be filtered either upon admixture, using a sterile, non-pyrogenic, low protein-binding 0.2/0.22μm or 5.0μm syringe filter, or upon administration, using an in-line, sterile, non-pyrogenic, low protein-binding 0.2μm or 0.22μm filter. Discard the unused portion at the end of the infusion period.

6. Although incompatibilities have not been shown with intravenous infusion fluids or commonly used cardiovascular drugs, it is recommended that ReoPro be administered in a separate intravenous line whenever possible and not mixed with other medications.

7. No incompatibilities have been observed with glass bottles or polyvinyl chloride bags or administration sets.

4.3 Contraindications

ReoPro should not be administered to patients with known sensitivity to abciximab, to any component of the product, or to murine monoclonal antibodies.

Because inhibition of platelet aggregation increases the risk of bleeding, ReoPro is contra-indicated in the following clinical situations: active internal bleeding; history of cerebrovascular accident within two years; recent (within two months) intracranial or intraspinal surgery or trauma; recent (within two months) major surgery; intracranial neoplasm, arteriovenous malformation or aneurysm; known bleeding diathesis or severe uncontrolled hypertension; pre-existing thrombocytopenia; vasculitis; hypertensive retinopathy; severe hepatic failure. Since there are only limited data available, use of ReoPro in severe renal failure patients requiring haemodialysis is contra-indicated (see also section 4.4).

4.4 Special warnings and special precautions for use

Careful assessment of risk:benefit should be made in individual patients before commencing therapy with ReoPro. A favourable risk:benefit has not been established in low risk patients $>$65 years of age.

Requirement for Specialist Facilities:

ReoPro should only be administered in conjunction with extensive specialist medical and nursing care. In addition, there must be availability of laboratory tests of haematology function and facilities for administration of blood products.

Concomitant Aspirin and Heparin Therapy:

ReoPro should be used as an adjunct to aspirin and heparin therapy.

Aspirin

Aspirin should be administered orally at a daily dose of approximately, but not less than, 300mg.

Heparin

1. Percutaneous Coronary Intervention

Heparin Bolus Pre-PTCA

If a patient's activated clotting time (ACT) is less than 200 seconds prior to the start of the PTCA procedure, an initial bolus of heparin should be given upon gaining arterial access according to the following algorithm:

ACT $<$150 seconds: Administer 70U/kg.

ACT 150-199 seconds: Administer 50U/kg.

The initial heparin bolus dose should not exceed 7,000U.

ACT should be checked a minimum of 2 minutes after the heparin bolus. If the ACT is $<$200 seconds, additional heparin boluses of 20U/kg may be administered. Should the ACT remain $<$200 seconds, additional 20U/kg boluses are to be given until an ACT $\geq$200 seconds is achieved.

Should a situation arise where higher doses of heparin are considered clinically necessary in spite of the possibility of a greater bleeding risk, it is recommended that heparin be carefully titrated using weight-adjusted boluses and that the target ACT not exceed 300 seconds.

Heparin Bolus During PTCA

During the PTCA procedure, ACT should be checked every 30 minutes. If ACT is $<$200 seconds, additional heparin boluses of 20U/kg may be administered. Should the ACT remain $<$200 seconds, additional 20U/kg boluses may be given until an ACT $\geq$200 seconds is achieved. ACT should be checked prior to, and a minimum of 2 minutes after, each heparin bolus.

As an alternative to giving additional boluses as described above, a continuous heparin infusion may be initiated after the initial heparin bolus doses achieve the ACT target

≥200 seconds at a rate of 7U/kg/hr and continued for the duration of the procedure.

Heparin Infusion After PTCA

Discontinuation of heparin immediately following completion of the procedure, with removal of the arterial sheath within 6 hours, is *strongly recommended*. In individual patients, if prolonged heparin therapy after PTCA or later sheath removal is used, then an initial infusion rate of 7U/kg/hr is recommended (see 'Bleeding Precautions: Femoral Artery Sheath Removal'). In all circumstances, heparin should be discontinued at least 2 hours prior to arterial sheath removal.

2. Stabilisation of Unstable Angina

Anticoagulation should be initiated with heparin to a target APTT of 60-85 seconds. The heparin infusion should be maintained during the ReoPro infusion. Following angioplasty, heparin management is outlined above under '1. Percutaneous Coronary Intervention'.

Bleeding Precautions:

Femoral Artery Access Site

ReoPro is associated with an increase in bleeding rate, particularly at the site of arterial access for femoral artery sheath placement. The following are specific recommendations for access site care:

Femoral Artery Sheath Insertion

- When appropriate, place only an arterial sheath for vascular access (avoid venous sheath placement).
- Puncture only the anterior wall of the artery or vein when establishing vascular access.
- The use of a through and through technique to identify the vascular structure is *strongly discouraged*.

While Femoral Artery Sheath Is In Place

- Check sheath insertion site and distal pulses of affected leg(s) every 15 minutes for 1 hour, then hourly for 6 hours.
- Maintain complete bed rest with head of bed ≤30°.
- Maintain affected leg(s) straight via sheet tuck method or soft restraint.
- Medicate for back/groin pain as necessary.
- Educate patient on post-PTCA care via verbal instructions.

Femoral Artery Sheath Removal

- Heparin should be discontinued at least 2 hours prior to arterial sheath removal.
- Check APTT or ACT prior to arterial sheath removal; do not remove sheath unless APTT ≤50 seconds or ACT ≤175 seconds.
- Apply pressure to access site for at least 30 minutes following sheath removal, using either manual compression or a mechanical device.
- Apply pressure dressing after haemostasis has been achieved.

After Femoral Artery Sheath Removal

- Check groin for bleeding/haematoma and distal pulses every 15 minutes for the first hour or until stable, then hourly for 6 hours following sheath removal.
- Continue complete bed rest with head of bed ≤30° and affected leg(s) straight for 6-8 hours following femoral artery sheath removal, 6-8 hours following discontinuation of ReoPro, or 4 hours following discontinuation of heparin, whichever is later.
- Remove pressure dressing prior to ambulation.
- Continue to medicate for discomfort.

Management of Femoral Access Site Bleeding/Haematoma Formation

In the event of groin bleeding, with or without haematoma formation, the following procedures are recommended:

- Lower head of bed to 0°.
- Apply manual pressure/compression device until haemostasis has been achieved.
- Any haematoma should be measured and monitored for enlargement.
- Change pressure dressing as needed.
- If heparin is being given, obtain APTT and adjust heparin as needed.
- Maintain intravenous access if sheath has been removed.

If groin bleed continues or the haematoma expands during ReoPro infusion, despite the above measures, the ReoPro infusion should be immediately discontinued and the arterial sheath removed according to the guidelines listed above. After sheath removal, intravenous access should be maintained until bleeding is controlled (see 'Overdose: Uncontrolled bleeding').

Potential Bleeding Sites

Careful attention should be paid to all potential bleeding sites, including arterial and venous puncture sites, catheter insertion sites, cutdown sites, and needle puncture sites.

Retroperitoneal Bleeding

ReoPro is associated with an increased risk of retroperitoneal bleeding in association with femoral vascular puncture. The use of venous sheaths should be minimised and only the anterior wall of the artery or vein should be punctured when establishing vascular access (see 'Bleeding Precautions: Femoral Artery Access Site').

Pulmonary (Mostly Alveolar) Haemorrhage

ReoPro has rarely been associated with pulmonary (mostly alveolar) haemorrhage. This can present with any or all of the following in close association with ReoPro administration: hypoxemia, alveolar infiltrates on chest x-ray, haemoptysis, or an unexplained drop in haemoglobin. If confirmed, ReoPro and all anticoagulant and other antiplatelet drugs should immediately be discontinued.

GI Bleeding Prophylaxis

In order to prevent spontaneous GI bleeding, it is recommended that patients are pretreated with H_2-histamine receptor antagonists or liquid antacids. Anti-emetics should be given as needed to prevent vomiting.

General Nursing Care

Unnecessary arterial and venous punctures, intramuscular injections, routine use of urinary catheters, nasotracheal intubation, nasogastric tubes, and automatic blood pressure cuffs should be avoided. When obtaining intravenous access, non-compressible sites (eg, subclavian or jugular veins) should be avoided. Saline or heparin locks should be considered for blood drawing. Vascular puncture sites should be documented and monitored. Gentle care should be provided when removing dressings.

Patient Monitoring

Before administration of ReoPro, platelet count, ACT, prothrombin time (PT), and APTT should be measured to identify pre-existing coagulation abnormalities. Additional platelet counts should be taken 2-4 hours following the bolus dose and at 24 hours. Haemoglobin and haematocrit measurements should be obtained prior to the ReoPro administration, at 12 hours following the ReoPro bolus injection, and again at 24 hours following the bolus injection. Twelve lead electrocardiograms (ECG) should be obtained prior to the bolus injection of ReoPro, and repeated once the patient has returned to the hospital ward from the catheterization laboratory, and at 24 hours after the bolus injection of ReoPro. Vital signs (including blood pressure and pulse) should be obtained hourly for the first 4 hours following the ReoPro bolus injection, and then at 6, 12, 18, and 24 hours following the ReoPro bolus injection.

Restoration of Platelet Function

Transfusion of donor platelets has been shown to restore platelet function following ReoPro administration in animal studies, and transfusions of fresh random donor platelets have been given empirically to restore platelet function in humans. In the event of serious uncontrolled bleeding or the need for emergency surgery, ReoPro should be discontinued. In the majority of patients, bleeding time returns to normal within 12 hours. If bleeding time remains prolonged and/or there is a marked inhibition of platelet function and/or if rapid haemostasis is required and/or in case(s) where haemostasis is not adequately restored, consideration should be given to seeking advice of a haematologist experienced in the diagnosis and management of bleeding disorders.

If rapid haemostasis is required, therapeutic doses of platelets may be administered (at least 5.5×10^{11} platelets). Redistribution of ReoPro from endogenous platelet receptors to platelets, which have been transfused, may take place. A single transfusion may be sufficient to reduce receptor blockade to 60% to 70%, at which level platelet function is restored. Repeat platelet transfusions may be required to maintain haemostasis.

Use of Thrombolytics, Anticoagulants, and Other Antiplatelet Agents:

Because ReoPro inhibits platelet aggregation, caution should be employed when used with other drugs affecting haemostasis, such as heparin, oral anticoagulants, such as warfarin, thrombolytics, and antiplatelet agents other than aspirin, such as dipyridamole, ticlopidine, or low molecular weight dextrans (see section 4.5).

Data in patients receiving thrombolytics suggest an increase in the risk of bleeding when ReoPro is administered to patients treated with thrombolytics at doses sufficient to produce a systemic fibrinolytic state. Therefore, the use of ReoPro therapy for rescue angioplasty in those patients that have received systemic thrombolytic therapy should only be considered after careful consideration of the risks and benefits for each patient. The risk of bleeding and ICH appears higher the sooner ReoPro is administered after the application of the thrombolytic.

The GUSTO V trial randomised 16,588 patients with acute myocardial infarction to treatment with combined ReoPro and half-dose reteplase or full dose reteplase alone. The incidence of moderate or severe non-intracranial bleeding was increased in those patients receiving ReoPro and half-dose reteplase versus those receiving reteplase alone (4.6% versus 2.3%, respectively).

If urgent intervention is required for refractory symptoms in a patient receiving ReoPro (or who has received the drug in the previous 48 hours), it is recommended that PTCA be attempted first to salvage the situation. Prior to further surgical interventions, the bleeding time should be determined and should be 12 minutes or less. Should PTCA and any other appropriate procedures fail, and should the angiographic appearance suggest that the aetiology is due to thrombosis, consideration may be given to the administration of adjunctive thrombolytic therapy via the intracoronary route. A systemic fibrinolytic state should be avoided if at all possible.

Thrombocytopenia:

To evaluate the possibility of thrombocytopenia, platelet counts should be monitored prior to treatment, 2 to 4 hours following the bolus dose of ReoPro, and at 24 hours. If a patient experiences an acute platelet decrease, additional platelet counts should be determined. These platelet counts should be drawn in three separate tubes containing ethylenediaminetetraacetic acid (EDTA), citrate, and heparin, respectively, to exclude pseudothrombocytopenia due to *in vitro* anticoagulant interaction. If true thrombocytopenia is verified, ReoPro should be immediately discontinued and the condition appropriately monitored and treated. A daily platelet count should be obtained until it returns to normal. If a patient's platelet count drops to 60,000 cells/μl, heparin and aspirin should be discontinued. If a patient's platelet count drops below 50,000 cells/μl, transfusion of platelets should be considered, especially if the patient is bleeding and/or invasive procedures are planned or ongoing. If the patient's platelet count drops below 20,000 cells/μl, platelets should be transfused. The decision to use platelet transfusion should be based upon clinical judgment on an individual basis.

Readministration:

Administration of ReoPro may result in the formation of human anti-chimeric antibody (HACA) that could potentially cause allergic or hypersensitivity reactions (including anaphylaxis), thrombocytopenia, or diminished benefit upon readministration. HACA formation appeared, generally as a low titre, in approximately 5% to 6% of patients after single administrations of ReoPro in Phase III trials (see section 4.8). Available evidence suggests that human antibodies to other monoclonal antibodies do not cross-react with ReoPro.

Readministration of ReoPro to patients undergoing PTCA was assessed in a registry that included 1,342 treatments in 1,286 patients. Most patients were receiving their second ReoPro exposure; 15% were receiving the third or subsequent exposure. The overall rate of HACA positivity prior to the readministration was 6% and increased to 27% post-readministration. There were no reports of serious allergic reactions or anaphylaxis. Thrombocytopenia was observed at higher rates in the readministration study than in the Phase III studies of first-time administration (see section 4.8), suggesting that readministration may be associated with an increased incidence and severity of thrombocytopenia.

Renal Disease:

Benefits may be reduced in patients with renal disease. The use of ReoPro in patients with severe renal failure should only be considered after careful appraisal of the risks and benefits. Because the potential risk of bleeding is increased in patients with severe renal disease, patients should be more frequently monitored for bleeding. In the event serious bleeding occurs, platelet transfusion should be considered (see 'Restoration of Platelet Function'). In addition, the bleeding precautions as described above should be taken into consideration.

Use of ReoPro in patients receiving dialysis is contra-indicated (see section 4.3).

Children or Age Over 80 Years:

Children or patients older than 80 years have not been studied.

4.5 Interaction with other medicinal products and other forms of Interaction

ReoPro has been formally studied as an adjunct to heparin and aspirin treatment. In the presence of ReoPro, heparin is associated with an increase in the incidence of bleeding. Limited experience with ReoPro in patients who have received thrombolytics suggests an increase in the risk of bleeding. Although there have been no formal studies of ReoPro with other commonly used cardiovascular drugs, in clinical studies there have been no adverse drug reactions associated with concomitant use of other medications used in the treatment of angina, myocardial infarction, or hypertension, nor with common intravenous infusion fluids. These medications have included warfarin (before and following but not during PTCA), beta-adrenergic receptor blockers, calcium-channel antagonists, angiotensin converting enzyme (ACE) inhibitors, and intravenous and oral nitrates.

4.6 Pregnancy and lactation

Animal reproduction studies have not been conducted with ReoPro. It is also not known whether ReoPro can cause foetal harm when administered to a pregnant woman or can affect reproduction capacity. ReoPro should be given to a pregnant woman only if clearly needed.

Breast-feeding of infants should be discontinued in nursing mothers, since the secretion of abciximab in animal or human breast milk has not been studied.

4.7 Effects on ability to drive and use machines

Not applicable.

4.8 Undesirable effects

In the EPIC trial, in which a non-weight-adjusted, standard heparin dose regimen was used, the most common complication during ReoPro therapy was bleeding during the first 36 hours. The incidences of major bleeding[1], minor bleeding[2], and transfusion of blood products were approximately doubled. In patients who had major bleeding, 67% had bleeding associated with the arterial access site in the groin.

[1]Decrease in haemoglobin >5g/dl.

[2]Spontaneous gross haematuria or haematemesis, or observed blood loss with a haemoglobin decrease >3g/dl or with a decrease in haemoglobin ⩾4g/dl with no observed blood loss.

In a subsequent clinical trial, EPILOG, using the heparin regimen, sheath removal and femoral access care guidelines outlined in section 4.4, the incidence of major bleeding not associated with CABG surgery in patients treated with ReoPro (1.1%) was not different from patients receiving placebo (1.1%) and there was no significant increase in the incidence of intracranial haemorrhage. The reduction in major bleeding observed in the EPILOG trial was achieved without loss of efficacy. Likewise, in the EPISTENT trial, the incidence of major bleeding not associated with CABG surgery in patients receiving ReoPro plus balloon angioplasty (0.6%) or ReoPro with stent placement (0.8%) was not significantly different from patients receiving placebo with stent placement (1.0%). In the CAPTURE trial, which did not use the low-dose heparin regimen, the incidence of major bleeding not associated with CABG surgery was higher in patients receiving ReoPro (3.8%) than in patients receiving placebo (1.9%).

Although data are limited, ReoPro treatment was not associated with excess major bleeding in patients who underwent CABG surgery. Some patients with prolonged bleeding times received platelet transfusions to correct the bleeding time prior to surgery. See 'Bleeding Precautions: Restoration of Platelet Function'.

Clinical trials suggest that adherence to the currently recommended weight-adjusted heparin regimen is associated with a lower risk of intracranial haemorrhage than previous (higher dose, non-weight-adjusted) protocols. The total incidence of intracranial haemorrhage and non-haemorrhagic stroke in all four pivotal trials was similar, 9/3,023 (0.30%) for placebo patients and 15/4,680 (0.32%) for ReoPro-treated patients. The incidence of intracranial haemorrhage was 0.10% in placebo patients and 0.15% in ReoPro patients.

Patients treated with ReoPro were more likely to experience thrombocytopenia (platelet counts less than 100,000 cells/μl) than placebo patients. The incidence in the EPILOG and EPISTENT trials using ReoPro with the recommended low-dose, weight-adjusted heparin regimen was 2.8% and 1.1% in placebo-treated patients. In a readministration registry study of patients receiving a second or subsequent exposure to ReoPro, the incidence of any degree of thrombocytopenia was 5%, with an incidence of profound thrombocytopenia of 2% (<20,000 cell/μl). Factors associated with an increased risk of thrombocytopenia were a history of thrombocytopenia on previous ReoPro exposure, readministration within 30 days, and a positive HACA assay prior to the readministration.

The most frequent adverse events are back pain, hypotension, nausea, chest pain, vomiting, headache pain, bradycardia, fever, puncture site pain, and thrombocytopenia. Cardiac tamponade, pulmonary (mostly alveolar) haemorrhage, and adult respiratory distress syndrome have been reported rarely. Human anti-chimeric antibody (HACA) appeared, generally as a low titre, in approximately 5% to 6% of patients 2 to 4 weeks after receiving a first exposure to ReoPro in the Phase III trials. Hypersensitivity or allergic reactions have been observed rarely following treatment with ReoPro. Nevertheless, anaphylaxis may potentially occur at any time during administration (see 'Administration Instructions').

4.9 Overdose

There has been no experience of adverse events associated with overdosage. However, in the event of acute allergic reactions, thrombocytopenia, or uncontrolled bleeding, the administration of ReoPro should be immediately discontinued. In the event of thrombocytopenia or uncontrolled bleeding, platelet transfusion is recommended.

Allergic reactions: See 'Administration Instructions'.

Thrombocytopenia: To evaluate the possibility of thrombocytopenia, platelet counts should be monitored prior to treatment, 2 to 4 hours following the bolus dose of ReoPro, and at 24 hours. If a patient experiences an acute platelet decrease, additional platelet counts should be determined. These platelet counts should be drawn in three separate tubes containing ethylenediaminetetraacetic acid (EDTA), citrate, and heparin, respectively, to exclude pseudothrombocytopenia due to *in vitro* anticoagulant interaction. If true thrombocytopenia is verified, ReoPro should be immediately discontinued and the condition appropriately monitored and treated. A daily platelet count should be obtained until it returns to normal. If a patient's platelet count drops to 60,000 cells/μl, heparin and aspirin should be discontinued. If a patient's platelet count drops below 50,000 cells/μl, platelets should be considered, especially if the patient is bleeding and/or invasive procedures are planned or ongoing. If the patient's platelet count drops below 20,000 cells/μl, platelets should be transfused. The decision to use platelet transfusion should be based upon clinical judgment on an individual basis.

Uncontrolled bleeding: (Specific guidelines for access site bleeding are given above under 'Bleeding Precautions: Femoral Artery Access Site'.) When considering the need to transfuse patients, the patient's intravascular volume should be assessed. If hypovolaemic, intravascular volume should be adequately restored with crystalloids. In asymptomatic patients, normovolaemic anaemia (haemoglobin 7-10g/dl) can be well tolerated; transfusion is not indicated unless a deterioration in vital signs is seen or unless the patient develops signs and symptoms. In symptomatic patients (eg, syncope, dyspnoea, postural hypotension, tachycardia), crystalloids should be used to replace intravascular volume. If symptoms persist, the patient should receive transfusions with packed red blood cells or whole blood on a unit-by-unit basis to relieve symptoms; one unit may be sufficient. Transfusion of donor platelets has been shown to restore platelet function following ReoPro administration in animal studies, and transfusions of fresh random donor platelets have been given empirically to restore platelet function in humans. In the event of serious uncontrolled bleeding or the need for emergency surgery, ReoPro should be discontinued. In the majority of patients, bleeding time returns to normal within 12 hours. If bleeding time remains prolonged and/or there is a marked inhibition of platelet function and/or if rapid haemostasis is required and/or in case(s) where haemostasis is not adequately restored, consideration should be given to seeking advice of a haematologist experienced in the diagnosis and management of bleeding disorders.

If rapid haemostasis is required, therapeutic doses of platelets may be administered (at least 5.5×10^{11} platelets). Redistribution of ReoPro from endogenous platelet receptors to platelets, which have been transfused, may take place. A single transfusion may be sufficient to reduce receptor blockade to 60% to 70%, at which level platelet function is restored. Repeat platelet transfusions may be required to maintain haemostasis.

5. PHARMACOLOGICAL PROPERTIES

5.1 Pharmacodynamic properties

ReoPro is the Fab fragment of the chimeric monoclonal antibody 7E3. It is directed against the glycoprotein (GP) IIb/IIIa ($\alpha_{IIb}\beta_3$) receptor located on the surface of human platelets. ReoPro inhibits platelet aggregation by preventing the binding of fibrinogen, von Willebrand factor, and other adhesive molecules to GPIIb/IIIa receptor sites on activated platelets. ReoPro also binds to the vitronectin ($\alpha_v\beta_3$) receptor found on platelets and endothelial cells. The vitronectin receptor mediates the pro-coagulant properties of platelets and proliferative properties of vessel wall endothelial and smooth muscle cells. Because of its dual specificity, ReoPro more effectively blocks the burst of thrombin generation that follows platelet activation than agents which inhibit GPIIb/IIIa alone.

In a Phase I trial, intravenous administration in humans of single bolus doses of ReoPro from 0.15mg/kg to 0.30mg/kg produced rapid dose-dependent inhibition of platelet function as measured by *ex vivo* platelet aggregation in response to adenosine diphosphate (ADP) or by prolongation of bleeding time. At the two highest doses (0.25 and 0.30mg/kg) at 2 hours post injection, over 80% of the GPIIb/IIIa receptors were blocked and platelet aggregation in response to 20μm ADP was almost abolished. Published data have shown that this level of platelet inhibition was established within 10 minutes of administration. In the Phase I trial, the median bleeding time increased to over 30 minutes at both doses compared with a baseline value of approximately 5 minutes. The 80% level of receptor blockade was selected as a target for pharmacological efficacy because animal models of severe coronary stenosis have shown that platelet inhibition associated with this degree of blockade prevents platelet thrombosis.

Intravenous administration in humans of a single bolus dose of 0.25mg/kg followed by a continuous infusion of 10 microgram/min for periods of 12 to 96 hours produced sustained high-grade GPIIb/IIIa receptor blockade (⩾80%) and inhibition of platelet function (*ex vivo* platelet aggregation in response to 20μm ADP less than 20% of baseline and bleeding time greater than 30 minutes) for the duration of the infusion in most patients. Equivalent results were obtained when a weight-adjusted infusion dose (0.125 microgram/kg/min to a maximum of 10 microgram/min) was used in patients up to 80kg. Results in patients who received the 0.25mg/kg bolus followed by a 5 microgram/min infusion for 24 hours showed a similar initial receptor blockade and inhibition of platelet aggregation, but the response was not maintained throughout the infusion period. Although low levels of GPIIb/IIIa receptor blockade are present for more than 10 days following cessation of the infusion, platelet function typically returned to normal over a period of 24 to 48 hours.

In clinical trials, ReoPro has demonstrated marked effects in reducing the thrombotic complications of coronary interventions such as balloon angioplasty, atherectomy, and stent placement. These effects were observed within hours of the intervention and sustained for 30 days in the EPIC, EPILOG, EPISTENT, and CAPTURE trials. In the EPIC trial, which enrolled high-risk angioplasty patients, and in the two intervention trials, which enrolled mainly high-risk angioplasty patients, EPILOG (36% low risk and 64% high risk) and EPISTENT (27% low risk and 73% high risk), the infusion dose was continued for 12 hours after the procedure and the reduction in the composite endpoint of death, MI, or repeat intervention was sustained for the period of follow-up, 3 years (EPIC), 1 year (EPILOG), and 1 year (EPISTENT), respectively. In the EPIC trial, the reduction in the composite endpoint was derived primarily from the effect on MI and both urgent and non-urgent revascularizations. In the EPILOG and EPISTENT trials, the reduction in the composite endpoint was derived primarily from the effect on non-Q-wave MI (identified by cardiac enzyme increases) and urgent revascularizations. In the CAPTURE trial, in patients with unstable angina not responding to medical therapy, ReoPro was administered as a bolus plus infusion starting up to 24 hours before the procedure until 1 hour after completion of the procedure. This regimen demonstrated stabilisation of patients prior to angioplasty, as shown, for example, by a reduction in MIs, and the reduction in thrombotic complications was sustained at the 30-day endpoint but not at 6 months.

5.2 Pharmacokinetic properties

Following intravenous bolus administration of ReoPro, free plasma concentrations decrease very rapidly, with an initial half-life of less than 10 minutes and a second phase half-life of about 30 minutes, probably related to rapid binding to the platelet GPIIb/IIIa receptors. Platelet function generally recovers over the course of 48 hours, although ReoPro remains in the circulation for 15 days or more in a platelet-bound state. Intravenous administration of a 0.25mg/kg bolus dose of ReoPro followed by continuous infusion of 10 microgram/min (or a weight-adjusted infusion of 0.125 microgram/kg/min to a maximum of 10 microgram/min) produces relatively constant free plasma concentrations throughout the infusion. At the termination of the infusion period, free plasma concentrations fall rapidly for approximately 6 hours then decline at a slower rate.

5.3 Preclinical safety data

No remarkable findings.

6. PHARMACEUTICAL PARTICULARS

6.1 List of excipients

Water for injection

Disodium phosphate dihydrate

Sodium dihydrogen phosphate monohydrate

Sodium chloride

Polysorbate 80

Trace amounts of papain, resulting from the production process, may be present.

6.2 Incompatibilities

No incompatibilities have been shown with intravenous infusion fluids or commonly used cardiovascular drugs. Nevertheless, it is recommended that ReoPro be administered in a separate intravenous line whenever possible and not mixed with other medications.

No incompatibilities have been observed with polyvinyl chloride bags or administration sets.

6.3 Shelf life

Three (3) years.

Chemical and physical in-use stability has been demonstrated for 24 hours at 25°C.

From a microbiological point of view, the product should be used immediately. If not used immediately, in-use storage times and conditions prior to use are the responsibility of the user and would not normally be longer than 24 hours at 2°C to 8°C, unless dilution has taken place in controlled and validated aseptic conditions.

6.4 Special precautions for storage

ReoPro should be stored at 2°C to 8°C. Do not freeze. Do not shake.

6.5 Nature and contents of container

ReoPro is supplied in Type I borosilicate glass vials with Teflon-coated rubber stoppers and aluminium crimps protected by a plastic cap.

Pack size: 10mg/5ml vial.

6.6 Instructions for use and handling

Do not shake vials. ReoPro does not contain a preservative and is for single use only. Unused portions should be discarded. For administration instructions see section 4.2 above.

ReoPro is for intravenous (IV) administration in adults.

Adults:

The recommended dose of ReoPro is a 0.25mg/kg intravenous bolus immediately followed by a 0.125μg/kg/min (to a maximum of 10μg/min) continuous intravenous infusion.

Instructions for dilution:

1. Parenteral drug products should be inspected visually for particulate matter prior to administration. Preparations of ReoPro containing visibly opaque particles should NOT be used.

2. As with all parenteral drug products, aseptic procedures should be used during the administration of ReoPro.

3. *Preparation of bolus injection:* Withdraw the necessary amount of ReoPro for the bolus injection into a syringe. Filter the bolus injection using a sterile, non-pyrogenic, low protein-binding 0.2/0.22μm or 5.0μm syringe filter. The bolus should be administered over one (1) minute.

4. *Preparation of IV infusion:* Withdraw the necessary amount of ReoPro for the continuous infusion into a syringe. Inject into an appropriate container of sterile 0.9% saline or 5% dextrose and infuse at the calculated rate via a continuous infusion pump. The continuous infusion should be filtered either upon admixture, using a sterile, non-pyrogenic, low protein-binding 0.2/0.22μm or 5.0μm syringe filter, or upon administration, using an in-line, sterile, non-pyrogenic, low protein-binding 0.2μm or 0.22μm filter. Discard the unused portion at the end of the infusion period.

5. Although incompatibilities have not been shown with intravenous infusion fluids or commonly used cardiovascular drugs, it is recommended that ReoPro be administered in a separate intravenous line whenever possible and not mixed with other medications.

6. No incompatibilities have been observed with glass bottles or polyvinyl chloride bags or administration sets.

7. MARKETING AUTHORISATION HOLDER

Centocor BV

Einsteinweg 101

2333 CB Leiden

The Netherlands

Distributor:

Eli Lilly and Company Limited

Lilly House

Priestley road

Basingstoke

Hampshire

RG24 9NL

England

8. MARKETING AUTHORISATION NUMBER(S)

PL 08563/0015 (UK)

PA 502/3/1 (RoI)

9. DATE OF FIRST AUTHORISATION/RENEWAL OF THE AUTHORISATION

Date of first authorisation:	23 March 1995 (UK)
Date of last renewal of authorisation:	22 March 2000 (UK)
Date of first authorisation:	12 July 1995 (RoI)
Date of last renewal of authorisation:	22 March 2000 (RoI)

10. DATE OF REVISION OF THE TEXT

September 2004 (UK)

November 2004 (RoI)

LEGAL CATEGORY

POM

*REOPRO (abciximab) is a trademark of Eli Lilly and Company.

RP13M

REPEVAX

(Sanofi Pasteur MSD)

1. NAME OF THE MEDICINAL PRODUCT

REPEVAX®▼

Diphtheria, Tetanus, Pertussis (Acellular, Component) and Poliomyelitis (Inactivated) Vaccine, adjuvanted.

Suspension for injection in prefilled syringes.

2. QUALITATIVE AND QUANTITATIVE COMPOSITION

Each dose (0.5 ml) contains:

Active Ingredients:	
Purified diphtheria toxoid	not less than 2 IU* (2 Lf)
Purified tetanus toxoid	not less than 20 IU* (5 Lf)
Pertussis antigens	
Purified pertussis toxoid (PT)	2.5 μg
Purified filamentous haemagglutinin (FHA)	5 μg
Purified fimbrial agglutinogens 2 + 3 (FIM)	5 μg
Purified pertactin (PRN)	3 μg
Inactivated poliomyelitis virus type 1	40 D antigen units**
Inactivated poliomyelitis virus type 2	8 D antigen units**
Inactivated poliomyelitis virus type 3	32 D antigen units**
Aluminium phosphate as adjuvant	0.33 mg (as aluminium)

For excipients, see section 6.1

* As lower confidence limit (p = 0.95) of activity measured according to the assay described in the European Pharmacopoeia.

** The inactivated polio vaccine is cultivated on Vero cells.

3. PHARMACEUTICAL FORM

Cloudy, white suspension for injection in prefilled syringes.

4. CLINICAL PARTICULARS

4.1 Therapeutic indications

REPEVAX® is indicated for active immunisation against diphtheria, tetanus, pertussis and poliomyelitis in persons from the age of three years (see Section 4.2) as a booster following primary immunisation.

REPEVAX® is not intended for primary immunisation.

The use of REPEVAX® should be determined on the basis of official recommendations.

4.2 Posology and method of administration

The same dosage, a single 0.5 ml dose, applies to all age groups.

REPEVAX® may be administered from the age of three years onwards. The use of REPEVAX® in children aged 3 to 5 years is based upon studies in which REPEVAX® was given as the fourth dose (first booster) of diptheria, tetanus, pertussis and poliomyelitis vaccines.

REPEVAX® should be administered in accordance with official recommendations and/or local practice regarding the use of vaccines that provide low-dose diphtheria toxoid plus tetanus toxoid in combination with pertussis and polio antigens.

Individuals with an incomplete, or no, history of a primary series of diphtheria and tetanus toxoids or polio vaccine should not be vaccinated with REPEVAX®. REPEVAX® is not precluded in subjects with an incomplete, or no, history of previous pertussis vaccination. However, a booster response will only be elicited in individuals who have been previously primed by vaccination or by natural infection. Repeat vaccination against diphtheria and tetanus should be performed at intervals as per official recommendations (generally 10 years). It is not necessary to re-commence primary vaccination, should the officially recommended inter-booster interval be exceeded.

There are currently no data upon which to base a recommendation for the optimal interval for administering subsequent booster doses with REPEVAX® to maintain antibody levels against pertussis. There are no data on the duration of protection against pertussis following vaccination with REPEVAX®.

REPEVAX® has not been studied in subjects with tetanus-prone injuries and should not be used in these circumstances.

Method of administration

REPEVAX® should be administered intramuscularly. The preferred site is into the deltoid muscle.

The intravascular or subcutaneous routes should not be used (for exception, see section 4.4). After insertion of the needle, aspirate to ensure that the needle has not entered a blood vessel.

4.3 Contraindications

REPEVAX® should not be administered to individuals who have previously had a hypersensitivity reaction to any vaccine containing diphtheria or tetanus toxoids, poliomyelitis viruses or pertussis (acellular or whole cell).

REPEVAX® should not be administered to individuals known to be hypersensitive to any component of the vaccine or residues carried over from manufacture (such as formaldehyde, streptomycin, neomycin and polymyxin B).

Vaccination should be deferred in the presence of any acute illness, including febrile illness. A minor afebrile illness such as mild upper respiratory infection is not usually a reason to defer immunisation.

REPEVAX® should not be administered to subjects who experienced an encephalopathy of unknown origin within 7 days of previous immunisation with a pertussis-containing vaccine, or to subjects who have experienced other neurological complications following previous immunisation with any of the antigens in REPEVAX®.

4.4 Special warnings and special precautions for use

As with all injectable vaccines, appropriate medical treatment and supervision should be readily available for immediate use in case of a rare anaphylactic reaction following the administration of the vaccine.

A persistent nodule at the site of injection may occur with all adsorbed vaccines, particularly if administered into the superficial layers of the subcutaneous tissue.

Intramuscular injections should be given with care in patients suffering from coagulation disorders, such as thrombocytopenia, because of the risk of haemorrhage. In these situations administration of REPEVAX® by deep subcutaneous injection may be considered, although there is a risk of increased local reactions.

The immunogenicity of the vaccine could be reduced by immunosuppressive treatment or immunodeficiency. It is recommended to postpone the vaccination until the end of such disease or treatment if practical. Nevertheless, vaccination of HIV-infected subjects or subjects with chronic immunodeficiency, such as AIDS, is recommended even if the antibody response might be limited.

4.5 Interaction with other medicinal products and other forms of Interaction

A clinical study has shown that REPEVAX® can be administered concomitantly with hepatitis B vaccine, using a separate limb for the site of injection. Interaction studies have not been carried out with other vaccines, biological products or therapeutic medications. However, in accordance with commonly accepted immunisation guidelines, since REPEVAX® is an inactivated product, there is no theoretical reason why it should not be administered concomitantly with other vaccines or immunoglobulins at separate sites.

In the case of immunosuppressive therapy please refer to Section 4.4, "Special warnings and precautions for use".

4.6 Pregnancy and lactation

The effect of REPEVAX® on embryo-foetal development has not been assessed. No teratogenic effect of vaccines containing diphtheria or tetanus toxoids, or inactivated poliovirus has been observed following use in pregnant women.

The use of this combined vaccine is not recommended during pregnancy.

It is preferable to avoid the use of this vaccine during breast-feeding.

4.7 Effects on ability to drive and use machines

The vaccine is unlikely to produce an effect on the ability to drive or operate machinery.

4.8 Undesirable effects

Adolescents and Adults (994 subjects)

In clinical studies in which REPEVAX® was administered to adolescents and adults, the most frequently reported adverse reactions occurring over all age groups during the first 24 hours after vaccination included the following:

Very common (>10%):	Injection site pain, erythema and swelling, headache, asthenia, nausea, rigors, myalgia, arthralgia or joint swelling
Common (1-10%):	Fever, diarrhoea, vomiting

There was a trend for higher rates of local and systemic reactions in adolescents than in adults. In both age groups, injection site pain was the most common adverse reaction.

Late-onset local adverse reactions (i.e. a local adverse reaction which had an onset or increase in severity 3 to 14 days post-immunisation), such as injection site pain, erythema and swelling occurred in less than 1.2%.

Children 5 to 6 years old (240 subjects)

In a clinical study, children were primed at 3, 5 and 12 months of age with a DTaP vaccine with no additional dose in the second year of life. These children received REPEVAX® at 5 to 6 years of age. The most frequently reported adverse reactions occurring during the first 24 hours included the following:

Very common (>10%):	Injection site pain and swelling; fatigue
Common (1-10%):	Injection site erythema and pruritus; fever $\geqslant$ 38°C
Uncommon (0.1-1%):	Diarrhoea, vomiting

The rates of general symptoms after the first day but within 10 days after vaccination were low; only fever ($\geqslant$38°C) and fatigue were reported in >10% of subjects. Transient severe swelling of the upper arm was reported in <1% of subjects.

Children 3 to 5 years old (150 subjects)

150 children primed at 2, 3, and 4 months of age with a DTwP vaccine (with no additional dose in the second year of life) received REPEVAX® at 3 to 5 years of age. The most frequently reported adverse reactions occurring during the first 7 days included the following:

Very common (>10%):	Injection site pain, erythema and swelling; fatigue, fever $\geqslant$37.5°C, irritability
Common (1-10%):	Injection site bruising and dermatitis; diarrhoea, vomiting and rash

4.9 Overdose

Not applicable.

5. PHARMACOLOGICAL PROPERTIES

5.1 Pharmacodynamic properties

Vaccine against diphtheria, tetanus, pertussis and poliomyelitis. (J07CA)

Immune responses of adults, adolescents and children 3 to 6 years of age one month post vaccination with REPEVAX® are shown in the table below.

IMMUNE RESPONSES 4 WEEKS AFTER VACCINATION

(see Table 1 on next page)

The safety and immunogenicity profile of REPEVAX® in adults and adolescents was shown to be comparable to that observed with a single booster dose of Td adsorbed or Td Polio adsorbed vaccines containing a similar amount of tetanus and diphtheria toxoids and inactivated poliovirus types 1, 2 and 3.

The lower response to diphtheria toxoid in adults probably reflected the inclusion of some participants with an uncertain or incomplete immunisation history.

Serological correlates for protection against pertussis have not been established. On comparison with data from the

Table 1 IMMUNE RESPONSES 4 WEEKS AFTER VACCINATION

Antigen	Criteria	Adults and adolescents* (n =994)	Children 5-6 years old† (n = 240)	Children 3-5 years old‡ (n = 148)
Diphtheria	≥0.1 IU/ml	92.8%	99.4%	100%
Tetanus	≥0.1 IU/ml§	100%	99.5%	100%
Pertussis				
PT	≥5 EU¶/ml	99.7%	91.2%	99.3%
FHA	≥5 EU¶/ml	99.9%	99.1%	99.3%
PRN	≥5 EU¶/ml	99.6%	100%	100%
FIM	≥5 EU¶/ml	99.8%	99.5%	100%
Polio 1	≥1:8 Dilution	99.9%	100%	100%
Polio 2	≥1:8 Dilution	100%	100%	100%
Polio 3	≥1:8 Dilution	100%	100%	100%

* From the age of 10 years onwards

† Primed with DTaP at 3 and 5 months with a booster at 12 months of age

‡ Primed with DTwP at 2, 3 and 4 months of age

§ Measured by ELISA

¶ EU = ELISA units: Antibody levels of >5 EU/mL were postulated as possible surrogate markers for protection against pertussis by Storsaeter J. et al, Vaccine 1998;16:1907-1916

two separate pertussis efficacy trials conducted in Sweden between 1992 and 1996, where primary immunisation with Aventis Pasteur Limited's acellular pertussis infant DTaP formulations conferred a protective efficacy of 85% against pertussis disease, it was considered that REPEVAX® had elicited protective immune responses.

Seroprotection rates 3 years post-vaccination with REPEVAX® in adults and adolescents are shown in the table below.

Antigen	Criteria	Adults and adolescents* (n = 251)
Diphtheria	≥0.01 IU/ml	95.6%
Tetanus	≥0.01 IU/ml†	100%
Pertussis		
PT	≥5 EU/ml	96.8%
FHA	≥5 EU/ml	100.0%
PRN	≥5 EU/ml	100.0%
FIM	≥5 EU/ml	98.0%
Polio 1	≥1:8 Dilution	100%
Polio 2	≥1:8 Dilution	100%
Polio 3	≥1:8 Dilution	100%

* From the age of 10 years onwards

† Measured by ELISA

There are currently no data available on the antibody levels to any of the antigens in REPEVAX® beyond four weeks post-vaccination in children. Studies are on-going to collect these data.

5.2 Pharmacokinetic properties

Not applicable.

5.3 Preclinical safety data

In animal studies, no specific risks were identified.

6. PHARMACEUTICAL PARTICULARS

6.1 List of excipients

2-phenoxyethanol (preservative)

Polysorbate 80

Water for injections

6.2 Incompatibilities

REPEVAX® must not be mixed with other medicinal products.

6.3 Shelf life

3 years. The vaccine must not be used after the expiry date indicated on the syringe label or carton.

6.4 Special precautions for storage

Store at 2°C to 8°C (in a refrigerator).

Do not freeze. Discard the vaccine if it has been frozen.

6.5 Nature and contents of container

Packs of 1, 10 or 20.

Single dose (0.5 ml) in prefilled syringe (type I glass) with a plunger-stopper (chlorobromobutyl) with attached needle and needle-guard (elastomer).

Single dose (0.5 ml) in prefilled syringe (type I glass) with a plunger-stopper (chlorobromobutyl) without needle and with a tip-cap (chlorobromobutyl). Up to 2 separate needles (for each syringe) may be included in the packs of 1 and 10 syringes.

Single dose (0.5 ml) in prefilled syringe (type I glass) with a plunger-stopper (butylisoprene siliconized) with attached needle and needle shield (grey natural rubber).

Not all pack sizes may be marketed.

6.6 Instructions for use and handling

For needle free syringes, the needle should be pushed firmly on to the end of the prefilled syringe and rotated through 90 degrees.

The vaccine's normal appearance is a cloudy white suspension which may sediment during storage. Shake the prefilled syringe well to distribute uniformly the suspension before administering the vaccine.

Parenteral biological products should be inspected visually for extraneous particulate matter and/or discolouration prior to administration. In the event of either being observed, discard the vaccine. Any unused product or waste material should be disposed of in accordance with local requirements.

7. MARKETING AUTHORISATION HOLDER

Sanofi Pasteur MSD Ltd
Mallards Reach
Bridge Avenue
Maidenhead
Berkshire
SL6 1QP

8. MARKETING AUTHORISATION NUMBER(S)

PL6745/0121

9. DATE OF FIRST AUTHORISATION/RENEWAL OF THE AUTHORISATION

02 November 2001

10. DATE OF REVISION OF THE TEXT

May 2005

Requip Tablets

(GlaxoSmithKline UK)

1. NAME OF THE MEDICINAL PRODUCT

Requip®

2. QUALITATIVE AND QUANTITATIVE COMPOSITION

Ropinirole hydrochloride equivalent to 0.25, 0.5, 1.0, 2.0 or 5.0 mg ropinirole free base.

3. PHARMACEUTICAL FORM

Film-coated, pentagonal-shaped tablets for oral administration. The tablet strengths are distinguished by colour; 0.25 mg (white), 0.5mg (yellow), 1.0 mg (green), 2.0 mg (pink) and 5.0 mg (blue).

4. CLINICAL PARTICULARS

4.1 Therapeutic indications

Treatment of idiopathic Parkinson's Disease:

Ropinirole may be used alone (without levodopa) in the treatment of idiopathic Parkinson's disease.

Addition of ropinirole to levodopa may be used to control "on-off" fluctuations and permit a reduction in the total daily dose of levodopa.

4.2 Posology and method of administration

Individual dose titration against efficacy and tolerability is recommended.

Ropinirole should be taken three times a day, preferably with meals to improve gastrointestinal tolerance.

Treatment initiation: The initial dose should be 0.25 mg t.i.d. A guide for the titration regimen for the first four weeks of treatment is given in the table below:

(see Table 1 below)

Therapeutic regimen: After the initial titration, weekly increments of up to 3 mg/day may be given. Ropinirole is usually given in divided doses three times per day.

If using the "Follow on Titration" pack, follow the proposed titration regime:

(see Table 2 on next page)

A therapeutic response may be seen between 3 and 9 mg/day, although adjunct therapy patients may require higher doses. If sufficient symptomatic control is not achieved, or maintained, the dose of ropinirole may be increased until an acceptable therapeutic response is established. Doses above 24 mg/day have not been investigated in clinical trials and this dose should not be exceeded.

When ropinirole is administered as adjunct therapy to L-dopa, the concurrent dose of L-dopa may be reduced gradually by around 20% in total.

When switching treatment from another dopamine agonist to ropinirole, the manufacturer's guidance on discontinuation should be followed before initiating ropinirole.

As with other dopamine agonists, ropinirole should be discontinued gradually by reducing the number of daily doses over the period of one week.

In parkinsonian patients with mild to moderate renal impairment (creatinine clearance 30-50 ml/min) no change in the clearance of ropinirole was observed, indicating that no dosage adjustment is necessary in this population

The use of ropinirole in patients with severe renal (creatinine clearance <30 ml/min) or hepatic impairment has not been studied. Administration of ropinirole to such patients is not recommended.

Elderly: The clearance of ropinirole is decreased in patients over 65 years of age, but the dose of ropinirole for elderly patients can be titrated in the normal manner.

Children: Parkinson's disease does not occur in children. The use of ropinirole in this population has therefore not been studied and it should not be given to children.

4.3 Contraindications

Hypersensitivity to ropinirole

In light of the results of animal studies and the lack of studies in human pregnancy, ropinirole is contra-indicated in pregnancy, lactation and in women of child-bearing potential unless adequate contraception is used.

4.4 Special warnings and special precautions for use

Due to the pharmacological action of ropinirole, patients with severe cardiovascular disease should be treated with caution.

Co-administration of ropinirole with anti-hypertensive and anti-arrhythmic agents has not been studied. As with other dopaminergic drugs, caution should be exercised when these compounds are given concomitantly with ropinirole because of the unknown potential for the occurrence of hypotension, bradycardias or other arrhythmias.

Patients with major psychotic disorders should only be treated with dopamine agonists if the potential benefits outweigh the risks (see also Section 4.5).

Ropinirole has been associated with somnolence and episodes of sudden sleep onset, particularly in patients with Parkinson's Disease. Sudden onset of sleep during daily activities, in some cases without awareness or warning signs, has been reported uncommonly. Patients must be informed of this and advised to exercise caution while driving or operating machines during treatment with ropinirole. Patients who have experienced somnolence and/or an episode of sudden sleep onset must refrain from driving

Table 1

	Week 1	2	3	4
Unit dose (mg)	0.25	0.5	0.75	1.0
Unit dose presentation (mg)	0.25	0.5	0.25, 0.5	1.0
Total daily dose (mg)	0.75	1.5	2.25	3.0

Table 2

	Week			
	5	6	7	8
Unit dose (mg) Unit dose presentation (mg)	1.5 0.5, 1.0	2.0 2.0	2.5 0.5, 2.0	3.0 1.0, 2.0
Total daily dose (mg)	4.5	6.0	7.5	9.0

Table 3

	Tablet strength (mg) and colour				
	0.25	0.5	1.0	2.0	5.0
Tablet Colour	White	Yellow	Green	Pink	Blue
Titanium Dioxide	√	√	√	√	√
Iron Oxide Yellow		√	√	√	
Iron Oxide Red		√		√	
Indigo Carmine Aluminium		√	√		√
Polysorbate 80	√				√

or operating machines. Furthermore, a reduction of dosage or termination of therapy may be considered.

4.5 Interaction with other medicinal products and other forms of Interaction

Neuroleptics and other centrally active dopamine antagonists, such as sulpiride or metoclopramide, may diminish the effectiveness of ropinirole and, therefore, concomitant use of these drugs with ropinirole should be avoided.

No pharmacokinetic interaction has been seen between ropinirole and L-dopa or domperidone which would necessitate dosage adjustment of either drug. No interaction has been seen between ropinirole and other drugs commonly used to treat Parkinson's disease but, as is common practice, care should be taken when adding a new drug to a treatment regimen. Other dopamine agonists may be used with caution.

In a study in parkinsonian patients receiving concurrent digoxin, no interaction was seen which would require dosage adjustment.

It has been established from in vitro experiments that ropinirole is metabolised by the cytochrome P450 enzyme CYP1A2. There is, therefore, the potential for an interaction between ropinirole and substrates (such as theophylline) or inhibitors (such as ciprofloxacin, fluvoxamine and cimetidine) of this enzyme. In patients already receiving ropinirole, the dose of ropinirole may need to be adjusted when these drugs are introduced or withdrawn.

Increased plasma concentrations of ropinirole have been observed in patients treated with high doses of oestrogens. In patients already receiving hormone replacement therapy (HRT), ropinirole treatment may be initiated in the normal manner. However, if HRT is stopped or introduced during treatment with ropinirole, dosage adjustment may be required.

No information is available on the potential for interaction between ropinirole and alcohol. As with other centrally active medications, patients should be cautioned against taking ropinirole with alcohol.

4.6 Pregnancy and lactation

Ropinirole should not be used during pregnancy. In animal studies, administration of ropinirole to pregnant rats at maternally toxic doses resulted in decreased foetal body weight at 60 mg/kg (approximately three times the AUC of the maximum dose in man), increased foetal death at 90 mg/kg (~x5) and digit malformations at 150 mg/kg (~x9). There was no teratogenic effect in the rat at 120 mg/kg (~x7) and no indication of an effect on development in the rabbit. There have been no studies of ropinirole in human pregnancy.

Ropinirole should not be used in nursing mothers as it may inhibit lactation.

4.7 Effects on ability to drive and use machines

Patients being treated with ropinirole and presenting with somnolence and/or sudden sleep episodes must be informed to refrain from driving or engaging in activities where impaired alertness may put themselves or others at risk of serious injury or death (e.g. operating machines) until such recurrent episodes and somnolence have resolved (see also Section 4.4).

4.8 Undesirable effects

The most common adverse experiences reported by early therapy patients receiving ropinirole in clinical trials, and not seen at an equivalent or greater incidence on placebo, were; nausea, somnolence, leg oedema, abdominal pain, vomiting and syncope.

Similarly, the most common adverse experiences reported in adjunct therapy clinical trials were; dyskinesia, nausea, hallucinations and confusion.

The incidence of postural hypotension, an event commonly associated with dopamine agonists, was not markedly different from placebo in clinical trials with ropinirole. However, decreases in systolic blood pressure have been noted; symptomatic hypotension and bradycardia, occasionally severe, may occur.

Ropinirole is associated with somnolence and has been associated uncommonly with excessive daytime somnolence and sudden sleep onset episodes.

4.9 Overdose

There have been no incidences of intentional overdose with ropinirole in clinical trials. It is anticipated that the symptoms of ropinirole overdose will be related to its dopaminergic activity.

5. PHARMACOLOGICAL PROPERTIES

5.1 Pharmacodynamic properties

Ropinirole is a non-ergoline dopamine agonist.

Parkinson's disease is characterised by a marked dopamine deficiency in the nigral striatal system. Ropinirole alleviates this deficiency by stimulating striatal dopamine receptors.

Ropinirole acts in the hypothalamus and pituitary to inhibit the secretion of prolactin.

5.2 Pharmacokinetic properties

Oral absorption of ropinirole is rapid and essentially complete. Bioavailability of ropinirole is approximately 50% and average peak concentrations of the drug are achieved at a median time of 1.5 hours post-dose. Wide inter-individual variability in the pharmacokinetic parameters has been seen but, overall, there is a proportional increase in the systemic exposure (C_{max} and AUC) to the drug with an increase in dose, over the therapeutic dose range. Consistent with its high lipophilicity, ropinirole exhibits a large volume of distribution (approx. 8 l/kg) and is cleared from the systemic circulation with an average elimination half-life of about six hours. Plasma protein binding of the drug is low (10-40%). Ropinirole is metabolised primarily by oxidative metabolism and ropinirole and its metabolites are mainly excreted in the urine. The major metabolite is at least 100 times less potent than ropinirole in animal models of dopaminergic function.

No change in the oral clearance of ropinirole is observed following single and repeated oral administration. As expected for a drug being administered approximately every half life, there is, on average, two-fold higher steady-state plasma concentrations of ropinirole following the recommended t.i.d. regimen compared to those observed following a single oral dose.

5.3 Preclinical safety data

General toxicology: Ropinirole is well tolerated in laboratory animals in the dose range of 15 to 50 mg/kg. The toxicology profile is principally determined by the pharmacological activity of the drug (behavioural changes, hypoprolactinaemia, decrease in blood pressure and heart rate, ptosis and salivation).

Genotoxicity: Genotoxicity was not observed in a battery of in vitro and in vivo tests.

Carcinogenicity: Two-year studies have been conducted in the mouse and rat at dosages up to 50 mg/kg. The mouse study did not reveal any carcinogenic effect. In the rat, the only drug-related lesions were Leydig cell hyperplasia/adenoma in the testis resulting from the hypoprolactinaemic effect of ropinirole. These lesions are considered to be a species specific phenomenon and do not constitute a hazard with regard to the clinical use of ropinirole.

6. PHARMACEUTICAL PARTICULARS

6.1 List of excipients

Tablet cores: hydrous lactose, microcrystalline cellulose, croscarmellose sodium, magnesium stearate.

The five tablet strengths of ropinirole are distinguished by colour. The composition of the film coat therefore varies. All film coats contain hydroxypropyl methylcellulose and polyethylene glycol. The variations are shown in the table below:

(see Table 3)

6.2 Incompatibilities

None known

6.3 Shelf life

Two years

6.4 Special precautions for storage

This product should be stored in a dry place at or below 25°C and protected from light.

6.5 Nature and contents of container

Opaque PVC/PVdC or PVC/Aclar blister starter pack of 105. (Each pack contains 42 ReQuip 0.25mg tablets, 42 ReQuip 0.5mg tablets and 21 ReQuip 1mg tablets.)

Opaque PVC/PVdC or PVC/Aclar blister follow on pack of 147. (Each pack contains 42 ReQuip 0.5mg tablets, 42 Requip 1mg tablets, 63 Requip 2mg tablets.)

Tablets 1 mg, in 60 ml HPDE bottle of 84.

Tablets 2 mg, in 60 ml HPDE bottle of 84.

Tablets 5 mg, in 60 ml HPDE bottle of 84.

6.6 Instructions for use and handling

None

Administrative Data

7. MARKETING AUTHORISATION HOLDER

SmithKline Beecham plc

Trading as:

GlaxoSmithKline UK,

Stockley Park West,

Uxbridge,

Middlesex UB11 1BT

8. MARKETING AUTHORISATION NUMBER(S)

Requip Tablets 0.25 mg 10592/0085

Requip Tablets 0.5 mg 10592/0086

Requip Tablets 1 mg 10592/0087

Requip Tablets 2 mg 10592/0088

Requip Tablets 5 mg 10592/0089

9. DATE OF FIRST AUTHORISATION/RENEWAL OF THE AUTHORISATION

2nd July 1996

10. DATE OF REVISION OF THE TEXT

2nd August 2002

11. Legal Status

POM

Resonium A

(sanofi-aventis)

1. NAME OF THE MEDICINAL PRODUCT

Resonium A.

2. QUALITATIVE AND QUANTITATIVE COMPOSITION

Contains Sodium Polystyrene Sulphonate 99.934% w/w.

3. PHARMACEUTICAL FORM

Buff coloured powder.

4. CLINICAL PARTICULARS

4.1 Therapeutic indications

Resonium A is an ion-exchange resin that is recommended for the treatment of hyperkalaemia associated with anuria or severe oliguria. It is also used to treat hyperkalaemia in patients requiring dialysis and in patients on regular haemodialysis or on prolonged peritoneal dialysis.

4.2 Posology and method of administration

Resonium A is for oral or rectal administration only.

The dosage recommendations detailed in this section are a guide only; the precise requirements should be decided on the basis of regular serum electrolyte determinations.

Adults, including the elderly:

Oral

The usual dose is 15g, three or four times a day. The resin is given by mouth in a little water, or it may be made into a paste with some sweetened vehicle.

Rectal

In cases where vomiting may make oral administration difficult, the resin may be given rectally as a suspension of 30g resin in 100ml 2% methylcellulose 450 BP (medium viscosity) and 100ml water, as a daily retention enema. In the initial stages administration by this route as well as orally may help to achieve a more rapid lowering of the serum potassium level.

The enema should if possible be retained for at least nine hours following which the colon should be irrigated to remove the resin. If both routes are used initially it is probably unnecessary to continue rectal administration once the oral resin has reached the rectum.

Children:

Oral

1g/kg body weight daily in divided doses for acute hyperkalaemia. Dosage may be reduced to 0.5g/kg of body weight daily in divided doses for maintenance therapy.

The resin is given orally, preferably with a drink (not a fruit squash because of the high potassium content) or a little jam or honey.

Rectal

When refused by mouth it should be given rectally, using a dose at least as great as that which would have been given orally, diluted in the same ratio as described for adults.

Following retention of the enema, the colon should be irrigated to ensure adequate removal of the resin.

Neonates:

Resonium A should not be given by the oral route. With rectal administration, the minimum effective dosage within the range 0.5g/kg to 1g/kg should be employed diluted as for adults and with adequate irrigation to ensure recovery of the resin.

4.3 Contraindications

• In patients with plasma potassium levels below 5mmol/litre.

• History of hypersensitivity to polystyrene sulphonate resins.

• Obstructive bowel disease.

• Resonium A should not be administered ***orally*** to neonates and is contraindicated in neonates with reduced gut motility (post-operatively or drug-induced).

4.4 Special warnings and special precautions for use

Hypokalaemia: The possibility of severe potassium depletion should be considered, and adequate clinical and biochemical control is essential during treatment, especially in patients on digitalis. Administration of the resin should be stopped when the serum potassium falls to 5mmol/litre.

Other electrolyte disturbances: Because the resin may bind calcium and magnesium ions, deficiencies of these electrolytes may occur. Accordingly, patients should be monitored for all applicable electrolyte disturbances.

Other risks: In the event of clinically significant constipation, treatment should be discontinued until normal bowel movement has resumed. Magnesium-containing laxatives should not be used (see section 4.5 Interactions).

The patient should be positioned carefully when ingesting the resin, in order to avoid aspiration, which may lead to bronchopulmonary complications.

Children and neonates: In neonates, sodium polystyrene sulphonate should not be given by the oral route. In children and neonates particular care is needed with rectal administration as excessive dosage or inadequate dilution could result in impaction of the resin. Due to the risk of digestive haemorrhage or colonic necrosis, particular care should be observed in premature infants or low birth weight infants.

Patients at risk from an increase in sodium load: Care should be taken when administering to patients in whom an increase in sodium load may be detrimental (i.e. congestive heart failure, hypertension, renal damage or oedema). In such cases, Calcium Resonium (calcium polystyrene sulphonate) may be used in place of Resonium A.

4.5 Interaction with other medicinal products and other forms of Interaction

Concomitant use not recommended

Sorbitol (oral or rectal): Concomitant use of sorbitol with sodium polystyrene sulphonate may cause colonic necrosis. Therefore concomitant administration is not recommended.

To be used with caution

• Cation-donating agents: may reduce the potassium binding effectiveness of Resonium A.

• Non-absorbable cation-donating antacids and laxatives: There have been reports of systemic alkalosis following concurrent administration of cation-exchange resins and non-absorbable cation-donating antacids and laxatives such as magnesium hydroxide and aluminium carbonate.

• Aluminium hydroxide: Intestinal obstruction due to concretions of aluminium hydroxide has been reported when aluminium hydroxide has been combined with the resin.

• Digitalis-like drugs: The toxic effects of digitalis on the heart, especially various ventricular arrhythmias and A-V nodal dissociation, are likely to be exaggerated if hypokalaemia is allowed to develop. (see 4.4 Special warnings and special precautions for use).

• Lithium: Possible decrease of lithium absorption.

• Levothyroxine: Possible decrease of levothyroxine absorption.

4.6 Pregnancy and lactation

No data are available regarding the use of polystyrene sulphonate resins in pregnancy and lactation. The administration of Resonium A in pregnancy and during breast feeding therefore, is not advised unless, in the opinion of the physician, the potential benefits outweigh any potential risks.

4.7 Effects on ability to drive and use machines

There are no specific warnings.

4.8 Undesirable effects

In accordance with its pharmacological actions, the resin may give rise to sodium retention, hypokalaemia and hypocalcaemia and their related clinical manifestations (see Warnings and Precautions and Overdosage).

• **Gastrointestinal disorders**

Gastric irritation, anorexia, nausea, vomiting, constipation and occasionally diarrhoea may occur. Faecal impaction following rectal administration particularly in children, and gastrointestinal concretions (bezoars) following oral administration have been reported. Intestinal obstruction has also been reported although this has been extremely rare and, possibly, a reflection of co-existing pathology or inadequate dilution of resin.

Gastro-intestinal tract ulceration or necrosis which could lead to intestinal perforation have been reported following administration of sodium polystyrene sulphonate.

• **Respiratory disorders**

Some cases of acute bronchitis and/or bronco-pneumonia associated with inhalation of particles of sodium polystyrene sulphonate have been described.

4.9 Overdose

Biochemical disturbances from overdosage may give rise to clinical signs of symptoms of hypokalaemia, including irritability, confusion, delayed thought processes, muscle weakness, hyporeflexia and eventual paralysis. Apnoea may be a serious consequence of this progression. Electrocardiographic changes may be consistent with hypokalaemia; cardiac arrhythmia may occur. Hypocalcaemic tetany may occur. Appropriate measures should be taken to correct serum electrolytes and the resin should be removed from the alimentary tract by appropriate use of laxatives or enemas.

5. PHARMACOLOGICAL PROPERTIES

5.1 Pharmacodynamic properties

Resonium A is a cation exchange resin for the treatment of hyperkalaemia.

5.2 Pharmacokinetic properties

Ion exchange resins with a particle size ranging from 5 - 10 micrometres (as in Resonium A) are not absorbed from the gastro-intestinal tract and are wholly excreted in the faeces.

5.3 Preclinical safety data

There are no pre-clinical data of relevance to the prescriber which are additional to that already included in other sections of the SPC.

6. PHARMACEUTICAL PARTICULARS

6.1 List of excipients

Resonium A also contains: saccharin and vanillin.

6.2 Incompatibilities

There are no specific incompatibilities.

6.3 Shelf life

60 months.

6.4 Special precautions for storage

None stated.

6.5 Nature and contents of container

Supplied in HDPE containers with LDPE tamper evident closures containing 454g Resonium A together with a plastic scoop, which, when filled level, contains approximately 15g.

6.6 Instructions for use and handling

Refer to 4.2. Posology and method of administration.

7. MARKETING AUTHORISATION HOLDER

Sanofi-Synthelabo

PO Box 597

Guildford

Surrey

8. MARKETING AUTHORISATION NUMBER(S)

11723/0070

9. DATE OF FIRST AUTHORISATION/RENEWAL OF THE AUTHORISATION

2 April 2003

10. DATE OF REVISION OF THE TEXT

February 2005

Legal category: P

Respontin Nebules

(Allen & Hanburys)

1. NAME OF THE MEDICINAL PRODUCT

Respontin™ Nebules™

2. QUALITATIVE AND QUANTITATIVE COMPOSITION

1ml or 2ml plastic ampoules containing 0.25mg/ml of Ipratropium Bromide Ph.Eur.

3. PHARMACEUTICAL FORM

Oral inhalation solution via a nebuliser.

4. CLINICAL PARTICULARS

4.1 Therapeutic indications

Respontin Nebules are indicated for the treatment of reversible airways obstruction.

4.2 Posology and method of administration

The recommended dose is:

Adults: 0.4 to 2ml solution (100-500 micrograms) up to four times daily.

Children (3 to 14 years): 0.4 to 2ml solution (100-500 micrograms) up to three times daily.

The volume of ipratropium bromide solution may need to be diluted in order to obtain a final volume suitable for the particular nebuliser used. If dilution is necessary use only sterile sodium chloride 0.9% solution.

There is no specific information on the use of the isotonic nebuliser solution in the elderly. Clinical trials with the previously available hypotonic formulation included patients over 65 years and no adverse reactions specific to this age group were reported.

4.3 Contraindications

Known hypersensitivity to any components of the formulation or to atropine.

4.4 Special warnings and special precautions for use

Use of the nebuliser solution should be subject to close medical supervision during initial dosing. There have been rare reports of paradoxical bronchospasm associated with the administration of ipratropium bromide nebuliser solution. The patient should be advised to seek medical advice should a reduced response become apparent.

Patients must be instructed in the correct administration of Respontin Nebules and warned not to allow the solution or mist to enter the eyes. Acute angle-closure glaucoma has been reported rarely when ipratropium bromide has been used in conjunction with nebulised β_2-agonist bronchodilators. Protection of the eyes appears to prevent any increase in intra-ocular pressure and patients who may be susceptible to glaucoma should be warned specifically of the need for ocular protection. Inhaled doses of ipratropium bromide up to 1mg have not been associated with elevation of intra-ocular pressure.

Use anticholinergic agents with caution in patients with prostatic hypertrophy.

4.5 Interaction with other medicinal products and other forms of Interaction

There is evidence that the concurrent administration of ipratropium bromide and sympathomimetic drugs produces a greater relief of bronchospasm than either drug given alone. Ipratropium bromide has been shown to produce effective bronchodilatation in patients receiving β-adrenergic blocking agents.

4.6 Pregnancy and lactation

Ipratropium bromide has been in general use for several years and there is no definite evidence of ill-consequence during pregnancy. Animal studies have shown no hazard. Nevertheless, medicines should not be used in pregnancy, especially during the first trimester, unless the expected benefit is thought to outweigh any possible risk to the fetus.

4.7 Effects on ability to drive and use machines

None stated.

4.8 Undesirable effects

Anticholinergic side-effects are unlikely at therapeutic doses, but some patients may experience a dry mouth. Urinary retention and constipation have only rarely been reported with ipratropium bromide. There is no evidence that in the therapeutic dose range, ipratropium bromide has any adverse effect on bronchial secretion.

4.9 Overdose

Inhaled doses of 5mg produce an increase in heart rate and palpitation but single doses at 2mg have been given to adults and 1mg to children without causing side-effects. Single doses of ipratropium bromide 30mg by mouth cause anticholinergic side effects but these are not severe and do not require specific reversal.

5. PHARMACOLOGICAL PROPERTIES

5.1 Pharmacodynamic properties

Ipratropium bromide is an anticholinergic bronchodilater which affects airways function primarily through its neural effects on the parasympathetic nervous system. Ipratropium bromide blocks the acetylcholine receptors on smooth muscle in the lung. Stimulation of these receptors normally produces contraction and depending on the degree of activation, bronchoconstriction. Thus ipratropium bromide will cause bronchodilatation.

5.2 Pharmacokinetic properties

Ipratropium bromide is a quaternary ammonium compound which is poorly absorbed from the gastro-intestinal tract, and is slow to cross mucous membranes and the blood/brain barrier. Following, inhalation, uptake into the plasma is minimal, a peak blood concentration is obtained 1½ to 3 hours after inhalation. Excretion is chiefly via the kidneys.

5.3 Preclinical safety data
There are no pre-clinical data of relevance to the prescriber which are additional to that already included in other sections of the SmPC.

6. PHARMACEUTICAL PARTICULARS

6.1 List of excipients

Sodium Chloride	Ph.Eur
Diluted Phosphoric Acid	Ph.Eur
Purified Water	Ph.Eur

6.2 Incompatibilities
None stated.

6.3 Shelf life
24 months.

6.4 Special precautions for storage
Store below 25°C. Protect from light.

This product contains no preservative. A new Nebule should be used for each dose. A Nebule should be opened immediately before administration and any remaining solution should be discarded. Any unused Nebules should be discarded four weeks after opening the foil pack.

6.5 Nature and contents of container
1 or 2 ml low density polyethylene ampoules in boxes of 20 in strips of 5 or 10.

6.6 Instructions for use and handling
The nebulised solution may be inhaled through a face mask, T-piece or via an endotracheal tube. Intermittent positive pressure ventilation (IPPV) may be used but is rarely necessary. When there is a risk of anoxia through hypoventilation, oxygen should be added to the inspired air.

As many nebulisers operate on a continuous flow basis, it is likely that some nebulised drug will be released into the local environment. Ipratropium bromide should therefore be administered in a well-ventilated room, particularly in hospitals where several patients may be using nebulisers at the same time. Do not allow the solution or mist to enter the eyes.

Administrative Data

7. MARKETING AUTHORISATION HOLDER
Glaxo Wellcome UK Limited, trading as Allen & Hanburys,
Stockley Park West,
Uxbridge,
Middlesex,
UB11 1BT.

8. MARKETING AUTHORISATION NUMBER(S)
PL10949/0275

9. DATE OF FIRST AUTHORISATION/RENEWAL OF THE AUTHORISATION
15th April 2003

10. DATE OF REVISION OF THE TEXT
September 1997

11. Legal Status
POM.

Retin-A Cream 0.025%

(Janssen-Cilag Ltd)

1. NAME OF THE MEDICINAL PRODUCT
RETIN-A® 0.025% Cream

2. QUALITATIVE AND QUANTITATIVE COMPOSITION
Tretinoin 0.025% w/w

3. PHARMACEUTICAL FORM
Cream

4. CLINICAL PARTICULARS

4.1 Therapeutic indications
Acne vulgaris.

Retin-A® Cream is suitable for use on dry skin.

4.2 Posology and method of administration
For cutaneous use.

RETIN-A should be applied once or twice daily to the area of skin where the acne lesions occur.

Only apply sufficient to cover the affected areas lightly, using a gauze swab, cotton wool or the tips of clean fingers. Avoid over-saturation to the extent that excess medication could run into the eyes, angles of the nose or other areas where treatment is not intended.

Initial application may cause transitory stinging and a feeling of warmth. The correct frequency of administration should produce a slight erythema similar to that of mild sunburn.

If RETIN-A is applied excessively, no more rapid or better results will be obtained and marked redness, peeling or discomfort may occur. Should this occur accidentally or through over enthusiastic use, application should be discontinued for a few days.

Patience is needed in this treatment, since the therapeutic effects will not usually be observed until after 6-8 weeks of treatment. During the early weeks of treatment, an apparent exacerbation of inflammatory lesions may occur. This is due to the action of the medication on deep, previously unseen comedones and papules.

Once the acne lesions have responded satisfactorily, it should be possible to maintain the improvement with less frequent applications.

Moisturisers and cosmetics may be used during treatment with RETIN-A but should not be applied to the skin at the same time. The skin should be thoroughly washed before application of RETIN-A. Astringent toiletries should be avoided.

4.3 Contraindications
RETIN-A® Cream is contraindicated in patients with:

- A history of sensitivity/hypersensitivity reactions to any of the components
- Pregnancy
- Personal or familial history of cutaneous epithelioma
- Acute eczemas (as tretinoin has been reported to cause severe irritation on eczematous skin)
- Rosacea and perioral dermatitis.

4.4 Special warnings and special precautions for use
<u>Local irritation</u>
The presence of cutaneous irritative signs (eg erythema, peeling, pruritus, sunburn, etc) should prohibit initiation or recommencement of treatment with RETIN-A until the symptoms resolve.

In certain sensitive individuals, topical use may induce severe local erythema, swelling, pruritus, warmth, burning or stinging, blistering, crusting and/or peeling at the site of application. If the degree of local irritation warrants, the patient should be directed to apply the medication less frequently or discontinue its use temporarily. If a patient experiences severe or persistent irritation, the patient should be advised to discontinue application of RETIN-A completely and, if necessary, consult a physician.

Weather extremes, such as wind or cold, also may be irritating to patients being treated with RETIN-A.

<u>Exposure to sunlight</u>
Exposure to sunlight, including ultraviolet sunlamps, should be avoided or minimised during the use of tretinoin. Patients with sunburn should be advised not to use the product until fully recovered because of potential severe irritation to skin. A patient who experiences considerable sun exposure due to occupational duties and/or anyone inherently sensitive to the sun should exercise particular caution. When exposure to sunlight cannot be avoided, use of sunscreen products and protective clothing over treated areas is recommended.

<u>General precautions for use:</u>
Before application of RETIN-A, areas to be treated should be cleansed thoroughly.

Abstain from washing the treated area frequently: twice daily is sufficient. Use of mild soap is recommended. Dry skin without rubbing.

Avoid contact with eyes, eyelids, nostrils, mouth and mucous membranes. If contact in these areas occurs, careful washing with water is recommended.

<u>Warning</u>
The weight of evidence indicates that topical tretinoin is not carcinogenic. In a lifetime study of CD-1 mice, a low incidence of skin tumours was seen at 100 and 200 times the estimated clinical dose but, although no such tumours were seen in the study controls, the incidence in these treated animals was within the historic control range for CD-1 mice. Studies in hairless albino mice suggest that tretinoin may accelerate the tumorigenic potential of UVB light from a solar simulator. In other studies, when lightly pigmented hairless mice treated with tretinoin were exposed to carcinogenic doses of UVB light, photocarcinogenic effects of tretinoin were not observed. Due to significantly different experimental conditions, no strict comparison of these disparate data is possible. Although the significance of these studies in man is not clear, patients should avoid or minimise exposure to sunlight.

The weight of evidence indicates that topical tretinoin is not mutagenic. The mutagenic potential of tretinoin was evaluated in the Ames assay and the *in vivo* mouse micronucleus assay, both of which showed negative findings.

4.5 Interaction with other medicinal products and other forms of Interaction
RETIN-A should be used with caution in the presence of:

– concomitant topical medications

– toiletry preparations having a strong drying, abrasive or desquamative effect.

Following prolonged use of a peeling agent it is advisable to "rest" a patient's skin until the effects of the peeling agent subside before use of RETIN-A is begun. When RETIN-A and peeling agents are alternated, contact dermatitis may result and the frequency of application may have to be reduced.

4.6 Pregnancy and lactation
The topical human dose used in a 50 kg adult applying a maximum volume of 500 mg of 0.05% RETIN-A cream is 0.005 mg/kg. In animal reproductive studies, oral tretinoin is known to be teratogenic and has been shown to be foetotoxic in rats when given in doses 500 times the topical human dose. In reproduction studies in rats and rabbits, topical tretinoin, when used at doses 500 and 320 times the topical human dose, respectively, induced minor skeletal abnormalities, eg irregularly contoured or partially ossified skull bones. These changes may be considered variants of normal development and are usually corrected after weaning. RETIN-A should not be used during pregnancy.

It is not known whether tretinoin is excreted in human milk, therefore caution should be exercised when RETIN-A is administered to a nursing mother.

4.7 Effects on ability to drive and use machines
RETIN-A is administered topically and is unlikely to have an effect on one's ability to drive or operate machinery.

4.8 Undesirable effects
Local reactions frequently reported during therapy included: dry or peeling skin, burning, stinging, warmth, erythema, pruritus, rash and temporary hypo- and hyper-pigmentation. These skin reactions were usually mild to moderate and were generally well-tolerated. They usually occurred early in therapy and, except for dry or peeling skin which persisted during therapy, generally decreased over the course of therapy. Rarely reported undesirable effects are blistering and crusting of the skin, eye irritation and oedema.

True contact allergy to topical tretinoin is rarely encountered. Heightened susceptibility to either sunlight or other sources of UVB light has been reported.

4.9 Overdose
Excessive application of RETIN-A does not improve the results of treatment and may induce marked irritation, e.g., erythema, peeling, pruritus, etc. Oral ingestion of RETIN-A may lead to the same effects associated with excessive oral intake of Vitamin A (eg pruritus, dry skin, arthralgias, anorexia, vomiting). In the event of accidental ingestion, if the ingestion is recent, an appropriate method of gastric emptying should be used as soon as possible.

5. PHARMACOLOGICAL PROPERTIES

5.1 Pharmacodynamic properties
Tretinoin (β-*all trans* retinoic acid, Vitamin A acid) produces profound metabolic changes in keratinising epithelia. Tretinoin increases the proliferative activity of epidermal cells in *in vivo* and *in vitro* studies, and cellular differentiation (keratinisation and cornification) is also altered.

5.2 Pharmacokinetic properties
Topical administration of RETIN-A products produces dose-dependent erythema, peeling and irritation, and excessive use of the products should be avoided. 0.1% w/w RETIN-A did not produce an allergic response when tested in 160 subjects by the Draize test. The percutaneous absorption of 0.1% w/w ^{14}C labelled retinoic acid was studied in 6 adult male volunteers; between 0.3% and 2.18% of the retinoic acid was absorbed through the skin following a single topical application of the ^{14}C retinoic acid formulation. No systemic toxic effects have been reported following topical application of RETIN-A formulations.

5.3 Preclinical safety data
No relevant information other than that contained elsewhere in the Summary of Product Characteristics.

6. PHARMACEUTICAL PARTICULARS

6.1 List of excipients
Butylated hydroxytoluene
Isopropyl myristate
Polyoxyl 40 stearate
Sorbic acid
Stearic acid
Stearyl alcohol
Xanthan gum
Purified water

6.2 Incompatibilities
Avoid or minimise exposure of RETIN-A treated areas to sunlight or sunlamps during the course of treatment.

6.3 Shelf life
24 months.

6.4 Special precautions for storage
Do not store above 25°C.

6.5 Nature and contents of container
Aluminium tube lined with epoxy resin or epoxy resin with wax. Tube cap of polyethylene or urea resin.

Available in tube sizes of: 10 g, 15 g, 20 g and 60 g

(Not all pack sizes are marketed.)

6.6 Instructions for use and handling
Not applicable

7. MARKETING AUTHORISATION HOLDER
Janssen-Cilag Ltd
Saunderton
High Wycombe
Buckinghamshire
HP14 4HJ
UK

8. MARKETING AUTHORISATION NUMBER(S)
PL 00242/0266

9. DATE OF FIRST AUTHORISATION/RENEWAL OF THE AUTHORISATION
2 October 1998 / 21 May 2003

10. DATE OF REVISION OF THE TEXT
Legal category POM

Retin-A Gel 0.01%

(Janssen-Cilag Ltd)

1. NAME OF THE MEDICINAL PRODUCT
Retin-A™ Gel 0.01%.

2. QUALITATIVE AND QUANTITATIVE COMPOSITION
Tretinoin 0.01% w/w.

3. PHARMACEUTICAL FORM
Gel.

4. CLINICAL PARTICULARS
4.1 Therapeutic indications
Treatment of acne vulgaris. Suitable for use on oily skin.

4.2 Posology and method of administration
Retin-A should be applied once or twice daily to the area of skin where acne lesions occur.

Only apply sufficient to cover the affected areas lightly, using a gauze swab, cotton wool or the tips of clean fingers. Avoid over-saturation to the extent that excess medication could run into the eyes, angles of the nose or other areas where treatment is not intended.

Initial application may cause transitory stinging and a feeling of warmth. The correct frequency of administration should produce a slight erythema similar to that of mild sunburn.

If Retin-A is applied excessively, no more rapid or better results will be obtained and marked redness, peeling or discomfort may occur. Should this occur accidentally or through over enthusiastic use, application should be discontinued for a few days.

Patience is needed in this treatment, since the therapeutic effects will not usually be observed until after 6- 8 weeks of treatment. During the early weeks of treatment, an apparent exacerbation of inflammatory lesions may occur. This is due to the action of the medication on deep, previously unseen comedones and papules.

Once the acne lesions have responded satisfactorily, it should be possible to maintain the improvement with less frequent applications.

Moisturisers and cosmetics may be used during treatment with Retin-A but should not be applied to the skin at the same time. The skin should be thoroughly washed before application of Retin-A. Astringent toiletries should be avoided.

Method of administration

For cutaneous administration

4.3 Contraindications
RETIN-A® Gel is contraindicated in patients with:

- A history of sensitivity/hypersensitivity reactions to any of the components

- Pregnancy

- Personal or familial history of cutaneous epithelioma

- Acute eczemas (as tretinoin has been reported to cause severe irritation on eczematous skin)

- Rosacea and perioral dermatitis.

4.4 Special warnings and special precautions for use
Local irritation

The presence of cutaneous irritative signs (eg erythema, peeling, pruritus, sunburn, etc) should prohibit initiation or recommencement of treatment with Retin-A until the symptoms resolve.

In certain sensitive individuals, topical use may induce severe local erythema, swelling, pruritus, warmth, burning or stinging, blistering, crusting and/or peeling at the site of application. If the degree of local irritation warrants, the patient should be directed to apply the medication less frequently or discontinue its use temporarily. If a patient experiences severe or persistent irritation, the patient should be advised to discontinue application of Retin-A completely and, if necessary, consult a physician.

Weather extremes, such as wind or cold, also may be irritating to patients being treated with Retin-A.

Exposure to sunlight
Exposure to sunlight, including ultraviolet sunlamps, should be avoided or minimised during the use of tretinoin. Patients with sunburn should be advised not to use the product until fully recovered because of potential severe irritation to skin. A patient who experiences considerable sun exposure due to occupational duties and/or anyone inherently sensitive to the sun should exercise particular caution. When exposure to sunlight cannot be avoided, use of sunscreen products and protective clothing over treated areas is recommended.

General precautions for use

Before application of Retin-A, areas to be treated should be cleansed thoroughly.

Abstain from washing the treated area frequently: twice daily is sufficient. Use of mild soap is recommended. Dry skin without rubbing.

Avoid contact with eyes, eyelids, nostrils, mouth and mucous membranes. If contact in these areas occurs, careful washing with water is recommended.

Warning

The weight of evidence indicates that topical tretinoin is not carcinogenic. In a lifetime study of CD-1 mice, a low incidence of skin tumours was seen at 100 and 200 times the estimated clinical dose but, although no such tumours were seen in the study controls, the incidence in these treated animals was within the historic control range for CD-1 mice.

Studies in hairless albino mice suggest that tretinoin may accelerate the tumorigenic potential of UVB light from a solar simulator. In other studies, when lightly pigmented hairless mice treated with tretinoin were exposed to carcinogenic doses of UVB light, the photocarcinogenic effects of tretinoin were not observed. Due to significantly different experimental conditions, no strict comparison of this disparate data is possible. Although the significance of these studies in man is not clear, patients should avoid or minimise exposure to sunlight.

The weight of evidence indicates that topical tretinoin is not mutagenic. The mutagenic potential of tretinoin was evaluated in the Ames assay and the *in vivo* mouse micronucleus assay, both of which showed negative findings.

4.5 Interaction with other medicinal products and other forms of Interaction
Retin-A should be used with caution in the presence of:

– concomitant topical medications

– toiletry preparations having a strong drying, abrasive or desquamative effect.

Following prolonged use of a peeling agent it is advisable to 'rest' a patient's skin until the effects of the peeling agent subside before the use of Retin-A is begun. When Retin-A and peeling agents are alternated contact dermatitis may result and the frequency of application may have to be reduced.

4.6 Pregnancy and lactation
The topical human dose used in a 50 kg adult applying a maximum volume of 500 mg of 0.05% Retin-A cream is 0.005 mg/kg. In animal reproductive studies, oral tretinoin is known to be teratogenic and has been shown to be foetotoxic in rats when given in doses 500 times the topical human dose. In reproduction studies in rats and rabbits, topical tretinoin, when used at doses 500 and 320 times the topical human dose, respectively, induced minor skeletal abnormalities, eg irregularly contoured or partially ossified skull bones. These changes may be considered variants of normal development and are usually corrected after weaning. Retin-A should not be used during pregnancy.

It is not known whether tretinoin is excreted in human milk, therefore caution should be exercised when Retin-A is administered to a nursing mother.

4.7 Effects on ability to drive and use machines
Retin-A is administered topically and is unlikely to have an effect on one's ability to drive or operate machinery.

4.8 Undesirable effects
Local reactions frequently reported during therapy included: dry or peeling skin, burning, stinging, warmth, erythema, pruritus, rash and temporary hypo- and hyperpigmentation. These skin reactions were usually mild to moderate and were generally well-tolerated. They usually occurred early in therapy and, except for dry or peeling skin which persisted during therapy, generally decreased over the course of therapy.

Rarely reported undesirable effects are blistering and crusting of the skin, eye irritation and oedema.

True contact allergy to topical tretinoin is rarely encountered. Heightened susceptibility to either sunlight or other sources of UVB light has been reported.

4.9 Overdose
Excessive application of Retin-A does not improve the results of treatment and may induce marked irritation, eg erythema, peeling, pruritus, etc. Oral ingestion of Retin-A may lead to the same effects associated with excessive oral intake of vitamin A (eg pruritus, dry skin, arthralgias, anorexia, vomiting). In the event of accidental ingestion, if the ingestion is recent an appropriate method of gastric emptying should be used as soon as possible.

5. PHARMACOLOGICAL PROPERTIES
5.1 Pharmacodynamic properties
Tretinoin (*β-all trans* retinoic acid, vitamin A acid) produces profound metabolic changes in keratinizing epithelia. Tretinoin increases the proliferative activity of epidermal cells in *in vivo* and *in vitro* studies, and cellular differentiation (keratinization and cornification) is also altered.

5.2 Pharmacokinetic properties
Topical administration of Retin-A products produces dose-dependent erythema, peeling and irritation and excessive use of the products should be avoided. Retin-A 0.1% w/w did not produce an allergic response when tested in 160 subjects by the Draize test. The percutaneous absorption of 0.1% w/w C^{14} labelled retinoic acid was studied in 6 adult male volunteers; between 0.3% and 2.18% of the retinoic acid was absorbed through the skin following a single topical application of the ^{14}C retinoic acid formulation. No systemic toxic effects have been reported following topical application of Retin-A formulations.

5.3 Preclinical safety data
See Sections 4.4 (Special warnings and precautions) and 4.6 (Pregnancy and lactation).

6. PHARMACEUTICAL PARTICULARS
6.1 List of excipients
Butylated hydroxytoluene

Hydroxypropyl cellulose

Undenatured ethanol

6.2 Incompatibilities
Avoid or minimise exposure of Retin-A areas to sunlight or sunlamps during the course of treatment.

6.3 Shelf life
36 months.

6.4 Special precautions for storage
Do not store above 25°C.

6.5 Nature and contents of container
Aluminium tube lined with epoxy resin or epoxy resin with wax. Tube cap of polyethylene or urea resin.

Aluminium tube may contain 20 or 60 gm of gel per pack.

(Not all pack sizes are marketed.)

6.6 Instructions for use and handling
Not applicable.

7. MARKETING AUTHORISATION HOLDER
Janssen-Cilag Ltd

Saunderton

High Wycombe

Buckinghamshire

HP14 4HJ

UK

8. MARKETING AUTHORISATION NUMBER(S)
PL 00242/0265

9. DATE OF FIRST AUTHORISATION/RENEWAL OF THE AUTHORISATION
1 September 1995/ November 2004

10. DATE OF REVISION OF THE TEXT
Legal category POM.

Retin-A Gel 0.025%

(Janssen-Cilag Ltd)

1. NAME OF THE MEDICINAL PRODUCT
RETIN-A™ Gel 0.025% w/w

2. QUALITATIVE AND QUANTITATIVE COMPOSITION
Tretinoin BP 0.025% w/w

3. PHARMACEUTICAL FORM
Gel.

4. CLINICAL PARTICULARS
4.1 Therapeutic indications
Treatment of acne vulgaris.

Retin-A® Gel is suitable for use on oily skin.

4.2 Posology and method of administration
Retin-A should be applied once or twice daily to the area of skin where acne lesions occur.

Only apply sufficient to cover the affected areas lightly, using a gauze swab, cotton wool or the tips of clean fingers. Avoid over-saturation to the extent that excess medication could run into the eyes, angles of the nose or other areas where treatment is not intended.

Initial application may cause transitory stinging and a feeling of warmth. The correct frequency of administration should produce a slight erythema similar to that of mild sunburn.

If Retin-A is applied excessively, no more rapid or better results will be obtained and marked redness, peeling or discomfort may occur. Should this occur accidentally or through over enthusiastic use, application should be discontinued for a few days.

Patience is needed in this treatment, since the therapeutic effects will not usually be observed until after 6- 8 weeks of treatment. During the early weeks of treatment, an apparent exacerbation of inflammatory lesions may occur. This is due to the action of the medication on deep, previously unseen comedones and papules.

Once the acne lesions have responded satisfactorily, it should be possible to maintain the improvement with less frequent applications.

Moisturisers and cosmetics may be used during treatment with Retin-A but should not be applied to the skin at the same time. The skin should be thoroughly washed before application of Retin-A. Astringent toiletries should be avoided.

Method of Administration

Cutaneous use.

4.3 Contraindications

Retin-A is contraindicated in patients with:

- A history of sensitivity/hypersensitivity reactions to any of the components
- Pregnancy
- Personal or familial history of cutaneous epithelioma
- Acute eczemas (as tretinoin has been reported to cause severe irritation on eczematous skin)
- Rosacea and perioral dermatitis.

4.4 Special warnings and special precautions for use

Local irritation

The presence of cutaneous irritative signs (eg erythema, peeling, pruritus, sunburn etc) should prohibit initiation or recommencement of treatment with Retin-A until the symptoms resolve.

In certain sensitive individuals, topical use may induce severe local erythema, swelling, pruritus, warmth, burning or stinging, blistering, crusting and/or peeling at the site of application. If the degree of local irritation warrants, the patient should be directed to apply the medication less frequently or discontinue its use temporarily. If a patient experiences severe or persistent irritation, the patient should be advised to discontinue application of Retin-A completely and, if necessary, consult a physician.

Weather extremes, such as wind or cold, also may be irritating to patients being treated with Retin-A.

Exposure to sunlight, including ultraviolet sunlamps, should be avoided or minimised during the use of tretinoin. Patients with sunburn should be advised not to use the product until fully recovered because of potential severe irritation to skin. A patient who experiences considerable sun exposure due to occupational duties and/or anyone inherently sensitive to the sun should exercise particular caution. When exposure to sunlight cannot be avoided, use of sunscreen products and protective clothing over treated areas is recommended.

General precautions for use:

Before application of Retin-A, areas to be treated should be cleansed thoroughly.

Abstain from washing the treated area frequently: twice daily is sufficient. Use of mild soap is recommended. Dry skin without rubbing.

Avoid contact with eyes, eyelids, nostrils, mouth and mucous membranes. If contact in these areas occurs, careful washing with water is recommended.

Warning:

The weight of evidence indicates that topical tretinoin is not carcinogenic. In a lifetime study of CD-1 mice, a low incidence of skin tumours was seen at 100 and 200 times the estimated clinical dose but, although no such tumours were seen in the study controls, the incidence in these treated animals was within the historic control range for CD-1 mice.

Studies in hairless albino mice suggest that tretinoin may accelerate the tumorigenic potential of UVB light from a solar simulator. In other studies, when lightly pigmented hairless mice treated with tretinoin were exposed to carcinogenic doses of UVB light, the photocarcinogenic effects of tretinoin were not observed. Due to significantly different experimental conditions, no strict comparison of this disparate data is possible. Although the significance of these studies in man is not clear, patients should avoid or minimise exposure to sunlight.

The weight of evidence indicates that topical tretinoin is not mutagenic. The mutagenic potential of tretinoin was evaluated in the Ames assay and the *in-vivo* mouse micronucleus assay, both of which showed negative findings.

4.5 Interaction with other medicinal products and other forms of Interaction

Retin-A should be used with caution in the presence of:

– concomitant topical medications

– toiletry preparations having a strong drying, abrasive or desquamative effect.

Following prolonged use of a peeling agent it is advisable to 'rest' a patients skin until the effects of the peeling agent subside before the use of Retin-A is begun. When Retin-A and peeling agents are alternated contact dermatitis may result and the frequency of application may have to be reduced.

4.6 Pregnancy and lactation

The topical human dose used in a 50 kg adult applying a maximum volume of 500 mg of 0.05% Retin-A cream is 0.005 mg/kg. In animal reproductive studies, oral tretinoin is known to be teratogenic and has been shown to be foetotoxic in rats when given in doses 500 times the topical human dose. In reproduction studies in rats and rabbits, topical tretinoin, when used at doses 500 and 320 times the topical human dose, respectively, induced minor skeletal abnormalities, eg irregularly contoured or partially ossified skull bones. These changes may be considered variants of normal development and are usually corrected after weaning. Retin-A should not be used during pregnancy.

It is not known whether tretinoin is excreted in human milk, therefore caution should be exercised when Retin-A is administered to a nursing mother.

4.7 Effects on ability to drive and use machines

Retin-A is administered topically and is unlikely to have an effect on one's ability to drive or operate machinery.

4.8 Undesirable effects

Local reactions frequently reported during therapy included: dry or peeling skin, burning, stinging, warmth, erythema, pruritus, rash and temporary hypo- and hyperpigmentation. These skin reactions were usually mild to moderate and were generally well-tolerated. They usually occurred early in therapy and, except for dry or peeling skin which persisted during therapy, generally decreased over the course of therapy.

Rarely reported undesirable effects are blistering and crusting of the skin, eye irritation and oedema.

True contact allergy to topical tretinoin is rarely encountered. Heightened susceptibility to either sunlight or other sources of UVB light has been reported.

4.9 Overdose

Excessive application of Retin-A does not improve the results of treatment and may induce marked irritation, e.g., erythema, peeling, pruritus etc. Oral ingestion of Retin-A may lead to the same effects associated with excessive oral intake of vitamin A (eg pruritus, dry skin, arthralgias, anorexia, vomiting). In the event of accidental ingestion, if the ingestion is recent an appropriate method of gastric emptying should be used as soon as possible.

5. PHARMACOLOGICAL PROPERTIES

5.1 Pharmacodynamic properties

Tretinoin (β-All trans retinoic acid, vitamin A acid) produces profound metabolic changes in keratinizing epithelia. Tretinoin increases the proliferative activity of epidermal cells in *in vivo* and *in vitro* studies, and cellular differentiation (keratinization and cornification) is also altered.

5.2 Pharmacokinetic properties

Topical administration of Retin-A products produces dose-dependent erythema, peeling and irritation and excessive use of the products should be avoided. Retin-A 0.025% w/w did not produce an allergic response when tested in 160 subjects by the Draize test. The percutaneous absorption of 0.1% w/w C^{14} labelled Retinoic Acid was studied in 6 adult male volunteers; between 0.3% and 2.18% of the retinoic acid was absorbed through the skin following a single topical application of the ^{14}C retinoic acid formulation. No systemic toxic effects have been reported following topical application of Retin-A formulations.

5.3 Preclinical safety data

See Sections 4.4 (Special warnings and precautions) and 4.6 (Pregnancy and lactation).

6. PHARMACEUTICAL PARTICULARS

6.1 List of excipients

Butylated hydroxytoluene

Hydroxypropyl cellulose

Undenatured ethanol

6.2 Incompatibilities

None known.

6.3 Shelf life

24 months.

6.4 Special precautions for storage

Do not store above 25°C.

6.5 Nature and contents of container

Aluminium tube lined with epoxy resin or epoxy resin with wax. Tube cap of polyethylene or urea resin.

Aluminium tube may contain 10, 15, 20 or 60 mg of gel per pack.

6.6 Instructions for use and handling

Not applicable.

7. MARKETING AUTHORISATION HOLDER

Janssen-Cilag Limited

Saunderton

High Wycombe

Buckinghamshire

HP14 4HJ

UK

8. MARKETING AUTHORISATION NUMBER(S)

PL 0242/0268

9. DATE OF FIRST AUTHORISATION/RENEWAL OF THE AUTHORISATION

1 September 1995/21 May 2003

10. DATE OF REVISION OF THE TEXT

26 August 2004

Legal category POM.

Retin-A Lotion

(Janssen-Cilag Ltd)

1. NAME OF THE MEDICINAL PRODUCT

RETIN-A® Lotion

2. QUALITATIVE AND QUANTITATIVE COMPOSITION

Tretinoin 0.025 w/w.

3. PHARMACEUTICAL FORM

Cutaneous solution

4. CLINICAL PARTICULARS

4.1 Therapeutic indications

Acne vulgaris. Suitable for use on very oily skin.

4.2 Posology and method of administration

For cutaneous use.

RETIN-A should be applied once or twice daily to the area of skin where the acne lesions occur.

Only apply sufficient to cover the affected areas lightly, using a gauze swab, cotton wool or the tips of clean fingers. Avoid over-saturation to the extent that excess medication could run into the eyes, angles of the nose or other areas where treatment is not intended.

Initial application may cause transitory stinging and a feeling of warmth. The correct frequency of administration should produce a slight erythema similar to that of mild sunburn.

If RETIN-A is applied excessively, no more rapid or better results will be obtained and marked redness, peeling or discomfort may occur. Should this occur accidentally or through over enthusiastic use, application should be discontinued for a few days.

Patience is needed in this treatment, since the therapeutic effects will not usually be observed until after 6-8 weeks of treatment. During the early weeks of treatment, an apparent exacerbation of inflammatory lesions may occur. This is due to the action of the medication on deep, previously unseen comedones and papules.

Once the acne lesions have responded satisfactorily, it should be possible to maintain the improvement with less frequent applications.

Moisturisers and cosmetics may be used during treatment with RETIN-A but should not be applied to the skin at the same time. The skin should be thoroughly washed before application of RETIN-A. Astringent toiletries should be avoided.

4.3 Contraindications

RETIN-A® Lotion is contraindicated in patients with:

- A history of sensitivity/hypersensitivity reactions to any of the components
- Pregnancy
- Personal or familial history of cutaneous epithelioma
- Acute eczemas (as tretinoin has been reported to cause severe irritation on eczematous skin)
- Rosacea and perioral dermatitis.

4.4 Special warnings and special precautions for use

Local irritation

The presence of cutaneous irritative signs (eg erythema, peeling, pruritus, sunburn, etc) should prohibit initiation or recommencement of treatment with RETIN-A until the symptoms resolve.

In certain sensitive individuals, topical use may induce severe local erythema, swelling, pruritus, warmth, burning or stinging, blistering, crusting and/or peeling at the site of application. If the degree of local irritation warrants, the patient should be directed to apply the medication less frequently or discontinue its use temporarily. If a patient experiences severe or persistent irritation, the patient should be advised to discontinue application of RETIN-A completely and, if necessary, consult a physician.

Weather extremes, such as wind or cold, also may be irritating to patients being treated with RETIN-A.

Exposure to sunlight

Exposure to sunlight, including ultraviolet sunlamps, should be avoided or minimised during the use of tretinoin. Patients with sunburn should be advised not to use the product until fully recovered because of potential severe irritation to skin. A patient who experiences considerable sun exposure due to occupational duties and/or anyone inherently sensitive to the sun should exercise particular caution. When exposure to sunlight cannot be avoided, use of sunscreen products and protective clothing over treated areas is recommended.

General precautions for use:

Before application of RETIN-A, areas to be treated should be cleansed thoroughly.

Abstain from washing the treated area frequently: twice daily is sufficient. Use of mild soap is recommended. Dry skin without rubbing.

Avoid contact with eyes, eyelids, nostrils, mouth and mucous membranes. If contact in these areas occurs, careful washing with water is recommended.

Warning

The weight of evidence indicates that topical tretinoin is not carcinogenic. In a lifetime study of CD-1 mice, a low incidence of skin tumours was seen at 100 and 200 times the estimated clinical dose but, although no such tumours were seen in the study controls, the incidence in these treated animals was within the historic control range for CD-1 mice. Studies in hairless albino mice suggest that tretinoin may accelerate the tumorigenic potential of UVB light from a solar simulator. In other studies, when lightly pigmented hairless mice treated with tretinoin were exposed to carcinogenic doses of UVB light, photocarcinogenic effects of tretinoin were not observed. Due to significantly different experimental conditions, no strict comparison of these disparate data is possible. Although the significance of these studies in man is not clear, patients should avoid or minimise exposure to sunlight.

The weight of evidence indicates that topical tretinoin is not mutagenic. The mutagenic potential of tretinoin was evaluated in the Ames assay and the *in vivo* mouse micronucleus assay, both of which showed negative findings.

4.5 Interaction with other medicinal products and other forms of Interaction
RETIN-A should be used with caution in the presence of:

- concomitant topical medications

- toiletry preparations having a strong drying, abrasive or desquamative effect.

Following prolonged use of a peeling agent it is advisable to 'rest' a patient's skin until the effects of the peeling agent subside before the use of RETIN-A is begun. When RETIN-A and peeling agents are alternated, contact dermatitis may result and the frequency of application may have to be reduced.

4.6 Pregnancy and lactation
The topical human dose used in a 50 kg adult applying a maximum volume of 500 mg of 0.5% RETIN-A cream is 0.005 mg/kg. In animal reproductive studies, oral tretinoin is known to be teratogenic and has been shown to be foetotoxic in rats when given in doses 500 times the typical human dose. In reproduction studies in rats and rabbits, topical tretinoin, when used at doses 500 and 320 times the topical human dose, respectively, induced minor skeletal abnormalities, eg irregularly contoured or partially ossified skull bones. These changes may be considered variants of normal development and are usually corrected after weaning. RETIN-A should not be used during pregnancy.

It is not known whether tretinoin is excreted in human milk, therefore caution should be exercised when RETIN-A is administered to a nursing mother.

4.7 Effects on ability to drive and use machines
RETIN-A is administered topically and is unlikely to have an effect on one's ability to drive or operate machinery.

4.8 Undesirable effects
Local reactions frequently reported during therapy included: dry or peeling skin, burning, stinging, warmth, erythema, pruritus, rash and temporary hypo- and hyper-pigmentation. These skin reactions were usually mild to moderate and were generally well-tolerated. They usually occurred early in therapy and, except for dry or peeling skin which persisted during therapy, generally decreased over the course of therapy. Rarely reported undesirable effects are blistering and crusting of the skin, eye irritation and oedema.
True contact allergy to topical tretinoin is rarely encountered. Heightened susceptibility to either sunlight or other sources of UVB light has been reported.

4.9 Overdose
Excessive application of RETIN-A does not improve the results of treatment and may induce marked irritation eg erythema, peeling, pruritus, etc. Oral ingestion of RETIN-A may lead to the same effects associated with excessive oral intake of Vitamin A (eg pruritus, dry skin, arthralgias, anorexia, vomiting). In the event of accidental ingestion, if the ingestion is recent, an appropriate method of gastric emptying should be used as soon as possible.

5. PHARMACOLOGICAL PROPERTIES
5.1 Pharmacodynamic properties
Tretinoin (β*-all trans* retinoic acid, Vitamin A acid) produces profound metabolic changes in keratinising epithelia, tretinoin increases the proliferative activity of epidermal cells in *in vivo* and *in vitro* studies, and cellular differentiation (keratinisation and cornification) is also altered.

5.2 Pharmacokinetic properties
Topical administration of RETIN-A products produces dose-dependent erythema, peeling and irritation, and excessive use of the products should be avoided. 0.1% RETIN-A did not produce an allergic response when tested in 160 subjects by the Draize test, the percutaneous absorption of 0.1% w/w ^{14}C labelled retinoic acid was studied in 6 adult male volunteers; between 0.3% and 2.18% of the retinoic acid was absorbed through the skin following a single topical application of the ^{14}C retinoic acid formulation. No systemic toxic effects have been reported following topical application of RETIN-A formulations.

5.3 Preclinical safety data
No relevant information other than that contained elsewhere in the Summary of Product Characteristics.

6. PHARMACEUTICAL PARTICULARS
6.1 List of excipients
Butylated hydroxytoluene

Ethanol pharma

Undenatured polyethylene glycol 400

6.2 Incompatibilities
Avoid or minimise exposure of RETIN-A treated areas to sunlight or sunlamps during the course of treatment.

6.3 Shelf life
24 months.

6.4 Special precautions for storage
Do not store above 25°C. Protect from light.

6.5 Nature and contents of container
80 ml and 100 ml amber glass bottles.

(Not all pack sizes are marketed.)

6.6 Instructions for use and handling
Not applicable

7. MARKETING AUTHORISATION HOLDER
Janssen-Cilag Limited

Saunderton

High Wycombe

Buckinghamshire

HP14 4HJ

UK

8. MARKETING AUTHORISATION NUMBER(S)
PL 00242/0269

9. DATE OF FIRST AUTHORISATION/RENEWAL OF THE AUTHORISATION
1st September 1995/ 2nd September 2003

10. DATE OF REVISION OF THE TEXT
Legal category POM

Retinova

(Janssen-Cilag Ltd)

1. NAME OF THE MEDICINAL PRODUCT
RETINOVA®

2. QUALITATIVE AND QUANTITATIVE COMPOSITION
RETINOVA® contains the active ingredient tretinoin 0.05% w/w in a water-in-oil emulsion for topical use only.

3. PHARMACEUTICAL FORM
Emollient Cream.

4. CLINICAL PARTICULARS
4.1 Therapeutic indications
For the topical treatment of mottled hyperpigmentation, roughness and fine wrinkling of photodamaged skin due to chronic sun exposure.

4.2 Posology and method of administration
Retinova should be applied to affected areas once at night daily. Only sufficient quantity to cover the areas lightly should be used. Application of Retinova may cause transitory stinging and a feeling of warmth. The correct frequency of administration normally produces a slight transient erythema similar to that of mild sunburn. No more rapid or better results will be obtained with excessive use of Retinova and local side effects such as redness, peeling or discomfort may occur. Should this occur treatment should be discontinued for a few days (See 4.4.1 Local Irritation).

Care should be taken to avoid contact with the eyes, nostrils, mouth or other areas where treatment is not intended.

Duration of Treatment: Improvements in the signs of photodamage with Retinova are not immediate but occur gradually over the course of therapy, hence patience is needed during this treatment. Onset of visible improvements varied across clinical studies, however, in general, effects emerged within 3-4 months of commencing treatment. Six months of treatment may be required before definite beneficial effects are seen.

Once the maximum beneficial effects have been achieved, they can be maintained with application of Retinova once to thrice weekly. If maintenance therapy is not used, the beneficial effect achieved will diminish over time.

Moisturisers and cosmetics may be used during treatment with Retinova but should not be applied to the skin at the same time. The skin should be thoroughly washed before application of Retinova (See 4.4 Special Warnings and Special Precautions for use). Patients should be advised on the importance of sun avoidance, use of sunscreens, moisturising products and protective clothing.

4.3 Contraindications
History of sensitivity/hypersensitivity reactions to any of the components, pregnancy, personal or familial history of cutaneous epithelioma.

4.4 Special warnings and special precautions for use
4.4.1. Local irritation:

The presence of cutaneous irritative signs (eg erythema, peeling, pruritus, sunburn, etc) should prohibit initiation or recommencement of treatment with Retinova until the symptoms resolve.

In certain sensitive individuals, topical use may induce severe local erythema, swelling, pruritus, warmth, burning or stinging, blistering, crusting and/or peeling at the site of application. If the degree of local irritation warrants, the patient should be directed to apply the medication less frequently or discontinue its use temporarily. If a patient experiences severe or persistent irritation, the patient should be advised to discontinue application of Retinova completely and, if necessary, consult a physician (see 4.2 Posology and Method of Administration).

Caution should be exercised during concomitant therapy with other local irritants, especially those having an abrasive, drying or desquamative effect (see 4.5 Interaction with Other Medicaments and other Forms of Interaction).

Weather extremes, such as wind or cold, also may be irritating to patients being treated with Retinova (also see 4.4.2 Exposure to Sunlight).

Tretinoin has been reported to cause severe irritation on eczematous skin and should be used with utmost caution in patients with this condition.

4.4.2 Exposure to sunlight:

Exposure to sunlight, including ultraviolet sunlamps, should be avoided or minimised during the use of tretinoin. Patients with sunburn should be advised not to use the product until fully recovered because of potential severe irritation to skin. A patient who experiences considerable sun exposure due to occupational duties and/or anyone inherently sensitive to the sun should exercise particular caution. When exposure to sunlight cannot be avoided, use of sunscreen products and protective clothing over treated areas is recommended.

4.4.3 General precautions for use:

Before application of Retinova, areas to be treated should be cleansed thoroughly.

Abstain from washing the treated area frequently: twice daily is sufficient. Use of a mild soap is recommended. Dry skin without rubbing.

Avoid contact with eyes, eyelids, nostrils, mouth and mucous membranes. If contact in these areas occurs, careful washing with water is recommended.

4.4.4 Warning:

The weight of evidence indicates that topical tretinoin is not carcinogenic. In a lifetime study of CD-1 mice, a low incidence of skin tumours was seen at 100 and 200 times the estimated clinical dose but, although no such tumours were seen in the study controls, the incidence in these treated animals was within the historic control range for CD-1 mice. Studies in hairless albino mice suggest that tretinoin may accelerate the tumorigenic potential of UVB light from a solar simulator. In other studies, when lightly pigmented hairless mice treated with tretinoin were exposed to carcinogenic doses of UVB light, the photocarcinogenic effects of tretinoin were not observed. Due to significantly different experimental conditions, no strict comparison of this disparate data is possible. Although the significance of these studies in man is not clear, patients should avoid or minimise exposure to sunlight (see 4.4.2 Exposure to Sunlight).

The weight of evidence indicates that topical tretinoin is not mutagenic. The mutagenic potential of tretinoin was evaluated in the Ames assay and the *in vivo* mouse micronucleus assay, both of which showed negative findings.

4.4.5 Paediatric Use:

Safety and effectiveness of Retinova in children have not been established.

4.5 Interaction with other medicinal products and other forms of Interaction
Use Retinova with caution in the presence of:

– concomitant topical medications;

– toiletry preparations having a strong drying, abrasive or desquamative effect.

4.6 Pregnancy and lactation
In clinical trials with Retinova, the topical human dose used in a 50 kg adult applying a maximum volume of 500 mg of 0.05% cream was 0.005 mg/kg. In animal reproductive studies, oral tretinoin is known to be teratogenic and has been shown to be foetotoxic in rats when given in doses 500 times the topical human dose. In reproduction studies in rats and rabbits, topical tretinoin, when used at doses 500 and 320 times the topical human dose, respectively, induced minor skeletal abnormalities, eg irregularly contoured or partially ossified skull bones. These changes may be considered variants of normal development and are usually corrected after weaning.

Retinova should not be used during pregnancy.

It is not known whether tretinoin is excreted in human milk, therefore caution should be exercised when Retinova is administered to a nursing mother.

4.7 Effects on ability to drive and use machines
Retinova is administered topically and is unlikely to have an effect on one's ability to drive or operate machinery.

4.8 Undesirable effects
Local reactions frequently reported during therapy included: dry or peeling skin, burning, stinging, warmth, erythema and pruritus and temporary hypo-pigmentation and hyper-pigmentation. These skin reactions were usually mild to moderate and were generally well-tolerated. They usually occurred early in therapy and, except for dry or peeling skin which persisted during therapy, generally decreased over the course of therapy (see 4.4.1 Local Irritation)

Clinical studies with Retinova showed no incidence of true allergic contact sensitivity. Heightened susceptibility to either sunlight or other sources of UVB light has been reported.

4.9 Overdose
Excessive application of Retinova does not improve the results of treatment and may induce marked irritation, eg erythema, peeling, pruritus, etc. Oral ingestion of Retinova may lead to the same side effects associated with excessive oral intake of vitamin A (eg pruritus, dry skin, arthralgias, anorexia, vomiting).

5. PHARMACOLOGICAL PROPERTIES

5.1 Pharmacodynamic properties
The mechanism of action of topical tretinoin as a treatment for photodamage is not completely understood. However, it is known that tretinoin activates gene transcription for many important proteins by binding to specific retinoid receptors in the cell nucleus. Studies employing light microscopy show an increase in Type 1 collagen, while ultrastructural studies show an increased number of anchoring fibrils in the papillary dermis of tretinoin-treated photodamaged skin. These molecular events, coupled with the characteristic histologic effects of tretinoin, ie increased epidermal and granular layer thickness with changes in stratum corneum morphology, indicate a specific effect rather than one induced by irritation, as has been previously suggested.

5.2 Pharmacokinetic properties
Upon topical application of Retinova, tretinoin penetrates both the epidermis and dermis. Percutaneous absorption of tretinoin in an emollient cream formulation was assessed in healthy male subjects after a single application and after repeated daily applications. The mean percutaneous absorption was less than 2% and endogenous concentrations of tretinoin and its major metabolites were unaltered.

5.3 Preclinical safety data
See Sections 4.4.4, 'Warning' and 4.6, 'Pregnancy and Lactation'.

6. PHARMACEUTICAL PARTICULARS

6.1 List of excipients
Light Mineral Oil
Sorbitol Solution (E420)
Hydroxyoctacosanyl Hydroxystearate
Methoxy PEG-22/Dodecyl Glycol Copolymer
PEG-45/Dodecyl Glycol Copolymer
Stearoxytrimethylsilane and Stearyl Alcohol
Dimethicone 50 cs
Fragrance
Methylparahydroxybenzoate (E218)
Edetate Disodium
Quaternium-15
Butylated Hydroxytoluene (E321)
Citric Acid (monohydrate)
Purified Water

6.2 Incompatibilities
None pertinent.

6.3 Shelf life
24 months.

6.4 Special precautions for storage
Store at or below 25°C (77°F). **DO NOT FREEZE.**

6.5 Nature and contents of container
Blind ended, lined aluminium tubes with opaque white polyethylene caps. Tubes will be supplied in 5, 15, 20, 30, 40 and 5 gm sizes.

6.6 Instructions for use and handling
Discard any remaining medicine upon completion of treatment.

7. MARKETING AUTHORISATION HOLDER
Janssen-Cilag Limited
Saunderton
High Wycombe
Buckinghamshire
HP14 4HJ

8. MARKETING AUTHORISATION NUMBER(S)
0242/0264

9. DATE OF FIRST AUTHORISATION/RENEWAL OF THE AUTHORISATION
15 January 1997 / 16 December 1999

10. DATE OF REVISION OF THE TEXT
16 December 1999

Legal category POM.

Retrovir 100 mg/10 ml, oral solution

(GlaxoSmithKline UK)

1. NAME OF THE MEDICINAL PRODUCT
Retrovir® 100 mg/10 ml, oral solution

2. QUALITATIVE AND QUANTITATIVE COMPOSITION
10 ml of solution contains:
Zidovudine 100 mg
For excipients see section 6.1

3. PHARMACEUTICAL FORM
Retrovir 100mg/10ml oral solution/syrup:

A clear, pale yellow, strawberry-flavoured, sugar-free oral solution.

The pack contains an oral-dosing syringe which should be fitted to the bottle before use.

4. CLINICAL PARTICULARS

4.1 Therapeutic indications
Retrovir oral formulations are indicated in anti-retroviral combination therapy for Human Immunodeficiency Virus (HIV) infected adults and children.

Retrovir chemoprophylaxis, is indicated for use in HIV-positive pregnant women (over 14 weeks of gestation) for prevention of maternal-foetal HIV transmission and for primary prophylaxis of HIV infection in newborn infants.

4.2 Posology and method of administration

Dosage in adults:
The usual recommended dose of Retrovir in combination with other anti-retroviral agents is 500 or 600 mg/day in two or three divided doses.

Dosage in children:
3 months - 12 years:

The recommended dose of Retrovir is 360 to 480 mg/m^2 per day, in 3 or 4 divided doses in combination with other antiretroviral agents. The maximum dosage should not exceed 200 mg every 6 hours.

<3 months:

The limited data available are insufficient to propose specific dosage recommendations (See below -maternal foetal transmission and section 5.2).

Dosage in the prevention of maternal-foetal transmission:
Although the optimal dosage schedule has not been identified the following dosage regimen has been shown to be effective. Pregnant women (over 14 weeks of gestation) should be given 500 mg/day orally (100 mg five times per day) until the beginning of labour. During labour and delivery Retrovir should be administered intravenously at 2 mg/kg bodyweight given over one hour followed by a continuous intravenous infusion at 1 mg/kg/h until the umbilical cord is clamped.

The newborn infants should be given 2 mg/kg bodyweight orally every 6 hours starting within 12 hours after birth and continuing until 6 weeks old (e.g. a 3 kg neonate would require a 0.6 ml dose of oral solution every 6 hours).

Due to the small volumes of oral solution required, care should be taken when calculating neonate doses. To facilitate dosing precision a 1 ml syringe is included in the neonate pack.

Infants unable to receive oral dosing should be given Retrovir intravenously at 1.5 mg/kg bodyweight infused over 30 minutes every 6 hours.

In case of planned caesarean, the infusion should be started 4 hours before the operation. In the event of a false labour, the Retrovir infusion should be stopped and oral dosing restarted.

Dosage adjustments in patients with haematological adverse reactions:
Dosage reduction or interruption of Retrovir therapy may be necessary in patients whose haemoglobin level falls to between 7.5 g/dl (4.65 mmol/l) and 9 g/dl (5.59 mmol/l) or whose neutrophil count falls to between 0.75 × 10^9/l and 1.0 × 10^9/l (see sections 4.3 and 4.4).

Dosage in the elderly:
Zidovudine pharmacokinetics have not been studied in patients over 65 years of age and no specific data are available. However, since special care is advised in this age group due to age-associated changes such as the decrease in renal function and alterations in haematological parameters, appropriate monitoring of patients before and during use of Retrovir is advised.

Dosage in renal impairment:
In patients with severe renal impairment, apparent zidovudine clearance after oral zidovudine administration was approximately 50% of that reported in healthy subjects with normal renal function. Therefore a dosage reduction to 300-400mg daily is recommended for patients with severe renal impairment with creatinine clearance -$\leq$ 10 ml/min. Haematological parameters and clinical response may influence the need for subsequent dosage adjustment.

Haemodialysis and peritoneal dialysis have no significant effect on zidovudine elimination whereas elimination of the glucuronide metabolite is increased.

Dosage in hepatic impairment:
Data in patients with cirrhosis suggest that accumulation of zidovudine may occur in patients with hepatic impairment because of decreased glucuronidation. Dosage reductions may be necessary but, as there is only limited data available, precise recommendations cannot be made. If monitoring of plasma zidovudine levels is not feasible, physicians will need to monitor for signs of intolerance, such as the development of haematological adverse reactions (anaemia, leucopenia, neutropenia) and reduce the dose and/or increase the interval between doses as appropriate (see section 4.4).

4.3 Contraindications
Retrovir Oral Formulations are contra-indicated in patients known to be hypersensitive to zidovudine, or to any of the components of the formulations.

Retrovir Oral Formulations should not be given to patients with abnormally low neutrophil counts (less than 0.75 × 10^9/litre) or abnormally low haemoglobin levels (less than 7.5 g/decilitre or 4.65 mmol/litre).

Retrovir is contra-indicated in new born infants with hyperbilirubinaemia requiring treatment other than phototherapy, or with increased transaminase levels of over five times the upper limit of normal.

4.4 Special warnings and special precautions for use
Retrovir is not a cure for HIV infection and patients remain at risk of developing illnesses which are associated with immune suppression, including opportunistic infections and neoplasms. Whilst it has been shown to reduce the risks of opportunistic infections, data on the development of neoplasms, including lymphomas, are limited. The available data on patients treated for advanced HIV disease indicate that the risk of lymphoma development is consistent with that observed in untreated patients. In patients with early HIV disease on long-term treatment the risk of lymphoma development is unknown.

Retrovir should be administered under the supervision of a doctor with experience of treating patients with HIV infection or AIDS. An appropriate treatment procedure requires access to suitable facilities eg. for performing haematological monitoring investigations, including determination of viral load, CD4 lymphocytes and for provision of blood transfusions if necessary.

The concomitant use of rifampicin, ribavirin or stavudine with zidovudine should be avoided (see section 4.5).

Haematological Adverse Reactions: Anaemia (usually not observed before six weeks of Retrovir therapy but occasionally occurring earlier), neutropenia (usually not observed before four weeks' therapy but sometimes occurring earlier) and leucopenia (usually secondary to neutropenia) can be expected to occur in patients receiving Retrovir; These occurred more frequently at higher dosages (1200-1500 mg/day) and in patients with poor bone marrow reserve prior to treatment, particularly with advanced HIV disease.

Haematological parameters should be carefully monitored. For patients with advanced symptomatic HIV disease it is generally recommended that blood tests are performed at least every two weeks for the first three months of therapy and at least monthly thereafter. In patients with early HIV disease (where bone marrow reserve is generally good), haematological adverse reactions are infrequent. Depending on the overall condition of the patient, blood tests may be performed less often, for example every 1 to 3 months.

If the haemoglobin level falls to between 7.5 g/dl (4.65 mmol/l) and 9 g/dl (5.59 mmol/l) or the neutrophil count falls to between 0.75 × 10^9/l and 1.0 × 10^9/l, the daily dosage may be reduced until there is evidence of marrow recovery; alternatively, recovery may be enhanced by brief (2-4 weeks) interruption of Retrovir therapy. Marrow recovery is usually observed within 2 weeks after which time Retrovir therapy at a reduced dosage may be reinstituted. In patients with significant anaemia, dosage adjustments do not necessarily eliminate the need for transfusions (see section 4.3).

Lactic acidosis: lactic acidosis usually associated with hepatomegaly and hepatic steatosis has been reported with the use of nucleoside analogues. Early symptoms (symptomatic hyperlactatemia) include benign digestive symptoms (nausea, vomiting and abdominal pain), non-specific malaise, loss of appetite, weight loss, respiratory symptoms (rapid and/or deep breathing) or neurological symptoms (including motor weakness).

Lactic acidosis has a high mortality and may be associated with pancreatitis, liver failure, or renal failure.

Lactic acidosis generally occurred after a few or several months of treatment.

Treatment with nucleoside analogues should be discontinued in the setting of symptomatic hyperlactataemia and metabolic/lactic acidosis, progressive hepatomegaly, or rapidly elevating aminotransferase levels.

Caution should be exercised when administering nucleoside analogues to any patient (particularly obese women) with hepatomegaly, hepatitis or other known risk factors for liver disease and hepatic steatosis (including certain medicinal products and alcohol). Patients co-infected with hepatitis C and treated with alpha interferon and ribavirin may constitute a special risk.

Patients at increased risk should be followed closely.

Mitochondrial toxicity: Nucleoside and nucleotide analogues have been demonstrated *in vitro* and *in vivo* to cause a variable degree of mitochondrial damage. There have been reports of mitochondrial dysfunction in HIV-negative infants exposed *in utero* and/or post-natally to nucleoside analogues. The main adverse events reported are haematological disorders (anaemia, neutropenia), metabolic disorders (hyperlactataemia, hyperlipasaemia). These events are often transitory. Some late-onset neurological disorders have been reported (hypertonia, convulsion, abnormal behaviour). Whether the neurological disorders are transient or permanent is currently unknown. Any child exposed *in utero* to nucleoside and nucleotide analogues, even HIV-negative children, should have clinical and laboratory follow-up and should be fully investigated for possible mitochondrial dysfunction in case of relevant signs or symptoms. These findings do not affect current recommendations to use antiretroviral therapy in pregnant women to prevent vertical transmission of HIV.

Lipodystrophy: Combination antiretroviral therapy has been associated with the redistribution of body fat (lipodystrophy) in HIV patients. The long-term consequences of these events are currently unknown. Knowledge about the mechanism is incomplete. A connection between visceral lipomatosis and PIs and lipoatrophy and NRTIs has been hypothesised. A higher risk of lipodystrophy has been associated with individual factors such as older age, and with drug related factors such as longer duration of antiretroviral treatment and associated metabolic disturbances. Clinical examination should include evaluation for physical signs of fat redistribution. Consideration should be given to the measurement of fasting serum lipids and blood glucose. Lipid disorders should be managed as clinically appropriate (see section 4.8).

Liver disease: The safety and efficacy of zidovudine has not been established in patients with significant underlying liver disorders.

Patients with chronic hepatitis B or C and treated with combination antiretroviral therapy are at an increased risk of severe and potentially fatal hepatic adverse events. In case of concomitant antiviral therapy for hepatitis B or C, please also refer to the relevant product information for these medicinal products.

Patients with pre-existing liver dysfunction, including chronic active hepatitis, have an increased frequency of liver function abnormalities during combination antiretroviral therapy and should be monitored according to standard practice. If there is evidence of worsening liver disease in such patients, interruption or discontinuation of treatment must be considered (see section 4.2).

Immune Reactivation Syndrome: In HIV-infected patients with severe immune deficiency at the time of institution of combination antiretroviral therapy (CART), an inflammatory reaction to asymptomatic or residual opportunistic pathogens may arise and cause serious clinical conditions, or aggravation of symptoms. Typically, such reactions have been observed within the first few weeks or months of initiation of CART. Relevant examples are cytomegalovirus retinitis, generalized and/or focal mycobacterial infections and *Pneumocystis carinii* pneumonia. Any inflammatory symptoms should be evaluated and treatment instituted when necessary.

Patients should be cautioned about the concomitant use of self-administered medications (see section 4.5).

Patients should be advised that Retrovir therapy has not been proven to prevent the transmission of HIV to others through sexual contact or blood contamination.

Use in Elderly and in Patients with Renal or Hepatic Impairment: see section 4.2.

4.5 Interaction with other medicinal products and other forms of Interaction

Limited data suggests that co-administration of zidovudine with rifampicin decreases the AUC (area under the plasma concentration curve) of zidovudine by 48% ± 34%. This may result in a partial loss or total loss of efficacy of zidovudine (see section 4.4).

Zidovudine in combination with either ribavirin or stavudine are antagonistic in vitro. The concomitant use of either ribavirin or stavudine with zidovudine should be avoided (see section 4.4).

Probenecid increases the AUC of zidovudine by 106% (range 100 to 170%). Patients receiving both drugs should be closely monitored for haematological toxicity.

A modest increase in C_{max} (28%) was observed for zidovudine when administered with lamivudine, however overall exposure (AUC) was not significantly altered. Zidovudine has no effect on the pharmacokinetics of lamivudine.

Phenytoin blood levels have been reported to be low in some patients receiving Retrovir, while in one patient a high level was noted. These observations suggest that phenytoin levels should be carefully monitored in patients receiving both drugs.

In a pharmacokinetic study co-administration of zidovudine and atovaquone showed a decrease in zidovudine clearance after oral dosing leading to a 35%±23% increase in plasma zidovudine AUC. Given the limited data available the clinical significance of this is unknown.

Valproic acid, fluconazole or methadone when co-administered with zidovudine have been shown to increase the AUC with a corresponding decrease in its clearance. As only limited data are available the clinical significance of these findings is unclear but if zidovudine is used concurrently with either valproic acid, fluconazole or methadone, patients should be monitored closely for potential toxicity of zidovudine.

Concomitant treatment, especially acute therapy, with potentially nephrotoxic or myelosuppressive drugs (eg. systemic pentamidine, dapsone, pyrimethamine, co-trimoxazole, amphotericin, flucytosine, ganciclovir, interferon, vincristine, vinblastine and doxorubicin) may also increase the risk of adverse reactions to zidovudine. If concomitant therapy with any of these drugs is necessary then extra care should be taken in monitoring renal function and haematological parameters and, if required, the dosage of one or more agents should be reduced.

Since some patients receiving zidovudine may continue to experience opportunistic infections, concomitant use of prophylactic antimicrobial therapy may have to be considered. Such prophylaxis has included co-trimoxazole, aerosolised pentamidine, pyrimethamine and aciclovir. Limited data from clinical trials do not indicate a significantly increased risk of adverse reactions to zidovudine with these drugs at doses used in prophylaxis.

Clarithromycin tablets reduce the absorption of zidovudine.

4.6 Pregnancy and lactation

Pregnancy:

The use of Retrovir in pregnant women over 14 weeks of gestation, with subsequent treatment of their newborn infants, has been shown to significantly reduce the rate of maternal-foetal transmission of HIV based on viral cultures in infants.

The results from the pivotal U.S. placebo-controlled study indicated that Retrovir reduced maternal-foetal transmission by approximately 70%. In this study, pregnant women had CD4 cell counts of 200 to 1818/mm^3 (median in treated group 560/ mm^3) and began treatment therapy between weeks 14 and 34 of gestation and had no clinical indications for Retrovir therapy; their newborn infants received Retrovir until 6-weeks old.

A decision to reduce the risk of maternal transmission of HIV should be based on the balance of potential benefits and potential risk. Pregnant women considering the use of Retrovir during pregnancy for prevention of HIV transmission to their infants should be advised that transmission may still occur in some cases despite therapy.

The efficacy of zidovudine to reduce the maternal-foetal transmission in women with previously prolonged treatment with zidovudine or other antiretroviral agents or women infected with HIV strains with reduced sensitivity to zidovudine is unknown.

It is unknown whether there are any long-term consequences of in-utero and infant exposure to Retrovir.

Based on the animal carcinogenicity/mutagenicity findings a carcinogenic risk to humans cannot be excluded (see section 5.3). The relevance of these findings to both infected and uninfected infants exposed to Retrovir is unknown. However, pregnant women considering using Retrovir during pregnancy should be made aware of these findings.

Given the limited data on the general use of Retrovir in pregnancy, Retrovir should only be used prior to the 14th week of gestation when the potential benefit to the mother and foetus outweigh the risks. Studies in pregnant rats and rabbits given zidovudine orally at dosage levels up to 450 and 500 mg/kg/day respectively during the major period of organogenesis have revealed no evidence of teratogenicity. There was, however, a statistically significant increase in foetal resorptions in rats given 150 to 450 mg/kg/day and in rabbits given 500 mg/kg/day.

A separate study, reported subsequently, found that rats given a dosage of 3000 mg/kg/day, which is very near the oral median lethal dose (3683 mg/kg), caused marked maternal toxicity and an increase in the incidence of foetal malformations. No evidence of teratogenicity was observed in this study at the lower dosages tested (600 mg/kg/day or less).

Fertility:

Zidovudine did not impair male or female fertility in rats given oral doses of up to 450 mg/kg/day. There are no data on the effect of Retrovir on human female fertility. In men, Retrovir has not been shown to affect sperm count, morphology or motility.

Lactation:

Health experts recommend that women infected with HIV do not breast feed their infants in order to avoid the transmission of HIV. After administration of a single dose of 200 mg zidovudine to HIV-infected women, the mean concentration of zidovudine was similar in human milk and serum. Therefore, since the drug and the virus pass into breast milk it is recommended that mothers taking Retrovir do not breast feed their infants.

4.7 Effects on ability to drive and use machines

There have been no studies to investigate the effect of Retrovir on driving performance or the ability to operate machinery. Furthermore, a detrimental effect on such activities cannot be predicted from the pharmacology of the drug. Nevertheless, the clinical status of the patient and the adverse event profile of Retrovir should be borne in mind when considering the patient's ability to drive or operate machinery.

4.8 Undesirable effects

The adverse event profile appears similar for adults and children. The most serious adverse reactions include anaemia (which may require transfusions), neutropenia and leucopenia. These occurred more frequently at higher dosages (1200-1500 mg/day) and in patients with advanced HIV disease (especially when there is poor bone marrow reserve prior to treatment), and particularly in patients with CD4 cell counts less than 100/mm^3. Dosage reduction or cessation of therapy may become necessary (see section 4.4).

The incidence of neutropenia was also increased in those patients whose neutrophil counts, haemoglobin levels and serum vitamin B_{12} levels were low at the start of Retrovir therapy.

Cases of lactic acidosis, sometimes fatal, usually associated with severe hepatomegaly and hepatic steatosis, have been reported with the use of nucleoside analogues (see section 4.4).

Combination antiretroviral therapy has been associated with redistribution of body fat (lipodystrophy) in HIV patients including the loss of peripheral and facial subcutaneous fat, increased intra-abdominal and visceral fat, breast hypertrophy and dorsocervical fat accumulation (buffalo hump).

Combination antiretroviral therapy has been associated with metabolic abnormalities such as hypertriglyceridaemia, hypercholesterolaemia, insulin resistance, hyperglycaemia and hyperlactataemia (see section 4.4).

In HIV-infected patients with severe immune deficiency at the time of initiation of combination antiretroviral therapy (CART), an inflammatory reaction to asymptomatic or residual opportunistic infections may arise (see section 4.4).

The following events have been reported in patients treated with Retrovir. They may also occur as part of the underlying disease process or in association with other drugs used in the management of HIV disease. The relationship between these events and use of Retrovir is therefore difficult to evaluate, particularly in the medically complicated situations which characterise advanced HIV disease. A reduction in dose or suspension of Retrovir therapy may be warranted in the management of these conditions.

The adverse events considered at least possibly related to the treatment are listed below by body system, organ class and absolute frequency. Frequencies are defined as Very common (greater than 10%), Common (1- 10%), Uncommon (0.1-1%), Rare (0.01-0.1%) and Very rare (less than 0.01%).

Blood and lymphatic system disorders

Common: Anaemia, neutropenia and leucopenia.

Uncommon: Thrombocytopenia and pancytopenia with marrow hypoplasia

Rare: Pure red cell aplasia

Very rare: Aplastic anaemia

Metabolism and nutrition disorders

Rare: Anorexia and lactic acidosis in the absence of hypoxaemia

Psychiatric disorders

Rare: Anxiety and depression

Nervous system disorders

Very common: Headache

Common: Dizziness

Rare: Insomnia, paraesthesia, somnolence, loss of mental acuity, convulsions

Cardiac disorders

Rare: Cardiomyopathy

Respiratory, thoracic and mediastinal disorders

Uncommon: Dyspnoea

Rare: Cough

Gastrointestinal disorders

Very common: Nausea

Common: Vomiting, abdominal pain, and diarrhoea

Uncommon: Flatulence

Rare: Oral mucosa pigmentation, taste disturbance and dyspepsia. Pancreatitis.

Hepatobiliary disorders

Common: Raised blood levels of liver enzymes and bilirubin

Rare: Liver disorders such as severe hepatomegaly with steatosis

Skin and subcutaneous tissue disorders

Uncommon: Rash and pruritis

Rare: Nail and skin pigmentation, urticaria and sweating

Musculoskeletal and connective tissue disorders

Common: Myalgia

Uncommon: Myopathy

Renal and urinary disorders

Rare: Urinary frequency

Reproductive system and breast disorders

Rare: Gynaecomastia

General disorders and administration site disorders:

Common: Malaise

Uncommon: Fever, generalised pain and asthenia

Rare: Chills, chest pain and influenza-like syndrome

The available data from both placebo-controlled and open-label studies indicate that the incidence of nausea and other frequently reported clinical adverse events consistently decreases over time during the first few weeks of therapy with Retrovir.

Adverse reactions with Retrovir for the prevention of maternal-foetal transmission:

In a placebo-controlled trial, overall clinical adverse events and laboratory test abnormalities were similar for women in the Retrovir and placebo groups. However, there was a trend for mild and moderate anaemia to be seen more commonly prior to delivery in the zidovudine treated women.

In the same trial, haemoglobin concentrations in infants exposed to Retrovir for this indication were marginally lower than in infants in the placebo group, but transfusion was not required. Anaemia resolved within 6 weeks after completion of Retrovir therapy. Other clinical adverse events and laboratory test abnormalities were similar in the Retrovir and placebo groups. It is unknown whether there are any long-term consequences of *in utero* and infant exposure to Retrovir.

4.9 Overdose

Symptoms and signs:

No specific symptoms or signs have been identified following acute overdose with zidovudine apart from those listed as undesirable effects such as fatigue, headache, vomiting, and occasional reports of haematological disturbances. Following a report where a patient took an unspecified quantity of zidovudine with serum levels consistent with an overdose of greater than 17 g there were no short term clinical, biochemical or haematological sequelae identified.

Treatment:

Patients should be observed closely for evidence of toxicity (see section 4.8) and given the necessary supportive therapy.

Haemodialysis and peritoneal dialysis appear to have a limited effect on elimination of zidovudine but enhance the elimination of the glucuronide metabolite.

5. PHARMACOLOGICAL PROPERTIES

5.1 Pharmacodynamic properties

Pharmacotherapeutic group – nucleoside analogue – ATC Code J05A F01

Mode of action:

Zidovudine is an antiviral agent which is highly active *in vitro* against retroviruses including the Human Immunodeficiency Virus (HIV).

Zidovudine is phosphorylated in both infected and uninfected cells to the monophosphate (MP) derivative by cellular thymidine kinase. Subsequent phosphorylation of zidovudine-MP to the diphosphate (DP), and then the triphosphate (TP) derivative is catalysed by cellular thymidylate kinase and non-specific kinases respectively. Zidovudine-TP acts as an inhibitor of and substrate for the viral reverse transcriptase. The formation of further proviral DNA is blocked by incorporation of zidovudine-MP into the chain and subsequent chain termination. Competition by zidovudine-TP for HIV reverse transcriptase is approximately 100-fold greater than for cellular DNA polymerase alpha.

Clinical virology:

The relationships between *in vitro* susceptibility of HIV to zidovudine and clinical response to therapy remain under investigation. *In vitro* sensitivity testing has not been standardised and results may therefore vary according to methodological factors. Reduced *in vitro* sensitivity to zidovudine has been reported for HIV isolates from patients who have received prolonged courses of Retrovir therapy. The available information indicates that for early HIV disease, the frequency and degree of reduction of *in vitro* sensitivity is notably less than for advanced disease.

The reduction of sensitivity with the emergence of zidovudine resistant strains limits the usefulness of zidovudine monotherapy clinically. In clinical studies, clinical endpoint data indicate that zidovudine, particularly in combination with lamivudine, and also with didanosine or zalcitabine results in a significant reduction in the risk of disease progression and mortality. The use of a protease inhibitor in a combination of zidovudine and lamivudine, has been shown to confer additional benefit in delaying disease progression, and improving survival compared to the double combination on its own.

The anti-viral effectiveness *in vitro* of combinations of antiretroviral agents are being investigated. Clinical and *in vitro* studies of zidovudine in combination with lamivudine indicate that zidovudine-resistant virus isolates can become zidovudine sensitive when they simultaneously acquire resistance to lamivudine. Furthermore there is clinical evidence that zidovudine plus lamivudine delays the emergence of zidovudine resistance in anti-retroviral naive patients.

In some *in vitro* studies zidovudine has been shown to act additively or synergistically with a number of anti-HIV agents, such as lamivudine, didanosine, and interferon-alpha, inhibiting the replication of HIV in cell culture. However, *in vitro* studies with triple combinations of nucleoside analogues or two nucleoside analogues and a protease inhibitor have been shown to be more effective in inhibiting HIV-1 induced cytopathic effects than one or two drug combinations.

Resistance to thymidine analogues (of which zidovudine is one) is well characterised and is conferred by the stepwise accumulation of up to six specific mutations in the HIV reverse transcriptase at codons 41, 67, 70, 210, 215 and 219. Viruses acquire phenotypic resistance to thymidine analogues through the combination of mutations at codons 41 and 215 or by the accumulation of at least four of the six mutations. These thymidine analogue mutations alone do not cause high-level cross-resistance to any of the other nucleosides, allowing for the subsequent use of any of the other approved reverse transcriptase inhibitors.

Two patterns of multi-drug resistance mutations, the first characterised by mutations in the HIV reverse transcriptase at codons 62, 75, 77, 116 and 151 and the second involving a T69S mutation plus a 6-base pair insert at the same position, result in phenotypic resistance to AZT as well as to the other approved nucleoside reverse transcriptase inhibitors. Either of these two patterns of multinucleoside resistance mutations severely limits future therapeutic options.

In the US ACTG076 trial, Retrovir was shown to be effective in reducing the rate of maternal-foetal transmission of HIV-1 (23% infection rate for placebo versus 8% for zidovudine) when administered (100 mg five times a day) to HIV-positive pregnant women (from 14-34of pregnancy) and their newborn infants (2 mg/kg every 6 hours) until 6 weeks of age. In the shorter duration 1998 Thailand CDC study, use of oral Retrovir therapy only (300 mg twice daily), from week 36 of pregnancy until delivery, also reduced the rate of maternal-foetal transmission of HIV (19% infection rate for placebo versus 9% for zidovudine). These data, and data from a published study comparing zidovudine regimens to prevent maternal-foetal HIV transmission have shown that short maternal treatments (from week 36 of pregnancy) are less efficacious than longer maternal treatments (from week 14-34 of pregnancy) in the reduction of perinatal HIV transmission.

5.2 Pharmacokinetic properties

Pharmacokinetics in adults:

Zidovudine is well absorbed from the gut and, at all dose levels studied, the bioavailability was 60-70%. From a bioequivalence study, steady-state mean (CV%) C[ss]max, C[ss]min, and AUC[ss] values in 16 patients receiving zidovudine 300 mg tablets twice daily were 8.57 (54%) microM (2.29 μg/ml), 0.08 (96%) microM (0.02 μg/ml), and 8.39 (40%) h*microM (2.24 h*μg/ml), respectively.

From studies with intravenous Retrovir, the mean terminal plasma half-life was 1.1 hours, the mean total body clearance was 27.1 ml/min/kg and the apparent volume of distribution was 1.6 Litres/kg. Renal clearance of zidovudine greatly exceeds creatinine clearance, indicating that significant tubular secretion takes place.

Zidovudine is primarily eliminated by hepatic conjugation to an inactive glucoronidated metabolite. The 5'-glucuronide of zidovudine is the major metabolite in both plasma and urine, accounting for approximately 50-80% of the administered dose eliminated by renal excretion. 3'-amino-3'-deoxythymidine (AMT) has been identified as a metabolite of zidovudine following intravenous dosing.

There are limited data on the pharmacokinetics of zidovudine in patients with renal or hepatic impairment (see section 4.2). No specific data are available on the pharmacokinetics of zidovudine in the elderly.

Pharmacokinetics in children:

In children over the age of 5-6 months, the pharmacokinetic profile of zidovudine is similar to that in adults. Zidovudine is well absorbed from the gut and, at all dose levels studied, its bioavailability was 60-74% with a mean of 65%. C^{ss}max levels were 4.45μM (1.19μg/ml) following a dose of 120mg Retrovir (in solution)/m^2 body surface area and 7.7μM (2.06μg/ml) at 180mg/m^2 body surface area. Dosages of 180 mg/m^2 four times daily in children produced similar systemic exposure (24 hour AUC 40.0 hr μM or 10.7 hr μg/ml) as doses of 200 mg six times daily in adults (40.7 hr μM or 10.9 hr μg/ml).

With intravenous dosing, the mean terminal plasma half-life and total body clearance were 1.5 hours and 30.9ml/min/kg respectively. The major metabolite is 5'-glucuronide. After intravenous dosing, 29% of the dose was recovered unchanged in the urine and 45% excreted as the glucuronide. Renal clearance of zidovudine greatly exceeds creatinine clearance indicating that significant tubular secretion takes place.

The data available on the pharmacokinetics in neonates and young infants indicate that glucuronidation of zidovudine is reduced with a consequent increase in bioavailability, reduction in clearance and longer half-life in infants less than 14 days old but thereafter the pharmacokinetics appear similar to those reported in adults.

Pharmacokinetics in pregnancy:

The pharmacokinetics of zidovudine has been investigated in a study of eight women during the third trimester of pregnancy. As pregnancy progressed, there was no evidence of drug accumulation. The pharmacokinetics of zidovudine was similar to that of non-pregnant adults. Consistent with passive transmission of the drug across the placenta, zidovudine concentrations in infant plasma at birth were essentially equal to those in maternal plasma at delivery.

Distribution:

In adults, the average cerebrospinal fluid/plasma zidovudine concentration ratio 2 to 4 hours after dosing was found to be approximately 0.5. Data indicate that zidovudine crosses the placenta and is found in amniotic fluid and foetal blood. Zidovudine has also been detected in semen and milk.

In children the mean cerebrospinal fluid/plasma zidovudine concentration ratio ranged from 0.52-0.85, as determined during oral therapy 0.5 to 4 hours after dosing and was 0.87 as determined during intravenous therapy 1-5 hours after a 1 hour infusion. During continuous intravenous infusion, the mean steady-state cerebrospinal fluid/plasma concentration ratio was 0.24.

Plasma protein binding is relatively low (34 to 38%) and drug interactions involving binding site displacement are not anticipated.

5.3 Preclinical safety data

Mutagenicity:

No evidence of mutagenicity was observed in the Ames test. However, zidovudine was weakly mutagenic in a mouse lymphoma cell assay and was positive in an *in vitro* cell transformation assay. Clastogenic effects were observed in an *in vitro* study in human lymphocytes and in *in vivo* oral repeat dose micronucleus studies in rats and mice. An *in vivo* cytogenetic study in rats did not show chromosomal damage. A study of the peripheral blood lymphocytes of eleven AIDS patients showed a higher chromosome breakage frequency in those who had received Retrovir than in those who had not. A pilot study has demonstrated that zidovudine is incorporated into leukocyte nuclear DNA of adults, including pregnant women, taking zidovudine as treatment for HIV-1 infection, or for the prevention of mother to child viral transmission. Zidovudine was also incorporated into DNA from cord blood leukocytes of infants from zidovudine-treated mothers. A transplacental genotoxicity study conducted in monkeys compared zidovudine alone with the combination of zidovudine and lamivudine at human-equivalent exposures. The study demonstrated that foetuses exposed *in utero* to the combination sustained a higher level of nucleoside analogue-DNA incorporation into multiple foetal organs, and showed evidence of more telomere shortening than in those exposed to zidovudine alone. The clinical significance of these findings is unknown.

Carcinogenicity:

In oral carcinogenicity studies with zidovudine in mice and rats, late appearing vaginal epithelial tumours were observed. A subsequent intravaginal carcinogenicity study confirmed the hypothesis that the vaginal tumours were the result of long term local exposure of the rodent vaginal epithelium to high concentrations of unmetabolised zidovudine in urine. There were no other drug-related tumours observed in either sex of either species.

In addition, two transplacental carcinogenicity studies have been conducted in mice. One study, by the US National Cancer Institute, administered zidovudine at maximum tolerated doses to pregnant mice from day 12 to 18 of gestation. One year post-natally, there was an increase in the incidence of tumours in the lung, liver and female reproductive tract of offspring exposed to the highest dose level (420 mg/kg term body weight).

In a second study, mice were administered zidovudine at doses up to 40 mg/kg for 24 months, with exposure beginning prenatally on gestation day 10. Treatment related findings were limited to late-occurring vaginal epithelial tumours, which were seen with a similar incidence and time of onset as in the standard oral carcinogenicity study. The second study thus provided no evidence that zidovudine acts as a transplacental carcinogen.

It is concluded that the transplacental carcinogenicity data from the first study represents a hypothetical risk, whereas the reduction in risk of maternal transfection of HIV to the uninfected child by the use of zidovudine in pregnancy has been well proven.

6. PHARMACEUTICAL PARTICULARS

6.1 List of excipients

Maltitol solution

Glycerol

Citric Acid

E211 Sodium Benzoate

Saccharin Sodium

Flavour Strawberry

Flavour White Sugar

Purified Water.

6.2 Incompatibilities

In the absence of compatibility studies, this medicinal product must not be mixed with other medicinal products.

6.3 Shelf life

2 years. Discard oral solution 1 month after first opening bottle.

6.4 Special precautions for storage

Do not store above 30°C. Store the bottle in the original outer carton.

6.5 Nature and contents of container

Retrovir Oral Solution/Syrup:

200 ml amber glass bottle with a plastic cap and polyethylene wad. A 10 ml oral-dosing syringe is included in the pack, with an adaptor, which should be fitted to the bottle before use.

Retrovir Oral Solution/Syrup (Neonate Pack):

200 ml amber glass bottle with a plastic cap and polyethylene wad. A 1 ml oral-dosing syringe is included in the pack, with an adaptor, which should be fitted to the bottle before use.

6.6 Instructions for use and handling

No special requirements

Administrative Data

7. MARKETING AUTHORISATION HOLDER

United Kingdom

The Wellcome Foundation Limited

trading as:

Glaxo Wellcome and/or GlaxoSmithKline UK

Stockley Park West

Uxbridge

Middlesex

UB11 1BT

8. MARKETING AUTHORISATION NUMBER(S)

PL 00003/0288

9. DATE OF FIRST AUTHORISATION/RENEWAL OF THE AUTHORISATION

16/08/1991

10. DATE OF REVISION OF THE TEXT

26 July 2005

Retrovir 100mg Capsules

(GlaxoSmithKline UK)

1. NAME OF THE MEDICINAL PRODUCT

Retrovir® 100 mg, capsule, hard

2. QUALITATIVE AND QUANTITATIVE COMPOSITION

Each capsules contains:

Zidovudine 100 mg

For excipients see section 6.1

3. PHARMACEUTICAL FORM

Retrovir 100 mg capsule, hard:

Hard gelatin capsules with opaque white cap and body and a central dark-blue band, printed "Wellcome", "100" and coded Y9C.

4. CLINICAL PARTICULARS

4.1 Therapeutic indications

Retrovir oral formulations are indicated in anti-retroviral combination therapy for Human Immunodeficiency Virus (HIV) infected adults and children.

Retrovir chemoprophylaxis, is indicated for use in HIV-positive pregnant women (over 14 weeks of gestation) for prevention of maternal-foetal HIV transmission and for primary prophylaxis of HIV infection in newborn infants.

4.2 Posology and method of administration

Dosage in adults:

The usual recommended dose of Retrovir in combination with other anti-retroviral agents is 500 or 600 mg/day in two or three divided doses.

Dosage in children:

3 months - 12 years:

The recommended dose of Retrovir is 360 to 480 mg/m^2 per day, in 3 or 4 divided doses in combination with other antiretroviral agents. The maximum dosage should not exceed 200 mg every 6 hours.

<3 months:

The limited data available are insufficient to propose specific dosage recommendations (See below -maternal foetal transmission and section 5.2).

Dosage in the prevention of maternal-foetal transmission:

Although the optimal dosage schedule has not been identified the following dosage regimen has been shown to be effective. Pregnant women (over 14 weeks of gestation) should be given 500 mg/day orally (100 mg five times per day) until the beginning of labour. During labour and delivery Retrovir should be administered intravenously at 2 mg/kg bodyweight given over one hour followed by a continuous intravenous infusion at 1 mg/kg/h until the umbilical cord is clamped.

The newborn infants should be given 2 mg/kg bodyweight orally every 6 hours starting within 12 hours after birth and continuing until 6 weeks old (e.g. a 3 kg neonate would require a 0.6 ml dose of oral solution every 6 hours). Infants unable to receive oral dosing should be given Retrovir intravenously at 1.5 mg/kg bodyweight infused over 30 minutes every 6 hours.

In case of planned caesarean, the infusion should be started 4 hours before the operation. In the event of a false labour, the Retrovir infusion should be stopped and oral dosing restarted.

Dosage adjustments in patients with haematological adverse reactions:

Dosage reduction or interruption of Retrovir therapy may be necessary in patients whose haemoglobin level falls to between 7.5 g/dl (4.65 mmol/l) and 9 g/dl (5.59 mmol/l) or whose neutrophil count falls to between 0.75 × 10^9/l and 1.0 × 10^9/l (see sections 4.3 and 4.4)

Dosage in the elderly:

Zidovudine pharmacokinetics have not been studied in patients over 65 years of age and no specific data are available. However, since special care is advised in this age group due to age-associated changes such as the decrease in renal function and alterations in haematological parameters, appropriate monitoring of patients before and during use of Retrovir is advised.

Dosage in renal impairment:

In patients with severe renal impairment, apparent zidovudine clearance after oral zidovudine administration was approximately 50% of that reported in healthy subjects with normal renal function. Therefore a dosage reduction to 300-400 mg daily is recommended for patients with severe renal impairment with creatinine clearance -≤ 10 ml/min. Haematological parameters and clinical response may influence the need for subsequent dosage adjustment.

Haemodialysis and peritoneal dialysis have no significant effect on zidovudine elimination whereas elimination of the glucuronide metabolite is increased.

Dosage in hepatic impairment:

Data in patients with cirrhosis suggest that accumulation of zidovudine may occur in patients with hepatic impairment because of decreased glucuronidation. Dosage reductions may be necessary but, as there is only limited data available, precise recommendations cannot be made. If monitoring of plasma zidovudine levels is not feasible, physicians will need to monitor for signs of intolerance, such as the development of haematological adverse reactions (anaemia, leucopenia, neutropenia) and reduce the dose and/or increase the interval between doses as appropriate (see section 4.4).

4.3 Contraindications

Retrovir Oral Formulations are contra-indicated in patients known to be hypersensitive to zidovudine, or to any of the components of the formulations.

Retrovir Oral Formulations should not be given to patients with abnormally low neutrophil counts (less than 0.75 × 10^9/litre) or abnormally low haemoglobin levels (less than 7.5 g/decilitre or 4.65 mmol/litre).

Retrovir is contra-indicated in new born infants with hyperbilirubinaemia requiring treatment other than phototherapy, or with increased transaminase levels of over five times the upper limit of normal.

4.4 Special warnings and special precautions for use

Retrovir is not a cure for HIV infection and patients remain at risk of developing illnesses which are associated with immune suppression, including opportunistic infections and neoplasms. Whilst it has been shown to reduce the risks of opportunistic infections, data on the development of neoplasms, including lymphomas, are limited. The available data on patients treated for advanced HIV disease indicate that the risk of lymphoma development is consistent with that observed in untreated patients. In patients with early HIV disease on long-term treatment the risk of lymphoma development is unknown.

Retrovir should be administered under the supervision of a doctor with experience of treating patients with HIV infection or AIDS. An appropriate treatment procedure requires access to suitable facilities eg. for performing haematological monitoring investigations, including determination of viral load, CD4 lymphocytes and for provision of blood transfusions if necessary.

The concomitant use of rifampicin, ribavirin or stavudine with zidovudine should be avoided (see section 4.5).

Haematological Adverse Reactions: Anaemia (usually not observed before six weeks of Retrovir therapy but occasionally occurring earlier), neutropenia (usually not observed before four weeks' therapy but sometimes occurring earlier) and leucopenia (usually secondary to neutropenia) can be expected to occur in patients receiving Retrovir; These occurred more frequently at higher dosages (1200-1500 mg/day) and in patients with poor bone marrow reserve prior to treatment, particularly with advanced HIV disease.

Haematological parameters should be carefully monitored. For patients with advanced symptomatic HIV disease it is generally recommended that blood tests are performed at least every two weeks for the first three months of therapy and at least monthly thereafter. In patients with early HIV disease (where bone marrow reserve is generally good), haematological adverse reactions are infrequent. Depending on the overall condition of the patient, blood tests may be performed less often, for example every 1 to 3 months.

If the haemoglobin level falls to between 7.5 g/dl (4.65 mmol/l) and 9 g/dl (5.59 mmol/l) or the neutrophil count falls to between 0.75 × 10^9/l and 1.0 × 10^9/l, the daily dosage may be reduced until there is evidence of marrow recovery; alternatively, recovery may be enhanced by brief (2-4 weeks) interruption of Retrovir therapy. Marrow recovery is usually observed within 2 weeks after which time Retrovir therapy at a reduced dosage may be reinstituted. In patients with significant anaemia, dosage adjustments do not necessarily eliminate the need for transfusions (see section 4.3).

Lactic acidosis: lactic acidosis usually associated with hepatomegaly and hepatic steatosis has been reported with the use of nucleoside analogues. Early symptoms (symptomatic hyperlactatemia) include benign digestive symptoms (nausea, vomiting and abdominal pain), non-specific malaise, loss of appetite, weight loss, respiratory symptoms (rapid and/or deep breathing) or neurological symptoms (including motor weakness).

Lactic acidosis has a high mortality and may be associated with pancreatitis, liver failure, or renal failure.

Lactic acidosis generally occurred after a few or several months of treatment.

Treatment with nucleoside analogues should be discontinued in the setting of symptomatic hyperlactataemia and metabolic/lactic acidosis, progressive hepatomegaly, or rapidly elevating aminotransferase levels.

Caution should be exercised when administering nucleoside analogues to any patient (particularly obese women) with hepatomegaly, hepatitis or other known risk factors for liver disease and hepatic steatosis (including certain medicinal products and alcohol). Patients co-infected with hepatitis C and treated with alpha interferon and ribavirin may constitute a special risk.

Patients at increased risk should be followed closely.

Mitochondrial toxicity: Nucleoside and nucleotide analogues have been demonstrated *in vitro* and *in vivo* to cause a variable degree of mitochondrial damage. There have been reports of mitochondrial dysfunction in HIV-negative infants exposed *in utero* and/or post-natally to nucleoside analogues. The main adverse events reported are haematological disorders (anaemia, neutropenia), metabolic disorders (hyperlactataemia, hyperlipasaemia). These events are often transitory. Some late-onset neurological disorders have been reported (hypertonia, convulsion, abnormal behaviour). Whether the neurological disorders are transient or permanent is currently unknown. Any child exposed *in utero* to nucleoside and nucleotide analogues, even HIV-negative children, should have clinical and laboratory follow-up and should be fully investigated for possible mitochondrial dysfunction in case of relevant signs or symptoms. These findings do not affect current recommendations to use antiretroviral therapy in pregnant women to prevent vertical transmission of HIV.

Lipodystrophy: Combination antiretroviral therapy has been associated with the redistribution of body fat (lipodystrophy) in HIV patients. The long-term consequences of these events are currently unknown. Knowledge about the mechanism is incomplete. A connection between visceral lipomatosis and PIs and lipoatrophy and NRTIs has been hypothesised. A higher risk of lipodystrophy has been associated with individual factors such as older age, and with drug related factors such as longer duration of antiretroviral treatment and associated metabolic disturbances. Clinical examination should include evaluation for physical signs of fat redistribution. Consideration should be given to the measurement of fasting serum lipids and blood glucose. Lipid disorders should be managed as clinically appropriate (see section 4.8).

Liver disease: The safety and efficacy of zidovudine has not been established in patients with significant underlying liver disorders.

Patients with chronic hepatitis B or C and treated with combination antiretroviral therapy are at an increased risk of severe and potentially fatal hepatic adverse events. In case of concomitant antiviral therapy for hepatitis B or C, please also refer to the relevant product information for these medicinal products.

Patients with pre-existing liver dysfunction, including chronic active hepatitis, have an increased frequency of liver function abnormalities during combination antiretroviral therapy and should be monitored according to standard practice. If there is evidence of worsening liver disease in such patients, interruption or discontinuation of treatment must be considered (see section 4.2).

Immune Reactivation Syndrome: In HIV-infected patients with severe immune deficiency at the time of institution of combination antiretroviral therapy (CART), an inflammatory reaction to asymptomatic or residual opportunistic pathogens may arise and cause serious clinical conditions, or aggravation of symptoms. Typically, such reactions have been observed within the first few weeks or months of initiation of CART. Relevant examples are cytomegalovirus retinitis, generalized and/or focal mycobacterial infections and *Pneumocystis carinii* pneumonia. Any inflammatory symptoms should be evaluated and treatment instituted when necessary.

Patients should be cautioned about the concomitant use of self-administered medications (see section 4.5).

Patients should be advised that Retrovir therapy has not been proven to prevent the transmission of HIV to others through sexual contact or blood contamination.

Use in Elderly and in Patients with Renal or Hepatic Impairment: see section 4.2.

4.5 Interaction with other medicinal products and other forms of Interaction

Limited data suggests that co-administration of zidovudine with rifampicin decreases the AUC (area under the plasma concentration curve) of zidovudine by 48% ± 34%. This may result in a partial loss or total loss of efficacy of zidovudine (see section 4.4).

Zidovudine in combination with either ribavirin or stavudine are antagonistic in vitro. The concomitant use of either ribavirin or stavudine with zidovudine should be avoided (see section 4.4).

Probenecid increases the AUC of zidovudine by 106% (range 100 to 170%). Patients receiving both drugs should be closely monitored for haematological toxicity.

A modest increase in C_{max} (28%) was observed for zidovudine when administered with lamivudine, however overall exposure (AUC) was not significantly altered. Zidovudine has no effect on the pharmacokinetics of lamivudine.

Phenytoin blood levels have been reported to be low in some patients receiving Retrovir, while in one patient a high level was noted. These observations suggest that phenytoin levels should be carefully monitored in patients receiving both drugs.

In a pharmacokinetic study co-administration of zidovudine and atovaquone showed a decrease in zidovudine clearance after oral dosing leading to a 35%±23% increase in plasma zidovudine AUC. Given the limited data available the clinical significance of this is unknown.

Valproic acid, fluconazole or methadone when co-administered with zidovudine have been shown to increase the AUC with a corresponding decrease in its clearance. As only limited data are available the clinical significance of these findings is unclear but if zidovudine is used concurrently with either valproic acid, fluconazole or methadone, patients should be monitored closely for potential toxicity of zidovudine.

Concomitant treatment, especially acute therapy, with potentially nephrotoxic or myelosuppressive drugs (eg. systemic pentamidine, dapsone, pyrimethamine, co-trimoxazole, amphotericin, flucytosine, ganciclovir, interferon, vincristine, vinblastine and doxorubicin) may also increase the risk of adverse reactions to zidovudine. If concomitant therapy with any of these drugs is necessary then extra care should be taken in monitoring renal function and haematological parameters and, if required, the dosage of one or more agents should be reduced.

Since some patients receiving zidovudine may continue to experience opportunistic infections, concomitant use of prophylactic antimicrobial therapy may have to be considered. Such prophylaxis has included co-trimoxazole, aerosolised pentamidine, pyrimethamine and aciclovir. Limited data from clinical trials do not indicate a significantly increased risk of adverse reactions to zidovudine with these drugs at doses used in prophylaxis.

Clarithromycin tablets reduce the absorption of zidovudine.

4.6 Pregnancy and lactation

Pregnancy:

The use of Retrovir in pregnant women over 14 weeks of gestation, with subsequent treatment of their newborn infants, has been shown to significantly reduce the rate of maternal-foetal transmission of HIV based on viral cultures in infants.

The results from the pivotal U.S. placebo-controlled study indicated that Retrovir reduced maternal-foetal transmission by approximately 70%. In this study, pregnant women had CD4 cell counts of 200 to 1818/mm^3 (median in treated group 560/mm^3) and began treatment therapy between weeks 14 and 34 of gestation and had no clinical indications for Retrovir therapy; their newborn infants received Retrovir until 6-weeks old.

A decision to reduce the risk of maternal transmission of HIV should be based on the balance of potential benefits and potential risk. Pregnant women considering the use of Retrovir during pregnancy for prevention of HIV transmission to their infants should be advised that transmission may still occur in some cases despite therapy.

The efficacy of zidovudine to reduce the maternal-foetal transmission in women with previously prolonged treatment with zidovudine or other antiretroviral agents or women infected with HIV strains with reduced sensitivity to zidovudine is unknown.

It is unknown whether there are any long-term consequences of in utero and infant exposure to Retrovir.

Based on the animal carcinogenicity/mutagenicity findings a carcinogenic risk to humans cannot be excluded (see section 5.3). The relevance of these findings to both infected and uninfected infants exposed to Retrovir is unknown. However, pregnant women considering using Retrovir during pregnancy should be made aware of these findings.

Given the limited data on the general use of Retrovir in pregnancy, Retrovir should only be used prior to the 14th week of gestation when the potential benefit to the mother and foetus outweigh the risks. Studies in pregnant rats and rabbits given zidovudine orally at dosage levels up to 450 and 500 mg/kg/day respectively during the major period of organogenesis have revealed no evidence of teratogenicity. There was, however, a statistically significant increase in foetal resorptions in rats given 150 to 450 mg/kg/day and in rabbits given 500 mg/kg/day.

A separate study, reported subsequently, found that rats given a dosage of 3000 mg/kg/day, which is very near the oral median lethal dose (3683 mg/kg), caused marked maternal toxicity and an increase in the incidence of foetal malformations. No evidence of teratogenicity was observed in this study at the lower dosages tested (600 mg/kg/day or less).

Fertility:

Zidovudine did not impair male or female fertility in rats given oral doses of up to 450 mg/kg/day. There are no data on the effect of Retrovir on human female fertility. In men, Retrovir has not been shown to affect sperm count, morphology or motility.

Lactation:

Health experts recommend that women infected with HIV do not breast feed their infants in order to avoid the transmission of HIV. After administration of a single dose of 200 mg zidovudine to HIV-infected women, the mean concentration of zidovudine was similar in human milk and serum. Therefore, since the drug and the virus pass into breast milk it is recommended that mothers taking Retrovir do not breast feed their infants.

4.7 Effects on ability to drive and use machines

There have been no studies to investigate the effect of Retrovir on driving performance or the ability to operate machinery. Furthermore, a detrimental effect on such activities cannot be predicted from the pharmacology of the drug. Nevertheless, the clinical status of the patient and the adverse event profile of Retrovir should be borne in mind when considering the patient's ability to drive or operate machinery.

4.8 Undesirable effects

The adverse event profile appears similar for adults and children. The most serious adverse reactions include anaemia (which may require transfusions), neutropenia and leucopenia. These occurred more frequently at higher dosages (1200-1500 mg/day) and in patients with advanced HIV disease (especially when there is poor bone marrow reserve prior to treatment), and particularly in patients with CD4+ cell counts less than 100/mm^3. Dosage reduction or cessation of therapy may become necessary (see section 4.4).

The incidence of neutropenia was also increased in those patients whose neutrophil counts, haemoglobin levels and serum vitamin B_{12} levels were low at the start of Retrovir therapy.

Cases of lactic acidosis, sometimes fatal, usually associated with severe hepatomegaly and hepatic steatosis, have been reported with the use of nucleoside analogues (see section 4.4).

Combination antiretroviral therapy has been associated with redistribution of body fat (lipodystrophy) in HIV patients including the loss of peripheral and facial subcutaneous fat, increased intra-abdominal and visceral fat, breast hypertrophy and dorsocervical fat accumulation (buffalo hump).

Combination antiretroviral therapy has been associated with metabolic abnormalities such as hypertriglyceridaemia, hypercholesterolaemia, insulin resistance, hyperglycaemia and hyperlactataemia (see section 4.4).

In HIV-infected patients with severe immune deficiency at the time of initiation of combination antiretroviral therapy (CART), an inflammatory reaction to asymptomatic or residual opportunistic infections may arise (see section 4.4).

The following events have been reported in patients treated with Retrovir. They may also occur as part of the underlying disease process or in association with other drugs used in the management of HIV disease. The relationship between these events and use of Retrovir is therefore difficult to evaluate, particularly in the medically complicated situations which characterise advanced HIV disease. A reduction in dose or suspension of Retrovir therapy may be warranted in the management of these conditions.

The adverse events considered at least possibly related to the treatment are listed below by body system, organ class and absolute frequency. Frequencies are defined as Very common (greater than 10%), Common (1 - 10%), Uncommon (0.1-1%), Rare (0.01-0.1%) and Very rare (less than 0.01%).

Blood and lymphatic system disorders

Common:Anaemia, neutropenia and leucopenia

Uncommon: Thrombocytopenia and pancytopenia with marrow hypoplasia

Rare: Pure red cell aplasia

Very rare: Aplastic anaemia

Metabolism and nutrition disorders

Rare: Anorexia and lactic acidosis in the absence of hypoxaemia

Psychiatric disorders

Rare: Anxiety and depression

Nervous system disorders

Very common: Headache

Common: Dizziness

Rare: Insomnia, paraesthesia, somnolence, loss of mental acuity, convulsions

Cardiac disorders

Rare: Cardiomyopathy

Respiratory, thoracic and mediastinal disorders

Uncommon: Dyspnoea

Rare: Cough

Gastrointestinal disorders

Very common: Nausea

Common: Vomiting, abdominal pain, and diarrhoea

Uncommon:Flatulence

Rare: Oral mucosa pigmentation, taste disturbance and dyspepsia. Pancreatitis.

Hepatobiliary disorders

Common:Raised blood levels of liver enzymes and bilirubin

Rare: Liver disorders such as severe hepatomegaly with steatosis

Skin and subcutaneous tissue disorders

Uncommon: Rash and pruritis

Rare: Nail and skin pigmentation, urticaria and sweating

Musculoskeletal and connective tissue disorders

Common: Myalgia

Uncommon: Myopathy

Renal and urinary disorders

Rare: Urinary frequency

Reproductive system and breast disorders

Rare: Gynaecomastia

General disorders and administration site disorders :

Common:Malaise

Uncommon: Fever, generalised pain and asthenia

Rare: Chills, chest pain and influenza-like syndrome

The available data from both placebo-controlled and open-label studies indicate that the incidence of nausea and other frequently reported clinical adverse events consistently decreases over time during the first few weeks of therapy with Retrovir.

Adverse reactions with Retrovir for the prevention of maternal-foetal transmission:

In a placebo-controlled trial, overall clinical adverse events and laboratory test abnormalities were similar for women in the Retrovir and placebo groups. However, there was a trend for mild and moderate anaemia to be seen more commonly prior to delivery in the zidovudine treated women.

In the same trial, haemoglobin concentrations in infants exposed to Retrovir for this indication were marginally lower than in infants in the placebo group, but transfusion was not required. Anaemia resolved within 6 weeks after completion of Retrovir therapy. Other clinical adverse events and laboratory test abnormalities were similar in the Retrovir and placebo groups. It is unknown whether there are any long-term consequences of *in utero* and infant exposure to Retrovir.

4.9 Overdose

Symptoms and signs:

No specific symptoms or signs have been identified following acute overdose with zidovudine apart from those listed as undesirable effects such as fatigue, headache, vomiting, and occasional reports of haematological disturbances. Following a report where a patient took an unspecified quantity of zidovudine with serum levels consistent with an overdose of greater than 17 g there were no short term clinical, biochemical or haematological sequelae identified.

Treatment:

Patients should be observed closely for evidence of toxicity (see section 4.8) and given the necessary supportive therapy.

Haemodialysis and peritoneal dialysis appear to have a limited effect on elimination of zidovudine but enhance the elimination of the glucuronide metabolite.

5. PHARMACOLOGICAL PROPERTIES

5.1 Pharmacodynamic properties

Pharmacotherapeutic group – nucleoside analogue – ATC Code J05A F01

Mode of action:

Zidovudine is an antiviral agent which is highly active *in vitro* against retroviruses including the Human Immunodeficiency Virus (HIV).

Zidovudine is phosphorylated in both infected and uninfected cells to the monophosphate (MP) derivative by cellular thymidine kinase. Subsequent phosphorylation of zidovudine-MP to the diphosphate (DP), and then the triphosphate (TP) derivative is catalysed by cellular thymidylate kinase and non-specific kinases respectively. Zidovudine-TP acts as an inhibitor of and substrate for the viral reverse transcriptase. The formation of further proviral DNA is blocked by incorporation of zidovudine-MP into the chain and subsequent chain termination. Competition by zidovudine-TP for HIV reverse transcriptase is approximately 100-fold greater than for cellular DNA polymerase alpha.

Clinical virology:

The relationships between *in vitro* susceptibility of HIV to zidovudine and clinical response to therapy remain under investigation. *In vitro* sensitivity testing has not been standardised and results may therefore vary according to methodological factors Reduced *in vitro* sensitivity to zidovudine has been reported for HIV isolates from patients who have received prolonged courses of Retrovir therapy. The available information indicates that for early HIV disease, the frequency and degree of reduction of *in vitro* sensitivity is notably less than for advanced disease.

The reduction of sensitivity with the emergence of zidovudine resistant strains limits the usefulness of zidovudine monotherapy clinically. In clinical studies, clinical endpoint data indicate that zidovudine, particularly in combination with lamivudine, and also with didanosine or zalcitabine results in a significant reduction in the risk of disease progression and mortality. The use of a protease inhibitor in a combination of zidovudine and lamivudine, has been shown to confer additional benefit in delaying disease progression, and improving survival compared to the double combination on its own.

The anti-viral effectiveness *in vitro* of combinations of antiretroviral agents are being investigated. Clinical and *in vitro* studies of zidovudine in combination with lamivudine indicate that zidovudine-resistant virus isolates can become zidovudine sensitive when they simultaneously acquire resistance to lamivudine. Furthermore there is clinical evidence that zidovudine plus lamivudine delays the emergence of zidovudine resistance in anti-retroviral naive patients.

In some *in vitro* studies zidovudine has been shown to act additively or synergistically with a number of anti-HIV agents, such as lamivudine, didanosine, and interferon-alpha, inhibiting the replication of HIV in cell culture. However, *in vitro* studies with triple combinations of nucleoside analogues or two nucleoside analogues and a protease inhibitor have been shown to be more effective in inhibiting HIV-1 induced cytopathic effects than one or two drug combinations.

Resistance to thymidine analogues (of which zidovudine is one) is well characterised and is conferred by the stepwise accumulation of up to six specific mutations in the HIV reverse transcriptase at codons 41, 67, 70, 210, 215 and 219. Viruses acquire phenotypic resistance to thymidine analogues through the combination of mutations at codons 41 and 215 or by the accumulation of at least four of the six mutations. These thymidine analogue mutations alone do not cause high-level cross-resistance to any of the other nucleosides, allowing for the subsequent use of any of the other approved reverse transcriptase inhibitors.

Two patterns of multi-drug resistance mutations, the first characterised by mutations in the HIV reverse transcriptase at codons 62, 75, 77, 116 and 151 and the second involving a T69S mutation plus a 6-base pair insert at the same position, result in phenotypic resistance to AZT as well as to the other approved nucleoside reverse transcriptase inhibitors. Either of these two patterns of multinucleoside resistance mutations severely limits future therapeutic options.

In the US ACTGO76 trial, Retrovir was shown to be effective in reducing the rate of maternal-foetal transmission of HIV-1 (23% infection rate for placebo versus 8% for zidovudine) when administered (100 mg five times a day) to HIV-positive pregnant women (from week 14-34 of pregnancy) and their newborn infants (2 mg/kg every 6 hours) until 6 weeks of age. In the shorter duration 1998 Thailand CDC study, use of oral Retrovir therapy only (300 mg twice daily), from week 36 of pregnancy until delivery, also reduced the rate of maternal-foetal transmission of HIV (19% infection rate for placebo versus 9% for zidovudine). These data, and data from a published study comparing zidovudine regimens to prevent maternal-foetal HIV transmission have shown that short maternal treatments (from week 36 of pregnancy) are less efficacious than longer maternal treatments (from week 14-34 of pregnancy) in the reduction of perinatal HIV transmission.

5.2 Pharmacokinetic properties

Pharmacokinetics in adults:

Zidovudine is well absorbed from the gut and, at all dose levels studied, the bioavailability was 60-70%. From a bioequivalence study, steady-state mean (CV%) C[ss]max, C[ss]min, and AUC[ss] values in 16 patients receiving zidovudine 300mg tablets twice daily were 8.57 (54%) microM (2.29 μg/ml), 0.08 (96%) microM (0.02 μg/ml), and 8.39 (40%) h*microM (2.24 h*μg/ml), respectively.

From studies with intravenous Retrovir, the mean terminal plasma half-life was 1.1 hours, the mean total body clearance was 27.1 ml/min/kg and the apparent volume of distribution was 1.6 Litres/kg. Renal clearance of zidovudine greatly exceeds creatinine clearance, indicating that significant tubular secretion takes place.

Zidovudine is primarily eliminated by hepatic conjugation to an inactive glucoronidated metabolite. The 5'-glucuronide of zidovudine is the major metabolite in both plasma and urine, accounting for approximately 50-80% of the administered dose eliminated by renal excretion. 3'-amino-3'-deoxythymidine (AMT) has been identified as a metabolite of zidovudine following intravenous dosing.

There are limited data on the pharmacokinetics of zidovudine in patients with renal or hepatic impairment (see section 4.2). No specific data are available on the pharmacokinetics of zidovudine in the elderly.

Pharmacokinetics in children:

In children over the age of 5-6 months, the pharmacokinetic profile of zidovudine is similar to that in adults. Zidovudine is well absorbed from the gut and, at all dose levels studied, its bioavailability was 60-74% with a mean of 65%. C^{ss}max levels were 4.45μM (1.19 μg/ml) following a dose of 120 mg Retrovir (in solution)/m^2 body surface area and 7.7 μM (2.06 μg/ml) at 180 mg/m^2 body surface area. Dosages of 180 mg/m^2 four times daily in children produced similar systemic exposure (24 hour AUC 40.0 hr μM or 10.7 hr μg/ml) as doses of 200 mg six times daily in adults (40.7 hr μM or 10.9 hr μg/ml).

With intravenous dosing, the mean terminal plasma half-life and total body clearance were 1.5 hours and 30.9 ml/min/kg respectively. The major metabolite is 5'-glucuronide. After intravenous dosing, 29% of the dose was recovered unchanged in the urine and 45% excreted as the glucuronide. Renal clearance of zidovudine greatly exceeds creatinine clearance indicating that significant tubular secretion takes place.

The data available on the pharmacokinetics in neonates and young infants indicate that glucuronidation of zidovudine is reduced with a consequent increase in bioavailability, reduction in clearance and longer half-life in infants less than 14 days old but thereafter the pharmacokinetics appear similar to those reported in adults.

Pharmacokinetics in pregnancy:

The pharmacokinetics of zidovudine has been investigated in a study of eight women during the third trimester of pregnancy. As pregnancy progressed, there was no evidence of drug accumulation. The pharmacokinetics of zidovudine was similar to that of non-pregnant adults. Consistent with passive transmission of the drug across the placenta, zidovudine concentrations in infant plasma at birth were essentially equal to those in maternal plasma at delivery.

Distribution:

In adults, the average cerebrospinal fluid/plasma zidovudine concentration ratio 2 to 4 hours after dosing was found to be approximately 0.5. Data indicate that zidovudine crosses the placenta and is found in amniotic fluid and foetal blood. Zidovudine has also been detected in semen and milk.

In children the mean cerebrospinal fluid/plasma zidovudine concentration ratio ranged from 0.52-0.85, as determined during oral therapy 0.5 to 4 hours after dosing and was 0.87 as determined during intravenous therapy 1-5 hours after a 1 hour infusion. During continuous intravenous infusion, the mean steady-state cerebrospinal fluid/plasma concentration ratio was 0.24.

Plasma protein binding is relatively low (34 to 38%) and drug interactions involving binding site displacement are not anticipated.

5.3 Preclinical safety data

Mutagenicity:

No evidence of mutagenicity was observed in the Ames test. However, zidovudine was weakly mutagenic in a mouse lymphoma cell assay and was positive in an *in vitro* cell transformation assay. Clastogenic effects were observed in an *in vitro* study in human lymphocytes and in *in vivo* oral repeat dose micronucleus studies in rats and mice. An *in vivo* cytogenetic study in rats did not show chromosomal damage. A study of the peripheral blood lymphocytes of eleven AIDS patients showed a higher chromosome breakage frequency in those who had received Retrovir than in those who had not. A pilot study has demonstrated that zidovudine is incorporated into leukocyte nuclear DNA of adults, including pregnant women, taking zidovudine as treatment for HIV-1 infection, or for the prevention of mother to child viral transmission. Zidovudine was also incorporated into DNA from cord blood leukocytes of infants from zidovudine-treated mothers. A transplacental genotoxicity study conducted in monkeys compared zidovudine alone with the combination of zidovudine and lamivudine at human-equivalent exposures. The study demonstrated that foetuses exposed *in utero* to the combination sustained a higher level of nucleoside analogue-DNA incorporation into multiple foetal organs, and showed evidence of more telomere shortening than in those exposed to zidovudine alone. The clinical significance of these findings is unknown.

Carcinogenicity:

In oral carcinogenicity studies with zidovudine in mice and rats, late appearing vaginal epithelial tumours were observed. A subsequent intravaginal carcinogenicity study confirmed the hypothesis that the vaginal tumours were the result of long term local exposure of the rodent vaginal epithelium to high concentrations of unmetabolised zidovudine in urine. There were no other drug-related tumours observed in either sex of either species.

In addition, two transplacental carcinogenicity studies have been conducted in mice. One study, by the US National Cancer Institute, administered zidovudine at maximum tolerated doses to pregnant mice from day 12 to 18 of gestation. One year post-natally, there was an increase in the incidence of tumours in the lung, liver and female reproductive tract of offspring exposed to the highest dose level (420 mg/kg term body weight).

In a second study, mice were administered zidovudine at doses up to 40 mg/kg for 24 months, with exposure beginning prenatally on gestation day 10. Treatment related findings were limited to late-occurring vaginal epithelial tumours, which were seen with a similar incidence and time of onset as in the standard oral carcinogenicity study. The second study thus provided no evidence that zidovudine acts as a transplacental carcinogen.

It is concluded that the transplacental carcinogenicity data from the first study represents a hypothetical risk, whereas the reduction in risk of maternal transfection of HIV to the uninfected child by the use of zidovudine in pregnancy has been well proven.

6. PHARMACEUTICAL PARTICULARS

6.1 List of excipients

Capsule core:

Maize starch

Microcrystalline Cellulose

Sodium Starch Glycollate

Magnesium Stearate.

Capsule coating:

E171 Titanium dioxide

Gelatin

Indigo carmine E132

Polysorbate 80

Printing ink:

Opacode S-IR-8100 HV Black (contains Black Iron Oxide E172)

6.2 Incompatibilities

Not applicable.

6.3 Shelf life

5 years

6.4 Special precautions for storage

Do not store above 30°C. Store in the original package.

6.5 Nature and contents of container

HDPE or glass bottle containing 100 capsules.

PVC/aluminium foil blister pack containing 100 capsules.

6.6 Instructions for use and handling

No special requirements

Administrative Data

7. MARKETING AUTHORISATION HOLDER

United Kingdom

The Wellcome Foundation Limited

trading as:

Glaxo Wellcome and/or GlaxoSmithKline UK

Stockley Park West

Uxbridge

Middlesex

UB11 1BT

8. MARKETING AUTHORISATION NUMBER(S)

PL 00003/0239

9. DATE OF FIRST AUTHORISATION/RENEWAL OF THE AUTHORISATION

03/03/1987

10. DATE OF REVISION OF THE TEXT

26 July 2005

Retrovir 250mg Capsules

(GlaxoSmithKline UK)

1. NAME OF THE MEDICINAL PRODUCT

Retrovir® 250 mg, capsule, hard

2. QUALITATIVE AND QUANTITATIVE COMPOSITION

Each capsule contains:

Zidovudine 250 mg

For excipients see section 6.1

3. PHARMACEUTICAL FORM

Retrovir 250 mg capsule, hard:

Hard gelatin capsules with opaque blue cap, opaque white body and a central dark-blue band, printed "Wellcome", "250" and coded H2F.

4. CLINICAL PARTICULARS

4.1 Therapeutic indications

Retrovir oral formulations are indicated in anti-retroviral combination therapy for Human Immunodeficiency Virus (HIV) infected adults and children.

Retrovir chemoprophylaxis is indicated for use in HIV-positive pregnant women (over 14 weeks of gestation) for prevention of maternal-foetal HIV transmission and for primary prophylaxis of HIV infection in newborn infants.

4.2 Posology and method of administration

Dosage in adults:

The usual recommended dose of Retrovir in combination with other anti-retroviral agents is 500 or 600 mg/day in two or three divided doses.

Dosage in children:

3 months - 12 years:

The recommended dose of Retrovir is 360 to 480 mg/m^2 per day, in 3 or 4 divided doses in combination with other antiretroviral agents. The maximum dosage should not exceed 200 mg every 6 hours.

<3 months:

The limited data available are insufficient to propose specific dosage recommendations (See below -maternal foetal transmission and section).

Dosage in the prevention of maternal-foetal transmission:

Although the optimal dosage schedule has not been identified the following dosage regimen has been shown to be effective. Pregnant women (over 14 weeks of gestation) should be given 500 mg/day orally (100 mg five times per day) until the beginning of labour. During labour and delivery Retrovir should be administered intravenously at 2 mg/kg bodyweight given over one hour followed by a continuous intravenous infusion at 1 mg/kg/h until the umbilical cord is clamped.

The newborn infants should be given 2 mg/kg bodyweight orally every 6 hours starting within 12 hours after birth and continuing until 6 weeks old (e.g. a 3 kg neonate would require a 0.6 ml dose of oral solution every 6 hours). Infants unable to receive oral dosing should be given Retrovir intravenously at 1.5 mg/kg bodyweight infused over 30 minutes every 6 hours.

In case of planned caesarean, the infusion should be started 4 hours before the operation. In the event of a false labour, the Retrovir infusion should be stopped and oral dosing restarted.

Dosage adjustments in patients with haematological adverse reactions:

Dosage reduction or interruption of Retrovir therapy may be necessary in patients whose haemoglobin level falls to between 7.5 g/dl (4.65 mmol/l) and 9 g/dl (5.59 mmol/l) or whose neutrophil count falls to between 0.75 × 10^9/l and 1.0 × 10^9/l (see sections 4.3 and 4.4)

Dosage in the elderly:

Zidovudine pharmacokinetics have not been studied in patients over 65 years of age and no specific data are available. However, since special care is advised in this age group due to age-associated changes such as the decrease in renal function and alterations in haematological parameters, appropriate monitoring of patients before and during use of Retrovir is advised.

Dosage in renal impairment:

In patients with severe renal impairment, apparent zidovudine clearance after oral zidovudine administration was approximately 50% of that reported in healthy subjects with normal renal function. Therefore a dosage reduction to 300-400 mg daily is recommended for patients with severe renal impairment with creatinine clearance -≤ 10ml/min. Haematological parameters and clinical response may influence the need for subsequent dosage adjustment.

Haemodialysis and peritoneal dialysis have no significant effect on zidovudine elimination whereas elimination of the glucuronide metabolite is increased.

Dosage in hepatic impairment:

Data in patients with cirrhosis suggest that accumulation of zidovudine may occur in patients with hepatic impairment because of decreased glucuronidation. Dosage reductions may be necessary but, as there is only limited data available, precise recommendations cannot be made. If monitoring of plasma zidovudine levels is not feasible, physicians will need to monitor for signs of intolerance, such as the development of haematological adverse reactions (anaemia, leucopenia, neutropenia) and reduce the dose and/or increase the interval between doses as appropriate (see section 4.4).

4.3 Contraindications

Retrovir Oral Formulations are contra-indicated in patients known to be hypersensitive to zidovudine, or to any of the components of the formulations.

Retrovir Oral Formulations should not be given to patients with abnormally low neutrophil counts (less than 0.75 × 10^9/litre) or abnormally low haemoglobin levels (less than 7.5 g/decilitre or 4.65 mmol/litre).

Retrovir is contra-indicated in new born infants with hyperbilirubinaemia requiring treatment other than phototherapy, or with increased transaminase levels of over five times the upper limit of normal.

4.4 Special warnings and special precautions for use

Retrovir is not a cure for HIV infection and patients remain at risk of developing illnesses which are associated with immune suppression, including opportunistic infections and neoplasms. Whilst it has been shown to reduce the risks of opportunistic infections, data on the development of neoplasms, including lymphomas, are limited. The available data on patients treated for advanced HIV disease indicate that the risk of lymphoma development is consistent with that observed in untreated patients. In patients with early HIV disease on long-term treatment the risk of lymphoma development is unknown.

Retrovir should be administered under the supervision of a doctor with experience of treating patients with HIV infection or AIDS. An appropriate treatment procedure requires access to suitable facilities eg. for performing haematological monitoring investigations, including determination of viral load, CD4 lymphocytes and for provision of blood transfusions if necessary.

The concomitant use of rifampicin, ribavirin or stavudine with zidovudine should be avoided (see section 4.5).

Haematological Adverse Reactions: Anaemia (usually not observed before six weeks of Retrovir therapy but occasionally occurring earlier), neutropenia (usually not observed before four weeks' therapy but sometimes occurring earlier) and leucopenia (usually secondary to neutropenia) can be expected to occur in patients receiving Retrovir; These occurred more frequently at higher dosages (1200-1500 mg/day) and in patients with poor bone marrow reserve prior to treatment, particularly with advanced HIV disease.

Haematological parameters should be carefully monitored. For patients with advanced symptomatic HIV disease it is generally recommended that blood tests are performed at least every two weeks for the first three months of therapy and at least monthly thereafter. In patients with early HIV disease (where bone marrow reserve is generally good), haematological adverse reactions are infrequent. Depending on the overall condition of the patient, blood tests may be performed less often, for example every 1 to 3 months.

If the haemoglobin level falls to between 7.5 g/dl (4.65 mmol/l) and 9 g/dl (5.59 mmol/l) or the neutrophil count falls to between 0.75 × 10^9/l and 1.0 × 10^9/l, the daily dosage may be reduced until there is evidence of marrow recovery; alternatively, recovery may be enhanced by brief (2-4 weeks) interruption of Retrovir therapy. Marrow recovery is usually observed within 2 weeks after which time Retrovir therapy at a reduced dosage may be reinstituted. In patients with significant anaemia, dosage adjustments do not necessarily eliminate the need for transfusions (see section 4.3).

Lactic acidosis: lactic acidosis usually associated with hepatomegaly and hepatic steatosis has been reported with the use of nucleoside analogues. Early symptoms (symptomatic hyperlactatemia) include benign digestive symptoms (nausea, vomiting and abdominal pain), non-specific malaise, loss of appetite, weight loss, respiratory symptoms (rapid and/or deep breathing) or neurological symptoms (including motor weakness).

Lactic acidosis has a high mortality and may be associated with pancreatitis, liver failure, or renal failure.

Lactic acidosis generally occurred after a few or several months of treatment.

Treatment with nucleoside analogues should be discontinued in the setting of symptomatic hyperlactataemia and metabolic/lactic acidosis, progressive hepatomegaly, or rapidly elevating aminotransferase levels.

Caution should be exercised when administering nucleoside analogues to any patient (particularly obese women) with hepatomegaly, hepatitis or other known risk factors for liver disease and hepatic steatosis (including certain medicinal products and alcohol). Patients co-infected with hepatitis C and treated with alpha interferon and ribavirin may constitute a special risk.

Patients at increased risk should be followed closely.

Mitochondrial toxicity: Nucleoside and nucleotide analogues have been demonstrated *in vitro* and *in vivo* to cause a variable degree of mitochondrial damage. There have been reports of mitochondrial dysfunction in HIV-negative infants exposed *in utero* and/or post-natally to nucleoside analogues. The main adverse events reported are haematological disorders (anaemia, neutropenia), metabolic disorders (hyperlactataemia, hyperlipasaemia). These events are often transitory. Some late-onset neurological disorders have been reported (hypertonia, convulsion, abnormal behaviour). Whether the neurological disorders are transient or permanent is currently unknown. Any child exposed *in utero* to nucleoside and nucleotide analogues, even HIV-negative children, should have clinical and laboratory follow-up and should be fully investigated for possible mitochondrial dysfunction in case of relevant signs or symptoms. These findings do not affect current recommendations to use antiretroviral therapy in pregnant women to prevent vertical transmission of HIV.

Lipodystrophy: Combination antiretroviral therapy has been associated with the redistribution of body fat (lipodystrophy) in HIV patients. The long-term consequences of these events are currently unknown. Knowledge about the mechanism is incomplete. A connection between visceral lipomatosis and PIs and lipoatrophy and NRTIs has been hypothesised. A higher risk of lipodystrophy has been associated with individual factors such as older age, and with drug related factors such as longer duration of antiretroviral treatment and associated metabolic disturbances. Clinical examination should include evaluation for physical signs of fat redistribution. Consideration should be given to the measurement of fasting serum lipids and blood glucose. Lipid disorders should be managed as clinically appropriate (see section 4.8).

Liver disease: The safety and efficacy of zidovudine has not been established in patients with significant underlying liver disorders.

Patients with chronic hepatitis B or C and treated with combination antiretroviral therapy are at an increased risk of severe and potentially fatal hepatic adverse events. In case of concomitant antiviral therapy for hepatitis B or C, please also refer to the relevant product information for these medicinal products.

Patients with pre-existing liver dysfunction, including chronic active hepatitis, have an increased frequency of liver function abnormalities during combination antiretroviral therapy and should be monitored according to standard practice. If there is evidence of worsening liver disease in such patients, interruption or discontinuation of treatment must be considered (see section 4.2).

Immune Reactivation Syndrome: In HIV-infected patients with severe immune deficiency at the time of institution of combination antiretroviral therapy (CART), an inflammatory reaction to asymptomatic or residual opportunistic pathogens may arise and cause serious clinical conditions, or aggravation of symptoms. Typically, such reactions have been observed within the first few weeks or months of initiation of CART. Relevant examples are cytomegalovirus retinitis, generalized and/or focal mycobacterial infections and *Pneumocystis carinii* pneumonia. Any inflammatory symptoms should be evaluated and treatment instituted when necessary.

Patients should be cautioned about the concomitant use of self-administered medications (see section 4.5).

Patients should be advised that Retrovir therapy has not been proven to prevent the transmission of HIV to others through sexual contact or blood contamination.

Use in Elderly and in Patients with Renal or Hepatic Impairment: see sectionn 4.2.

4.5 Interaction with other medicinal products and other forms of Interaction

Limited data suggests that co-administration of zidovudine with rifampicin decreases the AUC (area under the plasma concentration curve) of zidovudine by 48% ± 34%. This may result in a partial loss or total loss of efficacy of zidovudine (see section 4.4).

Zidovudine in combination with either ribavirin or stavudine are antagonistic in vitro. The concomitant use of either ribavirin or stavudine with zidovudine should be avoided (see section 4.4).

Probenecid increases the AUC of zidovudine by 106% (range 100 to 170%). Patients receiving both drugs should be closely monitored for haematological toxicity.

A modest increase in C_{max} (28%) was observed for zidovudine when administered with lamivudine, however overall exposure (AUC) was not significantly altered. Zidovudine has no effect on the pharmacokinetics of lamivudine.

Phenytoin blood levels have been reported to be low in some patients receiving Retrovir, while in one patient a high level was noted. These observations suggest that phenytoin levels should be carefully monitored in patients receiving both drugs.

In a pharmacokinetic study co-administration of zidovudine and atovaquone showed a decrease in zidovudine clearance after oral dosing leading to a 35%±23% increase in plasma zidovudine AUC. Given the limited data available the clinical significance of this is unknown.

Valproic acid, fluconazole or methadone when co-administered with zidovudine have been shown to increase the AUC with a corresponding decrease in its clearance. As only limited data are available the clinical significance of these findings is unclear but if zidovudine is used concurrently with either valproic acid, fluconazole or methadone, patients should be monitored closely for potential toxicity of zidovudine.

Concomitant treatment, especially acute therapy, with potentially nephrotoxic or myelosuppressive drugs (eg. systemic pentamidine, dapsone, pyrimethamine, co-trimoxazole, amphotericin, flucytosine, ganciclovir, interferon, vincristine, vinblastine and doxorubicin) may also increase the risk of adverse reactions to zidovudine. If concomitant therapy with any of these drugs is necessary then extra care should be taken in monitoring renal function and haematological parameters and, if required, the dosage of one or more agents should be reduced.

Since some patients receiving zidovudine may continue to experience opportunistic infections, concomitant use of prophylactic antimicrobial therapy may have to be considered. Such prophylaxis has included co-trimoxazole, aerosolised pentamidine, pyrimethamine and aciclovir. Limited data from clinical trials do not indicate a significantly increased risk of adverse reactions to zidovudine with these drugs at doses used in prophylaxis.

Clarithromycin tablets reduce the absorption of zidovudine

4.6 Pregnancy and lactation

Pregnancy:

The use of Retrovir in pregnant women over 14 weeks of gestation, with subsequent treatment of their newborn infants, has been shown to significantly reduce the rate of maternal-foetal transmission of HIV based on viral cultures in infants.

The results from the pivotal U.S. placebo-controlled study indicated that Retrovir reduced maternal-foetal transmission by approximately 70%. In this study, pregnant women had CD4 cell counts of 200 to 1818/mm^3 (median in treated group 560/ mm^3) and began treatment therapy between weeks 14 and 34 of gestation and had no clinical indications for Retrovir therapy; their newborn infants received Retrovir until 6-weeks old.

A decision to reduce the risk of maternal transmission of HIV should be based on the balance of potential benefits and potential risk. Pregnant women considering the use of Retrovir during pregnancy for prevention of HIV transmission to their infants should be advised that transmission may still occur in some cases despite therapy.

The efficacy of zidovudine to reduce the maternal-foetal transmission in women with previously prolonged treatment with zidovudine or other antiretroviral agents or women infected with HIV strains with reduced sensitivity to zidovudine is unknown.

It is unknown whether there are any long-term consequences of *in utero* and infant exposure to Retrovir.

Based on the animal carcinogenicity/mutagenicity findings a carcinogenic risk to humans cannot be excluded (see section 5.3). The relevance of these findings to both infected and uninfected infants exposed to Retrovir is unknown. However, pregnant women considering using Retrovir during pregnancy should be made aware of these findings.

Given the limited data on the general use of Retrovir in pregnancy, Retrovir should only be used prior to the 14th week of gestation when the potential benefit to the mother and foetus outweigh the risks. Studies in pregnant rats and rabbits given zidovudine orally at dosage levels up to 450 and 500 mg/kg/day respectively during the major period of organogenesis have revealed no evidence of teratogenicity. There was, however, a statistically significant increase in foetal resorptions in rats given 150 to 450 mg/kg/day and in rabbits given 500 mg/kg/day.

A separate study, reported subsequently, found that rats given a dosage of 3000 mg/kg/day, which is very near the oral median lethal dose (3683 mg/kg), caused marked maternal toxicity and an increase in the incidence of foetal malformations. No evidence of teratogenicity was observed in this study at the lower dosages tested (600 mg/kg/day or less).

Fertility:

Zidovudine did not impair male or female fertility in rats given oral doses of up to 450 mg/kg/day. There are no data on the effect of Retrovir on human female fertility. In men, Retrovir has not been shown to affect sperm count, morphology or motility.

Lactation:

Health experts recommend that women infected with HIV do not breast feed their infants in order to avoid the transmission of HIV. After administration of a single dose of 200 mg zidovudine to HIV-infected women, the mean concentration of zidovudine was similar in human milk and serum. Therefore, since the drug and the virus pass into breast milk it is recommended that mothers taking Retrovir do not breast feed their infants.

4.7 Effects on ability to drive and use machines

There have been no studies to investigate the effect of Retrovir on driving performance or the ability to operate machinery. Furthermore, a detrimental effect on such activities cannot be predicted from the pharmacology of the drug. Nevertheless, the clinical status of the patient and the adverse event profile of Retrovir should be borne in mind when considering the patient's ability to drive or operate machinery.

4.8 Undesirable effects

The adverse event profile appears similar for adults and children. The most serious adverse reactions include anaemia (which may require transfusions), neutropenia and leucopenia. These occurred more frequently at higher dosages (1200-1500 mg/day) and in patients with advanced HIV disease (especially when there is poor bone marrow reserve prior to treatment), and particularly in patients with CD4 cell counts less than 100/mm^3. Dosage reduction or cessation of therapy may become necessary (see section 4.4).

The incidence of neutropenia was also increased in those patients whose neutrophil counts, haemoglobin levels and serum vitamin B_{12} levels were low at the start of Retrovir therapy.

Cases of lactic acidosis, sometimes fatal, usually associated with severe hepatomegaly and hepatic steatosis, have been reported with the use of nucleoside analogues (see section 4.4).

Combination antiretroviral therapy has been associated with redistribution of body fat (lipodystrophy) in HIV patients including the loss of peripheral and facial subcutaneous fat, increased intra-abdominal and visceral fat, breast hypertrophy and dorsocervical fat accumulation (buffalo hump).

Combination antiretroviral therapy has been associated with metabolic abnormalities such as hypertriglyceridaemia, hypercholesterolaemia, insulin resistance, hyperglycaemia and hyperlactataemia (see section 4.4).

In HIV-infected patients with severe immune deficiency at the time of initiation of combination antiretroviral therapy (CART), an inflammatory reaction to asymptomatic or residual opportunistic infections may arise (see section 4.4).

The following events have been reported in patients treated with Retrovir. They may also occur as part of the underlying disease process or in association with other drugs used in the management of HIV disease. The relationship between these events and use of Retrovir is therefore difficult to evaluate, particularly in the medically complicated situations which characterise advanced HIV disease. A reduction in dose or suspension of Retrovir therapy may be warranted in the management of these conditions.

The adverse events considered at least possibly related to the treatment are listed below by body system, organ class and absolute frequency. Frequencies are defined as Very common (greater than 10%), Common (1 - 10%), Uncommon (0.1-1%), Rare (0.01-0.1%) and Very rare (less than 0.01%).

Blood and lymphatic system disorders

Common: Anaemia, neutropenia and leucopenia.

Uncommon: Thrombocytopenia and pancytopenia with marrow hypoplasia

Rare: Pure red cell aplasia

Very rare: Aplastic anaemia

Metabolism and nutrition disorders

Rare: Anorexia and lactic acidosis in the absence of hypoxaemia

Psychiatric disorders

Rare: Anxiety and depression

Nervous system disorders

Very common: Headache

Common: Dizziness

Rare: Insomnia, paraesthesia, somnolence, loss of mental acuity, convulsions

Cardiac disorders

Rare: Cardiomyopathy

Respiratory, thoracic and mediastinal disorders

Uncommon: Dyspnoea

Rare: Cough

Gastrointestinal disorders

Very common: Nausea

Common: Vomiting, abdominal pain, and diarrhoea

Uncommon: Flatulence

Rare: Oral mucosa pigmentation, taste disturbance and dyspepsia. Pancreatitis.

Hepatobiliary disorders

Common: Raised blood levels of liver enzymes and bilirubin

Rare: Liver disorders such as severe hepatomegaly with steatosis

Skin and subcutaneous tissue disorders

Uncommon: Rash and pruritis

Rare: Nail and skin pigmentation, urticaria and sweating

Musculoskeletal and connective tissue disorders

Common: Myalgia

Uncommon: Myopathy

Renal and urinary disorders

Rare: Urinary frequency

Reproductive system and breast disorders

Rare: Gynaecomastia

General disorders and administration site disorders :

Common: Malaise

Uncommon: Fever, generalised pain and asthenia

Rare: Chills, chest pain and influenza-like syndrome

The available data from both placebo-controlled and open-label studies indicate that the incidence of nausea and other frequently reported clinical adverse events consistently decreases over time during the first few weeks of therapy with Retrovir.

Adverse reactions with Retrovir for the prevention of maternal-foetal transmission:

In a placebo-controlled trial, overall clinical adverse events and laboratory test abnormalities were similar for women in the Retrovir and placebo groups. However, there was a trend for mild and moderate anaemia to be seen more commonly prior to delivery in the zidovudine treated women.

In the same trial, haemoglobin concentrations in infants exposed to Retrovir for this indication were marginally lower than in infants in the placebo group, but transfusion was not required. Anaemia resolved within 6 weeks after completion of Retrovir therapy. Other clinical adverse events and laboratory test abnormalities were similar in the Retrovir and placebo groups. It is unknown whether there are any long-term consequences of *in utero* and infant exposure to Retrovir.

4.9 Overdose

Symptoms and signs:

No specific symptoms or signs have been identified following acute overdose with zidovudine apart from those listed as undesirable effects such as fatigue, headache, vomiting, and occasional reports of haematological disturbances. Following a report where a patient took an unspecified quantity of zidovudine with serum levels consistent with an overdose of greater than 17 g there were no short term clinical, biochemical or haematological sequelae identified.

Treatment:

Patients should be observed closely for evidence of toxicity (see section 4.8) and given the necessary supportive therapy.

Haemodialysis and peritoneal dialysis appear to have a limited effect on elimination of zidovudine but enhance the elimination of the glucuronide metabolite.

5. PHARMACOLOGICAL PROPERTIES

5.1 Pharmacodynamic properties

Pharmacotherapeutic group – nucleoside analogue – ATC Code J05A F01

Mode of action:

Zidovudine is an antiviral agent which is highly active *in vitro* against retroviruses including the Human Immunodeficiency Virus (HIV).

Zidovudine is phosphorylated in both infected and uninfected cells to the monophosphate (MP) derivative by cellular thymidine kinase. Subsequent phosphorylation of zidovudine-MP to the diphosphate (DP), and then the triphosphate (TP) derivative is catalysed by cellular thymidylate kinase and non-specific kinases respectively. Zidovudine-TP acts as an inhibitor of and substrate for the viral reverse transcriptase. The formation of further proviral DNA is blocked by incorporation of zidovudine-MP into the chain and subsequent chain termination. Competition by zidovudine-TP for HIV reverse transcriptase is approximately 100-fold greater than for cellular DNA polymerase alpha.

Clinical virology:

The relationships between *in vitro* susceptibility of HIV to zidovudine and clinical response to therapy remain under investigation. *In vitro* sensitivity testing has not been standardised and results may therefore vary according to methodological factors. Reduced *in vitro* sensitivity to zidovudine has been reported for HIV isolates from patients who have received prolonged courses of Retrovir therapy. The available information indicates that for early HIV disease, the frequency and degree of reduction of *in vitro* sensitivity is notably less than for advanced disease.

The reduction of sensitivity with the emergence of zidovudine resistant strains limits the usefulness of zidovudine monotherapy clinically. In clinical studies, clinical endpoint data indicate that zidovudine, particularly in combination with lamivudine, and also with didanosine or zalcitabine results in a significant reduction in the risk of disease progression and mortality. The use of a protease inhibitor in a combination of zidovudine and lamivudine, has been shown to confer additional benefit in delaying disease progression, and improving survival compared to the double combination on its own.

The anti-viral effectiveness *in vitro* of combinations of antiretroviral agents are being investigated. Clinical and *in vitro* studies of zidovudine in combination with lamivudine indicate that zidovudine-resistant virus isolates can become zidovudine sensitive when they simultaneously acquire resistance to lamivudine. Furthermore there is clinical evidence that zidovudine plus lamivudine delays the emergence of zidovudine resistance in anti-retroviral naive patients.

In some *in vitro* studies zidovudine has been shown to act additively or synergistically with a number of anti-HIV agents, such as lamivudine, didanosine, and interferon-alpha, inhibiting the replication of HIV in cell culture. However, *in vitro* studies with triple combinations of nucleoside analogues or two nucleoside analogues and a protease inhibitor have been shown to be more effective in inhibiting HIV-1 induced cytopathic effects than one or two drug combinations.

Resistance to thymidine analogues (of which zidovudine is one) is well characterised and is conferred by the stepwise accumulation of up to six specific mutations in the HIV reverse transcriptase at codons 41, 67, 70, 210, 215 and 219. Viruses acquire phenotypic resistance to thymidine analogues through the combination of mutations at codons 41 and 215 or by the accumulation of at least four of the six mutations. These thymidine analogue mutations alone do not cause high-level cross-resistance to any of the other nucleosides, allowing for the subsequent use of any of the other approved reverse transcriptase inhibitors.

Two patterns of multi-drug resistance mutations, the first characterised by mutations in the HIV reverse transcriptase at codons 62, 75, 77, 116 and 151 and the second involving a T69S mutation plus a 6-base pair insert at the same position, result in phenotypic resistance to AZT as well as to the other approved nucleoside reverse transcriptase inhibitors. Either of these two patterns of multinucleoside resistance mutations severely limits future therapeutic options.

In the US ACTG076 trial, Retrovir was shown to be effective in reducing the rate of maternal-foetal transmission of HIV-1 (23% infection rate for placebo versus 8% for zidovudine) when administered (100 mg five times daily) to HIV-positive pregnant women (from week 14-34 of pregnancy) and their newborn infants (2 mg/kg every 6 hours) until 6 weeks of age. In the shorter duration 1998 Thailand CDC study, use of oral Retrovir therapy only (300 mg twice daily), from week 36 of pregnancy until delivery, also reduced the rate of maternal-foetal transmission of HIV (19% infection rate for placebo versus 9% for zidovudine). These data, and data from a published study comparing zidovudine regimes to prevent maternal-foetal HIV transmission have shown that short maternal treatments (from week 36 of pregnancy) are less efficacious than longer maternal treatments (from week 14-34 of pregnancy) in the reduction of perinatal HIV transmission.

5.2 Pharmacokinetic properties

Pharmacokinetics in adults:

Zidovudine is well absorbed from the gut and, at all dose levels studied, the bioavailability was 60-70%. From a bioequivalence study, steady-state mean (CV%) C[ss]max, C[ss]min, and AUC[ss] values in 16 patients receiving zidovudine 300mg tablets twice daily were 8.57 (54%) microM (2.29 μg/ml), 0.08 (96%) microM (0.02 μg/ml), and 8.39 (40%) h*microM (2.24 h*μg/ml), respectively.

From studies with intravenous Retrovir, the mean terminal plasma half-life was 1.1 hours, the mean total body clearance was 27.1 ml/min/kg and the apparent volume of distribution was 1.6 Litres/kg. Renal clearance of zidovudine greatly exceeds creatinine clearance, indicating that significant tubular secretion takes place.

Zidovudine is primarily eliminated by hepatic conjugation to an inactive glucoronidated metabolite. The 5'-glucuronide of zidovudine is the major metabolite in both plasma and urine, accounting for approximately 50-80% of the administered dose eliminated by renal excretion. 3'-amino-3'-deoxythymidine (AMT) has been identified as a metabolite of zidovudine following intravenous dosing.

There are limited data on the pharmacokinetics of zidovudine in patients with renal or hepatic impairment (see section 4.2). No specific data are available on the pharmacokinetics of zidovudine in the elderly.

Pharmacokinetics in children:

In children over the age of 5-6 months, the pharmacokinetic profile of zidovudine is similar to that in adults. Zidovudine is well absorbed from the gut and, at all dose levels studied, its bioavailability was 60-74% with a mean of 65%. C^{ss}max levels were 4.45 μM (1.19μg/ml) following a dose of 120 mg Retrovir (in solution)/m^2 body surface area and 7.7μM (2.06μg/ml) at 180 mg/m^2 body surface area. Dosages of 180 mg/m^2 four times daily in children produced similar systemic exposure (24 hour AUC 40.0 hr μM or 10.7 hr μg/ml) as doses of 200 mg six times daily in adults (40.7 hr μM or 10.9 hr μg/ml).

With intravenous dosing, the mean terminal plasma half-life and total body clearance were 1.5 hours and 30.9ml/min/kg respectively. The major metabolite is 5'-glucuronide. After intravenous dosing, 29% of the dose was recovered unchanged in the urine and 45% excreted as the glucuronide. Renal clearance of zidovudine greatly exceeds creatinine clearance indicating that significant tubular secretion takes place.

The data available on the pharmacokinetics in neonates and young infants indicate that glucuronidation of zidovudine is reduced with a consequent increase in bioavailability, reduction in clearance and longer half-life in infants less than 14 days old but thereafter the pharmacokinetics appear similar to those reported in adults.

Pharmacokinetics in pregnancy:

The pharmacokinetics of zidovudine has been investigated in a study of eight women during the third trimester of pregnancy. As pregnancy progressed, there was no evidence of drug accumulation. The pharmacokinetics of zidovudine was similar to that of non-pregnant adults. Consistent with passive transmission of the drug across the placenta, zidovudine concentrations in infant plasma at birth were essentially equal to those in maternal plasma at delivery.

Distribution:

In adults, the average cerebrospinal fluid/plasma zidovudine concentration ratio 2 to 4 hours after dosing was found to be approximately 0.5. Data indicate that zidovudine crosses the placenta and is found in amniotic fluid and foetal blood. Zidovudine has also been detected in semen and milk.

In children the mean cerebrospinal fluid/plasma zidovudine concentration ratio ranged from 0.52-0.85, as determined during oral therapy 0.5 to 4 hours after dosing and was 0.87 as determined during intravenous therapy 1-5 hours after a 1 hour infusion. During continuous intravenous infusion, the mean steady-state cerebrospinal fluid/plasma concentration ratio was 0.24.

Plasma protein binding is relatively low (34 to 38%) and drug interactions involving binding site displacement are not anticipated.

5.3 Preclinical safety data

Mutagenicity:

No evidence of mutagenicity was observed in the Ames test. However, zidovudine was weakly mutagenic in a mouse lymphoma cell assay and was positive in an *in vitro* cell transformation assay. Clastogenic effects were observed in an *in vitro* study in human lymphocytes and in *in vivo* oral repeat dose micronucleus studies in rats and mice. An *in vivo* cytogenetic study in rats did not show chromosomal damage. A study of the peripheral blood lymphocytes of eleven AIDS patients showed a higher chromosome breakage frequency in those who had received Retrovir than in those who had not. A pilot study has demonstrated that zidovudine is incorporated into leukocyte nuclear DNA of adults, including pregnant women, taking zidovudine as treatment for HIV-1 infection, or for the prevention of mother to child viral transmission. Zidovudine was also incorporated into DNA from cord blood leukocytes of infants from zidovudine-treated mothers. A transplacental genotoxicity study conducted in monkeys compared zidovudine alone with the combination of zidovudine and lamivudine at human-equivalent exposures. The study demonstrated that foetuses exposed *in utero* to the combination sustained a higher level of nucleoside analogue-DNA incorporation into multiple foetal organs, and showed evidence of more telomere shortening than in those exposed to zidovudine alone. The clinical significance of these findings is unknown.

Carcinogenicity:

In oral carcinogenicity studies with zidovudine in mice and rats, late appearing vaginal epithelial tumours were observed. A subsequent intravaginal carcinogenicity study confirmed the hypothesis that the vaginal tumours were the result of long term local exposure of the rodent vaginal epithelium to high concentrations of unmetabolised zidovudine in urine. There were no other drug-related tumours observed in either sex of either species.

In addition, two transplacental carcinogenicity studies have been conducted in mice. One study, by the US National Cancer Institute, administered zidovudine at maximum tolerated doses to pregnant mice from day 12 to 18 of gestation. One year post-natally, there was an increase in the incidence of tumours in the lung, liver and female reproductive tract of offspring exposed to the highest dose level (420 mg/kg term body weight).

In a second study, mice were administered zidovudine at doses up to 40 mg/kg for 24 months, with exposure beginning prenatally on gestation day 10. Treatment related findings were limited to late-occurring vaginal epithelial tumours, which were seen with a similar incidence and time of onset as in the standard oral carcinogenicity study. The second study thus provided no evidence that zidovudine acts as a transplacental carcinogen.

It is concluded that the transplacental carcinogenicity data from the first study represents a hypothetical risk, whereas the reduction in risk of maternal transfection of HIV to the uninfected child by the use of zidovudine in pregnancy has been well proven.

6. PHARMACEUTICAL PARTICULARS

6.1 List of excipients

Capsule core:

Maize starch

Microcrystalline Cellulose

Sodium Starch Glycollate

Magnesium Stearate.

Capsule coating:

E171 Titanium dioxide

Gelatin

Indigo carmine E132

Polysorbate 80

Printing ink:

Opacode S-IR-8100 HV Black (contains Black Iron Oxide E172)

6.2 Incompatibilities

Not applicable.

6.3 Shelf life

5 years

6.4 Special precautions for storage

Do not store above 30°C. Store in the original package.

6.5 Nature and contents of container

PVC/aluminium foil blister pack containing 40 capsules.

6.6 Instructions for use and handling

No special requirements

Administrative Data

7. MARKETING AUTHORISATION HOLDER

United Kingdom

The Wellcome Foundation Limited

trading as:

Glaxo Wellcome and/or GlaxoSmithKline UK

Stockley Park West

Uxbridge

Middlesex

UB11 1BT

8. MARKETING AUTHORISATION NUMBER(S)

PL 00003/0240

9. DATE OF FIRST AUTHORISATION/RENEWAL OF THE AUTHORISATION

03/03/1987

10. DATE OF REVISION OF THE TEXT

26 July 2005

Retrovir10 mg/ml IV for Infusion

(GlaxoSmithKline UK)

1. NAME OF THE MEDICINAL PRODUCT

Retrovir® 10 mg/ml IV for Infusion

2. QUALITATIVE AND QUANTITATIVE COMPOSITION

Vials containing Zidovudine 200 mg in 20ml solution (10 mg zidovudine/ml)

For excipients, see section 6.1.

3. PHARMACEUTICAL FORM

Concentrate for solution for infusion.

Retrovir IV for Infusion is a clear, nearly colourless, sterile aqueous solution with a pH of approximately 5.5.

4. CLINICAL PARTICULARS

4.1 Therapeutic indications

Retrovir IV for Infusion is indicated for the short-term management of serious manifestations of Human Immunodeficiency Virus (HIV) infection in patients with Acquired Immune Deficiency Syndrome (AIDS) who are unable to take Retrovir oral formulations. If at all possible Retrovir IV should not be used as monotherapy for this indication (see section 5.1).

Retrovir chemoprophylaxis, is indicated for use in HIV-positive pregnant women (over 14 weeks of gestation) for prevention of maternal-foetal HIV transmission and for primary prophylaxis of HIV infection in newborn infants. Retrovir IV should only be used when oral treatment is not possible (except during labour and delivery – see section 4.2).

4.2 Posology and method of administration

The required dose of Retrovir IV for Infusion must be administered by slow intravenous infusion of the diluted product over a one-hour period.

Retrovir IV for Infusion must **NOT** be given intramuscularly.

Dilution

Retrovir IV for Infusion **must** be diluted prior to administration (see section 6.6).

Dosage in adults:

A dose for Retrovir IV for Infusion of 1 or 2 mg zidovudine/kg bodyweight every 4 hours provides similar exposure (AUC) to an oral dose of 1.5 or 3.0 mg zidovudine/kg every 4 hours (600 or 1200 mg/day for a 70 kg patient). The current recommended oral dose of Retrovir is 500-600 mg/day in two or three divided doses. This current dose is used as part of a multi-drug treatment regimen.

Patients should receive Retrovir IV for Infusion only until oral therapy can be administered.

Dosage in children:

Limited data are available on the use of Retrovir IV for Infusion in children. A range of intravenous dosages between 80-160 mg/m^2 every 6 hours (320-640 mg/ m^2/day) have been used. Exposure following the 120 mg/ m^2 dose every 6 hours approximately corresponds to an oral dose of 180 mg/m^2 every 6 hours. The current recommended oral dose of Retrovir as part of a multi-drug treatment regimen is 360 to 480 mg/m^2 per day in 3 or 4 divided doses, which approximately corresponds to an intravenous dose of 240-320 mg/m^2/day in 3 or 4 divided doses.

Dosage in the prevention of maternal-foetal transmission:

Although the optimal dosage schedule has not been identified the following dosage regimen has been shown to be effective. Pregnant women (over 14 weeks of gestation) should be given 500 mg/day orally (100 mg five times per day) until the beginning of labour. During labour and delivery Retrovir should be administered intravenously at 2 mg/kg bodyweight given over one hour followed by a continuous intravenous infusion at 1 mg/kg/h until the umbilical cord is clamped.

The newborn infants should be given 2 mg/kg bodyweight orally every 6 hours starting within 12 hours after birth and continuing until 6 weeks-old (e.g. a 3 kg neonate would require a 0.6 ml dose of oral solution every 6 hours). Infants unable to receive oral dosing should be given Retrovir intravenously at 1.5 mg/kg bodyweight infused over 30 minutes every 6 hours.

In case of planned caesarean, the infusion should be started 4 hours before the operation. In the event of a false labour, the Retrovir infusion should be stopped and oral dosing restarted.

Dosage adjustments in patients with haematological adverse reactions:

Dosage reduction or interruption of Retrovir therapy may be necessary in patients whose haemoglobin level falls to between 7.5 g/dl (4.65 mmol/l) and 9 g/dl (5.59 mmol/l) or whose neutrophil count falls to between 0.75 × 10^9/l and 1.0 × 10^9/l (see sections 4.3 and 4.4)

Dosage in the elderly:

Zidovudine pharmacokinetics have not been studied in patients over 65 years of age and no specific data are available. However, since special care is advised in this age group due to age-associated changes such as the decrease in renal function and alterations in haematological parameters, appropriate monitoring of patients before and during use of Retrovir is advised.

Dosage in renal impairment:

Compared to healthy subjects, patients with advanced renal failure have a 50% higher peak plasma concentration after oral administration. Systemic exposure (measured as area under the zidovudine concentration time curve) is increased 100%; the half-life is not significantly altered. In renal failure there is substantial accumulation of the major glucuronide metabolite but this does not appear to cause toxicity.

In patients with severe renal impairment, the recommended IV dosage is 1 mg/kg 3-4 times daily. This is equivalent to the current recommended oral daily dosage for this patient group of 300 – 400 mg allowing for oral bioavailability of 60-70%. Haematological parameters and clinical response, may influence the need for subsequent dosage adjustment.

Haemodialysis and peritoneal dialysis have no significant effect on zidovudine elimination whereas elimination of the glucuronide metabolite is increased.

Dosage in hepatic impairment:

Data in patients with cirrhosis suggest that accumulation of zidovudine may occur in patients with hepatic impairment because of decreased glucuronidation. Dosage reductions may be necessary but, as there is only limited data available precise recommendations cannot be made. If monitoring of plasma zidovudine levels is not feasible, physicians will need to monitor for signs of intolerance, such as the development of haematological adverse reactions (anaemia, leucopenia, neutropenia) and reduce the dose and/or increase the interval between doses as appropriate (see section 4.4).

4.3 Contraindications

Retrovir IV for Infusion is contra-indicated in patients known to be hypersensitive to zidovudine, or to any of the components of the formulation.

Retrovir IV for infusion should not be given to patients with abnormally low neutrophil counts (less than 0.75 × 10^9/l) or abnormally low haemoglobin levels (less than 7.5 g/dl or 4.65 mmol/l).

Retrovir is contra-indicated in newborn infants with hyperbilirubinaemia requiring treatment other than phototherapy, or with increased transaminase levels of over five times the upper limit of normal.

4.4 Special warnings and special precautions for use

Retrovir is not a cure for HIV infection and patients remain at risk of developing illnesses which are associated with immune suppression, including opportunistic infections and neoplasms. Whilst it has been shown to reduce the risk of opportunistic infections, data on the development of neoplasms, including lymphomas, are limited. The available data on patients treated for advanced HIV disease indicate that the risk of lymphoma development is consistent with that observed in untreated patients. In patients with early HIV disease on long term treatment the risk of lymphoma development is unknown.

Retrovir should be administered under the supervision of a doctor with experience of treating patients with HIV infection or AIDS. An appropriate treatment procedure requires access to suitable facilities e.g. for performing haematological monitoring investigations, including determination of viral load, CD4 lymphocytes and for provision of blood transfusions if necessary.

The concomitant use of rifampicin, ribavirin or stavudine with zidovudine should be avoided (see section 4.5).

Haematological Adverse Reactions: Anaemia (usually not observed before six weeks of Retrovir therapy but occasionally earlier), neutropenia (usually not observed before four weeks therapy but sometimes earlier) and leucopenia (usually secondary to neutropenia) can be expected to occur in patients receiving Retrovir IV for Infusion. These occurred more frequently at high dosages (1200-1500 mg/day orally) and in patients with poor bone marrow reserve prior to treatment, particularly with advanced HIV disease.

Haematological parameters should be carefully monitored. It is recommended that blood tests are performed at least weekly in patients receiving Retrovir IV for Infusion.

If the haemoglobin level falls to between 7.5 g/dl (4.65 mmol/l) and 9 g/dl (5.59 mmol/l) or the neutrophil count falls to between 0.75 × 10^9/l and 1.0 × 10^9/l, the daily dosage may be reduced until there is evidence of marrow recovery; alternatively, recovery may be enhanced by brief (2-4 weeks) interruption of Retrovir therapy. Marrow recovery is usually observed within 2 weeks after which time Retrovir therapy at a reduced dosage may be reinstituted. Data on the use of intravenous Retrovir for periods in excess of 2 weeks are limited. In patients with significant anaemia, dosage adjustments do not necessarily eliminate the need for transfusions (see section 4.3).

Lactic acidosis: lactic acidosis usually associated with hepatomegaly and hepatic steatosis has been reported with the use of nucleoside analogues. Early symptoms (symptomatic hyperlactatemia) include benign digestive symptoms (nausea, vomiting and abdominal pain), non-specific malaise, loss of appetite, weight loss, respiratory symptoms (rapid and/or deep breathing) or neurological symptoms (including motor weakness).

Lactic acidosis has a high mortality and may be associated with pancreatitis, liver failure, or renal failure.

Lactic acidosis generally occurred after a few or several months of treatment.

Treatment with nucleoside analogues should be discontinued in the setting of symptomatic hyperlactataemia and metabolic/lactic acidosis, progressive hepatomegaly, or rapidly elevating aminotransferase levels.

Caution should be exercised when administering nucleoside analogues to any patient (particularly obese women) with hepatomegaly, hepatitis or other known risk factors for liver disease and hepatic steatosis (including certain medicinal products and alcohol). Patients co-infected with hepatitis C and treated with alpha interferon and ribavirin may constitute a special risk.

Patients at increased risk should be followed closely.

Mitochondrial toxicity: Nucleoside and nucleotide analogues have been demonstrated *in vitro* and *in vivo* to cause a variable degree of mitochondrial damage. There have been reports of mitochondrial dysfunction in HIV-negative infants exposed *in utero* and/or post-natally to nucleoside analogues. The main adverse events reported are haematological disorders (anaemia, neutropenia), metabolic disorders (hyperlactataemia, hyperlipasaemia). These events are often transitory. Some late-onset neurological disorders have been reported (hypertonia, convulsion, abnormal behaviour). Whether the neurological disorders are transient or permanent is currently unknown. Any child exposed *in utero* to nucleoside and nucleotide analogues, even HIV-negative children, should have clinical and laboratory follow-up and should be fully investigated for possible mitochondrial dysfunction in case of relevant signs or symptoms. These findings do not affect current recommendations to use antiretroviral therapy in pregnant women to prevent vertical transmission of HIV.

Lipodystrophy: Combination antiretroviral therapy has been associated with the redistribution of body fat (lipodystrophy) in HIV patients. The long-term consequences of these events are currently unknown. Knowledge about the mechanism is incomplete. A connection between visceral lipomatosis and PIs and lipoatrophy and NRTIs has been hypothesised. A higher risk of lipodystrophy has been associated with individual factors such as older age, and with drug related factors such as longer duration of antiretroviral treatment and associated metabolic disturbances. Clinical examination should include evaluation for physical signs of fat redistribution. Consideration should be given to the measurement of fasting serum lipids and blood glucose. Lipid disorders should be managed as clinically appropriate (see section 4.8).

Liver disease: The safety and efficacy of zidovudine has not been established in patients with significant underlying liver disorders.

Patients with chronic hepatitis B or C and treated with combination antiretroviral therapy are at an increased risk of severe and potentially fatal hepatic adverse events. In case of concomitant antiviral therapy for hepatitis B or C, please also refer to the relevant product information for these medicinal products.

Patients with pre-existing liver dysfunction, including chronic active hepatitis, have an increased frequency of liver function abnormalities during combination antiretroviral therapy and should be monitored according to standard practice. If there is evidence of worsening liver disease in such patients, interruption or discontinuation of treatment must be considered (see section 4.2).

Immune Reactivation Syndrome: In HIV-infected patients with severe immune deficiency at the time of institution of combination antiretroviral therapy (CART), an inflammatory reaction to asymptomatic or residual opportunistic pathogens may arise and cause serious clinical conditions, or aggravation of symptoms. Typically, such reactions have been observed within the first few weeks or months of initiation of CART. Relevant examples are cytomegalovirus retinitis, generalized and/or focal mycobacterial infections and *Pneumocystis carinii* pneumonia. Any inflammatory symptoms should be evaluated and treatment instituted when necessary.

Patients should be cautioned about the concomitant use of self-administered medications (see section 4.5).

Patients should be advised that Retrovir therapy has not been proven to prevent the transmission of HIV to others through sexual contact or blood contamination.

4.5 Interaction with other medicinal products and other forms of Interaction

Limited data suggests that co-administration of zidovudine with rifampicin decreases the AUC (area under the plasma concentration curve) of zidovudine by 48% ± 34%. This may result in a partial loss or total loss of efficacy of zidovudine (see section 4.4).

Zidovudine in combination with either ribavirin or stavudine are antagonistic in vitro. The concomitant use of either ribavirin or stavudine with zidovudine should be avoided (see section 4.4).

Probenecid increases the AUC of zidovudine by 106% (range 100 to 170%). Patients receiving both drugs should be closely monitored for haematological toxicity.

A modest increase in C_{max} (28%) was observed for zidovudine when administered with lamivudine, however overall exposure (AUC) was not significantly altered. Zidovudine has no effect on the pharmacokinetics of lamivudine.

Phenytoin blood levels have been reported to be low in some patients receiving Retrovir, while in one patient a high level was noted. These observations suggest that phenytoin levels should be carefully monitored in patients receiving both drugs.

In a pharmacokinetic study co-administration of zidovudine and atovaquone showed a decrease in zidovudine clearance after oral dosing leading to a 35%±23% increase in plasma zidovudine AUC. Given the limited data available the clinical significance of this is unknown.

Valproic acid, fluconazole or methadone when co-administered with zidovudine have been shown to increase the AUC with a corresponding decrease in its clearance. As only limited data are available the clinical significance of these findings is unclear but if zidovudine is used concurrently with either valproic acid, fluconazole or methadone, patients should be monitored closely for potential toxicity of zidovudine.

Concomitant therapy especially acute therapy with potentially nephrotoxic or myelosuppressive drugs (e.g. systemic pentamidine, dapsone, pyrimethamine, co-trimoxazole, amphotericin, flucytosine, ganciclovir, interferon, vincristine, vinblastine and doxorubicin) may also increase the risk of adverse reactions with zidovudine. If concomitant therapy with any of these drugs is necessary then extra care should be taken in monitoring renal function and haematological parameters and if required, the dosage of one or more agents should be reduced.

Since some patients receiving zidovudine may continue to experience opportunistic infections, concomitant use of prophylactic antimicrobial therapy may have to be considered. Such therapy has included co-trimoxazole, aerosolised pentamidine, pyrimethamine and aciclovir. Limited data from controlled clinical trials do not indicate a significantly increased risk of adverse reactions to zidovudine with these drugs at doses used in prophylaxis.

4.6 Pregnancy and lactation

Pregnancy:

The use of Retrovir in pregnant women over 14 weeks of gestation, with subsequent treatment of their newborn infants, has been shown to significantly reduce the rate of maternal-foetal transmission of HIV based on viral cultures in infants.

The results from the pivotal US placebo-controlled study indicated that Retrovir reduced maternal-foetal transmission by approximately 70%. In this study, pregnant women had CD4 cell counts of 200 to 1818/mm^3 (median in treated group 560/mm^3) and began treatment therapy between weeks 14 and 34 of gestation and had no clinical indications for Retrovir therapy; their newborn infants received Retrovir until 6-weeks old.

A decision to reduce the risk of maternal transmission of HIV should be based on the balance of potential benefits and potential risk. Pregnant women considering the use of Retrovir during pregnancy for prevention of HIV transmission to their infants should be advised that transmission may still occur in some cases despite therapy.

The efficacy of zidovudine to reduce the maternal-foetal transmission in women with previously prolonged treatment with zidovudine or other antiretroviral agents or women infected with HIV strains with reduced sensitivity to zidovudine is unknown.

It is unknown whether there are any long-term consequences of *in utero* and infant exposure to Retrovir.

Based on the animal carcinogenicity/mutagenicity findings a carcinogenic risk to humans cannot be excluded (see section 5.3). The relevance of these findings to both infected and uninfected infants exposed to Retrovir is unknown. However, pregnant women considering using Retrovir during pregnancy should be made aware of these findings.

Given the limited data on the general use of Retrovir in pregnancy, Retrovir should only be used prior to the 14th week of gestation when the potential benefit to the mother and foetus outweigh the risks. Studies in pregnant rats and rabbits given zidovudine orally at dosage levels up to 450 and 500 mg/kg/day respectively during the major period of organogenesis have revealed no evidence of teratogenicity. There was, however, a statistically significant increase in foetal-resorptions in rats given 150 to 450 mg/kg/day and in rabbits given 500 mg/kg/day.

A separate study, reported subsequently, found that rats given a dosage of 3000 mg/kg/day, which is very near the oral median lethal dose (3683 mg/kg), caused marked maternal toxicity and an increase in the incidence of foetal malformations. No evidence of teratogenicity was observed in this study at the lower dosages tested (600 mg/kg/day or less).

Fertility:

Zidovudine did not impair male or female fertility in rats given oral dosages of up to 450 mg/kg/day. There are no data on the effect of Retrovir on human female fertility. In men, Retrovir has not been shown to affect sperm count, morphology or motility.

Lactation:

Health experts recommend that women infected with HIV do not breast feed their infants in order to avoid the transmission of HIV. After administration of a single dose of 200 mg zidovudine to HIV-infected women, the mean concentration of zidovudine was similar in human milk and serum. Therefore, since the drug and the virus pass into breast milk it is recommended that mothers taking Retrovir do not breast feed their infants.

4.7 Effects on ability to drive and use machines

Retrovir IV for Infusion is generally used in an in-patient hospital population and information on ability to drive and use machinery is not usually relevant. There have been no studies to investigate the effect of Retrovir on driving performance or the ability to operate machinery. Further, a detrimental effect on such activities cannot be predicted from the pharmacology of the drug. Nevertheless, the clinical status of the patient and the adverse events profile of Retrovir should be borne in mind when considering the patient's ability to drive or operate machinery.

4.8 Undesirable effects

The adverse event profile appears similar for adults and children. The most serious adverse reactions include anaemia (which may require transfusions), neutropenia and leucopenia. These occur more frequently at higher doses (1200-1500 mg/day) and in patients with advanced HIV disease (especially when there is poor bone marrow reserve prior to treatment), and particularly in patients with CD4 cell counts less than 100/mm^3. Dosage reduction or cessation of therapy may become necessary (see section 4.4).

The incidence of neutropenia was also increased in those patients whose neutrophil counts, haemoglobin levels and vitamin B_{12} levels were low at the start of Retrovir therapy.

Cases of lactic acidosis, sometimes fatal, usually associated with severe hepatomegaly and hepatic steatosis, have been reported with the use of nucleoside analogues (see section 4.4).

Combination antiretroviral therapy has been associated with redistribution of body fat (lipodystrophy) in HIV patients including the loss of peripheral and facial subcutaneous fat, increased intra-abdominal and visceral fat, breast hypertrophy and dorsocervical fat accumulation (buffalo hump).

Combination antiretroviral therapy has been associated with metabolic abnormalities such as hypertriglyceridaemia, hypercholesterolaemia, insulin resistance, hyperglycaemia and hyperlactataemia (see section 4.4).

In HIV-infected patients with severe immune deficiency at the time of initiation of combination antiretroviral therapy (CART), an inflammatory reaction to asymptomatic or residual opportunistic infections may arise (see section 4.4).

The following events have been reported in patients treated with Retrovir. They may also occur as part of the underlying disease process in association with other drugs used in the management of HIV disease. The relationship between these events and use of Retrovir is therefore difficult to evaluate, particularly in the medically complicated situations which characterise advanced HIV disease. A reduction in dose or suspension of Retrovir therapy may be warranted in the management of these conditions.

The adverse events considered at least possibly related to the treatment are listed below by body system, organ class and absolute frequency. Frequencies are defined as Very common (greater than 10%), Common (1-10%), Uncommon (0.1-1%), Rare (0.01-0.1%) and Very rare (less than 0.01%).

Blood and lymphatic system disorders

Common:Anaemia, neutropenia and leucopenia

Uncommon: Thrombocytopenia and pancytopenia with marrow hypoplasia

Rare: Pure red cell aplasia

Very rare: Aplastic anaemia

Metabolism and nutrition disorders

Rare: Anorexia and lactic acidosis in the absence of hypoxaemia

Psychiatric disorders

Rare: Anxiety and depression

Nervous system disorders

Very common: Headache

Common: Dizziness

Rare: Insomnia, paraesthesia, somnolence, loss of mental acuity, convulsions

Cardiac disorders

Rare: Cardiomyopathy

Respiratory, thoracic and mediastinal disorders

Uncommon: Dyspnoea

Rare: Cough

Gastrointestinal disorders

Very common: Nausea

Common: Vomiting, abdominal pain, and diarrhoea

Uncommon: Flatulence

Rare: Oral mucosa pigmentation, taste disturbance and dyspepsia. Pancreatitis.

Hepatobiliary disorders

Common: Raised blood levels of liver enzymes and bilirubin

Rare: Liver disorders such as severe hepatomegaly with steatosis

Skin and subcutaneous tissue disorders

Uncommon: Rash and pruritis

Rare: Nail and skin pigmentation, urticaria and sweating

Musculoskeletal and connective tissue disorders

Common: Myalgia

Uncommon: Myopathy

Renal and urinary disorders

Rare: Urinary frequency

Reproductive system and breast disorders

Rare: Gynaecomastia

General disorders and administration site disorders :

Common: Malaise

Uncommon: Fever, generalised pain and asthenia

Rare: Chills, chest pain and influenza-like syndrome

Experience with Retrovir IV for Infusion treatment for periods in excess of two weeks is limited, although some patients have received treatment for up to 12 weeks. The most frequent adverse events were anaemia, neutropenia and leucopenia. Local reactions were infrequent.

The available data from studies of Retrovir Oral Formulations indicate that the incidence of nausea and other frequently reported clinical adverse events consistently decreased over time during the first few weeks of therapy with Retrovir.

Adverse reactions with Retrovir for the prevention of maternal-foetal transmission:

In a placebo-controlled trial, overall clinical adverse events and laboratory test abnormalities were similar for women in the Retrovir and placebo groups. However, there was a trend for mild and moderate anaemia to be seen more commonly prior to delivery in the zidovudine treated women.

In the same trial, haemoglobin concentrations in infants exposed to Retrovir for this indication were marginally lower than in infants in the placebo group, but transfusion was not required. Anaemia resolved within six weeks after completion of Retrovir therapy. Other clinical adverse events and laboratory test abnormalities were similar in the Retrovir and placebo groups. It is unknown whether there are any long-term consequences of *in utero* and infant exposure to Retrovir.

4.9 Overdose

Symptoms and signs:

Dosages as high as 7.5 mg/kg by infusion every four hours for two weeks have been administered to five patients. One patient experienced an anxiety reaction while the other four had no untoward effects.

No specific symptoms or signs have been identified following acute oral overdose with zidovudine, apart from those listed as undesirable effects such as fatigue, headache, vomiting, and occasional reports of haematological disturbances. Following a report where a patient took an unspecified quantity of zidovudine with serum levels consistent with an overdose of greater than 17 g there were no short term clinical, biochemical or haematological sequelae identified.

Treatment:

Patients should be observed closely for evidence of toxicity (see section 4.8) and given the necessary supportive therapy.

Haemodialysis and peritoneal dialysis appear to have a limited effect on elimination of zidovudine but enhances the elimination of the glucuronide metabolite.

5. PHARMACOLOGICAL PROPERTIES

5.1 Pharmacodynamic properties

Pharmacotherapeutic group - nucleoside analogue - ATC Code J05A F01

Mode of Action: Zidovudine is an antiviral agent which is highly active *in vitro* against retroviruses including the Human Immunodeficiency Virus (HIV).

Zidovudine is phosphorylated in both infected and uninfected cells to the monophosphate (MP) derivative by cellular thymidine kinase. Subsequent phosphorylation of zidovudine-MP to the diphosphate (DP), and then the triphosphate (TP) derivative is catalysed by cellular thymidylate kinase and non-specific kinases respectively. Zidovudine-TP acts as an inhibitor of and substrate for the viral reverse transcriptase. The formation of further proviral DNA is blocked by incorporation of zidovudine-MP into the chain and subsequent chain termination. Competition by zidovudine-TP for HIV reverse transcriptase is approximately 100-fold greater than for cellular DNA polymerase alpha.

Clinical virology: The relationships between *in vitro* susceptibility of HIV to zidovudine and clinical response to therapy remain under investigation. *In vitro* sensitivity testing has not been standardised and results may therefore vary according to methodological factors. Reduced *in vitro* sensitivity to zidovudine has been reported for HIV isolates from patients who have received prolonged courses of Retrovir therapy. The available information indicates that for early HIV disease, the frequency and the degree of reduction of *in vitro* sensitivity is notably less than for advanced disease.

The reduction of sensitivity with the emergence of zidovudine resistant strains limits the usefulness of zidovudine monotherapy clinically. In clinical studies, clinical endpoint data indicate that zidovudine, particularly in combination with lamivudine, and also with didanosine or zalcitabine results in a significant reduction in the risk of disease progression and mortality. The use of a protease inhibitor in a combination of zidovudine and lamivudine, has been shown to confer additional benefit in delaying disease progression, and improving survival compared to the double combination on its own.

The anti-viral effectiveness *in vitro* of combinations of antiretroviral agents are being investigated. Clinical and *in vitro* studies of zidovudine in combination with lamivudine indicate that zidovudine-resistant virus isolates can become zidovudine sensitive when they simultaneously acquire resistance to lamivudine. Furthermore there is clinical evidence that zidovudine plus lamivudine delays the emergence of zidovudine resistance in anti-retroviral naive patients.

In some *in vitro* studies zidovudine has been shown to act additively or synergistically with a number of anti-HIV agents, such as lamivudine, didanosine, and interferon-alpha, inhibiting the replication of HIV in cell culture. However, studies *in vitro* indicate that triple combinations of nucleoside analogues or two nucleoside analogues and a protease inhibitor are more effective in inhibiting HIV-1 induced cytopathic effects than one or two drug combinations.

Resistance to thymidine analogues (of which zidovudine is one) is well characterised and is conferred by the stepwise accumulation of up to six specific mutations in the HIV reverse transcriptase at codons 41, 67, 70, 210, 215 and 219. Viruses acquire phenotypic resistance to thymidine analogues through the combination of mutations at codons 41 and 215 or by the accumulation of at least four of the six mutations. These thymidine analogue mutations alone do not cause high-level cross-resistance to any of the other nucleosides, allowing for the subsequent use of any of the other approved reverse transcriptase inhibitors.

Two patterns of multi-drug resistance mutations, the first characterised by mutations in the HIV reverse transcriptase at codons 62, 75, 77, 116 and 151 and the second involving a T69S mutation plus a 6-base pair insert at the same position, result in phenotypic resistance to AZT as well as to the other approved nucleoside reverse transcriptase inhibitors. Either of these two patterns of multinucleoside resistance mutations severely limits future therapeutic options.

In the US ACTG076 trial, Retrovir was shown to be effective in reducing the rate of maternal-foetal transmission of HIV-1 (23% infection rate for placebo versus 8% for zidovudine) when administered (100 mg five times a day) to HIV-positive pregnant women (from week 14-34 of pregnancy) and their newborn infants (2 mg/kg every 6 hours) until 6 weeks of age. In the shorter duration 1998 Thailand CDC study, use of oral Retrovir therapy only (300 mg twice daily), from week 36 of pregnancy until delivery, also reduced the rate of maternal-foetal transmission of HIV (19% infection rate for placebo versus 9% for zidovudine). These data, and data from a published study comparing zidovudine regimes to prevent maternal-foetal HIV transmission have shown that short maternal treatments (from week 36 of pregnancy) are less efficacious than longer maternal treatments (from week 14-34 of pregnancy) in the reduction of perinatal HIV transmission.

5.2 Pharmacokinetic properties

Pharmacokinetics in adults:

Dose-independent kinetics were observed in patients receiving one-hour infusions of 1 to 5 mg/kg 3 to 6 times daily. Mean steady state peak ($C^{ss}max$) and trough ($C^{ss}min$) plasma concentrations in adults following a one-hour infusion of 2.5 mg/kg every 4 hours were 4.0 and 0.4 μM, respectively (or 1.1 and 0.1 μg/ml).

The mean terminal plasma half-life was 1.1 hours, the mean total body clearance was 27.1 ml/min/kg and the apparent volume of distribution was 1.6 litres/kg. Renal clearance of zidovudine greatly exceeds creatinine clearance, indicating significant tubular secretion takes place.

Zidovudine is primarily eliminated by hepatic conjugation to an inactive glucoronidated metabolite. The 5'-glucuronide of zidovudine is the major metabolite in both plasma and urine accounting for approximately 50-80% of the administered dose eliminated by renal excretion. 3'-amino-3'-deoxythymidine (AMT) has been identified as a metabolite of zidovudine following intravenous dosing.

There are limited data concerning the pharmacokinetics of zidovudine in patients with renal or hepatic impairment (see section 4.2). No specific data are available on the pharmacokinetics of zidovudine in the elderly.

Pharmacokinetics in children:

In children over the age of 5-6 months, the pharmacokinetic profile of zidovudine is similar to that in adults. $C^{ss}max$ levels were 1.46 μg/ml following an intravenous dose of 80 mg zidovudine/m^2 body surface area, 2.26 μg/ml following 120 mg/m^2 and 2.96 μg/ml following 160 mg/m^2.

With intravenous dosing, the mean terminal plasma half-life and total body clearance were 1.5 hours and 30.9 ml/min/kg respectively. The major metabolite is the 5'-glucuronide. After intravenous dosing, 29% of the dose was recovered unchanged in the urine and 45% excreted as the glucuronide. Renal clearance of zidovudine greatly exceeds creatinine clearance indicating that significant tubular secretion takes place.

The data available on the pharmacokinetics in neonates and young infants indicate that glucuronidation of zidovudine is reduced with a consequent increase in bioavailability, reduction in clearance and longer half-life in infants less than 14 days-old but thereafter the pharmacokinetics appear similar to those reported in adults.

Pharmacokinetics in pregnancy:

The pharmacokinetics of zidovudine has been investigated in a study of eight women during the last trimester of pregnancy. As pregnancy progressed, there was no evidence of drug accumulation. The pharmacokinetics of zidovudine was similar to that of non-pregnant adults. Consistent with passive transmission of the drug across the placenta, zidovudine concentrations in infant plasma at birth were essentially equal to those in maternal plasma at delivery.

Distribution:

In adults the average cerebrospinal fluid/plasma zidovudine concentration ratio 2 to 4 hours after chronic intermittent oral dosing was found to be approximately 0.5. Data indicate that zidovudine crosses the placenta and is found in amniotic fluid and foetal blood. Zidovudine has also been detected in semen and milk.

In children the mean cerebrospinal fluid/plasma zidovudine concentration ratio ranged from 0.52-0.85 as determined during oral therapy 0.5 to 4 hours after dosing and was 0.87 as determined during intravenous therapy 1-5 hours after a 1 hour infusion. During continuous intravenous infusion the mean steady-state cerebrospinal fluid/plasma concentration ratio was 0.24.

Plasma protein binding is relatively low (34 to 38%) and drug interactions involving binding site displacement are not anticipated.

5.3 Preclinical safety data

Mutagenicity:

No evidence of mutagenicity was observed in the Ames test. However, zidovudine was weakly mutagenic in a mouse lymphoma cell assay and was positive in an *in vitro* cell transformation assay. Clastogenic effects (chromosome damage) were observed in an *in vitro* study in human lymphocytes and in *in vivo* oral repeat dose micronucleus studies in rats and mice. An *in vivo* cytogenetic study in rats did not show chromosomal damage. A study of peripheral blood lymphocytes of eleven AIDS patients showed a higher chromosome breakage frequency in those who had received Retrovir than in those who had not. A pilot study has demonstrated that zidovudine is incorporated into leukocyte nuclear DNA of adults, including pregnant women, taking zidovudine as treatment for HIV-1 infection, or for the prevention of mother to child viral transmission. Zidovudine was also incorporated into DNA from cord blood leukocytes of infants from zidovudine-treated mothers. A transplacental genotoxicity study conducted in monkeys compared zidovudine alone with the combination of zidovudine and lamivudine at human-equivalent exposures. The study demonstrated that foetuses exposed *in utero* to the combination sustained a higher level of nucleoside analogue-DNA incorporation into multiple foetal organs, and showed evidence of more telomere shortening than in those exposed to zidovudine alone. The clinical significance of these findings is unknown.

Carcinogenicity:

In oral carcinogenicity studies with zidovudine in mice and rats, late appearing vaginal epithelial tumours were observed. A subsequent intravaginal carcinogenicity study confirmed the hypothesis that the vaginal tumours were the result of long term local exposure of the rodent vaginal epithelium to high concentrations of unmetabolised zidovudine in urine. There were no other drug-related tumours observed in either sex of either species.

In addition, two transplacental carcinogenicity studies have been conducted in mice. One study, by the US National Cancer Institute, administered zidovudine at maximum tolerated doses to pregnant mice from day 12 to 18 of gestation. One year post-natally, there was an increase in the incidence of tumours in the lung, liver and female reproductive tract of offspring exposed to the highest dose level (420 mg/kg term body weight).

In a second study, mice were administered zidovudine at doses up to 40 mg/kg for 24 months, with exposure beginning prenatally on gestation day 10. Treatment related findings were limited to late-occurring vaginal epithelial tumours, which were seen with a similar incidence and time of onset as in the standard oral carcinogenicity study. The second study thus provided no evidence that zidovudine acts as a transplacental carcinogen.

It is concluded that the transplacental carcinogenicity data from the first study represents a hypothetical risk, whereas the reduction in risk of maternal transfection of HIV to the uninfected child by the use of zidovudine in pregnancy has been well proven.

6. PHARMACEUTICAL PARTICULARS

6.1 List of excipients

Hydrochloric acid

Sodium hydroxide

Water for injection

6.2 Incompatibilities

In the absence of compatibility studies, this medicinal product must not be mixed with other medicinal products

6.3 Shelf life

3 years. (Refer to Section 6.6 for shelf life after opening)

6.4 Special precautions for storage

Do not store above 30°C. Store the vial in the original outer carton.

6.5 Nature and contents of container

5 Amber glass vials containing 20 ml.

6.6 Instructions for use and handling

Retrovir I.V. for Infusion must be diluted prior to administration. Since no antimicrobial preservative is included, dilution must be carried out under full aseptic conditions, preferably immediately prior to administration, and any unused portion of the vial should be discarded.

The required dose should be added to and mixed with Glucose Intravenous Infusion 5% w/v to give a final zidovudine concentration of either 2 mg/ml or 4 mg/ml. These dilutions are chemically and physically stable for up to 48 hours at both 5°C and 25°C. Should any visible turbidity appear in the product either before or after dilution or during infusion, the preparation should be discarded.

Administrative Data

7. MARKETING AUTHORISATION HOLDER

United Kingdom

The Wellcome Foundation Limited

trading as:

Glaxo Wellcome and/or GlaxoSmithKline UK

Stockley Park West

Uxbridge

Middlesex

UB11 1BT

8. MARKETING AUTHORISATION NUMBER(S)

PL 00003/0332

9. DATE OF FIRST AUTHORISATION/RENEWAL OF THE AUTHORISATION

A positive opinion was given by the CPMP at the December 1992 meeting.

Date of national authorisation – 20th April 1993

10. DATE OF REVISION OF THE TEXT

26 July 2005

REVAXIS

(Sanofi Pasteur MSD)

1. NAME OF THE MEDICINAL PRODUCT

REVAXIS® ▼

Suspension for injection in pre-filled syringe

Diphtheria, tetanus and poliomyelitis (inactivated) vaccine (adsorbed)

2. QUALITATIVE AND QUANTITATIVE COMPOSITION

Each dose (0.5 ml) contains:

Active ingredients:

Purified diphtheria toxoid not less than 2 IU* (5 Lf)

Purified tetanus toxoid not less than 20 IU* (10 Lf)

Inactivated poliomyelitis virus type 1 40 D antigen units**

Inactivated poliomyelitis virus type 2 8 D antigen units**

Inactivated poliomyelitis virus type 3 32 D antigen units**

aluminium hydroxide as adsorbant 0.35 mg (as aluminium)

For excipients, see section 6.1

*As lower confidence limit (p = 0.95) of activity measured according to the assay described in the European Pharmacopoeia.

**Or equivalent antigenic quantity determined by a suitable immunochemical method

The inactivated polio vaccine is cultivated on Vero cells.

3. PHARMACEUTICAL FORM

Suspension for injection in pre-filled syringe.

The vaccine has a cloudy white appearance.

4. CLINICAL PARTICULARS

4.1 Therapeutic indications

REVAXIS® is indicated for active immunisation against diphtheria, tetanus and poliomyelitis in children from six years of age, adolescents and adults as a booster following primary vaccination.

REVAXIS® is not intended for primary immunisation.

4.2 Posology and method of administration

Posology

The dose for children from the age of six years, adolescents and adults is 0.5 ml.

REVAXIS® should be administered in accordance with official recommendations and/or local practice regarding the use of vaccines that provide low (adult) dose diphtheria toxoid plus tetanus toxoid in combination with inactivated poliomyelitis viruses.

REVAXIS® may be used as a booster following primary immunisation with inactivated or oral poliomyelitis vaccines (IPV or OPV). There are no clinical data available regarding the use of REVAXIS® in individuals with an incomplete, or no, history of a primary series of diphtheria and tetanus toxoids or of vaccinations against poliomyelitis.

Although REVAXIS® has not been studied in subjects with tetanus-prone injuries, studies have shown that it induces similar tetanus antitoxin titres to Td vaccine. REVAXIS® may therefore be used in subjects with tetanus-prone injuries if concomitant vaccination against diphtheria and poliomyelitis is desirable.

Method of Administration

REVAXIS® is for intramuscular injection only. The recommended injection site is the deltoid region.

REVAXIS® must not be administered by intradermal or intravascular routes.

Under certain conditions (e.g. bleeding disorders) REVAXIS® may be administered as a deep subcutaneous injection.

4.3 Contraindications

Hypersensitivity to diphtheria, tetanus or poliomyelitis vaccines or to any other ingredient of the vaccine.

Hypersensitivity to neomycin, streptomycin or polymyxin B. These are used during production and traces may remain in the vaccine.

Acute severe febrile illness. The presence of a minor infection is not a contraindication.

Neurological complications following an earlier immunisation against diphtheria and/or tetanus.

4.4 Special warnings and special precautions for use

As for all vaccines, appropriate medical treatment should be readily available for immediate use in case of an anaphylactic reaction following vaccination.

The immunogenicity of the vaccine could be reduced in immunosuppressed subjects. Where possible, vaccination should be postponed until immune function has recovered. However, vaccination of subjects with chronic immunodeficiency, such as AIDS, is recommended even if the antibody response might be limited.

REVAXIS® must be administered with caution to subjects with thrombocytopenia or a bleeding disorder since bleeding may occur following an intramuscular administration to such subjects.

In order to minimise the risk of adverse events, REVAXIS® should not be administered to subjects who completed a primary vaccination course or received a booster of a vaccine containing diphtheria or tetanus toxoids within the previous five years.

4.5 Interaction with other medicinal products and other forms of Interaction

REVAXIS® may be administered at the same time as other vaccines or immunoglobulins provided that the injections are made at separate site.

Subjects who are taking immunosuppressive agents may not respond to REVAXIS®.

4.6 Pregnancy and lactation

The effect of REVAXIS® on embryo-foetal development has not been assessed in animals. No teratogenic effect of vaccines containing diphtheria or tetanus toxoids, or inactivated poliovirus has been observed following use in pregnant women. However, this vaccine should not be administered to pregnant women unless it is considered urgent to boost immunity.

REVAXIS® may be administered to breastfeeding women.

4.7 Effects on ability to drive and use machines

Vertigo has been reported following vaccination.

4.8 Undesirable effects

The adverse events are ranked under headings of frequency using the following convention:

Very common: $\geqslant$ 10%

Common: $\geqslant$ 1% and $<$ 10%

Uncommon: $\geqslant$ 0.1% and $<$ 1%

Rare: $\geqslant$ 0.01% and $<$ 0.1%

Very rare: $<$ 0.01%, including isolated reports

In clinical studies, the most common events occurring after vaccine administration were local injection site reactions (pain, erythema, induration and oedema) reported by 65 to 80% of subjects in each trial. These usually had their onset within the 48 hours following vaccination and persisted for 1 to 2 days. These reactions are sometimes accompanied by injection site nodules.

Blood and lymphatic system disorders:

Uncommon: lymphadenopathy

Ear and labyrinth disorders:

Common: vertigo

Gastro-intestinal system disorders:

Common: nausea / vomiting

General disorders and administration site conditions:

Very common: local reactions (injection site pain, injection site erythema, injection site induration, injection site oedema and injection site nodule)

Common: pyrexia

Uncommon: malaise

Musculo-skeletal and connective tissue disorders:
Uncommon: myalgia
Rare: arthralgia
Nervous system disorders:
Common: headache

Data from post-marketing surveillance:

Based on spontaneous reporting, the following additional adverse events have been reported during the commercial use of REVAXIS®.

These events have been very rarely reported, however exact incidence rates cannot precisely be calculated.

General disorders and administration site conditions:

asthenia, usually occurring and resolving within a few days

influenza-like symptoms, mostly the same day as the vaccination

Immune system disorders:

systemic allergic / anaphylactic reactions

Skin and subcutaneous tissue disorders:

allergic-type reactions such as urticaria, various types of rash, and face oedema

Potential adverse events:

Guillain-Barré-Syndrome has been reported after vaccination with tetanus-toxoid containing vaccines.

4.9 Overdose
Not documented.

5. PHARMACOLOGICAL PROPERTIES
5.1 Pharmacodynamic properties
VACCINE AGAINST DIPHTHERIA, TETANUS AND POLIOMYELITIS

J07C Bacterial and viral vaccines, combined.

During clinical studies, the immunogenicity of REVAXIS® was evaluated in 661 healthy subjects aged six to 78 years. In subjects vaccinated within ten years of a previous dose of diphtheria/tetanus/poliomyelitis vaccine, more than 99% achieved protective antibody levels for diphtheria, tetanus and poliomyelitis (types 1, 2 and 3) one month after receiving REVAXIS®.

In a clinical study carried out in 113 healthy subjects aged 40 to 78 years who received their last vaccination against diphtheria, tetanus and poliomyelitis more than ten years ago, REVAXIS® elicited a satisfactory booster response.

Antibody persistence over a two-year period was assessed in 113 healthy adults. Two years after receiving a dose of REVAXIS® the proportions of subjects with protective titres against diphtheria, tetanus and poliomyelitis (types 1, 2 and 3) were 100%, 94.7% and 100% respectively. In a clinical study in 151 healthy children aged six to nine years, antibody titres at one month after a dose of REVAXIS® were approximately three-fold higher than those seen in the healthy adults at two years post-dose. Therefore, it may be anticipated that antibody levels in children would be at least as good as those observed in adults at two years post-dose.

5.2 Pharmacokinetic properties
Evaluation of pharmacokinetic properties is not required for vaccines.

5.3 Preclinical safety data
Preclinical data reveal no special hazard for humans based on conventional studies of safety, specific toxicity and compatibility of ingredients.

6. PHARMACEUTICAL PARTICULARS
6.1 List of excipients
For adjuvant, see section 2.
2-Phenoxyethanol
Formaldehyde
Medium 199*
Water for injections

* Medium 199 is a complex medium of amino acids, mineral salts, vitamins, polysorbate 80 and other substances diluted in water for injections.

6.2 Incompatibilities
In the absence of compatibility studies, the vaccine must not be mixed with other medicinal products.

6.3 Shelf life
3 years.

6.4 Special precautions for storage
Store in a refrigerator (2°C to 8°C).
Do not freeze. Discard the vaccine if it has been frozen.

6.5 Nature and contents of container
0.5 ml of suspension in pre-filled syringe (0.5 ml, type I glass) with a plunger-stopper (chlorobromobutyl elastomer) and attached needle and needle-guard (natural rubber or polyisoprene elastomer).

0.5 ml of suspension in pre-filled syringe (0.5 ml, type I glass) with a plunger-stopper (chlorobromobutyl elastomer) and tip-cap (chlorobromobutyl elastomer), without needle.

Packs of 1, 10 and 20 syringes.

0.5 ml of suspension in pre-filled syringe (0.5 ml, type I glass) with a plunger-stopper (chlorobromobutyl elastomer) and tip-cap (chlorobromobutyl elastomer), with 1 or 2 separate needles (for each syringe).

Packs of 1 and 10 syringes.

Not all pack sizes and presentations may be marketed.

6.6 Instructions for use and handling
For needle free syringes, the needle should be pushed firmly on to the end of the pre-filled syringe and rotated through 90 degrees.

The vaccine's normal appearance is a cloudy white suspension that may sediment during storage. Shake the pre-filled syringe well to distribute uniformly the suspension before administering the vaccine.

Parenteral biological products should be inspected visually for extraneous particulate matter and/or discolouration prior to administration. In the event of either being observed, discard the vaccine. Any unused product or waste material should be disposed of in accordance with local requirements.

7. MARKETING AUTHORISATION HOLDER
SANOFI PASTEUR MSD Ltd, Mallards Reach, Bridge Avenue, Maidenhead, Berkshire, SL6 1QP

8. MARKETING AUTHORISATION NUMBER(S)
PL06745/0123

9. DATE OF FIRST AUTHORISATION/RENEWAL OF THE AUTHORISATION
3rd June 2003

10. DATE OF REVISION OF THE TEXT
May 2005

® Registered trademark
(TM) Trademark of Merck & Co., Inc.

Reyataz 100 mg, 150 mg and 200 mg Hard Capsules

(Bristol-Myers Squibb Pharmaceuticals Ltd)

1. NAME OF THE MEDICINAL PRODUCT
REYATAZ▼ 100 mg hard capsules
REYATAZ▼ 150 mg hard capsules
REYATAZ▼ 200 mg hard capsules

2. QUALITATIVE AND QUANTITATIVE COMPOSITION
Each capsule contains 100 mg, 150 mg or 200 mg of atazanavir (corresponding to 113.9 mg, 170.8 mg or 227.8 mg of atazanavir sulphate).

For excipients, see 6.1.

3. PHARMACEUTICAL FORM
Capsule, hard.

REYATAZ 100 mg capsules are opaque blue and white. They are printed with edible white and blue inks, with "BMS 100" on one half and with "3623" on the other half.

REYATAZ 150 mg capsules are opaque blue and powder blue. They are printed with edible white and blue inks, with "BMS 150" on one half and with "3624" on the other half.

REYATAZ 200 mg capsules are opaque blue. They are printed with edible white ink, with "BMS 200" on one half and with "3631" on the other half.

4. CLINICAL PARTICULARS
4.1 Therapeutic indications
REYATAZ is indicated for the treatment of HIV-1 infected, antiretroviral treatment experienced adults, in combination with other antiretroviral medicinal products.

In antiretroviral treatment experienced patients, the demonstration of efficacy is based on a study comparing REYATAZ 300 mg once daily in combination with ritonavir 100 mg once daily with lopinavir/ritonavir, each regimen in combination with tenofovir (see 4.8 and 5.1). Based on available virological and clinical data, no benefit is expected in patients with strains resistant to multiple protease inhibitors (> 4 PI mutations). The choice of REYATAZ should be based on individual viral resistance testing and the patient's treatment history (see 5.1).

4.2 Posology and method of administration
Therapy should be initiated by a physician experienced in the management of HIV infection.

Oral use.

Adults: the recommended dose of REYATAZ is 300 mg (REYATAZ is available as 100 mg, 150 mg and 200 mg hard capsules) once daily taken with ritonavir 100 mg once daily and with food. Ritonavir is used as a booster of atazanavir pharmacokinetics (see 4.5 and 5.1).

If REYATAZ with ritonavir is co-administered with didanosine, it is recommended that didanosine be taken 2 hours after REYATAZ with ritonavir taken with food (see 4.5).

Infants, toddlers, children, and adolescents: the efficacy and safety of REYATAZ have not been established in this population (see 5.2).

Patients with renal impairment: no dosage adjustment is needed (see 5.2).

Patients with hepatic impairment: REYATAZ with ritonavir should be used with caution in patients with mild hepatic insufficiency. REYATAZ should not be used in patients with moderate to severe hepatic insufficiency (see 4.3, 4.4, and 5.2). REYATAZ with ritonavir has not been studied in patients with hepatic insufficiency.

Method of administration: for oral administration. The capsules should be swallowed whole. REYATAZ oral powder is available for patients who are unable to swallow capsules (see Summary of Product Characteristics for REYATAZ oral powder).

4.3 Contraindications
Hypersensitivity to atazanavir or to any of the excipients (see 6.1).

Patients with moderate to severe hepatic insufficiency (see 4.2 and 4.4).

REYATAZ with ritonavir should not be used in combination with rifampicin (see 4.5).

REYATAZ with ritonavir should not be used in combination with medicinal products that are substrates of the CYP3A4 isoform of cytochrome P450 and have narrow therapeutic windows (e.g., astemizole, terfenadine, cisapride, pimozide, quinidine, bepridil, and ergot alkaloids, particularly, ergotamine, dihydroergotamine, ergonovine, methylergonovine) (see 4.5).

REYATAZ should not be administered with proton pump inhibitors due to an important reduction in atazanavir exposure (see 4.5).

REYATAZ should not be used in combination with products containing St. John's wort (*Hypericum perforatum*) (see 4.5).

4.4 Special warnings and special precautions for use
Patients should be advised that current antiretroviral therapy has not been proven to prevent the risk of transmission of HIV to others through blood or sexual contact. Appropriate precautions should continue to be employed.

There are insufficient data to recommend a dose in antiretroviral treatment-naive patients at present.

Co-administration of REYATAZ with ritonavir in doses greater than 100 mg once daily has not been clinically evaluated. The use of higher ritonavir doses might alter the safety profile of atazanavir (cardiac effects, hyperbilirubinemia) and therefore is not recommended.

Patients with coexisting conditions

Atazanavir is primarily hepatically metabolised and increased plasma concentrations were observed in patients with hepatic impairment (see 4.2 and 4.3). The safety and efficacy of REYATAZ has not been established in patients with significant underlying liver disorders. Patients with chronic hepatitis B or C and treated with combination antiretroviral therapy are at an increased risk for severe and potentially fatal hepatic adverse events. In case of concomitant antiviral therapy for hepatitis B or C, please refer also to the relevant Summary of Product Characteristics for these medicinal products (see 4.8).

Patients with pre-existing liver dysfunction, including chronic active hepatitis, have an increased frequency of liver function abnormalities during combination antiretroviral therapy and should be monitored according to standard practice. If there is evidence of worsening liver disease in such patients, interruption or discontinuation of treatment must be considered.

Dose related asymptomatic prolongations in PR interval with REYATAZ have been observed in clinical studies. Caution should be used with medicinal products known to induce PR prolongations. In patients with pre-existing conduction problems (second degree or higher atrioventricular or complex bundle-branch block), REYATAZ should be used with caution and only if the benefits exceed the risk (see 5.1).

There have been reports of increased bleeding, including spontaneous skin haematomas and haemarthroses, in type A and B haemophiliac patients treated with protease inhibitors. In some patients additional factor VIII was given. In more than half of the reported cases, treatment with protease inhibitors was continued or reintroduced if treatment had been discontinued. A causal relationship has been suggested, although the mechanism of action has not been elucidated. Haemophiliac patients should therefore be made aware of the possibility of increased bleeding.

Fat redistribution and metabolic disorders

Combination antiretroviral therapy has been associated with the redistribution of body fat (lipodystrophy) in HIV patients. The long-term consequences of these events are currently unknown. Knowledge about the mechanism is incomplete. A connection between visceral lipomatosis and protease inhibitors and lipoatrophy and nucleoside reverse transcriptase inhibitors has been hypothesised. A higher risk of lipodystrophy has been associated with individual factors such as older age, and with drug related factors such as longer duration of antiretroviral treatment and associated metabolic disturbances. Clinical examination should include evaluation for physical signs of fat redistribution.

Consideration should be given to the measurement of fasting serum lipids and blood glucose. Lipid disorders should be managed as clinically appropriate (see 4.8).

In clinical studies, REYATAZ (with or without ritonavir) has been shown to induce dyslipidemia to a lesser extent than comparators (see 5.1). However, the clinical impact of such findings has not been demonstrated in the absence of specific studies on cardiovascular risk.

Hyperglycaemia

New onset diabetes mellitus, hyperglycaemia, and exacerbation of existing diabetes mellitus have been reported in patients receiving protease inhibitors. In some of these, the hyperglycaemia was severe and in some cases also associated with ketoacidosis. Many patients had confounding medical conditions, some of which required therapy with medicinal products that have been associated with development of diabetes or hyperglycaemia.

Hyperbilirubinemia

Reversible elevations in indirect (unconjugated) bilirubin related to inhibition of UDP-glucuronosyl transferase (UGT) have occurred in patients receiving REYATAZ (see 4.8). Hepatic transaminase elevations that occur with elevated bilirubin in patients receiving REYATAZ should be evaluated for alternative etiologies. Alternative antiretroviral therapy to REYATAZ may be considered if jaundice or scleral icterus is unacceptable to a patient. Dose reduction of atazanavir is not recommended because it may result in a loss of therapeutic effect and development of resistance.

Indinavir is also associated with indirect (unconjugated) hyperbilirubinemia due to inhibition of UGT. Combinations of REYATAZ and indinavir have not been studied and co-administration of these medicinal products is not recommended (see 4.5).

Immune reactivation syndrome

In HIV-infected patients with severe immune deficiency at the time of institution of combination antiretroviral therapy (CART), an inflammatory reaction to asymptomatic or residual opportunistic pathogens may arise and cause serious clinical conditions, or aggravation of symptoms. Typically, such reactions have been observed within the first few weeks or months of initiation of CART. Relevant examples are cytomegalovirus retinitis, generalised and/or focal mycobacterial infections, and Pneumocystis carinii pneumonia. Any inflammatory symptoms should be evaluated and treatment instituted when necessary.

Lactose

Patients with rare hereditary problems of galactose intolerance, the Lapp lactase deficiency or glucose-galactose malabsorption should not take this medicinal product.

Interactions with other medicinal products

Co-administration of REYATAZ with simvastatin or lovastatin is not recommended (see 4.5).

Atazanavir is metabolised principally by CYP3A4. Co-administration of REYATAZ with ritonavir and medicinal products that induce CYP3A4 is not recommended (see 4.3 and 4.5).

The concomitant use of REYATAZ and oral contraceptives should be avoided (see 4.5).

4.5 Interaction with other medicinal products and other forms of Interaction

When REYATAZ and ritonavir are co-administered, the metabolic drug interaction profile for ritonavir may predominate because ritonavir is a more potent CYP3A4 inhibitor than atazanavir. The Summary of Product Characteristics for ritonavir must be consulted before initiation of therapy with REYATAZ and ritonavir.

Atazanavir is metabolised in the liver through CYP3A4. It inhibits CYP3A4. Therefore, REYATAZ with ritonavir is contraindicated with medicinal products that are substrates of CYP3A4 and have a narrow therapeutic index: astemizole, terfenadine, cisapride, pimozide, quinidine, bepridil and ergot alkaloids, particularly ergotamine and dihydroergotamine (see 4.3).

Antiretroviral agents

Nucleoside/nucleotide reverse transcriptase inhibitors (NRTIs):

Interaction studies with stavudine, lamivudine and zidovudine have been performed with REYATAZ without ritonavir. Based on data derived from these studies and because ritonavir is not expected to have a significant impact on the pharmacokinetics of NRTIs, the co-administration of REYATAZ and ritonavir with these medicinal products is not expected to significantly alter the exposure of the co-administered drugs. The same conclusion applies to the co-administration with abacavir. Considering that REYATAZ with ritonavir should be administered with food, didanosine should be taken 2 hours after REYATAZ with ritonavir.

Tenofovir disoproxil fumarate: atazanavir concentrations (AUC and C_{min}) are decreased when tenofovir is co-administered with REYATAZ (decrease of 25% and 40% of AUC and C_{min} respectively compared to atazanavir 400 mg). When ritonavir was added to atazanavir, the negative impact of tenofovir on atazanavir C_{min} was significantly reduced, whereas the decrease of AUC was of the same magnitude (decrease of 25% and 26% of AUC and C_{min} respectively compared to atazanavir/ritonavir 300/100 mg). The efficacy of REYATAZ with ritonavir in combination with tenofovir in treatment-experienced patients has been demonstrated in the clinical study 045 (see 4.8 and 5.1).

Non-nucleoside reverse transcriptase inhibitors (NNRTIs)

Efavirenz: if REYATAZ is to be co-administered with efavirenz, which decreases atazanavir exposure, it is recommended that REYATAZ 400 mg with ritonavir 100 mg be co-administered with efavirenz 600 mg (all as a single daily dose with food), as this combination is anticipated to result in atazanavir exposure that approximates the mean exposure to atazanavir produced by 300 mg of REYATAZ given with ritonavir 100 mg. No efficacy and safety data are available to support the co-administration of efavirenz and REYATAZ at the increased dose of 400 mg with ritonavir.

Nevirapine: the effects of co-administration of REYATAZ and nevirapine have not been studied. Nevirapine is a metabolic inducer of CYP3A4 and is expected to decrease atazanavir exposure. Therefore, in the absence of data regarding the expected interaction between REYATAZ with ritonavir and nevirapine, this co-administration is not recommended.

Protease inhibitors

Indinavir: indinavir is also associated with indirect (unconjugated) hyperbilirubinemia due to inhibition of UGT. Co-administration of REYATAZ and indinavir is not recommended (see 4.4).

Ritonavir: based on data in healthy volunteers, the addition of ritonavir 100 mg to atazanavir 300 mg has been shown to significantly increase the pharmacokinetic parameters of atazanavir (approximately, 2 fold increase of AUC and 7 fold increase of C_{min} in comparison to atazanavir 400 mg without ritonavir). In patients, the limited pharmacokinetic data currently available suggest that the impact of ritonavir might be less noticeable on the C_{min} (approximately, 3 fold increase).

The co-administration of REYATAZ with ritonavir and other protease inhibitors has not been studied, but would be expected to increase exposure to other protease inhibitors. Therefore, such co-administration is not recommended.

Other medicinal products

Antacids and medicinal products containing buffers: reduced plasma concentrations of atazanavir may be the consequence of increased gastric pH if antacids, including buffered medicinal products, are administered with REYATAZ with ritonavir. REYATAZ with ritonavir should be administered 2 hours before or 1 hour after buffered medicinal products.

Antiarrhythmics (amiodarone, systemic lidocaine, quinidine): concentrations may be increased when co-administered with REYATAZ with ritonavir. Caution is warranted and therapeutic concentration monitoring is recommended when available. The concomitant use of quinidine is contraindicated (see 4.3).

Antineoplastics: atazanavir inhibits UGT and may interfere with the metabolism of irinotecan, resulting in increased irinotecan toxicities.

Calcium channel blockers: co-administration of bepridil with REYATAZ is not recommended (see 4.3). Co-administration of diltiazem (180 mg once daily) with atazanavir (400 mg once daily) in healthy subjects resulted in a 2 to 3 fold increase in diltiazem and desacetyl-diltiazem exposure and no change in the pharmacokinetics of atazanavir. There was an increase in the maximum PR interval compared to atazanavir alone. Co-administration of diltiazem and REYATAZ with ritonavir has not been studied. An initial dose reduction of diltiazem by 50% is recommended, with subsequent titration as needed and ECG monitoring. Verapamil may also have its serum concentrations increased by REYATAZ with ritonavir; therefore, caution should be exercised when verapamil is co-administered with REYATAZ with ritonavir.

HMG-CoA reductase inhibitors (simvastatin, lovastatin, atorvastatin): simvastatin and lovastatin are highly dependent on CYP3A4 for their metabolism and co-administration with REYATAZ with ritonavir may result in increased concentrations. Concomitant use of simvastatin or lovastatin is not recommended due to an increased risk of myopathy including rhabdomyolysis. The risk of myopathy including rhabdomyolysis may also be increased when protease inhibitors, including REYATAZ with ritonavir, are used in combination with atorvastatin, which is also metabolised by CYP3A4. Caution should be exercised.

H_2-Receptor antagonists: the effects of H_2-receptor antagonists on REYATAZ have not been studied; however, reduced plasma concentrations of atazanavir may result due to increased gastric pH if these medicinal products are administered with REYATAZ with ritonavir. Caution should be exercised.

Immunosuppressants (cyclosporin, tacrolimus, sirolimus): concentrations of cyclosporin, tacrolimus, or sirolimus may be increased when co-administered with REYATAZ with ritonavir. More frequent therapeutic concentration monitoring of these medicinal products is recommended until plasma levels have been stabilised.

Macrolide antibiotics: co-administration of clarithromycin (500 mg twice daily) with atazanavir (400 mg once daily) resulted in a 2 fold increase in exposure to clarithromycin and a 70% decrease in exposure to 14-OH clarithromycin, with a 28% increase in the AUC of atazanavir. Dose reduction of clarithromycin may result in subtherapeutic concentrations of 14-OH clarithromycin. No recommendation regarding dose reduction can be made; therefore, caution should be exercised if REYATAZ plus ritonavir is co-administered with clarithromycin.

Oral contraceptives (ethinyl estradiol, norethindrone): the mean concentration of ethinyl estradiol, when co-administered as a 35-μg dose with atazanavir 400 mg once daily, was increased to a level between mean concentrations produced by a 35-μg and a 50-μg ethinyl estradiol dose, and the AUC of norethindrone was increased about 2 fold. In contrast, ritonavir may decrease ethinyl estradiol concentrations. The effects of co-administration of oral contraceptives and REYATAZ with ritonavir have not been studied. The concomitant use of REYATAZ and oral contraceptives should be avoided (see 4.4). Alternate reliable methods of contraception should be considered.

Proton pump inhibitors: Co-administration of omeprazole (40 mg once daily) with REYATAZ and ritonavir (300/100 mg once daily) resulted in a substantial reduction in atazanavir exposure (approximately 75% decrease in AUC, C_{max}, and C_{min}). Increasing the dose of REYATAZ/ritonavir to 400/100 mg did not compensate for the impact of omeprazole on atazanavir exposure. Thus, REYATAZ/ritonavir should not be co-administered with omeprazole. Although not studied, other daily doses of omeprazole may produce similar results and, therefore, co-administration of any dose of omeprazole is not recommended. In the absence of specific data, the recommendation against co-administration with REYATAZ should be extended to other proton pump inhibitors (see 4.3).

Rifabutin: simultaneous administration of 400 mg of atazanavir and 150 mg of rifabutin once daily for 14 days resulted in no clinically important change in the C_{max} or AUC for atazanavir. No dose adjustment is needed for REYATAZ. The rifabutin C_{max} for the 150-mg dose was 1.5 fold higher and the AUC was 2.3 fold higher than historical data for a standard 300-mg dose. A rifabutin dose reduction of up to 75% (e.g., 150 mg every other day or 3 times per week) is recommended when administered with REYATAZ with ritonavir.

Rifampicin: although the effect of rifampicin on REYATAZ has not been studied, rifampicin decreases plasma concentrations and AUC of most protease inhibitors by about 90%. This may result in loss of therapeutic effect and development of resistance. The concomitant use of REYATAZ and rifampicin is contraindicated (see 4.3).

Sildenafil: sildenafil is metabolised by CYP3A4. Co-administration with REYATAZ may result in increased concentrations of sildenafil and an increase in sildenafil-associated adverse events, including hypotension, visual changes, and priapism. Patients should be warned about these possible side effects.

Triazole antifungal agents: co-administration with ketoconazole has only been studied with REYATAZ without ritonavir. Co-administration of 200 mg of ketoconazole with 400 mg of atazanavir in healthy subjects resulted in negligible increases in atazanavir AUC and C_{max} (respectively 11% and 3%). Plasma levels of both atazanavir and ritonavir may be increased by ketoconazole and itraconazole. High doses of ketoconazole and itraconazole (> 200 mg/day) should be used cautiously with atazanavir and ritonavir, by assessing the risk versus the benefit of such a combination.

Warfarin: co-administration with REYATAZ with ritonavir has the potential to produce a decrease or, less often, an increase in INR (International Normalised Ratio). It is recommended that the INR be monitored carefully during treatment with REYATAZ and ritonavir, especially when commencing therapy.

St. John's wort (Hypericum perforatum): REYATAZ should not be used concomitantly with products containing St. John's wort since it may be expected to result in significant reduction in plasma levels of atazanavir. This effect may be due to an induction of CYP3A4. There is a risk of loss of therapeutic effect and development of resistance (see 4.3).

4.6 Pregnancy and lactation

There are no adequate and well-controlled studies in pregnant women. Studies in animals have not shown evidence of selective developmental toxicity or effects on reproductive function and fertility (see 5.3). REYATAZ should be used during pregnancy only if the potential benefit justifies the potential risk.

It is not known whether REYATAZ administered to the mother during pregnancy will exacerbate physiological hyperbilirubinemia and lead to kernicterus in neonates and infants. In the prepartum period, additional monitoring and alternative therapy to REYATAZ should be considered.

It is not known whether atazanavir is excreted in human milk. Studies in rats have demonstrated that atazanavir is excreted in the milk. It is therefore recommended that mothers being treated with REYATAZ not breast-feed their infants. As a general rule, it is recommended that HIV infected women not breast-feed their infants in order to avoid transmission of HIV.

4.7 Effects on ability to drive and use machines

There are no data to suggest that atazanavir affects the ability to drive or use machines. However, patients should be informed that dizziness has been reported during treatment with regimens containing REYATAZ (see 4.8).

4.8 Undesirable effects

Data on the safety and tolerability of REYATAZ 300 mg with ritonavir 100 mg once daily are limited, as this combination has only been evaluated in 119 patients in Study 045 in a regimen that also included tenofovir 300 mg once daily and a nucleoside reverse transcriptase inhibitor. Considering that tenofovir has been shown to decrease the plasma levels of atazanavir (with or without concomitant ritonavir), the safety data derived from this study may not fully reflect the safety profile of REYATAZ plus ritonavir when used in clinical practice within antiretroviral combinations that exclude tenofovir. An alteration of the safety profile of REYATAZ cannot be excluded in this context.

REYATAZ has been evaluated for safety and tolerability in combination therapy with other antiretroviral medicinal products in Phase II and III trials in 1,597 adult patients. The majority of patients (1,047) received REYATAZ 400 mg once daily without ritonavir. The median duration of treatment was 102 weeks in Phase II trials and 48 weeks in the Phase III trials. Adverse events were comparable between patients who received REYATAZ 300 mg with ritonavir 100 mg once daily and patients who received REYATAZ 400 mg once daily, except that jaundice and elevated total bilirubin levels were reported more frequently with REYATAZ plus ritonavir.

Among patients who received 400 mg once daily or 300 mg with ritonavir 100 mg once daily, the only adverse events of any severity reported very commonly with at least a possible relationship to regimens containing REYATAZ and one or more NRTIs were nausea (24%), headache (10%), and jaundice (10%). Among patients receiving REYATAZ 300 mg with ritonavir 100 mg, the frequency of jaundice was 16%. Jaundice was reported within a few days to a few months after the initiation of treatment (see 4.4).

Combination antiretroviral therapy has been associated with redistribution of body fat (lipodystrophy) in HIV patients, including loss of peripheral and facial subcutaneous fat, increased intra-abdominal and visceral fat, breast hypertrophy, and dorsocervical fat accumulation (buffalo hump).

Combination antiretroviral therapy has been associated with metabolic abnormalities such as hypertriglyceridaemia, hypercholesterolaemia, insulin resistance, hyperglycaemia, and hyperlactataemia (see 4.4 and 5.1).

Adult patients

The following adverse events of moderate intensity or greater with at least a possible relationship to regimens containing REYATAZ and one or more NRTIs have also been reported. The frequency of adverse reactions listed below is defined using the following convention: very common (≥ 1/10), common (≥ 1/100, < 1/10), uncommon (≥ 1/1,000, < 1/100), rare (≥ 1/10,000, < 1/1,000), or very rare (< 1/10,000).

Immune system disorders:	uncommon: allergic reaction
Metabolism and nutrition disorders:	common: lipodystrophy; uncommon: anorexia, appetite increased, weight decreased, weight gain
Psychiatric disorders:	uncommon: anxiety, depression, sleep disorder
Nervous system disorders:	common: headache, insomnia, peripheral neurologic symptoms; uncommon: abnormal dream, amnesia, confusion, dizziness, somnolence; rare: abnormal gait
Eye disorders:	common: scleral icterus
Cardiac disorders and vascular disorders:	uncommon: hypertension, syncope; rare: oedema, palpitation
Respiratory, thoracic and mediastinal disorders:	uncommon: dyspnea
Gastrointestinal disorders:	common: abdominal pain, diarrhoea, dyspepsia, nausea, vomiting; uncommon: dysgeusia, flatulence, gastritis, pancreatitis, stomatitis aphthous; rare: abdominal distension
Hepatobiliary disorders:	common: jaundice; uncommon: hepatitis; rare: hepatosplenomegaly
Skin and subcutaneous tissue disorders:	common: rash; uncommon: alopecia, pruritus, urticaria; rare: eczema, vasodilatation, vesiculobullous rash
Musculoskeletal and connective tissue disorders:	uncommon: arthralgia, muscle atrophy, myalgia; rare: myopathy
Renal and urinary disorders:	uncommon: hematuria, nephrolithiasis, pollakiuria, proteinuria; rare: kidney pain
Reproductive system and breast disorders:	uncommon: gynecomastia
General disorders and administration site conditions:	common: asthenia, fatigue; uncommon: chest pain, fever, malaise

In HIV-infected patients with severe immune deficiency at the time of initiation of combination antiretroviral therapy (CART), an inflammatory reaction to asymptomatic or residual opportunistic infections may arise (see section 4.4).

Laboratory abnormalities

The most frequently reported laboratory abnormality in patients receiving regimens containing REYATAZ and one or more NRTIs was elevated total bilirubin (84% Grade 1, 2, 3, or 4). Grade 3 or 4 elevation of total bilirubin was noted in 33% (28% Grade 3, 5% Grade 4, reported predominantly as elevated indirect [unconjugated] bilirubin). Among patients treated with REYATAZ 300 mg once daily with 100 mg ritonavir once daily, 49% had Grade 3-4 total bilirubin elevations (see 4.4).

Other marked clinical laboratory abnormalities (Grade 3 or 4) reported in ≥ 2% of patients receiving regimens containing REYATAZ and one or more NRTIs included: elevated amylase (12%), elevated creatine kinase (7%), elevated alanine aminotransferase/serum glutamic-pyruvic transaminase (ALT/SGPT) (5%), low neutrophils (5%), elevated aspartate aminotransferase/serum glutamic-oxaloacetic transaminase (AST/SGOT) (3%), and elevated lipase (3%).

One percent of patients treated with REYATAZ experienced concurrent Grade 3-4 ALT/AST and Grade 3-4 total bilirubin elevations.

Patients co-infected with hepatitis B and/or hepatitis C virus

Among 585 patients receiving atazanavir 400 mg once daily, 74 patients were co-infected with chronic hepatitis B or C, and among 119 patients receiving atazanavir 300 mg once daily with ritonavir 100 mg once daily, 20 were co-infected with chronic hepatitis B or C. Co-infected patients were more likely to have baseline hepatic transaminase elevations than those without chronic viral hepatitis. No differences in frequency of bilirubin elevations were observed between these patients and those without viral hepatitis. The frequency of treatment emergent hepatitis or transaminase elevations in co-infected patients was comparable between REYATAZ and comparator regimens (see 4.4).

4.9 Overdose

Human experience of acute overdose with REYATAZ is limited. Single doses up to 1,200 mg have been taken by healthy volunteers without symptomatic untoward effects. At high doses that lead to high drug exposures, jaundice due to indirect (unconjugated) hyperbilirubinemia (without associated liver function test changes) or PR interval prolongations may be observed (see 4.4 and 4.8).

Treatment of overdose with REYATAZ should consist of general supportive measures, including monitoring of vital signs and ECG, and observations of the patient's clinical status. If indicated, elimination of unabsorbed atazanavir should be achieved by emesis or gastric lavage. Administration of activated charcoal may also be used to aid removal of unabsorbed drug. There is no specific antidote for overdose with REYATAZ. Since atazanavir is extensively metabolised by the liver and is highly protein bound, dialysis is unlikely to be beneficial in significant removal of this medicinal product.

5. PHARMACOLOGICAL PROPERTIES

5.1 Pharmacodynamic properties

Pharmacotherapeutic group: protease inhibitor, ATC code: J05A E

Mechanism of action: atazanavir is an azapeptide HIV-1 protease inhibitor. The compound selectively inhibits the virus-specific processing of viral Gag-Pol proteins in HIV-1 infected cells, thus preventing formation of mature virions and infection of other cells.

Antiviral activityin vitro: atazanavir exhibits anti-HIV-1 activity (EC_{50} of 2 to 5 nM) against a variety of HIV isolates in the absence of human serum. Combinations of atazanavir with stavudine, didanosine, lamivudine, zidovudine, nelfinavir, indinavir, ritonavir, saquinavir, or amprenavir in HIV-infected peripheral blood mononuclear cells yielded additive antiviral effects and did not result in antagonistic anti-HIV activity or enhanced cytotoxic effects at the highest concentrations used for antiviral evaluation.

Cross-resistance in vitro in viruses resistant to other protease inhibitors: atazanavir susceptibility was evaluated in 943 clinical isolates from patients without prior atazanavir exposure and exhibited a wide array of genotypic and phenotypic patterns. *In vitro*, there was a clear trend toward decreased susceptibility to atazanavir as isolates exhibited high resistance levels to multiple protease inhibitors. In general, susceptibility to atazanavir was retained (83% of isolates displayed < 2.5 fold change in EC_{50}) among isolates resistant to no more than 2 protease inhibitors.

Eighteen percent of isolates had 4 or more of the following 6 mutations considered critical mutations for protease inhibitors: amino acid substitutions 10, 46, 54, 82, 84, and 90. These isolates expressed a median fold change in EC_{50} relative to wildtype of 12.0 for atazanavir. Therefore, viral isolates having at least 4 of these specific mutations would be considered resistant for atazanavir.

Resistance in vivo: in antiretroviral treatment naive patients, the I50L substitution, sometimes in combination with an A71V change, is the signature resistance mutation for atazanavir. An atazanavir resistance phenotype is expressed in all recombinant viral clones containing the I50L substitution in a variety of genetic backgrounds. Resistance levels ranged from 3.5- to 29-fold. There was no evidence of cross-resistance between atazanavir and amprenavir, with the presence of the I50L and I50V substitutions yielding selective resistance to atazanavir and amprenavir, respectively.

In antiretroviral treatment experienced patients, 100 isolates from patients designated as virological failures on therapy that included either atazanavir, atazanavir + ritonavir, or atazanavir + saquinavir were determined to have developed resistance to atazanavir. Of the 60 isolates from patients treated with either atazanavir or atazanavir + ritonavir, 18 (30%) displayed the I50L phenotype previously described in naive patients. The resistance in antiretroviral treatment experienced patients mainly occurs by accumulation of the primary and secondary resistance substitutions described previously to be involved in protease inhibitor resistance. These isolates developed higher levels of resistance to the other protease inhibitors.

Clinical experience: in antiretroviral treatment experienced patients, the benefit of REYATAZ is based only on Study 045 where REYATAZ 300 mg once daily was used with ritonavir 100 mg once daily and compared with lopinavir + ritonavir.

Study 045 is an ongoing, randomised, multicenter trial comparing REYATAZ (300 mg once daily) with ritonavir (100 mg once daily) to REYATAZ (400 mg once daily) with saquinavir soft gelatine capsules (1,200 mg once daily), and to lopinavir + ritonavir (400/100 mg fixed dose combination twice daily), each in combination with tenofovir (see 4.5 and 4.8) and one NRTI, in 347 (of 358 randomised) patients with virologic failure on two or more prior regimens containing at least one PI, NRTI, and NNRTI. For randomised patients, the mean time of prior antiretroviral exposure was 138 weeks for PIs, 281 weeks for NRTIs, and 85 weeks for NNRTIs. At baseline, 34% of patients were receiving a PI and 60% were receiving an NNRTI. Fifteen of 120 (13%) patients in the REYATAZ + ritonavir treatment arm and 17 of 123 (14%) patients in the lopinavir + ritonavir arm had four or more of the PI mutations 10, 46, 54, 82, 84, and 90. Thirty-two percent of patients in the study had a viral strain with fewer than two NRTI mutations. The mean baseline CD4 cell count was 337 cells/mm^3 (range: 14 to 1,543 cells/mm^3) and the mean baseline plasma HIV-1 RNA level was 4.4 $\log_{10}$ copies/ml (range: 2.6 to 5.9 $\log_{10}$ copies/ml). The population included in this study was moderately pretreated.

The primary endpoint was the time-averaged difference in change from baseline in HIV RNA through 48 weeks.

Through 48 weeks of treatment, the decreases from baseline in HIV RNA levels (primary endpoint) were 1.93 $\log_{10}$ copies/ml for REYATAZ + ritonavir and 1.87 $\log_{10}$ copies/ml for lopinavir + ritonavir. REYATAZ + ritonavir was similar (non-inferior) to lopinavir + ritonavir on this efficacy measure (time-averaged difference of 0.13, 97.5% confidence interval [-0.12, 0.39]). Consistent results were obtained with the last observation carried forward method of analysis (time-averaged difference of 0.11, 97.5% confidence interval [-0.15, 0.36]). The proportions of patients with HIV RNA < 400 copies/ml in the REYATAZ + ritonavir arm and the lopinavir + ritonavir arm were 53% and 54%, respectively, by intent-to-treat analysis, with missing values considered as failures. The proportions of patients with HIV RNA < 50 copies/ml in the REYATAZ + ritonavir arm and the lopinavir + ritonavir arm were 36% and 42%, respectively. By as-treated analysis, excluding missing values, the proportions of patients with HIV RNA < 400 copies/ml (< 50 copies/ml) in the REYATAZ + ritonavir arm and the lopinavir + ritonavir arm were 55% (40%) and 56% (46%), respectively. The mean increases from baseline in CD4 cell count were 110 cells/mm^3 and 121 cells/mm^3 in the REYATAZ + ritonavir and lopinavir + ritonavir arms, respectively.

Two types of analyses were performed based on baseline genotypic mutations. The first consisted in assessing the HIV RNA change from baseline in the subgroup of patients with < or ≥ of 4 of the following set of mutations: 10, 20, 24, 32, 33, 36, 46, 48, 50, 54, 63, 71, 73, 82, 84 and 90.

The second consisted in assessing the HIV RNA change from baseline in the subgroup of patients with < or ≥ of 4 of the following more specific set of mutations: 10, 46, 54, 82, 84, 90. In the analysis performed for patients with ≥ 4 protease gene mutations among the following set of mutations 10, 20, 24, 32, 33, 36, 46, 48, 50, 54, 63, 71, 73, 82, 84 and 90, the results significantly favoured the lopinavir + ritonavir arm. There were too few patients with ≥ 4 of the second more specific set of mutations (i.e. 10, 46, 54, 82, 84, 90) to assess the comparability of the REYATAZ + ritonavir and lopinavir + ritonavir regimens, but reduced virologic activity may be anticipated among patients with this resistance profile.

REYATAZ + saquinavir was shown to be inferior to lopinavir + ritonavir.

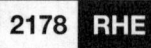

The data available on the lipid profile are described in the following table:

	Study -045 48 weeks	
	ATV/RTV	LPV/RTV
Total Cholesterol	-8%	6%
LDL Cholesterol	-10%	1%
HDL Cholesterol	-7%	2%
Triglycerides	-4%	30%

5.2 Pharmacokinetic properties

Limited data are available on the pharmacokinetics of atazanavir in association with low dose ritonavir. The pharmacokinetics of atazanavir were evaluated in healthy adult volunteers and in HIV-infected patients; no substantial differences were observed between the two groups. The pharmacokinetics of atazanavir exhibit a non-linear disposition and a high inter/intra-subject variability that is minimised with food. In healthy subjects, the AUC of atazanavir from the capsules and oral powder were similar. Therefore, HIV-infected patients can use the two formulations interchangeably.

Absorption: the pharmacokinetics of atazanavir boosted with ritonavir is currently supported by limited data in patients. In a pharmacokinetic study in HIV-positive patients (n= 10), multiple dosing of REYATAZ 300 mg once daily with ritonavir 100 mg once daily with a light meal for 2 weeks produced a mean steady-state C_{max} (SD) of 5,233 ng/ml (3,033), occurring approximately 3.0 hours (T_{max}) after administration, and a mean steady-state trough concentration (SD) of 862 ng/ml (838). The mean steady-state plasma AUC (SD) of atazanavir was 53,761 ng hr/ml (35,294).

Food effect: administration of atazanavir with either a light meal or a high fat meal decreased the coefficient of variation of AUC and C_{max} approximately one-half compared to the fasting state. A similar decrease in the coefficient of variation was noted when REYATAZ 300 mg once daily with ritonavir 100 mg once daily was administered with a light meal in healthy subjects. To enhance bioavailability and minimise variability, REYATAZ is to be taken with food.

Distribution: atazanavir was approximately 86% bound to human serum proteins over a concentration range of 100 to 10,000 ng/ml. Atazanavir binds to both alpha-1-acid glycoprotein (AAG) and albumin to a similar extent (89% and 86%, respectively, at 1,000 ng/ml). In a multiple-dose study in HIV-infected patients dosed with 400 mg of atazanavir once daily with a light meal for 12 weeks, atazanavir was detected in the cerebrospinal fluid and semen.

Metabolism: studies in humans and *in vitro* studies using human liver microsomes have demonstrated that atazanavir is principally metabolised by CYP3A4 isozyme to oxygenated metabolites. Metabolites are then excreted in the bile as either free or glucuronidated metabolites. Additional minor metabolic pathways consist of N-dealkylation and hydrolysis. Two minor metabolites of atazanavir in plasma have been characterised. Neither metabolite demonstrated *in vitro* antiviral activity.

Elimination: following a single 400-mg dose of ^{14}C-atazanavir, 79% and 13% of the total radioactivity was recovered in the faeces and urine, respectively. Unchanged drug accounted for approximately 20% and 7% of the administered dose in the faeces and urine, respectively. Mean urinary excretion of unchanged drug was 7% following 2 weeks of dosing at 800 mg once daily. The mean elimination half-life of atazanavir in HIV-infected adult patients (n= 10) was 8.6 hours at steady state following a dose of 300 mg daily with ritonavir 100 mg once daily with a light meal.

Special populations

Impaired renal function: in healthy subjects, the renal elimination of unchanged atazanavir was approximately 7% of the administered dose. There are no pharmacokinetic data available on patients with renal insufficiency (see 4.2); however, the impact of renal impairment on atazanavir elimination is anticipated to be minimal.

Impaired hepatic function: atazanavir is metabolised and eliminated primarily by the liver. The effects of hepatic impairment on the pharmacokinetics of atazanavir after a 300 mg dose with ritonavir have not been studied. Concentrations of atazanavir with or without ritonavir are expected to be increased in patients with moderately or severely impaired hepatic function (see 4.2, 4.3, and 4.4).

Age/Gender: a study of the pharmacokinetics of atazanavir was performed in 59 healthy male and female subjects (29 young, 30 elderly). There were no clinically important pharmacokinetic differences based on age or gender.

Race: a population pharmacokinetic analysis of samples from Phase II clinical trials indicated no effect of race on the pharmacokinetics of atazanavir.

Infants, toddlers, children, and adolescents: the pharmacokinetics of atazanavir is being studied after multiple doses in paediatric patients, stratified by age. There are insufficient data at this time to recommend a dose (see 4.2).

5.3 Preclinical safety data

In repeat-dose toxicity studies, conducted in mice, rats, and dogs, atazanavir-related findings were generally confined to the liver and included generally minimal to mild increases in serum bilirubin and liver enzymes, hepatocellular vacuolation and hypertrophy, and, in female mice only, hepatic single-cell necrosis. Systemic exposures of atazanavir in mice (males), rats, and dogs at doses associated with hepatic changes were at least equal to that observed in humans given 400 mg once daily. In female mice, atazanavir exposure at a dose that produced single-cell necrosis was 12 times the exposure in humans given 400 mg once daily. Serum cholesterol and glucose were minimally to mildly increased in rats but not in mice or dogs.

The cloned human cardiac potassium channel, hERG, was inhibited by 15% in an *in vitro* patch clamp assay at a concentration (30 μM) corresponding to 30-fold the free drug concentration at C_{max} in humans. Electrocardiographic changes (sinus bradycardia, prolongation of PR interval, prolongation of QT interval, and prolongation of QRS complex) were observed only in an initial 2-week oral toxicity study performed in dogs. Subsequent 2-week and 9-month oral toxicity studies in dogs showed no drug-related electrocardiographic changes. The clinical relevance of these preclinical data is unknown. Potential cardiac effects of this product in humans cannot be ruled out (see 4.4 and 4.8). The potential for PR prolongation should be considered in cases of overdose (see 4.9).

In a fertility and early embryonic development study in rats, atazanavir altered oestrus cycling with no effects on mating or fertility. No teratogenic effects were observed in rats or rabbits at maternally toxic doses. In pregnant rabbits, gross lesions of the stomach and intestines were observed in dead or moribund does at maternal doses 2 and 4 times the highest dose administered in the definitive embryo-development study. In the pre- and postnatal development assessment in rats, atazanavir produced a transient reduction in body weight in the offspring at a maternally toxic dose. Systemic exposure to atazanavir at doses that resulted in maternal toxicity was at least equal to or slightly greater than that observed in humans given 400 mg once daily.

Atazanavir was negative in an Ames reverse-mutation assay but did induce chromosomal aberrations *in vitro* in both the absence and presence of metabolic activation. In *in vivo* studies in rats, atazanavir did not induce micronuclei in bone marrow, DNA damage in duodenum (comet assay), or unscheduled DNA repair in liver at plasma and tissue concentrations exceeding those that were clastogenic *in vitro*.

In long-term carcinogenicity studies of atazanavir in mice and rats, an increased incidence of benign hepatic adenomas was seen in female mice only. The increased incidence of benign hepatic adenomas in female mice was likely secondary to cytotoxic liver changes manifested by single-cell necrosis and is considered to have no relevance for humans at intended therapeutic exposures. There were no tumorigenic findings in male mice or in rats.

Atazanavir increased opacity of bovine corneas in an *in vitro* ocular irritation study, indicating it may be an ocular irritant upon direct contact with the eye.

6. PHARMACEUTICAL PARTICULARS

6.1 List of excipients

Capsule contents:
Crospovidone
Lactose monohydrate
Magnesium stearate

Capsule shells:
Gelatine
Indigotin (E132)
Titanium dioxide (E171)

Blue ink containing:
Shellac
Dehydrated alcohol
Butyl alcohol
Propylene glycol
Ammonia solution
Indigotine aluminium lake (E132)

White ink containing:
Shellac
Titanium dioxide (E171)
Ammonium hydroxide
Propylene glycol
Simethicone

6.2 Incompatibilities

Not applicable.

6.3 Shelf life

2 years

6.4 Special precautions for storage

Do not store above 25°C.

6.5 Nature and contents of container

Each Alu/Alu blister card contains 6 capsules, 60 capsules per carton.

6.6 Instructions for use and handling

No special requirements.

7. MARKETING AUTHORISATION HOLDER

BRISTOL-MYERS SQUIBB PHARMA EEIG

141-149 Staines Road

Hounslow TW3 3JA

United Kingdom

8. MARKETING AUTHORISATION NUMBER(S)

REYATAZ 100 mg Hard Capsules - Blisters	EU/1/03/267/002
REYATAZ 150 mg Hard Capsules - Blisters	EU/1/03/267/004
REYATAZ 200 mg Hard Capsules - Blisters	EU/1/03/267/006

9. DATE OF FIRST AUTHORISATION/RENEWAL OF THE AUTHORISATION

02 March 2004

10. DATE OF REVISION OF THE TEXT

21 February 2005

Rheumatac Retard 75

(Sovereign Medical)

1. NAME OF THE MEDICINAL PRODUCT

Rheumatac Retard 75

2. QUALITATIVE AND QUANTITATIVE COMPOSITION

Rheumatac 75 Retard. Each tablet contains 75mg diclofenac sodium BP.

3. PHARMACEUTICAL FORM

Modified Release Tablets

4. CLINICAL PARTICULARS

4.1 Therapeutic indications

Rheumatoid arthritis, osteoarthritis, acute gout, low back pain, relief of pain in fractures, acute musculo-skeletal disorders and trauma including periarthritis (particularly frozen shoulder), bursitis, tendinitis, tenosynovitis, dislocations, sprains and strains, ankylosing spondylitis, and the control of pain and inflammation in orthopaedic, dental and other minor surgery.

4.2 Posology and method of administration

For oral administration. Tablets should be swallowed whole preferably with or after food.

Adults: One 75 mg tablet once or twice a day.

Children: Not suitable for use in children.

Elderly: Care should be used when treating patients who are frail or have a low body weight, as they will in general be more susceptible to adverse reactions. The elderly are at an increased risk of the serious consequences of adverse reactions. If an NSAID is considered necessary, the lowest effective dose should be used and for the shortest possible duration. The patient should be monitored regularly for GI bleeding during NSAID therapy.

4.3 Contraindications

Hypersensitivity to diclofenac sodium or any of the other constituents.

NSAIDs are contraindicated in patients who have previously shown hypersensitivity reactions (e.g. asthma, rhinitis, angioedema or urticaria) in response to ibuprofen, aspirin, or other non-steroidal anti-inflammatory drugs.

Severe hepatic, renal and cardiac failure (See section 4.4 – Special Warnings and Precautions for Use).

During the last trimester of pregnancy (See section 4.6 – Pregnancy and Lactation).

Active or previous peptic ulcer.

History of upper gastrointestinal bleeding or perforation, related to previous NSAIDs therapy.

Use with concomitant NSAIDs including cyclo-oxygenase-2 specific inhibitors (See section 4.5 - Interactions with other Medicaments and other forms of Interaction).

4.4 Special warnings and special precautions for use

In all patients:

Undesirable effects may be minimised by using the minimum effective dose for the shortest possible duration.

Monitoring of renal function, hepatic function (elevation of liver enzymes may occur) and blood counts should be performed on long-term NSAID patients, as a precautionary measure.

Elderly:

The elderly have an increased frequency of adverse reactions to NSAIDs especially gastrointestinal bleeding and perforation, which may be fatal (See section 4.2 – Posology and Method of Administration).

Respiratory disorders:

Caution is required if administered to patients suffering from, or with a previous history of, bronchial asthma since NSAIDs have been reported to precipitate bronchospasm in such patients.

Cardiovascular, Renal and Hepatic Impairment:

The administration of an NSAID may cause a dose dependent reduction in prostaglandin formation and precipitate renal failure. Patients at greatest risk of this reaction are those with impaired renal function, cardiac impairment, liver dysfunction, those taking diuretics, the elderly and those recovering from major surgery. Renal function should be monitored in these patients (Also see section 4.3 – Contra-Indications). On stopping diclofenac, effects on renal function are usually reversible.

Diclofenac must be stopped if liver function tests show abnormalities, which persist or worsen, or if liver disease develops or if other symptoms such as eosinophilia or rash occur.

Diclofenac may trigger an attack in patients with hepatic porphyria.

Caution in patients with a history of hypertension and/or heart failure as fluid retention and oedema have been reported in association with NSAID therapy.

Gastrointestinal bleeding, ulceration and perforation:

GI bleeding, ulceration or perforation, which can be fatal, has been reported with all NSAIDs at any time during treatment, with or without warning symptoms or a previous history of serious GI events.

Patients with a history of GI toxicity, particularly when elderly, should report any unusual abdominal symptoms (especially GI bleeding) particularly in the initial stages of treatment.

Caution should be advised in patients receiving concomitant medications which could increase the risk of gastrotoxicity or bleeding, such as corticosteroids, or anticoagulants such as warfarin or anti-platelet agents such as aspirin (See section 4.5 - Interactions with other Medicaments and other forms of Interaction).

When GI bleeding or ulceration occurs in patients receiving diclofenac, the treatment should be withdrawn.

NSAIDs should be given with care to patients with a history of gastrointestinal disease (ulcerative colitis, Crohn's disease) as these conditions may be exacerbated (See section 4.8 – Undesirable Effects). Patients with a history of haematemesis, or melaena, should be carefully observed.

Haematological disorders:

Care should be taken when treating patients with haematological abnormalities, or bleeding diathesis.

SLE and mixed connective tissue disease:

In patients with systemic lupus erythematosus (SLE) and mixed connective tissue disorders there may be an increased risk of aseptic meningitis (See section 4.8 – Undesirable Effects).

Female fertility:

The use of diclofenac may impair female fertility and is not recommended in women attempting to conceive. In women who have difficulties conceiving or who are undergoing investigation of infertility, withdrawal of diclofenac should be considered.

4.5 Interaction with other medicinal products and other forms of Interaction

Other analgesics: Avoid concomitant use of two or more NSAIDs (including aspirin) as this may increase the risk of adverse effects (See section 4.3 Contra-Indications).

If other systemic NSAIDs are given concomitantly with diclofenac the frequency of side effects may be increased.

Anti-hypertensives: Reduced anti-hypertensive effect.

Diuretics: Reduced diuretic effect. Diuretics can increase the risk of nephrotoxicity of NSAIDs. The activity of diuretics may be inhibited by some NSAIDs. Increased serum potassium levels may result when diclofenac is given concomitantly with potassium-sparing diuretics. Serum potassium levels should therefore be monitored.

Cardiac glycosides: NSAIDs may exacerbate cardiac failure, reduce GFR and increase plasma glycoside levels.

Lithium: Decreased elimination of lithium.

Methotrexate: Decreased elimination of methotrexate resulting in increased toxicity. Methotrexate and NSAIDs should only be administered within 24 hours of each other if given with extreme caution.

Ciclosporin: Increased risk of nephrotoxicity as a result of the effect of NSAIDs on renal prostaglandins.

Mifepristone: NSAIDs should not be used for 8-12 days after mifepristone administration as NSAIDs can reduce the effect of mifepristone.

Corticosteriods: Increased risk of GI bleeding (See section 4.4 – Special Warnings and Precautions for Use).

Anti-coagulants: NSAIDs may enhance the effects of anticoagulants, such as warfarin (See section 4.4 – Special Warnings and Precautions for Use). Monitoring is recommended to ensure the desired response to the anticoagulant is maintained, as there are rare reports of increased risk of haemorrhage with combined diclofenac and anticoagulant therapy.

Quinolone antibiotics: Animal data indicate that NSAIDs can increase the risk of convulsions associated with quinolone antibiotics. Patients taking NSAIDs and quinolones may have an increased risk of developing convulsions.

Tacrolimus: Possible increased risk of nephrotoxicity when NSAIDs are given with tacrolimus.

Anti-diabetics: It has been reported that hypo- and hyperglycaemic effects have occurred rarely when diclofenac and oral antidiabetic agents have been given together and adjustment of the hypoglycaemic may be required.

4.6 Pregnancy and lactation

Pregnancy:

Congenital abnormalities have been reported in association with NSAID administration in man; however, these are low in frequency and do not appear to follow any discernable pattern. In view of the known effects of NSAIDs on the foetal cardiovascular system (risk of closure of the ductus arteriosus), use in the last trimester of pregnancy is contraindicated. Theonset of labour maybe delayed and the duration increased with an increased bleeding tendency in both mother and child. (See section 4.3 Contra-Indications). NSAIDs should not be used during the first two trimesters of pregnancy or labour unless the potential benefit to the patient outweighs the potential risk to the foetus.

Lactation:

In limited studies so far available, NSAIDs can appear in breast milk in very low concentrations. NSAIDs should, if possible, be avoided when breastfeeding.

See section 4.4 - Special Warnings and Precautions for Use, regarding female fertility.

4.7 Effects on ability to drive and use machines

Undesirable effects such as dizziness, drowsiness, fatigue and visual disturbances are possible after taking NSAIDs. If affected, patients should not drive or operate machinery.

4.8 Undesirable effects

Gastrointestinal: The most commonly-observed adverse events are gastrointestinal in nature. Peptic ulcers, perforation or GI bleeding, sometimes fatal, particularly in the elderly, may occur (see section 4.4 - Special Warnings and Precautions for Use). Nausea, vomiting, diarrhoea, flatulence, constipation, dyspepsia, anorexia, abdominal pain, melaena, haematemesis, ulcerative stomatitis, exacerbation of colitis and Crohn's disease (See section 4.4 - Special Warnings and Precautions for Use) have been reported following administration. Less frequently, gastritis, glossitis, pancreatitis and oesophageal lesions have been observed.

Hypersensitivity: Hypersensitivity reactions have been reported following treatment with NSAIDs. These may consist of (a) non-specific allergic reactions and anaphylaxis (b) respiratory tract reactivity comprising asthma, aggravated asthma, bronchospasm or dyspnoea, or (c) assorted skin disorders, including rashes of various types, pruritus, urticaria, purpura, angiodema and more rarely, exfoliative and bullous dermatoses (including epidermal necrolysis and erythema multiforme).

Cardiovasular: Oedema has been reported in association with NSAID treatment. Hypertension, hypotension, chest pains and palpitations have been rarely reported.

Other adverse events reported less commonly include:

Renal: Nephrotoxicity in various forms, including interstitial nephritis, nephrotic syndrome and renal failure. Other occasional effects on the kidney include acute renal insufficiency, urinary abnormalities (e.g. haematuria, proteinuria), nephritic syndrome and papillary necrosis.

Hepatic: Abnormal liver function for example occasional reports of elevation of serum aminotransferase enzymes (ALT, AST), hepatitis and jaundice.

Neurological and special senses: Visual disturbances, optic nephritis, headaches, paraesthesia, reports of aseptic meningitis (especially in patients with existing autoimmune disorders, such as systemic lupus erythematosus, mixed connective tissue disease), with symptoms such as stiff neck, headache, nausea, vomiting, fever or disorientation (See section 4.4 – Special Warnings and Precautions for Use), depression, confusion, hallucinations, tinnitus, vertigo, dizziness, malaise, fatigue and drowsiness. Other isolated effects on the central nervous system include tiredness, impaired hearing, insomnia, convulsions, irritability, anxiety, psychotic reactions, tremor, memory disturbance, disturbance of sensation, nightmares and taste alterations.

Haematological: Thrombocytopenia, neutropenia, agranulocytosis, aplastic anaemia and haemolytic anaemia. Leucopenia has been rarely reported.

Dermatological: Photosensitivity, Stevens-Johnson syndrome, Lyell's syndrome, eczema, erythroderma, hair loss.

Other: Impotence has been reported rarely.

4.9 Overdose

Symptoms

Symptoms include headache, nausea, vomiting, epigastric pain, gastrointestinal bleeding, rarely diarrhoea, disorientation, excitation, coma, drowsiness, dizziness, tinnitus, fainting, occasionally convulsions. In cases of significant poisoning acute renal failure and liver damage are possible. Other complications that might be encountered include hypotension, respiratory depression, and gastrointestinal irritation.

b) Therapeutic measures

Patients should be treated symptomatically as required.

Within one hour of ingestion of a potentially toxic amount, activated charcoal should be considered. Alternatively, in adults, gastric lavage should be considered within one hour of ingestion of a potentially life-threatening overdose.

Good urine output should be ensured.

Renal and liver function should be closely monitored.

Patients should be observed for at least four hours after ingestion of potentially toxic amounts.

Frequent or prolonged convulsions should be treated with intravenous diazepam.

Other measures may be indicated by the patient's clinical condition.

5. PHARMACOLOGICAL PROPERTIES

5.1 Pharmacodynamic properties

Diclofenac sodium is a non-steroidal, anti-inflammatory drug (NSAID) with analgesic and antipyretic properties. It is an inhibitor of prostaglandin synthetase.

5.2 Pharmacokinetic properties

Diclofenac 75 Retard Tablets are extended release preparations designed to release diclofenac over a period of time. Following a pharmacokinetic study with the 100 mg tablet in volunteers it was found that the average time to reach maximum plasma concentration was 6.05 hours.

The average elimination half-life was found to be 6.75 hours. The average maximum plasma concentrations were found to be 262ng/ml.

<u>General characteristics of the active substance</u>

Diclofenac sodium is almost totally absorbed after oral administration and it is subject to significant first-pass metabolism with only approximately 60% of an oral dose reaching the systemic circulation.

Diclofenac sodium is highly protein bound (>99%). It is mainly excreted in the form of metabolites via the urine but also in the bile.

The main metabolite has minimal anti-inflammatory activity compared with the parent drug.

<u>Characteristics in patients</u>

Plasma concentration of unchanged diclofenac are not reported to be significantly affected by age, renal or hepatic impairment. The metabolite concentrations may be increased by severe renal impairment.

5.3 Preclinical safety data

No relevant information additional to that already included elsewhere in the SPC.

6. PHARMACEUTICAL PARTICULARS

6.1 List of excipients

Purified talc

Ethylcellulose

Magnesium Stearate

Povidine

Stearic acid

Hydroxypropylmethlcellulose

Ethylcellulose

Diethyl phthalate

Titanium dioxide E171

Polyethylene glycol 4000

6.2 Incompatibilities

Not applicable.

6.3 Shelf life

36 months.

6.4 Special precautions for storage

Do not store above 25°C. Protect from light.

6.5 Nature and contents of container

PVdC/PVC/aluminium/PVdC blister strip.

Number of tablets per carton 28, 30, 50, 56, 60, 84, 100, 250, 500, 1000

6.6 Instructions for use and handling

None stated.

7. MARKETING AUTHORISATION HOLDER

Waymade Healthcare Plc

t/a Sovereign Medical

Sovereign House

Miles Gray Road

Basildon

Essex, SS14 3FR

8. MARKETING AUTHORISATION NUMBER(S)

PL 06464/0505

9. DATE OF FIRST AUTHORISATION/RENEWAL OF THE AUTHORISATION

27 March 1998

10. DATE OF REVISION OF THE TEXT

January 2005

Rhinocort Aqua 64 micrograms, nasal spray

(AstraZeneca UK Limited)

1. NAME OF THE MEDICINAL PRODUCT
Rhinocort® Aqua, 64 micrograms, nasal spray.

2. QUALITATIVE AND QUANTITATIVE COMPOSITION
Each actuation contains: Budesonide 64 micrograms (1.28mg/ml).

For excipients, see 6.1.

3. PHARMACEUTICAL FORM
Nasal spray, suspension.

4. CLINICAL PARTICULARS
4.1 Therapeutic indications
Seasonal and perennial allergic rhinitis and vasomotor rhinitis. Treatment of nasal polyps.

4.2 Posology and method of administration
For nasal inhalation. Dosage should be individualised.

Rhinitis (Adults including elderly)

Recommended Start Dose	Once daily dosing	Twice daily dosing
256 micrograms per day	Two applications of 64 micrograms into each nostril each morning OR If good effect is achieved, one application of 64 micrograms.	One application of 64 micrograms into each nostril morning and evening.

Nasal Polyps (Adults including elderly)

Recommended Start Dose	Once daily dosing	Twice daily dosing
256 micrograms per day	Not applicable	One application of 64 micrograms into each nostril morning and evening.

Treatment can be continued for up to 3 months.

Patients should be reminded of the importance of taking this medicine regularly.

The dose should be titrated to the lowest dose at which effective control of symptoms is achieved.

Children: There are insufficient data to recommend the use of Rhinocort Aqua in children. However, it is unlikely that the risk/benefit ratio in children is different from that in adults.

4.3 Contraindications
Hypersensitivity to any of the ingredients.

4.4 Special warnings and special precautions for use
Special care is demanded in treatment of patients transferred from oral steroids to Rhinocort where disturbances of the hypothalamic-pituitary-adrenal (HPA) axis could be expected.

Special care is needed in patients with fungal and viral infections of the airways and in patients with lung tuberculosis.

The patient should be informed that the full effect of Rhinocort is not achieved until after a few days treatment. Treatment of seasonal rhinitis should, if possible, start before exposure to the allergens. Concomitant treatment may sometimes be necessary to counteract eye symptoms caused by the allergy. In continuous long-term treatment, the nasal mucosa should be inspected regularly e.g. every 6 months.

Systemic effects of nasal corticosteroids may occur, particularly at high doses prescribed for prolonged periods. Growth retardation has been reported in children receiving nasal corticosteroids at licensed doses.

It is recommended that the height of children receiving prolonged treatment with nasal corticosteroids is regularly monitored. If growth is slowed, therapy should be reviewed with the aim of reducing the dose of nasal corticosteroid, if possible, to the lowest dose at which effective control of symptoms is maintained. In addition, consideration should also be given to referring the patient to a paediatric specialist.

Treatment with higher than recommended doses may result in clinically significant adrenal suppression. If there is evidence for higher than recommended doses being used additional systemic corticosteroid cover should be considered during periods of stress or elective surgery.

In vivo studies have shown that oral administration of ketoconazole (a known inhibitor of CYP3A4 activity in the liver and in the intestinal mucosa, see also section 4.5 Interactions) may cause an increase in the systemic exposure to budesonide. This is of limited clinical importance for short-term (1-2 weeks) treatment with ketoconazole, but should be taken into consideration during long-term treatment.

4.5 Interaction with other medicinal products and other forms of Interaction
The metabolism of budesonide is primarily mediated by CYP3A4, a subfamily of cytochrome P450. Inhibitors of this enzyme, e.g. ketoconazole, can therefore increase systemic exposure to budesonide. However, the use of ketoconazole concomitant with Rhinocort Aqua for shorter periods is of limited importance, see section 4.4 Special warnings and precautions for use.

4.6 Pregnancy and lactation
Administration during pregnancy should be avoided unless there are compelling reasons. In pregnant animals administration of budesonide causes abnormalities of foetal development. The relevance of this to man has not been established. There is no information regarding the passage of budesonide into breast milk. Use in lactation requires that the therapeutic benefit to the mother be weighed against any potential risk to the neonate.

4.7 Effects on ability to drive and use machines
Rhinocort Aqua does not affect the ability to drive or operate machinery.

4.8 Undesirable effects
Occasionally sneezing, nasal stinging and dryness may follow immediately after the use of the spray. Slight haemorrhagic secretion/epistaxis may occur.

Hypersensitivity reactions including skin rashes and angioedema may occur in rare cases.

Rhinocort contains potassium sorbate (E202), an irritant which may cause dermatitis.

Ulceration of mucous membrane and nasal septal perforation has been reported following the use of intranasal aerosol corticosteroids, but these are extremely rare.

Rare cases of raised intraocular pressure or glaucoma have been reported following the use of intranasal steroid formulations.

Systemic effects of nasal corticosteroids may occur, particularly when prescribed at high doses for prolonged periods.

4.9 Overdose
Acute overdose with Rhinocort should not present clinical problems.

Inhalation of high doses of corticosteroids may lead to suppression of the hypothalamic- pituitary-adrenal (HPA) axis function.

5. PHARMACOLOGICAL PROPERTIES
5.1 Pharmacodynamic properties
Budesonide is a non-halogenated glucocorticosteroid with a high local anti-inflammatory action within the respiratory tract.

ATC code: R01A D05

5.2 Pharmacokinetic properties
Bioavailablity of oral budesonide in man is low (11-13%) due to an extensive first pass metabolism in the liver.

The systemic availability of budesonide from Rhinocort Aqua, with reference to the metered dose is 33%. In adults the maximal plasma concentration after administration of 256 micrograms budesonide from Rhinocort Aqua is 0.64 nM and is reached within 0.7 hours. The AUC after administration of 256 micrograms budesonide from Rhinocort Aqua is 2.7 nmolxh/L in adults.

5.3 Preclinical safety data
The acute toxicity of budesonide is low and of the same order of magnitude and type as that of the reference glucocorticoids studied (beclomethasone dipropionate, flucinolone acetonide). Results from subacute and chronic toxicity studies show that the systemic effects of budesonide are less severe than or similar to those observed after administration of the other glucocorticosteroids e.g. decreased body weight gain and atrophy of lymphoid tissues and adrenal cortex. An increased incidence of brain gliomas in male rats in a carcinogenicity study could not be verified in a repeat study, in which the incidence of gliomas did not differ between any of the groups on active treatment (budesonide, prednisolone, triamcinolone acetonide) and the control groups. Liver changes (primary hepatocellular neoplasms) found in male rats in the original carcinogenicity study were noted again in the repeat study with budesonide as well as with the reference glucocorticosteroids. These effects are most probably related to a receptor effect and thus represent a class effect.

Available clinical experience shows no indication that budesonide or other glucocorticosteroids induce brain gliomas or primary heptocellular neoplasms in man. Budesonide has been used successfully in the treatment of seasonal allergic rhinitis for several years.

6. PHARMACEUTICAL PARTICULARS
6.1 List of excipients
Disodium edetate,

Potassium sorbate (E202),

Glucose anhydrous,

Microcrystalline cellulose (E460),

Carboxymethylcellulose sodium (E466),

Polysorbate 80 (E433),

Hydrochloric acid

Purified water.

6.2 Incompatibilities
None known.

6.3 Shelf life
2 years.

6.4 Special precautions for storage
Use within 2 months of starting treatment.

Do not store above 30°C. Do not refrigerate or freeze.

6.5 Nature and contents of container
Rhinocort Aqua is an aqueous solution of budesonide in either a 10ml or 20ml amber/brown glass (type II) bottle. Each bottle is fitted with a spray pump and contains either 120 or 240 actuations. Not all pack sizes may be available in the UK.

6.6 Instructions for use and handling
Before using Rhinocort Aqua for the first time the nozzle must be primed (filled with the medicine.) To do this the bottle is shaken and the protective cap removed. The bottle is then held upright and the nozzle pumped up and down several times (5-10 times) spraying into the air, until an even mist is seen. The priming effect remains for approximately 24 hours. If a longer period of time passes before the next dose is taken, the nozzle must be loaded with medicine again. This time it is sufficient to spray just once into the air.

a. The patient is then instructed to blow their nose. Next the bottle needs to be shaken and the protective cap removed.

b. The bottle is then held upright with one finger held on either side of the nozzle.

c. The tip of the nozzle is inserted into the nostril and the nozzle pressed down once (or more as instructed by the doctor). The spray is then administered into the other nostril in the same way. Note: it is not necessary to inhale at the same time as spraying.

d. The nozzle needs to be wiped with a clean tissue after use and the protective cap replaced. The bottle should be stored in an upright position.

e. Keeping the Rhinocort Aqua Nozzle clean

The plastic nozzle of Rhinocort Aqua should be cleaned regularly and at any time the spray of medicine is not coming out as it should. If this happens, first the nozzle should be checked to ensure that it is primed with medicine (see earlier). If after the nozzle is primed again the pump is still not working, the nozzle should be cleaned by using the following instructions:

The plastic nozzle is removed with a clean tissue and washed in warm - not hot - water. The nozzle is then rinsed thoroughly, dried and then replaced onto the top of the bottle. The nozzle should not be unblocked with a pin or other sharp object. After cleaning, the nozzle must be primed (filled with medicine) again before use.

7. MARKETING AUTHORISATION HOLDER
AstraZeneca UK Ltd.

600 Capability Green

Luton

LU1 3LU

UK

8. MARKETING AUTHORISATION NUMBER(S)
PL 17901/0074

9. DATE OF FIRST AUTHORISATION/RENEWAL OF THE AUTHORISATION
12 December 2003

10. DATE OF REVISION OF THE TEXT

Riamet

(Novartis Pharmaceuticals UK Ltd)

1. NAME OF THE MEDICINAL PRODUCT
▼Riamet® 20/120mg tablets

2. QUALITATIVE AND QUANTITATIVE COMPOSITION
One tablet contains 20 mg artemether and 120 mg lumefantrine.

For excipients, see 6.1.

3. PHARMACEUTICAL FORM
Tablet.

Light yellow, round tablet with "NC" debossed on one side and "CG" on the other.

4. CLINICAL PARTICULARS

4.1 Therapeutic indications

Riamet is indicated for the treatment of acute uncomplicated *Plasmodium falciparum* malaria in patients of ⩾12 years of age and ⩾35 kg.

Consideration should be given to official guidance regarding the appropriate use of antimalarial agents.

4.2 Posology and method of administration

Tablets for oral administration

To increase absorption, Riamet should be taken with food. If patients are unable to tolerate food, Riamet should be administered, but the systemic exposure may be reduced. Patients who vomit within 1 hour of taking the medication should repeat the dose.

Adults

For patients of ⩾12 years of age and ⩾35 kg body weight, a course of treatment comprises six doses of four tablets i.e. total of 24 tablets, given over a period of 60 h as follows:

The first dose of four tablets, given at the time of initial diagnosis, should be followed by five further doses of four tablets given at 8, 24, 36, 48 and 60 hours thereafter.

Children

Due to inadequate data on which to base a dose recommendation, Riamet is not recommended for use in patients who are either less than 12 years of age and/or less than 35 kg body weight.

Elderly

Although no studies have been carried out in the elderly, no special precautions or dosage adjustments are considered necessary in such patients.

Renal or hepatic impairment

Caution is advised when administering Riamet to patients with severe renal or hepatic problems. In these patients, ECG and blood potassium monitoring is advised.

New infections

Data for a limited number of patients in a malaria endemic area show that new infections can be treated with a second course of Riamet. In the absence of carcinogenicity study data, and due to lack of clinical experience, more than two courses of Riamet cannot be recommended.

4.3 Contraindications

Riamet is contraindicated in:

- Patients with known hypersensitivity to the active substances or to any of the excipients.
- Patients with complicated malaria.
- Patients who are taking any drug which inhibits the cytochrome enzyme CYP3A4 (e.g. erythromycin, ketoconazole, itraconazole, cimetidine, HIV protease inhibitors).
- Patients who are taking any drug which is metabolised by the cytochrome enzyme CYP2D6 (e.g. flecainide, metoprolol, imipramine, amitryptyline, clomipramine).
- Patients with a family history of sudden death or of congenital prolongation of the QTc interval on electrocardiograms, or with any other clinical condition known to prolong the QTc interval.
- Patients with a history of symptomatic cardiac arythmias or with clinically relevant bradycardia or with congestive cardiac failure accompanied by reduced left ventricle ejection fraction.
- Patients with disturbances of electrolyte balance e.g. hypokalemia or hypomagnesemia
- Patients taking drugs that are known to prolong the QTc interval. These drugs include:-

Antiarrhythmics of classes IA and III

Neuroleptics, antidepressive agents

Certain antibiotics including some agents of the following classes: macrolides, fluoroquinolones, imidazole and triazole antifungal agents

Certain non-sedating antihistamines (terfenadine, astemizole)

Cisapride

4.4 Special warnings and special precautions for use

Riamet has not been evaluated for the treatment of complicated malaria, including cases of cerebral malaria or other severe manifestations such as pulmonary oedema or renal failure.

Riamet is not indicated for, and has not been evaluated in, the treatment of malaria due *to P. vivax*, *P. malariae* or *P. ovale*, although some patients in clinical studies had co-infection with *P. falciparum* and *P. vivax* at baseline. Riamet is active against blood stages of *Plasmodium vivax*, but is not active against hypnozoites. Therefore, sequential treatment with primaquine may be used to achieve hypnozoite eradication. Riamet is not indicated and has not been evaluated for prophylaxis.

Halofantrine, quinine and quinidine are known to cause QT interval prolongation. Asymptomatic prolongation of QTc intervals by >30 ms, with an actual QTc >450 ms in males and >470 ms in females, was observed in approximately 5% of patients treated with various dose regimens of Riamet in clinical trials. It is possible that these changes were disease related.

Concurrent administration of Riamet and other antimalarials, should be avoided (see Section 4.5).

Patients who remain averse to food during treatment should be closely monitored as the risk of recrudescence may be greater.

Caution is advised when administering Riamet to patients with severe renal, hepatic or cardiac problems (see Section 4.2).

4.5 Interaction with other medicinal products and other forms of Interaction

A drug interaction study with Riamet in man involved administration of a 6-dose regimen over 60 hours in healthy volunteers which was commenced at 12 h after completion of a 3-dose regimen of mefloquine or placebo. Plasma mefloquine concentrations from the time of addition of Riamet were not affected compared with a group which received mefloquine followed by placebo.

Pre-treatment with mefloquine had no effect on plasma concentrations of artemether or the artemether/dihydroartemisinin ratio but there was a significant reduction in plasma levels of lumefantrine, possibly due to lower absorption secondary to a mefloquine-induced decrease in bile production.

Both artemether and lumefantrine are metabolised by the cytochrome enzyme CYP3A4 but do not inhibit this enzyme at therapeutic concentrations. Due to the lack of clinical data, and unknown effects on safety, the co-administration of Riamet with drugs, that inhibit CYP3A4 is contraindicated. As grapefruit juice inhibits the metabolism of some drugs via the CYP3A4 cytochrome enzyme, it is advisable not to drink grapefruit juice while taking Riamet.

Whereas *in-vitro* studies with artemether at therapeutic concentrations revealed no significant interactions with cytochrome P450 enzymes, the artemisinins have some capacity to induce the production of the cytochrome enzyme CYP2C19, and perhaps also CYP3A4. It is possible that iso-enzyme induction could alter the therapeutic effects of drugs that are predominantly metabolised by these enzymes.

Lumefantrine was found to inhibit CYP2D6 *in vitro*. This may be of particular clinical relevance for compounds with a low therapeutic index. Co-administration of Riamet with drugs that are metabolised by this iso-enzyme is contra-indicated. *In-vitro* studies indicated that lumefantrine metabolism is inhibited by halofantrine and quinine.

Administration of Riamet is contra-indicated in patients taking drugs that are known to prolong the QT interval (see section 4.3).

In patients previously treated with halofantrine, Riamet should be dosed at least one month after the last halofantrine dose.

Due to the limited data on safety and efficacy, Riamet should not be given concurrently with any other antimalarial agent.

In addition, due to the propensity of some antimalarial agents to prolong the QT interval, caution is advised when administering Riamet to patients in whom there may still be detectable concentrations of these drugs in the plasma following prior treatments.

However, if a patient deteriorates whilst taking Riamet, alternative treatment for malaria should be commenced without delay. In such cases, monitoring of the ECG is recommended and steps should be taken to correct any electrolyte disturbances.

4.6 Pregnancy and lactation

Pregnancy

There are no adequate data from the use of artemether and lumefantrine in pregnant women. Reproductive studies in rats and rabbits have shown materno-, feto- and embryotoxicity with artemether. No evidence of teratogenicity for the combination or for the individual components lumefantrine and artemether has been reported, but results were unconclusive due to uncertain exposure (see section 5.3 Preclinical safety data). Riamet treatment should only be considered if the expected benefit to the mother outweighs the risk to the fetus.

Lactation

Animal data suggest excretion into breast milk but no data are available in humans. Riamet should not be taken by breast-feeding women. Due to the long elimination half-life of lumefantrine (4 to 6 days), it is recommended that breastfeeding should not resume until at least one week after the last dose of Riamet.

4.7 Effects on ability to drive and use machines

Patients receiving Riamet should be warned that dizziness or fatigue/asthenia may occur in which case they should not drive or use machines.

4.8 Undesirable effects

Adverse reactions are ranked under headings of frequency, the most frequent first, using the following convention: Very common (>1/10); common (>1/100, <1/10); uncommon (>1/1,000, <1/100); rare (>1/10,000, <1/1,000); very rare (<1/10,000), including isolated reports.

Table 1

Immune system disorders	
Very rare:	Hypersensitivity
Nervous system disorders	
Very common:	Headache, dizziness
Common:	Sleep disorder
Cardiac disorders	
Common:	Palpitation
Respiratory, thoracic and mediastinal disorders	
Common:	Cough
Gastrointestinal disorders	
Very common:	Abdominal pain, anorexia
Common:	Diarrhoea, vomiting, nausea
Skin and subcutaneous tissue disorders	
Common:	Pruritus, rash
Musculoskeletal and connective tissue disorders	
Common:	Arthralgia, myalgia
General disorders and administration site conditions	
Common:	Asthenia, fatigue

4.9 Overdose

In cases of suspected overdosage symptomatic and supportive therapy should be given as appropriate, which should include ECG and blood potassium monitoring.

5. PHARMACOLOGICAL PROPERTIES

5.1 Pharmacodynamic properties

Pharmacotherapeutic group

Antimalarials, Blood schizontocide (ATC code: P01BE52)

Pharmacodynamic effects

Riamet comprises a fixed ratio of 1:6 parts of artemether and lumefantrine, respectively. The site of antiparasitic action of both components is the food vacuole of the malarial parasite, where they are thought to interfere with the conversion of haem, a toxic intermediate produced during haemoglobin breakdown, to the nontoxic haemozoin, malaria pigment. Lumefantrine is thought to interfere with the polymerisation process, while artemether generates reactive metabolites as a result of the interaction between its peroxide bridge and haem iron. Both artemether and lumefantrine have a secondary action involving inhibition of nucleic acid- and protein synthesis within the malarial parasite.

The antimalarial activity of the combination of lumefantrine and artemether in Riamet is greater than that of either substance alone. In a double-blind comparative study in China, the 28-day cure rate of Riamet when given at 4 doses was 100 %, compared with 92 % for lumefantrine and 55 % for artemether when given as monotherapy.

In areas where multi-drug-resistant strains of *P. falciparum* malaria are common and in the resident population, 28-day cure rates with the 6-dose regimen (given over 60-96 h) were 97 % and 95 % for Riamet and 100 % for mefloquine/artesunate.

Patients of European origin were not included in trials with six-dose regimen. However, efficacy and safety was similar in European and Thai patients following a four-dose regimen. Thus, similar efficacy and safety profiles with the six-dose regimen would be expected in both populations.

In comparative clinical trials Riamet cleared gametocytes in less than one week and more rapidly than non-artemisinin antimalarials.

Riamet is active against blood stages of *Plasmodium vivax*, but is not active against hypnozoites. Therefore, sequential treatment with primaquine may be used to achieve hypnozoite eradication (see section 4.4).

5.2 Pharmacokinetic properties

Pharmacokinetic characterisation of Riamet is limited by the lack of an intravenous formulation, and the very high inter-and intrasubject variability of artemether and lumefantrine plasma concentrations and derived pharmacokinetic parameters (AUC, C_{max}).

Absorption

Artemether is absorbed fairly rapidly with peak plasma concentrations reached about 2 hours after dosing. Absorption of lumefantrine, a highly lipophilic compound, starts after a lag-time of up to 2 hours, with peak plasma concentration about 6-8 hours after dosing. Food enhances the absorption of both artemether and lumefantrine: in healthy volunteers the relative bioavailability of artemether was increased more than two-fold, and that of lumefantrine sixteen-fold compared with fasted conditions when Riamet was taken after a high-fat meal.

Food has also been shown to increase the absorption of lumefantrine in patients with malaria, although to a lesser extent (approximately two-fold), most probably due to the lower fat content of the food ingested by acutely ill patients. The food interaction data indicate that absorption of lumefantrine under fasted conditions is very poor (assuming 100 % absorption after a high-fat meal, the amount absorbed under fasted conditions would be <10 % of the dose). Patients should therefore be encouraged to take the medication with a normal diet as soon as food can be tolerated.

Distribution

Artemether and lumefantrine are both highly bound to human serum proteins *in vitro* (95.4 % and 99.9 %, respectively). Dihydroartemisinin is also bound to human serum proteins (47-76%).

Metabolism

Artemether is rapidly and extensively metabolised (substantial first-pass metabolism) both *in vitro* and in humans. Human liver microsomes metabolise artemether to the biologically active main metabolite dihydroartemisinin (demethylation), predominantly through the isoenzyme CYP3A4/5. This metabolite has also been detected in humans *in vivo*. The artemether/dihydroartemisinin AUC ratio is 1.2 after a single dose and 0.3 after 6 doses given over 3 days. *In-vivo* data indicate that artemisinins have some capacity to induce cytochrome isoenzymes CYP2C19 and CYP3A4. Dihydroartemisinin is further converted to inactive metabolites.

Lumefantrine is N-debutylated, mainly by CYP3A4, in human liver microsomes. *In vivo* in animals (dogs and rats), glucuronidation of lumefantrine takes place directly and after oxidative biotransformation. In humans, the kinetic profile of the metabolite desbutyl-lumefantrine, for which the in-vitro antiparasitic effect is 5 to 8 fold higher than lumefantrine, has not been documented. *In vitro,* lumefantrine significantly inhibits the activity of CYP2D6 at therapeutic plasma concentrations.

Elimination

Artemether and dihydroartemisinin are rapidly cleared from plasma with an elimination half-life of about 2 hours. Lumefantrine is eliminated very slowly with a terminal half-life of 2 - 3 days in healthy volunteers and 4 - 6 days in patients with falciparum malaria. Demographic characteristics such as sex and weight appear to have no clinically relevant effects on the pharmacokinetics of Riamet.

No urinary excretion data are available for humans. In rats and dogs unchanged artemether has not been detected in faeces and urine due to its rapid and high-first-pass metabolism, but several metabolites (unindentified) have been detected in both faeces and urine. Lumefantrine is eliminated via the bile in rats and dogs, with excretion primarily in the faeces. After oral dosing in rats and dogs qualitative and quantitative recovery of metabolites in bile and faeces was relatively low, most of the dose being recovered as parent drug.

5.3 Preclinical safety data

General toxicity

The main changes observed in repeat-dose toxicity studies were associated with the expected pharmacological action on erythrocytes, accompanied by responsive secondary haematopoiesis.

Mutagenicity

No evidence of Riamet mutagenicity was detected in *in vitro* or *in vivo* tests. In the micronucleus test myelotoxicity was seen at all dose levels (500, 1000 and 2000 mg/kg), but recovery was almost complete 48 hours after dosing.

Carcinogenicity

Carcinogenicity studies with Riamet were not conducted.

Reproductive toxicity studies

Reproductive toxicity studies with Riamet in rats showed both materno- and embryotoxic effects at doses of 60 to a 100 mg/kg but without evidence of teratogenicity. In rabbits, materno- and embryotoxicity were seen at 175 mg/kg, but not fetotoxicity or teratogenicity. A dose of 105 mg/kg was free of treatment-induced effects. Lumefantrine doses up to 1000 mg/kg showed no evidence to suggest materno-, embryo- or fetotoxicity or teratogenicity in rats and rabbits. Artemisinins are known to be embryotoxic in animals. Artemether showed no effects in rabbits at doses up to 25 mg/kg, but at 30 mg/kg, materno-, embryo- and fetotoxicity were observed. In rats materno-, embryo- and fetotoxicity were all noted at 10 mg/kg, but without evidence of teratogenicity at any dose level. Riamet was not embryotoxic in rats at doses of ⩽ 25 mg/kg.

Cardiovascular Pharmacology

In toxicity studies in dogs at doses ⩾ 600 mg/kg/day only, there was some evidence of prolongation of the QTc interval, at higher doses than intended for use in man. In an in vitro assay of HERG channels stably expressed in HEK293 cells, lumefrantrine and the main metabolite desbutyl-lumefantrine showed some inhibitory potential in one of the currents responsible for cardiac repolarization. The potency was lower than the other antimalarial drugs tested. From the estimated IC_{50} values, the order of potency of HERG current block was halofantrine (IC_{50} = 0.04 μM)> chloroquine (2.5 μM)> mefloquine 2.6 μM)> desbutyl-lumefantrine (5.5 μM)> lumefantrine (8.1 μM). In the absence of further clinical and pharmacokinetic data, the clinical significance of these findings is unclear (see sections 4.3 and 4.4).

6. PHARMACEUTICAL PARTICULARS

6.1 List of excipients

- Polysorbate 80
- Hypromellose
- Microcrystalline cellulose
- Colloidal anhydrous silica
- Croscarmellose sodium
- Magnesium stearate.

6.2 Incompatibilities

Not applicable.

6.3 Shelf life

2 years.

6.4 Special precautions for storage

Do not store above 30° C.

6.5 Nature and contents of container

PVC/PE/PVDC/Aluminium blisters containing 8 tablets in packs of, 24 or 400 tablets.

6.6 Instructions for use and handling

No special requirements.

7. MARKETING AUTHORISATION HOLDER

Novartis Pharmaceuticals UK Ltd.
Frimley Business Park
Frimley, Camberley
Surrey
GU16 7SR

8. MARKETING AUTHORISATION NUMBER(S)

PL 00101/0566

9. DATE OF FIRST AUTHORISATION/RENEWAL OF THE AUTHORISATION

Date of first authorisation: 30 November 1999

10. DATE OF REVISION OF THE TEXT

February 2005

LEGAL CATEGORY

POM

i

Ridaura Tiltab Tablets 3mg

(Astellas Pharma Limited)

1. NAME OF THE MEDICINAL PRODUCT

RIDAURA TILTAB TABLETS 3 MG

2. QUALITATIVE AND QUANTITATIVE COMPOSITION

Auranofin HSE 3mg

3. PHARMACEUTICAL FORM

Tablet

4. CLINICAL PARTICULARS

4.1 Therapeutic indications

Ridaura is an orally active gold preparation. It is indicated in the management of adults with active progressive rheumatoid arthritis only when non-steroidal anti-inflammatory drugs have been found to be inadequate alone to control the disease, i.e. when second-line therapy is required. In patients with adult rheumatoid arthritis Ridaura has been shown to reduce disease activity reflected by synovitis, associated symptoms, and appropriate laboratory parameters. Gold cannot reverse structural damage to joints caused by previous disease. Ridaura does not produce an immediate response and therapeutic effects may be seen after three to six months of treatment.

4.2 Posology and method of administration

For Adults and the Elderly only:

For Adults:

The usual starting dose is 6 mg daily as one 3 mg tablet twice a day, in the morning and the evening with meals. If this is well tolerated a single daily dose may be given as two 3 mg tablets with breakfast or with the evening meal.

Treatment should be continued for a minimum of three to six months to assess response, as Ridaura is a slow-acting drug. If the response is inadequate after six months an increase to 9 mg (one tablet three times a day) may be tolerated. If response remains inadequate after a three month trial of 9 mg daily, Ridaura therapy should be discontinued. Safety at dosages exceeding 9 mg daily has not been studied.

Absorption of gold from Ridaura tablets is rapid but incomplete. Although mean blood gold levels are proportional to dose, no correlation between blood gold levels and safety or efficacy has been established. Dosage adjustments should therefore depend on monitoring clinical response and adverse events rather than on monitoring blood gold concentrations.

Anti-inflammatory drugs and analgesics may be prescribed as necessary with Ridaura.

The Elderly:

Dosage as for adults. As with all drugs extra caution should be exercised in administration to the elderly.

4.3 Contraindications

Contraindicated in pregnancy.

Contraindicated where hypersensitivity to gold compounds or other heavy metals exists.

Although not necessarily reported in association with Ridaura, do not use in patients with a history of any of the following gold-induced disorders: necrotising enterocolitis, pulmonary fibrosis, exfoliate dermatitis, bone marrow aplasia, or other severe blood dyscrasias or toxicity to other heavy metals. Use should also be avoided in progressive renal disease or severe active hepatic disease and in systemic lupus erythromatosus.

4.4 Special warnings and special precautions for use

Use with caution in patients with any degree of renal impairment or hepatic dysfunction, inflammatory bowel disease, rash, or history of bone marrow depression.

Close monitoring is essential. Full blood count with differential and platelet counts (which should be plotted) and tests for urinary protein must be performed prior to Ridaura therapy and at least monthly thereafter, see also section 4.8. Ridaura should be withdrawn if the platelet count falls below 100,000 per ml or if signs and symptoms suggestive of thrombocytopenia, leucopenia and aplastic anaemia occur. The occurrence of purpura, ecchymoses or petechia would suggest the presence of thrombocytopenia and may indicate a need for additional platelet count determinations. Patients with gastrointestinal symptoms, with rash, with pruritus (which may precede rash), with stomatitis, or a metallic taste in the mouth (which might precede stomatitis), should also be closely monitored as such symptoms may indicate a need for modification of dosage or withdrawal, see also section 4.8. Pulmonary fibrosis may rarely occur and chest X-ray is recommended at least annually.

Prior to initiating treatment patients must be advised of the potential side effects associated with Ridaura. They should be warned to report promptly any unusual signs or symptoms during treatment such as pruritus, rash, metallic taste, sore throat or tongue, mouth ulceration, easy bruising, purpura, epistaxis, bleeding gums, menorrhagia, or diarrhoea.

Gold has been shown to be carcinogenic in rodents although there was no evidence of carcinogenicity in a 7-year dog study.

4.5 Interaction with other medicinal products and other forms of Interaction

None stated.

4.6 Pregnancy and lactation

Gold is teratogenic in some animal species. Ridaura should not be used in pregnancy. Women of child-bearing potential should not be treated with Ridaura without full consideration of the benefits of treatment against the potential risk of teratogenicity; they should practise effective contraception during treatment and for at least six months after. Patients should be fully informed of the teratogenic risk, and termination of any pregnancy occurring during treatment should be considered in view of the possibility of foetal malformation. If women are to be treated post-partum with Ridaura, breast-feeding should be avoided.

4.7 Effects on ability to drive and use machines

None stated.

4.8 Undesirable effects

Adverse reactions can occur throughout treatment with Ridaura, although the highest incidence can be expected during the first six months of treatment. The most common reaction to Ridaura is diarrhoea or loose stools, occurring in about 30% of patients according to the literature. Up to about one patient in twenty will be unable to tolerate Ridaura because of diarrhoea. Ulcerative enterocolitis has been very rarely reported (<0.01%), as with all gold containing drugs. Therefore patients with gastrointestinal symptoms should be carefully monitored for the appearance of gastrointestinal bleeding and treatment stopped if this occurs. See table.

Blood and lymphatic system	
Blood dyscrasias including leucopenia*, granulocytopenia and thrombocytopenia*, anaemia, eosinophilia	**Common** (>1/100, <1/10)
Agranulocytosis, aplastic anaemia*, red cell aplasia	**Very rare** (<1/10,000)
Nervous system disorders	
Headache	**Uncommon** (>1/1000, <1/100)
Peripheral neuropathy	**Very rare** (<1/10,000)

Eye disorders	
Conjunctivitis	**Common** (>1/100, <1/10)
Gold deposits in the lens/ corneas	**Very rare** (<1/10,000)
Respiratory, thoracic and Mediastinal disorders	
Interstitial pneumonitis	**Rare** (>1/10,000, <1/1,000)
Pulmonary fibrosis	**Very rare** (<1/10,000)
Gastrointestinal disorders	
Diarrhoea or loose stools	**Very Common** (>1/10)
Oral mucous membrane disorder and stomatitis, disturbed taste	**Uncommon** (>1/1000, <1/100)
Nausea and vomiting, abdominal pain	**Uncommon** (>1/1000, <1/100)
Ulcerative enterocolitis	**Very rare** (<1/10,000)
Skin and subcutaneous tissue disorders	
Rashes and pruritis	**Very Common** (>1/10)
Exfoliative dermatitis and alopecia	**Very rare** (<1/10,000)
Renal and urinary disorders	
Proteinuria	**Common** (>1/100, <1/10)
Glomerular disease/nephrotic syndrome/membranous glomerulonephritis	**Very rare** (<1/10,000)
Investigations	
Decrease in haemoglobin Decrease in haematocrit Changes in liver function Changes in renal function	**Common** (>1/100, <1/10)

* Please see section 4.4 for monitoring requirements and cessation of therapy

The frequencies are taken from adverse events reported in controlled studies and post-marketing experience.

Treatment with Ridaura should be stopped in cases of persistent rash, especially if accompanied by pruritus. In cases of clinically significant proteinuria treatment with Ridaura should be stopped promptly. Treatment may be restarted after the proteinuria has cleared, however, under close supervision in patients who have experienced only minimal proteinuria.

Transient decreases in haemoglobin or haematocrit early in treatment have been reported. Occasional decreases in white blood counts have been reported during auranofin treatment.

There have been some reports of gold deposits in the lens or corneas of patients treated with auranofin. These deposits have not led to any eye disorders or any degree of visual impairment.

4.9 Overdose
Ridaura overdosage experience is limited. One patient who took 27 mg daily for 10 days developed an encephalopathy and peripheral neuropathy. Ridaura was discontinued and the patient eventually recovered.

In case of acute overdosage, immediate induction of vomiting or gastric lavage and appropriate supportive therapy are recommended. Chelating agents such as BAL have been used in injectable gold overdosage, and may be considered, although there has been no specific experience with Ridaura.

5. PHARMACOLOGICAL PROPERTIES

5.1 Pharmacodynamic properties
Auranofin is a disease-modifying slow-acting immunomodulating agent.

5.2 Pharmacokinetic properties
About 20% to 30% of the gold in a dose of Ridaura is absorbed and, although there is considerable variation in absorption, this is less than that seen with parenteral gold. Steady state blood concentrations are achieved 8 to 12 weeks after starting and are on average 5 to 10 times less than those following parenteral gold, with no correlation with clinical response or adverse events. About 70% of the gold administered in Ridaura appears in the faeces during the first week following a single dose, and at six months after dosing, less than 1% of the gold administered remains in the body, in contrast to around 30% of gold given parenterally. In contrast to parenteral gold, which does not become cell-associated, 40% of the gold in the blood of Ridaura-treated patients is associated with blood cells.

The metabolism of Ridaura is not fully understood, although it is clear from both animal and in-vitro studies with human blood that both the sulphur and the phosphorus ligands of Ridaura are rapidly dissociated from the gold.

5.3 Preclinical safety data
No relevant pre-clinical safety data has been generated.

6. PHARMACEUTICAL PARTICULARS

6.1 List of excipients
Lactose

Microcrystalline cellulose

Maize starch

Sodium starch glycollate

Magnesium stearate

Hydroxypropylmethylcellulose

Propylene glycol

Opaspray M-1-6054

6.2 Incompatibilities
None

6.3 Shelf life
Five years

6.4 Special precautions for storage
None

6.5 Nature and contents of container
Standard SK&F polypropylene securitainers or HDPE containers with wadless polypropylene screw caps containing 60 tablets.

6.6 Instructions for use and handling
None

Administrative Data

7. MARKETING AUTHORISATION HOLDER
Yamanouchi Pharma Ltd

Yamanouchi House

Pyrford Road

West Byfleet

Surrey

KT14 6RA

8. MARKETING AUTHORISATION NUMBER(S)
0166/0176

9. DATE OF FIRST AUTHORISATION/RENEWAL OF THE AUTHORISATION
31/10/97

10. DATE OF REVISION OF THE TEXT
Date of partial revision = 18 November 2003.

11. Legal category
POM

Rifadin Capsules 150mg, 300mg, Syrup 100mg/5ml

(sanofi-aventis)

1. NAME OF THE MEDICINAL PRODUCT
Rifadin Capsules 150mg

Rifadin Capsules 300mg

Rifadin Syrup 100mg/5ml

2. QUALITATIVE AND QUANTITATIVE COMPOSITION
Rifadin Capsules150mg: Rifampicin Ph Eur 150 mg

Rifadin Capsules 300mg: Rifampicin Ph Eur 300 mg

Rifadin Syrup: Rifampicin Ph Eur 100 mg

3. PHARMACEUTICAL FORM
Rifadin Capsules 150mg: Blue and red hard gelatin capsules.

Rifadin Capsules 300mg: Red hard gelatin capsules.

Rifadin Syrup: Raspberry coloured and flavoured suspension.

4. CLINICAL PARTICULARS

4.1 Therapeutic indications
Indications for use

Tuberculosis: In combination with other active anti-tuberculosis drugs in the treatment of all forms of tuberculosis, including fresh, advanced, chronic and drug-resistant cases. Rifadin is also effective against most atypical strains of Mycobacteria.

Leprosy: In combination with at least one other active anti-leprosy drug in the management of multibacillary and paucibacillary leprosy to effect conversion of the infectious state to a non-infectious state.

Other Infections: In the treatment of Brucellosis, Legionnaires Disease, and serious staphylococcal infections. To prevent emergence of resistant strains of the infecting organisms, Rifadin should be used in combination with another antibiotic appropriate for the infection.

Prophylaxis of meningococcal meningitis: For the treatment of asymptomatic carriers of *N. meningitidis* to eliminate meningococci from the nasopharynx.

Haemophilus influenzae: For the treatment of asymptomatic carriers of *H.influenzae* and as chemoprophylaxis of exposed children, 4 years of age or younger.

4.2 Posology and method of administration
Recommended Dosage

For oral administration

The daily dose of Rifadin, calculated from the patient's body weight, should preferably be taken at least 30 minutes before a meal or 2 hours after a meal to ensure rapid and complete absorption.

Tuberculosis:

Rifadin should be given with other effective anti-tuberculosis drugs to prevent the possible emergence of rifampicin-resistant strains of Mycobacteria.

Adults: The recommended single daily dose in tuberculosis is 8-12 mg/kg.

Usual Daily dose: Patients weighing less than 50 kg - 450 mg. Patients weighing 50kg or more - 600 mg.

Children: In children, oral doses of 10-20 mg/kg body weight daily are recommended, although a total daily dose should not usually exceed 600 mg.

Leprosy:

600 mg doses of rifampicin should be given once per month. Alternatively, a daily regimen may be used. The recommended single daily dose is 10 mg/kg.

Usual daily dose: Patients weighing less than 50 kg - 450 mg. Patients weighing 50kg or more - 600 mg.

In the treatment of leprosy, rifampicin should always be used in conjunction with at least one other antileprosy drug.

Brucellosis, Legionnaires Disease or serious staphylococcal infections

Adults: The recommended daily dose is 600-1200 mg given in 2 to 4 divided doses, together with another appropriate antibiotic to prevent the emergence of resistant strains of the infecting organisms.

Prophylaxis of meningococcal meningitis

Adults: 600 mg twice daily for 2 days.

Children (1 - 12 years): 10 mg/kg twice daily for 2 days.

Children (3 months - 1 year): 5 mg/kg twice daily for 2 days.

Prophylaxis of Haemophilus influenzae

Adults and children: For members of households exposed to H. influenzae B disease when the household contains a child 4 years of age or younger, it is recommended that all members (including the child) receive rifampicin 20 mg/kg once daily (maximum daily dose 600 mg) for 4 days.

Index cases should be treated prior to discharge from hospital.

Neonates (1 month): 10 mg/kg daily for 4 days.

Impaired liver function:

A daily dose of 8 mg/kg should not be exceeded in patients with impaired liver function.

Use in the elderly:

In elderly patients, the renal excretion of rifampicin is decreased proportionally with physiological decrease of renal function; due to compensatory increase of liver excretion, the terminal half-life in serum is similar to that of younger patients. However, as increased blood levels have been noted in one study of rifampicin in elderly patients, caution should be exercised in using rifampicin in such patients, especially if there is evidence of impaired liver function.

4.3 Contraindications
Rifadin is contra-indicated in the presence of jaundice, and in patients who are hypersensitive to the rifamycins.

4.4 Special warnings and special precautions for use
Rifampicin should be given under the supervision of a respiratory or other suitably qualified physician.

Patients with impaired liver function should only be given rifampicin in cases of necessity, and then with caution and under close medical supervision. In these patients, lower doses of rifampicin are recommended and careful monitoring of liver function, especially serum glutamic pyruvic transaminase (SGPT) and serum glutamic oxaloacetic transaminase (SGOT) should initially be carried out prior to therapy, weekly for two weeks, then every two weeks for the next six weeks. If signs of hepatocellular damage occur, rifampicin should be withdrawn.

Rifampicin should also be withdrawn if clinically significant changes in hepatic function occur. The need for other forms of antituberculosis therapy and a different regimen should be considered. Urgent advice should be obtained from a specialist in the management of tuberculosis. If rifampicin is re-introduced after liver function has returned to normal, liver function should be monitored daily.

In patients with impaired liver function, elderly patients, malnourished patients, and possibly, children under two years of age, caution is particularly recommended when instituting therapeutic regimens in which isoniazid is to be used concurrently with Rifadin. If the patient has no evidence of pre-existing liver disease and normal pre-treatment liver function, liver function tests need only be repeated if fever, vomiting, jaundice or other deterioration in the patient's condition occur.

In some patients hyperbilirubinsemia can occur in the early days of treatment. This results from competition between rifampicin and bilirubin for hepatic excretion.

An isolated report showing a moderate rise in bilirubin and/or transaminase level is not in itself an indication for interrupting treatment; rather the decision should be made after repeating the tests, noting trends in the levels and considering them in conjunction with the patient's clinical condition.

All tuberculosis patients should have pre-treatment measurements of liver function.

Because of the possibility of immunological reaction (see side effects) occurring with intermittent therapy (less than 2 to 3 times per week) patients should be closely monitored. Patients should be cautioned against interrupting treatment.

Rifampicin has enzyme-inducing properties including induction of delta amino levulinic acid synthetase. Isolated reports have associated porphyria exacerbation with rifampicin administration.

4.5 Interaction with other medicinal products and other forms of Interaction

Rifampicin has been shown in animals and man to have liver enzyme inducing properties and may reduce the activity of anticoagulants, corticosteroids, cyclosporin, digitalis preparations, oral contraceptives, oral hypoglycaemic agents, dapsone, phenytoin, quinidine, narcotics and analgesics. It may be necessary to adjust the dosage of these drugs if they are given concurrently with Rifadin, particularly when it is initiated or withdrawn.

Patients on oral contraceptives should be advised to use alternative, non-hormonal methods of birth control during Rifadin therapy. Also diabetes may become more difficult to control.

If -aminosalicylic acid and rifampicin are both included in the treatment regimen, they should be given not less than eight hours apart to ensure satisfactory blood levels.

Therapeutic levels of rifampicin have been shown to inhibit standard microbiological assays for serum folate and Vitamin B12. Thus alternative assay methods should be considered. Transient elevation of BSP and serum bilirubin have been reported. Therefore, these tests should be performed before the morning dose of rifampicin.

4.6 Pregnancy and lactation

At very high doses in animals rifampicin has been shown to have teratogenic effects. There are no well controlled studies with rifampicin in pregnant women. Therefore, Rifadin should be used in pregnant women or in women of child bearing potential only if the potential benefit justifies the potential risk to the foetus. When Rifadin is administered during the last few weeks of pregnancy it may cause post-natal haemorrhages in the mother and infant for which treatment with Vitamin K1 may be indicated.

Rifampicin is excreted in breast milk, patients receiving rifampicin should not breast feed unless in the physician's judgement the potential benefit to the patient outweighs the potential risk to the infant.

4.7 Effects on ability to drive and use machines

None stated

4.8 Undesirable effects

Reactions occurring with either daily or intermittent dosage regimens include:

General hypersensitivity reactions involving the skin, exfoliative dermatitis, Lyells syndrome and pemphigoid reactions.

Cutaneous reactions which are mild and self-limiting and do not appear to be hypersensitivity reactions. Typically they consist of flushing and itching with or without a rash.

Gastrointestinal reactions consist of anorexia, nausea, vomiting, abdominal discomfort, and diarrhoea. Pseudomembranous colitis has been reported with rifampicin therapy.

Hepatitis can be caused by rifampicin and liver function tests should be monitored (see Precautions).

Thrombocytopenia with or without purpura may occur, usually associated with intermittent therapy, but is reversible if drug is discontinued as soon as purpura occurs. Cerebral haemorrhage and fatalities have been reported when rifampicin administration has been continued or resumed after the appearance of purpura.

Eosinophilia, leucopenia, oedema, muscle weakness and myopathy have been reported to occur in a small percentage of patients treated with rifampicin.

Reactions usually occurring with intermittent dosage regimens and probably of immunological origin include:

- 'Flu Syndrome' consisting of episodes of fever, chills, headache, dizziness, and bone pain appearing most commonly during the 3rd to the 6th monthly of therapy. The frequency of the syndrome varies but may occur in up to 50 % of patients given once-weekly regimens with a dose of rifampicin of 25 mg/kg or more.
- Shortness of breath and wheezing.
- Decrease in blood pressure and shock.
- Acute haemolytic anaemia.
- Acute renal failure usually due to acute tubular necrosis or acute interstitial nephritis.

If serious complications arise, e.g. renal failure, thrombocytopenia or haemolytic anaemia, rifampicin should be stopped and never restarted.

Occasional disturbances of the menstrual cycle have been reported in women receiving long-term anti-tuberculosis therapy with regimens containing rifampicin.

Rifampicin may produce a reddish discolouration of the urine, sputum and tears. The patient should be forewarned of this. Soft contact lenses may be permanently stained.

4.9 Overdose

In cases of overdose with Rifadin, gastric lavage should be performed as soon as possible. Intensive supportive measures should be instituted and individual symptoms treated as they arise.

5. PHARMACOLOGICAL PROPERTIES

5.1 Pharmacodynamic properties

Rifampicin is an active bactericidial antituberculosis drug which is particularly active against the rapidly growing extracellular organisms and also has bactericidial activity intracellularly. Rifampicin has activity against slow and intermittently-growing *M. Tuberculosis*.

Rifampicin inhibits DNA-dependent RNA polymerase activity in susceptible cells. Specifically, it interacts with bacterial RNA polymerase but does not inhibit the mammalian enzyme. Cross-resistance to rifampicin has only been shown with other rifamycins.

5.2 Pharmacokinetic properties

In normal subjects the biological half-life of rifampicin in serum averages about 3 hours after a 600 mg dose and increases to 5.1 hours after a 900 mg dose. With repeated administration, the half-life decreases and reaches average values of approximately 2-3 hours. If does not differ in patients with renal failure and consequently, no dosage adjustment is required.

Rifampicin is rapidly eliminated in the bile and an enterophepatic circulation ensues. During this process, rifampicin undergoes progressive deacetylation, so that nearly all the drug in the bile is in this form in about 6 hours. This metabolite retains essentially complete antibacterial activity. Intestinal absorption is reduced by deacetylation and elimination is facilitated. Up to 30 % of a dose is excreted in the urine, with about half of this being unchanged drug.

Rifampicin is widely distributed throughout the body. It is present in effective concentrations in many organs and body fluids, including cerebrospinal fluid. Rifampicin is about 80 % protein bound. Most of the unbound fraction is not ionized and therefore is diffused freely in tissues.

5.3 Preclinical safety data

Not applicable

6. PHARMACEUTICAL PARTICULARS

6.1 List of excipients

Rifadin Capsules

Corn starch Ph Eur

Magnesium stearate Ph Eur

Rifadin Syrup

Agar Ph Eur

Sucrose Ph Eur

Methyl-p-hydroxybenzoate Ph Eur

Propyl-p-hydroxybenzoate Ph Eur

Potassium sorbate Ph Eur

Sodium metabisulphite Ph Eur

Tween 80 Ph Eur

Raspberry essence HSE

Saccharin USNF

Diethanolamine USNF

Purified water Ph Eur

6.2 Incompatibilities

None stated

6.3 Shelf life

Rifadin Capsules: 4 years from date of manufacture

Rifadin Syrup: 3 years from date of manufacture

6.4 Special precautions for storage

Rifadin Capsules

Store below 25°C.

Protect from light and moisture.

Rifadin Syrup

Store below 30°C.

Do not dilute.

Dispense in clear or amber glass bottles.

6.5 Nature and contents of container

Rifadin Capsules

Blister packs of 100 capsules in cardboard cartons. Blister material is aluminium foil / PVDC (Aluminium 0.025 mm; PVDC 20 gsm) and transparent PVC / PVDC foil (PVC 0.25 mm; PVDC 60 gsm).

Rifadin Syrup

120ml in amber glass bottles

6.6 Instructions for use and handling

Not applicable

7. MARKETING AUTHORISATION HOLDER

Aventis Pharma Ltd

trading as Marion Merrell or Aventis Pharma

50 Kings Hill Avenue

Kings Hill

West Malling

ME19 4AH

UK

8. MARKETING AUTHORISATION NUMBER(S)

Rifadin 150mg Capsules: PL 04425/5915R

Rifadin 300mg Capsules: PL 04425/5916R

Rifadin Syrup: PL 04425/5917R

9. DATE OF FIRST AUTHORISATION/RENEWAL OF THE AUTHORISATION

Rifadin Capsules: 9th April 2005

Rifadin Syrup: 23rd March 2005

10. DATE OF REVISION OF THE TEXT

Rifadin Capsules: April 2005

Rifadin Syrup: March 2005

Legal Category

POM

Rifadin For Infusion 600mg

(sanofi-aventis)

1. NAME OF THE MEDICINAL PRODUCT

Rifadin for Infusion 600mg

2. QUALITATIVE AND QUANTITATIVE COMPOSITION

Rifampicin BP 600mg

3. PHARMACEUTICAL FORM

Lyophilisate (for reconstitution prior to use) and accompanying ampoule of solvent.

4. CLINICAL PARTICULARS

4.1 Therapeutic indications

Rifadin for Infusion is indicated for acutely ill patients who are unable to tolerate oral therapy e.g. post operative or comatose patients or patients in whom gastrointestinal absorption is impaired.

Tuberculosis: Rifadin, used in combination with other active anti-tuberculosis drugs, is indicated in the treatment of all forms of tuberculosis, including fresh, advanced, chronic and drug-resistant cases. Rifadin is also effective against most atypical strains of Mycobacteria.

Leprosy: Rifadin, used in combination with at least one other active anti-leprosy drug, is indicated in the management of multibacillary and paucibacillary leprosy to effect conversion of the infectious state to a non-infectious state.

Other infections: Rifadin is indicated in the treatment of Brucellosis, Legionnaires Disease, and serious staphylococcal infections. To prevent emergence of resistant strains of the infecting organisms, Rifadin should be used in combination with another antibiotic appropriate for the infection.

4.2 Posology and method of administration

Treatment with Rifadin for Infusion should include concomitant use of other appropriate antibacterials to prevent the emergence of resistant strains of the causative organism.

<u>Tuberculosis</u>:

Adults: A single daily administration of 600mg given by intravenous infusion over 2 to 3 hours has been found to be effective and well tolerated for adult patients. Serum concentrations following this dosage regimen are similar to those obtained after 600mg by mouth.

Children: The usual paediatric regimen is a single daily dose of up to 20mg/kg bodyweight; the total daily dose should not normally exceed 600mg.

<u>Leprosy</u>:

The recommended daily dose is 10 mg/kg.

Usual daily dose: Patients weighing less than 50 kg - 450 mg

Patients weighing 50 kg or more - 600 mg.

Alternatively, 600 mg doses of rifampicin may be given once per month.

In the treatment of leprosy, rifampicin should always be used in conjunction with at least one other antileprosy drug.

<u>Brucellosis, Legionnaires Disease or serious staphylococcal infections</u>:

Adults: The recommended daily dose is 600 - 1200mg given in 2 to 4 divided doses, together with another antibacterial agent with similar properties to prevent the emergence of resistant strains.

Impaired liver function:

A daily dose of 8mg/kg should not be exceeded in patients with impaired liver function.

Use in the elderly:

In elderly patients, the renal excretion of rifampicin is decreased proportionally with physiological decrease of renal function; due to compensatory increase of liver excretion, the serum terminal half-life is similar to that of younger patients. However, as increased blood levels have been noted in one study of rifampicin in elderly patients, caution should be exercised in using rifampicin in such patients, especially if there is evidence of liver function impairment.

When patients are able to accept oral medication, they should be transferred to Rifadin Capsules or Syrup (for further information on these products see their separate data sheets).

4.3 Contraindications

Rifadin for Infusion is contraindicated in patients who are hypersensitive to rifamycins.

Although not recommended for use in patients with jaundice, the therapeutic benefit of Rifadin for Infusion should be weighed against the possible risks.

4.4 Special warnings and special precautions for use

Rifampicin should be given under the supervision of a respiratory or other suitably qualified physician.

All tuberculosis patients should have pre-treatment measurements of liver function.

If the patient has no evidence of pre-existing liver disease and normal pre-treatment liver function, liver function tests need only be repeated if fever, vomiting, jaundice or other deterioration in the patient's condition occurs.

Patients with impaired liver function should only be given rifampicin in cases of necessity, and then with caution and under close medical supervision. In these patients, lower doses of rifampicin are recommended and careful monitoring of liver function, especially serum glutamic pyruvic transaminase (SGPT) and serum glutamic oxaloacetic transaminase (SGOT) should initially be carried out prior to therapy, weekly for two weeks, then every two weeks for the next six weeks. If signs of hepatocellular damage occur, rifampicin should be withdrawn.

Rifampicin should also be withdrawn if clinically significant changes in hepatic function occur. The need for other forms of antituberculosis therapy and a different regimen should be considered. Urgent advice should be obtained from a specialist in the management of tuberculosis. If rifampicin is re-introduced after liver function has returned to normal, liver function should be monitored daily.

In patients with impaired liver function, elderly patients, malnourished patients, and possibly, children under two years of age, caution is particularly recommended when instituting therapeutic regimens in which isoniazid is to be used concurrently with rifampicin.

In some patients hyperbilirubinemia can occur in the early days of treatment. This results from competition between rifampicin and bilirubin for hepatic excretion.

An isolated report showing a moderate rise in bilirubin and/or transaminase level is not in itself an indication for interrupting treatment; rather the decision should be made after repeating the tests, noting trends in the levels and considering them in conjunction with the patient's clinical condition.

Because of the possibility of immunological reaction (see 'undesirable effects') occurring with intermittent therapy (less than 2 to 3 times per week) patients should be closely monitored. Patients should be cautioned against interrupting treatment since these reactions may occur.

Rifampicin has enzyme-inducing properties including induction of delta amino levulinic acid synthetase. Isolated reports have associated porphyria exacerbation with rifampicin administration.

4.5 Interaction with other medicinal products and other forms of Interaction

Rifampicin has been shown in animals and man to have liver enzyme inducing properties and may reduce the activity of anticoagulants, corticosteroids, cyclosporin, digitalis preparations, oral contraceptives, oral hypoglycaemic agents, dapsone, phenytoin, quinidine, narcotics and analgesics. It may be necessary to adjust the dosage of these drugs if they are given concurrently with Rifadin, particularly when it is initiated or withdrawn.

Therapeutic levels of rifampicin have been shown to inhibit standard microbiological assays for serum folate and Vitamin B12. Thus alternative assay methods should be considered. Transient elevation of BSP and serum bilirubin have been reported. Therefore, these tests should be performed before the daily administration of Rifadin for Infusion.

4.6 Pregnancy and lactation

At very high doses in animals rifampicin has been shown to have teratogenic effects. There are no well controlled studies with rifampicin in pregnant women. Therefore, Rifadin for Infusion should be used in pregnant women or in women of child bearing potential only if the potential benefit justifies the potential risk to the foetus. When Rifadin is administered during the last few weeks of pregnancy it may cause post-natal haemorrhages in the mother and infant for which treatment with Vitamin K1 may be indicated.

Rifampicin is excreted in breast milk, patients receiving rifampicin should not breast feed unless in the physician's judgement the potential benefit to the patient outweighs the potential risk to the infant.

4.7 Effects on ability to drive and use machines

None known.

4.8 Undesirable effects

Rifadin for Infusion is generally well tolerated and accepted by patients, although hypersensitivity reactions have been described and occasionally patients have experienced fever, skin rashes and nausea/vomiting.

Occasional instances of phlebitis and pain at the infusion site have been reported.

Reactions occurring with either daily or intermittent dosage regimens include:

General hypersensitivity reactions involving the skin, exfoliative dermatitis, Lyells syndrome and pemphigoid reactions.

Cutaneous reactions which are mild and self-limiting may occur and do not appear to be hypersensitivity reactions. Typically they consist of flushing and itching with or without a rash.

Gastrointestinal reactions consist of anorexia, nausea, vomiting, abdominal discomfort, and diarrhoea. Pseudomembranous colitis has been reported with rifampicin therapy.

Hepatitis can be caused by rifampicin and liver function tests should be monitored (see 'Special Warnings and Special Precautions for Use').

Thrombocytopenia with or without purpura may occur, usually associated with intermittent therapy, but is reversible if drug is discontinued as soon as purpura occurs. Cerebral haemorrhage and fatalities have been reported when rifampicin administration has been continued or resumed after the appearance of purpura.

Eosinophilia, leucopenia, oedema, muscle weakness and myopathy have been reported to occur in a small percentage of patients treated with rifampicin.

Reactions usually occurring with intermittent dosage regimens and probably of immunological origin include:

- 'Flu Syndrome' consisting of episodes of fever, chills, headache, dizziness, and bone pain appearing most commonly during the 3rd to the 6th month of therapy. The frequency of the syndrome varies but may occur in up to 50 % of patients given once-weekly regimens with a dose of rifampicin of 25 mg/kg or more.
- Shortness of breath and wheezing.
- Decrease in blood pressure and shock.
- Acute haemolytic anaemia.
- Acute renal failure usually due to acute tubular necrosis or acute interstitial nephritis.

If serious complications arise, e.g. renal failure, thrombocytopenia or haemolytic anaemia, rifampicin should be stopped and never restarted.

Occasional disturbances of the menstrual cycle have been reported in women receiving long-term anti-tuberculosis therapy with regimens containing rifampicin.

Rifampicin may produce a reddish discolouration of the urine, sputum and tears. The patient should be forewarned of this. Soft contact lenses may be permanently stained.

4.9 Overdose

In cases of overdose with rifampicin, intensive supportive measures should be instituted and individual symptoms treated as they arise.

5. PHARMACOLOGICAL PROPERTIES

5.1 Pharmacodynamic properties

Rifampicin is an active bactericidal antituberculosis drug which is particularly active against the rapidly growing extracellular organisms and also has bactericidial activity intracellularly. Rifampicin has activity against slow and intermittently-growing *M. Tuberculosis*.

Rifampicin inhibits DNA-dependent RNA polymerase activity in susceptible cells. Specifically, it interacts with bacterial RNA polymerase but does not inhibit the mammalian enzyme. Cross-resistance to rifampicin has only been shown with other rifamycins.

5.2 Pharmacokinetic properties

In normal subjects the biological half-life of rifampicin in serum averages about 3 hours after a 600 mg dose and increases to 5.1 hours after a 900 mg dose. With repeated administration, the half-life decreases and reaches average values of approximately 2-3 hours. If does not differ in patients with renal failure and consequently, no dosage adjustment is required.

Rifampicin is rapidly eliminated in the bile and an enterohepatic circulation ensues. During this process, rifampicin undergoes progressive deacetylation, so that nearly all the drug in the bile is in this form in about 6 hours. This metabolite retains essentially complete antibacterial activity. Intestinal absorption is reduced by deacetylation and elimination is facilitated. Up to 30 % of a dose is excreted in the urine, with about half of this being unchanged drug.

Rifampicin is widely distributed throughout the body. It is present in effective concentrations in many organs and body fluids, including cerebrospinal fluid. Rifampicin is about 80 % protein bound. Most of the unbound fraction is not ionized and therefore is diffused freely in tissues.

5.3 Preclinical safety data

Not applicable

6. PHARMACEUTICAL PARTICULARS

6.1 List of excipients

Sodium sulfoxylate formaldehyde

Sodium hydroxide

Solvent

Polysorbate 81 (Tween 81)

Water for Injections.

6.2 Incompatibilities

Compatibilities: Rifadin for Infusion is compatible with the following infusion solutions for up to 6 hours: Mannitol 10% and 20%, Macrodex with Saline Solution, Macrodex with Glucose Solution, Rheomacrodex, Sodium Bicarbonate 1.4%, Laevulose 5% and 10%, Ringer Lactate, Ringer Acetate, Dextrose 5% and 10%, Saline Solution.

Incompatibilities: Rifadin for Infusion is incompatible with the following: Perfudex, Sodium Bicarbonate 5%, Sodium Lactate 0.167M, Ringer Acetate with Dextrose.

6.3 Shelf life

Unopened vial of lyophilisate: 48 months

Unopened ampoule of solvent: 60 months

Reconstituted Solution: 6 hours

6.4 Special precautions for storage

Store below 25°C.

6.5 Nature and contents of container

20ml clear neutral glass vial sealed with butyl rubber stopper and aluminium/plastic "flip-off" cap (colour coded blue) containing 600mg Rifampicin and 10ml clear glass ampoule containing solvent.

Pack size: combination of 1 vial of lyophilisate and 1 ampoule of solvent.

6.6 Instructions for use and handling

Not applicable.

Administrative Data

7. MARKETING AUTHORISATION HOLDER

Aventis Pharma Ltd

trading as Marion Merrell or Aventis Pharma

50 Kings Hill Avenue

Kings Hill

West Malling

ME19 4AH

UK

8. MARKETING AUTHORISATION NUMBER(S)

PL 04425/0051

9. DATE OF FIRST AUTHORISATION/RENEWAL OF THE AUTHORISATION

7th December 1982 / 9th April 2005

10. DATE OF REVISION OF THE TEXT

April 2005

Legal Category

POM

Rifater Tablets

(sanofi-aventis)

1. NAME OF THE MEDICINAL PRODUCT

Rifater ™ Tablets

2. QUALITATIVE AND QUANTITATIVE COMPOSITION

Rifampicin Ph Eur 120 mg

Isoniazid Ph Eur 50 mg

Pyrazinamide Ph Eur 300 mg

3. PHARMACEUTICAL FORM

Tablets

4. CLINICAL PARTICULARS

4.1 Therapeutic indications

Rifater is indicated in the treatment of pulmonary tuberculosis.

4.2 Posology and method of administration

Rifater is recommended in the initial intensive phase of the short-course treatment of pulmonary tuberculosis. During this phase, which lasts for 2 months, Rifater should be administered on a daily continuous basis. The concomitant administration of ethambutol or intramuscular streptomycin over the same period of time is advised.

Each Rifater tablet contains isoniazid (INH), pyrazinamide (Z) and rifampicin (RAMP) in such a ratio that the administration of 9-12mg/kg RAMP, 4-5mg/kg INH and

23-30mg/kg Z can be achieved by giving 3 tablets daily to patients weighing less than 40kg, 4 tablets to patients weighing 40-49kg, 5 tablets to patients weighing 50-64kg and 6 tablets to patients weighing 65kg or more.

Rifater should be given as a single dose and preferably on an empty stomach at least 30 minutes before a meal, or 2 hours after a meal to ensure rapid and complete absorption.

Once the initial intensive phase of treatment has been completed treatment can be continued with the combination rifampicin-isoniazid (Rifinah) always on a daily basis.

This regimen, if correctly applied, is 100% effective with very few, if any, relapses. The clinical evidence indicates that these occur generally in the first 6 months after stopping treatment with bacilli fully sensitive to the drugs employed, so that changes in the drugs to be utilised for further treatment are not required. The regimen has been found to be fully effective also in the presence of a bacillary population resistant to isoniazid, to streptomycin or to both drugs.

CHILDREN: The ratio of the three drugs in Rifater may not be appropriate in children (eg higher mg/kg doses of INH are usually given in children than in adults). Rifater can be used only in special cases, after careful consideration of the mg/kg dose of each component.

USE IN THE ELDERLY: Caution should be exercised in such patients, in view of the possible decrease of the excretory function of the kidney and of the liver.

4.3 Contraindications

Rifater is contra-indicated in patients who are hypersensitive to any one of the components of the combination. Rifater is contra-indicated in the presence of jaundice.

4.4 Special warnings and special precautions for use

The precautions for the use of Rifater are the same as those considered when a triple individual administration of rifampicin, isoniazid and pyrazinamide is required. Rifater should only be given under supervision. Each of these drugs has been associated with liver dysfunction.

Rifater should be given under the supervision of a respiratory or other suitably qualified physician.

All tuberculosis patients should have pre-treatment measurements of liver function.

Patients with impaired liver function should only be given Rifater in cases of necessity and then with caution and under strict medical supervision. In these patients, careful monitoring of liver function, especially serum glutamic pyruvic transaminase (SGPT) and serum glutamic oxaloacetic transaminase (SGOT) should be carried out prior to therapy and then every two to four weeks during therapy.

If signs of hepatocellular damage occur, Rifater should be withdrawn. The need for other forms of antituberculous therapy and a different regimen should be considered. Urgent advice should be obtained from a specialist in the management of tuberculosis. If rifampicin is reintroduced after liver function has been returned to normal, liver function should be monitored daily. Care should be exercised in the treatment of elderly or malnourished patients who may also require Vitamin B6 supplementation with the isoniazid therapy.

If the patient has no evidence of pre-existing liver disease and normal pretreatment liver function, liver function tests need only be repeated if fever, vomiting, jaundice or other deterioration in the patients' condition occurs.

In some cases hyperbilirubinaemia resulting from competition between rifampicin and bilirubin for excretory pathways of the liver at the cell level can occur in the early days of treatment. An isolated report showing a moderate rise in bilirubin and/or transaminase level is not in itself an indication for interrupting treatment; rather, the decision should be made after repeating the tests, noting trends in the levels and considering them in conjunction with the patient's clinical condition.

Rifater should be used with caution in patients with a history of gout. If hyperuricaemia accompanied by an acute gouty arthritis occurs, the patient should be transferred to a regimen not containing pyrazinamide (eg Rifinah 150 or 300).

The possibility of pyrazinamide having an adverse effect on blood clotting time or vascular integrity should be borne in mind in patients with haemoptysis.

Because of the possibility of immunological reaction (see 'Side-Effects') occurring with intermittent rifampicin therapy (less than 2 or 3 per week) patients should be closely monitored. Patients should be cautioned against interruption of dosage regimens since these reactions may occur.

4.5 Interaction with other medicinal products and other forms of Interaction

Rifater has liver enzyme-inducing properties and may reduce the activity of a number of drugs including antiarrhythmics (disopyramide, mexiletine, quinidine, tocainide), anticoagulants, anticonvulsants (e.g. phenytoin), antifungals (e.g. fluconazole, itraconazole, ketoconazole), antivirals, benzodiazepines (e.g. diazepam), beta-blockers, calcium channel blockers (diltiazem, nifedipine, verapamil), chloramphenicol, clarithromycin, dapsone, corticosteroids, cyclosporin, digitalis preparations, tricyclic antidepressants (e.g. amitriptyline, nortriptyline), oral contraceptives, oral hypoglycaemic agents, haloperidol, levothyroxine, analgesics, quinidine, tacrolimus and theophylline. It may be necessary to adjust the dosage of these drugs if they are given concurrently with Rifater.

Rifater may also reduce the plasma concentration of atovaquone.

Patients using oral contraceptives should be advised to change to non-hormonal methods of birth control during Rifater therapy. Also diabetes may become more difficult to control.

If p-aminosalicylic acid and rifampicin are both included in the treatment regimen, they should be given not less than eight hours apart to ensure satisfactory blood levels.

Therapeutic levels of rifampicin have been shown to inhibit standard microbiological assays for serum folate and Vitamin B12. Thus alternative assay methods should be considered. Transient elevation of BSP and serum bilirubin have been reported. Therefore, these tests should be performed before the morning dose of rifampicin.

Concomitant antacid administration may reduce the absorption of rifampicin.

The potential for hepatotoxicity is increased with anaesthetic.

Isoniazid may decrease the excretion of phenytoin and carbamazepine or may enhance its effects. Appropriate adjustment of the anticonvulsant dose should be made.

Pyrazinamide antagonizes the effects of probenecid and sulphinpyrazone.

4.6 Pregnancy and lactation

At very high doses in animals rifampicin has been shown to have teratogenic effects. There are no well controlled studies with Rifater in pregnant women. Therefore, Rifater should be used in pregnant women or in women of childbearing potential only if the potential benefit justifies the potential risk to the foetus. When administered during the last few weeks of pregnancy, Rifater may cause post-natal haemorrhages in the mother and infant, for which treatment with Vitamin K1 may be indicated.

Rifampicin and isoniazid are excreted in breast milk and infants should not be breast fed by a patient receiving Rifater unless in the physician's judgement the potential benefit to the patient outweighs the potential risk to the infant.

4.7 Effects on ability to drive and use machines

None stated.

4.8 Undesirable effects

Rifampicin: Reactions occurring with either daily or intermittent dosage regimens include:

General hypersensitivity reactions involving the skin, exfoliative dermatitis, Lyells syndrome and pemphigoid reactions.

CUTANEOUS REACTIONS which are mild and self-limiting may appear and do not appear to be hypersensitivity reactions. Typically they consist of flushing and itching with or without a rash.

GASTRO-INTESTINAL REACTIONS consist of anorexia, nausea, vomiting, abdominal discomfort, and diarrhoea. Pseudomembranous colitis has been reported with rifampicin therapy.

HEPATITIS can be caused by rifampicin and liver function tests should be monitored. (See 'Precautions').

THROMBOCYTOPENIA with or without purpura may occur, usually associated with intermittent therapy, but is reversible if drug is discontinued as soon as purpura occurs. Cerebral haemorrhage and fatalities have been reported when rifampicin administration has been continued or resumed after the appearance of purpura.

Eosinophilia, leucopenia, oedema, muscle weakness and myopathy have been reported to occur in a small percentage of patients treated with rifampicin.

Reactions usually occurring with intermittent dosage regimens and probably of immunological origin include:

- 'Flu Syndrome' consisting of episodes of fever, chills, headache, dizziness, and bone pain appearing most commonly during the 3rd to 6th month of therapy. The frequency of the syndrome varies but may occur in up to 50% of patients given once-weekly regimens with a dose of rifampicin of 25mg/kg or more.
- Shortness of breath and wheezing.
- Decrease in blood pressure and shock.
- Acute haemolytic anaemia.
- Acute renal failure usually due to acute tubular necrosis or to acute interstitial nephritis.

If serious complications arise, (renal failure, thrombocytopenia or haemolytic anaemia), Rifater should be stopped and never restarted.

Occasional disturbances of the menstrual cycle have been reported in women receiving long term anti-tuberculosis therapy with regimens containing rifampicin.

Rifampicin may produce a reddish discolouration of the urine, sputum and tears. The patient should be forewarned of this. Soft contact lenses may be permanently stained.

Isoniazid: Severe and sometimes fatal hepatitis may occur with isoniazid therapy. Hypersensitivity reactions including fever have been reported with isoniazid treatment. Polyneuritis associated with isoniazid, presenting as paraesthesia, muscle weakness, loss of tendon reflexes etc, is unlikely to occur with the recommended daily dose of Rifater. Various haematological disturbances have been identified during treatment with isoniazid, including eosinophilia, agranulocytosis, and anaemia. High doses of isoniazid can cause convulsions. The possibility that the frequency of seizures may be increased in patients with epilepsy should be borne in mind. Systemic lupus erythromatosus-like syndrome and pellagra have also been reported with isoniazid therapy.

Pyrazinamide: Adverse reactions, other than hepatic reactions, which have been attributed to pyrazinamide are active gout (pyrazinamide has been reported to reduce urate excretion), sideroblastic anaemia, arthralgia, anorexia, nausea and vomiting, dysuria, malaise, fever, urticaria and aggravation of peptic ulcer. The hepatic reaction is the most common adverse reaction and varies from a symptomless abnormality of hepatic cell function detected only through laboratory liver function tests, through a mild syndrome of fever, malaise and liver tenderness, to more serious reactions such as clinical jaundice and rare cases of acute yellow atrophy and death.

4.9 Overdose

In cases of overdosage with Rifater, gastric lavage should be instituted and individual symptoms treated as they arise. Parenteral pyridoxine (Vitamin B6) should be given. Symptoms are more likely to be related to isoniazid, including coma, respiratory distress, hyperglycaemia and metabolic ketoacidosis.

5. PHARMACOLOGICAL PROPERTIES

5.1 Pharmacodynamic properties

Rifampicin, isoniazid and pyrazinamide are all active bactericidal antituberculosis drugs. Rifampicin and isoniazid are particularly active against the rapidly growing extracellular organisms. Pyrazinamide is active against intracellular organisms, particularly in the acid pH environment of macrophages. Rifampicin and isoniazid also have bactericidal activity intracellularly. Rifampicin has activity against slow and intermittently-growing M tuberculosis. Thus, the three agents, rifampicin, isoniazid and pyrazinamide have activity against the three different bacterial populations.

Rifampicin inhibits DNA-dependent RNA polymerase activity in susceptible cells. Specifically, it interacts with bacterial RNA polymerase but does not inhibit the mammalian enzyme. Cross-resistance to rifampicin has only been shown after the development of resistance to other rifamycins.

5.2 Pharmacokinetic properties

Rifampicin

Rifampicin is readily absorbed from the stomach and the duodenum. Peak serum concentrations of the order of 10mcg/ml occur about 2-4 hours after a dose of 10mg/kg body weight on an empty stomach.

In normal subjects the biological half-life of rifampicin in serum averages about 3 hours after a 600mg dose and increases to 5.1 hours after 900mg dose. With repeated administration, the half-life decreases and reaches average values of approximately 2-3 hours. The half-life of rifampicin may be decreased when isoniazid is administered concurrently.

After absorption, rifampicin is rapidly eliminated in the bile and an enterohepatic circulation ensues. During this process, rifampicin undergoes progressive deacetylation, so that nearly all the drug in the bile is in this form in about 6 hours. This metabolite retains essentially complete antibacterial activity. Intestinal reabsorption is reduced by deacetylation and elimination is facilitated. Up to 30% of a dose is excreted in the urine with about half of this being unchanged drug. Absorption of rifampicin is reduced when the drug is ingested with food.

Rifampicin is widely distributed throughout the body. It is present in effective concentrations in many organs and body fluids, including cerebrospinal fluid. Rifampicin is about 80% protein bound. Most of the unbound fraction is not ionized and therefore is diffused freely in tissues.

Isoniazid

After oral administration, isoniazid produces peak blood levels within 1 to 2 hours, which decline to 50% or less within 6 hours. It diffuses readily into organs and excreta (saliva, sputum and faeces). The drug also passes through the placental barrier and into the milk in concentrations comparable to those in the plasma. From 50 to 70% of a dose of isoniazid is excreted in the urine in 24 hours.

Isoniazid is metabolised primarily by acetylation and dehydrazination. The rate of acetylation is genetically determined. Approximately 50% of Black and Europeans are 'slow inactivators', the majority of Asians are 'rapid inactivators'.

Pyridoxine deficiency (B_6) is sometimes observed in adults with high doses of isoniazid, probably due to its competition with pyridoxal phosphate of the enzyme apotryptophanase.

Pyrazinamide

Pyrazinamide is well absorbed from the gastrointestinal tract and rapidly distributed throughout the body, with peak plasma levels in 2 hours. It is hydrolyzed to pyrazinoic acid and then metabolised to 5-hydroxypyrazinoic acid.

Glomerular filtration is the primary route of excretion. It is bactericidal in acid pH, and has intracellular antibacterial activity against *M. tuberculosis*.

Pharmacokinetic studies in normal volunteers have shown that the three ingredients in Rifater have comparable bioavailability whether they are given together as individual dose forms or as Rifater.

5.3 Preclinical safety data
Not applicable.

6. PHARMACEUTICAL PARTICULARS

6.1 List of excipients
Polyvinylpyrrolidone
Sodium Carboxymethylcellulose
Sodium Lauryl Sulphate
Calcium Stearate
Sucrose
Acacia Gum
Talc
Light Magnesium Carbonate
Kaolin
Titanum Dioxide
Colloidal Silicon Dioxide
Aluminium Hydroxide Gel
Iron Oxide

6.2 Incompatibilities
None stated.

6.3 Shelf life
4 years from date of manufacture.

6.4 Special precautions for storage
Do not store above 25°C. Store in the original container.

6.5 Nature and contents of container
PDVC and PVC/PVDC aluminium foil blisters packed in cardboard cartons.

Pack size: 100 tablets.

6.6 Instructions for use and handling
Not applicable.

7. MARKETING AUTHORISATION HOLDER
Aventis Pharma Ltd
50 Kings Hill Avenue
Kings Hill
West Malling
Kent ME19 4AH
UK

8. MARKETING AUTHORISATION NUMBER(S)
PL 04425/0060

9. DATE OF FIRST AUTHORISATION/RENEWAL OF THE AUTHORISATION
27 April 1984/10 May 1995

10. DATE OF REVISION OF THE TEXT
July 2001

11. Legal Category
POM

Rifinah 150 and 300

(sanofi-aventis)

1. NAME OF THE MEDICINAL PRODUCT
Rifinah™ 150
Rifinah™ 300

2. QUALITATIVE AND QUANTITATIVE COMPOSITION
Rifinah 150: Rifampicin PhEur 150mg, Isoniazid PhEur 100mg

Rifinah 300: Rifampicin PhEur 300mg, Isoniazid PhEur 150mg

3. PHARMACEUTICAL FORM
Rifinah 150: Cyclamen, smooth, shiny, round, curved sugar coated tablet.

Rifinah 300: Orange, smooth, shiny capsule shaped sugar coated tablet.

4. CLINICAL PARTICULARS

4.1 Therapeutic indications
Rifinah is indicated in the treatment of all forms of tuberculosis, including fresh, advanced and chronic cases.

4.2 Posology and method of administration
For oral administration.

Another antituberculosis drug may be given concurrently with Rifinah until the susceptibility of the infecting organism to rifampicin and isoniazid has been confirmed.

Adults: Patients should be given the following single daily dose preferably on an empty stomach at least 30 minutes before a meal or 2 hours after a meal:

Rifinah 150: Patients weighing less than 50kg - 3 tablets.

Rifinah 300: Patients weighing 50kg or more - 2 tablets.

Use in the elderly: Caution should be exercised in such patients especially if there is evidence of liver impairment.

4.3 Contraindications
Rifinah is contraindicated in the presence of jaundice. Rifinah is contraindicated in patients who are hypersensitive to rifamycins or isoniazid.

4.4 Special warnings and special precautions for use
Rifinah is a combination of 2 drugs, each of which has been associated with liver dysfunction.

Rifampicin should be given under the supervision of a respiratory or other suitably qualified physician.

All tuberculosis patients should have pre-treatment measurements of liver function.

If the patient has no evidence of pre-existing liver disease and normal pre-treatment liver function, liver function tests need only be repeated if fever, vomiting, jaundice or other deterioration in the patient's condition occurs.

Patients with impaired liver function should only be given Rifampicin in cases of necessity, and then with caution and under close medical supervision. In these patients, lower doses of rifampicin are recommended and careful monitoring of liver function, especially serum glutamic pyruvic transaminase (SGPT) and serum glutamic oxaloacetic transaminase (SGOT) should initially be carried out prior to therapy, weekly for two weeks, then every two weeks for the next six weeks.

Rifampicin should also be withdrawn if clinically significant changes in hepatic function occur. The need for other forms of antituberculous therapy and a different regimen should be considered. Urgent advice should be obtained from a specialist in the management of tuberculosis. If rifampicin is re-introduced after liver function has returned to normal, liver function should be monitored daily.

In patients with impaired liver function, elderly patients, malnourished patients and possibly children under two years of age, caution is particularly recommended when instituting therapeutic regimens in which isoniazid is to be used concurrently with rifampicin.

In some patients hyperbilirubinaemia can occur in the early days of treatment. This results from competition between rifampicin and bilirubin for hepatic excretion. An isolated report showing a moderate rise in bilirubin and/or transaminase level is not in itself an indication for interrupting treatment; rather the decision should be made after repeating the tests, noting trends in the levels and considering them in conjunction with the patient's clinical condition.

Because of the possibility of immunological reaction (see "Undesirable Effects") occurring with intermittent therapy (less than 2 to 3 times per week) patients should be closely monitored. Patients should be cautioned against interruption of dosage regimens since these reactions may occur.

Rifampicin has enzyme-inducing properties including induction of delta amino levulinic acid synthetase. Isolated reports have associated porphyria exacerbation with rifampicin administration.

4.5 Interaction with other medicinal products and other forms of Interaction
Rifampicin has liver enzyme inducing properties and may reduce the activity of a number of drugs including anticoagulants, corticosteroids, cyclosporin, digitalis preparations, quinidine, oral contraceptives, oral hypoglycaemic agents, dapsone, narcotics and analgesics. It may be necessary to adjust the dosage of these drugs if they are given concurrently with Rifinah. Patients using oral contraceptives should be advised to change to non-hormonal methods of birth control during Rifinah therapy. Also, diabetes may become more difficult to control.

When rifampicin is taken with para-aminosalicylic acid (PAS), rifampicin levels in the serum may decrease. Therefore, the drugs should be taken at least eight hours apart. Therapeutic levels of rifampicin have been shown to inhibit standard microbiological assays for serum folate and Vitamin B12. Thus, alternative assay methods should be considered. Transient elevation of BSP and serum bilirubin have been reported. Therefore, these tests should be performed before the morning dose of rifampicin. Isoniazid may decrease the excretion of phenytoin or may enhance its effects. Appropriate adjustments of the anticonvulsant dose should be made.

4.6 Pregnancy and lactation
Rifampicin has been shown to be teratogenic in rodents when given in large doses. There are no well controlled studies with Rifinah in pregnant women. Therefore, Rifinah should be used in pregnant women or in women of child bearing potential only if the potential benefit justifies the potential risk to the foetus.

When administered during the last few weeks of pregnancy, rifampicin can cause post-natal haemorrhages in the mother and infant, for which treatment with Vitamin K1 may be indicated.

Rifampicin and isoniazid are excreted in breast milk and infants should not be breast fed by a patient receiving Rifinah unless in the physician's judgement the potential benefit to the patient outweighs the potential risk to the infant.

4.7 Effects on ability to drive and use machines
None stated.

4.8 Undesirable effects

Rifampicin

Reactions to rifampicin occurring with either daily or intermittent dosage regimens include:

General hypersensitivity reactions involving the skin, exfoliative dermatitis, Lyell's syndrome and pemphigoid reactions.

Cutaneous reactions which are mild and self-limiting may occur and do not appear to be hypersensitivity reactions. Typically they consist of flushing and itching with or without a rash. More serious hypersensitivity reactions occur but are uncommon.

Gastrointestinal reactions consist of anorexia, nausea, vomiting, abdominal discomfort, and diarrhoea. Pseudomembranous colitis has been reported with rifampicin therapy.

Hepatitis can be caused by rifampicin and liver function tests should be monitored (see "Special warnings and Special Precautions for Use").

Thrombocytopenia with or without purpura may occur, usually associated with intermittent therapy, but is reversible if drug is discontinued as soon as purpura occurs. Cerebral haemorrhage and fatalities have been reported when rifampicin administration has been continued or resumed after the appearance of purpura.

Eosinophilia, leucopenia, oedema, muscle weakness and myopathy have been reported to occur in a small percentage of patients treated with rifampicin.

Reactions usually occurring with intermittent dosage regimens and probably of immunological origin include:

- 'Flu Syndrome' consisting of episodes of fever, chills, headache, dizziness, and bone pain appearing most commonly during the 3rd to the 6th month of therapy. The frequency of the syndrome varies but may occur in up to 50 % of patients given once-weekly regimens with a dose of rifampicin of 25 mg/kg or more.
- Shortness of breath and wheezing.
- Decrease in blood pressure and shock.
- Acute haemolytic anaemia.
- Acute renal failure usually due to acute tubular necrosis or acute interstitial nephritis.

Agranulocytosis has been reported very rarely

If serious complications arise, e.g. renal failure, thrombocytopenia or haemolytic anaemia, rifampicin should be stopped and never restarted.

Occasional disturbances of the menstrual cycle have been reported in women receiving long-term antituberculosis therapy with regimens containing rifampicin.

Rifampicin may produce a reddish discolouration of the urine, sputum and tears. The patient should be forewarned of this. Soft contact lenses may be permanently stained.

Isoniazid

Severe and sometimes fatal hepatitis may occur with isoniazid therapy. Polyneuritis associated with isoniazid, presenting as paraesthesia, muscle weakness, loss of tendon reflexes etc, is unlikely to occur with the recommended daily dose of Rifinah. Various haematological disturbances have been identified during treatment with isoniazid, including eosinophilia, agranulocytosis, and anaemia. High doses of isoniazid can cause convulsions. The possibility that the frequency of seizures may be increased in patients with epilepsy should be borne in mind.

4.9 Overdose
In cases of overdosage with Rifinah, gastric lavage should be performed as soon as possible. Intensive supportive measures should be instituted and individual symptoms treated as they arise. Parenteral pyridoxine (Vitamin B_6) should be given. Symptoms are more likely to be related to isoniazid, including coma, respiratory distress, hyperglycaemia and metabolic ketoacidosis.

5. PHARMACOLOGICAL PROPERTIES

5.1 Pharmacodynamic properties
Rifampicin and isoniazid are active bactericidial antituberculosis drugs which are particularly active against the rapidly growing extracellular organisms and also have bactericidal activity intracellularly. Rifampicin has activity against slow- and intermittently-growing *M. Tuberculosis*.

Rifampicin inhibits DNA-dependent RNA polymerase activity in susceptible cells. Specifically, it interacts with bacterial RNA polymerase but does not inhibit the mammalian enzyme. Cross-resistance to rifampicin has only been shown with other rifamycins.

Isoniazid acts against actively growing tubercle bacilli.

5.2 Pharmacokinetic properties
Rifampicin

Rifampicin is readily absorbed from the stomach and the duodenum. Peak serum concentrations of the order of 10mcg/ml occur about 2-4 hours after a dose of 10mg/kg body weight on an empty stomach.

In normal subjects the biological half-life of rifampicin in serum averages about 3 hours after a 600mg dose and increases to 5.1 hours after a 900mg dose. With repeated administration, the half-life decreases and reaches average values of approximately 2-3 hours.

After absorption, rifampicin is rapidly eliminated in the bile and an enterohepatic circulation ensues. During this process, rifampicin undergoes progressive deacetylation, so that nearly all the drug in the bile is in this form in about 6 hours. This metabolite retains essentially complete antibacterial activity. Intestinal absorption is reduced by deacetylation and elimination is facilitated. Up to 30 % of a dose is excreted in the urine, with about half of this being unchanged drug. Absorption of rifampicin is reduced when the drug is ingested with food.

Rifampicin is widely distributed throughout the body. It is present in effective concentrations in many organs and body fluids, including cerebrospinal fluid. Rifampicin is about 80 % protein bound. Most of the unbound fraction is not ionized and therefore is diffused freely in tissues.

Isoniazid

After oral administration isoniazid produces peak blood levels within 1 to 2 hours which decline to 50% or less within 6 hours. It diffuses readily into all body fluids (cerebrospinal, pleural and ascitic fluids), tissues, organs and excreta (saliva, sputum and faeces). From 50 to 70% of a dose of isoniazid is excreted in the urine in 24 hours.

Isoniazid is metabolized primarily by acetylation and dehydration. The rate of acetylation is genetically determined.

Pharmacokinetic studies in normal volunteers have been shown that the two ingredients in Rifinah have comparable bioavailability whether they are given together as individual dose forms or as Rifinah.

5.3 Preclinical safety data
None stated.

6. PHARMACEUTICAL PARTICULARS

6.1 List of excipients
Sodium lauryl sulphate, calcium stearate, sodium carboxymethylcellulose, magnesium stearate, microcrystalline cellulose, acacia, gelatin, kaolin, magnesium carbonate - light, talc, titanium dioxide (E171), colloidal silicon dioxide, polyvinylpyrollidone K30, sucrose, carnauba wax, colophony, white beeswax, hard paraffin and erythrosine (E127) (Rifinah 150) or sunset yellow (E110) (Rifinah 300).

6.2 Incompatibilities
None stated.

6.3 Shelf life
48 months.

6.4 Special precautions for storage
Store below 25°C. If it proves necessary to open a blister pack, Rifinah should be dispensed in amber glass or plastic containers. Protect from moisture.

6.5 Nature and contents of container
Rifinah 150: Original packs of 84 tablets (4 weeks calendar packs).

Rifinah 300: Original packs of 56 tablets (4 weeks calendar packs).

6.6 Instructions for use and handling
None stated.

7. MARKETING AUTHORISATION HOLDER
Aventis Pharma Ltd
50 Kings Hill Avenue
Kings Hill
West Malling
Kent ME19 4AH

8. MARKETING AUTHORISATION NUMBER(S)
Rifinah 150: PL 04425/0041
Rifinah 300: PL 04425/0042

9. DATE OF FIRST AUTHORISATION/RENEWAL OF THE AUTHORISATION
19 April 1999

10. DATE OF REVISION OF THE TEXT
17 December 2003

11 LEGAL CLASSIFICATION
POM

Rilutek
(sanofi-aventis)

1. NAME OF THE MEDICINAL PRODUCT
RILUTEK 50 mg, film-coated tablets.

2. QUALITATIVE AND QUANTITATIVE COMPOSITION
Each film-coated tablet contains riluzole 50 mg

For excipients, see 6.1.

3. PHARMACEUTICAL FORM
Film-coated tablet

The tablets are capsule-shaped, white and engraved with "RPR 202" on one side.

4. CLINICAL PARTICULARS

4.1 Therapeutic indications
Riluzole is indicated to extend life or the time to mechanical ventilation for patients with amyotrophic lateral sclerosis (ALS).

Clinical trials have demonstrated that RILUTEK extends survival for patients with ALS (See 5.1 Pharmacodynamics properties). Survival was defined as patients who were alive, not intubated for mechanical ventilation and tracheotomy-free.

There is no evidence that riluzole exerts a therapeutic effect on motor function, lung function, fasciculations, muscle strength and motor symptoms. Riluzole has not been shown to be effective in the late stages of ALS.

Safety and efficacy of riluzole has only been studied in ALS. Therefore, riluzole should not be used in patients with any other form of motor neurone disease.

4.2 Posology and method of administration
Treatment with riluzole should only be initiated by specialist physicians with experience in the management of motor neurone diseases.

The recommended daily dose in adults or elderly is 100 mg (50 mg every 12 hours).

No significant increased benefit can be expected from higher daily doses.

Special populations:

Children: RILUTEK is not recommended for use in children, as the safety and effectiveness of riluzole in any neurodegenerative diseases occurring in children or adolescents have not been established (see 4.4. Special Warnings and Special Precautions for Use).

Patients with impaired renal function: RILUTEK is not recommended for use in patients with impaired renal function, as studies at repeated doses have not been conducted in this population (see 4.4. Special Warnings and Special Precautions for Use).

Elderly: Based on pharmacokinetic data, there are no special instructions for the use of RILUTEK in this population.

Patients with impaired hepatic function: (see 4.3. Contra-indications, 4.4. Special Warnings and Special Precautions for Use and 5.2. Pharmacokinetic properties).

4.3 Contraindications
Severe hypersensitivity to riluzole or any of excipients.

Hepatic disease or baseline transaminases greater than 3 times the upper limit of normal.

Patients who are pregnant or lactating.

4.4 Special warnings and special precautions for use
Liver impairment:

Riluzole should be prescribed with care in patients with a history of abnormal liver function, or in patients with slightly elevated serum transaminases (ALT/SGPT; AST/SGOT up to 3 times the upper limit of the normal range (ULN)), bilirubin and/or gamma-glutamyl transferase (GGT) levels. Baseline elevations of several liver function tests (especially elevated bilirubin) should preclude the use of riluzole (see 4.8. Undesirable Effects).

It is recommended that serum transaminases, including ALT, be measured before and during therapy with riluzole. ALT should be measured every month during the first 3 months of treatment, every 3 months during the remainder of the first year, and periodically thereafter. ALT levels should be measured more frequently in patients who develop elevated ALT levels.

Riluzole should be discontinued if the ALT levels increase to 5 times the ULN. There is no experience with dose reduction or rechallenge in patients who have developed an increase of ALT to 5 times ULN. Readministration of riluzole to patients in this situation cannot be recommended.

Neutropenia:

Patients should be warned to report any febrile illness to their physicians. The report of a febrile illness should prompt physicians to check white blood cell counts and to discontinue riluzole in case of neutropenia (see 4.8. Undesirable Effects).

Children:

The safety and effectiveness of riluzole in any neurodegenerative process occurring in children or adolescents have not been studied (see 4.2. Posology and Method of Administration).

Patients with impaired renal function:

Studies at repeated doses have not been conducted in this population (see 4.2. Posology and Method of Administration).

4.5 Interaction with other medicinal products and other forms of Interaction
There have been no clinical studies to evaluate the interactions of riluzole with other medicinal products.

In vitro studies using human liver microsomal preparations suggest that CYP 1A2 is the principal isozyme involved in the initial oxidative metabolism of riluzole. Inhibitors of CYP 1A2 (e.g. caffeine, diclofenac, diazepam, nicergoline, clomipramine, imipramine, fluvoxamine, phenacetin, theophylline, amitriptyline and quinolones) could potentially decrease the rate of riluzole elimination, while inducers of CYP 1A2 (e.g. cigarette smoke, charcoal-broiled food, rifampicin and omeprazole) could increase the rate of riluzole elimination.

4.6 Pregnancy and lactation
Pregnancy:

Riluzole must not be used in pregnant women. In the pregnant rat, the transfer of ^{14}C- riluzole across the placenta to the foetus has been detected. In rats, riluzole decreased the pregnancy rate and the number of implantations at exposure levels at least twice the systemic exposure of humans given clinical therapy. No malformations were seen in animal reproductive studies.

Clinical experience with riluzole in pregnant women is lacking.

Lactation:

Riluzole must not be used in lactating women. In lactating rats, ^{14}C -riluzole was detected in milk. It is not known whether riluzole is excreted in human milk.

4.7 Effects on ability to drive and use machines
Patients should be warned about the potential for dizziness or vertigo, and advised not to drive or operate machinery if these symptoms occur.

4.8 Undesirable effects
Anaphylactoid reaction, angioedema and pancreatitis have been reported very rarely. In phase III studies conducted in Europe and North America, the most frequent side-effects related to riluzole were asthenia, nausea and elevations in liver function tests. Elevations of alanine-aminotransferase (ALT) levels to more than 3 times the ULN were observed in about 11 % of the patients treated with riluzole compared to 4.2 % in the placebo group; levels increased to more than 5 times the ULN in 3.8% of the patients treated with riluzole compared to 1.7 % of the placebo treated patients. The increases in ALT usually appeared within 3 months after the start of therapy with riluzole; they were usually transient and levels returned to below twice the ULN after 2 to 6 months while treatment was continued. These increases were rarely associated with jaundice. In patients with increases in ALT to more than 5 times the ULN, treatment was discontinued and the levels returned to less than 2 times the ULN within 2 to 4 months (see 4.4. Special Warnings and Special Precautions for Use).

The listing that follows describes all the adverse events that occurred at a frequency of 1% or more among ALS patients receiving riluzole 100 mg/day and were greater than placebo by 1%, or were serious adverse events with frequency greater than placebo.

Adverse Events Occurring in Placebo-Controlled Clinical Trials
Percentage of patients reporting events*

Adverse Event*	Riluzole 100 mg/day (N=395)	Placebo (N=406)
Asthenia	17.5	11.3
Nausea	14.2	9.1
Headache	6.8	5.7
Abdominal pain	5.1	3.7
Pain	4.8	2.0
Vomiting	3.8	1.5
Dizziness	3.3	2.2
Tachycardia	3.0	1.5
Somnolence	2.0	1.0
Circumoral paraesthesia	1.3	0.0

* Where riluzole incidence is greater than placebo by 1%.

Among approximately 5000 patients given riluzole for ALS, there were three cases of marked neutropenia (absolute neutrophil count less than 500/mm^3), all seen within the first 2 months of riluzole treatment. In one case, neutrophil counts rose on continued treatment. In a second case, counts rose after therapy was stopped. A third case was associated with marked anaemia (see 4.4. Special Warnings and Special Precautions for Use).

4.9 Overdose
There has been one significant case of overdose reported with riluzole. In an apparent suicide attempt, a patient ingested up to 30 times the recommended 100 mg daily dose. The patient developed methaemoglobinaemia that abated quickly after an infusion of methylene blue.

In case of overdose, treatment is symptomatic and supportive.

5. PHARMACOLOGICAL PROPERTIES

5.1 Pharmacodynamic properties
Pharmacotherapeutic group: other nervous system drugs, ATC code N07XX02.

Although the pathogenesis of ALS is not completely elucidated, it is suggested that glutamate (the primary excitatory neurotransmitter in the central nervous system) plays a role for cell death in the disease.

Riluzole is proposed to act by inhibiting glutamate processes. The mode of action is unclear.

Clinical trials:

In a trial, 155 patients were randomised to riluzole 100 mg/day (50 mg twice daily) or placebo and were followed-up for 12 to 21 months. Survival, as defined in the second paragraph of section 4.1., was significantly extended for patients who received riluzole as compared to patients who received placebo. The median survival time was

17.7 months versus 14.9 months for riluzole and placebo, respectively.

In a dose-ranging trial, 959 patients with ALS were randomised to one of four treatment groups: riluzole 50, 100, 200 mg/day, or placebo and were followed-up for 18 months. In patients treated with riluzole 100 mg/day, survival was significantly higher compared to patients who received placebo. The effect of riluzole 50 mg/day was not statistically significant compared to placebo and the effect of 200 mg/day was essentially comparable to that of 100 mg/day. The median survival time approached 16.5 months versus 13.5 months for riluzole 100 mg/day and placebo, respectively.

In a parallel group study designed to assess the efficacy and safety of riluzole in patients at a late stage of the disease, survival time and motor function under riluzole did not differ significantly from that of placebo. In this study the majority of patients had a vital capacity less than 60%.

In a double-blind placebo-controlled trial designed to assess the efficacy and safety of riluzole in Japanese patients, 204 patients were randomised to riluzole 100 mg/day (50 mg twice daily) or placebo and were followed-up for 18 months. In this study, the efficacy was assessed on inability to walk alone, loss of upper limb function, tracheostomy, need for artificial ventilation, gastric tube feeding or death. Tracheostomy-free survival in patients treated with riluzole did not differ significantly from placebo. However, the power of this study to detect differences between treatment groups was low. Meta-analysis including this study and those described above showed a less striking effect on survival for riluzole as compared to placebo although the differences remained statistically significant.

5.2 Pharmacokinetic properties

The pharmacokinetics of riluzole have been evaluated in healthy male volunteers after single oral administration of 25 to 300 mg and after multiple-dose oral administration of 25 to 100 mg bid. Plasma levels increase linearly with the dose and the pharmacokinetic profile is dose-independent.

With multiple dose administration (10 day-treatment at 50 mg riluzole bid), unchanged riluzole accumulates in plasma by about 2 fold and steady-state is reached in less than 5 days.

Absorption:

Riluzole is rapidly absorbed after oral administration with maximal plasma concentrations occurring within 60 to 90 minutes (C_{max} = 173 ± 72 (sd) ng/ml). About 90% of the dose is absorbed and the absolute bioavailability is 60 ± 18%.

The rate and extent of absorption is reduced when riluzole is administered with high-fat meals (decrease in C_{max} of 44%, decrease in AUC of 17%).

Distribution:

Riluzole is extensively distributed throughout the body and has been shown to cross the blood brain barrier. The volume of distribution of riluzole is about 245 ± 69 l (3.4 l/kg). Riluzole is about 97% protein bound and it binds mainly to serum albumin and to lipoproteins.

Metabolism:

Unchanged riluzole is the main component in plasma and is extensively metabolised by cytochrome P450 and subsequent glucuronidation. In vitro studies using human liver preparations demonstrated that cytochrome P450 1A2 is the principal isoenzyme involved in the metabolism of riluzole. The metabolites identified in urine are three phenolic derivatives, one ureido-derivative and unchanged riluzole.

The primary metabolic pathway for riluzole is initial oxidation by cytochrome P450 1A2 producing N-hydroxy-riluzole (RPR112512), the major active metabolite of riluzole. This metabolite is rapidly glucuronoconjugated to O- and N-glucuronides.

Elimination:

The elimination half-life ranges from 9 to 15 hours. Riluzole is eliminated mainly in the urine.

The overall urinary excretion accounts for about 90% of the dose. Glucuronides accounted for more than 85% of the metabolites in the urine. Only 2% of a riluzole dose was recovered unchanged in the urine.

Special populations

Patients with impaired renal function: There is no significant difference in pharmacokinetic parameters between patients with moderate or severe chronic renal insufficiency (creatinine clearance between 10 and 50 $ml.min^{-1}$) and healthy volunteers after a single oral dose of 50 mg riluzole.

Elderly: The pharmacokinetic parameters of riluzole after multiple dose administration (4.5 days of treatment at 50 mg riluzole bid) are not affected in the elderly > 70 years).

Patients with impaired hepatic function: The AUC of riluzole after a single oral dose of 50 mg increases by about 1.7 fold in patients with mild chronic liver insufficiency and by about 3 fold in patients with moderate chronic liver insufficiency.

5.3 Preclinical safety data

Riluzole did not show any carcinogenicity potential in either rats or mice.

Standard tests for genotoxicity performed with riluzole were negative. Tests on the major active metabolite of riluzole gave positive results in two in vitro tests. Intensive testing in seven other standard *in vitro* or *in vivo* assays did not show any genotoxic potential of the metabolite. On the basis of these data, and taking into consideration the negative studies on the carcinogenesis of riluzole in the mouse and rat, the genotoxic effect of this metabolite is not considered to be of relevance in humans.

Reductions in red blood cell parameters and/or alterations in liver parameters were noted inconsistently in subacute and chronic toxicity studies in rats and monkeys. In dogs, haemolytic anaemia was observed.

In a single toxicity study, the absence of corpora lutea was noted at a higher incidence in the ovary of treated compared to control female rats. This isolated finding was not noted in any other study or species.

All these findings were noted at doses which were 2-10 times higher than the human dose of 100 mg/day.

Fertility studies in rats revealed slight impairment of reproductive performance and fertility at doses of 15 mg/kg/day (which is higher than the therapeutic dose), probably due to sedation and lethargy.

6. PHARMACEUTICAL PARTICULARS

6.1 List of excipients

Core:

Dibasic calcium phosphate, anhydrous

Micro crystalline cellulose

Colloidal silica, anhydrous

Magnesium stearate

Croscarmellose sodium

Coating:

Hypromellose

Macrogol 6000

Titanium dioxide (E171)

6.2 Incompatibilities

Not applicable.

6.3 Shelf life

3 years

6.4 Special precautions for storage

No special precautions for storage.

6.5 Nature and contents of container

Tablets are packaged in opaque pvc/aluminium blister cards.

Each package contains 56 tablets (4 blister cards of 14 tablets each).

6.6 Instructions for use and handling

Not applicable.

7. MARKETING AUTHORISATION HOLDER

Aventis Pharma S.A.

20 avenue Raymond Aron

F-92165 Antony Cedex

France

8. MARKETING AUTHORISATION NUMBER(S)

EU/1/96/010/001

9. DATE OF FIRST AUTHORISATION/RENEWAL OF THE AUTHORISATION

10.06.1996/ 11.07.2001

10. DATE OF REVISION OF THE TEXT

May 2004

Legal category: POM

Rinatec Nasal Spray 0.03%

(Boehringer Ingelheim Limited)

1. NAME OF THE MEDICINAL PRODUCT

RINATEC Nasal Spray 0.03%

2. QUALITATIVE AND QUANTITATIVE COMPOSITION

RINATEC Nasal Spray 0.03% is an aqueous formulation (adjusted to pH 4.0 - 5.0) available as a 15 ml (180 metered doses) and 30 ml (380 metered doses) pump spray. Each valve actuation delivers 70 μl of solution containing 21 micrograms of ipratropium bromide.

3. PHARMACEUTICAL FORM

Nasal Spray, solution

4. CLINICAL PARTICULARS

4.1 Therapeutic indications

RINATEC Nasal Spray 0.03% is indicated for the symptomatic relief of rhinorrhoea in allergic and non-allergic rhinitis.

4.2 Posology and method of administration

Adults: Two sprays (42 μg) in each nostril administered 2 - 3 times a day.

Children: The use of RINATEC Nasal Spray 0.03% has not been evaluated in children, and therefore is not recommended for use in patients below the age of 12 years.

Administration

To obtain the best results from your nasal spray follow the simple instructions given below. If you are unclear about how to use the nasal spray ask your doctor or pharmacist to explain.

1. Remove the dust cap.

2. The nasal spray pump must be primed before RINATEC Nasal Spray is used for the first time. To prime the pump, hold the bottle with your thumb at the base and your index and middle fingers on the white shoulder area. Make sure the bottle points upright and away from your eyes. Press your thumb firmly and quickly against the bottle seven times. The pump is now primed and can be used. Your pump will hold its prime for up to 24 hours. If you have not used your pump for more than 24 hours, you will need to prime it again before use. Reprime the pump as before, but this time only two sprays are required. If you have not used your pump for more than 7 days reprime using 7 sprays.

3. Blow your nose to clear your nostrils if necessary.

4. Close one nostril by gently placing your fingers against the side of your nose. Tilt your head slightly forward and, keeping the bottle upright, insert the nasal tip into the other nostril. Point the tip toward the back and outer side of the nose.

Press firmly and quickly upwards with the thumb at the base while holding the white shoulder portion of the pump between your index and middle fingers. Following each spray, sniff deeply and breathe out through your mouth.

After spraying the nostril and removing the unit, tilt your head backwards for a few seconds to let the spray spread over the back of the nose.

5. Repeat step 4 in the other nostril.

6. Replace the cap.

Avoid spraying RINATEC Nasal Spray in or around your eye. Should this occur, immediately flush your eye with cold tap water for several minutes. If you accidently spray RINATEC Nasal Spray in your eyes, you may experience a temporary blurring of vision and increased sensitivity to light, which may last a few hours. Follow your doctor's instructions about when and how to take your medicine and always read the label.

If the nasal tip becomes clogged, remove the clear plastic dust cap. Hold the nasal tip under warm running water for about a minute. Dry the nasal tip, reprime the nasal spray pump and replace the plastic dust cap.

4.3 Contraindications

RINATEC Nasal Spray 0.03% is contraindicated in patients known to be hypersensitive to atropine or its derivatives or to any other component of the product.

4.4 Special warnings and special precautions for use

Caution is advocated in the use of anticholinergic agents in patients with narrow-angle glaucoma, or with prostatic hyperplasia or bladder-outflow obstruction.

As patients with cystic fibrosis may be prone to gastro-intestinal motility disturbances, RINATEC, as with other anticholinergics, should be used with caution in these patients.

Immediate hypersensitivity reactions following the use of RINATEC have been demonstrated by rare cases of urticaria, angioedema, rash, bronchospasm, oropharyngeal oedema and anaphylaxis.

There have been isolated reports of ocular complications (i.e. mydriasis, increased intraocular pressure, narrow-angle glaucoma, eye pain) when aerosolised ipratropium bromide, either alone or in combination with an adrenergic $beta_2$-agonist, has come into contact with the eyes. Thus, patients must be instructed in the correct administration of RINATEC Nasal Spray 0.03%.

Eye pain or discomfort, blurred vision, visual halos or coloured images in association with red eyes from conjunctival congestion and corneal oedema may be signs of acute narrow-angle glaucoma. Should any combination of these symptoms develop, treatment with miotic drops should be initiated and specialist advice sought immediately.

4.5 Interaction with other medicinal products and other forms of Interaction

The concomitant use of RINATEC Nasal Spray 0.03% with other drugs commonly prescribed for perennial rhinitis i.e. antihistamines, decongestants or nasal steroids does not increase the incidence of nasal or non-nasal side-effects.

Ipratropium bromide is minimally absorbed into the systemic circulation; nonetheless, there is some potential for additive interaction with other concomitantly administered anticholinergic medications, including ipratropium bromide-containing aerosols for oral inhalation.

4.6 Pregnancy and lactation

The safety of RINATEC during human pregnancy has not been established. The benefits of using RINATEC during a confirmed or suspected pregnancy must be weighed against the possible hazards to the unborn child. Preclinical studies have shown no embryotoxic or teratogenic effects following inhalation or intranasal application at doses considerably higher than those recommended in man.

It is not known whether ipratropium bromide is excreted into breast milk. It is unlikely that ipratropium bromide would reach the infant to an important extent, however caution should be exercised when RINATEC Nasal Spray 0.03% is administered to nursing mothers.

4.7 Effects on ability to drive and use machines
None known.

4.8 Undesirable effects
The most frequent local undesirable effects reported are nasal reactions including epistaxis, dryness of the nose and nasal irritation. These effects may necessitate reduced frequency of administration. Pharyngitis and sinusitis may also occur.

Headache and nausea may occur as nonspecific reactions in association with use of RINATEC Nasal Spray. Potential systemic anticholinergic effects are dry mouth and dry throat. Ocular side effects (see Special Warnings and Special Precautions for Use), increase of heart rate and palpitations, urinary retention and gastrointestinal motility disturbances have been reported in isolated patients in association with use of ipratropium bromide either intranasally or after oral inhalation.

Allergic-type reactions such as skin rash, angioedema of tongue, lips and face, urticaria, laryngospasm and anaphylactic reactions may occur.

After oral inhalation of ipratropium bromide in patients suffering from COPD/Asthma supraventricular tachycardia and atrial fibrillation have been reported.

4.9 Overdose
No symptoms specific to overdosage have been encountered. In view of the wide therapeutic window and topical administration of RINATEC, no serious anticholinergic symptoms are to be expected. As with other anticholinergics, dry mouth, visual accommodation disturbances and tachycardia would be the expected symptoms and signs of overdose.

5. PHARMACOLOGICAL PROPERTIES

5.1 Pharmacodynamic properties
Ipratropium bromide, a quaternary ammonium derivative of atropine is an anticholinergic drug. Ipratropium bromide administered intranasally has a localised parasympathetic blocking action, which reduces watery hypersecretion from mucosal glands in the nose.

5.2 Pharmacokinetic properties
Ipratropium bromide is a quaternary amine that is rapidly absorbed from the nasal mucosa, however to a low extent. In normal volunteers, in patients with experimentally induced cold or in perennial rhinitis patients, approximately 10% of a nasally given dose (single or multiple administration) is absorbed, as estimated from the renal excretion of ipratropium bromide over 24 hours.

Kinetic parameters describing the distribution of ipratropium bromide were calculated from plasma concentrations after i.v. administration.

A rapid biphasic decline in plasma concentrations is observed. The volume of distribution (V_β) is 338 L (≙ 4.6 L/kg). The drug is minimally (less then 20%) bound to plasma proteins. The ipratropium ion does not cross the blood-brain barrier, consistent with the ammonium structure of the molecule.

The half-life of the terminal elimination phase is about 1.6 hours.

The mean total clearance of the drug is determined to be 2.3 L/min. The major portion of approximately 60% of the systemic available dose is eliminated by metabolic degradation, probably in the liver. The main urinary metabolites bind poorly to the muscarinic receptor and have to be regarded as ineffective.

A portion of approximately 40% of the systemic available dose is cleared via urinary excretion corresponding to an experimental renal clearance of 0.9 L/min. A study with radiolabelled material showed that approximately 10% of orally administered ipratropium bromide was absorbed from the gastro-intestinal tract and metabolised. Less than 1% of an oral dose is renally excreted as parent compound.

In excretion balance studies after intravenous administration of a radioactive dose, less than 10% of the drug-related radioactivity (including parent compound and all metabolites) is excreted via the biliary-faecal route. The dominant excretion of drug-related radioactivity occurs via the kidneys.

5.3 Preclinical safety data
The toxicity of ipratropium bromide has been investigated extensively in the following types of studies: acute, sub-chronic and chronic toxicity, carcinogenicity, reproductive toxicity and mutagenicity via oral, intravenous, subcutaneous, intranasal and/or inhalation routes. Based on these toxicity studies, the probability of systemic anticholinergic side effects decreases in the following order:

intravenous > subcutaneous > oral > inhalation > intranasal.

Pre-clinically, ipratropium bromide was found to be well-tolerated. Two-year carcinogenicity studies in rats and mice have revealed no carcinogenic activity at doses up to approximately 1,200 times the maximum recommended human daily dose for RINATEC Nasal Spray 0.03%. Results of various mutagenicity tests were negative.

6. PHARMACEUTICAL PARTICULARS

6.1 List of excipients
Sodium chloride
Benzalkonium chloride
Disodium edetate
Purified water
Hydrochloric acid and sodium hydroxide are used for pH adjustment.

6.2 Incompatibilities
None known

6.3 Shelf life
2 years
In-use: 6 months

6.4 Special precautions for storage
Do not store above 25°C.

6.5 Nature and contents of container
RINATEC Nasal Spray 0.03% is a clear colourless aqueous solution adjusted to the optimum pH 4.0-5.0. The solution is filled into either 15 ml or 30 ml amber glass bottles (Type I glass) fitted with 70μL manually activated nasal pump/closures.

6.6 Instructions for use and handling
None stated.

7. MARKETING AUTHORISATION HOLDER
Boehringer Ingelheim Limited
Ellesfield Avenue
Bracknell
Berkshire
RG12 8YS

8. MARKETING AUTHORISATION NUMBER(S)
PL 00015/0196

9. DATE OF FIRST AUTHORISATION/RENEWAL OF THE AUTHORISATION
20 March 1996

10. DATE OF REVISION OF THE TEXT
June 2004

11. Legal Category
POM
R3a/UK/SPC/9

Risperdal Consta 25 mg, 37.5 mg, 50 mg.

(Janssen-Cilag Ltd)

1. NAME OF THE MEDICINAL PRODUCT
Risperdal® Consta™▼ 25 mg, 37.5 mg, 50 mg.

2. QUALITATIVE AND QUANTITATIVE COMPOSITION
Each vial contains 25 mg, 37.5 mg or 50 mg risperidone.
For excipients see 6.1.

3. PHARMACEUTICAL FORM
Prolonged-release powder and solvent for suspension for injection, for intramuscular use.

Consisting of

Vial with powder: White to off-white free-flowing powder.

Pre-filled syringe of solvent: Clear, colourless aqueous solution.

4. CLINICAL PARTICULARS

4.1 Therapeutic indications
Risperdal Consta is indicated for the treatment of schizophrenic psychoses and other psychotic conditions, in which positive symptoms (such as hallucinations, delusions, thought disturbances, hostility, suspiciousness), and/or negative symptoms (such as blunted affect, emotional and social withdrawal, poverty of speech) are prominent. Risperdal Consta also alleviates affective symptoms (such as depression, guilt feelings, anxiety) associated with schizophrenia.

Risperdal Consta is also effective in maintaining the clinical improvement during continuation therapy in patients who have shown an initial treatment response to oral risperidone or another antipsychotic drug.

Risperdal Consta is not licensed for the treatment of behavioural symptoms of dementia (see section 4.4).

4.2 Posology and method of administration
Risperdal Consta should be administered every two weeks by deep intramuscular gluteal injection using the enclosed safety needle. Injections should alternate between the buttocks. Do not administer intravenously.

For instructions for use see 6.6.

Adults

As with all anti-psychotic medications it is good clinical practice to maintain patients on the lowest effective dose which in the case of Risperdal Consta is 25 mg (intramuscular injection) every two weeks. The maximum dose should not exceed 50 mg every two weeks.

Where patients are not stabilised on oral risperidone the recommended dose is 25 mg Risperdal Consta every two weeks. Should a dosage adjustment be required, see paragraph 4 for guidance on dose increments. Patients with no previous history of risperidone use should be pre-treated with oral Risperdal for several days as clinically feasible, to assess tolerability before the first injection.

For those patients stabilised on a fixed dose of oral risperidone for two weeks or more, the following conversion scheme should be considered. Patients treated with a dosage of 4 mg or less oral risperidone should receive 25 mg Risperdal Consta, patients treated with higher oral doses should be considered for the higher Risperdal Consta dose of 37.5 mg.

Dose increments from 25 mg to 37.5 mg or from 37.5 mg to 50 mg should be considered after a minimum of four weeks after the previous dose adjustment.

The effect of this dosage adjustment on the patient's clinical status should not be anticipated earlier than 3 weeks after the first injection with the higher dose.

Supplementation with oral risperidone, where appropriate, with the previously used dose, should be provided during the first three weeks after the first injection with Risperdal Consta to ensure coverage until the main release phase of risperidone from the injection site has begun.

After the first three weeks of Risperdal Consta treatment, oral risperidone should be discontinued. However, if clinically appropriate, oral risperidone up to 4 mg/day can be temporarily added to the treatment with Risperdal Consta while establishing an individual patient's optimal dose. The clinical value of adding oral risperidone should be routinely reassessed and, if there is continuing need for oral supplementation, consideration should be given to increasing the dose of Risperdal Consta.

Elderly (>65 years)

The only recommended dose for this age group is 25 mg intramuscularly every two weeks. Sufficient oral risperidone cover should be ensured for at least three weeks during the lag period following the first Risperdal Consta injection (see also 5.2. for pharmacokinetic properties).

Children and adolescents

Risperdal Consta has not been studied in children and adolescents younger than 18 years.

Hepatic and renal impairment

Risperdal Consta has not been studied in hepatically and renally impaired patients, and should therefore be used with caution. If hepatically or renally impaired patients require treatment with Risperdal Consta, a starting dose of 0.5 mg b.i.d. oral risperidone is recommended during the first week. In the second week 1 mg b.i.d. or 2 mg o.d. can be given. If an oral dose of at least 2 mg daily is well tolerated, an injection of 25 mg Risperdal Consta can be administered every 2 weeks.

4.3 Contraindications
Risperdal Consta is contraindicated in patients with a known hypersensitivity to the product or the diluent (see 6.1 List of excipients).

4.4 Special warnings and special precautions for use
Risperdal Consta is not recommended for the treatment of behavioural symptoms of dementia because of an increased risk of cerebrovascular adverse events (including cerebrovascular accidents and transient ischaemic attacks).

Data from randomised clinical trials conducted in elderly >65 years) patients with dementia indicate that there is an approximately 3-fold increased risk of cerebrovascular adverse events (including cerebrovascular accidents and transient ischaemic attacks) with oral risperidone, compared with placebo. Cerebrovascular adverse events occurred in 3.3% (33/989) of patients treated with risperidone and 1.2% (8/693) of patients treated with placebo. The Odds Ratio (95% exact confidence interval) was 2.96 (1.33, 7.45).

Physicians should consider carefully the risk of cerebrovascular adverse events with Risperdal (given the observations in elderly patients with dementia detailed above) before treating any patient with a previous history of CVA/TIA. Consideration should also be given to other risk factors for cerebrovascular disease including hypertension, diabetes, current smoking, atrial fibrillation, etc.

In all patients, the tolerability to oral Risperdal should have been established prior to initiation of treatment with Risperdal Consta.

Due to the alpha-blocking activity of risperidone, orthostatic hypotension can occur, especially during initiation of treatment. The risk benefit of further treatment with Risperdal Consta should be assessed if clinically relevant hypotension persists.

Risperidone should be used with caution in patients with known cardiovascular disease including those associated with prolongation of the QT interval. In clinical trials, risperidone was not associated with an increase in QTc intervals. As with other antipsychotics, caution is advised when prescribing with medications known to prolong the QT interval.

If further sedation is required, an additional drug (such as a benzodiazepine) should be administered rather than increasing the dose of Risperdal Consta.

Drugs with dopamine receptor antagonistic properties have been associated with the induction of tardive dyskinesia, characterised by rhythmical involuntary movements, predominantly of the tongue and/or face. It has been reported that the occurrence of extrapyramidal symptoms is a risk factor for the development of tardive dyskinesia. However, in patients treated with oral Risperdal for a minimum of 1 year, the overall severity of extrapyramidal symptoms, as well as the occurrence of new onset tardive dyskinesia was reduced compared with patients treated with classic neuroleptics. If signs and symptoms of tardive dyskinesia appear, the discontinuation of all antipsychotic drugs should be considered.

Neuroleptic malignant syndrome, characterised by hyperthermia, muscle rigidity, autonomic instability, altered consciousness and elevated CPK levels, has been reported to occur with neuroleptics. In this event all antipsychotic drugs including risperidone should be discontinued.

Caution should also be exercised when prescribing risperidone to patients with Parkinson's disease since, theoretically, it may cause a deterioration of the disease.

Hyperglycaemia or exacerbation of pre-existing diabetes has been reported in very rare cases during treatment with Risperdal. Appropriate clinical monitoring is advisable in diabetic patients and in patients with risk factors for the development of diabetes mellitus (see also section 4.8 Undesirable effects).

Classical neuroleptics are known to lower the seizure threshold. Caution is recommended when treating patients with epilepsy.

As with other antipsychotics, patients should be advised of the potential for weight gain.

Acute withdrawal symptoms, including nausea, vomiting, sweating, and insomnia have very rarely been described after abrupt cessation of high doses of antipsychotic drugs. Recurrence of psychotic symptoms may also occur, and the emergence of involuntary movement disorders (such as akathisia, dystonia and dyskinesia) has been reported. Therefore gradual withdrawal is advisable.

Risperdal Consta has not been studied in children and adolescents younger than 18 years of age.

4.5 Interaction with other medicinal products and other forms of Interaction

Possible interactions of risperidone with other drugs have not been systematically evaluated. Given the primary CNS effects of risperidone it should be used with caution in combination with other centrally acting drugs, including alcohol.

Risperidone may antagonise the effect of levodopa and other dopamine agonists.

Carbamazepine has been shown to decrease the plasma levels of the antipsychotic fraction of risperidone. A similar effect might be anticipated with other drugs which stimulate metabolising enzymes in the liver. On initiation of carbamazepine or other hepatic enzyme-inducing drugs, the dosage of risperidone should be re-evaluated and increased if necessary. Conversely, on discontinuation of such drugs, the dosage of risperidone should be re-evaluated and decreased if necessary.

Phenothiazines, tricyclic antidepressants and some beta-blockers may increase the plasma concentrations of risperidone but not those of the active antipsychotic fraction. Fluoxetine and paroxetine, CYP2D6 inhibitors, may increase the plasma concentration of risperidone but less so of the active antipsychotic fraction. When concomitant fluoxetine or paroxetine is initiated or discontinued, the physician should re-evaluate the dosing of Risperdal. Based on *in vitro* studies, the same interaction may occur with haloperidol. Amitriptyline does not affect the pharmacokinetics of risperidone or the active antipsychotic fraction. Cimetidine and ranitidine increase the bioavailability of risperidone, but only marginally that of the active antipsychotic fraction. Erythromycin, a CYP 3A4 inhibitor, does not change the pharmacokinetics of risperidone and the active antipsychotic fraction. The cholinesterase inhibitor galantamine does not show a clinically relevant effect on the pharmacokinetics of risperidone and the active antipsychotic fraction. A study of donepezil in non-elderly healthy volunteers also showed no clinically relevant effect on the pharmacokinetics of risperidone and the antipsychotic fraction.

When risperidone is taken together with other highly protein-bound drugs, there is no clinically relevant displacement of either drug from the plasma proteins.

Risperdal does not show a clinically relevant effect on the pharmacokinetics of valproate. In patients on long-term lithium and older/typical neuroleptic therapy, no significant change occurred in the pharmacokinetics of lithium after substitution of the concomitant neuroleptic with risperidone.

Risperidone does not affect the pharmacokinetic parameters of lithium and valproate.

4.6 Pregnancy and lactation

Pregnancy

Although, in experimental animals, risperidone did not show direct reproductive toxicity, some indirect, prolactin- and CNS-mediated effects were observed, typically delayed oestrus and changes in mating and nursing behaviour in rats. No teratogenic effect of risperidone was noted in any study. The safety of risperidone for use during human pregnancy has not been established. Therefore, risperidone should only be used during pregnancy if the benefits outweigh the risks.

Lactation

In animal studies, risperidone and 9-hydroxyrisperidone are excreted in the milk. It has been demonstrated that risperidone and 9-hydroxyrisperidone are also excreted in human breast milk. Therefore, women receiving risperidone should not breast feed.

4.7 Effects on ability to drive and use machines

Risperidone may interfere with activities requiring mental alertness. Therefore, patients should be advised not to drive or operate machinery until their individual susceptibility is known.

4.8 Undesirable effects

In the clinical trials the following undesirable effects associated with Risperdal Consta at doses within the therapeutic range have been reported:

Common (>1/100):

Weight gain, depression, fatigue and extrapyramidal symptoms. In a 1-year trial, patients who most frequently received 50 mg of Risperdal Consta once every 2 weeks had the largest average weight gain of 2.7 kg. The incidence of extrapyramidal symptoms in patients administered Risperdal Consta at doses up to 50 mg was comparable to that in the placebo group from a pooled analysis including non-randomised studies. Only the following EPS-related symptoms: extrapyramidal disorder, hyperkinesia, hypokinesia, bradykinesia, hyporeflexia, and tremor were reported at a higher incidence in the 50 mg dose group compared with the placebo group.

Uncommon (>0.1/100):

Weight decrease, nervousness, sleep disorder, apathy, impaired concentration, abnormal vision, hypotension, syncope, rash, pruritus, peripheral oedema, injection site reaction. Symptoms of hyperprolactinaemia such as non-puerperal lactation, amenorrhoea, abnormal sexual function, ejaculation failure, decreased libido and impotence.

The following have occasionally been reported: tardive dyskinesia and seizures.

Hematological variations such as increased or decreased white blood cell count have been found, likewise in some patients, increases in hepatic enzymes have been reported.

In addition, the following undesirable effects have been reported with oral risperidone; constipation, abdominal pain, rhinitis, urinary incontinence, priapism, somnolence, dizziness, insomnia, agitation, anxiety, headache, dyspepsia, nausea/vomiting, body temperature dysregulation, hyponatraemia with normal or excess body water due to either polydipsia or the syndrome of inappropriate secretion of antidiuretic hormone (SIADH). Cerebrovascular accidents have been observed during treatment with risperidone. (see Section 4.4 Special warnings and precautions for use).

Hyperglycemia and exacerbation of pre-existing diabetes have been reported in very rare cases during risperidone treatment.

Withdrawal reactions have been reported in association with antipsychotic drugs (see 4.4 Special warnings and special precautions for use).

4.9 Overdose

While overdosage is less likely to occur with parenteral than with oral medication, information pertaining to oral is presented.

Symptoms:

In general, reported signs and symptoms have been those resulting from an exaggeration of the drug's known pharmacological effects. These include drowsiness and sedation, tachycardia and hypotension, and extrapyramidal symptoms. In overdose, rare cases of QT-prolongation have been reported. In case of acute overdosage, the possibility of multiple drug involvement should be considered.

Treatment:

Establish and maintain a clear airway, and ensure adequate oxygenation and ventilation. Cardiovascular monitoring should commence immediately and should include continuous electrocardiographic monitoring to detect possible arrhythmias.

There is no specific antidote to Risperdal. Therefore appropriate supportive measures should be instituted. Hypotension and circulatory collapse should be treated with appropriate measures such as intravenous fluids and/or sympathomimetic agents. In case of severe extrapyramidal symptoms, anticholinergic medication should be administered. Close medical supervision and monitoring should continue until the patient recovers.

5. PHARMACOLOGICAL PROPERTIES

5.1 Pharmacodynamic properties

Pharmacotherapeutic group:

Risperdal Consta: antipsychotic drugs: ATC code: N05AX08.

Solvent for Risperdal Consta: solvents and diluting agents: ATC code: V07AB

Risperidone is a potent D_2 antagonist which is considered a selective monoaminergic antagonist with unique properties. It has a high affinity for serotoninergic 5-HT_2 and dopaminergic D_2 receptors. Risperidone binds also to α_1-adrenergic receptors, and, with lower affinity, to H_1-histaminergic and α_2-adrenergic receptors. Risperidone has no affinity for cholinergic receptors. Although risperidone is a potent D_2 antagonist, that is considered to improve the positive symptoms of schizophrenia, it causes less depression of motor activity and induction of catalepsy than classical neuroleptics. Balanced central serotonin and dopamine antagonism may reduce extrapyramidal side effect liability and extend the therapeutic activity to the negative and affective symptoms of schizophrenia.

Further information on clinical trials

The effectiveness of Risperdal Consta (25 mg and 50 mg) in the management of the manifestations of psychotic disorders (schizophrenia/schizoaffective) was established in one 12-week, placebo-controlled trial in adult psychotic inpatients and outpatients who met the DSM-IV criteria for schizophrenia.

In a 12-week comparative trial in stable patients with schizophrenia, Risperdal Consta was shown to be as effective as the oral tablet formulation (Figure 1). The long-term (50 weeks) safety and efficacy of Risperdal Consta was also evaluated in an open-label trial of stable psychotic inpatients and outpatients who met the DSM-IV criteria for schizophrenia or schizoaffective disorder. Over time efficacy was maintained with Risperdal Consta. The safety information is available in the safety section (Figure 2).

Figure 1.Mean total PANSS (Positive and Negative Syndrome Scale) score over time (12 weeks) (LOCF- Last Observation Carried Forward) in patients with schizophrenia (n=283)

(see Figure 1 below)

Figure 1 Mean total PANSS (Positive and Negative Syndrome Scale) score over time (12 weeks) (LOCF- Last Observation Carried Forward) in patients with schizophrenia (n= 283)

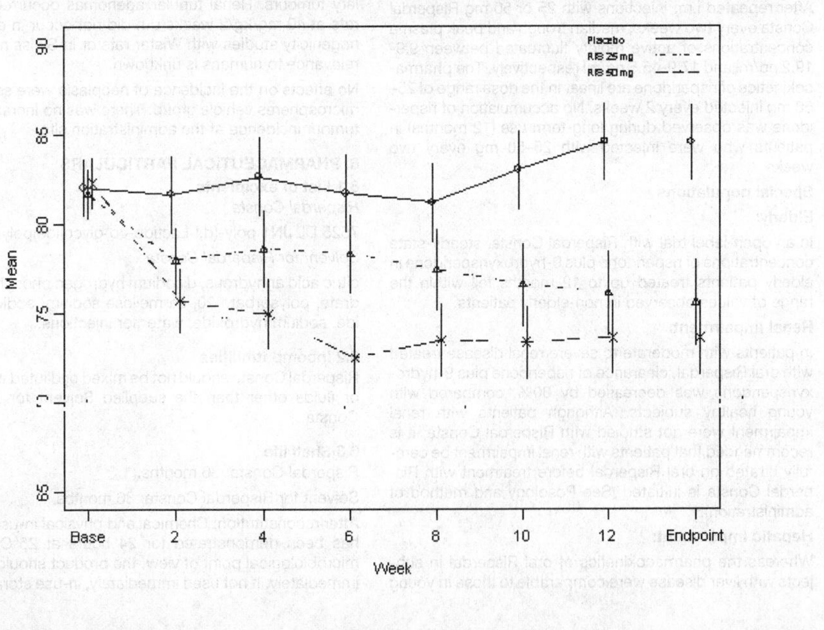

Figure 2 Mean change from baseline in total PANSS score for pooled data from patients treated with 25, 50, or 75 mg in the 50-week open-label trial (n= 667)

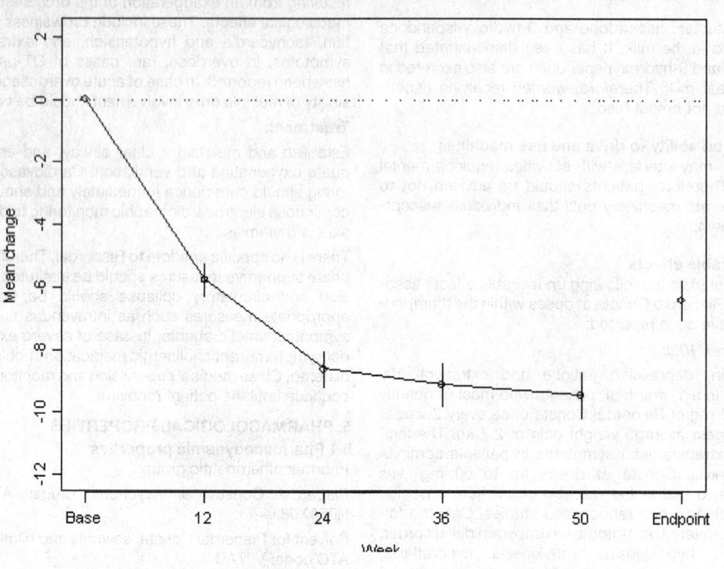

Negative changes indicate improvement

Figure 2. Mean change from baseline in total PANSS score for pooled data from patients treated with 25, 50, or 75 mg in the 50-week open-label trial (n= 667)

(see Figure 2 above)

5.2 Pharmacokinetic properties

Risperidone is metabolised by cytochrome CYP2D6 to 9-hydroxyrisperidone which has a similar pharmacological activity as risperidone. Risperidone plus 9-hydroxyrisperidone form the active antipsychotic fraction. Another metabolic pathway of risperidone is N-dealkylation.

General characteristics of risperidone after administration of Risperdal Consta in patients

After a single i.m. injection with Risperdal Consta the release profile consists of a small initial release of drug (<1% of the dose), followed by a lag time of 3 weeks. Following i.m. injection the main release of drug starts from 3 weeks onwards, is maintained from 4 to 6 weeks and subsides by week 7. Antipsychotic supplementation should therefore be given during the first 3 weeks of Risperdal Consta treatment (see section 4.2).

The combination of the release profile and the dosage regimen (i.m. injection every two weeks) result in sustained therapeutic plasma concentrations. Therapeutic plasma concentrations remain until 4 to 6 weeks after the last Risperdal Consta injection. The elimination phase is complete approximately 7 to 8 weeks after the last injection.

The absorption of risperidone from Risperdal Consta is complete.

Risperidone is rapidly distributed. The volume of distribution is 1-2 l/kg. In plasma, risperidone is bound to albumin and α_1-acid glycoprotein. The plasma protein binding of risperidone is 90 %, that of 9-hydroxyrisperidone is 77%.

Active moiety and risperidone clearances were 5.0 and 13.7 L/h in extensive metabolisers, and 3.2 and 3.3 L/h in poor metabolisers according to the CYP2D6 metabolic phenotype, respectively.

After repeated i.m. injections with 25 or 50 mg Risperdal Consta every two weeks, median trough and peak plasma concentrations of active moiety fluctuated between 9.9-19.2 ng/ml and 17.9-45.5 ng/ml respectively. The pharmacokinetics of risperidone are linear in the dose range of 25–50 mg injected every 2 weeks. No accumulation of risperidone was observed during long-term use (12 months) in patients who were injected with 25–50 mg every two weeks.

Special populations

Elderly:

In an open-label trial with Risperdal Consta, steady-state concentrations of risperidone plus 9-hydroxyrisperidone in elderly patients treated up to 12 months fell within the range of values observed in non-elderly patients.

Renal Impairment:

In patients with moderate to severe renal disease treated with oral Risperdal, clearance of risperidone plus 9-hydroxyrisperidone was decreased by 60%, compared with young healthy subjects. Although patients with renal impairment were not studied with Risperdal Consta, it is recommended that patients with renal impairment be carefully titrated on oral Risperdal before treatment with Risperdal Consta is initiated (See Posology and method of administration).

Hepatic Impairment:

Whereas the pharmacokinetics of oral Risperdal in subjects with liver disease were comparable to those in young healthy subjects, the mean free fraction of risperidone in plasma was increased by about 35% because of the diminished concentration of both albumin and α_1-acid glycoprotein. Although patients with hepatic impairment were not studied with Risperdal Consta, it is recommended that patients with hepatic impairment be carefully titrated on oral Risperdal before treatment with Risperdal Consta is initiated (See POSOLOGY AND METHOD OF ADMINISTRATION).

Pharmacokinetic/ pharmacodynamic relationship

There was no relationship between the plasma concentrations of the active moiety and the change in total PANSS (Positive and Negative Syndrome Scale) and total ESRS (Extrapyramidal Symptom Rating Scale) scores across the assessment visits in any of the phase-III trials where efficacy and safety was examined.

5.3 Preclinical safety data

Apart from local irritation at high volumes, the Risperdal Consta formulation has a similar toxicological profile when compared to the oral formulation.

In the (sub)chronic toxicity studies (up to 12 months of oral administration) in rats and dogs, the major effects were prolactin-mediated mammary gland stimulation and male and female genital tract changes, and central nervous system (CNS) effects, related to the pharmacodynamic activity of risperidone.

There was no evidence of mutagenic potential.

As expected for a potent dopamine D_2-antagonist, in an intramuscular carcinogenicity study in Wistar Han rats (doses of 5 and 40 mg/kg every two weeks), prolactin-mediated increased incidences of endocrine pancreas, pituitary gland and adrenal medullary neoplasia were observed at 40 mg/kg, while mammary gland neoplasia were present at 5 and 40 mg/kg.

Hypercalcaemia observed in both dose groups may have contributed to the increased incidence of adrenal medullary tumours. Renal tubular adenomas occurred in male rats at 40 mg/kg/2 weeks but did not occur in oral carcinogenicity studies with Wistar rats or in Swiss mice; their relevance to humans is unknown.

No effects on the incidence of neoplasia were seen in the microspheres vehicle group. There was no increase in the tumour incidence at the administration site.

6. PHARMACEUTICAL PARTICULARS

6.1 List of excipients

Risperdal Consta

7525 DL JN1 poly-(d,l-Lactide-co-glycolide)polymer

Solvent for Risperdal Consta

citric acid anhydrous, disodium hydrogen phosphate dihydrate, polysorbate 20, carmellose sodium, sodium chloride, sodium hydroxide, water for injections.

6.2 Incompatibilities

Risperdal Consta should not be mixed or diluted with drugs or fluids other than the supplied Solvent for Risperdal Consta.

6.3 Shelf life

Risperdal Consta: 36 months.

Solvent for Risperdal Consta: 36 months.

After reconstitution: Chemical and physical in-use stability has been demonstrated for 24 hours at 25°C. From a microbiological point of view, the product should be used immediately. If not used immediately, in-use storage times and conditions prior to use are the responsibility of the user and would normally not be longer than 6 hours at 25°C, unless reconstitution has taken place in controlled and validated aseptic conditions.

6.4 Special precautions for storage

The entire pack should be stored in a refrigerator. Store at 2°C to 8°C. Keep containers in the outer carton. It should not be exposed to temperatures above 25°C.

If refrigeration is unavailable, Risperdal Consta can be stored at temperatures not exceeding 25°C for no more than 7 days prior to administration.

6.5 Nature and contents of container

Risperdal Consta is packaged in the following container/closure configuration:

- One vial containing Risperdal Consta powder for suspension for injection.
- One prefilled syringe containing the Solvent for Risperdal Consta.
- Two Hypoint® 20G 2" TW needles for reconstitution.
- One Needle-Pro® needle for intramuscular injection (safety 20G 2" TW needle with needle protection device). (To be used with Risperdal Consta only).

6.6 Instructions for use and handling

Risperdal® Consta(TM) powder may **only** be suspended in the Solvent for Risperdal Consta supplied in the dose pack and must be administered with the needles supplied in the dose pack.

1. Remove the dose pack of Risperdal Consta from the refrigerator and allow it to come to room temperature prior to reconstitution.

2. Flip off the plastic coloured cap from the vial of Risperdal Consta.

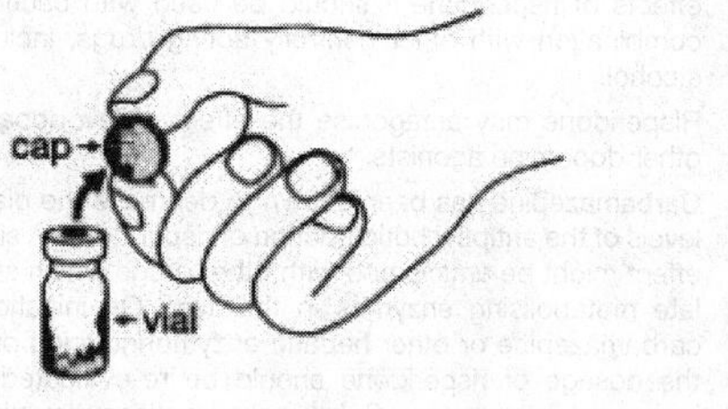

3. Open the syringe by breaking the seal of the white cap and remove the white cap together with the rubber tip cap inside.

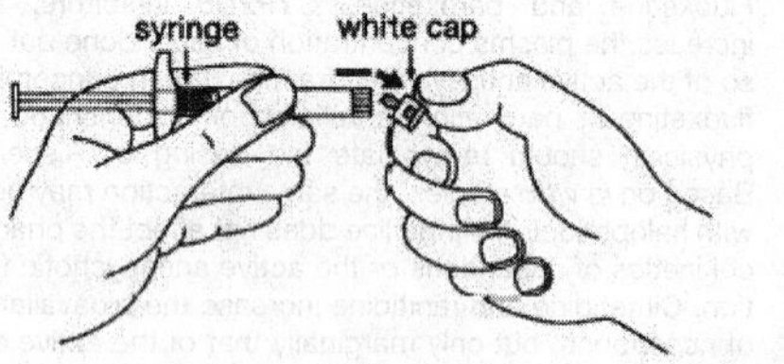

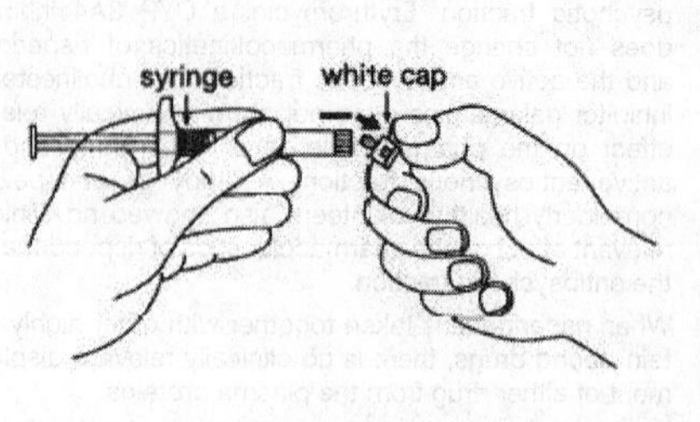

4. Attach one of the Hypoint(TM) needles with an easy clockwise twisting motion to the luer connection of the syringe.

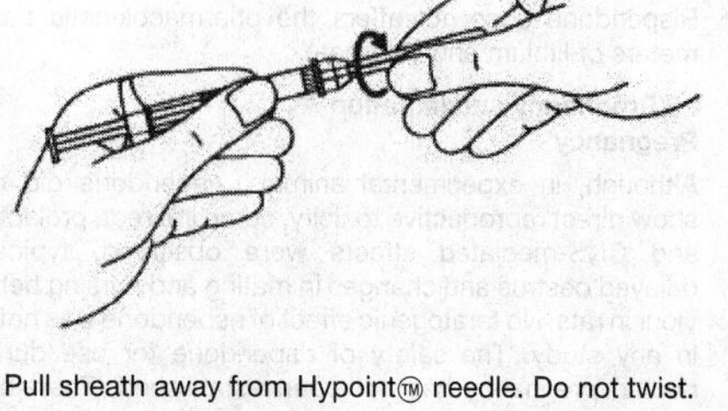

5. Pull sheath away from Hypoint(TM) needle. Do not twist.

6. Inject the entire content of the syringe with diluent into the vial.

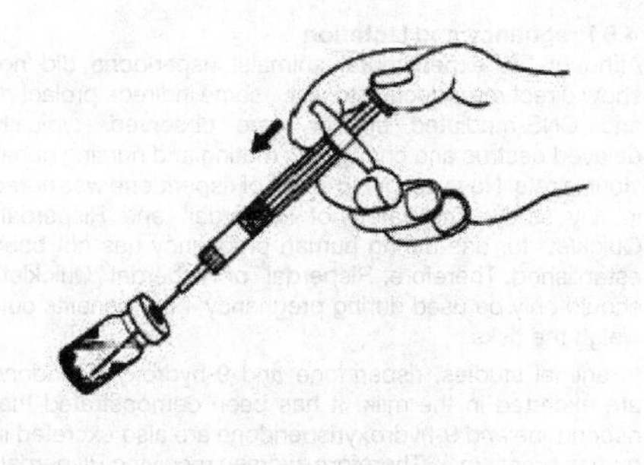

7. Withdraw the syringe with the Hypoint® needle from the vial.

8. Unscrew the Hypoint® needle from the syringe and discard the needle appropriately.

9. Before shaking the vial, attach the second Hypoint® needle with an easy clockwise twisting motion to the luer connection of the syringe. DO NOT REMOVE THE SHEATH FROM THE NEEDLE AT THIS STAGE.

10. Shake the vial vigorously for at least 10 seconds. Mixing is complete when the suspension appears uniform, thick, and milky in colour, and all the powder is fully dispersed.

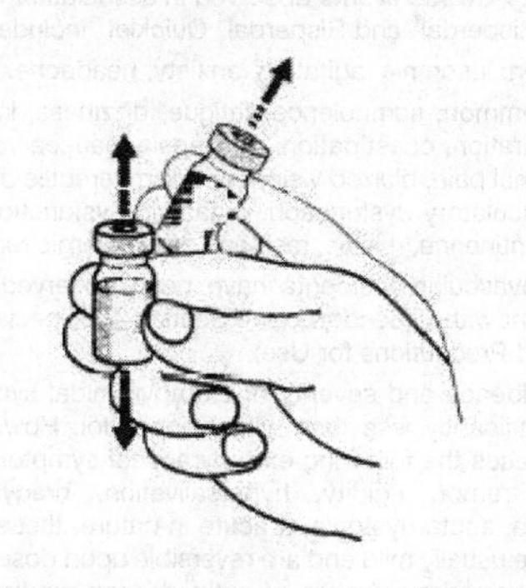

11. Do not store the vial after reconstitution or the suspension may settle.

12. Take the syringe and pull sheath away from the Hypoint® needle. Do not twist.

13. Insert the Hypoint® needle into the upright vial.

14. Slowly withdraw the suspension from the vial in an upright position as indicated in the diagram to ensure that the entire content is drawn up into the syringe.

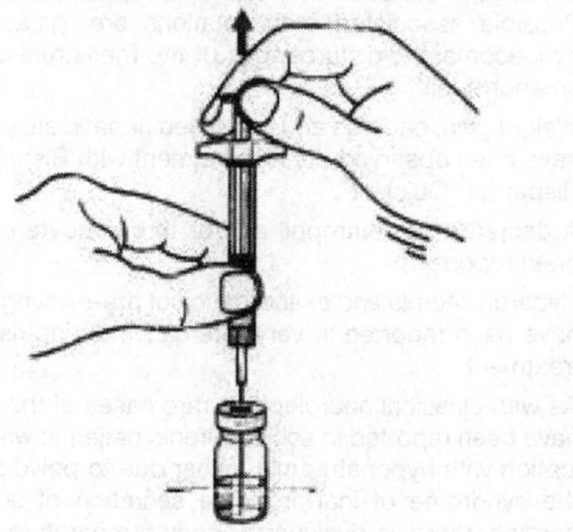

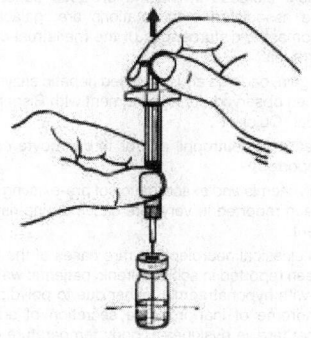

15. Withdraw the syringe with the Hypoint® needle from the vial.

16. Unscrew the Hypoint® needle from the syringe and discard the needle appropriately.

17. Peel the blister pouch of the Needle-Pro® device open half way.

Grasp sheath using the plastic peel pouch.

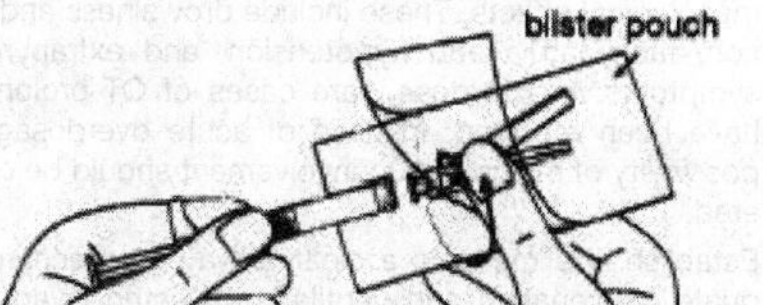

18. Attach the luer connection of the Needle- Pro® device with an easy clockwise twisting motion, to the syringe. Seat the needle firmly on the Needle-Pro® device with a push and clockwise twist.

19. Prepare the patient for injection.

20. Resuspension of Risperdal Consta will be necessary prior to administration as settling will occur over time once product is reconstituted. Shake vigorously for as long as it takes to resuspend.

21. Pull sheath away from the needle. Do not twist sheath as needle may be loosened from Needle-Pro® device.

22. Tap the syringe gently to make any air bubbles rise to the top.

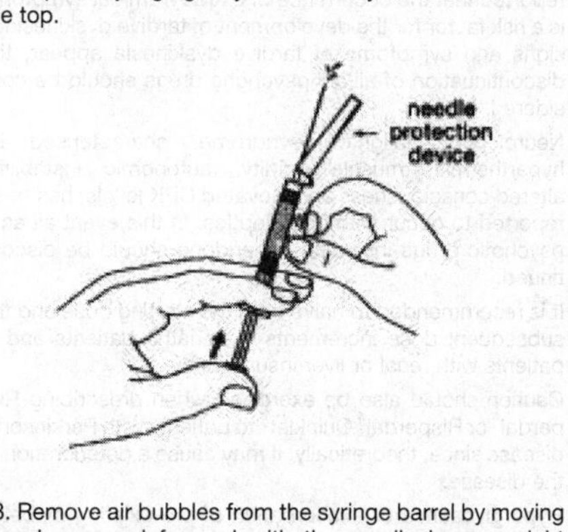

23. Remove air bubbles from the syringe barrel by moving the plunger rod forward with the needle in an upright position. Inject the entire content of the syringe intramuscularly into the buttock of the patient.

24. WARNING:

To avoid a needle stick injury with a contaminated needle, do not:

- intentionally disengage the Needle- Pro® device
- attempt to straighten the needle or engage Needle- Pro® device if the needle is bent or damaged
- mishandle the needle protection device that could lead to protrusion of the needle from the needle protector sheath.

25. After procedure is completed, press the needle into the sheath using a one-handed technique. Perform a one-handed technique by GENTLY pressing the sheath against a flat surface. As the sheath is pressed, the needle is firmly engaged into the sheath.

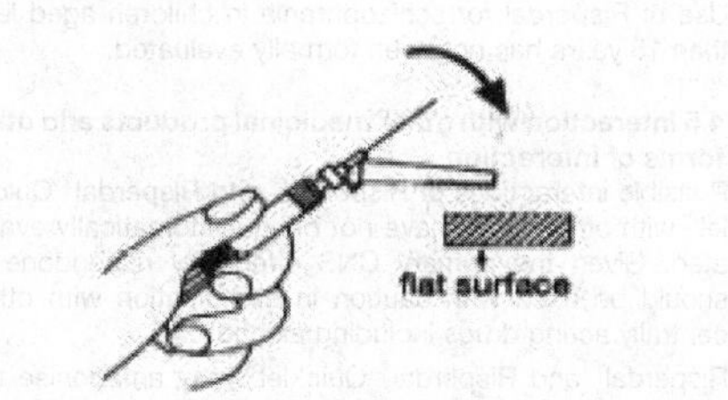

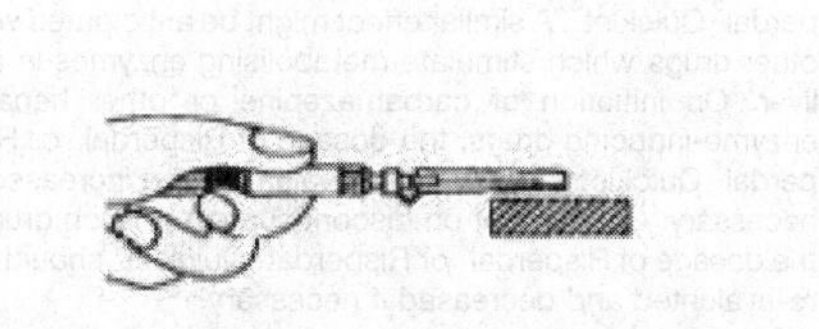

26. Visually confirm that the needle is fully engaged into the needle protection sheath.

27. Immediately discard appropriately.

ADMINISTRATION DETAILS

7. MARKETING AUTHORISATION HOLDER

Janssen-Cilag Ltd
Saunderton
High Wycombe
Buckinghamshire
HP14 4HJ
UK

8. MARKETING AUTHORISATION NUMBER(S)

Risperdal Consta 25 mg, 37.5 mg, 50 mg PL 00242 0375, 6, 7

Solvent for Risperdal Consta[T] PL 00242/0382

9. DATE OF FIRST AUTHORISATION/RENEWAL OF THE AUTHORISATION

8 August 2002

10. DATE OF REVISION OF THE TEXT

16 March 2005

11. LEGAL CATEGORY

POM

TM trademark

® registered trademark

Risperdal Tablets, Liquid & Quicklet

(Janssen-Cilag Ltd)

1. NAME OF THE MEDICINAL PRODUCT

Risperdal®

Risperdal® Quicklet® orodispersible tablets

2. QUALITATIVE AND QUANTITATIVE COMPOSITION

Risperdal® Tablets: risperidone 0.5, 1, 2, 3, 4 and 6 mg.

Risperdal® Liquid: risperidone 1 mg/ml.

Risperdal® Quicklet® orodispersible tablets: risperidone 0.5 mg, 1 mg and 2 mg

For excipients please see section 6.1

3. PHARMACEUTICAL FORM

Coated tablets:

0.5 mg: Brownish-red, oblong tablets, marked Ris|0.5.

1 mg: White, oblong tablets, marked Ris|1.

2 mg: Pale orange, oblong tablets, marked Ris|2.

3 mg: Yellow, oblong tablets, marked Ris|3.

4 mg: Green, oblong tablets, marked Ris|4.

6 mg: Yellow, circular tablets, marked Ris|6.

Oral solution

The solution is clear and colourless.

Orodispersible tablets

0.5 mg:Light coral, round, biconvex tablets, etched "R 0.5"

1 mg: Light coral, square, biconvex tablets, etched "R1"

2 mg: Light coral, round, biconvex tablets, etched "R2"

4. CLINICAL PARTICULARS

4.1 Therapeutic indications

Risperdal® Tablets and Liquid and Risperdal® Quicklet® are indicated for the treatment of acute and chronic schizophrenic psychoses, and other psychotic conditions, in which positive symptoms (such as hallucinations, delusions, thought disturbances, hostility, suspiciousness), and/or negative symptoms (such as blunted affect, emotional and social withdrawal, poverty of speech) are prominent. Risperdal® and Risperdal® Quicklet® also alleviate affective symptoms (such as depression, guilt feelings, anxiety) associated with schizophrenia.

Risperdal® and Risperdal® Quicklet® are also effective in maintaining the clinical improvement during continuation therapy in patients who have shown an initial treatment response.

Risperdal® and Risperdal® Quicklet are indicated for the treatment of mania in bipolar disorder. These episodes are characterized by symptoms such as elevated, expansive or irritable mood, inflated self-esteem, decreased need for sleep, pressured speech, racing thoughts, distractibility, or poor judgment, including disruptive or aggressive behaviours.

Risperdal® and Risperdal® Quicklet are not licensed for the treatment of behavioural symptoms of dementia (see section 4.4).

4.2 Posology and method of administration

Risperdal Liquid:

1 ml of Risperdal liquid contains 1 mg risperidone. If necessary Risperdal liquid may be diluted with mineral water, orange juice or black coffee. When diluted in this way, the product should be used immediately. The liquid should not be mixed with tea.

(See Section 6. Pharmaceutical Particulars).

4.2. a Schizophrenia:

Switching from other antipsychotics: where medically appropriate, gradual discontinuation of the previous treatment while Risperdal® or Risperdal® Quicklet® therapy is initiated is recommended. Where medically appropriate when switching patients from depot antipsychotics, consider initiating Risperdal® or Risperdal® Quicklet® therapy in place of the next scheduled injection. The need for continuing existing antiparkinson medication should be re-evaluated periodically.

Adults

Risperdal® or Risperdal® Quicklet® may be given once or twice daily. All patients, whether acute or chronic, should start with 2 mg/day Risperdal® or Risperdal® Quicklet®. The dosage may be increased to 4 mg/day on the second day. Some patients, such as first episode patients, may benefit from a slower rate of titration. From then on the dosage can be maintained unchanged, or further individualised, if needed. Most patients will benefit from daily doses between 4 and 6 mg/day although in some, an optimal response may be obtained at lower doses.

Doses above 10 mg/day generally have not been shown to provide additional efficacy to lower doses and may increase the risk of extrapyramidal symptoms. Doses above 10 mg/day should only be used in individual patients if the benefit is considered to outweigh the risk. Doses above 16 mg/day have not been extensively evaluated for safety and therefore should not be used.

Elderly

A starting dose of 0.5 mg bd is recommended. This dosage can be individually adjusted with 0.5 mg bd increments to 1 to 2 mg bd.

Children

Use of Risperdal for schizophrenia in children aged less than 15 years has not been formally evaluated.

Renal and liver disease

A starting dose of 0.5 mg bd is recommended. This dosage can be individually adjusted with 0.5 mg bd increments to 1 to 2 mg bd.

Risperdal® and Risperdal® Quicklet® should be used with caution in this group of patients until further experience is gained.

4.2. b Bipolar Mania:

Adults

Risperidone should be administered on a once daily schedule, starting with 2 mg. Dosage adjustments, if indicated, should occur at intervals of not less than 24 hours and in dosage increments of 1 mg per day. A dosing range between 1 and 6 mg per day is recommended.

As with all symptomatic treatments, the continued use of Risperdal must be evaluated and justified on an ongoing basis.

Elderly

A starting dose of 0.5 mg bd is recommended. This dosage can be individually adjusted with 0.5 mg bd increments to 1 to 2 mg bd.

Renal and liver disease

A starting dose of 0.5 mg bd is recommended. This dosage can be individually adjusted with 0.5 mg bd increments to 1 to 2 mg bd.

Risperdal should be used with caution in this group of patients until further experience is gained.

Combined use with mood stabilisers

There is limited information on the combined use of Risperdal with carbamazepine in bipolar mania. Carbamazepine has been shown to induce the metabolism of risperidone producing lower plasma levels of the antipsychotic fraction of Risperdal (see Section 4.5). It is therefore not recommended to co-administer Risperdal with carbamazepine in bipolar mania patients until further experience is gained. The combined use with lithium or valproate does not require any adjustment of the dose of Risperdal.

Method of administration

Oral use.

Risperdal® Quicklet®:

The Risperdal® Quicklet® tablet should be placed on the tongue. It begins disintegrating in the mouth within seconds and can be swallowed subsequently with or without water. The mouth should be empty before placing the tablet on the tongue.

As the tablets are fragile, they should not be pushed through the foil as this will cause damage. Open blister by pulling up the edge of the foil and peeling it off, then tip the tablet out. After removal from its blister, the Risperdal® Quicklet® tablet should be consumed immediately as it cannot be stored once removed. Risperdal® Quicklet® tablets begin disintegrating within seconds when placed on the tongue and the use of water is unnecessary. No attempt should be made to split the tablet.

4.3 Contraindications

Risperdal® and Risperdal® Quicklet® are contraindicated in patients with a known hypersensitivity to risperidone or any other ingredients in the product.

Risperdal® Quicklet® contains aspartame and therefore should not be taken by patients with phenylketonuria.

4.4 Special warnings and special precautions for use

Risperdal® and Risperdal® Quicklet® are not recommended for the treatment of behavioural symptoms of dementia because of an increased risk of cerebrovascular adverse events (including cerebrovascular accidents and transient ischaemic attacks). Treatment of acute psychoses in patients with a history of dementia should be limited to short term only and should be under specialist advice.

Data from randomised clinical trials conducted in elderly >65 years) patients with dementia indicate that there is an approximately 3-fold increased risk of cerebrovascular adverse events (including cerebrovascular accidents and transient ischaemic attacks) with risperidone, compared with placebo. Cerebrovascular adverse events occurred in 3.3% (33/989) of patients treated with risperidone and 1.2% (8/693) of patients treated with placebo. The Odds Ratio (95% exact confidence interval) was 2.96 (1.33, 7.45).

Physicians should consider carefully the risk of cerebrovascular adverse events with Risperdal (given the observations in elderly patients with dementia detailed above) before treating any patient with a previous history of CVA/TIA. Consideration should also be given to other risk factors for cerebrovascular disease including hypertension, diabetes, current smoking, atrial fibrillation, etc.

Due to the alpha-blocking activity of Risperdal® and Risperdal® Quicklet®, orthostatic hypotension can occur, especially during the initial dose-titration period. A dose reduction should be considered if hypotension occurs.

Risperdal® and Risperdal® Quicklet® should be used with caution in patients with known cardiovascular disease including those associated with prolongation of the QT interval and the dose should be gradually titrated. In clinical trials, Risperdal® was not associated with an increase in QTc intervals. As with other antipsychotics, caution is advised when prescribing with medications known to prolong the QT interval.

If further sedation is required, an additional drug (such as a benzodiazepine) should be administered rather than increasing the dose of Risperdal® or Risperdal® Quicklet®.

Drugs with dopamine receptor antagonistic properties have been associated with the induction of tardive dyskinesia, characterised by rhythmical involuntary movements, predominantly of the tongue and/or face. It has been reported that the occurrence of extrapyramidal symptoms is a risk factor for the development of tardive dyskinesia. If signs and symptoms of tardive dyskinesia appear, the discontinuation of all antipsychotic drugs should be considered.

Neuroleptic malignant syndrome, characterised by hyperthermia, muscle rigidity, autonomic instability, altered consciousness and elevated CPK levels, has been reported to occur with neuroleptics. In this event all antipsychotic drugs including risperidone should be discontinued.

It is recommended to halve both the starting dose and the subsequent dose increments in geriatric patients and in patients with renal or liver insufficiency.

Caution should also be exercised when prescribing Risperdal® or Risperdal® Quicklet® to patients with Parkinson's disease since, theoretically, it may cause a deterioration of the disease.

Hyperglycaemia or exacerbation of pre-existing diabetes has been reported in very rare cases during treatment with Risperdal. Appropriate clinical monitoring is advisable in diabetic patients and in patients with risk factors for the development of diabetes mellitus (see also section 4.8 Undesirable effects).

Classical neuroleptics are known to lower the seizure threshold. Caution is recommended when treating patients with epilepsy.

As with other antipsychotics, patients should be advised of the potential for weight gain.

Acute withdrawal symptoms, including nausea, vomiting, sweating, and insomnia have very rarely been described after abrupt cessation of high doses of antipsychotic drugs. Recurrence of psychotic symptoms may also occur, and the emergence of involuntary movement disorders (such as akathisia, dystonia and dyskinesia) has been reported. Therefore, gradual withdrawal is advisable.

Use of Risperdal for schizophrenia in children aged less than 15 years has not been formally evaluated.

4.5 Interaction with other medicinal products and other forms of Interaction

Possible interactions of Risperdal® and Risperdal® Quicklet® with other drugs have not been systematically evaluated. Given the primary CNS effects of risperidone, it should be used with caution in combination with other centrally acting drugs including alcohol.

Risperdal® and Risperdal® Quicklet® may antagonise the effect of levodopa and other dopamine-agonists.

Carbamazepine has been shown to decrease the plasma levels of the antipsychotic fraction of Risperdal® and Risperdal® Quicklet®. A similar effect might be anticipated with other drugs which stimulate metabolising enzymes in the liver. On initiation of carbamazepine or other hepatic enzyme-inducing drugs, the dosage of Risperdal® or Risperdal® Quicklet® should be re-evaluated and increased if necessary. Conversely, on discontinuation of such drugs, the dosage of Risperdal® or Risperdal® Quicklet® should be re-evaluated and decreased if necessary.

Phenothiazines, tricyclic antidepressants and some betablockers may increase the plasma concentrations of risperidone but not those of the active antipsychotic fraction. Fluoxetine and paroxetine, CYP2D6 inhibitors, may increase the plasma concentration of risperidone but less so of the active antipsychotic fraction. When concomitant fluoxetine or paroxetine is initiated or discontinued, the physician should re-evaluate the dosing of Risperdal. Based on *in vitro* studies, the same interaction may occur with haloperidol. Amitriptyline does not affect the pharmacokinetics of risperidone or the active antipsychotic fraction. Cimetidine and ranitidine increase the bioavailability of risperidone, but only marginally that of the active antipsychotic fraction. Erythromycin, a CYP 3A4 inhibitor, does not change the pharmacokinetics of risperidone and the active antipsychotic fraction. The cholinesterase inhibitor galantamine does not show a clinically relevant effect on the pharmacokinetics of risperidone and the active antipsychotic fraction. A study of donepezil in non-elderly healthy volunteers also showed no clinically relevant effect on the pharmacokinetics of risperidone and the antipsychotic fraction.

When Risperdal® or Risperdal® Quicklet® is taken together with other highly protein-bound drugs, there is no clinically relevant displacement of either drug from the plasma proteins.

Risperdal does not show a clinically relevant effect on the pharmacokinetics of valproate. In patients on long-term lithium and older/typical neuroleptic therapy, no significant change occurred in the pharmacokinetics of lithium after substitution of the concomitant neuroleptic with risperidone.

Food does not affect the absorption of risperidone from the stomach. The effect of food particles in the mouth on absorption from Risperdal® Quicklet® has not been studied.

4.6 Pregnancy and lactation

Although, in experimental animals, risperidone did not show direct reproductive toxicity, some indirect, prolactin- and CNS-mediated effects were observed, typically delayed oestrus and changes in mating and nursing behaviour in rats. No teratogenic effect of risperidone was noted in any study. The safety of Risperdal® and Risperdal® Quicklet® for use during human pregnancy has not been established. Therefore, Risperdal® or Risperdal® Quicklet® should only be used during pregnancy if the benefits outweigh the risks.

In animal studies, risperidone and 9-hydroxyrisperidone are excreted in the milk. It has been demonstrated that risperidone and 9-hydroxyrisperidone are also excreted in human breast milk. Therefore, women receiving Risperdal® or Risperdal® Quicklet® should not breast feed.

4.7 Effects on ability to drive and use machines

Risperdal® and Risperdal® Quicklet® may interfere with activities requiring mental alertness. Therefore, patients should be advised not to drive or operate machinery until their individual susceptibility is known.

4.8 Undesirable effects

Risperdal® and Risperdal® Quicklet® are generally well tolerated and in many instances it has been difficult to differentiate adverse events from symptoms of the underlying disease. Adverse events observed in association with the use of Risperdal® and Risperdal® Quicklet® include:

Common: insomnia, agitation, anxiety, headache.

Less common: somnolence, fatigue, dizziness, impaired concentration, constipation, dyspepsia, nausea/vomiting, abdominal pain, blurred vision, priapism, erectile dysfunction, ejaculatory dysfunction, orgasmic dysfunction, urinary incontinence, rhinitis, rash and other allergic reactions.

Cerebrovascular accidents have been observed during treatment with risperidone (see Section 4.4 Special warnings and Precautions for Use).

The incidence and severity of extrapyramidal symptoms are significantly less than with haloperidol. However, in some cases the following extrapyramidal symptoms may occur: tremor, rigidity, hypersalivation, bradykinesia, akathisia, acute dystonia. If acute in nature, these symptoms are usually mild and are reversible upon dose reduction and/or administration of antiparkinson medication, if necessary. In clinical trials in patients with acute mania risperidone treatment resulted in an incidence of EPS > 10%. This is lower than the incidence observed in patients treated with classical neuroleptics.

Occasionally, orthostatic dizziness, hypotension including orthostatic, tachycardia including reflex tachycardia and hypertension have been observed following administration of Risperdal® and Risperdal® Quicklet®.

Risperdal® and Risperdal® Quicklet® can induce a dose-dependent increase in plasma prolactin concentration. Possible associated manifestations are: galactorrhoea, gynaecomastia, disturbances of the menstrual cycle and amenorrhoea.

Weight gain, oedema and increased hepatic enzyme levels have been observed during treatment with Risperdal® and Risperdal® Quicklet®.

A decrease in neutrophil and/or thrombocyte count has been reported.

Hyperglycaemia and exacerbation of pre-existing diabetes have been reported in very rare cases during risperidone treatment.

As with classical neuroleptics, rare cases of the following have been reported in schizophrenic patients: water intoxication with hyponatraemia, either due to polydipsia or to the syndrome of inappropriate secretion of antidiuretic hormone; tardive dyskinesia, body temperature dysregulation and seizures.

Sedation has been reported more frequently in children and adolescents than in adults. In general, sedation is mild and transient.

Withdrawal reactions have been reported in association with antipsychotic drugs (see 4.4 Special warnings and special precautions for use).

4.9 Overdose

In general, reported signs and symptoms have been those resulting from an exaggeration of the drug's known pharmacological effects. These include drowsiness and sedation, tachycardia and hypotension, and extrapyramidal symptoms. In overdose, rare cases of QT-prolongation have been reported. In case of acute overdosage, the possibility of multiple drug involvement should be considered.

Establish and maintain a clear airway, and ensure adequate oxygenation and ventilation. Gastric lavage (after intubation, if the patient is unconscious) and administration of activated charcoal together with a laxative should be considered. Cardiovascular monitoring should commence immediately and should include continuous electrocardiographic monitoring to detect possible arrhythmias.

There is no specific antidote to Risperdal® or Risperdal® Quicklet®. Therefore appropriate supportive measures should be instituted. Hypotension and circulatory collapse should be treated with appropriate measures such as intravenous fluids and/or sympathomimetic agents. In case of severe extrapyramidal symptoms, anticholinergic medication should be administered. Close medical supervision and monitoring should continue until the patient recovers.

5. PHARMACOLOGICAL PROPERTIES

5.1 Pharmacodynamic properties

Risperidone is a novel antipsychotic belonging to a new class of antipsychotic agents, the benzisoxazole-derivatives.

Risperidone is a selective monoaminergic antagonist with a high affinity for both serotonergic 5-HT_2 and dopaminergic D_2 receptors. Risperidone binds also to alpha$_1$-adrenergic receptors and, with lower affinity, to H_1-histaminergic and alpha$_2$-adrenergic receptors. Risperidone has no affinity for cholinergic receptors. Although risperidone is a potent D_2 antagonist, that is considered to improve the positive symptoms of schizophrenia, it causes less depression of motor activity and induction of catalepsy than classical neuroleptics. Balanced central serotonin and dopamine antagonism may reduce the tendency to cause extrapyramidal side effects, and extend the therapeutic activity to the negative and affective symptoms of schizophrenia.

5.2 Pharmacokinetic properties

Risperidone is completely absorbed after oral administration, reaching peak plasma concentrations within 1 to 2 hours. Food does not affect the absorption of risperidone from the stomach. The effect of food particles in the mouth on absorption has not been studied.

The most important route of metabolism of risperidone is hydroxylation by cytochrome CYP 2D6 to 9-hydroxy-risperidone which has a similar pharmacological activity to risperidone. This hydroxylation is subject to debrisoquine-type genetic polymorphism but this does not affect the active antipsychotic fraction since this consists of risperidone and its active metabolite 9-hydroxyrisperidone. After oral administration, the elimination half-life of the active antipsychotic fraction is 24 hours.

A single-dose study showed higher active plasma concentrations and a slower elimination of risperidone in the elderly and in patients with renal insufficiency. Risperidone plasma concentrations were normal in patients with liver insufficiency.

Risperdal oro-dispersible tablets and oral solution are bioequivalent to Risperdal oral tablets.

5.3 Preclinical safety data

There are no preclinical data of relevance to the prescriber other than those already provided in other sections of the SPC.

6. PHARMACEUTICAL PARTICULARS

6.1 List of excipients

Risperdal® Tablets: All tablet strengths contain the following excipients.

Lactose
Maize starch
Microcrystalline cellulose
Hypromellose 2910 5 mPa.s
Magnesium stearate
Colloidal anhydrous silica
Sodium lauryl sulphate
Propylene glycol
Purified water*

* not present in the final product.

In addition, the tablets also contain the following excipients:

0.5 mg
Hypromellose 2910 15 mPa.s
Titanium dioxide (E171)
Talc
Red ferric oxide (E172)

1 mg
Hypromellose 2910 15 mPa.s

2 mg
Hypromellose 2910 15 mPa.s
Titanium dioxide (E171)
Talc
Orange yellow S (E110) aluminium lake

3 mg
Hypromellose 2910 15 mPa.s
Titanium dioxide (E171)
Talc
Quinoline yellow (E104)

4 mg
Hypromellose 2910 15 mPa.s
Titanium dioxide (E171)
Talc
Quinoline yellow (E104)
Indigotine disulphonate (E132) aluminium lake

6 mg
Titanium dioxide (E171)
Talc
Quinoline yellow (E104)
Orange yellow S (E110)

Risperdal®
Liquid
Tartaric acid
Benzoic acid
Sodium hydroxide
Purified water

Risperdal® Quicklet®:

Polacrilex resin (methacrylic acid polymer with divinylbenzene)
Gelatin type A
Mannitol
Glycine
Simethicone
Carbomer 34, 499cps
Sodium hydroxide
Aspartame
Red ferric oxide (E172)
Peppermint oil

6.2 Incompatibilities

Risperdal® tablets and Risperdal® Quicklet®: No incompatibilities known.

Risperdal® Liquid: Risperdal® Liquid should only be diluted with those beverages listed in Posology and method of administration (see section 4.2).

6.3 Shelf life

Risperdal® 1, 2, 3 and 4 mg Tablets: 36 months.

0.5, 6 mg Tablets: 24 months.

Liquid: The unopened bottles have a shelf life of 36 months. Once opened, the contents of the bottle should be used within 3 months.

Risperdal® Quicklet®: 36 months

6.4 Special precautions for storage

Risperdal® Tablets: Do not store above 30°C.

Risperdal® Liquid: Do not store above 30°C. Do not refrigerate.

Risperdal® Quicklet®: Do not store above 30°C. Store in the original container.

6.5 Nature and contents of container

Risperdal® Tablets: Blister strips consisting of 200 μm polyvinylchloride (PVC)/25 μm low density polyethylene (LDPE)/90 g/m^2 polyvinylidene chloride (PVDC) and 20 μm aluminium foil. The strips are packed in cardboard cartons to contain either 20 (0.5, 1 mg tablets only), 60 tablets (1, 2, 3 and 4 mg tablets) or 28 tablets (6 mg tablets) per pack.

Risperdal® Liquid: Amber glass bottle with a plastic child-resistant and tamper-evident cap. Each bottle contains 100 ml.

Risperdal® Quicklet: Blister strips consisting of polychlorotrifluoroethylene/polyvinylchloride/polyethylene film and aluminium foil (film/foil) or aluminium foil and aluminium foil (foil/foil). The strips are packed in cardboard cartons to contain 28 tablets per pack.

6.6 Instructions for use and handling

Risperdal® Tablets: Not applicable.

Risperdal® Liquid: A special dosing pipette is supplied with each pack of Risperdal

Instructions for using the pipette with Risperdal liquid

Fig. 1

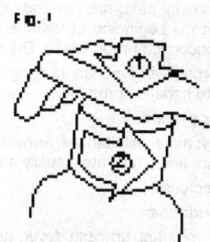

1. Remove the child-resistant cap from the bottle by pushing down on the cap while turning it anti-clockwise (Fig. 1).
2. Place the bottle on a flat surface.

Fig.2

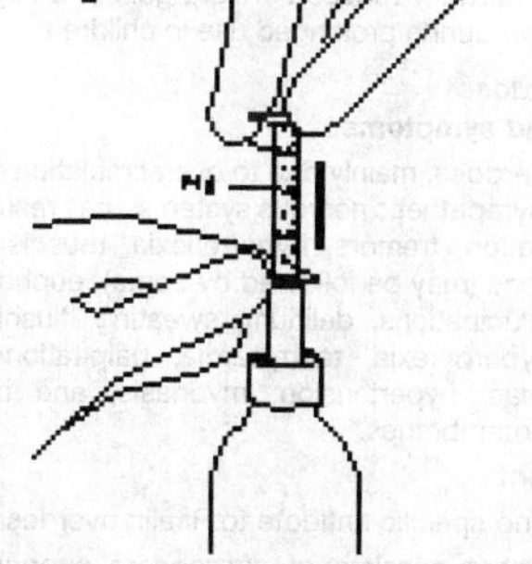

3. Insert the pipette into the liquid in the bottle.
4. While holding the lower ring, pull the top ring upwards until the mark that matches the number of mg or ml to be taken is just visible (Fig. 2).
5. Holding the lower ring, remove the whole pipette from the bottle (Fig. 3).

Fig.3

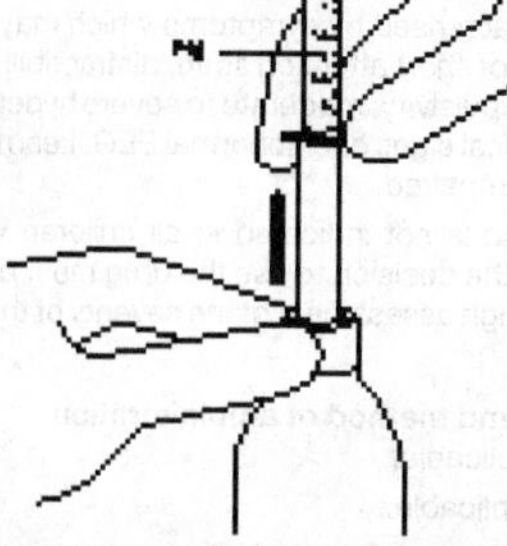

6. To empty the pipette, push down on the top ring while still holding the lower ring.
7. The contents of the pipette may be emptied directly into the mouth or into a drink of mineral water, orange juice or black coffee.
8. Rinse the pipette with some water.
9. Replace the child-resistant cap on the bottle by screwing it down clockwise until it locks fully.

Risperdal® Quicklet®: Please refer to Section 4.2. Posology and Method of Administration.

7. MARKETING AUTHORISATION HOLDER

Janssen-Cilag Ltd
Saunderton
High Wycombe
Buckinghamshire
HP14 4HJ
UK

8. MARKETING AUTHORISATION NUMBER(S)

Risperdal®:

0.5 mg tablets: PL 0242/0347
1 mg tablets: PL 0242/0186
2 mg tablets: PL 0242/0187
3 mg tablets: PL 0242/0188
4 mg tablets: PL 0242/0189
6 mg tablets: PL 0242/0317
1 mg/ml liquid: PL 0242/0199

Risperdal® Quicklet®:

0.5 mg:PL 0242/0378
1 mg: PL 0242/0379
2 mg: PL 0242/0380

9. DATE OF FIRST AUTHORISATION/RENEWAL OF THE AUTHORISATION

Risperdal®:

0.5 mg tablets: 30 June 2000/ 28 February 2004

1, 2, 3 and 4 mg tablets: 8 December 1992/8 December 1998/ 28 February 2004

6 mg tablets: 15 July 1997/ 28 February 2004

Liquid: 21 November 1995/ 28 February 2004

Risperdal® Quicklet®:

7 January 2003/ 28 February 2004

10. DATE OF REVISION OF THE TEXT

23 May 2005

LEGAL CATEGORY

POM

Ritalin

(Cephalon UK Limited)

1. NAME OF THE MEDICINAL PRODUCT

Ritalin®

2. QUALITATIVE AND QUANTITATIVE COMPOSITION

The active ingredient is Methylphenidate (INN for α-Phenyl-2-piperidineacetic acid methyl ester hydrochloride).

One tablet contains 10mg methylphenidate hydrochloride.

3. PHARMACEUTICAL FORM

Tablets.

4. CLINICAL PARTICULARS

4.1 Therapeutic indications

Ritalin is indicated as a part of a comprehensive treatment programme for attention-deficit hyperactivity disorder (ADHD) where remedial measures alone prove insufficient. Treatment must be under the supervision of a specialist in childhood behavioural disorders. Diagnosis should be made according to DSM-IV criteria or the guidelines in ICD-10.

Additional information on the safe use of the product: ADHD is also known as attention-deficit disorder (ADD). Other terms used to describe this behavioural syndrome include: hyperkinetic disorder, minimal brain damage, minimal brain dysfunction in children, minor cerebral dysfunction and psycho-organic syndrome of children.

A part of a comprehensive treatment programme, typically includes psychological, educational and social measures and is aimed at stabilising children with a behavioural syndrome characterised by symptoms which may include chronic history of short attention span, distractibility, emotional lability, impulsivity, moderate to severe hyperactivity, minor neurological signs and abnormal EEG. Learning may or may not be impaired.

Ritalin treatment is not indicated in all children with this syndrome and the decision to use the drug must be based on a very thorough assessment of the severity of the child's symptoms.

4.2 Posology and method of administration
Adults: Not applicable.

Elderly: Not applicable.

Children: (over 6 years). Begin with 5mg once or twice daily (e.g. at breakfast and lunch), increasing the dose and frequency of administration if necessary by weekly increments of 5-10mg in the daily dose. Doses above 60mg daily are not recommended. The total daily dose should be administered in divided doses. Ritalin is not indicated in children less than 6 years of age.

If the effect of the drug wears off too early in the evening, disturbed behaviour and/or inability to go to sleep may recur. A small evening dose may help to solve this problem.

Note: If improvement of symptoms is not observed after appropriate dosage adjustment over a one-month period, the drug should be discontinued. Ritalin should be discontinued periodically to assess the child's condition. Drug treatment is usually discontinued during or after puberty.

4.3 Contraindications
The presence of marked anxiety, agitation or tension is a contra-indication to the use of Ritalin as it may aggravate these symptoms.

Ritalin is also contra-indicated in patients with motor tics, tics in siblings, or a family history or diagnosis of Tourette's syndrome.

It is also contra-indicated in patients with hyperthyroidism, severe angina pectoris, cardiac arrhythmias, glaucoma, thyrotoxicosis, or known sensitivity to methylphenidate or to any of the excipients in Ritalin.

4.4 Special warnings and special precautions for use
Warnings

Ritalin should not be used in children under 6 years of age, since safety and efficacy in this age group have not been established.

Ritalin should not be used to treat severe exogenous or endogenous depression.

Clinical experience suggests that Ritalin may exacerbate symptoms of behavioural disturbance and thought disorder in psychotic children.

Available clinical evidence indicates that treatment during childhood does not increase the likelihood of addiction in later life.

Chronic abuse of Ritalin can lead to marked tolerance and psychological dependence with varying degrees of abnormal behaviour. Frank psychotic episodes may occur, especially with parenteral abuse.

Females of child-bearing potential (females post-menarche) should not use Ritalin unless clearly necessary (See Section 4.6, Pregnancy and Lactation and Section 5.3, Preclinical Safety Data).

Precautions

Treatment with Ritalin is not indicated in all cases of Attention-Deficit-Hyperactivity disorders, and should be considered only after detailed history-taking and evaluation. The decision to prescribe Ritalin should depend on an assessment of the severity of symptoms and their appropriateness to the child's age and not simply on the presence of one or more abnormal behavioural characteristics. Where these symptoms are associated with acute stress reactions, treatment with Ritalin is usually not indicated.

Moderately reduced weight gain and slight growth retardation have been reported with the long-term use of stimulants in children, although a causal relationship has not been confirmed. Careful monitoring of growth is recommended during extended treatment with Ritalin.

Blood pressure should be monitored at appropriate intervals in all patients taking Ritalin, especially those with hypertension.

Caution is called for in emotionally unstable patients, such as those with a history of drug dependence or alcoholism, because such patients may increase the dosage on their own initiative.

Ritalin should be used with caution in patients with epilepsy as clinical experience has shown that it can cause an increase in seizure frequency in a small number of such patients. If seizure frequency increases, Ritalin should be discontinued.

The long-term safety and efficacy profiles of Ritalin are not fully known. Patients requiring long-term therapy should therefore be carefully monitored and complete and differential blood counts and a platelet count performed periodically.

Careful supervision is required during drug withdrawal, since this may unmask depression as well as chronic over-activity. Some patients may require long-term follow-up.

4.5 Interaction with other medicinal products and other forms of Interaction
Human pharmacological studies have shown that Ritalin may inhibit the metabolism of coumarin anticoagulants, some anticonvulsants (e.g. phenobarbitone, phenytoin, primidone), phenylbutazone and tricyclic antidepressants. The dosage of these drugs may have to be reduced. Ritalin should be used cautiously in patients being treated with pressor agents and MAO inhibitors.

Ritalin may reduce the antihypertensive effects of guanethidine.

Alcohol may exacerbate the adverse CNS effect of psychoactive drugs, including Ritalin. It is therefore advisable for patients to abstain from alcohol during treatment.

4.6 Pregnancy and lactation
There are no adequate data from the use of Ritalin in pregnancy.

Studies in animals have shown reproductive toxicity (See Section 5.3, Preclinical Safety Data). The potential risk for humans is unknown.

Ritalin should not be used during pregnancy unless clearly necessary.

It is not known whether the active substance of Ritalin and/or its metabolites passes into breast milk, but for safety reasons breast-feeding mothers should not use Ritalin.

4.7 Effects on ability to drive and use machines
Ritalin may cause dizziness and drowsiness. It is therefore advisable to exercise caution when driving, operating machinery, or engaging in other potentially hazardous activities.

4.8 Undesirable effects
Frequency estimate: very common $\geqslant$ 10%; common $\geqslant$ 1% to $<$ 10%; uncommon $\geqslant$ 0.1% to $<$ 1%; rare $\geqslant$ 0.01% to $<$ 0.1%; very rare $<$ 0.01%.

Nervousness and insomnia are very common adverse reactions occurring at the beginning of treatment, but can usually be controlled by reducing the dosage and/or omitting the afternoon or evening dose.

Decreased appetite is also common but usually transient.

Central and peripheral nervous system:

Common: Headache, drowsiness, dizziness, dyskinesia.

Rare: Difficulties in visual accommodation, and blurred vision.

Very rare: Hyperactivity, convulsions, muscle cramps, choreo-athetoid movements, tics or exacerbation of existing tics, and Tourette's syndrome, toxic psychosis (sometimes with visual and tactile hallucinations), transient depressed mood, cerebral arteritis and/or occlusion.

Very rare reports of poorly documented neuroleptic malignant syndrome (NMS) have been received. In most of these reports patients were also receiving other medications. It is uncertain what role Ritalin played in these cases.

Gastro-intestinal tract:

Common: Abdominal pain, nausea and vomiting. These usually occur at the beginning of treatment and may be alleviated by concomitant food intake. Dry mouth.

Very rare: Abnormal liver function, ranging from transaminase elevation to hepatic coma.

Cardiovascular system:

Common: Tachycardia, palpitations, arrhythmias, changes in blood pressure and heart rate (usually an increase).

Rare: Angina pectoris.

Skin and appendages:

Common: Rash, pruritus, urticaria, fever, arthralgia, scalp hair loss.

Very rare: Thrombocytopenic purpura, exfoliative dermatitis, and erythema multiforme.

Blood:

Very rare: Leucopenia, thrombocytopenia, anaemia.

Miscellaneous:

Rare: Moderately reduced weight gain and slight growth retardation during prolonged use in children.

4.9 Overdose
Signs and symptoms

Acute overdose, mainly due to overstimulation of the central and sympathetic nervous systems, may result in vomiting, agitation, tremors, hyperreflexia, muscle twitching, convulsions (may be followed by coma), euphoria, confusion, hallucinations, delirium, sweating, flushing, headache, hyperpyrexia, tachycardia, palpitations, cardiac arrhythmias, hypertension, mydriasis, and dryness of mucous membranes.

Treatment

There is no specific antidote to Ritalin overdosage.

Management consists of appropriate supportive measures, preventing self-injury and protecting the patient from external stimuli that would aggravate over-stimulation already present. If the signs and symptoms are not too severe and the patient is conscious, gastric contents may be evacuated by induction of vomiting or gastric lavage. In the presence of severe intoxication, a carefully titrated dose of a short-acting barbiturate should be given before performing gastric lavage.

Intensive care must be provided to maintain adequate circulation and respiratory exchange; external cooling procedures may be required to reduce hyperpyrexia.

Efficacy of peritoneal dialysis or extracorporeal haemodialysis for overdose of Ritalin has not been established.

5. PHARMACOLOGICAL PROPERTIES
5.1 Pharmacodynamic properties
Mode of action: Ritalin is a mild CNS stimulant with more prominent effects on mental than on motor activities. Its mode of action in man is not completely understood but its effects are thought to be due to cortical stimulation and possibly to stimulation of the reticular activating system.

The mechanism by which Ritalin exerts its mental and behavioural effects in children is not clearly established, nor is there conclusive evidence showing how these effects relate to the condition of the central nervous system.

5.2 Pharmacokinetic properties
Absorption:

The active substance methylphenidate hydrochloride is rapidly and almost completely absorbed from the tablets. Owing to extensive first-pass metabolism its systemic availability amounts to only 30% (11-51%) of the dose. Ingestion together with food accelerates its absorption, but has no influence on the amount absorbed. Peak plasma concentrations of approximately 40nmol/litres (11ng/ml) are attained, on average, 1-2 hours after administration of 0.30mg/kg. The peak plasma concentrations, however, show considerable intersubject variability. The area under the plasma concentration curve (AUC), as well as the peak plasma concentration (Cmax), are proportional to the dose.

Distribution:

In the blood, methylphenidate and its metabolites become distributed in the plasma (57%) and the erythrocytes (43%). Methylphenidate and its metabolites have a low plasma protein-binding rate (10-33%). The apparent distribution volume has been calculated as 13.1 litres/kg.

Biotransformation

Biotransformation of methylphenidate is rapid and extensive. Peak plasma concentrations of α-phenyl-2-piperidyl acetic acid (PPAA) are attained approximately 2 hours after administration of methylphenidate and are 30-50 times higher than those of the unchanged substance. The half-life of PPAA is roughly twice as long as that of methylphenidate, and the mean systemic clearance is 0.17 litres/h/kg. Only small amounts of hydroxylated metabolites (e.g. hydroxymethylphenidate and hydroxyritalinic acid) are detectable. Therapeutic activity seems to be principally due to the parent compound.

Elimination:

Methylphenidate is eliminated from the plasma with a mean half-life of 2 hours, and the calculated mean systemic clearance is 10 litres/h/kg. Within 48-96 hours 78-97% of the dose administered is excreted in the urine and 1-3% in the faeces in the form of metabolites. Unchanged methylphenidate appears in the urine only in small quantities (<1%). The bulk of the dose is excreted in the urine as PPAA, (60-86%).

Characteristics in patients:

There are no apparent differences in the pharmacokinetic behaviour of methylphenidate in hyperactive children and healthy adult volunteers.

Elimination data from patients with normal renal function suggest that renal excretion of the unchanged methylphenidate would hardly be diminished at all in the presence of impaired renal function. However, renal excretion of PPAA may be reduced.

5.3 Preclinical safety data
There is evidence that methylphenidate may be a teratogen in two species. Spina bifida and limb malrotations have been reported in rabbits whilst in the rat, equivocal evidence of induction of abnormalities of the vertebrae was found.

Methylphenidate did not affect reproductive performance or fertility at low multiples of the clinical dose.

In life-time rat and mouse carcinogenicity studies, increased numbers of malignant liver tumours were noted in male mice only. The significance of this finding to humans is unknown.

The weight of evidence from geneotoxicity studies reveals no special hazard for humans.

6. PHARMACEUTICAL PARTICULARS
6.1 List of excipients
The tablets also contain calcium phosphate tribasic special, lactose, wheat starch, gelatin, magnesium stearate and talc.

6.2 Incompatibilities
None known.

6.3 Shelf life
Two years.

6.4 Special precautions for storage
Do not store above 25°C. Store in the original package.

Medicines should be kept out of reach of children.

6.5 Nature and contents of container

The tablets are available in blister packs of 30 tablets.

6.6 Instructions for use and handling

None

7. MARKETING AUTHORISATION HOLDER

Novartis Pharmaceuticals UK Limited

Trading as Ciba Laboratories

Frimley Business Park

Frimley

Camberley

Surrey

GU16 7SR.

8. MARKETING AUTHORISATION NUMBER(S)

PL 00101/0539

9. DATE OF FIRST AUTHORISATION/RENEWAL OF THE AUTHORISATION

31 October 1997 / 20 April 2004

10. DATE OF REVISION OF THE TEXT

26 July 2005

Legal Category

POM

Rivotril Ampoules

(Roche Products Limited)

1. NAME OF THE MEDICINAL PRODUCT

Rivotril Ampoules 1mg/ml

2. QUALITATIVE AND QUANTITATIVE COMPOSITION

Each ampoule contains 1mg of the active ingredient clonazepam.

For excipients, see 6.1.

3. PHARMACEUTICAL FORM

Concentrate for solution for injection or infusion.

Clear, colourless to slightly green-yellow solution.

4. CLINICAL PARTICULARS

4.1 Therapeutic indications

Administered intravenously, Rivotril quickly controls status epilepticus in all clinical forms.

4.2 Posology and method of administration

Rivotril ampoules are for intravenous administration. For the treatment of status epilepticus, the dose and rate of administration are governed by the response of the patient.

Adults

1mg (one ampoule of active substance mixed with one ampoule of diluent) by slow intravenous injection.

Elderly

Care should be taken with the elderly.

Children

0.5mg (equivalent to half an ampoule of active substance mixed with half an ampoule of diluent) by slow intravenous injection.

Special dosage instructions

Rivotril can be administered with one or several other antiepileptic agents, in which case the dosage of each drug must be adjusted to achieve optimum effect.

As with all antiepileptic agents, treatment with Rivotril must not be stopped abruptly, but must be reduced in a stepwise fashion (see section *4.8 Undesirable effects*).

Mode of administration

Rivotril must be diluted prior to administration in order to avoid irritation of the veins, see section *6.6 Instructions for use/handling*.

Intravenous injection of Rivotril should be into a large vein of the antecubital fossa. The injection should be given slowly - in adults, the rate of injection must not exceed 0.25mg – 0.5mg (0.5 – 1.0ml of the prepared solution) per minute – and should be administered with continuous monitoring of EEG, respiration and blood pressure. This will greatly diminish the rare possibility of hypotension or apnoea occurring. Nevertheless, facilities for resuscitation should always be available. A total dose of 20mg should not be exceeded.

Rivotril ampoule solution may be diluted when given in intravenous infusions of saline or glucose, such as are customary in the treatment of status epilepticus, see section *6.6 Instructions for use/handling*.

4.3 Contraindications

Patients with known sensitivity to benzodiazepines or any of the drugs excipients; acute pulmonary insufficiency, severe respiratory insufficiency, sleep apnoea syndrome, myasthenia gravis, severe hepatic insufficiency.

Rivotril ampoules contain benzyl alcohol. Since there have been reports of permanent neuropsychiatric deficits and multiple system organ failure associated with benzyl alcohol, administration to neonates, and especially to premature infants, must be avoided.

4.4 Special warnings and special precautions for use

Rivotril should be used with caution in patients with chronic pulmonary insufficiency, or with impairment of renal or hepatic function, and in the elderly or the debilitated. In these cases dosage should generally be reduced.

As with all other anti-epileptic drugs, treatment with Rivotril even if of short duration, must not be abruptly interrupted, but must be withdrawn by gradually reducing the dose in view of the risk of precipitating status epilepticus. This precaution must also be taken when withdrawing another drug while the patient is still receiving Rivotril therapy.

Rivotril may be used only with particular caution in patients with spinal or cerebellar ataxia, in the event of acute intoxication with alcohol or drugs and in patients with severe liver damage (e.g. cirrhosis of the liver).

Benzodiazepines should be used with extreme caution in patients with a history of alcohol or drug abuse.

In infants and small children Rivotril may cause increased production of saliva and bronchial secretion. Therefore special attention must be paid to maintaining patency of the airways.

The dosage of Rivotril must be carefully adjusted to individual requirements in patients with pre-existing disease of the respiratory system (e.g. chronic obstructive pulmonary disease) or liver and in patients undergoing treatment with other centrally acting medications or anticonvulsant (antiepileptic) agents (see section *4.5 Interaction with other medicaments and other forms of interaction*).

Like all drugs of this type, Rivotril may, depending on dosage, administration and individual susceptibility, modify the patients reactions (e.g. driving ability, behaviour in traffic).

Patients with a history of depression and/or suicide attempts should be kept under close supervision.

In cases of loss or bereavement, psychological adjustment may be inhibited by benzodiazepines.

During I.V. administration, a vein of sufficient caliber must be chosen and the injection administered very slowly, with continuous monitoring of respiration and blood pressure. If the injection is rapid or the caliber of the vein is insufficient, there is a risk of thrombophlebitis, which may in turn lead to thrombosis.

4.5 Interaction with other medicinal products and other forms of Interaction

Since alcohol can provoke epileptic seizures, irrespective of therapy, patients must under no circumstances drink alcohol while under treatment. In combination with Rivotril, alcohol may modify the effects of the drug, compromise the success of therapy or give rise to unpredictable side-effects.

When Rivotril is used in conjunction with other anti-epileptic drugs, side-effects such as sedation and apathy, and toxicity may be more evident, particularly with hydantoins or phenobarbitone and combinations including them. This requires extra care in adjusting dosage in the initial stages of treatment. The combination of Rivotril and sodium valproate has, rarely, been associated with the development of absence status epilepticus. Although some patients tolerate and benefit from this combination of drugs, this potential hazard should be borne in mind when its use is considered.

Known inhibitors of hepatic enzymes, e.g. cimetidine, have been shown to reduce the clearance of benzodiazepines and may potentiate their action and known inducers of hepatic enzymes, e.g. rifampicin, may increase the clearance of benzodiazepines.

In concurrent treatment with phenytoin or primidone, a change, usually a rise in the serum concentration of these two substances has occasionally been observed.

Concurrent use of Rivotril and other centrally acting medications, e.g. other anticonvulsant (antiepileptic) agents, anaesthetics, hypnotics, psychoactive drugs and some analgesics as well as muscle-relaxants may result in mutual potentiation of drug effects. This is especially true in the presence of alcohol. In combination therapy with centrally-acting medications, the dosage of each drug must be adjusted to achieve the optimum effect.

4.6 Pregnancy and lactation

Preclinical studies in animals have shown reproductive toxicity (see section *5.3 Preclinical safety data*). From epidemiological evaluations there is evidence that anticonvulsant drugs act as teratogens.

Rivotril has harmful pharmacological effects on pregnancy and the foetus/newborn child. Administration of high doses in the last trimester of pregnancy or during labour can cause irregularities in the heart beat of the unborn child and hypothermia, hypotonia, mild respiratory depression and poor sucking in the neonate. Infants born to mothers who took benzodiazepines chronically during the later stages of pregnancy may have developed physical dependence and may be at some risk for developing withdrawal symptoms in the post-natal period. Therefore Rivotril should not be used in pregnancy unless clearly necessary.

The active ingredient of Rivotril has been found to pass into the maternal milk in small amounts. Therefore Rivotril should not be used in mothers who breastfeed unless clearly necessary.

4.7 Effects on ability to drive and use machines

As a general rule, epileptic patients are not allowed to drive. Even when adequately controlled on Rivotril, it should be remembered that any increase in dosage or alteration in timings of dosage may modify patients' reactions, depending on individual susceptibility. Even if taken as directed, clonazepam can slow reactions to such an extent that the ability to drive a vehicle or operate machinery is impaired. This effect is aggravated by consumption of alcohol. Driving, operating machinery and other hazardous activities should therefore be avoided altogether or at least during the first few days of treatment. The decision on this question rests with the patients physician and should be based on the patient's response to treatment and the dosage involved.

4.8 Undesirable effects

The side-effects observed consist of fatigue, muscle weakness, dizziness, ataxia, light-headedness, somnolence, occasional muscular hypotonia and co-ordination disturbances. Such effects are usually transitory and disappear spontaneously as treatment continues or with dosage reduction. They tend to occur early in treatment and can be greatly reduced, if not avoided, by commencing with low dosages followed by progressive increases.

Poor concentration, restlessness, confusion and disorientation have been observed. Anterograde amnesia may occur using benzodiazepines at therapeutic dosage, the risk increasing at higher dosages. Amnestic effects may be associated with inappropriate behaviour.

Depression may occur in patients treated with Rivotril, but it may be also associated with the underlying disease.

In rare cases, urticaria, pruritus, transient hairloss, pigmentation changes, nausea, gastrointestinal symptoms, headache, decrease in sexual drive (loss of libido), impotence and urinary incontinence may occur. Isolated cases of reversible development of premature secondary sex characteristics in children (incomplete precocious puberty) have been reported. Allergic reactions and a very few cases of anaphylaxis and angioedema have been reported to occur with benzodiazepines.

Particularly in long-term or high-dose treatment, reversible disorders such as a slowing or slurring of speech (dysarthria), reduced co-ordination of movements and gait (ataxia) and disorders of vision (double vision, nystagmus) may occur.

Rarely respiratory depression may occur with intravenous Rivotril, particularly if other depressant drugs have been administered. As a rule, this effect can be avoided by careful adjustment of the dose in individual requirements.

Use of benzodiazepines may lead to the development of physical and psychological dependence upon these products. The risk of dependence increases with dose and duration of treatment and is particularly pronounced in predisposed patients with a history of alcoholism or drug abuse.

Once physical dependence has developed, abrupt termination of treatment will be accompanied by withdrawal symptoms. During long-term treatment, withdrawal symptoms may develop, especially with high doses or if the daily dose is reduced rapidly or abruptly discontinued. The symptoms include tremor, sweating, agitation, sleep disturbances and anxiety, headaches, muscle pain, extreme anxiety, tension, restlessness, confusion, irritability and epileptic seizures which may be associated with the underlying disease. In severe cases the following symptoms may occur: derealisation, depersonalisation, hyperacusis, numbness and tingling of the extremities, hypersensitivity to light, noise and physical contact or hallucinations. Since the risk of withdrawal symptoms is greater after abrupt discontinuation of treatment, abrupt withdrawal of the drug should therefore be avoided and treatment - even if only of short duration - should be terminated by gradually reducing the daily dose.

In infants and small children, and particularly those with a degree of mental impairment, Rivotril may give rise to salivary or bronchial hypersecretion with drooling. Supervision of the airway may be required.

With certain forms of epilepsy, an increase in the frequency of seizures during long-term treatment is possible.

As with other benzodiazepines, isolated cases of blood dyscrasias and abnormal liver function tests have been reported.

Rivotril generally has a beneficial effect on behaviour disturbances in epileptic patients. In certain cases, paradoxical effects such as aggressiveness, excitability, nervousness, hostility, anxiety, sleep disturbances, nightmares, vivid dreams, irritability, agitation, psychotic disorders and activation of new types of seizures may be precipitated. If these occur, the benefit of continuing the drug should be weighed against the adverse effect. The addition to the regimen of another suitable drug may be necessary or, in some cases, it may be advisable to discontinue Rivotril therapy.

Although Rivotril has been given uneventfully to patients with porphyria, rarely it may induce convulsions in these patients.

During IV administration, a vein of sufficient caliber must be chosen and the injection administered very slowly, with continuous monitoring of respiration and blood pressure. In adults, the rate of injection must not exceed 0.25 – 0.5mg (0.5 – 1ml of the prepared solution) per minute (see section *4.2 Posology and method of administration*). If the injection is rapid or the caliber of the vein is insufficient, there is a risk of thrombophlebitis, which may in turn lead to thrombosis.

4.9 Overdose

As with other benzodiazepine drugs, overdosage should not present undue problems of management or threat to life. Patients have recovered from overdoses in excess of 60mg without special treatment. Severe somnolence with muscle hypotonia will be present. Treatment is symptomatic and may include the need to maintain an airway. Gastric lavage may be useful if performed soon after ingestion.

The symptoms of overdosage or intoxication vary greatly from person to person depending on age, bodyweight and individual response. They range from drowsiness and light-headedness to ataxia, somnolence and stupor, and finally to coma with respiratory depression and circulatory collapse. Serious sequelae are rare unless other drugs or alcohol have been taken concomitantly.

In the management of overdose it should be borne in mind, that multiple agents may have been taken. In addition to monitoring of respiration, pulse rate and blood pressure, IV fluid replacement with general supportive measures is indicated. Hypotension may be treated with sympathomimetic agents.

The value of dialysis has not been determined.

Overdosage in non-epileptic patients may be treated with flumazenil, a specific IV antidote for use in emergency situations. Patients requiring such intervention should be monitored closely in hospital (see separate prescribing information).

Warning

The use of flumazenil is not recommended in epileptic patients who have been receiving benzodiazepine treatment for a prolonged period. Although flumazenil exerts a slight intrinsic anticonvulsant effect, its abrupt suppression of the protective effect of a benzodiazepine agonist can give rise to convulsions in epileptic patients.

If excitation occurs, barbiturates should not be used.

5. PHARMACOLOGICAL PROPERTIES

5.1 Pharmacodynamic properties

Clonazepam exhibits pharmacological properties which are common to benzodiazepines and include anticonvulsive, sedative, muscle relaxing and anxiolytic effects. Animal data and electroencephalographic investigations in man have shown that clonazepam rapidly suppresses many types of paroxysmal activity including the spike and wave discharge in absences seizures (petit mal), slow spike wave, generalised spike wave, spikes with temporal or other locations as well as irregular spikes and waves.

Generalised EEG abnormalities are more readily suppressed by clonazepam than are focal EEG abnormalities such as focal spikes. Clonazepam has beneficial effects in generalised and focal epilepsies.

5.2 Pharmacokinetic properties

Absorption

Clonazepam is quickly and completely absorbed after oral administration of Rivotril. Peak plasma concentrations are reached in most cases within 1 - 4 hours after an oral dose. Bioavailability is 90% after oral administration.

Routine monitoring of plasma concentrations of Rivotril is of unproven value since this does not appear to correlate well with either therapeutic response or side-effects.

Distribution

The mean volume of distribution of clonazepam is estimated at about 3 l/kg. Clonazepam must be assumed to cross the placental barrier and has been detected in maternal milk.

Metabolism

The biotransformation of clonazepam involves oxidative hydroxylation and reduction of the 7-nitro group by the liver with formation of 7-amino or 7-acetylamino compounds, with trace amounts of 3-hydroxy derivatives of all three compounds, and their glucuronide and sulphate conjugates. The nitro compounds are pharmacologically active, whereas the amino compounds are not.

Within 4 - 10 days 50 - 70% of the total radioactivity of a radiolabeled oral dose of clonazepam is excreted in the urine and 10 - 30% in the faeces, almost exclusively in the form of free or conjugated metabolites. Less than 0.5% appears as unchanged clonazepam in the urine.

Elimination

The elimination half-life is between 20 and 60 hours (mean 30 hours).

Pharmacokinetics in special clinical situations

Based on kinetic criteria no dose adjustment is required in patients with renal failure.

5.3 Preclinical safety data

In pre-clinical murine studies there was at least a two fold increase in teratogenic birth defects at dose levels of 3, 9 and 18 times the human therapeutic dose compared to the controls.

6. PHARMACEUTICAL PARTICULARS

6.1 List of excipients

Active substance ampoule: Ethanol absolute, glacial acetic acid, benzyl alcohol, propylene glycol, nitrogen pure.

Diluent ampoule: Water for injections.

6.2 Incompatibilities

It is recommended that Rivotril is only diluted in accordance with instructions given under section *4.2 Posology and method of administration* and section *6.6 Instructions for use/handling*.

6.3 Shelf life

60 months.

6.4 Special precautions for storage

Rivotril ampoules (active and diluent) should be protected from light and stored below 30°C.

6.5 Nature and contents of container

Each pack either contains five amber glass ampoules containing 1mg clonazepam (active) and five amber glass ampoules containing 1ml Water for Injections Ph. Eur. (diluent) or ten amber glass ampoules containing 1mg clonazepam (active) and ten amber glass ampoules containing 1ml Water for Injections Ph. Eur. (diluent).

6.6 Instructions for use and handling

Preparation of Rivotril intravenous injection:

The contents of the diluent ampoule, which contains 1ml Water for Injection Ph. Eur., *must* be added to the contents of the other ampoule, which contains 1mg clonazepam in 1ml, *immediately* before injection.

Preparation of Rivotril intravenous infusion:

Up to 3mg (3 ampoules) in 250ml of the following solutions is permissible:

Sodium chloride intravenous infusion 0.9% w/v BP

Glucose intravenous infusion BP 5% and 10%

Sodium chloride and Glucose intravenous infusion BP (0.45% sodium chloride and 2.5% glucose)

Do not prepare Rivotril infusions using sodium bicarbonate solution, as otherwise precipitation of the solution may occur.

From a chemical and physical stability point of view the product is stable for up to 12 hours. However, it should be used immediately after dilution in order to reduce the possibility of microbial contamination unless it is diluted under validated aseptic conditions.

The active ingredient clonazepam can be absorbed on PVC. It is therefore recommended either glass containers be used or, if PVC infusion bags are used, that the mixture be infused straight-away over a period of no longer than 2 hours.

Maintenance of stability cannot be guaranteed when Rivotril ampoule solution is diluted.

7. MARKETING AUTHORISATION HOLDER

Roche Products Limited
40 Broadwater Road
Welwyn Garden City
Hertfordshire
AL7 3AY

8. MARKETING AUTHORISATION NUMBER(S)

PL 0031/0078R

9. DATE OF FIRST AUTHORISATION/RENEWAL OF THE AUTHORISATION

20 February 1991/24 September 1996

10. DATE OF REVISION OF THE TEXT

July 2005

Rivotril is a registered trade mark

Rivotril Tablets

(Roche Products Limited)

1. NAME OF THE MEDICINAL PRODUCT

Rivotril 0.5mg Tablets

Rivotril 2mg Tablets

2. QUALITATIVE AND QUANTITATIVE COMPOSITION

Rivotril 0.5mg Tablets: Each tablet contains 0.5mg clonazepam.

Rivotril 2mg Tablets: Each tablet contains 2mg clonazepam.

For excipients, see 6.1.

3. PHARMACEUTICAL FORM

Tablets.

Rivotril 0.5mg Tablets: Round, dull pinkish-buff tablets with Roche 0.5 imprinted on one face and two break bars on the other

Rivotril 2mg Tablets: Round, white tablets with Roche 2 imprinted on one face and two break bars on the other.

4. CLINICAL PARTICULARS

4.1 Therapeutic indications

Tablets: All clinical forms of epileptic disease and seizures in infants, children and adults, especially absence seizures (petit mal) including atypical absence; primary or secondarily generalised tonic-clonic (grand mal), tonic or clonic seizures; partial (focal) seizures with elementary or complex symptomatology; various forms of myoclonic seizures, myoclonus and associated abnormal movements.

4.2 Posology and method of administration

The cross-scored 0.5mg tablets facilitate the administration of lower daily doses in the initial stages of treatment.

Adults

Initial dosage should not exceed 1mg/day. The maintenance dosage for adults normally falls within the range 4 to 8mg.

Elderly

The elderly are particularly sensitive to the effects of centrally depressant drugs and may experience confusion. It is recommended that the initial dosage of Rivotril should not exceed 0.5mg/day.

These are total daily dosages which should be divided into 3 or 4 doses taken at intervals throughout the day. If necessary, larger doses may be given at the discretion of the physician, up to a maximum of 20mg daily. The maintenance dose should be attained after 2 to 4 weeks of treatment.

Infants and children

To ensure optimum dosage adjustment, children should be given the 0.5mg tablets.

Initial dosage should not exceed 0.25mg/day for infants and small children (1 to 5 years) and 0.5mg/day for older children. The maintenance dosage normally falls within the ranges:

School children (5 to 12 years) 3 to 6mg

Small children (1 to 5 years) 1 to 3mg

Infants (0 to 1 year) 0.5 to 1mg

In some forms of childhood epilepsy, certain patients may cease to be adequately controlled by Rivotril. Control may be re-established by increasing the dose, or interrupting treatment with Rivotril for 2 or 3 weeks. During the interruption in therapy, careful observation and other drugs may be needed.

Mode of administration

Treatment should be started with low doses. The dose may be increased progressively until the maintenance dose suited to the individual patient has been found.

The dosage of Rivotril must be adjusted to the needs of each individual and depends on the individual response to therapy. The maintenance dosage must be determined according to clinical response and tolerance.

The daily dose should be divided into 3 equal doses. If doses are not equally divided, the largest dose should be given before retiring. Once the maintenance dose level has been reached, the daily amount may be given in a single dose in the evening.

Simultaneous administration of more than one antiepileptic drug is a common practice in the treatment of epilepsy and may be undertaken with Rivotril. The dosage of each drug may be required to be adjusted to obtain the optimum effect. If status epilepticus occurs in a patient receiving oral Rivotril, intravenous Rivotril may still control the status. Before adding Rivotril to an existing anticonvulsant regimen, it should be considered that the use of multiple anticonvulsants may result in an increase of undesired effects.

4.3 Contraindications

Patients with known sensitivity to benzodiazepines; or any of the drugs excipients; acute pulmonary insufficiency; severe respiratory insufficiency, sleep apnoea syndrome, myasthenia gravis, severe hepatic insufficiency.

4.4 Special warnings and special precautions for use

Rivotril should be used with caution in patients with chronic pulmonary insufficiency, or with impairment of renal or hepatic function, and in the elderly or the debilitated. In these cases dosage should generally be reduced.

As with all other antiepileptic drugs, treatment with Rivotril even if of short duration, must not be abruptly interrupted, but must be withdrawn by gradually reducing the dose in view of the risk of precipitating status epilepticus. This precaution must also be taken when withdrawing another drug while the patient is still receiving Rivotril therapy.

Prolonged use of benzodiazepines may result in dependence development with withdrawal symptoms on cessation of use.

Rivotril may be used only with particular caution in patients with spinal or cerebellar ataxia, in the event of acute intoxication with alcohol or drugs and in patients with severe liver damage (e.g. cirrhosis of the liver).

Benzodiazepines should be used with extreme caution in patients with a history of alcohol or drug abuse.

In infants and small children Rivotril may cause increased production of saliva and bronchial secretion. Therefore special attention must be paid to maintaining patency of the airways.

The dosage of Rivotril must be carefully adjusted to individual requirements in patients with pre-existing disease of the respiratory system (e.g. chronic obstructive pulmonary disease) or liver and in patients undergoing treatment with other centrally acting medications or anticonvulsant (antiepileptic) agents (see *Section 4.5 Interaction with other medicinal products and other forms of interaction*).

Like all drugs of this type, Rivotril may, depending on dosage, administration and individual susceptibility, modify the patients reactions (e.g. driving ability, behaviour in traffic).

Patients with a history of depression and/or suicide attempts should be kept under close supervision.

In cases of loss or bereavement, psychological adjustment may be inhibited by benzodiazepines.

4.5 Interaction with other medicinal products and other forms of Interaction

Since alcohol can provoke epileptic seizures, irrespective of therapy, patients must under no circumstances drink alcohol while under treatment. In combination with Rivotril, alcohol may modify the effects of the drug, compromise the success of therapy or give rise to unpredictable side-effects.

When Rivotril is used in conjunction with other antiepileptic drugs, side-effects such as sedation and apathy, and toxicity may be more evident, particularly with hydantoins or phenobarbital and combinations including them. This requires extra care in adjusting dosage in the initial stages of treatment. The combination of Rivotril and sodium valproate has, rarely, been associated with the development of absence status epilepticus. Although some patients tolerate and benefit from this combination of drugs, this potential hazard should be borne in mind when its use is considered.

Known inhibitors of hepatic enzymes, e.g. cimetidine, have been shown to reduce the clearance of benzodiazepines and may potentiate their action and known inducers of hepatic enzymes, e.g. rifampicin, may increase the clearance of benzodiazepines.

In concurrent treatment with phenytoin or primidone, a change, usually a rise in the serum concentration of these two substances has occasionally been observed.

Concurrent use of Rivotril and other centrally acting medications, e.g. other anticonvulsant (antiepileptic) agents, anaesthetics, hypnotics, psychoactive drugs and some analgesics as well as muscle-relaxants may result in mutual potentiation of drug effects. This is especially true in the presence of alcohol. In combination therapy with centrally-acting medications, the dosage of each drug must be adjusted to achieve the optimum effect.

4.6 Pregnancy and lactation

Preclinical studies in animals have shown reproductive toxicity (see *section 5.3 Preclinical safety data*). From epidemiological evaluations there is evidence that anticonvulsant drugs act as teratogens.

Rivotril has harmful pharmacological effects on pregnancy and the foetus/newborn child. Administration of high doses in the last trimester of pregnancy or during labour can cause irregularities in the heart beat of the unborn child and hypothermia, hypotonia, mild respiratory depression and poor sucking in the neonate. Infants born to mothers who took benzodiazepines chronically during the later stages of pregnancy may have developed physical dependence and may be at some risk for developing withdrawal symptoms in the post-natal period. Therefore Rivotril should not be used in pregnancy unless clearly necessary.

The active ingredient of Rivotril has been found to pass into the maternal milk in small amounts. Therefore Rivotril should not be used in mothers who breastfeed unless clearly necessary.

4.7 Effects on ability to drive and use machines

As a general rule, epileptic patients are not allowed to drive. Even when adequately controlled on Rivotril, it should be remembered that any increase in dosage or alteration in timings of dosage may modify patients' reactions, depending on individual susceptibility. Even if taken as directed, clonazepam can slow reactions to such an extent that the ability to drive a vehicle or operate machinery is impaired. This effect is aggravated by consumption of alcohol. Driving, operating machinery and other hazardous activities should therefore be avoided altogether or at least during the first few days of treatment. The decision on this question rests with the patients physician and should be based on the patient's response to treatment and the dosage involved.

4.8 Undesirable effects

The side-effects observed consist of fatigue, muscle weakness, dizziness, ataxia, light-headedness, somnolence, occasional muscular hypotonia and co-ordination disturbances. Such effects are usually transitory and disappear spontaneously as treatment continues or with dosage reduction. They tend to occur early in treatment and can be greatly reduced, if not avoided, by commencing with low dosages followed by progressive increases.

Poor concentration, restlessness, confusion and disorientation have been observed. Anterograde amnesia may occur using benzodiazepines at therapeutic dosage, the risk increasing at higher dosages. Amnestic effects may be associated with inappropriate behaviour.

Depression may occur in patients treated with Rivotril, but it may be also associated with the underlying disease.

In rare cases, urticaria, pruritus, transient hairloss, pigmentation changes, nausea, gastrointestinal symptoms, headache, decrease in sexual drive (loss of libido), impotence and urinary incontinence may occur. Isolated cases of reversible development of premature secondary sex characteristics in children (incomplete precocious puberty) have been reported. Allergic reactions and a very few cases of anaphylaxis and angioedema have been reported to occur with benzodiazepines.

Particularly in long-term or high-dose treatment, reversible disorders such as a slowing or slurring of speech (dysarthria), reduced co-ordination of movements and gait (ataxia) and disorders of vision (double vision, nystagmus) may occur.

Rarely respiratory depression may occur with intravenous Rivotril, particularly if other depressant drugs have been administered. As a rule, this effect can be avoided by careful adjustment of the dose in individual requirements.

Use of benzodiazepines may lead to the development of physical and psychological dependence upon these products. The risk of dependence increases with dose and duration of treatment and is particularly pronounced in predisposed patients with a history of alcoholism or drug abuse.

Once physical dependence has developed, abrupt termination of treatment will be accompanied by withdrawal symptoms. During long-term treatment, withdrawal symptoms may develop, especially with high doses or if the daily dose is reduced rapidly or abruptly discontinued. The symptoms include tremor, sweating, agitation, sleep disturbances and anxiety, headaches, muscle pain, extreme anxiety, tension, restlessness, confusion, irritability and epileptic seizures which may be associated with the underlying disease. In severe cases the following symptoms may occur: derealisation, depersonalisation, hyperacusis, numbness and tingling of the extremities, hypersensitivity to light, noise and physical contact or hallucinations. Since the risk of withdrawal symptoms is greater after abrupt discontinuation of treatment, abrupt withdrawal of the drug should therefore be avoided and treatment - even if only of short duration - should be terminated by gradually reducing the daily dose.

In infants and small children, and particularly those with a degree of mental impairment, Rivotril may give rise to salivary or bronchial hypersecretion with drooling. Supervision of the airway may be required.

With certain forms of epilepsy, an increase in the frequency of seizures during long-term treatment is possible.

As with other benzodiazepines, isolated cases of blood dyscrasias and abnormal liver function tests have been reported.

Rivotril generally has a beneficial effect on behaviour disturbances in epileptic patients. In certain cases, paradoxical effects such as aggressiveness, excitability, nervousness, hostility, anxiety, sleep disturbances, nightmares, vivid dreams, irritability, agitation, psychotic disorders and activation of new types of seizures may be precipitated. If these occur, the benefit of continuing the drug should be weighed against the adverse effect. The addition to the regimen of another suitable drug may be necessary or, in some cases, it may be advisable to discontinue Rivotril therapy.

Although Rivotril has been given uneventfully to patients with porphyria, rarely it may induce convulsions in these patients.

4.9 Overdose

As with other benzodiazepine drugs, overdosage should not present undue problems of management or threat to life. Patients have recovered from overdoses in excess of 60mg without special treatment. Severe somnolence with muscle hypotonia will be present. Treatment is symptomatic and may include the need to maintain an airway. Gastric lavage may be useful if performed soon after ingestion.

The symptoms of overdosage or intoxication vary greatly from person to person depending on age, bodyweight and individual response. They range from drowsiness and light-headedness to ataxia, somnolence and stupor, and finally to coma with respiratory depression and circulatory collapse. Serious sequelae are rare unless other drugs or alcohol have been taken concomitantly.

In the management of overdose it should be borne in mind, that multiple agents may have been taken. In addition to monitoring of respiration, pulse rate and blood pressure, IV fluid replacement with general supportive measures is indicated. Hypotension may be treated with sympathomimetic agents.

The value of dialysis has not been determined.

Overdosage in non-epileptic patients may be treated with Anexate, a specific IV antidote for use in emergency situations. Patients requiring such intervention should be monitored closely in hospital (*see separate prescribing information*).

Warning

The use of Anexate is not recommended in epileptic patients who have been receiving benzodiazepine treatment for a prolonged period. Although Anexate exerts a slight intrinsic anticonvulsant effect, its abrupt suppression of the protective effect of a benzodiazepine agonist can give rise to convulsions in epileptic patients.

If excitation occurs, barbiturates should not be used.

5. PHARMACOLOGICAL PROPERTIES

5.1 Pharmacodynamic properties

Clonazepam exhibits pharmacological properties which are common to benzodiazepines and include anticonvulsive, sedative, muscle relaxing and anxiolytic effects. Animal data and electroencephalographic investigations in man have shown that clonazepam rapidly suppresses many types of paroxysmal activity including the spike and wave discharge in absence seizures (petit mal), slow spike wave, generalised spike wave, spikes with temporal or other locations as well as irregular spikes and waves.

Generalised EEG abnormalities are more readily suppressed by clonazepam than are focal EEG abnormalities such as focal spikes. Clonazepam has beneficial effects in generalised and focal epilepsies.

5.2 Pharmacokinetic properties

Absorption

Clonazepam is quickly and completely absorbed after oral administration of Rivotril. Peak plasma concentrations are reached in most cases within 1 - 4 hours after an oral dose. Bioavailability is 90% after oral administration.

Routine monitoring of plasma concentrations of Rivotril is of unproven value since this does not appear to correlate well with either therapeutic response or side-effects.

Distribution

The mean volume of distribution of clonazepam is estimated at about 3 l/kg. Clonazepam must be assumed to cross the placental barrier and has been detected in maternal milk.

Metabolism

The biotransformation of clonazepam involves oxidative hydroxylation and reduction of the 7-nitro group by the liver with formation of 7-amino or 7-acetylamino compounds, with trace amounts of 3-hydroxy derivatives of all three compounds, and their glucuronide and sulphate conjugates. The nitro compounds are pharmacologically active, whereas the amino compounds are not.

Within 4 - 10 days 50 - 70% of the total radioactivity of a radiolabelled oral dose of clonazepam is excreted in the urine and 10 - 30% in the faeces, almost exclusively in the form of free or conjugated metabolites. Less than 0.5% appears as unchanged clonazepam in the urine.

Elimination

The elimination half-life is between 20 and 60 hours (mean 30 hours).

Pharmacokinetics in special clinical situations

Based on kinetic criteria no dose adjustment is required in patients with renal failure.

5.3 Preclinical safety data

In preclinical murine studies there was at least a two fold increase in teratogenic birth defects at dose levels of 3, 9 and 18 times the human therapeutic dose compared to the controls.

6. PHARMACEUTICAL PARTICULARS

6.1 List of excipients

Rivotril 0.5mg tablets:

Lactose (monohydrate)

Maize starch

Pregelatinised potato starch

Talc

Magnesium stearate

Deionised water

Dye iron oxide red E172

Dye iron oxide yellow E172.

Rivotril 2mg tablets:

Lactose (anhydrous)

Pregelatinised maize starch

Magnesium stearate

Microcrystalline cellulose.

6.2 Incompatibilities

Not applicable.

6.3 Shelf life

Blisters:

Rivotril 0.5mg Tablets: 60 months

Rivotril 2mg Tablets: 36 months

Bottles:

Rivotril 0.5mg Tablets: 60 months

Rivotril 2mg Tablets: 60 months

6.4 Special precautions for storage

Store in the original container and in the outer carton

6.5 Nature and contents of container

Rivotril tablets are available in plastic HDPE bottles with polyethylene snap closures, or amber glass bottles with aluminium screw closures, containing either 100 or 500 tablets and PVC blister packs containing 100 tablets.

6.6 Instructions for use and handling

There are no special instructions.

7. MARKETING AUTHORISATION HOLDER

Roche Products Limited

40 Broadwater Road

Welwyn Garden City

Hertfordshire

AL7 3AY.

8. MARKETING AUTHORISATION NUMBER(S)

Rivotril 0.5mg Tablets: PL 00031/0076R

Rivotril 2mg Tablets: PL 00031/0077R

9. DATE OF FIRST AUTHORISATION/RENEWAL OF THE AUTHORISATION
26 July 1983/27 May 2005

10. DATE OF REVISION OF THE TEXT
May 2005
Rivotril is a registered trade mark

Roaccutane

(Roche Products Limited)

1. NAME OF THE MEDICINAL PRODUCT
Roaccutane 5 mg soft capsules

Roaccutane 20 mg soft capsules

2. QUALITATIVE AND QUANTITATIVE COMPOSITION
Each soft capsule contains 5 mg or 20 mg of isotretinoin

For excipients, see 6.1.

3. PHARMACEUTICAL FORM
Capsules, soft

5mg capsule: Oval, opaque, pale red-violet and white capsules imprinted with R5 in black ink.

20mg capsule: Oval, opaque, pale red-violet and white capsules imprinted with R20 in black ink.

4. CLINICAL PARTICULARS

4.1 Therapeutic indications
Severe forms of acne (such as nodular or conglobate acne or acne at risk of permanent scarring) resistant to adequate courses of standard therapy with systemic antibacterials and topical therapy.

4.2 Posology and method of administration
Isotretinoin should only be prescribed by or under the supervision of physicians with expertise in the use of systemic retinoids for the treatment of severe acne and a full understanding of the risks of isotretinoin therapy and monitoring requirements.

The capsules should be taken with food once or twice daily.

Adults including adolescents and the elderly:

Isotretinoin therapy should be started at a dose of 0.5 mg/kg daily. The therapeutic response to isotretinoin and some of the adverse effects are dose-related and vary between patients. This necessitates individual dosage adjustment during therapy. For most patients, the dose ranges from 0.5-1.0 mg/kg per day.

Long-term remission and relapse rates are more closely related to the total dose administered than to either duration of treatment or daily dose. It has been shown that no substantial additional benefit is to be expected beyond a cumulative treatment dose of 120-150 mg/kg. The duration of treatment will depend on the individual daily dose. A treatment course of 16-24 weeks is normally sufficient to achieve remission.

In the majority of patients, complete clearing of the acne is obtained with a single treatment course. In the event of a definite relapse a further course of isotretinoin therapy may be considered using the same daily dose and cumulative treatment dose. As further improvement of the acne can be observed up to 8 weeks after discontinuation of treatment, a further course of treatment should not be considered until at least this period has elapsed.

Patients with severe renal insufficiency

In patients with severe renal insufficiency treatment should be started at a lower dose (e.g. 10 mg/day). The dose should then be increased up to 1 mg/kg/day or until the patient is receiving the maximum tolerated dose (see section 4.4).

Children

Isotretinoin is not indicated for the treatment of prepubertal acne and is not recommended in patients less than 12 years of age.

Patients with intolerance

In patients who show severe intolerance to the recommended dose, treatment may be continued at a lower dose with the consequences of a longer therapy duration and a higher risk of relapse. In order to achieve the maximum possible efficacy in these patients the dose should normally be continued at the highest tolerated dose.

4.3 Contraindications
Isotretinoin is contraindicated in women who are pregnant or breastfeeding. (see section 4.6).

Isotretinoin is contraindicated in women of childbearing potential unless all of the conditions of the Pregnancy Prevention Programme are met (see section 4.4).

Isotretinoin is also contraindicated in patients with hypersensitivity to isotretinoin or to any of the excipients. Roaccutane contains arachis oil (peanut oil), soya oil, partially hydrogenated soya oil, and hydrogenated soya oil. Therefore, Roaccutane is contraindicated in patients allergic to peanut or soya.

Isotretinoin is also contraindicated in patients

- With hepatic insufficiency
- With excessively elevated blood lipid values
- With hypervitaminosis A
- Receiving concomitant treatment with tetracyclines (see section 4.5)

4.4 Special warnings and special precautions for use
Pregnancy Prevention Programme

This medicinal product is TERATOGENIC

Isotretinoin is contraindicated in women of childbearing potential unless all of the following conditions of the Pregnancy Prevention Programme are met:

- She has severe acne (such as nodular or conglobate acne or acne at risk of permanent scarring) resistant to adequate courses of standard therapy with systemic antibacterials and topical therapy (see section 4.1).
- She understands the teratogenic risk.
- She understands the need for rigorous follow-up, on a monthly basis.
- She understands and accepts the need for effective contraception, without interruption, 1 month before starting treatment, throughout the duration of treatment and 1 month after the end of treatment. At least one and preferably two complementary forms of contraception including a barrier method should be used.
- Even if she has amenorrhea she must follow all of the advice on effective contraception.
- She should be capable of complying with effective contraceptive measures.
- She is informed and understands the potential consequences of pregnancy and the need to rapidly consult if there is a risk of pregnancy.
- She understands the need and accepts to undergo pregnancy testing before, during and 5 weeks after the end of treatment.
- She has acknowledged that she has understood the hazards and necessary precautions associated with the use of isotretinoin.

These conditions also concern women who are not currently sexually active unless the prescriber considers that there are compelling reasons to indicate that there is no risk of pregnancy.

The prescriber must ensure that:

- The patient complies with the conditions for pregnancy prevention as listed above, including confirmation that she has an adequate level of understanding.
- The patient has acknowledged the aforementioned conditions.
- The patient has used at least one and preferably two methods of effective contraception including a barrier method for at least 1 month prior to starting treatment and is continuing to use effective contraception throughout the treatment period and for at least 1 month after cessation of treatment.
- Negative pregnancy test results have been obtained before, during and 5 weeks after the end of treatment. The dates and results of pregnancy tests should be documented.

Contraception

Female patients must be provided with comprehensive information on pregnancy prevention and should be referred for contraceptive advice if they are not using effective contraception.

As a minimum requirement, female patients at potential risk of pregnancy must use at least one effective method of contraception. Preferably the patient should use two complementary forms of contraception including a barrier method. Contraception should be continued for at least 1 month after stopping treatment with isotretinoin, even in patients with amenorrhea.

Pregnancy testing

According to local practice, medically supervised pregnancy tests with a minimum sensitivity of 25mIU/mL are recommended to be performed in the first 3 days of the menstrual cycle, as follows.

Prior to starting therapy:

In order to exclude the possibility of pregnancy prior to starting contraception, it is recommended that an initial medically supervised pregnancy test should be performed and its date and result recorded. In patients without regular menses, the timing of this pregnancy test should reflect the sexual activity of the patient and should be undertaken approximately 3 weeks after the patient last had unprotected sexual intercourse. The prescriber should educate the patient about contraception.

A medically supervised pregnancy test should also be performed during the consultation when isotretinoin is prescribed or in the 3 days prior to the visit to the prescriber, and should have been delayed until the patient had been using effective contraception for at least 1 month. This test should ensure the patient is not pregnant when she starts treatment with isotretinoin.

Follow-up visits

Follow-up visits should be arranged at 28 day intervals. The need for repeated medically supervised pregnancy tests every month should be determined according to local practice including consideration of the patient's sexual activity and recent menstrual history (abnormal menses, missed periods or amenorrhea). Where indicated, follow-up pregnancy tests should be performed on the day of the prescribing visit or in the 3 days prior to the visit to the prescriber.

End of treatment

Five weeks after stopping treatment, women should undergo a final pregnancy test to exclude pregnancy.

Prescribing and dispensing restrictions

Prescriptions of isotretinoin for women of childbearing potential should be limited to 30 days of treatment and continuation of treatment requires a new prescription. Ideally, pregnancy testing, issuing a prescription and dispensing of isotretinoin should occur on the same day. Dispensing of isotretinoin should occur within a maximum of 7 days of the prescription.

Male patients:

There is no evidence to suggest that the fertility or offspring of male patients will be affected by them taking isotretinoin. However, male patients should be reminded that they must not share their medication with anyone, particularly not females.

Additional precautions

Patients should be instructed never to give this medicinal product to another person and to return any unused capsules to their pharmacist at the end of treatment.

Patients should not donate blood during therapy and for 1 month following discontinuation of isotretinoin because of the potential risk to the foetus of a pregnant transfusion recipient.

Educational material

In order to assist prescribers, pharmacists and patients in avoiding foetal exposure to isotretinoin the Marketing Authorisation Holder will provide educational material to reinforce the warnings about the teratogenicity of isotretinoin, to provide advice on contraception before therapy is started and to provide guidance on the need for pregnancy testing.

Full patient information about the teratogenic risk and the strict pregnancy prevention measures as specified in the Pregnancy Prevention Programme should be given by the physician to all patients, both male and female.

Psychiatric disorders

Depression, depression aggravated, anxiety, aggressive tendencies, mood alterations, psychotic symptoms, and very rarely, suicidal ideation, suicide attempts and suicide have been reported in patients treated with isotretinoin (see section 4.8). Particular care needs to be taken in patients with a history of depression and all patients should be monitored for signs of depression and referred for appropriate treatment if necessary. However, discontinuation of isotretinoin may be insufficient to alleviate symptoms and therefore further psychiatric or psychological evaluation may be necessary.

Skin and subcutaneous tissues disorders

Acute exacerbation of acne is occasionally seen during the initial period but this subsides with continued treatment, usually within 7 - 10 days, and usually does not require dose adjustment.

Exposure to intense sunlight or to UV rays should be avoided. Where necessary a sun-protection product with a high protection factor of at least SPF 15 should be used.

Aggressive chemical dermabrasion and cutaneous laser treatment should be avoided in patients on isotretinoin for a period of 5-6 months after the end of the treatment because of the risk of hypertrophic scarring in atypical areas and more rarely post inflammatory hyper or hypopigmentation in treated areas. Wax depilation should be avoided in patients on isotretinoin for at least a period of 6 months after treatment because of the risk of epidermal stripping.

Concurrent administration of isotretinoin with topical keratolytic or exfoliative anti-acne agents should be avoided as local irritation may increase.

Patients should be advised to use a skin moisturising ointment or cream and a lip balm from the start of treatment as isotretinoin is likely to cause dryness of the skin and lips.

Eye disorders

Dry eyes, corneal opacities, decreased night vision and keratitis usually resolve after discontinuation of therapy. Dry eyes can be helped by the application of a lubricating eye ointment or by the application of tear replacement therapy. Intolerance to contact lenses may occur which may necessitate the patient to wear glasses during treatment.

Decreased night vision has also been reported and the onset in some patients was sudden (see section 4.7). Patients experiencing visual difficulties should be referred for an expert ophthalmological opinion. Withdrawal of isotretinoin may be necessary.

Musculo-skeletal and connective tissue disorders

Myalgia, arthralgia and increased serum creatine phosphokinase values have been reported in patients receiving isotretinoin, particularly in those undertaking vigorous physical activity (see section 4.8).

Bone changes including premature epiphyseal closure, hyperostosis, and calcification of tendons and ligaments have occurred after several years of administration at very high doses for treating disorders of keratinisation. The dose levels, duration of treatment and total cumulative dose in these patients generally far exceeded those recommended for the treatment of acne.

Benign intracranial hypertension

Cases of benign intracranial hypertension have been reported, some of which involved concomitant use of tetracyclines (see section 4.3 and section 4.5). Signs and symptoms of benign intracranial hypertension include headache, nausea and vomiting, visual disturbances and papilloedema. Patients who develop benign intracranial hypertension should discontinue isotretinoin immediately.

Hepatobiliary disorders

Liver enzymes should be checked before treatment, 1 month after the start of treatment, and subsequently at 3 monthly intervals unless more frequent monitoring is clinically indicated. Transient and reversible increases in liver transaminases have been reported. In many cases these changes have been within the normal range and values have returned to baseline levels during treatment. However, in the event of persistent clinically relevant elevation of transaminase levels, reduction of the dose or discontinuation of treatment should be considered.

Renal insufficiency

Renal insufficiency and renal failure do not affect the pharmacokinetics of isotretinoin. Therefore, isotretinoin can be given to patients with renal insufficiency. However, it is recommended that patients are started on a low dose and titrated up to the maximum tolerated dose (see section 4.2).

Lipid Metabolism

Serum lipids (fasting values) should be checked before treatment, 1 month after the start of treatment, and subsequently at 3 monthly intervals unless more frequent monitoring is clinically indicated. Elevated serum lipid values usually return to normal on reduction of the dose or discontinuation of treatment and may also respond to dietary measures.

Isotretinoin has been associated with an increase in plasma triglyceride levels. Isotretinoin should be discontinued if hypertriglyceridaemia cannot be controlled at an acceptable level or if symptoms of pancreatitis occur (see section 4.8). Levels in excess of 800mg/dL or 9mmol/L are sometimes associated with acute pancreatitis, which may be fatal.

Gastrointestinal disorders

Isotretinoin has been associated with inflammatory bowel disease (including regional ileitis) in patients without a prior history of intestinal disorders. Patients experiencing severe (hemorrhagic) diarrhoea should discontinue isotretinoin immediately.

Allergic reactions

Anaphylactic reactions have been rarely reported, in some cases after previous topical exposure to retinoids. Allergic cutaneous reactions are reported infrequently. Serious cases of allergic vasculitis, often with purpura (bruises and red patches) of the extremities and extracutaneous involvement have been reported. Severe allergic reactions necessitate interruption of therapy and careful monitoring.

Fructose intolerance

Roaccutane contains sorbitol. Patients with rare hereditary problems of fructose intolerance should not take this medicine.

High Risk Patients

In patients with diabetes, obesity, alcoholism or a lipid metabolism disorder undergoing treatment with isotretinoin, more frequent checks of serum values for lipids and/or blood glucose may be necessary. Elevated fasting blood sugars have been reported, and new cases of diabetes have been diagnosed during isotretinoin therapy.

4.5 Interaction with other medicinal products and other forms of Interaction

Patients should not take vitamin A as concurrent medication due to the risk of developing hypervitaminosis A.

Cases of benign intracranial hypertension (pseudotumor cerebri) have been reported with concomitant use of isotretinoin and tetracyclines. Therefore, concomitant treatment with tetracyclines must be avoided (see section 4.3 and section 4.4).

4.6 Pregnancy and lactation

Pregnancy is an <u>absolute</u> contraindication to treatment with isotretinoin (see section 4.3). If pregnancy does occur in spite of these precautions during treatment with isotretinoin or in the month following, there is a great risk of very severe and serious malformation of the foetus.

The foetal malformations associated with exposure to isotretinoin include central nervous system abnormalities (hydrocephalus, cerebellar malformation/abnormalities, microcephaly), facial dysmorphia, cleft palate, external ear abnormalities (absence of external ear, small or absent external auditory canals), eye abnormalities (microphthalmia), cardiovascular abnormalities (conotruncal malformations such as tetralogy of Fallot, transposition of great vessels, septal defects), thymus gland abnormality and parathyroid gland abnormalities. There is also an increased incidence of spontaneous abortion.

If pregnancy occurs in a woman treated with isotretinoin, treatment must be stopped and the patient should be referred to a physician specialised or experienced in teratology for evaluation and advice.

<u>Lactation</u>:

Isotretinoin is highly lipophilic, therefore the passage of isotretinoin into human milk is very likely. Due to the potential for adverse effects in the mother and exposed child, the use of isotretinoin is contraindicated in nursing mothers.

4.7 Effects on ability to drive and use machines

A number of cases of decreased night vision have occurred during isotretinoin therapy and in rare instances have persisted after therapy (see section 4.4 and section 4.8). Because the onset in some patients was sudden, patients should be advised of this potential problem and warned to be cautious when driving or operating machines.

4.8 Undesirable effects

The following symptoms are the most commonly reported undesirable effects with isotretinoin: dryness of the mucosa e.g. of the lips, cheilitis, the nasal mucosa, epistaxis, and the eyes, conjunctivitis, dryness of the skin. Some of the side effects associated with the use of isotretinoin are dose-related. The side effects are generally reversible after altering the dose or discontinuation of treatment, however some may persist after treatment has stopped.

Infections:	
Very Rare (≤ 1/10 000)	Gram positive (mucocutaneous) bacterial infection
Blood and lymphatic system disorders:	
Very common (≥ 1/10)	Anaemia, red blood cell sedimentation rate increased, thrombocytopenia, thrombocytosis
Common (≥ 1/100, < 1/10)	Neutropenia
Very Rare (≤ 1/10 000)	Lymphadenopathy
Immune system disorders:	
Rare (≥ 1/10 000, < 1/1000)	Allergic skin reaction, anaphylactic reactions, hypersensitivity
Metabolism and nutrition disorders:	
Very Rare (≤ 1/10 000)	Diabetes mellitus, hyperuricaemia
Psychiatric disorders:	
Rare (≥ 1/10 000, < 1/1000)	Depression, depression aggravated, aggressive tendencies, anxiety, mood alterations.
Very Rare (≤ 1/10 000)	Abnormal behaviour, psychotic disorder, suicidal ideation suicide attempt, suicide
Nervous system disorders:	
Common (≥ 1/100, < 1/10)	Headache
Very Rare (≤ 1/10 000)	Benign intracranial hypertension, convulsions, drowsiness
Eye disorders:	
Very common (≥ 1/10)	Blepharitis, conjunctivitis, dry eye, eye irritation
Very Rare (≤ 1/10 000)	blurred vision, cataract, colour blindness (colour vision deficiencies), contact lens intolerance, corneal opacity, decreased night vision, keratitis, papilloedema (as sign of benign intracranial hypertension), photophobia
Ear and labyrinth disorders:	
Very Rare (≤ 1/10 000)	Hearing impaired
Vascular disorders:	
Very Rare (≤ 1/10 000)	Vasculitis (for example Wegener's granulomatosis, allergic vasculitis)
Respiratory, thoracic and mediastinal disorders:	
Common (≥ 1/100, < 1/10)	Epistaxis, nasal dryness, nasopharyngitis
Very Rare (≤ 1/10 000)	Bronchospasm (particularly in patients with asthma), hoarseness
Gastrointestinal disorders:	
Very Rare (≤ 1/10 000)	Colitis, ileitis, dry throat, gastrointestinal haemorrhage, haemorrhagic diarrhoea and inflammatory bowel disease, nausea, pancreatitis (see section 4.4)
Hepatobiliary disorders:	
Very common (≥ 1/10)	Transaminase increased (see section 4.4)
Very Rare (≤ 1/10 000)	Hepatitis
Skin and subcutaneous tissues disorders:	
Very common (≥ 1/10)	Cheilitis, dermatitis, dry skin, localised exfoliation, pruritus, rash erythematous, skin fragility (risk of frictional trauma)
Rare (≥ 1/10 000, < 1/1000)	Alopecia
Very Rare (≤ 1/10 000)	Acne fulminans, acne aggravated (acne flare), erythema (facial), exanthema, hair disorders, hirsutism, nail dystrophy, paronychia, photosensitivity reaction, pyogenic granuloma, skin hyperpigmentation, sweating increased
Musculo-skeletal and connective tissue disorders:	
Very common (≥ 1/10)	Arthralgia, myalgia, back pain (particularly adolescent patients)
Very Rare (≤ 1/10 000)	arthritis, calcinosis (calcification of ligaments and tendons), epiphyses premature fusion, exostosis, (hyperostosis), reduced bone density, tendonitis
Renal and urinary disorders:	
Very Rare (≤ 1/10 000)	Glomerulonephritis
General disorders and administration site conditions:	
Very Rare (≤ 1/10 000)	Granulation tissue (increased formation of), malaise
Investigations:	
Very common (≥ 1/10)	Blood triglycerides increased, high density lipoprotein decreased
Common (≥ 1/100, < 1/10)	Blood cholesterol increased, blood glucose increased, haematuria, proteinuria
Very Rare (≤ 1/10 000)	Blood creatine phosphokinase increased

The incidence of the adverse events was calculated from pooled clinical trial data involving 824 patients and from post-marketing data.

4.9 Overdose

Isotretinoin is a derivative of vitamin A. Although the acute toxicity of isotretinoin is low, signs of hypervitaminosis A could appear in cases of accidental overdose. Manifestations of acute vitamin A toxicity include severe headache, nausea or vomiting, drowsiness, irritability and pruritus. Signs and symptoms of accidental or deliberate overdosage with isotretinoin would probably be similar. These symptoms would be expected to be reversible and to subside without the need for treatment.

5. PHARMACOLOGICAL PROPERTIES

5.1 Pharmacodynamic properties

Pharmacotherapeutic group: anti-acne preparations for systemic use

ATC code: D10B A01

Mechanism of action

Isotretinoin is a stereoisomer of all-trans retinoic acid (tretinoin). The exact mechanism of action of isotretinoin has not yet been elucidated in detail, but it has been established that the improvement observed in the clinical picture of severe acne is associated with suppression of sebaceous gland activity and a histologically demonstrated reduction in the size of the sebaceous glands. Furthermore, a dermal anti-inflammatory effect of isotretinoin has been established.

Efficacy

Hypercornification of the epithelial lining of the pilosebaceous unit leads to shedding of corneocytes into the duct and blockage by keratin and excess sebum. This is followed by formation of a comedone and, eventually, inflammatory lesions. Isotretinoin inhibits proliferation of sebocytes and appears to act in acne by re-setting the orderly program of differentiation. Sebum is a major substrate for the growth of Propionibacterium acnes so that reduced sebum production inhibits bacterial colonisation of the duct.

5.2 Pharmacokinetic properties

Absorption

The absorption of isotretinoin from the gastro-intestinal tract is variable and dose-linear over the therapeutic range. The absolute bioavailability of isotretinoin has not been determined, since the compound is not available as an intravenous preparation for human use, but extrapolation from dog studies would suggest a fairly low and variable systemic bioavailability. When isotretinoin is taken with food, the bioavailability is doubled relative to fasting conditions.

Distribution

Isotretinoin is extensively bound to plasma proteins, mainly albumin (99.9 %). The volume of distribution of isotretinoin in man has not been determined since isotretinoin is not available as an intravenous preparation for human use. In humans little information is available on the distribution of isotretinoin into tissue. Concentrations of isotretinoin in the epidermis are only half of those in serum. Plasma concentrations of isotretinoin are about 1.7 times those of whole blood due to poor penetration of isotretinoin into red blood cells.

Metabolism

After oral administration of isotretinoin, three major metabolites have been identified in plasma: 4-oxo-isotretinoin, tretinoin, (all-trans retinoic acid), and 4-oxo-tretinoin. These metabolites have shown biological activity in several in vitro tests. 4-oxo-isotretinoin has been shown in a clinical study to be a significant contributor to the activity of isotretinoin (reduction in sebum excretion rate despite no effect on plasma levels of isotretinoin and tretinoin). Other minor metabolites includes glucuronide conjugates. The major metabolite is 4-oxo-isotretinoin with plasma concentrations at steady state, that are 2.5 times higher than those of the parent compound.

Isotretinoin and tretinoin (all-trans retinoic acid) are reversibly metabolised (interconverted), and the metabolism of tretinoin is therefore linked with that of isotretinoin. It has been estimated that 20-30 % of an isotretinoin dose is metabolised by isomerisation.

Enterohepatic circulation may play a significant role in the pharmacokinetics of isotretinoin in man. In vitro metabolism studies have demonstrated that several CYP enzymes are involved in the metabolism of isotretinoin to 4-oxo-isotretinoin and tretinoin. No single isoform appears to have a predominant role. Isotretinoin and its metabolites do not significantly affect CYP activity.

Elimination

After oral administration of radiolabelled isotretinoin approximately equal fractions of the dose were recovered in urine and faeces. Following oral administration of isotretinoin, the terminal elimination half-life of unchanged drug in patients with acne has a mean value of 19 hours. The terminal elimination half-life of 4-oxo-isotretinoin is longer, with a mean value of 29 hours.

Isotretinoin is a physiological retinoid and endogenous retinoid concentrations are reached within approximately two weeks following the end of isotretinoin therapy.

Pharmacokinetics in special populations

Since isotretinoin is contraindicated in patients with hepatic impairment, limited information on the kinetics of isotretinoin is available in this patient population. Renal failure does not significantly reduce the plasma clearance of isotretinoin or 4-oxo-isotretinoin.

5.3 Preclinical safety data

Acute toxicity

The acute oral toxicity of isotretinoin was determined in various animal species. LD50 is approximately 2000 mg/kg in rabbits, approximately 3000 mg/kg in mice, and over 4000 mg/kg in rats.

Chronic toxicity

A long-term study in rats over 2 years (isotretinoin dosage 2, 8 and 32 mg/kg/d) produced evidence of partial hair loss and elevated plasma triglycerides in the higher dose groups. The side effect spectrum of isotretinoin in the rodent thus closely resembles that of vitamin A, but does not include the massive tissue and organ calcifications observed with vitamin A in the rat. The liver cell changes observed with vitamin A did not occur with isotretinoin.

All observed side effects of hypervitaminosis A syndrome were spontaneously reversible after withdrawal of isotretinoin. Even experimental animals in a poor general state had largely recovered within 1–2 weeks.

Teratogenicity

Like other vitamin A derivatives, isotretinoin has been shown in animal experiments to be teratogenic and embryotoxic.

Due to the teratogenic potential of isotretinoin there are therapeutic consequences for the administration to women of a childbearing age (see section 4.3, section 4.4, and section 4.6).

Fertility

Isotretinoin, in therapeutic dosages, does not affect the number, motility and morphology of sperm and does not jeopardise the formation and development of the embryo on the part of the men taking isotretinoin.

Mutagenicity

Isotretinoin has not been shown to be mutagenic nor carcinogenic in *in vitro* or *in vivo* animal tests respectively.

6. PHARMACEUTICAL PARTICULARS

6.1 List of excipients

Capsule filling:

Beeswax, yellow;

Soya-bean oil, refined;

Soya-bean oil, hydrogenated,

Soya-bean oil, partially hydrogenated

Capsule shell:

Gelatin;

Glycerol;

Karion 83 containing sorbitol, mannitol, hydrogenated hydrolysed starch;

Titanium dioxide E171;

Canthaxanthin pigment E161, containing gelatin, arachis oil (peanut oil), canthaxanthin, ascorbyl palmitate, α-tocopherol and silica

Printing ink:

Shellac, refined;

Black iron oxide E172.

6.2 Incompatibilities

Not applicable.

6.3 Shelf life

3 years

6.4 Special precautions for storage

Aluminium-aluminium blisters:

Do not store above 30 °C.

Store in the original package in order to protect from moisture and light.

6.5 Nature and contents of container

Aluminium-aluminium blister packs containing 30 capsules

6.6 Instructions for use and handling

Return any unused Roaccutane capsules to the Pharmacist

7. MARKETING AUTHORISATION HOLDER

Roche Products Limited,

40 Broadwater Road,

Welwyn Garden City,

Hertfordshire

AL7 3AY

8. MARKETING AUTHORISATION NUMBER(S)

PL 00031/0158

PL 00031/0160

9. DATE OF FIRST AUTHORISATION/RENEWAL OF THE AUTHORISATION

July 2002

10. DATE OF REVISION OF THE TEXT

December 2004

Robaxin 750

(Shire Pharmaceuticals Limited)

1. NAME OF THE MEDICINAL PRODUCT

Robaxin-750

2. QUALITATIVE AND QUANTITATIVE COMPOSITION

Each white, capsule-shaped tablet contains 750 mg methocarbamol.

3. PHARMACEUTICAL FORM

Film coated tablet.

4. CLINICAL PARTICULARS

4.1 Therapeutic indications

As a short-term adjunct to the symptomatic treatment of acute musculoskeletal disorders associated with painful muscle spasms.

4.2 Posology and method of administration

For oral use.

Dosage:

Adults: The usual dose is 2 tablets four times daily but therapeutic response has been achieved with doses as low as 1 tablet three times daily.

Elderly: Half the maximum dose or less may be sufficient to produce a therapeutic response.

Children: Not recommended.

Hepatically impaired: In patients with chronic hepatic disease the elimination half-life may be prolonged. Therefore, consideration should be given to increasing the dose level.

4.3 Contraindications

Hypersensitivity to methocarbamol or any of the other excipients in Robaxin-750. Coma or pre-coma states. Known brain damage or epilepsy. Myasthenia gravis.

4.4 Special warnings and special precautions for use

Robaxin should be used with caution in patients with renal and hepatic insufficiency.

4.5 Interaction with other medicinal products and other forms of Interaction

This product may potentiate the effects of other central nervous system depressants and stimulants including alcohol, barbiturates, anaesthetics and appetite suppressants. The effects of anticholinergics, e.g. atropine and some psychotropic drugs may be potentiated by methocarbamol. Methocarbamol may inhibit the effect of pyridostigmine bromide. Therefore methocarbamol should be used with caution in patients with myasthenia gravis receiving anticholinesterase agents. Little is known about the possibility of interactions with other drugs.

Methocarbamol may cause colour interference in certain screening tests for 5-hydroxyindolacetic acid (5-HIAA) using nitrosoaphthol reagent and in screening tests for urinary vanillymandelic acid (VMA) using the Gitlow method.

4.6 Pregnancy and lactation

Animal reproductive studies have not been conducted with methocarbamol. It is also not known whether methocarbamol can cause foetal harm when administered to a pregnant woman or can affect reproduction capacity.

Safe use of methocarbamol has not been established with regard to possible adverse effects upon foetal development. There have been very rare reports of foetal and congenital abnormalities following in utero exposure to methocarbamol. Therefore methocarbamol tablets should not be used in women who are or may become pregnant and particularly during early pregnancy unless in the judgement of the physician the potential benefits outweigh the possible hazards.

Methocarbamol and/or its metabolites are excreted in the milk of dogs: however, it is not known whether methocarbamol or its metabolites are excreted in human milk. Because many drugs are excreted in human milk, caution should be exercised when Robaxin-750 is administered to a nursing woman.

4.7 Effects on ability to drive and use machines

This product may cause drowsiness and patients receiving it should not drive nor operate machinery unless their physical and mental capabilities remain unaffected - especially if other medication capable of causing drowsiness is also being taken.

4.8 Undesirable effects

Adverse reactions reported coincident with the administration of methocarbamol include

Body as a whole: Angioneurotic oedema, anaphylactic reaction, fever, headache.

Cardiovascular system: Bradycardia, flushing, hypotension, syncope.

Digestive system: Dyspepsia, jaundice (including cholestatic jaundice), nausea and vomiting.

Blood and lymphatic system: Leucopenia.

Nervous system: Restlessness, anxiety, tremor, amnesia, confusion, diplopia, dizziness or light-headedness, vertigo, drowsiness, insomnia, mild muscular incoordination, nystagmus, seizures (including grand mal).

Skin and special senses: Blurred vision, conjunctivitis with nasal congestion, metallic taste, pruritus, rash, urticaria.

4.9 Overdose

Limited information is available on the acute toxicity of methocarbamol. Overdose of methocarbamol is frequently in conjunction with alcohol or other CNS depressants and includes the following symptoms: nausea, drowsiness, blurred vision, hypotension, seizures and coma. One adult survived the deliberate ingestion of 22 to 30 grams of methocarbamol without serious toxicity. Another adult survived a dose of 30 to 50 grams. The principal symptom in both cases was extreme drowsiness. Treatment was symptomatic and recovery was uneventful. However, there have been cases of fatal overdose.

Management of overdose includes symptomatic and supportive treatment. Supportive measures include maintenance of an adequate airway, monitoring urinary output and vital signs, and administration of intravenous fluids if necessary. The usefulness of haemodialysis in managing overdose is unknown.

5. PHARMACOLOGICAL PROPERTIES

5.1 Pharmacodynamic properties

Robaxin 750 is used as a short-term adjunct to the symptomatic treatment of acute musculoskeletal disorders associated with painful muscle spasms.

The mechanism of action of methocarbamol in humans has not been established, but may be due to general central nervous system depression. It has no direct action on the contractile mechanism of striated muscle, the motor end plate or the nerve fibre.

5.2 Pharmacokinetic properties

Methocarbamol is absorbed from the gastro-intestinal tract and produces peak plasma concentrations after about 1-3 hours. Its activity derives from the intact molecule and only a small proportion is converted to guaiphenesin.

Renally impaired

The clearance of methocarbamol in renally-impaired patients on maintenance haemodialysis was reduced about 40% compared to a normal population, although the mean elimination half-life in these two groups was similar (1.2 versus 1.1 hours, respectively).

Hepatically impaired

In patients with cirrhosis secondary to alcohol abuse, the mean total clearance of methocarbamol was reduced approximately 70% compared to a normal population (11.9 L/hr), and the mean elimination half-life was extended to approximately 3.4 hours. The fraction of methocarbamol bound to plasma proteins was decreased to approximately 40 to 45% compared to 46 to 50% in an age- and weight-matched normal population.

5.3 Preclinical safety data

Nothing of note to the prescriber.

6. PHARMACEUTICAL PARTICULARS

6.1 List of excipients

Alginic acid, maize starch, povidone, sodium lauryl sulphate, gelatin, magnesium stearate, talc, sepifilm 002, sepisperse white AP 7001, potable mains water.

6.2 Incompatibilities

Not applicable.

6.3 Shelf life

HDPE bottles with HDPE child resistant caps: 60 months

6.4 Special precautions for storage

No special storage conditions are necessary.

6.5 Nature and contents of container

HDPE bottles with HDPE child resistant caps containing 100 tablets.

6.6 Instructions for use and handling

None

7. MARKETING AUTHORISATION HOLDER

Shire Pharmaceutical Contracts Ltd

Hampshire International Business Park

Chineham

Basingstoke

Hampshire

RG24 8EP

UK

8. MARKETING AUTHORISATION NUMBER(S)

PL 08081/0035

9. DATE OF FIRST AUTHORISATION/RENEWAL OF THE AUTHORISATION

26th August 2003

10. DATE OF REVISION OF THE TEXT

29th October 2003

LEGAL CATEGORY

POM

Robitussin Chesty Cough Medicine

(Wyeth Consumer Healthcare)

1. NAME OF THE MEDICINAL PRODUCT

Robitussin Chesty Cough Medicine

2. QUALITATIVE AND QUANTITATIVE COMPOSITION

Each 5ml contains

Guaiphenesin PhEur 100mg

3. PHARMACEUTICAL FORM

Liquid for oral administration.

4. CLINICAL PARTICULARS

4.1 Therapeutic indications

Expectorant for the treatment of coughs.

4.2 Posology and method of administration

Adults, the elderly and children over 12 years: One10 ml measure four times daily

Children

6-12 years: One 5ml measure four times daily

1-6 years: One 2.5ml measure four times daily

Under 1 year: Not recommended

4.3 Contraindications

Hypersensitivity to any of the ingredients

4.4 Special warnings and special precautions for use

1. If symptoms persist consult your doctor.

2. Keep out of the reach of children.

4.5 Interaction with other medicinal products and other forms of Interaction

None stated.

4.6 Pregnancy and lactation

Evidence of safety of guaiphenesin products in pregnancy and lactation is at present incomplete. However wide usage for many years has shown no apparent ill consequence.

4.7 Effects on ability to drive and use machines

None stated.

4.8 Undesirable effects

None stated

4.9 Overdose

Symptoms: Nausea and vomiting

Treatment: Gastric lavage together with appropriate supportive therapy dependent upon individual response to the preparation.

5. PHARMACOLOGICAL PROPERTIES

5.1 Pharmacodynamic properties

For the treatment of coughs, Robitussin Chesty Cough contains an expectorant

(Guaiphenesin).

Guaiphenesin

Guaiphenesin has an expectorant action which increases the output of respiratory tract fluid by reducing adhesiveness and surface tension. The increased flow of less viscid secretion promotes ciliary action and facilitates the removal of mucus. This changes a dry, unproductive cough to a cough that is more productive and less frequent.

5.2 Pharmacokinetic properties

Robitussin Chesty Cough is a liquid preparation containing the active ingredient:

Guaiphenesin 100mg/5ml.

Guaiphenesin

Guaiphenesin is absorbed from the gastro-intestinal tract. It is metabolised and excreted in the urine.

5.3 Preclinical safety data

As a well established and widely used product, the preclinical safety of the active is well documented.

6. PHARMACEUTICAL PARTICULARS

6.1 List of excipients

Glycerol, Sodium Carboxymethyl Cellulose, Sodium Benzoate, Sodium Cyclamate, Ethanol, Levomenthol, maltitol, Sorbitol Solution 70%, Natural Cherry Flavouring, Citric Acid Anhydrous, Caramel (E150), Acesulfame Potassium and Purified Water.

6.2 Incompatibilities

None stated

6.3 Shelf life

36 months.

6.4 Special precautions for storage

Store at a temperature not exceeding 25°C.

6.5 Nature and contents of container

Amber glass bottles fitted with LDPE tamper evident screw caps or jaycaps with LDPE liner, 100ml and 200m

PET bottles containing 100ml with PVdC lined PP screw caps

A clear polypropylene measuring cap also included

6.6 Instructions for use and handling

Not applicable

7. MARKETING AUTHORISATION HOLDER

Whitehall Laboratories Ltd trading as

Wyeth Consumer Healthcare

Huntercombe Lane South

Taplow

Berkshire

SL6 OPH

8. MARKETING AUTHORISATION NUMBER(S)

PL 00165/0097

9. DATE OF FIRST AUTHORISATION/RENEWAL OF THE AUTHORISATION

1 September 1993

10. DATE OF REVISION OF THE TEXT

August 2004

Robitussin Chesty Cough with Congestion

(Wyeth Consumer Healthcare)

1. NAME OF THE MEDICINAL PRODUCT

Robitussin Chesty Cough with Congestion

2. QUALITATIVE AND QUANTITATIVE COMPOSITION

Each 5ml contains

Guaiphenesin PhEur, 100mg

Pseudoephedrine Hydrochloride BP, 30mg

3. PHARMACEUTICAL FORM

Liquid for oral administration.

4. CLINICAL PARTICULARS

4.1 Therapeutic indications

Nasal decongestant and expectorant for the symptomatic relief of respiratory tract disorders.

4.2 Posology and method of administration

Oral Administration

Adults the elderly and children over 12 years: One 10ml measure up to four times daily

Children:

6-12 years: One 5ml measure up to four times daily

2-6 years: One 2.5ml measure up to four times daily

Under 2 years Not recommended

4.3 Contraindications

- Hypersensitivity to any of the ingredients
- Use in patients with ischaemic heart disease, thyrotoxicosis, glaucoma, diabetes, enlargement of the prostate or urinary retention.
- Patients currently receiving or who have within two weeks received, monoamine oxidase inhibitors
- Patients receiving tricyclic antidepressants.
- Patients receiving other sympathomimetic drugs.

4.4 Special warnings and special precautions for use

1. If symptoms persist consult your doctor.

2. Not to be taken by patients taking either cardiac glycosides or anti-hypertensive agents, except on a doctors advice.

3. Keep out of the reach of children.

4. Do not exceed the stated dose.

4.5 Interaction with other medicinal products and other forms of Interaction

1. An increased risk of cardiac arrhythmias may occur if sympathomimetics (such as pseudoephedrine hydrochloride) are given to patients receiving cardiac glycosides.

2. Sympathomimetics (such as pseudoephedrine hydrochloride) may increase blood pressure and therefore special care is advisable in patients receiving antihypertensive therapy.

4.6 Pregnancy and lactation

This product should not be used during pregnancy unless directed by a physician.

4.7 Effects on ability to drive and use machines

None stated.

4.8 Undesirable effects

May act as a cerebral stimulant in children and occasionally adults.

4.9 Overdose

Symptoms:

Guaiphenesin overdose: nausea and vomiting.

Pseudoephedrine overdose: CNS stimulation leading to excitement, restlessness, rapid speech, hallucinations, hypertonicity and hyperreflexia, dilated pupils and tachycardia.

Treatment:

Gastric lavage together with appropriate supportive therapy dependent upon individual response to the various constituents of the preparation.

5. PHARMACOLOGICAL PROPERTIES

5.1 Pharmacodynamic properties

Guaiphenesin

Guaiphenesin has an expectorant action which increases the output of respiratory tract fluid by reducing adhesiveness and surface tension. The increased flow of less viscid secretion promotes ciliary action and facilitates the removal of mucus. This changes a dry unproductive cough to a cough that is more productive and less frequent.

Pseudoephedrine Hydrochloride

Pseudoephedrine is a stereoisomer of ephedrine and has a similar action, but has been stated to have less pressor activity and central nervous system effects.

It is a sympathomimetic agent with indirect and direct effects on adrenergic receptors. It has Alpha- and Beta-Adrenergic activity and has pronounced stimulating effects on the central nervous system. In therapeutic doses it raises the blood pressure by increasing cardiac output and also by inducing peripheral vasoconstriction.

5.2 Pharmacokinetic properties

Guaiphenesin

Guaiphenesin is absorbed from the gastro-intestinal tract. It is metabolised and excreted in the urine.

Pseudoephedrine Hydrochloride

Pseudoephedrine is absorbed from the gastro-intestinal tract. It is resistant to metabolism by monoamine oxidase and is largely excreted unchanged (55-75%) in the urine together with small amounts of its hepatic metabolite. It has a half-life of several hours; elimination is enhanced and half-life accordingly shorter in acid urine.

5.3 Preclinical safety data

As well established and widely used product, the preclinical safety of the actives are well documented.

6. PHARMACEUTICAL PARTICULARS

6.1 List of excipients

Glycerol, Sodium Carboxymethyl Cellulose, Disodium Edetate, Sodium Benzoate, Sodium Cyclamate, Amaranth (E123), Ethanol, Levomenthol, Maltitol, Sorbitol Solution 70%, Natural Cherry Flavouring, Citric Acid Anhydrous, Caramel E150, Acesulfame Potassium and Purified Water.

6.2 Incompatibilities

None stated

6.3 Shelf life

36 months

6.4 Special precautions for storage

Do not store above 25°C

6.5 Nature and contents of container

Amber glass bottles fitted with LDPE tamper evident screw cap or jaycaps with LDPE liners, 30, 100, 200, 500 and 2000ml

PET bottles containing 100ml with PVdC lined PP screw caps

A clear polypropylene measuring cap also included

6.6 Instructions for use and handling

Not applicable

7. MARKETING AUTHORISATION HOLDER

Whitehall Laboratories Ltd *trading as*

Wyeth Consumer Healthcare

Huntercombe Lane South

Taplow

Berkshire

SL6 OPH

8. MARKETING AUTHORISATION NUMBER(S)

PL 00165/0098

9. DATE OF FIRST AUTHORISATION/RENEWAL OF THE AUTHORISATION

1 September 1993

10. DATE OF REVISION OF THE TEXT

August 2004

Robitussin Dry Cough Medicine

(Wyeth Consumer Healthcare)

1. NAME OF THE MEDICINAL PRODUCT

Robitussin Dry Cough Medicine

2. QUALITATIVE AND QUANTITATIVE COMPOSITION

Active Ingredient

Dextromethorphan Hydrobromide Ph Eur 7.5mg per 5ml

3. PHARMACEUTICAL FORM

Liquid for oral administration.

4. CLINICAL PARTICULARS

4.1 Therapeutic indications

For the relief of persistent dry irritant coughs.

4.2 Posology and method of administration

Adults: 10ml three or four times daily

Children 6-12 years: 5ml three or four times daily

Children under 6 years: Not recommended

4.3 Contraindications

Hypersensitivity to any of the constituents.

4.4 Special warnings and special precautions for use

Use with caution in patients with hepatic dysfunction.

4.5 Interaction with other medicinal products and other forms of Interaction

Use with caution in patients receiving monoamine oxidase inhibitors, or within two weeks of stopping treatment.

4.6 Pregnancy and lactation

Although dextromethorphan has been in wide spread use for many years without apparent ill-consequence, there are no specific data on their use during pregnancy. Caution should therefore be exercised by balancing the potential benefit of treatment against any possible hazards. It is not known whether dextromethorphan or its metabolites are excreted in human milk.

4.7 Effects on ability to drive and use machines

Dextromethorphan hydrobromide has no adverse effects on the patients ability to drive and to use machines.

4.8 Undesirable effects

Adverse effects with dextromethorphan hydrobromide are rare and may rarely cause dizziness and gastrointestinal upset.

4.9 Overdose

Gastric lavage and general supportive measures should be used.

5. PHARMACOLOGICAL PROPERTIES

5.1 Pharmacodynamic properties

Dextromethorphan hydrobromide is a cough suppressant which has a central action on the cough centre in the medulla. It has no analgesic properties and little sedative activity.

5.2 Pharmacokinetic properties

Dextromethorphan hydrobromide is well absorbed from the gastro-intestinal tract. It is metabolised in the liver and excreted in the urine as unchanged dextromethorphan and demethylated metabolites including dextrorphan, which has some cough suppressant activity.

5.3 Preclinical safety data

None stated.

6. PHARMACEUTICAL PARTICULARS

6.1 List of excipients

Glycerol Ph Eur

Sodium Carboxymethyl Cellulose Ph Eur

Sodium Benzoate Ph Eur

Disodium Edetate Ph Eur

Maltitol

Ethanol (96%) BP

Citric Acid Anhydrous Ph Eur

Amaranth E123

Caramel E150

Levomenthol Ph Eur

Cherry/Grenadine Flavour

Sorbitol Solution 70% Ph Eur

Sodium Cyclamate Ph Eur

Acesulfame Potassium Salt

Purified Water Ph Eur

6.2 Incompatibilities

None stated.

6.3 Shelf life

36 months.

6.4 Special precautions for storage

No special precautions required.

6.5 Nature and contents of container

Amber glass bottles fitted with low density polyethylene tamper evident J-caps or screw caps with low density polyethylene liners. 100ml and 200ml.

· PET bottles containing 100ml with PVdC lined PP screw caps

A clear polypropylene measuring cap also included

6.6 Instructions for use and handling

Not applicable.

7. MARKETING AUTHORISATION HOLDER

Whitehall Laboratories Ltd trading as *Wyeth Consumer Healthcare*

Huntercombe Lane South

Taplow

Maidenhead

Berkshire SL6 0PH

8. MARKETING AUTHORISATION NUMBER(S)

PL 0165/0100

9. DATE OF FIRST AUTHORISATION/RENEWAL OF THE AUTHORISATION

1 September 1993

10. DATE OF REVISION OF THE TEXT

August 2004

Robitussin Soft Pastilles for Dry Cough

(Wyeth Consumer Healthcare)

1. NAME OF THE MEDICINAL PRODUCT

Robitussin soft pastilles for dry cough

2. QUALITATIVE AND QUANTITATIVE COMPOSITION

Active Ingredient

Dextromethorphan Hydrobromide 7.5mg per pastille

For excipients see section 6.1

3. PHARMACEUTICAL FORM

Pastille

Soft round red gelatin pastille

4. CLINICAL PARTICULARS

4.1 Therapeutic indications

For the relief of persistent dry irritant coughs

4.2 Posology and method of administration

Adults: 2 pastilles three or four times daily

Children 6-12 years: 1 pastille three or four times daily

Children under 6 years: Not recommended

4.3 Contraindications

Hypersensitivity to any of the constituents

4.4 Special warnings and special precautions for use

Use with caution in-patients with hepatic dysfunction.

This product contains Amaranth (E123) which may cause allergic reactions.

Sorbitol containing products can cause stomach upset and diarrhoea.

4.5 Interaction with other medicinal products and other forms of Interaction

Use with caution in patients receiving monoamine oxidase inhibitors, or within two weeks of stopping treatment.

4.6 Pregnancy and lactation

Although dextromethorphan has been in wide spread use for many years without apparent ill-consequence, there are no specific data on their use during pregnancy. Caution should therefore be exercised by balancing the potential benefit of treatment against any possible hazards. It is not known whether dextromethorphan or its metabolites are excreted in human milk.

4.7 Effects on ability to drive and use machines

Dextromethorphan hydrobromide has no adverse effects on the patient's ability to drive and to use machines.

4.8 Undesirable effects

Adverse effects with dextromethorphan hydrobromide are rare and may rarely cause dizziness and gastrointestinal upset.

4.9 Overdose

Gastric lavage and general supportive measures should be used.

5. PHARMACOLOGICAL PROPERTIES

5.1 Pharmacodynamic properties

Dextromethorphan hydrobromide is a cough suppressant which has a central action on the cough centre in the medulla. It has no analgesic properties and little sedative activity.

5.2 Pharmacokinetic properties

Dextromethorphan hydrobromide is well absorbed from the gastro-intestinal tract. It is metabolised in the liver and excreted in the urine as unchanged dextromethorphan and demethylated metabolites including dextromethorphan, which has some cough suppressant activity.

5.3 Preclinical safety data

None stated

6. PHARMACEUTICAL PARTICULARS

6.1 List of excipients

Levomenthol, Acesulphame Potassium, Cherry Flavour, Natural Flavours, Propylene Glycol, Vegetable Oil, Beeswax, Purified Water, Gelatin, Dimethyl Siloxane, Mono and Di glycerides, Methylcellulose, Polyethylene Glycol Stearate, Xanthan Gum, Benzoic Acid (E210), Polyethylene Glycol, Sorbic Acid, Maltitol (E965), Sorbitol (E420), Amaranth (E123)

6.2 Incompatibilities

Not Applicable

6.3 Shelf life

2 years

6.4 Special precautions for storage

Do not store above 25°C

Store in the original package

6.5 Nature and contents of container

Foil blister packs contained in a carton. Each carton contains 20 pastilles

250 micron PVC/40gsm PVdC blisters on 20 micron hard tempered aluminum foil.

Each blister contains 10 pastilles, 2 Blisters per carton.

6.6 Instructions for use and handling

Not applicable.

7. MARKETING AUTHORISATION HOLDER

Whitehall Laboratories Ltd

Huntercombe Lane South

Taplow

Maidenhead

Berkshire SL6 0PH

8. MARKETING AUTHORISATION NUMBER(S)

PL0165/0151

9. DATE OF FIRST AUTHORISATION/RENEWAL OF THE AUTHORISATION

8 May 2003

10. DATE OF REVISION OF THE TEXT

August 2003

Rocaltrol

(Roche Products Limited)

1. NAME OF THE MEDICINAL PRODUCT

Rocaltrol® Capsules 0.25mcg.

Rocaltrol® Capsules 0.5mcg.

2. QUALITATIVE AND QUANTITATIVE COMPOSITION

Each capsule contains either 0.25 or 0.5 micrograms of calcitriol.

3. PHARMACEUTICAL FORM

Soft capsules.

0.25mcg: One length brown-red to orange-grey opaque and the other white to grey-yellow or grey-orange opaque.

0.5mcg: Both lengths brown-red to orange-grey opaque.

4. CLINICAL PARTICULARS

4.1 Therapeutic indications

Rocaltrol is indicated for the correction of the abnormalities of calcium and phosphate metabolism in patients with renal osteodystrophy.

Rocaltrol is also indicated for the treatment of established post-menopausal osteoporosis.

4.2 Posology and method of administration

The dose of Rocaltrol should be carefully adjusted for each patient according to the biological response so as to avoid hypercalcaemia.

The effectiveness of treatment depends in part on an adequate daily intake of calcium, which should be augmented by dietary changes or supplements if necessary. The capsules should be swallowed with a little water.

Oral intermittent (pulse) therapy with Rocaltrol two or three times weekly has been shown to be effective in patients with osteodystrophy refractory to continuous therapy.

Adults

Renal Osteodystrophy

The initial daily dose is 0.25mcg of Rocaltrol. In patients with normal or only slightly reduced calcium levels, doses of 0.25mcg every other day are sufficient. If no satisfactory response in the biochemical parameters and clinical manifestations of the disease is observed within 2 - 4 weeks, the dosage may be increased by 0.25mcg daily at 2 - 4 week intervals. During this period, serum calcium levels should be determined at least twice weekly. Should the serum calcium levels rise to 1mg/100ml (250μmol/l) above normal (9 to 11mg/100ml or 2250 - 2750μmol/l), or serum creatinine rises to $>$ 120μmol/l, treatment with Rocaltrol should be stopped immediately until normocalcaemia ensues. Most patients respond to between 0.5mcg and 1.0mcg daily. Higher doses may be necessary if barbiturates or anticonvulsant drugs are administered simultaneously.

Post-menopausal Osteoporosis

The recommended dose of Rocaltrol is 0.25mcg twice daily.

Serum calcium and creatinine levels should be determined at 4 weeks, 3 and 6 months and at 6 monthly intervals thereafter.

Elderly

Clinical experience with Rocaltrol in elderly patients indicates that the dosage recommended for use in younger adults may be given without apparent ill-consequence.

Children

Dosage in children has not been established.

Rocaltrol capsules are for oral administration only.

4.3 Contraindications

Rocaltrol should not be given to patients with hypercalcaemia or evidence of metastatic calcification. The use of Rocaltrol in patients with known hypersensitivity to calcitriol (or drugs of the same class) and any of the constituent excipients is contra-indicated.

Rocaltrol is contra-indicated if there is evidence of vitamin D toxicity.

4.4 Special warnings and special precautions for use

All other vitamin D compounds and their derivatives, including proprietary compounds or foodstuffs which may be "fortified" with vitamin D, should be withheld during treatment with Rocaltrol.

Treatment does not obviate the need to control plasma phosphate with phosphate-binding agents. Since Rocaltrol affects phosphate transport in the gut and bone, the dose of phosphate-binding agent may need to be modified.

4.5 Interaction with other medicinal products and other forms of Interaction

None stated.

4.6 Pregnancy and lactation

The safety of Rocaltrol during pregnancy has not been established. Studies of reproductive toxicology in animals have not yielded unequivocal findings, and no controlled studies on the effect of exogenous calcitriol on pregnancy and foetal development have been performed in human subjects. Consequently Rocaltrol should be given only when the potential benefit has been weighed against the possible hazard to the foetus. The usual caution in prescribing any drug for women of childbearing age should be observed.

It should be assumed that exogenous calcitriol passes into breast milk. Mothers may breastfeed while taking Rocaltrol, provided that the serum calcium levels of the mother and infant are monitored.

4.7 Effects on ability to drive and use machines

Not applicable.

4.8 Undesirable effects

The number of adverse effects reported from clinical use of Rocaltrol over a period of 15 years in all indications is very low with each individual effect, including hypercalcaemia, occurring rarely.

Hypercalcaemia and hypercalcuria are the major side effects of Rocaltrol and indicate excessive dosage. Patients with tertiary hyperparathyroidism, renal failure, or on regular haemodialysis are particularly prone to develop hypercalcaemia. The clinical features of hypercalcaemia include anorexia, constipation, nausea, vomiting, headache, weakness, apathy and somnolence. More severe manifestations may include thirst, dehydration, polyuria, nocturia, abdominal pain, paralytic ileus and cardiac arrhythmias. Rarely, overt psychosis and metastatic calcification may occur. The relatively short biological half-life of Rocaltrol permits rapid elimination of the compound when treatment is stopped and hypercalcaemia will recede within 2 - 7 days. This rate of reversal of biological effects is more rapid than when other vitamin D derivatives are used.

In patients with normal renal function, chronic hypercalcaemia may be associated with an increase in serum creatinine.

Mild, non-progressive and reversible elevations in levels of liver enzymes (SGOT, SGPT) have been noted in a few patients treated with Rocaltrol, but no pathological changes in the liver have been reported.

Hypersensitivity reactions may occur in susceptible individuals.

4.9 Overdose

In acute overdosage gastric lavage should be considered as soon after ingestion as possible provided that the drug was taken within the previous 6 - 8 hours.

Should hypercalcaemia occur, Rocaltrol should be discontinued until plasma calcium levels have returned to normal. A low-calcium diet will speed this reversal. Rocaltrol can then be restarted at a lower dose or given in the same dose but at less frequent intervals than previously. Severe hypercalcaemia may be treated by ensuring adequate hydration, inducing a diuresis where practicable and by general supportive measures. Calcitonin may increase the rate of fall of serum calcium when bone resorption is increased.

In patients treated by intermittent haemodialysis, a low concentration of calcium in the dialysate may also be used.

5. PHARMACOLOGICAL PROPERTIES

5.1 Pharmacodynamic properties

Calcitriol has the greatest biological activity of the known vitamin D metabolites and is normally formed in the kidneys from its immediate precursor, 25-hydroxycholecalciferol. In physiological amounts it augments the intestinal absorption of calcium and phosphate and plays a significant part in the regulation of bone mineralisation. The defective production of calcitriol in chronic renal failure contributes to the abnormalities of mineral metabolism found in that disorder.

Rocaltrol is a synthetic preparation of calcitriol. Oral administration of Rocaltrol to patients with chronic renal failure compensates for impaired endogenous production of calcitriol which is decreased when the glomerular filtration rate falls below 30ml/min. Consequently, intestinal malabsorption of calcium and phosphate and the resulting hypocalcaemia are improved, thereby reversing the signs and symptoms of bone disease.

In patients with established post-menopausal osteoporosis, Rocaltrol increases calcium absorption, elevates circulating levels of calcitriol and reduces vertebral fracture frequency.

The onset and reversal of the effects of Rocaltrol are more rapid than those of other compounds with vitamin D activity and adjustment of the dose can be achieved sooner and more precisely. The effects of inadvertent overdosage can also be reversed more readily.

5.2 Pharmacokinetic properties

Rocaltrol is efficiently absorbed following an oral dose, and peak serum levels are reached after 4 - 6 hours. Calcitriol concentrations return to the basal level with a half-life of 3 - 6 hours, although the duration of pharmacological activity is approximately 3 - 5 days. Following oral administration of 1mcg radiolabelled calcitriol to normal individuals, approximately 10% of the total radioactivity appears in the urine within 24 hours. Biliary excretion and enterohepatic recirculation also occur.

5.3 Preclinical safety data

None stated.

6. PHARMACEUTICAL PARTICULARS

6.1 List of excipients

Content

Butylated hydroxyanisole

Butylated hydroxytoluene

Triglycerides, medium chain

Shell

Gelatin

Glycerol

Sorbitol

Titanium dioxide E171

Canthaxanthin E161

6.2 Incompatibilities

None.

6.3 Shelf life

3 years.

6.4 Special precautions for storage

Glass bottles

Do not store above 30°C.

Blisters

Do not store above 25°C. Store in original container.

6.5 Nature and contents of container

Amber glass bottles with plastic screw caps containing 100 capsules and PVC opaque blisters containing 100 capsules (5 strips of 20 capsules).

Due to the use of a natural colouring agent, discolouration of the capsule may occur. This does not affect the quality of the medicine.

6.6 Instructions for use and handling

Not applicable.

7. MARKETING AUTHORISATION HOLDER

Roche Products Limited, 40 Broadwater Road, Welwyn Garden City, Hertfordshire, AL7 3AY.

8. MARKETING AUTHORISATION NUMBER(S)

Rocaltrol 0.25 microgram Capsules: PL 0031/0122

Rocaltrol 0.5 microgram Capsules: PL 0031/0123

9. DATE OF FIRST AUTHORISATION/RENEWAL OF THE AUTHORISATION

15 April 1996

10. DATE OF REVISION OF THE TEXT

July 2001

Rocaltrol is a registered trade mark

Rocephin

(Roche Products Limited)

1. NAME OF THE MEDICINAL PRODUCT

Rocephin® 250mg vials.

Rocephin® 1g vials.

Rocephin® 2g vials.

2. QUALITATIVE AND QUANTITATIVE COMPOSITION

Each 250mg vial contains 250mg ceftriaxone as 298.3mg hydrated disodium ceftriaxone.

Each 1g vial contains 1g ceftriaxone as 1.19g hydrated disodium ceftriaxone.

Each 2g vial contains 2g ceftriaxone as 2.39g hydrated disodium ceftriaxone.

3. PHARMACEUTICAL FORM

Powder for solution for injection.

Powder for solution for injection.

Powder for solution for injection/infusion.

4. CLINICAL PARTICULARS

4.1 Therapeutic indications

Ceftriaxone is indicated for the treatment of the following infections when known or likely to be due to one or more susceptible micro-organisms (see section *5.1*) and when parenteral therapy is required:

Pneumonia.

Septicaemia.

Meningitis.

Bone, skin and soft tissue infections.

Infections in neutropenic patients.

Gonorrhoea.

Peri-operative prophylaxis of infections associated with surgery.

Treatment may be started before the results of susceptibility tests are known.

Consideration should be given to official guidance on the appropriate use of antibacterial agents.

4.2 Posology and method of administration

Rocephin may be administered by deep intramuscular injection, slow intravenous injection, or as a slow intravenous infusion, after reconstitution of the solution according to the directions given below. Dosage and mode of administration should be determined by the severity of the infection, susceptibility of the causative organism and the patient's condition. Under most circumstances a once-daily dose - or, in the specified indications, a single dose - will give satisfactory therapeutic results.

Adults and children 12 years and over

Standard therapeutic dosage: 1g once daily.

Severe infections: 2 - 4g daily, normally as a single dose every 24 hours.

The duration of therapy varies according to the course of the disease. As with antibiotic therapy in general, administration of Rocephin should be continued for a minimum of 48 to 72 hours after the patient has become afebrile or evidence of bacterial eradication has been obtained.

Acute, uncomplicated gonorrhoea: A single dose of 250mg intramuscularly should be administered. Simultaneous administration of probenecid is not indicated.

Peri-operative prophylaxis: Usually 1g as a single intramuscular or slow intravenous dose. In colorectal surgery, 2g should be given intramuscularly, by slow intravenous injection or by slow intravenous infusion, in conjunction with a suitable agent against anaerobic bacteria.

Elderly

These dosages do not require modification in elderly patients provided that renal and hepatic function are satisfactory (see below).

Neonates, infants and children up to 12 years

The following dosage schedules are recommended for once daily administration:

Neonates

A daily dose of 20 - 50mg/kg body weight, not to exceed 50mg/kg. In the neonate, the intravenous dose should be given over 60 minutes to reduce the displacement of bilirubin from albumin, thereby reducing the potential risk of bilirubin encephalopathy (see section *4.4*).

Infants and children of up to 12 years

Standard therapeutic dosage: 20 - 50mg/kg body weight once daily.

In severe infections up to 80mg/kg body weight daily may be given. For children with body weights of 50kg or more, the usual adult dosage should be used. Doses of 50mg/kg or over should be given by slow intravenous infusion over at least 30 minutes. Doses greater than 80mg/kg body weight should be avoided because of the increased risk of biliary precipitates.

Renal and hepatic impairment

In patients with impaired renal function, there is no need to reduce the dosage of Rocephin provided liver function is intact. Only in cases of pre-terminal renal failure (creatinine clearance < 10ml per minute) should the daily dosage be limited to 2g or less.

In patients with liver damage there is no need for the dosage to be reduced provided renal function is intact.

In severe renal impairment accompanied by hepatic insufficiency, the plasma concentration of Rocephin should be determined at regular intervals and dosage adjusted.

In patients undergoing dialysis, no additional supplementary dosing is required following the dialysis. Serum concentrations should be monitored, however, to determine whether dosage adjustments are necessary, since the elimination rate in these patients may be reduced.

4.3 Contraindications

Hypersensitivity to ceftriaxone or to any of the cephalosporins.

Previous immediate and/or severe hypersensitivity reaction to a penicillin or to any other type of beta-lactam drug.

Rocephin should not be given to neonates with jaundice or to those who are hypoalbuminaemic or acidotic or have other conditions, such as prematurity, in which bilirubin binding is likely to be impaired.

4.4 Special warnings and special precautions for use

Before therapy with ceftriaxone is instituted, careful inquiry should be made to determine whether the patient has had any previous hypersensitivity reactions to ceftriaxone, any other cephalosporin, or to any penicillin or other beta-lactam drug. Ceftriaxone is contraindicated in patients who have had a previous hypersensitivity reaction to any cephalosporin. It is also contraindicated in patients who have had a previous immediate and/or any severe hypersensitivity reaction to any penicillin or to any other beta-lactam drug. Ceftriaxone should be given with caution to patients who have had any other type of hypersensitivity reaction to a penicillin or any other beta-lactam drug.

Ceftriaxone should be given with caution to patients who have other allergic diatheses.

Antibiotic-associated diarrhoea, colitis and pseudomembranous colitis have all been reported with the use of ceftriaxone. These diagnoses should be considered in any patient who develops diarrhoea during or shortly after treatment. Ceftriaxone should be discontinued if severe and/or bloody diarrhoea occurs during treatment and appropriate therapy instituted.

Ceftriaxone should be used with caution in individuals with a previous history of gastro-intestinal disease, particularly colitis.

As with other cephalosporins, prolonged use of ceftriaxone may result in the overgrowth of non-susceptible organisms, such as *enterococci* and *Candida spp.*

In severe renal impairment accompanied by hepatic insufficiency, dosage reduction is required as outlined under section *4.2*.

In vivo and *in vitro* studies have shown that ceftriaxone, like some other cephalosporins, can displace bilirubin from serum albumin. Clinical data obtained in neonates have confirmed this finding. Rocephin should therefore not be used in jaundiced new-borns or in those who are hypoalbuminaemic or acidotic, in whom bilirubin binding is likely to be impaired. Particular caution should be exercised in babies born prematurely.

Rocephin may precipitate in the gallbladder and then be detectable as shadows on ultrasound (see section *4.8*). This can happen in patients of any age, but is more likely in infants and small children who are usually given a larger dose of Rocephin on a body weight basis. In children, doses greater than 80mg/kg body weight should be avoided because of the increased risk of biliary precipitates. There is no clear evidence of gallstones or of acute cholecystitis developing in children or infants treated with Rocephin, and conservative management of ceftriaxone precipitate in the gallbladder is recommended.

Cephalosporins as a class tend to be absorbed onto the surface of the red cell membranes and react with antibodies directed against the drug to produce a positive Coombs' test and occasionally a rather mild haemolytic anaemia. In this respect, there may be some cross-reactivity with penicillins.

Cases of pancreatitis, possibly of biliary obstruction aetiology, have been rarely reported in patients treated with Rocephin. Most patients presented with risk factors for biliary stasis and biliary sludge, e.g. preceding major therapy, severe illness and total parenteral nutrition. A trigger or cofactor role of Rocephin-related biliary precipitation can not be ruled out.

The stated dosage should not be exceeded.

Each gram of Rocephin contains approximately 3.6mmol sodium. To be taken into consideration by patients on a controlled sodium diet.

4.5 Interaction with other medicinal products and other forms of Interaction

No impairment of renal function has been observed in man after simultaneous administration of Rocephin with diuretics.

No interference with the action or increase in nephrotoxicity of aminoglycosides has been observed during simultaneous administration with Rocephin.

The ceftriaxone molecule does not contain the N-methylthio-tetrazole substituent which has been associated with a disulfiram-like effect when alcohol is taken during therapy with certain cephalosporins.

In vitro, chloramphenicol has been shown to be antagonistic with respect to ceftriaxone and other cephalosporins. The clinical relevance of this finding is unknown, but caution is advised if concurrent administration of ceftriaxone with chloramphenicol is proposed.

In patients treated with Rocephin, the Coombs' test may rarely become false-positive. Rocephin, like other antibiotics, may result in false-positive tests for galactosaemia. Likewise, non-enzymatic methods for glucose determination in urine may give false-positive results. For this reason, urine-glucose determination during therapy with Rocephin should be done enzymatically.

Ceftriaxone may adversely affect the efficacy of oral hormonal contraceptives. Consequently, it is advisable to use supplementary (non-hormonal) contraceptive measures during treatment and in the month following treatment.

4.6 Pregnancy and lactation

Pregnancy

For ceftriaxone, limited clinical data on exposed pregnancies are available. Ceftriaxone crosses the placental barrier. Reproductive studies in animals have shown no evidence of embryotoxicity, foetotoxicity, teratogenicity or adverse effects on male or female fertility, birth or perinatal and postnatal development. In primates, no embryotoxicity or teratogenicity has been observed. Since safety in human pregnancy is not established ceftriaxone should not be used unless absolutely indicated.

Lactation

Low concentrations of ceftriaxone are excreted in human milk. Caution should be exercised when ceftriaxone is administered to a nursing woman.

4.7 Effects on ability to drive and use machines

Not applicable.

4.8 Undesirable effects

The most frequently reported adverse events for ceftriaxone are diarrhoea, nausea and vomiting. Other reported adverse events include hypersensitivity reactions such as allergic skin reactions and anaphylactic reactions, secondary infections with yeast, fungi or resistant organisms as well as changes in blood cell counts.

Infections and infestations

Rare (⩾ 0.01 % - < 0.1 %): Mycosis of the genital tract.

Superinfections of various sites with yeasts, fungi or other resistant organisms are possible.

Blood and lymphatic system disorders

Rare (⩾ 0.01 % - < 0.1 %): Neutropenia, leucopenia, eosinophilia, thrombocytopenia, anaemia (including haemolytic anaemia), slight prolongation of prothrombin time.

Very rare (< 0.01 %) including isolated reports: Positive Coombs' test, coagulation disorders, agranulocytosis (< 500/m^3), mostly after 10 days of treatment and following total doses of 20g ceftriaxone and more.

Immune system disorders

Rare (⩾ 0.01 % - < 0.1 %): Anaphylactic (e.g. bronchospasm) and anaphylactoid reactions (see section *4.4*)

Nervous system disorders

Rare (⩾ 0.01 % - < 0.1 %): Headache, dizziness.

Gastrointestinal disorders

Common (⩾ 1% - < 10%): Loose stools or diarrhoea, nausea, vomiting.

Rare (⩾ 0.01 % - < 0.1 %): Stomatitis, glossitis. These side effects are usually mild and commonly disappear during treatment or after discontinuation of treatment.

Very rare (< 0.01 %) including isolated reports: Pseudomembranous colitis (mostly caused by *Clostridium difficile*), pancreatitis (possibly caused by obstruction of bile ducts).

Hepato-biliary disorders

Rare (⩾ 0.01 % - < 0.1 %): Increase in serum liver enzymes (AST, ALT, alkaline phosphatase).

Precipitation of ceftriaxone calcium salt in the gallbladder has been observed (see section *4.4*), mostly in patients treated with doses higher than the recommended standard dose. In rare cases, the precipitations have been accompanied by clinical symptoms such as pain. Symptomatic treatment is recommended in these cases. Discontinuation of ceftriaxone may also be considered.

Skin and subcutaneous tissue disorders

Uncommon (⩾ 0.1 % - < 1 %): Allergic skin reactions such as maculopapular rash or exanthema, urticaria, dermatitis, pruritis, oedema.

Very rare (< 0.01 %) including isolated reports: Erythema multiforme, Stevens Johnson Syndrome, Lyell's Syndrome/toxic epidermal necrolysis.

Renal and urinary disorders

Rare (⩾ 0.01 % - < 0.1 %): Increase in serum creatinine, oliguria, glycosuria, haematuria.

Very rare (< 0.01 %) including isolated reports: Renal precipitation, mostly in children older than 3 years who have been treated with either high daily doses (80 mg/kg/day and more) or total doses exceeding 10g and with other risk factors such as dehydration or immobilisation. Renal precipitation is reversible upon discontinuation of ceftriaxone. Anuria and renal impairment have been reported in association.

General disorders and administration site conditions

Rare (⩾ 0.01 % - < 0.1 %): Phlebitis and injection site pain following intravenous administration. This can be minimised by slow injection over at least 2-4 minutes. Rigors, pyrexia.

An intramuscular injection without lidocaine is painful.

4.9 Overdose

In the case of overdosage, drug concentrations would not be reduced by haemodialysis or peritoneal dialysis. There is no specific antidote. Treatment should be symptomatic.

5. PHARMACOLOGICAL PROPERTIES

5.1 Pharmacodynamic properties

General properties

ATC classification

Pharmacotherapeutic group: cephalosporins and related substances, ATC code: J01DA13

Mode of action

Ceftriaxone has bactericidal activity resulting from the inhibition of bacterial cell wall synthesis ultimately leading to cell death. Ceftriaxone is stable to a broad range of bacterial β-lactamases and is active against a broad spectrum of bacterial pathogens including both Gram-positive and Gram-negative species.

Mechanism of resistance

Ceftriaxone is stable to a wide range of both Gram-positive and Gram-negative beta-lactamases, including those which are able to hydrolyse advanced generation penicillin derivatives and other cephalosporins. Resistance to ceftriaxone is encoded mainly by the production of some beta-lactam hydrolysing enzymes (including carbapenemases and some ESBLs) especially in Gram-negative organisms. For Gram-positive organisms such as *S. aureus* and *S. pneumoniae*, acquired resistance is mainly encoded by cell wall target site alterations. Outside of the advanced generation parenteral cephalosporins, cross-resistance to other drug classes is generally not encountered.

Breakpoints

Current MIC breakpoints used to interpret ceftriaxone susceptibility data are shown below. The use of NCCLS breakpoints predominate and are the breakpoints used in data presented in the Table. Values quoted comprise mg/L

(MIC testing) or mm (disk diffusion testing) using a 30mg/L drug concentration.

National Committee for Clinical Laboratory Standards (NCCLS) (M100-S12) – 2002

(see Table 1 opposite)

Susceptibility

The prevalence of acquired resistance may vary geographically and with time for selected species and local information on resistance is desirable, particularly when treating severe infections. As necessary, expert advice should be sought when the local prevalence of resistance is such that the utility of the agent in at least some types of infections is questionable.

Ceftriaxone susceptibility among Gram-positive and Gram-negative bacterial species in Europe from January 1999-December 2001:

Commonly susceptible species (i.e. resistance < 10% in all EU Member States)

Gram-Positive aerobes:
MS[a] coagulase negative *Staphylococcus* spp. (including *S. epidermis*)*
MS[b] *Staphylococcus aureus**
Group B (*Streptococcus agalactiae*)
Streptococcus bovis
*Streptococcus pneumoniae**
Group A *Streptococcus (Streptococcus pyogenes)**
*Streptococcus viridans**

Gram-Negative aerobes:
Citrobacter spp. (including *C.freundii*)
*Escherichia coli**
Haemophilus influenzae
(including beta-lactamase positive isolates)[c]*
*Haemophilus para-influenzae**
Klebsiella spp. (including *K. pneumoniae* and *K. oxytoca*)*
*Moraxella catarrhalis**
*Morganella morganii**
Neisseria gonorrhea (including penicillin-resistant isolates)*
*Neisseria meningitidis**
Proteus spp. (including *P. mirabilis* and *P. vulgaris*)*
Salmonella spp. (including *S. typhimurium*)
Serratia spp. (including *Serratia marsescens*)*
Shigella spp.

Anaerobes:
Clostridium spp.*

Species for which acquired resistance may be a problem (i.e. resistance ⩾ 10% in at least one EU Member State)

Gram-Negative aerobes:
Pseudomonas aeruginosa +
Enterobacter spp. (including *E. aerogenes* and *E. cloacae*)*+ *Acinetobacter* spp. (including *A. baumanii* and *A. calcoaceticus*)*+

Anaerobes:
Bacteroides spp.*
Peptostreptococcus spp.*

Inherently resistant organisms

Gram-Positive aerobes:
MR[d] coagulase negative *Staphylococcus* spp. (including *S. epidermidis*)
MR[e] *Staphylococcus aureus*
Enterococcus spp.

Gram-Negative aerobes:
Listeria monocytogenes
Mycoplasma spp.
Stenotrophomonas maltophilia
Ureaplasma urealyticum

Others:
Chlamydia spp.

[a]Methicillin-susceptible Coagulase-Negative *Staphylococcus*

[b]Methicillin-susceptible *Staphylococcus aureus*

[c]Non-susceptible range (no resistant breakpoints defined)

[d]Methicillin-resistant Coagulase-Negative *Staphylococcus*

[e]Methicillin-resistant *Staphylococcus aureus*

* Species for which the efficacy of ceftriaxone has been demonstrated both in vitro and in vivo

+ Species for which high rates of resistance have been observed in one or more regions within the EU

The table above comprises current levels of susceptibility according to routinely produced susceptibility test results in France, Germany, Greece, Italy, the Netherlands, Spain, and the United Kingdom. All data is presented using contemporary NCCLS derived susceptibility breakpoints except France (CA-SFM). Data is derived from The Surveillance Network® (TSN) Databases in each respective region. The prevalence of resistance may vary geographically and with time for selected species and local information on resistance is desirable, particularly when treating severe infections. This information gives only approximate guidance on probabilities whether microorganisms will be susceptible to ceftriaxone or not.

Table 1 National Committee for Clinical Laboratory Standards (NCCLS) (M100-S12) – 2002

	Susceptible	Intermediate	Resistant
Enterobacteriaceae, P. aeruginosa and other non-Enterobacteriaceae, Staphylococcus spp.	⩽8 Disk: ≤ 13	16-32 Disk: 14 – 20	⩾64 Disk: ≥ 21
Haemophilus spp.	⩽2 Disk: ⩾ 26	-	-
Neisseria spp.	⩽0.25 Disk: ⩾ 35	-	-
Streptococcus pneumoniae *	⩽0.5	1	⩾2
Other *Streptococcus* spp.**	Beta strep ⩽0.5 Disk: ≥24 Viridans group: ≤0.5 Disk: ≥27	- Viridans group: 1 Disk: 25-26	- Viridans group: ≥2 Disk: ≤24

* Recent 2002 *S. pneumoniae* breakpoints (NCCLS M100-S12) defined as ⩽1 (Sensitive), 2 (Intermediate) and ⩾4 (Resistant) for non-meningitis specimens and ≤ 0.5 (Sensitive), 1 (Intermediate), and ≥ 2 (Resistant) for meningitis specimens.

** Recent 2002 *Streptococcus viridans* group breakpoints (NCCLS M100-S12) defined ≤1 (Sensitive), 2 (Intermediate), and ≥4 (Resistant)

5.2 Pharmacokinetic properties

The pharmacokinetics of Rocephin are largely determined by its concentration-dependent binding to serum albumin. The plasma free (unbound) fraction of the drug in man is approximately 5% over most of the therapeutic concentration range, increasing to 15% at concentrations of 300mg/l. Owing to the lower albumin content, the proportion of free ceftriaxone in interstitial fluid is correspondingly higher than in plasma.

Plasma concentrations: Mean peak concentrations after bolus intravenous injection are about 120mg/l following a 500mg dose and about 200mg/l following a 1g dose; mean levels of 250mg/l are achieved after infusion of 2g over 30 minutes. Intramuscular injection of 500mg Rocephin in 1.06% Lidocaine produces mean peak plasma concentrations of 40 - 70mg/l within 1 hour. Bioavailability after intramuscular injection is 100%.

Excretion: Rocephin is eliminated mainly as unchanged ceftriaxone, approximately 60% of the dose being excreted in the urine (almost exclusively by glomerular filtration) and the remainder via the biliary and intestinal tracts. The total plasma clearance is 10 - 22ml/min. The renal clearance is 5 - 12ml/min. The elimination half-life in adults is about 8 hours. The half-life is not significantly affected by the dose, the route of administration or by repeated administration.

Pharmacokinetics in special clinical situations

In the first week of life, 80% of the dose is excreted in the urine; over the first month, this falls to levels similar to those in the adult.

In elderly persons aged over 75 years, the average elimination half-life is usually 2 to 3 times longer than in the young adult group. As with all cephalosporins, a decrease in renal function in the elderly may lead to an increase in half-life. Evidence gathered to date with ceftriaxone however, suggests that no modification of the dosage regimen is needed.

In patients with *renal* or *hepatic dysfunction*, the pharmacokinetics of ceftriaxone are only minimally altered and the elimination half-life is only slightly increased. If kidney function alone is impaired, biliary elimination of ceftriaxone is increased; if liver function alone is impaired, renal elimination is increased.

Cerebrospinal fluid: Rocephin crosses non-inflamed and inflamed meninges, attaining concentrations 4 - 17% of the simultaneous plasma concentration.

5.3 Preclinical safety data

There are no preclinical data of relevance to the prescriber which are additional to that already included in other sections of the SPC.

6. PHARMACEUTICAL PARTICULARS

6.1 List of excipients

None.

6.2 Incompatibilities

Solutions containing Rocephin should not be mixed with or added to solutions containing other agents. In particular, Rocephin is not compatible with calcium-containing solutions such as Hartmann's solution and Ringer's solution. Based on literature reports, ceftriaxone is not compatible with amsacrine, vancomycin, fluconozole, aminoglycosides and labetalol.

6.3 Shelf life

3 years.

For shelf life of diluted product see section *6.6*.

6.4 Special precautions for storage

Do not store above 25°C.

For shelf life of diluted product see section *6.6*.

6.5 Nature and contents of container

Rocephin 250mg and 1g: Type 1 Ph. Eur 15ml glass vial with teflonised rubber stopper and aluminium cap, containing a sterile, white to yellowish-orange crystalline powder. Packs of 1 vial.

Rocephin 2g: Type II Ph. Eur 50ml glass vial with teflonised rubber stopper and aluminium cap, containing a sterile, white to yellowish-orange crystalline powder. Packs of 1 vial.

Each gram of Rocephin contains approximately 3.6mmol sodium.

6.6 Instructions for use and handling

Preparation of solutions for injection and infusion

The use of freshly prepared solutions is recommended. These maintain potency for at least 6 hours at or below 25°C in daylight, or 24 hours at 2-8°C.

Rocephin should not be mixed in the same syringe with any drug other than 1.06% Lidocaine Hydrochloride BP solution (for intramuscular injection only).

Intramuscular injection: 250mg Rocephin should be dissolved in 1ml of 1.06% Lidocaine Hydrochloride BP solution, or 1g in 3.5ml of 1.06% Lidocaine Hydrochloride BP solution. The solution should be administered by deep intramuscular injection. Dosages greater than 1g should be divided and injected at more than one site.

Solutions in Lidocaine should not be administered intravenously.

Intravenous injection: 250mg Rocephin should be dissolved in 5ml of Water for Injections BP or 1g in 10ml of Water for Injections BP. The injection should be administered over at least 2 - 4 minutes, directly into the vein or via the tubing of an intravenous infusion.

Intravenous infusion: 2g of Rocephin should be dissolved in 40ml of one of the following calcium-free solutions: Dextrose Injection BP 5% or 10%, Sodium Chloride Injection BP, Sodium Chloride and Dextrose Injection BP (0.45% Sodium Chloride and 2.5% Dextrose), Dextran 6% in Dextrose Injection BP 5%, Hydroxyethyl Starch 6 - 10% infusions. The infusion should be administered over at least 30 minutes.

The displacement value of 250mg of Rocephin is 0.194ml.

7. MARKETING AUTHORISATION HOLDER

Roche Products Limited, 40 Broadwater Road, Welwyn Garden City, Hertfordshire, AL7 3AY.

8. MARKETING AUTHORISATION NUMBER(S)

Vials 250mg	PL 0031/0169
Vials 1g	PL 0031/0171
Vials 2g	PL 0031/0172

9. DATE OF FIRST AUTHORISATION/RENEWAL OF THE AUTHORISATION

23 October 2003

10. DATE OF REVISION OF THE TEXT

December 2003

P738215/304

Roferon Cartridge

(Roche Products Limited)

1. NAME OF THE MEDICINAL PRODUCT

Roferon-A 18MIU/0.6ml.

Cartridges containing solution for injection.

2. QUALITATIVE AND QUANTITATIVE COMPOSITION
Roferon-A is supplied in cartridges as a ready-to-use solution for injection.

Each cartridge contains 18 Million International Units interferon alfa-2a per 0.6 millilitres* (18MIU/0.6ml).

* Contains volume overages.

Recombinant interferon alfa-2a produced by genetic engineering from Escherichia coli.

For excipients see section *6.1*

3. PHARMACEUTICAL FORM
Cartridges containing solution for injection.

Solution is clear and colourless to light yellow.

4. CLINICAL PARTICULARS
4.1 Therapeutic indications
Roferon-A is indicated for the treatment of:

- Hairy cell leukaemia.

- AIDS patients with progressive, asymptomatic Kaposi's sarcoma who have a CD4 count > 250/mm^3.

- Chronic phase Philadelphia-chromosome positive chronic myelogenous leukaemia. Roferon-A is not an alternative treatment for CML patients who have an HLA-identical relative and for whom allogeneic bone marrow transplantation is planned or possible in the immediate future. It is still unknown whether Roferon-A can be considered as a treatment with a curative potential in this indication.

- Cutaneous T-cell lymphoma. Interferon alfa-2a (Roferon-A) may be active in patients who have progressive disease and who are refractory to, or unsuitable for, conventional therapy.

- Adult patients with histologically proven chronic hepatitis B who have markers for viral replication, i.e., those who are positive for HBV-DNA or HBeAg.

- Adult patients with histologically proven chronic hepatitis C who are positive for HCV antibodies or HCV RNA and have elevated serum alanine aminotransferase (ALT) without liver decompensation.

The efficacy of interferon alfa-2a in the treatment of hepatitis C is enhanced when combined with ribavirin. Roferon-A should be given alone mainly in case of intolerance or contra-indication to ribavirin.

- Follicular non-Hodgkin's lymphoma.

- Advanced renal cell carcinoma.

- Patients with AJCC Stage II malignant melanoma (Breslow tumour thickness > 1.5mm, no lymph node involvement or cutaneous spread) who are free of disease after surgery.

4.2 Posology and method of administration
Not all available Roferon-A strengths can be used for all indications mentioned in section *4.1 Therapeutic indications.* The prescribed strength should correspond with the recommended dose for each individual indication.

- HAIRY CELL LEUKAEMIA

Initial dosage:

Three million IU daily, given by subcutaneous injection for 16 – 24 weeks. If intolerance develops, either the daily dose should be lowered to 1.5 million IU or the schedule changed to three times per week, or both.

Maintenance dosage:

Three million IU, given three times per week by subcutaneous injection. If intolerance develops, the dose should be lowered to 1.5 million IU three times per week.

Duration of treatment:

Patients should be treated for approximately six months before the physician decides whether to continue treatment in responding patients or to discontinue treatment in non-responding patients. Patients have been treated for up to 20 consecutive months. The optimal duration of Roferon-A treatment for hairy cell leukaemia has not been determined.

The minimum effective dose of Roferon-A in hairy cell leukaemia has not been established.

- AIDS-RELATED KAPOSI'S SARCOMA

Roferon-A is indicated for the treatment of AIDS patients with progressive, asymptomatic Kaposi's sarcoma who have a CD4 count > 250/mm^3. AIDS patients with CD4 counts < 250/mm^3, or those with a history of opportunistic infections or constitutional symptoms, are unlikely to respond to Roferon-A therapy and therefore should not be treated. The optimal posology has not yet been well established.

Roferon-A should not be used in conjunction with protease inhibitors. With the exception of zidovudine, there is a lack of safety data for the combination of Roferon-A with reverse transcriptase inhibitors.

Initial dosage:

Roferon-A should be given by subcutaneous injection, and escalated to at least 18 million IU daily and if possible to 36 million IU daily for a total of ten to twelve weeks in patients of 18 years or older. The recommended escalation schedule is as follows:

Days 1 – 3	3 million IU daily
Days 4 – 6	9 million IU daily
Days 7 – 9	18 million IU daily - and, if tolerated, increase to:
Days 10 – 84	36 million IU daily

Maintenance dosage:

Roferon-A should be given by subcutaneous injection three times per week at the maximum dose which is acceptable to the patient, but not exceeding 36 million IU.

Patients with AIDS-related Kaposi's sarcoma treated with 3 million IU of Roferon-A given daily showed a lower response rate than those treated with the recommended dosage.

Duration of treatment:

The evolution of lesions should be documented to determine response to therapy. Patients should be treated for a minimum of ten weeks and preferably for at least twelve weeks before the physician decides whether to continue treatment in responding patients or to discontinue treatment in non-responding patients. Patients generally showed evidence of response after approximately three months of therapy. Patients have been treated for up to 20 consecutive months. If a response to treatment occurs, treatment should continue at least until there is no further evidence of tumour. The optimal duration of Roferon-A treatment for AIDS-related Kaposi's sarcoma has not been determined.

Note:

Lesions of Kaposi's sarcoma frequently reappear when Roferon-A treatment is discontinued.

- CHRONIC MYELOGENOUS LEUKAEMIA

Roferon-A is indicated for the treatment of patients with chronic phase Philadelphia-chromosome positive chronic myelogenous leukaemia. Roferon-A is not an alternative treatment for CML patients who have an HLA-identical relative and for whom allogeneic bone marrow transplantation is planned or possible in the immediate future.

Roferon-A produces haematological remissions in 60% of patients with chronic phase CML, independent of prior treatment. Two thirds of these patients have complete haematological responses which occur as late as 18 months after treatment start.

In contrast to cytotoxic chemotherapy, interferon alfa-2a is able to generate sustained, ongoing cytogenetic responses beyond 40 months. It is still unkown whether Roferon-A can be considered as a treatment with a curative potential in this indication.

Dosage:

It is recommended that Roferon-A should be given by subcutaneous injection for eight to twelve weeks to patients 18 years or more. The recommended schedule is:

Days 1 – 3	3 million IU daily
Days 4 – 6	6 million IU daily
Days 7 – 84	9 million IU daily

Duration of treatment:

Patients should be treated for a minimum of eight weeks, preferably for at least twelve weeks before the physician decides whether or not to continue treatment in responding patients or to discontinue treatment in patients not showing any changes in haematological parameters. Responding patients should be treated until complete haematological response is achieved or for a maximum of 18 months. All patients with complete haematologic responses should continue treatment with 9 million IU daily (optimum) or 9 million IU three times a week (minimum) in order to achieve a cytogenetic response in the shortest possible time. The optimal duration of Roferon-A treatment for chronic myelogenous leukaemia has not been determined, although cytogenetic responses have been observed two years after treatment start.

The safety, efficacy and optimal dosage of Roferon-A in children with CML has not yet been established.

– CUTANEOUS T-CELL LYMPHOMA (CTCL)

Interferon alfa-2a (Roferon-A) may be active in patients with progressive cutaneous T-cell lymphoma and who are refractory to, or unsuitable for, conventional therapy.

The optimal dosage has not been established.

Initial dosage:

Roferon-A should be given by subcutaneous injection, and escalated to 18 million IU daily for a total of twelve weeks in patients of 18 years or older. The recommended escalation schedule is as follows:

Days 1 – 3	3 million IU daily
Days 4 – 6	9 million IU daily
Days 7 – 84	18 million IU daily

Maintenance dosage:

Roferon-A should be given by subcutaneous injection three times per week at the maximum dose which is acceptable to the patient, but not exceeding 18 million IU.

Duration of treatment:

Patients should be treated for a minimum of eight weeks and preferably for at least twelve weeks before the physician decides whether to continue treatment in responding patients or to discontinue treatment in non-responding patients. Minimum treatment duration in responding patients should be twelve months in order to maximise the chance to achieve a complete response and improve the chance for a prolonged response. Patients have been treated for up to 40 consecutive months. The optimal duration of Roferon-A treatment for cutaneous T-cell lymphoma has not been determined.

Warning:

Objective tumour responses have not been observed in approximately 40% of patients with CTCL. Partial responses are usually seen within three months and complete responses within six months, although it may occasionally take more than one year to reach the best response.

– CHRONIC HEPATITIS B

Roferon-A is indicated for the treatment of adult patients with histologically proven chronic hepatitis B who have markers for viral replication, i.e., those who are positive for HBV-DNA or HBeAg.

Dosage recommendation:

The optimal schedule of treatment has not been established yet. The dose is usually in the range of 2.5 million IU to 5.0 million IU/m^2 body surface administered subcutaneously three times per week for a period of four to six months.

The dosage may be adjusted according to the patient's tolerance to the medication. If no improvement has been observed after three to four months of treatment, discontinuation of therapy should be considered.

Children: up to 10 million IU/m^2 has been safely administered to children with chronic hepatitis B. However efficacy of therapy has not been demonstrated.

– CHRONIC HEPATITIS C

ROFERON-A IN COMBINATION WITH RIBAVIRIN

RELAPSED PATIENTS

Roferon-A is given in combination with ribavirin for adult patients with chronic hepatitis C who have previously responded to interferon alpha monotherapy, but who have relapsed after treatment was stopped.

Dosage:

Roferon-A: 4.5 MIU three times per week by subcutaneous injection for a period of six months.

Dosage of Ribavirin:

Ribavirin dose: 1000 mg to 1200 mg/day in two divided doses (once in the morning with breakfast and once with the evening meal). Please refer to the SmPC for ribavirin for further details on the posology and method of administration of ribavirin.

NAÏVE PATIENTS

The efficacy of interferon alfa-2a in the treatment of hepatitis C is enhanced when combined with ribavirin. Roferon-A should be given alone mainly in case of intolerance or contra-indication to ribavirin.

Dosage:

Roferon-A: 3 to 4.5 MIU three times per week by subcutaneous injection for a period of at least six months. Treatment should be continued for an additional six months in patients who have negative HCV RNA at month six, and are infected with genotype 1 and have high pre-treatment viral load.

Dosage of Ribavirin: see above.

Other negative prognostic factors (age > 40 years, male gender, bridging fibrosis) should be taken into account in order to extend therapy to twelve months.

Patients who failed to show a virologic response after six months of treatment (HCV-RNA below lower limit of detection) do generally not become sustained virologic responders (HCV-RNA below lower limit of detection six months after withdrawal of treatment).

Roferon-A monotherapy:

Roferon-A monotherapy should be given mainly in case of intolerance or contra-indication to ribavirin.

Initial dosage:

Roferon-A should be administered at a dose of 3 to 6 million IU by subcutaneous injection three times a week for six months as induction therapy, patient tolerance permitting. In patients who fail to respond after three to four months of treatment, discontinuation of Roferon-A should be considered.

Maintenance dosage:

Patients whose serum ALT has normalised and/or HCV RNA has become undetectable require maintenance therapy with 3 million IU Roferon-A three times a week for an additional six months or longer to consolidate the complete response. The optimal duration of treatment has not yet been determined but a therapy of at least twelve months is advised.

Note:

The majority of patients who relapse after adequate treatment with Roferon-A alone do so within four months of the end of treatment.

- FOLLICULAR NON-HODGKINS LYMPHOMA

Roferon-A prolongs disease-free and progression-free survival when used as adjunctive treatment to CHOP-like chemotherapy regimens in patients with advanced (high tumour burden) follicular non-Hodgkin's lymphoma.

However, the efficacy of adjunctive interferon alfa-2a treatment on overall long-term survival of these patients has not yet been established.

Dosage recommendation:

Roferon-A should be administered concomitantly to a conventional chemotherapy regimen (such as the combination of cyclophosphamide, prednisone, vincristine and doxorubicin) according to a schedule such as 6 million IU/m^2 given subcutaneously from day 22 to day 26 of each 28-day cycle.

- ADVANCED RENAL CELL CARCINOMA

Therapy with Roferon-A in combination with vinblastine induces overall response rates of approximately 17 – 26%, delays disease progression, and prolongs overall survival in patients with advanced renal cell carcinoma.

Dosage recommendation:

Roferon-A should be given by subcutaneous injection at a dose of 3 million IU three times weekly for one week, 9 million IU three times weekly for the following week and 18 million IU three times weekly thereafter. Concomitantly vinblastine should be given intravenously according to the manufacturer's instructions at a dose of 0.1mg/kg once every three weeks.

If the Roferon-A dosage of 18 million IU three times per week is not tolerated the dose may be reduced to 9 million IU three times per week.

Treatment should be given for a minimum of three months, up to a maximum of twelve months or until the development of progressive disease. Patients who achieve a complete response may stop treatment three months after the response is established.

- SURGICALLY RESECTED MALIGNANT MELANOMA

Adjuvant therapy with a low dose of Roferon-A prolongs disease-free interval in patients with no nodal or distant metastases following resection of a melanoma (tumour thickness > 1.5mm).

Dosage recommendation:

Roferon-A should be administered subcutaneously or intramuscularly at a dose of 3 million IU three times a week for 18 months, starting no later than six weeks post surgery. If intolerance develops, the dose should be lowered to 1.5 million IU three times a week.

4.3 Contraindications

Roferon-A is contra-indicated in patients with:

1. a history of hypersensitivity to recombinant interferon alfa-2a or to any of the excipients,

2. severe pre-existing cardiac disease or with any history of cardiac illness. No direct cardiotoxic effect has been demonstrated, but it is likely that acute, self-limiting toxicities (i.e., fever, chills) frequently associated with administration of Roferon-A may exacerbate pre-existing cardiac conditions,

3. severe renal, hepatic or myeloid dysfunction,

4. uncontrolled seizure disorders and/or compromised central nervous system function (see section *4.4*),

5. chronic hepatitis with advanced, decompensated hepatic disease or cirrhosis of the liver,

6. chronic hepatitis who are being or have recently been treated with immunosuppressive agents.

7. Benzyl alcohol which is an excipient in Roferon-A solution for injection has on rare occasions been associated with potentially fatal toxicities and anaphylactoid reactions in children up to three years old. Therefore, Roferon-A solution for injection should not be used in premature babies, neonates, infants or young children. Roferon-A solution contains 10 mg/ml benzyl alcohol.

Combination therapy with ribavirin: Also see ribavirin labelling if interferon alfa-2a is to be administered in combination with ribavirin in patients with chronic hepatitis C.

4.4 Special warnings and special precautions for use

Roferon-A should be administered under the supervision of a qualified physician experienced in the management of the respective indication. Appropriate management of the therapy and its complications is possible only when adequate diagnostic and treatment facilities are readily available.

Patients should be informed not only of the benefits of therapy but also that they will probably experience adverse reactions.

Hypersensitivity: If a hypersensitivity reaction occurs during treatment with Roferon-A or in the combination therapy with ribavirin, treatment has to be discontinued and appropriate medical therapy has to be instituted immediately. Transient rashes do not necessitate interruption of treatment.

In transplant patients (e.g., kidney or bone marrow transplant) therapeutic immunosuppression may be weakened because interferons also exert an immunostimulatory action.

Psychiatric: Severe psychiatric adverse reactions may manifest in patients receiving therapy with interferons, including Roferon-A. Depression, suicidal ideation, suicidal attempt, and suicide may occur in patients with and without previous psychiatric illness. Physicians should monitor all patients treated with Roferon-A for evidence of depression. Physicians should inform patients of the possible development of depression prior to initiation of therapy, and patients should report any sign or symptom of depression immediately. Psychiatric intervention and/or drug discontinuation should be considered in such cases.

Ophthalmologic: As with other interferons, retinopathy including retinal haemorrhages, cotton wool spots, papilloedema, retinal artery or vein thrombosis and optic neuropathy which may result in loss of vision, have been reported after treatment with Roferon-A. Any patient complaining of decrease or loss of vision must have an eye examination. Because these ocular events may occur in conjunction with other disease states, a visual examination prior to initiation of Roferon-A monotherapy or in the combination therapy with ribavirin is recommended in patients with diabetes mellitus or hypertension. Roferon-A monotherapy or the combination therapy with ribavirin should be discontinued in patients who developed new or worsening ophthalmologic disorders.

Endocrine: Hyperglycaemia has been observed rarely in patients treated with Roferon-A. All patients who develop symptoms of hyperglycaemia should have their blood glucose measured and followed-up accordingly. Patients with diabetes mellitus may require adjustment of their antidiabetic regimen.

When mild to moderate renal, hepatic or myeloid dysfunction is present, close monitoring of these functions is required.

Hepatic function: In rare cases interferon alpha has been suspected of causing an exacerbation of an underlying autoimmune disease in hepatitis patients. Therefore, when treating hepatitis patients with a history of autoimmune disease caution is recommended. If a deterioration in liver function in these patients develops a determination of autoimmune antibodies should be considered. If necessary treatment should be discontinued.

Bone marrow suppression: Extreme caution should be exercised when administering Roferon-A to patients with severe myelosuppression as it has a suppressive effect on the bone marrow, leading to a fall in the white blood count, particularly granulocytes, platelet count and, less commonly, haemoglobin concentration. This can lead to an increased risk of infection or of haemorrhage. It is important to monitor closely these events in patients and periodic complete blood counts should be performed during the course of Roferon-A treatment, both prior to therapy and at appropriate periods during therapy.

Autoimmune: The development of different auto-antibodies has been reported during treatment with alfa interferons. Clinical manifestations of autoimmune disease during interferon therapy occur more frequently in subjects predisposed to the development of autoimmune disorders. In patients with an underlying or clinical history of autoimmune disorders, monitoring of symptoms suggestive of these disorders, as well as measurement of auto-antibodies and TSH level, is recommended.

The use of Roferon-A in children is not recommended as the safety and effectiveness of Roferon-A in children have not been established.

Efficacy in patients with chronic hepatitis B or C who are on haemodialysis or have haemophilia or are co-infected with human immunodeficiency virus has not been demonstrated.

This product contains less than 1 mmol sodium (23 mg) per 0.5 ml, i.e, essentially 'sodium free'.

Combination therapy with ribavirin: Also see ribavirin labelling if interferon alfa-2a is to be administered in combination with ribavirin in patients with chronic hepatitis C.

Patients co-infected with HIV and receiving Highly Active Anti-Retroviral Therapy (HAART) may be at increased risk of developing lactic acidosis. Caution should be used when adding Roferon-A and ribavirin to HAART therapy (see ribavirin SPC).

Co-infected patients with advanced cirrhosis receiving HAART may be at increased risk of hepatic decompensation and death. Adding treatment with alfa interferons alone or in combination with ribavirin may increase the risk in this patient subset.

4.5 Interaction with other medicinal products and other forms of Interaction

Since alfa-interferons alter cellular metabolism, the potential to modify the activity of other drugs exists. In a small study, Roferon-A was shown to have an effect on specific microsomal enzyme systems. The clinical relevance of these findings is unknown.

Alfa-interferons may affect the oxidative metabolic process; this should be borne in mind when prescribing concomitant therapy with drugs metabolised by this route. However, as yet no specific information is available.

Roferon-A has been reported to reduce the clearance of theophylline.

As Roferon-A may affect central nervous system functions, interactions could occur following concurrent administration of centrally-acting drugs. The neurotoxic, haematotoxic or cardiotoxic effects of previously or concurrently administered drugs may be increased by interferons.

Combination therapy with ribavirin: Also see ribavirin labelling if interferon alfa-2a is to be administered in combination with ribavirin in patients with chronic hepatitis C.

4.6 Pregnancy and lactation

Men and women receiving Roferon-A should practise effective contraception. There are no adequate data on the use of Roferon-A in pregnant women. When doses greatly in excess of the recommended clinical dose were administered to pregnant rhesus monkeys in the early to mid-foetal period, an abortifacient effect was observed (see section 5.3). Although animal tests do not indicate that Roferon-A is a teratogen, harm to the foetus from use during pregnancy cannot be excluded. In pregnancy, Roferon-A should be administered only if the benefit to the woman justifies the potential risk to the foetus.

It is not known whether this drug is excreted in human milk. A decision must be taken whether to suspend breast feeding or to discontinue the drug, taking into account the importance of the drug to the mother.

Combination therapy with ribavirin: Also see ribavirin labelling if interferon alfa-2a is to be administered in combination with ribavirin in patients with chronic hepatitis C.

4.7 Effects on ability to drive and use machines

Depending on dose and schedule as well as the sensitivity of the individual patient, Roferon-A may have an effect on the speed of reaction which could impair certain operations, e.g., driving, operation of machinery etc.

4.8 Undesirable effects

Combination therapy with ribavirin: Also see ribavirin labelling if interferon alfa-2a is to be administered in combination with ribavirin in patients with chronic hepatitis C.

The following data on adverse reactions are based on information derived from the treatment of cancer patients with a wide variety of malignancies and often refractory to previous therapy and suffering from advanced disease, patients with chronic hepatitis B, and patients with chronic hepatitis C.

Approximately two thirds of cancer patients experienced anorexia and one half nausea. Cardiovascular and pulmonary disorders were seen in about one fifth of cancer patients and consisted of transient hypotension, hypertension, oedema, cyanosis, arrhythmias, palpitations and chest pain.

Most cancer patients received doses that were significantly higher than the dose now recommended and may explain the higher frequency and severity of adverse reactions in this patient group compared with patients with hepatitis B where adverse reactions are usually transient, and patients return to pre-treatment status within 1 to 2 weeks after the end of therapy. Cardiovascular disorders were very rarely seen in patients with hepatitis B. In hepatitis B patients, changes in transaminases usually signal an improvement in the clinical state of the patient.

The majority of the patients experienced flu-like symptoms such as fatigue, pyrexia, rigors, decreased appetite, myalgia, headache, arthralgia and diaphoresis. These acute side-effects can usually be reduced or eliminated by concurrent administration of paracetamol and tend to diminish with continued therapy or dose modification although continuing therapy can lead to lethargy, asthenia and fatigue.

Infections & Infestations:

Rare: pneumonia, herpes simplex (including exacerbations of herpes labialis)

Blood & Lymphatic System Disorders:

Very Common: leukopenia

Common: thrombocytopenia, anaemia

Rare: agranulocytosis, haemolytic anaemia

Very Rare: idiopathic thrombocytopenia purpura

In myelosuppressed patients, thrombocytopenia and decreased haemoglobin occurred more frequently. Recovery of severe haematological deviations to pre-treatment levels usually occurred within seven to ten days after discontinuing Roferon-A/Roceron-A/Roféron-A treatment.

Immune System Disorders:

Rare: autoimmune disorder, acute hypersensitivity reactions (e.g. urticaria, angioedema, bronchospasm and anaphylaxis)

Very Rare: sarcoidosis

Endocrine Disorders:

Rare: hyperthyroidism, hypothyroidism, thyroid dysfunction

Metabolism & Nutrition Disorders:

Very Common: anorexia, nausea, inconsequential hypocalcaemia

Uncommon: electrolyte imbalance, dehydration

Rare: hyperglycaemia

Very Rare: diabetes mellitus, hypertriglyceridaemia

Psychiatric Disorders:

Uncommon: depression, anxiety, mental status changes, confusional state, abnormal behaviour, nervousness, memory impairment, sleep disorder

Rare: suicide, suicide attempt, suicidal ideation

Nervous System Disorders:

Very Common: headache

Uncommon: neuropathy, dizziness, somnolence, dysgeusia, paraesthesia, hypoesthisia, tremor

Rare: coma, cerebrovascular accident, convulsions, transient erectile dysfunction

Eye Disorders:

Uncommon: conjunctivitis, visual disturbance

Rare: ischaemic retinopathy

Very Rare: optic neuropathy, retinal artery thrombosis, retinal vein thrombosis, retinopathy, retinal haemorrhage, papilloedema, retinal exudates

Ear & Labyrinth Disorders:

Uncommon: vertigo

Cardiac Disorders:

Uncommon: arrhythmias, including atrioventricular block, palpitations

Rare: cardiorespiratory arrest, myocardial infarction, congestive heart failure, pulmonary oedema, cyanosis

Vascular Disorders:

Uncommon: hypertension, hypotension

Rare: vasculitis

Respiratory, Thoracic & Mediastinal Disorders:

Rare: dyspnoea, cough

Gastrointestinal Disorders:

Very Common: diarrhoea

Common: nausea/vomiting

Uncommon: abdominal pain, dry mouth

Rare: intestinal hypermotility, constipation, dyspepsia, flatulence, pancreatitis

Very Rare: reactivation of peptic ulcer, non-life threatening gastrointestinal bleeding

Hepatobiliary Disorders:

Rare: hepatic failure, hepatitis, hepatic dysfunction

Skin & Subcutaneous Tissue Disorders:

Very Common: alopecia (reversible upon discontinuation; increased hair loss may continue for several weeks after end of treatment), sweating increased

Uncommon: exacerbation of, or provocation of, psoriasis, pruritus

Rare: rash, dry skin, epistaxis, mucosal dryness, rhinorrhoea

Musculoskeletal & Connective Tissue Disorders:

Very Common: myalgia, arthralgia

Rare: systemic lupus erythematosus, arthritis

Renal & Urinary Disorders:

Uncommon: proteinuria **and increased cell count in urine**

Rare: acute renal failure (mainly in cancer patients with renal disease), renal impairment

General Disorders & Administration Site Conditions:

Very Common: flu-like illness, fatigue, pyrexia, rigors, appetite decreased

Uncommon: chest pain, oedema

Very Rare: injection site necrosis, injection site reaction

Investigations:

Uncommon: increases in ALT, blood alkaline phosphatase, and transaminase, weight loss

Rare: increases in blood LDH, blood bilirubin, blood creatinine, blood uric acid, blood urea increased

Neutralising antibodies to interferons may form in some patients. In certain clinical conditions (cancer, systemic lupus erythematosus, herpes zoster) antibodies to human leucocyte interferon may also occur spontaneously in patients who have never received exogenous interferons. The clinical significance of the development of antibodies has not been fully clarified.

In clinical trials where lyophilised Roferon-A which had been stored at 25°C was used, neutralising antibodies to Roferon-A have been detected in approximately one fifth of patients. In patients with hepatitis C, a trend for responding patients who develop neutralising antibodies to lose response while still on treatment and to lose it earlier than patients who do not develop such antibodies, has been seen. No other clinical sequelae of the presence of antibodies to Roferon-A have been documented. The clinical significance of the development of antibodies has not been fully clarified.

No data on neutralising antibodies yet exist from clinical trials in which lyophilised Roferon-A or Roferon-A solution for injection which is stored at 4°C has been used. In a mouse model, the relative immunogenicity of lyophilised Roferon-A increases with time when the material is stored at 25°C - no such increase in immunogenicity is observed when lyophilised Roferon-A is stored at 4°C, the recommended storage conditions.

4.9 Overdose

There are no reports of overdosage but repeated large doses of interferon can be associated with profound lethargy, fatigue, prostration and coma. Such patients should be hospitalised for observation and appropriate supportive treatment given.

Patients who experience severe reactions to Roferon-A will usually recover within days after discontinuation of therapy, given appropriate supportive care. Coma has been observed in 0.4% of cancer patients in clinical trials.

5. PHARMACOLOGICAL PROPERTIES

5.1 Pharmacodynamic properties

Pharmacotherapeutic group:	Cytokines and immunomodulators, *Interferons*
	ATC Code L03AB04

Roferon-A has been shown to possess many of the activities of the so-called natural human alfa-interferon preparations. Roferon-A exerts its antiviral effects by inducing a state of resistance to viral infections in cells and by modulating the effector arm of the immune system to neutralise viruses or eliminate virus infected cells. The essential mechanism for the anti-tumour action of Roferon-A is not yet known. However, several changes are described in human tumoural cells treated with Roferon-A: HT 29 cells show a significant reduction of DNA, RNA and protein synthesis. Roferon-A has been shown to exert antiproliferative activity against a variety of human tumours *in vitro* and to inhibit the growth of some human tumour xenografts in nude mice. A limited number of human tumour cell lines grown *in vivo* in immunocompromised nude mice has been tested for the susceptibility to Roferon-A. *In vivo* antiproliferative activity of Roferon-A has been studied on tumours including breast mucoid carcinoma, adenocarcinoma of the caecum, colon carcinoma and prostatic carcinoma. The degree of antiproliferative activity is variable.

Unlike other human proteins, many of the effects of interferon alfa-2a are partially or completely suppressed when it is tested in other animal species. However, significant antivaccinia virus activity was induced in rhesus monkeys pretreated with interferon alfa-2a.

Clinical Trials

Hairy Cell Leukaemia

The therapeutic efficacy of Roferon-A in the treatment of hairy cell leukaemia has been demonstrated in a large trial of 218 patients, of whom 174 were evaluable for efficacy after 16 – 24 weeks of therapy. Response was observed in 88% of patients (complete response 33%, partial response 55%).

AIDS-related Kaposi's Sarcoma

The efficacy of Roferon-A in the treatment of Kaposi's sarcoma was assessed in 364 patients receiving of 3 to 54 MIU per day. Objective response rates were dose-related, ranging from 14% to 50%, with a daily dose of 36 MIU producing the best overall therapeutic benefit (13.3% complete response, 12.2% partial response). High baseline CD4 lymphocyte count was a favourable prognostic factor for response, with 46% of patients with a CD4 count > 400/mm^3 responding to Roferon-A. Response to Roferon-A therapy was the strongest prognostic factor for survival.

Chronic Myelogenous Leukaemia (CML)

The efficacy of Roferon-A was assessed in 226 patients with chronic phase CML, and compared with 109 patients receiving chemotherapy (hydroxyurea or busulfan). Both groups had favourable features at diagnosis (less than 10% blasts in the blood) and treatment was initiated with interferon within six months of diagnosis. Treatment of patients with CML in the chronic phase leads to the same proportion of patients (85 – 90%) achieving a haematologic response as treatment with the standard chemotherapy regimens. In addition patients treated with Roferon-A resulted in 8% complete cytogenetic response and 38% partial cytogenetic response versus 9% partial cytogenetic response during chemotherapy. Time to progression from the chronic phase of leukaemia to an accelerated or a blastic phase was longer in the Roferon-A group (69 months) than in the conventional chemo-therapy group (46 months) ($p < 0.001$) as was median overall survival (72.8 months versus 54.5 months, $p = 0.002$).

Cutaneous T-cell Lymphoma (CTCL)

The efficacy of Roferon-A was assessed in 169 patients with CTCL, the majority of whom (78%) were resistant to, or had relapsed on, standard therapy. Among the 85 patients evaluable, overall response to treatment was 58% (20% complete response, 38% partial response). Patients with all stages of disease responded to therapy. Median duration of complete response from start of treatment was 22 months, with 94% of complete responders remaining in remission at 9 months.

Chronic Hepatitis B

The efficacy of Roferon-A in the treatment of chronic hepatitis B was assessed in trials involving over 900 patients. In the pivotal controlled study 238 patients were randomised into four groups: patients received either 2.5 MIU / m^2, 5.0 MIU / m^2, 10 MIU / m^2, tiw of Roferon-A or no treatment. Treatment duration was 12 – 24 weeks depending on response i.e. clearance of HBeAg and HBV DNA from serum. Patients were followed for up to twelve months after treatment was discontinued. There was a statistically significant difference in sustained response [clearance of hepatitis Be antigen (HBeAg)] and hepatitis B viral DNA (HBV DNA) between treated and untreated patients (37% versus 13%). Response differences between various dose groups did not reach statistical significance (33%, 34% and 43% for the 2.5, 5.0 and 10.0 MIU / m^2 groups). Serological and virological responses were associated with marked improvement in liver histology after twelve months of treatment free-follow up.

Chronic Hepatitis C

The efficacy of Roferon-A in the treatment of chronic hepatitis C has been assessed in 1701 patients, with 130 untreated or placebo treated controls. At recommended doses, Roferon-A induces complete biochemical response in up to 85% of patients, with response rates maintained for at least six months after treatment ranging from 11 to 44% depending on pre-treatment disease characteristics, IFN dose and treatment duration. Biochemical response to Roferon-A is associated with significant improvement of liver disease as shown by evaluation of pre-and post-liver biopsies. For those patients who have a sustained response three to six months after end of therapy, response has been reported to be maintained for up to four years.

The therapeutic efficacy of Interferon alfa-2a alone and in combination with ribavirin was compared in a double-blind randomised clinical trial in naïve (previously untreated) and relapsed patients with virologically, biochemically and histologically documented chronic hepatitis C. Six months after end of treatment sustained biochemical and virological response as well as histological improvement were assessed.

A statistically significant ten fold increase (from 4% to 43%; $p < 0.01$) in sustained virological and biochemical response was observed in relapsed patients. The favourable profile of the combination therapy was also reflected in the response rates relative to HCV genotype or baseline viral load. Although the sustained response rates in patients with HCV genotype-1 were lower than in the overall population (approx. 30% versus 0% in the monotherapy arm) the relative benefit of ribavirin in combination with interferon alfa-2a is particularly significant in this group of patients. In addition the histological improvement favoured the combination therapy.

Supportive favourable results from a small study in naïve patients were reported using interferon alfa-2a (3 MIU three times per week) with ribavirin.

For other information on pharmacodynamic properties please refer to the SmPC for Ribavirin.

Follicular Non-Hodgkin's lymphoma

The efficacy of Roferon-A in addition to cytotoxic chemotherapy (CHOP-like regimen of cyclophosphamide, vincristine, prednisone and doxorubicin) was assessed in 122 patients with clinically aggressive low-grade or intermediate-grade non-Hodgkin's lymphoma and compared with 127 controls receiving the same chemotherapy regimen. The two regimens produced comparable objective responses, but the regimen including Roferon-A had a greater effect in prolonging the time to treatment failure ($p < 0.001$), the duration of complete response ($p < 0.003$).

Renal Cell Carcinoma

The efficacy of Roferon-A, given in combination with vinblastine, was compared with vinblastine alone. The combination of Roferon-A plus vinblastine is superior to vinblastine alone in the treatment of patients with locally advanced or metastatic renal cell carcinoma. Median survival was 67.8 weeks for the 79 patients receiving Roferon-A plus vinblastine and 37.8 weeks for the 81 patients treated with vinblastine ($p = 0.0049$). Overall response rates were 16.5 % for patients treated with Roferon-A, plus vinblastine and 2.5% for patients treated with vinblastine alone ($p = 0.0025$).

Surgically Resected Malignant Melanoma

The efficacy of Roferon-A in patients with primary cutaneous melanoma thicker than 1.5 mm and without clinically detectable node metastasis was assessed in a large randomised study involving 253 patients receiving Roferon-A at a dose of 3 MIU three times a week for 18 months, compared with 246 untreated controls. After a median follow-up of 4.4 years a significant extension of relapse-free interval ($p = 0.035$) but no statistically significant difference in overall survival ($p = 0.059$) in Roferon-A treated patients compared with controls have been shown. The overall treatment effect was a 25% reduction in the risk of relapse.

5.2 Pharmacokinetic properties

The serum concentrations of interferon alfa-2a reflected a large intersubject variation in both healthy volunteers and patients with disseminated cancer. The pharmacokinetics of Roferon-A in animals (monkey, dog and mouse) were similar to those seen in man. The pharmacokinetics of Roferon-A in man were linear over a 3 million to 198 million IU dose range. In healthy man, interferon alfa-2a exhibited an elimination half-life of 3.7 – 8.5 hours (mean: 5.1 hours), a volume of distribution at steady state of 0.223 – 0.748 l/kg (mean: 0.4 l/kg) and a total body clearance of 2.14 – 3.62ml/min/kg (mean: 2.79ml/min/kg) after a 36 million IU intravenous infusion. After intramuscular administration of 36 million IU, peak serum concentrations ranged from 1500 to 2580pg/ml (mean: 2020pg/ml) at a mean time to peak of 3.8 hours, and after subcutaneous administration of 36 million IU from 1250 to 2320pg/ml (mean: 1730pg/ml) at a mean time to peak of 7.3 hours.

The apparent fraction of the dose absorbed after intramuscular or subcutaneous injection is greater than 80%.

The pharmacokinetics of interferon alfa-2a after single intramuscular doses to patients with disseminated cancer and chronic hepatitis B were similar to those found in healthy volunteers. Dose-proportional increases in serum concentrations were observed after single doses up to 198 million IU. There were no changes in the distribution or elimination of interferon alfa-2a during twice daily (0.5 – 36 million IU), once daily (1 - 54 million IU), or three times weekly (1 – 136 million IU) dosing regimens up to 28 days of dosing. Renal catabolism is the major pathway for Roferon-A elimination. Biliary excretion and liver metabolism are considered to be minor pathways of elimination of Roferon-A.

Intramuscular administration of Roferon-A one or more times daily for up to 28 days to some patients with disseminated cancer resulted in peak plasma concentrations of two to four times greater than those seen after single doses. However, multiple dosing caused no changes in its distribution or elimination parameters during several dosage regimens studied.

For other information on pharmacokinetic properties please refer to the SmPC for Ribavirin.

5.3 Preclinical safety data

Because of species specificity of human interferon, only limited toxicological studies have been carried out with Roferon-A. The acute parenteral toxicity of Roferon-A has been studied in mice, rats, rabbits and ferrets at doses up to 30 million IU/kg intravenously, and 500 million IU/kg intramuscularly. No treatment-related mortality was noted in any species studied given Roferon-A by any of the routes of administration. With doses greatly exceeding the recommended clinical dose no significant adverse effects were observed except for an abortifacient effect when administered to pregnant rhesus monkeys in the early to mid-foetal period and transient menstrual cycle irregularities including prolonged menstrual periods in non-pregnant monkeys. The relevance of these findings in man has not been established.

Mutagenic effects of Roferon-A have not been observed experimentally.

For other information on preclinical safety data please refer to the SmPC for Ribavirin.

6. PHARMACEUTICAL PARTICULARS

6.1 List of excipients

Ammonium acetate

Sodium Chloride

Benzyl alcohol

Polysorbate 80

Glacial Acetic acid

Sodium Hydroxide Solution

Water for Injections

6.2 Incompatibilities

Not applicable.

6.3 Shelf life

2 years.

After the first dose, Roferon-A cartridges may be stored at room temperature (below 25°C) for up to 28 days.

6.4 Special precautions for storage

Store cartridges at 2°C -8°C. Do not freeze. Keep container in the outer carton.

The 18MIU/0.6ml solution for injection is suitable for multiple-dose use.

6.5 Nature and contents of container

Cartridge barrel (0.6ml) composed of Type I flint glass Ph. Eur., PTFE laminated plunger stopper, aluminium crimp cap with PTFE laminated butyl rubber inner seal.

Pack sizes: Pack of 1, 3 and 6. Not all pack sizes may be marketed.

6.6 Instructions for use and handling

Roferon-A cartridges are for multi-dose and single patient use only and should be used exclusively with the Roferon-Pen. A new, sterile needle must be used for every injection.

Each Roferon-Pen is provided with a user manual which fully describes the use of the pen/cartridge combination. Penfine® needles are recommended for use with Roferon-Pen. However, a limited range of other needle types can also be used.

After each injection the Roferon-Pen/cartridge combination should be returned to the fridge. However, cartridges can be stored continually below 25°C for a maximum period of 28 days with no deterioration in quality.

Always discard cartridges containing residual drug after expiry of the in-use shelf life. Needles should be discarded safely after use.

7. MARKETING AUTHORISATION HOLDER

Roche Products Limited, 40 Broadwater Road, Welwyn Garden City, Hertfordshire AL7 3AY, England.

8. MARKETING AUTHORISATION NUMBER(S)

MA 0031/0510

PA 50/68/24

9. DATE OF FIRST AUTHORISATION/RENEWAL OF THE AUTHORISATION

Date of first Authorisation:

PL 0031/0510 22 July 1999

PA 50/68/24 15 September 2000

Date of last Renewal: 22 July 2004

10. DATE OF REVISION OF THE TEXT

25 July 2005

LEGAL STATUS

POM

Roferon-A is a registered trade mark

Roferon-A 18MIU/1ml Solution for Injection

(Roche Products Limited)

1. NAME OF THE MEDICINAL PRODUCT

Roferon-A® 18MIU/1ml

Vials containing solution for injection

2. QUALITATIVE AND QUANTITATIVE COMPOSITION

Roferon-A is supplied in vials as a ready-to-use solution for injection.

Each vial contains 18 Million International Units interferon alfa-2a* per millilitre (18MIU/1ml).

*Contains volume overages of 10% and manufacturing overages.

Recombinant interferon alfa-2a produced by genetic engineering from Escherichia coli.

For excipients, see *6.1*.

3. PHARMACEUTICAL FORM

Vials containing solution for injection.

Solution is clear and colourless to light yellow.

4. CLINICAL PARTICULARS

4.1 Therapeutic indications

Roferon-A is indicated for the treatment of:

- Hairy cell leukaemia.

- AIDS patients with progressive, asymptomatic Kaposi's sarcoma who have a CD4 count > 250/mm³.

- Chronic phase Philadelphia-chromosome positive chronic myelogenous leukaemia. Roferon-A is not an alternative treatment for CML patients who have an HLA-identical relative and for whom allogeneic bone marrow transplantation is planned or possible in the immediate future. It is still unknown whether Roferon-A can be considered as a treatment with a curative potential in this indication.

- Cutaneous T-cell lymphoma. Interferon alfa-2a (Roferon-A) may be active in patients who have progressive disease and who are refractory to, or unsuitable for, conventional therapy.

- Adult patients with histologically proven chronic hepatitis B who have markers for viral replication, i.e., those who are positive for HBV DNA or HBeAg.

- Adult patients with histologically proven chronic hepatitis C who are positive for HCV antibodies or HCV RNA and have elevated serum alanine aminotransferase (ALT) without liver decompensation.

The efficacy of interferon alfa-2a in the treatment of hepatitis C is enhanced when combined with ribavirin. Roferon-A should be given alone mainly in case of intolerance or contra-indication to ribavirin.

- Follicular non-Hodgkin's lymphoma.

- Advanced renal cell carcinoma.

- Patients with AJCC stage II malignant melanoma (Breslow tumour thickness > 1.5 mm, no lymph node involvement or cutaneous spread) who are free of disease after surgery.

4.2 Posology and method of administration

Not all available Roferon-A strengths can be used for all indications mentioned in section *4.1 Therapeutic indications*. The prescribed strength should correspond with the recommended dose for each individual indication.

- HAIRY CELL LEUKAEMIA

Initial dosage:

Three million IU daily, given by subcutaneous or intramuscular injection for 16 – 24 weeks. If intolerance develops, either the daily dose should be lowered to 1.5 million IU or the schedule changed to three times per week, or both.

Maintenance dosage:

Three million IU, given three times per week by subcutaneous or intramuscular injection. If intolerance develops, the dose should be lowered to 1.5 million IU three times per week.

Duration of treatment:

Patients should be treated for approximately six months before the physician decides whether to continue treatment in responding patients or to discontinue treatment in non-responding patients. Patients have been treated for up to 20 consecutive months. The optimal duration of Roferon-A treatment for hairy cell leukaemia has not been determined.

Note:

Subcutaneous administration is recommended for thrombocytopenic patients (platelet count less than 50 × 10⁹/l) or patients at risk of bleeding.

The minimum effective dose of Roferon-A in hairy cell leukaemia has not been established.

- AIDS-RELATED KAPOSI'S SARCOMA

Roferon-A is indicated for the treatment of AIDS patients with progressive, asymptomatic Kaposi's sarcoma who have a CD4 count > 250/mm³. AIDS patients with CD4 counts < 250/mm³, or those with a history of opportunistic infections or constitutional symptoms, are unlikely to respond to Roferon-A therapy and therefore should not be treated. The optimal posology has not yet been well established.

Roferon-A should not be used in conjunction with protease inhibitors. With the exception of zidovudine, there is a lack of safety data for the combination of Roferon-A with reverse transcriptase inhibitors.

Initial dosage:

Roferon-A should be given by subcutaneous or intramuscular injection, and escalated to at least 18 million IU daily and if possible to 36 million IU daily for a total of ten to twelve weeks in patients of 18 years or older. The recommended escalation schedule is as follows:

Days 1 – 3	3 million IU daily
Days 4 – 6	9 million IU daily
Days 7 – 9	18 million IU daily - and, if tolerated, increase to:
Days 10 – 84	36 million IU daily

Maintenance dosage:

Roferon-A should be given by subcutaneous or intramuscular injection three times per week at the maximum dose which is acceptable to the patient, but not exceeding 36 million IU.

Patients with AIDS-related Kaposi's sarcoma treated with 3 million IU of Roferon-A given daily showed a lower response rate than those treated with the recommended dosage.

Duration of treatment:

The evolution of lesions should be documented to determine response to therapy. Patients should be treated for a minimum of ten weeks and preferably for at least twelve weeks before the physician decides whether to continue treatment in responding patients or to discontinue treatment in non-responding patients. Patients generally showed evidence of response after approximately three months of therapy. Patients have been treated for up to 20 consecutive months. If a response to treatment occurs, treatment should continue at least until there is no further evidence of tumour. The optimal duration of Roferon-A treatment for AIDS-related Kaposi's sarcoma has not been determined.

Note:

Lesions of Kaposi's sarcoma frequently reappear when Roferon-A treatment is discontinued.

- CHRONIC MYELOGENOUS LEUKAEMIA

Roferon-A is indicated for the treatment of patients with chronic phase Philadelphia-chromosome positive chronic myelogenous leukaemia. Roferon-A is not an alternative treatment for CML patients who have an HLA-identical relative and for whom allogeneic bone marrow transplantation is planned or possible in the immediate future.

Roferon-A produces haematological remissions in 60% of patients with chronic phase CML, independent of prior treatment. Two thirds of these patients have complete haematological responses which occur as late as 18 months after treatment start.

In contrast to cytotoxic chemotherapy, interferon alfa-2a is able to generate sustained, ongoing cytogenetic responses beyond 40 months. It is still unknown whether Roferon-A can be considered as a treatment with a curative potential in this indication.

Dosage:

It is recommended that Roferon-A should be given by subcutaneous or intramuscular injection for eight to twelve weeks to patients 18 years or more. The recommended schedule is:

Days 1 – 3	3 million IU daily
Days 4 – 6	6 million IU daily
Days 7 – 84	9 million IU daily

Duration of treatment:

Patients should be treated for a minimum of eight weeks, preferably for at least twelve weeks before the physician decides whether or not to continue treatment in responding patients or to discontinue treatment in patients not showing any changes in haematological parameters. Responding patients should be treated until complete haematological response is achieved or for a maximum of 18 months. All patients with complete haematologic responses should continue treatment with 9 million IU daily (optimum) or 9 million IU three times a week (minimum) in order to achieve a cytogenetic response in the shortest possible time. The optimal duration of Roferon-A treatment for chronic myelogenous leukaemia has not been determined, although cytogenetic responses have been observed two years after treatment start.

The safety, efficacy and optimal dosage of Roferon-A in children with CML has not yet been established.

- **CUTANEOUS T-CELL LYMPHOMA (CTCL)**

Interferon alfa-2a (Roferon-A) may be active in patients with progressive cutaneous T-cell lymphoma and who are refractory to, or unsuitable for conventional therapy.

The optimal dosage has not been established.

Initial dosage:

Roferon-A should be given by subcutaneous or intramuscular injection, and escalated to 18 million IU daily for a total of twelve weeks in patients of 18 years or older. The recommended escalation schedule is as follows:

Days 1 – 3 3 million IU daily

Days 4 – 6 9 million IU daily

Days 7 – 84 18 million IU daily

Maintenance dosage:

Roferon-A should be given by subcutaneous or intramuscular injection three times per week at the maximum dose which is acceptable to the patient, but not exceeding 18 million IU.

Duration of treatment:

Patients should be treated for a minimum of eight weeks and preferably for at least twelve weeks before the physician decides whether to continue treatment in responding patients or to discontinue treatment in non-responding patients. Minimum treatment duration in responding patients should be twelve months in order to maximise the chance to achieve a complete response and improve the chance for a prolonged response. Patients have been treated for up to 40 consecutive months. The optimal duration of Roferon-A treatment for cutaneous T-cell lymphoma has not been determined.

Warning:

Objective tumour responses have not been observed in approximately 40% of patients with CTCL. Partial responses are usually seen within three months and complete responses within six months, although it may occasionally take more than one year to reach the best response.

- **CHRONIC HEPATITIS B**

Roferon-A is indicated for the treatment of adult patients with histologically proven chronic hepatitis B who have markers for viral replication, i.e., those who are positive for HBV DNA or HBeAg.

Dosage recommendation:

The optimal schedule of treatment has not been established yet. The dose is usually in the range of 2.5 million IU to 5.0 million IU/m^2 body surface administered subcutaneously three times per week for a period of four to six months.

The dosage may be adjusted according to the patient's tolerance to the medication. If no improvement has been observed after three to four months of treatment, discontinuation of therapy should be considered.

Children: up to 10 million IU/m^2 has been safely administered to children with chronic hepatitis B. However efficacy of therapy has not been demonstrated.

– **CHRONIC HEPATITIS C**

ROFERON-A IN COMBINATION WITH RIBAVIRIN

RELAPSED PATIENTS

Roferon-A is given in combination with ribavirin for adult patients with chronic hepatitis C who have previously responded to interferon alpha monotherapy, but who have relapsed after treatment was stopped.

Dosage:

Roferon-A 4.5MIU three times per week by subcutaneous or intramuscular injection for a period of six months.

Dosage of Ribavirin:

Ribavirin dose: 1000mg to 1200mg/day in two divided doses (once in the morning with breakfast and once with the evening meal). Please refer to the SmPC for ribavirin for further details on the posology and method of administration of ribavirin.

NAÏVE PATIENTS

The efficacy of interferon alfa-2a in the treatment of hepatitis C is enhanced when combined with ribavirin. Roferon-A should be given alone mainly in case of intolerance or contra-indication to ribavirin.

Dosage:

Roferon-A 3 to 4.5MIU three times per week by subcutaneous or intramuscular injection for a period of at least six months. Treatment should be continued for an additional six months in patients who have negative HCV RNA at month six, and are infected with genotype 1 and have high pre-treatment viral load.

Dosage of Ribavirin: see above.

Other negative prognostic factors (age > 40 years, male gender, bridging fibrosis) should be taken into account in order to extend therapy to twelve months.

Patients who failed to show a virologic response after six months of treatment (HCV-RNA below lower limit of detection) do generally not become sustained virologic responders (HCV-RNA below lower limit of detection six months after withdrawal of treatment).

Roferon-A monotherapy

Roferon-A monotherapy should be given mainly in case of intolerance or contra-indication to ribavirin.

Initial dosage:

Roferon-A should be administered at a dose of 3 to 6 million IU by subcutaneous or intramuscular injection three times a week for six months as induction therapy, patient tolerance permitting. In patients who fail to respond after three to four months of treatment, discontinuation of Roferon-A should be considered.

Maintenance dosage:

Patients whose serum ALT has normalised and/or HCV RNA has become undetectable require maintenance therapy with 3 million IU Roferon-A three times a week for an additional six months or longer to consolidate the complete response. The optimal duration of treatment has not yet been determined but a therapy of at least twelve months is advised.

Note:

The majority of patients who relapse after adequate treatment with Roferon-A alone do so within four months of the end of treatment.

- **FOLLICULAR NON-HODGKINS LYMPHOMA**

Roferon-A prolongs disease-free and progression-free survival when used as adjunctive treatment to CHOP-like chemotherapy regimens in patients with advanced (high tumour burden) follicular non-Hodgkin's lymphoma. However, the efficacy of adjunctive interferon alfa-2a treatment on overall long-term survival of these patients has not yet been established.

Dosage recommendation:

Roferon-A should be administered concomitantly to a conventional chemotherapy regimen (such as the combination of cyclophosphamide, prednisone, vincristine and doxorubicin) according to a schedule such as 6 million IU/m^2 given subcutaneously or intramuscularly from day 22 to day 26 of each 28-day cycle.

- **ADVANCED RENAL CELL CARCINOMA**

Therapy with Roferon-A in combination with vinblastine induces overall response rates of approximately 17 - 26%, delays disease progression, and prolongs overall survival in patients with advanced renal cell carcinoma.

Dosage recommendation:

Roferon-A should be given by subcutaneous or intramuscular injection at a dose of 3 million IU three times weekly for one week, 9 million IU three times weekly for the following week and 18 million IU three times weekly thereafter. Concomitantly vinblastine should be given intravenously according to the manufacturer's instructions at a dose of 0.1mg/kg once every three weeks.

If the Roferon-A dosage of 18 million IU three times per week is not tolerated the dose may be reduced to 9 million IU three times per week.

Treatment should be given for a minimum of three months, up to a maximum of twelve months or until the development of progressive disease. Patients who achieve a complete response may stop treatment three months after the response is established.

- **SURGICALLY RESECTED MALIGNANT MELANOMA**

Adjuvant therapy with a low dose of Roferon-A prolongs disease-free interval in patients with no nodal or distant metastases following resection of a melanoma (tumour thickness > 1.5 mm).

Dosage recommendation:

Roferon-A should be administered subcutaneously or intramuscularly at a dose of 3 million IU three times a week for 18 months, starting no later than six weeks post surgery. If intolerance develops, the dose should be lowered to 1.5 million IU three times a week.

4.3 Contraindications

Roferon-A is contra-indicated in patients with:

1. a history of hypersensitivity to recombinant interferon alfa-2a or to any of the excipients,

2. severe pre-existing cardiac disease or with any history of cardiac illness. No direct cardiotoxic effect has been demonstrated, but it is likely that acute, self-limiting toxicities (i.e., fever, chills) frequently associated with administration of Roferon-A may exacerbate pre-existing cardiac conditions,

3. severe renal, hepatic or myeloid dysfunction,

4. uncontrolled seizure disorders and/or compromised central nervous system function (see section *4.4 Special warnings and precautions for use*),

5. chronic hepatitis with advanced, decompensated hepatic disease or cirrhosis of the liver,

6. chronic hepatitis who are being or have recently been treated with immunosuppressive agents.

7. Benzyl alcohol which is an excipient in Roferon-A solution for injection has on rare occasions been associated with potentially fatal toxicities in children up to three years old. Therefore, Roferon-A solution for injection should not be used in infants or young children.

Combination therapy with ribavirin: Also see ribavirin labelling if interferon alfa-2a is to be administered in combination with ribavirin in patients with chronic hepatitis C.

4.4 Special warnings and special precautions for use

Roferon-A should be administered under the supervision of a qualified physician experienced in the management of the respective indication. Appropriate management of the therapy and its complications is possible only when adequate diagnostic and treatment facilities are readily available.

Patients should be informed not only of the benefits of therapy but also that they will probably experience adverse reactions.

When mild to moderate renal, hepatic or myeloid dysfunction is present, close monitoring of these functions is required.

In rare cases interferon alpha has been suspected of causing an exacerbation of an underlying autoimmune disease in hepatitis patients. Therefore, when treating hepatitis patients with a history of autoimmune disease caution is recommended. If a deterioration in liver function in these patients develops a determination of autoimmune antibodies should be considered. If necessary treatment should be discontinued.

Severe psychiatric adverse reactions may manifest in patients receiving therapy with interferons, including Roferon-A. Depression, suicidal ideation, and suicidal attempt may occur in patients with and without previous psychiatric illness. Physicians should monitor all patients treated with Roferon-A for evidence of depression. Physicians should inform patients of the possible development of depression prior to initiation of therapy, and patients should report any sign or symptom of depression immediately. Psychiatric intervention and/or drug discontinuation should be considered in such cases.

Extreme caution should be exercised when administering Roferon-A to patients with severe myelosuppression as it has a suppressive effect on the bone marrow, leading to a fall in the white blood count, particularly granulocytes, platelet count and, less commonly, haemoglobin concentration. This can lead to an increased risk of infection or of haemorrhage. It is important to monitor closely these events in patients and periodic complete blood counts should be performed during the course of Roferon-A treatment, both prior to therapy and at appropriate periods during therapy.

In transplant patients (e.g., kidney or bone marrow transplant) therapeutic immunosuppression may be weakened because interferons also exert an immunostimulatory action.

Use of alfa interferon has been rarely associated with exacerbation or provocation of psoriasis.

In rare cases, severe hepatic dysfunction and liver failure have been reported after treatment with alfa interferon.

Hyperglycaemia has been observed rarely in patients treated with Roferon-A. All patients who develop symptoms of hyperglycaemia should have their blood glucose measured and followed-up accordingly. Patients with diabetes mellitus may require adjustment of their anti-diabetic regimen.

The development of different auto-antibodies has been reported during treatment with alfa interferons. Clinical manifestations of autoimmune disease during interferon therapy occur more frequently in subjects predisposed to the development of autoimmune disorders. Autoimmune phenomena such as vasculitis, arthritis, haemolytic anaemia, thyroid dysfunction and lupus erythaematosus syndrome have been observed rarely in patients receiving Roferon-A. In patients with an underlying or clinical history of autoimmune disorders, monitoring of symptoms suggestive of these disorders, as well as measurement of auto-antibodies and TSH level, is recommended.

The use of Roferon-A in children is not recommended as the safety and effectiveness of Roferon-A in children have not been established.

Efficacy in patients with chronic hepatitis B or C who are on haemodialysis or have haemophilia or are co-infected with human immunodeficiency virus has not been demonstrated.

Combination therapy with ribavirin: Also see ribavirin labelling if interferon alfa-2a is to be administered in combination with ribavirin in patients with chronic hepatitis C.

4.5 Interaction with other medicinal products and other forms of Interaction

Since alfa-interferons alter cellular metabolism, the potential to modify the activity of other drugs exists. In a small study, Roferon-A was shown to have an effect on specific microsomal enzyme systems. The clinical relevance of these findings is unknown.

Alfa-interferons may affect the oxidative metabolic process; this should be borne in mind when prescribing concomitant therapy with drugs metabolised by this route. However, as yet no specific information is available.

Roferon-A has been reported to reduce the clearance of theophylline.

As Roferon-A may affect central nervous system functions, interactions could occur following concurrent administration of centrally-acting drugs. The neurotoxic, haematotoxic or cardiotoxic effects of previously or concurrently administered drugs may be increased by interferons.

Combination therapy with ribavirin: Also see ribavirin labelling if interferon alfa-2a is to be administered in combination with ribavirin in patients with chronic hepatitis C.

4.6 Pregnancy and lactation

Men and women receiving Roferon-A should practise effective contraception. In pregnancy, Roferon-A should be administered only if the benefit to the woman justifies the potential risk to the foetus. Although animal tests do not indicate that Roferon-A is a teratogen, harm to the foetus from use during pregnancy cannot be excluded. When doses greatly in excess of the recommended clinical dose were administered to pregnant rhesus monkeys in the early to mid-foetal period, an abortifacient effect was observed.

It is not known whether this drug is excreted in human milk. A decision must be taken whether to suspend breast feeding or to discontinue the drug, taking into account the importance of the drug to the mother.

Combination therapy with ribavirin: Also see ribavirin labelling if interferon alfa-2a is to be administered in combination with ribavirin in patients with chronic hepatitis C.

4.7 Effects on ability to drive and use machines

Depending on dose and schedule as well as the sensitivity of the individual patient, Roferon-A may have an effect on the speed of reaction which could impair certain operations, e.g., driving, operation of machinery etc.

4.8 Undesirable effects

The following data on adverse reactions are based on information derived from the treatment of cancer patients with a wide variety of malignancies and often refractory to previous therapy and suffering from advanced disease, patients with chronic hepatitis B and patients with chronic hepatitis C. Most cancer patients received doses that were significantly higher than the dose now recommended and this probably explains the higher frequency and severity of adverse reactions in this patient group compared with patients with hepatitis B where adverse reactions are usually transient, and patients return to pre-treatment status within one to two weeks after the end of therapy.

General symptoms: The majority of the patients experienced flu-like symptoms such as fatigue, fever, chills, appetite loss, myalgia, headache, arthralgia and diaphoresis. These acute side-effects can usually be reduced or eliminated by concurrent administration of paracetamol and tend to diminish with continued therapy or dose moderation although continuing therapy can lead to lethargy, weakness and fatigue. Reactions at injection sites, including, very rarely, necrotic site reactions have occurred in patients.

Gastrointestinal tract: About two thirds of cancer patients experienced anorexia and one half nausea. Emesis, taste alterations, mouth dryness, weight loss, diarrhoea and mild or moderate abdominal pain were less frequently observed. Constipation, flatulence, hypermotility or heartburn occurred rarely, and reactivation of peptic ulcer and non-life-threatening gastrointestinal bleeding, increase of pancreatic enzymes i.e. amylase/lipase with or without abdominal pain, reversible after drug discontinuation, have been reported in isolated cases.

Alterations of hepatic function shown by an elevation particularly of ALT, but also of alkaline phosphatase, LDH and bilirubin have been observed and generally did not require dose adjustment. In rare cases hepatitis was reported. In hepatitis B patients, changes in transaminases usually signal an improvement in the clinical state of the patient.

Central nervous system: Dizziness, vertigo, visual disturbances, decreased mental status, forgetfulness, depression, drowsiness, confusion, behavioural disturbances such as anxiety and nervousness, and sleep disturbances were uncommon. Suicidal ideation, suicide attempt and suicide, severe somnolence, convulsions, coma, cerebrovascular adverse events, transient impotence and ischemic retinopathy were rare complications.

Peripheral nervous system: Paraesthesia, numbness, neuropathy, itching and tremor occasionally occurred.

Cardiovascular and pulmonary systems: Disorders were seen in about one fifth of cancer patients and consisted of transient hypotensive and hypertensive episodes, oedema, cyanosis, arrhythmias, palpitations and chest pain. Coughing and mild dyspnoea were rarely observed. Rare cases of pulmonary oedema, pneumonia, congestive heart failure, cardiorespiratory arrest and myocardial infarction have been reported. Cardiovascular problems are very rarely seen in patients with hepatitis B.

Skin, mucous membranes and adnexa: Re-exacerbation of herpes labialis, rash, pruritus, dryness of skin and mucous membranes, rhinorrhea and epistaxis were reported rarely. Mild to moderate alopecia occurred in up to one fifth of patients, but this was reversible on discontinuation of treatment. Increased hair loss may continue for several weeks after treatment ends.

Renal and urinary system: In rare instances, decreased renal function has occurred. Electrolyte disturbances have been seen, generally in association with anorexia or dehydration. Disorders consisted primarily of proteinuria and increased cell count in sediment. Elevation of BUN, serum creatinine and uric acid has been observed in rare cases. Rare cases of acute renal failure have been reported, mainly in cancer patients with renal disease and/or nephrotoxic co-medications as concomitant risk factors.

Haematopoietic system: Transient leucopenia occurred variably in about one third to over one half of the patients, but rarely required restriction of dosage. In non-myelosuppressed patients, thrombocytopenia was less frequently seen, and decrease of haemoglobin and haematocrit occurred rarely. In myelosuppressed patients, thrombocytopenia and decreased haemoglobin occurred more frequently. Recovery of severe haematological deviations to pre-treatment levels usually occurred within seven to ten days after discontinuing Roferon-A treatment.

Endocrine disorders: Inconsequential hypocalcaemia was reported in about one half of the patients. Hypothyroidism, hyperthyroidism and hyperglycaemia have been observed rarely in patients treated with Roferon-A.

Anti-interferon antibodies: Neutralising antibodies to proteins may be formed in some subjects following homologous administration. Antibodies to all interferons, whether natural or recombinant, are therefore likely to be found in a certain proportion of patients. In certain clinical conditions (cancer, systemic lupus erythaematosus, herpes zoster) antibodies to human leukocyte interferon may also occur spontaneously in patients who have never received exogenous interferons.

In clinical trials where lyophilised Roferon-A which had been stored at 25°C was used, neutralising antibodies to Roferon-A have been detected in approximately one fifth of patients. In patients with hepatitis C, a trend for responding patients who develop neutralising antibodies to lose response while still on treatment and to lose it earlier than patients who do not develop such antibodies, has been seen. No other clinical sequelae of the presence of antibodies to Roferon-A have been documented. The clinical significance of the development of antibodies has not been fully clarified.

No data on neutralising antibodies yet exist from clinical trials in which lyophilised Roferon-A or Roferon-A solution for injection which is stored at 4°C has been used. In a mouse model, the relative immunogenicity of lyophilised Roferon-A increases with time when the material is stored at 25°C - no such increase in immunogenicity is observed when lyophilised Roferon-A is stored at 4°C, the recommended storage conditions.

Combination therapy with ribavirin: Also see ribavirin labelling if interferon alfa-2a is to be administered in combination with ribavirin in patients with chronic hepatitis C.

4.9 Overdose

There are no reports of overdosage but repeated large doses of interferon can be associated with profound lethargy, fatigue, prostration and coma. Such patients should be hospitalised for observation and appropriate supportive treatment given.

Patients who experience severe reactions to Roferon-A will usually recover within days after discontinuation of therapy, given appropriate supportive care. Coma has been observed in 0.4% of cancer patients in clinical trials.

5. PHARMACOLOGICAL PROPERTIES

5.1 Pharmacodynamic properties

Pharmacotherapeutic group:	Cytokines and immunomodulators, *Interferons*
	ATC Code L03AB04

Roferon-A has been shown to possess many of the activities of the so-called natural human alfa-interferon preparations. Roferon-A exerts its antiviral effects by inducing a state of resistance to viral infections in cells and by modulating the effector arm of the immune system to neutralise viruses or eliminate virus infected cells. The essential mechanism for the anti-tumour action of Roferon-A is not yet known. However, several changes are described in human tumoural cells treated with Roferon-A: HT 29 cells show a significant reduction of DNA, RNA and protein synthesis. Roferon-A has been shown to exert antiproliferative activity against a variety of human tumours *in vitro* and to inhibit the growth of some human tumour xenografts in nude mice. A limited number of human tumour cell lines grown *in vivo* in immunocompromised nude mice has been tested for the susceptibility to Roferon-A. *In vivo* antiproliferative activity of Roferon-A has been studied on tumours including breast mucoid carcinoma, adenocarcinoma of the caecum, colon carcinoma and prostatic carcinoma. The degree of antiproliferative activity is variable.

Unlike other human proteins, many of the effects of interferon alfa-2a are partially or completely suppressed when it is tested in other animal species. However, significant antivaccinia virus activity was induced in rhesus monkeys pretreated with interferon alfa-2a.

Clinical Trials

Hairy Cell Leukaemia

The therapeutic efficacy of Roferon-A in the treatment of hairy cell leukaemia has been demonstrated in a large trial of 218 patients, of whom 174 were evaluable for efficacy after 16 – 24 weeks of therapy. Response was observed in 88% of patients (complete response 33%, partial response 55%).

AIDS-related Kaposi's Sarcoma

The efficacy of Roferon-A in the treatment of Kaposi's sarcoma was assessed in 364 patients receiving 3 to 54MIU per day. Objective response rates were dose-related, ranging from 14% to 50%, with a daily dose of 36MIU producing the best overall therapeutic benefit (13.3% complete response, 12.2% partial response). High baseline CD4 lymphocyte count was a favourable prognostic factor for response, with 46% of patients with a CD4 count > 400/mm^3 responding to Roferon-A. Response to Roferon-A therapy was the strongest prognostic factor for survival.

Chronic Myelogenous Leukaemia (CML)

The efficacy of Roferon-A was assessed in 226 patients with chronic phase CML, and compared with 109 patients receiving chemotherapy (hydroxyurea or busulfan). Both groups had favourable features at diagnosis (less than 10% blasts in the blood) and treatment was initiated with interferon within six months of diagnosis. Treatment of patients with CML in the chronic phase leads to the same proportion of patients (85 – 90%) achieving a haematologic response as treatment with the standard chemotherapy regimens. In addition patients treated with Roferon-A resulted in 8% complete cytogenetic response and 38% partial cytogenetic response versus 9% partial cytogenetic response during chemotherapy. Time to progression from the chronic phase of leukaemia to an accelerated or a blastic phase was longer in the Roferon-A group (69 months) than in the conventional chemotherapy group (46 months) ($p < 0.001$) as was median overall survival (72.8 months versus 54.5 months, p = 0.002).

Cutaneous T-cell Lymphoma (CTCL)

The efficacy of Roferon-A was assessed in 169 patients with CTCL, the majority of whom (78%) were resistant to, or had relapsed on, standard therapy. Among the 85 patients evaluable, overall response to treatment was 58% (20% complete response, 38% partial response). Patients with all stages of disease responded to therapy. Median duration of complete response from start of treatment was 22 months, with 94% of complete responders remaining in remission at 9 months.

Chronic Hepatitis B

The efficacy of Roferon-A in the treatment of chronic hepatitis B was assessed in trials involving over 900 patients. In the pivotal controlled study 238 patients were randomised into four groups: patients received either 2.5MIU/m^2, 5.0MIU/m^2, 10MIU/m^2, tiw of Roferon-A or no treatment. Treatment duration was 12 – 24 weeks depending on response i.e. clearance of HBeAg and HBV DNA from serum. Patients were followed for up to 12 months after treatment was discontinued. There was a statistically significant difference in sustained response [clearance of hepatitis Be antigen (HBeAg) and hepatitis B viral DNA (HBV DNA)] between treated and untreated patients (37% versus 13%). Response differences between various dose groups did not reach statistical significance (33%, 34% and 43% for the 2.5, 5.0 and 10.0MIU/m^2 groups). Serological and virological responses were associated with marked improvement in liver histology after 12 months of treatment-free follow up.

Chronic Hepatitis C

The efficacy of Roferon-A in the treatment of chronic hepatitis C has been assessed in 1701 patients, with 130 untreated or placebo treated controls. At recommended doses, Roferon-A induces complete biochemical response in up to 85% of patients, with response rates maintained for at least six months after treatment ranging from 11 to 44% depending on pre-treatment disease characteristics, IFN dose and treatment duration. Biochemical response to Roferon-A is associated with significant improvement of liver disease as shown by evaluation of pre- and post-liver biopsies. For those patients who have a sustained response three to six months after end of therapy, response has been reported to be maintained for up to four years.

The therapeutic efficacy of Interferon alfa-2a alone and in combination with ribavirin was compared in a double-blind randomised clinical trial in naïve (previously untreated) and relapsed patients with virologically, biochemically and histologically documented chronic hepatitis C. Six months after end of treatment sustained biochemical and virological response as well as histological improvement were assessed.

A statistically significant ten-fold increase (from 4% to 43%; $p < 0.01$) in sustained virological and biochemical response was observed in relapsed patients. The favourable profile of the combination therapy was also reflected in the response rates relative to HCV genotype or baseline viral load. Although the sustained response rates in patients with HCV genotype-1 were lower than in the overall population (approx. 30% versus 0% in the monotherapy arm) the relative benefit of ribavirin in combination with interferon alfa-2a is particularly significant in this group of patients. In addition the histological improvement favoured the combination therapy.

Supportive favourable results from a small study in naïve patients were reported using interferon alfa-2a (3MIU three times per week) with ribavirin.

For other information on pharmacodynamic properties please refer to the SmPC for Ribavirin.

Follicular Non-Hodgkin's lymphoma

The efficacy of Roferon-A in addition to cytotoxic chemotherapy (CHOP-like regimen of cyclophosphamide, vincristine, prednisone and doxorubicin) was assessed in 122 patients with clinically aggressive low-grade or intermediate-grade non-Hodgkin's lymphoma and compared with 127 controls receiving the same chemotherapy regimen. The two regimens produced comparable objective responses, but the regimen including Roferon-A had a greater effect in prolonging the time to treatment failure ($p < 0.001$), the duration of complete response ($p < 0.003$).

Renal Cell Carcinoma

The efficacy of Roferon-A given in combination with vinblastine, was compared with vinblastine alone. The combination of Roferon-A plus vinblastine is superior to vinblastine alone in the treatment of patients with locally advanced or metastatic renal cell carcinoma. Median survival was 67.8 weeks for the 79 patients receiving Roferon-A plus vinblastine and 37.8 weeks for the 81 patients treated with vinblastine ($p = .0049$). Overall response rates were 16.5% for patients treated with Roferon-A plus vinblastine and 2.5% for patients treated with vinblastine alone ($p = .0025$).

Surgically Resected Malignant Melanoma

The efficacy of Roferon-A in patients with primary cutaneous melanoma thicker than 1.5mm and without clinically detectable node metastasis was assessed in a large randomised study involving 253 patients receiving Roferon-A at a dose of 3MIU three times a week for 18 months, compared with 246 untreated controls. After a median follow-up of 4.4 years a significant extension of relapse-free interval ($p = 0.035$) but no statistically significant difference in overall survival ($p = 0.059$) in Roferon-A treated patients compared with controls have been shown. The overall treatment effect was a 25% reduction in the risk of relapse.

5.2 Pharmacokinetic properties

The serum concentrations of interferon alfa-2a reflected a large intersubject variation in both healthy volunteers and patients with disseminated cancer. The pharmacokinetics of Roferon-A in animals (monkey, dog and mouse) were similar to those seen in man. The pharmacokinetics of Roferon-A in man were linear over a 3 million to 198 million IU dose range. In healthy man, interferon alfa-2a exhibited an elimination half-life of 3.7 – 8.5 hours (mean: 5.1 hours), a volume of distribution at steady state of 0.223 – 0.748 l/kg (mean: 0.4 l/kg) and a total body clearance of 2.14 – 3.62ml/min/kg (mean: 2.79ml/min/kg) after a 36 million IU intravenous infusion. After intramuscular administration of 36 million IU, peak serum concentrations ranged from 1500 to 2580pg/ml (mean: 2020pg/ml) at a mean time to peak of 3.8 hours, and after subcutaneous administration of 36 million IU from 1250 to 2320pg/ml (mean: 1730 pg/ml) at a mean time to peak of 7.3 hours.

The apparent fraction of the dose absorbed after intramuscular or subcutaneous injection is greater than 80%.

The pharmacokinetics of interferon alfa-2a after single intramuscular doses to patients with disseminated cancer and chronic hepatitis B were similar to those found in healthy volunteers. Dose-proportional increases in serum concentrations were observed after single doses up to 198 million IU. There were no changes in the distribution or elimination of interferon alfa-2a during twice daily (0.5 – 36 million IU), once daily (1 – 54 million IU), or three times weekly (1 – 136 million IU) dosing regimens up to 28 days of dosing. Renal catabolism is the major pathway for Roferon-A elimination. Biliary excretion and liver metabolism are considered to be minor pathways of elimination of Roferon-A.

Intramuscular administration of Roferon-A one or more times daily for up to 28 days to some patients with disseminated cancer resulted in peak plasma concentrations of two to four times greater than those seen after single doses. However, multiple dosing caused no changes in its distribution or elimination parameters during several dosage regimens studied.

For other information on pharmacokinetic properties please refer to the SmPC for Ribavirin.

5.3 Preclinical safety data

Because of species specificity of human interferon, only limited toxicological studies have been carried out with Roferon-A. The acute parenteral toxicity of Roferon-A has been studied in mice, rats, rabbits and ferrets at doses up to 30 million IU/kg intravenously, and 500 million IU/kg intramuscularly. No treatment-related mortality was noted in any species studied given Roferon-A by any of the routes of administration. With doses greatly exceeding the recommended clinical dose no significant adverse effects were observed except for an abortifacient effect when administered to pregnant rhesus monkeys in the early to mid-foetal period and transient menstrual cycle irregularities including prolonged menstrual periods in non-pregnant monkeys. The relevance of these findings in man has not been established.

Mutagenic effects of Roferon-A have not been observed experimentally.

For other information on preclinical safety data please refer to the SmPC for Ribavirin.

6. PHARMACEUTICAL PARTICULARS

6.1 List of excipients

Ammonium acetate

Sodium Chloride

Benzyl alcohol

Polysorbate 80

Glacial acetic acid

Sodium Hydroxide Solution

Water for Injections

6.2 Incompatibilities

Not applicable.

6.3 Shelf life

2 years.

6.4 Special precautions for storage

Store vials at 2°C - 8°C. Do not freeze. Keep container in the outer carton.

The 18MIU/1ml solution for injection is for single dose use.

6.5 Nature and contents of container

– Vial 2ml (flint glass), butyl rubber stopper laminated with FPE, aluminium cap. Each vial contains 1ml of solution for injection.

Pack sizes: Pack of 1, 3, 6, 12 and 15 (vials). Not all pack sizes may be marketed.

– An injection kit (1 syringe 2ml, 1 needle for i.m. injection, 1 needle for s.c. injection) may be supplied with the product.

Pack sizes: Pack of 1, 3, 6, 12 and 15 (injection kits). Not all pack sizes may be marketed.

6.6 Instructions for use and handling

Plastic syringes are recommended for administration of Roferon-A solution for injection.

For single use only.

Any unused product or waste material should be disposed of in accordance with local requirements.

7. MARKETING AUTHORISATION HOLDER

Roche Products Limited, 40 Broadwater Road, Welwyn Garden City, Hertfordshire, AL7 3AY, UK.

8. MARKETING AUTHORISATION NUMBER(S)

PL 0031/0456

PA 50/68/19

9. DATE OF FIRST AUTHORISATION/RENEWAL OF THE AUTHORISATION

PL 0031/0456 September 2000

PA 50/68/19 September 2000

10. DATE OF REVISION OF THE TEXT

December 2002

Roferon-A is a registered trade mark

P739571/303

Roferon-A Pre-Filled Syringe

(Roche Products Limited)

1. NAME OF THE MEDICINAL PRODUCT

Roferon-A 3 MIU/0.5ml Pre-filled syringe containing solution for injection.

Roferon-A 4.5 MIU/0.5ml Pre-filled syringe containing solution for injection.

Roferon-A 6 MIU/0.5ml Pre-filled syringe containing solution for injection.

Roferon-A 9 MIU/0.5ml Pre-filled syringe containing solution for injection.

Roferon-A 18 MIU/0.5ml Pre-filled syringe containing solution for injection.

2. QUALITATIVE AND QUANTITATIVE COMPOSITION

Roferon-A 3 MIU/0.5ml Solution for injection:

Roferon-A is supplied in pre-filled syringes as a ready-to-use solution for injection.

Each pre-filled syringe contains 3 Million International Units interferon alfa-2a per 0.5 millilitres* (3 MIU/0.5ml).

Roferon-A 4.5 MIU/0.5ml Solution for injection:

Roferon-A is supplied in syringes as a ready-to-use solution for injection.

Each syringe contains 4.5 Million International Units interferon alfa-2a per 0.5 millilitres* (4.5 MIU/0.5ml).

Roferon-A 6 MIU/0.5ml Solution for injection:

Roferon-A is supplied in syringes as a ready-to-use solution for injection.

Each syringe contains 6 Million International Units interferon alfa-2a per 0.5 millilitres* (6 MIU/0.5ml).

Roferon-A 9 MIU/0.5ml Solution for injection:

Roferon-A is supplied in syringes as a ready-to-use solution for injection.

Each syringe contains 9 Million International Units interferon alfa-2a per 0.5 millilitres* (9 MIU/0.5 ml).

Roferon-A 18MIU/0.5ml Solution for injection:

Roferon-A is supplied in pre-filled syringes as a ready-to-use Solution for injection.

Each pre-filled syringe contains 18 Million International Units interferon alfa-2a per 0.5 millilitres* (18 MIU/0.5 ml)

*Contains volume overages.

Recombinant interferon alfa-2a produced by genetic engineering from Escherichia coli.

For excipients, see *6.1*.

3. PHARMACEUTICAL FORM

Pre-filled syringe containing solution for injection.

Solution is clear and colourless to light yellow.

4. CLINICAL PARTICULARS

4.1 Therapeutic indications

Roferon-A is indicated for the treatment of:

- Hairy cell leukaemia.

- AIDS patients with progressive, asymptomatic Kaposi's sarcoma who have a CD4 count > 250/mm^3.

- Chronic phase Philadelphia-chromosome positive chronic myelogenous leukaemia. Roferon-A is not an alternative treatment for CML patients who have an HLA-identical relative and for whom allogeneic bone marrow transplantation is planned or possible in the immediate future. It is still unknown whether Roferon-A can be considered as a treatment with a curative potential in this indication.

- Cutaneous T-cell lymphoma. Interferon alfa-2a (Roferon-A) may be active in patients who have progressive disease and who are refractory to, or unsuitable for, conventional therapy.

- Adult patients with histologically proven chronic hepatitis B who have markers for viral replication, i.e., those who are positive for HBV DNA or HBeAg.

- Adult patients with histologically proven chronic hepatitis C who are positive for HCV antibodies or HCV RNA and have elevated serum alanine aminotransferase (ALT) without liver decompensation.

The efficacy of interferon alfa-2a in the treatment of hepatitis C is enhanced when combined with ribavirin. Roferon-A should be given alone mainly in case of intolerance or contra-indication to ribavirin.

- Follicular non-Hodgkin's lymphoma.

- Advanced renal cell carcinoma.

- Patients with AJCC stage II malignant melanoma (Breslow tumour thickness > 1.5mm, no lymph node involvement or cutaneous spread) who are free of disease after surgery.

4.2 Posology and method of administration

Not all available Roferon-A strengths can be used for all indications mentioned in section *4.1 Therapeutic indications*. The prescribed strength should correspond with the recommended dose for each individual indication.

- HAIRY CELL LEUKAEMIA

Initial dosage:

Three million IU daily, given by subcutaneous injection for 16 – 24 weeks. If intolerance develops, either the daily dose should be lowered to 1.5 million IU or the schedule changed to three times per week, or both.

Maintenance dosage:

Three million IU, given three times per week by subcutaneous injection. If intolerance develops, the dose should be lowered to 1.5 million IU three times per week.

Duration of treatment:

Patients should be treated for approximately six months before the physician decides whether to continue treatment in responding patients or to discontinue treatment in non-responding patients. Patients have been treated for up to 20 consecutive months. The optimal duration of Roferon-A treatment for hairy cell leukaemia has not been determined.

The minimum effective dose of Roferon-A in hairy cell leukaemia has not been established.

- AIDS-RELATED KAPOSI'S SARCOMA

Roferon-A is indicated for the treatment of AIDS patients with progressive, asymptomatic Kaposi's sarcoma who have a CD4 count > 250/mm^3. AIDS patients with CD4 counts < 250/mm^3, or those with a history of opportunistic infections or constitutional symptoms, are unlikely to respond to Roferon-A therapy and therefore should not be treated. The optimal posology has not yet been well established.

Roferon-A should not be used in conjunction with protease inhibitors. With the exception of zidovudine, there is a lack of safety data for the combination of Roferon-A with reverse transcriptase inhibitors.

Initial dosage:

Roferon-A should be given by subcutaneous injection, and escalated to at least 18 million IU daily and if possible to 36 million IU daily for a total of ten to twelve weeks in patients of 18 years or older. The recommended escalation schedule is as follows:

Days 1 – 3	3 million IU daily
Days 4 – 6	9 million IU daily
Days 7 – 9	18 million IU daily - and, if tolerated, increase to:
Days 10 – 84	36 million IU daily

Maintenance dosage:

Roferon-A should be given by subcutaneous injection three times per week at the maximum dose which is acceptable to the patient, but not exceeding 36 million IU.

Patients with AIDS-related Kaposi's sarcoma treated with 3 million IU of Roferon-A given daily showed a lower response rate than those treated with the recommended dosage.

Duration of treatment:

The evolution of lesions should be documented to determine response to therapy. Patients should be treated for a minimum of ten weeks and preferably for at least twelve weeks before the physician decides whether to continue treatment in responding patients or to discontinue treatment in non-responding patients. Patients generally showed evidence of response after approximately three months of therapy. Patients have been treated for up to 20 consecutive months. If a response to treatment occurs, treatment should continue at least until there is no further evidence of tumour. The optimal duration of Roferon-A treatment for AIDS-related Kaposi's sarcoma has not been determined.

Note:

Lesions of Kaposi's sarcoma frequently reappear when Roferon-A treatment is discontinued.

- CHRONIC MYELOGENOUS LEUKAEMIA

Roferon-A is indicated for the treatment of patients with chronic phase Philadelphia-chromosome positive chronic myelogenous leukaemia. Roferon-A is not an alternative treatment for CML patients who have an HLA-identical relative and for whom allogeneic bone marrow transplantation is planned or possible in the immediate future.

Roferon-A produces haematological remissions in 60% of patients with chronic phase CML, independent of prior treatment. Two thirds of these patients have complete haematological responses which occur as late as 18 months after treatment start.

In contrast to cytotoxic chemotherapy, interferon alfa-2a is able to generate sustained, ongoing cytogenetic responses beyond 40 months. It is still unknown whether Roferon-A can be considered as a treatment with a curative potential in this indication.

Dosage:

It is recommended that Roferon-A should be given by subcutaneous injection for eight to twelve weeks to patients 18 years or more. The recommended schedule is:

Days 1 – 3	3 million IU daily
Days 4 – 6	6 million IU daily
Days 7 – 84	9 million IU daily

Duration of treatment:

Patients should be treated for a minimum of eight weeks, preferably for at least twelve weeks before the physician decides whether or not to continue treatment in responding patients or to discontinue treatment in patients not showing any changes in haematological parameters. Responding patients should be treated until complete haematological response is achieved or for a maximum of 18 months. All patients with complete haematologic responses should continue treatment with 9 million IU daily (optimum) or 9 million IU three times a week (minimum) in order to achieve a cytogenetic response in the shortest possible time. The optimal duration of Roferon-A treatment for chronic myelogenous leukaemia has not been determined, although cytogenetic responses have been observed two years after treatment start.

The safety, efficacy and optimal dosage of Roferon-A in children with CML has not yet been established.

- CUTANEOUS T-CELL LYMPHOMA (CTCL)

Interferon alfa-2a (Roferon-A) may be active in patients with progressive cutaneous T-cell lymphoma and who are refractory to, or unsuitable for conventional therapy.

The optimal dosage has not been established.

Initial dosage:

Roferon-A should be given by subcutaneous injection, and escalated to 18 million IU daily for a total of twelve weeks in patients of 18 years or older. The recommended escalation schedule is as follows:

Days 1 – 3	3 million IU daily
Days 4 – 6	9 million IU daily
Days 7 – 84	18 million IU daily

Maintenance dosage:

Roferon-A should be given by subcutaneous injection three times per week at the maximum dose which is acceptable to the patient, but not exceeding 18 million IU.

Duration of treatment:

Patients should be treated for a minimum of eight weeks and preferably for at least twelve weeks before the physician decides whether to continue treatment in responding patients or to discontinue treatment in non-responding patients. Minimum treatment duration in responding patients should be twelve months in order to maximise the chance to achieve a complete response and improve the chance for a prolonged response. Patients have been treated for up to 40 consecutive months. The optimal duration of Roferon-A treatment for cutaneous T-cell lymphoma has not been determined.

Warning:

Objective tumour responses have not been observed in approximately 40% of patients with CTCL. Partial responses are usually seen within three months and complete responses within six months, although it may occasionally take more than one year to reach the best response.

- CHRONIC HEPATITIS B

Roferon-A is indicated for the treatment of adult patients with histologically proven chronic hepatitis B who have markers for viral replication, i.e., those who are positive for HBV DNA or HBeAg.

Dosage recommendation:

The optimal schedule of treatment has not been established yet. The dose is usually in the range of 2.5 million IU to 5.0 million IU/m^2 body surface administered subcutaneously three times per week for a period of four to six months.

The dosage may be adjusted accordingto the patient's tolerance to the medication. If no improvement has been observed after three to four months of treatment, discontinuation of therapy should be considered.

Children: up to 10 million IU/m^2 has been safely administered to children with chronic hepatitis B. However efficacy of therapy has not been demonstrated.

- CHRONIC HEPATITIS C

ROFERON-A IN COMBINATION WITH RIBAVIRIN

RELAPSED PATIENTS

Roferon-A is given in combination with ribavirin for adult patients with chronic hepatitis C who have previously responded to interferon alpha monotherapy, but who have relapsed after treatment was stopped.

Dosage:

Roferon-A 4.5 MIU three times per week by subcutaneous injection for a period of six months.

Dosage of Ribavirin:

Ribavirin dose: 1000mg to 1200mg/day in two divided doses (once in the morning with breakfast and once with the evening meal). Please refer to the SmPC for ribavirin for further details on the posology and method of administration of ribavirin.

NAÏVE PATIENTS

The efficacy of interferon alfa-2a in the treatment of hepatitis C is enhanced when combined with ribavirin. Roferon-A should be given alone mainly in case of intolerance or contra-indication to ribavirin.

Dosage:

Roferon-A 3 to 4.5 MIU three times per week by subcutaneous injection for a period of at least six months. Treatment should be continued for an additional six months in patients who have negative HCV RNA at month six, and are infected with genotype 1 and have high pre-treatment viral load.

Dosage of Ribavirin: see above.

Other negative prognostic factors (age > 40 years, male gender, bridging fibrosis) should be taken into account in order to extend therapy to twelve months.

Patients who failed to show a virologic response after six months of treatment (HCV-RNA below lower limit of detection) do generally not become sustained virologic responders (HCV-RNA below lower limit of detection six months after withdrawal of treatment).

Roferon-A monotherapy

Roferon-A monotherapy should be given mainly in case of intolerance or contra-indication to ribavirin.

Initial dosage:

Roferon-A should be administered at a dose of 3 to6 million IU by subcutaneous injection three times a week for six months as induction therapy, patient tolerance permitting. In patients who fail to respond after three to four months of treatment, discontinuation of Roferon-A should be considered.

Maintenance dosage:

Patients whose serum ALT has normalised and/or HCV RNA has become undetectable require maintenance therapy with 3 million IU Roferon-A three times a week for an additional sixmonths or longer to consolidate the complete response. The optimal duration of treatment has not yet been determined but a therapy of at least twelve months is advised.

Note:

The majority of patients who relapse after adequate treatment with Roferon-A alonedo so within four months of the end of treatment.

- FOLLICULAR NON-HODGKINS LYMPHOMA

Roferon-A prolongs disease-free and progression-free survival when used as adjunctive treatment to CHOP-like chemotherapy regimens in patients with advanced (high tumour burden) follicular non-Hodgkin's lymphoma. However, the efficacy of adjunctive interferon alfa-2a treatment on overall long-term survival of these patients has not yet been established.

Dosage recommendation:

Roferon-A should be administered concomitantly to a conventional chemotherapy regimen (such as the combination of cyclophosphamide, prednisone, vincristine and doxorubicin) according to a schedule such as 6 million IU/m^2 given subcutaneously from day 22 to day 26 of each 28-day cycle.

- ADVANCED RENAL CELL CARCINOMA

Therapy with Roferon-A in combination with vinblastine induces overall response rates of approximately 17 – 26%, delays disease progression, and prolongs overall survival in patients with advanced renal cell carcinoma.

Dosage recommendation:

Roferon-A should be given by subcutaneous injection at a dose of 3 million IU three times weekly for one week, 9 million IU three times weekly for the following week and 18 million IU three times weekly thereafter. Concomitantly vinblastine should be given intravenously according to the manufacturer's instructions at a dose of 0.1mg/kg once every three weeks.

If the Roferon-A dosage of 18 million IU three times per week is not tolerated the dose may be reduced to 9 million IU three times per week.

Treatment should be given for a minimum of three months, up to a maximum of twelve months or until the development of progressive disease. Patients who achieve a complete response may stop treatment three months after the response is established.

- SURGICALLY RESECTED MALIGNANT MELANOMA

Adjuvant therapy with a low dose of Roferon-A prolongs disease-free interval in patients with no nodal or distant metastases following resection of a melanoma (tumour thickness > 1.5mm).

Dosage recommendation:

Roferon-A should be administered subcutaneously at a dose of 3 million IU three times a week for 18 months, starting no later than six weeks post surgery. If intolerance develops, the dose should be lowered to 1.5 million IU three times a week.

4.3 Contraindications

Roferon-A is contraindicated in patients with:

1. a history of hypersensitivity to recombinant interferon alfa-2a or to any of the excipients,

2. patients with severe pre-existing cardiac disease or with any history of cardiac illness. No direct cardiotoxic effect has been demonstrated, but it is likely that acute, self-limiting toxicities (i.e., fever, chills) frequently associated with administration of Roferon-A may exacerbate pre-existing cardiac conditions,

3. severe renal, hepatic or myeloid dysfunction,

4. uncontrolled seizure disorders and/or compromised central nervous system function (see section *4.4 Special warnings and precautions for use*),

5. chronic hepatitis with advanced, decompensated hepatic disease or cirrhosis of the liver,

6. chronic hepatitis who are being or have recently been treated with immunosuppressive agents.

7. Benzyl alcohol, which is an excipient in Roferon-A solution for injection has on rare occasions been associated with potentially fatal toxicities an anaphylactoid reactions in children up to three years old. Therefore, Roferon-A solution for injection should not be used in premature babies, neonates, infants or young children. Roferon-A solution contains 10mg/ml benzyl alcohol.

Combination therapy with ribavirin: Also see ribavirin labelling if interferon alfa-2a is to be administered in combination with ribavirin in patients with chronic hepatitis C.

4.4 Special warnings and special precautions for use

Roferon-A should be administered under the supervision of a qualified physician experienced in the management of the respective indication. Appropriate management of the therapy and its complications is possible only when adequate diagnostic and treatment facilities are readily available.

Patients should be informed not only of the benefits of therapy but also that they will probably experience adverse reactions.

Hypersensitivity: If a hypersensitivity reaction occurs during treatment with Roferon-A or in the combination therapy with ribavirin, treatment has to be discontinued and appropriate medical therapy has to be instituted immediately. Transient rashes do not necessitate interruption of treatment.

In transplant patients (e.g., kidney or bone marrow transplant) therapeutic immunosuppression may be weakened because interferons also exert an immunostimulatory action.

Psychiatric: Severe psychiatric adverse reactions may manifest in patients receiving therapy with interferons, including Roferon-A. Depression, suicidal ideation, suicidal attempt, and suicide may occur in patients with and without previous psychiatric illness. Physicians should monitor all patients treated with Roferon-A for evidence of depression. Physicians should inform patients of the possible development of depression prior to initiation of therapy, and patients should report any sign or symptom of depression immediately. Psychiatric intervention and/or drug discontinuation should be considered in such cases.

Ophthalmologic: As with other interferons, retinopathy including retinal haemorrhages, cotton wool spots, papilloedema, retinal artery or vein thrombosis and optic neuropathy which may result in loss of vision, have been reported after treatment with Roferon-A. Any patient complaining of decrease or loss of vision must have an eye examination.

Because these ocular events may occur in conjunction with other disease states, a visual examination prior to initiation of Roferon-A monotherapy or in the combination therapy with ribavirin is recommended in patients with diabetes mellitus or hypertension. Roferon-A monotherapy or the combination therapy with ribavirin should be discontinued in patients who developed new or worsening ophthalmologic disorders.

Endocrine: Hyperglycaemia has been observed rarely in patients treated with Roferon-A. All patients who develop symptoms of hyperglycaemia should have their blood glucose measured and followed-up accordingly. Patients with diabetes mellitus may require adjustment of their antidiabetic regimen.

When mild to moderate renal, hepatic or myeloid dysfunction is present, close monitoring of these functions is required.

Hepatic function: In rare cases interferon alpha has been suspected of causing an exacerbation of an underlying autoimmune disease in hepatitis patients. Therefore, when treating hepatitis patients with a history of autoimmune disease caution is recommended. If a deterioration in liver function in these patients develops a determination of autoimmune antibodies should be considered. If necessary treatment should be discontinued.

Bone marrow suppression: Extreme caution should be exercised when administering Roferon-A to patients with severe myelosuppression as it has a suppressive effect on the bone marrow, leading to a fall in the white blood count, particularly granulocytes, platelet count and, less commonly, haemoglobin concentration. This can lead to an increased risk of infection or of haemorrhage. It is important to monitor closely these events in patients and periodic complete blood counts should be performed during the course of Roferon-A treatment, both prior to therapy and at appropriate periods during therapy.

Autoimmune: The development of different auto-antibodies has been reported during treatment with alfa interferons. Clinical manifestations of autoimmune disease during interferon therapy occur more frequently in subjects predisposed to the development of autoimmune disorders. In patients with an underlying or clinical history of autoimmune disorders, monitoring of symptoms suggestive of these disorders, as well as measurement of auto-antibodies and TSH level, is recommended.

The use of Roferon-A in children is not recommended as the safety and effectiveness of Roferon-A in children have not been established.

Efficacy in patients with chronic hepatitis B or C who are on haemodialysis or have haemophilia or are co-infected with human immunodeficiency virus has not been demonstrated. This product contains less than 1mmol sodium (23mg) per 0.5ml, ie, essentially 'sodium-free'.

Combination therapy with ribavirin: Also see ribavirin labelling if interferon alfa-2a is to be administered in combination with ribavirin in patients with chronic hepatitis C.

Patients co-infected with HIV and receiving Highly Active Anti-Retroviral Therapy (HAART) may be at increased risk of developing lactic acidosis. Caution should be used when adding Roferon-A and ribavirin to HAART therapy (see ribavirin SPC).

Co-infected patients with advanced cirrhosis receiving HAART may be at increased risk of hepatic decompensation and death. Adding treatment with alfa interferons alone or in combination with ribavirin may increase the risk in this patient subset.

4.5 Interaction with other medicinal products and other forms of Interaction

Since alfa-interferons alter cellular metabolism, the potential to modify the activity of other drugs exists. In a small study, Roferon-A was shown to have an effect on specific microsomal enzyme systems. The clinical relevance of these findings is unknown.

Alfa-interferons may affect the oxidative metabolic process; this should be borne in mind when prescribing concomitant therapy with drugs metabolised by this route. However, as yet no specific information is available.

Roferon-A has been reported to reduce the clearance of theophylline.

As Roferon-A may affect central nervous system functions, interactions could occur following concurrent administration of centrally-acting drugs. The neurotoxic, haematotoxic or cardiotoxic effects of previously or concurrently administered drugs may be increased by interferons.

Combination therapy with ribavirin: Also see ribavirin labelling if interferon alfa-2a is to be administered in combination with ribavirin in patients with chronic hepatitis C.

4.6 Pregnancy and lactation

Men and women receiving Roferon-A should practise effective contraception. There are no adequate data on the use of Roferon-A in pregnant women. When doses greatly in excess of the recommended clinical dose were administered to pregnant rhesus monkeys in the early to mid-foetal period, an abortifacient effect was observed (see section 5.3). Although animal tests do not indicate that Roferon-A is a teratogen, harm to the foetus from use during pregnancy cannot be excluded. In pregnancy, Roferon-A should be administered only if the benefit to the woman justifies the potential risk to the foetus.

It is not known whether this drug is excreted in human milk. A decision must be taken whether to suspend breast feeding or to discontinue the drug, taking into account the importance of the drug to the mother.

Combination therapy with ribavirin: Also see ribavirin labelling if interferon alfa-2a is to be administered in combination with ribavirin in patients with chronic hepatitis C.

4.7 Effects on ability to drive and use machines

Depending on dose and schedule as well as the sensitivity of the individual patient, Roferon-A may have an effect on the speed of reaction which could impair certain operations, e.g., driving, operation of machinery etc.

4.8 Undesirable effects

Combination therapy with ribavirin: Also see ribavirin labelling if interferon alfa-2a is to be administered in combination with ribavirin in patients with chronic hepatitis C.

The following data on adverse reactions are based on information derived from the treatment of cancer patients with a wide variety of malignancies and often refractory to previous therapy and suffering from advanced disease, patients with chronic hepatitis B, and patients with chronic hepatitis C.

Approximately two thirds of cancer patients experienced anorexia and one half nausea. Cardiovascular and pulmonary disorders were seen in about one fifth of cancer patients and consisted of transient hypotension, hypertension, oedema, cyanosis, arrhythmias, palpitations and chest pain. Most cancer patients received doses that were significantly higher than the dose now recommended and may explain the higher frequency and severity of adverse reactions in this patient group compared with patients with hepatitis B where adverse reactions are usually transient, and patients return to pre-treatment status within 1 to 2 weeks after the end of therapy. Cardiovascular disorders were very rarely seen in patients with hepatitis B. In hepatitis B patients, changes in transaminases usually signal an improvement in the clinical state of the patient.

The majority of the patients experienced 'flu-like symptoms such as fatigue, pyrexia, rigors, decreased appetite, myalgia, headache, arthralgia and diaphoresis. These acute side-effects can usually be reduced or eliminated by concurrent administration of paracetamol and tend to diminish with continued therapy or dose modification although continuing therapy can lead to lethargy, asthenia and fatigue.

Infections & Infestations:

Rare: pneumonia, herpes simplex (including exacerbations of herpes labialis)

Blood & Lymphatic System Disorders:

Very Common: leukopenia

Common: thrombocytopenia, anaemia

Rare: agranulocytosis, haemolytic anaemia

Very Rare: idiopathic thrombocytopenia purpura

In myelosuppressed patients, thrombocytopenia and decreased haemoglobin occurred more frequently. Recovery of severe haematological deviations to pre-treatment levels usually occurred within seven to ten days after discontinuing Roferon-A treatment.

Immune System Disorders:

Rare: autoimmune disorder, acute hypersensitivity reactions (eg urticaria, angioedema, bronchospasm and anaphylaxis)

Very Rare: sarcoidosis

Endocine Disorders:

Rare: hyperthyroidism, hypothyroidism, thyroid dysfunction

Metabolism & Nutrition Disorders:

Very Common: anorexia, nausea, inconsequential hypocalcaemia

Uncommon: electrolyte imbalance, dehydration

Rare: hyperglycaemia

Very Rare: diabetes mellitus, hypertriglyceridaemia

Psychiatric Disorders:

Uncommon: depression, anxiety, mental status changes, confusional state, abnormal behaviour, nervousness, memory impairment, sleep disorder

Rare: suicide, suicide attempt, suicidal ideation

Nervous System Disorders:

Very Common: headache

Uncommon: neuropathy, dizziness, somnolence, dysgeusia, paraesthesia, hypoaesthesia, tremor

Rare: coma, cerebrovascular accident, convulsions, transient erectile dysfunction

Eye Disorders:

Uncommon: conjunctivitis, visual disturbance

Rare: ischaemic retinopathy

Very Rare: optic neuropathy, retinal artery thrombosis, retinal vein thrombosis, retinopathy, retinal haemorrhage, papilloedema, retinal exudates

Ear & Labyrinth Disorders:

Uncommon: vertigo

Cardiac Disorders:

Uncommon: arrhythmias, including atrioventricular block, palpitations

Rare: cardiorespiratory arrest, myocardial infarction, congestive heart failure, pulmonary oedema, cyanosis

Vascular Disorders:

Uncommon: hypertension, hypotension

Rare: vasculitis

Respiratory, Thoracic & Mediastinal Disorders:

Rare: dyspnoea, cough

Gastrointestinal Disorders:

Very Common: diarrhoea

Common: nausea/vomiting

Uncommon: abdominal pain, dry mouth

Rare: intestinal hypermotility, constipation, dyspepsia, flatulence, pancreatitis

Very Rare: reactivation of peptic ulcer, non-life-threatening gastrointestinal bleeding

Hepatobiliary Disorders:

Rare: hepatic failure, hepatitis, hepatic dysfunction

Skin & Subcutaneous Tissue Disorders:

Very Common: alopecia (reversible upon discontinuation; increased hair loss may continue for several weeks after end of treatment), sweating increased

Uncommon: exacerbation of, or provocation of, psoriasis, pruritus

Rare: rash, dry skin, epistaxis, mucosal dryness, rhinorrhoea

Musculoskeletal & Connective Tissue Disorders:

Very Common: myalgia, arthralgia

Rare: systemic lupus erythematosus, arthritis

Renal & Urinary Disorders:

Uncommon: proteinuria and increased cell count in urine

Rare: acute renal failure (mainly in cancer patients with renal disease), renal impairment

General Disorders & Administration Site Conditions:

Very Common: 'flu-like illness, fatigue, pyrexia, rigors, appetite decreased

Uncommon: chest pain, oedema

Very Rare: injection site necrosis, injection site reaction

Investigations:

Uncommon: Increases inALT, blood alkaline phosphatase, and transaminase, weight loss

Rare: Increases inblood LDH, blood bilirubin, blood creatinine, blood uric acid, blood urea increased

Neutralising antibodies to interferons may form in some patients. In certain clinical conditions (cancer, systemic lupus erythematosus, herpes zoster) antibodies to human leukocyte interferon may also occur spontaneously in patients who have never received exogenous interferons. The clinical significance of the development of antibodies has not been fully clarified.

In clinical trials where lyophilised Roferon-A which had been stored at 25°C was used, neutralising antibodies to Roferon-A have been detected in approximately one fifth of patients. In patients with hepatitis C, a trend for responding patients who develop neutralising antibodies to lose response while still on treatment and to lose it earlier than patients who do not develop such antibodies, has been seen. No other clinical sequelae of the presence of antibodies to Roferon-A have been documented. The clinical significance of the development of antibodies has not been fully clarified.

No data on neutralising antibodies yet exist from clinical trials in which lyophilised Roferon-A or Roferon-A solution for injection which is stored at 4°C has been used. In a mouse model, the relative immunogenicity of lyophilised Roferon-A increases with time when the material is stored at 25°C - no such increase in immunogenicity is observed when lyophilised Roferon-A is stored at 4°C, the recommended storage conditions.

4.9 Overdose

There are no reports of overdosage but repeated large doses of interferon can be associated with profound lethargy, fatigue, prostration and coma. Such patients should be hospitalised for observation and appropriate supportive treatment given.

Patients who experience severe reactions to Roferon-A will usually recover within days after discontinuation of therapy, given appropriate supportive care. Coma has been observed in 0.4% of cancer patients in clinical trials.

5. PHARMACOLOGICAL PROPERTIES

5.1 Pharmacodynamic properties

Pharmacotherapeutic group:	Cytokines and immunomodulators, *Interferons*
	ATC Code L03AB04

Roferon-A has been shown to possess many of the activities of the so-called natural human alfa-interferon preparations. Roferon-A exerts its antiviral effects by inducing a state of resistance to viral infections in cells and by modulating the effector arm of the immune system to neutralise viruses or eliminate virus infected cells. The essential mechanism for the anti-tumour action of Roferon-A is not yet known. However, several changes are described in human tumoural cells treated with Roferon-A: HT 29 cells show a significant reduction of DNA, RNA and protein synthesis. Roferon-A has been shown to exert antiproliferative activity against a variety of human tumours *in vitro* and to inhibit the growth of some human tumour xenografts in nude mice. A limited number of human tumour cell lines grown *in vivo* in immunocompromised nude mice has been tested for the susceptibility to Roferon-A. *In vivo* antiproliferative activity of Roferon-A has been studied on tumours including breast mucoid carcinoma, adenocarcinoma of the caecum, colon carcinoma and prostatic carcinoma. The degree of antiproliferative activity is variable.

Unlike other human proteins, many of the effects of interferon alfa-2a are partially or completely suppressed when it is tested in other animal species. However, significant anti-vaccinia virus activity was induced in rhesus monkeys pre-treated with interferon alfa-2a.

Clinical Trials

Hairy Cell Leukaemia

The therapeutic efficacy of Roferon-A in the treatment of hairy cell leukaemia has been demonstrated in a large trial of 218 patients, of whom 174 were evaluable for efficacy after 16 - 24 weeks of therapy. Response was observed in 88% of patients (complete response 33%, partial response 55%).

AIDS-related Kaposi's Sarcoma

The efficacy of Roferon-A in the treatment of Kaposi's sarcoma was assessed in 364 patients receiving 3 to 54 MIU per day. Objective response rates were dose-related, ranging from 14% to 50%, with a daily dose of 36 MIU producing the best overall therapeutic benefit (13.3% complete response, 12.2% partial response). High baseline CD4 lymphocyte count was a favourable prognostic factor for response, with 46% of patients with a CD4 count > 400/mm^3 responding to Roferon-A. Response to Roferon-A therapy was the strongest prognostic factor for survival.

Chronic Myelogenous Leukaemia (CML)

The efficacy of Roferon-A was assessed in 226 patients with chronic phase CML, and compared with 109 patients receiving chemotherapy (hydroxyurea or busulfan). Both groups had favourable features at diagnosis (less than 10% blasts in the blood) and treatment was initiated with interferon within six months of diagnosis. Treatment of patients with CML in the chronic phase leads to the same proportion of patients (85 - 90%) achieving a haematologic response as treatment with the standard chemotherapy regimens. In addition patients treated with Roferon-A resulted in 8% complete cytogenetic response and 38% partial cytogenetic response versus 9% partial cytogenetic response during chemotherapy. Time to progression from the chronic phase of leukaemia to an accelerated or a blastic phase was longer in the Roferon-A group (69 months) than in the conventional chemotherapy group (46 months) ($p < 0.001$) as was median overall survival (72.8 months versus 54.5 months, $p = 0.002$).

Cutaneous T-cell Lymphoma (CTCL)

The efficacy of Roferon-A was assessed in 169 patients with CTCL, the majority of whom (78%) were resistant to, or had relapsed on, standard therapy. Among the 85 patients evaluable, overall response to treatment was 58% (20% complete response, 38% partial response). Patients with all stages of disease responded to therapy. Median duration of complete response from start of treatment was 22 months, with 94% of complete responders remaining in remission at 9 months.

Chronic Hepatitis B

The efficacy of Roferon-A in the treatment of chronic hepatitis B was assessed in trials involving over 900 patients. In the pivotal controlled study 238 patients were randomised into four groups: patients received either 2.5 MIU/m^2, 5.0 MIU/m^2, 10 MIU/m^2, tiw of Roferon-A or no treatment. Treatment duration was 12 - 24 weeks depending on response i.e. clearance of HBeAg and HBV DNA from serum. Patients were followed for up to 12 months after treatment was discontinued. There was a statistically significant difference in sustained response [clearance of hepatitis Be antigen (HBeAg) and hepatitis B viral DNA (HBV DNA)] between treated and untreated patients (37% versus 13%). Response differences between various dose groups did not reach statistical significance (33%, 34% and 43% for the 2.5, 5.0 and 10.0 MIU/m^2 groups). Serological and virological responses were associated with marked improvement in liver histology after 12 months of treatment-free follow up.

Chronic Hepatitis C

The efficacy of Roferon-A in the treatment of chronic hepatitis C has been assessed in 1701 patients, with 130 untreated or placebo treated controls. At recommended doses, Roferon-A induces complete biochemical response in up to 85% of patients, with response rates maintained for at least six months after treatment ranging from 11 to 44% depending on pre-treatment disease characteristics, IFN dose and treatment duration. Biochemical response to Roferon-A is associated with significant improvement of liver disease as shown by evaluation of pre- and post-liver biopsies. For those patients who have a sustained response three to six months after end of therapy, response has been reported to be maintained for up to four years. The therapeutic efficacy of Interferon alfa-2a alone and in combination with ribavirin was compared in a double-blind randomised clinical trial in naïve (previously untreated) and relapsed patients with virologically, biochemically and histologically documented chronic hepatitis C. Six months after end of treatment sustained biochemical and virological response as well as histological improvement were assessed.

A statistically significant ten-fold increase (from 4% to 43%; $p < 0.01$) in sustained virological and biochemical response was observed in relapsed patients. The favourable profile of the combination therapy was also reflected in the response rates relative to HCV genotype or baseline viral load. Although the sustained response rates in patients with HCV genotype-1 were lower than in the overall population (approx. 30% versus 0% in the monotherapy arm) the relative benefit of ribavirin in combination with interferon alfa-2a is particularly significant in this group of patients. In addition the histological improvement favoured the combination therapy.

Supportive favourable results from a small study in naïve patients were reported using interferon alfa-2a (3 MIU three times per week) with ribavirin.

For other information on pharmacodynamic properties please refer to the SmPC for Ribavirin.

Follicular Non-Hodgkin's lymphoma

The efficacy of Roferon-A in addition to cytotoxic chemotherapy (CHOP-like regimen of cyclophosphamide, vincristine, prednisone and doxorubicin) was assessed in 122 patients with clinically aggressive low-grade or intermediate-grade non-Hodgkin's lymphoma and compared with 127 controls receiving the same chemotherapy regimen. The two regimens produced comparable objective responses, but the regimen including Roferon-A had a greater effect in prolonging the time to treatment failure ($p < 0.001$), the duration of complete response ($p < 0.003$).

Renal Cell Carcinoma

The efficacy of Roferon-A given in combination with vinblastine, was compared with vinblastine alone. The combination of Roferon-A plus vinblastine is superior to vinblastine alone in the treatment of patients with locally advanced or metastatic renal cell carcinoma. Median survival was 67.8 weeks for the 79 patients receiving Roferon-A plus vinblastine and 37.8 weeks for the 81 patients treated with vinblastine ($p = 0.0049$). Overall response rates were 16.5% for patients treated with Roferon-A plus vinblastine and 2.5% for patients treated with vinblastine alone ($p = 0.0025$).

Surgically Resected Malignant Melanoma

The efficacy of Roferon-A in patients with primary cutaneous melanoma thicker than 1.5mm and without clinically detectable node metastasis was assessed in a large randomised study involving 253 patients receiving Roferon-A at a dose of 3 MIU three times a week for 18 months, compared with 246 untreated controls. After a median follow-up of 4.4 years a significant extension of relapse-free interval ($p = 0.035$) but no statistically significant difference in overall survival ($p = 0.059$) in Roferon-A treated patients compared with controls have been shown. The overall treatment effect was a 25% reduction in the risk of relapse.

5.2 Pharmacokinetic properties

The serum concentrations of interferon alfa-2a reflected a large intersubject variation in both healthy volunteers and patients with disseminated cancer. The pharmacokinetics of Roferon-A in animals (monkey, dog and mouse) were similar to those seen in man. The pharmacokinetics of Roferon-A in man were linear over a 3 million to 198 million IU dose range. In healthy man, interferon alfa-2a exhibited an elimination half-life of 3.7 - 8.5 hours (mean: 5.1 hours), a volume of distribution at steady state of 0.223 - 0.748 l/kg (mean: 0.4 l/kg) and a total body clearance of 2.14 - 3.62ml/min/kg (mean: 2.79ml/min/kg) after a 36 million IU intravenous infusion. After intramuscular administration of 36 million IU, peak serum concentrations ranged from 1500 to 2580pg/ml (mean: 2020pg/ml) at a mean time to peak of 3.8 hours, and after subcutaneous administration of 36 million IU from 1250 to 2320pg/ml (mean: 1730pg/ml) at a mean time to peak of 7.3 hours.

The apparent fraction of the dose absorbed after intramuscular or subcutaneous injection is greater than 80%.

The pharmacokinetics of interferon alfa-2a after single intramuscular doses to patients with disseminated cancer and chronic hepatitis B were similar to those found in healthy volunteers. Dose-proportional increases in serum concentrations were observed after single doses up to 198 million IU. There were no changes in the distribution or elimination of interferon alfa-2a during twice daily (0.5 - 36 million IU), once daily (1 - 54 million IU), or three times weekly (1 - 136 million IU) dosing regimens up to 28 days of dosing. Renal catabolism is the major pathway for Roferon-A elimination. Biliary excretion and liver metabolism are considered to be minor pathways of elimination of Roferon-A.

Intramuscular administration of Roferon-A one or more times daily for up to 28 days to some patients with disseminated cancer resulted in peak plasma concentrations of two to four times greater than those seen after single doses. However, multiple dosing caused no changes in its distribution or elimination parameters during several dosage regimens studied.

For other information on pharmacokinetic properties please refer to the SmPC for Ribavirin.

5.3 Preclinical safety data

Because of species specificity of human interferon, only limited toxicological studies have been carried out with Roferon-A. The acute parenteral toxicity of Roferon-A has been studied in mice, rats, rabbits and ferrets at doses up to 30 million IU/kg intravenously, and 500 million IU/kg intramuscularly. No treatment-related mortality was noted in any species studied given Roferon-A by any of the routes of administration. With doses greatly exceeding the recommended clinical dose no significant adverse effects were observed except for an abortifacient effect when administered to pregnant rhesus monkeys in the early to mid-foetal period and transient menstrual cycle irregularities including prolonged menstrual periods in non-pregnant monkeys. The relevance of these findings in man has not been established.

Mutagenic effects of Roferon-A have not been observed experimentally.

For other information on preclinical safety data please refer to the SmPC for Ribavirin.

6. PHARMACEUTICAL PARTICULARS

6.1 List of excipients

Ammonium acetate

Sodium Chloride

Benzyl alcohol

Polysorbate 80

Glacial Acetic acid

Sodium Hydroxide Solution

Water for Injection

6.2 Incompatibilities

Not applicable.

6.3 Shelf life

2 years.

6.4 Special precautions for storage

Store pre-filled syringes at 2°C - 8°C. Do not freeze. Keep container in the outer carton.

6.5 Nature and contents of container

Syringe barrel 1ml (flint glass), butyl rubber stopper laminated with PTFE (fluororesin D-3), tip cap of butyl rubber and laminated with ETFE (fluororesin D), plastic plunger rod, injection needle for subcutaneous injection made of stainless steel, needle hub made of polypropylene. Injection swabs may be supplied with the product.

Each pre-filled syringe contains 3, 4.5, 6, 9 or 18 MIU interferon alpha-2a in 0.5ml of ready-to-use solution for injection.

Pack sizes: Pack of 1, 5, 6, 12 and 30. Not all pack sizes may be marketed.

6.6 Instructions for use and handling

For single use only.

Any unused product or waste material should be disposed of in accordance with local requirements.

7. MARKETING AUTHORISATION HOLDER

Roche Products Limited, 40 Broadwater Road, Welwyn Garden City, Hertfordshire, AL7 3AY, UK.

8. MARKETING AUTHORISATION NUMBER(S)

Roferon-A 3 MIU/0.5ml Solution for injection:

PL 0031/0485; PA 50/68/20

Roferon-A 4.5 MIU/0.5ml Solution for injection:

PL 0031/0486; PA 50/68/21

Roferon-A 6 MIU/0.5ml Solution for injection:

PL 0031/0487; PA 50/68/22

Roferon-A 9 MIU/0.5ml Solution for injection:

PL 0031/0488; PA 50/68/23

Roferon-A 18 MIU/0.5ml Solution for injection:

PL 0031/0602; PA 50/68/25

9. DATE OF FIRST AUTHORISATION/RENEWAL OF THE AUTHORISATION

Date of First Authorisation:

PL 0031/0485 - 0488	29 July 1996
PA 50/68/20 - 23	1 October 1999
PL 0031/0602	18 July 2002
PA 50/68/25	24 Jan 2003

Date of last renewal: 22 July 2004

10. DATE OF REVISION OF THE TEXT

25 July 2005

LEGAL STATUS

POM

Roferon-A is a registered trade mark

P739574/204

Rogitine Ampoules 10mg

(Alliance Pharmaceuticals)

1. NAME OF THE MEDICINAL PRODUCT
Rogitine® ampoules 10mg

2. QUALITATIVE AND QUANTITATIVE COMPOSITION
Phentolamine mesylate PhEur 10mg.

3. PHARMACEUTICAL FORM
Colourless to pale yellow solution in 1ml Water for Injections PhEur

4. CLINICAL PARTICULARS

4.1 Therapeutic indications
Management of hypertensive episodes that may occur in patients with phaeochromocytoma, for example during pre-operative preparation and surgical manipulation.

Diagnosis of phaeochromocytoma by Rogitine blocking test if other more specific tests are not available.

4.2 Posology and method of administration

Adults

Management of hypertensive episodes in patients with phaeochromocytoma

For the management of hypertensive crises that arise during the pre-operative phase or during induction of anaesthesia, intubation, or surgical removal of the tumour, 2 to 5mg of Rogitine is injected intravenously and repeated if necessary. The blood pressure response should be monitored.

Diagnosis of phaeochromocytoma - Rogitine blocking test

The test is most reliable in detecting phaeochromocytoma in patients with sustained hypertension and least reliable in those with paroxysmal hypertension. False-positive tests may occur in patients with hypertension without phaeochromocytoma.

Preparation for the test:

Sedatives, analgesics and all other medications except those that might be deemed essential (such as digitalis and insulin) are withheld for at least 24 hours, and preferably 48 to 72 hours, prior to the test. Antihypertensive drugs are withheld until blood pressure returns to the untreated, hypertensive level. This test is not performed on a patient who is normotensive.

Procedure: (intravenous) The patient is kept at rest in the supine position throughout the test, preferably in a quiet, darkened room. Injection of Rogitine is delayed until blood pressure is stabilised, as evidenced by blood pressure readings taken every 10 minutes for at least 30 minutes.

The dose for adults is 5mg. The syringe needle is inserted into the vein and injection delayed until the pressor response to venepuncture has subsided.

Rogitine is injected rapidly. Blood pressure is recorded immediately after injection, at 30-second intervals for the first 3 minutes, and at 60-second intervals for the next 7 minutes.

Interpretation: A positive response, suggestive of phaeochromocytoma, is indicated when the blood pressure is reduced by more than 35mmHg systolic and by 25mmHg diastolic. A typical positive response is a reduction in pressure of 60mmHg systolic and 25mmHg diastolic. Usually, the maximal effect is evident within 2 minutes after injection. A return to preinjection pressure commonly occurs within 15 to 20 minutes but may occur more rapidly.

If blood pressure decreases to a dangerous level, the patient should be treated as outlined under Section 4.9 "Overdose".

A negative response is indicated when the blood pressure is elevated, unchanged, or reduced by less than 35mmHg systolic and 25mmHg diastolic after injection of Rogitine. A negative response to this test does not exclude the diagnosis of phaeochromocytoma, especially in patients with paroxysmal hypertension, in whom the incidence of false-negative responses is high.

Procedure: (intramuscular) A dose of 5mg is administered intramuscularly.

Interpretation: Blood pressure is recorded every 5 minutes for 30 to 45 minutes following injection. A positive response is indicated when the blood pressure is reduced by 35mmHg systolic and by 25mmHg diastolic, or more, within 20 minutes following injection.

Children:

Management of hypertensive episodes in patients with phaeochromocytoma*:* The dosage is 1mg given intravenously.

Diagnosis of phaeochromocytoma - Rogitine blocking test*:* The dosage is 1mg given intravenously or 3mg given intramuscularly.

Elderly: In elderly patients, it is advisable to use the lowest dose or a low infusion rate in case of undiagnosed coronary insufficiency, (see Section 4.3 "Contra-indications").

Patients with renal impairment: Since no pharmacokinetic studies with Rogitine have been performed in patients with renal impairment, use caution in administering Rogitine to these patients.

4.3 Contraindications
Known hypersensitivity to phentolamine and related compounds. Known hypersensitivity to sulphites. Hypotension. Myocardial infarction, history of myocardial infarction, coronary insufficiency, angina, or other evidence of coronary artery disease.

4.4 Special warnings and special precautions for use
Monitoring of the blood pressure is necessary for appropriate selection of patient, dosage, and duration of therapy. Myocardial infarction, cerebrovascular spasm, and cerebrovascular occlusion have been reported following the administration of Rogitine, usually in association with marked hypotensive episodes.

The presence of sulphites in Rogitine ampoules can lead to isolated hypersensitivity reactions especially in patients with bronchial asthma, which may become manifest as an acute asthma attack, shock, or clouding of consciousness.

For screening tests in patients with hypertension, the generally available urinary assay of catecholamines or other biochemical assays have largely replaced the Rogitine blocking test and other pharmacological tests for reasons of accuracy and safety. Therefore the Rogitine blocking test is not the procedure of choice and should be used only when these other specific tests are not available.

Tachycardia and cardiac arrhythmias may occur with the use of Rogitine.

Due to its stimulatory effect on the gastro-intestinal tract, including gastric secretion, Rogitine should be used with caution in patients with gastritis and peptic ulcer. Excessive cardiac stimulation and hypertensive crisis may occur during surgical removal of a tumour due to manipulation of the phaeochromocytoma, despite the fact that phentolamine had been given as pre-medication to prevent such an occurrence. In the event of this complication, use a $_1$-selective, -adrenergic blocking agent in slow i.v. injection.

4.5 Interaction with other medicinal products and other forms of Interaction
Rogitine may augment the hypotensive effect of other antihypertensive agents. Antipsychotics may enhance the hypotensive effect of -adrenergic blocking agents.

4.6 Pregnancy and lactation
Experience with Rogitine in pregnant women is not available. Do not use in pregnancy unless treatment is considered essential.

No information is available as to whether phentolamine passes into breast milk. For safety reasons, it is not recommended to use Rogitine during lactation.

4.7 Effects on ability to drive and use machines
Patients should be warned of the potential hazards of driving or operating machinery if they experience side effects such as dizziness and sedation.

4.8 Undesirable effects
Cardiovascular system: Frequent: Orthostatic hypotension and tachycardia. Occasional: Acute or prolonged hypotensive episodes (flushing, sweating and feelings of apprehension). Myocardial infarction, cerebrospasm, and cerebrovascular occlusion may occur under these circumstances. Rare: Anginal pain and cardiac arrhythmias.

Central nervous system: Occasional: Dizziness and weakness.

Gastro-intestinal tract: Occasional: Nausea, vomiting and diarrhoea.

Other organ systems: Occasional: Nasal stuffiness and flushing. Rare: Chest pain.

4.9 Overdose
Symptoms: Arterial hypotension, reflex tachycardia, cardiac stimulation, arrhythmia, increase of systemic venous capacity, and possibly shock. These effects may be accompanied by headache, hyperexcitability and disturbances of vision, sweating, increased gastric motility, vomiting and diarrhoea, hypoglycaemia.

Treatment: *Hypotension, excessive peripheral vasodilation*: noradrenaline, in cautiously titrated continuous i.v. infusion, can be considered the physiological antagonist; the effect of Rogitine may wear off in a short time, and administration of noradrenaline may have to be adjusted accordingly. When a pressor agent is used, ECG should be monitored, as major arrhythmias may occur. Alternative measures such as keeping the patient's legs raised and administering a plasma expander should be implemented concomitantly. Do not use adrenaline since this may cause a further fall of blood pressure under the given conditions.

Disturbances of cardiac rhythm: adjust treatment to the nature of the arrhythmia.

Hypoglycaemia: Provide glucose iv until reaction is compensated.

5. PHARMACOLOGICAL PROPERTIES

5.1 Pharmacodynamic properties
Phentolamine is a competitive non-selective $_1$ and $_2$-adrenergic receptor blocker of relatively short duration. It causes vasodilation and a fall in blood pressure which is based upon the blockade of both postjunctional vascular $_1$ and $_2$-adrenoceptors. It also antagonises the vasoconstrictor response to noradrenaline and adrenaline infusions. Enhanced neural release of noradrenaline due to presynaptic $_2$-blockade may contribute to the positive inotropic and chronotropic effects of Rogitine on cardiac muscle.

The administration of Rogitine intravenously to man produces transient declines in mean systemic vascular resistance and mean systemic arterial pressure as a result of dilatation in the arterial as well as in the venous vascular bed. These effects of Rogitine are accompanied by tachycardia, triggered by the baroreceptor reflex system and the autonomic nervous system.

5.2 Pharmacokinetic properties
The elimination of phentolamine from blood is rapid and does not follow first order kinetics. After two to four hours the concentration has fallen to about 15% of the peak value. At concentrations of 0.02 to 109μg/ml, 54% of phentolamine is bound to human serum proteins. Phentolamine is extensively metabolised, on average about 13% of a dose given by intravenous infusion is excreted unchanged in the urine. Phentolamine metabolism is more pronounced following oral administration than after intravenous administration.

5.3 Preclinical safety data
According to the experimental data available, phentolamine did not reveal either a mutagenic or a teratogenic potential. Long-term carcinogenicity studies have not been conducted with phentolamine.

6. PHARMACEUTICAL PARTICULARS

6.1 List of excipients
Water, sodium metabisulphite and glucose.

6.2 Incompatibilities
Rogitine should not be mixed with alkaline solutions.

6.3 Shelf life
5 Years

6.4 Special precautions for storage
Store ampoules in the outer carton at 2 to 8°C. Do not freeze.

6.5 Nature and contents of container
Glass ampoules in boxes of 5.

6.6 Instructions for use and handling
None

Administrative Data

7. MARKETING AUTHORISATION HOLDER
Alliance Pharmaceuticals Ltd
Avonbridge House
Bath Road
Chippenham
Wiltshire
SN15 2BB

8. MARKETING AUTHORISATION NUMBER(S)
PL16853/0012

9. DATE OF FIRST AUTHORISATION/RENEWAL OF THE AUTHORISATION
25 June 1998

10. DATE OF REVISION OF THE TEXT
October 2003

11. Legal Status
POM

Alliance, Alliance Pharmaceuticals and associated devices are registered Trademarks of Alliance Pharmaceuticals Ltd.

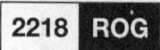

Rozex Cream

(Galderma (U.K.) Ltd)

1. NAME OF THE MEDICINAL PRODUCT
Rozex Cream

2. QUALITATIVE AND QUANTITATIVE COMPOSITION
Metronidazole Ph. Eur 0.75% w/w

3. PHARMACEUTICAL FORM
Cream

4. CLINICAL PARTICULARS

4.1 Therapeutic indications
Indicated in the treatment of inflammatory papules, pustules and erythema of rosacea

4.2 Posology and method of administration
For topical administration only.

The average period of treatment is three to four months. If a clear benefit has been demonstrated, continued therapy for a further three to four months period may be considered by the prescribing physician depending on the severity of the condition. In clinical studies, topical metronidazole therapy for rosacea has been continued for up to 2 years. In the absence of a clear clinical improvement, therapy should be stopped.

Adults: A pea-size amount of cream is applied to the affected areas of the skin, twice daily, morning and evening. Areas to be treated should be washed with a mild cleanser before application. Patients may use non-comedogenic and non-astringent cosmetics after application of Rozex Cream.

Elderly: The dosage recommended in the elderly is the same as that recommended in adults.

Children: Not recommended. Safety and efficacy have not been established.

4.3 Contraindications

Contraindicated in individuals with a history of hypersensitivity to Metronidazole, or other ingredients of the formulation.

4.4 Special warnings and special precautions for use

Rozex Cream has been reported to cause lacrimation of the eyes, therefore, contact with the eyes should be avoided. If a reaction suggesting local irritation occurs patients should be directed to use the medication less frequently, discontinue use temporarily or discontinue use until further instructions. Metronidazole is a nitroimidazole and should be used with care in patients with evidence of, or history of, blood dyscrasia. Exposure of treated sites to ultraviolet or strong sunlight should be avoided during use of metronidazole. Unnecessary and prolonged use of this medication should be avoided.

4.5 Interaction with other medicinal products and other forms of Interaction

Interaction with systemic medication is unlikely because absorption of metronidazole following cutaneous application of Rozex Cream is low. Oral metronidazole has been reported to potentiate the effect of warfarinand other coumarin anticoagulants, resulting in a prolongation of prothrombin time. The effect of topical metronidazole on prothrombin is not known. However, very rare cases of modification of the INR values have been reported with concomitant use of Rozex and coumarin anticoagulants.

4.6 Pregnancy and lactation

There is no experience to date with the use of Rozex Cream in pregnancy. Metronidazole crosses the placental barrier and rapidly enters the foetal circulation. There is inadequate evidence of the safety of Metronidazole in human pregnancy. In animals, Metronidazole was not teratogenic or embryotoxic unless administered at extremely high doses. Rozex Cream should only be used in pregnancy when there is no safer alternative.

After oral administration, Metronidazole is excreted in breast milk in concentrations similar to those found in the plasma. Even though Metronidazole blood levels from topical administration are significantly lower than those achieved after oral administration, in nursing mothers a decision should be made to discontinue nursing or to discontinue the drug, taking into account the importance of the drug to the mother.

4.7 Effects on ability to drive and use machines

Not applicable

4.8 Undesirable effects

Because of the minimal absorption of metronidazole and consequently its insignificant plasma concentration after topical administration, the adverse experiences reported with the oral form of the drug have not been reported with Rozex Cream. Adverse reactions reported with Rozex Cream have been only local and mild, and include skin discomfort (burning and stinging), erythema, pruritis, skin irritation, worsening of rosacea, nausea, metallic taste and tingling or numbness of the extremities, and watery eyes if applied too closely to this area.

4.9 Overdose

No data exists about overdosage in humans. Acute oral toxicity studies with a topical gel formulation containing 0.75% w/w metronidazole in rats have shown no toxic action with doses of up to 5 g of finished product per kilogram body weight, the highest dose used. This dose is equivalent to the oral intake of 12 tubes of 30g packaging Rozex Cream for an adult weighing 72 kg, and 2 tubes of Cream for a child weighing 12 kg.

5. PHARMACOLOGICAL PROPERTIES

5.1 Pharmacodynamic properties

Metronidazole is an antiprotozoal and antibacterial agent which is active against a wide range of pathogenic microorganisms. The mechanisms of action of metronidazole in rosacea are unknown but available evidence suggests that the effects may be antibacterial and/or anti-inflammatory.

5.2 Pharmacokinetic properties

Metronidazole is rapidly and nearly totally absorbed after oral administration. The drug is not significantly bound to serum proteins and distributes well to all body compartments with the lowest concentration found in the fat. Metronidazole is excreted primarily in the urine as parent drug, oxidative metabolites and conjugates.

Bioavailability studies with a topical 1g application of Rozex Cream to the face of normal subjects resulted in mean maximum serum concentrations of 32.9ng/ml (range 14.8 to 54.4ng/ml) which is approximately 100 times less than those attained after a single oral dose of 250 mg (mean Cmax = 7248ng/ml; range 4270 – 13970ng/ml). The peak concentration occurred between 0.25 – 4 hours after oral dosing, and 6 to 24 hours after cutaneous application of Rozex Cream.

Following topical application of Rozex Cream, serum concentrations of the major metabolite (the hydroxymetabolite 2-hydroxymethylmetronidazole) were below the quantifiable limit of the assay (<9.6ng/ml) at most of the time points, ranging to a maximum of 17.5ng/ml peak concentration between 8 and 24 hours after application. In comparison, the peak concentration following a 250mg oral dose ranged from 626 to 1788ng/ml between 4 and 12 hours after dosing.

The extent of exposure (Area under the curve, AUC) from a 1g application of metronidazole administered topically was 1.36% of the AUC of a single oral 250mg metronidazole dose (mean + 912.7ng.hr/ml and approximately 67207ng.ml/hr respectively).

5.3 Preclinical safety data

No evidence for a primary dermal irritation was observed in rabbits following a single 24-hour cutaneous application of Rozex Cream to abraded and non-abraded skin, under occlusion.

Metronidazole has shown mutagenic activity in several in vitro bacterial assay systems. In addition, a dose-response increase in the frequency of micronuclei was observed in mice after intraperitoneal injection and an increase in chromosome aberrations have been reported in patients with Crohn's disease who were treated with 200 to 1200mg/day of oral metronidazole for 1 to 24 months. However, the preponderance of evidence from these studies suggests that although metronidazole has a potential for producing mutations, this should not occur in well oxygenated mammalian cells, i.e., under normal aerobic conditions.

The carcinogenicity of metronidazole by the oral route of administration has been evaluated in rats, mice and hamsters. These studies showed that oral metronidazole caused an increased incidence of pulmonary tumours in mice and possibly other tumours, including liver tumours, in the rat. Conversely, two lifetime studies in hamsters produced negative results. Moreover, one study showed a significant enhancement of UV-induced skin tumours in hairless mice treated with metronidazole intraperitoneally (15μg per g body weight and per day for 28 weeks).

Although the significance of these results to the cutaneous use of metronidazole for the treatment of rosacea is unclear, patients should be advised to avoid or minimise exposure of metronidazole cream-treated sites to sun. After several decades of systemic use, no evidence has been published to suggest that metronidazole is associated with carcinogenic potential in humans.

6. PHARMACEUTICAL PARTICULARS

6.1 List of excipients

Emulsifying Wax, Benzyl alcohol, Isopropyl palmitate, Glycerol, Sorbitol 70% (non-crystallising), lactic acid and/or Sodium Hydroxide, Purified Water.

6.2 Incompatibilities

None known

6.3 Shelf life

Rozex Cream has a shelf life when unopened of 36 months

6.4 Special precautions for storage

Store at a temperature not exceeding 25°C. Do not refrigerate.

6.5 Nature and contents of container

Aluminium tubes with epoxy phenolic lining, fitted with white polypropylene screw caps;

pack sizes: 30g & 40g

6.6 Instructions for use and handling

Replace cap tightly after use.

7. MARKETING AUTHORISATION HOLDER

Galderma (UK.) Limited

Galderma House

Church Lane

Kings Langley

Herts, WD4 8JP

United Kingdom

8. MARKETING AUTHORISATION NUMBER(S)

PL 10590/0028

9. DATE OF FIRST AUTHORISATION/RENEWAL OF THE AUTHORISATION

18th June 1997

10. DATE OF REVISION OF THE TEXT

May 2004

Rozex Gel

(Galderma (U.K.) Ltd)

1. NAME OF THE MEDICINAL PRODUCT

Rozex Gel

2. QUALITATIVE AND QUANTITATIVE COMPOSITION

Metronidazole Ph. Eur 0.75% w/w

3. PHARMACEUTICAL FORM

Gel

4. CLINICAL PARTICULARS

4.1 Therapeutic indications

Indicated in the treatment of inflammatory papules, pustules and erythema of rosacea

4.2 Posology and method of administration

For topical administration only.

Adults: Apply and rub in a film of Gel twice daily, morning and evening, to entire affected area after washing.

Elderly: The dosage recommended in the elderly is the same as that recommended in adults.

Children: Not recommended

4.3 Contraindications

Contraindicated in individuals with a history of hypersensitivity to Metronidazole, or other ingredients of the formulation.

4.4 Special warnings and special precautions for use

Rozex Gel has been reported to cause lacrimation of the eyes, therefore, contact with the eyes should be avoided. If a reaction suggesting local irritation occurs patients should be directed to use the medication less frequently, discontinue use temporarily or discontinue use until further instructions. Metronidazole is a nitroimidazole and should be used with care in patients with evidence of, or history of, blood dyscrasia. Exposure of treated sites to ultraviolet or strong sunlight should be avoided during use of metronidazole. Unnecessary and prolonged use of this medication should be avoided.

4.5 Interaction with other medicinal products and other forms of Interaction

Interaction with systemic medication is unlikely because absorption of metronidazole following cutaneous application of Rozex Gel is low. Oral metronidazole has been reported to potentiate the effect of warfarin and other coumarin anticoagulants, resulting in a prolongation of prothrombin time. The effect of topical metronidazole on prothrombin is not known. However, very rare cases of modification of the INR values have been reported with concomitant use of Rozex and coumarin anticoagulants.

4.6 Pregnancy and lactation

There is no experience to date with the use of Rozex Gel in pregnancy. Metronidazole crosses the placental barrier and rapidly enters the foetal circulation. There is inadequate evidence of the safety of Metronidazole in human pregnancy. In animals, Metronidazole was not teratogenic or embryotoxic unless administered at extremely high doses. Rozex Gel should only be used in pregnancy where there is no safer alternative.

After oral administration, Metronidazole is excreted in breast milk in concentrations similar to those found in the plasma, Metronidazole blood levels from topical administration are significantly lower than those achieved after oral administration. A decision should be made to discontinue nursing or to discontinue the drug, taking into account the importance of the drug to the mother.

4.7 Effects on ability to drive and use machines

Not applicable

4.8 Undesirable effects

Because of the minimal absorption of metronidazole and consequently its insignificant plasma concentration after topical administration, the adverse experiences reported with the oral form of the drug have not been reported with Rozex Gel. Adverse reactions reported with Rozex Gel have been only local and mild, and include skin discomfort (burning and stinging), erythema, pruritis, skin irritation, worsening of rosacea, nausea, metallic taste and tingling or numbness of the extremities, and watery eyes if applied too closely to this area.

4.9 Overdose

No data exists about overdosage in humans. Acute oral toxicity studies with a topical gel formulation containing 0.75% w/w metronidazole in rats have shown no toxic action with doses of up to 5 g of finished product per kilogram body weight, the highest dose used. This dose is equivalent to the oral intake of 12 tubes of 30g packaging Rozex Gel for an adult weighing 72 kg, and 2 tubes of Gel for a child weighing 12 kg.

5. PHARMACOLOGICAL PROPERTIES

5.1 Pharmacodynamic properties

Metronidazole is an antiprotozoal and antibacterial agent which is active against a wide range of pathogenic microorganisms. The mechanisms of action of metronidazole in rosacea are unknown but available evidence suggests that the effects may be antibacterial and/or anti-inflammatory.

5.2 Pharmacokinetic properties

Metronidazole is rapidly and nearly totally absorbed after oral administration. The drug is not significantly bound to serum proteins and distributes well to all body compartments with the lowest concentration found in the fat. Metronidazole is excreted primarily in the urine as parent drug, oxidative metabolites and conjugates.

Bioavailability studies with Rozex Gel in rosacea patients treated with 7.5 mg metronidazole applied topically to the face resulted in maximum serum concentrations of 66 ng/ml which is approximately 100 times less than those attained after a single oral dose of 250 mg. In most patients at most time points after Rozex Gel application, serum concentrations of metronidazole were below the detectable limits of the assay (25 ng/ml).

5.3 Preclinical safety data

The toxicity studies conducted with the Metronidazole 0.75% Topical Gel formulation demonstrate that the product is non-toxic in rats after acute oral administration 5g/kg and produced no ocular irritation in rabbit eyes. The formulation produced no observable effects in rabbits after dermal application of 13 mg /kg for 90 days.

No compound-related dermal or systemic effects were observed in a 13-week cutaneous route toxicity study, in which Rozex gel containing Metronidazole 0.75% w/w was applied daily to rabbits at doses ranging between 0.13 and 13 mg/kg.

Metronidazole has shown evidence of carcinogenic activity in a number of studies involving chronic, oral administration in mice and rats but not in studies involving hamsters.

One study showed a significant enhancement of UV induced skin tumours in hairless mice treated with Metronidazole intraperitoneally (15μg per g body weight and per day for 28 weeks). Although the significance of these studies to man is not clear, patients should be advised to avoid or minimise exposure of metronidazole treated sites to sun.

Metronidazole has shown mutagenic activity in several in vitro bacterial assay systems. In addition, a dose-response increase in the frequency of micronuclei was observed in mice after intraperitoneal injection and an increase in chromosome aberrations have been reported in patients with Crohn's disease who were treated with 200 to 1200mg/day of metronidazole for 1 to 24 months. However, no excess chromosomal aberrations in circulating human lymphocytes have been observed in patients treated for 8 months.

6. PHARMACEUTICAL PARTICULARS

6.1 List of excipients

Carbomer 940 (Carbopol 980) Ph. Eur

Disodium Edetate Ph. Eur.

Methyl Hydroxybenzoate Ph. Eur.

Propyl Hydroxybenzoate Ph. Eur.

Propylene Glycol Ph. Eur.

Sodium Hydroxide Ph. Eur.

Purified Water Ph. Eur.

6.2 Incompatibilities

None known

6.3 Shelf life

Rozex Gel has a shelf life when unopened of 36 months

6.4 Special precautions for storage

Store at a temperature not exceeding 25°C, away from direct heat. Do not freeze.

6.5 Nature and contents of container

Aluminium tubes with epoxy phenolic lining, and white polypropylene or polyethylene screw caps;

pack sizes: 30g & 40g.

6.6 Instructions for use and handling

Not applicable

7. MARKETING AUTHORISATION HOLDER

Galderma (UK.) Limited

Galderma House

Church Lane

Kings Langley

Hertfordshire, WD4 8JP

England

8. MARKETING AUTHORISATION NUMBER(S)

PL 10590/0016

9. DATE OF FIRST AUTHORISATION/RENEWAL OF THE AUTHORISATION

4th January 1995

10. DATE OF REVISION OF THE TEXT

May 2004

Rynacrom 4% Nasal Spray

(sanofi-aventis)

1. NAME OF THE MEDICINAL PRODUCT

Rynacrom 4% Nasal Spray

2. QUALITATIVE AND QUANTITATIVE COMPOSITION

Sodium Cromoglicate BP 4% w/v

3. PHARMACEUTICAL FORM

Rynacrom 4% Nasal Spray is presented as an aqueous solution, containing 4% w/v sodium cromoglicate in a metered dose spray pack, for nasal administration.

4. CLINICAL PARTICULARS

4.1 Therapeutic indications

Rynacrom 4% Nasal Spray is indicated for the preventative treatment of allergic rhinitis (seasonal and perennial).

4.2 Posology and method of administration

For nasal administration

Adults (including the Elderly) and Children:

One spray into each nostril two to four times daily.

Each actuation of the pump unit delivers approximately 5.2mg of sodium cromoglicate.

Since therapy is essentially preventative, regular doses, distinct from using the drug intermittently to relieve symptoms, should be observed.

4.3 Contraindications

Rynacrom 4% Nasal Spray is contraindicated in patients with known sensitivity to sodium cromoglicate, or any of the ingredients.

4.4 Special warnings and special precautions for use

None known.

4.5 Interaction with other medicinal products and other forms of Interaction

There are no known interactions between sodium cromoglicate and other drugs. A reduction in concomitant antihistamine therapy will often be possible during treatment with Rynacrom 4% Nasal Spray.

4.6 Pregnancy and lactation

Cumulative experience with sodium cromoglicate suggests that it has no effect on foetal development. It should only be used in pregnancy if there is a clear need.

On the basis of animal studies and its physico-chemical properties, sodium cromoglicate is unlikely to pass into human breast milk. There is no evidence to suggest that the use of sodium cromoglicate by nursing mothers has any undesirable effects on the baby.

4.7 Effects on ability to drive and use machines

None known.

4.8 Undesirable effects

Occasional irritation of the nasal mucosa may occur during the first days of use. In rare cases wheezing or tightness of the chest have been reported by patients.

4.9 Overdose

No action other than medical supervision should be necessary.

5. PHARMACOLOGICAL PROPERTIES

5.1 Pharmacodynamic properties

Sodium cromoglicate inhibits the release of mediators of the allergic reaction from sensitised mast cells. In the nose, the inhibition of mediator release prevents the symptoms of rhinitis.

5.2 Pharmacokinetic properties

After instillation of Rynacrom 4% Nasal Spray into the nose, less than 7% of the total dose administered is absorbed via the nasal mucosa. This fraction is excreted unchanged in the bile and urine. The remainder of the dose is expelled from the nose, or swallowed and excreted via the alimentary tract.

5.3 Preclinical safety data

There are no pre-clinical safety data of relevance to the prescriber which are additional to those already included in other sections of the Summary of Product Characteristics.

6. PHARMACEUTICAL PARTICULARS

6.1 List of excipients

Disodium edetate

Benzalkonium chloride

Purified water

6.2 Incompatibilities

None known.

6.3 Shelf life

36 months.

6.4 Special precautions for storage

Store below 25°C. Protect from direct sunlight.

6.5 Nature and contents of container

Rynacrom 4% Nasal Spray is presented as a transparent, colourless to pale yellow liquid in a 22ml high density polyethylene bottle, fitted with a metered dose pump unit, protected by a polypropylene cover.

6.6 Instructions for use and handling

A patient information leaflet is included in each pack.

7. MARKETING AUTHORISATION HOLDER

Aventis Pharma Limited

50 Kings Hill Avenue

Kings Hill

West Malling

Kent, ME19 4AH

Inted Kingdom

8. MARKETING AUTHORISATION NUMBER(S)

PL 04425/0371

9. DATE OF FIRST AUTHORISATION/RENEWAL OF THE AUTHORISATION

1st May 2005

10. DATE OF REVISION OF THE TEXT

11. LEGAL CATEGORY

P

Rythmodan Capsules

(sanofi-aventis)

1. NAME OF THE MEDICINAL PRODUCT

Rythmodan 100mg Capsules.

Rythmodan 150mg Capsules

2. QUALITATIVE AND QUANTITATIVE COMPOSITION

Capsule containing Disopyramide BP 100mg.

Capsule containing Disopyramide BP 150mg

3. PHARMACEUTICAL FORM

Capsule.

4. CLINICAL PARTICULARS

4.1 Therapeutic indications

Rythmodan is used in the treatment of cardiac arrhythmias as follows:-

1. The prevention and treatment of arrhythmias occurring after myocardial infarction.

2. Maintenance of normal rhythm following electroconversion eg atrial fibrillation, atrial flutter.

3. Persistent ventricular extrasystoles.

4. Control of arrhythmias following the use of digitalis or similar glycosides.

5. Suppression of arrhythmias during surgical procedures eg cardiac catheterisation.

6. The prevention of paraxysmal supraventricular tachycardia.

7. Other types of arrhythmias e.g. atrial extrasystoles, Wolff-Parkinson-White Syndrome.

4.2 Posology and method of administration

Route of administration

Oral

300 mg to 800mg daily in divided doses.

Children:

Not recommended as insufficient data available.

Elderly

A dose reduction due to reduced renal and hepatic function in the elderly (especially elderly non-smokers) should be considered (see section 4.4)

4.3 Contraindications

Disopyramide is contra-indicated in un-paced second or third degree atrioventricular block; bundle-branch block associated with first-degree atrioventricular block; unpaced bifasicular block; pre-existing long QT syndromes; severe sinus node dysfunction; severe heart failure, unless of secondary to cardiac arrhythmia; hypersensitivity to disopyramide. It is also contra-indicated in concomitant administration with other anti-arrhythmics or other drugs liable to provoke ventricular arrythmias, especially Torsade de Pointes (see section 4.5). The sustained release formulation is contra-indicated in patients with renal or hepatic impairment.

4.4 Special warnings and special precautions for use

In view of the serious nature of many of the conditions being treated it is suggested that Rythmodan Injection should only be used when facilities exist for cardiac monitoring or defibrillation, should the need arise.

Antiarrhythmic drugs belonging to the class 1c (Vaughan Williams Classification) were included in the Cardiac Arrhythmia Suppression Trial (CAST), a long term multi-centre randomised, double blind study in patients with asymptomatic non life-threatening ventricular arrhythmia who have had a myocardial infarction more than six days but less than two years previously. A significant increase in mortality and non-fatal cardiac arrest rate was seen in patients treated with class 1c antiarrhythmic drugs when compared with a matched placebo group. The applicability of the CAST results to other antiarrhythmics and other populations (eg. those without recent infarction) is uncertain. At present, it is best to assume that the risk extends to other antiarrhythmic agents for patients with structural heart disease.

There is no evidence that prolonged suppression of ventricular premature contractions with antiarrhythmic drugs prevents sudden death.

All antiarrhythmic drugs can produce unwanted effects when they are used to treat symptomatic but not life threatening arrhythmia; the expected benefits should be balanced against their risks.

In patients with structural heart disease, proarrhythmia and cardiac decompensation are special risks associated with antiarrhythmic drugs. Special caution should be exercised when prescribing in this context.

Disopyramide should not be used in patients with uncompensated congestive heart failure, unless this heart failure is secondary to cardiac arrhythmia. If disopyramide is to be given under these circumstances, special care and monitoring are essential.

Haemodynamically significant arrhythmias are difficult to treat and affected patients have a high mortality risk. Treatment of these arrhythmias, by whatever modality, must be initiated in hospital.

Owing to its negative inotropic effect, disopyramide should be used with caution in patients suffering from significant cardiac failure. This group may be specially sensitive to the negative inotropic properties of disopyramide. Such patients should be fully digitalised or controlled with other therapy before treatment with disopyramide is commenced.

Aggravation of existing arrhythmia, or emergence of a new type of arrhythmia, demands urgent review of disopyramide treatment.

Similarly, if an atrioventricular block or a bifasicular block occurs during treatment, the use of disopyramide should be reviewed.

There have been reports of ventricular tachycardia, ventricular fibrillation and Torsade de Pointes in patients receiving disopyramide. These have usually, but not always, been associated with significant widening of the QRS complex or prolonged QT interval. The QT interval and QRS duration must be monitored and disopyramide should be stopped if these are increased by more than 25%. If these changes or arrhythmias develop the drug should be discontinued. Disopyramide should be used only with caution in patients with atrial flutter or atrial tachycardia with block as conversion of a partial AV block to a 1:1 response may occur, leading to a potentially more serious tachyarrhythmia.

The occurrence of hypotension following disopyramide administration requires prompt discontinuation of the drug. This has been observed especially in patients with cardiomyopathy or uncompensated congestive heart failure. Any resumption of therapy should be at a lower dose with close patient monitoring. Disopyramide should be used with caution in the treatment of digitalis intoxication.

Potassium imbalance: Antiarrhythmic drugs may be hazardous in patients with potassium imbalance, as potassium abnormalities can induce arrhythmias.

During treatment with disopyramide, potassium levels should be checked regularly. Patients treated with diuretics or stimulant laxatives are at particular risk of hypokalaemia.

Renal insufficiency: In renal insufficiency, the dosage of disopyramide should be reduced by adjusting the interval between administrations.

Hepatic insufficiency: Hepatic impairment causes an increase in the plasma half-life of Rythmodan and a reduced dosage may be required.

Hypoglycaemia: Hypoglycaemia has been reported in association with disopyramide administration. Patients at particular risk are the elderly, the malnourished, or diabetics. The risk of hypoglycaemia occurring is increased with impaired renal function or cardiac failure. Blood glucose should be monitored in all patients. Strict adherence to the dosing recommendations is advised. If hypoglycaemia occurs then treatment with disopyramide should be stopped.

Atropine–like effects: There is a risk of:

– ocular hypertension in patients with narrow–angle glaucoma,

– acute urinary retention in patients with prostatic enlargement,

– aggravation of myasthenia gravis.

4.5 Interaction with other medicinal products and other forms of Interaction

Combination with other antiarrhythmic drugs: Combinations of antiarrhythmic drugs are not well researched and their effect may be unpredictable. Thus, antiarrhythmic combination should be avoided except under certain circumstances, eg. beta–blockers for angina pectoris; digoxin with beta–blocker and verapamil for the control of atrial fibrillation, when defined as effective for an individual.

Interaction with drugs associated with risk of Torsade de Pointes, such as

– tricyclic and tetracyclic antidepressants

– All macrolide antibiotics (e.g. erythromycin, clarithromycin, azithromycin etc)

– astemizole; cisapride; pentamidine; pimozide; sparfloxacin; terfenadine and thioridazone.

The concomitant use of these medications whilst undergoing treatment with disopyramide increases the chance of cardiac arrhythmia.

There is some evidence that disopyramide is metabolised by hepatic CYP3A. Concomitant administration of significant inhibitors of this isozyme (e.g. certain macrolide or azole antifungal antibiotics) may therefore increase the serum levels of disopyramide. On the other hand, inducers of CYP3A (e.g. rifampicin and certain anticonvulsants such as phenytoin, primidone and phenobarbital) may reduce disopyramide and increase MN–disopyramide serum levels. Since the magnitude of such potential effects is not foreseeable, such drug combinations are not recommended.

When prescribing a drug metabolised by CYP3A [such as theophylline, HIV protease inhibitors (e.g. ritonavir, indinavir, saquinavir), cyclosporin A, warfarin] it should be kept in mind that disopyramide is probably also a substrate of this isozyme and thus competitive inhibition of metabolism might occur, possibly increasing serum levels of these drugs.

Interactions with hypokalaemia inducing drugs: Concomitant use with drugs can induce hypokalaemia such as: diuretics, amphotericin B, tetracosactrin (corticotrophin analogue), gluco and mineralo–corticoids may reduce the action of the drug, or potentiate proarrhythmic effects. Stimulant laxatives are not recommended to be given concomitantly, due to their potassium lowering potential.

Other drug interactions:

Atropine and other anticholinergic drugs, including phenothiazines, may potentiate the atropine–like effects of disopyramide.

4.6 Pregnancy and lactation

Pregnancy: Although Rythmodan has undergone animal tests for teratogenicity without evidence of any effect on the developing foetus, its safety in human pregnancy has not been established. Rythmodan has been reported to stimulate contractions of the pregnant uterus. The drug should only be used during pregnancy if benefits clearly outweigh the possible risks to the mother and foetus.

Lactation: Studies have shown that oral Rythmodan is secreted in breast milk, although no adverse effects to the infant have been noted. However, clinical experience is limited and Rythmodan should only be used in lactation if, in the clinician's judgement, it is essential for the welfare of the patient. The infant should be closely supervised, particularly for anticholinergic effects and drug levels determined if necessary. Ideally, if the drug is considered essential, an alternative method of feeding should be used.

4.7 Effects on ability to drive and use machines

Some adverse reactions may impair the patients ability to concentrate and react, and hence the ability to drive or operate machinery. (See section 4.8).

4.8 Undesirable effects

Cardiac: It is accepted that the arrhythmogenic potential of disopyramide is weak. However, as with all antiarrhythmic drugs, disopyramide may worsen or provoke arrhythmias. This proarrhythmic effect is more likely to occur in the presence of hypokalemia with the associated use of antiarrhythmic drugs, in patients with severe structural heart disease with prolongation of the QT interval.

Intra–cardiac conduction abnormalities may occur: QT interval prolongation, widening of the QRS complex, atrioventricular block and bundle–branch block.

Other types of arrhythmia have been reported: Bradycardia, sinus block, ventricular fibrillation, ventricular tachycardia and torsades de pointes.

Episodes of severe heart failure or even cardiogenic shock have also been described particularly in patients with severe structural heart disease. The resulting low cardiac output can cause hypotension, renal insufficiency and/or acute hepatic ischemia.

Other adverse reactions include:

Atropine like: Urinary (dysuria; acute urinary retention); ocular (disorders of accommodation; diplopia); gastrointestinal - (dry mouth; abdominal pain; nausea, voimting, anorexia, diarrhoea; constipation); impotence; psychiatric disorders.

Skin reactions: very rarely, rashes; isolated reports of anaphylactic–type reactions possibly culminating in shock (only reported in association with the injectable formulation).

Rarely:– Hypoglycaemia

Very rarely: cholestatic jaundice, headache, dizzy sensation, neutropenia.

Rapid infusion may cause profuse sweating.

4.9 Overdose

There is no specific antidote for disopyramide. Prostigmine derivatives can be used to treat anticholinergic effects. Symptomatic supportive measures may include: early gastric lavage; administration of a cathartic followed by activated charcoal by mouth or stomach tube; IV administration of isoprenaline, other vasopressors and/or positive inotropic agents; if needed - infusion of lactate and/or magnesium, electro–systolic assistance, cardioversion, insertion of an intra–aortic balloon for counterpulsion and mechanically assisted ventilation. Haemodialysis, haemofiltration or haemoperfusion with activated charcoal has been employed to lower the serum concentrations of the drug.

5. PHARMACOLOGICAL PROPERTIES

5.1 Pharmacodynamic properties

Class 1 anti-arrhythmic agent.

It decreases membrane responsiveness, prolongs the effective refractory period (ERP) and slows automaticity in cells with augmented automaticity. Effective refractory period of the atrium is lengthened, ERP of the A-V node is shortened and conduction in accessory pathways is prolonged.

Disopyramide is a myocardial depressant and has anticholinergic effects.

5.2 Pharmacokinetic properties

Elimination phase of plasma t1/2: 5-8 hours. Increased in hepatic impairment, cardiac and hepatic disease.

Protein binding : 50 - 60%. Saturable and concentration dependent.

Volume of distribution : Variable according to method of determination.

Metabolism : Approximately 25% of a dose metabolised to a mono-N-dealkylated derivative. Additional 10% as other matebolites.

Excretion : 75% unchanged drug via urine, remainder in faeces mono-N-dealkylated metabolite 25% in urine, 64% via faeces.

5.3 Preclinical safety data

Not applicable.

6. PHARMACEUTICAL PARTICULARS

6.1 List of excipients

The capsules contain maize starch, magnesium stearate, STA-RX 1500 and talc.

The 100mg capsule shell consists of an opaque green body (indigo carmine, iron oxide and titanium dioxide) and an opaque beige body (iron oxide and titanium dioxide).

The 150mg capsule shell consists of a white body and cap containing gelatin and titanium dioxide.

6.2 Incompatibilities

Not known.

6.3 Shelf life

PVC Blister: 5 years

6.4 Special precautions for storage

None.

6.5 Nature and contents of container

PVC Blister containing 84 capsules.

6.6 Instructions for use and handling

None.

7. MARKETING AUTHORISATION HOLDER

Hoechst Marion Roussel Ltd.

Broadwater Park

Denham

Uxbridge

Middlesex UB9 5HP

UK

8. MARKETING AUTHORISATION NUMBER(S)

Rythmodan 100mg capsules: PL 13402/0113

Rythmodan 150mg capsules: PL 13402/0114

9. DATE OF FIRST AUTHORISATION/RENEWAL OF THE AUTHORISATION

June 1998/March 2003

10. DATE OF REVISION OF THE TEXT

February 2004

Legal Category: POM

Rythmodan Injection

(sanofi-aventis)

1. NAME OF THE MEDICINAL PRODUCT

Rythmodan Injection.

2. QUALITATIVE AND QUANTITATIVE COMPOSITION

Each glass ampoule contains 12.88mg disopyramide phosphate (equivalent to 10mg of disopyramide) per 1ml of solution.

3. PHARMACEUTICAL FORM

Intravenous.

4. CLINICAL PARTICULARS

4.1 Therapeutic indications

Conversion of ventricular and supraventricular arrythmias after myocardial infarction, including patients not responding to lignocaine or other intravenous treatment.

Control of ventricular and atrial extrasystoles, supraventricular tachycardia, and Wolff–Parkinson–White syndrome.

Control of arrhythmias following digitalis or similar glycosides when Rythmodan cannot be given orally.

4.2 Posology and method of administration

Route of Administration: Rythmodan Injection is intended for intravenous use only.

Adults

The recommended dosage can be given by two different regimes:

1. An initial direct intravenous injection of 2mg/kg (but not exceeding 150mg (15ml) irrespective of body weight) should be given slowly over not less than five minutes, ie, the rate of injection must not exceed 30mg (3ml) per minute in order to reduce or avoid unwanted haemodynamic effects. If conversion occurs during this time the injection should be stopped. If the arrhythmia is to respond to Rythmodan it will usually do so within 10–15 minutes after completion of the injection.

If conversion is achieved by intravenous Rythmodan but the arrhythmia subsequently recurs, a further slow direct intravenous injection over not less than five minutes may be administered cautiously and preferably under ECG control. The total administration by the intravenous route should not exceed 4mg/kg (maximum 300mg) in the first hour, nor should the combined administration by the intravenous and oral routes exceed 800mg in 24 hours.

2. An initial direct intravenous injection as above, ie over not less than five minutes, maintained by intravenous infusion by drip of 20–30mg/hour (or 0.4mg/kg/hour) up to a maximum of 800mg daily. This regime should be employed if the patient is unable to take oral medication or in particularly serious arrhythmias being treated in coronary care units.

Children

Not applicable.

Rythmodan Injection is not intended for use in children.

Elderly

A dose reduction due to reduced renal and hepatic function in the elderly (especially elderly non-smokers) should be considered (see section 4.4).

4.3 Contraindications

Disopyramide is contra–indicated in un–paced second or third degree atrioventricular block; bundle–branch block associated with first degree atrioventricular block; unpaced bifasicular block; pre-existing long QT syndromes; severe sinus node dysfunction; severe heart failure, unless secondary to cardiac arrhythmia; and hypersensitivity to disopyramide. It is also contra–indicated in concomitant administration with other anti–arrhythmics or other drugs liable to provoke ventricular arrythmias, especially Torsade de Pointes (see section 4.5). The sustained release formulation is contra–indicated in patients with renal or hepatic impairment.

4.4 Special warnings and special precautions for use

In view of the serious nature of many of the conditions being treated it is suggested that Rythmodan Injection should only be used when facilities exist for cardiac monitoring or defibrillation, should the need arise.

Antiarrhythmic drugs belonging to the class 1c (Vaughan Williams Classification) were included in the Cardiac Arrhythmia Suppression Trial (CAST), a long term multicentre randomised, double blind study in patients with asymptomatic non life–threatening ventricular arrhythmia who had a myocardial infarction more than six days but less than two years previously. A significant increase in mortality and non–fatal cardiac arrest rate was seen in patients treated with class 1c antiarrhythmic drugs when compared with a matched placebo group. The applicability of the CAST results to other antiarrhythmics and other populations (eg. those without recent infarction) is uncertain. At present, it is best to assume that the risk extends to other antiarrhythmic agents for patients with structural heart disease.

There is no evidence that prolonged suppression of ventricular premature contractions with antiarrhythmic drugs prevents sudden death.

All antiarrhythmic drugs can produce unwanted effects when they are used to treat symptomatic but not life threatening arrhythmia; the expected benefits should be balanced against their risks.

In patients with structural heart disease, proarrhythmia and cardiac decompensation are special risks associated with antiarrhythmic drugs. Special caution should be exercised when prescribing in this taken context.

Disopyramide should not be used in patients with uncompensated congestive heart failure, unless this heart failure is secondary to cardiac arrhythmia. If disopyramide is to be given under these circumstances, special care and monitoring are essential.

Haemodynamically significant arrhythmias are difficult to treat and affected patients have a high mortality risk. Treatment of these arrhythmias, by whatever modality, must be initiated in hospital.

Owing to its negative inotropic effect, disopyramide should be used with caution in patients suffering from significant cardiac failure. This group may be specially sensitive to the negative inotropic properties of disopyramide. Such patients should be fully digitalised or controlled with other therapy before treatment with disopyramide is commenced.

Aggravation of existing arrhythmia, or emergence of a new type of arrhythmia, demands urgent review of disopyramide treatment.

Similarly, if an atrioventricular block or a bifasicular block occurs during treatment, the use of disopyramide should be reviewed.

There have been reports of ventricular tachycardia, ventricular fibrillation and Torsade de Pointes in patients receiving disopyramide. These have usually, but not always, been associated with significant widening of the QRS complex or prolonged QT interval. The QT interval and QRS duration must be monitored and disopyramide should be stopped if these are increased by more than 25%. If these changes or arrhythmias develop the drug should be discontinued. Disopyramide should be used with caution in patients with atrial flutter or atrial tachycardia with block as conversion of a partial AV block to a 1:1 response may occur, leading to a potentially more serious tachyarrhythmia.

The occurrence of hypotension following disopyramide administration, requires prompt discontinuation of the drug. This has been observed especially in patients with cardiomyopathy or uncompensated congestive heart failure. Any resumption of therapy should be at a lower dose with close patient monitoring. Disopyramide should be used with caution in the treatment of digitalis intoxication.

<u>Potassium imbalance:</u> Antiarrhythmic drugs may be hazardous in patients with potassium imbalance, as potassium abnormalities can induce arrhythmias.

During treatment with disopyramide, potassium levels should be checked regularly. Patients treated with diuretics or stimulant laxatives are at particular risk of hypokalaemia.

<u>Renal insufficiency:</u> In renal insufficiency, the dosage of disopyramide should be reduced by adjusting the interval between administrations.

<u>Hepatic insufficiency:</u> Hepatic impairment causes an increase in the plasma half–life of Rythmodan and a reduced dosage may be required.

<u>Hypoglycaemia:</u> Hypoglycaemia has been reported in association with disopyramide administration. Patients at particular risk are the elderly, the malnourished, or diabetics. The risk of hypoglycaemia occurring is increased with impaired renal function or cardiac failure. Blood glucose should be monitored in all patients. Strict adherence to the dosing recommendations is advised. If hypoglycaemia occurs then treatment with disopyramide should be stopped.

<u>Atropine–like effect:</u> There is a risk of:

- ocular hypertension in patients with narrow–angle glaucoma,

- acute urinary retention in patients with prostatic enlargement,

- aggravation of myasthenia gravis.

4.5 Interaction with other medicinal products and other forms of Interaction

<u>Combination with other antiarrhythmic drugs:</u> Combinations of antiarrhythmic drugs are not well researched and their effect may be unpredictable. Thus, antiarrhythmic combination should be avoided except under certain circumstances, eg. beta–blockers for angina pectoris; digoxin with beta–blocker and/or verapamil for the control of atrial fibrillation, when defined as effective for an individual.

<u>Interaction with drugs associated with risk of Torsade de Pointes, such as:</u>

– tricyclic and tetracyclic antidepressants

– All macrolide antibiotics (e.g. erythromycin, clarithromycin, azithromycin etc)

– astemizole; cisapride; pentamidine; pimozide; sparfloxacin; terfenadine and thioridazone.

The concomitant use of these medications whilst undergoing treatment with disopyramide increases the chance of cardiac arrhythmia.

There is some evidence that disopyramide is metabolised by hepatic CYP3A. Concomitant administration of significant inhibitors of this isozyme (e.g. certain macrolide or azole antifungal antibiotics) may therefore increase the serum levels of disopyramide. On the other hand, inducers of CYP3A (e.g. rifampicin and certain anticonvulsants such as phenytoin, primidone and phenobarbital) may reduce disopyramide and increase MN–disopyramide serum levels. Since the magnitude of such potential effects is not foreseeable, such drug combinations are not recommended.

When prescribing a drug metabolised by CYP3A [such as theophylline, HIV protease inhibitors (e.g. ritonavir, indinavir, saquinavir), cyclosporin A, warfarin] it should be kept in mind that disopyramide is probably also a substrate of this isozyme and thus competitive inhibition of metabolism might occur, possibly increasing serum levels of these drugs.

<u>Interactions with hypokalaemia inducing drugs:</u> Concomitant use with drugs that can induce hypokalaemia such as: diuretics, amphotericin B, tetracosactrin (corticotrophin analogue), gluco and mineralo–corticoids may reduce the action of the drug, or potentiate proarrhythmic effects. Stimulant laxatives are not recommended to be given concomitantly, due to their potassium lowering potential.

<u>Other drug interactions:</u>

Atropine and other anticholinergic drugs, including phenothiazines, may potentiate the atropine–like effects of disopyramide.

4.6 Pregnancy and lactation

Pregnancy: Although Rythmodan has undergone animal tests for teratogenicity without evidence of any effect on the developing foetus, its safety in human pregnancy has not been established. Rythmodan has been reported to stimulate contractions of the pregnant uterus. The drug should only be used during pregnancy if benefits clearly outweigh the possible risks to the mother and foetus.

Lactation: No data for Rythmodan Injection, but studies have shown that oral disopyramide is secreted in breast milk, although no adverse effects to the infant have been noted. However, clinical experience is limited and disopyramide should only be used in lactation if, in the clinician's judgement, it is essential for the welfare of the patient. The infant should be closely supervised, particularly for anticholinergic effects and drug levels determined if necessary. Ideally, if the drug is considered essential, an alternative method of feeding should be used.

4.7 Effects on ability to drive and use machines

Some adverse reactions may impair the patients' ability to concentrate and react, and hence the ability to drive or operate machinery. (See section 4.8).

4.8 Undesirable effects

<u>Cardiac:</u> It is accepted that the arrhythmogenic potential of disopyramide is weak. However, as with all antiarrhythmic drugs, disopyramide may worsen or provoke arrhythmias. This proarrhythmic effect is more likely to occur in the presence of hypokalaemia with the associated use of antiarrhythmic drugs, in patients with severe structural heart disease or prolongation of the QT interval.

Intra–cardiac conduction abnormalities may occur: QT interval prolongation, widening of the QRS complex, atrioventricular block and bundle–branch block.

Other types of arrhythmia have been reported: Bradycardia, sinus block, ventricular fibrillation, ventricular tachycardia and torsades de pointes.

Episodes of severe heart failure or even cardiogenic shock have also been described particularly in patients with severe structural heart disease. The resulting low cardiac output can cause hypotension, renal insufficiency and/or acute hepatic ischemia.

Other adverse reactions include:

Atropine like: Urinary (dysuria; acute urinary retention); ocular (disorders of accommodation; diplopia); gastrointestinal - (dry mouth; abdominal pain; nausea, vomiting, anorexia, diarrhoea; constipation); impotence; psychiatric disorders.

Skin reactions: very rarely, rashes; isolated reports of anaphylactic–type reactions possibly culminating in shock (only reported in association with the injectable formulation).

Rarely: Hypoglycaemia

Very rarely: cholestatic jaundice, headache, dizzy sensation, neutropenia.

Rapid infusion may cause profuse sweating.

4.9 Overdose

There is no specific antidote for disopyramide. Prostigmine derivatives can be used to treat anticholinergic effects. Symptomatic supportive measures may include: early gastric lavage; administration of a cathartic followed by activated charcoal by mouth or stomach tube; IV administration of isoprenaline, other vasopressors and/or positive inotropic agents; if needed - infusion of lactate and/or magnesium, electro–systolic assistance, cardioversion, insertion of an intra–aortic balloon for counterpulsion and mechanically assisted ventilation. Haemodialysis, haemofiltration or haemoperfusion with activated charcoal has been employed to lower the serum concentration of the drug.

5. PHARMACOLOGICAL PROPERTIES

5.1 Pharmacodynamic properties

Class 1 antiarrhythmic agent.

5.2 Pharmacokinetic properties

Following intravenous administration, disopyramide is rapidly distributed. Doses of 1.5–2mg/kg produce plasma levels of about 10microg/ml, declining rapidly to 3.8–4.2microg/ml at 5 minutes and to less than 3microg/ml at 15 minutes.

In multidose studies, direct slow intravenous injection of 2mg/kg followed by an infusion of 20mg/hr, maintained plasma levels of disopyramide between 2.5 and 2.8microg/ml from the first hour onwards.

<u>*Distribution T1/2*</u>: 2–4 minutes in healthy volunteers. Longer (15 minutes) in patients with acute myocardial infarct.

<u>*Elimination Phase Of Plasma T1/2*</u>: 5–8 hours. Increased in renal impairment, cardiac and hepatic disease.

<u>*Protein Binding*</u>: 50–60%. Saturable and concentration dependent.

<u>*Volume Of Distribution*</u>: Variable according to method of determination

<u>*Metabolism*</u>: Approximately 25% of a dose metabolised to a mono–n–dealkylated derivative. Additional 10% as other metabolites.

<u>*Excretion*</u>: 75% unchanged drug via urine, remainder in faeces. Mono–n–dealkylated metabolite 25% in urine, 64% via faeces.

5.3 Preclinical safety data

Not applicable.

6. PHARMACEUTICAL PARTICULARS

6.1 List of excipients

Benzyl Alcohol, Sorbitol and Water for Injection.

6.2 Incompatibilities

Not applicable.

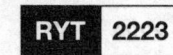

6.3 Shelf life
60 months.

6.4 Special precautions for storage
Store below 25°C

6.5 Nature and contents of container
Colourless neutral glass ampoules are available as 5ml.

6.6 Instructions for use and handling
Not Applicable.

7. MARKETING AUTHORISATION HOLDER
Hoechst Marion Roussel Ltd

Broadwater Park

Denham

Uxbridge

Middlesex UB9 5HP

UK

8. MARKETING AUTHORISATION NUMBER(S)
PL 13402/0112

9. DATE OF FIRST AUTHORISATION/RENEWAL OF THE AUTHORISATION
15th June 1998

10. DATE OF REVISION OF THE TEXT
August 2003

Rythmodan Retard

(sanofi-aventis)

1. NAME OF THE MEDICINAL PRODUCT
Rythmodan Retard.

2. QUALITATIVE AND QUANTITATIVE COMPOSITION
Tablets containing Disopyramide Phosphate 322.5mg (equivalent to 250mg base).

3. PHARMACEUTICAL FORM
Modified release tablet.

4. CLINICAL PARTICULARS

4.1 Therapeutic indications
Properties:

Prevention and control of a wide variety of cardiac arrhythmias, probably by slowing conduction in the his-Purkinje system and by increasing the effective refractory period of the atria and ventricles.

Indications:

1. Maintenance of normal rhythm following conversion by Rythmodan injection, other parenteral drugs or electroconversion.

2. Prevention of arrhythmias after myocardial infarction.

3. Treatment of persistent ventricular and atrial extrasystoles, paroxysmal supra ventricular tachycardia, Wolff-Parkinson-White syndrome.

4. Suppression of arrhythmias during surgical procedures.

5. Control of arrhythmias following the use of digitalis or similar glycosides.

4.2 Posology and method of administration
Route of administration

Oral:

Recommended dose for stabilised patients or those receiving Rythmodan for the first time is one to one and a half tablets (250-375mg) twice daily. Patients being transferred from intravenous therapy with Rythmodan should be stabilised on standard Rythmodan capsules for the first 24 hours. Tablets should be swallowed and not crushed or chewed.

Children:

There are insufficient data to recommend the use of Rythmodan in children.

Elderly:

A dose reduction due to reduced renal and hepatic function in the elderly (especially elderly non-smokers) should be considered (see section 4.4).

4.3 Contraindications
Disopyramide is contra–indicated in un–paced second or third degree atrioventricular block; bundle–branch block associated with first–degree atrioventricular block; un-paced bifasicular block; pre-existing long QT syndromes; severe sinus node dysfunction; severe heart failure, unless secondary to cardiac arrhythmia; hypersensitivity to disopyramide. It is also contra–indicated in concomitant administration with other anti–arrhythmics or other drugs liable to provoke ventricular arrhythmias, especially Torsade de Pointes (see section 4.5). The sustained release formulation is contra–indicated in patients with renal or hepatic impairment.

4.4 Special warnings and special precautions for use
In view of the serious nature of many of the conditions being treated it is suggested that Rythmodan Injection should only be used when facilities exist for cardiac monitoring or defibrillation, should the need arise.

Antiarrhythmic drugs belonging to the class 1c (Vaughan Williams Classification) were included in the Cardiac Arrhythmia Suppression Trial (CAST), a long term multi-centre randomised, double blind study in patients with asymptomatic non life–threatening ventricular arrhythmia who have had a myocardial infarction more than six days but less than two years previously. A significant increase in mortality and non–fatal cardiac arrest rate was seen in patients treated with class 1c antiarrhythmic drugs when compared with a matched placebo group. The applicability of the CAST results to other antiarrhythmics and other populations (eg. those without recent infarction) is uncertain. At present, it is best to assume that the risk extends to other antiarrhythmic agents for patients with structural heart disease.

There is no evidence that prolonged suppression of ventricular premature contractions with antiarrhythmic drugs prevents sudden death.

All antiarrhythmic drugs can produce unwanted effects when they are used to treat symptomatic but not life threatening arrhythmia; the expected benefits should be balanced against their risks.

In patients with structural heart disease, proarrhythmia and cardiac decompensation are special risks associated with antiarrhythmic drugs. Special caution should be exercised when prescribing in this context.

Disopyramide should not be used in patients with uncompensated congestive heart failure, unless this heart failure is secondary to cardiac arrhythmia. If disopyramide is to be given under these circumstances, special care and monitoring are essential.

Haemodynamically significant arrhythmias are difficult to treat and affected patients have a high mortality risk. Treatment of these arrhythmias, whatever modality, must be initiated in hospital.

Owing to its negative inotropic effect, disopyramide should be used with caution in patients suffering from significant cardiac failure. This group may be especially sensitive to the negative inotropic properties of disopyramide. Such patients should be fully digitalised or controlled with other therapy before treatment with disopyramide is commenced.

Aggravation of existing arrhythmia, or emergence of a new type of arrhythmia, demands an urgent review of disopyramide treatment.

Similarly, if an atrioventricular block or a bifasicular block occurs during treatment, the use of disopyramide should be reviewed.

There have been reports of ventricular tachycardia, ventricular fibrillation and Torsade de Pointes in patients receiving disopyramide. These have usually, but not always, been associated with significant widening of the QRS complex or prolonged QT interval. The QT interval and QRS duration must be monitored and disopyramide should be stopped if these are increased by more than 25%. If these changes or arrhythmias develop the drug should be discontinued. Disopyramide should be used only with caution in patients with atrial flutter or atrial tachycardia with block as conversion of a partial AV block to a 1:1 response may occur, leading to a potentially more serious tachyarrhythmia.

The occurrence of hypotension following disopyramide administration requires prompt discontinuation of the drug. This has been observed especially in patients with cardiomyopathy or uncompensated congestive heart failure. Any resumption of therapy should be at a lower dose with close patient monitoring. Disopyramide should be used with caution in the treatment of digitalis intoxication.

Potassium imbalance: Antiarrhythmic drugs may be hazardous in patients with potassium imbalance, as potassium abnormalities can induce arrhythmias.

During treatment with disopyramide, potassium levels should be checked regularly. Patients treated with diuretics or stimulant laxatives are at particular risk of hypokalaemia.

Renal insufficiency: In renal insufficiency the dosage of disopyramide should be reduced by adjusting the interval between administrations.

Hepatic insufficiency: Hepatic impairment causes an increase in the plasma half–life of Rythmodan and a reduced dosage may be required.

Hypoglycaemia:Hypoglycaemia has been reported in association with disopyramide administration. Patients at particular risk are the elderly, the malnourished, or diabetics. The risk of hypoglycaemia occurring is increased with impaired renal function or cardiac failure. Blood glucose should be monitored in all patients. Strict adherence to the dosing recommendations is advised. If hypoglycaemia occurs, then treatment with disopyramide should be stopped.

Atropine–like effects: There is a risk of:

– ocular hypertension in patients with narrow–angle glaucoma,

– acute urinary retention in patients with prostatic enlargement,

– aggravation of myasthenia gravis.

4.5 Interaction with other medicinal products and other forms of Interaction
Combination with other antiarrhythmic drugs: Combinations of antiarrhythmic drugs are not well researched and their effect may be unpredictable. Thus, antiarrhythmic combination should be avoided except under certain circumstances, eg. beta–blockers for angina pectoris; digoxin with beta–blocker and/or verapamil for the control of atrial fibrillation, when defined as effective for an individual.

Interaction with drugs associated with risk of Torsade de Pointes, such as

– tricyclic and tetracyclic antidepressants

– all macrolide antibiotics (e.g. erythromycin, clarithromycin, azithromycin etc)

– astemizole; cisapride; pentamidine; sparfloxacin; terfenadine; pimozide and thioridazine

The concomitant use of these medications whilst undergoing treatment with disopyramide increases the chance of cardiac arrhythmia.

There is some evidence that disopyramide is metabolised by hepatic CYP3A. Concomitant administration of significant inhibitors of this isozyme (e.g. macrolide or azole antifungal antibiotics) may therefore increase the serum levels of disopyramide. On the other hand, inducers of CYP3A (e.g. rifampicin and certain anticonvulsants such as phenytoin, primidone and phenobarbital) may reduce disopyramide and increase MN–disopyramide serum levels. Since the magnitude of such potential effects is not foreseeable, such drug combinations are not recommended.

When prescribing a drug metabolised by CYP3A [such as theophylline, HIV protease inhibitors (e.g. ritonavir, indinavir, saquinavir), cyclosporin A, warfarin] it should be kept in mind that disopyramide is probably also a substrate of this isozyme and thus competitive inhibition of metabolism might occur, possibly increasing serum levels of these drugs.

Interactions with hypokalaemia inducing drugs: Concomitant use with drugs that can induce hypokalaemia such as: diuretics, amphotericin B, tetracosactrin (corticotrophin analogue), gluco and mineralo–corticoids may reduce the action of the drug, or potentiate proarrhythmic effects. Stimulant laxatives are not recommended to be given concomitantly, due to their potassium lowering potential.

Other drug interactions:

Atropine and other anticholinergic drugs, including phenothiazines, may potentiate the atropine–like effects of disopyramide.

4.6 Pregnancy and lactation
Pregnancy: Although Rythmodan has undergone animal tests for teratogenicity without evidence of any effect on the developing foetus, its safety in human pregnancy has not been established. Rythmodan has been reported to stimulate contractions of the pregnant uterus. The drug should only be used during pregnancy if benefits clearly outweigh the possible risks to the mother and foetus.

Lactation: No data for Rythmodan Retard, but studies have shown that oral Rythmodan is secreted in breast milk, although no adverse effects to the infant have been noted. However, clinical experience is limited and Rythmodan should only be used in lactation if, in the clinician's judgement, it is essential for the welfare of the patient. The infant should be closely supervised, particularly for anticholinergic effects and drug levels determined if necessary. Ideally, if the drug is considered essential, an alternative method of feeding should be used.

4.7 Effects on ability to drive and use machines
Some adverse reactions may impair the patients' ability to concentrate and react, and hence the ability to drive or operate machinery. (See section 4.8).

4.8 Undesirable effects
Cardiac: It is accepted that the arrhythmogenic potential of disopyramide is weak. However, as with all antiarrhythmic drugs, disopyramide may worsen or provoke arrhythmias. This proarrhythmic effect is more likely to occur in the presence of hypokalaemia with the associated use of antiarrhythmic drugs, in patients with severe structural heart disease or prolongation of the QT interval.

Intra-cardiac conduction abnormalities may occur: QT interval prolongation, widening of the QRS complex, atrioventricular block and bundle–branch block.

Other types of arrhythmia have been reported: Bradycardia, sinus block, ventricular fibrillation, ventricular tachycardia and torsades de pointes.

Episodes of severe heart failure or even cardiogenic shock have also been described particularly in patients with severe structural heart disease. The resulting low cardiac output can cause hypotension, renal insufficiency and/or acute hepatic ischemia.

Other adverse reactions include:

Atropine like: Urinary (dysuria; acute urinary retention); ocular (disorders of accommodation; diplopia); gastrointestinal - (dry mouth; abdominal pain; nausea, vomiting, anorexia, diarrhoea; constipation); impotence; psychiatric disorders.

Skin reactions:– very rarely, rashes; isolated reports of anaphylactic–type reactions possibly culminating in shock (only reported in association with the injectable formulation).

Rarely:– Hypoglycaemia

Very rarely: cholestatic jaundice, headache, dizzy sensation, neutropenia.

4.9 Overdose

There is no specific antidote for disopyramide. Prostigmine derivatives can be used to treat anticholinergic effects. Symptomatic supportive measures may include: early gastric lavage; administration of a cathartic followed by activated charcoal by mouth or stomach tube; IV administration of isoprenaline, other vasopressors and/or positive inotropic agents; if needed - infusion of lactate and/or magnesium, electro–systolic assistance, cardioversion, insertion of an intra–aortic balloon for counterpulsion and mechanically assisted ventilation. Haemodialysis, haemofiltration or haemoperfusion with activated charcoal has been employed to lower the serum concentration of the drug.

5. PHARMACOLOGICAL PROPERTIES

5.1 Pharmacodynamic properties

Disopyramide is a Class 1 antiarrhythmic agent with a depressant action on the heart similar to that of quinidine and is used for the prevention and treatment of a wide variety of cardiac arrhythmias.

5.2 Pharmacokinetic properties

The dissolution characteristics of Rythmodan Retard are designed to release 250mg disopyramide over 12 hours. The dissolution profile is matched to the drug half-life of 6-8 hours with good therapeutic levels followed by steady release of disopyramide to sustain therapeutic effect. The sustained release mechanism is based on the matrix principle, adapted for disopyramide. Reliable release is achieved by strict control of particle size.

5.3 Preclinical safety data

Not applicable.

6. PHARMACEUTICAL PARTICULARS

6.1 List of excipients

The tablets contain glyceryl monostearate, castor sugar, povidone and magnesium stearate.

The film coating consists of hydroxypropyl methylcellulose, propylene glycol, sorbitan monolaurate and titanium dioxide E171.

6.2 Incompatibilities

Not known.

6.3 Shelf life

PVC Blister: 1 year

6.4 Special precautions for storage

PVC Blister: Do not store above 25°C

6.5 Nature and contents of container

PVC Blister containing 56 tablets

6.6 Instructions for use and handling

None.

7. MARKETING AUTHORISATION HOLDER

Hoechst Marion Roussel Ltd.
Broadwater Park
Denham
Uxbridge
Middlesex
UB9 5HP
UK

8. MARKETING AUTHORISATION NUMBER(S)

PL 13402/0115

9. DATE OF FIRST AUTHORISATION/RENEWAL OF THE AUTHORISATION

15th June 1998/April 2002

10. DATE OF REVISION OF THE TEXT

April 2002

Legal Category: POM

Sabril Sachets 0.5g and Tablets 500mg

(sanofi-aventis)

1. NAME OF THE MEDICINAL PRODUCT

Sabril™ Sachets 0.5g and Tablets 500mg.

For excipients, see 6.1

2. QUALITATIVE AND QUANTITATIVE COMPOSITION

Each sachet or tablet contains: Vigabatrin 500mg

3. PHARMACEUTICAL FORM

Powder or film coated tablets.

4. CLINICAL PARTICULARS

4.1 Therapeutic indications

Treatment in combination with other anti-epileptic drugs for patients with resistant partial epilepsy with or without secondary generalisation; that is, where all other appropriate drug combinations have proved inadequate or have not been tolerated.

Monotherapy in the treatment of infantile spasms (West's syndrome).

4.2 Posology and method of administration

Sabril treatment may only be initiated by a specialist in epileptology, neurology or paediatric neurology. Follow-up should be arranged under supervision of a specialist in epileptology, neurology or paediatric neurology.

Sabril is for oral administration once or twice daily and may be taken before or after meals. Sachet contents may be placed in beverage (e.g. water, fruit juice or milk) immediately before oral administration.

If the control of epilepsy is not clinically significantly improved after an adequate trial, vigabatrin treatment should not be continued. Vigabatrin should be gradually withdrawn under close medical supervision.

Adults

Maximal efficacy is usually seen in the 2-3g/day range. A starting dose of 1g daily should be added to the patient's current anti-epileptic drug regimen. The daily dose should then be titrated in 0.5g increments at weekly intervals depending on clinical response and tolerability. The highest recommended dose is 3g/day.

No direct correlation exists between the plasma concentration and the efficacy. The duration of the effect of the drug is dependent on the rate of GABA transaminase resynthesis rather than the concentration of the drug in the plasma (see also Sections 5.1 Pharmacodynamic properties and 5.2 Pharmacokinetic properties).

Children

The recommended starting dose in children is 40mg/kg/day. Maintenance recommendations in relation to bodyweight are:

Bodyweight:

10 to 15kg: 0.5-1g/day

15 to 30kg: 1-1.5g/day

30 to 50kg: 1.5-3g/day

>50kg: 2-3g/day

The maximum recommended dose in each of these categories should not be exceeded.

Infants - Monotherapy for infantile spasms (West's Syndrome). The recommended starting dose is 50mg/kg/day. This may be titrated over a period of one week if necessary. Doses of up to 150mg/kg/day have been used with good tolerability.

Elderly and Patients with Renal Impairment

Since vigabatrin is eliminated via the kidney, caution should be exercised when administering the drug to the elderly and more particularly in patients with creatinine clearance less than 60ml/min. Adjustment of dose or frequency of administration should be considered. Such patients may respond to a lower maintenance dose. Patients should be monitored for undesirable effects such as sedation or confusion (see Sections 4.4 Special warnings and special precautions for use, and 4.8 Undesirable effects).

4.3 Contraindications

Hypersensitivity to vigabatrin or to any excipient in the medicinal product.

4.4 Special warnings and special precautions for use

Except for the treatment of infantile spasms, Sabril should not be initiated as monotherapy.

Visual field defects have been reported in patients receiving vigabatrin with a high prevalence (about 1/3 of patients). The onset is usually after months to years of vigabatrin therapy. The degree of visual field restriction may be severe and this may have practical consequences for the patient. Most of the patients with perimetry-confirmed defects have been asymptomatic. Hence, this undesirable effect can only be reliably detected by systematic perimetry which is usually possible only in patients with a developmental age of more than 9 years. A specifically developed method based on field specific Visual Evoked Potentials (VEP) is available from the company on request to test the presence of peripheral vision in children aged 3 years and above. At present this method has not been validated in the detection of vigabatrin attributed visual field defects. Electroretinography may be useful but should be used only in adults who are unable to cooperate with perimetry or in the very young (see Visual Field Defects).

Available data suggests that visual field defects are irreversible even after discontinuation of vigabatrin.

Therefore, vigabatrin should only be used after a careful assessment of the balance of benefits and risk compared with alternatives.

Vigabatrin is not recommended for use in patients with any pre-existing clinically significant visual field defect.

Patients should undergo systematic screening examination when starting vigabatrin and at regular intervals for detection of visual field defects. Visual field testing should continue at 6 month intervals for the whole duration of treatment (see Visual Field Defects).

Visual Field Defects (VFD)

Based on available data, the usual pattern is a concentric constriction of the visual field of both eyes, which is generally more marked nasally than temporally. In the central visual field (within 30 degree of eccentricity), frequently an annular nasal defect is seen. Central visual acuity is not impaired. However, the VFDs reported in patients receiving vigabatrin have ranged from mild to severe. Severe cases are potentially disabling.

Most patients with perimetry-confirmed defects had not previously spontaneously noticed any symptoms, even in cases where a severe defect was observed in perimetry. Available evidence suggests that the VFD is irreversible even after discontinuation of vigabatrin.

Pooled data from prevalence surveys suggest that as many as 1/3 of patients receiving vigabatrin therapy have VFDs. Males may be at greater risk than females.

All patients should have ophthalmological consultation with visual field examination before the initiation of vigabatrin treatment.

Appropriate visual field testing (perimetry) by using a standardised static perimetry (Humphrey or Octopus) or kinetic perimetry (Goldmann) must be performed before treatment initiation and at six month intervals for the whole duration of treatment. Static perimetry is the preferred method for detecting vigabatrin associated visual field defect.

Electroretinography may be useful but should only be used in adults who are unable to cooperate with perimetry. Based on the available data the first oscillatory potential and 30 Hz flicker responses of the electroretinogram appear to be correlated with a vigabatrin associated VFD. These responses are delayed and reduced beyond the normal limits. Such changes have not been seen in vigabatrin treated patients without a VFD.

The patient and/or caregiver must be given a thorough description of the frequency and implications of the development of VFD during vigabatrin treatment. Patients should be instructed to report any new visual problems and symptoms which may be associated with visual field constriction. If visual symptoms develop, the patient should be referred to an ophthalmologist.

If a visual field constriction is observed during follow-up, consideration should be given to gradual discontinuation of vigabatrin. If the decision to continue treatment is made, consideration should be given to more frequent follow-up (perimetry) in order to detect progression or sight threatening defects.

Vigabatrin should not be used concomitantly with other retinotoxic drugs.

Children

Perimetry is seldom possible in children less than 9 years of developmental age. The risks of treatment must be very carefully weighed against possible benefit in children. Currently, there is no established method to diagnose or exclude visual field defects in children in whom a standardised perimetry cannot be performed. A specifically developed method based on field specific Visual Evoked Potentials (VEP) is available from the company on request to test the presence of peripheral vision in children aged 3 years and above. At present this method has not been validated in the detection of vigabatrin attributed visual field defects. If the method reveals normal central visual field response but an absent peripheral response, benefit-risk of vigabatrin must be reviewed and consideration given to gradual discontinuation. The presence of peripheral vision does not exclude the possibility of developing VFD. Electroretinography may be useful but should be used only in children less than 3 years of age.

Neurological and psychiatric conditions

In view of the results of the animal safety studies (see Section 5.3 Preclinical safety data), it is recommended that patients treated with vigabatrin are closely observed for adverse effects on neurological function.

Rare reports of encephalopathic symptoms such as marked sedation, stupor and confusion in association with non-specific slow wave activity on electroencephalogram have been described soon after the initiation of vigabatrin treatment. Risk factors for the development of these reactions include higher than recommended starting dose, faster dose escalation at higher steps than recommended, and renal failure. These events have been reversible following dose reduction or discontinuation of vigabatrin. (See Section 4.8 Undesirable effects).

As with other antiepileptic drugs some patients may experience an increase in seizure frequency or the onset of new types of seizures with vigabatrin (see Section 4.8 Undesirable effects). These phenomena may also be the consequence of an overdosage, a decrease in plasma concentrations of concomitant antiepileptic treatment, or a paradoxical effect.

As with other antiepileptic drugs, abrupt withdrawal may lead to rebound seizures. If a patient is to be withdrawn from vigabatrin treatment, it is recommended that this is done by gradual dose reduction over a 2- to 4-week period.

Vigabatrin should be used with caution in patients with a history of psychosis, depression or behavioural problems. Psychiatric events (e.g., agitation, depression, abnormal thinking, paranoid reactions) have been reported during vigabatrin treatment. These events occurred in patients with and without a psychiatric history, and were usually reversible when vigabatrin doses were reduced or gradually discontinued.

Elderly and patients with renal impairment

Since vigabatrin is eliminated via the kidney, caution should be exercised in patients with a creatinine clearance of less than 60ml/min and in elderly patients. These patients should be monitored closely for undesirable effects such as sedation and confusion. (See Section 4.2 Posology and method of administration).

4.5 Interaction with other medicinal products and other forms of Interaction

As vigabatrin is neither metabolised, nor protein bound and is not an inducer of hepatic cytochrome P450 drug metabolising-enzymes, interactions with other drugs are unlikely. However, during controlled clinical studies, a gradual reduction of 16-33% in the plasma concentration of phenytoin has been observed. The exact nature of this interaction is presently not understood, however, in the majority of cases it is unlikely to be of therapeutic significance.

The plasma concentrations of carbamazepine, phenobarbitone, and sodium valproate have also been monitored during controlled clinical trials and no clinically significant interactions have been detected.

Vigabatrin may lead to a decrease in measured plasma activity of alanine aminotransferase (ALT) and to a lesser extent, aspartate aminotransferase (AST). The magnitude of suppression for ALT has been reported to vary between 30% and 100%. Therefore, these liver tests may be quantitatively unreliable in patients taking vigabatrin. (See Section 4.8 Undesirable effects)

Vigabatrin may increase the amount of amino acids in the urine possibly leading to a false positive test for certain rare genetic metabolic disorders (eg, alpha aminoadipic aciduria).

4.6 Pregnancy and lactation

Data on a limited number (n=192) of exposed pregnancies are available. Congenital anomalies were reported in 14.5% of exposed pregnancies. Of these, 64.3% were major malformations. Spontaneous abortion was reported in 10.9% of exposed pregnancies. No definite conclusion can be drawn as to whether vigabatrin produces an increased risk of malformation when taken during pregnancy because of limited data, epilepsy itself, and the presence of concomitant antiepilepsy medicinal products during each reported pregnancy. There is no information on the possible occurrence of visual field defect in children who have been exposed to vigabatrin *in utero*.

Studies in animals have shown reproductive toxicity (see Section 5.3 Preclinical safety data). The relevance of these data for humans is unknown.

If a patient becomes or wishes to become pregnant, treatment should be reviewed. Sudden interruption of effective antiepileptic treatment may lead to aggravation of the condition in the mother that is detrimental to the foetus.

Vigabatrin should only be used during pregnancy if clearly necessary.

Vigabatrin is excreted into breast milk. Breast feeding is not recommended during vigabatrin treatment.

4.7 Effects on ability to drive and use machines
As a general rule, patients with uncontrolled epilepsy are not allowed to drive or handle potentially dangerous machinery. In view of the fact that drowsiness has been observed in clinical trials with Sabril, patients should be warned of this possibility at the start of treatment.

Visual field defects which can significantly affect the ability to drive and use machines have been frequently reported in association with Sabril. Patients should be evaluated for the presence of visual field defect (see also Section 4.4 Special Warnings and special precautions for use). Special care should be taken by patients driving, operating machinery or performing any hazardous task.

4.8 Undesirable effects
Visual field defects ranging from mild to severe have been reported frequently in patients receiving vigabatrin. Severe cases are potentially disabling. The onset is usually after months to years of vigabatrin therapy. Pooled data from prevalence surveys suggest that as many as 1/3 of patients receiving vigabatrin therapy develop visual field defects (see also Section 4.4 Special warnings and special precautions for use).

Approximately 50% of patients in controlled clinical studies have experienced undesirable effects during vigabatrin treatment. In adults, these were mostly central nervous system related such as sedation, drowsiness, fatigue and impaired concentration. However, in children excitation or agitation is frequent. The incidence of these undesirable effects is generally higher at the beginning of treatment and decreases with time.

As with other antiepileptic drugs, some patients may experience an increase in seizure frequency, including status epilepticus with vigabatrin. Patients with myoclonic seizures may be particularly liable to this effect. New onset myoclonus and exacerbation of existing myoclonus may occur in rare cases.

Very rare cases of hepatic reactions (including hepatitis) have been reported.

Very common (>1/10)	*General disorders*: Somnolence, fatigue *Psychiatric disorders**: Excitation and agitation (children) *Eye disorders*: Visual field defect
Common (>1/100, <1/10)	*General disorders*: Headache, weight gain, tremor, oedema *Nervous system disorders*: Dizziness, paraesthesia, disturbance of concentration and memory *Psychiatric disorders**: Agitation, agression, nervousness, irritability, depression, thought disturbance, paranoid reaction *Gastrointestinal disorders*: Nausea, abdominal pain *Eye disorders*: Blurred vision, diplopia, nystagmus
Uncommon (>1/1,000, <1/100)	*Nervous system disorders*: Ataxia *Psychiatric disorders**: Hypomania, mania, psychosis Skin disorders: Rash
Rare (<1/1,000)	*General disorders*: Angioedema, urticaria *Nervous system disorders*: Encephalopathic symptoms** *Psychiatric disorders*: Suicide attempt *Eye disorders*: Retinal disorder (such as peripheral retinal atrophy)
Very rare (<1/10,000)	*Eye disorders*: Optic neuritis, optic atrophy *Psychiatric disorders*: Hallucinations

*Psychiatric reactions have been reported during vigabatrin therapy. These reactions occurred in patients with and without a psychiatric history and were usually reversible when vigabatrin doses were reduced or gradually discontinued (see Section 4.4 Special warnings and special precautions for use). Depression was a common psychiatric reaction in clinical trials but seldom required discontinuation of vigabatrin.

**Rare reports of encephalopathic symptoms such as marked sedation, stupor and confusion in association with non-specific slow wave activity on electroencephalogram have been described soon after the initiation of vigabatrin treatment. Such reactions have been fully reversible following dose reduction or discontinuation of vigabatrin (see Section 4.4 Special warnings and special precautions for use).

Laboratory data indicate that vigabatrin treatment does not lead to renal or hepatic toxicity. Decreases in ALT and AST, which are considered to be a result of inhibition of these aminotransferases by vigabatrin, have been observed. Chronic treatment with vigabatrin may be associated with a slight decrease in haemoglobin which rarely attains clinical significance.

4.9 Overdose
Symptoms
Vigabatrin overdose has been reported. When provided, doses most commonly were between 7.5 to 30g; however, ingestions up to 90g have been reported. Nearly half of the cases involved multiple drug ingestions. When reported, the most common symptoms included drowsiness or coma. Other less frequently reported symptoms included vertigo, headache, psychosis, respiratory depression or apnoea, bradycardia, hypotension, agitation, irritability, confusion, abnormal behaviour, and speech disorder. None of the overdoses resulted in death.

Management
There is no specific antidote. The usual supportive measures should be employed. Measures to remove unabsorbed drug should be considered. Activated charcoal has been shown to not significantly adsorb vigabatrin in an in vitro study. The effectiveness of haemodialysis in the treatment of vigabatrin overdose is unknown. In isolated case reports in renal failure patients receiving therapeutic doses of vigabatrin, haemodialysis reduced vigabatrin plasma concentrations by 40% to 60%.

5. PHARMACOLOGICAL PROPERTIES
5.1 Pharmacodynamic properties
Pharmaco-therapeutic group: Antiepileptics, ATC code: N03AG04

Vigabatrin is an antiepileptic drug with a clearly defined mechanism of action. Treatment with vigabatrin leads to an increase in the concentration of GABA (gamma aminobutyric acid), the major inhibitory neurotransmitter in the brain. This is because vigabatrin was designed rationally as a selective irreversible inhibitor of GABA-transaminase, the enzyme responsible for the breakdown of GABA.

Controlled and long-term clinical trials have shown that vigabatrin is an effective anticonvulsant agent when given as add-on therapy in patients with epilepsy not controlled satisfactorily by conventional therapy. This efficacy is particularly marked in patients with seizures of partial origin.

5.2 Pharmacokinetic properties
Vigabatrin is a water soluble compound and it is rapidly and completely absorbed from the gastrointestinal tract. Food administration does not alter the extent of vigabatrin absorption. The drug is widely distributed with an apparent volume of distribution slightly greater than total body water. Plasma and cerebrospinal fluid concentrations are linearly related to dose over the recommended dose range.

There is no direct correlation between plasma concentration and efficacy. The duration of the effect of the drug is dependent on the GABA transaminase re-synthesis rate.

Vigabatrin is eliminated from the plasma with a terminal half-life of 5-8 hours with approximately 70% of a single oral dose being recovered as unchanged drug in the urine in the first 24 hours post-dose. No metabolites have been identified.

Vigabatrin does not induce the hepatic cytochrome P450 enzymes nor is it metabolised or protein bound. Therefore drug interactions are unlikely.

5.3 Preclinical safety data
Animal safety studies carried out in the rat, mouse, dog and monkey have indicated that vigabatrin has no significant adverse effects on the liver, kidney, lung, heart or gastrointestinal tract.

In the brain, microvacuolation has been observed in white matter tracts of rat, mouse and dog at doses of 30-50mg/kg/day. In the monkey these lesions are minimal or equivocal. This effect is caused by a separation of the outer lamellar sheath of myelinated fibres, a change characteristic of intramyelinic oedema. In both rat and dog the intramyelinic oedema was reversible on stopping vigabatrin treatment and even with continued treatment histologic regression was observed. However, in rodents, minor residual changes consisting of swollen axons (eosinophilic spheroids) and mineralised microbodies have been observed. In the dog, the results of an electrophysiological study indicate that intramyelinic oedema is associated with an increase in the latency of the somatosensory evoked potential which is reversible when the drug is withdrawn.

In humans, there is no evidence of intramyelinic oedema. Tests done to confirm lack of significant adverse effect on neurological function include evoked potentials, CAT scans, magnetic resonance imaging, CSF analyses and in a small number of cases, neuropathological examinations of brain specimens.

Vigabatrin-associated retinotoxicity has only been observed in albino rats, but not in pigmented rats, dogs or monkeys. The retinal changes in albino rats were characterised as focal or multifocal disorganisation of the outer nuclear layer with displacement of nuclei into the rod and cone area. The other layers of retina were not affected. These lesions were observed in 80-100% of animals at the dose of 300mg/kg/day orally. The histologic appearance of these lesions was similar to that found in albino rats following excessive exposure to light. However, the retinal changes may also represent a direct drug-induced effect.

Animal experiments have shown that vigabatrin has no negative influence on fertility or pup development. No teratogenicity was seen in rats in doses up to 150mg/kg (3 times the human dose) or in rabbits in doses up to 100mg/kg. However, in rabbits, a slight increase in the incidence of cleft palate at doses of 150-200mg/kg was seen.

Studies with vigabatrin revealed no evidence of mutagenic or carcinogenic effects.

6. PHARMACEUTICAL PARTICULARS
6.1 List of excipients
Sachets: Povidone.

Tablets: Povidone, microcrystalline cellulose, sodium starch glycollate, magnesium stearate, hydroxypropyl methylcellulose, titanium dioxide, polyethylene glycol 8000, deionised water.

6.2 Incompatibilities
Not applicable

6.3 Shelf life
Sachets: 3 years.

Tablets: 5 years.

6.4 Special precautions for storage
None stated.

6.5 Nature and contents of container
Sachets:

Container(s): Sachets (paper, polythene/aluminium foil/polythene laminated) packed in cardboard cartons.

Pack size: 50 sachets.

Tablets:

Container(s): PVC/Aluminium foil blister packs in cardboard cartons.

Pack size: 100 tablets.

6.6 Instructions for use and handling
Not applicable.

7. MARKETING AUTHORISATION HOLDER
Aventis Pharma Limited

50 Kings Hill Avenue

Kings Hill

West Malling

Kent

ME19 4AH

8. MARKETING AUTHORISATION NUMBER(S)
Sachets: PL 04425/0170

Tablets: PL 04425/0171

9. DATE OF FIRST AUTHORISATION/RENEWAL OF THE AUTHORISATION
Sachets: 26 January 2001

Tablets: 26 January 2001

10. DATE OF REVISION OF THE TEXT
May 2004

11. LEGAL CLASSIFICATION
POM

Saizen 1.33mg

(Serono Ltd)

1. NAME OF THE MEDICINAL PRODUCT
SAIZEN® 1.33mg, powder and solvent for solution for injection

2. QUALITATIVE AND QUANTITATIVE COMPOSITION
Each vial of SAIZEN® 1.33 mg contains Somatropin (recombinant human growth hormone).

For excipients, see 6.1.

3. PHARMACEUTICAL FORM
Powder and solvent for solution for injection.

4. CLINICAL PARTICULARS
4.1 Therapeutic indications
SAIZEN® is indicated in the treatment of:

- growth failure in children caused by decreased or absent secretion of endogenous growth hormone.
- growth failure in girls with gonadal dysgenesis (Turner Syndrome), confirmed by chromosomal analysis.
- growth failure in prepubertal children due to chronic renal failure (CRF).
- replacement therapy in adults with pronounced growth hormone deficiency as diagnosed by a single dynamic test

for growth hormone deficiency. Patients must also fulfil the following criteria:

Childhood Onset:

Patients who were diagnosed as growth hormone deficient during childhood, must be retested and their growth hormone deficiency confirmed before replacement therapy with Saizen is started.

Adult Onset:

Patients must have growth hormone deficiency as a result of hypothalamic or pituitary disease and at least one other hormone deficiency diagnosed (except for prolactin) and adequate replacement therapy instituted, before replacement therapy using growth hormone may begin.

4.2 Posology and method of administration

SAIZEN® 1.33 mg is intended for single-use.

SAIZEN® dosage should be individualised for each patient based on body surface area (BSA) or on body weight (BW).

It is recommended that SAIZEN® be administered at bedtime according to the following dosage:

Growth failure due to inadequate endogenous growth hormone secretion:

0.7-1.0 mg/m^2 body surface area (BSA) per day or 0.025-0.035 mg/kg body weight (BW) per day by subcutaneous or intramuscular administration.

Growth failure in girls due to gonadal dysgenesis (Turner Syndrome)

1.4 mg/m^2 body surface area (BSA) per day or 0.045-0.050 mg/kg body weight (BW) per day by subcutaneous administration.

Concomitant therapy with non-androgenic anabolic steroids in patients with Turner Syndrome can enhance the growth response.

Growth failure in prepubertal children due to chronic renal failure (CRF):

1.4 mg/m^2 body surface area (BSA), approximately equal to 0.045-0.050 mg/kg body weight (BW), per day by subcutaneous administration.

Duration of treatment

Treatment should be discontinued when the patient has reached a satisfactory adult height, or the epiphyses are fused.

Growth Hormone Deficiency in adults:

At the start of somatropin therapy, low doses of 0.15-0.3mg are recommended, given as a daily subcutaneous injection. The dose should be adjusted stepwise, controlled by Insulin-like Growth Factor 1 (IGF-1) values. The recommended final GH dose seldom exceeds 1.0mg/day. In general the lowest efficacious dose should be administered. In older or overweight patients, lower doses may be necessary.

4.3 Contraindications

SAIZEN® should not be used in children in whom epiphyseal fusion occurred.

SAIZEN® is contraindicated in patients known to be hypersensitive to Somatropin and any of the excipients in the powder for solution for injection or the solvent.

SAIZEN® is contraindicated in patients with active neoplasia. Any anti-tumor therapy must be completed prior to starting treatment with Somatropin.

SAIZEN® should not be used in cases with evidence of any progression or recurrence of an underlying intra-cranial lesion.

Growth hormone treatment should be discontinued in critically ill patients.

4.4 Special warnings and special precautions for use

Treatment should be carried out under the regular guidance of a physician who is experienced in the diagnosis and management of patients with growth hormone deficiency.

Hypothyroidism may become apparent during SAIZEN® therapy. Thyroid function tests should be performed periodically during SAIZEN® administration. The possible appearance of hypothyroidism in the course of the therapy with growth hormone should be corrected with thyroid hormone in order to obtain a sufficient treatment effect.

Patients with an intra or extracranial neoplasia in remission who are receiving treatment with growth hormone should be examined carefully and at regular intervals by the physician.

In patients with endocrine disorders, including growth hormone deficiency, slipped capital femoral epiphyses may occur more frequently.

Patients with growth failure due to chronic renal failure should be examined periodically for evidence of progression of renal osteodystrophy. Slipped capital femoral epiphysis or avascular necrosis of the femoral head may be seen in children with advanced renal osteodystrophy and it is uncertain whether these problems are affected by growth hormone therapy. X-rays of the hip should be obtained prior to initiating therapy. Physicians and parents should be alert to the development of a limp or complaints of hip or knee pain patients treated with SAIZEN®.

In children with chronic renal failure, renal function should have decreased to below 50% of normal before therapy is instituted. To verify the growth disturbance, growth should have been followed for a year before institution of therapy. Conservative treatment for renal insufficiency (which includes control of acidosis, hyperparathyroidism and nutritional status for one year prior to the treatment) should have been established and should be maintained during treatment. Treatment should be discontinued at the time of renal transplantation.

Patients with growth hormone deficiency secondary to an intracranial tumour should be examined frequently for progression or recurrence of the underlying disease process.

Some cases of leukaemia have been reported in growth hormone deficient children, untreated as well as treated with growth hormone, and might possibly represent a slightly increased incidence compared with non-growth hormone deficient children. A causal relationship to growth hormone therapy has not been established.

In case of severe or recurrent headache, visual problems, nausea and/or vomiting, funduscopy for papilloedema is recommended. If papilloedema is confirmed a diagnosis of benign intracranial hypertension (or pseudotumor cerebri) should be considered and SAIZEN® treatment should be discontinued. At present there is insufficient evidence to guide clinical decision-making in patients with resolved intracranial hypertension. If growth hormone treatment is restarted, careful monitoring for symptoms of intracranial hypertension is necessary and treatment should be discontinued if intracraneal hypertension recurs.

Growth Hormone administration is followed by a transient phase of hypoglycemia of approximately 2 hours, then from 2-4 hours onward by an increase in blood glucose levels despite high insulin concentrations. To detect insulin resistance, patients should be monitored for evidence of glucose intolerance.

SAIZEN® should be used with caution in patients with diabetes mellitus or with a family history of diabetes mellitus. Patients with diabetes mellitus may require adjustment of their antidiabetic therapy.

In all patients developing acute critical illness, the possible benefit of treatment with growth hormone must be weighed against the potential risk involved.

The injection site should be varied to prevent lipoatrophy.

In case of persistent oedema or severe paraesthesia the dosage should be decreased in order to avoid the development of carpal tunnel syndrome.

Growth Hormone Deficiency in the Adult is a lifelong condition and should be treated accordingly, however experience with patients over sixty years and experience with prolonged treatment is limited

4.5 Interaction with other medicinal products and other forms of Interaction

Concomitant corticosteroid therapy may inhibit the response to SAIZEN®.

4.6 Pregnancy and lactation

Pregnancy: Clinical experience with growth hormone in pregnant women is limited. Animal studies do not indicate direct or indirect harmful effects with respect to pregnancy, embryo-fetal development, parturition or postnatal development (see Section 5.3). Caution should be exercised when prescribing to pregnant women.

Lactation: It is not known if exogenous peptide hormones are excreted into breast milk but absorption of intact protein from the gastrointestinal tract of the infant is unlikely.

4.7 Effects on ability to drive and use machines

SAIZEN® does not interfere with the patient's ability to drive or use machinery.

4.8 Undesirable effects

Up to 10 % of patients may experience redness and itching at the site of injection, particularly when the subcutaneous route is used.

Antibodies to Somatropin can form in some patients; the clinical significance of these antibodies is unknown, though to date the antibodies have been of low binding capacity and have not been associated with growth attenuation except in patients with gene deletions. In very rare instances, where short stature is due to deletion of the growth hormone gene complex, treatment with growth hormone may induce growth attenuating antibodies.

Epiphysiolysis at the site of the hip joint may occur. A child with an unexplained limp should be examined.

Oedema, muscle pain, joint pain, and joint disorders were reported to occur in up to 10 % of adult patients receiving growth hormone replacement therapy. These side effects occurred primarily early in therapy and tended to be transient.

Adult patients with growth hormone deficiency, following diagnosis of growth hormone deficiency in childhood, reported side-effects less frequently than those with adult onset growth hormone deficiency.

4.9 Overdose

No cases of acute overdosage have been reported. However, exceeding the recommended doses can cause side effects. Overdosage can lead to hypoglycaemia and subsequently to hyperglycaemia. Long term overdosage could result in signs and symptoms of gigantism and/or acromegaly, consistent with the known effects of excess human growth hormone.

5. PHARMACOLOGICAL PROPERTIES

5.1 Pharmacodynamic properties

Pharmaco-therapeutic group: Anterior pituitary lobe hormones and analogues, ATC code: HO1A.

SAIZEN® contains recombinant human growth hormone produced by genetically engineered mammalian cells.

It is a peptide of 191 amino acids identical to human pituitary growth hormone with respect to aminoacid sequence and composition as well as peptide map, isoelectric point, molecular weight, isomeric structure and bioactivity.

Growth hormone is synthesised in a transformed murine cell line that has been modified by the addition of the gene for pituitary growth hormone.

SAIZEN® is an anabolic and anticatabolic agent which exerts effects not only on growth but also on body composition and metabolism. It interacts with specific receptors on a variety of cell types including myocytes, hepatocytes, adipocytes, lymphocytes and hematopoietic cells. Some, but not all of its effects are mediated through another class of hormones known as somatomedins (IGF-1 and IGF-2).

Depending on the dose, the administration of SAIZEN® elicits a rise in IGF-1, IGFBP-3, non-esterified fatty acids and glycerol, a decrease in blood urea, and decreases in urinary nitrogen, sodium and potassium excretion. The duration of the increase in GH levels may play a role in determining the magnitude of the effects. A relative saturation of the effects of SAIZEN® at high doses is probable. This is not the case for glycemia and urinary C-peptide excretion, which are significantly elevated only after high doses (20 mg).

5.2 Pharmacokinetic properties

The pharmacokinetics of SAIZEN® are linear at least up to doses of 8 IU (2.67 mg). At higher doses (60 IU/20 mg) some degree of non-linearity cannot be ruled out, however with no clinical relevance.

Following IV administration in healthy volunteers the volume of distribution at steady-state is around 7 L, total metabolic clearance is around 15 L/h while the renal clearance is negligible, and the drug exhibits an elimination half-life of 20 to 35 min.

Following single-dose SC and IM administration of SAIZEN®, the apparent terminal half-life is much longer, around 2 to 4 hours. This is due to a rate limiting absorption process.

Maximum serum growth hormone (GH) concentrations are reached after approximatively 4 hours and serum GH levels return to baseline within 24 hours, indicating that no accumulation of GH will occur during repeated administrations.

The absolute bioavailability of both routes is 70-90 %.

5.3 Preclinical safety data

Preclinical data reveal no special hazard for humans based on conventional studies of safety pharmacology, repeated dose toxicity and genotoxicity. Reproductive toxicology studies do not indicate any adverse effect on fertility and reproduction, despite administration of doses sufficiently high to produce some pharmacological effects on growth.

6. PHARMACEUTICAL PARTICULARS

6.1 List of excipients

Powder for solution for injection

Mannitol, Disodium phosphate dihydrate, Sodium dihydrogen phosphate monohydrate, Sodium Chloride

Solvent for parenteral use

0.9% w/v sodium chloride in water for injections

6.2 Incompatibilities

No incompatibilities of SAIZEN® with other pharmaceutical preparations are known at present.

6.3 Shelf life

2 years.

After reconstitution: Immediate usage is recommended. However, stability has been demonstrated up to 24 hours.

6.4 Special precautions for storage

Store at 2°C to 8°C in the original package.

Store the reconstituted product at 2°C to 8°C in the original package.

Do not freeze.

6.5 Nature and contents of container

The 5 ml vials of SAIZEN® 1.33 mg and the 2 ml ampoules containing 1 ml of the solvent are of neutral glass (Type I).

SAIZEN® 1.33 mg is available in the following pack sizes:

1 vial of SAIZEN® 1.33 mg product and 1 ampoule of solvent

5 vials of SAIZEN® 1.33 mg product and 5 ampoules of solvent.

10 vials of SAIZEN® 1.33 mg product and 10 ampoules of solvent.

6.6 Instructions for use and handling

Reconstitution:

The powder for solution for injection should be used with the enclosed solvent for parenteral use. The reconstituted solution for injection should be clear with no particles. If the solution contains particles, it must not be injected.

Use with a syringe:

To reconstitute SAIZEN®, inject 0.5 – 1ml of the solvent into the vial of SAIZEN® 1.33 mg aiming the liquid against the glass wall. Swirl the vial with a GENTLE rotary motion until the content is dissolved completely. Avoid vigorous shaking.

7. MARKETING AUTHORISATION HOLDER

Serono Pharmaceuticals Ltd.
Bedfont Cross, Stanwell Road
Feltham, Middlesex.
TW14 8NX
Telephone: +44(0)20 8818 7200

8. MARKETING AUTHORISATION NUMBER(S)

Product Licence Numbers

SAIZEN® 1.33 mg PL 03400/0023

Sodium chloride injection PL 03400/0024

Product Authorisation Number

SAIZEN® 1.33 mg PA 285/5/1

9. DATE OF FIRST AUTHORISATION/RENEWAL OF THE AUTHORISATION

First authorisationin the UK: 10th November 1989 Renewed 3rd April 1999

10. DATE OF REVISION OF THE TEXT

July 2001

LEGAL STATUS

POM*

NAME AND ADDRESS OF DISTRIBUTOR IN IRELAND

Allphar Service Limited
Pharmaceutical Agents and Distributors
Belgard Road
Tallaght
Dublin 24
Telephone: (01) 404 1600
*UK Status

Saizen 3.33mg

(Serono Ltd)

1. NAME OF THE MEDICINAL PRODUCT

SAIZEN® 3.33 mg, powder and solvent for solution for injection

2. QUALITATIVE AND QUANTITATIVE COMPOSITION

Each vial of SAIZEN® 3.33 mg contains Somatropin (recombinant human growth hormone).

For excipients, see 6.1.

3. PHARMACEUTICAL FORM

Powder and solvent for solution for injection

4. CLINICAL PARTICULARS

4.1 Therapeutic indications

SAIZEN® is indicated in the treatment of:

- growth failure in children caused by decreased or absent secretion of endogenous growth hormone.
- growth failure in girls with gonadal dysgenesis (Turner Syndrome), confirmed by chromosomal analysis.
- growth failure in prepubertal children due to chronic renal failure (CRF).
- replacement therapy in adults with pronounced growth hormone deficiency as diagnosed by a single dynamic test for growth hormone deficiency. Patients must also fulfil the following criteria:

Childhood Onset:

Patients who were diagnosed as growth hormone deficient during childhood, must be retested and their growth hormone deficiency confirmed before replacement therapy with Saizen is started.

Adult Onset:

Patients must have growth hormone deficiency as a result of hypothalamic or pituitary disease and at least one other hormone deficiency diagnosed (except for prolactin) and adequate replacement therapy instituted, before replacement therapy using growth hormone may begin.

4.2 Posology and method of administration

SAIZEN® 3.33 mg is intended for multiple dose use.

SAIZEN® dosage should be individualised for each patient based on body surface area (BSA) or on body weight (BW).

It is recommended that SAIZEN® be administered at bedtime according to the following dosage:

Growth failure due to inadequate endogenous growth hormone secretion:

0.7-1.0 mg/m² body surface area (BSA) per day or 0.025-0.035 mg/kg body weight (BW) per day by subcutaneous or intramuscular administration.

Growth failure in girls due to gonadal dysgenesis (Turner Syndrome)

1.4 mg/m² body surface area (BSA) per day or 0.045-0.050 mg/kg body weight (BW) per day by subcutaneous administration.

Concomitant therapy with non-androgenic anabolic steroids in patients with Turner Syndrome can enhance the growth response.

Growth failure in prepubertal children due to chronic renal failure (CRF):

1.4 mg/m² body surface area (BSA), approximately equal to 0.045-0.050 mg/kg body weight (BW), per day by subcutaneous administration.

Duration of treatment

Treatment should be discontinued when the patient has reached a satisfactory adult height, or the epiphyses are fused.

Growth Hormone Deficiency in adults:

At the start of somatropin therapy, low doses of 0.15-0.3mg are recommended, given as a daily subcutaneous injection. The dose should be adjusted stepwise, controlled by Insulin-like Growth Factor 1 (IGF-1) values. The recommended final GH dose seldom exceeds 1.0mg/day. In general the lowest efficacious dose should be administered. In older or overweight patients, lower doses may be necessary.

4.3 Contraindications

SAIZEN® should not be used in children in whom epiphyseal fusion occurred.

SAIZEN® is contraindicated in patients known to be hypersensitive to Somatropin and any of the excipients in the powder for solution for injection or the solvent.

SAIZEN® is contraindicated in patients with active neoplasia Any anti-tumor therapy must be completed prior to starting treatment with Somatropin.

SAIZEN® should not be used in cases with evidence of any progression or recurrence of an underlying intra-cranial lesion.

Growth hormone treatment should be discontinued in critically ill patients.

4.4 Special warnings and special precautions for use

Treatment should be carried out under the regular guidance of a physician who is experienced in the diagnosis and management of patients with growth hormone deficiency.

Hypothyroidism may become apparent during SAIZEN® therapy. Thyroid function tests should be performed periodically during SAIZEN® administration. The possible appearance of hypothyroidism in the course of the therapy with growth hormone should be corrected with thyroid hormone in order to obtain a sufficient treatment effect.

Patients with an intra or extracranial neoplasia in remission who are receiving treatment with growth hormone should be examined carefully and at regular intervals by the physician.

In patients with endocrine disorders, including growth hormone deficiency, slipped capital femoral epiphyses may occur more frequently.

Patients with growth failure due to chronic renal failure should be examined periodically for evidence of progression of renal osteodystrophy. Slipped capitalfemoral epiphysis or avascular necrosis of the femoral head may be seen in children with advanced renal osteodystrophy and it is uncertain whether these problems are affected by growth hormone therapy. X-rays of the hip should be obtained prior to initiating therapy. Physicians and parents should be alert to the development of a limp or complaints of hip or knee pain patients treated with SAIZEN®.

In children with chronic renal failure, renal function should have decreased to below 50% of normal before therapy is instituted. To verify the growth disturbance, growth should have been followed for a year before institution of therapy. Conservative treatment for renal insufficiency (which includes control of acidosis, hyperparathyroidism and nutritional status for one year prior to the treatment) should have been established and should be maintained during treatment. Treatment should be discontinued at the time of renal transplantation.

Patients with growth hormone deficiency secondary to an intracranial tumour should be examined frequently for progression or recurrence of the underlying disease process.

Some cases of leukaemia have been reported in growth hormone deficient children, untreated as well as treated with growth hormone, and might possibly represent a slightly increased incidence compared with non-growth hormone deficient children. A causal relationship to growth hormone therapy has not been established.

In case of severe or recurrent headache, visual problems, nausea and/or vomiting, funduscopy for papilloedema is recommended. If papilloedema is confirmed a diagnosis of benign intracranial hypertension (or pseudotumor cerebri) should be considered and SAIZEN® treatment should be discontinued. At present there is insufficient evidence to guide clinical decision-making in patients with resolved intracranial hypertension. If growth hormone treatment is restarted, careful monitoring for symptoms of intracranial hypertension is necessary and treatment should be discontinued if intracranial hypertension recurs.

Growth Hormone administration is followed by a transient phase of hypoglycemia of approximately 2 hours, then from 2-4 hours onward by an increase in blood glucose levels despite high insulin concentrations. To detect insulin resistance, patients should be monitored for evidence of glucose intolerance.

SAIZEN® should be used with caution in patients with diabetes mellitus or with a family history of diabetes mellitus. Patients with diabetes mellitus may require adjustment of their antidiabetic therapy.

In all patients developing acute critical illness, the possible benefit of treatment with growth hormone must be weighed against the potential risk involved.

The injection site should be varied to prevent lipoatrophy.

Benzylalcohol as a preservative in bacteriostatic sodiumchloride solution for injection has been associated with toxicity in children under 2 years of age. SAIZEN® may be reconstituted with Sodium Chloride Injection BP or Sterile Water for Injections for immediate use when administering to children under 2 years of age.

In case of persistent oedema or severe paraesthesia the dosage should be decreased in order to avoid the development of carpal tunnel syndrome.

Growth Hormone Deficiency in the Adult is a lifelong condition and should be treated accordingly, however experience with patients over sixty years and experience with prolonged treatment is limited

4.5 Interaction with other medicinal products and other forms of Interaction

Concomitant corticosteroid therapy may inhibit the response to SAIZEN®.

4.6 Pregnancy and lactation

Pregnancy: Clinical experience with growth hormone in pregnant women is limited. Animal studies do not indicate direct or indirect harmful effects with respect to pregnancy, embryo-fetal development, parturition or postnatal development (see Section 5.3). Caution should be exercised when prescribing to pregnant women.

Lactation: It is not known if exogenous peptide hormones are excreted into breast milk but absorption of intact protein from the gastrointestinal tract of the infant is unlikely.

4.7 Effects on ability to drive and use machines

SAIZEN® does not interfere with the patient's ability to drive or use machinery.

4.8 Undesirable effects

Up to 10 % of patients may experience redness and itching at the site of injection, particularly when the subcutaneous route is used.

Antibodies to Somatropin can form in some patients; the clinical significance of these antibodies is unknown, though to date the antibodies have been of low binding capacity and have not been associated with growth attenuation except in patients with gene deletions. In very rare instances, where short stature is due to deletion of the growth hormone gene complex, treatment with growth hormone may induce growth attenuating antibodies.

Epiphysiolysis at the site of the hip joint may occur. A child with an unexplained limp should be examined.

Oedema, muscle pain, joint pain, and joint disorders were reported to occur in up to 10 % of adult patients receiving growth hormone replacement therapy. These side effects occurred primarily early in therapy and tended to be transient.

Adult patients with growth hormone deficiency, following diagnosis of growth hormone deficiency in childhood, reported side-effects less frequently than those with adult onset growth hormone deficiency.

4.9 Overdose

No cases of acute overdosage have been reported. However, exceeding the recommended doses can cause side effects. Overdosage can lead to hypoglycaemia and subsequently to hyperglycaemia. Long term overdosage could result in signs and symptoms of gigantism and/or acromegaly, consistent with the known effects of excess human growth hormone.

5. PHARMACOLOGICAL PROPERTIES

5.1 Pharmacodynamic properties

Pharmaco-therapeutic group: Anterior pituitary lobe hormones and analogues, ATC code: HO1A.

SAIZEN contains recombinant human growth hormone produced by genetically engineered mammalian cells.

It is a peptide of 191 amino acids identical to human pituitary growth hormone with respect to aminoacid sequence and composition as well as peptide map, isoelectric point, molecular weight, isomeric structure and bioactivity.

Growth hormone is synthesised in a transformed murine cell line that has been modified by the addition of the gene for pituitary growth hormone.

SAIZEN® is an anabolic and anticatabolic agent which exerts effects not only on growth but also on body composition and metabolism. It interacts with specific receptors on a variety of cell types including myocytes, hepatocytes, adipocytes, lymphocytes and hematopoietic cells. Some, but not all of its effects are mediated through another class of hormones known as somatomedins (IGF-1 and IGF-2).

Depending on the dose, the administration of SAIZEN® elicits a rise in IGF-1, IGFBP-3, non-esterified fatty acids and glycerol, a decrease in blood urea, and decreases in urinary nitrogen, sodium and potassium excretion. The duration of the increase in GH levels may play a role in determining the magnitude of the effects. A relative saturation of the effects of SAIZEN® at high doses is probable. This is not the case for glycemia and urinary C-peptide excretion, which are significantly elevated only after high doses (20 mg).

5.2 Pharmacokinetic properties

The pharmacokinetics of SAIZEN® are linear at least up to doses of 8 IU (2.67 mg). At higher doses (60 IU/20 mg) some degree of non-linearity cannot be ruled out, however with no clinical relevance.

Following IV administration in healthy volunteers the volume of distribution at steady-state is around 7 L, total metabolic clearance is around 15 L/h while the renal clearance is negligible, and the drug exhibits an elimination half-life of 20 to 35 min.

Following single-dose SC and IM administration of SAIZEN®, the apparent terminal half-life is much longer, around 2 to 4 hours. This is due to a rate limiting absorption process.

Maximum serum growth hormone (GH) concentrations are reached after approximately 4 hours and serum GH levels return to baseline within 24 hours, indicating that no accumulation of GH will occur during repeated administrations.

The absolute bioavailability of both routes is 70-90 %.

5.3 Preclinical safety data

Preclinical data reveal no special hazard for humans based on conventional studies of safety pharmacology, repeated dose toxicity and genotoxicity. Reproductive toxicology studies do not indicate any adverse effect on fertility and reproduction, despite administration of doses sufficiently high to produce some pharmacological effects on growth.

6. PHARMACEUTICAL PARTICULARS

6.1 List of excipients

Powder for solution for injection

Mannitol, Disodium phosphate dihydrate, Sodium dihydrogen phosphate monohydrate

Solvent for parenteral use

0.9 % w/v sodium chloride in water for injections and 0.9 % w/v benzylalcohol

6.2 Incompatibilities

No incompatibilities of SAIZEN® with other pharmaceutical preparations are known at present.

6.3 Shelf life

2 years.

The reconstituted solution for injection is stable for 7 days.

6.4 Special precautions for storage

Store at 2°C to 8°C in the original package.

Store the reconstituted product at 2°C to 8°C in the original package.

Do not freeze.

6.5 Nature and contents of container

The 10 ml vials of SAIZEN® 3.33 mg and the 5 ml vials containing 5 ml of the solvent are of neutral glass (Type I).

SAIZEN® 3.33 mg is available in the following pack sizes:

1 vial of SAIZEN® 3.33 mg product and 1 vial of bacteriostatic solvent

5 vials of SAIZEN® 3.33 mg product and 5 vials of bacteriostatic solvent

6.6 Instructions for use and handling

Reconstitution:

The powder for solution for injection should be used with the enclosed solvent for parenteral use. The reconstituted solution for injection should be clear with no particles. If the solution contains particles, it must not be injected.

Use with a syringe:

To reconstitute SAIZEN®, inject 1 ml of the bacteriostatic solvent into the vial of SAIZEN® 3.33 mg aiming the liquid against the glass wall. Swirl the vial with a GENTLE rotary motion until the content is dissolved completely. Avoid vigorous shaking.

7. MARKETING AUTHORISATION HOLDER

Serono Ltd.

Bedfont Cross, Stanwell Road

Feltham, Middlesex.

TW14 8NX

Telephone: +44(0)20 8818 7200

8. MARKETING AUTHORISATION NUMBER(S)

Product Licence Numbers

SAIZEN® 3.33 mg PL 03400/0034

Bacteriostatic solvent PL 03400/0035

Product Authorisation Number

SAIZEN® 3.33 mg PA 285/5/2

9. DATE OF FIRST AUTHORISATION/RENEWAL OF THE AUTHORISATION

First authorisation in UK: 27th August 1991 Ireland: 18th August 1992

Renewed: 3rd April 1999

10. DATE OF REVISION OF THE TEXT

December 2002

LEGAL STATUS

POM*

NAME AND ADDRESS OF DISTRIBUTOR IN IRELAND

Allphar Service Limited

Pharmaceutical Agents and Distributors

Belgard Road

Tallaght

Dublin 24

Telephone: (01) 404 1600

*UK Status

Saizen 8mg click.easy

(Serono Ltd)

1. NAME OF THE MEDICINAL PRODUCT

Saizen® 8 mg click.easy(TM), powder and solvent for solution for injection

2. QUALITATIVE AND QUANTITATIVE COMPOSITION

Each vial of Saizen® 8 mg click.easy(TM) contains Somatropin (recombinant human growth hormone).

Reconstitution with the contents of the bacteriostatic solvent cartridge gives a concentration of 5.83 mg per ml.

For excipients, see 6.1.

3. PHARMACEUTICAL FORM

Powder and solvent for solution for injection.

4. CLINICAL PARTICULARS

4.1 Therapeutic indications

Saizen® is indicated in the treatment of:

• growth failure in children caused by decreased or absent secretion of endogenous growth hormone.

• growth failure in girls with gonadal dysgenesis (Turner Syndrome), confirmed by chromosomal analysis.

• growth failure in prepubertal children due to chronic renal failure (CRF).

• replacement therapy in adults with pronounced growth hormone deficiency as diagnosed by a single dynamic test for growth hormone deficiency. Patients must also fulfil the following criteria:

Childhood Onset:

Patients who were diagnosed as growth hormone deficient during childhood, must be retested and their growth hormone deficiency confirmed before replacement therapy with Saizen is started.

Adult Onset:

Patients must have growth hormone deficiency as a result of hypothalamic or pituitary disease and at least one other hormone deficiency diagnosed (except for prolactin) and adequate replacement therapy instituted, before replacement therapy using growth hormone may begin.

4.2 Posology and method of administration

Saizen® 8 mg click.easy(TM) is intended for multiple dose use.

Saizen® dosage should be individualised for each patient based on body surface area (BSA) or on body weight (BW).

It is recommended that Saizen® be administered at bedtime according to the following dosage:

Growth failure due to inadequate endogenous growth hormone secretion:

0.7-1.0 mg/m^2 body surface area (BSA) per day or 0.025-0.035 mg/kg body weight (BW) per day by subcutaneous administration.

Growth failure in girls due to gonadal dysgenesis (Turner Syndrome):

1.4 mg/m^2 body surface area (BSA) per day or 0.045-0.050 mg/kg body weight (BW) per day by subcutaneous administration.

Concomitant therapy with non-androgenic anabolic steroids in patients with Turner Syndrome can enhance the growth response.

Growth failure in prepubertal children due to chronic renal failure (CRF):

1.4 mg/m^2 body surface area (BSA), approximately equal to 0.045-0.050 mg/kg body weight (BW), per day by subcutaneous administration.

Duration of treatment

Treatment should be discontinued when the patient has reached a satisfactory adult height, or the epiphyses are fused.

Growth Hormone Deficiency in adults:

At the start of somatropin therapy, low doses of 0.15-0.3mg are recommended, given as a daily subcutaneous injection. The dose should be adjusted stepwise, controlled by Insulin-like Growth Factor 1 (IGF-1) values. The recommended final GH dose seldom exceeds 1.0mg/day. In general the lowest efficacious dose should be administered. In older or overweight patients, lower doses may be necessary.

Method of administration

For administration of the reconstituted solution for injection of Saizen® 8 mg click.easy(TM), follow the instructions given in the package leaflet and in the instruction manual provided with each one.click™ auto-injector or cool.click(TM) needle-free auto-injector. See also section 6.6 for instructions for use/handling.

4.3 Contraindications

Saizen® should not be used in children in whom epiphyseal fusion occurred.

Saizen® is contraindicated in patients known to be hypersensitive to Somatropin and any of the excipients in the powder for solution for injection or the solvent.

Saizen® is contraindicated in patients with active neoplasia. Any anti-tumor therapy must be completed prior to starting treatment with Somatropin.

Saizen® should not be used in cases with evidence of any progression or recurrence of an underlying intra-cranial lesion.

Growth hormone treatment should be discontinued in critically ill patients.

4.4 Special warnings and special precautions for use

Treatment should be carried out under the regular guidance of a physician who is experienced in the diagnosis and management of patients with growth hormone deficiency.

Hypothyroidism may become apparent during Saizen® therapy. Thyroid function tests should be performed periodically during Saizen® administration. The possible appearance of hypothyroidism in the course of the therapy with growth hormone should be corrected with thyroid hormone in order to obtain a sufficient treatment effect.

Patients with an intra or extracranial neoplasia in remission who are receiving treatment with growth hormone should be examined carefully and at regular intervals by the physician.

In patients with endocrine disorders, including growth hormone deficiency, slipped capital femoral epiphyses may occur more frequently.

Patients with growth failure due to chronic renal failure should be examined periodically for evidence of progression of renal osteodystrophy. Slipped capital femoral epiphysis or avascular necrosis of the femoral head may be seen in children with advanced renal osteodystrophy and it is uncertain whether these problems are affected by growth hormone therapy. X-rays of the hip should be obtained prior to initiating therapy. Physicians and parents should be alert to the development of a limp or complaints of hip or knee pain in patients treated with Saizen®.

In children with chronic renal failure, renal function should have decreased to below 50% of normal before therapy is instituted. To verify the growth disturbance, growth should have been followed for a year before institution of therapy. Conservative treatment for renal insufficiency (which includes control of acidosis, hyperparathyroidism and nutritional status for one year prior to the treatment) should have been established and should be maintained during treatment. Treatment should be discontinued at the time of renal transplantation.

Patients with growth hormone deficiency secondary to an intracranial tumour should be examined frequently for progression or recurrence of the underlying disease process.

Some cases of leukaemia have been reported in growth hormone deficient children, untreated as well as treated with growth hormone, and might possibly represent a slightly increased incidence compared with non-growth hormone deficient children. A causal relationship to growth hormone therapy has not been established.

In case of severe or recurrent headache, visual problems, nausea and/or vomiting, funduscopy for papilloedema is recommended. If papilloedema is confirmed a diagnosis of benign intracranial hypertension (or pseudotumor cerebri) should be considered and Saizen® treatment should be discontinued. At present there is insufficient evidence to guide clinical decision-making in patients with resolved intracranial hypertension. If growth hormone treatment is restarted, careful monitoring for symptoms of intracranial hypertension is necessary and treatment should be discontinued if intracranial hypertension recurs.

Growth Hormone administration is followed by a transient phase of hypoglycemia of approximately 2 hours, then from 2-4 hours onward by an increase in blood glucose levels despite high insulin concentrations. To detect insulin resistance, patients should be monitored for evidence of glucose intolerance.

Saizen® should be used with caution in patients with diabetes mellitus or with a family history of diabetes mellitus. Patients with diabetes mellitus may require adjustment of their antidiabetic therapy.

In all patients developing acute critical illness, the possible benefit of treatment with growth hormone must be weighed against the potential risk involved.

The injection site should be varied to prevent lipoatrophy.

In case of persistent oedema or severe paraesthesia the dosage should be decreased in order to avoid the development of carpal tunnel syndrome.

Growth Hormone Deficiency in the Adult is a lifelong condition and should be treated accordingly, however experience with patients over sixty years and experience with prolonged treatment is limited

4.5 Interaction with other medicinal products and other forms of Interaction

Concomitant corticosteroid therapy may inhibit the response to Saizen®.

4.6 Pregnancy and lactation

Pregnancy: Clinical experience with growth hormone in pregnant women is limited. Animal studies do not indicate direct or indirect harmful effects with respect to pregnancy, embryo-fetal development, parturition or postnatal development (see Section 5.3). Caution should be exercised when prescribing to pregnant women.Lactation: It is not known if exogenous peptide hormones are excreted into breast milk but absorption of intact protein from the gastrointestinal tract of the infant is unlikely.

4.7 Effects on ability to drive and use machines

Saizen® does not interfere with the patient's ability to drive or use machinery.

4.8 Undesirable effects

Up to 10 % of patients may experience redness and itching at the site of injection, particularly when the subcutaneous route is used.

Antibodies to Somatropin can form in some patients; the clinical significance of these antibodies is unknown, though to date the antibodies have been of low binding capacity and have not been associated with growth attenuation except in patients with gene deletions. In very rare instances, where short stature is due to deletion of the growth hormone gene complex, treatment with growth hormone may induce growth attenuating antibodies.

Epiphysiolysis at the site of the hip joint may occur. A child with an unexplained limp should be examined.

Oedema, muscle pain, joint pain, and joint disorders were reported to occur in up to 10 % of adult patients receiving growth hormone replacement therapy. These side effects occurred primarily early in therapy and tended to be transient.

Adult patients with growth hormone deficiency, following diagnosis of growth hormone deficiency in childhood, reported side-effects less frequently than those with adult onset growth hormone deficiency.

4.9 Overdose

No cases of acute overdose have been reported. However, exceeding the recommended doses can cause side effects. Overdosage can lead to hypoglycaemia and subsequently to hyperglycaemia. Long term overdosage could result in signs and symptoms of gigantism and/or acromegaly, constistent with the known effects of excess human growth hormone.

5. PHARMACOLOGICAL PROPERTIES

5.1 Pharmacodynamic properties

Pharmaco-therapeutic group: Anterior pituitary lobe hormones and analogues, ATC code: HO1A.

Saizen® contains recombinant human growth hormone produced by genetically engineered mammalian cells.

It is a peptide of 191 amino acids identical to human pituitary growth hormone with respect to aminoacid sequence and composition as well as peptide map, isoelectric point, molecular weight, isomeric structure and bioactivity.

Growth hormone is synthesised in a transformed murine cell line that has been modified by the addition of the gene for pituitary growth hormone.

Saizen® is an anabolic and anticatabolic agent which exerts effects not only on growth but also on body composition and metabolism. It interacts with specific receptors on a variety of cell types including myocytes, hepatocytes, adipocytes, lymphocytes and hematopoietic cells. Some, but not all of its effects are mediated through another class of hormones known as somatomedins (IGF-1 and IGF-2).

Depending on the dose, the administration of Saizen® elicits a rise in IGF-1, IGFBP-3, non-esterified fatty acids and glycerol, a decrease in blood urea, and decreases in urinary nitrogen, sodium and potassium excretion. The duration of the increase in GH levels may play a role in determining the magnitude of the effects. A relative saturation of the effects of Saizen® at high doses is probable. This is not the case for glycemia and urinary C-peptide excretion, which are significantly elevated only after high doses (20 mg).

5.2 Pharmacokinetic properties

The pharmacokinetics of Saizen® are linear at least up to doses of 8 IU (2.67 mg). At higher doses (60 IU/20 mg) some degree of non-linearity cannot be ruled out, however with no clinical relevance.

Following IV administration in healthy volunteers the volume of distribution at steady-state is around 7 L, total metabolic clearance is around 15 L/h while the renal clearance is negligible, and the drug exhibits an elimination half-life of 20 to 35 min.

Following single-dose SC and IM administration of Saizen®, the apparent terminal half-life is much longer, around 2 to 4 hours. This is due to a rate limiting absorption process.

Maximum serum growth hormone (GH) concentrations are reached after approximatively 4 hours and serum GH levels return to baseline within 24 hours, indicating that no accumulation of GH will occur during repeated administrations.

The absolute bioavailability of both routes is 70-90 %.

5.3 Preclinical safety data

The local tolerability of Saizen® solutions containing 0.3% metacresol when injected in animals was considered good and found suitable for SC or IM administration.

Preclinical data reveal no special hazard for humans based on conventional studies of safety pharmacology, repeated dose toxicity and genotoxicity. Reproductive toxicology studies do not indicate any adverse effect on fertility and reproduction, despite administration of doses sufficiently high to produce some pharmacological effects on growth.

6. PHARMACEUTICAL PARTICULARS

6.1 List of excipients

Powder for solution for injection

Sucrose

Phosphoric acid

Sodium Hydroxide

Solvent for parenteral use

Metacresol 0.3% (w/v) in water for injections

6.2 Incompatibilities

No incompatibilities of Saizen® with other pharmaceutical preparations are known at present.

6.3 Shelf life

3 years.

The reconstituted solution for injection is stable for 28 days.

6.4 Special precautions for storage

Do not store above 25°C. Store in the original package.

Store the reconstituted product at 2°C to 8°C in the cartridge.

Do not freeze.

6.5 Nature and contents of container

The DIN 2R 3 ml vials of Saizen® 8 mg click.easy™ and the cartridges of the solvent are of neutral glass (Type I).

Saizen® 8 mg click.easy™ is available in the following pack sizes:

1 vial of Saizen® 8 mg product and 1 cartridge of bacteriostatic solvent pre-assembled in 1 reconstitution device (click.easy™) comprising of 1 device housing and 1 sterile transfer cannula, 1 plunger rod.

5 vials of Saizen® 8 mg product and 5 cartridges of bacteriostatic solvent pre-assembled in 5 reconstitution devices (click.easy™) comprising each of 1 device housing and 1 sterile transfer cannula, 5 plunger rods.

Not all pack sizes may be marketed.

6.6 Instructions for use and handling

The cartridge containing the reconstituted solution of Saizen®

8 mg click.easy™ is for use only with the one.click™ auto-injector or the cool.click™ needle-free auto-injector.

For administration of Saizen® 8 mg click.easy™ follow the instructions given in the package leaflet and in the instruction manual provided with each one.click™ auto-injector or cool.click™ needle-free auto-injector.

The powder for solution for injection must be reconstituted with the enclosed bacteriostatic solvent (0.3% (w/v) metacresol in water for injections) for parenteral use, using the click.easy™ reconstitution device. The reconstituted solution for injection should be clear with no particles. If the solution contains particles, it must not be injected.

Any unused product or waste material should be disposed of in accordance with local requirements.

7. MARKETING AUTHORISATION HOLDER

Serono Ltd

Bedfont Cross, Stanwell Road

Feltham, Middlesex

TW14 8NX

Telephone: +44 (0)20 8818 7200

8. MARKETING AUTHORISATION NUMBER(S)

Product Licence Numbers

SAIZEN® 8 mg click.easy™ PL 03400/0079

Bacteriostatic Solvent cartridge PL 03400/0076

Product Authorisation Number

SAIZEN® 8 mg click.easy™ PA 285/5/4

9. DATE OF FIRST AUTHORISATION/RENEWAL OF THE AUTHORISATION

First authorisation in UK: 30th July 1998 Ireland: 2nd October 1998

Renewed: 3rd April 1999

10. DATE OF REVISION OF THE TEXT

December 2002

LEGAL STATUS

POM*

NAME AND ADDRESS OF DISTRIBUTOR IN IRELAND

Allphar Service Limited

Pharmaceutical Agents and Distributors

Belgard Road

Tallaght

Dublin 24

Telephone: (01) 404 1600

*UK Status

Salactol

(Dermal Laboratories Limited)

1. NAME OF THE MEDICINAL PRODUCT

SALACTOL™

2. QUALITATIVE AND QUANTITATIVE COMPOSITION

Salicylic Acid 16.7% w/w; Lactic Acid 16.7% w/w.

3. PHARMACEUTICAL FORM

Colourless or pale yellow/brown evaporative collodion paint.

4. CLINICAL PARTICULARS

4.1 Therapeutic indications

For the topical treatment of warts, verrucas, corns and calluses.

4.2 Posology and method of administration

For adults, children and the elderly. Salactol should be applied once daily usually at night. It can take up to twelve (12) weeks for resistant lesions to disappear, and it is necessary to persevere with the treatment. Soak the affected site in warm water and pat dry. Gently rub the surface of the wart, verruca, corn or callus with a pumice stone or manicure emery board to remove any hard skin. Using the applicator provided, carefully apply a few drops of Salactol to the lesion, allowing each drop to dry before applying the next one. Take care to localise the application to the affected area. Plantar warts should be covered with an adhesive plaster. Leave for 24 hours. Repeat the procedure daily, after first removing any plaster.

4.3 Contraindications

Not to be used on or near the face, intertriginous or anogenital regions or by diabetics or individuals with impaired peripheral blood circulation. Not to be used in cases of sensitivity to any of the ingredients. Not to be used on moles, birthmarks, hairy warts or on any other skin lesions for which Salactol is not indicated.

4.4 Special warnings and special precautions for use

Keep away from the eyes and mucous membranes. The gel should be applied carefully to the wart, verruca, corn or callus only, to avoid possible irritation of surrounding normal skin. Some mild, transient irritation may be expected, but in cases of more severe or persistent pain/irritation, the treatment should be suspended and/or discontinued. Extremely flammable. Avoid spillage. Avoid inhaling vapour. Replace cap tightly after use. For external use only.

4.5 Interaction with other medicinal products and other forms of Interaction

None known.

4.6 Pregnancy and lactation

No special precautions.

4.7 Effects on ability to drive and use machines

None known.

4.8 Undesirable effects

Salactol may be irritant in certain patients, which in rare instances may appear as a temporary blemish on the skin.

4.9 Overdose

Any excessive use of Salactol could cause irritation of the skin. If this occurs, Salactol should be used more sparingly or applied less frequently. Accidental oral ingestion should be treated immediately by gastric lavage with a 2 to 5% aqueous sodium bicarbonate solution. Fluid and electrolyte balance should be monitored and appropriate supportive measures should be provided. Symptoms include headache, nausea, vomiting, diarrhoea and respiratory depression.

5. PHARMACOLOGICAL PROPERTIES

5.1 Pharmacodynamic properties

The combination of salicylic acid and lactic acid in flexible collodion has been shown to be particularly efficacious in treating warts, verrucas, corns and calluses.

Salicylic acid has bacteriostatic and fungicidal actions as well as keratolytic properties. Its effectiveness for topical treatment of hyperkeratotic skin lesions is based on mild keratolytic action which produces slow and painless destruction of the epithelium. In the treatment of warts, a mild irritant reaction, which may render the virus more prone to immunologic stimulation or response, may add to the mechanical removal of infected cells. Apart from its antiseptic and caustic properties, lactic acid enhances the availability of salicylic acid from the dried collodion.

5.2 Pharmacokinetic properties

Salactol contains 16.7% salicylic acid and 16.7% lactic acid in flexible collodion. The bioavailability of salicylic acid is reduced as the collodion film dries on the skin due to entrapment of the drug which inhibits release. The addition of lactic acid to salicylic acid collodion provides more efficient release of the salicylic acid, since the non-volatile lactic acid remains in the film, thus permitting continued release of the keratolytic which may otherwise be entrapped within the dried collodion film. Systemic absorption of salicylic acid or lactic acid after application to small circumscribed areas is exceedingly unlikely.

5.3 Preclinical safety data

No special information.

6. PHARMACEUTICAL PARTICULARS

6.1 List of excipients

Pyroxylin; Colophony; Castor Oil; IMS; Ether.

6.2 Incompatibilities

None known.

6.3 Shelf life

36 months.

6.4 Special precautions for storage

Do not store above 25°C.

6.5 Nature and contents of container

Amber glass bottle containing 10 ml, incorporating a specially designed spatula for ease of application. This is supplied as an original pack (OP).

6.6 Instructions for use and handling

Not applicable.

7. MARKETING AUTHORISATION HOLDER

Dermal Laboratories

Tatmore Place, Gosmore

Hitchin, Herts SG4 7QR, UK.

8. MARKETING AUTHORISATION NUMBER(S)

0173/5006R.

9. DATE OF FIRST AUTHORISATION/RENEWAL OF THE AUTHORISATION

2 May 2001.

10. DATE OF REVISION OF THE TEXT

February 2002.

Salagen 5 mg Film Coated Tablets

(Novartis Pharmaceuticals UK Ltd)

1. NAME OF THE MEDICINAL PRODUCT

Salagen® 5 mg Film Coated Tablets

2. QUALITATIVE AND QUANTITATIVE COMPOSITION

Each film coated tablet contains 5 mg of pilocarpine hydrochloride.

For excipients, see 6.1.

3. PHARMACEUTICAL FORM

Film coated tablet.

Salagen Tablets for oral use are white, round biconvex tablets, marked " SAL " on one side and " 5 mg " on the other side.

4. CLINICAL PARTICULARS

4.1 Therapeutic indications

i. Alleviation of symptoms of salivary gland hypofunction in patients with severe xerostomia following irradiation for head and neck cancer.

ii. Treatment of symptoms of dry mouth and dry eyes in patients with Sjögren's syndrome.

4.2 Posology and method of administration

i. For head and neck cancer patients

The recommended initial dose for adults is 1 tablet of 5 mg three times daily. Tablets should be taken with a glass of water during or directly after meals. The last tablet should always be taken in conjunction with the evening meal. The maximal therapeutic effect is normally obtained after 4-8 weeks of therapy. For patients who have not responded sufficiently after 4 weeks and who tolerate the dose of 5 mg three times daily, doses of up to a maximum of 30 mg daily may be considered. However, higher daily doses are probably accompanied by an increase in drug-related adverse effects. Therapy should be discontinued if no improvement in xerostomia is noted after 2-3 months of therapy.

ii. For Sjögren's syndrome patients

The recommended dose for adults is one tablet of 5 mg four times daily. Tablets should be taken with a glass of water at meal times and bedtime. For patients who have not responded sufficiently to a dosage of 5 mg four times daily and who tolerate this dosage, increasing the dose up to a maximum of 30 mg daily, divided over the day may be considered. Therapy should be discontinued if no improvement in the symptoms of dry mouth and dry eyes is noted after 2-3 months.

Use in the elderly

There is no evidence to suggest that dosage should be different in the elderly.

Use in children

Safety and effectiveness of this drug in children have not been established.

Use in patients with impaired hepatic function

Patients with moderate and severe cirrhosis should commence treatment on a reduced daily dosage schedule. Depending on the safety and tolerability, the dosage may gradually be increased to the normal daily dosage schedule of 5 mg t.d.s.

4.3 Contraindications

Salagen is contraindicated in patients with clinically significant, uncontrolled cardio-renal disease, uncontrolled asthma and other chronic disease at risk for cholinergic agonists.

In addition, Salagen is contraindicated in patients with a known hypersensitivity to pilocarpine or to any of the excipients and when miosis is undesirable, such as in acute iritis.

4.4 Special warnings and special precautions for use

Pilocarpine has been reported to increase airway resistance in asthmatic patients. Also, patients with significant cardiovascular disease may be unable to compensate for transient changes in haemodynamics or heart rhythm induced by pilocarpine. Therefore, Salagen should be administered to patients with controlled asthma or significant cardiovascular disease only if the benefits are believed to outweigh the risks, and under close medical supervision.

Salagen should be used with caution in patients with the following illnesses/pathologies:

- chronic bronchitis and/or chronic obstructive pulmonary disease; these patients have hyperactive airways and may experience adverse effects due to increased bronchial smooth muscle tone and increased bronchial secretions.
- known or suspected cholelithiasis or biliary tract disease. Contractions of the gallbladder or biliary smooth muscle could precipitate complications including cholecystitis, cholangitis and biliary obstruction.
- peptic ulceration, due to the risk of increased acid secretion.
- underlying cognitive or psychiatric disturbances. Cholinergic agonists, like pilocarpine hydrochloride, may have dose-related central nervous system effects.
- renal insufficiency. Insufficient information is available to determine the importance of renal excretion of pilocarpine and its metabolites in relation to metabolic inactivation so as to recommend dosage adjustments for these patients. Pilocarpine may increase ureteral smooth muscle tone and could theoretically precipitate renal colic (or "ureteral reflux"), particularly in patients with nephrolithiasis.

Salagen should be administered with caution in patients with narrow-angle glaucoma.

Caution should be exercised in patients who are known or expected to sweat excessively and who cannot drink enough liquids, since dehydration could develop.

4.5 Interaction with other medicinal products and other forms of Interaction

Salagen should be administered with caution to patients taking beta-adrenergic antagonists because of the possibility of conduction disturbances.

Concurrent administration of Salagen and drugs with parasympathomimetic effects is expected to result in additive pharmacologic effects.

Pilocarpine might antagonise the anticholinergic effects of other drugs used concomitantly (e.g. atropine, inhaled ipratropium).

While no formal drug interaction studies have been performed, the following concomitant drugs were used in at least 10% of patients in either or both Sjögren's efficacy studies: acetylsalicylic acid, artificial tears, calcium, conjugated estrogens, hydroxychloroquine sulfate, ibuprofen, levothyroxine sodium, medroxyprogesterone acetate, methotrexate, multivitamins, naproxen, omeprazole, paracetamol, and prednisone. There were no reports of drug toxicities during either efficacy studies.

4.6 Pregnancy and lactation

Pregnancy

The safety of this medicinal product for use in human pregnancy has not been established. There are no known human data for the effects of pilocarpine on foetal survival and development. However, pre- and post-natal studies in rats have shown some toxicity (see Section 5.3 for details).

Salagen should not be given to a pregnant woman, unless the risks and benefit of the treatment have been carefully evaluated by the physician.

Nursing mothers

It is not known whether pilocarpine or its metabolites are secreted in human milk. Salagen should not be prescribed to a woman during lactation, unless the risk for the baby of continuing breast-feeding has been carefully evaluated by the physician.

Fertility

The effects of pilocarpine on male and female fertility are not known. Studies in rats have shown adverse effects on spermatogenesis and a possible impairment of female fertility (see Section 5.3 for details).

4.7 Effects on ability to drive and use machines

Ocular formulations of pilocarpine have been reported to cause impairment of depth perception and visual blurring. The latter may result in decreased visual acuity, especially at night and in patients with central lens changes. If this occurs, patients should be advised not to drive at night or perform hazardous activities in reduced lighting.

Patients who experience dizziness during Salagen treatment should be advised not to drive or operate machinery.

4.8 Undesirable effects

Most of the adverse experiences observed during Salagen treatment were a consequence of exaggerated parasympathetic stimulation. These adverse experiences were dose-dependent and usually mild and self-limited. However, severe adverse experiences might occasionally occur and, therefore, careful monitoring of the patient is recommended.

In controlled clinical trials the following adverse reactions were observed:

General Disorders

Very common (≥ 10%): flu syndrome

Common (1 - 10%): astheania, chills

Respiratory thoracic and mediastinal disorders

Common (1 - 10%): rhinitis

Skin and subcutaneous tissue disorders

Very common (≥ 10%): sweating

Common (1 –10%): allergic reactions, including rash, pruritus

Nervous System Disorders

Very common (≥ 10%): headache

Common (1 - 10%): dizziness

Renal and urinary disorders

Very common (≥ 10%): increased urinary frequency

Uncommon (0.1 – 1%): urinary urgency

Gastrointestinal adverse effects

Common (1 - 10%): dyspepsia; diarrhoea, abdominal pain, nausea, vomiting, constipation, increased salivation

Uncommon (0.1% - 1%): flatulence

Cardiovascular adverse effects

Common (1 - 10%): flushing (vasodilatation), hypertension, palpitations

Ocular adverse effects

Common (1 - 10%): lacrimation, blurred vision, abnormal vision, conjunctivitis, eye pain

There is no indication of a difference between older and younger patients, receiving Salagen, in reporting adverse experiences, except for dizziness, which was reported significantly more often by patients over 65 years.

The following adverse effects, which are due to the intrinsic pharmacological properties of pilocarpine, have been published in the medical literature:

- respiratory distress
- gastro-intestinal spasm
- atrio-ventricular block
- tachycardia
- bradycardia
- cardiac arrhythmia
- hypotension
- shock, tremors
- mental status changes including memory loss, hallucinations, lability of affect, confusion, agitation.

4.9 Overdose

Overdosage should be treated with atropine titration (0.5 mg to 1.0 mg given subcutaneously or intravenously) and supportive measures to maintain respiration and circulation. Adrenaline (0.3 mg to 1.0 mg, subcutaneously or intramuscularly) may also be of value in the presence of severe cardiovascular depression or bronchoconstrictor responses. It is not known if pilocarpine is dialysable. There is no safety information for doses greater than 10 mg t.d.s.

5. PHARMACOLOGICAL PROPERTIES

5.1 Pharmacodynamic properties

Pharmacotherapeutic group: Parasympathominetic

ATC code: N07A X01

Pilocarpine is a cholinergic parasympathomimetic agent exerting a broad spectrum of pharmacologic effects with predominant muscarinic action. Pilocarpine, in appropriate dosage, can increase secretion by exocrine glands such as the sweat, salivary, lacrimal, gastric, pancreatic and intestinal glands and the mucous cells of the respiratory tract.

Dose-related smooth muscle stimulation of the intestinal tract may cause increased tone, increased motility, spasm and tenesmus. Bronchial smooth muscle tone may increase. The tone and motility of urinary tract, gallbladder and biliary duct smooth muscle may be enhanced.

Pilocarpine may have paradoxical effects on the cardiovascular system. The expected effect of a muscarinic agonist is vasodepression, but administration of pilocarpine may produce hypertension after a brief episode of hypotension. Bradycardia and tachycardia have both been reported with use of pilocarpine.

In a study in healthy male volunteers an increase in salivary flow following single 5 and 10 mg doses of Salagen was noted 20 minutes after administration and lasted for 3 to 5 hours with a peak at 1 hour.

i. For head and neck cancer patients:

In two 12-week randomized, double-blind, placebo-controlled clinical studies in patients with xerostomia resulting from irradiation to the head and neck for cancer, Salagen treatment reduced dryness of the mouth; in one of these studies this did not occur until after 12 weeks of treatment. Also, Salagen treatment increased salivary flow. The greatest improvement in dryness was noted in patients with no measurable salivary flow at baseline.

In both studies, some patients noted improvement in the overall condition of xerostomia, speaking without drinking liquids and mouth comfort and there was reduced use of concomitant therapy (i.e., artificial saliva) for dry mouth.

ii. For Sjögren's syndrome patients:

Two separate 12-week randomized, double-blind, placebo-controlled clinical studies were conducted in patients diagnosed with primary or secondary Sjögren's syndrome. In both studies, the majority of patients best fit the European criteria for having primary Sjögren's syndrome. The ability of Salagen to stimulate saliva production was assessed. Relative to placebo, an increase in the amount of saliva being produced was observed following the first dose and was maintained throughout the duration of the trials in an approximate dose response fashion.

Compared to placebo, a statistically significant global improvement for both dry mouth and dry eyes was observed.

Efficacy of Salagen has not been established in patients with the Sjögren's syndrome during long term treatment > 12 weeks).

5.2 Pharmacokinetic properties

In a multiple-dose, pharmacokinetic study in volunteers given 5 or 10 mg of pilocarpine hydrochloride t.d.s. for two days, the T_{max} after the final dose was approximately 1 hour, the elimination T½ was approximately 1 hour, and the mean C_{maxs} were 15 ng/ml and 41 ng/ml for the 5 and 10 mg doses, respectively.

Pharmacokinetics in elderly male volunteers were comparable to those in younger subjects. In a small number of healthy, elderly, female volunteers the mean C_{max} and AUC were approximately twice that of elderly and young male volunteers, due to smaller volumes of distribution. However, the observed difference in pharmacokinetics was not reflected in the incidence of adverse events between young and elderly female patients.

When taken with a high fat meal by healthy, male volunteers, there was a decrease in the rate of absorption of pilocarpine from Salagen tablets. Mean T_{maxs} were 1.47 and 0.87 hours and mean C_{maxs} were 51.8 and 59.2 ng/ml for fed and fasted volunteers, respectively.

In a study with male albino rats, which were administered single s.c. injections at doses in the range of the median lethal dose (200 - 1000 mg/kg in rat), pilocarpine hydrochloride was found to cross the blood-brain barrier.

There is limited information available concerning the metabolism and elimination of pilocarpine in humans. Inactivation of pilocarpine is thought to occur at neuronal synapses and probably in plasma.

A single dose pharmacokinetic study in humans showed that an average of 30% of the orally administered dose of 10 mg pilocarpine could be detected in the urine after 12 hours, of which 14% was recovered as pilocarpic acid. No other metabolites were detected in the urine. It is expected that the remaining 70% is excreted via other routes and/or metabolised to unknown metabolites.

An *in-vitro* study showed that pilocarpine does not bind to plasma proteins.

5.3 Preclinical safety data

Genotoxicity and carcinogenicity

Preclinical data revealed no special hazard for humans based on conventional studies of genotoxicity and carcinogenic potential.

Reproductive toxicity

Two studies were conducted in rats in which males and females were exposed to pilocarpine before and after mating. Dosing in the females continuing to 21 days after parturition. There was evidence that doses of 18 mg/kg per day and above for 28 days to male rats would affect fertility adversely, decrease sperm motility and increase incidence of abnormal sperm. In females at these doses there was evidence of decreased fertility index and prolonged dioestrus. Offspring survival was decreased.

For these changes to reproductive performance, 3 mg/kg per day was a No Effect dose.

The post-natal development of the surviving F1 generation was not affected by doses of up to 72 mg/kg per day to the dams and the F2 generation was normal.

There was no evidence of a teratogenic effect at any dose in these studies.

6. PHARMACEUTICAL PARTICULARS

6.1 List of excipients

Binder/diluent

Microcrystalline cellulose

Acidifier/lubricant

Stearic acid

Film coating

Opadry white

YS-1-7003, containing hypromellose

Macrogol 400

Polysorbate 80

Titanium dioxide (E 171)

Polish

Carnauba wax

Branding ink

Opacode black

S-1-8085, containing Shellac

Propylene glycol

Synthetic black iron oxide (E 172)

6.2 Incompatibilities

Not applicable

6.3 Shelf life

3 years

6.4 Special precautions for storage

Do not store above 25°C.

Store in the original package in order to protect from light and moisture.

6.5 Nature and contents of container

Salagen is distributed for sale in perforated Al/PVC/PVDC blisters.

Each blister contains 14 or 21 tablets.

A cardboard box contains 1, 2 or 6 of the 14-tablet blisters, or 1 or 4 of the 21-tablet blisters. Each cardboard box contains a patient package insert.

Not all pack sizes may be marketed.

6.6 Instructions for use and handling

No special requirements.

7. MARKETING AUTHORISATION HOLDER

Novartis Pharmaceuticals UK Ltd

Frimley Business Park

Frimley

Surrey, GU16 7SR

UK

8. MARKETING AUTHORISATION NUMBER(S)

PL 00101/0630

9. DATE OF FIRST AUTHORISATION/RENEWAL OF THE AUTHORISATION

18 April 2002

10. DATE OF REVISION OF THE TEXT

17 December 2004

LEGAL CATEGORY

POM

Salatac Gel

(Dermal Laboratories Limited)

1. NAME OF THE MEDICINAL PRODUCT

SALATAC® GEL

2. QUALITATIVE AND QUANTITATIVE COMPOSITION

Salicylic Acid 12.0% w/w; Lactic Acid 4.0% w/w.

3. PHARMACEUTICAL FORM

Clear, colourless, collodion-like wart gel.

4. CLINICAL PARTICULARS

4.1 Therapeutic indications

For the topical treatment of warts, verrucas, corns and calluses.

4.2 Posology and method of administration

For adults, children and the elderly. Salatac Gel should be applied once daily. The gel should be applied once every night. Treatment can take up to twelve (12) weeks for resistant lesions to disappear, and it is necessary to persevere with treatment.

1. Every night, soak the affected site in warm water for 2 to 3 minutes.

2. Dry thoroughly with the patient's own towel.

3. Carefully apply one or two drops of the gel to the lesion and allow to dry over its surface. Take care to avoid spreading on to surrounding normal skin. No adhesive plaster is necessary.

4. The following evening, carefully remove and discard the elastic film formed from the previous application, and reapply the gel. Occasionally, if removal of the elastic film proves difficult, carefully reapply the gel over it and allow to dry. This should help thicken the film to assist removal. If necessary, such re-application may be made on two or three successive days.

5. Once a week, gently rub away the treated surface using an emery board, as provided, or pumice stone used only for this purpose, before re-applying the gel.

6. The wart, verruca, corn or callus may take up to twelve (12) weeks to disappear and it is important to persevere with the treatment.

7. At the end of treatment, if the elastic film is difficult to remove, it may be allowed to remain on the skin until it sheds.

4.3 Contraindications

Not to be used on or near the face, intertriginous or anogenital regions, or by diabetics or individuals with impaired peripheral blood circulation. Not to be used on moles or on any other skin lesions for which the gel is not indicated. Not to be used in cases of sensitivity to any of the ingredients.

4.4 Special warnings and special precautions for use

Keep away from the eyes, mucous membranes and from cuts and grazes. The gel should be applied carefully to the wart, verruca, corn or callus only, to avoid possible irritation of surrounding normal skin. Do not use excessively. Some mild, transient irritation may be expected, but in cases of more severe or persistent pain/irritation, treatment should be suspended and/or discontinued. Avoid inhaling vapour, and keep cap firmly closed when not in use. Contact with clothing, fabrics, plastics and other materials may cause damage, and should be avoided. For external use only.

4.5 Interaction with other medicinal products and other forms of Interaction

None known.

4.6 Pregnancy and lactation

No special precautions.

4.7 Effects on ability to drive and use machines

None known.

4.8 Undesirable effects

Salatac Gel may be irritant in certain patients, which in rare instances may appear as a temporary blemish on the skin.

4.9 Overdose

Any excessive use of Salatac Gel could cause irritation of the skin. If this occurs, Salatac Gel should be used more sparingly or applied less frequently.

5. PHARMACOLOGICAL PROPERTIES

5.1 Pharmacodynamic properties

The active ingredients, salicylic acid and lactic acid, are well-established pharmacopoeial substances. In combination, they are routinely used in the treatment of verrucas, warts, corns and calluses for their keratolytic properties.

When applied topically, and in high enough concentrations, salicylic acid acts by achieving a slow, painless destruction of the thickened stratum corneum. It softens and destroys the stratum corneum of the affected tissue by reducing the adhesiveness of the corneocytes while causing the cornified epithelium to swell, soften, macerate and finally desquamate. In the treatment of warts, a mild irritant reaction, which may render the virus more prone to immunologic stimulation or response, may add to the mechanical removal of infected cells. The other active ingredient, lactic acid, enhances the availability of the salicylic acid from the dried collodion, in addition to having antiseptic and caustic properties.

5.2 Pharmacokinetic properties

Salatac Gel contains 12% salicylic acid and 4% lactic acid in an evaporative collodion-like gel which forms a cohesive and adhesive film on the skin.

The formulation is presented in a collapsible aluminium tube fitted with a special applicator nozzle allowing the formulation to be dispensed precisely to the affected areas only. This minimises the spread of the preparation onto the surrounding healthy skin which could otherwise lead to inflammation, irritation and poor patient compliance. The film-forming characteristics of the collodion-like gel vehicle also offer distinct advantages in clinical usage.

The gel quickly forms a surface film, well before it dries completely, thereby prolonging the period during which the keratolytic solution can properly infiltrate and achieve intimate contact with the surface layers of the thickened stratum corneum.

Furthermore, even when the film appears to have dried completely, the inclusion of the non-evaporative lactic acid ensures that a proportion of the salicylic acid remains in solution within the vehicle, thus permitting continued release of the keratolytic, which may otherwise be entrapped within the collodion-like film.

Systemic absorption of salicylic acid or lactic acid after application of the recommended daily dose of one or two drops of the preparation to small, circumscribed areas is exceedingly unlikely.

5.3 Preclinical safety data
No special information.

6. PHARMACEUTICAL PARTICULARS

6.1 List of excipients
Camphor; Pyroxylin; Ethanol (96%); Ethyl Acetate.

6.2 Incompatibilities
None known.

6.3 Shelf life
36 months.

6.4 Special precautions for storage
Highly flammable - keep away from flames. Do not store above 25°C.

6.5 Nature and contents of container
Collapsible tube containing 8 g, complete with special applicator, emery board and instructions. This is supplied as an original pack (OP).

6.6 Instructions for use and handling
Not applicable.

7. MARKETING AUTHORISATION HOLDER
Dermal Laboratories
Tatmore Place, Gosmore
Hitchin, Herts SG4 7QR, UK.

8. MARKETING AUTHORISATION NUMBER(S)
0173/0046.

9. DATE OF FIRST AUTHORISATION/RENEWAL OF THE AUTHORISATION
20 April 1999.

10. DATE OF REVISION OF THE TEXT
September 2001.

Salazopyrin En-Tabs

(Pharmacia Limited)

1. NAME OF THE MEDICINAL PRODUCT
Salazopyrin En-Tabs

2. QUALITATIVE AND QUANTITATIVE COMPOSITION
Sulfasalazine EP 500mg

3. PHARMACEUTICAL FORM
Yellow film-coated, ovoid gastro-resistant tablets embossed "Kph" on one side and "102" on the other.

4. CLINICAL PARTICULARS

4.1 Therapeutic indications
a) Induction and maintenance of remission of ulcerative colitis; treatment of active Crohn's Disease.

b) Treatment of rheumatoid arthritis which has failed to respond to non-steroidal anti-inflammatory drugs (NSAIDs).

4.2 Posology and method of administration
EN-Tablets should be used where there is gastro-intestinal intolerance of plain tablets. They should not be crushed or broken.

The dose is adjusted according to the severity of the disease and the patient's tolerance to the drug, as detailed below.

Elderly Patients: No special precautions are necessary.

a) Ulcerative colitis

Adults

Severe Attack: Salazopyrin 2-4 tablets four times a day may be given in conjunction with steroids as part of an intensive management regime. Rapid passage of the tablets may reduce effect of the drug.

Night-time interval between doses should not exceed 8 hours.

Moderate Attack: 2-4 tablets four times a day may be given in conjunction with steroids.

Mild Attack: 2 tablets four times a day with or without steroids.

Maintenance Therapy: With induction of remission reduce the dose gradually to 4 tablets per day. This dosage should be continued indefinitely, since discontinuance even several years after an acute attack is associated with a four fold increase in risk of relapse.

Children

The dose is reduced in proportion to body weight.

Acute Attack or relapse: 40- 60mg/kg per day

Maintenance Dosage: 20 - 30mg/kg per day

Salazopyrin Suspension may provide a more flexible dosage form.

b) Crohn 's Disease

In active Crohn's Disease, Salazopyrin should be administered as in attacks of ulcerative colitis (see above).

c) Rheumatoid Arthritis

Patients with rheumatoid arthritis, and those treated over a long period with NSAIDs, may have sensitive stomachs and for this reason enteric-coated Salazopyrin (EN-Tabs) are recommended for this disease, as follows:

The patient should start with one tablet daily, increasing his dosage by a tablet a day each week until one tablet four times a day, or two three times a day are reached, according to tolerance and response. Onset of effect is slow and a marked effect may not be seen for six weeks. A reduction in ESR and C-reactive protein should accompany an improvement in joint mobility. $NSAID_s$ may be taken concurrently with Salazopyrin.

4.3 Contraindications
i) Use in infants under the age of 2 years.

ii) Use in patients where there is a significant hypersensitivity to sulfasalazine, sulfonamides or salicylates.

iii) Acute intermittent porphyria.

4.4 Special warnings and special precautions for use
Precautions: Haematological and hepatic side effects may occur. Differential white cell, red cell and platelet counts should be performed initially and at least monthly for a minimum of the first three months of treatment. The patient should also be counselled to report immediately with any sore throat, fever, malaise or unexpected non-specific illness. Treatment should be stopped immediately if there is suspicion or laboratory evidence of a potentially serious blood dyscrasia.

Liver function tests should be carried out at monthly intervals for the first three months of treatment. Patients with liver disease should be treated with caution.

The kidney function should be checked initially and at regular intervals during the treatment. Since sulfasalazine may cause haemolytic anaemia, it should be used with caution in patients with G-6-PD deficiency.

Changes in the blood picture (e.g. macrocytosis and pancytopenia) due to folic acid deficiency can be normalised by administration of folic acid or folinic acid (leucovorin).

4.5 Interaction with other medicinal products and other forms of Interaction
Uptake of digoxin and folate may be reduced.

Adequate fluid intake and avoidance of acidification of the urine (such as with concomitant use of methenamine) may minimise crystalluria and stone formation.

Sulfonamides bear certain chemical similarities to some oral hypoglycemic agents. Hypoglycemia has occurred in patients receiving sulfonamides. Patients receiving sulfasalazine and hypoglycemic agents should be closely monitored.

Due to inhibition of thiopurine methyltransferase by salazopyrin, bone marrow suppression and leucopenia have been reported when the thiopurine 6-mercaptopurine or it's prodrug, azathioprine, and oral salazopyrin were used concomitantly.

4.6 Pregnancy and lactation
Long-term clinical usage and experimental studies have failed to reveal any teratogenic or icteric hazards. The amounts of drug present in the milk should not present a risk to a healthy infant.

4.7 Effects on ability to drive and use machines
No specific effects.

4.8 Undesirable effects
Overall, about 75% of ADRs occur within 3 months of starting therapy, and over 90% by 6 months. Some undesirable effects are dose-dependent and symptoms can often be alleviated by reduction of the dose.

General

Sulfasalazine is split by intestinal bacteria to sulfapyridine and 5-amino salicylate so ADRs to either sulfonamide or salicylate are possible. Patients with slow acetylator status are more likely to experience ADRs related to sulfapyridine. The most commonly encountered ADRs are nausea, headache, rash, loss of appetite and raised temperature.

Specific

The following reactions have been recorded in patients taking sulfasalazine:

Haematological. Potentially fatal leucopenia, neutropenia, agranulocytosis, aplastic anaemia and thrombocytopenia. Leucopenia, which is normally mild and transient, may occur in up to 1.5% of patients and agranulocytosis in up to one in 700 patients during the second month of therapy.

The risk of sulfasalazine associated blood disorders is substantially higher in patients treated for rheumatoid arthritis than it is for patients treated for inflammatory bowel disease.

Heinz body anaemia, methaemoglobinaemia, hypoprothrombinaemia, haemolytic anaemia, megaloblastic anaemia.

Hypersensitivity reactions

Generalised skin eruptions, Stevens-Johnson Syndrome, exfoliative dermatitis, epidermal necrolysis, pruritis, urticaria, photosensitisation, anaphylaxis, serum sickness, drug fever, lymphadenopathy, periorbital oedema, conjuctivial and scleral polyarteritis nodosa, LE-phenomenon and lung complications with dyspnoea, fever, cough, eosinophilia, fibrosing alveolitis, pericarditis, vasculitis, nephritis, alopecia.

Gastro-intestinal reactions

Stomatitis, parotitis, pancreatitis, hepatitis.

CNS Reactions

Vertigo, tinnitus, peripheral neuropathy, aseptic meningitis, ataxia, convulsions, insomnia, mental depression and hallucinations.

Fertility

Oligospermia, reversible on discontinuance of drug.

Renal Reactions

Crystalluria, haematuria, proteinuria and nephrotic syndrome.

4.9 Overdose
The drug has low acute per oral toxicity in the absence of hyper-sensitivity. There is no specific antidote and treatment should be supportive.

5. PHARMACOLOGICAL PROPERTIES

5.1 Pharmacodynamic properties
Pharmacological particulars: around 90% of a dose reaches the colon where bacteria split the drug into sulfapyridine (SP) and mesalazine (ME). These are also active, and the unsplit sulfasalazine (SASP) is also active on a variety of symptoms. Most SP is absorbed, hydroxylated or glucuronidated and a mix of unchanged and metabolised SP appears in the urine. Some ME is taken up and acetylated in the colon wall, such that renal excretion is mainly AC-ME. SASP is excreted unchanged in the bile and urine.

Overall the drug and its metablites exert immunimodulatory effects, antibacterial effects, effects on the arachidonic acid cascade and alteration of activity of certain enzymes. The net result clinically is a reduction in activity of the inflammatory bowel disease. In rheumatoid arthritis a disease modifying effect is evident in 1-3 months, with characteristics falls in CRP and other indicators of inflammation. ME is not believed to be responsible for this effect.

Radiographic studies show marked reduction in progression (larsen or sharp index) compared with placebo or hydroxychloroquine over two years in early patients. If drug is stopped the benefit appears to be maintained.

5.2 Pharmacokinetic properties
Pharmacokinetic particulars: studies with en-tabs show no statistically significant differences in main parameters compared with an equivalent dose of SASP powder, and the figures produced below relate to ordinary tablets. With regard to the use of Salazopyrin in bowel disease there is no evidence that systemic levels are of any relevance other than with regard to ADR incidence. Here levels of SP over about 50μg/ml are associated with a substantial risk of ADRS, especially in slow acetylators.

For SASP given as a single 3g oral dose, peak serum levels of SASP occured in 3-5 hours, elimination half life was 5.7±0.7 hours, lag time 1.5 hours. During maintenance therapy renal clearance of SASP was 7.3±1.7ml/min, for SP 9.9±1.9 and AC-ME 100±20. Free SP first appears in plasma in 4.3 hours after a single dose with an absorption half life of 2.7 hours. The elimination half life was calculated as 18 hours.

Turning to mesalazine, in urine only AC-ME (not free ME) was demonstrable, the acetylation probably largely achieved in the colon mucosa. After a 3g SASP dose lag time was 6.1±2.3 hours and plasma levels kept below 2μg/ml total ME. Urinary excretion half life was 6.0±3.1 hours and absorption half life based on these figures 3.0±1.5 hours. Renal clearance constant was 125ml/min corresponding to the GFR.

With regard to rheumatoid arthritis there is no data which suggests any differences from those above.

5.3 Preclinical safety data
In two-year carcinogenicity studies in rats and mice, sulfasalazine showed some evidence of carcinogenicity. In rats, there was a small increase in the incidence of transitional cell papillomas in the urinary bladder and kidney. The tumours were judged to be induced mechanically by calculi formed in the urine rather than through a direct genotoxic mechanism. In the mouse study, there was a significant increase in the incidence of hepatocellular adenoma or carcinoma. The mechanism of induction of hepatocellular neoplasia has been investigated and attributed to species-specific effects of sulfasalazine that are not relevant to humans.

Sulfasalazine did not show mutagenicity in the bacterial reverse mutation assay (Ames test) or in the L51784 mouse lymphoma cell assay at the HGPRT gene. It did not induce sister chromatid exchanges or chromosomal aberrations in cultured Chinese hamster ovary cells, and in vivo mouse bone marrow chromosomal aberration tests were negative. However, sulfasalazine showed positive or equivocal mutagenic responses in rat and mouse micronucleus assays, and in human lymphocyte sister chromatid exchange, chromosomal aberration and micronucleus assays. The ability of sulfasalazine to induce chromosome damage has been attributed to perturbation of folic acid levels rather than to a direct genotoxic mechanism.

Based on information from non-clinical studies, sulfasalazine is judged to pose no carcinogenic risk to humans. Sulfasalazine use has not been associated with the development of neoplasia in human epidemiology studies.

6. PHARMACEUTICAL PARTICULARS

6.1 List of excipients
Povidone; maize starch; magnesium stearate; colloidal silicon dioxide; cellulose acetate phthalate; propylene glycol; traces of beeswax, carnauba wax, glyceryl monostearate, talc.

6.2 Incompatibilities
Certain types of extended wear soft contact lenses may be permanently stained during therapy.

6.3 Shelf life
The tablets are stable for five years.

6.4 Special precautions for storage
Store in a dry place

6.5 Nature and contents of container
Polyolefin Square pot with screw cap. To contain 112 tablets

6.6 Instructions for use and handling
Take the tablets whole: Do not break

7. MARKETING AUTHORISATION HOLDER
Pharmacia Ltd
C/O Pfizer Limited
Ramsgate Road
Sandwich
Kent CT13 9NJ
United Kingdom

8. MARKETING AUTHORISATION NUMBER(S)
PL 00032/0387

9. DATE OF FIRST AUTHORISATION/RENEWAL OF THE AUTHORISATION
16 September 2002

10. DATE OF REVISION OF THE TEXT
21st December 2004

11. LEGAL CATEGORY
POM.

SZB1_0

Salazopyrin Suppositories

(Pharmacia Limited)

1. NAME OF THE MEDICINAL PRODUCT
Salazopyrin Suppositories

2. QUALITATIVE AND QUANTITATIVE COMPOSITION
Sulfasalazine EP 0.5 g

3. PHARMACEUTICAL FORM
Suppository

4. CLINICAL PARTICULARS

4.1 Therapeutic indications
Ulcerative colitis or Crohn's Disease affecting the rectum.

4.2 Posology and method of administration
The dose is adjusted according to the severity of the disease and the patient's tolerance of the drug.

Acute attack or relapse - Adults and the Elderly

Two suppositories are to be inserted in the morning and two at bedtime after defecation. After three weeks the dosage is gradually reduced as improvement occurs.

Adjustment to oral therapy - Adults and the Elderly

In severe generalised ulcerative colitis of the rectum or recto sigmoid, or in cases who are responding slowly to oral therapy, one or two suppositories may be given in the morning and at bedtime additional to oral therapy.

Children

The adult dose is reduced on the basis of body weight.

4.3 Contraindications

General

Because of lower absorption levels and shorter retention time in the body, Salazopyrin Suppositories give rise to fewer adverse events than equivalent treatment by mouth. However, because of the theoretical possibility that serious adverse events can arise from treatment from either route, the details below are based on adverse event reports to both oral and rectal treatment.

i) A history of allergy to sulfonamides or salicylates.

ii) Use in infants under two years old.

iii) Acute intermittent porphyria.

4.4 Special warnings and special precautions for use
Haematological and hepatic side effects may occur. Differential white cell, red cell and platelet counts should be performed initially and at least monthly for a minimum of the first three months of treatment. The patient should also be counselled to report immediately with any sore throat, fever, malaise or unexpected non-specific illness. Treatment should be stopped immediately if there is suspicion or laboratory evidence of a potentially serious blood dyscrasia.

Liver function tests should be carried out at monthly intervals for the first three months of treatment. Patients with liver disease should be treated with caution.

The kidney function should be checked initially and at regular intervals during the treatment. Since sulfasalazine may cause haemolytic anaemia, it should be used with caution in patients with G-6-PD deficiency.

Changes in the blood picture (e.g., macrocytosis and pancytopenia) due to folic acid deficiency can be normalised by administration of folic acid or folinic acid (leucovorin).

4.5 Interaction with other medicinal products and other forms of Interaction
There have been no adverse interactions reported, due to the drug largely remaining confined to the rectum. However, there is a potential for interaction as follows:

Adequate fluid intake and avoidance of acidification of the urine (such as with concomitant use of methenamine) may minimise crystalluria and stone formation.

Sulfonamides bear certain chemical similarities to some oral hypoglycemic agents. Hypoglycemia has occurred in patients receiving sulfonamides. Patients receiving sulfasalazine and hypoglycemic agents should be closely monitored.

Due to inhibition of thiopurine methyltransferase by salazopyrin, bone marrow suppression and leucopenia have been reported when the thiopurine 6-mercaptopurine or it's prodrug, azathioprine, and oral salazopyrin were used concomitantly.

4.6 Pregnancy and lactation
Long-term clinical usage and experimental studies have failed to reveal any teratogenic or icteric hazards. The amounts of drug present in the milk should not present a risk to a healthy infant.

4.7 Effects on ability to drive and use machines
No specific effects.

4.8 Undesirable effects
The following have been reported to sulfasalazine given orally or rectally. The drug rectally is well tolerated. Overall, about 75% of adverse drug reactions occur within three months of starting therapy and over 90% by six months. Some undesirable effects are dose-dependent and symptoms can often be alleviated by reduction of the dose.

General

Sulfasalazine is split by intestinal bacteria to sulfapyridine and 5-amino salicylate so adverse drugs reactions to either sulfonamide or salicylate are possible. Patients with slow acetylator status are more likely to experience adverse drug reactions related to sulfapyridine. The most commonly encountered adverse drugs reactions are nausea, headache, rash, loss of appetite and raised temperature.

Specific

The following reactions have been recorded in patients taking sulfasalazine:

Haematological

Potentially fatal leucopenia, neutropenia, agranulocytosis, aplastic anaemia and thrombocytopenia. Leucopenia which is normally mild and transient, may occur in up to 1.5% of patients and agranulocytosis in up to one in 700 patients during the second month of therapy.

Heinz body anaemia, methaemoglobinaemia, hypoprothrombinaemia, haemolytic anaemia, megaloblastic anaemia.

Hypersensitivity Reactions

Generalised skin eruptions, Stevens-Johnson syndrome, exfoliative dermatitis, epidermal necrolysis, pruritus, urticaria, photosensitisation, anaphylaxis, serum sickness, drug fever, lymphadenopathy, periorbital oedema, conjunctival and scleral injection, arthralgia, allergic myocarditis, polyarteritis nodosa, LE-phenomenon and lung complications with dyspnoea, fever, cough, eosinophilia, fibrosing alveolitis, pericarditis, vasculitis, nephritis, alopecia.

Gastro-intestinal Reactions

Stomatitis, parotitis, pancreatitis, hepatitis.

CNS Reactions

Vertigo, tinnitus, peripheral neuropathy, aseptic meningitis, ataxia, convulsions, insomnia, mental depression and hallucinations.

Fertility

Oligospermia, reversible on discontinuance of drug.

Renal Reactions

Crystalluria, haematuria, proteinuria and nephrotic syndrome.

4.9 Overdose
Overdose with suppositories is unlikely. In the event, evacuate the bowel and treat supportively. The toxicity of sulphasalazine is low in acute dosage. There is no specific antidote.

5. PHARMACOLOGICAL PROPERTIES

5.1 Pharmacodynamic properties
Therapeutic benefit of sulfasalazine in ulcerative colitis and Crohn's Disease appears to be due to a local action of the sulfasalazine and its split product 5-aminosalicylic acid on the mucous membrane and deeper colonic structures. Pharmacological actions noted for these compounds include inhibition of neutrophil activation, free radical scavenging, inhibition of superoxide production, inhibition of bacterial growth. Sulfasalazine inhibits 15-Prostaglandin dehydrogenase and slows prostaglandin metabolism. Lipoxygenase release in inflammatory cells is also depressed. NK cells and T cell proliferation are inhibited.

5.2 Pharmacokinetic properties
There are considerable individual differences in the retention time of suppositories in volunteer studies. Consequently uptake values vary widely also. Given that the effect of the drug is almost certainly due to a local effect pharmacokinetics becomes less relevant to therapeutic action than to possible adverse effects related to systemic levels.

A study of five volunteers over three days following insertion of 2 × 0.5 g suppositories gave the following results:

Retention time: mean 8.9 hours (s.d. 5.2), serum concentration at 10 hours: sulfasalazine 1.7 mcg/ml (s.d. 0.46), sulfapyridine less than 1 mcg/ml. Percentage renal excretion: 10.2 (s.d. 4.3). Uptake as reflected by excretion is much below that of the oral rate and may explain the good tolerance of the dose form.

5.3 Preclinical safety data
In two-year carcinogenicity studies in rats and mice, sulfasalazine showed some evidence of carcinogenicity. In rats, there was a small increase in the incidence of transitional cell papillomas in the urinary bladder and kidney. The tumours were judged to be induced mechanically by calculi formed in the urine rather than through a direct genotoxic mechanism. In the mouse study, there was a significant increase in the incidence of hepatocellular adenoma or carcinoma. The mechanism of induction of hepatocellular neoplasia has been investigated and attributed to species-specific effects of sulfasalazine that are not relevant to humans.

Sulfasalazine did not show mutagenicity in the bacterial reverse mutation assay (Ames test) or in the L51784 mouse lymphoma cell assay at the HGPRT gene. It did not induce sister chromatid exchanges or chromosomal aberrations in cultured Chinese hamster ovary cells, and in vivo mouse bone marrow chromosomal aberration tests were negative. However, sulfasalazine showed positive or equivocal mutagenic responses in rat and mouse micronucleus assays, and in human lymphocyte sister chromatid exchange, chromosomal aberration and micronucleus assays. The ability of sulfasalazine to induce chromosome damage has been attributed to perturbation of folic acid levels rather than to a direct genotoxic mechanism.

Based on information from non-clinical studies, sulfasalazine is judged to pose no carcinogenic risk to humans. Sulfasalazine use has not been associated with the development of neoplasia in human epidemiology studies.

6. PHARMACEUTICAL PARTICULARS

6.1 List of excipients
Povidone

Adepa Solidus

6.2 Incompatibilities
Certain types of extended wear soft contact lenses may be permanently stained during therapy.

6.3 Shelf life
Five years

6.4 Special precautions for storage
Store in a cool place (below 15C)

6.5 Nature and contents of container
PVC/Polyethylene laminate moulds

6.6 Instructions for use and handling
As the suppositories melt at body temperature they should be kept cool and handled as little as possible before insertion so that they are firm.

Sulfasalazine is an orange dye, and care should thus be taken with clothing, bedding etc with regard to seepage or spillage.

Insertion

Empty the bowel if possible. Push the suppository through the anus with a finger, as far as possible. The urge to expel them will pass in a few minutes, once they have melted.

7. MARKETING AUTHORISATION HOLDER
Pharmacia Laboratories Limited
Davy Avenue
Milton Keynes
MK5 8PH

8. MARKETING AUTHORISATION NUMBER(S)
PL 00022/0156

9. DATE OF FIRST AUTHORISATION/RENEWAL OF THE AUTHORISATION
17 January 1994 / 22 February 1996

10. DATE OF REVISION OF THE TEXT
21st December 2004

11. LEGAL CATEGORY
POM.
SZC1_0

Salazopyrin Suspension

(Pharmacia Limited)

1. NAME OF THE MEDICINAL PRODUCT
Salazopyrin Suspension.

2. QUALITATIVE AND QUANTITATIVE COMPOSITION
Sulfasalazine Ph.Eur., 250 mg in 5 mL.

3. PHARMACEUTICAL FORM
Oral suspension.

4. CLINICAL PARTICULARS

4.1 Therapeutic indications
Induction and maintenance of remission of ulcerative colitis and treatment of active Crohn's disease.

4.2 Posology and method of administration
The dose is adjusted according to the severity of the disease and the patient's tolerance of the drug, as detailed below.

Adults and the Elderly

Severe attacks: 20 to 40 ml four times a day may be given in conjunction with steroids as part of an intensive management regime. Rapid passage of the suspension may reduce the effect of the drug.

The night time interval between doses should not exceed 8 hours.

Moderate attacks: 20 ml four times a day may be taken with or without steroids.

Maintenance therapy: With induction of remission, reduce the dose gradually to 40 ml per day. This dosage should be continued indefinitely, since discontinuance even several years after an acute attack is associated with a four-fold increase in relapse.

Children

The dose is reduced in proportion to body weight.

Acute attack or relapse: 0.8 - 1.2 ml/kg/day.

Maintenance dosage: 0.4 - 0.6 ml/kg/day.

4.3 Contraindications
- Use in infants under the age of two years.
- Use in patients where there is a significant hypersensitivity to sulfasalazine, sulfonamides, salicylates or the sodium benzoate preservative.
- Acute intermittent porphyria.

4.4 Special warnings and special precautions for use
Haematological and hepatic side effects may occur. Differential white cell, red cell and platelet cells should be performed initially and at least monthly for a minimum of the first three months of treatment. The patient should also be counselled to report immediately with any sore throat, fever, malaise or unexpected non-specific illness. Treatment should be stopped immediately if there is a suspicion or laboratory evidence of a potentially serious blood dyscrasia.

Liver function tests should be carried out at monthly intervals for the first three months of treatment. Patients with liver disease should be treated with caution.

Kidney function should be checked initially and at regular intervals during the treatment. Since sulfasalazine may cause haemolytic anaemia, it should be used with caution in patients with glucose-6-phosphate dehydrogenase deficiency.

Changes in blood picture (e.g. macrocytosis and pancytopenia) can be normalised by the administration of folic acid or folinic acid (leucovorin).

Sulfasalazine may colour the urine orange-yellow.

4.5 Interaction with other medicinal products and other forms of Interaction
Certain types of extended wear soft contact lenses may be permanently stained during therapy.

Uptake of digoxin and folate may be reduced.

Adequate fluid intake and avoidance of acidification of the urine (such as with concomitant use of methenamine) may minimise crystalluria and stone formation.

Sulfonamides bear certain chemical similarities to some oral hypoglycemic agents. Hypoglycemia has occurred in patients receiving sulfonamides. Patients receiving sulfasalazine and hypoglycemic agents should be closely monitored.

Due to inhibition of thiopurine methyltransferase by salazopyrin, bone marrow suppression and leucopenia have been reported when the thiopurine 6-mercaptopurine or it's prodrug, azathioprine, and oral salazopyrin were used concomitantly.

4.6 Pregnancy and lactation
Long-term clinical usage and experimental studies have failed to reveal any teratogenic or icteric hazards. The amounts of drug circulating in breast milk should not present a risk to a healthy infant.

4.7 Effects on ability to drive and use machines
No specific effects.

4.8 Undesirable effects
Overall, about 75% of ADRs occur within three months of treatment and over 90% by six months. Some unwanted effects are dose-dependent and symptoms can often be alleviated by reduction of the dose.

General

Sulfasalazine is split by intestinal bacteria to sulfapyridine and 5-amino salicylate so ADRs to either sulfonamide or salicylate are possible. Patients with slow acetylator status are more likely to experience ADRs related to sulfapyridine. The most commonly encountered ADRs are nausea, headache, rash, loss of appetite and raised temperature.

Specific

The following reactions have been recorded in patients taking sulfasalazine:

Haematological

Potentially fatal leucopenia, neutropenia, agranulocytosis, aplastic anaemia and thrombocytopenia. Leucopenia, which is normally mild and transient, may occur in up to 1.5% of patients and agranulocytosis in up to one in 700 patients during the second month of therapy.

The risk of sulfasalazine-associated blood disorders is substantially higher in patients treated for rheumatoid arthritis than it is in patients treated for inflammatory bowel disease.

Heinz body anaemia, methaemoglobinaemia, hypoprothrombinaemia, haemolytic anaemia, megaloblastic anaemia.

Hypersensitivity reactions

Generalised skin eruptions, Stevens-Johnson Syndrome, exfoliative dermatitis, epidermal necrolysis, pruritis, urticaria, photosensitisation, anaphylaxis, serum sickness, drug fever, lymphadenopathy, periorbital oedema, conjunctival and scleral injection, arthralgia, allergic myocarditis, polyarteritis nodosa, LE-phenomenon and lung complications with dyspnoea, fever, cough, eosinophilia, fibrosing alveolitis, pericarditis, vasculitis, nephritis, alopecia.

Gastro-intestinal reactions

Stomatitis, parotitis, pacreatitis, hepatitis.

CNS reactions

Vertigo, tinnitus, peripheral neuropathy, aseptic meningitis, ataxia, convulsions, insomnia, mental depression and hallucinations.

Fertility

Oligospermia, reversible on discontinuance of drug.

Renal Reactions

Crystalluria, haematuria, proteinurea and nephrotic syndrome.

4.9 Overdose
The drug has low acute per oral toxicity in the absence of hypersensitivity. There is no specific antidote and treatment should be supportive.

5. PHARMACOLOGICAL PROPERTIES

5.1 Pharmacodynamic properties
Sulfasalazine has beneficial effects in the treatment of ulcerative colitis and maintenance of remission, and in the treatment of acute Crohn's disease. Around 90% of a dose reaches the colon where bacteria split the drug into sulpyapyridine and mesalazine. These are active, and the unsplit sulfasalazine is also active on a variety of systems. Most Sulfapyridine is absorbed, hydroxylated or glucuronidated and a mix of unchanged and metabolised sulfapyridine appears in the urine.

Some mesalazine is taken up and acetylated in the colon wall, such that renal excretion is mainly acetyl-mesalazine. Sulfasalazine is excreted unchanged in the bile and urine. Overall the drug and its metabolites exert immunomodulatory effects, antibacterial effects, effects on the arachidonic acid cascade and alteration of activity of certain enzymes. The net result clinically is a reduction in activity of the inflammatory bowel disease.

The enteric coated sulfasalazine is registered for the treatment of rheumatoid arthritis, where the effect resembles penicillamine or gold.

5.2 Pharmacokinetic properties
With regard to the use of Salazopyrin in bowel disease there is no evidence that systemic levels are of any relevance other than with regard to ADR incidence. Here levels of sulfapyridine over about 50μg/ml are associated with a substantial risk of ADRs, especially in slow acetylators.

For sulfasalazine given as a single 3g oral dose, peak serum levels of sulfasalazine occurred in 3-5 hours, elimination half life was 5.7 ±0.7 hours, lag time 1.5 hours. During maintenance therapy renal clearance of sulfasalazine was 7.3 ±1.7ml/min, for sulfapyridine 9.9 ±1.9 and acetyl-mesalazine 100 ±20. Free sulfasalazine first appears in plasma in 4.3 hours after a single dose with an absorption half life of 2.7 hours. The elimination half life was calculated as 18 hours. For mesalazine, only acetyl-mesalazine (not free mesalazine) was demonstrable, the acetylation probably largely achieved in the colon mucosa. After 3g sulfasalazine dose lag time was 6.1 ±2.3 hours and plasma levels kept below 2μg/ml. total mesalazine. Urinary excretion half life was 6.0 ±3.1 hours and absorption half life based on these figures 3.0 ±1.5 hours. Renal clearance constant was 125 ml/min corresponding to the GFR. Studies in volunteers suggest that sulfasalazine is handled in a similar manner whether given as suspension or tablets.

5.3 Preclinical safety data
In two-year carcinogenicity studies in rats and mice, sulfasalazine showed some evidence of carcinogenicity. In rats, there was a small increase in the incidence of transitional cell papillomas in the urinary bladder and kidney. The tumours were judged to be induced mechanically by calculi formed in the urine rather than through a direct genotoxic mechanism. In the mouse study, there was a significant increase in the incidence of hepatocellular adenoma or carcinoma. The mechanism of induction of hepatocellular neoplasia has been investigated and attributed to species-specific effects of sulfasalazine that are not relevant to humans.

Sulfasalazine did not show mutagenicity in the bacterial reverse mutation assay (Ames test) or in the L51784 mouse lymphoma cell assay at the HGPRT gene. It did not induce sister chromatid exchanges or chromosomal aberrations in cultured Chinese hamster ovary cells, and in vivo mouse bone marrow chromosomal aberration tests were negative. However, sulfasalazine showed positive or equivocal mutagenic responses in rat and mouse micronucleus assays, and in human lymphocyte sister chromatid exchange, chromosomal aberration and micronucleus assays. The ability of sulfasalazine to induce chromosome damage has been attributed to perturbation of folic acid levels rather than to a direct genotoxic mechanism.

Based on information from non-clinical studies, sulfasalazine is judged to pose no carcinogenic risk to humans. Sulfasalazine use has not been associated with the development of neoplasia in human epidemiology studies.

6. PHARMACEUTICAL PARTICULARS

6.1 List of excipients
Xanthan gum, sodium benzoate, polysorbate 80, orange/lemon flavour, microcrystalline cellulose, sucrose, purified water.

6.2 Incompatibilities
None relevant.

6.3 Shelf life
30 months

6.4 Special precautions for storage
Do not store at above 25°C.

6.5 Nature and contents of container
Natural HDPE bottle with a tamper evident cap or child resistant cap and containing 500 ml of suspension.

6.6 Instructions for use and handling
Take the suspension with food.

7. MARKETING AUTHORISATION HOLDER
Pharmacia Limited
Davy Avenue
Milton Keynes
MK5 8PH

8. MARKETING AUTHORISATION NUMBER(S)
PL 00032/0389

9. DATE OF FIRST AUTHORISATION/RENEWAL OF THE AUTHORISATION
15 January 1994 / 02 February 1998

10. DATE OF REVISION OF THE TEXT
21st December 2004

11. LEGAL CATEGORY
POM.
SZD1_0

Salazopyrin Tablets

(Pharmacia Limited)

1. NAME OF THE MEDICINAL PRODUCT
Salazopyrin Tablets

2. QUALITATIVE AND QUANTITATIVE COMPOSITION
Sulfasalazine EP 500 mg

3. PHARMACEUTICAL FORM
Yellow round tablets embossed "KPh" on one side and "101" and a score line on the other.

4. CLINICAL PARTICULARS

4.1 Therapeutic indications
Induction and maintenance of remission of ulcerative colitis; treatment of active Crohn's Disease.

4.2 Posology and method of administration
The dose is adjusted according to the severity of the disease and the patient's tolerance to the drug, as detailed below.

Elderly Patients

No special precautions are necessary.

A) Ulcerative colitis

Adults

Severe Attacks

Salazopyrin 2-4 tablets four times a day may be given in conjunction with steroids as part of an intensive management regime. Rapid passage of the tablets may reduce effect of the drug.

Night-time interval between doses should not exceed 8 hours.

Moderate Attack

2-4 tablets four times a day may be given in conjunction with steroids.

Maintenance Therapy

With induction of remission reduce the dose gradually to 4 tablets per day. This dosage should be continued indefinitely since discontinuance even several years after an acute attack is associated with a four fold increase in risk of relapse.

Children

The dose is reduced in proportion to body weight.

Acute Attack or Relapse

40-60mg/kg per day

Maintenance Dosage

20-30mg/kg per day

Salazopyrin Suspension may provide a more flexible dosage form.

B) Crohn's Disease

In active Crohn's Disease, Salazopyrin should be administered as in attacks of ulcerative colitis (see above).

4.3 Contraindications

i) Use in infants under the age of 2 years.

ii) Use in patients where there is a significant hypersensitivity to sulfasalazine, sufonamides or salicylates.

iii) Acute intermittent porphyria.

4.4 Special warnings and special precautions for use

Precautions

Haematological and hepatic side effects may occur. Differential white cell, red cell and platelet counts should be performed initially and at least monthly for a minimum of the first three months of treatment. The patient should also be counselled to report immediately with any sore throat, fever, malaise or unexpected non-specific illness. Treatment should be stopped immediately if there is suspicion or laboratory evidence of a potentially serious blood dyscrasia.

Liver function tests should be carried out at monthly intervals for the first three months of treatment. Patients with liver disease should be treated with caution.

The kidney function should be checked initially and at regular intervals during the treatment. Since sulfasalazine may cause haemolytic anaemia, it should be used with caution in patients with G-6-PD deficiency.

Changes in the blood picture (e.g. macrocytosis and pancytopenia) due to folic acid deficiency can be normalised by administration of folic acid or folinic acid (leucovorin).

4.5 Interaction with other medicinal products and other forms of Interaction

Uptake of digoxin and folate may be reduced.

Adequate fluid intake and avoidance of acidification of the urine (such as with concomitant use of methenamine) may minimise crystalluria and stone formation.

Sulfonamides bear certain chemical similarities to some oral hypoglycemic agents. Hypoglycemia has occurred in patients receiving sulfonamides. Patients receiving sulfasalazine and hypoglycemic agents should be closely monitored.

Due to inhibition of thiopurine methyltransferase by salazopyrin, bone marrow suppression and leucopenia have been reported when the thiopurine 6-mercaptopurine or it's prodrug, azathioprine, and oral salazopyrin were used concomitantly.

4.6 Pregnancy and lactation

Long-term clinical usage and experimental studies have failed to reveal any teratogenic or icteric hazards. The amounts of drug present in the milk should not present a risk to a healthy infant.

4.7 Effects on ability to drive and use machines

No specific effects.

4.8 Undesirable effects

Overall, about 75% of ADRs occur within 3 months of starting therapy, and over 90% by 6 months. Some undesirable effects are dose-dependent and symptoms can often be alleviated by reduction of the dose.

General

Sulfasalazine is split by intestinal bacteria to sulfapyridine and 5-amino salicylate so ADRs to either sulfonamide or salicylate are possible. Patients with slow acetylator status are more likely to experience ADRs related to sulfapyridine. The most commonly encountered ADRs are nausea, headache, rash, loss of appetite and raised temperature.

Specific

The following reactions have been recorded in patients taking sulfasalazine:

Haematological

Potentially fatal leucopenia, neutropenia, agranulocytosis, aplastic anaemia and thrombocytopenia Leucopenia, which is normally mild and transient, may occur in up to 1.5% of patients and agranulocytosis in up to one in 700 patients during the second month of therapy.

Heinz body anaemia, methaemoglobinaemia, hypoprothrombinaemia, haemolytic anaemia, megaloblastic anaemia.

Hypersensitivity Reactions

Generalised skin eruptions, Stevens-Johnson Syndrome, exfoliative dermatitis, epidermal necrolysis, pruritis, urticaria, photosensitisation, anaphylaxis, serum sickness, drug fever, lymphadenopathy, periorbital oedema, conjuctivial and scleral infection, arthralgia, allergic myocarditis, polyarteritis nodosa, LE-phenomenon and lung complications with dyspnoea, fever, cough, eosinophilia, fibrosing alveolitis, pericarditis, vasculitis, nephritis, alopecia.

Gastro-Intestinal Reactions

Stomatitis, parotitis, pancreatitis, hepatitis.

CNS Reactions

Vertigo, tinnitus, peripheral neuropathy, aseptic meningitis, ataxia, convulsions, insomnia, mental depression and hallucinations.

Fertility

Oligospermia, reversible on discontinuance of drug.

Renal Reactions

Crystalluria, haematuria, proteinuria and nephrotic syndrome.

4.9 Overdose

The drug has low acute per oral toxicity in the absence of hypersensitivity. There is no specific antidote and treatment should be supportive.

5. PHARMACOLOGICAL PROPERTIES

5.1 Pharmacodynamic properties

Around 90% of a dose reaches the colon where bacteria split the drug into sulfapyridine (SP) and mesalazine (ME). These are active, and the unsplit sulfasalazine (SASP) is also active on a variety of symptoms. Most SP is absorbed, hydroxylated or glucuronidated and a mix of unchanged and metabolised SP appears in the urine. Some ME is taken up and acetylated in the colon wall, such that renal excretion is mainly ac-me. SASP is excreted unchanged in the bile and urine. Overall the drug and its metabolites exert immunomodulatory effects, antibacterial effects, effects on the arachidonic acid cascade and alteration of activity of certain enzymes. The net result clinically is a reduction in activity of the inflammatory bowel disease. The enteric coated SASP is registered for the treatment of rheumatoid arthritis, where the effect resembles penicillamine or gold.

5.2 Pharmacokinetic properties

With regard to the use of salazopyrin in bowel disease there is no evidence that systemic levels are of any relevance other than with regard to ADR incidence. Here levels of SP over about 50μg/ml are associated with a substantial risk of ADRs, especially in slow acetylators. For SASP given as a single 3g oral dose, peak serum levels of SASP occurred in 3-5 hours, elimination half life was 5.7 ±0.7 hours, lag time 1.5 hours. During maintenance therapy renal clearance of SASP was 7.3 ±1.7ml/min, for SP 9.9 ±1.9 and AC-ME 100 ±20. Free SP first appears in plasma in 4.3 hours after a single dose with an absorption half life of 2.7 hours. The elimination half life was calculated as 18 hours. Turning to mesalazine, in urine only AC-ME (not free ME) was demonstrable, the acetylation probably largely achieved in the colon mucosa. After a 3g SASP dose lag time was 6.1 ±2.3 hours and plasma levels kept below 2μg/ml total ME. Urinary excretion half-life was 6.0 ±3.1 hours and absorption half life based on these figures 3.0 ±1.5 hours. Renal clearance constant was 125 ml/min corresponding to the GFR.

5.3 Preclinical safety data

In two-year carcinogenicity studies in rats and mice, sulfasalazine showed some evidence of carcinogenicity. In rats, there was a small increase in the incidence of transitional cell papillomas in the urinary bladder and kidney. The tumours were judged to be induced mechanically by calculi formed in the urine rather than through a direct genotoxic mechanism. In the mouse study, there was a significant increase in the incidence of hepatocellular adenoma or carcinoma. The mechanism of induction of hepatocellular neoplasia has been investigated and attributed to species-specific effects of sulfasalazine that are not relevant to humans.

Sulfasalazine did not show mutagenicity in the bacterial reverse mutation assay (Ames test) or in the L51784 mouse lymphoma cell assay at the HGPRT gene. It did not induce sister chromatid exchanges or chromosomal aberrations in cultured Chinese hamster ovary cells, and in vivo mouse bone marrow chromosomal aberration tests were negative. However, sulfasalazine showed positive or equivocal mutagenic responses in rat and mouse micronucleus assays, and in human lymphocyte sister chromatid exchange, chromosomal aberration and micronucleus assays. The ability of sulfasalazine to induce chromosome damage has been attributed to perturbation of folic acid levels rather than to a direct genotoxic mechanism.

Based on information from non-clinical studies, sulfasalazine is judged to pose no carcinogenic risk to humans. Sulfasalazine use has not been associated with the development of neoplasia in human epidemiology studies.

6. PHARMACEUTICAL PARTICULARS

6.1 List of excipients

Povidone; Maize starch; magnesium stearate; colloidal silicon dioxide.

6.2 Incompatibilities

Certain types of extended wear soft contact lenses may be permanently stained during therapy.

6.3 Shelf life

The tablets are stable for 5 years.

6.4 Special precautions for storage

None

6.5 Nature and contents of container

Square or rectangular HDPE jar with easy to open tamper-evisent polypropylene screw-cap. To contain 112 tablets.

6.6 Instructions for use and handling

Take with water

7. MARKETING AUTHORISATION HOLDER

Pharmacia Limited.

Davy Avenue

Milton Keynes

MK5 8PH

8. MARKETING AUTHORISATION NUMBER(S)

PL 00032/0390

9. DATE OF FIRST AUTHORISATION/RENEWAL OF THE AUTHORISATION

02/04/2002

10. DATE OF REVISION OF THE TEXT

21st September 2004

11. LEGAL CATEGORY

POM.

SZE1_0

Salofalk 1000mg Granules

(Dr Falk Pharma UK Limited)

1. NAME OF THE MEDICINAL PRODUCT

Salofalk 1000 mg gastro-resistant prolonged release granules in sachets

2. QUALITATIVE AND QUANTITATIVE COMPOSITION

Each sachet of Salofalk 1000 mg granules contains 1000 mg mesalazine.

For excipients, see 6.1

3. PHARMACEUTICAL FORM

Gastro-resistant prolonged release granules.

Description: Stick-formed or round, greyish white granules

4. CLINICAL PARTICULARS

4.1 Therapeutic indications

For the treatment of acute episodes and the maintenance of remission of ulcerative colitis

4.2 Posology and method of administration

For the treatment of acute episodes of ulcerative colitis:

Depending on the clinical requirements in the individual case, one sachet of Salofalk 500mg granules three times daily or one sachet of Salofalk 1000 mg granules three times daily (equivalent to 1.5 – 3.0 g mesalazine daily).

For the maintenance of remission of ulcerative colitis:

One sachet of Salofalk 500 mg granules three times daily (equivalent to 1.5 g mesalazine daily).

Children below 6 years of age:

Salofalk granules should not be used in children under 6 years of age because there is very limited experience with this age group. Children older than 6 years of age and adolescents.

In acute attacks, depending on disease severity, 30-50 mg mesalazine/kg/day should be given in 3 divided doses. For maintenance of remission, 15-30 mg mesalazine/kg/day may be given in 2 divided doses.

It is generally recommended that half the adult dose may be given to children up to a body weight of 40 kg; and the normal adult dose to those above 40 kg. The content of Salofalk 1000 mg granules should not be chewed. The content of the sachet of Salofalk 1000 mg granules should be taken in the morning, at lunchtime and in the evening. The granules should be taken on the tongue and swallowed, without chewing, with plenty of liquid. Both in the treatment of acute inflammatory episodes and during long term treatment, Salofalk 1000 mg granules should be used on a regular basis and consistently in order to achieve the desired therapeutic effects. In general, an acute episode of ulcerative colitis subsides after 8-12 weeks; the dosage can then, in most patients, be reduced to 1.5 g mesalazine/ day.

4.3 Contraindications
Salofalk 1000 mg granules are contraindicated in cases of:

pre-existing hypersensitivity to salicylic acid and its derivatives or to any of the other constituents

severe impairment of hepatic and renal function

pre-existing gastric or duodenal ulcer

haemorrhagic diathesis.

4.4 Special warnings and special precautions for use
Blood tests (differential blood count; liver function parameters like ALT or AST; serum creatinine) and urinary status (dip sticks) should be determined prior to and during treatment, at the discretion of the treating physician. As a guideline, controls are recommended 14 days after commencement of treatment, then a further two to three times at intervals of 4 weeks. If the findings are normal, control examinations should be carried out every 3 months. If additional symptoms occur, control examinations should be performed immediately. Caution is recommended in patients with impaired hepatic function. Salofalk is not recommended in patients with impaired renal function. Mesalazine-induced renal toxicity should be considered if renal function deteriorates during treatment. Patients with pulmonary disease, in particular asthma, should be very carefully monitored during a course of treatment with Salofalk granules. Patients with a history of adverse drug reactions to preparations containing sulphasalazine should be kept under close medical surveillance on commencement of a course of treatment with Salofalk granules. Should Salofalk granules cause acute intolerability reactions such as cramps, acute abdominal pain, fever, severe headache and rash, therapy should be discontinued immediately. In patients with phenylketonuria it should be kept in mind that Salofalk 1000mg granules contain aspartame as a sweetening agent, equivalent to 1.12 mg phenylalanine. Salofalk granules should not be used for the treatment of children below the age of 6 years.

4.5 Interaction with other medicinal products and other forms of Interaction
Specific interaction studies have not been performed.

Interactions may occur during treatment with Salofalk 1000 mg granules and concomitant administration of the following medicinal products. Most of these possible interactions are based on theoretical reasons:

Coumarin-type anticoagulants: possible potentiation of the anticoagulant effects (increasing the risk of gastrointestinal haemorrhage)

Glucocorticoids: Possible increase in undesirable gastric effects

Sulphonylureas: Possible increase in the blood glucose-lowering effects

Methotrexate: Possible increase in the toxic potential of methotrexate

Probenecid/sulphinpyrazone: Possible attenuation of the uricosuric effects

Spironolactone/frusemide: Possible attenuation of the diuretic effects

Rifampicin: Possible attenuation of the tuberculostatic effects

Lactulose or similar preparations, which lower stool pH: Possible reduction of mesalazine release from granules due to decreased pH caused by bacterial metabolism

In patients who are concomitantly treated with azathioprine or 6-mercaptopurine, possible enhanced myelosuppressive effects of azathioprine or 6-mercaptopurine should be taken into account.

4.6 Pregnancy and lactation
There are no adequate data from the use of Salofalk gastro-resistant prolonged releasegranules in pregnant woman. However, data on a limited number of exposed pregnancies indicate no adverse effect of mesalazine on pregnancy or on the health of the fetus/newborn child. To date no other relevant epidemiologic data are available. In one single case after long-term use of a high dose mesalazine (2-4 g, orally) during pregnancy, renal failure in a neonate was reported. Animal studies on oral mesalazine do not indicate direct or indirect harmful effects with respect to pregnancy, embryonal/ fetal development, parturition or postnatal development. Salofalk granules should only be used during pregnancy if the potential benefit outweighs the possible risk.N-acetyl-5-aminosalicylic acid and to a lesser degree mesalazine are excreted in breast milk. Only limited experience during lactation in woman is available to date. Hypersensitivity reactions like diarrhoea can not be excluded. Therefore, Salofalk granules should only be used during breast-feeding if the potential benefit outweighs the possible risk. If the suckling neonate develops diarrhoea, the breast-feeding should be discontinued.

4.7 Effects on ability to drive and use machines
No effects on ability to drive and use machines have been observed

4.8 Undesirable effects
Gastrointestinal undesirable effects (rare, 0.01% - <0.1%):

Abdominal pain, diarrhoea, flatulence, nausea, vomiting

CNS-related undesirable effects (rare, 0.01% - <0.1%):

Headache, dizziness.

Renal undesirable effects (very rare, <0.01%):

Impairment of renal function including acute and chronic interstitial nephritis and renal insufficiency

Hypersensitivity reactions (very rare, <0.01%):

Allergic exanthema, drug fever, bronchospasm, peri- and myocarditis, acute pancreatitis, allergic alveolitis, lupus erythematosus syndrome, pancolitis.

Musculoskeletal disorders (very rare, <0.01%):

Myalgia, arthralgia.

Blood and the lymphatic system disorders (very rare, <0.01%):

Altered blood counts (aplastic anaemia, agranulocytosis, pancytopenia, neutropenia, leukopenia, thrombocytopenia).

Hepato-biliary disorders (very rare, <0.01%):

Changes in hepatic function parameters (increase in transaminases), hepatitis

Skin and appendages disorders (very rare, < 0.01%):

Alopecia

4.9 Overdose
No cases of intoxication have been reported to date and no specific antidotes are known. If necessary, intravenous infusion of electrolytes (forced diuresis) should be considered in cases of overdose.

5. PHARMACOLOGICAL PROPERTIES

5.1 Pharmacodynamic properties
Pharmacotherapeutic group: Intestinal antiinflammatory agent.

ATC code: A07EC02

The mechanism of the anti-inflammatory action is unknown. The results of in vitro studies indicate that inhibition of lipoxygenase may play a role. Effects on prostaglandin concentrations in the intestinal mucosa have also been demonstrated. Mesalazine (5-Aminosalicylic acid / 5-ASA) may also function as a radical scavenger of reactive oxygen compounds. Mesalazine, orally administered, acts predominantly locally at the gut mucosa and in the submucous tissue from the luminal side of the intestine. It is important, therefore, that mesalazine is available at the regions of inflammation. Systemic bioavailability / plasma concentrations of mesalazine therefore are of no relevance for therapeutic efficacy, but rather a factor for safety. In order to realise this, Salofalk granules are gastric juice resistant and release mesalazine in a pH dependent manner due to an Eudragit L coating, and prolonged manner due to the matrix granule structure.

5.2 Pharmacokinetic properties
General considerations of mesalazine:

Absorption:

Mesalazine absorption is highest in proximal gut regions and lowest in distal gut areas.

Biotransformation:

Mesalazine is metabolised both pre-systemically by the intestinal mucosa and the liver to the pharmacologically inactive N-acetyl-5-aminosalicylic acid (N-Ac-5-ASA). The acetylation seems to be independent of the acetylator phenotype of the patient. Some acetylation also occurs through the action of colonic bacteria. Protein binding of mesalazine and N-Ac-5-ASA is 43% and 78%, respectively.

Elimination:

Mesalazine and its metabolite N-Ac-5-ASA are eliminated via the faeces (major part), renally (varies between 20 and 50 %, dependent on kind of application, pharmaceutical preparation and route of mesalazine release, respectively), and biliary (minor part). Renal excretion predominantly occurs as N-Ac-5-ASA. About 1 % of total orally administered mesalazine dose is excreted into the breast milk mainly as N-Ac-5-ASA.

Salofalk Granules specific:

Distribution:

Owing to the granule size of about 1 mm, transit from the stomach to the small intestine is fast. A combined pharmacoscintigraphic/pharmacokinetic study showed that the compound reaches the ileocaecal region within approx. 3 hours and the ascending colon within approx. 4 hours. The total transit time in the colon amounts to about 20 hours. Approximately 80 % of an administered oral dose is estimated to be available in the colon, sigmoid and rectum.

Absorption:

Mesalazine release from Salofalk granules starts after a lag phase of about 2-3 hours, peak plasma concentrations are reached at about 4-5 hours. The systemic bioavailability of mesalazine after oral administration is estimated to be approximately 15-25 %.

Food intake delays absorption for 1 to 2 hours but does not change the rate and extent of absorption.

Elimination:

From a 3 × 500 mg daily mesalazine dose, a total renal elimination of mesalazine and NAc-5-ASA under steady state condition was calculated to be about 25%. The unmetabolised excreted mesalazine part was less than 1 % of the oral dose. The elimination half-life in this study was 4.4 hours.

5.3 Preclinical safety data
Preclinical data reveal no special hazard for humans based on conventional studies of safety pharmacology, genotoxicity, carcinogenicity (rat) or toxicity to reproduction. Kidney toxicity (renal papillary necrosis and epithelial damage in the proximal convoluted tubule or the whole nephron) has been seen in repeat-dose toxicity studies with high oral doses of mesalazine. The clinical relevance of this finding is unknown.

6. PHARMACEUTICAL PARTICULARS

6.1 List of excipients
Aspartame, Carmellose sodium, Citric acid, Silica colloidal anhydrous, Hypromellose, Magnesium stearate, Methacrylic acid-methyl methacrylate copolymer (1:1) (Eudragit L 100), Methylcellulose, Microcrystalline cellulose, Polyacrylate dispersion 40 % (Eudragit NE Page 5 of 6 Salofalk 1000mg granules in sachets, SPC from the eMC 40 D containing 2 % Nonoxynol 100), Povidone K 25, Simethicone, Sorbic acid, Talc, Titanium dioxide (E 171), Triethyl citrate, Vanilla custard flavouring (containing propylene glycol)

6.2 Incompatibilities
Not applicable

6.3 Shelf life
3 years.

6.4 Special precautions for storage
No special precautions for storage

6.5 Nature and contents of container
Container: Polyester/ Aluminium/ Polyethylene-Foil

Package sizes: 50 sachets, 100 sachets or 150 sachets Salofalk 1000mg granules.

Not all pack sizes will be marketed.

6.6 Instructions for use and handling
No special requirements

7. MARKETING AUTHORISATION HOLDER
Dr. Falk Pharma GmbH

Leinenweberstr. 5,

P. O. Box 6529

79041 Freiburg

Germany

Tel: +49 (0)761 1514-0

8. MARKETING AUTHORISATION NUMBER(S)
PL 08637/0008

9. DATE OF FIRST AUTHORISATION/RENEWAL OF THE AUTHORISATION
1st September 2003

10. DATE OF REVISION OF THE TEXT
November 2003

Salofalk 250mg Tablets

(Dr Falk Pharma UK Limited)

1. NAME OF THE MEDICINAL PRODUCT
Salofalk Tablets

2. QUALITATIVE AND QUANTITATIVE COMPOSITION
Mesalazine 250mg

For excipients, see 6.1

3. PHARMACEUTICAL FORM
Enteric coated tablet.

4. CLINICAL PARTICULARS

4.1 Therapeutic indications
Treatment of mild to moderate acute exacerbations of ulcerative colitis and for the maintenance of remission of ulcerative colitis.

4.2 Posology and method of administration
Method of administration: Oral.

Adults: Acute treatment: six tablets daily in three divided doses.

Maintenance Treatment: three to six tablets daily in divided doses.

Elderly: As for adults.

4.3 Contraindications
Patients with an active peptic ulcer, blood clotting abnormalities, severe hepatic or severe renal impairment or where there is a pathological propensity to bleeding. Salofalk should not be used in babies and young children.

4.4 Special warnings and special precautions for use
Serious blood dyscrasias have been reported very rarely with mesalazine. Haematological investigations should be performed if the patient develops unexplained bleeding, bruising, purpura, anaemia, fever or sore throat. Reports of interstitial nephritis occurring with mesalazine treatment are uncommon, however it is advisable that renal function be monitored, with serum creatinine levels measured prior to treatment start, every 3 months for the first year, 6

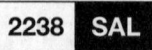

monthly for the next 4 years, and then annually thereafter. Use with extreme caution in patients with mild to moderate renal impairment (see section 4.3). If dehydration develops, normal electrolyte levels and fluid balance should be restored as soon as possible.

Treatment should be stopped if there is suspicion or evidence of blood dyscrasia or if renal function deteriorates.

4.5 Interaction with other medicinal products and other forms of Interaction

The hypoglycaemic action of sulphonylureas can be intensified, as can gastrointestinal haemorrhage cause by coumarins. The toxicity of methotrexate can be increased. The uricosuric action of probenecid and sulphinpyrazone can be decreased, as can the diuretic action of furosemide and the action of spironolactone. The antituberculosis action of rifampicin can also be diminished.

Concomitant use with other known nephrotoxic agents, such as NSAIDs and azathioprine may increase the risk of renal reactions (see section 4.4).

4.6 Pregnancy and lactation

Animal experiments with mesalazine have produced no evidence of embryonic effects. All competent authors recommend to continue treatment with sulphasalazine, the parent drug of mesalazine, during pregnancy. Up to now, they didn't see any untoward effect on its course or on the foetus. Therefore there is no reason to prohibit Salofalk treatment during pregnancy. No untoward effects were seen in the reproductive and fertility study with mesalazine in breast-fed rat pups. But up to now there is a limited experience in using mesalazine/sulphasalazine during the lactation period in man. Therefore, it should be stated that the experience with Salofalk 250 during lactation up to now is not sufficient. The acetylated form of mesalazine is found in the breast milk in slight amounts.

4.7 Effects on ability to drive and use machines

Salofalk is not expected to affect ability to drive and use machines.

4.8 Undesirable effects

Salofalk may cause hypersensitivity reactions. These are unrelated to dose. Mesalazine may be associated with an exacerbation of the symptoms of colitis in those patients who have previously had such problems with sulphasalazine. There have been rare reports of leucopenia, neutropenia, agranulocytosis, aplastic anaemia and thrombocytopenia, pancreatitis, abnormalities of hepatitic function and hepatitis, myocarditis and pericarditis, allergic lung reactions, lupus erythematosus-like reactions, bullous skin reactions including erythema multiforme, Stevens Johnson Syndrome and rash (including urticaria), interstitial nephritis and nephritic syndrome with oral mesalazine treatment, usually reversible on withdrawal. Renal failure has been reported. Mesalazine-induced nephrotoxicity should be suspected in patients developing renal dysfunction during treatment. Increased methaemoglobin levels may occur.

4.9 Overdose

Due to the enteric nature of the formulation of Salofalk tablets and the particular pharmacokinetic properties of mesalazine, only small amounts of the drug are available for systemic action. Consequently signs of intoxication are unlikely even after large doses. However, in principle, symptoms consistent with salicylate intoxication may occur (management of which is shown in brackets).

- Mixes Acidosis – Alkalosis (reinstatement of the acid-base balance to match the situation and electrolytic substitutions.
- Hyperventilation.
- Pulmonary Oedema
- Dehydration from perspiration and vomiting (fluid intake)
- Hypoglycaemia (glucose intake).

There is no specific antidote to mesalazine but in many cases of overdose, gastric lavage and intravenous transfusion of electrolytes to promote diuresis should be implemented.

5. PHARMACOLOGICAL PROPERTIES

5.1 Pharmacodynamic properties

The main site of action of mesalazine is the inflamed mucosa in the terminal ileum and colon. The pH dependent enteric coating applied to Salofalk tablets (Eudragit L) disintegrates above pH 6.0 ensuring that the drug is released at the site of action, where it is absorbed to a certain degree. The absorbed portion is acetylated and excreted predominantly in the acetylated form via the kidneys. A small portion (about 5% of the absorbed quantity) is excreted in the bile. In faces, mesalazine is found particularly in unchanged form and partially in acetylated form.

5.2 Pharmacokinetic properties

The elimination half-lives are 0.7 – 2.4 hours (mean 1.4 ± 0.6 hours). The plasma protein binding of mesalazine is 43% and of acetylated mesalazine 78%. The rapid acetylation is not reversible and, in contrast to sulfapyridine, there is no difference between slow and rapid acetylation.

5.3 Preclinical safety data

None stated.

6. PHARMACEUTICAL PARTICULARS

6.1 List of excipients

Sodium carbonate, glycine, polyvidone, microcrystalline cellulose (E460), colloidal anhydrous silica. Calcium stearate, hydroxypropylmethylcellulose (E464), methacrylic acid copolymer (Eudragit L), dibutyl phthalate talc, titanium dioxide (E171), iron oxide (E172), polyethylene glycol, polymethacrylate (Eudragit E).

6.2 Incompatibilities

None stated.

6.3 Shelf life

Three years

6.4 Special precautions for storage

None.

6.5 Nature and contents of container

Orange PVC/PVDC/A1 blister strips packed in cartons containing 10†, 100 or 300† tablets.

† not currently marketed.

6.6 Instructions for use and handling

Salofalk tablets should be swallowed whole and not chewed.

7. MARKETING AUTHORISATION HOLDER

Interfalk UK Ltd

Thames House

Wellington Street

London

SE18 6NZ

8. MARKETING AUTHORISATION NUMBER(S)

PL 10341/0004

9. DATE OF FIRST AUTHORISATION/RENEWAL OF THE AUTHORISATION

13 September 1991

10. DATE OF REVISION OF THE TEXT

March 2004

11. LEGAL CATEGORY

POM

Salofalk 500mg Granules

(Dr Falk Pharma UK Limited)

1. NAME OF THE MEDICINAL PRODUCT

Salofalk 500 mg gastro-resistant prolonged release granules in sachets

2. QUALITATIVE AND QUANTITATIVE COMPOSITION

Each sachet of Salofalk 500 mg granules contains 500 mg mesalazine.

For excipients, see 6.1

3. PHARMACEUTICAL FORM

Gastro-resistant prolonged release granules.

Description: Stick-formed or round, greyish white granules

4. CLINICAL PARTICULARS

4.1 Therapeutic indications

For the treatment of acute episodes and the maintenance of remission of ulcerative colitis

4.2 Posology and method of administration

For the treatment of acute episodes of ulcerative colitis:

Depending on the clinical requirements in the individual case, one sachet of Salofalk 500mg granules three times daily or one sachet of Salofalk 1000 mg granules three times daily (equivalent to 1.5 – 3.0 g mesalazine daily).

For the maintenance of remission of ulcerative colitis:

One sachet of Salofalk 500 mg granules three times daily (equivalent to 1.5 g mesalazine daily).

Children below 6 years of age:

Salofalk granules should not be used in children under 6 years of age because there is very limited experience with this age group.

Children older than 6 years of age and adolescents. In acute attacks, depending on disease severity, 30-50 mg mesalazine/kg/day should be given in 3 divided doses. For maintenance of remission, 15-30 mg mesalazine/kg/day may be given in 2 divided doses.

It is generally recommended that half the adult dose may be given to children up to a body weight of 40 kg; and the normal adult dose to those above 40 kg. The content of Salofalk 500 mg granules should not be chewed. The content of the sachet of Salofalk 500mg granules should be taken in the morning, at lunchtime and in the evening. The granules should be taken on the tongue and swallowed, without chewing, with plenty of liquid. Both in the treatment of acute inflammatory episodes and during long term treatment, Salofalk 500 mg granules should be used on a regular basis and consistently in order to achieve the desired therapeutic effects. In general, an acute episode of ulcerative colitis subsides after 8-12 weeks; the dosage can then, in most patients, be reduced to 1.5g mesalazine/day.

4.3 Contraindications

Salofalk 500 mg granules are contraindicated in cases of:

Pre-existing hypersensitivity to salicylic acid and its derivatives or to any of the other constituents

Severe impairment of hepatic and renal function

Pre-existing gastric or duodenal ulcer

Haemorrhagic diathesis.

4.4 Special warnings and special precautions for use

Blood tests (differential blood count; liver function parameters like ALT or AST; serum creatinine) and urinary status (dip sticks) should be determined prior to and during treatment, at the discretion of the treating physician. As a guideline, controls are recommended 14 days after commencement of treatment, then a further two to three times at intervals of 4 weeks. If the findings are normal, control examinations should be carried out every 3 months. If additional symptoms occur, control examinations should be performed immediately.

Caution is recommended in patients with impaired hepatic function. Salofalk is not recommended in patients with impaired renal function. Mesalazine-induced renal toxicity should be considered if renal function deteriorates during treatment. Patients with pulmonary disease, in particular asthma, should be very carefully monitored during a course of treatment with Salofalk granules. Patients with a history of adverse drug reactions to preparations containing sulphasalazine should be kept under close medical surveillance on commencement of a course of treatment with Salofalk granules. Should Salofalk granules cause acute intolerability reactions such as cramps, acute abdominal pain, fever, severe headache and rash, therapy should be discontinued immediately. In patients with phenylketonuria it should be kept in mind that Salofalk 500 mg granules contain aspartame as a sweetening agent, equivalent to 0.56 mg phenylalanine. Salofalk granules should not be used for the treatment of children below the age of 6 years.

4.5 Interaction with other medicinal products and other forms of Interaction

Specific interaction studies have not been performed.

Interactions may occur during treatment with Salofalk 500 mg granules and concomitant administration of the following medicinal products. Most of these possible interactions are based on theoretical reasons:

Coumarin-type anticoagulants:

Possible potentiation of the anticoagulant effects (increasing the risk of gastrointestinal haemorrhage).

Glucocorticoids:

Possible increase in undesirable gastric effects

Sulphonylureas:

Possible increase in the blood glucose-lowering effects

Methotrexate:

Possible increase in the toxic potential of methotrexate

Probenecid/sulphinpyrazone:

Possible attenuation of the uricosuric effects

Spironolactone/frusemide:

Possible attenuation of the diuretic effects

Rifampicin:

Possible attenuation of the tuberculostatic effects

Lactulose or similar preparations, which lower stool pH:

Possible reduction of mesalazine release from granules due to decreased pH caused by bacterial metabolism.

In patients who are concomitantly treated with azathioprine or 6-mercaptopurine, possible enhanced myelosuppressive effects of azathioprine or 6-mercaptopurine should be taken into account.

4.6 Pregnancy and lactation

There are no adequate data from the use of Salofalk gastro-resistant prolonged release granules in pregnant women.

However, data on a limited number of exposed pregnancies indicate no adverse effect of mesalazine on pregnancy or on the health of the fetus/newborn child. To date no other relevant epidmiologic data are available.

In one single case after long-term use of a high dose mesalazine (2-4 g, orally) during pregnancy, renal failure in a neonate was reported. Animal studies on oral mesalazine do not indicate direct or indirect harmful effects with respect to pregnancy, embryonal/ fetal development, parturition or postnatal development. Salofalk granules should only be used during pregnancy if the potential benefit outweighs the possible risk. N-acetyl-5- aminosalicylic acid and to a lesser degree mesalazine are excreted in breast milk. Only limited experience during lactation in woman is available to date. Hypersensivity reactions like diarrhoea can not be excluded. Therefore, Salofalk granules should only be used during breast-feeding if the potential benefit outweighs the possible risk. If the suckling neonate develops diarrhoea, the breast-feeding should be discontinued.

4.7 Effects on ability to drive and use machines

No effects on ability to drive and use machines have been observed.

4.8 Undesirable effects

Gastrointestinal undesirable effects (rare, 0.01% - <0.1%):

Abdominal pain, diarrhoea, flatulence, nausea, vomiting

CNS-related undesirable effects (rare, 0.01% - <0.1%):

Headache, dizziness.

Renal undesirable effects (very rare, <0.01%):

Impairment of renal function including acute and chronic interstitial nephritis and renal insufficiency

Hypersensitivity reactions (very rare, <0.01%):

Allergic exanthema, drug fever, bronchospasm, peri- and myocarditis, acute pancreatitis, allergic alveolitis, lupus erythematosus syndrome, pancolitis.

Musculoskeletal disorders (very rare, <0.01%):

Myalgia, arthralgia.

Blood and the lymphatic system disorders (very rare, <0.01%):

Altered blood counts (aplastic anaemia, agranulocytosis, pancytopenia, neutropenia, leukopenia, thrombocytopenia).

Hepato-biliary disorders (very rare, <0.01%):

Changes in hepatic function parameters (increase in transaminases), hepatitis

Skin and appendages disorders (very rare, < 0.01%):

Alopecia

4.9 Overdose

No cases of intoxication have been reported to date and no specific antidotes are known. If necessary, intravenous infusion of electrolytes (forced diuresis) should be considered in cases of overdose.

5. PHARMACOLOGICAL PROPERTIES

5.1 Pharmacodynamic properties

Pharmacotherapeutic group: Intestinal antiinflammatory agent

ATC code: A07EC02

The mechanism of the anti-inflammatory action is unknown. The results of in vitro studies indicate that inhibition of lipoxygenase may play a role. Effects on prostaglandin concentrations in the intestinal mucosa have also been demonstrated. Mesalazine (5-Aminosalicylic acid / 5-ASA) may also function as a radical scavenger of reactive oxygen compounds. Mesalazine, orally administered, acts predominantly locally at the gut mucosa and in the submucous tissue from the luminal side of the intestine. It is important, therefore, that mesalazine is available at the regions of inflammation. Systemic bioavailability / plasma concentrations of mesalazine therefore are of no relevance for therapeutic efficacy, but rather a factor for safety. In order to realise this, Salofalk granules are gastric juice resistant and release mesalazine in a pH dependent manner due to an Eudragit L coating, and prolonged manner due to the matrix granule structure.

5.2 Pharmacokinetic properties

General considerations of mesalazine:

Absorption:

Mesalazine absorption is highest in proximal gut regions and lowest in distal gut areas.

Biotransformation:

Mesalazine is metabolised both pre-systemically by the intestinal mucosa and the liver to the pharmacologically inactive N-acetyl-5-aminosalicylic acid (N-Ac-5-ASA). The acetylation seems to be independent of the acetylator phenotype of the patient. Some acetylation also occurs through the action of colonic bacteria. Protein binding of mesalazine and N-Ac-5-ASA is 43% and 78%, respectively.

Elimination:

Mesalazine and its metabolite N-Ac-5-ASA are eliminated via the faeces (major part), renally (varies between 20 and 50 %, dependent on kind of application, pharmaceutical preparation and route of mesalazine release, respectively), and biliary (minor part). Renal excretion predominantly occurs as N-Ac-5-ASA. About 1 % of total orally administered mesalazine dose is excreted into the breast milk mainly as N-Ac-5-ASA.

Salofalk Granules specific:

Distribution:

Owing to the granule size of about 1 mm, transit from the stomach to the small intestine is fast. A combined pharmacoscintigraphic/pharmacokinetic study showed that the compound reaches the ileocaecal region within approx. 3 hours and the ascending colon within approx. 4 hours. The total transit time in the colon amounts to about 20 hours.

Approximately 80 % of an administered oral dose is estimated to be available in the colon, sigmoid and rectum.

Absorption:

Mesalazine release from Salofalk granules starts after a lag phase of about 2-3 hours, peak plasma concentrations are reached at about 4-5 hours. The systemic bioavailability of mesalazine after oral administration is estimated to be approximately 15-25 %. Food intake delays absorption for 1 to 2 hours but does not change the rate and extent of absorption.

Elimination:

From a 3 × 500 mg daily mesalazine dose, a total renal elimination of mesalazine and NAc-5-ASA under steady state condition was calculated to be about 25%. The unmetabolised excreted mesalazine part was less than 1 % of the oral dose. The elimination half-life in this study was 4.4 hours.

5.3 Preclinical safety data

Preclinical data reveal no special hazard for humans based on conventional studies of safety pharmacology, genotoxicity, carcinogenicity (rat) or toxicity to reproduction. Kidney toxicity (renal papillary necrosis and epithelial damage in the proximal convoluted tubule or the whole nephron) has been seen in repeat-dose toxicity studies with high oral doses of mesalazine. The clinical relevance of this finding is unknown.

6. PHARMACEUTICAL PARTICULARS

6.1 List of excipients

Aspartame, Carmellose sodium, Citric acid, Silica colloidal anhydrous, Hypromellose, Magnesium stearate, Methacrylic acid-methyl methacrylate copolymer (1:1) (Eudragit L 100), Methylcellulose, Microcrystalline cellulose, Polyacrylate dispersion 40 % (Eudragit NE 40 D containing 2 % Nonoxynol 100), Povidone K 25, Simethicone, Sorbic acid, Talc, Titanium dioxide (E 171), Triethyl citrate, Vanilla custard flavouring (containing propylene glycol)

6.2 Incompatibilities

Not applicable

6.3 Shelf life

3 years.

6.4 Special precautions for storage

No special precautions for storage

6.5 Nature and contents of container

Container: Polyester/ Aluminium/ Polyethylene-Foil Package sizes: 50 sachets, 100 sachets or 300 sachets Salofalk 500mg granules.

Not all pack sizes will be marketed.

6.6 Instructions for use and handling

No special requirements

7. MARKETING AUTHORISATION HOLDER

Dr. Falk Pharma GmbH

Leinenweberstr. 5

P. O. Box 6529

79041 Freiburg

Germany

8. MARKETING AUTHORISATION NUMBER(S)

PL 08637/0007

9. DATE OF FIRST AUTHORISATION/RENEWAL OF THE AUTHORISATION

1st September 2003

10. DATE OF REVISION OF THE TEXT

November 2003

Salofalk Enema 2g

(Dr Falk Pharma UK Limited)

1. NAME OF THE MEDICINAL PRODUCT

Salofalk Enema 2g.

2. QUALITATIVE AND QUANTITATIVE COMPOSITION

Each enema contains the following active ingredient:

Mesalazine 2g in 59 ml of suspension.

3. PHARMACEUTICAL FORM

Enema.

4. CLINICAL PARTICULARS

4.1 Therapeutic indications

Therapy and prophylaxis of acute attacks of mild ulcerative colitis, especially in the rectum and sigmoid colon and also in the descending colon.

4.2 Posology and method of administration

Method of administration: Rectal

Adults and the Elderly: 1 enema once a day at bedtime. The action of Salofalk is enhanced if the patient lies on the left side when introducing the enema. The dosage should be adjusted to suit the progress of the condition. Do not discontinue treatment suddenly.

Children: There is no recommended dose for children. Mesalazine should not be used in babies and infants.

4.3 Contraindications

Severe renal and hepatic function disturbances. Active gastrointestinal ulcers.

Hypersensitivity to salicylates.

4.4 Special warnings and special precautions for use

The drug should not be prescribed for infants.

Serious blood dyscrasias have been reported very rarely with mesalazine.

Haematological investigations including methaemoglobin values should be performed regularly during the course of therapy and if the patient develops unexplained bleeding, bruising, purpura, anaemia, fever or sore throat. Treatment should be stopped if there is suspicion or evidence of blood dyscrasia or if renal function deteriorates.

Sulphite component as excipient in enema preparation may cause hypersensitivity reactions in patients suffering from bronchial asthma.

Reports of interstitial nephritis occurring with mesalazine treatment are uncommon, however, ipatients on oral forms may require renal monitoring. Use with extreme caution in patients with mild to moderate renal impairment (see section 4.3) and if dehydration develops normal electrolyte levels and fluid balance should be restored as soon as possible.

4.5 Interaction with other medicinal products and other forms of Interaction

Although the following interactions are theoretically possible, owing to the low degree of absorption of the rectally administered mesalazine, the risk of their onset is extremely low: mesalazine may potentiate the actions of sulphonylureas. Interactions with coumarin, methotrexate, probenecid, sulphinpyrazone, spironolactone, frusemide and rifampicin cannot be excluded. Mesalazine can theoretically potentiate the side effects of glucocorticoids on the stomach. Concurrent use with other known nephrotoxic agents such as NSAID's and azathioprine may increase the risk of renal reactions (see section 4.4).

4.6 Pregnancy and lactation

Animal experiments on mesalazine have produced no evidence of embryonic effects.

No untoward effects were seen in a reproductive and fertility study with mesalazine in breast-fed rat pups. Mesalazine is acetylated in the body and passes in this form into breast milk. Limited use of mesalazine in pregnancy has shown no untoward effect on the foetus. However, it should not be used during the first trimester. It can be used with caution during pregnancy and only if the potential benefits outweigh the potential risks.

4.7 Effects on ability to drive and use machines

Salofalk Enema is not expected to affect ability to drive and use machines. If dizziness develops, the patient should not drive or operate machinery.

4.8 Undesirable effects

Rectal Salofalk may cause acute intolerance (sensitivity reactions). This is characterised by abdominal pain, bloody diarrhoea, fever, pruritis and rash. These are unrelated to dose. The most common adverse effects following treatment with rectal mesalazine are:

General symptoms such as dizziness, malaise, paraesthesia, arthralgia and pyrexia may develop following rectal administration of sulphasalazine.

GI effects: abdominal pain, flatulence, nausea, worsening or development of diarrhoea.

CNS effects: Headache, malaise, dizziness and peripheral neuropathy.

Sensitivity reactons: Mesalazine may be associated with an exacerbation of the symptoms of colitis in those patients who have previously had such problems with sulphasalazine. Allergic skin reactions such as rash, bullous skin reactions including erythema multiforme and Stevens-Johnson syndrome.

Other adverse effects: Fever, arthralgia, pericarditis, myocarditis, pancreatitis.

Other adverse effects were reported following oral administration of mesalazine.

There have been rare reports of leucopenia, neutropenia, agranulocytosis, aplastic anaemia and thrombocytopenia, abnormalities of hepatic function, hepatitis, allergic lung reactions, interstitial nephritis and nephritic syndrome with oral mesalazine treatment, usually reversible on withdrawal. Renal failure has been reported.

Mesalazine-induced nephrotoxicity should be suspected in patients developing renal dysfunction during treatment. Increased methaemoglobin levels may occur. Headache and digestive disturbances such as nausea and diarrhoea may occur. Isolated cases of hair loss have been reported.

4.9 Overdose

There have been no reported cases of over dosage

5. PHARMACOLOGICAL PROPERTIES

5.1 Pharmacodynamic properties

Mesalazine is the biologically active metabolite of salicylazosulphapyridine that is used in the treatment of certain chronic inflammatory conditions of the intestine.

5.2 Pharmacokinetic properties

Following rectal administration the major fraction is recovered from the faeces, a small percentage (approximately 15%) is absorbed; the absorbed mesalazine is excreted mainly in the urine, bilary excretion is secondary. The acetylated and the non-acetylated forms of mesalazine bind slightly to plasma proteins.

5.3 Preclinical safety data

None stated.

6. PHARMACEUTICAL PARTICULARS

6.1 List of excipients

Salofalk Enema 2g contain the following excipients:

Carbomer

Disodium edentate

Potassium acetate

Potassium metabisulphite

Purified water

Sodium benzoate

Xanthan gum

6.2 Incompatibilities

None known.

6.3 Shelf life

24 months.

6.4 Special precautions for storage

Store at room temperature (15-25°C) and protect from light.

6.5 Nature and contents of container

Low density concertina shaped polythene bottle with a low density polythene application nozzle packed in cartons contained seven individually blister packed bottles.

6.6 Instructions for use and handling

None

7. MARKETING AUTHORISATION HOLDER

Dr Falk Pharma UK Limited

Unit K

Bourne End Business Park

Cores End Road

Bourne End

Bucks

SL8 5AS

United Kingdom

8. MARKETING AUTHORISATION NUMBER(S)

PI 10341/0008

9. DATE OF FIRST AUTHORISATION/RENEWAL OF THE AUTHORISATION

31st December 2004

10. DATE OF REVISION OF THE TEXT

Salofalk Rectal Foam 1g

(Dr Falk Pharma UK Limited)

1. NAME OF THE MEDICINAL PRODUCT

Salofalk 1g/actuation Rectal Foam.

2. QUALITATIVE AND QUANTITATIVE COMPOSITION

1 actuation contains:

Mesalazine 1.0g

For excipients see 6.1

3. PHARMACEUTICAL FORM

Rectal foam.

White-greyish to slightly reddish-violet, creamy firm foam.

4. CLINICAL PARTICULARS

4.1 Therapeutic indications

Treatment of active, mild ulcerative colitis of the sigmoid colon and rectum.

4.2 Posology and method of administration

Method of Administration: rectal.

Adults and adolescents above 12 years of age:

2 administrations once a day at bedtime. The canister is first fitted with an applicator and then shaken for about 15 seconds before the applicator is inserted into the rectum as far as comfortable. To administer a dose of Salofalk®, the pump dome is fully pushed down and released. Note that the spray will only work properly when held with the pump dome pointing down. Following the first or second activation depending upon need (see below) the applicator should be held in position for 10-15 seconds before being withdrawn from the rectum. If the patient has difficulty in holding this amount of foam, the foam can also be administered in divided doses: one at bedtime and the other during the night (after evacuation of the first single dose) or in the early morning. If the normal dose does not provide the required effect, the dosage may be doubled (2 administrations at bedtime and 2 administrations in the early morning). The best results are obtained when the intestine is evacuated prior to administration of Salofalk®.

In general, an acute episode of a mild ulcerative colitis subsides after 4-6 weeks. It is recommended to continue the maintenance therapy with an oral mesalazine preparation e.g. Salofalk gastro-resistant prolonged release granules at a dosage recommended for this preparation.

Children below 12 years of age:

Salofalk should not be used in children below 12 years of age because of insufficient experience with this age group.

4.3 Contraindications

Salofalk® is contraindicated in cases of:

- pre-existing hypersensitivity to salicylic acid and its derivatives or to any of the other constituents.
- severe impairment of hepatic and renal function
- pre-existing gastric or duodenal ulcers
- haemorrhagic diathesis

Salofalk should not be used for the treatment of children below the age of 12 years.

Caution:

Asthmatics should be treated with care with Salofalk® since sulphite contained in the foam may cause hypersensitivity reactions.

4.4 Special warnings and special precautions for use

Blood tests (differential blood counts; liver function parameters like ALT or AST; serum creatinine) and urinary status (dip sticks) should be determined prior to and during treatment, at the discretion of the treating physician. As a guideline, controls are recommended 14 days after commencement of treatment, then a further two to three times at intervals of 4 weeks.

If the findings are normal, control examinations should be carried out every 3 months. If additional symptoms occur, control examinations should be performed immediately. Caution is recommended in patients with impaired hepatic function. Salofalk is not recommended in patients with impaired renal function. Mesalazine-induced renal toxicity should be considered if renal function deteriorates during treatment.

Patients with pulmonary disease, in particular asthma, should be very carefully monitored during a course of treatment with Salofalk.

Patients with a history of adverse drug reactions to preparations containing sulphasalazine should be kept under close medical surveillance on commencement of a course of treatment with Salofalk. Should Salofalk cause acute intolerability reactions such as cramps, acute abdominal pain, fever, severe headache and rash, therapy should be discontinued immediately.

Special notes:

In isolated cases hypersensitivity reactions principally in the form of respiratory problems may be experienced also by non-asthmatics due to the content of sulphite. This medicine contains propylene glycol that may cause lactic acidosis, hyperosmolality, haemolysis and CNS depression. Slight to mild skin irritation due to propylene glycol may occur. This medicine contains cetostearyl alcohol that may cause local skin reactions (e.g contact dermatitis).

4.5 Interaction with other medicinal products and other forms of Interaction

Specific interaction studies have not been performed.

Interactions may occur during treatment with Salofalk and concomitant administration of the following medicinal products. Most of these possible interactions are based on theoretical reasons:

- *Coumarin-type Anticoagulants:* possible potentiation of the anticoagulant effects (increasing the risk of gastro-intestinal haemorrhage)
- *Glucocorticoids:* possible increase in undesirable gastric effects
- *Sulphonylureas:* possible increase in the blood glucose-lowering effects.
- *Methotrexate:* possible increase in the toxic potential of methotrexate.
- *Probenecid/Sulphinpyrazone:* possible attenuation of the uricosuric effects.
- *Spironolactone/frusemide:* possible attenuation of the diuretic effects.
- *Rifampicin:* possible attenuation of the tuberculostatic effects.

In patients who are concomitantly treated with azathioprine or 6-mercaptopurine, possible enhanced myelosuppresive effects of azathioprine or 6-mercaptopurine should be taken into account.

4.6 Pregnancy and lactation

There are no adequate data from the use of Salofalk rectal foam in pregnant women.

No animal reproductive studies with Salofalk® foam have been performed. Previous animal studies on oral mesalazine do not indicate direct or indirect harmful effects with respect to pregnancy, embryonal/fetal development, parturition or postnatal development. Salofalk should not be used during pregnancy unless the potential benefit outweighs the possible risk. N-Acetyl-mesalazine (N-Ac-5-ASA) and to a lesser degree mesalazine are excreted in breast milk. Salofalk Foam administration is not recommended in breastfeeding women. If treatment is necessary, breast-feeding should be discontinued.

4.7 Effects on ability to drive and use machines

No effects on ability to drive and use machines have been observed.

4.8 Undesirable effects

Gastrointestinal undesirable effects (rare; 0.01% - < 0.1%):

Abdominal pain, diarrhoea, flatulence, nausea, vomiting.

CNS-related undesirable effects (rare 0.01% - < 0.1%):

headache, dizziness.

Renal undesirable effects (very rare < 0.01%);

Impairment of renal function including acute and chronic interstitial nephritis and renal insufficiency.

Hypersensitivity reactions (very rare < 0.01%):

Allergic exanthema, drug fever, bronchospasm, peri- and myocarditis, acute pancreatitis, allergic alveolitis, lupus erythematosus syndrome, pancolitis.

Musculoskeletal disorders (very rare < 0.01%);

Myalgia, arthralgia.

Blood and the lymphatic system disorders (very rare < 0.01%):

Altered blood counts (aplastic anaemia, agranulocytosis, pancytopenia, neutropenia, leukopenia, thrombocytopenia).

Hepato-biliary disorders (very rare < 0.01%)

Changes in hepatic function parameters (increase in transaminases), hepatitis.

Skin and appendage disorders (very rare < 0.01%)

Alopecia.

Special note:

Care should be taken when administering Salofalk to patients with diminished renal function. In a clinical study, a mild to moderate perianal/anal burning has been reported in few cases, and in one case in addition meteorism.

4.9 Overdose

No cases of intoxication have been reported to date and no specific antidotes are known. If necessary, intravenous infusion of electrolytes (forced diuresis) should be considered in cases of overdose.

5. PHARMACOLOGICAL PROPERTIES

5.1 Pharmacodynamic properties

Pharmacotherapeutic group:

Aminosalicylic acid and similar agents mesalazine ATC Code: A07EC02.

The mechanism of the anti-inflammatory action is unknown. The results of *in vitro* studies indicate that inhibition of lipoxygenase may play a role. Effects on prostaglandin concentrations in the intestinal mucosa have also been demonstrated. Mesalazine may also function as a radical scavenger of reactive oxygen compounds. Mesalazine acts predominantly locally at the gut mucosa and in the submucus tissue from the luminal side of the intestine. It is important therefore that mesalazine is available at the regions of inflammation. Systemic bioavailability / plasma concentrations of mesalazine therefore are of no relevance for therapeutic efficacy, but rather a factor for safety.

5.2 Pharmacokinetic properties

General considerations of mesalazine:

Absorption:

Mesalazine absorption is highest in the proximal gut regions and lowest in distal gut areas.

Biotransformation:

Mesalazine is metabolised both pre-systemically by the intestinal mucosa and the liver tothe pharmacologically inactive N-acetyl-5-aminosalicylic acid (N-Ac-5-ASA). The acetylation seems to be independent of the acetylator phenotype of the patient. Some acetylation also occurs through the action of colonic bacteria. Protein binding of mesalazine and N-Ac-5-ASA is 43% and 78% respectively.

Elimination:

Mesalazine and its metabolite N-Ac-5-ASA are eliminated via the faeces (major part), renally (varies between 20 and 50%, dependant on kind of application, pharmaceutical preparation and route of mesalazine release, respectively), and biliary (minor part). Renal excretion predominantly occurs as N-Ac-5-ASA. About 1% of total orally administered mesalazine dose is excreted into the breast milk mainly as N-Ac-5-ASA.

Salofalk Foam Specific:

Distribution:

A combined pharmacoscintigraphic / pharmacokinetic study showed that spreading of Salofalk Foam is homogeneous and fast, and is almost complete within 1 hour. It reaches the gut regions rectum, sigmoid colon, and left-sided colon in dependence of extension of inflammation.

Absorption:

Absorption of mesalazine is fast, and peak plasma concentrations for mesalazine and its metabolite N-Ac-5-ASA are reached at about 4 hours. However, plasma concentrations of a 2g mesalazine dose of foam are about comparable with an 250mg oral dose mesalazine, reaching maximum concentrations of about 0.4μg/ml. Pre-systemic metabolisation is fast, and N-Ac-5-ASA reaches its maximum plasma concentrations also at about 4 hours, like mesalazine, but plasma concentrations are about 4-5 times higher, about 2μg/ml.

5.3 Preclinical safety data

With the exception of a local tolerance study in dogs, which showed good rectal tolerance, no preclinical studies have been performed with Salofalk Foam.

Preclinical data reveal no special hazard for humans based on conventional studies of safety pharmacology, genotoxicity, carcinogenicity (rat) or toxicity to reproduction. Kidney toxicity (renal papillary necrosis and epithelial damage in the proximal convoluted tubule or the whole nephron) has been seen in repeat-dose toxicity studies with high oral doses of mesalazine. The clinical relevance of this finding is unknown.

6. PHARMACEUTICAL PARTICULARS

6.1 List of excipients
Sodium metabisulphite (E223),

cetostearyl alcohol,

polysorbate 60,

disodium edetate,

propylene glycol,

Propellants:

propane,

n-butane,

isobutane.

6.2 Incompatibilities
Not applicable

6.3 Shelf life
3 years.

After first actuation: 12 weeks.

6.4 Special precautions for storage
Do not store above 25°C. Do not refrigerate or freeze. This is a pressurised container, containing 3.75% by mass of inflammable propellant. It should be kept away from any flames or sparks, including cigarettes. It should be protected from direct sunlight and must not be pierced or burned even when empty.

6.5 Nature and contents of container
Aluminium pressurised container with metering valve containing 80g (14 actuations) of suspension together with 14 PVC applicators coated with white soft paraffin and liquid paraffin for administration of the foam.

6.6 Instructions for use and handling
No special requirements

7. MARKETING AUTHORISATION HOLDER
Dr. Falk Pharma GmbH

Leinenweberstr. 5

D-79108 Freiburg

Germany

8. MARKETING AUTHORISATION NUMBER(S)
08637/0003

9. DATE OF FIRST AUTHORISATION/RENEWAL OF THE AUTHORISATION
1 October 2001

10. DATE OF REVISION OF THE TEXT
September 2003

Salofalk Suppositories 500mg

(Dr Falk Pharma UK Limited)

1. NAME OF THE MEDICINAL PRODUCT
Salofalk Suppositories 500mg.

2. QUALITATIVE AND QUANTITATIVE COMPOSITION
Each suppository contains the following active ingredient:

Mesalazine 500mg.

3. PHARMACEUTICAL FORM
Suppository.

4. CLINICAL PARTICULARS

4.1 Therapeutic indications
Management of mild and moderate attacks of ulcerative colitis, especially in the rectum and sigmoid colon and also in the descending colon.

4.2 Posology and method of administration
Method of administration: Rectal

Adults and the Elderly: 1 to 2 suppositories, 2 to 3 times daily. The action of Salofalk is enhanced if the patient lies on the left side when introducing the suppository. The dosage should be adjusted to suit the progress of the condition. Do not discontinue treatment suddenly.

Children: There is no recommended dose for children. Mesalazine should not be used in babies and infants.

4.3 Contraindications
Severe renal and hepatic function disturbances. Active gastrointestinal ulcers. Hypersensitivity to salicylates.

4.4 Special warnings and special precautions for use
The drug should not be prescribed for infants.

Serious blood dyscrasias have been reported very rarely with mesalazine.

Haematological investigations including methaemoglobin values should be performed regularly during the course of therapy and if the patient develops unexplained bleeding, bruising, purpura, anaemia, fever or sore throat. Treatment should be stopped if there is suspicion or evidence of blood dyscrasia or if renal function deteriorates. Reports of interstitial nephritis occurring with mesalazine treatment are uncommon. However, patients on oral formulations may require renal monitoring.

Use with extreme caution in patients with mild to moderate renal impairment (see section 4.4) and if dehydration develops normal electrolyte levels and fluid balance should be restored as soon as possible.

4.5 Interaction with other medicinal products and other forms of Interaction
Although the following interactions are theoretically possible, owing to the low degree of absorption of the rectally administered mesalazine, the risk of their onset is extremely low: mesalazine may potentiate the actions of sulphonylureas. Interactions with coumarin, methotrexate, probenecid, sulphinpyrazone, spironolactone, frusemide and rifampicin cannot be excluded. Mesalazine can theoretically potentiate the side effects of glucocorticoids on the stomach.

Concurrent use with other known nephrotoxic agents such as NSAID's and azathioprine may increase the risk of renal reactions (see section 4.4).

4.6 Pregnancy and lactation
Animal experiments on mesalazine have produced no evidence of embryonic effects.

No untoward effects were seen in a reproductive and fertility study with mesalazine in breast-fed rat pups. Mesalazine is acetylated in the body and passes in this form into breast milk. Limited use of mesalazine in pregnancy has shown no untoward effect on the foetus. However, it should not be used in the first trimester. It can be used with caution during pregnancy and only if the potential benefits outweigh the potential risks.

4.7 Effects on ability to drive and use machines
Salofalk suppositories are not expected to affect ability to drive and use machines. If dizziness develops, the patient should not drive or operate machinery.

4.8 Undesirable effects
Rectal Salofalk may cause acute intolerance (sensitivity reactions). This is characterised by abdominal pain, bloody diarrhoea, fever, pruritis and rash. These are unrelated to dose. The most common adverse effects following treatment with rectal mesalazine are:

General symptoms such as dizziness, malaise, paraesthesia, arthralgia and pyrexia may develop following rectal administration of sulphasalazine.

GI effects: abdominal pain, flatulence, nausea, worsening or development of diarrhoea.

CNS effects: Headache, malaise, dizziness and peripheral neuropathy.

Sensitivity reactons: Mesalazine may be associated with an exacerbation of the symptoms of colitis in those patients who have previously had such problems with sulphasalazine. Allergic skin reactions such as rash, bullous skin reactions including erythema multiforme and Stevens-Johnson syndrome.

Other adverse effects: Fever, arthralgia, pericarditis, myocarditis, pancreatitis.

Other adverse effects were reported following oral administration of mesalazine.

There have been rare reports of leucopenia, neutropenia, agranulocytosis, aplastic anaemia and thrombocytopenia, abnormalities of hepatic function, hepatitis, allergic lung reactions, interstitial nephritis and nephrotic syndrome with oral mesalazine treatment, usually reversible on withdrawal. Renal failure has been reported.

Mesalazine-induced nephrotoxicity should be suspected in patients developing renal dysfunction during treatment. Increased methaemoglobin levels may occur. Headache and digestive disturbances such as nausea and diarrhoea may occur. Isolated cases of hair loss have been reported.

4.9 Overdose
There have been no reported cases of over dosage

5. PHARMACOLOGICAL PROPERTIES

5.1 Pharmacodynamic properties
Mesalazine is the biologically active metabolite of salicylazosulphapyridine that is used in the treatment of certain chronic inflammatory conditions of the intestine.

5.2 Pharmacokinetic properties
Following rectal administration the major fraction is recovered from the faeces, a small percentage (approximately 15%) is absorbed; the absorbed mesalazine is excreted mainly in the urine, bilary excretion is secondary. The acetylated and the non-acetylated forms of mesalazine bind slightly to plasma proteins.

5.3 Preclinical safety data
None stated.

6. PHARMACEUTICAL PARTICULARS

6.1 List of excipients
Salofalk Suppositories 500mg contain the following excipients:

Hard Fat

Docusate sodium

Cetyl alcohol

6.2 Incompatibilities
None known.

6.3 Shelf life
36 months.

6.4 Special precautions for storage
Store at room temperature (15-25°C) and protect from light.

6.5 Nature and contents of container
Cartons of ten or thirty suppositories in white, opaque PVC/PE moulded strips.

Each strip contains five suppositories.

6.6 Instructions for use and handling
None

7. MARKETING AUTHORISATION HOLDER
Dr Falk Pharma UK Limited

Unit K

Bourne End Business Park

Cores End Road

Bourne End

Bucks

SL8 5AS

United Kingdom

8. MARKETING AUTHORISATION NUMBER(S)
PI 10341/0009

9. DATE OF FIRST AUTHORISATION/RENEWAL OF THE AUTHORISATION
31st December 2004

10. DATE OF REVISION OF THE TEXT

Sandimmun Concentrate for Infusion 50mg/ml

(Novartis Pharmaceuticals UK Ltd)

1. NAME OF THE MEDICINAL PRODUCT
SANDIMMUN Concentrate for Infusion 50mg/ml.

2. QUALITATIVE AND QUANTITATIVE COMPOSITION
Ciclosporin 50mg in 1ml.

3. PHARMACEUTICAL FORM
Concentrate for iv infusion.

4. CLINICAL PARTICULARS

4.1 Therapeutic indications
Organ transplantation

Prevention of graft rejection following kidney, liver, heart, combined heart-lung, lung or pancreas transplants.

Treatment of transplant rejection in patients previously receiving other immunosuppressive agents.

Bone marrow transplantation

Prevention of graft rejection following bone marrow transplantation and prophylaxis of graft-versus-host disease (GVHD).

Treatment of established graft-versus-host disease (GVHD).

4.2 Posology and method of administration
Organ transplantation

Initially, a single oral dose of 10-15mg/kg body weight, should be given 4-12 hours before transplantation. As a general rule, treatment should continue at a dose of 10-15mg/kg/day for 1-2 weeks post-operatively. Dosage should then be gradually reduced until a maintenance dose of 2-6mg/kg/day is reached. Dosage should be adjusted by monitoring ciclosporin blood levels and kidney function. When SANDIMMUN is given with other immunosuppressants (e.g. with corticosteroids or as part of a triple or quadruple drug therapy) lower doses (e.g. 3-6mg/kg/day orally initially) may be used.

The use of the concentrate for intravenous infusion is recommended in organ transplant patients who are unable to take SANDIMMUN orally (e.g. shortly after surgery) or in whom the absorption of the oral forms might be impaired during episodes of gastrointestinal disturbances. In such cases the intravenous dose is one third of the recommended oral dose. It is recommended, however, that patients are transferred to oral therapy as soon as the given circumstances allow.

Bone marrow transplantation/prevention and treatment of graft-versus-host disease (GVHD)

SANDIMMUN Concentrate for Intravenous Infusion is usually preferred for initiation of therapy, although the oral forms may be used. The recommended dosage by the intravenous route is 3-5mg/kg/day, starting on the day before transplantation and continuing during the immediate post-transplant period of up to two weeks until oral maintenance therapy begins.

Treatment with SANDIMMUN should continue using the oral forms at a dosage of 12.5mg/kg/day for at least three and preferably six months before tailing off to zero. In some cases higher oral doses or the use of i.v. therapy may be necessary in the presence of gastrointestinal disturbances which might decrease absorption. If oral treatment is used to initiate therapy the recommended dose is 12.5-15mg/kg/day starting on the day before transplantation.

If GVHD develops after SANDIMMUN is withdrawn it should respond to reinstitution of therapy. Low doses should be used for mild, chronic GVHD.

Intravenous administration

When SANDIMMUN is administered by the intravenous route, the intravenous dose is one third of the recommended oral dose.

SANDIMMUN concentrate should be diluted 1:20 to 1:100 with normal saline or 5% glucose before use and given by slow intravenous infusion over 2-6 hours.

Use in the elderly

Experience in the elderly is limited but no particular problems have been reported following the use of the drug at the recommended dose. However, factors sometimes associated with ageing, in particular impaired renal function, make careful supervision essential and may necessitate dosage adjustment.

Use in children

Experience with SANDIMMUN in young children is still limited. Transplant recipients from three months of age have received the drug at the recommended dosage with no particular problems, although at dosages above the upper end of the recommended range, children seem to be more susceptible to fluid retention, convulsions and hypertension. This responds to dosage reduction.

4.3 Contraindications

Known hypersensitivity to ciclosporin.

Concomitant use of tacrolimus is specifically contraindicated.

SANDIMMUN Concentrate for Intravenous Infusion should not be used in patients known to be hypersensitive to polyethoxylated castor oils.

4.4 Special warnings and special precautions for use

SANDIMMUN can impair renal function. Close monitoring of serum creatinine and urea is required and dosage adjustment may be necessary. Increases in serum creatinine and urea occurring during the first few weeks of SANDIMMUN therapy are generally dose-dependent and reversible and usually respond to dosage reduction. During long-term treatment, some patients may develop structural changes in the kidney (e.g. interstitial fibrosis) which, in renal transplant recipients, must be distinguished from chronic rejection.

SANDIMMUN may also affect liver function and dosage adjustment, based on the results of bilirubin and liver enzyme monitoring, may be necessary.

Regular monitoring of blood pressure is required during SANDIMMUN therapy. If hypertension develops, appropriate antihypertensive treatment must be instituted.

Ciclosporin enhances the risk of hyperkalaemia, especially in patients with renal dysfunction. Caution is also required when ciclosporin is co-administered with potassium sparing diuretics, angiotensin converting enzyme inhibitors, angiotensin II receptor antagonists and potassium containing drugs as well as in patients on a potassium rich diet. Control of potassium levels in these situations is advisable.

Ciclosporin enhances the clearance of magnesium. This can lead to symptomatic hypomagnesaemia, especially in the peri-transplant period. Control of serum magnesium levels is therefore recommended in the peri-transplant period, particularly in the presence of neurological symptom/signs. If considered necessary, magnesium supplementation should be given.

Caution is required in treating patients with hyperuricaemia because SANDIMMUN can aggravate this condition (see 4.8 Undesirable effects).

Ciclosporin increases the risk of malignancies including lymphomas, skin and other tumours. The increased risk appears to be related to the degree and duration of immunosuppression rather than to the specific use of ciclosporin. Hence a treatment regimen containing immunosuppressants should be used with caution as this could lead to lymphoproliferative disorders and solid organ tumours, some with reported fatalities.

Ciclosporin predisposes patients to infection with a variety of pathogens including bacteria, parasites, viruses and other opportunistic pathogens. This appears to be related to the degree and duration of immunosuppression rather than to the specific use of ciclosporin. As this can lead to a fatal outcome, effective pre-emptive and therapeutic strategies should be employed particularly in patients on multiple long-term immunosuppressive therapy.

In SANDIMMUN-treated renal transplant recipients, a machine perfusion time of more than 24 hours and a reanastomosis time of more than 45 minutes can have a significant effect on graft function. Both factors appear to increase the incidence of acute tubular necrosis.

The concentrate for intravenous infusion contains polyethoxylated castor oil, which has been reported to cause anaphylactoid reactions. These reactions can consist of flushing of face and upper thorax, acute respiratory distress with dyspnoea and wheezing and non-cardiogenic pulmonary oedema; blood pressure changes and tachycardia. Special caution is therefore necessary in patients who have previously received intravenous injections or intravenous infusions containing polyethoxylated castor oil, or in patients with an allergic predisposition.

Thus patients receiving SANDIMMUN i.v. should be under continuous observation for at least the first 30 minutes following start of the infusion and at frequent intervals thereafter. If anaphylaxis occurs, the infusion should be discontinued and the patient managed in accordance with common clinical practice.

SANDIMMUN can induce a reversible increase in blood lipids. It is therefore advisable to perform lipid determinations before treatment and thereafter as appropriate.

Ciclosporin may increase the risk of Benign Intracranial Hypertension. Patients presenting with signs of raised intracranial pressure should be investigated and if Benign Intracranial Hypertension is diagnosed, ciclosporin should be withdrawn due to the possible risk of permanent visual loss.

4.5 Interaction with other medicinal products and other forms of Interaction

Food interactions

The concomitant intake of a fat-rich meal or grapefruit juice has been reported to increase the bioavailability of ciclosporin.

Drug interactions

Of the many drugs reported to interact with ciclosporin, those for which the interactions are adequately substantiated and considered to have clinical implications are listed below.

Various agents are known to either increase or decrease plasma or whole blood ciclosporin levels usually by inhibition or induction of enzymes involved in the metabolism of ciclosporin, in particular cytochrome P450.

Drugs that decrease ciclosporin levels:

Barbiturates, carbamazepine, phenytoin; rifampicin; octreotide; orlistat; hypericum perforatum (St John's Wort); ticlopidine.

Drugs that increase ciclosporin levels:

Macrolide antibiotics (mainly erythromycin and clarithromycin); ketoconazole, fluconazole, itraconazole; diltiazem, nicardipine, verapamil; metoclopramide; oral contraceptives; danazol; methylprednisolone (high dose); allopurinol; amiodarone; ursodeoxycholic acid; protease inhibitors.

Other relevant drug interactions

Care should be taken when using ciclosporin together with other drugs that exhibit nephrotoxic synergy: aminoglycosides (including gentamicin, tobramycin), amphotericin B, ciprofloxacin, vancomycin, trimethoprim (+ sulfamethoxazole); non-steroidal anti-inflammatory drugs (including diclofenac, naproxen, sulindac); melphalan.

During treatment with ciclosporin, vaccination may be less effective; the use of live-attenuated vaccines should be avoided.

The concurrent administration of nifedipine with ciclosporin may result in an increased rate of gingival hyperplasia compared with that observed when ciclosporin is given alone.

The concomitant use of diclofenac and ciclosporin has been found to result in a significant increase in the bioavailability of diclofenac, with the possible consequence of reversible renal function impairment. The increase in the bioavailability of diclofenac is most probably caused by a reduction of its first-pass effect. If non-steroidal anti-inflammatory drugs with a low first-pass effect (e.g. acetylsalicylic acid) are given together with ciclosporin, no increase in their bioavailability is to be expected.

Ciclosporin may also reduce the clearance of digoxin thereby causing digoxin toxicity.

Ciclosporin has also been reported to reduce the clearance of prednisolone.

Administration of ciclosporin may enhance the potential of HMG-CoA reductase inhibitors and colchicine to induce muscular toxicity eg muscle pain and weakness, myositis and occasionally rhabdomyolysis.

Recommendations

If the concomitant use of drug known to interact with ciclosporin cannot be avoided, the following basic recommendations should be observed.

During the concomitant use of a drug that may exhibit nephrotoxic synergy, close monitoring of renal function (in particular serum creatinine) should be performed. If a significant impairment of renal function occurs, the dosage of the co-administered drug should be reduced or alternative treatment considered.

Drugs known to reduce or increase the bioavailability of ciclosporin: in transplant patients frequent measurement of ciclosporin levels and, if necessary, ciclosporin dosage adjustment are required, particularly during the introduction or withdrawal of the co-administered drug. In non-transplant patients the value of ciclosporin blood level monitoring is questionable, as in these patients the relationship between blood level and clinical effect is less well established. If drugs known to increase ciclosporin levels are given concomitantly, frequent assessment of renal function and careful monitoring for ciclosporin related side-effects may be more appropriate than blood level measurement.

The concomitant use of nifedipine should be avoided in patients in whom gingival hyperplasia develops as a side effect of ciclosporin.

Non-steroidal anti-inflammatory drugs known to undergo strong first-pass metabolism (e.g. diclofenac) should be given at doses lower than those that would be used in patients not receiving ciclosporin. When diclofenac is given concomitantly with ciclosporin the dose of diclofenac should be reduced by approximately half (see Section 4.2 Posology and Administration).

If digoxin, colchicine or HMG-CoA reductase inhibitors are used concurrently with ciclosporin, close clinical observation is required in order to enable early detection of toxic manifestations of the drug, followed by reduction of its dosage or its withdrawal.

4.6 Pregnancy and lactation

Ciclosporin is not teratogenic in animals. As the safety of SANDIMMUN in human pregnancy has not been fully established, it should only be used in pregnancy if the benefit outweighs any potential risks.

Ciclosporin passes into the breast milk and mothers receiving treatment with SANDIMMUN should not therefore, breast feed their infants.

4.7 Effects on ability to drive and use machines

No data exist on the effects of SANDIMMUN on the ability to drive and to use machines.

4.8 Undesirable effects

Many side effects associated with ciclosporin therapy are dose-dependent and responsive to dose reduction.

Frequency estimate: very common $\geqslant$ 10%, common $\geqslant$ 1% to $<$10%, Uncommon $\geqslant$ 0.1% to $<$1%, rare $\geqslant$ 0.01% to $<$0.1%, very rare $<$0.01%.

Blood and the lymphatic system disorders:

Uncommon: anaemia, thrombocytopenia

Rare: micro-angiopathic haemolytic anaemia, haemolytic uraemic syndrome

Endocrine disorders:

Rare: menstrual disturbances, gynaecomastia

Metabolism and nutrition disorders:

Very common: hyperlipidaemia

Common: hyperuricaemia, hyperkalaemia, hypomagnesaemia

Rare: hyperglycaemia

Nervous system disorders:

Very common: tremor, headache

Common: paraesthesia

Uncommon: signs of encephalopathy or demyelination, especially in liver transplant patients, such as convulsions, confusion, disorientation, decreased responsiveness, agitation, insomnia, visual disturbances, cortical blindness, coma, paresis, cerebellar ataxia.

Rare: motor polyneuropathy

Very rare: optic disc oedema including papilloedema with possible visual impairment secondary to Benign Intracranial Hypertension.

Cardiovascular disorders:

Very common: hypertension

Gastrointestinal disorders:

Common: anorexia, nausea, vomiting, abdominal pain, diarrhoea, gingival hyperplasia,

Hepato-biliary disorders:

Common: hepatic dysfunction

Rare: pancreatitis.

Skin and subcutaneous tissue disorders:

Common: hypertrichosis

Uncommon: allergic rashes

Musculoskeletal, connective tissue and bone disorders:

Common: muscle cramps, myalgia

Rare: muscle weakness, myopathy

Renal and urinary disorders:

Very common: renal dysfunction (see 4.4 'Special Warnings and special precautions for use')

General disorders and administration site conditions:

Common: fatigue

Uncommon: oedema, weight increase

The increased risk of developing malignancies and lymphoproliferative disorders appears to be related to the degree and duration of immunosuppression rather than to the use of specific agents (refer to Section 4.4 "Special Warnings and Precautions").

4.9 Overdose

Little experience is available with overdosage. Symptomatic treatment and general supportive measures should be followed in all cases of overdosage.

Signs of nephrotoxicity might occur which would be expected to resolve following drug withdrawal. SANDIMMUN is not dialysable to any great extent nor is it well cleared by charcoal haemoperfusion. Hypertension and convulsions have been reported in some patients receiving SANDIMMUN therapy at doses above the recommended range and in others with high trough blood levels of ciclosporin. This might, therefore, be expected as a feature of overdosage.

5. PHARMACOLOGICAL PROPERTIES

5.1 Pharmacodynamic properties

Pharmacotherapeutic group: selective immunosuppressive agents (ATC code L04A A01)

Ciclosporin A is a cyclic undecapeptide with immunosuppressant properties. Studies suggest that ciclosporin A inhibits the development of cell-mediated reactions, including allograft immunity, delayed cutaneous hypersensitivity, experimental allergic encephalomyelitis, Freund's adjuvant arthritis, graft-verus-host disease and also T-cell dependent antibody production. It also inhibits lymphokine production and release, including interleukin 2 or T-cell growth factor (TCGF). Ciclosporin appears to block the resting lymphocytes in the G_0 or G_1 phase of the cell cycle.

All available evidence suggests that ciclosporin acts specifically and reversibly on lymphocytes. Unlike cytostatic agents it does not depress haemopoeisis and has no effect on the function of phagocytic cells.

5.2 Pharmacokinetic properties

SANDIMMUN Concentrate for Intravenous Infusion has been shown to be bioequivalent to SANDIMMUN oral solution.

Absolute bioavailability is 25-50% at steady state and peak blood concentrations are achieved within 1-6 hours.

Ciclosporin A is distributed largely outside the blood volume. Within blood, 33-47% is present in plasma, 4-9% in lymphocytes, 5-12% in granulocytes and 41-58% in erythrocytes. In plasma, approximately 90% is bound to protein, mainly lipoproteins.

Ciclosporin is extensively biotransformed to approximately 15 metabolites, there being no single major metabolic pathway. Elimination is primarily biliary, with only 6% of the oral dose excreted in the urine; only 0.1% is excreted in the urine as unchanged drug. The terminal elimination half-life from blood is approximately 19 hours, irrespective of the dose or route of administration.

6. PHARMACEUTICAL PARTICULARS

6.1 List of excipients

Absolute ethanol and polyethoxylated castor oil.

6.2 Incompatibilities

Sandimmun concentrate for i.v. infusion contains polyoxyethylated castor oil, which can cause phthalate stripping from PVC. If available, glass containers should be used for infusion. Plastic bottles should be used only if they conform to the requirements for "Sterile plastic containers for human blood and blood components". If polyvinyl chloride bags are used, they should comply with the requirements for "Empty sterile containers of plasticised poly (vinyl chloride) for human blood and blood components" of the current European Pharmacopoeia. Containers and stoppers should be free of silicon oil and fatty substances.

6.3 Shelf life

4 years.

6.4 Special precautions for storage

Store below 30°C.

6.5 Nature and contents of container

SANDIMMUN concentrate for infusion is available in 1ml and 5ml uncoloured glass ampoules.

6.6 Instructions for use and handling

Not stated.

7. MARKETING AUTHORISATION HOLDER

Novartis Pharmaceuticals UK Limited

Trading as SANDOZ PHARMACEUTICALS

Frimley Business Park

Frimley

Camberley

Surrey

GU16 7SR

8. MARKETING AUTHORISATION NUMBER(S)

PL 00101/0153.

9. DATE OF FIRST AUTHORISATION/RENEWAL OF THE AUTHORISATION

17 February 1983/17 February 1998.

10. DATE OF REVISION OF THE TEXT

18 December 2004

Legal Category

POM

Sandocal 400 & 1000

(Novartis Consumer Health)

1. NAME OF THE MEDICINAL PRODUCT

SANDOCAL 400

SANDOCAL 1000

2. QUALITATIVE AND QUANTITATIVE COMPOSITION

SANDOCAL 400: Each effervescent tablet contains 930.8 mg calcium lactate gluconate and 700 mg calcium carbonate

SANDOCAL 1000: Each effervescent tablet contains 2.327 g calcium lactate gluconate and 1.75 g calcium carbonate

3. PHARMACEUTICAL FORM

Effervescent tablets.

4. CLINICAL PARTICULARS

4.1 Therapeutic indications

1. As an adjunct to conventional therapy in the arrest or slowing down of bone demineralisation in osteoporosis.

2. In the arrest or slowing down of bone demineralisation in osteoporosis where other effective treatment is contra-indicated.

3. As a supplemental source of calcium in the correction of dietary deficiencies or when normal requirements are high.

4.2 Posology and method of administration

Treatment of therapeutic supplementation should aim to restore or maintain normal levels of calcium (2.25 to 2.75 mmol/l or 4.5 to 5.5 meq/l).

Indication	Daily Dose	
Adults Osteoporosis	SANDOCAL 400 3 to 4 tablets/ day	SANDOCAL 1000 1 to 2 tablets/ day
Therapeutic supplement (dose dependent upon severity)	1 to 4 tablets/ day	1 to 2 tablets/ day
Children Calcium deficiency.	1 to 2 tablets/ day	1 tablet/day
Dietary supplementation	1 tablet/day	not applicable

Elderly

No evidence exists that tolerance is directly affected by advanced age. Elderly patients should be supervised, as factors sometimes associated with aging, such as poor diet or renal function may indirectly affect tolerance and may require dosage adjustment.

Route of administration

Oral.

4.3 Contraindications

Hypercalcaemia (e.g. in hyperparathyroidism, vitamin D overdosage, decalcifying tumours such as plasmocytoma, severe renal failure, bone metastases), severe hypercalciuria and renal calculi.

4.4 Special warnings and special precautions for use

In mild hypercalciuria exceeding 300 mg (7.5 mmol) per 24 hours, or renal failure, or where there is evidence of stone formation in the urinary tract, adequate checks must be kept on urinary calcium excretion; if necessary the dosage should be reduced or calcium therapy discontinued.

4.5 Interaction with other medicinal products and other forms of Interaction

High vitamin D intake should be avoided during calcium therapy, unless especially indicated (see Overdosage section). Thiazide diuretics reduce urinary calcium excretion so the risk of hypercalcaemia should be considered.

Oral calcium supplementation is aimed at restoring normal serum calcium levels. Although it is extremely unlikely that high enough levels will be achieved to adversely affect digitalised patients, this theoretical possibility should be considered.

Oral calcium administration may reduce the absorption of oral tetracycline or fluoride preparations. An interval of 3 hours should be observed if the two are to be given.

4.6 Pregnancy and lactation

The likelihood of hypercalcaemia is increased in pregnant women in whom calcium and Vitamin D are co-administered. Epidemiological studies with calcium have shown no increase in the teratogenic hazard to the foetus if used in the doses recommended. Although supplemental calcium may be excreted in breast milk, the concentration is unlikely to be sufficient to produce an adverse effect on the neonate.

4.7 Effects on ability to drive and use machines

None stated.

4.8 Undesirable effects

Mild gastrointestinal disturbances (e.g. constipation, diarrhoea) have occurred rarely. Although hypercalcaemia would not be expected in patients unless their renal function were impaired, the following symptoms could indicate the possibility of hypercalcaemia: nausea, vomiting, anorexia, constipation, abdominal pain, bone pain, thirst, polyuria, muscle weakness, drowsiness or confusion.

4.9 Overdose

The amount of calcium absorbed following overdosage with will depend on the individual's calcium status. Deliberate overdosage with effervescent preparations is unlikely and acute overdosage has not been reported. It might cause gastrointestinal disturbance but would not be expected to cause hypercalcaemia except in patients treated with excessive doses of vitamin D. Treatment should be aimed at lowering serum calcium levels, e.g. administration of oral phosphates.

5. PHARMACOLOGICAL PROPERTIES

5.1 Pharmacodynamic properties

Calcium is an endogenous ion of the body essential for the maintenance of a number of physiologic processes. It participates as an integral factor in the maintenance of the functional integrity of the nervous system, in the contractile mechanisms of muscle tissue, in the clotting of blood, and in the formation of the major structural material of the skeleton.

A dynamic equilibrium occurs between blood calcium and skeletal calcium, homeostasis being mainly regulated by the parathyroid hormone, by calcitonin and by vitamin D. Variations in the concentration of ionised calcium are responsible for the symptoms of hyper/hypocalcaemia. Soluble calcium salts are commonly used in the treatment of calcium deficiency and may be given by mouth or injection.

5.2 Pharmacokinetic properties

Concentrations of plasma calcium are determined chiefly by gastrointestinal absorption, bone metabolism and renal excretion, and levels are closely regulated within the normal limits of 4.5 to 5.5 meq/l (2.25 to 2.75 mmol/l) of which 50 to 60% is present in ionised form. Up to 105 is present as diffusible complexes with organic acids; the remainder is present as non-diffusible complexes with proteins. More than 99% of the body calcium is deposited in bone as hydroxyapatite crystals which are available for exchange with calcium in the extracellular fluids. In bone as a whole, about 1% of calcium is in a readily exchangable pool. Bone therefore functions as the main reservoir of these ions from which they may be readily mobilised if the plasma concentration falls, or in which they may be deposited if the plasma level rises.

5.3 Preclinical safety data

None stated.

6. PHARMACEUTICAL PARTICULARS

6.1 List of excipients

Citric acid, polyethylene glycol 4000, orange flavour and aspartame.

6.2 Incompatibilities

None.

6.3 Shelf life

36 months.

6.4 Special precautions for storage

Store below 30°C. Protect from humidity.

6.5 Nature and contents of container

SANDOCAL 400: The tablets are whitish, round and flat with a slightly rough surface and come in propylene tubes with polyethylene caps. Each tube contains 20 tablets. Five tubes are packed into a carton.

SANDOCAL 1000: The tablets are whitish, round and flat with a slightly rough surface and come in propylene tubes with polyethylene caps. Each tube contains 10 tablets. Three tubes are packed into a carton.

6.6 Instructions for use and handling

None.

7. MARKETING AUTHORISATION HOLDER

Novartis Consumer Health UK Ltd

Wimblehurst Road

Horsham

West Sussex

RH12 4AB

UK

Trading style: Novartis Consumer Health

8. MARKETING AUTHORISATION NUMBER(S)

SANDOCAL 400: PL 00030/0178

SANDOCAL 1000: PL 00030/0179

9. DATE OF FIRST AUTHORISATION/RENEWAL OF THE AUTHORISATION

4 September 2000

10. DATE OF REVISION OF THE TEXT

September 2000

Additional information

Legal category: P

Sando-K

(HK Pharma Limited)

1. NAME OF THE MEDICINAL PRODUCT

SANDO-K®

2. QUALITATIVE AND QUANTITATIVE COMPOSITION
Effervescent Tablets containing 0.6g potassium chloride Ph.Eur., 0.4g potassium bicarbonate USP

3. PHARMACEUTICAL FORM
Flat, round, white effervescent tablet with a slightly rough surface, weighing 2.4g and of 22mm diameter and 4.25mm thick

4. CLINICAL PARTICULARS

4.1 Therapeutic indications
Prevention and treatment of hypokalaemic states such as those associated with:

i) Use of drugs which can induce potassium depletion eg. frusemide, thiazide diuretics, corticosteroids, carbenoxolone and cardiac glycosides, especially in combination with diuretics;

ii) Potassium loss resulting from severe diarrhoea, vomiting or fistulas;

iii) Acid-base disturbances e.g. alkalosis, renal tubular acidosis, states in which there is aldosterone excess, Cushing syndrome;

iv) Decreased intake of potassium e.g. malnutrition, alcoholism, some elderly patients with deficient diets;

v) Since SANDO-K Effervescent Tablets contain Cl^- they may be used in the treatment of hypokalaemia associated with hypochloraemic alkalosis.

4.2 Posology and method of administration
Oral administration, after dissolution of the tablet in water. May be taken with food if preferred.

Adults and children: Dosage is dependent upon the clinical conditions and diet of the patient, however the administration of 2 to 4 tablets daily (24 to 48 mmol K^+) is likely to provide an adequate prophylactic or therapeutic dose in most patients. Large doses may be indicated in more severe hypokalaemic conditions when the dose should be regulated by the patient's response as determined by serum electrolyte levels and acid-base studies.

Dosage guidelines: A drop in serum potassium level of 1 mmol/l represents a loss of about 100-200 mmol of potassium from body stores. While serum potassium levels below 2 mmol/l may warrant intravenous replacement therapy, following are approximate guidelines in less severe potassium depletion:

For serum levels between 2-3 mmol/l, a maximum daily dose of 100-200 mmol K^+ (8-16 tablets) and for serum levels between 3-4 mmol/l, a maximum daily dose of 50-100 mmol K^+ (4-8 tablets) should be considered.

Elderly: No evidence exists that elderly patients require different dosages or show different side-effects than younger patients. However, such patients should be carefully supervised as factors sometimes associated with ageing, such as poor diet or impaired renal function, may indirectly affect the dosage or tolerability.

4.3 Contraindications
Severe renal impairment with oliguria, inadequately treated Addison's disease, hyperkalaemia from any cause, crush injuries and acute dehydration.

4.4 Special warnings and special precautions for use
Periodic evaluation of the patient's clinical status, serum electrolytes and the ECG should be carried out when replacement therapy is undertaken. This is particularly important in patients with cardiac disease and in those receiving digitalis. Care should be taken to avoid dosage in excess of requirements for patients with impaired renal function. Caution is also necessary in patients receiving potassium-sparing diuretics and ACE-inhibitors, and in patients with myotonia congenita or severe haemolysis. In patients with acidosis, the acid-base balance should be monitored. In patients with hypertension, it should be remembered that correction of hypokalaemia may lower blood pressure.

4.5 Interaction with other medicinal products and other forms of Interaction
If co-administered with potassium-sparing diuretics and ACE-inhibitors, the risk of hyperkalaemia must be considered.

4.6 Pregnancy and lactation
No clinical problems have been encountered during pregnancy and lactation. Nevertheless, the benefit of treatment should be considered in relation to the risks before SANDO-K is given to pregnant or nursing women.

4.7 Effects on ability to drive and use machines
No effects known

4.8 Undesirable effects
Abdominal discomfort, diarrhoea, nausea and vomiting may occur. If there are any signs of gastric irritancy, SANDO-K, in common with all other potassium salts, should be given with or after food. Gastric irritancy has occurred but this is rare since the tablets dissolve in water and are taken in solution, thus preventing high local concentrations. A moderate hyperkalaemia may be asymptomatic; if suspected reference to the section on overdosage is recommended.

4.9 Overdose
Hyperkalaemia. Poisoning is usually minimal below 6.5 mmol per litre but may be severe above 8 mmol per litre. However, comparatively low doses may cause adverse effects when excretion is delayed as in renal insufficiency. The absolute toxicity is dependent on other electrolytes and acid-base levels.

Hyperkalaemic symptoms include paraesthesia of the extremities, listlessness, mental confusion, weakness, paralysis, hypotension, cardiac arrhythmias, heart block and cardiac arrest.

Hyperkalaemia is often asymptomatic. However, increasing serum potassium levels can be detected by changes in the ECG; initially the appearance of tall, peaked T waves, followed by a widening of the QRS complex bending into the abnormal T waves. P-wave voltage decreases and the PR interval is prolonged.

Severe cardiac toxicity may be treated with calcium gluconate (10-20ml of a 10% injection given over 1-5 minutes with ECG monitoring). The effect may be transient and the injection may need to be repeated.

Raised serum potassium levels respond to administration of dextrose (300-500ml/hr of 10 or 25% solution), dextrose and insulin (as for dextrose with 10 units of insulin per 20g dextrose), or sodium bicarbonate solution.

Cation exchange resins may be used, or in severe cases peritoneal dialysis or haemodialysis may be necessary.

Caution should be exercised in patients who are digitalised and who may experience acute digitalis intoxication in the course of potassium removal.

5. PHARMACOLOGICAL PROPERTIES

5.1 Pharmacodynamic properties
The potassium ion is essential to the maintenance of body function, being involved in the synthesis of protein, metabolism of carbohydrate and storage of energy reserves. It interacts with sodium in the operation of the trans- membrane pump and at the site of exchange in the kidney, exchanges with sodium ion to maintain body homeostasis. A close relationship between potassium ion and magnesium ion has also been noted; a deficit in one ion has been associated with low levels of the other.

The diet of a healthy adult will provide an adequate intake of potassium (considered to be 20.5 to 33.3 mmol potassium daily) from a total intake of 60-100 mmol potassium. Total body potassium in an adult is about 3,500 mmol depending on the non-fat body tissues. A deficient intake or failure to conserve potassium leads to symptoms of hypokalaemia.

5.2 Pharmacokinetic properties
Unless a deficiency is present, requiring a supplement, sufficient potassium is taken into the body through the daily diet. The chloride salt of potassium is readily absorbed from the gastro-intestinal tract. Potassium enters the intracellular fluid to maintain a concentration of about 150 mEq/l and the normal range of concentration of potassium in the plasma is considered to be 3.5 - 5 mEq/l. Excretion of potassium is mainly by the distal tubules of the kidney, by the faeces (5 to 10 mmol/day) and a smaller amount in perspiration.

Metabolic, drug induced, or dietary deficiencies in potassium intake may require administration of a supplement.

5.3 Preclinical safety data
SANDO-K Effervescent Tablets contain potassium chloride and postassium bicarbonate (both of which are the subject of pharmacopoeial monographs). The physiological, pharmacological and clinical toxicity of potassium salts are well documented and limited animal data are therefore available

6. PHARMACEUTICAL PARTICULARS

6.1 List of excipients
Dioctyle sodium sulphosuccinate BPC, Colloidal anhydrous silica EP, Talc (acid washed) EP, Sodium saccharin BP, Icing sugar, CP HSE, Pulverised sugar, EP, Citric acid anhydrous 30/60 EP, Polyethylene glycol 4000 EP, Purified water EP

6.2 Incompatibilities
Not applicable

6.3 Shelf life
36 months

6.4 Special precautions for storage
Do not store above 25°C. Store in the original container. Keep the container tightly closed.

6.5 Nature and contents of container
High density polypropylene tube with polyethylene bellowed stopper containing integral silica gel dessicant capsule. Pack size 20.

6.6 Instructions for use and handling
Not applicable

7. MARKETING AUTHORISATION HOLDER
HK Pharma
PO Box 105
Hitchin
Herts SG5 2DE

8. MARKETING AUTHORISATION NUMBER(S)
PL 16784/0002

9. DATE OF FIRST AUTHORISATION/RENEWAL OF THE AUTHORISATION
28 April 1998

10. DATE OF REVISION OF THE TEXT
November 2002

Sandostatin 0.05mg/ml, 0.1 mg/ml, 0.5 mg/ml Ampoules and Multidose Vial 1 mg/5 ml

(Novartis Pharmaceuticals UK Ltd)

1. NAME OF THE MEDICINAL PRODUCT
Sandostatin® Ampoules 0.05 mg/ml

Sandostatin ® Ampoules 0.1 mg/ml

Sandostatin ® Ampoules 0.5 mg/ml

Sandostatin ®MULTIDOSE VIALS 1 mg/5 ml

2. QUALITATIVE AND QUANTITATIVE COMPOSITION
0.05 mg octreotide (INN) per ml.

0.1 mg octreotide (INN) per ml.

0.5 mg octreotide (INN) per ml.

0.2 mg octreotide (INN) per ml.

3. PHARMACEUTICAL FORM
Ampoules: 1 ml ampoules containing clear colourless solution for injection.

Multidose vials: 5 ml vials containing clear colourless solution for injection.

4. CLINICAL PARTICULARS

4.1 Therapeutic indications

GEP tumours

For the relief of symptoms associated with functional gastroenteropancreatic endocrine tumours including:

- carcinoid tumours with features of carcinoid syndrome
- VIPomas
- glucagonomas

Sandostatin is not antitumour therapy and is not curative in these patients.

Acromegaly

For symptomatic control and reduction of growth hormone and somatomedin c plasma levels in patients with acromegaly:

- in short term treatment, prior to pituitary surgery, or
- in long term treatment in those who are inadequately controlled by pituitary surgery, radiotherapy, or in the interim period until radiotherapy becomes effective.

Sandostatin is indicated for acromegalic patients for whom surgery is inappropriate.

Evidence from short term studies demonstrate that tumour size is reduced in some patients (prior to surgery); further tumour shrinkage however cannot be expected as a feature of continued long term treatment.

Prevention of complications following pancreatic surgery

Route of administration

Subcutaneous or intravenous use.

4.2 Posology and method of administration

GEP tumours

Initially 0.05 mg once or twice daily by s.c. injection. Depending on response, dosage can be gradually increased to 0.2 mg three times daily. Under exceptional circumstances, higher doses may be required. Maintenance doses are variable.

The recommended route of administration is subcutaneous, however, in instances where a rapid response is required, e.g. carcinoid crises, the initial recommended dose of Sandostatin may be administered by the intravenous route, diluted and given as a bolus, whilst monitoring the cardiac rhythm.

In carcinoid tumours, if there is no beneficial effect within a week, continued therapy is not recommended.

Acromegaly

0.1 – 0.2 mg three times daily by s.c. injection. Dosage adjustment should be based on monthly assessment of GH and IGF-1 levels (target: GH less than 2.5ng/ml, 5mU/l; IGF-1 within normal range) and clinical symptoms, and on tolerability. For patients on a stable dose of Sandostatin, assessment of GH should be made every 12 months. Six-monthly monitoring may be necessary in those patients whose clinical and biochemical control is adequate.

If no relevant reduction of growth hormone levels and no improvement of clinical symptoms have been achieved within three months of starting treatment, therapy should be discontinued.

For the prevention of complications following pancreatic surgery

0.1 mg three times daily by subcutaneous injection for 7 consecutive days, starting on the day of operation at least one hour before laparotomy.

Use in patients with impaired renal function

Impaired renal function did not affect the total exposure (AUC; area under the curve) to octreotide when administered s.c. therefore, no dose adjustment of Sandostatin is necessary.

Use in patients with impaired hepatic function

In a study with Sandostatin administered s.c. and i.v. it was shown that the elimination capacity maybe reduced in patients with liver cirrhosis, but not in patients with fatty liver disease. In patients with liver cirrhosis, an adjustment of the maintenance dose may therefore be necessary.

Use in the elderly

In elderly patients treated with Sandostatin, there is no evidence for reduced tolerability or altered dosage requirements.

Use in children

Experience with Sandostatin in children is very limited.

4.3 Contraindications

Known hypersensitivity to octreotide or to any component of the formulations (see 6.1 List of excipients).

4.4 Special warnings and special precautions for use

As growth hormone secreting pituitary tumours may sometimes expand, causing serious complications (e.g. visual field defects), it is essential that all patients be carefully monitored. If evidence of tumour expansion appears, alternative procedures may be advisable.

Sudden escape of gastroenteropancreatic endocrine tumours from symptomatic control by Sandostatin may occur infrequently, with rapid recurrence of severe symptoms.

Octreotide may increase the depth and duration of hypoglycaemia in patients with insulinoma. This is because it is relatively more potent in inhibiting growth hormone and glucagon secretion than in inhibiting insulin and because its duration of insulin inhibition is shorter. If Sandostatin is given to a patient with insulinoma, close monitoring is necessary on introduction of therapy and at each change of dosage. Marked fluctuations of blood glucose may be reduced by more frequent administration of Sandostatin.

Sandostatin may reduce insulin or oral hypoglycaemic requirements in patients with type I diabetes mellitus. In non-diabetics and type II diabetics with particularly intact insulin reserves, Sandostatin administration can result in prandial increases in glycaemia.

Thyroid function should be monitored in patients receiving long-term Sandostatin therapy.

Sandostatin exerts an inhibiting effect on gallbladder motility, bile acid secretion and bile flow and there is an acknowledged association with the development of gallstones. The incidence of gallstone formation with Sandostatin treatment is estimated to be between 15 - 30 %.

Ultrasonic examination of the gallbladder, before and at about 6 to 12 month intervals during Sandostatin therapy is therefore recommended. If gallstones do occur, they are usually asymptomatic; symptomatic stones should be treated in the normal manner with due attention to abrupt withdrawal of the drug.

In patients with cirrhosis, dosage adjustment may be necessary (see Section 4.2 Posology and Method of Administration).

4.5 Interaction with other medicinal products and other forms of Interaction

Octreotide has been reported to reduce the intestinal absorption of cyclosporin and to delay that of cimetidine.

Concomitant administration of octreotide and bromocriptine increases the availability of bromocriptine.

Limited published data indicate that somatostatin analogs might decrease the metabolic clearance of compounds known to be metabolized by cytochrome P450 enzymes, which may be due to the suppression of growth hormone. Since it cannot be excluded that octreotide may have this effect, other drugs mainly metabolised by CYP3A4 and which have a low therapeutic index should therefore be used with caution (e.g. carbamazepine, digoxin, warfarin and terfenadine).

4.6 Pregnancy and lactation

Experience with octreotide in pregnant or nursing women is very limited, and they should therefore be given the drug only under compelling circumstances.

Women receiving treatment with Sandostatin should not breastfeed their infants.

4.7 Effects on ability to drive and use machines

No data exists on the effects of Sandostatin on the ability to drive and use machines.

4.8 Undesirable effects

The main side-effects are local and gastrointestinal.

Body as a whole

Rare: hypersensitivity skin reactions; hair loss and isolated reports of anaphylactic reactions have been observed.

Cardiovascular system

Isolated cases of bradycardia.

Gastrointestinal system

Anorexia, nausea, vomiting, abdominal pain, abdominal bloating, flatulence, loose stools, diarrhoea and steatorrhea. Although measured faecal fate excretion may increase, there is no evidence to date that long-term treatment with octreotide has led to nutritional deficiency due to malabsorption. In rare instances, gastrointestinal side-effects may resemble acute intestinal obstruction with progressive abdominal distension, severe epigastric pain, abdominal tenderness and guarding. Occurrrence of gastrointestinal side-effects may be reduced by avoiding meals around the time of octreotide administration, that is, by injecting between meals or on retiring to bed.

Heptobiliary

Prolonged use of octreotide may result in gallstone formation (see 4.4 Special warnings and precautions for use), and there have been isolated cases of biliary colic following the abrupt withdrawal of the drug in acromegalic patients in whom biliary sludge or gallstones had developed.

There have been isolated reports of hepatic dysfunctions associated with octreotide administration. These consist of

- acute hepatitis, without cholestasis, where transaminase values have normalised on withdrawal of octreotide, or
- slow development of hyperbilirubinaemia in association with elevation of alkaline phosphatase, gamma-glutamyl transferase and, to a lesser extent, transaminases.

Pancreas

Because of its inhibitory action on growth hormone, glucagon, and insulin release, octreotide may affect glucose regulation. Postprandial glucose tolerance may be impaired and, in some instances, the state of persistent hyperglycaemia may be induced as a result of chronic administration. Hypoglycaemia has also been observed within the first hours or days of Sandostatin treatment and resolves on withdrawal of the drug. In addition, cholelithiasis-induced pancreatitis has been reported for patients on long-term Sandostatin treatment.

Local reactions

Pain or a sensation of stinging, tingling or burning at the site of s.c. injection, with redness and swelling, rarely lasting more than 15 minutes. Local discomfort may be reduced by allowing the solution to reach room temperature before injection.

4.9 Overdose

Doses of up to 2000 microgrammes octreotide given as subcutaneous tid for several months have been well tolerated.

No life-threatening reactions have been reported after acute overdosage. The maximum single dose so far given to an adult so far has been 1 mg by intravenous bolus injection. The observed signs and symptoms were a brief drop in heart rate, facial flushing, abdominal cramps, diarrhoea, an empty feeling in the stomach and nausea, which resolved in 24 hours of drug administration.

One patient has been reported to have received an accidental overdosage of Sandostatin by continuous infusion (250 microgrammes per hour for forty eight hours instead of 25 microgrammes per hour). He experienced no side-effects.

The management of overdosage is symptomatic.

5. PHARMACOLOGICAL PROPERTIES

5.1 Pharmacodynamic properties

Pharmacotherapeutic group: Antigrowth hormones (ATC code H01BC02).

Octreotide is a synthetic octapeptide derivative of naturally occurring somatostatin with similar pharmacological effects, but with a longer duration of action. It inhibits pathologically increased secretion of growth hormone and of peptides and serotonin produced within the gastroenteropancreatic endocrine (GEP) system.

In animals, octreotide is a more potent inhibitor of growth hormone, glucagon and insulin release than somatostatin with greater selectivity for growth hormone and glucagon suppression.

In normal healthy subjects octreotide, like somatostatin, has been shown to inhibit

- release of growth hormone stimulated by arginine, exercise and insulin-induced hypoglycaemia
- postprandial release of insulin, glucagon, gastrin other peptides of the gastroenteropancreatic system; arginine-stimulated release of insulin and glucagon and
- thyrotropin-releasing hormone (TRH) - stimulated release of thyroid stimulating hormone (TSH).

Unlike somatostatin, octreotide inhibits growth hormone preferentially over insulin and its administration is not followed by rebound hypersecretion of hormones (i.e. growth hormone in patients with acromegaly).

For patients undergoing pancreatic surgery, the peri and post-operative administration of Sandostatin reduces the incidence of typical post-operative complications (e.g. pancreatic fistula, abscess and subsequent sepsis, post-operative acute pancreatitis).

In patients with acromegaly, Sandostatin consistently lowers GH and normalises IGF-1 serum concentrations in the majority of patients. In most patients, Sandostatin markedly reduces the clinical symptoms of the disease, such as headache, perspiration, paresthesia, fatigue, osteoarthralgia and carpal tunnel syndrome. In individual patients with GH-secreting pituitary adenoma, Sandostatin was reported to lead to shrinkage of the tumour mass.

For patients with functional tumours of the gastroenteropancreatic endocrine system, treatment with octreotide provides continuous control of symptoms related to the underlying disease. The effect of octreotide in different types of gastroenteropancreatic tumours are as follows:

Carcinoid tumours

Administration of octreotide may result in improvement of symptoms, particularly of flushing and diarrhoea. In many cases, this is accompanied by a falling plasma serotonin and reduced urinary excretion of 5-hydroxyindole acetic acid.

VIPomas

The biochemical characteristics of these tumours is overproduction of vasoactive intestinal peptide (VIP). In most cases, administration of octreotide results in alleviation of the severe secretory diarrhoea typical of the condition, with consequent improvement in quality of life. This is accompanied by an improvement in associated electrolyte abnormalities, e.g. hypokalaemia, enabling enteral and parenteral fluid and electrolyte supplementation to be withdrawn. Clinical improvement is usually accompanied by a reduction in plasma VIP levels, which may fall into the normal reference range.

Glucagonomas

Administration of octreotide results in most cases in substantial improvement of the necrolytic migratory rash which is characteristic of the condition. The effect of octreotide on the state of mild diabetes mellitus which frequently occurs is not marked and, in general, does not result in a reduction of requirements for insulin or oral hypoglycaemic agents. Octreotide produces improvement of diarrhoea, and hence weight gain, in those patients affected. Although administration of octreotide often leads to an immediate reduction in plasma glucagon levels, this decrease is generally not maintained over a prolonged period of administration, despite continued symptomatic improvement.

5.2 Pharmacokinetic properties

Absorption

After subcutaneous injection, Sandostatin is rapidly and completely absorbed. Peak plasma concentrations are reached within 30 minutes.

Distribution

The volume of distribution is 0.27 l/kg and the total body clearance 160 ml/min. Plasma protein binding amounts to 65 %. The amount of octreotide bound to blood cells is negligible.

Elimination

The elimination half-life after subcutaneous administrations is 100 minutes. After intravenous injection the elimination is biphasic with half-lives of 10 and 90 minutes respectively. About 32 % is excreted unchanged into the urine.

5.3 Preclinical safety data

Preclinical data reveal no specific hazard for humans based on conventional studies of safety pharmacology, repeated dose toxicity, genotoxicity and carcinogenic potential.

Studies in animals showed transient growth retardation of offspring, possibly consequent upon the specific endocrine profiles of the species tested, but there was no evidence of foetotoxic, teratogenic, or other reproduction effects.

6. PHARMACEUTICAL PARTICULARS

6.1 List of excipients

Sandostatin Ampoules and Multidose vials:

Lactic acid, phenol (multidose vials only), mannitol, sodium hydrogen carbonate, water for injections.

6.2 Incompatibilities

None known

6.3 Shelf life

Ampoules: 5 years

Multidose vials: 4 years unopened. Opened vials may be stored for 2 weeks at room temperature for day to day use.

6.4 Special precautions for storage

For prolonged storage Sandostatin Ampoules and Multidose vials should be stored between 2°C and 8°C. For day-to-day use they may be stored at room temperature for up to two weeks. Protect from light. Do not freeze.

6.5 Nature and contents of container

Ampoules:

1 ml vial of uncoloured glass containing clear colourless solution.

Boxes of 5 ampoules.

Multidose vials:

5 ml vial of uncoloured glass containing clear colourless solution.

Boxes of 1 vial.

6.6 Instructions for use and handling

For i.v. use Sandostatin should be diluted with normal saline to a ratio of not less than 1 vol: 1 vol and not more than 1 vol: 9 vol. Dilution of Sandostatin with glucose solution is not recommended.

If Sandostatin has been diluted, the prepared solution may be kept at room temperature but should be administered within 8 hours of preparation.

To prevent contamination, it is recommended to puncture the cap of the vial not more than 10 times (Multidose vials only).

To reduce local discomfort, let the solution reach room temperature before injection. Avoid multiple injections at short intervals at the same site.

7. MARKETING AUTHORISATION HOLDER

Novartis Pharmaceuticals UK Limited

Trading as Sandoz Pharmaceuticals

Frimley Business Park

Frimley

Camberley

Surrey, GU16 7SR

8. MARKETING AUTHORISATION NUMBER(S)

Sandostatin Ampoules 0.05 mg/ml - PL 00101/0212

Sandostatin Ampoules 0.1 mg/ml - PL 00101/0213

Sandostatin Ampoules 0.5 mg/ml - PL 00101/0214

Sandostatin Multidose Vials 1 mg/5 ml - PL 00101/0300

9. DATE OF FIRST AUTHORISATION/RENEWAL OF THE AUTHORISATION

Ampoules: 03 April 1989 / 12 August 1994

Multidose vials: 20 October 1990 / 12 September 1995

10. DATE OF REVISION OF THE TEXT

31 March 2004

LEGAL CATEGORY

POM

Sandostatin Lar

(Novartis Pharmaceuticals UK Ltd)

1. NAME OF THE MEDICINAL PRODUCT

Sandostatin® LAR®

2. QUALITATIVE AND QUANTITATIVE COMPOSITION

One vial containing: Microspheres for suspension for injection

Active: Octreotide* free peptide, 10, 20 or 30 mg (present as octreotide acetate) 4.65% of nominal fill weight.

Other: Poly(DL-lactide-co-glycolide) 78.35% of nominal fill weight. Sterile mannitol 17.0% of nominal fill weight.

Each vial is filled with an overage of microspheres which ensures the correct dosage can be administered.

Two needles [40mm (1.5 inch), 19 gauge].

* INN rec.

3. PHARMACEUTICAL FORM

Sandostatin LAR is a long-acting depot injection form of octreotide. Microspheres to be suspended in a vehicle immediately prior to i.m. injection.

4. CLINICAL PARTICULARS

4.1 Therapeutic indications

Treatment of patients with acromegaly:

For symptomatic control and reduction of growth hormone and IGF-1 levels in patients with acromegaly

- who are adequately controlled on s.c. treatment with Sandostatin; in whom surgery or radiotherapy is inappropriate or ineffective, or in the interim period until radiotherapy becomes fully effective.
- in short term treatment (3-12 months) prior to pituitary surgery (see also Section 5.1 Pharmacological properties).

GEP tumours:

For the relief of symptoms associated with gastroenteropancreatic tumours including:

- Carcinoid tumours with features of carcinoid syndrome
- VIPomas
- Glucagonomas in patients whose symptoms are adequately controlled on s.c. treatment with Sandostatin. Sandostatin is not antitumour therapy and is not curative in these patients.

4.2 Posology and method of administration

Sandostatin LAR may only be administered by deep intragluteal injection. The site of repeat intragluteal injections should be alternated between the left and right gluteal muscle (see 6.6 Instructions for use/handling).

Acromegaly

For patients who have not received prior treatment with subcutaneous Sandostatin, a test dose of s.c. Sandostatin (50-100mcg) is recommended to assess any adverse reaction to octreotide prior to initiating treatment with Sandostatin LAR.

For *de novo* patients who have received a test dose and for patients who are adequately controlled with s.c. Sandostatin, treatment should be started with 20mg Sandostatin LAR intramuscularly at 4-week intervals for 3 months. Treatment with Sandostatin LAR can be started on the day after the last dose of s.c. Sandostatin. Subsequent dosage adjustment should be based on serum growth hormone (GH) and insulin-like growth factor I (IGF 1)/somatomedin C concentrations and clinical symptoms.

For patients in whom clinical symptoms and biochemical parameters (GH; IGF 1) are not fully controlled (GH concentrations still above 2.5μg/L{5mU/L}), the dose may be increased to 30mg every 4 weeks.

For patients whose GH concentrations are consistently below 1μg/L (2mU/L), whose IGF 1 serum concentrations have normalised, and in whom most reversible signs/symptoms of acromegaly have disappeared after 3 months of treatment with 20mg, the dose may be reduced to 10mg every 4 weeks. However, in this group of patients serum GH and IGF 1 concentrations, and clinical signs/symptoms should be monitored particularly closely.

In order to permit successful endocrine testing of the completeness of tumour removal 5-6 weeks post surgery, the last injection of Sandostatin LAR should be administered at least 3-4 weeks prior to surgery.

Gastroenteropancreatic tumours

After adequate control has been established with Sandostatin s.c., treatment should be started with 20mg Sandostatin LAR intramuscularly at 4-week intervals. Treatment with Sandostatin s.c. should be continued at the previously effective dosage for 2 weeks after the first injection of Sandostatin LAR. Response should be assessed after 3 months of treatment.

For patients in whom symptoms are only partially controlled after 3 months of treatment, the dose may be increased to 30mg Sandostatin LAR every 4 weeks.

For patients in whom symptoms and biological markers are well controlled after 3 months of treatment, the dose may be reduced to 10mg Sandostatin LAR every 4 weeks.

For days when symptoms associated with gastroenteropancreatic tumours may increase during treatment with Sandostatin LAR, additional administration of s.c. Sandostatin is recommended at the dose used prior to the Sandostatin LAR treatment.

Use in patients with impaired renal function

Impaired renal function did not affect the total exposure (AUC; area under the curve) to octreotide when administered s.c. as Sandostatin. Therefore, no dose adjustment of Sandostatin LAR is necessary.

Use in patients with impaired hepatic function

In a study with Sandostatin administered s.c. and i.v. it was shown that the elimination capacity may be reduced in patients with liver cirrhosis, but not in patients with fatty liver disease. Due to the wide therapeutic window of octreotide, no dose adjustment of Sandostatin LAR is necessary in patients with liver cirrhosis.

Use in elderly patients

In a study with Sandostatin administered s.c., no dose adjustment was necessary in patients ⩾ 65 years of age. Therefore, no dose adjustment is necessary in this group with Sandostatin LAR.

Use in children

There is very limited experience with use of Sandostatin LAR in children.

4.3 Contraindications

Hypersensitivity to octreotide or any components of the formulation.

4.4 Special warnings and special precautions for use

As GH-secreting pituitary tumours may sometimes expand, causing serious complications (eg. visual field defects), it is essential that all patients be carefully monitored. If evidence of tumour expansion appears, alternative procedures are advisable.

Development of gallstones has been reported in 10 to 20% of long-term recipients of s.c. Sandostatin. Long term exposure to Sandostatin LAR of patients with acromegaly or gastroenteropancreatic tumours suggests that treatment with Sandostatin LAR does not increase the incidence of gallstone formation, compared with s.c. treatment. Ultrasonic examination of the gallbladder before and at about 6 monthly intervals during Sandostatin LAR therapy is, however, recommended. If gallstones do occur, they are usually asymptomatic; symptomatic stones should be treated either by dissolution therapy with bile acids or by surgery.

In patients with concomitant diabetes mellitus, Sandostatin LAR may impair insulin secretion. It is, therefore, recommended to monitor glucose tolerance and antidiabetic treatment.

In patients with insulinomas, octreotide, because of its greater relative potency in inhibiting the secretion of GH and glucagon than that of insulin, and because of the shorter duration of the inhibitory action on insulin, may increase the depth and prolong the duration of hypoglycaemia. These patients should be closely monitored.

4.5 Interaction with other medicinal products and other forms of Interaction

Octreotide has been found to reduce the intestinal absorption of cyclosporin and to delay that of cimetidine.

Concomitant administration of octreotide and bromocriptine increases the bioavailability of bromocriptine.

Limited published data indicate that somatostatin analogs might decrease the metabolic clearance of compounds known to be metabolized by cytochrome P450 enzymes, which may be due to the suppression of growth hormone. Since it cannot be excluded that octreotide may have this effect, caution should be exercised during co-administration of octreotide and drugs mainly metabolized by CYP3A4, which have a low therapeutic index (e.g. carbamazepine, digoxin, warfarin and terfenadine).

4.6 Pregnancy and lactation

Experience with octreotide in pregnant or nursing women is not available and they should, therefore, be given the drug only under compelling circumstances.

4.7 Effects on ability to drive and use machines

No data exist on the effects of Sandostatin LAR on the ability to drive and use machines.

4.8 Undesirable effects

The main side effects encountered with Sandostatin LAR administration are local and gastrointestinal.

Gallbladder

Prolonged use of Sandostatin LAR may result in gallstone formation (see 4.4 Special warnings and special precautions for use).

Gastrointestinal System

Gastrointestinal side effects include anorexia, nausea, vomiting, crampy abdominal pain, abdominal bloating, flatulence, loose stools, diarrhoea and steatorrhoea. Although measured faecal fat excretion may increase, there is no evidence to date that long-term treatment with octreotide has led to nutritional deficiency due to malabsorption. In rare instances, gastrointestinal side-effects may resemble acute intestinal obstruction, with progressive abdominal distension, severe epigastric pain, abdominal tenderness and guarding.

Pancreas

Because of its inhibitory action on growth hormone, glucagon and insulin release, Sandostatin LAR may affect glucose regulation. Post-prandial glucose tolerance may be impaired. As reported for patients treated with s.c. Sandostatin, in some instances a state of persistent hyperglycaemia may be induced as a result of chronic administration. Hypoglycaemia has also been observed.

In rare instances, acute pancreatitis has been reported within the first hours or days of s.c. Sandostatin treatment. In addition, cholelithiasis-induced pancreatitis has been reported for patients on long-term s.c. Sandostatin treatment.

Liver

There have been isolated reports of hepatic dysfunction associated with s.c. Sandostatin administration. These concern:

- acute hepatitis without cholestasis, where there has been normalisation of transaminase values on withdrawal of s.c. Sandostatin
- the slow development of hyperbilirubinaemia in association with elevation of alkaline phosphatase, -glutamyl transferase and, to a lesser extent, transaminases.

Local reactions

Local injection site reactions to Sandostatin LAR may occur, and are usually mild and of short duration. They include local pain and, rarely, swelling and rash.

Body as a whole

Rarely, transient hair loss has been reported in patients receiving Sandostatin LAR treatment.

Very rarely, cases of hypersensitivity have been reported.

4.9 Overdose

To date no data are available on overdosage with Sandostatin LAR. However, no unexpected adverse events have been reported with doses up to 90mg Sandostatin LAR administered to cancer patients every 2 weeks. The signs and symptoms observed after a single dose of 1.0mg octreotide given as an i.v. bolus injection to an adult patient were a brief drop in heart rate, facial flushing, abdominal cramps, diarrhoea, an empty feeling in the stomach and nausea, all of which resolved within 24 hours of drug administration.

The management of overdosage is symptomatic.

5. PHARMACOLOGICAL PROPERTIES

5.1 Pharmacodynamic properties

Octreotide is a synthetic octapeptide derivative of naturally occurring somatostatin, with similar pharmacological effects, but with a considerably prolonged duration of action. It inhibits pathologically increased secretion of GH and of peptides and serotonin produced within the gastroenteropancreatic (GEP) endocrine system.

In animals, octreotide is a more potent inhibitor of GH, glucagon and insulin release than somatostatin, with greater selectivity for GH and glucagon suppression.

In healthy subjects octreotide, like somatostatin, has been shown to inhibit

- release of GH stimulated by arginine, exercise and insulin-induced hypoglycaemia;
- post-prandial release of insulin, glucagon, gastrin, other peptides of the GEP system, and arginine-stimulated release of insulin and glucagon;
- thyrotropin-releasing hormone (TRH)-stimulated release of thyroid- stimulating hormone (TSH).

Unlike somatostatin, octreotide inhibits GH preferentially over insulin and its administration is not followed by rebound hypersecretion of hormones (i.e. GH in patients with acromegaly).

In patients with acromegaly, Sandostatin LAR, a galenical formulation of octreotide suitable for repeated administration at intervals of 4 weeks, delivers consistent and therapeutic octreotide serum concentrations, thus consistently lowering GH and normalising IGF 1 serum concentrations in the majority of patients. In most patients, Sandostatin LAR markedly reduces the clinical symptoms of the disease, such as headache, perspiration, paraesthesia, fatigue, osteoarthralgia and carpal tunnel syndrome.

In individual patients with GH-secreting pituitary adenoma, Sandostatin LAR was reported to lead to shrinkage of the tumour mass (prior to surgery). However, progression to surgery should not be delayed. Further tumour shrinkage cannot be expected as a feature of continued long term treatment.

For patients with functional tumours of the gastroenteropancreatic endocrine system, treatment with Sandostatin LAR provides continuous control of symptoms related to the underlying disease. The effect of octreotide in different types of gastroenteropancreatic tumours are as follows:

Carcinoid tumours:

Administration of octreotide may result in improvement of symptoms, particularly of flushing and diarrhoea. In many cases, this is accompanied by a falling plasma serotonin and reduced urinary excretion of 5-hydroxyindole acetic acid.

VIPomas:

The biochemical characteristics of these tumours is overproduction of vasoactive intestinal peptide (VIP). In most cases, administration of octreotide results in alleviation of the severe secretory diarrhoea typical of the condition, with consequent improvement in quality of life. This is accompanied by an improvement in associated electrolyte abnormalities, e.g. hypokalaemia, enabling enteral and parenteral fluid and electrolyte supplementation to be withdrawn. Clinical improvement is usually accompanied by a reduction in plasma VIP levels, which may fall into the normal reference range.

Glucagonomas:

Administration of octreotide results in most cases in substantial improvement of the necrolytic migratory rash which is characteristic of the condition. The effect of octreotide on the state of mild diabetes mellitus which frequently occurs is not marked and, in general, does not result in a reduction of requirements for insulin or oral hypoglycaemic agents. Octreotide produces improvement of diarrhoea, and hence weight gain, in those patients affected. Although administration of octreotide often leads to an immediate reduction in plasma glucagon levels, this decrease is generally not maintained over a prolonged period of administration, despite continued symptomatic improvement.

5.2 Pharmacokinetic properties

After single i.m. injections of Sandostatin LAR, the octreotide concentration reaches a transient initial peak within 1 hour after administration, followed by a progressive decrease to a low undetectable octreotide level within 24 hours. After this peak on day 1, octreotide remains at subtherapeutic levels in the majority of the patients for the following 7 days.

Thereafter, octreotide concentrations increase again, reach plateau concentrations at around day 14 and remain relatively constant during the following 3 to 4 weeks. The peak level during day 1 is lower than levels during the plateau phase, and no more than 0.5% of the total drug release occurs during day 1. After about day 42, the octreotide concentration decreases slowly, concomitant with the terminal degradation phase of the polymer matrix of the dosage form.

In patients with acromegaly, mean plateau octreotide concentrations after single doses of 10mg, 20mg and 30mg of Sandostatin LAR amount to 358ng/L, 926ng/L and 1710ng/L, respectively. Steady-state serum octreotide concentrations, reached after 3 injections at 4-week intervals, are higher by a factor of approximately 1.6 to 1.8 and amount to 1557ng/L, and 2384ng/L after multiple injections of 20mg and 30mg of Sandostatin LAR, respectively.

In patients with carcinoid tumours, the mean (and median) steady-state serum concentrations of octreotide after multiple injections of 10mg, 20mg and 30mg of Sandostatin LAR given a 4-week intervals also increase linearly with dose and were 1231 (894) ng/L, 2620 (2270) ng/L, and 3928 (3010) ng/L respectively.

No accumulation of octreotide beyond that expected from overlapping release profiles occurred over a duration of up to 28 monthly injections of Sandostatin LAR.

The pharmacokinetic profile of octreotide after injection of Sandostatin LAR reflects the release profile from the polymer matrix and its biodegradation. Once released into the systemic circulation, octreotide distributes according to its known pharmacokinetic properties, as described for s.c. administration. The volume of distribution of octreotide at steady state is 0.27 L/kg and the total body clearance is 160 ml/min. Plasma protein binding amounts to 65% and essentially no drug is bound to blood cells.

5.3 Preclinical safety data

Acute toxicity

Acute toxicity studies of octreotide in mice revealed LD_{50} values of 72mg/kg by the i.v. route and of 470mg/kg by the s.c. route. The acute i.v. LD_{50} value of octreotide in rats was determined at 18mg/kg. Octreotide acetate was well tolerated by dogs receiving up to 1mg/kg body weight by i.v. bolus injection.

Repeated dose toxicity

In a repeat dose study performed in rats by i.m. injection of 2.5mg Sandostatin LAR in 50mg microspheres every 4 weeks for 21 weeks, with necropsy at 26 weeks, no drug-related necropsy findings were observed. The only histopathological findings considered to be of significance were at the injection site in treated and control animals, where the microspheres had provoked a reversible granulomatous myositis. After a single i.m. injection of Sandostatin LAR in rats and rabbits, biodegradation of microspheres was complete by day 75 after injection in both species.

Mutagenicity

Octreotide and/or its metabolites were devoid of mutagenic potential when investigated *in vitro* in validated bacterial and mammalian cell test systems. Increased frequencies of chromosomal changes were observed in V79 Chinese hamster cells *in vitro*, albeit at high and cytotoxic concentrations only. Chromosomal aberrations were, however, not increased in human lymphocytes incubated with octreotide acetate *in vitro. In vivo*, no clastogenic activity was observed in the bone marrow of mice treated with octreotide i.v. (micronucleus test) and no evidence of genotoxicity was obtained in male mice using a DNA repair assay of sperm heads. The microspheres were devoid of mutagenic potential when tested in a validated *in vitro* bacterial assay.

Carcinogenicity/chronic toxicity

In studies in rats in which s.c. Sandostatin at daily doses up to 1.25mg/kg body weight were administered, fibrosarcomas were observed, predominantly in a number of male animals, at the s.c. injection site after 52, 104 and 113/116 weeks. Local tumours occurred also in the control rats, however, development of these tumours was attributed to disordered fibroplasia produced by sustained irritant effects at the injection sites, enhanced by the acidic lactic acid/mannitol vehicle. This non-specific tissue reaction appeared to be particular to rats.

Neoplastic lesions were observed neither in mice receiving daily s.c. injections of Sandostatin at doses up to 2mg/kg for 98 weeks, nor in dogs which were treated with daily s.c. doses of the drug for 52 weeks.

The 116-week carcinogenicity study in rats with s.c. Sandostatin also revealed uterine endometrial adenocarcinomas, their incidence reaching statistical significance at the highest s.c. dose level of 1.25mg/kg per day. The finding was associated with an increased incidence of endometritis, a decreased number of ovarian corpora lutea, a reduction in mammary adenomas and the presence of uterine glandular and luminal dilation, suggesting a state of hormonal imbalance. The available information clearly indicates that the findings of endocrine-mediated tumours in rats are species-specific and are not relevant for the use of the drug in humans.

Reproduction toxicity

Fertility as well as pre-, peri- and post-natal studies in female rats revealed no adverse effects on reproductive performance and development of the offspring, when s.c. doses up to 1mg/kg body weight per day were administered. Some retardation of the physiological growth noted in pups was transient and attributable to GH inhibition brought about by excessive pharmacodynamic activity.

6. PHARMACEUTICAL PARTICULARS

6.1 List of excipients

Poly (DL-lactide-co-glycolide); mannitol.

6.2 Incompatibilities

Sandostatin LAR microspheres for injection is to be used as a single dose container, without any dilution with other products. Therefore, no compatibility data with other products have been generated.

6.3 Shelf life

36 months.

6.4 Special precautions for storage

Store at 2 to 8°C, protect from light. Sandostatin LAR can remain at room temperature on the day of injection. However, the suspension must only be prepared immediately prior to i.m. injection.

6.5 Nature and contents of container

The microspheres are packaged in 5ml glass vials (Type I, Ph Eur), with a PTFE-faced rubber stopper and sealed with an aluminium flip-off seal.

6.6 Instructions for use and handling

Instructions for i.m. injection of Sandostatin LAR for deep intragluteal injection only

Remove the cap from vial containing Sandostatin LAR. Assure that the powder is settled at the bottom of the vial by lightly tapping the vial. Remove the cap from the vehicle syringe. Attach one of the supplied needles to the vehicle syringe.

Insert needle through centre of rubber stopper of the Sandostatin LAR vial.

Without disturbing the Sandostatin LAR powder, gently inject the vehicle into the vial by running the vehicle down the inside wall of the vial. Do not inject the vehicle directly into the powder. Withdraw any excess air present in the vial.

Do not disturb the vial until the vehicle has wetted the Sandostatin LAR powder for suspension. Once complete wetting (approximately 2-5 minutes) has occurred, the vial should be moderately swirled until a uniform suspension is achieved. Do not vigorously shake the vial.

Immediately draw 2ml of air into the syringe and re-insert the needle through the rubber stopper. Inject the 2ml of air into the vial and then, with the bevel down and the vial tipped at approximately 45 degree angle, slowly draw the entire contents of the vial containing the suspension into the syringe. Immediately change the needle (supplied).

Gently invert the syringe as needed to maintain a uniform suspension. Eliminate air from syringe and disinfect the injection site. Insert needle into right or left gluteus and draw back to ensure that no blood vessel has been penetrated. Immediately inject i.m. by deep intragluteal injection.

Sandostatin LAR must be given only by intragluteal injection, never i.v. If a blood vessel has been penetrated, select another injection site.

7. MARKETING AUTHORISATION HOLDER

Novartis Pharmaceuticals UK Limited

(Trading as Sandoz Pharmaceuticals)

Frimley Business Park

Frimley

Camberley

Surrey

GU16 7SR

United Kingdom

8. MARKETING AUTHORISATION NUMBER(S)

Sandostatin LAR 10mg: PL 00101/0511

Sandostatin LAR 20mg: PL 00101/0512

Sandostatin LAR 30mg: PL 00101/0513

9. DATE OF FIRST AUTHORISATION/RENEWAL OF THE AUTHORISATION

29 April 1998

10. DATE OF REVISION OF THE TEXT

3 June 2004

Legal Category

POM

SANOMIGRAN 0.5mg Tablets

(Novartis Pharmaceuticals UK Ltd)

1. NAME OF THE MEDICINAL PRODUCT

SANOMIGRAN Tablets 0.5mg

2. QUALITATIVE AND QUANTITATIVE COMPOSITION

The active ingredient is: 4-(1-methyl-4-piperidylidene)-9,10-dihydro-4H-benzo-[4,5]cyclohepta [1,2-b] thiophene hydrogen malate (=pizotifen hydrogen malate).

Each tablet contains 0.725mg pizotifen hydrogen malate BP.

3. PHARMACEUTICAL FORM

Coated tablets.

4. CLINICAL PARTICULARS

4.1 Therapeutic indications

Prophylactic treatment of recurrent vascular headaches, including classical migraine, common migraine and cluster headaches (periodic migrainous neuralgia).

It is not effective in relieving migraine attacks once in progress.

4.2 Posology and method of administration

Adults

Usually 1.5mg daily. This may be taken as a single dose at night or in three divided doses. Dosage should be adjusted to individual patient requirements up to a maximum of 4.5mg daily. Up to 3mg may be given as a single dose.

Children (aged over 2 years)

Up to 1.5mg daily, usually as a divided dose, although up to 1mg has been given as a single dose at night.

Use in the elderly

Clinical work with SANOMIGRAN has not shown elderly patients to require different dosages from younger patients.

Method of administration

Oral.

4.3 Contraindications

Known hypersensitivity to pizotifen or any of the excipients (see ' 6.1. List of excipients').

4.4 Special warnings and special precautions for use

Although the anticholinergic activity of SANOMIGRAN is relatively weak, caution is required in the presence of closed angle glaucoma and in patients with a predisposition to urinary retention. Dosage adjustment may be necessary in patients with kidney insufficiency.

4.5 Interaction with other medicinal products and other forms of Interaction

The central effects of sedatives, hypnotics, antihistamines (including certain common cold preparations) and alcohol may be enhanced by SANOMIGRAN.

4.6 Pregnancy and lactation
As clinical data with SANOMIGRAN in pregnancy are very limited it should only be administered during pregnancy under compelling circumstances.

Although the concentrations of SANOMIGRAN measured in the milk of treated mothers are not likely to affect the infant, its use in nursing mothers is not recommended.

4.7 Effects on ability to drive and use machines
Patients should be cautioned about the possibility of drowsiness and informed of its significance in the driving of vehicles and the operation of machinery.

4.8 Undesirable effects
The most commonly occurring side-effects are drowsiness and an increased appetite which may lead to an increase in body weight. Other side-effects such as dizziness, dry mouth, nausea, constipation, hallucinations and paraesthesia have been reported infrequently. Rare instances of sleep disorders, depression and other mood disturbances such as anxiety and aggression have occurred. In children CNS stimulation may occur. Rare cases of hypersensitivity reaction such as rash, facial oedema and urticaria have been reported.

4.9 Overdose
Symptoms of overdosage may include drowsiness, dizziness, hypotension, dryness of the mouth, confusion, excitatory states (in children), ataxia, nausea, vomiting, dyspnoea, cyanosis, tachycardia, convulsions (particularly in children), coma and respiratory paralysis. Treatment: Administration of activated charcoal is recommended; in case of very recent uptake, gastric lavage may be considered. Severe hypotension must be corrected (CAVE: adrenaline may produce paradoxical effects). If necessary, symptomatic treatment including monitoring of the cardiovascular and respiratory systems. Excitory states or convulsions may be treated with short acting benzodiazepines.

5. PHARMACOLOGICAL PROPERTIES

5.1 Pharmacodynamic properties
Pharmacodynamic studies demonstrate pizotifen to have powerful anti-serotonin and anti-tryptaminic properties, marked anti-histaminic effects and some antagonistic activity against kinins. It also possesses weak anti-cholinergic effects and sedative properties.

Pizotifen also possesses appetite-stimulating properties.

The prophylactic effect of SANOMIGRAN in migraine is associated with its ability to modify the humoral mechanisms of headache.

It inhibits the permeability-increasing effect of serotonin and histamine on the affected cranial vessels, thereby checking the transudation of plasmakinin so that the pain threshold of the receptors is maintained at 'normal' levels. In the sequence of events leading to migraine attack, depletion of plasma serotonin contributes to loss of tone in the extracranial vessels. Pizotifen inhibits serotonin reuptake by the platelets, thus maintaining plasma serotonin and preventing the loss of tone and passive distension of the extracranial arteries.

5.2 Pharmacokinetic properties

Absorption

Absorption of pizotifen is fast (absorption half life 0.5 to 0.8 hours) and nearly complete (80%).

Biotransformation

Pizotifen is metabolised with a half life of about 1 hour. The main metabolite (N-glucuronide) is eliminated with a half life of approximately 23 hours.

Distribution

Protein binding amounts to 91% and distribution volume to 485 litres.

Elimination

Less than 1% of the administered dose is excreted unchanged in the urine, whereas 55% is excreted as metabolites.

5.3 Preclinical safety data
There are no pre-clinical data of relevance to the prescriber which are additional to that already included in other sections of the SPC.

6. PHARMACEUTICAL PARTICULARS

6.1 List of excipients
The tablet contains lactose, maize starch, polyvinylpyrrolidone, magnesium stearate, talc (acid washed), The coating constituents are sugar (granulated no.2), talc, gum acacia, titanium dioxide, iron oxide yellow, carnauba wax, printing wax, colloidal anhydrous silica and purified water.

6.2 Incompatibilities
None.

6.3 Shelf life
60 months.

6.4 Special precautions for storage
Protect from direct light.

6.5 Nature and contents of container
The tablets are ivory, circular, biconvex printed SMG on one side and come in PVC/PVDC opaque blister packs containing 60 tablets.

6.6 Instructions for use and handling
None.

7. MARKETING AUTHORISATION HOLDER
Novartis Pharmaceuticals UK Limited

(trading as Sandoz Pharmaceuticals)

Frimley Business Park

Frimley

Camberley

Surrey

GU16 7SR

8. MARKETING AUTHORISATION NUMBER(S)
PL 0101/0036.

9. DATE OF FIRST AUTHORISATION/RENEWAL OF THE AUTHORISATION
15 March 1974

10. DATE OF REVISION OF THE TEXT
26 November 2003

Legal Category
POM

SANOMIGRAN 1.5mg Tablets

(Novartis Pharmaceuticals UK Ltd)

1. NAME OF THE MEDICINAL PRODUCT
SANOMIGRAN Tablets 1.5mg

2. QUALITATIVE AND QUANTITATIVE COMPOSITION
Each tablet contains 2.175mg pizotifen hydrogen malate BP.

3. PHARMACEUTICAL FORM
Coated tablets.

4. CLINICAL PARTICULARS

4.1 Therapeutic indications
Prophylactic treatment of recurrent vascular headaches, including classical migraine, common migraine and cluster headaches (periodic migrainous neuralgia).

It is not effective in relieving migraine attacks once in progress.

4.2 Posology and method of administration

Adults

Usually 1.5mg daily. This may be taken as a single dose at night or in three divided doses. Dosage should be adjusted to individual patient requirements up to a maximum of 4.5mg daily. Up to 3mg may be given as a single dose.

Children (aged over 2 years)

Use of 1.5mg SANOMIGRAN Tablets is not recommended. The appropriate paediatric doses may be given using the 0.5mg SANOMIGRAN Tablets or SANOMIGRAN Elixir.

For children SANOMIGRAN is available in an elixir form.

Use in the elderly

Clinical work with SANOMIGRAN has not shown elderly patients to require different dosages from younger patients.

Method of administration

Oral.

4.3 Contraindications
Known hypersensitivity to pizotifen or any of the excipients (see ' 6.1. List of excipients').

4.4 Special warnings and special precautions for use
Although the anticholinergic activity of SANOMIGRAN is relatively weak, caution is required in the presence of closed angle glaucoma and in patients with a predisposition to urinary retention. Dosage adjustment may be necessary in patients with kidney insufficiency.

4.5 Interaction with other medicinal products and other forms of Interaction
The central effects of sedatives, hypnotics, antihistamines (including certain common cold preparations) and alcohol may be enhanced by SANOMIGRAN.

4.6 Pregnancy and lactation
As clinical data with SANOMIGRAN in pregnancy are very limited it should only be administered under compelling circumstances.

Although the concentrations of SANOMIGRAN measured in the milk of treated mothers are not likely to affect the infant, its use in nursing mothers is not recommended.

4.7 Effects on ability to drive and use machines
Patients should be cautioned about the possibility of drowsiness and informed of its significance in the driving of vehicles and the operation of machinery.

4.8 Undesirable effects
The most commonly occurring side-effects are drowsiness and an increased appetite which may lead to an increase in body weight. Other side-effects such as dizziness, dry mouth, nausea and constipation, hallucinations and paraesthesia have been reported infrequently. Rare instances of sleep disorders, depression and other mood disturbances such as anxiety and aggression have occurred. In children CNS stimulation may occur. Rare cases of hypersensitivity reaction such as rash, facial oedema and urticaria have been reported.

4.9 Overdose
Symptoms of overdosage may include drowsiness, dizziness, hypotension, dryness of the mouth, confusion, excitatory states (in children), ataxia, nausea, vomiting, dyspnoea, cyanosis, tachycardia, convulsions (particularly in children), coma and respiratory paralysis. Treatment: Administration of activated charcoal is recommended; in case of very recent uptake, gastric lavage may be considered. Severe hypotension must be corrected (CAVE: adrenaline may produce paradoxical effects). If necessary, symptomatic treatment including monitoring of the cardiovascular and respiratory systems. Excitory states or convulsions may be treated with short acting benzodiazepines.

5. PHARMACOLOGICAL PROPERTIES

5.1 Pharmacodynamic properties
Pharmacodynamic studies demonstrate pizotifen to have powerful anti-serotonin and anti-tryptaminic properties, marked anti-histaminic effects and some antagonistic activity against kinins. It also possesses weak anti-cholinergic effects and sedative properties.

Pizotifen also possesses appetite-stimulating properties.

The prophylactic effect of SANOMIGRAN in migraine is associated with its ability to modify the humoral mechanisms of headache.

It inhibits the permeability-increasing effect of serotonin and histamine on the affected cranial vessels, thereby checking the transudation of plasmakinin so that the pain threshold of the receptors is maintained at 'normal' levels. In the sequence of events leading to migraine attack, depletion of plasma serotonin contributes to loss of tone in the extracranial vessels. Pizotifen inhibits serotonin reuptake by the platelets, thus maintaining plasma serotonin and preventing the loss of tone and passive distension of the extracranial arteries.

5.2 Pharmacokinetic properties

Absorption

Absorption of pizotifen is fast (absorption half life 0.5 to 0.8 hours) and nearly complete (80%).

Biotransformation

The substance is metabolised with a half life of about 1 hour. The main metabolite (N-glucuronide) is eliminated with a half life of approximately 23 hours.

Distribution

Protein binding amounts to 91% and distribution volume to 485 litres.

Elimination

Less than 1% of the administered dose is excreted unchanged in the urine, whereas 55% is excreted as metabolites.

5.3 Preclinical safety data
There are no pre-clinical data of relevance to the prescriber which are additional to that already included in other sections of the SPC.

6. PHARMACEUTICAL PARTICULARS

6.1 List of excipients
The tablets contain lactose, maize starch, polyvinylpyrrolidone, magnesium stearate, talc (acid washed). The coating constituents are sugar (granulated no.2), talc, gum acacia, titanium dioxide, iron oxide yellow, carnauba wax, printing wax, colloidal anhydrous silica and purified water.

6.2 Incompatibilities
None.

6.3 Shelf life
60 months.

6.4 Special precautions for storage
Protect from direct light.

6.5 Nature and contents of container
The tablets are ivory, circular, biconvex printed SMG 1.5 on one side and come in PVDC opaque blister packs containing 28 tablets.

6.6 Instructions for use and handling
None.

7. MARKETING AUTHORISATION HOLDER
Novartis Pharmaceuticals UK Limited

(trading as Sandoz Pharmaceuticals)

Frimley Business Park

Frimley

Camberley

Surrey

GU16 7SR

8. MARKETING AUTHORISATION NUMBER(S)
PL 00101/0129.

9. DATE OF FIRST AUTHORISATION/RENEWAL OF THE AUTHORISATION
28 April 1981/3 September 2007

10. DATE OF REVISION OF THE TEXT
26 November 2003

Legal Category
POM

SANOMIGRAN Elixir

(Novartis Pharmaceuticals UK Ltd)

1. NAME OF THE MEDICINAL PRODUCT
SANOMIGRAN Elixir 0.25mg/5ml

2. QUALITATIVE AND QUANTITATIVE COMPOSITION
The active ingredient is: 4-(1-methyl-4-piperidylidene)-9,10-dihydro-4H-benzo-[4,5]cyclohepta [1,2-b] thiophene hydrogen maleate (= pizotifen hydrogen malate).

The syrup contains 0.365mg of pizotifen hydrogen malate B.P. in every 5mls.

3. PHARMACEUTICAL FORM
Syrup

4. CLINICAL PARTICULARS
4.1 Therapeutic indications
Prophylactic treatment of recurrent vascular headaches, including classical migraine, common migraine and cluster headaches (periodic migrainous neuralgia).

It is not effective in relieving migraine attacks once in progress.

4.2 Posology and method of administration
Adults
Usually 1.5mg daily. This may be taken as a single dose at night or in three divided doses. Dosage should be adjusted to individual patient requirements up to a maximum of 4.5mg daily. Up to 3mg may be given as a single dose.
Children (aged over 2 years)
Up to 1.5mg daily, usually as a divided dose, although up to 1mg has been given as a single dose at night.
Use in the elderly
Clinical work with SANOMIGRAN has not shown elderly patients to require different dosages from younger patients.
Method of administration
Oral.

4.3 Contraindications
Known hypersensitivity to pizotifen or any of the excipients (see 6.1 List of Excipients).

4.4 Special warnings and special precautions for use
SANOMIGRAN Elixir does not contain sucrose nor tartrazine. The sweetening agent in SANOMIGRAN Elixir is maltitol liquid at a concentration of 4g in 5ml. Maltitol liquid contains 45% readily absorbable carbohydrate. This should be considered if prescribing the drug for diabetic patients.

Although the anticholinergic activity of SANOMIGRAN is relatively weak, caution is required in the presence of closed angle glaucoma and in patients with a predisposition to urinary retention. Dosage adjustment may be necessary in patients with kidney insufficiency.

4.5 Interaction with other medicinal products and other forms of Interaction
The central effects of sedatives, hypnotics, antihistamines (including certain common cold preparations) and alcohol may be enhanced by SANOMIGRAN.

4.6 Pregnancy and lactation
As clinical data with SANOMIGRAN in pregnancy are very limited it should only be administered during pregnancy under compelling circumstances.

Although the concentrations of SANOMIGRAN measured in the milk of treated mothers are not likely to affect the infant, its use in nursing mothers is not recommended.

4.7 Effects on ability to drive and use machines
Patients should be cautioned about the possibility of drowsiness and informed of its significance in the driving of vehicles and the operation of machinery.

4.8 Undesirable effects
The most commonly occurring side-effects are drowsiness and an increased appetite which may lead to an increase in body weight. Other side-effects such as dizziness, dry mouth, nausea and constipation have been reported infrequently. Rare instances of sleep disorders, depression and other mood disturbances such as anxiety and aggression have occurred. In children CNS stimulation may occur. Rare cases of hypersensitivity reaction such as rash, facial oedema and urticaria have been reported.

4.9 Overdose
Symptoms of overdosage may include drowsiness, dizziness, hypotension, dryness of the mouth, confusion, excitatory states (in children), ataxia, nausea, vomiting, dyspnoea, cyanosis, tachycardia, convulsions (particularly in children), coma and respiratory paralysis.

Treatment: Administration of activated charcoal is recommended; in case of very recent uptake, gastric lavage may be considered. Severe hypotension must be corrected (CAVE: adrenaline may produce paradoxical effects). If necessary, symptomatic treatment including monitoring of the cardiovascular and respiratory systems. Excitory states or convulsions may be treated with short acting benzodiazepines.

5. PHARMACOLOGICAL PROPERTIES
5.1 Pharmacodynamic properties
Pharmacodynamic studies demonstrate pizotifen to have powerful anti-serotonin and anti-tryptaminic properties, marked anti-histaminic effects and some antagonistic activity against kinins. It also possesses weak anti-cholinergic effects and sedative properties.

Pizotifen also possesses appetite-stimulating properties.

The prophylactic effect of SANOMIGRAN in migraine is associated with its ability to modify the humoral mechanisms of headache.

It inhibits the permeability-increasing effect of serotonin and histamine on the affected cranial vessels, thereby checking the transudation of plasmakinin so that the pain threshold of the receptors is maintained at 'normal' levels. In the sequence of events leading to migraine attack, depletion of plasma serotonin contributes to loss of tone in the extracranial vessels. Pizotifen inhibits serotonin re-uptake by the platelets, thus maintaining plasma serotonin and preventing the loss of tone and passive distension of the extracranial arteries.

5.2 Pharmacokinetic properties
Absorption
Absorption of pizotifen is fast (absorption half life 0.5 to 0.8 hours) and nearly complete (80%).
Biotransformation
The substance is metabolised with a half life of about 1 hour. The main metabolite (N-glucuronide) is eliminated with a half life of approximately 23 hours.
Distribution
Protein binding amounts to 91% and distribution volume to 485 litres.
Elimination
Less than 1% of the administered dose is excreted unchanged in the urine, whereas 55% is excreted as metabolites.

5.3 Preclinical safety data
There are no pre-clinical data of relevance to the prescriber which are additional to that already included in other sections of the SPC.

6. PHARMACEUTICAL PARTICULARS
6.1 List of excipients
The syrup contains raspberry flavour 50969, maraschino flavour, methyl hydroxybenzoate, propyl hydroxybenzoate, citric acid (anhydrous), disodium phosphate (anhydrous), maltitol liquid, ethanol 96% and purified water.

6.2 Incompatibilities
None.

6.3 Shelf life
60 months.

6.4 Special precautions for storage
None.

6.5 Nature and contents of container
The syrup is clear, colourless liquid, with a fruity odour and taste and comes in amber glass bottles with a polypropylene closure (polythene wad faced with PP, PVDC or PET lining) in a 300ml pack size.

6.6 Instructions for use and handling
None.

7. MARKETING AUTHORISATION HOLDER
Novartis Pharmaceuticals UK Limited
(trading as Sandoz Pharmaceuticals)
Frimley Business Park
Frimley
Camberley
Surrey
GU16 7SR

8. MARKETING AUTHORISATION NUMBER(S)
PL 00101/0163

9. DATE OF FIRST AUTHORISATION/RENEWAL OF THE AUTHORISATION
06 June 1983 / 28 June 2001

10. DATE OF REVISION OF THE TEXT
26 November 2003

Legal Category
POM

Scopoderm TTS

(Novartis Consumer Health)

1. NAME OF THE MEDICINAL PRODUCT
SCOPODERM TTS

2. QUALITATIVE AND QUANTITATIVE COMPOSITION
Each patch contains 1.5mg hyoscine U.S.P.

3. PHARMACEUTICAL FORM
Scopoderm TTS is a transdermal therapeutic system. Each patch is a flat system of laminates, sealed around the edge, containing a clear oily filling. The system is a thin circular disc, tan coloured and fitted with a transparent, hexagonal protective liner which projects over the edge of the disc. Viewed through the liner, the system appears silver in colour. Each system has a contact surface area measuring 2.5cm^2 and hyoscine content of 1.5mg. The average amount of hyoscine absorbed from each system in 72 hours is 1mg.

4. CLINICAL PARTICULARS
4.1 Therapeutic indications
For the prevention of symptoms of motion sickness such as nausea, vomiting and vertigo.

4.2 Posology and method of administration
Route of Administration
Transdermal
Dosage and Administration
Adults
To achieve the optimum protective effect, one system should be applied about 5-6 hours before embarking on a journey (or on the evening before). The system should be placed onto a clean, dry, hairless area of skin behind the ear, taking care to avoid any cuts or irritation. One system can provide protection for up to 72 hours. Should protection be required for longer periods of time, a fresh system should be placed behind the other ear after 72 hours. (No more than one system should be used at a time). Conversely, if protection is only required for shorter periods of time, the system should be removed at the end of the journey.

Patients should wash their hands thoroughly after handling the system. In addition, after removal of the system, the site of application should also be washed. These precautions are necessary to minimise any chance of hyoscine accidentally being transferred to the eyes (see side-effects).

Limited contact with water (i.e. during bathing or swimming), should not affect the system, although it should be kept as dry as possible.

If the Scopoderm TTS becomes accidentally detached, it should be replaced by a fresh system.
Use in Elderly
Scopoderm TTS may be used in the elderly (see dosage recommendations for adults) although the elderly may be more prone to suffer from the side-effects of hyoscine (see precautions).
Use in Children
Scopoderm TTS can be used in children age 10 years or over (see dosage recommendations for adults). Insufficient data are available to recommend the use of Scopoderm TTS for younger children.

4.3 Contraindications
Scopoderm TTS is contra-indicated in patients with glaucoma or with a history of the condition, and in patients with known hypersensitivity to hyoscine.

4.4 Special warnings and special precautions for use
Scopoderm TTS should be used with caution in patients with pyloric stenosis, those who have bladder outflow obstruction, or in patients with intestinal obstruction.

Patients should not consume alcohol whilst using Scopoderm TTS.

Scopoderm TTS should also be used with caution in elderly patients, and in patients with impaired hepatic or renal function.

In rare cases, confusional states and visual hallucinations may occur. In such cases, Scopoderm TTS should be removed immediately. If severe symptoms persist, appropriate therapeutic measures should be taken
(see overdosage section).

Idiosyncratic reactions may occur with ordinary therapeutic doses of hyoscine.

In isolated cases an increase in seizure frequency in epileptic patients has been reported.

Care should be taken after removal of the system as side-effects may persist for up to 24 hours or longer.

4.5 Interaction with other medicinal products and other forms of Interaction
Scopoderm TTS should be used with caution in patients being treated with drugs that act on the central nervous system (including alcohol) or drugs with anticholinergic properties.

4.6 Pregnancy and lactation
Teratogenic studies have been performed in pregnant rats and rabbits with hyoscine administered by daily intravenous injection. No adverse effects were noted in rats. In rabbits, the drug had a marginal embryotoxic effect at a high dose (at drug plasma levels approximately 100 times those observed in humans using Scopoderm TTS).

Scopoderm TTS should only be used during pregnancy if the expected benefits to the mother outweigh the potential risks to the foetus.

It is not known if hyoscine passes into the breast milk. Therefore nursing mothers should refrain from breast feeding their infants whilst using Scopoderm TTS.

4.7 Effects on ability to drive and use machines
Scopoderm TTS may cause drowsiness, dizziness, confusion or visual disturbance in certain individuals. Patients using the system must not drive, operate machinery, pilot an aircraft, dive or engage in any other activities in which such symptoms could be dangerous (see side-effects).

4.8 Undesirable effects
The following side-effects may occur:

Eyes

In isolated cases pupillary dilatation may precipitate acute glaucoma, particularly narrow angle glaucoma

(see Contra-Indications).

Occasional: Irritation of the eyelids

If traces of hyoscine on the hands enter the eyes, transient cycloplegia and pupillary dilatation (occasionally unilateral) frequently occur.

Mouth

Frequent: Transient dryness of the mouth.

Central Nervous System

Occasional: Drowsiness.

Rare: Impairment of memory and concentration, restlessness, dizziness, disorientation, confusion and visual hallucinations. (see precautions).

Skin

Occasional: Local irritation

In isolated cases: A generalised skin rash

Urogenital system

Rare: Disturbances of micturition (i.e. urine retention)

Side-effects after removal of Scopoderm TTS

Rare: Unwanted effects, including headache, nausea, vomiting and disturbance of balance, occurring after removal of the system. These symptoms have occurred most often in patients who have used the system for several days. In such cases, patients should not drive or engage in other activities requiring concentration

(see warnings).

4.9 Overdose
Symptoms

Initially, restlessness, excitation and confusion may be observed. In response to higher doses, delirium, hallucinations and convulsions set in. At very high doses, coma and respiratory paralysis may occur.

Treatment

If symptoms of overdosage occur, the system(s) should be removed immediately. Physostigmine is the most effective antidote. Depending on the severity of poisoning, physostigmine should be given by slow intravenous injection in doses of 1-4mg (0.5mg in children). Repeated injections may be necessary since physostigmine is rapidly metabolised. Diazepam may be used to counter excitation and convulsions although at higher doses it may cause respiratory depression. In severe cases, artificial respiration may be necessary. If hyperthermia occurs, immediate action should be taken to dissipate heat.

5. PHARMACOLOGICAL PROPERTIES
5.1 Pharmacodynamic properties
The transdermal therapeutic system (TTS) is a novel form of drug delivery designed to achieve a continuous release of hyoscine through the intact skin to the systemic circulation for up to 72 hours.

Hyoscine has anticholinergic properties. It acts as a competitive antagonist to acetylchloline and other parasympathomimetic agents. Its mechanism of action in the central nervous system in preventing motion sickness has yet to be elucidated. Hyoscine produces classical symptoms of parasympathetic blockade.

5.2 Pharmacokinetic properties
Following Scopoderm TTS administration, measurement of the urinary excretion has shown the equilibrium between absorption and elimination to be reached within about 6 hours. Steady plasma concentrations of hyoscine in the range of 0.17-0.33nmol/litre are produced. Provided the system is not removed, this equilibrium is maintained and plasma hyoscine levels are within this therapeutic range for up to 72 hours.

After removal of Scopoderm TTS, the plasma concentration diminishes slowly to approximately one third over the following 24 hours because hyoscine in the skin continues to enter the blood stream.

5.3 Preclinical safety data
None stated

6. PHARMACEUTICAL PARTICULARS
6.1 List of excipients
The patches contain light mineral oil and polyisobutylene which are contained in both the drug reservoir and in the adhesive.

6.2 Incompatibilities
None stated

6.3 Shelf life
36 months

6.4 Special precautions for storage
Store below 25°C. Do not freeze.

6.5 Nature and contents of container
Scopoderm TTS - Individually packed into sealed paper laminated aluminium foil pouches. Outer cardboard carton containing two patches.

6.6 Instructions for use and handling
Patients should wash their hands thoroughly after handling the system. In addition, after removal of the system, the site of application should also be washed. These precautions are necessary to minimise any chance of hyoscine accidentally being transferred to the eyes (see side-effects).

Administrative Data
7. MARKETING AUTHORISATION HOLDER
Novartis Consumer Health UK Limited

Trading as: Novartis Consumer Health

Wimblehurst Road

Horsham

West Sussex

RH12 5AB

UK

8. MARKETING AUTHORISATION NUMBER(S)
00030/0180

9. DATE OF FIRST AUTHORISATION/RENEWAL OF THE AUTHORISATION
30 March 2001

10. DATE OF REVISION OF THE TEXT
30 March 2001

Other information

Legal category: Prescription only medicine

Sea-Legs Tablets

(SSL International plc)

1. NAME OF THE MEDICINAL PRODUCT
Sea-Legs Tablets.

2. QUALITATIVE AND QUANTITATIVE COMPOSITION
Meclozine Hydrochloride BP 12.5mg.

3. PHARMACEUTICAL FORM
Tablets for oral administration.

4. CLINICAL PARTICULARS
4.1 Therapeutic indications
For the prevention and treatment of motion sickness.

4.2 Posology and method of administration
For oral administration. Adults and children over 12 years: Two tablets (25mg) per 24 hours. The tablets may be taken one hour prior to commencement of journey or, as Sea-Legs can remain active for 24 hours after one dose, the previous night. Children 6-12 years: One tablet (12.5mg) per 24 hours. Children 2-6 years: Half a tablet (6.25mg) per 24 hours.

4.3 Contraindications
Pregnancy.

4.4 Special warnings and special precautions for use
Avoid alcoholic drink.

4.5 Interaction with other medicinal products and other forms of Interaction
None known.

4.6 Pregnancy and lactation
Contraindicated in pregnancy.

4.7 Effects on ability to drive and use machines
May cause drowsiness. If affected, do not drive or operate machinery. Avoid alcoholic drink.

4.8 Undesirable effects
None known.

4.9 Overdose
No specific statement.

5. PHARMACOLOGICAL PROPERTIES
5.1 Pharmacodynamic properties
Meclozine hydrochloride is a piperazine derivative with the properties of antihistamines. It is used for its anti-emetic action that may last for up to 24 hours. Sedative effects are not marked. It is used for the prevention and treatment of motion sickness.

5.2 Pharmacokinetic properties
In general, antihistamines are readily absorbed from the gastrointestinal tract, metabolised in the liver and excreted usually mainly as metabolites in the urine.

5.3 Preclinical safety data
None stated.

6. PHARMACEUTICAL PARTICULARS
6.1 List of excipients
Lactose Ph Eur; Maize Starch Ph Eur; Sodium Starch Glycolate BP; Magnesium Stearate Ph Eur; Povidone Powder Ph Eur; Industrial Methylated Spirits BP; Purified Water Ph Eur.

6.2 Incompatibilities
None known.

6.3 Shelf life
36 months.

6.4 Special precautions for storage
Do not store above 25°C

6.5 Nature and contents of container
A cellulose/aluminium foil/polythene laminate carrying 12 tablets overwrapped with a cardboard envelope; or Purelay-Pharm 100E white opaque (polypropylene) and Purelay-Lid (polypropylene).

6.6 Instructions for use and handling
Not applicable.

7. MARKETING AUTHORISATION HOLDER
Seton Products Limited, Tubiton House, Oldham, OL1 3HS.

8. MARKETING AUTHORISATION NUMBER(S)
PL 11314/0011.

9. DATE OF FIRST AUTHORISATION/RENEWAL OF THE AUTHORISATION
16th February 1994 / 9th December 2004

10. DATE OF REVISION OF THE TEXT
December 2004

Sebomin MR

(Alpharma Limited)

1. NAME OF THE MEDICINAL PRODUCT
Sebomin 100mg MR Capsules.

2. QUALITATIVE AND QUANTITATIVE COMPOSITION
Each capsule contains 100mg anhydrous minocycline (as the hydrochloride).

For excipients, see 6.1

3. PHARMACEUTICAL FORM
Prolonged-release capsule, hard.

Orange, opaque, hard gelatin capsules (size 2) printed "C" and "MR" in white.

4. CLINICAL PARTICULARS
4.1 Therapeutic indications
The treatment of acne.

4.2 Posology and method of administration
Dosage:

Adults: One 100mg capsule every 24 hours.

Children over 12 years: One 100mg capsule every 24 hours.

Children under 12 years: Sebomin MR is not recommended.

Elderly: No special dosing requirements.

Treatment of acne should be continued for a minimum of 6 weeks. If there is no satisfactory response to Sebomin MR after six months, the treatment should be discontinued and other therapies considered. If Sebomin MR is to be continued for longer than six months, patients should be monitored at least three monthly thereafter for signs and symptoms of hepatitis or SLE (see Special warnings and precautions for use).

Administration:

The capsules should be swallowed whole with plenty of fluid, while sitting or standing in order to reduce the risk of oesophageal irritation and ulceration. They should not be taken with food as this affects the absorption of minocycline.

4.3 Contraindications
- Known hypersensitivity to tetracyclines
- Pregnancy
- Lactation
- Children under the age of 12 years
- Complete renal failure.

4.4 Special warnings and special precautions for use
Minocycline should be used with caution in patients with hepatic dysfunction and in conjunction with alcohol and other hepatotoxic drugs. It is recommended that alcohol consumption should remain within the Government's recommended limits.

Rare cases of auto-immune hepatotoxicity and isolated cases of systemic lupus erythematosus (SLE) and also exacerbation of pre-existing SLE have been reported. If patients develop signs or symptoms of SLE or hepatotoxicity, or suffer exacerbation of pre-existing SLE, minocycline should be discontinued.

Clinical studies have shown that in patients with renal impairment there is no significant drug accumulation when they are treated with minocycline in the recommended doses. However, reduction of dosage and monitoring of renal function may be required in cases of severe renal insufficiency.

Cross-resistance between tetracyclines may develop in micro-organisms and cross-sensitisation in patients. Minocycline should be discontinued if there are signs/symptoms of overgrowth of resistant organisms, e.g. enteritis, glossitis, stomatitis, vaginitis, pruritus ani or staphylococcal enteritis.

Patients taking oral contraceptives should be warned that there is a possibility of contraceptive failure if diarrhoea or breakthrough bleeding occurs.

Minocycline may cause hyperpigmentation at various body sites. Hyperpigmentation may be present regardless of dose or duration of treatment but develops more commonly during long term treatment. Patients should be advised to report any unusual pigmentation without delay and minocycline should be discontinued.

If a photosensitivity reaction occurs, patients should be warned to avoid direct exposure to natural or artificial light and to discontinue therapy at the first sign of skin discomfort.

The capsule shell contains sunset yellow (E110), which can cause allergic - type reactions including asthma. Allergy is more common in those people who are allergic to aspirin.

Use in children:

The use of tetracyclines during tooth development in children under the age of 12 years may cause permanent discolouration. Enamel hypoplasia has also been reported.

4.5 Interaction with other medicinal products and other forms of Interaction

Minocycline should not be used with penicillins. Tetracyclines depress plasma prothrombin activity and reduced doses of concomitant anticoagulants may be necessary.

Absorption of minocycline is impaired by the concomitant administration of antacids, iron, calcium, magnesium, aluminium and zinc salts. It is recommended that any indigestion remedies, vitamins, or other supplements containing these salts are taken at least 3 hours before or after a dose of minocycline. The capsules should not be taken with food as this affects the absorption of minocycline.

4.6 Pregnancy and lactation

Pregnancy:

Results of animal studies indicate that tetracyclines cross the placenta, are found in foetal tissues and can have toxic effects on the developing foetus (often related to retardation of skeletal development). Evidence of embryotoxicity has also been noted in animals treated early in pregnancy. Minocycline therefore, should not be used in pregnancy unless considered essential.

The use of drugs of the tetracycline class during tooth development (last half of pregnancy) may cause permanent discolouration of the teeth (yellow-grey-brown). This adverse reaction has been observed following repeated short term courses however it is more common during long term use of the drug. Enamel hypoplasia has also been reported.

Lactation:

Tetracyclines have been found in the milk of lactating women who are taking a drug in this class. Permanent tooth discolouration may occur in the developing infant and enamel hypoplasia has been reported.

4.7 Effects on ability to drive and use machines

Minocycline has been associated with headache, lightheadedness, dizziness and vertigo and rarely impaired hearing. Patients should be warned about the possible hazards of driving or operating machinery during treatment.

4.8 Undesirable effects

Common

As with other tetracyclines, gastrointestinal disturbances including nausea, anorexia, vomiting and diarrhoea may occur. Dermatological reactions such as erythema multiforme, erythema nodosum, Stevens Johnson syndrome, exfoliative dermatitis, hair loss and photosensitivity have been reported, as well as maculopapular and erythematous rashes. Hypersensitivity reactions can include urticaria, fever, arthralgia, myalgia, arthritis, pulmonary infiltration, wheezing, angioneurotic oedema, anaphylaxis and anaphylactoid purpura.

Cases of systemic lupus erythematosus (SLE) and also exacerbation of pre-existing SLE have been reported (see also Special warnings and precautions for use).

In common with other tetracyclines, bulging fontanelles in infants and benign intracranial hypertension in juveniles and adults have been reported. If evidence of raised intracranial pressure develops, treatment should cease.

Blood haemolytic anaemia, thrombocytopenia, neutropenia and eosinophilia have been reported with tetracyclines.

As with other tetracyclines, transient increases in liver function test values have been reported. Some hepatic reactions have an auto-immune basis, and may occur after several months of minocycline treatment (see Posology and method of administration). When given over prolonged periods, tetracyclines have been reported to produce brown-black microscopic discolouration of thyroid tissue.

Uncommon

There have been isolated incidences of pancreatitis.

Hyperpigmentation of skin, nails or discolouration of teeth and buccal mucosa have been reported occasionally. These are generally reversible on cessation of therapy.

There are isolated cases of discolouration of conjunctiva, lacrimal secretions, breast secretions and perspiration.

Rare

Hepatitis and acute liver failure have been reported.

Fixed drug eruptions have been observed.

Pericarditis, myocarditis, vasculitis and renal failure including interstitial nephritis have been reported.

Bone discolouration has been observed.

(See also Pregnancy and Lactation).

4.9 Overdose

No specific antidote. Gastric lavage plus appropriate supportive treatment.

5. PHARMACOLOGICAL PROPERTIES

5.1 Pharmacodynamic properties

Pharmacotherapeutic group: Tetracycline, ATC code: J01A A08

Sebomin MR contain the active ingredient minocycline as minocycline hydrochloride, a semi-synthetic derivative of tetracycline.

Minocycline has a long serum half-life and can be administered at 12 hour intervals, the modified release form can be given once daily.

Minocycline interferes with the third stage of bacterial protein synthesis. After amino acids are activated and attached to t-RNA (transfer RNA), the resulting amino acyl-t-RNA migrates to the bacterial ribosome for synthesis of proteins. Minocycline binds to the 30s subunit on the ribosome and inhibits binding of the aminoacyl-t-RNA molecules.

There is also evidence that minocycline may cause alterations in the cytoplasmic membrane, thereby allowing leakage of nucleotides and other compounds from the cell. This would explain the rapid inhibition of DNA replication that ensues when cells are exposed to concentrations of minocycline greater than that needed to inhibit protein synthesis.

In higher concentration, minocycline inhibits mammalian protein synthesis and may aggravate pre-existing renal functional impairment. The drug may interfere with parenteral nutrition in post operative patients by inhibiting utilization of amino acids for protein synthesis.

Minocycline is reported to be active against both Gram negative and Gram positive organisms.

5.2 Pharmacokinetic properties

Absorption

Oral bioavailability for minocycline has been reported to be 90%.

One report has demonstrated that food did not significantly affect the absorption of minocycline following 50 mg oral doses. However, another study reported that minocycline absorption was decreased by 77%, 27% and 13% when given with iron, milk and food.

Distribution

Total protein binding of minocycline has been reported to be in the order of 76%.

Other sites of distribution of minocycline include the following:

AQUEOUS HUMOR

Minocycline administered orally with a loading dose of 200 mg followed by 2 doses of 100 mg 12 hours apart produce adequate drug concentration in the aqueous humor of noninflamed eyes. The plasma to aqueous humor ratio was approximately 2:1.

CEREBROSPINAL FLUID

Minocycline has been reported to cross the blood/brain barrier to a higher degree than doxycycline. However, passage of either drug has been shown to be significantly decreased in patients with uninflamed meninges.

GINGIVAL FLUID

The mean gingival crevicular fluid drug concentration of 8.03 +/- 1.64 mcg/ml was reported after 7 days of oral minocycline 200 mg in patients with moderate to severe periodontal disease. Mean serum concentration was 2.58 +/- 0.32 mcg/ml.

JOINT FLUID CONCENTRATIONS

Following 200 mg oral doses of minocycline, joint fluid levels 3 to 12 hours following the dose were 0.43 to 0.88 mcg/ml.

SALIVA/TEARS

Minocycline achieved significant levels in saliva and tears sufficient to inhibit most strains of meningococci. Following oral doses of 100 mg every 12 hours for 5 days, the concentration of drug in saliva and tear equalled or was greater than the average MIC for meningococci for up to 12 hours after the dose. Two hours following an oral dose, concentrations of minocycline in saliva and tears were at 0.3 mcg/mL and 0.4 mcg/mL, respectively.

SINUS SECRETIONS

Following a dose of 100 mg twice daily for 4 days in patients with sinusitis a sinus level of 1.06 mcg/5 mL was found. The mean minocycline serum level was 3.16 mcg/ml, giving a sinus secretion to serum level ratio of 0.34:1.

Metabolism

An inactive metabolite, 9-hydroxyminocycline has been isolated.

Elimination

Minocycline has a very low renal clearance as compared to other tetracyclines. However, urinary concentrations approximating 10 times that of serum are attained for the first 4 to 6 hours following an oral dose.

Minocycline is excreted 19% in the faeces, this level is much lower than most other tetracyclines.

5.3 Preclinical safety data

There are no preclinical data of relevance to the prescriber which are additional to that already included in other sections of the SPC.

6. PHARMACEUTICAL PARTICULARS

6.1 List of excipients

glycerol monostearate 40-55,

microcrystalline cellulose 101 (E460(i)),

povidone K-30 (E1201),

purified talc (E553b).

Capsule shell

gelatin,

purified water,

titanium dioxide (E171),

sunset yellow (E110),

quinoline yellow (E104).

Printing ink

shellac (E904),

ethyl alcohol,

isopropyl alcohol,

propylene glycol,

butyl alcohol,

povidone (E1201),

sodium hydroxide,

titanium dioxide (E171).

6.2 Incompatibilities

Not applicable.

6.3 Shelf life

24 months.

6.4 Special precautions for storage

Do not store above 30°C.

Polypropylene container - store in the original container,

PVC/aluminium blister pack - keep container in the outer carton.

6.5 Nature and contents of container

PVC/aluminium blister pack in outer cardboard container

28, 30, 56, 60, 84, 90

Polypropylene container with polyethylene cap

100, 112, 120, 200, 250, 500

Not all pack sizes may be marketed.

6.6 Instructions for use and handling

No special requirements.

7. MARKETING AUTHORISATION HOLDER

Alpharma Limited (Trading style: Alpharma, Cox Pharmaceuticals)

Whiddon Valley

Barnstaple

North Devon

EX32 8NS

United Kingdom

8. MARKETING AUTHORISATION NUMBER(S)

PL 00142/0526

9. DATE OF FIRST AUTHORISATION/RENEWAL OF THE AUTHORISATION

20 June 2003

10. DATE OF REVISION OF THE TEXT

January 2004

Seconal Sodium

(Flynn Pharma Ltd)

1. NAME OF THE MEDICINAL PRODUCT

SECONAL SODIUM

2. QUALITATIVE AND QUANTITATIVE COMPOSITION

Each 50mg capsule contains 50mg of Secobarbital Sodium BP

Each 100mg capsule contains 100mg of Secobarbital Sodium BP

3. PHARMACEUTICAL FORM

Capsule

4. CLINICAL PARTICULARS

4.1 Therapeutic indications

For the short term treatment of severe, intractable insomnia in patients already taking barbiturates. New patients should not be started on this preparation. Attempts should be made to wean patients off this preparation by gradual reduction of the dose over a period of days or weeks (*see drug abuse and dependence).* Abrupt discontinuation should be avoided as this may precipitate withdrawal effects *(see warnings).*

4.2 Posology and method of administration

For oral administration to adults only. Normal dosage is 100 mg at bedtime.

THE ELDERLY

Seconal Sodium is not recommended for use in elderly or debilitated patients.

CHILDREN

Seconal should not be administered to children or young adults.

In studies, secobarbitone sodium has been found to lose most of its effectiveness for both inducing and maintaining sleep by the end of two weeks of continued drug administration, even with the use of multiple doses.

4.3 Contraindications

Hypersensitivity to barbiturates, a history of manifest or latent porphyria, marked impairment of liver function or respiratory disease in which dyspnoea or obstruction is evident.

Barbiturates should not be administered to children, young adults, patients with a history of drug or alcohol addiction or abuse, the elderly and the debilitated.

4.4 Special warnings and special precautions for use

Addiction potential: secobarbitone sodium may be habit forming. Tolerance and psychological and physical dependence may occur with continued use. Patients who have psychological dependence on barbiturates may increase the dosage or decrease the dosage interval without consulting a doctor and, subsequently, may develop a physical dependence on barbiturates.

To minimise the possibility of overdsoage or development of dependence, the amount prescribed should be limited to that required for the interval until the next appointment.

Withdrawal symptoms occur after long term normal use (and particularly after abuse) on rapid cessation of barbiturate treatment. Symptoms include nightmares, irritability and insomnia and, in severe cases, tremors, delirium, convulsions and death.

Barbiturates should be withdrawn gradually from any patient known to be taking excessive doses over long periods.

Caution should be exercised when barbiturates are administered in the presence of acute or chronic pain, because paradoxical excitement could be induced or important symptoms could be masked.

Information for patients: The following information should be given to patients receiving secobarbitone:

1 The use of secobarbitone carries with it an associated risk of psychological and/or physical dependence. The patient should be warned against increasing the dose of the drug without consulting a doctor.

2 Secobarbitone may impair the mental and/or physical abilities required for the performance of potentially hazardous tasks, such as driving a car or operating machinery. The patient should be cautioned accordingly.

3 Alcohol should not be consumed while taking secobarbitone. The concurrent use of secobarbitone with other CNS depressants (eg alcohol, narcotics, tranquillisers and antihistamines) may result in additional CNS depressant effects.

Drug abuse and dependence: Barbiturates may be habit forming; tolerance, psychological and physical dependence may occur especially following prolonged use of high doses. Daily administration in excess of 400 mg secobarbitone, for approximately 90 days, is likely to produce some degree of physical dependence.

A dosage of 600 - 800 mg, for at least 35 days, is sufficient to produce withdrawal seizures. The average daily dose for the barbiturate addict is usually about 1.5g.

As tolerance to barbiturates develops, the amount needed to maintain the same level of intoxication increases; tolerance to a fatal dosage, however, does not increase more than twofold. As this occurs, the margin between intoxicating dosage and fatal dosage becomes smaller. The lethal dose of a barbiturate is far less if alcohol is also ingested.

Symptoms of acute intoxication include unsteady gait, slurred speech and sustained nystagmus. Mental signs of chronic intoxication include confusion, poor judgement, irritability, insomnia and somatic complaints.

The symptoms of barbiturate withdrawal can be severe and may cause death. Minor withdrawal symptoms may appear 8 to 12 hours after the last dose of a barbiturate. These symptoms usually appear in the following order: anxiety, muscle twitching, tremor of hands and fingers, progressive weakness, dizziness, distortion in visual perception, nausea, vomiting, insomnia and orthostatic hypotension. Major withdrawal symptoms (convulsions and delirium) may occur within 16 hours and last up to five days after abrupt cessation of barbiturates. Intensity of withdrawal symptoms gradually declines over a period of approximately 15 days. Individuals susceptible to barbiturate abuse and dependence include alcoholics and opiate abusers, as well as other sedative-hypnotic and amphetamine abusers.

Dependence on barbiturates arises from repeated administration on a continuous basis, generally in amounts exceeding therapeutic dose levels. Treatment of dependence consists of cautious and gradual withdrawal of the drug. Barbiturate-dependent patients can be withdrawn by using a number of withdrawal regimens. In all cases, withdrawal takes an extended period. One method involves substituting a 30 mg dose of phenobarbitone for each 100 - 200 mg dose of barbiturate that the patient has been taking. The total daily amount of phenobarbitone is then administered in three or four divided doses, not to exceed 600 mg daily. Should signs of withdrawal occur on the first day of treatment, a loading dose of 100 to 200 mg of phenobarbitone may be administered intramuscularly in addition to the oral dose. After stabilisation on phenobarbitone, the total daily dose is decreased by 30 mg a day as long as withdrawal is proceeding smoothly. A modification of this regimen involves initiating treatment at the patient's regular dosage level and decreasing the daily dosage by 10% as tolerated by the patient.

Infants that are physically dependent on barbiturates may be given phenobarbitone, 3 to 10 mg/kg/day. After withdrawal symptoms (hyperactivity, disturbed sleep, tremors and hyperreflexia) are relieved, the dosage of phenobarbitone should be gradually decreased and completely withdrawn over a two week period.

Carcinogenesis: Animal data show that phenobarbitone can be carcinogenic after lifetime administration.

Human data: In a 29 year epidemiological study of 9136 patients who were treated on an anticonvulsant protocol that included phenobarbitone, results indicated a higher than normal incidence of hepatic carcinoma. Previously some of these patients had been treated with thorotrast, a drug that is known to produce hepatic carcinomas. Thus, this study did not provide sufficient evidence that phenobarbitone is carcinogenic in humans.

A retrospective study of 84 children with brain tumours, matched to 73 normal controls and 78 cancer controls (malignant disease other than brain tumours), suggested an association between exposure to barbiturates prenatally and an increased incidence of brain tumours.

Barbiturates should be administered with caution, if at all, to patients who are mentally depressed or have suicidal tendencies. They should also be used with great caution and at reduced dosage in those with hepatic disease, marked renal dysfunction, shock or respiratory depression.

Elderly or debilitated patients may react to barbiturates with marked excitement, depression or confusion (see 'Contra-indications'). In some persons, barbiturates repeatedly produce excitement rather than depression.

Barbiturates should not be administered to patients showing the premonitory signs of hepatic coma(see 'Contra-indications').

A cumulative effect may occur with the barbiturates leading to features of chronic poisoning including headache, depression and slurred speech.

Automatism may follow the use of a hypnotic dose of barbiturate

Laboratory tests: Prolonged therapy with barbiturates should be accompanied by periodic evaluation of, for example, the haematopoietic, renal and hepatic systems (but see 'Uses).

4.5 Interaction with other medicinal products and other forms of Interaction

Toxic effects and fatalities have occurred following overdoses of secobarbitone alone and in combination with other CNS depressants. Caution should be exercised in prescribing unnecessarily large amounts of secobarbitone for patients who have a history of emotional disturbances or suicidal ideation or who have misused alcohol or other CNS drugs.

Anticoagulants, Antivirals, Calcium-channel Blockers, Ciclosporin, Levothyroxine, Theophylline : Barbiturates cause induction of the liver microsomal enzymes responsible for metabolising many other drugs. In particular they may result in increased metabolism, reduced plasma concentrations and decreased clinical response to: Oral anticoagulants (eg warfarin); antivirals (eg indinavir, nelfinavir, saquinavir); calcium-channel blockers (eg diltiazem, felodipine, isradipine, nicardipine, nifedipine, verapamil); ciclosporin; levothyroxine (thyroxine); theophylline. Patients stabilised on any of these therapies may require dosage adjustments if barbiturates are added to, or withdrawn from, their regimen.

Corticosteroids: Barbiturates appear to enhance the metabolism of exogenous corticosteroids and steroid dosage may also need adjustment.

Griseofulvin: Barbiturates may interfere with the absorption of oral griseofulvin, thus decreasing its blood level. Concomitant administration should be avoided if possible.

Doxycycline: Barbiturates may shorten the half-life of doxycycline for as long as two weeks after the barbiturate is discontinued. If administered concomitantly the clinical response to doxycycline should be monitored closely.

Phenytoin, Sodium Valproate, Valproic Acid: The effect of barbiturates on phenytoin metabolism is variable. Phenytoin and barbiturate blood levels should be monitored more frequently if administered concomitantly. Sodium valproate and valproic acid increase secobarbitone serum levels. Therefore these levels should be monitored and dosage adjustments made as clinically indicated.

CNS Depressants: Concomitant use of other CNS depressants, including other sedatives or hypnotics, antihistamines, tranquillisers or alcohol, may produce additive depressant effects.

Monoamine Oxidase Inhibitors (MAOIS): Prolong the effects of barbiturates.

Oestradiol, oestrone, progesterone and other steroidal hormones: There have been reports of patients treated with antiepileptic drugs (eg phenobarbitone) who became pregnant while taking oral contraceptives. Barbiturates may decrease the effect of oestradiol. An alternative contraceptive method might be suggested to women taking barbiturates.

4.6 Pregnancy and lactation

Usage in Pregnancy: Barbiturates are contraindicated during pregnancy since they can cause foetal harm. A higher than expected incidence of foetal abnormalities may be connected with maternal consumption of barbiturates. Barbiturates readily cross the placental barrier and are distributed throughout foetal tissues with highest concentrations in placenta, foetal liver and brain. Withdrawal symptoms occur in infants born to women who receive barbiturates during the last trimester of pregnancy. If a patient becomes pregnant whilst taking this drug, she should be told of the potential hazard to the foetus.

Reports of infants suffering from long term barbiturate exposure *in utero* included the acute withdrawal syndrome of seizures and hyper-irritability from birth to a delayed onset of up to 14 days.

Labour and Delivery: Respiratory depression has been noted in infants born following the use of barbiturates during labour. Premature infants are particularly susceptible. Resuscitation equipment should be available.

Nursing Mothers: Small amounts of barbiturates are excreted in the milk and they are therefore contraindicated for the nursing mother.

4.7 Effects on ability to drive and use machines

Secobarbitone may impair the mental and/or physical abilities required for the performance of potentially hazardous tasks such as driving a car or operating machinery. The patient should be cautioned accordingly

4.8 Undesirable effects

The following adverse reactions and their incidences were compiled from surveillance of thousands of hospitalised patients who received barbiturates. As such patients may be less aware of certain of the milder adverse effects of barbiturates, the incidence of these reactions may be somewhat higher in fully ambulatory patients.

More than 1 in 100 patients: The most common adverse reaction, estimated to occur at a rate of 1 to 3 patients per 100, is the following:

NERVOUS SYSTEM: Somnolence

LESS THAN 1 IN 100 PATIENTS: Adverse reactions estimated to occur at a rate of less than 1 in 100 patients are listed below grouped by organ system and by decreasing frequency:

NEUROLOGICAL: Agitation, confusion, hyperkinesia, ataxia, CNS depression, nightmares, nervousness, psychiatric disturbance, hallucinations, insomnia, anxiety, dizziness, abnormal thinking.

RESPIRATORY: Hypoventilation, apnoea.

CARDIOVASCULAR: Bradycardia, hypotension, syncope.

DIGESTIVE: Nausea, vomiting, constipation

OTHER: Headache, hypersensitivity reactions (angioneurotic oedema, rashes, exfoliative dermatitis), fever, liver damage. Hypersensitivity is more likely to occur in patients with asthma, urticaria or angioneurotic oedema. Megaloblastic anaemia has followed chronic phenobarbitone use.

4.9 Overdose

The toxic dose of barbiturates varies considerably. In general, an oral dose of 1g of most barbiturates produces serious poisoning in an adult. Death commonly occurs after 2 to 10g of ingested barbiturate. The sedative, therapeutic blood levels of secobarbitone range between 0.5 and 5 mg/l; the usual lethal blood level ranges from 15 to 40 mg/l. Barbiturate intoxication may be confused with alcoholism, bromide intoxication and various neurological disorders. Potential tolerance must be considered when evaluating significance of dose and plasma concentration.

In extreme overdose, all electrical activity in the brain may cease, in which case a "flat" EEG normally equated with clinical death cannot be accepted. This effect is fully reversible unless hypoxic damage occurs. Consideration should be given to the possibility of barbiturate intoxication even in situations that appear to involve trauma.

SIGNS AND SYMPTOMS: Symptoms of oral overdose may occur within 15 minutes and begin with CNS depression, absent or sluggish reflexes, underventilation, hypotension and hypothermia, which may progress to pulmonary oedema and death. Haemorrhagic blisters may develop, especially at pressure points.

Complications such as pneumonia, pulmonary oedema, cardiac arrhythmias, congestive heart failure and renal failure may occur. Uraemia may increase CNS sensitivity to barbiturates if renal function is impaired. Differential diagnosis should include hypoglycaemia, head trauma, cerebrovascular accidents, convulsive states and diabetic coma.

TREATMENT OF OVERDOSAGE

General management should consist of symptomatic and supportive therapy. Activated charcoal may be more effective than emesis or lavage. Diuresis and peritoneal dialysis are of little value. Haemodialysis and haemoperfusion enhance drug clearance and should be considered in serious poisoning. If the patient has chronically abused sedatives, withdrawal reactions may be manifest following acute overdose.

5. PHARMACOLOGICAL PROPERTIES

5.1 Pharmacodynamic properties

Seconal Sodium (secobarbitone sodium), a short acting barbiturate, is a CNS depressant. In ordinary doses the drug acts as a sedative and hypnotic.

Barbiturates are capable of producing all levels of CNS mood alteration, from excitation to mild sedation, hypnosis and deep coma. Overdosage can product death. Barbiturates depress the sensory cortex, decrease motor activity, alter cerebellar function and produce drowsiness, sedation and hypnosis.

Barbiturate-induced sleep differs from physiologic sleep. Sleep laboratory studies have demonstrated that barbiturates reduce the amount of time spent in the rapid eye movement (REM) phase of sleep, or dreaming stage. Also stages III and IV sleep are decreased. Following abrupt cessation of barbiturates used regularly, patients may experience markedly increased dreaming, nightmares and/or insomnia. Therefore, withdrawal of a single therapeutic dose over five or six days has been recommended to lessen the REM rebound and disturbed sleep which contribute to drug withdrawal syndrome (for example, decrease the dose from 3 to 2 doses a day for 1 week).

5.2 Pharmacokinetic properties

Barbiturates are weak acids that are absorbed and rapidly distributed to all tissues and fluids, with high concentrations in the brain, liver and kidneys. Lipid solubility of the barbiturates is the dominant factor in their distribution within the body. Barbiturates are bound to plasma and tissue proteins; the degree of binding increases as a function of lipid solubility. The onset of action of Seconal Sodium is from 10 to 15 minutes and the duration of action ranges from 3 to 4 hours. The plasma half life of Seconal Sodium is 15 - 40 hours.

Secobarbitone sodium has a high lipid solubility, plasma protein binding, brain protein binding, a short delay in onset of activity and a short duration of action.

Seconal is metabolised primarily by the hepatic microsomal enzyme system and the metabolic products are excreted in the urine and, less commonly, in the faeces. Seconal is detoxified in the liver.

5.3 Preclinical safety data

Carcinogenesis: Animal data show that phenobarbitone can be carcinogenic after lifetime administration.

6. PHARMACEUTICAL PARTICULARS

6.1 List of excipients

Starch, Silicone, Erythrosine, Quinoline yellow, Gelatin, Black Iron Oxide, Shellac

6.2 Incompatibilities

Not applicable

6.3 Shelf life

60 months

6.4 Special precautions for storage

Store below 25°C. Keep lid tightly closed.

6.5 Nature and contents of container

High density polyethylene bottles with screw caps containing 100 capsules.

6.6 Instructions for use and handling

Not applicable

7. MARKETING AUTHORISATION HOLDER

Flynn Pharma Ltd.

Alton House,

4 Herbert Street

Dublin 2,

Republic of Ireland

8. MARKETING AUTHORISATION NUMBER(S)

Seconal Sodium 50mg PL 13621/0002

Seconal Sodium 100mg PL 13621/0003

9. DATE OF FIRST AUTHORISATION/RENEWAL OF THE AUTHORISATION

1995

10. DATE OF REVISION OF THE TEXT

January 2001

Sectral Capsules and Tablets

(sanofi-aventis)

1. NAME OF THE MEDICINAL PRODUCT

Sectral Capsules 100mg

Sectral Capsules 200mg

Sectral Tablets 400mg

2. QUALITATIVE AND QUANTITATIVE COMPOSITION

in terms of the active ingredient (INN) name

The active component of Sectral Capsules 100mg is: Acebutolol hydrochloride 111.0mg (equivalent to 100mg of base).

The active component of Sectral Capsules 200mg is: Acebutolol hydrochloride 222.0mg (equivalent to 200mg of base).

Sectral Tablets 400mg: Acebutolol hydrochloride 443.40mg (equivalent to 400mg of base).

3. PHARMACEUTICAL FORM

Sectral Capsules 100: Hard gelatin capsules, the bodies being opaque yellowish-buff and the caps opaque white in colour. Length approximately 17mm, diameter of body approximately 6mm. Both body and cap are printed in black: Sectral 100

Sectral Capsules 200: Hard gelatin capsules, the bodies being opaque yellowish-buff and the caps opaque pink in colour. Length approximately 17mm, diameter of body approximately 6mm. Both body and cap are printed in black: Sectral 200

The capsules contain a white or almost white powder.

Sectral Tablets 400mg: White to off-white, circular, biconvex, film-coated tablets with bevel edges, one face impressed 'SECTRAL 400'. Plain reverse.

4. CLINICAL PARTICULARS

4.1 Therapeutic indications

Sectral is indicated for the following:

The management of all grades of hypertension, angina pectoris and the control of tachyarrhythmias.

4.2 Posology and method of administration

Hypertension: Initial dosage of 400mg orally once daily at breakfast or 200mg orally twice daily. If response is not adequate within two weeks, dosage may be increased up to 400mg orally twice daily; if the hypertension is still not adequately controlled consideration should be given to adding a second antihypertensive agent such as the calcium antagonist nifedipine or small doses of a thiazide diuretic.

Angina pectoris: Initial dosage of 400mg orally once daily at breakfast or 200mg twice daily. In severe forms up to 300mg three times daily may be required. Up to 1200mg daily has been used.

Cardiac Arrhythmias: When given orally, an initial dose of 200mg is recommended. The daily dose requirement for long term anti arrhythmic activity should lie between 400 and 1200mg daily. The dose can be gauged by response, and better control may be achieved by divided doses rather than single doses. It may take up to three hours for maximal anti-arrhythmic effect to become apparent.

Elderly: There are no specific dosage recommendations for the elderly with normal glomerular filtration rate. Dose reduction is necessary if moderate to severe renal impairment is present (see Section 4.4)

Children: Paediatric dose has not been established.

For all indications, it is advised that the lowest recommended dosage be used initially.

4.3 Contraindications

Cardiogenic shock is an absolute contraindication. Extreme caution is required in patients with blood pressures of the order of 100/60 mmHg or below.

Sectral is also contraindicated in patients with second and third degree heart block, sick sinus syndrome, marked bradycardia (< 45-50 bpm), uncontrolled heart failure, metabolic acidosis, severe.peripheral circulatory disorders, hypersensitivity to acebutolol, any of the excipients or to beta blockers, and untreated phaeochromocytoma

4.4 Special warnings and special precautions for use

Renal impairment is not a contraindication to the use of Sectral which has both renal and non-renal excretory pathways. Some caution should be exercised when administering high doses to patients with severe renal failure as accumulation could possibly occur in these circumstances.

The dosage frequency should not exceed once daily in patients with renal impairment. As a guide, the dosage should be reduced by 50% when glomerular filtration rates are between 25-50ml/min and by 75% when they are below 25ml/min (see Section 4.2).

Drug-induced bronchospasm is usually at least partially reversible by the use of a suitable agonist.

Although cardio-selective beta blockers may have less effect on lung function than non-selective beta blockers as with all beta-blockers they should be avoided in patients with obstructive airways disease unless there are compelling clinical reasons for their use. Where such reasons exist, cardio-selective β-blockers should be used with the utmost care (from Section 4.3).

Beta-blockers may induce bradycardia. In such cases, the dosage should be reduced.

They may be used with care in patients with controlled heart failure (see 4.3).

Use with caution in patients with Prinzmetal's angina.

Beta blockers may aggravate peripheral circulatory disorders. They may mask signs of thyrotoxicosis and hypoglycaemia. They should only be used in patients with phaeochromocytoma with comcomitant alpha-adrenoceptor therapy

Patients with known psoriasis should take beta-blockers only after careful consideration.

Beta-blockers may increase both the sensitivity towards allergens and the seriousness of anaphylactic reactions.

Withdrawal of treatment by beta blockers should be achieved by gradual dosage reduction; this is especially important in patients with ischaemic heart disease

When it has been decided to interrupt beta-blockade prior to surgery, therapy should be discontinued for at least 24 hours. Continuation of therapy reduces the risk of arrhythmias but the risk of hypertension may be increased. If treatment is continued, caution should be observed with the use of certain anaesthetic drugs. The patient may be protected against vagal reactions by intravenous administration of atropine.

4.5 Interaction with other medicinal products and other forms of Interaction

Sectral should not be used with verapamil or within several days of verapamil therapy (and vice versa). Use with great care with any other calcium antagonists, particularly diltiazem.

Class I anti-arrhythmic drugs (such as disopyramide) and amiodarone may increase atrial conduction time and induce negative inotropic effects when used concomitantly with beta-blockers.

In patients with labile and insulin-dependent diabetes, the dosage of the hypoglycaemic agent (ie insulin or oral diabetic drugs) may need to be reduced. However beta-blockers have also been known to blunt the effect of glibenclamide. Beta-adrenergic blockade may also prevent the appearance of signs of hypoglycaemia (tachycardia, see Section 4.4).

Cross reactions due to displacement of other drugs from plasma protein binding sites are unlikely due to the low degree of plasma protein binding exhibited by acebutolol and diacetolol.

If a beta-blocker is used concurrently with clonidine the latter should not be withdrawn until several days after the former is discontinued.

Acebutolol may antagonize the effect of sympathomimetic and xanthine bronchodilators.

Concurrent use of digoxin and beta blockers may occasionally induce serious bradycardia. The anti-hypertensive effects of beta blockers may be attenuated by non-steroidal anti-inflammatory agents.

Concomitant administration of tricyclic antidepressants, barbiturates and phenothiazines as well as other anti-hypertensive agent- may increase the blood pressure lowering effect of beta-blockers.

There is a theoretical risk that concurrent administration of monoamine oxidase inhibitors and high doses of beta-blockers, even if they are cardio-selective can produce hypertension.

Sectral therapy should be brought to the attention of the anaesthetist prior to general anaesthesia (see Section 4.4). If treatment is continued, special care should be taken when using anaesthetic agents causing myocardial depression such as ether, cyclopropane and trichlorethylene.

4.6 Pregnancy and lactation

Pregnancy: Sectral should not be administered to female patients during the first trimester of pregnancy unless the physician considers it essential. In such cases the lowest possible dose should be used.

Beta blockers administered in late pregnancy may give rise to bradycardia, hypoglycaemia and cardiac or pulmonary complications in the foetus/neonate.

Beta-blockers can reduce placental perfusion, which may result in intrauterine foetal death, immature and premature deliveries

Animal studies have shown no teratogenic hazard.

Lactation: Acebutolol and its active metabolite are excreted in breast milk and the half life of acebutolol in the neonate is double that in adults. The risks of hypoglycaemia and bradycardia occurring in the nursing infant have not been evaluated. Therefore, breast-feeding is not recommended during treatment.

4.7 Effects on ability to drive and use machines

As with all beta-blockers, dizziness or fatigue may occur occasionally. This should be taken into account when driving or operating machinery.

4.8 Undesirable effects

Sectral possesses antihypertensive effects but these are unlikely to be noted in normotensive subjects. The side-effects common to beta-blockade include: bradycardia, heart failure, a slowing of AV conduction or increase of an existing AV block, hypotension, gastrointestinal effects (such as nausea, vomiting and diarrhoea), cold and cyanotic extremities, paraesthesia, Raynaud's syndrome, intermittent claudication, confusion, dizziness, impaired vision, headaches, shortness of breath, nightmares, hallucinations, psychoses and depression, loss of libido and lethargy. The low lipid solubility and lack of accumulation in CNS tissues of acebutolol and its active metabolite reduce the likelihood of sleep disturbances, depression or other central effects and such occurrences are rare.

Pulmonary infiltration and pneumonitis appear to be rare but potentially serious complications of beta-blockade therapy. Cases of pneumonitis have been reported with acebutolol.

There have been reports of skin rashes and/or dry eyes associated with the use of beta-adrenoceptor blocking drugs. The reported incidence is small and in most cases the symptoms have cleared when treatment was withdrawn. Discontinuation of the drug should be considered in such cases.

Cessation of therapy with a beta-blocker should be gradual. (see Section 4.4)

Although some patients have developed anti-nuclear factor titres, the incidence of associated clinical symptoms is rare and when present, these clear promptly on discontinuation of treatment. Rare cases of a Lupus-like syndrome have been reported.

Bronchospasm has occurred rarely during treatment with acebutolol.

4.9 Overdose

In the event of excessive bradycardia or hypotension, 1mg atropine sulphate administered intravenously should be given without delay. If this is insufficient it should be followed by a slow intravenous injection of isoprenaline (5mcg per minute) with constant monitoring until a response occurs. In severe cases of self-poisoning with circulatory collapse unresponsive to atropine and catecholamines the intravenous injection of glucagon 10-20mg may produce a dramatic improvement. Cardiac pacing may be employed if bradycardia becomes severe.

Judicious use of vasopressors, diazepam, phenytoin, lidocaine, digoxin and bronchodilators should be considered depending on the presentation of the patient. Acebutolol can be removed from blood by haemodialysis. Other symptoms and signs of overdosage include cardiogenic shock, AV block, conduction defects, pulmonary oedema, depressed level of consciousness, bronchospasm, hypoglycaemia and rarely hyperkalaemia.

5. PHARMACOLOGICAL PROPERTIES

5.1 Pharmacodynamic properties

Mode of action: Sectral is a beta adrenoceptor antagonist which is cardioselective, i.e. acts preferentially on beta-1 adrenergic receptors in the heart. Its principal effects are to reduce heart rate especially on exercise and to lower blood pressure in hypertensive subjects. Sectral and its equally active metabolite, diacetolol have anti-arrhythmic activity, the combined plasma half-life of the active drug and metabolite being 7-10 hours. Both have partial agonist activity (PAA) also known as intrinsic sympathomimetic activity (ISA). This property ensures that some degree of stimulation of beta receptors is maintained. Under conditions of rest, this tends to balance the negative chronotropic and negative inotropic effects. Sectral blocks the effects of excessive catecholamine stimulation resulting from stress.

5.2 Pharmacokinetic properties

After oral administration, acebutolol is rapidly and almost completely absorbed. Absorption appears to be unaffected by the presence of food in the gut. There is rapid formation of a major equiactive metabolite, diacetolol, which possesses a similar pharmacological profile to acebutolol. Peak plasma concentrations of active material (i.e. acebutolol plus diacetolol) are achieved within 2-4 hours and the terminal plasma elimination half-life is around 8-10 hours. Because of biliary excretion and direct transfer across the gut wall from the systemic circulation to the gut lumen, more than 50% of an oral dose of Sectral is recovered in the faeces with acebutolol and diacetolol in equal proportions; the rest of the dose is recovered in the urine, mainly as diacetolol. Both acebutolol and diacetolol are hydrophilic and exhibit poor penetration of the CNS.

5.3 Preclinical safety data

No particulars.

6. PHARMACEUTICAL PARTICULARS

6.1 List of excipients

Sectral Capsules contain: Starch Potato, Aerosil (Silicon dioxide E551), Magnesium Stearate (E572), Opadry OY-L-28900 (Contains Titanium dioxide (E171) Ph. Eur, Lactose Ph. Eur., HPMC 2910 15cP (E464) Ph. Eur., Polyethylene Glycol 4000 NF).

Sectral Capsules 100mg Capsule Shell: Yellow iron oxide (E172), Titanium dioxide (E171), Gelatin BP, Ink:Opacode S-24-8109 Black

Sectral Capsules 200mg Capsule Shell: Yellow iron oxide (E172), Titanium dioxide (E171), Gelatin BP, Red iron oxide (E172), Ink: Opacode S-24-8109 Black

Sectral Tablets 400mg: Lactose, Maize starch, French chalk powdered (E553b), Aerosil (silicon dioxide E551), Povidone K30, Magnesium stearate (E572), Opadry OY-L-28900 (Contains Titanium dioxide (E171) Ph. Eur., Lactose Ph. Eur, HPMC 2910 15cP (E464) Ph. Eur, Polyethylene Glycol 4000 NF))

6.2 Incompatibilities

Not applicable

6.3 Shelf life

The shelf-life of Sectral Capsules is 60 months.

The shelf-life of Sectral Tablets 400mg is 36 months

6.4 Special precautions for storage

Sectral Capsules:Store in a dry place below 25°C. Protect from light

Sectral Tablets: None

6.5 Nature and contents of container

Sectral Capsules 100mg:Aluminium foil/UPVC blister strip packs of 84 tablets.

Sectral Capsules 200mg:Aluminium foil/UPVC blister strip packs of 56 tablets.

Sectral Tablets 400mg: Aluminium foil/PVC blister strip packs of 28 tablets.

6.6 Instructions for use and handling

None

7. MARKETING AUTHORISATION HOLDER

Aventis Pharma Ltd

50 Kings Hill Avenue

Kings Hill

West Malling

Kent

ME19 4AH

United Kingdom

8. MARKETING AUTHORISATION NUMBER(S)

Sectral Capsules 100mg: PL 4425/0262

Sectral Capsules 200mg: PL 4425/0263

Sectral Tablets 400mg: PL 4425/0264

9. DATE OF FIRST AUTHORISATION/RENEWAL OF THE AUTHORISATION

13th July 2001

10. DATE OF REVISION OF THE TEXT

January 2005

Legal category: POM

Securon 120 mg Tablets

(Abbott Laboratories Limited)

1. NAME OF THE MEDICINAL PRODUCT

Securon 120 mg Tablets

2. QUALITATIVE AND QUANTITATIVE COMPOSITION

Each tablet contains Verapamil Hydrochloride Ph Eur 120 mg

3. PHARMACEUTICAL FORM

White, film-coated tablets impressed with Securon 120 on one side and Knoll above the scoreline on the other.

4. CLINICAL PARTICULARS

4.1 Therapeutic indications

Securon is indicated for:

- The treatment of mild to moderate hypertension;

- The treatment and prophylaxis of chronic stable angina, vasospastic angina and unstable angina;

- The treatment and prophylaxis of paroxysmal supraventricular tachycardia and the reduction of ventricular rate in atrial flutter/fibrillation (note, however, that Securon should not be used when atrial flutter/fibrillation complicates Wolff-Parkinson-White syndrome; see section 4.4 'Special Warnings and Precautions for Use').

4.2 Posology and method of administration

For oral administration.

Adults

Hypertension:

Initially 120 mg b.d., increasing to 160 mg b.d., if necessary. In some cases, dosages of up to 480 mg daily in divided doses have been used. A further reduction in blood pressure may be obtained by combining Securon with other antihypertensive agents, in particular diuretics. For concomitant administration with beta-blockers, see section 4.4 'Special Warnings and Precautions for Use'.

Angina:

120 mg t.d.s. is recommended. 80 mg t.d.s. can be completely satisfactory in some patients with angina of effort. Less than 120 mg t.d.s. is not likely to be effective in variant angina.

Supraventricular tachycardias:

40-120 mg t.d.s. according to the severity of the condition.

Children

Up to 2 years: 20 mg, two to three times a day.

2 years and above: 40-120 mg, two to three times a day, according to age and effectiveness.

Elderly

The adult dose is recommended unless liver or renal function is impaired (see section 4.4 'Special Warnings and Precautions for Use').

4.3 Contraindications

Cardiogenic shock; acute myocardial infarction complicated by bradycardia, marked hypotension or left ventricular failure; second or third degree atrioventricular (AV) block; sino-atrial block; sick sinus syndrome; uncompensated heart failure; bradycardia of less than 50 beats/minute; hypotension of less than 90 mmHg systolic.

Concomitant ingestion of grapefruit juice.

4.4 Special warnings and special precautions for use

Since verapamil is extensively metabolised in the liver, careful dose titration of Securon is required in patients with liver disease. The disposition of verapamil in patients with renal impairment has not been fully established and therefore careful patient monitoring is recommended. Verapamil is not removed during dialysis.

Verapamil may affect impulse conduction and Securon should therefore be used with caution in patients with first degree AV block. Patients with atrial flutter/fibrillation in association with an accessory pathway (e.g. Wolff-Parkinson-White syndrome) may develop increased conduction across the anomalous pathway and ventricular tachycardia may be precipitated. Verapamil may affect left ventricular contractility; this effect is small and normally not important but cardiac failure may be precipitated or aggravated. In patients with incipient cardiac failure, therefore, Securon should be given only after such cardiac failure has been controlled with appropriate therapy.

4.5 Interaction with other medicinal products and other forms of Interaction

Verapamil has been shown to increase the serum concentration of digoxin and caution should be exercised with regard to digitalis toxicity. The digitalis level should be determined and the glycoside dose reduced, if required.

The combination of verapamil and beta-blockers, anti-arrhythmic agents or inhaled anaesthetics may lead to additive cardiovascular effects (*e.g.* AV block, bradycardia, hypotension, heart failure). Intravenous beta-blockers should not be given to patients under treatment with verapamil. The effects of verapamil may be additive to other hypotensive agents.

Interactions between verapamil and the following medications have been reported:

Carbamazepine, cyclosporin and theophylline: Use of verapamil has resulted in increased serum levels of these medications. This could lead to increased side effects.

Rifampicin, phenytoin and phenobarbital: Serum levels of verapamil reduced.

Lithium: Serum levels of lithium may be reduced (pharmacokinetic effect); there may be increased sensitivity to lithium causing enhanced neurotoxicity (pharmacodynamic effect).

Cimetidine: Increase in verapamil serum level is possible.

Neuromuscular blocking agents employed in anaesthesia: The effects may be potentiated.

Grapefruit juice: Increase in verapamil serum level has been reported.

4.6 Pregnancy and lactation

Although animal studies have not shown any teratogenic effects, verapamil should not be given during the first trimester of pregnancy unless, in the clinician's judgement, it is essential for the welfare of the patient.

Verapamil is excreted into the breast milk in small amounts and is unlikely to be harmful. However, rare hypersensitivity reactions have been reported with verapamil. For this reason, it should only be used during lactation if, in the clinician's judgement, it is essential for the welfare of the patient.

4.7 Effects on ability to drive and use machines

Depending on individual susceptibility, the patient's ability to drive a vehicle or operate machinery may be impaired. This is particularly true in the initial stages of treatment, or when changing over from another drug. Verapamil has been shown to increase the blood levels of alcohol and slow its elimination. Therefore, the effects of alcohol may be exaggerated.

4.8 Undesirable effects

Particularly when given in high doses or in the presence of previous myocardial damage, some cardiovascular effects of verapamil may occasionally be greater than therapeutically desired: bradycardic arrhythmias such as sinus bradycardia, sinus arrest with asystole, second and third degree AV block, bradyarrhythmia in atrial fibrillation, hypotension, development or aggravation of heart failure.

Securon is generally well tolerated. Side effects are usually mild and transient and discontinuation of therapy is rarely necessary. Constipation may occur. Flushing is observed occasionally and there have been rare reports of headache, nausea, vomiting, dizziness, fatigue and ankle oedema. Allergic reactions (e.g. erythema, pruritus) are very rarely seen. A reversible impairment of liver function, characterised by an increase in transaminase and/or alkaline phosphatase may occur on very rare occasions during verapamil treatment and is most probably a hypersensitivity reaction.

On very rare occasions, gynaecomastia has been observed in elderly male patients under long-term verapamil treatment, which was fully reversible in all cases when the drug was discontinued. Gingival hyperplasia may very rarely occur when the drug is administered over prolonged periods, and is fully reversible when the drug is discontinued.

4.9 Overdose

The symptoms of overdosage include hypotension, shock, loss of consciousness, first and second degree AV block (frequently as Wenckebach's phenomenon with or without escape rhythms), total AV block with total AV dissociation, escape rhythm, asystole, sinus bradycardia, sinus arrest.

Treatment of overdosage depends on the type and severity of symptoms. The specific antidote is calcium, *e.g.* 10-20 ml of 10% calcium gluconate solution i.v. (2.25-4.5 mmol) if necessary by repeated injection or continuous infusion (*e.g.* 5 mmol/hour). Gastric lavage, taking the usual precautionary measures, may be appropriate.

The usual emergency measures for acute cardiovascular collapse should be applied and followed by intensive care. Similarly, in the case of second or third degree AV block, atropine, isoprenaline and if required, pacemaker therapy should be considered. If there are signs of myocardial insufficiency, dopamine, dobutamine, cardiac glycosides or calcium gluconate (10-20 ml of a 10% solution) should be administered.

In the case of hypotension, after appropriately positioning the patient, dopamine, dobutamine or noradrenaline may be given.

5. PHARMACOLOGICAL PROPERTIES

5.1 Pharmacodynamic properties

Verapamil is a calcium antagonist.

5.2 Pharmacokinetic properties

Orally administered Securon is rapidly and completely absorbed. Gastrointestinal absorption ranged from 92 to 100%. Verapamil is subject to extensive first-pass hepatic metabolism resulting in a bioavailability ranging from 10 to 35%. Peak serum levels occur about 2 hours after ingestion and are proportional to the dose administered. Mean serum concentrations of verapamil after chronic administration of 240, 320 and 480 mg/day to 20 patients were 141 ng/ml, 206 ng/ml and 323 ng/ml, respectively. Chronic oral administration of 120 mg Securon every 6 hours resulted in plasma levels of verapamil ranging from 125 to 400 ng/ml, with higher values reported occasionally.

Verapamil is widely distributed throughout the body. Binding of verapamil to plasma proteins was found to be about 90%. This binding was not concentration-dependent over the range 10-2000 ng/ml. Neither renal insufficiency, cardiac catheterisation nor the addition of warfarin significantly altered verapamil protein binding.

Verapamil undergoes extensive hepatic metabolism. Twelve metabolites have been identified. Approximately 70% of a verapamil dose is excreted as metabolites in the urine and 16% in the faeces. About 3 to 4% is excreted in the urine as unchanged drug. In single dose studies, the elimination half-life of verapamil ranged from 2.8 to 7.4 hours. Elimination half-lives measured from the terminal slope of the verapamil concentration curves in plasma were similar after simultaneous intravenous and oral administration to the same subjects. After 6 to 10 consecutive oral doses, the half-life increased to a range of 4.5 to 12 hours. Elimination half-life is prolonged and volume of distribution increased in patients with liver dysfunction. Plasma clearance is reduced to about 30% of normal.

5.3 Preclinical safety data

Not applicable.

6. PHARMACEUTICAL PARTICULARS

6.1 List of excipients

Lactose, maize starch, microcrystalline cellulose, talc, gelatin, polyethylene glycol, hydroxypropylmethylcellulose, sodium starch glycolate, titanium dioxide, magnesium stearate, sodium lauryl sulphate.

6.2 Incompatibilities

None stated.

6.3 Shelf life

60 months.

6.4 Special precautions for storage

Do not store above 25°C.

Blister pack: Store in the original package.

Plastic container: Keep the container tightly closed.

6.5 Nature and contents of container

Blister pack containing 60 tablets.

Plastic container containing 100 tablets.

6.6 Instructions for use and handling

None.

7. MARKETING AUTHORISATION HOLDER

Abbott Laboratories Ltd.

Queenborough

Kent

ME11 5EL

United Kingdom

8. MARKETING AUTHORISATION NUMBER(S)

PL 0037/0366

9. DATE OF FIRST AUTHORISATION/RENEWAL OF THE AUTHORISATION

18 March 2003

10. DATE OF REVISION OF THE TEXT

28 August 2003

Securon I.V.

(Abbott Laboratories Limited)

1. NAME OF THE MEDICINAL PRODUCT

Securon IV

2. QUALITATIVE AND QUANTITATIVE COMPOSITION

Verapamil Hydrochloride BP 2.5 mg/ml

3. PHARMACEUTICAL FORM

Aqueous solution for intravenous injection.

4. CLINICAL PARTICULARS

4.1 Therapeutic indications

Securon IV is indicated for the treatment of paroxysmal supraventricular tachycardia and the reduction of ventricular rate in atrial flutter/fibrillation.

4.2 Posology and method of administration

For slow intravenous injection.

Adults: 5-10 mg by slow intravenous injection over a period of 2 minutes. The patient should be observed continuously, preferably under ECG and blood pressure control. If necessary, *e.g.* in paroxysmal tachycardia, a further 5 mg may be given after 5 to 10 minutes.

Children: Securon IV must always be administered under ECG monitoring in young patients.

0-1 year: 0.1-0.2 mg/kg bodyweight (usual single dose range: 0.75-2 mg).

1-15 years: 0.1-0.3 mg/kg bodyweight (usual single dose range: 2-5 mg).

The dose may be repeated after 30 minutes if necessary. Many cases are controlled by doses at the lower end of the range. The injection should be stopped at the onset of the desired effect.

Elderly: The dosage should be administered over 3 minutes to minimise the risk of adverse effects.

Dosage in impaired liver and renal function: Significant hepatic and renal impairment should not increase the effects of a single intravenous dose but may prolong its duration of action.

For use with beta-blocker therapy, see 'Contra-indications' and 'Special Warnings and Precautions for Use'.

4.3 Contraindications

Cardiogenic shock; acute myocardial infarction complicated by bradycardia, marked hypotension or left ventricular failure; second or third degree AV block; sino-atrial block; sick sinus syndrome; uncompensated heart failure; bradycardia of less than 50 beats/minute; hypotension of less than 90 mmHg systolic; simultaneous administration of intravenous beta-blockers.

Patients with atrial flutter/fibrillation in the presence of an accessory pathway (*e.g.* WPW syndrome) may develop increased conduction across the anomalous pathway and ventricular tachycardia may be precipitated.

4.4 Special warnings and special precautions for use

Verapamil may affect impulse conduction. For this reason, Securon IV should be used with caution in patients with first degree AV block. Verapamil may affect left ventricular contractility; this effect is small and normally not important but cardiac failure may be precipitated or aggravated. In patients with poor ventricular function, therefore, Securon IV should only be given after cardiac failure has been controlled with appropriate therapy, *e.g.* digitalis.

4.5 Interaction with other medicinal products and other forms of Interaction

Verapamil has been shown to increase the serum concentration of digoxin and caution should be exercised with regard to digitalis toxicity. The digitalis level should be determined and the glycoside dose reduced, if required.

The combination of Securon IV and beta-blockers, anti-arrhythmic agents or inhaled anaesthetics may lead to additive cardiovascular effects (*e.g.* AV block, bradycardia, hypotension, heart failure). Securon IV should not be given in combination with intravenous beta-blocker therapy and care must be exercised if Securon IV is combined with oral beta-blocker therapy or anti-arrhythmic agents by any route.

The effects of Securon IV may be additive to other hypotensive agents.

Interactions between verapamil and the following have been reported:

Carbamazepine, cyclosporin and theophylline: Use of verapamil has resulted in increased serum levels of these medications. This could lead to increased side effects.

Rifampicin: Serum levels of verapamil reduced.

Lithium: Serum levels of lithium may be reduced (pharmacokinetic effect); there may be increased sensitivity to lithium causing enhanced neurotoxicity (pharmacodynamic effect).

Neuromuscular blocking agents employed in anaesthesia: The effects may be potentiated.

4.6 Pregnancy and lactation

Although animal studies have not shown any teratogenic effects, verapamil should not be given during the first trimester of pregnancy unless, in the clinician's judgement, it is essential for the welfare of the patient.

Verapamil is excreted into the breast milk in small amounts and is unlikely to be harmful. However, rare hypersensitivity reactions have been reported with verapamil. For this reason, it should only be used during lactation if, in the clinician's judgement, it is essential for the welfare of the patient.

4.7 Effects on ability to drive and use machines

None stated.

4.8 Undesirable effects

Securon IV is generally well tolerated but due to the drug's mode of action, undesired cardiovascular effects may occur, particularly at high doses and in patients with AV block and/or impaired myocardial function. Decreased heart rate, hypotension and decreased myocardial contractility have been reported. On rare occasions, second or third degree AV block may occur and in extreme cases, this may lead to asystole. The asystole is usually of short duration and cardiac action returns spontaneously after a few seconds, usually in the form of sinus rhythm. If necessary, the procedures for the treatment of overdosage should be followed as described below.

A slight transient fall in blood pressure, due to a reduction in peripheral resistance, may be seen. In rare cases, this may lead to severe hypotension.

On rare occasions, dizziness, headache, nausea, vomiting, nervousness and flushing have been reported. Allergic reactions (erythema, pruritus, urticaria, bronchospasm) are extremely rare. A reversible impairment of liver function, characterised by an increase of transaminase and/or alkaline phosphatase may occur on very rare occasions during verapamil treatment and is most probably a hypersensitivity reaction.

On very rare occasions, gynaecomastia has been observed in elderly male patients under long-term verapamil treatment; this was fully reversible in all cases when the drug was discontinued. Gingival hyperplasia may occur very rarely when the drug is administered over prolonged periods, and is fully reversible when the drug is discontinued.

4.9 Overdose

The symptoms of overdosage include hypotension, shock, loss of consciousness, first and second degree AV block (frequently as Wenckebach's phenomenon with or without escape rhythms), total AV block with total AV dissociation, escape rhythm, asystole, sinus bradycardia, sinus arrest.

Treatment of overdosage depends on the type and severity of symptoms. The specific antidote is calcium, *e.g.* 10-20 ml of 10% calcium gluconate solution i.v. (2.25-4.5 mmol) if necessary by repeated injection or continuous infusion (*e.g.* 5 mmol/hour). The usual emergency measures for acute cardiovascular collapse should be applied and followed by intensive care. Similarly, in the case of second or third degree AV block, atropine, orciprenaline, isoprenaline and if required, pacemaker therapy should be considered. If there are signs of myocardial insufficiency, dopamine, dobutamine, cardiac glycosides or calcium gluconate (10-20 ml of a 10% solution) can be administered.

In the case of hypotension, after appropriately positioning the patient, dopamine, dobutamine or noradrenaline may be given.

5. PHARMACOLOGICAL PROPERTIES

5.1 Pharmacodynamic properties

Verapamil is a calcium antagonist which blocks the inward movement of calcium ions in cardiac muscle cells, in smooth muscle cells of the coronary and systemic arteries and in cells of the intracardiac conduction system. Because of its effect on the movement of calcium in the intracardiac conduction system, verapamil reduces automaticity, decreases conduction velocity and increases the refractory period.

5.2 Pharmacokinetic properties

Following intravenous infusion in man, verapamil is eliminated bi-exponentially with a rapid distribution phase (half-life about 4 minutes) and a slower terminal elimination phase (half-life 2-5 hours).

5.3 Preclinical safety data

Not applicable.

6. PHARMACEUTICAL PARTICULARS

6.1 List of excipients

Water for injections, sodium chloride (8.5 mg/ml), hydrochloric acid as pH adjuster.

6.2 Incompatibilities

Securon IV is incompatible with alkaline solutions.

6.3 Shelf life

Ampoule: 60 months.

Syringe: 36 months.

6.4 Special precautions for storage

Store at room temperature. Protect from light.

6.5 Nature and contents of container

2 ml glass ampoule (hydrolytic type 1) containing 5 mg verapamil. Pack size:

5 × 2 ml ampoules.

2 ml pre-filled glass syringe (borosilicate type 1) with tip cap and butyl rubber stopper and polystyrene plunger. Pack size: 5 × 2 ml syringes.

6.6 Instructions for use and handling

None.

7. MARKETING AUTHORISATION HOLDER

Abbott Laboratories Ltd

Queenborough

Kent

ME11 5EL

United Kingdom

8. MARKETING AUTHORISATION NUMBER(S)

PL 00037/0367

9. DATE OF FIRST AUTHORISATION/RENEWAL OF THE AUTHORISATION

17 June 2003

10. DATE OF REVISION OF THE TEXT

Securon SR 240 mg & Half Securon SR 120 mg Tablets

(Abbott Laboratories Limited)

1. NAME OF THE MEDICINAL PRODUCT

Securon SR 240 mg Tablets

Half Securon SR 120 mg Tablets

2. QUALITATIVE AND QUANTITATIVE COMPOSITION

Securon SR: Verapamil Hydrochloride Ph Eur - 240 mg

Half Securon SR: Verapamil Hydrochloride Ph Eur - 120 mg

3. PHARMACEUTICAL FORM

Modified-release tablets.

Securon SR tablets are oblong, pale green, scored and embossed with two Knoll logos (triangles) on one side.

Half Securon SR tablets are round, white, biconvex and embossed with the word 'Knoll' on the one side, and '120 SR' on the reverse.

4. CLINICAL PARTICULARS

4.1 Therapeutic indications

Securon SR and Half Securon SR are indicated for:

The treatment of mild to moderate hypertension.

The treatment and prophylaxis of angina pectoris.

Secondary prevention of re-infarction after an acute myocardial infarction in patients without heart failure, and not receiving diuretics (apart from low-dose diuretics when used for indications other than heart failure), and where beta-blockers are not appropriate. Treatment is to be started at least one week after an acute myocardial infarction.

4.2 Posology and method of administration

Securon SR 240 mg & 120 mg tablets should not be chewed. Securon SR 240 mg tablets are scored and may be halved without damaging the sustained release formulation.

Adults

Hypertension: One tablet of Securon SR 240 mg daily. For patients new to verapamil therapy, the physician should consider halving the initial dose to 120 mg (Half Securon SR 120 mg). Most patients respond to 240 mg daily (one tablet Securon SR 240 mg) given as a single dose. If control is not achieved after a period of at least one week, the dosage may be increased to a maximum of two Securon SR 240 mg tablets daily (one in the morning and one in the evening at an interval of about twelve hours). A further reduction in blood pressure may be achieved by combining Securon SR with other antihypertensive agents, in particular diuretics.

Angina pectoris: One tablet of Securon SR 240 mg twice daily. A small number of patients respond to a lower dose and where indicated, adjustment down to one tablet of Securon SR 240 mg daily could be made. Securon SR 120 mg may be used for dose titration purposes.

Secondary prevention of reinfarction after an acute myocardial infarction in patients without heart failure, and not receiving diuretics (apart from low-dose diuretics when used for indications other than heart failure), and where beta-blockers are not appropriate: Treatment is to be started at least one week after an acute myocardial infarction. 360 mg/day in divided doses, to be taken either as one Half Securon SR (120 mg) tablet three times daily, or as one Securon SR (240 mg) tablet in the morning and one Half Securon SR (120 mg) tablet in the evening, on a daily basis.

<u>Children</u>

Securon SR 240 mg & 120 mg tablets are not recommended for children.

<u>Elderly patients</u>

The adult dose is recommended unless liver or renal function is impaired (see Precautions).

4.3 Contraindications

Cardiogenic shock; acute myocardial infarction complicated by bradycardia, marked hypotension or left ventricular failure; second or third degree atrioventricular (AV) block; sino-atrial block; sick sinus syndrome; uncompensated heart failure; bradycardia of less than 50 beats/minute; hypotension of less than 90 mm Hg systolic.

Concomitant ingestion of grapefruit juice.

4.4 Special warnings and special precautions for use

Since verapamil is extensively metabolised in the liver, careful dose titration is required in patients with liver disease. The disposition of verapamil in patients with renal impairment has not been fully established and therefore careful patient monitoring is recommended. Verapamil is not removed during dialysis.

Verapamil may affect impulse conduction and should therefore be used with caution in patients with first degree AV block. Patients with atrial flutter/fibrillation in association with an accessory pathway (e.g. WPW-syndrome) may develop increased conduction across the anomalous pathway and ventricular tachycardia may be precipitated. Verapamil may affect left ventricular contractility; this effect is small and normally not important but cardiac failure may be precipitated or aggravated. In patients with incipient cardiac failure, therefore, verapamil should be given only after such cardiac failure has been controlled with appropriate therapy, e.g. digitalis.

When treating hypertension with verapamil, monitoring of the patient's blood pressure at regular intervals is required.

4.5 Interaction with other medicinal products and other forms of Interaction

Verapamil has been shown to increase the serum concentration of digoxin and caution should be exercised with regard to digitalis toxicity. The digitalis level should be determined and the glycoside dose reduced, if required. The combination of verapamil and beta-blockers, antiarrhythmic agents or inhaled anaesthetics may lead to additive cardiovascular effects (e.g. AV block, bradycardia, hypotension, heart failure). Intravenous beta-blockers should not be given to patients under treatment with verapamil. The effects of verapamil may be additive to other hypotensive agents.

Interactions between verapamil and the following medications have been reported:

Carbamazepine, Cyclosporin and Theophylline - Use of verapamil has resulted in increased serum levels of these medications, which could lead to increased side effects.

Rifampicin, Phenytoin and Phenobarbital - Serum levels of verapamil reduced.

Lithium - Serum levels of lithium may be reduced (pharmacokinetic effect); there may be increased sensitivity to lithium causing enhanced neurotoxicity (pharmacodynamic effect).

Cimetidine - Increase in verapamil serum level is possible.

Neuromuscular blocking agents employed in anaesthesia - The effects may be potentiated.

Grapefruit juice – Increase in verapamil serum level has been reported.

Alcohol –Increase in blood alcohol has been reported.

4.6 Pregnancy and lactation

Although animal studies have not shown any teratogenic effects, verapamil should not be given during the first trimester of pregnancy unless, in the clinician's judgement, it is essential for the welfare of the patient.

Verapamil is excreted into the breast milk in small amounts and is unlikely to be harmful.

However, rare hypersensitivity reactions have been reported with verapamil and therefore it should only be used during lactation if, in the clinician's judgement, it is essential for the welfare of the patient.

4.7 Effects on ability to drive and use machines

Depending on individual susceptibility, the patient's ability to drive a vehicle or operate machinery may be impaired. This is particularly true in the initial stages of treatment, or when changing over from another drug. Like many other common medicines, verapamil has been shown to increase the blood levels of alcohol and slow its elimination. Therefore, the effects of alcohol may be exaggerated.

4.8 Undesirable effects

Particularly when given in high doses or in the presence of previous myocardial damage, some cardiovascular effects of verapamil may occasionally be greater than therapeutically desired: bradycardic arrhythmias such as sinus bradycardia, sinus arrest with asystole, second and third degree AV block, bradyarrhythmia in atrial fibrillation, hypotension, development or aggravation of heart failure.

Securon SR 240 mg & 120 mg tablets are generally well tolerated. Side effects are usually mild and transient and discontinuation of therapy is rarely necessary. Constipation may occur. There have been rare reports of flushing, headache, nausea, vomiting, dizziness, fatigue and ankle oedema. Allergic reactions (e.g. erythema, pruritus, urticaria, Quincke's oedema, Stevens-Johnson syndrome) are very rarely seen. A reversible impairment of liver function, characterised by an increase in transaminase and/or alkaline phosphatase may occur on very rare occasions during verapamil treatment and is most probably a hypersensitivity reaction.

On very rare occasions, gynaecomastia has been observed in elderly male patients under long-term verapamil treatment, which was fully reversible in all cases when the drug was discontinued. Gingival hyperplasia may very rarely occur when the drug is administered over prolonged periods, and is fully reversible when the drug is discontinued.

Erythromelalgia and paraesthesia may occur. In very rare cases, there may be myalgia and arthralgia. Rises in prolactin levels have been reported.

4.9 Overdose

The course of symptoms in verapamil intoxication depends on the amount taken, the point in time at which detoxification measures are taken and myocardial contractility (age-related). The main symptoms are as follows: blood pressure fall (at times to values not detectable), shock symptoms, loss of consciousness, 1st and 2nd degree AV block (frequently as Wenckebach's phenomenon with or without escape rhythms), total AV block with total AV dissociation, escape rhythm, asystole, sinus bradycardia, sinus arrest.

The therapeutic measures to be taken depend on the point in time at which verapamil was taken and the type and severity of intoxication symptoms. In intoxications with large amounts of slow-release preparations

(Securon SR 240 mg & 120 mg tablets), it should be noted that the release of the active drug and the absorption in the intestine may take more than 48 hours. Depending on the time of ingestion, it should be taken into account that there may be some lumps of incompletely dissolved tablets along the entire length of the gastrointestinal tract, which function as active drug depots.

General measures to be taken: Gastric lavage with the usual precautions, even later than 12 hours after ingestion, if no gastrointestinal motility (peristaltic sounds) is detectable. Where intoxication by Securon SR 240 mg & 120 mg tablets is suspected, extensive elimination measures are indicated, such as induced vomiting, removal of the contents of the stomach and the small intestine under endoscopy, intestinal lavage, laxative, high enemas. The usual intensive resuscitation measures apply, such as extrathoracic heart massage, respiration, defibrillation and/or pacemaker therapy.

Specific measures to be taken: Elimination of cardiodepressive effects, hypotension or bradycardia. The specific antidote is calcium, e.g. 10 - 20 ml of a 10% calcium gluconate solution administered intravenously (2.25 - 4.5 mmol), repeated if necessary or given as a continuous drip infusion (e.g. 5 mmol/hour).

The following measures may also be necessary: In case of 2nd or 3rd degree AV block, sinus bradycardia, asystole - atropine, isoprenaline, orciprenaline or pacemaker therapy. In case of hypotension - dopamine, dobutamine, noradrenaline. If there are signs of continuing myocardial failure - dopamine, dobutamine, if necessary repeated calcium injections.

5. PHARMACOLOGICAL PROPERTIES

5.1 Pharmacodynamic properties

Verapamil, a phenylalkylamine calcium antagonist, has a balanced profile of cardiac and peripheral effects. It lowers heart rate, increases myocardial perfusion and reduces coronary spasm. In a clinical study in patients after myocardial infarction, verapamil reduced total mortality, sudden cardiac death and reinfarction rate.

Verapamil reduces total peripheral resistance and lowers high blood pressure by vasodilation, without reflex tachycardia. Because of its use-dependent action on the voltage-operated calcium channel, the effects of verapamil are more pronounced on high than on normal blood pressure.

As early as day one of treatment, blood pressure falls; the effect is found to persist also in long-term therapy. Verapamil is suitable for the treatment of all types of hypertension: for monotherapy in mild to moderate hypertension; combined with other antihypertensives in particular with diuretics and, according to more recent findings, with ACE inhibitors - in more severe types of hypertension. In hypertensive diabetic patients with nephropathy verapamil in combination with ACE inhibitors led to a marked reduction of albuminuria and to an improvement of creatinine clearance.

5.2 Pharmacokinetic properties

Absorption: More than 90% of an orally-administered dose of verapamil is absorbed. Due to an intensive hepatic first-pass metabolism, the absolute bioavailability is about 22%

with a variability of about 10 - 35%. Under multiple dosing, bioavailability increases by about 30%. Bioavailability is not affected by food consumption.

Distribution, biotransformation and elimination: Plasma concentrations reach their peak 4 - 8 hours after drug intake. Plasma protein binding of verapamil is more than 90%. The elimination half-life is about 5 - 8 hours. The mean residence time of modified-release verapamil is 13 hours. After repeated single daily doses, steady-state conditions are reached between 3 - 4 days.

Within 5 days, approximately 70% of an orally-administered dose is excreted in the urine and about 16% with the faeces. Only 3 - 4 % is eliminated renally as unchanged drug. Norverapamil, one of the 12 metabolites identified in urine, which represents about 6% of the dose eliminated, has 10 - 20% of the activity of verapamil. Norverapamil can reach steady-state plasma concentrations approximately equal to those of verapamil itself. Renal insufficiency does not affect the kinetics of verapamil.

At-risk patients: In patients with liver cirrhosis, bioavailability is increased and elimination half-life is prolonged. In patients with compensated hepatic insufficiency, no influence on the kinetics of verapamil was observed. Renal function has no influence on the elimination of verapamil.

5.3 Preclinical safety data
None stated.

6. PHARMACEUTICAL PARTICULARS

6.1 List of excipients

Securon SR:

Cellulose Microcrystalline, Hypromellose, Sodium Alginate, Povidone, Magnesium Stearate, Purified water, Macrogol 400, Macrogol 6000, Talc, Titanium Dioxide E171, Sicopharm green lake [quinoline yellow (E104) and indigo carmine (E132)], Montan Glycol Wax.

Half Securon SR:

Microcrystalline cellulose, sodium alginate, povidone, magnesium stearate, purified water, hydroxypropyl methylcellulose, polyethylene glycol 400, polyethylene glycol 6000, talc, titanium dioxide (E171), montan glycol wax.

6.2 Incompatibilities
None stated.

6.3 Shelf life
5 years

6.4 Special precautions for storage
Do not store above 25°C and store in the original package - blister pack.

Do not store above 25°C and keep the container tightly closed - bottle pack.

6.5 Nature and contents of container
PVC/PVDC blister packs, in a cardboard outer container, 28 tablets.

Polypropylene bottle with polyethylene stopper. Pack size: 100 tablets.

6.6 Instructions for use and handling
There are no specific instructions for use/handling. The tablets should not be chewed, but may be halved without affecting the modified-release form.

7. MARKETING AUTHORISATION HOLDER
Abbott Laboratories Limited
Queenborough
Kent
ME11 5EL
United Kingdom

8. MARKETING AUTHORISATION NUMBER(S)
Securon SR 240 mg Tablets - PL 00037/0369
Half Securon SR 120 mg Tablets - PL 00037/0370

9. DATE OF FIRST AUTHORISATION/RENEWAL OF THE AUTHORISATION
14 March 2002

10. DATE OF REVISION OF THE TEXT

Selexid Tablets

(Leo Laboratories Limited)

1. NAME OF THE MEDICINAL PRODUCT
Selexid® Tablets

2. QUALITATIVE AND QUANTITATIVE COMPOSITION
Pivmecillinam hydrochloride 200mg

3. PHARMACEUTICAL FORM
Tablets.

4. CLINICAL PARTICULARS

4.1 Therapeutic indications
Treatment of infections due to mecillinam sensitive organisms, including:

- urinary tract infections
- salmonellosis

Preliminary experience in a small number of patients suggests that Selexid may be a useful alternative antibiotic in the treatment of acute typhoid fever and in some carriers of salmonellae when antibiotic treatment is considered essential.

4.2 Posology and method of administration
Route of administration is oral. The tablets must be taken with at least half a glass of water and preferably taken with or immediately after a meal.

Adults and children weighing more than 40 kg:
Urinary tract infections:

- acute uncomplicated cystitis: 72 hour course of 2 tablets immediately followed by 1 tablet 3 times daily to a total of 10 tablets.
- Chronic or recurrent bacteriuria: 2 tablets 3 to 4 times daily.

Salmonellosis:

- Enteric fever: 1.2 - 2.4g daily for 14 days.
- Salmonella carriers: 1.2 - 2.4 g daily for 2-4 weeks.

Children weighing less than 40 kg:

- Urinary tract infections: 20-40 mg/kg body weight, daily, in 3 to 4 divided doses.
- Salmonellosis: 30-60 mg/kg body weight, daily, in 3 to 4 divided doses.

Dosage in the elderly:
Renal excretion of mecillinam is delayed in the elderly, but significant accumulation of the drug is not likely at the recommended adult dosage of Selexid.

4.3 Contraindications
Penicillin and cephalosporin hypersensitivity. Selexid is contra-indicated in patients with known carnitine deficiency and infants under 3 months. Oesophageal strictures and/or obstructive changes in the gastrointestinal tract.

4.4 Special warnings and special precautions for use
During long term use, it is advisable to carry out routine liver and kidney function tests.

As with other antibiotics which are excreted mainly by the kidneys, raised blood levels of mecillinam may occur if repeated doses are given to patients with impaired renal function.

Selexid should be used with caution for long-term or frequently-repeated treatment, due to the possibility of carnitine depletion.

Concurrent treatment with valproic acid, valproate or other medication liberating pivalic acid should be avoided.

4.5 Interaction with other medicinal products and other forms of Interaction
Clearance of methotrexate from the body can be reduced by concurrent use of penicillins. The methotrexate dose may need to be adjusted.

Probenecid reduces the excretion of penicillins and hence increases blood levels of the antibiotic.

4.6 Pregnancy and lactation
The drug, as mecillinam, crosses the placenta. Although tests in two animal species have shown no teratogenic effects, in keeping with current practice, use during pregnancy should be avoided.

4.7 Effects on ability to drive and use machines
Not stated.

4.8 Undesirable effects
Upper gastrointestinal disturbances such as nausea, vomiting and indigestion have occurred, more frequently when a dose has been given on an empty stomach.

Other side effects reported are diarrhoea and urticarial rash.

Reduction in serum and total body carnitine has been reported.

Anaphylactic reactions are rare.

4.9 Overdose
There has been no experience of overdosage with Selexid. However, excessive doses are likely to induce nausea, vomiting and gastritis. Treatment should be restricted to symptomatic and supportive measures.

5. PHARMACOLOGICAL PROPERTIES

5.1 Pharmacodynamic properties
Selexid is an orally active antibiotic. Chemically it is the pivaloyloxymethylester of the amidinopenicillanic acid, mecillinam. On oral administration it is well absorbed and subsequently hydrolysed in the body to mecillinam, the active antibacterial agent, by non-specific esterases present in blood, gastro-intestinal mucosa and other tissues.

Selexid is highly active against most enterobacteriaceae, including *E. coli*, Klebsiella, Proteus, Enterobacter, Serratia, Salmonella, Shigella and Yersina.

Selexid is less active against gram positive bacteria and organisms such as *Pseudomonas aeruginosa* and *Streptococcus faecalis* are practically resistant to mecillinam.

Whilst Selexid, like the penicillins and cephalosporins, interferes with the biosynthesis of the bacterial cell wall, the target of the inhibition is different. This different mode of action is probably responsible for the synergistic action which has been found, both *in vitro* and *in vivo*, between Selexid and various penicillins and cephalosporins.

5.2 Pharmacokinetic properties
Peak serum levels of mecillinam averaging 5 microgram/ml are reached after 1 hour following a dose of 10 mg/kg body weight in children and 400 mg in adults.

The serum half-life is 1.2 hours. The protein binding amounts to 5-10%. Approximately 50% of the administered dose is excreted as mecillinam in the urine within the first six hours. Mecillinam is partly excreted with bile, giving rise to biliary concentrations about 3 times the serum levels. Concurrent administration of probenecid delays the renal excretion of mecillinam, producing more sustained serum levels. The absorption of Selexid is practically unaffected by taking the tablets with food.

5.3 Preclinical safety data
There are no pre-clinical data of relevance to the prescriber which are additional to that already included in other sections of the SPC.

6. PHARMACEUTICAL PARTICULARS

6.1 List of excipients
Cellulose microcrystalline, hydroxypropyl cellulose, magnesium stearate, hydroxypropyl methylcellulose.

6.2 Incompatibilities
Not applicable.

6.3 Shelf life
3 years.

6.4 Special precautions for storage
Store below 25°C in a dry place.

6.5 Nature and contents of container
PVC/AL blisters of 10 tablets with polyamide-coated aluminium cover.

6.6 Instructions for use and handling
None.

7. MARKETING AUTHORISATION HOLDER
Leo Laboratories Limited,
Longwick Road
Princes Risborough
Bucks. HP27 9RR, UK.

8. MARKETING AUTHORISATION NUMBER(S)
0043/0048

9. DATE OF FIRST AUTHORISATION/RENEWAL OF THE AUTHORISATION
20 May 1977 / 20 May 1992

10. DATE OF REVISION OF THE TEXT
August 1999

LEGAL CATEGORY
POM

Semprex Capsules

(GlaxoSmithKline UK)

1. NAME OF THE MEDICINAL PRODUCT
Semprex Capsules
SEMPREX CAPSULES

2. QUALITATIVE AND QUANTITATIVE COMPOSITION
Acrivastine 8mg per capsule

3. PHARMACEUTICAL FORM
Capsule

4. CLINICAL PARTICULARS

4.1 Therapeutic indications
Semprex is indicated for the symptomatic relief of allergic rhinitis, including hay fever. Semprex is also indicated for chronic idiopathic urticaria, symptomatic dermographism, cholinergic urticaria and idiopathic acquired cold urticaria.

4.2 Posology and method of administration
Route of administration
Oral

Adults, and children over 12 years:
One 8 mg capsule three times a day.

Use in the elderly:
As yet, no specific studies have been carried out in the elderly. Until further information is available, Semprex should not be given to elderly patients.

4.3 Contraindications
Semprex is contra-indicated in individuals with known hypersensitivity to acrivastine or triprolidine. Renal excretion is the principal route of elimination of acrivastine. Until specific studies have been carried out Semprex should not be given to patients with significant renal impairment.

4.4 Special warnings and special precautions for use
The following statements will appear on the pack:

Store below 30°C. Protect from light. Keep dry. Keep out of the reach of children.

4.5 Interaction with other medicinal products and other forms of Interaction
It is usual to advise patients not to undertake tasks requiring mental alertness whilst under the influence of alcohol and other C.N.S. depressants. Concomitant administration

of acrivastine may, in some individuals, produce additional impairment.

4.6 Pregnancy and lactation
No information is available on the administration of Semprex during human pregnancy or lactation. Acrivastine like most medicines, should not be used during pregnancy or lactation unless the potential benefit of treatment to the mother outweighs any possible risk to the developing foetus/nursing infant.

Systemic administration of acrivastine in animal reproductive studies did not produce embryotoxic or teratogenic effects and did not impair fertility.

There is no information on the levels of acrivastine, which may appear in human breast milk after administration of Semprex.

4.7 Effects on ability to drive and use machines
Most patients do not experience drowsiness with Semprex. Nevertheless, as there is individual variation in response to all medication, it is sensible to caution all patients about engaging in activities requiring mental alertness, such as driving a car or operating machinery, until patients are familiar with their own response to the drug.

4.8 Undesirable effects
Reports of drowsiness directly attributable to Semprex are extremely rare. Indeed for the great majority of patients, treatment with Semprex is not associated with clinically significant anticholinergic or sedative side-effects.

4.9 Overdose
There is no experience of overdosage with Semprex. Appropriate supportive therapy, including gastric lavage, should be initiated if indicated.

5. PHARMACOLOGICAL PROPERTIES

5.1 Pharmacodynamic properties
Acrivastine provides symptomatic relief in conditions believed to depend wholly or partly upon the triggered release of histamine.

It is a potent competitive histamine H_1 antagonist which lacks significant anticholinergic effects, and has a low potential to penetrate the central nervous system.

After oral administration of a single dose of 8 mg acrivastine to adults, the onset of action, as determined by the ability to antagonise histamine-induced weals and flares in the skin, is within 1 hour. Peak effects occur at 2 hours, and although activity declines slowly thereafter, significant inhibition of histamine-induced weals and flares still occurs 8 hours after dose.

In patients, relief from the symptoms of allergic rhinitis is apparent within 1 hour after the systemic administration of the drug.

5.2 Pharmacokinetic properties
Acrivastine is well absorbed from the gut. In healthy adult volunteers, the peak plasma concentration (Cmax) is approximately 150 nanogram/ml, occurring at about 1.5 hours (Tmax) after the administration of 8 mg acrivastine. The plasma half-life is approximately 1.5 hours. In multiple dose studies over 6 days, no accumulation of acrivastine was observed. Renal excretion is the principal route of elimination of acrivastine.

5.3 Preclinical safety data
There are no preclinical data of relevance to the prescriber, which are additional to that in other sections of the SPC.

6. PHARMACEUTICAL PARTICULARS

6.1 List of excipients
Lactose EP
Sodium starch glycollate EP
Magnesium stearate EP

Capsule shell
Gelatin EP
Purified water EP
Titanium dioxide EP

6.2 Incompatibilities
None known.

6.3 Shelf life
60 months.

6.4 Special precautions for storage
Store below 30°C.
Keep dry.
Protect from light.

6.5 Nature and contents of container
PVC/aluminium foil blisters. Pack sizes: 7, 12, 21, 24 and 84.

Polypropylene containers with LDPE snap-on lids. Pack size: 100

6.6 Instructions for use and handling
No special instructions.

Administrative Data

7. MARKETING AUTHORISATION HOLDER
The Wellcome Foundation Ltd
Glaxo Wellcome House
Berkeley Avenue
Greenford
Middlesex
UB6 ONN

8. MARKETING AUTHORISATION NUMBER(S)
PL 00003/0254

9. DATE OF FIRST AUTHORISATION/RENEWAL OF THE AUTHORISATION
MAA: 23.09.88
Renewal: 13.05.94

10. DATE OF REVISION OF THE TEXT
22 January 1999

Legal Status
POM

Septrin for Infusion

(GlaxoSmithKline UK)

1. NAME OF THE MEDICINAL PRODUCT
Septrin for Infusion

2. QUALITATIVE AND QUANTITATIVE COMPOSITION

Sulfamethoxazole	EP	400mg
Trimethoprim	EP	80mg

per 5ml

3. PHARMACEUTICAL FORM
Solution for Infusion

4. CLINICAL PARTICULARS

4.1 Therapeutic indications
In general, the indications for the use of Septrin for Infusion are the same as those for oral presentations.

It is intended that Septrin for Infusion should be used only during such a period as the patient is unable to accept oral therapy, where initiation of treatment is particularly urgent or for convenience if the patient is already receiving intravenous fluids. Although intravenous co-trimoxazole is useful in critically ill patients, there may be no therapeutic advantage over the oral preparation.

Septrin should only be used where, in the judgement of the physician, the benefits of treatment outweigh any possible risks; consideration should be given to the use of a single effective antibacterial agent.

The *in vitro* susceptibility of bacteria varies geographically and with time; the local situation should always be considered when selecting antibiotic therapy.

Septrin for Infusion has been investigated clinically in the following indications amongst others:

Urinary tract infections:

Treatment of acute uncomplicated urinary tract infections. It is recommended that initial episodes of uncomplicated urinary tract infections be treated with a single effective antibacterial agent rather than a combination.

Treatment and prevention of *Pneumocystis jiroveci (P. carinii)* pneumonia (PCP) (see 4.2 Posology and Method of Administration and 4.8 Undesirable Effects).

Treatment and prophylaxis of toxoplasmosis, treatment of nocardiosis.

4.2 Posology and method of administration
Septrin for Infusion is for administration only by the intravenous route and must be diluted before administration.

Dilution should be carried out immediately before use. After adding Septrin for Infusion to the infusion solution, shake thoroughly to ensure complete mixing. If visible turbidity or crystallisation appears at any time before or during an infusion, the mixture should be discarded.

It is recommended that Septrin for Infusion is diluted according to the following schedules:

One ampoule (5 ml) to 125 ml infusion solution.

Two ampoules (10 ml) to 250 ml infusion solution.

Three ampoules (15 ml) to 500 ml infusion solution.

Septrin for Infusion is known to be compatible, when diluted as recommended above, with the following fluids:

Glucose Intravenous Infusion BP (5% w/v and 10% w/v).

Sodium Chloride Intravenous Infusion BP (0.9% w/v).

Sodium Chloride (0.18% w/v) and Glucose (4% w/v) Intravenous Infusion BP.

Dextran 70 Injection BP (6% w/v) in glucose (5% w/v) or normal saline.

Dextran 40 Injection BP (10% w/v) in glucose (5% w/v) or normal saline.

Ringer's Solution for Injection BPC 1959.

No other substance should be mixed with the infusion.

The duration of the infusion should be approximately one to one and a half hours, but this should be balanced against the fluid requirements of the patient.

When fluid restriction is necessary, Septrin for Infusion may be administered at a higher concentration, 5 ml diluted with 75 ml of glucose 5% w/v in water. The resultant solution, whilst being clear to the naked eye, may on occasion exceed the BP limits set for particulate matter in large volume parenterals. The solution should be infused over a period not exceeding one hour. Discard any unused solution.

<u>Acute Infections</u>

<u>Adults and children over 12 years:</u>

Standard dosage: 2 ampoules (10 ml) every 12 hours.

<u>Children aged 12 years and under:</u>

The recommended dosage is approximately 6 mg trimethoprim and 30 mg sulfamethoxazole per kg bodyweight per 24 hours, given in two equally divided doses. As a guide the following schedules may be used diluted as described above.

6 weeks to 5 months:	1.25 ml every 12 hours
6 months to 5 years:	2.5 ml every 12 hours
6 to 12 years:	5.0 ml every 12 hours

For severe infections in all age groups, dosage may be increased by 50%.

Treatment should be continued until the patient has been symptom free for two days; the majority will require treatment for at least 5 days.

<u>Special Dosage Recommendations</u>

<u>Impaired renal function:</u>

Adults and children over 12 years (no information is available for children under 12 years of age):

Creatinine Clearance (ml/min)	Recommended Dosage
More than 30	STANDARD DOSAGE
15-30	Half the STANDARD DOSAGE
Less than 15	Not recommended

Measurements of plasma concentrations of sulfamethoxazole at intervals of 2 to 3 days are recommended in samples obtained 12 hours after administration of Septrin for Infusion. If the concentration of total sulfamethoxazole exceeds 150 micrograms/ml then treatment should be interrupted until the value falls below 120 micrograms/ml.

<u>*Pneumocystis jiroveci(P. carinii)* pneumonia:</u>

<u>Treatment</u>

20 mg trimethoprim and 100 mg sulfamethoxazole per kg of bodyweight per day in two or more divided doses. Therapy should be changed to the oral route as soon as possible and continued for a total treatment period of two weeks. The aim is to obtain peak plasma or serum levels of trimethoprim of greater than or equal to 5 microgram/ml (verified in patients receiving 1-hour infusions of intravenous Septrin). (See 4.8 Undesirable Effects)

<u>Prevention</u>

Standard dosage (i.v. or oral as appropriate) for the duration of the period at risk.

Nocardiosis: There is no consensus on the most appropriate dosage. Adult doses of 6 to 8 tablets daily for up to 3 months have been used (one tablet contains 400 mg sulfamethoxazole and 80 mg trimethoprim).

Toxoplasmosis: There is no consensus on the most appropriate dosage for the treatment or prophylaxis of this condition. The decision should be based on clinical experience. For prophylaxis, however, the dosages suggested for prevention of PCP may be appropriate.

<u>Use in the elderly:</u>

See Special warnings and Precautions for Use.

4.3 Contraindications
Septrin for Infusion should not be given to patients with a history of hypersensitivity to sulphonamides, trimethoprim, co-trimoxazole or any excipients of Septrin.

Septrin for Infusion is contra-indicated in patients showing marked liver parenchymal damage.

Except under careful supervision Septrin for Infusion should not be given to patients with serious haematological disorders (see 4.8 Undesirable Effects). Co-trimoxazole has been given to patients receiving cytotoxic therapy with little or no additional effect on the bone marrow or peripheral blood.

Septrin for Infusion is contra-indicated in severe renal insufficiency where repeated measurements of the plasma concentration cannot be performed.

Septrin for Infusion should not be given to premature babies nor to full-term infants during the first six weeks of life except for the treatment/prophylaxis of PCP in infants 4 weeks of age or greater.

4.4 Special warnings and special precautions for use

Fatalities, although very rare, have occurred due to severe reactions including Stevens-Johnson syndrome, Lyell's syndrome (toxic epidermal necrolysis), fulminant hepatic necrosis, agranulocytosis, aplastic anaemia, other blood dyscrasias and hypersensitivity of the respiratory tract.

Septrin for Infusion should be discontinued at the first appearance of a skin rash (see 4.8 Undesirable Effects).

Septrin for Infusion contains sulphite. This may cause allergic-type reactions including anaphylactic symptoms and life-threatening or less severe asthmatic episodes in susceptible individuals.

Fluid overload is possible, especially when very high doses are being administered to patients with underlying cardiopulmonary disease.

An adequate urinary output should be maintained at all times. Evidence of crystalluria *in vivo* is rare, although sulphonamide crystals have been noted in cooled urine from treated patients. In patients suffering from malnutrition the risk may be increased.

For patients with known renal impairment special measures should be adopted (See 4.2 Posology and Method of Administration).

Regular monthly blood counts are advisable when Septrin is given for long periods since there exists a possibility of asymptomatic changes in haematological laboratory indices due to lack of available folate. These changes may be reversed by administration of folinic acid (5 to 10 mg/day) without interfering with the antibacterial activity.

Particular care is always advisable when treating elderly patients because, as a group, they are more susceptible to adverse reactions and more likely to suffer serious side effects as a result, particularly when complicating conditions exist, e.g. impaired kidney and/or liver function and/or concomitant drugs.

Special care should be exercised in treating elderly or suspected folate-deficient patients; folate supplementation should be considered.

A folate supplement should also be considered with prolonged high dosage of Septrin (see 4.5 Interaction with other Medicaments and 4.8 Undesirable Effects).

In glucose-6-phosphate dehydrogenase-deficient (G-6-PD) patients, haemolysis may occur.

Septrin should be given with caution to patients with severe allergy or bronchial asthma.

Septrin should not be used in the treatment of streptococcal pharyngitis due to Group A beta-haemolytic streptococci. Eradication of these organisms from the oropharynx is less effective than with penicillin.

Trimethoprim has been noted to impair phenylalanine metabolism but this is of no significance in phenylketonuric patients on appropriate dietary restriction.

The administration of Septrin to patients known or suspected to be at risk of acute porphyria should be avoided. Both trimethoprim and sulphonamides (although not specifically sulfamethoxazole) have been associated with clinical exacerbation of porphyria.

Close monitoring of serum potassium is warranted in patients at risk of hyperkalaemia.

4.5 Interaction with other medicinal products and other forms of Interaction

In elderly patients concurrently receiving diuretics, mainly thiazides, there appears to be an increased risk of thrombocytopenia with or without purpura.

Occasional reports suggest that patients receiving pyrimethamine as malarial prophylaxis at doses in excess of 25 mg weekly may develop megaloblastic anaemia should co-trimoxazole be prescribed concurrently.

In some situations, concomitant treatment with zidovudine may increase the risk of haematological adverse reactions to co-trimoxazole. If concomitant treatment is necessary, consideration should be given to monitoring of haematological parameters.

Administration of trimethoprim/sulfamethoxazole 160mg/800mg (co-trimoxazole) causes a 40% increase in lamivudine exposure because of the trimethoprim component. Lamivudine has no effect on the pharmacokinetics of trimethoprim or sulfamethoxazole.

Co-trimoxazole has been shown to potentiate the anticoagulant activity of warfarin via stereo-selective inhibition of its metabolism. Sulfamethoxazole may displace warfarin from plasma-albumin protein-binding sites *in vitro*. Careful control of the anticoagulant therapy during treatment with Septrin is advisable.

Co-trimoxazole prolongs the half-life of phenytoin and if co-administered the prescriber should be alert for excessive phenytoin effect. Close monitoring of the patient's condition and serum phenytoin levels is advisable.

Interaction with sulphonylurea hypoglycaemic agents is uncommon but potentiation has been reported.

Concurrent use of rifampicin and Septrin results in a shortening of the plasma half-life of trimethoprim after a period of about one week. This is not thought to be of clinical significance.

Reversible deterioration in renal function has been observed in patients treated with co-trimoxazole and ciclosporin following renal transplantation.

When trimethoprim is administered simultaneously with drugs that form cations at physiological pH, and are also partly excreted by active renal secretion (e.g. procainamide, amantadine), there is the possibility of competitive inhibition of this process which may lead to an increase in plasma concentration of one or both of the drugs.

Concomitant use of trimethoprim with digoxin has been shown to increase plasma digoxin levels in a proportion of elderly patients.

Caution should be exercised in patients taking any other drugs that can cause hyperkalaemia.

Co-trimoxazole may increase the free plasma levels of methotrexate.

If Septrin is considered appropriate therapy in patients receiving other anti-folate drugs such as methotrexate, a folate supplement should be considered

Trimethoprim interferes with assays for serum methotrexate when dihydrofolate reductase from *Lactobacillus casei* is used in the assay. No interference occurs if methotrexate is measured by radioimmuno assay.

Trimethoprim may interfere with the estimation of serum/plasma creatinine when the alkaline picrate reaction is used. This may result in overestimation of serum/plasma creatinine of the order of 10%. The creatinine clearance is reduced: the renal tubular secretion of creatinine is decreased from 23% to 9% whilst the glomerular filtration remains unchanged.

4.6 Pregnancy and lactation

Trimethoprim and sulfamethoxazole cross the placenta and their safety in human pregnancy has not been established. Trimethoprim is a folate antagonist and, in animal studies, both agents have been shown to cause foetal abnormalities (see 5.3 Preclinical Safety Data). Case-control studies have shown that there may be an association between exposure to folate antagonists and birth defects in humans. Therefore, co-trimoxazole should be avoided in pregnancy, particularly in the first trimester, unless the potential benefit to the mother outweighs the potential risk to the foetus; folate supplementation should be considered if co-trimoxazole is used in pregnancy.

Sulfamethoxazole competes with bilirubin for binding to plasma albumin. As significantly maternally derived drug levels persist for several days in the newborn, there may be a risk of precipitating or exacerbating neonatal hyperbilirubinaemia, with an associated theoretical risk of kernicterus, when Septrin is administered to the mother near the time of delivery. This theoretical risk is particularly relevant in infants at increased risk of hyperbilirubinaemia, such as those who are preterm and those with glucose-6-phosphate dehydrogenase deficiency.

Trimethoprim and sulfamethoxazole are excreted in breast milk. Administration of co-trimoxazole should be avoided in late pregnancy and in lactating mothers where the mother or infant has, or is at particular risk of developing, hyperbilirubinaemia. Additionally, administration of co-trimoxazole should be avoided in infants younger than eight weeks in view of the predisposition of young infants to hyperbilirubinaemia.

4.7 Effects on ability to drive and use machines

None known.

4.8 Undesirable effects

The frequency categories associated with the adverse events below are estimates. For most events, suitable data for estimating incidence were not available. In addition, adverse events may vary in their incidence depending on the indication.

Data from large published clinical trials were used to determine the frequency of very common to rare adverse events. Very rare adverse events were primarily determined from post-marketing experience data and therefore refer to reporting rate rather than a "true" frequency.

The following convention has been used for the classification of adverse events in terms of frequency:- Very common $\geqslant 1/10$, common $\geqslant 1/100$ and $< 1/10$, uncommon $\geqslant 1/1000$ and $< 1/100$, rare $\geqslant 1/10{,}000$ and $< 1/1000$, very rare $< 1/10{,}000$.

Infections and Infestations

Common: Monilial overgrowth

Blood and lymphatic system disorders

Very rare: Leucopenia, neutropenia, thrombocytopenia, agranulocytosis, megaloblastic anaemia, aplastic anaemia, haemolytic anaemia, methaemoglobinaemia, eosinophilia, purpura, haemolysis in certain susceptible G-6-PD deficient patients

The majority of haematological changes are mild and reversible when treatment is stopped. Most of the changes cause no clinical symptoms although they may become severe in isolated cases, especially in the elderly, in those with hepatic or renal dysfunction or in those with poor folate status. Fatalities have been recorded in at-risk patients and these patients should be observed carefully (see 4.3 Contra-indications).

Immune system disorders

Very rare: Serum sickness, anaphylaxis, allergic myocarditis, angioedema, drug fever, allergic vasculitis resembling Henoch-Schoenlein purpura, periarteritis nodosa, systemic lupus erythematosus

lMetabolism and nutrition disorders

Very common: Hyperkalaemia

Very rare: Hypoglycaemia, hyponatraemia, anorexia

Close supervision is recommended when co-trimoxazole is used in elderly patients or in patients taking high doses of co-trimoxazole as these patients may be more susceptible to hyperkalaemia and hyponatraemia.

Psychiatric disorders

Very rare: Depression, hallucinations

Nervous system disorders

Common: Headache

Very rare: Aseptic meningitis, convulsions, peripheral neuritis, ataxia, vertigo, tinnitus, dizziness

Aseptic meningitis was rapidly reversible on withdrawal of the drug, but recurred in a number of cases on re-exposure to either co- trimoxazole or to trimethoprim alone.

Respiratory, thoracic and mediastinal disorders

Very rare: Cough, shortness of breath, pulmonary infiltrates

Cough, shortness of breath and pulmonary infiltrates may be early indicators of respiratory hypersensitivity which, while very rare, has been fatal.

Gastrointestinal disorders

Common: Nausea, diarrhoea

Uncommon: Vomiting

Very rare: Glossitis, stomatitis, pseudomembranous colitis, pancreatitis

Hepatobiliary disorders

Very rare: Elevation of serum transaminases, elevation of bilirubin levels, cholestatic jaundice, hepatic necrosis

Cholestatic jaundice and hepatic necrosis may be fatal.

Skin and subcutaneous tissue disorders

Common: Skin rashes

Very rare: Photosensitivity, exfoliative dermatitis, fixed drug eruption, erythema multiforme, Stevens-Johnson syndrome, Lyell's syndrome (toxic epidermal necrolysis)

Lyell's syndrome carries a high mortality.

Musculoskeletal and connective tissue disorders

Very rare: Arthralgia, myalgia

Renal and urinary disorders

Very rare: Impaired renal function (sometimes reported as renal failure), interstitial nephritis

Effects associated with *Pneumocystis jiroveci(P. carinii)* Pneumonitis (PCP) management

Very rare: Severe hypersensitivity reactions, rash, fever, neutropenia, thrombocytopenia, raised liver enzymes, hyperkalaemia, hyponatraemia

At the high dosages used for PCP management severe hypersensitivity reactions have been reported, necessitating cessation of therapy. If signs of bone marrow depression occur, the patient should be given calcium folinate supplementation (5-10 mg/day). Severe hypersensitivity reactions have been reported in PCP patients on re-exposure to co-trimoxazole, sometimes after a dosage interval of a few days.

4.9 Overdose

The maximum tolerated dose in humans is unknown.

Nausea, vomiting, dizziness and confusion are likely symptoms of overdosage. Bone marrow depression has been reported in acute trimethoprim overdosage.

In cases of known, suspected or accidental overdosage, stop therapy.

Dependent on the status of renal function, administration of fluids is recommended if urine output is low.

Both trimethoprim and active sulfamethoxazole are dialysable by renal dialysis. Peritoneal dialysis is not effective.

5. PHARMACOLOGICAL PROPERTIES

5.1 Pharmacodynamic properties

In vitro activity: Sulfamethoxazole competitively inhibits the utilisation of para-aminobenzoic acid in the synthesis of dihydrofolate by the bacterial cell resulting in bacteriosis. Trimethoprim reversibly inhibits bacterial dihydrofolate to tetrahydrofolate. Depending on the conditions the effect may be bactericidal. Thus trimethoprim and sulfamethoxazole block two consecutive steps in the biosynthesis of purines and therefore nucleic acids essential to many bacteria. This action produces marked potentiation of activity *in vitro* between the two agents.

Trimethoprim binds to plasmodial DHFR but less tightly than to bacterial enzyme. Its affinity for mammalian DHFR is some 50,000 times less than for the corresponding bacterial enzyme.

Many common pathogenic bacteria are sensitive *in vitro* to trimethoprim and sulfamethoxazole at concentrations well below those reached in blood, tissue fluids and urine after the administration of recommended doses. In common with other antibiotics, however, *in vitro* activity does not necessarily imply that clinical efficacy has been demonstrated and it must be noted that satisfactory sensitivity testing is achieved only with recommended media free from inhibitory substances, especially thymidine and thymine.

5.2 Pharmacokinetic properties

Peak plasma levels of trimethoprim and sulfamethoxazole are higher and achieved more rapidly after one hour of intravenous infusion of Septrin for Infusion than after oral administration of an equivalent dose of a Septrin oral presentation. Plasma concentrations, elimination half-life and urinary excretion rates show no significant differences following either the oral or intravenous route of administration.

Trimethoprim is a weak base with a pKa of 7.3. It is lipophilic. Tissue levels of trimethoprim are generally higher than corresponding plasma levels, the lungs and kidneys showing especially high concentrations. Trimethoprim concentrations exceed those in plasma in the case of bile, prostatic fluid and tissue, sputum, and vaginal secretions. Levels in the aqueous humor, breast milk, cerebrospinal fluid, middle ear fluid, synovial fluid and tissue (interstitial) fluid are adequate for antibacterial activity. Trimethoprim passes into amniotic fluid and fetal tissues reaching concentrations approximating those of maternal serum.

Approximately 50% of trimethoprim in the plasma is protein bound. The half-life in man is in the range 8.6 to 17 hours in the presence of normal renal function. It is increased by a factor of 1.5 to 3.0 when the creatinine clearance is less than 10 ml/minute. There appears to be no significant difference in the elderly compared with young patients.

The principal route of excretion of trimethoprim is renal and approximately 50% of the dose is excreted in the urine within 24 hours as unchanged drug. Several metabolites have been identified in the urine. Urinary concentrations of trimethoprim vary widely.

Sulfamethoxazole is a weak acid with a pKa of 6.0. The concentration of active sulfamethoxazole in amniotic fluid, aqueous humor, bile, cerebrospinal fluid, middle ear fluid, sputum, synovial fluid and tissue (interstitial) fluid is of the order of 20 to 50% of the plasma concentration. Approximately 66% of sulfamethoxazole in the plasma is protein bound. The half-life in man is approximately 9 to 11 hours in the presence of normal renal function. There is no change in the half-life of active sulfamethoxazole with a reduction in renal function but there is prolongation of the half-life of the major, acetylated metabolite when the creatinine clearance is below 25 ml/minute.

The principal route of excretion of sulfamethoxazole is renal; between 15% and 30% of the dose recovered in the urine is in the active form. In elderly patients there is a reduced renal clearance of sulfamethoxazole.

5.3 Preclinical safety data

Reproductive toxicology: At doses in excess of recommended human therapeutic dose, trimethoprim and sulfamethoxazole have been reported to cause cleft palate and other foetal abnormalities in rats, findings typical of a folate antagonist. Effects with trimethoprim were preventable by administration of dietary folate. In rabbits, foetal loss was seen at doses of trimethoprim in excess of human therapeutic doses.

6. PHARMACEUTICAL PARTICULARS

6.1 List of excipients

Propylene Glycol	Ph Eur
Tromethamine	USP
Sodium Hydroxide	BP
Sodium Metabisulphite	BP
Ethanol	BP
Water for Injections	Ph Eur

6.2 Incompatibilities

None known.

6.3 Shelf life

36 months

6.4 Special precautions for storage

Store below 30°C. Protect from light.

6.5 Nature and contents of container

Neutral glass ampoules (5ml nominal fill volume)

Pack size: 10 × 5ml ampoules

6.6 Instructions for use and handling

None

Administrative Data

7. MARKETING AUTHORISATION HOLDER

The Wellcome Foundation Ltd.,
Glaxo Wellcome House,
Berkeley Avenue,
Greenford,
Middlesex
Trading as
GlaxoSmithKline UK
Stockley Park West
Uxbridge
Middlesex UB11 1BT

8. MARKETING AUTHORISATION NUMBER(S)

PL00003/0095R

9. DATE OF FIRST AUTHORISATION/RENEWAL OF THE AUTHORISATION

11/02/98

10. DATE OF REVISION OF THE TEXT

23 June 2005

11. Legal Status

POM

Septrin Oral Products

(GlaxoSmithKline UK)

1. NAME OF THE MEDICINAL PRODUCT

Septrin Forte Tablets
Septrin Tablets
Septrin Paediatric Suspension
Septrin Adult Suspension

2. QUALITATIVE AND QUANTITATIVE COMPOSITION

Septrin Forte Tablets:
Sulfamethoxazole 800mg Ph Eur
Trimethoprim 160mg Ph Eur
Septrin Tablets:
Sulfamethoxazole 400mg Ph Eur
Trimethoprim 80mg Ph Eur
Septrin Paediatric Suspension:
Sulfamethoxazole 200mg Ph Eur
Trimethoprim 40mg Ph Eur
Septrin Adult Suspension:
Sulfamethoxazole 400 mg
Trimethoprim 80 mg

3. PHARMACEUTICAL FORM

Tablet
Suspension

4. CLINICAL PARTICULARS

4.1 Therapeutic indications

Septrin should only be used where, in the judgement of the physician, the benefits of treatment outweigh any possible risks; consideration should be given to the use of a single effective antibacterial agent.

The *in vitro* susceptibility of bacteria to antibiotics varies geographically and with time; the local situation should always be considered when selecting antibiotic therapy.

Treatment and prevention of *Pneumocystis jiroveci (P. carinii)* pneumonitis (See 4.2 Posology and Method of Administration and 4.8 Undesirable Effects *)*.

Treatment and prophylaxis of toxoplasmosis, treatment of nocardiosis.

Urinary tract infections: Acute uncomplicated urinary tract infections: Treatment of urinary tract infections where there is bacterial evidence of sensitivity to co-trimoxazole and good reason to prefer this combination to a single antibiotic.

Respiratory tract infections: Otitis media: Acute treatment of otitis media, where there is good reason to prefer co-trimoxazole to a single antibiotic.

Treatment of acute exacerbations of chronic bronchitis, where there is bacterial evidence of sensitivity to co-trimoxazole and good reason to prefer this combination to a single antibiotic.

4.2 Posology and method of administration

Method of administration: oral.

It may be preferable to take Septrin with some food or drink to minimise the possibility of gastrointestinal disturbances.

Acute infections: Adults and children over 12 years:

STANDARD DOSAGE (TABLETS)

Forte Tablets:	1 every 12 hours
Tablets:	2 every 12 hours.

Children aged 12 years and under:

STANDARD DOSAGE (PAEDIATRIC SUSPENSION)

Age	
6 to 12 years	10 ml every 12 hours
6 months to 5 years	5 ml every 12 hours
6 weeks to 5 months	2.5 ml every 12 hours

STANDARD DOSAGE (ADULT SUSPENSION)

10 ml every 12 hours

This dosage approximates to 6 mg trimethoprim and 30 mg sulfamethoxazole per kilogram body weight per 24 hours.

Treatment should be continued until the patient has been symptom free for two days; the majority will require treatment for at least 5 days. If clinical improvement is not evident after 7 days' therapy, the patient should be reassessed.

As an alternative to STANDARD DOSAGE for acute uncomplicated lower urinary tract infections, short-term therapy of 1 to 3 days' duration has been shown to be effective.

Use in the elderly: Particular care is *always* advisable when treating elderly patients because, as a group, they are more susceptible to adverse reactions and more likely to suffer serious effects as a result particularly when complicating conditions exist, e.g. impaired kidney and/or liver function and/or concomitant use of other drugs.

Special dosage recommendations: Unless otherwise specified *standard dosage* applies.

Where dosage is expressed as "tablets" this refers to the adult tablet, i.e. 80 mg Trimethoprim BP and 400 mg Sulfamethoxazole BP. If other formulations are to be used appropriate adjustment should be made.

Impaired renal function:Adults and children over 12 years: (no information is available for children under 12 years of age).

Creatinine Clearance (ml/min)	Recommended Dosage
>30	STANDARD DOSAGE
15 to 30	Half the STANDARD DOSAGE
<15	Not recommended

Measurements of plasma concentration of sulfamethoxazole at intervals of 2 to 3 days are recommended in samples obtained 12 hours after administration of Septrin. If the concentration of total sulfamethoxazole exceeds 150 microgram/ml then treatment should be interrupted until the value falls below 120 microgram/ml.

Pneumocystis jiroveci (P.carinii) pneumonitis: Treatment: A higher dosage is recommended using 20 mg trimethoprim and 100 mg sulfamethoxazole per kg of body weight per day in two or more divided doses for two weeks. The aim is to obtain peak plasma or serum levels of trimethoprim of greater than or equal to 5 microgram/ml (verified in patients receiving 1-hour infusions of intravenous Septrin). (See 4.8 Undesirable Effects).

Prevention:

Adults: The following dose schedules may be used:

160 mg trimethoprim/800 mg sulfamethoxazole daily 7 days per week.

160 mg trimethoprim/800 mg sulfamethoxazole three times per week on alternative days.

320 mg trimethoprim/1600 mg sulfamethoxazole per day in two divided doses three times per week on alternative days.

Children:

The following dose schedules may be used for the duration of the period at risk (see Acute Infections subsection 4.2)

– Standard dosage taken in two divided doses, seven days per week

– Standard dosage taken in two divided doses, three times per week on alternate days

– Standard dosage taken in two divided doses, three times per week on consecutive days

– Standard dosage taken as a single dose, three times per week on consecutive days

The daily dose given on a treatment day approximates to 150 mg trimethoprim/m^2/day and 750 mg sulfamethoxazole/m^2/day. The total daily dose should not exceed 320 mg trimethoprim and 1600 mg sulfamethoxazole.

Nocardiosis: There is no consensus on the most appropriate dosage. Adult doses of 6 to 8 tablets daily for up to 3 months have been used.

Toxoplasmosis: There is no consensus on the most appropriate dosage for the treatment or prophylaxis of this condition. The decision should be based on clinical experience. For prophylaxis, however, the dosages suggested for prevention of PCP may be appropriate.

4.3 Contraindications

Septrin should not be given to patients with a history of hypersensitivity to sulphonamides, trimethoprim, co-trimoxazole or any excipients of Septrin.

Contra-indicated in patients showing marked liver parenchymal damage.

Contra-indicated in severe renal insufficiency where repeated measurements of the plasma concentration cannot be performed.

Except under careful supervision Septrin should not be given to patients with serious haematological disorders (see 4.8 Undesirable Effects). Co-trimoxazole has been given to patients receiving cytotoxic therapy with little or no additional effect on the bone marrow or peripheral blood.

Septrin should not be given to premature babies nor to full-term infants during the first 6 weeks of life except for the treatment/prophylaxis of PCP in infants 4 weeks of age or greater.

4.4 Special warnings and special precautions for use

Fatalities, although very rare, have occurred due to severe reactions including Stevens-Johnson syndrome, Lyell's syndrome (toxic epidermal necrolysis), fulminant hepatic necrosis, agranulocytosis, aplastic anaemia, other blood dyscrasias and hypersensitivity of the respiratory tract.

Septrin should be discontinued at the first appearance of skin rash. (See 4.8 Undesirable Effects).

Particular care is *always* advisable when treating elderly patients because, as a group, they are more susceptible to adverse reactions and more likely to suffer serious effects as a result particularly when complicating conditions exist, e.g. impaired kidney and/or liver function and/or concomitant use of other drugs.

Special care should be exercised in treating elderly or suspected folate-deficient patients; folate supplementation should be considered.

An adequate urinary output should be maintained at all times. Evidence of crystalluria *in vivo* is rare, although sulphonamide crystals have been noted in cooled urine from treated patients. In patients suffering from malnutrition the risk may be increased.

Regular monthly blood counts are advisable when Septrin is given for long periods since there exists a possibility of asymptomatic changes in haematological laboratory indices due to lack of available folate. These changes may be reversed by administration of folinic acid (5 to 10 mg/day) without interfering with the antibacterial activity.

A folate supplement should also be considered with prolonged high dosage of Septrin (see 4.5 Interaction with other Medicaments and 4.8 Undesirable Effects).

In glucose-6-phosphate dehydrogenase (G-6-PD) deficient patients haemolysis may occur.

Septrin should be given with caution to patients with severe allergy or bronchial asthma.

Septrin should not be used in the treatment of streptococcal pharyngitis due to Group A beta-haemolytic streptococci; eradication of these organisms from the oropharynx is less effective than with penicillin.

Trimethoprim has been noted to impair phenylalanine metabolism but this is of no significance in phenylketonuric patients on appropriate dietary restriction.

The administration of Septrin to patients known or suspected to be at risk of acute porphyria should be avoided. Both trimethoprim and sulphonamides (although not specifically sulfamethoxazole) have been associated with clinical exacerbation of porphyria.

Close monitoring of serum potassium is warranted in patients at risk of hyperkalaemia.

4.5 Interaction with other medicinal products and other forms of Interaction

In elderly patients concurrently receiving diuretics, mainly thiazides, there appears to be an increased risk of thrombocytopenia with or without purpura.

Occasional reports suggest that patients receiving pyrimethamine at doses in excess of 25 mg weekly may develop megaloblastic anaemia should co-trimoxazole be prescribed concurrently.

In some situations, concomitant treatment with zidovudine may increase the risk of haematological adverse reactions to co-trimoxazole. If concomitant treatment is necessary, consideration should be given to monitoring of haematological parameters.

Administration of trimethoprim/sulfamethoxazole 160mg/800mg (co-trimoxazole) causes a 40% increase in lamivudine exposure because of the trimethoprim component. Lamivudine has no effect on the pharmacokinetics of trimethoprim or sulfamethoxazole.

Reversible deterioration in renal function has been observed in patients treated with co-trimoxazole and ciclosporin following renal transplantation.

Co-trimoxazole has been shown to potentiate the anticoagulant activity of warfarin via stereo-selective inhibition of its metabolism. Sulfamethoxazole may displace warfarin from plasma-albumin protein-binding sites *in vitro*. Careful control of the anticoagulant therapy during treatment with Septrin is advisable.

Co-trimoxazole prolongs the half-life of phenytoin and if co-administered could result in excessive phenytoin effect. Close monitoring of the patient's condition and serum phenytoin levels are advisable.

Interaction with sulphonylurea hypoglycaemic agents is uncommon but potentiation has been reported.

Concurrent use of rifampicin and Septrin results in a shortening of the plasma half-life of trimethoprim after a period of about one week. This is not thought to be of clinical significance.

When trimethoprim is administered simultaneously with drugs that form cations at physiological pH, and are also partly excreted by active renal secretion (e.g. procainamide, amantadine), there is the possibility of competitive inhibition of this process which may lead to an increase in plasma concentration of one or both of the drugs.

Concomitant use of trimethoprim with digoxin has been shown to increase plasma digoxin levels in a proportion of elderly patients.

Caution should be exercised in patients taking any other drugs that can cause hyperkalaemia.

Co-trimoxazole may increase the free plasma levels of methotrexate.

If Septrin is considered appropriate therapy in patients receiving other anti-folate drugs such as methotrexate, a folate supplement should be considered.

4.6 Pregnancy and lactation

Trimethoprim and sulfamethoxazole cross the placenta and their safety in human pregnancy has not been established. Trimethoprim is a folate antagonist and, in animal studies, both agents have been shown to cause foetal abnormalities (see 5.3 Preclinical Safety Data). Case-control studies have shown that there may be an association between exposure to folate antagonists and birth defects in humans. Therefore, co-trimoxazole should be avoided in pregnancy, particularly in the first trimester, unless the potential benefit to the mother outweighs the potential risk to the foetus; folate supplementation should be considered if co-trimoxazole is used in pregnancy.

Sulfamethoxazole competes with bilirubin for binding to plasma albumin. As significantly maternally derived drug levels persist for several days in the newborn, there may be a risk of precipitating or exacerbating neonatal hyperbilirubinaemia, with an associated theoretical risk of kernicterus, when Septrin is administered to the mother near the time of delivery. This theoretical risk is particularly relevant in infants at increased risk of hyperbilirubinaemia, such as those who are preterm and those with glucose-6-phosphate dehydrogenase deficiency.

Trimethoprim and sulfamethoxazole are excreted in breast milk. Administration of co-trimoxazole should be avoided in late pregnancy and in lactating mothers where the mother or infant has, or is at particular risk of developing, hyperbilirubinaemia. Additionally, administration of co-trimoxazole should be avoided in infants younger than eight weeks in view of the predisposition of young infants to hyperbilirubinaemia.

4.7 Effects on ability to drive and use machines

There have been no studies to investigate the effect of Septrin on driving performance or the ability to operate machinery. Further a detrimental effect on such activities cannot be predicted from the pharmacology of the drug. Nevertheless the clinical status of the patient and the adverse events profile of Septrin should be borne in mind when considering the patients ability to operate machinery.

4.8 Undesirable effects

The frequency categories associated with the adverse events below are estimates. For most events, suitable data for estimating incidence were not available. In addition, adverse events may vary in their incidence depending on the indication.

Data from large published clinical trials were used to determine the frequency of very common to rare adverse events. Very rare adverse events were primarily determined from post-marketing experience data and therefore refer to reporting rate rather than a "true" frequency.

The following convention has been used for the classification of adverse events in terms of frequency:- Very common $\geqslant 1/10$, common $\geqslant 1/100$ and $< 1/10$, uncommon $\geqslant 1/1000$ and $< 1/100$, rare $\geqslant 1/10{,}000$ and $< 1/1000$, very rare $< 1/10{,}000$.

<u>Infections and Infestations</u>

Common: Monilial overgrowth

<u>Blood and lymphatic system disorders</u>

Very rare: Leucopenia, neutropenia, thrombocytopenia, agranulocytosis, megaloblastic anaemia, aplastic anaemia, haemolytic anaemia, methaemoglobinaemia, eosinophilia, purpura, haemolysis in certain susceptible G-6-PD deficient patients

The majority of haematological changes are mild and reversible when treatment is stopped. Most of the changes cause no clinical symptoms although they may become severe in isolated cases, especially in the elderly, in those with hepatic or renal dysfunction or in those with poor folate status. Fatalities have been recorded in at-risk patients and these patients should be observed carefully (see 4.3 Contra-indications).

<u>Immune system disorders</u>

Very rare: Serum sickness, anaphylaxis, allergic myocarditis, angioedema, drug fever, allergic vasculitis resembling Henoch-Schoenlein purpura, periarteritis nodosa, systemic lupus erythematosus

<u>Metabolism and nutrition disorders</u>

<u>Very common: Hyperkalaemia</u>

Very rare: Hypoglycaemia, hyponatraemia, anorexia

Close supervision is recommended when co-trimoxazole is used in ederly patients or in patients taking high doses of co-trimoxazole as these patients may be more susceptible to hyperkalaemia and hyponatraemia.

<u>Psychiatric disorders</u>

Very rare: Depression, hallucinations

<u>Nervous system disorders</u>

Common: Headache

Very rare: Aseptic meningitis, convulsions, peripheral neuritis, ataxia, vertigo, tinnitus, dizziness

Aseptic meningitis was rapidly reversible on withdrawal of the drug, but recurred in a number of cases on re-exposure to either co- trimoxazole or to trimethoprim alone.

<u>Respiratory, thoracic and mediastinal disorders</u>

Very rare: Cough, shortness of breath, pulmonary infiltrates

Cough, shortness of breath and pulmonary infiltrates may be early indicators of respiratory hypersensitivity which, while very rare, has been fatal.

<u>Gastrointestinal disorders</u>

Common: Nausea, diarrhoea

Uncommon: Vomiting

Very rare: Glossitis, stomatitis, pseudomembranous colitis, pancreatitis

<u>Hepatobiliary disorders</u>

Very rare: Elevation of serum transaminases, elevation of bilirubin levels, cholestatic jaundice, hepatic necrosis

Cholestatic jaundice and hepatic necrosis may be fatal.

<u>Skin and subcutaneous tissue disorders</u>

Common: Skin rashes

Very rare: Photosensitivity, exfoliative dermatitis, fixed drug eruption, erythema multiforme, Stevens-Johnson syndrome, Lyell's syndrome (toxic epidermal necrolysis)

Lyell's syndrome carries a high mortality.

<u>Musculoskeletal and connective tissue disorders</u>

Very rare: Arthralgia, myalgia

<u>Renal and urinary disorders</u>

Very rare: Impaired renal function (sometimes reported as renal failure), interstitial nephritis

<u>Effects associated with *Pneumocystis jiroveci(P. carinii)* Pneumonitis (PCP) management</u>

Very rare: Severe hypersensitivity reactions, rash, fever, neutropenia, thrombocytopenia, raised liver enzymes, hyperkalaemia, hyponatraemia

At the high dosages used for PCP management severe hypersensitivity reactions have been reported, necessitating cessation of therapy. If signs of bone marrow depression occur, the patient should be given calcium folinate supplementation (5-10 mg/day). Severe hypersensitivity reactions have been reported in PCP patients on re-exposure to co-trimoxazole, sometimes after a dosage interval of a few days.

4.9 Overdose

Nausea, vomiting, dizziness and confusion are likely signs/symptoms of overdosage. Bone marrow depression has been reported in acute trimethoprim overdosage.

If vomiting has not occurred, induction of vomiting may be desirable. Gastric lavage may be useful, though absorption from the gastrointestinal tract is normally very rapid and complete within approximately two hours. This may not be the case in gross overdosage. Dependent on the status of renal function administration of fluids is recommended if urine output is low.

Both trimethoprim and active sulfamethoxazole are moderately dialysable by haemodialysis. Peritoneal dialysis is not effective.

5. PHARMACOLOGICAL PROPERTIES

5.1 Pharmacodynamic properties

Sulfamethoxazole competitively inhibits the utilisation of para-aminobenzoic acid in the synthesis of dihydrofolate by the bacterial cell resulting in bacteriostasis. Trimethoprim reversibly inhibits bacterial dihydrofolate reductase (DHFR), an enzyme active in the folate metabolic pathway converting dihydrofolate to tetrahydrofolate. Depending on the conditions the effect may be bactericidal. Thus trimethoprim and sulfamethoxazole block two consecutive steps in the biosynthesis of purines and therefore nucleic acids essential to many bacteria. This action produces marked potentiation of activity *in vitro* between the two agents.

Trimethoprim binds to plasmodial DHFR but less tightly than to the bacterial enzyme. Its affinity for mammalian DHFR is some 50,000 times less than for the corresponding bacterial enzyme.

Many of common pathogenic bacteria are sensitive *in vitro* to trimethoprim and sulphamethoxazole at concentrations well below those reached in blood, tissue fluids and urine after the administration of recommended doses.In common with other antibiotics, however, *in vitro* activity does not necessarily imply that clinical efficacy has been demonstrated and it must be noted that satisfactory sensitivity testing is achieved only with recommended media free from inhibitory substances especially thymidine and thymine.

5.2 Pharmacokinetic properties

After oral administration trimethoprim and sulfamethoxazole are rapidly and nearly completely absorbed. The presence of food does not appear to delay absorption. Peak levels in the blood occur between one and four hours after ingestion and the level attained is dose related. Effective levels persist in the blood for up to 24 hours after a therapeutic dose. Steady state levels in adults are reached after dosing for 2-3 days. Neither component has an appreciable effect on the concentrations achieved in the blood by the other.

Trimethoprim is a weak base with a pKa of 7.4. It is lipophilic. Tissue levels of trimethoprim are generally higher than corresponding plasma levels, the lungs and kidneys showing especially high concentrations. Trimethoprim concentrations exceed those in plasma in the case of bile, prostatic fluid and tissue, saliva, sputum and vaginal secretions. Levels in the aqueous humor, breast milk, cerebrospinal fluid, middle ear fluid, synovial fluid and tissue (intestinal) fluid are adequate for antibacterial activity. Trimethoprim passes into amniotic fluid and foetal tissues reaching concentrations approximating those of maternal serum.

Approximately 50% of trimethoprim in the plasma is protein bound. The half-life in man is in the range 8.6 to 17 hours in the presence of normal renal function. It is increased by a factor of 1.5 to 3.0 when the creatinine clearance is less than 10 ml/minute. There appears to be no significant difference in the elderly compared with young patients.

The principal route of excretion of trimethoprim is renal and approximately 50% of the dose is excreted in the urine within 24 hours as unchanged drug. Several metabolites have been identified in the urine. Urinary concentrations of trimethoprim vary widely.

Sulfamethoxazole is a weak acid with a pKa of 6.0. The concentration of active sulfamethoxazole in a variety of body fluids is of the order of 20 to 50% of the plasma concentration.

Approximately 66% of sulfamethoxazole in the plasma is protein bound. The half-life in man is approximately 9 to 11 hours in the presence of normal renal function. There is no change in the half-life of active sulfamethoxazole with a reduction in renal function but there is prolongation of the half-life of the major, acetylated metabolite when the creatinine clearance is below 25 ml/minute.

The principal route of excretion of sulfamethoxazole is renal; between 15% and 30% of the dose recovered in the urine is in the active form. In elderly patients there is a reduced renal clearance of sulfamethoxazole.

5.3 Preclinical safety data

Reproductive toxicology: At doses in excess of recommended human therapeutic dose, trimethoprim and sulfamethoxazole have been reported to cause cleft palate and other foetal abnormalities in rats, findings typical of a folate antagonist. Effects with trimethoprim were preventable by administration of dietary folate. In rabbits, foetal loss was seen at doses of trimethoprim in excess of human therapeutic doses.

6. PHARMACEUTICAL PARTICULARS

6.1 List of excipients

Forte Tablets:

Povidone Ph Eur

Sodium Starch Glycollate BP

Magnesium Stearate Ph Eur

Docusate Sodium BP

Tablets:

Sodium starch glycollate

Povidone

*Dioctyl sodium sulphosuccinate

*Docusate sodium

Magnesium stearate

*alternative ingredients

Paediatric Suspension:

Sorbitol solution 70% (non crystallising) Glycerol

Dispersible Cellulose

Sodium Carmellose

Polysorbate 80 Methyl Hydroxybenzoate Sodium Benzoate

Saccharin sodium Ethanol (96%)

Flavour, Banana 81.605P HSE

Flavour, Vanilla 407 HSE

Purified Water to 5 ml Ph Eur

Adult Suspension:

Syrup or sucrose

Glycerol

Dispersible Cellulose

Sodium carboxymethylcellulose

Methyl hydroxybenzoate

Saccharin sodium

Ammonium glycyrrhizinate

Anise Oil

Ethanol (96%)

Flavour, vanilla 407

Polysorbate 80

Purified Water

6.2 Incompatibilities

None Known

6.3 Shelf life

Tablets: 60 months

Paediatric Suspension: 36 months

Adult Suspension: 48 months

6.4 Special precautions for storage

Tablets and Suspension:

Do not store above 25° C

Keep container in the outer carton

Paediatric Suspension

Store below 25° C

Protect from light

6.5 Nature and contents of container

Forte Tablets:

Polypropylene container with polyethylene snap-fit closure or PVC/Al foil blister packs

Pack Size: 100

Round enamelled tin

Pack Size: 2000

PVC/Aluminium foil blister pack (sample pack)

Pack Size: 5

Tablets:

Amber glass bottles with low density polyethylene snap-fit closures and PVL/Al foil blister pack.

Pack size: 100

Round enamelled tin with lever lids

Pack Size: 5000

Paediatric Suspension:

Amber Glass bottles with metal roll-on closures.

Pack Size: 100 ml and 30mL

A double-ended 5mL/2.5mL measuring spoon is included.

Paper/Aluminium foil/ionomer resin sachet

Pack size: 5ml

Adult Suspension;

Amber glass bottles with metal roll on pilfer proof caps or polypropylene child resistant caps.

Pack size: 100 ml

Septrin Adult Suspensioncomes with a double-ended polypropylene measuring spoon.

6.6 Instructions for use and handling

Trimethoprim interferes with assays for serum methotrexate when dihydrofolate reductase from *Lactobacillus casei* is used in the assay. No interference occurs if methotrexate is measured by radioimmuno assay.

Trimethoprim may interfere with the estimation of serum/plasma creatinine when the alkaline picrate reaction is used. This may result in overestimation of serum/plasma creatinine of the order of 10%. Functional inhibition of the renal tubular secretion of creatinine may produce a spurious fall in the estimated rate of creatinine clearance.

Septrin Adult Suspension: may be diluted with Syrup BP. Although they may show some sedimentation such dilutions remain stable for at least a month. Shake thoroughly before use.

Administrative Data

7. MARKETING AUTHORISATION HOLDER

The Wellcome Foundation Ltd

Glaxo Wellcome House

Berkeley Avenue

Greenford,

Middlesex, UB6 ONN

Trading as:

GlaxoSmithKline UK

Stockley Park West

Uxbridge

Middlesex UB11 1BT

8. MARKETING AUTHORISATION NUMBER(S)

Forte Tablets: 0003/0121R

Tablets: 0003/0109R

Paediatric Suspension: 0003/5222R

Adult Suspension: 0003/5223R

9. DATE OF FIRST AUTHORISATION/RENEWAL OF THE AUTHORISATION

Forte Tablets:

Date of first authorisation: 14 April 1997

Renewed: 15 July 2003

Tablets:

Date of first authorisation: 30 October 1986

Date of last renewal: 8 July 2003

Paediatric Suspension:

Date of authorisation: 1 September 1972

Date of last renewal: 30 March 1998.

Adult Suspension:

Date of authorisation: 30 October 1986

Date of last renewal: 15 December 1999

10. DATE OF REVISION OF THE TEXT

22 June 2005

11. Legal Status

POM

Seractil 300mg Film-Coated Tablets

(Genus Pharmaceuticals)

1. NAME OF THE MEDICINAL PRODUCT

Seractil ▼300 mg film-coated tablets

2. QUALITATIVE AND QUANTITATIVE COMPOSITION

Each film-coated tablet contains 300 mg of dexibuprofen. For excipients, see 6.1.

3. PHARMACEUTICAL FORM

Film-coated tablet

White, round, unscored film-coated tablet.

4. CLINICAL PARTICULARS

4.1 Therapeutic indications

Symptomatic treatment for the relief of pain and inflammation associated with osteoarthritis.

Acute symptomatic treatment of pain during menstrual bleeding (primary dysmenorrhoea).

Symptomatic treatment of other forms of mild to moderate pain, such as muscular-skeletal pain or dental pain.

4.2 Posology and method of administration

The dosage should be adjusted to the severity of the disorder and the complaints of the patient. During chronic administration, the dosage should be adjusted to the lowest maintenance dose that provides adequate control of symptoms.

For individual dosage film-coated tablets with 200, 300 and 400 mg dexibuprofen are available.

The recommended dosage is 600 to 900 mg dexibuprofen daily, divided in up to three single doses.

For the treatment of mild to moderate pain, initially single doses of 200 mg dexibuprofen and daily doses of 600 mg dexibuprofen are recommended.

The maximum single dose is 400 mg dexibuprofen.

The dose may be temporarily increased up to 1200 mg dexibuprofen per day in patients with acute conditions or exacerbations. The maximum daily dose is 1200 mg.

For dysmenorrhoea a daily dose of 600 to 900 mg dexibuprofen, divided in up to three single doses, is recommended. The maximum single dose is 300 mg, the maximum daily dose is 900 mg.

Dexibuprofen has not been studied in children and adolescents (< 18 years): Safety and efficacy have not been established and therefore it is not recommended in these age groups.

In elderly patients it is recommended to start the therapy at the lower end of the dosage range. The dosage may be increased to that recommended for general population only after good general tolerance has been ascertained.

Hepatic dysfunction: Patients with mild to moderate hepatic dysfunction should start therapy at reduced doses and be closely monitored. Dexibuprofen should not be used in patients with severe hepatic dysfunction (see 4.3. Contraindications).

Renal dysfunction: The initial dosage should be reduced in patients with mild to moderate impaired renal function. Dexibuprofen should not be used in patients with severe renal dysfunction (see 4.3. Contraindications).

The film coated tablets can be taken with or without a meal (see 5.2.). In general NSAIDs (non-steroidal anti-inflammatory drugs) are preferably taken with food to reduce gastrointestinal irritation, particularly during chronic use. However, a later onset of action in some patientsmay be anticipated when the tablets are taken with or directly after a meal.

The score in the 200 and 400 mg tablets makes it possible to divide the tablets before administration so as to assist with swallowing.

Dividing the tablets will not provide an exact "half" dose.

4.3 Contraindications

Dexibuprofen must not be administered in the following cases:

- Patients previously sensitive to dexibuprofen, to any other NSAID, or to any of the excipients of the product.

- Patients in whom substances with a similar action (e.g. aspirin or other NSAIDs)

precipitate attacks of asthma, bronchospasm, acute rhinitis, or cause nasal polyps, urticaria or angioneurotic oedema.

- Patients with active or suspected gastrointestinal ulcer or history of recurrent gastrointestinal ulcer.

- Patients who have gastrointestinal bleeding or other active bleedings or bleeding disorders.

- Patients with active Crohn's disease or active ulcerative colitis.

- Patients with severe heart failure.

- Patients with severe renal dysfunction (GFR < 30ml/min).

- Patients with severely impaired hepatic function.

- Patients with haemorrhagic diathesis and other coagulation disorders, or patients receiving anticoagulant therapy.

- From the beginning of 6th month of pregnancy (see 4.6).

4.4 Special warnings and special precautions for use

Care is recommended in conditions that predispose patients to the gastrointestinal adverse effects of NSAIDs such as dexibuprofen, including existing gastrointestinal disorders, previous gastric or duodenal ulcer, ulcerative colitis, Crohn's disease and alcoholism.

These patients should be closely monitored for digestive disturbances, especially gastrointestinal bleeding, when taking dexibuprofen or any other NSAID.

Gastrointestinal bleeding or ulceration/perforation have in general more serious consequences in the elderly. They can occur at any time during treatment with or without warning symptoms or a previous history of serious gastrointestinal events.

In the rare instances where gastrointestinal bleeding or ulceration occurs in patients receiving dexibuprofen, treatment should be immediately discontinued (see 4.3. Contraindications).

As with other NSAIDs, allergic reactions, including anaphylactic/anaphylactoid reactions, can also occur without earlier exposure to the drug.

In the treatment of patients with heart failure, hypertension, renal or hepatic disease, especially during concomitant diuretic treatment, the risk of fluid retention and a deterioration in renal function must be taken into account. If used in these patients, the dose of dexibuprofen should be kept as low as possible and renal function should be regularly monitored.

Caution must be exercised in the treatment of elderly patients, who generally have a greater tendency to experience side effects to NSAIDs.

Dexibuprofen should only be given with care to patients with systemic lupus erythematosus and mixed connective tissue disease, because such patients may be predisposed to NSAID-induced CNS and renal side effects.

Caution is required in patients suffering from, or with a previous history of, bronchial asthma since NSAIDs can cause bronchospasm in such patients (see 4.3 Contraindications).

NSAIDs may mask the symptoms of infections.

As with all NSAIDs, dexibuprofen can increase plasma urea nitrogen and creatinine. As with other inhibitors of NSAIDs, dexibuprofen can be associated with adverse effects on the renal system, which can lead to glomerular nephritis, interstitial nephritis, renal papillary necrosis, nephrotic syndrome and acute renal failure (see 4.2. Posology, 4.3. Contraindications and 4.5 Interactions).

As with other NSAIDs, dexibuprofen can cause transient small increases in some liver parameters, and also significant increases in SGOT and SGPT. In case of a relevant increase in such parameters, therapy must be discontinued (see 4.2. Posology and 4.3. Contraindications).

In common with other NSAIDs dexibuprofen may reversibly inhibit platelet aggregation and function and prolong bleeding time. Caution should be exercised when dexibuprofen is given concurrently with oral anticoagulants (see section 4.5).

Patients receiving long-term treatment with dexibuprofen should be monitored as a precautionary measure (renal, hepatic functions and haematologic function/blood counts).

During long-term, high dose, off-label treatment with analgesic drugs, headaches can occur which must not be treated with higher doses of the medicinal product.

In general the habitual use of analgesics, especially the combination of different analgesic drug substances, can lead to lasting renal lesions with the risk of renal failure (analgesic nephropathy). Thus combinations with racemic ibuprofen or other NSAIDs (including OTC products) should be avoided.

The use of dexibuprofen, as with any other drug known to inhibit cyclooxygenase / prostaglandin synthesis, may impair fertility reversibly and is not recommended in women attempting to conceive. In women who have difficulty conceiving or who are undergoing investigation of infertility, withdrawal of Seractil should be considered.

Data of preclinical studies indicate that inhibition of platelet aggregation by low-dose acetylsalicylic acid may be impaired if ibuprofen is administrated concurrently;

this interaction could reduce the cardiovascular-protective effect. Therefore if concomitant administration of low-dose acetylsalicylic acid is indicated special precaution is required if duration of treatment exceeds short term use.

4.5 Interaction with other medicinal products and other forms of Interaction

The information in this section is based upon previous experience with racemic ibuprofen and other NSAIDs.

In general, NSAIDs should be used with caution with other drugs that can increase the risk of gastrointestinal ulceration or gastrointestinal bleeding or renal impairment.

Concomitant use not recommended:

Anticoagulants: The effects of anticoagulants on bleeding time can be potentiated by NSAIDs. If concomitant treatment can not be avoidedblood coagulation tests (INR, bleeding time) should be performed during the initiation of dexibuprofen treatment and the dosage of the anticoagulant should be adjusted if necessary (see section 4.4).

Methotrexate used at doses of 15 mg/week or more: If NSAIDs and methotrexate are given within 24 hours of each other plasma levels of methotrexate may increase, via a reduction in its renal clearance thus increasing the potential for methotrexate toxicity. Therefore, in patients receiving high-dose treatment with methotrexate, the concomitant use of dexibuprofen is not recommended (see section 4.4).

Lithium: NSAIDs can increase the plasma levels of lithium, by reducing its renal clearance. The combination is not recommended (see section 4.4). Frequent lithium monitoring should be performed. The possibility of reducing the dose of lithium should be considered.

Other NSAIDs and salicylates (acetylsalicylic acid at doses above those used for anti-thrombotic treatment, approximately 100 mg/day): The concomitant use with other NSAIDs should be avoided, since simultanous administration of different NSAIDs can increase the risk of gastrointestinal ulceration and haemorrhage.

Precautions:

Acetylsalicylic acid: Concomitant administration of ibuprofen may impair inhibition of platelet aggregation by low-dose acetylsalicylic acid.

Antihypertensives: NSAIDs may reduce the efficacy of beta-blockers, possibly due to inhibition of the formation of vasodilatory prostaglandins.

The concomitant use of NSAIDs and ACE inhibitors or angiotensin-II receptor antagonists may be associated with an increased risk of acute renal failure, especially in patients with pre-existing impairment of renal function. When given to the elderly and/or dehydrated patients, such a combination can lead to acute renal failure by acting directly on glomerular filtration. At the beginning of the treatment, a careful monitoring of renal function is recommended.

Furthermore, chronic administration of NSAIDs can theoretically reduce the antihypertensive effect of angiotensin-II receptor antagonists, as reported with ACE inhibitors. Therefore, caution is required when using such a combination and at the start of treatment, renal function should be carefully monitored (and patients should be encouraged to maintain adequate fluid intake).

Ciclosporin, tacrolimus: Concomitant administration with NSAIDs may increase the risk of nephrotoxicity on account of reduced synthesis of prostaglandins in the kidney. During combination treatment renal function must be closely monitored, especially in the elderly.

Corticosteroids: The risk of gastrointestinal ulceration may be increased by the concomitant administration of NSAIDs and corticosteroids.

Digoxin: NSAIDs can increase the plasma levels of digoxin and increase the risk of digoxin toxicity.

Methotrexate used at doses lower than 15 mg/week: Ibuprofen has been reported to increase methotrexate levels. If dexibuprofen is used in combination with low doses of methotrexate, then the patient's blood count should be monitored carefully, particularly during the first weeks of coadministration. *An* increased surveillance is required in the presence of even mildly impaired renal function, notably in the elderly, and renal function should be monitored to anticipate any reductions in the clearance of methotrexate.

Phenytoin: Ibuprofen may displace phenytoin from protein-binding sites, possibly leading to increased phenytoin serum levels and toxicity. Although clinical evidence for this interaction is limited, phenytoin dosage adjustment, based on monitoring of plasma concentrations and/or observed signs of toxicity, is recommended.

Thiazides, thiazide-related substances, loop diuretics and potassium-sparing diuretics: Concurrent use of an NSAID and a diuretic may increase the risk of renal failure secondary to a reduction in renal blood flow.

Drugs increasing potassium plasma levels:

As with other NSAIDs, concomitant treatment with drugs increasing potassium plasma levels, like potassium-sparing diuretics, ACE inhibitors, angiotensin-II receptors antagonists, immunosuppressants like cyclosporin or tacrolimus, trimethoprime, heparins, etc... may be associated with increased serum potassium levels; hence serum potassium levels should be monitored.

Thrombolytics, ticlopidine and antiplatelet agents: Dexibuprofen inhibits platelet aggregation via inhibition of platelet cyclooxygenase. Therefore, caution is required when dexibuprofen is combined with thrombolytics, ticlopidine and other antiplatelet agents, because of the risk of increased antiplatelet effect.

4.6 Pregnancy and lactation

Pregnancy:

For dexibuprofen, no clinical data on exposed pregnancies are available. Animal studies with ibuprofen and other NSAIDs have shown reproductive toxicity (see 5.3 Preclinical Safety Data).

Inhibition of prostaglandin synthesis may adversely affect the pregnancy and/or the embryo/fetal development, and as the consequences of inhibiting the synthesis of prostaglandins are not fully known, dexibuprofen, like other drugs of this class, should only be administered in the first 5 months of pregnancy if clearly needed, in the lowest effective dose and as short as possible.

During the third trimester of pregnancy, all prostaglandin synthesis inhibitors may expose the fetus to:

- cardiopulmonary toxicity (with premature closure of the ductus arteriosus and pulmonary hypertension),

- renal dysfunction, which may progress to renal failure with oligo-hydroamniosis, the mother and the neonate, at the end of pregnancy, to:

- possible prolongation of bleeding time,

- inhibition of uterine contractions resulting in delayed or prolonged labour.

Therefore, from the beginning of the 6th month of pregnancy onward dexibuprofen is contraindicated.

The use of dexibuprofen, as with any drug substance known to inhibit cyclooxygenase / prostaglandin synthesis is not recommended in women attempting to conceive (see 4.4).

Lactation:

Ibuprofen is slightly excreted in human milk. Breast-feeding is possible with dexibuprofen if dosage is low and the treatment period is short.

4.7 Effects on ability to drive and use machines

During treatment with dexibuprofen the patient's reaction capacity may be reduced when dizziness or fatigue appear as side effects. This should be taken into consideration when increased alertness is required, e.g. when driving or operating machinery. For a single or short term use of Dexibuprofen no special precautions are necessary.

4.8 Undesirable effects

Clinical experience has shown that the risk of undesirable effects induced by dexibuprofen is comparable to that of racemic ibuprofen. The most common adverse events are gastrointestinal in nature.

It should be noted that the adverse events listed below include those reported predominantly for racemic ibuprofen, even though in some cases the adverse event has either not yet been observed with dexibuprofen or has not yet been reported in the frequency mentioned.

Gastrointestinal:

Very common (>1/10): Dyspepsia, diarrhoea.

Common (>1/100, <1/10): Nausea, vomiting, abdominal pain.

Uncommon (>1/1,000, <1/100): Gastrointestinal ulcers and bleeding, ulcerative stomatitis.

Rare (>1/10,000, <1/1,000): Gastrointestinal perforation, flatulence, constipation, esophagitis, esophageal strictures. Exacerbation of diverticular disease, unspecific haemorrhagic colitis, colitis ulcerosa or Crohn's disease.

If gastrointestinal blood loss occurs, this may cause anaemia and haematemesis.

Skin and hypersensitivity reaction:

Common: Rash.

Uncommon: Urticaria, pruritus, purpura (including allergic purpura), angiooedema, rhinitis, bronchospasm.

Rare: Anaphylactic reaction

Very rare (<1/10,000): Erythema multiforme, epidermal necrolysis, systemic lupus erythematosus, alopecia, photosensitivity reactions, severe skin reactions like Stevens-Johnson-Syndrome, acute toxic epidermal necrolysis (Lyell-Syndrome) and allergic vasculitis.

Generalized hypersensitivity reactions have not yet been reported with dexibuprofen but their occurrence cannot be excluded considering the clinical experience with racemic ibuprofen. The symptoms may include fever with rash, abdominal pain, headache, nausea and vomiting, signs of liver injury and even aseptic meningitis. In the majority of cases in which aseptic meningitis has been reported with ibuprofen, some form of underlying auto-immune disease (such as systemic lupus erythematosus or other collagen diseases) was present as a risk factor. In case of a severe generalized hypersensitivity reaction swelling of face, tongue and larynx, bronchospasm, asthma, tachycardia, hypotension and shock can occur.

Central nervous system:

Common: Fatigue or drowsiness, headache, dizziness, vertigo.

Uncommon: Insomnia, anxiety, restlessness, visual disturbances, tinnitus.

Rare: Psychotic reaction, agitation, irritability, depression, confusion or disorientation, reversible toxic amblyopia, impaired hearing.

Very rare: Aseptic meningitis (see hypersensitivity reactions).

Haematological:

Bleeding time may be prolonged. Rare cases of blood disorders include: Thrombocytopenia, leucopenia, granulocytopenia, pancytopenia, agranulocytosis, aplastic anemia or haemolytic anaemia.

Cardiovascular:

Peripheral oedema has been reported in association with dexibuprofen treatment.

Patients with hypertension or renal impairment seem to be predisposed to fluid retention.

Hypertension or cardiac failure (especially in the elderly) may occur.

Renal:

According to the experience with NSAIDs in general, interstitial nephritis, nephrotic syndrome or renal failure cannot be excluded.

Hepatic:

Rare cases of abnormal liver function, hepatitis and jaundice have been observed with racemic ibuprofen.

Others:

In very rare cases infection related inflammation may be aggravated.

4.9 Overdose

Dexibuprofen has a low acute toxicity and patients have survived after single doses as high as 54 g of racemic ibuprofen. Most overdoses have been asymptomatic. There is a risk of symptoms at doses>80 - 100 mg/kg racemic ibuprofen.

The onset of symptoms usually occurs within 4 hours. Mild symptoms are most common, including abdominal pain, nausea, vomiting, lethargy, drowsiness, headache, nystagmus, tinnitus and ataxia. Rarely, moderate or severe symptoms include gastrointestinal bleeding, hypotension, hypothermia, metabolic acidosis, seizures, impaired kidney function, coma, adult respiratory distress syndrome and transient episodes of apnea (in very young children following large ingestions).

Treatment is symptomatic, and there is no specific antidote. Amounts not likely to produce symptoms (less than 50 mg/kg dexibuprofen) may be diluted with water to minimize gastrointestinal upset. In case of ingestion of a significant amount, activated charcoal should be administered.

Emptying of the stomach by emesis may only be considered if the procedure can be undertaken within 60 minutes of ingestion. Gastric lavage should not be considered unless a patient has ingested a potentially life-threatening amount of the drug and the procedure can be undertaken within 60 minutes of ingestion. Forced diuresis, hemodialysis or hemoperfusion are unlikely to be of assistance because dexibuprofen is strongly bound to plasma proteins.

5. PHARMACOLOGICAL PROPERTIES

Pharmacotherapeutic group: Antiinflammatory and antirheumatic products, non-steroids, propionic acid derivatives.

ATC code: M01AE14

5.1 Pharmacodynamic properties

Dexibuprofen (= S(+)-ibuprofen) is considered to be the pharmacologically active enantiomer of racemic ibuprofen. Racemic ibuprofen is a non-steroidal substance with anti-inflammatory and analgesic effects. Its mechanism of action is thought to be due to inhibition of prostaglandin synthesis. Bridging studies in order to compare the efficacy of racemic ibuprofen and dexibuprofen in osteoarthritis over a treatment period of 15 days and in dysmenorrhea, including symptoms of pain, have demonstrated at least non-inferiority of dexibuprofen versus racemic ibuprofen at the recommended dosage.

5.2 Pharmacokinetic properties

Dexibuprofen is absorbed primarily from the small intestine. After metabolic transformation in the liver (hydroxylation, carboxylation), the pharmacologically inactive metabolites are completely excreted, mainly by the kidneys (90%), but also in the bile. The elimination half-life is 1.8 – 3.5 hours; the plasma protein binding is about 99 %. Maximum plasma levels are reached about 2 hours after oral administration.

The administration of dexibuprofen with a meal delays the time to reach maximum concentrations (from 2.1 hours after fasting conditions to 2.8 hours after non-fasting conditions) and decreases the maximum plasma concentrations (from 20.6 to 18.1 μg/ml, which is of no clinical relevance), but has no effect on the extent of absorption.

5.3 Preclinical safety data

Bridging studies on single and repeated dose toxicity, reproduction toxicity and mutagenicity have shown that the toxicological profile of dexibuprofen is comparable to that of racemic ibuprofen.

Racemic ibuprofen inhibited ovulation in the rabbit and impaired implantation in different animal species (rabbit, rat, mouse). Administration of prostaglandin synthesis inhibitors including ibuprofen (mostly in doses higher than used therapeutically) to pregnant animals has been shown to result in increased pre- and postimplantation loss, embryo-fetal lethality and increased incidences of malformations.

6. PHARMACEUTICAL PARTICULARS

6.1 List of excipients

Tablet core: Hypromellose, microcrystalline cellulose, carmellose calcium, colloidal anhydrous silica, talc.

Film-coating material: Hypromellose, titanium dioxide (E171), glycerol triacetate, talc, macrogol 6000.

6.2 Incompatibilities

Not applicable.

6.3 Shelf life

3 years (PVC/PVDC/aluminium blisters)

18 months (PE jars)

6.4 Special precautions for storage

Do not store above 25 °C.

6.5 Nature and contents of container

10, 20, 30, 50, 60, 90, 100, 100x1 and 500x1 film-coated tablets in PVC/PVDC/aluminium blisters.

150 film-coated tablets in PE jars with dosing hole and hinged closure.

Not all pack sizes may be marketed.

6.6 Instructions for use and handling

No special requirements.

7. MARKETING AUTHORISATION HOLDER

Gebro Pharma GmbH, A-6391 Fieberbrunn
Austria

8. MARKETING AUTHORISATION NUMBER(S)

PL 04536/0006

9. DATE OF FIRST AUTHORISATION/RENEWAL OF THE AUTHORISATION

31 October 2000

10. DATE OF REVISION OF THE TEXT

April 2004

11. Legal Category

POM

Seractil 400mg Film-Coated Tablets

(Genus Pharmaceuticals)

1. NAME OF THE MEDICINAL PRODUCT

Seractil▼ 400 mg film-coated tablets

2. QUALITATIVE AND QUANTITATIVE COMPOSITION

Each film-coated tablet contains 400 mg of dexibuprofen. For excipients, see 6.1.

3. PHARMACEUTICAL FORM

Film-coated tablet

White, oblong, both-sided scored film-coated tablet.

4. CLINICAL PARTICULARS

4.1 Therapeutic indications

Symptomatic treatment for the relief of pain and inflammation associated with osteoarthritis.

Acute symptomatic treatment of pain during menstrual bleeding (primary dysmenorrhoea).

Symptomatic treatment of other forms of mild to moderate pain, such as muscular-skeletal pain or dental pain.

4.2 Posology and method of administration

The dosage should be adjusted to the severity of the disorder and the complaints of the patient. During chronic administration, the dosage should be adjusted to the lowest maintenance dose that provides adequate control of symptoms.

For individual dosage film-coated tablets with 200, 300 and 400 mg dexibuprofen are available.

The recommended dosage is 600 to 900 mg dexibuprofen daily, divided in up to three single doses.

For the treatment of mild to moderate pain, initially single doses of 200 mg dexibuprofen and daily doses of 600 mg dexibuprofen are recommended.

The maximum single dose is 400 mg dexibuprofen.

The dose may be temporarily increased up to 1200 mg dexibuprofen per day in patients with acute conditions or exacerbations. The maximum daily dose is 1200 mg.

For dysmenorrhoea a daily dose of 600 to 900 mg dexibuprofen, divided in up to three single doses, is recommended. The maximum single dose is 300 mg, the maximum daily dose is 900 mg.

Dexibuprofen has not been studied in children and adolescents (< 18 years): Safety and efficacy have not been established and therefore it is not recommended in these age groups.

In elderly patients it is recommended to start the therapy at the lower end of the dosage range. The dosage may be increased to that recommended for general population only after good general tolerance has been ascertained.

Hepatic dysfunction: Patients with mild to moderate hepatic dysfunction should start therapy at reduced doses and be closely monitored. Dexibuprofen should not be used in patients with severe hepatic dysfunction (see 4.3. Contraindications).

Renal dysfunction: The initial dosage should be reduced in patients with mild to moderate impaired renal function. Dexibuprofen should not be used in patients with severe renal dysfunction (see 4.3. Contraindications).

The film coated tablets can be taken with or without a meal (see 5.2.). In general NSAIDs (non-steroidal anti-inflammatory drugs) are preferably taken with food to reduce gastrointestinal irritation, particularly during chronic use. However, a later onset of action in some patients may be anticipated when the tablets are taken with or directly after a meal.

The score in the 200 and 400 mg tablets makes it possible to divide the tablets before administration so as to assist with swallowing.

Dividing the tablets will not provide an exact "half" dose.

4.3 Contraindications

Dexibuprofen must not be administered in the following cases:

- Patients previously sensitive to dexibuprofen, to any other NSAID, or to any of the excipients of the product.
- Patients in whom substances with a similar action (e.g. aspirin or other NSAIDs)

precipitate attacks of asthma, bronchospasm, acute rhinitis, or cause nasal polyps, urticaria or angioneurotic oedema.

- Patients with active or suspected gastrointestinal ulcer or history of recurrent gastrointestinal ulcer.
- Patients who have gastrointestinal bleeding or other active bleedings or bleeding disorders.
- Patients with active Crohn's disease or active ulcerative colitis.
- Patients with severe heart failure.
- Patients with severe renal dysfunction (GFR < 30ml/min).
- Patients with severely impaired hepatic function.
- Patients with haemorrhagic diathesis and other coagulation disorders, or patients receiving anticoagulant therapy.
- From the beginning of 6th month of pregnancy (see 4.6).

4.4 Special warnings and special precautions for use

Care is recommended in conditions that predispose patients to the gastrointestinal adverse effects of NSAIDs such as dexibuprofen, including existing gastrointestinal disorders, previous gastric or duodenal ulcer, ulcerative colitis, Crohn's disease and alcoholism.

These patients should be closely monitored for digestive disturbances, especially gastrointestinal bleeding, when taking dexibuprofen or any other NSAID.

Gastrointestinal bleeding or ulceration/perforation have in general more serious consequences in the elderly. They can occur at any time during treatment with or without warning symptoms or a previous history of serious gastrointestinal events.

In the rare instances where gastrointestinal bleeding or ulceration occurs in patients receiving dexibuprofen, treatment should be immediately discontinued (see 4.3. Contraindications).

As with other NSAIDs, allergic reactions, including anaphylactic/anaphylactoid reactions, can also occur without earlier exposure to the drug.

In the treatment of patients with heart failure, hypertension, renal or hepatic disease, especially during concomitant diuretic treatment, the risk of fluid retention and a deterioration in renal function must be taken into account. If used in these patients, the dose of dexibuprofen should be kept as low as possible and renal function should be regularly monitored.

Caution must be exercised in the treatment of elderly patients, who generally have a greater tendency to experience side effects to NSAIDs.

Dexibuprofen should only be given with care to patients with systemic lupus erythematosus and mixed connective tissue disease, because such patients may be predisposed to NSAID-induced CNS and renal side effects.

Caution is required in patients suffering from, or with a previous history of, bronchial asthma since NSAIDs can cause bronchospasm in such patients (see 4.3 Contraindications).

NSAIDs may mask the symptoms of infections.

As with all NSAIDs, dexibuprofen can increase plasma urea nitrogen and creatinine. As with other NSAIDs, dexibuprofen can be associated with adverse effects on the renal system, which can lead to glomerular nephritis, interstitial nephritis, renal papillary necrosis, nephrotic syndrome and acute renal failure (see 4.2. Posology, 4.3. Contraindications and 4.5 Interactions).

As with other NSAIDs, dexibuprofen can cause transient small increases in some liver parameters, and also significant increases in SGOT and SGPT. In case of a relevant increase in such parameters, therapy must be discontinued (see 4.2. Posology and 4.3. Contraindications).

In common with other NSAIDs dexibuprofen may reversibly inhibit platelet aggregation and function and prolong bleeding time. Caution should be exercised when dexibuprofen is given concurrently with oral anticoagulants (see section 4.5).

Patients receiving long-term treatment with dexibuprofen should be monitored as a precautionary measure (renal, hepatic functions and haematologic function/blood counts).

During long-term, high dose, off-label treatment with analgesic drugs, headaches can occur which must not be treated with higher doses of the medicinal product.

In general the habitual use of analgesics, especially the combination of different analgesic drug substances, can lead to lasting renal lesions with the risk of renal failure (analgesic nephropathy). Thus combinations with racemic ibuprofen or other NSAIDs (including OTC products) should be avoided.

The use of dexibuprofen, as with any other drug known to inhibit cyclooxygenase / prostaglandin synthesis, may impair fertility reversibly and is not recommended in women attempting to conceive. In women who have difficulty conceiving or who are undergoing investigation of infertility, withdrawal of Seractil should be considered.

Data of preclinical studies indicate that inhibition of platelet aggregation by low-dose acetylsalicylic acid may be impaired if ibuprofen is administrated concurrently;

this interaction could reduce the cardiovascular-protective effect. Therefore if concomitant administration of low-dose acetylsalicylic acid is indicated special precaution is required if duration of treatment exceeds short term use.

4.5 Interaction with other medicinal products and other forms of Interaction

The information in this section is based upon previous experience with racemic ibuprofen and other NSAIDs.

In general, NSAIDs should be used with caution with other drugs that can increase the risk of gastrointestinal ulceration or gastrointestinal bleeding or renal impairment.

Concomitant use not recommended:

Anticoagulants: The effects of anticoagulants on bleeding time can be potentiated by NSAIDs. If concomitant treatment can not be avoided blood coagulation tests (INR, bleeding time) should be performed during the initiation of dexibuprofen treatment and the dosage of the anticoagulant should be adjusted if necessary (see section 4.4).

Methotrexate used at doses of 15 mg/week or more: If NSAIDs and methotrexate are given within 24 hours of each other plasma levels of methotrexate may increase, via a reduction in its renal clearance thus increasing the potential for methotrexate toxicity. Therefore, in patients receiving high-dose treatment with methotrexate, the concomitant use of dexibuprofen is not recommended (see section 4.4).

Lithium: NSAIDs can increase the plasma levels of lithium, by reducing its renal clearance. The combination is not recommended (see section 4.4). Frequent lithium monitoring should be performed. The possibility of reducing the dose of lithium should be considered.

Other NSAIDs and salicylates (acetylsalicylic acid at doses above those used for anti-thrombotic treatment, approximately 100 mg/day): The concomitant use with other NSAIDs should be avoided, since simultanous administration of different NSAIDs can increase the risk of gastrointestinal ulceration and haemorrhage.

Precautions:

Acetylsalicylic acid: Concomitant administration of ibuprofen may impair inhibition of platelet aggregation by low-dose acetylsalicylic acid.

Antihypertensives: NSAIDs may reduce the efficacy of beta-blockers, possibly due to inhibition of the formation of vasodilatory prostaglandins.

The concomitant use of NSAIDs and ACE inhibitors or angiotensin-II receptor antagonists may be associated with an increased risk of acute renal failure, especially in patients with pre-existing impairment of renal function. When given to the elderly and/or dehydrated patients, such a combination can lead to acute renal failure by acting directly on glomerular filtration. At the beginning of the treatment, a careful monitoring of renal function is recommended.

Furthermore, chronic administration of NSAIDs can theoretically reduce the antihypertensive effect of angiotensin-II receptor antagonists, as reported with ACE inhibitors. Therefore, caution is required when using such a combination and at the start of treatment, renal function should be carefully monitored (and patients should be encouraged to maintain adequate fluid intake).

Ciclosporin, tacrolimus: Concomitant administration with NSAIDs may increase the risk of nephrotoxicity on account of reduced synthesis of prostaglandins in the kidney. During combination treatment renal function must be closely monitored, especially in the elderly.

Corticosteroids: The risk of gastrointestinal ulceration may be increased by the concomitant administration of NSAIDs and corticosteroids.

Digoxin: NSAIDs can increase the plasma levels of digoxin and increase the risk of digoxin toxicity.

Methotrexate used at doses lower than 15 mg/week: Ibuprofen has been reported to increase methotrexate levels. If dexibuprofen is used in combination with low doses of methotrexate, then the patient's blood count should be monitored carefully, particularly during the first weeks of coadministration. An increased surveillance is required in the presence of even mildly impaired renal function, notably in the elderly, and renal function should be monitored to anticipate any reductions in the clearance of methotrexate.

Phenytoin: Ibuprofen may displace phenytoin from protein-binding sites, possibly leading to increased phenytoin serum levels and toxicity. Although clinical evidence for this interaction is limited, phenytoin dosage adjustment, based on monitoring of plasma concentrations and/or observed signs of toxicity, is recommended.

Thiazides, thiazide-related substances, loop diuretics and potassium-sparing diuretics: Concurrent use of an NSAID and a diuretic may increase the risk of renal failure secondary to a reduction in renal blood flow.

Drugs increasing potassium plasma levels:

As with other NSAIDs, concomitant treatment with drugs increasing potassium plasma levels, like potassium-sparing diuretics, ACE inhibitors, angiotensin-II receptors antagonists, immunosuppressants like cyclosporin or tacrolimus, trimethoprime, heparins, etc... may be associated with increased serum potassium levels; hence serum potassium levels should be monitored.

Thrombolytics, ticlopidine and antiplatelet agents: Dexibuprofen inhibits platelet aggregation via inhibition of platelet cyclooxygenase. Therefore, caution is required when dexibuprofen is combined with thrombolytics, ticlopidine and other antiplatelet agents, because of the risk of increased antiplatelet effect.

4.6 Pregnancy and lactation

Pregnancy:

For dexibuprofen, no clinical data on exposed pregnancies are available. Animal studies with ibuprofen and other NSAIDs have shown reproductive toxicity (see 5.3 Preclinical Safety Data).

Inhibition of prostaglandin synthesis may adversely affect the pregnancy and/or the embryo/fetal development, and as the consequences of inhibiting the synthesis of prostaglandins are not fully known, dexibuprofen, like other drugs of this class, should only be administered in the first 5 months of pregnancy if clearly needed, in the lowest effective dose and as short as possible.

During the third trimester of pregnancy, all prostaglandin synthesis inhibitors may expose the fetus to:

- cardiopulmonary toxicity (with premature closure of the ductus arteriosus and pulmonary hypertension),
- renal dysfunction, which may progress to renal failure with oligo-hydroamniosis, the mother and the neonate, at the end of pregnancy, to:
- possible prolongation of bleeding time,
- inhibition of uterine contractions resulting in delayed or prolonged labour.

Therefore, from the beginning of the 6th month of pregnancy onward dexibuprofen is contraindicated.

The use of dexibuprofen, as with any drug substance known to inhibit cyclooxygenase / prostaglandin synthesis is not recommended in women attempting to conceive (see 4.4).

Lactation:

Ibuprofen is slightly excreted in human milk. Breast-feeding is possible with dexibuprofen if dosage is low and the treatment period is short.

4.7 Effects on ability to drive and use machines

During treatment with dexibuprofen the patient's reaction capacity may be reduced when dizziness or fatigue appear as side effects. This should be taken into consideration when increased alertness is required, e.g. when driving or operating machinery. For a single or short term use of Dexibuprofen no special precautions are necessary.

4.8 Undesirable effects

Clinical experience has shown that the risk of undesirable effects induced by dexibuprofen is comparable to that of racemic ibuprofen. The most common adverse events are gastrointestinal in nature.

It should be noted that the adverse events listed below include those reported predominantly for racemic ibuprofen, even though in some cases the adverse event has either not yet been observed with dexibuprofen or has not yet been reported in the frequency mentioned.

Gastrointestinal:

Very common (> 1/10): Dyspepsia, diarrhoea.

Common (> 1/100, < 1/10): Nausea, vomiting, abdominal pain.

Uncommon (> 1/1,000, < 1/100): Gastrointestinal ulcers and bleeding, ulcerative stomatitis.

Rare (> 1/10,000, < 1/1,000): Gastrointestinal perforation, flatulence, constipation, esophagitis, esophageal strictures. Exacerbation of diverticular disease, unspecific haemorrhagic colitis, colitis ulcerosa or Crohn's disease.

If gastrointestinal blood loss occurs, this may cause anaemia and haematemesis.

Skin and hypersensitivity reaction:

Common: Rash.

Uncommon: Urticaria, pruritus, purpura (including allergic purpura), angiooedema, rhinitis, bronchospasm.

Rare: Anaphylactic reaction

Very rare (< 1/10,000): Erythema multiforme, epidermal necrolysis, systemic lupus erythematosus, alopecia, photosensitivity reactions, severe skin reactions like Stevens-Johnson-Syndrome, acute toxic epidermal necrolysis (Lyell-Syndrome) and allergic vasculitis.

Generalized hypersensitivity reactions have not yet been reported with dexibuprofen but their occurrence cannot be excluded considering the clinical experience with racemic ibuprofen. The symptoms may include fever with rash, abdominal pain, headache, nausea and vomiting, signs of liver injury and even aseptic meningitis. In the majority of cases in which aseptic meningitis has been reported with ibuprofen, some form of underlying auto-immune disease (such as systemic lupus erythematosus or other collagen diseases) was present as a risk factor. In case of a severe generalized hypersensitivity reaction swelling of face, tongue and larynx, bronchospasm, asthma, tachycardia, hypotension and shock can occur.

Central nervous system:

Common: Fatigue or drowsiness, headache, dizziness, vertigo.

Uncommon: Insomnia, anxiety, restlessness, visual disturbances, tinnitus.

Rare: Psychotic reaction, agitation, irritability, depression, confusion or disorientation, reversible toxic amblyopia, impaired hearing.

Very rare: Aseptic meningitis (see hypersensitivity reactions).

Haematological:

Bleeding time may be prolonged. Rare cases of blood disorders include: Thrombocytopenia, leucopenia, granulocytopenia, pancytopenia, agranulocytosis, aplastic anemia or haemolytic anaemia.

Cardiovascular:

Peripheral oedema has been reported in association with dexibuprofen treatment.

Patients with hypertension or renal impairment seem to be predisposed to fluid retention.

Hypertension or cardiac failure (especially in the elderly) may occur.

Renal:

According to the experience with NSAIDs in general, interstitial nephritis, nephrotic syndrome or renal failure cannot be excluded.

Hepatic:

Rare cases of abnormal liver function, hepatitis and jaundice have been observed with racemic ibuprofen.

Others:

In very rare cases infection related inflammation may be aggravated.

4.9 Overdose

Dexibuprofen has a low acute toxicity and patients have survived after single doses as high as 54 g of racemic ibuprofen. Most overdoses have been asymptomatic. There is a risk of symptoms at doses > 80 - 100 mg/kg racemic ibuprofen.

The onset of symptoms usually occurs within 4 hours. Mild symptoms are most common, including abdominal pain, nausea, vomiting, lethargy, drowsiness, headache, nystagmus, tinnitus and ataxia. Rarely, moderate or severe symptoms include gastrointestinal bleeding, hypotension, hypothermia, metabolic acidosis, seizures, impaired kidney function, coma, adult respiratory distress syndrome and transient episodes of apnea (in very young children following large ingestions).

Treatment is symptomatic, and there is no specific antidote. Amounts not likely to produce symptoms (less than 50 mg/kg dexibuprofen) may be diluted with water to minimize gastrointestinal upset. In case of ingestion of a significant amount, activated charcoal should be administered.

Emptying of the stomach by emesis may only be considered if the procedure can be undertaken within 60 minutes of ingestion. Gastric lavage should not be considered unless a patient has ingested a potentially life-threatening amount of the drug and the procedure can be undertaken within 60 minutes of ingestion. Forced diuresis, hemodialysis or hemoperfusion are unlikely to be of assistance because dexibuprofen is strongly bound to plasma proteins.

5. PHARMACOLOGICAL PROPERTIES
Pharmacotherapeutic group: Antiinflammatory and antirheumatic products, non-steroids, propionic acid derivatives.

ATC code: M01AE14

5.1 Pharmacodynamic properties
Dexibuprofen (= S(+)-ibuprofen) is considered to be the pharmacologically active enantiomer of racemic ibuprofen. Racemic ibuprofen is a non-steroidal substance with antiinflammatory and analgesic effects. Its mechanism of action is thought to be due to inhibition of prostaglandin synthesis. Bridging studies in order to compare the efficacy of racemic ibuprofen and dexibuprofen in osteoarthritis over a treatment period of 15 days and in dysmenorrhea, including symptoms of pain, have demonstrated at least non-inferiority of dexibuprofen versus racemic ibuprofen at the recommended dosage.

5.2 Pharmacokinetic properties
Dexibuprofen is absorbed primarily from the small intestine. After metabolic transformation in the liver (hydroxylation, carboxylation), the pharmacologically inactive metabolites are completely excreted, mainly by the kidneys (90%), but also in the bile. The elimination half-life is 1.8 – 3.5 hours; the plasma protein binding is about 99 %. Maximum plasma levels are reached about 2 hours after oral administration.

The administration of dexibuprofen with a meal delays the time to reach maximum concentrations (from 2.1 hours after fasting conditions to 2.8 hours after non-fasting conditions) and decreases the maximum plasma concentrations (from 20.6 to 18.1 μg/ml, which is of no clinical relevance), but has no effect on the extent of absorption.

5.3 Preclinical safety data
Bridging studies on single and repeated dose toxicity, reproduction toxicity and mutagenicity have shown that the toxicological profile of dexibuprofen is comparable to that of racemic ibuprofen.

Racemic ibuprofen inhibited ovulation in the rabbit and impaired implantation in different animal species (rabbit, rat, mouse). Administration of prostaglandin synthesis inhibitors including ibuprofen (mostly in doses higher than used therapeutically) to pregnant animals has been shown to result in increased pre- and postimplantation loss, embryo-fetal lethality and increased incidences of malformations.

6. PHARMACEUTICAL PARTICULARS

6.1 List of excipients
Tablet core: Hypromellose, microcrystalline cellulose, carmellose calcium, colloidal anhydrous silica, talc.

Film-coating material: Hypromellose, titanium dioxide (E171), glycerol triacetate, talc, macrogol 6000.

6.2 Incompatibilities
Not applicable.

6.3 Shelf life
3 years (PVC/PVDC/aluminium blisters)

18 months (PE jars)

6.4 Special precautions for storage
Do not store above 25 °C.

6.5 Nature and contents of container
10, 20, 30, 50, 60, 90, 100, 100x1 and 500x1 film-coated tablets in PVC/PVDC/aluminium blisters.

150 film-coated tablets in PE jars with dosing hole and hinged closure.

Not all pack sizes may be marketed.

6.6 Instructions for use and handling
No special requirements.

7. MARKETING AUTHORISATION HOLDER
Gebro Pharma GmbH, A-6391 Fieberbrunn
Austria

8. MARKETING AUTHORISATION NUMBER(S)
PL 04536/0007

9. DATE OF FIRST AUTHORISATION/RENEWAL OF THE AUTHORISATION
31 October 2000

10. DATE OF REVISION OF THE TEXT
April 2004

11. Legal Category
POM

Seretide 100, 250, 500 Accuhaler

(Allen & Hanburys)

1. NAME OF THE MEDICINAL PRODUCT
Seretide 100 Accuhaler

Seretide 250 Accuhaler

Seretide 500 Accuhaler

2. QUALITATIVE AND QUANTITATIVE COMPOSITION
Each single dose of Seretide provides:

50 micrograms of salmeterol (as salmeterol xinafoate) and 100, 250 or 500 micrograms of fluticasone propionate.

For excipients, see 6.1.

3. PHARMACEUTICAL FORM
Inhalation powder, pre-dispensed.

4. CLINICAL PARTICULARS

4.1 Therapeutic indications
Asthma

Seretide is indicated in the regular treatment of asthma where use of a combination product (long-acting beta-2-agonist and inhaled corticosteroid) is appropriate:

- patients not adequately controlled with inhaled corticosteroids and 'as needed' inhaled short acting beta-2-agonist

or

- patients already adequately controlled on both inhaled corticosteroid and long-acting beta-2-agonist.

Note: Seretide 50/100 microgram strength is not appropriate in adults and children with severe asthma.

Chronic Obstructive Pulmonary Disease (COPD)

Seretide is indicated for the symptomatic treatment of patients with severe COPD (FEV1 <50% predicted normal) and a history of repeated exacerbations, who have significant symptoms despite regular bronchodilator therapy.

4.2 Posology and method of administration
Seretide Accuhaler is for inhalation use only.

Patients should be made aware that Seretide Accuhaler must be used daily for optimum benefit, even when asymptomatic.

Patients should be regularly reassessed by a doctor, so that the strength of Seretide they are receiving remains optimal and is only changed on medical advice. The dose should be titrated to the lowest dose at which effective control of symptoms is maintained. Where the control of symptoms is maintained with the lowest strength of the combination given twice daily then the next step could include a test of inhaled corticosteroid alone. As an alternative, patients requiring a long acting beta-2-agonist could be titrated to Seretide given once daily if, in the opinion of the prescriber, it would be adequate to maintain disease control. In the event of once daily dosing when the patient has a history of nocturnal symptoms the dose should be given at night and when the patient has a history of mainly day-time symptoms the dose should be given in the morning.

Patients should be given the strength of Seretide containing the appropriate fluticasone propionate dosage for the severity of their disease. Prescribers should be aware that, in patients with asthma, fluticasone propionate is as effective as other inhaled steroids at approximately half the microgram daily dose. For example, 100mcg of fluticasone propionate is approximately equivalent to 200mcg of beclomethasone dipropionate (CFC containing) or budesonide. If an individual patient should require dosages outside the recommended regimen, appropriate doses of beta-agonist and/or corticosteroid should be prescribed.

Recommended Doses:

Asthma

Adults and adolescents 12 years and older:

One inhalation of 50 micrograms salmeterol and 100 micrograms fluticasone propionate twice daily.

or

One inhalation of 50 micrograms salmeterol and 250 micrograms fluticasone propionate twice daily.

or

One inhalation of 50 micrograms salmeterol and 500 micrograms fluticasone propionate twice daily.

Children 4 years and older:

One inhalation of 50 micrograms salmeterol and 100 micrograms fluticasone propionate twice daily.

The maximum licensed dose of fluticasone propionate delivered by Seretide Accuhaler in children 100mcg twice daily.

There are no data available for use of Seretide in children aged under 4 years.

COPD

Adults:

One inhalation of 50 micrograms salmeterol and 500 micrograms fluticasone propionate twice daily.

Special patient groups:

There is no need to adjust the dose in elderly patients or in those with renal impairment. There are no data available for use of Seretide in patients with hepatic impairment.

Using the Accuhaler:

The device is opened and primed by sliding the lever. The mouthpiece is then placed in the mouth and the lips closed round it. The dose can then be inhaled and the device closed.

4.3 Contraindications
Seretide is contraindicated in patients with hypersensitivity (allergy) to any of the active substances or to the excipient. (see 6.1 List of Excipients)

4.4 Special warnings and special precautions for use
The management of asthma should normally follow a stepwise programme and patient response should be monitored clinically and by lung function tests.

Seretide Accuhaler should not be used to treat acute asthma symptoms for which a fast and short acting bronchodilator is required. Patients should be advised to have their medicinal product to be used for relief in an acute asthma attack available at all times. Seretide Accuhaler is not intended for the initial management of asthma until the need for and approximate dosage of corticosteroids has been established.

Increasing use of short-acting bronchodilators to relieve symptoms indicates deterioration of control and patients should be reviewed by a physician.

Sudden and progressive deterioration in control of asthma is potentially life threatening and the patient should undergo urgent medical assessment. Consideration should be given to increasing corticosteroid therapy. The patient should also be medically reviewed where the current dosage of Seretide has failed to give adequate control of asthma. For patients with asthma or COPD, consideration should be given to additional corticosteroid therapies.

Treatment with Seretide should not be stopped abruptly in patients with asthma due to risk of exacerbation. Therapy should be down-titrated under physician supervision. For patients with COPD cessation of therapy may also be associated with symptomatic decompensation and should be supervised by a physician.

As with all inhaled medication containing corticosteroids, Seretide should be administered with caution in patients with pulmonary tuberculosis.

Seretide should be administered with caution in patients with severe cardiovascular disorders, including heart rhythm abnormalities, diabetes mellitus, untreated hypokalaemia or thyrotoxicosis.

There have been very rare reports of increases in blood glucose levels (See 4.8 'Undesirable Effects') and this should be considered when prescribing to patients with a history of diabetes mellitus.

Potentially serious hypokalaemia may result from systemic beta-2-agonist therapy but following inhalation at therapeutic doses plasma levels of salmeterol are very low.

As with other inhalation therapy paradoxical bronchospasm may occur with an immediate increase in wheezing after dosing. Seretide Accuhaler should be discontinued immediately, the patient assessed and alternative therapy instituted if necessary.

Seretide contains lactose up to 12.5 milligram /dose. This amount does not normally cause problems in lactose intolerant people.

Care should be taken when transferring patients to Seretide therapy, particularly if there is any reason to suppose that adrenal function is impaired from previous systemic steroid therapy.

Systemic effects may occur with any inhaled corticosteroid, particularly at high doses prescribed for long periods. These effects are much less likely to occur than with oral corticosteroids. Possible systemic effects include Cushing's syndrome, Cushingoid features, adrenal suppression, growth retardation in children and adolescents, decrease in bone mineral density, cataract and glaucoma. **It is important, therefore, that the patient is reviewed regularly the dose of inhaled corticosteroid is reduced to the lowest dose at which effective control of asthma is maintained.**

It is recommended that the height of children receiving prolonged treatment with inhaled corticosteroid is regularly monitored.

Prolonged treatment of patients with high doses of inhaled corticosteroids may result in adrenal suppression and acute adrenal crisis. Children and adolescents <16years taking high doses of fluticasone (typically ≥ 1000mcg/day) may be at particular risk. Very rare cases of adrenal suppression and acute adrenal crisis have also been described with doses of fluticasone propionate between 500 and less than 1000mcg. Situations, which could potentially trigger acute adrenal crisis in patients, include trauma, surgery, infection or any rapid reduction in dosage. Presenting symptoms are typically vague and may include anorexia, abdominal pain, weight loss, tiredness, headache, nausea, vomiting, hypotension, decreased level of consciousness, hypoglycaemia, and seizures.

Additional systemic corticosteroid cover should be considered during periods of stress or elective surgery.

The benefits of inhaled fluticasone propionate therapy should minimise the need for oral steroids, but patients transferring from oral steroids may remain at risk of impaired adrenal reserve for a considerable time. Patients who have required high dose emergency corticosteroid therapy in the past may also be at risk. This possibility of residual impairment should always be borne in mind in emergency and elective situations likely to produce stress, and appropriate corticosteroid treatment must be considered. The extent of the adrenal impairment may require specialist advice before elective procedures.

Ritonavir can greatly increase the concentration of fluticasone propionate in plasma. Therefore, concomitant use should be avoided, unless the potential benefit to the patient outweighs the risk of systemic corticosteroid side-effects. There is also an increased risk of systemic side effects when combining fluticasone propionate with other potent CYP3A inhibitors (see 4.5 Interaction with Other Medicinal Products and Other Forms of Interaction).

4.5 Interaction with other medicinal products and other forms of Interaction

Both non-selective and selective beta-blockers should be avoided unless there are compelling reasons for their use.

Concomitant use of other beta-adrenergic containing drugs can have a potentially additive effect.

Under normal circumstances, low plasma concentrations of fluticasone propionate are achieved after inhaled dosing, due to extensive first pass metabolism and high systemic clearance mediated by cytochrome P450 3A4 in the gut and liver. Hence, clinically significant drug interactions mediated by fluticasone propionate are unlikely.

In an interaction study in healthy subjects with intranasal fluticasone propionate, ritonavir (a highly potent cytochrome P450 3A4 inhibitor) 100 mg b.i.d. increased the fluticasone propionate plasma concentrations several hundred fold, resulting in markedly reduced serum cortisol concentrations. Information about this interaction is lacking for inhaled fluticasone propionate, but a marked increase in fluticasone propionate plasma levels is expected. Cases of Cushing's syndrome and adrenal suppression have been reported. The combination should be avoided unless the benefit outweighs the increased risk of systemic glucocorticoid side-effects.

In a small study in healthy volunteers, the slightly less potent CYP3A inhibitor ketoconazole increased the exposure of fluticasone propionate after a single inhalation by 150%. This resulted in a greater reduction of plasma cortisol as compared with fluticasone propionate alone. Co-treatment with other potent CYP3A inhibitors, such as itraconazole, is also expected to increase the systemic fluticasone propionate exposure and the risk of systemic side-effects. Caution is recommended and long-term treatment with such drugs should if possible be avoided.

4.6 Pregnancy and lactation

There are insufficient data on the use of salmeterol and fluticasone propionate during pregnancy and lactation in man to assess the possible harmful effects. In animal studies foetal abnormalities occur after administration of beta-2-adrenoreceptor agonists and glucocorticosteroids (see 5.3 'Preclinical Safety Data').

Administration of Seretide to pregnant women should only be considered if the expected benefit to the mother is greater than any possible risk to the foetus.

The lowest effective dose of fluticasone propionate needed to maintain adequate asthma control should be used in the treatment of pregnant women.

There are no data available for human breast milk. Both salmeterol and fluticasone propionate are excreted into breast milk in rats. Administration of Seretide to women who are breastfeeding should only be considered if the expected benefit to the mother is greater than any possible risk to the child.

4.7 Effects on ability to drive and use machines

No studies of the effect on the ability to drive and use machines have been performed.

4.8 Undesirable effects

As Seretide contains salmeterol and fluticasone propionate, the type and severity of adverse reactions associated with each of the compounds may be expected. There is no incidence of additional adverse events following concurrent administration of the two compounds.

Adverse events which have been associated with salmeterol/fluticasone propionate are given below, listed by system organ class and frequency. Frequencies are defined as: very common (≥1/10), common (≥1/100 and <1/10), uncommon (≥1/1000 and <1/100), and very rare (<1/10,000) including isolated reports. Very common, common and uncommon events were derived from clinical trial data. The incidence in placebo was not taken into account. Very rare events were derived from post-marketing spontaneous data.

System Organ Class	Adverse Event	Frequency
Infections & Infestations	Candidiasis of the mouth and throat	Common
Immune System Disorders	Hypersensitivity reactions with the following manifestations:	
	Cutaneous hypersensitivity reactions	Uncommon
	Angioedema (mainly facial and oropharyngeal oedema), Respiratory symptoms (dyspnoea and/or bronchospasm), Anaphylactic reactions	Very Rare
Endocrine Disorders	Cushing's syndrome, Cushingoid features, Adrenal suppression, Growth retardation in children and adolescents, Decreased bone mineral density, Cataract, Glaucoma	Very Rare
Metabolism & Nutrition Disorders	Hyperglycaemia	Very Rare
Psychiatric Disorders	Anxiety, sleep disorders and behavioural changes, including hyperactivity and irritability (predominantly in children)	Very Rare
Nervous System Disorders	Headache	*Very Common
	Tremor	Common
Cardiac Disorders	Palpitations	Common
	Tachycardia	Uncommon
	Cardiac arrhythmias (including atrial fibrillation, supraventricular tachycardia and extrasystoles).	Very Rare
Respiratory, Thoracic & Mediastinal Disorders	Throat irritation	Common
	Hoarseness/ dysphonia	Common
	Paradoxical bronchospasm	Very Rare
Musculoskeletal & Connective Tissue Disorders	Muscle cramps	Common
	Arthralgia	Very Rare
	Myalgia	Very Rare

*Reported commonly in placebo

The pharmacological side effects of beta-2-agonist treatment, such as tremor, palpitations and headache, have been reported, but tend to be transient and reduce with regular therapy.

Due to the fluticasone propionate component, hoarseness and candidiasis (thrush) of the mouth and throat can occur in some patients. Both hoarseness and incidence of candidiasis may be relieved by gargling with water after using the product. Symptomatic candidiasis can be treated with topical anti-fungal therapy whilst still continuing with the Seretide Accuhaler.

Possible systemic effects include Cushing's syndrome, Cushingoid features, adrenal suppression, growth retardation in children and adolescents, decrease in bone mineral density, cataract and glaucoma (see 4.4 'Special Warnings and Precautions For Use').

There have been very rare reports of hyperglycaemia (see 4.4 'Special Warnings and Precautions for Use').

As with other inhalation therapy, paradoxical bronchospasm may occur (see 4.4 'Special Warnings and Precautions for Use').

4.9 Overdose

There are no data available from clinical trials on overdose with Seretide, however data on overdose with both drugs are given below:

The signs and symptoms of salmeterol overdose are tremor, headache and tachycardia. The preferred antidotes are cardioselective beta-blocking agents, which should be used with caution in patients with a history of bronchospasm. If Seretide therapy has to be withdrawn due to overdose of the beta agonist component of the drug, provision of appropriate replacement steroid therapy should be considered. Additionally, hypokalaemia can occur and potassium replacement should be considered.

Acute: Acute inhalation of fluticasone propionate doses in excess of those recommended may lead to temporary suppression of adrenal function. This does not need emergency action as adrenal function is recovered in a few days, as verified by plasma cortisol measurements.

Chronic overdose of inhaled fluticasone propionate: Refer to section 4.4: risk of adrenal suppression. Monitoring of adrenal reserve may be necessary. In cases of fluticasone propionate overdose Seretide therapy may still be continued at a suitable dosage for symptom control.

5. PHARMACOLOGICAL PROPERTIES

5.1 Pharmacodynamic properties

Pharmacotherapeutic Group: Adrenergics and other anti-asthmatics.

ATC Code: R03AK06

Seretide Asthma clinical trials

A twelve month study (Gaining Optimal Asthma ControL, GOAL), in 3416 adult and adolescent patients with persistent asthma, compared the safety and efficacy of Seretide versus inhaled corticosteroid (Fluticasone Propionate) alone to determine whether the goals of asthma management were achievable. Treatment was stepped up every 12 weeks until **Total control was achieved or the highest dose of study drug was reached. GOAL showed more patients treated with Seretide achieved asthma control than patients treated with ICS alone. In general these effects were observed earlier with Seretide compared to inhaled corticosteroid alone and at a lower inhaled corticosteroid dose.

The overall study results showed:

(see Table 1 below)

Two further studies in adult and adolescent patients with mild to moderate asthma have shown that control of asthma symptoms may be maintained at a lower inhaled corticosteroid dose with Seretide compared to treatment with inhaled corticosteroid alone.

Seretide COPD clinical trials

Placebo-controlled clinical trials, over 6 and 12 months, have shown that regular use of (invented name) 50/500 micrograms improves lung function and reduces breathlessness and the use of relief medication. Over a 12 month period the risk of COPD exacerbations was reduced from 1.42 per year to 0.99 per year compared with placebo and the risk of exacerbations requiring oral corticosteroids was

Table 1 Percentage of Patients Attaining *Well Controlled (WC) and **Totally Controlled (TC) Asthma over 12 months

Pre-Study Treatment	Salmeterol/FP		FP	
	WC	TC	WC	TC
No ICS (SABA alone)	78%	50%	70%	40%
Low dose ICS (≤500mcg BDP or equivalent/day)	75%	44%	60%	28%
Medium dose ICS >500-1000mcg BDP or equivalent/day)	62%	29%	47%	16%
Pooled results across the 3 treatment levels	71%	41%	59%	28%

*Well controlled asthma; occasional symptoms or SABA use or less than 80% predicted lung function plus no night-time awakenings, no exacerbations and no side effects enforcing a change in therapy

**Total control of asthma; no symptoms, no SABA use, greater than or equal to 80% predicted lung function, no night-time awakenings, no exacerbations and no side effects enforcing a change in therapy

significantly reduced from 0.81 to 0.47 per year compared with placebo.

Mechanism of action:

Seretide contains salmeterol and fluticasone propionate which have differing modes of action. The respective mechanisms of action of both drugs are discussed below:

Salmeterol:

Salmeterol is a selective long-acting (12 hour) beta-2-adrenoceptor agonist with a long side chain which binds to the exo-site of the receptor.

Salmeterol produces a longer duration of bronchodilation, lasting for at least 12 hours, than recommended doses of conventional short-acting beta-2-agonists.

Fluticasone propionate:

Fluticasone propionate given by inhalation at recommended doses has a glucocorticoid anti-inflammatory action within the lungs, resulting in reduced symptoms and exacerbations of asthma, without the adverse effects observed when corticosteroids are administered systemically.

5.2 Pharmacokinetic properties

When salmeterol and fluticasone propionate were administered in combination by the inhaled route, the pharmacokinetics of each component were similar to those observed when the drugs were administered separately. For pharmacokinetic purposes therefore each component can be considered separately.

Salmeterol:

Salmeterol acts locally in the lung therefore plasma levels are not an indication of therapeutic effects. In addition there are only limited data available on the pharmacokinetics of salmeterol because of the technical difficulty of assaying the drug in plasma due to the low plasma concentrations at therapeutic doses (approximately 200 picogram /ml or less) achieved after inhaled dosing.

Fluticasone propionate:

The absolute bioavailability of inhaled fluticasone propionate in healthy subjects varies between approximately 10-30% of the nominal dose depending on the inhalation device used. In patients with asthma or COPD a lesser degree of systemic exposure to inhaled fluticasone propionate has been observed.

Systemic absorption occurs mainly through the lungs and is initially rapid then prolonged. The remainder of the inhaled dose may be swallowed but contributes minimally to systemic exposure due to the low aqueous solubility and pre-systemic metabolism, resulting in oral availability of less than 1%. There is a linear increase in systemic exposure with increasing inhaled dose.

The disposition of fluticasone propionate is characterised by high plasma clearance (1150ml/min), a large volume of distribution at steady-state (approximately 300l) and a terminal half-life of approximately 8 hours.

Plasma protein binding is 91%.

Fluticasone propionate is cleared very rapidly from the systemic circulation. The main pathway is metabolism to an inactive carboxylic acid metabolite, by the cytochrome P450 enzyme CYP3A4. Other unidentified metabolites are also found in the faeces.

The renal clearance of fluticasone propionate is negligible. Less than 5% of the dose is excreted in urine, mainly as metabolites. The main part of the dose is excreted in faeces as metabolites and unchanged drug.

5.3 Preclinical safety data

The only safety concerns for human use derived from animal studies of salmeterol xinafoate and fluticasone propionate given separately were effects associated with exaggerated pharmacological actions.

In animal reproduction studies, glucocorticosteroids have been shown to induce malformations (cleft palate, skeletal malformations). However, these animal experimental results do not seem to be relevant for man given recommended doses. Animal studies with salmeterol xinafoate have shown embryofoetal toxicity only at high exposure levels. Following co-administration, increased incidences of transposed umbilical artery and incomplete ossification of occipital bone were found in rats at doses associated with known glucocorticoid-induced abnormalities.

6. PHARMACEUTICAL PARTICULARS

6.1 List of excipients

Lactose monohydrate (which contains milk proteins).

6.2 Incompatibilities

Not applicable.

6.3 Shelf life

18 months.

6.4 Special precautions for storage

Do not store above 30°C.

6.5 Nature and contents of container

The inhalation powder is contained in blisters held on a formed PVC coated base, with a peelable laminate lid. The strip is contained in a moulded plastic device.

One Accuhaler delivers 28 or 60 doses.

Not all pack sizes may be marketed.

6.6 Instructions for use and handling

The Accuhaler releases a powder which is inhaled into the lungs.

A dose indicator on the Accuhaler indicates the number of doses left.

For detailed instructions for use see the Patient Information Leaflet.

Administrative Data

7. MARKETING AUTHORISATION HOLDER

Glaxo Wellcome UK Ltd, trading as Allen & Hanburys,
Stockley Park West,
Uxbridge,
Middlesex, UB11 1BT

8. MARKETING AUTHORISATION NUMBER(S)

Seretide 100 Accuhaler PL10949/0314

Seretide 250 Accuhaler PL10949/0315

Seretide 500 Accuhaler PL10949/0316

9. DATE OF FIRST AUTHORISATION/RENEWAL OF THE AUTHORISATION

1 February 1999

10. DATE OF REVISION OF THE TEXT

3rd August 2005

Seretide 50, 125, 250 Evohaler

(Allen & Hanburys)

1. NAME OF THE MEDICINAL PRODUCT

Seretide 50 Evohaler

Seretide 125 Evohaler

Seretide 250 Evohaler

2. QUALITATIVE AND QUANTITATIVE COMPOSITION

Each single actuation of Seretide provides:

25 micrograms of salmeterol (as salmeterol xinafoate) and 50, 125 or 250 micrograms of fluticasone propionate (delivered from the valve). This is equivalent to 21 micrograms of salmeterol and 44, 110 or 220 micrograms of fluticasone propionate delivered from the actuator (delivered dose).

For excipients, see 6.1.

3. PHARMACEUTICAL FORM

Pressurised inhalation, suspension.

4. CLINICAL PARTICULARS

4.1 Therapeutic indications

Seretide is indicated in the regular treatment of asthma where use of a combination product (long-acting beta-2-agonist and inhaled corticosteroid) is appropriate:

- patients not adequately controlled with inhaled corticosteroids and 'as needed' inhaled short acting beta-2-agonist

or

- patients already adequately controlled on both inhaled corticosteroid and long-acting beta-2-agonist.

4.2 Posology and method of administration

Seretide Evohaler is for inhalation use only.

Patients should be made aware that Seretide Evohaler must be used daily for optimum benefit, even when asymptomatic.

Patients should be regularly reassessed by a doctor, so that the strength of Seretide they are receiving remains optimal and is only changed on medical advice. The dose should be titrated to the lowest dose at which effective control of symptoms is maintained. Where the control of symptoms is maintained with the lowest strength of the combination given twice daily then the next step could include a test of inhaled corticosteroid alone. As an alternative, patients requiring a long acting beta-2-agonist could be titrated to Seretide given once daily if, in the opinion of the prescriber, it would be adequate to maintain disease control. In the event of once daily dosing when the patient has a history of nocturnal symptoms the dose should be given at night and when the patient has a history of mainly day-time symptoms the dose should be given in the morning.

Patients should be given the strength of Seretide containing the appropriate fluticasone propionate dosage for the severity of their disease. Note: Seretide 25/50 microgram strength is not appropriate in adults and children with severe asthma. Prescribers should be aware that, in patients with asthma, fluticasone propionate is as effective as other inhaled steroids at approximately half the microgram daily dose. For example, 100mcg of fluticasone propionate is approximately equivalent to 200mcg of beclomethasone dipropionate (CFC containing) or budesonide. If an individual patient should require dosages outside the recommended regimen, appropriate doses of beta-agonist and/or corticosteroid should be prescribed.

Recommended Doses:

Adults and adolescents 12 years and older:

Two inhalations of 25 micrograms salmeterol and 50 micrograms fluticasone propionate twice daily.

or

Two inhalations of 25 micrograms salmeterol and 125 micrograms fluticasone propionate twice daily.

or

Two inhalations of 25 micrograms salmeterol and 250 micrograms fluticasone propionate twice daily.

Children 4 years and older:

Two inhalations of 25 micrograms salmeterol and 50 micrograms fluticasone propionate twice daily.

The maximum licensed dose of fluticasone propionate delivered by Seretide inhaler in children is 100mcg twice daily.

There are no data available for use of Seretide inhaler in children aged under 4 years.

The use of a spacer device with the inhaler in order to derive greater therapeutic benefit is recommended for patients (in particular young children) who have difficulty co-ordinating inhalation with actuation (see section 4.4 Special Warnings and Precautions for use)

Special patient groups:

There is no need to adjust the dose in elderly patients or in those with renal impairment. There are no data available for use of Seretide in patients with hepatic impairment.

Testing the inhaler:

Before using for the first time remove the mouthpiece cover by gently squeezing the sides of the cover, shake the inhaler well, and release puffs into the air until the counter reads 120 to make sure that it works. If the inhaler has not been used for a week or more remove themouthpiece cover, shake the inhaler well and release two puffs into the air. Each time the inhaler is activated the number on the counter will count down by one.

4.3 Contraindications

Seretide is contraindicated in patients with hypersensitivity to any of the active substances or to the excipient.

4.4 Special warnings and special precautions for use

The management of asthma should normally follow a stepwise programme and patient response should be monitored clinically and by lung function tests.

Seretide Evohaler should not be used to treat acute asthma symptoms for which a fast and short acting bronchodilator is required. Patients should be advised to have their medicinal product to be used for relief in an acute asthma attack available at all times.Seretide Evohaler is not intended for the initial management of asthma until the need for and approximate dosage of corticosteroids has been established.

Increasing use of short-acting bronchodilators to relieve asthma symptoms indicates deterioration of asthma control and patients should be reviewed by a physician.

Sudden and progressive deterioration in control of asthma is potentially life-threatening and the patient should undergo urgent medical assessment.Consideration should be given to increasing corticosteroid therapy. The patient should also be medically reviewed where the current dosage of Seretide has failed to give adequate control of asthma. Consideration should be given to additional corticosteroid therapies.

Treatment with Seretide should not be stopped abruptly.

As with all inhaled medication containing corticosteroids, Seretide should be administered with caution in patients with pulmonary tuberculosis.

Seretide should be administered with caution in patients with severe cardiovascular disorders, including heart rhythm abnormalities, diabetes mellitus, untreated hypokalaemia or thyrotoxicosis.

There have been very rare reports of increases in blood glucose levels (See 4.8 'Undesirable Effects') and this should be considered when prescribing to patients with a history of diabetes mellitus.

Potentially serious hypokalaemia may result from systemic beta-2-agonist therapy, but following inhalation at therapeutic doses plasma levels of salmeterol are very low.

As with other inhalation therapy paradoxical bronchospasm may occur with an immediate increase in wheezing after dosing. Seretide Evohaler should be discontinued immediately, the patient assessed and alternative therapy instituted if necessary.

Care should be taken when transferring patients to Seretide therapy, particularly if there is any reason to suppose that adrenal function is impaired from previous systemic steroid therapy.

Systemic effects may occur with any inhaled corticosteroid, particularly at high doses prescribed for long periods. These effects are much less likely to occur than with oral corticosteroids. Possible systemic effects include Cushing's syndrome, Cushingoid features, adrenal suppression, growth retardation in children and adolescents, decrease in bone mineral density, cataract and glaucoma. **It is important, therefore, that the patient is reviewed regularly and the dose of inhaled corticosteroid is reduced to the lowest dose at which effective control of asthma is maintained.**

It is recommended that the height of children receiving prolonged treatment with inhaled corticosteroid is regularly monitored.

Prolonged treatment of patients with high doses of inhaled corticosteroids may result in adrenal suppression and acute adrenal crisis. Children and adolescents < 16years taking high doses of fluticasone (typically ≥ 1000mcg/day) may be at particular risk. Very rare cases of adrenal suppression and acute adrenal crisis have also been described with doses of fluticasone propionate between 500 and less than 1000mcg. Situations, which could potentially trigger acute adrenal crisis, include trauma, surgery, infection or any rapid reduction in dosage. Presenting symptoms are typically vague and may include anorexia, abdominal pain, weight loss, tiredness, headache, nausea, vomiting, hypotension, decreased level of consciousness, hypoglycaemia, and seizures. Additional systemic corticosteroid cover should be considered during periods of stress or elective surgery.

As systemic absorption is largely through the lungs, the use of a spacer plus metered dose inhaler may increase drug delivery to the lungs. It should be noted that this could potentially lead to an increase in the risk of systemic adverse effects.

The benefits of inhaled fluticasone propionate therapy should minimise the need for oral steroids, but patients transferring from oral steroids may remain at risk of impaired adrenal reserve for a considerable time. Patients who have required high dose emergency corticosteroid therapy in the past may also be at risk. This possibility of residual impairment should always be borne in mind in emergency and elective situations likely to produce stress, and appropriate corticosteroid treatment must be considered. The extent of the adrenal impairment may require specialist advice before elective procedures.

Ritonavir can greatly increase the concentration of fluticasone propionate in plasma. Therefore, concomitant use should be avoided, unless the potential benefit to the patient outweighs the risk of systemic corticosteroid side-effects. There is also an increased risk of systemic side effects when combining fluticasone propionate with other potent CYP3A inhibitors (see 4.5 Interaction with Other Medicinal Products and Other Forms of Interaction).

4.5 Interaction with other medicinal products and other forms of Interaction

Both non-selective and selective beta-blockers should be avoided in patients with asthma, unless there are compelling reasons for their use.

Concomitant use of other beta-adrenergic containing drugs can have a potentially additive effect.

Under normal circumstances, low plasma concentrations of fluticasone propionate are achieved after inhaled dosing, due to extensive first pass metabolism and high systemic clearance mediated by cytochrome P450 3A4 in the gut and liver. Hence, clinically significant drug interactions mediated by fluticasone propionate are unlikely.

In an interaction study in healthy subjects with intranasal fluticasone propionate, ritonavir (a highly potent cytochrome P450 3A4 inhibitor) 100 mg b.i.d. increased the fluticasone propionate plasma concentrations several hundred fold, resulting in markedly reduced serum cortisol concentrations. Information about this interaction is lacking for inhaled fluticasone propionate, but a marked increase in fluticasone propionate plasma levels is expected. Cases of Cushing's syndrome and adrenal suppression have been reported. The combination should be avoided unless the benefit outweighs the increased risk of systemic glucocorticoid side-effects.

In a small study in healthy volunteers, the slightly less potent CYP3A inhibitor ketoconazole increased the exposure of fluticasone propionate after a single inhalation by 150%. This resulted in a greater reduction of plasma cortisol as compared with fluticasone propionate alone. Co-treatment with other potent CYP3A inhibitors, such as itraconazole, is also expected to increase the systemic fluticasone propionate exposure and the risk of systemic side-effects. Caution is recommended and long-term treatment with such drugs should if possible be avoided.

4.6 Pregnancy and lactation

There are insufficient data on the use of salmeterol and fluticasone propionate during pregnancy and lactation in man to assess the possible harmful effects. In animal studies foetal abnormalities occur after administration of beta-2-adrenoreceptor agonists and glucocorticosteroids (see 5.3 'Preclinical Safety Data').

Administration of Seretide to pregnant women should only be considered if the expected benefit to the mother is greater than any possible risk to the foetus.

The lowest effective dose of fluticasone propionate needed to maintain adequate asthma control should be used in the treatment of pregnant women.

There are no data available for human breast milk. Both salmeterol and fluticasone propionate are excreted into breast milk in rats. Administration of Seretide to women who are breastfeeding should only be considered if the expected benefit to the mother is greater than any possible risk to the child.

4.7 Effects on ability to drive and use machines

No studies of the effect on the ability to drive and use machines have been performed.

4.8 Undesirable effects

As Seretide contains salmeterol and fluticasone propionate, the type and severity of adverse reactions associated with each of the compounds may be expected. There is no incidence of additional adverse events following concurrent administration of the two compounds.

Adverse events which have been associated with salmeterol/fluticasone propionate are given below, listed by system organ class and frequency. Frequencies are defined as: very common (≥ 1/10), common (≥ 1/100 and < 1/10), uncommon (≥ 1/1000 and < 1/100), and very rare (< 1/10,000) including isolated reports. Very common, common and uncommon events were derived from clinical trial data. The incidence in placebo was not taken into account. Very rare events were derived from post-marketing spontaneous data.

System Organ Class	Adverse Event	Frequency
Infections & Infestations	Candidiasis of the mouth and throat	Common
Immune System Disorders	Hypersensitivity reactions with the following manifestations:	
	Cutaneous hypersensitivity reactions	Uncommon
	Angioedema (mainly facial and oropharyngeal oedema), Respiratory symptoms (dyspnoea and/or bronchospasm), Anaphylactic reactions	Very Rare
Endocrine Disorders	Cushing's syndrome, Cushingoid features, Adrenal suppression, Growth retardation in children and adolescents, Decreased bone mineral density, Cataract, Glaucoma	Very Rare
Metabolism & Nutrition Disorders	Hyperglycaemia	Very Rare
Psychiatric Disorders	Anxiety, sleep disorders and behavioural changes, including hyperactivity and irritability (predominantly in children)	Very Rare
Nervous System Disorders	Headache	Very Common
	Tremor	Common
Cardiac Disorders	Palpitations	Common
	Tachycardia	Uncommon
	Cardiac arrhythmias (including atrial fibrillation, supraventricular tachycardia and extrasystoles).	Very Rare
Respiratory, Thoracic & Mediastinal Disorders	Throat irritation	Common
	Hoarseness/ dysphonia	Common
	Paradoxical bronchospasm	Very Rare
Musculoskeletal & Connective Tissue Disorders	Muscle cramps	Common
	Arthralgia	Very Rare
	Myalgia	Very Rare

*Reported commonly in placebo

The pharmacological side effects of beta-2-agonist treatment, such as tremor, palpitations and headache, have been reported, but tend to be transient and reduce with regular therapy.

Due to the fluticasone propionate component, hoarseness and candidiasis (thrush) of the mouth and throat can occur in some patients.Both hoarseness and incidence of candidiasis may be relieved by gargling with water after using the product. Symptomatic candidiasis can be treated with topical anti-fungal therapy whilst still continuing with the Seretide Evohaler.

Possible systemic effects include Cushing's syndrome, Cushingoid features, adrenal suppression, growth retardation in children and adolescents, decrease in bone mineral density, cataract and glaucoma (see 4.4 'Special Warnings and Precautions For Use').

There have been very rare reports of hyperglycaemia (see 4.4 'Special Warnings and Precautions for Use').

As with other inhalation therapy, paradoxical bronchospasm may occur (see 4.4 'Special Warnings and Precautions for Use').

4.9 Overdose

There are no data available from clinical trials on overdose with Seretide, however data on overdose with both drugs are given below:

The signs and symptoms of salmeterol overdose are tremor, headache and tachycardia. The preferred antidotes are cardioselective beta-blocking agents, which should be used with caution in patients with a history of bronchospasm. If Seretide therapy has to be withdrawn due to overdose of the beta agonist component of the drug, provision of appropriate replacement steroid therapy should be considered. Additionally, hypokalaemia can occur and potassium replacement should be considered.

Acute: Acute inhalation of fluticasone propionate doses in excess of those recommended may lead to temporary suppression of adrenal function. This does not need emergency action as adrenal function is recovered in a few days, as verified by plasma cortisol measurements.

Chronic overdose of inhaled fluticasone propionate: Refer to section 4.4: risk of adrenal suppression. Monitoring of adrenal reserve may be necessary. In cases of fluticasone propionate overdose Seretide therapy may still be continued at a suitable dosage for symptom control.

5. PHARMACOLOGICAL PROPERTIES

5.1 Pharmacodynamic properties

Pharmacotherapeutic Group: Adrenergics and other anti-asthmatics.

ATC Code: R03AK06

Seretide Asthma clinical trials

A twelve month study (Gaining Optimal Asthma ControL, GOAL), in 3416 adult and adolescent patients with persistent asthma, compared the safety and efficacy of Seretide versus inhaled corticosteroid (Fluticasone Propionate) alone to determine whether the goals of asthma management were achievable. Treatment was stepped up every 12 weeks until **Total control was achieved or the highest dose of study drug was reached. GOAL showed more patients treated with Seretide achieved asthma control than patients treated with ICS alone. In general these effects were observed earlier with Seretide compared to inhaled corticosteroid alone and at a lower inhaled corticosteroid dose.

The overall study results showed:

(see Table 1 on next page)

Two further studies in adult and adolescent patients with mild to moderate asthma have shown that control of asthma symptoms may be maintained at a lower inhaled corticosteroid dose with Seretide compared to treatment with inhaled corticosteroid alone.

Mechanism of action:

Seretide contains salmeterol and fluticasone propionate which have differing modes of action.

The respective mechanisms of action of both drugs are discussed below.

Salmeterol:

Salmeterol is a selective long-acting (12 hour) beta-2-adrenoceptor agonist with a long side chain which binds to the exo-site of the receptor.

Salmeterol produces a longer duration of bronchodilation, lasting for at least 12 hours, than recommended doses of conventional short-acting beta-2-agonists.

Fluticasone propionate:

Fluticasone propionate given by inhalation at recommended doses has a glucocorticoid anti-inflammatory action within the lungs, resulting in reduced symptoms and exacerbations of asthma, with less adverse effects than when corticosteroids are administered systemically.

5.2 Pharmacokinetic properties

When salmeterol and fluticasone propionate were administered in combination by the inhaled route, the pharmacokinetics of each component were similar to those observed when the drugs were administered separately. For pharmacokinetic purposes therefore each component can be considered separately.

Table 1 Percentage of Patients Attaining *Well Controlled (WC) and **Totally Controlled (TC) Asthma over 12 months

Pre-Study Treatment	Salmeterol/FP		FP	
	WC	TC	WC	TC
No ICS (SABA alone)	78%	50%	70%	40%
Low dose ICS (≤500mcg BDP or equivalent/day)	75%	44%	60%	28%
Medium dose ICS >500-1000mcg BDP or equivalent/day)	62%	29%	47%	16%
Pooled results across the 3 treatment levels	71%	41%	59%	28%

*Well controlled asthma; occasional symptoms or SABA use or less than 80% predicted lung function plus no night-time awakenings, no exacerbations and no side effects enforcing a change in therapy

**Total control of asthma; no symptoms, no SABA use, greater than or equal to 80% predicted lung function, no night-time awakenings, no exacerbations and no side effects enforcing a change in therapy

Salmeterol:

Salmeterol acts locally in the lung therefore plasma levels are not an indication of therapeutic effects. In addition there are only limited data available on the pharmacokinetics of salmeterol because of the technical difficulty of assaying the drug in plasma due to the low plasma concentrations at therapeutic doses (approximately 200 picogram/ml or less) achieved after inhaled dosing.

Fluticasone propionate:

The absolute bioavailability of inhaled fluticasone propionate in healthy subjects varies between approximately 10-30% of the nominal dose depending on the inhalation device used. In patients with asthma a lesser degree of systemic exposure to inhaled fluticasone propionate has been observed.

Systemic absorption occurs mainly through the lungs and is initially rapid then prolonged. The remainder of the inhaled dose may be swallowed but contributes minimally to systemic exposure due to the low aqueous solubility and pre-systemic metabolism, resulting in oral availability of less than 1%. There is a linear increase in systemic exposure with increasing inhaled dose.

The disposition of fluticasone propionate is characterised by high plasma clearance (1150ml/min), a large volume of distribution at steady-state (approximately 300l) and a terminal half-life of approximately 8 hours.

Plasma protein binding is 91%.

Fluticasone propionate is cleared very rapidly from the systemic circulation. The main pathway is metabolism to an inactive carboxylic acid metabolite, by the cytochrome P450 enzyme CYP3A4. Other unidentified metabolites are also found in the faeces.

The renal clearance of fluticasone propionate is negligible. Less than 5% of the dose is excreted in urine, mainly as metabolites. The main part of the dose is excreted as faeces as metabolites and unchanged drug.

5.3 Preclinical safety data

The only safety concerns for human use derived from animal studies of salmeterol xinafoate and fluticasone propionate given separately were effects associated with exaggerated pharmacological actions.

In animal reproduction studies, glucocorticosteroids have been shown to induce malformations (cleft palate, skeletal malformations). However, these animal experimental results do not seem to be relevant for man given recommended doses. Animal studies with salmeterol xinafoate have shown embryofoetal toxicity only at high exposure levels. Following co-administration, increased incidences of transposed umbilical artery and incomplete ossification of occipital bone were found in rats at doses associated with known glucocorticoid-induced abnormalities.

The non-CFC propellant, Norflurane, has been shown to have no toxic effect at very high vapour concentrations, far in excess of those likely to be experienced by patients, in a wide range of animal species exposed daily for periods of two years.

6. PHARMACEUTICAL PARTICULARS

6.1 List of excipients

Norflurane (HFA 134a).

6.2 Incompatibilities

Not applicable.

6.3 Shelf life

1 year.

6.4 Special precautions for storage

Do not store above 25° C.

6.5 Nature and contents of container

The suspension is contained in an internally lacquered, 8ml aluminium alloy pressurised container sealed with a metering valve. The containers are fitted into plastic actuators incorporating an atomising mouthpiece and fitted with dustcaps. The canister has a counter attached to it, which shows how many actuations of medicine are left. The number will show through a window in the back of the plastic actuator. One pressurised container delivers 120 actuations.

The devices are available in cardboard containers, which hold

1 × 120 actuations Inhaler

or 3 × 120 actuations Inhaler

or 10 × 120 actuations Inhaler - hospital/pharmacy use only (for dispensing purposes)

Not all pack sizes may be marketed.

6.6 Instructions for use and handling

Patients should be carefully instructed in the proper use of their inhaler (see Patient Information Leaflet).

As with most inhaled medicinal products in pressurised containers, the therapeutic effect of this medicinal product may decrease when the container is cold.

The container should not be punctured, broken or burnt even when apparently empty.

DO NOT PUT THE METAL CONTAINER IN WATER.

Administrative Data

7. MARKETING AUTHORISATION HOLDER

Glaxo Wellcome UK Limited
Trading as Allen & Hanburys
Stockley Park West
Uxbridge
Middlesex UB11 1BT.

8. MARKETING AUTHORISATION NUMBER(S)

Seretide 50 Evohaler PL10949/00337
Seretide 125 Evohaler PL10949/0338
Seretide 250 Evohaler PL10949/0339

9. DATE OF FIRST AUTHORISATION/RENEWAL OF THE AUTHORISATION

16 June 2000

10. DATE OF REVISION OF THE TEXT

3rd August 2005

Serevent Accuhaler

(Allen & Hanburys)

1. NAME OF THE MEDICINAL PRODUCT

Serevent™ Accuhaler™

2. QUALITATIVE AND QUANTITATIVE COMPOSITION

Serevent Accuhaler is a moulded plastic device containing a foil strip with regularly spaced blisters each containing 50 micrograms of salmeterol (as xinafoate).

For excipients, see 6.1

3. PHARMACEUTICAL FORM

Inhalation powder.

4. CLINICAL PARTICULARS

4.1 Therapeutic indications

Salmeterol is a selective β_2-agonist indicated for reversible airways obstruction in patients with asthma and chronic obstructive pulmonary disease (COPD).

In asthma (including nocturnal asthma and exercise induced symptoms) it is indicated for those treated with inhaled corticosteroids who require a long-acting beta agonist in accordance with current treatment guidelines.

Serevent Accuhaler is not a replacement for inhaled or oral corticosteroids which should be continued at the same dose, and not stopped or reduced, when treatment with Serevent Accuhaler is initiated.

4.2 Posology and method of administration

Serevent Accuhaler is for inhalation use only.

Serevent Accuhaler should be used regularly. The full benefits of treatment will be apparent after several doses of the drug.

In reversible airways obstruction such as asthma

Adults (including the elderly): One inhalation (50 micrograms) twice daily, increasing to two inhalations (2 × 50 micrograms) twice daily if required.

Children 4 years and over: One inhalation (50 micrograms) twice daily.

The dosage or frequency of administration should only be increased on medical advice.

There are insufficient clinical data to recommend the use of Serevent Accuhaler in children under the age of four.

In chronic obstructive pulmonary disease

Adults (including the elderly): One inhalation (50 micrograms) twice daily.

Children: Not appropriate.

Special patient groups: There is no need to adjust the dose in patients with impaired renal function.

4.3 Contraindications

Hypersensitivity to any ingredient of the preparation (see Pharmaceutical Particulars – List of Excipients 6.1)

4.4 Special warnings and special precautions for use

Serevent Accuhaler should not be initiated in patients with significantly worsening or acutely deteriorating asthma.

Sudden and progressive deterioration in asthma control is potentially life-threatening and consideration should be given to starting or increasing corticosteroid therapy. Under these circumstances, daily peak flow monitoring may be advisable. For maintenance treatment of asthma Serevent should be given in combination with inhaled or oral corticosteroids.

Serevent Accuhaler is not a replacement for inhaled or oral corticosteroids (see *Therapeutic indications*). Patients with asthma must be warned not to stop steroid therapy, and not to reduce it without medical advice, even if they feel better on Serevent Accuhaler.

With its relatively slow onset of action Serevent Accuhaler should not be used to relieve acute asthma symptoms, for which an inhaled short-acting bronchodilator is required. Patients should be advised to have such rescue medication available.

Long-acting bronchodilators should not be the only or the main treatment in maintenance asthma therapy (*see Therapeutic Indications*).

Increasing use of bronchodilators, in particular short-acting inhaled β_2-agonists to relieve symptoms, indicates deterioration of asthma control. The patient should be instructed to seek medical advice if short-acting relief bronchodilator treatment becomes less effective, or more inhalations than usual are required. In this situation the patient should be assessed and consideration given to the need for increased anti-inflammatory therapy (e.g. higher doses of inhaled corticosteroid or a course of oral corticosteroid). Severe exacerbations of asthma must be treated in the normal way.

Salmeterol should be administered with caution in patients with thyrotoxicosis.

Potentially serious hypokalaemia may result from β_2-agonist therapy. Particular caution is advised in acute severe asthma as this effect may be potentiated by hypoxia and by concomitant treatment with xanthine derivatives, steroids and diuretics. Serum potassium levels should be monitored in such situations.

Patients should be instructed in proper use and their technique checked to ensure that the drug is reaching the target areas within the lungs.

4.5 Interaction with other medicinal products and other forms of Interaction

Both non-selective and selective β-blockers should be avoided in patients with reversible obstructive airways disease, unless there are compelling reasons for their use.

4.6 Pregnancy and lactation

In animal studies, some effects on the fetus, typical for a β_2-agonist, occurred at exposure levels substantially higher than those that occur with therapeutic use. Extensive experience with other β_2-agonists has provided no evidence that such effects are relevant for women receiving clinical doses. As yet, experience of the use of salmeterol during pregnancy is limited. As with any medicine, use during pregnancy should be considered only if the expected benefit to the mother is greater than any possible risk to the fetus.

Plasma levels of salmeterol after inhaled therapeutic doses are negligible, and therefore levels in milk should be correspondingly low. Nevertheless, as there is limited experience of the use of salmeterol in nursing mothers, its use in such circumstances should only be considered if the expected benefit to the mother is greater than any possible risk to the infant.

Studies in lactating animals support the view that salmeterol is likely to be secreted in only very small amounts into breast milk.

4.7 Effects on ability to drive and use machines

None reported.

4.8 Undesirable effects

As with other inhalation therapy, paradoxical bronchospasm may occur with an immediate increase in wheezing and drop in peak expiratory flow rate (PEFR) after dosing.

This responds to a fast-acting inhaled bronchodilator. Serevent Accuhaler should be discontinued immediately, the patient assessed, and if necessary an alternative presentation or therapy should be instituted.

The pharmacological side effects of β_2-agonist treatment, such as tremor, subjective palpitations and headache, have been reported, but tend to be transient and to reduce with regular therapy. Tachycardia may occur in some patients. In common with other β_2 agonists, cardiac arrhythmias (including atrial fibrillation, supraventricular tachycardia and extrasystoles) have been reported in association with the use of salmeterol, usually in susceptible patients.

Potentially serious hypokalaemia may result from β_2-agonist therapy.

There have been reports of the following: hypersensitivity reactions such as rash and oedema including angioedema; muscle cramps, non-specific chest pain, arthralgia, nausea, dizziness, nervousness, insomnia and oropharyngeal irritation.

4.9 Overdose
The symptoms and signs of salmeterol overdosage are tremor, headache and tachycardia. Hypokalaemia may occur. Monitor serum potassium levels. The preferred antidote for overdosage with Serevent Accuhaler is a cardioselective β-blocking agent. Cardioselective β-blocking drugs should be used with caution in patients with a history of bronchospasm.

5. PHARMACOLOGICAL PROPERTIES

5.1 Pharmacodynamic properties
Salmeterol is a selective long-acting (usually 12 hours) β_2-adrenoceptor agonist with a long side-chain which binds to the exo-site of the receptor. These pharmacological properties of salmeterol offer more effective protection against histamine-induced bronchoconstriction and produce a longer duration of bronchodilatation, lasting for at least 12 hours, than recommended doses of conventional short-acting β_2-agonists. *In vitro* tests have shown that salmeterol is a potent and long-lasting inhibitor of the release from the human lung of mast cell mediators, such as histamine, leukotrienes and prostaglandin D2. In man, salmeterol inhibits the early and late phase response to inhaled allergen; the latter persisting for over 30 hours after a single dose when the bronchodilator effect is no longer evident. Single dosing with salmeterol attenuates bronchial hyper-responsiveness. These properties indicate that salmeterol has additional non-bronchodilator activity, but the full clinical significance is not yet clear. The mechanism is different from the anti-inflammatory effect of corticosteroids, which should not be stopped or reduced when Serevent Accuhaler is prescribed.

Salmeterol has been studied in the treatment of conditions associated with COPD, and has been shown to improve symptoms and pulmonary function, and quality of life. Salmeterol acts as a β_2-agonist on the reversible component of the disease. *In vitro* salmeterol has also been shown to increase cilial beat frequency of human bronchial epithelial cells, and also reduce a ciliotoxic effect of *Pseudomonas* toxin on the bronchial epithelium of patients with cystic fibrosis.

5.2 Pharmacokinetic properties
Salmeterol acts locally in the lung, therefore plasma levels are not predictive of therapeutic effects. In addition there are only limited data available on the pharmacokinetics of salmeterol because of the technical difficulty of assaying the drug in plasma because of the very low plasma concentrations at therapeutic doses (approximately 200 pg/ml or less) achieved after inhaled dosing. After regular dosing with salmeterol xinafoate, xinafoic acid can be detected in the systemic circulation, reaching steady state concentrations of approximately 100 ng/ml. These concentrations are up to 1000-fold lower than steady state levels observed in toxicity studies. These concentrations in long term regular dosing (more than 12 months) in patients with airways obstruction, have been shown to produce no ill effects.

5.3 Preclinical safety data
In reproduction studies in animals, some effects on the fetus, typical of a β_2-agonist, have been observed at very high doses.

Salmeterol xinafoate produced no genetic toxicity in a range of studies using either prokaryotic or eukaryotic cell systems *in vitro* or *in vivo* in the rat.

Long term studies with salmeterol xinafoate, induced class-related benign tumours of smooth muscle in the mesovarium of rats and the uterus of mice. The scientific literature and our own pharmacological studies provide good evidence that these effects are species-specific and have no relevance for clinical use.

6. PHARMACEUTICAL PARTICULARS

6.1 List of excipients
Lactose (which contains milk protein).

6.2 Incompatibilities
None reported.

6.3 Shelf life
24 months when not stored above 30°C for moderate climates.

18 months when not stored above 30°C for tropical climates.

6.4 Special precautions for storage
Do not store above 30°C.

Store in the original package.

6.5 Nature and contents of container
The powder mix of salmeterol xinafoate and lactose is filled into a blister strip consisting of a formed base foil with a peelable foil laminate lid. The foil strip is contained within the Accuhaler device. Pack sizes 28 or 60. Not all pack sizes may be marketed.

6.6 Instructions for use and handling
The powdered medicine is inhaled through the mouth into the lungs.

The Accuhaler device contains the medicine in individual blisters which are opened as the device is manipulated.

For detailed instructions for use refer to the Patient Information Leaflet in every pack.

Administrative Data

7. MARKETING AUTHORISATION HOLDER
Glaxo Wellcome UK Ltd

Trading as Allen & Hanburys

Stockley Park West

Uxbridge

Middlesex UB11 1BT.

8. MARKETING AUTHORISATION NUMBER(S)
10949/0214

9. DATE OF FIRST AUTHORISATION/RENEWAL OF THE AUTHORISATION
13 July 2000

10. DATE OF REVISION OF THE TEXT
4 February 2004

11. Legal Status
POM

Serevent Diskhaler

(Allen & Hanburys)

1. NAME OF THE MEDICINAL PRODUCT
SereventTM DiskhalerTM

2. QUALITATIVE AND QUANTITATIVE COMPOSITION
Disks comprising four regularly spaced double-foil blisters each delivering a mixture of 50 micrograms salmeterol (as xinafoate) and lactose used in a Diskhaler device.

For excipients, see 6.1

3. PHARMACEUTICAL FORM
Inhalation powder.

4. CLINICAL PARTICULARS

4.1 Therapeutic indications
Salmeterol is a selective β2-agonist indicated for reversible airways obstruction in patients with asthma and chronic obstructive pulmonary disease (COPD).

In asthma (including nocturnal asthma and exercise induced symptoms) it is indicated for those treated with inhaled corticosteroids who require a long-acting beta agonist in accordance with current treatment guidelines.

Serevent Diskhaler is not a replacement for inhaled or oral corticosteroids which should be continued at the same dose, and not stopped or reduced, when treatment with Serevent Diskhaler is initiated.

4.2 Posology and method of administration
Serevent Diskhaler is for inhalation use only.

Serevent Diskhaler should be used regularly. The full benefits of treatment will be apparent after several doses of the drug.

<u>In reversible airways obstruction such as asthma</u>

Adults (including the elderly): One blister (50 micrograms) twice daily, increasing to two blisters (2 × 50 micrograms) twice daily if required.

Children 4 years and over: One blister (50 micrograms) twice daily.

The dosage or frequency of administration should only be increased on medical advice.

There are insufficient clinical data to recommend the use of Serevent Diskhaler in children under the age of four.

<u>In chronic obstructive pulmonary disease</u>

Adults (including the elderly): One blister (50 micrograms) twice daily.

Children: Not appropriate.

Special patient groups: There is no need to adjust the dose in patients with impaired renal function.

4.3 Contraindications
Hypersensitivity to any ingredient of the preparation (see Pharmaceutical Particulars – List of Excipients 6.1)

4.4 Special warnings and special precautions for use
Serevent Diskhaler should not be initiated in patients with significantly worsening or acutely deteriorating asthma.

Sudden and progressive deterioration in asthma control is potentially life-threatening and consideration should be given to starting or increasing corticosteroid therapy. Under these circumstances, regular peak flow monitoring may be advisable. For maintenance treatment of asthma Serevent should be given in combination with inhaled or oral corticosteroids.

Serevent Diskhaler is not a replacement for inhaled or oral corticosteroids (see *Therapeutic indications*). Patients with asthma must be warned not to stop steroid therapy, and not to reduce it without medical advice, even if they feel better on Serevent Diskhaler.

With its relatively slow onset of action Serevent Diskhaler should not be used to relieve acute asthma symptoms, for which an inhaled short-acting bronchodilator is required. Patients should be advised to have such rescue medication available.

Long-acting bronchodilators should not be the only or the main treatment in maintenance asthma therapy (*see Therapeutic Indications*).

Increasing use of bronchodilators, in particular short-acting inhaled β2-agonists to relieve symptoms, indicates deterioration of asthma control. The patient should be instructed to seek medical advice if short-acting relief bronchodilator treatment becomes less effective, or more inhalations than usual are required. In this situation the patient should be assessed and consideration given to the need for increased anti-inflammatory therapy (e.g. higher doses of inhaled corticosteroid or a course of oral corticosteroid). Severe exacerbations of asthma must be treated in the normal way.

Salmeterol should be administered with caution in patients with thyrotoxicosis.

Potentially serious hypokalaemia may result from β2-agonist therapy. Particular caution is advised in acute severe asthma as this effect may be potentiated by hypoxia and by concomitant treatment with xanthine derivatives, steroids and diuretics. Serum potassium levels should be monitored in such situations.

4.5 Interaction with other medicinal products and other forms of Interaction
Both non-selective and selective β-blockers should be avoided in patients with reversible obstructive airways disease, unless there are compelling reasons for their use.

4.6 Pregnancy and lactation
In animal studies, some effects on the fetus, typical for a β2-agonist, occurred at exposure levels substantially higher than those that occur with therapeutic use. Extensive experience with other β2-agonists has provided no evidence that such effects are relevant for women receiving clinical doses. As yet, experience of the use of salmeterol during pregnancy is limited. As with any medicine, use during pregnancy should be considered only if the expected benefit to the mother is greater than any possible risk to the fetus.

Plasma levels of salmeterol after inhaled therapeutic doses are negligible, and therefore levels in milk should be correspondingly low. Nevertheless, as there is limited experience of the use of salmeterol in nursing mothers, its use in such circumstances should only be considered if the expected benefit to the mother is greater than any possible risk to the infant.

Studies in lactating animals support the view that salmeterol is likely to be secreted in only very small amounts into breast milk.

4.7 Effects on ability to drive and use machines
None reported.

4.8 Undesirable effects
As with other inhalation therapy, paradoxical bronchospasm may occur with an immediate increase in wheezing and drop in peak expiratory flow rate (PEFR) after dosing. This responds to a fast-acting inhaled bronchodilator. Serevent Diskhaler should be discontinued immediately, the patient assessed, and if necessary an alternative presentation or therapy should be instituted.

The pharmacological side-effects of β2-agonist treatment, such as tremor, subjective palpitations and headache, have been reported, but tend to be transient and to reduce with regular therapy. Tachycardia may occur in some patients. In common with other β2 agonists, cardiac arrhythmias (including atrial fibrillation, supraventricular tachycardia and extrasystoles) have been reported in association with the use of salmeterol, usually in susceptible patients.

Potentially serious hypokalaemia may result from β2-agonist therapy.

There have been reports of the following: hypersensitivity reactions such as rash and oedema including angioedema; muscle cramps, non-specific chest pain, arthralgia, nausea, dizziness, nervousness, insomnia and oropharyngeal irritation.

4.9 Overdose
The symptoms and signs of salmeterol overdosage are tremor, headache and tachycardia. Hypokalaemia may occur. Monitor serum potassium levels. The preferred antidote for overdosage with Serevent Diskhaler is a cardioselective β-blocking agent. Cardioselective β-blocking drugs should be used with caution in patients with a history of bronchospasm.

5. PHARMACOLOGICAL PROPERTIES

5.1 Pharmacodynamic properties

Salmeterol is a selective long-acting (usually 12 hours) β2-adrenoceptor agonist with a long side-chain which binds to the exo-site of the receptor. These pharmacological properties of salmeterol offer more effective protection against histamine-induced bronchoconstriction and produce a longer duration of bronchodilatation, lasting for at least 12 hours, than recommended doses of conventional short-acting β2-agonists. *In vitro* tests have shown that salmeterol is a potent and long-lasting inhibitor of the release from the human lung of mast cell mediators, such as histamine, leukotrienes and prostaglandin D2. In man, salmeterol inhibits the early and late phase response to inhaled allergen; the latter persisting for over 30 hours after a single dose when the bronchodilator effect is no longer evident. Single dosing with salmeterol attenuates bronchial hyper-responsiveness. These properties indicate that salmeterol has additional non-bronchodilator activity, but the full clinical significance is not yet clear. The mechanism is different from the anti-inflammatory effect of corticosteroids, which should not be stopped or reduced when Serevent Diskhaler is prescribed.

Salmeterol has been studied in the treatment of conditions associated with COPD, and has been shown to improve symptoms and pulmonary function, and quality of life. Salmeterol acts as a β2-agonist on the reversible component of the disease. *In vitro* salmeterol has also been shown to increase cilial beat frequency of human bronchial epithelial cells, and also reduce a ciliotoxic effect of *Pseudomonas* toxin on the bronchial epithelium of patients with cystic fibrosis.

5.2 Pharmacokinetic properties

Salmeterol acts locally in the lung, therefore plasma levels are not predictive of therapeutic effect. In addition there are only limited data available on the pharmacokinetics of salmeterol because of the technical difficulty of assaying the drug in plasma because of the very low plasma concentrations (approximately 200 pg/ml or less) achieved after inhaled dosing. After regular dosing with salmeterol xinafoate, xinafoic acid can be detected in the systemic circulation, reaching steady state concentrations of approximately 100 ng/ml. These concentrations are up to 1000-fold lower than steady state levels observed in toxicity studies. These concentrations in long term regular dosing (more than 12 months) in patients with airways obstruction, have been shown to produce no ill effects.

5.3 Preclinical safety data

In reproduction studies in animals, some effects on the fetus, typical of a β2-agonist, have been observed at very high doses.

Salmeterol xinafoate produced no genetic toxicity in a range of studies using either prokaryotic or eukaryotic cell systems *in vitro* or *in vivo* in the rat.

Long-term studies with salmeterol xinafoate, induced class-related benign tumours of smooth muscle in the mesovarium of rats and the uterus of mice. The scientific literature and our own pharmacological studies provide good evidence that these effects are species-specific and have no relevance for clinical use.

6. PHARMACEUTICAL PARTICULARS

6.1 List of excipients

Lactose (which contains milk protein).

6.2 Incompatibilities

None reported.

6.3 Shelf life

2 years when not stored above 25°C.

6.4 Special precautions for storage

Do not store above 25°C.

A disk may be kept in the Diskhaler device but the blisters must only be pierced immediately prior to use.

6.5 Nature and contents of container

A circular double-foil disk with four blisters containing the powder mix of salmeterol (as xinafoate) and lactose. The foil disk is inserted into the Diskhaler device.

The following packs are registered: 5, 7, 10, 14, 15 disks alone or with a Diskhaler. Starter pack consisting of a Diskhaler pre-loaded with one disk (with or without a spare disk, peak flow meter and diary card).

The following packs are available: 14 disks alone or with a Diskhaler. 5 disks with a Diskhaler (Hospital only).

6.6 Instructions for use and handling

The powdered medicine is inhaled through the mouth into the lungs. The Diskhaler device is loaded with a disk which contains the medicine in individual blisters which are opened as the device is manipulated.

For detailed instructions for use refer to the Patient Information Leaflet in every pack.

Administrative Data

7. MARKETING AUTHORISATION HOLDER

Glaxo Wellcome UK Ltd, trading as Allen & Hanburys

Stockley Park West,

Uxbridge, Middlesex, UB11 1BT

8. MARKETING AUTHORISATION NUMBER(S)

10949/0069

9. DATE OF FIRST AUTHORISATION/RENEWAL OF THE AUTHORISATION

14 October 1996

10. DATE OF REVISION OF THE TEXT

4 February 2004

11. Legal Category

POM.

Diskhaler and Serevent are trade marks of the Glaxo Wellcome Group of Companies.

Serevent Inhaler

(Allen & Hanburys)

1. NAME OF THE MEDICINAL PRODUCT

Serevent™ Inhaler

2. QUALITATIVE AND QUANTITATIVE COMPOSITION

Each metered dose actuation delivers 25 micrograms salmeterol (as xinafoate).

Each canister delivers 60/120 actuations.

For excipients, see 6.1

3. PHARMACEUTICAL FORM

Pressurised metered-dose aerosol.

4. CLINICAL PARTICULARS

4.1 Therapeutic indications

Salmeterol is a selective β2-agonist indicated for reversible airways obstruction in patients with asthma and chronic obstructive pulmonary disease (COPD).

In asthma (including nocturnal asthma and exercise induced symptoms) it is indicated for those treated with inhaled corticosteroids who require a long-acting beta agonist in accordance with current treatment guidelines.

Serevent Inhaler is not a replacement for inhaled or oral corticosteroids which should be continued at the same dose, and not stopped or reduced, when treatment with Serevent Inhaler is initiated.

4.2 Posology and method of administration

Serevent Inhaler is for inhalation use only. A Volumatic™ spacer device may be used in patients who find it difficult to synchronise aerosol actuation with inspiration of breath.

Serevent Inhaler should be used regularly. The full benefits of treatment will be apparent after several doses of the drug.

<u>In reversible airways obstruction such as asthma</u>

Adults (including the elderly): Two inhalations (2 × 25 micrograms) twice daily, increasing to four inhalations (4 × 25 micrograms) twice daily if required.

Children aged 4 years and over: Two inhalations (2 × 25 micrograms) twice daily.

The dosage or frequency of administration should only be increased on medical advice.

There are insufficient clinical data to recommend the use of Serevent Inhaler in children under the age of four.

<u>In chronic obstructive pulmonary disease</u>

Adults (including the elderly): Two inhalations (2 × 25 micrograms) twice daily.

Children: Not appropriate.

Special patient groups: There is no need to adjust the dose in patients with impaired renal function.

4.3 Contraindications

Hypersensitivity to any ingredient of the preparation (see Pharmaceutical Particulars – List of Excipients 6.1).

4.4 Special warnings and special precautions for use

Serevent Inhaler should not be initiated in patients with significantly worsening or acutely deteriorating asthma.

Sudden and progressive deterioration in asthma control is potentially life-threatening and consideration should be given to starting or increasing corticosteroid therapy. Under these circumstances, regular peak flow monitoring may be advisable. For maintenance treatment of asthma Serevent should be given in combination with inhaled or oral corticosteroids.

Serevent Inhaler is not a replacement for inhaled or oral corticosteroids (see *Therapeutic indications*). Patients with asthma must be warned not to stop steroid therapy and not to reduce it without medical advice, even if they feel better on Serevent Inhaler.

With its relatively slow onset of action Serevent Inhaler should not be used to relieve acute asthma symptoms, for which an inhaled short-acting bronchodilator is required. Patients should be advised to have such rescue medication available.

Long-acting bronchodilators should not be the only or the main treatment in maintenance asthma therapy (*see Therapeutic Indications*

Increasing use of bronchodilators, in particular short-acting inhaled β2-agonists to relieve symptoms, indicates deterioration of asthma control. The patient should be instructed to seek medical advice if short-acting relief bronchodilator treatment becomes less effective, or more inhalations than usual are required. In this situation the patient should be assessed and consideration given to the need for increased anti-inflammatory therapy (e.g. higher doses of inhaled corticosteroid or a course of oral corticosteroid). Severe exacerbations of asthma must be treated in the normal way.

Salmeterol should be administered with caution in patients with thyrotoxicosis.

Potentially serious hypokalaemia may result from β2-agonist therapy. Particular caution is advised in acute severe asthma as this effect may be potentiated by hypoxia and by concomitant treatment with xanthine derivatives, steroids and diuretics. Serum potassium levels should be monitored in such situations.

4.5 Interaction with other medicinal products and other forms of Interaction

Both non-selective and selective β-blockers should be avoided in patients with reversible obstructive airways disease, unless there are compelling reasons for their use.

4.6 Pregnancy and lactation

In animal studies, some effects on the foetus, typical for a β2-agonist, occurred at exposure levels substantially higher than those that occur with therapeutic use. Extensive experience with other β2-agonists has provided no evidence that such effects are relevant for women receiving clinical doses. As yet, experience of the use of salmeterol during pregnancy is limited. As with any medicine, use during pregnancy should be considered only if the expected benefit to the mother is greater than any possible risk to the foetus.

Plasma levels of salmeterol after inhaled therapeutic doses are negligible, and therefore levels in milk should be correspondingly low. Nevertheless, as there is limited experience of the use of salmeterol in nursing mothers, its use in such circumstances should only be considered if the expected benefit to the mother is greater than any possible risk to the infant.

Studies in lactating animals support the view that salmeterol is likely to be secreted in only very small amounts into breast milk.

4.7 Effects on ability to drive and use machines

None reported.

4.8 Undesirable effects

As with other inhalation therapy, paradoxical bronchospasm may occur with an immediate increase in wheezing and drop in peak expiratory flow rate (PEFR) after dosing. This responds to a fast-acting inhaled bronchodilator. Serevent Inhaler should be discontinued immediately, the patient assessed, and if necessary an alternative presentation (e.g. Serevent Diskhaler™) or therapy should be instituted.

In a study involving 11,000 patients a very low percentage (1.1%) of patients experienced a drop of 20% or more in PEFR whilst taking Serevent Inhaler. This occurred most frequently in patients over 60 and those with a poor baseline peak flow. This drop in PEFR occurred in a similar percentage in a control group of patients taking placebo.

The pharmacological side-effects of β2-agonist treatment, such as tremor, subjective palpitations and headache, have been reported, but tend to be transient and to reduce with regular therapy. Tachycardia may occur in some patients. In common with other β2 agonists, cardiac arrhythmias (including atrial fibrillation, supraventricular tachycardia and extrasystoles) have been reported in association with the use of salmeterol, usually in susceptible patients.

Potentially serious hypokalaemia may result from β2-agonist therapy.

There have been reports of the following: hypersensitivity reactions such as rash and oedema including angioedema; muscle cramps, non-specific chest pain, arthralgia, nausea, dizziness, nervousness, insomnia and oropharyngeal irritation.

4.9 Overdose

The symptoms and signs of salmeterol overdosage are tremor, headache and tachycardia. Hypokalaemia may occur. Monitor serum potassium levels. The preferred antidote for overdosage with Serevent Inhaler is a cardioselective β-blocking agent. Cardioselective β-blocking drugs should be used with caution in patients with a history of bronchospasm.

5. PHARMACOLOGICAL PROPERTIES

5.1 Pharmacodynamic properties

Salmeterol is a selective long-acting (usually 12 hours) β2-adrenoceptor agonist with a long side-chain which binds to the exo-site of the receptor. These pharmacological properties of salmeterol offer more effective protection against histamine-induced bronchoconstriction and produce a longer duration of bronchodilatation, lasting for at least 12 hours, than recommended doses of conventional short-acting β2-agonists. *In vitro* tests have shown that salmeterol is a potent and long-lasting inhibitor of the release from the human lung of mast cell mediators, such as histamine, leukotrienes and prostaglandin D2. In man, salmeterol inhibits the early and late phase response to inhaled allergen; the latter persisting for over 30 hours after a single dose when the bronchodilator effect is no longer evident. Single dosing with salmeterol attenuates bronchial hyper-responsiveness. These properties indicate that salmeterol has additional non-bronchodilator activity, but the full clinical significance is not yet clear. The mechanism is different from the anti-inflammatory effect of corticosteroids, which should not be stopped or reduced when Serevent Inhaler is prescribed.

Salmeterol has been studied in the treatment of conditions associated with COPD, and has been shown to improve symptoms and pulmonary function, and quality of life. Salmeterol acts as a β2-agonist on the reversible component of the disease. *In vitro* salmeterol has also been shown to increase cilial beat frequency of human bronchial epithelial cells, and also reduce a ciliotoxic effect of *Pseudomonas* toxin on the bronchial epithelium of patients with cystic fibrosis.

5.2 Pharmacokinetic properties

Salmeterol acts locally in the lung, therefore plasma levels are not predictive of therapeutic effect. In addition there are only limited data available on the pharmacokinetics of salmeterol because of the technical difficulty of assaying the drug in plasma because of the very low plasma concentrations (approximately 200 pg/ml or less) achieved after inhaled dosing. After regular dosing with salmeterol xinafoate, xinafoic acid can be detected in the systemic circulation, reaching steady state concentrations of approximately 100 ng/ml. These concentrations are up to 1000-fold lower than steady state levels observed in toxicity studies. These concentrations in long term regular dosing (more than 12 months) in patients with airways obstruction, have been shown to produce no ill effects.

5.3 Preclinical safety data

In reproduction studies in animals, some effects on the foetus, typical of a β2-agonist, have been observed at very high doses.

Salmeterol xinafoate produced no genetic toxicity in a range of studies using either prokaryotic or eukaryotic cell systems *in vitro* or *in vivo* in the rat.

Long-term studies with salmeterol xinafoate, induced class-related benign tumours of smooth muscle in the mesovarium of rats and the uterus of mice. The scientific literature and our own pharmacological studies provide good evidence that these effects are species-specific and have no relevance for clinical use.

6. PHARMACEUTICAL PARTICULARS

6.1 List of excipients

Soya lecithin.

Dichlorodifluoromethane.

Trichlorofluoromethane.

6.2 Incompatibilities

None reported.

6.3 Shelf life

2 years when not stored above 30°C.

6.4 Special precautions for storage

Salmeterol Inhaler should not be stored above 30°C.

As with most inhaled medications in aerosol canisters, the therapeutic effect of this medication may decrease when the canister is cold.

The canister should not be broken, punctured or burnt, even when apparently empty.

6.5 Nature and contents of container

An inhaler comprising an aluminium alloy can fitted with a metering valve, actuator and dust cap. Each canister contains 120 (Hospital packs 60) metered actuations of 25 micrograms salmeterol (as xinafoate).

6.6 Instructions for use and handling

The aerosol spray is inhaled through the mouth into the lungs. After shaking the inhaler, the mouthpiece is placed in the mouth and the lips closed around it. The actuator is depressed to release a spray, which must coincide with inspiration of breath.

For detailed instructions for use refer to the Patient Information Leaflet in every pack.

Administrative Data

7. MARKETING AUTHORISATION HOLDER

Glaxo Wellcome UK Limited, trading as

Allen & Hanburys,

Stockley Park West,

Uxbridge, Middlesex, UB11 1BT

8. MARKETING AUTHORISATION NUMBER(S)

10949/0068

9. DATE OF FIRST AUTHORISATION/RENEWAL OF THE AUTHORISATION

14 October 1996

10. DATE OF REVISION OF THE TEXT

4 February 2004

11. Legal Category

POM.

Diskhaler, Serevent and Volumatic are trade marks of the Glaxo Wellcome Group of Companies

Seroquel

(AstraZeneca UK Limited)

1. NAME OF THE MEDICINAL PRODUCT

SEROQUEL®

2. QUALITATIVE AND QUANTITATIVE COMPOSITION

25mg tablet: Each tablet contains 25 mg (as 28.78 mg quetiapine fumarate).

100mg tablet: Each tablet contains 100 mg (as 115.13 mg quetiapine fumarate).

150mg tablet: Each tablet contains 150 mg (as 172.69 mg quetiapine fumarate).

200mg tablet: Each tablet contains 200 mg (as 230.26 mg quetiapine fumarate).

300mg tablet: Each tablet contains 300 mg (as fumarate).

For excipients, see Section 6.1

3. PHARMACEUTICAL FORM

Film-coated tablet.

4. CLINICAL PARTICULARS

4.1 Therapeutic indications

Treatmentof schizophrenia.

Treatment of manic episodes associated with bipolar disorder.

4.2 Posology and method of administration

SEROQUEL should be administered twice daily, with or without food.

Adults

For the treatment of schizophrenia: the total daily dose for the first 4 days of therapy is 50 mg (Day 1), 100 mg (Day 2), 200 mg (Day 3) and 300 mg (Day 4).

From Day 4 onwards, the dose should be titrated to the usual effective dose range of 300 to 450 mg/day. Depending on the clinical response and tolerability of the individual patient, the dose may be adjusted within the range 150 to 750 mg/day.

For the treatment of manic episodes associated with bipolar disorder: as monotherapy or as adjunct therapy tomood stabilizers, the total daily dose for the first four days of therapy is 100 mg (Day 1), 200 mg (Day 2), 300 mg (Day 3) and 400 mg (Day 4). Further dosage adjustments up to 800 mg per day by Day 6 should be in increments of no greater than 200 mg per day.

The dose may be adjusted depending on clinical response and tolerability of the individual patient, within the range of 200 to 800 mg per day. The usual effective dose is in the range of 400 to 800 mg per day.

Elderly

As with other antipsychotics, SEROQUEL should be used with caution in the elderly, especially during the initial dosing period. Elderly patients should be started on SEROQUEL 25 mg/day. The dose should be increased daily, in increments of 25 to 50 mg, to an effective dose, which is likely to be lower than that in younger patients.

Children and adolescents

The safety and efficacy of SEROQUEL have not been evaluated in children and adolescents.

Renal and hepatic impairment

The oral clearance of quetiapine is reduced by approximately 25% in patients with renal or hepatic impairment. Quetiapine is extensively metabolised by the liver, and therefore should be used with caution in patients with known hepatic impairment.

Patients with renal or hepatic impairment should be started on SEROQUEL 25 mg/day. The dose should be increased daily, in increments of 25 to 50 mg, to an effective dose.

4.3 Contraindications

SEROQUEL is contra-indicated in patients who are hypersensitive to any component of this product.

4.4 Special warnings and special precautions for use

Cardiovascular disease

SEROQUEL should be used with caution in patients with known cardiovascular disease, cerebrovascular disease, or other conditions predisposing to hypotension.

SEROQUEL may induce orthostatic hypotension, especially during the initial dose-titration period; this is more common in elderly patients than in younger patients.

In clinical trials, quetiapine was not associated with a persistent increase in QT_c interval. However, as with other antipsychotics, caution should be exercised when quetiapine is prescribed with drugs known to prolong the QT_c interval, especially in the elderly.

Seizures

In controlled clinical trials there was no difference in the incidence of seizures in patients treated with SEROQUEL or placebo. As with other antipsychotics, caution is recommended when treating patients with a history of seizures.

Tardive dyskinesia

As with other antipsychotics, there is a potential for SEROQUEL to cause tardive dyskinesia after long-term treatment. If signs and symptoms of tardive dyskinesia appear, dose reduction or discontinuation of SEROQUEL should be considered.

Neuroleptic malignant syndrome

Neuroleptic malignant syndrome has been associated with antipsychotic treatment, including SEROQUEL (see Section 4.8).Clinical manifestations include hyperthermia, altered mental status, muscular rigidity, autonomic instability, and increased creatine phosphokinase. In such an event, SEROQUEL should be discontinued and appropriate medical treatment given.

Acute withdrawal reactions

Acute withdrawal symptoms including nausea, vomiting and insomnia have very rarely been described after abrupt cessation of high doses of antipsychotic drugs. Recurrence of psychotic symptoms may also occur, and the emergence of involuntary movement disorders (such as akathisia, dystonia and dyskinesia) has been reported. Therefore, gradual withdrawal is advisable.

Interactions

See also *Section 4.5 Interactions with other medicinal products and other forms of interaction*

Concomitant use of SEROQUEL with hepatic enzyme inducers such as carbamazepine may substantially decrease systemic exposure to quetiapine. Depending on clinical response, higher doses of SEROQUEL may need to be considered if SEROQUEL is used concomitantly with a hepatic enzyme inducer.

During concomitant administration of drugs which are potent CYP3A4 inhibitors (such as azole antifungals and macrolide antibiotics), plasma concentrations of quetiapine can be significantly higher than observed in patients in clinical trials. (See also *Section 5.2 Pharmacokinetics*.) As a consequence of this, lower doses of SEROQUEL should be used. Special consideration should be given in elderly and debilitated patients. The risk-benefit ratio needs to be considered on an individual basis in all patients.

Hyperglycaemia

Hyperglycaemia or exacerbation of pre-existing diabetes has been reported in very rare cases during treatment with quetiapine. Appropriate clinical monitoring is advisable in diabetic patients and in patients with risk factors for the development of diabetes mellitus (see also section 4.8 Undesirable effects).

4.5 Interaction with other medicinal products and other forms of Interaction

Given the primary central nervous system effects of quetiapine SEROQUEL should be used with caution in combination with other centrally acting drugs and alcohol.

The pharmacokinetics of lithium was not altered when co-administered with SEROQUEL.

The pharmacokinetics of valproic acid and quetiapine were not altered to a clinically relevant extent when co-administered as valproate semisodium (also known as divalproex sodium (USAN)) and SEROQUEL (quetiapine fumarate). Valproate semisodium is a stable coordination compound comprised of sodium valproate and valproic acid in a 1:1 molar relationship.

The pharmacokinetics of quetiapine was not significantly altered following co-administration with the antipsychotics risperidone or haloperidol. However co-administration of SEROQUEL and thioridazine caused increases in the clearance of quetiapine.

Quetiapine did not induce the hepatic enzyme systems involved in the metabolism of antipyrine. However, in a multiple dose trial in patients to assess the pharmacokinetics of quetiapine given before and during treatment with carbamazepine (a known hepatic enzyme inducer), co-administration of carbamazepine significantly increased the clearance of quetiapine. This increase in clearance reduced systemic quetiapine exposure (as measured by AUC) to an average of 13% of the exposure during administration of quetiapine alone; although a greater effect was seen in some patients. As a consequence of this interaction, lower plasma concentrations can occur, and hence, in each patient, consideration for a higher dose of SEROQUEL, depending on clinical response, should be considered. It should be noted that the recommended maximum daily dose of SEROQUEL is 750mg/day for the treatment of schizophrenia and 800mg/day for the treatment of manic episodes associated with bipolar disorder. Continued treatment at higher doses should only be considered as a result of careful consideration of the benefit risk assessment for an individual patient. Co-administration of SEROQUEL with another microsomal enzyme inducer, phenytoin, also caused increases in the clearance of quetiapine. Increased doses of SEROQUEL may be required to maintain control of psychotic symptoms in patients co-administered SEROQUEL and phenytoin and other hepatic enzyme inducers (e.g., barbiturates, rifampicin etc.). The dose of SEROQUEL may need to be reduced if phenytoin or carbamazepine or other hepatic enzyme inducers are withdrawn and replaced with a non-inducer (e.g., sodium valproate).

CYP3A4 is the primary enzyme responsible for cytochrome P450 mediated metabolism of quetiapine. The pharmacokinetics of quetiapine was not altered following co-administration with cimetidine, a known P450 enzyme inhibitor. The pharmacokinetics of quetiapine were not significantly altered following co-administration with the antidepressants imipramine (a known CYP2D6 inhibitor) or fluoxetine (a known CYP3A4 and CYP2D6 inhibitor). However, caution is recommended when SEROQUEL is co-administered with potent CYP3A4 inhibitors (such as azole antifungals and macrolide antibiotics). (See also *Section 4.4 Special Warnings & Special Precautions for Use* and *Section 5.2 Pharmacokinetics).*

4.6 Pregnancy and lactation

The safety and efficacy of SEROQUEL during human pregnancy have not been established (see *Section 5.3 Preclinical safety data, Reproduction studies,* for animal reproductive toxicology data). Therefore, SEROQUEL should only be used during pregnancy if the benefits justify the potential risks.

The degree to which quetiapine is excreted into human milk is unknown. Women who are breast feeding should therefore be advised to avoid breast feeding while taking SEROQUEL.

4.7 Effects on ability to drive and use machines

Because SEROQUEL may cause somnolence, patients should be cautioned about operating hazardous machines, including motor vehicles.

4.8 Undesirable effects

The most commonly reported Adverse Drug Reactions (ADRs) with SEROQUEL are somnolence, dizziness, dry mouth, mild asthenia, constipation, tachycardia, orthostatic hypotension, and dyspepsia.

As with other antipsychotics, syncope, neuroleptic malignant syndrome, leucopenia, neutropenia and peripheral edema, have been associated with SEROQUEL.

The incidences of ADRs associated with SEROQUEL therapy, are tabulated below according to the format recommended by the Council for International Organizations of Medical Sciences (CIOMS III Working Group; 1995).

Frequency	System Organ Class	Event
Very Common (≥10%)	*Nervous system disorders*	Dizziness [1, 6] Somnolence [2]
Common (≥ 1% - < 10 %)	*Blood and lymphatic system disorders*	Leucopenia [3]
	Cardiac disorders	Tachycardia [1, 6]
	Gastrointestinal disorders	Dry mouth Constipation Dyspepsia
	General disorders and administration site conditions	Mild asthenia Peripheral edema
	Investigations	Weight gain [4] Elevations in serum transaminases (ALT, AST) [5]
	Nervous system disorders	Syncope [1, 6]
	Respiratory, thoracic, and mediastinal disorders	Rhinitis
	Vascular disorders	Orthostatic hypotension [1, 6]
Uncommon (≥ 0.1% - < 1%)	*Blood and lymphatic system disorders*	Eosinophilia
	Immune system disorders	Hypersensitivity
	Investigations	Elevations in gamma-GT levels [5] Elevations in non-fasting serum triglyceride levels Elevations in total cholesterol
	Nervous system disorders	Seizure [1]
Rare (0.01% - < 0.1%)	*General disorders and administration site conditions*	Neuroleptic malignant syndrome [1]
	Reproductive system and breast disorders	Priapism
Very rare (< 0.01%)	*Blood and lymphatic system disorders*	Neutropenia [3]
	Metabolism and Nutritional Disorders	Hyperglycaemia [1, 7] Diabetes Mellitus [1, 7]

(1) See section 4.4 Special Warnings and Special Precautions for Use.

(2) Somnolence may occur, usually during the first two weeks of treatment and generally resolves with the continued administration of SEROQUEL.

(3) There were no cases of persistent severe neutropenia or agranulocytosis reported in controlled clinical trials with SEROQUEL. During post-marketing experience, resolution of leukopenia and/or neutropenia has followed cessation of therapy with SEROQUEL. Possible risk factors for leukopenia and/or neutropenia include pre-existing low white cell count and history of drug induced leukopenia and/or neutropenia.

(4) Occurs predominantly during the early weeks of treatment.

(5) Asymptomatic elevations in serum transaminase (ALT, AST) or gamma-GT-levels have been observed in some patients administered SEROQUEL. These elevations were usually reversible on continued SEROQUEL treatment.

(6) As with other antipsychotics with alpha1 adrenergic blocking activity, SEROQUEL may induce orthostatic hypotension, associated with dizziness, tachycardia and, in some patients, syncope, especially during the initial dose-titration period.

(7) Hyperglycaemia or exacerbation of pre-existing diabetes has been reported in very rare cases.

SEROQUEL treatment was associated with small dose-related decreases in thyroid hormone levels, particularly total T_4 and free T_4. The reduction in total and free T_4 was maximal within the first two to four weeks of SEROQUEL treatment, with no further reduction during long-term treatment. In nearly all cases, cessation of SEROQUEL treatment was associated with a reversal of the effects on total and free T_4, irrespective of the duration of treatment. Smaller decreases in total T_3 and reverse T_3 were seen only at higher doses. Levels of TBG were unchanged and in general, reciprocal increases in TSH were not observed, with no indication that SEROQUEL causes clinically relevant hypothyroidism.

Hyperglycemia and exacerbation of pre-existing diabetes have been reported in very rare cases during quetiapine treatment.

As with other antipsychotics, Seroquel may be associated with weight gain, predominantly during the early weeks of treatment.

As with other antipsychotics, SEROQUEL may cause prolongation of the QTc interval, but in clinical trials, this was not associated with a persistent increase (see *Section 4.4 Special warnings and special precautions for use*).

Acute withdrawal reactions have been reported (see Section 4.4 Special warnings and special precautions for use).

4.9 Overdose

In clinical trials, experience with SEROQUEL in overdosage is limited. Estimated doses of SEROQUEL up to 20 g have been taken; no fatalities were reported and patients recovered without sequelae. In postmarketing experience, there have been very rare reports of overdose of SEROQUEL alone resulting in death or coma or QT-prolongation.

In general, reported signs and symptoms were those resulting from an exaggeration of the drug's known pharmacological effects, i.e., drowsiness and sedation, tachycardia and hypotension.

There is no specific antidote to quetiapine. In cases of severe intoxication, the possibility of multiple drug involvement should be considered, and intensive care procedures are recommended, including establishing and maintaining a patent airway, ensuring adequate oxygenation and ventilation, and monitoring and support of the cardiovascular system.

Close medical supervision and monitoring should be continued until the patient recovers.

5. PHARMACOLOGICAL PROPERTIES

5.1 Pharmacodynamic properties

Pharmacotherapeutic group:Antipsychotics

Therapeutic classification: N05A H

Mechanism of action

Quetiapine is an atypical antipsychotic agent which interacts with a broad range of neurotransmitter receptors. Quetiapine exhibits a higher affinity for serotonin ($5HT_2$) receptors in the brain than it does for dopamine D_1 and D_2 receptors in the brain. Quetiapine also has high affinity at histaminergic and adrenergic α_1 receptors, with a lower affinity at adrenergic α_2 receptors, but no appreciable affinity at cholinergic muscarinic or benzodiazepine receptors. Quetiapine is active in tests for antipsychotic activity, such as conditioned avoidance.

Pharmacodynamic effects

The results of animal studies predictive of EPS liability revealed that quetiapine causes only weak catalepsy at effective dopamine D_2 receptor blocking doses, that quetiapine causes selective reduction in the firing of mesolimbic A10 dopaminergic neurones versus the A9 nigrostriatal neurones involved in motor function, and that quetiapine exhibits minimal dystonic liability in neuroleptic-sensitised monkeys.

Clinical Efficacy

The results of three placebo-controlled clinical trials, including one that used a dose range of SEROQUEL of 75 to 750 mg/day, identified no difference between SEROQUEL and placebo in the incidence of EPS or use of concomitant anticholinergics.

In four controlled trials, evaluating doses of SEROQUEL up to 800 mg for the treatment of bipolar mania, two each in monotherapy and as adjunct therapy to lithium or valproate semisodium, there were no differences between the SEROQUEL and placebo treatment groups in the incidence of EPS or concomitant use of anticholinergics.

SEROQUEL does not produce sustained elevations in prolactin. In a multiple fixed-dose clinical trial, there were no differences in prolactin levels at study completion between SEROQUEL, across the recommended dose range, and placebo.

In clinical trials, SEROQUEL has been shown to be effective in the treatment of both positive and negative symptoms of schizophrenia. In one trial against chlorpromazine, and two against haloperidol, SEROQUEL showed similar short-term efficacy.

In clinical trials, SEROQUEL has been shown to be effective as monotherapy or as adjunct therapy in reducing manic symptoms in patients with bipolar mania. The mean last week median dose of SEROQUEL in responders, was approximately 600 mg and approximately 85% of the responders were in the dose range of 400 to 800 mg per day.

5.2 Pharmacokinetic properties

Quetiapine is well absorbed and extensively metabolised following oral administration. The principal human plasma metabolites do not have significant pharmacological activity.

The bioavailability of quetiapine is not significantly affected by administration with food. The elimination half-life of quetiapine is approximately 7 hours. Quetiapine is approximately 83% bound to plasma proteins.

Clinical trials have demonstrated that SEROQUEL is effective when given twice a day. This is further supported by data from a positron emission tomography (PET) study which identified that $5HT_2$ and D_2 receptor occupancy are maintained for up to 12 hours after dosing with quetiapine.

The pharmacokinetics of quetiapine are linear, and do not differ between men and women.

The mean clearance of quetiapine in the elderly is approximately 30 to 50% lower than that seen in adults aged 18 to 65 years.

The mean plasma clearance of quetiapine was reduced by approximately 25% in subjects with severe renal impairment (creatinine clearance less than 30 ml/min/1.73m^2) and in subjects with hepatic impairment (stable alcoholic cirrhosis), but the individual clearance values are within the range for normal subjects.

Quetiapine is extensively metabolised, with parent compound accounting for less than 5% of unchanged drug-related material in the urine or faeces, following the administration of radiolabelled quetiapine. Approximately 73% of the radioactivity is excreted in the urine and 21% in the faeces.

In vitro investigations established that CYP3A4 is the primary enzyme responsible for cytochrome P450 mediated metabolism of quetiapine.

In a multiple-dose trial in healthy volunteers to assess the pharmacokinetics of quetiapine given before and during treatment with ketoconazole, co-administration of ketoconazole resulted in an increase in mean C_{max} and AUC of quetiapine of 235% and 522%, respectively, with a corresponding decrease in mean oral clearance of 84%. The mean half-life of quetiapine increased from 2.6 to 6.8 hours, but the mean t_{max} was unchanged.

Quetiapine and several of its metabolites were found to be weak inhibitors of human cytochrome P450 1A2, 2C9, 2C19, 2D6 and 3A4 activities, but only at concentrations at least 10- to 50-fold higher than those observed in the usual effective dose range of 300 to 450mg/day in humans. Based on these *in vitro* results, it is unlikely that co-administration of quetiapine with other drugs will result in clinically significant drug inhibition of cytochrome P450 mediated metabolism of the other drug.

5.3 Preclinical safety data

Acute toxicity studies

Quetiapine has low acute toxicity. Findings in mice and rats after oral (500 mg/kg) or intraperitoneal (100 mg/kg) dosing were typical of an effective neuroleptic agent and included decreased motor activity, ptosis, loss of righting reflex, fluid around the mouth and convulsions.

Repeat-dose toxicity studies

In multiple-dose studies in rats, dogs and monkeys, anticipated central nervous system effects of an antipsychotic drug were observed with quetiapine (eg, sedation at lower doses and tremor, convulsions or prostration at higher exposures).

Hyperprolactinaemia, induced through the dopamine D_2 receptor antagonist activity of quetiapine or its metabolites, varied between species but was most marked in the rat, and a range of effects consequent to this were seen in the 12-month study, including mammary hyperplasia, increased pituitary weight, decreased uterine weight and enhanced growth of females.

Reversible morphological and functional effects on the liver, consistent with hepatic enzyme induction, were seen in mouse, rat and monkey.

Thyroid follicular cell hypertrophy and concomitant changes in plasma thyroid hormone levels occurred in rat and monkey.

Pigmentation of a number of tissues, particularly the thyroid, was not associated with any morphological or functional effects.

Transient increases in heart rate, unaccompanied by an effect on blood pressure, occurred in dogs.

Posterior triangular cataracts seen after 6 months in dogs at 100 mg/kg/day were consistent with inhibition of cholesterol biosynthesis in the lens. No cataracts were observed in Cynomolgus monkeys dosed up to 225 mg/kg/day, nor in rodents. Monitoring in clinical studies did not reveal drug-related corneal opacities in man.

No evidence of neutrophil reduction or agranulocytosis was seen in any of the toxicity studies.

Carcinogenicity studies

In the rat study (doses 0, 20, 75 and 250 mg/kg/day) the incidence of mammary adenocarcinomas was increased at all doses in female rats, consequential to prolonged hyperprolactinaemia.

In male rat (250 mg/kg/day) and mouse (250 and 750 mg/kg/day), there was an increased incidence of thyroid follicular cell benign adenomas, consistent with known rodent-specific mechanisms resulting from enhanced hepatic thyroxine clearance.

Reproduction studies

Effects related to elevated prolactin levels (marginal reduction in male fertility and pseudopregnancy, protracted periods of diestrus, increased precoital interval and reduced pregnancy rate) were seen in rats, although these are not directly relevant to humans because of species differences in hormonal control of reproduction.

Quetiapine had no teratogenic effects.

Mutagenicity studies

Genetic toxicity studies with quetiapine show that it is not a mutagen or clastogen.

6. PHARMACEUTICAL PARTICULARS

6.1 List of excipients

Core	Coating
Povidone (Ph. Eur.)	Hypromellose (Ph. Eur.)
Calcium Hydrogen Phosphate (Ph. Eur.)	Macrogol 400 (Ph. Eur.) Titanium Dioxide (Ph. Eur., E171)
Microcrystalline Cellulose (Ph. Eur.)	Ferric Oxide, Yellow (Ph. Fr., E172) (25mg, 100mg and 150mg tablets)
Sodium Starch Glycollate Type A (Ph. Eur.)	Ferric Oxide, Red (Ph. Fr., E172) (25mg tablets)
Lactose Monohydrate (Ph. Eur.)	
Magnesium Stearate (Ph. Eur.)	

6.2 Incompatibilities

None known

6.3 Shelf life

36 months.

6.4 Special precautions for storage

Do not store above 30°C. Store in the original package.

6.5 Nature and contents of container

25mg tablet: The tablets are round, 6mm, peach coloured, bi-convex and film-coated.

100mg tablet: The tablets are round, 8.5 mm, yellow coloured, bi-convex and film-coated.

150mg tablet: The tablets are round, 100mm, pale yellow coloured, biconvex and film-coated.

200mg tablets: The tablets are round, 11mm, white, bi-convex and film-coated.

300mg tablets: The tablets are capsule-shaped, white and film-coated.

The tablets are packed into PVC aluminium foil blister strips. The blister strips are themselves packed into cartons.

Tablet strength	Carton (pack) contents	Strips/blisters
25mg tablets	6 tablets 20 tablets 30 tablets 60 tablets 50 tablets 100 tablets	1 strip of 6 blisters 2 strips of 10 blisters 3 strips of 10 blisters 6 strips of 10 blisters 10 strips of 5 blisters 10 strips of 10 blisters
100 mg, 150mg, 200mg and 300mg tablets	20 tablets 30 tablets 60 tablets 90 tablets 50 tablets	2 strips of 10 blisters 3 strips of 10 blisters 6 strips of 10 blisters 9 strips of 10 blisters 10 strips of 5 blisters

Tablet strength	Carton (pack) contents	Strips/blisters
	50 tablets 100 tablets	5 strips of 10 blisters 10 strips of 10 blisters (100 mg, 150 mg and 200 mg tablets only)
Mixed pack	10 tablets	1 strip containing 6 × 25 mg, 2 × 100 mg tablets and 2 × 150 mg tablets

6.6 Instructions for use and handling

None stated.

7. MARKETING AUTHORISATION HOLDER

AstraZeneca UK Limited

600 Capability Green,

Luton, LU1 3LU, UK.

8. MARKETING AUTHORISATION NUMBER(S)

25 mg tablet PL 17901/0038

100 mg tablet PL 17901/0039

150 mg tablet PL 17901/0041

200 mg tablet PL 17901/0040

300 mg tablet PL 17901/0088

9. DATE OF FIRST AUTHORISATION/RENEWAL OF THE AUTHORISATION

25th June 2000 / 18th Sept 2003

10. DATE OF REVISION OF THE TEXT

23rd June 2005

Seroxat Tablets 20mg, 30mg, Liquid 20mg/10ml

(GlaxoSmithKline UK)

1. NAME OF THE MEDICINAL PRODUCT

Seroxat® 20 mg tablets

Seroxat® 30 mg tablets

Seroxat® 20 mg/10ml liquid

2. QUALITATIVE AND QUANTITATIVE COMPOSITION

Each film-coated tablet contains 20 mg or 30 mg paroxetine.

Each ml of oral suspension contains 2mg of paroxetine.

3. PHARMACEUTICAL FORM

Film-coated tablet

Oral suspension

4. CLINICAL PARTICULARS

4.1 Therapeutic indications

Treatment of

- Major Depressive Episode
- Obsessive Compulsive Disorder
- Panic Disorder with and without agoraphobia
- Social Anxiety Disorders/Social phobia
- Generalised Anxiety Disorder
- Post-traumatic Stress Disorder

4.2 Posology and method of administration

It is recommended that paroxetine is administered once daily in the morning with food.

The tablet should be swallowed rather than chewed. For paroxetine liquid, shake the bottle before use.

MAJOR DEPRESSIVE EPISODE

The recommended dose is 20 mg daily. In general, improvement in patients starts after one week but may only become evident from the second week of therapy.

As with all antidepressant medicinal products, dosage should be reviewed and adjusted if necessary within 3 to 4 weeks of initiation of therapy and thereafter as judged clinically appropriate. In some patients, with insufficient response to 20 mg, the dose may be increased gradually up to a maximum of 50 mg a day in 10 mg steps according to the patient's response.

Patients with depression should be treated for a sufficient period of at least 6 months to ensure that they are free from symptoms.

OBSESSIVE COMPULSIVE DISORDER

The recommended dose is 40 mg daily. Patients should start on 20 mg/day and the dose may be increased gradually in 10 mg increments to the recommended dose. If after some weeks on the recommended dose insufficient response is seen some patients may benefit from having their dose increased gradually up to a maximum of 60 mg/day.

Patients with OCD should be treated for a sufficient period to ensure that they are free from symptoms. This period may be several months or even longer. (see section 5.1 Pharmacodynamic properties)

PANIC DISORDER

The recommended dose is 40 mg daily. Patients should be started on 10 mg/day and the dose gradually increased in 10 mg steps according to the patient's response up to the recommended dose. A low initial starting dose is recommended to minimise the potential worsening of panic symptomatology, which is generally recognised to occur early in the treatment of this disorder. If after some weeks on the recommended dose insufficient response is seen some patients may benefit from having their dose increased gradually up to a maximum of 60 mg/day.

Patients with panic disorder should be treated for a sufficient period to ensure that they are free from symptoms. This period may be several months or even longer (see section 5.1 Pharmacodynamic properties)

SOCIAL ANXIETY DISORDER/SOCIAL PHOBIA

The recommended dose is 20 mg daily.If after some weeks on the recommended dose insufficient response is seen some patients may benefit from having their dose increased gradually in 10 mg steps up to a maximum of 50 mg/day.Long-term use should be regularly evaluated (see section 5.1 Pharmacodynamic properties).

GENERALISED ANXIETY DISORDER

The recommended dose is 20 mg daily.If after some weeks on the recommended dose insufficient response is seen some patients may benefit from having their dose increased gradually in 10 mg steps up to a maximum of 50 mg/day.Long-term use should be regularly evaluated (see section 5.1 Pharmacodynamic properties).

POST-TRAUMATIC STRESS DISORDER

The recommended dose is 20 mg daily.If after some weeks on the recommended dose insufficient response is seen some patients may benefit from having their dose increased gradually in 10 mg steps up to a maximum of 50 mg/day.Long-term use should be regularly evaluated (see section 5.1 Pharmacodynamic properties).

GENERAL INFORMATION

WITHDRAWAL SYMPTOMS SEEN ON DISCONTINUATION OF PAROXETINE

Abrupt discontinuation should be avoided (see sections 4.4 Special Warnings and Precautions for Use & 4.8 Undesirable Effects). The taper phase regimen used in clinical trials involved decreasing the daily dose by 10 mg at weekly intervals. If intolerable symptoms occur following a decrease in the dose or upon discontinuation of treatment, then resuming the previously prescribed dose may be considered. Subsequently, the physician may continue decreasing the dose, but at a more gradual rate.

Special populations:

- Elderly

Increased plasma concentrations of paroxetine occur in elderly subjects, but the range of concentrations overlaps with that observed in younger patients. Dosing should commence at the adult starting dose. Increasing the dose might be useful in some patients, but the maximum dose should not exceed 40 mg daily.

- Children and adolescents (7-17 years)

Paroxetine should not be used for the treatment of children and adolescents as controlled clinical trials have found paroxetine to be associated with increased risk for suicidal behaviour and hostility. In addition, in these trials efficacy has not been adequately demonstrated (see section 4.4 Special warnings and special precautions for use and section 4.8 Undesirable effects).

- Children aged below 7 years

The use of paroxetine has not been studied in children less than 7 years. Paroxetine should not be used, as long as safety and efficacy in this age group have not been established.

- Renal/hepatic impairment

Increased plasma concentrations of paroxetine occur in patients with severe renal impairment (creatinine clearance less than 30 ml/min) or in those with hepatic impairment. Therefore, dosage should be restricted to the lower end of the dosage range.

4.3 Contraindications

Known hypersensitivity to paroxetine or any of the excipients.

Paroxetine is contraindicated in combination with monoamine oxidase inhibitors (MAOIs). Treatment with paroxetine can be initiated:

- two weeks after discontinuation of an irreversible MAOI, or

- at least 24hrs after discontinuation of a reversible MAOI (e.g. moclobemide).

At least one week should elapse between discontinuation of paroxetine and initiation of therapy with any MAOI.

Paroxetine should not be used in combination with thioridazine because, as with other drugs which inhibit the hepatic enzyme CYP450 2D6, paroxetine can elevate plasma levels of thioridazine (see Section 4.5, Interactions with other medicinal products and other forms of interaction). Administration of thioridazine alone can lead to QTc interval prolongation with associated serious ventricular arrhythmia such as torsades de pointes, and sudden death.

4.4 Special warnings and special precautions for use

Treatment with paroxetine should be initiated cautiously two weeks after terminating treatment with an irreversible MAOI or 24 hours after terminating treatment with a reversible MAO inhibitor. Dosage of paroxetine should be increased gradually until an optimal response is reached (see section 4.3 Contraindications and section 4.5 Interactions with other medicinal products and other forms of interaction).

Children and adolescents (7-17 years)

Paroxetine should not be used in the treatment of children and adolescents under the age of 18 years. In clinical trials increased suicidal related behaviours (suicide attempts and suicidal thoughts) and hostility (predominantly aggression, oppositional behaviour and anger) were more frequently observed in children and adolescents treated with paroxetine compared to those treated with placebo. In addition, in these trials efficacy has not been adequately demonstrated and long-term safety data in children and adolescents concerning growth, maturation and cognitive and behavioural development are lacking (see section 4.8 Undesirable effects).

Suicide/suicidal ideation

Depression is associated with an increased risk of suicidal thoughts, self harm and suicide. This risk persists until significant remission occurs. As improvement may not occur during the first few weeks or more of treatment, patients should be closely monitored until such improvement occurs. It is general clinical experience with all antidepressant therapies that the risk of suicide may increase in the early stages of recovery.

Other psychiatric conditions for which paroxetine is prescribed can also be associated with an increased risk of suicidal behaviour. In addition, these conditions may be co-morbid with major depressive disorder. The same precautions observed when treating patients with major depressive disorder should therefore be observed when treating patients with other psychiatric disorders.

Patients with a history of suicidal behaviour or thoughts, or those exhibiting a significant degree of suicidal ideation prior to commencement of treatment, are at a greater risk of suicidal thoughts or suicide attempts, and should receive careful monitoring during treatment.

There is a possibility of an increased risk of suicide related behaviour in young adults ages 18-29.

Young adults should therefore be monitored carefully throughout treatment.

There are insufficient data concerning the risk of suicide related behaviour in treatment naïve patients, but careful monitoring might be warranted.

Patients, (and caregivers of patients) should be alerted about the need to monitor for the emergence of suicidal ideation/behaviour or thoughts of harming themselves and to seek medical advice immediately if these symptoms present.

Akathisia

The use of paroxetine has been associated with the development of akathisia, which is characterized by an inner sense of restlessness and psychomotor agitation such as an inability to sit or stand still usually associated with subjective distress. This is most likely to occur within the first few weeks of treatment. In patients who develop these symptoms, increasing the dose may be detrimental.

Serotonin syndrome/neuroleptic malignant syndrome

On rare occasions development of a serotonin syndrome or neuroleptic malignant syndrome-like events may occur in association with treatment of paroxetine, particularly when given in combination with other serotonergic and/or neuroleptic drugs. As these syndromes may result in potentially life-threatening conditions, treatment with paroxetine should be discontinued if such events (characterised by clusters of symptoms such as hyperthermia, rigidity, myoclonus, autonomic instability with possible rapid fluctuations of vital signs, mental status changes including confusion, irritability, extreme agitation progressing to delirium and coma) occur and supportive symptomatic treatment should be initiated. Paroxetine should not be used in combination with serotonin-precursors (such as L-tryptophan, oxitriptan) due to the risk of serotonergic syndrome.

(See Sections 4.3 Contraindications and 4.5 Interactions with other medicinal products and other forms of interaction).

Mania

As with all antidepressants, paroxetine should be used with caution in patients with a history of mania. Paroxetine should be discontinued in any patient entering a manic phase.

Renal/hepatic impairment

Caution is recommended in patients with severe renal impairment or in those with hepatic impairment. (see section 4.2 Posology and method of administration)

Diabetes

In patients with diabetes, treatment with an SSRI may alter glycaemic control. Insulin and/or oral hypoglycaemic dosage may need to be adjusted.

Epilepsy

As with other antidepressants, paroxetine should be used with caution in patients with epilepsy.

Seizures

Overall the incidence of seizures is less than 0.1% in patients treated with paroxetine. The drug should be discontinued in any patient who develops seizures.

ECT

There is little clinical experience of concurrent administration of paroxetine with ECT.

Glaucoma

As with other SSRI's, paroxetine infrequently causes mydriasis and should be used with caution in patients with narrow angle glaucoma or history of glaucoma.

Cardiac conditions

The usual precautions should be observed in patients with cardiac conditions.

Hyponatraemia

Hyponatraemia has been reported rarely, predominantly in the elderly. Caution should also be exercised in those patients at risk of hyponatraemia e.g. from concomitant medications and cirrhosis. The hyponatraemia generally reverses on discontinuation of paroxetine.

Haemorrhage

There have been reports of cutaneous bleeding abnormalities such as ecchymoses and purpura with SSRIs. Other haemorrhagic manifestations e.g. gastrointestinal haemorrhage have been reported. Elderly patients may be at an increased risk.

Caution is advised in patients taking SSRI's concomitantly with oral anticoagulants, drugs known to affect platelet function or other drugs that may increase risk of bleeding (e.g. atypical antipsychotics such as clozapine, phenothiazines, most TCA's, acetylsalicylic acid, NSAID's, COX-2 inhibitors) as well as in patients with a history of bleeding disorders or conditions which may predispose to bleeding.

Parabens

Paroxetine oral suspension contains methyl and propyl hydroxybenzoate (parabens), which are known to cause urticaria; generally delayed type reactions, such as contact dermatitis, but rarely immediate reaction with bronchospasm.

Withdrawal symptoms seen on discontinuation of paroxetine treatment

Withdrawal symptoms when treatment is discontinued are common, particularly if discontinuation is abrupt (see section 4.8 Undesirable effects). In clinical trials adverse events seen on treatment discontinuation occurred in 30% of patients treated with paroxetine compared to 20% of patients treated with placebo. The occurrence of withdrawal symptoms is not the same as the drug being addictive or dependence producing.

The risk of withdrawal symptoms may be dependent on several factors including the duration and dose of therapy and the rate of dose reduction.

Dizziness, sensory disturbances (including paraesthesia and electric shock sensations), sleep disturbances (including intense dreams), agitation or anxiety, nausea, tremor, confusion, sweating, headache, diarrhoea, palpitations, emotional instability, irritability, and visual disturbances have been reported. Generally these symptoms are mild to moderate, however, in some patients they may be severe in intensity. They usually occur within the first few days of discontinuing treatment, but there have been very rare reports of such symptoms in patients who have inadvertently missed a dose. Generally these symptoms are self-limiting and usually resolve within 2 weeks, though in some individuals they may be prolonged (2-3 months or more). It is therefore advised that paroxetine should be gradually tapered when discontinuing treatment over a period of several weeks or months, according to the patient's needs (see "Withdrawal Symptoms Seen on Discontinuation of Paroxetine", Section 4.2 Posology and method of administration).

4.5 Interaction with other medicinal products and other forms of Interaction

Serotonergic drugs

As with other SSRIs, co-administration with serotonergic drugs (including MAOIs, L-tryptophan, triptans, tramadol, linezolid, SSRIs, lithium and St. John's Wort – Hypericum perforatum – preparations) may lead to an incidence of 5-HT associated effects (serotonin syndrome: see Section 4.3 Contraindications and Section 4.4 Special warnings and special precautions for use).

Caution should be advised and a closer clinical monitoring is required when these drugs are combined with paroxetine.

Drug metabolising enzyme

The metabolism and pharmacokinetics of paroxetine may be affected by the induction or inhibition of drug metabolising enzymes.

When paroxetine is to be co-administered with a known drug metabolising enzyme inhibitor, consideration should be given to using paroxetine doses at the lower end of the range.

No initial dosage adjustment is considered necessary when it is to be co-administered with known drug metabolising enzyme inducers (e.g. carbamazepine, rifampicin, phenobarbital, phenytoin). Any subsequent dosage adjustment should be guided by clinical effect (tolerability and efficacy).

Procyclidine

Daily administration of paroxetine increases significantly the plasma levels of procyclidine. If anti-cholinergic effects are seen, the dose of procyclidine should be reduced.

Anticonvulsants

Carbamazepine, phenytoin, sodium valproate. Concomitant administration does not seem to show any effect on pharmacokinetic/dynamic profile in epileptic patients.

CYP2D6 inhibitory potency of paroxetine

As with other antidepressants, including other SSRIs, paroxetine inhibits the hepatic cytochrome P450 enzyme CYP2D6. Inhibition of CYP2D6 may lead to increased plasma concentrations of co-administered drugs metabolised by this enzyme. These include certain tricyclic antidepressants (e.g. clomipramine, nortriptyline, and desipramine), phenothiazine neuroleptics (e.g. perphenazine and thioridazine see section 4.3 Contraindications), risperidone, Type 1c antiarrhythmics (e.g. propafenone and flecainide) and metoprolol. It is not recommended to use paroxetine in combination with metoprolol when given in cardiac insufficiency, because of the narrow therapeutic index of metoprolol in this indication.

Alcohol

As with other psychotropic drugs patients should be advised to avoid alcohol use while taking paroxetine

Oral anticoagulants

A pharmacodynamic interaction between paroxetine and oral anticoagulants may occur. Concomitant use of paroxetine and oral anticoagulants can lead to an increased anticoagulant activity and haemorrhagic risk. Therefore, paroxetine should therefore be used with caution in patients who are treated with oral anticoagulants. (see section 4.4 Special warnings and special precautions for use)

NSAIDs and acetylsalicylic acid, and other antiplatelet agents

A pharmacodynamic interaction between paroxetine and NSAIDs/acetylsalicylic acid may occur. Concomitant use of paroxetine and NSAIDs/acetylsalicylic acid can lead to an increased haemorrhagic risk. (see section 4.4 Special warnings and Special Precautions for use)

Caution is advised in patients taking SSRI's, concomitantly with oral anticoagulants, drugs known to affect platelet function or increase risk of bleeding (e.g. atypical antipsychotics such as clozapine, phenothiazines, most TCA's, acetylsalicylic acid, NSAID's, COX-2 inhibitors) as well as in patients with a history of bleeding disorders or conditions which may predispose to bleeding.

4.6 Pregnancy and lactation

Pregnancy

Data on a limited number of exposed pregnancies provide no indication of an increased risk of congenital malformations in the newborn.

Paroxetine should only be used during pregnancy when strictly indicated. Women planning a pregnancy and those becoming pregnant during therapy should be asked to consult their physician. Abrupt discontinuation should be avoided during pregnancy (see "Withdrawal Symptoms Seen on Discontinuation of Paroxetine", section 4.2 Posology and method of administration).

Neonates should be observed if maternal use of paroxetine continues into the later stages of pregnancy, particularly the third trimester.

The following symptoms may occur in the neonate after maternal paroxetine use in later stages of pregnancy: respiratory distress, cyanosis, apnoea, seizures, temperature instability, feeding difficulty, vomiting, hypoglycaemia, hypertonia, hypotonia, hyperreflexia, tremor, jitteriness, irritability, lethargy, constant crying, somnolence and difficulty in sleeping. These symptoms could be due to either serotonergic effects or withdrawal symptoms. In a majority of instances the complications begin immediately or soon (<24 hours) after delivery.

Animal studies showed reproductive toxicity, but did not indicate direct harmful effects with respect to pregnancy, embryonal/foetal development, parturition or postnatal development (see Section 5.3 Preclinical safety data).

Lactation

Small amounts of paroxetine are excreted in breast milk. In published studies, serum concentrations in breast-fed infants were undetectable (<2 ng/ml) or very low (<4 ng/ml). No signs of drug effects were observed in these infants. Nevertheless, paroxetine should not be used during lactation unless the expected benefits to the mother justify the potential risks for the infant.

4.7 Effects on ability to drive and use machines

Clinical experience has shown that therapy with paroxetine is not associated with impairment of cognitive or psychomotor function. However, as with all psychoactive drugs, patients should be cautioned about their ability to drive a car and operate machinery. Although paroxetine does not increase the mental and motor skill impairments caused by alcohol, the concomitant use of paroxetine and alcohol is not advised.

4.8 Undesirable effects

Some of the adverse drug reactions listed below may decrease in intensity and frequency with continued treatment and do not generally lead to cessation of therapy.Adverse drug reactions are listed below by system organ class and frequency. Frequencies are defined as: very common (≥1/10), common (≥1/100, <1/10), uncommon (≥1/1,000, <1/100), rare (≥1/10,000, <1/1,000), very rare (<1/10,000), including isolated reports.

Blood and lymphatic system disorders

Uncommon: abnormal bleeding, predominantly of the skin and mucous membranes (mostly ecchymosis).

Very rare: thrombocytopenia.

Immune system disorders

Very rare: allergic reactions (including urticaria and angioedema).

Endocrine disorders

Very rare: syndrome of inappropriate anti-diuretic hormone secretion (SIADH).

Metabolism & nutrition disorders

Common: decreased appetite

Rare: hyponatraemia.

Hyponatraemia has been reported predominantly in elderly patients and is sometimes due to the syndrome of inappropriate anti-diuretic hormone secretion (SIADH).

Psychiatric disorders

Common: somnolence, insomnia.

Uncommon: confusion, hallucinations

Rare: manic reactions, agitation, anxiety, depersonalisation, panic attacks, akathisia (see section 4.4 Special Warnings and Special Precautions for use).

These symptoms may also be due to the underlying disease.

Nervous system disorders

Common: dizziness, tremor.

Uncommon: extrapyramidal disorders.

Rare: convulsions.

Very rare: serotonin syndrome (symptoms may include agitation, confusion, diaphoresis, hallucinations, hyperreflexia, myoclonus, shivering, tachycardia and tremor).

Reports of extrapyramidal disorders including oro-facial dystonia have been received in patients sometimes with underlying movement disorders or who were using neuroleptic medication.

Eye disorders

Common: blurred vision.

Very rare: acute glaucoma.

Cardiac disorders

Uncommon: sinus tachycardia.

Rare: bradycardia.

Vascular disorders

Uncommon: transient increases or decreases in blood pressure.

Transient increases or decreases of blood pressure have been reported following treatment with paroxetine, usually in patients with pre-existing hypertension or anxiety.

Respiratory, thoracic and mediastinal disorders

Common: yawning.

Gastrointestinal disorders

Very common: nausea.

Common: constipation, diarrhoea, dry mouth.

Very rare: gastrointestinal bleeding.

Hepato-biliary disorders

Rare: elevation of hepatic enzymes.

Very rare: hepatic events (such as hepatitis, sometimes associated with jaundice and/or liver failure).

Elevation of hepatic enzymes have been reported. Post-marketing reports of hepatic events (such as hepatitis, sometimes associated with jaundice and/or liver failure) have also been received very rarely. Discontinuation of paroxetine should be considered if there is prolonged elevation of liver function test results.

Skin & subcutaneous tissue disorders

Common: sweating.

Uncommon: skin rashes, pruritus.

Very rare: photosensitivity reactions.

Renal & urinary disorders

Uncommon: urinary retention.

Reproductive system & breast disorders

Very common: sexual dysfunction

Rare: hyperprolactinaemia/galactorrhoea.

Very rare: priapism.

Musculoskeletal disorders

Very rare: arthralgia, myalgia.

General disorders & administration site conditions

Common: asthenia, body weight gain.

Very rare: peripheral oedema.

WITHDRAWAL SYMPTOMS SEEN ON DISCONTINUATION OF PAROXETINE TREATMENT

Common: Dizziness, sensory disturbances, sleep disturbances, anxiety, headache.

Uncommon: Agitation, nausea, tremor, confusion, sweating, emotional instability, visual disturbances, palpitations, diarrhoea, irritability.

Discontinuation of paroxetine (particularly when abrupt) commonly leads to withdrawal symptoms. Dizziness, sensory disturbances (including paraesthesia and electric shock sensations), sleep disturbances (including intense dreams), agitation or anxiety, nausea, tremor, confusion, sweating, headache, diarrhoea, palpitations, emotional instability, irritability, and visual disturbances have been reported.

Generally these events are mild to moderate and are self-limiting, however, in some patients they may be severe and/or prolonged. It is therefore advised that when paroxetine treatment is no longer required, gradual discontinuation by dose tapering be carried out (see sections 4.2 Posology and Method of Administration and, 4.4 Special warnings and precautions for use).

Adverse events from paediatric clinical trials

In short term (up to 10-12 weeks) clinical trials in children and adolescents, the following adverse events were observed in paroxetine treated patients at a frequency of at least 2% of patients and occurred at a rate of at least twice that of placebo were: increased suicidal related behaviours (including suicide attempts and suicidal thoughts), self-harm behaviours and increased hostility. Suicidal thoughts and suicide attempts were mainly observed in clinical trials of adolescents with Major Depressive Disorder. Increased hostility occurred particularly in children with obsessive compulsive disorder, and especially in younger children less than 12 years of age. Additional events that were more often seen in the paroxetine compared to placebo group were: decreased appetite, tremor, sweating, hyperkinesia, hostility, agitation, emotional lability (including crying and mood fluctuations).

In studies that used a tapering regimen, symptoms reported during the taper phase or upon discontinuation of paroxetine at a frequency of at least 2% of patients and that occurred at a rate of at least twice that of placebo were: emotional lability (including crying, mood fluctuations, self-harm, suicidal thoughts and attempted suicide), nervousness, dizziness, nausea and abdominal pain (see section 4.4 Special warnings and special precautions for use)

4.9 Overdose

Symptoms and signs

A wide margin of safety is evident from available overdose information on paroxetine.

Experience of paroxetine in overdose has indicated that, in addition to those symptoms mentioned under section 4.8 'Undesirable Effects', vomiting, dilated pupils, fever, blood pressure changes, headache, involuntary muscle contractions, agitation, anxiety and tachycardia have been reported.

Patients have generally recovered without serious sequelae even when doses of up to 2000 mg have been taken alone. Events such as coma or ECG changes have occasionally been reported and, very rarely a fatal outcome, but generally when paroxetine was taken in conjunction with other pyschotropic drugs, with or without alcohol.

Treatment

No specific antidote is known.

Treatment should consist of those general measures employed in the management of overdose with any antidepressant. Where appropriate, the stomach should be emptied either by the induction of emesis, lavage or both. Following evacuation, 20 to 30 g of activated charcoal may be administered every 4 to 6 h during the first 24 h after ingestion. Supportive care with frequent monitoring of vital signs and careful observation is indicated.

5. PHARMACOLOGICAL PROPERTIES

5.1 Pharmacodynamic properties

Pharmacotherapeutic group: Antidepressants – selective serotonin reuptake inhibitors, ATC code: N06A B05

Mechanism of Action

Paroxetine is a potent and selective inhibitor of 5-hydroxytryptamine (5-HT, serotonin) reuptake and its antidepressant action and efficacy in the treatment of OCD, Social Anxiety disorder/Social Phobia, General Anxiety Disorder, Post-traumatic Stress Disorder and panic disorder is thought to be related to its specific inhibition of 5-HT reuptake in brain neurones.

Paroxetine is chemically unrelated to the tricyclic, tetracyclic and other available antidepressants.

Paroxetine has low affinity for muscarinic cholinergic receptors and animal studies have indicated only weak anticholinergic properties.

In accordance with this selective action, *in vitro* studies have indicated that, in contrast to tricyclic antidepressants, paroxetine has little affinity for alpha1, alpha2 and beta-adrenoceptors, dopamine (D2), 5-HT1 like, 5-HT2 and histamine (H1) receptors. This lack of interaction with post-synaptic receptors *in vitro* is substantiated by *in vivo* studies which demonstrate lack of CNS depressant and hypotensive properties.

Pharmacodynamic Effects

Paroxetine does not impair psychomotor function and does not potentiate the depressant effects of ethanol.

As with other selective 5-HT uptake inhibitors, paroxetine causes symptoms of excessive 5-HT receptor stimulation when administered to animals previously given monoamine oxidase (MAO) inhibitors or tryptophan.

Behavioural and EEG studies indicate that paroxetine is weakly activating at doses generally above those required to inhibit 5-HT uptake. The activating properties are not "amphetamine-like" in nature.

Animal studies indicate that paroxetine is well tolerated by the cardiovascular system. Paroxetine produces no clinically significant changes in blood pressure, heart rate and ECG after administration to healthy subjects.

Studies indicate that, in contrast to antidepressants which inhibit the uptake of noradrenaline, paroxetine has a much reduced propensity to inhibit the antihypertensive effects of guanethidine.

In the treatment of depressive disorders, paroxetine exhibits comparable efficacy to standard antidepressants.

There is also some evidence that paroxetine may be of therapeutic value in patients who have failed to respond to standard therapy.

Morning dosing with paroxetine does not have any detrimental effect on either the quality or duration of sleep. Moreover, patients are likely to experience improved sleep as they respond to paroxetine therapy.

Dose response

In the fixed dose studies there is a flat dose response curve, providing no suggestion of advantage in terms of efficacy for using higher than the recommended doses. However, there are some clinical data suggesting that up-titrating the dose might be beneficial for some patients.

Long-term efficacy

The long-term efficacy of paroxetine in depression has been demonstrated in a 52 week maintenance study with relapse prevention design: 12% of patients receiving paroxetine (20-40mg daily) relapsed, versus 28% of patients on placebo.

The long-term efficacy of paroxetine in treating obsessive compulsive disorder has been examined in three 24 week maintenance studies with relapse prevention design. One of the three studies achieved a significant difference in the proportion of relapsers between paroxetine (38%) compared to placebo (59%).

The long-term efficacy of paroxetine in treating panic disorder has been demonstrated in a 24 week maintenance study with relapse prevention design: 5% of patients receiving paroxetine (10-40mg daily) relapsed, versus 30% of patients on placebo. This was supported by a 36 week maintenance study.

The long-term efficacy of paroxetine in treating social anxiety disorder and generalised anxiety disorder and Post-traumatic Stress Disorderhas not been sufficiently demonstrated.

5.2 Pharmacokinetic properties

Absorption

Paroxetine is well absorbed after oral dosing and undergoes first-pass metabolism. Due to first-pass metabolism, the amount of paroxetine available to the systemic circulation is less than that absorbed from the gastrointestinal tract. Partial saturation of the first-pass effect and reduced plasma clearance occur as the body burden increases with higher single doses or on multiple dosing. This results in disproportionate increases in plasma concentrations of paroxetine and hence pharmacokinetic parameters are not constant, resulting in non-linear kinetics. However, the non-linearity is generally small and is confined to those subjects who achieve low plasma levels at low doses.

Steady state systemic levels are attained by 7 to 14 days after starting treatment with immediate or controlled release formulations and pharmacokinetics do not appear to change during long-term therapy.

Distribution

Paroxetine is extensively distributed into tissues and pharmacokinetic calculations indicate that only 1% of the paroxetine in the body resides in the plasma.

Approximately 95% of the paroxetine present is protein bound at therapeutic concentrations.

No correlation has been found between paroxetine plasma concentrations and clinical effect (adverse experiences and efficacy).

Transfer to human breast milk, and to the foetuses of laboratory animals, occurs in small amounts.

Metabolism

The principal metabolites of paroxetine are polar and conjugated products of oxidation and methylation which are readily cleared. In view of their relative lack of pharmacological activity, it is most unlikely that they contribute to paroxetine's therapeutic effects.

Metabolism does not compromise paroxetine's selective action on neuronal 5-HT uptake.

Elimination

Urinary excretion of unchanged paroxetine is generally less than 2% of dose whilst that of metabolites is about 64% of dose. About 36% of the dose is excreted in faeces, probably via the bile, of which unchanged paroxetine represents less than 1% of the dose. Thus paroxetine is eliminated almost entirely by metabolism.

Metabolite excretion is biphasic, being initially a result of first-pass metabolism and subsequently controlled by systemic elimination of paroxetine.

The elimination half-life is variable but is generally about 1 day.

Special patient populations

Elderly and renal/hepatic impairment

Increased plasma concentrations of paroxetine occur in elderly subjects and in those subjects with severe renal impairment or in those with hepatic impairment, but the range of plasma concentrations overlaps that of healthy adult subjects.

5.3 Preclinical safety data

Toxicology studies have been conducted in rhesus monkeys and albino rats; in both, the metabolic pathway is similar to that described for humans. As expected with lipophilic amines, including tricyclic antidepressants, phospholipidosis was detected in rats. Phospholipidosis was not observed in primate studies of up to one-year duration at doses that were 6 times higher than the recommended range of clinical doses.

Carcinogenesis: In two-year studies conducted in mice and rats, paroxetine had no tumorigenic effect.

Genotoxicity: Genotoxicity was not observed in a battery of *in vitro* and *in vivo* tests.

Reproduction toxicity studies in rats have shown that paroxetine affects male and female fertility. In rats, increased pup mortality and delayed ossification were observed. The latter effects were likely related to maternal toxicity and are not considered a direct effect on the foetus/neonate.

6. PHARMACEUTICAL PARTICULARS

6.1 List of excipients

Tablet cores: Calcium phosphate (E341), sodium starch glycollate, magnesium stearate (E572).

Tablet film-coat: Hydroxypropyl methylcellulose (E464), titanium dioxide (E171), polyethylene glycol and polysorbate 80 (E433). The coating of the 30 mg tablets also contains indigo carmine (E132).

Liquid: Polacrilin potassium, dispersible cellulose (E460), propylene glycol, glycerol, (E422), sorbitol (E420), methyl parahydroxybenzoate (E218), propyl parahydroxybenzoate (E216), sodium citrate (E331), citric acid (E330), sodium saccharin (E954), natural orange flavour, natural lemon flavour, yellow colouring (E110), simethicone emulsion, purified water.

6.2 Incompatibilities

Not applicable

6.3 Shelf life

Tablets: Three years

Liquid: Two years

6.4 Special precautions for storage

Tablets: No special storage precautions are required.

Liquid: Do not store above 25 °C

6.5 Nature and contents of container

Tablets: Available in Original Packs of 30 (three PVC/aluminium or PVC/PVdC aluminium blister strips of 10 tablets).

Liquid: Bottles containing 150 ml with a child-resistant closure and cup

6.6 Instructions for use and handling

None.

Administrative Data

7. MARKETING AUTHORISATION HOLDER

SmithKline Beecham plc
Great West Road
Brentford
Middlesex TW8 9GS.
trading as:
SmithKline Beecham Pharmaceuticals
Welwyn Garden City
Hertfordshire AL7 1EY
And/or
GlaxoSmithKline UK,
Stockley Park West,
Uxbridge,
Middlesex UB11 1BT

8. MARKETING AUTHORISATION NUMBER(S)

Seroxat 20 mg tablets: 10592/0001

Seroxat 30 mg tablets: 10592/0002

Seroxat Liquid: 10592/0092

9. DATE OF FIRST AUTHORISATION/RENEWAL OF THE AUTHORISATION

Seroxat 20 mg tablets: 09.01.98

Seroxat 30 mg tablets: 09.01.98

Seroxat Liquid: 09.01.02

10. DATE OF REVISION OF THE TEXT

8th April 2005

11. LEGAL STATUS

POM

Sevoflurane

(Abbott Laboratories Limited)

1. NAME OF THE MEDICINAL PRODUCT

Sevoflurane

2. QUALITATIVE AND QUANTITATIVE COMPOSITION

The finished product is comprised only of the active ingredient (Sevoflurane).

3. PHARMACEUTICAL FORM

Sevoflurane is a nonflammable volatile liquid. Sevoflurane is administered via inhalation of the vaporised liquid.

4. CLINICAL PARTICULARS

4.1 Therapeutic indications

Sevoflurane is indicated for induction and maintenance of general anaesthesia in adult and paediatric patients for inpatient and outpatient surgery.

4.2 Posology and method of administration

Sevoflurane should be delivered via a vaporiser specifically calibrated for use with Sevoflurane so that the concentration delivered can be accurately controlled. MAC (minimum alveolar concentration) values for Sevoflurane decrease with age and with the addition of nitrous oxide. The table below indicates average MAC values for different age groups.

EFFECT OF AGE ON MAC OF SEVOFLURANE

Age of Patient (years)	Sevoflurane in Oxygen	Sevoflurane in 65% N_2O/35% O_2*
<3	3.3 - 2.6%	2.0%
3 - <5	2.5%	Not available
5 - 12	2.4%	Not available
25	2.5%	1.4%
35	2.2%	1.2%
40	2.05%	1.1%
50	1.8%	0.98%
60	1.6%	0.87%
80	1.4%	0.70%

* In paediatric patients, 60% N_2O/40% O_2 was used.

Induction:

Dosage should be individualised and titrated to the desired effect according to the patient's age and clinical status. A short acting barbiturate or other intravenous induction agent may be administered followed by inhalation of sevoflurane. Induction with sevoflurane may be achieved in oxygen or in combination with oxygen-nitrous oxide mixtures. In adults inspired concentrations of up to 5% Sevoflurane usually produce surgical anaesthesia in less than 2 minutes. In children, inspired concentrations of up to 7% Sevoflurane usually produce surgical anaesthesia in less than 2 minutes. Alternatively, for induction of anaesthesia in unpremedicated patients, inspired concentrations of up to 8% Sevoflurane may be used.

Maintenance:

Surgical levels of anaesthesia may be sustained with concentrations of 0.5 - 3% Sevoflurane with or without the concomitant use of nitrous oxide.

Elderly: As with other inhalation agents, lesser concentrations of Sevoflurane are normally required to maintain surgical anaesthesia.

Emergence:

Emergence times are generally short following Sevoflurane anaesthesia. Therefore, patients may require early post operative pain relief.

4.3 Contraindications

Sevoflurane should not be used in patients with known sensitivity to Sevoflurane. Sevoflurane is also contraindicated in patients with known or suspected genetic susceptibility to malignant hyperthermia.

4.4 Special warnings and special precautions for use

Sevoflurane should be administered only by persons trained in the administration of general anaesthesia. Facilities for maintenance of a patent airway, artificial ventilation, oxygen enrichment and circulatory resuscitation must be immediately available. Sevoflurane should be delivered via a vaporiser specifically calibrated for use with Sevoflurane so that the concentration delivered can be accurately controlled. Hypotension and respiratory depression increase as anaesthesia is deepened.

During the maintenance of anaesthesia, increasing the concentration of Sevoflurane produces dose-dependent decreases in blood pressure. Excessive decrease in blood pressure may be related to depth of anaesthesia and in such instances may be corrected by decreasing the inspired concentration of Sevoflurane. The recovery from general anaesthesia should be assessed carefully before patients are discharged from the recovery room.

Malignant Hyperthermia: In susceptible individuals, potent inhalation anaesthetic agents may trigger a skeletal muscle hypermetabolic state leading to high oxygen demand and the clinical syndrome known as malignant hyperthermia. Treatment includes discontinuation of triggering agents (e.g. Sevoflurane), administration of intravenous dantrolene sodium, and application of supportive therapy. Renal failure may appear later, and urine flow should be monitored and sustained if possible.

Because of the small number of patients with renal insufficiency (baseline serum creatinine greater than 133μmol/litre) studied, the safety of Sevoflurane administration in this group has not been fully established. Therefore, Sevoflurane should be used with caution in patients with renal insufficiency.

Sevoflurane produces low levels of Compound A (pentafluoroisopropenyl fluoromethyl ether (PIFE)) and trace amounts of Compound B (pentafluoromethoxy isopropyl fluoromethyl ether (PMFE)), when in direct contact with CO_2 absorbents. Levels of Compound A increase with:- increase in canister temperature; increase in anaesthetic concentration; decrease in gas flow rate and increase more with the use of Baralyme rather than Soda lime. (See also Pharmaceutical Particulars.)

In some studies in rats, nephrotoxicity was seen in animals exposed to levels of Compound A in excess of those usually seen in routine clinical practice. The mechanism of this renal toxicity in rats is unknown and its relevance to man has not been established. (See Section 5.3, Preclinical Safety Data for further details.)

The exothermic reaction that occurs with inhalational agents, including Sevoflurane and

CO_2 absorbents, is increased when the CO_2 absorbent becomes desiccated (dried out),

such as after an extended period of dry gas flow through the CO_2 absorbent canisters.

Rare cases of excessive heat production, smoke and/or fire in the anaesthetic machine have been reported during Sevoflurane use in conjunction with the use of desiccated CO_2

absorbent. An unusually delayed rise or unexpected decline of inspired Sevoflurane concentration compared to the vaporiser setting may inidicate excessive heating of the CO_2 absorbent canister.

When a clinician suspects that the CO_2 absorbent may be desiccated, it should be replaced. The colour indicator of most CO_2 absorbents does not necessarily change as a result of desiccation. Therefore, the lack of significant colour change should not be taken as an assurance of adequate hydration. CO_2 absorbents should be replaced routinely regardless of the state of the colour indicator.

Experience with repeat exposure to Sevoflurane is very limited. However, there were no obvious differences in adverse events between first and subsequent exposures.

4.5 Interaction with other medicinal products and other forms of Interaction

The action of non-depolarising muscle relaxants is potentiated with Sevoflurane, therefore, when administered with Sevoflurane, dosage adjustments of these agents should be made.

Sevoflurane is similar to isoflurane in the sensitisation of the myocardium to the arrhythmogenic effect of exogenously administered adrenaline.

MAC values for Sevoflurane decrease with the addition of nitrous oxide as indicated in the table on 'Effect of Age on MAC of Sevoflurane' (see Dosage and Method of Administration).

As with other agents, lesser concentrations of Sevoflurane may be required following use of an intravenous anaesthetic e.g. propofol.

The metabolism of Sevoflurane may be increased by known inducers of CYP2E1 (e.g. isoniazid and alcohol), but it is not inducible by barbiturates.

4.6 Pregnancy and lactation

With the exception of one study in Caesarean Section there are no other studies in pregnant women, including in labour and delivery. Experience in Caesarean section is limited to one trial in a small number of patients.

Reproduction studies have been performed in rats and rabbits at doses up to 1 MAC.

No effects on male and female reproductive capabilities were observed. Reduced foetal body weights concomitant with increased skeletal variations were noted in rats only at maternally toxic concentrations. No adverse foetal effects were observed in rabbits. Sevoflurane was not teratogenic.

Therefore, Sevoflurane should be used during pregnancy only if clearly needed.

It is not known whether Sevoflurane is excreted in human milk therefore caution should be exercised when Sevoflurane is administered to a nursing woman.

4.7 Effects on ability to drive and use machines

As with other agents, patients should be advised that performance of activities requiring mental alertness, such as operating hazardous machinery, may be impaired for some time after general anaesthesia.

Patients should not be allowed to drive for a suitable period after Sevoflurane anaesthesia.

4.8 Undesirable effects

As with all potent inhaled anaesthetics, Sevoflurane may cause dose-dependent cardio-respiratory depression. Most adverse events are mild to moderate in severity and are transient. Nausea and vomiting are commonly observed in the post-operative period, at a similar incidence to those found with other inhalation anaesthetics. These effects are common sequelae of surgery and general anaesthesia which may be due to the inhalational anaesthetic, other agents administered intra-operatively or post-operatively and to the patient's response to the surgical procedure.

Adverse event data are derived from controlled clinical trials conducted in the United States and Europe in over 3,200 patients. The type, severity and frequency of adverse events in Sevoflurane patients were comparable to adverse events in patients treated with other inhalation anaesthetics.

The most frequent adverse events associated with Sevoflurane overall were nausea (24%) and vomiting (17%). Agitation occurred frequently in children (23%).

Other frequent adverse events ($\geq$10%) associated with Sevoflurane administration overall were: increased cough and hypotension.

In addition to nausea and vomiting, other frequent adverse events ($\geq$10%) by age listings were: in adults, hypotension; in elderly, hypotension and bradycardia; in children, agitation and increased cough.

Less frequent adverse events (1-<10% overall) associated with Sevoflurane administration were: agitation, somnolence, chills, bradycardia, dizziness, increased salivation, respiratory disorder, hypertension, tachycardia, laryngismus, fever, headache, hypothermia, increased SGOT.

Occasional (<1% overall) adverse events occurring during clinical trials included: arrhythmias, increased LDH, increased SGPT, hypoxia, apnoea, leukocytosis, ventricular extrasystoles, supraventricular extrasystoles, asthma, confusion, increased creatinine, urinary retention, glycosuria, atrial fibrillation, complete AV block, bigeminy, leucopenia

Malignant hyperthermia and acute kidney failure have been reported very rarely.

Rare reports of allergic reactions, such as rash, urticaria, pruritus, bronchospasm, anaphylactic or anaphylactoid reactions have been reported.

Rare reports of post-operative hepatitis exist, but with an uncertain relationship to Sevoflurane.

Convulsions may occur extremely rarely following Sevoflurane administration, particularly in children.

There have been very rare reports of pulmonary oedema.

As with other anaesthetic agents, cases of twitching and jerking movements with spontaneous resolution have been reported in children receiving Sevoflurane for induction of anaesthesia with an uncertain relationship to Sevoflurane.

Laboratory findings:

Transient elevations in glucose and white blood cell count may occur as with use of other anaesthetic agents.

Occasional cases of transient changes in hepatic function tests were reported with Sevoflurane.

4.9 Overdose

In the event of overdosage, the following action should be taken: Stop drug administration, establish a clear airway and initiate assisted or controlled ventilation with pure oxygen and maintain adequate cardiovascular function.

5. PHARMACOLOGICAL PROPERTIES

5.1 Pharmacodynamic properties

Changes in the clinical effects of Sevoflurane rapidly follow changes in the inspired concentration.

Cardiovascular Effects

As with all other inhalation agents Sevoflurane depresses cardiovascular function in a dose related fashion. In one volunteer study, increases in Sevoflurane concentration resulted in decrease in mean arterial pressure, but there was no change in heart rate. Sevoflurane did not alter plasma noradrenaline concentrations in this study.

Nervous System Effects

No evidence of seizure was observed during the clinical development programme.

In patients with normal intracranial pressure (ICP), Sevoflurane had minimal effect on ICP and preserved CO_2 responsiveness. The safety of Sevoflurane has not been investigated in patients with a raised ICP. In patients at risk for elevations of ICP, Sevoflurane should be administered cautiously in conjunction with ICP-reducing manoeuvres such as hyperventilation.

5.2 Pharmacokinetic properties

The low solubility of Sevoflurane in blood should result in alveolar concentrations which rapidly increase upon induction and rapidly decrease upon cessation of the inhaled agent.

In humans <5% of the absorbed Sevoflurane is metabolised. The rapid and extensive pulmonary elimination of Sevoflurane minimises the amount of anaesthetic available for metabolism. Sevoflurane is defluorinated via cytochrome p450(CYP)2E1 resulting in the production of hexafluoroisopropanol (HFIP) with release of inorganic fluoride and carbon dioxide (or a one carbon fragment). HFIP is then rapidly conjugated with glucuronic acid and excreted in the urine.

The metabolism of Sevoflurane may be increased by known inducers of CYP2E1 (e.g. isoniazid and alcohol), but it is not inducible by barbiturates.

Transient increases in serum inorganic fluoride levels may occur during and after Sevoflurane anaesthesia. Generally, concentrations of inorganic fluoride peak within 2 hours of the end of Sevoflurane anaesthesia and return within 48 hours to pre-operative levels.

5.3 Preclinical safety data

Animal studies have shown that hepatic and renal circulation are well maintained with Sevoflurane.

Sevoflurane decreases the cerebral metabolic rate for oxygen ($CMRO_2$) in a fashion analogous to that seen with isoflurane. An approximately 50% reduction of $CMRO_2$ is observed at concentrations approaching 2.0 MAC. Animal studies have demonstrated that Sevoflurane does not have a significant effect on cerebral blood flow.

In animals, Sevoflurane significantly suppresses electroencephalographic (EEG) activity comparable to equipotent doses of isoflurane. There is no evidence that Sevoflurane is associated with epileptiform activity during normocapnia or hypocapnia. In contrast to enflurane, attempts to elicit seizure-like EEG activity during hypocapnia with rhythmic auditory stimuli have been negative.

Compound A was minimally nephrotoxic at concentrations of 50-114 ppm for 3 hours in a range of studies in rats. The toxicity was characterised by sporadic single cell necrosis of the proximal tubule cells. The mechanism of this renal toxicity in rats is unknown and its relevance to man has not been established. Comparable human thresholds for Compound A-related nephrotoxicity would be predicted to be 150-200 ppm. The concentrations of Compound A found in routine clinical practice are on average 19 ppm in adults (maximum 32 ppm) with use of Soda lime as the CO_2 absorbent.

6. PHARMACEUTICAL PARTICULARS

6.1 List of excipients

None.

6.2 Incompatibilities

Sevoflurane is chemically stable. No discernible degradation occurs in the presence of strong acids or heat. The only known degradation reaction in the clinical setting is through direct contact with CO_2 absorbents (Soda lime and Baralyme) producing low levels of Compound A (pentafluoroisopropenyl fluoromethyl ether (PIFE)), and trace amounts of Compound B (pentafluoromethoxy isopropyl fluoromethyl ether, (PMFE)). The interaction with CO_2 absorbents is not unique to Sevoflurane. The production of degradants in the anaesthesia circuit results from the extraction of the acidic proton in the presence of a strong base (KOH and/or NaOH) forming an alkene (Compound A) from Sevoflurane, similar to formation of 2-bromo-2-chloro-1,1-difluoro ethylene (BCDFE) from halothane. No dose adjustment or change in clinical practice is necessary when rebreathing circuits are used.

Higher levels of Compound A are obtained when using Baralyme rather than Soda lime.

6.3 Shelf life

The recommended shelf life is 24 months.

6.4 Special precautions for storage

Do not store above 25°C. Do not refrigerate. Keep cap tightly closed.

6.5 Nature and contents of container

100ml and 250ml amber polyethylene napthalate (PEN) or glass bottles.

6.6 Instructions for use and handling

Sevoflurane should be administered via a vaporiser calibrated specifically for Sevoflurane using a key filling system designed for Sevoflurane specific vaporisers or other appropriate Sevoflurane specific vaporiser filling systems.

Carbon dioxide absorbents should not be allowed to dry out when inhalational anaesthetics are being administered. Some halogenated anaesthetics have been reported to interact with dry carbon dioxide absorbent to form carbon monoxide. However, in order to minimise the risk of formation of carbon monoxide in re-breathing circuits and the possibility of elevated carboxyhaemoglobin levels, CO_2 absorbents should not be allowed to dry out. There have been rare cases of excessive heat production, smoke and fire in the anaesthetic machine when Sevoflurane has been used in conjunction with a desiccated (dried out) CO_2 absorbent. If the CO_2 absorbent is suspected to be desiccated it should be replaced.

Administrative Data

7. MARKETING AUTHORISATION HOLDER

Abbott Laboratories Ltd

Queenborough

Kent

ME11 5EL, UK.

8. MARKETING AUTHORISATION NUMBER(S)

PL 0037/0258

9. DATE OF FIRST AUTHORISATION/RENEWAL OF THE AUTHORISATION

1 September 1995

10. DATE OF REVISION OF THE TEXT

November 2003

Sevredol tablets 10 mg, 20 mg, 50 mg.

(Napp Pharmaceuticals Limited)

1. NAME OF THE MEDICINAL PRODUCT

SEVREDOL® tablets 10 mg, 20 mg, 50 mg.

2. QUALITATIVE AND QUANTITATIVE COMPOSITION

Morphine Sulphate 10 mg, 20 mg, 50 mg.

For excipients see section 6.1.

3. PHARMACEUTICAL FORM

Film-coated tablet.

10 mg

Blue, film-coated, capsule-shaped, biconvex tablet with a score line on one side. "IR" is marked on the left side and "10" on the right.

20 mg

Pink, film-coated, capsule-shaped, biconvex tablet with a score line on one side. "IR" is marked on the left side and "20" on the right.

50 mg

Pale, green film-coated, capsule-shaped, biconvex tablet with a score line on one side. "IR" is marked on the left side and "50" on the right.

4. CLINICAL PARTICULARS

4.1 Therapeutic indications

SEVREDOL tablets are indicated for the relief of severe pain.

4.2 Posology and method of administration

Route of administration

Oral.

Adults and children over 12 years:

The dosage of SEVREDOL tablets is dependent on the severity of pain and the patient's previous history of analgesic requirements. One tablet to be taken every four hours or as directed by a physician. Increasing severity of pain or tolerance to morphine will require increased dosage of SEVREDOL tablets using 10 mg, 20 mg or 50 mg alone or in combination to achieve the desired relief.

Patients receiving SEVREDOL tablets in place of parenteral morphine should be given a sufficiently increased dosage to compensate for any reduction in analgesic effects associated with oral administration. Usually such increased requirement is of the order of 100%. In such patients individual dose adjustments are required.

Elderly:

A reduction in adult dosage may be advisable.

Children 3 -12 years of age:

Only SEVREDOL 10 mg and 20 mg tablets are suitable for children:-

3 - 5 years	5 mg, 4-hourly
6 -12 years	5 -10 mg, 4-hourly

SEVREDOL tablets 50 mg are not recommended for children.

4.3 Contraindications
Hypersensitivity to any of the constituents, respiratory depression, head injury, obstructive airways disease, paralytic ileus, acute abdomen, delayed gastric emptying, known morphine sensitivity, acute hepatic disease, concurrent administration of monoamine oxidase inhibitors or within two weeks of discontinuation of their use. Not recommended during pregnancy.

Not recommended for children below 3 years of age.

4.4 Special warnings and special precautions for use
As with all narcotics a reduction in dosage may be advisable in the elderly, in hypothyroidism and in patients with significantly impaired renal or hepatic function. Use with caution in opiate dependent patients and in patients with raised intracranial pressure, hypotension with hypovolaemia, diseases of the biliary tract, pancreatitis, inflammatory bowel disorders, prostatic hypertrophy, adrenocortical insufficiency, acute alcoholism and patients with compulsive disorders.

Should paralytic ileus be suspected or occur during use, SEVREDOL tablets should be discontinued immediately. As with all morphine preparations, patients who are about to undergo cordotomy or other pain relieving procedures should not receive SEVREDOL tablets for 4 hours prior to surgery.

As with all morphine preparations, SEVREDOL tablets should be used with caution post-operatively, and following abdominal surgery as morphine impairs intestinal motility and should not be used until the physician is assured of normal bowel function.

Patients with rare hereditary problems of galactose intolerance, the Lapp lactase deficiency or glucose-galactose malabsorption should not take this medicine.

4.5 Interaction with other medicinal products and other forms of Interaction
Morphine potentiates the effects of tranquillisers, anaesthetics, hypnotics, sedatives, alcohol, muscle relaxants and antihypertensives. Cimetidine inhibits the metabolism of morphine. Monoamine oxidase inhibitors are known to interact with narcotic analgesics producing CNS excitation or depression with hyper- or hypotensive crisis. Mixed agonist/antagonist opioid analgesics (e.g. buprenorphine, nalbuphine, pentazocine) should not be administered to a patient who has received a course of therapy with a pure opioid agonist analgesic.

4.6 Pregnancy and lactation
SEVREDOL tablets are not recommended during pregnancy and labour due to the risk of neonatal respiratory depression. Administration to nursing mothers is not recommended as morphine is excreted in breast milk. Withdrawal symptoms may be observed in the new born of mothers undergoing chronic treatment.

4.7 Effects on ability to drive and use machines
Treatment with SEVREDOL tablets may cause sedation and it is not recommended that patients drive or use machines if they experience drowsiness.

4.8 Undesirable effects
In normal doses, the commonest side effects of morphine are nausea, vomiting, constipation and drowsiness. With chronic therapy, nausea and vomiting are unusual with SEVREDOL tablets but should they occur the tablets can be readily combined with an anti-emetic if required. Constipation may be treated with appropriate laxatives.

Other adverse reactions include:

Cardiovascular: Palpitations and rarely, clinically relevant reductions in blood pressure and heart rate have been observed.

Central Nervous System: Headache, disorientation, vertigo, mood changes, hallucinations and myoclonus. Overdose may produce respiratory depression.

Respiratory: Bronchospasm.

Gastrointestinal: Dry mouth, biliary spasm and colic may occur in a few patients. Paralytic ileus may be associated with opioid usage.

Genitourinary: Decreased libido, ureteric spasm and micturition may be difficult.

Dermatological: Rash, morphine has histamine releasing effects which may be responsible in part for reactions such as urticaria and pruritus.

General: Sweating, facial flushing and miosis.

The effects of morphine have led to its abuse and dependence may develop with regular, inappropriate use. This is not a major concern in the treatment of patients with severe pain.

4.9 Overdose
Signs of morphine toxicity and overdosage are pin-point pupils, respiratory depression and hypotension. Circulatory failure and deepening coma may occur in more severe cases. Rhabdomyolysis progressing to renal failure has been reported in opioid overdosage.

Treatment of morphine overdosage

Primary attention should be given to the establishment of a patent airway and institution of assisted or controlled ventilation.

In the case of massive overdosage, administer naloxone 0.8 mg intravenously. Repeat at 2-3 minute intervals as necessary, or by an infusion of 2 mg in 500 ml of normal saline or 5% dextrose (0.004 mg/ml).

The infusion should be run at a rate related to the previous bolus doses administered and should be in accordance with the patient's response. However, because the duration of action of naloxone is relatively short, the patient must be carefully monitored until spontaneous respiration is reliably re-established.

For less severe overdosage, administer naloxone 0.2 mg intravenously followed by increments of 0.1 mg every 2 minutes if required.

Naloxone should not be administered in the absence of clinically significant respiratory or circulatory depression secondary to morphine overdosage. Naloxone should be administered cautiously to persons who are known, or suspected, to be physically dependent on morphine. In such cases, an abrupt or complete reversal of opioid effects may precipitate an acute withdrawal syndrome.

Gastric contents may need to be emptied as this can be useful in removing unabsorbed drug.

5. PHARMACOLOGICAL PROPERTIES

5.1 Pharmacodynamic properties
Pharmacotherapeutic group: Natural opium alkaloid

ATC Code: N02A 01

Morphine acts as an agonist at opiate receptors in the CNS, particularly mu and to a lesser extent, kappa receptors. Mu receptors are thought to mediate supraspinal analgesia, respiratory depression, and euphoria, and kappa receptors, spinal analgesia, miosis and sedation. Morphine also has a direct action on the bowel wall nerve, causing constipation.

5.2 Pharmacokinetic properties
Morphine is well absorbed from SEVREDOL tablets, however first-pass metabolism does occur. Apart from the liver, metabolism also occurs in the kidney and intestinal mucosa. The major urinary metabolite is morphine-3-glucuronide but morphine-6-glucuronide is also formed. The half-life for morphine in the plasma is approximately 2.5 - 3.0 hours.

5.3 Preclinical safety data
There are no pre-clinical data of relevance to the prescriber which are additional to that already included in other sections of the SPC.

6. PHARMACEUTICAL PARTICULARS

6.1 List of excipients
Tablet core

Lactose (anhydrous)

Pregelatinised maize starch

Povidone

Purified water

Magnesium stearate

Talc

Film coat

10 mg tablet:	Opadry (blue) 06B20843 containing Macrogol 400, E464, E133, E171 Purified water
20 mg tablet:	Hypromellose (5 cps) Hypromellose (15 cps) Macrogol 400 Opaspray (pink) M-1-5503 containing E171, E127, E110 Purified water
50 mg tablet:	Opadry OY-21037 Green (containing hypromellose E464, titanium dioxide E171, macrogol 400, quinoline yellow E104, indigo carmine E132, iron oxide yellow E172)

6.2 Incompatibilities
None known.

6.3 Shelf life
3 years.

6.4 Special precautions for storage
Do not store above 30°C.

6.5 Nature and contents of container
PVdC coated PVC blister packs containing 56 tablets.

6.6 Instructions for use and handling
None.

Administrative Data

7. MARKETING AUTHORISATION HOLDER
Napp Pharmaceuticals Limited
Cambridge Science Park
Milton Road
Cambridge CB4 0GW

8. MARKETING AUTHORISATION NUMBER(S)
PL16950/0063-0065

9. DATE OF FIRST AUTHORISATION/RENEWAL OF THE AUTHORISATION
1 May 1999/22 March 2003

10. DATE OF REVISION OF THE TEXT
April 2005

11. Legal Category
CD (Sch 2), POM

® The Napp device and SEVREDOL are Registered Trade Marks.

Silkis 3 micrograms per g ointment

(Galderma (U.K.) Ltd)

1. NAME OF THE MEDICINAL PRODUCT
Silkis 3 micrograms per g ointment ▼

2. QUALITATIVE AND QUANTITATIVE COMPOSITION
One gram of ointment contains 3 micrograms of calcitriol (INN).

For excipients, see 6.1

3. PHARMACEUTICAL FORM
Ointment

White, translucent ointment

4. CLINICAL PARTICULARS

4.1 Therapeutic indications
Topical treatment of mild to moderately severe plaque psoriasis (psoriasis vulgaris) with up to 35% of body surface area involvement.

4.2 Posology and method of administration
Silkis Ointment should be applied to the psoriasis affected areas twice per day, once in the morning and once in the evening before retiring and after washing. It is recommended that not more than 35% of the body surface be exposed to daily treatment. Not more than 30 g of ointment should be used per day. There is limited clinical experience available for the use of this dosage regimen of more than 6 weeks.

There is no experience of the use of Silkis in children (see 4.4. Special Warnings and Precautions for Use). Patients with kidney or liver dysfunction should not use Silkis (see also 4.3. Contra-indications).

4.3 Contraindications
Patients on systemic treatment of calcium homeostasis.

Patients with kidney or liver dysfunction.

Patients with hypercalcaemia and patients known to suffer from abnormal calcium metabolism.

Silkis must not be used in patients known to be hypersensitive to the active substance or to any of the excipients.

4.4 Special warnings and special precautions for use
The ointment can be applied to the face with caution, as there is an increased risk of irritation in this area. Contact with the eyes should be avoided. The hands should be washed after applying the ointment in order to avoid unintentional application to non lesional areas. Not more than 35% of the body surface should be exposed to daily treatment. Not more than 30g of ointment should be used per day.

Due to potential effects on calcium metabolism, substances which stimulate absorption must not be added to the ointment, and the ointment must not be covered with an occlusive dressing.

In case of severe irritation or contact allergy, the treatment with Silkis should be discontinued and the patient should obtain medical advice. If contact allergy is demonstrated this discontinuation is definitive.

In view of the particular sensitivity of neonatal versus adult rodents to the toxic effects of calcitriol, exposure of children to calcitriol ointment should be avoided (see also 4.2. Posology and Method of administration)

Although no clinically significant hypercalcaemia was observed in clinical studies with a dosage under 30 g/day of Silkis ointment, some absorption of calcitriol through the skin does occur and excessive use of the ointment can lead to systemic side-effects, such as an increase in urine and serum calcium levels.

There is no information about the use of Silkis in other clinical forms of psoriasis (other than plaque psoriasis) *i.e.* Psoriasis guttata acuta, pustular psoriasis, psoriasis erythrodermica and rapid progressive plaque psoriasis.

4.5 Interaction with other medicinal products and other forms of Interaction
Silkis must be used with caution in patients receiving medications known to increase the serum calcium level, such as thiazide diuretics. Caution must also be exercised in patients receiving calcium supplements or high doses of vitamin D. There is no experience of the concurrent use of calcitriol and other medications for the treatment of psoriasis.

Information of interaction of systemic medications after the use of calcitriol ointment is limited. As no relevant elevation of plasma level is seen after the use of calcitriol on the skin, interaction with systemic medication is unlikely.

Silkis Ointment has a slight irritant potential, and therefore, it is possible that concomitant use of peeling agents, astringents or irritants products may produce additive irritant effects.

4.6 Pregnancy and lactation
Use during Pregnancy:

There are no adequate data from the use of Silkis in pregnant women. Studies in animals have shown developmental toxicity at doses which caused maternal toxicity (see section 5.3). The potential risk for humans is unknown.

Silkis should only be used during pregnancy in restricted amounts when clearly necessary. Calcium levels should be monitored.

Use during Lactation:

Calcitriol has been found in milk of lactating dams. Due to the lack of human data, it should not be used during breastfeeding.

4.7 Effects on ability to drive and use machines
No effects on ability to drive and use machines have been observed.

4.8 Undesirable effects
Skin irritation (reddening, itching), usually temporary, has been reported. In case of severe irritation or contact allergy, the treatment with Silkis should be discontinued and the patient should obtain medical advice. If contact allergy is demonstrated this discontinuation is definitive.

During clinical studies, no clinically significant hypercalcaemia was observed at the maximal dose of 30 g of ointment per day.

4.9 Overdose
The most common symptoms which may occur after accidental administration are anorexia, nausea, vomiting, constipation, hypotonia and depression. Lethargy and coma are occasionally observed. If hypercalcaemia or hypercalciuria occurs, the use of Silkis should be discontinued until the serum or urinary calcium levels have returned to normal.

If the medication is applied excessively no more rapid or better results will be obtained and marked redness, peeling or discomfort may occur.

5. PHARMACOLOGICAL PROPERTIES
5.1 Pharmacodynamic properties
ATC code: D 05AX03

Calcitriol inhibits the proliferation and stimulates differentiation of keratinocytes. Calcitriol inhibits proliferation of T-cells and normalises the production of various inflammation factors.

Topical administration of Silkis Ointment to patients with plaque psoriasis results in an improvement of the skin lesions. This effect is noted from 4 weeks after the start of treatment.

5.2 Pharmacokinetic properties
The mean absorption of calcitriol is estimated at around 10%. Following absorption, both unchanged calcitriol and metabolites have been demonstrated in plasma. The effect of the metabolites on calcium homeostasis is negligible. In most patients, circulating levels of exogenous calcitriol are below the level of detection (2pg/ml).

In clinical trials, no relevant increase in plasma calcitriol levels after treatment of large body surface areas of up to 6000 cm^2 (35% body surface area) was noted.

5.3 Preclinical safety data
Animal studies show that repeated excessive exposure to calcitriol leads to renal failure and tissue calcification due to hypervitaminosis D associated with hypercalciuria, hypercalcaemia, and hyperphosphataemia.

No indication of teratogenicity was observed in embryo-foetal toxicity studies designed to assess the teratogenic potential of calcitriol. Some evidence of developmental toxicity was obtained in a cutaneous rabbit study at doses which caused maternal toxicity. No such effect was found in rats.

Local toxicity studies in animals with Calcitriol showed slight skin and eye irritation.

6. PHARMACEUTICAL PARTICULARS
6.1 List of excipients
Liquid paraffin, white soft paraffin and alpha- tocopherol.

6.2 Incompatibilities
There are no relevant data on the compatibility of Silkis with other medicinal products. Therefore, Silkis should be used according to the posology and method of administration provided above (Section 4.2), and should not be mixed with other medicinal products.

6.3 Shelf life
3 years

6.4 Special precautions for storage
No special precautions for storage

6.5 Nature and contents of container
The product is packaged in collapsible aluminium tubes coated internally with an epoxy - phenolic resin and fitted with a white high density polyethylene or polypropylene screw cap. Tubes contain either 30 or 100g of ointment.

6.6 Instructions for use and handling
None.

7. MARKETING AUTHORISATION HOLDER
Galderma (UK) Ltd
Galderma House
Church Lane
Kings Langley
Herts
WD4 8JP
United Kingdom

8. MARKETING AUTHORISATION NUMBER(S)
PL 10590/0047

9. DATE OF FIRST AUTHORISATION/RENEWAL OF THE AUTHORISATION
12 December 2001

10. DATE OF REVISION OF THE TEXT
March 2004

Simulect 10mg and 20mg powder and solvent for solution for injection or infusion

(Novartis Pharmaceuticals UK Ltd)

1. NAME OF THE MEDICINAL PRODUCT
Simulect 10 mg powder and solvent for solution for injection or infusion

Simulect 20 mg powder and solvent for solution for injection or infusion.

2. QUALITATIVE AND QUANTITATIVE COMPOSITION
Each vial contains 10mg or 20 mg basiliximab.

One ml of the reconstituted solution contains 4 mg basiliximab.

For excipients, see section 6.1.

3. PHARMACEUTICAL FORM
Powder and solvent for solution for injection or infusion.

White powder

4. CLINICAL PARTICULARS
4.1 Therapeutic indications
Simulect is indicated for the prophylaxis of acute organ rejection in *de novo* allogeneic renal transplantation in adult and paediatric patients (see section 4.2). It is to be used concomitantly with ciclosporin for microemulsion- and corticosteroid-based immunosuppression, in patients with panel reactive antibodies less than 80%, or in a triple maintenance immunosuppressive regimen containing ciclosporin for microemulsion, corticosteroids and either azathioprine or mycophenolate mofetil.

4.2 Posology and method of administration
Simulect should be prescribed only by physicians who are experienced in the use of immunosuppressive therapy following organ transplantation. Simulect should be administered under qualified medical supervision.

Simulect is to be used concomitantly with ciclosporin for microemulsion- and corticosteroid-based immunosuppression. It can be used in a ciclosporin for microemulsion- and corticosteroid-based triple immunosuppressive regimen including azathioprine or mycophenolate mofetil.

Recommended dose

Adults

The standard total dose is 40 mg, given in two doses of 20 mg each. The first 20 mg dose should be given within 2 hours prior to transplantation surgery. Simulect must not be administered unless it is absolutely certain that the patient will receive the graft and concomitant immunosuppression. The second 20 mg dose should be given 4 days after transplantation. The second dose should be withheld if a severe hypersensitivity reaction to Simulect or graft loss occurs (see section 4.4)

Children and adolescents (1-17 years)

In paediatric patients weighing less than 35 kg, the recommended total dose is 20 mg, given in two doses of 10 mg each. In paediatric patients weighing 35 kg or more, the recommended dose is the adult dose, i.e. a total dose of 40 mg, given in two doses of 20 mg each. Simulect must not be administered unless it is absolutely certain that the patient will receive the graft and concomitant immunosuppression. The first dose should be given within 2 hours prior to transplantation surgery. The second dose should be given 4 days after transplantation. The second dose should be withheld if post-operative complications such as graft loss occur (see section 4.4)

Use in the elderly (⩾ 65 years)

There are limited data available on the use of Simulect in the elderly, but there is no evidence that elderly patients require a different dosage from younger adult patients.

Method of administration

Reconstituted Simulect can be administered as an intravenous bolus injection or as an intravenous infusion over 20–30 minutes.

For information on reconstituting Simulect, see section 6.6.

4.3 Contraindications
Hypersensitivity to the active substance or to any of the excipients (see section 6.1).

Simulect is contraindicated during pregnancy and lactation.

4.4 Special warnings and special precautions for use
Patients receiving Simulect must be managed in facilities equipped and staffed with adequate laboratory and supportive medical resources, including medications for the treatment of severe hypersensitivity reactions.

Severe acute (less than 24 hours) hypersensitivity reactions have been observed both on initial exposure to Simulect and on re-exposure to a subsequent course of therapy. These included anaphylactoid-type reactions such as urticaria, pruritus, sneezing, hypotension, tachycardia, dyspnoea, bronchospasm, pulmonary oedema and respiratory failure. There have been rare reports of such reactions in patients receiving Simulect (<1/1,000 patients). If a severe hypersensitivity reaction occurs, therapy with Simulect must be permanently discontinued and no further dose be administered.

Caution should be exercised when patients previously given Simulect are re-exposed to a subsequent course of therapy with this medicine.

There is accumulating evidence that a subgroup of patients is at an increased risk of developing hypersensitivity reactions. These are patients in whom, following the initial administration of Simulect, the concomitant immunosuppression was discontinued prematurely due, for example, to abandoned transplantation or early loss of the graft. Acute hypersensitivity reactions were observed on re-administration of Simulect for a subsequent transplantation in some of these patients.

Patients on immunosuppressive therapy following transplantation are at an increased risk of developing lymphoproliferative disorders (LPDs) and opportunistic infections. While Simulect is an immunosuppressive medicinal product, to date no increase in LPDs or opportunistic infections has been observed in patients treated with Simulect. No differences were found in the incidence of malignancies and LPDs between Simulect and placebo in a pooled analysis of two five-year extension studies (see section 4.8)

4.5 Interaction with other medicinal products and other forms of Interaction
Because Simulect is an immunoglobulin, no metabolic drug-drug interactions are to be expected.

In addition to ciclosporin for microemulsion, steroids, azathioprine and mycophenolate mofetil, other concomitant medications routinely administered in organ transplantation have been administered in clinical trials without any incremental adverse reactions. These concomitant medications include systemic antiviral, antibacterial and antimycotic medications, analgesics, antihypertensive medications such as beta-blocking agents or calcium channel blockers, and diuretics.

Human antimurine antibody (HAMA) responses were reported in a clinical trial of 172 patients treated with Simulect, without predictive value for clinical tolerability. The incidence was 2/138 in patients not exposed to muromonab-CD3 and 4/34 in patients who received muromonab-CD3 concomitantly. The use of Simulect does not preclude subsequent treatment with murine antilymphocyte antibody preparations.

In the original phase 3 studies during the first 3 months post-transplantation, 14% of patients in the Simulect group and 27% of patients in the placebo group had an acute rejection episode treated with antibody therapy (OKT 3 or ATG/ALG), with no increase in adverse events or infections in the Simulect group as compared to placebo.

Three clinical trials have investigated Simulect use in combination with a triple therapy regimen which included either azathioprine or mycophenolate mofetil. The total body clearance of Simulect was reduced by an average 22 % when azathioprine was added to a regimen consisting of ciclosporin for microemulsion and corticosteroids. The total body clearance of Simulect was reduced by an average 51 % when mycophenolate mofetil was added to a regimen consisting of ciclosporin for microemulsion and corticosteroids. The use of Simulect in a triple therapy regimen including azathioprine or mycophenolate mofetil did not increase adverse events or infections in the Simulect group as compared to placebo (see section 4.8).

4.6 Pregnancy and lactation
Simulect is contraindicated (see section 4.3) in pregnancy and lactation. Basiliximab has potentially hazardous pharmacological effects with respect to the course of gestation and the suckling neonate exposed to basiliximab in breast milk. This concern is based on basiliximab's immunosuppressive action. Women of childbearing potential have to use effective contraception during (and up to 16 weeks after) treatment.

There is no animal or human data available concerning excretion of basiliximab into breast milk. However, based on the IgG1 nature of basiliximab, excretion into milk should be expected. Breast-feeding must therefore be avoided.

4.7 Effects on ability to drive and use machines
No studies on the effects on the ability to drive and use machines have been performed.

4.8 Undesirable effects

Simulect has been tested in four randomized, double-blind, placebo-controlled studies in renal transplant recipients: in two studies patients were concomitantly treated with ciclosporin for microemulsion and corticosteroids (346 and 380 patients), in one study patients were concomitantly treated with ciclosporin for microemulsion, azathioprine and corticosteroids (340 patients), in one study patients were concomitantly treated with ciclosporin for microemulsion, mycophenolate mofetil and corticosteroids (123 patients). Safety data in paediatric patients have been obtained from one open-label pharmacokinetic and pharmacodynamic study in renal transplant recipients (41 patients).

Incidence of Adverse Events:

Simulect did not appear to add to the background of adverse events seen in organ transplantation patients as a consequence of their underlying disease and the concurrent administration of immunosuppressants and other medications. In the four placebo-controlled trials, the pattern of adverse events in 590 patients treated with the recommended dose of Simulect was indistinguishable from that in 595 patients treated with placebo. Simulect did not increase the incidence of serious adverse events observed when compared to placebo. The overall incidence of treatment-related adverse events among all patients in the individual studies was not significantly different between the Simulect (7.1 % - 40 %) and the placebo (7.6 % - 39 %) treatment groups.

Adult experience

The most commonly reported (> 20 %) events following dual or triple therapy in both treatment groups (Simulect vs. placebo) were constipation, urinary tract infections, pain, nausea, peripheral oedema, hypertension, anaemia, headache, hyperkalaemia, hypercholesterolaemia, surgical wound complication, weight increase, increased serum creatinine, hypophosphataemia, diarrhoea and upper respiratory tract infection.

Paediatric experience

The most commonly reported (> 20 %) events following dual therapy in both (< 35 kg vs. ⩾ 35 kg weight) cohorts were urinary tract infections, hypertrichosis, rhinitis, fever, hypertension, upper respiratory tract infection, viral infection, sepsis and constipation.

Incidence of Malignancies:

The overall incidence of malignancies among all patients in the individual studies was similar between the Simulect and the comparator treatment groups. Overall, lymphoma/lymphoproliferative disease occurred in 0.1 % (1/701) of patients in the Simulect group compared with 0.3 % (2/595) of placebo patients. Other malignancies were reported among 1.0 % (7/701) of patients in the Simulect group compared with 1.2 % (7/595) of placebo patients. In a pooled analysis of two five-year extension studies, the incidence of LPDs and cancer was found to be equal with Simulect 7% (21/295) and placebo 7% (21/291).

Incidence of Infectious Episodes:

The overall incidence and profile of infectious episodes among dual and triple therapy patients was similar between the Simulect and the placebo treatment groups (Simulect = 75.9 %, placebo = 75.6 %); the incidence of serious infections was 26.1 % in the Simulect group and 24.8 % in the comparator group. The incidence of CMV-infections was similar in both groups (14.6 % vs. 17.3 %), following either dual or triple therapy regimen.

The incidence and causes of deaths following dual or triple therapy were similar in Simulect (2.9 %) and placebo groups (2.6 %), with the most common cause of deaths in both treatment groups being infections (Simulect = 1.3 %, placebo = 1.4 %). In a pooled analysis of two five-year extension studies the incidence and cause of death remained similar in both treatment groups, (Simulect 15%, placebo 11%), the primary cause of death being cardiac-related disorders (Simulect 5%, placebo 4%).

Rare cases (< 1/1,000) of hypersensitivity/anaphylactoid-type reactions such as rash, urticaria, sneezing, wheezing, bronchospasm, pulmonary oedema, cardiac failure, respiratory failure and capillary leak syndrome, as well as individual cases of suspected cytokine release syndrome, have been reported during post-marketing experience with Simulect (see section 4.4).

4.9 Overdose

In clinical studies Simulect has been administered to humans in single doses of up to 60 mg and multiple doses of up to 150 mg over 24 days with no untoward acute effects.

In a 4-week study in rhesus monkeys, the no observable effect level was 5 mg/kg twice weekly, leading to a serum C_{max} of 170 μg/ml. Levels in humans are generally < 10 μg/ml with the recommended regimen.

5. PHARMACOLOGICAL PROPERTIES

5.1 Pharmacodynamic properties

Pharmacotherapeutic group: specific immunosuppressant; ATC code: L04AA09.

Simulect is a murine/human chimeric monoclonal antibody ($IgG_{1\kappa}$) that is directed against the interleukin-2 receptor α-chain (CD25 antigen), which is expressed on the surface of T-lymphocytes in response to antigenic challenge. Simulect specifically binds with high affinity (K_D-value 0.1 nM) to the CD25 antigen on activated T-lymphocytes expressing the high affinity interleukin-2 receptor and thereby prevents binding of interleukin-2, the signal for T-cell proliferation. Complete and consistent blocking of the interleukin-2 receptor is maintained as long as serum basiliximab levels exceed 0.2 μg/ml (which was 4–6 weeks). As concentrations fall below this level, expression of the CD25 antigen returns to pretherapy values within 1–2 weeks. Simulect does not cause myelosuppression.

Soluble IL-2R serum concentrations increase over the first 2–3 weeks following the administration of Simulect, reaching a plateau at levels of 80–120 ng/ml. These levels are maintained while IL-2R sites are saturated by basiliximab. When IL-2R sites are no longer saturated, soluble IL-2R levels fall to pretransplant levels over the following 1–2 weeks.

Clinical studies

The efficacy of Simulect in prophylaxis of organ rejection in *de novo* renal transplantation has been demonstrated in double-blind placebo-controlled studies. Results from two pivotal 12-month multicentre studies comparing Simulect with placebo show that Simulect, used concomitantly with ciclosporin for microemulsion and corticosteroids, significantly reduces the incidence of acute rejection episodes both within 6 (31 % vs. 45 %, p < 0.001) and 12 (33 % vs. 48 %, p < 0.001) months after transplantation. There was no significant difference between Simulect and placebo treated patients in graft survival after 6 and 12 months (at 12 months 32 graft losses on Simulect (9%) and 37 graft losses on placebo (10%)). The incidence of acute rejection episode was substantially lower in patients receiving Simulect and a triple drug immunosuppressive regimen.

Results from two multicentre double-blind studies comparing Simulect with placebo show that Simulect significantly reduces the incidence of acute rejection episodes within 6 months after transplantation when used concomitantly with ciclosporin for microemulsion, corticosteroids, and either azathioprine (21 % vs. 35 %) or mycophenolate mofetil (15 % vs. 27 %). Graft loss occurred in 6 % of Simulect and 10 % of placebo patients by 6 months. The adverse event profile remained comparable between treatment groups.

In a pooled analysis of two five-year open-label extension studies (586 patients total) the combined graft and patient survival rates were not statistically different for the Simulect and placebo groups. Extension studies also showed that patients who experienced an acute rejection episode during the first year after transplantation experienced more graft losses and deaths over the five-year follow-up period than patients who had no rejection. These events were not influenced by Simulect.

Simulect was used concomitantly with ciclosporin for microemulsion and steroids in an uncontrolled study in paediatric *de novo* renal transplant recipients. Acute rejection occurred in 14.6 % of patients by 6 months post-transplantation, and in 24.3 % by 12 months. Overall the adverse event profile was consistent with general clinical experience in the paediatric renal transplantation population and with the profile in the controlled adult transplantation studies.

Of 339 renal transplant patients treated with Simulect and tested for anti-idiotype antibodies, 4 (1.2 %) developed an anti-idiotype antibody response. In a clinical trial with 172 patients receiving Simulect, the incidence of human anti-murine antibody (HAMA) in renal transplantation patients treated with Simulect was 2/138 in patients not exposed to muromonab-CD3 and 4/34 in patients who received muromonab-CD3 concomitantly. The available clinical data on the use of muromonab-CD3 in patients previously treated with Simulect suggest that subsequent use of muromonab-CD3 or other murine anti-lymphocytic antibody preparations is not precluded.

5.2 Pharmacokinetic properties

Adults

Single-dose and multiple-dose pharmacokinetic studies have been conducted in adult patients undergoing kidney transplantation. Cumulative doses ranged from 20 mg up to 60 mg. Peak serum concentration following intravenous infusion of 20 mg over 30 minutes is 7.1 ± 5.1 mg/l. There is a proportional increase in C_{max} and AUC from 20 mg to 60 mg, the range of single-dose administrations tested. The volume of distribution at steady state was 8.6 ± 4.1 l. The extent and degree of distribution to various body compartments have not been fully studied. *In vitro* studies using human tissues indicate that Simulect binds only to activated lymphocytes and macrophages/monocytes. The terminal half-life was 7.2 ± 3.2 days. Total body clearance was 41 ± 19 ml/h.

No clinically relevant influence of body weight or gender on distribution volume or clearance has been observed in adult patients. Elimination half-life was not influenced by age, gender, or race.

Paediatrics

The pharmacokinetics of Simulect were assessed in 39 paediatric *de novo* renal transplantation patients. In infants and children (age 1–11 years, n = 25), the steady-state distribution volume was 4.8 ± 2.1 l, half-life was 9.5 ± 4.5 days and clearance was 17 ± 6 ml/h. Distribution volume and clearance are reduced by about 50% compared to adult renal transplantation patients. Disposition parameters were not influenced to a clinically relevant extent by age (1 – 11 years), body weight (9 – 37 kg) or body surface area (0.44 – 1.20 m^2) in this age group. In adolescents (age 12 – 16 years, n = 14), the steady-state distribution volume was 7.8 ± 5.1 l, half-life was 9.1 ± 3.9 days and clearance was 31 ± 19 ml/h. Disposition in adolescents was similar to that in adult renal transplantation patients. The relationship between serum concentration and receptor saturation was assessed in 13 patients and was similar to that characterised in adult renal transplantation patients.

5.3 Preclinical safety data

No toxicity was observed when rhesus monkeys received intravenous doses of up to 5 mg/kg basiliximab twice weekly for 4 weeks, resulting in approximately 20 times the systemic exposure (C_{max}) observed in patients given the recommended clinical dose together with concomitant immunosuppressive therapy.

No maternal toxicity, embryotoxicity, or teratogenicity was observed in cynomolgous monkeys following injections of up to 5 mg/kg basiliximab administered twice weekly during the organogenesis period.

No mutagenic potential was observed *in vitro*.

6. PHARMACEUTICAL PARTICULARS

6.1 List of excipients

Potassium dihydrogen phosphate

Disodium phosphate, anhydrous

Sodium chloride

Sucrose

Mannitol

Glycine

Water for injections

6.2 Incompatibilities

This medicinal product must not be mixed with other medicinal products except those mentioned in section 6.6.

6.3 Shelf life

Powder: 3 years

After reconstitution the solution may be stored at 2 °C – 8 °C for 24 hours or at room temperature for 4 hours.

6.4 Special precautions for storage

Store and transport refrigerated (2 ° C – 8 ° C).

6.5 Nature and contents of container

Simulect powder

Colourless glass vial, hydrolytic glass type I, grey fluor-resin coated butyl rubber stopper, held in place by a flanged aluminium band, blue polypropylene flip-off cap.

Water for injections

Colourless glass ampoule, hydrolytic glass type I.

Simulect is available in vials with 10mg or 20mg basiliximab.

6.6 Instructions for use and handling

Simulect 10 mg powder and solvent for solution for injection or infusion

To prepare the solution for infusion or injection, take 2.5 ml of water for injections out of the accompanying 5 ml-ampoule aseptically and add this 2.5 ml of water for injections aseptically to the vial containing the Simulect powder. Shake the vial gently to dissolve the powder. It is recommended that after reconstitution the colourless, clear to opalescent solution should be used immediately. After reconstitution it may be stored at 2 ° C – 8 ° C for 24 hours or at room temperature for 4 hours.

Discard the reconstituted solution if not used within 24 hours.

The reconstituted solution is isotonic and may be given as a bolus injection or diluted to a volume of 25 ml or greater with normal saline or dextrose 5% for infusion.

Simulect 20 mg powder and solvent for solution for injection or infusion:

To prepare the solution for infusion or injection, add 5 ml of water for injections from the accompanying ampoule aseptically to the vial containing the Simulect powder. Shake the vial gently to dissolve the powder. It is recommended that after reconstitution the colourless, clear to opalescent solution should be used immediately. After reconstitution it may be stored at 2 ° C – 8 ° C for 24 hours or at room temperature for 4 hours.

Discard the reconstituted solution if not used within 24 hours.

The reconstituted solution is isotonic and may be given as a bolus injection or diluted to a volume of 50 ml or greater with normal saline or dextrose 5% for infusion.

Since no data are available on the compatibility of Simulect with other intravenous substances, Simulect should not be mixed with other medications/substances and should always be given through a separate infusion line.

Compatibility with a number of infusion sets has been verified.

7. MARKETING AUTHORISATION HOLDER

Novartis Europharm Limited

Wimblehurst Road

Horsham

West Sussex, RH12 5AB

UNITED KINGDOM

8. MARKETING AUTHORISATION NUMBER(S)

Simulect 10 mg powder and solvent for solution for injection or infusion: EU/1/98/084/002

Simulect 20 mg powder and solvent for solution for injection or infusion: EU/1/98/084/001

9. DATE OF FIRST AUTHORISATION/RENEWAL OF THE AUTHORISATION

Simulect 10 mg powder and solvent for solution for injection or infusion: 07.03.2003/20.10.2003

Simulect 20 mg powder and solvent for solution for injection or infusion: 09.10.1998/20.10.2003

10. DATE OF REVISION OF THE TEXT

8 July 2005

Legal Category

POM

Sinemet 62.5, 110, Plus and 275 Tablets

(Bristol-Myers Squibb Pharmaceuticals Ltd)

1. NAME OF THE MEDICINAL PRODUCT

SINEMET® 62.5 Tablets

SINEMET® 110 Tablets

SINEMET® Plus Tablets

SINEMET® 275 Tablets

2. QUALITATIVE AND QUANTITATIVE COMPOSITION

Each tablet of Sinemet-62.5 contains 13.5 mg carbidopa (equivalent to 12.5 mg of anhydrous carbidopa) and 50 mg levodopa.

Each tablet of Sinemet-110 contains 10.8 mg carbidopa (equivalent to 10 mg of anhydrous carbidopa) and 100 mg levodopa.

Each tablet of Sinemet-Plus contains 27.0 mg carbidopa (equivalent to 25 mg of anhydrous carbidopa) and 100 mg levodopa.

Each tablet of Sinemet-275 contains 27.0 mg carbidopa (equivalent to 25 mg of anhydrous carbidopa) and 250 mg levodopa.

3. PHARMACEUTICAL FORM

Tablets.

Sinemet-62.5: yellow, oval-shaped tablets, one side scored and the other marked '520'.

Sinemet-110: dapple blue, oval-shaped tablets, one side plain and the other scored and marked '647'.

Sinemet-Plus: yellow, oval-shaped tablets, one side plain and the other scored and marked '650'.

Sinemet-275: dapple blue, oval-shaped tablets, one side plain and the other scored and marked '654'.

For excipients see 6.1.

4. CLINICAL PARTICULARS

4.1 Therapeutic indications

Antiparkinsonian agent.

For treatment of Parkinson's disease and syndrome.

4.2 Posology and method of administration

To be taken orally.

The optimum daily dosage of Sinemet must be determined by careful titration in each patient.

Sinemet Tablets are available in a ratio of 1:4 or 1:10 of carbidopa to levodopa to provide facility for fine dosage titration for each patient.

General Considerations

Studies show that the peripheral dopa-decarboxylase is fully inhibited (saturated) by carbidopa at doses between 70 and 100 mg a day. Patients receiving less than this amount of carbidopa are more likely to experience nausea and vomiting.

Standard antiparkinsonian drugs, other than levodopa alone, may be continued while Sinemet is being administered, although their dosage may have to be adjusted.

Because both therapeutic and adverse effects are seen more rapidly with Sinemet than with levodopa, patients should be carefully monitored during the dosage adjustment period. Involuntary movements, particularly blepharospasm, are a useful early sign of excess dosage in some patients.

Patients not receiving levodopa

Dosage may be best initiated with one tablet of Sinemet-Plus three times a day. This dosage schedule provides 75 mg of carbidopa per day. Dosage may be increased by one tablet of Sinemet-62.5 or Sinemet-Plus every day or every other day, as necessary, until a dosage equivalent of eight tablets of Sinemet-Plus a day is reached.

If Sinemet-110 or Sinemet-62.5 is used, dosage may be initiated with one tablet three or four times a day. Titration upward may be required in some patients to achieve optimum dosage of carbidopa. The dosage may be increased by one tablet every day or every other day until a total of eight tablets (two tablets q.d.s.) is reached.

For patients starting with Sinemet-275, the initial dose is one-half tablet taken once or twice daily. However, this may not provide the optimal amount of carbidopa needed by many patients. If necessary, add one-half tablet every day or every other day until optimal response is reached.

Response has been observed in one day, and sometimes after one dose. Fully effective doses usually are reached within seven days as compared to weeks or months with levodopa alone.

Sinemet-62.5 or Sinemet-110 may be used to facilitate dosage titration according to the needs of the individual patient.

Patients receiving levodopa

Discontinue levodopa at least 12 hours (24 hours for slow-release preparations) before starting therapy with Sinemet. The easiest way to do this is to give Sinemet as the first morning dose after a night without any levodopa. The dose of Sinemet should be approximately 20% of the previous daily dosage of levodopa.

Patients taking less than 1,500 mg levodopa a day should be started on one tablet of Sinemet-Plus three or four times a day dependent on patient need. The suggested starting dose for most patients taking more than 1,500 mg levodopa a day is one tablet of Sinemet-275 three or four times a day.

Maintenance

Therapy with Sinemet should be individualised and adjusted gradually according to response. When a greater proportion of carbidopa is required, each tablet of Sinemet-110 may be replaced with a tablet of Sinemet-Plus or Sinemet-62.5.

When more levodopa is required, Sinemet-275 should be substituted at a dosage of one tablet three or four times a day. If necessary, the dosage of Sinemet-275 may be increased by half to one tablet every other day to a maximum of eight tablets a day. Experience with a total daily dosage greater than 200 mg carbidopa is limited.

Patients receiving levodopa with another decarboxylase inhibitor

When transferring a patient to Sinemet from levodopa combined with another decarboxylase inhibitor, discontinue dosage at least 12 hours before Sinemet is started. Begin with a dosage of Sinemet that will provide the same amount of levodopa as contained in the other levodopa/decarboxylase inhibitor combination.

Patients receiving other antiparkinsonian agents

Current evidence indicates that other antiparkinsonian agents may be continued when Sinemet is introduced, although dosage may have to be adjusted in line with manufacturers recommendations.

Use in children

The safety of Sinemet in patients under 18 years of age has not been established and its use in patients below the age of 18 is not recommended.

Use in the elderly

There is wide experience in the use of this product in elderly patients. The recommendations set out above reflect the clinical data derived from this experience.

4.3 Contraindications

Nonselective monoamine oxidase (MAO) inhibitors are contraindicated for use with Sinemet. These inhibitors must be discontinued at least two weeks before starting Sinemet. Sinemet may be administered concomitantly with the manufacturer's recommended dose of an MAO inhibitor with selectivity for MAO type B (e.g. selegiline hydrochloride). (See 4.5 'Interaction with other medicinal products and other forms of interaction'.)

Sinemet is contraindicated in patients with narrow-angle glaucoma and in patients with known hypersensitivity to any component of this medication.

Since levodopa may activate a malignant melanoma, it should not be used in patients with suspicious undiagnosed skin lesions or a history of melanoma.

Use in patients with severe psychoses.

See also 4.6 'Pregnancy and lactation'.

4.4 Special warnings and special precautions for use

Sinemet is not recommended for the treatment of drug-induced extrapyramidal reactions.

Sinemet should be administered cautiously to patients with severe cardiovascular or pulmonary disease, bronchial asthma, renal, hepatic or endocrine disease, or history of peptic ulcer disease (because of the possibility of upper gastro-intestinal haemorrhage).

Care should be exercised when Sinemet is administered to patients with a history of myocardial infarction who have residual atrial nodal, or ventricular arrhythmias. Cardiac function should be monitored with particular care in such patients during the period of initial dosage adjustment.

Levodopa has been associated with somnolence and episodes of sudden sleep onset. Sudden onset of sleep during daily activities, in some cases without awareness or warning signs, has been reported very rarely. Patients must be informed of this and advised to exercise caution while driving or operating machines during treatment with levodopa. Patients who have experienced somnolence and/or an episode of sudden sleep onset must refrain from driving or operating machines. Furthermore a reduction of dosage or termination of therapy may be considered.

All patients should be monitored carefully for the development of mental changes, depression with suicidal tendencies, and other serious antisocial behaviour. Patients with current psychoses should be treated with caution.

Dyskinesias may occur in patients previously treated with levodopa alone because carbidopa permits more levodopa to reach the brain and, thus, more dopamine to be formed. The occurrence of dyskinesias may require dosage reduction.

As with levodopa, Sinemet may cause involuntary movements and mental disturbances. Patients with a history of severe involuntary movements or psychotic episodes when treated with levodopa alone should be observed carefully when Sinemet is substituted. These reactions are thought to be due to increased brain dopamine following administration of levodopa, and use of Sinemet may cause a recurrence. A syndrome resembling the neuroleptic malignant syndrome including muscular rigidity, elevated body temperature, mental changes and increased serum creatine phosphokinase has been reported with the abrupt withdrawal of antiparkinsonian agents. Therefore, any abrupt dosage reduction or withdrawal of Sinemet should be carefully observed, particularly in patients who are also receiving neuroleptics.

Concomitant administration of psycho-active drugs such as phenothiazines or butyrophenones should be carried out with caution, and the patient carefully observed for loss of antiparkinsonian effect. Patients with a history of convulsions should be treated with caution.

As with levodopa, periodic evaluation of hepatic, haematopoetic, cardiovascular and renal function are recommended during extended therapy.

Patients with chronic wide-angle glaucoma may be treated cautiously with Sinemet, provided the intra-ocular pressure is well controlled and the patient monitored carefully for changes in intra-ocular pressure during therapy.

If general anaesthesia is required, therapy with Sinemet may be continued for as long as the patient is permitted to take fluids and medication by mouth. If therapy has to be stopped temporarily, Sinemet may be restarted as soon as oral medication can be taken at the same daily dosage as before.

Laboratory Tests

Commonly, levels of blood urea nitrogen, creatinine, and uric acid are lower during administration of Sinemet than with levodopa. Transient abnormalities include elevated levels of blood urea, AST (SGOT), ALT (SGPT), LDH, bilirubin, and alkaline phosphatase.

Decreased haemoglobin, haematocrit, elevated serum glucose and white blood cells, bacteria and blood in the urine have been reported.

Positive Coombs' tests have been reported, both with Sinemet and levodopa alone.

Sinemet may cause a false positive result when a dipstick is used to test for urinary ketone; and this reaction is not altered by boiling the urine. The use of glucose oxidase methods may give false negative results for glycosuria.

4.5 Interaction with other medicinal products and other forms of Interaction

Caution should be exercised when the following drugs are administered concomitantly with Sinemet.

Antihypertensive agents

Postural hypotension can occur when Sinemet is added to the treatment of patients already receiving antihypertensive drugs. Dosage adjustment of the antihypertensive agent may be required.

Antidepressants

Rarely, reactions including hypertension and dyskinesia have been reported with the concomitant use of tricyclic antidepressants. (See first paragraph of 4.3 Contraindications for patients receiving MAOIs).

Anticholinergics

Anticholinergics may affect the absorption and thus the patient's response.

Iron

Studies demonstrate a decrease in the bioavailability of carbidopa and/or levodopa when it is ingested with ferrous sulphate or ferrous gluconate.

Other drugs

To date there has been no indication of interactions that would preclude concurrent use of standard antiparkinsonian drugs.

Dopamine D_2 receptor antagonists (e.g. phenothiazines, butyrophenones, and risperidone) and isoniazid, may reduce the therapeutic effects of levodopa. The beneficial effects of levodopa in Parkinson's disease have been reported to be reversed by phenytoin and papaverine. Patients taking these drugs with Sinemet should be carefully observed for loss of therapeutic response.

Concomitant therapy with selegiline and carbidopa-levodopa may be associated with severe orthostatic hypotension not attributable to carbidopa-levodopa alone (See 4.3 'Contraindications')

Since levodopa competes with certain amino acids, the absorption of Sinemet may be impaired in some patients on a high protein diet.

The effect of simultaneous administration of antacids with Sinemet on the bioavailability of levodopa has not been studied.

Sinemet may be given to patients with Parkinson's disease and syndrome who are taking vitamin preparations that contain pyridoxine hydrochloride (Vitamin B6).

4.6 Pregnancy and lactation

Pregnancy

Although the effects of Sinemet on human pregnancy are unknown, both levodopa and combinations of carbidopa and levodopa have caused visceral and skeletal malformations in rabbits. Therefore, the use of Sinemet in women of childbearing potential requires that the anticipated benefits of the drug be weighed against possible hazards should pregnancy occur.

Breast-feeding mothers

It is not known whether carbidopa or levodopa is excreted in human milk. In a study of one nursing mother with Parkinson's disease, excretion of levodopa in human breast milk was reported. Because many drugs are excreted in human milk and because of the potential for serious adverse reactions in infants, a decision should be made whether to discontinue breast-feeding or discontinue the use of Sinemet, taking into account the importance of the drug to the mother.

4.7 Effects on ability to drive and use machines

Individual responses to medication may vary and certain side effects that have been reported with Sinemet may affect some patients' ability to drive or operate machinery. Patients treated with levodopa and presenting with somnolence and/or sudden sleep episodes must be informed to refrain from driving or engaging in activities where impaired alertness may put themselves or others at risk of serious injury or death (e.g. operating machines), until such recurrent episodes and somnolence have resolved (see also section 4.4 'Special warnings and precautions for use').

4.8 Undesirable effects

Side effects that occur frequently with Sinemet are those due to the central neuropharmacological activity of dopamine. These reactions can usually be diminished by dosage reduction. The most common are dyskinesias including choreiform, dystonic and other involuntary movements and nausea. Muscle twitching and blepharospasm may be taken as early signs to consider dosage reduction.

Other side effects reported in clinical trials or in post-marketing experience include:

Body as a whole: syncope, chest pain, anorexia.

Cardiovascular: cardiac irregularities and/or palpitations, orthostatic effects including hypotensive episodes, hypertension, phlebitis.

Gastrointestinal: vomiting, gastrointestinal bleeding, development of duodenal ulcer, diarrhoea, dark saliva.

Haemotologic: leucopenia, haemolytic and non-haemolytic anaemia, thrombocytopenia, agranulocytosis.

Hypersensitivity: angioedema, urticaria, pruritus, Henoch-Schonlein purpura.

Nervous System/Psychiatric: neuroleptic malignant syndrome (see 4.3 'Contraindications'), bradykinetic episodes (the "on-off" phenomenon), dizziness, paraesthesia, psychotic episodes including delusions, hallucinations and paranoid ideation, depression with or without development of suicidal tendencies, dementia, dream abnormalities, agitation, confusion, increased libido. Levodopa is associated with somnolence and has been associated very rarely with excessive daytime somnolence and sudden sleep onset episodes.

Respiratory: dyspnoea.

Skin: alopecia, rash, dark sweat.

Urogenital: dark urine.

Rarely convulsions have occurred; however, a causal relationship with Sinemet has not been established.

Other side effects that have been reported with levodopa or levodopa/carbidopa combinations and may be potential side effects with Sinemet include:

Gastro-intestinal: dyspepsia, dry mouth, bitter taste, sialorrhoea, dysphagia, bruxism, hiccups, abdominal pain and distress, constipation, flatulence, burning sensation of the tongue.

Metabolic: weight gain or loss, oedema.

Nervous System/Psychiatric: asthenia, decreased mental acuity, disorientation, ataxia, numbness, increased hand tremor, muscle cramp, trismus, activation of latent Horner's syndrome, insomnia, anxiety, euphoria, falling and gait abnormalities.

Skin: flushing, increased sweating,

Special senses: diplopia, blurred vision, dilated pupils, oculogyric crises.

Urogenital: urinary retention, urinary incontinence, priapism.

Miscellaneous: weakness, faintness, fatigue, headache, hoarseness, malaise, hot flushes, sense of stimulation, bizarre breathing patterns, malignant melanoma (see 4.3 'Contraindications').

4.9 Overdose

Treatment

Management of acute overdosage with Sinemet is basically the same as management of acute overdosage with levodopa; however pyridoxine is not effective in reversing the actions of Sinemet. ECG monitoring should be instituted, and the patient carefully observed for the possible development of arrhythmias; if required, appropriate anti-arrhythmic therapy should be given. The possibility that the patient may have taken other drugs as well as Sinemet should be taken into consideration. To date, no experience has been reported with dialysis, and hence its value in the treatment of overdosage is not known.

The terminal half-life of levodopa is about two hours in the presence of carbidopa.

5. PHARMACOLOGICAL PROPERTIES

5.1 Pharmacodynamic properties

Levodopa is a precursor of dopamine, and is given as replacement therapy in Parkinson's disease.

Carbidopa is a peripheral dopa decarboxylase inhibitor. It prevents metabolism of levodopa to dopamine in the peripheral circulation, ensuring that a higher proportion of the dose reaches the brain, where dopamine acts. A lower dose of levodopa can be used, reducing the incidence and severity of side effects.

Sinemet is useful in relieving many of the symptoms of parkinsonism, particularly rigidity and bradykinesia. It is frequently helpful in the management of tremor, dysphagia, sialorrhoea, and postural instability associated with Parkinson's disease and syndrome.

When response to levodopa alone is irregular, and signs and symptoms of Parkinson's disease are not controlled evenly throughout the day, substitution of Sinemet usually reduces fluctuations in response. By reducing some of the adverse reactions produced by levodopa alone, Sinemet permits more patients to obtain adequate relief from the symptoms of Parkinson's disease.

5.2 Pharmacokinetic properties

Following oral dosing levodopa, in the absence of decarboxylase inhibitor, is rapidly but variably absorbed from the gastrointestinal tract. It has a plasma half life of about 1 hour and is mainly converted by decarboxylation to dopamine, a proportion of which is converted to noradrenaline. Up to 30 % is converted to 3-O-methyldopa which has a half life of 9 to 22 hours. About 80 % of levodopa is excreted in the urine within 24 hours mainly as homovanillic acid and dihydroxyphenylactic acid. Less than 1 % is excreted unchanged.

Once in the circulation it competes with other neutral amino acids for transport across the blood brain barrier. Once it has entered the striatal neurones it is decarboxylated to dopamine, stored and released from presynaptic neurones. Because levodopa is so rapidly decarboxylated in the gastrointestinal tract and the liver, very little unchanged drug is available for transport into the brain. The peripheral decarboxylation reduces the therapeutic effectiveness of levodopa but is responsible for many of its side effects. For this reason levodopa is usually administered together with a peripheral decarboxylase inhibitor such as carbidopa, so that lower doses may be given to achieve the same therapeutic effect.

Carbidopa in the absence of levodopa, is rapidly but incompletely absorbed from the gastrointestinal tract following oral dosing. Following an oral dose approximately 50% is recorded in the urine, with about 30 % of this as unchanged drug. It does not cross the blood brain barrier but crosses the placenta and is excreted in breast milk. Turnover of the drug is rapid and virtually all unchanged drug appears in the urine within 7 hours.

Carbidopa inhibits the peripheral decarboxylation of levodopa to dopamine but as it does not cross the blood brain barrier, effective brain levels of dopamine get produced with lower levels of levodopa therapy reducing the peripheral side effects, noticeably nausea and vomiting and cardiac arrhythmias.

5.3 Preclinical safety data

Sinemet is well established in medical use. Preclinical data is broadly consistent with clinical experience. (For reproductive toxicity, see section 4.6 'Pregnancy and Lactation'.)

6. PHARMACEUTICAL PARTICULARS

6.1 List of excipients

Sinemet-62.5 and Sinemet-Plus tablets contain quinoline yellow (E104), maize starch, pregelatinised maize starch, microcrystalline cellulose, magnesium stearate.

Sinemet-110 and Sinemet-275 tablets contain indigo carmine (E132), maize starch pregelatinised maize starch, microcrystalline cellulose, magnesium stearate.

6.2 Incompatibilities

Not applicable.

6.3 Shelf life

36 months

6.4 Special precautions for storage

Do not store above 25°C. Store in the original package.

6.5 Nature and contents of container

PVC/Al blister packs of 90 tablets.

6.6 Instructions for use and handling

Not applicable.

7. MARKETING AUTHORISATION HOLDER

Merck Sharp & Dohme Limited

Hertford Road

Hoddesdon

Hertfordshire EN11 9BU, UK.

Distributed by:

Bristol-Myers Squibb Pharmaceuticals Limited

Hounslow TW3 3JA, United Kingdom.

8. MARKETING AUTHORISATION NUMBER(S)

Sinemet-62.5 PL 0025/0226

Sinemet-110 PL 0025/0084

Sinemet-Plus PL 0025/0150

Sinemet-275 PL 0025/0085

9. DATE OF FIRST AUTHORISATION/RENEWAL OF THE AUTHORISATION

Sinemet-62.5 11 February 1988/13 March 2002

Sinemet-110 23 October 1973/13 March 2002

Sinemet-Plus 11 June 1981/13 March 2002

Sinemet-275 23 October 1973/13 March 2002

10. DATE OF REVISION OF THE TEXT

April 2004

11. LEGAL CATEGORY

Prescription only medicine

®Registered trademark of Merck & Co., Inc., Whitehouse Station, New Jersey, USA

Sinemet CR and Half Sinemet CR

(Bristol-Myers Squibb Pharmaceuticals Ltd)

1. NAME OF THE MEDICINAL PRODUCT

SINEMET®CR

HALF SINEMET®CR

2. QUALITATIVE AND QUANTITATIVE COMPOSITION

Each tablet of Sinemet CR contains carbidopa (equivalent to 50 mg of anhydrous carbidopa) and 200 mg levodopa.

Each tablet of Half Sinemet CR contains carbidopa (equivalent to 25 mg of anhydrous carbidopa) and 100 mg levodopa.

3. PHARMACEUTICAL FORM

Modified-release tablets.

Sinemet CR: peach-coloured, oval shaped, biconvex tablets, plain one side and the other scored and marked '521'.

Half Sinemet CR: pink-coloured, oval-shaped, biconvex tablets, plain one side and the other marked '601'.

4. CLINICAL PARTICULARS

4.1 Therapeutic indications

Antiparkinson agent.

Idiopathic Parkinson's disease, in particular to reduce off-period in patients who previously have been treated with levodopa/decarboxylase inhibitors, or with levodopa alone and who have experienced motor fluctuations. The experience is limited with Sinemet CR and Half Sinemet CR in patients who have not been treated with levodopa before.

4.2 Posology and method of administration

Sinemet CR and Half Sinemet CR tablets contain a 1:4 ratio of carbidopa to levodopa (Sinemet CR: carbidopa 50 mg/levodopa 200 mg, Half Sinemet CR 25mg/100mg per tablet). The daily dosage of Sinemet CR must be determined by careful titration. Patients should be monitored closely during the dose adjustment period, particularly with regard to appearance or worsening of nausea or abnormal involuntary movements, including dyskinesias, chorea and dystonia.

Route of administration: oral

Sinemet CR and Half Sinemet CR may only be administered as whole tablets. So that the controlled release properties of the product can be maintained, tablets should not be chewed, crushed, or halved.

Standard antiparkinson drugs, other than levodopa alone, may be continued while Sinemet CR or Half Sinemet CR are being administered, although their dosage may have to be adjusted. Since carbidopa prevents the reversal of levodopa effects caused by pyridoxine, Sinemet CR or Half Sinemet CR can be given to patients receiving supplemental pyridoxine (vitamin B_6).

Initial Dose

Patients currently treated with conventional levodopa/decarboxylase inhibitor combinations

Dosage with Sinemet CR should be substituted initially at an amount that provides no more than approximately 10% more levodopa per day when higher dosages are given (more than 900 mg per day). The dosing interval between doses should be prolonged by 30 to 50% at intervals ranging from 4 to 12 hours. It is recommended to give the smaller dose, if divided doses are not equal, at the end of the day. The dose needs to be titrated further depending on clinical response, as indicated below under 'Titration'. Dosages that provide up to 30% more levodopa per day may be necessary.

A guide for substitution of Sinemet CR treatment for conventional levodopa/decarboxylase inhibitor combinations is shown in the table below:

Guideline for Conversion from Sinemet to Sinemet CR

Sinemet	Sinemet CR	Dosage Regimen
Daily Dosage Levodopa (mg)	Daily Dosage Levodopa (mg)	
300-400	400	1 tablet 2 × daily
500-600	600	1 tablet 3 × daily
700-800	800	4 tablets in 3 or more divided doses
900-1000	1000	5 tablets in 3 or more divided doses
1100-1200	1200	6 tablets in 3 or more divided doses
1300-1400	1400	7 tablets in 3 or more divided doses
1500-1600	1600	8 tablets in 3 or more divided doses

Half Sinemet CR is available to facilitate titration when 100 mg steps are required.

Patients currently treated with levodopa alone

Levodopa must be discontinued at least eight hours before therapy with Sinemet CR is started. In patients with mild to moderate disease, the initial recommended dose is one tablet of Sinemet CR twice daily.

Patients not receiving levodopa

In patients with mild to moderate disease, the initial recommended dose is one tablet of Sinemet CR twice daily. Initial dosages should not exceed 600 mg per day of levodopa, nor be given at intervals of less than six hours.

Titration

Following initiation of therapy, doses and dosing intervals may be increased or decreased, depending upon therapeutic response. Most patients have been adequately treated with two to eight tablets per day of Sinemet CR administered as divided doses at intervals ranging from four to twelve hours during the waking day. Higher doses (up to 12 tablets) and shorter intervals (less than four hours) have been used, but are not usually recommended.

When doses of Sinemet CR are given at intervals of less than 4 hours, or if the divided doses are not equal, it is recommended that the smaller doses be given at the end of the day. In some patients the onset of effect of the first morning dose may be delayed for up to one hour compared with the response usually obtained from the first morning dose of Sinemet.

An interval of at least three days between dosage adjustments is recommended.

Maintenance

Because Parkinson's disease is progressive, periodic clinical evaluations are recommended and adjustment of the dosage regimen of Sinemet CR or Half Sinemet CR may be required.

Addition of other antiparkinson medication

Anticholinergic agents, dopamine agonists and amantadine can be given with Sinemet CR or Half Sinemet CR. Dosage adjustment of Sinemet CR or Half Sinemet CR may be necessary when these agents are added to an existing treatment regimen for Sinemet CR or Half Sinemet CR.

Interruption of therapy

Patients should be observed carefully if abrupt reduction or discontinuation of Sinemet CR or Half Sinemet CR is required, especially if the patient is receiving antipsychotics (see 4.4 'Special warnings and special precautions for use').

Use in Children

Safety and effectiveness of Sinemet CR or Half Sinemet CR in infants and children have not been established, and its use in patients below the age of 18 is not recommended.

4.3 Contraindications

Sinemet CR or Half Sinemet CR should not be given when administration of a sympathomimetic amine is contraindicated.

Nonselective monoamine oxidase (MAO) inhibitors are contraindicated for use with Sinemet CR or Half Sinemet CR. These inhibitors must be discontinued at least two weeks prior to initiating therapy with Sinemet CR or Half Sinemet CR. Sinemet CR or Half Sinemet CR may be administered concomitantly with the manufacturer's recommended dose of an MAO inhibitor with selectivity for MAO type B (e.g. selegiline hydrochloride) (See 4.5 'Interactions with other medicaments and other forms of interaction').

Sinemet CR or Half Sinemet CR is contraindicated in patients with known hypersensitivity to any component of this medication, and in patients with narrow-angle glaucoma.

Because levodopa may activate a malignant melanoma, Sinemet CR or Half Sinemet CR should not be used in patients with suspicious undiagnosed skin lesions or a history of melanoma.

Use in patients with severe psychoses.

4.4 Special warnings and special precautions for use

When patients are receiving levodopa monotherapy, levodopa must be discontinued at least eight hours before therapy with Sinemet CR or Half Sinemet CR is started (at least 12 hours if slow-release levodopa has been administered).

Dyskinesias may occur in patients previously treated with levodopa alone because carbidopa permits more levodopa to reach the brain and, thus, more dopamine to be formed. The occurrence of dyskinesias may require dosage reduction.

Sinemet CR and Half Sinemet CR are not recommended for the treatment of drug-induced extrapyramidal reactions or for the treatment of Huntingdon's chorea.

Based on the pharmacokinetic profile of Sinemet CR the onset of effect in patients with early morning dyskinesias may be slower than with conventional Sinemet. The incidence of dyskinesias is slightly higher during treatment with Sinemet CR than with conventional Sinemet (16.5% vs 12.2%) in advanced patients with motor fluctuations.

Sinemet CR or Half Sinemet CR should be administered cautiously to patients with severe cardiovascular or pulmonary disease, bronchial asthma, renal, hepatic or endocrine disease, or with a history of peptic ulcer disease or of convulsions.

Care should be exercised in administering Sinemet CR or Half Sinemet CR to patients with a history of recent myocardial infarction who have residual atrial, nodal, or ventricular arrhythmia. In such patients, cardiac function should be monitored with particular care during the period of initial dosage administration and titration.

Levodopa has been associated with somnolence and episodes of sudden sleep onset. Sudden onset of sleep during daily activities, in some cases without awareness or warning signs, has been reported very rarely. Patients must be informed of this and advised to exercise caution while driving or operating machines during treatment with Levodopa. Patients who have experienced somnolence and/or an episode of sudden sleep onset must refrain from driving or operating machines. Furthermore a reduction of dosage or termination of therapy may be considered.

As with levodopa, Sinemet CR or Half Sinemet CR may cause involuntary movements and mental disturbances. Patients with a history of severe involuntary movements or psychotic episodes when treated with levodopa alone or levodopa/decarboxylase inhibitor combination should be observed carefully when Sinemet CR or Half Sinemet CR is substituted. These reactions are thought to be due to increased brain dopamine following administration of levodopa and use of Sinemet CR or Half Sinemet CR may cause recurrence. Dosage reduction may be required. All patients should be observed carefully for the development of depression with concomitant suicidal tendencies. Patients with past or current psychoses should be treated with caution.

A symptom complex resembling the neuroleptic malignant syndrome including muscular rigidity, elevated body temperature, mental changes, and increased serum creatine phosphokinase has been reported when antiparkinsonian agents were withdrawn abruptly. Therefore, patients should be observed carefully when the dosage of carbidopa-levodopa combinations is reduced abruptly or discontinued, especially if the patient is receiving antipsychotics.

Patients with chronic wide-angle glaucoma may be treated cautiously with Sinemet CR or Half Sinemet CR, provided the intraocular pressure is well controlled and the patient monitored carefully for changes in intraocular pressure during therapy.

Periodic evaluations of hepatic, haematopoietic, cardiovascular and renal function are recommended during extended therapy.

If general anaesthesia is required, Sinemet CR or Half Sinemet CR may be continued as long as the patient is permitted to take oral medication. If therapy is interrupted temporarily, the usual dosage should be administered as soon as the patient is able to take oral medicine.

Laboratory Tests

Abnormalities in various laboratory tests have occurred with carbidopa-levodopa preparations and may occur with Sinemet CR or Half Sinemet CR. These include elevations of liver function tests such as alkaline phosphatase, SGOT (AST), SGPT (ALT), LDH, bilirubin, blood urea nitrogen, creatinine, uric acid and positive Coombs' test.

Carbidopa-levodopa preparations may cause a false-positive reaction for urinary ketone bodies when a test tape is used for determination of ketonuria. This reaction will not be altered by boiling the urine specimen. False-negative tests may result with the use of glucose-oxidase methods of testing for glycosuria.

Decreased haemoglobin and haematocrit, elevated serum glucose and white blood cells, bacteria and blood in the urine have been reported with standard Sinemet.

4.5 Interaction with other medicinal products and other forms of Interaction

Caution should be exercised when the following drugs are administered concomitantly with Sinemet CR or Half Sinemet CR:

Antihypertensive agents

Symptomatic postural hypotension has occurred when levodopa/decarboxylase inhibitor combinations were added to the treatment of patients receiving some antihypertensive drugs. Therefore when therapy with Sinemet CR or Half Sinemet CR is started, dosage adjustment of the antihypertensive drug may be required.

Antidepressants

There have been rare reports of adverse reactions, including hypertension and dyskinesia, resulting from the concomitant use of tricyclic antidepressants and carbidopa-levodopa preparations. (For patients receiving monomine oxidase inhibitors, see 4.3 'Contraindications').

Anticholinergics

Anticholinergics may affect the absorption and thus the patient's response.

Iron

Studies demonstrate a decrease in the bioavailability of carbidopa and/or levodopa when it is ingested with ferrous sulphate or ferrous gluconate.

Other drugs

Dopamine D_2 receptor antagonists (e.g. phenothiazines, butyrophenones and risperidone) and isoniazid may reduce the therapeutic effects of levodopa. The beneficial effects of levodopa in Parkinson's disease have been reported to be reversed by phenytoin and papaverine. Patients taking these drugs with Sinemet CR or Half Sinemet CR should be observed carefully for loss of therapeutic response.

Concomitant therapy with selegiline and carbidopa-levodopa may be associated with severe orthostatic hypotension not attributable to carbidopa-levodopa alone (See 4.3 Contraindications).

Since levodopa competes with certain amino acids, the absorption of levodopa may be impaired in some patients on a high protein diet.

The effect of simultaneous administration of antacids with Sinemet CR or Half Sinemet CR on the bioavailability of levodopa has not been studied.

4.6 Pregnancy and lactation

There are insufficient data to evaluate the possible harmfulness of this substance when used in human pregnancy. (See 5.3 'Preclinical Safety Data'). It is not known whether carbidopa or levodopa is excreted in human milk.) In a study of one nursing mother with Parkinson's disease, excretion of levodopa in human breast milk was reported. Sinemet CR or Half Sinemet CR should not be given during pregnancy and to nursing mothers.

4.7 Effects on ability to drive and use machines

Individual responses to medication may vary. Certain side effects that have been reported with Sinemet CR may affect some patients' ability to drive or operate machinery. Patients treated with Levodopa and presenting with somnolence and/or sudden sleep episodes must be informed to refrain from driving or engaging in activities where impaired alertness may put themselves or other at risk of serious injury or death (e.g. operating machines) until such recurrent episodes and somnolence have resolved (see also section 4.4 'Special warnings and precautions for use').

4.8 Undesirable effects

In controlled clinical trials in patients with moderate to severe motor fluctuations Sinemet CR did not produce side-effects which were unique to the modified-release formulation.

The side-effect reported most frequently was dyskinesia (a form of abnormal involuntary movements). A greater incidence of dyskinesias was seen with Sinemet CR than with Sinemet.

Other side-effects that also were reported frequently (above 2%) were: nausea, hallucinations, confusion, dizziness, chorea and dry mouth.

Side effects occurring less frequently (1-2%) were: dream abnormalities, dystonia, somnolence, insomnia, depression, asthenia, vomiting and anorexia.

Other side effects reported in clinical trials or in post-marketing experience include:

Body as a whole: chest pain, syncope.

Cardiovascular: palpitation, orthostatic effects including hypotensive episodes.

Gastrointestinal: constipation, diarrhoea, dyspepsia, gastrointestinal pain, dark saliva.

Hypersensitivity: angioedema, urticaria, pruritus.

Metabolic: weight loss.

Nervous System/Psychiatric: neuroleptic malignant syndrome (see 4.3 Contraindications), agitation, anxiety, decreased mental acuity, paraesthesia, disorientation, fatigue, headache, extrapyramidal and movement disorders, falling, gait abnormalities, muscle cramps, on-off phenomenon, increased libido, psychotic episodes including delusions and paranoid ideation. Levodopa is associated with somnolence and has been associated very rarely with excessive daytime somnolence and sudden sleep onset episodes.

Respiratory: dyspnoea

Skin: flushing, alopecia, rash, dark sweat.

Special Senses: blurred vision.

Urogenital: dark urine.

Other side effects that have been reported with levodopa or levodopa/carbidopa combinations and may be potential side-effects with Sinemet CR are listed below:

Cardiovascular: cardiac irregularities, hypertension, phlebitis.

Gastrointestinal: bitter taste, sialorrhoea, dysphagia, bruxism, hiccups, gastrointestinal bleeding, flatulence, burning sensation of tongue, development of duodenal ulcer.

Haematologic: leucopenia, haemolytic and non-haemolytic anaemia, thrombocytopenia, agranulocytosis.

Nervous system/Psychiatric: ataxia, numbness, increased hand tremor, muscle twitching, blepharospasm, trismus, activation of latent Horner's syndrome, euphoria, and dementia, depression with suicidal tendencies.

Skin: increased sweating.

Special senses: diplopia, dilated pupils, oculogyric crises.

Urogenital: urinary retention, urinary incontinence, priapism.

Miscellaneous: weight gain, oedema, weakness, faintness, hoarseness, malaise, hot flashes, sense of stimulation, bizarre breathing patterns, malignant melanoma (see 4.3 Contraindications), Henoch-Schonlein purpura.

Convulsions have occurred; however, a causal relationship with levodopa or levodopa/carbidopa combinations has not been established.

4.9 Overdose

Management of acute overdosage with Sinemet CR or Half Sinemet CR is basically the same as management of acute overdosage with levodopa; however, pyridoxine is not effective in reversing the actions of Sinemet CR or Half Sinemet CR.

Electrocardiographic monitoring should be instituted and the patient observed carefully for the development of arrhythmias; if required, appropriate antiarrhythmic therapy should be given. The possibility that the patient may have taken other drugs as well as Sinemet CR or Half Sinemet CR should be taken into consideration. To date, no experience has been reported with dialysis; hence, its value in overdosage is not known.

5. PHARMACOLOGICAL PROPERTIES

5.1 Pharmacodynamic properties

Sinemet CR and Half Sinemet CR are a combination of carbidopa, an aromatic amino acid decarboxylase inhibitor, and levodopa, the metabolic precursor of dopamine, in a polymer-based controlled-release tablet formulation, for use in the treatment of Parkinson's disease. Sinemet CR and Half Sinemet CR are particularly useful to reduce 'off' time in patients treated previously with a conventional levodopa/decarboxylase inhibitor combination who have had dyskinesias and motor fluctuations.

Patients with Parkinson's disease treated with preparations containing levodopa may develop motor fluctuations characterised by end-of-dose failure, peak dose dyskinesia, and akinesia. The advanced form of motor fluctuations ('on-off' phenomenon) is characterised by unpredictable swings from mobility to immobility. Although the causes of the motor fluctuations are not completely understood, it has been demonstrated that they can be attenuated by treatment regimens that produce steady plasma levels of levodopa.

Levodopa relieves the symptoms of Parkinson's disease by being decarboxylated to dopamine in the brain. Carbidopa, which does not cross the blood-brain barrier, inhibits only the extracerebral decarboxylation of levodopa, making more levodopa available for transport to the brain and subsequent conversion to dopamine. This normally obviates the necessity for large doses of levodopa at frequent intervals. The lower dosage reduces or may help eliminate gastrointestinal and cardiovascular side-effects, especially those which are attributed to dopamine being formed in extracerebral tissues.

Sinemet CR and Half Sinemet CR are designed to release their active ingredients over a four-six hour period. With this formulation there is less variation in plasma levodopa levels and the peak plasma level is 60% lower than with conventional Sinemet, as established in healthy volunteers.

In clinical trials, patients with motor fluctuations experienced reduced 'off'-time with Sinemet CR when compared with Sinemet. The reduction of the 'off'-time is rather small (about 10%) and the incidence of dyskinesias increases slightly after administration of Sinemet CR compared to standard Sinemet. Global ratings of improvement and activities of daily living in the 'on' and 'off' state, as assessed by both patient and physician, were better during therapy with Sinemet CR than with Sinemet. Patients considered Sinemet CR to be more helpful for their clinical fluctuations, and preferred it over Sinemet. In patients without motor fluctuations, Sinemet CR under controlled conditions, provided the same therapeutic benefit with less frequent dosing than with Sinemet. Generally, there was no further improvement of other symptoms of Parkinson's disease.

5.2 Pharmacokinetic properties

The pharmacokinetics of levodopa following administration of Sinemet CR were studied in young and elderly healthy volunteers. The mean time to peak plasma levodopa level after Sinemet CR was approximately two hours compared to 0.75 hours with Sinemet. The mean peak plasma levodopa levels were 60 percent lower with Sinemet CR than with Sinemet. The in vivo absorption of levodopa following administration of Sinemet CR was continuous for 4 to 6 hours. In these studies, as with patients, plasma levodopa concentrations fluctuated in a narrower range than with Sinemet. Because the bioavailability of levodopa from Sinemet CR relative to Sinemet is approximately 70 percent, the daily dosage of levodopa in the controlled release formulation will usually be higher that with conventional formulations. There was no evidence that Sinemet CR released its ingredients in a rapid or uncontrolled fashion.

The pharmacokinetics of levodopa following administration of Half Sinemet CR were studied in patients with Parkinson's disease. Chronic three month, open-label, twice daily dosing with Half Sinemet CR (range: 50 mg carbidopa, 200 mg levodopa up to 150 mg carbidopa, 600 mg levodopa per day) did not result in accumulation of plasma levodopa. The dose-adjusted bioavailability for one Half Sinemet CR tablet was equivalent to that for one Sinemet CR tablet. The mean peak concentration of levodopa following administration of one Half Sinemet CR tablet was greater than 50% of that following one Sinemet CR tablet. Mean time-to-peak plasma levels may be slightly less for Half Sinemet CR than for Sinemet CR.

It is not known whether or not or to what extent the absorption is influenced by a protein rich diet. The bioavailability may be influenced by drugs which affect the gastrointestinal propulsion.

5.3 Preclinical safety data

The medicine has appeared harmful in animal trials (visceral and skeletal malformations in rabbits). For reproductive toxicity, see section 4.6 'Pregnancy and Lactation'.

6. PHARMACEUTICAL PARTICULARS

6.1 List of excipients

Hydroxypropylcellulose

Magnesium Stearate

Poly (Vinyl Acetate-Crotonic Acid) Copolymer

Quinoline Yellow 10 Aluminium Lake E104 (Sinemet CR only)

Red Iron Oxide E172

6.2 Incompatibilities

Not applicable

6.3 Shelf life

36 months

6.4 Special precautions for storage

Avoid storage above 30°C.

6.5 Nature and contents of container

All aluminium blister pack of 60 tablets.

6.6 Instructions for use and handling

Not applicable.

7. MARKETING AUTHORISATION HOLDER

Merck Sharp & Dohme Limited

Hertford Road, Hoddesdon, Hertfordshire, EN11 9BU, UK.

Distributed by

Bristol-Myers Squibb Pharmaceuticals Limited, 141-149 Staines Road, Hounslow TW3 3JA, United Kingdom.

8. MARKETING AUTHORISATION NUMBER(S)

Sinemet CR PL 0025/0269

Half Sinemet CR PL 0025/0287

9. DATE OF FIRST AUTHORISATION/RENEWAL OF THE AUTHORISATION

Sinemet CR 5 September 1991/Renewed 24 April 2002

Half Sinemet CR 7 October 1992/Renewed 24 April 2002

10. DATE OF REVISION OF THE TEXT

April 2004

11. LEGAL CATEGORY

Prescription only medicine

®Registered trademark of Merck & Co., Inc., Whitehouse Station, New Jersey, USA

Sinequan

(Pfizer Limited)

1. NAME OF THE MEDICINAL PRODUCT

SINEQUAN® Capsules

2. QUALITATIVE AND QUANTITATIVE COMPOSITION

Active Ingredient: Doxepin Hydrochloride BP

The capsules contain Doxepin Hydrochloride BP equivalent to 10, 25, 50 or 75mg doxepin.

3. PHARMACEUTICAL FORM

Capsules for oral administration.

4. CLINICAL PARTICULARS

4.1 Therapeutic indications

Symptoms of depressive illness, especially where sedation is required.

4.2 Posology and method of administration

The optimum oral dose depends on the severity of the condition and the individual patient's response. The dose varies from 30-300mg daily. Doses up to 100mg daily may be given on a divided or once daily schedule. Should doses over 100mg daily be required, they should be administered in three divided doses daily. 100mg is the maximum dose recommended at any one time. This dose may be given at bedtime.

For the majority of patients with moderate or severe symptoms, it is recommended that treatment commences with an initial dose of 75mg daily. Many of these patients will respond satisfactorily at this dose level. For patients who do not, the dosage may be adjusted according to individual response. In more severely ill patients, it may be necessary to administer a dose of up to 300mg in divided doses daily, to obtain a clinical response.

In patients where insomnia is a troublesome symptom, it is recommended that the total daily dose be divided so that a higher proportion is given for the evening dose; similarly, if drowsiness is experienced as a side effect of treatment, Sinequan may be administered by this regimen or the dosage may be reduced. It is often possible, having once obtained a satisfactory therapeutic response, to reduce the dose for maintenance therapy.

The optimal anti-depressant effect may not be evident for two to three weeks.

Use in children The use of Sinequan in children under 12 years is not recommended because safe conditions for its use have not been established.

Use in the elderly In general, lower doses are recommended. Where the presenting symptoms are mild in nature, it is advisable to initiate treatment at a dose of 10-50mg daily. A satisfactory clinical response is obtained in many of these patients at a daily dose of 30-50mg. The dosage may be adjusted according to the individual response.

Use in hepatic impairment Dosage reduction may be required in patients with hepatic impairment (see 'Special warnings and special precautions for use').

Use in renal impairment (see 'Special warnings and special precautions for use').

4.3 Contraindications

Doxepin is contra-indicated in individuals who have shown hypersensitivity to tricyclic antidepressants (TCAs), doxepin, or any of the inactive ingredients.

Doxepin is also contra-indicated in patients with mania, severe liver disease, lactation, glaucoma, tendency to urinary retention.

4.4 Special warnings and special precautions for use

The once-a-day dosage regimen of Sinequan in patients with intercurrent illness or patients taking other medications should be carefully adjusted. This is especially important in patients receiving other medications with anticholinergic effects.

The use of Sinequan on a once-a-day dosage regimen in geriatric patients should be adjusted carefully on the basis of the patient's condition. The elderly are particularly liable to experience toxic effects, especially agitation, confusion and postural hypotension. The initial dose should be increased with caution under close supervision. Half the normal maintenance dose may be sufficient to produce a satisfactory clinical response.

Patients should be warned that drowsiness may occur with the use of Sinequan. Patients should also be cautioned that their response to alcohol may be potentiated.

Although Sinequan carries less risk than other tricyclic antidepressants, caution should be observed in the treatment of patients with severe cardiovascular disease, including patients with heart block, cardiac arrhythmia and those who have experienced a recent myocardial infarction.

Use in hepatic/renal impairment Use with caution in patients with hepatic and/or renal impairment.

Use in patients with epilepsy Use with caution in patients with a history of epilepsy.

Since suicide is an inherent risk in any depressed patient until significant improvement has occurred, patients should be closely supervised during early therapy.

Patients with benign prostatic hyperplasia may experience an increase in associated urinary retention (see 'Undesirable effects').

4.5 Interaction with other medicinal products and other forms of Interaction

Sinequan, like other tricyclic antidepressants (TCAs), is metabolised by cytochrome P450 (CYP) 2D6. Inhibitors or substrates of CYP2D6 (e.g quinidine, selective serotonin reuptake inhibitors [SSRIs]) may increase the plasma concentration of TCAs when administered concomitantly. The extent of interaction depends on the variability of effect on CYP2D6 and the therapeutic index of the TCA. The clinical significance of this interaction with doxepin has not been systematically evaluated.

Combined use with other anti-depressants, alcohol or anti-anxiety agents should be undertaken with due recognition of the possibility of potentiation. It is known, for example, that monoamine oxidase inhibitors may potentiate other drug effects, therefore Sinequan should not be given concurrently, or within two weeks of cessation of therapy, with monoamine oxidase inhibitors.

Cimetidine has been reported to produce clinically significant fluctuations in steady-state serum concentrations of Sinequan.

Sinequan should not be given with sympathomimetic agents such as ephedrine, isoprenaline, noradrenaline, phenylephrine and phenylpropanolamine.

General anaesthetics and local anaesthetics (containing sympathomimetics) given during tricyclic or tetracyclic anti-depressant therapy may increase the risk of arrhythmias and hypotension, or hypertension. If surgery is necessary, the anaesthetist should be informed that a patient is being so treated.

Sinequan may decrease the anti-hypertensive effect of agents such as debrisoquine, bethanidine, guanethidine and possibly clonidine. It usually requires daily doses of Sinequan in excess of 150mg before any effect on the action of guanethidine is seen. It would be advisable to review all anti-hypertensive therapy during treatment with tricyclic anti-depressants.

Barbiturates may increase the rate of metabolism of Sinequan.

Sinequan may reduce the effect of sublingual nitrates owing to dry mouth.

The dose of thyroid hormone medication may need reducing if Sinequan is being given concurrently.

4.6 Pregnancy and lactation
Doxepin crosses the placenta. Reproduction studies have been performed in rats, rabbits and monkeys and there was no evidence of harm to the animal foetus. The relevance to humans is not known. Since there is insufficient experience in pregnant women who have received this drug, its safety in pregnancy has not been established.

Doxepin and its active metabolite desmethyldoxepin are excreted in breast milk. There has been a report of apnoea and drowsiness occurring in a nursing infant whose mother was taking doxepin. The use of Sinequan is contraindicated during lactation.

4.7 Effects on ability to drive and use machines
Since drowsiness may occur with the use of Sinequan, patients should be warned of the possibility and cautioned against driving a car or operating machinery while taking this drug.

4.8 Undesirable effects
Sinequan is well tolerated. Most side-effects are mild and generally disappear with continued treatment, or if necessary a reduction in dose.

Note Some of the side-effects noted below have not been specifically reported with Sinequan. However, due to the close pharmacological similarities amongst the tricyclics, the reactions should be considered when prescribing Sinequan.

The most common side-effects to Sinequan are drowsiness, dry mouth and constipation. For further details see below under central nervous system and anti-cholinergic effects.

Anti-cholinergic effects Anti-cholinergic effects are relatively common and may occur immediately following the first dose of a tricyclic anti-depressant. Dry mouth and constipation are the most common anti-cholinergic effects. Blurred vision and sweating occur occasionally. Urinary retention is rare except in predisposed males who have an enlarged prostate gland. Tolerance is often achieved if treatment is continued. If these undesirable effects do not subside with continued therapy, or if they become severe, it may be necessary to reduce the dosage.

Central nervous system effects Drowsiness is the most commonly noticed side effect. This tends to disappear as therapy is continued. Insomnia and nightmares have also been reported. Other infrequently reported CNS side effects are confusion, disorientation, agitation, numbness or paraesthesiae, tremor (which is usually mild). But at high doses, in susceptible individuals (particularly the elderly) other extrapyramidal symptoms may occur including tardive dyskinesia. Rarely reported are hallucinations, ataxia (generally where mixtures of CNS drugs have been given), and convulsions. Convulsions are unlikely except in people predisposed to seizure activity by brain damage or alcohol and drug abuse.

Psychotic manifestations, including mania and paranoid delusions may be exacerbated during treatment with tricyclic anti-depressants.

Cardiovascular Cardiovascular effects including postural hypotension, and tachycardia have been reported occasionally and changes in ECG parameters (widening of the QRS and PR interval) very rarely (see 'Special warnings and special precautions for use').

Allergic Allergic reactions to tricyclic anti-depressants are uncommon. They include skin rash, facial oedema, photosensitisation, pruritus and urticaria.

Haematological Rare cases of eosinophilia and bone marrow depression manifesting as agranulocytosis, leucopenia, thrombocytopenia and purpura. Haemolytic anaemia.

Gastro-intestinal Nausea, vomiting, indigestion, taste disturbances, diarrhoea, anorexia and aphthous stomatitis have been reported (see 'Anti-cholinergic effects').

Endocrine Occasional reports of raised or lowered libido, testicular swelling, raised or lowered blood sugar levels. Rarely the syndrome of inappropriate anti-diuretic hormone secretion, gynaecomastia, enlargement of breasts and galactorrhoea in the female.

Other Dizziness, weight gain, chills, fatigue, weakness, flushing, alopecia, headache, exacerbation of asthma and hyperpyrexia (in association with chlorpromazine) have been occasionally observed. Rare reports of jaundice and of tinnitus.

Withdrawal Withdrawal symptoms may occur on abrupt cessation of tricyclic anti-depressant therapy and include insomnia, irritability and excessive perspiration. Withdrawal symptoms in neonates whose mothers received tricyclic anti-depressants during the third trimester have also been reported and include respiratory depression, convulsions and "jitteriness" (hyper-reflexia).

4.9 Overdose
Signs and symptoms
Mild: drowsiness, stupor, blurred vision, excessive dryness of mouth.

Severe: respiratory depression, hypotension, coma, convulsions, cardiac arrhythmias and tachycardias.

Also urinary retention (bladder atony), decreased gastro-intestinal motility (paralytic ileus), hyperthermia (or hypothermia), hypertension, dilated pupils, hyperactive reflexes.

Deaths have been reported involving overdoses of doxepin. The reported cases involved doxepin alone and in combination with other drugs and/or alcohol.

Management and treatment
Mild: observation and supportive therapy is all that is usually necessary.

Severe: medical management of severe Sinequan overdosage consists of aggressive supportive therapy. If the patient is conscious, gastric lavage with appropriate precautions to prevent pulmonary aspiration should be performed even though Sinequan is rapidly absorbed. The use of activated charcoal has been recommended, as has been continuous gastric lavage with saline for 24 hours or more. An adequate airway should be established in comatose patients and assisted ventilation used if necessary. ECG monitoring may be required for several days, since relapse after apparent recovery has been reported. Arrhythmias should be treated with the appropriate anti-arrhythmic agent. It has been reported that many of the cardiovascular and CNS symptoms of tricyclic anti-depressant poisoning in adults may be reversed by the slow intravenous administration of 1mg to 3mg of physostigmine salicylate.

Because physostigmine is rapidly metabolised, the dosage should be repeated as required. Convulsions may respond to standard anti-convulsant therapy. However, barbiturates may potentiate any respiratory depression. Dialysis and forced diuresis generally are not of value in the management of overdosage due to high tissue and protein binding of Sinequan.

5. PHARMACOLOGICAL PROPERTIES
5.1 Pharmacodynamic properties
The mechanism of action of Sinequan is not definitely known. It is not a central nervous system stimulant nor a monoamine oxidase inhibitor. The current hypothesis is that the clinical effects are due, at least in part, to influences on the adrenergic activity at the synapses so that deactivation of noradrenaline by reuptake into the nerve terminals is prevented. In animal studies anti-cholinergic, anti-serotonergic and anti-histaminergic effects on smooth muscle have been demonstrated. At higher than usual clinical doses, adrenaline response was potentiated in animals. This effect was not demonstrated in humans.

5.2 Pharmacokinetic properties
Doxepin is well absorbed from the gastro-intestinal tract. Approximately 55%-87% of orally administered doxepin undergoes first pass metabolism in the liver, forming the primary active metabolite desmethyldoxepin.

In healthy volunteers, a single oral dose of 75mg resulted in peak plasma concentrations for doxepin ranging from 8.8-45.8 ng/ml (mean 26.1 ng/ml). Peak levels were reached between 2 and 4 hours (mean 2.9 hours) after administration. Peak levels for the primary metabolite desmethyldoxepin ranged from 4.8-14.5 ng/ml (mean 9.7 ng/ml) and were achieved between 2 and 10 hours after administration. The mean apparent volume of distribution for doxepin is approximately 20 l/kg. The protein binding for doxepin is approximately 76%. In healthy volunteers the plasma elimination half-life of doxepin ranged from 8 to 24 hours (mean 17 hours). The half-life of desmethyldoxepin ranged from 33-80 hours (mean 51 hours). Mean plasma clearance for doxepin is approximately 0.84 1/kg/hr. Paths of metabolism of doxepin include demethylation, N-oxidation, hydroxylation and glucuronide formation. Doxepin is excreted primarily in the urine, mainly as its metabolites, either free or in conjugate form.

6. PHARMACEUTICAL PARTICULARS
6.1 List of excipients
Sinequan 10mg capsule: lactose, magnesium stearate, maize starch dried, sodium lauryl sulphate; capsule shell constituents: amaranth (E123), erythrosine (E127), gelatin, sunset yellow (E110) and titanium dioxide (E171).

Sinequan 25mg capsule: lactose, magnesium stearate, maize starch dried, sodium lauryl sulphate; capsule shell constituents: amaranth (E123), erythrosine (E127), gelatin, patent blue V(E131), sunset yellow (E110) and titanium dioxide (E171).

Sinequan 50mg capsule: lactose, magnesium stearate, maize starch dried, sodium lauryl sulphate; capsule shell constituents: erythrosine (E127), gelatin, patent blue V (E131) and titanium dioxide (E171).

Sinequan 75mg capsule: magnesium stearate, maize starch dried, sodium lauryl sulphate; capsule shell constituents: erythrosine (E127), gelatin, patent blue V (E131), quinoline yellow (E104), and titanium dioxide (E171).

Sinequan capsules are free of gluten and sucrose.

6.2 Incompatibilities
None known.

6.3 Shelf life
3 years.

6.4 Special precautions for storage
Store below 25°C.

6.5 Nature and contents of container
Sinequan 10mg capsules are available as:

Packs of 56 capsules. Aluminium/PVC blister strips; 2 rows of 7 capsules per strip, 4 strips in a carton box.

Sinequan 25mg capsules are available as:

Packs of 28 capsules. Aluminium/PVC blister strips; 2 rows of 7 capsules per strip, 2 strips in a carton box.

Sinequan 50mg capsules are available as:

Packs of 28 capsules. Aluminium/PVC blister strips; 2 rows of 7 capsules per strip, 2 strips in a carton box.

Sinequan 75mg capsules are available as:

Packs of 28 capsules. Aluminium/PVC blister strips; 2 rows of 7 capsules per strip, 2 strips in a carton box.

6.6 Instructions for use and handling
No special requirements.

7. MARKETING AUTHORISATION HOLDER
Pfizer Limited

Ramsgate Road

Sandwich

Kent CT13 9NJ

United Kingdom

8. MARKETING AUTHORISATION NUMBER(S)
Sinequan capsules 10mg PL 0057/5032R

Sinequan capsules 25mg PL 0057/5033R

Sinequan capsules 50mg PL 0057/5034R

Sinequan capsules 75mg PL 0057/0133

9. DATE OF FIRST AUTHORISATION/RENEWAL OF THE AUTHORISATION
Sinequan capsules 10mg PL 0057/5032R 30/09/96

Sinequan capsules 25mg PL 0057/5033R 30/09/96

Sinequan capsules 50mg PL 0057/5034R 30/09/96

Sinequan capsules 75mg PL 0057/0133 12/09/96

10. DATE OF REVISION OF THE TEXT
July 2004

LEGAL CATEGORY
POM

Ref: SQ2_3

SINGULAIR 10 mg Tablets/4 and 5 mg Paediatric Tablets

(Merck Sharp & Dohme Limited)

1. NAME OF THE MEDICINAL PRODUCT
SINGULAIR® 10 mg Tablets

SINGULAIR® Paediatric 5 mg Chewable Tablets

SINGULAIR® Paediatric 4 mg Chewable Tablets

2. QUALITATIVE AND QUANTITATIVE COMPOSITION
10 mg tablet:

One film-coated tablet contains montelukast sodium, which is equivalent to 10 mg of montelukast.

5 mg chewable tablet:

One chewable tablet contains montelukast sodium, which is equivalent to 5 mg montelukast.

4 mg chewable tablet:

One chewable tablet contains montelukast sodium, which is equivalent to 4 mg montelukast.

For excipients, see 6.1.

3. PHARMACEUTICAL FORM

10 mg film-coated tablet:

Beige, rounded square, film-coated (size 7.9 mm by 7.9 mm) with 'SINGULAIR' engraved on one side, 'MSD 117' on the other.

5 mg chewable tablet:

Pink, round, biconvex (diameter 9.5 mm), with 'SINGULAIR' engraved on one side, 'MSD 275' on the other.

4 mg chewable tablet:

Pink, oval, biconvex-shaped, 'SINGULAIR' engraved on one side, 'MSD 711' on the other.

4. CLINICAL PARTICULARS

4.1 Therapeutic indications

'Singulair' is indicated in the treatment of asthma as add-on therapy in those patients with mild to moderate persistent asthma who are inadequately controlled on inhaled corticosteroids and in whom 'as-needed' short-acting β-agonists provide inadequate clinical control of asthma.

10 mg tablet ONLY: In those asthmatic patients in whom 'Singulair' is indicated in asthma, 'Singulair' can also provide symptomatic relief of seasonal allergic rhinitis.

'Singulair' is also indicated in the prophylaxis of asthma in which the predominant component is exercise-induced bronchoconstriction.

4.2 Posology and method of administration

10 mg tablet:

The dosage for adults 15 years of age and older with asthma, or with asthma and concomitant seasonal allergic rhinitis, is one 10 mg tablet daily to be taken in the evening.

5 mg chewable tablet:

The dosage for paediatric patients 6-14 years of age is one 5 mg chewable tablet daily to be taken in the evening. If taken in connection with food, 'Singulair' should be taken 1 hour before or 2 hours after food. No dosage adjustment within this age group is necessary.

4 mg chewable tablet:

The dosage for paediatric patients 2-5 years of age is one 4 mg chewable tablet daily to be taken in the evening. If taken in connection with food, 'Singulair' should be taken 1 hour before or 2 hours after food. No dosage adjustment within this age group is necessary. Experience in the paediatric population below 2 years of age is limited and use of montelukast is not recommended until further data become available. Safety and efficacy have not yet been established in this age group.

General recommendations: The therapeutic effect of 'Singulair' on parameters of asthma control occurs within one day. 'Singulair' may be taken with or without food. Patients should be advised to continue taking 'Singulair' even if their asthma is under control, as well as during periods of worsening asthma. *10 mg tablet:* 'Singulair' should not be used concomitantly with other products containing the same active ingredient, montelukast.

No dosage adjustment is necessary for the elderly, or for patients with renal insufficiency, or mild to moderate hepatic impairment. There are no data on patients with severe hepatic impairment. The dosage is the same for both male and female patients.

Therapy with 'Singulair' in relation to other treatments for asthma.

'Singulair' can be added to a patient's existing treatment regimen.

β -agonist therapy: 'Singulair' can be added to the treatment regimen of patients who are not adequately controlled on 'as-needed' short-acting β-agonist. When a clinical response is evident (usually after the first dose), the patient may be able to decrease the use of 'as-needed' short-acting β-agonist.

Inhaled corticosteroids: Treatment with 'Singulair' can be used as add-on therapy in patients when other agents, such as inhaled corticosteroids provide inadequate clinical control. 'Singulair' should not be substituted for inhaled corticosteroids (*See Section 4.4*).

10 mg tablets are available for adults 15 years of age and older.

5 mg chewable tablets are available for paediatric patients 6 to14 years of age.

4 mg chewable tablets are available for paediatric patients 2 to 5 years of age.

4.3 Contraindications

Hypersensitivity to the active substance or to any of the excipients.

4.4 Special warnings and special precautions for use

Patients should be advised never to use oral montelukast to treat acute asthma attacks and to keep their usual appropriate rescue medication for this purpose readily available. If an acute attack occurs, a short-acting inhaled β-agonist should be used. Patients should seek their doctor's advice as soon as possible if they need more inhalations of short-acting β-agonists than usual.

Montelukast should not be substituted for inhaled or oral corticosteroids.

There are no data demonstrating that oral corticosteroids can be reduced when montelukast is given concomitantly.

In rare cases, patients on therapy with anti-asthma agents including montelukast may present with systemic eosinophilia, sometimes presenting with clinical features of vasculitis consistent with Churg-Strauss syndrome, a condition which is often treated with systemic corticosteroid therapy. These cases usually, but not always, have been associated with the reduction or withdrawal of oral corticosteroid therapy. The possibility that leukotriene receptor antagonists may be associated with emergence of Churg-Strauss syndrome can neither be excluded nor established. Physicians should be alert to eosinophilia, vasculitic rash, worsening pulmonary symptoms, cardiac complications, and/or neuropathy presenting in their patients. Patients who develop these symptoms should be reassessed and their treatment regimens evaluated.

10 mg tablet:

Treatment with montelukast does not alter the need for patients with aspirin-sensitive asthma to avoid taking aspirin and other non-steroidal anti-inflammatory drugs.

Patients with rare hereditary problems of galactose intolerance, the Lapp lactase deficiency or glucose-galactose malabsorption should not take this medicine.

5 mg chewable tablet:

'Singulair' contains aspartame, a source of phenylalanine. Patients with phenylketonuria should take into account that each 5 mg chewable tablet contains phenylalanine in an amount equivalent to 0.842 mg phenylalanine per dose.

4 mg chewable tablet:

Safety and efficacy have not yet been established in the paediatric population below 2 years of age.

'Singulair' contains aspartame, a source of phenylalanine. Patients with phenylketonuria should take into account that each 4 mg chewable tablet contains phenylalanine in an amount equivalent to 0.674 mg phenylalanine per dose.

4.5 Interaction with other medicinal products and other forms of Interaction

Montelukast may be administered with other therapies routinely used in the prophylaxis and chronic treatment of asthma. In drug-interactions studies, the recommended clinical dose of montelukast did not have clinically important effects on the pharmacokinetics of the following drugs: theophylline, prednisone, prednisolone, oral contraceptives (ethinyl oestradiol/norethindrone 35/1), terfenadine, digoxin and warfarin.

The area under the plasma concentration curve (AUC) for montelukast was decreased approximately 40% in subjects with co-administration of phenobarbital. Since montelukast is metabolised by CYP 3A4, caution should be exercised, particularly in children, when montelukast is co-administered with inducers of CYP 3A4, such as phenytoin, phenobarbital and rifampicin.

4.6 Pregnancy and lactation

Since there are no controlled studies in pregnant or nursing women, montelukast should not be used during pregnancy or in nursing mothers unless it is considered to be clearly essential. (*See Section 5.3*).

4.7 Effects on ability to drive and use machines

Montelukast is not expected to affect a patient's ability to drive a car or operate machinery. However, in very rare cases, individuals have reported drowsiness.

4.8 Undesirable effects

Montelukast has been evaluated in clinical studies as follows:

- 10 mg film-coated tablets in approximately 4,000 adult asthmatic patients 15 years of age and older.
- 10 mg film-coated tablets in approximately 400 adult asthmatic patients with seasonal allergic rhinitis 15 years of age and older
- 5-mg chewable tablets in approximately 1,100 paediatric asthmatic patients 6 to 14 years of age, and
- 4 mg chewable tablets in 573 paediatric patients 2 to 5 years of age.

The following drug-related adverse reactions in placebo-controlled clinical studies were reported commonly >1/100, <1/10) in asthmatic patients treated with montelukast and at a greater incidence than in patients treated with placebo.

(see Table 1 above)

Table 1

Body System Class	Adult Patients 15 years and older (two 12-week studies; n=795)	Paediatric Patients 6 to 14 years old (one 8-week study; n=201)	Paediatric Patients 2 to 5 years old (one 12-week study; n=461)
Body as a whole	abdominal pain		
Digestive system disorders			thirst
Nervous system/psychiatric	headache	headache	

With prolonged treatment in clinical trials with a limited number of patients for up to 2 years for adults, and up to 6 months for paediatric patients 6 to 14 years of age, the safety profile did not change.

Cumulatively, 502 paediatric patients 2 to 5 years of age were treated with montelukast for at least 3 months, 338 for 6 months or longer, and 256 patients for 12 months or longer. With prolonged treatment, the safety profile did not change in these patients either.

The following adverse reactions have been reported in post-marketing use very rarely:

Body as whole: asthenia/fatigue, malaise, oedema, hypersensitivity reactions including anaphylaxis, angioedema, urticaria, pruritus, rash and one isolated report of hepatic eosinophilic infiltration

Nervous system/psychiatric: dizziness, dream abnormalities including nightmares, hallucinations, drowsiness, insomnia, paraesthesia/hypoesthesia, irritability, agitation including aggressive behaviour, restlessness, seizure

Musculo-skeletal disorders: arthralgia, myalgia including muscle cramps

Digestive system disorders: diarrhoea, dry mouth, dyspepsia, nausea, vomiting.

Hepato-biliary disorders: elevated levels of serum transaminases (ALT, AST), cholestatic hepatitis.

Cardiovascular disorders: increased bleeding tendency, bruising, palpitations.

Very rare cases of Churg-Strauss Syndrome (CSS) have been reported during montelukast treatment in asthmatic patients. (See Section 4.4).

4.9 Overdose

No specific information is available on the treatment of overdosage with montelukast. In chronic asthma studies, montelukast has been administered at doses up to 200 mg/day to patients for 22 weeks and in short-term studies, up to 900 mg/day to patients for approximately one week without clinically important adverse experiences.

There have been reports of acute overdosage in children in post-marketing experience and clinical studies of up to at least 150 mg/day with montelukast. The clinical and laboratory findings observed were consistent with the safety profile in adults and older paediatric patients. There were no adverse experiences reported in the majority of overdosage reports. The most frequent adverse experiences observed were thirst, somnolence, mydriasis, hyperkinesia, and abdominal pain.

It is not known whether montelukast is dialysable by peritoneal- or haemo-dialysis.

5. PHARMACOLOGICAL PROPERTIES

5.1 Pharmacodynamic properties

Pharmacotherapeutic group: Anti-Asthmatics for systemic use, Leukotriene receptor antagonist

ATC Code: RO3D CO3

The cysteinyl leukotrienes (LTC_4, LTD_4, LTE_4) are potent inflammatory eicosanoids released from various cells including mast cells and eosinophils. These important pro-asthmatic mediators bind to cysteinyl leukotriene (CysLT) receptors. The CysLT type-1 ($CysLT_1$) receptor is found in the human airway (including airway smooth muscle cells and airway macrophages) and on other pro-inflammatory cells (including eosinophils and certain myeloid stem cells). CysLTs have been correlated with the pathophysiology of asthma and allergic rhinitis. In asthma, leukotriene-mediated effects include bronchoconstriction, mucous secretion, vascular permeability, and eosinophil recruitment. In allergic rhinitis, CysLTs are released from the nasal mucosa after allergen exposure during both early- and late-phase reactions and are associated with symptoms of allergic rhinitis. Intranasal challenge with CySLTs has been shown to increase nasal airway resistance and symptoms of nasal obstruction.

Montelukast is an orally active compound which binds with high affinity and selectivity to the $CysLT_1$ receptor. In clinical studies, montelukast inhibits bronchoconstriction due to inhaled LTD_4 at doses as low as 5 mg. Bronchodilation was observed within two hours of oral administration. The bronchodilation effect caused by a β-agonist was additive to that caused by montelukast. Treatment with montelukast inhibited both early- and late-phase bronchoconstriction due to antigen challenge. Montelukast, compared with placebo, decreased peripheral blood eosinophils in adult and paediatric patients. In a separate study, treatment with montelukast significantly decreased eosinophils in the airways (as measured in sputum) and in peripheral blood while improving clinical asthma control. In adult and paediatric patients 2 to 14 years of age, montelukast, compared with placebo, decreased peripheral blood eosinophils while improving clinical asthma control.

In studies in adults, montelukast 10 mg once daily, compared with placebo, demonstrated significant improvements in morning FEV_1 (10.4% vs 2.7% change from baseline), AM peak expiratory flow rate (PEFR) (24.5 L/min vs 3.3 L/min change from baseline), and significant decrease in total β-agonist use (-26.1% vs -4.6% change from baseline). Improvement in patient-reported daytime and night-time asthma symptoms scores was significantly better than placebo.

Studies in adults demonstrated the ability of montelukast to add to the clinical effect of inhaled corticosteroid (% change from baseline for inhaled beclomethasone plus montelukast vs beclomethasone, respectively for FEV_1 : 5.43% vs 1.04%; β-agonist use: -8.70% vs 2.64%). Compared with inhaled beclomethasone (200 μg twice daily with a spacer device), montelukast demonstrated a more rapid initial response, although over the 12-week study, beclomethasone provided a greater average treatment effect (% change from baseline for montelukast vs beclomethasone, respectively for FEV_1 : 7.49% vs 13.3%; β-agonist use: -28.28% vs -43.89%). However, compared with beclomethasone, a high percentage of patients treated with montelukast achieved similar clinical responses (e.g. 50% of patients treated with beclomethasone achieved an improvement in FEV_1 of approximately 11% or more over baseline while approximately 42% of patients treated with montelukast achieved the same response).

10 mg tablets:

A clinical study was conducted to evaluate montelukast for the symptomatic treatment of seasonal allergic rhinitis in adult asthmatic patients 15 years of age and older with concomitant seasonal allergic rhinitis. In this study, montelukast 10-mg tablets administered once daily demonstrated a statistically significant improvement in the Daily Rhinitis Symptoms score, compared with placebo. The Daily Rhinitis Symptoms score is the average of the Daytime Nasal Symptoms score (mean of nasal congestion, rhinorrhea, sneezing, nasal itching) and the Nighttime Symptoms score (mean of nasal congestion upon awakening, difficulty going to sleep, and night-time awakenings scores). Global evaluations of allergic rhinitis by patients and physicians, were significantly improved, compared with placebo. The evaluation of asthma efficacy was not a primary objective of this study.

4 mg tablets:

In a 12-week, placebo-controlled study in paediatric patients 2 to 5 years of age, montelukast 4 mg once daily improved parameters of asthma control compared with placebo, irrespective of concomitant controller therapy (inhaled/nebulised corticosteroids or inhaled/nebulised sodium cromoglycate). 60% of patients were not on any other controller therapy. Montelukast improved daytime symptoms (including coughing, wheezing, trouble breathing and activity limitation) and night-time symptoms compared with placebo. Montelukast also decreased 'as needed' β-agonist use and corticosteroid rescue for worsening asthma compared with placebo. Patients receiving montelukast had more days without asthma than those receiving placebo. A treatment effect was achieved after the first dose.

In an 8-week study in paediatric patients 6 to 14 years of age, montelukast 5 mg once daily, compared with placebo, significantly improved respiratory function (FEV_1 8.71% vs 4.16% change from baseline; AM PEFR 27.9 L/min vs 17.8 L/min change from baseline) and decreased 'as-needed' β-agonist use (-11.7% vs +8.2% change from baseline).

Significant reduction of exercise-induced bronchoconstriction (EIB) was demonstrated in a 12-week study in adults (maximal fall in FEV_1 22.33% for montelukast vs 32.40% for placebo; time to recovery to within 5% of baseline FEV_1 44.22 min vs 60.64 min). This effect was consistent throughout the 12-week study period. Reduction in EIB was also demonstrated in a short term study in paediatric patients 6 to 14 years of age (maximal fall in FEV_1 18.27% vs 26.11%; time to recovery to within 5% of baseline FEV_1 17.76 min vs 27.98 min). The effect in both studies was demonstrated at the end of the once-daily dosing interval.

In aspirin-sensitive asthmatic patients receiving concomitant inhaled and/or oral corticosteroids, treatment with montelukast, compared with placebo, resulted in significant improvement in asthma control (FEV_1 8.55% vs -1.74% change from baseline and decrease in total β-agonist use -27.78% vs 2.09% change from baseline).

5.2 Pharmacokinetic properties

Absorption: Montelukast is rapidly absorbed following oral administration. For the 10 mg film-coated tablet, the mean peak plasma concentration (C_{max}) is achieved three hours (T_{max}) after administration in adults in the fasted state. The mean oral bioavailability is 64%. The oral bioavailability and C_{max} are not influenced by a standard meal. Safety and efficacy were demonstrated in clinical trials where the 10 mg film-coated tablet was administered without regard to the timing of food ingestion.

For the 5 mg chewable tablet, the C_{max} is achieved in two hours after administration in adults in the fasted state. The mean oral bioavailability is 73% and is decreased to 63% by a standard meal.

After administration of the 4 mg chewable tablet to paediatric patients 2 to 5 years of age in the fasted state, C_{max} is achieved 2 hours after administration. The mean C_{max} is 66% higher while mean C_{min} is lower than in adults receiving a 10 mg tablet.

Distribution: Montelukast is more than 99% bound to plasma proteins. The steady-state volume of distribution of montelukast averages 8-11 litres. Studies in rats with radiolabelled montelukast indicate minimal distribution across the blood-brain barrier. In addition, concentrations of radiolabelled material at 24 hours post-dose were minimal in all other tissues.

Biotransformation: Montelukast is extensively metabolised. In studies with therapeutic doses, plasma concentrations of metabolites of montelukast are undetectable at steady state in adults and children.

In vitro studies using human liver microsomes indicate that cytochromes P450 3A4, 2A6 and 2C9 are involved in the metabolism of montelukast. Based on further *in vitro* results in human liver microsomes, therapeutic plasma concentrations of montelukast do not inhibit cytochromes P450 3A4, 2C9, 1A2, 2A6, 2C19, or 2D6. The contribution of metabolites to the therapeutic effect of montelukast is minimal.

Elimination: The plasma clearance of montelukast averages 45 ml/min in healthy adults. Following an oral dose of radiolabelled montelukast, 86% of the radioactivity was recovered in 5-day faecal collections and <0.2% was recovered in urine. Coupled with estimates of montelukast oral bioavailability, this indicates that montelukast and its metabolites are excreted almost exclusively *via* the bile.

Characteristics in patients: No dosage adjustment is necessary for the elderly or mild to moderate hepatic insufficiency. Studies in patients with renal impairment have not been undertaken. Because montelukast and its metabolites are eliminated by the biliary route, no dose adjustment is anticipated to be necessary in patients with renal impairment. There are no data on the pharmacokinetics of montelukast in patients with severe hepatic insufficiency (Child-Pugh score>9).

With high doses of montelukast (20- and 60-fold the recommended adult dose), a decrease in plasma theophylline concentration was observed. This effect was not seen at the recommended dose of 10 mg once daily.

5.3 Preclinical safety data

In animal toxicity studies, minor serum biochemical alterations in ALT, glucose, phosphorus and triglycerides were observed which were transient in nature. The signs of toxicity in animals were increased excretion of saliva, gastro-intestinal symptoms, loose stools and ion imbalance. These occurred at dosages which provided>17-fold the systemic exposure seen at the clinical dosage. In monkeys, the adverse effects appeared at doses from 150 mg/kg/day (>232-fold the systemic exposure seen at the clinical dose). In animal studies, montelukast did not affect fertility or reproductive performance at systemic exposure exceeding the clinical systemic exposure by greater than 24-fold. A slight decrease in pup body weight was noted in the female fertility study in rats at 200 mg/kg/day (>69-fold the clinical systemic exposure). In studies in rabbits, a higher incidence of incomplete ossification, compared with concurrent control animals, was seen at systemic exposure>24-fold the clinical systemic exposure seen at the clinical dose. No abnormalities were seen in rats. Montelukast has been shown to cross the placental barrier and is excreted in breast milk of animals.

No deaths occurred following a single oral administration of montelukast sodium at doses up to 5000 mg/kg in mice and rats (15,000 mg/m^2 and 30,000 mg/m^2 in mice and rats, respectively) the maximum dose tested. This dose is equivalent to 25,000 times the recommended daily adult human dose (based on an adult patient weight of 50 kg).

Montelukast was determined not to be phototoxic in mice for UVA, UVB or visible light spectra at doses up to 500 mg/kg/day (approximately>200-fold based on systemic exposure).

Montelukast was neither mutagenic in *in vitro* and *in vivo* tests nor tumorigenic in rodent species.

6. PHARMACEUTICAL PARTICULARS

6.1 List of excipients

10 mg tablet:

Microcrystalline cellulose, lactose monohydrate (89.3 mg), croscarmellose sodium, hydroxypropyl cellulose, and magnesium stearate.

Film coating: hypromellose, hydroxypropyl cellulose, titanium dioxide (E171), red and yellow ferric oxide (E172) and carnauba wax.

5 mg and 4 mg chewable tablets:

Mannitol, microcrystalline cellulose, hydroxypropylcellulose, red ferric oxide (E172), croscarmellose sodium, cherry flavour, aspartame and magnesium stearate.

6.2 Incompatibilities

Not applicable

6.3 Shelf life

10 mg tablet:

3 years.

5 mg and 4 mg chewable tablets:

2 years

6.4 Special precautions for storage

Store in the original package.

6.5 Nature and contents of container

Packaged in polyamide/PVC/aluminium blister package in:

Blisters (with weekdays indicated), in packages of: 7, 14, 28, 56, 98 and 140 tablets.

Blisters (without weekdays indicated), in packages of: 10, 20, 28, 30, 50, 100 and 200 tablets.

Blisters (unit doses), in packages of: 49, 50 and 56 tablets.

Not all pack sizes may be marketed

6.6 Instructions for use and handling

No special requirements.

7. MARKETING AUTHORISATION HOLDER

Merck Sharp & Dohme Limited

Hertford Road, Hoddesdon, Hertfordshire EN11 9BU, UK

8. MARKETING AUTHORISATION NUMBER(S)

10 mg tablet: PL 0025/0358

5 mg chewable tablet: PL 0025/0357

4 mg chewable tablet: PL 0025/0412

9. DATE OF FIRST AUTHORISATION/RENEWAL OF THE AUTHORISATION

10 mg tablet UK: 15 January 1998/31 July 2002

5 mg chewable tablet UK: 15 January 1998/31 July 2002

4 mg chewable tablet UK: 24 January 2001/31 July 2002

10. DATE OF REVISION OF THE TEXT

November 2004

LEGAL CATEGORY

POM

MSD (logo)

Merck Sharp & Dohme Limited

Hertford Road, Hoddesdon, Hertfordshire EN11 9BU, UK

SPC.SGA.04.UK/IRL.1089 (W028&W029)

SINGULAIR PAEDIATRIC 4 mg GRANULES

(Merck Sharp & Dohme Limited)

1. NAME OF THE MEDICINAL PRODUCT

SINGULAIR® Paediatric 4 mg Granules

2. QUALITATIVE AND QUANTITATIVE COMPOSITION

One sachet of granules contains montelukast sodium, which is equivalent to 4 mg montelukast.

For excipients, see 6.1.

3. PHARMACEUTICAL FORM

Granules.

White granules.

4. CLINICAL PARTICULARS

4.1 Therapeutic indications

'Singulair' is indicated in the treatment of asthma as add-on therapy in those patients with mild to moderate persistent asthma who are inadequately controlled on inhaled corticosteroids and in whom 'as-needed' short acting β-agonists provide inadequate clinical control of asthma.

'Singulair' is also indicated in the prophylaxis of asthma in which the predominant component is exercise-induced bronchoconstriction.

4.2 Posology and method of administration

The dosage for paediatric patients 6 months to 5 years of age is one sachet of 4-mg granules daily to be taken in the evening. No dosage adjustment within this age group is necessary. The experience in use in paediatric patients 6 to 12 months of age is limited. Safety and efficacy below 6 months of age have not been established.

Administration of 'Singulair' granules

'Singulair' granules can be administered either directly in the mouth, or mixed with a spoonful of cold or room temperature soft food (e.g. applesauce, ice cream, carrots and rice). The sachet should not be opened until ready to use. After opening the sachet, the full dose of 'Singulair' granules must be administered immediately (within 15 minutes). If mixed with food, 'Singulair' granules must not be stored for future use. 'Singulair' granules are not intended to be dissolved in liquid for administration. However, liquids may be taken subsequent to administration. 'Singulair' granules can be administered without regard to the timing of food ingestion.

*General recommendations:*The therapeutic effect of 'Singulair' on parameters of asthma control occurs within one day. Patients should be advised to continue taking

'Singulair' even if their asthma is under control, as well as during periods of worsening asthma.

No dosage adjustment is necessary for patients with renal insufficiency, or mild to moderate hepatic impairment. There are no data on patients with severe hepatic impairment. The dosage is the same for both male and female patients.

Therapy with 'Singulair' in relation to other treatments for asthma.

'Singulair' can be added to a patient's existing treatment regimen.

β -agonist therapy: 'Singulair' can be added to the treatment regimen of patients who are not adequately controlled on 'as-needed' short acting *β*-agonist. When a clinical response is evident (usually after the first dose), the patient may be able to decrease the use of 'as-needed' short acting *β*-agonist.

Inhaled corticosteroids: Treatment with 'Singulair' can be used as add-on therapy in patients when other agents, such as inhaled corticosteroids, provide inadequate clinical control. 'Singulair' should not be substituted for inhaled corticosteroids. (See section 4.4 'Special warnings and precautions for use'.)

10-mg tablets are available for adults 15 years of age and older.

5-mg chewable tablets are available for paediatric patients 6 to 14 years of age.

4-mg chewable tablets are available as an alternative formulation for paediatric patients 2 to 5 years of age.

4.3 Contraindications

Hypersensitivity to the active substance or to any of the excipients.

4.4 Special warnings and special precautions for use

Patients should be advised never to use oral montelukast to treat acute asthma attacks and to keep their usual appropriate rescue medication for this purpose readily available. If an acute attack occurs, a short-acting inhaled *β*-agonist should be used. Patients should seek their doctors' advice as soon as possible if they need more inhalations of short-acting *β*-agonists than usual.

Montelukast should not be substituted for inhaled or oral corticosteroids.

There are no data demonstrating that oral corticosteroids can be reduced when montelukast is given concomitantly.

In rare cases, patients on therapy with anti-asthma agents including montelukast may present with systemic eosinophilia, sometimes presenting with clinical features of vasculitis consistent with Churg-Strauss syndrome, a condition which is often treated with systemic corticosteroid therapy. These cases usually, but not always, have been associated with the reduction or withdrawal of oral corticosteroid therapy. The possibility that leukotriene receptor antagonists may be associated with emergence of Churg-Strauss syndrome can neither be excluded nor established. Physicians should be alert to eosinophilia, vasculitic rash, worsening pulmonary symptoms, cardiac complications, and/or neuropathy presenting in their patients. Patients who develop these symptoms should be reassessed and their treatment regimens evaluated.

Safety and efficacy have not yet been established in the paediatric population below 6 months of age.

4.5 Interaction with other medicinal products and other forms of Interaction

Montelukast may be administered with other therapies routinely used in the prophylaxis and chronic treatment of asthma. In drug-interactions studies, the recommended clinical dose of montelukast did not have clinically important effects on the pharmacokinetics of the following drugs: theophylline, prednisone, prednisolone, oral contraceptives (ethinyl estradiol/norethindrone 35/1), terfenadine, digoxin and warfarin.

The area under the plasma concentration curve (AUC) for montelukast was decreased approximately 40% in subjects with co-administration of phenobarbital. Since montelukast is metabolised by CYP 3A4, caution should be exercised, particularly in children, when montelukast is coadministered with inducers of CYP 3A4, such as phenytoin, phenobarbital and rifampicin.

4.6 Pregnancy and lactation

Since there are no controlled studies in pregnant or nursing women, montelukast should not be used during pregnancy or in nursing mothers unless it is considered to be clearly essential. (See section 5.3 'Preclinical safety data'.)

4.7 Effects on ability to drive and use machines

Montelukast is not expected to affect a patient's ability to drive a car or operate machinery. However, in very rare cases, individuals have reported drowsiness.

4.8 Undesirable effects

Montelukast has been evaluated in clinical studies as follows:

- 10-mg film-coated tablets in approximately 4,000 adult patients 15 years of age and older
- 5-mg chewable tablets in approximately 1,100 paediatric patients 6 to 14 years of age.
- 4-mg chewable tablets in 573 paediatric patients 2 to 5 years of age, and
- 4-mg granules in 175 paediatric patients 6 months to 2 years of age.

The following drug-related adverse reactions in placebo-controlled clinical studies were reported commonly (>1/100, <1/10) in patients treated with montelukast and at a greater incidence than in patients treated with placebo:

(see Table 1)

With prolonged treatment in clinical trials with a limited number of patients for up to 2 years for adults, and up to 6 months for paediatric patients 6 to 14 years of age, the safety profile did not change.

Cumulatively, 502 paediatric patients 2 to 5 years of age were treated with montelukast for at least 3 months, 338 for 6 months or longer, and 256 patients for 12 months or longer. With prolonged treatment, the safety profile did not change in these patients either.

The safety profile in paediatric patients 6 months to 2 years of age did not change with treatment up to 3 months.

The following adverse reactions have been reported in post-marketing use very rarely:

Body as whole: asthenia/fatigue, malaise, oedema, hypersensitivity reactions including anaphylaxis, angioedema, urticaria, pruritus, rash and one isolated report of hepatic eosinophilic infiltration.

Nervous system/psychiatric: dizziness, dream abnormalities including nightmares, hallucinations, drowsiness, insomnia, paraesthesia/hypoesthesia, irritability, agitation including aggressive behaviour, restlessness, seizure.

Musculo-skeletal disorders: arthralgia, myalgia including muscle cramps.

Digestive system disorders: diarrhoea, dry mouth, dyspepsia, nausea, vomiting.

Hepato-biliary disorders: elevated levels of serum transaminases (ALT, AST), cholestatic hepatitis.

Cardiovascular disorders: increased bleeding tendency, bruising, palpitations.

Very rare cases of Churg-Strauss Syndrome (CSS) have been reported during montelukast treatment in asthmatic patients. (see Section 4.4 *'Special warnings and precautions for use'*).

4.9 Overdose

No specific information is available on the treatment of overdosage with montelukast. In chronic asthma studies, montelukast has been administered at doses up to 200 mg/day to adult patients for 22 weeks and in short term studies, up to 900 mg/day to patients for approximately one week without clinically important adverse experiences.

There have been reports of acute overdosage in children in post-marketing experience and clinical studies of up to at least 150 mg/day with montelukast. The clinical and laboratory findings observed were consistent with the safety profile in adults and older paediatric patients. There were no adverse experiences reported in the majority of overdosage reports. The most frequent adverse experiences observed were thirst, somnolence, mydriasis, hyperkinesia, and abdominal pain.

It is not known whether montelukast is dialysable by peritoneal- or haemo-dialysis.

5. PHARMACOLOGICAL PROPERTIES

5.1 Pharmacodynamic properties

Pharmacotherapeutic group: Anti-Asthmatics for systemic use, Leukotriene receptor antagonist

ATC-code: R03D C03

The cysteinyl leukotrienes (LTC_4, LTD_4, LTE_4) are potent inflammatory eicosanoids released from various cells including mast cells and eosinophils. These important pro-asthmatic mediators bind to cysteinyl leukotriene receptors (CysLT) found in the human airway and cause airway actions, including bronchoconstriction, mucous secretion, vascular permeability, and eosinophil recruitment.

Montelukast is an orally active compound which binds with high affinity and selectivity to the $CysLT_1$ receptor. In clinical studies, montelukast inhibits bronchoconstriction due to inhaled LTD_4 at doses as low as 5 mg. Bronchodilation was observed within 2 hours of oral administration. The bronchodilation effect caused by a *β*-agonist was additive to that caused by montelukast. Treatment with montelukast inhibited both early- and late-phase bronchoconstriction due to antigen challenge. Montelukast, compared with placebo, decreased peripheral blood eosinophils in adult and paediatric patients. In a separate study, treatment with montelukast significantly decreased eosinophils in the airways (as measured in sputum). In adult and paediatric patients 2 to 14 years of age, montelukast, compared with placebo, decreased peripheral blood eosinophils while improving clinical asthma control.

In studies in adults, montelukast, 10 mg once daily, compared with placebo, demonstrated significant improvements in morning FEV_1 (10.4% vs 2.7% change from baseline), AM peak expiratory flow rate (PEFR) (24.5 L/min vs 3.3 L/min change from baseline), and significant decrease in total *β*-agonist use (-26.1% vs -4.6% change from baseline). Improvement in patient-reported daytime and night-time asthma symptoms scores was significantly better than placebo.

Studies in adults demonstrated the ability of montelukast to add to the clinical effect of inhaled corticosteroid (% change from baseline for inhaled beclomethasone plus montelukast vs beclomethasone, respectively for FEV_1: 5.43% vs 1.04%; *β*-agonist use: -8.70% vs 2.64%). Compared with inhaled beclomethasone (200 μg twice daily with a spacer device), montelukast demonstrated a more rapid initial response, although over the 12-week study, beclomethasone provided a greater average treatment effect (% change from baseline for montelukast vs beclomethasone, respectively for FEV_1: 7.49% vs 13.3%; *β*-agonist use: -28.28% vs -43.89%). However, compared with beclomethasone, a high percentage of patients treated with montelukast achieved similar clinical responses (e.g. 50% of patients treated with beclomethasone achieved an improvement in FEV_1 of approximately 11% or more over baseline while approximately 42% of patients treated with montelukast achieved the same response).

In an 8-week study in paediatric patients 6 to 14 years of age, montelukast 5 mg once daily, compared with placebo, significantly improved respiratory function (FEV_1 8.71% vs 4.16% change from baseline; AM PEFR 27.9 L/min vs 17.8 L/min change from baseline) and decreased 'as-needed' *β*-agonist use (-11.7% vs +8.2% change from baseline).

In a 12-week, placebo-controlled study in paediatric patients 2 to 5 years of age, montelukast 4 mg once daily improved parameters of asthma control compared with placebo irrespective of concomitant controller therapy (inhaled/nebulised corticosteroids or inhaled/nebulised sodium cromoglycate). Sixty percent of patients were not on any other controller therapy. Montelukast improved daytime symptoms (including coughing, wheezing, trouble breathing and activity limitation) and night-time symptoms compared with placebo. Montelukast also decreased 'as-needed' *β*-agonist use and corticosteroid rescue for worsening asthma compared with placebo. Patients receiving montelukast had more days without asthma than those receiving placebo. A treatment effect was achieved after the first dose.

Efficacy of montelukast is supported in paediatric patients 6 months to 2 years of age by extrapolation from the demonstrated efficacy in patients 2 years of age and older with asthma, and is based on similar pharmacokinetic data, as well as the assumption that the disease course, pathophysiology and the drug's effect are substantially similar among these populations.

Significant reduction of exercise-induced bronchoconstriction (EIB) was demonstrated in a 12-week study in adults (maximal fall in FEV_1 22.33% for montelukast vs 32.40% for placebo; time to recovery to within 5% of baseline FEV_1 44.22 min vs 60.64 min). This effect was consistent throughout the 12-week study period. Reduction in EIB was also demonstrated in a short term study in paediatric patients 6 to 14 years of age (maximal fall in FEV_1 18.27% vs 26.11%; time to recovery to within 5% of baseline FEV_1 17.76 min vs 27.98 min). The effect in both studies was demonstrated at the end of the once-daily dosing interval.

Table 1

Body System Class	Adult Patients 15 years and older (two 12-week studies; n=795)	Paediatric Patients 6 to 14 years old (one 8-week study; n=201)	Paediatric Patients 2 to 5 years old (one 12-week study; n=461)	Paediatric Patients 6 months up to 2 years old (one 6-week study; n=175)
Body as a whole	abdominal pain,			
Digestive system disorders			thirst	diarrhoea
Nervous system/psychiatric	headache	headache		hyperkinesia
Respiratory system disorders				asthma
Skin/skin appendages disorder				eczematous dermatitis, rash

In aspirin-sensitive asthmatic patients receiving concomitant inhaled and/or oral corticosteroids, treatment with montelukast, compared with placebo, resulted in significant improvement in asthma control (FEV_1 8.55% vs -1.74% change from baseline and decrease in total β-agonist use -27.78% vs 2.09% change from baseline).

5.2 Pharmacokinetic properties

Absorption: Montelukast is rapidly absorbed following oral administration. For the 10-mg film-coated tablet, the mean peak plasma concentration (C_{max}) is achieved 3 hours (T_{max}) after administration in adults in the fasted state. The mean oral bioavailability is 64%. The oral bioavailability and C_{max} are not influenced by a standard meal. Safety and efficacy were demonstrated in clinical trials where the 10-mg film-coated tablet was administered without regard to the timing of food ingestion.

For the 5-mg chewable tablet, the C_{max} is achieved in 2 hours after administration in adults in the fasted state. The mean oral bioavailability is 73% and is decreased to 63% by a standard meal.

After administration of the 4-mg chewable tablet to paediatric patients 2 to 5 years of age in the fasted state, C_{max} is achieved 2 hours after administration. The mean C_{max} is 66% higher while mean C_{min} is lower than in adults receiving a 10-mg tablet.

The 4-mg granule formulation is bioequivalent to the 4-mg chewable tablet when administered to adults in the fasted state. In paediatric patients 6 months to 2 years of age, C_{max} is achieved 2 hours after administration of the 4-mg granules formulation. C_{max} is nearly 2-fold greater than in adults receiving a 10-mg tablet. The co-administration of applesauce or a high-fat standard meal with the granule formulation did not have a clinically meaningful effect on the pharmacokinetics of montelukast as determined by AUC (1225.7 vs 1223.1 ng·hr/mL with and without applesauce, respectively, and 1191.8 vs 1148.5 ng·hr/mL with and without a high-fat standard meal, respectively).

Distribution: Montelukast is more than 99% bound to plasma proteins. The steady-state volume of distribution of montelukast averages 8-11 litres. Studies in rats with radiolabeled montelukast indicate minimal distribution across the blood-brain barrier. In addition, concentrations of radiolabeled material at 24 hours post-dose were minimal in all other tissues.

Biotransformation: Montelukast is extensively metabolised. In studies with therapeutic doses, plasma concentrations of metabolites of montelukast are undetectable at steady state in adults and children.

In vitro studies using human liver microsomes indicate that cytochrome P450 3A4, 2A6 and 2C9 are involved in the metabolism of montelukast. Based on further *in vitro* results in human liver microsomes, therapeutic plasma concentrations of montelukast do not inhibit cytochromes P450 3A4, 2C9, 1A2, 2A6, 2C19, or 2D6. The contribution of metabolites to the therapeutic effect of montelukast is minimal.

Elimination: The plasma clearance of montelukast averages 45 ml/min in healthy adults. Following an oral dose of radiolabeled montelukast, 86% of the radioactivity was recovered in 5-day faecal collections and <0.2% was recovered in urine. Coupled with estimates of montelukast oral bioavailability, this indicates that montelukast and its metabolites are excreted almost exclusively *via* the bile.

Characteristics in patients: No dosage adjustment is necessary for the elderly or mild to moderate hepatic insufficiency. Studies in patients with renal impairment have not been undertaken. Because montelukast and its metabolites are eliminated by the biliary route, no dose adjustment is anticipated to be necessary in patients with renal impairment. There are no data on the pharmacokinetics of montelukast in patients with severe hepatic insufficiency (Child-Pugh score>9).

With high doses of montelukast (20- and 60-fold the recommended adult dose), a decrease in plasma theophylline concentration was observed. This effect was not seen at the recommended dose of 10 mg once daily.

5.3 Preclinical safety data

In animal toxicity studies, minor serum biochemical alterations in ALT, glucose, phosphorus and triglycerides were observed which were transient in nature. The signs of toxicity in animals were increased excretion of saliva, gastro-intestinal symptoms, loose stools and ion imbalance. These occurred at dosages which provided >17-fold the systemic exposure seen at the clinical dosage. In monkeys, the adverse effects appeared at doses from 150 mg/kg/day (>232-fold the systemic exposure seen at the clinical dose). In animal studies, montelukast did not affect fertility or reproductive performance at systemic exposure exceeding the clinical systemic exposure by greater than 24-fold. A slight decrease in pup body weight was noted in the female fertility study in rats at 200 mg/kg/day (>69-fold the clinical systemic exposure). In studies in rabbits, a higher incidence of incomplete ossification, compared with concurrent control animals, was seen at systemic exposure>24-fold the clinical systemic exposure seen at the clinical dose. No abnormalities were seen in rats. Montelukast has been shown to cross the placental barrier and is excreted in breast milk of animals.

No deaths occurred following a single oral administration of montelukast sodium at doses up to 5,000 mg/kg in mice and rats (15,000 mg/m^2 and 30,000 mg/m^2 in mice and rats, respectively) the maximum dose tested. This dose is equivalent to 25,000 times the recommended daily adult human dose (based on an adult patient weight of 50 kg).

Montelukast was determined not to be phototoxic in mice for UVA, UVB or visible light spectra at doses up to 500 mg/kg/day (approximately>200-fold based on systemic exposure).

Montelukast was neither mutagenic in *in vitro* and *in vivo* tests nor tumorigenic in rodent species.

6. PHARMACEUTICAL PARTICULARS

6.1 List of excipients

Mannitol, hydroxypropyl cellulose, and magnesium stearate.

6.2 Incompatibilities

Not applicable.

UK PAGE 10

6.3 Shelf life

2 years

6.4 Special precautions for storage

Store in the original package.

6.5 Nature and contents of container

Packaged in polyethylene/aluminum/polyester sachet in:

Cartons of 7, 20, 28 and 30 sachets.

Not all pack sizes may be marketed.

6.6 Instructions for use and handling

No special requirements.

7. MARKETING AUTHORISATION HOLDER

Merck Sharp & Dohme Limited

Hertford Road

Hoddesdon

Hertfordshire EN11 9BU

UK

8. MARKETING AUTHORISATION NUMBER(S)

PL 0025/0440

9. DATE OF FIRST AUTHORISATION/RENEWAL OF THE AUTHORISATION

14 February 2003.

UK Page 11

10. DATE OF REVISION OF THE TEXT

December 2003.

LEGAL CATEGORY

POM

® denotes registered trademark of Merck & Co., Inc., Whitehouse Station, NJ, USA.

SPC.SGA-OG.03.UK/IRL.0953 (W25)

IRL PAGE 10

Sinthrome Tablets 1mg

(Alliance Pharmaceuticals)

1. NAME OF THE MEDICINAL PRODUCT

Sinthrome® Tablets 1mg.

2. QUALITATIVE AND QUANTITATIVE COMPOSITION

Acenocoumarol BP 1mg.

3. PHARMACEUTICAL FORM

White, round, flat tablets with slightly bevelled edges, with one side bearing the imprint "CG", and the other the imprint "AA".

4. CLINICAL PARTICULARS

4.1 Therapeutic indications

Treatment and prevention of thromboembolic diseases.

4.2 Posology and method of administration

Sensitivity to anticoagulants varies from patient to patient and may also fluctuate during the course of treatment. Therefore, it is essential to perform regular coagulant tests and to adjust the patient's dosage accordingly. If this is not possible, Sinthrome should not be used.

Sinthrome should be given in a single oral dose at the same time every day.

Adults

Initial dosage: If the thromboplastin time is within the normal range before starting treatment, the following dosage schedule is recommended:

First day: 4 to 12mg (within this range, lower doses may be required if patients are receiving heparin).

Second day: 4 to 8mg.

If the initial thromboplastin time is abnormal, treatment should be instituted with caution.

Maintenance therapy: the maintenance dose of Sinthrome varies from patient to patient and must be determined on the basis of regular laboratory estimations of the patient's blood coagulation time.

Adjustment of the maintenance dose can only be made by monitoring the Quick value of international normalised ratio (INR) at regular intervals, ensuring that the dosage remains within the therapeutic range. Depending on the individual, the maintenance dose generally lies between 1 to 8mg daily.

Before the start of treatment, up to the time when the coagulation valency is stabilised within the optimum range, routine measurement of the thromboplastin time should be carried out daily in hospital. Blood samples for laboratory tests should always be taken at the same time of day.

The INR is the ratio of the patient's plasma thromboplastin time and the normal thromboplastin time raised to a power determined for a reference thromboplastin. As the Quick value decreases, the patient's thromboplastin time increases and the INR is greater. The therapeutic range generally lies between INR values of 2 to 4.5. Within this range, the majority of patients show no risk of severe haemorrhagic complications nor a recurrence of thrombosis.

Generally, after withdrawal of Sinthrome, there is usually no danger of reactive hypercoagulability and therefore it is not necessary to give gradually diminishing doses. However, in extremely rare cases, in some high risk patients (e.g. after myocardial infarction), withdrawal should be gradual.

Children: Not recommended.

Elderly: A dose lower than the recommended adult dose may be sufficient in elderly patients (see Section 4.4, " Special warnings and precautions for use").

4.3 Contraindications

Pregnancy. Known hypersensitivity to acenocoumarol and related coumarin derivatives or to the excipients of Sinthrome, and in patients unable to co-operate (e.g. unsupervised and senile patients, alcoholics and patients with psychiatric disorders).

All conditions where the risk of haemorrhage exceeds possible clinical benefit e.g. haemorrhagic diathesis and/or blood dyscrasia; immediately prior to, or after surgery on the central nervous system or eyes and traumatising surgery involving extensive exposure of the tissues; peptic ulceration or haemorrhage in the gastro-intestinal tract, urogenital tract or respiratory system; cerebrovascular haemorrhages; acute pericarditis; pericardial effusion; infective endocarditis; severe hypertension (due to occult risks); severe hepatic or renal disease; and in cases of increased fibrinolytic activity following operations on the lung, prostate or uterus.

4.4 Special warnings and special precautions for use

Strict medical supervision should be given in cases where the disease or condition may reduce the protein binding of Sinthrome (e.g. thyrotoxicosis, tumours, renal disease, infections and inflammation).

Particular care should be taken in patients with hepatic dysfunction since the synthesis of blood coagulation factors may be impaired. Disorders affecting gastro-intestinal absorption may alter the anticoagulant activity of Sinthrome. In severe heart failure, a very cautious dosage schedule must be adopted, since hepatic congestion may reduce the activation of γ-carboxylation of coagulation factors. However with reversal of the hepatic congestion, it may be necessary to raise the dosage.

In elderly patients, anticoagulant medication should be monitored with special care (see Sections 4.2 "Posology and method of administration" and 5.2 "Pharmacokinetic properties").

Since acenocoumarol is extensively metabolised by the liver, impaired renal function will not greatly affect the elimination of the drug, although care should be taken due to the possibility of underlying platelet dysfunction.

During treatment with anticoagulants, intramuscular injections may cause haematomas and should be avoided. Subcutaneous and intravenous injections may be given without such complications.

Meticulous care should be taken where it is necessary to shorten the thromboplastin time for diagnostic or therapeutic procedures (eg angiography, lumbar puncture, minor surgery, tooth extractions etc).

4.5 Interaction with other medicinal products and other forms of Interaction

There are many possible interactions between coumarins and other drugs; those of clinical relevance are given below. Many of these are isolated reports only or have been reported with warfarin rather than acenocoumarol; for completeness, all have been included. The mechanisms of these interactions include disturbances of absorption, inhibition or induction of liver microsomal enzyme systems and reduced availability of vitamin K_1, necessary for γ-carboxylation of coagulation factors. Every form of therapy may involve the risk of an interaction, although not all will be significant. Thus careful surveillance is important and frequent coagulation tests (e.g. twice weekly) should be carried out when initially prescribing any drug in combination with Sinthrome, or when withdrawing a concomitantly administered drug.

The anticoagulant effect may be potentiated by concomitant administration of the following drugs:

- allopurinol;
- anabolic steroids;
- androgens;
- anti-arrhythmic agents (e.g. amiodarone, quinidine);

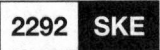

- antibiotics:
- broad spectrum antibiotics (e.g. amoxicillin, co-amoxiclav) macrolides (e.g. erythromycin, clarithromycin);
- cotrimoxazole;
- metronidazole;
- quinolones (e.g. ciprofloxacin, norfloxacin, ofloxacin);
- tetracyclines;
- neomycin;
- chloramphenicol.
- clofibric acid, its derivatives and structural analogues (e.g. fenofibrate, gemfibrozil);
- disulfiram;
- etacrynic acid;
- glucagon;
- H_2 antagonists (e.g. cimetidine);
- Imidazole derivatives, including topical administration (e.g. econazole, fluconazole, ketoconazole, miconazole);
- sulphonamides (including co-trimoxazole);
- oral antidiabetics (e.g. glibenclamide);
- thyroid hormones (including dextrothyroxine);
- sulfinpyrazone;
- statins (e.g. atorvastatin, fluvastatin, simvastatin);
- selective serotonin re-uptake inhibitors (e.g. fluoxetine, paroxetine)
- tamoxifen;
- 5-fluorouracil and analogues.

Drugs altering haemostasis may potentiate the anticoagulant activity of Sinthrome and thereby increase the risk of haemorrhage. Consequently, Sinthrome should not be prescribed with such drugs, which include:

- heparin (including low-molecular-weight heparin);
- platelet-aggregation inhibitors (e.g. dipyridamole, clopidogrel), salicylic acid and its derivatives, acetylsalicylic acid, para-aminosalicylic acid;
- diflunisal, phenylbutazone or other pyrazolone derivatives (e.g. sulfinpyrazone), and other non-steroidal anti-inflammatory drugs (NSAIDs).

The risk of gastrointestinal haemorrhage is increased if Sinthrome is prescribed in combination with NSAIDs, including selective COX-2 inhibitors. In the case of unavoidable concurrent use, coagulation tests should be performed more frequently.

The anticoagulant effect may be diminished by concomitant administration of the following drugs:

- aminoglutethimide;
- azathioprine;
- barbiturates;
- carbamazepine;
- colestyramine (see Section 4.9 "Overdose");
- griseofulvin;
- oral contraceptives;
- rifampicin;
- thiazide diuretics;
- St. John's Wort.

Unpredictable effect on anticoagulation, including both increase and decrease in anticoagulant activity have been reported with the following drugs:

- protease inhibitors (e.g. indinavir, nelfinavir, ritonavir, saquinavir).

Effects on the activity of concomitant medications have been reported with the following medications:

- phenytoin.

During concomitant treatment with hydantoin derivatives, the serum hydantoin concentration may rise.

Sinthrome may potentiate the hypoglycaemic effect of sulphonylurea derivatives e.g.:

- glibenclamide, glimepiride.

Patients being treated with Sinthrome (especially those suffering from hepatic dysfunction) should limit their alcohol intake, since it is not possible to predict the severity of any drug interactions, nor identify any early signs of such interactions.

Cranberry juice should be avoided in patients receiving Sinthrome due to a theoretical risk of enhanced anti-coagulation. Increased medical supervision and INR monitoring should be considered for any patient receiving Sinthrome and regularly drinking cranberry juice. It is not known whether other cranberry products, such as capsules or concentrates, might also interact with Sinthrome. Therefore similar caution should be observed with these products.

4.6 Pregnancy and lactation

Sinthrome, like other coumarin derivatives, may be associated with congenital malformations of the embryo, therefore Sinthrome is contra-indicated for use in pregnancy. Women of child-bearing potential should take contraceptive measures during treatment with Sinthrome.

Acenocoumarol passes into the breast milk of lactating mothers, but in quantities so small that no undesirable effects on the infant are to be expected. However, as a precaution, the infant should be given 1mg vitamin K_1 per week as a prophylactic measure.

4.7 Effects on ability to drive and use machines

None known.

4.8 Undesirable effects

Haemorrhage, in various organs, is the most common side-effect associated with Sinthrome; its occurrence is related to the dosage of the drug, the patient's age and the nature of the underlying disease (but not the duration of treatment). Fatalities have been reported. Possible sites of haemorrhage include the gastro-intestinal tract, brain, urogenital tract, uterus, liver, gall bladder and the eye. If haemorrhage occurs in a patient with a thromboplastin time within the therapeutic range, diagnosis of their condition must be clarified.

Rare effects noted with acenocoumarol and similar coumarin derivatives include gastro-intestinal disorders (loss of appetite, nausea, vomiting), allergic reactions (urticaria and other rashes, dermatitis and fever) and reversible alopecia. Isolated cases of haemorrhagic skin necrosis (usually associated with congenital protein C deficiency or its cofactor protein S), vasculitis and liver damage have also been reported.

4.9 Overdose

Clinical manifestations of overdosage are unlikely with large single doses, but more likely following prolonged use of daily doses exceeding those required therapeutically.

Symptoms:

The onset and severity of the symptoms are dependent on the individual's sensitivity to oral anticoagulants, the size of the overdose and the duration of treatment.

Haemorrhage is the prominent feature of an overdose and may occur within 1 to 5 days after ingestion. Nose-bleeds, haematemesis, haemoptysis, gastro-intestinal haemorrhage, vaginal bleeding, haematuria (with renal colic), cutaneous haemorrhages, gingival bleeding, and bleeding into the joints or menorrhagia may be experienced.

Further symptoms include tachycardia, hypotension, peripheral circulatory disorders due to loss of blood, nausea, vomiting, diarrhoea and abdominal pains.

Laboratory tests will show an extremely low Quick value (or high INR value), pronounced prolongation of the recalcification time or thromboplastin time and disturbed γ-carboxylation of factors II, VII, IX and X.

Treatment:

For patients who have not previously received anticoagulants, arriving within 1 hour of ingestion, who are not comatose or convulsing, and show no signs of bleeding from any source, then drug absorption may be reduced by emesis with syrup of ipecac and gastric lavage. (However, note that gastric lavage may provoke bleeding). This may then be followed by the administration of activated charcoal. For patients who are already anticoagulated, emesis should not be induced. It should also be noted that vitamin-K mediated reversal of anticoagulation may be dangerous for patients who require constant anticoagulation such as those with prosthetic heart valves. Colestyramine may markedly enhance the drug's elimination by inhibiting the enterohepatic circulation.

A temporary reduction of the dose of Sinthrome is often sufficient to control slight bleeding.

Vitamin K_1 (phytomenadione) may antagonise the effect of Sinthrome within 3 to 5 hours. In cases of moderate haemorrhage, 2 to 5 mg Vitamin K_1 should be given orally; in severe haemorrhage, 5 to 10mg Vitamin K_1 should be injected very slowly (at a rate less than 1mg/min) intravenously. Additional doses (up to a maximum dose of 40mg daily) should be given at 4-hour intervals. Vitamin K_1 should not be given by intramuscular injection.

Doses of Vitamin K_1 in excess of 5mg can cause resistance to further anticoagulant therapy for several days. If an anticoagulant is required, heparin may be used temporarily, although oral anticoagulant therapy should be resumed at the same time and heparin withdrawn once the therapeutic range has been reached.

In the case of life-threatening haemorrhage, intravenous transfusions of fresh frozen plasma or whole blood can abolish the effects of Sinthrome.

5. PHARMACOLOGICAL PROPERTIES

5.1 Pharmacodynamic properties

To initiate blood clotting, Vitamin K causes γ-carboxylation of certain glutamic acid molecules on the coagulation factors II, VII, IX and X, and of protein C and its cofactor protein S. Coumarin derivatives, such as Sinthrome, prevent γ-carboxylation of these proteins by Vitamin K, although the precise nature of this antagonism has yet to be established.

Depending on the initial dosage, Sinthrome prolongs the thromboplastin time within approximately 36 to 72 hours. Following withdrawal of Sinthrome, the thromboplastin time usually reverts to normal after a few days.

5.2 Pharmacokinetic properties

Absorption

Following oral administration, Sinthrome is rapidly absorbed; at least 60% of the administered dose is systemically available. Peak plasma concentrations are achieved within 1 to 3 hours after a single dose of 10mg and AUC values are proportional to the size of the dose over a dosage range of 8 to 16mg.

No correlation between plasma concentrations of acenocoumarol and the apparent prothombin levels can be established, due to the variation of plasma drug concentrations between patients.

Plasma drug concentrations are generally higher in patients of 70 years or over when compared with younger patients, after the same dose.

Distribution

Over 98% of acenocoumarol is protein-bound, mainly to albumin. The calculated apparent volume of distribution is 0.16-0.18 L/kg for the R(+) enantiomer and 0.22-0.34 L/kg for the S(-) enantiomer.

Metabolism

Acenocoumarol is extensively metabolised, although the metabolites appear to be pharmacologically inactive in man.

Elimination

The elimination half-life of acenocoumarol from the plasma is 8 to 11 hours. 29% is excreted in the faeces and 60% in the urine, with less than 0.2% of the dose renally excreted being unchanged.

5.3 Preclinical safety data

There are no other clinically relevant pre-clinical safety data in addition to those mentioned in other sections of the Summary of Product Characteristics.

6. PHARMACEUTICAL PARTICULARS

6.1 List of excipients

Aerosil 200 (silica aerogel), hydroxypropylmethylcellulose, lactose, magnesium stearate, maize starch and talc.

6.2 Incompatibilities

None stated.

6.3 Shelf life

3 years.

6.4 Special precautions for storage

None stated.

6.5 Nature and contents of container

Blister packs of 100 tablets.

6.6 Instructions for use and handling

None stated

Administrative Data

7. MARKETING AUTHORISATION HOLDER

Alliance Pharmaceuticals Ltd.

Avonbridge House

2 Bath Road

Chippenham

Wiltshire

SN15 2BB

8. MARKETING AUTHORISATION NUMBER(S)

PL16853/0013

9. DATE OF FIRST AUTHORISATION/RENEWAL OF THE AUTHORISATION

25 June 1998

10. DATE OF REVISION OF THE TEXT

July 2005

11. Legal Status

POM

Alliance, Alliance Pharmaceuticals and associated devices are registered Trademarks of Alliance Pharmaceuticals Ltd.

Skelid 200mg Tablet

(sanofi-aventis)

1. NAME OF THE MEDICINAL PRODUCT

SKELID 200mg Tablet

2. QUALITATIVE AND QUANTITATIVE COMPOSITION

Disodium tiludronate	240.00 mg
Quantity corresponding to tiludronic acid	200.00 mg
Sodium laurilsulphate	4.50 mg
Hypromellose	5.25 mg
Crospovidone	15.00 mg
Magnesium stearate	0.60 mg
Lactose monohydrate	34.65 mg

for one tablet of 300.00 mg

3. PHARMACEUTICAL FORM

Round, biconvex, white tablets with "SW" engraved on one side and "200" on the other.

4. CLINICAL PARTICULARS

4.1 Therapeutic indications

Treatment of Paget's disease

4.2 Posology and method of administration
Oral route

For adults only

Daily dosage: 400 mg (*i.e.* 2 tablets) as a single dose for three months (*i.e.* 12 weeks).

Most patients respond to treatment during the first three months regardless of whether or not they were previously treated with another bisphosphonate.

Serum alkaline phosphatase levels can continue to improve 18 months after withdrawal of treatment.

Treatment can be repeated if the biochemical markers (increase in serum alkaline phosphatase levels with or without elevated hydroxyprolinuria) or pain indicate a recurrence of the condition.

Allow a period of at least 6 months to elapse before administering a second course of treatment.

The tablets should be taken with the help of a glass of water on an empty stomach (at least two hours) before / after meals.

Foodstuffs, particularly those with a high calcium potents (e.g.milk and dairy products) and antacids providing gastric protection should be avoided for two hours pre and post-dose (see interactions).

4.3 Contraindications
- History of allergy to bisphosphonates
- Severe kidney failure (creatinine clearance less than 30 ml/min)
- Juvenile Paget's disease
- Pregnancy and lactation (see 4.6 pregnancy and lactation)

4.4 Special warnings and special precautions for use
- Tiludronate is not metabolised and is excreted unchanged via the kidneys. Tiludronate must be administered with caution to patients suffering from mild (creatinine clearance ranging from 60 to 90 ml/min) and moderately severe kidney failure (creatinine clearance between 30 and 60 ml/min) (kidney function monitored on a regular basis).
- Patients must have an adequate calcium and vitamin D intake. calcium metabolism disorders (hypocalcaemia, vitamin D deficiency) must be controlled before instituting treatment.

4.5 Interaction with other medicinal products and other forms of Interaction
- Combination therapy warranting precautions in use:

Allow over two hours between administration of tiludronate and consumption of:

. calcium salts, topical gastro-intestinal agents, oral antacids (reduced gastro-intestinal absorption of bisphosphonates).

. indomethacin (increased bioavailability of tiludronic acid).

- The pharmacokinetic parameters of tiludronate are not significantly changed by concomitant administration of aspirin or diclofenac.

- The pharmacokinetic parameters of digoxin are not significantly changed by concurrent administration of tiludronate.

- Tiludronate should not be combined with products likely to induce mineralisation disorders.

4.6 Pregnancy and lactation
Pregnancy

Administration is contraindicated during pregnancy (lack of data).

Although there is no evidence of any deleterious effects with tiludronate in reproduction studies, delayed skeletal and bone development in the fetus has been reported in animals experiments conducted with other bisphosphonates. The passage of tiludronate through human placenta has not been documented.

Lactation

Administration is contraindicated during lactation (lack of data).

4.7 Effects on ability to drive and use machines
Drivers and machine operators are not required to take any specific precautions.

4.8 Undesirable effects
- Gastro-intestinal tract:

Common: abdominal pain, nausea and diarrhoea. These events are of slight to moderate severity and their incidence is dose-related.

- Skin:

Uncommon: rash

- Central nervous system:

Rare: asthenia, dizziness, headache.

4.9 Overdose
Some patients may present with hypocalcaemia and kidney failure following a massive overdose. Gastric lavage may prove useful in order to evacuate any as yet unabsorbed tiludronate.

Symptomatic treatment of hypocalcaemia (intravenous administration of calcium salts such as calcium gluconate) and/or kidney failure should be instituted.

5. PHARMACOLOGICAL PROPERTIES

5.1 Pharmacodynamic properties
Used in the treatment of bone diseases.

(M05 BA bisphosphonates).

Like other bisphosphonates, tiludronate inhibits the bone absorption of osteoclasts.

Tiludronate slows down the bone remodelling of lesions due to Paget's disease, as manifested by the fall in serum alkaline phosphatase levels. Preliminary studies of Paget's disease involving a small number of biopsies showed that tiludronate reduces excessive remodelling due to this disease.

No clinical data on potential long-term mineralisation disorders are available. However, long-term administration (6 months to 1 year) of high daily doses did not cause osteomalacia in rats or baboons.

5.2 Pharmacokinetic properties
The absolute bioavailability of tiludronate is low (averaging 6 %) and variable (2 to 11 %). Plasma concentration peaks following repeated dosing with 400 mg per day were extremely variable (generally between 1 and 5 mg/L occurring 1 to 2 hours post-dose). Bioavailability is decreased when the product is administered during or after a meal and falls considerably in the presence of calcium.

Plasma protein binding is of the order of 91 % and is constant within the therapeutic concentration range. Albumin is the protein responsible for this phenomenon. Less than 5 % binds to red blood cells. Approximately half of the dose absorbed is bound to bone.

Tiludronate is excreted unchanged via the kidneys. 3.5 ≠ 1.9 % of excreted unchanged tiludronate are detected 48 hours after single oral administration.

The decrease in tiludronate plasma levels following treatment withdrawal occurs in two stages, the second of which is much slower and difficult to assess accurately due to the very low plasma concentrations (half-life of over 100 hours). This last phase is due to bone remodelling and to the very slow absorption of tiludronate from the bones.

5.3 Preclinical safety data
- Single dose toxicity: Acute moderate toxicity (LD50 of about 550 mg/kg) and low toxicity (LD50 ⩾ 1000 mg/kg) were observed in the rat and mouse respectively following oral administration. The principal target organs are the kidney, stomach and lungs.

- Repeated dose toxicity: gastritis and proximal renal tubulopathies were observed mainly in the rat and baboon following repeated oral dosing with ⩾50mg/kg/day for up to a year. These doses are considerably higher than the pharmacologically active daily dose levels of 5 to 10 mg/kg which lead to inhibition of bone resorption and increase the bone density of trabecular bone.

- Genotoxicity and carcinogenicity: in-vitro and in-vivo studies of gene mutation, chromosomal aberration and DNA repair processes did not reveal any signs of toxicity.

No evidence of carcinogenicity was detected in mice given up to 50 mg/kg/day for 80 weeks or in rats receiving up to 25 mg/kg/day for 2 years.

- Reproduction toxicity: orally administered doses of up to 375 mg/kg/day did not induce any direct teratogenic or embryotoxic effect in rats, mice or rabbits.

Neither fertility nor peri- and post-natal development were affected in the rat following administration of up to 75 mg/kg/day.

However, given the retarded skeletal and bone maturation observed in animal foetuses during studies with other bisphosphonates, and since no data are available on the passage of tiludronate through human placenta, this product is contraindicated during pregnancy.

6. PHARMACEUTICAL PARTICULARS

6.1 List of excipients

Sodium laurilsulphate	4.50 mg
Hypromellose	5.25 mg
Crospovidone	15.00 mg
Magnesium stearate	0.60 mg
Lactose monohydrate	34.65 mg

for a finished tablet of 300.00 mg

6.2 Incompatibilities
None.

6.3 Shelf life
Three years.

6.4 Special precautions for storage
No special precautions for storage.

6.5 Nature and contents of container
28 tablets in heat-formed blister packs (polyamide - aluminium - PVC/aluminium)

6.6 Instructions for use and handling
No special requirements

7. MARKETING AUTHORISATION HOLDER
Sanofi- Synthelabo

PO Box 597

Guildford

Surrey

8. MARKETING AUTHORISATION NUMBER(S)
PL 11723/0207

9. DATE OF FIRST AUTHORISATION/RENEWAL OF THE AUTHORISATION
6th February 1996

10. DATE OF REVISION OF THE TEXT
December 2001

Legal Category: POM

Slo-Phyllin 60mg, 125mg, 250mg, Capsules

(Merck Pharmaceuticals)

1. NAME OF THE MEDICINAL PRODUCT
Slo-Phyllin 60mg Capsules

Slo-Phyllin 125mg Capsules

Slo-Phyllin 250mg Capsules

2. QUALITATIVE AND QUANTITATIVE COMPOSITION
Slo-Phyllin 60mg Capsules each contain theophylline (anhydrous) EP 60mg

Slo-Phyllin 125mg Capsules each contain theophylline (anhydrous) EP 125mg

Slo-Phyllin 250mg Capsules each contain theophylline (anhydrous) EP 250mg

3. PHARMACEUTICAL FORM
Prolonged release capsule

4. CLINICAL PARTICULARS

4.1 Therapeutic indications
As a bronchodilator in the symptomatic and prophylactic treatment of asthma and for reversible bronchoconstriction associated with chronic bronchitis and bronchial asthma.

4.2 Posology and method of administration
Method of administration: Oral

Dosage

Children:

2 - 6 years (10 - 20kg): 60 - 120mg twice daily

6 - 12 years (20 - 35kg): 125 - 250mg twice daily

over 12 years: 250-500 mg twice daily

Adults: 250-500 mg twice daily

Elderly: There is a tendency for theophylline clearance to decrease with age leading to higher serum levels. A reduction of the adult dosage may therefore be necessary and close monitoring is advised.

Each patient should be titrated to a suitable dosage regimen by clinical assessment. It may also be necessary to measure plasma theophylline levels.

Initially the lowest dosage for each group is recommended. This may be increased gradually if optimal bronchodilator effects are not achieved. The total dosage should not normally exceed 24 mg/kg body weight for children and 13 mg/kg for adults. However the plasma theophylline level measured 4-8 hours after dosing and at least three days after any dosage adjustment, provides a more accurate assessment of the patients' dosage need, especially as significant variations in the rate of drug elimination can occur between individuals. The following table provides a guide:

Plasma level (mcg/ml)	Result	Directions (if clinically indicated)
Below 10	Too low	Increase dose by 25%
10-20	Correct	Maintain dose
20-25	Too high	Decrease dose by 10%
25-30	Too high	Miss next dose and decrease subsequent doses by 25%
Over 30	Too high	Miss next two doses and decrease subsequent doses by 50%

It is advisable to recheck the plasma level after dose adjustment and every 6-12 months.

It is not possible to ensure bioequivalence between different sustained release theophylline products. Once titrated to an effective dose, patients should not be changed from Slo-Phyllin to another sustained release xanthine preparation without re-titration and clinical assessment.

4.3 Contraindications
Hypersensitivity to theophylline or other xanthines. Concomitant use of theophylline and ephedrine in children.

4.4 Special warnings and special precautions for use
Smoking and alcohol consumption can increase the clearance of theophylline and a higher dose may be necessary.

Careful monitoring is recommended for patients with congestive heart failure, chronic alcoholism, hepatic dysfunction, or viral infections, as they may have a lower clearance of theophylline, which could lead to higher than normal plasma levels.

Caution should be exercised in patients with peptic ulcers, cardiac arrhythmias, other cardiovascular diseases, hyperthyroidism or hypertension. Slo-Phyllin should not be used concurrently with other preparations containing xanthines derivatives. If it is necessary to administer aminophylline to a patient who is already receiving Slo-Phyllin, plasma theophylline concentration should be monitored.

The use of alternative treatments is advised in patients with a history of seizures, as these may be exacerbated by theophylline.

4.5 Interaction with other medicinal products and other forms of Interaction

Theophylline has been reported to interact with a number of drugs. The following increase clearance and it may therefore be necessary to increase dosage to ensure therapeutic effect: barbiturates, carbamazepine, lithium, phenytoin, rifampicin and sulphinpyrazone.

The following reduce clearance and a reduced dosage may therefore be necessary to avoid side-effects: allopurinol, cimetidine, ciprofloxacin, corticosteroids, diltiazem, erythromycin, frusemide, isoprenaline, oral contraceptives, thiabendazole and verapamil. There is some evidence of an interaction between theophylline and influenza vaccine.

Xanthines can potentiate hypokalaemia resulting from $beta_2$ agonist therapy, steroids, diuretics and hypoxia. Particular caution is advised in severe asthma. It is recommended that serum potassium levels are monitored in such situations.

The concomitant use of theophylline and fluvoxamine should usually be avoided. Where this is not possible, patients should have their theophylline dose halved and plasma theophylline should be monitored closely.

Plasma concentrations of theophylline can be reduced by concomitant use of the herbal remedy St John's wort (Hypericum perforatum).

4.6 Pregnancy and lactation

Slo-Phyllin is not recommended since theophylline is known to cross the placenta and its safety in pregnancy has not been established.

Theophylline is distributed in breast milk and therefore Slo-Phyllin should be used with caution in nursing mothers.

4.7 Effects on ability to drive and use machines

None known

4.8 Undesirable effects

Side effects usually occur when theophylline blood levels exceed 20 micrograms/ml and include gastric irritation, nausea, vomiting, abdominal discomfort, palpitations, a fall in blood pressure, headache, occasional diarrhoea and insomnia. CNS stimulation and diuresis may also occur, especially in children.

4.9 Overdose

Signs and symptoms: Headache, nausea, vomiting, restlessness, hypotension, tachycardia, arrhythmias (usually supraventricular tachyarrhythmias), hypokalaemia, CNS depression, convulsions, dehydration and coma may occur. Massive overdosage may result in cardiac inhibition, circulatory and respiratory failure.

Treatment: The stomach should be emptied by gastric lavage and emesis. Repeated doses of activated charcoal should be considered. Blood glucose, electrolytes, arterial gases and pH should be monitored. Serum theophylline should be measured 4 hours after ingestion and at 4 to 12 hourly intervals thereafter if symptoms are severe. Intensive supportive therapy may be required to maintain respiration and cardiovascular function. Convulsions may be controlled by diazepam. Haemoperfusion may be necessary. Slo-Phyllin is a timed-release capsule and effects may be slow in onset and prolonged.

5. PHARMACOLOGICAL PROPERTIES

5.1 Pharmacodynamic properties

The mechanism of action of theophylline is unclear although a number of pharmacological actions have been implicated. The principal of these are:-

1) Inhibition of the enzyme phosphodiesterase leading to raised cyclic AMP levels.

2) Antagonism of adenosine receptors.

3) Inhibition of the intracellular release of calcium.

4) Stimulation of catecholamine release

5) Anti-inflammatory action possible involving the inhibition of submucosal action.

5.2 Pharmacokinetic properties

Following administration of Slo-Phyllin capsules at an appropriate twice daily dosage, peak levels occur 4-8 hours after dosing, and steady state is achieved in three days.

5.3 Preclinical safety data

No adverse effects can be predicted from animal toxicology studies other than those documented from human use of theophylline.

6. PHARMACEUTICAL PARTICULARS

6.1 List of excipients

The inactive ingredients are sucrose, maize starch, refined bleached lac and talc. The gelatine capsules contain the following shell colours: Slo-Phyllin 60mg E171; Slo-Phyllin 125mg E171 and E172; Slo-Phyllin 250mg E171, E127 and E132.

6.2 Incompatibilities

None stated.

6.3 Shelf life

Three years.

6.4 Special precautions for storage

Do not store above 25 degree C. Store in the original package.

6.5 Nature and contents of container

PVC/Foil blister packs of 56 tablets

Sample PVC/Foil blister packs of 8 tablets

Plastic container of 100 tablets.

6.6 Instructions for use and handling

Patients should be instructed not to chew or suck the capsules or pellets as this destroys the time release properties. However, for those who experience difficulty in swallowing capsules, the contents of a capsule may be sprinkled on to a spoonful of soft food, e.g. yoghurt.

7. MARKETING AUTHORISATION HOLDER

Rona Laboratories Ltd., Harrier House, High Street, West Drayton, Middlesex, UB7 7QG, UK

8. MARKETING AUTHORISATION NUMBER(S)

Slo-Phyllin 60mg capsules PL 0161/0021

Slo-Phyllin 125mg capsules PL 0161/0019

Slo-Phyllin 250mg capsules PL 0161/0020

9. DATE OF FIRST AUTHORISATION/RENEWAL OF THE AUTHORISATION

Year granted - 1977

10. DATE OF REVISION OF THE TEXT

14 March 2003

Slow Sodium

(HK Pharma Limited)

1. NAME OF THE MEDICINAL PRODUCT

®Slow Sodium

2. QUALITATIVE AND QUANTITATIVE COMPOSITION

The active ingredient is Sodium Chloride Ph.Eur. Sodium Chloride contains not less than 99.0 per cent and not more than 100.5 per cent of NaCl. One coated tablet contains 600 mg sodium chloride.

3. PHARMACEUTICAL FORM

Coated tablets.

4. CLINICAL PARTICULARS

4.1 Therapeutic indications

For the treatment and prophylaxis of sodium chloride deficiency.

4.2 Posology and method of administration

It is important that the tablets should be swallowed whole with water (approx. 70ml per tablet where kidney function is normal to avoid hypernatraemia), and not chewed.

Adults: For prophylaxis 4-8 tablets per day. For treatment dosage to be adjusted to individual needs up to a maximum of 20 tablets per day in cases of severe salt depletion. For control of muscle cramps during routine maintenance haemodialysis usually 10-16 tablets per dialysis. In some cases of chronic renal salt-wasting up to 20 tablets per day may be required with appropriate fluid intake.

Children: Dosage should be adjusted to individual needs.

Elderly: No special dosage adjustment.

4.3 Contraindications

Slow Sodium is contra-indicated in any situation where salt retention is undesirable, such as oedema, heart disease, cardiac decompensation and primary or secondary aldosteronism; or where therapy is being given to produce salt and water loss.

4.4 Special warnings and special precautions for use

Warnings: None

Precautions Use of Slow Sodium without adequate water supplementation can produce hypernatraemia. The matrix (ghost) is often eliminated intact and owing to the risk of obstruction Slow Sodium should not be given to patients suffering from Crohn's disease or any other intestinal condition where strictures or diverticula may form.

4.5 Interaction with other medicinal products and other forms of Interaction

In hypertensive patients with chronic renal failure Slow Sodium may tend to impair the efficacy of antihypertensive drugs.

4.6 Pregnancy and lactation

As with most medicines, consult your doctor first if you are pregnant or breastfeeding.

4.7 Effects on ability to drive and use machines

Nil

4.8 Undesirable effects

No side effects have been reported with Slow Sodium at the recommended dosage.

4.9 Overdose

Signs and symptoms. Excessive intake of sodium chloride can result in hypernatraemia. Symptoms of hypernatraemia include restlessness, weakness, thirst, reduced salivation and lachrymation, swollen tongue, flushing of the skin, pyrexia, dizziness, headache, oliguria, hypertension, tachycardia, delirium, hyperpnoea and respiratory arrest.

Treatment. Treatment requires the use of sodium-free liquids and the cessation of excessive sodium intake. In the event of a significant overdose serum sodium levels should be evaluated as soon as possible and appropriate steps taken to correct any abnormalities. The use of a loop diuretic e.g. frusemide (with potassium supplementation as required) may be appropriate in severe cases of hypernatraemia. Levels should be monitored until they return to normal.

5. PHARMACOLOGICAL PROPERTIES

5.1 Pharmacodynamic properties

Mode of action: Sodium chloride is the principle salt involved in maintaining the osmotic tension of blood and tissues, changes in osmotic tension influence the movement of fluids and diffusion of salts in cellular tissue.

Slow Sodium provides a source of sodium (in the form of sodium chloride) where a deficiency exists.

5.2 Pharmacokinetic properties

Sodium chloride is readily absorbed from the gastro-intestinal tract. It is present in all body fluids but specially in the extracellular fluid. The amount of sodium lost (as sweat) is normally small. Osmotic balance is maintained by excretion of surplus amounts in the urine.

5.3 Preclinical safety data

No information available.

6. PHARMACEUTICAL PARTICULARS

6.1 List of excipients

The coated tablets contain cetostearyl alcohol, gelatin, magnesium stearate, acacia, talc, titanium dioxide and polyethylene glycol.

6.2 Incompatibilities

None known.

6.3 Shelf life

Five years.

6.4 Special precautions for storage

Protect from moisture and store below 30°C. The tablets should be dispensed in moisture proof containers.

Medicines should be kept out of reach of children.

6.5 Nature and contents of container

The tablets are available in containers of 100 tablets.

6.6 Instructions for use and handling

None

7. MARKETING AUTHORISATION HOLDER

HK Pharma Ltd

PO Box 105

Hitchin

SG5 2GG

8. MARKETING AUTHORISATION NUMBER(S)

16784/0003

9. DATE OF FIRST AUTHORISATION/RENEWAL OF THE AUTHORISATION

28 April 1998

10. DATE OF REVISION OF THE TEXT

February 2001

SLOW TRASICOR Tablets 160 mg

(Amdipharm)

1. NAME OF THE MEDICINAL PRODUCT

SLOW TRASICOR Tablets 160 mg.

2. QUALITATIVE AND QUANTITATIVE COMPOSITION

Oxprenolol hydrochloride EP 160 mg.

3. PHARMACEUTICAL FORM

Tablets.

4. CLINICAL PARTICULARS

4.1 Therapeutic indications

Hypertension: As monotherapy or for use in combination with other antihypertensives, e.g. with a diuretic, peripheral vasodilator, calcium channel blocker or ACE inhibitor.

Angina Pectoris: For long-term prophylactic use (if necessary nitrates should be employed for alleviating acute attacks).

4.2 Posology and method of administration

The dosage should be individualised. Before raising the dosage, the heart rate at rest should always be checked. If it is 50-55 beats/min, the dosage should not be increased, see contraindications. The tablets should be swallowed with liquid.

If the maximum recommended dose is insufficient to produce the desired response appropriate combined therapy should be considered.

When discontinuing prolonged treatment with a beta-blocker, the medication should not be interrupted abruptly, but withdrawn gradually.

The sustained-release formulation provides a longer pharmacological action from a given dose, thus allowing once daily administration. When the dose is raised to more than one TRASICOR sustained-release tablet, it is usual for this to continue to be given once daily.

The sustained-release tablets should be swallowed whole with liquid. Oxprenolol is only gradually released from the sustained-release tablet, extending the duration of effect. The occurrence of high peak concentrations in the plasma is thus avoided.

Elderly

No special dosage regime is necessary but concurrent hepatic insufficiency should be taken into account.

Children

No adequate experience has been acquired on the use of SLOW TRASICOR in children.

Adults

Hypertension: 160mg once daily. If necessary, the dosage can be raised to 320mg.

Angina pectoris: 160mg once daily. If necessary, the dosage can be raised to 320mg.

4.3 Contraindications

SLOW TRASICOR is contraindicated in patients with

- Hypersensitivity to oxprenolol and related derivatives, cross-sensitivity to other beta-blockers or to any of the excipients.
- Cardiogenic shock.
- Second or third degree atrioventricular block.
- Uncontrolled heart failure.
- Sick-sinus syndrome.
- Bradycardia (< 45–50bpm).
- Hypotension.
- Untreated phaeochromocytoma.
- Severe peripheral arterial circulatory disturbances.
- History of bronchospasm and bronchial asthma. (A warning stating "Do not take this medicine if you have a history of wheezing or asthma" will appear on the label)
- Prinzmetal's angina (variant angina pectoris).
- Use of anaesthetics which are known to have a negative inotropic effect.
- Metabolic acidosis.

4.4 Special warnings and special precautions for use

Owing to the risk of bronchoconstriction, non-selective beta-blockers such as SLOW TRASICOR should be used with particular caution in patients with chronic obstructive lung disease. (see "Contra-indications").

As beta-blockers increase the AV conduction time, beta-blockers should only be given with caution to patients with first degree AV block.

Beta-blockers should not be used in patients with untreated congestive heart failure. This condition should first be stabilised.

If the patient develops increasing bradycardia less than 50-55 beats per minute at rest and the patient experiences symptoms related to bradycardia, the dosage should be reduced or gradually withdrawn (see "Contra-indications").

Beta-blockers are liable to affect carbohydrate metabolism. Diabetic patients, especially those dependent on insulin, should be warned that beta-blockers can mask symptoms of hypoglycaemia (e.g. tachycardia) (see "Interactions with other medicaments and other forms of interaction"). Hypoglycaemia, producing loss of consciousness in some cases, may occur in non-diabetic individuals who are taking beta-blockers, particularly those who undergo prolonged fasting or severe exercise. The concurrent use of beta-blockers and anti-diabetic medication should always be monitored to confirm that diabetic control is well maintained.

Beta-blockers may mask certain clinical signs (e.g. tachycardia) of hyperthyroidism and the patient should be carefully monitored.

Beta-blockers may reduce liver function and thus affect the metabolism of other drugs. Like many beta-blockers oxprenolol undergoes substantial first-pass hepatic metabolism. In the presence of liver cirrhosis the bioavailability of oxprenolol may be increased leading to higher plasma concentrations (see "Pharmacokinetic properties"). Patients with severe renal failure might be more susceptible to the effects of antihypertensive drugs due to haemodynamic effects. Careful monitoring is advisable (see "Pharmacokinetic properties").

In patients with peripheral circulatory disorders (e.g. Raynaud's disease or syndrome, intermittent claudication), beta-blockers should be used with great caution as aggravation of these disorders may occur (see "Contra-indications").

In patients with phaeochromocytoma a beta-blocker should only be given together with an alpha-blocker, (see "Contra-indications").

Owing to the danger of cardiac arrest, a calcium antagonist of the verapamil type must not be administered intravenously to the patient already receiving treatment with a beta-blocker. Furthermore, since beta-blockers may potentiate the negative-inotropic and dromotropic effects of calcium antagonists, like verapamil or diltiazem, any oral co-medication (e.g. in angina pectoris) requires close clinical control (see also "Interactions with other medicaments and other forms of interaction").

Anaphylactic reactions precipitated by other agents may be particularly severe in patients taking beta-blockers, especially non-selective drugs, and may require higher than normal doses of adrenaline for treatment. Whenever possible, beta-blockers should be discontinued in patients who are at increased risk for anaphylaxis.

Especially in patients with ischaemic heart disease, treatment should not be discontinued suddenly. The dosage should gradually be reduced, i.e. over 1-3 weeks, if necessary, at the same time initiating alternative therapy, to prevent exacerbation of angina pectoris.

If a patient receiving oxprenolol requires anaesthesia, the anaesthetist should be informed of the use of the medication prior to the use of general anaesthetic to permit him to take the necessary precautions. The anaesthetic selected should be one exhibiting as little inotropic activity as possible, e.g. halothane/nitrous oxide. If on the other hand, inhibition of sympathetic tone during the operation is regarded as undesirable, the beta-blocker should be withdrawn gradually at least 48 hours prior to surgery.

The full development of the "oculomucocutaneous syndrome", as previously described with practolol has not been reported with oxprenolol. However some features of this syndrome have been noted such as dry eyes alone or occasionally associated with skin rash. In most cases the symptoms cleared after withdrawal of the treatment. Discontinuation of oxprenolol should be considered, and a switch to another antihypertensive drug might be advisable, see advice on discontinuation above.

4.5 Interaction with other medicinal products and other forms of Interaction

Calcium channel blockers: e.g. verapamil, diltiazem: Potentiation of bradycardia, myocardial depression and hypotension; particularly after intravenous administration of verapamil in patients taking oral beta-blockers, the possibility of hypotension and cardiac arrhythmias cannot be excluded (see "Special Warnings and Precautions").

Class I anti-arrhythmic drugs and amiodarone: Drugs like disopyramide, quinidine and amiodarone may increase atrial-conduction time and induce negative inotropic effect when administered concomitantly with beta-blockers.

Sympathomimetic drugs: Non-cardioselective beta-blockers such as oxprenolol enhance the pressor response to sympathomimetic drugs such as adrenaline, noradrenaline, isoprenaline, ephedrine and phenylephrine (e.g. local anaesthetics in dentistry, nasal and ocular drops), resulting in hypertension and bradycardia.

Clonidine: When clonidine is used in conjunction with non-selective beta-blockers, such as oxprenolol, treatment with clonidine should be continued for some time after beta-blocker has been discontinued to reduce the danger of rebound hypertension.

Catecholamine-depleting drugs: e.g. guanethidine, reserpine, may have an additive effect when administered concomitantly with beta-blockers. Patients should be closely observed for hypotension.

Beta-blockers may modify blood glucose concentrations in patients being treated with insulin and oral antidiabetic drugs and may alter the response to hypoglycaemia by prolonging the recovery (blood glucose rise) from hypoglycaemia, causing hypotension and blocking tachycardia. In diabetic patients receiving beta-blockers hypoglycaemic episodes may not result in the expected tachycardia but hypoglycaemia-induced sweating will occur and may even be intensified and prolonged. (see "Special Warnings and Precautions).

Non-steroidal anti-inflammatory drugs (NSAIDs): Non-steroidal anti-inflammatory drugs (NSAIDs) can reduce the hypotensive effect of beta-blockade.

Cimetidine: Hepatic metabolism of beta-blockers may be reduced resulting in increased plasma levels of beta-blocker and prolonged serum half-life. Marked bradycardia may occur.

Ergot alkaloids: Concomitant administration with beta-blockers may enhance the vasoconstrictive action of ergot alkaloids.

Anaesthetic drugs: Beta-blockers and certain anaesthetics (e.g. halothane) are additive in their cardiodepressant effect. However, continuation of beta-blockers reduces the risk of arrhythmia during anaesthesia (see "Special Warnings and Precautions").

Digitalis glycosides: Beta-blockers and digitalis glycosides may be additive in their depressant effect on myocardial conduction, particularly through the atrioventricular node, resulting in bradycardia or heart block.

Lidocaine: Concomitant administration with beta-blockers may increase lidocaine blood concentrations and potential toxicity; patients should be closely monitored for increased lidocaine effects.

Alcohol and beta-blocker effects on the central nervous system have been observed to be additive and it is possible that symptoms such as dizziness may be exaggerated if alcohol and SLOW TRASICOR are taken together (see also "Special Warnings and Precautions").

4.6 Pregnancy and lactation

As in the case of any form of drug therapy, oxprenolol should be employed with caution during pregnancy, especially in the first 3 months.

Beta-blockers may reduce placental perfusion, which may result in intrauterine foetal death, immature and premature deliveries. Use the lowest possible dose. If possible, discontinue beta-blocker therapy at least 2 to 3 days prior to delivery to avoid the effects on uterine contractility and possible adverse effects, especially bradycardia and hypoglycaemia, in the foetus and neonate.

Oxprenolol is excreted into breast milk (see "Pharmacokinetic properties"). However, although the estimated daily infant dose derived from breast-feeding is likely to be very low, breast feeding is not recommended.

4.7 Effects on ability to drive and use machines

Patients receiving oxprenolol should be warned that dizziness, fatigue or visual disturbances (see "Undesirable Effects") may occur, in which case they should not drive, operate machinery or do anything else requiring alertness, particularly if they also consume alcohol.

4.8 Undesirable effects

Side-Effects: Frequency estimate: very common > 10%, common > 1% - < 10%, uncommon > 0.1% - < 1%, rare > 0.01% - < 0.1%, very rare < 0.01%.

Central nervous system:

Common: Fatigue, dizziness, headache, mental depression.

Uncommon: Sleep disturbances, nightmares.

Rare: Hallucinations, exertional tiredness.

Cardiovascular system:

Common: Hypotension, heart failure, peripheral vascular disorders (e.g. cold extremities, paraesthesia).

Uncommon: Bradycardia, disturbance of cardiac conduction.

Rare: Raynaud-like symptoms.

Gastro-intestinal tract:

Very common: Dry mouth, constipation.

Common: Nausea.

Uncommon: Diarrhoea, vomiting, flatulence.

Skin and appendages:

Uncommon: Allergic skin rash (e.g. urticarial, psoriasiform, eczematous, lichenoid).

Rare: Worsening of psoriasis.

Respiratory system:

Common: Dyspnoea, bronchoconstriction (see "Special Warnings and Precautions" and "Contra-indications").

Sense organs:

Uncommon: Visual disturbances ("blurred vision", "vision abnormal").

Rare: Dry eyes, keratoconjuctivitis.

Others:

Common: Disturbances of libido and potency.

Very rare: Thrombocytopenia.

4.9 Overdose

Signs and symptoms:

Poisoning due to an overdosage of beta-blocker may lead to pronounced hypotension, bradycardia, hypoglycaemia, heart failure, cardiogenic shock, conduction abnormalities (first or second degree block, complete heart block, asystole), or even cardiac arrest. In addition, dyspnoea, bronchospasm, vomiting, impairment of consciousness, and also generalised convulsions may occur.

The manifestations of poisoning with beta-blocker are dependent on the pharmacological properties of the ingested drug. Although the onset of action is rapid, effects of massive overdose may persist for several days despite declining plasma levels. Watch carefully for cardiovascular or respiratory deterioration in an intensive care setting, particularly in the early hours. Observe mild overdose cases for at least 4 hours for the development of signs of poisoning.

Treatment:

Patients who are seen soon after potentially life-threatening overdosage (within 4 hours) should be treated by gastric lavage and activated charcoal.

Treatment of symptoms is based on modern methods of intensive care, with continuous monitoring of cardiac function, blood gases, and electrolytes, and if necessary, emergency measures such as artificial respiration, resuscitation or cardiac pacemaker.

Significant bradycardia should be treated initially with atropine. Large doses of isoprenaline may be necessary for control of heart rate and hypotension. Glucagon has positive chronotropic and inotropic effects on the heart that are independent of interactions with beta-adrenergic receptors and it represents a useful alternative treatment for hypotension and heart failure.

For seizures, diazepam has been effective and is the drug of choice.

For bronchospasm, aminophylline, salbutamol or terbutaline ($beta_2$-agonist) are effective bronchodilator drugs. Monitor the patient for dysrhythmias during and after administration.

Patients who recover should be observed for signs of beta-blocker withdrawal phenomenon (see "Special Warnings and Precautions").

5. PHARMACOLOGICAL PROPERTIES

5.1 Pharmacodynamic properties

Oxprenolol, the active substance of TRASICOR, is a non-selective, lipophilic beta-blocker exerting a sympatholytic effect and displaying mild to modest partial agonistic activity (PAA), also known as intrinsic sympathomimetic activity (ISA).

Drugs like oxprenolol with PAA cause comparatively less slowing of the resting heart rate and a less marked negative-inotropic effect than those without PAA. The risk of substantial bradycardia at rest and heart failure is lessened.

The antiarrhythmic effect of oxprenolol is primarily due to suppression of the arrhythmogenic sympathetic influence of catecholamines. Evidence that increased sympathetic stimulation predisposes to many arrhythmias is strong. This is supported by the increased incidence of arrhythmias in man in situations associated with high sympathetic drive or myocardial sensitisation to catecholamines e.g. exercise, emotional stress, phaeochromocytoma, trauma, myocardial ischaemia, anaesthesia, hyperthyroidism.

Oxprenolol decreases cardiac impulse formation in the sinus node with resultant slowing of the sinus rate; it slightly prolongs the sino-atrial conduction time; both the atrioventricular (AV) conduction time and the AV node refractory periods are lengthened.

Some beta-blockers such as oxprenolol possess a membrane stabilising activity (MSA) on the cardiac action potential, also known as "quinidine-like" or "local anaesthetic" action, a property that tends to result in greater cardiac depression than is seen with beta-blockers which do not have this pharmacological characteristic. However, at normal therapeutic doses, this property is probably clinically irrelevant and it only becomes manifest after overdose.

In coronary artery disease, oxprenolol is beneficial in increasing exercise tolerance and decreasing the frequency and severity of anginal attacks.

Emotional stress and anxiety states, the symptoms of which are largely caused by increased sympathetic drive, are alleviated by the sympatholytic effect of oxprenolol.

The exact way in which beta-blockers exert their antihypertensive action is still not fully understood. Various modes of action have been postulated. During chronic therapy the antihypertensive effect of beta-blockers is associated with a decline in peripheral resistance.

Oxprenolol is effective in lowering elevated supine, standing and exercise blood pressure; postural hypotension is unlikely to occur.

5.2 Pharmacokinetic properties

Absorption:

Oxprenolol is rapidly and completely absorbed from the sustained release tablets, regardless of whether or not they are taken together with food. Peak plasma concentrations are attained after an average of approximately 3 hours.

During treatment with the sustained release forms, prolongation of the absorption phase enables therapeutically active plasma concentrations to be maintained over a longer period than when the same doses are given in conventional dosage forms and avoids high peak drug concentrations in the plasma.

Biotransformation:

Oxprenolol is subject to first-pass metabolism. Its systemic bioavailability is 20 – 70%.

Distribution:

Oxprenolol has a plasma-protein binding rate of approx. 80% and a calculated distribution volume of 1.2 l/kg.

Oxprenolol crosses the placental barrier. The concentration in the breast milk is equivalent to approx. 30% of that in the plasma.

Elimination:

Oxprenolol has an elimination half-life of 1 – 2 hours. Oxprenolol is extensively metabolised, direct O-glucuronidation being the major metabolic pathway and oxidative reactions minor ones. Oxprenolol is excreted chiefly in the urine (almost exclusively in the form of inactive metabolites). The drug is not likely to accumulate.

Characteristics in patients:

Age has no effect on the pharmacokinetics of oxprenolol.

In patients with acute or chronic inflammatory diseases an increase in the plasma levels of oxprenolol has been observed. The plasma levels may also increase in the presence of severe hepatic insufficiency associated with a reduced metabolism.

Impaired renal function generally leads to an increase in the blood levels of oxprenolol, but the concentrations measured remain within – although at the upper limit of – the concentration range recorded in subjects with healthy kidneys. In addition, in patients with renal failure the apparent elimination half-life for unchanged, i.e. active, oxprenolol is comparable with the corresponding half-life values determined in subjects with no renal disease. Hence, there is no need to readjust the dosage in the presence of impaired renal function.

5.3 Preclinical safety data

None stated.

6. PHARMACEUTICAL PARTICULARS

6.1 List of excipients

Lactose, silicon dioxide, calcium stearate, methacrylic acid copolymer, glyceryl palmitostearate, hydroxypropyl methylcellulose, magnesium stearate, polysorbate, talc and titanium dioxide.

6.2 Incompatibilities

None known.

6.3 Shelf life

60 months.

6.4 Special precautions for storage

None.

6.5 Nature and contents of container

PVC* Blister packs of 28 tablets *PVC 250micron, aluminium foil 20 micron.

6.6 Instructions for use and handling

None.

7. MARKETING AUTHORISATION HOLDER

Amdipharm plc

Regency House

Miles Gray Road

Basildon

Essex

SS14 3AF

UK

8. MARKETING AUTHORISATION NUMBER(S)

PL 20072/0017

9. DATE OF FIRST AUTHORISATION/RENEWAL OF THE AUTHORISATION

1st January 2005

10. DATE OF REVISION OF THE TEXT

Slow-K Tablets 600 mg

(Alliance Pharmaceuticals)

1. NAME OF THE MEDICINAL PRODUCT

Slow-K® Tablets 600mg

2. QUALITATIVE AND QUANTITATIVE COMPOSITION

Potassium chloride 600mg PhEur

3. PHARMACEUTICAL FORM

Pale orange, round, biconvex, polished, sugar-coated modified release tablets. Printed Slow-K in black on one side.

4. CLINICAL PARTICULARS

4.1 Therapeutic indications

The correction and/or prevention of hypokalaemia in those patients who cannot tolerate and/or refuse to take liquid or effervescent potassium chloride, or when there is a problem of compliance with these preparations.

4.2 Posology and method of administration

Slow-K is taken orally. It is important that the tablets should be swallowed whole, with fluid, during meals, whilst the patient is sitting upright.

Adults:

The dosage of Slow-K should be adapted to the cause, degree and duration of potassium depletion. 2 to 3 tablets daily are usually an adequate supplement. In states of severe potassium deficiency, a higher dose of 9 to 12 tablets daily may be needed.

If the dosage exceeds 16mmol K^+ (2 tablets) it should be taken in divided doses. Where intermittent diuretic therapy is being used, it is advisable to give Slow-K on intervening days between administration of the diuretic. The response to treatment should preferably be monitored by repeat determination of plasma potassium and Slow-K continued until the hypokalaemia has been corrected.

Children:

Not recommended.

Elderly:

No special dosage regime is usually necessary, but concurrent renal insufficiency should be taken into account (See Section 4.4 "Special warnings and precautions").

4.3 Contraindications

Hypersensitivity to potassium administration, eg hyperkalaemic periodic paralysis, congenital paramyotonia. Marked renal failure (even when not yet associated with manifest hyperkalaemia), untreated Addison's Disease, hyporeninaemic hypoaldosteronism, acute dehydration, hyperkalaemia and conditions involving extensive cell destruction (eg severe burns).

All solid forms of potassium medication are contra-indicated in the presence of obstructions in the digestive tract (eg resulting from compression of the oesophagus due to dilation of the left atrium or from stenosis of the gut).

In cases of metabolic acidosis, the hypokalaemia should be treated not with potassium chloride but with an alkaline potassium salt (eg potassium bicarbonate).

Concomitant treatment with potassium sparing diuretics (eg spironolactone, triamterene, amiloride).

4.4 Special warnings and special precautions for use

If a patient under treatment with Slow-K develops severe vomiting, severe abdominal pains or flatulence, or gastro-intestinal haemorrhage, the preparation should be withdrawn at once, because in the presence of an obstruction it could conceivably give rise to ulceration or perforation.

Oral potassium preparations should be prescribed with particular caution in patients with a history of peptic ulcer.

Caution should be exercised when prescribing solid oral potassium preparations, particularly in high dosage, in patients concurrently receiving anticholinergics, because of their potential to slow gastrointestinal motility.

Patients with ostomies may have altered intestinal transit times and are better treated with other forms of potassium salts.

In patients suffering from impaired renal function, special care should be exercised when prescribing potassium salts owing to the risk of their producing hyperkalaemia. Monitoring of the serum electrolytes is particularly necessary in patients with diseases of the heart or kidneys.

In some patients, diuretic-induced magnesium deficiency will prevent restoration of intracellular deficits of potassium, so that hypomagnesaemia should be corrected at the same time as hypokalaemia.

4.5 Interaction with other medicinal products and other forms of Interaction

Combined treatment with the following increase the risk of hyperkalaemia: ACE inhibitors, cyclosporin, NSAIDs, β-blockers, heparin, digoxin, potassium sparing diuretics (see Section 4.3 "Contra-indications").

4.6 Pregnancy and lactation

Because of gastrointestinal hypomotility associated with pregnancy, solid forms of oral potassium preparations should be given to pregnant women only if clearly needed.

The normal K^+ content of human milk is about 13mmol/litre. Since oral potassium becomes part of the body's potassium pool, provided this is not excessive, Slow-K can be expected to have little or no effect on the potassium level in human milk.

4.7 Effects on ability to drive and use machines

None known.

4.8 Undesirable effects

Side effects are rare with Slow-K, as any excess potassium is rapidly excreted in the urine.

Gastrointestinal tract:

Rare: oral potassium preparations may provoke gastrointestinal disturbances (nausea, vomiting, abdominal pains, diarrhoea) necessitating either a reduction in dosage or withdrawal of medication (see Section 4.4 "Special warnings and precautions for use"). Isolated cases: obstruction, bleeding and ulceration, with or without perforation of the upper or lower GIT, have been reported, usually associated with other factors known to predispose a patient to these effects (eg delayed GIT transit time, obstruction of GIT).

Skin:

Rare: Pruritus and/or skin rash, urticaria.

Electrolytes:

Hyperkalaemia may develop in patients having difficulty with either renal potassium excretion or potassium metabolism.

4.9 Overdose

Signs and symptoms:

Mainly cardiovascular (hypotension, shock, ventricular arrhythmias, bundle-branch block, ventricular fibrillation leading possibly to cardiac arrest) and neuromuscular (paraesthesiae, convulsions, areflexia, flaccid paralysis of striated muscle leading possibly to respiratory paralysis). Beside elevation of serum potassium concentration, typical ECG changes are also encountered (increasing amplitude and peaking of T waves, disappearance of P wave, widening of QRS complex and S-T segment depression).

Treatment:

Gastric lavage, administration of cation exchange agents, infusion of glucose and insulin, forced diuresis and possibly peritoneal dialysis or haemodialysis.

5. PHARMACOLOGICAL PROPERTIES

5.1 Pharmacodynamic properties

The potassium chloride in Slow-K is finely distributed in a neutral wax base, from which it is gradually released over a period of 3 to 6 hours during its passage through the digestive tract. This special form of potassium substitution therapy is designed to avoid high localised concentrations of potassium chloride which might irritate or damage the mucosa. The potassium chloride in Slow-K is completely absorbed in the intestinal tract.

5.2 Pharmacokinetic properties

The potassium chloride in Slow-K has been shown to be completely absorbed; occasionally patients may notice "ghost" tablet cores in the faeces, these do not contain any potassium.

Following a single dose of Slow-K, potassium chloride is released over a period of approximately 4 hours. Renal excretion of potassium chloride following ingestion of Slow-K occurs 30 to 60 minutes later than when the same dose is given in the form of a solution. In the presence of a normal potassium balance, 90% of the potassium supplied by Slow-K is excreted renally within 8 hours, and more than 98% by 24 hours.

5.3 Preclinical safety data

There are no pre-clinical data of relevance to the prescriber which are additional to those already included in other sections of the Summary of Product Characteristics.

6. PHARMACEUTICAL PARTICULARS

6.1 List of excipients

Cetostearyl alcohol, gelatin, magnesium stearate, acacia, titanium dioxide (E171), talc, sucrose, polyethylene glycol 6000, red iron oxide (E172), yellow iron oxide (E172) and printing ink (Opacode black S-1-27708 or Opacode black S-1-8015 consisting of methylated spirit, shellac, propylene glycol, vegetable carbon E153, water and dimethylpolysiloxane).

6.2 Incompatibilities

None known.

6.3 Shelf life

5 years.

6.4 Special precautions for storage

Do not store above 30°C. Keep the container tightly closed.

6.5 Nature and contents of container

Polypropylene Securitainer with polyethylene cap containing 100 tablets.

6.6 Instructions for use and handling

None.

7. MARKETING AUTHORISATION HOLDER

Alliance Pharmaceuticals Ltd

Avonbridge House

Bath Road

Chippenham

Wiltshire

SN15 2BB

8. MARKETING AUTHORISATION NUMBER(S)

PL16853/0014

9. DATE OF FIRST AUTHORISATION/RENEWAL OF THE AUTHORISATION

25 June 1998

10. DATE OF REVISION OF THE TEXT

November 1998

11. Legal Status

P

Alliance, Alliance Pharmaceuticals and associated devices are registered Trademarks of Alliance Pharmaceuticals Ltd.

Slozem 120mg, 180mg, 240mg, 300mg Capsules

(Merck Pharmaceuticals)

1. NAME OF THE MEDICINAL PRODUCT

Slozem 120mg Capsules

Slozem 180mg Capsules

Slozem 240mg Capsules

Slozem 300mg Capsules

2. QUALITATIVE AND QUANTITATIVE COMPOSITION

Slozem 120mg Capsules each contain 120mg diltiazem hydrochloride

Slozem 180mg Capsules each contain 180mg diltiazem hydrochloride

Slozem 240mg Capsules each contain 240mg diltiazem hydrochloride

Slozem 300mg Capsules each contain 300mg diltiazem hydrochloride

For excipients, see 6.1.

3. PHARMACEUTICAL FORM

Prolonged release capsule, hard.

Slozem 120mg Capsules have a natural transparent cap with a pink transparent body and contain white-grey to light yellow approximately spherical pellets.

Slozem 180mg Capsules have a natural transparent cap with a pink opaque body and contain white-grey to light yellow approximately spherical pellets.

Slozem 240mg Capsules have a natural transparent cap with a scarlet opaque body and contain white-grey to light yellow approximately spherical pellets.

Slozem 300mg Capsules have an opaque white cap with an opaque scarlet body and contain white-grey to light yellow approximately spherical pellets.

4. CLINICAL PARTICULARS

4.1 Therapeutic indications

Mild to moderate hypertension. Angina pectoris.

4.2 Posology and method of administration

Adults

Starting dose: 240mg once daily

Dosage titration in 60mg to 120mg steps at 2-weekly intervals may be required to obtain satisfactory clinical response (usually 240mg to 360mg daily will suffice). Dosage should be reduced in the presence of adverse reactions or if the pulse rate falls below 50 per minute.

Elderly and patients with impaired hepatic or renal function

Starting dose 120mg once daily.

Children

Not recommended

4.3 Contraindications

In pregnancy and in women of childbearing potential. Slozem depresses atrioventricular node conduction and is therefore contraindicated in patients with marked bradycardia, sick sinus syndrome, uncontrolled heart failure or second or third degree AV block. Hypersensitivity to diltiazem or any of the inactive ingredients.

4.4 Special warnings and special precautions for use

Slozem should be used with caution in patients with reduced left ventricular function. Patients with mild bradycardia, and/or having a prolonged PR interval, should be observed closely.

4.5 Interaction with other medicinal products and other forms of Interaction

In common with other calcium antagonists, when Slozem is used with drugs which may induce bradycardia (eg amiodarone and beta-blockers) or with other antihypertensive drugs the possibility of an additive effect should be borne in mind.

Diltiazem has been used safely in combination with beta-blockers, diuretics, ACE inhibitors and other antihypertensive agents. It is recommended that patients receiving these combinations should be regularly monitored. Concomitant use with alpha blockers such as prazosin should be strictly monitored because of the possible marked synergistic hypotensive effect of this combination. Case reports have suggested that blood levels of carbamazepine, cyclosporin and theophylline may be increased when given concurrently with diltiazem hydrochloride. Care should be exercised in patients taking these drugs. In common with other calcium antagonists diltiazem may cause small increases in plasma levels of digoxin.

In patients taking H_2 receptor antagonists concurrently with diltiazem increased levels of diltiazem may be produced.

Diltiazem hydrochloride treatment has been continued without problem during anaesthesia, but the anaesthetist should be informed that the patient is receiving a calcium antagonist.

4.6 Pregnancy and lactation

Diltiazem hydrochloride is teratogenic in some animal species. In the absence of adequate evidence of safety in human pregnancy Slozem should not be used in pregnancy or in women of child-bearing potential.

Nursing mothers:

Diltiazem hydrochloride is excreted in breast milk. One report suggests that concentrations in breast milk reach similar levels to those in serum. If use of Slozem is considered essential, an alternative method of infant feeding should be instituted.

4.7 Effects on ability to drive and use machines

None known

4.8 Undesirable effects

The following have been reported: ankle oedema, malaise, headache, hot flushes, gastro-intestinal disturbances and very rarely symptomatic bradycardia, sino-atrial block and atrio-ventricular block. Rashes and other cutaneous reactions have been reported in association with diltiazem. These reactions are generally mild and resolve on cessation of therapy, however there have been occasional reports of severe vascular skin reactions, and of erythema multiforme. Isolated cases of moderate and transient elevation of liver transaminases have been observed at the start of treatment. Isolated cases of clinical hepatitis have been reported which resolved on cessation of therapy.

The current literature suggests that the effects of vasodilation, particularly ankle oedema, are dose dependent and are more frequent in the elderly.

4.9 Overdose

Signs and symptoms:

Acute intoxication can lead to severe hypotension, bradycardia, first to third degree atrioventricular block and, on occasions, to cardiac arrest. Hyperglycaemia may require treatment. Onset of symptoms may be delayed for several hours after ingestion and have been described after as little as 900mg diltiazem.

Treatment:

Observation in a coronary or intensive care unit is advisable if a substantial overdose has been ingested. Soon after ingestion, gastric lavage followed by activated charcoal may reduce absorption. Profound hypotension requires plasma expanders, I V calcium gluconate and inotropic agents (e.g. dopamine, dobutamine or isoprenaline). Symptomatic bradycardia and heart block may respond to atropine, isoprenaline or, if necessary, cardiac pacing. Slozem capsules are extended release capsules and effects may be slow in onset and prolonged.

5. PHARMACOLOGICAL PROPERTIES

5.1 Pharmacodynamic properties

Diltiazem hydrochloride is a calcium antagonist. It selectively reduces calcium entry through voltage-dependent calcium channels into vascular smooth muscle cells and myocardial cells. This lowers the concentration of intracellular calcium which is available to active contractile proteins. In vascular tissue, diltiazem relaxes arterial smooth muscle, reducing systemic peripheral resistance and dilating the coronary arteries. In cardiac muscle diltiazem reduces contractility and slows the heart rate through its negative chronotropic and inotropic actions. Cardiac work and oxygen demand can therefore be reduced and high blood pressure lowered without reflex tachycardia.

5.2 Pharmacokinetic properties

Diltiazem is well absorbed from the gastrointestinal tract and is subject to an extensive first-pass effect, giving an absolute bioavailability (compared to intravenous administration) of about 40%.

Diltiazem in plasma is 80-85% protein bound. Plasma levels above 40-50ng/ml are associated with pharmacological activity.

Diltiazem is extensively metabolised by the liver, the plasma elimination half-life being on average 3-4.5 hours.

The two major active circulating metabolites, desacetyldiltiazem and N-monodesmethyl diltiazem possess coronary artery vasodilatory activity equivalent to about 50% of that of diltiazem. Only 0.2 to 4% diltiazem is found unchanged in the urine.

The prolonged release pellets in this presentation usually achieve maximum plasma diltiazem levels six to eight hours after dosing and have an apparent plasma half-life of approximately 7 hours, allowing once daily dosing

The bioavailability of diltiazem from the Slozem formulation given once a day is equivalent to that obtained from a conventional release tablet given three times a day, when the same total daily dose is administered.

Data from studies in patients and healthy volunteers have also demonstrated that trough plasma levels (i.e. 24 hours post dosing) can be maintained within the minimum therapeutic range by appropriate dose titration.

Plasma concentrations in elderly patients and in hepatic failure are in general higher than in young subjects, due to an increase in apparent bioavailability. In renal failure, a reduction in dosage is only necessary as a function of the clinical response

5.3 Preclinical safety data

There are no preclinical data of relevance to the prescriber which are additional to that already included in other sections of the SPC.

6. PHARMACEUTICAL PARTICULARS

6.1 List of excipients

Maize starch, sucrose, povidone, shellac, ethylcellulose, talc, gelatin, erythrosine (E127), indigo carmine (E132), black iron oxide (E172) and (180mg, 240mg and 300mg only) titanium dioxide (E171).

6.2 Incompatibilities

Not applicable

6.3 Shelf life

3 years.

6.4 Special precautions for storage

Slozem 120mg, 180mg and 240mg Capsules:

Store below 30 degree C in a dry place.

Slozem 300mg Capsules:

Do not store above 25 degree C.

6.5 Nature and contents of container

28 capsules in PVC/PVDC/Aluminium blisters enclosed in a cardboard carton.

6.6 Instructions for use and handling

None

7. MARKETING AUTHORISATION HOLDER

Merck Ltd. (t/a Merck Pharmaceuticals (A division of Merck Ltd.))

Harrier House

High Street

West Drayton

Middlesex UB7 7QG

8. MARKETING AUTHORISATION NUMBER(S)

Slozem 120mg Capsules PL 11648/0045

Slozem 180mg Capsules PL 11648/0046

Slozem 240mg Capsules PL 11648/0047

Slozem 300mg Capsules PL 11648/0042

9. DATE OF FIRST AUTHORISATION/RENEWAL OF THE AUTHORISATION
Slozem 120mg, 180mg and 240mg Capsules:

1 February 2001

Slozem 300mg Capsules:

15 January 2001

10. DATE OF REVISION OF THE TEXT
1 February 2001

LEGAL CATEGORY
POM

SNO Tears

(Chauvin Pharmaceuticals Ltd)

1. NAME OF THE MEDICINAL PRODUCT
Sno* tears

2. QUALITATIVE AND QUANTITATIVE COMPOSITION
Polyvinyl Alcohol 1.4% w/v.

3. PHARMACEUTICAL FORM
Multidose eye drops.

4. CLINICAL PARTICULARS

4.1 Therapeutic indications
Sno tears is used topically to provide tear-like lubrication for the symptomatic relief of dry eyes and eye irritation associated with deficient tear production (usually in cases of keratoconjunctivitis sicca and xerophthalmia).

Sno tears is also used as an ocular lubricant for artificial eyes.

4.2 Posology and method of administration
Adults (including the elderly) and children:

The dose depends on the need for lubrication. Usually one or more drops should be used as required, or as prescribed.

4.3 Contraindications
Hypersensitivity to any component of the preparation.

This product contains benzalkonium chloride, therefore, soft contact lenses should be removed during treatment with Sno tears.

4.4 Special warnings and special precautions for use
If irritation persists or worsens or headache, eye pain, vision changes or continued redness occurs, discontinue use and consult a physician.

4.5 Interaction with other medicinal products and other forms of Interaction
None known.

4.6 Pregnancy and lactation
There is no evidence of safety of the drug in human pregnancy, but it has been in widespread use for many years without apparent ill consequence. If any therapy is needed in pregnancy, this preparation can be used if recommended by a physician.

4.7 Effects on ability to drive and use machines
May cause transient blurring of vision on instillation. Do not drive or operate hazardous machinery until vision is clear.

4.8 Undesirable effects
May cause transient, mild stinging or temporarily blurred vision.

4.9 Overdose
Not applicable.

5. PHARMACOLOGICAL PROPERTIES

5.1 Pharmacodynamic properties
Polyvinyl alcohol is a wetting agent and as such enables the formation of a tear film to relieve the symptoms of dry eye.

5.2 Pharmacokinetic properties
There are not expected to be any systemic reactions occurring following the use of Sno tears.

5.3 Preclinical safety data
There are no preclinical data of relevance to the prescriber which are additional to that already included in other sections of the SPC.

6. PHARMACEUTICAL PARTICULARS

6.1 List of excipients
Benzalkonium Chloride

Disodium Edetate

Hydroxyethylcellulose

Sodium Chloride

Sodium Hydroxide

Purified Water

6.2 Incompatibilities
None known.

6.3 Shelf life
Unopened: 36 months

Opened: 1 month

6.4 Special precautions for storage
Store below 25°C.

6.5 Nature and contents of container
A 10ml polyethylene bottle fitted with a polyethylene plug and a tamper evident polystyrene or polyethylene pilfer proof cap.

6.6 Instructions for use and handling
Discard any remaining solution 1 month after first opening the container.

7. MARKETING AUTHORISATION HOLDER
Chauvin Pharmaceuticals Ltd

106 London Road

Kingston-upon-Thames

Surrey

KT2 6TN

England

8. MARKETING AUTHORISATION NUMBER(S)
PL 0033/0097

9. DATE OF FIRST AUTHORISATION/RENEWAL OF THE AUTHORISATION
15.2.83 \ 14.02.98

15.2.84

10. DATE OF REVISION OF THE TEXT
October 1997

November 2002

Sodiofolin 50 mg/ml, solution for injection

(medac GmbH)

1. NAME OF THE MEDICINAL PRODUCT
Sodiofolin 50 mg/ml, solution for injection

2. QUALITATIVE AND QUANTITATIVE COMPOSITION
Sodiofolin 50 mg/ml, solution for injection contains 54.65 mg/ml disodium folinate equivalent to 50 mg/ml folinic acid.

3. PHARMACEUTICAL FORM
Solution for injection or intravenous infusion

4. CLINICAL PARTICULARS

4.1 Therapeutic indications
I. Enhancement of fluorouracil cytotoxicity

In combination with fluorouracil, disodium folinate enhances the effect of fluorouracil in the palliative therapy of colorectal carcinomas.

II. Preventing the manifestations of intoxication in methotrexate therapy.

Disodium folinate is used to diminish the toxicity and counteract the action of folic acid antagonists such as methotrexate in cytotoxic therapy. This procedure is commonly known as folinate rescue.

Note:

Persistently high serum methotrexate levels may also be expected in low-dose methotrexate therapy particularly in pleural effusions, ascites, renal insufficiency and inadequate fluid intake during methotrexate therapy.

4.2 Posology and method of administration
Palliative treatment of colorectal carcinomas

The combined use of disodium folinate and fluorouracil is reserved for physicians experienced in the treatment of colorectal carcinoma.

The dosage schedules specified below have been tested in clinical studies carried out in large numbers of patients. They should therefore form the basis of a therapeutic decision, for it is not possible to state at present whether one or other of these regimes is superior to the remaining schedules.

<u>1. Weekly regime</u>

1.1 Moderately high-dose fluorouracil

500 mg/m^2 folinic acid (= 546.5 mg/m^2 disodium folinate) as i.v. infusion over a period of 2 hours plus 600 mg/m^2 fluorouracil as i.v. bolus injection 1 hour after the start of the disodium folinate infusion.

Repeat once a week for a total of 6 weeks (= 1 cycle).

Repeat the cycle after a 2-week treatment interval. The number of cycles will depend on the response of the tumour.

<u>Dose adjustment of fluorouracil</u>

The fluorouracil dosage should be adjusted in accordance with the toxicity observed:

Gastrointestinal toxicity WHO ≥ 1:	Reduction to 500 mg/m^2. Resumption of therapy only when findings have completely returned to normal.
Bone marrow toxicity WHO ≥ 1:	Reduction to 500 mg/m^2. Resumption of therapy only when the findings are as follows: Leukocytes > 3,000/µl; Thrombocytes > 100,000/µl

1.2 High-dose fluorouracil

500 mg/m^2 folinic acid (= 546.5 mg/m^2 disodium folinate) as i.v. infusion over a period of 1-2 hours and subsequently 2,600 mg/m^2 fluorouracil by continuous infusion over 24 hours.

Repeat once a week for a total of 6 weeks (= 1 cycle).

Repeat the cycle after a 2-week treatment interval. The number of cycles will depend on the response of the tumour.

<u>Dose adjustment of fluorouracil</u>

The fluorouracil dosage should be adjusted in accordance with the toxicity observed:

Life-threatening cardiotoxicity:	Termination of therapy
Bone marrow toxicity WHO ≥ 3:	Reduction by 20% Resumption of therapy only when the findings are as follows: Leukocytes > 3,000/µl; Thrombocytes > 100,000/µl
Gastrointestinal toxicity WHO ≥ 3:	Reduction by 20%

<u>2. Monthly regime</u>

2.1 Moderately high-dosed disodium folinate

200 mg/m^2 folinic acid (= 218.6 mg/m^2 disodium folinate) daily, followed by 370 mg/m^2 fluorouracil daily, both given as i.v. bolus injection. Repeat on 5 successive days (= 1 cycle).

Repeat the cycle after 4 weeks, 8 weeks and every 5 weeks after that. The number of cycles will depend on the response of the tumour.

<u>Dose adjustment of fluorouracil</u>

The dosage of fluorouracil should be adjusted in each subsequent cycle in accordance with the toxicity (WHO) observed, as follows:

WHO toxicity 0:	Increase daily dose by 30 mg/m^2
WHO toxicity 1:	Daily dose unchanged
WHO toxicity ≥ 2:	Reduce daily dose by 30 mg/m^2

2.2 Low-dose disodium folinate

20 mg/m^2 folinic acid (= 21.86 mg/m^2 disodium folinate) daily, followed by 425 mg/m^2 fluorouracil daily, both given as i.v. bolus injection. Repeat on 5 successive days (= 1 cycle).

Repeat the cycle after 4 weeks, 8 weeks and every 5 weeks after that. The number of cycles will depend on the response of the tumour.

<u>Dose adjustment of fluorouracil</u>

In the absence of toxicity (especially if no significant bone marrow toxicity and no non-haematological side-effects occur in the interval) it is recommended to increase the dosage of fluorouracil by 10% in each case.

Preventing the manifestations of intoxication in methotrexate therapy (folinate rescue):

Only physicians experienced in the use of high-dose methotrexate therapy should use prophylactic disodium folinate.

The prophylactic use of disodium folinate can only be achieved when plasma levels of methotrexate are available.

The use of a dose of methotrexate at ≥ 100 mg/m^2 (body surface) must be followed by the administration of disodium folinate. There are no uniform recommendations for the dosage and mode of use of disodium folinate as an antidote in high-dose methotrexate therapy. The following dosage recommendations are therefore given as examples:

Disodium folinate rescue following methotrexate (MTX) therapy:

MTX serum levels at 24-30 hours	Disodium folinate dose (equivalent to folinic acid)	Duration
1.0×10^{-8} mol/l to 1.5×10^{-6} mol/l	10 to 15 mg/m^2 body surface every 6 hours	48 hours
1.5×10^{-6} mol/l to 5.0×10^{-6} mol/l	30 mg/m^2 body surface every 6 hours	up to plasma level $< 5 \times 10^{-8}$ mol/l
$> 5.0 \times 10^{-6}$ mol/l	60 to 100 mg/m^2 body surface every 6 hours	up to plasma level $< 5 \times 10^{-8}$ mol/l

Disodium folinate is given intravenously.

Start of rescue

Not later than 18 to 30 hours after the start of methotrexate infusion.

End of rescue

72 hours after the start of methotrexate infusion at the earliest. On completion of the rescue, the methotrexate level should be below 10^{-7} mol/l, preferably below 10^{-8} mol/l.

An "over-rescue" may impair the efficacy of methotrexate. With inadequate rescue, considerable toxic side-effects are likely with high-dosed methotrexate therapy.

Administration

For i.v. injection or infusion.

For i.v. infusion the disodium folinate solution may be diluted with 0.9 % sodium chloride solution.

4.3 Contraindications

The combination of disodium folinate with fluorouracil for palliative treatment of colorectal carcinoma is not indicated in:

existing contraindications against fluorouracil and severe diarrhoea.

Therapy with disodium folinate combined with fluorouracil must not be initiated or continued in patients who have symptoms of gastrointestinal toxicity of any severity until those symptoms have completely resolved. Patients with diarrhoea must be monitored with particular care until the diarrhoea has resolved, as rapid clinical deterioration leading to death can occur (see also sections 4.2, 4.4 and 4.5).

Disodium folinate is not suitable for the treatment of pernicious anaemia or other anaemias due to Vitamin B_{12} deficiency. Although haematological remissions may occur, the neurological manifestations remain progressive.

4.4 Special warnings and special precautions for use

Disodium folinate should not be given simultaneously with an antineoplastic folic acid antagonist (e.g. methotrexate) to modify or abort clinical toxicity, as the therapeutic effect of the antagonist may be nullified except in the case of folic acid antagonist overdose - see below.

Concomitant disodium folinate will not however inhibit the antibacterial activity of other folic acid antagonists such as trimethoprim and pyrimethamine.

In the combination regimen with fluorouracil, the toxicity profile of fluorouracil may be enhanced or shifted by disodium folinate. The commonest manifestations are leucopenia, mucositis, stomatitis and/or diarrhoea which may be dose limiting. When disodium folinate and fluorouracil are used in the treatment of colorectal cancer, the fluorouracil dosage must be reduced more in cases of toxicity than when fluorouracil is used alone. Toxicities observed in patients treated with the combination are qualitatively similar to those observed in patients treated with fluorouracil alone. Gastrointestinal toxicities are observed more commonly and may be more severe or even life threatening (particularly stomatitis and diarrhoea). In severe cases, treatment is withdrawal of fluorouracil and disodium folinate, and supportive intravenous therapy. Patients should be instructed to consult their treating physician immediately if stomatitis (mild to moderate ulcers) and/or diarrhoea (watery stools or bowel movements) two times per day occur (see also section 4.2).

Particular care should be taken in the treatment of elderly or debilitated colorectal cancer patients, as these patients may be at increased risk of severe toxicity.

In the treatment of accidental overdosage of folic acid antagonists, disodium folinate should be administered as promptly as possible. As the time interval between antifolate administration (e.g. methotrexate) and disodium folinate rescue increases the effectiveness of disodium folinate in counteracting toxicity decreases. Monitoring of the serum methotrexate concentration is essential in determining the optimal dose and duration of treatment with disodium folinate. Delayed methotrexate excretion may be caused by third space fluid accumulation (i.e., ascites, pleural effusion), renal insufficiency or inadequate hydration. Under such circumstances, higher doses of disodium folinate or prolonged administration may be indicated.

Disodium folinate has no effect on non-haematological toxicities of methotrexate such as the nephrotoxicity resulting from drug and/or metabolite precipitation in the kidney.

When using methotrexate, an overdosage of disodium folinate may result in a decrease of efficacy of methotrexate ("over-rescue").

4.5 Interaction with other medicinal products and other forms of Interaction

Disodium folinate is an antidote of folic acid antagonists - e.g. methotrexate. Following the use of methotrexate, disodium folinate overdosage may lead to a loss of the effect of methotrexate therapy ("over-rescue").

Concomitant use of disodium folinate counteracts the antineoplastic activity of methotrexate and increases the cytotoxic effects of fluorouracil.

The following side-effects for disodium folinate used in conjunction with 5-fluorouracil were reported frequently: diarrhoea, stomatitis and leucopenia. Less commonly infections, thrombocytopenia, nausea, vomiting, constipation, malaise, alopecia, dermatitis and anorexia have been observed.

Life threatening diarrhoeas have been observed if 600 mg/m^2 of fluorouracil (i.v. bolus once weekly) is given together with disodium folinate. When disodium folinate and fluorouracil are used in the treatment of colorectal cancer, the fluorouracil dosage must be reduced more than when fluorouracil is used alone.

In epileptic seizures the effect of phenytoin, primidone and phenobarbital may be reduced and has been shown to increase the frequency of seizures in susceptible children.

4.6 Pregnancy and lactation

Methotrexate therapy is contra-indicated during pregnancy and lactation period. Therefore, prevention of consequences of a methotrexate therapy does not apply.

Combination therapy with disodium folinate and fluorouracil is contra-indicated during pregnancy and lactation period.

No information is available on the effects of folinic acid alone on fertility and general reproductive performance.

4.7 Effects on ability to drive and use machines

Disodium folinate is unlikely to affect the ability to drive or operate machines. The general condition of the patient is likely to be more significant than any drug-induced effects.

4.8 Undesirable effects

Adverse reactions to disodium folinate are rare but occasional pyrexial reactions have been reported following parenteral administration. Isolated case of allergic reactions - sensitisation, including anaphylactoid reactions and urticaria, can occur. At high dosage, gastrointestinal disorders, sleep disturbances, agitation and depression have been observed. In rare cases an increase in the frequency of epileptic attacks has been reported.

4.9 Overdose

Should overdosage of the combination of fluorouracil and Sodiofolin solution for injection occur, overdosage instructions for fluorouracil should be followed.

5. PHARMACOLOGICAL PROPERTIES

5.1 Pharmacodynamic properties

Folinic acid is the formyl derivative or active form of folic acid. It is involved in various metabolic processes including purine synthesis, pyrimidine nucleotide synthesis and amino acid metabolism.

Biochemical rationale for the combination of disodium folinate with fluorouracil:

fluorouracil inhibits *inter alia* DNA synthesis by binding thymidilate synthetase. The combination of disodium folinate with fluorouracil results in the formation of a stable ternary complex consisting of thymidilate synthetase, 5-fluorodeoxy-uridinemonophosphate and 5,10-methylene-tetrahydrofolate.

This leads to an extended blockade of thymidilate synthetase with enhanced inhibition of DNA biosynthesis, resulting in increased cytotoxicity as compared to fluorouracil monotherapy.

5.2 Pharmacokinetic properties

Bioequivalence

A pharmacokinetic study was performed to demonstrate the bioequivalence of disodium folinate in comparison with a licensed calcium folinate reference preparation. The bioequivalence criteria determined were fulfilled in respect of the pharmacokinetic parameters for D- and L-folinic acid and for the metabolite 5-methyltetrahydrofolic acid. Calcium folinate and disodium folinate solutions are bioequivalent and may be exchanged within the scope of any intended therapy.

Distribution

The distribution volume of folinic acid is not known. With i.v. application, peak serum levels of the parent substance (D/L-formyltetrahydrofolic acid, folinic acid) are obtained after 10 minutes.

Metabolism

The active isomeric form L-5-formyltetrahydrofolic acid is quickly metabolised to 5-methyltetrahydrofolic acid (folic acid) in the liver. It is assumed that this conversion is not linked to the presence of dihydrofolate reductase and occurs more quickly and more completely after oral application than after parenteral application.

Excretion

The inactive isomeric form D-5-formyltetrahydrofolic acid is excreted virtually completely unchanged via the kidneys. The active isomeric form L-5-formyltetra-hydrofolic acid is in part excreted unchanged via the kidneys, but is predominantly metabolised to folic acid.

5.3 Preclinical safety data

Toxicity tests on combined use with fluorouracil have not been carried out.

No further information is available of relevance to the prescriber which is not already included in other relevant sections of the SPC.

6. PHARMACEUTICAL PARTICULARS

6.1 List of excipients

Sodium hydroxide, hydrochloric acid, water for injection

6.2 Incompatibilities

Because of chemical incompatibilities, disodium folinate solutions should not be mixed with hydrogen carbonate-containing infusions.

6.3 Shelf life

36 months for 100, 200, 300, 350, 400, 500 and 900 mg in the closed container.

Once the container has been opened, any remainder should be discarded.

The solution for injection may be diluted with 0.9 % sodium chloride solution. This solution will be stable for 72 hours at room temperature (20-25 °C). Nonetheless, it must be considered that a risk of microbiological contamination can never be fully excluded even when the diluted infusion is prepared under aseptic conditions. Therefore, the storage time for the prepared dilutions should be as short as possible.

This medicinal product should not be used after its expiry date.

6.4 Special precautions for storage

Store at 2 - 8 °C. Protect from light.

6.5 Nature and contents of container

Colourless glass vial, rubber stopper with aluminium flip-off cap as seal.

Presentation:

Sodiofolin 50 mg/ml, solution for injection, 100 mg: 1 vial of 2 ml solution contains 109.3 mg disodium folinate equivalent to 100 mg folinic acid.

Sodiofolin 50 mg/ml, solution for injection, 200 mg: 1 vial of 4 ml solution contains 218.6 mg disodium folinate equivalent to 200 mg folinic acid.

Sodiofolin 50 mg/ml, solution for injection, 300 mg: 1 vial of 6 ml solution contains 327.9 mg disodium folinate equivalent to 300 mg folinic acid.

Sodiofolin 50 mg/ml, solution for injection, 350 mg: 1 vial of 7 ml solution contains 382.55 mg disodium folinate equivalent to 350 mg folinic acid.

Sodiofolin 50 mg/ml, solution for injection, 400 mg: 1 vial of 8 ml solution contains 437.2 mg disodium folinate equivalent to 400 mg folinic acid.

Sodiofolin 50 mg/ml, solution for injection, 500 mg: 1 vial of 10 ml solution contains 546.5 mg disodium folinate equivalent to 500 mg folinic acid.

Sodiofolin 50 mg/ml, solution for injection, 900 mg: 1 vial of 18 ml solution contains 983.7 mg disodium folinate equivalent to 900 mg folinic acid.

6.6 Instructions for use and handling

No special instructions for use are necessary.

7. MARKETING AUTHORISATION HOLDER

Name and permanent address of the holder of the marketing authorisation

medac

Gesellschaft fur klinische

Spezialpraeparate mbH

Fehlandtstrasse 3

D-20354 Hamburg

Germany

8. MARKETING AUTHORISATION NUMBER(S)

PL: 11587/0005

9. DATE OF FIRST AUTHORISATION/RENEWAL OF THE AUTHORISATION

2 August 2000

10. DATE OF REVISION OF THE TEXT

Dezember 2000

Sodium Amytal

(Flynn Pharma Ltd)

1. NAME OF THE MEDICINAL PRODUCT

SODIUM AMYTAL

2. QUALITATIVE AND QUANTITATIVE COMPOSITION

Each 60mg capsule contains 60mg of Amobarbital Sodium EP

Each 200mg capsule contains 200mg of Amobarbital Sodium EP

3. PHARMACEUTICAL FORM

Capsule

4. CLINICAL PARTICULARS

4.1 Therapeutic indications

For the short term treatment of severe, intractable insomnia for the short term treatment of severe, intractable insomnia in patients already taking barbiturates. New patients should not be started on this preparation. Attempts should be made to wean patients off this preparation by gradual reduction of the dose over a period of days or weeks (*see drug abuse and dependence*). Abrupt discontinuation should be avoided as this may precipitate withdrawal effects (*see Warnings*)

4.2 Posology and method of administration
For oral administration to adults only. Normal dosage is 60-200 mg at bedtime.

THE ELDERLY

Sodium Amytal is not recommended for use in elderly or debilitated patients.

CHILDREN

Amytal should not be administered to children or young adults.

Amylobarbitone sodium is expected to lose most of its effectiveness for both inducing and maintaining sleep by the end of two weeks of continued drug administration, even with the use of multiple doses.

4.3 Contraindications
Hypersensitivity to barbiturates, a history of manifest or latent porphyria, marked impairment of liver function or respiratory disease in which dyspnoea or obstruction is evident. Oral barbiturates should not be administered in the presence of acute or chronic pain, because paradoxical excitement may be induced or important symptoms may be masked.

Barbiturates should not be administered to children, young adults, patients with a history of drug or alcohol addiction or abuse, the elderly and the debilitated.

4.4 Special warnings and special precautions for use
Addiction potential: Barbiturates have a high addiction potential. Long-term use, or use of high dosage for short periods, may lead to tolerance and subsequently to physical and psychological dependence. Patients who have psychological dependence on barbiturates may increase the dosage or decrease the dosage interval without consulting a doctor and, subsequently, may develop a physical dependence on barbiturates.

To minimise the possibility of overdosage or development of dependence, the amount prescribed should be limited to that required for the interval until the next appointment.

Withdrawal symptoms occur after long term normal use (and particularly after abuse) on rapid cessation of barbiturate treatment. Symptoms include nightmares, irritability and insomnia and, in severe cases, tremors, delirium, convulsions and death.

Barbiturates should be withdrawn gradually from any patient known to be taking excessive doses over long periods.

Caution should be exercised when barbiturates are administered in the presence of acute or chronic pain, because paradoxical excitement could be induced or important symptoms could be masked.

Information for patients: The following information should be given to patients receiving amylobarbitone sodium:

1 The use of amylobarbitone carries with it an associated risk of psychological and/or physical dependence. The patient should be warned against increasing the dose of the drug without consulting a doctor.

2 Amylobarbitone may impair the mental and/or physical abilities required for the performance of potentially hazardous tasks, such as driving a car or operating machinery. The patient should be cautioned accordingly.

3 Alcohol should not be consumed while taking amylobarbitone. The concurrent use of amylobarbitone with other CNS depressants (eg alcohol, narcotics, tranquillisers and antihistamines) may result in additional CNS depressant effects.

Drug abuse and dependence: Barbiturates may be habit forming; tolerance, psychological and physical dependence may occur especially following prolonged use of high doses. Daily administration in excess of 400 mg secobarbitone, for approximately 90 days, is likely to produce some degree of physical dependence.

A dosage of 600 - 800 mg, for at least 35 days, is sufficient to produce withdrawal seizures. The average daily dose for the barbiturate addict is usually about 1.5g.

As tolerance to barbiturates develops, the amount needed to maintain the same level of intoxication increases; tolerance to a fatal dosage, however, does not increase more than twofold. As this occurs, the margin between intoxicating dosage and fatal dosage becomes smaller. The lethal dose of a barbiturate is far less if alcohol is also ingested.

Symptoms of acute intoxication include unsteady gait, slurred speech and sustained nystagmus. Mental signs of chronic intoxication include confusion, poor judgement, irritability, insomnia and somatic complaints.

The symptoms of barbiturate withdrawal can be severe and may cause death. Minor withdrawal symptoms may appear 8 to 12 hours after the last dose of a barbiturate. These symptoms usually appear in the following order: anxiety, muscle twitching, tremor of hands and fingers, progressive weakness, dizziness, distortion in visual perception, nausea, vomiting, insomnia and orthostatic hypotension. Major withdrawal symptoms (convulsions and delirium) may occur within 16 hours and last up to five days after abrupt cessation of barbiturates. Intensity of withdrawal symptoms gradually declines over a period of approximately 15 days. Individuals susceptible to barbiturate abuse and dependence include alcoholics and opiate abusers, as well as other sedative-hypnotic and amphetamine abusers.

Dependence on barbiturates arises from repeated administration on a continuous basis, generally in amounts exceeding therapeutic dose levels. Treatment of dependence consists of cautious and gradual withdrawal of the drug. Barbiturate-dependent patients can be withdrawn by using a number of withdrawal regimens. In all cases, withdrawal takes an extended period. One method involves substituting a 30 mg dose of phenobarbitone for each 100 - 200 mg dose of barbiturate that the patient has been taking. The total daily amount of phenobarbitone is then administered in three or four divided doses, not to exceed 600 mg daily. Should signs of withdrawal occur on the first day of treatment, a loading dose of 100 to 200 mg of phenobarbitone may be administered intramuscularly in addition to the oral dose. After stabilisation on phenobarbitone, the total daily dose is decreased by 30 mg a day as long as withdrawal is proceeding smoothly. A modification of this regimen involves initiating treatment at the patient's regular dosage level and decreasing the daily dosage by 10% as tolerated by the patient.

Infants that are physically dependent on barbiturates may be given phenobarbitone, 3 to 10 mg/kg/day. After withdrawal symptoms (hyperactivity, disturbed sleep, tremors and hyperreflexia) are relieved, the dosage of phenobarbitone should be gradually decreased and completely withdrawn over a two week period.

Carcinogenesis: Animal data show that phenobarbitone can be carcinogenic after lifetime administration.

Human data: In a 29 year epidemiological study of 9136 patients who were treated on an anticonvulsant protocol that included phenobarbitone, results indicated a higher than normal incidence of hepatic carcinoma. Previously some of these patients had been treated with thorotrast, a drug that is known to produce hepatic carcinomas. Thus, this study did not provide sufficient evidence that phenobarbitone is carcinogenic in humans.

A retrospective study of 84 children with brain tumours, matched to 73 normal controls and 78 cancer controls (malignant disease other than brain tumours), suggested an association between exposure to barbiturates prenatally and an increased incidence of brain tumours.

Barbiturates should be administered with caution, if at all, to patients who are mentally depressed or have suicidal tendencies. They should also be used with great caution and at reduced dosage in those with hepatic disease, marked renal dysfunction, shock or respiratory depression.

Elderly or debilitated patients may react to barbiturates with marked excitement, depression or confusion (see 'Contra-indications'). In some persons, barbiturates repeatedly produce excitement rather than depression.

Barbiturates should not be administered to patients showing the premonitory signs of hepatic coma (see 'Contra-indications').

A cumulative effect may occur with the barbiturates leading to features of chronic poisoning including headache, depression and slurred speech.

Automatism may follow the use of a hypnotic dose of barbiturate.

The systemic effects of exogenous and endogenous corticosteroids may be diminished by amylobarbitone. This product should therefore be administered with caution to patients with borderline hypoadrenal function, regardless of whether it is of pituitary or of primary adrenal origin.

Laboratory tests: Prolonged therapy with barbiturates should be accompanied by periodic evaluation of, for example, the haematopoietic, renal and hepatic systems (but see 'Uses).

4.5 Interaction with other medicinal products and other forms of Interaction
Toxic effects and fatalities have occurred following overdoses of amylobarbital alone and in combination with other CNS depressants. Caution should be exercised in prescribing unnecessarily large amounts of amylobarbitone for patients who have a history of emotional disturbances or suicidal ideation or who have misused alcohol or other CNS drugs.

Anticoagulants: Barbiturates cause induction of the liver microsomal enzymes responsible for metabolising many other drugs. In particular they may result in increased metabolism and decreased anticoagulant response of oral anticoagulants (eg warfarin). Patients stabilised on anticoagulant therapy may require dosage adjustments if barbiturates are added to or withdrawn from their regimen.

Corticosteroids: Barbiturates appear to enhance the metabolism of exogenous corticosteroids and steroid dosage may also need adjustment.

Griseofulvin: Barbiturates may interfere with the absorption of oral griseofulvin, thus decreasing its blood level. Concomitant administration should be avoided if possible.

Doxycycline: Barbiturates may shorten the half-life of doxycycline for as long as two weeks after the barbiturate is discontinued. If administered concomitantly the clinical response to doxycycline should be monitored closely.

Phenytoin, Sodium Valproate, Valproic Acid: The effect of barbiturates on phenytoin metabolism is variable. Phenytoin and barbiturate blood levels should be monitored more frequently if administered concomitantly. Sodium valproate and valproic acid increase amylobarbital serum levels. Therefore these levels should be monitored and dosage adjustments made as clinically indicated.

CNS Depressants: Concomitant use of other CNS depressants, including other sedatives or hypnotics, antihistamines, tranquillisers or alcohol, may produce additive depressant effects.

Monoamine Oxidase Inhibitors (MAOIS): Prolong the effects of barbiturates.

Oestradiol, oestrone, progesterone and other steroidal hormones: There have been reports of patients treated with antiepileptic drugs (eg phenobarbitone) who became pregnant while taking oral contraceptives. Barbiturates may decrease the effect of oestradiol. An alternative contraceptive method might be suggested to women taking barbiturates.

4.6 Pregnancy and lactation
Usage in Pregnancy: Barbiturates are contraindicated during pregnancy since they can cause foetal harm. A higher than expected incidence of foetal abnormalities may be connected with maternal consumption of barbiturates. Barbiturates readily cross the placental barrier and are distributed throughout foetal tissues with highest concentrations in placenta, foetal liver and brain. Withdrawal symptoms occur in infants born to women who receive barbiturates during the last trimester of pregnancy. If a patient becomes pregnant whilst taking this drug, she should be told of the potential hazard to the foetus.

Reports of infants suffering from long term barbiturate exposure *in utero* included the acute withdrawal syndrome of seizures and hyper-irritability from birth to a delayed onset of up to 14 days.

Labour and Delivery: Respiratory depression has been noted in infants born following the use of barbiturates during labour. Premature infants are particularly susceptible. Resuscitation equipment should be available.

Nursing Mothers: Small amounts of barbiturates are excreted in the milk and they are therefore contraindicated for the nursing mother.

4.7 Effects on ability to drive and use machines
Amylobarbitone may impair the mental and/or physical abilities required for the performance of potentially hazardous tasks such as driving a car or operating machinery. The patient should be cautioned accordingly

4.8 Undesirable effects
The following adverse reactions and their incidences were compiled from surveillance of thousands of hospitalised patients who received barbiturates. As such patients may be less aware of certain of the milder adverse effects of barbiturates, the incidence of these reactions may be somewhat higher in fully ambulatory patients.

More than 1 in 100 patients: The most common adverse reaction, estimated to occur at a rate of 1 to 3 patients per 100, is the following:

NERVOUS SYSTEM: Somnolence

LESS THAN 1 IN 100 PATIENTS: Adverse reactions estimated to occur at a rate of less than 1 in 100 patients are listed below grouped by organ system and by decreasing frequency:

NEUROLOGICAL: Agitation, confusion, hyperkinesia, ataxia, CNS depression, nightmares, nervousness, psychiatric disturbance, hallucinations, insomnia, anxiety, dizziness, abnormal thinking.

RESPIRATORY: Hypoventilation, apnoea.

CARDIOVASCULAR: Bradycardia, hypotension, syncope.

DIGESTIVE: Nausea, vomiting, constipation

OTHER: Headache, hypersensitivity reactions (angioneurotic oedema, rashes, exfoliative dermatitis), fever, liver damage. Hypersensitivity is more likely to occur in patients with asthma, urticaria or angioneurotic oedema. Megaloblastic anaemia has followed chronic phenobarbitone use.

4.9 Overdose
The toxic dose of barbiturates varies considerably. In general, an oral dose of 1g of most barbiturates produces serious poisoning in an adult. Death commonly occurs after 2 to 10g of ingested barbiturate. The sedative, therapeutic blood levels of amylobarbitone range between 2 and 10 mg/l; the usual lethal blood level ranges from 40 to 80 mg/l. Barbiturate intoxication may be confused with alcoholism, bromide intoxication and various neurological disorders. Potential tolerance must be considered when evaluating significance of dose and plasma concentration.

In extreme overdose, all electrical activity in the brain may cease, in which case a "flat" EEG normally equated with clinical death cannot be accepted. This effect is fully reversible unless hypoxic damage occurs. Consideration should be given to the possibility of barbiturate intoxication even in situations that appear to involve trauma.

SIGNS AND SYMPTOMS: Symptoms of oral overdose may occur within 15 minutes and begin with CNS depression, absent or sluggish reflexes, underventilation, hypotension and hypothermia, which may progress to pulmonary oedema and death. Haemorrhagic blisters may develop, especially at pressure points.

Complications such as pneumonia, pulmonary oedema, cardiac arrhythmias, congestive heart failure and renal failure may occur. Uraemia may increase CNS sensitivity to barbiturates if renal function is impaired. Differential diagnosis should include hypoglycaemia, head trauma, cerebrovascular accidents, convulsive states and diabetic coma.

TREATMENT OF OVERDOSAGE

General management should consist of symptomatic and supportive therapy. Activated charcoal may be more effective than emesis or lavage. Diuresis and peritoneal dialysis are of little value. Haemodialysis and haemoperfusion enhance drug clearance and should be considered in serious poisoning. If the patient has chronically abused sedatives, withdrawal reactions may be manifest following acute overdose.

5. PHARMACOLOGICAL PROPERTIES

5.1 Pharmacodynamic properties

Sodium Amytal (amylobarbitone sodium), a barbiturate of intermediate duration of action, is a CNS depressant. In ordinary doses the drug acts as a sedative and hypnotic.

Barbiturates are capable of producing all levels of CNS mood alteration, from excitation to mild sedation, hypnosis and deep coma. Overdosage can produce death. Barbiturates depress the sensory cortex, decrease motor activity, alter cerebellar function and produce drowsiness, sedation and hypnosis. In high enough therapeutic doses barbiturates induce anaesthesia.

Barbiturate-induced sleep differs from physiologic sleep. Sleep laboratory studies have demonstrated that barbiturates reduce the amount of time spent in the rapid eye movement (REM) phase of sleep, or dreaming stage. Also stages III and IV sleep are decreased. Following abrupt cessation of barbiturates used regularly, patients may experience markedly increased dreaming, nightmares and/or insomnia. Therefore, withdrawal of a single therapeutic dose over five or six days has been recommended to lessen the REM rebound and disturbed sleep which contribute to drug withdrawal syndrome (for example, decrease the dose from 3 to 2 doses a day for 1 week).

5.2 Pharmacokinetic properties

Barbiturates are weak acids that are absorbed and rapidly distributed to all tissues and fluids, with high concentrations in the brain, liver and kidneys. Lipid solubility of the barbiturates is the dominant factor in their distribution within the body. Barbiturates are bound to plasma and tissue proteins; the degree of binding increases as a function of lipid solubility. Amylobarbitone sodium is readily absorbed from the gastro-intestinal tract; its onset of action being from 30 to 45 minutes and its duration of action ranging from 6 to 8 hours. The rate of absorption is increased if taken on an empty stomach. Following absorption some 60% is bound to plasma proteins. It has a half-life of about 20 to 25 hours, which is considerably extended in neonates. It is metabolised in the liver; up to about 50% is excreted in the urine as 3'-hydroxyamylobarbitone and up to about 30% as *N*-hydroxyamylobarbitone. Less than 1% appears unchanged in urine and up to about 5% in faeces.

5.3 Preclinical safety data

Carcinogenesis: Animal data show that phenobarbitone can be carcinogenic after lifetime administration.

6. PHARMACEUTICAL PARTICULARS

6.1 List of excipients

Starch, Dimeticone, Patent Blue V, Gelatin, Black Iron Oxide, Shellac

6.2 Incompatibilities

Not applicable

6.3 Shelf life

60 months

6.4 Special precautions for storage

Store below 25°C. Keep lid tightly closed.

6.5 Nature and contents of container

High density polyethylene bottles with screw caps containing 100 capsules.

6.6 Instructions for use and handling

Not applicable

7. MARKETING AUTHORISATION HOLDER

Flynn Pharma Ltd.

Alton House

4 Herbert Street

Dublin 2,

Republic of Ireland

8. MARKETING AUTHORISATION NUMBER(S)

Sodium Amytal 60mg PL 13621/0005

Sodium Amytal 200mg PL 13621/0006

9. DATE OF FIRST AUTHORISATION/RENEWAL OF THE AUTHORISATION

1995

10. DATE OF REVISION OF THE TEXT

DECEMBER 1995

11. LEGAL CATEGORY

CD (Sch.3), POM

Sodium Bicarbonate Injection Bp Minijet 8.4%

(International Medication Systems (UK) Ltd)

1. NAME OF THE MEDICINAL PRODUCT

Sodium Bicarbonate Injection BP Minijet 8.4% w/v

2. QUALITATIVE AND QUANTITATIVE COMPOSITION

Sodium Bicarbonate BP 8.4% w/v

3. PHARMACEUTICAL FORM

Sterile aqueous solution for parenteral administration to humans.

4. CLINICAL PARTICULARS

4.1 Therapeutic indications

For the correction of metabolic acidosis associated with cardiac arrest after other resuscitative measures such as cardiac compression, ventilation, adrenaline and antiarrhythmic agents have been used.

4.2 Posology and method of administration

For intravenous administration only.

Adults: the usual dose is 1mmol/kg (2ml/kg 4.2% solution or 1ml/kg 8.4% solution) followed by 0.5mmol/kg (1ml/kg 4.2% solution or 0.5ml/kg 8.4% solution) given at 10 minute intervals.

Children: the usual dose is 1mmol/kg by slow iv injection.

In premature infants and neonates, the 4.2% solution should be used or the 8.4% solution should be diluted 1:1 with 5% dextrose.

Elderly: as for adults.

4.3 Contraindications

Administration of sodium bicarbonate is contraindicated in patients with renal failure, metabolic or respiratory alkalosis, hypertension, oedema, congestive heart failure, a history of urinary calculi and coexistent potassium depletion or hypocalcaemia, hypoventilation, chloride depletion or hypernatraemia.

4.4 Special warnings and special precautions for use

Whenever sodium bicarbonate is used intravenously, arterial blood gas analyses, in particular arterial/venous blood pH and carbon dioxide levels, should be performed before and during the course of treatment to minimise the possibility of overdosage and resultant alkalosis.

Accidental extravascular injection of hypertonic solutions may cause vascular irritation or sloughing. The use of scalp veins should be avoided.

Whenever respiratory acidosis is concomitant with metabolic acidosis, both pulmonary ventilation and perfusion must be adequately supported to get rid of excess CO_2.

4.5 Interaction with other medicinal products and other forms of Interaction

Caution should be used when administering sodium ions to patients receiving corticosteroids or corticotrophin.

Urinary alkalisation will increase the renal clearance of tetracyclines, especially doxycycline but it will increase the half life and duration of action of basic drugs such as quinidine, amphetamines, ephedrine and pseudoephedrine.

Hypochloraemic alkalosis may occur if sodium bicarbonate is used in conjunction with potassium depleting diuretics such as bumetanide, ethacrynic acid, frusemide and thiazides. Concurrent use in patients taking potassium supplements may reduce serum potassium concentration by promoting an intracellular ion shift.

4.6 Pregnancy and lactation

Safe use in pregnancy has not been established. The use of any drug in pregnant or lactating women requires that the expected benefit be carefully weighed against the possible risk to the mother and child.

Patients requiring i.v. sodium bicarbonate are unlikely to be fit enough to breast feed.

4.7 Effects on ability to drive and use machines

Not applicable; this preparation is intended for use only in emergencies.

4.8 Undesirable effects

Alkalosis and/or hypokalaemia may ensue as a result of prolonged use or over-correction of the bicarbonate deficit.

Hyperirritability or tetany may occur caused by rapid shifts of free ionised calcium or due to serum protein alterations arising from pH changes.

4.9 Overdose

Symptoms: metabolic alkalosis accompanied by compensatory hyperventilation, paradoxical acidosis of the cerebrospinal fluid, severe hypokalaemia, hyperirritability and tetany.

Treatment: discontinue the administration of sodium bicarbonate, rebreathe the expired air or, if more severe administer calcium gluconate especially if tetany is present. In severe alkalosis, an infusion of 2.14% ammonium chloride is recommended, except in patients with pe-existing hepatic disease. If hypokalaemia is present administer potassium chloride.

5. PHARMACOLOGICAL PROPERTIES

5.1 Pharmacodynamic properties

Sodium bicarbonate therapy increases plasma bicarbonate, buffers excess hydrogen ion concentration, raises blood pH and reverses clinical manifestations of metabolic acidosis.

5.2 Pharmacokinetic properties

Sodium bicarbonate is eliminated principally in the urine and effectively alkalises it.

5.3 Preclinical safety data

Not applicable since sodium bicarbonate has been used in clinical practice for many years and its effects in man are well known.

6. PHARMACEUTICAL PARTICULARS

6.1 List of excipients

Water for Injection USP

6.2 Incompatibilities

The addition of sodium bicarbonate to parenteral solutions containing calcium should be avoided except where compatibility has been previously established; precipitation or haze may result, should this occur, the solution should not be used.

6.3 Shelf life

36 months.

6.4 Special precautions for storage

Store below 25°C.

6.5 Nature and contents of container

The solution is contained in a USP type I glass vial with an elastomeric closure which meets all the relevant USP specifications.

The 8.4% w/v is available as 10 or 50ml.

6.6 Instructions for use and handling

The container is specially designed for use with the IMS Minijet injector.

Administrative Data

7. MARKETING AUTHORISATION HOLDER

International Medication Systems (UK) Limited

208 Bath Road

Slough

Berkshire

SL1 3WE

UK

8. MARKETING AUTHORISATION NUMBER(S)

PL 3265/0003R

9. DATE OF FIRST AUTHORISATION/RENEWAL OF THE AUTHORISATION

Date first granted: 28 February 1991

Date renewed: 29 November 1996

10. DATE OF REVISION OF THE TEXT

April 2001

POM

Sodium Bicarbonate Injection Minijet 4.2%

(International Medication Systems (UK) Ltd)

1. NAME OF THE MEDICINAL PRODUCT

Sodium Bicarbonate Injection BP Minijet 4.2% w/v

2. QUALITATIVE AND QUANTITATIVE COMPOSITION

Sodium Bicarbonate BP 4.2% w/v

3. PHARMACEUTICAL FORM

Sterile aqueous solution for parenteral administration to humans.

4. CLINICAL PARTICULARS

4.1 Therapeutic indications

For the correction of metabolic acidosis associated with cardiac arrest after other resuscitative measures such as cardiac compression, ventilation, adrenaline and antiarrhythmic agents have been used.

4.2 Posology and method of administration

For intravenous administration only.

Adults: the usual dose is 1mmol/kg (2ml/kg 4.2% solution or 1ml/kg 8.4% solution) followed by 0.5mmol/kg (1ml/kg 4.2% solution or 0.5ml/kg 8.4% solution) given at 10 minute intervals.

Children: the usual dose is 1mmol/kg by slow iv injection.

In premature infants and neonates, the 4.2% solution should be used or the 8.4% solution should be diluted 1:1 with 5% dextrose.

Elderly: as for adults.

4.3 Contraindications

Administration of sodium bicarbonate is contraindicated in patients with renal failure, metabolic or respiratory alkalosis, hypertension, oedema, congestive heart failure, a history of urinary calculi and coexistent potassium depletion or hypocalcaemia, hypoventilation, chloride depletion or hypernatraemia.

4.4 Special warnings and special precautions for use

Whenever sodium bicarbonate is used intravenously, arterial blood gas analyses, in particular arterial/venous blood pH and carbon dioxide levels, should be performed before and during the course of treatment to minimise the possibility of overdosage and resultant alkalosis.

Accidental extravascular injection of hypertonic solutions may cause vascular irritation or sloughing. The use of scalp veins should be avoided.

Whenever respiratory acidosis is concomitant with metabolic acidosis, both pulmonary ventilation and perfusion must be adequately supported to get rid of excess CO_2.

4.5 Interaction with other medicinal products and other forms of Interaction

Caution should be used when administering sodium ions to patients receiving corticosteroids or corticotrophin.

Urinary alkalisation will increase the renal clearance of tetracyclines, especially doxycycline but it will increase the half life and duration of action of basic drugs such as quinidine, amphetamines, ephedrine and pseudoephedrine.

Hypochloraemic alkalosis may occur if sodium bicarbonate is used in conjunction with potassium depleting diuretics such as bumetamide, ethacrynic acid, frusemide and thiazides. Concurrent use in patients taking potassium supplements may reduce serum potassium concentration by promoting an intracellular ion shift.

4.6 Pregnancy and lactation

Safe use in pregnancy has not been established. The use of any drug in pregnant or lactating women requires that the expected benefit be carefully weighed against the possible risk to the mother and child.

Patients requiring i.v. sodium bicarbonate are unlikely to be fit enough to breast feed.

4.7 Effects on ability to drive and use machines

Not applicable; this preparation is intended for use only in emergencies.

4.8 Undesirable effects

Alkalosis and/or hypokalaemia may ensue as a result of prolonged use or over-correction of the bicarbonate deficit.

Hyperirritability or tetany may occur caused by rapid shifts of free ionised calcium or due to serum protein alterations arising from pH changes.

4.9 Overdose

Symptoms: metabolic alkalosis accompanied by compensatory hyperventilation, paradoxical acidosis of the cerebrospinal fluid, severe hypokalaemia, hyperirritability and tetany.

Treatment: discontinue the administration of sodium bicarbonate, rebreathe expired air or, if more severe administer calcium gluconate especially if tetany is present. In severe alkalosis, an infusion of 2.14% ammonium chloride is recommended, except in patients with pe-existing hepatic disease. If hypokalaemia is present administer potassium chloride.

5. PHARMACOLOGICAL PROPERTIES

5.1 Pharmacodynamic properties

Sodium bicarbonate therapy increases plasma bicarbonate, buffers excess hydrogen ion concentration, raises blood pH and reverses clinical manifestations of metabolic acidosis.

5.2 Pharmacokinetic properties

Sodium bicarbonate is eliminated principally in the urine and effectively alkalises it.

5.3 Preclinical safety data

Not applicable since sodium bicarbonate has been used in clinical practice for many years and its effects in man are well known.

6. PHARMACEUTICAL PARTICULARS

6.1 List of excipients

Water for Injection USP

6.2 Incompatibilities

The addition of sodium bicarbonate to parenteral solutions containing calcium should be avoided except where compatibility has been previously established; precipitation or haze may result, should this occur, the solution should not be used.

6.3 Shelf life

36 months.

6.4 Special precautions for storage

Store below 25°C.

6.5 Nature and contents of container

The solution is contained in a USP type I glass vial with an elastomeric closure which meets all the relevant USP specifications.

The 4.2% w/v is available as 10ml.

6.6 Instructions for use and handling

The container is specially designed for use with the IMS Minijet injector.

Administrative Data

7. MARKETING AUTHORISATION HOLDER

International Medication Systems (UK) Limited

208 Bath Road

Slough

Berkshire

SL1 3WE

UK

8. MARKETING AUTHORISATION NUMBER(S)

PL 3265/0001R

9. DATE OF FIRST AUTHORISATION/RENEWAL OF THE AUTHORISATION

Date first granted: 28 February 1991

Date renewed: 29 November 1996

10. DATE OF REVISION OF THE TEXT

April 2001

POM

Sofradex Ear / Eye Drops

(sanofi-aventis)

1. NAME OF THE MEDICINAL PRODUCT

Sofradex Ear/Eye Drops.

2. QUALITATIVE AND QUANTITATIVE COMPOSITION

Each bottle contains 0.5% w/v of Framycetin Sulphate Ph.Eur., Dexamethasone Sodium Metasulphobenzoate (equivalent to 0.050% w/v of Dexamethasone) and 0.005% w/v of Gramicidin USP.

3. PHARMACEUTICAL FORM

Sterile clear colourless ear/eye drops.

4. CLINICAL PARTICULARS

4.1 Therapeutic indications

In the Eye: For the short term treatment of steroid responsive conditions of the eye when prophylactic antibiotic treatment is also required, after excluding the presence of fungal and viral disease.

In the Ear: Otitis Externa.

4.2 Posology and method of administration

DOSAGE

Adults (and the Elderly) and Children:

In the Eye: One or two drops applied to each affected eye up to six times daily or more frequently if required.

In the Ear: Two or three drops instilled into the ear three or four times daily.

ADMINISTRATION

Auricular and Ocular use.

4.3 Contraindications

Viral, fungal, tuberculous or purulent conditions of the eye. Use is contraindicated if glaucoma is present or herpetic keratitis (e.g. dendritic ulcer) is considered a possibility. Use of topical steroids in the latter condition can lead to extension of the ulcer and marked visual deterioration.

Otitis Externa should not be treated when the eardrum is perforated because of the risk of ototoxicity.

Hypersensitivity to the preparation.

4.4 Special warnings and special precautions for use

Topical corticosteroids should never be given for an undiagnosed red eye as inappropriate use is potentially blinding.

Treatment with corticosteroid/antibiotic combinations should not be continued for more than 7 days in the absence of any clinical improvement, since prolonged use may lead to occult extension of infections due to the masking effect of the steroid. Prolonged use may also lead to skin sensitisation and the emergence of resistant organisms.

Prolonged use may lead to the risk of adrenal suppression in infants.

Treatment with corticosteroid preparations should not be repeated or prolonged without regular review to exclude raised intraocular, pressure, cataract formation or unsuspected infections.

Aminoglycosides antibiotics may cause irreversible, partial or total deafness when given systemically or when applied topically to open wounds or damaged skin. This effect is dose related and is enhanced by renal or hepatic impairment. Although this effect has not been reported following ocular use, the possibility should be considered when high dose topical is given to small children or infants.

4.5 Interaction with other medicinal products and other forms of Interaction

None relevant to topical use

4.6 Pregnancy and lactation

Safety for use in pregnancy and lactation has not been established. There is inadequate evidence of safety in human pregnancy. Topical administration of corticosteroids to pregnant animals can cause abnormalities of foetal development including cleft palate and intrauterine growth retardation. There may therefore be a very small risk of such effects in the human foetus. There is a risk of foetal ototoxicity if aminoglycoside antibiotics preparations are administrated during pregnancy.

4.7 Effects on ability to drive and use machines

May cause transient blurring of vision on instillation. Warn patients not to drive or operate hazardous machinery unless vision is clear.

4.8 Undesirable effects

Hypersensitivity reactions, usually of the delayed type, may occur leading to irritation, burning, stinging, itching and dermatitis.

Topical steroid use may result in increased intraocular pressure leading to optic nerve damage, reduced visual acuity and visual field defects.

Intensive or prolonged use of topical corticosteroids may lead to formation of posterior subcapsular cataracts.

In those diseases causing thinning of the cornea or sclera, corticosteroid therapy may result in the thinning of the globe leading to perforation.

4.9 Overdose

Long-term intensive topical use may lead to systemic effects.

Oral ingestion of the contents of one bottle (up to 10ml) is unlikely to lead to any serious adverse effects.

5. PHARMACOLOGICAL PROPERTIES

5.1 Pharmacodynamic properties

Framycetin Sulphate is an aminoglycoside antibiotic with a spectrum of activity similar to that of neomycin, this includes Staph. aureus and most clinically significant gram negative organisms.

Gramicidin is an antimicrobial cyclic polypeptide active in vitro against many gram positive bacteria. It is used for the local treatment of susceptible infections, sometimes in combination with other antimicrobial agents and frequently with a corticosteroid.

Dexamethasone is a synthetic glucocorticoid and has the general properties as other corticosteroids.

5.2 Pharmacokinetic properties

Framycetin Sulphate absorption occurs from inflamed skin and wounds. Once absorbed it is rapidly excreted by the kidneys in active form. It has been reported to have a half life of 2-3 hours

Gramicidin has properties similar to those of Tyrothricin and is too toxic to be administered systemically.

Dexamethasone is readily absorbed from the gastro-intestinal tract. It has a biological half-life in plasma of about 190 minutes.

5.3 Preclinical safety data

Not applicable.

6. PHARMACEUTICAL PARTICULARS

6.1 List of excipients

The ear/eye drops contains Citric Acid BP, Sodium Citrate BP, Lithium Chloride, Phenylethyl Alcohol, Industrial Methylated Spirit BP, Polysorbate 80 BP, Purified Water BP.

6.2 Incompatibilities

None known.

6.3 Shelf life

24 Months.

Discard contents 28 days after opening.

6.4 Special precautions for storage

Store below 25°C, do not refrigerate.

6.5 Nature and contents of container

Glass bottle fitted with a special dropper attachment: Pack size of 8 or 10ml.

Plastic dropper bottle: Pack size of 5, 8 or 10ml.

6.6 Instructions for use and handling

Not applicable.

7. MARKETING AUTHORISATION HOLDER

Aventis Pharma Ltd

50 Kings Hill Avenue

Kings Hill

West Malling

Kent, ME19 4AH

United Kingdom

8. MARKETING AUTHORISATION NUMBER(S)

PL 04425/0210

9. DATE OF FIRST AUTHORISATION/RENEWAL OF THE AUTHORISATION

4th June 2005

10. DATE OF REVISION OF THE TEXT

June 2005

Legal Category: POM

Soframycin Eye Drops

(sanofi-aventis)

1. NAME OF THE MEDICINAL PRODUCT
Soframycin Eye Drops.

2. QUALITATIVE AND QUANTITATIVE COMPOSITION
Contains 0.5%w/v Framycetin Sulphate Ph.Eur.

3. PHARMACEUTICAL FORM
Eye Drops.

4. CLINICAL PARTICULARS

4.1 Therapeutic indications
The topical treatment of bacterial infections such as blepharitis, conjunctivitis, styes, infected corneal abrasions and burns of the eye caused by sensitive organisms.

It may also be used prophylactically in patients undergoing removal of ocular foreign bodies.

It may also be indicated for corneal ulcers.

4.2 Posology and method of administration
Adults (& Elderly) & Children:

For rapid effect, preferably during the daytime, one or two drops should be applied to each affected eye every one or two hours or more frequently if required.

Severe infections may require one or two drops every 15-20 minutes initially, reducing the frequency of instillation gradually as the infection is controlled.

4.3 Contraindications
Known hypersensitivity to framycetin or chemically related antibiotics or any of the other components in the preparation.

4.4 Special warnings and special precautions for use
1. Prolonged use of an anti-infective may result in the development of superinfection due to micro-organisms, including fungi, resistant to that anti-infective.

2. Contact lenses should be removed during the period of treatment.

3. Aminoglycosides have been reported to cause irreversible partial or total deafness when given systemically, topically to open wounds or broken skin, or intraperitoneally. These effects have not been reported with topical ocular administration of framycetin. However, the possibility should be considered when using high dose topical treatment in the elderly, small children, or those patients with renal or hepatic impairment.

4. In cases of severe infections the topical use of framycetin should be supplemented with appropriate systemic treatment.

4.5 Interaction with other medicinal products and other forms of Interaction
None relevant to topical use.

4.6 Pregnancy and lactation
There is inadequate evidence for the safety of framycetin in pregnancy and lactation, however, it has been used for many years with no direct evidence for ill consequences. Use should be only when considered essential by the physician.

4.7 Effects on ability to drive and use machines
Topical eye drop preparations may cause transient blurring of vision on instillation. Patients should be warned not to drive or operate hazardous machinery unless vision is clear.

4.8 Undesirable effects
Hypersensitivity reactions, usually of the delayed type, may occur with local treatment with framycetin (cross-sensitivity with other aminoglycoside antibiotics may occur). Irritation, stinging or burning, itching and dermatitis may sometimes occur.

4.9 Overdose
Not applicable.

5. PHARMACOLOGICAL PROPERTIES

5.1 Pharmacodynamic properties
Framycetin is an aminoglycoside antibiotic with a spectrum of activity similar to that of neomycin, this includes *Staph. aureus* and most clinically significant gram negative organisms.

It is not active against *Pseudomonas aeruginosa* and resistant strains of gram-negative bacteria which are more common than with gentamicin.

5.2 Pharmacokinetic properties
Absorption occurs from inflamed skin and wounds. Once absorbed it is rapidly excreted by the kidneys in active form. It has been reported to have a half life of 2-3 hours.

5.3 Preclinical safety data
Not applicable.

6. PHARMACEUTICAL PARTICULARS

6.1 List of excipients
The product contains citric acid, sodium citrate, sodium chloride, benzalkonium chloride solution, water for injection, sodium hydroxide and hydrochloric acid.

6.2 Incompatibilities
No major incompatibilities *in vivo* are known.

6.3 Shelf life
Finished Product: 36 months

After first opening the Container:

Discard contents 4 weeks after opening.

6.4 Special precautions for storage
Store below 25°C. Protect from light.

Avoid contamination during use.

6.5 Nature and contents of container
Polypropylene dropper bottle fitted with a plug and cap: Pack size of 5ml or 10ml.

6.6 Instructions for use and handling
Not applicable.

7. MARKETING AUTHORISATION HOLDER
Aventis Pharma Ltd.,

50 Kings Hill,

West Malling

Kent

ME19 4AH

United Kingdom

8. MARKETING AUTHORISATION NUMBER(S)
PL 04425/0331

9. DATE OF FIRST AUTHORISATION/RENEWAL OF THE AUTHORISATION
11 October 2002

10. DATE OF REVISION OF THE TEXT
30 June 2003

Solaraze 3%, gel

(Shire Pharmaceuticals Limited)

1. NAME OF THE MEDICINAL PRODUCT
Solaraze™ 3%, gel

2. QUALITATIVE AND QUANTITATIVE COMPOSITION
Each gram contains 30 mg diclofenac sodium (3% w/w).

For excipients, see section 6.1.

3. PHARMACEUTICAL FORM
Gel

A clear, transparent, colourless or pale yellow gel.

4. CLINICAL PARTICULARS

4.1 Therapeutic indications
For the treatment of actinic keratoses

4.2 Posology and method of administration
Use in Adults: Solaraze is applied locally to the skin 2 times daily and smoothed into the skin gently. The amount needed depends on the size of the lesion. Normally 0.5 grams (the size of a pea) of the gel is used on a 5 cm × 5 cm lesion site. The usual duration of therapy is from 60 to 90 days. Maximum efficacy has been observed with treatment duration towards the upper end of this range. Complete healing of the lesion(s) or optimal therapeutic effect may not be evident for up to 30 days following cessation of therapy. A maximum of 8 grams daily should not be exceeded. Long term efficacy has not been established.

Use in the Elderly: The usual adult dose may be used.

Use in Children: Dosage recommendations and indications for the use of Solaraze have not been established for use in children.

4.3 Contraindications
Solaraze is contraindicated in patients with a known hypersensitivity to diclofenac, benzyl alcohol, macrogol monomethyl ether 350 and/ or sodium hyaluronate.

Because of cross-reactions, the gel should not be used by patients who have experienced hypersensitivity reactions such as symptoms of asthma, allergic rhinitis or urticaria, to acetylsalicylic acid or other non-steroidal anti-inflammatory agents.

The use of Solaraze is contraindicated during the last trimester of pregnancy (see Section 4.6).

4.4 Special warnings and special precautions for use
The likelihood of systemic side effects occurring following the topical application of Solaraze is very small compared to the frequency of side effects with oral diclofenac, owing to low systemic absorption with Solaraze. This product should be used with caution in patients with a history of and/or active gastrointestinal ulceration or bleeding, or reduced heart, liver or renal function, since isolated cases of systemic adverse reactions consisting of renal affection, has been reported with topically administered antiphlogistics.

It is known that NSAIDs can interfere with platelet function. Although the likelihood of systemic side effects is very low, caution should be used in patients with intracranial haemorrhage and bleeding diathesis.

Direct sunlight, including solarium, should be avoided during treatment. If sensitivity skin reactions occur, discontinue use.

Solaraze should not be applied to skin wounds, infections or exfoliative dermatitis. It should not be allowed to come into contact with the eyes or mucous membranes.

4.5 Interaction with other medicinal products and other forms of Interaction
No drug interactions during treatment with Solaraze have been reported. After topical administration, systemic absorption is limited. Drug interactions applied to orally administered NSAIDs are improbable.

4.6 Pregnancy and lactation
Use in pregnancy: Solaraze is contraindicated during the last trimester of pregnancy (see Section 4.3) and should not be used during the first two trimesters of pregnancy unless clearly necessary. If used during pregnancy, Solaraze must not be applied to a large area of the skin (>30% of the body surface) and must not be used for long-term treatment (>3 weeks).

There are no adequate data from the use of diclofenac in pregnant women. Animals have shown reproductive toxicity (see section 5.3). The potential risk to humans is unknown.

The use of prostaglandin synthetase inhibitors in the second and third trimesters of pregnancy may result in:

- Functional renal injury in the foetus. From the 12th week: oligohydramnios (usually reversible after the end of treatment), or anamnios (particularly with prolonged exposure). After birth: kidney failure may persist (particularly with late and prolonged exposure).
- Pulmonary and cardiac toxicity in the foetus (pulmonary hypertension with preterm closing of the ductus arteriosus). The risk exists from the beginning of the 6th month and increases if administration is close to full term.
- Inhibition of the uterine contractions.
- Prolongation of pregnancy and labour.
- Increased risk of bleeding in the mother and child.
- Increased risk of oedema formation for the mother.

Use during lactation:- It is not expected that any measurable amount of diclofenac sodium would occur in breast milk following topical application. Solaraze can be used at the recommended therapeutic dose, however, Solaraze should not be applied to the breast area of nursing mothers.

4.7 Effects on ability to drive and use machines
Not applicable

4.8 Undesirable effects
Most frequently reported reactions include localised skin reactions such as contact dermatitis, erythema and rash or application site reactions such as inflammation, irritation, pain and blistering. In studies there appeared to be no age specific increase or pattern of reactions.

(see Table 1 on next page)

Patch testing of previously treated patients indicate a 2.18% probability of allergic contact dermatitis sensation (type IV) to diclofenac with as yet unknown clinical relevance. Cross-reactivity to other NSAIDs is not likely. Serum testing more than 100 patients indicated no presence of type I anti-diclofenac antibodies.

4.9 Overdose
Due to the low systemic absorption of Solaraze, overdosage is extremely unlikely as a result of topical use. However, the skin should be rinsed with water. There have been no clinical cases of ingestion of Solaraze inducing overdosage.

In the event of accidental ingestion resulting in significant systemic side effects, general therapeutic measures normally adopted to treat poisoning with non-steroidal anti-inflammatories should be used.

Supporting and symptomatic treatment should be given for complications such as renal failure, convulsions, gastrointestinal irritation and respiratory depression. Specific therapies such as forced diuresis and dialysis will probably not be therapeutic in eliminating NSAIDs due to their high rate of protein binding.

5. PHARMACOLOGICAL PROPERTIES

5.1 Pharmacodynamic properties
ATC-Code: D11 AX

Other Dermatologicals

Mechanisms of action: Diclofenac is a non-steroidal anti-inflammatory drug. The mechanism of action of diclofenac in actinic keratosis is not known but may be related to the inhibition of the cyclooxygenase pathway leading to reduced prostaglandin E_2 (PGE_2) synthesis. Efficacy of the treatment has only been demonstrated in placebo-controlled studies. Comparative studies with topical 5-fluorouracil have not been conducted. The long term beneficial effects of Solaraze has not been proven.

Pharmacodynamic Effects: Solaraze has been shown to clear AK lesions with maximum therapeutic effect seen 30 days after cessation of drug therapy.

5.2 Pharmacokinetic properties
Absorption: Mean absorption through the skin varies between <1-12% with large inter-individual variability.

Table 1

Organ system	Common (>1/100, <1/10)	Uncommon (>1/1000, < 1/100)	Rare (>1/10000, < 1/1000)	Isolated cases <1/10000
Eye disorders	Conjunctivitis	Eye pain, lacrimation disorder		
Gastrointestinal Disorders		Abdominal pain, diarrhoea, nausea		Gastrointestinal haemorrhage
General Disorders and Administration Site Conditions	Application site reactions (including inflammation, irritation, pain and tingling or blistering at the treatment site)			
Immune System Disorders	Topical application of large amounts may result in systemic effects including hypersensitivity			
Nervous System	Hyperesthesia, hypertonia, localised paraesthesia			
Renal and Urinary System Disorders				Renal failure
Skin and Subcutaneous Tissue Disorders	Contact dermatitis, dry skin, erythema, oedema, pruritus, rash, scaly rash, skin hypertrophy, skin ulcer, vesiculobullous rash	Alopecia, face oedema, maculopapular rash, photosensitivity reaction, seborrhoea		
Vascular Disorders		Haemorrhage		

Absorption is dependant on the amount of the topical dose applied and the site of application.

Distribution: Diclofenac binds highly to serum albumin.

Biotransformation: Biotransformation of diclofenac involves partly conjugation of the intact molecule, but mainly single and multiple hydroxylations resulting in several phenolic metabolites, most of which are converted to glucuronide conjugates. Two of these phenolic metabolites are biologically active, however to a much lesser extent than diclofenac. Metabolism of diclofenac following percutaneous and oral administration is similar.

Elimination: Diclofenac and its metabolites are excreted mainly in the urine. Systemic clearance of diclofenac from plasma is 263 ± 56 ml/min (mean value ± SD) following oral administration. Terminal plasma half-life is short (1-2 hours). For the metabolites also have short terminal half-lives of 1-3 hours.

Pharmacokinetics in special patient populations: After topical application, the absorption of diclofenac in normal and compromised epidermis are comparable although there is a large inter-individual variation. Systemic absorption of diclofenac is approximately 12% of the administered dose for compromised skin and 9% for intact skin.

5.3 Preclinical safety data

Published animal studies have shown that when given orally, the principal adverse effect is on the gastrointestinal tract. Diclofenac inhibited ovulation in the rabbit and impaired implantation, as well as the early embryonic development, in the rat. The embryo/foetal-toxic potential of diclofenac was evaluated in three animal species (rat, mouse and rabbit). Foetal death and growth retardation occurred at maternal toxic doses, however, on the basis of available data, diclofenac is not considered to be teratogenic. The gestation period and the duration of parturition were extended by diclofenac. Doses lower than maternal toxic ones did not affect the postnatal development. Results from extensive genotoxicity and carcinogenicity testing suggest that it is unlikely that diclofenac would pose a significant carcinogenic hazard to humans.

6. PHARMACEUTICAL PARTICULARS

6.1 List of excipients

Sodium hyaluronate, benzyl alcohol, macrogol monomethyl ether 350 and purified water

6.2 Incompatibilities

Not applicable.

6.3 Shelf life

3 years

6.4 Special precautions for storage

Do not store above 25°C.

6.5 Nature and contents of container

The product is supplied in an epoxy-phenolic lined sealed aluminium tube with a white polypropylene screw on cap with a pierced tip, in 25g and 50g sizes.

No all pack sizes may be marketed.

6.6 Instructions for use and handling

No special requirements.

Administrative Data

7. MARKETING AUTHORISATION HOLDER

Shire Pharmaceutical Contracts Ltd

Hampshire International Business Park

Chineham

Basingstoke

Hampshire RG24 8EP, UK

8. MARKETING AUTHORISATION NUMBER(S)

PL 08081/0034

9. DATE OF FIRST AUTHORISATION/RENEWAL OF THE AUTHORISATION

15 November 2002

10. DATE OF REVISION OF THE TEXT

October 2004

LEGAL CATEGORY

POM

Solian

(sanofi-aventis)

1. NAME OF THE MEDICINAL PRODUCT

SOLIAN 50

SOLIAN 100

SOLIAN 200

SOLIAN 400

Solian® Solution, 100mg/ml

2. QUALITATIVE AND QUANTITATIVE COMPOSITION

Active ingredient: Amisulpride (INN) 50 mg, 100 mg, 200 mg or 400 mg per tablet; Solian Solution: Amisulpride (INN) 100 mg/ml.

For excipients, see 6.1.

3. PHARMACEUTICAL FORM

Solian 50, 100, 200, 400: Tablet

Solian Solution: Oral Solution. A clear yellow liquid in appearance.

4. CLINICAL PARTICULARS

4.1 Therapeutic indications

Solian is indicated for the treatment of acute and chronic schizophrenic disorders, in which positive symptoms (such as delusions, hallucinations, thought disorders) and/or negative symptoms (such as blunted affect, emotional and social withdrawal) are prominent, including patients characterised by predominant negative symptoms.

4.2 Posology and method of administration

For acute psychotic episodes, oral doses between 400 mg/d and 800 mg/d are recommended. In individual cases, the daily dose may be increased up to 1200 mg/d. Doses above 1200 mg/d have not been extensively evaluated for safety and therefore should not be used. No specific titration is required when initiating the treatment with Solian. Doses should be adjusted according to individual response.

For patients with mixed positive and negative symptoms, doses should be adjusted to obtain optimal control of positive symptoms.

Maintenance treatment should be established individually with the minimally effective dose.

For patients characterised by predominant negative symptoms, oral doses between 50 mg/d and 300 mg/d are recommended. Doses should be adjusted individually.

Solian can be administered once daily at oral doses up to 300 mg, higher doses should be administered bid.

Elderly: Solian should be used with particular caution because of a possible risk of hypotension or sedation.

Children: Solian is contra-indicated in children under 15 years of age as its safety has not yet been established.

Renal insufficiency: Solian is eliminated by the renal route. In renal insufficiency, the dose should be reduced to half in patients with creatinine clearance (CR_{CL}) between 30-60 ml/min and to a third in patients with CR_{CL} between 10-30 ml/min.

As there is no experience in patients with severe renal impairment (CR_{CL} < 10 ml/min) particular care is recommended in these patients (see 4.4 Special warning and precautions for use)

Hepatic insufficiency: since the drug is weakly metabolised a dosage reduction should not be necessary.

4.3 Contraindications

- Hypersensitivity to the active ingredient or to other ingredients of the drug
- Concomitant prolactin-dependent tumours e.g. pituitary gland prolactinomas and breast cancer
- Phaeochromocytoma
- Children under 15 years of age
- Pregnancy or lactation
- Women of childbearing potential unless using adequate contraception
- Combination with the following medications which could induce torsades de pointes:

- Class Ia antiarrhythmic agents such as quinidine, disopyramide, procainamide.

- Class III antiarrhythmic agents such as amiodarone, sotalol.

- Others medications such as bepridil, cisapride, sultopride, thioridazine, IV erythromycin, IV vincamine, halofantrine, pentamidine, sparfloxacin.

- This list is not exhaustive.
- Combination with levodopa

(see 4.5 Interactions with other medical products and other forms of interaction)

4.4 Special warnings and special precautions for use

As with other neuroleptics, Neuroleptic Malignant Syndrome, characterized by hyperthermia, muscle rigidity, autonomic instability, altered consciousness and elevated CPK, may occur. In the event of hyperthermia, particularly with high daily doses, all antipsychotic drugs including Solian should be discontinued.

Solian is eliminated by the renal route. In cases of severe renal insufficiency, the dose should be decreased and intermittent treatment should be considered (see 4.2 Posology and method of administration).

Solian may lower the seizure threshold. Therefore patients with a history of epilepsy should be closely monitored during Solian therapy.

In elderly patients, Solian, like other neuroleptics, should be used with particular caution because of a possible risk of hypotension or sedation.

As with other antidopaminergic agents, caution should be also exercised when prescribing Solian to patients with Parkinson's disease since it may cause worsening of the disease. Solian should be used only if neuroleptic treatment cannot be avoided.

Acute withdrawal symptoms including nausea, vomiting and insomnia have very rarely been described after abrupt cessation of high doses of antipsychotic drugs. Recurrence of psychotic symptoms may also occur, and the emergence of involuntary movement disorders (such as akathisia, dystonia and dyskinesia) has been reported. Therefore, gradual withdrawal is advisable.

Prolongation of the QT interval

Amisulpride induces a dose-dependent prolongation of the QT interval. This effect, known to potentiate the risk of serious ventricular arrhythmias such as torsades de pointes is enhanced by the pre-existence of bradycardia, hypokalaemia, congenital or acquired long QT interval.

Hypokalaemia should be corrected.

Before any administration, and if possible according to the patient's clinical status, it is recommended to monitor factors which could favour the occurrence of this rhythm disorder:

- bradycardia less than 55 bpm,
- hypokalaemia,
- congenital prolongation of the QT interval.

- on-going treatment with a medication likely to produce pronounced bradycardia (< 55 bpm), hypokalaemia, decreased intracardiac conduction, or prolongation of the QTc interval (see 4.5 Interaction with other medicinal products and other forms of interaction).

4.5 Interaction with other medicinal products and other forms of Interaction

COMBINATIONS WHICH ARE CONTRAINDICATED

Medications which could induce torsades de pointes

- Class Ia antiarrhythmic agents such as quinidine, disopyramide, procainamide.

- Class III antiarrhythmic agents such as amiodarone, sotalol.

- Others medications such as bepridil, cisapride, sultopride, thioridazine, V erythromycin, IV vincamine, halofantrine, pentamidine, sparfloxacin.

This list is not exhaustive.

Levodopa: reciprocal antagonism of effects between levodopa and neuroleptics.

COMBINATIONS WHICH ARE NOT RECOMMENDED

Solian may enhance the central effects of alcohol.

COMBINATIONS WHICH REQUIRE PRECAUTIONS FOR USE

Medications which enhance the risk of torsades de pointes:

- Bradycardia-inducing medications such as beta-blockers, bradycardia- inducing calcium channel blockers such as diltiazem and verapamil, clonidine, guanfacine; digitalis.

- Medications which induce hypokalaemia: hypokalemic diuretics, stimulant laxatives, IV amphotericin B, glucocorticoids, tetracosactides.

- Neuroleptics such as pimozide, haloperidol; imipramine antidepressants; lithium

COMBINATIONS TO BE TAKEN INTO ACCOUNT

CNS depressants including narcotics, anaesthetics, analgesics, sedative H1 antihistamines, barbiturates, benzodiazepines and other anxiolytic drugs, clonidine and derivatives

Antihypertensive drugs and other hypotensive medications

Dopamine agonists (eg: levodopa) since it may attenuate their action

4.6 Pregnancy and lactation

Pregnancy

In animals, Solian did not show reproductive toxicity. A decrease in fertility linked to the pharmacological effects of the drug (prolactin mediated effect) was observed. No teratogenic effects of Solian were noted.

The safety of Solian during human pregnancy has not been established. Therefore, use of the drug is contraindicated during pregnancy and in women of child bearing potential unless using adequate contraception.

Lactation

It is not known whether Solian is excreted in breast milk, breast-feeding is therefore contra-indicated.

4.7 Effects on ability to drive and use machines

Even used as recommended, Solian may affect reaction time so that the ability to drive vehicles or operate machinery can be impaired.

4.8 Undesirable effects

The following adverse effects have been observed in controlled clinical trials. It should be noted that in some instances it can be difficult to differentiate adverse events from symptoms of the underlying disease.

Common adverse effects (5-10 %):

insomnia, anxiety, agitation

Less common adverse effects (0.1-5 %):

somnolence, gastrointestinal disorders such as constipation, nausea, vomiting, dry mouth.

As with other neuroleptics:

Solian causes an increase in plasma prolactin levels which is reversible after drug discontinuation. This may result in galactorrhoea, amenorrhoea, gynaecomastia, breast pain, orgasmic dysfunction and impotence.

Weight gain may occur under therapy with Solian.

Acute dystonia (spasm torticolis, oculogyric crisis, trismus) may appear. This is reversible without discontinuation of Solian upon treatment with an antiparkinsonian agent.

Extrapyramidal symptoms may occur: tremor, rigidity, hypokinesia, hypersalivation, akathisia. These symptoms are generally mild at optimal dosages and partially reversible without discontinuation of Solian upon administration of antiparkinsonian medication. The incidence of extrapyramidal symptoms which is dose related, remains very low in the treatment of patients with predominantly negative symptoms with doses of 50-300mg/day.

Tardive dyskinesia characterised by rhythmic, involuntary movements primarily of the tongue and/or face have been reported, usually after long term administration. Antiparkinsonian medication is ineffective or may induce aggravation of the symptoms.

Hypotension and bradycardia have been reported occasionally. Cases of QT prolongation and very rare cases of torsades de pointes have been reported.

Acute withdrawal reactions have very rarely been reported (see Section 4.4).

Allergic reactions, elevations of hepatic enzymes, mainly transaminases and cases of seizures have been very rarely reported.

Very rare cases of Neuroleptic Malignant Syndrome have been reported (see 4.4 Special warnings and precautions for use).

4.9 Overdose

Experience with Solian in overdosage is limited. Exaggeration of the known pharmacological effects of the drug have been reported. These include drowsiness and sedation, coma, hypotension and extrapyramidal symptoms.

In cases of acute overdosage, the possibility of multiple drug intake should be considered.

Since Solian is weakly dialysed, hemodialysis is of no use to eliminate the drug.

There is no specific antidote to Solian.

Appropriate supportive measures should therefore be instituted with close supervision of vital functions including continuous cardiac monitoring due to the risk of prolongation of the QT interval.

If severe extrapyramidal symptoms occur, anticholinergic agents should be administered.

5. PHARMACOLOGICAL PROPERTIES

5.1 Pharmacodynamic properties

Amisulpride binds selectively with a high affinity to human dopaminergic D_2/D_3 receptor subtypes whereas it is devoid of affinity for D_1, D_4 and D_5 receptor subtypes.

Unlike classical and atypical neuroleptics, amisulpride has no affinity for serotonin, $\propto$-adrenergic, histamine H_1 and cholinergic receptors. In addition, amisulpride does not bind to sigma sites.

In animal studies, at high doses, amisulpride blocks dopamine receptors located in the limbic structures in preference to those in the striatum.

At low doses it preferentially blocks pre-synaptic D_2/D_3 receptors, producing dopamine release responsible for its disinhibitory effects.

This pharmacological profile explains the clinical efficacy of Solian against both negative and positive symptoms of schizophrenia.

5.2 Pharmacokinetic properties

In man, amisulpride shows two absorption peaks: one which is attained rapidly, one hour post-dose and a second between 3 and 4 hours after administration. Corresponding plasma concentrations are 39 ± 3 and 54 ± 4 ng/ml after a 50 mg dose.

The volume of distribution is 5.8 l/kg, plasma protein binding is low (16%) and no drug interactions are suspected.

Absolute bioavailability is 48%. Amisulpride is weakly metabolised: two inactive metabolites, accounting for approximately 4% of the dose, have been identified. There is no accumulation of amisulpride and its pharmacokinetics remain unchanged after the administration of repeated doses. The elimination half-life of amisulpride is approximately 12 hours after an oral dose.

Amisulpride is eliminated unchanged in the urine. Fifty percent of an intravenous dose is excreted via the urine, of which 90% is eliminated in the first 24 hours. Renal clearance is in the order of 20 l/h or 330 ml/min.

A carbohydrate rich meal (containing 68% fluids) significantly decreases the AUCs, Tmax and Cmax of amisulpride but no changes were seen after a high fat meal. However, the significance of these findings in routine clinical use is not known.

Hepatic insufficiency: since the drug is weakly metabolised a dosage reduction should not be necessary in patients with hepatic insufficiency.

Renal insufficiency: The elimination half-life is unchanged in patients with renal insufficiency while systemic clearance is reduced by a factor of 2.5 to 3. The AUC of amisulpride in mild renal failure increased two fold and almost tenfold in moderate renal failure (see chapter 4.2). Experience is however limited and there is no data with doses greater than 50 mg.

Amisulpride is very weakly dialysed.

Limited pharmacokinetic data in elderly subjects > 65 years) show that a 10-30 % rise occurs in Cmax, T1/2 and AUC after a single oral dose of 50 mg. No data are available after repeat dosing.

5.3 Preclinical safety data

An overall review of the completed safety studies indicates that Solian is devoid of any general, organ-specific, teratogenic, mutagenic or carcinogenic risk. Changes observed in rats and dogs at doses below the maximum tolerated dose are either pharmacological effects or are devoid of major toxicological significance under these conditions. Compared with the maximum recommended dosages in man, maximum tolerated doses are 2 and 7 times greater in the rat (200 mg/kg/d) and dog (120 mg/kg/d) respectively in terms of AUC. No carcinogenic risk, relevant to man, was identified in the rat at up to 1.5 to 4.5 times the expected human AUC.

A mouse carcinogenicity study (120 mg/kg/d) and reproductive studies (160, 300 and 500 mg/kg/d respectively in rat, rabbit and mouse) were performed. The exposure of the animals to amisulpride during these latter studies was not evaluated.

6. PHARMACEUTICAL PARTICULARS

6.1 List of excipients

Solian 50mg,100mg & 200mg tablets

Sodium starch glycolate, lactose monohydrate, microcrystalline cellulose, hypromellose, magnesium stearate.

Solian 400mg tablets

Sodium starch glycollate, lactose monohydrate, microcrystalline cellulose, hypromellose, magnesium stearate, polyoxyl 40 stearate, titanium dioxide (E171).

Solian Solution

Saccharin sodium, sodium gluconate, glucono delta lactone, hydrochloric acid, methyl parahydroxybenzoate, propyl parahydroxybenzoate, potassium sorbate, caramel flavour (tonka beans extract, vanillin, benzaldehyde, acetyl methyl carbinol, gamma and delta decalactones, esters from acetic, butyric and 2 methyl utyric acid, esters from ethyl and cinnamyl alcohol, propylene glycol and ethyl alcohol), purified water.

6.2 Incompatibilities

None known.

6.3 Shelf life

Tablets:

3 years

Solution:

Shelf life of the medicinal product as packaged for sale: 3 years

Shelf life after first opening the container: 2 months

Dispose of within two months of opening.

6.4 Special precautions for storage

No special precautions.

6.5 Nature and contents of container

Tablets: PVC/aluminium foil blister packs containing 60 tablets

Solution: 60 ml brown glass bottle (type III) and child resistant cap with a PVDC/PE seal, with a 5ml graduated oral syringe.

6.6 Instructions for use and handling

No special precautions

7. MARKETING AUTHORISATION HOLDER

Sanofi-Synthelabo Limited

One Onslow Street

Guildford

Surrey

GU1 4YS

United Kingdom

8. MARKETING AUTHORISATION NUMBER(S)

50mg tablets: PL 11723/0308

100mg tablets: PL 11723/0355

200mg tablets: PL 11723/0309

400mg tablets: PL 11723/0356

Solution: PL 11723/0377

9. DATE OF FIRST AUTHORISATION/RENEWAL OF THE AUTHORISATION

50 mg tablets February 2001

100mg, 400mg tablets September 2000

200mg tablets January 2001

Solution May 2001

10. DATE OF REVISION OF THE TEXT

50mg, 100mg, 200mg: December 2004

400mg tablets: March 2004

Solution: October 2004

Legal Category: POM

Solpadol Capsules, Solpadol Effervescent Tablets, Solpadol Caplets

(sanofi-aventis)

1. NAME OF THE MEDICINAL PRODUCT

Solpadol Caplets Tablets.

Solpadol Capsules

Solpadol Effervescent Tablets

2. QUALITATIVE AND QUANTITATIVE COMPOSITION

Active Constituents

Paracetamol 500.0mg

Codeine Phosphate Hemihydrate 30.0mg

For excipients see 6.1.

3. PHARMACEUTICAL FORM

Tablets:

Solpadol Caplets are white capsule shaped tablets, marked SOLPADOL on one side.

Capsules:

Solpadol Capsules are grey and purple with SOLPADOL printed on them in black ink.

Effervescent Tablets:

Solpadol Effervescent Tablets are white bevelled-edge tablets scored on one face.

4. CLINICAL PARTICULARS

4.1 Therapeutic indications

For the relief of severe pain.

4.2 Posology and method of administration

Adults: Two tablets not more frequently than every 4 hours, up to a maximum of 8 tablets in any 24 hour period.

Elderly: As adults, however a reduced dose may be required. See warnings.

Children: Not recommended for children under 12 years of age.

Solpadol Caplets, Capsules and Effervescent tablets are for oral administration.

4.3 Contraindications

Hypersensitivity to paracetamol or codeine which is rare.

Hypersensitivity to any of the other constituents.

Conditions where morphine and opioids are contraindicated e.g:

- Acute asthma
- Respiratory depression
- Acute alcoholism
- Head injuries
- Raised intra-cranial pressure
- Following biliary tract surgery

Monoamine oxidase inhibitor therapy, concurrent or within 14 days.

4.4 Special warnings and special precautions for use

Care should be observed in administering the product to any patient whose condition may be exacerbated by opioids, particularly the elderly, who may be sensitive to their central and gastro-intestinal effects, those on concurrent CNS depressant drugs, those with prostatic hypertrophy and those with inflammatory or obstructive bowel disorders. Care should also be observed if prolonged therapy is contemplated.

Care is advised in the administration of paracetamol to patients with severe renal or severe hepatic impairment. The hazards of overdose are greater in those with alcoholic liver disease.

Patients should be advised not to exceed the recommended dose and not take other paracetamol containing products concurrently.

Patients should be advised to consult a doctor should symptoms persist and to keep the product out of the reach of children.

Solpadol Effervescent Tablets only:

Each effervescent tablet of the soluble formulation contains 388mg sodium (16.87mEquivalents). This sodium content should be taken into account when prescribing for patients in whom sodium restriction is indicated.

As the effervescent tablets contain sorbitol, patients with rare heretidary problems of fructose intolerance should not take this medicine.

4.5 Interaction with other medicinal products and other forms of Interaction

Paracetamol may increase the elimination half-life of chloramphenicol. Oral contraceptives may increase its rate of clearance. The speed of absorption of paracetamol may be increased by metoclopramide or domperidone and absorption reduced by colestyramine.

The anticoagulant effect of warfarin and other coumarins may be enhanced by prolonged regular use of paracetamol with increased risk of bleeding; occasional doses have no significant effect.

The effects of CNS depressants (including alcohol) may be potentiated by codeine.

4.6 Pregnancy and lactation

There is inadequate evidence of the safety of codeine in human pregnancy, but there is epidemiological evidence for the safety of paracetamol. Both substances have been used for many years without apparent ill consequences and animal studies have not shown any hazard. Nonetheless careful consideration should be given before prescribing the products for pregnant patients. Opioid analgesics may depress neonatal respiration and cause withdrawal effects in neonates of dependent mothers.

Paracetamol is excreted in breast milk but not in a clinically significant amount.

4.7 Effects on ability to drive and use machines

Patients should be advised not to drive or operate machinery if affected by dizziness or sedation.

4.8 Undesirable effects

Codeine can produce typical opioid effects including constipation, nausea, vomiting, dizziness, light-headedness, confusion, drowsiness and urinary retention. The frequency and severity are determined by dosage, duration of treatment and individual sensitivity. Tolerance and dependence can occur, especially with prolonged high dosage of codeine.

Adverse effects of paracetamol are rare but hypersensitivity including skin rash may occur. There have been reports of blood dyscrasias including thrombocytopenia and agranulocytosis, but these were not necessarily causally related to paracetamol.

4.9 Overdose

Codeine

The effects of Codeine overdosage will be potentiated by simultaneous ingestion of alcohol and psychotropic drugs.

Symptoms

Central nervous system depression, including respiratory depression, may develop but is unlikely to be severe unless other sedative agents have been co-ingested, including alcohol, or the overdose is very large. The pupils may be pin-point in size; nausea and vomiting are common. Hypotension and tachycardia are possible but unlikely.

Management

Management should include general symptomatic and supportive measures including a clear airway and monitoring of vital signs until stable. Consider activated charcoal if an adult presents within one hour of ingestion of more than 350 mg or a child more than 5 mg/kg.

Give naloxone if coma or respiratory depression is present. Naloxone is a competitive antagonist and has a short half-life so large and repeated doses may be required in a seriously poisoned patient. Observe for at least 4 hours after ingestion, or 8 hours if a sustained release preparation has been taken.

Paracetamol

Patients in whom oxidative liver enzymes have been induced, including alcoholics and those receiving barbiturates, and patients who are chronically malnourished, may be particularly sensitive to the toxic effects of paracetamol in overdose.

Symptoms

Symptoms of paracetamol overdosage in the first 24 hours are pallor, nausea, vomiting, anorexia and abdominal pain. Liver damage may become apparent 12 to 48 hours after ingestion. Abnormalities of glucose metabolism and metabolic acidosis may occur. In severe poisoning, hepatic failure may progress to encephalopathy, coma and death. Acute renal failure with acute tubular necrosis may develop even in the absence of severe liver damage. Cardiac arrhythmias and pancreatitis have been reported.

Liver damage is likely in adults who have taken 10g or more of paracetamol. It is considered that excess quantities of a toxic metabolite (usually adequately detoxified by glutathione when normal doses of paracetamol are ingested), become irreversibly bound to liver tissue.

Management

Immediate treatment is essential in the management of paracetamol overdose. Despite a lack of significant early symptoms, patients should be referred to hospital urgently for immediate medical attention and any patient who has ingested around 7.5g or more of paracetamol in the preceding 4 hours should undergo gastric lavage. Administration of oral methionine or intravenous N-acetylcysteine which may have a beneficial effect up to at least 48 hours after the overdose, may be required. General supportive measures must be available.

5. PHARMACOLOGICAL PROPERTIES

5.1 Pharmacodynamic properties

Pharmacotherapeutic group: Anilides, Paracetamol combinations

ATC Code: NO2B E51

Paracetamol is an analgesic which acts peripherally, probably by blocking impulse generation at the bradykinin sensitive chemo-receptors which evoke pain. Although it is a prostaglandin synthetase inhibitor, the synthetase system in the CNS rather than the periphery appears to be more sensitive to it. This may explain paracetamol's lack of appreciable anti-inflammatory activity. Paracetamol also exhibits antipyretic activity.

Codeine is a centrally acting analgesic which produces its effect by its action at opioid-binding sites (μ-receptors) within the CNS. It is a full agonist.

5.2 Pharmacokinetic properties

Following oral administration of two tablets (ie, a dose of paracetamol 1000mg and codeine 60mg) the mean maximum plasma concentrations of paracetamol and codeine were 15.96μg/ml and 212.4ng/ml respectively. The mean times to maximum plasma concentrations were 0.88 hours for paracetamol and 1.05 hours for codeine.

The mean AUC for the 9 hours following administration was 49.05μg.ml $^{-1}$.h for paracetamol and 885.0 ng/ml $^{-1}$.h for codeine.

The bioavailabilities of paracetamol and codeine when given as the combination are similar to those when they are given separately.

5.3 Preclinical safety data

There are no preclinical data of relevance which are additional to that already included in other sections of the SPC.

6. PHARMACEUTICAL PARTICULARS

6.1 List of excipients

Caplets:

Pregelatinised starch

Maize starch

Povidone

Potassium sorbate

Microcrystalline cellulose

Stearic acid

Talc

Magnesium stearate

Croscarmellose sodium (type A).

Capsules:

Maize starch

Magnesium stearate

Talc

Indigotine E132

Azorubine E122

Titanium dioxide E171

Gelatin

Black iron oxide E172

Shellac

Soya lecithin

Anti-foam DC 1510.

Effervescent Tablets:

Sodium bicarbonate

Anhydrous citric acid

Anhydrous sodium carbonate

Sorbitol powder

Saccharin sodium

Povidone

Dimeticone

Sodium lauril sulfate.

6.2 Incompatibilities

None known.

6.3 Shelf life

Caplets: 5 years.

Capsules: 3 years

Effervescent Tablets: 4 years in PPFP strips

6.4 Special precautions for storage

Store in the original package. Do not store above 25°C.

6.5 Nature and contents of container

Caplets:

PVC/aluminium foil (250μm/20μm) or PVC/aluminium foil (250μm/20μm) / PVC (15μm) blister packs. Pack sizes: 30 and 100 tablets.

Capsules:

White, opaque PVC (250μm)/aluminium foil (20μm) blister packs or White, opaque PVC (250μm)/aluminium foil (20μm)/ PVC (15μm) blister packs contained in cardboard cartons.

Pack sizes of 30 and 100 capsules.

Effervescent Tablets:

PPFP strips in cardboard containers.

Pack sizes: 30 and 100 tablets.

6.6 Instructions for use and handling

Caplets & Capsules: no special requirements.

Effervescent Tablets: should be dissolved in half a tumblerful of water before taking.

7. MARKETING AUTHORISATION HOLDER

Sanofi-Synthelabo

One Onslow Street

Guildford

Surrey

GU1 4YS

8. MARKETING AUTHORISATION NUMBER(S)

Solpadol Caplets: PL 11723/0071

Solpadol Capsules: PL 11723/0117

Solpadol Effervescent Tablets: PL 11723/0072

9. DATE OF FIRST AUTHORISATION/RENEWAL OF THE AUTHORISATION

Solpadol Caplets: 10 March 1997/ 2nd November 2004

Solpadol Capsules: 29th December 1994/ 2nd November 2004

Solpadol Effervescent Tablets: 11th March 1996/ 2nd November 2004

10. DATE OF REVISION OF THE TEXT

October 2004

Legal Category: POM

Soltamox 10mg/5ml

(Rosemont Pharmaceuticals Limited)

1. NAME OF THE MEDICINAL PRODUCT

Soltamox 10mg/5ml Oral Solution

2. QUALITATIVE AND QUANTITATIVE COMPOSITION

Each 5ml dose of oral solution contains tamoxifen 10mg (as tamoxifen citrate)

For excipients, see section 6.1.

3. PHARMACEUTICAL FORM

Oral Solution

A clear colourless liquid

4. CLINICAL PARTICULARS

4.1 Therapeutic indications

- Adjuvant treatment of breast cancer following primary therapy. Metastatic breast cancer

4.2 Posology and method of administration

Breast Cancer ***Adults (including elderly)***

The dosage range is 20mg to 40mg daily, given either in divided doses twice daily or as a single dose once daily. If high doses have to be taken, dividing the daily dose is recommended.

Therapy with tamoxifen is usually a long-term treatment that should be monitored by physicians experienced in oncology. Currently, a treatment duration of at least 5 years is recommended for the adjuvant treatment of hormone-receptor positive early breast cancer. The optimal duration is still under investigation.

Children: Not applicable.

4.3 Contraindications

Pregnancy

Use in children

Hypersensitivity to tamoxifen or to any of the excipients.

4.4 Special warnings and special precautions for use

Premenopausal patients must be carefully examined before treatment to exclude pregnancy.

Women should be informed of the potential risks to the foetus, should they become pregnant whilst taking tamoxifen; or within two months of cessation of therapy.

A number of secondary primary tumours, occurring at sites other than the endometrium and the opposite breast, have been reported in clinical trials, following the treatment of breast cancer patients with tamoxifen. No causal link has been established and the clinical significance of these observations remains unclear.

Menstruation is suppressed in a proportion of premenopausal women receiving tamoxifen for the treatment of breast cancer.

Any patients who have received tamoxifen therapy and have reported abnormal vaginal bleeding or patients presenting with menstrual irregularities, vaginal discharge and pelvic pressure or pain should undergo prompt investigationdue to the increased incidence of endometrial changes including hyperplasia, polyps, cancer and uterine sarcoma (mostly malignant mixed Mullerian tumours) which has been reported in association with tamoxifen treatment. The underlying mechanism is unknown, but may be related to the oestrogenic-like effect of tamoxifen. Before initiating tamoxifen a complete personal history should be taken. Physical examination (including pelvic examination) should be guided by the patients past medical history and by the 'contraindications' and 'special warnings and precautions for use' warnings for use for tamoxifen. During treatment periodic check-ups including gynaecological examination focussing on endometrial changes are recommended of a frequency and nature adapted to the individual woman and modified according to her clinical needs.

When starting tamoxifen therapy the patient should undergo an ophthalmological examination. If visual changes (cataracts and retinopathy) occur while on tamoxifen therapy it is urgent that an ophthalmological investigation be performed, because some of such changes may resolve after cessation of treatment if recognised at an early stage.

In cases of severe thrombocytopenia, leucocytopenia or hypercalcaemia, individual risk-benefit assessment and thorough medical supervision are necessary.

Venous thromboembolism

A 2-3-fold increase in the risk for VTE has been demonstrated in healthy tamoxifen-treated women (see section 4.8).

Prescribers should obtain careful histories with respect to the patient's personal and family history of VTE. If suggestive of a prothrombotic risk, patients should be screened for thrombophilic factors. Patients who test positive should be counselled regarding their thrombotic risk. The decision to use tamoxifen in these patients should be based on the overall risk to the patient. In selected patients, the use of tamoxifen with prophylactic anticoagulation may be justified (cross-reference section 4.5)

• The risk of VTE is further increased by severe obesity, increasing age and all other risk factors for VTE. The risks and benefits should be carefully considered for all patients before treatment with tamoxifen. This risk is also increased by concomitant chemotherapy (see section 4.5). Long-term anti-coagulant prophylaxis may be justified for some patients with breast cancer who have multiple risk factors for VTE.

• Surgery and immobility: Tamoxifen treatment should only be stopped if the risk of tamoxifen-induced thrombosis clearly outweighs the risks associated with interrupting treatment. All patients should receive appropriate thrombosis prophylactic measures and should include graduated compression stockings for the period of hospitalisation, early ambulation, if possible, and anti-coagulant treatment.

• If any patient presents with VTE, tamoxifen should be stopped immediately and appropriate anti-thrombosis measures initiated. The decision to re-start tamoxifen should be made with respect to the overall risk for the patient. In selected patients with breast cancer, the continued use of tamoxifen with prophylactic anticoagulation may be justified.

•All patients should be advised to contact their doctors immediately if they become aware of any symptoms of VTE.

The blood count including thrombocytes, liver function test and serum calcium should be controlled regularly.

Assessment of triglycerides in serum may be advisable because in most published cases of severe hypertriglyceridemia dyslipoproteinemia was the underlying disorder.

This product contains 19%v/v ethanol, i.e. up to 788mg per dose equivalent to 19ml of beer or 8ml of wine per dose. It is harmful for those suffering from alcoholism. It should be taken into account in pregnant or lactating women, children and high-risk groups such as patients with liver disease or epilepsy. It may modify or increase the effect of other medicines. The amount of alcohol in this product may impair the ability to drive or use machines.

This product contains glycerol which may cause headache, stomach upset and diarrhoea.

This product also contains sorbitol. Patients with rare hereditary problems of fructose intolerance should not take this medicine.

4.5 Interaction with other medicinal products and other forms of Interaction

Coumarin-type anti-coagulants:

When used in combination with tamoxifen solution a significant increase in anticoagulant effect may occur. In the case of concomitant treatment particularly during the initial phase thorough monitoring of the coagulation status is mandatory.

Thrombocyte aggregation inhibitors

In order to avoid bleeding during a possible thrombocytopenic interval thrombocyte aggregation inhibitors should not be combined with tamoxifen.

Cytotoxic agents:

When used in combination with tamoxifen solution there is increased risk of thromboembolic events occurring (see also Sections 4.4 and 4.8). Because of this increase in risk of VTE, thrombosis prophylaxis should be considered for these patients for the period of concomitant chemotherapy.

Tamoxifen and its metabolites have been found to be potent inhibitors of hepatic cytochrome p-450 mixed function oxidases. The effect of tamoxifen on metabolism and excretion of other antineoplastic drugs, such as cyclophosphamide and other drugs that require mixed function oxidases of activation, is not known.

Bromocriptine:

Tamoxifen increases the dopaminergic effect of bromocriptine.

Hormone preparations:

Hormone preparations, particularly oestrogens (e.g. oral contraceptives) should not be combined with tamoxifen because a mutual decrease in effect is possible.

As tamoxifen is metabolised by cytochrome P450 34A, care is required when co-administered with drugs known to induce this enzyme, such as rifampicin, as tamoxifen levels may be reduced. The clinical relevance of this reduction is unknown.

4.6 Pregnancy and lactation

Tamoxifen must not be taken during pregnancy. Pregnancy has to be excluded prior to prescribing tamoxifen. There have been a small number of reports of spontaneous abortions, birth defects and foetal deaths after women have taken tamoxifen, although no causal relationship has been established.

Women should be advised not to become pregnant whilst taking tamoxifen and within two months after stopping tamoxifen medication and should use barrier or other non-hormonal contraceptive methods if sexually active.

It is not known whether tamoxifen is excreted into breast milk and it is therefore not recommended for use in breast feeding mothers. The decision either to discontinue nursing or discontinue tamoxifen therapy should take into account the importance of the drug to the mother.

In rodent models of foetal reproductive tract development, tamoxifen was associated with changes similar to those caused by estradiol, ethinylestradiol, clomifene and diethylstilbestrol (DES). Although the clinical relevance of these changes is unknown, some of them, especially vaginal adenosis, are similar to those seen in young women who were exposed to DES in utero and who have a 1 in 1000 risk of developing clear-cell carcinoma of the vagina or cervix. Only a small number of pregnant women have been exposed to tamoxifen. Such exposure has not been reported to cause subsequent vaginal adenosis or clear cell carcinoma of the vagina or cervix in young women exposed in utero to tamoxifen.

Reproductive toxicology studies in rats, rabbits and monkeys have shown no teratogenic potential.

4.7 Effects on ability to drive and use machines

No studies on the effects of the ability to drive and use machines have been performed.

4.8 Undesirable effects

very common >1/10)	hot flushes, vaginal discharge, pruritus vulvae, vaginal bleeding
common >1/100, <1/10)	bone and tumour pain, fluid retention, increase in serum triglycerides, light-headedness, headache, corneal changes, cataracts and/or retinopathy, venous thromboembolic events (including deep vein thrombosis and pulmonary embolism), nausea, alopecia
uncommon >1/1000, <1/100)	hypercalcaemia, vomiting
rare >1/10,000, <1/1000)	temporary anaemia, temporary neutropenia, temporary thrombocytopenia, changes in liver enzymes, fatty liver, cholestasis and hepatitis Hypersensitivity, including angioneurotic oedema, skin rash, cystic ovarian swellings, uterine fibroids, endometrial changes, including hyperplasia and polyps, uterine sarcoma and cancer, suppression of menstruation
very rare (<1/10,000) including isolated reports.	severe neutropenia, pancytopenia, severe hypertriglyceridemia, pancreatitis, agranulocytosis, liver cell necrosis, erythema multiforme, Stevens-Johnson-syndrome, bullous pemphigoid, interstitial pneumonitis.

General

Hot flushes are very common partly due to the antioestrogenic effect of tamoxifen. Response to tamoxifen treatment is commonly accompanied by bone and tumour pain.

Blood and lymphatic system disorders

In breast cancer patients, temporary reductions in blood count such as temporary anaemia, neutropenia and temporary thrombocytopenia (usually to 80,000 - 90,000 per cu mm but occasionally lower) have been observed during tamoxifen treatment. Very rarely, severe neutropenia and pancytopenia were observed.

Endocrine disorders

Uncommonly, patients with bony metastases have developed hypercalcaemia on initiation of therapy.

Metabolism disorders

Fluid retention is common. Tamoxifen may commonly lead to an increase in serum triglycerides. Very rarely it may cause severe hypertriglyceridemia which may be partly combined with pancreatitis.

Nervous system disorders

Light-headedness and headache may occur.

Eye disorders

Commonly, cases of visual disturbances including corneal changes, cataracts and/or retinopathy that are only partly reversible have been reported. The risk for cataracts increases with the duration of tamoxifen treatment.

Vascular disorders

Venous thromboembolic events occur commonly. The risk of venous thromboembolic events including deep vein thrombosis and pulmonary embolism increases when tamoxifen is used in combination with cytotoxic agents.

Respiratory disorders

Very rarely, cases of interstitial pneumonitis have been reported.

Gastrointestinal disorders

Nausea was reported commonly and vomiting uncommonly.

Hepato-biliary disorders

Changes in liver enzyme levels, and rarely with more severe liver abnormalities including fatty liver, cholestasis and hepatitis. A single case of agranulocytosis and liver cell necrosis was reported.

Skin and Subcutaneous tissue disorders

Hypersensitivity, including angioneurotic oedema occurs rarely. Skin rash was observed and very rarely even erythema multiforme, Stevens-Johnson-syndrome or bullous pemphigoid.

Alopecia occurs commonly.

Gynaecological

Vaginal discharge, pruritus vulvae and vaginal bleeding are reported very commonly. An increased incidence in endometrial changes, including hyperplasia and polyps, endometrial cancer and uterine sarcoma (mostly malignant mixed Mullerian tumours) has been reported in association with tamoxifen. According to recent publications the risk for endometrial carcinoma increases with the duration of tamoxifen treatment to a frequency two- to four-fold higher compared with women not treated with tamoxifen. In a proportion of pre-menopausal women treated for breast cancer, there is a suppression of menstruation. Cystic ovarian swellings have occasionally been observed in pre-menopausal women. Uterine fibroids have been reported.

When undesirable events are severe it may be possible to control them by a simple reduction of dosage without loss of control of the disease. If undesirable events do not respond to this measure, it may be necessary to cease treatment.

4.9 Overdose

Little is known about overdoses in humans. At doses of 160mg/m^2 daily and higher, changes in ECG (QT-prolongation) and at doses of 300 mg/m^2 daily, neurotoxicity (tremor, hyperreflexia, gait disorders, and dizziness) occurred.

Overdosage of tamoxifen will increase the anti-oestrogenic effects. In animals, extremely high doses (over 100 times the recommended daily dosage) have caused oestrogenic effects.

There is no specific antidote to overdosage and treatment should therefore be symptomatic.

5. PHARMACOLOGICAL PROPERTIES

5.1 Pharmacodynamic properties

Pharmacotherapeutic group: Hormone antagonists and related agents

ATC Code: L02B A01

Tamoxifen is a non-steroidal anti-oestrogen and inhibits the effects of endogenous oestrogen, probably by binding with oestrogen receptors. Tamoxifen competes for the binding sites with estradiol and by occupying the receptor reduces the amount of receptor available for endogenous estradiol. Tamoxifen also prevents the normal feedback inhibition of oestrogen synthesis in the hypothalamus and in the pituitary.

Tamoxifen decreases cell division in oestrogen-dependent tissues. In metastatic breast cancer, partial or complete remissions were observed in 50-60% of cases, particularly in bone and soft tissue metastases if oestrogen-receptors were found in the tumour. In cases of negative hormone-receptor status, particularly of the metastases only approx. 10% showed objective remissions. Women with oestrogen receptor- positive tumours or tumours with unknown receptor status who received adjuvant treatment with tamoxifen experienced significantly less tumour recurrences and had a higher 10-year survival rate. The effect was greater after 5 years of adjuvant treatment compared with 1-2 years of treatment. The benefit appears to be independent of age, menopausal status, daily tamoxifen dose and additional chemotherapy.

5.2 Pharmacokinetic properties

After oral administration the compound is well-absorbed achieving maximum serum concentrations within 4 - 7 hours and is extensively metabolised. Elimination occurs, chiefly as conjugates with practically no unchanged drug, principally through the faeces and to a lesser extent through the kidneys.

Tamoxifen is highly protein bound to serum albumin >99%). Metabolism is by hydroxylation, demethylation and conjugation, giving rise to several metabolites which have a similar pharmacological profile to the parent compound and thus contribute to the therapeutic effect. Tamoxifen concentrations have been observed in lung, liver, adrenals, kidney, pancreas, uterus and mammary tissues. After four weeks of daily therapy, it was observed that steady state serum levels were achieved and an elimination half-life of seven days was calculated whereas that for N-desmethyltamoxifen, the principal circulating metabolite, is 14 days.

5.3 Preclinical safety data

Tamoxifen has proved to be effective in the treatment of some breast cancers. During this time, data has been generated relating to the safety of tamoxifen and its mode of action.

Reproductive toxicology studies in rats, rabbits and monkeys have shown no teratogenic potential.

Tamoxifen was not mutagenic in a range if *in vitro* and *in vivo* mutagenicity tests. Investigations in different in vivo and in vitro systems have shown that tamoxifen has a genotoxic potential following hepatic activation. Gonadal tumours in mice and liver tumours in rats receiving tamoxifen have been reported in long-term studies. The clinical relevance of these findings has not been established.

6. PHARMACEUTICAL PARTICULARS

6.1 List of excipients

Ethanol, glycerol, propylene glycol, sorbitol solution 70%, liquorice and aniseed flavours and purified water.

6.2 Incompatibilities

None known

6.3 Shelf life

2 years - unopened

After first opening - 3 months

6.4 Special precautions for storage

Do not store above 25°C. Store in the original package in order to protect from light.

6.5 Nature and contents of container

Bottle:Amber (Type III) glass

Closure:a) Aluminium, EPE wadded, roll-on pilfer-proof screw cap

b) HDPE, EPE wadded, tamper evident screw cap

c) HDPE, EPE wadded, tamper evident, child resistant closure.

Pack: 1 bottle with 150ml or 250ml oral solution

4 bottles with 250ml oral solution

Not all pack sizes may be marketed.

6.6 Instructions for use and handling

No special requirements.

Administrative Data

7. MARKETING AUTHORISATION HOLDER

Rosemont Pharmaceuticals Ltd, Rosemont House, Yorkdale Industrial Park, Braithwaite Street, Leeds, LS11 9XE, UK

8. MARKETING AUTHORISATION NUMBER(S)

00427/0121

9. DATE OF FIRST AUTHORISATION/RENEWAL OF THE AUTHORISATION

Date of first authorisation: 16 August 1999

Date of last renewal: 27 November 2004

10. DATE OF REVISION OF THE TEXT

November 2004

Soluble Prednisolone Tablets 5mg

(Sovereign Medical)

1. NAME OF THE MEDICINAL PRODUCT

Prednesol Tablets 5mg

Soluble Prednisolone Tablets 5mg

2. QUALITATIVE AND QUANTITATIVE COMPOSITION

Small, pink, soluble tablets engraved 'Pred 5 Sov' on one side and scored on the reverse. Each tablet contains 5mg prednisolone as the sodium phosphate ester.

3. PHARMACEUTICAL FORM

Tablet.

4. CLINICAL PARTICULARS

4.1 Therapeutic indications

A wide variety of diseases may sometimes require corticosteroid therapy. Some of the principal indications are:

- bronchial asthma, severe hypersensitivity reactions, anaphylaxis; rheumatoid arthritis, systemic lupus erythematosus, dermatomyositis, mixed connective tissue disease (excluding systemic sclerosis), polyarteritis nodosa;
- inflammatory skin disorders, including pemphigus vulgaris, bullous pemphigoid and pyoderma gangrenosum;
- minimal change nephrotic syndrome, acute interstitial nephritis;
- ulcerative colitis, Crohn's disease; sarcoidosis;
- rheumatic carditis;
- haemolytic anaemia (autoimmune), acute lymphoblastic and chronic lymphocytic leukaemia, malignant lymphoma, multiple myeloma, idiopathic thrombocytopenic purpura;
- immunosuppression in transplantation.

4.2 Posology and method of administration

Prednesol/Soluble Prednisolone Tablets are best taken dissolved in water, but they can be swallowed whole without difficulty.

The lowest dosage that will produce an acceptable result should be used (See precautions section); when it is possible to reduce the dosage, this must be accomplished by stages. During prolonged therapy any intercurrent illness, trauma or surgical procedure will require a temporary increase in dosage; if corticosteroids have been stopped following prolonged therapy they may need to be temporarily re-introduced.

Adults: The dose used will depend upon the disease, its severity, and the clinical response obtained. The following regimens are for guidance only. Divided dosage is usually employed.

Short-term treatment: 20 to 30mg daily for the first few days, subsequently reducing the daily dosage by 2.5 or 5mg every two to five days, depending upon the response.

Rheumatoid arthritis: 7.5 to 10mg daily. For maintenance therapy the lowest effective dosage is used.

Most other conditions: 10 to 100mg daily for one to three weeks, then reducing to the minimum effective dosage.

Children: Fractions of the adult dosage may be used (e.g. 75% at 12 years, 50% at 7 years and 25% at 1 year) but clinical factors must be given due weight.

Soluble Prednisolone Tablets may be given early in treatment of acute asthma attacks in children. For children over 5 years use a dose of 30-40 mg prednisolone. For children aged 2-5 years use a dose of 20 mg prednisolone. Those already receiving maintenance steroid tablets should receive 2 mg/kg prednisolone up to a maximum dose of 60 mg. The dose of prednisolone may be repeated for children who vomit; but intravenous steroids should be considered in children who are unable to retain orally ingested medication. Treatment for up to three days is usually sufficient, but the length of course should be tailored to the number of days necessary to bring about recovery. There is no need to taper the dose at the end of treatment.

For children under 2 years, Soluble Prednisolone Tablets can be used early in the management of moderate to severe episodes of acute asthma in the hospital setting, at a dose of 10 mg for up to three days.

4.3 Contraindications

Systemic infections, unless specific anti-infective therapy is employed. Live virus immunisation. Hypersensitivity to any component of the tablets.

4.4 Special warnings and special precautions for use

In patients who have received more than physiological doses of systemic corticosteroids (approximately 7.5mg prednisolone or equivalent) for greater than 3 weeks, withdrawal should not be abrupt. How dose reduction should be carried out depends largely on whether the disease is likely to relapse as the dose of systemic corticosteroids is reduced. Clinical assessment of disease activity may be needed during withdrawal. If the disease is unlikely to relapse on withdrawal of systemic corticosteroids but there is uncertainty about HPA suppression, the dose of systemic corticosteroid may be reduced rapidly to physiological doses. Once a daily dose equivalent to 7.5mg prednisolone is reached, dose reduction should be slower to allow the HPA-axis to recover.

Abrupt withdrawal of systemic corticosteroid treatment, which has continued up to 3 weeks is appropriate if it is considered that the disease is unlikely to relapse. Abrupt withdrawal of doses of up to 40mg daily of prednisolone, or equivalent for 3 weeks is unlikely to lead to clinically relevant HPA-axis suppression, in the majority of patients. In the following patient groups, gradual withdrawal of systemic corticosteroid therapy should be *considered* even after courses lasting 3 weeks or less:

- Patients who have had repeated courses of systemic corticosteroids, particularly if taken for greater than 3 weeks
- When a short course has been prescribed within one year of cessation of long-term therapy (months or years),
- Patients who may have reasons for adrenocortical insufficiency other than exogenous corticosteroid therapy,
- Patients receiving doses of systemic corticosteroid greater than 40mg daily of prednisolone (or equivalent),
- Patients repeatedly taking doses in the evening.

Patients should carry 'Steroid treatment' cards which give clear guidance on the precautions to be taken to minimise risk and which provide details of prescriber, drug, dosage and the duration of treatment.

Adrenal cortical atrophy develops during prolonged therapy and may persist for years after stopping treatment. Withdrawal of corticosteroids after prolonged therapy must therefore always be gradual to avoid acute adrenal insufficiency, being tapered off over weeks or months according to the dose and duration of treatment. During prolonged therapy any intercurrent illness, trauma or surgical procedure will require a temporary increase in dosage; if corticosteroids have been stopped following prolonged therapy they may need to be temporarily re-introduced.

Suppression of the HPA axis and other undesirable effects may be minimised by using the lowest effective dose for the minimum period, and by administering the daily requirement as a single morning dose or whenever possible as a single morning dose on alternate days. Frequent patient review is required to appropriately titrate the dose against disease activity. (See dosage section)

Suppression of the inflammatory response and immune function increases the susceptibility to infections and their severity. The clinical presentation may often be atypical and serious infections such as septicaemia and tuberculosis may be masked and may reach an advanced stage before being recognised.

Chickenpox is of particular concern since this normally minor illness may be fatal in immunosuppressed patients. Patients without a definite history of chickenpox should be advised to avoid close personal contact with chickenpox or herpes zoster and if exposed they should seek urgent medical attention. If the patient is a child parents must be given the above advice. Passive immunisation with varicella zoster immunoglobulin (VZIG) is needed by exposed non-immune patients who are receiving systemic corticosteroids or who have used them within the previous 3 months; this should be given within 10 days of exposure to chickenpox. If a diagnosis of chickenpox is confirmed, the illness warrants specialist care and urgent treatment. Corticosteroids should not be stopped and the dose may need to be increased.

Patients should be advised to take particular care to avoid exposure to measles and to seek immediate advice if exposure occurs. Prophylaxis with intramuscular normal immunoglobulin may be needed.

Live vaccines should not be given to individuals with impaired immune responsiveness. The antibody response to other vaccines may be diminished.

Because of the possibility of fluid retention, care must be taken when corticosteroids are administered to patients with renal insufficiency or hypertension or congestive heart failure.

Corticosteroids may worsen diabetes mellitus, osteoporosis, hypertension, glaucoma and epilepsy and therefore patients with these conditions or a family history of them should be monitored frequently.

Care is required and frequent patient monitoring necessary where there is a history of severe affective disorders (especially a previous history of steroid psychosis), previous steroid myopathy, peptic ulceration or patients with a history of tuberculosis.

In patients with liver failure, blood levels of corticosteroid may be increased, as with other drugs which are metabolised in the liver. Frequent patient monitoring is therefore necessary.

Use in Children: Corticosteroids cause dose-related growth retardation in infancy, childhood and adolescence, which may be irreversible.

Use in the Elderly: The common adverse effects of systemic corticosteroids may be associated with more serious consequences in old age, especially osteoporosis, hypertension, hypokalaemia, diabetes, susceptibility to infection and thinning of the skin. Close clinical supervision is required to avoid life-threatening reactions.

4.5 Interaction with other medicinal products and other forms of Interaction

Rifampicin, rifabutin, carbamazepine, phenobarbitone, phenytoin, primidone, ephedrine and aminoglutethimide enhance the metabolism of corticosteroids and its therapeutic effects may be reduced.

Mifepristone may reduce the effect of corticosteroids for 3-4 days.

Erythromycin and ketoconazole may inhibit the metabolism of some corticosteroids.

Ciclosporin increases plasma concentration of prednisolone. The same effect is possible with ritonavir.

Oestrogens and other oral contraceptives may potentiate the effects of glucocorticoids and dosage adjustments may be required if oral contraceptives are added to or withdrawn from a stable dose regimen.

The desired effects of hypoglycaemic agents (including insulin), anti-hypertensives and diuretics are antagonised by corticosteroids.

The growth promoting effect of somatotropin may be inhibited by the concomitant use of corticosteroids.

Steroids may reduce the effects of anticholinesterases in myasthenia gravis and cholecystographic x-ray media.

The efficacy of coumarin anticoagulants and warfarin may be enhanced by concurrent corticosteroid therapy and close monitoring of the INR or prothrombin time is required to avoid spontaneous bleeding.

Concomitant use of aspirin and Non Steroidal Anti-Inflammatory Drugs (NSAIDs) with corticosteroids increases the risk of gastro-intestinal bleeding and ulceration.

The renal clearance of salicylates is increased by corticosteroids and steroid withdrawal may result in salicylate intoxication.

The hypokalaemic effects of acetazolamide, loop diuretics, thiazide diuretics, and carbenoxolone, are enhanced by corticosteroids. The risk of hypokalaemia is increased with theophylline and amphotericin. Corticosteroids should not be given concomitantly with amphotericin, unless required to control reactions.

The risk of hypokalaemia also increases if high doses of corticosteroids are given with high doses of bambuterol, fenoterol, formoterol, ritodrine, salbutamol, salmeterol and terbutaline. The toxicity of cardiac glycosides is increased if hypokalaemia occurs with corticosteroids.

Concomitant use with methotrexate may increase the risk of haematological toxicity.

High doses of corticosteroids impair the immune response and so live vaccines should be avoided (see also warnings).

4.6 Pregnancy and lactation

The ability of corticosteroids to cross placenta varies between individual drugs, however, 88% of prednisolone is inactivated as it crosses the placenta.

Administration of corticosteroids to pregnant animals can cause abnormalities of foetal development including cleft palate, intra-uterine growth retardation and effects on brain growth and development. There is no evidence that corticosteroids result in an increased incidence of congenital abnormalities, such as cleft palate/lip in man. However, when administered for prolonged periods or repeatedly during pregnancy, corticosteroids may increase the risk of intra-uterine growth retardation.

Hypoadrenalism may, in theory, occur in the neonate following prenatal exposure to corticosteroids but usually resolves spontaneously following birth and is rarely clinically important. As with all drugs, corticosteroids should only be prescribed when the benefits to the mother and child outweigh the risks. When corticosteroids are essential however, patients with normal pregnancies may be treated as though they were in the non-gravid state.

Patients with pre-eclampsia or fluid retention require close monitoring.

Depression of hormone levels has been described in pregnancy but the significance of this finding is not clear.

Lactation:

Corticosteroids are excreted in small amounts in breast milk. However doses of up to 40mg daily of prednisolone are unlikely to cause systemic effects in the infant. Infants of mothers taking higher doses than this may have a degree of adrenal suppression but the benefits of breast feeding are likely to outweigh any theoretical risk.

4.7 Effects on ability to drive and use machines

None known.

4.8 Undesirable effects

The incidence of predictable undesirable effects, including hypothalamic-pituitary-adrenal suppression correlates with the relative potency of the drug, dosage, timing of administration and the duration of treatment. (See other special warnings and precautions)

Endocrine/metabolic:

Suppression of the hypothalamic-pituitary-adrenal axis, growth suppression in infancy, childhood and adolescence, menstrual irregularity and amenorrhoea. Cushingoid facies, hirsutism, weight gain, impaired carbohydrate tolerance with increased requirement for anti-diabetic therapy. Negative protein and calcium balance. Increased appetite.

Anti-inflammatory and Immunosuppressive effects:

Increased susceptibility and severity of infections with suppression of clinical symptoms and signs, opportunistic infections, recurrence of dormant tuberculosis (See other special warnings and precautions).

Musculoskeletal:

Osteoporosis, vertebral and long bone fractures, avascular osteonecrosis particularly of the femoral head may occur after prolonged corticosteroid therapy or after repeat short courses involving high doses, tendon rupture. Proximal myopathy.

Fluid and electrolyte disturbance:

Sodium and water retention, hypertension, potassium loss, hypokalaemic alkalosis.

Neuropsychiatric:

Euphoria, psychological dependence, depression, insomnia and aggravation of schizophrenia. Increased intra-cranial pressure with papilloedema in children (pseudotumour cerebri), usually after treatment withdrawal. Aggravation of epilepsy.

Ophthalmic:

Increased intra-ocular pressure, glaucoma, papilloedema, posterior subcapsular cataracts, corneal or scleral thinning, exacerbation of ophthalmic viral or fungal diseases.

Gastrointestinal:

Dyspepsia, peptic ulceration with perforation and haemorrhage, acute pancreatitis, candidiasis, nausea.

Dermatological:

Impaired healing, skin atrophy, bruising, telangiectasia, striae, acne.

Cardiovascular:

Myocardial rupture following recent myocardial infarction.

General:

Malaise, hiccups, leucocytosis, thromboembolism. Hypersensitivity including anaphylaxis, has been reported.

Withdrawal symptoms and signs

Too rapid a reduction of corticosteroid dosage following prolonged treatment can lead to acute adrenal insufficiency, hypotension and death. (See other special warnings and precautions)

A 'withdrawal syndrome' may also occur including, fever, myalgia, arthralgia, rhinitis, conjunctivitis, painful itchy skin nodules and loss of weight.

4.9 Overdose

Treatment is unlikely to be needed in cases of acute overdosage.

5. PHARMACOLOGICAL PROPERTIES

5.1 Pharmacodynamic properties

Prednesol/Soluble Prednisolone tablets contain the equivalent of 5mg of prednisolone in the form of the 21-disodium phosphate ester. Prednisolone sodium phosphate is a synthetic glucocorticoid with the same general properties as prednisolone itself and other compounds classified as corticosteroids. Prednisolone is four times as active as hydrocortisone on a weight for weight basis.

Prednisolone sodium phosphate is very soluble in water, and is therefore less likely to cause local gastric irritation than prednisolone alcohol, which is only slightly soluble. This is important when high dosages are required, as in immuno-suppressive therapy.

5.2 Pharmacokinetic properties

Absorption

Prednisolone is readily absorbed from the gastrointestinal tract with peak plasma concentrations achieved by 1-2 hours after an oral dose. Plasma prednisolone is mainly protein bound (70-90%), with binding to albumin and corticosteroid-binding globulin. The plasma half-life of prednisolone, after a single dose, is between 2.5-3.5 hours.

Distribution

The volume of distribution and clearance of total and unbound prednisolone are concentration dependent, and this has been attributed to saturable protein binding over the therapeutic plasma concentration range.

Metabolism

Prednisolone is extensively metabolised, mainly in the liver, but the metabolic pathways are not clearly defined.

Excretion

Over 90% of the prednisolone dose is excreted in the urine, with 7-30% as free prednisolone, and the remainder being recovered as a variety of metabolites.

5.3 Preclinical safety data

No additional data of relevance.

6. PHARMACEUTICAL PARTICULARS

6.1 List of excipients

Sodium Acid Citrate BP

Sodium Bicarbonate Ph.Eur

Saccharin Sodium BP

Povidone BP

Erythorine E127 HSE

Sodium Benzoate Ph.Eur

6.2 Incompatibilities

None known.

6.3 Shelf life

2 years.

6.4 Special precautions for storage

Store below 25°C.

Protect from light.

6.5 Nature and contents of container

The tablets are foil strip packed and supplied in cartons of 30 or 100 tablets.

6.6 Instructions for use and handling

For detailed instructions for use refer to the Patient Information Leaflet in every pack.

7. MARKETING AUTHORISATION HOLDER

Waymade PLC *trading as* Sovereign Medical

Sovereign House

Miles Gray Road

Basildon

Essex

SS14 3FR

8. MARKETING AUTHORISATION NUMBER(S)

PL 06464/0914

9. DATE OF FIRST AUTHORISATION/RENEWAL OF THE AUTHORISATION

16 December 1999

10. DATE OF REVISION OF THE TEXT

June 2003

Solu-Cortef

(Pharmacia Limited)

1. NAME OF THE MEDICINAL PRODUCT

Solu-Cortef® 100 mg or Hydrocortisone sodium succinate for injection BP 100 mg.

2. QUALITATIVE AND QUANTITATIVE COMPOSITION

Hydrocortisone sodium succinate 133.7 mg equivalent to hydrocortisone 100.0 mg.

3. PHARMACEUTICAL FORM

White, freeze dried powder for parenteral use.

4. CLINICAL PARTICULARS

4.1 Therapeutic indications

Anti-inflammatory agent.

Solu-Cortef is indicated for any condition in which rapid and intense corticosteroid effect is required such as:

1. Endocrine disorders

Primary or secondary adrenocortical insufficiency

2. Collagen diseases

Systemic lupus erythematosus

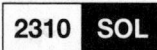

3. Dermatological diseases

Severe erythema multiforme (Stevens-Johnson syndrome)

4. Allergic states

Bronchial asthma, anaphylactic reactions

5. Gastro-intestinal diseases

Ulcerative colitis, Crohn's disease

6. Respiratory diseases

Aspiration of gastric contents

7. Medical emergencies

Solu-Cortef is indicated in the treatment of shock secondary to adrenocortical insufficiency or shock unresponsive to conventional therapy when adrenocortical insufficiency may be present.

4.2 Posology and method of administration

Solu-Cortef may be administered by intravenous injection, by intravenous infusion, or by intramuscular injection, the preferred method for initial emergency use being intravenous injection. Following the initial emergency period, consideration should be given to employing a longer-acting injectable preparation or an oral preparation.

Dosage usually ranges from 100 mg to 500 mg depending on the severity of the condition, administered by intravenous injection over a period of one to ten minutes. This dose may be repeated at intervals of 2, 4 or 6 hours as indicated by the patient's response and clinical condition.

In general high-dose corticosteroid therapy should be continued only until the patient's condition has stabilised - usually not beyond 48 to 72 hours. If hydrocortisone therapy must be continued beyond 48 to 72 hours hypernatraemia may occur, therefore it may be preferable to replace Solu-Cortef with a corticosteroid such as methylprednisolone sodium succinate as little or no sodium retention occurs. Although adverse effects associated with high dose, short-term corticoid therapy are uncommon, peptic ulceration may occur. Prophylactic antacid therapy may be indicated.

Patients subjected to severe stress following corticoid therapy should be observed closely for signs and symptoms of adrenocortical insufficiency.

Corticosteroid therapy is an adjunct to, and not a replacement for, conventional therapy.

Elderly patients: Solu-Cortef is primarily used in acute short-term conditions. There is no information to suggest that a change in dosage is warranted in the elderly. However, treatment of elderly patients should be planned bearing in mind the more serious consequences of the common side-effects of corticosteroids in old age and close clinical supervision is required (see Special warnings and special precautions for use).

Children: While the dose may be reduced for infants and children, it is governed more by the severity of the condition and response of the patient than by age or body weight but should not be less than 25 mg daily (see Special warnings and special precautions for use).

Preparation of solutions: For intravenous or intramuscular injection prepare the solution aseptically by adding not more than 2 ml of Sterile Water for Injections to the contents of one vial of Solu-Cortef 100 mg, shake and withdraw for use.

For intravenous infusion, first prepare the solution by adding not more than 2 ml of Sterile Water for Injections to the vial; this solution may then be added to 100 ml - 1000 ml (but not less than 100 ml) of 5% dextrose in water (or isotonic saline solution or 5% dextrose in isotonic saline solution if patient is not on sodium restriction).

When reconstituted as directed the pH of the solution will range from 7.0 to 8.0.

4.3 Contraindications

Solu-Cortef is contra-indicated where there is known hypersensitivity to components and in systemic fungal infection unless specific anti-infective therapy is employed.

Administration of live or live, attenuated vaccines is contra-indicated inpatients receiving immunosuppressive doses of corticosteroids.

4.4 Special warnings and special precautions for use

Warnings and Precautions:

1. A Patient Information Leaflet is provided in the pack by the manufacturer.

2. Undesirable effects may be minimised by using the lowest effective dose for the minimum period. Frequent patient review is required to appropriately titrate the dose against disease activity (see Posology and method of administration).

3. Adrenal cortical atrophy develops during prolonged therapy and may persist for months after stopping treatment. In patients who have received more than physiological doses of systemic corticosteroids (approximately 30 mg hydrocortisone) for greater than 3 weeks, withdrawal should not be abrupt. How dose reduction should be carried out depends largely on whether the disease is likely to relapse as the dose of systemic corticosteroids is reduced. Clinical assessment of disease activity may be needed during withdrawal. If the disease is unlikely to relapse on withdrawal of systemic corticosteroids, but there is uncertainty about HPA suppression, the dose of systemic corticosteroid may be reduced rapidly to physiological doses. Once a daily dose of 30 mg hydrocortisone is reached, dose reduction should be slower to allow the HPA-axis to recover.

Abrupt withdrawal of systemic corticosteroid treatment, which has continued up to 3 weeks is appropriate if it considered that the disease is unlikely to relapse. Abrupt withdrawal of doses up to 160 mg hydrocortisone for 3 weeks is unlikely to lead to clinically relevant HPA-axis suppression, in the majority of patients. In the following patient groups, gradual withdrawal of systemic corticosteroid therapy should be ***considered*** even after courses lasting 3 weeks or less:

- Patients who have had repeated courses of systemic corticosteroids, particularly if taken for greater than 3 weeks.
- When a short course has been prescribed within one year of cessation of long-term therapy (months or years).
- Patients who may have reasons for adrenocortical insufficiency other than exogenous corticosteroid therapy.
- Patients receiving doses of systemic corticosteroid greater than 160 mg hydrocortisone.
- Patients repeatedly taking doses in the evening.

4. Patients should carry 'Steroid Treatment' cards which give clear guidance on the precautions to be taken to minimise risk and which provide details of prescriber, drug, dosage and the duration of treatment.

5. Corticosteroids may mask some signs of infection, and new infections may appear during their use. Suppression of the inflammatory response and immune function increases the susceptibility to fungal, viral and bacterial infections and their severity. The clinical presentation may often be atypical and may reach an advanced stage before being recognised.

6. Chickenpox is of serious concern since this normally minor illness may be fatal in immunosuppressed patients. Patients (or parents of children) without a definite history of chickenpox should be advised to avoid close personal contact with chickenpox or herpes zoster and if exposed they should seek urgent medical attention. Passive immunization with varicella/zoster immunoglobin (VZIG) is needed by exposed non-immune patients who are receiving systemic corticosteroids or who have used them within the previous 3 months; this should be given within 10 days of exposure to chickenpox. If a diagnosis of chickenpox is confirmed, the illness warrants specialist care and urgent treatment. Corticosteroids should not be stopped and the dose may need to be increased.

7. Exposure to measles should be avoided. Medical advice should be sought immediately if exposure occurs. Prophylaxis with normal intramuscular immuneglobulin may be needed.

8. Live vaccines should not be given to individuals with impaired immune responsiveness. The antibody response to other vaccines may be diminished.

9 The use of Solu-Cortef in active tuberculosis should be restricted to those cases of fulminating or disseminated tuberculosis in which the corticosteroid is used for the management of the disease in conjunction with appropriate antituberculosis regimen. If corticosteroids are indicated in patients with latent tuberculosis or tuberculin reactivity, close observation is necessary as reactivation of the disease may occur. During prolonged corticosteroid therapy, these patients should receive chemoprophylaxis.

10. Rarely anaphylactoid reactions have been reported following parenteral Solu-Cortef therapy. Physicians using the drug should be prepared to deal with such a possibility. Appropriate precautionary measures should be taken prior to administration, especially when the patient has a history of drug allergy.

11. Care should be taken for patients receiving cardioactive drugs such as digoxin because of steroid induced electrolyte disturbance/potassium loss (see Undesirable effects).

12. Corticosteroids should not be used for the management of head injury or stroke because it is unlikely to be of benefit and may even be harmful.

Special precautions:

Particular care is required when considering the use of systemic corticosteroids in patients with the following conditions and frequent patient monitoring is necessary.

1. Osteoporosis (post-menopausal females are particularly at risk).
2. Hypertension or congestive heart failure.
3. Existing or previous history of severe affective disorders (especially previous steroid psychosis).
4. Diabetes mellitus (or a family history of diabetes).
5. History of tuberculosis.
6. Glaucoma (or a family history of glaucoma).
7. Previous corticosteroid-induced myopathy.
8. Liver failure or cirrhosis.
9. Renal insufficiency.
10. Epilepsy.
11. Peptic ulceration.
12. Fresh intestinal anastomoses.
13. Predisposition to thrombophlebitis.
14. Abscess or other pyogenic infections.
15. Ulcerative colitis.
16. Diverticulitis.
17. Myasthenia gravis.
18. Ocular herpes simplex, for fear of corneal perforation.
19. Hypothyroidism.
20. Recent myocardial infarction (myocardial rupture has been reported).
21. Kaposi's sarcoma has been reported to occur in patients receiving corticosteroid therapy. Discontinuation of corticosteroids may result in clinical remission.
22. Hydrocortisone can cause elevation of blood pressure, salt and water retention and increased excretion of potassium. Dietary salt restriction and potassium supplementation may be necessary. All corticosteroids increase calcium excretion.

Use in children: Corticosteroids cause growth retardation in infancy, childhood and adolescence, which may be irreversible. Treatment should be limited to the minimum dosage for the shortest possible time. The use of steroids should be restricted to the most serious indications.

Use in the elderly: The common adverse effects of systemic corticosteroids may be associated with more serious consequences in old age, especially osteoporosis, hypertension, hypokalaemia, diabetes, susceptibility to infection and thinning of the skin. Close clinical supervision is required to avoid life-threatening reactions.

4.5 Interaction with other medicinal products and other forms of Interaction

1. Convulsions have been reported with concurrent use of corticosteroids and cyclosporin. Since concurrent administration of these agents results in a mutual inhibition of metabolism, it is possible that convulsions and other adverse effects associated with the individual use of either drug may be more apt to occur.

2. Drugs that induce hepatic enzymes, such as rifampicin, rifabutin, carbamazepine, phenobarbitone, phenytoin, primidone, and aminoglutethimide enhance the metabolism of corticosteroids and its therapeutic effects may be reduced.

3. Drugs which inhibit the CYP3A4 enzyme, such as cimetidine, erythromycin, ketoconazole, itraconazole, diltiazem and mibefradil, may decrease the rate of metabolism of corticosteroids and hence increase the serum concentration.

4. Steroids may reduce the effects of anticholinesterases in myasthenia gravis. The desired effects of hypoglycaemic agents (including insulin), anti-hypertensives and diuretics are antagonised by corticosteroids, and the hypokalaemic effects of acetazolamide, loop diuretics, thiazide diuretics and carbenoxolone are enhanced.

5. The efficacy of coumarin anticoagulants may be enhanced by concurrent corticosteroid therapy and close monitoring of the INR or prothrombin time is required to avoid spontaneous bleeding.

6. The renal clearance of salicylates is increased by corticosteroids and steroid withdrawal may result in salicylate intoxication. Salicylates and non-steroidal anti-inflammatory agents should be used cautiously in conjunction with corticosteroids in hypothrombinaemia.

7. Steroids have been reported to interact with neuromuscular blocking agents such as pancuronium with partial reversal of the neuromuscular block.

4.6 Pregnancy and lactation

Pregnancy

The ability of corticosteroids to cross the placenta varies between individual drugs, however, hydrocortisone readily crosses the placenta.

Administration of corticosteroids to pregnant animals can cause abnormalities of foetal development including cleft palate, intra-uterine growth retardation and affects on brain growth and development. There is no evidence that corticosteroids result in an increased incidence of congenital abnormalities, such as cleft palate in man, however, when administered for long periods or repeatedly during pregnancy, corticosteroids may increase the risk of intra-uterine growth retardation. Hypoadrenalism may, in theory, occur in the neonate following prenatal exposure to corticosteroids but usually resolves spontaneously following birth and is rarely clinically important. As with all drugs, corticosteroids should only be prescribed when the benefits to the mother and child outweigh the risks. When corticosteroids are essential, however, patients with normal pregnancies may be treated as though they were in the non-gravid state.

Lactation

Corticosteroids are excreted in breast milk, although no data are available for hydrocortisone. Doses up to 160 mg daily of hydrocortisone are unlikely to cause systemic systemic effects in the infant. Infants of mothers taking higher doses than this may have a degree of adrenal suppression, but the benefits of breastfeeding are likely to outweigh any theoretical risk.

4.7 Effects on ability to drive and use machines

None stated.

4.8 Undesirable effects

Since Solu-Cortef is normally employed on a short-term basis it is unlikely that side-effects will occur; however, the possibility of side-effects attributable to corticosteroid therapy should be recognised (see Special warnings and special precautions for use). Such side-effects include:

PARENTERAL CORTICOSTEROID THERAPY - Anaphylactoid reaction e.g. bronchospasm, hypopigmentation or hyperpigmentation, subcutaneous and cutaneous atrophy, sterile abscess, laryngeal oedema and urticaria.

GASTRO-INTESTINAL - Dyspepsia, peptic ulceration with perforation and haemorrhage, abdominal distension, oesophageal ulceration, oesophageal candidiasis, acute pancreatitis, perforation of bowel, gastric haemorrhage.

Increases in alanine transaminase (ALT, SGPT) aspartate transaminase (AST, SGOT) and alkaline phosphatase have been observed following corticosteroid treatment. These changes are usually small, not associated with any clinical syndrome and are reversible upon discontinuation.

ANTI-INFLAMMATORY AND IMMUNOSUPPRESSIVE EFFECTS - Increased susceptibility and severity of infections with suppression of clinical symptoms and signs, opportunistic infections, may suppress reactions to skin tests, recurrence of dormant tuberculosis (see Special warnings and special precautions for use).

MUSCULOSKELETAL - Proximal myopathy, osteoporosis, vertebral and long bone fractures, avascular osteonecrosis, tendon rupture, aseptic necrosis, muscle weakness.

FLUID AND ELECTROLYTE DISTURBANCE - Sodium and water retention, potassium loss, hypertension, hypokalaemic alkalosis, congestive heart failure in susceptible patients.

DERMATOLOGICAL - Impaired healing, petechiae and ecchymosis, skin atrophy, bruising, striae, increased sweating, telangiectasia, acne. Kaposi's sarcoma has been reported to occur in patients receiving corticosteroid therapy. Discontinuation of corticosteroids may result in clinical remission.

ENDOCRINE/METABOLIC - Suppression of the hypothalamo-pituitary-adrenal axis; growth suppression in infancy, childhood and adolescence; menstrual irregularity and amenorrhoea, Cushingoid facies, hirsutism, weight gain, impaired carbohydrate tolerance with increased requirement for antidiabetic therapy, negative nitrogen and calcium balance. Increased appetite.

NEUROPSYCHIATRIC - Euphoria, psychological dependence, mood swings, depression, personality changes, insomnia, convulsions. Increased intra-cranial pressure with papilloedema in children (pseudotumour cerebri), usually after treatment withdrawal. Psychosis, aggravation of schizophrenia, seizures.

OPHTHALMIC - Increased intra-ocular pressure, glaucoma, papilloedema with possible damage to the optic nerve, cataracts, corneal or scleral thinning, exacerbation of ophthalmic viral or fungal disease, exophthalmos.

CARDIOVASCULAR – Myocardial rupture following a myocardial infarction.

GENERAL - Leucocytosis, hypersensitivity reactions including anaphylaxis, thrombo-embolism, nausea, malaise, persistent hiccups with high doses of corticosteroids.

WITHDRAWAL SYMPTOMS - Too rapid a reduction of corticosteroid dosage following prolonged treatment can lead to acute adrenal insufficiency, hypotension and death. However, this is more applicable to corticosteroids with an indication where continuous therapy is given (see Special warnings and special precautions for use).

A 'withdrawal syndrome' may also occur including, fever, myalgia, arthralgia, rhinitis, conjunctivitis, painful itchy skin nodules and loss of weight.

4.9 Overdose

There is no clinical syndrome of acute overdosage with Solu-Cortef. Hydrocortisone is dialysable.

5. PHARMACOLOGICAL PROPERTIES

5.1 Pharmacodynamic properties

Hydrocortisone sodium succinate has the same metabolic and anti-inflammatory actions as hydrocortisone. It is a glucocorticosteroid. Used in pharmacological doses, its actions supress the clinical manifestations of disease in a wide range of disorders.

5.2 Pharmacokinetic properties

Twelve normal subjects received 100, 200 or 400 mg Solu-Cortef intravenously. Radio-immunoassay results were as follows:-

DOSE (mg)	CMAX (mcg/100 ml)	TMAX (hr)	12-HR AUC (mG/100 ml × hr)
100	132.3	0.35	418.0
200	231.8	0.25	680.0
400	629.8	0.38	1024.0

In another study, a 1 mg/kg i.m. dose of Solu-Cortef peaked in 30-60 minutes, with a plasma cmax of 80 mg/100 ml.

In analysing hydrocortisone metabolism, a 25 mg IV dose resulted in higher plasma concentrations in females than in males.

6. PHARMACEUTICAL PARTICULARS

6.1 List of excipients

Sodium biphosphate, sodium phosphate.

6.2 Incompatibilities

None stated.

6.3 Shelf life

Shelf-life of the medicinal product as packaged for sale: 60 months.

After reconstitution with Sterile Water for Injections, use immediately, discard any remainder.

6.4 Special precautions for storage

Store below 25°C.

Refer to Section 4.2 Dosage and Administration. No diluents other than those referred to are recommended. Parenteral drug products should be inspected visually for particulate matter and discoloration prior to administration.

6.5 Nature and contents of container

Type I flint glass vials with a butyl rubber plug and metal seal. Each vial of Solu-Cortef 100 mg contains the equivalent of 100 mg hydrocortisone as the sodium succinate for reconstitution with 2 ml of Sterile Water for Injections.

6.6 Instructions for use and handling

No special requirements.

7. MARKETING AUTHORISATION HOLDER

Pharmacia Limited

Davy Avenue

Milton Keynes

MK5 8PH

UK

8. MARKETING AUTHORISATION NUMBER(S)

PL 0032/5019

9. DATE OF FIRST AUTHORISATION/RENEWAL OF THE AUTHORISATION

PL 0032/5019 date of first authorisation: 18 May 1990

Last renewal date: 7 December 1995

10. DATE OF REVISION OF THE TEXT

May 2005

Legal category

POM

SC1_1

Solu-Medrone 2 Gram

(Pharmacia Limited)

1. NAME OF THE MEDICINAL PRODUCT

Solu-Medrone® 2 gram or methylprednisolone sodium succinate for injection.

2. QUALITATIVE AND QUANTITATIVE COMPOSITION

Methylprednisolone sodium succinate 2.652 grams equivalent to 2 grams of methylprednisolone.

3. PHARMACEUTICAL FORM

Powder for injection.

4. CLINICAL PARTICULARS

4.1 Therapeutic indications

Solu-Medrone is indicated to treat any condition in which rapid and intense corticosteroid effect is required such as:

1. Dermatological disease

Severe erythema multiforme (Stevens-Johnson syndrome)

2. Allergic states

Bronchial asthma

Severe seasonal and perennial allergic rhinitis

Angioneurotic oedema

Anaphylaxis

3. Gastro-intestinal diseases

Ulcerative colitis

Crohn's disease

4. Respiratory diseases

Aspiration of gastric contents

Fulminating or disseminated tuberculosis (with appropriate antituberculous chemotherapy)

5. Neurological disorders

Cerebral oedema secondary to cerebral tumour

6. Miscellaneous

TB meningitis (with appropriate antituberculous chemotherapy)

Transplantation

7. Acute spinal cord injury. The treatment should begin within eight hours of injury.

4.2 Posology and method of administration

Solu-Medrone may be administered intravenously or intramuscularly, the preferred method for emergency use being intravenous injection given over a suitable time interval. When administering Solu-Medrone in high doses intravenously it should be given over a period of at least 30 minutes. Doses up to 250 mg should be given intravenously over a period of at least five minutes.

For intravenous infusion the initially prepared solution may be diluted with 5% dextrose in water, isotonic saline solution, or 5% dextrose in isotonic saline solution. To avoid compatibility problems with other drugs Solu-Medrone should be administered separately, only in the solutions mentioned.

Undesirable effects may be minimised by using the lowest effective dose for the minimum period (see Special warnings and special precautions for use).

Parenteral drug products should wherever possible be visually inspected for particulate matter and discoloration prior to administration.

Adults: Dosage should be varied according to the severity of the condition, initial dosage will vary from 10 to 500 mg. In the treatment of graft rejection reactions following transplantation, a dose of up to 1 g/day may be required. Although doses and protocols have varied in studies using methylprednisolone sodium succinate in the treatment of graft rejection reactions, the published literature supports the use of doses of this level, with 500 mg to 1 g most commonly used for acute rejection. Treatment at these doses should be limited to a 48-72 hour period until the patient's condition has stabilised, as prolonged high dose corticosteroid therapy can cause serious corticosteroid induced side-effects (see Undesirable effects and Special warnings and special precautions for use).

Children: In the treatment of high dose indications, such as haematological, rheumatic, renal and dermatological conditions, a dosage of 30 mg/kg/day to a maximum of 1 g/day is recommended. This dosage may be repeated for three pulses either daily or on alternate days. In the treatment of graft rejection reactions following transplantation, a dosage of 10 to 20 mg/kg/day for up to 3 days, to a maximum of 1 g/day, is recommended. In the treatment of status asthmaticus, a dosage of 1 to 4 mg/kg/day for 1-3 days is recommended.

Solu-Medrone is not recommended for use in spinal cord injury in children.

Elderly patients: Solu-Medrone is primarily used in acute short-term conditions. There is no information to suggest that a change in dosage is warranted in the elderly. However, treatment of elderly patients should be planned bearing in mind the more serious consequences of the common side-effects of corticosteroids in old age and close clinical supervision is required (see Special warnings and special precautions for use).

Detailed recommendations for adult dosage are as follows:

In anaphylactic reactions adrenaline or noradrenaline should be administered first for an immediate haemodynamic effect, followed by intravenous injection of Solu-Medrone (methylprednisolone sodium succinate) with other accepted procedures. There is evidence that corticosteroids through their prolonged haemodynamic effect are of value in preventing recurrent attacks of acute anaphylactic reactions.

In sensitivity reactions Solu-Medrone is capable of providing relief within one half to two hours. In patients with status asthmaticus Solu-Medrone may be given at a dose of 40 mg intravenously, repeated as dictated by patient response. In some asthmatic patients it may be advantageous to administer by slow intravenous drip over a period of hours.

In graft rejection reactions following transplantation doses of up to 1 g per day have been used to suppress rejection crises, with doses of 500 mg to 1 g most commonly used for acute rejection. Treatment should be continued only until the patient's condition has stabilised; usually not beyond 48-72 hours.

In cerebral oedema corticosteroids are used to reduce or prevent the cerebral oedema associated with brain tumours (primary or metastatic).

In patients with oedema due to tumour, tapering the dose of corticosteroid appears to be important in order to avoid a rebound increase in intracranial pressure. If brain swelling does occur as the dose is reduced (intracranial bleeding having been ruled out), restart larger and more frequent doses parenterally. Patients with certain malignancies may need to remain on oral corticosteroid therapy for months or even life. Similar or higher doses may be helpful to control oedema during radiation therapy.

The following are suggested dosage schedules for oedemas due to brain tumour.

(see Table 1 on next page)

Aim to discontinue therapy after a total of 10 days.

REFERENCES

1. Fox JL, MD. "Use of Methylprednisolone in Intracranial Surgery" Medical Annals of the District of Columbia, 34:261-265,1965.

2. Cantu RC, MD Harvard Neurological Service, Boston, Massachusetts. Letter on file, The Upjohn Company (February 1970).

For treatment of acute spinal cord injury, administer intravenously 30 mg methylprednisolone per kilogram of body weight in a bolus dose over a 15 minute period, followed by a 45 minute pause, and then a continuous infusion of 5.4 mg/kg per hour for 23 hours. There should

Table 1

Schedule A (1)	Dose (mg)	Route	Interval in hours	Days Duration
Pre-operative:	20	IM	3-6	
During Surgery:	20 to 40	IV	hourly	
Post operative:	20	IM	3	24 hours
	16	IM	3	24 hours
	12	IM	3	24 hours
	8	IM	3	24 hours
	4	IM	3	24 hours
	4	IM	6	24 hours
	4	IM	12	24 hours
Schedule B (2)	**Dose (mg)**	**Route**	**Interval in hours**	**Days Duration**
Pre-operative:	40	IM	6	2-3
Post-operative:	40	IM	6	3-5
	20	Oral	6	1
	12	Oral	6	1
	8	Oral	8	1
	4	Oral	12	1
	4	Oral		1

be a separate intravenous site for the infusion pump. The treatment should begin within eight hours of injury.

In other indications, initial dosage will vary from 10 to 500 mg depending on the clinical problem being treated. Larger doses may be required for short-term management of severe, acute conditions. The initial dose, up to 250 mg, should be given intravenously over a period of at least 5 minutes, doses exceeding 250 mg should be given intravenously over a period of at least 30 minutes. Subsequent doses may be given intravenously or intramuscularly at intervals dictated by the patient's response and clinical condition. Corticosteroid therapy is an adjunct to, and not replacement for, conventional therapy.

4.3 Contraindications

Solu-Medrone is contra-indicated where there is known hypersensitivity to components, in systemic fungal infections unless specific anti-infective therapy is employed and in cerebral oedema in malaria.

4.4 Special warnings and special precautions for use

Warnings and Precautions:

1. A Patient Information Leaflet is provided in the pack by the manufacturer.

2. Undesirable effects may be minimised by using the lowest effective dose for the minimum period. Frequent patient review is required to appropriately titrate the dose against disease activity (see Posology and method of administration).

3. Adrenal cortical atrophy develops during prolonged therapy and may persist for months after stopping treatment. In patients who have received more than physiological doses of systemic corticosteroids (approximately 6 mg methylprednisolone) for greater than 3 weeks, withdrawal should not be abrupt. How dose reduction should be carried out depends largely on whether the disease is likely to relapse as the dose of systemic corticosteroids is reduced. Clinical assessment of disease activity may be needed during withdrawal. If the disease is unlikely to relapse on withdrawal of systemic corticosteroids, but there is uncertainty about HPA suppression, the dose of systemic corticosteroid may be reduced rapidly to physiological doses. Once a daily dose of 6 mg methylprednisolone is reached, dose reduction should be slower to allow the HPA-axis to recover.

Abrupt withdrawal of systemic corticosteroid treatment, which has continued up to 3 weeks is appropriate if it considered that the disease is unlikely to relapse. Abrupt withdrawal of doses up to 32 mg daily of methylprednisolone for 3 weeks is unlikely to lead to clinically relevant HPA-axis suppression, in the majority of patients. In the following patient groups, gradual withdrawal of systemic corticosteroid therapy should be *considered* even after courses lasting 3 weeks or less:

• Patients who have had repeated courses of systemic corticosteroids, particularly if taken for greater than 3 weeks.

• When a short course has been prescribed within one year of cessation of long-term therapy (months or years).

• Patients who may have reasons for adrenocortical insufficiency other than exogenous corticosteroid therapy.

• Patients receiving doses of systemic corticosteroid greater than 32 mg daily of methylprednisolone.

• Patients repeatedly taking doses in the evening.

4. Patients should carry 'Steroid Treatment' cards which give clear guidance on the precautions to be taken to minimise risk and which provide details of prescriber, drug, dosage and the duration of treatment.

5. Although Solu-Medrone is not approved in the UK for use in any shock indication, the following warning statement should be adhered to. Data from a clinical study conducted to establish the efficacy of Solu-Medrone in septic shock, suggest that a higher mortality occurred in subsets of patients who entered the study with elevated serum creatinine levels or who developed a secondary infection after therapy began. Therefore this product should not be used in the treatment of septic syndrome or septic shock.

6. There have been a few reports of cardiac arrhythmias and/or circulatory collapse and/or cardiac arrest associated with the rapid intravenous administration of large doses of Solu-Medrone (greater than 500 mg administered over a period of less than 10 minutes). Bradycardia has been reported during or after the administration of large doses of methylprednisolone sodium succinate, and may be unrelated to the speed and duration of infusion.

7. Corticosteroids may mask some signs of infection, and new infections may appear during their use. Suppression of the inflammatory response and immune function increases the susceptibility to fungal, viral and bacterial infections and their severity. The clinical presentation may often be atypical and may reach an advanced stage before being recognised.

8. Chickenpox is of serious concern since this normally minor illness may be fatal in immunosuppressed patients. Patients (or parents of children) without a definite history of chickenpox should be advised to avoid close personal contact with chickenpox or herpes zoster and if exposed they should seek urgent medical attention. Passive immunisation with varicella/zoster immunoglobin (VZIG) is needed by exposed non-immune patients who are receiving systemic corticosteroids or who have used them within the previous 3 months; this should be given within 10 days of exposure to chickenpox. If a diagnosis of chickenpox is confirmed, the illness warrants specialist care and urgent treatment. Corticosteroids should not be stopped and the dose may need to be increased.

9. Exposure to measles should be avoided. Medical advice should be sought immediately if exposure occurs. Prophylaxis with normal intramuscular immuneglobulin may be needed.

10. Live vaccines should not be given to individuals with impaired immune responsiveness. The antibody response to other vaccines may be diminished.

11. The use of Solu-Medrone in active tuberculosis should be restricted to those cases of fulminating or disseminated tuberculosis in which the corticosteroid is used for the management of the disease in conjunction with an appropriate anti-tuberculous regimen. If corticosteroids are indicated in patients with latent tuberculosis or tuberculin reactivity, close observation is necessary as reactivation of the disease may occur. During prolonged corticosteroid therapy, these patients should receive chemoprophylaxis.

12. Rarely anaphylactoid reactions have been reported following parenteral Solu-Medrone therapy. Physicians using the drug should be prepared to deal with such a possibility. Appropriate precautionary measures should be taken prior to administration, especially when the patient has a history of drug allergy.

13. Care should be taken for patients receiving cardioactive drugs such as digoxin because of steroid induced electrolyte disturbance/potassium loss (see Undesirable effects).

14. Corticosteroids should not be used for the management of head injury or stroke because it is unlikely to be of benefit and may even be harmful.

Special precautions:

Particular care is required when considering the use of systemic corticosteroids in patients with the following conditions and frequent patient monitoring is necessary.

1. Osteoporosis (post-menopausal females are particularly at risk).

2. Hypertension or congestive heart failure.

3. Existing or previous history of severe affective disorders (especially previous steroid psychosis).

4. Diabetes mellitus (or a family history of diabetes).

5. History of tuberculosis.

6. Glaucoma (or a family history of glaucoma).

7. Previous corticosteroid-induced myopathy.

8. Liver failure or cirrhosis.

9. Renal insufficiency.

10. Epilepsy.

11. Peptic ulceration.

12. Fresh intestinal anastomoses.

13. Predisposition to thrombophlebitis.

14. Abscess or other pyogenic infections.

15. Ulcerative colitis.

16. Diverticulitis.

17. Myasthenia gravis.

18. Ocular herpes simplex, for fear of corneal perforation.

19. Hypothyroidism.

20. Recent myocardial infarction (myocardial rupture has been reported).

21. Kaposi's sarcoma has been reported to occur in patients receiving corticosteroid therapy. Discontinuation of corticosteroids may result in clinical remission.

Use in children: Corticosteroids cause growth retardation in infancy, childhood and adolescence, which may be irreversible. Treatment should be limited to the minimum dosage for the shortest possible time. In order to minimise suppression of the hypothalamo-pituitary-adrenal axis and growth retardation, treatment should be administered where possible as a single dose on alternate days.

Use in the elderly: The common adverse effects of systemic corticosteroids may be associated with more serious consequences in old age, especially osteoporosis, hypertension, hypokalaemia, diabetes, susceptibility to infection and thinning of the skin. Close clinical supervision is required to avoid life-threatening reactions.

4.5 Interaction with other medicinal products and other forms of Interaction

1. Convulsions have been reported with concurrent use of methylprednisolone and ciclosporin. Since concurrent administration of these agents results in a mutual inhibition of metabolism, it is possible that convulsions and other adverse events associated with the individual use of either drug may be more apt to occur.

2. Drugs that induce hepatic enzymes, such as rifampicin, rifabutin, carbamazepine, phenobarbitone, phenytoin, primidone, and aminoglutethimide enhance the metabolism of corticosteroids and its therapeutic effects may be reduced.

3. Drugs which inhibit the CYP3A4 enzyme, such as cimetidine, erythromycin, ketoconazole, itraconazole, diltiazem and mibefradil, may decrease the rate of metabolism of corticosteroids and hence increase the serum concentration.

4. Steroids may reduce the effects of anticholinesterases in myasthenia gravis. The desired effects of hypoglycaemic agents (including insulin), anti-hypertensives and diuretics are antagonised by corticosteroids, and the hypokalaemic effects of acetazolamide, loop diuretics, thiazide diuretics and carbenoxolone are enhanced.

5. The efficacy of coumarin anticoagulants may be enhanced by concurrent corticosteroid therapy and close monitoring of the INR or prothrombin time is required to avoid spontaneous bleeding.

6. The renal clearance of salicylates is increased by corticosteroids and steroid withdrawal may result in salicylate intoxication. Salicylates and non-steroidal anti-inflammatory agents should be used cautiously in conjunction with corticosteroids in hypothrombinaemia.

7. Steroids have been reported to interact with neuromuscular blocking agents such as pancuronium with partial reversal of the neuromuscular block.

4.6 Pregnancy and lactation

Pregnancy

The ability of corticosteroids to cross the placenta varies between individual drugs, however, methylprednisolone does cross the placenta.

Administration of corticosteroids to pregnant animals can cause abnormalities of foetal development including cleft palate, intra-uterine growth retardation and affects on brain growth and development. There is no evidence that corticosteroids result in an increased incidence of congenital abnormalities, such as cleft palate in man, however, when administered for long periods or repeatedly during pregnancy, corticosteroids may increase the risk of intra-uterine growth retardation. Hypoadrenalism may, in theory, occur in the neonate following prenatal exposure to corticosteroids but usually resolves spontaneously following birth and is rarely clinically important. As with all drugs, corticosteroids should only be prescribed when the benefits to the mother and child outweigh the risks. When corticosteroids are essential, however, patients with normal pregnancies may be treated as though they were in the non-gravid state.

Lactation

Corticosteroids are excreted in small amounts in breast milk, however, doses of up to 40 mg daily of methylprednisolone are unlikely to cause systemic effects in the infant.

Infants of mothers taking higher doses than this may have a degree of adrenal suppression, but the benefits of breastfeeding are likely to outweigh any theoretical risk.

4.7 Effects on ability to drive and use machines
None stated.

4.8 Undesirable effects
Under normal circumstances Solu-Medrone therapy would be considered as short-term. However, the possibility of side-effects attributable to corticosteroid therapy should be recognised, particularly when high-dose therapy is being used (see Special warnings and special precautions for use). Such side-effects include:

PARENTERAL CORTICOSTEROID THERAPY - Anaphylactic reaction with or without circulatory collapse, cardiac arrest, bronchospasm, cardiac arrhythmias, hypotension or hypertension, hypopigmentation or hyperpigmentation.

GASTRO-INTESTINAL - Dyspepsia, peptic ulceration with perforation and haemorrhage, abdominal distension, oesophageal ulceration, oesophageal candidiasis, acute pancreatitis, perforation of the bowel, gastric haemorrhage. Nausea, vomiting and bad taste in mouth may occur especially with rapid administration.

Increases in alanine transaminase (ALT, SGPT) aspartate transaminase (AST, SGOT) and alkaline phosphatase have been observed following corticosteroid treatment. These changes are usually small, not associated with any clinical syndrome and are reversible upon discontinuation.

ANTI-INFLAMMATORY AND IMMUNOSUPPRESSIVE EFFECTS - Increased susceptibility and severity of infections with suppression of clinical symptoms and signs, opportunistic infections, may suppress reactions to skin tests, recurrence of dormant tuberculosis (see Special warnings and special precautions for use).

MUSCULOSKELETAL - Proximal myopathy, osteoporosis, vertebral and long bone fractures, avascular osteonecrosis, tendon rupture.

FLUID AND ELECTROLYTE DISTURBANCE - Sodium and water retention, potassium loss, hypertension, hypokalaemic alkalosis, congestive heart failure in susceptible patients.

DERMATOLOGICAL - Impaired healing, petechiae and ecchymosis, skin atrophy, bruising, striae, telangiectasia, acne. Kaposi's sarcoma has been reported to occur in patients receiving corticosteroid therapy. Discontinuation of corticosteroids may result in clinical remission.

ENDOCRINE/METABOLIC - Suppression of the hypothalamo-pituitary-adrenal axis; growth suppression in infancy, childhood and adolescence; menstrual irregularity and amenorrhoea. Cushingoid facies, hirsutism, weight gain, impaired carbohydrate tolerance with increased requirement for antidiabetic therapy, negative nitrogen and calcium balance. Increased appetite.

NEUROPSYCHIATRIC - Euphoria, psychological dependence, mood swings, depression, personality changes, insomnia. Increased intra-cranial pressure with papilloedema in children (pseudotumour cerebri), usually after treatment withdrawal. Psychosis, aggravation of schizophrenia, seizures.

OPHTHALMIC - Increased intra-ocular pressure, glaucoma, papilloedema with possible damage to the optic nerve, cataracts, corneal or scleral thinning, exacerbation of ophthalmic viral or fungal disease.

CARDIOVASCULAR – Myocardial rupture following a myocardial infarction.

GENERAL - Leucocytosis, hypersensitivity including anaphylaxis, thrombo-embolism, malaise, persistent hiccups with high doses of corticosteroids.

WITHDRAWAL SYMPTOMS - Too rapid a reduction of corticosteroid dosage following prolonged treatment can lead to acute adrenal insufficiency, hypotension and death. However, this is more applicable to corticosteroids with an indication where continuous therapy is given (see Special warnings and special precautions for use).

A 'withdrawal syndrome' may also occur including, fever, myalgia, arthralgia, rhinitis, conjunctivitis, painful itchy skin nodules and loss of weight.

4.9 Overdose
There is no clinical syndrome of acute overdosage with Solu-Medrone. Methylprednisolone is dialysable. Following chronic overdosage the possibility of adrenal suppression should be guarded against by gradual diminution of dose levels over a period of time. In such event the patient may require to be supported during any further stressful episode.

5. PHARMACOLOGICAL PROPERTIES

5.1 Pharmacodynamic properties
Medrone is a corticosteroid with an anti-inflammatory activity at least five times that of hydrocortisone. An enhanced separation of glucocorticoid and mineralocorticoid effect results in a reduced incidence of sodium and water retention.

5.2 Pharmacokinetic properties
Methylprednisolone is extensively bound to plasma proteins, mainly to globulin and less so to albumin. Only unbound corticosteroid has pharmacological effects or is metabolised. Metabolism occurs in the liver and to a lesser extent in the kidney. Metabolites are excreted in the urine. Mean elimination half-life ranges from 2.4 to 3.5 hours in normal healthy adults and appears to be independent of the route of administration.

Total body clearance following intravenous or intramuscular injection of methylprednisolone to healthy adult volunteers is approximately 15-16l/hour. Peak methylprednisolone plasma levels of 33.67 micrograms/100 ml were achieved in 2 hours after a single 40 mg i.m. injection to 22 adult male volunteers.

6. PHARMACEUTICAL PARTICULARS

6.1 List of excipients
Sodium biphosphate and sodium phosphate.

6.2 Incompatibilities
None stated.

6.3 Shelf life
Shelf-life of the medicinal product as packaged for sale: 60 months.

After reconstitution with Sterile Water for Injections, use immediately, discard any remainder.

6.4 Special precautions for storage
Store below 25°C.

Refer to Section 4.2 Dosage and Administration. No diluents other than those referred to are recommended. Parenteral drug products should be inspected visually for particulate matter and discoloration prior to administration.

6.5 Nature and contents of container
Type I clear glass vial with butyl rubber plug and flip top seal. Each vial contains 2 grams of methylprednisolone as the sodium succinate for reconstitution with 31.2 ml of Sterile Water for Injections.

6.6 Instructions for use and handling
No special requirements.

7. MARKETING AUTHORISATION HOLDER
Pharmacia Limited
Davy Avenue
Milton Keynes
MK5 8PH
UK

8. MARKETING AUTHORISATION NUMBER(S)
PL 0032/0073

9. DATE OF FIRST AUTHORISATION/RENEWAL OF THE AUTHORISATION
PL 0032/0073 date of first authorisation: 20 February 1980
Last renewal dated: 17 October 1995

10. DATE OF REVISION OF THE TEXT
May 2005

Legal category
POM

Ref: SMB1_1

Solu-Medrone 40mg, 125mg, 500mg and 1 gram

(Pharmacia Limited)

1. NAME OF THE MEDICINAL PRODUCT
Solu-Medrone 40 mg
Solu-Medrone 125mg
Solu-Medrone 500mg
Solu-Medrone 1gram

2. QUALITATIVE AND QUANTITATIVE COMPOSITION
Solu-Medrone 40 mg: Methylprednisolone sodium succinate 53.0 mg equivalent to 40 mg of methylprednisolone.

Solu-Medrone 125mg: Methylprednisolone sodium succinate 165.8 mg equivalent to 125 mg of methylprednisolone.

Solu-Medrone 500mg: Methylprednisolone sodium succinate 663.0 mg equivalent to 500 mg of methylprednisolone.

Solu-Medrone 1g: Methylprednisolone sodium succinate 1.326 gm equivalent to 1.0 g of methylprednisolone.

3. PHARMACEUTICAL FORM
Powder for injection.

4. CLINICAL PARTICULARS

4.1 Therapeutic indications
Solu-Medrone is indicated to treat any condition in which rapid and intense corticosteroid effect is required such as:

1. Dermatological disease

Severe erythema multiforme (Stevens-Johnson syndrome)

2. Allergic states

Bronchial asthma

Severe seasonal and perennial allergic rhinitis

Angioneurotic oedema

Anaphylaxis

3. Gastro-intestinal diseases

Ulcerative colitis

Crohn's disease

4. Respiratory diseases

Aspiration of gastric contents

Fulminating or disseminated tuberculosis (with appropriate antituberculous chemotherapy)

5. Neurological disorders

Cerebral oedema secondary to cerebral tumour

Acute exacerbations of multiple sclerosis superimposed on a relapsing-remitting background.

6. Miscellaneous

T.B. meningitis (with appropriate antituberculous chemotherapy)

Transplantation

4.2 Posology and method of administration
Solu-Medrone may be administered intravenously or intramuscularly, the preferred method for emergency use being intravenous injection given over a suitable time interval. When administering Solu-Medrone in high doses intravenously it should be given over a period of at least 30 minutes. Doses up to 250 mg should be given intravenously over a period of at least five minutes.

For intravenous infusion the initially prepared solution may be diluted with 5% dextrose in water, isotonic saline solution, or 5% dextrose in isotonic saline solution. To avoid compatibility problems with other drugs Solu-Medrone should be administered separately, only in the solutions mentioned.

Undesirable effects may be minimised by using the lowest effective dose for the minimum period (see Other special warnings and precautions).

Parenteral drug products should wherever possible be visually inspected for particulate matter and discoloration prior to administration.

Adults: Dosage should be varied according to the severity of the condition, initial dosage will vary from 10 to 500 mg. In the treatment of graft rejection reactions following transplantation, a dose of up to 1 g/day may be required. Although doses and protocols have varied in studies using methylprednisolone sodium succinate in the treatment of graft rejection reactions, the published literature supports the use of doses of this level, with 500 mg to 1 g most commonly used for acute rejection. Treatment at these doses should be limited to a 48-72 hour period until the patient's condition has stabilised, as prolonged high dose corticosteroid therapy can cause serious corticosteroid induced side-effects (see Undesirable effects and Special warnings and special precautions for use).

Children: In the treatment of high dose indications, such as haematological, rheumatic, renal and dermatological conditions, a dosage of 30 mg/kg/day to a maximum of 1 g/day is recommended. This dosage may be repeated for three pulses either daily or on alternate days. In the treatment of graft rejection reactions following transplantation, a dosage of 10 to 20 mg/kg/day for up to 3 days, to a maximum of 1 g/day, is recommended. In the treatment of status asthmaticus, a dosage of 1 to 4 mg/kg/day for 1-3 days is recommended.

Elderly patients: Solu-Medrone is primarily used in acute short-term conditions. There is no information to suggest that a change in dosage is warranted in the elderly. However, treatment of elderly patients should be planned bearing in mind the more serious consequences of the common side-effects of corticosteroids in old age and close clinical supervision is required (see Special warnings and special precautions for use).

Detailed recommendations for adult dosage are as follows:

In anaphylactic reactions adrenaline or noradrenaline should be administered first for an immediate haemodynamic effect, followed by intravenous injection of Solu-Medrone (methylprednisolone sodium succinate) with other accepted procedures. There is evidence that corticosteroids through their prolonged haemodynamic effect are of value in preventing recurrent attacks of acute anaphylactic reactions.

In sensitivity reactions Solu-Medrone is capable of providing relief within one half to two hours. In patients with status asthmaticus Solu-Medrone may be given at a dose of 40 mg intravenously, repeated as dictated by patient response. In some asthmatic patients it may be advantageous to administer by slow intravenous drip over a period of hours.

In graft rejection reactions following transplantation doses of up to 1 g per day have been used to suppress rejection crises, with doses of 500 mg to 1 g most commonly used for acute rejection. Treatment should be continued only until the patient's condition has stabilised; usually not beyond 48-72 hours.

In cerebral oedema corticosteroids are used to reduce or prevent the cerebral oedema associated with brain tumours (primary or metastatic).

In patients with oedema due to tumour, tapering the dose of corticosteroid appears to be important in order to avoid a rebound increase in intracranial pressure. If brain swelling does occur as the dose is reduced (intracranial bleeding having been ruled out), restart larger and more frequent doses parenterally. Patients with certain malignancies may need to remain on oral corticosteroid therapy for months or even life. Similar or higher doses may be helpful to control oedema during radiation therapy.

The following are suggested dosage schedules for oedemas due to brain tumour.

(see Table 1 below)

Aim to discontinue therapy after a total of 10 days.

REFERENCES

1. Fox JL, MD. "Use of Methylprednisolone in Intracranial Surgery" Medical Annals of the District of Columbia, 34:261-265,1965.

2. Cantu RC, MD Harvard Neurological Service, Boston, Massachusetts. Letter on file, The Upjohn Company (February 1970).

In the treatment of **acute exacerbations of multiple sclerosis** in adults, the recommended dose is 1 g daily for 3 days. Solu-Medrone should be given as an intravenous infusion over at least 30 minutes.

In other indications, initial dosage will vary from 10 to 500 mg depending on the clinical problem being treated. Larger doses may be required for short-term management of severe, acute conditions. The initial dose, up to 250 mg, should be given intravenously over a period of at least 5 minutes, doses exceeding 250 mg should be given intravenously over a period of at least 30 minutes. Subsequent doses may be given intravenously or intramuscularly at intervals dictated by the patient's response and clinical condition. Corticosteroid therapy is an adjunct to, and not replacement for, conventional therapy.

4.3 Contraindications

Solu-Medrone is contra-indicated where there is known hypersensitivity to components, in systemic infection unless specific anti-infective therapy is employed and in cerebral oedema in malaria.

4.4 Special warnings and special precautions for use

Warnings and Precautions:

1. A Patient Information Leaflet is provided in the pack by the manufacturer.

2. Undesirable effects may be minimised by using the lowest effective dose for the minimum period. Frequent patient review is required to appropriately titrate the dose against disease activity (see Posology and method of administration).

3. Adrenal cortical atrophy develops during prolonged therapy and may persist for months after stopping treatment. In patients who have received more than physiological doses of systemic corticosteroids (approximately 6 mg methylprednisolone) for greater than 3 weeks, withdrawal should not be abrupt. How dose reduction should be carried out depends largely on whether the disease is likely to relapse as the dose of systemic corticosteroids is reduced. Clinical assessment of disease activity may be needed during withdrawal. If the disease is unlikely to relapse on withdrawal of systemic corticosteroids, but there is uncertainty about HPA suppression, the dose of systemic corticosteroid may be reduced rapidly to physiological doses. Once a daily dose of 6 mg methylprednisolone is reached, dose reduction should be slower to allow the HPA-axis to recover.

Abrupt withdrawal of systemic corticosteroid treatment, which has continued up to 3 weeks is appropriate if it considered that the disease is unlikely to relapse. Abrupt withdrawal of doses up to 32 mg daily of methylprednisolone for 3 weeks is unlikely to lead to clinically relevant HPA-axis suppression, in the majority of patients. In the following patient groups, gradual withdrawal of systemic corticosteroid therapy should be *considered* even after courses lasting 3 weeks or less:

- Patients who have had repeated courses of systemic corticosteroids, particularly if taken for greater than 3 weeks.
- When a short course has been prescribed within one year of cessation of long-term therapy (months or years).
- Patients who may have reasons for adrenocortical insufficiency other than exogenous corticosteroid therapy.
- Patients receiving doses of systemic corticosteroid greater than 32 mg daily of methylprednisolone.
- Patients repeatedly taking doses in the evening.

4. Patients should carry 'Steroid Treatment' cards which give clear guidance on the precautions to be taken to minimise risk and which provide details of prescriber, drug, dosage and the duration of treatment.

5. Although Solu-Medrone is not approved in the UK for use in any shock indication, the following warning statement should be adhered to. Data from a clinical study conducted to establish the efficacy of Solu-Medrone in septic shock, suggest that a higher mortality occurred in subsets of patients who entered the study with elevated serum creatinine levels or who developed a secondary infection after therapy began. Therefore this product should not be used in the treatment of septic syndrome or septic shock.

6. There have been a few reports of cardiac arrhythmias and/or circulatory collapse and/or cardiac arrest associated with the rapid intravenous administration of large doses of Solu-Medrone (greater than 500 mg administered over a period of less than 10 minutes). Bradycardia has been reported during or after the administration of large doses of methylprednisolone sodium succinate, and may be unrelated to the speed and duration of infusion.

7. Corticosteroids may mask some signs of infection, and new infections may appear during their use. Suppression of the inflammatory response and immune function increases the susceptibility to fungal, viral and bacterial infections and their severity. The clinical presentation may often be atypical and may reach an advanced stage before being recognised.

8. Chickenpox is of serious concern since this normally minor illness may be fatal in immunosuppressed patients. Patients (or parents of children) without a definite history of chickenpox should be advised to avoid close personal contact with chickenpox or herpes zoster and if exposed they should seek urgent medical attention. Passive immunization with varicella/zoster immunoglobin (VZIG) is needed by exposed non-immune patients who are receiving systemic corticosteroids or who have used them within the previous 3 months; this should be given within 10 days of exposure to chickenpox. If a diagnosis of chickenpox is confirmed, the illness warrants specialist care and urgent treatment. Corticosteroids should not be stopped and the dose may need to be increased.

9. Exposure to measles should be avoided. Medical advice should be sought immediately if exposure occurs. Prophylaxis with normal intramuscular immuneglobulin may be needed.

10. Live vaccines should not be given to individuals with impaired immune responsiveness. The antibody response to other vaccines may be diminished.

11. The use of Solu-Medrone in active tuberculosis should be restricted to those cases of fulminating or disseminated tuberculosis in which the corticosteroid is used for the management of the disease in conjunction with an appropriate anti-tuberculous regimen. If corticosteroids are indicated in patients with latent tuberculosis or tuberculin reactivity, close observation is necessary as reactivation of the disease may occur. During prolonged corticosteroid therapy, these patients should receive chemoprophylaxis.

12. Rarely anaphylactoid reactions have been reported following parenteral Solu-Medrone therapy. Physicians using the drug should be prepared to deal with such a possibility. Appropriate precautionary measures should be taken prior to administration, especially when the patient has a history of drug allergy.

13. Care should be taken for patients receiving cardioactive drugs such as digoxin because of steroid induced electrolyte disturbance/potassium loss (see Undesirable effects).

14. Corticosteroids should not be used for the management of head injury or stroke because it is unlikely to be of benefit and may even be harmful.

Special precautions:

Particular care is required when considering the use of systemic corticosteroids in patients with the following conditions and frequent patient monitoring is necessary.

1. Osteoporosis (post-menopausal females are particularly at risk).
2. Hypertension or congestive heart failure.
3. Existing or previous history of severe affective disorders (especially previous steroid psychosis).
4. Diabetes mellitus (or a family history of diabetes).
5. History of tuberculosis.
6. Glaucoma (or a family history of glaucoma).
7. Previous corticosteroid-induced myopathy.
8. Liver failure or cirrhosis.
9. Renal insufficiency.
10. Epilepsy.
11. Peptic ulceration.
12. Fresh intestinal anastomoses.
13. Predisposition to thrombophlebitis.
14. Abscess or other pyogenic infections.
15. Ulcerative colitis.
16. Diverticulitis.
17. Myasthenia gravis.
18. Ocular herpes simplex, for fear of corneal perforation.
19. Hypothyroidism.
20. Recent myocardial infarction (myocardial rupture has been reported).
21. Kaposi's sarcoma has been reported to occur in patients receiving corticosteroid therapy. Discontinuation of corticosteroids may result in clinical remission

Use in children: Corticosteroids cause growth retardation in infancy, childhood and adolescence, which may be irreversible. Treatment should be limited to the minimum dosage for the shortest possible time. In order to minimise suppression of the hypothalamo-pituitary-adrenal axis and growth retardation, treatment should be administered where possible as a single dose on alternate days.

Use in the elderly: The common adverse effects of systemic corticosteroids may be associated with more serious consequences in old age, especially osteoporosis, hypertension, hypokalaemia, diabetes, susceptibility to infection and thinning of the skin. Close clinical supervision is required to avoid life-threatening reactions.

4.5 Interaction with other medicinal products and other forms of Interaction

1. Convulsions have been reported with concurrent use of methylprednisolone and ciclosporin. Since concurrent administration of these agents results in a mutual inhibition of metabolism, it is possible that convulsions and other adverse events associated with the individual use of either drug may be more apt to occur.

2. Drugs that induce hepatic enzymes, such as rifampicin, rifabutin, carbamazepine, phenobarbitone, phenytoin, primidone, and aminoglutethimide enhance the metabolism of corticosteroids and its therapeutic effects may be reduced.

3. Drugs which inhibit the CYP3A4 enzyme, such as cimetidine, erythromycin, ketoconazole, itraconazole, diltiazem and mibefradil, may decrease the rate of metabolism of corticosteroids and hence increase the serum concentration.

4. Steroids may reduce the effects of anticholinesterases in myasthenia gravis. The desired effects of hypoglycaemic agents (including insulin), anti-hypertensives and diuretics are antagonised by corticosteroids, and the hypokalaemic effects of acetazolamide, loop diuretics, thiazide diuretics and carbenoxolone are enhanced.

5. The efficacy of coumarin anticoagulants may be enhanced by concurrent corticosteroid therapy and close monitoring of the INR or prothrombin time is required to avoid spontaneous bleeding.

6. The renal clearance of salicylates is increased by corticosteroids and steroid withdrawal may result in salicylate intoxication. Salicylates and non-steroidal anti-inflammatory agents should be used cautiously in conjunction with corticosteroids in hypothrombinaemia.

7. Steroids have been reported to interact with neuromuscular blocking agents such as pancuronium with partial reversal of the neuromuscular block.

4.6 Pregnancy and lactation

Pregnancy

The ability of corticosteroids to cross the placenta varies between individual drugs, however, methylprednisolone does cross the placenta.

Administration of corticosteroids to pregnant animals can cause abnormalities of foetal development including cleft

Table 1

Schedule A (1)	Dose (mg)	Route in hours	Interval	Duration
Pre-operative:	20	IM	3-6	
During Surgery:	20 to 40	IV	hourly	
Post operative:	20	IM	3	24 hours
	16	IM	3	24 hours
	12	IM	3	24 hours
	8	IM	3	24 hours
	4	IM	3	24 hours
	4	IM	6	24 hours
	4	IM	12	24 hours
Schedule B (2)	**Dose (mg)**	**Route in hours**	**Duration**	**Days**
Pre-operative:	40	IM	6	2-3
Post-operative:	40	IM	6	3-5
	20	Oral	6	1
	12	Oral	6	1
	8	Oral	8	1
	4	Oral	12	1
	4	Oral		1

palate, intra-uterine growth retardation and affects on brain growth and development. There is no evidence that corticosteroids result in an increased incidence of congenital abnormalities, such as cleft palate in man, however, when administered for long periods or repeatedly during pregnancy, corticosteroids may increase the risk of intra-uterine growth retardation. Hypoadrenalism may, in theory, occur in the neonate following prenatal exposure to corticosteroids but usually resolves spontaneously following birth and is rarely clinically important. As with all drugs, corticosteroids should only be prescribed when the benefits to the mother and child outweigh the risks. When corticosteroids are essential, however, patients with normal pregnancies may be treated as though they were in the non-gravid state.

Lactation

Corticosteroids are excreted in small amounts in breast milk, however, doses of up to 40 mg daily of methylprednisolone are unlikely to cause systemic effects in the infant. Infants of mothers taking higher doses than this may have a degree of adrenal suppression, but the benefits of breast-feeding are likely to outweigh any theoretical risk.

4.7 Effects on ability to drive and use machines
None stated.

4.8 Undesirable effects
Under normal circumstances Solu-Medrone therapy would be considered as short-term. However, the possibility of side-effects attributable to corticosteroid therapy should be recognised, particularly when high-dose therapy is being used (see Special warnings and special precautions for use). Such side-effects include:

PARENTERAL CORTICOSTEROID THERAPY - Anaphylactic reaction with or without circulatory collapse, cardiac arrest, bronchospasm, cardiac arrhythmias, hypotension or hypertension, hypopigmentation or hyperpigmentation.

GASTRO-INTESTINAL - Dyspepsia, peptic ulceration with perforation and haemorrhage, abdominal distension, oesophageal ulceration, oesophageal candidiasis, acute pancreatitis, perforation of the bowel, gastric haemorrhage. Nausea, vomiting and bad taste in mouth may occur especially with rapid administration.

Increases in alanine transaminase (ALT, SGPT) aspartate transaminase (AST, SGOT) and alkaline phosphatase have been observed following corticosteroid treatment. These changes are usually small, not associated with any clinical syndrome and are reversible upon discontinuation.

ANTI-INFLAMMATORY AND IMMUNOSUPPRESSIVE EFFECTS - Increased susceptibility and severity of infections with suppression of clinical symptoms and signs, opportunistic infections, may suppress reactions to skin tests, recurrence of dormant tuberculosis (see Special warnings and special precautions for use).

MUSCULOSKELETAL - Proximal myopathy, osteoporosis, vertebral and long bone fractures, avascular osteonecrosis, tendon rupture.

FLUID AND ELECTROLYTE DISTURBANCE - Sodium and water retention, potassium loss, hypertension, hypokalaemic alkalosis, congestive heart failure in susceptible patients.

DERMATOLOGICAL - Impaired healing, petechiae and ecchymosis, skin atrophy, bruising, striae, telangiectasia, acne. Kaposi's sarcoma has been reported to occur in patients receiving corticosteroid therapy. Discontinuation of corticosteroids may result in clinical remission.

ENDOCRINE/METABOLIC - Suppression of the hypothalamo-pituitary-adrenal axis, growth suppression in infancy, childhood and adolescence, menstrual irregularity and amenorrhoea. Cushingoid facies, hirsutism, weight gain, impaired carbohydrate tolerance with increased requirement for antidiabetic therapy, negative nitrogen and calcium balance. Increased appetite.

NEUROPSYCHIATRIC - Euphoria, psychological dependence, mood swings, depression, personality changes, insomnia. Increased intra-cranial pressure with papilloedema in children (pseudotumour cerebri), usually after treatment withdrawal. Psychosis, aggravation of schizophrenia, seizures.

OPHTHALMIC - Increased intra-ocular pressure, glaucoma, papilloedema with possible damage to the optic nerve, cataracts, corneal or scleral thinning, exacerbation of ophthalmic viral or fungal disease.

CARDIOVASCULAR – Myocardial rupture following a myocardial infarction.

GENERAL - Leucocytosis, hypersensitivity including anaphylaxis, thrombo-embolism, malaise, persistent hiccups with high doses of corticosteroids.

WITHDRAWAL SYMPTOMS - Too rapid a reduction of corticosteroid dosage following prolonged treatment can lead to acute adrenal insufficiency, hypotension and death. However, this is more applicable to corticosteroids with an indication where continuous therapy is given (see Special warnings and special precautions for use).

A 'withdrawal syndrome' may also occur including, fever, myalgia, arthralgia, rhinitis, conjunctivitis, painful itchy skin nodules and loss of weight.

4.9 Overdose
There is no clinical syndrome of acute overdosage with Solu-Medrone. Methylprednisolone is dialysable. Following chronic overdosage the possibility of adrenal suppression should be guarded against by gradual diminution of dose levels over a period of time. In such event the patient may require to be supported during any further stressful episode.

5. PHARMACOLOGICAL PROPERTIES

5.1 Pharmacodynamic properties
Medrone is a corticosteroid with an anti-inflammatory activity at least five times that of hydrocortisone. An enhanced separation of glucocorticoid and mineralocorticoid effect results in a reduced incidence of sodium and water retention.

5.2 Pharmacokinetic properties
Methylprednisolone is extensively bound to plasma proteins, mainly to globulin and less so to albumin. Only unbound corticosteroid has pharmacological effects or is metabolised. Metabolism occurs in the liver and to a lesser extent in the kidney. Metabolites are excreted in the urine.

Mean elimination half-life ranges from 2.4 to 3.5 hours in normal healthy adults and appears to be independent of the route of administration.

Total body clearance following intravenous or intramuscular injection of methylprednisolone to healthy adult volunteers is approximately 15-16l/hour. Peak methylprednisolone plasma levels of 33.67 mcg/100 ml were achieved in 2 hours after a single 40 mg i.m. injection to 22 adult male volunteers.

6. PHARMACEUTICAL PARTICULARS

6.1 List of excipients
Sodium biphosphate and sodium phosphate.

The 40 mg vial also contains lactose.

6.2 Incompatibilities
None stated.

6.3 Shelf life
Shelf-life of the medicinal product as packaged for sale: 60 months.

After reconstitution with Sterile Water for injections, use immediately, discard any remainder.

6.4 Special precautions for storage
Store below 25°C.

Refer to Section 4.2 Dosage and Administration. No diluents other than those referred to are recommended. Parenteral drug products should be inspected visually for particulate matter and discoloration prior to administration.

6.5 Nature and contents of container
Type I clear glass vial with butyl rubber plug and flip top seal.

Each vial of Solu-Medrone 40 mg contains the equivalent of 40 mg of methylprednisolone as the sodium succinate for reconstitution with 1 ml of Sterile Water for Injections.

Each vial of Solu-Medrone 125 mg contains the equivalent of 125 mg of methylprednisolone as the sodium succinate for reconstitution with 2 ml of Sterile Water for Injections.

Each vial of Solu-Medrone 500 mg contains the equivalent of 500 mg of methylprednisolone as the sodium succinate for reconstitution with 7.8 ml of Sterile Water for Injections.

Each vial of Solu-Medrone 1 g contains the equivalent of 1 g of methylprednisolone as the sodium succinate for reconstitution with 15.6 ml of Sterile Water for Injections.

6.6 Instructions for use and handling
No special requirements.

7. MARKETING AUTHORISATION HOLDER
Pharmacia Limited
Davy Avenue
Milton Keynes
MK5 8PH
UK

8. MARKETING AUTHORISATION NUMBER(S)

Solu- Medrone 40 mg	PL 0032/0033
Solu-Medrone 125mg	PL 0032/0034
Solu-Medrone 500mg	PL 0032/0035
Solu-Medrone 1g	PL 0032/0039

9. DATE OF FIRST AUTHORISATION/RENEWAL OF THE AUTHORISATION
PL 0032/0033: 21 February 1990
PL 0032/0034: 21 February 1990
PL 0032/0035: 21 February 1990
PL 0032/0039: 30 July 1990

10. DATE OF REVISION OF THE TEXT
May 2005

Legal category: POM

SM1_1

Solvazinc

(Provalis Healthcare)

1. NAME OF THE MEDICINAL PRODUCT
Solvazinc® Effervescent Tablets

2. QUALITATIVE AND QUANTITATIVE COMPOSITION
Each Solvazinc® tablet contains the following active ingredient:

Zinc sulphate monohydrate: 125mg (equivalent to 45mg elemental zinc).

For excipients, see 6.1

3. PHARMACEUTICAL FORM
Effervescent tablet.

4. CLINICAL PARTICULARS

4.1 Therapeutic indications
Zinc sulphate is a source of zinc which is an essential trace element and involved in a number of body enzyme systems.

Indications: For the treatment of zinc deficiency.

4.2 Posology and method of administration
Method of Administration: oral after dissolution in water.

Adults: One tablet, dissolved in water, once to three times daily after meals.

Children: More than 30kg: One tablet, dissolved in water, once to three times daily after meals.

10-30kg: ½ tablet, dissolved in water, once to three times daily after meals.

Less than 10kg: ½ tablet, dissolved in water, once daily after meals.

4.3 Contraindications
None.

4.4 Special warnings and special precautions for use
Accumulation of zinc may occur in cases of renal failure.

4.5 Interaction with other medicinal products and other forms of Interaction
Zinc may inhibit the absorption of concurrently administered tetracyclines;

when both are being given an interval of at least three hours should be allowed.

4.6 Pregnancy and lactation
The safety of this product in human pregnancy has not been established.

Zinc crosses the placenta and is present in breast milk.

4.7 Effects on ability to drive and use machines
Solvazinc® is not expected to affect ability to drive and use machines.

4.8 Undesirable effects
Zinc salts may cause abdominal pain and dyspepsia.

4.9 Overdose
Zinc sulphate is corrosive in overdosage. Symptoms are corrosion and inflammation of the mucous membrane of the mouth and stomach; ulceration of the stomach followed by perforation may occur. Gastric lavage and emesis should be avoided. Demulcents such as milk should be given. Chelating agents such as sodium calcium edetate may be useful.

5. PHARMACOLOGICAL PROPERTIES

5.1 Pharmacodynamic properties
Zinc is an essential trace element involved in many enzyme systems.

Severe deficiency causes skin lesion, alopecia, diarrhoea, increased susceptibility to infections and failure to thrive in children. Symptoms of less severe deficiency include distorted or absent perceptions of taste and smell and poor wound healing.

5.2 Pharmacokinetic properties
Zinc is absorbed from the gastrointestinal tract and distributed throughout the body. The highest concentrations occur in hair, eyes, male reproductive organs and bone. Lower levels are present in liver, kidney and muscle.

In blood 80% is found in erythrocytes. Plasma zinc levels range from 70 to 110μg/dL and about 50% of this is loosely bound to albumin.

About 7% is amino-acid bound and the rest is tightly bound to alpha 2-macroglobulins and other proteins.

5.3 Preclinical safety data
None Stated

6. PHARMACEUTICAL PARTICULARS

6.1 List of excipients
Solvazinc® contains the following excipients:

Sorbitol, mannitol, sodium hydrogen carbonate, citric acid, saccharin sodium, povidone K25, sodium citrate and sodium carbonate anhydrous.

6.2 Incompatibilities
None.

6.3 Shelf life
Three years.

6.4 Special precautions for storage
Store below 25°C, protect from moisture.

6.5 Nature and contents of container
Polypropylene containers with polyethylene caps and packed in cartons of three containers. Each tablet container contains 30 tablets. The tablet containers also contain a desiccant capsule.

6.6 Instructions for use and handling
None.

Administrative Data

7. MARKETING AUTHORISATION HOLDER
Provalis Healthcare Limited,
Newtech Square,
Deeside Industrial Park,
Deeside, Flintshire
CH5 2NT.

8. MARKETING AUTHORISATION NUMBER(S)
14658/0004.

9. DATE OF FIRST AUTHORISATION/RENEWAL OF THE AUTHORISATION
01 September 1998

10. DATE OF REVISION OF THE TEXT
January 04

Somatuline Autogel 60 mg, Somatuline Autogel 90 mg, Somatuline Autogel 120 mg

(Ipsen Ltd)

1. NAME OF THE MEDICINAL PRODUCT
SOMATULINE® AUTOGEL® 60 mg, solution for injection.
SOMATULINE® AUTOGEL® 90 mg, solution for injection.
SOMATULINE® AUTOGEL® 120 mg, solution for injection.

2. QUALITATIVE AND QUANTITATIVE COMPOSITION
Lanreotide (I.N.N.) 60 mg, 90 mg or 120 mg (as acetate).
For excipients, see 6.1.

3. PHARMACEUTICAL FORM
Solution for injection.
White to off-white, translucent and viscous supersaturated solution in a pre-filled syringe, ready for use.

4. CLINICAL PARTICULARS

4.1 Therapeutic indications
SOMATULINE AUTOGEL is indicated for the treatment of individuals with acromegaly when the circulating levels of Growth Hormone (GH) and/or Insulin-like Growth Factor-1 (IGF-1) remain abnormal after surgery and/or radiotherapy, or in patients who otherwise require medical treatment. The goal of treatment in acromegaly is to reduce GH and IGF-1 levels and where possible to normalise these values.

SOMATULINE AUTOGEL is also indicated for the treatment of symptoms associated with neuroendocrine (particularly carcinoid) tumours.

4.2 Posology and method of administration
• <u>**Posology**</u>

- Acromegaly

In patients receiving a somatostatin analogue for the first time, the recommended starting dose is 60 mg of SOMATULINE AUTOGEL administered every 28 days.

In patients previously treated with Somatuline LA 30 mg once every 14 days, the initial dose of SOMATULINE AUTOGEL should be 60 mg every 28 days; in patients previously treated with Somatuline LA 30 mg once every 10 days, the initial dose of SOMATULINE AUTOGEL should be 90 mg every 28 days; and in patients treated with Somatuline LA 30 mg once every 7 days, the initial dose of SOMATULINE AUTOGEL should be 120 mg every 28 days.

Thereafter, for all patients, the dose should be individualised according to the response of the patient (as judged by a reduction in symptoms and/or a reduction in GH and/or IGF1 levels).

If the desired response is not obtained, the dose may be increased.

If complete control is obtained (based on GH levels under 1 ng/ml, normalised IGF1 levels and/or disappearance of symptoms), the dose may be decreased.

Long term monitoring of symptoms, GH and IGF1 levels should be undertaken as clinically indicated.

- Neuroendocrine tumours:

The recommended starting dose is 60 to 120 mg administered every 28 days.

The dose should be adjusted according to the degree of symptomatic relief obtained.

<u>Hepatic/renal impairment and the elderly.</u>

Subjects with severe renal impairment show an approximately 2-fold decrease in total serum clearance of lanreotide, with a consequent increase in half-life and AUC. In hepatic impairment, an increase in volume of distribution and mean residence time are observed, but there is no difference in total clearance or AUC. Elderly subjects show an increase in half-life and mean residence time compared with healthy young subjects. Due to the wide therapeutic window of lanreotide, it is not necessary to alter the dose in these circumstances.

<u>Children.</u>

Currently there is no experience of administration of SOMATULINE AUTOGEL in children, therefore use of SOMATULINE AUTOGEL in children cannot be recommended.

• <u>**Method of administration**</u>

SOMATULINE AUTOGEL should be injected via the deep sub-cutaneous route in the superior external quadrant of the buttock. The skin should not be folded. The needle should be inserted rapidly to its full length, perpendicularly to the skin.

4.3 Contraindications
Hypersensitivity to lanreotide or related peptides.

4.4 Special warnings and special precautions for use
Pharmacological studies in animals and humans show that lanreotide, like somatostatin and its analogues, may produce a transient inhibition of the secretion of insulin and glucagon. Hence, diabetic patients treated by SOMATULINE AUTOGEL may experience a slight transient change in blood glucose levels. Blood glucose levels should be checked in order to determine whether anti-diabetic treatment needs to be adjusted.

Slight decreases in thyroid function have been seen during treatment with lanreotide in acromegalic patients, although clinical hypothyroidism is rare (<1%). Tests of thyroid function should be done where clinically indicated.

Lanreotide may reduce gall bladder motility and therefore, gall bladder echography may be advisable at the start of treatment and as clinically indicated thereafter. If gallstones do occur, they are generally asymptomatic. Symptomatic stones should be treated as medically indicated.

4.5 Interaction with other medicinal products and other forms of Interaction
The gastrointestinal effects of SOMATULINE AUTOGEL may reduce the intestinal absorption of co-administered drugs.

Concomitant administration of lanreotide injection with cyclosporin may decrease blood levels of cyclosporin, hence blood levels of cyclosporin should be monitored.

Interactions with highly plasma bound drugs are unlikely in view of the moderate binding of lanreotide to serum proteins (78 % mean serum binding).

4.6 Pregnancy and lactation
Reproductive studies in rats and rabbits at doses up to 33 times the human dose have failed to demonstrate a risk to the foetus; however there are no adequate and well-controlled studies in pregnant women. Because animal reproductive studies are not always predictive of human response, this drug should be used during pregnancy only if clearly needed.

Six pregnancies and one suspected pregnancy have been reported in patients who were being treated with lanreotide. Four pregnancies resulted in healthy, full term infants. One acromegalic patient delivered prematurely due to maternal complications. One patient with acromegaly had a first trimester miscarriage. One additional patient with acromegaly had a suspected first trimester miscarriage

There is no information available on the presence of lanreotide in human breast milk. SOMATULINE AUTOGEL should not be used during breast-feeding unless clearly necessary.

4.7 Effects on ability to drive and use machines
Therapy with SOMATULINE AUTOGEL is unlikely to impair patients' ability to drive or use machines.

4.8 Undesirable effects
• <u>**Clinical tolerance**</u>

The adverse reactions related to SOMATULINE AUTOGEL during clinical trials are consistent with those seen with other prolonged release formulations of lanreotide, and are predominantly gastrointestinal. In clinical trials of SOMATULINE AUTOGEL in acromegalic patients, 80% of patients experienced at least 1 adverse event. More than 50% of these adverse events were classified as gastrointestinal system disorders. The most commonly reported adverse reactions are diarrhoea, abdominal pain and nausea. These reactions are usually mild and transient.

Very common adverse reactions: the following adverse reactions occurred in more than 10% of patients: Diarrhoea, abdominal pain, nausea.

Common adverse reactions: the following adverse reactions occurred in greater than 5% but less than 10% of patients: constipation, flatulence, cholelithiasis, gall bladder sludge.

Less common adverse reactions: the following adverse reactions occurred in between 1 and 5% of patients: asthenia, fatigue, increased bilirubin.

Uncommon adverse reactions: the following adverse reactions occurred in less than 1% of patients. Injection site pain, skin nodule, hot flushes, leg pain, malaise, headache, tenesmus, vomiting, abnormal glucose tolerance, hyperglycaemia, decreased libido, somnolence, pruritus, increased sweating, skin disorder (not specified).

In rare instances, acute pancreatitis has been reported within a short time after the first administration of lanreotide in prolonged release formulations other than SOMATULINE AUTOGEL.

Cardiovascular effects including sinusal bradycardia, a myocardial infarction (ref. Section 4.9 "Overdose"), high blood pressure episodes and ventricular tachycardia have also been reported in exceptional cases with other prolonged release formulations of lanreotide.

• <u>**Local tolerance**</u>

Reactions at the injection site may occur after the deep subcutaneous injection of SOMATULINE AUTOGEL in the buttock. When specific enquiry was made, pain, redness, itching and induration were reported at the injection site 30 minutes after dosing in up to 8%, 5%, 5% and 19% of patients respectively. After 3 dosing intervals, these symptoms or signs were reduced to 6%, 2% 3% and 9% of patients or fewer. In all cases, the symptoms were described as mild.

4.9 Overdose
In clinical trials, lanreotide has been administered in doses up to 15 mg per day without serious adverse events related to the treatment. Human experience of overdose of prolonged release forms of lanreotide is limited to one unconfirmed case report of overdose where a patient was reported to have taken one intramuscular injection of the 30 mg prolonged release formulation daily for two months (instead of 1 injection every 7 to 14 days). One week after stopping therapy the 52 year-old man with a history of acromegaly, diabetes mellitus and arterial hypertension suffered a fatal cardiac infarction.

If overdosage occurs, symptomatic management is indicated.

5. PHARMACOLOGICAL PROPERTIES

5.1 Pharmacodynamic properties
Pharmacotherapeutic group: Antigrowth hormones, ATC code: H01C B03.

Lanreotide is an octapeptide analogue of natural somatostatin. Like somatostatin, lanreotide is an inhibitor of various endocrine, neuroendocrine, exocrine and paracrine functions. It shows high binding affinity for human somatostatin receptors (SSTR) 2, 3 and 5, and reduced affinity for human SSTR 1 and 4. Activity at SSTR 2 and 5 is the primary mechanism considered to be responsible for GH inhibition.

Lanreotide, like somatostatin, exhibits a general exocrine anti-secretory action. It inhibits the basal secretion of motilin, gastric inhibitory peptide and pancreatic polypeptide, but has no significant effect on fasting secretin or gastrin secretion. Lanreotide markedly inhibits meal-induced increases in superior mesenteric artery blood flow and portal venous blood flow. Lanreotide significantly reduces prostaglandin E1-stimulated jejunal secretion of water, sodium, potassium and chloride. Lanreotide reduces prolactin levels in acromegalic patients treated long term.

5.2 Pharmacokinetic properties
Pharmacokinetic parameters of lanreotide after intravenous administration in healthy volunteers indicated limited extravascular distribution, with a steady-state volume of distribution of 13 l. Total clearance was 20 l/h, terminal half-life was 2.5 hours and mean residence time was 0.68 hours.

After a single subcutaneous injection of SOMATULINE AUTOGEL 60 mg in healthy volunteers, a maximum serum concentration (Cmax) of 5.8 ± 4 ng/ml was reached after 6 hours, followed by a slow decrease (mean residence time: 30 ± 6 days, apparent half-life: 33 ± 14 days). The absolute bioavailability was 63 ± 10%.

After a single intramuscular injection of SOMATULINE AUTOGEL 60 mg in healthy volunteers, a maximum serum concentration (Cmax) of 6.8 ± 3 ng/ml was reached after 15 hours, followed by a slow decrease (mean residence time: 23 ± 11 days, apparent half-life: 23 ± 9 days). The absolute bioavailability was 79 ± 10%.

Therefore the route of administration (subcutaneous or intramuscular) does not show any marked influence on the lanreotide pharmacokinetic profile.

After a single intramuscular injection of SOMATULINE AUTOGEL 90 mg in healthy volunteers, a maximum serum concentration (Cmax) of 9.8 ± 5 ng/ml was reached after 10 hours, followed by a slow decrease (mean residence time: 26 ± 4 days, apparent half-life: 31 ± 16 days). The absolute bioavailability was 58 ± 10%.

After a single intramuscular injection of SOMATULINE AUTOGEL 120 mg in healthy volunteers, a maximum serum concentration (Cmax) of 12.8 ± 7 ng/ml was reached after 16 hours, followed by a slow decrease (mean residence time: 29 ± 3 days, apparent half-life: 28 ± 6 days). The absolute bioavailability was 55 ± 10%.

Therefore lanreotide serum concentration after intramuscular administration of SOMATULINE AUTOGEL 60, 90 and 120 mg shows an almost log-linear first order lanreotide release profile.

Trough lanreotide serum levels obtained after three deep subcutaneous injections of SOMATULINE AUTOGEL 60, 90 or 120 mg given every 28 days are similar to the steady-state trough lanreotide serum levels obtained in acromegalic patients previously treated with intramuscular administrations of lanreotide 30 mg prolonged release microparticles (Somatuline LA) every 14, 10 or 7 days respectively.

Lanreotide serum levels of 1 ng/ml are able to suppress GH to < 5 ng/ml in more than 60% of patients studied. Lanreotide serum levels of 2.5 ng/ml are able to suppress GH to < 5 ng/ml in more than 90% of patients studied.

5.3 Preclinical safety data

In vitro and animal toxicology studies have not shown any specific toxic potential for lanreotide. The observed effects are related to the pharmacological properties of lanreotide on the endocrine system.

6. PHARMACEUTICAL PARTICULARS

6.1 List of excipients

Water for injections

6.2 Incompatibilities

Not applicable.

6.3 Shelf life

24 months.

6.4 Special precautions for storage

Store in a refrigerator between + 2°C and + 8°C in its original package. Do not freeze.

6.5 Nature and contents of container

SOMATULINE AUTOGEL is supplied in a clear polypropylene pre-filled syringe with a stainless steel needle and a plunger stopper made from bromobutyl rubber coated with silicone.

Each pre-filled syringe is packed in a nylon / polyethylene / aluminium laminated bag.

Box of one individual 60mg dose in a 0.3ml syringe with a needle (1.2 mm × 20 mm).

Box of one individual 90mg dose in a 0.3ml syringe with a needle (1.2 mm × 20 mm).

Box of one individual 120mg dose in a 0.5ml syringe with a needle (1.4 mm × 20 mm).

6.6 Instructions for use and handling

The solution for injection in a pre-filled syringe is ready for use.

For immediate and single use following first opening.

7. MARKETING AUTHORISATION HOLDER

IPSEN Limited

190 Bath Road

Slough, Berkshire

SL1 3XE, UK.

8. MARKETING AUTHORISATION NUMBER(S)

PL 06958/0013 (SOMATULINE® AUTOGEL® 60 mg).

PL 06958/0014 (SOMATULINE® AUTOGEL® 90 mg).

PL 06958/0015 (SOMATULINE® AUTOGEL® 120 mg).

9. DATE OF FIRST AUTHORISATION/RENEWAL OF THE AUTHORISATION

16 October 2001.

10. DATE OF REVISION OF THE TEXT

August 2001.

Somatuline LA

(Ipsen Ltd)

1. NAME OF THE MEDICINAL PRODUCT

Somatuline LA

2. QUALITATIVE AND QUANTITATIVE COMPOSITION

Lanreotide (I.N.N., B.A.N.) 0.030 g*

*Each vial is filled with a quantity of microparticles of lanreotide acetate and co-polymers corresponding to 40 mg of lanreotide base, which ensures the actual injection of 30 mg of lanreotide.

3. PHARMACEUTICAL FORM

Powder for suspension for injection.

4. CLINICAL PARTICULARS

4.1 Therapeutic indications

Acromegaly:

Somatuline LA is indicated for the treatment of acromegaly when the circulating levels of growth hormone remain abnormal after surgery and/or radiotherapy.

Thyrotrophic Adenomas:

Somatuline LA is indicated for the treatment of thyrotrophic adenomas when the circulating level of thyroid stimulating hormone remains inappropriately high after surgery and/or radiotherapy.

Neuroendocrine Tumours:

Somatuline LA is also indicated for the relief of symptoms associated with neuroendocrine (particularly carcinoid) tumours.

4.2 Posology and method of administration

Acromegaly and Neuroendocrine Tumours:

Initially, one intramuscular injection should be given every 14 days. The frequency of subsequent injections may be varied in accordance with the individual patient's response (as judged by a reduction in symptoms and/or a reduction in GH and/or IGF-1 levels) such that injections can be given every 7 to 10 days as necessary.

Thyroid tumours:

Treatment should only be initiated and maintained by physicians experienced in the management of this condition.

Initially, one intra-muscular injection should be given every 14 days. In the case of an insufficient response, as judged by the levels of thyroid hormone and TSH, the frequency of injection may be increased to 1 every 10 days. Continued treatment should be guided by periodic measurement of thyroid hormone and TSH.

Elderly:

No dose modification is required in elderly patients.

Children:

As there is no experience of the use of the product in children, the use of Somatuline LA in children cannot be advised.

4.3 Contraindications

Somatuline LA should not be prescribed during pregnancy and lactation, nor in patients presenting with hypersensitivity to the peptide or related peptides.

4.4 Special warnings and special precautions for use

Pharmacological studies in animals and humans show that lanreotide, like somatostatin and its analogues, inhibit secretion of insulin and glucagon. Hence, patients treated with Somatuline LA may experience hypoglycaemia or hyperglycaemia. Blood glucose levels should be monitored when lanreotide treatment is initiated and treatment of diabetic patients should be accordingly adjusted (see Section 4.8).

Lanreotide may reduce gall bladder motility and therefore, gall bladder echography is advised at the start of treatment and every six months thereafter. If gallstones do occur, they are generally asymptomatic. Symptomatic stones should be treated as medically indicated.

Fat concentrations in stools may increase to levels high enough to result in steatorrhoea, requiring the use of appropriate corrective therapy.

In patients with hepatic/renal dysfunction, kidney and liver function should be regularly monitored and the dose interval adjusted if necessary.

4.5 Interaction with other medicinal products and other forms of Interaction

The gastrointestinal effects of Somatuline LA may reduce the intestinal absorption of co-administered drugs. As with other somatostatin analogues, Somatuline LA may reduce the intestinal absorption of cyclosporin A. Interactions with highly plasma bound drugs are unlikely in view of the moderate binding of lanreotide to serum proteins (78 % mean serum binding).

4.6 Pregnancy and lactation

Studies in animals showed transitory growth retardation of offspring prior to weaning. Although no teratogenic effects have been observed in animals, in the absence of clinical experience, lanreotide must not be administered to pregnant or lactating women.

4.7 Effects on ability to drive and use machines

Therapy with Somatuline LA is unlikely to impair a patient's ability to drive or use machinery.

4.8 Undesirable effects

Clinical tolerance

The side effects of Somatuline LA reported in the clinical trials are mainly local and gastrointestinal.

Local tolerance: moderate, transitory pain at the injection site is sometimes associated with local redness.

General tolerance: gastrointestinal side effects are the most common and include: diarrhoea or soft stools, abdominal pain, flatulence, anorexia, nausea and vomiting. In general, all these side effects are mild to moderate in intensity; in most cases the frequency and the intensity of such effects appear to diminish or to resolve with continued therapy.

Cases of asymptomatic and symptomatic gallbladder lithiasis have been reported in patients during prolonged treatment. A precautionary statement is included in section 4.4. In rare instances, acute pancreatitis has been reported within a short time after the first administration.

Biological tolerance

Altered glucose regulation has been reported in healthy volunteers. In non-diabetic patients both glucose intolerance and hyperglycaemia has been observed (See section 4.4).

4.9 Overdose

There is no human experience of overdosage. Animal data do not predict any effects other than those on insulin and glucagon secretion and the gastrointestinal system. If overdosage occurs, symptomatic management is indicated.

5. PHARMACOLOGICAL PROPERTIES

5.1 Pharmacodynamic properties

Like natural somatostatin, lanreotide is a peptide inhibitor of a number of endocrine, neuroendocrine, exocrine and paracrine functions. It shows good affinity for peripheral somatostatin receptors (anterior pituitary and pancreatic). In contrast, its affinity for central receptors is much lower. This profile confers a good specificity of action at the level of growth hormone and digestive hormone secretion.

Lanreotide shows a much longer duration of action than natural somatostatin. In addition, its marked selectivity for the secretion of growth hormone, compared to that of insulin, makes it a suitable candidate for the treatment of acromegaly. By inhibiting the synthesis of thyroid stimulating hormone (TSH), lanreotide also normalised thyroid function of patients with thyrotrophin secreting adenomas in 50% (8/16) of the per-protocol population treated for 6 months. There was no significant reduction in the size of the adenoma. Furthermore, the inhibitory action of lanreotide on intestinal exocrine secretion, digestive hormones and cellular proliferation mechanisms is suited to the symptomatic treatment of endocrine digestive tumours, especially carcinoids.

5.2 Pharmacokinetic properties

The plasma profile of lanreotide administered intramuscularly in healthy volunteers, is characterised by an initial rapid release phase (phase 1) followed by a prolonged slow release phase (phase 2). The first plasma peak (C_{max1}: 6.8 ± 3.8μg/l) occurs at 1.4 ± 0.8 hours and the second (C_{max2}: 2.5 ± 0.9μg/l) at 1.9 ± 1.8 days. The absolute bioavailability is 46.1 ± 16.7%. The mean residence time of 8.0 ± 1.0 days and the apparent half-life of 5.2 ± 2.5 days, confirm the prolonged release of the product.

After a single administration in acromegaly patients, a comparable pharmacokinetic profile is observed and the levels of growth hormone and IGF-1 are significantly reduced for a period of about 14 days. With repeated administration over several months, there is no evidence of accumulation of lanreotide.

5.3 Preclinical safety data

In vitro and animal toxicology studies have not shown any specific toxic potential for lanreotide. The observed effects are related to the pharmacological properties of lanreotide on the endocrine system. The resorption of Somatuline LA is complete in 45-60 days.

6. PHARMACEUTICAL PARTICULARS

6.1 List of excipients

Lactide-glycolide copolymer

Lactic-glycolic copolymer

Mannitol

Carmellose (Na)

Polysorbate 80

6.2 Incompatibilities

Somatuline LA must be made up immediately prior to use, using only the solution supplied in the package.

6.3 Shelf life

2 years

6.4 Special precautions for storage

Store at a temperature between +2°C and 8°C (in the refrigerator), do not freeze.

6.5 Nature and contents of container

Type I, clear, slightly tinted, glass vial containing sterile Somatuline LA.

Box of 1 vial, 1 ampoule (vehicle), 2 needles and 1 syringe.

Box of 2 vials, 2 ampoules (vehicle), 4 needles and 2 syringes.

Box of 6 vials, 6 ampoules (vehicle), 12 needles and 6 syringes.

6.6 Instructions for use and handling

Somatuline LA must be made up in the supplied solution immediately before injection, by shaking the vial, gently, 20 to 30 times, in order to obtain a homogenous suspension with a milky appearance. This must not be mixed with other medications.

NB: It is important that injection of this product is performed according to the instructions in the leaflet.

7. MARKETING AUTHORISATION HOLDER

IPSEN LIMITED

190 BATH ROAD

SLOUGH SL 1 3XE

8. MARKETING AUTHORISATION NUMBER(S)

Somatuline LA PL number: 06958 / 0018

9. DATE OF FIRST AUTHORISATION/RENEWAL OF THE AUTHORISATION

26 January 1998

10. DATE OF REVISION OF THE TEXT

4th August 2003

SOMAVERT 10mg, 15mg and 20mg

(Pfizer Limited)

1. NAME OF THE MEDICINAL PRODUCT

SOMAVERT▼ 10 mg powder and solvent for solution for injection.

SOMAVERT▼ 15 mg Powder and solvent for solution for injection.

SOMAVERT▼ 20 mg Powder and solvent for solution for injection.

2. QUALITATIVE AND QUANTITATIVE COMPOSITION

Presentations	
SOMAVERT 10mg	Each vial contains 10 mg of pegvisomant. After reconstitution, 1 ml of solution contains 10 mg pegvisomant.
SOMAVERT 15mg	Each vial contains 15 mg of pegvisomant. After reconstitution, 1 ml of solution contains 15 mg pegvisomant.
SOMAVERT 20mg	Each vial contains 20 mg of pegvisomant. After reconstitution, 1 ml of solution contains 20 mg pegvisomant.

Pegvisomant is produced by recombinant DNA technology in an *E.Coli* expression system.

For excipients, see 6.1.

3. PHARMACEUTICAL FORM

Powder and solvent for solution for injection.

The powder is white to slightly off-white.

4. CLINICAL PARTICULARS

4.1 Therapeutic indications

Treatment of patients with acromegaly who have had an inadequate response to surgery and/or radiation therapy and in whom an appropriate medical treatment with somatostatin analogues did not normalize IGF-I concentrations or was not tolerated.

4.2 Posology and method of administration

Treatment should be initiated under the supervision of a physician experienced in the treatment of acromegaly.

It should be considered whether to continue treatment with somatostatin analogues as the use in combination with SOMAVERT has not been studied.

For the different dosage regimens the following strengths are available: Somavert 10 mg, Somavert 15 mg and Somavert 20 mg.

A loading dose of 80 mg pegvisomant should be administered subcutaneously under medical supervision. Following this, SOMAVERT 10 mg reconstituted in 1 ml of water for injections should be administered once daily as a subcutaneous injection.

Dose adjustments should be based on serum IGF-I levels. Serum IGF-I concentrations should be measured every four to six weeks and appropriate dose adjustments made in increments of 5 mg/day in order to maintain the serum IGF-I concentration within the age-adjusted normal range and to maintain an optimal therapeutic response.

The maximum dose should not exceed 30 mg/day.

Elderly patients

No dose adjustment is required.

Paediatric patients

The safety and effectiveness of SOMAVERT in paediatric patients has not been established.

Patients with impaired hepatic or renal function

The safety and effectiveness of SOMAVERT in patients with renal or hepatic insufficiency has not been established.

Diabetic patients

Insulin sensitivity may increase following initiation of treatment with SOMAVERT. The risk of hypoglycaemia was observed in some diabetic patients treated by insulin or oral hypoglycaemic medicinal products while receiving SOMAVERT treatment. Therefore, in patients with diabetes mellitus, doses of insulin or oral hypoglycemic medicinal products may need to be decreased (see sections 4.4 and 4.5).

4.3 Contraindications

Hypersensitivity to pegvisomant or any of the excipients.

4.4 Special warnings and special precautions for use

Growth hormone-secreting pituitary tumours may sometimes expand, causing serious complications (for example, visual field defects). Treatment by SOMAVERT does not reduce tumour size. All patients with these tumours should be carefully monitored in order to avoid any eventual progression in tumour size under treatment.

SOMAVERT is a potent antagonist of growth hormone action. A growth hormone deficient state may result from SOMAVERT administration, despite the presence of elevated serum growth hormone levels. Serum IGF-I concentrations should be monitored and maintained within the age-adjusted normal range by adjustment of SOMAVERT dosing.

Serum concentrations of alanine aminotransferase (ALT) and aspartate transaminase (AST) should be monitored at four to six week intervals for the first six months of treatment with SOMAVERT, or at any time in patients exhibiting symptoms suggestive of hepatitis. Evidence of obstructive biliary tract disease should be ruled out in patients with elevations of ALT and AST or in patients with a prior history of treatment with any somatostatin analogue. Administration of SOMAVERT should be discontinued if signs of liver disease persist.

The study conducted with SOMAVERT in diabetic patients treated either by insulin or by oral hypoglycaemic medicinal products revealed the risk of hypoglycemia in this population. Therefore, in acromegalic patients with diabetes mellitus, doses of insulin or hypoglycaemic medicinal products may need to be decreased (see also sections 4.2 and 4.5).

The therapeutic benefits of a reduction in IGF-I concentration which results in improvement of the patient's clinical condition could potentially increase fertility in female patients. Patients should be advised to use adequate contraception if necessary. SOMAVERT is not recommended during pregnancy (see also section 4.6).

The use of SOMAVERT in combination with other medicinal products for the treatment of acromegaly has not been extensively investigated.

4.5 Interaction with other medicinal products and other forms of Interaction

Interactions between SOMAVERT and other medicinal products have not been evaluated in formal studies.

Patients receiving insulin or oral hypoglycaemic medicinal products may require dose reduction of these therapeutic agents due to the effect of pegvisomant on insulin sensitivity (see sections 4.2 and 4.4).

SOMAVERT has significant structural similarity to growth hormone which causes it to cross-react in commercially available growth hormone assays. Since serum concentrations of therapeutically-effective doses of SOMAVERT are generally 100 to 1000 times higher than the actual serum growth hormone concentrations seen in acromegalics, measurements of serum growth hormone concentrations will be spuriously reported in commercially available growth hormone assays. SOMAVERT treatment should therefore not be monitored or adjusted based on serum growth hormone concentrations reported from these assays.

4.6 Pregnancy and lactation

For pegvisomant no clinical data on exposed pregnancies are available.

Animal studies are insufficient with respect to effects on pregnancy, embryonal/foetal development, parturition or postnatal development (see section 5.3).

The potential risk for humans is unknown. Therefore SOMAVERT is not recommended during pregnancy (see also section 4.4).

Use during lactation

It is not known whether pegvisomant is excreted into breast milk. Therefore, SOMAVERT should not be used in breast-feeding women or breast-feeding should be discontinued.

4.7 Effects on ability to drive and use machines

No studies on the effect on the ability to drive and use machines have been performed.

4.8 Undesirable effects

The list below contains adverse reactions seen in clinical trials. Only events for which there is at least a reasonable suspicion of a causal relationship to SOMAVERT treatment are listed. In clinical studies, for patients treated with pegvisomant (n=160), the majority of adverse reactions to pegvisomant were of mild to moderate intensity, of limited duration and did not require discontinuation of treatment. The most commonly reported adverse events considered related to SOMAVERT occurring in ⩾ 5% of patients with acromegaly during the clinical trials were injection site reactions 11%, sweating 7%, headache 6% and asthenia 6%. Most injection site reactions characterised as localised erythemas and soreness, spontaneously resolved with local symptomatic treatment, while SOMAVERT therapy continued.

The development of isolated low-titre anti-growth hormone antibodies was observed in 16.9% of patients treated with SOMAVERT. The clinical significance of these antibodies is unknown.

Adverse reactions are listed according to the following categories:

Very common: ⩾10%

Common: ⩾1% and <10%

Uncommon: ⩾0.1% and <1%

<u>**Gastrointestinal disorders:**</u>

Common: Diarrhoea, constipation, nausea, vomiting, abdominal distension, dyspepsia, flatulence, elevated liver function tests

Uncommon: dry mouth, hemorrhoids, salivary hypersecretion, tooth disorder

<u>**General disorders:**</u>

Common: Influenza-like illness, fatigue, injection site bruising or bleeding, injection site reaction, injection site hypertrophy

Uncommon: oedema lower limb, pyrexia, weakness, asthenia, feeling abnormal, impaired healing, peripheral oedema

<u>**Musculoskeletal, connective tissue and bone disorders:**</u>

Common: arthralgia, myalgia, peripheral swelling

Uncommon: arthritis

<u>**Nervous system disorders:**</u>

Common: headache, dizziness, somnolence, tremor

Uncommon: hypoesthesia, dysgeusia, migraine, narcolepsy

<u>**Skin and subcutaneous tissue disorders:**</u>

Common: sweating, pruritis, rash

Uncommon: face oedema, dry skin, contusion, tendency to bruise, night sweats

<u>**Psychiatric disorders:**</u>

Common: abnormal dreams, sleep disorder

Uncommon: anger, apathy, confusion, increased libido, panic attack, short term memory loss

<u>**Metabolism and nutrition disorders:**</u>

Common: hypercholesterolemia, weight gain, hyperglycemia, hunger

Uncommon: hypertriglyceridemia, hypoglycemia

<u>**Respiratory, thoracic and mediastinal disorders:**</u>

Uncommon: dyspnea

<u>**Eye disorders:**</u>

Uncommon: asthenopia, eye pain

<u>**Renal and urinary disorders:**</u>

Uncommon: heamaturia, proteinuria, polyuria, renal impairment

<u>**Vascular disorders:**</u>

Common: hypertension

<u>**Ear and labyrinth disorders:**</u>

Uncommon: meniere's disease

<u>**Blood and lymphatic disorders:**</u>

Uncommon: thrombocytopenia, leukopenia, leukocytosis, bleeding tendency

4.9 Overdose

There is limited experience of overdosage with SOMAVERT. In the one reported incident of acute overdosage, where 80 mg/day was administered for 7 days, the patient experienced a slight increase in fatigue and dry mouth. In the week following discontinuation of treatment the adverse events noted were: insomnia, increased fatigue, a trace of foot oedema, fine tremor, and weight gain. Two weeks after stopping treatment, leukocytosis and moderate bleeding from injection and vein puncture sites was observed which were considered possibly related to SOMAVERT.

In cases of overdose, administration of SOMAVERT should be discontinued and not resumed until IGF-I levels return to within or above the normal range.

5. PHARMACOLOGICAL PROPERTIES

5.1 Pharmacodynamic properties

<u>Pharmacotherapeutic group:</u> ATC code: H01AX01

Pegvisomant is an analogue of human growth hormone that has been genetically modified to be a growth hormone receptor antagonist. Pegvisomant binds to growth hormone receptors on cell surfaces, where it blocks growth hormone binding, and thus interferes with intracellular growth hormone signal transduction. Pegvisomant is highly selective for the GH receptor, and does not cross-react with other cytokine receptors, including prolactin. Inhibition of growth hormone action with pegvisomant leads to decreased serum concentrations of insulin-like growth factor-I (IGF-I), as well as other growth hormone-responsive serum proteins such as free IGF-I, the acid-labile subunit of IGF-I (ALS), and insulin-like growth factor binding protein-3 (IGFBP-3).

Acromegalic patients (n=112) have been treated in a 12-week, randomised, double-blind, multicentre study comparing placebo and pegvisomant. Dose-dependent, statistically significant reductions in mean IGF-I ($p<0.0001$), free IGF-I ($p<0.05$), IGFBP-3 ($p<0.05$) and ALS ($p<0.05$) were observed at all post-baseline visits in the pegvisomant treatment groups. The serum IGF-1 was normalised at the end of the study (week 12) in 9.7%, 38.5%, 75% and 82% of subjects treated with placebo, 10 mg/day, 15 mg/day or 20 mg/day SOMAVERT respectively.

Statistically significant differences from placebo ($p<0.05$) were observed for improvements in the total signs and symptoms score for all dose groups compared to placebo.

A cohort of 38 acromegalic subjects has been followed in a long-term, open-label, dose-titration study for at least 12 consecutive months of daily dosing with pegvisomant (mean = 55 weeks). The mean IGF-I concentration in this cohort fell from 917 ng/ml to 299 ng/ml on pegvisomant, with 92% achieving a normal (age-adjusted) IGF-I concentration.

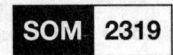

5.2 Pharmacokinetic properties

Absorption of pegvisomant following subcutaneous administration is slow and prolonged, and peak serum pegvisomant concentrations are not generally attained until 33-77 hours after administration. The mean extent of absorption of a subcutaneous dose was 57% relative to an intravenous dose.

The apparent volume of distribution of pegvisomant is relatively small (7-12 l). The mean total body systemic clearance of pegvisomant following multiple doses is estimated to be 28 ml/h for subcutaneous doses ranging from 10 to 20 mg/day. Renal clearance of pegvisomant is negligible and accounts for less than 1% of total body clearance. Pegvisomant is slowly eliminated from serum, with mean estimates of half-life generally ranging from 74 to 172 hours following either single or multiple-doses. The metabolism of pegvisomant is not studied.

After single subcutaneous pegvisomant administration no linearity is observed with rising doses of 10, 15 or 20 mg. Approximately linear pharmacokinetics is observed at steady state in the population pharmacokinetic studies. The data from 145 patients in two long-term studies who received daily doses of 10, 15, or 20 mg, demonstrate pegvisomant mean serum concentrations (± SD) of approximately 8800 ± 6300, 13200 ± 8000 and 15600 ± 10300 ng/ml, respectively.

The pharmacokinetics of pegvisomant are similar in normal healthy volunteers and acromegaly patients, although heavier individuals tend to have a higher total body clearance of pegvisomant than lighter individuals, and may thus require greater doses of pegvisomant.

No pharmacokinetic data in special populations (children, populations with renal and hepatic impairment) are available.

5.3 Preclinical safety data

Preclinical data revealed no special hazard for humans based on studies of repeated dose toxicity in rat and monkey. However, due to the marked pharmacological response in monkey, systemic exposures higher than those achieved in patients at therapeutic doses have not been studied. Except for one segment II test in the rabbit, no other reproductive toxicity studies were conducted.

No data on carcinogenic potential are available.

6. PHARMACEUTICAL PARTICULARS

6.1 List of excipients

Powder:

Glycine

Mannitol (E421)

Sodium phosphate dibasic anhydrous

Sodium phosphate monobasic monohydrate

Solvent: Water for Injections

6.2 Incompatibilities

This medicinal product must not be mixed with other medicinal products except those mentioned in section 6.6.

6.3 Shelf life

24 months

After reconstitution, the product should be used immediately.

6.4 Special precautions for storage

Store at 2°C – 8°C (in a refrigerator). Do not freeze. Keep the container in the outer carton in order to protect from light.

After reconstitution:

Use immediately.

6.5 Nature and contents of container

Powder in a 6 ml vial (type I glass) with a rubber stopper (butyl) and 8 ml solvent in a vial (type I) glass, with a rubber stopper (butyl).

Pack size: 30 vials of powder along with 30 vials of solvent. SOMAVERT 20 mg also available in pack size of 1 vial.

6.6 Instructions for use and handling

Reconstitute using 1 ml water for injections.

Add solvent to vial with powder for injection. Gently dissolve the powder with a slow, swirling motion. Do not shake vigorously, as this might cause denaturation of the active ingredient.

After reconstitution, if the solution is cloudy or contains particulate matter, the product must be discarded.

For single use only. Any unused product should be disposed of in accordance with local requirements.

7. MARKETING AUTHORISATION HOLDER

Pfizer Limited

Sandwich,

Kent CT13 9NJ,

United Kingdom

8. MARKETING AUTHORISATION NUMBER(S)

EU/1/02/240/001 - SOMAVERT 10 mg; pack size 30 vials

EU/1/02/240/002 - SOMAVERT 15 mg; pack size 30 vials

EU/1/02/240/003 - SOMAVERT 20 mg; pack size 30 vials

EU/1/02/240/004 - SOMAVERT 20 mg; pack size 1 vial

9. DATE OF FIRST AUTHORISATION/RENEWAL OF THE AUTHORISATION

13/11/2002

10. DATE OF REVISION OF THE TEXT

January 2005

11. LEGAL CATEGORY

POM

Ref: SV2_0

Somnite Suspension

(Norgine Limited)

1. NAME OF THE MEDICINAL PRODUCT

Nitrazepam Mixture BP (SOMNITE Suspension).

2. QUALITATIVE AND QUANTITATIVE COMPOSITION

Each 5 ml spoonful contains 2.5 mg Nitrazepam BP.

3. PHARMACEUTICAL FORM

Oral suspension.

4. CLINICAL PARTICULARS

4.1 Therapeutic indications

For the short term treatment of insomnia where daytime sedation is acceptable.

Benzodiazepines should be used to treat insomnia only when it is severe, disabling, or subjecting the individual to extreme distress.

4.2 Posology and method of administration

Nitrazepam is a long acting benzodiazepine, and the lowest dose which can control the symptoms should be used. If possible, treatment should be intermittent. The maximum dose should not be exceeded.

Adults: 5 mg (two 5 ml spoonfuls) before retiring to bed. This dose may, if necessary, be increased to 10 mg (four 5 ml spoonfuls).

Elderly and patients with impaired liver and/or renal function:

2.5 mg (one 5 ml spoonful) before retiring to bed. This dose may, if necessary, be increased to 5 mg (two 5 ml spoonfuls)

Children: Not recommended.

Generally the duration of treatment varies from a few days to two weeks with a maximum, including the tapering off process, of four weeks.

Patients who have taken benzodiazepines chronically may require a longer tapering off period. In certain cases extension beyond the maximum treatment period may be necessary; if so, it should not take place without re-evaluation of the patient's status.

4.3 Contraindications

Myasthenia gravis, hypersensitivity to benzodiazepines, severe respiratory insufficiency, sleep apnoea syndrome and severe hepatic insufficiency.

4.4 Special warnings and special precautions for use

Tolerance

Some loss of efficacy to the hypnotic effects of benzodiazepines may develop after repeated use for a few weeks.

Dependence

Use of benzodiazepines may lead to the development of physical and psychic dependence upon these products. The risk of dependence increases with dose and duration of treatment; it is also greater in patients with a history of alcohol or drug abuse.

Once physical dependence has developed, abrupt termination of treatment will be accompanied by withdrawal symptoms. These may consist of headaches, muscle pain, extreme anxiety, tension, restlessness, confusion and irritability.

In severe cases the following symptoms may occur:

derealization, depersonalisation, hyperacusis, numbness and tingling of the extremities, hypersensitivity to light, noise and physical contact, hallucinations or epileptic seizures.

Rebound insomnia and anxiety: a transient syndrome whereby the symptoms that led to treatment with a benzodiazepine recur in an enhanced form, may occur on withdrawal of treatment. It may be accompanied by other reactions including mood changes, anxiety or sleep disturbances and restlessness. Since the risk of withdrawal phenomena/rebound phenomena is greater after abrupt discontinuation of treatment, it is recommended that the dosage is decreased gradually.

Duration of treatment

The duration of treatment should be as short as possible (see Posology) depending on the indication, but should not exceed 4 weeks for insomnia. Extension beyond this period should not take place without re-evaluation of the situation.

It may be useful to inform the patient when treatment is started that it will be of limited duration and to explain precisely how the dosage will be progressively decreased. Moreover it is important that the patient should be aware of the possibility of rebound phenomena, thereby minimising anxiety over such symptoms should they occur while Somnite is being discontinued.

If a change is made to a benzodiazepine with a short duration of action, the patient should be warned that withdrawal symptoms may develop.

Amnesia

Benzodiazepines may induce anterograde amnesia. The condition occurs most often several hours after ingesting the product and therefore to reduce the risk patients should ensure that they will be able to have an uninterrupted sleep of 7-8 hours (see also Undesirable Effects).

Psychiatric and paradoxical reactions

Reactions like restlessness, agitation, irritability, aggressiveness, delusion, rages, nightmares, hallucinations, psychoses, inappropriate behaviour and other adverse behavioural effects are known to occur when using benzodiazepines. They may be quite severe and are more likely in children and the elderly. Should they occur, use of the medicinal product should be discontinued.

Specific patient groups

Benzodiazepines should not be given to children without careful assessment of the need to do so; the duration of treatment must be kept to a minimum. Elderly should be given a reduced dose (see Posology). A lower dose is also recommended for patients with chronic respiratory insufficiency due to the risk of respiratory depression. Benzodiazepines are not indicated to treat patients with severe hepatic insufficiency as they may precipitate encephalopathy.

Benzodiazepines are not recommended for the primary treatment of psychotic illness.

Benzodiazepines should not be used alone to treat depression or anxiety associated with depression (suicide may be precipitated in such patients).

Benzodiazepines should be used with extreme caution in patients with a history of alcohol or drug abuse.

4.5 Interaction with other medicinal products and other forms of Interaction

Not recommended: Concomitant intake with alcohol. The sedative effect may be enhanced when the product is used in combination with alcohol. This affects the ability to drive or use machines.

Take into account: Combination with CNS depressants

Enhancement of the central depressive effect may occur in cases of concomitant use with antipsychotics (neuroleptics), hypnotics, anxiolytics/sedatives, antidepressant agents, narcotic analgesics, anti-epileptic products, anaesthetics and sedative antihistamines.

In the case of narcotic analgesics enhancement of the euphoria may also occur leading to an increase in psychic dependence.

Compounds which inhibit certain hepatic enzymes (particularly cytochrome P450) may enhance the activity of benzodiazepines. To a lesser degree this also applies to benzodiazepines that are metabolised only by conjugation.

4.6 Pregnancy and lactation

If the product is prescribed to a woman of childbearing potential, she should be warned to contact her physician regarding discontinuance of the product if she intends to become or suspects that she is pregnant.

If, for compelling medical reasons, the product is administered during the late phase of pregnancy, or during labour at high doses, effects on the neonate, such as hypothermia, hypotonia and moderate respiratory depression, can be expected, due to the pharmacological action of the compound.

Moreover, infants born to mothers who took benzodiazepines chronically during the latter stages of pregnancy may have developed physical dependence and may be at some risk for developing withdrawal symptoms in the postnatal period.

Since benzodiazepines are found in the breast milk, benzodiazepines should not be given to breast feeding mothers.

4.7 Effects on ability to drive and use machines

Sedation, amnesia, impaired concentration and impaired muscular function may adversely affect the ability to drive or to use machines. If insufficient sleep duration occurs, the likelihood of impaired alertness may be increased (See also Interactions).

4.8 Undesirable effects

Drowsiness, numbed emotions, reduced alertness, confusion, fatigue, headache, dizziness, muscle weakness, ataxia or double vision. These phenomena occur predominantly at the start of therapy and usually disappear with repeated administration. Other side effects like gastrointestinal disturbances, changes in libido or skin reactions have been reported occasionally.

Amnesia

Anterograde amnesia may occur using therapeutic dosages, the risk increasing at higher dosages. Amnestic effect may be associated with inappropriate behaviour. (See *Special Warnings and Special Precautions for Use*).

Depression

Pre-existing depression may be unmasked during benzodiazepine use.

Psychiatric and Paradoxical Reactions

Psychiatric and paradoxical reactions are known to occur. (See *Special Warnings and Special Precautions for Use*).

Dependence

Use (even at therapeutic doses) may lead to the development of physical dependence: discontinuation of the therapy may result in withdrawal or rebound phenomena. (See *Special Warnings and Special Precautions for Use*). Psychic dependence may occur. Abuse of benzodiazepines has been reported.

4.9 Overdose

As with other benzodiazepines, overdose should not present a threat to life unless combined with other CNS depressants (including alcohol).

In the management of overdose with any medicinal product, it should be borne in mind that multiple agents may have been taken.

Following overdose with oral benzodiazepines, vomiting should be induced (within one hour) if the patient is conscious or gastric lavage undertaken with the airway protected if the patient is unconscious. If there is no advantage in emptying the stomach, activated charcoal should be given to reduce absorption. Special attention should be paid to respiratory and cardiovascular functions in intensive care.

Overdose of benzodiazepines is usually manifested by degrees of central nervous system depression ranging from drowsiness to coma. In mild cases, symptoms include drowsiness, mental confusion and lethargy; in more serious cases, symptoms may include ataxia, hypotonia, hypotension, respiratory depression, rarely coma and very rarely death. Flumazenil may be useful as an antidote.

5. PHARMACOLOGICAL PROPERTIES

5.1 Pharmacodynamic properties

Nitrazepam is a long acting benzodiazepine with anxiolytic, sedative and hypnotic characteristics.

5.2 Pharmacokinetic properties

SOMNITE is well absorbed from the GI tract with peak blood levels of nitrazepam being achieved within 2-3 hours of administration.

Half life is approximately 24 hours and plasma steady state levels are achieved after 5 days.

5.3 Preclinical safety data

Preclinical studies provide only limited evidence of safety. Nitrazepam has no significant systemic toxicity potential at the doses in clinical use with the exception of use in pregnancy and lactation for which evidence of safety is lacking.

6. PHARMACEUTICAL PARTICULARS

6.1 List of excipients

Sucrose, microcrystalline cellulose, carboxymethyl cellulose sodium, mixed esters of p-hydroxybenzoic acid, cherry flavour and water.

6.2 Incompatibilities

None known.

6.3 Shelf life

2 years.

6.4 Special precautions for storage

Do not store above 25°C. Protect from light. Do not freeze.

6.5 Nature and contents of container

Amber glass bottles containing 150 ml of suspension.

6.6 Instructions for use and handling

The bottle should be shaken before use.

7. MARKETING AUTHORISATION HOLDER

Norgine Limited

Chaplin House

Widewater Place

Moorhall Road

Harefield

UXBRIDGE

Middlesex, UB9 6NS

United Kingdom

8. MARKETING AUTHORISATION NUMBER(S)

PL 00322/0039

9. DATE OF FIRST AUTHORISATION/RENEWAL OF THE AUTHORISATION

26 February 1982/ 26 February 1992

10. DATE OF REVISION OF THE TEXT

July 1997.

11. LEGAL CATEGORY

Prescription only medicine

Sonata 5mg & 10mg Hard Capsules

(Wyeth Pharmaceuticals)

1. NAME OF THE MEDICINAL PRODUCT

Sonata 5 mg hard capsules

Sonata 10 mg hard capsules

2. QUALITATIVE AND QUANTITATIVE COMPOSITION

Each 5mg capsule contains 5 mg of zaleplon.

Each 10mg capsule contains 10 mg of zaleplon.

For excipients, see 6.1.

3. PHARMACEUTICAL FORM

Hard capsules.

5 mg capsules have an opaque white and opaque light brown hard shell with gold band, "W" and the strength "5 mg".

10 mg capsules have an opaque white hard shell with pink band, "W" and the strength "10 mg".

4. CLINICAL PARTICULARS

4.1 Therapeutic indications

Sonata is indicated for the treatment of patients with insomnia who have difficulty falling asleep. It is indicated only when the disorder is severe, disabling or subjecting the individual to extreme distress.

4.2 Posology and method of administration

Treatment should be as short as possible with a maximum duration of two weeks.

Sonata can be taken immediately before going to bed or after the patient has gone to bed and is experiencing difficulty falling asleep. Administration after food delays the time to maximal plasma concentration by approximately 2 hours, but the total extent of absorption is not altered.

For adults, the recommended dose is 10 mg.

Elderly patients may be sensitive to the effects of hypnotics; therefore, 5 mg is the recommended dose of Sonata.

The total daily dose of Sonata should not exceed 10 mg in any patient. Patients should be advised not to take a second dose within a single night.

No data are available in children (under 18 years of age) and thus prescribing Sonata for children is not recommended.

Hepatic insufficiency: as clearance is reduced, patients with mild to moderate hepatic impairment should be treated with Sonata 5 mg.

Renal insufficiency: no dosage adjustment is required in patients with mild to moderate renal insufficiency, because Sonata pharmacokinetics is not altered in such patients. Safety in patients with severe renal impairment has not been established (see section 4.4 and section 5.2).

4.3 Contraindications

Severe hepatic insufficiency

Hypersensitivity to the active substance or to any of the excipients, including indigo carmine (E132)

Sleep apnoea syndrome

Myasthenia gravis

Severe respiratory insufficiency

Children (under 18 years of age)

4.4 Special warnings and special precautions for use

Insomnia may represent an underlying physical or psychiatric disorder. Insomnia that persists or worsens after a short course of zaleplon treatment may indicate a need to re-evaluate the patient.

Due to zaleplon's short plasma half-life, alternative therapy should be considered if early morning awakening is experienced. Patients should be advised not to take a second dose within a single night.

Co-administration of Sonata with medicinal products known to influence CYP3A4 is expected to result in changes in zaleplon's plasma concentrations. (See section 4.5)

Patients with rare hereditary problems of galactose intolerance, the Lapp lactase deficiency or glucose-galactose malabsorption should not take this medicine.

Tolerance

Some loss of efficacy to the hypnotic effects of short-acting benzodiazepines and benzodiazepine-like agents may develop after repeated use for a few weeks.

Dependence

Use of benzodiazepines and benzodiazepine-like agents may lead to physical and psychic dependence. The risk of dependence increases with dose and duration of treatment and is greater with patients having a history of alcohol and drug abuse. Once physical dependence has developed, abrupt termination of treatment will be accompanied by withdrawal symptoms. These may consist of headaches, muscle pain, extreme anxiety, tension, restlessness, confusion and irritability. In severe cases the following symptoms may occur: unreality, depersonalisation, hyperacusis, numbness and tingling of the extremities, hypersensitivity to light, noise and physical contact, hallucinations or epileptic seizures.

Rebound insomnia and anxiety

A transient syndrome whereby the symptoms that led to the treatment with a benzodiazepine or benzodiazepine-like agent recur in an enhanced form, may occur on withdrawal of treatment. It may be accompanied by other reactions including mood changes, anxiety, or sleep disturbances and restlessness.

Duration of treatment

The duration of treatment should be as short as possible (see section 4.2), and should not exceed two weeks. Extension beyond these periods should not take place without clinical re-evaluation of the patient.

It may be useful to inform the patient when treatment is started that it will be of limited duration. It is important that patients be aware of the possibility of rebound phenomena, thereby minimising anxiety should such symptoms develop when the medicinal product is discontinued.

Memory and psychomotor impairment

Benzodiazepines and benzodiazepine-like agents may induce anterograde amnesia and psychomotor impairment. These occur most often up to several hours after ingesting the product. To reduce the risk, patients should not undertake activities requiring psychomotor co-ordination until 4 hours or more after taking Sonata (see section 4.7).

Psychiatric and "paradoxical" reactions

Reactions like restlessness, agitation, irritability, decreased inhibition, aggressiveness, abnormal thinking, delusion, rages, nightmares, depersonalisation, hallucinations, psychoses, inappropriate behaviour, extroversion that seems out of character and other behavioural effects are known to occur when using benzodiazepines or benzodiazepine-like agents. They may be drug-induced, spontaneous in origin, or a result of an underlying psychiatric or physical disorder. These reactions are more likely to occur in the elderly. Should this occur, use of this product should be discontinued. Any new behavioural sign or symptom requires careful and immediate evaluation.

Specific patient groups

Use in the elderly

Sonata can be administered to the elderly including those over 75 years of age. The pharmacokinetic profile of zaleplon is not significantly different in elderly men and women, including those over 75 years of age, from that in healthy young subjects.

As elderly patients may be sensitive to the effects of hypnotics, a 5 mg dose is recommended (section 4.2 and section 5.2).

Alcohol and drug abuse

Benzodiazepine and benzodiazepine-like agents should be used with extreme caution in patients with a history of alcohol or drug abuse.

Hepatic impairment

Benzodiazepine and benzodiazepine-like agents are not indicated to treat patients with severe hepatic insufficiency as they may precipitate encephalopathy (seesection 4.2). In patients with mild to moderate hepatic insufficiency, the bioavailability of zaleplon is increased because of reduced clearance, and the dose will therefore need to be modified in these patients.

Renal insufficiency

In patients with renal insufficiency, the pharmacokinetic profile of zaleplon is not significantly different than that in healthy subjects, but these patients are exposed to higher levels of zaleplon's inactive metabolites (see section 5.2).

Respiratory insufficiency

Caution should be observed when prescribing sedative medicinal products to patients with chronic respiratory insufficiency.

Psychosis

Benzodiazepine and benzodiazepine-like agents are not recommended for the primary treatment of psychotic illness.

Depression

Benzodiazepines and benzodiazepine-like agents should not be used alone to treat depression or anxiety associated with depression (suicide may be precipitated in such patients). Also, because of the increased risk for intentional overdose in patients with depression in general, the quantity of a medicinal product, including zaleplon, prescribed for such patients should be kept to the necessary minimum.

Children

No data are available in children (under 18 years of age) and thus prescribing Sonata for children is not recommended.

4.5 Interaction with other medicinal products and other forms of Interaction

Concomitant intake with alcohol is not recommended. The sedative effect may be enhanced when the product is used in combination with alcohol. This affects the ability to drive or use machines.

Combination with other CNS-acting compounds should be taken into account. Enhancement of the central sedation may occur in cases of concomitant use with antipsychotics (neuroleptics), hypnotics, anxiolytics/sedatives, antidepressant agents, narcotic analgesics, anti-epileptic medicinal products, anaesthetics, and sedative antihistamines.

Coadministration of a single zaleplon 10 mg dose and venlafaxine (extended release) 75 mg or 150 mg daily did not produce any interaction on memory (immediate and delayed word recall) or psychomotor performance (digit symbol substitution test). Additionally, there was no pharmacokinetic interaction between zaleplon and venlafaxine (extended release).

In the case of narcotic analgesics enhancement of the euphoria may occur leading to an increase in physiological dependence.

Cimetidine, a non-specific moderate inhibitor of several hepatic enzymes including both aldehyde oxidase and CYP3A4, produced an 85% increase in plasma concentrations of zaleplon because it inhibited both the primary (aldehyde oxidase) and secondary (CYP3A4) enzymes responsible for zaleplon's metabolism. Therefore caution is advisable in co-administering cimetidine and Sonata.

Co-administration of Sonata with a single 800 mg dose of erythromycin, a strong, selective CYP3A4 inhibitor, produced a 34% increase in zaleplon's plasma concentrations. A routine dosage adjustment of Sonata is not considered necessary, but patients should be advised that the sedative effects might be enhanced.

In contrast, rifampicin, a strong inducer of several hepatic enzymes, including CYP3A4 resulted in a four fold reduction in zaleplon plasma concentration. Co-administration of Sonata together with inducers of CYP3A4 such as rifampicin, carbamazepine and phenobarbitone, may result in a reduction of zaleplon's efficacy.

Sonata did not affect the pharmacokinetic and pharmacodynamic profiles of digoxin and warfarin, two compounds with a narrow therapeutic index. In addition, ibuprofen, as an example of compounds that alter renal excretion, showed no interaction with Sonata.

4.6 Pregnancy and lactation

Although animal studies have shown no teratogenic or embryotoxic effects, insufficient clinical data are available on Sonata to assess its safety during pregnancy and lactation. Use of Sonata is not recommended during pregnancy. If the medicinal product is prescribed to a woman of childbearing potential, she should be warned to contact her physician regarding discontinuance of the medicinal product if she intends to become or suspects that she is pregnant.

If for compelling medical reasons, the medicinal product is administered during the late phase of pregnancy, or during labour at high doses, effects on the neonate, such as hypothermia, hypotonia and moderate respiratory depression, can be expected, due to the pharmacological action of the compound.

Infants born to mothers who took benzodiazepine and benzodiazepine-like agents chronically during the latter stages of pregnancy may have developed physical dependence and may be at some risk for developing withdrawal symptoms in the postnatal period.

Because zaleplon is excreted in the breast milk, Sonata should not be administered to breast-feeding mothers.

4.7 Effects on ability to drive and use machines

Sedation, amnesia, impaired concentration and impaired muscular function may adversely affect the ability to drive or to use machines. If insufficient sleep duration occurs, the likelihood of impaired alertness may be increased (see section 4.5). Caution is recommended for patients performing skilled tasks.

4.8 Undesirable effects

Organ/System (Frequency)	**Adverse Reactions**
General disorders	
Uncommon (>1/1000, <1/100):	anorexia, asthenia, hypoaesthesia, malaise, photosensitivity reaction
Immune System Disorders	
Very rare (<1/10,000):	Anaphylactic/anaphylactoid reactions
Psychiatric and nervous system disorders	
Common (>1/100, <1/10):	amnesia, paraesthesia, somnolence
Uncommon (>1/1000, <1/100):	ataxia/incoordination, confusion, decreased concentration, apathy, depersonalisation, depression, dizziness, hallucinations; hyperacusis; parosmia; speech disorder (dysarthria, slurred speech); abnormal vision, diplopia

See also below under Amnesia, Depression and Psychiatric and "paradoxical" reactions.

Gastrointenstinal disorders	
Uncommon (>1/1000, <1/100):	nausea
Frequency undetermined:	hepatotoxicity (mostly described as increased transaminase levels)
Reproductive system disorders	
Common (>1/100, <1/10):	dysmenorrhea

Amnesia

Anterograde amnesia may occur using recommended therapeutic dosages, the risk increasing at higher dosages. Amnestic effects may be associated with inappropriate behaviour (see section 4.4).

Depression

Pre-existing depression may be unmasked during benzodiazepine or benzodiazepine-like agent use.

Psychiatric and "paradoxical" reactions

Reactions like restlessness, agitation, irritability, decreased inhibition, aggressiveness, abnormal thinking, delusions, rages, nightmares, depersonalisation, hallucinations, psychoses, inappropriate behaviour, extroversion that seems out of character, and other adverse behavioural effects are known to occur when using benzodiazepines or benzodiazepine-like agents. Such reactions are more likely to occur in the elderly.

Dependence

Use (even at therapeutic doses) may lead to the development of physical dependence: discontinuation of therapy may result in withdrawal or rebound phenomena (see section 4.4). Psychic dependence may occur. Abuse of benzodiazepines and benzodiazepine-like drugs has been reported.

4.9 Overdose

There is limited clinical experience with the effects of an acute overdose of Sonata, and overdose levels in humans have not been determined.

As with other benzodiazepines or benzodiazepine-like agents, overdose should not present a threat to life unless combined with other CNS depressants (including alcohol).

In the management of overdose with any medicinal product, it should be borne in mind that multiple agents may have been taken.

Following overdose with oral benzodiazepine or benzodiazepine-like agents, vomiting should be induced (within one hour) if the patient is conscious or gastric lavage undertaken with the airway protected if the patient is unconscious. If there is no advantage in emptying the stomach, activated charcoal should be given to reduce the absorption. Special attention should be paid to respiratory or cardiovascular functions in intensive care.

Overdose of benzodiazepine or benzodiazepine-like agents is usually manifested by degrees of central nervous system depression ranging from drowsiness to coma. In mild cases, symptoms include drowsiness, mental confusion, and lethargy, in more serious cases, symptoms may include ataxia, hypotonia, hypotension, respiratory depression, rarely coma and very rarely death.

Chromaturia (blue-green urine discolouration) has been reported with zaleplon overdose.

Flumazenil may be useful as an antidote. Animal studies suggest that flumazenil is an antagonist to zaleplon and should be considered in the management of Sonata overdose. However, there is no clinical experience with the use of flumazenil as an antidote to a Sonata overdose.

5. PHARMACOLOGICAL PROPERTIES

Zaleplon is a pyrazolopyrimidine hypnotic that is structurally different from benzodiazepines and other hypnotics. Zaleplon binds selectively to the benzodiazepine type I receptor.

5.1 Pharmacodynamic properties

Pharmacotherapeutic Group: Benzodiazepine Related Drugs, ATC Code N05CF03

Zaleplon's pharmacokinetic profile shows rapid absorption and elimination (see section 5.2). In combination with its subtype selective receptor-binding characteristics, with high selectivity and low affinity for the benzodiazepine type I receptor, these properties are responsible for the overall characteristics of Sonata.

Sonata's efficacy has been demonstrated in both sleep laboratory studies using objective polysomnography (PSG) measures of sleep and in outpatient studies using patient questionnaires to assess sleep. In these studies, patients were diagnosed with primary (psychophysiological) insomnia.

Sleep latency in outpatient studies was decreased for up to 4 weeks in non-elderly patients with Sonata 10 mg. In elderly patients, sleep latency was often significantly decreased with Sonata 5 mg and was consistently decreased with Sonata 10 mg compared with placebo in 2-week studies. This decreased sleep latency was significantly different from that observed with placebo. Results from the 2- and 4-week studies showed that no pharmacological tolerance developed with any dose of Sonata.

In Sonata studies using objective PSG measures, Sonata 10 mg was superior to placebo in decreasing sleep latency and increasing sleep duration during the first half of the night. Sonata has been shown to preserve sleep stages in controlled studies that measured the percentage of sleep time spent in each sleep stage.

5.2 Pharmacokinetic properties

Absorption

Zaleplon is rapidly and almost completely absorbed after oral administration, and peak concentrations are reached in approximately 1 hour. At least 71% of the orally-administered dose is absorbed. Zaleplon undergoes presystemic metabolism, resulting in an absolute bioavailability of approximately 30%.

Distribution

Zaleplon is lipophilic with a volume of distribution of about 1.4±0.3 l/kg following intravenous administration. The *in vitro* plasma protein binding is approximately 60%, suggesting little risk of drug interaction due to protein binding.

Metabolism

Zaleplon is primarily metabolised by aldehyde oxidase to form 5-oxo-zaleplon. Additionally, zaleplon is metabolised by CYP3A4 to form desethylzaleplon which is further metabolised by aldehyde oxidase to form 5-oxo-desethylzaleplon. The oxidative metabolites are further metabolised by conjugation via glucuronidation. All of zaleplon's metabolites are inactive in both animal behavioural models and *in vitro* activity assays.

Zaleplon plasma concentrations increased linearly with dose, and zaleplon showed no signs of accumulation following administration of up to 30 mg/day. The elimination half-life of zaleplon is approximately 1 hour.

Excretion

Zaleplon is excreted in the form of inactive metabolites, mainly in the urine (71%) and faeces (17%). Fifty-seven percent (57%) of the dose is recovered in urine in the form of 5-oxo-zaleplon and its glucuronide metabolite, an additional 9% is recovered as 5-oxo-desethylzaleplon and its glucuronide metabolite. The remainder of the urinary recovery consists of minor metabolites. The majority of the faecal recovery consists of 5-oxo-zaleplon.

Hepatic Impairment

Zaleplon is metabolised primarily by the liver and undergoes significant presystemic metabolism. Consequently, the oral clearance of zaleplon was reduced by 70% and 87% in compensated and decompensated cirrhotic patients, respectively, leading to marked increases in mean C_{max} and AUC (up to 4-fold and 7-fold in compensated and decompensated patients, respectively) relative to healthy subjects. The dose of zaleplon should be reduced in patients with mild to moderate hepatic impairment, and zaleplon is not recommended for use in patients with severe hepatic impairment.

Renal Impairment

The single dose pharmacokinetics of zaleplon were studied in patients with mild (creatinine clearance 40 to 89 ml/min) and moderate (20 to 39 ml/min) renal impairment, and in patients on dialysis. In patients with moderate impairment and those on dialysis there was a reduction of approximately 23% in peak plasma concentration compared to healthy volunteers. The extent of exposure to zaleplon was similar among all groups. Therefore, no dose adjustment is necessary in patients with mild to moderate renal impairment. Zaleplon has not been adequately studied in patients with severe renal impairment.

5.3 Preclinical safety data

Repeated oral administration of zaleplon to rats and dogs elicited increases in liver and adrenal weights; however, these increases occurred at high multiples of the maximum therapeutic dose, were reversible, were not associated with degenerative microscopic changes in liver or adrenal glands, and were consistent with effects in animals with other compounds that bind to benzodiazepine receptors. In a three month study in prepubescent dogs there was significant reduction in the weight of both prostate and testes at high multiples of the maximum therapeutic dose. Oral administration of zaleplon to rats for 104 consecutive weeks at dosage levels up to 20 mg/kg/day did not result in compound-related tumorigenicity. Oral administration of zaleplon to mice for 65 or 104 consecutive weeks at high dosage levels (≥100 mg/kg/day) elicited a statistically significant increase in benign but not in malignant liver tumors. The increased incidence of benign liver tumors in mice was likely an adaptive event.

Overall, the results of the preclinical studies do not suggest any significant safety hazard for use of Sonata at recommended doses in humans.

6. PHARMACEUTICAL PARTICULARS

6.1 List of excipients

Microcrystalline cellulose,

pregelatinised starch,

silicon dioxide,

sodium lauryl sulphate,

magnesium stearate,

lactose monohydrate,

indigo carmine (E132),

titanium dioxide (E171).

Sonata has been designed so that if the contents of the capsule are dissolved in a liquid, the liquid will change colour and become cloudy.

Ingredients of the 5mg capsule shell:
gelatin,
titanium dioxide (E171),
red iron oxide (E172),
yellow iron oxide (E172),
black iron oxide (E172),
sodium lauryl sulphate,
silicon dioxide.
Printing inks on the shell contain the following (gold ink S-13050):
shellac,
lecithin,
simethicone,
yellow iron oxide (E172).
Ingredients of the 10mg capsule shell:
gelatin,
titanium dioxide (E171),
sodium lauryl sulphate,
silicon dioxide.
Printing inks on the shell contain the following (pink ink SW-1105):
shellac,
titanium dioxide (E171),
ammonium hydroxide,
red iron oxide (E172),
yellow iron oxide (E172).

6.2 Incompatibilities
Not applicable

6.3 Shelf life
3 years.

6.4 Special precautions for storage
Do not store above 30° C.

6.5 Nature and contents of container
PVC / PVDC aluminium blister packages of 7, 10, 14 capsules and 100 × 1 capsules in perforated unit-dose blisters. Not all pack sizes may be marketed.

6.6 Instructions for use and handling
No special requirements

7. MARKETING AUTHORISATION HOLDER
Wyeth Europa Ltd.
Huntercombe Lane South
Taplow
Maidenhead
Berkshire
SL6 0PH
United Kingdom

8. MARKETING AUTHORISATION NUMBER(S)
5mg Capsules: EU/1/99/102/001-003 (7, 10, 14); EU/1/99/102/007 (100)
10mg Capsules: EU/1/99/102/004-006 (7, 10, 14); EU/1/99/102/008 (100)

9. DATE OF FIRST AUTHORISATION/RENEWAL OF THE AUTHORISATION
March 1999/March 2004

10. DATE OF REVISION OF THE TEXT
4 July 2005

Soothelip

(Alpharma Limited)

1. NAME OF THE MEDICINAL PRODUCT
SOOTHELIP
ACICLOVIR CREAM 5% FOR COLD SORES

2. QUALITATIVE AND QUANTITATIVE COMPOSITION
Contains 5% w/w Aciclovir PhEur.

3. PHARMACEUTICAL FORM
White to off-white cream.

4. CLINICAL PARTICULARS

4.1 Therapeutic indications
Treatment of cold sore infection (Herpes labialis).

4.2 Posology and method of administration
Soothelip should be applied to the lesion or impending lesion as early as possible after the start of an infection. It is particularly important to start treatment of recurrent episodes during the prodromal period or when lesions first appear.

Adults (*including elderly*): Soothelip should be applied five times daily at approximately four hourly intervals, omitting the night time application. Treatment should be continued for five days. If, after five days, healing is not complete then treatment can be continued for up to an additional five days. If the cold sore has not fully healed after 10 days or gets worse during treatment medical attention should be sought.

4.3 Contraindications
Hypersensitivity to aciclovir, cetyl alcohol, dimethicone, heavy liquid paraffin, polyethylene glycol - 5 glyceryl stearate, propylene glycol, sorbic acid, white soft paraffin or water; do not use in eyes.

4.4 Special warnings and special precautions for use
Patients with a severe infection should consult their doctor.

Patients should be advised to take the necessary steps to prevent transmission of the infection, such as:

- Washing the hands before and after using the cream
- Not rubbing the lesion
- Not sharing towels

In severely immunocompromised patients (*e.g.* AIDS patients or bone marrow transplant recipients) oral Aciclovir dosing should be considered. Such patients should be encouraged to consult a physician concerning the treatment of any infection. Soothelip is not recommended for application to mucous membranes such as in the mouth, eye or vagina, as it may be irritant. Particular care should be taken to avoid accidental introduction into the eye. The results of a wide range of mutagenicity tests *in vitro* and *in vivo* indicate that Soothelip does not pose a genetic risk to man. Soothelip was not found to be carcinogenic in long term studies in the rat and the mouse. Largely reversible adverse effects on spermatogenesis in association with overall toxicity in rats and dogs have been reported only at doses of Soothelip greatly in excess of those employed therapeutically. There has been no experience of the effect of Soothelip on human fertility. Two generation studies in mice did not reveal any effect of (orally administered) Soothelip on fertility. Aciclovir Tablets have been shown to have no definite effect upon sperm count, morphology or motility in man.

4.5 Interaction with other medicinal products and other forms of Interaction
Probenecid increases the mean half-life and area under the plasma concentration curve of systematically administered Soothelip. However, this is likely to be of little relevance to the topical application of Soothelip.

4.6 Pregnancy and lactation
Systemic administration of aciclovir in internationally accepted standard tests did not produce embryotoxic or teratogenic effects in rats, rabbits and mice. In a non-standard test in rats, foetal abnormalities were observed, but only following such high subcutaneous doses that maternal toxicity was produced. The clinical relevance of these findings is uncertain. Experience in humans is limited, so use of Soothelip should be considered only when the potential benefits outweigh the possibility of unknown risks. Limited human data show that the drug does pass into breast milk following systemic administration.

4.7 Effects on ability to drive and use machines
None known.

4.8 Undesirable effects
Transient burning or stinging following application of Aciclovir Cream may occur in some patients. Mild drying or flaking of the skin has occurred in 5% of patients. Erythema and itching has been reported in a small proportion of patients.

Contact dermatitis has been reported rarely following application. Where sensitivity tests have been conducted the reactive substances have most often been shown to be components of the cream base rather than aciclovir.

4.9 Overdose
No untoward effects would be expected if the entire contents of a Soothelip 10g tube containing 500mg of Aciclovir were ingested orally. Oral doses of 800mg five times daily (4g/daily), have been administered for seven days without adverse effects. Single intravenous doses of up to 80mg/kg have been inadvertently administered without adverse effects. Soothelip is dialysable.

5. PHARMACOLOGICAL PROPERTIES

5.1 Pharmacodynamic properties
Aciclovir is an antiviral agent which is highly active *in vitro* against herpes simplex virus (HSV) types I and II and varicella zoster virus. Toxicity to mammalian host cells is low.

Aciclovir is phosphorylated after entry into herpes infected cells to the active compound Aciclovir triphosphate. The first step in this process is dependant on the presence of the HSV-coded thymidine kinase. Aciclovir triphosphate acts as an inhibitor of, and substrate for, the herpes-specified DNA polymerase, preventing further viral DNA synthesis without affecting the normal cellular processes.

5.2 Pharmacokinetic properties
Aciclovir is excreted through the kidney by both glomerular filtration and tubular secretion. The terminal or beta-phase half-life is reported to be about 2 to 3 hours for adults without renal impairment. In chronic renal failure this value is increased and may be up to 19.5 hours in anuric patients. During haemodialysis and the half-life is reduced to 5.7 hours, with 60% of a dose of aciclovir being removed in 6 hours. Faecal excretion may account for about 2% of a dose. There is a wide distribution to various tissues, including the CSF where concentrations achieved are about 50% of those achieved in plasma. Protein binding is reported to range from 9-33%. Aciclovir crosses the placenta and is excreted in breast milk in concentrations approximately 3 times higher than those in maternal serum. Absorption of aciclovir is usually slight following topical application to intact skin, although it may be increased by changes in formulation.

5.3 Preclinical safety data
Not applicable.

6. PHARMACEUTICAL PARTICULARS

6.1 List of excipients
Also contains: cetyl alcohol, dimethicone, heavy liquid paraffin, polyethylene glycol - 5 glyceryl stearate, propylene glycol, sorbic acid, white soft paraffin and water.

6.2 Incompatibilities
None known.

6.3 Shelf life
Shelf-life
Three years from the date of manufacture.
Shelf-life after dilution/reconstitution
Not applicable.
Shelf-life after first opening
Not applicable.

6.4 Special precautions for storage
Do not store above 25°C.
Do not refrigerate or freeze.

6.5 Nature and contents of container
The product is supplied in aluminium tubes with screw caps in cartons.
Carton: White backed folding board
Tube: manufactured from 99.5% pure aluminium lacquered internally.
Cap: polythene or polypropylene.

6.6 Instructions for use and handling
Not applicable.

Administrative Data

7. MARKETING AUTHORISATION HOLDER
Alpharma Limited
(Trading styles: Alpharma, Cox Pharmaceuticals)
Whiddon Valley
BARNSTAPLE
N Devon
EX32 8NS

8. MARKETING AUTHORISATION NUMBER(S)
PL 0142/0462

9. DATE OF FIRST AUTHORISATION/RENEWAL OF THE AUTHORISATION
12 February 2002

10. DATE OF REVISION OF THE TEXT
February 2005

Legal Category
GSL

Sotacor Injection 10mg/ml

(Bristol-Myers Pharmaceuticals)

1. NAME OF THE MEDICINAL PRODUCT
SOTACOR INJECTION 10MG/ML

2. QUALITATIVE AND QUANTITATIVE COMPOSITION
Ampoules containing sotalol hydrochloride 40mg in each 4 ml of solution.

3. PHARMACEUTICAL FORM
Intravenous injection

4. CLINICAL PARTICULARS

4.1 Therapeutic indications
Termination of acute and life-threatening arrhythmias, including life-threatening ventricular tachyarrhythmias, symptomatic non-sustained ventricular arrhythmias;

Testing of drug efficacy during programmed electrical stimulation in patients with inducible ventricular and supraventricular tachyarrhythmias;

Transitory substitution for oral SOTACOR in patients temporarily unable to take oral medications.

4.2 Posology and method of administration
The initiation of treatment or changes in dosage with SOTACOR should follow an appropriate medical evaluation including ECG control with measurement of the corrected QT interval, and assessment of renal function, electrolyte balance, and concomitant medications (see 4.4 Warnings and precautions).

As with other antiarrhythmic agents, it is recommended that SOTACOR be initiated and doses increased in a facility capable of monitoring and assessing cardiac rhythm. The dosage must be individualized and based on the patient's response. Proarrhythmic events can occur not only at initiation of therapy, but also with each upward dosage adjustment.

In view of its β-adrenergic blocking properties, treatment with SOTACOR should not be discontinued suddenly, especially in patients with ischaemic heart disease (angina pectoris, prior acute myocardial infarction) or hypertension, to prevent exacerbation of the disease (see 4.4 Warnings).

The following dosing schedule can be recommended:

For the management of acute arrhythmias, dosage range is from 20-120 mg intravenously (0.5 mg to 1.5 mg/kg). The total calculated dose has been safely administered over a 10-minute period and can be repeated at 6-hour intervals if necessary. For high risk patients with acute myocardial infarction and/or congestive heart failure, careful monitoring for haemodynamic or electrocardiographic changes is recommended.

For programmed electrical stimulation, an initial bolus of 1.5 mg/kg should be given over 10 to 20 minutes, followed by maintenance infusion at a rate of between 0.2 and 0.5 mg/kg/hour.

For substitution in place of oral therapy, infusion of between 0.2 and 0.5 mg/kg/hour should be used with the total daily dose not exceeding 640 mg.

Children

SOTACOR is not intended for administration to children.

Dosage in renally impaired patients

Because SOTACOR is excreted mainly in urine, the dosage should be reduced when the creatinine clearance is less than 60 ml/min according to the following table:

Creatinine clearance (ml/min)	Adjusted doses
> 60	Recommended SOTACOR Dose
30-6 0	½ recommended SOTACOR Dose
10-30	¼ recommended SOTACOR Dose
< 10	Avoid

The creatinine clearance can be estimated from serum creatinine by the Cockroft and Gault formula:

Men:

$$\frac{(140 - age) \times weight\ (kg)}{72\ x\ serum\ creatinine\ (mg/dl)}$$

Women: idem × 0.85

When serum creatinine is given in μmol/l, divide the value by 88.4 (1mg/dl = 88.4 μmol/l).

Dosage in hepatically impaired patients

No dosage adjustment is required in hepatically impaired patients.

4.3 Contraindications

SOTACOR should not be used where there is evidence of sick sinus syndrome; second and third degree AV heart block unless a functioning pacemaker is present; congenital or acquired long QT syndromes; torsades de pointes; symptomatic sinus bradycardia; uncontrolled congestive heart failure; cardiogenic shock; anaesthesia that produces myocardial depression; untreated phaeochromocytoma; hypotension (except due to arrhythmia); Raynaud's phenomenon and severe peripheral circulatory disturbances; history of chronic obstructive airway disease or bronchial asthma; hypersensitivity to any of the components of the formulation; metabolic acidosis; renal failure (creatinine clearance < 10 ml/min).

4.4 Special warnings and special precautions for use

Abrupt Withdrawal Hypersensitivity to catecholamines is observed in patients withdrawn from beta-blocker therapy. Occasional cases of exacerbation of angina pectoris, arrhythmias, and in some cases, myocardial infarction have been reported after abrupt discontinuation of therapy. Patients should be carefully monitored when discontinuing chronically administered SOTACOR, particularly those with ischaemic heart disease. If possible the dosage should be gradually reduced over a period of one to two weeks, if necessary at the same time initiating replacement therapy. Abrupt discontinuation may unmask latent coronary insufficiency. In addition, hypertension may develop.

Proarrhythmias The most dangerous adverse effect of Class I and Class III antiarrhythmic drugs (such as sotalol) is the aggravation of pre-existing arrhythmias or the provocation of new arrhythmias. Drugs that prolong the QT-interval may cause torsades de pointes, a polymorphic ventricular tachycardia associated with prolongation of the QT-interval. Experience to date indicates that the risk of torsades de pointes is associated with the prolongation of the QT-interval, reduction of the heart rate, reduction in serum potassium and magnesium, high plasma sotalol concentrations and with the concomitant use of sotalol and other medications which have been associated with torsades de pointes (see 4.5: Interactions). Females may be at increased risk of developing torsades de pointes.

The incidence of torsades de pointes is dose dependent. Torsades de pointes usually occurs early after initiating therapy or escalation of the dose and can progress to ventricular fibrillation.

In clinical trials of patients with sustained VT/VF the incidence of severe proarrhythmia (torsades de pointes or new sustained VT/VF) was <2% at doses up to 320 mg. The incidence more than doubled at higher doses.

Other risk factors for torsades de pointes were excessive prolongation of the QT_C and history of cardiomegaly or congestive heart failure. Patients with sustained ventricular tachycardia and a history of congestive heart failure have the highest risk of serious proarrhythmia (7%). Proarrhythmic events must be anticipated not only on initiating therapy but with every upward dose adjustment. Initiating therapy at 80 mg with gradual upward dose titration thereafter reduces the risk of proarrhythmia. In patients already receiving SOTACOR caution should be used if the QT_C exceeds 500 msec whilst on therapy, and serious consideration should be given to reducing the dose or discontinuing therapy when the QT_C-interval exceeds 550 msec. Due to the multiple risk factors associated with torsades de pointes, however, caution should be exercised regardless of the QT_C-interval.

Electrolyte Disturbances SOTACOR should not be used in patients with hypokalaemia or hypomagnesaemia prior to correction of imbalance; these conditions can exaggerate the degree of QT prolongation, and increase the potential for torsades de pointes. Special attention should be given to electrolyte and acid-base balance in patients experiencing severe or prolonged diarrhoea or patients receiving concomitant magnesium- and/or potassium-depleting drugs.

Congestive Heart Failure Beta-blockade may further depress myocardial contractility and precipitate more severe heart failure. Caution is advised when initiating therapy in patients with left ventricular dysfunction controlled by therapy (i.e. ACE Inhibitors, diuretics, digitalis, etc); a low initial dose and careful dose titration is appropriate.

Recent MI In post-infarction patients with impaired left ventricular function, the risk versus benefit of sotalol administration must be considered. Careful monitoring and dose titration are critical during initiation and follow-up of therapy. SOTACOR should be avoided in patients with left ventricular ejection fractions ≤40% without serious ventricular arrhythmias.

Electrocardiographic Changes Excessive prolongation of the QT-interval, >500 msec, can be a sign of toxicity and should be avoided (see Proarrhythmias above). Sinus bradycardia has been observed very commonly in arrhythmia patients receiving sotalol in clinical trials. Bradycardia increases the risk of torsades de pointes. Sinus pause, sinus arrest and sinus node dysfunction occur in less than 1% of patients. The incidence of 2nd- or 3rd-degree AV block is approximately 1%.

Anaphylaxis Patients with a history of anaphylactic reaction to a variety of allergens may have a more severe reaction on repeated challenge while taking beta-blockers. Such patients may be unresponsive to the usual doses of adrenaline used to treat the allergic reaction.

Anaesthesia As with other beta-blocking agents, SOTACOR should be used with caution in patients undergoing surgery and in association with anaesthetics that cause myocardial depression, such as cyclopropane or trichloroethylene.

Diabetes Mellitus SOTACOR should be used with caution in patients with diabetes (especially labile diabetes) or with a history of episodes of spontaneous hypoglycaemia, since beta-blockade may mask some important signs of the onset of acute hypoglycaemia, e.g. tachycardia.

Thyrotoxicosis Beta-blockade may mask certain clinical signs of hyperthyroidism (e.g., tachycardia). Patients suspected of developing thyrotoxicosis should be managed carefully to avoid abrupt withdrawal of beta-blockade which might be followed by an exacerbation of symptoms of hyperthyroidism, including thyroid storm.

Renal Impairment As sotalol is mainly eliminated via the kidneys the dose should be adjusted in patients with renal impairment (see dosage).

Psoriasis Beta-blocking drugs have been reported rarely to exacerbate the symptoms of psoriasis vulgaris.

4.5 Interaction with other medicinal products and other forms of Interaction

Antiarrhythmics Class 1a antiarrhythmic drugs, such as disopyramide, quinidine and procainamide and other antiarrhythmic drugs such as amiodarone and bepridil are not recommended as concomitant therapy with SOTACOR, because of their potential to prolong refractoriness (see 4.4 Special Warnings and Precautions). The concomitant use of other beta-blocking agents with SOTACOR may result in additive Class II effects.

Other drugs prolonging the QT-interval SOTACOR should be given with extreme caution in conjunction with other drugs known to prolong the QT-interval such as phenothiazines, tricyclic antidepressants, terfenadine and astemizole. Other drugs that have been associated with an increased risk for torsades de pointes include, erythromycin IV, halofantrine, pentamidine, and quinolone antibiotics.

Floctafenine beta-adrenergic blocking agents may impede the compensatory cardiovascular reactions associated with hypotension or shock that may be induced by floctafenine.

Calcium channel blocking drugs Concurrent administration of beta-blocking agents and calcium channel blockers has resulted in hypotension, bradycardia, conduction defects, and cardiac failure. Beta-blockers should be avoided in combination with cardiodepressant calcium-channel blockers such as verapamil and diltiazem because of the additive effects on atrioventricular conduction, and ventricular function.

Potassium-Depleting Diuretics Hypokalaemia or hypomagnesaemia may occur, increasing the potential for torsades de pointes (see Special Warnings and Precautions for Use).

Other potassium-depleting drugs Amphotericin B (IV route), corticosteroids (systemic administration) and some laxatives may also be associated with hypokalaemia; potassium levels should be monitored and corrected appropriately during concomitant administration with SOTACOR.

Clonidine Beta-blocking drugs may potentiate the rebound hypertension sometimes observed after discontinuation of clonidine; therefore, the beta-blocker should be discontinued slowly several days before the gradual withdrawal of clonidine.

Digitalis glycosides Single and multiple doses of SOTACOR do not significantly affect serum digoxin levels. Proarrhythmic events were more common in sotalol treated patients also receiving digitalis glycosides; however, this may be related to the presence of CHF, a known risk factor for proarrhythmia, in patients receiving digitalis glycosides. Association of digitalis glycosides with beta-blockers may increase auriculo-ventricular conduction time.

Catecholamine-depleting agents Concomitant use of catecholamine-depleting drugs, such as reserpine, guanethidine or alpha methyldopa, with a beta-blocker may produce an excessive reduction of resting sympathetic nervous tone. Patients should be closely monitored for evidence of hypotension and/or marked bradycardia which may produce syncope.

Insulin and oral hypoglycaemics Hyperglycaemia may occur, and the dosage of antidiabetic drugs may require adjustment. Symptoms of hypoglycaemia (tachycardia) may be masked by beta-blocking agents.

Neuromuscular blocking agents like Tubocurarin The neuromuscular blockade is prolonged by beta-blocking agents.

Beta-2-receptor stimulants Patients in need of beta-agonists should not normally receive SOTACOR. However, if concomitant therapy is necessary beta-agonists may have to be administered in increased dosages.

Drug/Laboratory interaction The presence of sotalol in the urine may result in falsely elevated levels of urinary metanephrine when measured by photometric methods. Patients suspected of having phaeochromocytoma and who are treated with sotalol should have their urine screened utilizing the HPLC assay with solid phase extraction.

4.6 Pregnancy and lactation

Pregnancy Animal studies with sotalol hydrochloride have shown no evidence of teratogenicity or other harmful effects on the foetus. Although there are no adequate and well-controlled studies in pregnant women, sotalol hydrochloride has been shown to cross the placenta and is found in amniotic fluid. Beta-blockers reduce placental perfusion, which may result in intrauterine foetal death, immature and premature deliveries. In addition, adverse effects (especially hypoglycaemia and bradycardia) may occur in foetus and neonate. There is an increased risk of cardiac and pulmonary complications in the neonate in the postnatal period. Therefore, SOTACOR should be used in pregnancy only if the potential benefits outweigh the possible risk to the foetus. The neonate should be monitored very carefully for 48 - 72 hours after delivery if it was not possible to interrupt maternal therapy with SOTACOR 2-3 days before the birthdate.

Most beta-blockers, particularly lipophilic compounds, will pass into breast milk although to a variable extent. Breast feeding is therefore not recommended during administration of these compounds.

4.7 Effects on ability to drive and use machines

There are no data available, but the occasional occurrence of side-effects such as dizziness and fatigue should be taken into account (see 4.8 Undesirable effects).

4.8 Undesirable effects

The most frequent adverse effects of sotalol arise from its beta-blockade properties. Adverse effects are usually transient in nature and rarely necessitate interruption of, or withdrawal from treatment. If they do occur, they usually disappear when the dosage is reduced. The most significant adverse effects, however, are those due to proarrhythmia, including torsades de pointes (see Warnings).

The following are adverse events considered related to therapy, occuring in 1% or more of patients treated with SOTACOR.

Cardiovascular Bradycardia, dyspnoea, chest pain, palpitations, oedema, ECG abnormalities, hypotension, proarrhythmia, syncope, heart failure, presyncope.

Dermatologic Rash.

Gastro-intestinal Nausea/vomiting, diarrhoea, dyspepsia, abdominal pain, flatulence.

Musculoskeletal Cramps.

Nervous/psychiatric Fatigue, dizziness, asthenia, lightheadedness, headache, sleep disturbances, depression, paresthesia, mood changes, anxiety.

Urogenital Sexual dysfunction.

Special Senses Visual disturbances, taste abnormalities, hearing disturbances.

Body as a whole Fever.

In trials of patients with cardiac arrhythmia, the most common adverse events leading to discontinuation of SOTACOR were fatigue 4%, bradycardia (< 50 bpm) 3%, dyspnoea 3%, proarrhythmia 2%, asthenia 2%, and dizziness 2%.

Cold and cyanotic extremities, Raynaud's phenomenon, increase in existing intermittent claudication and dry eyes have been seen in association with other beta-blockers.

4.9 Overdose

Intentional or accidental overdosage with SOTACOR has rarely resulted in death. Haemodialysis results in a large reduction of plasma levels of sotalol.

Symptoms and treatment of overdosage: The most common signs to be expected are bradycardia, congestive heart failure, hypotension, bronchospasm and hypoglycaemia. In cases of massive intentional overdosage (2-16 g) of SOTACOR the following clinical findings were seen: hypotension, bradycardia, prolongation of QT-interval, premature ventricular complexes, ventricular tachycardia, torsades de pointes.

If overdosage occurs, therapy with SOTACOR should be discontinued and the patient observed closely. In addition, if required, the following therapeutic measures are suggested:

Bradycardia Atropine (0.5 to 2 mg IV), another anticholinergic drug, a beta-adrenergic agonist (isoprenaline, 5 microgram per minute, up to 25 microgram, by slow IV injection) or transvenous cardiac pacing.

Heart Block (second and third degree) Transvenous cardiac pacing.

Hypotension Adrenaline rather than isoprenaline or noradrenaline may be useful, depending on associated factors.

Bronchospasm Aminophylline or aerosol beta-2-receptor stimulant.

Torsades de pointes DC cardioversion, transvenous cardiac pacing, adrenaline, and/or magnesium sulphate.

5. PHARMACOLOGICAL PROPERTIES

5.1 Pharmacodynamic properties

D,l-sotalol is a non-selective hydrophilic -adrenergic receptor blocking agent, devoid of intrinsic sympathomimetic activity or membrane stabilizing activity.

SOTACOR has both beta-adrenoreceptor blocking (Vaughan Williams Class II) and cardiac action potential duration prolongation (Vaughan Williams Class III) antiarrhythmic properties. Sotalol has no known effect on the upstroke velocity and therefore no effect on the depolarisation phase.

Sotalol uniformly prolongs the action potential duration in cardiac tissues by delaying the repolarisation phase. Its major effects are prolongation of the atrial, ventricular and accessory pathway effective refractory periods.

The Class II and III properties may be reflected on the surface electrocardiogram by a lengthening of the PR, QT and QT_C (QT corrected for heart rate) intervals with no significant alteration in the QRS duration.

The d- and l-isomers of sotalol have similar Class III antiarrhythmic effects while the l-isomer is responsible for virtually all of the beta-blocking activity. Although significant beta-blockade may occur at oral doses as low as 25 mg, Class III effects are usually seen at daily doses of greater than 160 mg.

Its β-adrenergic blocking activity causes a reduction in heart rate (negative chronotropic effect) and a limited reduction in the force of contraction (negative inotropic effect). These cardiac changes reduce myocardial oxygen consumption and cardiac work. Like other -blockers, sotalol inhibits renin release. The renin-suppressive effect of sotalol is significant both at rest and during exercise. Like other beta adrenergic blocking agents, SOTACOR produces a gradual but significant reduction in both systolic and diastolic blood pressures in hypertensive patients. Twenty-four-hour control of blood pressure is maintained both in the supine and upright positions with a single daily dose.

5.2 Pharmacokinetic properties

The bioavailability of oral sotalol is essentially complete (greater than 90%). After oral administration, peak levels are reached in 2.5 to 4 hours, and steady-state plasma levels are attained within 2-3 days. The absorption is reduced by approximately 20% when administered with a standard meal, in comparison to fasting conditions. Over the dosage range 40-640 mg/day SOTACOR displays dose proportionality with respect to plasma levels. Distribution occurs to a central (plasma) and a peripheral compartment, with an elimination half-life of 10-20 hours. Sotalol does not bind to plasma proteins and is not metabolised. There is very little inter-subject variability in plasma levels. Sotalol crosses the blood brain barrier poorly, with cerebrospinal fluid concentrations only 10% of those in plasma. The primary route of elimination is renal excretion. Approximately 80 to 90% of a dose is excreted unchanged in the urine, while the remainder is excreted in the faeces. Lower doses are necessary in conditions of renal impairment (see Dosage and Administration in patients with renal dysfunction). Age does not significantly alter the pharmacokinetics, although impaired renal function in geriatric patients can decrease the excretion rate, resulting in increased drug accumulation.

5.3 Preclinical safety data

No further particulars.

6. PHARMACEUTICAL PARTICULARS

6.1 List of excipients

Glacial acetic acid, sodium chloride, sodium hydroxide, water.

6.2 Incompatibilities

There are no known incompatibilities.

6.3 Shelf life

Three years.

6.4 Special precautions for storage

Store between 15 and 30°C in a dry place, protected from light.

6.5 Nature and contents of container

SOTACOR injection is supplied as 40 mg sotalol hydrochloride in 4 ml ampoules, with 5 ampoules per box.

6.6 Instructions for use and handling

SOTACOR injection fluid can be administered as an intravenous infusion with 5% glucose intravenous infusion or 0.9% sodium chloride intravenous infusion. The final concentration should be between 0.01-2 mg/ml.

In concentrations of 0.01-2 mg/ml, dilution of SOTACOR injection fluid with 5% glucose intravenous infusion or 0.9% sodium chloride intravenous infusion, is chemically and physically stable during at least 4 days at room temperature (15-25 °C) and 3 weeks under refrigeration (2-8 °C).

As the formulation does not contain a preservative, the solutions of SOTACOR should be prepared in an aseptic manner. Prompt use of the solution is recommended.

7. MARKETING AUTHORISATION HOLDER

Bristol-Myers Squibb Holdings Limited

t/a Bristol-Myers Pharmaceuticals

Uxbridge Business Park

Sanderson Road

Uxbridge

Middlesex UB8 1DH

8. MARKETING AUTHORISATION NUMBER(S)

0125/0123

9. DATE OF FIRST AUTHORISATION/RENEWAL OF THE AUTHORISATION

25 January 1990

10. DATE OF REVISION OF THE TEXT

July 2005

Sotacor Tablets

(Bristol-Myers Pharmaceuticals)

1. NAME OF THE MEDICINAL PRODUCT

SOTACOR TABLETS

2. QUALITATIVE AND QUANTITATIVE COMPOSITION

Sotacor Tablets 80mg:

Each tablet containing 80mg sotalol hydrochloride.

Sotacor Tablets 160mg:

Each tablet containing 160mg sotalol hydrochloride.

3. PHARMACEUTICAL FORM

Sotacor Tablets 80mg:

Round, biconvex, white tablets scored on one side and engraved on the other side with "80".

Sotacor Tablets 160mg:

Round, biconvex, white tablets scored on one side and engraved on the other side with "160".

4. CLINICAL PARTICULARS

4.1 Therapeutic indications

SOTACOR tablets are indicated for:

Ventricular arrhythmias:

- Treatment of life-threatening ventricular tachyarrhythmias;
- Treatment of symptomatic non-sustained ventricular tachyarrhythmias;

Supraventricular arrhythmias:

- Prophylaxis of paroxysmal atrial tachycardia, paroxysmal atrial fibrillation, paroxysmal A-V nodal re-entrant tachycardia, paroxysmal A-V re-entrant tachycardia using accessory pathways, and paroxysmal supraventricular tachycardia after cardiac surgery;
- Maintenance of normal sinus rhythm following conversion of atrial fibrillation or atrial flutter.

4.2 Posology and method of administration

The initiation of treatment or changes in dosage with SOTACOR should follow an appropriate medical evaluation including ECG control with measurement of the corrected QT interval, and assessment of renal function, electrolyte balance and concomitant medications (See 4.4 Warnings and precautions).

As with other antiarrhythmic agents, it is recommended that SOTACOR be initiated and doses increased in a facility capable of monitoring and assessing cardiac rhythm. The dosage must be individualized and based on the patient's response. Proarrhythmic events can occur not only at initiation of therapy, but also with each upward dosage adjustment.

In view of its β-adrenergic blocking properties, treatment with SOTACOR should not be discontinued suddenly, especially in patients with ischaemic heart disease (angina pectoris, prior acute myocardial infarction) or hypertension, to prevent exacerbation of the disease (see 4.4 Warnings).

The following dosing schedule can be recommended:

The initial dose is 80 mg, administered either singly or as two divided doses.

Oral dosage of SOTACOR should be adjusted gradually allowing 2-3 days between dosing increments in order to attain steady-state, and to allow monitoring of QT intervals. Most patients respond to a daily dose of 160 to 320 mg administered in two divided doses at approximately 12 hour intervals. Some patients with life-threatening refractory ventricular arrhythmias may require doses as high as 480 - 640 mg/day. These doses should be used under specialist supervision and should only be prescribed when the potential benefit outweighs the increased risk of adverse events, particularly proarrhythmias (see 4.4 Warnings).

Children

SOTACOR is not intended for administration to children.

Dosage in renally impaired patients

Because SOTACOR is excreted mainly in urine, the dosage should be reduced when the creatinine clearance is less than 60 ml/min according to the following table:

Creatinine clearance (ml/min)	Adjusted doses
> 60	Recommended SOTACOR Dose
30-60	½ recommended SOTACOR Dose
10-30	¼ recommended SOTACOR Dose
< 10	Avoid

The creatinine clearance can be estimated from serum creatinine by the Cockroft and Gault formula:

Men:
$$\frac{(140 - age) \times weight\ (kg)}{72\ x\ serum\ creatinine\ (mg/dl)}$$

Women: as above × 0.85

When serum creatinine is given in μmol/l, divide the value by 88.4 (1mg/dl = 88.4 μmol/l).

Dosage in hepatically impaired patients

No dosage adjustment is required in hepatically impaired patients.

4.3 Contraindications

SOTACOR should not be used where there is evidence of sick sinus syndrome; second and third degree AV heart block unless a functioning pacemaker is present; congenital or acquired long QT syndromes; torsades de pointes; symptomatic sinus bradycardia; uncontrolled congestive heart failure; cardiogenic shock; anaesthesia that produces myocardial depression; untreated phaeochromocytoma; hypotension (except due to arrhythmia); Raynaud's phenomenon and severe peripheral circulatory disturbances; history of chronic obstructive airway disease or bronchial asthma (a warning will appear on the label); hypersensitivity to any of the components of the formulation; metabolic acidosis; renal failure (creatinine clearance < 10 ml/min).

4.4 Special warnings and special precautions for use

Abrupt Withdrawal Hypersensitivity to catecholamines is observed in patients withdrawn from beta-blocker therapy. Occasional cases of exacerbation of angina pectoris, arrhythmias, and in some cases, myocardial infarction have been reported after abrupt discontinuation of therapy.

Patients should be carefully monitored when discontinuing chronically administered SOTACOR, particularly those with ischaemic heart disease. If possible the dosage should be gradually reduced over a period of one to two weeks, if necessary at the same time initiating replacement therapy. Abrupt discontinuation may unmask latent coronary insufficiency. In addition, hypertension may develop.

Proarrhythmias The most dangerous adverse effect of Class I and Class III antiarrhythmic drugs (such as sotalol) is the aggravation of pre-existing arrhythmias or the provocation of new arrhythmias. Drugs that prolong the QT-interval may cause torsades de pointes, a polymorphic ventricular tachycardia associated with prolongation of the QT-interval. Experience to date indicates that the risk of torsades de pointes is associated with the prolongation of the QT-interval, reduction of the heart rate, reduction in serum potassium and magnesium, high plasma sotalol concentrations and with the concomitant use of sotalol and other medications which have been associated with torsades de pointes (see 4.5: Interactions). Females may be at increased risk of developing torsades de pointes.

The incidence of torsades de pointes is dose dependent. Torsades de pointes usually occurs early after initiating therapy or escalation of the dose and can progress to ventricular fibrillation.

In clinical trials of patients with sustained VT/VF the incidence of severe proarrhythmia (torsades de pointes or new sustained VT/VF) was <2% at doses up to 320 mg. The incidence more than doubled at higher doses.

Other risk factors for torsades de pointes were excessive prolongation of the QT_c and history of cardiomegaly or congestive heart failure. Patients with sustained ventricular tachycardia and a history of congestive heart failure have the highest risk of serious proarrhythmia (7%).

Proarrhythmic events must be anticipated not only on initiating therapy but with every upward dose adjustment. Initiating therapy at 80 mg with gradual upward dose titration thereafter reduces the risk of proarrhythmia. In patients already receiving SOTACOR caution should be used if the QT_c exceeds 500msec whilst on therapy, and serious consideration should be given to reducing the dose or discontinuing therapy when the QT_c-interval exceeds 550 msec. Due to the multiple risk factors associated with torsades de pointes, however, caution should be exercised regardless of the QT_c-interval.

Electrolyte Disturbances SOTACOR should not be used in patients with hypokalaemia or hypomagnesaemia prior to correction of imbalance; these conditions can exaggerate the degree of QT prolongation, and increase the potential for torsades de pointes. Special attention should be given to electrolyte and acid-base balance in patients experiencing severe or prolonged diarrhoea or patients receiving concomitant magnesium- and/or potassium-depleting drugs.

Congestive Heart Failure Beta-blockade may further depress myocardial contractility and precipitate more severe heart failure. Caution is advised when initiating therapy in patients with left ventricular dysfunction controlled by therapy (i.e. ACE Inhibitors, diuretics, digitalis, etc); a low initial dose and careful dose titration is appropriate.

Recent MI In post-infarction patients with impaired left ventricular function, the risk versus benefit of sotalol administration must be considered. Careful monitoring and dose titration are critical during initiation and follow-up of therapy. SOTACOR should be avoided in patients with left ventricular ejection fractions $\leq$40% without serious ventricular arrhythmias.

Electrocardiographic Changes Excessive prolongation of the QT-interval, >500 msec, can be a sign of toxicity and should be avoided (see Proarrhythmias above). Sinus bradycardia has been observed very commonly in arrhythmia patients receiving sotalol in clinical trials. Bradycardia increases the risk of torsades de pointes. Sinus pause, sinus arrest and sinus node dysfunction occur in less than 1% of patients. The incidence of 2nd- or 3rd-degree AV block is approximately 1%.

Anaphylaxis Patients with a history of anaphylactic reaction to a variety of allergens may have a more severe reaction on repeated challenge while taking beta-blockers. Such patients may be unresponsive to the usual doses of adrenaline used to treat the allergic reaction.

Anaesthesia As with other beta-blocking agents, SOTACOR should be used with caution in patients undergoing surgery and in association with anaesthetics that cause myocardial depression, such as cyclopropane or trichloroethylene.

Diabetes Mellitus SOTACOR should be used with caution in patients with diabetes (especially labile diabetes) or with a history of episodes of spontaneous hypoglycaemia, since beta-blockade may mask some important signs of the onset of acute hypoglycaemia, e.g. tachycardia.

Thyrotoxicosis Beta-blockade may mask certain clinical signs of hyperthyroidism (e.g., tachycardia). Patients suspected of developing thyrotoxicosis should be managed carefully to avoid abrupt withdrawal of beta-blockade which might be followed by an exacerbation of symptoms of hyperthyroidism, including thyroid storm.

Renal Impairment As sotalol is mainly eliminated via the kidneys the dose should be adjusted in patients with renal impairment (see dosage).

Psoriasis Beta-blocking drugs have been reported rarely to exacerbate the symptoms of psoriasis vulgaris.

4.5 Interaction with other medicinal products and other forms of Interaction

Antiarrhythmics Class 1a antiarrhythmic drugs, such as disopyramide, quinidine and procainamide and other antiarrhythmic drugs such as amiodarone and bepridil are not recommended as concomitant therapy with SOTACOR, because of their potential to prolong refractoriness (see 4.4 Special Warnings and Precautions). The concomitant use of other beta-blocking agents with SOTACOR may result in additive Class II effects.

Other drugs prolonging the QT-interval SOTACOR should be given with extreme caution in conjunction with other drugs known to prolong the QT-interval such as phenothiazines, tricyclic antidepressants, terfenadine and astemizole. Other drugs that have been associated with an increased risk for torsades de pointes include erythromycin IV, halofantrine, pentamidine, and quinolone antibiotics.

Floctafenine beta-adrenergic blocking agents may impede the compensatory cardiovascular reactions associated with hypotension or shock that may be induced by Floctafenine.

Calcium channel blocking drugs Concurrent administration of beta-blocking agents and calcium channel blockers has resulted in hypotension, bradycardia, conduction defects, and cardiac failure. Beta-blockers should be avoided in combination with cardiodepressant calcium-channel blockers such as verapamil and diltiazem because of the additive effects on atrioventricular conduction, and ventricular function.

Potassium-Depleting Diuretics Hypokalaemia or hypomagnesaemia may occur, increasing the potential for torsade de pointes (see Special Warnings and Precautions for Use).

Other potassium-depleting drugs Amphotericin B (IV route), corticosteroids (systemic administration), and some laxatives may also be associated with hypokalaemia; potassium levels should be monitored and corrected appropriately during concomitant administration with SOTACOR.

Clonidine Beta-blocking drugs may potentiate the rebound hypertension sometimes observed after discontinuation of clonidine; therefore, the beta-blocker should be discontinued slowly several days before the gradual withdrawal of clonidine.

Digitalis glycosides Single and multiple doses of SOTACOR do not significantly affect serum digoxin levels. Proarrhythmic events were more common in sotalol treated patients also receiving digitalis glycosides; however, this may be related to the presence of CHF, a known risk factor for proarrhythmia, in patients receiving digitalis glycosides. Association of digitalis glycosides with beta-blockers may increase auriculo-ventricular conduction time.

Catecholamine-depleting agents Concomitant use of catecholamine-depleting drugs, such as reserpine, guanethidine, or alpha methyldopa, with a beta-blocker may produce an excessive reduction of resting sympathetic nervous tone. Patients should be closely monitored for evidence of hypotension and/or marked bradycardia which may produce syncope.

Insulin and oral hypoglycaemics Hyperglycaemia may occur, and the dosage of antidiabetic drugs may require adjustment. Symptoms of hypoglycaemia (tachycardia) may be masked by beta-blocking agents.

Neuromuscular blocking agents like Tubocurarin The neuromuscular blockade is prolonged by beta-blocking agents.

Beta-2-receptor stimulants Patients in need of beta-agonists should not normally receive SOTACOR. However, if concomitant therapy is necessary beta-agonists may have to be administered in increased dosages.

Drug/Laboratory interaction The presence of sotalol in the urine may result in falsely elevated levels of urinary metanephrine when measured by photometric methods. Patients suspected of having phaeochromocytoma and who are treated with sotalol should have their urine screened utilizing the HPLC assay with solid phase extraction.

4.6 Pregnancy and lactation

Pregnancy Animal studies with sotalol hydrochloride have shown no evidence of teratogenicity or other harmful effects on the foetus. Although there are no adequate and well-controlled studies in pregnant women, sotalol hydrochloride has been shown to cross the placenta and is found in amniotic fluid. Beta-blockers reduce placental perfusion, which may result in intrauterine foetal death, immature and premature deliveries. In addition, adverse effects (especially hypoglycaemia and bradycardia) may occur in foetus and neonate. There is an increased risk of cardiac and pulmonary complications in the neonate in the postnatal period. Therefore, SOTACOR should be used in pregnancy only if the potential benefits outweigh the possible risk to the foetus. The neonate should be monitored very carefully for 48 - 72 hours after delivery if it was not possible to interrupt maternal therapy with SOTACOR 2-3 days before the birthdate.

Most beta-blockers, particularly lipophilic compounds, will pass into breast milk although to a variable extent. Breast feeding is therefore not recommended during administration of these compounds.

4.7 Effects on ability to drive and use machines

There are no data available, but the occasional occurrence of side-effects such as dizziness and fatigue should be taken into account (see 4.8 Undesirable effects).

4.8 Undesirable effects

The most frequent adverse effects of sotalol arise from its beta-blockade properties. Adverse effects are usually transient in nature and rarely necessitate interruption of, or withdrawal from treatment. If they do occur, they usually disappear when the dosage is reduced. The most significant adverse effects, however, are those due to proarrhythmia, including torsades de pointes (see Warnings).

The following are adverse events considered related to therapy, occurring in 1% or more of patients treated with SOTACOR.

Cardiovascular Bradycardia, dyspnoea, chest pain, palpitations, oedema, ECG abnormalities, hypotension, proarrhythmia, syncope, heart failure, presyncope.

Dermatologic Rash.

Gastro-intestinal Nausea/vomiting, diarrhoea, dyspepsia, abdominal pain, flatulence.

Musculoskeletal Cramps.

Nervous/psychiatric Fatigue, dizziness, asthenia, light-headedness, headache, sleep disturbances, depression, paraesthesia, mood changes, anxiety.

Urogenital Sexual dysfunction.

Special Senses Visual disturbances, taste abnormalities, hearing disturbances.

Body as a whole Fever.

In trials of patients with cardiac arrhythmia, the most common adverse events leading to discontinuation of SOTACOR were fatigue 4%, bradycardia (<50 bpm) 3%, dyspnoea 3%, proarrhythmia 2%, asthenia 2%, and dizziness 2%.

Cold and cyanotic extremities, Raynaud's phenomenon, increase in existing intermittent claudication and dry eyes have been seen in association with other beta-blockers.

4.9 Overdose

Intentional or accidental overdosage with SOTACOR has rarely resulted in death. Haemodialysis results in a large reduction of plasma levels of sotalol.

Symptoms and treatment of overdosage: The most common signs to be expected are bradycardia, congestive heart failure, hypotension, bronchospasm and hypoglycaemia. In cases of massive intentional overdosage (2-16 g) of SOTACOR the following clinical findings were seen: hypotension, bradycardia, prolongation of QT-interval, premature ventricular complexes, ventricular tachycardia, torsades de pointes.

If overdosage occurs, therapy with SOTACOR should be discontinued and the patient observed closely. In addition, if required, the following therapeutic measures are suggested:

Bradycardia Atropine (0.5 to 2 mg IV), another anticholinergic drug, a beta-adrenergic agonist (isoprenaline, 5 microgram per minute, up to 25 microgram, by slow IV injection) or transvenous cardiac pacing.

Heart Block (second and third degree) Transvenous cardiac pacing.

Hypotension Adrenaline rather than isoprenaline or noradrenaline may be useful, depending on associated factors.

Bronchospasm Aminophylline or aerosol beta-2-receptor stimulant.

Torsades de pointes DC cardioversion, transvenous cardiac pacing, adrenaline, and/or magnesium sulphate.

5. PHARMACOLOGICAL PROPERTIES

5.1 Pharmacodynamic properties

D,l-sotalol is a non-selective hydrophilic β-adrenergic receptor blocking agent, devoid of intrinsic sympathomimetic activity or membrane stabilizing activity.

SOTACOR has both beta-adrenoreceptor blocking (Vaughan Williams Class II) and cardiac action potential duration prolongation (Vaughan Williams Class III) antiarrhythmic properties. Sotalol has no known effect on the upstroke velocity and therefore no effect on the depolarisation phase.

Sotalol uniformly prolongs the action potential duration in cardiac tissues by delaying the repolarisation phase. Its major effects are prolongation of the atrial, ventricular and accessory pathway effective refractory periods.

The Class II and III properties may be reflected on the surface electrocardiogram by a lengthening of the PR, QT and QT_c (QT corrected for heart rate) intervals with no significant alteration in the QRS duration.

The d- and l-isomers of sotalol have similar Class III antiarrhythmic effects while the l-isomer is responsible for virtually all of the beta-blocking activity. Although significant beta-blockade may occur at oral doses as low as

25 mg, Class III effects are usually seen at daily doses of greater than 160 mg.

Its β-adrenergic blocking activity causes a reduction in heart rate (negative chronotropic effect) and a limited reduction in the force of contraction (negative inotropic effect). These cardiac changes reduce myocardial oxygen consumption and cardiac work. Like other β-blockers, sotalol inhibits renin release. The renin-suppressive effect of sotalol is significant both at rest and during exercise. Like other beta adrenergic blocking agents, SOTACOR produces a gradual but significant reduction in both systolic and diastolic blood pressures in hypertensive patients. Twenty-four-hour control of blood pressure is maintained both in the supine and upright positions with a single daily dose.

5.2 Pharmacokinetic properties

The bioavailability of oral sotalol is essentially complete (greater than 90%). After oral administration, peak levels are reached in 2.5 to 4 hours, and steady-state plasma levels are attained within 2-3 days. The absorption is reduced by approximately 20% when administered with a standard meal, in comparison to fasting conditions. Over the dosage range 40-640 mg/day SOTACOR displays dose proportionality with respect to plasma levels. Distribution occurs to a central (plasma) and a peripheral compartment, with an elimination half-life of 10-20 hours. Sotalol does not bind to plasma proteins and is not metabolised. There is very little inter-subject variability in plasma levels. Sotalol crosses the blood brain barrier poorly, with cerebrospinal fluid concentrations only 10% of those in plasma. The primary route of elimination is renal excretion. Approximately 80 to 90% of a dose is excreted unchanged in the urine, while the remainder is excreted in the faeces. Lower doses are necessary in conditions of renal impairment (see Dosage and Administration in patients with renal dysfunction). Age does not significantly alter the pharmacokinetics, although impaired renal function in geriatric patients can decrease the excretion rate, resulting in increased drug accumulation.

5.3 Preclinical safety data

No further particulars.

6. PHARMACEUTICAL PARTICULARS

6.1 List of excipients

Colloidal anhydrous silica, lactose, magnesium stearate, maize starch, micro-crystalline cellulose, stearic acid.

6.2 Incompatibilities

There are no known incompatibilities.

6.3 Shelf life

Three years.

6.4 Special precautions for storage

Do not store above 25°C. Protect from light.

6.5 Nature and contents of container

Original packs of 28 - blister strips of 14 tablets with 2 strips to a carton.

6.6 Instructions for use and handling

None.

7. MARKETING AUTHORISATION HOLDER

Bristol-Myers Squibb Holdings Limited

t/a Bristol-Myers Pharmaceuticals

Uxbridge Business Park

Sanderson Road

Uxbridge

Middlesex UB8 1DH

8. MARKETING AUTHORISATION NUMBER(S)

Sotacor Tablets 80mg: 0125/0076

Sotacor Tablets 160mg: 0125/0093

9. DATE OF FIRST AUTHORISATION/RENEWAL OF THE AUTHORISATION

Sotacor Tablets 80mg: 9th August 1989

Sotacor Tablets 160mg: 11th February 1992

10. DATE OF REVISION OF THE TEXT

July 2005

Spasmonal 60mg

(Norgine Limited)

1. NAME OF THE MEDICINAL PRODUCT

SPASMONAL 60 mg

2. QUALITATIVE AND QUANTITATIVE COMPOSITION

Each capsule contains 60mg alverine citrate.

3. PHARMACEUTICAL FORM

An opaque size 3 capsule with a grey cap and blue body, marked "SP 60".

4. CLINICAL PARTICULARS

4.1 Therapeutic indications

The relief of smooth muscle spasm, in conditions such as irritable bowel syndrome, painful diverticular disease of the colon and primary dysmenorrhoea

4.2 Posology and method of administration

Recommended dose and dosage schedules:

Adults (including the elderly): 1 or 2 capsules one to three times daily.

Children below the age of 12 years: not recommended.

4.3 Contraindications

Paralytic ileus or known hypersensitivity to any of the ingredients.

4.4 Special warnings and special precautions for use

Additional warnings to be included in the Patient Information Leaflet:

If this is the first time you have had these symptoms, consult your doctor before using any treatment.

If any of the following apply do not use SPASMONAL 60 mg; it may not be the right treatment for you. See your doctor as soon as possible if:

- you are aged 40 years or over
- you have passed blood from the bowel
- you are feeling sick or vomiting
- you have lost your appetite or lost weight
- you are looking pale and feeling tired
- you are suffering from severe constipation
- you have a fever
- you have recently travelled abroad
- you are or may be pregnant
- you have abnormal vaginal bleeding or discharge
- you have difficulty or pain passing urine.

Consult your doctor if you have developed new symptoms, or if your symptoms worsen, or if they do not improve after 2 weeks treatment.

4.5 Interaction with other medicinal products and other forms of Interaction

None stated.

4.6 Pregnancy and lactation

Although no teratogenic effects have been reported, use during pregnancy or lactation is not recommended as evidence of safety in preclinical studies is limited.

4.7 Effects on ability to drive and use machines

None.

4.8 Undesirable effects

Possible side effects may include nausea, headache, dizziness, itching, rash, and allergic reactions.

There have been isolated reports of jaundice due to hepatitis, which may have been immune-mediated; but this adverse reaction resolved on cessation of alverine treatment.

4.9 Overdose

Can produce hypotension and atropine-like toxic effects. Management is as for atropine poisoning with supportive therapy for hypotension.

5. PHARMACOLOGICAL PROPERTIES

5.1 Pharmacodynamic properties

Alverine citrate is a spasmolytic, which has a specific action on the smooth muscle of the alimentary tract and uterus, without affecting the heart, blood vessels and tracheal muscle at therapeutic doses.

5.2 Pharmacokinetic properties

After oral administration, alverine is rapidly converted to its primary active metabolite, which is then further converted to two secondary metabolites. There is a high renal clearance of all metabolites indicating that they are eliminated by active renal secretion. The peak plasma level of the most active metabolite occurs between 1 and 1½ hours after oral dosing.

5.3 Preclinical safety data

Preclinical studies provide evidence that alverine citrate has no significant systemic toxicity potential at the proposed dosage.

6. PHARMACEUTICAL PARTICULARS

6.1 List of excipients

Maize Starch

Magnesium Stearate

Capsule Shell:

Gelatin, E132, E171, E172

6.2 Incompatibilities

None stated.

6.3 Shelf life

3 years.

6.4 Special precautions for storage

Store in a dry place. Do not store above 25°C.

6.5 Nature and contents of container

Plastic containers of 20 or 100 capsules; foil/UPVC blister packs containing 3, 10, 12, 20, 90 or 100 capsules.

6.6 Instructions for use and handling

None.

7. MARKETING AUTHORISATION HOLDER

Norgine Limited

Chaplin House

Widewater Place

Moorhall Road

Harefield

UXBRIDGE

Middlesex UB9 6NS

United Kingdom

8. MARKETING AUTHORISATION NUMBER(S)

PL 00322/5014R

9. DATE OF FIRST AUTHORISATION/RENEWAL OF THE AUTHORISATION

June 1998

10. DATE OF REVISION OF THE TEXT

6th April 2004

Legal category: **P**

Spasmonal Forte 120mg

(Norgine Limited)

1. NAME OF THE MEDICINAL PRODUCT

SPASMONAL Forte 120 mg

2. QUALITATIVE AND QUANTITATIVE COMPOSITION

Each capsule contains 120 mg alverine citrate.

3. PHARMACEUTICAL FORM

An opaque, size 1 capsule with a grey cap and blue body, marked "SP120".

4. CLINICAL PARTICULARS

4.1 Therapeutic indications

The relief of smooth muscle spasm, in conditions such as irritable bowel syndrome, painful diverticular disease of the colon and primary dysmenorrhoea.

4.2 Posology and method of administration

Recommended dose and dosage schedules:

Adults (including the elderly): 1 capsule one to three times daily.

Children below the age of 12 years: not recommended.

4.3 Contraindications

Paralytic ileus or known hypersensitivity to any of the ingredients.

4.4 Special warnings and special precautions for use

Additional warnings to be included in the Patient Information Leaflet:

If this is the first time you have had these symptoms, consult your doctor before using any treatment.

If any of the following apply do not use SPASMONAL Forte 120 mg; it may not be the right treatment for you. See your doctor as soon as possible if:

- you are aged 40 years or over
- you have passed blood from the bowel
- you are feeling sick or vomiting
- you have lost your appetite or lost weight
- you are looking pale and feeling tired
- you are suffering from severe constipation
- you have a fever
- you have recently travelled abroad
- you are or may be pregnant
- you have abnormal vaginal bleeding or discharge
- you have difficulty or pain passing urine.

Consult your doctor if you have developed new symptoms, or if your symptoms worsen, or if they do not improve after 2 weeks treatment.

4.5 Interaction with other medicinal products and other forms of Interaction

None stated.

4.6 Pregnancy and lactation

Although no teratogenic effects have been reported, use during pregnancy or lactation is not recommended, as evidence of safety in preclinical studies is limited.

4.7 Effects on ability to drive and use machines

None.

4.8 Undesirable effects

Possible side effects may include nausea, headache, dizziness, itching, rash, and allergic reactions, including anaphylaxis.

There have been isolated reports of jaundice due to hepatitis, which may have been immune-mediated; but this adverse reaction resolved on cessation of alverine treatment.

4.9 Overdose

Can produce hypotension and atropine-like toxic effects. Management is as for atropine poisoning with supportive therapy for hypotension.

5. PHARMACOLOGICAL PROPERTIES

5.1 Pharmacodynamic properties

Alverine citrate is a spasmolytic, which has a specific action on the smooth muscle of the alimentary tract and uterus, without affecting the heart, blood vessels and tracheal muscle at therapeutic doses.

5.2 Pharmacokinetic properties

After oral administration, alverine is rapidly converted to its primary active metabolite, which is then further converted to two secondary metabolites. There is a high renal clearance of all metabolites indicating that they are eliminated by active renal secretion. The peak plasma level of the most active metabolite occurs between 1 and 1½ hours after oral dosing.

5.3 Preclinical safety data

Pre-clinical studies provide evidence that alverine citrate has no significant systemic toxicity potential at the proposed dosage.

6. PHARMACEUTICAL PARTICULARS

6.1 List of excipients

Maize Starch

Magnesium Stearate

Capsule Shell:

Gelatin, E132, E171, E172

6.2 Incompatibilities

None stated.

6.3 Shelf life

3 years.

6.4 Special precautions for storage

Store in a dry place. Do not store above 25°C.

6.5 Nature and contents of container

A box of aluminium foil/UPVC blister strip packs containing 2, 10, 20, 30, 60 or 90 capsules, in strips of 10 capsules as appropriate.

6.6 Instructions for use and handling

None.

7. MARKETING AUTHORISATION HOLDER

Norgine Limited

Chaplin House

Widewater Place

Moorhall Road

Harefield

UXBRIDGE

Middlesex, UB9 6NS

United Kingdom

8. MARKETING AUTHORISATION NUMBER(S)

PL 00322/0075

9. DATE OF FIRST AUTHORISATION/RENEWAL OF THE AUTHORISATION

October 1997

10. DATE OF REVISION OF THE TEXT

6th April 2004

Legal category: **P**

Spectraban Lotion 25

(Stiefel Laboratories (UK) Limited)

1. NAME OF THE MEDICINAL PRODUCT

SpectraBAN 25 Lotion

2. QUALITATIVE AND QUANTITATIVE COMPOSITION

Padimate 3.2% w/w

Para aminobenzoic Acid 5.0% w/w

3. PHARMACEUTICAL FORM

Solution for topical use.

4. CLINICAL PARTICULARS

4.1 Therapeutic indications

SpectraBAN 25 Lotion is a protective sunscreen lotion indicated in patients at risk from exposure to ultraviolet light within the wavelength range 290 - 320nm. It is this narrow waveband of ultraviolet light which is responsible for burning and tanning of the skin in man. Use of the product should allow fifteen times normal exposure to sunlight before burning.

SpectraBAN 25 Lotion is indicated in sun-sensitive conditions such as polymorphic light eruptions and solar urticaria, and any condition made worse by UVB light such as lupus erythematosus.

4.2 Posology and method of administration

The following dosages and schedules are applicable for adults, children and the elderly.

Apply evenly and liberally to areas to be exposed or protected only by light clothing. Allow 45 minutes before swimming or sweat producing exercise. A single application may give day-long protection, but the product should be reapplied during prolonged sunning after excessive sweating or swimming or as directed by a doctor.

4.3 Contraindications

Sunscreen preparations occasionally produce a sensitivity reaction. Although such occurrences are rare with SpectraBAN 25 Lotion, treatment should be discontinued if a skin rash or irritation develops.

4.4 Special warnings and special precautions for use

Avoid contact with the eyes. Avoid flame. Can stain clothing. Keep in a cool dark place.

4.5 Interaction with other medicinal products and other forms of Interaction

None.

4.6 Pregnancy and lactation

There is no evidence of the safety of the drug in human pregnancy, but it has been in wide use for many years with no apparent ill consequences.

4.7 Effects on ability to drive and use machines

None.

4.8 Undesirable effects

Sunscreen agents occasionally produce a sensitivity reaction and can cause contact dermatitis.

4.9 Overdose

Not applicable.

5. PHARMACOLOGICAL PROPERTIES

5.1 Pharmacodynamic properties

The sunscreen agents used in SpectraBAN 25 Lotion, Padimate O and Para aminobenzoic acid, exert their effect by absorption of ultraviolet light.

5.2 Pharmacokinetic properties

Not applicable.

5.3 Preclinical safety data

Not applicable.

6. PHARMACEUTICAL PARTICULARS

6.1 List of excipients

Denatured alcohol

Carbomer 941

Polyoxyethylene 15 cocoamine

Oleyl Alcohol

Carmoisine red

Essence A-3012

Purified Water.

6.2 Incompatibilities

None.

6.3 Shelf life

a) For the product as packaged for sale

Three years

b) After first opening the container

Comply with expiry date.

6.4 Special precautions for storage

Keep in a cool, dark place.

6.5 Nature and contents of container

High density polyethylene bottle containing 150ml.

6.6 Instructions for use and handling

None.

7. MARKETING AUTHORISATION HOLDER

Stiefel Laboratories (UK) Ltd

Holtspur Lane

Wooburn Green

High Wycombe

Bucks

HP10 0AU

8. MARKETING AUTHORISATION NUMBER(S)

PL 0174/0035.

9. DATE OF FIRST AUTHORISATION/RENEWAL OF THE AUTHORISATION

30th March 1978

10. DATE OF REVISION OF THE TEXT

September 2005.

Spiriva

(Boehringer Ingelheim Limited)

1. NAME OF THE MEDICINAL PRODUCT

▼SPIRIVA® 18 microgram inhalation powder, hard capsule

2. QUALITATIVE AND QUANTITATIVE COMPOSITION

Each capsule contains 22.5 microgram tiotropium bromide monohydrate equivalent to 18 microgram tiotropium.

The delivered dose (the dose that leaves the mouthpiece of the HandiHaler® device) is 10 microgram.

For excipients, see 6.1.

3. PHARMACEUTICAL FORM

Inhalation powder, hard capsule

Light green hard capsules, containing a white or yellowish white powder, with product code and company logo printed on the capsule.

4. CLINICAL PARTICULARS

4.1 Therapeutic indications

Tiotropium is indicated as a maintenance bronchodilator treatment to relieve symptoms of patients with chronic obstructive pulmonary disease (COPD).

4.2 Posology and method of administration

The recommended dosage of tiotropium bromide is inhalation of the contents of one capsule once daily with the HandiHaler device at the same time of day (for complete instructions for use see 6.6 Instructions for use and handling and disposal).

Tiotropium bromide should only be inhaled with the HandiHaler device.

The recommended dose should not be exceeded.

Tiotropium bromide capsules must not be swallowed.

Special Populations:

Geriatric patients can use tiotropium bromide at the recommended dose.

Renally impaired patients can use tiotropium bromide at the recommended dose. For patients with moderate to severe impairment (creatinine clearance ≤ 50 ml/min) see 4.4 Special warnings and special precautions for use and 5.2 Pharmacokinetic properties.

Hepatically impaired patients can use tiotropium bromide at the recommended dose (see 5.2 Pharmacokinetic properties).

Paediatric patients: Safety and effectiveness of tiotropium bromide inhalation powder in paediatric patients have not been established and therefore it should not be used in patients under 18 years of age.

4.3 Contraindications

Tiotropium bromide inhalation powder is contraindicated in patients with hypersensitivity to tiotropium bromide, atropine or its derivatives, e.g. ipratropium or oxitropium or to the excipient lactose monohydrate.

4.4 Special warnings and special precautions for use

Tiotropium bromide, as a once daily maintenance bronchodilator, should not be used for the initial treatment of acute episodes of bronchospasm, i.e. rescue therapy.

Immediate hypersensitivity reactions may occur after administration of tiotropium bromide inhalation powder.

As with other anticholinergic drugs, tiotropium bromide should be used with caution in patients with narrow-angle glaucoma, prostatic hyperplasia or bladder-neck obstruction.

Inhaled medicines may cause inhalation-induced bronchospasm.

As plasma concentration increases with decreased renal function in patients with moderate to severe renal impairment (creatinine clearance ≤ 50 ml/min) tiotropium bromide should be used only if the expected benefit outweighs the potential risk. There is no long term experience in patients with severe renal impairment (see 5.2 Pharmacokinetic properties).

Patients should be cautioned to avoid getting the drug powder into their eyes. They should be advised that this may result in precipitation or worsening of narrow-angle glaucoma, eye pain or discomfort, temporary blurring of vision, visual halos or coloured images in association with red eyes from conjunctival and corneal congestion. Patients should stop using tiotropium bromide and consult a physician immediately when signs and symptoms of narrow-angle glaucoma appear.

Dry mouth, which has been observed with anti-cholinergic treatment, may in the long term be associated with dental caries.

Tiotropium bromide should not be used more frequently than once daily (see section 4.9 Overdose).

4.5 Interaction with other medicinal products and other forms of Interaction

Although no formal drug interaction studies have been performed, tiotropium bromide inhalation powder has been used concomitantly with other drugs without adverse drug reactions. These include sympathomimetic bronchodilators, methylxanthines, oral and inhaled steroids, commonly used in the treatment of COPD.

The co-administration of tiotropium bromide with other anticholinergic-containing drugs has not been studied and is therefore not recommended.

4.6 Pregnancy and lactation

For tiotropium bromide, no clinical data on exposed pregnancies are available. Studies in animals have shown reproductive toxicity associated with maternal toxicity. See 5.3 Preclinical safety data.

Clinical data from nursing women exposed to tiotropium bromide are not available. Based on lactating rodent studies, a small amount of tiotropium bromide is excreted in milk.

Therefore, tiotropium bromide should not be used in pregnant or nursing women unless the expected benefit outweighs any possible risk to the unborn child or the infant.

4.7 Effects on ability to drive and use machines

No studies on the effects on the ability to drive and use machines have been performed. However, on the basis of the pharmacodynamic and reported undesirable effects profiles at the recommended dose, there is no evidence for a potential influence on the ability to drive and use machines.

4.8 Undesirable effects

a) General Description

In one-year studies of 906 patients receiving tiotropium bromide, the most commonly reported adverse drug reaction was dry mouth. Dry mouth occurred in approximately 14% of patients. Dry mouth was usually mild and often resolved with continued treatment.

b) Table of Adverse Reactions [1] based on reporting incidences in patients treated with tiotropium bromide in one year clinical trials (according to the WHO System Organ Class)

WHO Preferred Term	Frequency[2]
Body As A Whole:	
Allergic reaction[4]	Uncommon
Gastro-Intestinal System Disorders:	
Mouth Dry	Very common
Constipation	Common[3]
Heart Rate and Rhythm Disorders:	
Tachycardia	Uncommon
Palpitations	Uncommon
Resistance Mechanism Disorders:	
Moniliasis	Common[3]
Respiratory System Disorders:	
Sinusitis	Common[3]
Pharyngitis	Common[3]
Epistaxis	Common[3]
Urinary System Disorders:	
Urinary difficulty	Uncommon
Urinary retention	Uncommon

[1]based on possible causal association

[2]very common > 1/10; common> 1/100, < 1/10; uncommon > 1/1,000, < 1/100 according to frequency

[3]all events listed as common were reported with a frequency in excess of placebo between 1% and 2%.

[4]refer to section 4.8c

Post marketing experience:

Spontaneous reports have been received for nausea, hoarseness and dizziness.

c) Information Characterising Individual Serious and/or Frequently Occurring Adverse Reactions

The most common anticholinergic adverse reaction reported by COPD patients was dry mouth. Dry mouth was mild in the majority of cases. In general, dry mouth had an onset between 3 and 5 weeks. Dry mouth commonly resolved while patients continued to receive tiotropium bromide. Dry mouth led to discontinuation from the one-year studies by 3 of 906 patients (0.3% of the treated patients).

Isolated adverse reactions occurring in single cases reported as severe and consistent with anticholinergic effects in the one-year trials included constipation and urinary retention. Urinary retention was limited to elderly men with predisposing factors (e.g. prostatic hyperplasia).

Isolated adverse reactions of supraventricular tachycardia and atrial fibrillation were reported in association with the use of tiotropium bromide, usually in susceptible patients.

In common with all inhaled medications, tiotropium may cause inhalation-induced bronchospasm.

Allergic reactions observed from spontaneous reports include angioedema, rash, urticaria and pruritus.

d) Pharmacological Class - Adverse Reactions

Several organ systems and functions are under control of the parasympathetic nervous system and thus can be affected by anticholinergic agents. Possible adverse events attributable to systemic anticholinergic effects include dry mouth, dry throat, increased heart rate, blurred vision, glaucoma, urinary difficulty, urinary retention, and constipation. In addition, local upper airway irritant phenomena were observed in patients receiving tiotropium bromide. An increased incidence of dry mouth and constipation may occur with increasing age.

4.9 Overdose

High doses of tiotropium bromide may lead to anticholinergic signs and symptoms.

However, there were no systemic anticholinergic adverse effects following a single inhaled dose of up to 340 micrograms tiotropium bromide in healthy volunteers. Additionally, no relevant adverse effects, beyond dry mouth, were observed following 7 day dosing of up to 170 micrograms tiotropium bromide in healthy volunteers. In a multiple dose study in COPD patients with a maximum daily dose of 43 micrograms tiotropium bromide over four weeks no significant undesirable effects have been observed.

Acute intoxication by inadvertent oral ingestion of tiotropium bromide capsules is unlikely due to low oral bioavailability.

5. PHARMACOLOGICAL PROPERTIES

5.1 Pharmacodynamic properties

Pharmacotherapeutic group: Anticholinergics

ATC code: R03B B04

Tiotropium bromide is a long-acting, specific muscarinic receptor antagonist, in clinical medicine often called an anticholinergic. By binding to the muscarinic receptors in the bronchial smooth musculature, tiotropium bromide inhibits the cholinergic (bronchoconstrictive) effects of acetylcholine, released from parasympathetic nerve endings. It has similar affinity to the subtypes of muscarinic receptors, M_1 to M_5. In the airways, tiotropium bromide competitively and reversibly antagonises the M3 receptors, resulting in relaxation. The effect was dose dependent and lasted longer than 24h. The long duration is probably due to the very slow dissociation from the M_3 receptor, exhibiting a significantly longer dissociation half-life than ipratropium. As an N-quaternary anticholinergic, tiotropium bromide is topically (broncho-) selective when administered by inhalation, demonstrating an acceptable therapeutic range before systemic anticholinergic effects may occur. The bronchodilation is primarily a local effect (on the airways), not a systemic one.

Dissociation from M_2-receptors is faster than from M_3, which in functional in vitro studies, elicited (kinetically controlled) receptor subtype selectivity of M_3 over M_2. The high potency and slow receptor dissociation found its clinical correlate in significant and long-acting bronchodilation in patients with COPD.

The clinical development programme included four one-year and two six-month randomised, double-blind studies in 2663 patients (1308 receiving tiotropium bromide). The one-year programme consisted of two placebo-controlled trials and two trials with an active control (ipratropium). The two six-month trials were both, salmeterol and placebo controlled. These studies included lung function and health outcome measures of dyspnea, exacerbations and health-related quality of life.

In the aforementioned studies, tiotropium bromide, administered once daily, provided significant improvement in lung function (forced expiratory volume in one second, FEV_1 and forced vital capacity, FVC) within 30 minutes following the first dose which was maintained for 24 hours. Pharmacodynamic steady state was reached within one week with the majority of bronchodilation observed by the third day. Tiotropium bromide significantly improved morning and evening PEFR (peak expiratory flow rate) as measured by patient's daily recordings. The bronchodilator effects of tiotropium bromide were maintained throughout the one-year period of administration with no evidence of tolerance.

A randomised, placebo-controlled clinical study in 105 COPD patients demonstrated that bronchodilation was maintained throughout the 24 hour dosing interval in comparison to placebo regardless of whether the drug was administered in the morning or in the evening.

The following health outcome effect was demonstrated in the long term (6-month and one-year) trials:

Tiotropium bromide significantly improved dyspnea (as evaluated using the Transition Dyspnea Index). This improvement was maintained throughout the treatment period.

5.2 Pharmacokinetic properties

a) General Introduction

Tiotropium bromide is a non-chiral quaternary ammonium compound and is sparingly soluble in water. Tiotropium bromide is administered by dry powder inhalation. Generally with the inhaled route of administration, the majority of the delivered dose is deposited in the gastro-intestinal tract, and to a lesser extent in the intended organ of the lung. Many of the pharmacokinetic data described below were obtained with higher doses than recommended for therapy.

b) General Characteristics of the Active Substance After Administration of the Medicinal Product

Absorption: Following dry powder inhalation by young healthy volunteers, the absolute bioavailability of 19.5% suggests that the fraction reaching the lung is highly bioavailable. It is expected from the chemical structure of the compound (quaternary ammonium compound) and from in-vitro experiments that tiotropium bromide is poorly absorbed from the gastrointestinal tract (10-15%). Oral solutions of tiotropium bromide have an absolute bioavailability of 2-3%. Maximum tiotropium bromide plasma concentrations were observed five minutes after inhalation. Food is not expected to influence the absorption of this quaternary ammonium compound.

Distribution: The drug is bound by 72% to plasma proteins and shows a volume of distribution of 32 L/kg. At steady state, tiotropium bromide plasma levels in COPD patients at peak were 17 – 19 pg/ml when measured 5 minutes after dry powder inhalation of a 18 microgram dose and decreased rapidly in a multi-compartmental manner. Steady state trough plasma concentrations were 3-4 pg/ml. Local concentrations in the lung are not known, but the mode of administration suggests substantially higher concentrations in the lung. Studies in rats have shown that tiotropium bromide does not penetrate the blood-brain barrier to any relevant extent.

Biotransformation: The extent of biotransformation is small. This is evident from a urinary excretion of 74% of unchanged substance after an intravenous dose to young healthy volunteers. The ester tiotropium bromide is nonenzymatically cleaved to the alcohol (N-methylscopine) and acid compound (dithienylglycolic acid) that are inactive on muscarinic receptors. In-vitro experiments with human liver microsomes and human hepatocytes suggest that some further drug (< 20% of dose after intravenous administration) is metabolised by cytochrome P450 (CYP) dependent oxidation and subsequent glutathion conjugation to a variety of Phase II-metabolites.

In vitro studies in liver microsomes reveal that the enzymatic pathway can be inhibited by the CYP 2D6 (and 3A4) inhibitors, quinidine, ketoconazole and gestodene. Thus CYP 2D6 and 3A4 are involved in metabolic pathway that is responsible for the elimination of a smaller part of the dose. Tiotropium bromide even in supra-therapeutic concentrations does not inhibit CYP 1A1, 1A2, 2B6, 2C9, 2C19, 2D6, 2E1 or 3A in human liver microsomes.

Elimination: The terminal elimination half-life of tiotropium bromide is between 5 and 6 days following inhalation. Total clearance was 880 ml/min after an intravenous dose in young healthy volunteers with an interindividual variability of 22%. Intravenously administered tiotropium bromide is mainly excreted unchanged in urine (74%). After dry powder inhalation urinary excretion is 14% of the dose, the remainder being mainly non-absorbed drug in gut that is eliminated via the faeces. The renal clearance of tiotropium bromide exceeds the creatinine clearance, indicating secretion into the urine. After chronic once daily inhalation by COPD patients, pharmacokinetic steady state was reached after 2-3 weeks with no accumulation thereafter.

Linearity / Nonlinearity: Tiotropium bromide demonstrates linear pharmacokinetics in the therapeutic range after both intravenous administration and dry powder inhalation.

c) Characteristics in Patients

Geriatric Patients: As expected for all predominantly renally excreted drugs, advanced age was associated with a decrease of tiotropium bromide renal clearance (326 mL/min in COPD patients < 58 years to 163 mL/min in COPD patients> 70 years) which may be explained by decreased renal function. Tiotropium bromide excretion in urine after inhalation decreased from 14% (young healthy volunteers) to about 7% (COPD patients), however plasma concentrations did not change significantly with advancing age within COPD patients if compared to inter- and intraindividual variability (43% increase in AUC_{0-4h} after dry powder inhalation.

Renally Impaired Patients: In common with all other drugs that undergo predominantly renal excretion, renal impairment was associated with increased plasma drug concentrations and reduced renal drug clearance after both intravenous infusion and dry powder inhalations. Mild renal impairment (CL_{CR} 50-80 ml/min) which is often seen in elderly patients increased tiotropium bromide plasma concentrations slightly (39% increase in AUC_{0-4h} after intravenous infusion). In COPD patients with moderate to severe renal impairment (CL_{CR} < 50 ml/min) the intravenous administration of tiotropium bromide resulted in doubling of the plasma concentrations (82% increase in AUC_{0-4h}), which was confirmed by plasma concentrations after dry powder inhalation.

Hepatically Impaired Patients: Liver insufficiency is not expected to have any relevant influence on tiotropium bromide pharmacokinetics. Tiotropium bromide is predominantly cleared by renal elimination (74% in young healthy volunteers) and simple non-enzymatic ester cleavage to pharmacologically inactive products.

Paediatric Patients: See 4.2 Posology and Method of Administration

d) Pharmacokinetic / Pharmacodynamic Relationship(s)

There is no direct relationship between pharmacokinetics and pharmacodynamics.

5.3 Preclinical safety data

Many effects observed in conventional studies of safety pharmacology, repeated dose toxicity, and reproductive toxicity could be explained by the anticholinergic properties of tiotropium bromide. Typically in animals reduced food consumption, inhibited body weight gain, dry mouth and nose, reduced lacrimation and salivation, mydriasis and increased heart rate were observed. Other relevant effects noted in repeated dose toxicity studies were: mild irritancy of the respiratory tract in rats and mice evinced by rhinitis and epithelial changes of the nasal cavity and larynx, and prostatitis along with proteinaceous deposits and lithiasis in the bladder in rats.

Harmful effects with respect to pregnancy, embryonal/foetal development, parturition or postnatal development could only be demonstrated at maternally toxic dose levels. Tiotropium bromide was not teratogenic in rats or rabbits. The respiratory (irritation) and urogenital (prostatitis) changes and reproductive toxicity was observed at local or systemic exposures more than five-fold the therapeutic exposure. Studies on genotoxicity and carcinogenic potential revealed no special hazard for humans.

6. PHARMACEUTICAL PARTICULARS

6.1 List of excipients

Lactose monohydrate

6.2 Incompatibilities

Not applicable

6.3 Shelf life

2 years

After first opening of the blister: 9 days

6.4 Special precautions for storage

Do not store above 25°C

Do not freeze

6.5 Nature and contents of container

Type and material of the container in contact with the medicinal product: Aluminium / PVC / Aluminium blister strips containing 10 capsules

Package sizes and devices supplied:

- Cardboard box containing 30 capsules (3 blister strips)
- Cardboard box containing 60 capsules (6 blister strips)
- Cardboard box containing 90 capsules (9 blister strips)
- Cardboard box containing HandiHaler device
- Cardboard box containing HandiHaler device and 10 capsules (1 blister strip)
- Cardboard box containing HandiHaler device and 30 capsules (3 blister strips)
- Hospital pack: Bundle pack containing 5 cardboard boxes of 30 capsules plus HandiHaler device
- Hospital pack: Bundle pack containing 5 cardboard boxes of 60 capsules

Not all pack sizes may be marketed

6.6 Instructions for use and handling

The following are the instructions for the patient on how to inhale from the Spiriva capsule by means of the HandiHaler.

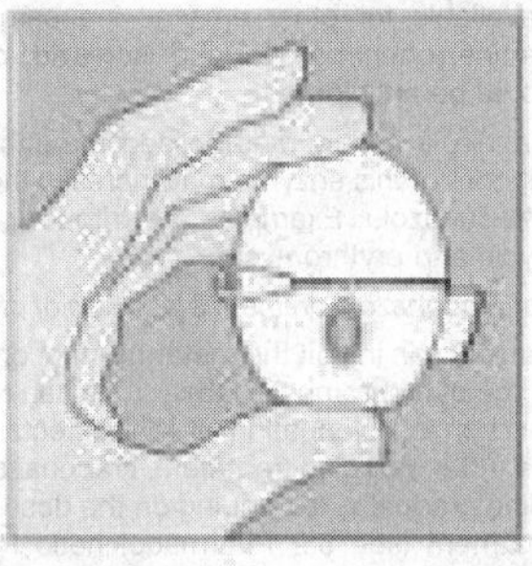

Remember to carefully follow your doctor's instructions for using Spiriva. The HandiHaler is especially designed for Spiriva. You must not use it to take any other medication. You can use your HandiHaler for up to one year to take your medication.

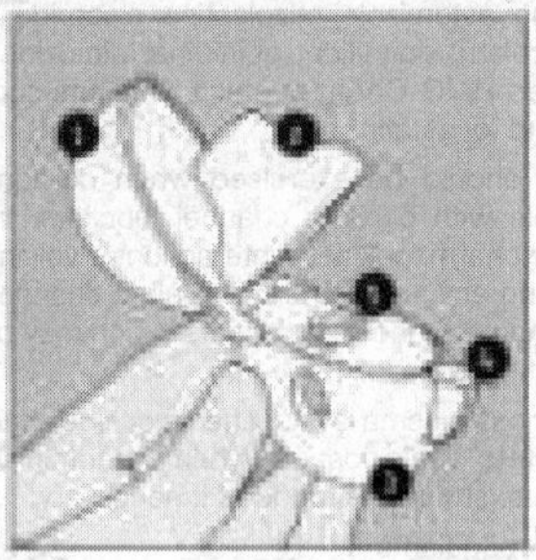

The HandiHaler

1 Dust cap

2 Mouthpiece

3 Base

4 Piercing button

5 Centre chamber

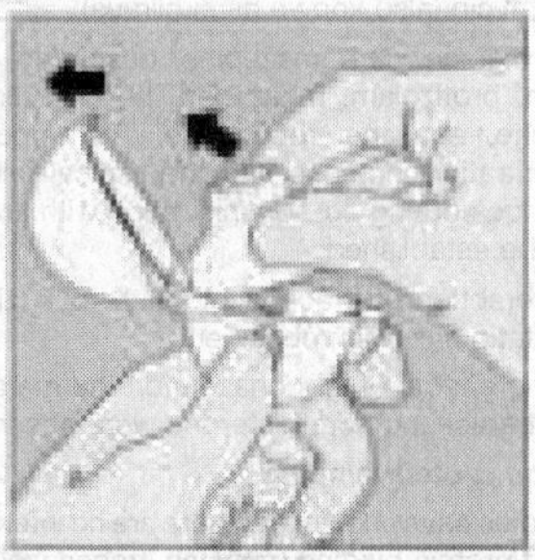

1. Open the dust cap by pulling it upwards. Then open the mouthpiece.

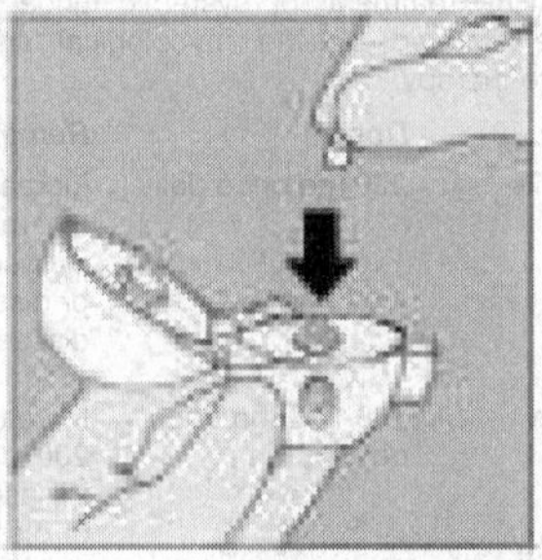

2. Remove a Spiriva capsule from the blister (only immediately before use) and place it in the centre chamber. Put the Spiriva capsule in the centre chamber (5), as illustrated. It does not matter which way the capsule is placed in the chamber.

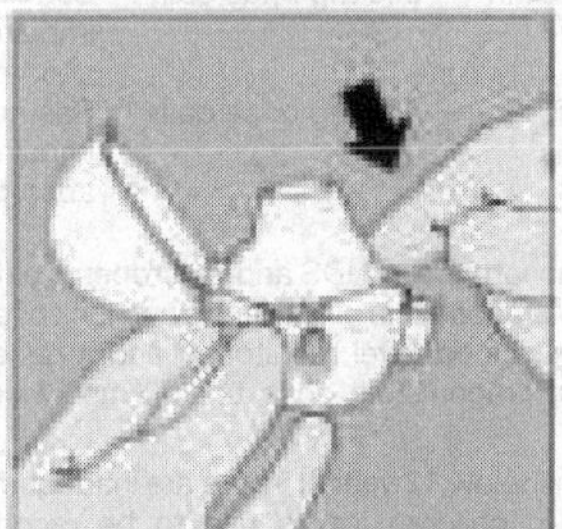

3. Close the mouthpiece firmly until you hear a click, leaving the dust cap open.

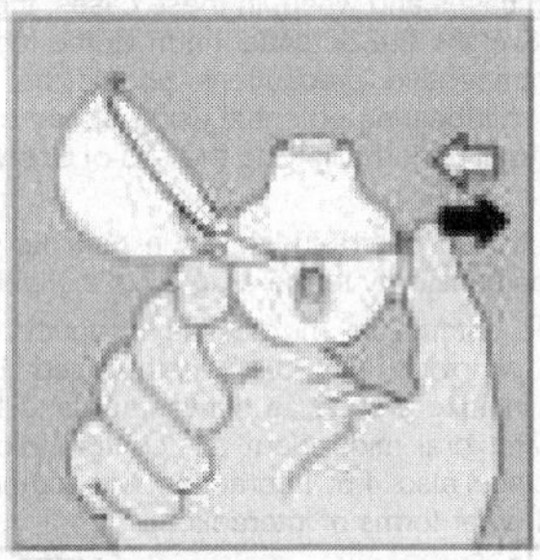

4. Hold the HandiHaler with the mouthpiece upwards and press the green button completely in once, and release. This makes holes in the capsule and allows the medication to be released when you breathe in.

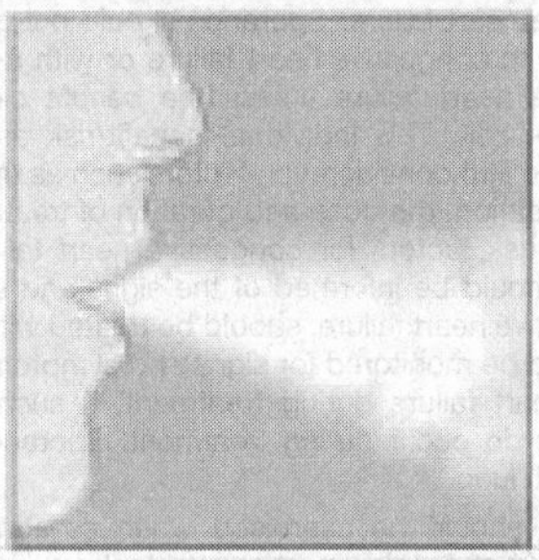

5. Breathe out completely. Important: Please avoid breathing into the mouthpiece at any time.

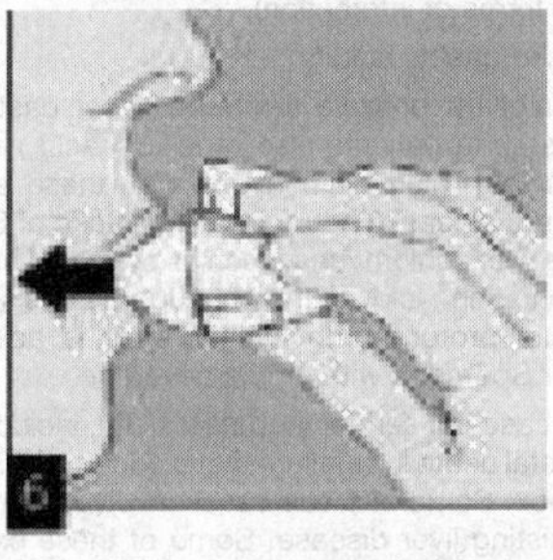

6. Raise the HandiHaler to your mouth and close your lips tightly around the mouthpiece. Keep your head in an upright position and breathe in slowly and deeply but at a rate sufficient to hear the capsule vibrate. Breathe until your lungs are full; then hold your breath as long as comfortable and at the same time take the HandiHaler out of your mouth. Resume normal breathing. Repeat step 5 and 6 once, this will empty the capsule completely.

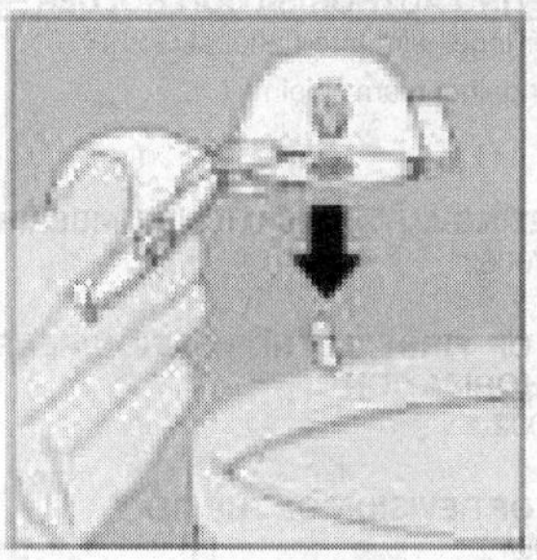

7. Open the mouthpiece again. Tip out the used capsule and dispose. Close the mouthpiece and dust cap for storage of your HandiHaler.

Cleaning your HandiHaler

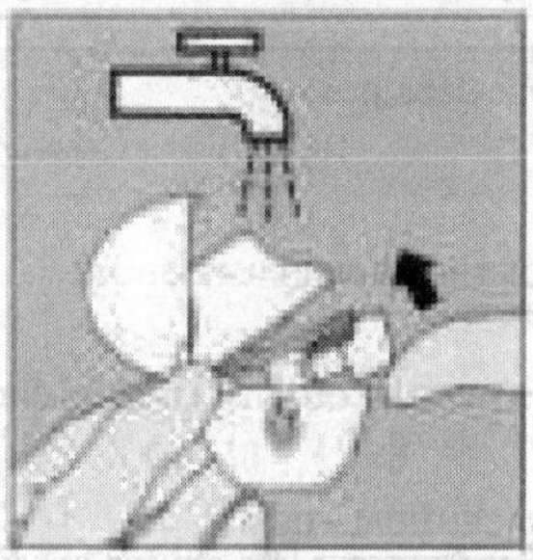

Clean the HandiHaler once a month. Open the dust cap and mouthpiece. Then open the base by lifting the piercing button. Rinse the complete inhaler with warm water to remove any powder. Dry the HandiHaler thoroughly by tipping excess of water out on a paper towel and air-dry afterwards, leaving the dust cap, mouthpiece and base open. It takes 24 hours to air dry, so clean it right after you used it and it will be ready for your next dose. If needed, the outside of the mouthpiece may be cleaned with a moist but not wet tissue.

Blister handling

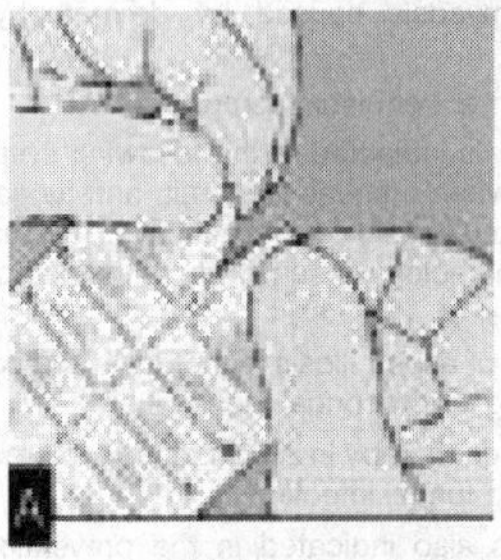

A. Separate the blister strips by tearing along the perforation

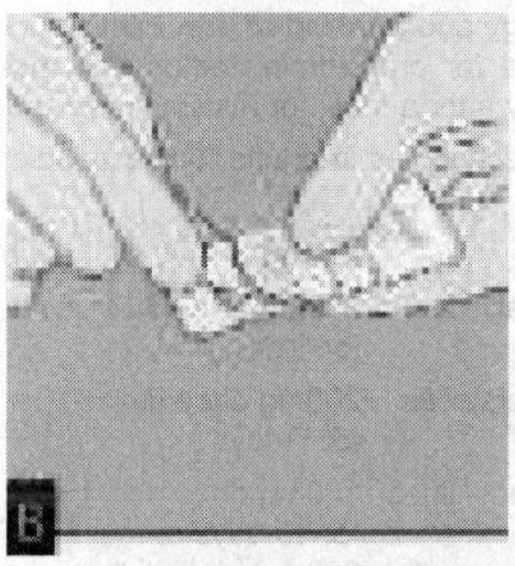

B. Peel back foil (only immediately before use) using the tab until one capsule is fully visible. In case a second capsule is exposed to air inadvertently this capsule has to be discarded.

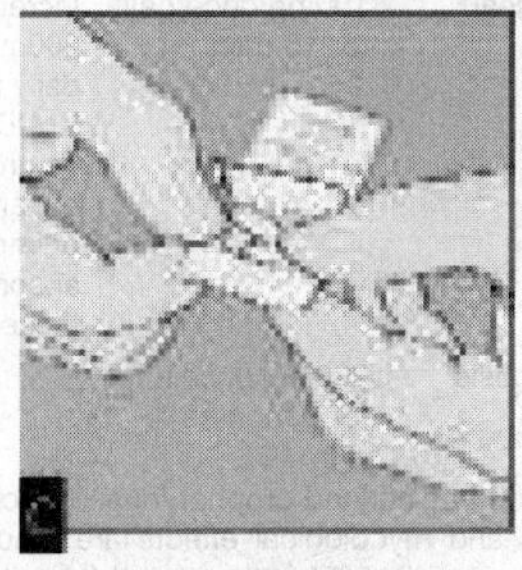

C. Remove capsule.

Spiriva® capsules contain only a small amount of powder so that the capsule is only partially filled.

7. MARKETING AUTHORISATION HOLDER
Boehringer Ingelheim International GmbH
D-55216 Ingelheim am Rhein
Germany

8. MARKETING AUTHORISATION NUMBER(S)
PL 14598/0062

9. DATE OF FIRST AUTHORISATION/RENEWAL OF THE AUTHORISATION
14 May 2002

10. DATE OF REVISION OF THE TEXT
August 2004

11 Legal Category
POM

S8/UK/SPC/8

Sporanox Capsules

(Janssen-Cilag Ltd)

1. NAME OF THE MEDICINAL PRODUCT
SPORANOX®.

2. QUALITATIVE AND QUANTITATIVE COMPOSITION
Itraconazole 100 mg.

3. PHARMACEUTICAL FORM
Capsule (Size 0): opaque blue cap and pink transparent body containing coated beads.

4. CLINICAL PARTICULARS
4.1 Therapeutic indications
1. Vulvovaginal candidosis.

2. Pityriasis versicolor.

3. Dermatophytoses caused by organisms susceptible to itraconazole *(Trichophyton spp., Microsporum spp., Epidermophyton floccosum)* e.g. tinea pedis, tinea cruris, tinea corporis, tinea manuum.

4. Oropharyngeal candidosis.

5. Onychomycosis caused by dermatophytes and/or yeasts.

6. The treatment of histoplasmosis.

7. Sporanox is indicated in the following systemic fungal conditions when first-line systemic anti-fungal therapy is inappropriate or has proved ineffective. This may be due to underlying pathology, insensitivity of the pathogen or drug toxicity.

- Treatment of aspergillosis, candidosis and cryptococcosis (including cryptococcal meningitis);

- Maintenance therapy in AIDS patients to prevent relapse of underlying fungal infection.

Sporanox is also indicated in the prevention of fungal infection during prolonged neutropenia when standard therapy is considered inappropriate.

4.2 Posology and method of administration
Sporanox is for oral administration and must be taken immediately after a meal for maximal absorption.

Treatment schedules in adults for each indication are as follows:

Indication	*Dose*	*Remarks*
Vulvovaginal candidosis	200mg twice daily for 1 day	
Pityriasis versicolor	200mg once daily for 7 days	
Tinea corporis, tinea cruris	100mg once daily for 15 days or 200mg once daily for 7 days	
Tinea pedis, tinea manuum	100mg once daily for 30 days	
Oropharyngeal candidosis	100mg once daily for 15 days	Increase dose to 200mg once daily for 15 days in AIDS or neutropenic patients because of impaired absorption in these groups.
Onychomycosis	200 mg once daily for 3 months	

For skin, vulvovaginal and oropharyngeal infections, optimal clinical and mycological effects are reached 1 - 4 weeks after cessation of treatment and for nail infections, 6 - 9 months after the cessation of treatment. This is because elimination of itraconazole from skin, nails and mucous membranes is slower than from plasma.

The length of treatment for systemic fungal infections should be dictated by the mycological and clinical response to therapy:

Indication	*Dose*	*Remarks*
Aspergillosis	200 mg once daily	Increase dose to 200 mg twice daily in case of invasive or disseminated disease
Candidosis	100-200 mg once daily	Increase dose to 200 mg twice daily in case of invasive or disseminated disease
Non-meningeal Cryptococcosis	200 mg once daily	
Cryptococcal meningitis	200 mg twice daily	
Histoplasmosis	200 mg once daily - 200 mg twice daily	
Maintenance in AIDS	200 mg once daily	See note on impaired absorption below
Prophylaxis in neutropenia	200 mg once daily	See note on impaired absorption below

Impaired absorption in AIDS and neutropenic patients may lead to low itraconazole blood levels and lack of efficacy. In such cases, blood level monitoring and if necessary, an increase in itraconazole dose to 200 mg twice daily, is indicated.

In Children (below 12 years): There are inadequate data on Sporanox in children for its use to be recommended, unless the potential benefits outweigh the risks.

In Elderly: As for use in children.

4.3 Contraindications
Sporanox should only be given to pregnant women in life-threatening cases and when, in these cases, the potential benefit outweighs the potential harm to the foetus. Adequate contraceptive precautions should be taken by women of childbearing potential using Sporanox until the next menstrual period following the end of Sporanox therapy.

Sporanox is also contra-indicated in patients who have shown hypersensitivity to the drug or its excipients.

Terfenadine, astemizole, mizolastine, cisapride, dofetilide, quinidine, pimozide, CYP3A4 metabolised HMG-CoA reductase inhibitors such as simvastatin and lovastatin, triazolam and oral midazolam are contra-indicated with Sporanox (see also 4.5: Interaction with other medicaments and other forms of interaction).

4.4 Special warnings and special precautions for use
• In a healthy volunteer study with Sporanox® IV, a transient asymptomatic decrease of the left ventricular ejection fraction was observed.

• Itraconazole has been shown to have a negative inotropic effect and Sporanox has been associated with reports of congestive heart failure. Sporanox should not be used in patients with congestive heart failure or with a history of congestive heart failure unless the benefit clearly outweighs the risk. This individual benefit/risk assessment should take into consideration factors such as the severity of the indication, the dose and duration of treatment, and individual risk factors for congestive heart failure. Such patients should be informed of the signs and symptoms of congestive heart failure, should be treated with caution, and should be monitored for signs and symptoms of congestive heart failure during treatment; if such signs or symptoms do occur during treatment, Sporanox should be discontinued.

• Caution should be exercised when co-administering itraconazole and calcium channel blockers (see section 4.5, Interactions with other medicinal products).

• Sporanox has a potential for clinically important drug interactions. (See 4.5: Interaction with other medicaments and other forms of interaction).

• Decreased gastric acidity:

Absorption of itraconazole is impaired when gastric acidity is decreased. In patients also receiving acid neutralising medicines (e.g. aluminium hydroxide), these should be administered at least 2 hours after the intake of Sporanox. In patients with achlorhydria, such as certain AIDS patients and patients on acid secretion suppressors (e.g. H_2 - antagonists, proton-pump inhibitors), it is advisable to administer Sporanox with a cola beverage.

Very rare cases of serious hepatotoxicity, including some cases of fatal acute liver failure, have occurred with the use of Sporanox. Some of these cases involved patients with no pre-existing liver disease. Some of these cases have been observed within the first month of treatment, including some within the first week. Liver function monitoring should be considered in patients receiving Sporanox treatment. Patients should be instructed to promptly report to their physician signs and symptoms suggestive of hepatitis such as anorexia, nausea, vomiting, fatigue, abdominal pain or dark urine. In these patients treatment should be stopped immediately and liver function testing conducted.

Most cases of serious hepatotoxicity involved patients who had pre-existing liver disease, were treated for systemic indications, had significant other medical conditions and/or were taking other hepatotoxic drugs. In patients with raised liver enzymes or active liver disease, or who have experienced liver toxicity with other drugs, treatment should not be started unless the expected benefit exceeds the risk of hepatic injury. In such cases liver enzyme monitoring is necessary.

• Hepatic impairment:

Itraconazole is predominantly metabolised in the liver. A slight decrease in oral bioavailability in cirrhotic patients has been observed, although this was not of statistical significance. The terminal half-life was however significantly increased. The dose should be adapted if necessary.

• Renal impairment:

The oral bioavailability of itraconazole may be lower in patients with renal insufficiency. Dose adaptation may be considered.

• If neuropathy occurs which may be attributable to Sporanox, treatment should be discontinued.

• There is no information regarding cross hypersensitivity between itraconazole and other azole antifungal agents. Caution should be used in prescribing Sporanox to patients with hypersensitivity to other azoles.

• In systemic candidosis, if fluconazole-resistant strains of *Candida* species are suspected, it cannot be assumed that these are sensitive to itraconazole, hence their sensitivity should be tested before the start of Sporanox therapy.

4.5 Interaction with other medicinal products and other forms of Interaction
1. Drugs affecting the metabolism of itraconazole:

Interaction studies have been performed with rifampicin, rifabutin and phenytoin. Since the bioavailability of itraconazole and hydroxy-itraconazole was decreased in these studies to such an extent that efficacy may be largely reduced, the combination of itraconazole with these potent enzyme inducers is not recommended. No formal study data are available for other enzyme inducers, such as carbamazepine, phenobarbital and isoniazid, but similar effects should be anticipated.

As itraconazole is mainly metabolised through CYP3A4, potent inhibitors of this enzyme may increase the bioavailability of itraconazole. Examples are: ritonavir, indinavir, clarithromycin and erythromycin.

2. Effects of itraconazole on the metabolism of other drugs:

2.1 Itraconazole can inhibit the metabolism of drugs metabolised by the cytochrome 3A family. This can result in an increase and/or a prolongation of their effects, including side effects. After stopping treatment, itraconazole plasma levels decline gradually, depending on the dose and duration of treatment (see 5.2 Pharmacokinetic Properties). This should be taken into account when the inhibitory effect of itraconazole on co-administered drugs is considered.

Examples are:

• Drugs which should not be used during treatment with itraconazole:

Terfenadine, astemizole, mizolastine, cisapride, triazolam, oral midazolam, dofetilide, quinidine, pimozide, CYP3A4 metabolised HMG-CoA reductase inhibitors such as simvastatin and lovastatin.

• Caution should be exercised when co-administering itraconazole with calcium channel blockers. In addition to possible pharmacokinetic interactions involving the drug metabolising enzyme CYP3A4, calcium channel blockers can have negative inotropic effects which may be additive to those of itraconazole.

• Drugs whose plasma levels, effects or side effects should be monitored. Their dosage, when co-administered with itraconazole, should be reduced if necessary:

§ Oral anticoagulants

§ HIV protease inhibitors such as ritonavir, indinavir, saquinavir

§ Certain antineoplastic agents such as vinca alkaloids, busulphan, docetaxel and trimetrexate

§ CYP3A4 metabolised calcium channel blockers such as dihydropyridines and verapamil

§ Certain immunosuppressive agents: ciclosporin, tacrolimus, rapamycin (also known as sirolimus)

§ Others: digoxin, carbamazepine, buspirone, alfentanil, alprazolam, brotizolam, midazolam IV, rifabutin, methylprednisolone, ebastine, reboxetine. The importance of the concentration increase and the clinical relevance of these changes during co-administration with itraconazole remain to be established.

2.2 No interaction of itraconazole with AZT (zidovudine) and fluvastatin has been observed.

No inducing effects of itraconazole on the metabolism of ethinyloestradiol and norethisterone were observed.

3. Effect on protein binding:

In vitro studies have shown that there are no interactions on the plasma protein binding between itraconazole and imipramine, propranolol, diazepam, cimetidine, indomethacin, tolbutamide or sulphadimidine.

4.6 Pregnancy and lactation

Pregnancy: When administered at high doses to pregnant rats (40 mg/kg/day or higher) and mice (80 mg/kg/day or higher), itraconazole was shown to increase the incidence of foetal abnormalities and did produce adverse effects on the embryo.Studies of the use of itraconazole in pregnant women are not available. Therefore, Sporanox should only be given in life-threatening cases of systemic mycosis and when in these cases the potential benefit outweighs the potential harm to the foetus.

Lactation: A very small amount of itraconazole is excreted in human milk. The expected benefits of Sporanox therapy should be weighed against the risks of breast feeding. In case of doubt, the patient should not breast feed.

4.7 Effects on ability to drive and use machines

None known.

4.8 Undesirable effects

Approximately 9% of patients can be expected to experience adverse reactions while taking itraconazole. In patients receiving prolonged (approximately 1 month) continuous treatment, the incidence of adverse events was higher (about 15%). The most frequently reported adverse experiences were of gastrointestinal, hepatic and dermatological origin. Within each system organ class, the adverse reactions are ranked under the headings of frequency, using the following convention: Rare $>1/10{,}000$, $<1/1{,}000$) and very rare ($<1/10{,}000$), including isolated reports. Based upon the post-marketing experience, the following adverse reactions have also been reported:

• Metabolism and Nutrition Disorders

• ***Very rare:*** *hypokalemia*

• Nervous System Disorders

• ***Very rare:*** *peripheral neuropathy, headache, and dizziness*

• Cardiac Disorders

• ***Very rare:*** *congestive heart failure*

• Respiratory, Thoracic and Mediastinal Disorders

• ***Very rare:*** *pulmonary oedema*

• Gastrointestinal Disorders

• ***Very rare:*** *abdominal pain, vomiting, dyspepsia, nausea, diarrhoea and constipation*

• Hepato-Biliary Disorders

• ***Very rare:*** *fatal acute liver failure, serious hepatotoxicity, hepatitis, and reversible increases in hepatic enzymes*

• Skin and Subcutaneous Tissue Disorders

• ***Very rare:*** *Stevens-Johnson syndrome, angio-oedema, urticaria, alopecia, rash, and pruritis*

• Reproductive System and Breast Disorders

• ***Very rare:*** *menstrual disorder*

• General Disorders and Administrative Site Conditions

• ***Very rare:*** *allergic reaction, and oedema*

4.9 Overdose

In the event of overdosage, patients should be treated symptomatically with supportive measures. Within the first hour after ingestion, gastric lavage may be performed. Activated charcoal may be given if considered appropriate. No specific antidote is available. Itraconazole cannot be removed by haemodialysis.

5. PHARMACOLOGICAL PROPERTIES

5.1 Pharmacodynamic properties

Itraconazole is a substituted triazole antimycotic with a broad spectrum of activity against Candida spp and other yeasts, dermatophytes and pathogenic fungi. It acts by impairing the synthesis of ergosterol in fungal cell membranes.

5.2 Pharmacokinetic properties

Peak plasma concentrations of itraconazole in the region of 1 mcg equiv/ml are reached 1.5-3 hrs after administration. In man the elimination half life is about 20 hrs. Oral intake immediately after a meal doubled the peak level 3-4 hrs after intake.

Peak concentrations of itraconazole in keratinous tissues, especially skin, are up to 3 times higher than in plasma. Therapeutic levels in the skin persist for up to 2-4 weeks after stopping treatment as elimination is related to epidermal regeneration, rather than redistribution into the systemic circulation.

Itraconazole is extensively metabolised by the liver to a large number of metabolites, which constitute 40% of the excreted dose. Faecal excretion of parent drug varies from 3-18% of the dose, and urinary excretion of unchanged drug is less than 0.03%.

5.3 Preclinical safety data

Not applicable.

6. PHARMACEUTICAL PARTICULARS

6.1 List of excipients

Sugar spheres

Hypromellose 2910 5mPa.s

Macrogol 20000

Capsule shell:

Titanium dioxide

Indigo carmine

Gelatin

Erythrosine

6.2 Incompatibilities

None known.

6.3 Shelf life

36 months.

6.4 Special precautions for storage

Protect from light. Store in a dry place. Store between 15°C and 30°C.

6.5 Nature and contents of container

Perlalux tristar blister - plastic foil consisting of 3 layers

* Polyvinylchloride on the outside;

* Low density polyethylene in the middle;

* Polyvinylidene chloride on the inside;

Aluminium foil (thickness 20μm) coated on the inner side with colourless heat-seal Lacquer: PVC mixed polymers with acrylates, 6 g/m^2.

or:

PVC blister consisting of -

Polyvinylchloride 'genotherm' glass clear, thickness 250μm;

Aluminium foil (thickness 20μm) coated on the inner side with a colourless heat-seal Lacquer: PVC mixed polymers with acrylates, 6g/m^2.

Pack sizes: 4, **6*not marketed**, 15, 60 capsules.

6.6 Instructions for use and handling

Not applicable.

7. MARKETING AUTHORISATION HOLDER

Janssen-Cilag Ltd
Saunderton
High Wycombe
Bucks
HP14 4HJ

8. MARKETING AUTHORISATION NUMBER(S)

0242/0142

9. DATE OF FIRST AUTHORISATION/RENEWAL OF THE AUTHORISATION

18/01/89, 11/01/95

10. DATE OF REVISION OF THE TEXT

November 2002

Legal category POM.

Sporanox IV

(Janssen-Cilag Ltd)

1. NAME OF THE MEDICINAL PRODUCT

Sporanox® I.V. 10 mg/ml concentrate and solvent for solution for infusion.

2. QUALITATIVE AND QUANTITATIVE COMPOSITION

Each ml of the concentrate contains 10 mg itraconazole.

One ampoule with 25 ml contains 250 mg itraconazole (itraconazole trihydrochloride salt formed *in situ*).

Each ml of the admixed solution contains 3.33 mg itraconazole.

One single dose of 200 mg itraconazole corresponds to 60 ml of the admixed solution.

For excipients, see 6.1.

3. PHARMACEUTICAL FORM

Concentrate and solvent for solution for infusion.

4. CLINICAL PARTICULARS

4.1 Therapeutic indications

Sporanox I.V. is indicated for the treatment of histoplasmosis.

Sporanox I.V. is indicated in the following systemic fungal conditions when first-line systemic anti-fungal therapy is inappropriate or has proved ineffective. (This may be due to underlying pathology, insensitivity of the pathogen or drug toxicity).

Treatment of aspergillosis, candidosis and cryptococcosis (including cryptococcal meningitis).

4.2 Posology and method of administration

Sporanox I.V. is given on the first two days in a loading dose twice daily, followed by once daily dosing.

Day 1 and 2 of the treatment: 1-hour infusion of 200 mg (60 ml of the admixed solution) Sporanox I.V. twice daily. See section 6.6.

From day 3 on: one 1-hour infusion of 200 mg (60 ml of the admixed solution) Sporanox I.V. each day. Safety for periods longer than 14 days has not been established.

Use in children: Since clinical data on the use of Sporanox I.V. in paediatric patients are unavailable, Sporanox I.V. should not be used in children unless the potential benefit outweighs the potential risk. See section 4.4. (Special warning and precautions for use).

Use in elderly: Since clinical data of the use of Sporanox I.V. in elderly patients are limited, it is advised to use Sporanox I.V. in these patients only if the potential benefit outweighs the potential risk. See section 4.4. (Special warning and precautions for use).

Use in patients with renal impairment: Hydroxypropyl-β-cyclodextrin, when administered intravenously, is eliminated through glomerular filtration. Therefore, patients with severe renal impairment defined as creatinine clearance below 30 ml/min should not be treated with Sporanox I.V. See section 4.4. (Special warning and precautions for use).

In patients with mild and moderate renal impairment, Sporanox I.V. should be used with caution. Serum creatinine levels should be closely monitored and, if renal toxicity is suspected, consideration should be given to changing to the oral capsule formulation. See sections 4.3 Contraindications and section 4.4. (Special warning and precautions for use).

Use in patients with hepatic impairment: Itraconazole is predominantly metabolised in the liver. The terminal half life of itraconazole in cirrhotic is somewhat prolonged. A dose adjustment may be considered. See section 4.4. (Special warning and precautions for use).

4.3 Contraindications

– Sporanox I.V. is contraindicated in patients with a known hypersensitivity to itraconazole or to any of the excipients.

– Sporanox I.V. cannot be used when administration of Sodium Chloride Injection is contraindicated.

– The excipient hydroxypropyl-β-cyclodextrin is eliminated through glomerular filtration. Therefore, Sporanox I.V. is contraindicated in patients with severe renal impairment (defined as creatinine clearance below 30 ml/min) See section 4.4 Special warning and precautions for use.

– Coadministration of CYP3A4 metabolised substrates that can prolong the QT-interval e.g., terfenadine, astemizole, mizolastine, cisapride, dofetilide, quinidine or pimozide with Sporanox I.V. is contraindicated since coadministration may result in increased plasma levels of these substrates which can lead to QTc prolongation and rare occurrences of *torsades de pointes* (see section 4.5).

– Coadministration of CYP3A4 metabolised HMG-CoA reductase inhibitors such as simvastatin, lovastatin and atorvastatin, triazolam and oral midazolam are contraindicated with Sporanox I.V. (see section 4.5).

– Sporanox I.V. must not be given during pregnancy (except for life-threatening cases) and lactation (see section 4.6).

4.4 Special warnings and special precautions for use

– Sporanox has a potential for clinically important drug interactions. (See 4.5: Interaction with other medicinal products and other forms of interaction).

– Paediatric use: Since clinical data on the use of Sporanox I.V. in paediatric patients are unavailable, Sporanox I.V. should not be used in children unless the potential benefit outweighs the potential risk.

– Use in elderly: Since clinical data of the use of Sporanox I.V. in elderly patients are limited, it is advised to use Sporanox I.V. in these patients only if the potential benefit outweighs the potential risk.

– Very rare cases of serious hepatotoxicity, including some cases of fatal acute liver failure, have occurred with the use of Sporanox. Some of these cases involved patients with no pre-existing liver disease. Some of these cases have been observed within the first month of treatment, including some within the first week. Liver function monitoring should be considered in patients receiving Sporanox treatment. Patients should be instructed to promptly report to their physician signs and symptoms suggestive of hepatitis such as anorexia, nausea, vomiting, fatigue, abdominal pain or dark urine. In these patients treatment should be stopped immediately and liver function testing should be conducted. Most cases of serious hepatotoxicity involved patients who had pre-existing liver disease, were treated for systemic indications, had significant other medical conditions and/or were taking other hepatotoxic drugs. In patients with raised liver enzymes or active liver disease, or who have experienced liver toxicity with other drugs, treatment should not be started unless the expected benefit exceeds the risk of hepatic injury. In such cases liver enzyme monitoring is necessary.

– Hepatic impairment: Itraconazole is predominantly metabolised in the liver. The terminal half life of itraconazole in cirrhotic patients is somewhat prolonged. A dose adjustment may be considered.

– Renal impairment: Hydroxypropyl-β-cyclodextrin, when administered intravenously, is eliminated through glomerular filtration. Therefore, patients with renal impairment defined as creatinine clearance below 30 ml/min should not be treated with Sporanox I.V. (see section 5.2).

– Sporanox I.V. should be used with caution in patients with a lesser degree of renal failure. In patients with mild and moderate renal impairment, serum creatinine levels should be closely monitored and, if renal toxicity is suspected, consideration should be given to changing to the oral capsule formulation. See section 4.4. Special warning and precautions for use.

– If neuropathy occurs that may be attributable to Sporanox I.V., the treatment should be discontinued.

– There is no information regarding cross hypersensitivity between itraconazole and other azole antifungal agents. Caution should be used in prescribing Sporanox I.V. to patients with hypersensitivity to other azoles.

– In a healthy volunteer study with Sporanox I.V., a transient asymptomatic decrease of the left ventricular ejection fraction was observed; this resolved before the next infusion. A similar investigation was not performed in the target patient population.

– Itraconazole has been shown to have a negative inotropic effect and Sporanox has been associated with reports of congestive heart failure. Sporanox should not be used in patients with congestive heart failure or with a history of congestive heart failure unless the benefit clearly outweighs the risk.

– Physicians should carefully review the risks and benefits of Sporanox therapy for patients with known risk factors for congestive heart failure. These risk factors include *cardiac disease, such as ischaemic and valvular disease; significant pulmonary disease, such as chronic obstructive pulmonary disease; and renal failure and other edematous disorders.* Such patients should be informed of the signs and symptoms of congestive heart failure, should be treated with caution, and should be monitored for signs and symptoms of congestive heart failure during treatment. If such signs or symptoms do occur during treatment, Sporanox should be discontinued.

– Caution should be exercised when co-administering itraconazole and calcium channel blockers (see section 4.5, Interactions with other medicinal products).

4.5 Interaction with other medicinal products and other forms of Interaction

1. Drugs affecting the metabolism of itraconazole:

Itraconazole is mainly metabolised through the cytochrome CYP3A4. Interaction studies have been performed with rifampicin, rifabutin and phenytoin, which are potent enzyme inducers of CYP3A4. Since the bioavailability of itraconazole and hydroxy-itraconazole was decreased in these studies to such an extent that efficacy may be largely reduced, the combination with these enzyme inducers is not recommended. No formal study data are available for other enzyme inducers, such as carbamazepine, *Hypericum perforatum* (St John's Wort), phenobarbital and isoniazid but similar effects should be anticipated.

Potent inhibitors of CYP3A4 may increase the bioavailability of itraconazole. Examples are: ritonavir, indinavir, clarithromycin and erythromycin.

2. Effect of itraconazole on the metabolism of other drugs:

Itraconazole can inhibit the metabolism of drugs metabolised by the cytochrome 3A family. This can result in an increase and/or a prolongation of their effects, including side effects. After stopping treatment, itraconazole plasma levels decline gradually, depending on the dose and duration of treatment (see 5.2. Pharmacokinetic Properties). This should be taken into account when the inhibitory effect of itraconazole on comedicated drugs is considered.

Drugs which are contraindicated with itraconazole:

Terfenadine, astemizole, mizolastine, cisapride, dofetilide, quinidine or pimozide are contraindicated with Sporanox I.V. since coadministration may result in increased plasma levels of these substrates which can lead to QTc prolongation and rare occurrences of *torsades de pointes* (see section 4.3).

Coadministration of CYP3A4 metabolised HMG-CoA reductase inhibitors such as simvastatin, lovastatin, atorvastatin, triazolam and oral midazolam are contraindicated with Sporanox I.V. (see section 4.3).

Caution should be exercised when co-administering itraconazole with calcium channel blockers. In addition to possible pharmacokinetic interactions involving the drug metabolising enzyme CYP3A4, calcium channel blockers can have negative inotropic effects which may be additive to those of itraconazole.

Drugs whose plasma levels, effects or side effects should be monitored. Their dosage, if co-administered with itraconazole, should be reduced if necessary.

– Oral anticoagulants;

– Anti-HIV Protease Inhibitors such as ritonavir, indinavir, saquinavir;

– Certain Antineoplastic Agents such as vinca alkaloids, busulphan, docetaxel and trimetrexate;

– CYP3A4 metabolised Calcium Channel Blockers such as dihydropyridines and verapamil;

– Certain CYP3A4 metabolised HMG-CoA reductase inhibitors such as cerivastatin (see also drugs which are contraindicated with itraconazole);

– Certain Immunosuppressive Agents: cyclosporine, tacrolimus, rapamycin (also known as sirolimus);

– Others: digoxin, carbamazepine, buspirone, alfentanil, alprazolam, brotizolam, midazolam I.V., rifabutin, methylprednisolone, ebastine and reboxetine. The importance of the concentration increase and clinical relevance of these changes during co-administration with itraconazole remain to be established.

No interaction of itraconazole with AZT (zidovudine) and fluvastatine has been observed.

No inducing effects of itraconazole on the metabolism of ethinyloestradiol and norethisterone were observed.

3. Effect on protein binding:

In vitro studies have shown that there are no interactions on the plasma protein binding between itraconazole and imipramine, propranolol, diazepam, cimetidine, indomethacin, tolbutamide and sulfamethazine.

4.6 Pregnancy and lactation

Pregnancy

In animal studies itraconazole shows reproduction toxicity (see section 5.3)

Itraconazole is contraindicated in pregnancy (see section 4.3) and should only be given to pregnant women in life threatening cases and when in these cases the potential benefit outweighs the potential harm to the foetus.

Adequate contraceptive precautions should be taken by women of childbearing potential using itraconazole until the next menstrual period following the end of itraconazole therapy.

Lactation

A very small amount of itraconazole is excreted in human milk and must not be administered to lactating women. Breast-feeding is to be discontinued prior to taking itraconazole.

4.7 Effects on ability to drive and use machines

No effects have been observed.

4.8 Undesirable effects

In clinical trials with intravenous itraconazole, the most frequently reported adverse experiences were of gastrointestinal, metabolic and nutritional, and hepato-biliary origin.

Based upon the post-marketing experience, the following adverse reactions have also been reported: within each system organ class, the adverse reactions are ranked under the headings of frequency, using the following convention: Very common >1/10); common >1/100, <1/10); uncommon >1/1,000, <1/100); rare >1/10,000, <1/1,000) and very rare (<1/10,000) including isolated reports.

Metabolism and Nutrition Disorders

Very rare:*hypokalemia and hyperglycaemia.*

Nervous System Disorders

Very rare:*peripheral neuropathy, headache, and dizziness.*

Cardiac Disorders

Very rare:*congestive heart failure and hypertension.*

Respiratory, Thoracic and Mediastinal Disorders

Very rare:*pulmonary oedema.*

Gastrointestinal Disorders

Very rare:*abdominal pain, vomiting, dyspepsia, nausea, diarrhoea and constipation.*

Hepato-Biliary Disorders

Very rare:*fatal acute liver failure, serious hepatotoxicity, hepatitis, jaundice, reversible increases in hepatic enzymes, and bilirubinaemia.*

Skin and Subcutaneous Tissue Disorders

Very rare:*Stevens-Johnson syndrome, angio-oedema, urticaria, alopecia, rash and pruritus.*

Reproductive system and Breast Disorders

Very rare:*menstrual disorder.*

General Disorders and Administrative Site Conditions

Very rare:*allergic reaction, and oedema.*

4.9 Overdose

In the event of accidental overdosage, supportive measures should be employed. Itraconazole cannot be removed by haemodialysis. No specific antidote is available.

5. PHARMACOLOGICAL PROPERTIES

5.1 Pharmacodynamic properties

Pharmacotherapeutic classification: (Antimycotics for systemic use, triazole derivatives).

ATC code: J02A C02

Itraconazole, a triazole derivate, has a broad spectrum of activity against Candida spp. and other yeasts, dermatophytes and pathogenic fungi.

In vitro studies have demonstrated that itraconazole impairs the synthesis of ergosterol in fungal cells. Ergosterol is a vital cell membrane component in fungi. Impairment of its synthesis ultimately results in an antifungal effect.

5.2 Pharmacokinetic properties

After single intravenous administration of 200 mg itraconazole, the mean plasma clearance is 312 ml/min, the mean volume of distribution Vd_{ss} is 561 l and the mean terminal half-life is 33 h. The kinetics of itraconazole are slightly disproportional: in the dose-range between 50 and 200 mg, the plasma clearance of itraconazole decreases by 20-25 %, each time the dose is doubled.

Plasma concentrations of itraconazole in patients with mild to moderate renal insufficiency (CL_{CR} ranging between 30 - 80 ml/min) were comparable to those obtained in healthy subjects. The majority of HP-β-CD was eliminated in urine during a 120 hour collection period. Following single IV dose of 200 mg to patients with severe renal impairment (CL_{CR} < 30 ml/min), clearance of HP-β-CD was reduced six-fold compared with subjects with normal renal function.

Pharmacokinetics of itraconazole in elderly patients after intravenous injection were not investigated. In general, treatment of elderly patients should be cautious. Taking into consideration the higher incidence of decreased hepatic and renal function, and of concomitant disease or other drug therapy. As it is known that the glomerular filtration rate changes in function of the age, increasing HP-β-CD levels may be expected with increasing age (see pharmacokinetics in patients with renal insufficiency).

Itraconazole is extensively metabolised by the liver into a large number of metabolites. The major enzyme involved in the overall metabolism of itraconazole is CYP3A4. One of the metabolites is hydroxy-itraconazole, which has *in vitro* a comparable antifungal activity to itraconazole. Faecal excretion of parent itraconazole varies between 3-18% of the dose. Renal excretion of itraconazole and hydroxy-itraconazole is less than 1% of the dose.

Using the intravenous dosing scheme of itraconazole 200 mg b.i.d. on days 1-2, followed by 200 mg o.d. from day 3 onwards, steady-state plasma concentrations of itraconazole and hydroxy-itraconazole are attained after 2 and 4 days, respectively. Predose plasma levels of hydroxy-itraconazole are about twice as high as those of itraconazole.

The plasma protein binding of itraconazole is 99.8%. Itraconazole is extensively distributed into tissues which are prone to fungal invasion. Concentrations in lung, kidney, liver, bone, stomach, spleen and muscle were found to be two to three times higher than the corresponding plasma concentration.

5.3 Preclinical safety data

The main target organs of itraconazole therapy were

- The adrenal cortex
- The liver
- The mononuclear phagosystem
- Disorders of the lipid metabolism presenting as xanthoma cells in various organs.

At high dosages, histological investigations of adrenal cortex showed a reversible swelling with cellular hypertrophy of the zona reticularis and fasciculata, which was sometimes associated with a thinning of the zona glomerulosa.

Reversible hepatic changes were found at high doses. Slight changes were observed in the sinusoidal cells and vacuolation of the hepatocytes, the latter indicating cellular dysfunction, but without visible hepatitis or hepatocellular necrosis.

Histological changes of the mononuclear phagosystem were mainly characterised by macrophages with increased proteinaceous material in various parenchymal tissues.

There are no indications of a mutagenic potential of itraconazole.

In male rats there was a higher incidence of soft-tissue sarcoma, which are attributed to the increase in non-neoplastic, chronic inflammatory reactions of the connective tissue as a consequence of raised cholesterol levels and cholesterosis in connective tissue.

Reproductive toxicity:

There is no evidence of a primary influence on fertility under treatment with itraconazole. Itraconazole was found to cause a dose-related increase in maternal toxicology, embryotoxicity, and teratogenicity in rats and mice at high doses. In rats the teratogenicity consisted of major skeletal defects; in mice, it consisted of encephaloceles and macroglossia.

In juvenile dogs a global lower bone mineral density was observed after chronic itraconazole administration.

In three toxicology studies using rats, itraconazole induced bone defects. The induced defects included reduced bone plate activity, thinning of the zona compacta of the large bones, and an increased bone fragility.

Hydroxypropyl- β-cyclodextrin (HP- β-CD)

Single and repeat dose toxicity studies in mice, rats and dogs indicate a wide safety margin after oral and intravenous administration of (HP-β-CD). Most effects were adaptive in nature (histological changes in urinary tract, softening of faeces related to the osmotic water retention in the large intestine, activation of the mononuclear phagocyte system) and showed good reversibility. Slight liver changes occurred at doses of about 30 times the proposed human dosage of HP-β-CD.

HP-β-CD has no antifertile, no direct embryotoxic and no teratogenic effect, and is not mutagenic.

In the rat carcinogenicity study, an increased incidence of neoplasms in the large intestine (at 5000 mg/kg/day) and in the exocrine pancreas (from 500 mg/kg/day) were seen.

Development of the pancreatic tumours is related to the mitogenic action of cholecystokinin in rats. This finding was not observed in the mouse carcinogenicity study, nor in a 12-month toxicity study in dogs or in a 2-year toxicity study in female cynomolgus monkeys. There is no evidence that cholecystokinin has a mitogenic action in man. Based on

Figure 1 Breaking the ampoule as shown

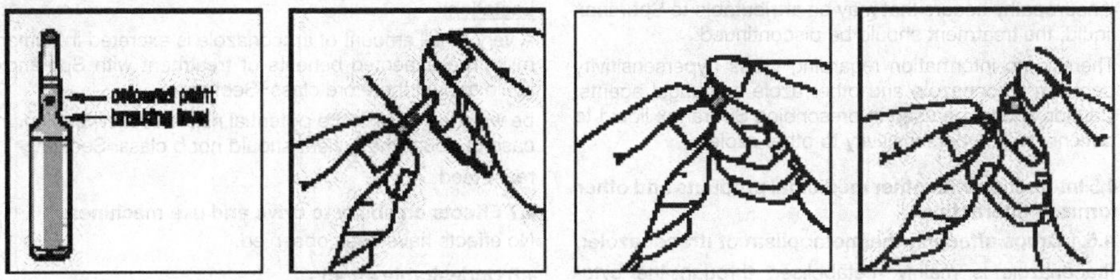

body surface comparisons, the exposure to humans of HP-β-CD at the recommended clinical dose of SPORANOX oral solution, is approximately equivalent to 1.7 times the exposure at the lowest dose in the rat study.

6. PHARMACEUTICAL PARTICULARS

6.1 List of excipients

Sporanox I.V.: Hydroxypropyl-β-cyclodextrin, propylene glycol, hydrochloric acid, sodium hydroxide, water for injections.

0.9% Sodium Chloride Injection: Sodium Chloride, water for Injection

6.2 Incompatibilities

Itraconazole has the potential to precipitate when Sporanox I.V. is diluted in solutions other than the 50ml 0.9% sodium chloride injection supplied.

6.3 Shelf life

Sporanox I.V.:

Shelf life as packaged:

2 years

0.9 % Sodium Chloride Injection:

2 years

Admixed Solution:

24 hours.

6.4 Special precautions for storage

Sporanox I.V.:

Do not store above 25°C. Store in the original container.

0.9 % Sodium Chloride Injection:

Do not store above 25°C. Do not freeze.

Admixed solution:

Protect from direct sunlight.

From a microbiological point of view, the product should be used immediately. If not used immediately, in-use storage times and conditions prior to use are the responsibility of the user and would not normally be longer than 24 hours at 2 to 8°C, unless the admixture has taken place in controlled and validated aseptic conditions.

6.5 Nature and contents of container

Sporanox I.V.:

25 ml siliconised type I glass ampoule with 25 ml containing 250 mg itraconazole.

0.9 % Sodium Chloride:

Flexible 100ml polyvinylchloride infusion bag, equipped with a flexible inlet and outlet port, and containing 52 to 56ml of 0.9% Sodium Chloride Injection.

Extension Line:

Polyvinylchloride tubing with 2-way stopcock and in-line filter.

6.6 Instructions for use and handling

0.9% Sodium Chloride Injection:

To open:

Tear outer wrap at notch and remove infusion bag. Some opacity of the plastic due to moisture absorption during the sterilisation process may be observed. This is normal and does not affect the solution quality or safety. The opacity will diminish gradually.

Using aseptic technique and an additive delivery needle of appropriate length, add the medication by puncturing the resealable additive port and inject. Withdraw needle after injecting medication.

Gently agitate the bag.

Push the pin of the infusion set in the flexible port of the infusion bag.

Close the rotary clamp.

Fill the drip chamber by squeezing (pumping) it.

Open the rotary clamp until all air has been expelled from the tubing.

Connect the infusion set to the venipuncture device.

Adjust the drip rate by means of the rotary clamp.

The solution is intended for single-dose infusion only. No administration should occur unless the solution is clear and the infusion bag undamaged.

Sporanox I.V.:

Itraconazole has the potential to precipitate when 25 ml of Sporanox I.V. are diluted in solutions other than 50 ml 0.9% Sodium Chloride Injection. The full amount of 25 ml of Sporanox I.V. from the ampoule must be diluted into the Sodium Chloride Infusion Bag, which is intended to be used exclusively in combination with Sporanox I.V. No other bag should be used. Use the dedicated Sporanox extension line. Sporanox I.V. cannot be co-administered with other drugs or fluids. See section 6.2. The concentrate, the solvent and the reconstituted solution for infusion are to be visually inspected prior to use. Only clear solutions without particles should be used.

Sporanox I.V. should be administered according to the following instructions:

- Opening ampoule:

- Break the ampoule as shown:

(see Figure 1 above)

- Flush procedure:

- First rinse the extension line with 5 to 10 ml 0.9% sodium chloride solution via the two way stop cock.

- Admixing Sporanox I.V. and 0.9% Sodium Chloride Injection:

- Each component must be at room temperature.

- Admix only in the **infusion bag** provided. Add the whole volume (25 ml) of **Sporanox I.V.** to the bag in a single action.

- Gently agitate the bag once the Sporanox I.V. is completely transferred to the bag.

The admixture should be used immediately and should be protected from direct sunlight: see section 6.3. (Shelf life) and section 6.4 (Special precautions for storage). Sporanox I.V. is for single use only and any unused solution should be discarded.

Aseptic technique must be used while preparing the admixture of Sporanox I.V. into the infusion bag and while handling the infusion line.

- Infusion:

- The infusion bag should now contain 25 ml Sporanox I.V. and 50 ml 0.9% Sodium Chloride Injection.

- Connect an infusion line to the two-way stop cock of the extension line.

- Adjust the infusion rate to 1 ml/min (approximatly 25 drops/min).

- Administer **60 ml** of the solution to the patient over approximately one hour.

- Stop the infusion when 60 ml is administered.

- Note that 200 mg of itraconazole has been administered.

- Flush procedure:

- After the infusion a complete flush procedure must be started to clean the I.V. line in the catheter and to avoid compatibility problems between residual amounts of itraconazole and other drugs which later could be administered through the same catheter.

Perform the flush in a continuous run of between 30 seconds to 15 minutes.

Flush the extension line with 15 – 20 ml 0.9% sodium chloride solution at the two-way stop cock, just before the 0.2 μm in-line filter. Remove the infusion line and the extension line.

Discard the infusion set after use. Do not re-sterilise or re-use.

- To avoid precipitation do not introduce comedication in the same bag or line as the itraconazole infusion.

- Other medication should only be administered after flushing of the lines-catheters or by using another lumen in case of multi-lumen I.V. catheters.

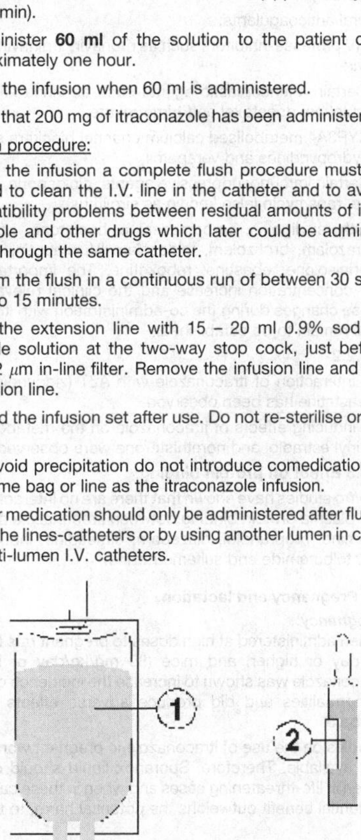

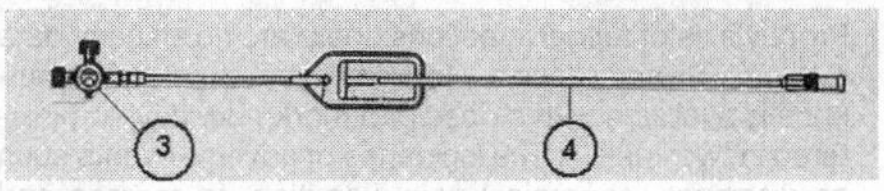

1. Sodium chloride bag
2. Sporanox I.V. ampoule
3. Two way stop cock
4. Extension line.

Administrative Data

7. MARKETING AUTHORISATION HOLDER

Janssen-Cilag Ltd.
Saunderton
High Wycombe
Bucks
HP14 4HJ
UK

8. MARKETING AUTHORISATION NUMBER(S)

PL 0242/0344

9. DATE OF FIRST AUTHORISATION/RENEWAL OF THE AUTHORISATION

22 July 1999 / 22nd July 2004

10. DATE OF REVISION OF THE TEXT

November 2004

Sporanox Liquid

(Janssen-Cilag Ltd)

1. NAME OF THE MEDICINAL PRODUCT

Sporanox® liquid 10mg/ml.

2. QUALITATIVE AND QUANTITATIVE COMPOSITION

1ml Sporanox liquid contains 10mg Itraconazole.

For excipients, see section 6.1.

3. PHARMACEUTICAL FORM

Oral solution.

Sporanox liquid is clear.

4. CLINICAL PARTICULARS

4.1 Therapeutic indications

Sporanox® liquid is indicated:

– For the treatment of oral and/or oesophageal candidosis in HIV-positive or other immunocompromised patients.

– As prophylaxis of deep fungal infections anticipated to be susceptible to itraconazole, when standard therapy is considered inappropriate, in patients with haematological malignancy or undergoing bone marrow transplant, and who are expected to become neutropenic (ie < 500 cells/μl). At present there are insufficient clinical efficacy data in the prevention of aspergillosis.

Consideration should be given to national and/or local guidance regarding the appropriate use of antifungal agents.

4.2 Posology and method of administration

For optimal absorption, Sporanox liquid should be taken without food (patients are advised to refrain from eating for at least 1 hour after intake).

For the treatment of oral and/or oesophageal candidosis, the liquid should be swished around the oral cavity (approx. 20 seconds) and swallowed. There should be no rinsing after swallowing.

Treatment of oral and/or oesophageal candidosis: 200 mg (2 measuring cups) per day preferably in two intakes, or alternatively in one intake, for 1 week. If there is no response after 1 week, treatment should be continued for another week.

Treatment of fluconazole resistant oral and/or oesophageal candidosis: 100 to 200 mg (1-2 measuring cups) twice daily for 2 weeks. If there is no response after 2 weeks, treatment should be continued for another 2 weeks. The 400mg daily dose should not be used for longer than 14 days if there are no signs of improvement.

Prophylaxis of fungal infections: 5 mg/kg per day administered in two intakes. In clinical trials, prophylaxis treatment was started immediately prior to the cytostatic treatment and generally one week before transplant procedure. Almost all proven deep fungal infections occurred in patients reaching neutrophil counts below 100 cells/μl. Treatment was continued until recovery of neutrophils (ie > 1000 cells/μl).

Pharmacokinetic parameters from clinical studies in neutropenic patients demonstrate considerable intersubject variation. Blood level monitoring should be considered particularly in the presence of gastrointestinal damage, diarrhoea and during prolonged courses of Sporanox liquid.

Use in children:

Since clinical data on the use of Sporanox liquid in paediatric patients is limited, its use in children is not recommended.

Prophylaxis of fungal infections: there are no efficacy data available in neutropenic children. Limited safety experience is available with a dose of 5 mg/kg per day administered in two intakes. The incidence of adverse events such as diarrhoea, abdominal pain, vomiting, fever, rash and mucositis was higher than in adults.

Use in elderly:

Since clinical data on the use of Sporanox liquid in elderly patients is limited, it is advised to use Sporanox liquid in these patients only if the potential benefit outweighs the potential risks.

Use in patients with hepatic impairment

Itraconazole is predominantly metabolised in the liver. The terminal half-life of itraconazole in cirrhotic patients is somewhat prolonged. A decrease in the oral bioavailability of itraconazole from Sporanox capsules was observed in cirrhotic patients. This can also be expected with Sporanox liquid. A dose adjustment may be considered.

Use in patients with renal impairment

A decrease in the oral bioavailability of itraconazole from Sporanox capsules was observed in some patients with renal insufficiency. This can also be expected with Sporanox liquid. A dose adjustment may be considered.

4.3 Contraindications

Sporanox liquid is contra-indicated in patients with a known hypersensitivity to the drug or its excipients.

Terfenadine, astemizole, mizolastine, cisapride, triazolam and oral midazolam, dofetilide, quinidine, pimozide, CYP3A4 metabolised HMG-CoA reductase inhibitors such as simvastatin, lovastatin and atorvastatin are contra-indicated with Sporanox liquid. (See section 4.5. Interaction with other medicinal products and other forms of interaction).

Sporanox liquid should only be given to pregnant women in life-threatening cases and when in these cases the potential benefit outweighs the potential harm to the foetus.

4.4 Special warnings and special precautions for use

In a healthy volunteer study with Sporanox® IV, a transient asymptomatic decrease of the left ventricular ejection fraction was observed.

Itraconazole has been shown to have a negative inotropic effect and Sporanox has been associated with reports of congestive heart failure. Sporanox liquid should not be used in patients with congestive heart failure or with a history of congestive heart failure unless the benefit clearly outweighs the risk. This individual benefit/risk assessment should take into consideration factors such as the severity of the indication, the dose and duration, and individual risk factors for congestive heart failure. Such patients should be informed of the signs and symptoms of congestive heart failure, should be treated with caution, and should be monitored for signs and symptoms of congestive heart failure during treatment; if such signs or symptoms do occur during treatment, Sporanox liquid should be discontinued.

Caution should be exercised when co-administering itraconazole and calcium channel blockers (see section 4.5, Interactions with other medicinal products).

Sporanox has a potential for clinically important drug interactions. (See Section 4.5.: Interaction with other medicinal products and other forms of interaction).

Very rare cases of serious hepatotoxicity, including some cases of fatal acute liver failure, have occurred with the use of Sporanox. Some of these cases involved patients with no pre-existing liver disease. Some of these cases have been observed within the first month of treatment, including some within the first week. Liver function monitoring should be considered in patients receiving Sporanox treatment. Patients should be instructed to promptly report to their physician signs and symptoms suggestive of hepatitis such as anorexia, nausea, vomiting, fatigue, abdominal pain or dark urine. In these patients treatment should be stopped immediately and liver function testing should be conducted. Most cases of serious hepatotoxicity involved patients who had pre-existing liver disease, were treated for systemic indications, had significant other medical conditions and/or were taking other hepatotoxic drugs. In patients with raised liver enzymes or active liver disease, or who have experienced liver toxicity with other drugs, treatment should not be started unless the expected benefit exceeds the risk of hepatic injury. In such cases liver enzyme monitoring is necessary.

Hepatic impairment: Itraconazole is predominantly metabolised in the liver. The terminal half-life of itraconazole in cirrhotic patients is somewhat prolonged. A decrease in the oral bioavailability of itraconazole from Sporanox capsules was observed in cirrhotic patients. This can also be expected with Sporanox liquid. A dose adjustment may be considered.

Renal impairment: A decrease in the oral bioavailability of itraconazole from Sporanox capsules was observed in some patients with renal insufficiency. This can also be expected with Sporanox liquid. A dose adjustment may be considered.

Prophylaxis in neutropenic patients: in clinical trials diarrhoea was the most frequent adverse event. This disturbance of the gastrointestinal tract may result in impaired absorption and may alter the microbiological flora potentially favouring fungal colonisation. Consideration should be given to discontinuing Sporanox liquid in these circumstances.

If neuropathy occurs that may be attributable to Sporanox liquid, the treatment should be discontinued.

There is no information regarding cross hypersensitivity between itraconazole and other azole antifungal agents. Caution should be used in prescribing Sporanox liquid to patients with hypersensitivity to other azoles.

4.5 Interaction with other medicinal products and other forms of Interaction

4.5.1 Drugs affecting the metabolism of itraconazole:

Itraconazole is mainly metabolised through the cytochrome CYP3A4. Interaction studies have been performed with rifampicin, rifabutin and phenytoin, which are potent enzyme inducers of CYP3A4. Since the bioavailability of itraconazole and hydroxy-itraconazole was decreased in these studies to such an extent that efficacy may be largely reduced, the combination with these enzyme inducers is not recommended. No formal study data are available for other enzyme inducers, such as carbamazepine, phenobarbital and isoniazid, but similar effects should be anticipated.

Potent inhibitors of this enzyme such as ritonavir, indinavir, clarithromycin and erythromycin may increase the bioavailability of itraconazole.

4.5.2 Effect of itraconazole on the metabolism of other drugs:

4.5.2.1 Itraconazole can inhibit the metabolism of drugs metabolised by the cytochrome 3A family. This can result in an increase and/or a prolongation of their effects, including side effects. After stopping treatment, itraconazole plasma levels decline gradually, depending on the dose and duration of treatment (See Section 5.2: Pharmacokinetic Properties). This should be taken into account when the inhibitory effect of itraconazole on comedicated drugs is considered.

Examples are:

Drugs which should not be used during treatment with itraconazole:

Terfenadine, astemizole, mizolastine, cisapride, triazolam oral midazolam, dofetilide, quinidine, pimozide, CYP3A4 metabolised HMG-CoA reductase inhibitors such as simvastatin, lovastatin and atorvastatin. (See section 4.3. Contra-indications.)

Caution should be exercised when co-administering itraconazole with calcium channel blockers. In addition to possible pharmacokinetic interactions involving the drug metabolising enzyme CYP3A4, calcium channel blockers can have negative inotropic effects which may be additive to those of itraconazole.

Drugs whose plasma levels, effects or side effects should be monitored.

Their dosage, if co-administered with itraconazole, should be reduced if

necessary.

- Oral anticoagulants;
- HIV protease inhibitors such as ritonavir, indinavir, saquinavir;
- Certain antineoplastic agents such as vinca alkaloids, busulphan, docetaxel and trimetrexate;
- CYP3A4 metabolised calcium channel blockers such as dihydropyridines and verapamil;
- Certain immunosuppressive agents: ciclosporin, tacrolimus, rapamycin (also known as sirolimus);
- Others: digoxin, carbamazepine, buspirone, alfentanil, alprazolam, brotizolam, midazolam IV, rifabutin, methylprednisolone, ebastine, reboxetine. The importance of the concentration increase and the clinical relevance of these changes during the co-administration with itraconazole remain to be established.

4.5.2.2

No interaction of itraconazole with AZT (zidovudine) and fluvastatine has been observed.

No inducing effects of itraconazole on the metabolism of ethinyl estradiol and norethisterone were observed.

4.5.3 Effect on protein binding:

In vitro studies have shown that there are no interactions on the plasma protein binding between itraconazole and imipramine, propranolol, diazepam, cimetidine, indomethacin, tolbutamide and sulfamethazine.

4.6 Pregnancy and lactation

Pregnancy:

When administered at high doses to pregnant rats (40 mg/kg/day or higher) and mice (80 mg/kg/day or higher), itraconazole was shown to increase the incidence of foetal abnormalities and did produce adverse effects on the embryo.

Studies on the use of itraconazole in pregnant women are not available. Therefore, Sporanox liquid should only be given in life-threatening cases and when in these cases the potential benefit outweighs the potential harm, to the foetus.

Women of child-bearing potential:

Adequate contraceptive precautions should be taken by women of child-bearing potential using Sporanox liquid until the next menstrual period following the end of Sporanox therapy.

Lactation:

A very small amount of itraconazole is excreted in human milk. The expected benefits of treatment with Sporanox liquid should therefore class=Section>

be weighed against the potential risk of breast-feeding. In case of doubt the patient should not b class=Section>

reast-feed.

4.7 Effects on ability to drive and use machines

No effects have been observed.

4.8 Undesirable effects

Approximately 9% of patients can be expected to experience adverse reactions while taking itraconazole. In patients receiving prolonged (approximately 1 month) continuous treatment especially, the incidence of adverse events was higher (about 15%). The most frequently reported adverse experiences were of gastrointestinal, hepatic and dermatological origin. Within each system organ class, the adverse reactions are ranked under the headings of frequency, using the following convention: Rare $>1/10,000$, $<1/1,000$) and very rare ($<1/10,000$), including isolated reports. Based upon the post-marketing experience, the following adverse reactions have also been reported:

- Metabolism and Nutrition Disorders
- ***Very rare:*** *hypokalemia*
- Nervous System Disorders
- ***Very rare:*** *peripheral neuropathy, headache, and dizziness*
- Cardiac Disorders
- ***Very rare:*** *congestive heart failure*
- Respiratory, Thoracic and Mediastinal Disorders
- ***Very rare:*** *pulmonary oedema*
- Gastrointestinal Disorders
- ***Very rare:*** *abdominal pain, vomiting, dyspepsia, nausea, diarrhoea and constipation*
- Hepato-Biliary Disorders
- ***Very rare:*** *fatal acute liver failure, serious hepatotoxicity, hepatitis, and reversible increases in hepatic enzymes*
- Skin and Subcutaneous Tissue Disorders
- ***Very rare:*** *Stevens-Johnson syndrome, angio-oedema, urticaria, alopecia, rash, and pruritis*
- Reproductive System and Breast Disorders
- ***Very rare:*** *menstrual disorder*
- General Disorders and Administrative Site Conditions
- ***Very rare:*** *allergic reaction, and oedema*

4.9 Overdose

Symptoms:

There are limited data on the outcomes of patients ingesting high doses of itraconazole. In patients taking either 1000 mg of Sporanox liquid or up to 3000 mg of Sporanox capsules, the adverse event profile was similar to that observed at recommended doses.

Treatment:

In the event of accidental overdosage, supportive measures should be employed. Within the first hour after ingestion, gastric lavage may be performed. Activated charcoal may be given if considered appropriate. Itraconazole cannot be removed by haemodialysis. No specific antidote is available.

5. PHARMACOLOGICAL PROPERTIES

5.1 Pharmacodynamic properties

Pharmacotherapeutic classification: J02A C02 (Antimycotics for systemic use, triazole derivatives)

In vitro studies demonstrate that itraconazole, a triazole derivative, inhibits the growth of a broad range of fungi pathogenic for humans at concentrations usually ranging from $\leqslant 0.025$ - 0.8 μg/ml. These include: *Candida albicans*, many *Candida non-albicans* spp., *Aspergillus* spp., *Trichosporon* spp., *Geotrichum* spp., *Cryptococcus neoformans*, dermatophytes and many dematiaceous fungi such as *Fonsecaea* spp., *Histoplasma* spp., *Pseudallescheria boydii* and *Penicullium marneffei*.

Candida glabrata and *Candida tropicalis* are generally the least susceptible Candida species, with some isolates showing unequivocal resistance to itraconazole *in vitro*.

The principal fungus types that are not inhibited by itraconazole are *Zygomycetes* (eg *Rhizopus* spp., *Rhizomucor* spp., *Mucor* spp. and *Absidia* spp.), *Fusarium* spp., *Scedosporium* spp. and *Scopulariopsis* spp.

In vitro studies have demonstrated that itraconazole impairs the synthesis of ergosterol in fungal cells. Ergosterol is a vital cell membrane component in fungi. Impairment of its synthesis ultimately results in an anti-fungal effect.

5.2 Pharmacokinetic properties

The oral bioavailability of itraconazole is maximal when Sporanox liquid is taken without food. During chronic administration, steady-state is reached after 1-2 weeks. Peak plasma levels are observed 2 hours (fasting for at least 2 hours) to 5 hours (with food) following the oral administration. After repeated once a day administration of itraconazole 200 mg in fasting condition, steady-state plasma concentrations of itraconazole fluctuated between 1 and 2 μg/ml (trough to peak). When the oral solution is taken with food, steady-state plasma concentrations of itraconazole are about 25% lower.

The plasma protein binding of itraconazole is 99.8%. Itraconazole is extensively distributed into tissues which are prone to fungal invasion. Concentrations in lung, kidney, liver, bone, stomach, spleen and muscle were found to be two to three times higher than the corresponding plasma concentration.

Itraconazole is extensively metabolised by the liver into a large number of metabolites. One of the metabolites is hydroxy-itraconazole, which has *in vitro* a comparable antifungal activity to itraconazole. Plasma levels of hydroxy-itraconazole are about twice as high as those of itraconazole.

After repeated oral administration, elimination of itraconazole from plasma is biphasic with a terminal half-life of 1.5 days. Faecal excretion of the parent drug varies between 3-18% of the dose. Renal excretion of the parent drug is less than 0.03% of the dose. About 35% of the dose is excreted as metabolites in the urine within 1 week.

Hepatic Insufficiency: A pharmacokinetic study using a single 100 mg dose of itraconazole (one 100 mg capsule) was conducted in 6 healthy and 12 cirrhotic subjects. No statistically significant differences in AUC_∞ were seen between these two groups. A statistically significant reduction in average C_{max} (47%) and a two fold increase in the elimination half-life (37 ± 17 versus 16 ±5 hours) of itraconazole were noted in cirrhotic subjects compared with healthy subjects. Patients with impaired hepatic function should be carefully monitored when taking itraconazole.

Renal Insufficiency: A pharmacokinetic study using a single 200 mg dose of itraconazole was conducted in three groups of patients with renal impairment (uremia: n=7; hemodialysis: n=7; and continuous ambulatory peritoneal: n=5). In uremic subjects with a mean creatinine clearance of 13 ml/min × 1.73m², the bioavailability was slightly reduced compared with normal subjects (AUC_∞: ↓20.5%; C_{max}: ↓27.7%). This study did not demonstrate any significant effect of hemodialysis or continuous ambulatory peritoneal dialysis on the pharmacokinetics of itraconazole.

5.3 Preclinical safety data

Hydroxypropyl- β-cyclodextrin (HP- β-CD)

Single and repeated dose toxicity studies in mice, rats and dogs indicate a wide safety margin after oral and intravenous administration of HP-β-CD. Most effects were adaptive in nature (histological changes in the urinary tract, softening of faeces related to the osmotic water retention in the large intestine, activation of the mononuclear phagocyte system) and showed good reversibility. Slight liver changes occurred at doses of about 30 times the proposed human dose of HP-β-CD.

HP-β-CD has no antifertile, no direct embryotoxic and no teratogenic effect, and is not mutagenic.

In the rat carcinogenicity study, an increased incidence of neoplasms in the large intestine (at 5000 mg/kg/day) and in the exocrine pancreas (from 500 mg/kg/day) were seen.

Development of the pancreatic tumours is related to the mitogenic action of cholecystokinin in rats. This finding was not observed in the mouse carcinogenicity study, nor in a 12-month toxicity study in dogs or in a 2-year toxicity study in female cynomolgus monkeys. There is no evidence that cholecystokinin has a mitogenic action in man. Based on body surface comparisons, the exposure to humans of HP-β-CD at the recommended clinical dose of Sporanox liquid, is approximately equivalent to 1.7 times the exposure at the lowest dose in the rat study.

6. PHARMACEUTICAL PARTICULARS

6.1 List of excipients

Hydroxypropyl-β-cyclodextrin, sorbitol, propylene glycol, hydrochloric acid, cherry flavour 1, cherry flavour 2, caramel, sodium saccharin, sodium hydroxide, purified water.

6.2 Incompatibilities

None known.

6.3 Shelf life

24months as packaged for sale.

1 month after first opening the container.

6.4 Special precautions for storage

Do not store above 25°C.

6.5 Nature and contents of container

150 ml amber glass bottle, with child resistant polypropylene screw cap and LDPE liner ring.

6.6 Instructions for use and handling

Sporanox liquid is supplied in bottles with a child-proof cap, and should be opened as follows: push the plastic screw cap down while turning it counter clockwise.

Administrative Data

7. MARKETING AUTHORISATION HOLDER

Janssen-Cilag Ltd

Saunderton

High Wycombe

Buckinghamshire

HP14 4HJ

8. MARKETING AUTHORISATION NUMBER(S)

0242/0307

9. DATE OF FIRST AUTHORISATION/RENEWAL OF THE AUTHORISATION

26 April 1996

10. DATE OF REVISION OF THE TEXT

June 2002

Legal category POM.

Sporanox -Pulse

(Janssen-Cilag Ltd)

1. NAME OF THE MEDICINAL PRODUCT

SPORANOX®-Pulse.

2. QUALITATIVE AND QUANTITATIVE COMPOSITION

Itraconazole 100 mg.

3. PHARMACEUTICAL FORM

Capsule (Size 0): opaque blue cap and pink transparent body containing coated beads.

4. CLINICAL PARTICULARS

4.1 Therapeutic indications

Onychomycosis caused by dermatophytes and/or yeasts.

Tinea pedis and/or tinea manuum.

4.2 Posology and method of administration

Sporanox-Pulse is for oral administration and must be taken immediately after a meal for maximal absorption.

Treatment schedules in adults are as follows:

Indication	Dose	Remarks
Tinea pedis and/ or tinea manuum	1 pulse treatment	A pulse treatment consists of 200 mg bd. for 7 days.
Onychomycosis – fingernails	2 pulse treatments	Pulse treatments are separated by a 3-week
Onychomycosis – toenails	3 pulse treatments	drug-free interval

Impaired absorption in AIDS and neutropenic patients may lead to low itraconazole blood levels and lack of efficacy. In such cases, blood level monitoring is indicated.

In Children (below 12 years):

There are inadequate data on Sporanox-Pulse in children for its use to be recommended, unless the potential benefits outweigh the risks.

In Elderly:

As for use in children.

4.3 Contraindications

Sporanox - Pulse is contra-indicated in pregnancy. Adequate contraceptive precautions should be taken by women of childbearing potential using Sporanox - Pulse until the next menstrual period following the end of Sporanox - Pulse therapy.

Sporanox - Pulse is also contra-indicated in patients who have shown hypersensitivity to the drug or its excipients.

Terfenadine, astemizole, mizolastine, cisapride, dofetilide, quinidine, pimozide, CYP3A4 metabolised HMG-CoA reductase inhibitors such as simvastatin and lovastatin, triazolam and oral midazolam are contra-indicated with Sporanox - Pulse (see also 4.5: Interaction with other Medicaments and other forms of Interaction).

4.4 Special warnings and special precautions for use

- In a healthy volunteer study with Sporanox® IV, a transient asymptomatic decrease of the left ventricular ejection fraction was observed.

- Itraconazole has been shown to have a negative inotropic effect and Sporanox has been associated with reports of congestive heart failure. Sporanox-Pulse should not be used in patients with congestive heart failure or with a history of congestive heart failure unless the benefit clearly outweighs the risk. This individual benefit/risk assessment should take into consideration factors such as the severity of the indication, the dose and duration of treatment, and individual risk factors for congestive heart failure. Such patients should be informed of the signs and symptoms of congestive heart failure, should be treated with caution, and should be monitored for signs and symptoms of congestive heart failure during treatment; if such signs or symptoms do occur during treatment, Sporanox-Pulse should be discontinued.

- Caution should be exercised when co-administering itraconazole and calcium channel blockers (see section 4.5, Interactions with other medicinal products).

- Sporanox - Pulse has a potential for clinically important drug interactions. (See section 4.5: Interactions with other medicaments and other forms of interaction).

- Decreased gastric acidity:

Absorption of itraconazole from Sporanox - Pulse is impaired when the gastric acidity is decreased. In patients also receiving acid neutralising medicines (eg aluminium hydroxide), these should be administered at least 2 hours after the intake of Sporanox-Pulse. In patients with achlorhydria such as certain AIDS patients and patients on secretion suppressors (eg H2-antagonists, proton-pump inhibitors), it is advisable to administer Sporanox-Pulse with a cola beverage.

Very rare cases of serious hepatotoxicity, including some cases of fatal acute liver failure, have occurred with the use of Sporanox. Some of these cases involved patients with no pre-existing liver disease. Some of these cases have been observed within the first month of treatment, including some within the first week. Liver function monitoring should be considered in patients receiving Sporanox treatment. Patients should be instructed to promptly report to their physician signs and symptoms suggestive of hepatitis such as anorexia, nausea, vomiting, fatigue, abdominal pain or dark urine. In these patients treatment should be stopped immediately and liver function testing conducted. Most cases of serious hepatotoxicity involved patients who had pre-existing liver disease, were treated for systemic indications, had significant other medical conditions and/ or were taking other hepatotoxic drugs. In patients with raised liver enzymes or active liver disease, or who have experienced liver toxicity with other drugs, treatment should not be started unless the expected benefit exceeds the risk of hepatic injury. In such cases liver enzyme monitoring is necessary.

- Hepatic impairment:

Itraconazole is predominantly metabolised in the liver. A slight decrease in oral bioavailability in cirrhotic patients has been observed, although this was not of statistical significance. The terminal half-life was however significantly increased. The dose should be adapted if necessary.

- Renal impairment:

The oral bioavailability of itraconazole may be lower in patients with renal insufficiency. Dose adaptation may be considered.

- If neuropathy occurs which may be attributable to Sporanox-Pulse, treatment should be discontinued.

- There is no information regarding cross hypersensitivity between itraconazole and other azole antifungal agents. Caution should be used in prescribing Sporanox to patients with hypersensitivity to other azoles.

4.5 Interaction with other medicinal products and other forms of Interaction

1. Drugs affecting the metabolism of itraconazole:

Interaction studies have been performed with rifampicin, rifabutin and phenytoin. Since the bioavailability of itraconazole and hydroxy-itraconazole was decreased in these studies to such an extent that efficacy may be largely reduced, the combination of itraconazole with these potent enzyme inducers is not recommended. No formal study data are available for other enzyme inducers, such as carbamazepine, phenobarbital and isoniazid, but similar effects should be anticipated.

As itraconazole is mainly metabolised through CYP3A4, potent inhibitors of this enzyme may increase the bioavailability of itraconazole. Examples are: ritonavir, indinavir, clarithromycin and erythromycin.

2. Effects of itraconazole on the metabolism of other drugs:

2.1 Itraconazole can inhibit the metabolism of drugs metabolised by the cytochrome 3A family. This can result in an increase and/or a prolongation of their effects, including side effects. After stopping treatment, itraconazole plasma levels decline gradually, depending on the dose and duration of treatment (see 5.2 Pharmacokinetic Properties). This should be taken into account when the inhibitory effect of itraconazole on co-administered drugs is considered.

Examples are:

- Drugs which should not be used during treatment with itraconazole:

– Terfenadine, astemizole, mizolastine, cisapride, triazolam, oral midazolam, dofetilide, quinidine, pimozide, CYP3A4 metabolised HMG-CoA reductase inhibitors such as simvastatin and lovastatin.

- Caution should be exercised when co-administering itraconazole with calcium channel blockers. In addition to possible pharmacokinetic interactions involving the drug metabolising enzyme CYP3A4, calcium channel blockers can have negative inotropic effects which may be additive to those of itraconazole.

- Drugs whose plasma levels, effects or side effects should be monitored. Their dosage, when co-administered with itraconazole, should be reduced if necessary:

§ Oral anticoagulants

§ HIV protease inhibitors such as ritonavir, indinavir, saquinavir

§ Certain antineoplastic agents such as vinca alkaloids, busulphan, docetaxel and trimetrexate

§ CYP3A4 metabolised calcium channel blockers such as dihydropyridines and verapamil

§ Certain immunosuppressive agents: ciclosporin, tacrolimus, rapamycin (also known as sirolimus)

§ Others: digoxin, carbamazepine, buspirone, alfentanil, alprazolam, brotizolam, midazolam IV, rifabutin, methylprednisolone, ebastine, reboxetine. The importance of the concentration increase and the clinical relevance of these changes during co-administration remain to be established.

2.2 No interaction of itraconazole with AZT (zidovudine) and fluvastatin has been observed.

No inducing effects of itraconazole on the metabolism of ethinyloestradiol and norethisterone were observed.

3. Effect on protein binding:

In vitro studies have shown that there are no interactions on the plasma protein binding between itraconazole and imipramine, propranolol, diazepam, cimetidine, indomethacin, tolbutamide or sulphadimidine.

4.6 Pregnancy and lactation

Pregnancy: Sporanox-Pulse is contra-indicated in pregnancy. When administered at high doses to pregnant rats (40 mg/kg/day or higher) and mice (80 mg/kg/day or higher), itraconazole was shown to cause abnormalities of foetal development. Studies of the use of itraconazole in pregnant women are not available. Adequate contraceptive precautions should be taken by women of childbearing potential using Sporanox - Pulse until the next menstrual period following the end of Sporanox - Pulse therapy.

Lactation: A very small amount of itraconazole is excreted in human milk. The expected benefits of Sporanox-Pulse therapy should be weighed against the risks of breast feeding. In case of doubt, the patient should not breast feed.

4.7 Effects on ability to drive and use machines

None known.

4.8 Undesirable effects

Approximately 9% of patients can be expected to experience adverse reactions while taking itraconazole. In patients receiving prolonged (approximately 1 month) continuous treatment, the incidence of adverse events was higher (about 15%). The most frequently reported adverse experiences were of gastrointestinal, hepatic and dermatological origin. Within each system organ class, the adverse reactions are ranked under the headings of frequency, using the following convention: Rare $>1/10,000$, $<1/1,000$) and very rare ($<1/10,000$), including isolated reports. Based upon the post-marketing experience, the following adverse reactions have also been reported:

- Metabolism and Nutrition Disorders
- ***Very rare:*** *hypokalemia*
- Nervous System Disorders
- ***Very rare:*** *peripheral neuropathy, headache, and dizziness*
- Cardiac Disorders
- ***Very rare:*** *congestive heart failure*
- Respiratory, Thoracic and Mediastinal Disorders
- ***Very rare:*** *pulmonary oedema*
- Gastrointestinal Disorders
- ***Very rare:*** *abdominal pain, vomiting, dyspepsia, nausea, diarrhoea and constipation*
- Hepato-Biliary Disorders
- ***Very rare:*** *fatal acute liver failure, serious hepatotoxicity, hepatitis, and reversible increases in hepatic enzymes*
- Skin and Subcutaneous Tissue Disorders
- ***Very rare:*** *Stevens-Johnson syndrome, angio-oedema, urticaria, alopecia, rash, and pruritis*
- Reproductive System and Breast Disorders
- ***Very rare:*** *menstrual disorder*
- General Disorders and Administrative Site Conditions
- ***Very rare:*** *allergic reaction, and oedema*

4.9 Overdose

In the event of overdosage, patients should be treated symptomatically with supportive measures. Within the first hour after ingestion, gastric lavage may be performed. Activated charcoal may be given if considered appropriate. No specific antidote is available. Itraconazole cannot be removed by haemodialysis.

5. PHARMACOLOGICAL PROPERTIES

5.1 Pharmacodynamic properties

Itraconazole is a substituted triazole antimycotic with a broad spectrum of activity against Candida spp and other yeasts, dermatophytes and pathogenic fungi. It acts by impairing the synthesis of ergosterol in fungal cell membranes.

5.2 Pharmacokinetic properties

Peak plasma concentrations of itraconazole in the region of 1 mcg equiv./ml are reached 1.5-3 hrs after administration. In man the elimination half life is about 20 hrs. Oral intake immediately after a meal doubled the peak level 3-4 hrs after intake.

Peak concentrations of itraconazole in keratinous tissues, especially skin, are up to 3 times higher than in plasma. Therapeutic levels in the skin persist for up to 2-4 weeks after stopping treatment as elimination is related to dermal regeneration, rather than redistribution into the systemic circulation.

Itraconazole is extensively metabolised by the liver to a large number of metabolites, which constitute 40% of the excreted dose. Faecal excretion of parent drug varies from 3-18% of the dose, and urinary excretion of unchanged drug is less than 0.03%.

5.3 Preclinical safety data

No relevant information additional to that contained elsewhere in the Summary of Product Characteristics.

6. PHARMACEUTICAL PARTICULARS

6.1 List of excipients

Sugar spheres NF

Hypromellose 2910 5mPa.s PhEur.

Macrogol 20000 NF

Capsule shell:

Titanium dioxide E171

Indigotin carmine E132

Gelatin PhEur.

Erythrosine E127

6.2 Incompatibilities

None known.

6.3 Shelf life

36 months.

6.4 Special precautions for storage

Protect from light. Store in a dry place. Store between 15°C and 30°C.

6.5 Nature and contents of container

Tristar blister - plastic foil consisting of 3 layers

- polyvinylchloride on the outside
- low density polyethylene in the middle
- polyvinylidene chloride on the inside

Aluminium foil (thickness 20 μm) coated on the inner side with colourless heatseal lacquer: PVC mixed polymers with acrylates 6 g/m^2

or:

PVC blister consisting of:-

Polyvinylchloride "genotherm" glass clear, thickness 250 μm

Aluminium foil (thickness 20 μm) coated on the inner side with a colourless heatseal lacquer: PVC mixed polymers with acrylates 6 g/m^2

Pack size: 28 capsules.

6.6 Instructions for use and handling

Not applicable.

Administrative Data

7. MARKETING AUTHORISATION HOLDER

Janssen-Cilag Ltd

Saunderton

High Wycombe

Buckinghamshire

HP14 4HJ

UK

8. MARKETING AUTHORISATION NUMBER(S)

0242/0334

9. DATE OF FIRST AUTHORISATION/RENEWAL OF THE AUTHORISATION

26 March 1997

10. DATE OF REVISION OF THE TEXT

November 2002

Legal category POM.

Stalevo

(Orion Pharma (UK) Limited)

1. NAME OF THE MEDICINAL PRODUCT

Stalevo▼ 50 mg/12.5 mg/200 mg film-coated tablet

Stalevo▼ 100 mg/25 mg/200 mg film-coated tablet

Stalevo▼ 150 mg/37.5 mg/200 mg film-coated tablet

2. QUALITATIVE AND QUANTITATIVE COMPOSITION

Each Stalevo 50 mg/12.5 mg/200 mg tablet contains 50 mg of levodopa, 12.5 mg of carbidopa and 200 mg of entacapone.

Each Stalevo 100 mg/25 mg/200 mg tablet contains 100 mg of levodopa, 25 mg of carbidopa and 200 mg of entacapone.

Each Stalevo 150 mg/37.5 mg/200 mg tablet contains 150 mg of levodopa, 37.5 mg of carbidopa and 200 mg of entacapone.

For excipients, see 6.1.

3. PHARMACEUTICAL FORM

Brownish- or greyish-red film-coated tablets.

Stalevo 50 mg/12.5 mg/200 mg: Round, biconvex tablets marked with 'LCE 50' on one side.

Stalevo 100 mg/25 mg/200 mg: Oval tablets marked with 'LCE 100' on one side.

Stalevo 150 mg/37.5 mg/200 mg: Elongated ellipse-shaped tablets marked with 'LCE 150' on one side.

4. CLINICAL PARTICULARS

4.1 Therapeutic indications

Stalevo is indicated for the treatment of patients with Parkinson's disease and end-of-dose motor fluctuations not stabilised on levodopa/dopa decarboxylase (DDC) inhibitor treatment.

4.2 Posology and method of administration

Each tablet is to be taken orally either with or without food (see section 5.2). One tablet contains one treatment dose and the tablet may only be administered as whole tablets.

The optimum daily dosage must be determined by careful titration of levodopa in each patient. The daily dose should be preferably optimised using one of the three available tablet strengths (50/12.5/200 mg, 100/25/200 mg, or 150/37.5/200 mg levodopa/carbidopa/entacapone).

Patients should be instructed to take only one Stalevo tablet per dose administration. Patients receiving less than 70-100 mg carbidopa a day are more likely to experience nausea and vomiting. While the experience with total daily dosage greater than 200 mg carbidopa is limited, the maximum recommended daily dose of entacapone is 2000 mg and therefore the maximum Stalevo dose is 10 tablets per day.

Usually Stalevo is to be used in patients who are currently treated with corresponding doses of standard release levodopa/DDC inhibitor and entacapone.

How to transfer patients taking levodopa/ DDC inhibitor (carbidopa or benserazide) preparations and entacapone tablets to Stalevo

a. Patients who are currently treated with entacapone and with standard release levodopa/carbidopa in doses equal to Stalevo tablet strengths can be directly transferred to corresponding Stalevo tablets.

For example, a patient taking one tablet of 50/12.5 mg of levodopa/carbidopa with one tablet of entacapone 200 mg four times daily can take one 50/12.5/200 mg Stalevo tablet four times daily in place of their usual levodopa/carbidopa and entacapone doses. A patient taking one tablet of 100/25 mg of levodopa/carbidopa with one tablet of entacapone 200 mg four times daily can take one 100/25/200 mg Stalevo tablet four times daily in place of their usual levodopa/carbidopa and entacapone doses. A patient taking one tablet of 150/37.5 mg of levodopa/carbidopa with one tablet of entacapone 200 mg four times daily can take one 150/37.5/200 mg Stalevo tablet four times daily in place of their usual levodopa/carbidopa and entacapone doses.

b. When initiating Stalevo therapy for patients currently treated with entacapone and levodopa/carbidopa in doses not equal to Stalevo 50/12.5/200 mg, (or 100/25/200 mg, or 150/37.5/200 mg) tablets, Stalevo dosing should be carefully titrated for optimal clinical response. At the initiation, Stalevo should be adjusted to correspond as closely as possible to the total daily dose of levodopa currently used.

c. When initiating Stalevo in patients currently treated with entacapone and levodopa/benserazide in a standard release formulation, discontinue dosing of levodopa/benserazide the previous night and start Stalevo the next morning. Begin with a dosage of Stalevo that will provide either the same amount of levodopa or slightly (5-10 %) more.

How to transfer patients not currently treated with entacapone to Stalevo

Initiation of Stalevo may be considered at corresponding doses to current treatment in some patients with Parkinson's disease and end-of-dose motor fluctuations, who are not stabilised on their current standard release levodopa/DDC inhibitor treatment. However, a direct switch from levodopa/DDC inhibitor to Stalevo is not recommended for patients who have dyskinesias or whose daily levodopa dose is above 800 mg. In such patients it is advisable to introduce entacapone treatment as a separate medication (entacapone tablets) and adjust the levodopa dose if necessary, before switching to Stalevo.

Entacapone enhances the effects of levodopa. It may therefore be necessary, particularly in patients with dyskinesia, to reduce levodopa dosage by 10-30% within the first days to first weeks after initiating Stalevo treatment. The daily dose of levodopa can be reduced by extending the dosing intervals and/or by reducing the amount of levodopa per dose, according to the clinical condition of the patient.

Dosage adjustment during the course of the treatment

When more levodopa is required, an increase in the frequency of doses and/or the use of an alternative strength of Stalevo should be considered, within the dosage recommendations.

When less levodopa is required, the total daily dosage of Stalevo should be reduced either by decreasing the frequency of administration by extending the time between doses, or by decreasing the strength of Stalevo at an administration.

If other levodopa products are used concomitantly with a Stalevo tablet, the maximum dosage recommendations should be followed.

Discontinuation of Stalevo therapy: If Stalevo treatment (levodopa/carbidopa/entacapone) is discontinued and the patient is transferred to levodopa/DDC inhibitor therapy without entacapone, it is necessary to adjust the dosing of other antiparkinsonian treatments, especially levodopa, to achieve a sufficient level of control of the parkinsonian symptoms.

Children and adolescents: Safety and efficacy of Stalevo in patients under 18 years of age has not been established. Therefore the use of the medicinal product in patients under the age of 18 cannot be recommended.

Elderly: No dosage adjustment of Stalevo is required for elderly patients.

Hepatic impairment: It is advised that Stalevo should be administered cautiously to patients with mild to moderate hepatic impairment. Dose reduction may be needed (see Section 5.2.b).

Renal insufficiency: Renal insufficiency does not affect the pharmacokinetics of entacapone. No particular studies are reported on the pharmacokinetics of levodopa and carbidopa in patients with renal insufficiency, therefore Stalevo therapy should be administered cautiously to patients in severe renal impairment including those receiving dialysis therapy (see Section 5.2.b).

4.3 Contraindications

- Known hypersensitivity to the active substances or to any of the excipients.
- Severe hepatic impairment.
- Narrow-angle glaucoma.
- Pheochromocytoma.
- Concomitant use of Stalevo with non-selective monoamine oxidase (MAO-A and MAO-B) inhibitors (e.g. phenelzine, tranylcypromine).
- Concomitant use of a selective MAO-A inhibitor and a selective MAO-B inhibitor (see section 4.5).
- A previous history of Neuroleptic Malignant Syndrome (NMS) and/or non-traumatic rhabdomyolysis.

4.4 Special warnings and special precautions for use

- Stalevo is not recommended for the treatment of drug-induced extrapyramidal reactions.
- Stalevo therapy should be administered cautiously to patients with severe cardiovascular or pulmonary disease, bronchial asthma, renal, hepatic or endocrine disease, or history of peptic ulcer disease or of convulsions.
- In patients with a history of myocardial infarction who have residual atrial nodal, or ventricular arrhythmias, cardiac function should be monitored with particular care during the period of initial dosage adjustments.
- All patients treated with Stalevo should be monitored carefully for the development of mental changes, depression with suicidal tendencies, and other serious antisocial behaviour. Patients with past or current psychosis should be treated with caution.
- Concomitant administration of antipsychotics with dopamine receptor-blocking properties, particularly D_2 receptor antagonists should be carried out with caution, and the patient carefully observed for loss of antiparkinsonian effect or worsening of parkinsonian symptoms.
- Patients with chronic wide-angle glaucoma may be treated with Stalevo with caution, provided the intra-ocular pressure is well controlled and the patient is monitored carefully for changes in intra-ocular pressure.
- Stalevo may induce orthostatic hypotension. Therefore Stalevo should be given cautiously to patients who are taking other medicinal products which may cause orthostatic hypotension.
- Entacapone in association with levodopa has been associated with somnolence and episodes of sudden sleep onset in patients with Parkinson's disease and caution should therefore be exercised when driving or operating machines (see also section 4.7).
- In clinical studies, undesirable dopaminergic effects, e.g dyskinesia, were more common in patients who received entacapone and dopamine agonists (such as bromocriptine), selegiline or amantadine compared to those who received placebo with this combination. The doses of other antiparkinsonian medicinal products may need to be adjusted when Stalevo treatment is substituted for a patient currently not treated with entacapone.
- Rhabdomyolysis secondary to severe dyskinesias or Neuroleptic Malignant Syndrome (NMS) has been observed rarely in patients with Parkinson's disease. Therefore, any abrupt dosage reduction or withdrawal of levodopa should be carefully observed, particularly in patients who are also receiving neuroleptics. NMS, including rhabdomyolysis and hyperthermia, is characterised by motor symptoms (rigidity, myoclonus, tremor), mental status changes (e.g., agitation, confusion, coma), hyperthermia, autonomic dysfunction (tachycardia, labile blood pressure) and elevated serum creatine phosphokinase. In individual cases, only some of these symptoms and/or findings may be evident. The early diagnosis is important for the appropriate management of NMS. A syndrome resembling the neuroleptic malignant syndrome including muscular rigidity, elevated body temperature, mental changes and increased serum creatine phosphokinase has been reported with the abrupt withdrawal of antiparkinsonian agents. Neither NMS nor rhabdomyolysis have been reported in association with entacapone treatment from controlled trials in which entacapone was discontinued abruptly. Since the introduction of entacapone into the market, a rare number of cases with some similar signs and symptoms have been reported. Prescribers should exercise caution when substituting levodopa/DDC inhibitor therapy without entacapone in a patient currently treated with Stalevo. When considered necessary, the replacement of Stalevo with levodopa and DDC inhibitor without entacapone should proceed slowly and an increase in levodopa dosage may be necessary.
- If general anaesthesia is required, therapy with Stalevo may be continued for as long as the patient is permitted to take fluids and medication by mouth. If therapy has to be stopped temporarily, Stalevo may be restarted as soon as oral medication can be taken at the same daily dosage as before.
- Periodic evaluation of hepatic, haematopoietic, cardiovascular and renal function is recommended during extended therapy with Stalevo.

4.5 Interaction with other medicinal products and other forms of Interaction

Other antiparkinsonian medicinal products: To date there has been no indication of interactions that would preclude concurrent use of standard antiparkinsonian medicinal products with Stalevo therapy. Entacapone in high doses may affect the absorption of carbidopa. However, no interaction with carbidopa has been observed with the recommended treatment schedule (200 mg of entacapone up to 10 times daily). Interactions between entacapone and selegiline have been investigated in repeated dose studies in Parkinson's disease patients treated with levodopa/DDC inhibitor and no interaction was observed. When used with Stalevo, the daily dose of selegiline should not exceed 10 mg.

Caution should be exercised when the following active substances are administered concomitantly with levodopa therapy.

Antihypertensives: Symptomatic postural hypotension may occur when levodopa is added to the treatment of patients already receiving antihypertensives. Dosage adjustment of the antihypertensive agent may be required.

Antidepressants: Rarely, reactions including hypertension and dyskinesia have been reported with the concomitant use of tricyclic antidepressants and levodopa/carbidopa. Interactions between entacapone and imipramine and between entacapone and moclobemide have been investigated in single dose studies in healthy volunteers. No pharmacodynamic interactions were observed. A significant number of Parkinson's disease patients have been treated with the combination of levodopa, carbidopa and entacapone with several active substances including MAO-A inhibitors, tricyclic antidepressants, noradrenaline reuptake inhibitors such as desipramine, maprotiline and venlafaxine and medicinal products that are metabolised by COMT (e.g. catechol-structured compounds, paroxetine). No pharmacodynamic interactions have been observed. However, caution should be exercised when these medicinal products are used concomitantly with Stalevo (see also section 4.3 and section 4.4).

Other active substances: Dopamine receptor antagonists (e.g. some antipsychotics and antiemetics), phenytoin and papaverine may reduce the therapeutic effect of levodopa. Patients taking these medicinal products with Stalevo should be carefully observed for loss of therapeutic response.

Due to entacapone's affinity to cytochrome P450 2C9 *in vitro* (see section 5.2), Stalevo may potentially interfere with active substances whose metabolism is dependent on this isoenzyme, such as S-warfarin. However, in an interaction study with healthy volunteers, entacapone did not change the plasma levels of S-warfarin, while the AUC for R-warfarin increased on average by 18 % [CI_{90} 11-26 %]. The INR values increased on average by 13 % [CI_{90} 6-19 %]. Thus, a control of INR is recommended when Stalevo is initiated for patients receiving warfarin.

Other forms of interactions: Since levodopa competes with certain amino acids, the absorption of Stalevo may be impaired in some patients on high protein diet.

Levodopa and entacapone may form chelates with iron in the gastrointestinal tract. Therefore, Stalevo and iron preparations should be taken at least 2-3 hours apart (see section 4.8).

Stalevo may be given to patients with Parkinson's disease who are taking vitamin preparations that contain pyridoxine hydrochloride (Vitamin B6).

In vitro data: Entacapone binds to human albumin binding site II which also binds several other medicinal products, including diazepam and ibuprofen. According to *in vitro* studies, significant displacement is not anticipated at therapeutic concentrations of the medicinal products. Accordingly, to date there has been no indication of such interactions.

4.6 Pregnancy and lactation

There are no adequate data from the use of the combination of levodopa/carbidopa/entacapone in pregnant women. Studies in animals have shown reproductive toxicity of the separate compounds (see section 5.3). The potential risk for humans is unknown. Stalevo should not be used during pregnancy unless the benefits for the mother outweigh the possible risks to the foetus.

Levodopa is excreted in human breast milk. There is evidence that lactation is suppressed during treatment with levodopa. Carbidopa and entacapone were excreted in milk in animals but is not known whether they are excreted in human breast milk. The safety of levodopa, carbidopa or entacapone in the infant is not known. Women should not breast-feed during treatment with Stalevo.

4.7 Effects on ability to drive and use machines

Levodopa, carbidopa and entacapone together may cause dizziness and symptomatic orthostatism. Therefore, caution should be exercised when driving or using machines.

Patients being treated with Stalevo and presenting with somnolence and/or sudden sleep onset episodes must be instructed to refrain from driving or engaging in activities where impaired alertness may put themselves or others at risk of serious injury or death (e.g. operating machines) until such recurrent episodes have resolved (see also section 4.4).

4.8 Undesirable effects

The following section describes the undesirable effects reported for levodopa/carbidopa and for entacapone used in combination with levodopa/DDC inhibitor.

Levodopa / carbidopa

Undesirable effects that occur frequently with levodopa/carbidopa are those due to central neuropharmacological activity of dopamine. These reactions can usually be diminished by levodopa dosage reduction. The most common undesirable effects are dyskinesias including choreiform, dystonic and other involuntary movements. Muscle twitching and blepharospasm may be taken as early signs to consider levodopa dosage reduction. Nausea, also related to enhanced central dopaminergic activity, is a common adverse effect of levodopa/carbidopa.

Other undesirable effects associated with levodopa/carbidopa therapy are mental changes, including paranoid ideation and psychotic episodes; depression, with or without development of suicidal tendencies; and cognitive dysfunction. Adding of entacapone to levodopa/DDC inhibitor therapy (carbidopa or benserazide), i.e. initiation of Stalevo treatment in an entacapone naive patient, may aggravate some of these mental changes.

Less frequent undesirable effects of levodopa/carbidopa therapy are irregular heart rhythm and/or palpitations, orthostatic hypotensive episodes, bradykinetic episodes (the 'on-off' phenomenon), anorexia, vomiting, dizziness, and somnolence.

Gastro-intestinal bleeding, development of duodenal ulcer, hypertension, phlebitis, leucopenia, haemolytic and non-haemolytic anaemia, thrombocytopenia, agranulocytosis, chest pain, dyspnoea and paraesthesia have occurred rarely with levodopa/carbidopa.

Convulsions have occurred rarely with levodopa/carbidopa; however a causal relationship to levodopa/carbidopa therapy has not been established.

Other undesirable effects that have been reported with levodopa and may, therefore, be potential undesirable effects of Stalevo as well, include:

Metabolism and nutrition disorders: Weight gain or loss, oedema.

Psychiatric disorders: Confusion, insomnia, nightmares, hallucinations, delusions, agitation, anxiety, euphoria.

Nervous system disorders: Ataxia, numbness, increased hand tremor, muscle twitching, muscle cramp, trismus, activation of latent Horner's syndrome. Also falling and gait abnormalities are potential undesirable effects.

Eye disorders: Diplopia, blurred vision, dilated pupils, oculogyric crises.

Gastro-intestinal disorders: Dry mouth, bitter taste, sialorrhoea, dysphagia, bruxism, hiccups, abdominal pain and distress, constipation, diarrhoea, flatulence, burning sensation of the tongue.

Skin and subcutaneous tissue disorders: Flushing, increased sweating, dark sweat, rash, hair loss.

Renal and urinary disorders: Urinary retention, urinary incontinence, dark urine, priapism.

Miscellaneous: Weakness, faintness, fatigue, headache, hoarseness, malaise, hot flushes, sense of stimulation, bizarre breathing patterns, neuroleptic malignant syndrome, malignant melanoma.

Entacapone

The most frequent adverse reactions caused by entacapone relate to the increased dopaminergic activity and occur most commonly at the beginning of the treatment. Reduction of levodopa dosage decreases the severity and frequency of the reactions. The other major class of adverse reactions are gastrointestinal symptoms, including e.g. nausea, vomiting, abdominal pain, constipation and diarrhoea. Urine may be discoloured reddish-brown by entacapone, but this is a harmless phenomenon.

The following adverse reactions, listed in Table 1, have been accumulated both from clinical studies with entacapone and since the introduction of entacapone into the market for the combination use of entacapone with levodopa/DDC inhibitor.

Table 1. Adverse reactions

Psychiatric disorders

Common: Insomnia, hallucinations, confusion, paroniria

Very rare: Agitation

Central & peripheral nervous system disorders

Very common: Dyskinesia

Common: Parkinsonism aggravated, dizziness, dystonia, hyperkinesia

Gastrointestinal system disorders

Very common: Nausea

Common: Diarrhoea, abdominal pain, mouth dry, constipation, vomiting

Liver and biliary system disorders

Rare: Hepatic function tests abnormal

Skin and appendages disorders

Rare: Erythematous or maculopapular rash

Very rare: Urticaria

Urinary system disorders

Very common: Urine discolouration

Body as a whole - general disorders

Common: Fatigue, sweating increased

Secondary terms - events

Common: Fall

*Adverse reactions are ranked under headings of frequency, the most frequent first, using the following convention: Very common (>1/10); common (>1/100, <1/10); uncommon (>1/1,000, <1/100); rare (>1/10,000, <1/1,000), very rare (<1/10,000), including isolated reports.

Isolated cases of hepatitis with cholestatic features have been reported.

Entacapone in association with levodopa has been associated with isolated cases of excessive daytime somnolence and sudden sleep onset episodes.

Laboratory tests:

The following laboratory abnormalities have been reported with levodopa/carbidopa treatment and should, therefore, be acknowledged when treating patients with Stalevo:

Commonly, levels of blood urea nitrogen, creatinine, and uric acid are lower during administration of levodopa/carbidopa than with levodopa alone. Transient abnormalities include elevated values of blood urea, AST (SGOT), ALT (SGPT), LDH, bilirubin, and alkaline phosphatase.

Decreased haemoglobin, haematocrit, elevated serum glucose and white blood cells, bacteria and blood in the urine have been reported.

Positive Coombs' tests have been reported, both for levodopa/carbidopa and for levodopa alone, but haemolytic anaemia is extremely rare.

Levodopa/carbidopa may cause false positive result when a dipstick is used to test for urinary ketone; and this reaction is not altered by boiling the urine sample. The use of glucose oxidase methods may give false negative results for glycosuria.

4.9 Overdose

No case of overdose has been reported.

Management of acute overdosage with Stalevo therapy is similar to acute overdosage with levodopa. Pyridoxine, however, is not effective in reversing the actions of Stalevo. Hospitalisation is advised and general supportive measures should be employed with immediate gastric lavage and repeated doses of charcoal over time. This may hasten the elimination of entacapone in particular by decreasing its absorption/reabsorption from the GI tract. The adequacy of the respiratory, circulatory and renal systems should be carefully monitored and appropriate supportive measures employed. ECG monitoring should be started and the patient carefully monitored for the possible development of arrhythmias. If required, appropriate, anti-arrhythmic therapy should be given. The possibility that the patient has taken other active substances in addition to Stalevo should be taken into consideration. The value of dialysis in the treatment of overdosage is not known.

5. PHARMACOLOGICAL PROPERTIES

5.1 Pharmacodynamic properties

Pharmacotherapeutic group: Anti-parkinsonian dopaminergic medicinal product.

ATC code: N04BA03

According to the current understanding, the symptoms of Parkinson's disease are related to depletion of dopamine in the corpus striatum. Dopamine does not cross the blood-brain barrier. Levodopa, the precursor of dopamine, crosses the blood brain barrier and relieves the symptoms of the disease. As levodopa is extensively metabolised in the periphery only a small portion of a given dose reaches the central nervous system when levodopa is administered without metabolic enzyme inhibitors.

Carbidopa and benserazide are peripheral DDC inhibitors which reduce the peripheral metabolism of levodopa to dopamine and, thus, more levodopa is available to the brain. When decarboxylation of levodopa is reduced with the co-administration of a DDC inhibitor, a lower dose of levodopa can be used and the incidence of undesirable effects such as nausea is reduced.

With inhibition of the decarboxylase by a DDC inhibitor, COMT becomes the major peripheral metabolic pathway catalyzing the conversion of levodopa to 3-O-methyldopa (3-OMD), a potentially harmful metabolite of levodopa. Entacapone is a reversible, specific and mainly peripherally acting COMT inhibitor designed for concomitant administration with levodopa. Entacapone slows the clearance of levodopa from the bloodstream resulting in an increased area under the curve (AUC) in the pharmacokinetic profile of levodopa. Consequently the clinical response to each dose of levodopa is enhanced and prolonged.

The evidence of the therapeutic effects of Stalevo is based on two phase III double-blind studies, in which 376 Parkinson's disease patients with end-of-dose motor fluctuations received either entacapone or placebo with each levodopa/DDC inhibitor dose. Daily ON time with and without entacapone was recorded in home-diaries by patients. In the first study, entacapone increased the mean daily ON time by 1 h 20 min ($CI_{95\%}$ 45 min, 1h 56min) from baseline. This corresponded to an 8.3% increase in the proportion of daily ON time. Correspondingly, the decrease in daily OFF time was 24% in the entacapone group and 0 % in the placebo group. In the second study, the mean proportion of daily ON time increased by 4.5% ($CI_{95\%}$ 0.93%, 7.97 %) from baseline. This is translated to a mean increase of 35 min in the daily ON time. Correspondingly, the daily OFF time decreased by 18% on entacapone and by 5% on placebo. Because the effects of Stalevo tablets are equivalent with entacapone 200 mg tablet administered concomitantly with the commercially available standard release carbidopa/levodopa preparations in corresponding doses these results are applicable to describe the effects of Stalevo as well.

5.2 Pharmacokinetic properties

a) General characteristics of the active substances

Absorption/Distribution: There are substantial inter- and intra-individual variations in the absorption of levodopa, carbidopa and entacapone. Both levodopa and entacapone are rapidly absorbed and eliminated. Carbidopa is absorbed and eliminated slightly slower compared with levodopa. When given separately without the two other active substances, the bioavailability for levodopa is 15 - 33 %, for carbidopa 40 - 70 % and for entacapone 35 % after a 200 mg oral dose. Meals rich in large neutral amino acids may delay and reduce the absorption of levodopa. Food does not significantly affect the absorption of entacapone. The distribution volume of both levodopa (Vd 0.36 - 1.6 l/kg) and entacapone (Vd_{ss} 0.27 l/kg) is moderately small while no data for carbidopa are available.

Levodopa is bound to plasma protein only to a minor extent of about 10-30 % and carbidopa is bound approximately 36 %, while entacapone is extensively bound to plasma proteins (about 98 %), mainly to serum albumin. At therapeutic concentrations, entacapone does not displace other extensively bound active substances (e.g. warfarin, salicylic acid, phenylbutazone, or diazepam), nor is it displaced to any significant extent by any of these substances at therapeutic or higher concentrations.

Metabolism and Elimination: Levodopa is extensively metabolised to various metabolites, decarboxylation by dopa decarboxylase (DDC) and O-methylation by catechol-O-methyltransferase (COMT) being the most important pathways.

Carbidopa is metabolized to two main metabolites which are excreted in the urine as glucuronides and unconjugated compounds. Unchanged carbidopa accounts for 30 % of the total urinary excretion.

Entacapone is almost completely metabolized prior to excretion via urine (10 to 20%) and bile/faeces (80 to 90%). The main metabolic pathway is glucuronidation of entacapone and its active metabolite, the cis-isomer, which accounts for about 5 % of plasma total amount.

Total clearance for levodopa is in the range of 0.55 - 1.38 l/kg/h and for entacapone is in the range of 0.70 l/kg/h. The elimination half-life ($t_{1/2}$) is 0.6 - 1.3 hours for levodopa, 2 - 3 hours for carbidopa and 0.4 - 0.7 h for entacapone, each given separately.

Due to short elimination half-lives, no true accumulation of levodopa or entacapone occurs on repeated administration.

Data from *in vitro* studies using human liver microsomal preparations indicate that entacapone inhibits cytochrome P450 2C9 (IC50 ~ 4 μM). Entacapone showed little or no inhibition of other types of P450 isoenzymes (CYP1A2, CYP2A6, CYP2D6, CYP2E1, CYP3A and CYP2C19) see section 4.5.

b) Characteristics in patients

Elderly: When given without carbidopa and entacapone, the absorption of levodopa is greater and elimination is slower in elderly than in young subjects. However, after combination of carbidopa with levodopa, the absorption of levodopa is similar between the elderly and the young, but the AUC is still 1.5 fold greater in the elderly due to decreased DDC activity and lower clearance by aging. There are no significant differences in the AUC of carbidopa or entacapone between younger (45 – 64 years) and elderly subjects (65 – 75 years).

Gender: Bioavailability of levodopa is significantly higher in women than in men. In the pharmacokinetic studies with Stalevo the bioavailability of levodopa is higher in women than in men, primarily due to the difference in body weight, while there is no gender difference with carbidopa and entacapone.

Hepatic impairment: The metabolism of entacapone is slowed in patients with mild to moderate hepatic impairment (Child-Pugh Class A and B) leading to an increased plasma concentration of entacapone both in the absorption and elimination phases (see sections 4.2 and 4.3). No particular studies on the pharmacokinetics of carbidopa and levodopa in patients with hepatic impairment are reported, however, it is advised that Stalevo should be administered cautiously to patients with mild or moderate hepatic impairment.

Renal impairment: Renal impairment does not affect the pharmacokinetics of entacapone. No particular studies are reported on the pharmacokinetics of levodopa and carbidopa in patients with renal impairment. However, a longer dosing interval of Stalevo may be considered for patients who are receiving dialysis therapy (see section 4.2).

5.3 Preclinical safety data

Preclinical data of levodopa, carbidopa and entacapone tested alone or in combination revealed no special hazard for humans based on conventional studies of safety pharmacology, repeated dose toxicity, genotoxicity, and carcinogenic potential. In repeated dose toxicity studies with entacapone, anaemia most likely due to iron chelating properties of entacapone was observed. Regarding reproduction toxicity of entacapone, decreased foetal weight and a slightly delayed bone development were noticed in rabbits treated at systemic exposure levels in the therapeutic range. Both levodopa and combinations of carbidopa and levodopa have caused visceral and skeletal malformations in rabbits.

6. PHARMACEUTICAL PARTICULARS

6.1 List of excipients

Tablet core:

Croscarmellose sodium

Magnesium stearate

Maize starch

Mannitol (E 421)

Povidone K30 (E1201)

Film-coating:

Glycerol 85 % (E 422)

Hypromellose

Magnesium stearate

Polysorbate 80

Red iron oxide (E 172)

Sucrose

Titanium dioxide (E 171)

Yellow iron oxide (E 172)

6.2 Incompatibilities

Not applicable.

6.3 Shelf life

3 years

6.4 Special precautions for storage

No special precautions for storage

6.5 Nature and contents of container

HDPE bottles with PP-closure

Pack sizes:

10, 30, 100 and 250 tablets.

Not all pack sizes may be marketed.

6.6 Instructions for use and handling

No special requirements.

7. MARKETING AUTHORISATION HOLDER

Orion Corporation

Orionintie 1

FIN-02200 Espoo

FINLAND

8. MARKETING AUTHORISATION NUMBER(S)

EU/1/03/260/001-012

9. DATE OF FIRST AUTHORISATION/RENEWAL OF THE AUTHORISATION

17.10.03

10. DATE OF REVISION OF THE TEXT

Stamaril

(Sanofi Pasteur MSD)

1. NAME OF THE MEDICINAL PRODUCT

STAMARIL®

Yellow Fever Vaccine (Live) Ph.Eur.

2. QUALITATIVE AND QUANTITATIVE COMPOSITION
Each 0.5 millilitre dose contains:

Injectable, freeze-dried suspension in stabiliser of the 17 D strain of live yellow fever virus, propagated in specific pathogen-free chick embryos, in particular free from avian leucosis viruses. ....not less than 1000 mouse LD50 units.

3. PHARMACEUTICAL FORM
A lyophilised powder for injection after suspension with sodium chloride solution.

4. CLINICAL PARTICULARS
4.1 Therapeutic indications
Prevention of yellow fever, the vaccination is recommended for:

Adults and children aged 9 months and over, travelling through, or living in, infected areas and those travelling outside urban areas of countries in the yellow fever endemic zone (even if these countries have not officially reported the disease and do not require evidence of immunisation on entry).

• Travellers requiring an International Certificate of Vaccination for entry into a country.

• Laboratory workers handling infected material.

In order to comply with vaccine regulations and to be officially recognised, Stamaril® vaccination must be administered at a designated vaccination centre and registered on an International Certificate. The International Certificate is valid for ten years from the tenth day after immunisation and immediately after re-immunisation.

Vaccination for children aged under 9 months is not recommended.

4.2 Posology and method of administration
After reconstitution of the vaccine by completely dissolving the freeze-dried preparation in the diluent, a single dose should be given by deep subcutaneous injection.

The vaccination schedule is identical for adults and children.

For vaccine association, see paragraph 4.5 in relation to interactions with other drugs and other forms of interactions.

Revaccination every ten years is recommended for patients at risk of infection.

4.3 Contraindications
The usual contra-indications to live virus vaccines should be observed:

All patients currently being treated for malignant disease with chemotherapy or generalised radiotherapy, or within 6 months of terminating such treatment.

All patients who have received an organ transplant and/or are currently on immunosuppressive treatment (children who receive prednisolone, orally or rectally, at a daily dose of 2 milligrams/kilogram/day for at least one week or 1 milligram/kilogram/day for one month; and adults receiving 40 milligrams or more of prednisolone per day for more than one week should be considered immunosuppressed).

Patients who, within the previous six months, have received a bone marrow transplant.

Patients with evidence of impaired cell mediated immunity such as symptomatic HIV infection, Severe Combined Immunodeficiency Syndrome, Di George Syndrome and other combined immunodeficiency syndromes.

The yellow fever vaccine should also not be given to:

Those suffering from fever or acute disease.

Pregnant women, because of the theoretical risk of foetal infection. However the Prescriber should consider the use of the vaccine where the benefit of its use outweighs the associated risk.

Persons with known hypersensitivity to a yellow fever vaccine, or any of its components.

Persons known to have had an anaphylactic reaction to egg. A letter stating immunisation is contra-indicated on these grounds may be acceptable in some countries although advice should be sought from the relevant Embassies.

HIV positive individuals, whether symptomatic or asymptomatic, since there is insufficient evidence as to the safety of its use. Travellers should be told of this uncertainty and advised not to be immunised unless there are compelling reasons.

Patients suffering from malignant conditions such as lymphoma, leukaemia, Hodgkin's disease or other tumours of the reticulo-endothelial system, or where the immunological mechanism may be impaired as in hypogammaglobulinaemia.

Infants under 9 months should only be immunised if the risk of yellow fever is unavoidable as there is a very small risk of encephalitis in this age group.

Normal human immunoglobulin is unlikely to contain antibody to the yellow fever virus; travellers may therefore be given the vaccine at the same time as an injection of immunoglobulin.

4.4 Special warnings and special precautions for use
Do not inject intravenously: make sure that the needle does not penetrate a blood vessel.

Not for intradermal injection (except as described below).

A tolerance test is indicated for subjects where there is a suspicion but no evidence of true allergy to a vaccine component: intradermal injection of 0.1 millilitre of vaccine followed, in absence of a reaction within 10 to 15 minutes, by deep subcutaneous injection of the rest of the dose, i.e. 0.4 millilitre.

In some cases, the yellow fever vaccination can be given to patients undergoing immunosuppressive treatment; it is advisable to only carry out the vaccination one month after the treatment is stopped and to make sure that biological parameters are normal.

Although anaphylaxis is rare, facilities for its management should always be available during vaccination.

Very rare reports of systemic infection have been associated with yellow fever vaccination, especially in the debilitated and elderly. Yellow fever vaccine should only be given to the elderly and debilitated if it is considered that there is a notable risk of yellow fever infection during travel.

4.5 Interaction with other medicinal products and other forms of Interaction
In case of immunosuppressive therapy or of corticosteroid therapy, refer to paragraph 4.3 related to the contra-indications.

The concomitant administration of injectable cholera vaccine or whole cell paratyphoid vaccine is incompatible as lower immunogenic responses are seen. A period of 3 weeks is recommended between yellow fever vaccination and these other vaccinations. If other live virus vaccines are required, they should either be given at different sites at the same time or with an interval of three weeks between them.

The association with other vaccines, such as vaccines against hepatitis A, meningococcal meningitis A and C, measles vaccine or Vi capsular polysaccharide vaccine against typhoid fever have given satisfactory results regarding the immunogenicity and tolerance of the different components.

4.6 Pregnancy and lactation
As with all live vaccines, pregnancy normally constitutes a contra-indication (see paragraph 4.3).

4.7 Effects on ability to drive and use machines
Not applicable.

4.8 Undesirable effects
Local reactions at the injection site may occur.

The following systemic reactions may also occur: fever, headache, myalgia, asthenia, rash, urticaria and lymphadenopathy.

A reaction may occur between the 4th and the 7th days in the form of stiffness with fever, tiredness and headaches. In this case, symptomatic treatment is advisable.

Very rare cases of neurological disorders such as meningitis, encephalitis or meningoencephalitis have also been reported.

Anaphylactoid reactions have also occurred very rarely.

Very rarely, causes of yellow fever-like illness have been reported after certain yellow fever vaccinations, some of which have been fatal. The pathophysiological mechanism for this has not been determined.

4.9 Overdose
Not applicable.

5. PHARMACOLOGICAL PROPERTIES
5.1 Pharmacodynamic properties
Stamaril® is a live stabilised vaccine for the prevention of yellow fever. Immunity appears 7 to 10 days after injection and revaccination every ten years is recommended for patients at risk of infection.

5.2 Pharmacokinetic properties
None stated.

5.3 Preclinical safety data
None stated.

6. PHARMACEUTICAL PARTICULARS
6.1 List of excipients
Stabilising medium:

Lactose, sorbitol, L-histidine hydrochloride, L-alanine, sodium chloride, potassium chloride, disodium phosphate, monopotassium phosphate, calcium chloride, magnesium sulphate, sodium hydroxide.

Diluent:

Sodium chloride, Water for Injections.

6.2 Incompatibilities
Do not admix with other medicinal products.

6.3 Shelf life
36 months when stored between +2°C and +8°C (in a refrigerator).

6.4 Special precautions for storage
Store between +2°C and +8°C (in a refrigerator). Do not freeze. In case of cold chain interruption, several studies have demonstrated that Stamaril® is not modified after 6 months storage at a temperature between +20°C and +25°C; or after 2 weeks storage at +37°C. Storage at temperatures above +2°C to +8°C cannot be recommended due to the difficulty in monitoring the exact temperature and monitoring repeated exposures to time out of refrigeration.

6.5 Nature and contents of container
• Containers in type I glass:

- Lyophilisate: one vial
- Diluent: one dose syringe (0.5 millilitre)

• Closure:

- Vial: chlorobutyl lyophilisation stopper with flip-off plastic cap
- Syringe: elastomer plunger stopper

6.6 Instructions for use and handling
Rehydrate carefully the content of each lyophilisate vial with the syringe of diluent. After complete dissolution, the vaccine should be drawn into the syringe and is ready for injection. The vaccine must be used within the hour following the reconstitution.

7. MARKETING AUTHORISATION HOLDER
Sanofi Pasteur MSD Limited
Mallards Reach
Bridge Avenue
Maidenhead
Berkshire
SL6 1QP

8. MARKETING AUTHORISATION NUMBER(S)
PL 6745/0087 (Lyophilised Vaccine)
PL 6745/0088 (Diluent)

9. DATE OF FIRST AUTHORISATION/RENEWAL OF THE AUTHORISATION
13 October 1998

10. DATE OF REVISION OF THE TEXT
May 2005

11. LEGAL CATEGORY
POM
® Registered trademark

Staril Tablets

(E. R. Squibb & Sons Limited)

1. NAME OF THE MEDICINAL PRODUCT
Staril Tablets 10mg
Staril Tablets 20mg

2. QUALITATIVE AND QUANTITATIVE COMPOSITION
Staril tablets contain 10mg or 20mg fosinopril sodium.

3. PHARMACEUTICAL FORM
Tablets.

4. CLINICAL PARTICULARS
4.1 Therapeutic indications
Hypertension:
Staril is indicated in the treatment of hypertension. Staril may be used alone as initial therapy or in combination with other antihypertensive agents. The antihypertensive effects of Staril and diuretics used concomitantly are approximately additive.

Heart Failure:
Staril is indicated for the treatment of heart failure in combination with a diuretic. In these patients, Staril improves symptoms and exercise tolerance, reduces severity of heart failure and decreases the frequency of hospitalisation for heart failure.

4.2 Posology and method of administration
ADULTS

Hypertensive patients not being treated with diuretics:
The dose range is 10 to 40mg per day administered in a single dose and without regard to meals. The normal starting dose for patients is 10mg once a day. Dosage may need to be adjusted after approximately 4 weeks according to blood pressure response. No additional blood pressure lowering is achieved with doses greater than 40mg daily. If blood pressure is not adequately controlled with Staril alone, a diuretic can be added.

Hypertensive patients being treated with concomitant diuretic therapy:
The diuretic should preferably be discontinued for several days prior to beginning therapy with Staril to reduce the risk of an excessive hypotensive response. If blood pressure is inadequately controlled after an observation period of approximately 4 weeks, diuretic therapy may be resumed. Alternatively, if diuretic therapy cannot be discontinued, an initial dose of 10 mg of Staril should be used with careful medical supervision for several hours, until blood pressure has stabilised. In diuretic treated hypertensive patients, mean cerebral blood flow is maintained between 4 and 24 hours after Staril, despite significant reduction in blood pressure.

Heart Failure:
The recommended initial dose is 10mg once daily, initiated under close medical supervision. If the initial dose is well tolerated patients should then be titrated to a dose of up to

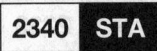

40mg once daily. The appearance of hypotension after the initial dose should not preclude careful dose titration of Staril, following effective management of the hypotension. Staril should be used in conjunction with a diuretic.

Heart Failure - High Risk Patients

It is recommended that treatment is initiated in hospital for patients with severe cardiac failure (NYHA IV) and those at particular risk of first dose hypotension, i.e. patients on multiple or high dose diuretics (e.g. > 80mg frusemide), patients with hypovolaemia, hyponatraemia (serum sodium < 130 meq/l), preexisting hypotension (systolic blood pressure <90 mmHg), patients with unstable cardiac failure and those on high-dose vasodilator therapy.

CHILDREN AND ADOLESCENTS

Use in this age group is not recommended.

There is limited clinical trial experience of the use of fosinopril in hypertensive children aged 6 years and above (see Section 5.1, 5.2 and 4.8). The optimum dosage has not been determined in children of any age. An appropriate dose strength is not available for children weighing less than 50 kg.

ELDERLY

No dosage reduction is necessary in patients with clinically normal renal and hepatic function as no significant differences in the pharmacokinetic parameters or antihypertensive effect of fosinoprilat have been found compared with younger subjects.

IMPAIRED HEPATIC FUNCTION

Treatment should be initiated at a dose of 10mg. Although the rate of hydrolysis may be slowed, the extent of hydrolysis is not appreciably reduced in patients with hepatic impairment. In this group of patients, there is evidence of reduced hepatic clearance of fosinoprilat with compensatory increase in renal excretion.

RENAL IMPAIRMENT

Treatment should be initiated at a dose of 10mg. Depending on the response, the dose should then be titrated to achieve the desired therapeutic effect.

Absorption, bioavailability, protein binding, biotransformation and metabolism are not appreciably altered by reduced renal function. In patients with impaired renal function, the total body clearance of fosinoprilat is approximately 50% slower than that in patients with normal renal function. However, since hepatobiliary elimination compensates at least partially for diminished renal elimination, the body clearance of fosinoprilat is not appreciably different over a wide range of renal insufficiency (creatinine clearances ranging from <10 to 80 ml/min/1.73m^2, i.e. including end-stage renal failure).

Clearance of fosinoprilat by haemodialysis and peritoneal dialysis averages 2% and 7%, respectively, of urea clearances.

4.3 Contraindications

A history of hypersensitivity to fosinopril or any of the tablet excipients.

Pregnancy: Staril is contraindicated in pregnancy. It has been shown to be lethal to rabbit foetuses at doses that were maternally toxic. Oligohydramnios and neonatal hypotension and/or anuria have been reported following use of ACE inhibitors in the second and third trimester of pregnancy.

Nursing mothers: Staril should not be given to nursing mothers as fosinoprilat has been detected in human breast milk.

4.4 Special warnings and special precautions for use

WARNING

Hypotension: As with all ACE inhibitors, a hypotensive response may be observed. If this occurs it is usually associated with the first dose and in most instances, symptoms are relieved simply by the patient lying down. A transient, hypotensive episode is not a contraindication to continuing therapy once the patient's blood pressure has been stabilised.

As with other ACE inhibitors, patients at risk of an excessive hypotensive response, sometimes associated with renal dysfunction, include those with: congestive heart failure, renovascular hypertension, renal dialysis, or volume and/or salt depletion of any aetiology. In patients with any one of these risk factors, it may be prudent to discontinue or reduce the dose of diuretic therapy or take other measures to ensure adequate hydration prior to initiating fosinopril treatment. Treatment of these high risk patients should be initiated under careful medical supervision and they should be followed closely, particularly if it becomes necessary to resume or increase the dose of diuretic or STARIL.

Impaired Renal Function: When treated with ACE inhibitors, patients with pre- existing congestive heart failure, renovascular hypertension (especially renal artery stenosis), and salt or volume depletion of any aetiology are at increased risk of developing findings indicative of renal dysfunction, including: increases in BUN and serum creatinine and potassium; proteinuria; changes in urine volume (including oliguria/anuria); and an abnormal urinalysis. Dosage reduction and/or discontinuation of diuretic and/ or fosinopril may be required.

Anaphylactoid-like Reactions: Recent clinical observations have shown a high incidence of anaphylactoid-like reactions during haemodialysis with high-flux dialysis membranes (e.g. AN69) in patients receiving ACE inhibitors. Therefore, this combination should be avoided. Similar reactions during LDL apheresis with dextran sulphate absorption have been observed. Rare instances of anaphylactoid reactions during desensitisation treatment (hymenoptera venom) have been recorded with other ACE inhibitors.

Idiosyncratic: Angioedema involving the extremities, face, lips, mucous membranes, tongue, glottis or larynx has been seen in patients treated with ACE inhibitors. If such symptoms occur during treatment with STARIL, therapy should be discontinued.

Liver Function: Rare potentially fatal cases of cholestatic jaundice and hepatocellular injury have been reported with ACE inhibitors. Patients who develop jaundice or marked elevations of hepatic enzymes should discontinue ACE inhibitor treatment.

Hyperkalaemia: When treated with ACE inhibitors, patients at risk of developing hyperkalaemia include those with renal insufficiency, diabetes mellitus, and those using concomitant potassium-sparing diuretics, potassium supplements and/or potassium- containing salt substitutes.

Neutropenia: ACE inhibitors have been reported rarely to cause agranulocytosis and bone marrow depression; these occur more frequently in patients with renal impairment, especially if they also have a collagen-vascular disease such as systemic lupus erythematosus or scleroderma. Monitoring of white blood cell counts should be considered in such patients.

Surgery/Anaesthesia: ACE inhibitors may augment the hypotensive effects of anaesthetics and analgesics. If hypotension occurs in patients undergoing surgery/anaesthesia and concomitantly receiving ACE inhibitors, it can usually be corrected by intravenous administration of fluid.

PRECAUTIONS

Pretreatment assessment of renal function: Evaluation of the hypertensive patient should include assessment of renal function prior to initiation of therapy and during treatment where appropriate.

4.5 Interaction with other medicinal products and other forms of Interaction

Potassium supplements and potassium-sparing diuretics:

Fosinopril can attenuate potassium loss caused by a thiazide diuretic. Potassium-sparing diuretics or potassium supplements can increase the risk of hyperkalaemia. Therefore, if concomitant use of such agents is indicated, they should be given with caution and the patient's serum potassium should be monitored frequently.

Antacids:

Antacids may impair absorption of fosinopril. Administration of STARIL and antacids should be separated by at least 2 hours.

N.S.A.I.D.s:

Non-steroidal anti-inflammatory drugs may interfere with the antihypertensive effect. However, the concomitant use of fosinopril and NSAIDs (including aspirin) is not associated with an increase in clinically significant adverse reactions.

Lithium:

Concomitant therapy with lithium may increase the serum lithium concentration.

Other Anti-Hypertensive Agents:

Combination with other anti-hypertensive agents such as beta blockers, methyldopa, calcium antagonists, and diuretics may increase the anti-hypertensive efficacy.

Other Drugs:

In pharmacokinetic studies with nifedipine, propranolol, cimetidine, metoclopramide and propantheline the bioavailability of fosinoprilat was not altered by coadministration of Staril with any one of these drugs.

Staril has been used concomitantly with paracetamol, antihistamines, hypoglycaemic agents, insulin, lipid-lowering agents or oestrogen without evidence of clinically important adverse events.

Laboratory tests: Staril may cause a false low measurement of serum digoxin levels with assays using the charcoal absorption method for digoxin. Other kits which use the antibody coated-tube method may be used.

4.6 Pregnancy and lactation

See Contraindications.

4.7 Effects on ability to drive and use machines

Not applicable.

4.8 Undesirable effects

In placebo controlled studies, there were no significant differences in clinical adverse experiences.

The most commonly reported side effects with Staril were dizziness, cough, upper respiratory symptoms, nausea / vomiting, diarrhoea and abdominal pain, palpitations/chest pain, rash/pruritus, musculoskeletal pain/paraesthesia, fatigue and taste disturbance.

As with other ACE-inhibitors, hypotension, including orthostatic hypotension, has been reported in Staril heart failure trials. Pancreatitis has been reported rarely in patients treated with ACE Inhibitors; in some cases this has proved fatal.

The incidence and type of side effects did not differ between elderly and younger patients.

Laboratory test findings showed some modest, usually transient, decreases in haemoglobin and haematocrit values and, infrequently, small increases in blood urea.

In a randomised clinical trial of children and adolescents aged 6 to 16 years, the adverse experience profile was similar to that seen in adult patients with hypertension. However, the long-term effects of fosinopril on growth, puberty and general development have not been studied.

4.9 Overdose

Blood pressure should be monitored and if hypotension develops, volume expansion is the treatment of choice. Fosinoprilat cannot be removed from the body by dialysis.

5. PHARMACOLOGICAL PROPERTIES

5.1 Pharmacodynamic properties

Fosinopril, {(4S)-4-Cyclohexyl-1-[(RS)-2-methyl-1-(propionyloxy)propoxy] (4- phenylbutyl) =phosphinoylacetyl} -L-proline; sodium salt, is the ester prodrug of an angiotensin converting enzyme (ACE) inhibitor, fosinoprilat. Angiotensin converting enzyme is a peptidyl dipeptidase enzyme that catalyses a number of peptide conversions. These include the conversion of decapeptide Angiotensin I to the octapeptide, Angiotensin II. Staril also inhibits kininase, the enzyme that degrades bradykinin.

Reduction of blood pressure with low (0.1 mg/kg), medium (0.3 mg/kg) and high (0.6 mg/kg) target doses of once-daily fosinopril was evaluated in a randomised double-blind study of 252 children and adolescents aged 6 to 16 years of age with hypertension or high-normal blood pressure. At the end of the four weeks of treatment, the mean reduction from baseline in trough systolic blood pressure was similar for children treated with low, medium and high dose fosinopril.

5.2 Pharmacokinetic properties

The absolute absorption of fosinopril averaged 36% of an oral dose, and was not affected by the presence of food. Rapid and complete hydrolysis to active fosinoprilat occurs in the gastrointestinal mucosa and liver.

The time to reach C_{max} is independent of dose, achieved in approximately three hours and consistent with peak inhibition of the angiotensin I pressor response 3 to 6 hours following administration.

In hypertensive patients with normal renal and hepatic function who received repeated doses of fosinopril, the effective T½ for accumulation of fosinoprilat averaged 11.5 hours. In patients with heart failure, the effective T½ was 14 hours. Fosinoprilat is highly protein bound > 95%), has a relatively small volume of distribution and negligible binding to cellular components in blood. The elimination of fosinopril is by both hepatic and renal routes. Unlike other ACE-inhibitors, there is compensatory excretion by the alternative route in patients with renal or hepatic insufficiency.

In a single dose pharmacokinetic study in children from 6-16 years of age who received 0.3 mg/kg solution of fosinopril, the AUC and Cmax values of fosinoprilat (active form of fosinopril) were comparable to those seen in adults receiving a solution of 20 mg of fosinopril. The terminal elimination half-life for fosinoprilat was 11-13 hours and similar at all stages studied.

5.3 Preclinical safety data

Animal studies indicate a toxicity profile which is an extension of the pharmacological effects of fosinopril. It has shown no evidence of carcinogenicity in rodent studies and no potential for mutagenicity in either *in vitro* or *in vivo* tests.

6. PHARMACEUTICAL PARTICULARS

6.1 List of excipients

Staril Tablets 10 mg: White, flat end, diamond tablets each containing fosinopril sodium 10 mg. Engraved with Squibb and unilog number 158 on one face and a star design on the other.

Staril Tablets 20 mg: White, round biconvex tablets each containing fosinopril sodium 20 mg. Engraved with Squibb and unilog number 609 on one face and a star design on the other.

Other ingredients: Crospovidone, lactose, sodium stearyl fumarate, microcrystalline cellulose, povidone.

6.2 Incompatibilities

None known.

6.3 Shelf life

36 months.

6.4 Special precautions for storage

Store below 30°C in a dry place.

6.5 Nature and contents of container

Cartons containing blister packs of 28 tablets.

6.6 Instructions for use and handling

No special handling instructions.

7. MARKETING AUTHORISATION HOLDER

E.R. Squibb & Sons Limited
Uxbridge Business Park
Sanderson Road
Uxbridge
Middlesex UB8 1DH

8. MARKETING AUTHORISATION NUMBER(S)

Staril Tablets 10mg PL 0034/0293
Staril Tablets 20mg PL 0034/0294

9. DATE OF FIRST AUTHORISATION/RENEWAL OF THE AUTHORISATION

3rd July 1990 / 30th August 2001

10. DATE OF REVISION OF THE TEXT

June 2005

Starlix 60mg, 120mg, 180mg film coated tablets

(Novartis Pharmaceuticals UK Ltd)

1. NAME OF THE MEDICINAL PRODUCT

Starlix® 60 mg film-coated tablets.
Starlix® 120 mg film-coated tablets.
Starlix® 180 mg film-coated tablets.

2. QUALITATIVE AND QUANTITATIVE COMPOSITION

Each Starlix 60 mg film-coated tablet contains 60 mg nateglinide.

Each Starlix 120 mg film-coated tablet contains 120 mg nateglinide

Each Starlix 180 mg film-coated tablet contains 180 mg nateglinide

For excipients, see 6.1.

3. PHARMACEUTICAL FORM

Film-coated tablet

60 mg pink, round, bevelled-edge tablets with "STARLIX" marked on one side and "60" on the other.

120 mg yellow, ovaloid tablets with "STARLIX" marked on one side and "120" on the other.

180 mg red, ovaloid tablets with "STARLIX" marked on one side and "180" on the other.

4. CLINICAL PARTICULARS

4.1 Therapeutic indications

Nateglinide is indicated for combination therapy with metformin in type 2 diabetic patients inadequately controlled despite a maximally tolerated dose of metformin alone.

4.2 Posology and method of administration

Nateglinide should be taken within 1 to 30 minutes before meals (usually breakfast, lunch and dinner).

The dosage of nateglinide should be determined by the physician according to the patient's requirements.

The recommended starting dose is 60 mg three times daily before meals, particularly in patients who are near goal HbA_{1c}. This may be increased to 120 mg three times daily.

Dose adjustments should be based on periodic glycosylated haemoglobin (HbA_{1c}) measurements. Since the primary therapeutic effect of Starlix is to reduce mealtime glucose, (a contributor to HbA_{1c}), the therapeutic response to Starlix may also be monitored with 1–2 hour post-meal glucose.

The recommended maximum single daily dose is 180 mg taken before the three main meals. The total maximum daily dose should not exceed 180 mg before three main meals.

Specific patient groups

Elderly

The clinical experience in patients over 75 years of age is limited.

Children and adolescents

There are no data available on the use of nateglinide in patients under 18 years of age, and therefore its use in this age group is not recommended.

Patients with hepatic impairment

No dose adjustment is necessary for patients with mild to moderate hepatic impairment. As patients with severe liver disease were not studied, nateglinide is contraindicated in this group.

Patients with renal impairment

No dose adjustment is necessary in patients with mild to moderate renal impairment.

Although there is a 49 % decrease in C_{max} of nateglinide in dialysis patients, the systemic availability and half-life in diabetic subjects with moderate to severe renal insufficiency (creatinine clearance 15–50 ml/min) was comparable between renal subjects requiring haemodialysis and healthy subjects. Although safety was not compromised in this population dose adjustment may be required in view of low C_{max}.

Others

In debilitated or malnourished patients the initial and maintenance dosage should be conservative and careful titration is required to avoid hypoglycaemic reactions.

4.3 Contraindications

Starlix is contraindicated in patients with:

- Hypersensitivity to the active substance or to any of the excipients
- Type 1 diabetes (insulin-dependent diabetes mellitus, C-peptide negative)
- Diabetic ketoacidosis, with or without coma
- Pregnancy and breast-feeding (see section 4.6, "Pregnancy and lactation")
- Severe hepatic impairment

4.4 Special warnings and special precautions for use

General

Nateglinide should not be used in monotherapy.

Like other insulin secretagogues, nateglinide is capable of producing hypoglycaemia.

Hypoglycaemia has been observed in patients with type 2 diabetes on diet and exercise, and in those treated with oral antidiabetic agents (see section 4.8, "Undesirable effects"). Elderly, malnourished patients and those with adrenal or pituitary insufficiency or severe renal impairment are more susceptible to the glucose-lowering effect of these treatments. The risk of hypoglycaemia in type 2 diabetic patients may be increased by strenuous physical exercise, or ingestion of alcohol.

Symptoms of hypoglycaemia (unconfirmed by blood glucose levels) were observed in patients whose baseline HbA_{1C} was close to the therapeutic target ($HbA_{1C} < 7.5\%$).

Combination with metformin is associated with an increased risk of hypoglycaemia compared to monotherapy.

Hypoglycaemia may be difficult to recognise in subjects receiving beta-blockers.

When a patient stabilised on any oral hypoglycaemic agent is exposed to stress such as fever, trauma, infection or surgery, a loss of glycaemic control may occur. At such times, it may be necessary to discontinue oral hypoglycaemic treatment and replace it with insulin on a temporary basis.

Specific patient groups

Nateglinide should be used with caution in patients with moderate hepatic impairment.

No clinical studies have been conducted in patients with severe hepatic impairment or children and adolescents. Treatment is, therefore, not recommended in these patient groups.

4.5 Interaction with other medicinal products and other forms of Interaction

A number of medicinal products influence glucose metabolism and possible interactions should, therefore, be taken into account by the physician:

The following agents may enhance the hypoglycaemic effect of nateglinide: angiotensin-converting enzyme inhibitors (ACEI).

The following agents may reduce the hypoglycaemic effect of nateglinide: diuretics, corticosteroids, and beta2 agonists.

When these medicinal products are administered to or withdrawn from patients receiving nateglinide, the patient should be observed closely for changes in glycaemic control.

Data available from both *in vitro* and *in vivo* experiments indicate that nateglinide is predominantly metabolised by CYP2C9 with involvement of CYP3A4 to a smaller extent.

In an interaction trial with sulfinpyrazone, a CYP2C9 inhibitor, a modest increase in nateglinide AUC (~28 %) was observed in healthy volunteers, with no changes in the mean C_{max} and elimination half-life. A more prolonged effect and possibly a risk of hypoglycaemia cannot be excluded in patients when nateglinide is co-administered with CYP2C9 inhibitors.

Particular caution is recommended when nateglinide is co-administered with other more potent inhibitors of CYP2C9, e.g. fluconazole or gemfibrozil, or in patients known to be poor metabolisers for CYP2C9.

Interaction studies with a 3A4 inhibitor have not been carried out *in vivo*.

In vivo, nateglinide has no clinically relevant effect on the pharmacokinetics of medicinal products metabolised by CYP 2C9 and CYP 3A4. The pharmacokinetics of warfarin (a substrate for CYP 3A4 and CYP 2C9), diclofenac (a substrate for CYP 2C9) and digoxin were unaffected by coadministration with nateglinide. Conversely, these medicinal products had no effect on the pharmacokinetics of nateglinide. Thus, no dosage adjustment is required for digoxin, warfarin or other drugs that are CYP 2C9 or CYP 3A4 substrates upon coadministration with Starlix. Similarly, there was no clinically significant pharmacokinetic interaction of Starlix with other oral antidiabetic agents such as metformin or glibenclamide.

Nateglinide has shown a low potential for protein displacement in *in vitro* studies.

4.6 Pregnancy and lactation

Studies in animals have shown developmental toxicity (see section 5.3).

There is no experience in pregnant women, therefore the safety of Starlix in pregnant women cannot be assessed. Starlix, like other oral antidiabetic agents, is not recommended for use in pregnancy.

Nateglinide is excreted in the milk following a peroral dose to lactating rats. Although it is not known whether nateglinide is excreted in human milk, the potential for hypoglycaemia in breast-fed infants may exist and, therefore, nateglinide should not be used in lactating women.

4.7 Effects on ability to drive and use machines

Patients should be advised to take precautions to avoid hypoglycaemia whilst driving or operating machinery. This is particularly important in those who have reduced or absent awareness of the warning signs of hypoglycaemia or have frequent episodes of hypoglycaemia. The advisability of driving should be considered in these circumstances.

4.8 Undesirable effects

Based on the experience with nateglinide and with other hypoglycaemic agents, the following adverse reactions have been seen.

Frequencies are defined as:
common ($> 1/100$, $< 1/10$)
uncommon $> 1/1000$, $< 1/100$)
rare ($> 1/10,000$, $< 1/1,000$)
very rare ($< 1/10,000$).

Hypoglycaemia

As with other antidiabetic agents, symptoms suggestive of hypoglycaemia have been observed after administration of nateglinide. These symptoms included sweating, trembling, dizziness, increased appetite, palpitations, nausea, fatigue and weakness. These were generally mild in nature and easily handled by intake of carbohydrates when necessary. In completed clinical trials, symptoms of hypoglycaemia were reported in 10.4% with nateglinide monotherapy, 14.5% with nateglinide+metformin combination, 6.9% with metformin alone, 19.8% with glibenclamide alone, and 4.1% with placebo.

Immune system disorders

Rare: Hypersensitivity reactions such as rash, itching and urticaria.

Metabolism and nutrition disorders

Common: Symptoms suggestive of hypoglycaemia.

Hepato-biliary disorders

Rare: Elevations in liver enzymes.

Other events

Other adverse events observed in clinical studies were of a similar incidence in Starlix-treated and placebo-treated patients. They include gastrointestinal complaints (e.g. abdominal pain, dyspepsia, diarrhoea), headache and events consistent with concomitant conditions likely to be present in these patient populations, such as respiratory infections.

4.9 Overdose

In a clinical study in patients, Starlix was administered in increasing doses up to 720 mg a day for 7 days and was well tolerated. There is no experience of an overdose of Starlix in clinical trials. However, an overdose may result in an exaggerated glucose-lowering effect, with the development of hypoglycaemic symptoms. Hypoglycaemic symptoms without loss of consciousness or neurological findings should be treated with oral glucose and adjustments in dosage and/or meal patterns. Severe hypoglycaemic reactions with coma, seizure or other neurological symptoms should be treated with intravenous glucose. As nateglinide is highly protein-bound, dialysis is not an efficient means of removing it from the blood.

5. PHARMACOLOGICAL PROPERTIES

5.1 Pharmacodynamic properties

Pharmacotherapeutic group: D-phenylalanine derivative

ATC code: A10 BX 03

Nateglinide is an amino acid (phenylalanine) derivative, which is chemically and pharmacologically distinct from other antidiabetic agents. Nateglinide is a rapid, short-acting oral insulin secretagogue. Its effect is dependent on functioning beta cells in the pancreas islets.

Early insulin secretion is a mechanism for the maintenance of normal glycaemic control. Nateglinide, when taken before a meal, restores early or first phase insulin secretion, which is lost in patients with type 2 diabetes, resulting in a reduction in post-meal glucose and HbA_{1c}.

Nateglinide closes ATP-dependent potassium channels in the beta-cell membrane with characteristics that distinguish it from other sulphonylurea receptor ligands. This depolarises the beta cell and leads to an opening of the calcium channels. The resulting calcium influx enhances insulin secretion. Electrophysiological studies demonstrate that nateglinide has 45-300 fold selectivity for pancreatic beta cell versus cardiovascular K^{+}_{ATP} channels.

In type 2 diabetic patients, the insulinotropic response to a meal occurs within the first 15 minutes following an oral dose of nateglinide. This results in a blood-glucose-lowering effect throughout the meal period. Insulin levels return to baseline within 3 to 4 hours, reducing post-meal hyperinsulinaemia.

Nateglinide-induced insulin secretion by pancreatic beta cells is glucose-sensitive, such that less insulin is secreted as glucose levels fall. Conversely, the coadministration of food or a glucose infusion results in an enhancement of insulin secretion.

In combination with metformin, which mainly affected fasting plasma glucose, the effect of nateglinide on HbA_{1c} was additive compared to either agent alone.

Nateglinide efficacy was inferior to that of metformin in monotherapy (decrease in HbA_{1c} (%) with metformin 500 mg three times daily monotherapy: –1.23 [95% CI: –1.48;–0.99] and with nateglinide 120 mg three times daily monotherapy –0.90 [95% CI: –1.14;–0.66]).

The efficacy of nateglinide in combination with metformin has not been compared to the combination of sulphonylurea plus metformin.

An outcome study has not been conducted with nateglinide, therefore the long-term benefits associated with improved glycaemic control have not been demonstrated.

5.2 Pharmacokinetic properties
Absorption and bioavailability

Nateglinide is rapidly absorbed following oral administration of Starlix tablets prior to a meal, with mean peak drug concentration generally occurring in less than 1 hour. Nateglinide is rapidly and almost completely (⩾ 90 %) absorbed from an oral solution. Absolute oral bioavailability is estimated to be 72 %. In type 2 diabetic patients given Starlix over the dose range 60 to 240 mg before three meals per day for one week, nateglinide showed linear pharmacokinetics for both AUC and C_{max}, and t_{max} was independent of dose.

Distribution

The steady-state volume of distribution of nateglinide based on intravenous data is estimated to be approximately 10 litres. *In vitro* studies show that nateglinide is extensively bound (97-99 %) to serum proteins, mainly serum albumin and to a lesser extent alpha$_1$-acid glycoprotein. The extent of serum protein binding is independent of drug concentration over the test range of 0.1-10 μg Starlix/ml.

Metabolism

Nateglinide is extensively metabolised. The main metabolites found in humans result from hydroxylation of the isopropyl side-chain, either on the methine carbon, or one of the methyl groups; activity of the main metabolites is about 5-6 and 3 times less potent than nateglinide, respectively. Minor metabolites identified were a diol, an isopropene and acyl glucuronide(s) of nateglinide; only the isopropene minor metabolite possesses activity, which is almost as potent as nateglinide. Data available from both *in vitro* and *in vivo* experiments indicate that nateglinide is predominantly metabolised by CYP2C9 with involvement of CYP3A4 to a smaller extent.

Excretion

Nateglinide and its metabolites are rapidly and completely eliminated. Most of the [^{14}C] nateglinide is excreted in the urine (83 %), with an additional 10 % eliminated in the faeces. Approximately 75 % of the administered [^{14}C] nateglinide is recovered in the urine within six hours post-dose. Approximately 6-16 % of the administered dose was excreted in the urine as unchanged drug. Plasma concentrations decline rapidly and the elimination half-life of nateglinide typically averaged 1.5 hours in all studies of Starlix in volunteers and type 2 diabetic patients. Consistent with its short elimination half-life, there is no apparent accumulation of nateglinide upon multiple dosing with up to 240 mg three times daily.

Food effect

When given post-prandially, the extent of nateglinide absorption (AUC) remains unaffected. However, there is a delay in the rate of absorption characterised by a decrease in C_{max} and a delay in time to peak plasma concentration (t_{max}). It is recommended that Starlix be administered prior to meals. It is usually taken immediately (1 minute) before a meal but may be taken up to 30 minutes before meals.

Sub-populations

Elderly

Age did not influence the pharmacokinetic properties of nateglinide.

Hepatic impairment

The systemic availability and half-life of nateglinide in non-diabetic subjects with mild to moderate hepatic impairment did not differ to a clinically significant degree from those in healthy subjects.

Renal impairment

The systemic availability and half-life of nateglinide in diabetic patients with mild, moderate (creatinine clearance 31–50 ml/min) and severe (creatinine clearance 15–30 ml/min) renal impairment (not undergoing dialysis) did not differ to a clinically significant degree from those in healthy subjects. There is a 49 % decrease in C_{max} of nateglinide in dialysis-dependent diabetic patients. The systemic availability and half-life in dialysis-dependent diabetic patients was comparable with healthy subjects. Although safety was not compromised in this population dose adjustment may be required in view of low C_{max}.*Gender* No clinically significant differences in nateglinide pharmacokinetics were observed between men and women.

5.3 Preclinical safety data

Preclinical data revealed no special hazard for humans based on conventional studies of safety pharmacology, repeated dose toxicity, genotoxicity, carcinogenic potential and toxicity to fertility and post-natal development. Nateglinide was not teratogenic in rats. In rabbits, at maternally toxic doses, a higher incidence of foetuses with no gallbladder was observed

6. PHARMACEUTICAL PARTICULARS

6.1 List of excipients

Starlix 60 mg film-coated tablet

Lactose monohydrate, cellulose microcrystalline, povidone, croscarmellose sodium, magnesium stearate, iron oxide (red, E172), hypromellose, titanium dioxide (E171), talc, macrogol, silica, colloidal anhydrous.

Starlix 120 mg film-coated tablet

Lactose monohydrate, cellulose microcrystalline, povidone, croscarmellose sodium, magnesium stearate, iron oxide (yellow, E172), hypromellose, titanium dioxide (E171), talc, macrogol, silica, colloidal anhydrous.

Starlix 180 mg film-coated tablet

Lactose monohydrate, cellulose microcrystalline, povidone, croscarmellose sodium, magnesium stearate, iron oxide (red, E172), hypromellose, titanium dioxide (E171), talc, macrogol, silica, colloidal anhydrous.

6.2 Incompatibilities

Not applicable

6.3 Shelf life

3 years

6.4 Special precautions for storage

Do not store above 30°C.

Store in the original package.

6.5 Nature and contents of container

Blisters: PVC/PE/PVDC moulded foil with aluminium lidding foil.

Packs contain 84 tablets.

6.6 Instructions for use and handling

No special requirements

7. MARKETING AUTHORISATION HOLDER

Novartis Europharm Limited

Wimblehurst Road

Horsham

West Sussex, RH12 5AB

United Kingdom

8. MARKETING AUTHORISATION NUMBER(S)

Starlix 60 mg film-coated tablet – EU/1/01/174/005

Starlix 120 mg film-coated tablet – EU/1/01/174/012

Starlix 180 mg film-coated tablet - EU/1/01/174/019

9. DATE OF FIRST AUTHORISATION/RENEWAL OF THE AUTHORISATION

3 April 2001

10. DATE OF REVISION OF THE TEXT

2 August 2004

LEGAL CATEGORY

POM

Stemetil Eff

(sanofi-aventis)

1. NAME OF THE MEDICINAL PRODUCT

Stemetil Eff

2. QUALITATIVE AND QUANTITATIVE COMPOSITION

The active component of Stemetil Eff is prochlorperazine mesilate 5 mg equivalent to 3.3 mg prochlorperazine base.

3. PHARMACEUTICAL FORM

White effervescent granular powder which dissolves in water to give a lemon flavoured effervescent solution.

4. CLINICAL PARTICULARS

4.1 Therapeutic indications

Prevention of nausea and vomiting. Treatment of nausea and vomiting. Treatment of vertigo and Meniere's syndrome. Adjunct in the short-term management of anxiety.

4.2 Posology and method of administration

Adults

For oral administration.

Indication	Dosage
Prevention of nausea and vomiting	5 to 10 mg b.d. or t.d.s.
Treatment of nausea and vomiting	20 mg stat, followed if necessary by 10 mg two hours later.
Vertigo and Meniere's syndrome	5 mg t.d.s. increasing if necessary to a total of 30 mg daily. After several weeks dosage may be reduced gradually to 5-10 mg daily.
Adjunct in the short-term management of anxiety	15-20 mg daily in divided doses initially but this may be increased if necessary to a maximum of 40 mg daily in divided doses.

Children

Not recommended.

Elderly

A lower dose is recommended. Please see Special Warnings and Precautions for Use.

4.3 Contraindications

Known hypersensitivity to prochlorperazine or to any of the other ingredients.

4.4 Special warnings and special precautions for use

Stemetil should be avoided in patients with liver or renal dysfunction, Parkinson's disease, hypothyroidism, cardiac failure, phaeochromocytoma, myasthenia gravis, prostate hypertrophy. It should be avoided in patients known to be hypersensitive to phenothiazines or with a history of narrow angle glaucoma or agranulocytosis.

Close monitoring is required in patients with epilepsy or a history of seizures, as phenothiazines may lower the seizure threshold.

As agranulocytosis has been reported, regular monitoring of the complete blood count is recommended. The occurrence of unexplained infections or fever may be evidence of blood dyscrasia (see section 4.8 below), and requires immediate haematological investigation.

It is imperative that treatment be discontinued in the event of unexplained fever, as this may be a sign of neuroleptic malignant syndrome (pallor, hyperthermia, autonomic dysfunction, altered consciousness, muscle rigidity). Signs of autonomic dysfunction, such as sweating and arterial instability, may precede the onset of hyperthermia and serve as early warning signs. Although neuroleptic malignant syndrome may be idiosyncratic in origin, dehydration and organic brain disease are predisposing factors.

Acute withdrawal symptoms, including nausea, vomiting and insomnia, have very rarely been reported following the abrupt cessation of high doses of neuroleptics. Relapse may also occur, and the emergence of extrapyramidal reactions has been reported. Therefore, gradual withdrawal is advisable.

As with other neuroleptics, cases of QT interval prolongation have been reported with prochlorperazine very rarely (see section 4.8, below). The risk-benefit should be fully assessed before Stemetil treatment is commenced, and patients with predisposing factors for ventricular arrhythmias, (e.g. cardiac disease; metabolic abnormalities such as hypokalaemia, hypocalcaemia or hypomagnesaemia; starvation; alcohol abuse; concomitant therapy with other drugs known to prolong the QT interval) should be carefully monitored (biochemical status and ECG), particularly during the initial phase of treatment.

As with all antipsychotic drugs, Stemetil should not be used alone where depression is predominant.

Because of the risk of photosensitisation, patients should be advised to avoid exposure to direct sunlight.

To prevent skin sensitisation in those frequently handling preparations of phenothiazines, the greatest care must be taken to avoid contact of the drug with the skin (see section 4.8, below).

Due to its aspartame content, Stemetil Eff should not be given to patients with phenylketonuria.

It should be used with caution in the elderly, particularly during very hot or very cold weather (risk of hyper-, hypothermia).

The elderly are particularly susceptible to postural hypotension.

Stemetil should be used cautiously in the elderly owing to their susceptibility to drugs acting on the central nervous system and a lower initial dosage is recommended. There is an increased risk of drug-induced Parkinsonism in the elderly particularly after prolonged use. Care should also be taken not to confuse the adverse effects of Stemetil, e.g. orthostatic hypotension, with the effects due to the underlying disorder.

4.5 Interaction with other medicinal products and other forms of Interaction

Adrenaline must not be used in patients overdosed with Stemetil (see section 4.9, below).

The CNS depressant actions of neuroleptic agents may be intensified (additively) by alcohol, barbiturates and other sedatives. Respiratory depression may occur.

Anticholinergic agents may reduce the antipsychotic effect of neuroleptics and the mild anticholinergic effect of neuroleptics may be enhanced by other anticholinergic drugs, possibly leading to constipation, heat stroke, etc.

Some drugs interfere with absorption of neuroleptic agents: antacids, anti-Parkinson drugs and lithium.

Where treatment for neuroleptic-induced extrapyramidal symptoms is required, anticholinergic antiparkinsonian agents should be used in preference to levodopa, since neuroleptics antagonise the antiparkinsonian action of dopaminergics.

High doses of neuroleptics reduce the response to hypoglycaemic agents, the dosage of which might have to be raised.

The hypotensive effect of most antihypertensive drugs especially alpha adrenoceptor blocking agents may be exaggerated by neuroleptics.

The action of some drugs may be opposed by phenothiazine neuroleptics; these include amfetamine, levodopa, clonidine, guanethidine, adrenaline.

Increases or decreases in the plasma concentrations of a number of drugs, e.g. propranolol, phenobarbital have been observed but were not of clinical significance.

Simultaneous administration of desferrioxamine and prochlorperazine has been observed to induce transient metabolic encephalopathy characterised by loss of consciousness for 48-72 hours.

There is an increased risk of arrhythmias when neuroleptics are used concurrently with drugs which prolong the QT interval, including certain antiarrhythmics, antidepressants, and other antipsychotics (see section 4.8, below).

There is an increased risk of agranulocytosis when neuroleptics are used concurrently with drugs with myelosuppressive potential, such as carbamazepine or certain antibiotics and cytotoxics.

In patients treated concurrently with neuroleptics and lithium, there have been rare reports of neurotoxicity.

4.6 Pregnancy and lactation

There is inadequate evidence of safety in pregnancy. There is evidence of harmful effects in animals. Stemetil should be avoided in pregnancy unless the physician considers it essential. Neuroleptics may occasionally prolong labour and at such time should be withheld until the cervix is dilated 3-4 cm. Possible adverse effects on the neonate include lethargy or paradoxical hyperexcitability, tremor and low apgar score.

Phenothiazines may be excreted in milk, therefore breast feeding should be suspended during treatment.

4.7 Effects on ability to drive and use machines

Patients should be warned about drowsiness during the early days of treatment and advised not to drive or operate machinery.

4.8 Undesirable effects

Generally, adverse reactions occur at a low frequency; the most common reported adverse reactions are nervous system disorders.

Adverse effects:

Blood and lymphatic system disorders: A mild leukopenia occurs in up to 30% of patients on prolonged high dosage. Agranulocytosis may occur rarely: it is not dose related (see section 4.4, above).

Endocrine: Hyperprolactinaemia which may result in galactorrhoea, gynaecomastia, amenorrhoea; impotence.

Nervous system disorders: Acute dystonia or dyskinesias, usually transitory are commoner in children and young adults, and usually occur within the first 4 days of treatment or after dosage increases.

Akathisia characteristically occurs after large initial doses.

Parkinsonism is more common in adults and the elderly. It usually develops after weeks or months of treatment. One or more of the following may be seen: tremor, rigidity, akinesia or other features of Parkinsonism. Commonly just tremor.

Tardive dyskinesia: If this occurs it is usually, but not necessarily, after prolonged or high dosage. It can even occur after treatment has been stopped. Dosage should therefore be kept low whenever possible.

Insomnia and agitation may occur.

Eye disorders: Ocular changes and the development of metallic greyish-mauve coloration of exposed skin have been noted in some individuals mainly females, who have received chlorpromazine continuously for long periods (four to eight years). This could possibly happen with Stemetil

Cardiac disorders: Cardiac arrhythmias, including atrial arrhythmia, A-V block, ventricular tachycardia and fibrillation have been reported during neuroleptic therapy, possibly related to dosage. Pre-existing cardiac disease, old age, hypokalemia and concurrent tricyclic antidepressants may predispose. ECG changes, usually benign, include widened QT interval, ST depression, U-waves and T-wave changes (see section 4.4, above).

Vascular disorders: Hypotension, usually postural, commonly occurs. Elderly or volume depleted subjects are particularly susceptible; it is more likely to occur after intramuscular injection.

Gastrointestinal disorders: dry mouth may occur.

Respiratory, thoracic and mediastinal disorders: Respiratory depression is possible in susceptible patients. Nasal stuffiness may occur.

Hepato-biliary disorders: Jaundice, usually transient, occurs in a very small percentage of patients taking neuroleptics. A premonitory sign may be sudden onset of fever after one to three weeks of treatment followed by the development of jaundice. Neuroleptic jaundice has the biochemical and other characteristics of obstructive jaundice and is associated with obstruction of the canaliculi by bile thrombi; the frequent presence of an accompanying eosinphilia indicates the allergic nature of this phenomenon. Treatment should be withheld on the development of jaundice (see section 4.4, above).

Skin and subcutaneous tissue disorders: Contact skin sensitisation may occur rarely in those frequently handling preparations of certain phenothiazines (see section 4.4, above). Skin rashes of various kinds may also be seen in patients treated with the drug. Patients on high dosage should be warned that they may develop photosensitivity in sunny weather and should avoid exposure to direct sunlight.

General disorders and administration site conditions: Neuroleptic malignant syndrome (hyperthermia, rigidity, autonomic dysfunction and altered consciousness) may occur with any neuroleptic (see section 4.4, above).

4.9 Overdose

Symptoms of phenothiazine overdosage include drowsiness or loss of consciousness, hypotension, tachycardia, ECG changes, ventricular arrhythmias and hypothermia. Severe extrapyramidal dyskinesias may occur.

If the patient is seen sufficiently soon (up to 6 hours) after ingestion of a toxic dose, gastric lavage may be attempted. Pharmacological induction of emesis is unlikely to be of any use. Activated charcoal should be given. There is no specific antidote. Treatment is supportive.

Generalised vasodilatation may result in circulatory collapse; raising the patient's legs may suffice. In severe cases, volume expansion by intravenous fluids may be needed; infusion fluids should be warmed before administration in order not to aggravate hypothermia.

Positive inotropic agents such as dopamine may be tried if fluid replacement is insufficient to correct the circulatory collapse. Peripheral vasoconstrictor agents are not generally recommended. Avoid the use of adrenaline.

Ventricular or supraventricular tachy-arrhythmias usually respond to restoration of normal body temperature and correction of circulatory or metabolic disturbances. If persistent or life threatening, appropriate anti-arrhythmic therapy may be considered. Avoid lidocaine and, as far as possible, long acting anti-arrhythmic drugs.

Pronounced central nervous system depression requires airway maintenance or, in extreme circumstances, assisted respiration. Severe dystonic reactions usually respond to procyclidine (5-10 mg) or orphenadrine (20-40 mg) administered intramuscularly or intravenously. Convulsions should be treated with intravenous diazepam.

Neuroleptic malignant syndrome should be treated with cooling. Dantrolene sodium may be tried.

5. PHARMACOLOGICAL PROPERTIES

5.1 Pharmacodynamic properties

Prochlorperazine (PCP) is a dopamine and histamine antagonist. The mechanism of the anti-emetic effect is due predominantly to blockade of the histamine H_1 and dopamine D_2 neurotransmitter receptors in the chemoreceptor trigger zone and vomiting centre. It also has weak anticholinergic effect and prevents acid reflux by increasing the tone of the lower oesphangeal sphincter.

5.2 Pharmacokinetic properties

Peak prochlorperazine (PCP) concentrations of approximately 1.1 ng/ml were reached at 2.8 hours after oral administration of an aqueous solution of prochlorperazine mesilate (Stemetil syrup) to healthy volunteers.

PCP was rapidly metabolised to the S-oxide due to a first pass effect during absorption, thus producing peak metabolite concentrations of 17 ng/ml at 0.5 hour. The AUC values for the S-oxide indicate that PCP is well absorbed orally, compared with i.m. injection. Plasma concentrations of PCP and the S-oxide fell with half-lives of 6.2 and 8.5 hours, respectively.

PCP is widely distributed throughout the body and diffuses rapidly across the placenta. It is excreted in the urine and faeces mainly as metabolites.

5.3 Preclinical safety data

There are no preclinical data of relevance to the prescriber which are additional to that already included in other sections of the SPC.

6. PHARMACEUTICAL PARTICULARS

6.1 List of excipients

Tartaric acid (E334), Povidone K30, sodium bicarbonate (E500), fresh lemon juice (Flav-O-Lok 610406E), citric acid anhydrous (E330), ascorbic acid (E300), sodium carbonate dried 1968 C (E500), aspartame (E951).

6.2 Incompatibilities

None stated.

6.3 Shelf life

36 months.

6.4 Special precautions for storage

Store below 25°C.

6.5 Nature and contents of container

Stemetil Eff is available in sealed sachets consisting of paper/foil/polyethylene laminate in cartons of 21.

6.6 Instructions for use and handling

None stated.

Administrative Data

7. MARKETING AUTHORISATION HOLDER

Castlemead Healthcare Limited

20 Clanwilliam Terrace

Dublin 2

Ireland

8. MARKETING AUTHORISATION NUMBER(S)

PL 16946/0002

9. DATE OF FIRST AUTHORISATION/RENEWAL OF THE AUTHORISATION

1 July 1998

10. DATE OF REVISION OF THE TEXT

September 2004

Legal category: POM

Stemetil Injection

(sanofi-aventis)

1. NAME OF THE MEDICINAL PRODUCT

Stemetil injection 1.25% w/v

2. QUALITATIVE AND QUANTITATIVE COMPOSITION

Each 1 ml of Stemetil injection contains 12.5 mg prochlorperazine mesilate.

3. PHARMACEUTICAL FORM

Colourless sterile solution.

4. CLINICAL PARTICULARS

4.1 Therapeutic indications

Stemetil is a potent phenothiazine neuroleptic.

Uses: The treatment of nausea and vomiting and in schizophrenia (particularly the chronic stage) and acute mania.

4.2 Posology and method of administration

Adults

For deep intramuscular injection.

Indication	Dosage
Treatment of nausea and vomiting	12.5 mg by deep i.m. injection followed by oral medication 6 hours later if necessary.
Schizophrenia and other psychotic disorders	12.5 mg to 25 mg b.i.d. or t.d.s. by deep i.m. injection until oral treatment becomes possible.

Children

Intramuscular Stemetil should not be given to children.

Elderly

A lower dose is recommended. Please see Special Warnings and Precautions for Use.

4.3 Contraindications

Known hypersensitivity to prochlorperazine or to any of the other ingredients.The use of Stemetil injection is contraindicated in children as it has been associated with dystonic reactions after the cumulative dose of 0.5 mg/kg.

4.4 Special warnings and special precautions for use

Stemetil should be avoided in patients with liver or renal dysfunction, Parkinson's disease, hypothyroidism, cardiac failure, phaeochromocytoma, myasthenia gravis, prostate hypertrophy. It should be avoided in patients known to be hypersensitive to phenothiazines or with a history of narrow angle glaucoma or agranulocytosis.

Close monitoring is required in patients with epilepsy or a history of seizures, as phenothiazines may lower the seizure threshold.

As agranulocytosis has been reported, regular monitoring of the complete blood count is recommended. The occurrence of unexplained infections or fever may be evidence of blood dyscrasia (see section 4.8 below), and requires immediate haematological investigation.

It is imperative that treatment be discontinued in the event of unexplained fever, as this may be a sign of neuroleptic malignant syndrome (pallor, hyperthermia, autonomic dysfunction, altered consciousness, muscle rigidity). Signs of autonomic dysfunction, such as sweating and arterial instability, may precede the onset of hyperthermia and serve as early warning signs. Although neuroleptic malignant syndrome may be idiosyncratic in origin, dehydration and organic brain disease are predisposing factors.

Acute withdrawal symptoms, including nausea, vomiting and insomnia, have very rarely been reported following the abrupt cessation of high doses of neuroleptics. Relapse may also occur, and the emergence of extrapyramidal reactions has been reported. Therefore, gradual withdrawal is advisable.

In schizophrenia, the response to neuroleptic treatment may be delayed. If treatment is withdrawn, the recurrence of symptoms may not become apparent for some time.

As with other neuroleptics, cases of QT interval prolongation have been reported with prochlorperazine very rarely (see section 4.8, below). The risk-benefit should be fully assessed before Stemetil treatment is commenced, and patients with predisposing factors for ventricular arrhythmias, (e.g. cardiac disease; metabolic abnormalities such as hypokalaemia, hypocalcaemia or hypomagnesaemia; starvation; alcohol abuse; concomitant therapy with other drugs known to prolong the QT interval) should be carefully monitored (biochemical status and ECG), particularly during the initial phase of treatment.

As with all antipsychotic drugs, Stemetil should not be used alone where depression is predominant. However, it may be combined with antidepressant therapy to treat those conditions in which depression and psychosis coexist.

Because of the risk of photosensitisation, patients should be advised to avoid exposure to direct sunlight.

To prevent skin sensitisation in those frequently handling preparations of phenothiazines, the greatest care must be taken to avoid contact of the drug with the skin (see section 4.8, below).

Postural hypotension with tachycardia as well as local pain or nodule formation may occur after i.m. administration.

It should be used with caution in the elderly, particularly during very hot or very cold weather (risk of hyper-, hypothermia).

The elderly are particularly susceptible to postural hypotension.

Stemetil should be used cautiously in the elderly owing to their susceptibility to drugs acting on the central nervous system and a lower initial dosage is recommended. There is an increased risk of drug-induced Parkinsonism in the elderly particularly after prolonged use. Care should also be taken not to confuse the adverse effects of Stemetil, e.g. orthostatic hypotension, with the effects due to the underlying disorder.

4.5 Interaction with other medicinal products and other forms of Interaction

Adrenaline must not be used in patients overdosed with Stemetil (see section 4.9, below).

The CNS depressant actions of neuroleptic agents may be intensified (additively) by alcohol, barbiturates and other sedatives. Respiratory depression may occur.

Anticholinergic agents may reduce the antipsychotic effect of neuroleptics and the mild anticholinergic effect of neuroleptics may be enhanced by other anticholinergic drugs, possibly leading to constipation, heat stroke, etc.

Some drugs interfere with absorption of neuroleptic agents: antacids, anti-Parkinson drugs and lithium.

Where treatment for neuroleptic-induced extrapyramidal symptoms is required, anticholinergic antiparkinsonian agents should be used in preference to levodopa, since neuroleptics antagonise the antiparkinsonian action of dopaminergics.

High doses of neuroleptics reduce the response to hypoglycaemic agents, the dosage of which might have to be raised.

The hypotensive effect of most antihypertensive drugs especially alpha adrenoceptor blocking agents may be exaggerated by neuroleptics.

The action of some drugs may be opposed by phenothiazine neuroleptics; these include amfetamine, levodopa, clonidine, guanethidine, adrenaline.

Increases or decreases in the plasma concentrations of a number of drugs, e.g. propranolol, phenobarbital have been observed but were not of clinical significance.

Simultaneous administration of desferrioxamine and prochlorperazine has been observed to induce transient metabolic encephalopathy characterised by loss of consciousness for 48-72 hours.

There is an increased risk of arrhythmias when neuroleptics are used concurrently with drugs which prolong the QT interval, including certain antiarrhythmics, antidepressants, and other antipsychotics (see section 4.8, below).

There is an increased risk of agranulocytosis when neuroleptics are used concurrently with drugs with myelosuppressive potential, such as carbamazepine or certain antibiotics and cytotoxics.

In patients treated concurrently with neuroleptics and lithium, there have been rare reports of neurotoxicity.

4.6 Pregnancy and lactation

There is inadequate evidence of safety in pregnancy. There is evidence of harmful effects in animals. Stemetil should be avoided in pregnancy unless the physician considers it essential. Neuroleptics may occasionally prolong labour and at such time should be withheld until the cervix is dilated 3-4 cm. Possible adverse effects on the neonate include lethargy or paradoxical hyperexcitability, tremor and low apgar score.

Phenothiazines may be excreted in milk, therefore breast feeding should be suspended during treatment.

4.7 Effects on ability to drive and use machines

Patients should be warned about drowsiness during the early days of treatment and advised not to drive or operate machinery.

4.8 Undesirable effects

Generally, adverse reactions occur at a low frequency; the most common reported adverse reactions are nervous system disorders.

Adverse effects:

Blood and lymphatic system disorders: A mild leukopenia occurs in up to 30% of patients on prolonged high dosage. Agranulocytosis may occur rarely: it is not dose related (see section 4.4, above).

Endocrine: Hyperprolactinaemia which may result in galactorrhoea, gynaecomastia, amenorrhoea; impotence.

Nervous system disorders: Acute dystonia or dyskinesias, usually transitory are commoner in children and young adults, and usually occur within the first 4 days of treatment or after dosage increases.

Akathisia characteristically occurs after large initial doses.

Parkinsonism is more common in adults and the elderly. It usually develops after weeks or months of treatment. One or more of the following may be seen: tremor, rigidity, akinesia or other features of Parkinsonism. Commonly just tremor.

Tardive dyskinesia: If this occurs it is usually, but not necessarily, after prolonged or high dosage. It can even occur after treatment has been stopped. Dosage should therefore be kept low whenever possible.

Insomnia and agitation may occur.

Eye disorders: Ocular changes and the development of metallic greyish-mauve coloration of exposed skin have been noted in some individuals mainly females, who have received chlorpromazine continuously for long periods (four to eight years). This could possibly happen with Stemetil.

Cardiac disorders: Cardiac arrhythmias, including atrial arrhythmia, A-V block, ventricular tachycardia and fibrillation have been reported during neuroleptic therapy, possibly related to dosage. Pre-existing cardiac disease, old age, hypokalemia and concurrent tricyclic antidepressants may predispose. ECG changes, usually benign, include widened QT interval, ST depression, U-waves and T-wave changes (see section 4.4, above).

Vascular disorders: Hypotension, usually postural, commonly occurs. Elderly or volume depleted subjects are particularly susceptible; it is more likely to occur after intramuscular injection.

Gastrointestinal disorders: dry mouth may occur.

Respiratory, thoracic and mediastinal disorders: Respiratory depression is possible in susceptible patients. Nasal stuffiness may occur.

Hepato-biliary disorders: Jaundice, usually transient, occurs in a very small percentage of patients taking neuroleptics. A premonitory sign may be sudden onset of fever after one to three weeks of treatment followed by the development of jaundice. Neuroleptic jaundice has the biochemical and other characteristics of obstructive jaundice and is associated with obstruction of the canaliculi by bile thrombi; the frequent presence of an accompanying eosinphilia indicates the allergic nature of this phenomenon. Treatment should be withheld on the development of jaundice (see section 4.4, above).

Skin and subcutaneous tissue disorders: Contact skin sensitisation may occur rarely in those frequently handling preparations of certain phenothiazines (see section 4.4, above). Skin rashes of various kinds may also be seen in patients treated with the drug. Patients on high dosage should be warned that they may develop photosensitivity in sunny weather and should avoid exposure to direct sunlight.

General disorders and administration site conditions: Neuroleptic malignant syndrome (hyperthermia, rigidity, autonomic dysfunction and altered consciousness) may occur with any neuroleptic (see section 4.4, above).

4.9 Overdose

Symptoms of phenothiazine overdosage include drowsiness or loss of consciousness, hypotension, tachycardia, ECG changes, ventricular arrhythmias and hypothermia. Severe extrapyramidal dyskinesias may occur.

If the patient is seen sufficiently soon (up to 6 hours) after ingestion of a toxic dose, gastric lavage may be attempted. Pharmacological induction of emesis is unlikely to be of any use. Activated charcoal should be given. There is no specific antidote. Treatment is supportive.

Generalised vasodilatation may result in circulatory collapse; raising the patient's legs may suffice. In severe cases, volume expansion by intravenous fluids may be needed; infusion fluids should be warmed before administration in order not to aggravate hypothermia.

Positive inotropic agents such as dopamine may be tried if fluid replacement is insufficient to correct the circulatory collapse. Peripheral vasoconstrictor agents are not generally recommended. Avoid the use of adrenaline.

Ventricular or supraventricular tachy-arrhythmias usually respond to restoration of normal body temperature and correction of circulatory or metabolic disturbances. If persistent or life threatening, appropriate anti-arrhythmic therapy may be considered. Avoid lidocaine and, as far as possible, long acting anti-arrhythmic drugs.

Pronounced central nervous system depression requires airway maintenance or, in extreme circumstances, assisted respiration. Severe dystonic reactions usually respond to procyclidine (5-10 mg) or orphenadrine (20-40 mg) administered intramuscularly or intravenously. Convulsions should be treated with intravenous diazepam.

Neuroleptic malignant syndrome should be treated with cooling. Dantrolene sodium may be tried.

5. PHARMACOLOGICAL PROPERTIES

5.1 Pharmacodynamic properties

Stemetil is a potent phenothiazine neuroleptic.

5.2 Pharmacokinetic properties

There is little information about blood levels, distribution and excretion in humans. The rate of metabolism and excretion of phenothiazines decreases in old age.

5.3 Preclinical safety data

There are no preclinical data of relevance to the prescriber which are additional to that already included in other sections of the SPC.

6. PHARMACEUTICAL PARTICULARS

6.1 List of excipients

Stemetil injection also contains the following excipients: sodium sulphite anhydrous (E221), sodium metabisulphite powder (E223), sodium chloride, ethanolamine and water for injections (non-sterilised).

6.2 Incompatibilities

None stated.

6.3 Shelf life

60 months.

6.4 Special precautions for storage

Protect from light. Discoloured solutions should not be used.

6.5 Nature and contents of container

Stemetil injection is supplied in colourless glass ampoules in packs of 10 × 1ml.

6.6 Instructions for use and handling

None.

7. MARKETING AUTHORISATION HOLDER

Castlemead Healthcare Limited

20 Clanwilliam Terrace

Dublin 2

Ireland

8. MARKETING AUTHORISATION NUMBER(S)

PL 16946/0003

9. DATE OF FIRST AUTHORISATION/RENEWAL OF THE AUTHORISATION

1 July 1998

10. DATE OF REVISION OF THE TEXT

April 2005

Legal category: POM

Stemetil Suppositories

(sanofi-aventis)

1. NAME OF THE MEDICINAL PRODUCT

STEMETIL SUPPOSITORIES

2. QUALITATIVE AND QUANTITATIVE COMPOSITION

Each Stemetil 5 mg suppository contains 0.32% w/w prochlorperazine base, equivalent to 5 mg prochlorperazine maleate. Each Stemetil 25 mg suppository contains 0.78% w/w prochlorperazine base, equivalent to 25 mg prochlorperazine maleate

3. PHARMACEUTICAL FORM

Cream, smooth, torpedo-shaped suppositories.

4. CLINICAL PARTICULARS

4.1 Therapeutic indications

Stemetil is a potent phenothiazine neuroleptic.

Stemetil 5mg suppository: The treatment of nausea and vomiting, the prevention of post-operative vomiting. The management of nausea and vomiting and in schizophrenia (particularly the chronic stage) and acute mania.

Stemetil 25mg suppository: The treatment of nausea and vomiting and in the management of schizophrenia (particularly the chronic stage) and acute mania.

4.2 Posology and method of administration

Adults

Route of administration: Rectal.

Indication	Dosage
Treatment of nausea and vomiting	25 mg followed by oral medication 6 hours later if necessary.
For the management of nausea and vomiting due to migraine	One 5 mg suppository three times a day. In acute cases an intramuscular injection may be administered followed by the use of suppositories.

Prevention of post-operative vomiting	Two 5 mg suppositories before operation followed by two every five hours for up to 20 hours thereafter.
Schizophrenia and other psychotic disorders	25 mg b.d. or t.d.s. until oral treatment becomes possible.

Children

Stemetil suppositories should not be given to children.

Elderly

A lower dose is recommended. Please see Special Warnings and Precautions for Use.

4.3 Contraindications

Children under 12 years of age. Known hypersensitivity to prochlorperazine or to any of the other ingredients.

4.4 Special warnings and special precautions for use

Stemetil should be avoided in patients with liver or renal dysfunction, Parkinson's disease, hypothyroidism, cardiac failure, phaeochromocytoma, myasthenia gravis, prostate hypertrophy. It should be avoided in patients known to be hypersensitive to phenothiazines or with a history of narrow angle glaucoma or agranulocytosis.

Close monitoring is required in patients with epilepsy or a history of seizures, as phenothiazines may lower the seizure threshold.

As agranulocytosis has been reported, regular monitoring of the complete blood count is recommended.

It is imperative that treatment be discontinued in the event of unexplained fever, as this may be a sign of neuroleptic malignant syndrome (pallor, hyperthermia, autonomic dysfunction, altered consciousness, muscle rigidity). Signs of autonomic dysfunction, such as sweating and arterial instability, may precede the onset of hyperthermia and serve as early warning signs. Although neuroleptic malignant syndrome may be idiosyncratic in origin, dehydration and organic brain disease are predisposing factors.

The occurrence of unexplained infections or fever may be evidence of blood dyscrasia (see section 4.8 below), and requires immediate haematological investigation.

Acute withdrawal symptoms, including nausea, vomiting and insomnia, have very rarely been reported following the abrupt cessation of high doses of neuroleptics. Relapse may also occur, and the emergence of extrapyramidal reactions has been reported. Therefore, gradual withdrawal is advisable.

In schizophrenia, the response to neuroleptic treatment may be delayed. If treatment is withdrawn, the recurrence of symptoms may not become apparent for some time.

As with other neuroleptics, cases of QT interval prolongation have been reported with prochlorperazine very rarely (see section 4.8, below). The risk-benefit should be fully assessed before Stemetil treatment is commenced, and patients with predisposing factors for ventricular arrhythmias, (e.g. cardiac disease; metabolic abnormalities such as hypokalaemia, hypocalcaemia or hypomagnesaemia; starvation; alcohol abuse; concomitant therapy with other drugs known to prolong the QT interval) should be carefully monitored (biochemical status and ECG), particularly during the initial phase of treatment.

As with all antipsychotic drugs, Stemetil should not be used alone where depression is predominant. However, it may be combined with antidepressant therapy to treat those conditions in which depression and psychosis coexist.

Because of the risk of photosensitisation, patients should be advised to avoid exposure to direct sunlight.

To prevent skin sensitisation in those frequently handling preparations of phenothiazines, the greatest care must be taken to avoid contact of the drug with the skin (see section 4.8, below).

It should be used with caution in the elderly, particularly during very hot or very cold weather (risk of hyper-, hypothermia).

The elderly are particularly susceptible to postural hypotension.

Stemetil should be used cautiously in the elderly owing to their susceptibility to drugs acting on the central nervous system and a lower initial dosage is recommended. There is an increased risk of drug-induced Parkinsonism in the elderly particularly after prolonged use. Care should also be taken not to confuse the adverse effects of Stemetil, e.g. orthostatic hypotension, with the effects due to the underlying disorder.

4.5 Interaction with other medicinal products and other forms of Interaction

Adrenaline must not be used in patients overdosed with Stemetil (see section 4.9, below).

The CNS depressant actions of neuroleptic agents may be intensified (additively) by alcohol, barbiturates and other sedatives. Respiratory depression may occur.

Anticholinergic agents may reduce the antipsychotic effect of neuroleptics and the mild anticholinergic effect of neuroleptics may be enhanced by other anticholinergic drugs, possibly leading to constipation, heat stroke, etc.

Some drugs interfere with absorption of neuroleptic agents: antacids, anti-Parkinson drugs and lithium.

Where treatment for neuroleptic-induced extrapyramidal symptoms is required, anticholinergic antiparkinsonian agents should be used in preference to levodopa, since neuroleptics antagonise the antiparkinsonian action of dopaminergics.

High doses of neuroleptics reduce the response of to hypoglycaemic agents, the dosage of which might have to be raised.

The hypotensive effect of most antihypertensive drugs especially alpha adrenoceptor blocking agents may be exaggerated by neuroleptics.

The action of some drugs may be opposed by phenothiazine neuroleptics; these include amphetamine, levodopa, clonidine, guanethidine, adrenaline.

Increases or decreases in the plasma concentrations of a number of drugs, e.g. propranolol, phenobarbitone have been observed but were not of clinical significance.

Simultaneous administration of desferrioxamine and prochlorperazine has been observed to induce transient metabolic encephalopathy characterised by loss of consciousness for 48-72 hours.

There is an increased risk of arrhythmias when neuroleptics are used concurrently with drugs which prolong the QT interval, including certain antiarrhythmics, antidepressants, and other antipsychotics (see section 4.8, below).

There is an increased risk of agranulocytosis when neuroleptics are used concurrently with drugs with myelosuppressive potential, such as carbamazepine or certain antibiotics and cytotoxics.

In patients treated concurrently with neuroleptics and lithium, there have been rare reports of neurotoxicity.

4.6 Pregnancy and lactation

There is inadequate evidence of safety in pregnancy. There is evidence of harmful effects in animals. Stemetil should be avoided in pregnancy unless the physician considers it essential. Neuroleptics may occasionally prolong labour and at such time should be withheld until the cervix is dilated 3-4 cm. Possible adverse effects on the neonate include lethargy or paradoxical hyperexcitability, tremor and low apgar score.

Phenothiazines may be excreted in milk, therefore breast feeding should be suspended during treatment.

4.7 Effects on ability to drive and use machines

Patients should be warned about drowsiness during the early days of treatment and advised not to drive or operate machinery.

4.8 Undesirable effects

Generally, adverse reactions occur at a low frequency; the most common reported adverse reactions are nervous system disorders.

Adverse effects:

Blood and lymphatic system disorders: A mild leukopenia occurs in up to 30% of patients on prolonged high dosage. Agranulocytosis may occur rarely: it is not dose related (see section 4.4, above).

Endocrine: Hyperprolactinaemia which may result in galactorrhoea, gynaecomastia, amenorrhoea; impotence.

Nervous system disorders: Acute dystonia or dyskinesias, usually transitory are commoner in children and young adults, and usually occur within the first 4 days of treatment or after dosage increases.

Akathisia characteristically occurs after large initial doses.

Parkinsonism is more common in adults and the elderly. It usually develops after weeks or months of treatment. One or more of the following may be seen: tremor, rigidity, akinesia or other features of Parkinsonism. Commonly just tremor.

Tardive dyskinesia: If this occurs it is usually, but not necessarily, after prolonged or high dosage. It can even occur after treatment has been stopped. Dosage should therefore be kept low whenever possible.

Insomnia and agitation may occur.

Eye disorders: Ocular changes and the development of metallic greyish-mauve coloration of exposed skin have been noted in some individuals mainly females, who have received chlorpromazine continuously for long periods (four to eight years). This could possibly happen with Stemetil.

Cardiac disorders: Cardiac arrhythmias, including atrial arrhythmia, A-V block, ventricular tachycardia and fibrillation have been reported during neuroleptic therapy, possibly related to dosage. Pre-existing cardiac disease, old age, hypokalemia and concurrent tricyclic antidepressants may predispose. ECG changes, usually benign, include widened QT interval, ST depression, U-waves and T-wave changes (see section 4.4, above).

Vascular disorders: Hypotension, usually postural, commonly occurs. Elderly or volume depleted subjects are particularly susceptible; it is more likely to occur after intramuscular injection.

Gastrointestinal disorders: dry mouth may occur.

Respiratory, thoracic and mediastinal disorders: Respiratory depression is possible in susceptible patients. Nasal stuffiness may occur.

Hepato-biliary disorders: Jaundice, usually transient, occurs in a very small percentage of patients taking neuroleptics. A premonitory sign may be sudden onset of fever after one to three weeks of treatment followed by the development of jaundice. Neuroleptic jaundice has the biochemical and other characteristics of obstructive jaundice and is associated with obstruction of the canaliculi by bile thrombi; the frequent presence of an accompanying eosinphilia indicates the allergic nature of this phenomenon. Treatment should be withheld on the development of jaundice (see section 4.4, above).

Skin and subcutaneous tissue disorders: Contact skin sensitisation may occur rarely in those frequently handling preparations of certain phenothiazines (see section 4.4, above). Skin rashes of various kinds may also be seen in patients treated with the drug. Patients on high dosage should be warned that they may develop photosensitivity in sunny weather and should avoid exposure to direct sunlight.

General disorders and administration site conditions: Neuroleptic malignant syndrome (hyperthermia, rigidity, autonomic dysfunction and altered consciousness) may occur with any neuroleptic (see section 4.4, above).

4.9 Overdose

Symptoms of phenothiazine overdosage include drowsiness or loss of consciousness, hypotension, tachycardia, ECG changes, ventricular arrhythmias and hypothermia. Severe extrapyramidal dyskinesias may occur.

If the patient is seen sufficiently soon (up to 6 hours) after ingestion of a toxic dose, gastric lavage may be attempted. Pharmacological induction of emesis is unlikely to be of any use. Activated charcoal should be given. There is no specific antidote. Treatment is supportive.

Generalised vasodilatation may result in circulatory collapse; raising the patient's legs may suffice. In severe cases, volume expansion by intravenous fluids may be needed; infusion fluids should be warmed before administration in order not to aggravate hypothermia.

Positive inotropic agents such as dopamine may be tried if fluid replacement is insufficient to correct the circulatory collapse. Peripheral vasoconstrictor agents are not generally recommended. Avoid the use of adrenaline.

Ventricular or supraventricular tachy-arrhythmias usually respond to restoration of normal body temperature and correction of circulatory or metabolic disturbances. If persistent or life threatening, appropriate anti-arrhythmic therapy may be considered. Avoid lignocaine and, as far as possible, long acting anti-arrhythmic drugs.

Pronounced central nervous system depression requires airway maintenance or, in extreme circumstances, assisted respiration. Severe dystonic reactions usually respond to procyclidine (5-10 mg) or orphenadrine (20-40 mg) administered intramuscularly or intravenously. Convulsions should be treated with intravenous diazepam.

Neuroleptic malignant syndrome should be treated with cooling. Dantrolene sodium may be tried.

5. PHARMACOLOGICAL PROPERTIES

5.1 Pharmacodynamic properties

Stemetil is a potent phenothiazine neuroleptic.

5.2 Pharmacokinetic properties

There is little information about blood levels, distribution and excretion in humans. The rate of metabolism and excretion of phenothiazines decreases in old age.

5.3 Preclinical safety data

There are no preclinical data of relevance to the prescriber which are additional to that already included in other sections of the SPC.

6. PHARMACEUTICAL PARTICULARS

6.1 List of excipients

Stemetil suppositories also contain suppository base E75 and suppository base W35.

6.2 Incompatibilities

None stated.

6.3 Shelf life

36 months.

6.4 Special precautions for storage

Store below 25°C. Protect from light.

6.5 Nature and contents of container

Suppositories enclosed automatically during filling in preformed strips of PVC and polyethylene being the inner surface in contact with the product. Sealing of bandolier effected by the action of heat and pressure. Stemetil suppositories are available in packs of 10.

6.6 Instructions for use and handling

None stated.

Administrative Data

7. MARKETING AUTHORISATION HOLDER

Castlemead Healthcare Limited

20 Clanwilliam Terrace

Dublin 2

Ireland

8. MARKETING AUTHORISATION NUMBER(S)
Suppositories 5mg PL 16946/0004

Suppositories 25mg PL 16946/0005

9. DATE OF FIRST AUTHORISATION/RENEWAL OF THE AUTHORISATION
1 July 1998

10. DATE OF REVISION OF THE TEXT
July 2002

11. Legal Classification
POM

Stemetil Syrup

(sanofi-aventis)

1. NAME OF THE MEDICINAL PRODUCT
Stemetil Syrup

2. QUALITATIVE AND QUANTITATIVE COMPOSITION
The active component of the Stemetil syrup is prochlorperazine mesilate 5 mg per 5 ml.

3. PHARMACEUTICAL FORM
A dark straw coloured syrup.

4. CLINICAL PARTICULARS
4.1 Therapeutic indications
Vertigo due to Meniere's Syndrome, labyrinthitis and other causes, and for nausea and vomiting from whatever cause including that associated with migraine. It may also be used for schizophrenia (particularly in the chronic stage), acute mania and as an adjunct to the short-term management of anxiety.

4.2 Posology and method of administration
Adults

Indication	**Dosage**
Prevention of nausea and vomiting	5 to 10 mg b.d. or t.d.s.
Treatment of nausea and vomiting	20 mg stat, followed if necessary by 10 mg two hours later.
Vertigo and Meniere's syndrome	5 mg t.d.s. increasing if necessary to a total of 30 mg daily. After several weeks dosage may be reduced gradually to 5-10 mg daily.
Adjunct in the short term management of anxiety	15-20 mg daily in divided doses initially but this may be increased if necessary to a maximum of 40 mg daily in divided doses.
Schizophrenia and other psychotic disorders	Usual effective daily oral dosage is in the order of 75-100 mg daily. Patients vary widely in response. The following schedule is suggested: Initially 12.5 mg twice daily for 7 days, the daily amount being subsequently increased by 12.5 mg at 4 to 7 days interval until a satisfactory response is obtained. After some weeks at the effective dosage, an attempt should be made reduce this dosage. Total daily amounts as small as 50 mg or even 25 mg have sometimes been found to be effective.

Children

Indication	**Dosage**
Prevention and treatment of nausea and vomiting	If it is considered unavoidable to use Stemetil for a child, the dosage is 0.25 mg/kg bodyweight two or three **times** a day. Stemetil is not recommended for children weighing less than 10 kg or below 1 year of age.

Elderly
A lower dose is recommended - please see Special Warnings and Precautions for Use.

4.3 Contraindications
Known hypersensitivity to prochlorperazine or to any of the other ingredients.

4.4 Special warnings and special precautions for use
Stemetil should be avoided in patients with liver or renal dysfunction, Parkinson's disease, hypothyroidism, cardiac failure, phaeochromocytoma, myasthenia gravis, prostate hypertrophy. It should be avoided in patients known to be hypersensitive to phenothiazines or with a history of narrow angle glaucoma or agranulocytosis.

Close monitoring is required in patients with epilepsy or a history of seizures, as phenothiazines may lower the seizure threshold.

As agranulocytosis has been reported, regular monitoring of the complete blood count is recommended. The occurrence of unexplained infections or fever may be evidence of blood dyscrasia (see section 4.8 below), and requires immediate haematological investigation.

It is imperative that treatment be discontinued in the event of unexplained fever, as this may be a sign of neuroleptic malignant syndrome (pallor, hyperthermia, autonomic dysfunction, altered consciousness, muscle rigidity). Signs of autonomic dysfunction, such as sweating and arterial instability, may precede the onset of hyperthermia and serve as early warning signs. Although neuroleptic malignant syndrome may be idiosyncratic in origin, dehydration and organic brain disease are predisposing factors.

Acute withdrawal symptoms, including nausea, vomiting and insomnia, have very rarely been reported following the abrupt cessation of high doses of neuroleptics. Relapse may also occur, and the emergence of extrapyramidal reactions has been reported. Therefore, gradual withdrawal is advisable.

In schizophrenia, the response to neuroleptic treatment may be delayed. If treatment is withdrawn, the recurrence of symptoms may not become apparent for some time.

As with other neuroleptics, cases of QT interval prolongation have been reported with prochlorperazine very rarely (see section 4.8, below). The risk-benefit should be fully assessed before Stemetil treatment is commenced, and patients with predisposing factors for ventricular arrhythmias, (e.g. cardiac disease; metabolic abnormalities such as hypokalaemia, hypocalcaemia or hypomagnesaemia; starvation; alcohol abuse; concomitant therapy with other drugs known to prolong the QT interval) should be carefully monitored (biochemical status and ECG), particularly during the initial phase of treatment.

As with all antipsychotic drugs, Stemetil should not be used alone where depression is predominant. However, it may be combined with antidepressant therapy to treat those conditions in which depression and psychosis coexist.

Because of the risk of photosensitisation, patients should be advised to avoid exposure to direct sunlight.

To prevent skin sensitisation in those frequently handling preparations of phenothiazines, the greatest care must be taken to avoid contact of the drug with the skin (see section 4.8, below).

It should be used with caution in the elderly, particularly during very hot or very cold weather (risk of hyper-, hypothermia).

The elderly are particularly susceptible to postural hypotension.

Stemetil should be used cautiously in the elderly owing to their susceptibility to drugs acting on the central nervous system and a lower initial dosage is recommended. There is an increased risk of drug-induced Parkinsonism in the elderly particularly after prolonged use. Care should also be taken not to confuse the adverse effects of Stemetil, e.g. orthostatic hypotension, with the effects due to the underlying disorder.

Children: Stemetil has been associated with dystonic reactions particularly after a cumulative dosage of 0.5 mg/kg. It should therefore be used cautiously in children.

4.5 Interaction with other medicinal products and other forms of Interaction
Adrenaline must not be used in patients overdosed with Stemetil (see section 4.9, below).

The CNS depressant actions of neuroleptic agents may be intensified (additively) by alcohol, barbiturates and other sedatives. Respiratory depression may occur.

Anticholinergic agents may reduce the antipsychotic effect of neuroleptics and the mild anticholinergic effect of neuroleptics may be enhanced by other anticholinergic drugs, possibly leading to constipation, heat stroke, etc.

Some drugs interfere with absorption of neuroleptic agents: antacids, anti-Parkinson drugs and lithium.

Where treatment for neuroleptic-induced extrapyramidal symptoms is required, anticholinergic antiparkinsonian agents should be used in preference to levodopa, since neuroleptics antagonise the antiparkinsonian action of dopaminergics.

High doses of neuroleptics reduce the response to hypoglycaemic agents, the dosage of which might have to be raised.

The hypotensive effect of most antihypertensive drugs especially alpha adrenoceptor blocking agents may be exaggerated by neuroleptics.

The action of some drugs may be opposed by phenothiazine neuroleptics; these include amfetamine, levodopa, clonidine, guanethidine, adrenaline.

Increases or decreases in the plasma concentrations of a number of drugs, e.g. propranolol, phenobarbital have been observed but were not of clinical significance.

Simultaneous administration of desferrioxamine and prochlorperazine has been observed to induce transient metabolic encephalopathy characterised by loss of consciousness for 48-72 hours.

There is an increased risk of arrhythmias when neuroleptics are used concurrently with drugs which prolong the QT interval, including certain antiarrhythmics, antidepressants, and other antipsychotics (see section 4.8, below).

There is an increased risk of agranulocytosis when neuroleptics are used concurrently with drugs with myelosuppressive potential, such as carbamazepine or certain antibiotics and cytotoxics.

In patients treated concurrently with neuroleptics and lithium, there have been rare reports of neurotoxicity.

4.6 Pregnancy and lactation
There is inadequate evidence of safety in pregnancy. There is evidence of harmful effects in animals. Stemetil should be avoided in pregnancy unless the physician considers it essential. Neuroleptics may occasionally prolong labour and at such time should be withheld until the cervix is dilated 3-4 cm. Possible adverse effects on the neonate include lethargy or paradoxical hyperexcitability, tremor and low apgar score.

Phenothiazines may be excreted in milk, therefore breast feeding should be suspended during treatment.

4.7 Effects on ability to drive and use machines
Patients should be warned about drowsiness during the early days of treatment and advised not to drive or operate machinery.

4.8 Undesirable effects
Generally, adverse reactions occur at a low frequency; the most common reported adverse reactions are nervous system disorders.

Adverse effects:

Blood and lymphatic system disorders: A mild leukopenia occurs in up to 30% of patients on prolonged high dosage. Agranulocytosis may occur rarely: it is not dose related (see section 4.4, above).

Endocrine: Hyperprolactinaemia which may result in galactorrhoea, gynaecomastia, amenorrhoea; impotence.

Nervous system disorders: Acute dystonia or dyskinesias, usually transitory are commoner in children and young adults, and usually occur within the first 4 days of treatment or after dosage increases.

Akathisia characteristically occurs after large initial doses.

Parkinsonism is more common in adults and the elderly. It usually develops after weeks or months of treatment. One or more of the following may be seen: tremor, rigidity, akinesia or other features of Parkinsonism. Commonly just tremor.

Tardive dyskinesia: If this occurs it is usually, but not necessarily, after prolonged or high dosage. It can even occur after treatment has been stopped. Dosage should therefore be kept low whenever possible.

Insomnia and agitation may occur.

Eye disorders: Ocular changes and the development of metallic greyish-mauve coloration of exposed skin have been noted in some individuals mainly females, who have received chlorpromazine continuously for long periods (four to eight years). This could possibly happen with Stemetil.

Cardiac disorders: Cardiac arrhythmias, including atrial arrhythmia, A-V block, ventricular tachycardia and fibrillation have been reported during neuroleptic therapy, possibly related to dosage. Pre-existing cardiac disease, old age, hypokalemia and concurrent tricyclic antidepressants may predispose. ECG changes, usually benign, include widened QT interval, ST depression, U-waves and T-wave changes (see section 4.4, above).

Vascular disorders: Hypotension, usually postural, commonly occurs. Elderly or volume depleted subjects are particularly susceptible; it is more likely to occur after intramuscular injection.

Gastrointestinal disorders: dry mouth may occur.

Respiratory, thoracic and mediastinal disorders: Respiratory depression is possible in susceptible patients. Nasal stuffiness may occur.

Hepato-biliary disorders: Jaundice, usually transient, occurs in a very small percentage of patients taking neuroleptics. A premonitory sign may be sudden onset of fever after one to three weeks of treatment followed by the development of jaundice. Neuroleptic jaundice has the biochemical and other characteristics of obstructive jaundice and is associated with obstruction of the canaliculi by bile thrombi; the frequent presence of an accompanying eosinphilia indicates the allergic nature of this phenomenon. Treatment should be witheld on the development of jaundice (see section 4.4, above).

Skin and subcutaneous tissue disorders: Contact skin sensitisation may occur rarely in those frequently handling preparations of certain phenothiazines (see section 4.4, above). Skin rashes of various kinds may also be seen in patients treated with the drug. Patients on high dosage should be warned that they may develop photosensitivity in sunny weather and should avoid exposure to direct sunlight.

General disorders and administration site conditions: Neuroleptic malignant syndrome (hyperthermia, rigidity, autonomic dysfunction and altered consciousness) may occur with any neuroleptic (see section 4.4, above).

4.9 Overdose

Symptoms of phenothiazine overdosage include drowsiness or loss of consciousness, hypotension, tachycardia, ECG changes, ventricular arrhythmias and hypothermia. Severe extrapyramidal dyskinesias may occur.

If the patient is seen sufficiently soon (up to 6 hours) after ingestion of a toxic dose, gastric lavage may be attempted. Pharmacological induction of emesis is unlikely to be of any use. Activated charcoal should be given. There is no specific antidote. Treatment is supportive.

Generalised vasodilatation may result in circulatory collapse; raising the patient's legs may suffice. In severe cases, volume expansion by intravenous fluids may be needed; infusion fluids should be warmed before administration in order not to aggravate hypothermia.

Positive inotropic agents such as dopamine may be tried if fluid replacement is insufficient to correct the circulatory collapse. Peripheral vasoconstrictor agents are not generally recommended. Avoid the use of adrenaline.

Ventricular or supraventricular tachy-arrhythmias usually respond to restoration of normal body temperature and correction of circulatory or metabolic disturbances. If persistent or life threatening, appropriate anti-arrhythmic therapy may be considered. Avoid lidocaineand, as far as possible, long acting anti-arrhythmic drugs.

Pronounced central nervous system depression requires airway maintenance or, in extreme circumstances, assisted respiration. Severe dystonic reactions usually respond to procyclidine (5-10 mg) or orphenadrine (20-40 mg) administered intramuscularly or intravenously. Convulsions should be treated with intravenous diazepam.

Neuroleptic malignant syndrome should be treated with cooling. Dantrolene sodium may be tried.

5. PHARMACOLOGICAL PROPERTIES

5.1 Pharmacodynamic properties

Stemetil is a potent phenothiazine neuroleptic.

5.2 Pharmacokinetic properties

There is little information about blood levels, distribution and excretion in humans. The rate of metabolism and excretion of phenothiazines decreases in old age.

5.3 Preclinical safety data

There are no preclinical data of relevance to the prescriber which are additional to that already included in other sections of the SPC.

6. PHARMACEUTICAL PARTICULARS

6.1 List of excipients

Sucrose, Tween 80. (E433), Zimm banana 504, caramel HT (E150a), citric acid anhydrous (E330), sodium citrate gran. (E331), sodium benzoate (E211), sodium sulphite anhydrous (E221), sodium metabisulphite powder(E223), ascorbic acid L(+) (E300) and demineralised water.

6.2 Incompatibilities

None stated.

6.3 Shelf life

36 months.

6.4 Special precautions for storage

Store protected from light.

6.5 Nature and contents of container

Stemetil Syrup is available in amber glass bottles containing 100 and 125 ml. Rolled on pilfer proof aluminium cap and a PVDC emulsion coated wad or HDPE/ Polypropylene child resistant cap with a tamper evident band.

6.6 Instructions for use and handling

None.

7. MARKETING AUTHORISATION HOLDER

Castlemead Healthcare Limited

20 Clanwilliam Terrace

Dublin 2

Ireland

8. MARKETING AUTHORISATION NUMBER(S)

PL 16946/0008

9. DATE OF FIRST AUTHORISATION/RENEWAL OF THE AUTHORISATION

1 July 1998

10. DATE OF REVISION OF THE TEXT

September 2004

Legal Category: POM

Stemetil Tablets 25mg

(sanofi-aventis)

1. NAME OF THE MEDICINAL PRODUCT

Stemetil tablets 25 mg

2. QUALITATIVE AND QUANTITATIVE COMPOSITION

The active component of the Stemetil tablets is prochlorperazine maleate BP 25 mg.

3. PHARMACEUTICAL FORM

Off-white to pale cream coloured circular tablets for oral use. The tablets are marked on one face 'STEMETIL' around a centrally impressed '25', a breakline on the reverse.

4. CLINICAL PARTICULARS

4.1 Therapeutic indications

Schizophrenia (particularly in the chronic stage) and acute mania.

4.2 Posology and method of administration

Adults

Indication	Dosage
Schizophrenia and other psychotic disorders	Usual effective daily oral dosage is in the order of 75-100 mg daily. Patients vary widely in response. The following schedule is suggested: Initially 12.5 mg twice daily for 7 days, the daily amount being subsequently increased by 12.5 mg at 4 to 7 days interval until a satisfactory response is obtained. After some weeks at the effective dosage, an attempt should be made reduce this dosage. Total daily amounts as small as 50 mg or even 25 mg have sometimes been found to be effective.

Elderly

A lower dose is recommended - please see Special Warnings and Precautions for Use.

4.3 Contraindications

Known hypersensitivity to prochlorperazine or to any of the other ingredients.

4.4 Special warnings and special precautions for use

Stemetil should be avoided in patients with liver or renal dysfunction, Parkinson's disease, hypothyroidism, cardiac failure, phaeochromocytoma, myasthenia gravis, prostate hypertrophy. It should be avoided in patients known to be hypersensitive to phenothiazines or with a history of narrow angle glaucoma or agranulocytosis.

Close monitoring is required in patients with epilepsy or a history of seizures, as phenothiazines may lower the seizure threshold.

As agranulocytosis has been reported, regular monitoring of the complete blood count is recommended. The occurrence of unexplained infections or fever may be evidence of blood dyscrasia (see section 4.8 below), and requires immediate haematological investigation.

It is imperative that treatment be discontinued in the event of unexplained fever, as this may be a sign of neuroleptic malignant syndrome (pallor, hyperthermia, autonomic dysfunction, altered consciousness, muscle rigidity). Signs of autonomic dysfunction, such as sweating and arterial instability, may precede the onset of hyperthermia and serve as early warning signs. Although neuroleptic malignant syndrome may be idiosyncratic in origin, dehydration and organic brain disease are predisposing factors.

Acute withdrawal symptoms, including nausea, vomiting and insomnia, have very rarely been reported following the abrupt cessation of high doses of neuroleptics. Relapse may also occur, and the emergence of extrapyramidal reactions has been reported. Therefore, gradual withdrawal is advisable.

In schizophrenia, the response to neuroleptic treatment may be delayed. If treatment is withdrawn, the recurrence of symptoms may not become apparent for some time.

As with other neuroleptics, cases of QT interval prolongation have been reported with prochlorperazine very rarely (see section 4.8, below). The risk-benefit should be fully assessed before Stemetil treatment is commenced, and patients with predisposing factors for ventricular arrhythmias, (e.g. cardiac disease; metabolic abnormalities such as hypokalaemia, hypocalcaemia or hypomagnesaemia; starvation; alcohol abuse; concomitant therapy with other drugs known to prolong the QT interval) should be carefully monitored (biochemical status and ECG), particularly during the initial phase of treatment.

As with all antipsychotic drugs, Stemetil should not be used alone where depression is predominant. However, it may be combined with antidepressant therapy to treat those conditions in which depression and psychosis coexist.

Because of the risk of photosensitisation, patients should be advised to avoid exposure to direct sunlight.

To prevent skin sensitisation in those frequently handling preparations of phenothiazines, the greatest care must be taken to avoid contact of the drug with the skin (see section 4.8, below).

It should be used with caution in the elderly, particularly during very hot or very cold weather (risk of hyper-, hypothermia).

The elderly are particularly susceptible to postural hypotension.

Stemetil should be used cautiously in the elderly owing to their susceptibility to drugs acting on the central nervous system and a lower initial dosage is recommended. There is an increased risk of drug-induced Parkinsonism in the elderly particularly after prolonged use. Care should also be taken not to confuse the adverse effects of Stemetil, e.g. orthostatic hypotension, with the effects due to the underlying disorder.

4.5 Interaction with other medicinal products and other forms of Interaction

Adrenaline must not be used in patients overdosed with Stemetil (see section 4.9, below).

The CNS depressant actions of neuroleptic agents may be intensified (additively) by alcohol, barbiturates and other sedatives. Respiratory depression may occur.

Anticholinergic agents may reduce the antipsychotic effect of neuroleptics andthe mild anticholinergic effect of neuroleptics may be enhanced by other anticholinergic drugs, possibly leading to constipation, heat stroke, etc.

Some drugs interfere with absorption of neuroleptic agents: antacids, anti-Parkinson drugs and lithium.

Where treatment for neuroleptic-induced extrapyramidal symptoms is required, anticholinergic antiparkinsonian agents should be used in preference to levodopa, since neuroleptics antagonise the antiparkinsonian action of dopaminergics.

High doses of neuroleptics reduce the response to hypoglycaemic agents, the dosage of which might have to be raised.

The hypotensive effect of most antihypertensive drugs especially alpha adrenoceptor blocking agents may be exaggerated by neuroleptics.

The action of some drugs may be opposed by phenothiazine neuroleptics; these include amphetamine, levodopa, clonidine, guanethidine, adrenaline.

Increases or decreases in the plasma concentrations of a number of drugs, e.g. propranolol, phenobarbitone have been observed but were not of clinical significance.

Simultaneous administration of desferrioxamine and prochlorperazine has been observed to induce transient metabolic encephalopathy characterised by loss of consciousness for 48-72 hours.

There is an increased risk of arrhythmias when neuroleptics are used concurrently with drugs which prolong the QT interval, including certain antiarrhythmics, antidepressants, and other antipsychotics (see section 4.8, below).

There is an increased risk of agranulocytosis when neuroleptics are used concurrently with drugs with myelosuppressive potential, such as carbamazepine or certain antibiotics and cytotoxics.

In patients treated concurrently with neuroleptics and lithium, there have been rare reports of neurotoxicity.

4.6 Pregnancy and lactation

There is inadequate evidence of safety in pregnancy. There is evidence of harmful effects in animals. Stemetil should be avoided in pregnancy unless the physician considers it essential. Neuroleptics may occasionally prolong labour and at such time should be withheld until the cervix is dilated 3-4 cm. Possible adverse effects on the neonate include lethargy or paradoxical hyperexcitability, tremor and low apgar score.

Phenothiazines may be excreted in milk, therefore breast feeding should be suspended during treatment.

4.7 Effects on ability to drive and use machines

Patients should be warned about drowsiness during the early days of treatment and advised not to drive or operate machinery.

4.8 Undesirable effects

Generally, adverse reactions occur at a low frequency; the most common reported adverse reactions are nervous system disorders.

Adverse effects:

Blood and lymphatic system disorders: A mild leukopenia occurs in up to 30% of patients on prolonged high dosage. Agranulocytosis may occur rarely: it is not dose related (see section 4.4, above).

Endocrine: Hyperprolactinaemia which may result in galactorrhoea, gynaecomastia, amenorrhoea; impotence.

Nervous system disorders: Acute dystonia or dyskinesias, usually transitory are commoner in children and young adults, and usually occur within the first 4 days of treatment or after dosage increases.

Akathisia characteristically occurs after large initial doses.

Parkinsonism is more common in adults and the elderly. It usually develops after weeks or months of treatment. One or more of the following may be seen: tremor, rigidity, akinesia or other features of Parkinsonism. Commonly just tremor.

Tardive dyskinesia: If this occurs it is usually, but not necessarily, after prolonged or high dosage. It can even occur after treatment has been stopped. Dosage should therefore be kept low whenever possible.

Insomnia and agitation may occur.

Eye disorders: Ocular changes and the development of metallic greyish-mauve coloration of exposed skin have been noted in some individuals mainly females, who have received chlorpromazine continuously for long periods (up four to eight years). This could possibly happen with Stemetil.

Cardiac disorders: Cardiac arrhythmias, including atrial arrhythmia, A-V block, ventricular tachycardia and fibrillation have been reported during neuroleptic therapy, possibly related to dosage. Pre-existing cardiac disease, old age, hypokalemia and concurrent tricyclic antidepressants may predispose. ECG changes, usually benign, include widened QT interval, ST depression, U-waves and T-wave changes (see section 4.4, above).

Vascular disorders: Hypotension, usually postural, commonly occurs. Elderly or volume depleted subjects are particularly susceptible; it is more likely to occur after intramuscular injection.

Gastrointestinal disorders: dry mouth may occur.

Respiratory, thoracic and mediastinal disorders: Respiratory depression is possible in susceptible patients. Nasal stuffiness may occur.

Hepato-biliary disorders: Jaundice, usually transient, occurs in a very small percentage of patients taking neuroleptics. A premonitory sign may be sudden onset of fever after one to three weeks of treatment followed by the development of jaundice. Neuroleptic jaundice has the biochemical and other characteristics of obstructive jaundice and is associated with obstruction of the canaliculi by bile thrombi; the frequent presence of an accompanying eosinphilia indicates the allergic nature of this phenomenon. Treatment should be withheld on the development of jaundice (see section 4.4, above).

Skin and subcutaneous tissue disorders: Contact skin sensitisation may occur rarely in those frequently handling preparations of certain phenothiazines (see section 4.4, above).Skin rashes of various kinds may also be seen in patients treated with the drug. Patients on high dosage should be warned that they may develop photosensitivity in sunny weather and should avoid exposure to direct sunlight.

General disorders and administration site conditions: Neuroleptic malignant syndrome (hyperthermia, rigidity, autonomic dysfunction and altered consciousness) may occur with any neuroleptic (see section 4.4, above).

4.9 Overdose

Symptoms of phenothiazine overdosage include drowsiness or loss of consciousness, hypotension, tachycardia, ECG changes, ventricular arrhythmias and hypothermia. Severe extrapyramidal dyskinesias may occur.

If the patient is seen sufficiently soon (up to 6 hours) after ingestion of a toxic dose, gastric lavage may be attempted. Pharmacological induction of emesis is unlikely to be of any use. Activated charcoal should be given. There is no specific antidote. Treatment is supportive.

Generalised vasodilatation may result in circulatory collapse; raising the patient's legs may suffice. In severe cases, volume expansion by intravenous fluids may be needed; infusion fluids should be warmed before administration in order not to aggravate hypothermia.

Positive inotropic agents such as dopamine may be tried if fluid replacement is insufficient to correct the circulatory collapse. Peripheral vasoconstrictor agents are not generally recommended. Avoid the use of adrenaline.

Ventricular or supraventricular tachy-arrhythmias usually respond to restoration of normal body temperature and correction of circulatory or metabolic disturbances. If persistent or life threatening, appropriate anti-arrhythmic therapy may be considered. Avoid lignocaine and, as far as possible, long acting anti-arrhythmic drugs.

Pronounced central nervous system depression requires airway maintenance or, in extreme circumstances, assisted respiration. Severe dystonic reactions usually respond to procyclidine (5-10 mg) or orphenadrine (20-40 mg) administered intramuscularly or intravenously. Convulsions should be treated with intravenous diazepam.

Neuroleptic malignant syndrome should be treated with cooling. Dantrolene sodium may be tried.

5. PHARMACOLOGICAL PROPERTIES

5.1 Pharmacodynamic properties

Stemetil is a potent phenothiazine neuroleptic.

5.2 Pharmacokinetic properties

There is little information about blood levels, distribution and excretion in humans. The rate of metabolism and excretion of phenothiazines decreases in old age.

5.3 Preclinical safety data

There are no preclinical data of relevance to the prescriber which are additional to that already included in other sections of the SPC.

6. PHARMACEUTICAL PARTICULARS

6.1 List of excipients

Stemetil tablets also contain the following excipients: lactose BP, starch maize BP, aerosil (E551) and magnesium stearate BP.

6.2 Incompatibilities

None stated.

6.3 Shelf life

60 months.

6.4 Special precautions for storage

Store protected from light.

6.5 Nature and contents of container

Stemetil tablets 25 mg are available in PVDC coated UPVC/aluminium foil blisters containing 56 tablets.

6.6 Instructions for use and handling

None.

7. MARKETING AUTHORISATION HOLDER

Castlemead Healthcare Limited
20 Clanwilliam Terrace
Dublin 2
Ireland

8. MARKETING AUTHORISATION NUMBER(S)

PL 16946/0007

9. DATE OF FIRST AUTHORISATION/RENEWAL OF THE AUTHORISATION

1 July 1998

10. DATE OF REVISION OF THE TEXT

July 2002

Legal category: POM

Stemetil Tablets 5mg

(sanofi-aventis)

1. NAME OF THE MEDICINAL PRODUCT

Stemetil tablets 5mg

2. QUALITATIVE AND QUANTITATIVE COMPOSITION

The active component of the Stemetil tablets is prochlorperazine maleate BP 5 mg

3. PHARMACEUTICAL FORM

Stemetil tablets 5 mg: Off-white to pale cream coloured circular tablets for oral use. The tablets are marked on one face 'STEMETIL' around a centrally impressed '5', reverse face plain.

4. CLINICAL PARTICULARS

4.1 Therapeutic indications

Vertigo due to Meniere's Syndrome, labyrinthis and other causes, and for nausea and vomiting from whatever cause including that associated with migraine. It may also be used for schizophrenia (particularly in the chronic stage), acute mania and as an adjunct to the short-term management of anxiety.

4.2 Posology and method of administration

Adults

Indication	Dosage
Prevention of nausea and vomiting	5 to 10 mg b.d. or t.d.s.
Treatment of nausea and vomiting	20 mg stat, followed if necessary by 10 mg two hours later.
Vertigo and Meniere's syndrome	5 mg t.d.s. increasing if necessary to a total of 30 mg daily. After several weeks dosage may be reduced gradually to 5-10 mg daily.
Adjunct in the short term management of anxiety	15-20 mg daily in divided doses initially but this may be increased if necessary to a maximum of 40 mg daily in divided doses.
Schizophrenia and other psychotic disorders	Usual effective daily oral dosage is in the order of 75-100 mg daily. Patients vary widely in response. The following schedule is suggested: Initially 12.5 mg twice daily for 7 days, the daily amount being subsequently increased 12.5 mg at 4 to 7 days interval until a satisfactory response is obtained. After some weeks at the effective dosage, an attempt should be made reduce this dosage. Total daily amounts as small as 50 mg or even 25 mg have sometimes been found to be effective.

Children

Indication	Dosage
Prevention and treatment of nausea and vomiting	If it is considered unavoidable to use Stemetil for a child, the dosage is 0.25 mg/kg bodyweight two or three a day. Stemetil is not recommended for children weighing less than 10 Kg or below 1 year of age.

Elderly

A lower dose is recommended. Please see Special Warnings and Special Precautions for Use.

4.3 Contraindications

Known hypersensitivity to prochlorperazine or to any of the other ingredients.

4.4 Special warnings and special precautions for use

Stemetil should be avoided in patients with liver or renal dysfunction, Parkinson's disease, hypothyroidism, cardiac failure, phaeochromocytoma, myasthenia gravis, prostate hypertrophy. It should be avoided in patients known to be hypersensitive to phenothiazines or with a history of narrow angle glaucoma or agranulocytosis.

Close monitoring is required in patients with epilepsy or a history of seizures, as phenothiazines may lower the seizure threshold.

As agranulocytosis has been reported, regular monitoring of the complete blood count is recommended. The occurrence of unexplained infections or fever may be evidence of blood dyscrasia (see section 4.8 below), and requires immediate haematological investigation.

It is imperative that treatment be discontinued in the event of unexplained fever, as this may be a sign of neuroleptic malignant syndrome (pallor, hyperthermia, autonomic dysfunction, altered consciousness, muscle rigidity). Signs of autonomic dysfunction, such as sweating and arterial instability, may precede the onset of hyperthermia and serve as early warning signs. Although neuroleptic malignant syndrome may be idiosyncratic in origin, dehydration and organic brain disease are predisposing factors.

Acute withdrawal symptoms, including nausea, vomiting and insomnia, have very rarely been reported following the abrupt cessation of high doses of neuroleptics. Relapse may also occur, and the emergence of extrapyramidal reactions has been reported. Therefore, gradual withdrawal is advisable.

In schizophrenia, the response to neuroleptic treatment may be delayed. If treatment is withdrawn, the recurrence of symptoms may not become apparent for some time.

As with other neuroleptics, cases of QT interval prolongation have been reported with prochlorperazine very rarely (see section 4.8, below). The risk-benefit should be fully assessed before Stemetil treatment is commenced, and patients with predisposing factors for ventricular arrhythmias, (e.g. cardiac disease; metabolic abnormalities such as hypokalaemia, hypocalcaemia or hypomagnesaemia; starvation; alcohol abuse; concomitant therapy with other drugs known to prolong the QT interval) should be carefully monitored (biochemical status and ECG), particularly during the initial phase of treatment.

As with all antipsychotic drugs, Stemetil should not be used alone where depression is predominant. However, it may be combined with antidepressant therapy to treat those conditions in which depression and psychosis coexist.

Because of the risk of photosensitisation, patients should be advised to avoid exposure to direct sunlight.

To prevent skin sensitisation in those frequently handling preparations of phenothiazines, the greatest care must be taken to avoid contact of the drug with the skin (see section 4.8, below).

It should be used with caution in the elderly, particularly during very hot or very cold weather (risk of hyper-, hypothermia).

The elderly are particularly susceptible to postural hypotension.

Stemetil should be used cautiously in the elderly owing to their susceptibility to drugs acting on the central nervous system and a lower initial dosage is recommended. There is an increased risk of drug-induced Parkinsonism in the elderly particularly after prolonged use. Care should also be taken not to confuse the adverse effects of Stemetil, e.g. orthostatic hypotension, with the effects due to the underlying disorder.

Children: Stemetil has been associated with dystonic reactions particularly after a cumulative dosage of 0.5 mg/kg. It should therefore be used cautiously in children.

4.5 Interaction with other medicinal products and other forms of Interaction

Adrenaline must not be used in patients overdosed with Stemetil (see section 4.9, below).

The CNS depressant actions of neuroleptic agents may be intensified (additively) by alcohol, barbiturates and other sedatives. Respiratory depression may occur.

Anticholinergic agents may reduce the antipsychotic effect of neuroleptics and the mild anticholinergic effect of neuroleptics may be enhanced by other anticholinergic drugs, possibly leading to constipation, heat stroke, etc.

Some drugs interfere with absorption of neuroleptic agents: antacids, anti-Parkinson drugs and lithium.

Where treatment for neuroleptic-induced extrapyramidal symptoms is required, anticholinergic antiparkinsonian agents should be used in preference to levodopa, since neuroleptics antagonise the antiparkinsonian action of dopaminergics.

High doses of neuroleptics reduce the response to hypoglycaemic agents, the dosage of which might have to be raised.

The hypotensive effect of most antihypertensive drugs especially alpha adrenoceptor blocking agents may be exaggerated by neuroleptics.

The action of some drugs may be opposed by phenothiazine neuroleptics; these include amphetamine, levodopa, clonidine, guanethidine, adrenaline.

Increases or decreases in the plasma concentrations of a number of drugs, e.g. propranolol, phenobarbitone have been observed but were not of clinical significance.

Simultaneous administration of desferrioxamine and prochlorperazine has been observed to induce transient metabolic encephalopathy characterised by loss of consciousness for 48-72 hours.

There is an increased risk of arrhythmias when neuroleptics are used concurrently with drugs which prolong the QT interval, including certain antiarrhythmics, antidepressants, and other antipsychotics (see section 4.8, below).

There is an increased risk of agranulocytosis when neuroleptics are used concurrently with drugs with myelosuppressive potential, such as carbamazepine or certain antibiotics and cytotoxics.

In patients treated concurrently with neuroleptics and lithium, there have been rare reports of neurotoxicity.

4.6 Pregnancy and lactation

There is inadequate evidence of safety in pregnancy. There is evidence of harmful effects in animals. Stemetil should be avoided in pregnancy unless the physician considers it essential. Neuroleptics may occasionally prolong labour and at such time should be withheld until the cervix is dilated 3-4 cm. Possible adverse effects on the neonate include lethargy or paradoxical hyperexcitability, tremor and low apgar score.

Phenothiazines may be excreted in milk, therefore breast feeding should be suspended during treatment.

4.7 Effects on ability to drive and use machines

Patients should be warned about drowsiness during the early days of treatment and advised not to drive or operate machinery.

4.8 Undesirable effects

Generally, adverse reactions occur at a low frequency; the most common reported adverse reactions are nervous system disorders.

Adverse effects:

Blood and lymphatic system disorders: A mild leukopenia occurs in up to 30% of patients on prolonged high dosage. Agranulocytosis may occur rarely: it is not dose related (see section 4.4, above).

Endocrine: Hyperprolactinaemia which may result in galactorrhoea, gynaecomastia, amenorrhoea; impotence.

Nervous system disorders: Acute dystonia or dyskinesias, usually transitory are commoner in children and young adults, and usually occur within the first 4 days of treatment or after dosage increases.

Akathisia characteristically occurs after large initial doses.

Parkinsonism is more common in adults and the elderly. It usually develops after weeks or months of treatment. One or more of the following may be seen: tremor, rigidity, akinesia or other features of Parkinsonism. Commonly just tremor.

Tardive dyskinesia: If this occurs it is usually, but not necessarily, after prolonged or high dosage. It can even occur after treatment has been stopped. Dosage should therefore be kept low whenever possible.

Insomnia and agitation may occur.

Eye disorders: Ocular changes and the development of metallic greyish-mauve coloration of exposed skin have been noted in some individuals mainly females, who have received chlorpromazine continuously for long periods (four to eight years). This could possibly happen with Stemetil.

Cardiac disorders: Cardiac arrhythmias, including atrial arrhythmia, A-V block, ventricular tachycardia and fibrillation have been reported during neuroleptic therapy, possibly related to dosage. Pre-existing cardiac disease, old age, hypokalemia and concurrent tricyclic antidepressants may predispose. ECG changes, usually benign, include widened QT interval, ST depression, U-waves and T-wave changes (see section 4.4, above).

Vascular disorders: Hypotension, usually postural, commonly occurs. Elderly or volume depleted subjects are particularly susceptible; it is more likely to occur after intramuscular injection.

Gastrointestinal disorders: dry mouth may occur.

Respiratory, thoracic and mediastinal disorders: Respiratory depression is possible in susceptible patients. Nasal stuffiness may occur.

Hepato-biliary disorders: Jaundice, usually transient, occurs in a very small percentage of patients taking neuroleptics. A premonitory sign may be sudden onset of fever after one to three weeks of treatment followed by the development of jaundice. Neuroleptic jaundice has the biochemical and other characteristics of obstructive jaundice and is associated with obstruction of the canaliculi by bile thrombi; the frequent presence of an accompanying eosinphilia indicates the allergic nature of this phenomenon. Treatment should be withheld on the development of jaundice (see section 4.4, above).

Skin and subcutaneous tissue disorders: Contact skin sensitisation may occur rarely in those frequently handling preparations of certain phenothiazines (see section 4.4, above). Skin rashes of various kinds may also be seen in patients treated with the drug. Patients on high dosage should be warned that they may develop photosensitivity in sunny weather and should avoid exposure to direct sunlight.

General disorders and administration site conditions: Neuroleptic malignant syndrome (hyperthermia, rigidity, autonomic dysfunction and altered consciousness) may occur with any neuroleptic (see section 4.4, above).

4.9 Overdose

Symptoms of phenothiazine overdosage include drowsiness or loss of consciousness, hypotension, tachycardia, ECG changes, ventricular arrhythmias and hypothermia. Severe extrapyramidal dyskinesias may occur.

If the patient is seen sufficiently soon (up to 6 hours) after ingestion of a toxic dose, gastric lavage may be attempted. Pharmacological induction of emesis is unlikely to be of any use. Activated charcoal should be given. There is no specific antidote. Treatment is supportive.

Generalised vasodilatation may result in circulatory collapse; raising the patient's legs may suffice. In severe cases, volume expansion by intravenous fluids may be needed; infusion fluids should be warmed before administration in order not to aggravate hypothermia.

Positive inotropic agents such as dopamine may be tried if fluid replacement is insufficient to correct the circulatory collapse. Peripheral vasoconstrictor agents are not generally recommended. Avoid the use of adrenaline.

Ventricular or supraventricular tachy-arrhythmias usually respond to restoration of normal body temperature and correction of circulatory or metabolic disturbances. If persistent or life threatening, appropriate anti-arrhythmic therapy may be considered. Avoid lignocaine and, as far as possible, long acting anti-arrhythmic drugs.

Pronounced central nervous system depression requires airway maintenance or, in extreme circumstances, assisted respiration. Severe dystonic reactions usually respond to procyclidine (5-10 mg) or orphenadrine (20-40 mg) administered intramuscularly or intravenously. Convulsions should be treated with intravenous diazepam.

Neuroleptic malignant syndrome should be treated with cooling. Dantrolene sodium may be tried.

5. PHARMACOLOGICAL PROPERTIES

5.1 Pharmacodynamic properties

Stemetil is a potent phenothiazine neuroleptic

5.2 Pharmacokinetic properties

There is little information about blood levels, distribution and excretion in humans. The rate of metabolism and excretion of phenothiazines decreases in old age.

5.3 Preclinical safety data

There are no pre-clinical data of relevance to the prescriber which are additional to that already included in other sections of the SPC.

6. PHARMACEUTICAL PARTICULARS

6.1 List of excipients

Stemetil tablets also contain the following excipients: lactose BP, starch maize BP, aerosil (E551), and magnesium stearate BP.

6.2 Incompatibilities

None stated.

6.3 Shelf life

60 months.

6.4 Special precautions for storage

Store protected from light.

6.5 Nature and contents of container

Stemetil tablets 5mg are available in PVDC coated UPVC/aluminium foil blisters containing 84 tablets.

6.6 Instructions for use and handling

None

7. MARKETING AUTHORISATION HOLDER

Castlemead Healthcare Limited

20 Clanwilliam Terrace

Dublin 2

Ireland

8. MARKETING AUTHORISATION NUMBER(S)

PL 16946/0006

9. DATE OF FIRST AUTHORISATION/RENEWAL OF THE AUTHORISATION

1 July 1998

10. DATE OF REVISION OF THE TEXT

July 2002

Legal category: POM

Sterets H Pre-Injection Swabs

(Medlock Medical Ltd)

1. NAME OF THE MEDICINAL PRODUCT

Sterets H Pre-Injection Swabs.

2. QUALITATIVE AND QUANTITATIVE COMPOSITION

Isopropyl Alcohol BP 70% v/v; Chlorhexidine Acetate BP 0.5% w/v.

3. PHARMACEUTICAL FORM

Sachets containing viscose swab impregnated with isopropyl alcohol and chlorhexidine acetate.

4. CLINICAL PARTICULARS

4.1 Therapeutic indications

To be used for pre-injection site cleansing.

4.2 Posology and method of administration

Topical. There are no differences in use between adults, the elderly and children. Use the wipe to cleanse the injection site.

4.3 Contraindications

None stated.

4.4 Special warnings and special precautions for use

Avoid contact with eyes or broken skin.

4.5 Interaction with other medicinal products and other forms of Interaction

Alcohol should not be brought into contact with some vaccines and skin test injections (patch tests). If in doubt, consult the vaccine manufacturers' literature.

4.6 Pregnancy and lactation

No special precautions required.

4.7 Effects on ability to drive and use machines

Not applicable.

4.8 Undesirable effects

Normally without side effects although minor skin reactions have been attributed to chlorhexidine and to isopropyl alcohol (infrequent, minor).

4.9 Overdose

Not applicable.

5. PHARMACOLOGICAL PROPERTIES

5.1 Pharmacodynamic properties

Isopropyl alcohol has disinfectant properties. Chlorhexidine is a disinfectant that is effective against a wide range of vegetative Gram-positive and Gram-negative bacteria. A 0.5% solution of chlorhexidine acetate in 70% isopropyl alcohol is used for pre-operative disinfection of the skin. The solution is appropriate for swabbing on to cleanse and lower the skin bacteriological count prior to injections.

5.2 Pharmacokinetic properties

There is little absorption of isopropyl alcohol through intact skin. Chlorhexidine acetate is adsorbed on to the skin surface but there is minimal further absorption. Pharmacokinetic particulars are not applicable.

5.3 Preclinical safety data

Not applicable.

6. PHARMACEUTICAL PARTICULARS

6.1 List of excipients

Purified water.

6.2 Incompatibilities

None stated.

6.3 Shelf life

60 months unopened.

6.4 Special precautions for storage

Store in a cool dry place, away from direct sunlight. Flammable contents. Flash point 24°C. Product/contents should be kept away from a naked flame.

6.5 Nature and contents of container

100 sachets per box. Printed aluminium foil laminated sachets (laminates of coated paper/polyethylene/aluminium foil/surlyn, the surlyn layer innermost).

6.6 Instructions for use and handling

None stated.

7. MARKETING AUTHORISATION HOLDER

Seton Prebbles Limited, St Johns Road, Bootle, L20 8NJ.

8. MARKETING AUTHORISATION NUMBER(S)

PL 0303/0013R.

9. DATE OF FIRST AUTHORISATION/RENEWAL OF THE AUTHORISATION

14th March 1990 / 9th May 2002.

10. DATE OF REVISION OF THE TEXT

May 2002.

Sterets Pre-Injection Swabs

(Medlock Medical Ltd)

1. NAME OF THE MEDICINAL PRODUCT

Sterets Pre-injection Swabs.

2. QUALITATIVE AND QUANTITATIVE COMPOSITION

Isopropyl Alcohol BP 70% v/v.

3. PHARMACEUTICAL FORM

Sachets containing viscose swab impregnated with isopropyl alcohol.

4. CLINICAL PARTICULARS

4.1 Therapeutic indications

To be used for pre-injection site cleansing.

4.2 Posology and method of administration
For topical administration. There are no differences in use between adults, children and the elderly.

4.3 Contraindications
No contraindications known for clinical conditions.

4.4 Special warnings and special precautions for use
Avoid contact with eyes or broken skin.

4.5 Interaction with other medicinal products and other forms of Interaction
Alcohol should not be brought into contact with some vaccines and skin test injections (patch tests). If in doubt, consult the vaccine manufacturers' literature.

4.6 Pregnancy and lactation
No special precautions required.

4.7 Effects on ability to drive and use machines
Not applicable.

4.8 Undesirable effects
Normally without side effects although minor skin reactions have occasionally been attributed to the application of isopropyl alcohol (infrequent, minor).

4.9 Overdose
Not applicable.

5. PHARMACOLOGICAL PROPERTIES

5.1 Pharmacodynamic properties
70% isopropyl alcohol has disinfectant properties and is appropriate for swabbing on to cleanse and lower the skin bacteriological count prior to injections.

5.2 Pharmacokinetic properties
There is little absorption of isopropyl alcohol through intact skin. Pharmacokinetic particulars are not applicable.

5.3 Preclinical safety data
None stated.

6. PHARMACEUTICAL PARTICULARS

6.1 List of excipients
Purified water; absorbent viscose pad.

6.2 Incompatibilities
None known.

6.3 Shelf life
60 months unopened.

6.4 Special precautions for storage
Flammable contents, flash point 24°C. Product/contents should be kept away from a naked flame. The product should be stored in a cool dry place, away from direct sunlight.

6.5 Nature and contents of container
Printed aluminium foil laminated sachets (laminates of coated paper/polyethylene/aluminium foil/surlyn, the surlyn layer innermost). The sachets are in strips of two, separated by serrations. 100 sachets are packed per carton.

6.6 Instructions for use and handling
Not applicable.

7. MARKETING AUTHORISATION HOLDER
Seton Prebbles Limited, Tubiton House, Oldham. OL1 3HS.

8. MARKETING AUTHORISATION NUMBER(S)
PL 0303/0012R.

9. DATE OF FIRST AUTHORISATION/RENEWAL OF THE AUTHORISATION
2nd August 1990 / 29th August 2003.

10. DATE OF REVISION OF THE TEXT
August 2003.

Sterets Tisept

(Medlock Medical Ltd)

1. NAME OF THE MEDICINAL PRODUCT
Sterets Tisept Sachets.

2. QUALITATIVE AND QUANTITATIVE COMPOSITION
Chlorhexidine Gluconate Solution 20% equivalent to Chlorhexidine Gluconate 0.015% w/v; Cetrimide 0.15% w/v.

3. PHARMACEUTICAL FORM
Cutaneous solution

4. CLINICAL PARTICULARS

4.1 Therapeutic indications
A broad spectrum antiseptic with detergent properties for swabbing in obstetrics and during dressing changes. For disinfecting and cleansing traumatic and surgical wounds and burns.

4.2 Posology and method of administration
Use without further dilution. For topical administration only.

4.3 Contraindications
Sterets Tisept should not come into contact with the brain, eyes, meninges or middle ear and is contraindicated for persons who have previously shown a hypersensitivity to chlorhexidine.

4.4 Special warnings and special precautions for use
For external use only. Not for injection. When used in aseptic procedures, the outside of the sachet should be disinfected before opening. Discard any surplus immediately after use. Do not use within body cavities.

4.5 Interaction with other medicinal products and other forms of Interaction
Hypochlorite bleaches may cause brown stains to develop in fabrics that have previously been in contact with Sterets Tisept solution.

4.6 Pregnancy and lactation
Although there are no adverse reports for this product in pregnant and lactating mothers, as with all medicines, care should be exercised when administering the product to pregnant or lactating women.

4.7 Effects on ability to drive and use machines
None known.

4.8 Undesirable effects
Idiosyncratic skin reactions and generalized allergenic reactions to chlorhexidine can occur, but these are rare.

4.9 Overdose
Treatment of accidental ingestion: Gastric lavage should be carried out with milk, egg white, gelatin or mild soap.

5. PHARMACOLOGICAL PROPERTIES

5.1 Pharmacodynamic properties
Chlorhexidine is a disinfectant which is effective against a wide range of vegetative Gram-positive and Gram-negative bacteria; it is more effective against Gram-positive than Gram-negative bacteria, some species of Pseudomonas and Proteus being less susceptible. The wide range of organisms against which chlorhexidine is active explains the rationale for presenting it in a solution for swabbing wounds and burns and in obstetrics. Cetrimide is a quaternary ammonium disinfectant with properties and uses typical of cationic surfactants. It is used in Sterets Tisept for its surfactant and bactericidal properties.

5.2 Pharmacokinetic properties
The British Pharmacopoeia 1993 contains monographs for both Chlorhexidine Gluconate solution 20% w/v and Cetrimide. The pharmacokinetics of the compounds when applied to the skin are well described in the literature.

5.3 Preclinical safety data
Not applicable.

6. PHARMACEUTICAL PARTICULARS

6.1 List of excipients
Sunset Yellow E110; Sodium hydroxide; purified water.

6.2 Incompatibilities
Sterets Tisept is incompatible with anionic agents.

6.3 Shelf life
36 months unopened.

6.4 Special precautions for storage
Store in a cool, dark place. Store sachets in outer container.

6.5 Nature and contents of container
Nylon/ethylene propylene copolymer laminate sachets containing either 25 or 100ml of product, overwrapped in heat sealed polythene/nylon and/or polythene/polyester pouches.

6.6 Instructions for use and handling
Not applicable.

7. MARKETING AUTHORISATION HOLDER
Seton Prebbles Limited, St Johns Road, Bootle, L20 8NJ.

8. MARKETING AUTHORISATION NUMBER(S)
PL 0303/0017.

9. DATE OF FIRST AUTHORISATION/RENEWAL OF THE AUTHORISATION
23rd April 1987 / 8th November 2004.

10. DATE OF REVISION OF THE TEXT
November 2004.

Sterets Unisept

(Medlock Medical Ltd)

1. NAME OF THE MEDICINAL PRODUCT
Sterets Unisept.

2. QUALITATIVE AND QUANTITATIVE COMPOSITION
Chlorhexidine Gluconate Solution 20% w/v BP 0.05% w/v.

3. PHARMACEUTICAL FORM
Sterile aqueous solution.

4. CLINICAL PARTICULARS

4.1 Therapeutic indications
Chlorhexidine gluconate is a potent antibacterial agent for general antiseptic purposes. It is bactericidal to a broad spectrum of organisms. Sterets Unisept is recommended for use in obstetrics and for swabbing burns and wounds.

4.2 Posology and method of administration
There is no distinction between adults, the elderly and children in terms of the use of this product. Sterets Unisept should be used without further dilution for topical administration only.

4.3 Contraindications
Sterets Unisept should not come into contact with the brain, eyes, meninges or middle ear. The use of Sterets Unisept is also contraindicated in patients who have shown hypersensitivity to chlorhexidine gluconate. However, such reactions are rare.

4.4 Special warnings and special precautions for use
For external use only. Not for injection. When Sterets Unisept is used in aseptic procedures, the outside of the sachet should be disinfected before opening. Discard any surplus immediately after use.

4.5 Interaction with other medicinal products and other forms of Interaction
Hypochlorite bleaches may cause brown stains to develop in fabrics which have previously been in contact with Sterets Unisept solution.

4.6 Pregnancy and lactation
Although there are no adverse reports for this product in pregnant and lactating mothers, as with all medicines, care should be exercised when administering the product to pregnant or lactating women.

4.7 Effects on ability to drive and use machines
None known.

4.8 Undesirable effects
Idiosyncratic skin reactions can occur as can generalized allergenic reactions to chlorhexidine gluconate, but these are rare occurrences.

4.9 Overdose
Treatment: Accidental ingestion - gastric lavage should be carried out with milk, egg white, gelatine or mild soap.

5. PHARMACOLOGICAL PROPERTIES

5.1 Pharmacodynamic properties
Chlorhexidine is a disinfectant which is effective against a wide range of vegetative Gram-positive and Gram-negative bacteria: it is more effective against Gram-positive than Gram-negative bacteria, some species of Pseudomonas and Proteus being less susceptible. The wide range of organisms against which chlorhexidine is active explains the rationale for presenting it in a solution for swabbing wounds and burns and in obstetrics.

5.2 Pharmacokinetic properties
The British Pharmacopoeia 1993 contains a monograph for Chlorhexidine Gluconate Solution 20% w/v. The pharmacokinetics of the compound when applied to the skin as a topical antiseptic are well understood and described in the literature.

5.3 Preclinical safety data
Not applicable.

6. PHARMACEUTICAL PARTICULARS

6.1 List of excipients
Nonoxynol 10; sodium hydroxide; Carmoisine Red E122; purified water.

6.2 Incompatibilities
Sterets Unisept is incompatible with anionic agents.

6.3 Shelf life
36 months.

6.4 Special precautions for storage
Store in a cool dark place. Store sachets in the outer containers.

6.5 Nature and contents of container
Nylon-ethylene-propylene copolymer laminate sachets containing either 25 ml or 100 ml of product overwrapped in heat sealed polythene/nylon and / or polythene/polyester pouches.

6.6 Instructions for use and handling
Not applicable.

7. MARKETING AUTHORISATION HOLDER
Seton Prebbles Limited, St Johns Road, Bootle, L20 8NJ.

8. MARKETING AUTHORISATION NUMBER(S)
PL 00303/0016.

9. DATE OF FIRST AUTHORISATION/RENEWAL OF THE AUTHORISATION
24th April 1987 / 8th November 2004.

10. DATE OF REVISION OF THE TEXT
November 2004.

Sterile Dopamine Concentrate BP Selectajet

(International Medication Systems (UK) Ltd)

1. NAME OF THE MEDICINAL PRODUCT
Sterile Dopamine Concentrate BP Selectajet

2. QUALITATIVE AND QUANTITATIVE COMPOSITION
Dopamine Hydrochloride 40 mg/ml

3. PHARMACEUTICAL FORM
Solution for injection.

4. CLINICAL PARTICULARS
4.1 Therapeutic indications
For the correction of haemodynamic imbalances present in the shock syndrome due to myocardial infarction, trauma, endotoxic septicaemia, cardiac surgery, renal failure and chronic cardiac decompensation as in congestive failure.

4.2 Posology and method of administration
Adults, elderly and children over 12 years old:

Begin infusion at between 1 - 5 mcg/kg/min. Increase dose by 1 - 5 mcg/kg/min, as required every 10 - 30 minutes, up to 20 - 50 mcg/kg/min. Most patients can be maintained at 20mcg/kg/min or less. Doses in excess of 50mcg/kg/min have been used in advanced states of circulatory decompensation.

Patients with severe refractory chronic congestive heart failure should be started on 0.5 - 2mcg/kg/min and the dose increased by 1 - 3 mcg/kg/min as urinary output increases.

ECG, blood pressure and urine output should be monitored. Cardiac output and pulmonary wedge pressure should be monitored if possible.

Children under 12 years:

The safety and efficacy of dopamine in children has not been established.

4.3 Contraindications
Dopamine should not be used in patients with phaeochromocytoma, uncorrected tachyarrhythmias, or ventricular fibrillation.

4.4 Special warnings and special precautions for use
Correct hypovolaemia, before administering dopamine if possible.

Administer dilute solution through as large a vein as possible, to minimise the risk of extravasation. A metering chamber or device should be used to accurately control dosage in drops/minute.

Dopamine infusion should be withdrawn gradually, to avoid unnecessary hypotension.

Patients with a history of occlusive vascular disease (e.g. atherosclerosis, arterial embolism, Raynaud's disease, cold injury, diabetic endarteritis and Buerger's disease) should be closely monitored for any changes in colour or temperature of the skin in the extremities. If ischaemia occurs and is thought to be the result of vasoconstriction, the benefits of continued dopamine infusion should be weighed against the risk of possible necrosis. This condition may be reversed by either decreasing the rate or discontinuing the infusion. IV administration of phentolamine mesylate 5-10 mg may reverse the ischaemia.

If excessive vasoconstriction (as indicated by a disproportionate rise in diastolic pressure and a marked decrease in pulse pressure) is observed, the infusion rate should be decreased or suspended and the patient observed closely.

As the effect of dopamine on impaired renal and hepatic function is not known, close monitoring is advised.

4.5 Interaction with other medicinal products and other forms of Interaction
The action of dopamine is potentiated by monoamine oxidase inhibitors (MAOI's). In patients who have received MAOI's within the previous 2-3 weeks, the initial dopamine dose should be no greater than 10% of the usual dose.

The concurrent administration of cyclopropane or halogenated hydrocarbon anaesthetics may cause ventricular arrhythmias.

The cardiac effects of dopamine are antagonised by beta-adrenergic blocking agents such as propranolol and metoprolol.

The ergot alkaloids should be avoided because of the possibility of excessive vasoconstriction. Tricyclic antidepressants and guanethidine may potentiate the pressor response to dopamine.

Hypotension and bradycardia have been observed in patients receiving phenytoin.

Dopamine may increase the effect of diuretic agents.

Peripheral vasoconstriction may be antagonised by alpha-adrenergic blocking agents, such as phentolamine. Other vasodilators may also be useful in patients with heart failure, allowing greater inotropic and renal effects without the associated vasoconstriction. Care must be taken to avoid hypotension.

4.6 Pregnancy and lactation
The use of any drug in pregnant women or women of child-bearing potential requires that the expected benefit be carefully weighed against the possible risk to mother and child. Animal studies have shown no evidence of teratogenic effect. It is not known whether dopamine crosses the placenta or enters breast milk.

4.7 Effects on ability to drive and use machines
This drug is intended for use in life threatening situations.

4.8 Undesirable effects
Extravasation of dopamine into the tissues may cause local necrosis. The area should be infiltrated with 5-10mg phentolamine in 10-15mL saline.

The most frequent adverse reactions include ectopic beats, nausea, vomiting, tachycardia, anginal pain, palpitations, dyspnoea, headache, hypotension, hypertension and vasoconstriction. Other less frequent adverse reactions are aberrant ventricular conduction, bradycardia, piloerection, mydriasis, widened QRS complex, azotaemia and elevated blood pressure. Peripheral ischaemic gangrene in patients with pre-existing vascular disease. Fatal ventricular arrhythmias have been reported on rare occasions.

4.9 Overdose
In case of accidental overdosage, as evidenced by excessive blood pressure elevation, reduce the rate of administration or temporarily discontinue dopamine until the patients condition stabilises. Since the duration of action of dopamine is quite short, no additional measures are usually necessary. If these measures fail to stabilise the patient's condition, use of the short-acting alpha- adrenergic blocking agent such as phentolamine should be considered.

5. PHARMACOLOGICAL PROPERTIES
5.1 Pharmacodynamic properties
Dopamine is a catecholamine. It is an agonist for specific dopamine receptors in the CNS, renal and other vascular beds (vasodilation) and for b_1 adrenoceptors in the heart (positive inotrope). At high doses it activates a-adrenoceptors (vasoconstriction).

5.2 Pharmacokinetic properties
The half life of an iv bolus of dopamine is about 2 minutes, thus it is given by continuous infusion. Steady state is reached within 5 - 10 minutes. On termination of the infusion, dopamine is cleared from the plasma with a half life of about 9 minutes.

Dopamine is widely distributed throughout the body, but does not cross the blood/brain barrier. Dopamine like all catecholamines is metabolised by monoamine oxidase (MAO) and catechol-O-methyl transerase (COMT), in the liver, kidney and plasma. A small amount of unchanged drug plus its main metabolites, homovanillic acid (HVA) and 3,4-dihydroxyphenyl acetic acid (DOPAC) are excreted in the urine.

5.3 Preclinical safety data
The LD_{50} values for IV dopamine hydrochloride have been determined as 290 mg/kg in mice and 38.8 mg/kg in rats; the animals suffered massive internal bleeding and pulmonary congestion.

Subacute toxicity tests in rats revealed prostatic hypertrophy with associated bladder distension and hydronephrosis. In animals given higher doses (570 mg/kg daily) weights of heart, kidneys and lung were significantly higher than in controls, the weight of the spleen was significantly lower. Dogs given dopamine continuously for two weeks suffered intractable vomiting. Subsequent examination showed an increase in weight of the adrenal glands in all animals and an increase in weight of the prostate gland in dogs given the higher doses, some of which also had small areas of myocardial necrosis.

6. PHARMACEUTICAL PARTICULARS
6.1 List of excipients
Sodium bisulphite

Water for Injection USP

6.2 Incompatibilities
Do not add dopamine to any alkaline diluent solution e.g. sodium bicarbonate, since the drug is inactivated by these solutions.

6.3 Shelf life
36 months.

6.4 Special precautions for storage
Store below 25°C. Protect from light.

6.5 Nature and contents of container
The solution is contained in a USP type I glass vial with an elastomeric closure which meets all the relevant USP specifications. The product is available as 5 ml, 10 ml and 20ml.

6.6 Instructions for use and handling
Dopamine must be diluted before use. Appropriate diluents include 5% dextrose, sodium chloride 0.9% or compound sodium lactate. Incompatible with sodium bicarbonate or any other alkali solution.

Dopamine is stable for about 24 hours in sodium chloride or dextrose. It should be used as soon as possible after mixing.

The container is specially designed for use with the IMS Select-A-Jet injector.

7. MARKETING AUTHORISATION HOLDER
International Medication Systems (UK) Ltd.

208 Bath Road

Slough

Berkshire

SL1 3WE

UK

8. MARKETING AUTHORISATION NUMBER(S)
PL 03265/0027

9. DATE OF FIRST AUTHORISATION/RENEWAL OF THE AUTHORISATION
Date first granted: 16.07.79

Date renewed: 29.03.00

10. DATE OF REVISION OF THE TEXT
April 2001

POM

Sterile Saline Solution (0.9%)

(GlaxoSmithKline UK)

1. NAME OF THE MEDICINAL PRODUCT
Sterile Saline Solution (0.9%)

2. QUALITATIVE AND QUANTITATIVE COMPOSITION
None

3. PHARMACEUTICAL FORM
Diluent containing sterile solution for the reconstitution of lyophilised vaccine preparations.

4. CLINICAL PARTICULARS
4.1 Therapeutic indications
For reconstitution of lyophilised vaccines.

4.2 Posology and method of administration
Subcutaneous or intramuscular injection.

4.3 Contraindications
As for the product to be reconstituted.

4.4 Special warnings and special precautions for use
As for the product to be reconstituted.

4.5 Interaction with other medicinal products and other forms of Interaction
As for the product to be reconstituted.

4.6 Pregnancy and lactation
As for the product to be reconstituted.

4.7 Effects on ability to drive and use machines
As for the product to be reconstituted.

4.8 Undesirable effects
As for the product to be reconstituted.

4.9 Overdose
As for the product to be reconstituted.

5. PHARMACOLOGICAL PROPERTIES
5.1 Pharmacodynamic properties
Not applicable.

5.2 Pharmacokinetic properties
Not applicable.

5.3 Preclinical safety data
Not applicable.

6. PHARMACEUTICAL PARTICULARS
6.1 List of excipients
Sodium Chloride

Water for Injection

6.2 Incompatibilities
As for the product to be reconstituted.

6.3 Shelf life
60 months.

6.4 Special precautions for storage
Protect from light, store between 2°C and 8°C. Do not freeze.

6.5 Nature and contents of container
Type I, Ph Eur glass syringes with or without needles, fitted with rubber stoppers. The stoppers are attached to a polypropylene or polystyrene plunger.

This diluent is for use with the following vaccines:

Hiberix PL 10592/0120

AC Vax PL 10592/0013

ACWY Vax PL 10592/0014

6.6 Instructions for use and handling
As for the product to be reconstituted.

Administrative Data
7. MARKETING AUTHORISATION HOLDER
Smith Kline & French Laboratories Limited

Great West Road, Brentofrd, Middlesex TW8 9GS

Trading as:

GlaxoSmithKline UK,

Stockley Park West,

Uxbridge,

Middlesex, UB11 1BT

8. MARKETING AUTHORISATION NUMBER(S)
PL 00002/0236

9. DATE OF FIRST AUTHORISATION/RENEWAL OF THE AUTHORISATION
15 May 1998

10. DATE OF REVISION OF THE TEXT
15th October 2002

Steripaste Medicated Paste Bandage

(Medlock Medical Ltd)

1. NAME OF THE MEDICINAL PRODUCT
Steripaste Medicated Paste Bandage.

2. QUALITATIVE AND QUANTITATIVE COMPOSITION
Zinc Oxide BP 15% w/w.

3. PHARMACEUTICAL FORM
Sterile, open wove bleached cotton bandage impregnated with the paste formulation.

4. CLINICAL PARTICULARS

4.1 Therapeutic indications
For the treatment of venous ulcers.

4.2 Posology and method of administration
For topical administration only. Adults, the elderly, and children: Not applicable: the product is a medicated paste bandage. Frequency of dressing changes is at the discretion of the responsible physician. (Differentiation between patients of differing age groups is less important when considering the dosage regime than the apparent healing rate of the wound/condition.)

4.3 Contraindications
Hypersensitivity to an ingredient of the paste, and acute eczematous lesions.

4.4 Special warnings and special precautions for use
Avoid use on grossly macerated skin. One of the functions of occlusive bandages is to increase absorption. Care should be taken, therefore, if it is decided to apply topical steroid preparations under these bandages as their absorption may be significantly increased.

4.5 Interaction with other medicinal products and other forms of Interaction
None known.

4.6 Pregnancy and lactation
No special precautions required.

4.7 Effects on ability to drive and use machines
Not applicable.

4.8 Undesirable effects
None known.

4.9 Overdose
Not applicable.

5. PHARMACOLOGICAL PROPERTIES

5.1 Pharmacodynamic properties
The product is a paste bandage with the active constituent presented in an aqueous/oil based emulsion paste, spread onto a cotton bandage. Zinc Oxide as a zinc salt has astringent properties and has been shown to play a role in wound healing. Much of the therapeutic action of paste bandages is attributable to the bandaging technique, the physical support and protection provided and to the maintenance of moist wound healing conditions.

5.2 Pharmacokinetic properties
The pharmacokinetics of the active ingredient are those relevant to topical application of the substances through whole or broken skin.

5.3 Preclinical safety data
Not applicable.

6. PHARMACEUTICAL PARTICULARS

6.1 List of excipients
Glycerol; fractionated coconut oil; aluminium magnesium silicate; xanthan gum; polysorbate 80; sorbitan mono-oleate; synthetic spermacetti; purified water; open-wove cotton bandage.

6.2 Incompatibilities
None known.

6.3 Shelf life
Three years.

6.4 Special precautions for storage
Store in a dry place at or below 25°C.

6.5 Nature and contents of container
Individually wrapped in waxed paper within a sealed aluminium foil/polythene bag, and cardboard carton. 12 cartons packed per corrugated cardboard carton.

6.6 Instructions for use and handling
Not applicable.

7. MARKETING AUTHORISATION HOLDER
Seton Healthcare Group plc, Tubiton House, Oldham, OL1 3HS.

8. MARKETING AUTHORISATION NUMBER(S)
PL 00223/0031.

9. DATE OF FIRST AUTHORISATION/RENEWAL OF THE AUTHORISATION
7th July 1994 / 7th July 1999.

10. DATE OF REVISION OF THE TEXT
July 1999.

Ster-Zac Bath Concentrate

(Medlock Medical Ltd)

1. NAME OF THE MEDICINAL PRODUCT
Ster-Zac Bath Concentrate.

2. QUALITATIVE AND QUANTITATIVE COMPOSITION
Triclosan 2% w/v.

3. PHARMACEUTICAL FORM
Clear liquid.

4. CLINICAL PARTICULARS

4.1 Therapeutic indications
This product has an antibacterial effect in water and is intended for the prevention of cross infection and secondary infection.

4.2 Posology and method of administration
For bathing: Add 28.5ml of Ster-Zac Bath Concentrate to a bathful of water (approximately 140 litres) immediately prior to the patient entering the water. For washing: Add 1ml of Ster-Zac Bath Concentrate to 5 litres of water, prior to use. No specific dosage recommendations are made for administration to the elderly or children.

4.3 Contraindications
Not to be used on pregnant women.

4.4 Special warnings and special precautions for use
For external use only. Avoid contact with the eyes. Keep out of the reach of children.

4.5 Interaction with other medicinal products and other forms of Interaction
None stated.

4.6 Pregnancy and lactation
Not to be used on pregnant women.

4.7 Effects on ability to drive and use machines
None stated.

4.8 Undesirable effects
Erythema may arise in some patients with allergy problems.

4.9 Overdose
If erythema or other skin rashes occur, rinse thoroughly with water. Seek medical advice if the condition worsens.

5. PHARMACOLOGICAL PROPERTIES

5.1 Pharmacodynamic properties
Triclosan is a bactericide.

5.2 Pharmacokinetic properties
None stated.

5.3 Preclinical safety data
None stated.

6. PHARMACEUTICAL PARTICULARS

6.1 List of excipients
Industrial methylated spirit; isopropyl alcohol; dioctyl sodium sulphosuccinate 60%; trisodium edetate; triethanolamide; purified water.

6.2 Incompatibilities
None stated.

6.3 Shelf life
3 years.

6.4 Special precautions for storage
Store in a cool place.

6.5 Nature and contents of container
High density polyethylene container with either a polypropylene cap or a compression moulded screw cap with a steran faced liner, containing 28.5 ml or 500ml.

6.6 Instructions for use and handling
Not applicable.

7. MARKETING AUTHORISATION HOLDER
Medlock Medical Limited, Tubiton House, Medlock Street, Oldham, OL1 3HS.

8. MARKETING AUTHORISATION NUMBER(S)
PL 21248/0031.

9. DATE OF FIRST AUTHORISATION/RENEWAL OF THE AUTHORISATION
14th March 2005

10. DATE OF REVISION OF THE TEXT
March 2005.

Stesolid Rectal Tubes 10mg

(Alpharma Limited)

1. NAME OF THE MEDICINAL PRODUCT
Stesolid® rectal tubes 10 mg.

2. QUALITATIVE AND QUANTITATIVE COMPOSITION
Diazepam 4 mg/ml.

3. PHARMACEUTICAL FORM
Enema.

4. CLINICAL PARTICULARS

4.1 Therapeutic indications
Diazepam has anticonvulsant, sedative, and muscle relaxant properties. It is used in the treatment of severe anxiety and tension states, as a sedative and premedication, in the control of muscle spasm, and in the management of alcohol withdrawal symptoms.

Stesolid rectal tubes 10 mg may be used in acute severe anxiety and agitation, epileptic and febrile convulsions, tetanus, as a sedative in minor surgical and dental procedures, or in other circumstances in which a rapid effect is required but where intravenous injection is impracticable or undesirable.

Stesolid rectal tubes 10 mg may be of particular value for the immediate treatment of convulsions in infants and children.

4.2 Posology and method of administration
Sensitivity to diazepam varies with age.

Children above 1 year of age: 0.5 mg/kg body weight

Adults: 0.5 mg/kg body weight

Elderly patients: 0.25 mg/kg body weight

A maximum dose of 30 mg diazepam is recommended, unless adequate medical supervision and monitoring are available.

4.3 Contraindications
Myasthenia gravis, hypersensitivity to benzodiazepines, severe respiratory insufficiency, sleep apnoea syndrome, severe hepatic insufficiency.

4.4 Special warnings and special precautions for use
Tolerance

Some loss of efficacy to the hypnotic effects of diazepam may develop after repeated use for a few weeks.

Dependence

Use of benzodiazepines may lead to development of physical and psychic dependence upon these products. The risk of dependence increases with dose and duration of treatment; it is also greater in patients with a history of alcohol or drug abuse.

Once physical dependence has developed, abrupt termination of treatment will be accompanied by withdrawal symptoms. These may consist of headaches, muscle pain, extreme anxiety, tension, restlessness, confusion and irritability. In severe cases the following symptoms may occur: derealisation, depersonalisation, hyperacusis, numbness and tingling of the extremities, hypersensitivity to light, noise and physical contact, hallucinations or epileptic seizures.

Rebound insomnia and anxiety: a transient syndrome whereby the symptoms that led to treatment with a benzodiazepine recur in an enhanced form may occur on withdrawal of treatment. It may be accompanied by other reactions including mood changes, anxiety or sleep disturbances and restlessness. Since the risk of withdrawal phenomena/rebound phenomena is greater after abrupt discontinuation of treatment, it is recommended that the dosage is decreased gradually.

Psychiatric and paradoxical reactions

Reactions like restlessness, agitation, irritability, aggressiveness, delusion, rages, nightmares, hallucinations, psychosis, inappropriate behaviour and other adverse behavioural effects are known to occur when using benzodiazepines. Should this occur, use of the medicinal product should be discontinued.

They are more likely to occur in children and the elderly.

Specific patient groups

Benzodiazepines should not be given to children without careful assessment of the need to do so; the duration of treatment must be kept to a minimum. Elderly should be given a reduced dose (see Posology). A lower dose is also recommended for patients with chronic respiratory insufficiency due to the risk of respiratory depression. Benzodiazepines are not indicated to treat patients with severe hepatic insufficiency as they may precipitate encephalopathy.

Benzodiazepines are not recommended for the primary treatment of psychotic illness.

Benzodiazepines should not be used alone to treat depression or anxiety associated with depression (suicide may be precipitated in such patients).

In common with other benzodiazepines, the use of diazepam may be associated with amnesia and should not be used in cases of loss or bereavement as psychological adjustment may be inhibited.

Stesolid rectal tubes 10 mg should not be used in phobic or obsessional states, as there is insufficient evidence of efficacy and safety in such conditions.

Benzodiazepines should be used with extreme caution in patients with a history of alcohol or drug abuse.

4.5 Interaction with other medicinal products and other forms of Interaction
- Not recommended: concomitant intake with alcohol.

The sedative effects may be enhanced when the product is used in combination with alcohol. This affects the ability to drive or use machines.

- Take into account: combination with CNS depressants.

Enhancement of the central depressive effect may occur in cases of concomitant use with antipsychotics (neuroleptics), hypnotics, anxiolytics/sedatives, antidepressant agents, narcotic analgesics, anti-epileptic products, anaesthetics and sedative antihistamines.

In the case of narcotic analgesics enhancement of the euphoria may also occur leading to an increase in psychic dependence.

Compounds which inhibit certain hepatic enzymes (particularly cytochrome P450) may enhance the activity of benzodiazepines. To a lesser degree this also applies to benzodiazepines that are metabolised only by conjugation.

4.6 Pregnancy and lactation

There is no evidence as to the safety of diazepam in human pregnancy. It should not be used, especially during the first and last trimesters, unless the benefit is considered to outweigh the potential risk.

In labour, high single doses or repeated low doses have been reported to produce hypotonia, poor sucking, and hyperthermia in the neonate, and irregularities in the foetal heart.

If benzodiazepines are prescribed to a woman of child-bearing potential, she should be warned to contact her physician regarding discontinuance of the product if she intends to become or suspects that she is pregnant.

If, for compelling medical reasons, the product is administered during the late phase of pregnancy, or during labour at high doses, effects on neonate, such as hypothermia, hypotonia and moderate respiratory depression, can be expected, due to the pharmacological action of the compound.

Infants born to mothers who took benzodiazepines chronically during the later states of pregnancy may have developed physical dependence and may be at some risk for developing withdrawal symptoms in the postnatal period.

Since benzodiazepines are found in breast milk, benzodiazepines should not be given to breast feeding mothers.

4.7 Effects on ability to drive and use machines

Sedation, amnesia, impaired muscular function may adversely affect the ability to drive or use machines. If insufficient sleep occurs, the likelihood of impaired alertness may be increased (see also Interactions).

4.8 Undesirable effects

The side effects of diazepam are usually mild and infrequent.

The most common side effects are drowsiness, light-headedness, unsteadiness, and ataxia. Elderly patients are particularly susceptible to these effects.

Rare side effects include hypotension, apnoea, gastrointestinal and visual disturbances, skin rashes, urinary retention, headache, confusion, vertigo, changes in libido, blood dyscrasias, and jaundice.

Paradoxical reactions to the benzodiazepines, provoking excitement instead of sedation, have been reported.

4.9 Overdose

As with other benzodiazepines, overdose should not present a threat to life unless combined with other CNS depressants (including alcohol).

In the management of overdose with any medical product, it should be borne in mind that multiple agents might have been taken.

Overdose of benzodiazepines is usually manifested by degrees of central nervous system depression ranging from drowsiness to coma. In mild cases, symptoms include drowsiness, mental confusion and lethargy, in more serious cases, symptoms may include ataxia, hypotonia, hypotension, respiratory depression, rarely coma and very rarely death.

Emergency procedure is gastric lavage and adequate airway maintenance. Otherwise, the treatment is symptomatic. Intravenous fluids may be administered and Flumazenil may be useful as an antidote.

5. PHARMACOLOGICAL PROPERTIES

5.1 Pharmacodynamic properties

Pharmacotherapeutic group: Diazepam has anticonvulsant, sedative, and muscle relaxant properties.

5.2 Pharmacokinetic properties

Absorption: Diazepam is quickly absorbed from the rectal mucosa. The maximum serum concentration is reached within 17 minutes. Absorption is 100% compared with that of intravenous injection of diazepam.

5.3 Preclinical safety data

Not applicable.

6. PHARMACEUTICAL PARTICULARS

6.1 List of excipients

Benzoic acid

Ethanol

Propylene glycol

Sodium benzoate

Benzyl alcohol

Purified water.

6.2 Incompatibilities

None known.

6.3 Shelf life

30 months at 25°C.

6.4 Special precautions for storage

The storage temperature must not exceed 25°C.

6.5 Nature and contents of container

Carton containing sealed low density polyethylene tubes, single packed in aluminium laminated bags.

Package size: 5 × 2.5 ml

6.6 Instructions for use and handling

Not applicable.

Administrative Data

7. MARKETING AUTHORISATION HOLDER

Dumex Ltd.

Whiddon Valley

Barnstaple

Devon EX32 8NS

England

8. MARKETING AUTHORISATION NUMBER(S)

PL 10183/0004

9. DATE OF FIRST AUTHORISATION/RENEWAL OF THE AUTHORISATION

3 February 1992

10. DATE OF REVISION OF THE TEXT

12 October 1999

Stesolid Rectal Tubes 5mg

(Alpharma Limited)

1. NAME OF THE MEDICINAL PRODUCT

Stesolid® rectal tubes 5 mg.

2. QUALITATIVE AND QUANTITATIVE COMPOSITION

Diazepam 2 mg/ml.

3. PHARMACEUTICAL FORM

Enema.

4. CLINICAL PARTICULARS

4.1 Therapeutic indications

Diazepam has anticonvulsant, sedative, and muscle relaxant properties. It is used in the treatment of severe anxiety and tension states, as a sedative and premedication, in the control of muscle spasm, and in the management of alcohol withdrawal symptoms.

Stesolid rectal tubes 5 mg may be used in acute severe anxiety and agitation, epileptic and febrile convulsions, tetanus, as a sedative in minor surgical and dental procedures, or in other circumstances in which a rapid effect is required but where intravenous injection is impracticable or undesirable.

Stesolid rectal tubes 5 mg may be of particular value for the immediate treatment of convulsions in infants and children.

4.2 Posology and method of administration

Sensitivity to diazepam varies with age.

Children above 1 year of age: 0.5 mg/kg body weight

Adults: 0.5 mg/kg body weight

Elderly patients: 0.25 mg/kg body weight

A maximum dose of 30 mg diazepam is recommended, unless adequate medical supervision and monitoring are available.

4.3 Contraindications

Myasthenia gravis, hypersensitivity to benzodiazepines, severe respiratory insufficiency, sleep apnoea syndrome, severe hepatic insufficiency.

4.4 Special warnings and special precautions for use

Tolerance

Some loss of efficacy to the hypnotic effects of diazepam may develop after repeated use for a few weeks.

Dependence

Use of benzodiazepines may lead to development of physical and psychic dependence upon these products. The risk of dependence increases with dose and duration of treatment; it is also greater in patients with a history of alcohol or drug abuse.

Once physical dependence has developed, abrupt termination of treatment will be accompanied by withdrawal symptoms. These may consist of headaches, muscle pain, extreme anxiety, tension, restlessness, confusion and irritability. In severe cases the following symptoms may occur: derealisation, depersonalisation, hyperacusis, numbness and tingling of the extremities, hypersensitivity to light, noise and physical contact, hallucinations or epileptic seizures.

Rebound insomnia and anxiety: a transient syndrome whereby the symptoms that led to treatment with a benzodiazepine recur in an enhanced form may occur on withdrawal of treatment. It may be accompanied by other reactions including mood changes, anxiety or sleep disturbances and restlessness. Since the risk of withdrawal phenomena/rebound phenomena is greater after abrupt discontinuation of treatment, it is recommended that the dosage is decreased gradually.

Psychiatric and paradoxical reactions

Reactions like restlessness, agitation, irritability, aggressiveness, delusion, rages, nightmares, hallucinations, psychosis, inappropriate behaviour and other adverse behavioural effects are known to occur when using benzodiazepines. Should this occur, use of the medicinal product should be discontinued.

They are more likely to occur in children and the elderly.

Specific patient groups

Benzodiazepines should not be given to children without careful assessment of the need to do so; the duration of treatment must be kept to a minimum. Elderly should be given a reduced dose (see posology). A lower dose is also recommended for patients with chronic respiratory insufficiency due to the risk of respiratory depression. Benzodiazepines are not indicated to treat patients with severe hepatic insufficiency as they may precipitate encephalopathy.

Benzodiazepines are not recommended for the primary treatment of psychotic illness.

Benzodiazepines should not be used alone to treat depression or anxiety associated with depression (suicide may be precipitated in such patients).

In common with other benzodiazepines, the use of diazepam may be associated with amnesia and should not be used in cases of loss or bereavement as psychological adjustment may be inhibited.

Stesolid rectal tubes 5 mg should not be used in phobic or obsessional states, as there is insufficient evidence of efficacy and safety in such conditions.

Benzodiazepines should be used with extreme caution in patients with a history of alcohol or drug abuse.

4.5 Interaction with other medicinal products and other forms of Interaction

- Not recommended: concomitant intake with alcohol.

The sedative effects may be enhanced when the product is used in combination with alcohol. This affects the ability to drive or use machines.

- Take into account: combination with CNS depressants.

Enhancement of the central depressive effect may occur in cases of concomitant use with antipsychotics (neuroleptics), hypnotics, anxiolytics/sedatives, antidepressant agents, narcotic analgesics, anti-epileptic products, anaesthetics and sedative antihistamines.

In the case of narcotic analgesics enhancement of the euphoria may also occur leading to an increase in psychic dependence.

Compounds which inhibit certain hepatic enzymes (particularly cytochrome P450) may enhance the activity of benzodiazepines. To a lesser degree this also applies to benzodiazepines that are metabolised only by conjugation.

4.6 Pregnancy and lactation

There is no evidence as to the safety of diazepam in human pregnancy. It should not be used, especially during the first and last trimesters, unless the benefit is considered to outweigh the potential risk.

In labour, high single doses or repeated low doses have been reported to produce hypotonia, poor sucking, and hyperthermia in the neonate, and irregularities in the foetal heart.

If benzodiazepines are prescribed to a woman of child-bearing potential, she should be warned to contact her physician regarding discontinuance of the product if she intends to become or suspects that she is pregnant.

If, for compelling medical reasons, the product is administered during the late phase of pregnancy, or during labour at high doses, effects on neonate, such as hypothermia, hypotonia and moderate respiratory depression, can be expected, due to the pharmacological action of the compound.

Infants born to mothers who took benzodiazepines chronically during the later states of pregnancy may have developed physical dependence and may be at some risk for developing withdrawal symptoms in the postnatal period.

Since benzodiazepines are found in breast milk, benzodiazepines should not be given to breast feeding mothers.

4.7 Effects on ability to drive and use machines

Sedation, amnesia, impaired muscular function may adversely affect the ability to drive or use machines. If insufficient sleep occurs, the likelihood of impaired alertness may be increased (see also Interactions).

4.8 Undesirable effects

The side effects of diazepam are usually mild and infrequent.

The most common side effects are drowsiness, light-headedness, unsteadiness, and ataxia. Elderly patients are particularly susceptible to these effects.

Rare side effects include hypotension, apnoea, gastrointestinal and visual disturbances, skin rashes, urinary retention, headache, confusion, vertigo, changes in libido, blood dyscrasias, and jaundice.

Paradoxical reactions to the benzodiazepines, provoking excitement instead of sedation, have been reported.

4.9 Overdose
As with other benzodiazepines, overdose should not present a threat to life unless combined with other CNS depressants (including alcohol).

In the management of overdose with any medical product, it should be borne in mind that multiple agents might have been taken.

Overdose of benzodiazepines is usually manifested by degrees of central nervous system depression ranging from drowsiness to coma. In mild cases, symptoms include drowsiness, mental confusion and lethargy, in more serious cases, symptoms may include ataxia, hypotonia, hypotension, respiratory depression, rarely coma and very rarely death.

Emergency procedure is gastric lavage and adequate airway maintenance. Otherwise, the treatment is symptomatic. Intravenous fluids may be administered and Flumazenil may be useful as an antidote.

5. PHARMACOLOGICAL PROPERTIES
5.1 Pharmacodynamic properties
Pharmacotherapeutic group: Diazepam has anticonvulsant, sedative, and muscle relaxant properties.

5.2 Pharmacokinetic properties
Absorption: Diazepam is quickly absorbed from the rectal mucosa. The maximum serum concentration is reached within 17 minutes. Absorption is 100% compared with that of intravenous injection of diazepam.

5.3 Preclinical safety data
Not applicable.

6. PHARMACEUTICAL PARTICULARS
6.1 List of excipients
Benzoic acid
Ethanol
Propylene glycol
Sodium benzoate
Benzyl alcohol
Purified water.

6.2 Incompatibilities
None known.

6.3 Shelf life
30 months at 25°C.

6.4 Special precautions for storage
The storage temperature must not exceed 25°C.

6.5 Nature and contents of container
Carton containing sealed low density polyethylene tubes, single packed in aluminium laminated bags.

Package size: 5 × 2.5 ml

6.6 Instructions for use and handling
Not applicable.

Administrative Data
7. MARKETING AUTHORISATION HOLDER
Dumex Ltd.
Whiddon Valley
Barnstaple
Devon EX32 8NS
England

8. MARKETING AUTHORISATION NUMBER(S)
PL 10183/0003

9. DATE OF FIRST AUTHORISATION/RENEWAL OF THE AUTHORISATION
3 February 1992

10. DATE OF REVISION OF THE TEXT
12 October 1999

Stiemycin
(Stiefel Laboratories (UK) Limited)

1. NAME OF THE MEDICINAL PRODUCT
Stiemycin 2.0% w/w.

2. QUALITATIVE AND QUANTITATIVE COMPOSITION
Erythromycin Base EP 2.46 w/w.

3. PHARMACEUTICAL FORM
Solution for topical use.

4. CLINICAL PARTICULARS
4.1 Therapeutic indications
Stiemycin is indicated for use in the treatment of acne vulgaris.

4.2 Posology and method of administration
To be applied to the affected area twice daily after washing with soap and water.

4.3 Contraindications
Stiemycin is contraindicated in patients with known sensitivity to any of the ingredients.

4.4 Special warnings and special precautions for use
Avoid contact with eyes and other mucous membranes. Concomitant topical acne therapy should be used with caution because a cumulative irritant effect may occur.

4.5 Interaction with other medicinal products and other forms of Interaction
None known.

4.6 Pregnancy and lactation
There is no evidence of hazard from erythromycin in human pregnancy. It has been in wide use for many years without apparent ill consequence.

4.7 Effects on ability to drive and use machines
None.

4.8 Undesirable effects
None.

4.9 Overdose
Not applicable.

5. PHARMACOLOGICAL PROPERTIES
5.1 Pharmacodynamic properties
Erythromycin suppresses *Propionibacterium acnes*, a resident bacterial of sebaceous follicles, and as a result of this organism's role in the hydrolysis of triglycerides to free fatty acids, administration decreases fatty acid formation. This is thought to be responsible for its effectiveness in reducing acne lesion counts and the fatty acid to fatty ester ratios in acne patients.

5.2 Pharmacokinetic properties
Not applicable.

5.3 Preclinical safety data
None.

6. PHARMACEUTICAL PARTICULARS
6.1 List of excipients
Propylene Glycol
Ethanol Absolute
Laureth 4 (BRIJ 30).

6.2 Incompatibilities
None

6.3 Shelf life
36 months

6.4 Special precautions for storage
Store in a cool place

6.5 Nature and contents of container
Amber glass screw capped bottle of 50ml.

6.6 Instructions for use and handling
There are no special instructions for use or handling of Stiemycin.

7. MARKETING AUTHORISATION HOLDER
Stiefel Laboratories (UK) Ltd
Holtspur Lane,
Wooburn Green,
High Wycombe,
Bucks HP10 0AU

8. MARKETING AUTHORISATION NUMBER(S)
PL 0174/0047

9. DATE OF FIRST AUTHORISATION/RENEWAL OF THE AUTHORISATION
21 June 1988

10. DATE OF REVISION OF THE TEXT
September 2005.

Stilnoct 5mg, Stilnoct 10mg
(sanofi-aventis)

1. NAME OF THE MEDICINAL PRODUCT
Stilnoct 5mg/zolpidem tartrate 5mg tablets
Stilnoct 10mg/zolpidem tartrate 10mg tablets

2. QUALITATIVE AND QUANTITATIVE COMPOSITION
Stilnoct 5mg/Zolpidem tartrate 5mg Tablets:

Round white film coated tablets containing 5mg zolpidem tartrate.

Stilnoct 10mg/Zolpidem tartrate 10mg Tablets:

White to off-white film-coated oblong tablet, scored and engraved SN 10 on one side, containing 10mg zolpidem tartrate.

3. PHARMACEUTICAL FORM
Coated tablets for oral administration.

4. CLINICAL PARTICULARS
4.1 Therapeutic indications
The short-term treatment of insomnia in situations where the insomnia is debilitating or is causing severe distress for the patient.

4.2 Posology and method of administration
Route of administration: Oral

Zolpidem tartrate acts rapidly and therefore should be taken immediately before retiring, or in bed.

The recommended daily dose for adults is 10 mg. Elderly or debilitated patients may be especially sensitive to the effects of zolpidem tartrate therefore a 5mg dose is recommended. These recommended doses should not be exceeded.

As clearance and metabolism of zolpidem tartrate is reduced in hepatic impairment, dosage should begin at 5mg with particular caution being exercised in elderly patients. In adults (under 65 years) dosage may be increased to 10mg only where the clinical response is inadequate and the drug is well tolerated.

The duration of treatment should usually vary from a few days to two weeks with a maximum of four weeks including tapering off where clinically appropriate.

As with all hypnotics, long-term use is not recommended and a course of treatment should not exceed four weeks.

Zolpidem tartrate should not be used in children.

4.3 Contraindications
Zolpidem tartrate is contraindicated in patients with a hypersensitivity to zolpidem tartrate, obstructive sleep apnoea, myasthenia gravis, severe hepatic insufficiency, acute and/or severe respiratory depression. In the absence of data, zolpidem tartrate should not be prescribed for children or patients with psychotic illness.

4.4 Special warnings and special precautions for use
The cause of insomnia should be identified wherever possible and the underlying factors treated before a hypnotic is prescribed. The failure of insomnia to remit after a 7-14 day course of treatment may indicate the presence of a primary psychiatric or physical disorder, and the patient should be carefully re-evaluated at regular intervals.

4.4.1 Specific patient groups
Elderly: See dose recommendations.

Depression: As with other sedative/hypnotic drugs, zolpidem tartrate should be administered with caution in patients exhibiting symptoms of depression. Suicidal tendencies may be present therefore the least amount of drug that is feasible should be supplied to these patients because of the possibility of intentional overdosage by the patient.

Use in patients with a history of drug or alcohol abuse: Extreme caution should be exercised when prescribing for patients with a history of drug or alcohol abuse. These patients should be under careful surveillance when receiving zolpidem tartrate or any other hypnotic, since they are at risk of habituation and psychological dependence.

4.4.2 General information
General information relating to effects seen following administration of benzodiazepines and other hypnotic agents which should be taken into account by the prescribing physician are described below.

Tolerance
Some loss of efficacy to the hypnotic effects of short-acting benzodiazepines and benzodiazepine-like agents may develop after repeated use for a few weeks.

Dependence
Use of benzodiazepines or benzodiazepine-like agents may lead to the development of physical and psychological dependence. The risk of dependence increases with dose and duration of treatment; it is also greater in patients with a history of psychiatric disorders and/or alcohol or drug abuse.

These patients should be under careful surveillance when receiving hypnotics.

Once physical dependence has developed, abrupt termination of treatment will be accompanied by withdrawal symptoms. These may consist of headaches or muscle pain, extreme anxiety and tension, restlessness, confusion and irritability. In severe cases the following symptoms may occur: derealisation, depersonalisation, hyperacusis, numbness and tingling of the extremities, hypersensitivity to light, noise and physical contact, hallucinations or epileptic seizures.

Rebound insomnia
A transient syndrome whereby the symptoms that led to treatment with a benzodiazepine or benzodiazepine-like agent recur in an enhanced form, may occur on withdrawal of hypnotic treatment. It may be accompanied by other reactions including mood changes, anxiety and restlessness.

It is important that the patient should be aware of the possibility of rebound phenomena, thereby minimising anxiety over such symptoms should they occur when the medicinal product is discontinued. Since the risk of withdrawal phenomena or rebound has been shown to be greater after abrupt discontinuation of treatment, it is recommended that the dosage is decreased gradually where clinically appropriate.

There are indications that, in the case of benzodiazepines and benzodiazepine-like agents with a short duration of action, withdrawal phenomena can become manifest within the dosage interval, especially when the dosage is high.

Amnesia
Benzodiazepines or benzodiazepine-like agents may induce anterograde amnesia. The condition occurs most often several hours after ingesting the product and

therefore to reduce the risk patients should ensure that they will be able to have an uninterrupted sleep of 7-8 hours.

Psychiatric and "paradoxical" reactions

Reactions like restlessness, aggravated insomnia, agitation, irritability, aggressiveness, delusion, rages, nightmares, hallucinations, psychoses, inappropriate behaviour and other adverse behavioural effects are known to occur when using benzodiazepines or benzodiazepine-like agents. Should this occur, use of the product should be discontinued. These reactions are more likely to occur in the elderly.

4.5 Interaction with other medicinal products and other forms of Interaction

- **Not recommended**: Concomitant intake with alcohol.

The sedative effect may be enhanced when the product is used in combination with alcohol. This affects the ability to drive or use machines.

- **Take into account**: Combination with CNS depressants.

Enhancement of the central depressive effect may occur in cases of concomitant use with antipsychotics (neuroleptics), hypnotics, anxiolytics/sedatives, antidepressant agents, narcotic analgesics, antiepileptic drugs, anaesthetics and sedative antihistamines.

Zolpidem tartrate appears to interact with sertraline. This interaction may cause increased drowsiness. Also, isolated cases of visual hallucinations were reported

In the case of narcotic analgesics enhancement of euphoria may also occur leading to an increase in psychological dependence.

Compounds which inhibit certain hepatic enzymes (particularly cytochrome P450) may enhance the activity of benzodiazepines and benzodiazepine-like agents.

Zolpidem tartrate is metabolised via several hepatic cytochrome P450 enzymes, the main enzyme being CYP3A4 with the contribution of CYP1A2. The pharmacodynamic effect of zolpidem tartrate is decreased when it is administered with rifampicin (a CYP3A4 inducer).

However when zolpidem tartrate was administered with itraconazole (a CYP3A4 inhibitor) its pharmacokinetics and pharmacodynamics were not significantly modified. The clinical relevance of these results is unknown.

Since CYP3A4 plays an important role in zolpidem tartrate metabolism, possible interactions with drugs that are substrates or inducers of CYP3A4 should be considered.

Others: When zolpidem tartrate was administered with ranitidine or cimetidine, no significant pharmacokinetic interactions were observed.

4.6 Pregnancy and lactation

Although animal studies have shown no teratogenic or embryotoxic effects, safety in pregnancy has not been established. As with all drugs zolpidem tartrate should be avoided in pregnancy particularly during the first trimester.

If the product is prescribed to a woman of childbearing potential, she should be warned to contact her physician about stopping the product if she intends to become or suspects that she is pregnant.

If, for compelling medical reasons, zolpidem tartrate is administered during the late phase of pregnancy, or during labour, effects on the neonate, such as hypothermia, hypotonia and moderate respiratory depression, can be expected due to the pharmacological action of the product.

Infants born to mothers who took benzodiazepines or benzodiazepine-like agents chronically during the latter stages of pregnancy may have developed physical dependence and may be at some risk of developing withdrawal symptoms in the postnatal period.

Small quantities of zolpidem tartrate appear in breast milk. The use of zolpidem tartrate in nursing mothers is therefore not recommended.

4.7 Effects on ability to drive and use machines

Vehicle drivers and machine operators should be warned that, as with other hypnotics, there may be a possible risk of drowsiness the morning after therapy. In order to minimise this risk a resting period of 7 to 8 hours is recommended between taking zolpidem tartrate and driving.

4.8 Undesirable effects

There is evidence of a dose-relationship for adverse effects associated with zolpidem tartrate use, particularly for certain CNS and gastrointestinal events. As recommended in section 4.2 Posology and method of administration, they should in theory be less if zolpidem tartrate is taken immediately before retiring, or in bed. They occur most frequently in elderly patients.

Daytime drowsiness, reduced alertness, confusion, fatigue, headache, dizziness, muscle weakness, gait disturbances or diplopia. These phenomena usually occur predominantly at the start of therapy.

Other effects like gastrointestinal disturbances, changes in libido or skin reactions have been reported occasionally.

Amnesia – anterograde amnesia may occur using therapeutic dosages, the risk increasing at higher dosages. Amnestic effects may be associated with inappropriate behaviour.

Psychiatric and paradoxical reactions - reactions like restlessness, agitation, irritability, aggressiveness, delusion, rages, nightmares, hallucinations, psychoses, inappropriate behaviour, somnambulism and other adverse behavioural effects are known to occur when using zolpidem tartrate. Such reactions are more likely to occur in the elderly.

Depression – pre-existing depression may be unmasked during use of zolpidem tartrate. Since insomnia may be a symptom of depression, the patient should be re-evaluated if insomnia persists.

4.9 Overdose

In reports of overdose with zolpidem tartrate alone, impairment of consciousness has ranged from somnolence to light coma. Individuals have fully recovered from zolpidem tartrate overdoses up to 400mg.

Overdose cases involving zolpidem tartrate among multiple CNS-depressant agents (including alcohol), have resulted in more severe symptomatology, including fatal outcomes.

General symptomatic and supportive measures should be used. If there is no advantage in emptying the stomach, activated charcoal should be given to reduce absorption. Sedating drugs should be withheld even if excitation occurs.

Use of flumazenil may be considered where serious symptoms are observed.

Flumazenil is reported to have an elimination half-life of about 40 to 80 minutes. Patients should be kept under close observation because of this short duration of action; further doses of flumazenil may be necessary. However, flumazenil administration may contribute to the appearance of neurological symptoms (convulsions).

In the management of overdose with any medicinal product, it should be borne in mind that multiple agents may have been taken.

5. PHARMACOLOGICAL PROPERTIES

5.1 Pharmacodynamic properties

(GABA-A receptor modulator selective for omega-1 receptor subtype hypnotic agent).

Zolpidem tartrate is an imidazopyridine which preferentially binds the omega-1 receptor subtype (also known as the benzodiazepine-1 subtype) which corresponds to GABA-A receptors containing the alpha-1 sub-unit, whereas benzodiazepines non-selectively bind both omega-1 and omega-2 subtypes. The modulation of the chloride anion channel via this receptor leads to the specific sedative effects demonstrated by zolpidem tartrate. These effects are reversed by the benzodiazepine antagonist flumazenil.

In animals: The selective binding of zolpidem tartrate to omega-1 receptors may explain the virtual absence at hypnotic doses of myorelaxant and anti-convulsant effects in animals which are normally exhibited by benzodiazepines which are not selective for omega-1 sites.

In man: zolpidem tartrate decreases sleep latency and the number of awakenings, and increases sleep duration and sleep quality. These effects are associated with a characteristic EEG profile, different from that of the benzodiazepines. In studies that measured the percentage of time spent in each sleep stage, zolpidem tartrate has generally been shown to preserve sleep stages. At the recommended dose, zolpidem tartrate has no influence on the paradoxical sleep duration (REM). The preservation of deep sleep (stages 3 and 4 - slow-wave sleep) may be explained by the selective omega-1 binding by zolpidem tartrate. All identified effects of zolpidem tartrate are reversed by the benzodiazepine antagonist flumazenil.

5.2 Pharmacokinetic properties

Zolpidem tartrate has both a rapid absorption and onset of hypnotic action. Bioavailability is 70% following oral administration and demonstrates linear kinetics in the therapeutic dose range. Peak plasma concentration is reached at between 0.5 and 3 hours.

The elimination half-life is short, with a mean of 2.4 hours (± 0.2 h) and a duration of action of up to 6 hours.

Protein binding amounts to 92.5% ± 0.1%. First pass metabolism by the liver amounts to approximately 35%. Repeated administration has been shown not to modify protein binding indicating a lack of competition between zolpidem tartrate and its metabolites for binding sites.

The distribution volume in adults is 0.54 ± 0.02 L/kg and decreases to 0.34 ± 0.05 L/kg in the very elderly.

All metabolites are pharmacologically inactive and are eliminated in the urine (56%) and in the faeces (37%).

Zolpidem tartrate has been shown in trials to be non-dialysable.

Plasma concentrations in elderly subjects and those with hepatic impairment are increased. In patients with renal insufficiency, whether dialysed or not, there is a moderate reduction in clearance. The other pharmacokinetic parameters are unaffected.

Zolpidem tartrate is metabolised via several hepatic cytochrome P450 enzymes, the main enzyme being CYP3A4 with the contribution of CYP1A2. Since CYP3A4 plays an important role in zolpidem tartrate metabolism, possible interactions with drugs that are substrates or inducers of CYP3A4 should be considered.

5.3 Preclinical safety data

No data of therapeutic relevance.

6. PHARMACEUTICAL PARTICULARS

6.1 List of excipients

Tablet core: Lactose monohydrate, Microcrystalline cellulose, Hypromellose, Sodium starch glycollate, Magnesium stearate.

Film coating: Hypromellose, Titanium dioxide (E171), Macrogol 400 (Stilnoct 10mg only), Polyethylene glycol 400 (Stilnoct 5mg only)

6.2 Incompatibilities

None known

6.3 Shelf life

Stilnoct 5mg: 3 years

Stilnoct 10mg: 4 years

6.4 Special precautions for storage

Stilnoct 5mg: Store in a dry place below 30°C

Stilnoct 10mg: No special precautions

6.5 Nature and contents of container

Stilnoct 5mg: Cartons of 28 tablets in PVC/foil blister strips.

Stilnoct 10mg: Cartons of 28 tablets in PVC/foil blister strips.

6.6 Instructions for use and handling

Please consult the package insert before use. Do not use after the stated expiry date on the carton and blister.

KEEP OUT OF THE REACH OF CHILDREN

Administrative Data

7. MARKETING AUTHORISATION HOLDER

Sanofi-Synthelabo Limited

One Onslow Street

Guildford

Surrey

GU1 4YS

UK

Trading as Lorex Synthelabo or Sanofi-Synthelabo

PO Box 597

Guildford

Surrey

8. MARKETING AUTHORISATION NUMBER(S)

Stilnoct 5mg: PL11723/0323

Stilnoct 10mg: PL 11723/0324

9. DATE OF FIRST AUTHORISATION/RENEWAL OF THE AUTHORISATION

1st February 2003

10. DATE OF REVISION OF THE TEXT

Stilnoct 5mg: February 2004

Stilnoct 10mg: July 2004

Legal Category: POM

Strattera 10mg, 18mg, 25mg, 40mg, or 60mg hard capsules.

(Eli Lilly and Company Limited)

1. NAME OF THE MEDICINAL PRODUCT

Strattera*▼ 10mg, 18mg, 25mg, 40mg, or 60mg hard capsules.

2. QUALITATIVE AND QUANTITATIVE COMPOSITION

The active substance is atomoxetine hydrochloride. Each Strattera 10mg, 18mg, 25mg, 40mg, or 60mg capsule contains atomoxetine hydrochloride equivalent to 10mg, 18mg, 25mg, 40mg, or 60mg of atomoxetine.

For excipients, see section 6.1.

3. PHARMACEUTICAL FORM

Hard capsules.

Strattera 10mg capsules are opaque white, imprinted with 'Lilly 3227' on the cap and '10mg' on the body in black ink.

Strattera 18mg capsules are gold (cap) and opaque white (body), imprinted with 'Lilly 3238' on the cap and '18mg' on the body in black ink.

Strattera 25mg capsules are opaque blue (cap) and opaque white (body), imprinted with 'Lilly 3228' on the cap and '25mg' on the body in black ink.

Strattera 40mg capsules are opaque blue, imprinted with 'Lilly 3229' on the cap and '40mg' on the body in black ink.

Strattera 60mg capsules are opaque blue (cap) and gold (body), imprinted with 'Lilly 3239' on the cap and '60mg' on the body in black ink.

4. CLINICAL PARTICULARS

4.1 Therapeutic indications

Strattera is indicated for the treatment of Attention-Deficit/Hyperactivity Disorder (ADHD) in children of 6 years and older and in adolescents as part of a comprehensive treatment programme. Diagnosis should be made according to DSM-IV criteria or the guidelines in ICD-10.

Additional information for the safe use of this product: A comprehensive treatment programme typically includes psychological, educational, and social measures and is aimed at stabilising children with a behavioural syndrome characterised by symptoms which may include chronic history of short attention span, distractibility, emotional lability, impulsivity, moderate to severe hyperactivity, minor neurological signs, and abnormal EEG. Learning may or may not be impaired.

Pharmacological treatment is not indicated in all children with this syndrome and the decision to use the drug must be based on a very thorough assessment of the severity of the child's symptoms in relation to the child's age and the persistence of symptoms.

4.2 Posology and method of administration

For oral use. Strattera can be administered as a single daily dose in the morning, with or without food. Patients who do not achieve a satisfactory clinical response (tolerability or efficacy) when taking Strattera as a single daily dose might benefit from taking it as twice daily evenly divided doses in the morning and late afternoon or early evening.

Dosing of children/adolescents up to 70 kg body weight: Strattera should be initiated at a total daily dose of approximately 0.5mg/kg. The initial dose should be maintained for a minimum of 7 days prior to upward dose titration according to clinical response and tolerability. The recommended maintenance dose is approximately 1.2mg/kg/day (depending on the patient's weight and available dosage strengths of atomoxetine). No additional benefit has been demonstrated for doses higher than 1.2mg/kg/day. The safety of single doses over 1.8mg/kg/day and total daily doses above 1.8mg/kg have not been systematically evaluated. In some cases it might be appropriate to continue treatment into adulthood.

Dosing of children/adolescents over 70 kg body weight: Strattera should be initiated at a total daily dose of 40mg. The initial dose should be maintained for a minimum of 7 days prior to upward dose titration according to clinical response and tolerability. The recommended maintenance dose is 80mg. No additional benefit has been demonstrated for doses higher than 80mg (see section 5.1). The maximum recommended total daily dose is 100mg. The safety of single doses over 120mg and total daily doses above 150mg have not been systematically evaluated. In some cases it might be appropriate to continue treatment into adulthood.

Additional information for the safe use of this product: Treatment must be initiated by or under the supervision of a physician with appropriate knowledge and experience in treating ADHD.

In the study programme, no distinct withdrawal symptoms have been described. In cases of significant adverse effects, atomoxetine may be stopped abruptly; otherwise the drug may be tapered off over a suitable time period.

In adolescents whose symptoms persist into adulthood and who have shown clear benefit from treatment, it may be appropriate to continue treatment into adulthood. However, start of treatment with Strattera in adults is not appropriate.

Special Populations

Hepatic insufficiency: For patients with moderate hepatic insufficiency (Child-Pugh class B), initial and target doses should be reduced to 50% of the usual dose. For patients with severe hepatic insufficiency (Child-Pugh class C), initial dose and target doses should be reduced to 25% of usual dose.

Renal insufficiency: Subjects with end stage renal disease had higher systemic exposure to atomoxetine than healthy subjects (about a 65% increase), but there was no difference when exposure was corrected for mg/kg dose. Strattera can therefore be administered to ADHD patients with end stage renal disease or lesser degrees of renal insufficiency using the usual dosing regimen. Atomoxetine may exacerbate hypertension in patients with end stage renal disease.

The safety and efficacy of Strattera in children under 6 years of age have not been established. Therefore, Strattera should not be used in children under 6 years of age.

Elderly patients: Not applicable.

4.3 Contraindications

Hypersensitivity to atomoxetine or to any of the excipients.

Atomoxetine should not be used in combination with monoamine oxidase inhibitors (MAOIs). Atomoxetine should not be used within a minimum of 2 weeks after discontinuing therapy with a MAOI. Treatment with a MAOI should not be initiated within 2 weeks after discontinuing atomoxetine.

Atomoxetine should not be used in patients with narrow angle glaucoma, as in clinical trials the use of atomoxetine was associated with an increased incidence of mydriasis.

4.4 Special warnings and special precautions for use

Possible allergic events: Although uncommon, allergic reactions, including rash, angioneurotic oedema, and urticaria, have been reported in patients taking atomoxetine.

Many patients taking atomoxetine experience a modest increase in pulse (mean <10 bpm) and/or increase in blood pressure (mean <5 mmHg) (see section 4.8). For most patients, these changes are not clinically important. Atomoxetine should be used with caution in patients with hypertension, tachycardia, or cardiovascular or cerebrovascular disease. Pulse and blood pressure should be measured periodically while on therapy. Orthostatic hypotension has also been reported. Use with caution in any condition that may predispose patients to hypotension.

Strattera should be discontinued in patients with jaundice or laboratory evidence of liver injury, and should not be restarted. Very rarely, liver toxicity, manifested by elevated hepatic enzymes and bilirubin with jaundice, has been reported.

Growth and development should be monitored during treatment with atomoxetine. Patients requiring long-term therapy should be monitored and consideration should be given to dose reduction or interrupting therapy in patients who are not growing or gaining weight satisfactorily.

Clinical data do not suggest a deleterious effect of atomoxetine on cognition or sexual maturation, however, the amount of available long-term data is limited. Therefore, patients requiring long-term therapy should be carefully monitored.

Suicide related behaviour (suicide attempts and suicidal ideation) has been reported in patients treated with atomoxetine. In double-blind clinical trials, suicide related behaviours occurred at a frequency of 0.44% in atomoxetine-treated patients (6 out of 1,357 patients treated, one case of suicide attempt and five of suicidal ideation). There were no events in the placebo group (n = 851). The age range of children experiencing these events was 7 to 12 years. It should be noted that the number of adolescent patients included in the clinical trials was low.

Hostility (predominantly aggression, oppositional behaviour, and anger) and emotional lability were more frequently observed in clinical trials among children and adolescents treated with Strattera compared to those treated with placebo.

Patients who are being treated for ADHD should be carefully monitored for the appearance or worsening of suicide related behaviour, hostility, and emotional lability. As with other psychotropic medication, the possibility of rare, serious psychiatric adverse effects cannot be excluded.

Strattera is not indicated for the treatment of major depressive episodes and/or anxiety, as the results of clinical trials that were conducted in adults did not show any effect compared to placebo and therefore were negative.

4.5 Interaction with other medicinal products and other forms of Interaction

Effects of Other Drugs on Atomoxetine

MAOIs: Atomoxetine should not be used with MAOIs (see section 4.3).

CYP2D6 inhibitors (eg, fluoxetine, paroxetine): Atomoxetine is primarily metabolised by the CYP2D6 pathway to 4-hydroxyatomoxetine. In CYP2D6 extensive metaboliser patients, selective inhibitors of CYP2D6 may increase atomoxetine steady-state plasma concentrations to exposures similar to those observed in CYP2D6 poor metaboliser patients. *In vitro* studies suggest that co-administration of cytochrome P450 inhibitors to CYP2D6 poor metabolisers will not increase the plasma concentrations of atomoxetine. Slower titration of atomoxetine may be necessary in those patients who are also taking CYP2D6 inhibitor drugs.

Salbutamol: Atomoxetine should be administered with caution to patients being treated with high dose nebulised or systemically administered (oral or intravenous) salbutamol (or other $beta_2$ agonists) because the action of salbutamol on the cardiovascular system can be potentiated.

Pressor agents: Because of possible effects on blood pressure, atomoxetine should be used cautiously with pressor agents.

Drugs that affect noradrenaline: Drugs that affect noradrenaline should be used cautiously when co-administered with atomoxetine because of the potential for additive or synergistic pharmacological effects. Examples include antidepressants, such as imipramine, venlafaxine, and mirtazapine, or the decongestants pseudoephedrine or phenylephrine.

Drugs that affect gastric pH: Drugs that elevate gastric pH (magnesium hydroxide/aluminium hydroxide, omeprazole) had no effect on atomoxetine bioavailability.

Drugs highly bound to plasma protein:In vitro drug-displacement studies were conducted with atomoxetine and other highly bound drugs at therapeutic concentrations. Warfarin, acetylsalicylic acid, phenytoin, or diazepam did not affect the binding of atomoxetine to human albumin. Similarly, atomoxetine did not affect the binding of these compounds to human albumin.

Effects of Atomoxetine on Other Drugs

Cytochrome P450 enzymes: Atomoxetine did not cause clinically significant inhibition or induction of cytochrome P450 enzymes, including CYP1A2, CYP3A, CYP2D6, and CYP2C9.

4.6 Pregnancy and lactation

For atomoxetine, no clinical data on exposed pregnancies are available.

Animal studies in general do not indicate direct or indirect harmful effects with respect to pregnancy, embryonal/foetal development, parturition, or postnatal development (see section 5.3).

Atomoxetine should not be used during pregnancy unless the potential benefit justifies the potential risk to the foetus.

Atomoxetine and/or its metabolites were excreted in the milk of rats. It is not known if atomoxetine is excreted in human milk. Because of the lack of data, atomoxetine should be avoided during breast-feeding.

4.7 Effects on ability to drive and use machines

No studies on the effects on the ability to drive and use machines have been performed. Atomoxetine was associated with increased rates of fatigue relative to placebo. In paediatric patients only, atomoxetine was associated with increased rates of somnolence relative to placebo. Patients should be advised to use caution when driving a car or operating hazardous machinery until they are reasonably certain that their performance is not affected by atomoxetine.

4.8 Undesirable effects

Children and adolescents: Abdominal pain and decreased appetite are the adverse events most commonly associated with atomoxetine, and are reported by about 18% and 16% of patients, respectively, but seldom lead to drug discontinuation (discontinuation rates are 0.3% for abdominal pain and 0.0% for decreased appetite). These effects are usually transient.

Associated with decreased appetite, some patients lost weight early in therapy (average about 0.5 kg), and effects were greatest at the highest doses. After an initial decrease in weight, patients treated with atomoxetine showed a mean increase in weight during long-term treatment. Growth rates (weight and height) after 2 years of treatment are near normal (see section 4.4).

Nausea or vomiting can occur in about 9% and 11% of patients, respectively, particularly during the first month of therapy. However, these episodes were usually mild to moderate in severity and transient, and did not result in a significant number of discontinuations from therapy (discontinuation rate 0.5%).

In paediatric placebo-controlled trials, patients taking atomoxetine experienced a mean increase in heart rate of about 6 beats/minute and mean increases in systolic and diastolic blood pressure of about 2 mmHg compared with placebo. In adult placebo-controlled trials, patients taking atomoxetine experienced a mean increase in heart rate of 6 beats/minute and mean increases in systolic (about 3 mmHg) and diastolic (about 1 mmHg) blood pressures compared with placebo.

Because of its effect on noradrenergic tone, orthostatic hypotension (0.2%; n = 7) and syncope (0.8%; n = 26) have been reported in patients taking atomoxetine. Atomoxetine should be used with caution in any condition that may predispose patients to hypotension.

The following table of undesirable effects is based on adverse event reporting and laboratory investigations from clinical trials in child and adolescent patients:

Infections and Infestations *Common (1-10%):* Influenza (ie, cold/flu symptoms).
Metabolism and Nutrition Disorders *Very common (>10%):* Appetite decreased. *Common (1-10%):* Anorexia (loss of appetite).
Psychiatric Disorders *Common (1-10%):* Early morning awakening, irritability, mood swings.
Nervous System Disorders *Common (1-10%):* Dizziness, somnolence.
Eye Disorders *Common (1-10%):* Mydriasis.
Cardiac Disorders *Uncommon (0.1-1%):* Palpitations, sinus tachycardia.
Gastro-intestinal Disorders *Very common (>10%):* Abdominal pain, vomiting. *Common (1-10%):* Constipation, dyspepsia, nausea.
Skin and Subcutaneous Tissue Disorders *Common (1-10%):* Dermatitis, pruritus, rash.
General Disorders and Administration Site Conditions *Common (1-10%):* Fatigue.
Investigations *Common (1-10%):* Weight decreased.

The following adverse events occurred in at least 2% of CYP2D6 poor metaboliser (PM) patients and were either twice as frequent or statistically significantly more frequent in PM patients compared with CYP2D6 extensive metaboliser (EM) patients: appetite decreased (24.1% of PMs, 17.0% of EMs); insomnia (10.5% of PMs, 6.8% of EMs); middle insomnia (3.8% of PMs, 1.5% of EMs); enuresis (3.0% of PMs, 1.2% of EMs); depressed mood (3.0% of PMs, 1.0% of EMs); tremor (5.1% of PMs, 1.1% of EMs); early morning awakening (3.0% of PMs, 1.1% of EMs);

conjunctivitis (3.0% of PMs, 1.5% of EMs); syncope (2.1% of PMs, 0.7% of EMs); mydriasis (2.5% of PMs, 0.7% of EMs). The following events did not meet the above criteria but were reported by more PM patients than EM patients: anxiety (2.5% of PMs, 2.2% of EMs); depression (2.5% of PMs, 1.9% of EMs). In addition, in trials lasting up to 10 weeks, weight loss was more pronounced in PM patients (mean of 0.6 kg in EM and 1.1 kg in PM).

Adults: In adults, the adverse events reported most frequently with atomoxetine treatment were gastro-intestinal or genitourinary. A complaint of urinary retention or urinary hesitancy in adults should be considered potentially related to atomoxetine. No serious safety concerns were observed during acute or long-term treatment. The following table of undesirable effects is based on adverse event reporting and laboratory investigations from clinical trials in adult patients:

Metabolism and Nutrition Disorders *Very common (>10%):* Appetite decreased.
Psychiatric Disorders *Common (1-10%):* Early morning awakening, libido decreased, sleep disorder.
Nervous System Disorders *Very common (>10%):* Insomnia. *Common (1-10%):* Dizziness, middle insomnia, sinus headache.
Cardiac Disorders *Common (1-10%):* Palpitations, tachycardia.
Vascular Disorders *Common (1-10%):* Hot flushes. *Uncommon (0.1-1%):* Peripheral coldness.
Gastro-intestinal Disorders *Very common (>10%):* Dry mouth, nausea. *Common (1-10%):* Abdominal pain, constipation, dyspepsia, flatulence.
Skin and Subcutaneous Tissue Disorders *Common (1-10%):* Dermatitis, sweating increased.
Renal and Urinary Disorders *Common (1-10%):* Difficulty in micturition, urinary hesitation, urinary retention.
Reproductive System and Breast Disorders *Common (1-10%):* Dysmenorrhoea, ejaculation disorder, ejaculation failure, erectile disturbance, impotence, menstruation irregular, orgasm abnormal, prostatitis.
General Disorders and Administration Site Conditions *Common (1-10%):* Fatigue, lethargy, rigors.
Investigations *Common (1-10%):* Weight decreased.

Post-marketing experience: Suicide-related events have been reported (see section 4.4).

The following events have been reported very rarely: abnormal liver function tests, jaundice, and hepatitis.

4.9 Overdose

Signs and symptoms: There is limited clinical trial experience with atomoxetine overdose and no fatalities were observed.

During post-marketing, there have been reports of non-fatal acute and chronic overdoses of atomoxetine. The most commonly reported symptoms accompanying acute and chronic overdoses were somnolence, agitation, hyperactivity, abnormal behaviour, and gastro-intestinal symptoms. All events were mild to moderate. Signs and symptoms consistent with mild to moderate sympathetic nervous system activation (eg, mydriasis, tachycardia, dry mouth) have also been observed. All patients recovered from these events.

Management of overdose: An airway should be established. Monitoring of cardiac and vital signs is recommended, along with appropriate symptomatic and supportive measures. Gastric lavage may be indicated if performed soon after ingestion. Activated charcoal may be useful in limiting absorption. Because atomoxetine is highly protein-bound, dialysis is not likely to be useful in the treatment of overdose.

5. PHARMACOLOGICAL PROPERTIES

5.1 Pharmacodynamic properties

Pharmacotherapeutic group: Centrally acting sympathomimetics. *ATC code:* N06BA09.

Atomoxetine is a highly selective and potent inhibitor of the pre-synaptic noradrenaline transporter, its presumed mechanism of action, without directly affecting the serotonin or dopamine transporters. Atomoxetine has minimal affinity for other noradrenergic receptors or for other neurotransmitter transporters or receptors. Atomoxetine has two major oxidative metabolites: 4-hydroxyatomoxetine and N-desmethylatomoxetine. 4-hydroxyatomoxetine is equipotent to atomoxetine as an inhibitor of the noradrenaline transporter but, unlike atomoxetine, this metabolite also exerts some inhibitory activity at the serotonin transporter. However, any effect on this transporter is likely to be minimal, as the majority of 4-hydroxyatomoxetine is further metabolised such that it circulates in plasma at much lower concentrations (1% of atomoxetine concentration in EMs and 0.1% of atomoxetine concentration in PMs). N-desmethylatomoxetine has substantially less pharmacological activity compared with atomoxetine. It circulates in plasma at lower concentrations in extensive metabolisers and at comparable concentrations to the parent drug in poor metabolisers at steady-state.

Atomoxetine is not a psychostimulant and is not an amphetamine derivative. In a randomised, double-blind, placebo-controlled, abuse-potential study in adults comparing effects of atomoxetine and placebo, atomoxetine was not associated with a pattern of response that suggested stimulant or euphoriant properties.

Strattera has been studied in trials involving over 4,000 children and adolescents with ADHD. The acute efficacy of Strattera in the treatment of ADHD was established in six randomised, double-blind, placebo-controlled trials of six to nine weeks duration. Signs and symptoms of ADHD were evaluated by a comparison of mean change from baseline to endpoint for Strattera-treated and placebo-treated patients. In each of the six trials, atomoxetine was statistically significantly superior to placebo in reducing ADHD signs and symptoms.

Additionally, the efficacy of atomoxetine in maintaining symptom response was demonstrated in a 1 year, placebo-controlled trial with over 400 patients, primarily conducted in Europe (approximately 3 months of open-label acute treatment followed by 9 months of double-blind, placebo-controlled maintenance treatment). The proportion of patients relapsing after 1 year was 18.7% and 31.4% (atomoxetine and placebo, respectively). After 1 year of atomoxetine treatment, patients who continued atomoxetine for 6 additional months were less likely to relapse or to experience partial symptom return compared with patients who discontinued active treatment and switched to placebo (2% versus 12%, respectively). For children and adolescents, periodic assessment of the value of ongoing treatment during long-term treatment should be performed.

Strattera was effective as a single daily dose and as a divided dose administered in the morning and late afternoon/early evening. Strattera administered once daily demonstrated statistically significantly greater reduction in severity of ADHD symptoms compared with placebo, as judged by teachers and parents.

Atomoxetine does not worsen tics in patients with ADHD and comorbid chronic motor tics or Tourette's disorder.

536 adult patients with ADHD were enrolled in 2 randomised, double-blind, placebo-controlled clinical studies of 10 weeks duration.

Patients received Strattera twice daily titrated according to clinical response in a range of 60 to 120mg/day. The mean final dose of Strattera for both studies was approximately 95mg/day. In both studies, ADHD symptoms were statistically significantly improved on Strattera, as measured on the ADHD Symptom score from the CAARS scale. Magnitude of symptom improvement in adults was less than that observed in children. Long-term maintenance of effect in adults has not been shown.

5.2 Pharmacokinetic properties

The pharmacokinetics of atomoxetine in children and adolescents are similar to those in adults. The pharmacokinetics of atomoxetine have not been evaluated in children under 6 years of age.

Absorption: Atomoxetine is rapidly and almost completely absorbed after oral administration, reaching mean maximal observed plasma concentration (C_{max}) approximately 1 to 2 hours after dosing. The absolute bioavailability of atomoxetine following oral administration ranged from 63% to 94%, depending upon inter-individual differences in the modest first pass metabolism. Atomoxetine can be administered with or without food.

Distribution: Atomoxetine is widely distributed and is extensively (98%) bound to plasma proteins, primarily albumin.

Biotransformation: Atomoxetine undergoes biotransformation primarily through the cytochrome P450 2D6 (CYP2D6) enzymatic pathway. The major oxidative metabolite formed is 4-hydroxyatomoxetine that is rapidly glucuronidated. 4-hydroxyatomoxetine is equipotent to atomoxetine but circulates in plasma at much lower concentrations. Although 4-hydroxyatomoxetine is primarily formed by CYP2D6, in individuals that lack CYP2D6 activity, 4-hydroxyatomoxetine can be formed by several other cytochrome P450 enzymes, but at a slower rate. Atomoxetine does not inhibit or induce CYP2D6 at therapeutic doses.

Elimination: The mean elimination half-life of atomoxetine after oral administration is 3.6 hours in extensive metabolisers and 21 hours in poor metabolisers. Atomoxetine is excreted primarily as 4-hydroxyatomoxetine-O-glucuronide, mainly in the urine.

Linearity/non-linearity: Pharmacokinetics of atomoxetine are linear over the range of doses studied in both extensive and poor metabolisers.

5.3 Preclinical safety data

Preclinical data revealed no special hazard for humans based on conventional studies of safety pharmacology, repeated dose toxicity, genotoxicity, carcinogenicity, or reproduction and development.

A study was conducted in young rats to evaluate the effects of atomoxetine on growth and neurobehavioural and sexual development. Slight delays in onset of vaginal patency (all doses) and preputial separation (≥10mg/kg/day), and slight decreases in epididymal weight and sperm number (≥10mg/kg/day) were seen; however, there were no effects on fertility or reproductive performance. The significance of these findings to humans is unknown.

Pregnant rabbits were treated with up to 100mg/kg/day of atomoxetine by gavage throughout the period of organogenesis. At this dose, in 1 of 3 studies, decrease in live foetuses, increase in early resorption, slight increases in the incidences of atypical origin of carotid artery and absent subclavian artery were observed. These findings were observed at doses that caused slight maternal toxicity. The incidence of these findings is within historical control values. The no-effect dose for these findings was 30mg/kg/day. Exposure (AUC) to unbound atomoxetine in rabbits, at 100mg/kg/day, was approximately 3.3-times (CYP2D6 extensive metabolisers) and 0.4-times (CYP2D6 poor metabolisers) those in humans at the maximum daily dose of 1.4mg/kg/day. The findings in one of three rabbit studies were equivocal and the relevance to man is unknown.

6. PHARMACEUTICAL PARTICULARS

6.1 List of excipients

The capsules contain:

Starch, pregelatinised (maize)

Dimeticone

Capsule shell:

Sodium laurilsulfate

Gelatin

Edible black ink SW-9008 or edible black ink SW-9010 (containing shellac and black iron oxide E172)

Capsule shell cap colourants:

10mg: Titanium dioxide E171

18mg: Yellow iron oxide E172

25mg, 40mg, and 60mg: FD&C Blue 2 (indigo carmine) E132 and titanium dioxide E171

Capsule shell body colourants:

10mg, 18mg, and 25mg: Titanium dioxide E171

40mg: FD&C Blue 2 (indigo carmine) E132 and titanium dioxide E171

60mg: Yellow iron oxide E172

6.2 Incompatibilities

Not applicable.

6.3 Shelf life

3 years.

6.4 Special precautions for storage

Do not store above 25°C.

6.5 Nature and contents of container

Polyvinyl chloride (PVC)/polyethylene (PE)/polychlorotrifluoroethylene (PCTFE) blister sealed with aluminium foil lid.

Available in pack sizes of 7, 14, 28, and 56 capsules. Not all pack sizes may be marketed.

6.6 Instructions for use and handling

No special requirements.

7. MARKETING AUTHORISATION HOLDER

Eli Lilly and Company Limited

Kingsclere Road

Basingstoke

Hampshire

RG21 6XA

United Kingdom

8. MARKETING AUTHORISATION NUMBER(S)

Strattera 10mg hard capsules:	PL 00006/0375
Strattera 18mg hard capsules:	PL 00006/0376
Strattera 25mg hard capsules:	PL 00006/0377
Strattera 40mg hard capsules:	PL 00006/0378
Strattera 60mg hard capsules:	PL 00006/0379

9. DATE OF FIRST AUTHORISATION/RENEWAL OF THE AUTHORISATION

Date of first authorisation: 27 May 2004

10. DATE OF REVISION OF THE TEXT

27 September 2005

LEGAL CATEGORY

POM

*STRATTERA (atomoxetine) is a trademark of Eli Lilly and Company.

Stugeron 15mg

(Janssen-Cilag Ltd)

1. NAME OF THE MEDICINAL PRODUCT
Stugeron® 15 mg.

2. QUALITATIVE AND QUANTITATIVE COMPOSITION
Each tablet contains 15 mg cinnarizine.

3. PHARMACEUTICAL FORM
White circular tablet with S/15 on one side and Janssen on the other side.

4. CLINICAL PARTICULARS

4.1 Therapeutic indications
Stugeron is for the control of vestibular disorders such as vertigo, tinnitus, nausea and vomiting such as is seen in Meniere's Disease.

Stugeron is also effective in the control of motion sickness.

4.2 Posology and method of administration
Route of administration
Oral. The tablets may be chewed, sucked or swallowed whole.

Dosage
Stugeron should preferably be taken after meals.

Vestibular symptoms
Adults, elderly and children over 12 years: 2 tablets three times a day.

Children 5 to 12 years: One half the adult dose.

These doses should not be exceeded.

Motion sickness
Adults, elderly and children over 12 years: 2 tablets 2 hours before you travel and 1 tablet every 8 hours during your journey.

Children 5 to 12 years: One half the adult dose.

4.3 Contraindications
Stugeron should not be given to patients with known hypersensitivity to cinnarizine.

4.4 Special warnings and special precautions for use
As with other antihistamines, Stugeron may cause epigastric discomfort; taking it after meals may diminish the gastric irritation.

In patients with Parkinson's Disease, Stugeron should only be given if the advantages outweigh the possible risk of aggravating this disease.

4.5 Interaction with other medicinal products and other forms of Interaction
Concurrent use of alcohol, CNS depressants or tricyclic antidepressants may potentiate the sedative effects of either these drugs or of Stugeron.

Because of its antihistamine effect, Stugeron may prevent an otherwise positive reaction to dermal reactivity indicators if used within 4 days prior to testing.

4.6 Pregnancy and lactation
The safety of Stugeron in human pregnancy has not been established although studies in animals have not demonstrated teratogenic effects. As with other drugs it is not advisable to administer Stugeron in pregnancy.

There are no data on the excretion of Stugeron in human breast milk. Use of Stugeron is not recommended in nursing mothers.

4.7 Effects on ability to drive and use machines
Stugeron may cause drowsiness, especially at the start of treatment; patients affected in this way should not drive or operate machinery.

4.8 Undesirable effects
For all indications: Drowsiness and gastro-intestinal disturbances may occur. These are usually transient.

In rare cases, headache, dry mouth, perspiration or allergic reactions may occur.

For long term treatment, i.e. vestibular symptoms: Rare cases of weight gain and very rare cases of lichen planus, lupus-like skin reactions and cholestatic jaundice have been reported. Rare cases of aggravation or appearance of extrapyramidal symptoms (sometimes associated with depressive feelings) have been described, predominantly in elderly people during prolonged therapy. The treatment should be discontinued in such cases.

4.9 Overdose
Vomiting, drowsiness, coma, tremor and hypotonia may occur.

There is no specific antidote to Stugeron but in the event of overdosage, gastric lavage and the administration of activated charcoal may help.

5. PHARMACOLOGICAL PROPERTIES

5.1 Pharmacodynamic properties
Cinnarizine has been shown to be a non-competitive antagonist of the smooth muscle contractions caused by various vasoactive agents including histamine.

Cinnarizine also acts on vascular smooth muscle by selectively inhibiting the calcium influx into depolarised cells, thereby reducing the availability of free Ca^{2+} ions for the induction and maintenance of contraction.

Vestibular eye reflexes induced by caloric stimulation of the labyrinth in guinea pigs are markedly depressed by cinnarizine.

Cinnarizine has been shown to inhibit nystagmus.

5.2 Pharmacokinetic properties
In animals, cinnarizine is extensively metabolised, N-dealkylation being the major pathway. Approx. two thirds of the metabolites are excreted with the faeces, the rest in the urine, mainly during the first five days after a single dose.

In man, after oral administration, absorption is relatively slow, peak serum concentrations occurring after 2.5 to 4 hours.

Cinnarizine undergoes extensive metabolism but there is considerable interindividual variation in the extent of metabolism. The drug is excreted in the urine unchanged as metabolites and glucuronide conjugates. The terminal elimination half life is about 3 hours.

5.3 Preclinical safety data
No relevant information additional to that contained elsewhere in the Summary of Product Characteristics.

6. PHARMACEUTICAL PARTICULARS

6.1 List of excipients
Lactose monohydrate

Maize starch

Sucrose

Talc

Magnesium stearate

Polyvidone K90

6.2 Incompatibilities
None known.

6.3 Shelf life
5 years

6.4 Special precautions for storage
None.

6.5 Nature and contents of container
PVC/Aluminium foil blisters

or

Polystyrene tubs with polyethylene caps

Each pack containing 100 tablets.

6.6 Instructions for use and handling
The tablets may be chewed, sucked or swallowed whole.

7. MARKETING AUTHORISATION HOLDER
Janssen-Cilag Limited
Saunderton
High Wycombe
Buckinghamshire
HP14 4HJ
UK

8. MARKETING AUTHORISATION NUMBER(S)
PL 0242/5009R

9. DATE OF FIRST AUTHORISATION/RENEWAL OF THE AUTHORISATION
Date of First Authorisation: 14/09/89

Renewal of Authorisation: 23/03/95

10. DATE OF REVISION OF THE TEXT
July 2001

Legal category P

Stugeron Forte 75mg

(Janssen-Cilag Ltd)

1. NAME OF THE MEDICINAL PRODUCT
Stugeron® Forte 75 mg Capsules

2. QUALITATIVE AND QUANTITATIVE COMPOSITION
Each capsule contains cinnarizine 75 mg.

3. PHARMACEUTICAL FORM
Orange and yellow capsule.

4. CLINICAL PARTICULARS

4.1 Therapeutic indications
Long term management of symptoms of peripheral arterial disease, including intermittent claudication, rest pain, muscular cramps and vasospastic disorders, eg Raynaud's disease.

4.2 Posology and method of administration
For oral administration.

Stugeron Forte should preferably be taken after meals.

Adults:

Starting dose: One capsule three times daily.

Maintenance dose: Once capsule two or three times daily, according to response.

These doses should not be exceeded.

Peripheral arterial disease is slow to improve with any form of drug treatment. Maximum benefit with Stugeron Forte will not be felt until after several weeks of continuous treatment, although significant improvement in blood flow has frequently been demonstrated after one week.

Elderly:

As for adults.

Children:

Not recommended.

4.3 Contraindications
Stugeron Forte should not be given to patients with known hypersensitivity to cinnarizine.

4.4 Special warnings and special precautions for use
Stugeron Forte has not been found to reduce blood pressure significantly. However, the drug should be used with reasonable caution in hypotensive patients.

As with other antihistamines, Stugeron Forte may cause epigastric discomfort; taking it after meals may diminish gastric irritation.

In patients with Parkinson's disease, Stugeron Forte should only be given if the advantages outweigh the possible risk of aggravating this disease.

4.5 Interaction with other medicinal products and other forms of Interaction
Concurrent use of alcohol, CNS depressants or tricyclic antidepressants may potentiate the sedative effects of either these drugs or of Stugeron Forte.

Because of its antihistamine effect, Stugeron Forte may prevent an otherwise positive reaction to dermal reactivity indicators if used within 4 days prior to testing.

4.6 Pregnancy and lactation
The safety of Stugeron Forte in human pregnancy has not been established although studies in animals have not demonstrated teratogenic effects. As with other drugs, it is not advisable to administer Stugeron Forte in pregnancy.

There are no data on the excretion of Stugeron Forte in human breast milk. Use of Stugeron Forte is not recommended in nursing mothers.

4.7 Effects on ability to drive and use machines
Stugeron Forte may cause drowsiness, especially at the start of treatment. Patients affected in this way should not drive or operate machinery.

4.8 Undesirable effects
Drowsiness and gastro-intestinal disturbances may occur. These are usually transient.

Rare cases of weight gain, headache, dry mouth, perspiration or allergic reactions may occur.

Very rare cases of lichen planus, lupus-like skin reactions and cholestatic jaundice have been reported.

Rare cases of aggravation or appearance of extrapyramidal symptoms (sometimes associated with depressive feelings) have been described, predominantly in elderly people during prolonged treatment. The treatment should be discontinued in such cases.

4.9 Overdose
Vomiting, drowsiness, coma, tremor and hypotonia may occur.

There is no specific antidote to Stugeron Forte but in the event of overdosage, gastric lavage and the administration of activated charcoal may help.

5. PHARMACOLOGICAL PROPERTIES

5.1 Pharmacodynamic properties
Cinnarizine's actions in the treatment of peripheral vascular disease are due to its anti-vasoconstrictor properties, its action on blood hyperviscosity and its anti-ischaemic effect. Anti-vasoconstriction is thought to be through a calcium blocker mechanism, and is evident selectively in vascular smooth muscle. Increased peripheral muscle blood flow may be mediated by prevention of calcium entry into ischaemic erythrocytes, thereby preserving flexibility.

5.2 Pharmacokinetic properties
After a single 75 mg dose of cinnarizine, peak plasma levels of

160 ± 130 ng/ml occurred after a mean time of 3.4 hours. Plasma concentrations declined with a half life of 3.04 hours. The mean area under the curve was 925 ± 603 μg/ml/hr. Absorption may be varied between subjects - the highest peak concentrations being 19 times the lowest value in one study. Less than 20% of isotopically labelled cinnarizine appears in the urine and about 40% in the faeces.

5.3 Preclinical safety data
No relevant information additional to that contained elsewhere in the Summary of Product Characteristics.

6. PHARMACEUTICAL PARTICULARS

6.1 List of excipients
Lactose, hydrous PhEur

Corn starch PhEur

Talc PhEur

Magnesium stearate PhEur

Capsule cap:

Titanium dioxide (E171) PhEur

Orange yellow S (E110) PhEur

Erythrosine (E127) FP

Gelatin PhEur

Capsule body:

Titanium dioxide (E171) PhEur

Yellow ferric oxide (E172) NF

Gelatin PhEur

6.2 Incompatibilities
None known.

6.3 Shelf life
60 months.

6.4 Special precautions for storage
None.

6.5 Nature and contents of container
Blisters consisting of:

Aluminium foil hermatalu, thickness 20 μm

Perlalux tristar, PVC 200 μm, LDPE 25 μm and PVDC 90 g/m^2

containing 100 capsules.

6.6 Instructions for use and handling
Not applicable.

7. MARKETING AUTHORISATION HOLDER
Janssen-Cilag Ltd

Saunderton

High Wycombe

Buckinghamshire

HP14 4HJ

UK

8. MARKETING AUTHORISATION NUMBER(S)
PL/0242/0008

9. DATE OF FIRST AUTHORISATION/RENEWAL OF THE AUTHORISATION
17 June 1977/18 February 2002

10. DATE OF REVISION OF THE TEXT
Legal category P.

Ⓣ trademark

Sublimaze

(Janssen-Cilag Ltd)

1. NAME OF THE MEDICINAL PRODUCT
SublimazeⓉ

2. QUALITATIVE AND QUANTITATIVE COMPOSITION
Fentanyl citrate 78.5 micrograms equivalent to 50 micrograms per ml fentanyl base.

3. PHARMACEUTICAL FORM
Injection.

4. CLINICAL PARTICULARS

4.1 Therapeutic indications
Sublimaze is an opioid analgesic used:

a. In low doses to provide analgesia during short surgical procedures.

b. In high doses as an analgesic/respiratory depressant in patients requiring assisted ventilation.

c. In combination with a neuroleptic in the technique of neuroleptanalgesia.

d. In the treatment of severe pain, such as the pain of myocardial infarction.

4.2 Posology and method of administration
Route of administration

Intravenous administration either as a bolus or by infusion.

Intramuscular administration.

Sublimaze, by the intravenous route, can be administered to both adults and children. The dose of Sublimaze should be individualised according to age, body weight, physical status, underlying pathological condition, use of other drugs and type of surgery and anaesthesia.

The usual dosage regimen is as follows:

(see Table 1)

Table 1

	Adults		Children	
	Initial	Supplemental	Initial	Supplemental
Spontaneous Respiration	50-200 mcg	50 mcg	3-5 mcg/kg	1 mcg/kg
Assisted Ventilation	300-3500 mcg	100-200 mcg	15 mcg/kg	1-3 mcg/kg

Doses in excess of 200 mcg are for use in anaesthesia only. As a premedicant, 1-2 ml Sublimaze may be given intramuscularly 45 minutes before induction of anaesthesia.

After intravenous administration in unpremedicated adult patients, 2 ml Sublimaze may be expected to provide sufficient analgesia for 10-20 minutes in surgical procedures involving low pain intensity. 10 ml Sublimaze injected as a bolus gives analgesia lasting about one hour. The analgesia produced is sufficient for surgery involving moderately painful procedures. Giving a dose of 50 mcg/kg Sublimaze will provide intense analgesia for some four to six hours, for intensely stimulating surgery.

Sublimaze may also be given as an infusion. In ventilated patients, a loading dose of Sublimaze may be given as a fast infusion of approximately 1 mcg/kg/min for the first 10 minutes followed by an infusion of approximately 0.1 mcg/kg/min. Alternatively the loading dose of Sublimaze may be given as a bolus. Infusion rates should be titrated to individual patient response; lower infusion rates may be adequate. Unless it is planned to ventilate post-operatively, the infusion should be terminated at about 40 minutes before the end of surgery.

Lower infusion rates, eg 0.05-0.08 mcg/kg/minute are necessary if spontaneous ventilation is to be maintained. Higher infusion rates (up to 3 mcg/kg/minute) have been used in cardiac surgery.

Sublimaze is chemically incompatible with the induction agents thiopentone and methohexitone because of wide differences in pH.

Use in elderly and debilitated patients: It is wise to reduce the dosage in the elderly and debilitated patients. The effect of the initial dose should be taken into account in determining supplemental doses.

4.3 Contraindications
Respiratory depression, obstructive airways disease. Concurrent administration with monoamine oxidase inhibitors, or within 2 weeks of their discontinuation. Known intolerance to fentanyl or other morphinomimetics.

4.4 Special warnings and special precautions for use
Warnings:

Tolerance and dependence may occur. Following intravenous administration of fentanyl, a transient fall in blood pressure may occur, especially in hypovolaemic patients. Appropriate measures to maintain a stable arterial pressure should be taken.

Significant respiratory depression will occur following the administration of fentanyl in doses in excess of 200 mcg. This, and the other pharmacological effects of fentanyl, can be reversed by specific narcotic antagonists (eg naloxone). Additional doses of the latter may be necessary because the respiratory depression may last longer than the duration of action of the opioid antagonist.

Bradycardia and possibly asystole can occur in non-atropinised patients, and can be antagonised by atropine.

Muscular rigidity (morphine-like effect) may occur.

Rigidity, which may also involve the thoracic muscles, can be avoided by the following measures:

– slow iv injection (usually sufficient for lower doses);

– premedication with benzodiazepines;

– use of muscle relaxants.

Precautions:

As with all opioid analgesics, care should be observed when administering fentanyl to patients with myasthenia gravis.

It is wise to reduce dosage in the elderly and debilitated patients.

In hypothyroidism, pulmonary disease, decreased respiratory reserve, alcoholism and liver or renal impairment the dosage should be titrated with care and prolonged monitoring may be required.

Patients on chronic opioid therapy or with a history of opioid abuse may require higher doses.

Administration in labour may cause respiratory depression in the new born infant.

As with all potent opioids, profound analgesia is accompanied by marked respiratory depression, which may persist into or recur in the early postoperative period. Care should be taken after large doses or infusions of fentanyl to ensure that adequate spontaneous breathing has been established and maintained before discharging the patient from the recovery area.

Resuscitation equipment and opioid antagonists should be readily available. Hyperventilation during anaesthesia may alter the patients response to CO_2, thus affecting respiration postoperatively.

The use of rapid bolus injections of opioids should be avoided in patients with compromised intracerebral compliance; in such patients the transient decrease in the mean arterial pressure has occasionally been accompanied by a transient reduction of the cerebral perfusion pressure.

4.5 Interaction with other medicinal products and other forms of Interaction
The use of opioid premedication, barbiturates, benzodiazepines, neuroleptics, halogenic gases and other non-selective CNS depressants (eg alcohol) may enhance or prolong the respiratory depression of fentanyl.

When patients have received CNS-depressants, the dose of fentanyl required will be less than usual. Likewise, following the administration of fentanyl the dose of other CNS-depressant drugs should be reduced.

Fentanyl, a high clearance drug, is rapidly and extensively metabolised mainly by CYP3A4. Itraconazole (a potent CYP3A4 inhibitor) at 200 mg/day given orally for 4 days had no significant effect on the pharmacokinetics of iv fentanyl.

Oral ritonavir (one of the most potent CYP3A4 inhibitors) reduced the clearance of iv fentanyl by two thirds; however, peak plasma concentrations after a single dose of iv fentanyl were not affected.

When fentanyl is used in a single dose, the concomitant use of potent CYP3A4 inhibitors such as ritonavir requires special patient care and observation. With continuous treatment, dose reduction of fentanyl may be required to avoid accumulation of fentanyl, which may increase the risk of prolonged or delayed respiratory depression.

Bradycardia and possibly asystole can occur when fentanyl is combined with non-vagolytic muscle relaxants.

The concomitant use of droperidol can result in a higher incidence of hypotension.

4.6 Pregnancy and lactation
Although no teratogenic or acute embryotoxic effects have been observed in animal experiments, insufficient data are available to evaluate any harmful effects in humans. As with other drugs, possible risks should be weighed against potential benefits to the patient.

Administration during childbirth (including Caesarean section) is not recommended because fentanyl crosses the placenta and the foetal respiratory centre is particularly sensitive to opioids. If fentanyl is nevertheless administered, an antidote for the child should always be at hand.

Fentanyl may enter the maternal milk. It is therefore recommended that breast feeding is not initiated within 24 hours of treatment.

4.7 Effects on ability to drive and use machines
Where early discharge is envisaged, patients should be advised not to drive or operate machinery for 24 hours following administration.

4.8 Undesirable effects
The side effects are those associated with intravenous opioids eg respiratory depression, apnoea, muscular rigidity (which may also involve the thoracic muscles), myoclonic movements, bradycardia, transient hypotension, nausea, vomiting, dizziness, insomnia and sexual dysfunction (eg decreased libido).

Other less frequently reported adverse reactions are:

– laryngospasm;

– allergic reactions (eg anaphylaxis, bronchospasm, pruritus, urticaria) and asystole although it is uncertain whether there is a causal relationship as several drugs were co-administered;

– secondary rebound respiratory depression has rarely been reported.

When a neuroleptic such as droperidol is used with fentanyl, the following adverse reactions may be observed: chills and/or shivering, restlessness, post-operative hallucinatory episodes and extrapyramidal symptoms.

4.9 Overdose
Symptoms:

The manifestations of fentanyl overdosage are generally an extension of its pharmacological action. Depending on the individual sensitivity, the clinical picture is determined primarily by the degree of respiratory depression, which varies from bradypnoea to apnoea.

Treatment:

Hypoventilation or apnoea:	O_2 administration, assisted or controlled respiration.
Respiratory depression:	Specific narcotic antagonist (eg naloxone). This does not preclude the use of immediate countermeasures.
Muscular rigidity:	Intravenous neuromuscular blocking agent.

The patient should be carefully observed; body warmth and adequate fluid intake should be maintained. If hypotension is severe or if it persists, the possibility of hypovolaemia should be considered and, if present, it should be controlled with appropriate parenteral fluid administration.

5. PHARMACOLOGICAL PROPERTIES

5.1 Pharmacodynamic properties

Fentanyl is a synthetic opiate with a clinical potency of 50 to 100 times that of morphine. Its onset of action is rapid and its duration of action is short. In man, a single iv dose of 0.5-1 mg/70 kg body weight immediately produces a pronounced state of surgical analgesia, respiratory depression, bradycardia and other typical morphine-like effects. The duration of action of the peak effects is about 30 minutes. All potent morphine-like drugs produce relief from pain, ventilatory depression, emesis, constipation, physical dependence, certain vagal effects and varying degrees of sedation. Fentanyl, however, differs from morphine not only by its short duration of action but also by its lack of emetic effect and minimal hypotensive activity in animals.

5.2 Pharmacokinetic properties

Some pharmacokinetic parameters for fentanyl are as follows:

Urinary excretion = 8%

Bound in plasma = 80%

Clearance (ml/min/kg) = 13±2

Volume of distribution (litres/kg) = 4.0±0.4

Estimates of terminal half-life range from 141 to 853 minutes.

5.3 Preclinical safety data

No relevant information additional to that contained elsewhere in the Summary of Product Characteristics.

6. PHARMACEUTICAL PARTICULARS

6.1 List of excipients

Sodium chloride

Water for injections

6.2 Incompatibilities

The product is chemically incompatible with the induction agents thiopentone and methohexitone because of the wide differences in pH.

6.3 Shelf life

60 months.

6.4 Special precautions for storage

Protect from light.

Do not store above 30°C.

Keep container in the outer carton.

Keep out of reach and sight of children.

6.5 Nature and contents of container

Colourless glass ampoules (PhEur, USP Type I).

Pack size: packs of 10 **and 50*** of 2 ml and **5 ml*** ampoules; packs of 5 and **10*** of 10 ml ampoules.

*** not marketed**

6.6 Instructions for use and handling

Not applicable (store as a CD).

7. MARKETING AUTHORISATION HOLDER

Janssen-Cilag Ltd

Saunderton

High Wycombe

Buckinghamshire

HP14 4HJ

UK

8. MARKETING AUTHORISATION NUMBER(S)

0242/5001R

9. DATE OF FIRST AUTHORISATION/RENEWAL OF THE AUTHORISATION

26 February 1980

10. DATE OF REVISION OF THE TEXT

5 June 2003

Legal category POM/CD

SUBUTEX 0.4mg, 2mg and 8mg sublingual tablets

(Schering-Plough Ltd)

1. NAME OF THE MEDICINAL PRODUCT

SUBUTEX 0.4mg, 2mg and 8mg sublingual tablets.

2. QUALITATIVE AND QUANTITATIVE COMPOSITION

Buprenorphine hydrochloride equivalent to buprenorphine base: 0.4mg, 2mg or 8mg.

3. PHARMACEUTICAL FORM

Sublingual tablet

4. CLINICAL PARTICULARS

4.1 Therapeutic indications

Substitution treatment for opioid drug dependence, within a framework of medical, social and psychological treatment.

4.2 Posology and method of administration

Treatment with SUBUTEX sublingual tablets is intended for use in adults and children age 16 years or over who have agreed to be treated for addiction.

When initiating SUBUTEX treatment, the physician should be aware of the partial agonist profile of buprenorphine and that it can precipitate withdrawal in opioid-dependent patients. Buprenorphine binds to the μ and κ opiate receptors.

Administration is sublingual. Physicians must advise patients that the sublingual route is the only effective and safe route of administration for this drug. The tablet should be kept under the tongue until dissolved, which usually occurs within 5 to 10 minutes.

- **Induction therapy**: the initial dose is from 0.8mg to 4mg, administered as a single daily dose.

• **for opioid-dependent drug addicts who have not undergone withdrawal:** one dose of SUBUTEX tablet(s) administered sublingually at least 4 hours after the last use of the opioid, or when the first signs of craving appear.

• **For patients receiving methadone**: before beginning SUBUTEX therapy, the dose of methadone should be reduced to a maximum of 30mg/day. SUBUTEX may precipitate symptoms of withdrawal in patients dependent upon methadone.

- **Dosage adjustment and maintenance**: the dose of SUBUTEX should be increased progressively according to the clinical effect of the individual patient and should not exceed a maximum single daily dose of 32 mg. The dosage is titrated according to reassessment of the clinical and psychological status of the patient.

- **Dosage reduction and termination of treatment**: after a satisfactory period of stabilisation has been achieved, the dosage may be reduced gradually to a lower maintenance dose; when deemed appropriate, treatment may be discontinued in some patients. The availability of the sublingual tablet in doses of 0.4 mg, 2 mg and 8 mg, respectively, allows for a downward titration of dosage. Patients should be monitored following termination of buprenorphine treatment because of the potential for relapse.

4.3 Contraindications

- Hypersensitivity to buprenorphine or any other component of the tablet
- Children less than 16 years of age
- Severe respiratory insufficiency
- Severe hepatic insufficiency
- Acute alcoholism or delirium tremens
- Breast feeding

4.4 Special warnings and special precautions for use

• **Warnings**

SUBUTEX sublingual tablets are recommended only for the treatment of opioid drug dependence.

- Respiratory Depression: some cases of death due to respiratory depression have been reported, particularly when used in combination with benzodiazepines (see **4.5 Interaction with other medicaments and other forms of interaction**) or when buprenorphine was not used according to labelling.

Hepatitis, hepatic events: hepatic necrosis and hepatitis with jaundice, which generally have resolved favourably, have been reported in patients who use buprenorphine. Causality has not been clearly established. When a hepatic event is suspected and the causality is unknown, further evaluation is required. If SUBUTEX is suspected to be the cause of hepatic necrosis or jaundice, it must be discontinued as rapidly as the patient's clinical condition permits. All patients should have liver function tests performed at regular intervals.

- This product can cause opioid withdrawal symptoms if administered to an addicted patient less than 4 hours after the last use of the drug (see **4.2 Posology and method of administration**.)

- This product can cause drowsiness, which may be exacerbated by other centrally acting agents, such as: alcohol, tranquillisers, sedatives, hypnotics (see **4.5 Interactions with other medicaments and other forms of interaction**.)

- This product can cause orthostatic hypotension.

- Studies in animals, as well as clinical experience, have demonstrated that buprenorphine may produce a low level of dependence.

- Athletes should be aware that this medicine may cause a positive reaction to "anti-doping tests."

• **Paediatric Use**

No data are available in children less than 16 years of age; therefore, SUBUTEX should not be used in children under the age of 16.

• **Precautions for use**

This product should be used with care in patients with:

- asthma or respiratory insufficiency (cases of respiratory depression have been reported with buprenorphine);

- renal insufficiency (20% of the administered dose is eliminated by the renal route; thus, renal elimination may be prolonged);

- hepatic insufficiency (hepatic metabolism of buprenorphine may be altered).

4.5 Interaction with other medicinal products and other forms of Interaction

SUBUTEX should not be taken together with alcoholic drinks or medications containing alcohol. Alcohol increases the sedative effect of buprenorphine (see 4.7. Effects on the ability to drive vehicles or operate machinery.)

SUBUTEX should be used cautiously together with:

- Benzodiazepines: This combination may potentiate respiratory depression of central origin, with risk of death; therefore, dosages must be individually titrated and the patient monitored carefully. The risk of drug abuse should also be considered (see **4.4 Special warnings and special precautions for use**).

- Other central nervous system depressants; other opioid derivatives (analgesics and antitussives); certain antidepressants, sedative H_1-receptor antagonists, barbiturates, anxiolytics other than benzodiazepines, neuroleptics, clonidine and related substances. This combination increases central nervous system depression.

- Monoamine oxidase inhibitors (MAOI): Possible exaggeration of the effects of opioids, based on experience with morphine.

- To date, no notable interaction has been observed with cocaine, the agent most frequently used by multi-drug abusers in association with opioids.

A suspected interaction between buprenorphine injection and phenprocoumon, resulting in purpura, has been reported.

An interaction study of buprenorphine with ketoconazole (a potent inhibitor of CYP3A4) resulted in increased Cmax and AUC of buprenorphine (approximately 70% and 50% respectively) and, to a lesser extent, of the metabolite, norbuprenorphine. Patients receiving Subutex should be closely monitored and the dose of buprenorphine should be halved when starting treatment with ketoconazole.

Further titration of Subutex should be made as clinically indicated. Although no data from clinical trials are available, the use of other inhibitors of CYP3A4 (e.g. gestodene, troleandoymycin, the HIV protease inhibitors ritonavir, indinavir and saquinavir) may also increase exposure levels to buprenorphine and norbuprenorphine and a similar dose-reduction should be considered when initiating treatment.

The interaction of buprenorphine with CYP 3A4 inducers has not been investigated, therefore it is recommended that patients receiving Subutex should be closely monitored if enzyme inducers (e.g. phenobarbital, carbamazepine, phenytoin, rifampicin) are co-administered. Use of these medications may increase the metabolism of buprenorphine and the dose of buprenorphine should be increased appropriately if patients complain of decreased benefit from buprenorphine or if there is re-emergence of craving for illicit drugs.

4.6 Pregnancy and lactation

Pregnancy

Studies in rats and rabbits have evidenced foetotoxicity including post-implantation loss. In addition, maternal oral administration at high doses during gestation and lactation resulted in a slight delay in the development of some neurological functions (surface righting reflex and startle response) in neonatal rats.

In humans, there is currently not sufficient data to evaluate potential malformative or foetotoxic effects of buprenorphine when administered during pregnancy.

At the end of pregnancy, high doses, even for a short duration of time, may induce respiratory depression in neonates. During the last three months of pregnancy, chronic use of buprenorphine may be responsible for a withdrawal syndrome in neonates. Consequently, the use of buprenorphine is not recommended during pregnancy.

Breast-feeding

As evidenced in rats, buprenorphine has the potential to inhibit lactation or milk production. In addition, because buprenorphine passes into the mother's milk, breast-feeding is contra-indicated.

4.7 Effects on ability to drive and use machines

SUBUTEX may cause drowsiness, particularly when taken together with alcohol or central nervous system depressants. Therefore, patients should be warned against driving or operating machinery (see **4.5 Interaction with other medicaments and other forms of interaction**.)

4.8 Undesirable effects

The onset of side effects depends on the patient's tolerance threshold, which is higher in drug addicts than in the general population.

The symptoms most frequently observed with buprenorphine administration are:

- constipation
- headaches
- insomnia
- asthenia
- drowsiness
- nausea and vomiting
- fainting and dizziness

- orthostatic hypotension
- sweating

Other side effects that have been reported are:

- respiratory depression (see **4.4 Special warnings and special precautions for use**, and **4.5 Interaction with other medicaments and other forms of interaction**).
- hepatic necrosis and hepatitis (see **4.4 Special warnings and special precautions for use**)
- hallucinations

Cases of bronchospasm, angioneurotic oedema and anaphylactic shock have also been reported.

In patients presenting with marked drug dependence, initial administration of buprenorphine can produce a withdrawal effect similar to that associated with naloxone.

4.9 Overdose

In the event of accidental overdose, general supportive measures should be instituted, including close monitoring of respiratory and cardiac status of the patient. The major symptom requiring intervention is respiratory depression, which could lead to respiratory arrest and death. If the patient vomits, care must be taken to prevent aspiration of the vomitus.

Treatment: Symptomatic treatment of respiratory depression, following standard intensive care measures, should be instituted. A patient airway and assisted or controlled ventilation must be assured. The patient should be transferred to an environment within which full resuscitation facilities are available. Use of an opioid antagonist (i.e., naloxone) is recommended, despite the modest effect it may have in reversing the respiratory symptoms of buprenorphine compared with its effects on full agonist opioid agents.

The long duration of action of SUBUTEX should be taken into consideration when determining length of treatment needed to reverse the effects of an overdose.

5. PHARMACOLOGICAL PROPERTIES

5.1 Pharmacodynamic properties

OPIOID ANALGESIC

(N: central nervous system)

Buprenorphine is an opioid partial agonist/antagonist which attaches itself to the μ (mu) and κ (kappa) receptors of the brain. Its activity in opioid maintenance treatment is attributed to its slowly reversible link with the μ receptors which, over a prolonged period, minimises the need of the addicted patient for drugs.

During clinical pharmacologic studies in opiate-dependent subjects, buprenorphine demonstrated a ceiling effect on a number of parameters, including positive mood, "good effect", and respiratory depression.

5.2 Pharmacokinetic properties

Absorption

When taken orally, buprenorphine undergoes first-pass hepatic metabolism with N-dealkylation and glucuroconjugation in the small intestine. The use of this medication by the oral route is therefore inappropriate.

Peak plasma concentrations are achieved 90 minutes after sublingual administration and the maximal dose-concentration relationship is linear, between 2 mg and 16 mg.

Distribution

The absorption of buprenorphine is followed by a rapid distribution phase and a half-life of 2 to 5 hours.

Metabolism and elimination

Buprenorphine is oxidatively metabolised by 14-N-dealkylation to N-desalkyl-buprenorphine (also known as norbuprenorphine) via cytochrome P450 CYP3A4 and by glucuroconjugation of the parent molecule and the dealkylated metabolite. Norbuprenorphine is a μ (mu) agonist with weak intrinsic activity.

Elimination of buprenorphine is bi- or tri- exponential, with a long terminal elimination phase of 20 to 25 hours, due in part to reabsorption of buprenorphine after intestinal hydrolysis of the conjugated derivative, and in part to the highly lipophilic nature of the molecule.

Buprenorphine is essentially eliminated in the faeces by biliary excretion of the glucuroconjugated metabolites (80%), the rest being eliminated in the urine.

5.3 Preclinical safety data

Acute toxicity of buprenorphine was determined in the mouse and rat following oral and parenteral administration. The median lethal doses (LD_{50}) in the mouse were 26, 94 and 261 mg/kg for intravenous, intraperitoneal and oral administration, respectively. The LD_{50} values in the rat were 35, 243, and 600 mg/kg for intravenous, intraperitoneal and oral administration, respectively.

When beagles were dosed continuously subcutaneously for one month, rhesus monkeys orally for one month and rats and baboons intramuscularly for six months, buprenorphine showed remarkably low tissue and biochemical toxicities.

From teratology studies in rats and rabbits, it was concluded that buprenorphine is not embryotoxic or teratogenic, and it does not have any marked effects on weaning potential. There were no adverse effects on fertility or general reproductive function in rats, although at the highest intramuscular dose (5mg/kg/day) the mothers experienced some difficulty in parturition and there was a high neonatal mortality.

Minimal to moderate hyperplasia of the bile duct with associated peribiliary fibrosis occurred in dogs following 52 weeks of oral dosing of 75mg/kg/day.

6. PHARMACEUTICAL PARTICULARS

6.1 List of excipients

Monohydrated lactose, mannitol, maize starch, povidone excipient K30, citric acid, sodium citrate and magnesium stearate

6.2 Incompatibilities

None known

6.3 Shelf life

3 years

6.4 Special precautions for storage

Do not store above 30°C. Store in the original package.

6.5 Nature and contents of container

7 or 28 tablets in PVC/PVdC/Aluminium blister packs

6.6 Instructions for use and handling

Not applicable

Administrative Data

7. MARKETING AUTHORISATION HOLDER

Schering-Plough Ltd
Shire Park
Welwyn Garden City
Hertfordshire
AL7 1TW
UK

8. MARKETING AUTHORISATION NUMBER(S)

Subutex 0.4mg, sublingual tablets:	PL 00201/0241
Subutex 2mg, sublingual tablets:	PL 00201/0242
Subutex 8mg, sublingual tablets:	PL 00201/0243

9. DATE OF FIRST AUTHORISATION/RENEWAL OF THE AUTHORISATION

February 1998 (UK)

10. DATE OF REVISION OF THE TEXT

April 2004

Legal Category

CD (Sch 3), POM

Subutex/UK/4-04/6

Sudafed Plus Tablets

(Pfizer Consumer Healthcare)

1. NAME OF THE MEDICINAL PRODUCT

SUDAFED Plus Tablets

2. QUALITATIVE AND QUANTITATIVE COMPOSITION

SUDAFED Plus Tablets contain 60 mg of pseudoephedrine hydrochloride and 2.5 mg of triprolidine hydrochloride in each tablet.

For excipients, see 6.1.

3. PHARMACEUTICAL FORM

Tablet

4. CLINICAL PARTICULARS

4.1 Therapeutic indications

Symptomatic relief of allergic rhinitis.

4.2 Posology and method of administration

Adults and children over 12 years

Oral: One tablet every 4 - 6 hours up to 4 times a day.

Use in the elderly

No specific studies have been carried out in the elderly, but triprolidine and pseudoephedrine have been widely used in older people.

Hepatic dysfunction

Caution should be exercised when administering SUDAFED Plus Tablets to patients with severe hepatic impairment.

Renal dysfunction

Caution should be exercised when administering SUDAFED Plus Tablets to patients with moderate to severe renal impairment.

4.3 Contraindications

SUDAFED Plus is contraindicated in individuals with known hypersensitivity to pseudoephedrine or triprolidine.

SUDAFED Plus is contraindicated in individuals who are taking or have taken monoamine oxidase inhibitors within the preceding two weeks. The concomitant use of pseudoephedrine and this type of product may occasionally cause a rise in blood pressure.

SUDAFED Plus is contraindicated in patients with severe hypertension or severe coronary artery disease.

The antibacterial agent furazolidone is known to cause a dose-related inhibition of monoamine oxidase. Although there are no reports of hypertensive crises caused by the concurrent administration of SUDAFED Plus and furazolidone, they should not be taken together.

4.4 Special warnings and special precautions for use

SUDAFED Plus may cause drowsiness and impair performance in tests of auditory vigilance. Patients should not drive or operate machinery until they have determined their own response.

Although there are no objective data, users of SUDAFED Plus should avoid the concomitant use of alcohol or other centrally acting sedatives.

Although pseudoephedrine has virtually no pressor effects in patients with normal blood pressure, SUDAFED Plus should be used with caution in patients taking antihypertensive agents, tricyclic antidepressants, other sympathomimetic agents, such as decongestants, appetite suppressants and amfetamine-like psychostimulants. The effects of a single dose on the blood pressure of these patients should be observed before recommending repeated or unsupervised treatment.

As with other sympathomimetic agents, caution should be exercised in patients with uncontrolled diabetes, hyperthyroidism, elevated intraocular pressure and prostatic enlargement.

There have been no specific studies of SUDAFED Plus in patients with hepatic and/or renal dysfunction. Caution should be exercised in the presence of severe renal or hepatic impairment.

There is insufficient information available to determine whether triprolidine or pseudoephedrine have mutagenic or carcinogenic potential.

Patients with rare hereditary problems of galactose intolerance, the Lapp lactose deficiency or glucose-galactose malaborption should not take this medicine.

4.5 Interaction with other medicinal products and other forms of Interaction

Concomitant use of SUDAFED Plus with sympathomimetic agents such as decongestants, tricyclic antidepressants, appetite suppressants and amfetamine-like psychostimulants or with monoamine oxidase inhibitors, which interfere with the catabolism of sympathomimetic amines, may occasionally cause a rise in blood pressure.

Because of its pseudoephedrine content, SUDAFED Plus may partially reverse the hypotensive action of drugs which interfere with sympathetic activity including bretylium betanidine, guanethedine, debrisoquine, methyldopa, alpha and beta-adrenergic blocking agents.

4.6 Pregnancy and lactation

Although pseudoephedrine and triprolidine have been in widespread use for many years without apparent ill consequence, there are no specific data on their use during pregnancy. Caution should therefore be exercised by balancing the potential benefit of treatment, to the mother against any possible hazards to the developing foetus.

In rats and rabbits systemic administration of triprolidine up to 75 times the human dose did not produce teratogenic effects. Systemic administration of pseudoephedrine, up to 50 times the human dose in rats and up to 35 times the human dose in rabbits, did not produce teratogenic effects.

No studies have been conducted in animals to determine whether triprolidine or pseudoephedrine have potential to impair fertility. There is no information on the effect of SUDAFED Plus on human fertility.

Pseudoephedrine and triprolidine are excreted in breast milk in small amounts but the effect of this on breast fed infants is not known. It has been estimated that 0.5 - 0.7% of a single dose of pseudoephedrine ingested by a mother will be excreted in the breast milk over 24 hours.

4.7 Effects on ability to drive and use machines

SUDAFED Plus may cause drowsiness and impair performance in tests of auditory vigilance. Patients should not drive a vehicle or operate machinery until they have determined their own response.

4.8 Undesirable effects

Central nervous system (CNS) depression or excitation may occur, drowsiness being reported most frequently. Sleep disturbance and, rarely, hallucinations have been reported.

Skin rashes with or without irritation, tachycardia, dryness of mouth, nose and throat have occasionally been reported. Urinary retention has been reported occasionally in men receiving pseudoephedrine, prostatic enlargement could have been an important predisposing factor.

4.9 Overdose

The effects of acute toxicity from SUDAFED Plus Tablets may include drowsiness, lethargy, dizziness, ataxia, weakness, hypotonicity, respiratory depression, dryness of the skin and mucous membranes, tachycardia, hypertension, hyperpyrexia, hyperactivity, irritability, convulsions and difficulty with micturition.

Necessary measures should be taken to maintain and support respiration and control convulsions. Gastric lavage should be performed up to 3 hours after ingestion if indicated. Catheterisation of the bladder may be necessary. If desired, the elimination of pseudoephedrine can be accelerated by acid diuresis or by dialysis.

5. PHARMACOLOGICAL PROPERTIES

5.1 Pharmacodynamic properties

Pseudoephedrine has a direct and indirect sympathomimetic activity and is an orally effective upper respiratory tract decongestant. Pseudoephedrine is substantially less potent than ephedrine in producing both tachycardia and elevation in systolic blood pressure and considerably less potent in causing stimulation of the central nervous system.

Triprolidine provides antihistamine activity by antagonising H_1 receptors.

5.2 Pharmacokinetic properties

Pseudoephedrine is rapidly and completely absorbed after oral administration. After an oral dose of 180 mg to man, peak plasma concentrations of 500-900 ng/ml were obtained about 2 hours post dose. The plasma half life was approximately 5.5 hours and was increased in subjects with alkaline urine and decreased in subjects with acid urine. The only metabolism was n-demethylation which occurred to a small extent. Excretion was mainly via the urine.

In common with other antihistamines, triprolidine hydrochloride is rapidly absorbed, peak plasma levels being observed 2 hours after an oral dose, metabolised in the liver and excreted, mainly as metabolites in the urine. The plasma half life is approximately 3.2 hours.

5.3 Preclinical safety data

The active ingredients of Sudafed Plus are well known constituents of medicinal products and their safety profiles are well documented. The results of pre-clinical studies do not add anything of relevance for therapeutic purposes.

6. PHARMACEUTICAL PARTICULARS

6.1 List of excipients

Lactose

Starches

Povidone

Magnesium Stearate

Purified Water

6.2 Incompatibilities

None known

6.3 Shelf life

36 months unopened.

6.4 Special precautions for storage

Do not store above 25°C.

Store in the original package.

6.5 Nature and contents of container

6, 12, 21, 84 - PVC/PVDC/aluminium foil blister packs (The six tablet pack is a starter pack).

100 –Polypropylene containers with polyethylene snap-on lids, or, high density polyethylene (HDPE) containers with low density polyethylene (LDPE) snap-fit, tamper-evident caps, or, amber glass bottles with low density polyethylene snap-fit closures.

6.6 Instructions for use and handling

Not applicable

7. MARKETING AUTHORISATION HOLDER

Pfizer Consumer Healthcare

Alternative Trading Style:

Warner-Lambert Consumer Healthcare

Walton Oaks

Dorking Road

Walton-on-the-Hill

Surrey, KT20 7NS

United Kingdon

8. MARKETING AUTHORISATION NUMBER(S)

PL 15513/0029

9. DATE OF FIRST AUTHORISATION/RENEWAL OF THE AUTHORISATION

28 March 1997

10. DATE OF REVISION OF THE TEXT

October 2004

Sudocrem Antiseptic Healing Cream

(Forest Laboratories UK Limited)

1. NAME OF THE MEDICINAL PRODUCT

Sudocrem Antiseptic Healing Cream

2. QUALITATIVE AND QUANTITATIVE COMPOSITION

	% w/w
Zinc oxide, EP	15.25
Benzyl alcohol, BP	0.39
Benzyl benzoate, BP	1.01
Benzyl cinnamate	0.15
Lanolin (hypoallergenic)	4.00

3. PHARMACEUTICAL FORM

Emulsified water in oil cream

4. CLINICAL PARTICULARS

4.1 Therapeutic indications

In the treatment of:

1. Napkin rash
2. Eczema
3. Bedsores
4. Acne
5. Minor burns
6. Surface wounds
7. Sunburn
8. Chilblains

4.2 Posology and method of administration

Apply a thin layer with suitable covering where necessary. Renew application as required. No distinction is required between indications or between adults, children and the elderly.

Topical cream for external use only.

4.3 Contraindications

Hypersensitivity to any of the ingredients.

4.4 Special warnings and special precautions for use

For external use only and should not be allowed to come into contact with the eyes and the mucous membranes.

4.5 Interaction with other medicinal products and other forms of Interaction

None known

4.6 Pregnancy and lactation

There are no known contraindications.

4.7 Effects on ability to drive and use machines

Not applicable

4.8 Undesirable effects

Side effects include local hypersensitivity occasionally.

4.9 Overdose

No cases of overdose have been reported. If large amounts are swallowed accidentally, this may cause vomiting, diarrhoea, CNS stimulation and convulsions. Symptomatic treatment should be provided.

5. PHARMACOLOGICAL PROPERTIES

5.1 Pharmacodynamic properties

Zinc oxide:

A dermatological agent with astringent, soothing and protective properties.

Benzyl alcohol:

A local anaesthetic with disinfectant properties.

Benzyl benzoate:

An acaricide and has been used as a pediculicide, insect repellent and pharmaceutical solubilising agent. It is a constituent of many natural balsams and is one of the principal esters of Peru Balsam.

Benzyl cinnamate:

This is the other principal ester of Peru Balsam BPC 1973. It is synthesised from benzyl alcohol and cinnamic acid which has antibacterial and antifungal properties. Peru Balsam is categorised as having a mild antiseptic action because of cinnamic acid and its derivatives present.

Lanolin:

Resembles the sebaceous secretions of human skin. The grade (hypoallergenic) used is manufactured so as to exclude many sensitising substances present in the lanolin.

5.2 Pharmacokinetic properties

Not applicable.

5.3 Preclinical safety data

Not applicable

6. PHARMACEUTICAL PARTICULARS

6.1 List of excipients

Purified Water

Sodium Benzoate

Paraffin wax

Microcrystalline wax

Heavy Liquid Paraffin

Synthetic Beeswax

Sorbitan sesquioleate

Propylene glycol

Antioxidant (formulation consisting of butylated hydroxyanisole (BHA), citric acid and propylene glycol)

Linalyl acetate

Lavender

6.2 Incompatibilities

None known

6.3 Shelf life

Not exceeding 5 years from date of manufacture.

6.4 Special precautions for storage

No special precautions for storage.

6.5 Nature and contents of container

			Pack size (g)
a)	Polypropylene jars with polyethylene tamper-evident caps	(1)	60
		(2)	125
		(3)	250
		(4)	400
		(5)	750
		(6)	1000
b)	Polypropylene jars with polyethylene caps	(1)	15
		(2)	25
c)	Aluminium or laminated plastic aluminium tubes with aluminium membrane and plastic caps	(1)	30
		(2)	50

6.6 Instructions for use and handling

Not applicable

7. MARKETING AUTHORISATION HOLDER

Marketing Authorisation Holder	UK Distributor
Forest Tosara Limited	Forest Laboratories UK Limited
Unit 146 Baldoyle Industrial Estate	Bourne Road
Baldoyle	Bexley
Dublin 13	Kent DA5 1NX
Republic of Ireland	UK

8. MARKETING AUTHORISATION NUMBER(S)

PL 06166/0003

9. DATE OF FIRST AUTHORISATION/RENEWAL OF THE AUTHORISATION

5 March 2004

10. DATE OF REVISION OF THE TEXT

Legal Category

GSL

Suleo-M Lotion

(SSL International plc)

1. NAME OF THE MEDICINAL PRODUCT

Suleo-M Lotion.

2. QUALITATIVE AND QUANTITATIVE COMPOSITION

Malathion 0.5% w/v.

3. PHARMACEUTICAL FORM

Lotion.

4. CLINICAL PARTICULARS

4.1 Therapeutic indications

For the eradication of head lice infestation.

4.2 Posology and method of administration

Adults, the elderly and children aged 6 months and over: For topical external use only.

Rub the lotion gently into the scalp until all the hair and scalp is thoroughly moistened. Allow to dry naturally in a well ventilated room. Do not use a hairdryer or other artificial heat. Live lice will be eradicated after a minimum treatment period of two hours. However, the lotion should be left on the head for a further period of 8-10 hours to ensure that all lice eggs are totally eradicated. Shampoo in the normal manner. Rinse and comb the hair whilst wet to remove the dead lice. In the event of early reinfestation, Suleo-M Lotion may be applied again provided 7 days have elapsed since the first application. Residual protective effect is variable of short duration and should not be relied upon. Not to be used on children under the age of 6 months, except on medical advice.

4.3 Contraindications

Not to be used on infants less than 6 months old except under medical supervision. Known sensitivity to malathion.

4.4 Special warnings and special precautions for use

Avoid contact with the eyes. Do not cover the head until the hair has dried completely. It is advisable that nursing staff involved in repeated applications should wear rubber gloves when carrying out treatment. Suleo-M Lotion is for external use only and should be kept out of the reach of children. Keep away from exposed flame or lighted objects (for example, cigarettes, gas and electric fires) during application and while hair is wet. Continued prolonged treatment with Suleo-M Lotion should be avoided. It should be used not more than once a week for three weeks at a time. Alcohol based skin products may cause a stinging sensation on patients with sensitive skin.

4.5 Interaction with other medicinal products and other forms of Interaction

None stated.

4.6 Pregnancy and lactation
No known effects in pregnancy and lactation. However, as with all medicines, use with caution.

4.7 Effects on ability to drive and use machines
None stated.

4.8 Undesirable effects
Very rarely skin irritation has been reported with malathion products.

4.9 Overdose
In the event of deliberate or accidental ingestion, empty stomach contents by gastric lavage. Atropine and pralidoxime may be required to counteract cholinesterase inhibition.

5. PHARMACOLOGICAL PROPERTIES

5.1 Pharmacodynamic properties
Suleo-M Lotion contains malathion, a widely used organophosphorus insecticide which is active by cholinesterase inhibition. It is effective against a wide range of insects, but is one of the least toxic organophosphorus insecticides since it is rapidly detoxified by plasma carboxylesterases.

5.2 Pharmacokinetic properties
Suleo-M Lotion is applied topically to the affected area.

5.3 Preclinical safety data
None stated.

6. PHARMACEUTICAL PARTICULARS

6.1 List of excipients
Isopropyl Alcohol; D-Limonene 17449; Terpineol 18689; Perfume Loxol P6160; Citric Acid; Shellsol T.

6.2 Incompatibilities
None stated.

6.3 Shelf life
Two years.

6.4 Special precautions for storage
Store at or below 25°C. Protect from sunlight.

6.5 Nature and contents of container
Cartoned, clear or amber glass bottles with low density polyethylene caps and high density polypropylene sprinkler inserts containing either 50 or 200 ml of product.

6.6 Instructions for use and handling
None stated.

7. MARKETING AUTHORISATION HOLDER
Seton Products Limited, Tubiton House, Oldham, OL1 3HS.

8. MARKETING AUTHORISATION NUMBER(S)
11314/0055.

9. DATE OF FIRST AUTHORISATION/RENEWAL OF THE AUTHORISATION
14th November 1995 / 26th March 2001.

10. DATE OF REVISION OF THE TEXT
March 2001.

Sulpitil

(Pharmacia Limited)

1. NAME OF THE MEDICINAL PRODUCT
Sulpitil™

2. QUALITATIVE AND QUANTITATIVE COMPOSITION
Each tablet contains 200 mg sulpiride

3. PHARMACEUTICAL FORM
Round, white tablet with bevelled edge, marked 'L113' on one side and scored on the reverse.

4. CLINICAL PARTICULARS

4.1 Therapeutic indications
For the treatment of acute and chronic schizophrenia.

4.2 Posology and method of administration
For oral administration.

Adult dose: In mild cases, 400 mg to 800 mg daily given as one or two tablets twice daily. In severe cases, a maximum dosage of 1200 mg to 1800 mg per day may be given. A maintenance dose of 400 mg to 800 mg is recommended.

Children: 3 - 5 mg/kg body weight daily is recommended. Clinical experience in children under the age of 14 years is insufficient to permit specific recommendations.

Dosage in the elderly: Elderly patients are usually more sensitive to all centrally-acting drugs, therefore an initial dose of 50 mg to 100 mg is recommended, increasing gradually to the normal adult dose. Reduced dosage should be used in patients with renal impairment.

4.3 Contraindications
Phaeochromocytoma. Severe hepatic, renal or blood disease. Alcoholic intoxication and other disorders which depress CNS function.

4.4 Special warnings and special precautions for use
Sulpiride should be given with caution to patients suffering from extrapyramidal disturbances, hypertension, and to patients with tumours.

As with all drugs, of which the kidney is a major elimination pathway, the usual precautions should be taken in cases of renal failure.

Patients should be warned against taking alcohol with sulpiride as reaction capacity may be impaired.

Increased motor agitation has been reported at high doses in a small number of patients, i.e. in excessively agitated or excited phases of the disease process, this drug may aggravate symptoms. Care should be exercised when hypomania is present. If warranted, reduction in dosage or anti-parkinsonian medication is sufficient.

As with all neuroleptic drugs, the presence of unexpalined hyperthermia could indicate the neuroleptic malignant syndrome (NMS).

Acute withdrawal symptoms including nausea, vomiting, sweating, and insomnia have been described after abrupt cessation of antipsychotic drugs. Recurrence of psychotic symptoms may also occur, and the emergence of involuntary movement disorders (such as akathisia, dystonia and dyskinesia) have been reported. Therefore gradual withdrawal is advisable.

4.5 Interaction with other medicinal products and other forms of Interaction
Although no drug interactions are known, unnecessary polypharmacy should be avoided. Patients should be warned against taking alcohol with sulpiride, as reaction capacity may be impaired. Sulpiride has no anticholinergic or significant cardiovascular activity.

4.6 Pregnancy and lactation
Despite the negative results of teratogenicity studies in animals sensitive to the effects of thalidomide and the lack of teratogenic effect during widespread clinical use in other countries, this drug should not be considered an exception to the general principle of avoiding drug treatment during pregnancy, particularly during the first sixteen weeks, with potential benefits being weighed against probable hazards.

4.7 Effects on ability to drive and use machines
Patients should be advised not to drive or operate machinery if they experience symptoms of slowing of reaction time or loss of concentration.

4.8 Undesirable effects
Extrapyramidal symptoms can occur: tremor, tardive dyskinesia (rare), akathisia, dystonia (including oculogyric crises). Insomnia and other sleep disturbances have been reported.

As is usual with neuroleptic and psychotropic drugs, sulpiride increases serum prolactin levels, sometimes causing gynaecomastia and galactorrhoea. Amenorrhoea has also been reported.

Sulpiride has a low toxicity and, unlike other neuroleptics, does not produce serious adverse effects on the autonomic nervous system.

Cases of convulsions, sometimes in patients with no previous history, have been reported.

Hepatic reactions have been reported.

There have been rare reports of cardiac arrhythmia including QT prolongation leading to torsade de pointes.

As with other neuroleptics, rare cases of neuroleptic malignant syndrome, characterised by hyperthermia, muscle rigidity, autonomic instability, altered consciousness and elevated CPK levels, have been reported. In such an event, all antipsychotic drugs, including Sulpitil, should be discontinued.

4.9 Overdose
Overdosage may be treated with alkaline osmotic diuresis and anti-parkinsonian drugs to treat any extrapyramidal symptoms. An overdose of more than 7 g may cause coma which has been observed to last for up to four days and which should receive suitable treatment.

5. PHARMACOLOGICAL PROPERTIES

5.1 Pharmacodynamic properties
Sulpiride belongs to a new class of neuroleptics, the benzamides, and has both antidepressant and neuroleptic properties. In high doses it controls florid positive symptoms but in lower doses it has an alerting effect on apathetic withdrawn schizophrenics; further reductions in dosage increase this alerting effect.

5.2 Pharmacokinetic properties
The plasma half-life of sulpiride is 8 - 9 hours.

5.3 Preclinical safety data
In long-term animal studies with neuroleptic drugs, including sulpiride, an increased incidence of various endocrine tumours, some of which have been malignant, has been found in some, but not all, strains of rats and mice studied. The significance of these findings to man is not known. There is no current evidence of an association between neuroleptic use and tumour risk in man.

6. PHARMACEUTICAL PARTICULARS

6.1 List of excipients
Microcrystalline cellulose Ph. Eur
Maize starch Ph. Eur
Lactose Ph. Eur
Gelatin BP
Talc Ph. Eur
Sodium stearyl fumarate (PRUV) HSE

6.2 Incompatibilities
None stated.

6.3 Shelf life
60 months.

6.4 Special precautions for storage
Store in a dry place below 25°C.

6.5 Nature and contents of container
Polyethylene containers each fitted with a tamper-evident strip closure and enclosed within a printed cardboard carton, containing either 28 or 112 tablets.

6.6 Instructions for use and handling
None stated.

Administrative Data

7. MARKETING AUTHORISATION HOLDER
Pharmacia Limited
Davy Avenue
Milton Keynes
MK5 8PH
United Kingdom

8. MARKETING AUTHORISATION NUMBER(S)
PL 00032/0326

9. DATE OF FIRST AUTHORISATION/RENEWAL OF THE AUTHORISATION
28 April 2003

10. DATE OF REVISION OF THE TEXT

Sulpor

(Rosemont Pharmaceuticals Limited)

1. NAME OF THE MEDICINAL PRODUCT
Sulpor.

2. QUALITATIVE AND QUANTITATIVE COMPOSITION
Sulpiride 200mg/5ml.

3. PHARMACEUTICAL FORM
A colourless to slightly yellow oral solution.

4. CLINICAL PARTICULARS

4.1 Therapeutic indications
Acute and chronic schizophrenia.

4.2 Posology and method of administration
For oral administration only.

Adults:

A starting dose of 400mg to 800mg daily, given in two divided doses (morning and early evening) is recommended.

Predominantly positive symptoms (formal thought disorder, hallucinations, delusions, incongruity of affect) respond to higher doses, and a starting dose of at least 400mg twice daily is recommended, increasing if necessary up to a suggested maximum of 1200mg twice daily. Increasing the dose beyond this level has not been shown to produce further improvement. Predominantly negative symptoms (flattening of affect, poverty of speech, anergia, apathy), as well as depression, respond to doses below 800mg daily; therefore, a starting dose of 400mg twice daily is recommended. Reducing this dose towards 200mg twice daily will normally increase the alerting effect of sulpiride.

Patients with mixed positive and negative symptoms, with neither predominating, will normally respond to dosage of 400-600mg twice daily.

Children:

Clinical experience in children under the age of 14 years of age is insufficient to permit specific recommendations.

Elderly:

The same dose ranges may be required in the elderly, but should be reduced if there is evidence of renal impairment.

4.3 Contraindications
Phaeochromocytoma. Acute porphyria. Hypersensitivity to any of the ingredients in this product. Severe renal, haematological or hepatic disease. Alcoholic intoxication and other disorders which depress CNS function.

4.4 Special warnings and special precautions for use
Increased motor agitation has been reported at high dosage in a small number of patients: in aggressive, agitated or excited phases of the disease process, low doses of sulpiride may aggravate symptoms. Care should be exercised where hypomania is present.

If extrapyramidal reactions occur, a reduction in dosage of sulpiride or initiation of anti-parkinsonian medication may be necessary.

As with all neuroleptic drugs, the presence of unexplained hyperthermia could indicate the neuroleptic malignant syndrome (NMS). In this event sulpiride and any associated neuroleptic treatment should be discontinued until the origin of the fever has been determined.

Although sulpiride only induces slight EEG modifications, caution is advised in prescribing it for patients with unstable epilepsy. Patients requiring sulpiride who are receiving anti-convulsant therapy should continue unchanged on the latter medication. Cases of convulsions, sometimes in patients with no previous history, have been reported.

Sulpiride has no significant anticholinergic or cardiovascular activity.

As with all drugs for which the kidney is the major elimination pathway, the usual precautions should be taken in cases of renal failure.

Patients should be warned against taking alcohol with sulpiride as reaction capacity may be impaired.

Abrupt cessation of treatment in some patients may produce a withdrawal response.

The product contains liquid maltitol. Patients with rare hereditary problems of fructose intolerance should not take this medicine.

4.5 Interaction with other medicinal products and other forms of Interaction
While no drug interactions are known, unnecessary polypharmacy should be avoided. As with other psychotropic compounds, sulpiride may increase the effect of antihypertensives and CNS depressants or stimulants.

The bioavailability of sulpiride is reduced by concomitant administration with sucralfate and antacids and should not, therefore, be taken at the same time.

Also concurrent use with lithium may cause extrapyramidal symptoms to develop.

4.6 Pregnancy and lactation
Despite the negative results of teratogenicity studies in animals and the lack of teratogenic effects during widespread clinical use in other countries, sulpiride should not be considered an exception to the general principle of avoiding drug treatment in pregnancy, particularly during the first 16 weeks, with potential benefits being weighed against possible hazards.

Sulpiride has been found in low concentrations in breast milk. It is, therefore, recommended that the use of sulpiride be avoided in patients who are breast feeding.

4.7 Effects on ability to drive and use machines
Patients should be advised not to drive or operate machinery if they experience symptoms of slowing of reaction time, drowsiness or loss of concentration.

4.8 Undesirable effects
Sulpiride is very well tolerated and usually only minor side-effects occur, if at all, at the recommended doses.

Extrapyramidal reactions, principally akathisia, tremor and tardive dyskinesia have been reported in a small number of cases.

Insomnia has been reported.

Hepatic reactions including jaundice and hepatitis have been reported.

As is usual with neuroleptics and psychotic drugs, sulpiride raises serum prolactin levels, which may be associated with galactorrhoea, oligomenorrhoea and amenorrhoea, and less frequently with gynaecomastia. Sexual function may also be increased or decreased.

A mild laxative effect or diarrhoea may be caused by the liquid maltitol in the formulation.

4.9 Overdose
The range of single toxic doses is 1 to 16g but no death has occurred even at the 16g dose.

The clinical manifestations of poisoning vary depending upon the size of the dose taken. After single doses of 1 to 3g restlessness and clouding of consciousness have been reported and (rarely) extrapyramidal symptoms.

Doses of 3 to 7g may produce a degree of agitation, confusion and extrapyramidal symptoms; more than 7g can cause, in addition, coma and low blood pressure.

The duration of intoxication is generally short, the symptoms disappearing within a few hours. Comas which have occurred after large doses have lasted up to four days. There are no specific complications from overdose. In particular no haematological or hepatic toxicity has been reported.

Overdose may be treated with alkaline osmotic diuresis and, if necessary, anti-parkinsonian drugs. Coma needs appropriate nursing. Emetic drugs are unlikely to be effective in sulpiride overdosage.

5. PHARMACOLOGICAL PROPERTIES

5.1 Pharmacodynamic properties
One of the characteristics of sulpiride is its bimodal activity, as it has both antidepressant and neuroleptic properties. Schizophrenia characterised by a lack of social contact can benefit strikingly. Mood elevation is observed after a few days treatment, followed by disappearance of the florid schizophrenic symptoms. The sedation and lack of effect characteristically associated with classical neuroleptics of the phenothiazine or butyrophenone type are not features of sulpiride therapy.

Sulpiride is a member of the group of substituted benzamides, which are structurally distinct from the phenothiazines, butyrophenones and thioxanthenes. Current evidence suggests that the actions of sulpiride hint at an important distinction between different types of dopamine receptors or receptor mechanisms in the brain.

Behaviourally and biochemically, sulpiride shares with these classical neuroleptics a number of properties indicative of cerebral dopamine receptor antagonism. Essential and intriguing differences include lack of catalepsy at doses active in other behavioural tests, lack of effect in the dopamine sensitive adenylate cyclase systems, lack of effect upon noradrenaline or 5HT turnover, negligible anticholinesterase activity, no effect on muscarinic or GABA receptor binding, and a radical difference in the binding of tritiated sulpiride to striatal preparations in-vitro, compared to ^{3}H-spiperone and ^{3}H-haloperidol. These findings indicate a major differentiation between sulpiride and classical neuroleptics which lack such specificity.

5.2 Pharmacokinetic properties
Peak sulpiride serum levels are reached 3-6 hours after an oral dose. The plasma half-life in man is approximately 8 hours. Approximately 40% sulpiride is bound to plasma proteins. 95% of the compound is excreted in the urine and faeces as unchanged sulpiride.

5.3 Preclinical safety data
In long-term animal studies with neuroleptic drugs, including sulpiride, an increased incidence of various endocrine tumours (some of which have occasionally been malignant) has been seen in some but not all strains of rats and mice studied. The significance of these findings to man is not known; there is no current evidence of any association between neuroleptic use and tumour risk in man. However, when prescribing neuroleptics to patients with existing mammary neoplasia or a history of this disease, possible risks should be weighed against benefits of therapy.

6. PHARMACEUTICAL PARTICULARS

6.1 List of excipients
Methyl parahydroxybenzoate, propyl parahydroxybenzoate, propylene glycol, citric acid monohydrate, liquid maltitol, lemon flavour, aniseed flavour and purified water.

6.2 Incompatibilities
None known.

6.3 Shelf life
36 months – unopened

3 months - opened

6.4 Special precautions for storage
Do not store above 25°C.

6.5 Nature and contents of container
Bottle: 150ml amber (Type III) glass.

Closure: a) Aluminium, EPE wadded, roll-on pilfer-proof screw cap.

b) HDPE, EPE wadded, tamper evident screw cap.

c) HDPE, EPE wadded, tamper evident, child resistant closure.

6.6 Instructions for use and handling
The date of opening should be entered on the label next to the "use within 3 months of opening" statement.

7. MARKETING AUTHORISATION HOLDER
Rosemont Pharmaceuticals Ltd, Rosemont House, Yorkdale Industrial Park, Braithwaite Street, Leeds, LS11 9XE, UK.

8. MARKETING AUTHORISATION NUMBER(S)
PL 00427/0129

9. DATE OF FIRST AUTHORISATION/RENEWAL OF THE AUTHORISATION
08/08/01

10. DATE OF REVISION OF THE TEXT
11/11/03

Sultrin Triple Sulfa Cream

(Janssen-Cilag Ltd)

1. NAME OF THE MEDICINAL PRODUCT
Sultrin® Triple Sulfa Cream

2. QUALITATIVE AND QUANTITATIVE COMPOSITION
Sulphabenzamide 3.7% w/w

Sulphacetamide 2.86% w/w

Sulphathiazole 3.42% w/w

3. PHARMACEUTICAL FORM
White to off-white cream.

4. CLINICAL PARTICULARS

4.1 Therapeutic indications
Treatment of infections caused by *Haemophilus vaginalis.*

4.2 Posology and method of administration
For intravaginal administration.

One applicatorful intravaginally twice daily for ten days. The dosage may then be reduced to once a day, if necessary.

4.3 Contraindications
Sulphonamide sensitivity.

Kidney disease.

Known hypersensitivity to peanuts.

Throughout pregnancy and during the nursing period because sulphonamides cross the placenta, are excreted in breast milk and may cause kernicterus.

4.4 Special warnings and special precautions for use
The safety and effectiveness for use in children have not been established.

Caution should be used in prescribing the product to elderly patients who potentially may have impaired renal function.

Patients should be observed for skin rash or evidence of systemic toxicity and, if these develop, the medication should be discontinued.

Sultrin Triple Sulfa Cream contains arachis oil (peanut oil) and should not be applied by patients known to be allergic to peanut (See Section 4.3 Contra-indications). As there is a possible relationship between allergy to peanut and allergy to Soya, patients with Soya allergy should also avoid Sultrin Triple Sulfa Cream.

4.5 Interaction with other medicinal products and other forms of Interaction
Contact should be avoided between contraceptive diaphragms or latex condoms and Sultrin Triple Sulfa Cream, since the rubber may be damaged.

4.6 Pregnancy and lactation
The safe use of sulphonamides in pregnancy has not been established. The teratogenic potential of most sulphonamides has not been thoroughly investigated in either animals or humans. However, a significant increase in the incidence of cleft palate and other bony abnormalities of offspring has been observed when certain sulphonamides of the short, intermediate and long-acting types were given to pregnant rats and mice at high oral doses (7 to 25 times the human therapeutic dose).

Because sulphonamides are excreted in breast milk and may cause serious adverse reactions in breast feeding infants, a decision should be made whether to discontinue breast feeding or to discontinue Sultrin, depending on the importance of the drug to the mother.

See 4.3 Contra-indications

4.7 Effects on ability to drive and use machines
None.

4.8 Undesirable effects
Local irritation and/or allergy have occasionally been reported. As sulphonamides may be absorbed from the vaginal mucosa, the following adverse effects associated with such compounds should be borne in mind:

– Hypersensitivity reactions: Skin rashes; severe and potentially fatal skin reactions such as toxic epidermal necrolysis (Lyell's Syndrome) and erythema multiforme bullosa (Stevens-Johnson Syndrome).

– Blood dyscrasias: Including agranulocytosis and aplastic anaemia.

– Renal failure.

4.9 Overdose
If accidental ingestion of large quantities of the product occurs, an appropriate method of gastric emptying may be used if considered desirable. Elimination of sulphonamides in the urine may be assisted by giving alkalis, such as sodium bicarbonate, and increasing fluid intake.

5. PHARMACOLOGICAL PROPERTIES

5.1 Pharmacodynamic properties
Sulphonamides are structural analogues and competitive antagonists of para-aminobenzoic acid (PABA) and prevent normal bacterial utilisation of PABA for the synthesis of folic acid. Sulphonamides are competitive inhibitors of the bacterial enzyme responsible for the incorporation of PABA into dihydropteroic acid, the immediate precursor of folic acid. The three sulphonamides exert optimal bacteriostatic action at different pH levels, as follows:

- Sulphathiazole pH 7.0
- Sulphacetamide pH 5.2
- Sulphabenzamide pH 4.6

5.2 Pharmacokinetic properties
Studies with sulphacetamide and sulphathiazole have indicated that sulphonamides are absorbed in low and variable amounts from the vagina. Once absorbed, sulphonamides become distributed throughout the tissues and pass the placental barrier.

Elimination occurs partly as unchanged drug and partly as metabolites with the major route of elimination via the urine. Small amounts are excreted in the faeces, bile and milk.

5.3 Preclinical safety data
No relevant information additional to that contained elsewhere in the Summary of Product Characteristics.

6. PHARMACEUTICAL PARTICULARS

6.1 List of excipients

Arachis oil
Cetyl alcohol
Cholesterol
Clearate(TM) paste (lecithin)
Tegacid(TM) Regular (glyceryl monostearate) (E471)
Wool fat (anhydrous lanolin)
Methyl parahydroxybenzoate (E218)
Phosphoric acid (E338)
Propylene glycol
Propyl parahydroxybenzoate (E216)
Stearic acid (E570)
Diethylaminoethyl stearamide
Urea
Purified water

6.2 Incompatibilities

None known.

6.3 Shelf life

36 months.

6.4 Special precautions for storage

Store at room temperature (not exceeding 25°C).

6.5 Nature and contents of container

Tube of epoxy resin lacquered aluminium, with polyethylene cap, containing 80 g cream.

6.6 Instructions for use and handling

Not applicable.

7. MARKETING AUTHORISATION HOLDER

Janssen-Cilag Limited
Saunderton
High Wycombe
Buckinghamshire
HP14 4HJ

8. MARKETING AUTHORISATION NUMBER(S)

PL 00242/0273

9. DATE OF FIRST AUTHORISATION/RENEWAL OF THE AUTHORISATION

1 September 1995

10. DATE OF REVISION OF THE TEXT

March 2003

Legal category POM.

Supralip 160mg

(Fournier Pharmaceuticals Limited)

1. NAME OF THE MEDICINAL PRODUCT

Supralip® 160 mg, film-coated tablet.

2. QUALITATIVE AND QUANTITATIVE COMPOSITION

Each tablet contains 160.0 mg fenofibrate.

For excipients, see 6.1.

3. PHARMACEUTICAL FORM

Film coated tablet.

White, oblong, film-coated tablets engraved "160" on one side and "Fournier logo" on the other side.

4. CLINICAL PARTICULARS

4.1 Therapeutic indications

Hypercholesterolaemia and hypertriglyceridaemia alone or combined (types IIa, IIb, IV dyslipidaemias, as well as types III and V dyslipidaemias although only a few patients have been treated during clinical trials) in patients unresponsive to dietary and other non-drug therapeutic measures (e.g. weight reduction or increased physical activity), particularly when there is evidence of associated risk factors.

The treatment of secondary hyperlipoproteinaemias is indicated if the hyperlipoproteinaemia persists despite effective treatment of the underlying disease (e.g. dyslipidaemia in diabetes mellitus).

Dietary measures initiated before therapy should be continued.

4.2 Posology and method of administration

Posology:

Adults: The recommended dose is one tablet containing 160 mg fenofibrate taken once daily. Patients currently taking one Lipantil Micro 200mg capsule can be changed to one Supralip 160 mg tablet without further dose adjustment.

Elderly patients: The usual adult dose is recommended.

Patients with renal impairment: Dosage reduction is required in patients with renal impairment. The use of dosage forms containing a lower dose of active ingredient (67 mg micronised fenofibrate capsules or 100 mg standard fenofibrate capsules) is recommended in these patients.

Children: The use of the 160 mg dosage form is contra-indicated in children.

Hepatic disease: Patients with hepatic disease have not been studied.

Dietary measures initiated before therapy should be continued.

If after several months of fenofibrate administration (e.g. 3 months) serum lipid levels have not been reduced satisfactorily, complementary or different therapeutic measures should be considered.

Method of administration: Tablet should be swallowed whole during a meal.

4.3 Contraindications

– hepatic insufficiency (including biliary cirrhosis),
– renal insufficiency,
– children,
– hypersensitivity to fenofibrate or any component of this medication,
– known photoallergy or phototoxic reaction during treatment with fibrates or ketoprofen,
– gallbladder disease.

Use during pregnancy and lactation: see section 4.6.

Supralip 160mg should not be taken in patients allergic to peanut or arachis oil or soya lecithin or related products due to the risk of hypersensitivity reactions.

4.4 Special warnings and special precautions for use

Liver function: As with other lipid lowering agents, increases have been reported in transaminase levels in some patients. In the majority of cases these elevations were transient, minor and asymptomatic. It is recommended that transaminase levels be monitored every 3 months during the first 12 months of treatment. Attention should be paid to patients who develop increase in transaminase levels and therapy should be discontinued if ASAT and ALAT levels increase to more than 3 times the upper limit of the normal range or 100 IU.

Pancreatitis: Pancreatitis has been reported in patients taking fenofibrate. This occurrence may represent a failure of efficacy in patients with severe hypertriglyceridemia, a direct drug effect, or a secondary phenomenon mediated through biliary tract stone or sludge formation, resulting in the obstruction of the common bile duct.

Muscle: Muscle toxicity, including very rare cases of rhabdomyolysis, has been reported with administration of fibrates and other lipid-lowering agents. The incidence of this disorder increases in cases of hypoalbuminaemia and previous renal insufficiency. Muscle toxicity should be suspected in patients presenting diffuse myalgia, myositis, muscular cramps and weakness and/or marked increases in CPK (levels exceeding 5 times the normal range). In such cases treatment with fenofibrate should be stopped.

Patients with pre-disposing factors for myopathy and/or rhabdomyolysis, including age above 70 years old, personal or familial history of hereditary muscular disorders, renal impairment, hypothyroidism and high alcohol intake, may be at an increased risk of developing rhabdomyolysis. For these patients, the putative benefits and risks of fenofibrate therapy should be carefully weighed up.

The risk of muscle toxicity may be increased if the drug is administered with another fibrate or an HMG-CoA reductase inhibitor, especially in cases of pre-existing muscular disease. Consequently, the co-prescription of fenofibrate with a statin should be reserved to patients with severe combined dyslipidaemia and high cardiovascular risk without any history of muscular disease. This combination therapy should be used with caution and patients should be monitored closely for signs of muscle toxicity.

For hyperlipidaemic patients taking oestrogens or contraceptives containing oestrogens it should be ascertained whether the hyperlipidaemia is of primary or secondary nature (possible elevation of lipid values caused by oral oestrogen).

This medicinal product contains lactose. Therefore patients with rare hereditary problems of galactose intolerance, the Lapp lactase deficiency or glucose-galactose malabsorptionshould nottake this medicine.

Renal function: Treatment should be interrupted in case of an increase in creatinine levels > 50% ULN (upper limit of normal).

It is recommended that creatinine measurement may be considered during the first three months after initiation of treatment.

4.5 Interaction with other medicinal products and other forms of Interaction

Oral anticoagulants: Fenofibrate enhances oral anticoagulant effect and may increase risk of bleeding. It is recommended that the dose of anticoagulants is reduced by about one third at the start of treatment and then gradually adjusted if necessary according to INR (International Normalised Ratio) monitoring. Therefore, this combination is not recommended.

Cyclosporin: Some severe cases of reversible renal function impairment have been reported during concomitant administration of fenofibrate and cyclosporin. The renal function of these patients must therefore be closely monitored and the treatment with fenofibrate stopped in the case of severe alteration of laboratory parameters.

HMG-CoA reductase inhibitors and other fibrates: The risk of serious muscle toxicity is increased if fenofibrate is used concomitantly with HMG-CoA reductase inhibitors or other fibrates. Such combination therapy should be used with caution and patients monitored closely for signs of muscle toxicity (See section 4.4.).

4.6 Pregnancy and lactation

There are no adequate data from the use of fenofibrate in pregnant women. Animal studies have not demonstrated any teratogenic effects. Embryotoxic effects have been shown at doses in the range of maternal toxicity (see section 5.3). The potential risk for humans is unknown. Therefore, Supralip 160mg film-coated tablet should only be used during pregnancy after a careful benefit/riskassessment.

There are no data on the excretion of fenofibrate and/or its metabolites into breast milk.

Consequently Supralip 160mg film-coated tablet should not be used in nursing mother.

4.7 Effects on ability to drive and use machines

No effect noted.

4.8 Undesirable effects

The frequencies of adverse events are ranked according to the following: Very common (>1/10); Common (>1/100, (<1/10); Uncommon (>1/1,000, <1/100); Rare (>1/10,000, <1/1,000); Very rare (<1/10,000), including isolated reports.

Gastrointestinal disorders:

Common: Digestive, gastric or intestinal disorders (abdominal pain, nausea, vomiting, diarrhoea, and flatulence) moderate in severity

Very rare: cases of pancreatitis have been reported during treatment with fenofibrate

Hepato-biliary disorders:

Common: Moderately elevated levels of serum transaminases (see Special precautions for use)

Uncommon: Development of gallstones

Very rare: episodes of hepatitis. When symptoms (e.g. jaundice, pruritus) indicative of hepatitis occur, laboratory tests are to be conducted for verification and fenofibrate discontinued, if applicable (see Special warnings)

Skin and subcutaneous tissue disorders:

Uncommon: rashes, pruritus, urticaria or photosensitivity reactions

Rare: alopecia

Very rare: cutaneous photosensitivity with erythema, vesiculation or nodulation on parts of the skin exposed to sunlight or artificial UV light (e.g. sunlamp) in individual cases (even after many months of uncomplicated use)

Musculoskeletal, connective tissue and bone disorders:

Rare: diffuse myalgia, myositis, muscular cramps and weakness

Very rare: rhabdomyolysis

Blood and lymphatic system disorders:

Rare: decrease in haemoglobin and leukocytes

Nervous system disorders:

Rare: sexual asthenia

Respiratory, thoracic and mediastinal disorders:

Very rare: interstitial pneumopathies

Investigation:

Uncommon: Increases in serum creatinine and urea.

4.9 Overdose

No case of overdosage has been reported. No specific antidote is known. If an overdose is suspected, treat symptomatically and institute appropriate supportive measures as required. Fenofibrate cannot be eliminated by haemodialysis.

5. PHARMACOLOGICAL PROPERTIES

5.1 Pharmacodynamic properties

Serum Lipid Reducing Agents / Cholesterol and Triglycerides Reducers / Fibrates.

ATC code: C10 AB 05

Fenofibrate is a fibric acid derivative whose lipid modifying effects reported in humans are mediated via activation of Peroxisome Proliferator Activated Receptor type alpha (PPARα).

Through activation of PPARα, fenofibrate increases the lipolysis and elimination of atherogenic triglyceride-rich particles from plasma by activating lipoprotein lipase and reducing production of apoprotein CIII. Activation of PPARα also induces an increase in the synthesis of apoproteins AI and AII.

The above stated effects of fenofibrate on lipoproteins lead to a reduction in very low- and low density fractions (VLDL and LDL) containing apoprotein B and an increase in the high density lipoprotein fraction (HDL) containing apoprotein AI and AII.

In addition, through modulation of the synthesis and the catabolism of VLDL fractions fenofibrate increases the LDL clearance and reduces small dense LDL, the levels of which are elevated in the atherogenic lipoprotein phenotype, a common disorder in patients at risk for coronary heart disease.

During clinical trials with fenofibrate, total cholesterol was reduced by 20 to 25%, triglycerides by 40 to 55% and HDL cholesterol was increased by 10 to 30%.

In hypercholesterolaemic patients, where LDL cholesterol levels are reduced by 20 to 35%, the overall effect on cholesterol results in a decrease in the ratios of total cholesterol to HDL cholesterol, LDL cholesterol to HDL cholesterol, or Apo B to Apo AI, all of which are markers of atherogenic risk.

Because of its significant effect on LDL cholesterol and triglycerides, treatment with fenofibrate should be beneficial in hypercholesterolaemic patients with or without hypertriglyceridaemia, including secondary hyperlipoproteinaemia such as type 2 diabetes mellitus.

At the present time, no results of long-term controlled clinical trials are available to demonstrate the efficacy of fenofibrate in the primary or secondary prevention of atherosclerotic complications.

Extravascular deposits of cholesterol (tendinous and tuberous xanthoma) may be markedly reduced or even entirely eliminated during fenofibrate therapy.

Patients with raised levels of fibrinogen treated with fenofibrate have shown significant reductions in this parameter, as have those with raised levels of Lp(a). Other inflammatory markers such as C Reactive Protein are reduced with fenofibrate treatment.

The uricosuric effect of fenofibrate leading to reduction in uric acid levels of approximately 25% should be of additional benefit in those dyslipidaemic patients with hyperuricaemia.

Fenofibrate has been shown to possess an anti-aggregatory effect on platelets in animals and in a clinical study, which showed a reduction in platelet aggregation induced by ADP, arachidonic acid and epinephrine.

5.2 Pharmacokinetic properties
Supralip 160 mg is a film-coated tablet containing 160 mg of micronised fenofibrate and is suprabioavailable (larger bioavailability) compared to the previous formulations.

Absorption: Maximum plasma concentrations (Cmax) occur within 4 to 5 hours after oral administration. Plasma concentrations are stable during continuous treatment in any given individual.

The absorption of fenofibrate is increased when administered with food.

Distribution: Fenofibric acid is strongly bound to plasma albumin (more than 99%).

Plasma half-life: The plasma elimination half-life of fenofibric acid is approximately 20 hours.

Metabolism and excretion: No unchanged fenofibrate can be detected in the plasma where the principal metabolite is fenofibric acid. The drug is excreted mainly in the urine. Practically all the drug is eliminated within 6 days. Fenofibrate is mainly excreted in the form of fenofibric acid and its glucuronide conjugate. In elderly patients, the fenofibric acid apparent total plasma clearance is not modified.

Kinetic studies following the administration of a single dose and continuous treatment have demonstrated that the drug does not accumulate. Fenofibric acid is not eliminated by haemodialysis.

5.3 Preclinical safety data
Chronic toxicity studies have yielded no relevant information about specific toxicity of fenofibrate.

Studies on mutagenicity of fenofibrate have been negative.

In rats and mice, liver tumours have been found at high dosages, which are attributable to peroxisome proliferation. These changes are specific to small rodents and have not been observed in other animal species. This is of no relevance to therapeutic use in man.

Studies in mice, rats and rabbits did not reveal any teratogenic effect. Embryotoxic effects were observed at doses in the range of maternal toxicity. Prolongation of the gestation period and difficulties during delivery were observed at high doses. No sign of any effect on fertility has been detected.

6. PHARMACEUTICAL PARTICULARS

6.1 List of excipients
Sodium laurilsulfate, lactose monohydrate, povidone, crospovidone, microcrystalline cellulose, silica colloidal anhydrous, sodium stearyl fumarate.

Composition of the coating

Opadry®: polyvinyl alcohol, titanium dioxide (E171), talc, soybean lecithin, xanthan gum.

6.2 Incompatibilities
Not applicable.

6.3 Shelf life
2 years.

6.4 Special precautions for storage
Store in the original package in order to protect from moisture.

Do not store above 30°C.

6.5 Nature and contents of container
Thermoformed blister strips (PVC/PE/PVDC) of 14 tablets each.

Pack of 28 tablets.

Not all pack sizes may be marketed.

6.6 Instructions for use and handling
No special requirements.

7. MARKETING AUTHORISATION HOLDER
Fournier Pharmaceuticals Ltd

19-20 Progress Business Centre

Whittle Parkway

Slough SL1 6DQ

Berkshire, UK

8. MARKETING AUTHORISATION NUMBER(S)
PL 12509/0017

9. DATE OF FIRST AUTHORISATION/RENEWAL OF THE AUTHORISATION
Date of first authorisation: September 2000

Date of last renewal: 4th November 2004

10. DATE OF REVISION OF THE TEXT

11. Legal category
POM

Suprax Powder for Paediatric Oral Suspension

(sanofi-aventis)

1. NAME OF THE MEDICINAL PRODUCT
Suprax Powder for Paediatric Oral Suspension

2. QUALITATIVE AND QUANTITATIVE COMPOSITION
Each 5mL of reconstituted suspension contains 100 mg cefixime (anhydrous).

3. PHARMACEUTICAL FORM
For oral administration.

Bottles of powder for the preparation of suspension. When reconstituted, each 5 ml volume contains 100 mg of cefixime. The suspension contains 2.5 g of sucrose in 5 ml.

4. CLINICAL PARTICULARS

4.1 Therapeutic indications
Suprax is an orally active cephalosporin antibiotic which has marked *in vitro* bactericidal activity against a wide variety of Gram-positive and Gram-negative organisms.

It is indicated for the treatment of the following acute infections when caused by susceptible micro-organisms:

Upper Respiratory Tract Infections (URTI): e.g. otitis media; and other URTI where the causative organism is known or suspected to be resistant to other commonly used antibiotics, or where treatment failure may carry significant risk.

Lower Respiratory Tract Infection: e.g. bronchitis.

Urinary Tract Infections: e.g. cystitis, cystourethritis, uncomplicated pyelonephritis.

Clinical efficacy has been demonstrated in infections caused by commonly occuring pathogens including *Streptococcus pneumoniae, Streptococcus pyogenes, Escherichia coli, Proteus mirabilis, Kliebsiella* species, *Haemophilus influenzae* (beta-lactamase positive and negative), *Branhamella catarrhalis* (beta-lactamase positive and negative) and *Enterobacter* species. Suprax is highly stable in the presence of beta-lactamase enzymes.

Most strains of enterococci (*Streptococcus faecalis*, group D Streptococci) and Staphylococci (including coagulase positive and negative strains and methicillin-resistant strains) are resistant to Suprax. In addition, most strains of *Pseudomonas, Bacteriodes fragalis, Listeria monocytogenes* and *Clostridia* are resistant to Suprax.

4.2 Posology and method of administration
Route of Administration: Oral

Absorption of Suprax is not significantly modified by the presence of food. The usual course of treatment is 7 days. This may be continued for up to 14 days if required.

Adults and Children over 10 Years: The recommended adult dosage is 200-400 mg daily according to the severity of infection, given either as a single dose or in two divided doses.

The Elderly: Elderly patients may be given the same dose as recommended for adults. Renal function should be assessed and dosage should be adjusted in severe renal impairment (See "Dosage in Renal Impairment").

Children (Use Paediatric Oral Suspension): The recommended dosage for children is 8 mg/kg/day administered as a single dose or in two divided doses. As a general guide for prescribing in children the following daily doses in terms of volume of Paediatric Oral Suspension are suggested:

6 months up to 1 year: 3.75 ml daily

Children 1-4 years: 5 ml daily

Children 5-10 years: 10 ml daily

(A spoon is supplied to aid correct dosing - see "Nature and Contents of Container").

Children weighing more than 50 kg or older than 10 years should be treated with the recommended adult dose (200 - 400 mg daily depending on the severity of infection).

The safety and efficacy of cefixime has not been established in children less than 6 months.

Dosage In Renal Impairment: Suprax may be administered in the presence of impaired renal function. Normal dose and schedule may be given in patients with creatinine clearances of 20 ml/min or greater. In patients whose creatinine clearance is less than 20 ml/min, it is recommended that a dose of 200 mg once daily should not be exceeded. The dose and regimen for patients who are maintained on chronic ambulatory peritoneal dialysis or haemodialysis should follow the same recommendation as that for patients with creatinine clearances of less than 20 ml/min.

4.3 Contraindications
Patients with known hypersensitivity to cephalosporin antibiotics.

4.4 Special warnings and special precautions for use
Suprax should be given with caution to patients who have shown hypersensitivity to other drugs. Cephalosporins should be given with caution to penicillin-sensitive patients, as there is some evidence of partial cross-allergenicity between the penicillins and cephalosporins.

Patients have had severe reactions (including anaphylaxis) to both classes of drugs. If an allergic effect occurs with Suprax, the drug should be discontinued and the patient treated with appropriate agents if necessary.

Suprax should be administered with caution in patients with markedly impaired renal function (See "Dosage in Renal Impairment").

Treatment with broad spectrum antibiotics alters the normal flora of the colon and may permit overgrowth of clostridia. Studies indicate that a toxin produced by *Clostridium difficile* is a primary cause of antibiotic-associated diarrhoea. Pseudomembranous colitis is associated with the use of broad-spectrum antibiotics (including macrolides, semi-synthetic penicillins, lincosamides and cephalosporins); it is therefore important to consider its diagnosis in patients who develop diarrhoea in association with the use of antibiotics. Symptoms of pseudomembranous colitis may occur during or after antibiotic treatment.

Management of pseudomembranous colitis should include sigmoidoscopy, appropriate bacteriologic studies, fluids, electrolytes and protein supplementation. If the colitis does not improve after the drug has been discontinued, or if the symptoms are severe, oral vancomycin is the drug of choice for antibiotic-associated pseudomembranous colitis produced by *C. difficile*. Other causes of colitis should be excluded.

4.5 Interaction with other medicinal products and other forms of Interaction
A false positive reaction for glucose in the urine may occur with Benedict's or Fehling's solutions or with copper sulphate test tablets, but not with tests based on enzymatic glucose oxidase reactions.

A false positive direct Coombs test has been reported during treatment with cephalosporin antibiotics, therefore it should be recognised that a positive Coombs test may be due to the drug.

In common with other cephalosporins, increases in prothrombin times have been noted in a few patients. Care should therefore be taken in patients receiving anticoagulation therapy.

4.6 Pregnancy and lactation
Reproduction studies have been performed in mice and rats at doses up to 400 times the human dose and have revealed no evidence of impaired fertility or harm to the foetus due to cefixime. In the rabbit, at doses up to 4 times the human dose, there was no evidence of a teratogenic effect; there was a high incidence of abortion and maternal death which is an expected consequence of the known sensitivity of rabbits to antibiotic-induced changes in the population of the microflora of the intestine. There are no adequate and well-controlled studies in pregnant women. Suprax should therefore not be used in pregnancy or in nursing mothers unless considered essential by the physician.

4.7 Effects on ability to drive and use machines
None.

4.8 Undesirable effects
Suprax is generally well tolerated. The majority of adverse reactions observed in clinical trials were mild and self-limiting in nature.

Gastrointestinal Disturbances: The most frequent side effects seen with Suprax are diarrhoea and stool changes; diarrhoea has been more commonly associated with higher doses. Some cases of moderate to severe diarrhoea have been reported; this has occasionally warranted cessation of therapy. Suprax should be discontinued if marked diarrhoea occurs. Other gastrointestinal side effects seen less frequently are nausea, abdominal pain, dyspepsia, vomiting and flatulence. Pseudomembranous colitis has been reported (see above).

Central Nervous System: Headache and dizziness.

Hypersensitivity Reactions: Allergies in the form of rash, pruritus, urticaria, drug fever and arthralgia have been observed. These reactions usually subsided upon discontinuation of therapy. Rarely, erythema multiforme,

Stevens-Johnson syndrome and toxic epidermal necrolysis have been reported.

Haematological and Clinical Chemistry: Thrombocytopenia, leukopenia and eosinophilia have been reported. These reactions were infrequent and reversible. Mild transient changes in liver and renal function tests have been observed.

Miscellaneous: Other possible reactions include genital pruritus and vaginitis.

4.9 Overdose

There is no experience with overdoses with Suprax.

Adverse reactions seen at dose levels up to 2 g Suprax in normal subjects did not differ from the profile seen in patients treated at the recommended doses. Gastric lavage may be indicated in overdosage. No specific antidote exists. Cefixime is not removed from the circulation in significant quantities by dialysis.

5. PHARMACOLOGICAL PROPERTIES

5.1 Pharmacodynamic properties

Cefixime is an oral third generation cephalosporin which has marked *in vitro* bactericidal activity against a wide variety of Gram-positive and Gram-negative organisms.

Clinical efficacy has been demonstrated in infections caused by commonly occurring pathogens including *Streptococcus pneumoniae, Streptococcus pyogenes, Escherichia coli, Proteus mirabilis, Klebsiella* species, *Haemophilus influenzae* (beta-lactamase positive and negative), *Branhamella catarrhalis* (beta-lactamase positive and negative) and *Enterobacter* species. It is highly stable in the presence of beta-lactamase enzymes.

Most strains of enterococci (*Streptococcus faecalis*, group D Streptococci) and Staphylococci (including coagulase positive and negative strains and methicillin-resistant strains) are resistant to cefixime. In addition, most strains of *Pseudomonas, Bacteroides fragilis, Listeria monocytogenes* and *Clostridia* are resistant to cefixime.

5.2 Pharmacokinetic properties

The absolute oral bioavailability of cefixime is in the range of 22-54%. Absorption is not significantly modified by the presence of food. Cefixime may therefore be given without regard to meals.

From *in vitro* studies, serum or urine concentrations of 1 mcg/ml or greater were considered to be adequate for most common pathogens against which cefixime is active. Typically, the peak serum levels following the recommended adult or paediatric doses are between 1.5 and 3 mcg/ml. Little or no accumulation of cefixime occurs following multiple dosing.

The pharmacokinetics of cefixime in healthy elderly (age > 64 years) and young volunteers (11-35) compared the administration of 400 mg doses once daily for 5 days. Mean C_{max} and AUC values were slightly greater in the elderly. Elderly patients may be given the same dose as the general population.

Cefixime is predominantly eliminated as unchanged drug in the urine. Glomerular filtration is considered the predominant mechanism. Metabolites of cefixime have not been isolated from human serum or urine.

Serum protein binding is well characterised for human and animal sera; cefixime is almost exclusively bound to the albumin fraction, the mean free fraction being approximately 30%. Protein binding of cefixime is only concentration dependent in human serum at very high concentrations which are not seen following clinical dosing.

Transfer of ^{14}C-labelled cefixime from lactating rats to their nursing offspring through breast milk was quantitatively small (approximately 1.5% of the mothers' body content of cefixime in the pup). No data are available on secretion of cefixime in human breast milk. Placetal transfer of cefixime was small in pregnant rats dosed with labelled cefixime.

5.3 Preclinical safety data

There are no pre-clinical data of relevance to the prescriber which are additional to that already included in other sections of the Summary of Product Characteristics.

6. PHARMACEUTICAL PARTICULARS

6.1 List of excipients

Sucrose, xantham gum, sodium benzoate and strawberry flavour.

6.2 Incompatibilities

None.

6.3 Shelf life

2 years unopened.

2 weeks after reconstitution.

6.4 Special precautions for storage

Do not store unreconstituted product above 25°C.

Bottled product: To reconstitute, add 33 ml of water (50 ml bottle) or 66 ml of water (100 ml bottle) in two portions shaking after each addition. After reconstitution, the suspension may be stored at room temperature (below 25° C) for 14 days without significant loss of potency. Do not freeze. Keep bottles tightly closed and shake well before use. Discard any unused portion after 14 days. Dilution of the suspension is not recommended.

6.5 Nature and contents of container

Type III amber glass screw necked bottle with child resistant push/turn closure with white polyethylene cap with polyethylene film seal on expanded low density polyethylene. Bottles are supplied with a single ended transparent polypropylene (plastic) spoon capable of measuring 3.75 and 5.0ml of the suspension. Pack sizes of 50 and 100 ml.

6.6 Instructions for use and handling

None stated.

7. MARKETING AUTHORISATION HOLDER

May & Baker Limited

trading as Rhône-Poulenc Rorer or Aventis Pharma

50 Kings Hill Avenue

Kings Hill

West Malling

Kent ME19 4AH

8. MARKETING AUTHORISATION NUMBER(S)

PL 00012/0318

9. DATE OF FIRST AUTHORISATION/RENEWAL OF THE AUTHORISATION

14 October 1998

10. DATE OF REVISION OF THE TEXT

April 2004

11 LEGAL CLASSIFICATION

POM

Suprax Tablets

(sanofi-aventis)

1. NAME OF THE MEDICINAL PRODUCT

Suprax™ Tablets 200mg

2. QUALITATIVE AND QUANTITATIVE COMPOSITION

Each tablet contains 200mg cefixime (anhydrous).

3. PHARMACEUTICAL FORM

Convex, off-white, film-coated tablets engraved with 'ORO' on one side.

For oral administration.

4. CLINICAL PARTICULARS

4.1 Therapeutic indications

Suprax is an orally active cephalosporin antibiotic which has marked *in vitro* bactericidal activity against a wide variety of Gram-positive and Gram-negative organisms.

It is indicated for the treatment of the following acute infections when caused by susceptible micro-organisms:

UPPER RESPIRATORY TRACT INFECTIONS (URTI): e.g. otitis media; and other URTI where the causative organism is known or suspected to be resistant to other commonly used antibiotics, or where treatment failure may carry significant risk.

LOWER RESPIRATORY TRACT INFECTION: e.g. bronchitis.

URINARY TRACT INFECTIONS: e.g. cystitis, cystourethritis, uncomplicated pyelonephritis.

Clinical efficacy has been demonstrated in infections caused by commonly occuring pathogens including *Streptococcus pneumoniae, Streptococcus pyogenes, Escherichia coli, Proteus mirabilis, Klebsiella* species, *Haemophilus influenzae* (beta-lactamase positive and negative), *Branhamella catarrhalis* (beta-lactamase positive and negative) and *Enterobacter* species. Suprax is highly stable in the presence of beta-lactamase enzymes.

Most strains of enterococci (*Streptococcus faecalis*, group D Streptococci) and Staphylococci (including coagulase positive and negative strains and methicillin-resistant strains) are resistant to Suprax. In addition, most strains of *Pseudomonas, Bacteriodes fragalis, Listeria monocytogenes* and *Clostridia* are resistant to Suprax.

4.2 Posology and method of administration

Absorption of Suprax is not significantly modified by the presence of food. The usual course of treatment is 7 days. This may be continued for up to 14 days if required.

ADULTS AND CHILDREN OVER 10 YEARS: The recommended adult dosage is 200-400 mg daily according to the severity of infection, given either as a single dose or in two divided doses.

THE ELDERLY: Elderly patients may be given the same dose as recommended for adults. Renal function should be assessed and dosage should be adjusted in severe renal impairment (See ''Dosage in Renal Impairment'').

CHILDREN (Use Paediatric Oral Suspension): The recommended dosage for children is 8 mg/kg/day administered as a single dose or in two divided doses. As a general guide for prescribing in children the following daily doses in terms of volume of Paediatric Oral Suspension are suggested:

6 months up to 1 year: 3.75 mL daily

Children 1-4 years: 5 mL daily

Children 5-10 years: 10 mL daily

Children weighing more than 50 kg or older than 10 years should be treated with the recommended adult dose (200 - 400 mg daily depending on the severity of infection).

The safety and efficacy of cefixime has not been established in children less than 6 months.

DOSAGE IN RENAL IMPAIRMENT: Suprax may be administered in the presence of impaired renal function. Normal dose and schedule may be given in patients with creatinine clearances of 20 mL/min or greater. In patients whose creatinine clearance is less than 20 mL/min, it is recommended that a dose of 200 mg once daily should not be exceeded. The dose and regimen for patients who are maintained on chronic ambulatory peritoneal dialysis or haemodialysis should follow the same recommendation as that for patients with creatinine clearances of less than 20 mL/min.

4.3 Contraindications

Patients with known hypersensitivity to cephalosporin antibiotics.

4.4 Special warnings and special precautions for use

Suprax should be given with caution to patients who have shown hypersensitivity to other drugs. Cephalosporins should be given with caution to penicillin-sensitive patients, as there is some evidence of partial cross-allergenicity between the penicillins and cephalosporins.

Patients have had severe reactions (including anaphylaxis) to both classes of drugs. If an allergic effect occurs with Suprax, the drug should be discontinued and the patient treated with appropriate agents if necessary.

Suprax should be administered with caution in patients with markedly impaired renal function (See ''Dosage in Renal Impairment'').

Treatment with broad spectrum antibiotics alters the normal flora of the colon and may permit overgrowth of clostridia. Studies indicate that a toxin produced by *Clostridium difficile* is a primary cause of antibiotic-associated diarrhoea. Pseudomembranous colitis is associated with the use of broad-spectrum antibiotics (including macrolides, semi-synthetic penicillins, lincosamides and cephalosporins); it is therefore important to consider its diagnosis in patients who develop diarrhoea in association with the use of antibiotics. Symptoms of pseudomembranous colitis may occur during or after antibiotic treatment.

Management of pseudomembranous colitis should include sigmoidoscopy, appropriate bacteriologic studies, fluids, electrolytes and protein supplementation. If the colitis does not improve after the drug has been discontinued, or if the symptoms are severe, oral vancomycin is the drug of choice for antibiotic-associated pseudomembranous colitis produced by *C. difficile*. Other causes of colitis should be excluded.

4.5 Interaction with other medicinal products and other forms of Interaction

A false positive reaction for glucose in the urine may occur with Benedict's or Fehling's solutuions or with copper sulphate test tablets, but not with tests based on enzymatic glucose oxidase reactions.

A false positive direct Coombs test has been reported during treatment with cephalosporin antibiotics, therefore it should be recognised that a positive Coombs test may be due to the drug.

In common with other cephalosporins, increases in prothrombin times have been noted in a few patients. Care should therefore be taken in patients receiving anticoagulation therapy.

4.6 Pregnancy and lactation

Reproduction studies have been performed in mice and rats at doses up to 400 times the human dose and have revealed no evidence of impaired fertility or harm to the foetus due to cefixime. In the rabbit, at doses up to 4 times the human dose, there was no evidence of a teratogenic effect; there was a high incidence of abortion and maternal death which is an expected consequence of the known sensitivity of rabbits to antibiotic-induced changes in the population of the microflora of the intestine. There are no adequate and well-controlled studies in pregnant women. Suprax should therefore not be used in pregnancy or in nursing mothers unless considered essential by the physician.

4.7 Effects on ability to drive and use machines

None.

4.8 Undesirable effects

Suprax is generally well tolerated. The majority of adverse reactions observed in clinical trials were mild and self-limiting in nature.

GASTROINTESTINAL DISTURBANCES: The most frequent side effects seen with cefixime are diarrhoea and stool changes; diarrhoea has been more commonly associated with higher doses. Some cases of moderate to severe diarrhoea have been reported; this has occasionally warranted cessation of therapy. Suprax should be discontinued if marked diarrhoea occurs. Other gastrointestinal side effects seen less frequently are nausea, abdominal pain, dyspepsia, vomiting and flatulence. Pseudomembranous colitis has been reported (see above).

CENTRAL NERVOUS SYSTEM: Headache and dizziness.

HYPERSENSITIVITY REACTIONS:Allergies in the form of rash, pruritus, urticaria, drug fever and arthralgia have been observed. These reactions usually subsided upon discontinuation of therapy. Rarely, erythema multiforme, Stevens-Johnson syndrome and toxic epidermal necrolysis have been reported.

HAEMATOLOGICAL AND CLINICAL CHEMISTRY: Thrombocytopenia, leukopenia and eosinophilia have been reported. These reactions were infrequent and reversible. Mild transient changes in liver and renal function tests have been observed.

HEPATIC DISORDERS: Transient rises in liver transaminases, alkaline phosphatase and jaundice can also occur.

MISCELLANEOUS: Other possible reactions include genital pruritus and vaginitis.

4.9 Overdose

There is no experience with overdoses with Suprax.

Adverse reactions seen at dose levels up to 2 g Suprax in normal subjects did not differ from the profile seen in patients treated at the recommended doses. Gastric lavage may be indicated in overdosage. No specific antidote exists. Cefixime is not removed from the circulation in significant quantities by dialysis.

5. PHARMACOLOGICAL PROPERTIES

5.1 Pharmacodynamic properties

Cefixime is an oral third generation cephalosporin which has marked *in vitro* bactericidal activity against a wide variety of Gram-positive and Gram-negative organisms.

Clinical efficacy has been demonstrated in infections caused by commonly occurring pathogens including *Streptococcus pneumoniae, Streptococcus pyogenes, Escherichia coli, Proteus mirabilis, Klebsiella* species, *Haemophilus influenzae* (beta-lactamase positive and negative), *Branhamella catarrhalis* (beta-lactamase positive and negative) and *Enterobacter* species. It is highly stable in the presence of beta-lactamase enzymes.

Most strains of enterococci (*Streptococcus faecalis*, group D Streptococci) and Staphylococci (including coagulase positive and negative strains and methicillin-resistant strains) are resistant to cefixime. In addition, most strains of *Pseudomonas, Bacteroides fragilis, Listeria monocytogenes* and *Clostridia* are resistant to cefixime.

5.2 Pharmacokinetic properties

The absolute oral bioavailability of cefixime is in the range of 22-54%. Absorption is not significantly modified by the presence of food. Cefixime may therefore be given without regard to meals.

From *in vitro* studies, serum or urine concentrations of 1 mcg/mL or greater were considered to be adequate for most common pathogens against which cefixime is active. Typically, the peak serum levels following the recommended adult or paediatric doses are between 1.5 and 3 mcg/mL. Little or no accumulation of cefixime occurs following multiple dosing.

The pharmacokinetics of cefixime in healthy elderly (age> 64 years) and young volunteers (11-35) compared the administration of 400 mg doses once daily for 5 days. Mean C_{max} and AUC values were slightly greater in the elderly. Elderly patients may be given the same dose as the general population.

Cefixime is predominantly eliminated as unchanged drug in the urine. Glomerular filtration is considered the predominant mechanism. Metabolites of cefixime have not been isolated from human serum or urine.

Serum protein binding is well characterised for human and animal sera; cefixime is almost exclusively bound to the albumin fraction, the mean free fraction being approximately 30%. Protein binding of cefixime is only concentration dependent in human serum at very high concentrations which are not seen following clinical dosing.

Transfer of ^{14}C-labelled cefixime from lactating rats to their nursing offspring through breast milk was quantitatively small (approximately 1.5% of the mothers' body content of cefixime in the pup). No data are available on secretion of cefixime in human breast milk. Placental transfer of cefixime was small in pregnant rats dosed with labelled cefixime.

5.3 Preclinical safety data

There are no pre-clinical data of relevance to the prescriber which are additional to that already included in other sections of the Summary of Product Characteristics.

6. PHARMACEUTICAL PARTICULARS

6.1 List of excipients

Tablet cores: microcrystalline cellulose, pregelatinised starch, calcium hydrogen phosphate dihydrate and magnesium stearate.

Tablet coating: hypromellose, Macrogol 6000 and titanium dioxide.

6.2 Incompatibilities

None.

6.3 Shelf life

24 months.

6.4 Special precautions for storage

Do not store above 25° C.

6.5 Nature and contents of container

PVC/aluminium foil blister packs - packs of 7.

6.6 Instructions for use and handling

None stated.

7. MARKETING AUTHORISATION HOLDER

Rhone-Poulenc Rorer

RPR House

50 Kings Hill Avenue

Kings Hill

West Malling

Kent

ME19 4AH

8. MARKETING AUTHORISATION NUMBER(S)

PL 00012/0316

9. DATE OF FIRST AUTHORISATION/RENEWAL OF THE AUTHORISATION

12 August 1998

10. DATE OF REVISION OF THE TEXT

August 1999

11. Legal Category

POM

Suprecur Injection

(sanofi-aventis)

1. NAME OF THE MEDICINAL PRODUCT

Suprecur Injection

2. QUALITATIVE AND QUANTITATIVE COMPOSITION

Suprecur injection contains 1.00 mg buserelin as buserelin acetate in 1 ml aqueous solution.

1.00 mg buserelin is equivalent to 1.05 buserelin acetate.

3. PHARMACEUTICAL FORM

Solution for Injection.

4. CLINICAL PARTICULARS

4.1 Therapeutic indications

Pituitary desensitisation in preparation for ovulation induction regimens using gonadotrophins

4.2 Posology and method of administration

The total daily dose is usually in the range 200 - 500 microgram (μg) given as a single injection by the subcutaneous route. Treatment should start in the early follicular phase (day 1) or, provided the existence of an early pregnancy has been excluded, in the midluteal phase (day 21). It should continue at least until down-regulation is achieved e.g. serum oestradiol <180pmol/l and serum progesterone <3nmol/l. This will usually take about 1 - 3 weeks. Doses may have to be adjusted for individuals. Occasionally, patients may require up to 500 μg twice daily in order to achieve down-regulation. When down-regulation is achieved, stimulation with gonadotropin is commenced while the dosage of buserelin is maintained. At the appropriate stage of follicular development, gonadotropin and buserelin are stopped and hCG is given to induce ovulation.

Treatment monitoring, oocyte transfer and fertilisation techniques are performed according to the normal practice of the individual clinic.

Luteal support with hCG or progesterone should be given as appropriate.

4.3 Contraindications

Hypersensitivity to buserelin, LHRH, or to any of the excipients; pregnancy, lactation, undiagnosed vaginal bleeding; hormone-dependant neoplasms.

4.4 Special warnings and special precautions for use

Suprecur injection is for subcutaneous administration ONLY

Patients known to suffer from depression should be carefully monitored during treatment with Suprecur.

In patients with hypertension, blood pressure must be monitored regularly.

In diabetic patients, blood glucose levels must be checked regularly.

Whenever the treatment is self-administered, it is strongly recommended that initial doses should be administered under close medical supervision due to the possibility of hypersensitivity reactions. Patients should cease injections and seek medical attention should any adverse event occur which may represent an allergic reaction.

Treatment with Suprecur should be initiated only under the supervision of a specialist with experience of the indication.

Induction of ovulation should be carried out under close medical supervision. Risks specific to IVF/ET and related assisted reproduction procedures such as increase in ectopic and multiple pregnancies are unaltered under adjunctive use of buserelin. However, follicle recruitment may be increased especially in patients with polycystic ovarian disorder (PCOD).

Combined use of buserelin with gonadotrophins may bear a higher risk of ovarian hyperstimulation syndrome (OHSS) than the use of gonadotrophins alone. The stimulation cycle should be monitored carefully to identify patients at risk of developing OHSS. hCG should be withheld if necessary.

Possible clinical signs of ovarian hyperstimulation syndrome (OHSS) include: abdominal pain, feeling of abdominal tension, increased abdominal girth, occurrence of ovarian cysts, nausea, vomiting, as well as massive enlargement of the ovaries, dyspnoea, diarrhoea, oligurea, haemoconcentration, hypercoagulability. Pedicle tension or rupture of the ovary may lead to an acute abdomen. Severe thromboembolic events may also occur. Fatal outcome is possible.

Ovarian cysts have been observed in the initial phase of buserelin treatment. No impact on the stimulation cycle has been reported so far.

4.5 Interaction with other medicinal products and other forms of Interaction

During treatment with Suprecur, the effect of antidiabetic agents may be attenuated.

4.6 Pregnancy and lactation

Pregnancy must be excluded before starting buserelin and the medication should be stopped on the day of administration of hCG. Buserelin must not be administered to lactating mothers; detectable levels of drug are found in milk.

4.7 Effects on ability to drive and use machines

Certain adverse effects (e.g. dizziness) may impair the ability to concentrate and react, and therefore constitute a risk in situations where these abilities are of special importance (e.g. operating a vehicle or machinery).

4.8 Undesirable effects

After administration of the injection, pain or local reaction at the injection site is possible. Hypersensitivity reactions may also occur. These may become manifest for example as reddening of the skin, itching, skin rashes (including urticaria) and allergic asthma with dyspnoea as well as, in isolated cases, anaphylactic/anaphylactoid shock.

Side-effects consequent upon the suppression of hormone production occur in most patients. Hot flushes, increased sweating and loss of libido generally occur some weeks after starting treatment and may be severe in some patients. Dryness of the vagina may also be noticed.

Changes in bone density: a decrease in bone mineral, the magnitude of which relates to the duration of therapy, occurs during treatment with buserelin alone. The evidence available indicates that six months treatment is associated with a decrease in bone mineral density of the spine of 3.5 %. These changes are similar to those seen with other agonists. Increased levels of serum alkaline phosphatase may occur.

Combined use of buserelin with gonadotrophins may bear a higher risk of ovarian hyperstimulation syndrome (OHSS) than the use of gonadotrophins alone (see section 4.4).

Very rare cases of pituitary adenomas were reported during treatment with LH-RH agonists, including buserelin.

Other adverse effects may include:

Frequent: Vaginal discharge, increase or decrease in breast size, breast tenderness, dry skin, acne, increase or decrease in scalp hair, headache, palpitations, nervousness, sleep disturbances, tiredness, drowsiness, dizziness, emotional instability, lower abdominal pain, stomach ache, nausea, vomiting, diarrhoea, constipation, increase or decrease in weight, musculoskeletal discomfort and pain (including shoulder pain/stiffness).

Occasional: dry eyes (possibly leading to eye irritations in women who wear contact lenses), impaired vision (eg blurred vision), feeling of pressure behind the eyes, splitting nails, increase or decrease in body hair, lactation, oedema (of face and extremities), disturbances of memory and concentration, anxiety, depression or worsening of existing depression, increase thirst, changes in appetite, paraesthesia, increase in serum liver enzyme levels (e.g. transaminases), increase in serum bilirubin.

Rare: increase or decrease in blood lipid levels, tinnitus, hearing disorders.

Very rare: deterioration of blood pressure levels in patients with hypertension, reduction in glucose tolerance which may lead to worsening of metabolic control in diabetics, thrombocytopenia, leucopenia.

Isolated cases: severe hypersensitivity reactions with shock.

4.9 Overdose

Overdose may lead to signs and symptoms such as asthenia, headache, nervousness, hot flushes, dizziness, nausea, abdominal pain, oedemas of the lower extremities, and mastodynia. Treatment should be symptomatic.

5. PHARMACOLOGICAL PROPERTIES

5.1 Pharmacodynamic properties

Buserelin is a synthetic peptide. It is a superactive analogue of natural gonadotrophin releasing hormone (gonadorelin, LHRH or GNRH). After an initial stimulation of gonadotrophin release, it down-regulates the hypothalamic-pituitary-gonadal (HPO) axis such that a decrease in ovarian steroid secretion into the post-menopausal range occurs. The time taken to achieve these levels varies between individuals and with the regimen of administration, so that close monitoring of circulating levels of oestradiol and progesterone should be performed during treatment. This effect provides an appropriate setting for the administration of follicle-stimulating therapy and reduces the incidence of premature ovulation by inhibition of surges in LH.

5.2 Pharmacokinetic properties
The bioavailability of buserelin after subcutaneous injection is 100%. C_{max} occurs at about 1 hour post-injection. The half-life after injection is about 80 minutes.

Buserelin accumulates preferentially in the liver, kidneys and in the anterior pituitary lobe, the biological target organ. Buserelin circulates in serum predominantly in the intact, active form. Protein binding is about 15 %.

Buserelin is inactivated by peptidases (pyrogutamyl peptidase and chymotrypsin-like endopeptidases) in the liver and kidneys. In the pituitary gland, receptor-bound buserelin is inactivated by membrane-located enzymes. Buserelin and inactive buserelin metabolites are excreted via the renal and the biliary route.

5.3 Preclinical safety data
No signs of toxicity or histopathological changes were detected in long-term pharmacology and toxicology studies with buserelin in rats, dogs, and monkeys; the endocrine effects observed were restricted to the gonads. Pituitary adenoma occurred during long-term treatment in rats, this phenomenon has not been found in dogs and monkeys. There are no indications of a mutagenic or carcinogenic potential.

6. PHARMACEUTICAL PARTICULARS

6.1 List of excipients
sodium chloride Ph.Eur.

sodium dihydrogen phosphate BP.

sodium hydroxide BP.

benzyl alcohol BP.

Water for Injections Ph. Eur.

6.2 Incompatibilities
Not applicable.

6.3 Shelf life
Unopened: 36 months

(see section 6.6).

6.4 Special precautions for storage
Store between 2°C and 25°C. Do not freeze. Protect from light.

6.5 Nature and contents of container
Box of 2 × 5.5 ml multidose vials each containing 1.05 mg buserelin acetate per 1 ml, corresponding to 1.00 mg buserelin per 1 ml.

6.6 Instructions for use and handling
Each vial contains enough material for 10 doses. After finishing the course of treatment the vial should be disposed of and a new vial started for the next treatment. Do not use if the contents of the vial are cloudy or discoloured. Patients should be instructed on the correct handling of the vial (aseptic technique) by a doctor or nurse.

7. MARKETING AUTHORISATION HOLDER
Aventis Pharma Ltd

50, Kings Hill Avenue

Kings Hill

West Malling

Kent

ME19 4AH

8. MARKETING AUTHORISATION NUMBER(S)
PL 04425/0278

9. DATE OF FIRST AUTHORISATION/RENEWAL OF THE AUTHORISATION
23 April 2002

10. DATE OF REVISION OF THE TEXT
29 August 2003

Legal category: POM

Suprecur Nasal Spray

(sanofi-aventis)

1. NAME OF THE MEDICINAL PRODUCT
SUPRECUR NASAL SPRAY

2. QUALITATIVE AND QUANTITATIVE COMPOSITION
Suprecur nasal spray contains 150 micrograms buserelin, as buserelin acetate, in one spray dose.

1.50 mg buserelin is equivalent to 1.575 mg buserelin acetate.

3. PHARMACEUTICAL FORM
Nasal Spray

4. CLINICAL PARTICULARS

4.1 Therapeutic indications
The treatment of endometriosis in cases that do not require surgery as primary therapy.

Pituitary desensitisation in preparation for ovulation induction regimens using gonadotrophins.

4.2 Posology and method of administration
Endometriosis: The total daily dose is 900 micrograms buserelin, administered as one spray dose in each nostril in the morning, at mid-day and in the evening. The product may be used before or after meals or at other times, provided that uniform intervals are maintained between doses.

The usual duration of treatment is six months and this should not be exceeded. Only a single course of treatment is recommended.

Pituitary desensitisation prior to ovulation induction: The total daily intranasal dose for this indication is 600 micrograms buserelin, given in four divided dosages of 150 micrograms (one application in one nostril) spread over the waking hours. Treatment should start in the early follicular phase (day 1) or, provided the existence of an early pregnancy has been excluded in the midluteal phase (day 21). It should continue at least until down-regulation is achieved e.g. serum oestradiol <50 ng/l and serum progesterone <1 microgram/l. This will usually take about 2–3 weeks. In some patients, dosages up to 4 × 300 micrograms may be required to achieve these levels. When down-regulation is achieved, stimulation with gonadotropin is commenced while the dosage of buserelin is maintained. At the appropriate stage of follicular development, gonadotropin and buserelin are stopped and hCG is given to induce ovulation.

Treatment monitoring, oocyte transfer and fertilisation techniques are performed according to the normal practice of the individual clinic.

Luteal support with hCG or progesterone should be given as appropriate.

If used correctly, reliable absorption of the active ingredient takes place via nasal mucous membranes. The drug is absorbed even if the patient has a cold; however, in such cases the nose should be blown thoroughly before administration.

If nasal decongestants are being used concurrently, they should be administered at least 30 minutes after the buserelin.

Children: Suprecur is not suitable for use in children.

Elderly: Suprecur is not suitable for use in post-menopausal women.

4.3 Contraindications
Pregnancy, lactation, undiagnosed vaginal bleeding, hormone dependent neoplasms, hypersensitivity to buserelin acetate, LHRH or benzalkonium chloride.

4.4 Special warnings and special precautions for use
Patients known to suffer from depression should be carefully monitored during treatment with Suprecur.

In patients with hypertension, blood pressure must be checked regularly.

In diabetic patients blood glucose levels must be checked regularly.

Endometriosis: Patients should discontinue oral contraceptives before starting treatment. Where appropriate, alternative, non-hormonal methods of contraception should be used. If treatment is interrupted even for only a few days, ovulation may occur and there is a risk of pregnancy.

Suprecur treatment should be started on the first or second day of menstruation in order to exclude pre-existing pregnancy as far as possible. A pregnancy test is advisable if there is any doubt.

A menstruation-like bleed usually occurs during the first few weeks of treatment. Breakthrough bleeding may also occur during continuing courses of treatment in some patients. Recovery of pituitary-gonadal function usually occurs within 8 weeks of discontinuing treatment.

In the initial treatment with buserelin, ovarian cysts may develop.

Pituitary desensitisation prior to ovulation induction: Induction of ovulation should be carried out under close medical supervision. Risks specific to IVF/ET and related assisted reproduction procedures such as increase in miscarriages, ectopic and multiple pregnancies are unaltered under adjunctive use of buserelin. In addition, follicle recruitment may be increased especially in patients with PCOD.

Combined use of buserelin with gonadotrophins may bear a higher risk of ovarian hyperstimulation syndrome (OHSS) than the use of gonadotrophins alone. The stimulation cycle should be monitored carefully to identify patients at risk of developing OHSS. hCG should be withheld if necessary.

Possible clinical signs of ovarian hyperstimulation syndrome (OHSS) include: abdominal pain, feeling of abdominal tension, increased abdominal girth, occurrence of ovarian cysts, nausea, vomiting, as well as massive enlargement of the ovaries, dyspnoea, diarrhoea, oligurea, haemoconcentration, hypercoagulability. Pedicle tension or rupture of the ovary may lead to an acute abdomen. Severe thromboembolic events may also occur. Fatal outcome is possible.

Ovarian cysts have been observed in the initial phase of buserelin treatment. No impact on the stimulation cycle has been reported so far.

Treatment with Suprecur should be initiated only under the supervision of a specialist with experience of the indication.

4.5 Interaction with other medicinal products and other forms of Interaction
During treatment with buserelin, the effect of antidiabetic agents may be attenuated.

In concomitant treatment with sexual hormones ("add back"), the dosage is to be selected so as to ensure that the overall therapeutic effect is not affected

4.6 Pregnancy and lactation
Suprecur is contraindicated in pregnancy and lactation. In rats, fetal malformations have been seen after very high doses.

In endometriosis: It is unlikely that pregnancy will occur in the later stages of treatment if the recommended doses are taken regularly. However, if treatment is interrupted even for only a few days, ovulation may occur and the patient may become pregnant. In this event, Suprecur must be withdrawn immediately (see also precautions).

In pituitary desensitisation prior to ovulation induction: Pregnancy should be excluded before starting Suprecur, and the medication should be stopped on the day of administration of hCG.

Buserelin, in small quantities, is excreted in milk. Suprecur should not be prescribed to lactating mothers, although no effects on the child have been observed so far.

4.7 Effects on ability to drive and use machines
Certain adverse effects (e.g. dizziness) may impair the patients ability to concentrate and react, and therefore, constitute a risk in those situations where these abilities are of special importance (e.g. operating a vehicle or machinery).

4.8 Undesirable effects
As evidence of the biological response to hormone deprivation, patients may experience menopausal-like symptoms and withdrawal bleeding, which are directly related to the pharmacological action of the drug. Symptoms such as hot flushes, increased sweating, dry vagina, dyspareunia, loss of libido occur some weeks after starting treatment and may be severe in some patients. Withdrawal bleeding may occur during the first few weeks of treatment. Breakthrough bleeding may occur during continuing treatment.

Changes in bone density: A decrease in bone mineral, the magnitude of which relates to the duration of therapy, occurs during treatment with buserelin alone. The evidence available indicates that six months' treatment is associated with a decrease in bone mineral density of the spine of 3.5%. These changes are similar to those seen with other agonists. Increased levels of serum alkaline phosphatase may occur. These are reversible on discontinuing treatment.

Other adverse events not directly attributable to the pharmacological effect have been observed. These are changes in breast size (increase/decrease), breast tenderness, splitting nails, acne, dry skin and occasionally vaginal discharge and oedema of the face and extremities (arms and legs).

In addition, vomiting, lactation, stomach ache, lower abdominal pain, paraesthesia may occur, as may dryness of the eyes, leading to eye irritation in wearers of contact lenses.

Very rare cases of pituitary adenomas were reported during treatment with LH-RH agonists, including buserelin.

Buserelin treatment may also lead to:

- changes in scalp and body hair (alopecia, hirsutism)

- deterioration in blood pressure levels in patients with hypertension.

- hypersensitivity reactions, such as reddening of the skin, itching, skin rashes (including urticaria), and allergic asthma with dyspnoea, as well as in isolated cases leading to anaphylactic/anphylactoid shock.

- reduction in glucose tolerance.

- changes in blood lipids, increase in serum levels of liver enzymes (transaminases) increase in bilirubin; thrombopenia and leucopenia.

- headache (of migranous type in rare instances), palpitations, nervousness, sleep disturbances, fatigue (asthenia), drowsiness, disturbances of memory and concentration, emotional instability, feelings of anxiety. In rare cases depression may develop or existing depression may worsen.

- dizziness, tinnitus, hearing disorders, impaired vision (e.g. blurred vision), feeling of pressure behind the eyes.

- nausea, increased thirst, diarrhoea, constipation, changes in appetite, weight changes (increase or decrease).

- musculoskeletal discomfort and pain (including shoulder pain/stiffness).

The nasal spray may irritate the nasal mucosa. This may lead to nosebleeds and hoarseness as well as to disturbances of smell and taste.

4.9 Overdose
Overdose may lead to signs and symptoms such as asthenia, headache, nervousness, hot flushes, dizziness, nausea, abdominal pain, oedema of the lower extremities and mastodynia. Treatment should be symptomatic.

5. PHARMACOLOGICAL PROPERTIES
5.1 Pharmacodynamic properties
Buserelin is a synthetic peptide. It is a superactive analogue of natural gonadotrophin releasing hormone (gonadorelin, LHRH or GNRH). After an initial stimulation of gonadotrophin release, it down-regulates the hypothalamic-pituitary-gonadal axis.

5.2 Pharmacokinetic properties
The intra-nasal absorption rate of buserelin is about 3%. Metabolic inactivation by peptides occurs in the liver and kidney. The drug is also inactivated by pituitary membrane enzymes. After intra-nasal administration to humans, buserelin is excreted for more than 8 hours in the urine. Virtually all the serum fraction, and half the urine fraction of buserelin, are present as the parent drug.

The bioavailability of buserelin after nasal administration is not adversely influenced by the presence of rhinitis.

5.3 Preclinical safety data
None of clinical relevance.

6. PHARMACEUTICAL PARTICULARS
6.1 List of excipients
The nasal spray also contains citric acid, sodium citrate, sodium chloride and benzalkonium chloride in aqueous solution.

6.2 Incompatibilities
None

6.3 Shelf life
3 years. 5 weeks after first opening.

6.4 Special precautions for storage
Store between 2 and 25°C. Do not freeze.

6.5 Nature and contents of container
Cartons containing two bottles and two metered-dose pumps (nebulisers). Each bottle contains 10g solution.

6.6 Instructions for use and handling
How to use the spray bottle:

1. Remove screw cap from bottle.

2. Remove metered-dose nebulizer from transparent plastic container and take off both protective caps.

3. Screw nebulizer on to bottle.

4. Before first application only, pump 5-8 times, holding bottle vertical, until the solution has filled the system and a uniform spray is emitted. The preliminary pumping is for the purpose of filling the system and testing the spray. It must not be repeated after the first use, in order to avoid wasting the contents.

5. Keeping bottle vertical and bending head over it slightly, spray solution into nose. If necessary, the nose should be cleaned before applying the solution.

6. After use leave nebulizer on bottle. After replacing protective cap, spray bottle is best stored in its transparent container in an upright position.

7. MARKETING AUTHORISATION HOLDER
Aventis Pharma Ltd
50 Kings Hill Avenue
Kings Hill
West Malling
Kent
ME19 4AH

8. MARKETING AUTHORISATION NUMBER(S)
PL 04425/0277

9. DATE OF FIRST AUTHORISATION/RENEWAL OF THE AUTHORISATION
23 April 2002

10. DATE OF REVISION OF THE TEXT
29 August 2003

Legal category: POM

Suprefact Injection

(sanofi-aventis)

1. NAME OF THE MEDICINAL PRODUCT
Suprefact® Injection

2. QUALITATIVE AND QUANTITATIVE COMPOSITION
Suprefact injection contains 1.00 mg buserelin as buserelin acetate in 1ml aqueous solution.

1.00 mg buserelin is equivalent to 1.05 mg buserelin acetate.

3. PHARMACEUTICAL FORM
Injection

4. CLINICAL PARTICULARS
4.1 Therapeutic indications
For the treatment of advanced prostatic carcinoma (stage C or stage D according to the classification of Murphy *et al*, in Cancer 45, p1889-95, 1980) in which suppression of testosterone is indicated. Buserelin acts by blockade and subsequent down-regulation of pituitary LHRH receptor synthesis. Gonadotrophin release is consequently inhibited. As a result of this inhibition there is reduced stimulation of testosterone secretion and serum testosterone levels fall to castration range. Before inhibition occurs there is a brief stimulatory phase during which testosterone levels may rise.

4.2 Posology and method of administration
Initiation of therapy: is most conveniently carried out in hospital; 0.5ml Suprefact injection should be injected subcutaneously at 8 hourly intervals for 7 days.

Maintenance therapy: on the 8th day of treatment the patient is changed to intranasal administration of Suprefact. (see literature for dosage).

4.3 Contraindications
Suprefact should not be used if the tumour is found to be insensitive to hormone manipulation or after surgical removal of the testes. It should not be used in pregnancy. It is contraindicated in cases of known hypersensitivity to benzyl alcohol (injection) or buserelin.

4.4 Special warnings and special precautions for use
Patients known to suffer from depression should be carefully monitored during treatment with Suprefact.

Prostatic carcinoma: Monitoring of the effect of clinical effect of Suprefact is carried out by methods generally used in prostatic carcinoma. Initially serum testosterone levels rise and a clinical effect will not be seen until levels start to fall into therapeutic (castration) range. Disease flare (temporary deterioration of the patient's condition) has been reported at the beginning of the treatment. The incidence is variable, but of the order of the 10%. Symptoms are usually confined to transient increase in pain, but the exact nature depends on the site of the lesions. Neurological sequelae have been reported where secondary deposits impinge upon the spinal cord or CNS. Disease flare is prevented by the prophylactic use of an anti-androgen, e.g. cyproterone acetate, 300 mg daily. It is recommended that the treatment should be started at least 3 days before the first dose of Suprefact and continued for at least 3 weeks after commencement of the Suprefact therapy.

Once testosterone levels have started to fall below their baseline concentration clinical improvement should start to become apparent. If testosterone levels do not reach the therapeutic range within 4 weeks (6 weeks at the latest) the dose schedule should be checked to be sure that it is being followed exactly. It is unlikely that a patient who is taking the full dose will not show a suppression of testosterone to the therapeutic range. If this is the case, alternative therapy should be considered.

After the initial determination, testosterone levels should be monitored at 3-monthly intervals. A proportion of patients will have tumours that are not sensitive to hormone manipulation. Absence of clinical improvement in the face of adequate testosterone suppression is diagnostic of this condition, which will not benefit from further therapy with buserelin.

In patients with hypertension, blood pressure must be monitored regularly.

In diabetic patients blood glucose levels must be checked regularly.

4.5 Interaction with other medicinal products and other forms of Interaction
During treatment with Suprefact, the effect of antidiabetic agents may be attenuated.

4.6 Pregnancy and lactation
Not applicable.

4.7 Effects on ability to drive and use machines
Certain adverse effects (eg.dizziness) may impair the ability to concentrate and react, and therefore constitute a risk in situations where these abilities are of special importance (eg. Operating a vehicle or machinery).

4.8 Undesirable effects
At the beginning of treatment, a transient rise in the serum testosterone level usually develops and may lead to temporary activation of the tumour with secondary reactions such as:

- occurrence of exacerbation of bone pain in patients with metastases.

- signs of neurological deficit due to tumour compression with eg. muscle weakness in the legs.

- impaired micturition, hydronephrosis or lymphostasis.

- thrombosis with pulmonary embolism.

Such reactions can be largely avoided when an anti-androgen is given concomitantly in the initial phase of buserelin treatment (see Precautions and Warnings). However, even with concomitant anti-androgen therapy, a mild but transient increase in tumour pain as well as a deterioration in general well being may develop in some patients.

Additionally, in most patients, hot flushes and loss of potency or libido (result of hormone deprivation); painless gynaecomastia (occasionally) as well as mild oedemas of the ankles and lower legs may occur.

Very rare cases of pituitary adenomas were reported during treatment with LHRH agonists, including buserelin.

Buserelin treatment may also lead to:

- changes in scalp or body hair (increase or decrease);

- deterioration in blood pressure levels in patients with hypertension.

- hypersensitivity reactions. These may become manifest as, eg.reddening of the skin, itching, skin rashes (including urticaria) and allergic asthma with dyspnoea as well as, in isolated cases leading to anaphylactic/anaphylactoid shock.

- reduction in glucose tolerance. This may in diabetic patients lead to a deterioration in metabolic control.

- changes in blood lipids, increase in serum levels of liver enzymes (eg transaminases) increase in bilirubin, thrombopenia and leucopenia.

- headaches, palpitations, nervousness, sleep disturbances, tiredness, drowsiness, disturbances of memory and concentration, emotional instability, feelings of anxiety. In rare cases, depression may develop or existing depression worsen.

- dizziness, tinnitus, hearing disorders, impaired vision (eg. blurred vision), feeling pressure behind the eyes

- nausea, vomiting, increased thirst, diarrhoea, constipation, changes in appetite, weight changes (increase or decrease).

- Paraesthesia, musculoskeletal discomfort and pain.

After administration of the injection, pain or local reaction at the injection site is possible.

4.9 Overdose
Overdose may lead to signs and symptoms such as asthenia, headache, nervousness, hot flushes, dizziness, nausea, abdominal pain, oedemas of the lower extremities, and mastodynia. Treatment should be symptomatic.

5. PHARMACOLOGICAL PROPERTIES
5.1 Pharmacodynamic properties
Buserelin is a synthetic peptide. It is a superactive analogue of natural gonadotrophin releasing hormone (gonadorelin, LHRH or GNRH). After an initial stimulation of gonadotrophin release, it down-regulates the hypothalamic-pituitary-gonadal axis.

5.2 Pharmacokinetic properties
Metabolic inactivation by peptidases occurs in the liver and kidney. The drug is also inactivated by pituitary membrane enzymes.

5.3 Preclinical safety data
None stated

6. PHARMACEUTICAL PARTICULARS
6.1 List of excipients
Sodium Chloride
Sodium Dihydrogen Phosphate
Sodium Hydroxide
Benzyl Alcohol
Water for injections

6.2 Incompatibilities
Not applicable

6.3 Shelf life
3 years

6.4 Special precautions for storage
Store between 2° and 25°C. Protect from light.

6.5 Nature and contents of container
Box of 1 × 5.5 ml multidose vial containing 1.05 mg buserelin acetate per 1ml, corresponding to 1.00mg buserelin per 1 ml.

Pack size: 2 individual cardboard boxes are wrapped together in a clear plastic outer.

6.6 Instructions for use and handling
No special instructions

7. MARKETING AUTHORISATION HOLDER
Aventis Pharma Ltd
50 Kings Hill Avenue
Kings Hill
West Malling
Kent
ME19 4AH

8. MARKETING AUTHORISATION NUMBER(S)
PL 04425/0268

9. DATE OF FIRST AUTHORISATION/RENEWAL OF THE AUTHORISATION
28 August 2002

10. DATE OF REVISION OF THE TEXT
13 February 2004

Legal category: POM

Suprefact Nasal Spray

(sanofi-aventis)

1. NAME OF THE MEDICINAL PRODUCT

SUPREFACT NASAL SPRAY

2. QUALITATIVE AND QUANTITATIVE COMPOSITION

Suprefact nasal spray contains 100 micrograms buserelin as buserelin acetate in 1 spray dose (100mg) of aqueous solution containing benzalkonium chloride as preservative.

1.00 mg buserelin is equivalent to 1.05 mg buserelin acetate.

3. PHARMACEUTICAL FORM

Nasal spray

4. CLINICAL PARTICULARS

4.1 Therapeutic indications

For the treatment of advanced prostatic carcinoma (stage C or stage D according to the classification of Murphy *et al*. in Cancer, 45, p 1889–95, 1980) in which suppression of testosterone is indicated. Buserelin acts by blockade and subsequent down-regulation of pituitary LHRH receptor synthesis. Gonadotrophin release is consequently inhibited. As a result of this inhibition there is reduced stimulation of testosterone secretion and serum testosterone levels fall to the castration range. Before inhibition occurs there is a brief stimulatory phase during which testosterone levels may rise.

4.2 Posology and method of administration

Initiation of therapy: is most conveniently carried out in hospital; 0.5 ml Suprefact injection should be injected subcutaneously at 8 hourly intervals for 7 days.

Maintenance therapy: on the 8th day of treatment the patient is changed to intranasal administration of Suprefact. One spray dose is introduced into each nostril 6 times a day according to the following schedule:

1st dose before breakfast

2nd dose after breakfast

3rd and 4th doses before and after midday meal

5th and 6th doses before and after evening meal.

This dosage regimen is to ensure adequate absorption of the material and to distribute the dose throughout the day.

If used correctly, reliable absorption of the active ingredient takes place via nasal mucous membranes. Suprefact nasal spray is absorbed even if the patient has a cold.

If nasal decongestants are being used concurrently, they should be administered at least 30 minutes after buserelin.

4.3 Contraindications

Suprefact should not be used if the tumour is found to be insensitive to hormone manipulation or after surgical removal of the testes. It should not be used in pregnancy. It is contra-indicated in cases of known hypersensitivity to benzalkonium chloride or buserelin.

4.4 Special warnings and special precautions for use

Patients known to suffer from depression should be carefully monitored during treatment with Suprefact.

Monitoring of the clinical effect of Suprefact is carried out by the methods generally used in prostatic carcinoma. Initially serum testosterone levels rise and a clinical effect will not be seen until levels start to fall into the therapeutic (castration) range. Disease flare (temporary deterioration of patient's condition) has been reported at the beginning of treatment. The incidence is variable, but of the order of 10%. Symptoms are usually confined to transient increase in pain, but the exact nature depends on the site of the lesions. Neurological sequelae have been reported where secondary deposits impinge upon the spinal cord or CNS. Disease flare is prevented by the prophylactic use of an anti-androgen, e.g. cyproterone acetate, 300 mg daily. It is recommended that treatment should be started at least 3 days before the first dose of Suprefact and continued for at least 3 weeks after commencement of Suprefact therapy.

Once testosterone levels have started to fall below their baseline concentration clinical improvement should start to become apparent. If testosterone levels do not reach the therapeutic range within 4 weeks (6 weeks at the latest) the dose schedule should be checked to be sure that it is being followed exactly. It is unlikely that a patient who is taking the full dose will not show a suppression of testosterone to the therapeutic range. If this is the case, alternative therapy should be considered.

After the initial determination, testosterone levels should be monitored at 3–monthly intervals. A proportion of patients will have tumours that are not sensitive to hormone manipulation. Absence of clinical improvement in the face of adequate testosterone suppression is diagnostic of this condition, which will not benefit from further therapy with buserelin.

In patients with hypertension, blood pressure must be monitored regularly.

In diabetic patients blood glucose levels must be checked regularly.

4.5 Interaction with other medicinal products and other forms of Interaction

During treatment with Suprefact, the effect of antidiabetic agents may be attenuated.

4.6 Pregnancy and lactation

Not applicable.

4.7 Effects on ability to drive and use machines

Certain adverse effects (eg dizziness) may impair the ability to concentrate and react, and therefore constitute a risk in situations where these abilities are of special importance (eg operating a vehicle or machinery).

4.8 Undesirable effects

At the beginning of treatment, a transient rise in the serum testosterone level usually develops and may lead to temporary activation of the tumour with secondary reactions such as:

- occurence or exacerbation of bone pain in patients with metastases.
- signs of neurological deficit due to tumour compression with eg. muscle weakness in the legs.
- impaired micturition, hydronephrosis or lymphostasis.
- thrombosis with pulmonary embolism.

Such reactions can be largely avoided when an anti-androgen is given concomitantly in the initial phase of buserelin treatment (see Precautions and Warnings). However, even with concomitant anti-androgen therapy, a mild but transient increase in tumour pain as well as a deterioration in general well-being may develop in some patients.

Additionally, in most patients, hot flushes and loss of potency or libido (result of hormone deprivation); painless gynaecomastia (occasionally) as well as mild oedemas of the ankles and lower legs may occur.

Very rare cases of pituitary adenomas were reported during treatment with LHRH agonists, including buserelin.

Suprefact treatment may also lead to:

- changes in scalp or body hair (increase or decrease);
- deterioration in blood pressure levels in patients with hypertension
- hypersensitivity reactions. These may become manifest as, eg. reddening of the skin, itching, skin rashes (including urticaria) and allergic asthma with dyspnoea as well as, in isolated cases leading to anaphylactic/anaphylactoid shock.
- reduction in glucose tolerance. This may in diabetic patients, lead to a deterioration of metabolic control.
- changes in blood lipids, increase in serum levels of liver enzymes (eg. transaminases) increase in bilirubin, thrombopenia and leucopenia.
- headaches, palpitations, nervousness, sleep disturbances, tiredness, drowsiness, disturbances of memory and concentration, emotional instability, feelings of anxiety. In rare cases, depression may develop or existing depression worsen
- dizziness, tinnitus, hearing disorders, impaired vision (eg. blurred vision), feeling of pressure behind the eyes.
- nausea, vomiting, increased thirst, diarrhoea, constipation, changes in appetite, weight changes (increase or decrease).
- Paraesthesia, musculoskeletal discomfort and pain.

Administration of the nasal spray, may irritate the mucosa in the nasopharynx. This may lead to nosebleeds and hoarseness as well as to disturbances of taste and smell.

4.9 Overdose

Overdose may lead to signs and symptoms such as asthenia, headache, nervousness, hot flushes, dizziness, nausea, abdominal pain, oedemas of the lower extremities, and mastodynia. Treatment should be symptomatic.

5. PHARMACOLOGICAL PROPERTIES

5.1 Pharmacodynamic properties

Buserelin is a synthetic peptide. It is a superactive analogue of natural gonadotrophin releasing hormone (gonadorelin, LHRH or GNRH). After an initial stimulation of gonadotrophin release, it down-regulates the hypothalamic-pituitary-gonadal axis.

5.2 Pharmacokinetic properties

The intra-nasal absorption rate of buserelin is about 3%. Metabolic inactivation by peptidases occurs in the liver and kidney. The drug is also inactivated by pituitary membrane enzymes. After intra-nasal administration to humans, buserelin is excreted for more than 8 hours in the urine. Virtually all the serum fraction, and half the urine fraction of buserelin, are present as the parent drug.

The bioavailability of buserelin after nasal administration is not adversely influenced by the presence of rhinitis.

5.3 Preclinical safety data

None stated

6. PHARMACEUTICAL PARTICULARS

6.1 List of excipients

Sodium Chloride

Citric Acid Monohydrate

Sodium Citrate Dihydrate

Benzalkonium Chloride

Water for Injections

6.2 Incompatibilities

Not applicable.

6.3 Shelf life

2½ years.

6.4 Special precautions for storage

Store below 25°C. The spray solution should last for 1 week of treatment. Any residual material after this time should be discarded.

6.5 Nature and contents of container

Box of 4 bottles each containing 10g solution and 4 spray pumps

6.6 Instructions for use and handling

How to use the spray bottle.

1. Remove spray cap from bottle.
2. Remove metered dose nebulizer from transparent plastic container and take off both protective caps.
3. Screw nebuliser on to bottle.
4. Before first application only, pump 5-8 times, holding bottle vertical, until the solution has filled the system and a uniform spray is emitted. The preliminary pumping is for the purpose of filling the system and testing the spray. It must not be repeated after the first use, in order to avoid wasting the contents.
5. Keeping the bottle vertical and bending head over it slightly, spray solution into nose. If necessary the nose should be cleaned before applying the solution.
6. After use leave nebulizer on bottle. After replacing protective cap, spray bottle is best stored in its transparent container in an upright position.

7. MARKETING AUTHORISATION HOLDER

Aventis Pharma Ltd

50 Kings Hill Avenue

Kings Hill

West Malling

Kent

ME19 4AH

8. MARKETING AUTHORISATION NUMBER(S)

PL 04425/0279

9. DATE OF FIRST AUTHORISATION/RENEWAL OF THE AUTHORISATION

24 June 2002

10. DATE OF REVISION OF THE TEXT

13 February 2004

Legal category: POM

Surgam 300mg

(sanofi-aventis)

1. NAME OF THE MEDICINAL PRODUCT

Surgam Tablets 300 mg.

2. QUALITATIVE AND QUANTITATIVE COMPOSITION

Each tablet contains 300 mg Tiaprofenic Acid.

3. PHARMACEUTICAL FORM

Tablets

4. CLINICAL PARTICULARS

4.1 Therapeutic indications

Rheumatoid arthritis, osteoarthritis, ankylosing spondylitis, low back pain, musculo-skeletal disorders such as fibrositis, capsulitis, epicondylitis and other soft-tissue inflammatory conditions, sprains and strains, post-operative inflammation and pain and other soft tissue injuries.

4.2 Posology and method of administration

For oral administration.

To be swallowed whole.

Adults:

600 mg daily in divided doses

300 mg twice a day

Alternatively 200 mg three times a day

Elderly:

As for adults (see Section 4.4, Special Warnings and Precautions). NSAIDs should be used with particular caution in older patients who generally are more prone to adverse reactions.

In cases of renal, cardiac or hepatic impairment, the dosage should be kept as low as possible. It is suggested that in such cases, the dosage be reduced to 200 mg twice daily.

Elderly patients should receive the lowest dose and be monitored for gastrointestinal bleeding for 4 weeks following initiation of NSAID therapy

Children:

There are insufficient data to recommend use of Surgam in children.

4.3 Contraindications

- Active gastroduodenal ulceration or history of gastroduodenal ulceration.
- Active bladder or prostatic disease or symptoms.
- History of recurrent urinary tract disorders.

- Hypersensitivity to tiaprofenic acid and to any of the ingredients in the drug.
- History of asthma, rhinitis or urticaria whether or not induced by aspirin and other NSAIDs.
- Pregnancy (see Section 4.6, Pregnancy and Lactation)
- Severe renal or hepatic insufficiency.

4.4 Special warnings and special precautions for use

Undesirable effects may be reduced by using the minimum effective dose for the shortest possible duration. Patients treated with NSAIDs long-term should undergo regular medical supervision to monitor for adverse events.

As with other NSAIDs, Surgam should be used with care in the elderly, patients with a history of gastrointestinal disease and in patients with renal, cardiac or hepatic insufficiency as the use of these drugs may result in the deterioration of renal function. The dose should be kept as low as possible and renal function should be monitored. Renal function should also be monitored in patients on diuretics. Tiaprofenic acid should be used with caution in patients with a history of heart failure or with arterial hypertension.

Tiaprofenic acid can cause cystitis which may become severe if the treatment is continued after the onset of urinary symptoms. If urinary symptoms such as frequency, urgency, dysuria, nocturia or haematuria occur, tiaprofenic acid should be stopped immediately and urinalysis and urine culture performed. Patients should be warned about the onset of urinary symptoms which may suggest cystitis and are advised to stop taking the drug and seek medical advice if these occur.

Because of the risk of serious gastrointestinal side effects, especially in patients on anticoagulant treatment, special attention should be paid to the appearance of any gastrointestinal symptoms; treatment should be stopped immediately in the event of gastrointestinal haemorrhage.

There is a risk of cross-sensitivity among aspirin and NSAIDs, including the group to which tiaprofenic acid belongs. These pseudo-allergic reactions may include rash, urticaria and angioedema or more potentially severe manifestations (e.g. laryngeal oedema, bronchoconstriction and shock). The risk of pseudo-allergic reactions is greater in patients with recurrent rhino-sinusitis, nasal polyposis or chronic urticaria. Asthmatic patients are particularly at risk of dangerous reactions. Therefore tiaprofenic acid must not be administered to patients with a history of asthma.

As NSAIDs can interfere with platelet function, they should be used with caution in patients with intracranial haemorrhage and bleeding diathesis.

4.5 Interaction with other medicinal products and other forms of Interaction

Since Surgam is highly protein-bound, it is not recommended for co-administration with other highly protein-bound drugs such as heparin. Modification of the dosage may be necessary with hypoglycaemic agents, phenytoin and diuretics. With oral hypoglycaemic agents, an inhibition of metabolism of sulphonylurea drugs, prolonged half-life and increased risk of hypoglycaemia has been reported. It is considered unsafe to take NSAIDs in combination with warfarin or heparin unless under direct medical supervision.

Concomitant use of Surgam with corticosteroids and other NSAIDs (including high-dose salicylates) should be avoided due to an increased risk of gastrointestinal disorders such as bleeding.

Caution should be exercised when Surgam is administered with cardiac glycosides and sulphonamides. With cardiac glycosides, NSAIDs may exacerbate cardiac failure, reduce GFR and increase plasma cardiac glycoside levels.

Concomitant use of Surgam with methotrexate causes a decreased elimination of methotrexate. Concomitant use with high dose methotrexate should be avoided. Use with caution with low dose methotrexate.

NSAIDs have been reported to increase steady state plasma levels of lithium and it is, therefore, recommended that these levels are monitored in patients receiving Surgam therapy.

The use of aspirin and other NSAIDs should be avoided for at least 8-12 days after mifepristone.

NSAIDs may cause some sodium and fluid retention and may interfere with the natriuretic action of diuretic agents and reduce the effect of these. Diuretics can increase the risk of nephrotoxicity of NSAIDs.

NSAIDs also interact with antihypertensive drugs (e.g. beta-blockers, ACE inhibitors and anti-angiotensin II receptor antagonists) and cause an increased risk of renal impairment and an increased risk of hyperkalaemia. This should be borne in mind in patients with incipient or actual congestive heart failure and/or hypertension.

The risk of nephrotoxicity may be increased if NSAIDs are given with cyclosporins. Convulsions may occur due to an interaction with quinolone antibiotics.

Care should also be taken if Surgam is concomitantly administered with aminoglycosides or probenecid. Aminoglycosides may interact with NSAIDs to cause a reduction in renal function in susceptible individuals, decreased elimination of aminoglycoside and increased plasma concentrations. A reduction in metabolism and elimination of NSAID and metabolites has been observed with probenecid.

4.6 Pregnancy and lactation

Pregnancy: Tiaprofenic acid crosses the placental barrier. Although animal studies have not revealed evidence of teratogenicity, safety in human pregnancy and lactation cannot be assumed and, in common with other NSAIDs, administration during the first trimester should be avoided. In view of the known effects of NSAIDs on the foetal cardiovascular system (a closure of ductus arteriosus), use in late pregnancy should be avoided.

Lactation: The level of Surgam in mother's milk has been studied and the total daily exposure is very small; approximately 0.2% of the administered dose and is unlikely to be of pharmacological significance. Breast feeding or treatment of the mother should be stopped as necessary.

4.7 Effects on ability to drive and use machines

None known.

4.8 Undesirable effects

Gastrointestinal Tract:

Reported reactions include dyspepsia, nausea, vomiting, abdominal pain, anorexia, indigestion, heartburn, constipation, gastritis, flatulence and diarrhoea. In common with other NSAIDs, gastroduodenal ulcers, perforation and overt or occult gastrointestinal haemorrhage resulting in anaemia have occasionally been reported and in exceptional case may have been associated with fatalities.

Muco-cutaneous:

Rash, urticaria, pruritus, purpura, alopecia and very rarely erythema multiforme and bullous eruptions (Stevens Johnson Syndrome or, exceptionally, toxic epidermal necrolysis) have been reported.Very rarely photosensitivity reactions and aphthous stomatitis.

Hypersensitivity Reactions:

Non-specific allergic reactions, asthmatic attacks, especially in subjects allergic to aspirin and other NSAIDs, bronchospasm, dyspnoea, angio-oedema. Anaphylactic shock has also been reported.

Haemotological:

Thrombocytopenia, prolongation of bleeding time may occur.

Nervous system:

Headaches, dizziness, tinnitus and drowsiness.

Urinary System:

Bladder pain, dysuria, frequency and cystitis have been reported with tiaprofenic acid and other NSAIDs. On the basis of spontaneous reports, tiaprofenic acid appears to have a greater propensity than other NSAIDs to cause urinary disorders. Although generally reversible, in some cases where tiaprofenic acid has continued after the onset of urinary symptoms and an association with tiaprofenic acid not recognised, serious consequences requiring surgical intervention have resulted. Therefore, treatment with tiaprofenic acid should be discontinued immediately if urinary disorders develop.

Renal:

Sodium and water retention (see Section 4.4, Special Warnings and Precautions).

NSAIDs have been reported to cause nephrotoxicity in various forms. As with other NSAIDs, isolated cases of acute interstitial nephritis, nephrotic syndrome and renal failure have also been reported with tiaprofenic acid.

Hepatic:

Liver test abnormalities, hepatitis, jaundice.

Other side-effects that have been reported with NSAIDS but not specifically with Surgam are:

Neurological & special senses – Visual disturbances, optic neuritis, paraesthesia, depression, confusion, hallucinations, vertigo, malaise, fatigue.

Haematological – Neutropenia, agranulocytosis, aplastic anaemia, haemolytic anaemia.

4.9 Overdose

In the event of overdosage with Surgam, supportive and symptomatic therapy is indicated.

5. PHARMACOLOGICAL PROPERTIES

5.1 Pharmacodynamic properties

Non-steroidal anti-inflammatory drug.

Further Information:

The effects of tiaprofenic acid on articular cartilage have been investigated in *in vitro* experiments and in *ex vivo* studies using different animal models of arthritis. *Ex vivo* experiments on human chondrocyte cultures have also been conducted. In these experiments, tiaprofenic acid, in concentrations equivalent to the therapeutic dose, did not depress the biosynthesis of proteoglycans and did not alter the differentiation of proteoglycans secreted. The degradation of proteoglycan aggregates was inhibited. These results suggest a neutral or possibly beneficial effect of tiaprofenic acid on joint cartilage under experimental conditions. The clinical significance of these findings has been studied in a long term double-blind controlled study, in which tiaprofenic acid did not significantly increase the rate of radiological deterioration of joint space in patients with osteoarthritis of the knee.

5.2 Pharmacokinetic properties

Single dose studies: Following oral administration (max. at 90 mins). Plasma level zero at 24 hours. $t\frac{1}{2}$ = 1.5 to 2 hours.

Repeat dose studies: Surgam is rapidly eliminated and there is no accumulation after repeated doses of 600mg/day in divided doses. Steady state after first day. No impairment of absorption in patients with RA undergoing long term therapy. There is no evidence of different pharmacokinetics in the elderly.

Protein Binding = 97 - 98%

Plasma clearance = 6 litres/hour

Elimination = 60% of urine remainder in bile

Metabolites = there two main metabolites which account for about 10% of urinary excretion and have low pharmacological activity. The parent compound is excreted mostly in the form of acylglucuronide.

5.3 Preclinical safety data

Not applicable

6. PHARMACEUTICAL PARTICULARS

6.1 List of excipients

Maize starch, pluronic F68, magnesium stearate and talc.

6.2 Incompatibilities

None known

6.3 Shelf life

60 months

6.4 Special precautions for storage

Store below 25°C. Protect from light.

6.5 Nature and contents of container

Polyethylene bottles with screw cap, amber glass bottles with polyethylene caps or blister packs sealed with aluminium foil in a cardboard carton in packs of 10, 12, 14, 20, 28, 30, 56 or 60.

6.6 Instructions for use and handling

Not applicable.

7. MARKETING AUTHORISATION HOLDER

Aventis Pharma Ltd
50 Kings Hill Avenue
Kings Hill
West Malling
Kent ME19 4AH
United Kingdom

8. MARKETING AUTHORISATION NUMBER(S)

PL 04425/0318

9. DATE OF FIRST AUTHORISATION/RENEWAL OF THE AUTHORISATION

31 March 2003

10. DATE OF REVISION OF THE TEXT

Surgam SA

(sanofi-aventis)

1. NAME OF THE MEDICINAL PRODUCT

Surgam SA Capsule

2. QUALITATIVE AND QUANTITATIVE COMPOSITION

Each capsule contains 300 mg tiaprofenic acid.

3. PHARMACEUTICAL FORM

Capsules containing a pellet formulation providing sustained release.

4. CLINICAL PARTICULARS

4.1 Therapeutic indications

Rheumatoid arthritis, osteoarthritis, ankylosing spondylitis, low back pain, musculo-skeletal disorders such as fibrositis, capsulitis, epicondylitis and other soft-tissue inflammatory conditions, sprains and strains, post-operative inflammation and pain and other soft tissue injuries.

4.2 Posology and method of administration

For oral administration. Capsules to be swallowed whole.

Adults:

Two capsules (600 mg tiaprofenic acid) once daily.

Elderly:

As for adults (see Section 4.4 Special Warnings and Precautions). NSAIDs should be used with particular caution in older patients who generally are more prone to adverse reactions.

In cases of renal, cardiac or hepatic impairment, the dosage should be kept as low as possible. It is suggested that in such cases, the dosage be reduced to 200 mg twice daily.

Elderly patients should receive the lowest dose and be monitored for gastrointestinal bleeding for 4 weeks following initiation of NSAID therapy

Children

There are insufficient data to recommend use of Surgam in children.

4.3 Contraindications

- Active gastroduodenal ulceration or history of gastroduodenal ulceration.

- Active bladder or prostatic disease or symptoms.
- History of recurrent urinary tract disorders.
- Hypersensitivity to tiaprofenic acid and to any of the ingredients in the drug.
- History of asthma, rhinitis or urticaria whether or not induced by aspirin and other NSAIDs.
- Pregnancy (see Section 4.6, Pregnancy and Lactation)
- Severe renal or hepatic insufficiency.

4.4 Special warnings and special precautions for use

Undesirable effects may be reduced by using the minimum effective dose for the shortest possible duration. Patients treated with NSAIDs long-term should undergo regular medical supervision to monitor for adverse events.

As with other NSAIDs, Surgam should be used with care in the elderly, patients with a history of gastrointestinal disease and in patients with renal, cardiac or hepatic insufficiency as the use of these drugs may result in the deterioration of renal function. The dose should be kept as low as possible and renal function should be monitored. Renal function should also be monitored in patients on diuretics. Tiaprofenic acid should be used with caution in patients with a history of heart failure or with arterial hypertension.

Tiaprofenic acid can cause cystitis which may become severe if the treatment is continued after the onset of urinary symptoms. If urinary symptoms such as frequency, urgency, dysuria, nocturia or haematuria occur, tiaprofenic acid should be stopped immediately and urinalysis and urine culture performed. Patients should be warned about the onset of urinary symptoms which may suggest cystitis and are advised to stop taking the drug and seek medical advice if these occur.

Because of the risk of serious gastrointestinal side effects, especially in patients on anticoagulant treatment, special attention should be paid to the appearance of any gastrointestinal symptoms; treatment should be stopped immediately in the event of gastrointestinal haemorrhage.

As NSAIDs can interfere with platelet function, they should be used with caution in patients with intracranial haemorrhage and bleeding diathesis.

There is a risk of cross-sensitivity among aspirin and NSAIDs, including the group to which tiaprofenic acid belongs. These pseudo-allergic reactions may include rash, urticaria and angioedema or more potentially severe manifestations (e.g. laryngeal oedema, bronchoconstriction and shock). The risk of pseudo-allergic reactions is greater in patients with recurrent rhino-sinusitis, nasal polyposis or chronic urticaria. Asthmatic patients are particularly at risk of dangerous reactions. Therefore tiaprofenic acid must not be administered to patients with a history of asthma.

4.5 Interaction with other medicinal products and other forms of Interaction

Since Surgam is highly protein-bound, it is not recommended for co-administration with other highly protein-bound drugs. Modification of the dosage may be necessary with hypoglycaemic agents, phenytoin and diuretics. With oral hypoglycaemic agents, an inhibition of metabolism of sulphonylurea drugs, prolonged half-life and increased risk of hypoglycaemia has been reported. It is considered unsafe to take NSAIDs in combination with warfarin or heparin unless under direct medical supervision.

Concomitant use of Surgam with corticosteroids and other NSAIDs (including high-dose salicylates) should be avoided due to an increased risk of gastrointestinal disorders such as bleeding.

Caution should be exercised when Surgam is administered with cardiac glycosides and sulphonamides. With cardiac glycosides, NSAIDs may exacerbate cardiac failure, reduce GFR and increase plasma cardiac glycoside levels.

Concomitant use of Surgam with methotrexate causes a decreased elimination of methotrexate. Concomitant use with high dose methotrexate should be avoided. Use with caution with low dose methotrexate.

NSAIDs have been reported to increase steady state plasma levels of lithium and it is, therefore, recommended that these levels are monitored in patients receiving Surgam therapy.

The use of aspirin and other NSAIDs should be avoided for at least 8-12 days after mifepristone.

NSAIDs may cause some sodium and fluid retention and may interfere with the natriuretic action of diuretic agents and reduce the effect of these. Diuretics can increase the risk of nephrotoxicity of NSAIDs.

NSAIDs also interact with antihypertensive drugs (e.g. beta-blockers, ACE inhibitors and anti-angiotensin II receptor antagonists) and cause an increased risk of renal impairment and an increased risk of hyperkalaemia. This should be borne in mind in patients with incipient or actual congestive heart failure and/or hypertension.

The risk of nephrotoxicity may be increased if NSAIDs are given with cyclosporins. Convulsions may occur due to an interaction with quinolone antibiotics.

Care should also be taken if Surgam is concomitantly administered with aminoglycosides or probenecid. Aminoglycosides may interact with NSAIDs to cause a reduction in renal function in susceptible individuals, decreased elimination of aminoglycoside and increased plasma concentrations. A reduction in metabolism and elimination of NSAID and metabolites has been observed with probenecid.

4.6 Pregnancy and lactation

Pregnancy: Tiaprofenic acid crosses the placental barrier. Although animal studies have not revealed evidence of teratogenicity, safety in human pregnancy and lactation cannot be assumed and, in common with other NSAIDs, administration during the first trimester should be avoided. In view of the known effects of NSAIDs on the foetal cardiovascular system (a closure of ductus arteriosus), use in late pregnancy should be avoided.

Lactation: The level of Surgam in mother's milk has been studied and the total daily exposure is very small, approximately 0.2% of the administered dose, and is unlikely to be of pharmacological significance. Breast feeding or treatment of the mother should be stopped as necessary.

4.7 Effects on ability to drive and use machines

None known.

4.8 Undesirable effects

Gastrointestinal Tract:

Reported reactions include dyspepsia, nausea, vomiting, abdominal pain, anorexia, indigestion, heartburn, constipation, gastritis, flatulence and diarrhoea. In common with other NSAIDs, gastroduodenal ulcers, perforation and overt or occult gastrointestinal haemorrhage resulting in anaemia have occasionally been reported and in exceptional case may have been associated with fatalities.

Muco-cutaneous:

Rash, urticaria, pruritus, purpura, alopecia and very rarely erythema multiforme and bullous eruptions (Stevens Johnson Syndrome or, exceptionally, toxic epidermal necrolysis) have been reported.Very rarely photosensitivity reactions and aphthous stomatitis.

Hypersensitivity Reactions:

Non-specific allergic reactions, asthmatic attacks, especially in subjects allergic to aspirin and other NSAIDs, bronchospasm, dyspnoea, angio-oedema, anaphylactic shock has also been reported.

Haemotological:

Thrombocytopenia, prolongation of bleeding time may occur.

Nervous system:

Headaches, dizziness, tinnitus and drowsiness.

Urinary System:

Bladder pain, dysuria, frequency and cystitis have been reported with tiaprofenic acid and other NSAIDs. On the basis of spontaneous reports, tiaprofenic acid appears to have a greater propensity than other NSAIDs to cause urinary disorders. Although generally reversible, in some cases where tiaprofenic acid has continued after the onset of urinary symptoms and an association with tiaprofenic acid not recognised, serious consequences requiring surgical intervention have resulted. Therefore, treatment with tiaprofenic acid should be discontinued immediately if urinary disorders develop

Renal:

Sodium and water retention (see Section 4.4, Special Warnings and Precautions).

NSAIDs have been reported to cause nephrotoxicity in various forms. As with other NSAIDs, isolated cases of acute interstitial nephritis, nephrotic syndrome and renal failure have also been reported with tiaprofenic acid.

Hepatic:

Liver test abnormalities, hepatitis, jaundice.

Other side-effects that have been reported with NSAIDS but not specifically with Surgam are:

Neurological & special senses – Visual disturbances, optic neuritis, paraesthesia, depression, confusion, hallucinations, vertigo, malaise, fatigue.

Haematological – Neutropenia, agranulocytosis, aplastic anaemia, haemolytic anaemia.

4.9 Overdose

In the event of overdosage with Surgam, supportive and symptomatic therapy is indicated.

5. PHARMACOLOGICAL PROPERTIES

5.1 Pharmacodynamic properties

Tiaprofenic acid is a propionic acid derivative having anti-inflammatory and analgesic properties.

5.2 Pharmacokinetic properties

Surgam SA (600mg) gives a Cmax of 28.1mg/l which is not significantly different from 300mg conventional Surgam (37.3mg/l).

The plasma concentration remains above 10mg/l for 6-8 hours, against 2 to 3 hours with the conventional tablet.

Despite these differences in profile, there was no significant difference in the amount of Tiaprofenic acid absorbed as measured by areas under the plasma concentration curve and quantities eliminated in the urine.

5.3 Preclinical safety data

Not applicable

6. PHARMACEUTICAL PARTICULARS

6.1 List of excipients

Pellets

Glyceryl monostearate

Microcrystalline Cellulose

Purified Talc

Capsule Shell - CAP

Erythrosine E127

Titanium Dioxide E171

Indigo carmine E132

Capsule Shell - BODY

Erythrosine E127

Indigo carmine E132

Gelatin

6.2 Incompatibilities

None known

6.3 Shelf life

60 months from date of manufacture.

6.4 Special precautions for storage

Store below 25°C in a dry place and protect from light.

6.5 Nature and contents of container

Blister packs of 8, 20 or 56 capsules manufactured from 250 μm PVC/20 μm aluminium foil.

Polyethylene bottle with screw-neck fitted with a polyethylene cap. Contains a pack size of 60 capsules.

6.6 Instructions for use and handling

Not applicable.

7. MARKETING AUTHORISATION HOLDER

Aventis Pharma Ltd

Aventis House

50 Kings Hill Avenue

Kings Hill

West Malling

Kent ME19 4AH

United Kingdom

8. MARKETING AUTHORISATION NUMBER(S)

04425/0304

9. DATE OF FIRST AUTHORISATION/RENEWAL OF THE AUTHORISATION

14 September 2002

10. DATE OF REVISION OF THE TEXT

Surmontil 10mg and 25mg Tablets

(sanofi-aventis)

1. NAME OF THE MEDICINAL PRODUCT

Surmontil 10mg Tablets

Surmontil 25mg Tablets

2. QUALITATIVE AND QUANTITATIVE COMPOSITION

In terms of the active ingredient (BAN rINN if appropriate)

Trimipramine Maleate EP 14 mg equivalent to 10 mg trimipramine per tablet

Trimipramine Maleate EP 34.9mg equivalent to 25 mg trimipramine per tablet

3. PHARMACEUTICAL FORM

Film-coated tablet

4. CLINICAL PARTICULARS

4.1 Therapeutic indications

Surmontil has a potent antidepressant action similar to that of other tricyclic antidepressants. It also possesses pronounced sedative action. It is, therefore, indicated in the treatment of depressive illness, especially where sleep disturbance, anxiety or agitation are presenting symptoms. Sleep disturbance is controlled within 24 hours and true antidepressant action follows within 7 to 10 days.

4.2 Posology and method of administration

Adults

For depression 50-75 mg/day initially increasing to 150-300 mg/day in divided doses or one dose at night. The maintenance dose is 75-150 mg/day.

Elderly

10-25 mg three times a day initially. The initial dose should be increased with caution under close supervision. Half the normal maintenance dose may be sufficient to produce a satisfactory clinical response.

Children

Not recommended.

Route of administration is oral.

4.3 Contraindications

Recent myocardial infarction. Any degree of heart block or other cardiac arrhythmias. Mania. Severe liver disease. During breast feeding.

4.4 Special warnings and special precautions for use

The elderly are particularly liable to experience adverse reactions, especially agitation, confusion and postural hypotension.

Avoid if possible in patients with narrow angle glaucoma, symptoms suggestive of prostatic hypertrophy and a history of epilepsy.

Patients posing a high suicidal risk require close initial supervision. Tricyclic antidepressants potentiate the central nervous depressant action of alcohol.

Anaesthetics given during tri/tetracyclic antidepressant therapy may increase the risk of arrhythmias and hypotension. If surgery is necessary, the anaesthetist should be informed that a patient is being so treated.

It may be advisable to monitor liver function in patients on long term treatment with Surmontil.

Patients with rare hereditary problems of galactose intolerance, the Lapp lactase deficiency or glucose-galactose malabsorption should not take this medicine.

4.5 Interaction with other medicinal products and other forms of Interaction

Trimipramine should not be given concurrently with, or within 2 weeks of cessation of, therapy with monoamine oxidase inhibitors. Trimipramine may decrease the antihypertensive effect of guanethidine, debrisoquine, bethanidine and possibly clonidone. It would be advisable to review all antihypertensive therapy during treatment with tricyclic antidepressants.

Trimipramine should not be given with sympathomimetic agents such as adrenaline, ephedrine, isoprenaline, noradrenaline, phenylephrine and phenylpropanolamine.

Barbiturates may increase the rate of metabolism.

Surmontil should be administered with care in patients receiving therapy for hyperthyrodism.

4.6 Pregnancy and lactation

Do not use in pregnancy especially during the first and last trimesters unless there are compelling reasons. There is no evidence from animal work that it is free from hazard.

Trimipramine is contraindicated during lactation.

4.7 Effects on ability to drive and use machines

Trimipramine may initially impair alertness. Patients should be warned of the possible hazard when driving or operating machinery.

4.8 Undesirable effects

Cardiac arrhythmias and severe hypotension are likely to occur with high dosage or in deliberate overdosage. They may also occur in patients with pre-existing heart disease taking normal dosage.

The following adverse effects, although not necessarily all reported with trimipramine, have occurred with other tricyclic antidepressants.

Atropine-like side effects including dry mouth, disturbance of accommodation, tachycardia, constipation and hesitancy of micturation are common early in treatment but usually lessen.

Other common adverse effects include drowsiness, sweating, postural hypotension, tremor and skin rashes. Interference with sexual function may occur.

Serious adverse effects are rare; the following have been reported: depression of bone marrow, including agranularcytosis, cholestatic jaundice, hypomania, convulsions and peripheral neuropathy. Psychotic manifestations including mania and paranoid delusions, may be exacerbated during treatment with tricyclic antidepressants. Withdrawal symptoms may occur on abrupt cessation of therapy and include insomnia, irritability and excessive perspiration.

Adverse effects such as withdrawal symptoms, respiratory depression and agitation have been reported in neonates whose mothers had taken trimipramine during the last trimester of pregnancy.

4.9 Overdose

Acute overdosage may be accompanied by hypotensive collapse, convulsions and coma. Provided coma is not present, gastric lavage should be carries out without delay even though some time may have passed since the drug was ingested. Patients in coma should have an endotracheal tube passed before gastric lavage is started. Absorption of trimipramine is slow but, as cardiac effects may appear soon after the drug is absorbed, a saline purge should be given. Electrocardiography monitoring is essential.

It is important to treat acidosis as soon as it appears with, for example, 20 ml per kg of M/6 sodium lactate injection by slow intravenous injection. Intubation is necessary and the patient should be ventilated before convulsions develop. Convulsions should be treated with diazepam administered intravenously.

Ventricular tachycardia or fibrillation should be treated by electrical defibrillation. If supraventricular tachycardia develops, pyridostigmine bromide 1 mg (adults) intravenously or propranolol 1mg (adults) should be administered at intervals as required.

Treatment should be continued for at least three days even if the patient appears to have recovered.

5. PHARMACOLOGICAL PROPERTIES

5.1 Pharmacodynamic properties

Trimipramine is a tricyclic antidepressant. It has marked sedative properties.

5.2 Pharmacokinetic properties

Trimipramine undergoes high first-pass hepatic clearance, with a mean value for bioavailability of about 41% after oral administration.

The absolute volume of distribution is 31 litres/kg and total metabolic clearance is 16 ml/min/kg.

Plasma protein binding of trimipramine is about 95%. The plasma elimination half-life is around 23 hours. Trimipramine is largely metabolised by demethylation prior to conjugation yielding a glucuronide.

5.3 Preclinical safety data

No additional pre-clinical data of relevance to the prescriber.

6. PHARMACEUTICAL PARTICULARS

6.1 List of excipients

Calcium Hydrogen Phosphate
Starch Potato
Magnesium Stearate
Talc
Coat
Opadry OY-L-28900 *

* Opadry OY-L-28900 contains: Lactose Monohydrate Hypromellose, Titanium Dioxide, Macrogol.

6.2 Incompatibilities

None known

6.3 Shelf life

60 months

6.4 Special precautions for storage

Protect from light

6.5 Nature and contents of container

Surmontil 10mg tablets; Cartons containing PVDC/coated UPVC/aluminium foil blister packs of 84 or 28 tablets.

Surmontil 25mg tablets; Cardboard cartons containing blisters of 84 or 28 tablets.

6.6 Instructions for use and handling

None stated.

7. MARKETING AUTHORISATION HOLDER

Aventis Pharma Limited

50 Kings Hill Avenue

Kings Hill

West Malling

Kent

ME19 4AH

United Kingdom

8. MARKETING AUTHORISATION NUMBER(S)

Surmontil 10mg tablets; PL 04425/0266

Surmontil 25mg tablets; PL 04425/0267

9. DATE OF FIRST AUTHORISATION/RENEWAL OF THE AUTHORISATION

13th July, 2001

10. DATE OF REVISION OF THE TEXT

February 2005

Legal Category: POM

Surmontil Capsules 50mg

(sanofi-aventis)

1. NAME OF THE MEDICINAL PRODUCT

Surmontil Capsules 50mg

Trimipramine 50mg Capsules

2. QUALITATIVE AND QUANTITATIVE COMPOSITION

In terms of the active ingredient (BAN rINN if appropriate)

Trimipramine Maleate EP 69.75 mg per capsule

3. PHARMACEUTICAL FORM

Capsule

4. CLINICAL PARTICULARS

4.1 Therapeutic indications

Surmontil has a potent antidepressant action similar to that of other tricyclic antidepressants. It also possesses pronounced sedative action. It is, therefore, indicated in the treatment of depressive illness, especially where sleep disturbance, anxiety or agitation are presenting symptoms. Sleep disturbance is controlled within 24 hours and true antidepressant action follows within 7 to 10 days.

4.2 Posology and method of administration

Adults

For depression 50-75 mg/day initially increasing to 150-300 mg/day in divided doses or one dose at night. The maintenance dose is 75-150 mg/day.

Elderly

10-25 mg three times a day initially. The initial dose should be increased with caution under close supervision. Half the normal maintenance dose may be sufficient to produce a satisfactory clinical response.

Children

Not recommended.

Route of administration is oral.

4.3 Contraindications

Recent myocardial infarction. Any degree of heart block or other cardiac arrhythmias. Mania. Severe liver disease. During breast feeding.

4.4 Special warnings and special precautions for use

The elderly are particularly liable to experience adverse reactions, especially agitation, confusion and postural hypotension.

Avoid if possible in patients with narrow angle glaucoma, symptoms suggestive of prostatic hypertrophy and a history of epilepsy.

Patients posing a high suicidal risk require close initial supervision. Tricyclic antidepressants potentiate the central nervous depressant action of alcohol.

Anaesthetics given during tri/tetracyclic antidepressant therapy may increase the risk of arrhythmias and hypotension. If surgery is necessary, the anaesthetist should be informed that a patient is being so treated.

It may be advisable to monitor liver function in patients on long term treatment with Surmontil.

4.5 Interaction with other medicinal products and other forms of Interaction

Trimipramine should not be given concurrently with, or within 2 weeks of cessation of, therapy with monoamine oxidase inhibitors. Trimipramine may decrease the antihypertensive effect of guanethidine, debrisoquine, bethanidine and possibly clonidone. It would be advisable to review all antihypertensive therapy during treatment with tricyclic antidepressants.

Trimipramine should not be given with sympathomimetic agents such as adrenaline, ephedrine, isoprenaline, noradrenaline, phenylephrine and phenylpropanolamine.

Barbiturates may increase the rate of metabolism. Surmontil should be administered with care in patients receiving therapy for hyperthyroidism.

4.6 Pregnancy and lactation

Do not use in pregnancy especially during the first and last trimesters unless there are compelling reasons. There is no evidence from animal work that it is free from hazard.

Trimipramine is contraindicated during lactation.

4.7 Effects on ability to drive and use machines

Trimipramine may initially impair alertness. Patients should be warned of the possible hazard when driving or operating machinery.

4.8 Undesirable effects

Cardiac arrhythmias and severe hypotension are likely to occur with high dosage or in deliberate overdosage. They may also occur in patients with pre-existing heart disease taking normal dosage.

The following adverse effects, although not necessarily all reported with trimipramine, have occurred with other tricyclic antidepressants.

Atropine-like side effects including dry mouth, disturbance of accommodation, tachycardia, constipation and hesitancy of micturition are common early in treatment but usually lessen.

Other common adverse effects include drowsiness, sweating, postural hypotension, tremor and skin rashes. Interference with sexual function may occur.

Serious adverse effects are rare. The following have been reported: depression of the bone marrow, including agranulocytosis, cholestatic jaundice, hypomania, convulsions and peripheral neuropathy. Psychotic manifestations including mania and paranoid delusions, may be exacerbated during treatment with tricyclic antidepressants.

Withdrawal symptoms may occur on abrupt cessation of therapy and include insomnia, irritability and excessive perspiration.

Adverse effects such as withdrawal symptoms, respiratory depression and agitation have been reported in neonates whose mothers had taken trimipramine during the last trimester of pregnancy.

4.9 Overdose

Acute overdosage may be accompanied by hypotensive collapse, convulsions and coma. Provided coma is not present, gastric lavage should be carries out without delay even though some time may have passed since the drug was ingested. Patients in coma should have an endotracheal tube passed before gastric lavage is started. Absorption of trimipramine is slow but, as cardiac effects may appear soon after the drug is absorbed, a saline purge should be given. Electrocardiography monitoring is essential.

It is important to treat acidosis as soon as it appears with, for example, 20 ml per kg of M/6 sodium lactate injection by slow intravenous injection. Intubation is necessary and the patient should be ventilated before convulsions develop. Convulsions should be treated with diazepam administered intravenously.

Ventricular tachycardia or fibrillation should be treated by electrical defibrillation. If supraventricular tachycardia develops, pyridostigmine bromide 1 mg (adults) intravenously or propranolol 1mg (adults) should be administered at intervals as required.

Treatment should be continued for at least three days even if the patient appears to have recovered.

5. PHARMACOLOGICAL PROPERTIES

5.1 Pharmacodynamic properties

Trimipramine is a tricyclic antidepressant. It has marked sedative properties.

5.2 Pharmacokinetic properties

Trimipramine undergoes high first-pass hepatic clearance, with a mean value for bioavailability of about 41% after oral administration.

The absolute volume of distribution is 31 litres/kg.

The metabolic clearance is 16 ml/min/kg.

Plasma protein binding of trimipramine is about 95%. The plasma elimination half-life is around 23 hours. Trimipramine is largely metabolised by demethylation prior to conjugation yielding a glucuronide.

5.3 Preclinical safety data

No additional pre-clinical data of relevance to the prescriber.

6. PHARMACEUTICAL PARTICULARS

6.1 List of excipients

Starch Maize	BP
Microcrystalline cellulose E460	BP
Magnesium stearate	BP
Colloidal Silicon dioxide	HSE

Capsule shell:

Titanium dioxide E171

Indigo Carmine E132

Iron Oxide Yellow E172

Gelatin BP/USNF

Ink Iron Oxide black E172

6.2 Incompatibilities

None known

6.3 Shelf life

36 months

6.4 Special precautions for storage

Store in a dry place below 25°C and protect from light.

6.5 Nature and contents of container

HDPE bottles or Securitainers of 50 capsules. Cartons containing PVC/aluminium blisters of 28.

6.6 Instructions for use and handling

None stated.

7. MARKETING AUTHORISATION HOLDER

Aventis Pharma Limited
50 Kings Hill Avenue
Kings Hill
West Malling
Kent, ME19 4AH, United Kingdom

8. MARKETING AUTHORISATION NUMBER(S)

PL 04425/0265

9. DATE OF FIRST AUTHORISATION/RENEWAL OF THE AUTHORISATION

13 July 2001

10. DATE OF REVISION OF THE TEXT

May 2002

11. LEGAL CLASSIFICATION

POM

Survanta

(Abbott Laboratories Limited)

1. NAME OF THE MEDICINAL PRODUCT

Survanta

2. QUALITATIVE AND QUANTITATIVE COMPOSITION

Each ml contains Beractant equivalent to:

Phospholipids 25 mg/ml

(including disaturated phosphatidylcholines 11.0 - 15.5 mg/ml)

Triglycerides 0.5 - 1.75 mg/ml

Free Fatty Acids 1.4 - 3.5 mg/ml

Protein 0.1 - 1.0 mg/ml

3. PHARMACEUTICAL FORM

Sterile suspension for intratracheal administration

4. CLINICAL PARTICULARS

4.1 Therapeutic indications

Survanta is indicated for treatment of Respiratory Distress Syndrome (RDS) (hyaline membrane disease) in new born premature infants with a birth weight of 700g or greater and who are intubated and are receiving mechanical ventilation.

Survanta is also indicated for the prophylactic treatment of premature infants <32 weeks gestational age at risk of developing RDS.

4.2 Posology and method of administration

Dosage In Infants

100 mg phosholipid/kg birth weight in a volume not exceeding 4ml/kg.

Treatment: Survanta should be administered early in the course of RDS, i.e. preferably less than 8 hours of age. Depending on clinical course, this dose may be repeated within 48 hours at intervals of at least six hours for up to 4 doses.

Prophylaxis: The first dose of Survanta should be administered as soon as possible after birth, preferably within 15 minutes. Depending on clinical course, this dose may be repeated within 48 hours at intervals of at least six hours for up to 4 doses.

Method of Administration:

Survanta should be administered by intratracheal administration (i.e. drug should be conducted into the lungs via an endotracheal tube) using a 5 Fr catheter. The tip of the catheter should lie at the end of the endotracheal tube. Infants should not be intubated solely for the administration of Survanta.

Survanta should be warmed to room temperature before administration (see Precautions).

Before administering Survanta to infants on mechanical ventilation, set the respiratory frequency at 60/minute - with inspiration time 0.5s and F_{I2} at 1.0. Inspiratory pressure needs no change at this point.

To ensure distribution of Survanta throughout the lungs, each dose is divided into fractional doses. Each dose can be administered as either two half-doses or four quarter-doses. Each fractional dose is administered with the infant in different positions as given below. Between each position the infant should be ventilated for 30 seconds.

For Four quarter-doses, the recommended positions are:

Right Lateral Position with the head lowered (i.e. head and body slanting down at an angle of approximately 15°).

Left Lateral Position with the head lowered (i.e. head and body slanting down at an angle of approximately 15°).

Right Lateral Position with head elevated (i.e. head and body slanting up at an angle of approximately 15°).

Left Lateral Position with head elevated (i.e. head and body slanting up at an angle of approximately 15°).

For administration of each quarter dose, the ventilator is disconnected, the catheter inserted, the dose administered then the ventilator reconnected. Between each quarter dose the infant is ventilated for 30 seconds.

For two half-doses, the recommended positions are:

With infant supine, the head and body turned approximately 45° to the right.

With infant supine, the head and body turned approximately 45° to the left.

When two half-doses of Survanta are being administered there are 2 alternative methods of administration:

Installation with disconnection from the ventilator

Each half dose is administered by disconnecting the endotracheal tube from the ventilator, inserting the catheter and administering the half dose. Between the half doses, the ventilator is reconnected for 30 seconds.

Alternatively,

Instillation without disconnection from the ventilator (through a suction port connector).

The first half dose is administered by inserting the catheter through a suction port connector without disconnection from the ventilator. There should be at least 30 seconds between the half doses during which time the catheter is retracted from the endotracheal tube but not removed from the connector. The catheter is then reinserted into the endotracheal tube and the second half dose administered. The catheter is then withdrawn completely.

Dosage in Adults

Not applicable.

Dosage in Elderly

Not applicable.

4.3 Contraindications

No specific contraindications for Survanta have been defined by the clinical studies.

4.4 Special warnings and special precautions for use

Survanta should only be administered with adequate facilities for ventilation and monitoring of babies with RDS.

Marked improvements in oxygenation may occur within minutes of the administration of Survanta. Therefore, frequent and careful monitoring of systemic oxygenation is essential to avoid hyperoxia. Following Survanta administration, monitoring of the arterial blood gases, the fraction of inspired oxygen and ventilatory change is required to ensure appropriate adjustments.

During the dosing procedure, transient episodes of bradycardia and/or oxygen desaturation have been reported. If these occur, dosing should be stopped and appropriate measures to alleviate the condition should be initiated. After stabilisation, the dosing procedure should be resumed.

Survanta is stored refrigerated (2-8°C). Before administration, Survanta should be warmed by standing at room temperature for 20 minutes or warmed in the hand for 8 minutes. ARTIFICIAL WARMING METHODS SHOULD NOT BE USED. Discard each vial if not used within 8 hours of rewarming to room temperature. Vials should not be returned to the refrigerator once warmed.

Each vial of Survanta is for single use only. Used vials with residual drug should be discarded.

Survanta should be inspected visually for discolouration prior to administration. The colour of Survanta is off-white to light brown. Some settling may occur during storage. If this occurs, gently invert the vial several times (DO NOT SHAKE) to redisperse.

4.5 Interaction with other medicinal products and other forms of Interaction

None known to date.

4.6 Pregnancy and lactation

Not applicable.

4.7 Effects on ability to drive and use machines

Not applicable.

4.8 Undesirable effects

Intracranial haemorrhage has been observed in patients who received either Survanta or placebo. The incidence of intracranial haemorrhage in all patients is similar to that reported in the literature in this patient population. Pulmonary haemorrhage has also been reported. No other serious adverse reactions have been reported. No antibody production to Survanta proteins has been observed. Blockage of the endotracheal tube by mucous secretions has been reported.

4.9 Overdose

If an excessively large dose of Survanta is given, observe the infant for signs of acute airway obstruction. Treatment should be symptomatic and supportive. Rales and moist breath sounds can transiently occur after Survanta is given, and do not indicate overdosage. Endotracheal suction or other remedial action is not required unless clear-cut signs of airway obstruction are present.

5. PHARMACOLOGICAL PROPERTIES

5.1 Pharmacodynamic properties

The mode of action of Survanta is biophysical rather than biochemical, i.e. it reduces surface tension and concomitantly increases lung compliance.

Intratracheally administered Survanta distributes rapidly to the alveolar surfaces and stabilises the alveoli against collapse during respiration thereby increasing alveolar ventilation.

In clinical studies of premature infants with Respiratory Distress Syndrome (RDS), a significant improvement in oxygenation was demonstrated after treatment with a single dose of Survanta.

These infants showed a decreased need for supplemental oxygen and an increase in the arterial/alveolar oxygen ratio (a/ApO_2). Significantly decreased need for respiratory support, as indicated by a lower mean airway pressure, was also observed. In most cases these effects were maintained for at least 72 hours after the administration of the single dose of Survanta.

5.2 Pharmacokinetic properties

In preclinical studies using radiolabelled phosphatidylcholine, the clearance rate of Survanta in the lung of three day old rabbits has been shown to be similar to that of natural calf and sheep surfactants (approximately 13% within 24 hours). In addition some re-uptake and secretion of Survanta was shown, implying its entry into a metabolically active surfactant pool.

Since an exogenous preparation of Survanta is delivered directly to the lung, classical clinical pharmocokinetic parameters (blood levels, plasma half-life etc.) have not been studied.

5.3 Preclinical safety data

There are no pre-clinical data of relevance to the prescriber which are additional to that already included in other sections of the SPC.

6. PHARMACEUTICAL PARTICULARS

6.1 List of excipients

Sodium chloride and water for injection.

6.2 Incompatibilities

None experienced to date, as product administration is unique.

6.3 Shelf life
18 months

6.4 Special precautions for storage
Store under refrigerated conditions (2-8°C) protected from light.

6.5 Nature and contents of container
21ml glass bottle with a 20mm rubber stopper and a 20mm aluminium seal finish containing 8ml of product.

Pack sizes: 1, 3 and 10

6.6 Instructions for use and handling
Do not freeze. Any inadvertently frozen product should be discarded.

Administrative Data

7. MARKETING AUTHORISATION HOLDER
Abbott Laboratories Limited

Queenborough

Kent

ME11 5EL

8. MARKETING AUTHORISATION NUMBER(S)
PL 0037 / 0218

9. DATE OF FIRST AUTHORISATION/RENEWAL OF THE AUTHORISATION
13th October 1998

10. DATE OF REVISION OF THE TEXT
August 2004

Suscard Buccal Tablets

(Forest Laboratories UK Limited)

1. NAME OF THE MEDICINAL PRODUCT
SUSCARD BUCCAL TABLETS 2MG

SUSCARD BUCCAL TABLETS 3MG

SUSCARD BUCCAL TABLETS 5MG

2. QUALITATIVE AND QUANTITATIVE COMPOSITION
Each tablet contains 2mg, 3mg or 5mg glyceryl trinitrate as Diluted Nitroglycerin USP.

3. PHARMACEUTICAL FORM
Prolonged release muco-adhesive buccal tablet.

4. CLINICAL PARTICULARS

4.1 Therapeutic indications
Management and treatment of angina pectoris. This product may also be of benefit in the in-patient management of unstable angina.

Acute and congestive cardiac failure.

4.2 Posology and method of administration
For buccal administration

Dosage

Adults and Elderly Patients:

Angina:

Administration of Suscard Tablets should start with the 2mg strength. If angina occurs while the tablet is in place, the dosage strength used should be increased to 3mg where necessary. The 5mg dosage strength should be reserved for patients with severe angina pectoris refractory to treatment with the lower dosage strengths.

Suggested dosage frequency in angina:

A) For patients suffering only occasional angina pectoris – the tablets may be administered on a p.r.n. basis to relieve the acute attack.

B) For patients suffering angina pectoris in response to known stimuli - the tablet may be administered a few minutes prior to encountering the angina-precipitating stimulus.

C) For patients in whom chronic therapy is indicated - the tablet should be administered on a thrice daily basis or as dictated by the dissolution rate of the tablet in an individual patient. If angina occurs during the period between the disappearance of one tablet and the time the next tablet is due to be put in place, dosage frequency should be increased.

Note that if an acute attack of angina pectoris is suffered while a tablet is in place, an additional tablet may be positioned on the opposite side of the mouth.

Unstable Angina:

Dosage should be rapidly titrated upwards in order to relieve and prevent symptoms. Suscard Tablets may be used in addition to pre-existing anti-anginal therapy, where considered appropriate.

As indicated in the above section the higher 5mg dosage strength may be required to achieve a satisfactory therapeutic response in patients exhibiting severe symptoms. Unstable angina is a serious condition managed under hospitalised conditions and involving continuous monitoring of ECG changes with frequent monitoring of appropriate haemodynamic variables. In common with other nitrate therapy a fall in systolic blood pressure, of 10-15mm hg may occur.

Acute heart failure:

Administer 5mg, repeated as indicated by the patient response until the symptoms abate.

Congestive cardiac failure:

Dosage should commence with the 5mg strength, administered three times daily. In moderately severe or severe cases, particularly where patients have not responded to standard therapy (digitalis/diuretics), the dosage may need to be increased to 10mg (2 × 5mg tablets) t.i.d. over a period of three or four days. In such instances one tablet should be placed between the upper lip and the gum, on each side of the front teeth.

Method of Administration

Suscard is for buccal administration. The Suscard tablet is placed high up between the upper lip and gum to either side of the front teeth.

The onset of action of Suscard tablets is extremely rapid and the tablets may be substituted for sublingual glyceryl trinitrate tablets in the treatment of acute angina pectoris. The duration of action of the Suscard Tablet, once in place correlates with the dissolution time of the tablet. This is normally 3-5 hours. However, the first few doses may dissolve more rapidly until the patient is used to the presence of the tablet.

During the dissolution period the tablet will soften and adhere to the gum; in practice the presence of the tablet is not noticeable to the patient after a short time.

Patients should be instructed as to the correct placement of the tablet and should note the following points

A) The tablet should not be moved about the mouth with the tongue, as this will cause it to dissolve more rapidly.

B) A slight stinging sensation (as for sublingual glyceryl trinitrate) may be felt for a few minutes after placement of the tablet.

C) If a tablet is accidentally swallowed it may be replaced by a further tablet.

D) In patients who wear dentures, the tablet may be placed in any comfortable position between the lip and the gum.

E) The patient may alternate the placement of successive tablets on the right and left sides of the front teeth.

The tablets should not be placed under the tongue, chewed or intentionally swallowed.

4.3 Contraindications
As for glyceryl trinitrate. Suscard Tablets should not be used in patients with marked anaemia, head trauma, cerebral haemorrhage or close angle glaucoma.

Sildenafil has been shown to potentiate the hypotensive effects of nitrates, and its co-administration with nitrates or nitric oxide donors is therefore contraindicated.

4.4 Special warnings and special precautions for use
Rarely, prolonged use in susceptible individuals with poor dental hygiene and associated plaque may lead to an increased risk of dental caries. Patients should, therefore be instructed to alternate the site of application and careful attention should be paid to dental hygiene, particularly in those areas where the tablet is applied. In conditions where xerostomia (dry mouth) may occur, e.g. during concomitant medication with drugs having anticholinergic effects, patients should be instructed to moisten the buccal mucosa with the tongue, or with a little water, prior to insertion of Suscard.

4.5 Interaction with other medicinal products and other forms of Interaction
The hypotensive effects of nitrates are potentiated by concurrent administration of sildenafil.

4.6 Pregnancy and lactation
There is no information on the safety of nitrates in pregnancy and lactation. Nitrates should not be administered to pregnant women and nursing mothers unless considered essential by the physician.

4.7 Effects on ability to drive and use machines
None known

4.8 Undesirable effects
Side effects are predominantly headache, dizziness, facial flushing and postural hypotension. In the unlikely event of severe side effects, the tablet may simply be removed from the mouth.

4.9 Overdose
Toxic effects of glyceryl trinitrate include vomiting, restlessness, cyanosis, methaemoglobinaemia and syncope. Overdosage (i.e. if large numbers of tablets have been swallowed) should be treated with gastric aspiration and lavage plus attention to the respiratory and circulatory systems.

5. PHARMACOLOGICAL PROPERTIES

5.1 Pharmacodynamic properties
The principal action of glyceryl trinitrate is relaxation of vascular smooth muscle producing a vasodilator effect on both peripheral arteries and veins. Dilation of the post-capillary vessels, including large veins, promotes peripheral pooling of blood and decreases venous return to the heart, thereby reducing left ventricular end-diastolic pressure (preload). Arteriolar relaxation reduces systemic vascular resistance and arterial pressure (afterload). Myocardial oxygen consumption or demand for a given level of exercise is decreased by both the arterial and venous effects of nitroglycerin. Dilatation of the large epicardial coronary arteries by nitroglycerin contributes to the relief of exertional angina.

5.2 Pharmacokinetic properties
Bioavailability:

relative to sublingual GTN 107%.

Mean plasma levels:

0.7ng/ml obtained with 5mg Buccal Tablet over 5 hours compared with 0.4ng/ml over 30 minutes with 0.4mg sublingual GTN.

Maximum plasma concentration:

1.7ng/ml following 5mg Buccal compared with 0.9ng/ml following 0.4mg sublingual GTN.

Time to maximum plasma concentration:

1.52 hours following Buccal GTN compared with 6 minutes following sublingual GTN.

Apparent elimination half-life:

1.30 hours for Buccal GTN compared with an elimination half-life of 5 minutes following sublingual GTN.

Pharmacodynamic studies have shown a dose-related response with a rapid onset equivalent to sublingual GTN together with a prolonged duration of activity of 4-5 hours.

5.3 Preclinical safety data
There are no preclinical data of relevance to the prescriber which are additional to that already included in other sections of the SPC.

6. PHARMACEUTICAL PARTICULARS

6.1 List of excipients
Lactose hydrous

Buccal Synchron consisting of: Hydroxypropyl methylcellulose

Purified Water

Peppermint flavour

Spearmint flavour

Stearic acid

Silica gel

6.2 Incompatibilities
None stated

6.3 Shelf life
3 years

6.4 Special precautions for storage
Do not store above 25°C

6.5 Nature and contents of container
Aluminium foil blister strips in cartons of 30, 50, 60, 90 and 100 tablets.

Professional sample pack size of 10 tablets.

6.6 Instructions for use and handling
None stated.

7. MARKETING AUTHORISATION HOLDER
Forest Laboratories UK Limited

Bourne Road

Bexley

Kent DA5 1NX

8. MARKETING AUTHORISATION NUMBER(S)
Suscard Buccal Tablets 2mg: 0108/0069

Suscard Buccal Tablets 3mg: 0108/0073

Suscard Buccal Tablets 5mg: 0108/0071

9. DATE OF FIRST AUTHORISATION/RENEWAL OF THE AUTHORISATION
Suscard Buccal Tablets 2mg, 5mg: 15 March 1982 / 26 June 1997

Suscard Buccal Tablets 3mg: 7 October 1982 / 26 November 1997

10. DATE OF REVISION OF THE TEXT
Suscard 2mg and 5mg tablets: June 1997

Suscard 3mg tablets: November 1997

11. Legal Category
P

Sustiva 30 mg/ml Oral Solution

(Bristol-Myers Squibb Pharmaceuticals Ltd)

1. NAME OF THE MEDICINAL PRODUCT
SUSTIVA 30 mg/ml oral solution

2. QUALITATIVE AND QUANTITATIVE COMPOSITION
Each millilitre contains 30 mg efavirenz

For excipients, see section 6.1.

3. PHARMACEUTICAL FORM
Oral solution

SUSTIVA 30 mg/ml oral solution is a colourless to slightly yellow clear liquid.

4. CLINICAL PARTICULARS

4.1 Therapeutic indications

SUSTIVA oral solution is indicated in antiviral combination treatment of HIV-1 infected adults, adolescents and children 3 years of age and older, who are unable to swallow the hard capsules.

SUSTIVA has not been adequately studied in patients with advanced HIV disease, namely in patients with CD4 counts < 50 cells/mm^3, or after failure of protease inhibitor (PI) containing regimens. Although cross-resistance of efavirenz with PIs has not been documented, there are at present insufficient data on the efficacy of subsequent use of PI based combination therapy after failure of regimens containing SUSTIVA.

For a summary of clinical and pharmacodynamic information, see section 5.1.

4.2 Posology and method of administration

Concomitant antiretroviral therapy: SUSTIVA must be given in combination with other antiretroviral medications (see section 4.5).

SUSTIVA may be taken with or without food (see section 5.2).

In order to improve the tolerability of nervous system undesirable effects, bedtime dosing is recommended during the first two to four weeks of therapy and in patients who continue to experience these symptoms (see section 4.8).

Therapy should be initiated by a physician experienced in the management of HIV infection.

Adults: the recommended dosage of SUSTIVA in combination with nucleoside analogue reverse transcriptase inhibitors (NRTIs) with or without a PI (see section 4.5) is 24 ml orally, once daily.

Adolescents and children (3 to 17 years): the recommended dose of SUSTIVA in combination with a PI and/or NRTIs for patients between 3 and 17 years of age is described in Table 1. SUSTIVA hard capsules must only be administered to children who are able to reliably swallow hard capsules. SUSTIVA has not been studied in children under the age of 3 years or children weighing less than 13 kg.

Table 1

Paediatric dose to be administered once daily

Body Weight kg	SUSTIVA oral solution (30 mg/ml) Dose (ml)	
	Children 3 - < 5 years	Adults and children aged 5 years or more
13 to < 15	12	9
15 to < 20	13	10
20 to < 25	15	12
25 to < 32.5	17	15
32.5 to < 40	-	17
⩾ 40	-	24

SUSTIVA oral solution is less bioavailable than the hard capsule on a mg per mg basis. The dose recommendations in Table 1 have been adjusted to take into account the difference in bioavailability (see section 5.2).

Renal insufficiency: the pharmacokinetics of efavirenz have not been studied in patients with renal insufficiency; however, less than 1% of an efavirenz dose is excreted unchanged in the urine, so the impact of renal impairment on efavirenz elimination should be minimal (see section 4.4).

Liver disease: patients with mild to moderate liver disease may be treated with their normally recommended dose of efavirenz. Patients should be monitored carefully for dose-related adverse events, especially nervous system symptoms (see sections 4.3 and 4.4).

4.3 Contraindications

SUSTIVA is contraindicated in patients with clinically significant hypersensitivity to the active substance or to any of the excipients.

Efavirenz must not be used in patients with severe hepatic impairment (Child Pugh Grade C) (see section 5.2).

Efavirenz must not be administered concurrently with terfenadine, astemizole, cisapride, midazolam, triazolam, pimozide, bepridil, or ergot alkaloids (for example, ergotamine, dihydroergotamine, ergonovine, and methylergonovine) because competition for CYP3A4 by efavirenz could result in inhibition of metabolism and create the potential for serious and/or life-threatening undesirable effects [for example, cardiac arrhythmias, prolonged sedation or respiratory depression] (see section 4.5).

Herbal preparations containing St. John's wort *(Hypericum perforatum)* must not be used while taking efavirenz due to the risk of decreased plasma concentrations and reduced clinical effects of efavirenz (see section 4.5).

SUSTIVA must not be administered concurrently with voriconazole because efavirenz significantly decreases voriconazole plasma concentrations while voriconazole also significantly increases efavirenz plasma concentrations (see section 4.5).

4.4 Special warnings and special precautions for use

Efavirenz must not be used as a single agent to treat HIV or added on as a sole agent to a failing regimen. As with all other non-nucleoside reverse transcriptase inhibitors (NNRTIs), resistant virus emerges rapidly when efavirenz is administered as monotherapy. The choice of new antiretroviral agent(s) to be used in combination with efavirenz should take into consideration the potential for viral cross-resistance (see section 5.1).

When prescribing medicinal products concomitantly with SUSTIVA, physicians should refer to the corresponding Summary of Product Characteristics.

Patients should be advised that current antiretroviral therapy, including efavirenz, has not been proven to prevent the risk of transmission of HIV to others through sexual contact or blood contamination. Appropriate precautions should continue to be employed.

If any antiretroviral medicinal product in a combination regimen is interrupted because of suspected intolerance, serious consideration should be given to simultaneous discontinuation of all antiretroviral medicinal products. The antiretroviral medicinal products should be restarted at the same time upon resolution of the intolerance symptoms. Intermittent monotherapy and sequential reintroduction of antiretroviral agents is not advisable because of the increased potential for selection of resistant virus.

Rash: mild-to-moderate rash has been reported in clinical studies with efavirenz and usually resolves with continued therapy. Appropriate antihistamines and/or corticosteroids may improve the tolerability and hasten the resolution of rash. Severe rash associated with blistering, moist desquamation or ulceration has been reported in less than 1% of patients treated with efavirenz. The incidence of erythema multiforme or Stevens-Johnson syndrome was approximately 0.1%. Efavirenz must be discontinued in patients developing severe rash associated with blistering, desquamation, mucosal involvement or fever. If therapy with efavirenz is discontinued, consideration should also be given to interrupting therapy with other antiretroviral agents to avoid development of resistant virus (see section 4.8).

Rash was reported in 26 of 57 children (46%) treated with efavirenz during a 48-week period and was severe in three patients. Prophylaxis with appropriate antihistamines prior to initiating therapy with efavirenz in children may be considered.

Patients who discontinued treatment with other NNRTIs due to rash may be at higher risk of developing rash during treatment with efavirenz.

Psychiatric symptoms: psychiatric adverse experiences have been reported in patients treated with efavirenz. Patients with a prior history of psychiatric disorders appear to be at greater risk of these serious psychiatric adverse experiences. In particular, severe depression was more common in those with a history of depression. There have also been post-marketing reports of severe depression, death by suicide, delusions and psychosis-like behaviour. Patients should be advised that if they experience symptoms such as severe depression, psychosis or suicidal ideation, they should contact their doctor immediately to assess the possibility that the symptoms may be related to the use of efavirenz, and if so, to determine whether the risks of continued therapy outweigh the benefits (see section 4.8).

Nervous system symptoms: symptoms including, but not limited to, dizziness, insomnia, somnolence, impaired concentration and abnormal dreaming are frequently reported undesirable effects in patients receiving efavirenz 600 mg daily in clinical studies (see section 4.8). Nervous system symptoms usually begin during the first one or two days of therapy and generally resolve after the first 2 - 4 weeks. Patients should be informed that if they do occur, these common symptoms are likely to improve with continued therapy and are not predictive of subsequent onset of any of the less frequent psychiatric symptoms.

Cholesterol: monitoring of cholesterol should be considered in patients treated with efavirenz (see section 4.8).

Immune Reactivation Syndrome: in HIV infected patients with severe immune deficiency at the time of institution of combination antiretroviral therapy (CART), an inflammatory reaction to asymptomatic or residual opportunistic pathogens may arise and cause serious clinical conditions, or aggravation of symptoms. Typically, such reactions have been observed within the first few weeks or months of initiation of CART. Relevant examples are cytomegalovirus retinitis, generalised and/or focal mycobacterial infections, and *Pneumocystis carinii* pneumonia. Any inflammatory symptoms should be evaluated and treatment instituted when necessary.

Lipodystrophy and metabolic abnormalities: combination antiretroviral therapy has been associated with the redistribution of body fat (lipodystrophy) in HIV patients. The long-term consequences of these events are currently unknown. Knowledge about the mechanism is incomplete. A connection between visceral lipomatosis and PIs and lipoatrophy and NRTIs has been hypothesised. A higher risk of lipodystrophy has been associated with individual factors such as older age, and with drug related factors such as longer duration of antiretroviral treatment and associated metabolic disturbances. Clinical examination should include evaluation for physical signs of fat redistribution. Consideration should be given to the measurement of fasting serum lipids and blood glucose. Lipid disorders should be managed as clinically appropriate (see section 4.8).

Special populations:

Liver disease: because of the extensive cytochrome P450-mediated metabolism of efavirenz and limited clinical experience in patients with chronic liver disease, caution must be exercised in administering efavirenz to patients with mild-to-moderate liver disease. Patients should be monitored carefully for dose-related adverse events, especially nervous system symptoms. Laboratory tests should be performed to evaluate their liver disease at periodic intervals (see section 4.2).

The safety and efficacy of efavirenz has not been established in patients with significant underlying liver disorders. Efavirenz is contraindicated in patients with severe hepatic impairment (see section 4.3). Patients with chronic hepatitis B or C and treated with combination antiretroviral therapy are at increased risk for severe and potentially fatal hepatic adverse events. Patients with pre-existing liver dysfunction including chronic active hepatitis have an increased frequency of liver function abnormalities during combination antiretroviral therapy and should be monitored according to standard practice. If there is evidence of worsening liver disease or persistent elevations of serum transaminases to greater than 5 times the upper limit of the normal range, the benefit of continued therapy with efavirenz needs to be weighed against the potential risks of significant liver toxicity. In such patients, interruption or discontinuation of treatment must be considered (see section 4.8).

In patients treated with other medicinal products associated with liver toxicity, monitoring of liver enzymes is also recommended. In case of concomitant antiviral therapy for hepatitis B or C, please refer also to the relevant product information for these medicinal products.

Renal insufficiency: the pharmacokinetics of efavirenz have not been studied in patients with renal insufficiency; however, less than 1% of an efavirenz dose is excreted unchanged in the urine, so the impact of renal impairment on efavirenz elimination should be minimal (see section 4.2). There is no experience in patients with severe renal failure and close safety monitoring is recommended in this population.

Elderly: insufficient numbers of elderly patients have been evaluated in clinical studies to determine whether they respond differently than younger patients.

Children: efavirenz has not been evaluated in children below 3 years of age or who weigh less than 13 kg. Evidence exists indicating that efavirenz may have altered pharmacokinetics in very young children. For this reason, efavirenz oral solution should not be given to children less than 3 years of age.

Seizures: convulsions have been observed rarely in patients receiving efavirenz, generally in the presence of known medical history of seizures. Patients who are receiving concomitant anticonvulsant medicinal products primarily metabolised by the liver, such as phenytoin, carbamazepine and phenobarbital, may require periodic monitoring of plasma levels. Caution must be taken in any patient with a history of seizures.

4.5 Interaction with other medicinal products and other forms of Interaction

Efavirenz is an inducer of CYP3A4 and an inhibitor of some CYP isozymes including CYP3A4 (see section 5.2). Other compounds that are substrates of CYP3A4 may have decreased plasma concentrations when co-administered with efavirenz. Efavirenz exposure may also be altered when given with medicinal products or food (for example, grapefruit juice) which affect CYP3A4 activity.

Efavirenz must not be administered concurrently with terfenadine, astemizole, cisapride, midazolam, triazolam, pimozide, bepridil, or ergot alkaloids (for example, ergotamine, dihydroergotamine, ergonovine, and methylergonovine) since inhibition of their metabolism may lead to serious, life-threatening events (see section 4.3).

Concomitant antiretroviral agents

Protease Inhibitors:

Amprenavir: although efavirenz has been seen to decrease the C_{max}, AUC and C_{min} of amprenavir by approximately 40% in adults, when amprenavir is combined with ritonavir, the effect of efavirenz is compensated by the pharmacokinetic booster effect of ritonavir. Therefore, if efavirenz is given in combination with amprenavir (600 mg twice daily) and ritonavir (100 or 200 mg twice daily), no dosage adjustment is necessary.

Further, if efavirenz is given in combination with amprenavir and nelfinavir, no dosage adjustment is necessary for any of the medicinal products. Treatment with efavirenz in combination with amprenavir and saquinavir is not recommended, as the exposure to both PIs is expected to be significantly decreased. No dose recommendation can be given for the co-administration of amprenavir with another PI and efavirenz in children and patients with renal impairment. Such combinations should be avoided in patients with hepatic impairment.

Indinavir: when indinavir (800 mg every 8 hours) was given with efavirenz (200 mg every 24 hours), the indinavir AUC and C_{trough} were decreased by approximately 31% and 40% respectively. When indinavir at an increased dose (1,000 mg every 8 hours) was given with efavirenz (600 mg once daily) in uninfected volunteers, the indinavir AUC and C_{trough} were decreased on average by 33 - 46% and 39 - 57%, respectively (ranges represent diurnal variation), compared to when indinavir was given alone at the standard dose (800 mg every 8 hours). Similar differences in indinavir AUC and C_{trough} were also observed in HIV-infected patients who received indinavir (1,000 mg every 8 hours) with efavirenz (600 mg once daily) compared to indinavir given alone (800 mg every 8 hours). While the clinical significance of decreased indinavir concentrations has not been established, the magnitude of the observed pharmacokinetic interaction should be taken into consideration when choosing a regimen containing both efavirenz and indinavir.

When efavirenz 600 mg once daily was given with indinavir/ritonavir 800/100 mg twice daily in uninfected volunteers (n = 14), the indinavir AUC, C_{min}, and C_{max} were decreased by approximately 25%, 50% and 17%, respectively, compared to when indinavir/ritonavir 800/100 mg twice daily were given without efavirenz. The geometric mean C_{min} for indinavir (0.33 mg/l) when given with ritonavir and efavirenz was higher than the mean historical C_{min} (0.15 mg/l) when indinavir was given alone at 800 mg every 8 hours. The pharmacokinetics of efavirenz given in combination with indinavir/ritonavir were comparable to efavirenz alone (600 mg once daily).

When efavirenz 600 mg once daily was given with indinavir/ritonavir 800/100 mg twice daily in HIV-1 infected patients (n = 6), the pharmacokinetics of indinavir and efavirenz were generally comparable to these uninfected volunteer data.

No adjustment of the dose of efavirenz is necessary when given with indinavir or indinavir/ritonavir.

Lopinavir/ritonavir: when used in combination with efavirenz and two NRTIs, 533/133 mg lopinavir/ritonavir twice daily yielded similar lopinavir plasma concentrations as compared to lopinavir/ritonavir 400/100 mg twice daily without efavirenz (historical data). When co-administered with efavirenz, an increase of the lopinavir/ritonavir doses by 33% should be considered (4 capsules/~6.5 ml twice daily instead of 3 capsules/5 ml twice daily). Caution is warranted since this dosage adjustment might be insufficient in some patients.

Nelfinavir: the AUC and C_{max} of nelfinavir are increased by 20% and 21%, respectively when given with efavirenz. The combination was generally well tolerated and no dose adjustment is necessary when nelfinavir is administered in combination with efavirenz.

Ritonavir: when efavirenz was given with ritonavir 500 mg or 600 mg twice daily, the combination was not well tolerated (for example, dizziness, nausea, paraesthesia and elevated liver enzymes occurred). Data on the tolerability of efavirenz with low-dose ritonavir (100 mg twice daily) alone are not available.

Saquinavir: when saquinavir (1,200 mg given 3 times a day, soft capsule formulation) was given with efavirenz, the saquinavir AUC and C_{max} were decreased by 62% and 50% respectively. Use of efavirenz in combination with saquinavir as the sole PI is not recommended.

Saquinavir/ritonavir: no data are available on the potential interactions of efavirenz with the combination of saquinavir and ritonavir.

NRTIs: studies of the interaction between efavirenz and the combination of zidovudine and lamivudine were performed in HIV-infected patients. No clinically significant pharmacokinetic interactions were observed. Specific interaction studies have not been performed with efavirenz and other NRTIs. Clinically significant interactions would not be expected since the NRTIs are metabolised via a different route than efavirenz and would be unlikely to compete for the same metabolic enzymes and elimination pathways.

NNRTIs: no studies have been performed with efavirenz in combination with other NNRTIs and the potential for pharmacokinetic or pharmacodynamic interactions is unknown.

Antimicrobial agents:

Rifamycins: rifampicin reduced efavirenz AUC by 26% and C_{max} by 20% in uninfected volunteers. The dose of efavirenz must be increased to 800 mg/day when taken with rifampicin. No dose adjustment of rifampicin is recommended when given with efavirenz. In one study in uninfected volunteers, efavirenz induced a reduction in rifabutin C_{max} and AUC by 32% and 38% respectively. Rifabutin had no significant effect on the pharmacokinetics of efavirenz. These data suggest that the daily dose of rifabutin should be increased by 50% when administered with efavirenz and that the rifabutin dose may be doubled for regimens in which rifabutin is given two or three times a week in combination with efavirenz.

Macrolide antibiotics:

Azithromycin: co-administration of single doses of azithromycin and multiple doses of efavirenz in uninfected volunteers did not result in any clinically significant pharmacokinetic interaction. No dosage adjustment is necessary when azithromycin is given in combination with efavirenz.

Clarithromycin: co-administration of 400 mg of efavirenz once daily with clarithromycin given as 500 mg every 12 hours for seven days resulted in a significant effect of efavirenz on the pharmacokinetics of clarithromycin. The AUC and C_{max} of clarithromycin decreased 39% and 26%, respectively, while the AUC and C_{max} of the active clarithromycin hydroxymetabolite were increased 34% and 49%, respectively, when used in combination with efavirenz. The clinical significance of these changes in clarithromycin plasma levels is not known. In uninfected volunteers 46% developed rash while receiving efavirenz and clarithromycin. No dose adjustment of efavirenz is recommended when given with clarithromycin. Alternatives to clarithromycin may be considered.

Other macrolide antibiotics, such as erythromycin, have not been studied in combination with efavirenz.

Antifungal agents:

Voriconazole: co-administration of efavirenz (400 mg orally once daily) with voriconazole (200 mg orally every 12 hours) in uninfected volunteers resulted in a 2-way interaction. The steady state AUC and C_{max} of voriconazole decreased by on average 77% and 61%, respectively, while the steady state AUC and C_{max} of efavirenz increased by on average 44% and 38%, respectively. Co-administration of efavirenz and voriconazole is contraindicated (see section 4.3).

No clinically significant pharmacokinetic interactions were seen when fluconazole and efavirenz were co-administered to uninfected volunteers. The potential for interactions with efavirenz and other imidazole and triazole antifungals, such as itraconazole and ketoconazole, has not been studied.

Other interactions

Antacids/famotidine: neither aluminium/magnesium hydroxide antacids nor famotidine altered the absorption of efavirenz in uninfected volunteers. These data suggest that alteration of gastric pH by other medicinal products would not be expected to affect efavirenz absorption.

Oral contraceptives: only the ethinyloestradiol component of oral contraceptives has been studied. The AUC following a single dose of ethinyloestradiol was increased (37%) after multiple dosing of efavirenz. No significant changes were observed in C_{max} of ethinyloestradiol. The clinical significance of these effects is not known. No effect of a single dose of ethinyloestradiol on efavirenz C_{max} or AUC was observed. Because the potential interaction of efavirenz with oral contraceptives has not been fully characterised, a reliable method of barrier contraception must be used in addition to oral contraceptives.

Anticonvulsants: no data are available on the potential interactions of efavirenz with phenytoin, carbamazepine or phenobarbital, or other anticonvulsants. When efavirenz is administered concomitantly with these agents, there is a potential for reduction or increase in the plasma concentrations of each agent; therefore, periodic monitoring of plasma levels should be conducted.

Methadone: in a study of HIV-infected IV drug users, co-administration of efavirenz with methadone resulted in decreased plasma levels of methadone and signs of opiate withdrawal. The methadone dose was increased by a mean of 22% to alleviate withdrawal symptoms. Patients should be monitored for signs of withdrawal and their methadone dose increased as required to alleviate withdrawal symptoms.

St. John's wort *(Hypericum perforatum)*: plasma levels of efavirenz can be reduced by concomitant use of the herbal preparation St. John's wort (*Hypericum perforatum)*. This is due to induction of drug metabolising enzymes and/or transport proteins by St. John's wort. Herbal preparations containing St. John's wort must not be used concomitantly with SUSTIVA. If a patient is already taking St. John's wort, stop St. John's wort, check viral levels and if possible efavirenz levels. Efavirenz levels may increase on stopping St. John's wort and the dose of SUSTIVA may need adjusting. The inducing effect of St. John's wort may persist for at least 2 weeks after cessation of treatment (see section 4.3).

Antidepressants: there were no clinically significant effects on pharmacokinetic parameters when paroxetine and efavirenz were co-administered. No dose adjustments are necessary for either efavirenz or paroxetine when these drugs are co-administered. Since fluoxetine shares a similar metabolic profile with paroxetine, i.e. a strong CYP2D6 inhibitory effect, a similar lack of interaction would be expected for fluoxetine. Sertraline, a CYP3A4 substrate, did not significantly alter the pharmacokinetics of efavirenz. Efavirenz decreased sertraline C_{max}, C24 and AUC by 28.6 to 46.3%. Sertraline dose increases should be guided by clinical response.

Cetirizine: the H1-antihistamine, cetirizine, had no clinically significant effect on efavirenz pharmacokinetic parameters. Efavirenz decreased cetirizine C_{max} by 24% but did not alter cetirizine AUC. These changes are not considered to be clinically significant. No dose adjustments are necessary for either efavirenz or cetirizine when these drugs are co-administered.

Lorazepam: efavirenz increased lorazepam C_{max} and AUC by 16.3% and 7.3% respectively. These changes are not considered to be clinically significant. No dose adjustments are necessary for either efavirenz or lorazepam when these drugs are co-administered.

4.6 Pregnancy and lactation

Pregnancy should be avoided in women treated with efavirenz. Barrier contraception should always be used in combination with other methods of contraception (for example, oral or other hormonal contraceptives). Women of childbearing potential should undergo pregnancy testing before initiation of efavirenz. Efavirenz should not be used during pregnancy unless there are no other appropriate treatment options.

There are no adequate and well-controlled studies of efavirenz in pregnant women. In postmarketing experience through an antiretroviral pregnancy registry, more than 200 pregnancies with first-trimester exposure to efavirenz as part of a combination antiretroviral regimen have been reported with no specific malformation pattern. Retrospectively in this registry, a small number of cases of neural tube defects, including meningomyelocele, have been reported but causality has not been established. Studies in animals have shown reproductive toxicity including marked teratogenic effects (see section 5.3).

Studies in rats have demonstrated that efavirenz is excreted in milk reaching concentrations much higher than those in maternal plasma. It is not known whether efavirenz is excreted in human milk. Since animal data suggest that the substance may be passed into breast milk, it is recommended that mothers taking efavirenz do not breast feed their infants. It is recommended that HIV infected women do not breast feed their infants under any circumstances in order to avoid transmission of HIV.

4.7 Effects on ability to drive and use machines

Efavirenz has not been specifically evaluated for possible effects on the ability to drive a car or operate machinery. Efavirenz may cause dizziness, impaired concentration, and/or somnolence. Patients should be instructed that if they experience these symptoms they should avoid potentially hazardous tasks such as driving or operating machinery.

4.8 Undesirable effects

Efavirenz has been studied in over 9,000 patients. In a subset of 1,008 adult patients who received 600 mg efavirenz daily in combination with PIs and/or NRTIs in controlled clinical studies, the most frequently reported treatment-related undesirable effects of at least moderate severity reported in at least 5% of patients were rash (11.6%), dizziness (8.5%), nausea (8.0%), headache (5.7%) and fatigue (5.5%). The most notable undesirable effects associated with efavirenz are rash and nervous system symptoms (see section 4.4).

The long-term safety profile of efavirenz-containing regimens was evaluated in a controlled trial (006) in which patients received efavirenz + zidovudine + lamivudine (n = 412, median duration 180 weeks), efavirenz + indinavir (n = 415, median duration 102 weeks), or indinavir + zidovudine + lamivudine (n = 401, median duration 76 weeks). Long-term use of efavirenz in this study was not associated with any new safety concerns.

Rash: in clinical studies, 26% of patients treated with 600 mg of efavirenz experienced skin rash compared with 17% of patients treated in control groups. Skin rash was considered treatment related in 18% of patients treated with efavirenz. Severe rash occurred in less than 1% of patients treated with efavirenz, and 1.7% discontinued therapy because of rash. The incidence of erythema multiforme or Stevens-Johnson syndrome was approximately 0.1%.

Rashes are usually mild-to-moderate maculopapular skin eruptions that occur within the first two weeks of initiating therapy with efavirenz. In most patients rash resolves with continuing therapy with efavirenz within one month. Efavirenz can be reinitiated in patients interrupting therapy because of rash. Use of appropriate antihistamines and/or corticosteroids is recommended when efavirenz is restarted.

Experience with efavirenz in patients who discontinued other antiretroviral agents of the NNRTI class is limited. Nineteen patients who discontinued nevirapine because of rash have been treated with efavirenz. Nine of these patients developed mild-to-moderate rash while receiving therapy with efavirenz, and two discontinued because of rash.

Psychiatric symptoms: serious psychiatric adverse experiences have been reported in patients treated with efavirenz. In controlled trials of 1,008 patients treated with regimens containing efavirenz for an average of 1.6 years and 635 patients treated with control regimens for an average of 1.3 years, the frequency of specific serious psychiatric events are detailed hereafter:

	Efavirenz regimen	Control regimen
- severe depression	1.6%	0.6%
- suicidal ideation	0.6%	0.3%
- non-fatal suicide attempts	0.4%	0%
- aggressive behaviour	0.4%	0.3%
- paranoid reactions	0.4%	0.3%
- manic reactions	0.1%	0%

Patients with a history of psychiatric disorders appear to be at greater risk of these serious psychiatric adverse experiences with the frequency of each of the above events ranging from 0.3% for manic reactions to 2.0% for both severe depression and suicidal ideation. There have also been post-marketing reports of death by suicide, delusions and psychosis-like behaviour.

Nervous system symptoms: in clinical controlled trials, frequently reported undesirable effects in patients receiving 600 mg efavirenz with other antiretroviral agents included, but were not limited to: dizziness, insomnia, somnolence, impaired concentration and abnormal dreaming. Nervous system symptoms of moderate-to-severe intensity were experienced by 19.4% of patients compared to 9.0% of patients receiving control regimens. These symptoms were severe in 2.0% of patients receiving efavirenz 600 mg daily and in 1.3% of patients receiving control regimens. In clinical studies 2.1% of patients treated with 600 mg of efavirenz discontinued therapy because of nervous system symptoms.

Nervous system symptoms usually begin during the first one or two days of therapy and generally resolve after the first 2 - 4 weeks. In one clinical study, the monthly prevalence of nervous system symptoms of at least moderate severity between weeks 4 and 48, ranged from 5% - 9% in patients treated with regimens containing efavirenz and 3% - 5% in patients treated with the control regimen. In a study of uninfected volunteers, a representative nervous system symptom had a median time to onset of 1 hour post-dose and a median duration of 3 hours. Nervous system symptoms may occur more frequently when efavirenz is taken concomitantly with meals possibly due to increased efavirenz plasma levels (see section 5.2). Dosing at bedtime seems to improve the tolerability of these symptoms and can be recommended during the first weeks of therapy and in patients who continue to experience these symptoms (see section 4.2). Dose reduction or splitting the daily dose has not been shown to provide benefit.

Analysis of long-term data from study 006 (median follow-up 180 weeks, 102 weeks, and 76 weeks for patients treated with efavirenz + zidovudine + lamivudine, efavirenz + indinavir, and indinavir + zidovudine + lamivudine, respectively) showed that, beyond 24 weeks of therapy, the incidences of new-onset nervous system symptoms among efavirenz-treated patients were generally similar to those in the control arm.

Adverse reactions of moderate or greater severity with at least possible relationship to treatment regimen (based on investigator attribution) reported in clinical trials of efavirenz at the recommended dose in combination therapy (n = 1,008) are listed below. Frequency is defined using the following convention: very common ($\geq$ 1/10); common ($\geq$ 1/100, $<$ 1/10); uncommon ($\geq$ 1/1,000, $<$ 1/100); rare ($\geq$ 1/10,000, $<$ 1/1,000); very rare ($<$ 1/10,000).

Immune system disorders

uncommon: hypersensitivity

Psychiatric disorders

common: anxiety, depression

uncommon: affect lability, aggression, euphoric mood, hallucination, mania, paranoia, suicide attempt, suicide ideation

Nervous system disorders

common: abnormal dreams, disturbance in attention, dizziness, headache, insomnia, somnolence

uncommon: agitation, amnesia, ataxia, coordination abnormal, confusional state, convulsions, thinking abnormal

Eye disorders

uncommon: vision blurred

Ear and labyrinth disorders

uncommon: vertigo

Gastrointestinal disorders

common: abdominal pain, diarrhoea, nausea, vomiting

uncommon: pancreatitis acute

Hepatobiliary disorders

uncommon: hepatitis acute

Skin and subcutaneous tissue disorders

very common: rash

common: pruritus

uncommon: erythema multiforme

General disorders and administration site conditions

common: fatigue

Immune Reactivation Syndrome: in HIV infected patients with severe immune deficiency at the time of initiation of combination antiretroviral therapy (CART), an inflammatory reaction to asymptomatic or residual opportunistic infections may arise (see section 4.4).

Lipodystrophy and metabolic abnormalities: combination antiretroviral therapy has been associated with redistribution of body fat (lipodystrophy) in HIV patients including the loss of peripheral and facial subcutaneous fat, increased intra-abdominal and visceral fat, breast hypertrophy and dorsocervical fat accumulation (buffalo hump).

Combination antiretroviral therapy has been associated with metabolic abnormalities such as hypertriglyceridaemia, hypercholesterolaemia, insulin resistance, hyperglycaemia and hyperlactataemia (see section 4.4).

Laboratory test abnormalities:

Liver enzymes: elevations of aspartate aminotransferase (AST) and alanine aminotransferase (ALT) to greater than five times the upper limit of the normal range (ULN) were seen in 3% of 1,008 patients treated with 600 mg of efavirenz (5-8% after long-term treatment in study 006). Similar elevations were seen in patients treated with control regimens (5% after long-term treatment). Elevations of gamma-glutamyltransferase (GGT) to greater than five times ULN were observed in 4% of all patients treated with 600 mg of efavirenz and 1.5-2% of patients treated with control regimens (7% of efavirenz-treated patients and 3% of control-treated patients after long-term treatment). Isolated elevations of GGT in patients receiving efavirenz may reflect enzyme induction. In the long-term study (006), 1% of patients in each treatment arm discontinued because of liver or biliary system disorders.

In the long-term data set from study 006, 137 patients treated with efavirenz-containing regimens (median duration of therapy, 68 weeks) and 84 treated with a control regimen (median duration, 56 weeks) were seropositive at screening for hepatitis B (surface antigen positive) and/or C (hepatitis C antibody positive). Among these co-infected patients, elevations in AST to greater than five times ULN developed in 13% of patients in the efavirenz arms and 7% of those in the control arm, and elevations in ALT to greater than five times ULN developed in 20% of patients in the efavirenz arms and 7% of the patients in the control arm. Among co-infected patients, 3% of those treated with efavirenz -containing regimens and 2% in the control arm discontinued from the study because of liver or biliary system disorders. Reasons for discontinuation among co-infected recipients of efavirenz included abnormalities in hepatic enzymes; there were no discontinuations reported in this study for cholestatic hepatitis, hepatic failure, or fatty liver (see section 4.4).

Amylase: in the clinical trial subset of 1,008 patients, asymptomatic increases in serum amylase levels greater than 1.5 times the upper limit of normal were seen in 10% of patients treated with efavirenz and 6% of patients treated with control regimens. The clinical significance of asymptomatic increases in serum amylase is unknown.

Lipids: increases in total cholesterol of 10 - 20% have been observed in some uninfected volunteers receiving efavirenz. Increases in non-fasting total cholesterol and HDL of approximately 20% and 25%, respectively, were observed in patients treated with efavirenz + zidovudine + lamivudine and of approximately 40% and 35%, in patients treated with efavirenz + indinavir. The effects of efavirenz on triglycerides and LDL were not well characterised. The clinical significance of these findings is unknown (see section 4.4).

Cannabinoid test interaction: efavirenz does not bind to cannabinoid receptors. False positive urine cannabinoid test results have been reported in uninfected volunteers who received efavirenz. False positive test results have only been observed with the CEDIA DAU Multi-Level THC assay, which is used for screening, and have not been observed with other cannabinoid assays tested including tests used for confirmation of positive results.

Postmarketing experience with efavirenz has shown the following additional adverse events to occur in association with efavirenz-containing antiretroviral treatment regimens: delusion, gynaecomastia, hepatic failure, neurosis, photoallergic dermatitis, psychosis and completed suicide.

Adolescents and children: undesirable effects in children were generally similar to those of adult patients. Rash was reported more frequently in children (in a clinical study including 57 children who received efavirenz during a 48-week period, rash was reported in 46%) and was more often of higher grade than in adults (severe rash was reported in 5.3% of children). Prophylaxis with appropriate antihistamines prior to initiating therapy with efavirenz in children may be considered. Although nervous system symptoms are difficult for young children to report, they appear to be less frequent in children and were generally mild. In the study of 57 children, 3.5% of patients experienced nervous system symptoms of moderate intensity, predominantly dizziness. No child had severe symptoms or had to discontinue because of nervous system symptoms. Diarrhoea occurred in six of nineteen (32%) children, aged 3 - 8 years, who took efavirenz oral solution in combination with nelfinavir (20 - 30 mg/kg given three times a day) and one or more NRTIs.

4.9 Overdose

Some patients accidentally taking 600 mg twice daily have reported increased nervous system symptoms. One patient experienced involuntary muscle contractions.

Treatment of overdose with efavirenz should consist of general supportive measures, including monitoring of vital signs and observation of the patient's clinical status. Administration of activated charcoal may be used to aid removal of unabsorbed efavirenz. There is no specific antidote for overdose with efavirenz. Since efavirenz is highly protein bound, dialysis is unlikely to remove significant quantities of it from blood.

5. PHARMACOLOGICAL PROPERTIES

5.1 Pharmacodynamic properties

Pharmacotherapeutic group: HIV-1 specific NNRTI.

ATC code: J05A G03

Mechanism of action: efavirenz is a NNRTI of HIV-1. Efavirenz is a non-competitive inhibitor of HIV-1 reverse transcriptase (RT) and does not significantly inhibit HIV-2 RT or cellular DNA polymerases (α, β, γ or δ).

Antiviral activity: the free concentration of efavirenz required for 90 to 95% inhibition of wild type or zidovudine-resistant laboratory and clinical isolates *in vitro* ranged from 0.46 to 6.8 nM in lymphoblastoid cell lines, peripheral blood mononuclear cells (PBMCs) and macrophage/monocyte cultures.

Resistance: the potency of efavirenz in cell culture against viral variants with amino acid substitutions at positions 48, 108, 179, 181 or 236 in RT or variants with amino acid substitutions in the protease was similar to that observed against wild type viral strains. The single substitutions which led to the highest resistance to efavirenz in cell culture correspond to a leucine-to-isoleucine change at position 100 (L100I, 17 to 22-fold resistance) and a lysine-to-asparagine at position 103 (K103N, 18 to 33-fold resistance). Greater than 100-fold loss of susceptibility was observed against HIV variants expressing K103N in addition to other amino acid substitutions in RT.

K103N was the most frequently observed RT substitution in viral isolates from patients who experienced a significant rebound in viral load during clinical studies of efavirenz in combination with indinavir or zidovudine + lamivudine. This mutation was observed in 90% of patients receiving efavirenz with virological failure. Substitutions at RT positions 98, 100, 101, 108, 138, 188, 190 or 225 were also observed, but at lower frequencies, and often only in combination with K103N. The pattern of amino acid substitutions in RT associated with resistance to efavirenz was independent of the other antiviral medications used in combination with efavirenz.

Cross resistance: cross resistance profiles for efavirenz, nevirapine and delavirdine in cell culture demonstrated that the K103N substitution confers loss of susceptibility to all three NNRTIs. Two of three delavirdine-resistant clinical isolates examined were cross-resistant to efavirenz and contained the K103N substitution. A third isolate which carried a substitution at position 236 of RT was not cross-resistant to efavirenz.

Viral isolates recovered from PBMCs of patients enrolled in efavirenz clinical studies who showed evidence of treatment failure (viral load rebound) were assessed for susceptibility to NNRTIs. Thirteen isolates previously characterised as efavirenz-resistant were also resistant to nevirapine and delavirdine. Five of these NNRTI-resistant isolates were found to have K103N or a valine-to-isoleucine substitution at position 108 (V108I) in RT. Three of the efavirenz treatment failure isolates tested remained sensitive to efavirenz in cell culture and were also sensitive to nevirapine and delavirdine.

The potential for cross resistance between efavirenz and PIs is low because of the different enzyme targets involved. The potential for cross-resistance between efavirenz and NRTIs is low because of the different binding sites on the target and mechanism of action.

Pharmacodynamic effects

Efavirenz has not been studied in controlled studies in patients with advanced HIV disease, namely with CD4 counts $<$ 50 cells/mm^3, or in PI or NNRTI experienced patients. Clinical experience in controlled studies with combinations including didanosine or zalcitabine is limited.

Two controlled studies (006 and ACTG 364) of approximately one year duration with efavirenz in combination with NRTIs and/or PIs, have demonstrated reduction of viral load below the limit of quantification of the assay and increased CD4 lymphocytes in antiretroviral therapy-naïve and NRTI-experienced HIV-infected patients. Study 020 showed similar activity in NRTI-experienced patients over 24 weeks. In these studies the dose of efavirenz was 600 mg once daily; the dose of indinavir was 1,000 mg every 8 hours when used with efavirenz and 800 mg every 8 hours when used without efavirenz. The dose of nelfinavir was 750 mg given three times a day. The standard doses of NRTIs given every 12 hours were used in each of these studies.

Study 006, a randomized, open-label trial, compared efavirenz + zidovudine + lamivudine or efavirenz + indinavir with indinavir + zidovudine + lamivudine in 1,266 patients who were required to be efavirenz-, lamivudine-, NNRTI-, and PI-naive at study entry. The mean baseline CD4 cell count was 341 cells/mm3 and the mean baseline HIV-RNA level was 60,250 copies/ml. Efficacy results for study 006 on a subset of 614 patients who had been enrolled for at least 48 weeks are found in Table 2. In the analysis of responder rates (the non-completer equals failure analysis [NC = F]), patients who terminated the study early for any reason, or who had a missing HIV-RNA measurement that was either preceded or followed by a measurement above the limit of assay quantification were considered to have HIV-RNA above 50 or above 400 copies/ml at the missing time points.

Table 2 Efficacy results for study 006

Treatment Regimen[d]	n	Responder rates (NC = F[a]) Plasma HIV-RNA < 400 copies/ml (95% C.I.[b]) 48 weeks	< 50 copies/ml (95% C.I.[b]) 48 weeks	Mean change from baseline-CD4 cell count cells/mm^3 (S.E.M.[c]) 48 weeks
EFV + ZDV + 3TC	202	67% (60%, 73%)	62% (55%, 69%)	187 (11.8)
EFV + IDV	206	54% (47%, 61%)	48% (41%, 55%)	177 (11.3)
IDV + ZDV + 3TC	206	45% (38%, 52%)	40% (34%, 47%)	153 (12.3)

[a] NC = F, noncompleter = failure.
[b] C.I., confidence interval.
[c] S.E.M., standard error of the mean.
[d] EFV, efavirenz; ZDV, zidovudine; 3TC, lamivudine; IDV, indinavir.

Table 2: Efficacy results for study 006
(see Table 2 above)

Long-term results at 168 weeks of study 006 (160 patients completed study on treatment with EFV+IDV, 196 patients with EFV+ZDV+3TC and 127 patients with IDV+ZDV+3TC, respectively), suggest durability of response in terms of proportions of patients with HIV RNA < 400 copies/ml, HIV RNA < 50 copies/ml and in terms of mean change from baseline CD4 cell count.

Efficacy results for studies ACTG 364 and 020 are found in Table 3. Study ACTG 364 enrolled 196 patients who had been treated with NRTIs but not with PIs or NNRTIs. Study 020 enrolled 327 patients who had been treated with NRTIs but not with PIs or NNRTIs. Physicians were allowed to change their patient's NRTI regimen upon entry into the study. Responder rates were highest in patients who switched NRTIs.

Table 3: Efficacy results for studies ACTG 364 and 020
(see Table 3 below)

Paediatric trial: ACTG 382 is an ongoing uncontrolled study of 57 NRTI-experienced paediatric patients (3 - 16 years) which characterises the pharmacokinetics, antiviral activity and safety of efavirenz in combination with nelfinavir (20 - 30 mg/kg given three times a day) and one or more NRTIs. The starting dose of efavirenz was the equivalent of a 600 mg dose (adjusted from calculated body size based on weight). The response rate, based on the NC = F analysis of the percentage of patients with plasma HIV-RNA < 400 copies/ml at 48 weeks was 60% (95%, C.I. 47, 72), and 53% (C.I. 40, 66) based on percentage of patients with plasma HIV-RNA < 50 copies/ml. The mean CD4 cell counts were increased by 63 ± 34.5 cells/mm^3 from baseline. The durability of the response was similar to that seen in adult patients.

5.2 Pharmacokinetic properties

Absorption: peak efavirenz plasma concentrations of 1.6 - 9.1 μM were attained by 5 hours following single oral doses of 100 mg to 1,600 mg administered to uninfected volunteers. Dose related increases in C_{max} and AUC were seen for doses up to 1,600 mg; the increases were less than proportional suggesting diminished absorption at higher doses. Time to peak plasma concentrations (3 - 5 hours) did not change following multiple dosing and steady-state plasma concentrations were reached in 6 - 7 days.

In HIV infected patients at steady state, mean C_{max}, mean C_{min}, and mean AUC were linear with 200 mg, 400 mg, and 600 mg daily doses. In 35 patients receiving efavirenz 600 mg once daily, steady state C_{max} was 12.9 ± 3.7 μM (29%) [mean ± S.D. (% C.V.)], steady state C_{min} was 5.6 ± 3.2 μM (57%), and AUC was 184 ± 73 μM·h (40%).

In uninfected adult volunteers, the C_{max} and AUC of a 240 mg dose of SUSTIVA oral solution were 78% and 97%, respectively, of the values measured when SUSTIVA was given as a 200 mg hard capsule.

Effect of food: the AUC and C_{max} of a single 240 mg dose of efavirenz oral solution in uninfected adult volunteers was increased by 30% and 43%, respectively, when given with a high-fat meal, relative to fasted conditions.

Distribution: efavirenz is highly bound (approximately 99.5 - 99.75%) to human plasma proteins, predominantly albumin. In HIV-1 infected patients (n = 9) who received efavirenz 200 to 600 mg once daily for at least one month, cerebrospinal fluid concentrations ranged from 0.26 to 1.19% (mean 0.69%) of the corresponding plasma concentration. This proportion is approximately 3-fold higher than the non-protein-bound (free) fraction of efavirenz in plasma.

Biotransformation: studies in humans and *in vitro* studies using human liver microsomes have demonstrated that efavirenz is principally metabolised by the cytochrome P450 system to hydroxylated metabolites with subsequent glucuronidation of these hydroxylated metabolites. These metabolites are essentially inactive against HIV-1. The *in vitro* studies suggest that CYP3A4 and CYP2B6 are the major isozymes responsible for efavirenz metabolism and that it inhibited P450 isozymes 2C9, 2C19, and 3A4. In *in vitro* studies efavirenz did not inhibit CYP2E1 and inhibited CYP2D6 and CYP1A2 only at concentrations well above those achieved clinically.

Efavirenz has been shown to induce P450 enzymes, resulting in the induction of its own metabolism. In uninfected volunteers, multiple doses of 200 - 400 mg per day for 10 days resulted in a lower than predicted extent of accumulation (22 - 42% lower) and a shorter terminal half-life of 40 - 55 hours (single dose half-life 52 - 76 hours).

Elimination: efavirenz has a relatively long terminal half-life of 52 to 76 hours after single doses and 40 - 55 hours after multiple doses. Approximately 14 - 34% of a radiolabelled dose of efavirenz was recovered in the urine and less than 1% of the dose was excreted in urine as unchanged efavirenz.

In the single patient studied with severe hepatic impairment (Child Pugh Grade C), half life was doubled indicating a potential for a much greater degree of accumulation.

Paediatric pharmacokinetics: the equivalent of a 600 mg dose of efavirenz was given as hard capsules (dose adjusted from calculated body size based on weight) to 49 paediatric patients. The pharmacokinetics of efavirenz in paediatric patients were similar to adults. Steady state C_{max} was 14.1 μM, steady state C_{min} was 5.6 μM, and AUC was 216 μM·h. In 17 paediatric patients receiving an investigational oral solution similar to the commercial formulation adjusted on the basis of body size to be equivalent to an adult 600 mg capsule dose, the steady-state C_{max} was 11.8 μM, steady state C_{min} was 5.2 μM, and AUC was 188 μM·h. In the subset of 6 children aged 3 - 5 who were compliant with their drug regimen, the mean AUC was 147 μM·h, which was 23% lower than expected. Therefore, the dosage recommendation provided in Table 1 incorporates a higher dose of efavirenz oral solution for these younger children.

Gender, race, elderly: pharmacokinetics of efavirenz in patients appear to be similar between men and women and among the racial groups studied. Although limited data suggest that Asian and Pacific Island patients may have higher exposure to efavirenz, they do not appear to be less tolerant of efavirenz. Pharmacokinetic studies have not been performed in the elderly.

5.3 Preclinical safety data

Efavirenz was not mutagenic or clastogenic in conventional genotoxicity assays.

Efavirenz induced foetal resorptions in rats. Malformations were observed in 3 of 20 foetuses/ newborns from efavirenz-treated cynomolgus monkeys given doses resulting in plasma efavirenz concentrations similar to those seen in humans. Anencephaly and unilateral anophthalmia with secondary enlargement of the tongue were observed in one foetus, microophthalmia was observed in another foetus, and cleft palate was observed in a third foetus. No malformations were observed in foetuses from efavirenz-treated rats and rabbits.

Biliary hyperplasia was observed in cynomolgus monkeys given efavirenz for ⩾ 1 year at a dose resulting in mean AUC values approximately 2-fold greater than those in humans given the recommended dose. The biliary hyperplasia regressed upon cessation of dosing. Biliary fibrosis has been observed in rats. Non-sustained convulsions were observed in some monkeys receiving efavirenz for ⩾ 1 year, at doses yielding plasma AUC values 4- to 13-fold greater than those in humans given the recommended dose (see sections 4.4 and 4.8).

Carcinogenicity studies showed an increased incidence of hepatic and pulmonary tumours in female mice, but not in male mice. The mechanism of tumour formation and the potential relevance for humans are not known.

Carcinogenicity studies in male mice, male and female rats were negative. While the carcinogenic potential in humans is unknown, these data suggest that the clinical benefit of efavirenz outweighs the potential carcinogenic risk to humans.

6. PHARMACEUTICAL PARTICULARS

6.1 List of excipients

Medium chain triglycerides, benzoic acid (E210) and strawberry/mint flavour.

6.2 Incompatibilities

Not applicable.

6.3 Shelf life

3 years.

The oral solution should be used within one month of first opening the bottle.

6.4 Special precautions for storage

No special precautions for storage.

6.5 Nature and contents of container

HDPE bottles with a child-resistant polypropylene closure containing 180 ml of oral solution. An oral syringe with a push-in bottle-neck adapter is included in the carton.

6.6 Instructions for use and handling

No special requirements.

7. MARKETING AUTHORISATION HOLDER

Bristol-Myers Squibb Pharma EEIG
141 - 149 Staines Road
Hounslow TW3 3JA
United Kingdom

8. MARKETING AUTHORISATION NUMBER(S)

EU/1/99/110/005 - bottle

9. DATE OF FIRST AUTHORISATION/RENEWAL OF THE AUTHORISATION

Date of first authorisation: 18 October 2001

Date of last renewal: 29 April 2004

10. DATE OF REVISION OF THE TEXT

August 2005

Table 3 Efficacy results for studies ACTG 364 and 020

Study Number/ Treatment Regimens[b]	n	Responder rates (NC = F[a]) Plasma HIV-RNA %	(95% C.I.[c])	%	(95% C.I.)	Mean change from baseline-CD4 cell count cells/mm^3	(S.E.M.[d])
Study ACTG 364 48 weeks		< 500 copies/ml		< 50 copies/ml			
EFV + NFV + NRTIs	65	70	(59, 82)	—	—	107	(17.9)
EFV + NRTIs	65	58	(46, 70)	—	—	114	(21.0)
NFV + NRTIs	66	30	(19, 42)	—	—	94	(13.6)
Study 020 24 weeks		< 400 copies/ml		< 50 copies/ml			
EFV + IDV + NRTIs	157	60	(52, 68)	49	(41, 58)	104	(9.1)
IDV + NRTIs	170	51	(43, 59)	38	(30, 45)	77	(9.9)

[a] NC = F, noncompleter = failure.
[b] EFV, efavirenz; ZDV, zidovudine; 3TC, lamivudine; IDV, indinavir; NRTI, nucleoside reverse transcriptase inhibitor; NFV, nelfinavir.
[c] C.I., confidence interval for proportion of patients in response.
[d] S.E.M., standard error of the mean.
—, not performed.

Sustiva 50 mg, 100 mg and 200 mg Hard Capsules

(Bristol-Myers Squibb Pharmaceuticals Ltd)

1. NAME OF THE MEDICINAL PRODUCT

SUSTIVA® 50 mg, 100mg and 200mg hard capsules

2. QUALITATIVE AND QUANTITATIVE COMPOSITION

Each capsule contains 50 mg, 100mg or 200mg efavirenz

For excipients, see section 6.1.

3. PHARMACEUTICAL FORM

Hard capsule

SUSTIVA 50 mg hard capsules are dark yellow and white, printed with "SUSTIVA" on the dark yellow cap and "50 mg" on the white body.

SUSTIVA 100 mg hard capsules are white, printed with "SUSTIVA" on the body and "100 mg" on the cap.

SUSTIVA 200 mg hard capsules are dark yellow, printed with "SUSTIVA" on the body and "200 mg" on the cap.

4. CLINICAL PARTICULARS

4.1 Therapeutic indications

SUSTIVA is indicated in antiviral combination treatment of HIV-1 infected adults, adolescents and children 3 years of age and older.

SUSTIVA has not been adequately studied in patients with advanced HIV disease, namely in patients with CD4 counts < 50 cells/mm^3, or after failure of protease inhibitor (PI) containing regimens. Although cross-resistance of efavirenz with PIs has not been documented, there are at present insufficient data on the efficacy of subsequent use of PI based combination therapy after failure of regimens containing SUSTIVA.

For a summary of clinical and pharmacodynamic information, see section 5.1.

4.2 Posology and method of administration

Concomitant antiretroviral therapy: SUSTIVA must be given in combination with other antiretroviral medications (see section 4.5).

SUSTIVA may be taken with or without food (see section 5.2).

In order to improve the tolerability of nervous system undesirable effects, bedtime dosing is recommended during the first two to four weeks of therapy and in patients who continue to experience these symptoms (see section 4.8).

Therapy should be initiated by a physician experienced in the management of HIV infection.

Adults: the recommended dosage of SUSTIVA in combination with nucleoside analogue reverse transcriptase inhibitors (NRTIs) with or without a PI (see section 4.5) is 600 mg orally, once daily.

Adolescents and children (3 to 17 years): the recommended dose of SUSTIVA in combination with a PI and/or NRTIs for patients between 3 and 17 years of age is described in Table 1. SUSTIVA hard capsules must only be administered to children who are able to reliably swallow hard capsules. SUSTIVA has not been studied in children under the age of 3 years or children weighing less than 13 kg.

Table 1

Paediatric dose to be administered once daily

Body Weight	**SUSTIVA**
kg	**Dose (mg)**
13 to < 15	200
15 to < 20	250
20 to < 25	300
25 to < 32.5	350
32.5 to < 40	400
⩾ 40	600

Renal insufficiency: the pharmacokinetics of efavirenz have not been studied in patients with renal insufficiency; however, less than 1% of an efavirenz dose is excreted unchanged in the urine, so the impact of renal impairment on efavirenz elimination should be minimal (see section 4.4).

Liver disease: patients with mild to moderate liver disease may be treated with their normally recommended dose of efavirenz. Patients should be monitored carefully for dose-related adverse events, especially nervous system symptoms (see sections 4.3 and 4.4).

4.3 Contraindications

SUSTIVA is contraindicated in patients with clinically significant hypersensitivity to the active substance or to any of the excipients.

Efavirenz must not be used in patients with severe hepatic impairment (Child Pugh Grade C) (see section 5.2).

Efavirenz must not be administered concurrently with terfenadine, astemizole, cisapride, midazolam, triazolam, pimozide, bepridil, or ergot alkaloids (for example, ergotamine, dihydroergotamine, ergonovine, and methylergonovine) because competition for CYP3A4 by efavirenz could result in inhibition of metabolism and create the potential for serious and/or life-threatening undesirable effects [for example, cardiac arrhythmias, prolonged sedation or respiratory depression] (see section 4.5).

Herbal preparations containing St. John's wort *(Hypericum perforatum)* must not be used while taking efavirenz due to the risk of decreased plasma concentrations and reduced clinical effects of efavirenz (see section 4.5).

SUSTIVA must not be administered concurrently with voriconazole because efavirenz significantly decreases voriconazole plasma concentrations while voriconazole also significantly increases efavirenz plasma concentrations (see section 4.5).

4.4 Special warnings and special precautions for use

Efavirenz must not be used as a single agent to treat HIV or added on as a sole agent to a failing regimen. As with all other non-nucleoside reverse transcriptase inhibitors (NNRTIs), resistant virus emerges rapidly when efavirenz is administered as monotherapy. The choice of new antiretroviral agent(s) to be used in combination with efavirenz should take into consideration the potential for viral cross-resistance (see section 5.1).

When prescribing medicinal products concomitantly with SUSTIVA, physicians should refer to the corresponding Summary of Product Characteristics.

Patients should be advised that current antiretroviral therapy, including efavirenz, has not been proven to prevent the risk of transmission of HIV to others through sexual contact or blood contamination. Appropriate precautions should continue to be employed.

If any antiretroviral medicinal product in a combination regimen is interrupted because of suspected intolerance, serious consideration should be given to simultaneous discontinuation of all antiretroviral medicinal products. The antiretroviral medicinal products should be restarted at the same time upon resolution of the intolerance symptoms. Intermittent monotherapy and sequential reintroduction of antiretroviral agents is not advisable because of the increased potential for selection of resistant virus.

Rash: mild-to-moderate rash has been reported in clinical studies with efavirenz and usually resolves with continued therapy. Appropriate antihistamines and/or corticosteroids may improve the tolerability and hasten the resolution of rash. Severe rash associated with blistering, moist desquamation or ulceration has been reported in less than 1% of patients treated with efavirenz. The incidence of erythema multiforme or Stevens-Johnson syndrome was approximately 0.1%. Efavirenz must be discontinued in patients developing severe rash associated with blistering, desquamation, mucosal involvement or fever. If therapy with efavirenz is discontinued, consideration should also be given to interrupting therapy with other antiretroviral agents to avoid development of resistant virus (see section 4.8).

Rash was reported in 26 of 57 children (46%) treated with efavirenz during a 48-week period and was severe in three patients. Prophylaxis with appropriate antihistamines prior to initiating therapy with efavirenz in children may be considered.

Patients who discontinued treatment with other NNRTIs due to rash may be at higher risk of developing rash during treatment with efavirenz.

Psychiatric symptoms: psychiatric adverse experiences have been reported in patients treated with efavirenz. Patients with a prior history of psychiatric disorders appear to be at greater risk of these serious psychiatric adverse experiences. In particular, severe depression was more common in those with a history of depression. There have also been post-marketing reports of severe depression, death by suicide, delusions and psychosis-like behaviour. Patients should be advised that if they experience symptoms such as severe depression, psychosis or suicidal ideation, they should contact their doctor immediately to assess the possibility that the symptoms may be related to the use of efavirenz, and if so, to determine whether the risks of continued therapy outweigh the benefits (see section 4.8).

Nervous system symptoms: symptoms including, but not limited to, dizziness, insomnia, somnolence, impaired concentration and abnormal dreaming are frequently reported undesirable effects in patients receiving efavirenz 600 mg daily in clinical studies (see section 4.8). Nervous system symptoms usually begin during the first one or two days of therapy and generally resolve after the first 2 - 4 weeks. Patients should be informed that if they do occur, these common symptoms are likely to improve with continued therapy and are not predictive of subsequent onset of any of the less frequent psychiatric symptoms.

Effect of food: the administration of SUSTIVA with food may increase efavirenz exposure (see section 5.2) and may lead to an increase in the frequency of undesirable effects. This effect may be more evident for the film-coated tablets than for the hard capsules. It is recommended that SUSTIVA be taken on an empty stomach, preferably at bedtime.

Cholesterol: monitoring of cholesterol should be considered in patients treated with efavirenz (see section 4.8).

Immune Reactivation Syndrome: in HIV infected patients with severe immune deficiency at the time of institution of combination antiretroviral therapy (CART), an inflammatory reaction to asymptomatic or residual opportunistic pathogens may arise and cause serious clinical conditions, or aggravation of symptoms. Typically, such reactions have been observed within the first few weeks or months of initiation of CART. Relevant examples are cytomegalovirus retinitis, generalised and/or focal mycobacterial infections, and *Pneumocystis carinii* pneumonia. Any inflammatory symptoms should be evaluated and treatment instituted when necessary.

Lipodystrophy and metabolic abnormalities: combination antiretroviral therapy has been associated with the redistribution of body fat (lipodystrophy) in HIV patients. The long-term consequences of these events are currently unknown. Knowledge about the mechanism is incomplete. A connection between visceral lipomatosis and PIs and lipoatrophy and NRTIs has been hypothesised. A higher risk of lipodystrophy has been associated with individual factors such as older age, and with drug related factors such as longer duration of antiretroviral treatment and associated metabolic disturbances. Clinical examination should include evaluation for physical signs of fat redistribution. Consideration should be given to the measurement of fasting serum lipids and blood glucose. Lipid disorders should be managed as clinically appropriate (see section 4.8).

Lactose: this medicinal product contains 342 mg of lactose in each 600-mg daily dose. This quantity is not likely to induce symptoms of lactose intolerance.

Efavirenz capsules are unsuitable for individuals with the rare hereditary disorders of galactosaemia or glucose/galactose malabsorption syndrome. Individuals with these conditions may take efavirenz oral solution, which is free from lactose.

Special populations:

Liver disease: because of the extensive cytochrome P450-mediated metabolism of efavirenz and limited clinical experience in patients with chronic liver disease, caution must be exercised in administering efavirenz to patients with mild-to-moderate liver disease. Patients should be monitored carefully for dose-related adverse events, especially nervous system symptoms. Laboratory tests should be performed to evaluate their liver disease at periodic intervals (see section 4.2).

The safety and efficacy of efavirenz has not been established in patients with significant underlying liver disorders. Efavirenz is contraindicated in patients with severe hepatic impairment (see section 4.3). Patients with chronic hepatitis B or C and treated with combination antiretroviral therapy are at increased risk for severe and potentially fatal hepatic adverse events. Patients with pre-existing liver dysfunction including chronic active hepatitis have an increased frequency of liver function abnormalities during combination antiretroviral therapy and should be monitored according to standard practice. If there is evidence of worsening liver disease or persistent elevations of serum transaminases to greater than 5 times the upper limit of the normal range, the benefit of continued therapy with efavirenz needs to be weighed against the potential risks of significant liver toxicity. In such patients, interruption or discontinuation of treatment must be considered (see section 4.8).

In patients treated with other medicinal products associated with liver toxicity, monitoring of liver enzymes is also recommended. In case of concomitant antiviral therapy for hepatitis B or C, please refer also to the relevant product information for these medicinal products.

Renal insufficiency: the pharmacokinetics of efavirenz have not been studied in patients with renal insufficiency; however, less than 1% of an efavirenz dose is excreted unchanged in the urine, so the impact of renal impairment on efavirenz elimination should be minimal (see section 4.2). There is no experience in patients with severe renal failure and close safety monitoring is recommended in this population.

Elderly: insufficient numbers of elderly patients have been evaluated in clinical studies to determine whether they respond differently than younger patients.

Children: efavirenz has not been evaluated in children below 3 years of age or who weigh less than 13 kg.

Seizures: convulsions have been observed rarely in patients receiving efavirenz, generally in the presence of known medical history of seizures. Patients who are receiving concomitant anticonvulsant medicinal products primarily metabolised by the liver, such as phenytoin, carbamazepine and phenobarbital, may require periodic monitoring of plasma levels. Caution must be taken in any patient with a history of seizures.

4.5 Interaction with other medicinal products and other forms of Interaction

Efavirenz is an inducer of CYP3A4 and an inhibitor of some CYP isozymes including CYP3A4 (see section 5.2). Other compounds that are substrates of CYP3A4 may have decreased plasma concentrations when co-administered with efavirenz. Efavirenz exposure may also be altered when given with medicinal products or food (for example, grapefruit juice) which affect CYP3A4 activity.

Efavirenz must not be administered concurrently with terfenadine, astemizole, cisapride, midazolam, triazolam, pimozide, bepridil, or ergot alkaloids (for example, ergotamine, dihydroergotamine, ergonovine, and methylergonovine) since inhibition of their metabolism may lead to serious, life-threatening events (see section 4.3).

Concomitant antiretroviral agents

Protease Inhibitors:

Amprenavir: although efavirenz has been seen to decrease the C_{max}, AUC and C_{min} of amprenavir by approximately 40% in adults, when amprenavir is combined with ritonavir, the effect of efavirenz is compensated by the pharmacokinetic booster effect of ritonavir. Therefore, if efavirenz is given in combination with amprenavir (600 mg twice daily) and ritonavir (100 or 200 mg twice daily), no dosage adjustment is necessary.

Further, if efavirenz is given in combination with amprenavir and nelfinavir, no dosage adjustment is necessary for any of the medicinal products. Treatment with efavirenz in combination with amprenavir and saquinavir is not recommended, as the exposure to both PIs is expected to be significantly decreased. No dose recommendation can be given for the co-administration of amprenavir with another PI and efavirenz in children and patients with renal impairment. Such combinations should be avoided in patients with hepatic impairment.

Indinavir: when indinavir (800 mg every 8 hours) was given with efavirenz (200 mg every 24 hours), the indinavir AUC and C_{trough} were decreased by approximately 31% and 40% respectively. When indinavir at an increased dose (1,000 mg every 8 hours) was given with efavirenz (600 mg once daily) in uninfected volunteers, the indinavir AUC and C_{trough} were decreased on average by 33 - 46% and 39 - 57%, respectively (ranges represent diurnal variation), compared to when indinavir was given alone at the standard dose (800 mg every 8 hours). Similar differences in indinavir AUC and C_{trough} were also observed in HIV-infected patients who received indinavir (1,000 mg every 8 hours) with efavirenz (600 mg once daily) compared to indinavir given alone (800 mg every 8 hours). While the clinical significance of decreased indinavir concentrations has not been established, the magnitude of the observed pharmacokinetic interaction should be taken into consideration when choosing a regimen containing both efavirenz and indinavir.

When efavirenz 600 mg once daily was given with indinavir/ritonavir 800/100 mg twice daily in uninfected volunteers (n = 14), the indinavir AUC, C_{min}, and C_{max} were decreased by approximately 25%, 50% and 17%, respectively, compared to when indinavir/ritonavir 800/100 mg twice daily were given without efavirenz. The geometric mean C_{min} for indinavir (0.33 mg/l) when given with ritonavir and efavirenz was higher than the mean historical C_{min} (0.15 mg/l) when indinavir was given alone at 800 mg every 8 hours. The pharmacokinetics of efavirenz given in combination with indinavir/ritonavir were comparable to efavirenz alone (600 mg once daily).

When efavirenz 600 mg once daily was given with indinavir/ritonavir 800/100 mg twice daily in HIV-1 infected patients (n = 6), the pharmacokinetics of indinavir and efavirenz were generally comparable to these uninfected volunteer data.

No adjustment of the dose of efavirenz is necessary when given with indinavir or indinavir/ritonavir.

Lopinavir/ritonavir: when used in combination with efavirenz and two NRTIs, 533/133 mg lopinavir/ritonavir twice daily yielded similar lopinavir plasma concentrations as compared to lopinavir/ritonavir 400/100 mg twice daily without efavirenz (historical data). When co-administered with efavirenz, an increase of the lopinavir/ritonavir doses by 33% should be considered (4 capsules/~6.5 ml twice daily instead of 3 capsules/5 ml twice daily). Caution is warranted since this dosage adjustment might be insufficient in some patients.

Nelfinavir: the AUC and C_{max} of nelfinavir are increased by 20% and 21%, respectively when given with efavirenz. The combination was generally well tolerated and no dose adjustment is necessary when nelfinavir is administered in combination with efavirenz.

Ritonavir: when efavirenz was given with ritonavir 500 mg or 600 mg twice daily, the combination was not well tolerated (for example, dizziness, nausea, paraesthesia and elevated liver enzymes occurred). Data on the tolerability of efavirenz with low-dose ritonavir (100 mg twice daily) alone are not available.

Saquinavir: when saquinavir (1,200 mg given 3 times a day, soft capsule formulation) was given with efavirenz, the saquinavir AUC and C_{max} were decreased by 62% and 50% respectively. Use of efavirenz in combination with saquinavir as the sole PI is not recommended.

Saquinavir/ritonavir: no data are available on the potential interactions of efavirenz with the combination of saquinavir and ritonavir.

NRTIs: studies of the interaction between efavirenz and the combination of zidovudine and lamivudine were performed in HIV-infected patients. No clinically significant pharmacokinetic interactions were observed. Specific interaction studies have not been performed with efavirenz and other NRTIs. Clinically significant interactions would not be expected since the NRTIs are metabolised via a different route than efavirenz and would be unlikely to compete for the same metabolic enzymes and elimination pathways.

NNRTIs: no studies have been performed with efavirenz in combination with other NNRTIs and the potential for pharmacokinetic or pharmacodynamic interactions is unknown.

Antimicrobial agents:

Rifamycins: rifampicin reduced efavirenz AUC by 26% and C_{max} by 20% in uninfected volunteers. The dose of efavirenz must be increased to 800 mg/day when taken with rifampicin. No dose adjustment of rifampicin is recommended when given with efavirenz. In one study in uninfected volunteers, efavirenz induced a reduction in rifabutin C_{max} and AUC by 32% and 38% respectively. Rifabutin had no significant effect on the pharmacokinetics of efavirenz. These data suggest that the daily dose of rifabutin should be increased by 50% when administered with efavirenz and that the rifabutin dose may be doubled for regimens in which rifabutin is given two or three times a week in combination with efavirenz.

Macrolide antibiotics:

Azithromycin: co-administration of single doses of azithromycin and multiple doses of efavirenz in uninfected volunteers did not result in any clinically significant pharmacokinetic interaction. No dosage adjustment is necessary when azithromycin is given in combination with efavirenz.

Clarithromycin: co-administration of 400 mg of efavirenz once daily with clarithromycin given as 500 mg every 12 hours for seven days resulted in a significant effect of efavirenz on the pharmacokinetics of clarithromycin. The AUC and C_{max} of clarithromycin decreased 39% and 26%, respectively, while the AUC and C_{max} of the active clarithromycin hydroxymetabolite were increased 34% and 49%, respectively, when used in combination with efavirenz. The clinical significance of these changes in clarithromycin plasma levels is not known. In uninfected volunteers 46% developed rash while receiving efavirenz and clarithromycin. No dose adjustment of efavirenz is recommended when given with clarithromycin. Alternatives to clarithromycin may be considered.

Other macrolide antibiotics, such as erythromycin, have not been studied in combination with efavirenz.

Antifungal agents:

Voriconazole: co-administration of efavirenz (400 mg orally once daily) with voriconazole (200 mg orally every 12 hours) in uninfected volunteers resulted in a 2-way interaction. The steady state AUC and C_{max} of voriconazole decreased by on average 77% and 61%, respectively, while the steady state AUC and C_{max} of efavirenz increased by on average 44% and 38%, respectively. Co-administration of efavirenz and voriconazole is contraindicated (see section 4.3).

No clinically significant pharmacokinetic interactions were seen when fluconazole and efavirenz were co-administered to uninfected volunteers. The potential for interactions with efavirenz and other imidazole and triazole antifungals, such as itraconazole and ketoconazole, has not been studied.

Other interactions

Antacids/famotidine: neither aluminium/magnesium hydroxide antacids nor famotidine altered the absorption of efavirenz in uninfected volunteers. These data suggest that alteration of gastric pH by other medicinal products would not be expected to affect efavirenz absorption.

Oral contraceptives: only the ethinyloestradiol component of oral contraceptives has been studied. The AUC following a single dose of ethinyloestradiol was increased (37%) after multiple dosing of efavirenz. No significant changes were observed in C_{max} of ethinyloestradiol. The clinical significance of these effects is not known. No effect of a single dose of ethinyloestradiol on efavirenz C_{max} or AUC was observed. Because the potential interaction of efavirenz with oral contraceptives has not been fully characterised, a reliable method of barrier contraception must be used in addition to oral contraceptives.

Anticonvulsants: no data are available on the potential interactions of efavirenz with phenytoin, carbamazepine or phenobarbital, or other anticonvulsants. When efavirenz is administered concomitantly with these agents, there is a potential for reduction or increase in the plasma concentrations of each agent; therefore, periodic monitoring of plasma levels should be conducted.

Methadone: in a study of HIV-infected IV drug users, co-administration of efavirenz with methadone resulted in decreased plasma levels of methadone and signs of opiate withdrawal. The methadone dose was increased by a mean of 22% to alleviate withdrawal symptoms. Patients should be monitored for signs of withdrawal and their methadone dose increased as required to alleviate withdrawal symptoms.

St. John's wort *(Hypericum perforatum)*: plasma levels of efavirenz can be reduced by concomitant use of the herbal preparation St. John's wort (*Hypericum perforatum)*. This is due to induction of drug metabolising enzymes and/or transport proteins by St. John's wort. Herbal preparations containing St. John's wort must not be used concomitantly with SUSTIVA. If a patient is already taking St. John's wort, stop St. John's wort, check viral levels and if possible efavirenz levels. Efavirenz levels may increase on stopping St. John's wort and the dose of SUSTIVA may need adjusting. The inducing effect of St. John's wort may persist for at least 2 weeks after cessation of treatment (see section 4.3).

Antidepressants: there were no clinically significant effects on pharmacokinetic parameters when paroxetine and efavirenz were co-administered. No dose adjustments are necessary for either efavirenz or paroxetine when these drugs are co-administered. Since fluoxetine shares a similar metabolic profile with paroxetine, i.e. a strong CYP2D6 inhibitory effect, a similar lack of interaction would be expected for fluoxetine. Sertraline, a CYP3A4 substrate, did not significantly alter the pharmacokinetics of efavirenz. Efavirenz decreased sertraline C_{max}, C24 and AUC by 28.6 to 46.3%. Sertraline dose increases should be guided by clinical response.

Cetirizine: the H1-antihistamine, cetirizine, had no clinically significant effect on efavirenz pharmacokinetic parameters. Efavirenz decreased cetirizine C_{max} by 24% but did not alter cetirizine AUC. These changes are not considered to be clinically significant. No dose adjustments are necessary for either efavirenz or cetirizine when these drugs are co-administered.

Lorazepam: efavirenz increased lorazepam C_{max} and AUC by 16.3% and 7.3% respectively. These changes are not considered to be clinically significant. No dose adjustments are necessary for either efavirenz or lorazepam when these drugs are co-administered.

4.6 Pregnancy and lactation

Pregnancy should be avoided in women treated with efavirenz. Barrier contraception should always be used in combination with other methods of contraception (for example, oral or other hormonal contraceptives). Women of childbearing potential should undergo pregnancy testing before initiation of efavirenz. Efavirenz should not be used during pregnancy unless there are no other appropriate treatment options.

There are no adequate and well-controlled studies of efavirenz in pregnant women. In postmarketing experience through an antiretroviral pregnancy registry, more than 200 pregnancies with first-trimester exposure to efavirenz as part of a combination antiretroviral regimen have been reported with no specific malformation pattern. Retrospectively in this registry, a small number of cases of neural tube defects, including meningomyelocele, have been reported but casuality has not been established. Studies in animals have shown reproductive toxicity including marked teratogenic effects (see section 5.3).

Studies in rats have demonstrated that efavirenz is excreted in milk reaching concentrations much higher than those in maternal plasma. It is not known whether efavirenz is excreted in human milk. Since animal data suggest that the substance may be passed into breast milk, it is recommended that mothers taking efavirenz do not breast feed their infants. It is recommneded that HIV infected women do not breast feed their infants under any circumstances in order to avoid transmission of HIV.

4.7 Effects on ability to drive and use machines

Efavirenz has not been specifically evaluated for possible effects on the ability to drive a car or operate machinery. Efavirenz may cause dizziness, impaired concentration, and/or somnolence. Patients should be instructed that if they experience these symptoms they should avoid potentially hazardous tasks such as driving or operating machinery.

4.8 Undesirable effects

Efavirenz has been studied in over 9,000 patients. In a subset of 1,008 adult patients who received 600 mg efavirenz daily in combination with PIs and/or NRTIs in controlled clinical studies, the most frequently reported treatment-related undesirable effects of at least moderate severity reported in at least 5% of patients were rash (11.6%), dizziness (8.5%), nausea (8.0%), headache (5.7%) and fatigue (5.5%). The most notable undesirable effects associated with efavirenz are rash and nervous system symptoms. The administration of SUSTIVA with food may increase efavirenz exposure and may lead to an increase in the frequency of undesirable effects (see section 4.4).

The long-term safety profile of efavirenz-containing regimens was evaluated in a controlled trial (006) in which patients received efavirenz + zidovudine + lamivudine (n = 412, median duration 180 weeks), efavirenz + indinavir (n = 415, median duration 102 weeks), or indinavir + zidovudine + lamivudine (n = 401, median duration 76 weeks). Long-term use of efavirenz in this study was not associated with any new safety concerns.

Rash: in clinical studies, 26% of patients treated with 600 mg of efavirenz experienced skin rash compared with 17% of patients treated in control groups. Skin rash was considered treatment related in 18% of patients treated with efavirenz. Severe rash occurred in less than 1% of patients treated with efavirenz, and 1.7% discontinued therapy because of rash. The incidence of erythema multiforme or Stevens-Johnson syndrome was approximately 0.1%.

Rashes are usually mild-to-moderate maculopapular skin eruptions that occur within the first two weeks of initiating therapy with efavirenz. In most patients rash resolves with continuing therapy with efavirenz within one month. Efavirenz can be reinitiated in patients interrupting therapy because of rash. Use of appropriate antihistamines and/or corticosteroids is recommended when efavirenz is restarted.

Experience with efavirenz in patients who discontinued other antiretroviral agents of the NNRTI class is limited. Nineteen patients who discontinued nevirapine because of rash have been treated with efavirenz. Nine of these patients developed mild-to-moderate rash while receiving therapy with efavirenz, and two discontinued because of rash.

Psychiatric symptoms: serious psychiatric adverse experiences have been reported in patients treated with efavirenz. In controlled trials of 1,008 patients treated with regimens containing efavirenz for an average of 1.6 years and 635 patients treated with control regimens for an average of 1.3 years, the frequency of specific serious psychiatric events are detailed hereafter:

	Efavirenz regimen	Control regimen
- severe depression	1.6%	0.6%
- suicidal ideation	0.6%	0.3%
- non-fatal suicide attempts	0.4%	0%
- aggressive behaviour	0.4%	0.3%
- paranoid reactions	0.4%	0.3%
- manic reactions	0.1%	0%

Patients with a history of psychiatric disorders appear to be at greater risk of these serious psychiatric adverse experiences with the frequency of each of the above events ranging from 0.3% for manic reactions to 2.0% for both severe depression and suicidal ideation. There have also been post-marketing reports of death by suicide, delusions and psychosis-like behaviour.

Nervous system symptoms: in clinical controlled trials, frequently reported undesirable effects in patients receiving 600 mg efavirenz with other antiretroviral agents included, but were not limited to: dizziness, insomnia, somnolence, impaired concentration and abnormal dreaming. Nervous system symptoms of moderate-to-severe intensity were experienced by 19.4% of patients compared to 9.0% of patients receiving control regimens. These symptoms were severe in 2.0% of patients receiving efavirenz 600 mg daily and in 1.3% of patients receiving control regimens. In clinical studies 2.1% of patients treated with 600 mg of efavirenz discontinued therapy because of nervous system symptoms.

Nervous system symptoms usually begin during the first one or two days of therapy and generally resolve after the first 2 - 4 weeks. In one clinical study, the monthly prevalence of nervous system symptoms of at least moderate severity between weeks 4 and 48, ranged from 5% - 9% in patients treated with regimens containing efavirenz and 3% - 5% in patients treated with the control regimen. In a study of uninfected volunteers, a representative nervous system symptom had a median time to onset of 1 hour post-dose and a median duration of 3 hours. Nervous system symptoms may occur more frequently when efavirenz is taken concomitantly with meals possibly due to increased efavirenz plasma levels (see section 5.2). Dosing at bedtime seems to improve the tolerability of these symptoms and can be recommended during the first weeks of therapy and in patients who continue to experience these symptoms (see section 4.2). Dose reduction or splitting the daily dose has not been shown to provide benefit.

Analysis of long-term data from study 006 (median follow-up 180 weeks, 102 weeks, and 76 weeks for patients treated with efavirenz + zidovudine + lamivudine, efavirenz + indinavir, and indinavir + zidovudine + lamivudine, respectively) showed that, beyond 24 weeks of therapy, the incidences of new-onset nervous system symptoms among efavirenz-treated patients were generally similar to those in the control arm.

Adverse reactions of moderate or greater severity with at least possible relationship to treatment regimen (based on investigator attribution) reported in clinical trials of efavirenz at the recommended dose in combination therapy (n = 1,008) are listed below. Frequency is defined using the following convention: very common (⩾ 1/10); common (⩾ 1/100, < 1/10); uncommon (⩾ 1/1,000, < 1/100); rare (⩾ 1/10,000, < 1/1,000); very rare (< 1/10,000).

<u>Immune system disorders</u>

uncommon: hypersensitivity

<u>Psychiatric disorders</u>

common: anxiety, depression

uncommon: affect lability, aggression, euphoric mood, hallucination, mania, paranoia, suicide attempt, suicide ideation

<u>Nervous system disorders</u>

common: abnormal dreams, disturbance in attention, dizziness, headache, insomnia, somnolence

uncommon: agitation, amnesia, ataxia, coordination abnormal, confusional state, convulsions, thinking abnormal

<u>Eye disorders</u>

uncommon: vision blurred

<u>Ear and labyrinth disorders</u>

uncommon: vertigo

<u>Gastrointestinal disorders</u>

common: abdominal pain, diarrhoea, nausea, vomiting

uncommon: pancreatitis acute

<u>Hepatobiliary disorders</u>

uncommon: hepatitis acute

<u>Skin and subcutaneous tissue disorders</u>

very common: rash

common: pruritus

uncommon: erythema multiforme

<u>General disorders and administration site conditions</u>

common: fatigue

Immune Reactivation Syndrome: in HIV infected patients with severe immune deficiency at the time of initiation of combination antiretroviral therapy (CART), an inflammatory reaction to asymptomatic or residual opportunistic infections may arise (see section 4.4).

Lipodystrophy and metabolic abnormalities: combination antiretroviral therapy has been associated with redistribution of body fat (lipodystrophy) in HIV patients including the loss of peripheral and facial subcutaneous fat, increased intra-abdominal and visceral fat, breast hypertrophy and dorsocervical fat accumulation (buffalo hump).

Combination antiretroviral therapy has been associated with metabolic abnormalities such as hypertriglyceridaemia, hypercholesterolaemia, insulin resistance, hyperglycaemia and hyperlactataemia (see section 4.4).

Laboratory test abnormalities:

<u>Liver enzymes</u>: elevations of aspartate aminotransferase (AST) and alanine aminotransferase (ALT) to greater than five times the upper limit of the normal range (ULN) were seen in 3% of 1,008 patients treated with 600 mg of efavirenz (5-8% after long-term treatment in study 006). Similar elevations were seen in patients treated with control regimens (5% after long-term treatment). Elevations of gamma-glutamyltransferase (GGT) to greater than five times ULN were observed in 4% of all patients treated with 600 mg of efavirenz and 1.5-2% of patients treated with control regimens (7% of efavirenz-treated patients and 3% of control-treated patients after long-term treatment). Isolated elevations of GGT in patients receiving efavirenz may reflect enzyme induction. In the long-term study (006), 1% of patients in each treatment arm discontinued because of liver or biliary system disorders.

In the long-term data set from study 006, 137 patients treated with efavirenz-containing regimens (median duration of therapy, 68 weeks) and 84 treated with a control regimen (median duration, 56 weeks) were seropositive at screening for hepatitis B (surface antigen positive) and/or C (hepatitis C antibody positive). Among these co-infected patients, elevations in AST to greater than five times ULN developed in 13% of patients in the efavirenz arms and 7% of those in the control arm, and elevations in ALT to greater than five times ULN developed in 20% of patients in the efavirenz arms and 7% of the patients in the control arm. Among co-infected patients, 3% of those treated with efavirenz-containing regimens and 2% in the control arm discontinued from the study because of liver or biliary system disorders. Reasons for discontinuation among co-infected recipients of efavirenz included abnormalities in hepatic enzymes; there were no discontinuations reported in this study for cholestatic hepatitis, hepatic failure, or fatty liver (see section 4.4).

<u>Amylase</u>: in the clinical trial subset of 1,008 patients, asymptomatic increases in serum amylase levels greater than 1.5 times the upper limit of normal were seen in 10% of patients treated with efavirenz and 6% of patients treated with control regimens. The clinical significance of asymptomatic increases in serum amylase is unknown.

<u>Lipids</u>: increases in total cholesterol of 10 - 20% have been observed in some uninfected volunteers receiving efavirenz. Increases in non-fasting total cholesterol and HDL of approximately 20% and 25%, respectively, were observed in patients treated with efavirenz + zidovudine + lamivudine and of approximately 40% and 35%, in patients treated with efavirenz + indinavir. The effects of efavirenz on triglycerides and LDL were not well characterised. The clinical significance of these findings is unknown (see section 4.4).

<u>Cannabinoid test interaction</u>: efavirenz does not bind to cannabinoid receptors. False positive urine cannabinoid test results have been reported in uninfected volunteers who received efavirenz. False positive test results have only been observed with the CEDIA DAU Multi-Level THC assay, which is used for screening, and have not been observed with other cannabinoid assays tested including tests used for confirmation of positive results.

Postmarketing experience with efavirenz has shown the following additional adverse events to occur in association with efavirenz-containing antiretroviral treatment regimens: delusion, gynaecomastia, hepatic failure, neurosis, photoallergic dermatitis, psychosis and completed suicide.

Adolescents and children: undesirable effects in children were generally similar to those of adult patients. Rash was reported more frequently in children (in a clinical study including 57 children who received efavirenz during a 48-week period, rash was reported in 46%) and was more often of higher grade than in adults (severe rash was reported in 5.3% of children). Prophylaxis with appropriate antihistamines prior to initiating therapy with efavirenz in children may be considered. Although nervous system symptoms are difficult for young children to report, they appear to be less frequent in children and were generally mild. In the study of 57 children, 3.5% of patients experienced nervous system symptoms of moderate intensity, predominantly dizziness. No child had severe symptoms or had to discontinue because of nervous system symptoms.

4.9 Overdose

Some patients accidentally taking 600 mg twice daily have reported increased nervous system symptoms. One patient experienced involuntary muscle contractions.

Treatment of overdose with efavirenz should consist of general supportive measures, including monitoring of vital signs and observation of the patient's clinical status. Administration of activated charcoal may be used to aid removal of unabsorbed efavirenz. There is no specific antidote for overdose with efavirenz. Since efavirenz is highly protein bound, dialysis is unlikely to remove significant quantities of it from blood.

5. PHARMACOLOGICAL PROPERTIES

5.1 Pharmacodynamic properties

Pharmacotherapeutic group: HIV-1 specific NNRTI.

ATC code: J05A G03

Mechanism of action: efavirenz is a NNRTI of HIV-1. Efavirenz is a non-competitive inhibitor of HIV-1 reverse transcriptase (RT) and does not significantly inhibit HIV-2 RT or cellular DNA polymerases (α, β, γ or δ).

Antiviral activity: the free concentration of efavirenz required for 90 to 95% inhibition of wild type or zidovudine-resistant laboratory and clinical isolates *in vitro* ranged from 0.46 to 6.8 nM in lymphoblastoid cell lines, peripheral blood mononuclear cells (PBMCs) and macrophage/monocyte cultures.

Resistance: the potency of efavirenz in cell culture against viral variants with amino acid substitutions at positions 48, 108, 179, 181 or 236 in RT or variants with amino acid substitutions in the protease was similar to that observed against wild type viral strains. The single substitutions which led to the highest resistance to efavirenz in cell culture correspond to a leucine-to-isoleucine change at position 100 (L100I, 17 to 22-fold resistance) and a lysine-to-asparagine at position 103 (K103N, 18 to 33-fold resistance). Greater than 100-fold loss of susceptibility was observed against HIV variants expressing K103N in addition to other amino acid substitutions in RT.

K103N was the most frequently observed RT substitution in viral isolates from patients who experienced a significant rebound in viral load during clinical studies of efavirenz in combination with indinavir or zidovudine + lamivudine. This mutation was observed in 90% of patients receiving efavirenz with virological failure. Substitutions at RT positions 98, 100, 101, 108, 138, 188, 190 or 225 were also observed, but at lower frequencies, and often only in combination with K103N. The pattern of amino acid substitutions in RT associated with resistance to efavirenz was independent of the other antiviral medications used in combination with efavirenz.

Cross resistance: cross resistance profiles for efavirenz, nevirapine and delavirdine in cell culture demonstrated that the K103N substitution confers loss of susceptibility to all three NNRTIs. Two of three delavirdine-resistant clinical isolates examined were cross-resistant to efavirenz and contained the K103N substitution. A third isolate which carried a substitution at position 236 of RT was not cross-resistant to efavirenz.

Viral isolates recovered from PBMCs of patients enrolled in efavirenz clinical studies who showed evidence of treatment failure (viral load rebound) were assessed for susceptibility to NNRTIs. Thirteen isolates previously characterised as efavirenz-resistant were also resistant to nevirapine and delavirdine. Five of these NNRTI-resistant isolates were found to have K103N or a valine-to-isoleucine substitution at position 108 (V108I) in RT. Three of the efavirenz treatment failure isolates tested remained sensitive to efavirenz in cell culture and were also sensitive to nevirapine and delavirdine.

The potential for cross resistance between efavirenz and PIs is low because of the different enzyme targets involved. The potential for cross-resistance between efavirenz and NRTIs is low because of the different binding sites on the target and mechanism of action.

Pharmacodynamic effects

Efavirenz has not been studied in controlled studies in patients with advanced HIV disease, namely with CD4 counts < 50 cells/mm^3, or in PI or NNRTI experienced patients. Clinical experience in controlled studies with combinations including didanosine or zalcitabine is limited.

Two controlled studies (006 and ACTG 364) of approximately one year duration with efavirenz in combination with NRTIs and/or PIs, have demonstrated reduction of viral load below the limit of quantification of the assay and increased CD4 lymphocytes in antiretroviral therapy-naïve and NRTI-experienced HIV-infected patients. Study 020 showed similar activity in NRTI-experienced patients over 24 weeks. In these studies the dose of efavirenz was 600 mg once daily; the dose of indinavir was 1,000 mg every 8 hours when used with efavirenz and 800 mg every 8 hours when used without efavirenz. The dose of nelfinavir was 750 mg given three times a day. The standard doses of NRTIs given every 12 hours were used in each of these studies.

Table 2 Efficacy results for study 006

		Responder rates (NC = F[a]) Plasma HIV-RNA		Mean change from baseline-CD4 cell count
		< 400 copies/ml (95% C.I.[b])	< 50 copies/ml (95% C.I.[b])	cells/mm^3 (S.E.M.[c])
Treatment Regimen[d]	n	48 weeks	48 weeks	48 weeks
EFV + ZDV + 3TC	202	67% (60%, 73%)	62% (55%, 69%)	187 (11.8)
EFV + IDV	206	54% (47%, 61%)	48% (41%, 55%)	177 (11.3)
IDV + ZDV + 3TC	206	45% (38%, 52%)	40% (34%, 47%)	153 (12.3)

[a] NC = F, noncompleter = failure.

[b] C.I., confidence interval.

[c] S.E.M., standard error of the mean.

[d] EFV, efavirenz; ZDV, zidovudine; 3TC, lamivudine; IDV, indinavir.

Study 006, a randomized, open-label trial, compared efavirenz + zidovudine + lamivudine or efavirenz + indinavir with indinavir + zidovudine + lamivudine in 1,266 patients who were required to be efavirenz-, lamivudine-, NNRTI-, and PI-naive at study entry. The mean baseline CD4 cell count was 341 cells/mm3 and the mean baseline HIV-RNA level was 60,250 copies/ml. Efficacy results for study 006 on a subset of 614 patients who had been enrolled for at least 48 weeks are found in Table 2. In the analysis of responder rates (the non-completer equals failure analysis [NC = F]), patients who terminated the study early for any reason, or who had a missing HIV-RNA measurement that was either preceded or followed by a measurement above the limit of assay quantification were considered to have HIV-RNA above 50 or above 400 copies/ml at the missing time points.

Table 2: Efficacy results for study 006

(see Table 2 above)

Long-term results at 168 weeks of study 006 (160 patients completed study on treatment with EFV+IDV, 196 patients with EFV+ZDV+3TC and 127 patients with IDV+ZDV+3TC, respectively), suggest durability of response in terms of proportions of patients with HIV RNA < 400 copies/ml, HIV RNA < 50 copies/ml and in terms of mean change from baseline CD4 cell count.

Efficacy results for studies ACTG 364 and 020 are found in Table 3. Study ACTG 364 enrolled 196 patients who had been treated with NRTIs but not with PIs or NNRTIs. Study 020 enrolled 327 patients who had been treated with NRTIs but not with PIs or NNRTIs. Physicians were allowed to change their patient's NRTI regimen upon entry into the study. Responder rates were highest in patients who switched NRTIs.

Table 3: Efficacy results for studies ACTG 364 and 020

(see Table 3 below)

Paediatric trial: ACTG 382 is an ongoing uncontrolled study of 57 NRTI-experienced paediatric patients (3 - 16 years) which characterises the pharmacokinetics, antiviral activity and safety of efavirenz in combination with nelfinavir (20 - 30 mg/kg given three times a day) and one or more NRTIs. The starting dose of efavirenz was the equivalent of a 600 mg dose (adjusted from calculated body size based on weight). The response rate, based on the NC = F analysis of the percentage of patients with plasma HIV-RNA < 400 copies/ml at 48 weeks was 60% (95%, C.I. 47, 72), and 53% (C.I. 40, 66) based on percentage of patients with plasma HIV-RNA < 50 copies/ml. The mean CD4 cell counts were increased by 63 ± 34.5 cells/mm^3 from baseline. The durability of the response was similar to that seen in adult patients.

5.2 Pharmacokinetic properties

Absorption: peak efavirenz plasma concentrations of 1.6 - 9.1 μM were attained by 5 hours following single oral doses of 100 mg to 1,600 mg administered to uninfected volunteers. Dose related increases in C_{max} and AUC were seen for doses up to 1,600 mg; the increases were less than proportional suggesting diminished absorption at higher doses. Time to peak plasma concentrations (3 - 5 hours) did not change following multiple dosing and steady-state plasma concentrations were reached in 6 - 7 days.

In HIV infected patients at steady state, mean C_{max}, mean C_{min}, and mean AUC were linear with 200 mg, 400 mg, and 600 mg daily doses. In 35 patients receiving efavirenz 600 mg once daily, steady state C_{max} was 12.9 ± 3.7 μM (29%) [mean ± S.D. (% C.V.)], steady state C_{min} was 5.6 ± 3.2 μM (57%), and AUC was 184 ± 73 μM·h (40%).

The effect of food: the bioavailability of a single 600 mg dose of efavirenz in uninfected volunteers was increased 22% and 17%, respectively, when given with a meal of high fat or normal composition, relative to the bioavailability of a 600 mg dose given under fasted conditions (see section 4.4).

Distribution: efavirenz is highly bound (approximately 99.5 - 99.75%) to human plasma proteins, predominantly albumin. In HIV-1 infected patients (n = 9) who received efavirenz 200 to 600 mg once daily for at least one month, cerebrospinal fluid concentrations ranged from 0.26 to 1.19% (mean 0.69%) of the corresponding plasma concentration. This proportion is approximately 3-fold higher than the non-protein-bound (free) fraction of efavirenz in plasma.

Table 3 Efficacy results for studies ACTG 364 and 020

		Responder rates (NC = F[a]) Plasma HIV-RNA				Mean change from baseline-CD4 cell count	
Study Number/ Treatment Regimens[b]	n	%	(95% C.I.[c])	%	(95% C.I.)	cells/mm^3	(S.E.M.[d])
Study ACTG 364 48 weeks		< 500 copies/ml		< 50 copies/ml			
EFV + NFV + NRTIs	65	70	(59, 82)	—	—	107	(17.9)
EFV + NRTIs	65	58	(46, 70)	—	—	114	(21.0)
NFV + NRTIs	66	30	(19, 42)	—	—	94	(13.6)
Study 020 24 weeks		< 400 copies/ml		< 50 copies/ml			
EFV + IDV + NRTIs	157	60	(52, 68)	49	(41, 58)	104	(9.1)
IDV + NRTIs	170	51	(43, 59)	38	(30, 45)	77	(9.9)

[a] NC = F, noncompleter = failure.

[b] EFV, efavirenz; ZDV, zidovudine; 3TC, lamivudine; IDV, indinavir; NRTI, nucleoside reverse transcriptase inhibitor; NFV, nelfinavir.

[c] C.I., confidence interval for proportion of patients in response.

[d] S.E.M., standard error of the mean.

—, not performed.

Biotransformation: studies in humans and *in vitro* studies using human liver microsomes have demonstrated that efavirenz is principally metabolised by the cytochrome P450 system to hydroxylated metabolites with subsequent glucuronidation of these hydroxylated metabolites. These metabolites are essentially inactive against HIV-1. The *in vitro* studies suggest that CYP3A4 and CYP2B6 are the major isozymes responsible for efavirenz metabolism and that it inhibited P450 isozymes 2C9, 2C19, and 3A4. In *in vitro* studies efavirenz did not inhibit CYP2E1 and inhibited CYP2D6 and CYP1A2 only at concentrations well above those achieved clinically.

Efavirenz has been shown to induce P450 enzymes, resulting in the induction of its own metabolism. In uninfected volunteers, multiple doses of 200 - 400 mg per day for 10 days resulted in a lower than predicted extent of accumulation (22 - 42% lower) and a shorter terminal half-life of 40 - 55 hours (single dose half-life 52 - 76 hours).

Elimination: efavirenz has a relatively long terminal half-life of 52 to 76 hours after single doses and 40 - 55 hours after multiple doses. Approximately 14 - 34% of a radiolabelled dose of efavirenz was recovered in the urine and less than 1% of the dose was excreted in urine as unchanged efavirenz.

In the single patient studied with severe hepatic impairment (Child Pugh Grade C), half life was doubled indicating a potential for a much greater degree of accumulation.

Paediatric pharmacokinetics: in 49 paediatric patients receiving the equivalent of a 600 mg dose of efavirenz (dose adjusted from calculated body size based on weight), steady state C_{max} was 14.1 μM, steady state C_{min} was 5.6 μM, and AUC was 216 μM·h. The pharmacokinetics of efavirenz in paediatric patients were similar to adults.

Gender, race, elderly: pharmacokinetics of efavirenz in patients appear to be similar between men and women and among the racial groups studied. Although limited data suggest that Asian and Pacific Island patients may have higher exposure to efavirenz, they do not appear to be less tolerant of efavirenz. Pharmacokinetic studies have not been performed in the elderly.

5.3 Preclinical safety data

Efavirenz was not mutagenic or clastogenic in conventional genotoxicity assays.

Efavirenz induced foetal resorptions in rats. Malformations were observed in 3 of 20 foetuses/ newborns from efavirenz-treated cynomolgus monkeys given doses resulting in plasma efavirenz concentrations similar to those seen in humans. Anencephaly and unilateral anophthalmia with secondary enlargement of the tongue were observed in one foetus, microophthalmia was observed in another foetus, and cleft palate was observed in a third foetus. No malformations were observed in foetuses from efavirenz-treated rats and rabbits.

Biliary hyperplasia was observed in cynomolgus monkeys given efavirenz for ⩾ 1 year at a dose resulting in mean AUC values approximately 2-fold greater than those in humans given the recommended dose. The biliary hyperplasia regressed upon cessation of dosing. Biliary fibrosis has been observed in rats. Non-sustained convulsions were observed in some monkeys receiving efavirenz for ⩾ 1 year, at doses yielding plasma AUC values 4- to 13-fold greater than those in humans given the recommended dose (see sections 4.4 and 4.8).

Carcinogenicity studies showed an increased incidence of hepatic and pulmonary tumours in female mice, but not in male mice. The mechanism of tumour formation and the potential relevance for humans are not known.

Carcinogenicity studies in male mice, male and female rats were negative. While the carcinogenic potential in humans is unknown, these data suggest that the clinical benefit of efavirenz outweighs the potential carcinogenic risk to humans.

6. PHARMACEUTICAL PARTICULARS

6.1 List of excipients

Sodium laurilsulfate, lactose monohydrate, magnesium stearate and sodium starch glycolate.

Capsule shell:

50 mg Capsules: gelatine, sodium laurilsulfate, yellow iron oxide (E172), titanium dioxide (E171) and silicon dioxide.

100 mg Capsules: gelatine, sodium laurilsulfate, titanium dioxide (E171) and silicon dioxide.

200 mg Capsules: gelatine, sodium laurilsulfate, yellow iron oxide (E172) and silicon dioxide.

Printing ink: cochineal carminic acid (E120), indigo carmine (E132) and titanium dioxide (E171).

6.2 Incompatibilities

Not applicable.

6.3 Shelf life

3 years.

6.4 Special precautions for storage

No special precautions for storage.

6.5 Nature and contents of container

SUSTIVA 50 mg or SUSTIVA 100 mg capsules - HDPE bottles with a child-resistant polypropylene closure. Bottles of 30 hard capsules.

SUSTIVA 200 mg - HDPE bottles with a child-resistant polypropylene closure. Bottles of 90 hard capsules.

6.6 Instructions for use and handling

No special requirements.

7. MARKETING AUTHORISATION HOLDER

Bristol-Myers Squibb Pharma EEIG

141 - 149 Staines Road

Hounslow TW3 3JA

United Kingdom

8. MARKETING AUTHORISATION NUMBER(S)

SUSTIVA 50 mg hard capsules, bottle of 30 hard capsules EU/1/99/110/001

SUSTIVA 100 mg hard capsules, bottle of 30 hard capsules EU/1/99/110/002

SUSTIVA 200 mg hard capsules, bottle of 90 hard capsules EU/1/99/110/003

9. DATE OF FIRST AUTHORISATION/RENEWAL OF THE AUTHORISATION

Date of first authorisation: 28 May 1999

Date of last renewal: 29 April 2004

10. DATE OF REVISION OF THE TEXT

August 2005

Sustiva 600 mg Film-Coated Tablets

(Bristol-Myers Squibb Pharmaceuticals Ltd)

1. NAME OF THE MEDICINAL PRODUCT

SUSTIVA 600 mg film-coated tablets

2. QUALITATIVE AND QUANTITATIVE COMPOSITION

Each film-coated tablet contains 600 mg efavirenz.

For excipients, see section 6.1.

3. PHARMACEUTICAL FORM

Film-coated tablet

SUSTIVA 600 mg film-coated tablets are dark yellow, capsule-shaped, printed with "SUSTIVA" on both sides.

4. CLINICAL PARTICULARS

4.1 Therapeutic indications

SUSTIVA is indicated in antiviral combination treatment of HIV-1 infected adults, adolescents and children 3 years of age and older.

SUSTIVA has not been adequately studied in patients with advanced HIV disease, namely in patients with CD4 counts < 50 cells/mm^3, or after failure of protease inhibitor (PI) containing regimens. Although cross-resistance of efavirenz with PIs has not been documented, there are at present insufficient data on the efficacy of subsequent use of PI based combination therapy after failure of regimens containing SUSTIVA.

For a summary of clinical and pharmacodynamic information, see section 5.1.

4.2 Posology and method of administration

Concomitant antiretroviral therapy: SUSTIVA must be given in combination with other antiretroviral medications (see section4.5).

It is recommended that SUSTIVA be taken on an empty stomach. The increased efavirenz concentrations observed following administration of SUSTIVA with food may lead to an increase in frequency of adverse events (see sections 4.4 and 5.2).

In order to improve the tolerability of nervous system undesirable effects, bedtime dosing is recommended (see section4.8).

Therapy should be initiated by a physician experienced in the management of HIV infection.

Adults and adolescents over 40 kg: the recommended dosage of SUSTIVA in combination with nucleoside analogue reverse transcriptase inhibitors (NRTIs) with or without a PI (see section 4.5) is 600 mg orally, once daily.

Efavirenz film-coated tablets are not suitable for children weighing less than 40 kg. Efavirenz hard capsules are available for these patients.

Renal insufficiency: the pharmacokinetics of efavirenz have not been studied in patients with renal insufficiency; however, less than 1% of an efavirenz dose is excreted unchanged in the urine, so the impact of renal impairment on efavirenz elimination should be minimal (see section 4.4).

Liver disease: patients with mild to moderate liver disease may be treated with their normally recommended dose of efavirenz. Patients should be monitored carefully for dose-related adverse events, especially nervous system symptoms (see sections 4.3 and 4.4).

4.3 Contraindications

SUSTIVA is contraindicated in patients with clinically significant hypersensitivity to the active substance or to any of the excipients.

Efavirenz must not be used in patients with severe hepatic impairment (Child Pugh Grade C) (see section 5.2).

Efavirenz must not be administered concurrently with terfenadine, astemizole, cisapride, midazolam, triazolam, pimozide, bepridil, or ergot alkaloids (for example, ergotamine, dihydroergotamine, ergonovine, and methylergonovine) because competition for CYP3A4 by efavirenz could result in inhibition of metabolism and create the potential for serious and/or life-threatening undesirable effects [for example, cardiac arrhythmias, prolonged sedation or respiratory depression] (see section4.5).

Herbal preparations containing St. John's wort (*Hypericum perforatum)* must not be used while taking efavirenz due to the risk of decreased plasma concentrations and reduced clinical effects of efavirenz (see section 4.5).

SUSTIVA must not be administered concurrently with voriconazole because efavirenz significantly decreases voriconazole plasma concentrations while voriconazole also significantly increases efavirenz plasma concentrations (see section 4.5).

4.4 Special warnings and special precautions for use

Efavirenz must not be used as a single agent to treat HIV or added on as a sole agent to a failing regimen. As with all other non-nucleoside reverse transcriptase inhibitors (NNRTIs), resistant virus emerges rapidly when efavirenz is administered as monotherapy. The choice of new antiretroviral agent(s) to be used in combination with efavirenz should take into consideration the potential for viral cross-resistance (see section 5.1).

When prescribing medicinal products concomitantly with SUSTIVA, physicians should refer to the corresponding Summary of Product Characteristics.

Patients should be advised that current antiretroviral therapy, including efavirenz, has not been proven to prevent the risk of transmission of HIV to others through sexual contact or blood contamination. Appropriate precautions should continue to be employed.

If any antiretroviral medicinal product in a combination regimen is interrupted because of suspected intolerance, serious consideration should be given to simultaneous discontinuation of all antiretroviral medicinal products. The antiretroviral medicinal products should be restarted at the same time upon resolution of the intolerance symptoms. Intermittent monotherapy and sequential reintroduction of antiretroviral agents is not advisable because of the increased potential for selection of resistant virus.

Rash: mild-to-moderate rash has been reported in clinical studies with efavirenz and usually resolves with continued therapy. Appropriate antihistamines and/or corticosteroids may improve the tolerability and hasten the resolution of rash. Severe rash associated with blistering, moist desquamation or ulceration has been reported in less than 1% of patients treated with efavirenz. The incidence of erythema multiforme or Stevens-Johnson syndrome was approximately 0.1%. Efavirenz must be discontinued in patients developing severe rash associated with blistering, desquamation, mucosal involvement or fever. If therapy with efavirenz is discontinued, consideration should also be given to interrupting therapy with other antiretroviral agents to avoid development of resistant virus (see section4.8).

Rash was reported in 26 of 57 children (46%) treated with efavirenz during a 48-week period and was severe in three patients. Prophylaxis with appropriate antihistamines prior to initiating therapy with efavirenz in children may be considered.

Patients who discontinued treatment with other NNRTIs due to rash may be at higher risk of developing rash during treatment with efavirenz.

Psychiatric symptoms: psychiatric adverse experiences have been reported in patients treated with efavirenz. Patients with a prior history of psychiatric disorders appear to be at greater risk of these serious psychiatric adverse experiences. In particular, severe depression was more common in those with a history of depression. There have also been post-marketing reports of severe depression, death by suicide, delusions and psychosis-like behaviour. Patients should be advised that if they experience symptoms such as severe depression, psychosis or suicidal ideation, they should contact their doctor immediately to assess the possibility that the symptoms may be related to the use of efavirenz, and if so, to determine whether the risks of continued therapy outweigh the benefits (see section4.8).

Nervous system symptoms: symptoms including, but not limited to, dizziness, insomnia, somnolence, impaired concentration and abnormal dreaming are frequently reported undesirable effects in patients receiving efavirenz 600 mg daily in clinical studies (see section 4.8). Nervous system symptoms usually begin during the first one or two days of therapy and generally resolve after the first 2 - 4 weeks. Patients should be informed that if they do occur, these common symptoms are likely to improve with continued therapy and are not predictive of subsequent onset of any of the less frequent psychiatric symptoms.

Effect of food: the administration of SUSTIVA with food may increase efavirenz exposure (see section 5.2) and may lead to an increase in the frequency of undesirable effects. This effect may be more evident for the film-coated tablets than for the hard capsules. It is recommended that SUSTIVA be taken on an empty stomach, preferably at bedtime.

Cholesterol: monitoring of cholesterol should be considered in patients treated with efavirenz (see section 4.8).

Immune Reactivation Syndrome: in HIV infected patients with severe immune deficiency at the time of institution of combination antiretroviral therapy (CART), an inflammatory reaction to asymptomatic or residual opportunistic pathogens may arise and cause serious clinical conditions, or aggravation of symptoms. Typically, such reactions have been observed within the first few weeks or months of initiation of CART. Relevant examples are cytomegalovirus retinitis, generalised and/or focal mycobacterial infections, and *Pneumocystis carinii* pneumonia. Any inflammatory symptoms should be evaluated and treatment instituted when necessary.

Lipodystrophy and metabolic abnormalities: combination antiretroviral therapy has been associated with the redistribution of body fat (lipodystrophy) in HIV patients. The long-term consequences of these events are currently unknown. Knowledge about the mechanism is incomplete. A connection between visceral lipomatosis and PIs and lipoatrophy and NRTIs has been hypothesised. A higher risk of lipodystrophy has been associated with individual factors such as older age, and with drug related factors such as longer duration of antiretroviral treatment and associated metabolic disturbances. Clinical examination should include evaluation for physical signs of fat redistribution. Consideration should be given to the measurement of fasting serum lipids and blood glucose. Lipid disorders should be managed as clinically appropriate (see section 4.8).

Lactose: this medicinal product contains 250 mg of lactose in each 600-mg daily dose. This quantity is not likely to induce symptoms of lactose intolerance.

Efavirenz film-coated tablets are unsuitable for individuals with the rare hereditary disorders of galactosaemia or glucose/galactose malabsorption syndrome. Individuals with these conditions may take efavirenz oral solution, which is free from lactose.

Special populations:

Liver disease: because of the extensive cytochrome P450-mediated metabolism of efavirenz and limited clinical experience in patients with chronic liver disease, caution must be exercised in administering efavirenz to patients with mild-to-moderate liver disease. Patients should be monitored carefully for dose-related adverse events, especially nervous system symptoms. Laboratory tests should be performed to evaluate their liver disease at periodic intervals (see section 4.2).

The safety and efficacy of efavirenz has not been established in patients with significant underlying liver disorders. Efavirenz is contraindicated in patients with severe hepatic impairment (see section 4.3). Patients with chronic hepatitis B or C and treated with combination antiretroviral therapy are at increased risk for severe and potentially fatal hepatic adverse events. Patients with pre-existing liver dysfunction including chronic active hepatitis have an increased frequency of liver function abnormalities during combination antiretroviral therapy and should be monitored according to standard practice. If there is evidence of worsening liver disease or persistent elevations of serum transaminases to greater than 5 times the upper limit of the normal range, the benefit of continued therapy with efavirenz needs to be weighed against the potential risks of significant liver toxicity. In such patients, interruption or discontinuation of treatment must be considered (see section 4.8).

In patients treated with other medicinal products associated with liver toxicity, monitoring of liver enzymes is also recommended. In case of concomitant antiviral therapy for hepatitis B or C, please refer also to the relevant product information for these medicinal products.

Renal insufficiency: the pharmacokinetics of efavirenz have not been studied in patients with renal insufficiency; however, less than 1% of an efavirenz dose is excreted unchanged in the urine, so the impact of renal impairment on efavirenz elimination should be minimal (see section 4.2). There is no experience in patients with severe renal failure and close safety monitoring is recommended in this population.

Elderly: insufficient numbers of elderly patients have been evaluated in clinical studies to determine whether they respond differently than younger patients.

Children: efavirenz has not been evaluated in children below 3 years of age or who weigh less than 13 kg.

Seizures: convulsions have been observed rarely in patients receiving efavirenz, generally in the presence of known medical history of seizures. Patients who are receiving concomitant anticonvulsant medicinal products primarily metabolised by the liver, such as phenytoin, carbamazepine and phenobarbital, may require periodic monitoring of plasma levels. Caution must be taken in any patient with a history of seizures.

4.5 Interaction with other medicinal products and other forms of Interaction

Efavirenz is an inducer of CYP3A4 and an inhibitor of some CYP isozymes including CYP3A4 (see section 5.2). Other compounds that are substrates of CYP3A4 may have decreased plasma concentrations when co-administered with efavirenz. Efavirenz exposure may also be altered when given with medicinal products or food (for example, grapefruit juice) which affect CYP3A4 activity.

Efavirenz must not be administered concurrently with terfenadine, astemizole, cisapride, midazolam, triazolam, pimozide, bepridil, or ergot alkaloids (for example, ergotamine, dihydroergotamine, ergonovine, and methylergonovine) since inhibition of their metabolism may lead to serious, life-threatening events (see section 4.3).

Concomitant antiretroviral agents

Protease Inhibitors:

Amprenavir: although efavirenz has been seen to decrease the C_{max}, AUC and C_{min} of amprenavir by approximately 40% in adults, when amprenavir is combined with ritonavir, the effect of efavirenz is compensated by the pharmacokinetic booster effect of ritonavir. Therefore, if efavirenz is given in combination with amprenavir (600 mg twice daily) and ritonavir (100 or 200 mg twice daily), no dosage adjustment is necessary.

Further, if efavirenz is given in combination with amprenavir and nelfinavir, no dosage adjustment is necessary for any of the medicinal products. Treatment with efavirenz in combination with amprenavir and saquinavir is not recommended, as the exposure to both PIs is expected to be significantly decreased. No dose recommendation can be given for the co-administration of amprenavir with another PI and efavirenz in children and patients with renal impairment. Such combinations should be avoided in patients with hepatic impairment.

Indinavir: when indinavir (800 mg every 8 hours) was given with efavirenz (200 mg every 24 hours), the indinavir AUC and C_{trough} were decreased by approximately 31% and 40% respectively. When indinavir at an increased dose (1,000 mg every 8 hours) was given with efavirenz (600 mg once daily) in uninfected volunteers, the indinavir AUC and C_{trough} were decreased on average by 33 - 46% and 39 - 57%, respectively (ranges represent diurnal variation), compared to when indinavir was given alone at the standard dose (800 mg every 8 hours). Similar differences in indinavir AUC and C_{trough} were also observed in HIV-infected patients who received indinavir (1,000 mg every 8 hours) with efavirenz (600 mg once daily) compared to indinavir given alone (800 mg every 8 hours). While the clinical significance of decreased indinavir concentrations has not been established, the magnitude of the observed pharmacokinetic interaction should be taken into consideration when choosing a regimen containing both efavirenz and indinavir.

When efavirenz 600 mg once daily was given with indinavir/ritonavir 800/100 mg twice daily in uninfected volunteers (n = 14), the indinavir AUC, C_{min}, and C_{max} were decreased by approximately 25%, 50% and 17%, respectively, compared to when indinavir/ritonavir 800/100 mg twice daily were given without efavirenz. The geometric mean C_{min} for indinavir (0.33 mg/l) when given with ritonavir and efavirenz was higher than the mean historical C_{min} (0.15 mg/l) when indinavir was given alone at 800 mg every 8 hours. The pharmacokinetics of efavirenz given in combination with indinavir/ritonavir were comparable to efavirenz alone (600 mg once daily).

When efavirenz 600 mg once daily was given with indinavir/ritonavir 800/100 mg twice daily in HIV-1 infected patients (n = 6), the pharmacokinetics of indinavir and efavirenz were generally comparable to these uninfected volunteer data.

No adjustment of the dose of efavirenz is necessary when given with indinavir or indinavir/ritonavir.

Lopinavir/ritonavir: when used in combination with efavirenz and two NRTIs, 533/133 mg lopinavir/ritonavir twice daily yielded similar lopinavir plasma concentrations as compared to lopinavir/ritonavir 400/100 mg twice daily without efavirenz (historical data). When co-administered with efavirenz, an increase of the lopinavir/ritonavir doses by 33% should be considered (4 capsules/~6.5 ml twice daily instead of 3 capsules/5 ml twice daily). Caution is warranted since this dosage adjustment might be insufficient in some patients.

Nelfinavir: the AUC and C_{max} of nelfinavir are increased by 20% and 21%, respectively when given with efavirenz. The combination was generally well tolerated and no dose adjustment is necessary when nelfinavir is administered in combination with efavirenz.

Ritonavir: when efavirenz was given with ritonavir 500 mg or 600 mg twice daily, the combination was not well tolerated (for example, dizziness, nausea, paraesthesia and elevated liver enzymes occurred). Data on the tolerability of efavirenz with low-dose ritonavir (100 mg twice daily) alone are not available.

Saquinavir: when saquinavir (1,200 mg given 3 times a day, soft capsule formulation) was given with efavirenz, the saquinavir AUC and C_{max} were decreased by 62% and 50% respectively. Use of efavirenz in combination with saquinavir as the sole PI is not recommended.

Saquinavir/ritonavir: no data are available on the potential interactions of efavirenz with the combination of saquinavir and ritonavir.

NRTIs: studies of the interaction between efavirenz and the combination of zidovudine and lamivudine were performed in HIV-infected patients. No clinically significant pharmacokinetic interactions were observed. Specific interaction studies have not been performed with efavirenz and other NRTIs. Clinically significant interactions would not be expected since the NRTIs are metabolised via a different route than efavirenz and would be unlikely to compete for the same metabolic enzymes and elimination pathways.

NNRTIs: no studies have been performed with efavirenz in combination with other NNRTIs and the potential for pharmacokinetic or pharmacodynamic interactions is unknown.

Antimicrobial agents:

Rifamycins: rifampicin reduced efavirenz AUC by 26% and C_{max} by 20% in uninfected volunteers. The dose of efavirenz must be increased to 800 mg/day when taken with rifampicin. No dose adjustment of rifampicin is recommended when given with efavirenz. In one study in uninfected volunteers, efavirenz induced a reduction in rifabutin C_{max} and AUC by 32% and 38% respectively. Rifabutin had no significant effect on the pharmacokinetics of efavirenz. These data suggest that the daily dose of rifabutin should be increased by 50% when administered with efavirenz and that the rifabutin dose may be doubled for regimens in which rifabutin is given two or three times a week in combination with efavirenz.

Macrolide antibiotics:

Azithromycin: co-administration of single doses of azithromycin and multiple doses of efavirenz in uninfected volunteers did not result in any clinically significant pharmacokinetic interaction. No dosage adjustment is necessary when azithromycin is given in combination with efavirenz.

Clarithromycin: co-administration of 400 mg of efavirenz once daily with clarithromycin given as 500 mg every 12 hours for seven days resulted in a significant effect of efavirenz on the pharmacokinetics of clarithromycin. The AUC and C_{max} of clarithromycin decreased 39% and 26%, respectively, while the AUC and C_{max} of the active clarithromycin hydroxymetabolite were increased 34% and 49%, respectively, when used in combination with efavirenz. The clinical significance of these changes in clarithromycin plasma levels is not known. In uninfected volunteers 46% developed rash while receiving efavirenz and clarithromycin. No dose adjustment of efavirenz is recommended when given with clarithromycin. Alternatives to clarithromycin may be considered.

Other macrolide antibiotics, such as erythromycin, have not been studied in combination with efavirenz.

Antifungal agents:

Voriconazole: co-administration of efavirenz (400 mg orally once daily) with voriconazole (200 mg orally every 12 hours) in uninfected volunteers resulted in a 2-way interaction. The steady state AUC and C_{max} of voriconazole decreased by on average 77% and 61%, respectively, while the steady state AUC and C_{max} of efavirenz increased by on average 44% and 38%, respectively. Co-administration of efavirenz and voriconazole is contraindicated (see section 4.3).

No clinically significant pharmacokinetic interactions were seen when fluconazole and efavirenz were co-administered to uninfected volunteers. The potential for interactions with efavirenz and other imidazole and triazole antifungals, such as itraconazole and ketoconazole, has not been studied.

Other interactions

Antacids/famotidine: neither aluminium/magnesium hydroxide antacids nor famotidine altered the absorption of efavirenz in uninfected volunteers. These data suggest that alteration of gastric pH by other medicinal products would not be expected to affect efavirenz absorption.

Oral contraceptives: only the ethinyloestradiol component of oral contraceptives has been studied. The AUC following a single dose of ethinyloestradiol was increased (37%) after multiple dosing of efavirenz. No significant changes were observed in C_{max} of ethinyloestradiol. The clinical significance of these effects is not known. No effect of a single dose of ethinyloestradiol on efavirenz C_{max} or AUC was observed. Because the potential interaction of efavirenz with oral contraceptives has not been fully characterised, a reliable method of barrier contraception must be used in addition to oral contraceptives.

Anticonvulsants: no data are available on the potential interactions of efavirenz with phenytoin, carbamazepine or phenobarbital, or other anticonvulsants. When efavirenz is administered concomitantly with these agents, there is the potential for reduction or increase in the plasma concentrations of each agent; therefore, periodic monitoring of plasma levels should be conducted.

Methadone: in a study of HIV-infected IV drug users, co-administration of efavirenz with methadone resulted in decreased plasma levels of methadone and signs of opiate withdrawal. The methadone dose was increased by a mean of 22% to alleviate withdrawal symptoms. Patients should be monitored for signs of withdrawal and their methadone dose increased as required to alleviate withdrawal symptoms.

St. John's wort *(Hypericum perforatum)*: plasma levels of efavirenz can be reduced by concomitant use of the herbal preparation St. John's wort (*Hypericum perforatum*). This is due to induction of drug metabolising enzymes and/or transport proteins by St. John's wort. Herbal preparations containing St. John's wort must not be used concomitantly with SUSTIVA. If a patient is already taking St. John's wort, stop St. John's wort, check viral levels and if possible efavirenz levels. Efavirenz levels may increase on stopping St. John's wort and the dose of SUSTIVA may need adjusting. The inducing effect of St. John's wort may persist for at least 2 weeks after cessation of treatment (see section 4.3).

Antidepressants: there were no clinically significant effects on pharmacokinetic parameters when paroxetine and efavirenz were co-administered. No dose adjustments are necessary for either efavirenz or paroxetine when these drugs are co-administered. Since fluoxetine shares a similar metabolic profile with paroxetine, i.e. a strong CYP2D6 inhibitory effect, a similar lack of interaction would be expected for fluoxetine. Sertraline, a CYP3A4 substrate, did not significantly alter the pharmacokinetics of efavirenz. Efavirenz decreased sertraline C_{max}, C24 and AUC by 28.6 to 46.3%. Sertraline dose increases should be guided by clinical response.

Cetirizine: the H1-antihistamine, cetirizine, had no clinically significant effect on efavirenz pharmacokinetic parameters. Efavirenz decreased cetirizine C_{max} by 24% but did not alter cetirizine AUC. These changes are not considered to be clinically significant. No dose adjustments are necessary for either efavirenz or cetirizine when these drugs are co-administered.

Lorazepam: efavirenz increased lorazepam C_{max} and AUC by 16.3% and 7.3% respectively. These changes are not considered to be clinically significant. No dose adjustments are necessary for either efavirenz or lorazepam when these drugs are co-administered.

4.6 Pregnancy and lactation

Pregnancy should be avoided in women treated with efavirenz. Barrier contraception should always be used in combination with other methods of contraception (for example, oral or other hormonal contraceptives). Women of childbearing potential should undergo pregnancy testing before initiation of efavirenz. Efavirenz should not be used during pregnancy unless there are no other appropriate treatment options.

There are no adequate and well-controlled studies of efavirenz in pregnant women. In postmarketing experience through an antiretroviral pregnancy registry, more than 200 pregnancies with first-trimester exposure to efavirenz as part of a combination antiretroviral regimen have been reported with no specific malformation pattern. Retrospectively in this registry, a small number of cases of neural tube defects, including meningomyelocele, have been reported but causality has not been established. Studies in animals have shown reproductive toxicity including marked teratogenic effects (see section5.3).

Studies in rats have demonstrated that efavirenz is excreted in milk reaching concentrations much higher than those in maternal plasma. It is not known whether efavirenz is excreted in human milk. Since animal data suggest that the substance may be passed into breast milk, it is recommended that mothers taking efavirenz do not breast feed their infants. It is recommended that HIV infected women do not breast feed their infants under any circumstances in order to avoid transmission of HIV.

4.7 Effects on ability to drive and use machines

Efavirenz has not been specifically evaluated for possible effects on the ability to drive a car or operate machinery. Efavirenz may cause dizziness, impaired concentration, and/or somnolence. Patients should be instructed that if they experience these symptoms they should avoid potentially hazardous tasks such as driving or operating machinery.

4.8 Undesirable effects

Efavirenz has been studied in over 9,000 patients. In a subset of 1,008 adult patients who received 600 mg efavirenz daily in combination with PIs and/or NRTIs in controlled clinical studies, the most frequently reported treatment-related undesirable effects of at least moderate severity reported in at least 5% of patients were rash (11.6%), dizziness (8.5%), nausea (8.0%), headache (5.7%) and fatigue (5.5%). The most notable undesirable effects associated with efavirenz are rash and nervous system symptoms. The administration of SUSTIVA with food may increase efavirenz exposure and may lead to an increase in the frequency of undesirable effects (see section4.4).

The long-term safety profile of efavirenz-containing regimens was evaluated in a controlled trial (006) in which patients received efavirenz + zidovudine + lamivudine (n = 412, median duration 180 weeks), efavirenz + indinavir (n = 415, median duration 102 weeks), or indinavir + zidovudine + lamivudine (n = 401, median duration 76 weeks). Long-term use of efavirenz in this study was not associated with any new safety concerns.

Rash: in clinical studies, 26% of patients treated with 600 mg of efavirenz experienced skin rash compared with 17% of patients treated in control groups. Skin rash was considered treatment related in 18% of patients treated with efavirenz. Severe rash occurred in less than 1% of patients treated with efavirenz, and 1.7% discontinued therapy because of rash. The incidence of erythema multiforme or Stevens-Johnson syndrome was approximately 0.1%.

Rashes are usually mild-to-moderate maculopapular skin eruptions that occur within the first two weeks of initiating therapy with efavirenz. In most patients rash resolves with continuing therapy with efavirenz within one month. Efavirenz can be reinitiated in patients interrupting therapy because of rash. Use of appropriate antihistamines and/or corticosteroids is recommended when efavirenz is restarted.

Experience with efavirenz in patients who discontinued other antiretroviral agents of the NNRTI class is limited. Nineteen patients who discontinued nevirapine because of rash have been treated with efavirenz. Nine of these patients developed mild-to-moderate rash while receiving therapy with efavirenz, and two discontinued because of rash.

Psychiatric symptoms: serious psychiatric adverse experiences have been reported in patients treated with efavirenz. In controlled trials of 1,008 patients treated with regimens containing efavirenz for an average of 1.6 years and 635 patients treated with control regimens for an average of 1.3 years, the frequency of specific serious psychiatric events are detailed hereafter:

	Efavirenz regimen	Control regimen
- severe depression	1.6%	0.6%
- suicidal ideation	0.6%	0.3%
- non-fatal suicide attempts	0.4%	0%
- aggressive behaviour	0.4%	0.3%
- paranoid reactions	0.4%	0.3%
- manic reactions	0.1%	0%

Patients with a history of psychiatric disorders appear to be at greater risk of these serious psychiatric adverse experiences with the frequency of each of the above events ranging from 0.3% for manic reactions to 2.0% for both severe depression and suicidal ideation. There have also been post-marketing reports of death by suicide, delusions and psychosis-like behaviour.

Nervous system symptoms: in clinical controlled trials, frequently reported undesirable effects in patients receiving 600 mg efavirenz with other antiretroviral agents included, but were not limited to: dizziness, insomnia, somnolence, impaired concentration and abnormal dreaming. Nervous system symptoms of moderate-to-severe intensity were experienced by 19.4% of patients compared to 9.0% of patients receiving control regimens. These symptoms were severe in 2.0% of patients receiving efavirenz 600 mg daily and in 1.3% of patients receiving control regimens. In clinical studies 2.1% of patients treated with 600 mg of efavirenz discontinued therapy because of nervous system symptoms.

Nervous system symptoms usually begin during the first one or two days of therapy and generally resolve after the first 2 - 4 weeks. In one clinical study, the monthly prevalence of nervous system symptoms of at least moderate severity between weeks 4 and 48, ranged from 5% - 9% in patients treated with regimens containing efavirenz and 3% - 5% in patients treated with the control regimen. In a study of uninfected volunteers, a representative nervous system symptom had a median time to onset of 1 hour post-dose and a median duration of 3 hours. Nervous system symptoms may occur more frequently when efavirenz is taken concomitantly with meals possibly due to increased efavirenz plasma levels (see section 5.2). Dosing at bedtime seems to improve the tolerability of these symptoms and can be recommended during the first weeks of therapy and in patients who continue to experience these symptoms (see section 4.2). Dose reduction or splitting the daily dose has not been shown to provide benefit.

Analysis of long-term data from study 006 (median follow-up 180 weeks, 102 weeks, and 76 weeks for patients treated with efavirenz + zidovudine + lamivudine, efavirenz + indinavir, and indinavir + zidovudine + lamivudine, respectively) showed that, beyond 24 weeks of therapy, the incidences of new-onset nervous system symptoms among efavirenz-treated patients were generally similar to those in the control arm.

Adverse reactions of moderate or greater severity with at least possible relationship to treatment regimen (based on investigator attribution) reported in clinical trials of efavirenz at the recommended dose in combination therapy (n = 1,008) are listed below. Frequency is defined using the following convention: very common (⩾ 1/10); common (⩾ 1/100, < 1/10); uncommon (⩾ 1/1,000, < 1/100); rare (⩾ 1/10,000, < 1/1,000); very rare (< 1/10,000).

Immune system disorders

uncommon: hypersensitivity

Psychiatric disorders

common: anxiety, depression

uncommon: affect lability, aggression, euphoric mood, hallucination, mania, paranoia, suicide attempt, suicide ideation

Nervous system disorders

common: abnormal dreams, disturbance in attention, dizziness, headache, insomnia, somnolence

uncommon: agitation, amnesia, ataxia, coordination abnormal, confusional state, convulsions, thinking abnormal

Eye disorders

uncommon: vision blurred

Ear and labyrinth disorders

uncommon: vertigo

Gastrointestinal disorders

common: abdominal pain, diarrhoea, nausea, vomiting

uncommon: pancreatitis acute

Hepatobiliary disorders

uncommon: hepatitis acute

Skin and subcutaneous tissue disorders

very common: rash

common: pruritus

uncommon: erythema multiforme

General disorders and administration site conditions

common: fatigue

Immune Reactivation Syndrome: in HIV infected patients with severe immune deficiency at the time of initiation of combination antiretroviral therapy (CART), an inflammatory reaction to asymptomatic or residual opportunistic infections may arise (see section 4.4).

Lipodystrophy and metabolic abnormalities: combination antiretroviral therapy has been associated with redistribution of body fat (lipodystrophy) in HIV patients including the loss of peripheral and facial subcutaneous fat, increased intra-abdominal and visceral fat, breast hypertrophy and dorsocervical fat accumulation (buffalo hump).

Combination antiretroviral therapy has been associated with metabolic abnormalities such as hypertriglyceridaemia, hypercholesterolaemia, insulin resistance, hyperglycaemia and hyperlactataemia (see section 4.4).

Laboratory test abnormalities:

Liver enzymes: elevations of aspartate aminotransferase (AST) and alanine aminotransferase (ALT) to greater than five times the upper limit of the normal range (ULN) were seen in 3% of 1,008 patients treated with 600 mg of efavirenz (5-8% after long-term treatment in study 006). Similar elevations were seen in patients treated with control regimens (5% after long-term treatment). Elevations of gamma-glutamyltransferase (GGT) to greater than five times ULN were observed in 4% of all patients treated with 600 mg of efavirenz and 1.5-2% of patients treated with control regimens (7% of efavirenz-treated patients and 3% of control-treated patients after long-term treatment). Isolated elevations of GGT in patients receiving efavirenz may reflect enzyme induction. In the long-term study (006), 1% of patients in each treatment arm discontinued because of liver or biliary system disorders.

In the long-term data set from study 006, 137 patients treated with efavirenz-containing regimens (median duration of therapy, 68 weeks) and 84 treated with a control regimen (median duration, 56 weeks) were seropositive at screening for hepatitis B (surface antigen positive) and/or C (hepatitis C antibody positive). Among these co-infected patients, elevations in AST to greater than five times ULN developed in 13% of patients in the efavirenz arms and 7% of those in the control arm, and elevations in ALT to greater than five times ULN developed in 20% of patients in the efavirenz arms and 7% of the patients in the control arm. Among co-infected patients, 3% of those treated with efavirenz-containing regimens and 2% in the control arm discontinued from the study because of liver or biliary system disorders. Reasons for discontinuation among co-infected recipients of efavirenz included abnormalities in hepatic enzymes; there were no discontinuations reported in this study for cholestatic hepatitis, hepatic failure, or fatty liver (see section 4.4).

Amylase: in the clinical trial subset of 1,008 patients, asymptomatic increases in serum amylase levels greater than 1.5 times the upper limit of normal were seen in 10% of patients treated with efavirenz and 6% of patients treated with control regimens. The clinical significance of asymptomatic increases in serum amylase is unknown.

Lipids: increases in total cholesterol of 10 - 20% have been observed in some uninfected volunteers receiving efavirenz. Increases in non-fasting total cholesterol and HDL of approximately 20% and 25%, respectively, were observed in patients treated with efavirenz + zidovudine + lamivudine and of approximately 40% and 35%, in patients treated with efavirenz + indinavir. The effects of efavirenz on triglycerides and LDL were not well-characterised. The clinical significance of these findings is unknown (see section 4.4).

Cannabinoid test interaction: efavirenz does not bind to cannabinoid receptors. False positive urine cannabinoid test results have been reported in uninfected volunteers who received efavirenz. False positive test results have only been observed with the CEDIA DAU Multi-Level THC assay, which is used for screening, and have not been observed with other cannabinoid assays tested including tests used for confirmation of positive results.

Postmarketing experience with efavirenz has shown the following additional adverse events to occur in association with efavirenz-containing antiretroviral treatment regimens: delusion, gynaecomastia, hepatic failure, neurosis, photoallergic dermatitis, psychosis and completed suicide.

Adolescents and children: undesirable effects in children were generally similar to those of adult patients. Rash was reported more frequently in children (in a clinical study including 57 children who received efavirenz during a 48-week period, rash was reported in 46%) and was more often of higher grade than in adults (severe rash was reported in 5.3% of children). Prophylaxis with appropriate antihistamines prior to initiating therapy with efavirenz in children may be considered. Although nervous system symptoms are difficult for young children to report, they appear to be less frequent in children and were generally mild. In the study of 57 children, 3.5% of patients experienced nervous system symptoms of moderate intensity, predominantly dizziness. No child had severe symptoms or had to discontinue because of nervous system symptoms.

4.9 Overdose

Some patients accidentally taking 600 mg twice daily have reported increased nervous system symptoms. One patient experienced involuntary muscle contractions.

Treatment of overdose with efavirenz should consist of general supportive measures, including monitoring of vital signs and observation of the patient's clinical status. Administration of activated charcoal may be used to aid removal of unabsorbed efavirenz. There is no specific antidote for overdose with efavirenz. Since efavirenz is highly protein bound, dialysis is unlikely to remove significant quantities of it from blood.

5. PHARMACOLOGICAL PROPERTIES

5.1 Pharmacodynamic properties

Pharmacotherapeutic group: HIV-1 specific NNRTI.

ATC code: J05A G03

Mechanism of action: efavirenz is a NNRTI of HIV-1. Efavirenz is a non-competitive inhibitor of HIV-1 reverse transcriptase (RT) and does not significantly inhibit HIV-2 RT or cellular DNA polymerases (α, β, γ or δ).

Antiviral activity: the free concentration of efavirenz required for 90 to 95% inhibition of wild type or zidovudine-resistant laboratory and clinical isolates *in vitro* ranged from 0.46 to 6.8 nM in lymphoblastoid cell lines, peripheral blood mononuclear cells (PBMCs) and macrophage/monocyte cultures.

Resistance: the potency of efavirenz in cell culture against viral variants with amino acid substitutions at positions 48, 108, 179, 181 or 236 in RT or variants with amino acid substitutions in the protease was similar to that observed against wild type viral strains. The single substitutions which led to the highest resistance to efavirenz in cell culture correspond to a leucine-to-isoleucine change at position 100 (L100I, 17 to 22-fold resistance) and a lysine-to-asparagine at position 103 (K103N, 18 to 33-fold resistance). Greater than 100-fold loss of susceptibility was observed against HIV variants expressing K103N in addition to other amino acid substitutions in RT.

K103N was the most frequently observed RT substitution in viral isolates from patients who experienced a significant rebound in viral load during clinical studies of efavirenz in combination with indinavir or zidovudine + lamivudine. This mutation was observed in 90% of patients receiving efavirenz with virological failure. Substitutions at RT positions 98, 100, 101, 108, 138, 188, 190 or 225 were also observed, but at lower frequencies, and often only in combination with K103N. The pattern of amino acid substitutions in RT associated with resistance to efavirenz was independent of the other antiviral medications used in combination with efavirenz.

Cross resistance: cross resistance profiles for efavirenz, nevirapine and delavirdine in cell culture demonstrated that the K103N substitution confers loss of susceptibility to all three NNRTIs. Two of three delavirdine-resistant clinical isolates examined were cross-resistant to efavirenz and contained the K103N substitution. A third isolate which carried a substitution at position 236 of RT was not cross-resistant to efavirenz.

Viral isolates recovered from PBMCs of patients enrolled in efavirenz clinical studies who showed evidence of treatment failure (viral load rebound) were assessed for susceptibility to NNRTIs. Thirteen isolates previously characterised as efavirenz-resistant were also resistant to nevirapine and delavirdine. Five of these NNRTI-resistant isolates were found to have K103N or a valine-to-isoleucine substitution at position 108 (V108I) in RT. Three of the efavirenz treatment failure isolates tested remained sensitive to efavirenz in cell culture and were also sensitive to nevirapine and delavirdine.

The potential for cross resistance between efavirenz and PIs is low because of the different enzyme targets involved. The potential for cross-resistance between efavirenz and NRTIs is low because of the different binding sites on the target and mechanism of action.

Table 1 Efficacy results for study 006

		Responder rates (NC = F[a]) Plasma HIV-RNA		Mean change from baseline-CD4 cell count
		< 400 copies/ml (95% C.I.[b])	< 50 copies/ml (95% C.I.[b])	cells/mm^3 (S.E.M.[c])
Treatment Regimen[d]	n	48 weeks	48 weeks	48 weeks
EFV + ZDV + 3TC	202	67% (60%, 73%)	62% (55%, 69%)	187 (11.8)
EFV + IDV	206	54% (47%, 61%)	48% (41%, 55%)	177 (11.3)
IDV + ZDV + 3TC	206	45% (38%, 52%)	40% (34%, 47%)	153 (12.3)

[a] NC = F, noncompleter = failure.
[b] C.I., confidence interval.
[c] S.E.M., standard error of the mean.
[d] EFV, efavirenz; ZDV, zidovudine; 3TC, lamivudine; IDV, indinavir.

Pharmacodynamic effects

Efavirenz has not been studied in controlled studies in patients with advanced HIV disease, namely with CD4 counts < 50 cells/mm^3, or in PI or NNRTI experienced patients. Clinical experience in controlled studies with combinations including didanosine or zalcitabine is limited.

Two controlled studies (006 and ACTG 364) of approximately one year duration with efavirenz in combination with NRTIs and/or PIs, have demonstrated reduction of viral load below the limit of quantification of the assay and increased CD4 lymphocytes in antiretroviral therapy-naïve and NRTI-experienced HIV-infected patients. Study 020 showed similar activity in NRTI-experienced patients over 24 weeks. In these studies the dose of efavirenz was 600 mg once daily; the dose of indinavir was 1,000 mg every 8 hours when used with efavirenz and 800 mg every 8 hours when used without efavirenz. The dose of nelfinavir was 750 mg given three times a day. The standard doses of NRTIs given every 12 hours were used in each of these studies.

Study 006, a randomized, open-label trial, compared efavirenz + zidovudine + lamivudine or efavirenz + indinavir with indinavir + zidovudine + lamivudine in 1,266 patients who were required to be efavirenz-, lamivudine-, NNRTI-, and PI-naive at study entry. The mean baseline CD4 cell count was 341 cells/mm3 and the mean baseline HIV-RNA level was 60,250 copies/ml. Efficacy results for study 006 on a subset of 614 patients who had been enrolled for at least 48 weeks are found in Table 1. In the analysis of responder rates (the non-completer equals failure analysis [NC = F]), patients who terminated the study early for any reason, or who had a missing HIV-RNA measurement that was either preceded or followed by a measurement above the limit of assay quantification were considered to have HIV-RNA above 50 or above 400 copies/ml at the missing time points.

Table 1: Efficacy results for study 006

(see Table 1 above)

Long-term results at 168 weeks of study 006 (160 patients completed study on treatment with EFV+IDV, 196 patients with EFV+ZDV+3TC and 127 patients with IDV+ZDV+3TC, respectively), suggest durability of response in terms of proportions of patients with HIV RNA < 400 copies/ml, HIV RNA < 50 copies/ml and in terms of mean change from baseline CD4 cell count.

Efficacy results for studies ACTG 364 and 020 are found in Table 2. Study ACTG 364 enrolled 196 patients who had been treated with NRTIs but not with PIs or NNRTIs. Study 020 enrolled 327 patients who had been treated with NRTIs but not with PIs or NNRTIs. Physicians were allowed to change their patient's NRTI regimen upon entry into the study. Responder rates were highest in patients who switched NRTIs.

Table 2: Efficacy results for studies ACTG 364 and 020

(see Table 2 below)

Paediatric trial: ACTG 382 is an ongoing uncontrolled study of 57 NRTI-experienced paediatric patients (3 - 16 years) which characterises the pharmacokinetics, antiviral activity and safety of efavirenz in combination with nelfinavir (20 - 30 mg/kg given three times a day) and one or more NRTIs. The starting dose of efavirenz was the equivalent of a 600 mg dose (adjusted from calculated body size based on weight). The response rate, based on the NC = F analysis of the percentage of patients with plasma HIV-RNA < 400 copies/ml at 48 weeks was 60% (95%, C.I. 47, 72), and 53% (C.I. 40, 66) based on percentage of patients with plasma HIV-RNA < 50 copies/ml. The mean CD4 cell counts were increased by 63 ± 34.5 cells/mm^3 from baseline. The durability of the response was similar to that seen in adult patients.

5.2 Pharmacokinetic properties

Absorption: peak efavirenz plasma concentrations of 1.6 - 9.1 μM were attained by 5 hours following single oral doses of 100 mg to 1,600 mg administered to uninfected volunteers. Dose related increases in C_{max} and AUC were seen for doses up to 1,600 mg; the increases were less than proportional suggesting diminished absorption at higher doses. Time to peak plasma concentrations (3 - 5 hours) did not change following multiple dosing and steady-state plasma concentrations were reached in 6 - 7 days.

In HIV infected patients at steady state, mean C_{max}, mean C_{min}, and mean AUC were linear with 200 mg, 400 mg, and 600 mg daily doses. In 35 patients receiving efavirenz 600 mg once daily, steady state C_{max} was 12.9 ± 3.7 μM (29%) [mean ± S.D. (% C.V.)], steady state C_{min} was 5.6 ± 3.2 μM (57%), and AUC was 184 ± 73 μM·h (40%).

Effect of food: the AUC and C_{max} of a single 600 mg dose of efavirenz film-coated tablets in uninfected volunteers was increased by 28% (90% CI: 22-33%) and 79% (90% CI: 58-102%), respectively, when given with a high fat meal, relative to when given under fasted conditions (see section 4.4).

Distribution: efavirenz is highly bound (approximately 99.5 - 99.75%) to human plasma proteins, predominantly albumin. In HIV-1 infected patients (n = 9) who received efavirenz 200 to 600 mg once daily for at least one month, cerebrospinal fluid concentrations ranged from 0.26 to 1.19% (mean 0.69%) of the corresponding plasma concentration. This proportion is approximately 3-fold higher than the non-protein-bound (free) fraction of efavirenz in plasma.

Biotransformation: studies in humans and *in vitro* studies using human liver microsomes have demonstrated that efavirenz is principally metabolised by the cytochrome P450 system to hydroxylated metabolites with subsequent glucuronidation of these hydroxylated metabolites. These metabolites are essentially inactive against HIV-1. The *in vitro* studies suggest that CYP3A4 and CYP2B6 are the major isozymes responsible for efavirenz metabolism and that it inhibited P450 isozymes 2C9, 2C19, and 3A4. In *in vitro* studies efavirenz did not inhibit CYP2E1 and inhibited CYP2D6 and CYP1A2 only at concentrations well above those achieved clinically.

Efavirenz has been shown to induce P450 enzymes, resulting in the induction of its own metabolism. In uninfected volunteers, multiple doses of 200 - 400 mg per day for 10 days resulted in a lower than predicted extent of accumulation (22 - 42% lower) and a shorter terminal half-life of 40 - 55 hours (single dose half-life 52 - 76 hours).

Elimination: efavirenz has a relatively long terminal half-life of 52 to 76 hours after single doses and 40 - 55 hours after multiple doses. Approximately 14 - 34% of a radiolabelled dose of efavirenz was recovered in the urine and less than 1% of the dose was excreted in urine as unchanged efavirenz.

In the single patient studied with severe hepatic impairment (Child Pugh Grade C), half life was doubled indicating a potential for a much greater degree of accumulation.

Paediatric pharmacokinetics: in 49 paediatric patients receiving the equivalent of a 600 mg dose of efavirenz (dose adjusted from calculated body size based on weight), steady state C_{max} was 14.1 μM, steady state C_{min} was 5.6 μM, and AUC was 216 μM·h. The pharmacokinetics of efavirenz in paediatric patients were similar to adults.

Gender, race, elderly: pharmacokinetics of efavirenz in patients appear to be similar between men and women and among the racial groups studied. Although limited data suggest that Asian and Pacific Island patients may have higher exposure to efavirenz, they do not appear to be less tolerant of efavirenz. Pharmacokinetic studies have not been performed in the elderly.

5.3 Preclinical safety data

Efavirenz was not mutagenic or clastogenic in conventional genotoxicity assays.

Efavirenz induced foetal resorptions in rats. Malformations were observed in 3 of 20 foetuses/ newborns from efavirenz-treated cynomolgus monkeys given doses resulting in plasma efavirenz concentrations similar to those seen in humans. Anencephaly and unilateral anophthalmia with secondary enlargement of the tongue were observed in one foetus, microophthalmia was observed in another foetus, and cleft palate was observed in a third foetus. No malformations were observed in foetuses from efavirenz-treated rats and rabbits.

Biliary hyperplasia was observed in cynomolgus monkeys given efavirenz for ⩾ 1 year at a dose resulting in mean AUC values approximately 2-fold greater than those in humans given the recommended dose. The biliary hyperplasia regressed upon cessation of dosing. Biliary fibrosis has been observed in rats. Non-sustained convulsions were observed in some monkeys receiving efavirenz for ⩾ 1 year, at doses yielding plasma AUC values 4- to 13-fold greater than those in humans given the recommended dose (see sections 4.4 and 4.8).

Carcinogenicity studies showed an increased incidence of hepatic and pulmonary tumours in female mice, but not in male mice. The mechanism of tumour formation and the potential relevance for humans are not known.

Carcinogenicity studies in male mice, male and female rats were negative. While the carcinogenic potential in humans is unknown, these data suggest that the clinical benefit of efavirenz outweighs the potential carcinogenic risk to humans.

6. PHARMACEUTICAL PARTICULARS

6.1 List of excipients

Tablet core: croscarmellose sodium, microcrystalline cellulose, sodium laurilsulfate, hydroxypropylcellulose, lactose monohydrate and magnesium stearate.

Film coating: hypromellose (E464), titanium dioxide (E171), macrogol 400, yellow iron oxide (E172) and carnauba wax.

Printing ink: hypromellose (E464), propylene glycol, cochineal carminic acid (E120), indigo carmine (E132) and titanium dioxide (E171).

6.2 Incompatibilities

Not applicable.

6.3 Shelf life

2 years.

6.4 Special precautions for storage

No special precautions for storage.

6.5 Nature and contents of container

Packs of 30 × 1 film-coated tablets in aluminium/PVC perforated unit dose blisters.

6.6 Instructions for use and handling

No special requirements.

Table 2 Efficacy results for studies ACTG 364 and 020

		Responder rates (NC = F[a]) Plasma HIV-RNA				Mean change from baseline-CD4 cell count	
Study Number/ Treatment Regimens[b]	n	%	(95% C.I.[c])	%	(95% C.I.)	cells/mm^3	(S.E.M.[d])
Study ACTG 364 48 weeks		< 500 copies/ml		< 50 copies/ml			
EFV + NFV + NRTIs	65	70	(59, 82)	—	—	107	(17.9)
EFV + NRTIs	65	58	(46, 70)	—	—	114	(21.0)
NFV + NRTIs	66	30	(19, 42)	—	—	94	(13.6)
Study 020 24 weeks		< 400 copies/ml		< 50 copies/ml			
EFV + IDV + NRTIs	157	60	(52, 68)	49	(41, 58)	104	(9.1)
IDV + NRTIs	170	51	(43, 59)	38	(30, 45)	77	(9.9)

[a] NC = F, noncompleter = failure.
[b] EFV, efavirenz; ZDV, zidovudine; 3TC, lamivudine; IDV, indinavir; NRTI, nucleoside reverse transcriptase inhibitor; NFV, nelfinavir.
[c] C.I., confidence interval for proportion of patients in response.
[d] S.E.M., standard error of the mean.
—, not performed.

7. MARKETING AUTHORISATION HOLDER
Bristol-Myers Squibb Pharma EEIG
141 - 149 Staines Road
Hounslow TW3 3JA
United Kingdom

8. MARKETING AUTHORISATION NUMBER(S)
EU/1/99/110/009 - blister

9. DATE OF FIRST AUTHORISATION/RENEWAL OF THE AUTHORISATION
Date of first authorisation: 22 August 2002
Date of last renewal: 29 April 2004

10. DATE OF REVISION OF THE TEXT
August 2005

Symbicort 200/6 Turbohaler Inhalation powder

(AstraZeneca UK Limited)

1. NAME OF THE MEDICINAL PRODUCT
Symbicort® 200/6 Turbohaler®, Inhalation powder.

2. QUALITATIVE AND QUANTITATIVE COMPOSITION
Each delivered dose (the dose that leaves the mouthpiece) contains: budesonide 160 micrograms/inhalation and formoterol fumarate dihydrate 4.5 micrograms/inhalation.

Symbicort 200/6 Turbohaler delivers the same amount of budesonide and formoterol as the corresponding Turbohaler monoproducts, i.e. budesonide 200 micrograms/ inhalation (metered dose) and formoterol 6 micrograms/ inhalation (metered dose) alternatively labelled as 4.5 micrograms/inhalation (delivered dose).

For excipients, see 6.1.

3. PHARMACEUTICAL FORM
Inhalation powder.
White powder.

4. CLINICAL PARTICULARS
4.1 Therapeutic indications
Asthma

Symbicort Turbohaler is indicated in the regular treatment of asthma where use of a combination (inhaled corticosteroid and long acting beta-agonist) is appropriate:

- patients not adequately controlled with inhaled corticosteroids and "as needed" inhaled short acting $beta_2$-agonists.

or

- patients already adequately controlled on both inhaled corticosteroids and long acting $beta_2$-agonists.

COPD

Symptomatic treatment of patients with severe COPD (FEV1 < 50% predicted normal) and a history of repeated exacerbations, who have significant symptoms despite regular therapy with long-acting bronchodilators.

4.2 Posology and method of administration
Asthma

Symbicort Turbohaler is not intended for the initial management of asthma. The dosage of the components of Symbicort Turbohaler is individual and should be adjusted to the severity of the disease. This should be considered not only when treatment with combination products is initiated but also when the dose is adjusted. If an individual patient should require a combination of doses other than those available in the combination inhaler, appropriate doses of beta-agonist and/or corticosteroids by individual inhalers should be prescribed.

Recommended doses:

Adults (18 years and older): 1-2 inhalations twice daily. Some patients may require up to a maximum of 4 inhalations twice daily.

Adolescents (12 – 17 years and older): 1-2 inhalations twice daily.

Patients should be regularly reassessed by a doctor, so that the dosage of Symbicort Turbohaler remains optimal. The dose should be titrated to the lowest dose at which effective control of symptoms is maintained. When control of symptoms is maintained with the lowest recommended dosage, then the next step could include a test of inhaled corticosteroid alone.

In usual practice when control of symptoms is achieved with the twice daily regimen, titration to the lowest effective dose could include Symbicort Turbohaler given once daily, when in the opinion of the prescriber, a long acting bronchodilator would be required to maintain control.

Children (6 years and older): A lower strength is available for children 6-11 years.

COPD

Adults: 2 inhalations twice daily

Special patient groups: There is no need to adjust the dose in elderly patients. There are no data available for use of Symbicort Turbohaler in patients with hepatic or renal impairment. As budesonide and formoterol are primarily eliminated via hepatic metabolism, an increased exposure can be expected in patients with severe liver cirrhosis.

Instructions for correct use of Turbohaler:

Turbohaler is inspiratory flow-driven, which means that when the patient inhales through the mouthpiece, the substance will follow the inspired air into the airways.

Note: It is important to instruct the patient

- To carefully read the instructions for use in the patient information leaflet which is packed together with each inhaler
- To breathe in forcefully and deeply through the mouthpiece to ensure that an optimal dose is delivered to the lungs
- Never to breathe out through the mouthpiece
- To rinse the mouth out with water after inhaling the prescribed dose to minimise the risk of oropharyngeal thrush

The patient may not taste or feel any medication when using Symbicort Turbohaler due to the small amount of drug dispensed.

4.3 Contraindications
Hypersensitivity (allergy) to budesonide, formoterol or inhaled lactose.

4.4 Special warnings and special precautions for use
It is recommended that the dose is tapered when the treatment is discontinued and should not be stopped abruptly.

If patients find the treatment ineffective, or exceed the current dose of the fixed combination, medical attention must be sought. Increasing use of rescue bronchodilators indicates a worsening of the underlying condition and warrants a reassessment of the asthma therapy. Sudden and progressive deterioration in control of asthma or COPD is potentially life threatening and the patient should undergo urgent medical assessment. In this situation, consideration should be given to the need for increased therapy with corticosteroids or addition of systemic anti-inflammatory therapy, such as a course of oral corticosteroids, or antibiotic treatment if an infection is present.

There are no data available on the use of Symbicort Turbohaler in the treatment of an acute asthma attack. Patients should be advised to have their rapid acting bronchodilator available at all times.

Patients should be reminded to take Symbicort Turbohaler daily as prescribed even when asymptomatic.

Therapy should not be initiated during an exacerbation.

As with other inhalation therapy, paradoxical bronchospasm may occur, with an immediate increase in wheezing after dosing. Symbicort Turbohaler should then be discontinued; treatment should be re-assessed and alternative therapy instituted if necessary.

Systemic effects may occur with any inhaled corticosteroid, particularly at high doses prescribed for long periods. These effects are much less likely to occur with inhalation treatment than with oral corticosteroids. Possible systemic effects include adrenal suppression, growth retardation in children and adolescents, decrease in bone mineral density, cataract and glaucoma.

It is recommended that the height of children receiving prolonged treatment with inhaled corticosteroids is regularly monitored. If growth is slowed, therapy should be re-evaluated with the aim of reducing the dose of inhaled corticosteroid. The benefits of the corticosteroid therapy and the possible risks of growth suppression must be carefully weighed. In addition consideration should be given to referring the patient to a paediatric respiratory specialist.

Limited data from long-term studies suggest that most children and adolescents treated with inhaled budesonide will ultimately achieve their adult target height. However, an initial small but transient reduction in growth (approximately 1cm) has been observed. This generally occurs within the first year of treatment.

Potential effects on bone density should be considered, particularly in patients on high doses for prolonged periods that have coexisting risk factors for osteoporosis. Long-term studies with inhaled budesonide in children at mean daily doses of 400 micrograms (metered dose) or in adults at daily doses of 800 micrograms (metered dose) have not shown any significant effects on bone mineral density. No information regarding the effect of Symbicort at higher doses is available.

If there is any reason to suppose that adrenal function is impaired from previous systemic steroid therapy, care should be taken when transferring patients to Symbicort Turbohaler therapy.

The benefits of inhaled budesonide therapy would normally minimise the need for oral steroids, but patients transferring from oral steroids may remain at risk of impaired adrenal reserve for a considerable time. Patients who have required high dose emergency corticosteroid therapy in the past or prolonged treatment with high doses of inhaled corticosteroids may also be at risk. Additional systemic corticosteriod cover should be considered during periods of stress or elective surgery.

To minimise the risk of oropharyngeal candida infection, the patient should be instructed to rinse the mouth with water after each dosing occasion.

Concomitant treatment with itraconazole and ritonavir or other potent CYP3A4 inhibitors should be avoided (see section 4.5). If this is not possible, the time interval between administration of the interacting drugs should be as long as possible.

Symbicort Turbohaler should be administered with caution in patients with thyrotoxicosis, phaeochromocytoma, diabetes mellitus, untreated hypokalaemia, hypertrophic obstructive cardiomyopathy, idiopathic subvalvular aortic stenosis, severe hypertension, aneurysm or other severe cardiovascular disorders, such as ischaemic heart disease, tachyarrhythmias or severe heart failure.

Caution should be observed when treating patients with prolongation of the QTc-interval. Formoterol itself may induce prolongation of the QTc-interval.

The need for, and dose of, inhaled corticosteroids should be re-evaluated in patients with active or quiescent pulmonary tuberculosis, fungal and viral infections in the airways.

Potentially serious hypokalaemia may result from high doses of $beta_2$-agonists. Concomitant treatment of $beta_2$-agonists with drugs which can induce hypokalaemia or potentiate a hypokalaemic effect, e.g xanthine-derivatives, steroids and diuretics, may add to a possible hypokalaemic effect of the $beta_2$-agonist. Particular caution is recommended in unstable asthma with variable use of rescue bronchodilators, in acute severe asthma as the associated risk may be augmented by hypoxia and in other conditions when the likelihood for hypokalaemia adverse effects is increased. It is recommended that serum potassium levels are monitored during these circumstances.

As for all $beta_2$-agonists, additional blood glucose controls should be considered in diabetic patients.

Symbicort Turbohaler contains lactose (<1 mg/inhalation). This amount does not normally cause problems in lactose intolerant people.

4.5 Interaction with other medicinal products and other forms of Interaction
Pharmacokinetic interactions

The metabolic conversion of budesonide is impeded by substances metabolized by CYP P450 3A4 (e.g. itraconazole, ritonavir). The concomitant administration of these potent inhibitors of CYP P450 3A4 may increase plasma levels of budesonide. The concomitant use of these drugs should be avoided unless the benefit outweighs the increased risk of systemic side-effects.

Pharmacodynamic interactions

Beta-adrenergic blockers can weaken or inhibit the effect of formoterol. Symbicort Turbohaler should therefore not be given together with beta-adrenergic blockers (including eye drops) unless there are compelling reasons.

Concomitant treatment with quinidine, disopyramide, procainamide, phenothiazines, antihistamines (terfenadine), monoamine oxidase inhibitors and tricyclic antidepressants can prolong the QTc-interval and increase the risk of ventricular arrhythmias.

In addition L-Dopa, L-thyroxine, oxytocin and alcohol can impair cardiac tolerance towards β_2-sympathomimetics.

Concomitant treatment with monoamine oxidase inhibitors, including agents with similar properties such as furazolidone and procarbazine, may precipitate hypertensive reactions.

There is an elevated risk of arrhythmias in patients receiving concomitant anaesthesia with halogenated hydrocarbons.

Concomitant use of other beta-adrenergic drugs can have a potentially additive effect.

Hypokalaemia may increase the disposition towards arrhythmias in patients who are treated with digitalis glycosides.

Budesonide has not been observed to interact with any other drugs used in the treatment of asthma.

4.6 Pregnancy and lactation
For Symbicort Turbohaler or the concomitant treatment with formoterol and budesonide, no clinical data on exposed pregnancies are available. Animal studies with respect to reproductive toxicity of the combination have not been performed.

There are no adequate data from use of formoterol in pregnant women. In animal studies formoterol has caused adverse effects in reproduction studies at very high systemic exposure levels (see section 5.3).

Data on approximately 2000 exposed pregnancies indicate no increased teratogenic risk associated with the use of inhaled budesonide. In animal studies glucocorticosteroids have been shown to induce malformations (see section 5.3). This is not likely to be relevant for humans given recommended doses.

Animal studies have also identified an involvement of excess prenatal glucocorticoids in increased risks for intrauterine growth retardation, adult cardiovascular disease and permanent changes in glucocorticoid receptor density, neurotransmitter turnover and behaviour at exposures below the teratogenic dose range.

During pregnancy, Symbicort Turbohaler should only be used when the benefits outweigh the potential risks. The lowest effective dose of budesonide needed to maintain adequate asthma control should be used.

It is not known whether formoterol or budesonide passes into human breast milk. In rats, small amounts of formoterol have been detected in maternal milk. Administration of Symbicort Turbohaler to women who are breastfeeding should only be considered if the expected benefit to the mother is greater than any possible risk to the child.

4.7 Effects on ability to drive and use machines

Symbicort Turbohaler has no or negligible influence on the ability to drive and use machines.

4.8 Undesirable effects

Since Symbicort Turbohaler contains both budesonide and formoterol, the same pattern of undesirable effects as reported for these substances may occur. No increased incidence of adverse reactions has been seen following concurrent administration of the two compounds. The most common drug related adverse reactions are pharmacologically predictable side-effects of $beta_2$-agonist therapy, such as tremor and palpitations. These tend to be mild and usually disappear within a few days of treatment. In a 3-year clinical trial with budesonide in COPD, skin bruises and pneumonia occurred at a frequency of 10% and 6%, respectively, compared with 4% and 3% in the placebo group ($p<0.001$ and $p<0.01$, respectively).

Adverse reactions, which have been associated with budesonide or formoterol, are given below, listed by system organ class and frequency. Frequency are defined as: very common (≥1/10), common (≥1/100 and <1/10), uncommon (≥1/1000 and <1/100), rare (≥1/10 000 and <1/1000) and very rare (<1/10 000).

Cardiac disorders	Common	Palpitations
	Uncommon	Tachycardia
	Rare	Atrial fibrillation, supraventricular tachycardia, extrasystoles
	Very rare	Angina pectoris
Endocrine disorders	Very rare	Signs or symptoms of systemic glucocorticosteroid effects (including hypofunction of the adrenal gland)
Gastrointestinal disorders	Uncommon	Nausea
Immune system disorders	Rare	Exanthema, urticaria, pruritus, dermatitis, angioedema
Infections and infestations	Common	Candida infections in the oropharynx
Metabolic and nutrition disorders	Rare	Hypokalemia
	Very rare	Hyperglycemia
Musculoskeletal, connective tissue and bone disorders	Uncommon	Muscle cramps
Nervous system disorders	Common	Headache, tremor
	Uncommon	Dizziness
	Very rare	Taste disturbances
Psychiatric disorders	Uncommon	Agitation, restlessness, nervousness, sleep disturbances
	Very rare	Depression, behavioural disturbances (mainly in children)
Respiratory, thoracic and mediastinal disorders	Common	Mild irritation in the throat, coughing, hoarseness
	Rare	Bronchospasm
Skin and subcutaneous tissue disorders	Uncommon	Bruises
Vascular disorders	Very rare	Variations in blood pressure

As with other inhalation therapy, paradoxical bronchospasm may occur in very rare cases (see section 4.4).

Systemic effects of inhaled corticosteroids may occur, particularly at high doses prescribed for prolonged periods.These may include adrenal suppression, growth retardation in children and adolescents, decrease in bone mineral density, cataract and glaucoma (see also 4.4).

Treatment with β2-agonists may result in an increase in blood levels of insulin, free fatty acids, glycerol and ketone bodies.

4.9 Overdose

An overdose of formoterol would likely lead to effects that are typical for $beta_2$-adrenergic agonists: tremor, headache, palpitations. Symptoms reported from isolated cases are tachycardia, hyperglycaemia, hypokalaemia, prolonged QTc-interval, arrhythmia, nausea and vomiting. Supportive and symptomatic treatment may be indicated. A dose of 90 micrograms administered during three hours in patients with acute bronchial obstruction raised no safety concerns.

Acute overdosage with budesonide, even in excessive doses, is not expected to be a clinical problem. When used chronically in excessive doses, systemic glucocorticosteroid effects, such as hypercorticism and adrenal suppression, may appear.

If Symbicort therapy has to be withdrawn due to overdose of the formoterol component of the drug, provision of appropriate inhaled corticosteroid therapy must be considered.

5. PHARMACOLOGICAL PROPERTIES

5.1 Pharmacodynamic properties

Pharmacotherapeutic group: Adrenergics and other drugs for obstructive airway diseases.

ATC-code: R03AK07

Mechanisms of action and pharmacodynamic effects

Symbicort Turbohaler contains formoterol and budesonide, which have different modes of action and show additive effects in terms of reduction of asthma exacerbations. The mechanisms of action of the two substances, respectively are discussed below.

Budesonide

Budesonide given by inhalation at recommended doses has a glucocorticoid antiinflammatory action within the lungs, resulting in reduced symptoms and exacerbations of asthma with less adverse effects than when corticosteroids are administered systemically. The exact mechanism responsible for this anti-inflammatory effect is unknown.

Formoterol

Formoterol is a selective $beta_2$-adrenergic agonist that produces relaxation of bronchial smooth muscle in patients with reversible airways obstruction. The bronchodilating effect sets in rapidly, within 1-3 minutes after inhalation, and has a duration of 12 hours after a single dose.

Symbicort Turbohaler

Asthma

In clinical trials in adults, the addition of formoterol to budesonide improved asthma symptoms and lung function, and reduced exacerbations.

In two12-week studies the effect on lung function of Symbicort Turbohaler in asthma was equal to that of the free combination of budesonide and formoterol, and exceeded that of budesonide alone. There was no sign of attenuation of the anti-asthmatic effect over time.

In a 12-week paediatric study 85 children aged 6-11 years were treated for asthma with Symbicort Turbohaler (2 inhalations of 80/4.5 micrograms/inhalations twice daily), which improved lung function and was well tolerated.

COPD

In two 12-month studies, the effects on lung function and the rate of exacerbation (defined as courses of oral steroids and/or course antibiotics and/or hospitalisations) in patients with severe COPD was evaluated. Median FEV_1 at inclusion in the trials was 36% of predicted normal. The mean number of exacerbations per year (as defined above) was significantly reduced with Symbicort as compared with treatment with formoterol alone or placebo (mean rate 1.4 compared with 1.8-1.9 in the placebo/formoterol group). The mean number of days on oral corticosteroids/ patients during the 12 months was slightly reduced in the Symbicort group (7-8 days/ patients/ year compared with 11-12 and 9-12 days in the placebo and formoterol groups, respectively). For changes in lung-function parameters, such as FEV_1, Symbicort was not superior to treatment with formoterol alone.

5.2 Pharmacokinetic properties

Absorption

Symbicort Turbohaler and the corresponding monoproducts have been shown to be bioequivalent with regard to systemic exposure of budesonide and formoterol, respectively. In spite of this, a small increase in cortisol suppression was seen after administration of Symbicort Turbohaler compared to the monoproducts. The difference is considered not to have an impact on clinical safety.

There was no evidence of pharmacokinetic interactions between budesonide and formoterol.

Pharmacokinetic parameters for the respective substances were comparable after the administration of budesonide and formoterol as monoproducts or as Symbicort Turbohaler. For budesonide, AUC was slightly higher, rate of absorption more rapid and maximal plasma concentration higher after administration of the fixed combination. For formoterol, maximal plasma concentration was similar after administration of the fixed combination. Inhaled budesonide is rapidly absorbed and the maximum plasma concentration is reached within 30 minutes after inhalation. In studies, mean lung deposition of budesonide after inhalation via Turbohaler ranged from 32 to 44% of the delivered dose. The systemic bioavailability is approximately 49% of the delivered dose.

Inhaled formoterol is rapidly absorbed and the maximum plasma concentration is reached within 10 minutes after inhalation. In studies the mean lung deposition of formoterol after inhalation via Turbohaler ranged from 28-49% of the delivered dose. The systemic bioavailability is about 61% of the delivered dose.

Distribution and metabolism

Plasma protein binding is approximately 50% for formoterol and 90% for budesonide. Volume of distribution is about 4 L/kg for formoterol and 3 L/kg for budesonide. Formoterol is inactivated via conjugation reactions (active O-demethylated and deformylated metabolites are formed, but they are seen mainly as inactivated conjugates). Budesonide undergoes an extensive degree (approx. 90%) of biotransformation on first passage through the liver to metabolites of low glucocorticosteroid activity. The glucocorticosteroid activity of the major metabolites, 6-beta-hydroxy-budesonide and 16-alfa-hydroxy-prednisolone, is less than 1% of that of budesonide. There are no indications of any metabolic interactions or any displacement reactions between formoterol and budesonide.

Elimination

The major part of a dose of formoterol is transformed by liver metabolism followed by renal elimination. After inhalation, 8-13% of the delivered dose of formoterol is excreted unmetabolised in the urine. Formoterol has a high systemic clearance (approximately 1.4 L/min) and the terminal elimination half-life averages 17 hours.

Budesonide is eliminated via metabolism mainly catalysed by the enzyme CYP3A4. The metabolites of budesonide are eliminated in urine as such or in conjugated form. Only negligible amounts of unchanged budesonide have been detected in the urine. Budesonide has a high systemic clearance (approximately 1.2 L/min) and the plasma elimination half-life after i.v. dosing averages 4 hours.

The pharmacokinetics of budesonide or formoterol in patients with renal failure is unknown. The exposure of budesonide and formoterol may be increased in patients with liver disease.

5.3 Preclinical safety data

The toxicity observed in animal studies with budesonide and formoterol, given in combination or separately, were effects associated with exaggerated pharmacological activity.

In animal reproduction studies, corticosteroids such as budesonide have been shown to induce malformations (cleft palate, skeletal malformations). However, these animal experimental results do not seem to be relevant in humans at the recommended doses. Animal reproduction studies with formoterol have shown a somewhat reduced fertility in male rats at high systemic exposure and implantation losses as well as decreased early postnatal survival and birth weight at considerably higher systemic exposures than those reached during clinical use. However, these animal experimental results do not seem to be relevant in humans.

6. PHARMACEUTICAL PARTICULARS

6.1 List of excipients

Lactose monohydrate (which contains milk proteins).

6.2 Incompatibilities

Not applicable.

6.3 Shelf life

2 years.

6.4 Special precautions for storage

Do not store above 30°C. Keep the container tightly closed.

6.5 Nature and contents of container

Symbicort Turbohaler is an inspiratory flow driven, multidose powder inhaler. The inhaler is white with a red turning grip. The inhaler is made of different plastic materials (PP, PC, HDPE, LDPE, LLDPE, PBT). Each inhaler contains 60 doses or 120 doses. In each secondary package there are 1, 2, 3, 10 or 18 inhalers. Not all pack-sizes may be marketed.

6.6 Instructions for use and handling

No special requirements.

7. MARKETING AUTHORISATION HOLDER

AstraZeneca UK Limited,

600 Capability Green,

Luton, LU1 3LU, UK.

8. MARKETING AUTHORISATION NUMBER(S)

PL 17901/0092

9. DATE OF FIRST AUTHORISATION/RENEWAL OF THE AUTHORISATION

Date of first authorisation: 15th May 2001

Date of last Renewal: 25th August 2005

10. DATE OF REVISION OF THE TEXT

25th August 2005

Symbicort 400/12 Turbohaler, Inhalation powder.

(AstraZeneca UK Limited)

1. NAME OF THE MEDICINAL PRODUCT

Symbicort® 400/12 Turbohaler®, Inhalation powder.

2. QUALITATIVE AND QUANTITATIVE COMPOSITION

Each delivered dose (the dose that leaves the mouthpiece) contains: budesonide 320 micrograms/inhalation and formoterol fumarate dihydrate 9 micrograms/inhalation.

Symbicort 400/12 Turbohaler delivers the same amount of budesonide and formoterol as the corresponding Turbohaler monoproducts, i.e. budesonide 400 micrograms/inhalation (metered dose) and formoterol 12 micrograms/inhalation (metered dose) alternatively labelled as 9 micrograms/inhalation (delivered dose).

For excipients, see 6.1.

3. PHARMACEUTICAL FORM

Inhalation powder,

White powder

4. CLINICAL PARTICULARS

4.1 Therapeutic indications

Asthma

Symbicort Turbohaler is indicated in the regular treatment of asthma where use of a combination (inhaled corticosteroid and long acting beta-agonist) is appropriate:

- patients not adequately controlled with inhaled corticosteroids and "as needed" inhaled short acting beta$_2$-agonists.

or

- patients already adequately controlled on both inhaled corticosteroids and long acting beta$_2$-agonists.

COPD

Symptomatic treatment of patients with severe COPD (FEV1 < 50% predicted normal) and a history of repeated exacerbations, who have significant symptoms despite regular therapy with long-acting bronchodilators.

4.2 Posology and method of administration

Asthma

Symbicort Turbohaler is not intended for the initial management of asthma. The dosage of the components of Symbicort Turbohaler is individual and should be adjusted to the severity of the disease. This should be considered not only when treatment with combination products is initiated but also when the dose is adjusted. If an individual patient should require a combination of doses other than those available in the combination inhaler, appropriate doses of beta-agonist and/or corticosteroids by individual inhalers should be prescribed.

Recommended doses:

Adults (18 years and older): 1 inhalation twice daily. Some patients may require up to a maximum of 2 inhalations twice daily.

Adolescents (12-17 years):1 inhalation twice daily.

Patients should be regularly reassessed by a doctor, so that the dosage of Symbicort Turbohaler remains optimal. The dose should be titrated to the lowest dose at which effective control of symptoms is maintained. When control of symptoms is maintained with the lowest recommended dosage, then the next step could include a test of inhaled corticosteroid alone.

In usual practice when control of symptoms is achieved with the twice daily regimen, titration to the lowest effective dose could include Symbicort Turbohaler given once daily, when in the opinion of the prescriber, a long acting bronchodilator would be required to maintain control.

Children under 12 years: Efficacy and safety have not been fully studied in children. (see section 5.1). Symbicort forte is not recommended for children under 12 years of age.

COPD

Adults:1 inhalation twice daily.

Special patient groups: There is no need to adjust the dose in elderly patients. There are no data available for use of Symbicort Turbohaler in patients with hepatic or renal impairment. As budesonide and formoterol are primarily eliminated via hepatic metabolism, an increased exposure can be expected in patients with severe liver cirrhosis.

Instructions for correct use of Turbohaler:

Turbohaler is inspiratory flow-driven, which means that when the patient inhales through the mouthpiece, the substance will follow the inspired air into the airways.

Note: It is important to instruct the patient

- To carefully read the instructions for use in the patient information leaflet which is packed together with each inhaler
- To breathe in forcefully and deeply through the mouthpiece to ensure that an optimal dose is delivered to the lungs
- Never to breathe out through the mouthpiece
- To rinse the mouth out with water after inhaling the prescribed dose to minimise the risk of oropharyngeal thrush

The patient may not taste or feel any medication when using Symbicort Turbohaler due to the small amount of drug dispensed.

4.3 Contraindications

Hypersensitivity (allergy) to budesonide, formoterol or inhaled lactose.

4.4 Special warnings and special precautions for use

It is recommended that the dose is tapered when the treatment is discontinued and should not be stopped abruptly.

If patients find the treatment ineffective, or exceed the current dose of the fixed combination, medical attention must be sought. Increasing use of rescue bronchodilators indicates a worsening of the underlying condition and warrants a reassessment of the asthma therapy. Sudden and progressive deterioration in control of asthma or COPD is potentially life threatening and the patient should undergo urgent medical assessment. In this situation consideration should be given to the need for increased therapy with corticosteroids or addition of systemic anti-inflammatory therapy, such as a course of oral corticosteroids, or antibiotic treatment if an infection is present.

There are no data available on the use of Symbicort Turbohaler in the treatment of an acute asthma attack. Patients should be advised to have their rapid acting bronchodilator available at all times.

Patients should be reminded to take Symbicort Turbohaler daily as prescribed even when asymptomatic.

Therapy should not be initiated during an exacerbation.

As with other inhalation therapy, paradoxical bronchospasm may occur, with an immediate increase in wheezing after dosing. Symbicort Turbohaler should then be discontinued; treatment should be re-assessed and alternative therapy instituted if necessary.

Systemic effects may occur with any inhaled corticosteroid, particularly at high doses prescribed for long periods. These effects are much less likely to occur with inhalation treatment than with oral corticosteroids. Possible systemic effects include adrenal suppression, growth retardation in children and adolescents, decrease in bone mineral density, cataract and glaucoma. It is recommended that the height of children receiving prolonged treatment with inhaled corticosteroids is regularly monitored. If growth is slowed, therapy should be re-evaluated with the aim of reducing the dose of inhaled corticosteroid. The benefits of the corticosteroid therapy and the possible risks of growth suppression must be carefully weighed. In addition consideration should be given to referring the patient to a paediatric respiratory specialist.

Limited data from long-term studies suggest that most children and adolescents treated with inhaled budesonide will ultimately achieve their adult target height. However, an initial small but transient reduction in growth (approximately 1cm) has been observed. This generally occurs within the first year of treatment.

Potential effects on bone density should be considered particularly in patients on high doses for prolonged periods that have coexisting risk factors for osteoperosis. Long-term studies with inhaled budesonide in children at mean daily doses of 400 micrograms (metered dose) or in adults at daily doses of 800 micrograms (metered dose) have not shown any significant effects on bone mineral density. No information regarding the effect of Symbicort at higher doses is available.

If there is any reason to suppose that adrenal function is impaired from previous systemic steroid therapy, care should be taken when transferring patients to Symbicort Turbohaler therapy.

The benefits of inhaled budesonide therapy would normally minimise the need for oral steroids, but patients transferring from oral steroids may remain at risk of impaired adrenal reserve for a considerable time. Patients who have required high dose emergency corticosteroid therapy in the past or prolonged treatment with high doses of inhaled corticosteroids may also be at risk. Additional systemic corticosteriod cover should be considered during periods of stress or elective surgery.

To minimise the risk of oropharyngeal candida infection the patient should be instructed to rinse the mouth with water after each dosing occasion.

Concomitant treatment with itraconazole and ritonavir or other potent CYP3A4 inhibitors should be avoided (see section 4.5). If this is not possible, the time interval between administration of the interacting drugs should be as long as possible.

Symbicort Turbohaler should be administered with caution in patients with thyrotoxicosis, phaeochromocytoma, diabetes mellitus, untreated hypokalaemia, hypertrophic obstructive cardiomyopathy, idiopathic subvalvular aortic stenosis, severe hypertension, aneurysm or other severe cardiovascular disorders, such as ischaemic heart disease, tachyarrhythmias or severe heart failure.

Caution should be observed when treating patients with prolongation of the QTc-interval. Formoterol itself may induce prolongation of the QTc-interval.

The need for, and dose of, inhaled corticosteroids should be re-evaluated in patients with active or quiescent pulmonary tuberculosis, fungal and viral infections in the airways.

Potentially serious hypokalaemia may result from high doses of beta$_2$-agonists. Concomitant treatment of beta$_2$-agonists with drugs which can induce hypokalaemia or potentiate a hypokalaemic effect, e.g xanthine-derivatives, steroids and diuretics, may add to a possible hypokalaemic effect of the beta$_2$-agonist. Particular caution is recommended in unstable asthma with variable use of rescue bronchodilators, in acute severe asthma as the associated risk may be augmented by hypoxia and in other conditions when the likelihood for hypokalaemia adverse effects is increased. It is recommended that serum potassium levels are monitored during these circumstances.

As for all beta$_2$-agonists, additional blood glucose controls should be considered in diabetic patients.

Symbicort 400/12 Turbohaler contains lactose (<1 mg/inhalation). This amount does not normally cause problems in lactose intolerant people.

4.5 Interaction with other medicinal products and other forms of Interaction

Pharmacokinetic interactions

The metabolic conversion of budesonide is impeded by substances metabolized by CYP P450 3A4 (e.g. itraconazole, ritonavir). The concomitant administration of these potent inhibitors of CYP P450 3A4 may increase plasma levels of budesonide. The concomitant use of these drugs should be avoided unless the benefit outweighs the increased risk of systemic side-effects.

Pharmacodynamic interactions

Beta-adrenergic blockers can weaken or inhibit the effect of formoterol. Symbicort Turbohaler should therefore not be given together with beta-adrenergic blockers (including eye drops) unless there are compelling reasons.

Concomitant treatment with quinidine, disopyramide, procainamide, phenothiazines, antihistamines (terfenadine), monoamine oxidase inhibitors and tricyclic anti-depressants can prolong the QTc-interval and increase the risk of ventricular arrhythmias.

In addition L-Dopa, L-thyroxine, oxytocin and alcohol can impair cardiac tolerance towards β_2-sympathomimetics.

Concomitant treatment with monoamine oxidase inhibitors, including agents with similar properties such as furazolidone and procarbazine, may precipitate hypertensive reactions.

There is an elevated risk of arrhythmias in patients receiving concomitant anaesthesia with halogenated hydrocarbons.

Concomitant use of other beta-adrenergic drugs can have a potentially additive effect.

Hypokalaemia may increase the disposition towards arrhythmias in patients who are treated with digitalis glycosides.

Budesonide has not been observed to interact with any other drugs used in the treatment of asthma.

4.6 Pregnancy and lactation

For Symbicort Turbohaler or the concomitant treatment with formoterol and budesonide, no clinical data on exposed pregnancies are available. Animal studies with respect to reproductive toxicity of the combination have not been performed.

There are no adequate data from use of formoterol in pregnant women. In animal studies formoterol has caused adverse effects in reproduction studies at very high systemic exposure levels (see section 5.3).

Data on approximately 2000 exposed pregnancies indicate no increased teratogenic risk associated with the use of inhaled budesonide. In animal studies glucocorticosteroids have been shown to induce malformations (see section 5.3). This is not likely to be relevant for humans given recommended doses.

Animal studies have also identified an involvement of excess prenatal glucocorticoids in increased risks for intrauterine growth retardation, adult cardiovascular disease and permanent changes in glucocorticoid receptor density, neurotransmitter turnover and behaviour at exposures below the teratogenic dose range.

During pregnancy, Symbicort Turbohaler should only be used when the benefits outweigh the potential risks. The lowest effective dose of budesonide needed to maintain adequate asthma control should be used.

It is not known whether formoterol or budesonide passes into human breast milk. In rats, small amounts of formoterol have been detected in maternal milk. Administration of Symbicort Turbohaler to women who are breast-feeding should only be considered if the expected benefit to the mother is greater than any possible risk to the child.

4.7 Effects on ability to drive and use machines

Symbicort Turbohaler has no or negligible influence on the ability to drive or use machines.

4.8 Undesirable effects

Since Symbicort Turbohaler contains both budesonide and formoterol, the same pattern of undesirable effects as reported for these substances may occur. No increased incidence of adverse reactions has been seen following concurrent administration of the two compounds. The most common drug related adverse reactions are pharmacologically predictable side-effects of beta$_2$-agonist therapy, such as tremor and palpitations. These tend to be mild and usually disappear within a few days of treatment. In a 3-year clinical trial with budesonide in COPD, skin bruises and pneumonia occurred at a frequency of 10% and 6%, respectively, compared with 4% and 3% in the placebo group ($p<0.001$ and $p<0.01$, respectively).

Adverse reactions, which have been associated with budesonide or formoterol, are given below, listed by system organ class and frequency. Frequency are defined as: very common (≥1/10), common (≥1/100 and <1/10), uncommon (≥1/1000 and <1/100), rare (≥1/10 000 and <1/1000) and very rare (<1/10 000).

Cardiac disorders	Common	Palpitations
	Uncommon	Tachycardia
	Rare	Atrial fibrillation, supraventricular tachycardia, extrasystoles
	Very rare	Angina pectoris
Endocrine disorders	Very rare	Signs or symptoms of systemic glucocorticosteroid effects (including hypofunction of the adrenal gland)
Gastrointestinal disorders	Uncommon	Nausea
Immune system disorders	Rare	Exanthema, urticaria, pruritus, dermatitis, angioedema
Infections and infestations	Common	Candida infections in the oropharynx
Metabolic and nutrition disorders	Rare	Hypokalemia
	Very rare	Hyperglycemia
Musculoskeletal, connective tissue and bone disorders	Uncommon	Muscle cramps
Nervous system disorders	Common	Headache, tremor
	Uncommon	Dizziness
	Very rare	Taste disturbances
Psychiatric disorders	Uncommon	Agitation, restlessness, nervousness, sleep disturbances
	Very rare	Depression, behavioural disturbances (mainly in children)
Respiratory, thoracic and mediastinal disorders	Common	Mild irritation in the throat, coughing, hoarseness
	Rare	Bronchospasm
Skin and subcutaneous tissue disorders	Uncommon	Bruises
Vascular disorders	Very rare	Variations in blood pressure

As with other inhalation therapy, paradoxical bronchospasm may occur in very rare cases (see section 4.4).

Systemic effects of inhaled corticosteroids may occur, particularly at high doses prescribed for prolonged periods.These may include adrenal suppression, growth retardation in children and adolescents, decrease in bone mineral density, cataract and glaucoma (see also 4.4).

Treatment with β2-agonists may result in an increase in blood levels of insulin, free fatty acids, glycerol and ketone bodies.

4.9 Overdose

An overdose of formoterol would likely lead to effects that are typical for beta$_2$-adrenergic agonists: tremor, headache, palpitations. Symptoms reported from isolated cases are tachycardia, hyperglycaemia, hypokalaemia, prolonged QTc-interval, arrhythmia, nausea and vomiting. Supportive and symptomatic treatment may be indicated. A dose of 90 micrograms administered during three hours in patients with acute bronchial obstruction raised no safety concerns.

Acute overdosage with budesonide, even in excessive doses, is not expected to be a clinical problem. When used chronically in excessive doses, systemic glucocorticosteroid effects, such as hypercorticism and adrenal suppression, may appear.

If Symbicort therapy has to be withdrawn due to overdose of the formoterol component of the drug, provision of appropriate inhaled corticosteroid therapy must be considered.

5. PHARMACOLOGICAL PROPERTIES

5.1 Pharmacodynamic properties

Pharmacotherapeutic group: Adrenergics and other drugs for obstructive airway diseases.

ATC-code: R03AK07

Mechanisms of action and pharmacodynamic effects

Symbicort Turbohaler contains formoterol and budesonide, which have different modes of action and show additive effects in terms of reduction of asthma exacerbations. The mechanisms of action of the two substances, respectively are discussed below.

Budesonide

Budesonide given by inhalation at recommended doses has a glucocorticoid anti-inflammatory action within the lungs, resulting in reduced symptoms and exacerbations of asthma with less adverse effects than when corticosteroids are administered systemically. The exact mechanism responsible for this anti-inflammatory effect is unknown.

Formoterol

Formoterol is a selective beta$_2$-adrenergic agonist that produces relaxation of bronchial smooth muscle in patients with reversible airways obstruction. The bronchodilating effect sets in rapidly, within 1-3 minutes after inhalation, and has a duration of 12 hours after a single dose.

Symbicort Turbohaler

Asthma

In clinical trials, the addition of formoterol to budesonide improved asthma symptoms and lung function, and reduced exacerbations.

In two 12-week studies, the effect on lung function of Symbicort Turbohaler in asthma was equal to that of the free combination of budesonide and formoterol, and exceeded that of budesonide alone. There was no sign of attenuation of the anti-asthmatic effect over time. No clinical studies have been performed with Symbicort 400/12 Turbohaler. Corresponding doses delivered with the lower strengths of Symbicort Turbohaler are efficacious and well tolerated.

In a 12-week paediatric study 85 children aged 6-11 years were treated for asthma with Symbicort Turbohaler (2 inhalations of 80/4.5 micrograms/inhalation twice daily), which improved lung function and was well tolerated.

COPD

In two 12-month studies, the effect on lung function and the rate of exacerbation (defined as courses of oral steroids and/or course antibiotics and/or hospitalisations) in patients with severe COPD was evaluated. Median FEV_1 at inclusion in the trials was 36% of predicted normal. The mean number of exacerbations per year (as defined above) was significantly reduced with Symbicort as compared with treatment with formoterol alone or placebo (mean rate 1.4 compared with 1.8-1.9 in the placebo/formoterol group). The mean number of days on oral corticosteroids/patients during the 12 months was slightly reduced in the Symbicort group (7-8 days/ patient/ year compared with 11-12 and 9-12 days in the placebo and formoterol groups, respectively). For changes in lung-function parameters, such as FEV_1, Symbicort was not superior to treatment with formoterol alone.

5.2 Pharmacokinetic properties

Absorption

Symbicort Turbohaler and the corresponding monoproducts have been shown to be bioequivalent with regard to systemic exposure of budesonide and formoterol, respectively. In spite of this, a small increase in cortisol suppression was seen after administration of Symbicort Turbohaler compared with the monoproducts. The difference is considered not to have an impact on clinical safety.

There was no evidence of pharmacokinetic interactions between budesonide and formoterol.

Pharmacokinetic parameters for the respective substances were comparable after the administration of budesonide and formoterol as monoproducts or as Symbicort Turbohaler. For budesonide, AUC was slightly higher, rate of absorption more rapid and maximal plasma concentration higher after administration of the fixed combination. For formoterol, maximal plasma concentration was similar after administration of the fixed combination. Inhaled budesonide is rapidly absorbed and the maximum plasma concentration is reached within 30 minutes after inhalation. In studies, mean lung deposition of budesonide after inhalation via Turbohaler ranged from 32 to 44% of the delivered dose. The systemic bioavailability is approximately 49% of the delivered dose.

Inhaled formoterol is rapidly absorbed and the maximum plasma concentration is reached within 10 minutes after inhalation. In studies the mean lung deposition of formoterol after inhalation via Turbohaler ranged from 28-49% of the delivered dose. The systemic bioavailability is about 61% of the delivered dose.

Distribution and metabolism

Plasma protein binding is approximately 50% for formoterol and 90% for budesonide. Volume of distribution is about 4 L/kg for formoterol and 3 L/kg for budesonide. Formoterol is inactivated via conjugation reactions (active O-demethylated and deformylated metabolites are formed, but they are seen mainly as inactivated conjugates). Budesonide undergoes an extensive degree (approx. 90%) of biotransformation on first passage through the liver to metabolites of low glucocorticosteroid activity. The glucocorticosteroid activity of the major metabolites, 6-beta-hydroxy-budesonide and 16-alfa-hydroxy-prednisolone, is less than 1% of that of budesonide. There are no indications of any metabolic interactions or any displacement reactions between formoterol and budesonide.

Elimination

The major part of a dose of formoterol is transformed by liver metabolism followed by renal elimination. After inhalation, 8-13% of the delivered dose of formoterol is excreted unmetabolised in the urine. Formoterol has a high systemic clearance (approximately 1.4 L/min) and the terminal elimination half-life averages 17 hours.

Budesonide is eliminated via metabolism mainly catalysed by the enzyme CYP3A4. The metabolites of budesonide are eliminated in urine as such or in conjugated form. Only negligible amounts of unchanged budesonide have been detected in the urine. Budesonide has a high systemic clearance (approximately 1.2 L/min) and the plasma elimination half-life after i.v. dosing averages 4 hours.

The pharmacokinetics of budesonide or formoterol in patients with renal failure is unknown. The exposure of budesonide and formoterol may be increased in patients with liver disease.

5.3 Preclinical safety data

The toxicity observed in animal studies with budesonide and formoterol, given in combination or separately, were effects associated with exaggerated pharmacological activity.

In animal reproduction studies, corticosteroids such as budesonide have been shown to induce malformations (cleft palate, skeletal malformations). However, these animal experimental results do not seem to be relevant in humans at the recommended doses. Animal reproduction studies with formoterol have shown a somewhat reduced fertility in male rats at high systemic exposure and implantation losses as well as decreased early postnatal survival and birth weight at considerably higher systemic exposures than those reached during clinical use. However, these animal experimental results do not seem to be relevant in humans.

6. PHARMACEUTICAL PARTICULARS

6.1 List of excipients

Lactose monohydrate (which contains milk proteins).

6.2 Incompatibilities

Not applicable.

6.3 Shelf life

2 years.

6.4 Special precautions for storage

Do not store above 30°C. Keep the container tightly closed.

6.5 Nature and contents of container

Symbicort Turbohaler is an inspiratory flow driven, multidose powder inhaler. The inhaler is white with a red turning grip. The inhaler is made of different plastic materials (PP, PC, HDPE, LDPE, LLDPE, PBT). Each inhaler contains 60 doses. In each secondary package there are 1, 2, 3, 10 or 18 inhalers. Not all pack sizes may be marketed.

6.6 Instructions for use and handling

No special requirements.

7. MARKETING AUTHORISATION HOLDER

AstraZeneca UK Limited

600 Capability Green

Luton

LU1 3LU

United Kingdom

8. MARKETING AUTHORISATION NUMBER(S)

PL 17901/0200

9. DATE OF FIRST AUTHORISATION/RENEWAL OF THE AUTHORISATION
Date of first authorisation: 20th March 2003

Date of last Renewal: 25th August 2005

10. DATE OF REVISION OF THE TEXT
25th August 2005

Symbicort Turbohaler 100/6, Inhalation powder.

(AstraZeneca UK Limited)

1. NAME OF THE MEDICINAL PRODUCT
Symbicort® 100/6 Turbohaler®, Inhalation powder.

2. QUALITATIVE AND QUANTITATIVE COMPOSITION
Each delivered dose (the dose that leaves the mouthpiece) contains: budesonide 80 micrograms/inhalation and formoterol fumarate dihydrate 4.5 micrograms/inhalation.

Symbicort 100/6 Turbohaler delivers the same amount of budesonide and formoterol as the corresponding Turbohaler monoproducts, i.e. budesonide 100 micrograms/inhalation (metered dose) and formoterol 6 micrograms/inhalation (metered dose) alternatively labelled as 4.5 micrograms/inhalation (delivered dose).

For excipients, see 6.1.

3. PHARMACEUTICAL FORM
Inhalation powder.

White powder.

4. CLINICAL PARTICULARS
4.1 Therapeutic indications
Symbicort Turbohaler is indicated in the regular treatment of asthma where use of a combination (inhaled corticosteroid and long acting beta-agonist) is appropriate:

- patients not adequately controlled with inhaled corticosteroids and "as needed" inhaled short acting $beta_2$-agonists.

or

- patients already adequately controlled on both inhaled corticosteroids and long acting $beta_2$-agonists.

Note: Symbicort Turbohaler (100/6 micrograms/inhalation) is not appropriate in patients with severe asthma.

4.2 Posology and method of administration
Symbicort Turbohaler is not intended for the initial management of asthma. The dosage of the components of Symbicort Turbohaler is individual and should be adjusted to the severity of the disease. This should be considered not only when treatment with combination products is initiated but also when the dose is adjusted. If an individual patient should require a combination of doses other than those available in the combination inhaler, appropriate doses of beta-agonist and/or corticosteroids by individual inhalers should be prescribed.

Recommended doses:

Adults (18 years and older): 1-2 inhalations twice daily. Some patients may require up to a maximum of 4 inhalations twice daily.

Adolescents (12 – 17 years): 1-2 inhalations twice daily.

Children (6 years and older): 2 inhalations twice daily.

Patients should be regularly reassessed by a doctor, so that the dosage of Symbicort Turbohaler remains optimal. The dose should be titrated to the lowest dose at which effective control of symptoms is maintained. When control of symptoms is maintained with the lowest recommended dosage, then the next step could include a test of inhaled corticosteroid alone.

In usual practice when control of symptoms is achieved with the twice daily regimen, titration to the lowest effective dose could include Symbicort Turbohaler given once daily, when in the opinion of the prescriber, a long acting bronchodilator would be required to maintain control.

Children under 6 years: Symbicort is not recommended for children under 6 years of age.

Special patient groups: There is no need to adjust the dose in elderly patients. There are no data available for use of Symbicort Turbohaler in patients with hepatic or renal impairment. As budesonide and formoterol are primarily eliminated via hepatic metabolism, an increased exposure can be expected in patients with severe liver cirrhosis.

Instructions for correct use of Turbohaler:

Turbohaler is inspiratory flow-driven, which means that when the patient inhales through the mouthpiece, the substance will follow the inspired air into the airways.

Note: It is important to instruct the patient

- To carefully read the instructions for use in the patient information leaflet which is packed together with each inhaler
- To breathe in forcefully and deeply through the mouthpiece to ensure that an optimal dose is delivered to the lungs
- Never to breathe out through the mouthpiece
- To rinse the mouth out with water after inhaling the prescribed dose to minimise the risk of oropharyngeal thrush

The patient may not taste or feel any medication when using Symbicort Turbohaler due to the small amount of drug dispensed.

4.3 Contraindications
Hypersensitivity (allergy) to budesonide, formoterol or inhaled lactose.

4.4 Special warnings and special precautions for use
It is recommended that the dose is tapered when the treatment is discontinued and should not be stopped abruptly.

If patients find the treatment ineffective, or exceed the current dose of the fixed combination, medical attention must be sought. Increasing use of rescue bronchodilators indicates a worsening of the underlying condition and warrants a reassessment of the asthma therapy. Sudden and progressive deterioration in control of asthma is potentially life threatening and the patient should undergo urgent medical assessment. In this situation consideration should be given to the need for increased therapy with corticosteroids or addition of systemic anti-inflammatory therapy, such as a course of oral corticosteroids, or antibiotic treatment if an infection is present.

There are no data available on the use of Symbicort Turbohaler in the treatment of an acute asthma attack. Patients should be advised to have their rapid acting bronchodilator available at all times.

Patients should be reminded to take Symbicort Turbohaler daily as prescribed even when asymptomatic.

Therapy should not be initiated during an exacerbation.

As with other inhalation therapy, paradoxical bronchospasm may occur, with an immediate increase in wheezing after dosing. Symbicort Turbohaler should then be discontinued; treatment should be re-assessed and alternative therapy instituted if necessary.

Systemic effects may occur with any inhaled corticosteroid, particularly at high doses prescribed for long periods. These effects are much less likely to occur with inhalation treatment than with oral corticosteroids. Possible systemic effects include adrenal suppression, growth retardation in children and adolescents, decrease in bone mineral density, cataract and glaucoma

It is recommended that the height of children receiving prolonged treatment with inhaled corticosteroids is regularly monitored. If growth is slowed, therapy should be re-evaluated with the aim of reducing the dose of inhaled corticosteroid. The benefits of the corticosteroid therapy and the possible risks of growth suppression must be carefully weighed. In addition consideration should be given to referring the patient to a paediatric respiratory specialist.

Limited data from long-term studies suggest that most children and adolescents treated with inhaled budesonide will ultimately achieve their adult target height. However, an initial small but transient reduction in growth (approximately 1cm) has been observed. This generally occurs within the first year of treatment.

Long-term studies with inhaled budesonide in children at mean daily doses of 400 micrograms (metered dose) or in adults at daily doses of 800 micrograms (metered dose) have not shown any significant effects on bone mineral density. No information regarding the effect of Symbicort at higher doses is available.

If there is any reason to suppose that adrenal function is impaired from previous systemic steroid therapy, care should be taken when transferring patients to Symbicort Turbohaler therapy.

The benefits of inhaled budesonide therapy would normally minimise the need for oral steroids, but patients transferring from oral steroids may remain at risk of impaired adrenal reserve for a considerable time. Patients who have required high dose emergency corticosteroid therapy in the past or prolonged treatment with high doses of inhaled corticosteroids, particularly higher than the recommended doses, may also be at risk. Additional systemic corticosteriod cover should be considered during periods of stress or elective surgery.

To minimise the risk of oropharyngeal candida infection the patient should be instructed to rinse the mouth with water after each dosing occasion.

Concomitant treatment with itraconazole and ritonavir or other potent CYP3A4 inhibitors should be avoided (see section 4.5). If this is not possible the time interval between administration of the interacting drugs should be as long as possible.

Symbicort Turbohaler should be administered with caution in patients with thyrotoxicosis, phaeochromocytoma, diabetes mellitus, untreated hypokalaemia, hypertrophic obstructive cardiomyopathy, idiopathic subvalvular aortic stenosis, severe hypertension, aneurysm or other severe cardiovascular disorders, such as ischaemic heart disease, tachyarrhythmias or severe heart failure.

Caution should be observed when treating patients with prolongation of the QTc-interval. Formoterol itself may induce prolongation of the QTc-interval.

The need for, and dose of, inhaled corticosteroids should be re-evaluated in patients with active or quiescent pulmonary tuberculosis, fungal and viral infections in the airways.

Potentially serious hypokalaemia may result from high doses of $beta_2$-agonists. Concomitant treatment of $beta_2$-agonists with drugs which can induce hypokalaemia or potentiate a hypokalaemic effect, e.g xanthine-derivatives, steroids and diuretics, may add to a possible hypokalaemic effect of the $beta_2$-agonist. Particular caution is recommended in unstable asthma with variable use of rescue bronchodilators, in acute severe asthma as the associated risk may be augmented by hypoxia and in other conditions when the likelihood for hypokalaemia adverse effects is increased. It is recommended that serum potassium levels are monitored during these circumstances.

As for all $beta_2$-agonists, additional blood glucose controls should be considered in diabetic patients.

Symbicort Turbohaler contains lactose ($<$1 mg/inhalation). This amount does not normally cause problems in lactose intolerant people.

4.5 Interaction with other medicinal products and other forms of Interaction
Pharmacokinetic interactions

The metabolic conversion of budesonide is impeded by substances metabolized by CYP P450 3A4 (e.g. itraconazole, ritonavir). The concomitant administration of these potent inhibitors of CYP P450 3A4 may increase plasma levels of budesonide. The concomitant use of these drugs should be avoided unless the benefit outweighs the increased risk of systemic side-effects.

Pharmacodynamic interactions

Beta-adrenergic blockers can weaken or inhibit the effect of formoterol. Symbicort Turbohaler should therefore not be given together with beta-adrenergic blockers (including eye drops) unless there are compelling reasons.

Concomitant treatment with quinidine, disopyramide, procainamide, phenothiazines, antihistamines (terfenadine), monoamine oxidase inhibitors and tricyclic antidepressants can prolong the QTc-interval and increase the risk of ventricular arrhythmias.

In addition L-Dopa, L-thyroxine, oxytocin and alcohol can impair cardiac tolerance towards β_2-sympathomimetics.

Concomitant treatment with monoamine oxidase inhibitors including agents with similar properties such as furazolidone and procarbazine may precipitate hypertensive reactions.

There is an elevated risk of arrhythmias in patients receiving concomitant anaesthesia with halogenated hydrocarbons.

Concomitant use of other beta-adrenergic drugs can have a potentially additive effect.

Hypokalaemia may increase the disposition towards arrhythmias in patients who are treated with digitalis glycosides.

Budesonide has not been observed to interact with any other drugs used in the treatment of asthma.

4.6 Pregnancy and lactation
For Symbicort Turbohaler or the concomitant treatment with formoterol and budesonide, no clinical data on exposed pregnancies are available. Animal studies with respect to reproductive toxicity of the combination have not been performed.

There are no adequate data from use of formoterol in pregnant women. In animal studies formoterol has caused adverse effects in reproduction studies at very high systemic exposure levels (see section 5.3).

Data on approximately 2000 exposed pregnancies indicate no increased teratogenic risk associated with the use of inhaled budesonide. In animal studies glucocorticosteroids have been shown to induce malformations (see section 5.3). This is not likely to be relevant for humans given recommended doses.

Animal studies have also identified an involvement of excess prenatal glucocorticoids in increased risks for intrauterine growth retardation, adult cardiovascular disease and permanent changes in glucocorticoid receptor density, neurotransmitter turnover and behaviour at exposures below the teratogenic dose range.

During pregnancy, Symbicort Turbohaler should only be used when the benefits outweigh the potential risks. The lowest effective dose of budesonide needed to maintain adequate asthma control should be used.

It is not known whether formoterol or budesonide passes into human breast milk. In rats, small amounts of formoterol have been detected in maternal milk. Administration of Symbicort Turbohaler to women who are breastfeeding should only be considered if the expected benefit to the mother is greater than any possible risk to the child.

4.7 Effects on ability to drive and use machines
Symbicort Turbohaler has no or negligible influence on the ability to drive and use machines.

4.8 Undesirable effects
Since Symbicort Turbohaler contains both budesonide and formoterol, the same pattern of undesirable effects as reported for these substances may occur. No increased incidence of adverse reactions has been seen following

concurrent administration of the two compounds. The most common drug related adverse reactions are pharmacologically predictable side-effects of $beta_2$-agonist therapy, such as tremor and palpitations. These tend to be mild and usually disappear within a few days of treatment.

Adverse reactions, which have been associated with budesonide or formoterol, are given below, listed by system organ class and frequency. Frequency are defined as: very common (≥1/10), common (≥1/100 and <1/10), uncommon (≥1/1000 and <1/100), rare (≥1/10 000 and <1/1000) and very rare (<1/10 000).

Cardiac disorders	Common	Palpitations
	Uncommon	Tachycardia
	Rare	Atrial fibrillation, supraventricular tachycardia, extrasystoles
	Very rare	Angina pectoris
Endocrine disorders	Very rare	Signs or symptoms of systemic glucocorticosteroid effects (including hypofunction of the adrenal gland)
Gastrointestinal disorders	Uncommon	Nausea
Immune system disorders	Rare	Exanthema, urticaria, pruritus, dermatitis, angioedema
Infections and infestations	Common	Candida infections in the oropharynx
Metabolic and nutrition disorders	Rare	Hypokalemia
	Very rare	Hyperglycemia
Musculoskeletal, connective tissue and bone disorders	Uncommon	Muscle cramps
Nervous system disorders	Common	Headache, tremor
	Uncommon	Dizziness
	Very rare	Taste disturbances
Psychiatric disorders	Uncommon	Agitation, restlessness, nervousness, sleep disturbances
	Very rare	Depression, behavioural disturbances (mainly in children)
Respiratory, thoracic and mediastinal disorders	Common	Mild irritation in the throat, coughing, hoarseness
	Rare	Bronchospasm
Skin and subcutaneous tissue disorders	Uncommon	Bruises
Vascular disorders	Very rare	Variations in blood pressure

As with other inhalation therapy, paradoxical bronchospasm may occur in very rare cases (see section 4.4).

Systemic effects of inhaled corticosteroids may occur, particularly at high doses prescribed for prolonged periods. These may include adrenal suppression, growth retardation in children and adolescents, decrease in bone mineral density, cataract and glaucoma (see also 4.4).

Treatment with β_2-agonists may result in an increase in blood levels of insulin, free fatty acids, glycerol and ketone bodies.

4.9 Overdose

An overdose of formoterol would likely lead to effects that are typical for $beta_2$-adrenergic agonists: tremor, headache, palpitations. Symptoms reported from isolated cases are tachycardia, hyperglycaemia, hypokalaemia, prolonged QTc-interval, arrhythmia, nausea and vomiting. Supportive and symptomatic treatment may be indicated. A dose of 90 micrograms administered during three hours in patients with acute bronchial obstruction raised no safety concerns.

Acute overdosage with budesonide, even in excessive doses, is not expected to be a clinical problem. When used chronically in excessive doses, systemic glucocorticosteroid effects, such as hypercorticism and adrenal suppression, may appear.

If Symbicort therapy has to be withdrawn due to overdose of the formoterol component of the drug, provision of appropriate inhaled corticosteroid therapy must be considered.

5. PHARMACOLOGICAL PROPERTIES

5.1 Pharmacodynamic properties

Pharmacotherapeutic group: Adrenergics and other drugs for obstructive airway diseases.

ATC-code: R03AK07

Mechanisms of action and pharmacodynamic effects

Symbicort Turbohaler contains formoterol and budesonide, which have different modes of action and show additive effects in terms of reduction of asthma exacerbations. The mechanisms of action of the two substances, respectively are discussed below.

Budesonide

Budesonide given by inhalation at recommended doses has a glucocorticoid antiinflammatory action within the lungs, resulting in reduced symptoms and exacerbations of asthma with less adverse effects than when corticosteroids are administered systemically. The exact mechanism responsible for this anti-inflammatory effect is unknown.

Formoterol

Formoterol is a selective $beta_2$-adrenergic agonist that produces relaxation of bronchial smooth muscle in patients with reversible airways obstruction. The bronchodilating effect sets in rapidly, within 1-3 minutes after inhalation, and has a duration of 12 hours after a single dose.

Symbicort Turbohaler

In clinical trials in adults, the addition of formoterol to budesonide improved asthma symptoms and lung function, and reduced exacerbations.

In two 12-week studies the effect on lung function of Symbicort Turbohaler was equal to that of the free combination of budesonide and formoterol, and exceeded that of budesonide alone. There was no sign of attenuation of the anti-asthmatic effect over time.

In a 12-week paediatric study 85 children aged 6-11 years were treated with Symbicort Turbohaler (2 inhalations of 80/4.5 micrograms/inhalations twice daily), which improved lung function and was well tolerated.

5.2 Pharmacokinetic properties

Absorption

Symbicort Turbohaler and the corresponding monoproducts have been shown to be bioequivalent with regard to systemic exposure of budesonide and formoterol, respectively. In spite of this, a small increase in cortisol suppression was seen after administration of Symbicort Turbohaler compared to the monoproducts. The difference is considered not to have an impact on clinical safety.

There was no evidence of pharmacokinetic interactions between budesonide and formoterol.

Pharmacokinetic parameters for the respective substances were comparable after the administration of budesonide and formoterol as monoproducts or as Symbicort Turbohaler. For budesonide, AUC was slightly higher, rate of absorption more rapid and maximal plasma concentration higher after administration of the fixed combination. For formoterol, maximal plasma concentration was similar after administration of the fixed combination. Inhaled budesonide is rapidly absorbed and the maximum plasma concentration is reached within 30 minutes after inhalation. In studies, mean lung deposition of budesonide after inhalation via Turbohaler ranged from 32 to 44% of the delivered dose. The systemic bioavailability is approximately 49% of the delivered dose. In children 6-16 years the lung deposition fall in the same range as in adults for the same given dose, the resulting plasma concentrations were not determined.

Inhaled formoterol is rapidly absorbed and the maximum plasma concentration is reached within 10 minutes after inhalation. In studies the mean lung deposition of formoterol after inhalation via Turbohaler ranged from 28-49% of the delivered dose. The systemic bioavailability is about 61% of the delivered dose.

Distribution and metabolism

Plasma protein binding is approximately 50% for formoterol and 90% for budesonide. Volume of distribution is about 4 L/kg for formoterol and 3 L/kg for budesonide. Formoterol is inactivated via conjugation reactions (active O-demethylated and deformylated metabolites are formed, but they are seen mainly as inactivated conjugates). Budesonide undergoes an extensive degree (approx. 90%) of biotransformation on first passage through the liver to metabolites of low glucocorticosteroid activity. The glucocorticosteroid activity of the major metabolites, 6-beta-hydroxy-budesonide and 16-alfa-hydroxy-prednisolone, is less than 1% of that of budesonide. There are no indications of any metabolic interactions or any displacement reactions between formoterol and budesonide.

Elimination

The major part of a dose of formoterol is transformed by liver metabolism followed by renal elimination. After inhalation, 8-13% of the delivered dose of formoterol is excreted unmetabolised in the urine. Formoterol has a high systemic clearance (approximately 1.4 L/min) and the terminal elimination half-life averages 17 hours.

Budesonide is eliminated via metabolism mainly catalysed by the enzyme CYP3A4. The metabolites of budesonide are eliminated in urine as such or in conjugated form. Only negligible amounts of unchanged budesonide have been detected in the urine. Budesonide has a high systemic clearance (approximately 1.2 L/min) and the plasma elimination half-life after i.v. dosing averages 4 hours.

The pharmacokinetics of formoterol in children have not been studied. The pharmacokinetics of budesonide and formoterol in patients with renal failure are unknown. The exposure of budesonide and formoterol may be increased in patients with liver disease.

5.3 Preclinical safety data

The toxicity observed in animal studies with budesonide and formoterol, given in combination or separately, were effects associated with exaggerated pharmacological activity.

In animal reproduction studies, corticosteroids such as budesonide have been shown to induce malformations (cleft palate, skeletal malformations). However, these animal experimental results do not seem to be relevant in humans at the recommended doses. Animal reproduction studies with formoterol have shown a somewhat reduced fertility in male rats at high systemic exposure and implantation losses as well as decreased early postnatal survival and birth weight at considerably higher systemic exposures than those reached during clinical use. However, these animal experimental results do not seem to be relevant in humans.

6. PHARMACEUTICAL PARTICULARS

6.1 List of excipients

Lactose monohydrate (which contains milk proteins).

6.2 Incompatibilities

Not applicable.

6.3 Shelf life

2 years.

6.4 Special precautions for storage

Do not store above 30°C. Keep the container tightly closed.

6.5 Nature and contents of container

Symbicort Turbohaler is an inspiratory flow driven, multidose powder inhaler. The inhaler is white with a red turning grip. The inhaler is made of different plastic materials (PP, PC, HDPE, LDPE, LLDPE, PBT). Each inhaler contains 60 doses or 120 doses. In each secondary package there are 1, 2, 3, 10 or 18 inhalers. Not all pack-sizes may be marketed.

6.6 Instructions for use and handling

No special requirements.

7. MARKETING AUTHORISATION HOLDER

AstraZeneca UK Limited,

600 Capability Green,

Luton, LU1 3LU, UK.

8. MARKETING AUTHORISATION NUMBER(S)

PL 17901/0091

9. DATE OF FIRST AUTHORISATION/RENEWAL OF THE AUTHORISATION

Date of first authorisation: 15th May 2001

Date of last Renewal: 25th August 2005

10. DATE OF REVISION OF THE TEXT

25th August 2005

Symmetrel Capsules

(Alliance Pharmaceuticals)

1. NAME OF THE MEDICINAL PRODUCT

Symmetrel® capsules 100mg

2. QUALITATIVE AND QUANTITATIVE COMPOSITION

Amantadine hydrochloride PhEur 100mg.

3. PHARMACEUTICAL FORM

Brownish-red, hard gelatin capsules imprinted SYMM in white on both cap and body.

4. CLINICAL PARTICULARS

4.1 Therapeutic indications

Parkinson's disease.

Herpes zoster. It is recommended that Symmetrel be given to elderly or debilitated patients in whom the physician suspects that a severe and painful rash could occur. Symmetrel can significantly reduce the proportion of patients experiencing pain of long duration.

4.2 Posology and method of administration

Parkinson's disease: Initially 100mg daily for the first week, increasing to 100mg twice daily. The dose can be titrated against signs and symptoms. Doses exceeding

200mg daily may provide some additional relief, but may also be associated with increasing toxicity. A dose of 400mg/day should not be exceeded. The dose should be increased gradually, at intervals of not less than 1 week. Since patients over 65 years of age tend to show lower renal clearance and consequently higher plasma concentrations, the lowest effective dose should be used.

Amantadine acts within a few days, but may appear to lose efficacy within a few months of continuous treatment. Its effectiveness may be prolonged by withdrawal for three to four weeks, which seems to restore activity. During this time, existing concomitant antiparkinsonian therapy should be continued, or low dose L-dopa treatment initiated if clinically necessary.

Symmetrel withdrawal should be gradual, e.g. half the dose at weekly intervals. Abrupt discontinuation may exacerbate Parkinsonism, regardless of the patient's response to therapy (see Section 4.4, "Special warnings and precautions for use"). *Combined treatment:* any antiparkinson drug already in use should be continued during initial Symmetrel treatment. It may then be possible to reduce the other drug gradually. If increased side effects occur, the dosage should be reduced more quickly. In patients receiving large doses of anticholinergic agents or L-dopa, the initial phase of Symmetrel treatment should be extended to 15 days.

Herpes zoster: 100mg twice daily for 14 days. Treatment should be started as soon as possible after diagnosis. If post-herpetic pain persists treatment can be continued for a further 14 days.

In patients with **renal impairment**: the dose of amantadine should be reduced. This can be achieved by either reducing the total daily dose, or by increasing the dosage interval in accordance with the creatinine clearance. For example,

Creatinine clearance ml/(min)	Dose
< 15	Symmetrel contra-indicated.
15 – 35	100mg every 2 to 3 days.
> 35	100mg every day

The above recommendations are for guidance only and physicians should continue to monitor their patients for signs of unwanted effects.

4.3 Contraindications

Known hypersensitivity to amantadine or any of the excipients. Individuals subject to convulsions. A history of gastric ulceration. Severe renal disease. Pregnancy.

4.4 Special warnings and special precautions for use

Symmetrel should be used with caution in patients with confusional or hallucinatory states or underlying psychiatric disorders, in patients with liver or kidney disorders, and those suffering from, or who have a history of, cardiovascular disorders. Caution should be applied when prescribing amantadine with other medications having an effect on the CNS (See section 4.5, Interactions with other medicaments and other forms of interaction).

Abrupt discontinuation of amantadine may result in worsening of Parkinsonism. Symmetrel should not be stopped abruptly in patients who are treated concurrently with neuroleptics. There have been isolated reports of precipitation or aggravation of neuroleptic malignant syndrome or neuroleptic-induced catatonia following the withdrawal of amantadine in patients taking neuroleptic agents. **A similar syndrome has also been reported rarely following withdrawal of amantadine and other anti-parkinson agents in patients who were not taking concurrent psychoactive medication.**

As some individuals have attempted suicide with amantadine, prescriptions should be written for the smallest quantity consistent with good patient management.

Peripheral oedema (thought to be due to an alteration in the responsiveness of peripheral vessels) may occur in some patients during chronic treatment (not usually before four weeks) with Symmetrel. This should be taken into account in patients with congestive heart failure.

4.5 Interaction with other medicinal products and other forms of Interaction

Concurrent administration of amantadine and anticholinergic agents or levodopa may increase confusion, hallucinations, nightmares, gastro-intestinal disturbances, or other atropine-like side effects (see Section 4.9 "Overdose"). Psychotic reactions have been observed in patients receiving amantadine and levodopa.

In isolated cases, worsening of psychotic symptoms has been reported in patients receiving amantadine and concomitant neuroleptic medication.

Concurrent administration of amantadine and drugs or substances (e.g. alcohol) acting on the CNS may result in additive CNS toxicity. Close observation is recommended (see Section 4.9 "Overdose").

There have been isolated reports of a suspected interaction between amantadine and combination diuretics (hydrochlorothiazide + potassium sparing diuretics). One or both of the components apparently reduce the clearance of amantadine, leading to higher plasma concentrations and toxic effects (confusion, hallucinations, ataxia, myoclonus).

4.6 Pregnancy and lactation

Amantadine-related complications during pregnancy have been reported. Symmetrel is contra-indicated during pregnancy and in women **trying** to become pregnant. Amantadine passes into breast milk. Undesirable effects have been reported in breast-fed infants. Nursing mothers should not take Symmetrel.

4.7 Effects on ability to drive and use machines

Patients should be warned of the potential hazards of driving or operating machinery if they experience side effects such as dizziness or blurred vision.

4.8 Undesirable effects

Amantadine's undesirable effects are often mild and transient, usually appearing within the first 2 to 4 days of treatment and promptly disappearing 24 to 48 hours after discontinuation. A direct relationship between dose and incidence of side effects has not been demonstrated, although there seems to be a tendency towards more frequent undesirable effects (particularly affecting the CNS) with increasing doses.

Side effects reported include:

Frequency estimates: frequent> 10%, occasional 1%-10%, rare 0.001%-1%, isolated cases < 0.001%.

Central nervous system: Occasional: anxiety, elevation of mood, lightheadedness, headache, lethargy, hallucinations, nightmares, ataxia, slurred speech, blurred vision, lossof concentration, nervousness, depression, insomnia, myalgia. Hallucinations, confusion and nightmares are more common when amantadine is administered concurrently with anticholinergic agents or when the patient has an underlying psychiatric disorder. Rare: confusion, disorientation, psychosis, tremor, dyskinesia, convulsions, **neuroleptic malignant-like syndrome.** Delirium, hypomanic state and mania have been reported but their incidence cannot be readily deduced from the literature. *Cardiovascular system:* Frequent: oedema of ankles, livedo reticularis (usually after very high doses or use over many months). Occasional: palpitations, orthostatic hypotension. Isolated cases: heart insufficiency/failure. *Blood*: Isolated cases: leucopenia, reversible elevation of liver enzymes. *Gastrointestinal tract:* Occasional: dry mouth, anorexia, nausea, vomiting, constipation. Rare: diarrhoea. *Skin and appendages:* Occasional: diaphoresis. Rare: exanthema. Isolated cases: photosensitisation. *Sense organs*: Rare: corneal lesions, e.g. punctate subepithelial opacities which might be associated with superficial punctate keratitis, corneal epithelial oedema, and markedly reduced visual acuity. *Urogenital tract:* Rare: urinary retention, urinary incontinence.

4.9 Overdose

Signs and symptoms: *Neuromuscular* disturbances and symptoms of acute psychosis are prominent. *Central nervous system:* Hyperreflexia, motor restlessness, convulsions, extrapyramidal signs, torsion spasms, dystonic posturing, dilated pupils, confusion, disorientation, delirium, visual hallucinations. *Respiratory system*: hyperventilation, pulmonary oedema, respiratory distress, including adult respiratory distress syndrome. *Cardiovascular system*: sinus tachycardia, arrhythmia. *Gastrointestinal system*: nausea, vomiting, dry mouth. *Renal function*: urine retention, renal dysfunction, including increase in BUN and decreased creatinine clearance.

Overdose from combined drug treatment: the effects of anticholinergic drugs are increased by amantadine. Acute psychotic reactions (which may be identical to those of atropine poisoning) may occur when large doses of anticholinergic agents are used. Where alcohol or central nervous stimulants have been taken at the same time, the signs and symptoms of acute poisoning with amantadine may be aggravated and/or modified.

Management: There is no specific antidote. Induction of vomiting and/or gastric aspiration (and lavage if patient is conscious), activated charcoal or saline cathartic may be used if judged appropriate. Since amantadine is excreted mainly unchanged in the urine, maintenance of renal function and copious diuresis (forced diuresis if necessary) are effective ways to remove it from the blood stream. Acidification of the urine favours its excretion. Haemodialysis does not remove significant amounts of amantadine.

Monitor the blood pressure, heart rate, ECG, respiration and body temperature, and treat for possible hypotension and cardiac arhythmias, as necessary. *Convulsions and excessive motor restlessness*: administer anticonvulsants such as diazepam iv, paraldehyde im or per rectum, or phenobarbital im. *Acute psychotic symptoms, delirium, dystonic posturing, myoclonic manifestations*: physostigmine by slow iv infusion (1mg doses in adults, 0.5mg in children) repeated administration according to the initial response and the subsequent need, has been reported. *Retention of urine*: bladder should be catheterised; an indwelling catheter can be left in place for the time required.

5. PHARMACOLOGICAL PROPERTIES

5.1 Pharmacodynamic properties

Herpes Zoster: The mechanism of action of Symmetrel in herpes zoster has not been fully characterised.

Parkinson's disease: Symmetrel is believed to enhance the release of dopamine and delay its reuptake into synaptic vesicles. It may also exert some anticholinergic activity. Whether administered alone or in combination, amantadine produces an improvement in the cardinal signs and symptoms of parkinsonism and improves functional capacity in about 60% of patients. The positive effect generally sets in two to five days after the start of treatment, particularly on akinesia, rigidity and tremor.

5.2 Pharmacokinetic properties

Absorption: Amantadine is absorbed slowly but almost completely. Peak plasma concentrations of approximately 250ng/ml and 500ng/ml are seen 3 to 4 hours after single oral administration of 100mg and 200mg amantadine, respectively. Following repeated administration of 200mg daily, the steady-state plasma concentration settles at 300ng/ml within 3 days.

Distribution: Amantadine accumulates after several hours in nasal secretions and crosses the blood-brain barrier (this has not been quantified). *In vitro*, 67% is bound to plasma proteins, with a substantial amount bound to red blood cells. The concentration in erythrocytes in normal healthy volunteers is 2.66 times the plasma concentration. The apparent volume of distribution is 5 to 10L/kg, suggesting extensive tissue binding. This declines with increasing doses. The concentrations in the lung, heart, kidney, liver and spleen are higher than in the blood.

Biotransformation: Amantadine is metabolised to a minor extent, principally by N-acetylation.

Elimination: The drug is eliminated in healthy young adults with a mean plasma elimination half-life of 15 hours (10 to 31 hours). The total plasma clearance is about the same as renal clearance (250ml/min). The renal amantadine clearance is much higher than the creatinine clearance, suggesting renal tubular secretion. After 4 to 5 days, 90% of the dose appears unchanged in urine. The rate is considerably influenced by urinary pH: a rise in pH brings about a fall in excretion.

Characteristics in special patient populations:

Elderly patients: compared with healthy young adults, the half-life may be doubled and renal clearance diminished. Tubular secretion diminishes more than glomerular filtration in the elderly. In elderly patients with renal impairment, repeated administration of 100mg daily for 14 days raised the plasma concentration into the toxic range.

Renal impairment: amantadine may accumulate in renal failure, causing severe side effects. The rate of elimination from plasma correlates to creatinine clearance divided by body surface area, although total renal elimination exceeds this value (possibly due to tubular secretion). The effects of reduced kidney function are dramatic: a reduction of creatinine clearance to 40ml/min may result in a five-fold increase in elimination half-life. The urine is the almost exclusive route of excretion, even with renal failure, and amantadine may persist in the plasma for several days. Haemodialysis does not remove significant amounts of amantadine, possibly due to extensive tissue binding.

5.3 Preclinical safety data

Reproductive toxicity studies were performed in rats and rabbits. In rat oral doses of 50 and 100 mg/kg proved to be teratogenic. The maximum recommended dose of 400mg is less than 6mg/kg.

There are no other pre-clinical data of relevance to the prescriber which are additional to those already included in other sections of the Summary of Product Characteristics.

6. PHARMACEUTICAL PARTICULARS

6.1 List of excipients

Lactose, polyvinylpyrrolidone, magnesium stearate, red iron oxide (E172), titanium dioxide (E171), gelatin and white printer's ink.

6.2 Incompatibilities

None known.

6.3 Shelf life

Five years.

6.4 Special precautions for storage

Protect from moisture. Medicines should be kept out of reach of children.

6.5 Nature and contents of container

Aluminium/PVdC blister packs of 56 capsules.

6.6 Instructions for use and handling

None.

7. MARKETING AUTHORISATION HOLDER

Alliance Pharmaceuticals Ltd
Avonbridge House
Bath Road
Chippenham
Wiltshire
SN15 2BB

8. MARKETING AUTHORISATION NUMBER(S)

PL16853/0015

9. DATE OF FIRST AUTHORISATION/RENEWAL OF THE AUTHORISATION

26 June 1998

10. DATE OF REVISION OF THE TEXT

October 2001

11. Legal Status
POM

Alliance, Alliance Pharmaceuticals and associated devices are registered Trademarks of Alliance Pharmaceuticals Ltd.

Symmetrel Syrup

(Alliance Pharmaceuticals)

1. NAME OF THE MEDICINAL PRODUCT
Symmetrel® syrup 50mg/5ml

2. QUALITATIVE AND QUANTITATIVE COMPOSITION
Amantadine hydrochloride PhEur 50mg/5 mL.

3. PHARMACEUTICAL FORM
Clear, citrus flavoured syrup with a lemon odour.

4. CLINICAL PARTICULARS
4.1 Therapeutic indications
Prophylaxis and treatment of signs and symptoms of infection caused by influenza A virus. It is suggested that Symmetrel be given to patients suffering from clinical influenza in which complications might be expected to occur. In addition, Symmetrel is recommended prophylactically in cases particularly at risk. This can include those with chronic respiratory disease or debilitating conditions, the elderly and those living in crowded conditions. It can also be used for individuals in families where influenza has already been diagnosed, for control of institutional outbreaks or for those in essential services who are unvaccinated or when vaccination is unavailable or contra-indicated.

Symmetrel does not completely prevent the host immune response to influenza A infection, so individuals who take this drug still develop immune responses to the natural disease or vaccination and may be protected when later exposed to antigenically related viruses. Symmetrel may also be used in post-exposure prophylaxis in conjunction with inactivated vaccine during an outbreak until protective antibodies develop, or in patients who are not expected to have a substantial antibody response (immunosuppression).

Parkinson's disease.
Herpes zoster.
It is recommended that Symmetrel be given to elderly or debilitated patients in whom the physician suspects that a severe and painful rash could occur. Symmetrel can significantly reduce the proportion of patients experiencing pain of long duration.

4.2 Posology and method of administration
Influenza A: Treatment:
It is advisable to start treating influenza as early as possible and to continue for 4 to 5 days. When amantadine is started within 48 hours of symptoms appearing, the duration of fever and other effects is reduced by one or two days and the inflammatory reaction of the bronchial tree that usually accompanies influenza resolves more quickly.

Prophylaxis:
Treat daily for as long as protection from infection is required. In most instances this is expected to be for 6 weeks. When used with inactivated influenza A vaccine, amantadine is continued for 2 to 3 weeks following inoculation.

Adults:
100mg daily for the recommended period.

Children aged 10-15 years:100mg daily for the recommended period.

Children under 10 years of age:
Dosage not established.

Adults over 65 years of age:
Plasma amantadine concentrations are influenced by renal function. In elderly patients, the elimination half-life is longer and renal clearance of the compound is diminished in comparison to young people. Therefore a daily dose of less than 100mg, or 100mg given at intervals of greater than one day, may be appropriate.

Parkinson's disease:
Initially 100mg daily for the first week, increasing to 100mg twice daily. The dose can be titrated against signs and symptoms. Doses exceeding 200mg daily may provide some additional relief, but may also be associated with increasing toxicity. A dose of 400mg/day should not be exceeded. The dose should be increased gradually, at intervals of not less than 1 week. Since patients over 65 years of age tend to show lower renal clearance and consequently higher plasma concentrations, the lowest effective dose should be used.

Amantadine acts within a few days, but may appear to lose efficacy within a few months of continuous treatment. Its effectiveness may be prolonged by withdrawal for three to four weeks, which seems to restore activity. During this time, existing concomitant antiparkinsonian therapy should be continued, or low dose L-dopa treatment initiated if clinically necessary.

Symmetrel withdrawal should be gradual, e.g. half the dose at weekly intervals. Abrupt discontinuation may exacerbate Parkinsonism, regardless of the patient's response to therapy (see Section 4.4, "Special warnings and precautions for use"). *Combined treatment:* any antiparkinson drug already in use should be continued during initial Symmetrel treatment. It may then be possible to reduce the other drug gradually. If increased side effects occur, the dosage should be reduced more quickly. In patients receiving large doses of anticholinergic agents or L-dopa, the initial phase of Symmetrel treatment should be extended to 15 days.

Herpes zoster:
100mg twice daily for 14 days. Treatment should be started as soon as possible after diagnosis. If post-herpetic pain persists treatment can be continued for a further 14 days.

In patients with **renal impairment** the dose of amantadine should be reduced. This can be achieved by either reducing the total daily dose, or by increasing the dosage interval in accordance with the creatinine clearance. For example,

Creatinine clearance ml/(min)	Dose
< 15	Symmetrel contra-indicated.
15 - 35	100mg every 2 to 3 days.
> 35	100mg every day

The above recommendations are for guidance only and physicians should continue to monitor their patients for signs of unwanted effects.

4.3 Contraindications
Known hypersensitivity to amantadine or any of the excipients. Individuals subject to convulsions. A history of gastric ulceration. Severe renal disease. Pregnancy.

4.4 Special warnings and special precautions for use
Symmetrel should be used with caution in patients with confusional or hallucinatory states or underlying psychiatric disorders, in patients with liver or kidney disorders, and those suffering from, or who have a history of, cardiovascular disorders. Caution should be applied when prescribing amantadine with other medications having an effect on the CNS (See section 4.5, Interactions with other medicaments and other forms of interaction).

Abrupt discontinuation of amantadine may result in worsening of Parkinsonism. Symmetrel should not be stopped abruptly in patients who are treated concurrently with neuroleptics. There have been isolated reports of precipitation or aggravation of neuroleptic malignant syndrome or neuroleptic-induced catatonia following the withdrawal of amantadine in patients taking neuroleptic agents.

Resistance to amantadine occurs during serial passage of influenza virus strains in vitro or in vivo in the presence of the drug. Apparent transmission of drug-resistant viruses may have been the cause of failure of prophylaxis and treatment in household contacts and in nursing-home patients. However, there is no evidence to date that the resistant virus produces a disease that is in any way different from that produced by sensitive viruses.

As some individuals have attempted suicide with amantadine, prescriptions should be written for the smallest quantity consistent with good patient management.

Peripheral oedema (thought to be due to an alteration in the responsiveness of peripheral vessels) may occur in some patients during chronic treatment (not usually before 4 weeks) with Symmetrel. This should be taken into account in patients with congestive heart failure.

4.5 Interaction with other medicinal products and other forms of Interaction
Concurrent administration of amantadine and anticholinergic agents or levodopa may increase confusion, hallucinations, nightmares, gastro-intestinal disturbances, or other atropine-like side effects (see Section 4.9 "Overdose"). Psychotic reactions have been observed in patients receiving amantadine and levodopa.

In isolated cases, worsening of psychotic symptoms has been reported in patients receiving amantadine and concomitant neuroleptic medication.

Concurrent administration of amantadine and drugs or substances (e.g. alcohol) acting on the CNS may result in additive CNS toxicity. Close observation is recommended (see Section 4.9 "Overdose").

There have been isolated reports of a suspected interaction between amantadine and combination diuretics (hydrochlorothiazide + potassium sparing diuretics). One or both of the components apparently reduce the clearance of amantadine, leading to higher plasma concentrations and toxic effects (confusion, hallucinations, ataxia, myoclonus).

4.6 Pregnancy and lactation
Amantadine-related complications during pregnancy have been reported. Symmetrel is contra-indicated during pregnancy and in women wishing to become pregnant. Amantadine passes into breast milk. Undesirable effects have been reported in breast-fed infants. Nursing mothers should not take Symmetrel.

4.7 Effects on ability to drive and use machines
Patients should be warned of the potential hazards of driving or operating machinery if they experience side effects such as dizziness or blurred vision.

4.8 Undesirable effects
Amantadine's undesirable effects are often mild and transient, usually appearing within the first 2 to 4 days of treatment and promptly disappearing 24 to 48 hours after discontinuation. A direct relationship between dose and incidence of side effects has not been demonstrated, although there seems to be a tendency towards more frequent undesirable effects (particularly affecting the CNS) with increasing doses.

The side effects reported after the pivotal clinical studies in influenza in over 1200 patients receiving amantadine at 100mg daily were mostly mild, transient, and equivalent to placebo. Only 7% of subjects reported adverse events, many being similar to the effects of influenza itself. The most commonly reported effects were gastro-intestinal disturbances (anorexia, nausea), CNS effects (loss of concentration, dizziness, agitation, nervousness, depression, insomnia, fatigue, weakness), or myalgia.

Side effects reported after higher doses or chronic use, in addition to those already stated, include:

Frequency estimates: frequent > 10%, occasional 1%-10%, rare 0.001%-1%, isolated cases < 0.001%.

Central nervous system:
Occasional: anxiety, elevation of mood, lightheadedness, headache, lethargy, hallucinations, nightmares, ataxia, slurred speech, blurred vision. Hallucinations, confusion and nightmares are more common when amantadine is administered concurrently with anticholinergic agents or when the patient has an underlying psychiatric disorder. Rare: confusion, disorientation, psychosis, tremor, dyskinesia, convulsions. Delirium, hypomanic state and mania have been reported but their incidence cannot be readily deduced from the literature.

Cardiovascular system:
Frequent: oedema of ankles, livedo reticularis (usually after very high doses or use over many months). Occasional: palpitations, orthostatic hypotension. Isolated cases: heart insufficiency/failure.

Blood:
Isolated cases: leucopenia, reversible elevation of liver enzymes.

Gastrointestinal tract:
Occasional: dry mouth, anorexia, nausea, vomiting, constipation. Rare: diarrhoea.

Skin and appendages:
Occasional: diaphoresis. Rare: exanthema. Isolated cases: photosensitisation.

Sense organs:
Rare: corneal lesions, e.g. punctate subepithelial opacities which might be associated with superficial punctate keratitis, corneal epithelial oedema, and markedly reduced visual acuity.

Urogenital tract:
Rare: urinary retention, urinary incontinence.

4.9 Overdose
Signs and symptoms:
Neuromuscular disturbances and symptoms of acute psychosis are prominent. Central nervous system: Hyperreflexia, motor restlessness, convulsions, extrapyramidal signs, torsion spasms, dystonic posturing, dilated pupils, confusion, disorientation, delirium, visual hallucinations. Respiratory system: hyperventilation, pulmonary oedema, respiratory distress, including adult respiratory distress syndrome. Cardiovascular system: sinus tachycardia, arrhythmia. Gastrointestinal system: nausea, vomiting, dry mouth. Renal function: urine retention, renal dysfunction, including increase in BUN and decreased creatinine clearance.

Overdose from combined drug treatment: the effects of anticholinergic drugs are increased by amantadine. Acute psychotic reactions (which may be identical to those of atropine poisoning) may occur when large doses of anticholinergic agents are used. Where alcohol or central nervous stimulants have been taken at the same time, the signs and symptoms of acute poisoning with amantadine may be aggravated and/or modified.

Management:
There is no specific antidote. Induction of vomiting and/or gastric aspiration (and lavage if patient is conscious), activated charcoal or saline cathartic may be used if judged appropriate. Since amantadine is excreted mainly unchanged in the urine, maintenance of renal function and copious diuresis (forced diuresis if necessary) are effective ways to remove it from the blood stream. Acidification of the urine favours its excretion. Haemodialysis does not remove significant amounts of amantadine.

Monitor the blood pressure, heart rate, ECG, respiration and body temperature, and treat for possible hypotension and cardiac arhythmias, as necessary. Convulsions and excessive motor restlessness: administer anticonvulsants such as diazepam iv, paraldehyde im or per rectum, or phenobarbital im. Acute psychotic symptoms, delirium, dystonic posturing, myoclonic manifestations: physostigmine by slow iv infusion (1mg doses in adults, 0.5mg in children) repeated administration according to the initial response and the subsequent need, has been reported. Retention of urine: bladder should be catheterised; an indwelling catheter can be left in place for the time required.

5. PHARMACOLOGICAL PROPERTIES

5.1 Pharmacodynamic properties

Influenza:
Amantadine specifically inhibits the replication of influenza A viruses at low concentrations. If using a sensitive plaque-reduction assay, human influenza viruses, including H_1N_1, H_2N_2 and H_3N_2 subtypes, are inhibited by $\leqslant$0.4g/ml of amantadine. Amantadine inhibits an early stage in viral replication by blocking the proton pump of the M_2 protein in the virus. This has two actions; it stops the virus uncoating and inactivates newly synthesised viral haemagglutinin. Effects on late replicative steps have been found for representative avian influenza viruses.

Data from tests with representative strains of influenza A virus indicate that Symmetrel is likely to be active against previously unknown strains, and could be used in the early stages of an epidemic, before a vaccine against the causative strain is generally available.

Herpes Zoster:
The mechanism of action of Symmetrel in herpes zoster has not been fully characterised.

Parkinson's disease:
Symmetrel is believed to enhance the release of dopamine and delay its reuptake into synaptic vesicles. It may also exert some anticholinergic activity. Whether administered alone or in combination, amantadine produces an improvement in the cardinal signs and symptoms of parkinsonism and improves functional capacity in about 60% of patients. The positive effect generally sets in two to five days after the start of treatment, particularly on akinesia, rigidity and tremor.

5.2 Pharmacokinetic properties

Absorption:
Amantadine is absorbed slowly but almost completely. Peak plasma concentrations of approximately 250ng/ml and 500ng/ml are seen 3 to 4 hours after single oral administration of 100mg and 200mg amantadine, respectively. Following repeated administration of 200mg daily, the steady-state plasma concentration settles at 300ng/ml within 3 days.

Distribution:
Amantadine accumulates after several hours in nasal secretions and crosses the blood-brain barrier (this has not been quantified). *In vitro*, 67% is bound to plasma proteins, with a substantial amount bound to red blood cells. The concentration in erythrocytes in normal healthy volunteers is 2.66 times the plasma concentration. The apparent volume of distribution is 5 to 10L/kg, suggesting extensive tissue binding. This declines with increasing doses. The concentrations in the lung, heart, kidney, liver and spleen are higher than in the blood.

Biotransformation:
Amantadine is metabolised to a minor extent, principally by N-acetylation.

Elimination:
The drug is eliminated in healthy young adults with a mean plasma elimination half-life of 15 hours (10 to 31 hours). The total plasma clearance is about the same as renal clearance (250ml/min). The renal amantadine clearance is much higher than the creatinine clearance, suggesting renal tubular secretion. After 4 to 5 days, 90% of the dose appears unchanged in urine. The rate is considerably influenced by urinary pH: a rise in pH brings about a fall in excretion.

Characteristics in special patient populations:
Elderly patients:
compared with healthy young adults, the half-life may be doubled and renal clearance diminished. Tubular secretion diminishes more than glomerular filtration in the elderly. In elderly patients with renal impairment, repeated administration of 100mg daily for 14 days raised the plasma concentration into the toxic range.

Renal impairment:
amantadine may accumulate in renal failure, causing severe side effects. The rate of elimination from plasma correlates to creatinine clearance divided by body surface area, although total renal elimination exceeds this value (possibly due to tubular secretion). The effects of reduced kidney function are dramatic: a reduction of creatinine clearance to 40ml/min may result in a five-fold increase in elimination half-life. The urine is the almost exclusive route of excretion, even with renal failure, and amantadine may persist in the plasma for several days. Haemodialysis does not remove significant amounts of amantadine, possibly due to extensive tissue binding.

5.3 Preclinical safety data
Reproductive toxicity studies were performed in rats and rabbits. In rat oral doses of 50 and 100 mg/kg proved to be teratogenic. This is 33-fold the recommended dose of 100mg for influenza. The maximum recommended dose, of 400mg in Parkinson's disease, is less than 6mg/kg.

There are no other pre-clinical data of relevance to the prescriber which are additional to those already included in other sections of the Summary of Product Characteristics.

6. PHARMACEUTICAL PARTICULARS

6.1 List of excipients
Methyl hydroxybenzoate, propyl hydroxybenzoate, sorbitol, disodium hydrogen citrate, lemon flavouring, strawberry flavouring and water.

6.2 Incompatibilities
None known.

6.3 Shelf life
Five years.

6.4 Special precautions for storage
Protect from heat and light. Keep container closed.

6.5 Nature and contents of container
150ml amber glass bottles with child proof closures.

6.6 Instructions for use and handling
None

7. MARKETING AUTHORISATION HOLDER
Alliance Pharmaceuticals Ltd

Avonbridge House

Bath Road

Chippenham

Wiltshire

SN15 2BB

8. MARKETING AUTHORISATION NUMBER(S)
PL16853/0016.

9. DATE OF FIRST AUTHORISATION/RENEWAL OF THE AUTHORISATION
25 June 1998

10. DATE OF REVISION OF THE TEXT
October 1999

11. Legal Status
POM

Alliance, Alliance Pharmaceuticals and associated devices are registered Trademarks of Alliance Pharmaceuticals Ltd.

Synacthen Ampoules 250mcg

(Alliance Pharmaceuticals)

1. NAME OF THE MEDICINAL PRODUCT
Synacthen® Ampoules 250mcg

2. QUALITATIVE AND QUANTITATIVE COMPOSITION
Tetracosactide acetate PhEur 250micrograms per ampoule.

3. PHARMACEUTICAL FORM
A clear colourless sterile solution in a clear glass ampoule.

4. CLINICAL PARTICULARS

4.1 Therapeutic indications
Diagnostic test for the investigation of adrenocortical insufficiency.

4.2 Posology and method of administration
Adults: This preparation of Synacthen is intended for administration for diagnostic purposes only as a single intramuscular or intravenous dose; it is not to be used for repeated therapeutic administration.

The 30-minute Synacthen diagnostic test: This test is based on measurement of the plasma cortisol concentration immediately before and exactly 30 minutes after an intramuscular or intravenous injection of 250micrograms (1ml) Synacthen. Adrenocortical function can be regarded as normal if the post-injection rise in plasma cortisol concentration amounts to at least 200nmol/litre (70micrograms/litre).

Where the 30-minute test has yielded inconclusive results, or where it is desired to determine the functional reserve of the adrenal cortex, a 5-hour test can be performed with Synacthen Depot (see separate Summary of Product Characteristics). Furthermore, a 3-day test with Synacthen Depot may be used to differentiate between primary and secondary adrenocortical insufficiency.

Children: An intravenous dose of 250micrograms/1.73m^2 body surface area has been suggested. Thus for children aged 5 to 7 years, approximately half the adult dose will be adequate. For more accurate dosing of other ages, standard body surface area tables should be consulted.

Elderly: There is no evidence to suggest that dosage should be different in the elderly.

4.3 Contraindications
History of hypersensitivity to ACTH, Synacthen or Synacthen Depot. Synacthen is contra-indicated in patients with allergic disorders (e.g. asthma).

4.4 Special warnings and special precautions for use
Before using Synacthen, the doctor should make every effort to find out whether the patient is suffering from, or has a history of, allergic disorders (see Section 4.3 "Contra-indications"). In particular, he should enquire whether the patient has previously experienced adverse reactions to ACTH, Synacthen or other drugs.

Synacthen should only be administered under the supervision of appropriate senior hospital medical staff (e.g. consultants).

If local or systemic hypersensitivity reactions occur after the injection (for example, marked redness and pain at the injection site, urticaria, pruritus, flushing, faintness or dyspnoea), Synacthen or other ACTH preparations should be avoided in the future. Hypersensitivity reactions tend to occur within 30 minutes of an injection. The patient should therefore be kept under observation during this time.

Preparation should be made in advance to combat any anaphylactic reaction that may occur after an injection of Synacthen. In the event of a serious anaphylactic reaction occurring, the following measures must be taken immediately: administer adrenaline (0.4 to 1ml of a 0.1% solution intramuscularly or 0.1 to 0.2ml of a 0.1% solution in 10ml physiological saline slowly intravenously) as well as a large intravenous dose of a corticosteroid (for example 100mg to 500mg hydrocortisone, three or four times in 24 hours), repeating the dose if necessary.

The hydrocortisone product information prepared by the manufacturer should also be consulted.

4.5 Interaction with other medicinal products and other forms of Interaction
None known.

4.6 Pregnancy and lactation
The Synacthen test should not be utilised during pregnancy and lactation unless there are compelling reasons for doing so.

4.7 Effects on ability to drive and use machines
Patients should be warned of the potential hazards of driving or operating machinery if they experience side effects such as dizziness.

4.8 Undesirable effects
Hypersensitivity reactions:

Synacthen may provoke hypersensitivity reactions. In patients suffering from, or susceptible to, allergic disorders (especially asthma) this may take the form of anaphylactic shock (see Section 4.3 "Contra-indications").

Hypersensitivity may be manifested as skin reactions at the injection site, dizziness, nausea, vomiting, urticaria, pruritus, flushing, malaise, dyspnoea, angioneurotic oedema and Quinke's oedema.

Other side effects are unlikely to be observed with short-term use of Synacthen as a diagnostic tool. Should information be required on the side effects reported with therapeutic use of tetracosactide acetate, see Synacthen Depot Summary of Product Characteristics.

4.9 Overdose
Overdosage is unlikely to be a problem when the product is used as a single dose for diagnostic purposes.

5. PHARMACOLOGICAL PROPERTIES

5.1 Pharmacodynamic properties
Tetracosactide acetate consists of the first 24 amino acids occurring in the natural corticotropic hormone (ACTH) sequence and displays the same physiological properties as ACTH. In the adrenal cortex, it stimulates the biosynthesis of glucocorticoids, mineralocorticoids, and, to a lesser extent androgens.

The site of action of ACTH is the plasma membrane of the adrenocortical cells, where it binds to a specific receptor. The hormone-receptor complex activates adenylate cyclase, stimulating the production of cyclic AMP (adenosine monophosphate) and so promoting the synthesis of pregnenolone from cholesterol. From pregnenolone the various corticosteroids are produced via different enzymatic pathways.

5.2 Pharmacokinetic properties
Following an intravenous injection, elimination of tetracosactide acetate from the plasma consists of 3 phases. The half-lives of these phases are approximately 7 minutes (0 to 1 hour), 37 minutes (1 to 2 hours) and 3 hours thereafter.

Tetracosactide acetate has an apparent volume of distribution of approximately 0.4L/kg.

In the serum, tetracosactide acetate is broken down by serum endopeptidases into inactive oligopeptides and then by aminopeptidases into free amino acids. The rapid elimination from plasma is probably not attributable to this relatively slow cleavage process, but rather to the rapid concentration of the active substance in the adrenal glands and kidneys.

Following an iv dose of ^{131}I-labelled tetracosactide acetate, 95 to 100% of the radioactivity is excreted in the urine within 24 hours.

5.3 Preclinical safety data
There are no pre-clinical data of relevance to the prescriber, which are additional to those already included in other sections of the Summary of Product Characteristics.

6. PHARMACEUTICAL PARTICULARS

6.1 List of excipients
Acetic acid, sodium acetate, sodium chloride and water.

6.2 Incompatibilities
None known.

6.3 Shelf life
5 years.

6.4 Special precautions for storage
Synacthen should be protected from light and stored in a refrigerator (2 - 8°C).

6.5 Nature and contents of container
The ampoules are colourless glass PhEur type I. Five ampoules are packed in a cardboard box.

6.6 Instructions for use and handling

Shake well before use.

Administrative Data

7. MARKETING AUTHORISATION HOLDER

Alliance Pharmaceuticals Ltd

Avonbridge House

Bath Road

Chippenham

Wiltshire

SN15 2BB

8. MARKETING AUTHORISATION NUMBER(S)

PL 16853/0017

9. DATE OF FIRST AUTHORISATION/RENEWAL OF THE AUTHORISATION

25 June 1998

10. DATE OF REVISION OF THE TEXT

February 2005

11. Legal Status

POM

Alliance, Alliance Pharmaceuticals and associated devices are registered Trademarks of Alliance Pharmaceuticals Ltd.

Synacthen Depot

(Alliance Pharmaceuticals)

1. NAME OF THE MEDICINAL PRODUCT

Synacthen Depot® Ampoules 1mg/ml

2. QUALITATIVE AND QUANTITATIVE COMPOSITION

Tetracosactide acetate PhEur 1mg/ml

3. PHARMACEUTICAL FORM

Tetracosactide acetate is absorbed on to zinc phosphate. A sterile, milky white suspension, which settles on standing, in a clear glass ampoule.

4. CLINICAL PARTICULARS

4.1 Therapeutic indications

Therapeutic use: Synacthen Depot should normally only be used for short-term therapy in conditions for which glucocorticoids are indicated in principle, for example, in ulcerative colitis and Crohn's disease, juvenile rheumatoid arthritis, or as adjunct therapy in patients with rheumatoid arthritis and osteoarthrosis. Synacthen Depot may be particularly useful in patients unable to tolerate oral glucocorticoid therapy or in patients where normal therapeutic doses of glucocorticoids have been ineffective.

Diagnostic use: As a diagnostic aid for the investigation of adrenocortical insufficiency.

4.2 Posology and method of administration

Synacthen Depot is intended for intramuscular injection. The ampoule should be shaken before use.

Therapeutic use: Initially, daily doses of Synacthen Depot should be given but after approximately 3 days, intermittent doses may be given.

Adults: Initially 1mg intramuscularly daily or 1mg every 12 hours in acute cases. After the acute symptoms of the disease have disappeared, treatment may be continued at a dose of 1mg every 2 to 3 days; in patients who respond well, the dosage may be reduced to 0.5mg every 2 to 3 days or 1mg per week.

Infants and children under 3 years: Not recommended due to the presence of benzyl alcohol in the formulation.

Children aged 3 to 5 years: Initially 0.25 to 0.5mg intramuscularly daily; the maintenance dose is 0.25 to 0.5mg every 2 to 8 days.

Children aged 5 to 12 years: Initially 0.25 to 1mg intramuscularly daily; the maintenance dose is 0.25 to 1mg every 2 to 8 days.

Elderly: There is no evidence to suggest that dosage should be different in the elderly.

Diagnostic use: In cases of suspected adrenocortical insufficiency, where the 30-minute diagnostic test with Synacthen ampoules (see Synacthen Summary of Product Characteristics) has yielded inconclusive results or where it is desired to determine the functional reserve of the adrenal cortex, a 5-hour test with Synacthen Depot may be performed.

Adults: This test is based on measurement of the plasma cortisol concentration before and exactly 30 minutes, 1, 2, 3, 4 and 5 hours after an intramuscular injection of 1mg Synacthen Depot. Adrenocortical function can be regarded as normal if the post-injection rise in plasma cortisol concentration increases 2-fold in the first hour, and continues to rise steadily. The values expected would be 600 to 1,250nmol/l in the first hour increasing slowly up to 1,000 to 1,800nmol/l by the fifth hour. Lower concentrations of plasma cortisol may be attributable to Addison's disease, secondary adrenocortical insufficiency due to a disorder of hypothalamo-pituitary function, or overdosage of corticosteroids.

A 3-day test with Synacthen Depot may be used to differentiate between primary and secondary adrenocortical insufficiency.

Children: No paediatric dosage has been established. Synacthen Depot is not recommended for children under 3 years of age due to the presence of benzyl alcohol in the formulation.

Elderly: There is no evidence to suggest that dosage should be different in the elderly.

4.3 Contraindications

History of hypersensitivity to ACTH, Synacthen or Synacthen Depot. Acute psychoses, infectious diseases, Cushing's syndrome, peptic ulcer, refractory heart failure, adrenogenital syndrome and for therapeutic use in adrenocortical insufficiency.

In view of the increased risk of anaphylactic reactions, Synacthen Depot should not be used in patients known to have asthma and/or other forms of allergy.

Synacthen Depot is contra-indicated for use in children under 3 years of age as it contains benzyl alcohol, which can cause severe poisoning and hypersensitivity reactions.

Therapeutic use is contra-indicated during pregnancy or lactation. Diagnostic use should only occur during pregnancy or lactation if there are compelling reasons.

Synacthen Depot must not be administered intravenously.

4.4 Special warnings and special precautions for use

Before using Synacthen Depot, the doctor should make every effort to find out whether the patient is suffering from, or has a history of, allergic disorders. In particular, he should enquire whether the patient has previously experienced adverse reactions to ACTH, Synacthen Depot or other drugs.

Synacthen Depot should only be administered under medical supervision.

If local or systemic hypersensitivity reactions occur during or after an injection (for example, marked redness and pain at the injection site, urticaria, pruritus, flushing, faintness or dyspnoea), Synacthen Depot or other ACTH preparations should be avoided in the future. Hypersensitivity reactions tend to occur within 30 minutes of the injection. The patient should therefore be kept under observation during this time.

In the event of a serious anaphylactic reaction occurring despite these precautions, the following measures must be taken immediately: administer adrenaline (0.4 to 1ml of a 0.1% solution intramuscularly or 0.1 to 0.2ml of a 0.1% solution in 10ml physiological saline slowly intravenously) as well as a large intravenous dose of a corticosteroid (for example 100 to 500mg hydrocortisone, three or four times in 24 hours) repeating the dose if necessary.

The hydrocortisone product information prepared by the manufacturer should also be consulted.

Synacthen Depot should not be used in the presence of active infectious or systemic diseases, when the use of live vaccine is contemplated or in the presence of a reduced immune response, unless adequate disease specific therapy is being given.

Use with care in patients with non-specific ulcerative colitis, diverticulitis, recent intestinal anastomosis, renal insufficiency, hypertension, thromboembolic tendencies, osteoporosis and myasthenia gravis.

The increased production of adrenal steroids may result in corticosteroid type effects:

- Salt and water retention can occur and may respond to a low salt diet. Potassium supplementation may be necessary during long term treatment.

- Psychological disturbances may be triggered or aggravated.

- Latent infections (e.g. amoebiasis, tuberculosis) may become activated.

- Ocular effects may be produced (e.g. glaucoma, cataracts).

- Provided the dose is chosen to meet the individual's needs, Synacthen Depot is unlikely to inhibit growth in children. Nevertheless, growth should be monitored in children undergoing long-term treatment. In infants and children aged up to 5 years, reversible myocardial hypertrophy may occur in rare cases following long-term treatment with high doses. Therefore echocardiographic recordings should be made regularly.

- Dosage adjustments may be necessary in patients being treated for diabetes or hypertension.

An enhanced effect of tetracosactide acetate therapy may occur in patients with hypothyroidism and in those with cirrhosis of the liver.

4.5 Interaction with other medicinal products and other forms of Interaction

Interactions are likely with drugs whose actions are affected by adrenal steroids (see Section 4.4 "Special warnings and precautions for use").

4.6 Pregnancy and lactation

Synacthen Depot is contra-indicated for therapeutic use during pregnancy and lactation. It should not be used as a diagnostic tool unless there are compelling reasons for doing so.

4.7 Effects on ability to drive and use machines

Patients should be warned of the potential hazards of driving or operating machinery if they experience side effects such as dizziness.

4.8 Undesirable effects

Since Synacthen Depot stimulates the adrenal cortex to increase the output of glucocorticoids and mineralocorticoids, side effects associated with excessive adrenocorticotropic activity may be encountered.

Hypersensitivity reactions: Synacthen Depot may provoke hypersensitivity reactions. In patients suffering from, or susceptible to, allergic disorders (especially asthma) this may take the form of anaphylactic shock. (see Section 4.3 "Contra-indications").

Hypersensitivity may be manifested as skin reactions at the injection site, dizziness, nausea, vomiting, urticaria, pruritus, flushing, malaise, dyspnoea, angioneurotic oedema and Quincke's oedema.

In rare cases, the benzyl alcohol in Synacthen Depot may provoke hypersensitivity reactions.

The following side effects have also been reported during corticotropin/corticosteroid therapy, although not necessarily observed during Synacthen Depot therapy:

Musculoskeletal system: Osteoporosis, muscle weakness, steroid myopathy, loss of muscle mass, vertebral compression fractures, aseptic necrosis of femoral and humeral heads, pathologic fracture of long bones and tendon rupture.

Gastro-intestinal tract: Peptic ulceration with possible perforation and haemorrhage, pancreatitis, abdominal distension and ulcerative oesophagitis.

Skin and appendages: Impaired wound healing, thin fragile skin, petechia and ecchymosis, facial erythema, increased sweating, suppression of skin test reactions, acne and skin pigmentation.

Central and peripheral nervous system: Convulsions, increased intracranial pressure with papilloedema (pseudotumour cerebri) usually after treatment, vertigo, headache and psychic changes.

Endocrine system: Sodium retention, fluid retention, potassium loss, hypokalaemic alkalosis and calcium loss. Menstrual irregularities, Cushing's syndrome, suppression of growth in children, secondary adrenocortical and pituitary unresponsiveness, particularly in times of stress, as in trauma, surgery or illness; decreased carbohydrate tolerance, hyperglycaemia, manifestations of latent diabetes mellitus, hirsutism.

Ophthalmic: Posterior subcapsular cataracts, increased intraocular pressure, glaucoma and exophthalmos.

Metabolism: Negative nitrogen balance due to protein catabolism.

Cardiovascular system: A rise in blood pressure, necrotising angiitis and congestive heart failure. In infants and small children treated over a prolonged period with high doses, reversible myocardial hypertrophy may occur in isolated cases.

Miscellaneous: Increased susceptibility to infection, abscess, thromboembolism, weight gain, increased appetite, leucocytosis.

4.9 Overdose

Relating to therapeutic usage of Synacthen Depot:

Overdosage may lead to fluid retention and signs of excessive adrenocorticotropic activity (Cushing's Syndrome). In such cases, Synacthen Depot should either be withdrawn temporarily, given in lower doses or the interval between injections should be prolonged (e.g. 5 to 7 days).

Treatment: There is no known antidote. Treatment should be symptomatic.

5. PHARMACOLOGICAL PROPERTIES

5.1 Pharmacodynamic properties

Tetracosactide acetate consists of the first 24 amino acids occurring in the natural corticotropic hormone (ACTH) sequence and displays the same physiological properties as ACTH. In the adrenal cortex, it stimulates the biosynthesis of glucocorticoids, mineralocorticoids, and, to a lesser extent, androgens, which explains its therapeutic effect in conditions responsive to glucocorticoid treatment.

However, its pharmacological activity is not comparable to that of corticosteroids, because under ACTH treatment (in contrast to treatment with a single glucocorticoid) the tissues are exposed to a physiological spectrum of corticosteroids.

The site of action of ACTH is the plasma membrane of the adrenocortical cells, where it binds to a specific receptor. The hormone-receptor complex activates adenylate cyclase, stimulating the production of cyclic AMP (adenosine monophosphate) and so promoting the synthesis of pregnenolone from cholesterol. From pregnenolone the various corticosteroids are produced via different enzymatic pathways.

5.2 Pharmacokinetic properties

Tetracosactide acetate is absorbed on to a zinc phosphate complex which ensures the sustained release of the active substance from the intramuscular injection site. After an intramuscular injection of 1mg Synacthen Depot, the radioimmunologically determined plasma concentrations of tetracosactide acetate range between 200 to 300pg/ml and are maintained for 12 hours.

Tetracosactide acetate has an apparent volume of distribution of approximately 0.4litres/kg.

In the serum, tetracosactide acetate is broken down by serum endopeptidases into inactive oligopeptides and then by aminopeptidases into free amino acids.

Following an intravenous dose of ^{131}I-labelled tetracosactide acetate, 95 to 100% of the radioactivity is excreted in the urine within 24 hours.

5.3 Preclinical safety data
There are no pre-clinical data of relevance to the prescriber which are additional to those already included in other sections of the Summary of Product Characteristics.

6. PHARMACEUTICAL PARTICULARS
6.1 List of excipients
Zinc chloride, disodium phosphate dodecahydrate, benzyl alcohol, sodium chloride, sodium hydroxide and water for injections.

6.2 Incompatibilities
None known

6.3 Shelf life
3 years

6.4 Special precautions for storage
Protect from light. Store in a refrigerator (2 to 8°C).

6.5 Nature and contents of container
1ml ampoules packed in boxes of 10.

6.6 Instructions for use and handling
None

Administrative Data
7. MARKETING AUTHORISATION HOLDER
Alliance Pharmaceuticals Ltd
Avonbridge House
Bath Road
Chippenham
Wiltshire
SN15 2BB

8. MARKETING AUTHORISATION NUMBER(S)
PL16853/0018

9. DATE OF FIRST AUTHORISATION/RENEWAL OF THE AUTHORISATION
25 June 1998

10. DATE OF REVISION OF THE TEXT
February 2004

11. Legal Status
POM

Alliance, Alliance Pharmaceuticals and associated devices are registered Trademarks of Alliance Pharmaceuticals Ltd.

Synagis

(Abbott Laboratories Limited)

1. NAME OF THE MEDICINAL PRODUCT
Synagis▼50 mg or 100mg powder and solvent for solution for injection

2. QUALITATIVE AND QUANTITATIVE COMPOSITION
One vial contains 50 mg or 100mg palivizumab, providing 100mg/ml of palivizumab when reconstituted as recommended.

For excipients, see section 6.1.

3. PHARMACEUTICAL FORM
Powder and solvent for solution for injection

4. CLINICAL PARTICULARS
4.1 Therapeutic indications
Synagis is indicated for the prevention of serious lower respiratory tract disease requiring hospitalisation caused by respiratory syncytial virus (RSV) in children at high risk for RSV disease:

- Children born at 35 weeks of gestation or less and less than 6 months of age at the onset of the RSV season
- Children less than 2 years of age and requiring treatment for bronchopulmonary dysplasia within the last 6 months.
- Children less than 2 years of age and with haemodynamically significant congenital heart disease.

4.2 Posology and method of administration
Recommended dose

The recommended dose of palivizumab is 15 mg/kg of body weight, given once a month during anticipated periods of RSV risk in the community. Where possible, the first dose should be administered prior to commencement of the RSV season. Subsequent doses should be administered monthly throughout the RSV season.

The majority of experience including the pivotal phase III clinical trials with palivizumab has been gained with 5 injections during one season (see section 5.1). Data, although limited, are available on greater than 5 doses (see section 4.8 and section 5.1), therefore the benefit in terms of protection beyond 5 doses has not been established.

To reduce risk of rehospitalisation, it is recommended that children receiving palivizumab who are hospitalised with RSV continue to receive monthly doses of palivizumab for the duration of the RSV season.

For children undergoing cardiac bypass, it is recommended that a 15 mg/kg injection of palivizumab be administered as soon as stable after surgery to ensure adequate palivizumab serum levels. Subsequent doses should resume monthly through the remainder of the RSV season for children that continue to be at high risk of RSV disease (see section 5.2).

Method of administration

Palivizumab is administered in a dose of 15 mg/kg once a month intramuscularly, preferably in the anterolateral aspect of the thigh. The gluteal muscle should not be used routinely as an injection site because of the risk of damage to the sciatic nerve. The injection should be given using standard aseptic technique. Injection volumes over 1 ml should be given as a divided dose.

For information on reconstituting Synagis, see section 6.6.

4.3 Contraindications
Palivizumab is contraindicated in patients with known hypersensitivity to palivizumab or any component of the formulation (see section 6.1), or other humanised monoclonal antibodies.

4.4 Special warnings and special precautions for use
Allergic reactions including very rare cases of anaphylaxis have been reported following palivizumab administration (see section 4.8).

Medications for the treatment of severe hypersensitivity reactions, including anaphylaxis, should be available for immediate use following administration of palivizumab.

A moderate to severe acute infection or febrile illness may warrant delaying the use of palivizumab, unless, in the opinion of the physician, withholding palivizumab entails a greater risk. A mild febrile illness, such as mild upper respiratory infection, is not usually reason to defer administration of palivizumab.

As with any intramuscular injection, palivizumab should be given with caution to patients with thrombocytopaenia or any coagulation disorder.

The efficacy of palivizumab when administered to patients as a second course of treatment during an ensuing RSV season has not been formally investigated in a study performed with this objective. The possible risk of enhanced RSV infection in the season following the season in which the patients were treated with palivizumab has not been conclusively ruled out by studies performed aiming at this particular point.

4.5 Interaction with other medicinal products and other forms of Interaction
No formal drug-drug interactions studies were conducted, however no interactions have been described to date. In the phase III IMpact-RSV study in the premature and bronchopulmonary dysplasia paediatric populations, the proportions of patients in the placebo and palivizumab groups who received routine childhood vaccines, influenza vaccine, bronchodilators or corticosteroids were similar and no incremental increase in adverse reactions was observed among patients receiving these agents.

Since the monoclonal antibody is specific for RSV, palivizumab is not expected to interfere with the immune response to vaccines.

4.6 Pregnancy and lactation
Not applicable.

4.7 Effects on ability to drive and use machines
Not applicable.

4.8 Undesirable effects
Adverse drug reactions (ADRs) reported in the prophylactic paediatric studies were similar in the placebo and palivizumab groups. The majority of ADRs were transient and mild to moderate in severity.

Adverse events at least possibly causally-related to palivizumab, both clinical and laboratory, are displayed by system organ class and frequency (common > 1/100 ≤ 1/10; uncommon > 1/1000 ≤ 1/100) in studies conducted in premature and bronchopulmonary dysplasia paediatric patients, and congenital heart disease patients (Tables 1 and 2, respectively).

Table 1
Undesirable Effects in Prophylactic Clinical Studies with Premature and Bronchopulmonary Dysplasia Paediatric Populations

Infections and infestations	Uncommon	Upper respiratory infection Viral infection
Blood and lymphatic system disorders	Uncommon	Leucopaenia
Psychiatric disorders	Common	Nervousness
Respiratory, thoracic and mediastinal disorders	Uncommon	Rhinitis Cough Wheeze
Gastrointestinal disorders	Uncommon	Diarrhoea Vomiting
Skin and subcutaneous tissue disorders	Uncommon	Rash
General disorders and administration site conditions	Common Uncommon	Fever Injection site reaction Pain
Investigations	Uncommon	AST increase Abnormal liver function test ALT increase

No medically important differences were observed during the prophylatic studies carried out in the premature and bronchopulmonary dysplasia paediatric populations in ADRs by body system or when evaluated in subgroups of children by clinical category, gender, age, gestational age, country, race/ethnicity or quartile serum palivizumab concentration. No significant difference in safety profile was observed between children without active RSV infection and those hospitalised for RSV. Permanent discontinuation of palivizumab due to ADRs was rare (0.2%). Deaths were balanced between the integrated placebo and palivizumab groups and were not drug-related.

Table 2
Undesirable Effects in the Prophylactic Paediatric Congenital Heart Disease Clinical Study

Infections and infestations	Uncommon	Upper respiratory infection Gasteroenteritis
Psychiatric disorders	Uncommon	Nervousness
Nervous System	Uncommon	Somnolence Hyperkinesia
Vascular disorders	Uncommon	Haemorrhage
Respiratory, thoracic and mediastinal disorders	Uncommon	Rhinitis
Gastrointestinal disorders	Uncommon	Diarrhoea Vomiting Constipation
Skin and subcutaneous tissue disorders	Uncommon	Rash Eczema
General disorders and administration site conditions	Common Uncommon	Injection site reaction Fever Asthenia

In the congenital heart disease study no medically important differences were observed in ADRs by body system or when evaluated in subgroups of children by clinical category. The incidence of serious adverse events was significantly lower in the palivizumab group compared to the placebo group. No serious adverse events related to palivizumab were reported. The incidences of cardiac surgeries classified as planned, earlier than planned or urgent were balanced between the groups. Deaths associated with RSV infection occurred in 2 patients in the palivizumab group and 4 patients in the placebo group and were not drug-related.

Post-marketing experience:

The following events were reported during post-marketing experience of palivizumab:

Rare ADRs > 1/10,000, < 1/1,000): apnoea

Very rare ADRs (< 1/10,000): anaphylaxis, urticaria

Post-marketing serious spontaneous adverse events reported during palivizumab treatment between 1998 and 2002 covering four RSV seasons were evaluated. A total of 1291 serious reports were received where palivizumab had been administered as indicated and the duration of therapy was within one season. The onset of the adverse event occurred after the sixth or greater dose in only 22 of these reports (15 after the sixth dose, 6 after the seventh doses and 1 after the eight dose). These events are similar in character to those after the initial five doses.

Palivizumab treatment schedule and adverse events were monitored in a group of nearly 20,000 infants tracked through a patient compliance registry between 1998 and 2000. Of this group 1250 enrolled infants had 6 injections, 183 infants had 7 injections, and 27 infants had either 8 or 9 injections. Adverse events observed in patients after a sixth or greater dose were similar in character and frequency to those after the initial 5 doses.

Human anti-human antibody (HAHA) response:

Antibody to palivizumab was observed in approximately 1% of patients in the IMpact-RSV during the first course of therapy. This was transient, low titre, resolved despite continued use (first and second season), and could not be detected in 55/56 infants during the second season (including 2 with titres during the first season). Therefore, HAHA responses appear to be of no clinical relevance.

Immunogenicity was not studied in the congenital heart disease study.

4.9 Overdose
In clinical studies, three children received an overdose of more than 15 mg/kg. These doses were 20.25 mg/kg, 21.1 mg/kg and 22.27 mg/kg. No medical consequences were identified in these instances.

5. PHARMACOLOGICAL PROPERTIES

5.1 Pharmacodynamic properties
Pharmacotherapeutic group: Immunoglobulins; ATC Code J06BB16

Palivizumab is a humanised $IgG_{1\kappa}$ monoclonal antibody directed to an epitope in the A antigenic site of the fusion protein of respiratory syncytial virus (RSV). This humanised monoclonal antibody is composed of human (95%) and murine (5%) antibody sequences. It has potent neutralising and fusion-inhibitory activity against both RSV subtype A and B strains.

Palivizumab serum concentrations of approximately 30 µg/ml have been shown to produce a 99% reduction in pulmonary RSV replication in the cotton rat model.

Clinical studies

In a placebo-controlled trial of RSV disease prophylaxis in (IMpact-RSV trial) 1502 high-risk children (1002 Synagis; 500 placebo), 5 monthly doses of 15 mg/kg reduced the incidence of RSV related hospitalisation by 55% (p = < 0.001). The RSV hospitalisation rate was 10.6% in the placebo group. On this basis, the absolute risk reduction (ARR) is 5.8% which means the number needed to treat (NNT) is 17 to prevent one hospitalisation. The severity of RSV disease in children hospitalised despite prophylaxis with palivizumab in terms of days in ICU stay per 100 children and days of mechanical ventilation per 100 children was not affected.

A total of 222 children were enrolled in two separate studies to examine the safety of palivizumab when it is administered for a second RSV season. One hundred and three (103) children received monthly palivizumab injections for the first time, and 119 children received palivizumab for two consecutive seasons. No difference between groups regarding immunogenicity was observed in either study. However, as the efficacy of palivizumab when administered to patients as a second course of treatment during an ensuing RSV season has not been formally investigated in a study performed with this objective, the relevance of these data in terms of efficacy is unknown.

In an open label prospective trial designed to evaluate pharmacokinetics, safety and immunogenicity after administration of 7 doses of palivizumab within a single RSV season, pharmacokinetic data indicated that adequate mean palivizumab levels were achieved in all 18 children enrolled. Transient, low levels of antipalivizumab antibody were observed in one child after the second dose of palivizumab that dropped to undetectable levels at the fifth and seventh dose.

In a placebo-controlled trial in 1287 patients ≤ 24 months of age with haemodynamically significant congenital heart disease (639 Synagis; 648 placebo), 5 monthly doses of 15 mg/kg Synagis reduced the incidence of RSV hospitalisations by 45% (p = 0.003) (congenital heart disease study). Groups were equally balanced between cyanotic and acyanotic patients. The RSV hospitalisation rate was 9.7% in the placebo group and 5.3% in the Synagis group. Secondary efficacy endpoints showed significant reductions in the Synagis group compared to placebo in total days of RSV hospitalisation (56% reduction, p = 0.003) and total RSV days with increased supplemental oxygen (73% reduction, p = 0.014) per 100 children.

5.2 Pharmacokinetic properties
In studies in adult volunteers, palivizumab had a pharmacokinetic profile similar to a human IgG_1 antibody with regard to volume of distribution (mean 57 ml/kg) and half-life (mean 18 days). In prophylactic studies in premature and bronchopulmonary dysplasia paediatric populations, the mean half-life of palivizumab was 20 days and monthly intramuscular doses of 15 mg/kg achieved mean 30 day trough serum drug concentrations of approximately 40 µg/ml after the first injection, approximately 60 µg/ml after the second injection, approximately 70 µg/ml after the third injection and fourth injection. In the congenital heart disease study, monthly intramuscular doses of 15 mg/kg achieved mean 30 day trough serum drug concentrations of approximately 55 µg/ml after the first injection and approximately 90 µg/ml after the fourth injection.

Among 139 children in the congenital heart disease study receiving palivizumab who had cardio-pulmonary bypass and for whom paired serum samples were available, the mean serum palivizumab concentration was approximately 100 µg/ml pre-cardiac bypass and declined to approximately 40 µg/ml after bypass.

5.3 Preclinical safety data
Single dose toxicology studies have been conducted in cynomolgus monkeys (maximum dose 30 mg/kg), rabbits (maximum dose 50 mg/kg) and rats (maximum dose 840 mg/kg). No significant findings were observed.

Studies carried out in rodents gave no indication of enhancement of RSV replication, or RSV-induced pathology or generation of virus escape mutants in the presence of palivizumab under the chosen experimental conditions.

6. PHARMACEUTICAL PARTICULARS

6.1 List of excipients
Powder:

Histidine, glycine, mannitol

Water for Injections

6.2 Incompatibilities
Palivizumab should not be mixed with any medications or diluents other than Water for Injections.

6.3 Shelf life
3 years.

After reconstitution according to the instructions: 3 hours

6.4 Special precautions for storage
Store in a refrigerator (2°C to 8°C). Do not freeze.

Store in the original container.

6.5 Nature and contents of container
Synagis powder: clear, colourless, type I glass vial with stopper and flip-off seal

Water for Injections: clear, colourless type I glass ampoule containing 1 ml water for injections

One vial of Synagis powder and one ampoule of Water for Injections per pack.

6.6 Instructions for use and handling
SLOWLY add 0.6 ml of Water for Injections for the 50mg vial or 1.0ml of Water for Injections for the 100mg vial along the inside wall of the vial to minimise foaming. After the water is added, tilt the vial slightly and gently rotate the vial for 30 seconds. DO NOT SHAKE VIAL. Palivizumab solution should stand at room temperature for a minimum of 20 minutes until the solution clarifies. Palivizumab solution does not contain a preservative and should be administered within 3 hours of preparation. Any remaining contents should be discarded after use.

When reconstituted as recommended, the final concentration is 100 mg/ml.

7. MARKETING AUTHORISATION HOLDER
Abbott Laboratories Limited

Queenborough, Kent ME11 5EL

United Kingdom

8. MARKETING AUTHORISATION NUMBER(S)
50mg vial: EU/1/99/117/001

100mg vial: EU/1/99/117/002

9. DATE OF FIRST AUTHORISATION/RENEWAL OF THE AUTHORISATION
13 August 1999

10. DATE OF REVISION OF THE TEXT
September 2004

Synarel Nasal Spray

(Pharmacia Limited)

1. NAME OF THE MEDICINAL PRODUCT
SYNAREL®

2. QUALITATIVE AND QUANTITATIVE COMPOSITION
Solution containing 2mg/ml of nafarelin (as acetate) supplied in bottles fitted with a metered spray pump that delivers 200 micrograms of nafarelin base per spray.

3. PHARMACEUTICAL FORM
Nasal spray

4. CLINICAL PARTICULARS

4.1 Therapeutic indications
The hormonal management of endometriosis, including pain relief and reduction of endometriotic lesions.

Use in controlled ovarian stimulation programmes prior to in-vitro fertilisation, under the supervision of an infertility specialist.

4.2 Posology and method of administration
Adult: Synarel is for administration by the intranasal route only.

Experience with the treatment of endometriosis has been limited to women 18 years of age and older.

Endometriosis: In the use of Synarel in endometriosis, the aim is to induce chronic pituitary desensitisation, which gives a menopause-like state maintained over many months.

The recommended daily dose of Synarel is 200 mcg taken twice daily as one spray (200 mcg of nafarelin) to one nostril in the morning and one spray into the other nostril in the evening (400 mcg/day). Treatment should be started between days 2 and 4 of the menstrual cycle. The recommended duration of therapy is six months; only one 6-month course is advised. In clinical studies the majority of women have only received up to six-months treatment with Synarel.

Controlled ovarian stimulation prior to in vitro fertilisation: In the use of Synarel associated with controlled ovarian stimulation prior to *in vitro* fertilisation, the long protocol should be employed, whereby Synarel is continued through a period of transient gonadotrophin stimulation lasting 10-15 days (the 'flare effect') through to pituitary desensitisation (down-regulation). Down-regulation may be defined as serum oestradiol ≤50pg/ml and serum progesterone ≤1ng/ml, and the majority of patients down-regulate within 4 weeks.

The recommended daily dose of Synarel is 400 mcg taken twice daily as one spray to each nostril in the morning, and one spray to each nostril in the evening (800 mcg/day).

Once down-regulation is achieved, controlled ovarian stimulation with gonadotrophins, e.g. hMG, is commenced, and the Synarel dosage maintained until the administration of hCG at follicular maturity (usually a further 8-12 days).

If patients do not down-regulate within 12 weeks of starting Synarel, it is recommended that Synarel therapy be discontinued and the cycle cancelled.

Treatment may begin in either the early follicular phase (day 2) or the mid-luteal phase (usually day 21).

If the use of a nasal decongestant is required at the time of nafarelin administration, it is recommended that the nasal decongestant be used at least 30 minutes after nafarelin dosing.

Sneezing during or immediately after dosing may impair absorption of Synarel. If sneezing occurs upon administration, repeating the dose may be advisable.

Bottles contain either 30 or 60 doses and should not be used for a greater number of doses. The 60 dose-unit bottle is sufficient for 30 days' treatment at 400mcg (2 sprays) per day, and 15 days treatment at 800mcg (4 sprays) per day.

The 30 dose-unit bottle is sufficient for 15 days' treatment at 400mcg (2 sprays) per day, and 7 days' treatment at 800mcg (4 sprays) per day. Patients should therefore be advised that continued use after this time may result in delivery of an insufficient amount of nafarelin.

4.3 Contraindications
A small loss of trabecula bone mineral content occurs during 6 months treatment with nafarelin. Although this is mostly reversible within 6 months of stopping treatment, there are no data on the effects of repeat courses on bone loss. Retreatment with Synarel or use for longer than 6 months is, therefore, not recommended. (See Side-effects section on 'Changes in bone density').

Synarel should not be administered to patients who:

1. are hypersensitive to GnRH, GnRH agonist analogues or any of the excipients in Synarel;
2. have undiagnosed vaginal bleeding;
3. are pregnant or may become pregnant whilst taking Synarel (see 'use in pregnancy and lactation');
4. are breast-feeding.

4.4 Special warnings and special precautions for use
When regularly used at the recommended dose, nafarelin inhibits ovulation. Patients should be advised to use non-hormonal, barrier methods of contraception. In the event of missed doses there may be breakthrough ovulation and a potential for conception. If a patient becomes pregnant during treatment, administration of the drug must be discontinued and the patient must be informed of a potential risk to fetal development. N.B. Synarel treatment will be stopped at least 3 days before fertilised embryos are placed in the uterine cavity.

As with other drugs in this class ovarian cysts have been reported to occur in the first two months of therapy with Synarel. Many, but not all, of these events occurred in patients with polycystic ovarian disease. These cystic enlargements may resolve spontaneously, generally by about four to six weeks of therapy, but in some cases may require discontinuation of drug and/or surgical intervention.

Controlled ovarian stimulation prior to in vitro fertilisation; Transient ovarian cyst formation is a recognised complication of GnRH agonist use. These cysts tend to regress spontaneously over a number of weeks and are more common when GnRH agonists are commenced in the follicular phase of the cycle.

There are no clinical data available on the use of Synarel in ovulation induction regimens involving patients with polycystic ovarian syndrome. Caution is advised in this patient group as they are at greater risk of excessive follicular recruitment when undergoing ovulation induction regimes.

Administration of nafarelin in therapeutic doses results in suppression of the pituitary-gonadal system. Normal function is usually restored within 8 weeks after treatment is discontinued. Diagnostic tests of pituitary-gonadal function conducted during the treatment and up to 8 weeks after discontinuation of nafarelin therapy may therefore be misleading.

4.5 Interaction with other medicinal products and other forms of Interaction

Nafarelin would not be expected to participate in pharmacokinetic-based drug-drug interactions because degradation of the compound is primarily by the action of peptidases not cytochrome P-450 enzymes. Additionally, because nafarelin is only about 80% bound to plasma proteins (albumin), drug interactions at the protein-binding level would not be expected to occur.

Rhinitis does not impair nasal absorption of nafarelin. Nasal decongestants used 30 minutes before nafarelin administration decrease absorption.

4.6 Pregnancy and lactation

When administered intramuscularly to rats on days 6-15 of pregnancy at doses of 0.4, 1.6 and 6.4 mcg/kg/day (0.6, 2.5 and 10.0 times the intranasal human dose of 400mcg per day), 4/80 fetuses in the highest dose group had major fetal abnormalities that were not seen in a repeat study in rats. Moreover, studies in mice and rabbits failed to demonstrate an increase in fetal abnormalities. In rats, there was a dose-related increase in fetal mortality, and a decrease in fetal weight with the highest dose. These effects on rat fetal mortality are logical consequences of the alterations in hormonal levels brought about by nafarelin in this species.

Use of nafarelin in human pregnancy has not been studied.

Synarel should not therefore be used during pregnancy or suspected pregnancy. Before starting treatment with Synarel pregnancy must be excluded. If a patient becomes pregnant during treatment, administration of the drug must be discontinued and the patient must be informed of a potential risk to fetal development.

Controlled ovarian stimulation prior to in vitro fertilisation: Pregnancy should be excluded before starting treatment with Synarel, and the medication should be stopped on the day of administration of hCG. Barrier methods of contraception should be employed whilst Synarel is being taken.

It is not known whether or to what extent nafarelin is excreted into human breast milk. The effects, if any on the breast-fed child have not been determined and therefore Synarel should not be used by breast-feeding women.

4.7 Effects on ability to drive and use machines

Not applicable.

4.8 Undesirable effects

In approximately 0.2% of adult patients, symptoms suggestive of drug sensitivity, such as shortness of breath, chest pain, urticaria, rash and pruritus have occurred.

As would be expected with a drug which lowers serum oestradiol levels to menopausal concentrations the most frequently reported adverse reactions are those related to hypo-oestrogenism.

In controlled studies of nafarelin 400mcg/day, adverse reactions that were most frequently reported are listed in order of decreasing frequency; hot flushes, changes in libido, vaginal dryness, headaches, emotional lability, acne, myalgia, decreased breast size and irritation of the nasal mucosa.

During post-marketing surveillance, depression, paraesthesia, alopecia, migraine, palpitations, blurred vision have been reported. Emotional lability and depression would be expected with a drug that towers serum oestradiol to post-menopausal levels.

Changes in bone density: After six months of Synarel treatment there was a reduction in vertebral trabecular bone density and total vertebral mass, averaging about 9% and 4%, respectively. There was very little, if any, decrease in the mineral content of compact bone of the distal radius and second metacarpal. Substantial recovery of bone occurred during the post-treatment period. Total vertebral bone mass, measured by dual photon absorptiometry (DPA), decreased by a mean of about 6% at the end of treatment. Mean total vertebral mass, re-examined by DPA six months after completion of treatment, was 1.4% below pretreatment levels. These changes are similar to those which occur during treatment with other GnRH agonists.

Carcinogenesis/mutagenesis: As seen with other GnRH agonists, nafarelin given parenterally in high doses to laboratory rodents for prolonged periods induced hyperplasia and neoplasia of endocrine organs, including the anterior pituitary (adenoma/carcinoma) of both mice and rats; tumours of the pancreatic islets, adrenal medulla, testes and ovaries occurred only in long-term studies in rats. No metastases of these tumours were observed. Monkeys treated with high doses of nafarelin for one year did not develop any tumours or proliferative changes. Experience in humans is limited but there is no evidence for tumorigenesis of GnRH analogues in human beings.

In vitro studies conducted in bacterial and mammalian systems provided no indication of a mutagenic potential for nafarelin.

Impairment of fertility: Reproduction studies in rats of both sexes have shown full reversibility of fertility suppression when drug treatment was discontinued after continuous administration for up to six months.

Laboratory values: Increased levels of SGOT/SGPT and serum alkaline phosphatase may rarely occur which are reversible on discontinuing treatment.

4.9 Overdose

In animals, subcutaneous administration of up to 60 times the recommended human dose (expressed on a mcg/kg basis) had no adverse effects. Orally-administered nafarelin is subject to enzymatic degradation in the gastrointestinal tract and is therefore inactive. At present there is no clinical experience with overdosage of nafarelin.

Based on studies in monkeys, nafarelin is not absorbed after oral administration.

5. PHARMACOLOGICAL PROPERTIES

5.1 Pharmacodynamic properties

Nafarelin is a potent agonistic analogue of gonadotrophin releasing hormone (GnRH). Given as a single dose, nafarelin stimulates release of the pituitary gonadotrophins, LH and FSH, with consequent increase of ovarian and testicular steroidogenesis. During repeated dosing this response to stimulation gradually diminishes. Within three to four weeks, daily administration leads to decreased pituitary gonadotrophin secretion and/or the secretion of gonadotrophin secretion and/or the secretion of gonadotrophins with lowered biological activity. There is a consequent suppression of gonadal steroidogenesis and inhibition of functions in tissues that depend on gonadal steroids for their maintenance.

5.2 Pharmacokinetic properties

Nafarelin is rapidly absorbed into the circulation after intranasal administration. Maximum plasma concentration is achieved 20 minutes after dosing and the plasma half-life is approximately 4 hours. Bioavailability of the intranasal dose averages 2.8% (range 1.2-5.6%).

5.3 Preclinical safety data

This is discussed in Section 4.8 undesirable effects.

6. PHARMACEUTICAL PARTICULARS

6.1 List of excipients

Synarel contains:

Sorbitol, benzalkonium chloride, glacial acetic acid and water.

Sodium hydroxide or hydrochloric acid to adjust pH.

6.2 Incompatibilities

None stated.

6.3 Shelf life

The shelf life of Synarel is 2 years.

6.4 Special precautions for storage

Store upright below 25°C. Avoid heat above 30°C. Protect from light and freezing.

6.5 Nature and contents of container

White, high density polyethylene bottles with a 0.1ml metered spray pump, containing 6.5ml or 10ml.

PVC-coated glass bottles with an internal conical reservoir in the base and a valois pump, with either an aluminium crimp-on cap or a polypropylene snap-on cap, containing 4ml or 8ml.

6.6 Instructions for use and handling

None.

7. MARKETING AUTHORISATION HOLDER

Pharmacia Limited

Davy Avenue

Milton Keynes

Bucks. MK5 8PH

United Kingdom

8. MARKETING AUTHORISATION NUMBER(S)

PL 00032/0421

9. DATE OF FIRST AUTHORISATION/RENEWAL OF THE AUTHORISATION

13 August 2003

10. DATE OF REVISION OF THE TEXT

February 2004

11. LEGAL CATEGORY

POM

Ref: SL1_0UK

Syndol Caplets

(SSL International plc)

1. NAME OF THE MEDICINAL PRODUCT

Syndol Caplets.

2. QUALITATIVE AND QUANTITATIVE COMPOSITION

Paracetamol BP 450.0mg, Codeine Phosphate BP 10.0mg, Doxylamine Succinate NF 5.0mg, Caffeine BP 30.0mg.

3. PHARMACEUTICAL FORM

Tablets.

4. CLINICAL PARTICULARS

4.1 Therapeutic indications

For the treatment of mild to moderate pain and as an antipyretic. Syndol Caplets are recommended for the symptomatic relief of headache, including muscle contraction or tension headache, migraine, neuralgia, toothache, sore throat, dysmenorrhoea, muscular and rheumatic aches and pains and for post-operative analgesia following surgical or dental procedures.

4.2 Posology and method of administration

For oral administration. Adults and children over 12 years: 1 or 2 tablets every four to six hours as needed for relief. Total dosage over a 24 hour period should not normally exceed 8 tablets.

Codeine should be used with caution in the elderly and debilitated patients, as they may be more susceptible to the respiratory depressant effects.

4.3 Contraindications

Hypersensitivity to paracetamol, codeine or other opioid analgesics, or any of the other constituents.

4.4 Special warnings and special precautions for use

Do not exceed the stated dose. Do not take concurrently with any other paracetamol or codeine containing compounds. Care is advised in the administration of this preparation to patients with impaired kidney or liver function and in those with hypertension, hypothyroidism, adrenocortical insufficiency, prostatic hypertrophy, shock, obstructive bowel disorders, acute abdominal conditions, recent gastrointestinal surgery, gallstones, myasthenia gravis, a history of cardiac arrhythmias or convulsions and in patients with a history of drug abuse or emotional instability.

Prolonged use of codeine may lead to dependence and should be avoided. Codeine may induce faecal impaction, producing incontinence, spurious diarrhoea, abdominal pain and rarely colonic obstruction. Elderly patients may metabolise or eliminate opioid analgesics more slowly than younger adults.

4.5 Interaction with other medicinal products and other forms of Interaction

The speed of absorption of paracetamol may be increased by metoclopramide or domperidone and absorption reduced by cholestyramine. The anticoagulant effect of warfarin and other coumarins may be enhanced by prolonged regular daily use of paracetamol with increased risk of bleeding; occasional doses have no significant effect.

The depressant effects of codeine are enhanced by depressants of the central nervous system such as alcohol, anaesthetics, hypnotics, sedatives, tricyclic antidepressants and phenothiazines. The hypotensive actions of diuretics and anti hypertensive agents may be potentiated when used concurrently with opioid analgesics. Concurrent use of hydroxyzine with codeine may result in increased analgesia as well as increased CNS depressant and hypotensive effects. Concurrent use of codeine with antidiarrhoeal and antiperistaltic agents such as loperamide and kaolin may increase the risk of severe constipation. Concomitant use of antimuscarinics or medications with antimuscarinic action may result in an increased risk of severe constipation that may lead to paralytic ileus and/or urinary retention. The respiratory depressant effect caused by neuromuscular blocking agents may be additive to the central respiratory depressant effects of opioid analgesics. CNS depression or excitation may occur if codeine is given to patients receiving monoamine oxidase inhibitors, or within two weeks of stopping treatment with them. Quinidine can inhibit the analgesic effect of codeine. Codeine may delay the absorption of mexiletine and thus reduce the antiarrhythmic effect of the latter. Codeine may antagonise the gastrointestinal effects of metoclopramide, cisapride and domperidone. Cimetidine inhibits the metabolism of opioid analgesics resulting in increased plasma concentrations. Naloxone antagonises the analgesic, CNS and respiratory depressant effects of opioid analgesics. Naltrexone also blocks the therapeutic effect of opioids.

Incompatibilities: Codeine has been reported to be incompatible with phenobarbitone sodium forming a codeine-phenobarbitone complex, and with potassium iodide, forming crystals of codeine periodide. Acetylation of codeine phosphate by aspirin has occurred in solid dosage forms containing the two drugs, even at low moisture levels.

Interference with laboratory tests: Opioid analgesics interfere with a number of laboratory tests including plasma amylase, lipase, bilirubin, alkaline phosphatase, lactate dehydrogenase, alanine aminotransferase and aspartate aminotransferase. Opioids may also interfere with gastric emptying studies as they delay gastric emptying and with hepatobiliary imaging-using technetium Tc 99m disofenin as opioid treatment may cause constriction of the sphincter of Oddi and increase biliary tract pressure.

4.6 Pregnancy and lactation

Epidemiological studies in human pregnancy have shown no ill effects due to paracetamol used in the recommended dosage, but patients should follow the advice of their doctor regarding its use. Codeine crosses the placenta. There is no adequate evidence of safety in human pregnancy and a possible association with respiratory and cardiac malformations has been reported. Regular use during pregnancy may cause physical dependence in the foetus leading to withdrawal symptoms in the neonate. Use during pregnancy should be avoided if possible.

Use of opioid analgesia during labour may cause respiratory depression in the neonate, especially the premature neonate. These agents should not be given during the delivery of a premature baby.

Codeine passes into breast milk in very small amounts that are considered to be compatible with breast feeding.

4.7 Effects on ability to drive and use machines

Not applicable.

4.8 Undesirable effects

Doxylamine succinate may cause drowsiness or dizziness in some patients.

Adverse effects of paracetamol are rare but hypersensitivity including skin rash may occur. There have been a few reports of blood dyscrasias including thrombocytopenia and agranulocytosis but these were not necessarily causally related to paracetamol.

The most frequent undesirable effects of codeine are constipation and drowsiness. Less frequent effects are nausea, vomiting, sweating, facial flushing, dry mouth, blurred or double vision, dizziness, orthostatic hypotension, malaise, tiredness, headache, anorexia, vertigo, bradycardia, palpitations, respiratory depression, dyspnoea, allergic reactions (itch, skin rash, facial oedema) and difficulties in micturition (dysuria, increased frequency, decrease in amount). Side effects that occur rarely include convulsions, hallucinations, nightmares, uncontrolled muscle movements, muscle rigidity, mental depression and stomach cramps. The euphoric activity of codeine may lead to its abuse and dependence.

4.9 Overdose

Symptoms of overdose in the first 24 hours are pallor, nausea, vomiting, anorexia, and abdominal pain. Liver damage may become apparent 12 to 48 hours after ingestion. Abnormalities of glucose metabolism and metabolic acidosis may occur. In severe poisoning, hepatic failure may progress to encephalopathy, coma and death. Acute renal failure with acute tubular necrosis may develop even in the absence of severe liver damage. Cardiac arrhythmias and pancreatitis have been reported. Liver damage is possible in adults who have taken 10g or more of paracetamol. It is considered that excess quantities of a toxic metabolite (usually adequately detoxified by glutathione when normal doses of paracetamol are ingested) become irreversibly bound to liver tissue. Immediate treatment is essential in the management of a paracetamol overdose. Despite a lack of significant early symptoms, patients should be referred to hospital urgently for immediate medical attention and any patient who has ingested around 7.5g or more of paracetamol in the preceding 4 hours should undergo gastric lavage. Administration of oral methionine or intravenous N-acetylcysteine which may have a beneficial effect up to at least 48 hours after the overdose, may be required. General supportive measures must be available.

While the dose of codeine phosphate in this preparation is relatively small and therefore less likely to prove a problem, symptoms of overdose include cold clammy skin, confusion, convulsions, dizziness, drowsiness, nervousness or restlessness, miosis, bradycardia, dyspnoea, unconsciousness and weakness. Codeine in large doses may produce respiratory depression, hypotension, circulatory failure and deepening coma. Death may occur from respiratory failure.

Initial treatment includes emptying the stomach by aspiration and lavage. Intensive support therapy may be required to correct respiratory failure and shock. In addition the specific narcotic antagonist, naloxone hydrochloride, may be used rapidly to counteract the severe respiratory depression and coma. A dose of 0.4-2 mg is given intravenously or intramuscularly to adults, this is repeated at intervals of 2-3 minutes; if necessary up to 10mg of naloxone may be given. In children doses of 5-10μg/kg body weight may be given intravenously or intramuscularly. Codeine is not dialysable.

5. PHARMACOLOGICAL PROPERTIES

5.1 Pharmacodynamic properties

Paracetamol - antipyretic, analgesic; codeine phosphate - analgesic; doxylamine succinate - antihistamine; caffeine - mild stimulant.

5.2 Pharmacokinetic properties

The pharmacokinetics of paracetamol, codeine phosphate and caffeine are widely published (see Goodman & Gilman's The Pharmacological Basis of Therapeutics, Seventh Edition, pp 693, 505 and 596 respectively). Doxylamine succinate is readily absorbed from the gastrointestinal tract. Following oral administration, the effects start within 15 to 30 minutes and peak within one hour. In humans, 60-80% of doxylamine given has been recovered in urine at 24 hours post-dose.

5.3 Preclinical safety data

None stated.

6. PHARMACEUTICAL PARTICULARS

6.1 List of excipients

Tablet Core: Povidone; Croscarmellose Sodium; Corn Starch; Magnesium Stearate; Talc; Purified water.

Coating: Opadry II Yellow (Lactose Monohydrate; Hydroxypropyl Methyl Cellulose (Methocel E15); Polyethylene Glycol 4000; Quinoline Yellow Aluminium Lake (E104); Sunset Yellow Aluminium Lake (E110); Titanium Dioxide)

6.2 Incompatibilities

Not applicable.

6.3 Shelf life

60 months.

6.4 Special precautions for storage

None stated.

6.5 Nature and contents of container

Blister strips: 250 micron UPVC/PVDC and aluminium foil 20 micron coated with lacquer. Blister strips are presented in cardboard cartons. Pack sizes are 10,20 or 30 tablets.

6.6 Instructions for use and handling

None.

7. MARKETING AUTHORISATION HOLDER

Seton Products Limited, Tubiton House, Oldham, OL1 3HS

8. MARKETING AUTHORISATION NUMBER(S)

PL 11314/0122.

9. DATE OF FIRST AUTHORISATION/RENEWAL OF THE AUTHORISATION

16th January 1999.

10. DATE OF REVISION OF THE TEXT

June 2002.

Synflex Tablets

(Roche Products Limited)

1. NAME OF THE MEDICINAL PRODUCT

Synflex Tablets

2. QUALITATIVE AND QUANTITATIVE COMPOSITION

Naproxen sodium 275mg (equivalent to naproxen 250mg).

3. PHARMACEUTICAL FORM

Pale blue, opaque film-coated tablet.

4. CLINICAL PARTICULARS

4.1 Therapeutic indications

Synflex is indicatedfor the treatment of musculoskeletal disorders (including sprains and strains, direct trauma, lumbo-sacral pain, cervical spondylitis, fibrositis, bursitis and tendinitis); uterine pain following IUCD insertion, post-operative (including orthopaedic) pain; post-partum pain, rheumatoid arthritis, osteoarthrosis, ankylosing spondylitis, acute gout and dysmenorrhoea.

Synflex is also indicated for the relief of migraine.

4.2 Posology and method of administration

Therapy should be started at the lowest recommended dose, especially in the elderly.

Adults

For musculoskeletal disorders and post-operative pain, post IUCD insertion, rheumatoid arthritis, osteoarthrosis and ankylosing spondylitis the recommended dosage is 550mg twice daily, not more than 1100mg being taken per day.

For post-partum pain a single dose of 550mg is recommended.

For dysmenorrhoea and acute gout the recommended dosage is 550mg initially, followed by 275mg at 6 - 8 hour intervals as needed. This represents a maximum dose on the first day of 1375mg and 1100mg per day thereafter.

For the relief of migraine, the recommended dose is 825mg at the first symptom of an impending attack. 275 - 550mg can be taken in addition throughout the day, if necessary, but not before half an hour after the initial dose. A total dose of 1375mg per day should not be exceeded.

Elderly

Studies indicate that although the total plasma concentration of naproxen is unchanged, the unbound plasma fraction of naproxen is increased in the elderly. The implication of this finding for Synflex dosing is unknown. As with other drugs used in the elderly it is prudent to use the lowest effective dose. For the effect of reduced elimination in the elderly, refer to the section *Use in patients with impaired renal function*.

Children

Synflex is not recommended for use in children under sixteen years of age.

4.3 Contraindications

Active or history of peptic ulceration or active gastrointestinal bleeding. Hypersensitivity to naproxen or naproxen sodium formulations. Since the potential exists for cross-sensitivity reactions, Synflex should not be given to patients in whom aspirin or other non-steroidal anti-inflammatory/analgesic drugs induce asthma, rhinitis or urticaria.

4.4 Special warnings and special precautions for use

Episodes of gastro-intestinal bleeding have been reported in patients with naproxen or naproxen sodium therapy. Synflex should therefore be given under close supervision to patients with a history of gastro-intestinal disease.

Serious gastro-intestinal adverse reactions can occur, at any time in patients on therapy with non-steroidal anti-inflammatory drugs. The risk of their occurrence does not seem to change with duration of therapy. Studies to date have not identified any subset of patients not at risk of developing peptic ulcer and bleeding, however, elderly and debilitated patients tolerate gastro-intestinal ulceration or bleeding less well than others. Most of the serious gastro-intestinal events associated with non-steroidal anti-inflammatory drugs occurred in this patient population.

The antipyretic and anti-inflammatory activities of Synflex may reduce fever and inflammation, thereby diminishing their usefulness as diagnostic signs.

Bronchospasm may be precipitated in patients suffering from, or with a history of, bronchial asthma or allergic disease.

Sporadic abnormalities in laboratory tests (e.g. liver function tests) have occurred in patients on naproxen or naproxen sodium therapy, but no definite trend was seen in any test indicating toxicity.

Naproxen decreases platelet aggregation and prolongs bleeding time. This effect should be kept in mind when bleeding times are determined.

Mild peripheral oedema has been observed in a few patients receiving naproxen or naproxen sodium. Although sodium retention has not been reported in metabolic studies, it is possible that patients with questionable or compromised cardiac function may be at a greater risk when taking Synflex.

Each Synflex tablet contains approximately 25mg of sodium (about 1m Eq). This should be considered in patients whose overall intake of sodium must be markedly restricted.

Use in patients with impaired renal function: As naproxen is eliminated to a large extent (95%) by urinary excretion via glomerular filtration, it should be used with great caution in patients with impaired renal function and the monitoring of serum creatinine and/or creatinine clearance is advised in these patients. Synflex is not recommended in patients having baseline creatinine clearance of less than 20ml/minute.

Certain patients, specifically those whose renal blood flow is compromised, such as in extracellular volume depletion, cirrhosis of the liver, sodium restriction, congestive heart failure, and pre-existing renal disease, should have renal function assessed before and during Synflex therapy. Some elderly patients in whom impaired renal function may be expected, as well as patients using diuretics, may also fall within this category. A reduction in daily dosage should be considered to avoid the possibility of excessive accumulation of naproxen metabolites in these patients.

Use in patients with impaired liver function: Chronic alcoholic liver disease and probably also other forms of cirrhosis reduce the total plasma concentration of naproxen, but the plasma concentration of unbound naproxen is increased. The implication of this finding for Synflex dosing is unknown but it is prudent to use the lowest effective dose.

Haematological

Patients who have coagulation disorders or are receiving drug therapy that interferes with haemostasis should be carefully observed if naproxen-containing products are administered.

Patients at high risk of bleeding or those on full anti-coagulation therapy (e.g. dicoumarol derivatives) may be at increased risk of bleeding if given naproxen-containing products concurrently.

Anaphylactic (anaphylactoid) reactions

Hypersensitivity reactions may occur in susceptible individuals. Anaphylactic (anaphylactoid) reactions may occur both in patients with and without a history of hypersensitivity or exposure to aspirin, other non-steroidal anti-inflammatory drugs or naproxen-containing products. They may also occur in individuals with a history of angioedema, bronchospastic reactivity (e.g. asthma), rhinitis and nasal polyps.

Anaphylactoid reactions, like anaphylaxis, may have a fatal outcome.

Steroids

If steroid dosage is reduced or eliminated during therapy, the steroid dosage should be reduced slowly and the patients must be observed closely for any evidence of adverse effects, including adrenal insufficiency and exacerbation of symptoms of arthritis.

Ocular effects

Studies have not shown changes in the eye attributable to naproxen administration. In rare cases, adverse ocular disorders including papillitis, retrobulbar optic neuritis and papilledema, have been reported in users of NSAIDs including naproxen, although a cause-and-effect relationship cannot be established; accordingly, patients who develop visual disturbances during treatment with naproxen-containing products should have an ophthalmological examination.

Combination with other NSAIDs

The combination of naproxen-containing products and other NSAIDs is not recommended, because of the cumulative risks of inducing serious NSAID-related adverse events.

4.5 Interaction with other medicinal products and other forms of Interaction

Concomitant administration of antacid or cholestyramine can delay the absorption of naproxen but does not affect its extent. Concomitant administration of food can delay the absorption of naproxen, but does not affect its extent.

Due to the high plasma protein binding of naproxen, patients simultaneously receiving hydantoins, anti-coagulants or a highly protein-bound sulfonamide should be observed for signs of overdosage of these drugs. No interactions have been observed in clinical studies with naproxen sodium or naproxen and anti-coagulants or sulfonylureas, but caution is nevertheless advised since interaction has been seen with other non-steroidal agents of this class.

The natriuretic effect of frusemide has been reported to be inhibited by some drugs of this class.

Inhibition of renal lithium clearance leading to increases in plasma lithium concentrations has also been reported.

Naproxen and other non-steroidal anti-inflammatory drugs can reduce the antihypertensive effect of propranolol and other beta-blockers and may increase the risk of renal impairment associated with the use of ACE-inhibitors.

Probenecid given concurrently increases naproxen plasma levels and extends its half-life considerably.

Caution is advised where methotrexate is given concurrently because of possible enhancement of its toxicity since naproxen, among other non-steroidal anti-inflammatory drugs, has been reported to reduce the tubular secretion of methotrexate in an animal model.

NSAIDs may exacerbate cardiac failure, reduce GFR and increase plasma cardiac glycoside levels when co-administered with cardiac glycosides.

As with all NSAIDs caution is advised when cyclosporin is co-administered because of the increased risk of nephrotoxicity.

NSAIDs should not be used for 8 - 12 days after mifepristone administration as NSAIDs can reduce the effects of mifepristone.

As with all NSAIDs, caution should be taken when co-administering with cortico-steroids because of the increased risk of bleeding.

Patients taking quinolones may have an increased risk of developing convulsions.

It is suggested that Synflex therapy be temporarily discontinued 48 hours before adrenal function tests are performed because naproxen may artifactually interfere with some tests for 17-ketogenic steroids. Similarly, naproxen may interfere with some assays of urinary 5-hydroxyindoleacetic acid.

4.6 Pregnancy and lactation

Teratology studies in rats and rabbits at dose levels equivalent on a human multiple basis to those which have produced foetal abnormality with certain other non-steroidal anti-inflammatory agents, e.g. aspirin, have not produced evidence of foetal damage with Synflex. As with other drugs of this type Synflex delays parturition in animals (the relevance of this finding to human patients is unknown) and also affects the human foetal cardiovascular system (closure of the ductus arteriosus). Good medical practice indicates minimal drug usage in pregnancy, and use of this class of therapeutic agent requires cautious balancing of possible benefit against potential risk to the mother and foetus especially in the first and third trimesters.

The use of Synflex should be avoided in patients who are breast-feeding.

4.7 Effects on ability to drive and use machines

Some patients may experience drowsiness, dizziness, vertigo, insomnia or depression with the use of Synflex. If patients experience these or similar undesirable effects, they should exercise caution in carrying out activities that require alertness.

4.8 Undesirable effects

Gastro-intestinal: The more frequent reactions are nausea, vomiting, abdominal discomfort and epigastric distress. More serious reactions which may occur occasionally are gastro-intestinal bleeding, peptic ulceration (sometimes with haemorrhage and perforation), non-peptic gastro-intestinal ulceration and colitis.

Dermatological: Skin rash, urticaria, angio-oedema. Alopecia, erythema multiforme, Stevens Johnson syndrome, epidermal necrolysis and photosensitivity reactions (including cases in which skin resembles porphyria cutanea tarda "pseudoporphyria") or epidermolysis bullosa may occur rarely.

Renal: Including, but not limited to, glomerular nephritis, interstitial nephritis, nephrotic syndrome, haematuria, renal papillary necrosis and renal failure.

CNS: Convulsions, headache, insomnia, inability to concentrate and cognitive dysfunction have been reported.

Haematological: Thrombocytopenia, granulocytopenia including agranulocytosis, aplastic anaemia and haemolytic anaemia may occur rarely.

Other: Tinnitus, hearing impairment, vertigo, mild peripheral oedema. Anaphylactic reactions to naproxen and naproxen sodium formulations have been reported in patients with, or without, a history of previous hypersensitivity reactions to NSAIDs. Jaundice, fatal hepatitis, visual disturbances, eosinophilic pneumonitis, vasculitis, aseptic meningitis, hyperkalaemia and ulcerative stomatitis have been reported rarely.

4.9 Overdose

Significant overdosage of the drug may be characterised by drowsiness, heartburn, indigestion, nausea or vomiting. A few patients have experienced seizures, but it is not clear whether these were naproxen-related or not. It is not known what dose of the drug would be life-threatening.

Should a patient ingest a large amount of Synflex accidentally or purposefully, the stomach may be emptied and usual supportive measures employed. Animal studies indicate that the prompt administration of activated charcoal in adequate amounts would tend to reduce markedly the absorption of the drug.

Haemodialysis does not decrease the plasma concentration of naproxen because of the high degree of protein binding. However, haemodialysis may still be appropriate in a patient with renal failure who has taken Synflex.

5. PHARMACOLOGICAL PROPERTIES

5.1 Pharmacodynamic properties

Synflex is a non-steroidal, anti-inflammatory agent. It has analgesic, anti-inflammatory and antipyretic properties.

5.2 Pharmacokinetic properties

The sodium salt of naproxen is absorbed more rapidly than naproxen leading to earlier and higher plasma levels of naproxen. This is particularly useful for analgesia, where early availability of the drug in circulation is advantageous.

Typical pharmacokinetic values for naproxen sodium and naproxen are as follows:

(see Table 1)

See also *Special warnings and special precautions for use* for certain patients, i.e. the elderly and those with impaired renal or liver function.

5.3 Preclinical safety data

None stated.

6. PHARMACEUTICAL PARTICULARS

6.1 List of excipients

Povidone BP, magnesium stearate BP, microcrystalline cellulose BP, purified water BP, talc BP and opadry.

6.2 Incompatibilities

None stated.

6.3 Shelf life

5 years.

6.4 Special precautions for storage

Protect from light and moisture.

6.5 Nature and contents of container

a. Opaque high density polyethylene container containing 100 tablets.

b. PVC/foil blister pack containing 60 tablets.

c. Polypropylene securitainers with high density polyethylene lid containing 2 or 4 tablets.

6.6 Instructions for use and handling

None stated.

Table 1

Parameter	2 × 275mg Naproxen-Na tablet	2 × 250mg Naproxen tablet	p. value
Biol T1/2 (hrs)	13.41	13.43	0.993
T max (min)	56.67	110.0	0.036
Cp max (mcg/ml)	74.67	65.58	0.007
AUC Total (mcg/ml × hr)	1050.9	1006.1	0.478

7. MARKETING AUTHORISATION HOLDER

Roche Products Limited, 40 Broadwater Road, Welwyn Garden City, Hertfordshire, AL7 3AY.

8. MARKETING AUTHORISATION NUMBER(S)

PL 0031/0478

9. DATE OF FIRST AUTHORISATION/RENEWAL OF THE AUTHORISATION

30 May 1996

10. DATE OF REVISION OF THE TEXT

October 1997

Synflex is a registered trade mark P835009/699

Synphase Tablets

(Pharmacia Limited)

1. NAME OF THE MEDICINAL PRODUCT

Synphase.

2. QUALITATIVE AND QUANTITATIVE COMPOSITION

Synphase consists of 7 blue tablets containing norethisterone 500 micrograms and ethinylestradiol 35 micrograms, marked 'BX' on one side and 'SEARLE' on the other; 9 white tablets containing norethisterone 1.0 milligram and ethinylestradiol 35 micrograms inscribed 'SEARLE' on one face and 'BX' on the other; 5 blue tablets containing norethisterone 500 micrograms and ethinylestradiol 35 micrograms, marked 'BX' on one side and 'SEARLE' on the other.

3. PHARMACEUTICAL FORM

Tablets for oral administration.

4. CLINICAL PARTICULARS

4.1 Therapeutic indications

Synphase is indicated for oral contraception, with the benefit of a low intake of oestrogen.

4.2 Posology and method of administration

Oral Administration: The dosage of Synphase for the initial cycle of therapy is 1 tablet taken at the same time each day from the first day of the menstrual cycle. For subsequent cycles, no tablets are taken for 7 days, then a new course is started of 1 tablet daily for the next 21 days. This sequence of 21 days on treatment, seven days off treatment is repeated for as long as contraception is required.

Patients unable to start taking Synphase tablets on the first day of the menstrual cycle may start treatment on any day up to and including the 5th day of the menstrual cycle.

Patients starting on day 1 of their period will be protected at once. Those patients delaying therapy up to day 5 may not be protected immediately and it is recommended that another method of contraception is used for the first 7 days of tablet-taking. Suitable methods are condoms, caps plus spermicides and intra-uterine devices.

The rhythm, temperature and cervical-mucus methods should not be relied upon.

Tablet omissions

Tablets must be taken daily in order to maintain adequate hormone levels and contraceptive efficacy.

If a tablet is missed within 12 hours of the correct dosage time then the missed tablet should be taken as soon as possible, even if this means taking 2 tablets on the same day, this will ensure that contraceptive protection is maintained. If one or more tablets are missed for more than 12 hours from the correct dosage time it is recommended that the patient takes the last missed tablet as soon as possible and then continues to take the rest of the tablets in the normal manner. In addition, it is recommended that extra contraceptive protection, such as a condom, is used for the next 7 days.

Patients who have missed one or more of the last 7 tablets in a pack should be advised to start the next pack of tablets as soon as the present one has finished (i.e. without the normal seven day gap between treatments). This reduces the risk of contraceptive failure resulting from tablets being missed close to a 7 day tablet free period.

Changing from another oral contraceptive

In order to ensure that contraception is maintained it is advised that the first dose of Synphase tablets is taken on the day immediately after the patient has finished the previous pack of tablets.

Use after childbirth, miscarriage or abortion

Providing the patient is not breast feeding the first dose of Synphase tablets should be taken on the 21st day after childbirth. This will ensure the patient is protected immediately. If there is any delay in taking the first dose, contraception may not be established until 7 days after the first tablet has been taken. In these circumstances patients should be advised that extra contraceptive methods will be necessary.

After a miscarriage or abortion patients can take the first dose of Synphase tablets on the next day; in this way they will be protected immediately.

Figure 1 Estimated cumulative numbers of breast cancers per 10,000 women diagnosed in 5 years of use and up to 10 years after stopping COCs, compared with numbers of breast cancers diagnosed in 10,000 women who had never used COCs

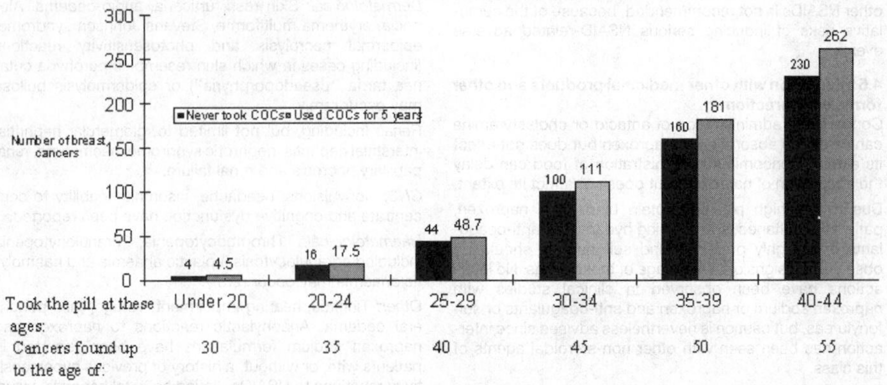

4.3 Contraindications

As with all combined progestogen/oestrogen oral contraceptives, the following conditions should be regarded as contra-indications:

i. History of confirmed venous thromboembolic disease (VTE), family history of idiopathic VTE and other known risk factors of VTE

ii. Thrombophlebitis, cerebrovascular disorders, coronary artery disease, myocardial infarction, angina, hyperlipidaemia or a history of these conditions.

iii. Acute or severe chronic liver disease, including liver tumours, Dubin-Johnson or Rotor syndrome.

iv. History during pregnancy of idiopathic jaundice, severe pruritus or pemphigoid gestationis.

v. Known or suspected breast or genital cancer.

vi. Known or suspected oestrogen-dependent neoplasia.

vii. Undiagnosed abnormal vaginal bleeding.

viii. A history of migraines classified as classical, focal or crescendo.

ix. Pregnancy.

4.4 Special warnings and special precautions for use

Assessment of women prior to starting oral contraceptives (and at regular intervals thereafter) should include a personal and family medical history of each woman. Physical examination should be guided by this and by the contra-indications (section 4.3) and warnings (section 4.4) for this product. The frequency and nature of these assessments should be based upon relevant guidelines and should be adapted to the individual woman, but should include measurement of blood pressure and, if judged appropriate by the clinician, breast, abdominal and pelvic examination including cervical cytology.

Women taking oral contraceptives require careful observation if they have or have had any of the following conditions: breast nodules; fibrocystic disease of the breast or an abnormal mammogram; uterine fibroids; a history of severe depressive states; varicose veins; sickle-cell anaemia; diabetes; hypertension; cardiovascular disease; migraine; epilepsy; asthma; otosclerosis; multiple sclerosis; porphyria; tetany; disturbed liver functions; gallstones; kidney disease; chloasma; any condition that is likely to worsen during pregnancy. The worsening or first appearance of any of these conditions may indicate that the oral contraceptive should be stopped. Discontinue treatment if there is a gradual or sudden, partial or complete loss of vision or any evidence of ocular changes, onset or aggravation of migraine or development of headache of a new kind which is recurrent, persistent or severe.

Gastro-intestinal upsets, such as vomiting and diarrhoea, may interfere with the absorption of the tablets leading to a reduction in contraceptive efficacy. Patients should continue to take Synphase, but they should also be encouraged to use another contraceptive method during the period of gastro-intestinal upset and for the next 7 days.

Progestogen oestrogen preparations should be used with caution in patients with a history of hepatic dysfunction or hypertension.

An increased risk of venous thromboembolic disease (VTE) associated with the use of oral contraceptives is well established but is smaller than that associated with pregnancy, which has been estimated at 60 cases per 100,000 pregnancies. Some epidemiological studies have reported a greater risk of VTE for women using combined oral contraceptives containing desogestrel or gestodene (the so-called 'third generation' pills) than for women using pills containing levonorgestrel or norethisterone (the so-called 'second generation' pills)

The spontaneous incidence of VTE in healthy non-pregnant women (not taking any oral contraceptive) is about 5 cases per 100,000 per year. The incidence in users of second generation pills is about 15 per 100,000 women per year of use. The incidence in users of third generation pills is about 25 cases per 100,000 women per year of use; this excess incidence has not been satisfactorily explained by bias or confounding. The level of all of these risks of VTE increases with age and is likely to be further increased in women with other known risk factors for VTE such as obesity. The excess risk of VTE is highest during the first year a woman ever uses a combined oral contraceptive.

Patients receiving oral contraceptives should be kept under regular surveillance, in view of the possibility of development of conditions such as thromboembolism.

The risk of coronary artery disease in women taking oral contraceptives is increased by the presence of other predisposing factors such as cigarette smoking, hypercholesterolaemia, obesity, diabetes, history of pre-eclamptic toxaemia and increasing age. After the age of thirty-five years, the patient and physician should carefully re-assess the risk/benefit ratio of using combined oral contraceptives as opposed to alternative methods of contraception.

Synphase should be discontinued at least four weeks before, and for two weeks following, elective operations and during immobilisation. Patients undergoing injection treatment for varicose veins should not resume taking Synphase until 3 months after the last injection.

Benign and malignant liver tumours have been associated with oral contraceptive use. The relationship between occurrence of liver tumours and use of female sex hormones is not known at present. These tumours may rupture causing intra-abdominal bleeding. If the patient presents with a mass or tenderness in the right upper quadrant or an acute abdomen, the possible presence of a tumour should be considered.

An increased risk of congenital abnormalities, including heart defects and limb defects, has been reported following the use of sex hormones, including oral contraceptives, in pregnancy. If the patient does not adhere to the prescribed schedule, the possibility of pregnancy should be considered at the time of the first missed period and further use of oral contraceptives should be withheld until pregnancy has been ruled out. It is recommended that for any patient who has missed two consecutive periods, pregnancy should be ruled out before continuing the contraceptive regimen. If pregnancy is confirmed the patient should be advised of the potential risks to the foetus and the advisability of continuing the pregnancy should be discussed in the light of these risks. It is advisable to discontinue Synphase three months before a planned pregnancy.

The risk of arterial thrombosis associated with combined oral contraceptives increases with age, and this risk is aggravated by cigarette smoking. The use of combined oral contraceptives by women in the older age group, especially those who are cigarette smokers, should therefore be discouraged and alternative methods advised.

The use of this product in patients suffering from epilepsy, migraine, asthma or cardiac dysfunction may result in exacerbation of these disorders because of fluid retention. Caution should also be observed in patients who wear contact lenses.

Decreased glucose tolerance may occur in diabetic patients on this treatment, and their control must be carefully supervised.

The use of oral contraceptives has also been associated with a possible increased incidence of gall bladder disease.

Women with a history of oligomenorrhoea or secondary amenorrhoea or young women without regular cycles may have a tendency to remain anovulatory or to become amenorrhoeic after discontinuation of oral contraceptives. Women with these pre-existing problems should be advised of this possibility and encouraged to use other contraceptive methods.

Numerous epidemiological studies have been reported on the risks of ovarian, endometrial, cervical and breast cancer in women using combined oral contraceptives. The evidence is clear that combined oral contraceptives offer substantial protection against both ovarian and endometrial cancer.

An increased risk of cervical cancer in long-term users of combined oral contraceptives has been reported in some studies, but there continues to be controversy about the extent to which this is attributable to the confounding effects of sexual behaviour and other factors.

A meta-analysis from 54 epidemiological studies reported that there is a slightly increased relative risk (RR = 1.24) of having breast cancer diagnosed in women who are currently using combined oral contraceptives (COCs). The observed pattern of increased risk may be due to an earlier diagnosis of breast cancer in COC users, the biological effects of COCs or a combination of both. The additional breast cancers diagnosed in current users of COCs or in women who have used COCs in the last ten years are more likely to be localised to the breast than those in women who never used COCs.

Breast cancer is rare among women under 40 years of age whether or not they take COCs. Whilst this background risk increases with age, the excess number of breast cancer diagnoses in current and recent COC users is small in relation to the overall risk of breast cancer (see bar chart).

The most important risk factor for breast cancer in COC users is the age women discontinue the COC; the older the age at stopping, the more breast cancers are diagnosed. Duration of use is less important and the excess risk gradually disappears during the course of the 10 years after stopping COC use such that by 10 years there appears to be no excess.

The possible increase in risk of breast cancer should be discussed with the user and weighed against the benefits of COCs taking into account the evidence that they offer substantial protection against the risk of developing certain other cancers (e.g. ovarian and endometrial cancer).

Estimated cumulative numbers of breast cancers per 10,000 women diagnosed in 5 years of use and up to 10 years after stopping COCs, compared with numbers of breast cancers diagnosed in 10,000 women who had never used COCs.

(see figure 1 above)

4.5 Interaction with other medicinal products and other forms of Interaction

The herbal remedy St John's wort (*Hypericum perforatum*) should not be taken concomitantly with this medicine as this could potentially lead to a loss of contraceptive effect.

Some drugs may modify the metabolism of Synphase reducing its effectiveness; these include certain sedatives, antibiotics, anti-epileptic and anti-arthritic drugs. During the time such agents are used concurrently, it is advised that mechanical contraceptives also be used.

The results of a large number of laboratory tests have been shown to be influenced by the use of oestrogen containing oral contraceptives, which may limit their diagnostic value. Among these are: biochemical markers of thyroid and liver function; plasma levels of carrier proteins, triglycerides, coagulation and fibrinolysis factors.

4.6 Pregnancy and lactation

Contra-indicated in pregnancy.

Patients who are fully breast-feeding should not take Synphase tablets since, in common with other combined oral contraceptives, the oestrogen component may reduce the amount of milk produced. In addition, active ingredients or their metabolites have been detected in the milk of mothers taking oral contraceptives. The effect of Synphase on breast-fed infants has not been determined.

4.7 Effects on ability to drive and use machines

Not applicable.

4.8 Undesirable effects

As with all oral contraceptives, there may be slight nausea at first, weight gain or breast discomfort, which soon disappear.

Other side-effects known or suspected to occur with oral contraceptives include gastro-intestinal symptoms, changes in libido and appetite, headache, exacerbation of existing uterine fibroid disease, depression, and changes in carbohydrate, lipid and vitamin metabolism.

Spotting or bleeding may occur during the first few cycles. Usually menstrual bleeding becomes light and occasionally there may be no bleeding during the tablet-free days.

Hypertension, which is usually reversible on discontinuing treatment, has occurred in a small percentage of women taking oral contraceptives.

4.9 Overdose

Overdosage may be manifested by nausea, vomiting, breast enlargement and vaginal bleeding. There is no specific antidote and treatment should be symptomatic. Gastric lavage may be employed if the overdose is large and the patient is seen sufficiently early (within four hours).

5. PHARMACOLOGICAL PROPERTIES

5.1 Pharmacodynamic properties

The mode of action of Synphase is similar to that of other progestogen/oestrogen oral contraceptives and includes the inhibition of ovulation, the thickening of cervical mucus so as to constitute a barrier to sperm and the rendering of the endometrium unreceptive to implantation. Such activity is exerted through a combined effect on one or more of the following: hypothalamus, anterior pituitary, ovary, endometrium and cervical mucus.

5.2 Pharmacokinetic properties
Norethisterone is rapidly and completely absorbed after oral administration, peak plasma concentrations occurring in the majority of subjects between 1 and 3 hours. Due to first-pass metabolism, blood levels after oral administration are 60% of those after i.v. administration. The half life of elimination varies from 5 to 12 hours, with a mean of 7.6 hours. Norethisterone is metabolised mainly in the liver. Approximately 60% of the administered dose is excreted as metabolites in urine and faeces.

Ethinylestradiol is rapidly and well absorbed from the gastro-intestinal tract but is subject to some first-pass metabolism in the gut-wall. Compared to many other oestrogens it is only slowly metabolised in the liver. Excretion is via the kidneys with some appearing also in the faeces.

5.3 Preclinical safety data
The toxicity of norethisterone is very low. Reports of teratogenic effects in animals are uncommon. No carcinogenic effects have been found even in long-term studies.

Long-term continuous administration of oestrogens in some animals increases the frequency of carcinoma of the breast, cervix, vagina and liver.

6. PHARMACEUTICAL PARTICULARS
6.1 List of excipients
Synphase tablets contain:

Maize starch, polyvidone, magnesium stearate and lactose. The blue tablets also contain E132.

6.2 Incompatibilities
None stated.

6.3 Shelf life
The shelf life of Synphase tablets is 5 years.

6.4 Special precautions for storage
Store in a dry place below 25°C away from direct sunlight.

6.5 Nature and contents of container
Synphase tablets are supplied in pvc/foil blister packs of 21 and 63 tablets.

6.6 Instructions for use and handling
None.

7. MARKETING AUTHORISATION HOLDER
Pharmacia Limited

Davy Avenue, Knowlhill,

Milton Keynes

MK5 8PH

8. MARKETING AUTHORISATION NUMBER(S)
PL 0032/0422

9. DATE OF FIRST AUTHORISATION/RENEWAL OF THE AUTHORISATION
May 10th 1996

10. DATE OF REVISION OF THE TEXT
December 2004

SY1_0

Syntocinon Ampoules 10 IU/ml

(Alliance Pharmaceuticals)

1. NAME OF THE MEDICINAL PRODUCT
Syntocinon® Ampoules 10 IU/ml

2. QUALITATIVE AND QUANTITATIVE COMPOSITION
Oxytocin PhEur 10 units in 1ml.

3. PHARMACEUTICAL FORM
A clear, colourless, sterile solution in 1ml clear glass ampoules.

4. CLINICAL PARTICULARS
4.1 Therapeutic indications
Induction of labour for medical reasons; stimulation of labour in hypotonic uterine inertia; during caesarean section, following delivery of the child; prevention and treatment of postpartum uterine atony and haemorrhage.

Early stages of pregnancy as a adjunctive therapy for the management of incomplete, inevitable, or missed abortion.

4.2 Posology and method of administration
Induction or enhancement of labour: Oxytocin should not be started for 6 hours following administration of vaginal prostaglandins. Syntocinon should be administered as an iv drip infusion or, preferably, by means of a variable-speed infusion pump. For drip infusion it is recommended that 5 IU of Syntocinon be added to 500ml of a physiological electrolyte solution. For patients in whom infusion of sodium chloride must be avoided, 5% dextrose solution may be used as the diluent (see Section 4.4 "Special warnings and precautions for use"). To ensure even mixing, the bottle or bag must be turned upside down several times before use.

The initial infusion rate should be set at 1 to 4mU/min (2 to 8 drops/min). It may be gradually increased at intervals not shorter than 20 min, until a contraction pattern similar to that of normal labour is established. In pregnancy near term this can often be achieved with an infusion of less than 10mU/min (20 drops/min), and the recommended maximum rate is 20mU/min (40 drops/min). In the unusual event that higher rates are required, as may occur in the management of foetal death *in utero* or for induction of labour at an earlier stage of pregnancy, when the uterus is less sensitive to oxytocin, it is advisable to use a more concentrated Syntocinon solution, e.g., 10 IU in 500ml.

When using a motor-driven infusion pump which delivers smaller volumes than those given by drip infusion, the concentration suitable for infusion within the recommended dosage range must be calculated according to the specifications of the pump.

The frequency, strength, and duration of contractions as well as the foetal heart rate must be carefully monitored throughout the infusion. Once an adequate level of uterine activity is attained, aiming for 3 to 4 contractions every 10 minutes, the infusion rate can often be reduced. In the event of uterine hyperactivity and/or foetal distress, the infusion must be discontinued immediately.

If, in women who are at term or near term, regular contractions are not established after the infusion of a total amount of 5 IU, it is recommended that the attempt to induce labour be ceased; it may be repeated on the following day, starting again from a rate of 1 to 4mU/min (see Section 4.3 "Contra-indications").

Caesarean section: 5 IU by slow iv injection immediately after delivery.

Prevention of postpartum uterine haemorrhage: The usual dose is 5 IU slowly iv after delivery of the placenta. In women given Syntocinon for induction or enhancement of labour, the infusion should be continued at an increased rate during the third stage of labour and for the next few hours thereafter.

Treatment of postpartum uterine haemorrhage: 5 IU slowly iv, followed in severe cases by iv infusion of a solution containing 5 to

20 IU of oxytocin in 500ml of a non-hydrating diluent, run at the rate necessary to control uterine atony.

Incomplete, inevitable, or missed abortion: 5 IU slowly iv, if necessary followed by iv infusion at a rate of 20 to 40mU/min or higher.

Children: Not applicable.

Elderly: Not applicable.

Route of administration: Intravenous infusion or intravenous injection.

4.3 Contraindications
Hypersensitivity to the drug. Hypertonic uterine contractions, mechanical obstruction to delivery, foetal distress. Any condition in which, for foetal or maternal reasons, spontaneous labour is inadvisable and/or vaginal delivery is contra-indicated: e.g., significant cephalopelvic disproportion; foetal malpresentation; placenta praevia and vasa praevia; placental abruption; cord presentation or prolapse; overdistension or impaired resistance of the uterus to rupture as in multiple pregnancy; polyhydramnios; grand multiparity and in the presence of a uterine scar resulting from major surgery including classical caesarean section.

Syntocinon should not be used for prolonged periods in patients with oxytocin-resistant uterine inertia, severe pre-eclamptic toxaemia or severe cardiovascular disorders.

4.4 Special warnings and special precautions for use
The induction of labour by means of oxytocin should be attempted only when strictly indicated for medical reasons. Administration should only be under hospital conditions and qualified medical supervision. When given for induction and enhancement of labour, Syntocinon must only be administered as an iv infusion and never by iv bolus injection. Careful monitoring of foetal heart rate and uterine motility (frequency, strength, and duration of contractions) is essential, so that the dosage may be adjusted to individual response.

When Syntocinon is given for induction or enhancement of labour, particular caution is required in the presence of borderline cephalopelvic disproportion, secondary uterine inertia, mild or moderate degrees of pregnancy-induced hypertension or cardiac disease, and in patients above 35 years of age or with a history of lower-uterine-segment caesarean section.

In the case of foetal death *in utero*, and/or in the presence of meconium-stained amniotic fluid, tumultous labour must be avoided, as it may cause amniotic fluid embolism.

Because oxytocin possesses slight antidiuretic activity, its prolonged iv administration at high doses in conjunction with large volumes of fluid, as may be the case in the treatment of inevitable or missed abortion or in the management of postpartum haemorrhage, may cause water intoxication associated with hyponatraemia. To avoid this rare complication, the following precautions must be observed whenever high doses of oxytocin are administered over a long time: an electrolyte-containing diluent must be used (not dextrose); the volume of infused fluid should be kept low (by infusing oxytocin at a higher concentration than recommended for the induction or enhancement of labour at term); fluid intake by mouth must be restricted; a fluid balance chart should be kept, and serum electrolytes should be measured when electrolyte imbalance is suspected.

When Syntocinon is used for prevention or treatment of uterine haemorrhage, rapid iv injection should be avoided, as it may cause an acute short-lasting drop in blood pressure.

4.5 Interaction with other medicinal products and other forms of Interaction
Since it has been found that prostaglandins potentiate the effect of oxytocin, it is not recommended that these drugs are used together. If used in sequence, the patient's uterine activity should be carefully monitored.

Some inhalation anaesthetics, e.g., cyclopropane or halothane, may enhance the hypotensive effect of oxytocin and reduce its oxytocic action. Their concurrent use with oxytocin has also been reported to cause cardiac rhythm disturbances.

When given during or after caudal block anaesthesia, oxytocin may potentiate the pressor effect of sympathomimetic vasoconstrictor agents.

4.6 Pregnancy and lactation
See Section 4.1 "Therapeutic indications".

4.7 Effects on ability to drive and use machines
None known.

4.8 Undesirable effects
As there is a wide variation in uterine sensitivity, uterine spasm may be caused in some instances by what are normally considered to be low doses. When oxytocin is used by iv infusion for the induction or enhancement of labour, administration at too high doses results in uterine overstimulation which may cause foetal distress, asphyxia, and death, or may lead to hypertonicity, tetanic contractions, soft tissue damage or rupture of the uterus.

Water intoxication associated with maternal and neonatal hyponatraemia has been reported in cases where high doses of oxytocin together with large amounts of electrolyte-free fluid have been administered over a prolonged period of time (see Section 4.4 "Special warnings and precautions for use"). Symptoms of water intoxication include:

1. Headache, anorexia, nausea, vomiting and abdominal pain.

2. Lethargy, drowsiness, unconsciousness and grand-mal type seizures.

3. Low blood electrolyte concentration.

Rapid iv bolus injection of oxytocin at doses amounting to several IU may result in acute short-lasting hypotension accompanied with flushing and reflex tachycardia.

Oxytocin may occasionally cause nausea, vomiting, haemorrhageor cardiac arrhythmias. In a few cases, skin rashes and anaphylactoid reactions associated with dyspnoea, hypotension, or shock have been reported.

4.9 Overdose
The fatal dose of Syntocinon has not been established. Syntocinon is subject to inactivation by proteolytic enzymes of the alimentary tract. Hence it is not absorbed from the intestine and is not likely to have toxic effects when ingested.

The symptoms and consequences of overdosage are those mentioned under Section 4.8 "Undesirable effects". In addition, as a result of uterine overstimulation, placental abruption and/or amniotic fluid embolism have been reported.

Treatment: When signs or symptoms of overdosage occur during continuous iv administration of Syntocinon, the infusion must be discontinued at once and oxygen should be given to the mother. In cases of water intoxication it is essential to restrict fluid intake, promote diuresis, correct electrolyte imbalance, and control convulsions that may eventually occur, by judicious use of diazepam. In the case of coma, a free airway should be maintained with routine measures normally employed in the nursing of the unconscious patient.

5. PHARMACOLOGICAL PROPERTIES
5.1 Pharmacodynamic properties
The active principle of Syntocinon is a synthetic nonapeptide identical with oxytocin, a hormone released by the posterior lobe of the pituitary. It exerts a stimulatory effect on the smooth musculature of the uterus, particularly towards the end of pregnancy, during labour, after delivery, and in the puerperium, i.e., at times when the number of specific oxytocin receptors in the myometrium is increased.

When given by low-dose iv infusion, Syntocinon elicits rhythmic uterine contractions that are indistinguishable in frequency, force, and duration from those observed during spontaneous labour. At higher infusion dosages, or when given by single injection, the drug is capable of causing sustained uterine contractions.

Being synthetic, Syntocinon does not contain vasopressin, but even in its pure form oxytocin possesses some weak intrinsic vasopressin-like antidiuretic activity.

Another pharmacological effect observed with high doses of oxytocin, particularly when administered by rapid iv bolus injection, consists of a transient direct relaxing effect on vascular smooth muscle, resulting in brief hypotension, flushing and reflex tachycardia.

5.2 Pharmacokinetic properties
The plasma half-life of oxytocin is of the order of five minutes, hence the need for continuous iv infusion. Elimination is via the liver, kidney, functional mammary gland and oxytocinase.

5.3 Preclinical safety data
There are no pre-clinical data of relevance to the prescriber which are additional to those already included in other sections of the Summary of Product Characteristics.

6. PHARMACEUTICAL PARTICULARS

6.1 List of excipients
Sodium acetate tri-hydrate, acetic acid, chlorobutanol, ethanol and water for injections.

6.2 Incompatibilities
Syntocinon should not be infused via the same apparatus as blood or plasma, because the peptide linkages are rapidly inactivated by oxytocin-inactivating enzymes. Syntocinon is incompatible with solutions containing sodium metabisulphite as a stabiliser.

6.3 Shelf life
Five years

6.4 Special precautions for storage
Store between 2°C and 8°C. May be stored up to 30°C for 3 months, but must then be discarded.

6.5 Nature and contents of container
Clear glass 1ml ampoules. Boxes of 5 ampoules.

6.6 Instructions for use and handling
Snap ampoules: no file required.

Syntocinon is compatible with the following infusion fluids, but due attention should be paid to the advisability of using electrolyte fluids in individual patients: sodium/potassium chloride (103mmol Na^+ and 51mmol K^+), sodium bicarbonate 1.39%, sodium chloride 0.9%, sodium lactate 1.72%, dextrose 5%, laevulose 20%, macrodex 6%, rheomacrodex 10%, Ringer's solution.

Administrative Data

7. MARKETING AUTHORISATION HOLDER
Alliance Pharmaceuticals Ltd
Avonbridge House
Bath Road
Chippenham
Wiltshire
SN15 2BB

8. MARKETING AUTHORISATION NUMBER(S)
PL 16853/0020

9. DATE OF FIRST AUTHORISATION/RENEWAL OF THE AUTHORISATION
25 June 1998

10. DATE OF REVISION OF THE TEXT
December 2004

11. LEGAL STATUS
POM

Alliance, Alliance Pharmaceuticals and associated devices are registered Trademarks of Alliance Pharmaceuticals Ltd.

Syntocinon Ampoules 5 IU/ml

(Alliance Pharmaceuticals)

1. NAME OF THE MEDICINAL PRODUCT
Syntocinon® Ampoules 5 IU/ml

2. QUALITATIVE AND QUANTITATIVE COMPOSITION
Oxytocin PhEur 5 units in 1ml.

3. PHARMACEUTICAL FORM
A clear, colourless, sterile solution in 1ml clear glass ampoules.

4. CLINICAL PARTICULARS

4.1 Therapeutic indications
Induction of labour for medical reasons; stimulation of labour in hypotonic uterine inertia; during caesarean section, following delivery of the child; prevention and treatment of postpartum uterine atony and haemorrhage.

Early stages of pregnancy as a adjunctive therapy for the management of incomplete, inevitable, or missed abortion.

4.2 Posology and method of administration
Induction or enhancement of labour: Oxytocin should not be started for 6 hours following administration of vaginal prostaglandins. Syntocinon should be administered as an iv drip infusion or, preferably, by means of a variable-speed infusion pump. For drip infusion it is recommended that 5 IU of Syntocinon be added to 500ml of a physiological electrolyte solution. For patients in whom infusion of sodium chloride must be avoided, 5% dextrose solution may be used as the diluent (see Section 4.4 "Special warnings and precautions for use"). To ensure even mixing, the bottle or bag must be turned upside down several times before use.

The initial infusion rate should be set at 1 to 4mU/min (2 to 8 drops/min). It may be gradually increased at intervals not shorter than 20 min, until a contraction pattern similar to that of normal labour is established. In pregnancy near term this can often be achieved with an infusion of less than 10mU/min (20 drops/min), and the recommended maximum rate is 20mU/min (40 drops/min). In the unusual event that higher rates are required, as may occur in the management of foetal death *in utero* or for induction of labour at an earlier stage of pregnancy, when the uterus is less sensitive to oxytocin, it is advisable to use a more concentrated Syntocinon solution, e.g., 10 IU in 500ml.

When using a motor-driven infusion pump which delivers smaller volumes than those given by drip infusion, the concentration suitable for infusion within the recommended dosage range must be calculated according to the specifications of the pump.

The frequency, strength, and duration of contractions as well as the foetal heart rate must be carefully monitored throughout the infusion. Once an adequate level of uterine activity is attained, aiming for 3 to 4 contractions every 10 minutes, the infusion rate can often be reduced. In the event of uterine hyperactivity and/or foetal distress, the infusion must be discontinued immediately.

If, in women who are at term or near term, regular contractions are not established after the infusion of a total amount of 5 IU, it is recommended that the attempt to induce labour be ceased; it may be repeated on the following day, starting again from a rate of 1 to 4mU/min (see Section 4.3 "Contra-indications").

Caesarean section: 5 IU by slow iv injection immediately after delivery.

Prevention of postpartum uterine haemorrhage: The usual dose is 5 IU slowly iv after delivery of the placenta. In women given Syntocinon for induction or enhancement of labour, the infusion should be continued at an increased rate during the third stage of labour and for the next few hours thereafter.

Treatment of postpartum uterine haemorrhage: 5 IU slowly iv, followed in severe cases by iv infusion of a solution containing 5 to 20 IU of oxytocin in 500ml of a non-hydrating diluent, run at the rate necessary to control uterine atony.

Incomplete, inevitable, or missed abortion: 5 IU slowly iv, if necessary followed by iv infusion at a rate of 20 to 40mU/min or higher.

Children: Not applicable.

Elderly: Not applicable.

Route of administration: Intravenous infusion or intravenous injection.

4.3 Contraindications
Hypersensitivity to the drug. Hypertonic uterine contractions, mechanical obstruction to delivery, foetal distress. Any condition in which, for foetal or maternal reasons, spontaneous labour is inadvisable and/or vaginal delivery is contra-indicated: e.g., significant cephalopelvic disproportion; foetal malpresentation; placenta praevia and vasa praevia; placental abruption; cord presentation or prolapse; overdistension or impaired resistance of the uterus to rupture as in multiple pregnancy; polyhydramnios; grand multiparity and in the presence of a uterine scar resulting from major surgery including classical caesarean section.

Syntocinon should not be used for prolonged periods in patients with oxytocin-resistant uterine inertia, severe pre-eclamptic toxaemia or severe cardiovascular disorders.

4.4 Special warnings and special precautions for use
The induction of labour by means of oxytocin should be attempted only when strictly indicated for medical reasons. Administration should only be under hospital conditions and qualified medical supervision. When given for induction and enhancement of labour, Syntocinon must only be administered as an iv infusion and never by iv bolus injection. Careful monitoring of foetal heart rate and uterine motility (frequency, strength, and duration of contractions) is essential, so that the dosage may be adjusted to individual response.

When Syntocinon is given for induction or enhancement of labour, particular caution is required in the presence of borderline cephalopelvic disproportion, secondary uterine inertia, mild or moderate degrees of pregnancy-induced hypertension or cardiac disease, and in patients above 35 years of age or with a history of lower-uterine-segment caesarean section.

In the case of foetal death *in utero*, and/or in the presence of meconium-stained amniotic fluid, tumultous labour must be avoided, as it may cause amniotic fluid embolism.

Because oxytocin possesses slight antidiuretic activity, its prolonged iv administration at high doses in conjunction with large volumes of fluid, as may be the case in the treatment of inevitable or missed abortion or in the management of postpartum haemorrhage, may cause water intoxication associated with hyponatraemia. To avoid this rare complication, the following precautions must be observed whenever high doses of oxytocin are administered over a long time: an electrolyte-containing diluent must be used (not dextrose); the volume of infused fluid should be kept low (by infusing oxytocin at a higher concentration than recommended for the induction or enhancement of labour at term); fluid intake by mouth must be restricted; a fluid balance chart should be kept, and serum electrolytes should be measured when electrolyte imbalance is suspected.

When Syntocinon is used for prevention or treatment of uterine haemorrhage, rapid iv injection should be avoided, as it may cause an acute short-lasting drop in blood pressure.

4.5 Interaction with other medicinal products and other forms of Interaction
Since it has been found that prostaglandins potentiate the effect of oxytocin, it is not recommended that these drugs are used together. If used in sequence, the patient's uterine activity should be carefully monitored.

Some inhalation anaesthetics, e.g., cyclopropane or halothane, may enhance the hypotensive effect of oxytocin and reduce its oxytocic action. Their concurrent use with oxytocin has also been reported to cause cardiac rhythm disturbances.

When given during or after caudal block anaesthesia, oxytocin may potentiate the pressor effect of sympathomimetic vasoconstrictor agents.

4.6 Pregnancy and lactation
See Section 4.1 "Therapeutic indications".

4.7 Effects on ability to drive and use machines
None known.

4.8 Undesirable effects
As there is a wide variation in uterine sensitivity, uterine spasm may be caused in some instances by what are normally considered to be low doses. When oxytocin is used by iv infusion for the induction or enhancement of labour, administration at too high doses results in uterine overstimulation which may cause foetal distress, asphyxia, and death, or may lead to hypertonicity, tetanic contractions, soft tissue damage or rupture of the uterus.

Water intoxication associated with maternal and neonatal hyponatraemia has been reported in cases where high doses of oxytocin together with large amounts of electrolyte-free fluid have been administered over a prolonged period of time (see Section 4.4 "Special warnings and precautions for use"). Symptoms of water intoxication include:

1. Headache, anorexia, nausea, vomiting and abdominal pain.

2. Lethargy, drowsiness, unconsciousness and grand-mal type seizures.

3. Low blood electrolyte concentration.

Rapid iv bolus injection of oxytocin at doses amounting to several IU may result in acute short-lasting hypotension accompanied with flushing and reflex tachycardia.

Oxytocin may occasionally cause nausea, vomiting, haemorrhage or cardiac arrhythmias. In a few cases, skin rashes and anaphylactoid reactions associated with dyspnoea, hypotension, or shock have been reported.

4.9 Overdose
The fatal dose of Syntocinon has not been established. Syntocinon is subject to inactivation by proteolytic enzymes of the alimentary tract. Hence it is not absorbed from the intestine and is not likely to have toxic effects when ingested.

The symptoms and consequences of overdosage are those mentioned under Section 4.8 "Undesirable effects". In addition, as a result of uterine overstimulation, placental abruption and/or amniotic fluid embolism have been reported.

Treatment: When signs or symptoms of overdosage occur during continuous iv administration of Syntocinon, the infusion must be discontinued at once and oxygen should be given to the mother. In cases of water intoxication it is essential to restrict fluid intake, promote diuresis, correct electrolyte imbalance, and control convulsions that may eventually occur, by judicious use of diazepam. In the case of coma, a free airway should be maintained with routine measures normally employed in the nursing of the unconscious patient.

5. PHARMACOLOGICAL PROPERTIES

5.1 Pharmacodynamic properties
The active principle of Syntocinon is a synthetic nonapeptide identical with oxytocin, a hormone released by the posterior lobe of the pituitary. It exerts a stimulatory effect on the smooth musculature of the uterus, particularly towards the end of pregnancy, during labour, after delivery, and in the puerperium, i.e., at times when the number of specific oxytocin receptors in the myometrium is increased.

When given by low-dose iv infusion, Syntocinon elicits rhythmic uterine contractions that are indistinguishable in frequency, force, and duration from those observed during spontaneous labour. At higher infusion dosages, or when given by single injection, the drug is capable of causing sustained uterine contractions.

Being synthetic, Syntocinon does not contain vasopressin, but even in its pure form oxytocin possesses some weak intrinsic vasopressin-like antidiuretic activity.

Another pharmacological effect observed with high doses of oxytocin, particularly when administered by rapid iv bolus injection, consists of a transient direct relaxing effect on vascular smooth muscle, resulting in brief hypotension, flushing and reflex tachycardia.

5.2 Pharmacokinetic properties

The plasma half-life of oxytocin is of the order of five minutes, hence the need for continuous iv infusion. Elimination is via the liver, kidney, functional mammary gland and oxytocinase.

5.3 Preclinical safety data

There are no pre-clinical data of relevance to the prescriber which are additional to those already included in other sections of the Summary of Product Characteristics.

6. PHARMACEUTICAL PARTICULARS

6.1 List of excipients

Sodium acetate tri-hydrate, acetic acid, chlorobutanol, ethanol and water for injections.

6.2 Incompatibilities

Syntocinon should not be infused via the same apparatus as blood or plasma, because the peptide linkages are rapidly inactivated by oxytocin-inactivating enzymes. Syntocinon is incompatible with solutions containing sodium metabisulphite as a stabiliser.

6.3 Shelf life

Five years

6.4 Special precautions for storage

Store between 2°C and 8°C. May be stored up to 30°C for 3 months, but must then be discarded.

6.5 Nature and contents of container

Clear glass 1ml ampoules. Boxes of 5 ampoules.

6.6 Instructions for use and handling

Snap ampoules: no file required.

Syntocinon is compatible with the following infusion fluids, but due attention should be paid to the advisability of using electrolyte fluids in individual patients: sodium/potassium chloride (103mmol Na^+ and 51mmol K^+), sodium bicarbonate 1.39%, sodium chloride 0.9%, sodium lactate 1.72%, dextrose 5%, laevulose 20%, macrodex 6%, rheomacrodex 10%, Ringer's solution.

Administrative Data

7. MARKETING AUTHORISATION HOLDER

Alliance Pharmaceuticals Ltd

Avonbridge House

Bath Road

Chippenham

Wiltshire

SN15 2BB

8. MARKETING AUTHORISATION NUMBER(S)

PL 16853/0019

9. DATE OF FIRST AUTHORISATION/RENEWAL OF THE AUTHORISATION

25 June 1998

10. DATE OF REVISION OF THE TEXT

March 2005

11. LEGAL STATUS

POM

Alliance, Alliance Pharmaceuticals and associated devices are registered Trademarks of Alliance Pharmaceuticals Ltd.

Syntometrine Ampoules

(Alliance Pharmaceuticals)

1. NAME OF THE MEDICINAL PRODUCT

Syntometrine® Ampoules

2. QUALITATIVE AND QUANTITATIVE COMPOSITION

Each 1ml ampoule contains 5IU oxytocin PhEur and 0.5mg ergometrine maleate PhEur.

3. PHARMACEUTICAL FORM

A clear colourless sterile liquid in a 1ml clear colourless glass ampoule.

4. CLINICAL PARTICULARS

4.1 Therapeutic indications

The active management of the third stage of labour, or routinely, following the birth of the placenta, to prevent or treat postpartum haemorrhage.

4.2 Posology and method of administration

Syntometrine is usually administered by intramuscular injection.

Adults:

Active management of third stage of labour: Intramuscular injection of 1ml after delivery of the anterior shoulder, or at the latest, immediately after delivery of the child. Expulsion of the placenta, which is normally separated by the first strong uterine contraction, should be assisted by gentle suprapubic pressure and controlled cord traction.

Prevention and treatment of postpartum haemorrhage: Intramuscular injection of 1ml following expulsion of the placenta, or when bleeding occurs.

Third stage of labour and postpartum haemorrhage: Syntometrine may also be administered by a slow intravenous injection in a dose of 0.5 to 1ml. This route of administration is not generally recommended.

Children: Not applicable.

Elderly: Not applicable.

4.3 Contraindications

Hypersensitivity to any of the components.

Pregnancy, first stage of labour, primary or secondary uterine inertia. Second stage of labour before crowning of the head.

Severe disorders of cardiac, liver or kidney functions; occlusive vascular disease, sepsis, severe hypertension, pre-eclampsia, eclampsia.

4.4 Special warnings and special precautions for use

When the intravenous route is employed, care should be exercised in patients of doubtful cardiac status.

In breech presentations and other abnormal presentations, Syntometrine should not be given until after delivery of the child, and in multiple births not until the last child has been delivered. In postpartum haemorrhage, if bleeding is not arrested by the injection of Syntometrine, the possibility of retained placental fragments, of soft tissue injury (cervical or vaginal laceration), or of a clotting defect, should be excluded before a further injection is given. Caution should be exercised in the presence of mild or moderate hypertension, or with mild or moderate degrees of cardiac, liver or kidney disease.

4.5 Interaction with other medicinal products and other forms of Interaction

Halothane anaesthesia may diminish the uterotonic effect of Syntometrine. Syntometrine may enhance the effects of vasoconstrictors and of prostaglandins.

4.6 Pregnancy and lactation

See Section 4.1 ''Therapeutic Indications''.

4.7 Effects on ability to drive and use machines

None known.

4.8 Undesirable effects

Nausea, vomiting, abdominal pain, headache, dizziness and skin rashes. On rare occasions hypertension, bradycardia, cardiac arrhythmias, chest pain or anaphylactoid reactions associated with dyspnoea, hypotension, collapse or shock.

4.9 Overdose

No case of maternal intoxication with Syntometrine has been reported to the company. If such a case were to occur the most likely symptoms would be those of ergometrine intoxication: nausea, vomiting, hypertension or hypotension, vasospastic reactions, respiratory depression, convulsions, coma. Treatment would have to be symptomatic.

Accidental administration to the newborn infant has been reported and has proved fatal. In these accidental neonatal overdosage cases, symptoms such as respiratory depression, convulsions and hypertonia, heart arrhythmia have been reported. Treatment has been symptomatic in most cases; respiratory and cardiovascular support have been required.

5. PHARMACOLOGICAL PROPERTIES

5.1 Pharmacodynamic properties

Syntometrine combines the known sustained oxytocic action of ergometrine with the more rapid action of oxytocin on the uterus.

5.2 Pharmacokinetic properties

Ergometrine is reported to be rapidly and completely absorbed after an intramuscular injection. Uterine stimulation occurs within 7 minutes of im injection and immediately after iv injection. Oxytocin is also rapidly absorbed and is rapidly metabolised by the liver and the kidneys.

5.3 Preclinical safety data

There are no pre-clinical data of relevance to the prescriber which are additional to those already included in other sections of the Summary of Product Characteristics.

6. PHARMACEUTICAL PARTICULARS

6.1 List of excipients

Sodium chloride, maleic acid, water for injections.

6.2 Incompatibilities

None.

6.3 Shelf life

3 years.

6.4 Special precautions for storage

For prolonged periods store between 2° and 8°C. Protect from light. Syntometrine may be stored up to 25°C for 2 months when protected from light, but must then be discarded.

6.5 Nature and contents of container

Uncoloured borosilicate glass Type I snap ampoule. Packs of 5 ampoules.

6.6 Instructions for use and handling

None

Administrative Data

7. MARKETING AUTHORISATION HOLDER

Alliance Pharmaceuticals Ltd

Avonbridge House

Bath Road

Chippenham

Wiltshire

SN15 2BB

8. MARKETING AUTHORISATION NUMBER(S)

PL16853/0021

9. DATE OF FIRST AUTHORISATION/RENEWAL OF THE AUTHORISATION

25 June 1998

10. DATE OF REVISION OF THE TEXT

January 1999

11. Legal Status

POM

Alliance, Alliance Pharmaceuticals and associated devices are registered Trademarks of Alliance Pharmaceuticals Ltd.

Syprol Oral Solution 10mg/5ml

(Rosemont Pharmaceuticals Limited)

1. NAME OF THE MEDICINAL PRODUCT

Propranolol Hydrochloride 10mg/5ml Oral Solution

Syprol 10mg/5ml

2. QUALITATIVE AND QUANTITATIVE COMPOSITION

Propranolol Hydrochloride 10mg/5ml

3. PHARMACEUTICAL FORM

Oral Solution

A clear colourless liquid with odour of orange/tangerine.

4. CLINICAL PARTICULARS

4.1 Therapeutic indications

Propranolol is indicated in:

- the control of hypertension
- the management of angina pectoris
- the long term prophylaxis against reinfarction after recovery from acute myocardial infarction
- the control of most forms of cardiac arrhythmia
- the prophylaxis of migraine
- the management of essential tremor
- relief of situational anxiety and generalised anxiety symptoms, particularly those of the somatic type
- prophylaxis of upper gastro-intestinal bleeding in patients with portal hypertension and oesophageal varices
- the adjunctive management of thyrotoxicosis and thyrotoxic crisis
- management of hypertrophic obstructive cardiomyopathy
- management of phaeochromocytoma perioperatively (with an alpha-adrenoceptor blocking drug).

4.2 Posology and method of administration

For oral administration only.

Adults:

Hypertension – A starting dose of 80mg twice a day may be increased at weekly intervals according to response. The usual dose range is 160 – 320mg per day. With concurrent diuretic or other antihypertensive drugs a further reduction of blood pressure is obtained.

Angina, migraine and essential tremor – A starting dose of 40mg two or three times daily may be increased by the same amount at weekly intervals according to patient response. An adequate response in migraine and essential tremor is usually seen in the range 80-160mg/day and in angina in the range 120-240mg/day.

Situational and generalised anxiety – A dose of 40mg daily may provide short term relief of acute situational anxiety. Generalised anxiety, requiring longer term therapy, usually responds adequately to 40mg twice daily which, in individual cases, may be increased to 40mg three times daily. Treatment should be continued according to response. Patients should be reviewed after six to twelve months treatment.

Arrhythmias, anxiety, tachycardia, hypertrophic obstructive cardiomyopathy and thyrotoxicosis – A dosage range of 10-40mg three or four times a day usually achieves the required response.

Post myocardial infarction - Treatment should start between days 5 and 21 after myocardial infarction with an initial dose of 40mg four times a day for 2 or 3 days. In order to improve compliance the total daily dosage may thereafter be given as 80mg twice daily.

Portal hypertension:

Dosage should be titrated to achieve approximately 25% reduction in resting heart rate. Dosage should begin with 40mg twice daily, increasing to 80mg twice daily depending on heart rate response. If necessary, the dose may be increased incrementally to a maximum of 160mg twice daily.

Phaeochromocytoma (Used only with an alpha-receptor blocking drug)

Pre-operative: 60mg daily for three days is recommended.

Non-operable malignant cases: 30mg daily.

Children

Arrhythmias, phaeochromocytoma, thyrotoxicosis – Dosage should be individually determined and the following is only a guide: 250 – 500 micrograms per Kilogram three or four times daily as required.

Migraine –

Under the age of 12: 20mg two or three times daily.

Over the age of 12: the adult dose.

Fallot's tetralogy – The value of propranolol in this condition is confined mainly to the relief of right-ventricular outflow tract shut-down. It is also useful for treatment of associated arrhythmias and angina. Dosage should be individually determined and the following is only a guide: Up to 1mg/Kg repeated three or four times a day as required.

Elderly

With regard to the elderly the optimum dose should be individually determined according to the clinical response.

4.3 Contraindications

Propranolol must not be used if there is a history of bronchial asthma or bronchospasm.

The product label states the following warning: "Do not take propranolol if you have a history of asthma or wheezing". A similar warning appears in the patient information leaflet.

Bronchospasm can usually be reversed by beta$_2$-agonist bronchodilators such as salbutamol. Large doses of the beta$_2$-agonist bronchodilator may be required to overcome the beta-blockade produced by propranolol and the dose should be titrated according to the clinical response; both intravenous and inhalational administration should be considered. The use of intravenous aminophylline and/or the use of ipratropium (given by nebuliser) may also be considered. Glucagon (1 to 2mg given intravenously) has also been reported to produce a bronchodilator effect in asthmatic patients. Oxygen or artificial ventilation may be required in severe cases.

Propranolol as with other beta-adrenoceptor blocking drugs must not be used in patients with any of the following:

hypersensitivity to propranolol hydrochloride or any of the ingredients; the presence of second or third degree heart block; in cardiogenic shock; metabolic acidosis; after prolonged fasting; bradycardia; hypotension; severe peripheral arterial circulatory disturbances; sick sinus syndrome; untreated phaeochromocytoma; uncontrolled heart failure or Prinzmetal's angina.

4.4 Special warnings and special precautions for use

Although contra-indicated in uncontrolled heart failure, propranolol may be used where the signs of heart failure have been controlled by the use of appropriate concomitant medication. Propranolol should be used with caution in patients whose cardiac reserve is poor.

Treatment should not be discontinued abruptly in patients with ischaemic heart disease. Either the equivalent dose of another beta-adrenoceptor blocking drug may be substituted or the withdrawal of propranolol should be gradual.

Propranolol may modify the tachycardia of hypoglycaemia (see interactions).

Although contra-indicated in severe peripheral arterial circulatory disturbances, propranolol may also aggravate less severe peripheral arterial circulatory disturbances.

One of the pharmacological actions of propranolol is to reduce the heart rate. Therefore the dosage should be reduced in those rare cases where symptoms are attributable to a slow heart rate.

Due to propranolol having a negative effect on conduction time, caution must be exercised if it is given to patients with first degree heart block.

Since the half life may be increased in patients with significant hepatic or renal impairment, caution must be exercised when starting treatment and selecting the initial dose.

In patients with portal hypertension, liver function may deteriorate and hepatic encephalopathy may develop. There have been reports suggesting that treatment with propranolol may increase the risk of developing hepatic encephalopathy.

Propranolol may cause a more severe reaction to a variety of allergens, when given to patients with a history of anaphylactic reaction to such allergens. Such patients may be unresponsive to the usual doses of adrenaline used to treat the allergic reactions.

Propranolol may mask the signs of thyrotoxicosis.

Propranolol must be used with caution in patients with decompensated cirrhosis.

Laboratory Tests: Propranolol has been reported to interfere with the estimation of serum bilirubin by the diazo method and with the determination of catecholamines by methods using fluorescence.

4.5 Interaction with other medicinal products and other forms of Interaction

Hypoglycaemic agents: Tachycardia associated with hypoglycaemia may be modified by propranolol. Use of propranolol alongside hypoglycaemic therapy in diabetic patients should be with caution since it may prolong the hypoglycaemic response to insulin.

Clonidine: Caution should be exercised when transferring patients from clonidine to beta-adrenoceptor blocking drugs. If propranolol and clonidine are given concurrently, clonidine should not be discontinued until several days after the withdrawal of the beta blocker. If replacing clonidine by beta-adrenoceptor blocking drug therapy, the introduction of the beta-adrenoceptor blocking drugs should be delayed for several days after clonidine administration has stopped.

Anti-arrhythmics: Care should be taken when prescribing a beta-adrenergic blocking drug with Class 1 anti-arrhythmic agents such as disopyramide.

Verapamil, Diltiazem: In patients with impaired ventricular function who are also taking verapamil or diltiazem, beta-blockers should be used with caution. The combination should not be given to patients with conduction abnormalities. Neither drug should be administered intravenously within 48 hours of discontinuing the other.

Anaesthesia: Caution must be exercised when using anaesthetic agents with propranolol. The anaesthetist should be informed and the choice of anaesthetic should be the agent with as little negative inotropic activity as possible. Use of beta-adrenoceptor blocking drugs with anaesthetic drugs may result in attenuation of the reflex tachycardia and increase the risk of hypotension. Anaesthetic agents causing myocardial depression are best avoided.

Sympathomimetic Agents and Parenteral Adrenaline: Concomitant use of sympathomimetic agents e.g. adrenaline, may counteract the effect of beta-adrenoceptor blocking drugs. Caution should be taken in the parenteral administration of preparations containing adrenaline to people taking beta-adrenoceptor blocking drugs as, in rare cases, vasoconstriction, hypertension and bradycardia may result.

Dihydropyridines: Concomitant therapy with dihydropyridines e.g. nifedipine, may increase the risk of hypotension, and cardiac failure may occur in patients with latent cardiac insufficiency.

Digitalis Glycosides: These preparations in association with beta-adrenoceptor blocking drugs, may increase atrio-ventricular conduction time.

Lignocaine: Administration of propranolol during infusion of lignocaine may increase the plasma concentration of lignocaine by approximately 30%. Patients already receiving propranolol tend to have higher lignocaine levels than controls. The combination should be avoided.

Ergotamine: Caution should be exercised if ergotamine, dihydroergotamine or related compounds are given in combination with propranolol since vasospastic reactions have been reported in a few patients.

Prostaglandin Synthetase Inhibiting Drugs: Concomitant use of these e.g. ibuprofen or indomethacin, may decrease the hypotensive effects of propranolol.

Chlorpromazine: Concomitant administration with propranolol may result in an increase in plasma levels of both drugs. This may lead to an enhanced antipsychotic effect for chlorpromazine and an increased antihypertensive effect for propranolol.

Cimetidine, hydralazine, alcohol: Concomitant use of cimetidine and hydralazine will increase, whereas concomitant use of alcohol will decrease, the plasma level of propranolol.

Pharmacokinetic studies have shown that the following agents may interact with propranolol due to effects on enzyme systems in the liver which metabolise propranolol and these agents: quinidine, propafenone, rifampicin, theophylline, warfarin, thioridazine and dihydropyridine calcium channel blockers such as nifedipine, nisoldipine, nicardipine, isradipine and lacidipine. Owing to the fact that blood concentrations of either agent may be affected, dosage adjustments may be needed according to clinical judgement. (See also the interaction above concerning the concomitant therapy with dihydropyridine calcium channel blockers).

4.6 Pregnancy and lactation

As with all drugs, propranolol should not be given in pregnancy unless absolutely essential. There is no evidence of teratogenicity with propranolol. However, beta adrenoceptor blocking agents reduce placenta perfusion, which may result in intra-uterine foetal death, immature and premature deliveries. In addition, adverse effects (especially hypoglycaemia and bradycardia in the neonate and bradycardia in the foetus) may occur. There is an increased risk of cardiac and pulmonary complications in the neonate in the post-natal period.

Most beta-adrenoceptor blocking drugs particularly lipophilic compounds, will pass into breast milk although to a variable extent. Breast feeding is therefore not recommended following administration of these compounds.

4.7 Effects on ability to drive and use machines

Use is unlikely to result in any impairment of the ability of patients to drive or operate machinery. However, it should be taken into account that occasionally dizziness or fatigue may occur.

4.8 Undesirable effects

Propranolol is usually well tolerated, however, listed below are the side effects that may occur:-

Cardiovascular: Bradycardia, heart failure deterioration, postural hypotension which may be associated with syncope, heart block and congestive cardiac failure, exacerbation of claudication, cold extremities, Raynaud's phenomenon.

Respiratory: Bronchospasm (especially in patients with a history of asthma)

Neurological and CNS: Confusion, dizziness, mood changes, nightmares, psychoses and hallucinations, sleep disturbances, paraesthesia especially of the hands.

Haematological: Purpura, thrombocytopenia.

Endocrine: Hypoglycaemia in children.

Gastro-intestinal: Gastro-intestinal disturbance, nausea, diarrhoea.

Integumentary: Alopecia, dry eyes, psoriasiform skin reactions and exacerbation of psoriasis, skin rashes.

Senses: Visual disturbances.

Others: Muscle fatigue, lassitude, insomnia, an increase in ANA (antinuclear antibodies) although the clinical relevance of this has not been established.

If these effects occur, thought should be given to withdrawing the drug. However, it should be withdrawn gradually.

Bradycardia and hypotension are usually a sign of overdosage but may be rarely linked to intolerance. If this occurs the drug should be withdrawn and overdosage treatment initiated.

4.9 Overdose

The symptoms of overdosage may include bradycardia, hypotension, acute cardiac insufficiency and bronchospasm.

General treatment should include: close supervision, treatment in an intensive care ward, the use of gastric lavage, activated charcoal and a laxative to prevent absorption of any drug still present in the gastrointestinal tract, the use of plasma or plasma substitutes to treat hypotension and shock.

Excessive bradycardia can be countered with atropine 1-2mg intravenously and/or a cardiac pacemaker. If necessary, this may be followed by a bolus dose of glucagon 10mg intravenously. If required, this may be repeated or followed by an intravenous infusion of glucagon 1-10mg/hour depending on response. If no response to glucagon occurs or if glucagon is unavailable, a beta-adrenoceptor stimulant such as dobutamine 2.5 to 10 micrograms/Kg/minute by intravenous infusion may be given. Dobutamine, because of its positive inotropic effect could also be used to treat hypotension and acute cardiac insufficiency. It is likely that these doses would be inadequate to reverse the cardiac effects of beta-blockade if a large overdose has been taken. The dose of dobutamine should therefore be increased if necessary to achieve the required response according to the clinical condition of the patient.

5. PHARMACOLOGICAL PROPERTIES

5.1 Pharmacodynamic properties

Propranolol is a competitive antagonist at both beta$_1$ and beta$_2$-adrenoceptors.

It has no agonist activity at the beta-adrenoceptor, but has membrane stabilising activity at concentrations exceeding 1-3mg/litre, though such concentrations are rarely achieved during oral therapy. Competitive beta-adrenoceptor blockade has been demonstrated in man by a parallel shift to the right in the dose-heart rate response curve to beta-agonists such as isoprenaline.

Propranolol, as with other beta-adrenoceptor blocking drugs, has negative inotropic effects, and is therefore contra-indicated in uncontrolled heart failure.

Propranolol is a racemic mixture and the active form is the S(-) isomer. With the exception of inhibition of the conversion of thyroxine to triiodothyronine it is unlikely that any additional ancillary properties possessed by R(+) propranolol, in comparison with the racemic mixture will give rise to different therapeutic effects.

Propranolol is effective and well tolerated in most ethnic populations, although the response may be less in black patients.

5.2 Pharmacokinetic properties

Following intravenous administration, the plasma half-life of propranolol is about 2 hours and the ratio of metabolites to parent drug in the blood is lower than after oral administration. In particular, 4-hydroxypropranolol is not present after intravenous administration. Propranolol is completely absorbed after oral administration and peak plasma concentrations occur 1-2 hours after dosing in fasting patients. The liver removes up to 90% of an oral dose with an elimination half-life of 3 to 6 hours. Propranolol is widely and rapidly distributed throughout the body with highest levels occurring in the lungs, liver, kidney, brain and heart. Propranolol is highly protein bound (80-95%).

5.3 Preclinical safety data
Propranolol is a drug on which extensive clinical experience has been obtained. Relevant information for the prescriber is provided elsewhere in the Summary of Product Characteristics.

6. PHARMACEUTICAL PARTICULARS

6.1 List of excipients
Citric acid monohydrate, methyl parahydroxybenzoate (E218), propyl parahydroxybenzoate (E216), propylene glycol, liquid maltitol, orange/tangerine flavour (including ethanol (0.12%v/v) and butylhydroxyanisol E320) and purified water.

6.2 Incompatibilities
None known.

6.3 Shelf life
24 months unopened

3 months opened.

6.4 Special precautions for storage
Do not store above 25°C. Do not refrigerate or freeze.

6.5 Nature and contents of container
Amber (Type III) glass bottles.

Closures: -

a) Aluminium, EPE wadded, roll-on pilfer-proof screw cap.
b) HDPE, EPE wadded, tamper evident screw cap.

c) HDPE, EPE wadded, tamper evident, child resistant closure.

Pack Size: 150ml

6.6 Instructions for use and handling
Not applicable.

Administrative Data

7. MARKETING AUTHORISATION HOLDER
Rosemont Pharmaceuticals Ltd, Rosemont House, Yorkdale Industrial Park, Braithwaite Street, Leeds, LS11 9XE, UK.

8. MARKETING AUTHORISATION NUMBER(S)
PL 00427/0123

9. DATE OF FIRST AUTHORISATION/RENEWAL OF THE AUTHORISATION
11 December 2000

10. DATE OF REVISION OF THE TEXT

Syprol Oral Solution 50mg/5ml

(Rosemont Pharmaceuticals Limited)

1. NAME OF THE MEDICINAL PRODUCT
Propranolol Hydrochloride 50mg/5ml Oral Solution

Syprol 50mg/5ml

2. QUALITATIVE AND QUANTITATIVE COMPOSITION
Propranolol Hydrochloride 50mg/5ml

3. PHARMACEUTICAL FORM
Oral Solution

A clear bright orange liquid with odour of orange/tangerine.

4. CLINICAL PARTICULARS

4.1 Therapeutic indications
Propranolol is indicated in:

- the control of hypertension
- the management of angina pectoris
- the long term prophylaxis against reinfarction after recovery from acute myocardial infarction
- the control of most forms of cardiac arrhythmia
- the prophylaxis of migraine
- the management of essential tremor
- relief of situational anxiety and generalised anxiety symptoms, particularly those of the somatic type.
- prophylaxis of upper gastro-intestinal bleeding in patients with portal hypertension and oesophageal varices.
- the adjunctive management of thyrotoxicosis and thyrotoxic crisis
- management of hypertrophic obstructive cardiomyopathy
- management of phaeochromocytoma perioperatively (with an alpha-adrenoceptor blocking drug).

4.2 Posology and method of administration
For oral administration only.

Adults:

Hypertension – A starting dose of 80mg twice a day may be increased at weekly intervals according to response. The usual dose range is 160 – 320mg per day. With concurrent diuretic or other antihypertensive drugs a further reduction of blood pressure is obtained.

Angina, migraine and essential tremor – A starting dose of 40mg two or three times daily may be increased by the same amount at weekly intervals according to patient response. An adequate response in migraine and essential tremor is usually seen in the range 80-160mg/day and in angina in the range 120-240mg/day.

Situational and generalised anxiety – A dose of 40mg daily may provide short term relief of acute situational anxiety. Generalised anxiety, requiring longer term therapy, usually responds adequately to 40mg twice daily which, in individual cases, may be increased to 40mg three times daily. Treatment should be continued according to response. Patients should be reviewed after six to twelve months treatment.

Arrhythmias, anxiety, tachycardia, hypertrophic obstructive cardiomyopathy and thyrotoxicosis – A dosage range of 10-40mg three or four times a day usually achieves the required response.

Post myocardial infarction - Treatment should start between days 5 and 21 after myocardial infarction with an initial dose of 40mg four times a day for 2 or 3 days. In order to improve compliance the total daily dosage may thereafter be given as 80mg twice daily.

Portal hypertension:

Dosage should be titrated to achieve approximately 25% reduction in resting heart rate. Dosage should begin with 40mg twice daily, increasing to 80mg twice daily depending on heart rate response. If necessary, the dose may be increased incrementally to a maximum of 160mg twice daily.

Phaeochromocytoma (Used only with an alpha-receptor blocking drug)- Pre-operative: 60mg daily for three days is recommended.

Non-operable malignant cases: 30mg daily.

Children

Arrhythmias, phaeochromocytoma, thyrotoxicosis – Dosage should be individually determined and the following is only a guide: 250 – 500 micrograms per Kilogram three or four times daily as required.

Migraine –

Under the age of 12: 20mg two or three times daily

Over the age of 12: the adult dose

Fallot's tetralogy – The value of propranolol in this condition is confined mainly to the relief of right-ventricular outflow tract shut-down. It is also useful for treatment of associated arrhythmias and angina. Dosage should be individually determined and the following is only a guide: Up to 1mg/Kg repeated three or four times a day as required.

Elderly

With regard to the elderly the optimum dose should be individually determined according to the clinical response.

4.3 Contraindications
Propranolol must not be used if there is a history of bronchial asthma or bronchospasm.

The product label states the following warning: "Do not take propranolol if you have a history of asthma or wheezing". A similar warning appears in the patient information leaflet.

Bronchospasm can usually be reversed by $beta_2$-agonist bronchodilators such as salbutamol. Large doses of the $beta_2$-agonist bronchodilator may be required to overcome the beta-blockade produced by propranolol and the dose should be titrated according to the clinical response; both intravenous and inhalational administration should be considered. The use of intravenous aminophylline and/or the use of ipratropium (given by nebuliser) may also be considered. Glucagon (1 to 2mg given intravenously) has also been reported to produce a bronchodilator effect in asthmatic patients. Oxygen or artificial ventilation may be required in severe cases.

Propranolol as with other beta-adrenoceptor blocking drugs must not be used in patients with any of the following:

hypersensitivity to propranolol hydrochloride or any of the ingredients; the presence of second or third degree heart block; in cardiogenic shock; metabolic acidosis; after prolonged fasting; bradycardia; hypotension; severe peripheral arterial circulatory disturbances; sick sinus syndrome; untreated phaeochromocytoma; uncontrolled heart failure or Prinzmetal's angina.

4.4 Special warnings and special precautions for use
Although contra-indicated in uncontrolled heart failure, propranolol may be used where the signs of heart failure have been controlled by the use of appropriate concomitant medication. Propranolol should be used with caution in patients whose cardiac reserve is poor.

Treatment should not be discontinued abruptly in patients with ischaemic heart disease. Either the equivalent dose of another beta-adrenoceptor blocking drug may be substituted or the withdrawal of propranolol should be gradual.

Propranolol may modify the tachycardia of hypoglycaemia (see interactions).

Although contra-indicated in severe peripheral arterial circulatory disturbances, propranolol may also aggravate less severe peripheral arterial circulatory disturbances.

One of the pharmacological actions of propranolol is to reduce the heart rate. Therefore the dosage should be reduced in those rare cases where symptoms are attributable to a slow heart rate.

Due to propranolol having a negative effect on conduction time, caution must be exercised if it is given to patients with first degree heart block.

Since the half life may be increased in patients with significant hepatic or renal impairment, caution must be exercised when starting treatment and selecting the initial dose.

In patients with portal hypertension, liver function may deteriorate and hepatic encephalopathy may develop. There have been reports suggesting that treatment with propranolol may increase the risk of developing hepatic encephalopathy.

Propranolol may cause a more severe reaction to a variety of allergens, when given to patients with a history of anaphylactic reaction to such allergens. Such patients may be unresponsive to the usual doses of adrenaline used to treat the allergic reactions.

Propranolol may mask the signs of thyrotoxicosis.

Propranolol must be used with caution in patients with decompensated cirrhosis.

Laboratory Tests: Propranolol has been reported to interfere with the estimation of serum bilirubin by the diazo method and with the determination of catecholamines by methods using fluorescence.

4.5 Interaction with other medicinal products and other forms of Interaction
Hypoglycaemic agents: Tachycardia associated with hypoglycaemia may be modified by propranolol. Use of propranolol alongside hypoglycaemic therapy in diabetic patients should be with caution since it may prolong the hypoglycaemic response to insulin.

Clonidine: Caution should be exercised when transferring patients from clonidine to beta-adrenoceptor blocking drugs. If propranolol and clonidine are given concurrently, clonidine should not be discontinued until several days after the withdrawal of the beta blocker. If replacing clonidine by beta-adrenoceptor blocking drug therapy, the introduction of the beta-adrenoceptor blocking drugs should be delayed for several days after clonidine administration has stopped.

Anti-arrhythmics: Care should be taken when prescribing a beta-adrenergic blocking drug with Class 1 anti-arrhythmic agents such as disopyramide.

Verapamil, Diltiazem: In patients with impaired ventricular function who are also taking verapamil or diltiazem, beta-blockers should be used with caution. The combination should not be given to patients with conduction abnormalities. Neither drug should be administered intravenously within 48 hours of discontinuing the other.

Anaesthesia: Caution must be exercised when using anaesthetic agents with propranolol. The anaesthetist should be informed and the choice of anaesthetic should be the agent with as little negative inotropic activity as possible. Use of beta-adrenoceptor blocking drugs with anaesthetic drugs may result in attenuation of the reflex tachycardia and increase the risk of hypotension. Anaesthetic agents causing myocardial depression are best avoided.

Sympathomimetic Agents and Parenteral Adrenaline: Concomitant use of sympathomimetic agents e.g. adrenaline, may counteract the effect of beta-adrenoceptor blocking drugs. Caution should be taken in the parenteral administration of preparations containing adrenaline to people taking beta-adrenoceptor blocking drugs as, in rare cases, vasoconstriction, hypertension and bradycardia may result.

Dihydropyridines: Concomitant therapy with dihydropyridines e.g. nifedipine, may increase the risk of hypotension, and cardiac failure may occur in patients with latent cardiac insufficiency.

Digitalis Glycosides: These preparations in association with beta-adrenoceptor blocking drugs, may increase atrio-ventricular conduction time.

Lidocaine: Administration of propranolol during infusion of lidocaine may increase the plasma concentration of lidocaine by approximately 30%. Patients already receiving propranolol tend to have higher lidocaine levels than controls. The combination should be avoided.

Ergotamine: Caution should be exercised if ergotamine, dihydroergotamine or related compounds are given in combination with propranolol since vasospastic reactions have been reported in a few patients.

Prostaglandin Synthetase Inhibiting Drugs: Concomitant use of these e.g. ibuprofen or indometacin, may decrease the hypotensive effects of propranolol.

Chlorpromazine: Concomitant administration with propranolol may result in an increase in plasma levels of both drugs. This may lead to an enhanced antipsychotic effect for chlorpromazine and an increased antihypertensive effect for propranolol.

Cimetidine, hydralazine, alcohol: Concomitant use of cimetidine and hydralazine will increase, whereas concomitant use of alcohol will decrease, the plasma level of propranolol.

Pharmacokinetic studies have shown that the following agents may interact with propranolol due to effects on enzyme systems in the liver which metabolise propranolol and these agents: quinidine, propafenone, rifampicin, theophylline, warfarin, thioridazine and dihydropyridine calcium channel blockers such as nifedipine, nisoldipine, nicardipine, isradipine and lacidipine. Owing to the fact that blood concentrations of either agent may be affected, dosage adjustments may be needed according to clinical judgement. (See also the interaction above concerning the concomitant therapy with dihydropyridine calcium channel blockers).

4.6 Pregnancy and lactation

As with all drugs, propranolol should not be given in pregnancy unless absolutely essential. There is no evidence of teratogenicity with propranolol. However, beta adrenoceptor blocking agents reduce placenta perfusion, which may result in intra-uterine foetal death, immature and premature deliveries. In addition, adverse effects (especially hypoglycaemia and bradycardia in the neonate and bradycardia in the foetus) may occur. There is an increased risk of cardiac and pulmonary complications in the neonate in the post-natal period.

Most beta-adrenoceptor blocking drugs particularly lipophilic compounds, will pass into breast milk although to a variable extent. Breast feeding is therefore not recommended following administration of these compounds.

4.7 Effects on ability to drive and use machines

Use is unlikely to result in any impairment of the ability of patients to drive or operate machinery. However, it should be taken into account that occasionally dizziness or fatigue may occur.

4.8 Undesirable effects

Propranolol is usually well tolerated, however, listed below are the side effects that may occur:-

Cardiovascular: Bradycardia, heart failure deterioration, postural hypotension which may be associated with syncope, heart block and congestive cardiac failure, exacerbation of claudication, cold extremities, Raynaud's phenomenon.

Respiratory: Bronchospasm (especially in patients with a history of asthma).

Neurological and CNS: Confusion, dizziness, mood changes, nightmares, psychoses and hallucinations, sleep disturbances, paraesthesia especially of the hands.

Haematological: Purpura, thrombocytopenia.

Endocrine: Hypoglycaemia in children.

Gastro-intestinal: Gastro-intestinal disturbance, nausea, diarrhoea.

Integumentary: Alopecia, dry eyes, psoriasiform skin reactions and exacerbation of psoriasis, skin rashes.

Senses: Visual disturbances.

Others: Muscle fatigue, lassitude, insomnia, an increase in ANA (antinuclear antibodies) although the clinical relevance of this has not been established.

If these effects occur, thought should be given to withdrawing the drug. However, it should be withdrawn gradually.

Bradycardia and hypotension are usually a sign of overdosage but may be rarely linked to intolerance. If this occurs the drug should be withdrawn and overdosage treatment initiated.

4.9 Overdose

The symptoms of overdosage may include bradycardia, hypotension, acute cardiac insufficiency and bronchospasm.

General treatment should include: close supervision, treatment in an intensive care ward, the use of gastric lavage, activated charcoal and a laxative to prevent absorption of any drug still present in the gastrointestinal tract, the use of plasma or plasma substitutes to treat hypotension and shock.

Excessive bradycardia can be countered with atropine 1-2mg intravenously and/or a cardiac pacemaker. If necessary, this may be followed by a bolus dose of glucagon 10mg intravenously. If required, this may be repeated or followed by an intravenous infusion of glucagon 1-10mg/hour depending on response. If no response to glucagon occurs or if glucagon is unavailable, a beta-adrenoceptor stimulant such as dobutamine 2.5 to 10 micrograms/Kg/minute by intravenous infusion may be given. Dobutamine, because of its positive inotropic effect could also be used to treat hypotension and acute cardiac insufficiency. It is likely that these doses would be inadequate to reverse the cardiac effects of beta-blockade if a large overdose has been taken. The dose of dobutamine should therefore be increased if necessary to achieve the required response according to the clinical condition of the patient.

5. PHARMACOLOGICAL PROPERTIES

5.1 Pharmacodynamic properties

Propranolol is a competitive antagonist at both $beta_1$ and $beta_2$-adrenoceptors.

It has no agonist activity at the beta-adrenoceptor, but has membrane stabilising activity at concentrations exceeding 1-3mg/litre, though such concentrations are rarely achieved during oral therapy. Competitive beta-adrenoceptor blockade has been demonstrated in man by a parallel shift to the right in the dose-heart rate response curve to beta-agonists such as isoprenaline.

Propranolol, as with other beta-adrenoceptor blocking drugs, has negative inotropic effects, and is therefore contra-indicated in uncontrolled heart failure.

Propranolol is a racemic mixture and the active form is the S(-) isomer. With the exception of inhibition of the conversion of thyroxine to triiodothyronine it is unlikely that any additional ancillary properties possessed by R(+) propranolol, in comparison with the racemic mixture will give rise to different therapeutic effects.

Propranolol is effective and well tolerated in most ethnic populations, although the response may be less in black patients.

5.2 Pharmacokinetic properties

Following intravenous administration, the plasma half-life of propranolol is about 2 hours and the ratio of metabolites to parent drug in the blood is lower than after oral administration. In particular, 4-hydroxypropranolol is not present after intravenous administration.

Propranolol is completely absorbed after oral administration and peak plasma concentrations occur 1-2 hours after dosing in fasting patients. The liver removes up to 90% of an oral dose with an elimination half-life of 3 to 6 hours. Propranolol is widely and rapidly distributed throughout the body with highest levels occurring in the lungs, liver, kidney, brain and heart.

Propranolol is highly protein bound (80-95%).

5.3 Preclinical safety data

Propranolol is a drug on which extensive clinical experience has been obtained. Relevant information for the prescriber is provided elsewhere in the Summary of Product Characteristics.

6. PHARMACEUTICAL PARTICULARS

6.1 List of excipients

Citric acid monohydrate, methyl parahydroxybenzoate (E218), propyl parahydroxybenzoate (E216), propylene glycol, liquid maltitol, sunset yellow E110, orange/tangerine flavour (including ethanol (0.12%v/v) and butylhydroxyanisol E320) and purified water.

6.2 Incompatibilities

None known.

6.3 Shelf life

24 months unopened

3 months opened.

6.4 Special precautions for storage

Do not store above 25°C. Do not refrigerate or freeze.

6.5 Nature and contents of container

Amber (Type III) glass bottles

Closures:

a) Aluminium, EPE wadded, roll-on pilfer-proof screw cap.

b) HDPE, EPE wadded, tamper evident screw cap.

c) HDPE, EPE wadded, tamper evident, child resistant closure.

Pack Size: 150ml

6.6 Instructions for use and handling

Not applicable.

Administrative Data

7. MARKETING AUTHORISATION HOLDER

Rosemont Pharmaceuticals Ltd, Rosemont House, Yorkdale Industrial Park, Braithwaite Street, Leeds, LS11 9XE, UK.

8. MARKETING AUTHORISATION NUMBER(S)

PL 00427/0124

9. DATE OF FIRST AUTHORISATION/RENEWAL OF THE AUTHORISATION

11 December 2000

10. DATE OF REVISION OF THE TEXT

April 2004

Syprol Oral Solution 5mg/5ml

(Rosemont Pharmaceuticals Limited)

1. NAME OF THE MEDICINAL PRODUCT

Propranolol Hydrochloride 5mg/5ml Oral Solution

Syprol 5mg/5ml

2. QUALITATIVE AND QUANTITATIVE COMPOSITION

Propranolol Hydrochloride 5mg/5ml

3. PHARMACEUTICAL FORM

Oral Solution

A clear colourless liquid with odour of orange/tangerine.

4. CLINICAL PARTICULARS

4.1 Therapeutic indications

Propranolol is indicated in:

- the control of hypertension
- the management of angina pectoris
- the long term prophylaxis against reinfarction after recovery from acute myocardial infarction
- the control of most forms of cardiac arrhythmia
- the prophylaxis of migraine
- the management of essential tremor
- relief of situational anxiety and generalised anxiety symptoms, particularly those of the somatic type.
- prophylaxis of upper gastro-intestinal bleeding in patients with portal hypertension and oesophageal varices.
- the adjunctive management of thyrotoxicosis and thyrotoxic crisis
- management of hypertrophic obstructive cardiomyopathy
- management of phaeochromocytoma perioperatively (with an alpha-adrenoceptor blocking drug).

4.2 Posology and method of administration

For oral administration only.

Adults:

Hypertension – A starting dose of 80mg twice a day may be increased at weekly intervals according to response. The usual dose range is 160 – 320mg per day. With concurrent diuretic or other antihypertensive drugs a further reduction of blood pressure is obtained.

Angina, migraine and essential tremor – A starting dose of 40mg two or three times daily may be increased by the same amount at weekly intervals according to patient response. An adequate response in migraine and essential tremor is usually seen in the range 80-160mg/day and in angina in the range 120-240mg/day.

Situational and generalised anxiety – A dose of 40mg daily may provide short term relief of acute situational anxiety. Generalised anxiety, requiring longer term therapy, usually responds adequately to 40mg twice daily which, in individual cases, may be increased to 40mg three times daily. Treatment should be continued according to response. Patients should be reviewed after six to twelve months treatment.

Arrhythmias, anxiety, tachycardia, hypertrophic obstructive cardiomyopathy and thyrotoxicosis – A dosage range of 10-40mg three or four times a day usually achieves the required response.

Post myocardial infarction - Treatment should start between days 5 and 21 after myocardial infarction with an initial dose of 40mg four times a day for 2 or 3 days. In order to improve compliance the total daily dosage may thereafter be given as 80mg twice daily.

Portal hypertension:

Dosage should be titrated to achieve approximately 25% reduction in resting heart rate. Dosage should begin with 40mg twice daily, increasing to 80mg twice daily depending on heart rate response. If necessary, the dose may be increased incrementally to a maximum of 160mg twice daily.

Phaeochromocytoma (Used only with an alpha-receptor blocking drug)

Pre-operative: 60mg daily for three days is recommended.

Non-operable malignant cases: 30mg daily.

Children

Arrhythmias, phaeochromocytoma, thyrotoxicosis – Dosage should be individually determined and the following is only a guide: 250 – 500 micrograms per Kilogram three or four times daily as required.

Migraine –

Under the age of 12: 20mg two or three times daily.

Over the age of 12: the adult dose.

Fallot's tetralogy – The value of propranolol in this condition is confined mainly to the relief of right-ventricular outflow tract shut-down. It is also useful for treatment of associated arrhythmias and angina. Dosage should be individually determined and the following is only a guide: Up to 1mg/Kg repeated three or four times a day as required.

Elderly

With regard to the elderly the optimum dose should be individually determined according to the clinical response.

4.3 Contraindications

Propranolol must not be used if there is a history of bronchial asthma or bronchospasm.

The product label states the following warning: "Do not take propranolol if you have a history of asthma or wheezing". A similar warning appears in the patient information leaflet.

Bronchospasm can usually be reversed by $beta_2$-agonist bronchodilators such as salbutamol. Large doses of the $beta_2$-agonist bronchodilator may be required to overcome the beta-blockade produced by propranolol and the dose should be titrated according to the clinical response; both intravenous and inhalational administration should be considered. The use of intravenous aminophylline and/or the use of ipratropium (given by nebuliser) may also be considered. Glucagon (1 to 2mg given intravenously) has also been reported to produce a bronchodilator effect in asthmatic patients. Oxygen or artificial ventilation may be required in severe cases.

Propranolol as with other beta-adrenoceptor blocking drugs must not be used in patients with any of the following:

hypersensitivity to propranolol hydrochloride or any of the ingredients; the presence of second or third degree heart block; in cardiogenic shock; metabolic acidosis; after prolonged fasting; bradycardia; hypotension; severe peripheral arterial circulatory disturbances; sick sinus syndrome; untreated phaeochromocytoma; uncontrolled heart failure or Prinzmetal's angina.

4.4 Special warnings and special precautions for use

Although contra-indicated in uncontrolled heart failure, propranolol may be used where the signs of heart failure have been controlled by the use of appropriate concomitant medication. Propranolol should be used with caution in patients whose cardiac reserve is poor.

Treatment should not be discontinued abruptly in patients with ischaemic heart disease. Either the equivalent dose of another beta-adrenoceptor blocking drug may be substituted or the withdrawal of propranolol should be gradual.

Propranolol may modify the tachycardia of hypoglycaemia (see interactions).

Although contra-indicated in severe peripheral arterial circulatory disturbances, propranolol may also aggravate less severe peripheral arterial circulatory disturbances.

One of the pharmacological actions of propranolol is to reduce the heart rate. Therefore the dosage should be reduced in those rare cases where symptoms are attributable to a slow heart rate.

Due to propranolol having a negative effect on conduction time, caution must be exercised if it is given to patients with first degree heart block.

Since the half life may be increased in patients with significant hepatic or renal impairment, caution must be exercised when starting treatment and selecting the initial dose.

In patients with portal hypertension, liver function may deteriorate and hepatic encephalopathy may develop. There have been reports suggesting that treatment with propranolol may increase the risk of developing hepatic encephalopathy.

Propranolol may cause a more severe reaction to a variety of allergens when given to patients with a history of anaphylactic reaction to such allergens. Such patients may be unresponsive to the usual doses of adrenaline used to treat the allergic reactions.

Propranolol may mask the signs of thyrotoxicosis.

Propranolol must be used with caution in patients with decompensated cirrhosis.

Laboratory Tests: Propranolol has been reported to interfere with the estimation of serum bilirubin by the diazo method and with the determination of catecholamines by methods using fluorescence.

4.5 Interaction with other medicinal products and other forms of Interaction

Hypoglycaemic agents: Tachycardia associated with hypoglycaemia may be modified by propranolol. Use of propranolol alongside hypoglycaemic therapy in diabetic patients should be with caution since it may prolong the hypoglycaemic response to insulin.

Clonidine: Caution should be exercised when transferring patients from clonidine to beta-adrenoceptor blocking drugs. If propranolol and clonidine are given concurrently, clonidine should not be discontinued until several days after the withdrawal of the beta blocker. If replacing clonidine by beta-adrenoceptor blocking drug therapy, the introduction of the beta-adrenoceptor blocking drugs should be delayed for several days after clonidine administration has stopped.

Anti-arrhythmics: Care should be taken when prescribing a beta-adrenergic blocking drug with Class 1 anti-arrhythmic agents such as disopyramide.

Verapamil, Diltiazem: In patients with impaired ventricular function who are also taking verapamil or diltiazem, beta-blockers should be used with caution. The combination should not be given to patients with conduction abnormalities. Neither drug should be administered intravenously within 48 hours of discontinuing the other.

Anaesthesia: Caution must be exercised when using anaesthetic agents with propranolol. The anaesthetist should be informed and the choice of anaesthetic should be the agent with as little negative inotropic activity as possible. Use of beta-adrenoceptor blocking drugs with anaesthetic drugs may result in attenuation of the reflex tachycardia and increase the risk of hypotension. Anaesthetic agents causing myocardial depression are best avoided.

Sympathomimetic Agents and Parenteral Adrenaline: Concomitant use of sympathomimetic agents e.g. adrenaline, may counteract the effect of beta-adrenoceptor blocking drugs. Caution should be taken in the parenteral administration of preparations containing adrenaline to people taking beta-adrenoceptor blocking drugs as, in rare cases, vasoconstriction, hypertension and bradycardia may result.

Dihydropyridines: Concomitant therapy with dihydropyridines e.g. nifedipine, may increase the risk of hypotension, and cardiac failure may occur in patients with latent cardiac insufficiency.

Digitalis Glycosides: These preparations in association with beta-adrenoceptor blocking drugs, may increase atrio-ventricular conduction time.

Lignocaine: Administration of propranolol during infusion of lignocaine may increase the plasma concentration of lignocaine by approximately 30%. Patients already receiving propranolol tend to have higher lignocaine levels than controls. The combination should be avoided.

Ergotamine: Caution should be exercised if ergotamine, dihydroergotamine or related compounds are given in combination with propranolol since vasospastic reactions have been reported in a few patients.

Prostaglandin Synthetase Inhibiting Drugs: Concomitant use of these e.g. ibuprofen or indomethacin, may decrease the hypotensive effects of propranolol.

Chlorpromazine: Concomitant administration with propranolol may result in an increase in plasma levels of both drugs. This may lead to an enhanced antipsychotic effect for chlorpromazine and an increased antihypertensive effect for propranolol.

Cimetidine, hydralazine, alcohol: Concomitant use of cimetidine and hydralazine will increase, whereas concomitant use of alcohol will decrease, the plasma level of propranolol.

Pharmacokinetic studies have shown that the following agents may interact with propranolol due to effects on enzyme systems in the liver which metabolise propranolol and these agents: quinidine, propafenone, rifampicin, theophylline, warfarin, thioridazine and dihydropyridine calcium channel blockers such as nifedipine, nisoldipine, nicardipine, isradipine and lacidipine. Owing to the fact that blood concentrations of either agent may be affected, dosage adjustments may be needed according to clinical judgement. (See also the interaction above concerning the concomitant therapy with dihydropyridine calcium channel blockers).

4.6 Pregnancy and lactation

As with all drugs, propranolol should not be given in pregnancy unless absolutely essential. There is no evidence of teratogenicity with propranolol. However, beta adrenoceptor blocking agents reduce placenta perfusion, which may result in intra-uterine foetal death, immature and premature deliveries. In addition, adverse effects (especially hypoglycaemia and bradycardia in the neonate and bradycardia in the foetus) may occur. There is an increased risk of cardiac and pulmonary complications in the neonate in the post-natal period.

Most beta-adrenoceptor blocking drugs particularly lipophilic compounds, will pass into breast milk although to a variable extent. Breast feeding is therefore not recommended following administration of these compounds.

4.7 Effects on ability to drive and use machines

Use is unlikely to result in any impairment of the ability of patients to drive or operate machinery. However, it should be taken into account that occasionally dizziness or fatigue may occur.

4.8 Undesirable effects

Propranolol is usually well tolerated, however, listed below are the side effects that may occur:-

Cardiovascular: Bradycardia, heart failure deterioration, postural hypotension which may be associated with syncope, heart block and congestive cardiac failure, exacerbation of claudication, cold extremities, Raynaud's phenomenon.

Respiratory: Bronchospasm (especially in patients with a history of asthma)

Neurological and CNS: Confusion, dizziness, mood changes, nightmares, psychoses and hallucinations, sleep disturbances, paraesthesia especially of the hands.

Haematological: Purpura, thrombocytopenia.

Endocrine: Hypoglycaemia in children.

Gastro-intestinal: Gastro-intestinal disturbance, nausea, diarrhoea

Integumentary: Alopecia, dry eyes, psoriasiform skin reactions and exacerbation of psoriasis, skin rashes.

Senses: Visual disturbances.

Others: Muscle fatigue, lassitude, insomnia, an increase in ANA (antinuclear antibodies) although the clinical relevance of this has not been established.

If these effects occur, thought should be given to withdrawing the drug. However, it should be withdrawn gradually.

Bradycardia and hypotension are usually a sign of overdosage but may be rarely linked to intolerance. If this occurs the drug should be withdrawn and overdosage treatment initiated.

4.9 Overdose

The symptoms of overdosage may include bradycardia, hypotension, acute cardiac insufficiency and bronchospasm.

General treatment should include: close supervision, treatment in an intensive care ward, the use of gastric lavage, activated charcoal and a laxative to prevent absorption of any drug still present in the gastrointestinal tract, the use of plasma or plasma substitutes to treat hypotension and shock.

Excessive bradycardia can be countered with atropine 1-2mg intravenously and/or a cardiac pacemaker. If necessary, this may be followed by a bolus dose of glucagon 10mg intravenously. If required, this may be repeated or followed by an intravenous infusion of glucagon 1-10mg/hour depending on response. If no response to glucagon occurs or if glucagon is unavailable, a beta-adrenoceptor stimulant such as dobutamine 2.5 to 10 micrograms/Kg/minute by intravenous infusion may be given. Dobutamine, because of its positive inotropic effect could also be used to treat hypotension and acute cardiac insufficiency. It is likely that these doses would be inadequate to reverse the cardiac effects of beta-blockade if a large overdose has been taken. The dose of dobutamine should therefore be increased if necessary to achieve the required response according to the clinical condition of the patient.

5. PHARMACOLOGICAL PROPERTIES

5.1 Pharmacodynamic properties

Propranolol is a competitive antagonist at both $beta_1$ and $beta_2$-adrenoceptors.

It has no agonist activity at the beta-adrenoceptor, but has membrane stabilising activity at concentrations exceeding 1-3mg/litre, though such concentrations are rarely achieved during oral therapy. Competitive beta-adrenoceptor blockade has been demonstrated in man by a parallel shift to the right in the dose-heart rate response curve to beta-agonists such as isoprenaline.

Propranolol, as with other beta-adrenoceptor blocking drugs, has negative inotropic effects, and is therefore contra-indicated in uncontrolled heart failure.

Propranolol is a racemic mixture and the active form is the S(-) isomer. With the exception of inhibition of the conversion of thyroxine to triiodothyronine it is unlikely that any additional ancillary properties possessed by R(+) propranolol, in comparison with the racemic mixture will give rise to different therapeutic effects.

Propranolol is effective and well tolerated in most ethnic populations, although the response may be less in black patients.

5.2 Pharmacokinetic properties

Following intravenous administration, the plasma half-life of propranolol is about 2 hours and the ratio of metabolites to parent drug in the blood is lower than after oral administration. In particular, 4-hydroxypropranolol is not present after intravenous administration.

Propranolol is completely absorbed after oral administration and peak plasma concentrations occur 1-2 hours after dosing in fasting patients. The liver removes up to 90% of an oral dose with an elimination half-life of 3 to 6 hours. Propranolol is widely and rapidly distributed throughout the body with highest levels occurring in the lungs, liver, kidney, brain and heart.

Propranolol is highly protein bound (80-95%).

5.3 Preclinical safety data

Propranolol is a drug on which extensive clinical experience has been obtained. Relevant information for the prescriber is provided elsewhere in the Summary of Product Characteristics.

6. PHARMACEUTICAL PARTICULARS

6.1 List of excipients

Citric acid monohydrate, methyl parahydroxybenzoate (E218), propyl parahydroxybenzoate (E216), propylene glycol, liquid maltitol, orange/tangerine flavour (including ethanol (0.12%v/v) and butylhydroxyanisol E320) and purified water.

6.2 Incompatibilities

None known.

6.3 Shelf life

24 months unopened

3 months opened.

6.4 Special precautions for storage

Do not store above 25°C. Do not refrigerate or freeze.

6.5 Nature and contents of container

Amber (Type III) glass bottles

Closures: -

a) Aluminium, EPE wadded, roll-on pilfer-proof screw cap

b) HDPE, EPE wadded, tamper evident screw cap

c) HDPE, EPE wadded, tamper evident, child resistant closure.

Pack Size: 150ml

6.6 Instructions for use and handling

Not applicable.

Administrative Data

7. MARKETING AUTHORISATION HOLDER

Rosemont Pharmaceuticals Ltd, Rosemont House, Yorkdale Industrial Park, Braithwaite Street, Leeds, LS11 9XE, UK.

8. MARKETING AUTHORISATION NUMBER(S)

PL 00427/0122

9. DATE OF FIRST AUTHORISATION/RENEWAL OF THE AUTHORISATION

11 December 2000

10. DATE OF REVISION OF THE TEXT

Sytron

(Link Pharmaceuticals Ltd)

1. NAME OF THE MEDICINAL PRODUCT

Sytron®

2. QUALITATIVE AND QUANTITATIVE COMPOSITION

Sodium feredetate 190mg (equivalent to 27.5mg of iron/5ml)

3. PHARMACEUTICAL FORM

Oral solution

4. CLINICAL PARTICULARS

4.1 Therapeutic indications

Iron deficiency anaemia, notably in paediatrics.

In pregnancy when other forms of oral iron may not be well tolerated.

Anaemias secondary to rheumatoid arthritis.

4.2 Posology and method of administration

For oral administration

Adults:	5ml increasing gradually to 10ml three times daily.
Elderly (over 65 years):	As for adults.
Infants(including premature infants) up to 1 year:	2.5ml twice daily; somewhat smaller doses should be used initially.
1 to 5 years:	2.5ml three times daily.
6 to 12 years:	5ml three times daily.

4.3 Contraindications

None known

4.4 Special warnings and special precautions for use

None known

4.5 Interaction with other medicinal products and other forms of Interaction

None known

4.6 Pregnancy and lactation

No adverse effects have been reported.

4.7 Effects on ability to drive and use machines

None known

4.8 Undesirable effects

Patients have occasionally complained of nausea or mild diarrhoea in the early stages of treatment. In such cases it has been found that if treatment is withdrawn for a short time, these symptoms quickly disappear and subsequently the patient will tolerate further doses, which should be on a somewhat reduced scale. Normal individuals have taken Sytron at twice the recommended dosage and some of these have experienced mild diarrhoea. This should be taken into account if dosage is increased much higher than the recommended scale.

4.9 Overdose

Initial symptoms of iron overdosage include nausea, vomiting, diarrhoea, abdominal pain, haematemesis, rectal bleeding, lethargy and circulatory collapse. Hyperglycaemia and metabolic acidosis may occur.

Treatment of overdosage

1. Administer an emetic.

2. Emesis should be followed by gastric lavage with desferrioxamine solution (2g/l). Desferrioxamine 5g in 50ml to 100ml water should be introduced into the stomach following gastric emptying.

3. Keep the patient under constant surveillance to detect possible aspiration of vomitus. Maintain suction apparatus and standby emergency oxygen in case of need.

4. In adults, a drink of mannitol or sorbitol should be given to induce small bowel emptying. Inducing diarrhoea in children may be dangerous and should not be undertaken in young children.

5. Severe poisoning: in the presence of shock and/or coma with high serum iron levels (adults $>142\mu$mol/l, children $>90\mu$mol/l), immediate supportive measures should be introduced. Desferrioxamine should be given by slow iv infusion (adults 5mg/kg/h, children 15mg/kg/h). The maximum dose is 80mg/kg/24h. Warning: hypotension may occur if the infusion rate is too rapid.

6. Less severe poisoning: im desferrioxamine should be administered (adults 50mg/kg to a maximum of 4g, children 1g 4 to 6 hourly).

7. Serum iron levels should be monitored throughout.

5. PHARMACOLOGICAL PROPERTIES

5.1 Pharmacodynamic properties

Iron preparations

ATC classification: B03A

After absorption, elemental iron is available for haemoglobin regeneration and reversal of anaemia associated with iron-deficient states.

5.2 Pharmacokinetic properties

Sodium feredetate is not an iron salt as it contains iron in an un-ionised form. In this compound the iron is ''insulated'' or ''sequestered'' with the sodium salt of ethylenediamine tetra-acetic acid (EDTA) to form a chelate. This accounts for the fact that Sytron is not astringent and does not discolour teeth. Studies using radioactive tracers have shown that the iron chelate is split within the gastro-intestinal tract, releasing elemental iron which is absorbed and rendered available for haemoglobin regeneration.

Iron absorption is enhanced in iron-deficiency states. Post-absorption distribution of elemental iron is as follows: 60% to 70% is incorporated into haemoglobin and most of the remainder is present in storage forms, either as ferritin or haemosiderin, in the reticulo-endothelial system and to a lesser extent, hepatocytes. A further 4% is present in myoglobin and haeme-containing enzymes, or bound to transferrin in plasma. Excretion is mainly in the faeces.

EDTA passes through the body unchanged. The compound is poorly absorbed, and that which reaches the bloodstream is eliminated by both glomerular filtration and tubular excretion.

5.3 Preclinical safety data

There are no pre-clinical data of relevance to the prescriber which are additional to that already included in other sections of the Summary of Product Characteristics.

6. PHARMACEUTICAL PARTICULARS

6.1 List of excipients

Methyl hydroxybenzoate, propyl hydroxybenzoate, citric acid monohydrate, saccharin sodium, glycerol, sorbitol solution, ethanol 96%, black cherry flavour 51-779A, Ponceau 4R (E124), potable water

6.2 Incompatibilities

None known

6.3 Shelf life

60 months

If this product has been diluted with water use within 14 days of preparation.

6.4 Special precautions for storage

Store below 30°C

6.5 Nature and contents of container

Sytron is supplied in round amber glass bottles with a ropp cap. Each bottle contains either 125ml or 500ml or 2250ml of Sytron.

6.6 Instructions for use and handling

Water is the recommended diluent for this product.

7. MARKETING AUTHORISATION HOLDER

Link Pharmaceuticals Limited, Bishops Weald House, Albion Way, Horsham, West Sussex, RH12 1AH

8. MARKETING AUTHORISATION NUMBER(S)

PL 12406/0005

9. DATE OF FIRST AUTHORISATION/RENEWAL OF THE AUTHORISATION

13 October 1993/11 November 1998

10. DATE OF REVISION OF THE TEXT

August 2003

11. Legal Category

P

® Sytron is a registered trade mark

Tagamet Injection

(GlaxoSmithKline UK)

1. NAME OF THE MEDICINAL PRODUCT
Tagamet® Injection

2. QUALITATIVE AND QUANTITATIVE COMPOSITION
Tagamet Injection contains 200 mg cimetidine in 2 ml.

3. PHARMACEUTICAL FORM
Ampoules containing 200 mg cimetidine in 2 ml solution.

4. CLINICAL PARTICULARS

4.1 Therapeutic indications
Tagamet is a histamine H_2-receptor antagonist which rapidly inhibits both basal and stimulated gastric secretion of acid and reduces pepsin output.

Tagamet is indicated in the treatment of duodenal and benign gastric ulceration, including that associated with non-steroidal anti-inflammatory agents, recurrent and stomal ulceration, oesophageal reflux disease and other conditions where reduction of gastric acid by Tagamet has been shown to be beneficial: persistent dyspeptic symptoms with or without ulceration, particularly meal-related upper abdominal pain, including such symptoms associated with non-steroidal anti-inflammatory agents; the prophylaxis of gastrointestinal haemorrhage from stress ulceration in seriously ill patients; before general anaesthesia in patients thought to be at risk of acid aspiration (Mendelson's) syndrome, particularly obstetric patients during labour; to reduce malabsorption and fluid loss in the short bowel syndrome; and in pancreatic insufficiency to reduce degradation of enzyme supplements. Tagamet is also recommended in the management of the Zollinger-Ellison syndrome.

4.2 Posology and method of administration
Tagamet is usually given orally, but parenteral dosing may be substituted for all or part of the recommended oral dose in cases where oral dosing is impracticable or considered inappropriate.

The total daily dose by any route should not normally exceed 2.4 g. Dosage should be reduced in patients with impaired renal function (see *Section 4.4*).

ADULTS

Tagamet may be given intramuscularly or intravenously.

The dose by intramuscular injection is normally 200 mg, which may be repeated at four- to six-hourly intervals.

The usual dosage for intravenous administration is 200 - 400 mg, which may be repeated four to six-hourly.

If direct intravenous injection cannot be avoided, 200 mg should be given *slowly* over at least five minutes, and may be repeated four to six-hourly. Rapid intravenous injection has been associated with cardiac arrest and arrhythmias. For critically ill patients and patients with cardiovascular impairment, or if a larger dose is needed, the dose should be diluted and given over at least 10 minutes. In such cases infusion is preferable.

For intermittent intravenous infusion, Tagamet may be given at a dosage of 200 mg to 400 mg every 4 to 6 hours.

If continuous intravenous infusion is required, Tagamet may be given at an average rate of 50 to 100 mg/hour over 24 hours.

In the prophylaxis of haemorrhage from stress ulceration in seriously ill patients, doses of 200 - 400 mg can be given every four to six hours by oral, nasogastric or parenteral routes. By direct intravenous injection a dose of 200 mg should not be exceeded: see above.

In patients thought to be at risk of acid aspiration syndrome an oral dose of 400 mg can be given 90 - 120 minutes before induction of general anaesthesia or, in obstetric practice, at the start of labour. While such a risk persists, a dose of up to 400 mg may be repeated (parenterally if appropriate) at four-hourly intervals as required up to the usual daily maximum of 2.4 g. The usual precautions to avoid acid aspiration should be taken.

To reduce degradation of pancreatic enzyme supplements, 800 - 1600 mg a day may be given according to response in four divided doses, one to one and a half hours before meals.

ELDERLY

The normal adult dosage may be used unless renal function is markedly impaired (see *Section 4.4*).

CHILDREN

Experience in children is less than that in adults. In children more than one year old, Tagamet 25 - 30 mg/kg body weight per day in divided doses may be administered.

The use of Tagamet in infants under one year old is not fully evaluated; 20 mg/kg body weight per day in divided doses has been used.

4.3 Contraindications
Hypersensitivity to cimetidine.

4.4 Special warnings and special precautions for use
Rapid intravenous injection of cimetidine (less than 5 minutes) should be avoided as there have been rare associations with cardiac arrest and arrhythmias. Transient hypotension has also been observed, particularly in critically ill patients (see dosage and administration)

Dosage should be reduced in patients with impaired renal function according to creatinine clearance. The following dosages are suggested: creatinine clearance of 0 to 15 ml per minute, 200 mg twice a day; 15 to 30 ml per minute, 200 mg three times a day; 30 to 50 ml per minute, 200 mg four times a day; over 50 ml per minute, normal dosage. Cimetidine is removed by haemodialysis, but not to any significant extent by peritoneal dialysis.

Clinical trials of over six years' continuous treatment and more than 15 years' widespread use have not revealed unexpected adverse reactions related to long-term therapy. The safety of prolonged use is not, however, fully established and care should be taken to observe periodically patients given prolonged treatment.

Tagamet treatment can mask the symptoms and allow transient healing of gastric cancer. The potential delay in diagnosis should particularly be borne in mind in patients of middle age and over with new or recently changed dyspeptic symptoms.

Care should be taken that patients with a history of peptic ulcer, particularly the elderly, being treated with Tagamet and a non-steroidal anti-inflammatory agent are observed regularly.

4.5 Interaction with other medicinal products and other forms of Interaction
Tagamet can prolong the elimination of drugs metabolised by oxidation in the liver. Although pharmacological interactions with a number of drugs (e.g. diazepam, propranolol) have been demonstrated, only those with oral anticoagulants, phenytoin, theophylline and intravenous lignocaine appear, to date, to be of clinical significance. Close monitoring of patients on Tagamet receiving oral anticoagulants or phenytoin is recommended and a reduction in the dosage of these drugs may be necessary.

In patients on drug treatment or with illnesses that could cause falls in blood cell count, the possibility that H_2-receptor antagonism could potentiate this effect should be borne in mind.

4.6 Pregnancy and lactation
Although tests in animals and clinical evidence have not revealed any hazards from the administration of Tagamet during pregnancy or lactation, both animal and human studies have shown that it does cross the placental barrier and is excreted in milk. As with most drugs, the use of Tagamet should be avoided during pregnancy and lactation unless essential.

4.7 Effects on ability to drive and use machines
Not applicable.

4.8 Undesirable effects
Over 56 million patients have been treated with Tagamet worldwide and adverse reactions have been infrequent. Diarrhoea, dizziness or rash, usually mild and transient, and tiredness have been reported. Gynaecomastia has been reported and is almost always reversible on discontinuing treatment. Biochemical or biopsy evidence of reversible liver damage has been reported occasionally, as have rare cases of hepatitis. Reversible confusional states have occurred, usually in elderly or already very ill patients, e.g. those with renal failure. Hallucination has been reported rarely; depression has been reported infrequently. Thrombocytopenia and leucopenia, including agranulocytosis (see *Section 4.4*), reversible on withdrawal of treatment, have been reported rarely; pancytopenia and aplastic anaemia have been reported very rarely. There have been very rare reports of interstitial nephritis, acute pancreatitis, fever, headache, myalgia, arthralgia, sinus bradycardia, tachycardia and heart block, all reversible on withdrawal of treatment. In common with other H_2-receptor antagonists, there have been very rare reports of anaphylaxis. Rare cases of hypersensitivity vasculitis have been reported. These usually cleared on withdrawal of the drug. Alopecia has been reported but no causal relationship has been established. Reversible impotence has also been very rarely reported but no causal relationship has been established at usual therapeutic doses. Isolated increases of plasma creatinine have been of no clinical significance.

4.9 Overdose
Acute over-dosage of up to 20 grams has been reported several times with no significant ill effects. Induction of vomiting and/or gastric lavage may be employed together with symptomatic and supportive therapy.

5. PHARMACOLOGICAL PROPERTIES

5.1 Pharmacodynamic properties
Cimetidine is a histamine H_2-receptor antagonist which rapidly inhibits both basal and stimulated gastric secretion of acid and reduces pepsin output.

5.2 Pharmacokinetic properties
Cimetidine is metabolised in the liver and excreted mainly through the kidney with a half-life of about two hours. The effects on acid secretion are of longer duration.

5.3 Preclinical safety data
Not applicable.

6. PHARMACEUTICAL PARTICULARS

6.1 List of excipients
The injection contains hydrochloric acid (E507) and water for injections.

6.2 Incompatibilities
Not applicable.

6.3 Shelf life
Five years.

6.4 Special precautions for storage
Store ampoules below 30°C, protected from light.

6.5 Nature and contents of container
2 ml clear glass ampoules in boxes of 20.

6.6 Instructions for use and handling
Tagamet is compatible with electrolyte and dextrose solutions commonly used for intravenous infusion.

Administrative Data

7. MARKETING AUTHORISATION HOLDER
Smith Kline & French Laboratories Ltd
Great West Road, Brentford, Middlesex TW8 9GS.
trading as:
GlaxoSmithKline UK,
Stockley Park West,
Uxbridge, Middlesex, UB11 1BT

8. MARKETING AUTHORISATION NUMBER(S)
PL 0002/0059R

9. DATE OF FIRST AUTHORISATION/RENEWAL OF THE AUTHORISATION
4 September 2002

10. DATE OF REVISION OF THE TEXT
15 October 2002

11. Legal Status
POM.

TAGAMET TABLETS & SYRUP

(Chemidex Pharma Ltd.)

1. NAME OF THE MEDICINAL PRODUCT
Tagamet 200mg, 400mg & 800mg Tablets
Tagamet Syrup

2. QUALITATIVE AND QUANTITATIVE COMPOSITION
Each tablet contains 200mg, 400mg or 800mg cimetidine per tablet

The syrup contains 200mg cimetidine in each 5ml dose.

3. PHARMACEUTICAL FORM
200mg Tablets: Pale green, circular, biconvex, film-coated tablets, embossed Tagamet on one side and 200 on reverse.

400mg Tablets: Pale green, oblong, film-coated tablets, embossed Tagamet on one side and 400 on reverse.

800mg Tablets: Pale green, oval, film-coated tablets, embossed Tagamet on one side and 800 on reverse.

Syrup: Clear, orange coloured, peach-flavoured syrup.

4. CLINICAL PARTICULARS

4.1 Therapeutic indications
Tagamet is a histamine H_2- receptor antagonist which rapidly inhibits both basal and stimulated gastric secretion of acid and reduces pepsin output.

Tagamet is indicated in the treatment of duodenal and benign gastric ulceration, including that associated with non-steroidal anti-inflammatory agents, recurrent and stomal ulceration, oesophageal reflux disease and other conditions where reduction of gastric acid by Tagamet has been shown to be beneficial: persistent dyspeptic symptoms with or without ulceration, particularly meal-related upper abdominal pain, including such symptoms associated with non-steroidal anti-inflammatory agents; the prophylaxis of gastrointestinal haemorrhage from stress ulceration in critically ill patients; before general anaesthesia in patients thought to be at risk of acid aspiration

(Mendelson's) syndrome, particularly obstetric patients during labour; to reduce malabsorption and fluid loss in the short bowel syndrome; and in pancreatic insufficiency to reduce degradation of enzyme supplements. Tagamet is also recommended in the management of the Zollinger-Ellison syndrome.

4.2 Posology and method of administration

The total daily dose should not normally exceed 2.4g. Dosage should be reduced in patients with impaired renal function (see Section 4.4).

Adults: For patients with duodenal or benign gastric ulceration, a single daily dose of 800mg at bedtime is recommended. Otherwise the usual dosage is 400mg twice a day with breakfast and at bedtime. Other effective regimens are 200mg three times a day with meals and 400mg at bedtime (1.0g/day) and, if inadequate, 400mg four times a day (1.6g/day) also with meals and at bedtime.

Treatment should be given initially for at least four weeks (six weeks in benign gastric ulcer), eight weeks in ulcer associated with continued non-steroidal anti-inflammatory agents even if symptomatic relief has been achieved sooner. Most ulcers will have healed by that stage, but those which have not usually do so after a further course of treatment.

Treatment may be continued for longer periods in those patients who may benefit from reduction of gastric secretion and the dosage may be reduced in those who have responded to treatment, for example to 400mg at bedtime or 400mg in the morning and at bedtime.

In patients with benign peptic ulcer disease who have responded to the initial course, relapse may be prevented by continued treatment, usually with 400mg at bedtime; 400mg in the morning and at bedtime has also been used.

In oesophageal reflux disease, 400mg four times a day, with meals and at bedtime, for four to eight weeks is recommended to heal oesophagitis and relieve associated symptoms.

In patients with very high gastric acid secretion (e.g. Zollinger-Ellison syndrome) it may be necessary to increase the dose to 400mg four times a day, or in occasional cases further.

Antacids can be made available to all patients until symptoms disappear.

In the prophylaxis of haemorrhage from stress ulceration in seriously ill patients, doses of 200-400mg can be given every four to six hours.

In patients thought to be at risk of acid aspiration syndrome an oral dose of 400mg can be given 90-120 minutes before induction of general anaesthesia or, in obstetric practice, at the start of labour. While such a risk persists, a dose of up to 400mg may be repeated at four hourly intervals as required up to the usual daily maximum of 2.4g. Tagamet Syrup should not be used. The usual precautions to avoid acid aspiration should be taken.

In the short bowel syndrome, e.g. following substantial resection for Crohn's disease, the usual dosage range (see above) can be used according to individual response.

To reduce degradation of pancreatic enzyme supplements, 800-1600mg a day may be given according to response in four divided doses, one to one and a half hours before meals.

Elderly: The normal adult dosage may be used unless renal function is markedly impaired (see Section 4.4).

Children: Experience in children is less than that in adults. In children more than one year old, Tagamet 25-30mg/kg body weight per day in divided doses may be administered.

The use of Tagamet in infants under one year old is not yet fully evaluated; 20mg/kg body weight per day in divided doses has been used.

Administration: Oral; the tablets should be swallowed with a drink of water.

4.3 Contraindications

Hypersensitivity to cimetidine.

4.4 Special warnings and special precautions for use

Dosage should be reduced in patients with impaired renal function according to creatinine clearance. The following dosages are suggested: creatinine clearance of 0-15ml per minute, 200mg twice a day; 15 to 30ml per minute, 200mg three times a day; 30 to 50ml per minute, 200mg four times a day; over 50ml per minute, normal dosage. Cimetidine is removed by haemodialysis, but not to any significant extent by peritoneal dialysis.

Clinical trials of over six years continuous treatment and more than 15 years' widespread use have not revealed unexpected adverse reactions related to long term therapy. The safety of prolonged use is not fully established and care should be taken to observe periodically patients given prolonged treatment.

Care should be taken that patients with a history of peptic ulcer, particularly the elderly, being treated with cimetidine and a non-steroidal anti-inflammatory agent are observed regularly.

Before initiating therapy with this preparation for any gastric ulceration, malignancy should be excluded by endoscopy and biopsy, if possible, because Tagamet can relieve the symptoms and help the superficial healing of the gastric cancer. The consequences of potential delay in diagnosis should be borne in mind especially in middle aged patients or over, with new or recently changed dyspeptic symptoms.

4.5 Interaction with other medicinal products and other forms of Interaction

Cimetidine can prolong the elimination of drugs metabolised by oxidation in the liver

Although pharmacological interactions between cimetidine and a number of drugs have been demonstrated e.g. diazepam and propranolol, only those with oral anticoagulants, phenytoin, theophylline and intravenous lidocaine appear, to date, to be of clinical significance. Close monitoring of patients on cimetidine receiving oral anticoagulants or phenytoin is recommended and a reduction in the dosage of these drugs may be necessary.

In patients on drug treatment or with illnesses that could cause falls in blood cell count, the possibility that H_2-receptor antagonism could potentiate this effect should be borne in mind.

4.6 Pregnancy and lactation

Although tests in animals and clinical evidence have not revealed any hazards from the administration of Tagamet during pregnancy or lactation, both animal and human studies have shown that it does cross the placental barrier and is excreted in milk. The use of this preparation during pregnancy and lactation should be avoided unless considered essential.

4.7 Effects on ability to drive and use machines

None known.

4.8 Undesirable effects

Over 56 million patients have been treated with cimetidine worldwide and adverse reactions have been infrequent. Diarrhoea, dizziness or rash, usually mild and transient, and tiredness have been reported. Gynaecomastia has been reported and is almost always reversible on discontinuing treatment. Biochemical or biopsy evidence of reversible liver damage has been reported occasionally, as have rare cases of hepatitis. Reversible confusional states have occurred, usually in elderly or already very ill patients e.g. those with renal failure. Hallucination has been reported rarely; depression has been reported infrequently. Thrombocytopenia and leucopenia, including agranulocytosis (see Section 4.4), reversible on withdrawal of treatment, have been reported rarely; pancytopenia and aplastic anaemia have been reported very rarely. There have been very rare reports of interstitial nephritis, acute pancreatitis, fever, headache, myalgia, arthralgia, sinus bradycardia, tachycardia and heart block, all reversible on withdrawal of treatment. In common with other H_2-receptor antagonists, there have been very rare reports of anaphylaxis. Rare cases of hypersensitivity vasculitis have been reported. These usually cleared on withdrawal of the drug. Alopecia has been reported but no causal relationship has been established. Reversible impotence has also been very rarely reported but no causal relationship has been established at usual therapeutic doses. Isolated increases of plasma creatinine have been of no clinical significance.

4.9 Overdose

Acute overdosage of up to 20g has been reported several times with no significant ill effects. Induction of vomiting and/or gastric lavage may be employed together with symptomatic and supportive therapy.

5. PHARMACOLOGICAL PROPERTIES

5.1 Pharmacodynamic properties

Cimetidine, one of the H2 blockers is a reversible, competitive antagonist of the actions of histamine on H2 receptors. It is highly selective in its action and is virtually without effect on H1 receptors or, indeed, on receptors for other autacoids or drugs. The most prominent of the effects of histamine that are mediated by H2 receptors is stimulation of gastric acid secretion and they interfere remarkably little with physiological functions other than gastric secretion.

Cimetidine inhibits gastric acid secretion elicited by histamine or other H2 agonists in a dose-dependent, competitive manner; the degree of inhibition parallels the plasma concentration of the drug over a wide range. In addition, the H2 blockers inhibit gastric secretion elicited by muscarinic agonists or by gastrin, although this effect is not always complete.

This breadth of inhibitory effect is not due to non-specific actions at the receptors for these other secretagogues. Rather, this effect, which is non-competitive and indirect, appears to indicate either that these two classes of secretagogues utilise histamine as the final common mediator or, more probably, that ongoing histaminergic stimulation of the parietal cell is important for amplification of the stimuli provided by ACh or gastrin when they act on their own discrete receptors. Receptors for all three secretagogues are present on the parietal cell. The ability of H2 blockers to suppress responses to all three physiological secretagogues makes them potent inhibitors of all phases of gastric acid secretion. Thus these drugs will inhibit basal (fasting) secretion and nocturnal secretion and also that stimulated by food, sham feeding, fundic distension, insulin, or caffeine. The H2 blockers reduce both the volume of gastric juice secreted and its hydrogen ion concentration. Output of pepsin, which is secreted by the chief cells of the gastric glands (mainly under cholinergic control), generally falls in parallel with the reduction in volume of the gastric juice. Secretion of intrinsic factor is also reduced, but it is normally secreted in great excess, and absorption of vitamin B12 is usually adequate even during long-term therapy with H2 blockers.

Concentrations of gastrin in plasma are not significantly altered under fasting conditions; however, the normal prandial elevation of gastrin concentration may be augmented, apparently as a consequence of a reduction in the negative feedback that is normally provided by acid.

5.2 Pharmacokinetic properties

Cimetidine is rapidly and virtually completely absorbed. Absorption is little impaired by food or by antacids. Peak concentrations in plasma are attained in about 1 to 2 hours. Hepatic first-pass metabolism results in bioavailabilities of about 60% for cimetidine. The elimination half-life is about 2 to 3 hours. Cimetidine is eliminated primarily by the kidneys, and 60% or more may appear in the urine unchanged; much of the rest is oxidation products. Small amounts are recovered in the stool.

5.3 Preclinical safety data

Not available.

6. PHARMACEUTICAL PARTICULARS

6.1 List of excipients

200 mg, 400mg & 800mg Tablets

Microcrystalline cellulose
Povidone 30
Sodium starch glycollate
Sodium lauryl sulphate
Colloidal anhydrous silica
Magnesium stearate
Hypromellose (E464)
Titanium dioxide (E171)
Macrogol 400
Indigo carmine aluminium lake (E132)
Iron oxide yellow (E172)
Quinoline yellow aluminium lake (E104)

Syrup

Saccharin sodium,
Hydrochloric acid (E507)
Ethyl alcohol
Methyl parahydroxybenzoate (E218)
Propyl parahydroxybenzoate (E216)
Propylene glycol,
Sodium chloride,
Disodium hydrogen phosphate (E339)
Sorbitol (E420)
Sucrose
FD&C Yellow No.6 (E110)
Peach flavour
Spearmint flavour
Mafco Magnasweet 180
Ethylene oxide and propylene oxide polymer
Water

The sodium content per 5ml of the syrup is 12.8mg

6.2 Incompatibilities

Not applicable

6.3 Shelf life

Tablets and syrup: 3 years

6.4 Special precautions for storage

Tablets:

Blister: Do not store above 25°C. Store in the original package. Keep blister in the outer carton.

Syrup: Store below 25°C

6.5 Nature and contents of container

Tablets

Blister packs consisting of 250μm clear PVC and 20μm hard temper aluminium foil contained in a carton.

200mg tablets: Pack sizes: 60 & 120 tablets

400mg tablets: Pack sizes 60 tablets

800mg tablets: Pack sizes: 30 tablets

Syrup

White opaque HDPE bottles containing 600ml

6.6 Instructions for use and handling

Not applicable

Administrative Data

7. MARKETING AUTHORISATION HOLDER

Chemidex Pharma Limited,
Chemidex House,
Egham Business Village,
Crabtree Road,
Egham,
Surrey TW20 8RB
United Kingdom

8. MARKETING AUTHORISATION NUMBER(S)
200mg tablets: PL 17736/0020
400mg tablets: PL 17736/0021
800mg tablets: PL 17736/0022
Syrup: PL 17736/0067

9. DATE OF FIRST AUTHORISATION/RENEWAL OF THE AUTHORISATION
Tablets: 23 December 2002
Syrup: 25 June 2004

10. DATE OF REVISION OF THE TEXT
Tablets: 25 June 2004

Tambocor 100mg Tablets

(3M Health Care Limited)

1. NAME OF THE MEDICINAL PRODUCT
Tambocor® 100 mg Tablets

2. QUALITATIVE AND QUANTITATIVE COMPOSITION
Each tablet contains flecainide acetate 100 mg.

3. PHARMACEUTICAL FORM
Tablet

4. CLINICAL PARTICULARS
Tambocor is a potent sodium channel blocking agent for the treatment of the conditions listed below:

The effect on the JT interval is insignificant at therapeutic levels.

4.1 Therapeutic indications
Tambocor tablets are indicated for:

a) AV nodal reciprocating tachycardia; arrhythmias associated with Wolff-Parkinson-White Syndrome and similar conditions with accessory pathways.

b) Paroxysmal atrial fibrillation in patients with disabling symptoms when treatment need has been established and in the absence of left ventricular dysfunction (see 4.4, Special warnings and special precautions for use). Arrhythmias of recent onset will respond more readily.

c) Symptomatic sustained ventricular tachycardia.

d) Premature ventricular contractions and/or non-sustained ventricular tachycardia which are causing disabling symptoms, where these are resistant to other therapy or when other treatment has not been tolerated.

Tambocor tablets can be used for the maintenance of normal rhythm following conversion by other means.

Tambocor tablets are for oral administration.

4.2 Posology and method of administration
Adults: Supraventricular arrhythmias: The recommended starting dosage is 50mg twice daily and most patients will be controlled at this dose. If required the dose may be increased to a maximum of 300mg daily.

Ventricular arrhythmias: The recommended starting dosage is 100mg twice daily. The maximum daily dose is 400mg and this is normally reserved for patients of large build or where rapid control of the arrhythmia is required.

After 3-5 days it is recommended that the dosage be progressively adjusted to the lowest level which maintains control of the arrhythmia. It may be possible to reduce dosage during long-term treatment.

Children: Tambocor is not recommended in children under 12, as there is insufficient evidence of its use in this age group.

Elderly Patients: The rate of flecainide elimination from plasma may be reduced in elderly people. This should be taken into consideration when making dose adjustments.

Plasma levels: Based on PVC suppression, it appears that plasma levels of 200-1000 ng/ml may be needed to obtain the maximum therapeutic effect. Plasma levels above 700-1000 ng/ml are associated with increased likelihood of adverse experiences.

Dosage in impaired renal function: In patients with significant renal impairment (creatinine clearance of 35ml/min/1.73 sq.m. or less) the maximum initial dosage should be 100mg daily (or 50mg twice daily).

When used in such patients, frequent plasma level monitoring is strongly recommended.

It is recommended that intravenous treatment with Tambocor should be initiated in hospital.

Treatment with oral Tambocor should be under direct hospital or specialist supervision for patients with:

a) AV nodal reciprocating tachycardia; arrhythmias associated with Wolff-Parkinson-White Syndrome and similar conditions with accessory pathways.

b) Paroxysmal atrial fibrillation in patients with disabling symptoms.

Treatment for patients with other indications should continue to be initiated in hospital.

4.3 Contraindications
Tambocor is contra-indicated in cardiac failure and in patients with a history of myocardial infarction who have either asymptomatic ventricular ectopics or asymptomatic non-sustained ventricular tachycardia.

It is also contra-indicated in patients with long standing atrial fibrillation in whom there has been no attempt to convert to sinus rhythm, and in patients with haemodynamically significant valvular heart disease.

Unless pacing rescue is available, Tambocor should not be given to patients with sinus node dysfunction, atrial conduction defects, second degree or greater atrio-ventricular block, bundle branch block or distal block.

4.4 Special warnings and special precautions for use
Electrolyte disturbances should be corrected before using Tambocor.

Since flecainide elimination from the plasma can be markedly slower in patients with significant hepatic impairment, flecainide should not be used in such patients unless the potential benefits clearly outweigh the risks. Plasma level monitoring is strongly recommended in these circumstances.

Tambocor is known to increase endocardial pacing thresholds - ie to decrease endocardial pacing sensitivity. This effect is reversible and is more marked on the acute pacing threshold than on the chronic. Tambocor should thus be used with caution in all patients with permanent pacemakers or temporary pacing electrodes, and should not be administered to patients with existing poor thresholds or non-programmable pacemakers unless suitable pacing rescue is available.

Generally, a doubling of either pulse width or voltage is sufficient to regain capture, but it may be difficult to obtain ventricular thresholds less than 1 Volt at initial implantation in the presence of Tambocor.

The minor negative inotropic effect of flecainide may assume importance in patients predisposed to cardiac failure. Difficulty has been experienced in defibrillating some patients. Most of the cases reported had pre-existing heart disease with cardiac enlargement, a history of myocardial infarction, arterio-sclerotic heart disease and cardiac failure.

Tambocor should be avoided in patients with structural organic heart disease or abnormal left ventricular function.

Tambocor should be used with caution in patients with acute onset of atrial fibrillation following cardiac surgery.

In a large scale, placebo-controlled clinical trial in post-myocardial infarction patients with asymptomatic ventricular arrhythmia, oral flecainide was associated with a 2.2 fold higher incidence of mortality or non-fatal cardiac arrest as compared with its matching placebo. In that same study, an even higher incidence of mortality was observed in flecainide-treated patients with more than one myocardial infarction. Comparable placebo-controlled clinical trials have not been done to determine if flecainide is associated with higher risk of mortality in other patient groups.

4.5 Interaction with other medicinal products and other forms of Interaction
Flecainide is a class I anti-arrhythmic and interactions are possible with other anti-arrhythmic drugs where additive effects may occur or where drugs interfere with the metabolism of flecainide. The following known categories of drugs may intereact with flecainide:

Cardiac glycosides; Flecainide can cause the plasma *digoxin* level to rise by about 15%, which is unlikely to be of clinical significance for patients with plasma levels in the therapeutic range. It is recommended that the *digoxin* plasma level in digitalised patients should be measured not less than six hours after any *digoxin* dose, before or after administration of flecainide.

Class II anti-arrhythmics; the possibility of additive negative inotropic effects of beta-blockers and other cardiac depressants with flecainide should be recognised

Class III anti-arrhythmics; when flecainide is given in the presence of *amiodarone*, the usual flecainide dosage should be reduced by 50% and the patient monitored closely for adverse effects. Plasma level monitoring is strongly recommended in these circumstances

Class IV anti-arrhythmics; use of flecainide with other sodium channel blockers is not recommended.

Anti-depressants; *fluoxetine* increases plasma flecainide concentration; increased risk of arrhythmias with *tricyclics*; manufacturer of *reboxetine* advises caution.

Anti-epileptics; limited data in patients receiving known enzyme inducers (*phenytoin, phenobarbital, carbamazepine*) indicate only a 30% increase in the rate of flecainide elimination.

Anti-psychotics: *clozapine* – increased risk of arrhythmias

Anti-histamines; increased risk of ventricular arrhythmias with *mizolastine* and *terfenadine* (avoid concomitant use)

Anti-malarials: *quinine* increases plasma concentration of flecainide.

Antivirals: plasma concentration increased by *ritonavir, lopinavar* and *indinavir* (increased risk of ventricular arrhythmias (avoid concomitant use)

Diuretics: Class effect due to hypokalaemia giving rise to cardiac toxicity.

Ulcer healing drugs: *cimetidine* inhibits metabolism of flecainide. In healthy subjects receiving *cimetidine* (1g daily) for one week, plasma flecainide levels increased by about 30% and the half-life increased by about 10%.

Anti-smoking aids: Co-administration of *bupropion* with drugs that are metabolized by CYP2D6 isoenzyme including flecainide, should be approached with caution and should be initiated at the lower end of the dose range of the concomitant medication. If *bupropion* is added to the treatment regimen of a patient already receiving flecainide, the need to decrease the dose of the original medication should be considered.

Treatment with Tambocor is compatible with use of oral anti-coagulants.

4.6 Pregnancy and lactation
There is no evidence as to drug safety in human pregnancy. In New Zealand White rabbits high doses of flecainide caused some foetal abnormalities, but these effects were not seen in Dutch Belted rabbits or rats. The relevance of these findings to humans has not been established. Data have shown that flecainide crosses the placenta to the foetus in patients taking flecainide during pregnancy.

Flecainide is excreted in human milk and appears in concentrations which reflect those in maternal blood. The risk of adverse effects to the nursing infant is very small.

4.7 Effects on ability to drive and use machines
No effect.

4.8 Undesirable effects
Body as a Whole: Asthenia, fatigue, fever, oedema

Cardiovascular: Pro-arrhythmic effects occur but are most likely in patients with structural heart disease and/or significant left ventricular impairement.

In patients with atrial flutter the use of Tambocor has been associated with

1:1 AV conduction following initial atrial slowing with resultant ventricular acceleration. This has been seen most commonly following the use of the injection for acute conversion. This effect is usually short lived and abates quickly following cessation of therapy.

The following adverse effects have also been reported.

AV block-second-degree and third degree, bradycardia, cardiac failure/congestive cardiac failure, chest pain, hypotension, myocardial infarction, palpitation and sinus pause or arrest and tachycardia (AT or VT).

Skin and Appendages: A range of allergic skin reactions have been reported including rashes, alopecia and rare but serious reports of urticaria. There have also been isolated cases of photosensitivity.

Immune System: A small number of cases of increases in anti-nuclear antibodies have been reported, with and without systemic inflammatory involvement.

Haematological: Reductions in red blood cells white blood cells and platelets have been occasionally reported. These changes are usually mild.

Psychiatric: Rarely, hallucinations, depression, confusion, amnesia. Anxiety and insomnia have been reported

Gastrointestinal: Occasionally nausea and vomiting. The following have also been reported: abdominal pain, anorexia, constipation, diarrhoea, dyspepsia and flatulence (bloating).

Liver and Bilary System: A number of cases of elevated liver enzymes and jaundice have been reported in association with Tambocor treatment. So far this has always been reversible on stopping treatment. Hepatic dysfunction has also been reported.

Neurological: Most commonly giddiness, dizziness and lightheadedness, which are usually transient. Rare instances of dyskinesia have been reported, which have improved on withdrawal of flecainide therapy. Rare instances of convulsions, and during long term therapy a few cases of peripheral neuropathy; paraesthesia and ataxia have been reported. There also have been reports of flushing, headache, hypoaesthesia, increased sweating, somnolence, syncope, tinnitus, tremor and vertigo.

Ophthalmological: Visual disturbances, such as double vision and blurring of vision may occur but these are usually transient and disappear upon continuing or reducing the dosage.

Extremely rare cases of corneal deposits have also been reported.

Respiratory: Dyspnoea and rare cases of pneumonitis have been reported.

4.9 Overdose
Overdosage with flecainide is a potentially life threatening medical emergency. No specific antidote is known. There is no known way of rapidly removing flecainide from the system, but forced acid diuresis may theoretically be helpful. Neither dialysis nor haemoperfusion is helpful and injections of anticholinergics are not recommended.

Treatment may include therapy with an inotropic agent, intravenous calcium, giving circulatory assistance (eg balloon pumping), mechanically assisting respiration, or temporarily inserting a transvenous pacemaker if there are severe conduction disturbances or the patient's left ventricular function is otherwise compromised.

5. PHARMACOLOGICAL PROPERTIES

5.1 Pharmacodynamic properties
Tambocor is a Class 1 anti-arrhythmic (local anaesthetic) agent.

Tambocor slows conduction through the heart, having its greatest effect on His Bundle conduction. It also acts selectively to increase anterograde and particularly retrograde accessory pathway refractoriness. Its actions may be reflected in the ECG by prolongation of the PR interval and widening of the QRS complex. The effect on the JT interval is insignificant.

5.2 Pharmacokinetic properties
Oral administration of flecainide results in extensive absorption, with bioavailability approaching 90 to 95%. Flecainide does not appear to undergo significant hepatic first-pass metabolism. In patients, 200 to 500 mg flecainide daily produced plasma concentrations within the therapeutic range of 200-1000 μg/L. Protein binding of flecainide is within the range 32 to 58%.

Recovery of unchanged flecainide in urine of healthy subjects was approximately 42% of a 200mg oral dose, whilst the two major metabolites (Meta-O-Dealkylated and Dealkylated Lactam Metabolites) accounted for a further 14% each. The elimination half-life was 12 to 27 hours.

5.3 Preclinical safety data
Not applicable

6. PHARMACEUTICAL PARTICULARS

6.1 List of excipients
Pregelatinised Starch, BP
Croscarmellose Sodium, USNF
Microcrystalline Cellulose, Ph Eur
Hydrogenated Vegetable Oil, USNF
Magnesium Stearate, Ph Eur

6.2 Incompatibilities
None known

6.3 Shelf life
5 years

6.4 Special precautions for storage
Store below 30°C. Protect from light.

6.5 Nature and contents of container
UPVC/PVDC blister packs containing 60 tablets

6.6 Instructions for use and handling
Not applicable

7. MARKETING AUTHORISATION HOLDER
3M Health Care Limited
3M House
Morley Street
Loughborough
Leics
LE11 1EP

8. MARKETING AUTHORISATION NUMBER(S)
00068/0102

9. DATE OF FIRST AUTHORISATION/RENEWAL OF THE AUTHORISATION
7 April 1983/15 December 1994

10. DATE OF REVISION OF THE TEXT
July 2003

Tambocor 10mg/ml Injection

(3M Health Care Limited)

1. NAME OF THE MEDICINAL PRODUCT
Tambocor® 10mg/ml Injection

2. QUALITATIVE AND QUANTITATIVE COMPOSITION
Each ampoule contains 15 ml of a solution of flecainide acetate 10 mg/ml.

3. PHARMACEUTICAL FORM
Solution for injection.

4. CLINICAL PARTICULARS

4.1 Therapeutic indications
Tambocor Injection is indicated when rapid control of the following arrhythmias is the main clinical requirement:

a) Ventricular tachyarrhythmias where these are resistant to other treatment.

b) AV nodal reciprocating tachycardia; arrhythmias associated with Wolff-Parkinson-White Syndrome and similar conditions with accessory pathways.

c) Paroxysmal atrial fibrillation in patients with disabling symptoms when treatment need has been established and in the absence of left ventricular dysfunction (see 4.4, Special warnings and special precautions for use). Arrhythmias of recent onset will respond more readily.

Tambocor Injection is for bolus injection or intravenous infusion.

4.2 Posology and method of administration
a) Bolus injection: Tambocor injection can be given in an emergency or for rapid effect by a slow injection of 2mg/kg over not less than ten minutes, or in divided doses. If preferred, the dose may be diluted with 5% dextrose and given as a mini-infusion.

Continuous ECG monitoring is recommended in all patients receiving the bolus dose. The injection should be stopped when there is control of the arrhythmia.

It is recommended that Tambocor injection should be administered more slowly to patients in sustained ventricular tachycardia, with careful monitoring of the electrocardiogram. Similar caution should apply to patients with a history of cardiac failure, who may become decompensated during the administration. For such patients it is recommended that the initial dose is given over 30 minutes. The maximum recommended bolus dose is 150 mg.

b) Intravenous infusion: When prolonged parenteral administration is required, it is recommended that therapy is initiated by slow injection of 2 mg/kg over 30 minutes and continued by intravenous infusion at the following rates:

First hour: 1.5 mg/kg per hour.

Second and later hours: 0.1 - 0.25 mg/kg per hour.

It is recommended that the infusion duration should not exceed 24 hours. However, where this is considered necessary, or for patients receiving the upper end of the dose range, plasma level monitoring is strongly recommended. The maximum cumulative dose given in the first 24 hours should not exceed 600 mg. In patients with severe renal impairment (creatinine clearance of less than 35 ml/min/1.73 sq.m.), each of the above dosage recommendations should be reduced by half.

Transition to oral dosing should be accomplished as soon as possible by stopping the infusion and administering the first required oral dose.

Oral maintenance is then continued as indicated in the relevant oral dosage instructions.

Children: Tambocor is not recommended in children under 12, as there is insufficient evidence of its use in this age group.

Elderly Patients: The rate of flecainide elimination from plasma may be reduced in elderly people. This should be taken into consideration when making dose adjustments.

4.3 Contraindications
Tambocor is contra-indicated in cardiac failure and in patients with a history of myocardial infarction who have either asymptomatic ventricular ectopics or asymptomatic non-sustained ventricular tachycardia.

It is also contra-indicated in patients with long standing atrial fibrillation in whom there has been no attempt to convert to sinus rhythm, and in patients with haemodynamically significant valvular heart disease.

Unless pacing rescue is available, Tambocor should not be given to patients with sinus node dysfunction, atrial conduction defects, second degree or greater atrio-ventricular block, bundle branch block or distal block.

4.4 Special warnings and special precautions for use
Electrolyte disturbances should be corrected before using Tambocor.

Since flecainide elimination from the plasma can be markedly slower in patients with significant hepatic impairment, flecainide should not be used in such patients unless the potential benefits clearly outweigh the risks. Plasma level monitoring is strongly recommended in these circumstances.

Tambocor is known to increase endocardial pacing thresholds - ie to decrease endocardial pacing sensitivity. This effect is reversible and is more marked on the acute pacing threshold than on the chronic.

Tambocor should thus be used with caution in all patients with permanent pacemakers or temporary pacing electrodes, and should not be administered to patients with existing poor thresholds or non-programmable pacemakers unless suitable pacing rescue is available.

Generally, a doubling of either pulse width or voltage is sufficient to regain capture, but it may be difficult to obtain ventricular thresholds less than 1 Volt at initial implantation in the presence of Tambocor.

The minor negative inotropic effect of flecainide may assume importance in patients predisposed to cardiac failure. Difficulty has been experienced in defibrillating some patients. Most of the cases reported had pre-existing heart disease with cardiac enlargement, a history of myocardial infarction, arterio-sclerotic heart disease and cardiac failure.

Tambocor should be avoided in patients with structural organic heart disease or abnormal left ventricular function.

Tambocor should be used with caution in patients with acute onset of atrial fibrillation following cardiac surgery.

In a large scale, placebo-controlled clinical trial in post-myocardial infarction patients with asymptomatic ventricular arrhythmia, oral flecainide was associated with a 2.2 fold higher incidence of mortality or non-fatal cardiac arrest as compared with its matching placebo. In that same study, an even higher incidence of mortality was observed in flecainide-treated patients with more than one myocardial infarction. Comparable placebo-controlled clinical trials have not been done to determine if flecainide is associated with higher risk of mortality in other patient groups.

4.5 Interaction with other medicinal products and other forms of Interaction
Flecainide is a class I anti-arrhythmic and interactions are possible with other anti-arrhythmic drugs where additive effects may occur or where drugs interfere with the metabolism of flecainide. The following known categories of drugs may intereact with flecainide:

Cardiac glycosides; Flecainide can cause the plasma *digoxin* level to rise by about 15%, which is unlikely to be of clinical significance for patients with plasma levels in the therapeutic range. It is recommended that the *digoxin* plasma level in digitalised patients should be measured not less than six hours after any *digoxin* dose, before or after administration of flecainide.

Class II anti-arrhythmics; the possibility of additive negative inotropic effects of beta-blockers and other cardiac depressants with flecainide should be recognised

Class III anti-arrhythmics; when flecainide is given in the presence of *amiodarone*, the usual flecainide dosage should be reduced by 50% and the patient monitored closely for adverse effects. Plasma level monitoring is strongly recommended in these circumstances

Class IV anti-arrhythmics; use of flecainide with other sodium channel blockers is not recommended.

Anti-depressants; *fluoxetine* increases plasma flecainide concentration; increased risk of arrhythmias with *tricyclics*; manufacturer of *reboxetine* advises caution.

Anti-epileptics; limited data in patients receiving known enzyme inducers (*phenytoin, phenobarbital, carbamazepine*) indicate only a 30% increase in the rate of flecainide elimination.

Anti-psychotics: *clozapine* – increased risk of arrhythmias

Anti-histamines; increased risk of ventricular arrhythmias with *mizolastine* and *terfenadine* (avoid concomitant use)

Anti-malarials: *quinine* increases plasma concentration of flecainide.

Antivirals: plasma concentration increased by *ritonavir, lopinavar* and *indinavir* (increased risk of ventricular arrhythmias) avoid concomitant use

Diuretics: Class effect due to hypokalaemia giving rise to cardiac toxicity.

Ulcer healing drugs: *cimetidine* inhibits metabolism of flecainide. In healthy subjects receiving *cimetidine* (1g daily) for one week, plasma flecainide levels increased by about 30% and the half-life increased by about 10%.

Anti-smoking aids: Co-administration of *bupropion* with drugs that are metabolized by CYP2D6 isoenzyme including flecainide, should be approached with caution and should be initiated at the lower end of the dose range of the concomitant medication. If *bupropion* is added to the treatment regimen of a patient already receiving flecainide, the need to decrease the dose of the original medication should be considered.

Treatment with Tambocor is compatible with use of oral anti-coagulants.

4.6 Pregnancy and lactation
There is no evidence as to drug safety in human pregnancy. In New Zealand White rabbits high doses of flecainide caused some foetal abnormalities, but these effects were not seen in Dutch Belted rabbits or rats. The relevance of these findings to humans has not been established. Data have shown that flecainide crosses the placenta to the foetus in patients taking flecainide during pregnancy.

Flecainide is excreted in human milk and appears in concentrations which reflect those in maternal blood. The risk of adverse effects to the nursing infant is very small.

4.7 Effects on ability to drive and use machines
No effect.

4.8 Undesirable effects
Body as a Whole: Asthenia, fatigue, fever, oedema

Cardiovascular: Pro-arrhythmic effects occur but are most likely in patients with structural heart disease and/or significant left ventricular impairment.

In patients with atrial flutter the use of Tambocor has been associated with 1:1 AV conduction following initial atrial slowing with resultant ventricular acceleration. This has been seen most commonly following the use of the injection for acute conversion. This effect is usually short lived and abates quickly following cessation of therapy.

The following adverse effects have also been reported.

AV block-second-degree and third degree, bradycardia, cardiac failure/congestive cardiac failure, chest pain, hypotension, myocardial infarction, palpitation, sinus pause or arrest and tachycardia (AT or VT).

Skin and Appendages: A range of allergic skin reactions have been reported including rashes and rare but serious reports of urticaria. There have also been isolated cases of photosensitivity.

Immune System: A small number of cases of increases in anti-nuclear antibodies have been reported, with and without systemic inflammatory involvement.

Haematological: Reductions in red blood cells, white blood cells and platelets have been occasionally reported. These changes are usually mild.

Psychiatric: Rarely, hallucinations, depression, confusion, amnesia, anxiety and insomnia have been reported.

Gastrointestinal: Occasionally nausea and vomiting. The following have been also reported: abdominal pain, anorexia, constipation, diarrhoea, dyspepsia and flatulence (bloating).

Liver and Bilary System: A number of cases of elevated liver enzymes and jaundice have been reported in association with Tambocor treatment. So far this has always been reversible on stopping treatment. Hepatic dysfunction has also been reported.

Neurological: Most commonly giddiness, dizziness and lightheadedness which are usually transient. Rare instances of dyskinesia have been reported, which have improved on withdrawal of flecainide therapy. Rare instances of convulsions, and during long term therapy a few cases of peripheral neuropathy, paraesthesia and ataxia have been reported. There also have been reports of flushing, headache, hypoaesthesia, increased sweating, somnolence, syncope, tinnitus, tremor and vertigo.

Ophthalmological: Visual disturbances, such as double vision and blurring of vision may occur but these are usually transient and disappear upon continuing or reducing the dosage.

Extremely rare cases of corneal deposits have also been reported.

Respiratory: Dyspnoea and rare cases of pneumonitis have been reported.

4.9 Overdose

Overdosage with flecainide is a potentially life threatening medical emergency. No specific antidote is known. There is no known way of rapidly removing flecainide from the system, but forced acid diuresis may theoretically be helpful. Neither dialysis nor haemoperfusion is helpful and injections of anticholinergics are not recommended.

Treatment may include therapy with an inotropic agent, intravenous calcium, giving circulatory assistance (eg balloon pumping), mechanically assisting respiration, or temporarily inserting a transvenous pacemaker if there are severe conduction disturbances or the patient's left ventricular function is otherwise compromised.

5. PHARMACOLOGICAL PROPERTIES

5.1 Pharmacodynamic properties

Tambocor is a Class 1 anti-arrhythmic (local anaesthetic) agent.

Tambocor slows conduction through the heart, having its greatest effect on His Bundle conduction. It also acts selectively to increase anterograde and particularly retrograde accessory pathway refractoriness. Its actions may be reflected in the ECG by prolongation of the PR interval and widening of the QRS complex. The effect on the JT interval is insignificant.

5.2 Pharmacokinetic properties

Intravenous administration of 0.5 - 2.0 mg/kg to healthy subjects resulted in plasma concentrations ranging from 70 - 340 mcg/l. Protein binding ranges from 32 to 58%. The volume of distribution in healthy subjects following intravenous infusion of 2 mg/kg averaged 512 litres.

The elimination half life after IV administration to patients was 7 to 19 hours.

5.3 Preclinical safety data

Not applicable

6. PHARMACEUTICAL PARTICULARS

6.1 List of excipients

Sodium Acetate PhEur.

Glacial Acetic Acid Ph Eur

Water for injections.

6.2 Incompatibilities

None known

6.3 Shelf life

3 years

6.4 Special precautions for storage

Do not store above 30°C. Do not freeze. Protect from light.

6.5 Nature and contents of container

Boxes containing 5 × 15 ml glass ampoules.

6.6 Instructions for use and handling

Dilution: When necessary Tambocor injection should be diluted with, or injected into, sterile solutions of 5% dextrose. If chloride containing solutions, such as sodium chloride or Ringer's lactate are used, the injection should be added to a volume of not less than 500 ml, otherwise a precipitate will form.

7. MARKETING AUTHORISATION HOLDER

3M Health Care Limited

1 Morley Street

Loughborough

Leics.

LE11 1EP

8. MARKETING AUTHORISATION NUMBER(S)

0068/ 0101

9. DATE OF FIRST AUTHORISATION/RENEWAL OF THE AUTHORISATION

7 April 1983 / 14 April 1999

10. DATE OF REVISION OF THE TEXT

July 2003

Tambocor 50mg Tablets

(3M Health Care Limited)

1. NAME OF THE MEDICINAL PRODUCT

Tambocor® 50mg Tablets

2. QUALITATIVE AND QUANTITATIVE COMPOSITION

Each tablet contains flecainide acetate 50mg

3. PHARMACEUTICAL FORM

Tablet

4. CLINICAL PARTICULARS

Tambocor is a potent sodium channel blocking agent for the treatment of the conditions listed below:

The effect on the JT interval is insignificant at therapeutic levels.

4.1 Therapeutic indications

Tambocor tablets are indicated for:

a) AV nodal reciprocating tachycardia; arrhythmias associated with Wolff-Parkinson-White Syndrome and similar conditions with accessory pathways.

b) Paroxysmal atrial fibrillation in patients with disabling symptoms when treatment need has been established and in the absence of left ventricular dysfunction (see 4.4, Special warnings and special precautions for use). Arrhythmias of recent onset will respond more readily.

c) Symptomatic sustained ventricular tachycardia.

d) Premature ventricular contractions and/or non-sustained ventricular tachycardia which are causing disabling symptoms, where these are resistant to other therapy or when other treatment has not been tolerated.

Tambocor tablets can be used for the maintenance of normal rhythm following conversion by other means.

Tambocor tablets are for oral administration.

4.2 Posology and method of administration

Adults: Supraventricular arrhythmias: The recommended starting dosage is 50mg twice daily and most patients will be controlled at this dose. If required the dose may be increased to a maximum of 300mg daily.

Ventricular arrhythmias: The recommended starting dosage is 100mg twice daily. The maximum daily dose is 400mg and this is normally reserved for patients of large build or where rapid control of the arrhythmia is required.

After 3-5 days it is recommended that the dosage be progressively adjusted to the lowest level which maintains control of the arrhythmia. It may be possible to reduce dosage during long-term treatment.

Children: Tambocor is not recommended in children under 12, as there is insufficient evidence of its use in this age group.

Elderly Patients: The rate of flecainide elimination from plasma may be reduced in elderly people. This should be taken into consideration when making dose adjustments.

Plasma levels: Based on PVC suppression, it appears that plasma levels of 200-1000 ng/ml may be needed to obtain the maximum therapeutic effect. Plasma levels above 700-1000 ng/ml are associated with increased likelihood of adverse experiences.

Dosage in impaired renal function: In patients with significant renal impairment (creatinine clearance of 35ml/min/1.73 sq.m. or less) the maximum initial dosage should be 100mg daily (or 50mg twice daily).

When used in such patients, frequent plasma level monitoring is strongly recommended.

It is recommended that intravenous treatment with Tambocor should be administered in hospitals.

Treatment with oral Tambocor should be under direct hospital or specialist supervision for patients with:

a) AV nodal reciprocating tachycardia; arrhythmias associated with Wolff-Parkinson-White Syndrome and similar conditions with accessory pathways

b) Paroxysmal atrial fibrillation in patients with disabling symptoms.

Treatment for patients with other indications should continue to be initiated in hospital.

4.3 Contraindications

Tambocor is contra-indicated in cardiac failure and in patients with a history of myocardial infarction who have either asymptomatic ventricular ectopics or asymptomatic non-sustained ventricular tachycardia.

It is also contra-indicated in patients with long standing atrial fibrillation in whom there has been no attempt to convert to sinus rhythm, and in patients with haemodynamically significant valvular heart disease.

Unless pacing rescue is available, Tambocor should not be given to patients with sinus node dysfunction, atrial conduction defects, second degree or greater atrio-ventricular block, bundle branch block or distal block.

4.4 Special warnings and special precautions for use

Electrolyte disturbances should be corrected before using Tambocor.

Since flecainide elimination from the plasma can be markedly slower in patients with significant hepatic impairment, flecainide should not be used in such patients unless the potential benefits clearly outweigh the risks. Plasma level monitoring is strongly recommended in these circumstances.

Tambocor is known to increase endocardial pacing thresholds - ie to decrease endocardial pacing sensitivity. This effect is reversible and is more marked on the acute pacing threshold than on the chronic. Tambocor should thus be used with caution in all patients with permanent pacemakers or temporary pacing electrodes, and should not be administered to patients with existing poor thresholds or non-programmable pacemakers unless suitable pacing rescue is available.

Generally, a doubling of either pulse width or voltage is sufficient to regain capture, but it may be difficult to obtain ventricular thresholds less than 1 Volt at initial implantation in the presence of Tambocor.

The minor negative inotropic effect of flecainide may assume importance in patients predisposed to cardiac failure. Difficulty has been experienced in defibrillating some patients. Most of the cases reported had pre-existing heart disease with cardiac enlargement, a history of myocardial infarction, arterio-sclerotic heart disease and cardiac failure.

Tambocor should be avoided in patients with structural organic heart disease or abnormal left ventricular function.

Tambocor should be used with caution in patients with acute onset of atrial fibrillation following cardiac surgery.

In a large scale, placebo-controlled clinical trial in post-myocardial infarction patients with asymptomatic ventricular arrhythmia, oral flecainide was associated with a 2.2 fold higher incidence of mortality or non-fatal cardiac arrest as compared with its matching placebo. In that same study, an even higher incidence of mortality was observed in flecainide-treated patients with more than one myocardial infarction. Comparable placebo-controlled clinical trials have not been done to determine if flecainide is associated with higher risk of mortality in other patient groups.

4.5 Interaction with other medicinal products and other forms of Interaction

Flecainide is a class I anti-arrhythmic and interactions are possible with other anti-arrhythmic drugs where additive effects may occur or where drugs interfere with the metabolism of flecainide. The following known categories of drugs may intereact with flecainide:

Cardiac glycosides; Flecainide can cause the plasma *digoxin* level to rise by about 15%, which is unlikely to be of clinical significance for patients with plasma levels in the therapeutic range. It is recommended that the *digoxin* plasma level in digitalised patients should be measured not less than six hours after any *digoxin* dose, before or after administration of flecainide.

Class II anti-arrhythmics; the possibility of additive negative inotropic effects of beta-blockers and other cardiac depressants with flecainide should be recognised

Class III anti-arrhythmics; when flecainide is given in the presence of *amiodarone*, the usual flecainide dosage should be reduced by 50% and the patient monitored closely for adverse effects. Plasma level monitoring is strongly recommended in these circumstances

Class IV anti-arrhythmics; use of flecainide with other sodium channel blockers is not recommended.

Anti-depressants; *fluoxetine* increases plasma flecainide concentration; increased risk of arrhythmias with *tricyclics*; manufacturer of *reboxetine* advises caution.

Anti-epileptics; limited data in patients receiving known enzyme inducers (*phenytoin, phenobarbital, carbamazepine*) indicate only a 30% increase in the rate of flecainide elimination.

Anti-psychotics: *clozapine* – increased risk of arrhythmias

Anti-histamines; increased risk of ventricular arrhythmias with *mizolastine* and *terfenadine* (avoid concomitant use)

Anti-malarials: *quinine* increases plasma concentration of flecainide.

Antivirals: plasma concentration increased by *ritonavir, lopinavar* and *indinavir* (increased risk of ventricular arrhythmias (avoid concomitant use)

Diuretics: Class effect due to hypokalaemia giving rise to cardiac toxicity.

Ulcer healing drugs: *cimetidine* inhibits metabolism of flecainide. In healthy subjects receiving *cimetidine* (1g daily) for one week, plasma flecainide levels increased by about 30% and the half-life increased by about 10%.

Anti-smoking aids: Co-administration of *bupropion* with drugs that are metabolized by CYP2D6 isoenzyme including flecainide, should be approached with caution and should be initiated at the lower end of the dose range of the concomitant medication. If *bupropion* is added to the treatment regimen of a patient already receiving flecainide, the need to decrease the dose of the original medication should be considered.

Treatment with Tambocor is compatible with use of oral anti-coagulants.

4.6 Pregnancy and lactation
There is no evidence as to drug safety in human pregnancy. In New Zealand White rabbits high doses of flecainide caused some foetal abnormalities, but these effects were not seen in Dutch Belted rabbits or rats. The relevance of these findings to humans has not been established. Data have shown that flecainide crosses the placenta to the foetus in patients taking flecainide during pregnancy.

Flecainide is excreted in human milk and appears in concentrations which reflect those in maternal blood. The risk of adverse effects to the nursing infant is very small.

4.7 Effects on ability to drive and use machines
No effect.

4.8 Undesirable effects
Body as a Whole: Asthenia, fatigue, fever, oedema.

Cardiovascular: Pro-arrhythmic effects occur but are most likely in patients with structural heart disease and/or significant left ventricular impairment.

In patients with atrial flutter the use of Tambocor has been associated with

1:1 AV conduction following initial atrial slowing with resultant ventricular acceleration. This has been seen most commonly following the use of the injection for acute conversion. This effect is usually short lived and abates quickly following cessation of therapy.

The following adverse effects have also been reported.

AV block-second-degree and third degree, bradycardia, cardiac failure/congestive cardiac failure, chest pain, hypotension, myocardial infarction, palpitation, sinus pause or arrest and tachycardia (AT or VT).

Skin and Appendages: A range of allergic skin reactions have been reported including rashes, alopecia and rare but serious reports of urticaria. There have also been isolated cases of photosensitivityand rash.

Immune System: A small number of cases of increases in anti-nuclear antibodies have been reported, with and without systemic inflammatory involvement.

Haematological: Reductions in red blood cells, white blood cells and platelets have been occasionally reported. These changes are usually mild.

Psychiatric: Rarely, hallucinations, depression, confusion, amnesia, anxiety and insomnia have been reported.

Gastrointestinal: Occasionally nausea and vomiting. The following have also been reported: abdominal pain, anorexia, constipation, diarrhoea, dyspepsia and flatulence (bloating)

Liver and Bilary System: A number of cases of elevated liver enzymes and jaundice have been reported in association with Tambocor treatment. So far this has always been reversible on stopping treatment. Hepatic dysfunction has also been reported.

Neurological: Most commonly giddiness, dizziness and lightheadedness which are usually transient. Rare instances of dyskinesia have been reported, which have improved on withdrawal of flecainide therapy. Rare instances of convulsions, and during long term therapy a few cases of peripheral neuropathy, paraesthesia and ataxia have been reported. There also have been reports of flushing, headache, hypoaesthesia, increased sweating, somnolence, syncope, tinnitus, tremor and vertigo.

Ophthalmological: Visual disturbances, such as double vision and blurring of vision may occur but these are usually transient and disappear upon continuing or reducing the dosage.

Extremely rare cases of corneal deposits have also been reported.

Respiratory: Dyspnoea and rare cases of pneumonitis have been reported.

4.9 Overdose
Overdosage with flecainide is a potentially life threatening medical emergency. No specific antidote is known. There is no known way of rapidly removing flecainide from the system, but forced acid diuresis may theoretically be helpful. Neither dialysis nor haemoperfusion is helpful and injections of anticholinergics are not recommended.

Treatment may include therapy with an inotropic agent, intravenous calcium, giving circulatory assistance (eg balloon pumping), mechanically assisting respiration, or temporarily inserting a transvenous pacemaker if there are severe conduction disturbances or the patient's left ventricular function is otherwise compromised.

5. PHARMACOLOGICAL PROPERTIES

5.1 Pharmacodynamic properties
Tambocor is a Class 1 anti-arrhythmic (local anaesthetic) agent.

Tambocor slows conduction through the heart, having its greatest effect on His Bundle conduction. It also acts selectively to increase anterograde and particularly retrograde accessory pathway refractoriness. Its actions may be reflected in the ECG by prolongation of the PR interval and widening of the QRS complex. The effect on the JT interval is insignificant.

5.2 Pharmacokinetic properties
Oral administration of flecainide results in extensive absorption, with bioavailability approaching 90 to 95%. Flecainide does not appear to undergo significant hepatic first-pass metabolism. In patients, 200 to 600 mg flecainide daily produced plasma concentrations within the therapeutic range of 200-

1000 μg/L. Protein binding of flecainide is within the range 32 to 58%.

Recovery of unchanged flecainide in urine of healthy subjects was approximately 42% of a 200mg oral dose, whilst the two major metabolites (Meta-O-Dealkylated and Dealkylated Lactam Metabolites) accounted for a further 14% each. The elimination half-life was 12 to 27 hours.

5.3 Preclinical safety data
Not applicable

6. PHARMACEUTICAL PARTICULARS

6.1 List of excipients
Pregelatinised Starch, USNF

Croscarmellose Sodium, USNF

Microcrystalline Cellulose, Ph Eur

Hydrogenated Vegetable Oil, USNF

Magnesium Stearate, Ph Eur

6.2 Incompatibilities
None known

6.3 Shelf life
5 years

6.4 Special precautions for storage
Do not store above 30°C. Keep container in the outer carton.

6.5 Nature and contents of container
UPVC/PVDC blister packs containing 60 tablets

6.6 Instructions for use and handling
Not applicable

7. MARKETING AUTHORISATION HOLDER
3M Health Care Limited

1 Morley Street

Loughborough

Leics.

LE11 1EP

8. MARKETING AUTHORISATION NUMBER(S)
0068/0152

9. DATE OF FIRST AUTHORISATION/RENEWAL OF THE AUTHORISATION
22 May 1997

10. DATE OF REVISION OF THE TEXT
July 2003

Tamiflu

(Roche Products Limited)

1. NAME OF THE MEDICINAL PRODUCT
Tamiflu▼ 75 mg capsule, hard.

2. QUALITATIVE AND QUANTITATIVE COMPOSITION
Each hard capsule contains 98.5 mg oseltamivir phosphate, corresponding to 75 mg of oseltamivir.

For excipients, see 6.1.

3. PHARMACEUTICAL FORM
Capsule, hard.

The hard capsule consists of a grey opaque body bearing the imprint "ROCHE" and a light yellow opaque cap bearing the imprint "75 mg". Imprints are blue.

4. CLINICAL PARTICULARS

4.1 Therapeutic indications
Treatment of influenza in adults and children one year of age or older who present with symptoms typical of influenza, when influenza virus is circulating in the community. Efficacy has been demonstrated when treatment is initiated within two days of first onset of symptoms. This indication is based on clinical studies of naturally occurring influenza in which the predominant infection was influenza A (see section 5.1).

-Prevention of influenza

- Post exposure prevention in adults and adolescents 13 years of age or older following contact with a clinically diagnosed influenza case when influenza virus is circulating in the community.

- The appropriate use of Tamiflu for prevention of influenza should be determined on a case by case basis by the circumstances and the population requiring protection. In exceptional situations (e.g. in case of a mismatch between the circulating and vaccine virus strains, and a pandemic situation) seasonal prevention could be considered in adults and adolescents 13 years of age or older.

Tamiflu is not a substitute for influenza vaccination.

The use of antivirals for the treatment and prevention of influenza should be determined on the basis of official recommendations taking into consideration variability of epidemiology and the impact of the disease in different geographical areas and patient populations.

4.2 Posology and method of administration
Tamiflu capsules and Tamiflu suspension are bioequivalent formulations, 75 mg doses can be administered as either one 75 mg capsule or by administering one 30 mg dose plus one 45 mg dose of suspension. Adults, adolescents or children (> 40 kg) who are unable to swallow capsules may receive appropriate doses of Tamiflu suspension.

Treatment of influenza

Treatment should be initiated as soon as possible within the first two days of onset of symptoms of influenza.

For adults and adolescents 13 years or older the recommended oral dose is 75 mg oseltamivir twice daily, for 5 days.

For children one year or older, Tamiflu oral suspension is available. For children with body weight above 40 kg, capsules may be prescribed at the adult dosage of 75 mg twice daily for 5 days.

The safety and efficacy of Tamiflu in children less than one year of age have not been established (Please see also Section 5.3 Preclinical Safety Data).

Prevention of influenza

Post exposure prevention in adults and adolescents 13 years or older: The recommended dose for prevention of influenza following close contact with an infected individual is 75 mg oseltamivir once daily for at least 7 days. Therapy should begin as soon as possible within two days of exposure to an infected individual.

Prevention during an influenza epidemic in the community: The recommended dose for prevention of influenza during a community outbreak is 75 mg oseltamivir once daily for up to six weeks.

The safety and efficacy of Tamiflu for the prevention of influenza in children 12 years or younger have not been established.

Special populations

Hepatic impairment

No dose adjustment is required either for treatment or for prevention, in patients with hepatic dysfunction.

Renal impairment

Treatment of influenza: Dose adjustment is recommended for adults with severe renal impairment. Recommended doses are detailed in the table below.

Creatinine clearance	Recommended dose for treatment
>30 (ml/min)	75 mg twice daily
>10 to ⩽30 (ml/min)	75 mg once daily or 30 mg suspension twice daily
⩽10 (ml/min)	Not recommended
dialysis patients	Not recommended

Prevention of influenza: Dose adjustment is recommended for adults with severe renal impairment as detailed in the table below

Creatinine clearance	Recommended dose for prevention
>30 (ml/min)	75 mg once daily
>10 to ⩽30 (ml/min)	75 mg every second day or 30 mg suspension once daily
⩽10 (ml/min)	Not recommended
dialysis patients	Not recommended

Elderly

No dose adjustment is required, unless there is evidence of severe renal impairment.

4.3 Contraindications
Hypersensitivity to oseltamivir phosphate or to any of the excipients.

4.4 Special warnings and special precautions for use
Oseltamivir is effective only against illness caused by influenza viruses. There is no evidence for efficacy of oseltamivir in any illness caused by agents other than influenza viruses.

The safety and efficacy of oseltamivir treatment of children of less than one year of age have not been established (Please see also Section 5.3 Preclinical Safety Data).

The safety and efficacy of oseltamivir for the prevention of influenza in children 12 years or younger have not been established.

No information is available regarding the safety and efficacy of oseltamivir in patients with any medical condition sufficiently severe or unstable to be considered at imminent risk of requiring hospitalisation.

The safety and efficacy of oseltamivir in either treatment or prevention of influenza in immunocompromised patients have not been established.

Efficacy of oseltamivir in the treatment of subjects with chronic cardiac disease and/or respiratory disease has not been established. No difference in the incidence of complications was observed between the treatment and placebo groups in this population (see section 5.1).

Tamiflu is not a substitute for influenza vaccination. Use of Tamiflu must not affect the evaluation of individuals for annual influenza vaccination. The protection against influenza lasts only as long as Tamiflu is administered. Tamiflu should be used for the treatment and prevention of influenza only when reliable epidemiological data indicate that influenza virus is circulating in the community.

Severe renal impairment

Dose adjustment is recommended for both treatment and prevention in adults with severe renal insufficiency. There are no data concerning the safety and efficacy of oseltamivir in children with renal impairment (see 4.2 Posology and method of administration and 5.2 Pharmacokinetic properties).

4.5 Interaction with other medicinal products and other forms of Interaction

Pharmacokinetic properties of oseltamivir, such as low protein binding and metabolism independent of the CYP450 and glucuronidase systems (See 5.2, Pharmacokinetic properties), suggest that clinically significant drug interactions via these mechanisms are unlikely.

No dose adjustment is required when co-administering with probenecid in patients with normal renal function. Co-administration of probenecid, a potent inhibitor of the anionic pathway of renal tubular secretion results in an approximate 2-fold increase in exposure to the active metabolite of oseltamivir.

Oseltamivir has no kinetic interaction with amoxicillin, which is eliminated via the same pathway suggesting that oseltamivir interaction with this pathway is weak.

Clinically important drug interactions involving competition for renal tubular secretion are unlikely, due to the known safety margin for most of these substances, the elimination characteristics of the active metabolite (glomerular filtration and anionic tubular secretion) and the excretion capacity of these pathways. However, care should be taken when prescribing oseltamivir in subjects when taking co-excreted agents with a narrow therapeutic margin (e.g. chlorpropamide, methotrexate, phenylbutazone).

No pharmacokinetic interactions between oseltamivir or its major metabolite have been observed when co-administering oseltamivir with paracetamol, acetyl-salicylic acid, cimetidine or with antacids (magnesium and aluminium hydroxides and calcium carbonates).

4.6 Pregnancy and lactation

There are no adequate data from the use of oseltamivir in pregnant women. Animal studies do not indicate direct or indirect harmful effects with respect to pregnancy, embryonal/foetal or postnatal development (see 5.3). Oseltamivir should not be used during pregnancy unless the potential benefit to the mother justifies the potential risk to the foetus.

In lactating rats, oseltamivir and the active metabolite are excreted in the milk. It is not known whether oseltamivir or the active metabolite are excreted in human milk. Oseltamivir should be used during lactation only if the potential benefit for the mother justifies the potential risk for the nursing infant.

4.7 Effects on ability to drive and use machines

Tamiflu has no known influence on the ability to drive and use machines.

4.8 Undesirable effects

Treatment of influenza in adults and adolescents: A total of 2107 patients participated in phase III studies in the treatment of influenza. The most frequently reported undesirable effects were nausea, vomiting and abdominal pain. The majority of these events were reported on a single occasion on either the first or second treatment day and resolved spontaneously within 1-2 days. All events that were reported commonly, (i.e. at an incidence of at least 1 %, irrespective of causality) in subjects receiving oseltamivir 75 mg twice daily, are included in the table below.

Treatment of influenza in elderly: In general, the safety profile in the elderly patients was similar to adults aged up to 65 years: the incidence of nausea was lower in oseltamivir treated elderly persons (6.7 %) than in those taking placebo (7.8 %) whereas the incidence of vomiting was higher in those who received oseltamivir (4.7 %) than among placebo recipients (3.1 %).

The adverse event profile in adolescents and in the patients with chronic cardiac and/or respiratory disease was qualitatively similar to that of healthy young adults.

Prevention of influenza In prevention studies, where the dosage of oseltamivir was 75 mg once daily for up to 6 weeks,, adverse events reported more commonly in subjects receiving oseltamivir compared to subjects receiving placebo (in addition to the events listed in the table below) were: Aches and pains, rhinorrhoea, dyspepsia and upper respiratory tract infection. There were no clinically relevant differences in the safety profile of the elderly subjects, who received oseltamivir or placebo, compared with the younger population.

Most Frequent Adverse Events in Studies in Naturally Acquired Influenza

(see Table 1)

Treatment of influenza in children: A total of 1032 children aged 1 to 12 years (including 695 otherwise healthy children aged 1 to 12 years and 334 asthmatic children aged 6 to 12 years) participated in phase III studies of oseltamivir given for the treatment of influenza. A total of 515 children received treatment with oseltamivir suspension. Adverse events occurring in greater than 1 % of children receiving oseltamivir are listed in the table below. The most frequently reported adverse event was vomiting. Other events reported more frequently by oseltamivir treated children included abdominal pain, epistaxis, ear disorder and conjunctivitis. These events generally occurred once, resolved despite continued dosing and did not cause discontinuation of treatment in the vast majority of cases.

Adverse Events occurring in greater than 1 % of children enrolled in Phase III studies of oseltamivir treatment of naturally acquired influenza.

(see Table 2)

In general, the adverse event profile in the children with asthma was qualitatively similar to that of otherwise healthy children.

Observed during clinical practice: The following adverse reactions have been reported during postmarketing use of oseltamivir: dermatitis, rash, eczema, urticaria, hypersensitivity reactions, including anaphylactic/anaphylactoid reactions, as well as very rare reports of severe skin reactions, including Stevens-Johnson Syndrome and erythema multiforme. Additionally, there are very rare reports of hepatic function disorders, including hepatitis and elevated liver enzymes in patients with influenza-like illness.

4.9 Overdose

There is no experience with overdose. However, the anticipated manifestations of acute overdose would be nausea, with or without accompanying vomiting, and dizziness. Patients should discontinue the treatment in the event of overdose. No specific antidote is known.

5. PHARMACOLOGICAL PROPERTIES

5.1 Pharmacodynamic properties

Pharmacotherapeutic group: Antiviral

ATC code: J05AH02

Oseltamivir is a pro-drug of the active metabolite (oseltamivir carboxylate). The active metabolite is a selective inhibitor of influenza virus neuraminidase enzymes, which are glycoproteins found on the virion surface. Viral neuraminidase enzyme activity is essential for the release of recently formed virus particles from infected cells and the further spread of infectious virus in the body.

Oseltamivir carboxylate inhibits influenza A and B neuraminidases *in vitro*. Oseltamivir given orally inhibits influenza A and B virus replication and pathogenicity *in vivo* in animal

Table 1 Most Frequent Adverse Events in Studies in Naturally Acquired Influenza

System Organ Class	Adverse Event	Treatment		Prevention	
		Placebo (N=1050)	Oseltamivir 75 mg twice daily (N=1057)	Placebo (N=1434)	Oseltamivir 75 mg once daily (N=1480)
Gastrointestinal Disorders	Vomiting [2]	3.0 %	8.0 %	1.0 %	2.1 %
	Nausea [1, 2]	5.7 %	7.9 %	3.9 %	7.0 %
	Diarrhoea	8.0 %	5.5 %	2.6 %	3.2 %
	Abdominal Pain	2.0 %	2.2 %	1.6 %	2.0 %
Infections and Infestations	Bronchitis	5.0 %	3.7 %	1.2 %	0.7 %
	Bronchitis acute	1.0 %	1.0 %	-	-
General Disorders	Dizziness	3.0 %	1.9 %	1.5 %	1.6 %
	Fatigue	0.7 %	0.8 %	7.5 %	7.9 %
Neurological Disorders	Headache Insomnia	1.5 % 1.0 %	1.6 % 1.0 %	17.5 % 1.0 %	20.1 % 1.2 %

[1] Subjects who experienced nausea alone; excludes subjects who experienced nausea in association with vomiting.

[2] The difference between the placebo and oseltamivir groups was statistically significant.

Table 2 Adverse Events occurring in greater than 1 % of children enrolled in Phase III studies of oseltamivir treatment of naturally acquired influenza

System Organ Class	Adverse Event	Treatment	
		Placebo (N = 517)	Oseltamivir 2 mg/kg (N = 515)
Gastrointestinal Disorders	Vomiting	9.3 %	15.0 %
	Diarrhoea	10.6 %	9.5 %
	Abdominal pain	3.9 %	4.7 %
	Nausea	4.3 %	3.3 %
Infections and Infestations	Otitis media	11.2 %	8.7 %
	Pneumonia	3.3 %	1.9 %
	Sinusitis	2.5 %	1.7 %
	Bronchitis	2.1 %	1.6 %
Respiratory Disorders	Asthma (incl. aggravated)	3.7 %	3.5 %
	Epistaxis	2.5 %	3.1 %
Disorders of the Ear and Labyrinth	Ear disorder	1.2 %	1.7 %
	Tympanic membrane disorder	1.2 %	1.0 %
Skin and Subcutaneous Disorders	Dermatitis	1.9 %	1.0 %
Disorders of the Blood and Lymphatic System	Lymphadenopathy	1.5 %	1.0 %
Vision disorders	Conjunctivitis	0.4 %	1.0 %

models of influenza infection at antiviral exposures similar to that achieved in man with 75 mg twice daily.

Antiviral activity of oseltamivir was supported for influenza A and B by experimental challenge studies in healthy volunteers.

Neuraminidase enzyme IC50 values for oseltamivir for clinically isolated influenza A ranged from 0.1 nM to 1.3 nM, and for influenza B was 2.6 nM. Higher IC50 values for influenza B, up to a median of 8.5 nM, have been observed in published trials.

Reduced sensitivity of viral neuraminidase: In clinical studies in naturally acquired infection, 0.34 % (4/1177) of adults and adolescents and 4.5 % (17/374) of children aged one to 12 years were found to transiently carry influenza A virus with decreased neuraminidase susceptibility to oseltamivir carboxylate. Neuraminidase from influenza B with reduced sensitivity has not been observed either in cell culture or in clinical studies.

Cross resistance between zanamivir-resistant influenza mutants and oseltamivir-resistant influenza mutants has been observed in vitro. Insufficient information is available to fully characterise the risk of emergence of oseltamivir resistance and cross-resistance in clinical use.

Treatment of influenza infection

Oseltamivir is effective only against illnesses caused by influenza virus. Statistical analyses are therefore presented only for influenza-infected subjects. In the pooled treatment study population which included both influenza-positive and-negative subjects (ITT) primary efficacy was reduced proportional to the number of influenza-negative individuals. In the overall treatment population influenza infection was confirmed in 67 % (range 46 % to 74 %) of the recruited patients. Of the elderly subjects, 64 % were influenza positive and of those with chronic cardiac and/or respiratory disease 62 % were influenza positive. In all phase III treatment studies, patients were recruited only during the period in which influenza was circulating in the local community.

Adults and adolescents aged 13 years and older:. Patients were eligible if they reported within 36 hours of onset of symptoms, had fever ⩾37.8 °C, accompanied by at least one respiratory symptom (cough, nasal symptoms or sore throat) and at least one systemic symptom (myalgia, chills/sweats, malaise, fatigue or headache). In a pooled analysis of all influenza-positive adults and adolescents (N = 2413) enrolled into treatment studies oseltamivir 75 mg twice daily for 5 days reduced the median duration of influenza illness by approximately one day from 5.2 days (95 % CI 4.9 – 5.5 days) in the placebo group to 4.2 days (95 % CI 4.0 – 4.4 days) (p ⩽ 0.0001).

The proportion of subjects who developed specified lower respiratory tract complications (mainly bronchitis) treated with antibiotics was reduced from 12.7 % (135/1063) in the placebo group to 8.6 % (116/1350) in the oseltamivir treated population (p = 0.0012).

Treatment of influenza in high risk populations:

The median duration of influenza illness in elderly subjects (⩾ 65 years) and in subjects with chronic cardiac and/or respiratory disease receiving oseltamivir 75 mg twice daily for 5 days was not reduced significantly. The total duration of fever was reduced by one day in the groups treated with oseltamivir. In the influenza-positive elderly, oseltamivir significantly reduced the incidence of specified lower respiratory tract complications (mainly bronchitis) treated with antibiotics, from 19 % (52/268) in the placebo group to 12 % (29/250) in the oseltamivir treated population (p = 0.0156).

In influenza-positive patients with chronic cardiac and/or respiratory disease the combined incidence of lower respiratory tract complications (mainly bronchitis) treated with antibiotics was 17% (22/133) in the placebo group and 14 % (16/118) in the oseltamivir treated population (p = 0.5976).

Treatment of influenza in children: In a study of otherwise healthy children (65 % influenza-positive), aged 1 to 12 years (mean age 5.3 years), who had fever (⩾37.8° C) plus either cough or coryza, 67 % of influenza-positive patients were infected with influenza A and 33 % with influenza B. Oseltamivir treatment, started within 48 hours of onset of symptoms, significantly reduced the time to freedom from illness (defined as the simultaneous return to normal health and activity and alleviation of fever, cough and coryza,) by 1.5 days (95 % CI 0.6 - 2.2 days, p < 0.0001) compared to placebo. Oseltamivir reduced the incidence of acute otitis media from 26.5 % (53/200) in the placebo group to 16 % (29/183) in the oseltamivir treated children (p = 0.013).

A second study was completed in 334 asthmatic children aged 6 to12 years old of which 53.6 % were influenza-positive. In the oseltamivir treated group the median duration of illness was not reduced significantly. By day 6 (the last day of treatment) FEV_1 had increased by 10.8 % in the oseltamivir treated group compared to 4.7 % on placebo (p = 0.0148) in this population.

Treatment of influenza B infection: Overall 15 % of the influenza-positive population were infected by influenza B, proportions ranging from 1 to 33 % in individual studies. The median duration of illness in influenza B infected subjects did not differ significantly between the treatment groups in individual studies. Data from 504 influenza B infected subjects were pooled across all studies for analysis. Oseltamivir reduced the time to alleviation of all symptoms by 0.7 days (95 % CI 0.1 – 1.6 days; p = 0.022) and the duration of fever (⩾37.8° C), cough and coryza by one day (95 % CI 0.4 – 1.7 days; p <0.001), compared to placebo.

Prevention of influenza

The efficacy of oseltamivir in preventing naturally occurring influenza illness has been demonstrated in a post-exposure prophylaxis study in households and two seasonal prophylaxis studies. The primary efficacy parameter for all of these studies was the incidence of laboratory confirmed influenza. The virulence of influenza epidemics is not predictable and varies within a region and from season to season, therefore the number needed to treat (NNT) in order to prevent one case of influenza illness varies.

Post-exposure prevention: A study in contacts (12.6 % vaccinated against influenza) of an index case of influenza, oseltamivir 75 mg once daily, was started within 2 days of onset of symptoms in the index case and continued for seven days. Influenza was confirmed in 163 out of 377 index cases. Oseltamivir significantly reduced the incidence of clinical influenza illness occurring in the contacts of confirmed influenza cases from 24/200 (12 %) in the placebo group to 2/205 (1 %) in the oseltamivir group (92 % reduction, (95 % CI 6 – 16), p ⩽ 0.0001). The NNT in contacts of true influenza cases was 10 (95 % CI 9 – 12) and was 16 (95 % CI 15 – 19) in the whole population (ITT) regardless of infection status in the index case.

Prevention during an influenza epidemic in the community: In a pooled analysis of two other studies conducted in unvaccinated otherwise healthy adults, oseltamivir 75 mg once daily given for 6 weeks significantly reduced the incidence of clinical influenza illness from 25/519 (4.8 %) in the placebo group to 6/520 (1.2 %) in the oseltamivir group (76 % reduction, (95 % CI 1.6 – 5.7); p = 0.0006) during a community outbreak of influenza. The NNT in this study was 28 (95 % CI 24 – 50).

A study in elderly residents of nursing homes, where 80 % of participants received vaccine in the season of the study, oseltamivir 75 mg once daily given for 6 weeks significantly reduced the incidence of clinical influenza illness from 12/272 (4.4 %) in the placebo group to 1/276 (0.4 %) in the oseltamivir group (92 % reduction, (95 % CI1.5 – 6.6); p = 0.0015. The NNT in this study was 25 (95 % CI 23 – 62).

Specific studies have not been conducted to assess of the reduction in the risk of complications.

5.2 Pharmacokinetic properties

Absorption

Oseltamivir is readily absorbed from the gastrointestinal tract after oral administration of oseltamivir phosphate (pro-drug) and is extensively converted by predominantly hepatic esterases to the active metabolite (oseltamivir carboxylate). At least 75 % of an oral dose reaches the systemic circulation as the active metabolite. Exposure to the pro-drug is less than 5 % relative to the active metabolite. Plasma concentrations of both pro-drug and active metabolite are proportional to dose and are unaffected by co-administration with food.

Distribution

The mean volume of distribution at steady state of the oseltamivir carboxylate is approximately 23 litres in humans, a volume equivalent to extracellular body fluid. Since neuraminidase activity is extracellular oseltamivir carboxylate distributes to all sites of influenza virus spread.

The binding of the oseltamivir carboxylate to human plasma protein is negligible (approximately 3 %).

Metabolism

Oseltamivir is extensively converted to oseltamivir carboxylate by esterases located predominantly in the liver. *In-vitro* studies demonstrated, that neither oseltamivir, nor the active metabolite is a substrate for, or an inhibitor of, the major cytochrome P450 isoforms. No phase 2 conjugates of either compound have been identified *in vivo*.

Elimination

Absorbed oseltamivir is primarily (>90 %) eliminated by conversion to oseltamivir carboxylate. It is not further metabolised and is eliminated in the urine. Peak plasma concentrations of oseltamivir carboxylate decline with a half-life of 6 to 10 hours in most subjects. The active metabolite is eliminated entirely by renal excretion. Renal clearance (18.8 l/h) exceeds glomerular filtration rate (7.5 l/h) indicating that tubular secretion occurs in addition to glomerular filtration. Less than 20 % of an oral radiolabelled dose is eliminated in faeces.

Renal impairment

Administration of 100 mg oseltamivir phosphate twice daily for 5 days to patients with various degrees of renal impairment showed that exposure to oseltamivir carboxylate is inversely proportional to declining renal function. For dosing, see 4.2 Posology and method of administration.

Hepatic impairment

In vitro studies have concluded that exposure to oseltamivir is not expected to be increased significantly nor is exposure to the active metabolite expected to be significantly decreased in patients with hepatic impairment (See 4.2 Posology and method of administration).

Elderly

Exposure to the active metabolite at steady state was 25 to 35 % higher in elderly (age 65 to 78 years) compared to adults less than 65 years of age, given comparable doses of oseltamivir. Half–lives observed in the elderly were similar to those seen in young adults. On the basis of drug exposure and tolerability, dosage adjustments are not required for elderly patients unless there is evidence of severe renal impairment (creatinine clearance below 30 ml/min) (See 4.2 Posology and method of administration).

Children

The pharmacokinetics of oseltamivir have been evaluated in single dose pharmacokinetic studies in children aged one to 16 years. Multiple dose pharmacokinetics were studied in a small number of children enrolled in a clinical efficacy study. Younger children cleared both the prodrug and its active metabolite faster than adults, resulting in a lower exposure for a given mg/kg dose. Doses of 2 mg/kg give oseltamivir carboxylate exposures comparable to those achieved in adults, receiving a single 75 mg dose (approximately 1 mg/kg). The pharmacokinetics of oseltamivir in children over 12 years of age are similar to those in adults.

5.3 Preclinical safety data

Preclinical data reveal no special hazard for humans based on conventional studies of safety pharmacology, repeated dose toxicity and genotoxicity. Results of the conventional rodent carcinogenicity studies showed a trend towards a dose-dependent increase in the incidence of some tumours that are typical for the rodent strains used. Considering the margins of exposure in relation to the expected exposure in the human use, these findings do not change the benefit-risk of Tamiflu in its adopted therapeutic indications.

Teratology studies have been conducted in rats and rabbits at doses of up to 1500 mg/kg/day and 500 mg/kg/day, respectively. No effects on foetal development were observed. A rat fertility study up to a dose of 1500 mg/kg/day demonstrated no adverse effects on either sex. In pre- / post-natal rat studies, prolonged parturition was noted at 1500 mg/kg/day: the safety margin between human exposure and the highest no-effect dose (500 mg/kg/day) in rats is 480-fold for oseltamivir and 44-fold for the active metabolite, respectively. Foetal exposure in the rats and rabbits was approximately 15 to 20 % of that of the mother.

In lactating rats, oseltamivir and the active metabolite are excreted in the milk. It is not known whether oseltamivir or the active metabolite are excreted in human milk, but extrapolation of the animal data provides estimates of 0.01 mg/day and 0.3 mg/day for the respective compounds.

A potential for skin sensitisation to oseltamivir was observed in a "maximisation" test in guinea pigs. Approximately 50 % of the animals treated with the unformulated active ingredient showed erythema after challenging the induced animals. Reversible irritancy of rabbits' eyes was detected.

In a two-week study in unweaned rats a single dose of 1000 mg/kg oseltamivir phosphate to 7-day old pups resulted in deaths associated with unusually high exposure to the pro-drug. However, at 2000 mg/kg in 14-day old unweaned pups, there were no deaths or other significant effects. No adverse effects occurred at 500 mg/kg/day administered from 7 to 21 days *post partum.* In a single-dose investigatory study of this observation in 7-, 14- and 24-day old rats, a dose of 1000 mg/kg resulted in brain exposure to the pro-drug that suggested, respectively, 1500-, 650-, and 2-fold the exposure found in the brain of adult (42-day old) rats.

6. PHARMACEUTICAL PARTICULARS

6.1 List of excipients

Pregelatinised starch (derived from maize starch), talc, povidone, croscarmellose sodium, and sodium stearyl fumarate. The capsule shell contains gelatin, yellow iron oxide (E172), red iron oxide (E172), black iron oxide (E172) and titanium dioxide (E171). The printing ink contains shellac, titanium dioxide (E171) and FD and C Blue 2 (indigo carmine, E132).

6.2 Incompatibilities

Not applicable.

6.3 Shelf life

5 years.

6.4 Special precautions for storage

No special precautions for storage.

6.5 Nature and contents of container

One box contains 10 capsules in a triplex blister pack (PVC/PE/PVDC, sealed with aluminium foil).

6.6 Instructions for use and handling

No special requirements.

7. MARKETING AUTHORISATION HOLDER

Roche Registration Limited

40 Broadwater Road

Welwyn Garden City

Hertfordshire, AL7 3AY

United Kingdom.

8. MARKETING AUTHORISATION NUMBER(S)
EU/1/02/222/001

9. DATE OF FIRST AUTHORISATION/RENEWAL OF THE AUTHORISATION
20 June 2002

10. DATE OF REVISION OF THE TEXT
24 February 2005

Tamiflu Suspension

(Roche Products Limited)

1. NAME OF THE MEDICINAL PRODUCT
Tamiflu▼ 12 mg/ml powder for oral suspension.

2. QUALITATIVE AND QUANTITATIVE COMPOSITION
Powder for oral suspension, containing 39.4 mg oseltamivir phosphate per 1 g filling mixture.

The reconstituted suspension contains 12 mg oseltamivir per ml.

For excipients, see 6.1.

3. PHARMACEUTICAL FORM
Powder for oral suspension.

The powder is a granulate or clumped granulate with a white to light yellow colour.

4. CLINICAL PARTICULARS

4.1 Therapeutic indications
Treatment of influenza in adults and children one year of age or older who present with symptoms typical of influenza, when influenza virus is circulating in the community. Efficacy has been demonstrated when treatment is initiated within two days of first onset of symptoms. This indication is based on clinical studies of naturally occurring influenza in which the predominant infection was influenza A (see section 5.1).

-Prevention of influenza

- Post exposure prevention in adults and adolescents 13 years of age or older following a contact with clinically diagnosed influenza case when influenza virus is circulating in the community.

- The appropriate use of Tamiflu for prevention of influenza should be determined on a case by case basis by the circumstances and the population requiring protection. In exceptional situations (e.g. in case of a mismatch between the circulating and vaccine virus strains, and a pandemic situation) seasonal prevention could be considered in adults and adolescents 13 years of age or older.

Tamiflu is not a substitute for influenza vaccination.

The use of antivirals for the treatment and prevention of influenza should be determined on the basis of official recommendations taking into consideration variability of epidemiology and the impact of the disease in different geographical areas and patient populations.

4.2 Posology and method of administration
Tamiflu suspension and Tamiflu capsules are bioequivalent formulations, 75 mg doses can be administered as either one 75 mg capsule or by administering one 30 mg dose plus one 45 mg dose of suspension. Adults, adolescents or children (>40 kg) who are able to swallow capsules may receive appropriate doses of Tamiflu capsules.

Treatment of influenza

Treatment should be initiated as soon as possible within the first two days of onset of symptoms of influenza.

For adults and adolescents 13 years or older the recommended oral dose is 75 mg oseltamivir twice daily, for 5 days.

For children of one to 12 years of age: The recommended dose of Tamiflu oral suspension is indicated in the table below. The following weight adjusted dosing regimens are recommended for children one year or older:

Body Weight	Recommended dose for 5 days
⩽ 15 kg	30 mg twice daily
>15 kg to 23 kg	45 mg twice daily
>23 kg to 40 kg	60 mg twice daily
>40 kg	75 mg twice daily

For dosing an oral dispenser with 30 mg, 45 mg, and 60 mg graduations is provided in the box. For accurate dosing the oral dispenser supplied should be used exclusively.

The safety and efficacy of Tamiflu in children less than one year of age have not been established (Please see also Section 5.3 Preclinical Safety Data).

Prevention of influenza

Post exposure prevention in adults and adolescents 13 years or older the recommended dose for prevention of influenza following close contact with an infected individual is 75 mg oseltamivir once daily for at least 7 days. Therapy should begin as soon as possible within two days of exposure to an infected individual.

Prevention during an influenza epidemic in the community: The recommended dose for prevention of influenza during a community outbreak is 75 mg oseltamivir once daily for up to six weeks.

The safety and efficacy of Tamiflu for the prevention of influenza in children 12 years or younger have not been established.

Special populations

Hepatic impairment

No dose adjustment is required either for treatment or for prevention, in patients with hepatic dysfunction.

Renal impairment

Treatment of influenza: Dose adjustment is recommended for adults with severe renal impairment. Recommended doses are detailed in the table below.

Creatinine clearance	Recommended dose for treatment
>30 (ml / min)	75 mg twice daily
>10 to ⩽ 30 (ml / min)	75 mg once daily or 30 mg suspension twice daily
⩽10 (ml / min)	Not recommended
dialysis patients	Not recommended

Prevention of influenza: Dose adjustment is recommended for adults with severe renal impairment as detailed in the table below.

Creatinine clearance	Recommended dose for prevention
>30 (ml / min)	75 mg once daily
>10 to ⩽ 30 (ml / min)	75 mg every second day or 30 mg suspension once daily
⩽10 (ml / min)	Not recommended
dialysis patients	Not recommended

Elderly

No dose adjustment is required, unless there is evidence of severe renal impairment.

4.3 Contraindications
Hypersensitivity to oseltamivir phosphate or to any of the excipients.

4.4 Special warnings and special precautions for use
Oseltamivir is effective only against illness caused by influenza viruses. There is no evidence for efficacy of oseltamivir in any illness caused by agents other than influenza viruses.

The safety and efficacy of oseltamivir treatment of children of less than one year of age have not been established (Please see also Section 5.3 Preclinical Safety Data).

The safety and efficacy of oseltamivir for the prevention of influenza in children 12 years or younger have not been established.

No information is available regarding the safety and efficacy of oseltamivir in patients with any medical condition sufficiently severe or unstable to be considered at imminent risk of requiring hospitalisation.

The safety and efficacy of oseltamivir in either treatment or prevention of influenza in immunocompromised patients have not been established.

Efficacy of oseltamivir in the treatment of subjects with chronic cardiac disease and/or respiratory disease has not been established. No difference in the incidence of complications was observed between the treatment and placebo groups in this population (see section 5.1).

Tamiflu is not a substitute for influenza vaccination. Use of Tamiflu must not affect the evaluation of individuals for annual influenza vaccination. The protection against influenza lasts only as long as Tamiflu is administered. Tamiflu should be used for the treatment and prevention of influenza only when reliable epidemiological data indicate that influenza virus is circulating in the community.

Severe renal impairment

Dose adjustment is recommended for both treatment and prevention in adults with severe renal insufficiency. There are no data concerning the safety and efficacy of oseltamivir in children with renal impairment (see 4.2 Posology and method of administration and 5.2 Pharmacokinetic properties).

This medicinal product contains 26 g of sorbitol. One dose of 45 mg oseltamivir administered twice daily delivers 2.6 g of sorbitol. For subjects with hereditary fructose intolerance this is above the recommended daily maximum limit of sorbitol.

4.5 Interaction with other medicinal products and other forms of Interaction
Pharmacokinetic properties of oseltamivir, such as low protein binding and metabolism independent of the CYP450 and glucuronidase systems (See 5.2, Pharmacokinetic properties), suggest that clinically significant drug interactions via these mechanisms are unlikely.

No dose adjustment is required when co-administering with probenecid in patients with normal renal function. Co-administration of probenecid, a potent inhibitor of the anionic pathway of renal tubular secretion results in an approximate 2-fold increase in exposure to the active metabolite of oseltamivir.

Oseltamivir has no kinetic interaction with amoxicillin, which is eliminated via the same pathway suggesting that oseltamivir interaction with this pathway is weak. Clinically important drug interactions involving competition for renal tubular secretion are unlikely, due to the known safety margin for most of these substances, the elimination characteristics of the active metabolite (glomerular filtration and anionic tubular secretion) and the excretion capacity of these pathways. However, care should be taken when prescribing oseltamivir in subjects when taking co-excreted agents with a narrow therapeutic margin (e.g. chlorpropamide, methotrexate, phenylbutazone).

No pharmacokinetic interactions between oseltamivir or its major metabolite have been observed when co-administering oseltamivir with paracetamol, acetyl-salicylic acid, cimetidine or with antacids (magnesium and aluminium hydroxides and calcium carbonates).

4.6 Pregnancy and lactation
There are no adequate data from the use of oseltamivir in pregnant women. Animal studies do not indicate direct or indirect harmful effects with respect to pregnancy, embryonal/foetal or postnatal development (see 5.3). Oseltamivir should not be used during pregnancy unless the potential benefit to the mother justifies the potential risk to the foetus.

In lactating rats, oseltamivir and the active metabolite are excreted in the milk. It is not known whether oseltamivir or the active metabolite are excreted in human milk. Oseltamivir should be used during lactation only if the potential benefit for the mother justifies the potential risk for the nursing infant.

4.7 Effects on ability to drive and use machines
Tamiflu has no known influence on the ability to drive and use machines.

4.8 Undesirable effects
Treatment of influenza in adults and adolescents: A total of 2107 patients participated in phase III studies in the treatment of influenza. The most frequently reported undesirable effects were nausea, vomiting and abdominal pain. The majority of these events were reported on a single occasion on either the first or second treatment day and resolved spontaneously within 1-2 days. All events that were reported commonly, (i.e. at an incidence of at least 1 %, irrespective of causality) in subjects receiving oseltamivir 75 mg twice daily, are included in the table below.

Treatment of influenza in elderly: In general, the safety profile in the elderly patients was similar to adults aged up to 65 years: the incidence of nausea was lower in oseltamivir treated elderly persons (6.7 %) than in those taking placebo (7.8 %) whereas the incidence of vomiting was higher in those who received oseltamivir (4.7 %) than among placebo recipients (3.1 %).

The adverse event profile in adolescents and in the patients with chronic cardiac and/or respiratory disease was qualitatively similar to that of healthy young adults.

Prevention of influenza. In prevention studies, where the dosage of oseltamivir was 75 mg once daily for up to 6 weeks, adverse events reported more commonly in subjects receiving oseltamivir compared to subjects receiving placebo (in addition to the events listed in the table below) were: Aches and pains, rhinorrhoea, dyspepsia and upper respiratory tract infection. There were no clinically relevant differences in the safety profile of the elderly subjects, who received oseltamivir or placebo, compared with the younger population.

Most Frequent Adverse Events in Studies in Naturally Acquired Influenza

(see Table 1 on next page)

Treatment of influenza in children: A total of 1032 children aged 1 to 12 years (including 695 otherwise healthy children aged 1 to 12 years and 334 asthmatic children aged 6 to 12 years) participated in phase III studies of oseltamivir given for the treatment of influenza. A total of 515 children received treatment with oseltamivir suspension. Adverse events occurring in greater 1 % of children receiving oseltamivir are listed in the table below. The most frequently reported adverse event was vomiting. Other events reported more frequently by oseltamivir treated children included abdominal pain, epistaxis, ear disorder and conjunctivitis. These events generally occurred once, resolved despite continued dosing and did not cause discontinuation of treatment in the vast majority of cases.

Adverse Events occurring in greater 1 % of children enrolled in Phase III studies of oseltamivir treatment of naturally acquired influenza.

(see Table 2 on next page)

In general, the adverse event profile in the children with asthma was qualitatively similar to that of otherwise healthy children.

Table 1 Most Frequent Adverse Events in Studies in Naturally Acquired Influenza

System Organ Class	Adverse Event	Treatment		Prevention	
		Placebo (N = 1050)	Oseltamivir 75 mg twice daily (N = 1057)	Placebo (N = 1434)	Oseltamivir 75 mg once daily (N = 1480)
Gastrointestinal Disorders	Vomiting [2]	3.0 %	8.0 %	1.0 %	2.1 %
	Nausea [1, 2]	5.7 %	7.9 %	3.9 %	7.0 %
	Diarrhoea	8.0 %	5.5 %	2.6 %	3.2 %
	Abdominal Pain	2.0 %	2.2 %	1.6 %	2.0 %
Infections and Infestations	Bronchitis	5.0 %	3.7 %	1.2 %	0.7 %
	Bronchitis acute	1.0 %	1.0 %		-
General Disorders	Dizziness	3.0 %	1.9 %	1.5 %	1.6 %
	Fatigue	0.7 %	0.8 %	7.5 %	7.9 %
Neurological Disorders	Headache	1.5 %	1.6 %	17.5 %	20.1 %
	Insomnia	1.0 %	1.0 %	1.0 %	1.2 %

[1] Subjects who experienced nausea alone; excludes subjects who experienced nausea in association with vomiting.
[2] The difference between the placebo and oseltamivir groups was statistically significant.

Table 2 Adverse Events occurring in greater 1 % of children enrolled in Phase III studies of oseltamivir treatment of naturally acquired influenza

System Organ Class	Adverse Event	Treatment	
		Placebo (N = 517)	Oseltamivir 2 mg/kg (N = 515)
Gastrointestinal Disorders	Vomiting	9.3 %	15.0 %
	Diarrhoea	10.6 %	9.5 %
	Abdominal pain	3.9 %	4.7 %
	Nausea	4.3 %	3.3 %
Infections and Infestations	Otitis media	11.2 %	8.7 %
	Pneumonia	3.3 %	1.9 %
	Sinusitis	2.5 %	1.7 %
	Bronchitis	2.1 %	1.6 %
Respiratory Disorders	Asthma (incl. aggravated)	3.7 %	3.5 %
	Epistaxis	2.5 %	3.1 %
Disorders of the Ear and Labyrinth	Ear disorder	1.2 %	1.7 %
	Tympanic membrane disorder	1.2 %	1.0 %
Skin and Subcutaneous Disorders	Dermatitis	1.9 %	1.0 %
Disorders of the Blood and Lymphatic System	Lymphadenopathy	1.5 %	1.0 %
Vision disorders	Conjunctivitis	0.4 %	1.0 %

Observed during clinical practice: The following adverse reactions have been reported during postmarketing use of oseltamivir: dermatitis, rash, eczema, urticaria, hypersensitivity reactions, including anaphylactic/anaphylactoid reactions, as well as very rare reports of severe skin reactions, including Stevens-Johnson Syndrome and erythema multiforme. Additionally, there are very rare reports of hepatic function disorders, including hepatitis and elevated liver enzymes in patients with influenza-like illness.

4.9 Overdose

There is no experience with overdose. However, the anticipated manifestations of acute overdose would be nausea, with or without accompanying vomiting, and dizziness. Patients should discontinue the treatment in the event of overdose. No specific antidote is known.

5. PHARMACOLOGICAL PROPERTIES

5.1 Pharmacodynamic properties

Pharmacotherapeutic group: Antiviral

ATC code: J05AH02

Oseltamivir is a pro-drug of the active metabolite (oseltamivir carboxylate). The active metabolite is a selective inhibitor of influenza virus neuraminidase enzymes, which are glycoproteins found on the virion surface. Viral neuraminidase enzyme activity is essential for the release of recently formed virus particles from infected cells and the further spread of infectious virus in the body.

Oseltamivir carboxylate inhibits influenza A and B neuraminidases *in vitro*. Oseltamivir given orally inhibits influenza A and B virus replication and pathogenicity *in vivo* in animal models of influenza infection at antiviral exposures similar to that achieved in man with 75 mg twice daily.

Antiviral activity of oseltamivir was supported for influenza A and B by experimental challenge studies in healthy volunteers.

Neuraminidase enzyme IC50 values for oseltamivir for clinically isolated influenza A ranged from 0.1nM to 1.3nM, and for influenza B was 2.6nM. Higher IC50 values for influenza B, up to a median of 8.5nM, have been observed in published trials.

Reduced sensitivity of viral neuraminidase In clinical studies in naturally acquired infection, 0.34 % (4/1177) of adults and adolescents and 4.5 % (17/374) of children aged one to 12 years were found to transiently carry influenza A virus with decreased neuraminidase susceptibility to oseltamivir carboxylate. Neuraminidase from influenza B with reduced sensitivity has not been observed either in cell culture or in clinical studies.

Cross resistance between zanamivir-resistant influenza mutants and oseltamivir-resistant influenza mutants has been observed in vitro. Insufficient information is available to fully characterise the risk of emergence of oseltamivir resistance and cross-resistance in clinical use.

Treatment of influenza infection

Oseltamivir is effective only against illnesses caused by influenza virus. Statistical analyses are therefore presented only for influenza-infected subjects. In the pooled treatment study population which included both influenza-positive and -negative subjects (ITT) primary efficacy was reduced proportional to the number of influenza negative individuals. In the overall treatment population influenza infection was confirmed in 67 % (range 46 % to 74 %) of the recruited patients. Of the elderly subjects, 64 % were influenza positive and of those with chronic cardiac and/or respiratory disease 62 % were influenza positive. In all phase III treatment studies, patients were recruited only during the period in which influenza was circulating in the local community.

Adults and adolescents aged 13 years and older: Patients were eligible if they reported within 36 hours of onset of symptoms, had fever ⩾37.8°C, accompanied by at least one respiratory symptom (cough, nasal symptoms or sore throat) and at least one systemic symptom (myalgia, chills/sweats, malaise, fatigue or headache). In a pooled analysis of all influenza-positive adults and adolescents (N = 2413) enrolled into treatment studies oseltamivir 75 mg twice daily for 5 days reduced the median duration of influenza illness by approximately one day from 5.2 days (95 % CI 4.9 – 5.5 days) in the placebo group to 4.2 days (95 % CI 4.0 – 4.4 days) ($p \leqslant 0.0001$).

The proportion of subjects who developed specified lower respiratory tract complications(mainly bronchitis) treated with antibiotics was reduced from 12.7 % (135/1063) in the placebo group to 8.6 % (116/1350) in the oseltamivir treated population ($p = 0.0012$).

Treatment of influenza in high risk populations:

The median duration of influenza illness in elderly subjects (⩾ 65 years) and in subjects with chronic cardiac and/or respiratory disease receiving oseltamivir 75 mg twice daily for 5 days was _not_ reduced significantly. The total duration of fever was reduced by one day in the groups treated with oseltamivir. In the influenza-positive elderly, oseltamivir significantly reduced the incidence of specified lower respiratory tract complications (mainly bronchitis) treated with antibiotics, from 19 % (52/268) in the placebo group to 12 % (29/250) in the oseltamivir treated population ($p = 0.0156$).

In influenza-positive patients with chronic cardiac and/or respiratory disease the combined incidence of lower respiratory tract complications (mainly bronchitis) treated with antibiotics was 17 % (22/133) in the placebo group and 14 % (16/118) in the oseltamivir treated population ($p = 0.5976$).

Treatment of influenza in children: In a study of otherwise healthy children (65% influenza-positive), aged 1 to 12 years (mean age 5.3 years), who had fever (⩾ 37.8°C) plus either cough or coryza, 67 % of influenza-positive patients were infected with influenza A and 33 % with influenza B. Oseltamivir treatment started within 48 hours of onset of symptoms, significantly reduced the duration of time to freedom from illness (defined as the simultaneous return to normal health and activity and alleviation of fever, cough and coryza) by 1.5 days (95 % CI 0.6 - 2.2 days, $p < 0.0001$) compared to placebo. Oseltamivir reduced the incidence of acute otitis media from 26.5 % (53/200) in the placebo group to 16 % (29/183) in the oseltamivir treated children ($p = 0.013$).

A second study was completed in 334 asthmatic children aged 6 to12 years old of which 53.6 % were influenza-positive. In the oseltamivir treated group the median duration of illness was _not_ reduced significantly. By day 6 (the last day of treatment) FEV_1 had increased by 10.8 % in the oseltamivir treated group compared to 4.7 % on placebo ($p = 0.0148$) in this population.

Treatment of influenza B infection: Overall 15 % of the influenza-positive population were infected by influenza B, proportions ranging from 1 to 33 % in individual studies. The median duration of illness in influenza B infected subjects did not differ significantly between the treatment groups in individual studies. Data from 504 influenza B infected subjects were pooled across all studies for analysis. Oseltamivir reduced the time to alleviation of all symptoms by 0.7 days (95 % CI 0.1 – 1.6 days; $p = 0.022$) and the duration of fever (⩾ 37.8° C), cough and coryza by one day (95 % CI 0.4 - 1.7 days; $p < 0.001$), compared to placebo.

Prevention of influenza

The efficacy of oseltamivir in preventing naturally occurring influenza illness has been demonstrated in a post-exposure prophylaxis study in households and two seasonal prophylaxis studies. The primary efficacy parameter for all of these studies was the incidence of laboratory confirmed influenza. The virulence of influenza epidemics is not predictable and varies within a region and from season to season, therefore the number needed to treat (NNT) in order to prevent one case of influenza illness varies.

Post-exposure prevention: A study in contacts (12.6 % vaccinated against influenza) of an index case of influenza, oseltamivir 75 mg once daily, was started within 2 days of onset of symptoms in the index case and continued for seven days. Influenza was confirmed in 163 out of 377 index cases. Oseltamivir significantly reduced the incidence of clinical influenza illness occurring in the contacts of confirmed influenza cases from 24/200 (12 %) in the placebo group to 2/205 (1 %) in the oseltamivir group (92 % reduction, (95% CI 6 – 16), p ⩽ 0.0001). The NNT in contacts of true influenza cases was 10 (95 % CI 9 – 12) and was 16 (95 % CI 15 – 19) in the whole population (ITT) regardless of infection status in the index case.

Prevention during an influenza epidemic in the community: In a pooled analysis of two other studies conducted in unvaccinated otherwise healthy adults, oseltamivir 75 mg once daily given for 6 weeks significantly reduced the incidence of clinical influenza illness from 25/519 (4.8 %) in the placebo group to 6/520 (1.2 %) in the oseltamivir group (76 % reduction, 95 % CI 1.6 – 5.7); p = 0.0006) during a community outbreak of influenza. The NNT in this study was 28 (95 % CI 24 – 50).

A study in elderly residents of nursing homes, where 80 % of participants received vaccine in the season of the study, oseltamivir 75 mg once daily given for 6 weeks significantly reduced the incidence of clinical influenza illness from 12/272 (4.4 %) in the placebo group to 1/276 (0.4 %) in the oseltamivir group (92 % reduction, (95 % CI 1.5 – 6.6); p = 0.0015). The NNT in this study was 25 (95 % CI 23 – 62).

Specific studies have not been conducted to assess of the reduction in the risk of complications.

5.2 Pharmacokinetic properties

Absorption

Oseltamivir is readily absorbed from the gastrointestinal tract after oral administration of oseltamivir phosphate (pro-drug) and is extensively converted by predominantly hepatic esterases to the active metabolite (oseltamivir carboxylate). At least 75 % of an oral dose reaches the systemic circulation as the active metabolite. Exposure to the pro-drug is less than 5 % relative to the active metabolite. Plasma concentrations of both pro-drug and active metabolite are proportional to dose and are unaffected by co-administration with food.

Distribution

The mean volume of distribution at steady state of the oseltamivir carboxylate is approximately 23 litres in humans, a volume equivalent to extracellular body fluid. Since neuraminidase activity is extracellular oseltamivir carboxylate distributes to all sites of influenza virus spread.

The binding of the oseltamivir carboxylate to human plasma protein is negligible (approximately 3 %).

Metabolism

Oseltamivir is extensively converted to oseltamivir carboxylate by esterases located predominantly in the liver. *In-vitro* studies demonstrated, that neither oseltamivir, nor the active metabolite is a substrate for, or an inhibitor of, the major cytochrome P450 isoforms. No phase 2 conjugates of either compound have been identified *in vivo*.

Elimination

Absorbed oseltamivir is primarily (>90 %) eliminated by conversion to oseltamivir carboxylate. It is not further metabolised and is eliminated in the urine. Peak plasma concentrations of oseltamivir carboxylate decline with a half-life of 6 to 10 hours in most subjects. The active metabolite is eliminated entirely by renal excretion. Renal clearance (18.8 l/h) exceeds glomerular filtration rate (7.5 l/h) indicating that tubular secretion occurs in addition to glomerular filtration. Less than 20 % of an oral radiolabelled dose is eliminated in faeces.

Renal impairment

Administration of 100 mg oseltamivir phosphate twice daily for 5 days to patients with various degrees of renal impairment showed that exposure to oseltamivir carboxylate is inversely proportional to declining renal function. For dosing, see 4.2 Posology and method of administration.

Hepatic impairment

In vitro studies have concluded that exposure to oseltamivir is not expected to be increased significantly nor is exposure to the active metabolite expected to be significantly decreased in patients with hepatic impairment (See 4.2 Posology and method of administration).

Elderly

Exposure to the active metabolite at steady state was 25 to 35 % higher in elderly (age 65 to 78 years) compared to adults less than 65 years of age, given comparable doses of oseltamivir. Half-lives observed in the elderly were similar to those seen in young adults. On the basis of drug exposure and tolerability, dosage adjustments are not required for elderly patients unless there is evidence of severe renal impairment (creatinine clearance below 30 ml/min) (See 4.2 Posology and method of administration).

Children

The pharmacokinetics of oseltamivir have been evaluated in single dose pharmacokinetic studies in children aged one to 16 years. Multiple dose pharmacokinetics were studied in a small number of children enrolled in a clinical efficacy study. Younger children cleared both the prodrug and its active metabolite faster than adults, resulting in a lower exposure for a given mg/kg dose. Doses of 2 mg/kg give oseltamivir carboxylate exposures comparable to those achieved in adults, receiving a single 75 mg dose (approximately 1 mg/kg). The pharmacokinetics of oseltamivir in children over 12 years of age are similar to those in adults.

5.3 Preclinical safety data

Preclinical data reveal no special hazard for humans based on conventional studies of safety pharmacology, repeated dose toxicity and genotoxicity. Results of the conventional rodent carcinogenicity studies showed a trend towards a dose-dependent increase in the incidence of some tumours that are typical for the rodent strains used. Considering the margins of exposure in relation to the expected exposure in the human use, these findings do not change the benefit-risk of Tamiflu in its adopted therapeutic indications.

Teratology studies have been conducted in rats and rabbits at doses of up to 1500 mg/kg/day and 500 mg/kg/day, respectively. No effects on foetal development were observed. A rat fertility study up to a dose of 1500 mg/kg/day demonstrated no adverse effects on either sex. In pre-/post-natal rat studies, prolonged parturition was noted at 1500 mg/kg/day: the safety margin between human exposure and the highest no-effect dose (500 mg/kg/day) in rats is 480-fold for oseltamivir and 44-fold for the active metabolite, respectively. Foetal exposure in the rats and rabbits was approximately 15 to 20 % of that of the mother.

In lactating rats, oseltamivir and the active metabolite are excreted in the milk. It is not known whether oseltamivir or the active metabolite are excreted in human milk, but extrapolation of the animal data provides estimates of 0.01 mg/day and 0.3 mg/day for the respective compounds.

A potential for skin sensitisation to oseltamivir was observed in a "maximisation" test in guinea pigs. Approximately 50 % of the animals treated with the unformulated active ingredient showed erythema after challenging the induced animals. Reversible irritancy of rabbits' eyes was detected.

In a two-week study in unweaned rats a single dose of 1000 mg/kg oseltamivir phosphate to 7-day old pups resulted in deaths associated with unusually high exposure to the pro-drug. However, at 2000 mg/kg in 14-day old unweaned pups, there were no deaths or other significant effects. No adverse effects occurred at 500 mg/kg/day administered from 7 to 21 days *post partum*. In a single-dose investigatory study of this observation in 7-, 14- and 24-day old rats, a dose of 1000 mg/kg resulted in brain exposure to the pro-drug that suggested, respectively, 1500-, 650-, and 2-fold the exposure found in the brain of adult (42-day old) rats.

6. PHARMACEUTICAL PARTICULARS

6.1 List of excipients

Sorbitol (E420), sodium dihydrogen citrate (E331(a)), xanthan gum (E415), sodium benzoate (E211), saccharin sodium (E954), titanium dioxide (E171) and tutti frutti flavour (including maltodextrins (maize), propylene glycol, arabic gum E414 and natural identical flavouring substances) (mainly consisting of banana, pineapple and peach flavour).

6.2 Incompatibilities

Not applicable.

6.3 Shelf life

2 years.

After reconstitution, the suspension should not be used for longer than 10 days.

6.4 Special precautions for storage

Do not store above 30°C.

After reconstitution, store the suspension at 2°C- 8°C (in a refrigerator).

6.5 Nature and contents of container

Carton containing a 100 ml amber glass bottle (with child-resistant plastic screw cap) with 30 g of powder for oral suspension, a plastic adapter, a plastic oral dispenser and a plastic measuring cup). After reconstitution with 52 ml of water, the usable volume of oral suspension allows for the retrieval of a total of 10 doses of 75 mg oseltamivir.

6.6 Instructions for use and handling

It is recommended that Tamiflu oral suspension should be reconstituted by the pharmacist prior to its dispensing to the patient.

Preparation of Oral Suspension

1. Tap the closed bottle gently several times to loosen the powder.

2. Measure 52 ml of water by filling the measuring cup to the indicated level (measuring cup included in the box).

3. Add all 52 ml of water into the bottle, recap the bottle and shake the closed bottle well for 15 seconds.

4. Remove the cap and push the bottle adapter into the neck of the bottle.

5. Close the bottle tightly with the cap (on the top of the bottle adapter). This will make sure that the bottle adapter fits in the bottle in the right position.

Tamiflu powder for suspension will appear as an opaque and white to light yellow suspension after reconstitution.

7. MARKETING AUTHORISATION HOLDER

Roche Registration Limited

40 Broadwater Road

Welwyn Garden City

Hertfordshire, AL7 3AY

United Kingdom.

8. MARKETING AUTHORISATION NUMBER(S)

EU/1/02/222/002

9. DATE OF FIRST AUTHORISATION/RENEWAL OF THE AUTHORISATION

20 June 2002

10. DATE OF REVISION OF THE TEXT

24 February 2005

Tamoxifen Tablets BP 10mg

(Wockhardt UK Ltd)

1. NAME OF THE MEDICINAL PRODUCT

Tamoxifen Tablets BP 10mg

2. QUALITATIVE AND QUANTITATIVE COMPOSITION

Tamoxifen Citrate BP 15.20mg, equivalent to 10mg of tamoxifen.

For excipients, see 6.1.

3. PHARMACEUTICAL FORM

Tablet - Oral

4. CLINICAL PARTICULARS

4.1 Therapeutic indications

Tamoxifen tablets are used for the treatment of breast carcinoma, particularly in oestrogen receptor positive patients and for the treatment of anovulatory infertility.

4.2 Posology and method of administration

Breast carcinoma: The recommended daily dose of tamoxifen is normally 20mg. No additional benefit, in terms of delayed recurrence or improved survival in patients, has been demonstrated with higher doses. Substantive evidence supporting the use of treatment with 30-40mg per day is not available, although these doses have been used in some patients with advanced disease.

Elderly patients: Similar dosage regimens of tamoxifen have been used in elderly patients with breast cancer and in some of these patients it has been used as sole therapy.

Anovulatory infertility: Before commencing any course of treatment, whether initial or subsequent, the possibility of pregnancy must be excluded. In women with regular menstruation but anovular cycles, treatment should be initiated with 20mg daily given on the second, third, fourth and fifth days of the menstrual cycle. If treatment is unsuccessful (unsatisfactory basal temperature records or poor pre-ovulatory cervical mucus), further courses may be given during subsequent menstrual periods, increasing the dosage to 40mg and then 80mg daily.

In women with irregular menstruation, treatment may be initiated on any day. If no signs of ovulation are apparent, a subsequent course of treatment may be commenced 45 days later with dosage increased as above. If the patient responds with menstruation, the next course of treatment should start on the second day of the cycle.

4.3 Contraindications

Tamoxifen must not be administered during pregnancy. Pre-menopausal patients must be carefully examined before treatment for breast cancer or infertility to exclude the possibility of pregnancy (see also Section 4.6).

Tamoxifen should not be given to patients who have experienced hypersensitivity to the product or any of its ingredients.

Treatment for infertility: Patients with a personal or family history of confirmed idiopathic venous thromboembolic events or a known genetic defect.

4.4 Special warnings and special precautions for use

Menstruation is suppressed in a proportion of pre-menopausal women receiving tamoxifen for the treatment of breast cancer.

An increased incidence of endometrial changes including hyperplasia, polyps, cancer and uterine sarcoma (mostly malignant mixed Mullerian tumours), has been reported in association with tamoxifen treatment. The underlying mechanism is unknown but may be related to the oestrogen-like properties of tamoxifen. Any patient receiving or having previously received tamoxifen who reports abnormal gynaecological symptoms, especially vaginal bleeding, or who presents with menstrual irregularities, vaginal discharge and symptoms such as pelvic pain or pressure should be promptly investigated.

A number of second primary tumours, occurring at sites other than the endometrium and the opposite breast, have been reported in clinical trials, following the treatment of breast cancer patients with tamoxifen. No causal link has been established and the clinical significance of these observations remains unclear.

Venous thromboembolism (VTE)

• A two- to three-fold increase in the risk for VTE has been demonstrated in healthy tamoxifen-treated women (see section 4.8).

• In patients with breast cancer, prescribers should obtain careful histories with respect to the patient's personal and family history of VTE. If suggestive of a prothrombotic risk, patients should be screened for thrombophilic factors. Patients who test positive should be counselled regarding their thrombotic risk. The decision to use tamoxifen in these patients should be based on the overall risk to the patient. In selected patients, the use of tamoxifen with prophylactic anticoagulation may be justified (see section 4.5)

• The risk of VTE is further increased by severe obesity, increasing age and all other risk factors for VTE. The risks and benefits should be carefully considered for all patients before treatment with tamoxifen. In patients with breast cancer, this risk is also increased by concomitant chemotherapy (see section 4.5). Long-term anti-coagulant prophylaxis may be justified for some patients with breast cancer who have multiple risk factors for VTE.

• Surgery and immobility: For patients being treated for infertility, tamoxifen should be stopped at least 6 weeks before surgery or long-term immobility (when possible) and re-started only when the patient is fully mobile. For patients with breast cancer, tamoxifen treatment should only be stopped if the risk of tamoxifen-induced thrombosis clearly outweighs the risks associated with interrupting treatment. All patients should receive appropriate thrombosis prophylactic measures and should include graduated compression stockings for the period of hospitalisation, early ambulation, if possible, and anti-coagulant treatment.

• If any patient presents with VTE, tamoxifen should be stopped immediately and appropriate anti-thrombosis measures initiated. In patients being treated for infertility, tamoxifen should not be re-started unless there is a compelling alternative explanation for their thrombotic event. In patients receiving tamoxifen for breast cancer, the decision to re-start tamoxifen should be made with respect to the overall risk for the patient. In selected patients with breast cancer, the continued use of tamoxifen with prophylactic anticoagulation may be justified.

•All patients should be advised to contact their doctors immediately if they become aware of any symptoms of VTE.

4.5 Interaction with other medicinal products and other forms of Interaction

When tamoxifen is used in combination with coumarin-type anticoagulants, a significant increase in anticoagulant effect may occur. Where such co-administration is initiated, careful monitoring of the patient is recommended.

When tamoxifen is used in combination with cytotoxic agents for the treatment of breast cancer, there is an increased risk of thromboembolic events occurring (see also Sections 4.4 and 4.8). Because of this increase in the risk of VTE, thrombosis prophylaxis should be considered for these patients for the period of concomitant chemotherapy.

As tamoxifen is metabolised by cytochrome P450 3A4, care is required when co-administering with drugs, such as rifampicin, known to induce thisenzyme, as tamoxifen levels may be reduced. The clinical relevance of this reduction is unknown.

4.6 Pregnancy and lactation

Pregnancy

Tamoxifen must not be administered during pregnancy. There have been a small number of reports of spontaneous abortions, birth defects and foetal deaths after women have taken tamoxifen, although no causal relationship has been established.

Reproductive toxicology studies in rats, rabbits and monkeys have shown no teratogenic potential.

In rodent models of foetal reproductive tract development, tamoxifen was associated with changes similar to those caused by oestradiol, ethynyloestradiol, clomiphene and diethylstilboestrol (DES). Although the clinical relevance of these changes is unknown, some of them, especially vaginal adenosis, are similar to those seen in young women who were exposed to DES in-utero and who have a 1 in 1000 risk of developing clear-cell carcinoma of the vagina or cervix. Only a small number of pregnant women have been exposed to tamoxifen. Such exposure has not been reported to cause subsequent vaginal adenosis or clear-cell carcinoma of the vagina or cervix in young women exposed in utero to tamoxifen.

Women should be advised not to become pregnant whilst taking tamoxifen and should use barrier or other non-hormonal contraceptive methods if sexually active. Pre-menopausal patients must be carefully examined before treatment to exclude pregnancy. Women should be informed of the potential risks to the foetus, should they become pregnant whilst taking tamoxifen or within two months of cessation of therapy.

Lactation

It is not known if tamoxifen is excreted in human milk and therefore the drug is not recommended during lactation. The decision either to discontinue nursing or discontinue tamoxifen should take into account the importance of the drug to the mother.

4.7 Effects on ability to drive and use machines

None

4.8 Undesirable effects

During long term treatment side-effects are generally mild.

Side effects can be classified as either due to the pharmacological action of the drug, e.g. hot flushes, vaginal bleeding, vaginal discharge, pruritus vulvae and tumour flare, or as more general side effects, e.g. gastrointestinal intolerance, headache, light-headedness and, occasionally, fluid retention andalopecia.

When side effects are severe, it may be possible to control them by a simple reduction of dosage (to not less than 20 mg/day) without loss of control of the disease. If side effects do not respond to this measure, it may be necessary to stop the treatment.

Skin rashes (including isolated reports of erythema multiforme, Stevens- Johnson syndrome and bullous pemphigoid) and rare hypersensitivity reactions, including angioedema, have been reported.

A small number of patients with bony metastases have developed hypercalcaemia on initiation of therapy.

Falls in platelet count, usually to 80,000-90,000 per cu mm but occasionally lower, have been reported in patients receiving tamoxifen for breast carcinoma.

A number of cases of visual disturbance including reports ofcorneal changesand retinopathyand an increased incidence of cataracts, have been described in patients receiving tamoxifen therapy.

Uterine fibroids, endometriosis and otherendometrial changes includinghyperplasia and polyps havebeen reported.

Cystic ovarian swellings have occasionally been observed in pre-menopausal women receiving tamoxifen.

Leucopenia has been observed following the administration of tamoxifen, sometimes in association with anaemia and/or thrombocytopenia. Neutropenia has been reported on rare occasions; this can sometimes be severe.

Cases of deep vein thrombosis and pulmonary embolism have been reported during tamoxifen therapy (see sections 4.3, 4.4 and 4.5). When tamoxifen is used in combination with cytotoxic agents, there is an increased risk of thrombo-embolic events.

Very rarely, cases of interstitial pneumonitis have been reported.

Tamoxifen has been associated with changes in liver enzyme levels and rarely with more severe liver abnormalities including fatty liver, cholestasis and hepatitis.

Rarely, elevation of serum triglyceride levels, in some cases with pancreatitis, may be associated with the use of tamoxifen.

An increased incidence of endometrial cancer and uterine sarcoma (mostly malignant mixed Mullerian tumours) has been reported in association with tamoxifen treatment.

4.9 Overdose

a) Symptoms

In theory, overdosage causes antioestrogenic side-effects. In animals extremely high doses (greater than 100 times the recommended dosage) have caused oestrogenic effects.

b) Treatment

Treatment is symptomatic, as there is no specific antidote.

5. PHARMACOLOGICAL PROPERTIES

5.1 Pharmacodynamic properties

Tamoxifen is a non-steroidal, triphenylethylene-based drug which displays a complex spectrum of oestrogen antagonist and oestrogen agonist-like pharmacological effects in different tissues. In breast cancer patients, at the tumour level, tamoxifen acts primarily as an antioestrogen, preventing oestrogen binding to the oestrogen receptor. However, clinical results have shown some benefit in oestrogen receptor negative tumours, which may indicate other mechanisms of action. In the clinical situation, it is recognised that tamoxifen leads to reductions in levels of blood total cholesterol and low density lipoproteins in postmenopausal women of the order of 10 - 20%. Tamoxifen does not adversely affect bone mineral density.

5.2 Pharmacokinetic properties

Peak plasma concentrations of tamoxifen occur four to seven hours after an oral dose. Steady state concentrations (about 300ng/ml) are achieved after four weeks of treatment with 40mg daily. It is extensively protein bound to serum albumin >99%). Metabolism is by hydroxylation, demethylation and conjugation, giving rise to several metabolites which have a similar pharmacological profile to the parent compound and thus contribute to the therapeutic effect. Excretion occurs primarily via the faeces and an elimination half-life of approximately seven days has been calculated for the drug itself, whereas that forN-desmethyltamoxifen, the principal circulating metabolite, is 14 days.

5.3 Preclinical safety data

A small number of cases of endometrial polyps and endometrial carcinoma have been reported in association with tamoxifen treatment. A definitive relationship to tamoxifen therapy has not been established.

Tamoxifen was not mutagenic in a range of in vitro and in vivo mutagenicity tests. Gonadal tumours in mice and liver tumours in rats receiving tamoxifen have been reported in long term studies. The clinical relevance of these findings has not been established.

6. PHARMACEUTICAL PARTICULARS

6.1 List of excipients

Lactose

Maize starch

Pregelatinised maize starch

Magnesium stearate

Water

Film Coat

Methylhydroxypropylcellulose

Propylene glycol

Opaspray M-1-7111B (E171, E464)

Water

6.2 Incompatibilities

None known

6.3 Shelf life

Three years.

6.4 Special precautions for storage

Do not store above 25°C.

Store in the original container in order to protect from light and moisture.

6.5 Nature and contents of container

Packs of tablets in polypropylene or polyethylene containers with child resistant closures or amber glass bottles.

Blister packs of white PVC and aluminium foil coated with PVC/PVDC film.

6.6 Instructions for use and handling

The tablets are administered orally. Take the tablets with a glass of water.

Administrative Data

7. MARKETING AUTHORISATION HOLDER

CP Pharmaceuticals Ltd

Ash Road North

Wrexham

LL13 9UF

UK

8. MARKETING AUTHORISATION NUMBER(S)

04543/0353

9. DATE OF FIRST AUTHORISATION/RENEWAL OF THE AUTHORISATION

27/2/95

10. DATE OF REVISION OF THE TEXT

February 2003

Tamoxifen Tablets BP 20mg

(Wockhardt UK Ltd)

1. NAME OF THE MEDICINAL PRODUCT

Tamoxifen Tablets BP 20mg

2. QUALITATIVE AND QUANTITATIVE COMPOSITION

Tamoxifen Citrate BP 30.40mg equivalent to 20mg of tamoxifen.

For excipients, see 6.1.

3. PHARMACEUTICAL FORM

Tablet - Oral

4. CLINICAL PARTICULARS

4.1 Therapeutic indications

Tamoxifen tablets are used for the treatment of breast carcinoma, particularly in oestrogen receptor positive patients and for the treatment of anovulatory infertility.

4.2 Posology and method of administration

Breast carcinoma: The recommended daily dose of tamoxifen is normally 20mg. No additional benefit, in terms of delayed recurrence or improved survival in patients, has been demonstrated with higher doses. Substantive evidence supporting the use of treatment with 30-40mg per day is not available, although these doses have been used in some patients with advanced disease.

Elderly patients: Similar dosage regimens of tamoxifen have been used in elderly patients with breast cancer and in some of these patients it has been used as sole therapy.

Anovulatory infertility: Before commencing any course of treatment, whether initial or subsequent, the possibility of pregnancy must be excluded. In women with regular menstruation but anovular cycles, treatment should be initiated with 20mg daily given on the second, third, fourth and fifth days of the menstrual cycle. If treatment is unsuccessful (unsatisfactory basal temperature records or poor pre-ovulatory cervical mucus), further courses may be given during subsequent menstrual periods, increasing the dosage to 40mg and then 80mg daily.

In women with irregular menstruation, treatment may be initiated on any day. If no signs of ovulation are apparent, a subsequent course of treatment may be commenced 45 days later with dosage increased as above. If the patient responds with menstruation, the next course of treatment should start on the second day of the cycle.

4.3 Contraindications

Tamoxifen must not be administered during pregnancy. Pre-menopausal patients must be carefully examined before treatment for breast cancer or infertility to exclude the possibility of pregnancy (see also Section 4.6).

Tamoxifen should not be given to patients who have experienced hypersensitivity to the product or any of its ingredients.

Treatment for infertility: Patients with a personal or family history of confirmed idiopathic venous thromboembolic events or a known genetic defect.

4.4 Special warnings and special precautions for use

Menstruation is suppressed in a proportion of pre-menopausal women receiving tamoxifen for the treatment of breast cancer.

An increased incidence of endometrial changes including hyperplasia, polyps, cancer and uterine sarcoma (mostly malignant mixed Mullerian tumours), has been reported in association with tamoxifen treatment. The underlying mechanism is unknown but may be related to the oestrogen-like properties of tamoxifen. Any patient receiving or having previously received tamoxifen who reports abnormal gynaecological symptoms, especially vaginal bleeding, or who presents with menstrual irregularities, vaginal discharge and symptoms such as pelvic pain or pressure should be promptly investigated.

A number of second primary tumours, occurring at sites other than the endometrium and the opposite breast, have been reported in clinical trials, following the treatment of breast cancer patients with tamoxifen. No causal link has been established and the clinical significance of these observations remains unclear.

Venous thromboembolism (VTE)

- A two- to three-fold increase in the risk for VTE has been demonstrated in healthy tamoxifen-treated women (see section 4.8).
- In patients with breast cancer, prescribers should obtain careful histories with respect to the patient's personal and family history of VTE. If suggestive of a prothrombotic risk, patients should be screened for thrombophilic factors. Patients who test positive should be counselled regarding their thrombotic risk. The decision to use tamoxifen in these patients should be based on the overall risk to the patient. In selected patients, the use of tamoxifen with prophylactic anticoagulation may be justified (see section 4.5)
- The risk of VTE is further increased by severe obesity, increasing age and all other risk factors for VTE. The risks and benefits should be carefully considered for all patients before treatment with tamoxifen. In patients with breast cancer, this risk is also increased by concomitant chemotherapy (see section 4.5). Long-term anti-coagulant prophylaxis may be justified for some patients with breast cancer who have multiple risk factors for VTE.
- Surgery and immobility: For patients being treated for infertility, tamoxifen should be stopped at least 6 weeks before surgery or long-term immobility (when possible) and re-started only when the patient is fully mobile. For patients with breast cancer, tamoxifen treatment should only be stopped if the risk of tamoxifen-induced thrombosis clearly outweighs the risks associated with interrupting treatment. All patients should receive appropriate thrombosis prophylactic measures and should include graduated compression stockings for the period of hospitalisation, early ambulation, if possible, and anti-coagulant treatment.
- If any patient presents with VTE, tamoxifen should be stopped immediately and appropriate anti-thrombosis measures initiated. In patients being treated for infertility, tamoxifen should not be re-started unless there is a compelling alternative explanation for their thrombotic event. In patients receiving tamoxifen for breast cancer, the decision to re-start tamoxifen should be made with respect to the overall risk for the patient. In selected patients with breast cancer, the continued use of tamoxifen with prophylactic anticoagulation may be justified.
- All patients should be advised to contact their doctors immediately if they become aware of any symptoms of VTE.

4.5 Interaction with other medicinal products and other forms of Interaction

When tamoxifen is used in combination with coumarin-type anticoagulants, a significant increase in anticoagulant effect may occur. Where such co-administration is initiated, careful monitoring of the patient is recommended.

When tamoxifen is used in combination with cytotoxic agents for the treatment of breast cancer, there is an increased risk of thromboembolic events occurring(see also Sections 4.4 and 4.8). Because of this increase in the risk of VTE, thrombosis prophylaxis should be considered for these patients for the period of concomitant chemotherapy.

As tamoxifen is metabolised by cytochrome P450 3A4, care is required when co-administering with drugs, such as rifampicin, known to induce this enzyme, as tamoxifen levels may be reduced. The clinical relevance of this reduction is unknown.

4.6 Pregnancy and lactation

Pregnancy

Tamoxifen must not be administered during pregnancy. There have been a small number of reports of spontaneous abortions, birth defects and foetal deaths after women have taken tamoxifen, although no causal relationship has been established.

Reproductive toxicology studies in rats, rabbits and monkeys have shown no teratogenic potential.

In rodent models of foetal reproductive tract development, tamoxifen was associated with changes similar to those caused by oestradiol, ethynyloestradiol, clomiphene and diethylstilboestrol (DES). Although the clinical relevance of these changes is unknown, some of them, especially vaginal adenosis, are similar to those seen in young women who were exposed to DES in-utero and who have a 1 in 1000 risk of developing clear-cell carcinoma of the vagina or cervix. Only a small number of pregnant women have been exposed to tamoxifen. Such exposure has not been reported to cause subsequent vaginal adenosis or clear-cell carcinoma of the vagina or cervix in young women exposed in utero to tamoxifen.

Women should be advised not to become pregnant whilst taking tamoxifen and should use barrier or other non-hormonal contraceptive methods if sexually active. Pre-menopausal patients must be carefully examined before treatment to exclude pregnancy. Women should be informed of the potential risks to the foetus, should they become pregnant whilst taking tamoxifen or within two months of cessation of therapy.

Lactation

It is not known if tamoxifen is excreted in human milk and therefore the drug is not recommended during lactation. The decision either to discontinue nursing or discontinue tamoxifen should take into account the importance of the drug to the mother.

4.7 Effects on ability to drive and use machines

None

4.8 Undesirable effects

During long term treatment side-effects are generally mild.

Side effects can be classified as either due to the pharmacological action of the drug, e.g. hot flushes, vaginal bleeding, vaginal discharge, pruritus vulvae and tumour flare, or as more general side effects, e.g. gastrointestinal intolerance, headache, light-headedness and, occasionally, fluid retention andalopecia.

When side effects are severe, it may be possible to control them by a simple reduction of dosage (to not less than 20 mg/day) without loss of control of thedisease. If side effects do not respond to this measure, it may be necessary to stop the treatment.

Skin rashes(including isolated reports of erythema multiforme, Stevens- Johnson syndrome and bullous pemphigoid) and rare hypersensitivity reactions, including angioedema, have been reported.

A small number of patients with bony metastases have developed hypercalcaemia on initiation of therapy.

Falls in platelet count, usually to 80,000-90,000 per cu mm but occasionally lower, have been reported in patients receiving tamoxifen for breast carcinoma.

A number of cases of visual disturbance including reports ofcorneal changesand retinopathyand an increased incidence of cataracts, have been described in patients receiving tamoxifen therapy.

Uterine fibroids, endometriosis and otherendometrial changes includinghyperplasia and polyps have been reported.

Cystic ovarian swellings have occasionally been observed in pre-menopausal women receiving tamoxifen.

Leucopenia has been observed following the administration of tamoxifen, sometimes in association with anaemia and/or thrombocytopenia. Neutropenia has been reported on rare occasions; this can sometimes be severe.

Cases of deep vein thrombosis and pulmonary embolism have been reported during tamoxifen therapy (see sections 4.3, 4.4 and 4.5). When tamoxifen is used in combination with cytotoxic agents, there is an increased risk of thrombo-embolic events.

Very rarely, cases of interstitial pneumonitis have been reported.

Tamoxifen has been associated with changes in liver enzyme levels and rarely with more severe liver abnormalities including fatty liver, cholestasis and hepatitis.

Rarely, elevation of serum triglyceride levels, in some cases with pancreatitis, may be associated with the use of tamoxifen.

An increased incidence of endometrial cancer and uterine sarcoma (mostly malignant mixed Mullerian tumours) has been reported in association with tamoxifen treatment.

4.9 Overdose

a) Symptoms

In theory, overdosage causes antioestrogenic side-effects. In animals extremely high doses (greater than 100 times the recommended dosage) have caused oestrogenic effects.

b) Treatment

Treatment is symptomatic, as there is no specific antidote.

5. PHARMACOLOGICAL PROPERTIES

5.1 Pharmacodynamic properties

Tamoxifen is a non-steroidal, triphenylethylene-based drug which displays a complex spectrum of oestrogen antagonist and oestrogen agonist-like pharmacological effects in different tissues. In breast cancer patients, at the tumour level, tamoxifen acts primarily as an antioestrogen, preventing oestrogen binding to the oestrogen receptor. However, clinical results have shown some benefit in oestrogen receptor negative tumours, which may indicate other mechanisms of action. In the clinical situation, it is recognised that tamoxifen leads to reductions in levels of blood total cholesterol and low density lipoproteins in postmenopausal women of the order of 10 - 20%. Tamoxifen does not adversely affect bone mineral density.

5.2 Pharmacokinetic properties

Peak plasma concentrations of tamoxifen occur four to seven hours after an oral dose. Steady state concentrations (about 300ng/ml) are achieved after four weeks of treatment with 40mg daily. It is extensively protein bound to serum albumin (>99%). Metabolism is by hydroxylation, demethylation and conjugation, giving rise to several metabolites which have a similar pharmacological profile to the parent compound and thus contribute to the therapeutic effect. Excretion occurs primarily via the faeces and an elimination half-life of approximately seven days has been calculated for the drug itself, whereas that forN-desmethyltamoxifen, the principal circulating metabolite, is 14 days.

5.3 Preclinical safety data

A small number of cases of endometrial polyps and endometrial carcinoma have been reported in association with tamoxifen treatment. A definitive relationship to tamoxifen therapy has not been established.

Tamoxifen was not mutagenic in a range of in vitro and in vivo mutagenicity tests. Gonadal tumours in mice and liver tumours in rats receiving tamoxifen have been reported in long term studies. The clinical relevance of these findings has not been established.

6. PHARMACEUTICAL PARTICULARS

6.1 List of excipients

Lactose

Maize starch

Pregelatinised maize starch

Magnesium stearate

Water

Film Coat

Methylhydroxypropylcellulose

Propylene glycol

Opaspray M-1-7111B (E171, E464)

Water

6.2 Incompatibilities

None known

6.3 Shelf life

Three years.

6.4 Special precautions for storage

Do not store above 25°C.

Store in the original container in order to protect from light and moisture.

6.5 Nature and contents of container

Packs of tablets in polypropylene or polyethylene containers with child resistant closures or amber glass bottles.

Blister packs of white PVC and aluminium foil coated with PVC/PVDC film.

6.6 Instructions for use and handling

The tablets are administered orally. Take the tablets with a glass of water.

Administrative Data

7. MARKETING AUTHORISATION HOLDER

CP Pharmaceuticals Ltd

Ash Road North

Wrexham

LL13 9UF

UK

8. MARKETING AUTHORISATION NUMBER(S)

4543/0354

9. DATE OF FIRST AUTHORISATION/RENEWAL OF THE AUTHORISATION

27/2/95

10. DATE OF REVISION OF THE TEXT

February 2003

Tamoxifen Tablets BP 40mg

(Wockhardt UK Ltd)

1. NAME OF THE MEDICINAL PRODUCT

Tamoxifen Tablets BP 40mg

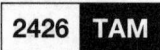

2. QUALITATIVE AND QUANTITATIVE COMPOSITION

Tamoxifen Citrate BP 60.8 mg equivalent to 40mg of tamoxifen.

For excipients, see 6.1.

3. PHARMACEUTICAL FORM

Tablet - Oral

4. CLINICAL PARTICULARS

4.1 Therapeutic indications

Tamoxifen tablets are used for the treatment of breast carcinoma, particularly in oestrogen receptor positive patients and for the treatment of anovulatory infertility.

4.2 Posology and method of administration

Breast carcinoma: The recommended daily dose of tamoxifen is normally 20mg. No additional benefit, in terms of delayed recurrence or improved survival in patients, has been demonstrated with higher doses. Substantive evidence supporting the use of treatment with 30-40mg per day is not available, although these doses have been used in some patients with advanced disease.

Elderly patients: Similar dosage regimens of tamoxifen have been used in elderly patients with breast cancer and in some of these patients it has been used as sole therapy.

Anovulatory infertility: Before commencing any course of treatment, whether initial or subsequent, the possibility of pregnancy must be excluded. In women with regular menstruation but anovular cycles, treatment should be initiated with 20mg daily given on the second, third, fourth and fifth days of the menstrual cycle. If treatment is unsuccessful (unsatisfactory basal temperature records or poor preovulatory cervical mucus), further courses may be given during subsequent menstrual periods, increasing the dosage to 40mg and then 80mg daily.

In women with irregular menstruation, treatment may be initiated on any day. If no signs of ovulation are apparent, a subsequent course of treatment may be commenced 45 days later with dosage increased as above. If the patient responds with menstruation, the next course of treatment should start on the second day of the cycle.

4.3 Contraindications

Tamoxifen must not be administered during pregnancy. Pre-menopausal patients must be carefully examined before treatment for breast cancer or infertility to exclude the possibility of pregnancy (see also Section 4.6).

Tamoxifen should not be given to patients who have experienced hypersensitivity to the product or any of its ingredients.

Treatment for infertility: Patients with a personal or family history of confirmed idiopathic venous thromboembolic events or a known genetic defect.

4.4 Special warnings and special precautions for use

Menstruation is suppressed in a proportion of pre-menopausal women receiving tamoxifen for the treatment of breast cancer.

An increased incidence of endometrial changes including hyperplasia, polyps, cancer and uterine sarcoma (mostly malignant mixed Mullerian tumours), has been reported in association with tamoxifen treatment. The underlying mechanism is unknown but may be related to the oestrogen-like properties of tamoxifen. Any patient receiving or having previously received tamoxifen who reports abnormal gynaecological symptoms, especially vaginal bleeding, or who presents with menstrual irregularities, vaginal discharge and symptoms such as pelvic pain or pressure should be promptly investigated.

A number of second primary tumours, occurring at sites other than the endometrium and the opposite breast, have been reported in clinical trials, following the treatment of breast cancer patients with tamoxifen. No causal link has been established and the clinical significance of these observations remains unclear.

Venous thromboembolism (VTE)

• A two- to three-fold increase in the risk for VTE has been demonstrated in healthy tamoxifen-treated women (see section 4.8).

• In patients with breast cancer, prescribers should obtain careful histories with respect to the patient's personal and family history of VTE. If suggestive of a prothrombotic risk, patients should be screened for thrombophilic factors. Patients who test positive should be counselled regarding their thrombotic risk. The decision to use tamoxifen in these patients should be based on the overall risk to the patient. In selected patients, the use of tamoxifen with prophylactic anticoagulation may be justified (see section 4.5)

• The risk of VTE is further increased by severe obesity, increasing age and all other risk factors for VTE. The risks and benefits should be carefullyconsidered for all patients before treatment with tamoxifen. In patients with breast cancer, this risk is also increased by concomitant chemotherapy (see section 4.5). Long-term anti-coagulant prophylaxis may be justified for some patients with breast cancer who have multiple risk factors for VTE.

• Surgery and immobility: For patients being treated for infertility, tamoxifen should be stopped at least 6 weeks before surgery or long-term immobility (when possible) and re-started only when the patient is fully mobile. For patients with breast cancer, tamoxifen treatment should only be stopped if the risk of tamoxifen-induced thrombosis clearly outweighs the risks associated with interrupting treatment. All patients should receive appropriate thrombosis prophylactic measures and should include graduated compression stockings for the period of hospitalisation, early ambulation, if possible, and anti-coagulant treatment.

• If any patient presents with VTE, tamoxifen should be stopped immediately and appropriate anti-thrombosis measures initiated. In patients being treated for infertility, tamoxifen should not be re-started unless there is a compelling alternative explanation for their thrombotic event. In patients receiving tamoxifen for breast cancer, the decision to re-start tamoxifen should be made with respect to the overall risk for the patient. In selected patients with breast cancer, the continued use of tamoxifen with prophylactic anticoagulation may be justified.

•All patients should be advised to contact their doctors immediately if they become aware of any symptoms of VTE.

4.5 Interaction with other medicinal products and other forms of Interaction

When tamoxifen is used in combination with coumarin-type anticoagulants, a significant increase in anticoagulant effect may occur. Where such co-administration is initiated, careful monitoring of the patient is recommended.

When tamoxifen is used in combination with cytotoxic agents for the treatment of breast cancer, there is an increased risk of thromboembolic events occurring(see also Sections 4.4 and 4.8). Because of this increase in the risk of VTE, thrombosis prophylaxis should be considered for these patients for the period of concomitant chemotherapy.

As tamoxifen is metabolised by cytochrome P450 3A4, care is required when co-administering with drugs, such as rifampicin, known to induce this enzyme, as tamoxifen levels may be reduced. The clinical relevance of this reduction is unknown.

4.6 Pregnancy and lactation

Pregnancy

Tamoxifen must not be administered during pregnancy. There have been a small number of reports of spontaneous abortions, birth defects and foetal deaths after women have taken tamoxifen, although no causal relationship has been established.

Reproductive toxicology studies in rats, rabbits and monkeys have shown no teratogenic potential.

In rodent models of foetal reproductive tract development, tamoxifen was associated with changes similar to those caused by oestradiol, ethynyloestradiol, clomiphene and diethylstilboestrol (DES). Although the clinical relevance of these changes is unknown, some of them, especially vaginal adenosis, are similar to those seen in young women who were exposed to DES in-utero and who have a 1 in 1000 risk of developing clear-cell carcinoma of the vagina or cervix. Only a small number of pregnant women have been exposed to tamoxifen. Such exposure has not been reported to cause subsequent vaginal adenosis or clear-cell carcinoma of the vagina or cervix in young women exposed in utero to tamoxifen.

Women should be advised not to become pregnant whilst taking tamoxifen and should use barrier or other non-hormonal contraceptive methods if sexually active. Premenopausal patients must be carefully examined before treatment to exclude pregnancy. Women should be informed of the potential risks to the foetus, should they become pregnant whilst taking tamoxifen or within two months of cessation of therapy.

Lactation

It is not known if tamoxifen is excreted in human milk and therefore the drug is not recommended during lactation. The decision either to discontinue nursing or discontinue tamoxifen should take into account the importance of the drug to the mother.

4.7 Effects on ability to drive and use machines

None

4.8 Undesirable effects

During long term treatment side-effects are generally mild.

Side effects can be classified as either due to the pharmacological action of the drug, e.g. hot flushes, vaginal bleeding, vaginal discharge, pruritus vulvae and tumour flare or as more general side effects, e.g. gastrointestinal intolerance, headache, light-headedness and, occasionally, fluid retention andalopecia.

When side effects are severe, it may be possible to control them by a simple reduction of dosage (to not less than 20 mg/day) without loss of control of the disease. If side effects do not respond to this measure, it may be necessary to stop the treatment.

Skin rashes(including isolated reports of erythema multiforme, Stevens- Johnson syndrome and bullous pemphigoid) and rare hypersensitivity reactions, including angioedema, have been reported.

A small number of patients with bony metastases have developed hypercalcaemia on initiation of therapy.

Falls in platelet count, usually to 80,000-90,000 per cu mm but occasionally lower, have been reported in patients receiving tamoxifen for breast carcinoma.

A number of cases of visual disturbance including reports ofcorneal changesand retinopathyand an increased incidence of cataracts, have been described in patients receiving tamoxifen therapy.

Uterine fibroids, endometriosis and otherendometrial changes includinghyperplasia and polyps havebeen reported.

Cystic ovarian swellings have occasionally been observed in pre-menopausal women receiving tamoxifen.

Leucopenia has been observed following the administration of tamoxifen, sometimes in association with anaemia and/or thrombocytopenia. Neutropenia has been reported on rare occasions; this can sometimes be severe.

Cases of deep vein thrombosis and pulmonary embolism have been reported during tamoxifen therapy (see sections 4.3, 4.4 and 4.5). When tamoxifen is used in combination with cytotoxic agents, there is an increased risk of thrombo-embolic events.

Very rarely, cases of interstitial pneumonitis have been reported.

Tamoxifen has been associated with changes in liver enzyme levels and rarely with more severe liver abnormalities including fatty liver, cholestasis and hepatitis.

Rarely, elevation of serum triglyceride levels, in some cases with pancreatitis, may be associated with the use of tamoxifen.

An increased incidence of endometrial cancer and uterine sarcoma (mostly malignant mixed Mullerian tumours) has been reported in association with tamoxifen treatment.

4.9 Overdose

a) Symptoms

In theory, overdosage causes antioestrogenic side-effects. In animals extremely high doses (greater than 100 times the recommended dosage) have caused oestrogenic effects.

b) Treatment

Treatment is symptomatic, as there is no specific antidote.

5. PHARMACOLOGICAL PROPERTIES

5.1 Pharmacodynamic properties

Tamoxifen is a non-steroidal, triphenylethylene-based drug which displays a complex spectrum of oestrogen antagonist and oestrogen agonist-like pharmacological effects in different tissues. In breast cancer patients, at the tumour level, tamoxifen acts primarily as an antioestrogen, preventing oestrogen binding to the oestrogen receptor. However, clinical results have shown some benefit in oestrogen receptor negative tumours, which may indicate other mechanisms of action. In the clinical situation, it is recognised that tamoxifen leads to reductions in levels of blood total cholesterol and low density lipoproteins in postmenopausal women of the order of 10 - 20%. Tamoxifen does not adversely affect bone mineral density.

5.2 Pharmacokinetic properties

Peak plasma concentrations of tamoxifen occur four to seven hours after an oral dose. Steady state concentrations (about 300ng/ml) are achieved after four weeks of treatment with 40mg daily. It is extensively protein bound to serum albumin (>99%). Metabolism is by hydroxylation, demethylation and conjugation, giving rise to several metabolites which have a similar pharmacological profile to the parent compound and thus contribute to the therapeutic effect. Excretion occurs primarily via the faeces and an elimination half-life of approximately seven days has been calculated for the drug itself, whereas that forN-desmethyltamoxifen, the principal circulating metabolite, is 14 days.

5.3 Preclinical safety data

A small number of cases of endometrial polyps and endometrial carcinoma have been reported in association with tamoxifen treatment. A definitive relationship to tamoxifen therapy has not been established.

Tamoxifen was not mutagenic in a range of in vitro and in vivo mutagenicity tests. Gonadal tumours in mice and liver tumours in rats receiving tamoxifen have been reported in long term studies. The clinical relevance of these findings has not been established.

6. PHARMACEUTICAL PARTICULARS

6.1 List of excipients

Lactose

Maize starch

Pregelatinised maize starch

Magnesium stearate

Water

Film Coat

Methylhydroxypropylcellulose

Propylene glycol

Opaspray M-1-7111B (E171, E464)

Water

6.2 Incompatibilities

None known

6.3 Shelf life

Three years.

6.4 Special precautions for storage

Do not store above 25°C.

Store in the original container in order to protect from light and moisture.

6.5 Nature and contents of container

Packs of tablets in polypropylene or polyethylene containers with child resistant closures or amber glass bottles.

Blister packs of white PVC and aluminium foil coated with PVC/PVDC film.

6.6 Instructions for use and handling
The tablets are administered orally. Take the tablets with a glass of water.

Administrative Data

7. MARKETING AUTHORISATION HOLDER
CP Pharmaceuticals Ltd
Ash Road North
Wrexham
LL13 9UF
UK

8. MARKETING AUTHORISATION NUMBER(S)
04543/0355

9. DATE OF FIRST AUTHORISATION/RENEWAL OF THE AUTHORISATION
27/2/95

10. DATE OF REVISION OF THE TEXT
February 2003

Tarceva 25mg, 100mg and 150mg Film-Coated Tablets

(Roche Products Limited)

1. NAME OF THE MEDICINAL PRODUCT
Tarceva ▼ 25 mg, 100 mg and 150 mg film-coated tablets

2. QUALITATIVE AND QUANTITATIVE COMPOSITION
One film-coated tablet of each strength contains 25 mg, 100 mg or 150 mg erlotinib (as erlotinib hydrochloride).

For excipients, see section 6.1.

3. PHARMACEUTICAL FORM
Film-coated tablet

White to yellowish, round, biconvex tablets with 'Tarceva 25' and logo printed in brownish yellow on one side.

White to yellowish, round, biconvex tablets with 'Tarceva 100' and logo printed in grey on one side.

White to yellowish, round, biconvex tablets with 'Tarceva 150' and logo printed in brown on one side.

4. CLINICAL PARTICULARS

4.1 Therapeutic indications
Tarceva is indicated for the treatment of patients with locally advanced or metastatic non-small cell lung cancer after failure of at least one prior chemotherapy regimen.

When prescribing Tarceva, factors associated with prolonged survival should be taken into account.

No survival benefit or other clinically relevant effects of the treatment have been demonstrated in patients with EGFR-negative tumours (see section 5.1).

4.2 Posology and method of administration
Tarceva treatment should be supervised by a physician experienced in the use of anticancer therapies.

The recommended daily dose of Tarceva is 150 mg taken at least one hour before or two hours after the ingestion of food.

When dose adjustment is necessary, reduce in 50 mg steps (see section 4.4).

Tarceva is available in strengths of 25 mg, 100 mg and 150 mg.

Concomitant use of CYP3A4 substrates and modulators may require dose adjustment (see section 4.5).

Hepatic impairment: Erlotinib is eliminated by hepatic metabolism and biliary excretion. The safety and efficacy of erlotinib has not been studied in patients with hepatic impairment. Therefore caution should be exercised when administering Tarceva to patients with hepatic impairment. Use of Tarceva in patients with severe hepatic impairment is not recommended (see section 5.2).

Renal impairment: The safety and efficacy of erlotinib has not been studied in patients with renal impairment (serum creatinine concentration >1.5 times the upper normal limit). Based on pharmacokinetic data no dose adjustments appear necessary in patients with mild or moderate renal impairment (see section 5.2). Use of Tarceva in patients with severe renal impairment is not recommended.

Paediatric use: The safety and efficacy of erlotinib has not been studied in patients under the age of 18 years. Use of Tarceva in paediatric patients is not recommended.

4.3 Contraindications
Severe hypersensitivity to erlotinib or to any of the excipients.

4.4 Special warnings and special precautions for use
Potent inducers of CYP3A4 may reduce the efficacy of erlotinib whereas potent inhibitors of CYP3A4 may lead to increased toxicity. Concomitant treatment with these types of agents should be avoided (see section 4.5).

Current smokers should be advised to stop smoking, as plasma concentrations could be reduced otherwise (see section 4.5).

Cases of interstitial lung disease (ILD), including fatalities, have been reported uncommonly in patients receiving Tarceva for treatment of non-small cell lung cancer (NSCLC) or other advanced solid tumours. In the pivotal study BR.21 in NSCLC, the incidence of ILD (0.8 %) was the same in both the placebo and Tarceva groups. The overall incidence in Tarceva-treated patients from all studies (including uncontrolled studies and studies with concurrent chemotherapy) is approximately 0.6 % compared to 0.2 % in patients on placebo. Reported diagnoses in patients suspected of having ILD included pneumonitis, interstitial pneumonia, interstitial lung disease, obliterative bronchiolitis, pulmonary fibrosis, Acute Respiratory Distress Syndrome (ARDS), and lung infiltration. Confounding or contributing factors such as concomitant or prior chemotherapy, prior radiotherapy, pre-existing parenchymal lung disease, metastatic lung disease, or pulmonary infections were frequent.

In patients who develop acute onset of new and/or progressive unexplained pulmonary symptoms such as dyspnoea, cough and fever, Tarceva therapy should be interrupted pending diagnostic evaluation. If ILD is diagnosed, Tarceva should be discontinued and appropriate treatment initiated as necessary (see section 4.8).

Diarrhoea has occurred in approximately 50 % of patients on Tarceva and moderate or severe diarrhoea should be treated with e.g. loperamide. In some cases dose reduction may be necessary. In the clinical studies doses were reduced by 50 mg steps. Dose reductions by 25 mg steps have not been investigated. In the event of severe or persistent diarrhoea, nausea, anorexia, or vomiting associated with dehydration, Tarceva therapy should be interrupted and appropriate measures should be taken to treat the dehydration (see section 4.8).

The tablets contain lactose and should not be administered to patients with rare hereditary problems of galactose intolerance, Lapp lactase deficiency or glucose-galactose malabsorption.

Erlotinib is characterised by a decrease in solubility at pH above 5. The effect of antacids, proton pump inhibitors and H2 antagonists on the absorption of erlotinib have not been investigated but absorption may be impaired, leading to lower plasma levels. Caution should be exercised when these medicinal products are combined with erlotinib.

4.5 Interaction with other medicinal products and other forms of Interaction
Erlotinib is a potent inhibitor of CYP1A1, and a moderate inhibitor of CYP3A4 and CYP2C8, as well as a strong inhibitor of glucuronidation by UGT1A1 *in vitro*.

The physiological relevance of the strong inhibition of CYP1A1 is unknown due to the very limited expression of CYP1A1 in human tissues.

The effects of CYP1A2 inhibitors on the pharmacokinetics of erlotinib have not been investigated and caution should be exercised when these inhibitors are combined with erlotinib.

No clinical interaction study with a CYP3A4 substrate has been performed as yet. Based on *in vitro* data, combination of erlotinib with CYP3A4 substrates should be conducted with caution. If such a combination is considered necessary a close clinical monitoring should be performed. In a clinical study, erlotinib was shown not to affect pharmacokinetics of the concomitantly administered CYP3A4/2C8 substrate paclitaxel.

The inhibition of glucuronidation may cause interactions with medicinal products which are substrates of UGT1A1 and exclusively cleared by this pathway. Patients with low expression levels of UGT1A1 or genetic glucuronidation disorders (e.g. Gilbert's disease) may exhibit increased serum concentrations of bilirubin and must be treated with caution.

Erlotinib is metabolised in the liver by the hepatic cytochromes in humans, primarily CYP3A4 and to a lesser extent by CYP1A2. Extrahepatic metabolism by CYP3A4 in intestine, CYP1A1 in lung, and CYP1B1 in tumour tissue also potentially contribute to the metabolic clearance of erlotinib. Potential interactions may occur with active substances which are metabolised by, or are inhibitors or inducers of, these enzymes.

Potent inhibitors of CYP3A4 activity decrease erlotinib metabolism and increase erlotinib plasma concentrations. In a clinical study, the concomitant use of erlotinib with ketoconazole (200 mg orally twice daily for 5 days), a potent CYP3A4 inhibitor, resulted in an increase of erlotinib exposure (86 % of AUC and 69 % of C_{max}). Therefore, caution should be used when erlotinib is combined with a potent CYP3A4 inhibitor, e.g. azole antifungals (i.e. ketoconazole, itraconazole, voriconazole), protease inhibitors, erythromycin or clarithromycin. If necessary the dose of erlotinib should be reduced, particularly if toxicity is observed.

Potent inducers of CYP3A4 activity increase erlotinib metabolism and significantly decrease erlotinib plasma concentrations. In a clinical study, the concomitant use of erlotinib and rifampicin (600 mg orally once daily for 7 days), a potent CYP3A4 inducer, resulted in a 69 % decrease in the median erlotinib AUC. The clinical relevance of this observation is unclear, but efficacy may be reduced. Reduced exposure may also occur with other inducers e.g. phenytoin, carbamazepine, barbiturates or St. Johns Wort (*hypericum perforatum*). Caution should be observed when these active substances are combined with erlotinib. Alternate treatments lacking potent CYP3A4 inducing activity should be considered when possible.

International Normalised Ratio (INR) elevations, and bleeding events including gastrointestinal bleeding have been reported in clinical studies, some associated with concomitant warfarin administration (see section 4.8) and some with concomitant NSAID administration. Patients taking warfarin or other coumarin-derivative anticoagulants should be monitored regularly for changes in prothrombin time or INR.

Based on the results of the population pharmacokinetic study, patients who are still smoking should be encouraged to stop smoking while taking Tarceva, as plasma concentrations could be reduced otherwise.

Erlotinib is a substrate for the P-glycoprotein active substance transporter. Concomitant administration of inhibitors of Pgp, e.g. cyclosporine and verapamil, may lead to altered distribution and/or altered elimination of erlotinib. The consequences of this interaction for e.g. CNS toxicity has not been established. Caution should be exercised in such situations.

Erlotinib is characterised by a decrease in solubility at pH above 5. The effect of antacids, proton pump inhibitors and H2 antagonists on the absorption of erlotinib have not been investigated but absorption may be impaired, leading to lower plasma levels. Caution should be exercised when these medicinal products are combined with erlotinib.

4.6 Pregnancy and lactation
There are no studies in pregnant women using erlotinib. Studies in animals have shown some reproductive toxicity (see section 5.3). The potential risk for humans is unknown. Women of childbearing potential must be advised to avoid pregnancy while on Tarceva. Adequate contraceptive methods should be used during therapy, and for at least 2 weeks after completing therapy. Treatment should only be continued in pregnant women if the potential benefit to the mother outweighs the risk to the foetus.

It is not known whether erlotinib is excreted in human milk. Because of the potential harm to the infant, mothers should be advised against breastfeeding while receiving Tarceva.

4.7 Effects on ability to drive and use machines
No studies on the effects on the ability to drive and use machines have been performed; however erlotinib is not associated with impairment of mental ability.

4.8 Undesirable effects
Rash (75 %) and diarrhoea (54 %) were the most commonly reported adverse drug reactions (ADRs). Most were Grade 1/2 in severity and manageable without intervention. Grade 3/4 rash and diarrhoea occurred in 9 % and 6 %, respectively in Tarceva-treated patients and each resulted in study discontinuation in 1 % of patients. Dose reduction for rash and diarrhoea was needed in 6 % and 1 % of patients, respectively. In study BR.21, the median time to onset of rash was 8 days, and the median time to onset of diarrhoea was 12 days.

Adverse events occurring more frequently (≥3 %) in Tarceva-treated patients than in the placebo group in the pivotal study BR.21, and in at least 10 % of patients in the Tarceva group, are summarised by National Cancer Institute-Common Toxicity Criteria (NCI-CTC) Grade in Table 1.

Table 1: Very common ADRs in study BR.21

(see Table 1 on next page)

Other Observations:

The primary safety population was defined as the 759 patients treated with at least one 150 mg dose of Tarceva monotherapy during Phase III study BR.21, Phase II study A248-1007, and three Phase II studies in populations other than NSCLC: 248-101 (ovarian cancer), A248-1003 (head and neck cancer), and OSI2288g (metastatic breast cancer) and the 242 patients who received placebo in study BR.21. The following common and uncommon adverse reactions have been observed in patients who received Tarceva monotherapy in the primary safety population.

The following terms are used to rank the undesirable effects by frequency: very common >1/10); common >1/100, <1/10); uncommon >1/1,000, <1/100); rare >1/10,000, <1/1000); very rare (<1/10,000) including isolated reports.

Gastrointestinal disorders:

Common: Gastrointestinal bleeding. In clinical studies, some cases have been associated with concomitant warfarin administration (see section 4.5) and some with concomitant NSAID administration.

Hepato-biliary disorders:

Common: Liver function test abnormalities (including increased alanine aminotransferase [ALT], aspartate aminotransferase [AST], bilirubin). These were mainly mild or moderate in severity, transient in nature or associated with liver metastases.

Eye disorders:

Common: Keratitis. One isolated case of corneal ulceration was reported in one patient receiving Tarceva with concurrent chemotherapy, as a complication of mucocutaneous inflammation.

Table 1 Very common ADRs in study BR.21

	Erlotinib N = 485			Placebo N = 242		
NCI-CTC Grade	**Any Grade**	**3**	**4**	**Any Grade**	**3**	**4**
MedDRA Preferred Term	**%**	**%**	**%**	**%**	**%**	**%**
Total patients with any AE	99	40	22	96	36	22
Infections and infestations						
Infection	24	4	0	15	2	0
Metabolism and nutrition disorders						
Anorexia	52	8	1	38	5	< 1
Eye disorders						
Conjunctivitis	12	< 1	0	2	< 1	0
Keratoconjunctivitis sicca	12	0	0	3	0	0
Respiratory, thoracic and mediastinal disorders						
Dyspnoea	41	17	11	35	15	11
Cough	33	4	0	29	2	0
Gastrointestinal disorders						
Diarrhoea	54	6	< 1	18	< 1	0
Nausea	33	3	0	24	2	0
Vomiting	23	2	< 1	19	2	0
Stomatitis	17	< 1	0	3	0	0
Abdominal pain	11	2	< 1	7	1	< 1
Skin and subcutaneous tissue disorders						
Rash	75	8	< 1	17	0	0
Pruritus	13	< 1	0	5	0	0
Dry skin	12	0	0	4	0	0
General disorders and administration site conditions						
Fatigue	52	14	4	45	16	4

Respiratory, thoracic and mediastinal disorders:

Uncommon: Serious interstitial lung disease (ILD), including fatalities, in patients receiving Tarceva for treatment of NSCLC or other advanced solid tumours (see section 4.4).

4.9 Overdose

Single oral doses of Tarceva up to 1000 mg erlotinib in healthy subjects, and up to 1600 mg in cancer patients have been tolerated. Repeated twice daily doses of 200 mg in healthy subjects were poorly tolerated after only a few days of dosing. Based on the data from these studies, severe adverse events such as diarrhoea, rash and possibly increased activity of liver aminotransferases may occur above the recommended dose of 150 mg. In case of suspected overdose, Tarceva should be withheld and symptomatic treatment initiated.

5. PHARMACOLOGICAL PROPERTIES

5.1 Pharmacodynamic properties

Pharmacotherapeutic group: antineoplastic agent, ATC code: L01XX34

Erlotinib is an epidermal growth factor receptor/ human epidermal growth factor receptor type 1 (EGFR also known as HER1) tyrosine kinase inhibitor. Erlotinib potently inhibits the intracellular phosphorylation of EGFR. EGFR is expressed on the cell surface of normal cells and cancer cells. In non-clinical models, inhibition of EGFR phosphotyrosine results in cell stasis and/or death.

Non-small cell lung cancer (NSCLC):

The efficacy and safety of Tarceva was demonstrated in a randomised, double-blind, placebo-controlled trial (BR.21), in 731 patients with locally advanced or metastatic NSCLC after failure of at least one chemotherapy regimen. Patients were randomised 2:1 to receive Tarceva 150 mg or placebo orally once daily. Study endpoints included overall survival, progression-free survival (PFS), response rate, duration of response, time to deterioration of lung cancer-related symptoms (cough, dyspnoea and pain), and safety. The primary end-point was survival.

Demographic characteristics were well balanced between the two treatment groups. About two-thirds of the patients were male and approximately one-third had a baseline ECOG performance status (PS) of 2, and 9 % had a baseline ECOG PS of 3. Ninety-three percent and 92 % of all patients in the Tarceva and placebo groups, respectively, had received a prior platinum-containing regimen and 36 % and 37 % of all patients, respectively, had received a prior taxane therapy.

The adjusted hazard ratio (HR) for death in the Tarceva group relative to the placebo group was 0.73 (95 % CI, 0.60 to 0.87) (p = 0.001). The percent of patients alive at 12 months was 31.2 % and 21.5 %, for the Tarceva and placebo groups respectively. The median overall survival was 6.7 months in the Tarceva group (95 % CI, 5.5 to 7.8 months) compared with 4.7 months in the placebo group (95 % CI, 4.1 to 6.3 months).

The effect on overall survival was explored across different patient subsets. The effect of Tarceva on overall survival was similar in patients with a baseline performance status (ECOG) of 2-3 (HR = 0.77, CI 0.6-1.0) or 0-1 (HR = 0.73, 0.6-0.9), male (HR = 0.76, CI 0.6-0.9) or female patients (HR = 0.80, CI 0.6-1.1), patients < 65 years of age (HR = 0.75, CI 0.6-0.9) or older patients (HR = 0.79, CI 0.6-1.0), patients with one prior regimen (HR = 0.76, CI 0.6-1.0) or more than one prior regimen (HR = 0.75, CI 0.6-1.0), Caucasian (HR = 0.79, CI 0.6-1.0) or Asian patients (HR = 0.61, 0.4-1.0), patients with adenocarcinoma (HR = 0.71, CI 0.6-0.9) or squamous cell carcinoma (HR = 0.67, CI 0.5-0.9), but not in patients with other histologies (HR 1.04, CI 0.7-1.5), patients with stage IV disease at diagnosis (HR = 0.92, CI 0.7-1.2) or < stage IV disease at diagnosis (HR = 0.65, 0.5-0.8). Patients who never smoked had a much greater benefit from erlotinib (survival HR = 0.42, CI 0.28-0.64) compared with current or ex-smokers (HR = 0.87, CI 0.71-1.05).

In the 45 % of patients with known EGFR-expression status, the hazard ratio was 0.68 (CI 0.49-0.94) for patients with EGFR-positive tumours and 0.93 (CI 0.63-1.36) for patients with EGFR-negative tumours (defined by IHC using EGFR pharmDx kit and defining EGFR-negative as less than 10% tumour cells staining). In the remaining 55 % of patients with unknown EGFR-expression status, the hazard ratio was 0.77 (CI 0.61-0.98).

The median PFS was 9.7 weeks in the Tarceva group (95 % CI, 8.4 to 12.4 weeks) compared with 8.0 weeks in the placebo group (95 % CI, 7.9 to 8.1 weeks).

The objective response rate by RECIST in the Tarceva group was 8.9 % (95 % CI, 6.4 to 12.0).

The first 330 patients were centrally assessed (response rate 6.2 %); 401 patients were investigator-assessed (response rate 11.2 %).

The median duration of response was 34.3 weeks, ranging from 9.7 to 57.6+ weeks. The proportion of patients who experienced complete response, partial response or stable disease was 44.0 % and 27.5 %, respectively, for the Tarceva and placebo groups (p = 0.004).

A survival benefit of Tarceva was also observed in patients who did not achieve an objective tumour response (by RECIST). This was evidenced by a hazard ratio for death of 0.82 (95% CI, 0.68 to 0.99) among patients whose best response was stable disease or progressive disease.

Tarceva resulted in symptom benefits by significantly prolonging time to deterioration in cough dyspnoea and pain, versus placebo.

5.2 Pharmacokinetic properties

Absorption: After oral administration, erlotinib peak plasma levels are obtained in approximately 4 hours after oral dosing. A study in normal healthy volunteers provided an estimate of the absolute bioavailability of 59 %. The exposure after an oral dose may be increased by food.

Distribution: Erlotinib has a mean apparent volume of distribution of 232 l and distributes into tumour tissue of humans. In a study of 4 patients (3 with non-small cell lung cancer [NSCLC], and 1 with laryngeal cancer) receiving 150 mg daily oral doses of Tarceva, tumour samples from surgical excisions on day 9 of treatment revealed tumour concentrations of erlotinib that averaged 1,185 ng/g of tissue. This corresponded to an overall average of 63 % (range 5-161 %) of the steady state observed peak plasma concentrations. The primary active metabolites were present in tumour at concentrations averaging 160 ng/g tissue, which corresponded to an overall average of 113 % (range 88-130 %) of the observed steady state peak plasma concentrations. Plasma protein binding is approximately 95 %. Erlotinib binds to serum albumin and alpha-1 acid glycoprotein (AAG).

Metabolism: Erlotinib is metabolised in the liver by the hepatic cytochromes in humans, primarily CYP3A4 and to a lesser extent by CYP1A2. Extrahepatic metabolism by CYP3A4 in intestine, CYP1A1 in lung, and 1B1 in tumour tissue potentially contribute to the metabolic clearance of erlotinib.

There are three main metabolic pathways identified: 1) O-demethylation of either side chain or both, followed by oxidation to the carboxylic acids; 2) oxidation of the acetylene moiety followed by hydrolysis to the aryl carboxylic acid; and 3) aromatic hydroxylation of the phenyl-acetylene moiety. The primary metabolites OSI-420 and OSI-413 of erlotinib produced by O-demethylation of either side chain have comparable potency to erlotinib in preclinical *in vitro* assays and *in vivo* tumour models. They are present in plasma at levels that are < 10 % of erlotinib and display similar pharmacokinetics as erlotinib.

Elimination: Erlotinib is excreted predominantly as metabolites via the faeces > 90 %) with renal elimination accounting for only a small amount (approximately 9 %) of an oral dose. Less than 2 % of the orally administered dose is excreted as parent substance. A population pharmacokinetic analysis in 591 patients receiving single agent Tarceva shows a mean apparent clearance of 4.47 l/hour with a median half-life of 36.2 hours. Therefore, the time to reach steady state plasma concentration would be expected to occur in approximately 7-8 days.

Pharmacokinetics in special populations:

Based on population pharmacokinetic analysis, no clinically significant relationship between predicted apparent clearance and patient age, bodyweight, gender and ethnicity were observed. Patient factors, which correlated with erlotinib pharmacokinetics, were serum total bilirubin, AAG and current smoking. Increased serum concentrations of total bilirubin and AAG concentrations were associated with a reduced erlotinib clearance. The clinical relevance of these differences is unclear. However, smokers had an increased rate of erlotinib clearance.

Based on the results of the population pharmacokinetic study, current smokers should be advised to stop smoking while taking Tarceva, as plasma concentrations could be reduced otherwise.

Based on population pharmacokinetic analysis, the presence of an opioid appeared to increase exposure by about 11 %

There have been no specific studies in paediatric or elderly patients.

Hepatic impairment: Erlotinib is primarily cleared by the liver. No data are currently available regarding the influence of hepatic dysfunction and/or hepatic metastases on the pharmacokinetics of erlotinib. In population pharmacokinetic analysis, increased serum concentrations of total bilirubin were associated with a slower rate of erlotinib clearance.

Renal impairment: Erlotinib and its metabolites are not significantly excreted by the kidney, as less than 9 % of a single dose is excreted in the urine. In population pharmacokinetic analysis, no clinically significant relationship was observed between erlotinib clearance and creatinine clearance, but there are no data available for patients with creatinine clearance < 15 ml/min.

5.3 Preclinical safety data

Chronic dosing effects observed in at least one animal species or study included effects on the cornea (atrophy, ulceration), skin (follicular degeneration and inflammation, redness, and alopecia), ovary (atrophy), liver (liver necrosis), kidney (renal papillary necrosis and tubular dilatation), and gastrointestinal tract (delayed gastric emptying and diarrhoea). Red blood cell parameters were decreased and white blood cells, primarily neutrophils, were increased. There were treatment-related increases in ALT, AST and bilirubin. These findings were observed at exposures well below clinically relevant exposures.

Based on the mode of action, erlotinib has the potential to be a teratogen. Data from reproductive toxicology tests in rats and rabbits at doses near the maximum tolerated dose and/or maternally toxic doses showed reproductive (embryotoxicity in rats, embryo resorption and foetotoxicity in rabbits) and developmental (decrease in pup growth and survival in rats) toxicity, but was not teratogenic and did not impair fertility. These findings were observed at clinically relevant exposures.

Erlotinib tested negative in conventional genotoxicity studies. Carcinogenicity studies have not been performed.

A mild phototoxic skin reaction was observed in rats after UV irradiation.

6. PHARMACEUTICAL PARTICULARS

6.1 List of excipients

Tablet core:

Lactose monohydrate

Cellulose, microcrystalline (E460)

Sodium starch glycolate Type A

Sodium laurilsulfate

Magnesium stearate (E470 b)

Tablet coat:

Hydroxypropyl cellulose (E463)

Titanium dioxide (E171)

Macrogol

Hypromellose (E464)

Printing ink:

Tarceva 25 mg: Shellac (E904), Iron oxide yellow (E172)

Tarceva 100 mg: Shellac (E904), Iron oxide yellow (E172), Iron oxide black (E172), Titanium dioxide (E171)

Tarceva 150 mg: Shellac (E904), Iron oxide yellow (E172), Iron oxide black (E172), Iron oxide red (E172)

6.2 Incompatibilities

Not applicable.

6.3 Shelf life

3 years.

6.4 Special precautions for storage

This medicinal product does not require any special storage conditions.

6.5 Nature and contents of container

PVC blister sealed with aluminium foil containing 30 tablets.

Not all strengths / pack sizes may be marketed.

6.6 Instructions for use and handling

No special requirements.

7. MARKETING AUTHORISATION HOLDER

Roche Registration Limited

40 Broadwater Road

Welwyn Garden City

Hertfordshire, AL7 3AY

United Kingdom

8. MARKETING AUTHORISATION NUMBER(S)

EU/1/05/311/001 – 25 mg film-coated tablets

EU/1/05/311/002 – 100 mg film-coated tablets

EU/1/05/311/003 – 150 mg film-coated tablets

9. DATE OF FIRST AUTHORISATION/RENEWAL OF THE AUTHORISATION

19 September 2005

10. DATE OF REVISION OF THE TEXT

Not applicable.

LEGAL STATUS

POM

Targocid 200mg & 400mg

(sanofi-aventis)

1. NAME OF THE MEDICINAL PRODUCT

Targocid 200mg

Targocid 400mg

2. QUALITATIVE AND QUANTITATIVE COMPOSITION

Teicoplanin 200mg

Teicoplanin 400mg

3. PHARMACEUTICAL FORM

Powder for Injection

4. CLINICAL PARTICULARS

4.1 Therapeutic indications

Targocid is indicated in potentially serious Gram-positive infections including those which cannot be treated with other antimicrobial drugs, eg. penicillins and cephalosporins.

Targocid is useful in the therapy of serious staphylococcal infections in patients who cannot receive or who have failed to respond to the penicillins and cephalosporins, or who have infections with staphylococci resistant to other antibiotics.

The effectiveness of teicoplanin has been documented in the following infections:-

Skin and soft tissue infections, urinary tract infections, lower respiratory tract infections, joint and bone infections, septicaemia, endocarditis and peritonitis related to continuous ambulatory peritoneal dialysis.

Targocid may be used for antimicrobial prophylaxis in orthopaedic surgery at risk of Gram-positive infection.

4.2 Posology and method of administration

Administration

The reconstituted Targocid injection may be administered directly either intravenously or intramuscularly. The intravenous injection may be administered either as a bolus or as a 30 minute infusion. Dosage is usually once daily but, in cases of severe infection, a second injection should be administered on the first day in order to reach more rapidly the required serum concentrations.

The majority of patients with infections caused by organisms sensitive to the antibiotic show a therapeutic response within 48-72 hours. The total duration of therapy is determined by the type and severity of the infection and the clinical response of the patient. In endocarditis and osteomyelitis, treatment for three weeks or longer is recommended.

Determination of teicoplanin serum concentrations may optimise therapy. In severe infections, trough serum concentrations should not be less than 10mg/L. Peak concentrations measured one hour after a 400mg intravenous dose are usually in the range of 20-50mg/L; peak serum concentrations of up to 250mg/L have been reported after intravenous doses of 25mg/kg. A relationship between serum concentration and toxicity has not been established.

Therapeutic dosage:

Adult or elderly patients with normal renal function

Prophylaxis: 400mg intravenously as a single dose at induction of anaesthesia

Moderate infections: Skin and soft tissue infection, urinary tract infection, lower respiratory tract infection

Loading dose: One single i.v. or i.m. injection of 400mg on the first day

Maintenance dose: A single i.v. or i.m. injection of 200mg daily

Severe infections: Joint and bone infection, septicaemia, endocarditis

Loading dose: Three 400mg i.v. injections, administered 12 hours apart

Maintenance dose: A single i.v. or i.m. injection of 400mg daily

1. Standard doses of 200 and 400mg equate respectively to mean doses of 3 and 6mg/kg. In patients weighing more than 85kg it is recommended to adapt the dosage to the weight following the same therapeutic schedule: moderate infection 3mg/kg, severe infection 6mg/kg.

2. In some clinical situations, such as infected, severely burned patients or Staphylococcus aureus endocarditis, unit maintenance doses of up to 12mg/kg have been administered (intravenously).

Children

Teicoplanin can be used to treat Gram-positive infections in children from the age of 2 months. For severe infections and neutropenic patients the recommended dose is 10mg/kg every 12 hours for the first three doses; thereafter a dose of 10mg/kg should be administered by either intravenous or intramuscular injection as a single dose each day.

For moderate infections the recommended dose is 10mg/kg every twelve hours for the first three doses; thereafter a dose of 6mg/kg should be administered by either intravenous or intramuscular injection as a single dose each day.

The recommended dosage regimen for neonates is a loading dose of 16mg/kg followed by a daily dose of 8mg/kg.

In continuous ambulatory periotoneal dialysis

after a single loading IV dose of 400mg of the patient is febrile, the recommended dosage is 20mg/L per bag in the first week, 20mg/L in alternate bags in the second week and 20mg/L in the overnight dwell bag only during the third week.

Adults and elderly patients with renal insufficiency

For patients with impaired renal function, reduction of dosage is not required until the fourth day of Targocid treatment. Measurement of the serum concentration of teicoplanin may optimise therapy (see section 'Administration').

From the fourth day of treatment

in mild renal insufficiency

creatinine clearance between 40 and 60ml/min, Targocid dose should be halved, either by administering the initial unit dose every two days, or by administering half of this dose once a day.

in severe renal insufficiency

creatinine clearance less than 40ml/min and in haemodialysed patients, Targocid dose should be one third of the normal either by administering the initial unit dose every third day, or by administering one third of this dose once a day. Teicoplanin is not removed by dialysis.

4.3 Contraindications

Teicoplanin is contra-indicated in patients who have exhibited previous hypersensitivity to the drug.

4.4 Special warnings and special precautions for use

Warnings:

Targocid should be administered with caution in patients known to be hypersensitive to vancomycin since cross hypersensitivity may occur. However, a history of the "Red Man Syndrome" that can occur with vancomycin is not a contra-indication to Targocid.

Thrombocytopenia has been reported with teicoplanin, especially at higher doses than those usually recommended. It is advisable for periodic haematological studies to be performed during treatment. Liver and renal function tests are advised during treatment.

Serial renal and auditory function tests should be undertaken in the following circumstances:

Prolonged treatment in patients with renal insufficiency.

Concurrent and sequential use of other drugs which may have neurotoxic and/or nephrotoxic properties. These include aminoglycosides, colistin, amphotericin B, cyclosporin, cisplatin, frusemide and ethacrynic acid.

However, there is no evidence of synergistic toxicity with combinations with Targocid.

Dosage must be adapted in patients with renal impairment (see 'Dosage').

Precautions:

Superinfection: as with other antibiotics, the use of teicoplanin, especially if prolonged, may result in overgrowth of non-susceptible organisms. Repeated evaluation of the patients condition is essential. If superinfection occurs during therapy, appropriate measures should be taken.

4.5 Interaction with other medicinal products and other forms of Interaction

Targocid should be used with care in conjunction with or sequentially with other drugs with known nephrotoxic or ototoxic potential. Of particular concern are streptomycin, neomycin, kanamycin, gentamicin, amikacin, tobramycin, cephaloridine, colistin.

In clinical trials teicoplanin has been administered to many patients already receiving various medications including other antibiotics, antihypertensives, anaesthetic agents, cardiac drugs and antidiabetic agents without evidence of adverse interaction.

Animal studies have shown lack of interaction with diazepam, thiopentone, morphine, neuromuscular blocking agents or halothane.

4.6 Pregnancy and lactation

Animal reproduction studies have not shown evidence of impairment of fertility or teratogenic effect. At high doses in rats there was an increased incidence of stillbirths and neonatal mortality. It is recommended that Targocid should not be used during confirmed or presumed pregnancy or during lactation unless a physician considers that the potential benefits outweigh a possible risk. There is no information about the excretion of teicoplanin in milk or placental transfer of the drug.

4.7 Effects on ability to drive and use machines

There is no indication to suggest an effect of teicoplanin on a patient's ability to drive or use machinery.

4.8 Undesirable effects

Targocid is generally well tolerated. Side-effects rarely require cessation of therapy and are generally mild and transient: serious side-effects are rare. The following adverse events have been reported:

Local reactions: erythema, local pain, thrombophlebitis, injection site abscess.

Hypersensitivity: rash, pruritis, fever, bronchospasm, anaphylactic reactions, anaphylactic shock, rigors, urticaria, angioedema, rare reports of exfolative dermatitis, toxic epidermal necrolysis, rare cases of erythema multiforme including Stevens-Johnson Syndrome. In addition, infusion-related events, such as erythema or flushing of the upper body, have been rarely reported in which the events occurred without a history of previous teicoplanin exposure and did not recur on re-exposure when the infusion rate was slowed and/or concentration decreased. These events were not specific to any concentration or rate of infusion.

Gastric-intestinal: nausea, vomiting, diarrhoea.

Blood: eosinophilia, leucopenia, thrombocytopenia, thrombocytosis, neutropenia, rare cases of reversible agranulocytosis.

Liver function: increases in serum transaminases and/or serum alkaline phosphatase.

Renal function: transient elevations of serum creatinine, renal failure.

Central nervous system: dizziness, headache.

Auditory/vestibular: mild hearing loss, tinnitus and vestibular disorder.

Other: Superinfection (overgrowth of non-susceptible organisms).

4.9 Overdose
Teicoplanin is not removed by haemodialysis. Treatment of overdosage should be symptomatic. Several overdoses of 100mg/kg/day have been administered in error to two neutropenic patients aged 4 and 8 years. Despite high plasma concentrations of teicoplanin up to 300mg/ml there were no symptoms or laboratory abnormalities.

5. PHARMACOLOGICAL PROPERTIES

5.1 Pharmacodynamic properties
Teicoplanin is a bactericidial, glycopeptide antibiotic, produced by fermentation of *Actinoplanes teichomyceticus*. It is active against both aerobic and anaerobic Gram-positive bacteria.

Species usually sensitive (MIC less than or equal to 16mg/1):

Staphylococcus aureus and coagulase negative staphylococci (sensitive or resistant to methicillin), streptococci, enterococci, *Listeria monocytogenes*, micrococci, *Eikenella corrodens*, group *JK corynebacteria* and Gram-positive anaerobes including *Clostridium difficile*, and peptococci.

Species usually resistant (MIC superior to 16mg/1):

Nocardia asteroides, Lactobacillus spp, Leuconostoc and all Gram-negative bacteria.

Bactericidal synergy has been demonstrated *in vitro* with aminoglycosides against group D streptococci and staphylococci. *In vitro* combinations of teicoplanin with rifampicin or fluorinated quinolones show primarily additive effects and sometimes synergy.

One-step resistance to teicoplanin could not be obtained *in vitro* and multi-step resistance was only reached *in vitro* after 11-14 passages.

Teicoplanin does not show cross-resistance with other classes of antibiotics.

The use of teicoplanin may result in overgrowth of non-susceptible organisms. If new infections due to bacteria or fungi appear during treatment appropriate measures should be taken.

Susceptibility testing:

Sensidiscs are charged with 30 micrograms of teicoplanin. Strains showing an inhibition zone diameter of 14mm or more are susceptible and those of 10mm or less are resistant.

5.2 Pharmacokinetic properties
Following injection teicoplanin rapidly penetrates into tissues, including skin, fat and bones and reaches the highest concentrations in the kidney, trachea, lungs and adrenals. Teicoplanin does not readily penetrate into the cerebrospinal fluid (CSF).

In man the plasma level profile after intravenous administration indicates a biphasic distribution (with a rapid distribution phase having a half-life of about 0.3 hours, followed by a more prolonged distribution phase having a half-life of about 3 hours), followed by slow elimination (with a terminal elimination half-life of about 150 hours). At 6mg/kg administered intravenously at 0, 12, 24 hours and every 24 hours thereafter as a 30 minute infusion, a predicted trough serum concentration of 10mg/L would be reached by Day 4. The steady state volume of distribution after 3 to 6mg/kg intravenously ranges from 0.94 L/kg to 1.4 L/kg. The volume of distribution in children is not substantially different from that in adults.

Approximately 90-95% teicoplanin is bound with weak affinity to plasma proteins. Teicoplanin penetrates readily into blister exudates and into joint fluid; it penetrates neutrophils and enhances their bactericidal activity; it does not penetrate red blood cells.

No metabolites of teicoplanin have been identified; more than 97% of the administered teicoplanin is excreted unchanged. The elimination of teicoplanin from the plasma is prolonged with a terminal half-life of elimination in man of about 150 hours. Teicoplanin is excreted mainly in the urine.

5.3 Preclinical safety data
Not Applicable

6. PHARMACEUTICAL PARTICULARS

6.1 List of excipients
Sodium chloride

6.2 Incompatibilities
Solutions of teicoplanin and aminoglycosides are incompatible when mixed directly and should not be mixed before injection.

6.3 Shelf life
3 years unopened.

24 hours after reconstitution.

6.4 Special precautions for storage
Finished Product:

Vials of dry Targocid should not be stored above 25°C.

Reconstituted Product:

In keeping with good clinical pharmaceutical practise reconstituted vials of Targocid should be used immediately and any unused portion discarded. On the few occasions when changing circumstances make this impractical reconstituted solutions should be kept at 2 - 8°C and discarded within 24 hours.

Do not store in a syringe.

6.5 Nature and contents of container
Colourless, BP, Type I glass vials, closed with a butyl rubber plug and combination aluminium/plastic "flip-off cap" (colour coded yellow).

Pack size: 1 vial

6.6 Instructions for use and handling
Preparation of Injection

The entire contents of the water ampoule should be slowly added to the vial of Targocid and the vial rolled gently until the powder is completely dissolved, taking care to avoid formation of foam. If the solution does become foamy then allow to stand for about 15 minutes for the foam to subside.

A calculated excess is included in each vial of Targocid so that, when prepared as described above, a full dose of 100mg, 200mg or 400mg (depending on the strength of the vial) will be obtained if all the reconstituted solution is withdrawn from the vial by a syringe. The concentration of teicoplanin in these injections will be 100mg in 1.5ml (from the 100mg and 200mg vials) and 400mg in 3ml (from the 400mg vial).

The reconstituted solution may be injected directly, or alternatively diluted with:

- 0.9% Sodium Chloride Injection
- Compound Sodium Lactate Injection (Ringer-Lactate Solution, Hartmanns Solution)
- 5% Dextrose Injection
- 0.18% Sodium Chloride and 4% Dextrose Injection
- Peritoneal dialysis solution containing 1.36% or 3.86% Dextrose.

7. MARKETING AUTHORISATION HOLDER
Aventis Pharma Limited

50 Kings Hill Avenue

Kings Hill

West Malling

Kent

ME19 4AH

8. MARKETING AUTHORISATION NUMBER(S)
TARGOCID 200MG: PL 04425/0088

TARGOCID 400MG: PL 04425/0089

WATER FOR INJECTIONS PL 04425/0090

9. DATE OF FIRST AUTHORISATION/RENEWAL OF THE AUTHORISATION
2 AUGUST 1989/7 MARCH 2001

10. DATE OF REVISION OF THE TEXT
JULY 2001

TARGRETIN CAPSULES

(Zeneus Pharma Ltd)

1. NAME OF THE MEDICINAL PRODUCT
Targretin▼ 75 mg capsules, soft

2. QUALITATIVE AND QUANTITATIVE COMPOSITION
Each capsule contains 75 mg of bexarotene

For excipients, see section 6.1

3. PHARMACEUTICAL FORM
Soft capsule

Off-white capsule, containing a liquid suspension and imprinted with "Targretin"

4. CLINICAL PARTICULARS

4.1 Therapeutic indications
Targretin capsules are indicated for the treatment of skin manifestations of advanced stage CTCL patients refractory to at least one systemic treatment.

4.2 Posology and method of administration
Bexarotene therapy should only be initiated and maintained by physicians experienced in the treatment of patients with CTCL. The recommended initial dose is 300 mg/m^2/day. Targretin capsules should be taken as a single oral daily dose with a meal (see 4.5). Initial dose calculations according to body surface area are as follows:

Initial dose level (300 mg/m^2/day)		Number of 75 mg Targretin capsules
Body Surface Area (m^2)	Total daily dose (mg/day)	
0.88 – 1.12	300	4
1.13 - 1.37	375	5
1.38 - 1.62	450	6
1.63 - 1.87	525	7
1.88 - 2.12	600	8
2.13 - 2.37	675	9
2.38 - 2.62	750	10

Dose modification guidelines: the 300 mg/m^2/day dose level may be adjusted to 200 mg/m^2/day then to 100 mg/m^2/day, or temporarily suspended, if necessitated by toxicity. When toxicity is controlled, doses may be carefully readjusted upward. With appropriate clinical monitoring, individual patients may benefit from doses above 300 mg/m^2/day. Doses greater than 650 mg/m^2/day have not been evaluated in patients with CTCL. In clinical trials, bexarotene was administered for up to 118 weeks to patients with CTCL. Treatment should be continued as long as the patient is deriving benefit.

Use in children and adolescents: the clinical safety and effectiveness of bexarotene in the paediatric population (below 18 years of age) have not been studied and this product should not be used in a paediatric population until further data become available.

Use in the elderly: of the total number of patients with CTCL in clinical studies, 61% were 60 years or older, while 30% were 70 years or older. No overall differences in safety were observed between patients 70 years or older and younger patients, but greater sensitivity of some older individuals to bexarotene cannot be ruled out. The standard dose should be used in the elderly.

Renal insufficiency: no formal studies have been conducted in patients with renal insufficiency. Clinical pharmacokinetic data indicate that urinary elimination of bexarotene and its metabolites is a minor excretory pathway for bexarotene. In all evaluated patients, the estimated renal clearance of bexarotene was less than 1 ml/minute. In view of the limited data, patients with renal insufficiency should be monitored carefully while on bexarotene therapy.

4.3 Contraindications
Known hypersensitivity to bexarotene or to any of the excipients of the product

Pregnancy and lactation

Women of child-bearing potential without effective birth-control measures

History of pancreatitis

Uncontrolled hypercholesterolaemia

Uncontrolled hypertriglyceridaemia

Hypervitaminosis A

Uncontrolled thyroid disease

Hepatic insufficiency

Ongoing systemic infection

4.4 Special warnings and special precautions for use
General: Targretin capsules should be used with caution in patients with a known hypersensitivity to retinoids. No clinical instances of cross-reactivity have been noted. Patients receiving bexarotene should not donate blood for transfusion.

Lipids: hyperlipidaemia has been identified as an effect associated with the use of bexarotene in clinical studies. Fasting blood lipid determinations (triglycerides and cholesterol) should be performed before bexarotene therapy is initiated and at weekly intervals until the lipid response to bexarotene is established, which usually occurs within two to four weeks, and then at intervals no less than monthly thereafter. Fasting triglycerides should be normal or normalised with appropriate intervention prior to bexarotene therapy. Every attempt should be made to maintain triglyceride levels below 4.52 mmol/l in order to reduce the risk of clinical sequelae. If fasting triglycerides are elevated or become elevated during treatment, institution of antilipaemic therapy is recommended, and if necessary, dose reductions (from 300 mg/m^2/day of bexarotene to 200 mg/m^2/day, and if necessary to 100 mg/m^2/day) or treatment discontinuation. Data from clinical studies indicate that bexarotene concentrations were not affected by concomitant administration of atorvastatin. However, concomitant administration of gemfibrozil resulted in substantial increases in plasma concentrations of bexarotene and therefore, concomitant administration of gemfibrozil with bexarotene is not recommended (see 4.5). Elevations of serum cholesterol should be managed according to current medical practice.

Pancreatitis: acute pancreatitis associated with elevations of fasting serum triglycerides has been reported in clinical studies. Patients with CTCL having risk factors for pancreatitis (e.g., prior episodes of pancreatitis, uncontrolled hyperlipidaemia, excessive alcohol consumption, uncontrolled diabetes mellitus, biliary tract disease, and medications known to increase triglyceride levels or to be associated with pancreatic toxicity) should not be treated with bexarotene, unless the potential benefit outweighs the risk.

Liver Function Test (LFT) abnormalities: LFT elevations associated with the use of bexarotene have been reported. Based on data from ongoing clinical trials, elevation of LFTs resolved within one month in 80% of patients following a decrease in dose or discontinuation of therapy. Baseline LFTs should be obtained, and LFTs should be carefully monitored weekly during the first month and then monthly thereafter. Consideration should be given to a suspension or discontinuation of bexarotene if test results reach greater than three times the upper limit of normal values for SGOT/AST, SGPT/ALT, or bilirubin.

Thyroid function test alterations: changes in thyroid function tests have been observed in patients receiving bexarotene, most often noted as a reversible reduction in thyroid hormone (total thyroxine [total T_4]) and thyroid-stimulating hormone (TSH) levels. Baseline thyroid function tests should be obtained and then monitored at least monthly during treatment and as indicated by the emergence of symptoms consistent with hypothyroidism. Patients with symptomatic hypothyroidism on bexarotene therapy have been treated with thyroid hormone supplements with resolution of symptoms.

Leucopenia: leucopenia associated with bexarotene therapy has been reported in clinical studies. The majority of cases resolved after dose reduction or discontinuation of treatment. Determination of white blood cell count with differential count should be obtained at baseline, weekly during the first month and then monthly thereafter.

Anaemia: anaemia associated with bexarotene therapy has been reported in clinical studies. Determination of haemoglobin should be obtained at baseline, weekly during the first month and then monthly thereafter. Decreases of haemoglobin should be managed according to current medical practice.

Lens opacities: following bexarotene treatment, some patients were observed to have previously undetected lens opacities or a change in pre-existing lens opacities unrelated to treatment duration or dose level of exposure. Given the high prevalence and natural rate of cataract formation in the older patient population represented in the clinical studies, there was no apparent association between the incidence of lens opacity formation and bexarotene administration. However, an adverse effect of long-term bexarotene treatment on lens opacity formation in humans has not been excluded. Any patient treated with bexarotene who experiences visual difficulties should have an appropriate ophthalmologic examination.

Vitamin A supplementation: because of the relationship of bexarotene to vitamin A, patients should be advised to limit vitamin A supplements to ≤15,000 IU/day to avoid potential additive toxic effects.

Patients with diabetes mellitus: caution should be exercised when administering bexarotene in patients using insulin, agents enhancing insulin secretion (e.g. sulfonylureas), or insulin-sensitisers (e.g. thiazolidinediones). Based on the known mechanism of action, bexarotene may potentially enhance the action of these agents, resulting in hypoglycaemia. No cases of hypoglycaemia associated with the use of bexarotene as monotherapy have been reported.

Photosensitivity: the use of some retinoids has been associated with photosensitivity. Patients should be advised to minimise exposure to sunlight and avoid sun lamps during therapy with bexarotene, as *in vitro* data indicate that bexarotene may potentially have a photosensitising effect.

Oral contraceptives: bexarotene can potentially induce metabolic enzymes and thereby theoretically reduce the efficacy of oestroprogestive contraceptives. Thus, if treatment with bexarotene is intended in a woman of child-bearing potential, a reliable, non-hormonal form of contraception is also required, because bexarotene belongs to a therapeutic class for which the human malformative risk is high.

4.5 Interaction with other medicinal products and other forms of Interaction

Drug interactions: effects of other substances on bexarotene: no formal studies to evaluate drug interactions with bexarotene have been conducted. On the basis of the oxidative metabolism of bexarotene by cytochrome P450 3A4 (CYP3A4), coadministration with other CYP3A4 substrates such as ketoconazole, itraconazole, protease inhibitors, clarithromycin and erythromycin may theoretically lead to an increase in plasma bexarotene concentrations. Furthermore, co-administration with CYP3A4 inducers such as rifampicin, phenytoin, dexamethasone or phenobarbital may theoretically cause a reduction in plasma bexarotene concentrations.

A population analysis of plasma bexarotene concentrations in patients with CTCL indicated that concomitant administration of gemfibrozil resulted in substantial increases in plasma concentrations of bexarotene. The mechanism of this interaction is unknown. Under similar conditions, bexarotene concentrations were not affected by concomitant administration of atorvastatin or levothyroxine. Concomitant administration of gemfibrozil with bexarotene is not recommended.

Drug interactions: effects of bexarotene on other substances: there are indications that bexarotene may induce CYP3A4. Therefore, repeated administration of bexarotene may result in an auto-induction of its own metabolism and, particularly at dose levels greater than 300 mg/m^2/day, may increase the rate of metabolism and reduce plasma concentrations of other substances metabolised by cytochrome P450 3A4, such as tamoxifen. For example bexarotene may reduce the efficacy of oral contraceptives (see 4.4 and 4.6).

Laboratory test interactions: CA125 assay values in patients with ovarian cancer may be accentuated with bexarotene therapy.

Food interactions: in all clinical trials, patients were instructed to take Targretin capsules with or immediately following a meal. In one clinical study, plasma bexarotene AUC and C_{max} values were substantially higher following the administration of a fat-containing meal versus those following the administration of a glucose solution. Because safety and efficacy data from clinical trials are based upon administration with food, it is recommended that Targretin capsules be administered with food.

On the basis of the oxidative metabolism of bexarotene by cytochrome P450 3A4, grapefruit juice may theoretically lead to an increase in plasma bexarotene concentrations.

4.6 Pregnancy and lactation

Pregnancy: there are no adequate data from the use of bexarotene in pregnant women. Studies in animals have shown reproductive toxicity. Based on the comparison of animal and patient exposures to bexarotene, a margin of safety for human teratogenicity has not been demonstrated (see 5.3). Bexarotene is contraindicated in pregnancy (see 4.3).

If this drug is used inadvertently during pregnancy, or if the patient becomes pregnant while taking this medicinal product, the patient should be informed of the potential hazard to the foetus.

Women of childbearing potential must use adequate birth-control measures when bexarotene is used. A negative, sensitive, pregnancy test (e.g. serum beta-human chorionic gonadotropin, beta-HCG) should be obtained within one week prior to bexarotene therapy. Effective contraception must be used from the time of the negative pregnancy test through the initiation of therapy, during therapy and for at least one month following discontinuation of therapy. Whenever contraception is required, it is recommended that two reliable forms of contraception be used simultaneously. Bexarotene can potentially induce metabolic enzymes and thereby theoretically reduce the efficacy of oestroprogestative contraceptives (see 4.5). Thus, if treatment with bexarotene is intended in a woman with child-bearing potential, a reliable, non-hormonal contraceptive method is also recommended. Male patients with sexual partners who are pregnant, possibly pregnant, or may potentially become pregnant must use condoms during sexual intercourse while taking bexarotene and for at least one month after the last dose.

Lactation: it is not known whether bexarotene is excreted in human milk. Bexarotene should not be used in nursing mothers.

4.7 Effects on ability to drive and use machines

No studies on the effects on the ability to drive and use machines have been performed. However, dizziness and visual difficulties have been reported in patients taking Targretin. Patients who experience dizziness or visual difficulties during therapy must not drive or operate machinery.

4.8 Undesirable effects

The safety of bexarotene has been examined in clinical studies of 193 patients with CTCL who received bexarotene for up to 118 weeks and in 420 non-CTCL cancer patients in other studies.

In 109 patients with CTCL treated at an initial dose of 300 mg/m^2/day, the most commonly reported adverse drug reactions were hyperlipaemia ((primarily elevated triglycerides) 74%), hypothyroidism (29%), hypercholesterolaemia (28%), headache (27%), leucopenia (20%), pruritus (20%), asthenia (19%), rash (16%), exfoliative dermatitis (15%), and pain (12%).

The following drug-related adverse reactions were reported during clinical studies in patients with CTCL (N=109) treated at an initial dose of 300 mg/m^2/day. The frequency of adverse reactions are classified as very common (>1/10), common (>1/100, <1/10), uncommon (>1/1,000, <1/100), rare (>1/10,000, <1/1,000), and very rare (<1/10,000).

Haemic & Lymphatic

Very common: leucopenia

Common: hypochromic anaemia, lymphadenopathy, lymphoma like reaction

Uncommon: anaemia, blood dyscrasia, coagulation disorder, increased coagulation time, eosinophilia, leukocytosis, lymphocytosis, purpura, thrombocythaemia, thrombocytopenia

Endocrine

Very common: hypothyroidism

Common: thyroid disorder

Uncommon: hyperthyroidism

Metabolic & Nutrition

Very common: hyperlipaemia, hypercholesterolaemia

Common: increased SGOT, increased SGPT, increased lactic dehydrogenase, increased creatinine, hypoproteinaemia, weight gain

Uncommon: bilirubinaemia, increased blood urea nitrogen, gout, decreased High Density Lipoprotein

Nervous system

Common: insomnia, dizziness, hypesthesia

Uncommon: agitation, ataxia, depression, hyperaesthesia, neuropathy, vertigo

Special senses

Common: dry eyes, deafness, eye disorder

Uncommon: abnormal vision, amblyopia, blepharitis, specified cataract, conjunctivitis, corneal lesion, ear disorder, visual field defect

Cardiovascular

Common: peripheral oedema

Uncommon: oedema, hemorrhage, hypertension, tachycardia, varicose vein, vasodilatation

Digestive

Common: nausea, diarrhoea, dry mouth, cheilitis, anorexia, constipation, flatulence, abnormal liver function tests, vomiting

Uncommon: gastrointestinal disorder, hepatic failure, pancreatitis

Skin & appendages

Very common: pruritus, rash, exfoliative dermatitis

Common: dry skin, skin disorder, alopecia, skin ulcer, acne, skin hypertrophy, skin nodule, sweating

Uncommon: hair disorder, herpes simplex, nail disorder, pustular rash, serous drainage, skin discoloration

Musculoskeletal

Common: arthralgia, bone pain, myalgia

Uncommon: myasthenia

Urogenital

Uncommon: albuminuria, abnormal kidney function

Body as a whole

Very common: headache, asthenia, pain

Common: altered hormone level, chills, abdominal pain, allergic reaction, infection

Uncommon: back pain, cellulitis, fever, parasitic infection, abnormal lab test, mucous membrane disorder, neoplasm

The following adverse reactions were noted with increased frequency when bexarotene was administered at a dose >300 mg/m^2/day (CTCL): anaemia, hypochromic anaemia, eosinophilia, bilirubinaemia, increased blood urea nitrogen, depression, abnormal vision, specified cataract, vasodilatation, diarrhoea, anorexia, pancreatitis, gastrointestinal disorder, alopecia, serous drainage, hair disorder, nail disorder, myasthenia, albuminuria, chills, altered hormone level, back pain and fever.

Additional adverse reactions were also noted when bexarotene was administered at a dose >300 mg/m^2/day (CTCL): abnormal white blood cells, increased gonadotrophic luteinizing hormone, weight loss, increased alkaline phosphatase, increased creatinine phosphokinase, somnolence, hypertonia, decreased libido, nervousness, lacrimation disorder, night blindness, tinnitus, dyspnoea, sinusitis, dyspepsia, maculopapular rash and flu syndrome.

In non-CTCL cancer patients the following adverse reactions were noted with increased frequency when bexarotene was administered at a dose of 300 mg/m^2/day: anaemia, increased coagulation time, leucocytosis, depression, abnormal vision, specified cataract, vasodilatation, cheilitis, dry mouth, dry skin, back pain and fever. The following additional reactions were also noted: paraesthesia, dyspnoea, pharyngitis, thirst, maculopapular rash and chest pain.

In non-CTCL cancer patients the following adverse reactions were noted with increased frequency when bexarotene was administered at a dose of >300 mg/m^2/day (compared to administration to CTCL patients at 300 mg/m^2/day): anaemia, increased coagulation time, thrombocytopenia, bilirubinaemia, depression, amblyopia, abnormal vision, specified cataract, conjunctivitis, vasodilatation, oedema, nausea, diarrhoea, dry mouth, pancreatitis, dry skin, nail disorder, skin discolouration, albuminuria, fever, back pain and mucous membrane disorder.

The following additional adverse reactions were also noted in non-CTCL cancer patients when bexarotene was administered at a dose >300 mg/m^2/day: decreased thromboplastin, ecchymosis, abnormal erythrocytes, petechia, abnormal white blood cells, increased alkaline phosphatase, weight loss, hypercalcaemia, increased creatine phosphokinase, increased lipase, dehydration, anxiety, confusion, paraesthesia, peripheral neuritis, nystagmus, nervousness, somnolence, emotional lability, taste perversion, migraine, arrhythmia, peripheral vascular disorder, dyspnoea, increased cough, haemoptysis, pharyngitis, mouth ulceration, stomatitis, abnormal stools, dyspepsia, dysphagia, eructation, oral moniliasis, maculopapular rash, vesicobullous rash, leg cramps, haematuria, chest pain, pelvic pain, body odour and generalised oedema.

At doses of 300 mg/m^2/day (non-CTCL) there were also isolated reports (single patient reports) of the following: abnormal white blood cells, increased creatine phosphokinase, hyponatraemia, weight loss, circumoral paraesthesia, taste perversion, palpitation, epistaxis, pneumonia, respiratory disorder, abnormal stools, dyspepsia, increased appetite, psoriasis and carcinoma.

With increased dosage (>300 mg/m^2/day, CTCL and non-CTCL), there were also isolated reports (single patient reports) of the following: bone marrow depression, decreased prothrombin, decreased gonadotrophic luteinizing hormone, dehydration, hypokalaemia, increased amylase, hyperuricaemia, hypocholesterolaemia, hypolipaemia, hypomagnesaemia, hyponatraemia, hypovolaemia, abnormal gait, confusion, stupor, abnormal thinking, decreased libido, subdural haematoma, taste perversion, eye pain, congestive heart failure, pallor, vascular anomaly, vascular disorder, laryngismus, pneumonia, rhinitis, lung disorder, pleural disorder, cholestatic jaundice, abnormal stools, dysphagia, eructation, jaundice, liver damage, cholecystitis, gingivitis, melaena, nausea and vomiting, tenesmus, thirst, herpes zoster, seborrhoea, contact dermatitis, furunculosis, lichenoid dermatitis, arthritis, joint disorder, leg cramps, polyuria, breast enlargement, impotence, nocturia, urinary retention, impaired urination, urine abnormality, malaise, viral infection, chest pain, generalized oedema, enlarged abdomen, face oedema and photosensitivity reaction.

The majority of adverse reactions were noted at a higher incidence at doses greater than 300 mg/m^2/day. Generally, these resolved without sequelae on dose reduction or drug withdrawal. However, among a total of 810 patients including those without malignancy treated with bexarotene, there were three serious adverse reactions with fatal outcome (acute pancreatitis, subdural haematoma and liver failure). Of these, liver failure, subsequently determined to be not related to bexarotene, was the only one to occur in a CTCL patient.

Hypothyroidism generally occurs 4-8 weeks after commencement of therapy. It may be asymptomatic and responds to treatment with thyroxine and resolves upon drug withdrawal.

Bexarotene has a different adverse reaction profile to other oral, non-retinoid X receptor (RXR) -selective retinoid drugs. Owing to its primarily RXR-binding activity, bexarotene is less likely to cause mucocutaneous, nail, and hair toxicities; arthralgia; and myalgia; which are frequently reported with retinoic acid receptor (RAR) -binding agents.

4.9 Overdose

No clinical experience with an overdose of Targretin capsules has been reported. Any overdose should be treated with supportive care for the signs and symptoms exhibited by the patient.

Doses up to 1000 mg/m^2/day of bexarotene have been administered in clinical studies with no acute toxic effects. Single doses of 1500 mg/kg (9000 mg/m^2) and 720 mg/kg (14,400 mg/m^2) were tolerated without significant toxicity in rats and dogs, respectively.

5. PHARMACOLOGICAL PROPERTIES

5.1 Pharmacodynamic properties

Pharmacotherapeutic Group: other antineoplastic agents ATC code: L01XX25

Bexarotene is a synthetic compound that exerts its biological action through selective binding and activation of the three RXRs: α, β, and γ. Once activated, these receptors function as transcription factors that regulate processes such as cellular differentiation and proliferation, apoptosis, and insulin sensitisation. The ability of the RXRs to form heterodimers with various receptor partners that are important in cellular function and in physiology indicates that the biological activities of bexarotene are more diverse than those of compounds that activate the RARs. *In vitro*, bexarotene inhibits the growth of tumour cell lines of haematopoietic and squamous cell origin. *In vivo*, bexarotene causes tumour regression in some animal models and prevents tumour induction in others. However, the exact mechanism of action of bexarotene in the treatment of cutaneous T-cell lymphoma (CTCL) is unknown.

Bexarotene capsules were evaluated in clinical trials of 193 patients with CTCL of whom 93 had advanced stage disease refractory to prior systemic therapy. Among the 61 patients treated at an initial dose of 300 mg/m^2/day, the overall response rate, according to a global assessment by the physician, was 51% (31/61) with a clinical complete response rate of 3%. Responses were also determined by a composite score of five clinical signs (surface area, erythema, plaque elevation, scaling and hypo/hyperpigmentation) which also considered all extracutaneous CTCL manifestations. The overall response rate according to this composite assessment was 31% (19/61) with a clinical complete response rate of 7% (4/61).

5.2 Pharmacokinetic properties

Absorption/dose proportionality: pharmacokinetics were linear up to a dose of 650 mg/m^2. Terminal elimination half-life values were generally between one and three hours. Following repeat once daily dose administration at dose levels $\geqslant$ 230 mg/m^2, C_{max} and AUC in some patients were less than respective single dose values. No evidence of prolonged accumulation was observed. At the recommended initial daily-dose level (300 mg/m^2), single-dose and repeated daily-dose bexarotene pharmacokinetic parameters were similar.

Protein binding/distribution: bexarotene is highly bound (>99%) to plasma proteins. The uptake of bexarotene by organs or tissues has not been evaluated.

Metabolism: bexarotene metabolites in plasma include 6- and 7-hydroxy-bexarotene and 6- and 7-oxo-bexarotene. *In vitro* studies suggest glucuronidation as a metabolic pathway, and that cytochrome P450 3A4 is the major cytochrome P450 isozyme responsible for formation of the oxidative metabolites. Based on the *in vitro* binding and the retinoid receptor activation profile of the metabolites, and on the relative amounts of individual metabolites in plasma, the metabolites have little impact on the pharmacological profile of retinoid receptor activation by bexarotene.

Excretion: neither bexarotene nor its metabolites are excreted in urine in any appreciable amounts. The estimated renal clearance of bexarotene is less than 1 ml/minute. Renal excretion is not a significant elimination pathway for bexarotene.

5.3 Preclinical safety data

Carcinogenesis, mutagenesis, impairment of fertility: bexarotene is not genotoxic. Carcinogenicity studies have not been conducted. Fertility studies have not been conducted; however, in sexually immature male dogs, reversible aspermatogenesis (28-day study) and testicular degeneration (91-day study) were seen. When bexarotene was administered for six months to sexually mature dogs, no testicular effects were seen. Effects on fertility cannot be excluded. Bexarotene, in common with the majority of retinoids, was teratogenic and embryotoxic in an animal test species at systemic exposures that are achievable clinically in humans. Irreversible cataracts involving the posterior area of the lens occurred in rats and dogs treated with bexarotene at systemic exposures that are achievable clinically in humans. The aetiology of this finding is unknown. An adverse effect of long-term bexarotene treatment on cataract formation in humans has not been excluded.

6. PHARMACEUTICAL PARTICULARS

6.1 List of excipients

Capsule content:

macrogol

polysorbate

povidone

butylated hydroxyanisole

Capsule shell:

gelatin

sorbitol special-glycerin blend (glycerin, sorbitol, sorbitol anhydrides (1,4-sorbitan), mannitol and water)

titanium dioxide (E171)

printing ink (shellac glaze-45% (20% esterified) in SD-45 alcohol, indigo carmine lake (E132) and simethicone)

6.2 Incompatibilities

Not applicable

6.3 Shelf life

2 years

6.4 Special precautions for storage

Do not store above 30°C.

Keep the bottle tightly closed.

6.5 Nature and contents of container

High-density polyethylene bottles with child-resistant closures containing 100 capsules

6.6 Instructions for use and handling

No special requirements

7. MARKETING AUTHORISATION HOLDER

Ligand Pharmaceuticals UK Limited

Innovis House

108 High Street

Crawley

West Sussex

RH10 1BB

United Kingdom

8. MARKETING AUTHORISATION NUMBER(S)

EU/1/01/178/001

9. DATE OF FIRST AUTHORISATION/RENEWAL OF THE AUTHORISATION

29 March 2001

10. DATE OF REVISION OF THE TEXT

14th June 2004

11. LEGAL CATEGORY

POM

Tarivid 200mg & 400mg Tablets

(sanofi-aventis)

1. NAME OF THE MEDICINAL PRODUCT

Tarivid 200 mg Tablets

Tarivid 400 mg Tablets

2. QUALITATIVE AND QUANTITATIVE COMPOSITION

Tarivid Tablets 200mg contain 200mg of ofloxacin

Tarivid Tablets 400mg contain 400mg of ofloxacin

3. PHARMACEUTICAL FORM

Film coated tablets

4. CLINICAL PARTICULARS

4.1 Therapeutic indications

Ofloxacin is a synthetic 4-fluoroquinolone antibacterial agent with bactericidal activity against a wide range of Gram-negative and Gram-positive organisms. It is indicated for the treatment of the following infections when caused by sensitive organisms: Upper and lower urinary tract infections; lower respiratory tract infections; uncomplicated urethral and cervical gonorrhoea; non-gonococcal urethritis and cervicitis, skin and soft tissue infections.

4.2 Posology and method of administration

General dosage recommendations: The dose of ofloxacin is determined by the type and severity of the infection. The dosage range for adults is 200mg to 800mg daily. Up to 400mg may be given as a single dose, preferably in the morning, larger doses should be given as two divided doses. Generally, individual doses are to be given at approximately equal intervals. Tarivid tablets should be swallowed with liquid; they should not be taken within two hours of magnesium/aluminium containing antacids, sucralfate or iron preparations since reduction of absorption of ofloxacin can occur.

Lower urinary tract infection: 200–400 mg daily.

Upper urinary tract infection: 200–400 mg daily increasing, if necessary, to 400 mg twice a day.

Lower respiratory tract infection: 400 mg daily increasing, if necessary, to 400 mg twice daily.

Uncomplicated urethral and cervical gonorrhoea: A single dose of 400 mg.

Non-gonococcal urethritis and cervicitis: 400 mg daily in single or divided doses.

Skin and soft tissue infections: 400 mg twice daily.

Impaired renal function: Following a normal initial dose, dosage should be reduced in patients with impairment of renal function. When creatinine clearance is 20–50 ml/minute (serum creatinine 1.5–5.0 mg/dl) the dosage should be reduced by half (100–200 mg daily). If creatinine clearance is less than 20 ml/minute (serum creatinine greater than 5 mg/dl) 100 mg should be given every 24 hours. In patients undergoing haemodialysis or peritoneal dialysis, 100 mg should be given every 24 hours.

Impaired liver function: The excretion of ofloxacin may be reduced in patients with severe hepatic dysfunction.

Elderly: No adjustment of dosage is required in the elderly, other than that imposed by consideration of renal or hepatic function.

Children: Ofloxacin is not indicated for use in children or growing adolescents.

Duration of treatment: Duration of treatment is dependent on the severity of the infection and the response to treatment. The usual treatment period is 5–10 days except in uncomplicated gonorrhoea, where a single dose is recommended.

Treatment should not exceed 2 months duration.

4.3 Contraindications

Ofloxacin should not be used in patients with known hypersensitivity to

4-quinolone antibacterials or any of the tablet excipients.

Ofloxacin should not be used in patients with a past history of tendinitis.

Ofloxacin, like other 4-quinolones, is contra-indicated in patients with a history of epilepsy or with a lowered seizure threshold. Ofloxacin is contra-indicated in children or growing adolescents, and in pregnant or breast-feeding women, since animal experiments do not entirely exclude the risk of damage to the cartilage of joints in the growing subject.

Patients with latent or actual defects in glucose-6-phosphate dehydrogenase activity may be prone to haemolytic reactions when treated with quinolone antibacterial agents.

4.4 Special warnings and special precautions for use

Patients being treated with ofloxacin should not expose themselves unnecessarily to strong sunlight and should avoid UV rays (sun lamps, solaria). Caution is recommended if the drug is to be used in psychotic patients or in patients with a history of psychiatric disease.

Administration of antibiotics, especially of prolonged, may lead to proliferation of resistant micro-organisms. The patient's condition must therefore be checked at regular intervals. If a secondary infection occurs, appropriate measures must be taken.

4.5 Interaction with other medicinal products and other forms of Interaction

Co-administered magnesium/aluminium antacids, sucralfate or iron preparations can reduce absorption. Therefore, ofloxacin should be taken 2 hours before such preparations. Prolongation of bleeding time has been reported during concomitant administration of Tarivid and anticoagulants.

There may be a further lowering of the cerebral seizure threshold when quinolones are given concurrently with other drugs which lower the seizure threshold, e.g. theophylline. However ofloxacin is not thought to cause a pharmacokinetic interaction with theophylline, unlike some other fluoroquinolones.

Further lowering of the cerebral seizure threshold may also occur with certain nonsteroidal anti-inflammatory drugs.

Ofloxacin may cause a slight increase in serum concentrations of glibenclamide administered concurrently; patients treated with this combination should be closely monitored.

With high doses of quinolones, impairment of excretion and an increase in serum levels may occur when co-administered with other drugs that undergo renal tubular secretion (e.g. probenecid, cimetidine, frusemide and methotrexate).

Interaction with laboratory tests: Determination of opiates or porphyrins in urine may give false-positive results during treatment with ofloxacin.

4.6 Pregnancy and lactation

The safety of this medicinal product for use in human pregnancy has not been established. Reproduction studies performed in rats and rabbits did not reveal any evidence of teratogenicity, impairment of fertility or impairment of peri- and post-natal development. However, as with other quinolones, ofloxacin has been shown to cause arthropathy in immature animals and therefore its use during pregnancy is not recommended. Studies in rats have indicated that ofloxacin is secreted in milk. It should therefore not be used during lactation.

4.7 Effects on ability to drive and use machines

Since there have been occasional reports of somnolence, impairment of skills, dizziness and visual disturbances, patients should know how they react to Tarivid before they drive or operate machinery. These effects may be enhanced by alcohol.

4.8 Undesirable effects

The overall frequency of adverse reactions from the clinical trial data base is about 7%. The commonest events involved the gastrointestinal system (about 5.0%) and the nervous system (about 2.0%).

The following provides a tabulation based on post marketing experience where occasional represents a frequency of 0.1 - 1.0%, rare <0.1%, very rare <0.01% and isolated cases <0.01%:

Digestive and Liver side effects:

Occasional: Nausea and vomiting, diarrhoea, abdominal pain, gastric symptoms. (Diarrhoea may sometimes be a symptom of enterocolitis which may, in some cases, be haemorrhagic).

Rare: Loss of appetite, increase in liver enzymes and/or bilirubin.

Very rare: cholestatic jaundice; hepatitis or severe liver damage may develop. A particular form of enterocolitis that can occur with antibiotics is pseudomembranous colitis (in most cases due to Clostridium difficile). Even if Clostridium difficile is only suspected, administration of ofloxacin should be discontinued immediately, and appropriate treatment given. Drugs that inhibit peristalsis should not be administered in such cases.

Central nervous system:

Occasional: Headache, dizziness, sleep disorders, restlessness.

Rare: Confusion, nightmares, anxiety, depression, hallucinations and psychotic reactions, drowsiness, unsteady gait and tremor (due to disorders of muscular co-ordination), neuropathy, numbness and paraesthesia or hypaesthesiae, visual disturbances, disturbances of taste and smell (including, in exceptional cases, loss of function), extrapyramidal symptoms.

Very rare: Convulsions, hearing disorders (including, in exceptional cases, loss of hearing).

These reactions have occurred in some patients after the first dose of ofloxacin. In such cases, discontinue treatment immediately.

Isolated cases: Psychotic reactions and depression with self-endangering behaviour including suicidal ideation or acts.

Cardiovascular system:

Tachycardia and a temporary decrease in blood pressure have been reported.

Rare: circulatory collapse (due to pronounced drop in blood pressure).

Haematological side effects:

Very rare: anaemia, leucopenia (including agranulocytosis), thrombocytopenia, pancytopenia.

Only in some cases are these due to bone marrow depression. In very rare cases, haemolytic anaemia may develop.

Renal side effects:

Rare: Disturbances of kidney function.

Isolated cases: Acute interstitial nephritis, or an increase in serum creatinine, which may progress to acute renal failure.

Allergic and skin side effects:

Occasional: Skin rash, itching.

Very rare: Rash on exposure to strong sunlight, other severe skin reactions. Hypersensitivity reactions, immediate or delayed, usually involving the skin (e.g. erythema multiforme, Stevens-Johnson syndrome, Lyell's syndrome, and vasculitis) may occur. In exceptional circumstances, vasculitis can lead to skin lesions including necrosis and may also involve internal organs. There are rarely other signs of anaphylaxis such as tachycardia, fever, dyspnoea, shock, angioneurotic oedema, vasculitic reactions, eosinophilia. In these cases treatment should be discontinued immediately and where appropriate, supportive treatment given.

Isolated cases: Pneumonitis.

Other side effects:

Rare: Malaise.

Very rare: Excessive rise or fall in blood-sugar levels. Weakness, joint and muscle pains (in isolated cases these may be symptoms of rhabdomyolysis).

Isolated cases: Tendon discomfort including inflammation and rupture of tendons (e.g. the Achilles tendon) particularly in patients treated concurrently with corticosteroids. In the event of signs of inflammation of a tendon, treatment with Tarivid must be halted immediately and appropriate treatment must be initiated for the affected tendon.

The possibility cannot be ruled out that ofloxacin may trigger an attack of porphyria in predisposed patients.

Except in very rare instances (e.g. isolated cases of smell, taste and hearing disorders) the adverse effects observed subsided after discontinuation of ofloxacin.

4.9 Overdose

The most important signs to be expected following acute overdosage are CNS symptoms such as confusion, dizziness, impairment of consciousness and convulsive seizures as well as gastrointestinal reactions such as nausea and mucosal erosions.

In the case of overdose steps to remove any unabsorbed ofloxacin eg gastric lavage, administration of adsorbants and sodium sulphate, if possible during the first 30 minutes, are recommended; antacids are recommended for protection of the gastric mucosa.

Elimination of ofloxacin may be increased by forced diuresis.

5. PHARMACOLOGICAL PROPERTIES

5.1 Pharmacodynamic properties

Ofloxacin is a quinolone-carboxylic acid derivative with a wide range of antibacterial activity against both gram negative and gram positive organisms. It is active after oral administration. It inhibits bacterial DNA replication by blocking DNA topo-isomerases, in particular DNA gyrase.

Therapeutic doses of ofloxacin are devoid of pharmacological effects on the voluntary or autonomic nervous systems.

Microbiological results indicate that the following pathogens may be regarded as sensitive: *Staphylococcus aureus* (including methicillin resistant staphylococci), *Staphylococcus epidermidis*, Neisseria species, *Escherichia coli*, Citrobacter, Klebsiella, Enterobacter, Hafnia, Proteus (indole-negative and indole-positive strains), *Haemophilus influenzae*, Chlamydiae, Legionella, Gardnerella.

Variable sensitivity is shown by Streptococci, *Serratia marcescens*, *Pseudomonas aeruginosa* and Mycoplasmas.

Anaerobic bacteria (e.g. Fusobacterium species, Bacteroides species, Eubacterium species, Peptococci, Peptostreptococci) are normally resistant.

Tarivid is not active against *Treponema pallidum*.

5.2 Pharmacokinetic properties

Ofloxacin is almost completely absorbed after oral administration. Maximal blood levels occur 1-3 hours after dosing and the elimination half-life is 4-6 hours. Ofloxacin is primarily excreted unchanged in the urine.

In renal insufficiency the dose should be reduced.

No clinically relevant interactions were seen with food and no interaction was found between ofloxacin and theophylline.

5.3 Preclinical safety data

Not Applicable

6. PHARMACEUTICAL PARTICULARS

6.1 List of excipients

Tarivid Tablets 200mg: Maize starch, lactose, hyprolose, carmellose NS300, magnesium stearate, hypromellose (2910), titanium dioxide (E171) talc, macrogol 8000.

Tarivid Tablets 400mg: Lactose, maize starch, sodium starch glycolate, hyprolose, magnesium stearate, hypromellose, macrogol 8000, talc, titanium dioxide (E171), yellow ferric oxide (E172), purified water.

6.2 Incompatibilities

None known

6.3 Shelf life

Tarivid Tablets 200mg: 5 years

Tarivid Tablets 400mg: 3 years

6.4 Special precautions for storage

Tarivid Tablets 200mg: No special conditions for storage

Tarivid Tablets 400mg: Store in a dry place

6.5 Nature and contents of container

Tarivid Tablets 200mg: Blister packs of 10, 20 and 100 tablets

Tarivid Tablets 400mg: Aluminium/PVC blister pack with aluminium foil 20μg and PVC (bluish clear) 250μg. Pack sizes: 5, 10 and 50 tablets

6.6 Instructions for use and handling

None

7. MARKETING AUTHORISATION HOLDER

Aventis Pharma Ltd
50 Kings Hill Avenue
Kings Hill
West Malling
Kent
ME19 4AH
United Kingdom

8. MARKETING AUTHORISATION NUMBER(S)

Tarivid Tablets 200mg: PL 04425/0216

Tarivid Tablets 400mg: PL 04425/0217

9. DATE OF FIRST AUTHORISATION/RENEWAL OF THE AUTHORISATION

Tarivid Tablets 200mg: April 2002

Tarivid Tablets 400mg: 1st January 2002

10. DATE OF REVISION OF THE TEXT

May 2005

Legal category: POM

Tarivid IV Infusion Solution

(sanofi-aventis)

1. NAME OF THE MEDICINAL PRODUCT

TarividTM IV Infusion Solution.

2. QUALITATIVE AND QUANTITATIVE COMPOSITION

Ofloxacin, 2 mg/ml.

3. PHARMACEUTICAL FORM

Solution for Infusion.

4. CLINICAL PARTICULARS

4.1 Therapeutic indications

Ofloxacin is a synthetic 4-fluoroquinolone antibacterial agent with bactericidal activity against a wide range of Gram-negative and Gram-positive organisms. It is indicated for the treatment of the following infections when caused by sensitive organisms:

Lower Respiratory Tract: Acute and chronic infections.

Upper and Lower Urinary Tract: Acute and chronic lower urinary tract infections; acute and chronic upper urinary tract infections (pyelonephritis). Septicaemia.

Skin and soft tissue infections.

Microbiological results indicate that the following pathogens may be regarded as sensitive: *Staphylococcus aureus* (including methicillin resistant staphylococci), *Staphylococcus epidermidis*, Neisseria species, *Escherichia coli*, Citrobacter, Klebsiella, Enterobacter, Hafnia, Proteus (indole-negative and indole-positive strains), Salmonella, Shigella, Acinetobacter, *Yersinia enterocolitica, Campylobacter jejuni,* Aeromonas, Plesiomonas, *Vibrio cholerae, Vibrio parahaemolyticus, Haemophilus influenzae*, Chlamydiae, Legionella, Gardenerella.

Variable sensitivity is shown by Streptococci, *Serratia marcescens*, *Pseudomonas aeruginosa*, Clostridium species and Mycoplasmas.

Anaerobic bacteria (e.g. Fusobacterium species, Bacteroides species, Eubacterium species, Peptococci, Peptostreptococci) are normally resistant.

Tarivid is not active against *Treponema pallidum.*

4.2 Posology and method of administration

General dosage recommendations: The dose of ofloxacin is determined by the type and severity of the infection.

Adults: The usual intravenous dosages in adults are:

Complicated urinary tract infection: 200 mg daily.

Lower respiratory tract infection: 200 mg twice daily.

Septicaemia: 200 mg twice daily.

Skin and soft tissue infections: 400 mg twice daily.

The infusion time for Tarivid IV should not be less than 30 minutes for 200 mg. Generally, individual doses are to be given at approximately equal intervals.

The dose may be increased to 400 mg twice daily in severe or complicated infections.

Impaired renal function: Following a normal initial dose, dosage should be reduced in patients with impairment of renal function. When creatinine clearance is 20–50 ml/minute (serum creatinine 1.5–5.0 mg/dl) the dosage should be reduced by half (100–200 mg daily). If creatinine clearance is less than 20 ml/minute (serum creatinine greater than 5 mg/dl) 100 mg should be given every 24 hours. In patients undergoing haemodialysis or peritoneal dialysis, 100 mg should be given every 24 hours.

Impaired liver function: The excretion of ofloxacin may be reduced in patients with severe hepatic dysfunction.

Children: Ofloxacin is not indicated for use in children or growing adolescents.

Elderly: No adjustment of dosage is required in the elderly, other than that imposed by consideration of renal or hepatic function.

Duration of treatment: The duration of treatment is determined according to the response of the causative organisms and the clinical picture. As with all antibacterial agents, treatment with Tarivid should be continued for at least 3 days after the body temperature has returned to normal and the symptoms have subsided.

In most cases of acute infection, a course of treatment lasting 7 to 10 days is sufficient. Once the patient's condition has improved, the mode of administration should be changed from parenteral to oral, normally at the same total daily dose.

Treatment should not exceed 2 months duration.

4.3 Contraindications

Ofloxacin should not be used in patients with known hypersensitivity to 4-quinolone antibacterials, or any of the excipients.

Ofloxacin should not be used in patients with a past history of tendinitis.

Ofloxacin, like other 4-quinolones, is contra-indicated in patients with a history of epilepsy or with a lowered seizure threshold. Ofloxacin is contra-indicated in children or growing adolescents, and in pregnant or breast-feeding women, since animal experiments do not entirely exclude the risk of damage to the cartilage of joints in the growing subject.

Patients with latent or actual defects in glucose-6-phosphate dehydrogenase activity may be prone to haemolytic reactions when treated with quinolone antibacterial agents.

4.4 Special warnings and special precautions for use

Patients being treated with ofloxacin should not expose themselves unnecessarily to strong sunlight and should avoid UV rays (sunlamps, solaria). Caution is recommended if the drug is to be used in psychotic patients or in patients with a history of psychiatric disease.

Sudden reductions in blood pressure may occur when Tarivid IV is administered with hypotensive agents. In such cases, or if the drug is given concomitantly with barbiturate anaesthetics, cardiovascular function should be monitored.

Administration of antibiotics, especially if prolonged, may lead to proliferation of resistant micro-organisms. The patient's condition must therefore be checked at regular intervals. If a secondary infection occurs, appropriate measures must be taken.

4.5 Interaction with other medicinal products and other forms of Interaction

Prolongation of bleeding time has been reported during concomitant administration of Tarivid and anticoagulants.

There may be a further lowering of the cerebral seizure threshold when quinolones are given concurrently with other drugs which lower the seizure threshold e.g. theophylline. However, ofloxacin is not thought to cause a pharmacokinetic interaction with theophylline, unlike some other fluoroquinolones.

Further lowering of the cerebral seizure threshold may also occur with certain nonsteroidal anti-inflammatory drugs.

Ofloxacin may cause a slight increase in serum concentrations of glibenclamide administered concurrently; patients treated with this combination should be closely monitored.

With high doses of quinolones, impairment of excretion and an increase in serum levels may occur when co-administered with other drugs that undergo renal tubular secretion (e.g. probenecid, cimetidine, frusemide and methotrexate).

Interactions with laboratory tests: Determination of opiates or porphyrins in urine may give false-positive results during treatment with ofloxacin.

4.6 Pregnancy and lactation

The safety of this medicinal product for use in human pregnancy has not been established. Reproduction studies performed in rats and rabbits did not reveal any evidence of teratogenicity, impairment of fertility or impairment of peri- and post-natal development. However, as with other quinolones, ofloxacin has been shown to cause arthropathy in immature animals and therefore its use during pregnancy is not recommended. Studies in rats have indicated that ofloxacin is secreted in milk. It should therefore not be used during lactation.

4.7 Effects on ability to drive and use machines

Since there have been occasional reports of somnolence, impairment of skills, dizziness and visual disturbances, patients should know how they react to Tarivid before they drive or operate machinery. These effects may be enhanced by alcohol.

4.8 Undesirable effects

In rare cases after i.v. infusion, a reduction in blood pressure may occur. If this effect is marked, the infusion should be stopped. Pain, reddening of the infusion site and thrombophlebitis have been reported in rare cases.

The overall frequency of adverse reactions from the clinical trial data base is about 7%. The commonest events involved the gastrointestinal system (about 5.0%) and the nervous system (about 2.0%).

The following provides a tabulation based on post marketing experience where occasional represents a frequency of 0.1-1.0%, rare <0.1%, very rare <0.01% and isolated cases <0.01%.

Digestive and liver side effects:

Occasional: Nausea and vomiting, diarrhoea, abdominal pain, gastric symptoms. (Diarrhoea may sometimes be a symptom of enterocolitis which may, in some cases, be haemorrhagic).

Rare: Loss of appetite, increase in liver enzymes and/or bilirubin.

Very rare: cholestatic jaundice, hepatitis or severe liver damage may develop. A particular form of enterocolitis that can occur with antibiotics is pseudomembranous colitis (in most cases due to *Clostridium difficile*). Even if *Clostridium difficile* is only suspected, administration of ofloxacin should be discontinued immediately, and appropriate treatment given. Drugs that inhibit peristalsis should not be administered in such cases.

Central nervous system:

Occasional: Headache, dizziness, sleep disorders, restlessness.

Rare: Confusion, nightmares, anxiety, depression, hallucinations and psychotic reactions, drowsiness, unsteady gait and tremor (due to disorders of muscular co-ordination), neuropathy, numbness and paraesthesia or hypaesthesiae, visual disturbances, disturbances of taste and smell (including, in exceptional cases, loss of function), extrapyramidal symptoms.

Very rare: Convulsions, hearing disorders (including, in exceptional cases, loss of hearing).

Isolated cases: Psychotic reactions and depression with self-endangering behaviour including suicidal ideation or acts.

These reactions have occurred in some patients after the first dose of ofloxacin. In such cases, discontinue treatment immediately.

Cardiovascular system:

Tachycardia and a temporary decrease in blood pressure have been reported.

Rare: circulatory collapse (due to pronounced drop in blood pressure).

Haematological side effects:

Very rare: anaemia, leucopenia (including agranulocytosis), thrombocytopenia, pancytopenia. Only in some cases are these due to bone marrow depression. In very rare cases, haemolytic anaemia may develop.

Renal side effects:

Rare: Disturbances of kidney function.

Isolated cases: Acute interstitial nephritis, or an increase in serum creatinine, which may progress to acute renal failure.

Allergic and skin side effects:

Occasional: Skin rash, itching.

Very rare: Rash on exposure to strong sunlight, other severe skin reactions. Hypersensitivity reactions, immediate or delayed, usually involving the skin (e.g. erythema multiforme, Stevens-Johnson syndrome, Lyell's syndrome and vasculitis) may occur. In exceptional circumstances, vasculitis can lead to skin lesions including necrosis and may also involve internal organs. There are rarely other signs of anaphylaxis such as tachycardia, fever, dyspnoea, shock, angioneurotic oedema, vasculitic reactions, eosinophilia. In these cases treatment should be discontinued immediately and where appropriate, supportive treatment given.

Isolated cases: Pneumonitis.

Other side effects:

Rare: Malaise.

Very rare: Excessive rise or fall in blood-sugar levels. Weakness, joint and muscle pains (in isolated cases these may be symptoms of rhabdomyolysis).

Isolated cases: Tendon discomfort, including inflammation and rupture of tendons (e.g. the Achilles tendon) particularly in patients treated concurrently with corticosteroids. In the event of signs of inflammation of a tendon, treatment with Tarivid must be halted immediately and appropriate treatment must be initiated for the affected tendon.

The possibility cannot be ruled out that ofloxacin may trigger an attack of porphyria in predisposed patients.

Except in very rare instances (e.g. isolated cases of smell, taste and hearing disorders) the adverse effects observed subsided after discontinuation of ofloxacin.

4.9 Overdose

The most important signs to be expected following acute overdosage are CNS symptoms such as confusion, dizziness, impairment of consciousness and convulsive seizures, as well as gastrointestinal reactions such as nausea and mucosal erosions.

Elimination of ofloxacin may be increased by forced diuresis.

5. PHARMACOLOGICAL PROPERTIES

5.1 Pharmacodynamic properties

Ofloxacin is a quinolone-carboxylic acid derivative with a wide range of antibacterial activity against both Gram-negative and Gram-positive organisms. It inhibits bacterial DNA replication by blocking DNA topo-isomerases, in particular DNA gyrase.

Therapeutic doses of ofloxacin are devoid of pharmacological effects on the voluntary or autonomic nervous systems.

5.2 Pharmacokinetic properties

Maximum plasma concentrations occur within five minutes of the end of the infusion. The plasma half life is about five hours. Ofloxacin is primarily excreted unchanged in the urine.

Urinary clearance is reduced in renal insufficiency.

5.3 Preclinical safety data

None stated.

6. PHARMACEUTICAL PARTICULARS

6.1 List of excipients

Sodium chloride, hydrochloric acid and water for injections.

6.2 Incompatibilities

Tarivid IV should be administered alone unless compatibility with other infusion fluids has been demonstrated. Compatible infusion solutions include isotonic sodium chloride, Ringer's solution and 5 % glucose solution. Heparin and ofloxacin are incompatible.

6.3 Shelf life

3 years.

6.4 Special precautions for storage

Tarivid IV presented in glass infusion bottles should be protected from light.

6.5 Nature and contents of container

Clear, colourless Type I glass vials with grey chlorobutyl rubber closures and aluminium caps containing 200 ml infusion solution.

6.6 Instructions for use and handling

None.

7. MARKETING AUTHORISATION HOLDER

Aventis Pharma Ltd

50 Kings Hill Avenue

Kings Hill

West Malling

Kent

ME19 4AH

United Kingdom

8. MARKETING AUTHORISATION NUMBER(S)

PL 04425/0215

9. DATE OF FIRST AUTHORISATION/RENEWAL OF THE AUTHORISATION

28/06/02

10. DATE OF REVISION OF THE TEXT

May 2005

Legal category: POM

Tarka 180/2 mg Capsules

(Abbott Laboratories Limited)

1. NAME OF THE MEDICINAL PRODUCT

Tarka® 180mg/2mg capsules

2. QUALITATIVE AND QUANTITATIVE COMPOSITION

Each Tarka capsule contains 180 mg of verapamil hydrochloride in a sustained-release form and 2 mg of trandolapril.

For excipients see also section 6.1 'List of excipients'.

3. PHARMACEUTICAL FORM

Capsules.

Pale pink opaque.

4. CLINICAL PARTICULARS

4.1 Therapeutic indications

Essential hypertension in patients whose blood pressure has been normalized with the individual components in the same proportion of doses.

4.2 Posology and method of administration

The usual dosage is one Tarka capsule once daily, taken in the morning before, with or after breakfast. The Tarka capsule should be swallowed whole.

Dosage in children: Tarka is contraindicated in children (see also section 4.3. 'Contra-Indications').

Dosage in the elderly: See section 4.4 'Special Warnings and Special Precautions for Use'.

4.3 Contraindications

- Known hypersensitivity to trandolapril or any other ACE inhibitor and/or verapamil.
- History of angioneurotic oedema associated with previous ACE inhibitor therapy.
- Hereditary/idiopathic angioneurotic oedema.
- Cardiogenic shock.
- Recent myocardial infarction with complications.
- Second- or third-degree AV block without pacemaker.
- SA block.
- Sick sinus syndrome.
- Congestive heart failure.
- Atrial flutter/fibrillation in association with an accessory pathway (e.g. WPW-syndrome)
- Severe renal impairment (creatinine clearance < 10 ml/min).
- Dialysis.
- Liver cirrhosis with ascites.
- Aortic or mitral stenosis, obstructive hypertrophic cardiomyopathy.
- Primary aldosteronism.
- Pregnancy.
- Lactation.
- Use in children.

4.4 Special warnings and special precautions for use

Symptomatic hypotension:

Under certain circumstances, Tarka may occasionally produce symptomatic hypotension. This risk is elevated in patients with a stimulated renin-angiotensin-aldosterone system (e.g., volume or salt depletion, due to the use of diuretics, a low-sodium diet, dialysis, diarrhoea or vomiting; decreased left ventricular function renovascular hypertension).

Such patients should have their volume or salt depletion corrected beforehand and therapy should preferably be initiated in a hospital setting. Patients experiencing hypotension during titration should lie down and may require volume expansion by oral fluid supply or intravenous administration of normal saline. Tarka therapy can usually be continued once blood volume and pressure have been effectively corrected.

Kidney function impairment: (see also section 4.3 'Contraindications'):

Patients with moderate renal impairment should have their kidney function monitored. Tarka may produce hyperkalaemia in patients with renal dysfunction.

Acute deterioration of kidney function (acute renal failure) may occur especially in patients with pre-existing kidney function impairment, or congestive heart failure. There is no sufficient experience with Tarka in secondary hypertension and particularly in renal vascular hypertension. Hence, Tarka should not be administered to these patients, especially since patients with bilateral renal artery stenosis or unilateral renal artery stenosis in individuals with a single functioning kidney (eg renal transplant patients) are endangered to suffer an acute loss of kidney function.

Proteinuria:

Proteinuria may occur particularly in patients with existing renal function impairment or on relatively high doses of ACE inhibitors.

Severe liver function impairment:

Since there is insufficient therapeutic experience in those patients, the use of Tarka cannot be recommended. Tarka is contraindicated in patients with liver cirrhosis with ascites.

Angioneurotic oedema:

Rarely, ACE inhibitors (such as trandolapril) may cause angioneurotic oedema that includes swelling of the face, extremities, tongue, glottis, and/or larynx. Patients experiencing angioneurotic oedema must immediately discontinue trandolapril therapy and be monitored until oedema resolves.

Angioneurotic oedema confined to the face will usually resolve spontaneously. Oedema involving not only the face but also the glottis may be life-threatening because of the risk of airway obstruction.

Compared to non-black patients a higher incidence of angiooedema has been reported in black patients treated with ACE inhibitors.

Angioneurotic oedema involving the tongue, glottis or larynx requires immediate sub-cutaneous administration of 0.3-0.5 ml of epinephrine solution (1:1000) along with other therapeutic measures as appropriate.

Caution must be exercised in patients with a history of idiopathic angioneurotic oedema, and Tarka is contraindicated if angioneurotic oedema was an adverse reaction to an ACE inhibitor (see also section 4.3 'Contraindications').

Neutropenia/agranulocytosis:

The risk of neutropenia appears to be dose-and type related and is dependant on patient's clinical status. It is rarely seen in uncomplicated patients but may occur in patients with some degree of renal impairment especially when it is associated with collagen vascular disease e.g. systemic lupus erythematosus, scleroderma and therapy with immunosuppressive agents. It is reversible after discontinuation of the ACE inhibitor.

Cough:

During treatment with an ACE inhibitor a dry and non-productive cough may occur which disappears after discontinuation.

Hyperkalaemia:

Hyperkalaemia may occur during treatment with an ACE inhibitor, especially in the presence of renal insufficiency and/or heart failure. Potassium supplements or potassium sparing diuretics are generally not recommended, since they may lead to significant increases in plasma potassium. If concomitant use of the above mentioned agents is deemed appropriate, they should be used with frequent monitoring of serum potassium.

Elderly:

Tarka has been studied in a limited number of elderly hypertensive patients only. Pharmacokinetic data show that the systemic availability of Tarka is higher in elderly compared to younger hypertensives. Some elderly patients might experience a more pronounced blood pressure lowering effect than others. Evaluation of renal function at the beginning of treatment is recommended.

Surgical patients:

In patients undergoing major surgery requiring general anaesthesia, ACE inhibitors may produce hypotension, which can be corrected by plasma volume expanders.

Conduction disturbances:

Tarka should be used with caution in patients with first degree atrioventricular block (see also section 4.3 'Contraindications').

Bradycardia:

Tarka should be used with caution in patients with bradycardia.

Diseases in which neuromuscular transmission is effected:

Tarka should be used with caution in patients with diseases in which neuromuscular transmission is effected (myasthenia gravis, Lambert-Eaton syndrome, advanced Duchenne muscular dystrophy).

Haemodialysis patients (see also section 4.3 Contra-Indicartions):

Patients on concurrent ACE inhibitor therapy and haemodialysis with polyacrylonitrile methallyl sulfonate high-flux membranes (e.g. "AN 69") have experienced anaphylactoid reactions. Such membranes should therefore not be used in these patients.

Desensitisation:

Anaphylactoid reactions (in some cases life threatening) may develop in patients receiving ACE inhibitor therapy and concomitant desensitisation against animal venoms.

LDL-apheresis:

Life threatening anaphylactoid reactions have been noted when patients on LDL-apheresis take ACE inhibitors at the same time.

Evaluation of the patients should include assessment of renal function prior to initiation of therapy and during treatment.

Blood pressure readings for evaluation of therapeutic response to Tarka should always be taken before the next dose.

4.5 Interaction with other medicinal products and other forms of Interaction

Not recommended association

- *Potassium sparing diuretics or potassium supplements:* ACE inhibitors attenuate diuretic induced potassium loss. Potassium sparing diuretics e.g. spironolactone, triamterene, or amiloride, potassium supplements, or potassium containing salt substitutes may lead to significant increases in serum potassium, particularly in the presence of renal function impairment. If concomitant use is indicated because of demonstrated hypokalaemia they should be used with caution and with frequent monitoring of serum potassium.

- The simultaneous use of verapamil with dantrolene is not recommended.

Precaution for use

- *Antihypertensive agents*: Increase in the hypotensive effect of Tarka.

- *Diuretics*: Patients on diuretics and especially those who are volume-and / or salt depleted may experience an excessive reduction of blood pressure after initiation of therapy with an ACE inhibitor. The possibility of hypotensive effects can be reduced by discontinuation of the diuretic, by increasing volume or salt intake prior to intake and by initiation of therapy with low doses. Further increases in dosage should be performed with caution.

- *Lithium*: There have been reports of both an increase and a reduction in the effects of lithium used concurrently with verapamil. The concomitant administration of ACE inhibitors with lithium may reduce the excretion of lithium. Serum lithium levels should be monitored frequently.

- *Anaesthetic drugs*: Tarka may enhance the hypotensive effects of certain anaesthetic drugs.

- *Narcotic drugs/Antipsychotics*: Postural hypotension may occur.

- *Allopurinol, cytostatic or immunosuppressive agents, systemic corticosteroids or procainamide*: Concomitant administration with ACE inhibitors may lead to an increased risk of leucopoenia.

- *Cardiodepressive drugs*: The concurrent use of verapamil and cardiodepressive drugs, i.e., drugs that inhibit cardiac impulse generation and conduction (e.g. beta-adrenergic blocking agents, antiarrhythmic drugs, inhalation anaesthetics), may produce undesirable additive effects.

- *Quinidine*: The concomitant use of quinidine and oral verapamil in patients with hypertrophic (obstructive) cardiomyopathy has resulted in hypotension and pulmonary oedema in a small number of cases.

- *Digoxin*: Concurrent use of digoxin and verapamil has been reported to result in 50-75% higher digoxin plasma concentrations, requiring reduction of the digoxin dosage.

- *Muscle relaxants*: The effects of muscle relaxants may be enhanced.

- *Tranquillisers/antidepressant agents*: As with all antihypertensive drugs, there is an elevated risk of orthostatic hypotension when combining Tarka with major tranquillisers or antidepressant medications containing imipramine.

Take into account

- *Non-steroidal anti-inflammatory drugs*: The administration of a non-steroidal anti-inflammatory agent may reduce the antihypertensive effect of an ACE inhibitor. Furthermore it has been described that NSAIDs and ACE inhibitors exert an additive effect on the increase in serum potassium, whereas renal function may decrease. These effects are in principle reversible, and occur especially in patients with compromised renal function.

- *Antacids:* Induce decreased bioavailability of ACE inhibitors.

- *Sympathomimetics:* May reduce the antihypertensive effects of ACE inhibitors; patient should be carefully monitored to confirm that the desired effect is being obtained.

- *Alcohol*: Enhances the hypotensive effect.

- Verapamil may increase the plasma concentrations of carbamazepine, cyclosporin, and theophylline.

- Rifampicin, phenytoin, and phenobarbital reduce the efficacy of verapamil, whereas cimetidine may increase the effect of verapamil.

- *Antidiabetics*: A dose adjustment of antidiabetics or of Tarka may be necessary in individual cases especially at the start of therapy due to increased reduction of blood glucose.

- Grapefruit juice has been shown to increase the plasma levels of verapamil, which is a component of Tarka. Grapefruit juice should therefore not be ingested with Tarka.

4.6 Pregnancy and lactation

Pregnancy

The safe use of Tarka in pregnant women is inadequately documented. However, there have been anecdotal reports of neonatal lung hypoplasia, intra-uterine growth retardation, persistent ductus arteriosus, and cranial hypoplasia following exposure of fetuses to ACE inhibitors. In addition, the pharmacologic activity of ACE inhibitors is compatible with the possibility of fetal hypotension, which may be associated with fetal/neonatal oliguria/anuria and oligohydramnios (see also section 5.3 'Preclinical Safety Data').

Teratogenic effects are primarily expected when ACE inhibitors are used in the second and third trimesters of pregnancy, and it is not known whether exposure of the embryo/fetus to an ACE inhibitor only in the first trimester is teratogenic or embryotoxic/fetotoxic. Women who wish to get pregnant or are pregnant must consult their doctor without delay, so an alternative pharmacologic treatment can be prescribed.

Women of child-bearing potential

Doctors should instruct women of child-bearing potential accordingly before prescribing an ACE inhibitor.

Lactation

Tarka is contrainidicated when breastfeeding.

4.7 Effects on ability to drive and use machines

While no effect on the ability to drive and use machinery has been established, impairment of alertness cannot be ruled out altogether, since Tarka may produce dizziness and fatigue.

4.8 Undesirable effects

The adverse drug reactions for Tarka are consistent with those known for its components or the respective class of drugs. The most commonly reported adverse drug reactions are cough increased, headache, constipation, vertigo, dizziness and hot flushes (see table below).

Adverse events either reported spontaneously or observed in clinical trials are depicted in the following table. Within each system organ class, the ADRs are ranked under headings of frequency, using the following convention: common (>1/100, <1/10), uncommon (>1/1,000, <1/100), rare (>1/10,000, <1/1,000), very rare (<1/10,000), including isolated reports.

System Organ Class	Frequency	Undesirable Effects
Blood and lymphatic system disorders	very rare	leucopoenia pancytopoenia thrombocytopoenia
Immune system disorders	uncommon	allergic reaction, unspecified
	very rare	increase in gammaglobulin hypersensitivity, unspecified
Metabolism and nutritional disorders	uncommon	hyperlipodaemia
	rare	anorexia
Psychiatric disorders	uncommon	somnolence
	very rare	aggression anxiety depression nervousness
Nervous system disorders	common	dizziness vertigo
	uncommon	tremor
	rare	collapse
	very rare	impaired balance insomnia paraesthesia or hyperaesthesia syncope or acute circulatory failures with loss of consciousness taste aberration weakness
Eye disorders	very rare	abnormal/blurred vision
Cardiac disorders/ vascular disorders	common	hot flushes
	uncommon	AV block, first degree Palpitation
	very rare	angina pectoris atrial fibrillation AV block, complete AV block, unspecified bradycardia cardiac arrest cerebral haemorrhage oedema, peripheral oedema, unspecified flushing heart failure hypotensive events including orthostasis or fluctuation of blood pressure (see also section 4.4) tachycardia
Respiratory, thoracic and mediastirial disorders	common	cough increased
	very rare	asthma bronchitis dyspnoea sinus congestion
Gastrointestinal disorders	common	constipation
	uncommon	abdominal pain diarrhoea gastrointestinal disorders unspecified nausea
	very rare	dry mouth/throat pancreatitis vomiting
Hepatobiliary disorders	very rare	cholestasis hepatitis increase in γGT increase in LDH increase in lipase jaundice
Skin and subcutaneous tissue disorders	uncommon	facial oedema pruritus rash sweating increased
	rare	alopecia herpes simplex skin disorders, unspecified
	very rare	angioneurotic oedema (see also section 4.4) erythema multiforme exanthema or dermatitis psoriasis urticaria
Musculoskeletal, connective tissue and bone disorders	very rare	arthralgia myalgia myasthenia
Renal and urinary disorders	uncommon	polyuria
	very rare	acute renal failure (see also section 4.4)
Reproductive system and breast disorders	very rare	gynaecomastia impotence
General disorders and administration site conditions	common	headache
	uncommon	chest pain
	very rare	fatigue or asthenia
Investigations	uncommon	liver function test, abnormal
	rare	bilirubinaemia
	very rare	increase in alkaline phosphatase increase in serum potassium increase in transaminases

The following adverse reaction have not yet been reported in relation to Tarka, but are generally accepted as being attributable to ACE inhibitors:

- *Blood and lymphatic system disorders*: decreases in haemoglobin and haematocrit, and in individual cases agranulocytosis. Isolated cases of haemolytic anemia have been reported in patients with congenital G-6-PDH deficiency.

- *Psychiatric disorders*: occasionally confusion.

- *Nervous system disorders*: rarely, sleep disorder.

- *Ear and labyrinth disorders*: rarely, problems with balance, tinnitus.

- *Cardiac disorders/vascular disorders*: Individual cases of arrhythmia, myocardial infarction and transient ischaemic attacks have been reported for ACE inhibitors in association with hypotension.

- *Respiratory, thoracic and mediastinal disorders*: Rarely, sinusitis, rhinitis, glossitis, and bronchospasm.

- *Gastrointestinal disorders*: occasionally indigestion. Individual cases of ileus.

- *Hepatobiliary disorders*: individual cases of cholestatic icterus.

- *Skin and subcutaneous tissue disorders*: occasionally allergic and hypersensitivity reactions such as Stevens-Johnson syndrome, toxic epidermic necrolysis. This can be accompanied by fever, myalgia, arthralgia, eosinophilia and/or increased ANA – titres.

- *Investigations*: increases in blood urea and plasma creatinine may occur especially in the presence of renal insufficiency, severe heart failure and renovascular hypertension. These increases are however reversible on discontinuation.

Symptomatic or severe hypotension has occasionally occurred after initiation of therapy with ACE inhibitors. This occurs especially in certain risk groups, such as patients with a stimulated renin-angiotensin-aldosterone system.

The following adverse reactions have not yet been reported in relation to Tarka, but are generally accepted as being attributable to phenylalkylamine calcium-channel blockers.

- *Nervous system disorders*: in some cases, there may be extrapyramidal symptoms (Parkinson's disease, choreoathetosis, dystonic syndrome). Experience so far has shown that these symptoms resolve once the medication is discontinued. There have been isolated reports of exacerbation of myasthenia gravis, Lambert-Eaton syndrome and advanced cases of Duchenne's muscular dystrophy.

- *Gastrointestinal disorders*: gingival hyperplasia following long-term treatment is extremely rare and reversible after discontinuation of therapy.

- *Skin and subcutaneous tissue disorders*: Stevens-Johnson syndrome and erythromelalgia have been described. In isolated cases allergic skin reactions like erythema.

- *Reproductive system and breast disorders*: Hyperprolactinaemia and galactorrhoea have been described.

Excessive hypotension in patients with angina pectoris or cerebrovascular disease treated with Verapamil may result in myocardial infarction or cerebrovascular accident.

4.9 Overdose

There have as yet been no reports of overdosage with the combination product.

The highest dose used in clinical trials was 16mg of trandolapril. This dose produced no signs or symptoms of intolerance.

The most important symptom to be expected after a significant overdose is hypotension. Administration of normal saline solution is recommended in this case.

The most important signs and symptoms of a verapamil overdose are due to the pharmacological activity of the drug in the cardiovascular system and include hypotension arising from peripheral vasodilation and a negative inotropic effect, depression of impulse generation in the sinus node and cardiac impulse conduction disturbances that may result in sinus bradycardia, sinus arrest, AV block, and asystole.

Following oral verapamil overdosage, the patient must be monitored and treated in an intensive care setting. Overdose management must be aimed at preventing the further absorption of verapamil from the gastrointestinal tract, providing symptomatic treatment of the toxic effects (see above), and compensating for the calcium-antagonistic effects of this drug. Further absorption of verapamil from the gastrointestinal tract can be prevented by gastric lavage, administration of adsorbent material (activated charcoal) and a cathartic (sodium sulphate). Apart from general supportive measure in response to severe hypotension (to the point of shock), i.e., maintenance of an adequate circulating blood volume by administering plasma or a plasma expander, it may be necessary to stimulate the heart muscle with such positive inotropic drugs as dopamine, dobutamine or isoproterenol.

Atropine (or methylatropine) may be useful in the management of sinus bradycardia. AV block should be treated with sympathomimetic drugs (isoproterenol or metaproterenol) or a pacemaker. Asystole should be handled by the usual measures including cardiopulmonary resuscitation, cardiac pacing, etc. The calcium-antagonistic effect can be offset by parenteral administration of calcium, for instance as calcium gluconate.

5. PHARMACOLOGICAL PROPERTIES

5.1 Pharmacodynamic properties

Tarka is a fixed combination of the heart-rate lowering calcium antagonist verapamil and the ACE inhibitor trandolapril (ATC-Code: CO8DA51).

Verapamil:

The pharmacological action of verapamil is due to inhibition of the influx of calcium ions through the slow channels of the cell membrane of vascular smooth muscle cells and of the conductile and contractile cells in the heart.

The mechanism of action of verapamil produces the following effects:

1. Arterial vasodilation.

Verapamil reduces arterial pressure both at rest and at a given level of exercise by dilating peripheral arterioles.

This reduction in total peripheral resistance (afterload) reduces myocardial oxygen requirements and energy consumption

2. Reduction of myocardial contractility.

The negative inotropic activity of verapamil can be compensated by the reduction in total peripheral resistance.

The cardiac index will not be decreased unless in patients with pre-existing left ventricular dysfunction.

Verapamil does not interfere with sympathetic regulation of the heart because it does not block the beta-adrenergic receptors.

Spastic bronchitis and similar conditions, therefore, are not contraindications to verapamil.

Trandolapril:

Trandolapril suppresses the plasma renin-angiotensin aldosterone system (RAS). Renin is an endogenous enzyme synthesised by the kidneys and released into the circulation where it converts angiotensinogen to angiotensin I a relatively inactive decapeptide. Angiotensin I is then converted by angiotensin converting enzyme, a peptidyldipeptidase, to angiotensin II. Angiotensin II is a potent vasoconstrictor responsible for arterial vasoconstriction and increased blood pressure, as well as for stimulation of the adrenal gland to secrete aldosterone. Inhibition of ACE results in decreased plasma angiotensin II, which leads to decreased vasopressor activity and to reduced aldosterone secretion. Although the latter decrease is small, small increase in serum potassium concentrations may occur, along with sodium and fluid loss. The cessation of the negative feedback of angiotensin II on the renin secretion results in an increase of the plasma renin activity.

Another function of the converting enzyme is to degrade the potent vasodilating kinin peptide, bradykinin to inactive metabolites. Therefore inhibition of ACE results in an increased activity of circulating and local kallikrein-kinin system which contributes to peripheral vasodilation by activating the prostaglandin system. It is possible that this mechanism is involved in the hypotensive effects of ACE inhibitors and is responsible for certain side effects. In patients with hypertension administration of ACE inhibitors results in a reduction of supine and standing blood pressure to about the same extent with no compensatory increase of the heart rate. Peripheral arterial resistance is reduced with either no change or an increase in cardiac output.

There is an increase in renal blood flow and glomerular filtration rate is usually unchanged. Achievement of optimal blood pressure reduction may require several weeks of therapy in some patients. The antihypertensive effects are maintained during long term therapy. Abrupt withdrawal of therapy has not been associated with a rapid increase in blood pressure.

The antihypertensive effect of trandolapril sets in one hour post-dose and lasts for at least 24 hours, but trandolapril does not interfere with the circadian blood pressure pattern.

Tarka:

Neither animal studies nor healthy volunteer studies could demonstrate pharmacokinetic or RAS interactions between verapamil and trandolapril. The observed synergistic activity of these two drugs must therefore be due to their complementary pharmacodynamic actions.

In clinical trials, Tarka was more effective in reducing high blood pressure than either drug alone. In long-term trials, Tarka proved to be safe and well tolerated.

5.2 Pharmacokinetic properties

Verapamil:

Absorption:

About 90% of orally administered verapamil is absorbed. The mean bioavailability is as low as 22% because of extensive hepatic first-pass extraction, and shows great variation (10-35%). The mean bioavailability following repeated administration may increase to 30%.

The presence of food has no effect on the bioavailability of verapamil.

Distribution and biotransformation:

The mean time to peak plasma concentration is 4 hours. The peak plasma concentration of norverapamil is attained about 6 hours post-dose.

Steady state after multiple once daily dosing is reached after 3-4 days.

Plasma protein binding of verapamil is about 90%.

Elimination:

The mean elimination half-life after repeated administration is 8 hours, 3-4% of a dose is excreted renally as unchanged drug. Metabolite excretion is in the urine (70%) and in the faeces (16%). Norverapamil is one of 12 metabolites identified in urine, has 10-20% of the pharmacologic activity of verapamil, and accounts for 6% of excreted drug. The steady-state plasma concentrations of norverapamil and verapamil are similar. Verapamil kinetics is not altered by renal function impairment.

The bioavailability and elimination half-life of verapamil are increased in patients with liver cirrhosis. Verapamil kinetics is, however, unchanged in patients with compensated hepatic dysfunction. Kidney function has no effect on verapamil elimination.

Trandolapril:

Absorption:

Orally administered trandolapril is absorbed rapidly. Absorption is 40-60% and independent of the presence of food.

The time to peak plasma concentration is about 30 minutes.

Distribution and biotransformation:

Trandolapril disappears very rapidly from plasma, and its half-life is less than one hour.

Trandolapril is hydrolysed in plasma to form trandolaprilat, a specific angiotensin converting enzyme (ACE) inhibitor. The amount of trandolaprilat formed is independent of food intake.

The time to peak plasma concentration of trandolaprilat is 4-6 hours.

Plasma protein binding of trandolaprilat is greater than 80%. Trandolaprilat binds with great affinity to ACE, and this is a saturable process. Most of circulating trandolaprilat binds to albumin in a nonsaturable process. Steady state after multiple once daily dosing is reached after about 4 days in healthy volunteers as well as in younger and elderly hypertensive patients.

The effective half-life calculated from accumulation is 16-24 hours.

Elimination:

10-15% of an administered trandolapril dose is excreted as unchanged trandolaprilat in urine. Following oral administration of radioactively labelled trandolapril, one third of radioactivity is recovered in urine and two thirds in faeces.

The renal clearance of trandolaprilat shows a linear correlation with creatinine clearance. The trandolaprilat plasma concentration is significantly higher in patients whose creatinine clearance is [≤] 30 ml/min. Following repeated administration to patients with chronic renal dysfunction, steady state is, however, also reached after four days, independently of the extent of kidney function impairment.

The trandolapril plasma concentration may be 10 times higher in patients with liver cirrhosis than in healthy volunteers. The plasma concentration and renal extraction of trandolaprilat are also increased in cirrhotic patients, albeit to a lesser extent. Trandolapril(at) kinetics are unchanged in patients with compensated hepatic dysfunction.

Tarka

As there are no known kinetic interactions between verapamil and trandolapril or trandolaprilat, the single-agent kinetic parameters of these two drugs apply to the combination product as well.

5.3 Preclinical safety data

General toxicity effects were observed in animals only at exposures that were sufficiently in excess of the maximum human exposure to make any concern for human safety negligible. Genotoxicity assays revealed no special hazard for humans.

Animal studies have shown that ACE inhibitors tend to have an adverse effect on late foetal development, resulting in foetal death and congenital abnormalities of the skull in particular. These cranial abnormalities are thought to be due to the pharmacological activity of these drugs and be related to ACE inhibitor-induced oligohydramnios.

6. PHARMACEUTICAL PARTICULARS

6.1 List of excipients

Tarka also contains:

Film-coated tablets:

- Microcrystalline cellulose,
- Povidone,
- Sodium alginate,
- Magnesium stearate,
- Hypromellose,
- Hydroxypropylcellulose,
- Macrogol 400 and 6000,
- Talc,
- Colloidal anhydrous silica,
- Docusate sodium,
- Titanium dioxide (E171),

Granules:

- Maize starch,
- Lactose monohydrate,
- Povidone,
- Sodium stearyl fumarate

Gelatin capsules:

- Titanium dioxide (E171),
- Iron oxide (E172),
- Gelatin,
- Sodium lauryl sulphate

6.2 Incompatibilities

Not applicable

6.3 Shelf life

3 years.

6.4 Special precautions for storage

Do not store above 25°C

6.5 Nature and contents of container

PVC/PVDC-aluminium blister strips

Calendar packs of 14, 28, 56, 98, 280 capsules in blister strips

Package of 20, 30, 50, 100 and 300 capsules in blister strips.

Not all pack sizes may be marketed.

6.6 Instructions for use and handling

No special requirements.

7. MARKETING AUTHORISATION HOLDER

Abbott Laboratories Limited
Queenborough
Kent
ME11 5EL
United Kingdom

8. MARKETING AUTHORISATION NUMBER(S)

PL 00037/0371

9. DATE OF FIRST AUTHORISATION/RENEWAL OF THE AUTHORISATION

4 September 2002

10. DATE OF REVISION OF THE TEXT

March 2002

Tasmar 100 mg Tablets

(Valeant Pharmaceuticals Ltd)

1. NAME OF THE MEDICINAL PRODUCT

Tasmar 100 mg film-coated tablets.▼

2. QUALITATIVE AND QUANTITATIVE COMPOSITION

Each film-coated tablet contains 100 mg tolcapone.

For excipients, see section 6.1

3. PHARMACEUTICAL FORM

Tasmar 100 mg is a pale to light yellow, hexagonal, biconvex, film-coated tablet. "TASMAR" and "100" are engraved on one side.

4. CLINICAL PARTICULARS

Since Tasmar should be used only in combination with levodopa/benserazide and levodopa/carbidopa, the prescribing information for these levodopa preparations is also applicable to their concomitant use with Tasmar.

4.1 Therapeutic indications

Tasmar is indicated in combination with levodopa/benserazide or levodopa/carbidopa for use in patients with levodopa-responsive idiopathic Parkinson's disease and motor fluctuations, who failed to respond to or are intolerant of other COMT inhibitors (see 5.1). Because of the risk of potentially fatal, acute liver injury, Tasmar should not be considered as a first-line adjunct therapy to levodopa/benserazide or levodopa/carbidopa (see 4.4 and 4.8). If substantial clinical benefits are not seen within 3 weeks of the initiation of the treatment, Tasmar should be discontinued.

4.2 Posology and method of administration

The administration of Tasmar is restricted to prescription and supervision by physicians experienced in the management of advanced Parkinson's disease.

Posology

The recommended dose of Tasmar is 100 mg three times daily, always as an adjunct to levodopa/benserazide or levodopa/carbidopa therapy. Only in exceptional circumstances, when the anticipated incremental clinical benefit justifies the increased risk of hepatic reactions, should the dose be increased to 200 mg three times daily. (See 4.4 and 4.8). If substantial clinical benefits are not seen within 3 weeks of the initiation of the treatment (regardless of dose) Tasmar should be discontinued.

The maximum therapeutic dose of 200 mg three times daily should not be exceeded, as there is no evidence of additional efficacy at higher doses.

Liver function should be checked before starting treatment with Tasmar and then monitored every 2 weeks for the first year of therapy, every 4 weeks for the next 6 months and every 8 weeks thereafter. If the dose is increased to 200 mg tid, liver enzyme monitoring should take place before increasing the dose and then be reinitiated following the same sequence of frequencies as above (See 4.4 and 4.8).

Tasmar treatment should also be discontinued if ALT (alanine amino transferase) and/or AST (aspartate amino transferase) exceed the upper limit of normal or symptoms or signs suggest the onset of hepatic failure (see 4.4).

Levodopa adjustments during Tasmar treatment:

As Tasmar decreases the breakdown of levodopa in the body, side effects due to increased levodopa concentrations may occur when beginning Tasmar treatment. In clinical trials, more than 70 % of patients required a decrease in their daily levodopa dose if their daily dose of levodopa was >600 mg or if patients had moderate or severe dyskinesias before beginning treatment.

The average reduction in daily levodopa dose was about 30 % in those patients requiring a levodopa dose reduction. When beginning Tasmar, all patients should be informed of the symptoms of excessive levodopa dosage and what to do if it occurs.

Levodopa adjustments when Tasmar is discontinued:

The following suggestions are based on pharmacological considerations and have not been evaluated in clinical trials. Levodopa dose should not be decreased when Tasmar therapy is being discontinued due to side effects related to too much levodopa. However, when Tasmar therapy is being discontinued for reasons other than too much levodopa, levodopa dosage may have to be increased to levels equal to or greater than before initiation of Tasmar therapy, especially if the patient had large decreases in levodopa when starting Tasmar. In all cases, patients should be educated on the symptoms of levodopa underdosage and what to do if it occurs. Adjustments in levodopa are most likely to be required within 1-2 days of Tasmar discontinuation.

Patients with impaired renal function (see 5.2): No dose adjustment of Tasmar is recommended for patients with mild or moderate renal impairment (creatinine clearance of 30 ml/min or greater).

Patients with hepatic impairment (see 4.3): Tasmar is contraindicated for patients with liver disease or increased liver enzymes.

Elderly patients: No dose adjustment of Tasmar is recommended for elderly patients.

Children: Tasmar should not be used in children as there are no data available. There is no identified potential use of tolcapone in paediatric patients.

Method of administration

Tasmar is administered orally three times daily. The first dose of the day of Tasmar should be taken together with the first dose of the day of a levodopa preparation, and the subsequent doses should be given approximately 6 and 12 hours later.

Tasmar may be taken with or without food (see 5.2).

Tasmar tablets are film-coated and should be swallowed whole because tolcapone has a bitter taste.

Tasmar can be combined with all pharmaceutical formulations of levodopa/benserazide and levodopa/carbidopa (see also 4.5).

4.3 Contraindications

Tasmar is contraindicated in patients with:

- Evidence of liver disease or increased liver enzymes
- Severe dyskinesia
- A previous history of Neuroleptic Malignant Syndrome Symptom Complex (NMS) and /or non-traumatic Rhabdomyolysis or Hyperthermia.

- Hypersensitivity to tolcapone or any of its other ingredients.
- Phaeochromocytoma.

4.4 Special warnings and special precautions for use

Tasmar therapy should only be initiated by physicians experienced in the management of advanced Parkinson's disease, to ensure an appropriate risk-benefit assessment. Tasmar should not be prescribed until there has been a complete informative discussion of the risks with the patient.

Tasmar should be discontinued if substantial clinical benefits are not seen within 3 weeks of the initiation of the treatment regardless of dose.

Liver Injury:

Because of the risk of rare but potentially fatal acute liver injury, Tasmar is only indicated for use in patients with levodopa-responsive idiopathic Parkinson's disease and motor fluctuations, who failed to respond to or are intolerant of other COMT inhibitors. Periodic monitoring of liver enzymes cannot reliably predict the occurrence of fulminant hepatitis. However, it is generally believed that early detection of medication-induced hepatic injury along with immediate withdrawal of the suspect medication enhances the likelihood for recovery. Liver injury has most often occurred between 1 month and 6 months after starting treatment with Tasmar.

It should also be noted that female patients may have a higher risk of liver injury (see 4.8).

Before starting treatment: If liver function tests are abnormal or there are signs of impaired liver function, Tasmar should not be prescribed. If Tasmar is to be prescribed, the patient should be informed about the signs and symptoms which may indicate liver injury, and to contact the physician immediately.

During treatment: Liver function should be monitored every 2 weeks for the first year of therapy, every 4 weeks for the next 6 months and every 8 weeks thereafter. If the dose is increased to 200 mg tid, liver enzyme monitoring should take place before increasing the dose and then be re-initiated following the sequence of frequencies as above. Treatment should be immediately discontinued if ALT and/or AST exceed the upper limit of normal or if symptoms or signs suggesting the onset of hepatic failure (persistent nausea, fatigue, lethargy, anorexia, jaundice, dark urine, pruritus, right upper quadrant tenderness) develop.

If treatment is discontinued: Patients who show evidence of acute liver injury while on Tasmar and are withdrawn from the drug may be at increased risk for liver injury if Tasmar is re-introduced. Accordingly, such patients should not be considered for re-treatment.

Neuroleptic Malignant Syndrome (NMS):

In Parkinson's patients, NMS tends to occur when discontinuing or stopping dopaminergic-enhancing medications. Therefore, if symptoms occur after discontinuing Tasmar, physicians should consider increasing the patient's levodopa dose (see 4.2).

Isolated cases consistent with NMS have been associated with Tasmar treatment. Symptoms have usually onset during Tasmar treatment or shortly after Tasmar has been discontinued. NMS is characterised by motor symptoms (rigidity, myoclonus and tremor), mental status changes (agitation, confusion, stupor and coma), elevated temperature, autonomic dysfunction (labile blood pressure, tachycardia) and elevated serum creatine phosphokinase (CPK) which may be a consequence of myolysis. A diagnosis of NMS should be considered even if not all the above findings are present. Under such a diagnosis Tasmar should be immediately discontinued and the patient should be followed up closely.

Before starting treatment: To reduce the risk of NMS, Tasmar should not be prescribed for patients with severe dyskinesia or a previous history of NMS including rhabdomyolysis or hyperthermia (see 4.3). Patients receiving multiple medications with effects on different CNS pathways (e.g. antidepressants, neuroleptics, anticholinergics) may be at greater risk of developing NMS.

Dyskinesia, nausea and other levodopa-associated adverse reactions: Patients may experience an increase in levodopa-associated adverse reactions. Reducing the dose of levodopa (see 4.2) may often mitigate these adverse reactions.

Diarrhoea: In clinical trials, diarrhoea developed in 16 % and 18 % of patients receiving Tasmar 100 mg tid and 200 mg tid respectively, compared to 8 % of patients receiving placebo. Diarrhoea associated with Tasmar usually began 2 to 4 months after initiation of therapy. Diarrhoea led to withdrawal of 5% and 6% of patients receiving Tasmar 100 mg tid and 200 mg tid respectively, compared to 1 % of patients receiving placebo.

Benserazide interaction: Due to the interaction between high dose benserazide and tolcapone (resulting in increased levels of benserazide), the prescriber should, until more experience has been gained, be observant of dose-related adverse events (see 4.5).

MAO inhibitors: Tasmar should not be given in conjunction with non-selective monoamine oxidase (MAO) inhibitors (e.g. phenelzine and tranylcypromine). The combination of MAO-A and MAO-B inhibitors is equivalent to non-selective MAO-inhibition, therefore they should not both be given concomitantly with Tasmar and levodopa preparations (see also 4.5). Selective MAO-B inhibitors should not be used at higher than recommended doses (e.g. selegiline 10 mg/day) when co-administered with Tasmar.

Warfarin: Since clinical information is limited regarding the combination of warfarin and tolcapone, coagulation parameters should be monitored when these drugs are co-administered.

Lactose intolerance: Each tablet contains 7.5 mg lactose; this quantity is probably not sufficient to induce symptoms of lactose intolerance.

Patients with rare hereditary problems of galactose intolerance, the Lapp lactase deficiency or glucose-galactose malabsorption should not take this medicine.

Special populations: Patients with severe renal impairment (creatinine clearance <30 ml/min) should be treated with caution. No information on the tolerability of tolcapone in these populations is available (see 5.2).

4.5 Interaction with other medicinal products and other forms of Interaction

Tasmar, as a COMT inhibitor, is known to increase the bioavailability of the co-adminstered levodopa. The consequent increase in dopaminergic stimulation can lead to the dopaminergic side effects observed after treatment with COMT inhibitors. The most common of these are increased dyskinesia, nausea, vomiting, abdominal pain, syncope, orthostatic complains, constipation, sleep disorders, somnolence, hallucination.

Levodopa has been associated with somnolence and episodes of sudden sleep onset. Sudden onset of sleep during daily activities, in some cases without awareness or warning signs, has been reported very rarely. Patients must be informed of this and advised to exercise caution while driving or operating machines during treatment with levodopa. Patients who have experienced somnolence and/or an episode of sudden sleep onset must refrain from driving or operating machines. Furthermore a reduction of levodopa dosage or termination of therapy may be considered.

Protein binding: Although tolcapone is highly protein bound, *in vitro* studies have shown that tolcapone did not displace warfarin, tolbutamide, digitoxin and phenytoin from their binding sites at therapeutic concentrations.

Catechols and other drugs metabolised by catechol-O-methyltransferase (COMT): Tolcapone may influence the pharmacokinetics of drugs metabolised by COMT. No effects were seen on the pharmacokinetics of the COMT substrate carbidopa. An interaction was observed with benserazide, which may lead to increased levels of benserazide and its active metabolite. The magnitude of the effect was dependent on the dose of benserazide. The plasma concentrations of benserazide observed after co-administration of tolcapone and benserazide-25 mg/levodopa were still within the range of values observed with levodopa/benserazide alone. On the other hand, after co-administration of tolcapone and benserazide-50 mg/levodopa the benserazide plasma concentrations could be increased above the levels usually observed with levodopa/benserazide alone. The effect of tolcapone on the pharmacokinetics of other drugs metabolised by COMT such as α-methyldopa, dobutamine, apomorphine, adrenaline and isoprenaline have not been evaluated. The prescriber should be observant of adverse effects caused by putative increased plasma levels of these drugs when combined with Tasmar.

Effect of tolcapone on the metabolism of other drugs: Due to its affinity for cytochrome *CYP2C9 in vitro*, tolcapone may interfere with drugs whose clearance is dependent on this metabolic pathway, such as tolbutamide and warfarin. In an interaction study, tolcapone did not change the pharmacokinetics of tolbutamide. Therefore, clinically relevant interactions involving cytochrome *CYP2C9* appear unlikely.

Since clinical information is limited regarding the combination of warfarin and tolcapone, coagulation parameters should be monitored when these drugs are co-administered.

Tolcapone did not change the pharmacokinetics of desipramine, even though both drugs share glucuronidation as their main metabolic pathway.

Drugs that increase catecholamines: Since tolcapone interferes with the metabolism of catecholamines, interactions with other drugs affecting catecholamine levels are theoretically possible.

Tolcapone did not influence the effect of ephedrine, an indirect sympathomimetic, on hemodynamic parameters or plasma catecholamine levels, either at rest or during exercise. Since tolcapone did not alter the tolerability of ephedrine, these drugs can be co-administered.

When Tasmar was given together with levodopa/carbidopa and desipramine, there was no significant change in blood pressure, pulse rate and plasma concentrations of desipramine. Overall, the frequency of adverse events increased slightly. These adverse events were predictable based on the known adverse reactions to each of the three drugs individually. Therefore, caution should be exercised when potent noradrenaline uptake inhibitors such as desipramine, maprotiline, or venlafaxine are administered to Parkinson's disease patients being treated with Tasmar and levodopa preparations.

In clinical trials, patients receiving Tasmar/levodopa preparations reported a similar adverse event profile independent of whether or not they were also concomitantly administered selegiline (a MAO-B inhibitor).

4.6 Pregnancy and lactation

Pregnancy: In rats and rabbits, embryo-foetal toxicity was observed after tolcapone administration (see 5.3). The potential risk for humans is unknown.

There are no adequate data from the use of tolcapone in pregnant women. Therefore, Tasmar should be used during pregnancy only if the potential benefit justifies the potential risk to the foetus.

Lactation: In animal studies, tolcapone was excreted into maternal milk.

The safety of tolcapone in infants is unknown; therefore, women should not breast-feed during treatment with Tasmar.

4.7 Effects on ability to drive and use machines

No studies on the effects of Tasmar on the ability to drive and use machines have been performed.

There is no evidence from clinical studies that Tasmar adversely influences a patient's ability to drive and use machines. However patients should be advised that their ability to drive and operate machines may be compromised due to their Parkinson's disease symptoms.

Tasmar, as a COMT inhibitor, is known to increase the bioavailability of the co-adminstered levodopa. The consequent increase in dopaminergic stimulation can lead to the dopaminergic side effects observed after treatment with COMT inhibitors. Patients being treated with Levodopa and presenting with somnolence and/or sudden sleep episodes must be informed to refrain from driving or engaging in activities where impaired alertness may put themselves or others at risk of serious injury or death (e.g. operating machines) until such recurrent episodes and somnolence have resolved (see also Section 4.4)

4.8 Undesirable effects

The most commonly observed adverse events associated with the use of Tasmar, occurring more frequently than in placebo-treated patients are listed in the table below. However, Tasmar, as a COMT inhibitor, is known to increase the bioavailability of the co-adminstered levodopa. The consequent increase in dopaminergic stimulation can lead to the dopaminergic side effects observed after treatment with COMT inhibitors. The most common of these are increased dyskinesia, nausea, vomiting, abdominal pain, syncope, orthostatic complains, constipation, sleep disorders, somnolence, hallucination.

The only adverse event commonly leading to discontinuation of Tasmar in clinical trials was diarrhoea (see 4.4).

Increases to more than three times the upper limit of normal (ULN) in alanine aminotransferase (ALT) occurred in 1 % of patients receiving Tasmar 100 mg three times daily, and 3 % of patients at 200 mg three times daily. Increases were approximately two times more likely in females. The increases usually appeared within 6 to 12 weeks of starting treatment, and were not associated with any clinical signs or symptoms. In about half the cases, transaminase levels returned spontaneously to baseline values whilst patients continued Tasmar treatment. For the remainder, when treatment was discontinued, transaminase levels returned to pre-treatment levels.

Rare cases of severe hepatocellular injury resulting in death have been reported during marketed use (see 4.4).

Isolated cases of patients with symptoms suggestive of Neuroleptic Malignant Syndrome Symptom Complex (see 4.4) have been reported following reduction or discontinuation of Tasmar and following introduction of Tasmar when this was accompanied by a significant reduction in other concomitant dopaminergic medications. In addition, rhabdomyolysis, secondary to NMS or severe dyskinesia, has been observed.

Urine discolouration: Tolcapone and its metabolites are yellow and can cause a harmless intensification in the colour of the patient's urine.

Experience with Tasmar obtained in parallel placebo-controlled randomised studies in patients with Parkinson's disease is shown in the following table, which lists adverse reactions with a potential relationship to Tasmar.

Summary of potentially Tasmar-related adverse reactions, with crude incidence rates for the phase III placebo-controlled studies:

(see Table 1 on next page)

4.9 Overdose

Isolated cases of either accidental or intentional overdose with tolcapone tablets have been reported. However clinical circumstances of these cases were so diverse, that no general conclusions can be drawn from the cases.

The highest dose of tolcapone administered to humans was 800 mg three times daily, with and without levodopa coadministration, in a one week study in healthy elderly volunteers. The peak plasma concentrations of tolcapone at this dose were on average 30 μg/ml (compared to 3 and

Table 1

Adverse Events	Placebo N=298 (%)	100 mg tid Tolcapone N=296 (%)	200 mg tid Tolcapone =298 (%)
Dyskinesia	19.8	41.9	51.3
Nausea	17.8	30.4	34.9
Sleep Disorder	18.1	23.6	24.8
Dystonia	17.1	18.6	22.1
Excessive Dreaming	17.1	21.3	16.4
Anorexia	12.8	18.9	22.8
Orthostatic Complaints	13.8	16.6	16.8
Somnolence	13.4	17.9	14.4
Diarrhoea	7.7	15.5	18.1
Dizziness	9.7	13.2	6.4
Confusion	8.7	10.5	10.4
Headache	7.4	9.8	11.4
Hallucination	5.4	8.4	10.4
Vomiting	3.7	8.4	9.7
Constipation	5.0	6.4	8.4
Upper Respiratory Tract Infection	3.4	4.7	7.4
Sweating Increased	2.3	4.4	7.4
Xerostomia	2.3	4.7	6.4
Abdominal Pain	2.7	4.7	5.7
Syncope	2.7	4.1	5.0
Urine Discoloration	0.7	2.4	7.4
Dyspepsia	1.7	4.1	3.0
Influenza	1.7	3.0	4.0
Chest Pain	1.3	3.4	1.0
Hypokinesia	0.7	0.7	2.7

6 μg/ml with 100 mg tid and 200 mg tid of tolcapone respectively). Nausea, vomiting and dizziness were observed, particularly in combination with levodopa.

Management of overdose: Hospitalisation is advised. General supportive care is indicated. Based on the physicochemical properties of the compound, hemodialysis is unlikely to be of benefit.

5. PHARMACOLOGICAL PROPERTIES

Tolcapone is an orally active, selective and reversible catechol-O-methyltransferase (COMT) inhibitor. Administered concomitantly with levodopa and an aromatic amino acid decarboxylase inhibitor (AADC-I), it leads to more stable plasma levels of levodopa by reducing metabolism of levodopa to 3-methoxy-4-hydroxy-L-phenylalanine (3-OMD).

High levels of plasma 3-OMD have been associated with poor response to levodopa in Parkinson's disease patients. Tolcapone markedly reduces the formation of 3-OMD.

5.1 Pharmacodynamic properties

Pharmaco-therapeutic group: Anti-Parkinson drug, ATC code: NO4BX01

Clinical pharmacology

Studies in healthy volunteers have shown that tolcapone reversibly inhibits human erythrocyte COMT activity after oral administration. The inhibition is closely related to plasma tolcapone concentration. With 200 mg tolcapone, maximum inhibition of erythrocyte COMT activity is, on average, greater than 80 %. During dosing with Tasmar 200 mg three times daily, erythrocyte COMT inhibition at trough is 30 % to 45 %, with no development of tolerance.

Transient elevation above pretreatment levels of erythrocyte COMT activity was observed after withdrawal of tolcapone. However, a study in Parkinson's patients confirmed that after treatment discontinuation there was no significant change in levodopa pharmacokinetics or in patient response to levodopa compared to pretreatment levels.

When Tasmar is administered together with levodopa, it increases the relative bioavailability (AUC) of levodopa approximately twofold. This is due to a decrease in clearance in L-dopa resulting in a prolongation of the terminal elimination half-life ($t_{1/2}$) of levodopa. In general, the average peak levodopa plasma concentration (C_{max}) and the time of its occurrence (t_{max}) were unaffected. The onset of effect occurs after the first administration. Studies in healthy volunteers and parkinsonian patients have confirmed that the maximum effect occurs with 100 – 200 mg tolcapone. Plasma levels of 3-OMD were markedly and dose-dependently decreased by tolcapone when given with levodopa/AADC-I (aromatic amino acid decarboxylase - inhibitor) (benserazide or carbidopa).

Tolcapone's effect on levodopa pharmacokinetics is similar with all pharmaceutical formulations of levodopa/benserazide and levodopa/carbidopa; it is independent of levodopa dose, levodopa/AADC-I (benserazide or carbidopa) ratio and the use of sustained-release formulations.

Clinical studies

Double blind placebo controlled clinical studies have shown a significant reduction of approximately 20 % to 30 % in OFF time and a similar increase in ON time, accompanied by reduced severity of symptoms in fluctuating patients receiving Tasmar. Investigator's global assessments of efficacy also showed significant improvement.

A double-blind trial compared Tasmar with entacapone in Parkinson's disease patients who had at least three hours of OFF time per day while receiving optimised levodopa therapy. The primary outcome was the proportion of patients with a 1 or more hour increase in ON time (see Table 1).

Tab. 2 Primary and Secondary Outcome of double-blind Trial

(see Table 2 below)

5.2 Pharmacokinetic properties

In the therapeutic range, tolcapone pharmacokinetics are linear and independent of levodopa/AADC-I (benserazide or carbidopa) coadministration.

Absorption: Tolcapone is rapidly absorbed with a t_{max} of approximately 2 hours. The absolute bioavailability of an oral administration is around 65 %. Tolcapone does not accumulate with three times daily dosing of 100 or 200 mg. At these doses, C_{max} is approximately 3 and 6 μg/ml, respectively. Food delays and decreases the absorption of tolcapone, but the relative bioavailability of a dose of tolcapone taken with a meal is still 80 % to 90 %.

Distribution: The volume of distribution (V_{ss}) of tolcapone is small (9 l). Tolcapone does not distribute widely into tissues due to its high plasma protein binding >99.9 %). *In vitro* experiments have shown that tolcapone binds mainly to serum albumin.

Metabolism/Elimination: Tolcapone is almost completely metabolised prior to excretion, with only a very small amount (0.5 % of dose) found unchanged in urine. The main metabolic pathway of tolcapone is conjugation to its inactive glucuronide. In addition, the compound is methylated by COMT to 3-O-methyl-tolcapone and metabolised by cytochromes *P450* 3A4 and *P450* 2A6 to a primary alcohol (hydroxylation of the methyl group), which is subsequently oxidised to the carboxylic acid. The reduction to a putative amine, as well as the subsequent *N*-acetylation, occurs to a minor extent. After oral administration, 60 % of drug-related material is excreted into urine and 40 % into faeces.

Tolcapone is a low-extraction-ratio drug (extraction ratio = 0.15), with a moderate systemic clearance of about 7 L/h. The $t_{1/2}$ of tolcapone is approximately 2 hours.

Hepatic impairment: Because of the risk of liver injury observed during post-marketing use, Tasmar is contra-indicated in patients with liver disease or increased liver enzymes. A study in patients with hepatic impairment has shown that moderate non-cirrhotic liver disease had no impact on the pharmacokinetics of tolcapone. However, in patients with moderate cirrhotic liver disease, clearance of unbound tolcapone was reduced by almost 50 %. This reduction may increase the average concentration of unbound drug two-fold.

Renal impairment: The pharmacokinetics of tolcapone have not been investigated in patients with renal impairment. However, the relationship of renal function and tolcapone pharmacokinetics has been investigated using population pharmacokinetics during clinical trials. The data of more than 400 patients have confirmed that over a wide range of creatinine clearance values (30-130 mL/min) the pharmacokinetics of tolcapone are unaffected by renal function. This could be explained by the fact that only a negligible amount of unchanged tolcapone is excreted in the urine, and the main metabolite, tolcapone-glucuronide, is excreted both in urine and in bile (faeces).

5.3 Preclinical safety data

Preclinical data reveal no special hazard for humans based on conventional studies of safety pharmacology, repeated dose toxicity, genotoxicity, carcinogenic potential, toxicity to reproduction.

Carcinogenesis, mutagenesis: 3 % and 5 % of rats in the mid- and high- dose groups, respectively, of the 24-month carcinogenicity study were shown to have renal epithelial tumours (adenomas or carcinomas). However, no evidence of renal toxicity was observed in the low-dose group. An increased incidence of uterine adenocarcinomas was seen in the high-dose group of the rat carcinogenicity study. There were no similar renal findings in the mouse or dogs carcinogenicity studies.

Mutagenesis: Tolcapone was shown not to be genotoxic in a complete series of mutagenicity studies.

Toxicity to reproduction: Tolcapone, when administered alone, was shown to be neither teratogenic nor to have any relevant effects on fertility.

6. PHARMACEUTICAL PARTICULARS

6.1 List of excipients

Tablet core:

Calcium hydrogen phosphate (anhydrous)

Microcrystalline cellulose

Polyvidone K30

Sodium starch glycollate

Lactose monohydrate

Talc

Magnesium stearate.

Film-coat:

Methylhydroxypropylcellulose,

Talc

Yellow iron oxide (E 172)

Ethylcellulose

Titanium dioxide (E 171)

Triacetin

Sodium lauryl sulfate

6.2 Incompatibilities

Not applicable

6.3 Shelf life

3 years

6.4 Special precautions for storage

This medicinal product does not require any special storage conditions

6.5 Nature and contents of container

Tasmar is available in PVC/PE/PVDC blisters (pack sizes of 30 and 60 film-coated tablets) and in glass bottles (pack sizes of 100 film-coated tablets).

Not all pack sizes may be marketed

Table 2 Primary and Secondary Outcome of double-blind Trial

	Entacapone N=75	Tolcapone N=75	p value	95 % CI
Primary Outcome				
Number (proportion) with ⩾1 hour ON time response	32 (43 %)	40 (53 %)	p=0.191	-5.2;26.6
Secondary Outcome				
Number (proportion) with moderate or marked improvement	19 (25 %)	29 (39 %)	p=0.080	-1.4;28.1
Number (proportion) improved on both primary and secondary outcome	13 (17 %)	24 (32 %)	NA	NA

6.6 Instructions for use and handling
No special requirements.

7. MARKETING AUTHORISATION HOLDER
Valeant Pharmaceuticals Ltd.

Cedarwood, Chineham Business Park

Crockford Lane

Basingstoke

Hampshire, RG24 8WD

United Kingdom

8. MARKETING AUTHORISATION NUMBER(S)
Tasmar 100 mg tablets: EU/1/97/044/001-3

9. DATE OF FIRST AUTHORISATION/RENEWAL OF THE AUTHORISATION
27 August 1997

10. DATE OF REVISION OF THE TEXT

Tavanic 250mg & 500mg Tablets

(sanofi-aventis)

1. NAME OF THE MEDICINAL PRODUCT
Tavanic 250 mg film-coated tablet

Tavanic 500 mg film-coated tablet

2. QUALITATIVE AND QUANTITATIVE COMPOSITION
Each film-coated tablet of Tavanic contains 250 mg of levofloxacin as active substance corresponding to 256.23 mg of levofloxacin hemihydrate.

Each film-coated tablet of Tavanic contains 500 mg of levofloxacin as active substance corresponding to 512.46 mg of levofloxacin hemihydrate.

For excipients, see 6.1

3. PHARMACEUTICAL FORM
Film-coated tablet.

Score line pale yellowish-white to reddish-white film-coated tablets

4. CLINICAL PARTICULARS
4.1 Therapeutic indications
In adults with infections of mild or moderate severity, Tavanic tablets are indicated for the treatment of the following infections when due to levofloxacin-susceptible microorganisms:

- Acute sinusitis
- Acute exacerbations of chronic bronchitis
- Community-acquired pneumonia
- Uncomplicated urinary tract infections
- Complicated urinary tract infections including pyelonephritis
- Chronic bacterial prostatitis.
- Skin and soft tissue infections.

Before prescribing Tavanic, consideration should be given to national and/or local guidance on the appropriate use of fluoroquinolones.

4.2 Posology and method of administration
Tavanic tablets are administered once or twice daily. The dosage depends on the type and severity of the infection and the sensitivity of the presumed causative pathogen.

Duration of treatment

The duration of therapy varies according to the course of the disease (see table below). As with antibiotic therapy in general, administration of Tavanic tablets should be continued for a minimum of 48 to 72 hours after the patient has become afebrile or evidence of bacterial eradication has been obtained.

Method of administration

Tavanic tablets should be swallowed without crushing and with sufficient amount of liquid. They may be divided at the score line to adapt the dosage. The tablets may be taken during meals or between meals. Tavanic tablets should be taken at least two hours before or after iron salts, antacids and sucralfate administration since reduction of absorption can occur (see 4.5: "Interactions").

The following dose recommendations can be given for Tavanic:

Dosage in patients with normal renal function(creatinine clearance > 50 ml/min)

Indication	**Daily dose regimen *(according to severity)***	**Duration of treatment**
Acute sinusitis	500 mg once daily	10 - 14 days
Acute exacerbations of chronic bronchitis	250 to 500 mg once daily	7 - 10 days
Community-acquired pneumonia	500 mg once or twice daily	7 - 14 days
Uncomplicated urinary tract infections	250 mg once daily	3 days
Complicated urinary tract infections including pyelonephritis	250 mg once daily	7 - 10 days
Chronic bacterial prostatitis.	500 mg once daily	28 days
Skin and soft tissue infections	250 mg once daily or 500 mg once or twice daily	7 - 14 days

Dosage in patients with impaired renal function (creatinine clearance ⩽ 50ml/min)

(see Table 1 below)

Dosage in patients with impaired liver function

No adjustment of dosage is required since levofloxacin is not metabolised to any relevant extent by the liver and is mainly excreted by the kidneys.

Dosage in elderly

No adjustment of dosage is required in the elderly, other than that imposed by consideration of renal function.

4.3 Contraindications
Tavanic tablets must not be used:

- in patients hypersensitive to levofloxacin or other quinolones or any of the excipients,
- in patients with epilepsy,
- in patients with history of tendon disorders related to fluoroquinolone administration,
- in children or growing adolescents,
- during pregnancy,
- in breast-feeding women.

4.4 Special warnings and special precautions for use
In the most severe cases of pneumococcal pneumonia Tavanic may not be the optimal therapy.

Nosocomial infections due to *P. aeruginosa* may require combination therapy.

Tendinitis and tendon rupture

Tendinitis may rarely occur. It most frequently involves the Achilles tendon and may lead to tendon rupture. The risk of tendinitis and tendon rupture is increased in the elderly and in patients using corticosteroids. Close monitoring of these patients is therefore necessary if they are prescribed Tavanic. All patients should consult their physician if they experience symptoms of tendinitis. If tendinitis is suspected, treatment with Tavanic must be halted immediately, and appropriate treatment (e.g. immobilisation) must be initiated for the affected tendon

Clostridium difficile-associated disease

Diarrhoea, particularly if severe, persistent and/or bloody, during or after treatment with Tavanic tablets, may be symptomatic of *Clostridium difficile*-associated disease, the most severe form of which is pseudomembranous colitis. If pseudomembranous colitis is suspected, Tavanic tablets must be stopped immediately and patients should be treated with supportive measures ± specific therapy without delay (e.g. oral vancomycin). Products inhibiting the peristalsis are contraindicated in this clinical situation.

Patients predisposed to seizures

Tavanic tablets are contraindicated in patients with a history of epilepsy and, as with other quinolones, should be used with extreme caution in patients predisposed to seizures, such as patients with pre-existing central nervous system lesions, concomitant treatment with fenbufen and similar non-steroidal anti-inflammatory drugs or with drugs which lower the cerebral seizure threshold, such as theophylline (see 4.5: "Interactions").

Patients with G-6- phosphate dehydrogenase deficiency

Patients with latent or actual defects in glucose-6-phosphate dehydrogenase activity may be prone to haemolytic reactions when treated with quinolone antibacterial agents, and so levofloxacin should be used with caution.

Patients with renal impairment

Since levofloxacin is excreted mainly by the kidneys, the dose of Tavanic should be adjusted in patients with renal impairment.

Prevention of photosensitisation

Although photosensitisation is very rare with levofloxacin, it is recommended that patients should not expose themselves unnecessarily to strong sunlight or to artificial UV rays (e.g. sunray lamp, solarium), in order to prevent photosensitisation.

Patients treated with Vitamin K antagonists

Due to possible increase in coagulation tests (PT/INR) and/or bleeding in patients treated with Tavanic in combination with a vitamin K antagonist (e.g. warfarin), coagulation tests should be monitored when these drugs are given concomitantly (see 4.5: Interactions With Other Medicinal Products)

4.5 Interaction with other medicinal products and other forms of Interaction

Iron salts, magnesium- or aluminium-containing antacids

Levofloxacin absorption is significantly reduced when iron salts, or magnesium- or aluminium-containing antacids are administered concomitantly with Tavanic tablets. It is recommended that preparations containing divalent or trivalent cations such as iron salts, or magnesium- or aluminium-containing antacids should not be taken 2 hours before or after Tavanic tablet administration. No interaction was found with calcium carbonate.

Sucralfate

The bioavailability of Tavanic tablets is significantly reduced when administered together with sucralfate. If the patient is to receive both sucralfate and Tavanic, it is best to administer sucralfate 2 hours after the Tavanic tablet administration.

Theophylline, fenbufen or similar non-steroidal anti-inflammatory drugs

No pharmacokinetic interactions of levofloxacin were found with theophylline in a clinical study. However a pronounced lowering of the cerebral seizure threshold may occur when quinolones are given concurrently with theophylline, non-steroidal anti-inflammatory drugs, or other agents which lower the seizure threshold.

Levofloxacin concentrations were about 13% higher in the presence of fenbufen than when administered alone.

Probenecid and cimetidine

Probenecid and cimetidine had a statistically significant effect on the elimination of levofloxacin. The renal clearance of levofloxacin was reduced by cimetidine (24%) and probenecid (34%). This is because both drugs are capable of blocking the renal tubular secretion of levofloxacin. However, at the tested doses in the study, the statistically significant kinetic differences are unlikely to be of clinical relevance.

Caution should be exercised when levofloxacin is coadministered with drugs that effect the tubular renal secretion such as probenecid and cimetidine, especially in renally impaired patients.

Cyclosporin

The half-life of cyclosporin was increased by 33% when coadministered with levofloxacin.

Vitamin K antagonists

Increased coagulation tests (PT/INR) and/or bleeding, which may be severe, have been reported in patients treated with levofloxacin in combination with a vitamin K antagonist (e.g. warfarin). Coagulation tests, therefore, should be monitored in patients treated with vitamin K antagonists

Meals

There is no clinically relevant interaction with food. Tavanic tablets may therefore be administered regardless of food intake.

Other relevant information

Clinical pharmacology studies were carried out to investigate possible pharmacokinetic interactions between levofloxacin and commonly prescribed drugs. The pharmacokinetics of levofloxacin were not affected to any clinically relevant extent when levofloxacin was administered together with the following drugs: calcium carbonate, digoxin, glibenclamide, ranitidine, warfarin.

4.6 Pregnancy and lactation
Pregnancy

Reproductive studies in animals did not raise specific concern. However in the absence of human data and due to the experimental risk of damage by fluoroquinolones to the weight-bearing cartilage of the growing organism, Tavanic tablets must not be used in pregnant women.

Table 1

	Dose regimen		
	250 mg/24 h	**500 mg/24 h**	**500 mg/12 h**
Creatinine clearance	*first dose:* 250 mg	*first dose:* 500 mg	*first dose:* 500 mg
50-20 ml/min	*then:* 125 mg/24 h	*then*: 250 mg/24 h	*then*: 250 mg/12 h
19-10 ml/min	*then:* 125 mg/48 h	*then*: 125 mg/24 h	*then*: 125 mg/12 h
< 10 ml/min (including haemodialysis and CAPD)[1]	then: 125 mg/48 h	then: 125 mg/24 h	then: 125 mg/24 h

[1] No additional doses are required after haemodialysis or continuous ambulatory peritoneal dialysis (CAPD).

Lactation

In the absence of human data and due to the experimental risk of damage by fluoroquinolones to the weight-bearing cartilage of the growing organism, Tavanic tablets must not be used in breast-feeding women.

4.7 Effects on ability to drive and use machines

Some undesirable effects (e.g. dizziness/vertigo, drowsiness, visual disturbances) may impair the patient's ability to concentrate and react, and therefore may constitute a risk in situations where these abilities are of special importance (e.g. driving a car or operating machinery).

4.8 Undesirable effects

The information given below is based on data from clinical studies in more than 5000 patients and on extensive post marketing experience.

The following frequency rating has been used:

Very common: more than 10%

Common: 1 % to 10 %

Uncommon 0.1 % to 1 %

Rare: 0.01 % to 0.1 %

Very rare: less than 0.01 %

Isolated cases:

Allergic reactions

Uncommon: pruritus, rash.

Rare: urticaria, bronchospasm / dyspnoea.

Very rare: angio-oedema, hypotension, anaphylactic-like shock, photosensitisation.

Isolated cases: severe bullous eruptions such as Stevens-Johnson syndrome, toxic epidermal necrolysis (Lyell's syndrome) and erythema exsudativum multiforme.

Muco-cutaneous, anaphylactic /-oid reactions may sometimes occur even after the first dose.

Gastro-intestinal, metabolism

Common: nausea, diarrhoea.

Uncommon: anorexia, vomiting, abdominal pain, dyspepsia.

Rare: bloody diarrhoea which in very rare cases may be indicative of enterocolitis, including pseudomembranous colitis.

Very rare: hypoglycaemia, particularly in diabetic patients.

Neurological

Uncommon: headache, dizziness/vertigo, drowsiness, insomnia.

Rare: paraesthesia, tremor, anxiety, depression, psychotic reactions, agitation, confusion, convulsion.

Very rare: hypoaesthesia, visual and auditory disturbances, disturbances of taste and smell, hallucinations.

Cardiovascular

Rare: tachycardia, hypotension.

Very rare: shock (anaphylactic-like).

Isolated cases: QT-interval prolongation (see section 4.9)

Musculo-skeletal

Rare: arthralgia, myalgia, tendon disorders incl. tendinitis (e.g. Achilles tendon), (see 4.4: Special Warnings And Special Precautions For Use).

Very rare: tendon rupture (e.g. Achilles tendon); this undesirable effect may occur within 48 hours of starting treatment and may be bilateral. (see 4.4: Special Warnings And Special Precautions For Use). Muscular weakness, which may be of special importance in patients with myasthenia gravis.

Isolated cases: rhabdomyolysis.

Liver, kidney

Common: increase in liver enzymes (e.g. ALT / AST).

Uncommon: increase in bilirubin, increase in serum creatinine.

Very rare: liver reactions such as hepatitis; acute kidney failure (e.g. due to interstitial nephritis).

Blood

Uncommon: eosinophilia, leukopenia.

Rare: neutropenia, thrombocytopenia.

Very rare: agranulocytosis.

Isolated cases: haemolytic anaemia, pancytopenia.

Others

Uncommon: asthenia, fungal overgrowth and proliferation of other resistant microorganisms.

Very rare: allergic pneumonitis, fever.

Other undesirable effects which have been associated with fluoroquinolone administration include:

- extrapyramidal symptoms and other disorders of muscular coordination,
- hypersensitivity vasculitis,
- attacks of porphyria in patients with porphyria.

4.9 Overdose

According to toxicity studies in animals or clinical pharmacology studies performed with supra-therapeutic doses, the most important signs to be expected following acute overdosage of Tavanic tablets are central nervous system symptoms such as confusion, dizziness, impairment of consciousness, and convulsive seizures, increases in QT interval as well as gastro-intestinal reactions such as nausea and mucosal erosions.

In the event of overdose, symptomatic treatment should be implemented. ECG monitoring should be undertaken, because of the possibility of QT interval prolongation. Antacids may be used for protection of gastric mucosa. Haemodialysis, including peritoneal dialysis and CAPD, are not effective in removing levofloxacin from the body. No specific antidote exists.

5. PHARMACOLOGICAL PROPERTIES

5.1 Pharmacodynamic properties

Levofloxacin is a synthetic antibacterial agent of the fluoroquinolone class (ATC code J01MA) and is the S (-) enantiomer of the racemic drug substance ofloxacin.

Mode of action

As a fluoroquinolone antibacterial agent, levofloxacin acts on the DNA-DNA-gyrase complex and topoisomerase IV.

Breakpoints

The preliminary NCCLS (US National Committee on Clinical Laboratory Standards) recommended MIC breakpoints for levofloxacin, separating susceptible from intermediately susceptible organisms and intermediately susceptible from resistant organisms are:

susceptible ⩽ 2 mg/L, resistant ⩾ 8 mg/L.

Antibacterial spectrum

The prevalence of resistance may vary geographically and with time for selected species and local information on resistance is desirable, particularly when treating severe infections. Therefore, the information presented provides only an approximate guidance on probabilities as to whether microorganisms will be susceptible to levofloxacin or not. Only microorganisms relevant to the given clinical indications are presented here.

(see Table 2)

Other information

The main mechanism of resistance is due to a *gyr-A* mutation. *In vitro* there is a cross-resistance between levofloxacin and other fluoroquinolones.

Acquired resistance with levofloxacin has recently been documented in 1997:

- *S. pneumoniae* France ⩽ 1%
- *H. influenzae:* rare.

Due to the mechanism of action, there is generally no cross-resistance between levofloxacin and other classes of antibacterial agents.

Nosocomial infections due to *P. aeruginosa* may require combination therapy.

5.2 Pharmacokinetic properties

Absorption

Orally administered levofloxacin is rapidly and almost completely absorbed with peak plasma concentrations being obtained within 1 h. The absolute bioavailability is approximately 100 %. Levofloxacin obeys linear pharmacokinetics over a range of 50 to 600 mg.

Food has little effect on the absorption of levofloxacin.

Distribution

Approximately 30 - 40 % of levofloxacin is bound to serum protein. 500 mg once daily multiple dosing with levofloxacin showed negligible accumulation. There is modest but predictable accumulation of levofloxacin after doses of 500 mg twice daily. Steady-state is achieved within 3 days.

Penetration into tissues and body fluids:

Penetration into Bronchial Mucosa, Epithelial Lining Fluid (ELF)

Maximum levofloxacin concentrations in bronchial mucosa and epithelial lining fluid after 500 mg p.o. were 8.3 μg/g and 10.8 μg/ml respectively. These were reached approximately one hour after administration.

Penetration into Lung Tissue

Maximum levofloxacin concentrations in lung tissue after 500 mg p.o. were approximately 11.3 μg/g and were reached between 4 and 6 hours after administration. The concentrations in the lungs consistently exceeded those in plasma.

Penetration into Blister Fluid

Maximum levofloxacin concentrations of about 4.0 and 6.7 μg/ml in the blister fluid were reached 2 - 4 hours after administration following 3 days dosing at 500 mg once or twice daily, respectively.

Penetration into Cerebro-Spinal Fluid

Levofloxacin has poor penetration into cerebro-spinal fluid.

Penetration into prostatic tissue

After administration of oral 500mg levofloxacin once a day for three days, the mean concentrations in prostatic tissue were 8.7 μg/g, 8.2 μg/g and 2.0 μg/g respectively after 2 hours, 6 hours and 24 hours; the mean prostate/plasma concentration ratio was 1.84.

Concentration in urine

The mean urine concentrations 8 -12 hours after a single oral dose of 150 mg, 300 mg or 500 mg levofloxacin were 44 mg/L, 91 mg/L and 200 mg/L, respectively.

Metabolism

Levofloxacin is metabolised to a very small extent, the metabolites being desmethyl-levofloxacin and levofloxacin N-oxide. These metabolites account for < 5 % of the dose excreted in urine. Levofloxacin is stereochemically stable and does not undergo chiral inversion.

Elimination

Following oral and intravenous administration of levofloxacin, it is eliminated relatively slowly from the plasma ($t_{½}$: 6 - 8 h). Excretion is primarily by the renal route > 85 % of the administered dose).

Table 2

In vitro **antibacterial spectrum - Category with European range of resistance where this is known to vary**

Susceptible			
Aerobic Gram-positive micro-organisms:			
Enterococcus faecalis[1]	10-35%	Streptococci, group C and G	
Staphylococcus aureus[1] methi-S		*Streptococcus agalactiae*	
Staphylococcus coagulase negative methi-S(1)	0-30%	*Streptococcus pneumoniae*[1] peni-I/S/R	
Staphylococcus saprophyticus		*Streptococcus pyogenes*[1]	
Aerobic Gram-negative micro-organisms:			
Acinetobacter baumannii[1]	40%	*Klebsiellapneumoniae*[1]	<5-10%
Citrobacter freundii[1]	7%	*Moraxella catarrhalis*[1] β+ / β-	
Eikenella corrodens		*Morganella morganii*[1]	5%
Enterobacter aerogenes	30%	*Pasteurella multocida*	
Enterobacter agglomerans		*Proteus mirabilis*[1]	0-15%
Enterobactercloacae[1]	7%	*Proteusvulgaris*	
Escherichia coli[1]	0-20%[2]	*Providencia rettgeri*	
Haemophilus influenzae[1] ampi-S/R		*Providencia stuartii*	35%
Haemophilus para-influenzae[1]		*Pseudomonas aeruginosa*[1]	10-50%
Klebsiella oxytoca		*Serratia marcescens*[1]	7%
Anaerobic micro-organisms:			
Bacteroides fragilis		Peptostreptococcus	
Clostridium perfringens			
Other micro-organisms:			
Chlamydia pneumoniae[1]		*Legionella pneumophila*[1]	
Chlamydia psittaci		*Mycoplasma pneumoniae*[1]	
Chlamydia trachomatis		*Mycoplasma hominis*	
		Ureaplasma urealyticum	
Intermediately susceptible			
Aerobic Gram-positive micro-organisms:		Aerobic Gram-negative micro-organisms:	
		Burkholderia cepacia	
Anaerobic micro-organisms:			
Bacteroides ovatus		Bacteroides vulgatus	
Bacteroides thetaiotamicron		*Clostridium difficile*	
Resistant			
Aerobic Gram-positive micro-organisms:			
Staphylococcus aureus methi-R		*Staphylococcus coagulase negative methi-R*	

[1] Clinical efficacy has been proven in clinical studies.

[2] (20% in Spain and Portugal)

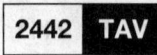

There are no major differences in the pharmacokinetics of levofloxacin following intravenous and oral administration, suggesting that the oral and intravenous routes are interchangeable.

Subjects with renal insufficiency

The pharmacokinetics of levofloxacin are affected by renal impairment. With decreasing renal function renal elimination and clearance are decreased, and elimination half-lives increased as shown in the table below:

Cl_{cr} [ml/min]	< 20	20 - 40	50 - 80
Cl_R [ml/min]	13	26	57
$t_{1/2}$ [h]	35	27	9

Elderly subjects

There are no significant differences in levofloxacin kinetics between young and elderly subjects, except those associated with differences in creatinine clearance.

Gender differences

Separate analysis for male and female subjects showed small to marginal gender differences in levofloxacin pharmacokinetics. There is no evidence that these gender differences are of clinical relevance.

5.3 Preclinical safety data

Acute toxicity

The median lethal dose (LD_{50}) values obtained in mice and rats after oral administration of levofloxacin were in the range 1500-2000 mg/kg.

Administration of 500 mg/kg p.o. to monkeys induced little effect apart from vomiting.

Repeated dose toxicity

Studies of one and six months duration by gavage have been carried out in the rat and monkey. Doses were 50, 200, 800 mg/kg/day and 20, 80, 320 mg/kg/day for 1 and 6 months in the rat and 10, 30, 100 mg/kg/day and 10, 25, 62.5 mg/kg/day for 1 and 6 months in the monkey.

Signs of reaction to treatment were minor in the rat with slight effects principally at 200 mg/kg/day and above in reducing food consumption and slightly altering haematological and biochemical parameters. The No Observed Adverse Effect Levels (NOELs) in these studies were concluded to be 200 and 20 mg/kg/day after 1 and 6 months respectively.

Toxicity after oral dosing in the monkey was minimal with reduced body weight at 100 mg/kg/day together with salivation, diarrhoea and decreased urinary pH in some animals at this dose. No toxicity was seen in the 6-month study. The NOELs were concluded to be 30 and 62.5 mg/kg/day after 1 and 6 months respectively.

The NOELs in the six-month studies were concluded to be 20 and 62.5 mg/kg/day in the rat and monkey respectively.

Reproductive toxicity

Levofloxacin caused no impairment of fertility or reproductive performance in rats at oral doses as high as 360 mg/kg/day or intravenous doses up to 100 mg/kg/day.

Levofloxacin was not teratogenic in rats at oral doses as high as 810 mg/kg/day, or at intravenous doses as high as 160 mg/kg/day. No teratogenicity was observed when rabbits were dosed orally with up to 50 mg/kg/day or intravenously with up to 25 mg/kg/day.

Levofloxacin had no effect on fertility and its only effect on foetuses was delayed maturation as a result of maternal toxicity.

Genotoxicity

Levofloxacin did not induce gene mutations in bacterial or mammalian cells but did induce chromosome aberrations in Chinese hamster lung cells *in vitro* at or above 100 μg/ml, in the absence of metabolic activation. *In vivo* tests (micronucleus, sister chromatid exchange, unscheduled DNA synthesis, dominant lethal tests) did not show any genotoxic potential.

Phototoxic potential

Studies in the mouse after both oral and intravenous dosing showed levofloxacin to have phototoxic activity only at very high doses. Levofloxacin did not show any genotoxic potential in a photomutagenicity assay, and it reduced tumour development in a photocarcinogenicity assay.

Carcinogenic potential

No indication of carcinogenic potential was seen in a two year study in the rat with dietary administration (0, 10, 30 and 100 mg/kg/day).

Toxicity to joints

In common with other fluoroquinolones, levofloxacin showed effects on cartilage (blistering and cavities) in rats and dogs. These findings were more marked in young animals.

6. PHARMACEUTICAL PARTICULARS

6.1 List of excipients

Tavanic 250 mg film-coated tablets contain the following excipients for a weight of 315 mg:

Tavanic 500 mg film-coated tablets contain the following excipients for a weight of 630 mg:

Tablet core:

Crospovidone, hypromellose, microcrystalline cellulose and sodium stearyl fumarate.

Tablet coating:

Hypromellose, titanium dioxide (E 171), talc, macrogol, yellow ferric oxide (E 172) and red ferric oxide (E 172).

6.2 Incompatibilities

Not applicable.

6.3 Shelf life

5 years.

6.4 Special precautions for storage

No special conditions for storage.

6.5 Nature and contents of container

PVC aluminium blisters containing film-coated tablets.

Pack sizes for 250mg tablets and 500mg tablets: 1, 5 or 10.

6.6 Instructions for use and handling

A score line allows adaptation of the dose in patients with impaired renal function.

7. MARKETING AUTHORISATION HOLDER

Hoechst Marion Roussel Ltd

Broadwater Park

Denham, Uxbridge

Middlesex

UB9 5HP

8. MARKETING AUTHORISATION NUMBER(S)

PL 13402/0011 250mg tablets

PL 13402/0012 500mg tablets

9. DATE OF FIRST AUTHORISATION/RENEWAL OF THE AUTHORISATION

6 June 1997/6 June 2002

10. DATE OF REVISION OF THE TEXT

October 2004

Tavanic i.v.

(sanofi-aventis)

1. NAME OF THE MEDICINAL PRODUCT

Tavanic 5 mg/ml solution for infusion

2. QUALITATIVE AND QUANTITATIVE COMPOSITION

Each 100 ml bottle of Tavanic 5 mg/ml solution for infusion contains 500 mg (5 mg/ml) of levofloxacin as active substance.

For excipients, see 6.1

3. PHARMACEUTICAL FORM

Solution for infusion.

Tavanic 5 mg/ml solution for infusion is a clear greenish-yellow solution

4. CLINICAL PARTICULARS

4.1 Therapeutic indications

In adults for whom intravenous therapy is considered to be appropriate, Tavanic solution for infusion is indicated for the treatment of the following infections when due to levofloxacin-susceptible microorganisms:

- Community-acquired pneumonia.
- Complicated urinary tract infections including pyelonephritis.
- Chronic bacterial prostatitis.
- Skin and soft tissue infections.

Before prescribing Tavanic, consideration should be given to national and/or local guidance on the appropriate use of fluoroquinolones.

4.2 Posology and method of administration

Tavanic solution is administered by slow intravenous infusion once or twice daily. The dosage depends on the type and severity of the infection and the sensitivity of the presumed causative pathogen. It is usually possible to switch from initial intravenous treatment to the oral route after a few days (Tavanic 250 or 500 mg tablets), according to the condition of the patient. Given the bioequivalence of the parenteral and oral forms, the same dosage can be used.

Duration of treatment

The duration of therapy varies according to the course of the disease. As with antibiotic therapy in general, administration of Tavanic (solution for infusion or tablets) should be continued for a minimum of 48 to 72 hours after the patient has become afebrile or evidence of bacterial eradication has been obtained.

Method of administration

Tavanic solution for infusion is only intended for slow intravenous infusion; it is administered once or twice daily. The infusion time must be at least 30 minutes for 250 mg or 60 minutes for 500 mg Tavanic solution for infusion (see 4.4: "Special Warnings"). It is possible to switch from an initial intravenous application to the oral route at the same dosage after a few days, according to the condition of the patient.

For incompatibilities see 6.2 and compatibility with other infusion solutions see 6.6.

The following dose recommendations can be given for Tavanic:

Dosage in patients with normal renal function(creatinine clearance > 50 ml/min)

Indication	**Daily dose regimen** *(according to severity)*
Community-acquired pneumonia	500 mg once or twice daily
Complicated urinary tract infections including pyelonephritis	250 mg[1] once daily
Chronic bacterial prostatitis.	500mg once daily
Skin and soft tissue infections	500 mg twice daily

[1] Consideration should be given to increasing the dose in cases of severe infection.

Dosage in patients with impaired renal function (creatinine clearance ⩽ 50ml/min)

(see Table 1 below)

Dosage in patients with impaired liver function

No adjustment of dosage is required since levofloxacin is not metabolised to any relevant extent by the liver and is mainly excreted by the kidneys.

Dosage in elderly

No adjustment of dosage is required in the elderly, other than that imposed by consideration of renal function.

4.3 Contraindications

Tavanic solution for infusion must not be used:

- in patients hypersensitive to levofloxacin or any other quinolone,
- in patients with epilepsy,
- in patients with history of tendon disorders related to fluoroquinolone administration,
- in children or growing adolescents,
- during pregnancy,
- in breast-feeding women.

4.4 Special warnings and special precautions for use

In the most severe cases of pneumococcal pneumonia Tavanic may not be the optimal therapy.

Nosocomial infections due to *P. aeruginosa* may require combination therapy.

Infusion Time

The recommended infusion time of at least 30 minutes for 250 mg or 60 minutes for 500mg Tavanic solution for infusion should be observed. It is known for ofloxacin, that during infusion tachycardia and a temporary decrease in blood pressure may develop. In rare cases, as a consequence of a profound drop in blood pressure, circulatory collapse may occur. Should a conspicuous drop in blood pressure occur during infusion of levofloxacin, (*l*-isomer of ofloxacin) the infusion must be halted immediately.

Tendinitis and tendon rupture

Tendinitis may rarely occur. It most frequently involves the Achilles tendon and may lead to tendon rupture. The risk of tendinitis and tendon rupture is increased in the elderly and in patients using corticosteroids. Close monitoring of these patients is therefore necessary if they are prescribed Tavanic. All patients should consult their physician if they experience symptoms of tendinitis. If tendinitis is suspected, treatment with Tavanic must be halted immediately, and appropriate treatment (e.g. immobilisation) must be initiated for the affected tendon

Clostridium difficile-associated disease

Diarrhoea, particularly if severe, persistent and/or bloody, during or after treatment with Tavanic solution for infusion, may be symptomatic of *Clostridium difficile*-associated disease, the most severe form of which is

Table 1

	Dose regimen		
	250 mg/24 h	**500 mg/24 h**	**500 mg/12 h**
Creatinine clearance	*first dose:* 250 mg	*first dose:* 500 mg	*first dose:* 500 mg
50 - 20 ml/min	*then:* 125 mg/24 h	*then:* 250 mg/24 h	*then:* 250 mg/12 h
19-10 ml/min	*then:* 125 mg/48 h	*then:* 125 mg/24 h	*then:* 125 mg/12 h
< 10 ml/min (including haemodialysis and CAPD) [1]	then: 125 mg/48 h	then: 125 mg/24 h	then: 125 mg/24 h

[1] No additional doses are required after haemodialysis or continuous ambulatory peritoneal dialysis (CAPD).

pseudomembranous colitis. If pseudomembranous colitis is suspected, Tavanic solution for infusion must be stopped immediately and patients should be treated with supportive measures ± specific therapy without delay (e.g. oral vancomycin). Products inhibiting the peristalsis are contraindicated in this clinical situation.

Patients predisposed to seizures

Tavanic solution for infusion is contraindicated in patients with a history of epilepsy and, as with other quinolones, should be used with extreme caution in patients predisposed to seizures, such as patients with pre-existing central nervous system lesions, concomitant treatment with fenbufen and similar non-steroidal anti-inflammatory drugs or with drugs which lower the cerebral seizure threshold, such as theophylline (see 4.5: "Interactions").

Patients with G-6- phosphate dehydrogenase deficiency

Patients with latent or actual defects in glucose-6-phosphate dehydrogenase activity may be prone to haemolytic reactions when treated with quinolone antibacterial agents, and so levofloxacin should be used with caution.

Patients with renal impairment

Since levofloxacin is excreted mainly by the kidneys, the dose of Tavanic should be adjusted in patients with renal impairment.

Prevention of photosensitisation

Although photosensitisation is very rare with levofloxacin, it is recommended that patients should not expose themselves unnecessarily to strong sunlight or to artificial UV rays (e.g. sunray lamp, solarium), in order to prevent photosensitisation.

Patients treated with Vitamin K antagonists

Due to possible increase in coagulation tests (PT/INR) and/or bleeding in patients treated with Tavanic in combination with a vitamin K antagonist (e.g. warfarin), coagulation tests should be monitored when these drugs are given concomittantly (see 4.5: Interactions With Other Medicinal Products)

4.5 Interaction with other medicinal products and other forms of Interaction

Theophylline, fenbufen or similar non-steroidal anti-inflammatory drugs

No pharmacokinetic interactions of levofloxacin were found with theophylline in a clinical study. However a pronounced lowering of the cerebral seizure threshold may occur when quinolones are given concurrently with theophylline, non-steroidal anti-inflammatory drugs, or other agents which lower the seizure threshold.

Levofloxacin concentrations were about 13% higher in the presence of fenbufen than when administered alone.

Probenecid and cimetidine

Probenecid and cimetidine had a statistically significant effect on the elimination of levofloxacin. The renal clearance of levofloxacin was reduced by cimetidine (24%) and probenecid (34%). This is because both drugs are capable of blocking the renal tubular secretion of levofloxacin. However, at the tested doses in the study, the statistically significant kinetic differences are unlikely to be of clinical relevance.

Caution should be exercised when levofloxacin is coadministered with drugs that effect the tubular renal secretion such as probenecid and cimetidine, especially in renally impaired patients.

Cyclosporin

The half-life of cyclosporin was increased by 33% when coadministered with levofloxacin.

Vitamin K antagonists

Increased coagulation tests (PT/INR) and/or bleeding, which may be severe, have been reported in patients treated with levofloxacin in combination with a vitamin K antagonist (e.g. warfarin). Coagulation tests, therefore, should be monitored in patients treated with vitamin K antagonists

Other relevant information

Clinical pharmacology studies were carried out to investigate possible pharmacokinetic interactions between levofloxacin and commonly prescribed drugs. The pharmacokinetics of levofloxacin were not affected to any clinically relevant extent when levofloxacin was administered together with the following drugs: calcium carbonate, digoxin, glibenclamide, ranitidine, warfarin.

4.6 Pregnancy and lactation

Pregnancy

Reproductive studies in animals did not raise specific concern. However in the absence of human data and due to the experimental risk of damage by fluoroquinolones to the weight-bearing cartilage of the growing organism, Tavanic must not be used in pregnant women.

Lactation

In the absence of human data and due to the experimental risk of damage by fluoroquinolones to the weight-bearing cartilage of the growing organism, Tavanic solution for infusion must not be used in breast-feeding women.

4.7 Effects on ability to drive and use machines

Some undesirable effects (e.g. dizziness/vertigo, drowsiness, visual disturbances) may impair the patient's ability to concentrate and react, and therefore may constitute a risk in situations where these abilities are of special importance (e.g. driving a car or operating machinery).

4.8 Undesirable effects

The information given below is based on data from clinical studies in more than 5000 patients and on extensive post marketing experience.

The following frequency rating has been used:

Very common: more than 10%

Common: 1 % to 10 %

Uncommon 0.1 % to 1 %

Rare: 0.01 % to 0.1 %

Very rare: less than 0.01 %

Isolated cases:

Allergic reactions

Uncommon: pruritus, rash.

Rare: urticaria, bronchospasm / dyspnoea.

Very rare: angio-oedema, hypotension, anaphylactic-like shock, photosensitisation.

Isolated cases: severe bullous eruptions such as Stevens-Johnson syndrome, toxic epidermal necrolysis (Lyell's syndrome) and erythema exsudativum multiforme.

Muco-cutaneous, anaphylactic /- oid reactions may sometimes occur even after the first dose.

Gastro-intestinal, metabolism

Common: nausea, diarrhoea.

Uncommon: anorexia, vomiting, abdominal pain, dyspepsia.

Rare: bloody diarrhoea which in very rare cases may be indicative of enterocolitis, including pseudomembranous colitis.

Very rare: hypoglycaemia, particularly in diabetic patients.

Neurological

Uncommon: headache, dizziness/vertigo, drowsiness, insomnia.

Rare: paraesthesia, tremor, anxiety, depression, psychotic reactions, agitation, confusion, convulsion.

Very rare: hypoaesthesia, visual and auditory disturbances, disturbances of taste and smell, hallucinations.

Cardiovascular

Rare: tachycardia, hypotension.

Very rare: shock (anaphylactic-like).

Isolated cases: QT-interval prolongation (see section 4.9)

Musculo-skeletal

Rare: arthralgia, myalgia, tendon disorders incl. tendinitis (e.g. Achilles tendon), (see 4.4: Special Warnings And Special Precautions For Use).

Very rare: tendon rupture (e.g. Achilles tendon); this undesirable effect may occur within 48 hours of starting treatment and may be bilateral. (see 4.4: Special Warnings And Special Precautions For Use). Muscular weakness, which may be of special importance in patients with myasthenia gravis.

Isolated cases: rhabdomyolysis.

Liver, kidney

Common: increase in liver enzymes (e.g. ALT / AST).

Uncommon: increase in bilirubin, increase in serum creatinine.

Very rare: liver reactions such as hepatitis; acute kidney failure (e.g. due to interstitial nephritis).

Blood

Uncommon: eosinophilia, leukopenia.

Rare: neutropenia, thrombocytopenia.

Very rare: agranulocytosis.

Isolated cases: haemolytic anaemia, pancytopenia.

Others

Common: pain, reddening of the infusion site and phlebitis.

Uncommon: asthenia, fungal overgrowth and proliferation of other resistant microorganisms.

Very rare: allergic pneumonitis, fever.

Other undesirable effects which have been associated with fluoroquinolone administration include:

- extrapyramidal symptoms and other disorders of muscular coordination,
- hypersensitivity vasculitis,
- attacks of porphyria in patients with porphyria.

4.9 Overdose

According to toxicity studies in animals or clinical pharmacology studies performed with supra-therapeutic doses, the most important signs to be expected following acute overdosage of Tavanic solution for infusion are central nervous system symptoms such as confusion, dizziness, impairment of consciousness, and convulsive seizures, increases in QT interval.

In the event of overdose, symptomatic treatment should be implemented. ECG monitoring should be undertaken, because of the possibility of QT interval prolongation. Haemodialysis, including peritoneal dialysis and CAPD, are not effective in removing levofloxacin from the body. No specific antidote exists.

5. PHARMACOLOGICAL PROPERTIES

5.1 Pharmacodynamic properties

Levofloxacin is a synthetic antibacterial agent of the fluoroquinolone class (ATC code J01MA) and is the S (-) enantiomer of the racemic drug substance ofloxacin.

Mode of action

As a fluoroquinolone antibacterial agent, levofloxacin acts on the DNA-DNA-gyrase complex and topoisomerase IV.

Breakpoints

The preliminary NCCLS (US National Committee on Clinical Laboratory Standards) recommended MIC breakpoints for levofloxacin, separating susceptible from intermediately susceptible organisms and intermediately susceptible from resistant organisms are:

susceptible $\leqslant$ 2 mg/L, resistant $\geqslant$ 8 mg/L.

Antibacterial spectrum

The prevalence of resistance may vary geographically and with time for selected species and local information on resistance is desirable, particularly when treating severe infections. Therefore, the information presented provides only an approximate guidance on probabilities as to whether microorganisms will be susceptible to levofloxacin or not. Only microorganisms relevant to the given clinical indications are presented here.

(see Table 2 on next page)

Other information

The main mechanism of resistance is due to a *gyr-A* mutation. *In vitro* there is a cross-resistance between levofloxacin and other fluoroquinolones.

Acquired resistance with levofloxacin has recently been documented in 1997:

- *S. pneumoniae* France $\leqslant$ 1%
- *H. influenzae:* rare.

Due to the mechanism of action, there is generally no cross-resistance between levofloxacin and other classes of antibacterial agents.

Nosocomial infections due to *P. aeruginosa* may require combination therapy.

5.2 Pharmacokinetic properties

Absorption

Orally administered levofloxacin is rapidly and almost completely absorbed with peak plasma concentrations being obtained within 1 h. The absolute bioavailability is approximately 100 %. Levofloxacin obeys linear pharmacokinetics over a range of 50 to 600 mg.

Food has little effect on the absorption of levofloxacin.

Distribution

Approximately 30 - 40 % of levofloxacin is bound to serum protein. 500 mg once daily multiple dosing with levofloxacin showed negligible accumulation. There is modest but predictable accumulation of levofloxacin after doses of 500 mg twice daily. Steady-state is achieved within 3 days.

Penetration into tissues and body fluids:

Penetration into Bronchial Mucosa, Epithelial Lining Fluid (ELF)

Maximum levofloxacin concentrations in bronchial mucosa and epithelial lining fluid after 500 mg po were 8.3 μg/g and 10.8 μg/ml respectively. These were reached approximately one hour after administration.

Penetration into Lung Tissue

Maximum levofloxacin concentrations in lung tissue after 500 mg po were approximately 11.3 μg/g and were reached between 4 and 6 hours after administration. The concentrations in the lungs consistently exceeded those in plasma.

Penetration into Blister Fluid

Maximum levofloxacin concentrations of about 4.0 and 6.7 μg/ml in the blister fluid were reached 2 - 4 hours after administration following 3 days dosing at 500 mg once or twice daily respectively.

Penetration into Cerebro-Spinal Fluid

Levofloxacin has poor penetration into cerebro-spinal fluid.

Penetration into prostatic tissue

After administration of oral 500mg levofloxacin once a day for three days, the mean concentrations in prostatic tissue were 8.7 μg/g, 8.2 μg/g and 2.0 μg/g respectively after 2 hours, 6 hours and 24 hours; the mean prostate/plasma concentration ratio was 1.84.

Concentration in urine

The mean urine concentrations 8 -12 hours after a single oral dose of 150 mg, 300 mg or 500 mg levofloxacin were 44 mg/L, 91 mg/L and 200 mg/L, respectively.

Metabolism

Levofloxacin is metabolised to a very small extent, the metabolites being desmethyl-levofloxacin and levofloxacin N-oxide. These metabolites account for $<$ 5 % of the dose excreted in urine. Levofloxacin is stereochemically stable and does not undergo chiral inversion.

Elimination

Following oral and intravenous administration of levofloxacin, it is eliminated relatively slowly from the plasma ($t_{½}$: 6 - 8 h). Excretion is primarily by the renal route $>$ 85 % of the administered dose).

Table 2

In vitro **antibacterial spectrum - Category with European range of resistance where this is known to vary**

Susceptible			
Aerobic Gram-positive micro-organisms:			
Enterococcus faecalis[1]	10-35%	Streptococci, group C and G	
Staphylococcus aureus[1] methi-S		*Streptococcus agalactiae*	
Staphylococcus coagulase negative methi-S(1)	0-30%	*Streptococcus pneumoniae*[1] peni-I/S/R	
Staphylococcus saprophyticus		*Streptococcus pyogenes*[1]	
Aerobic Gram-negative micro-organisms:			
Acinetobacter baumannii[1]	40%	*Klebsiellapneumoniae*[1]	<5-10%
Citrobacter freundii[1]	7%	*Moraxella catarrhalis*[1] β+ / β-	
Eikenella corrodens		*Morganella morganii*[1]	5%
Enterobacter aerogenes	30%	*Pasteurella multocida*	
Enterobacter agglomerans		*Proteus mirabilis*[1]	0-15%
Enterobactercloacae[1]	7%	*Proteusvulgaris*	
Escherichia coli[1]	0-20%[2]	*Providencia rettgeri*	
Haemophilus influenzae[1] ampi-S/R		*Providencia stuartii*	35%
Haemophilus para-influenzae[1]		*Pseudomonas aeruginosa*[1]	10-50%
Klebsiella oxytoca		*Serratia marcescens*[1]	7%
Anaerobic micro-organisms:			
Bacteroides fragilis		Peptostreptococcus	
Clostridium perfringens			
Other micro-organisms:			
Chlamydia pneumoniae[1]		*Legionella pneumophila*[1]	
Chlamydia psittaci		*Mycoplasma pneumoniae*[1]	
Chlamydia trachomatis		*Mycoplasma hominis*	
		Ureaplasma urealyticum	
Intermediately susceptible			
Aerobic Gram-positive micro-organisms:		Aerobic Gram-negative micro-organisms:	
		Burkholderia cepacia	
Anaerobic micro-organisms:			
Bacteroides ovatus		Bacteroides vulgatus	
Bacteroides thetaiotamicron		*Clostridium difficile*	
Resistant			
Aerobic Gram-positive micro-organisms:			
Staphylococcus aureus methi-R		*Staphylococcus coagulase negative methi-R*	

[1] Clinical efficacy has been proven in clinical studies.

[2] (20% in Spain and Portugal)

There are no major differences in the pharmacokinetics of levofloxacin following intravenous and oral administration, suggesting that the oral and intravenous routes are interchangeable.

Subjects with renal insufficiency

The pharmacokinetics of levofloxacin are affected by renal impairment. With decreasing renal function renal elimination and clearance are decreased, and elimination half-lives increased as shown in the table below:

Cl_{cr} [ml/min]	< 20	20 - 40	50 - 80
Cl_R [ml/min]	13	26	57
$t_{1/2}$ [h]	35	27	9

Elderly subjects

There are no significant differences in levofloxacin kinetics between young and elderly subjects, except those associated with differences in creatinine clearance.

Gender differences

Separate analysis for male and female subjects showed small to marginal gender differences in levofloxacin pharmacokinetics. There is no evidence that these gender differences are of clinical relevance.

5.3 Preclinical safety data

Acute toxicity

The median lethal dose (LD_{50}) values obtained in mice and rats after intravenous administration of levofloxacin were in the range 250-400 mg/kg; in dogs the LD_{50} value was approximately 200 mg/kg with one of two animals which received this dose dying.

Repeated dose toxicity

Studies of one month duration with intravenous administration have been carried out in the rat (20, 60, 180 mg/kg/day) and monkey (10, 25, 63 mg/kg/day) and a three-month study has also been carried in the rat (10, 30, 90 mg/kg/day).

The "No Observed Adverse Effect Levels" (NOEL) in the rat studies were concluded to be 20 and 30 mg/kg/day in the one-month and three-month studies respectively. Crystal deposits in urine were seen in both studies at doses of 20 mg/kg/day and above. High doses (180 mg/kg/day for 1 month or 30 mg/kg/day and above for 3 months) slightly decreased food consumption and body weight gain. Haematological examination showed reduced erythrocytes and increased leucocytes and reticulocytes at the end of the 1 month, but not the 3 months study.

The NOEL in the monkey study was concluded to be 63 mg/kg/day with only minor reduction in food and water consumption at this dose.

Reproductive toxicity

Levofloxacin caused no impairment of fertility or reproductive performance in rats at oral doses as high as 360 mg/kg/day or intravenous doses up to 100 mg/kg/day.

Levofloxacin was not teratogenic in rats at oral doses as high as 810 mg/kg/day, or at intravenous doses as high as 160 mg/kg/day. No teratogenicity was observed when rabbits were dosed orally with up to 50 mg/kg/day or intravenously with up to 25 mg/kg/day.

Levofloxacin had no effect on fertility and its only effect on fetuses was delayed maturation as a result of maternal toxicity.

Genotoxicity

Levofloxacin did not induce gene mutations in bacterial or mammalian cells but did induce chromosome aberrations in Chinese hamster lung (CHL) cells *in vitro* at or above 100 μg/ml, in the absence of metabolic activation. *In vivo* tests (micronucleus, sister chromatid exchange, unscheduled DNA synthesis, dominant lethal tests) did not show any genotoxic potential.

Phototoxic potential

Studies in the mouse after both intravenous and oral dosing showed levofloxacin to have phototoxic activity only at very high doses. Levofloxacin did not show any genotoxic potential in a photomutagenicity assay, and it reduced tumour development in a photocarcinogenicity assay.

Carcinogenic potential

No indication of carcinogenic potential was seen in a two-year study in the rat with dietary administration (0, 10, 30 and 100 mg/kg/day).

Toxicity to joints

In common with other fluoroquinolones, levofloxacin showed effects on cartilage (blistering and cavities) in rats and dogs. These findings were more marked in young animals.

6. PHARMACEUTICAL PARTICULARS

6.1 List of excipients

Tavanic 5 mg/ml solution for infusion contains the following excipients:

Sodium chloride, sodium hydroxide, hydrochloric acid *(qs: pH 4.8)* and water for injection. (Na $^{+}$ concentration: 154 mmol / L).

6.2 Incompatibilities

Tavanic 5 mg/ml solution for infusion should not be mixed with heparin or alkaline solutions (e.g. sodium hydrogen carbonate).

6.3 Shelf life

Shelf life as packaged for sale: 3 years

Shelf life after removal of the outer packaging: 3 days (under indoor light conditions).

Shelf life after perforation of the rubber stopper: (see 6.6).

6.4 Special precautions for storage

Keep container in the outer carton in order to protect from light

6.5 Nature and contents of container

100ml, type 1 glass vial with flanged aluminium cap, chlorobutyl rubber stopper and tear-off polypropylene lid. Each vial contains 100 ml solution. Pack of 1 vial is available.

6.6 Instructions for use and handling

Tavanic solution for infusion should be used immediately (within 3 hours) after perforation of the rubber stopper in order to prevent any bacterial contamination. No protection from light is necessary during infusion.

Mixture with other solutions for infusion:

Tavanic solution for infusion is compatible with the following solutions for infusion:

0.9 % sodium chloride solution USP.

5 % dextrose injection USP.

2.5 % dextrose in Ringer solution.

Combination solutions for parenteral nutrition (amino acids, carbohydrates, electrolytes).

See 6.2 for incompatibilities.

Inspect the vial before use. It must only be used if the solution is clear, greenish-yellow solution, practically free from particles.

7. MARKETING AUTHORISATION HOLDER

Hoechst Marion Roussel Limited

Broadwater Park

Denham

Uxbridge

Middlesex

UB9 5HP

United Kingdom

8. MARKETING AUTHORISATION NUMBER(S)

PL 13402/0013

9. DATE OF FIRST AUTHORISATION/RENEWAL OF THE AUTHORISATION

6 June 1997 / 6 June 2002

10. DATE OF REVISION OF THE TEXT

October 2004

Taxol 6mg/ml, Concentrate for Solution for Infusion

(Bristol-Myers Squibb Pharmaceuticals Ltd)

1. NAME OF THE MEDICINAL PRODUCT

Taxol® 6 mg/ml, concentrate for solution for infusion.

2. QUALITATIVE AND QUANTITATIVE COMPOSITION

Paclitaxel: 6 mg per 1 ml of concentrate for solution for infusion.

A vial of 5 ml contains 30 mg of paclitaxel.

A vial of 16.7 ml contains 100 mg of paclitaxel.

A vial of 25 ml contains 150 mg of paclitaxel.

A vial of 50 ml contains 300 mg of paclitaxel.

For excipients, see 6.1.

3. PHARMACEUTICAL FORM

Concentrate for solution for infusion.

Taxol® is a clear, colourless to slightly yellow viscous solution.

4. CLINICAL PARTICULARS

4.1 Therapeutic indications

Ovarian carcinoma: in the first-line chemotherapy of ovarian cancer, Taxol is indicated for the treatment of patients with advanced carcinoma of the ovary or with residual disease (> 1 cm) after initial laparotomy, in combination with cisplatin.

In the second-line chemotherapy of ovarian cancer, Taxol is indicated for the treatment of metastatic carcinoma of the ovary after failure of standard, platinum containing therapy.

Breast carcinoma: In the adjuvant setting, Taxol is indicated for the treatment of patients with node-positive breast carcinoma following anthracycline and cyclophosphamide (AC) therapy. Adjuvant treatment with Taxol should be regarded as an alternative to extended AC therapy.

Taxol is indicated for the initial treatment of locally advanced or metastatic breast cancer either in combination with an anthracycline in patients for whom anthracycline therapy is suitable, or in combination with trastuzumab, in patients who over-express HER-2 at a 3+ level as determined by immunohistochemistry and for whom an anthracycline is not suitable (see 4.4 and 5.1).

As a single agent, Taxol is indicated for the treatment of metastatic carcinoma of the breast in patients who have failed, or are not candidates for standard, anthracycline containing therapy.

Advanced non-small cell lung carcinoma: Taxol, in combination with cisplatin, is indicated for the treatment of non-small cell lung carcinoma (NSCLC) in patients who are not candidates for potentially curative surgery and/or radiation therapy.

AIDS-related Kaposi's sarcoma: Taxol is indicated for the treatment of patients with advanced AIDS-related Kaposi's sarcoma (KS) who have failed prior liposomal anthracycline therapy.

Limited efficacy data supports this indication, a summary of the relevant studies is shown in section 5.1.

4.2 Posology and method of administration

All patients must be premedicated with corticosteroids, antihistamines, and H_2 antagonists prior to Taxol, e.g.

Drug	Dose	Administration prior to Taxol
dexamethasone	20 mg oral* or IV	For oral administration: approximately 12 and 6 hours or for IV administration: 30 to 60 min
diphenhydramine**	50 mg IV	30 to 60 min
cimetidine or ranitidine	300 mg IV 50 mg IV	30 to 60 min

* 8-20 mg for KS patients

** or an equivalent antihistamine e.g. chlorpheniramine

Taxol should be administered through an in-line filter with a microporous membrane $\leqslant 0.22\ \mu m$ (see 6.6).

First-line chemotherapy of ovarian carcinoma: although other dosage regimens are under investigation, a combination regimen of Taxol and cisplatin is recommended. According to duration of infusion, two doses of Taxol are recommended: Taxol 175 mg/m^2 administered intravenously over 3 hours, followed by cisplatin at a dose of 75 mg/m^2 every three weeks or Taxol 135 mg/m^2, in a 24-hour infusion, followed by cisplatin 75 mg/m^2, with a 3 week interval between courses (see 5.1).

Second-line chemotherapy of ovarian carcinoma: the recommended dose of Taxol is 175 mg/m^2 administered over a period of 3 hours, with a 3 week interval between courses.

Adjuvant chemotherapy in breast carcinoma: the recommended dose of Taxol is 175 mg/m^2 administered over a period of 3 hours every 3 weeks for four courses, following AC therapy.

First-line chemotherapy of breast carcinoma: when used in combination with doxorubicin (50 mg/m^2), Taxol should be administered 24 hours after doxorubicin. The recommended dose of Taxol is 220 mg/m^2 administered intravenously over a period of 3 hours, with a 3-week interval between courses (see 4.5 and 5.1).

When used in combination with trastuzumab, the recommended dose of Taxol is 175 mg/m^2 administered intravenously over a period of 3 hours, with a 3-week interval between courses (see 5.1). Taxol infusion may be started the day following the first dose of trastuzumab or immediately after the subsequent doses of trastuzumab if the preceding dose of trastuzumab was well tolerated (for detailed trastuzumab posology see the Summary of Product Characteristics of Herceptin®).

Second-line chemotherapy of breast carcinoma: the recommended dose of Taxol is 175 mg/m^2 administered over a period of 3 hours, with a 3-week interval between courses.

Treatment of advanced NSCLC: the recommended dose of Taxol is 175 mg/m^2 administered over a period of 3 hours, followed by cisplatin 80 mg/m^2, with a 3 week interval between courses.

Treatment of AIDS-related KS: the recommended dose of Taxol is 100 mg/m^2 administered as a 3-hour intravenous infusion every two weeks.

Subsequent doses of Taxol should be administered according to individual patient tolerance.

Taxol should not be readministered until the neutrophil count is $\geqslant$ 1,500/mm^3 ($\geqslant$ 1,000/mm^3 for KS patients) and the platelet count is $\geqslant$ 100,000/mm^3 ($\geqslant$ 75,000/mm^3 for KS patients). Patients who experience severe neutropenia (neutrophil count $<$ 500/mm^3 for $\geqslant$ 7 days) or severe peripheral neuropathy should receive a dose reduction of 20% for subsequent courses (25% for KS patients) (see 4.4).

Patients with hepatic impairment: Inadequate data are available to recommend dosage alterations in patients with mild to moderate hepatic impairments (see 4.4 and 5.2). Patients with severe hepatic impairment should not be treated with paclitaxel.

4.3 Contraindications

Taxol is contraindicated in patients with severe hypersensitivity to paclitaxel or to any excipient, especially polyoxyethylated castor oil (see 4.4).

Taxol is contraindicated during pregnancy and lactation (see 4.6), and should not be used in patients with baseline neutrophils $<$ 1,500/mm^3 ($<$ 1,000/mm^3 for KS patients).

In KS, Taxol is also contraindicated in patients with concurrent, serious, uncontrolled infections.

4.4 Special warnings and special precautions for use

Taxol should be administered under the supervision of a physician experienced in the use of cancer chemotherapeutic agents. Since significant hypersensitivity reactions may occur, appropriate supportive equipment should be available.

Patients must be pretreated with corticosteroids, antihistamines and H_2 antagonists (see 4.2).

Taxol should be given before cisplatin when used in combination (see 4.5).

Significant hypersensitivity reactions characterised by dyspnoea and hypotension requiring treatment, angioedema and generalised urticaria have occurred in $<$ 1% of patients receiving Taxol after adequate premedication. These reactions are probably histamine-mediated. In the case of severe hypersensitivity reactions, Taxol infusion should be discontinued immediately, symptomatic therapy should be initiated and the patient should not be rechallenged with the drug.

Bone marrow suppression (primarily neutropenia) is the dose-limiting toxicity. Frequent monitoring of blood counts should be instituted. Patients should not be retreated until neutrophils recover to $\geqslant$ 1,500/mm^3 ($\geqslant$ 1,000/mm^3 for KS patients) and platelets recover to $\geqslant$ 100,000/mm^3 ($\geqslant$ 75,000/mm^3 for KS patients). In the KS clinical study, the majority of patients were receiving granulocyte colony stimulating factor (G-CSF).

Severe cardiac conduction abnormalities have been reported rarely with single agent Taxol. If patients develop significant conduction abnormalities during Taxol administration, appropriate therapy should be administered and continuous cardiac monitoring should be performed during subsequent therapy with Taxol. Hypotension, hypertension, and bradycardia have been observed during Taxol administration; patients are usually asymptomatic and generally do not require treatment. Frequent vital sign monitoring, particularly during the first hour of Taxol infusion, is recommended. Severe cardiovascular events were observed more frequently in patients with NSCLC than breast or ovarian carcinoma. A single case of heart failure related to paclitaxel was seen in the AIDS-KS clinical study.

When Taxol is used in combination with doxorubicin or trastuzumab for initial treatment of metastatic breast cancer, attention should be placed on the monitoring of cardiac function. When patients are candidates for treatment with Taxol in these combinations, they should undergo baseline cardiac assessment including history, physical examination, ECG, echocardiogram, and/or MUGA scan. Cardiac function should be further monitored during treatment (e.g. every three months). Monitoring may help to identify patients who develop cardiac dysfunction and treating physicians should carefully assess the cumulative dose (mg/m^2) of anthracycline administered when making decisions regarding frequency of ventricular function assessment. When testing indicates deterioration in cardiac function, even asymptomatic, treating physicians should carefully assess the clinical benefits of further therapy against the potential for producing cardiac damage, including potentially irreversible damage. If further treatment is administered, monitoring of cardiac function should be more frequent (e.g. every 1-2 cycles). For more details see Summary of Product Characteristics of Herceptin® or doxorubicin.

Although the occurrence of ***peripheral neuropathy***is frequent, the development of severe symptoms is rare. In severe cases, a dose reduction of 20% (25% for KS patients) for all subsequent courses of Taxol is recommended. In NSCLC patients and in ovarian cancer patients treated in the first-line setting, the administration of Taxol as a three hour infusion in combination with cisplatin, resulted in a greater incidence of severe neurotoxicity than both single agent Taxol and cyclophosphamide followed by cisplatin.

Patients with hepatic impairment may be at increased risk of toxicity, particularly grade III-IV myelosuppression. There is no evidence that the toxicity of Taxol is increased when given as a 3-hour infusion to patients with mildly abnormal liver function. When Taxol is given as a longer infusion, increased myelosuppression may be seen in patients with moderate to severe hepatic impairment. Patients should be monitored closely for the development of profound myelosuppression (see 4.2). Inadequate data are available to recommend dosage alterations in patients with mild to moderate hepatic impairments (see 5.2).

No data are available for patients with severe baseline cholestasis. Patients with severe hepatic impairment should not be treated with paclitaxel.

Since Taxol contains ethanol (396 mg/ml), consideration should be given to possible CNS and other effects.

Special care should be taken to avoid intra-arterial application of Taxol, since in animal studies testing for local tolerance severe tissue reactions were observed after intra-arterial application.

Pseudomembranous colitis has been rarely reported including cases in patients who have not been concomitantly treated with antibiotics. This reaction should be considered in the differential diagnosis of cases of severe or persistent diarrhoea occurring during or shortly after treatment with paclitaxel.

Taxol in combination with radiation of the lung, irrespective of their chronological order, may contribute to the development of ***interstitial pneumonitis***.

In KS patients, ***severe mucositis*** is rare. If severe reactions occur, the paclitaxel dose should be reduced by 25%.

4.5 Interaction with other medicinal products and other forms of Interaction

Paclitaxel clearance is not affected by cimetidine premedication.

The recommended regimen of Taxol administration for the first-line chemotherapy of ovarian carcinoma is for Taxol to be given <u>before</u> cisplatin. When Taxol is given <u>before</u> cisplatin, the safety profile of Taxol is consistent with that reported for single-agent use. When Taxol was given <u>after</u> cisplatin, patients showed a more profound myelosuppression and an approximately 20% decrease in paclitaxel clearance. Patients treated with Taxol and cisplatin may have an increased risk of renal failure as compared to cisplatin alone in gynecological cancers.

Since the elimination of doxorubicin and its active metabolites can be reduced when paclitaxel and doxorubicin are given closer in time, Taxol for initial treatment of metastatic breast cancer should be administered 24 hours after doxorubicin (see 5.2).

The metabolism of paclitaxel is catalysed, in part, by cytochrome P450 isoenzymes CYP2C8 and 3A4 (see 5.2). Clinical studies have demonstrated that CYP2C8-mediated metabolism of paclitaxel, to 6α-hydroxypaclitaxel, is the major metabolic pathway in humans. Concurrent administration of ketoconazole, a known potent inhibitor of CYP3A4, does not inhibit the elimination of paclitaxel in patients; thus, both medicinal products may be administered together without dosage adjustment. Further data on the potential of drug interactions between paclitaxel and other CYP3A4 substrates/inhibitors are limited. Therefore, caution should be exercised when administering paclitaxel concomitantly with medicines known to inhibit (e.g. erythromycin, fluoxetine, gemfibrozil) or induce (e.g. rifampicin, carbamazepine, phenytoin, phenobarbital, efavirenz, nevirapine) either CYP2C8 or 3A4.

Studies in KS patients, who were taking multiple concomitant medications, suggest that the systemic clearance of paclitaxel was significantly lower in the presence of nelfinavir and ritonavir, but not with indinavir. Insufficient information is available on interactions with other protease inhibitors. Consequently, paclitaxel should be administered with caution in patients receiving protease inhibitors as concomitant therapy.

4.6 Pregnancy and lactation

Taxol has been shown to be embryotoxic and foetotoxic in rabbits, and to decrease fertility in rats.

There is no information on the use of Taxol in pregnant women. As with other cytotoxic drugs, Taxol may cause foetal harm, and is therefore contraindicated during pregnancy. Women should be advised to avoid becoming pregnant during therapy with Taxol, and to inform the treating physician immediately should this occur.

It is not known whether paclitaxel is excreted in human milk. Taxol is contraindicated during lactation. Breastfeeding should be discontinued for the duration of therapy.

4.7 Effects on ability to drive and use machines

Taxol has not been demonstrated to interfere with this ability. However, it should be noted that Taxol does contain alcohol (see 4.4 and 6.1).

4.8 Undesirable effects

Unless otherwise noted, the following discussion refers to the overall safety database of 812 patients with solid tumours treated with single-agent Taxol in clinical studies. As the KS population is very specific, a special chapter based on a clinical study with 107 patients, is presented at the end of this section.

The frequency and severity of undesirable effects, unless otherwise mentioned, are generally similar between patients receiving Taxol for the treatment of ovarian carcinoma, breast carcinoma, or NSCLC. None of the observed toxicities were clearly influenced by age.

The most frequent significant undesirable effect was **bone marrow suppression**. Severe neutropenia ($<$ 500 cells/mm^3) occurred in 28% of patients, but was not associated with febrile episodes. Only 1% of patients experienced severe neutropenia for $\geqslant$ 7 days. Thrombocytopenia was reported in 11% of patients. Three percent of patients had a platelet count nadir $<$ 50,000/mm^3 at least once while on study. Anaemia was observed in 64% of patients, but was severe (Hb $<$ 5 mmol/l) in only 6% of patients. Incidence and severity of anaemia is related to baseline haemoglobin status.

Neurotoxicity, mainly **peripheral neuropathy**, appeared to be more frequent and severe with a 175 mg/m^2 3-hour infusion (85% neurotoxicity, 15% severe) than with a 135 mg/m^2 24-hour infusion (25% peripheral neuropathy, 3% severe) when Taxol was combined with cisplatin. In

NSCLC patients and in ovarian cancer patients treated with Taxol over 3 hours followed by cisplatin, there is an apparent increase in the incidence of severe neurotoxicity. Peripheral neuropathy can occur following the first course and can worsen with increasing exposure to Taxol. Peripheral neuropathy was the cause of Taxol discontinuation in a few cases. Sensory symptoms have usually improved or resolved within several months of Taxol discontinuation. Pre-existing neuropathies resulting from prior therapies are not a contraindication for Taxol therapy.

Arthralgia or myalgia affected 60% of patients and was severe in 13% of patients.

A significant hypersensitivity reaction with possible fatal outcome (defined as hypotension requiring therapy, angioedema, respiratory distress requiring bronchodilator therapy, or generalised urticaria) occurred in two (< 1%) of patients. Thirty-four percent of patients (17% of all courses) experienced minor hypersensitivity reactions. These minor reactions, mainly flushing and rash, did not require therapeutic intervention nor did they prevent continuation of Taxol therapy.

Injection site reactions during intravenous administration may lead to localised oedema, pain, erythema, and induration; on occasion, extravasation can result in cellulitis. Skin sloughing and/or peeling has been reported, sometimes related to extravasation. Skin discoloration may also occur. Recurrence of skin reactions at a site of previous extravasation following administration of Taxol at a different site, i.e. "recall", has been reported rarely. A specific treatment for extravasation reactions is unknown at this time.

The table below lists undesirable effects regardless of severity associated with the administration of single agent Taxol administered as a three hour infusion in the metastatic setting (812 patients treated in clinical studies) and as reported in the postmarketing surveillance* of Taxol.

The frequency of undesirable effects listed below is defined using the following convention:

very common (≥ 1/10); common (≥ 1/100, < 1/10); uncommon (≥ 1/1,000, < 1/100); rare (≥ 1/10,000, < 1/1,000); very rare (< 1/10,000).

Infections and infestations:	*Very common*: infection (mainly urinary tract and upper respiratory tract infections), with reported cases of fatal outcome *Uncommon*: septic shock *Rare**: pneumonia, peritonitis, sepsis
Blood and the lymphatic system disorders:	*Very common*: myelosuppression, neutropenia, anaemia, thrombocytopenia, leucopenia, bleeding *Rare**: febrile neutropenia *Very rare**: acute myeloid leukaemia, myelodysplastic syndrome
Immune system disorders:	*Very common*: minor hypersensitivity reactions (mainly flushing and rash) *Uncommon*: significant hypersensitivity reactions requiring therapy (e.g., hypotension, angioneurotic oedema, respiratory distress, generalised urticaria, chills, back pain, chest pain, tachycardia, abdominal pain, pain in extremities, diaphoresis and hypertension) *Rare**: anaphylactic reactions *Very rare**: anaphylactic shock
Metabolism and nutrition disorders:	*Very rare**: anorexia
Psychiatric disorders:	*Very rare**: confusional stage
Nervous system disorders:	*Very common*: neurotoxicity (mainly: peripheral neuropathy) *Rare**: motor neuropathy (with resultant minor distal weakness) *Very rare**: autonomic neuropathy (resulting in paralytic ileus and orthostatic hypotension), grand mal seizures, convulsions, encephalopathy, dizziness, headache, ataxia
Eye disorders:	*Very rare**: optic nerve and/or visual disturbances (scintillating scotomata), particularly in patients who have received higher doses than recommended
Ear and labyrinth disorders:	*Very rare**: ototoxicity, hearing loss, tinnitus, vertigo
Cardiac disorders:	*Common:* bradycardia *Uncommon:* cardiomyopathy, asymptomatic ventricular tachycardia, tachycardia with bigeminy, AV block and syncope, myocardial infarction *Very rare**: atrial fibrillation, supraventricular tachycardia
Vascular disorders:	*Very common*: hypotension *Uncommon*: hypertension, thrombosis, thrombophlebitis *Very rare**: shock
Respiratory, thoracic and mediastinal disorders:	*Rare**: dyspnoea, pleural effusion, interstitial pneumonia, lung fibrosis, pulmonary embolism, respiratory failure *Very rare**: cough
Gastrointestinal disorders:	*Very common*: nausea, vomiting, diarrhoea, mucosal inflammation *Rare**: bowel obstruction, bowel perforation, ischaemic colitis, pancreatitis *Very rare**: mesenteric thrombosis, pseudomembranous colitis, oesophagitis, constipation, ascites, neutropenic colitis
Hepato-biliary disorders:	*Very rare**: hepatic necrosis, hepatic encephalopathy (both with reported cases of fatal outcome)
Skin and subcutaneous tissue disorders:	*Very common*: alopecia *Common*: transient and mild nail and skin changes *Rare**: pruritus, rash, erythema *Very rare**: Stevens-Johnson syndrome, epidermal necrolysis, erythema multiforme, exfoliative dermatitis, urticaria, onycholysis (patients on therapy should wear sun protection on hands and feet)
Musculoskeletal, connective tissue and bone disorders:	*Very common*: arthralgia, myalgia
General disorders and administration site conditions:	*Common*: injection site reactions (including localised oedema, pain, erythema, induration, on occasion extravasation can result in cellulitis, skin fibrosis and skin necrosis) *Rare**: asthenia, pyrexia, dehydration, oedema, malaise
Investigations:	*Common*: severe elevation in AST (SGOT), severe elevation in alkaline phosphatase *Uncommon*: severe elevation in bilirubin *Rare**: increase in blood creatinine

Breast cancer patients who received Taxol in the adjuvant setting following AC experienced more neurosensory toxicity, hypersensitivity reactions, arthralgia/myalgia, anaemia, infection, fever, nausea/vomiting and diarrhoea than patients who received AC alone. However, the frequency of these events was consistent with the use of single agent Taxol, as reported above.

Combination treatment

The following discussion refers to two major trials for the first-line chemotherapy of ovarian carcinoma (Taxol + cisplatin: over 1050 patients); two phase III trials in the first line treatment of metastatic breast cancer: one investigating the combination with doxorubicin (Taxol + doxorubicin: 267 patients), another one investigating the combination with trastuzumab (planned subgroup analysis Taxol + trastuzumab: 188 patients) and two phase III trials for the treatment of advanced NSCLC (Taxol + cisplatin: over 360 patients) (see 5.1).

When administered as a three hour infusion for the first-line chemotherapy of ovarian cancer, neurotoxicity, arthralgia/myalgia, and hypersensitivity were reported as more frequent and severe by patients treated with Taxol followed by cisplatin than patients treated with cyclophosphamide followed by cisplatin. Myelosuppression appeared to be less frequent and severe with Taxol as a three hour infusion followed by cisplatin compared with cyclophosphamide followed by cisplatin.

For the first line chemotherapy of metastatic breast cancer, neutropenia, anaemia, peripheral neuropathy, arthralgia/myalgia, asthenia, fever, and diarrhoea were reported more frequently and with greater severity when Taxol (220 mg/m^2) was administered as a 3-hour infusion 24 hours following doxorubicin (50 mg/m^2) when compared to standard FAC therapy (5-FU 500 mg/m^2, doxorubicin 50 mg/m^2, cyclophosphamide 500 mg/m^2). Nausea and vomiting appeared to be less frequent and severe with the Taxol (220 mg/m^2) / doxorubicin (50 mg/m^2) regimen as compared to the standard FAC regimen. The use of corticosteroids may have contributed to the lower frequency and severity of nausea and vomiting in the Taxol/doxorubicin arm.

When Taxol was administered as a 3-hour infusion in combination with trastuzumab for the first line treatment of patients with metastatic breast cancer, the following events (regardless of relationship to Taxol or trastuzumab) were reported more frequently than with single agent Taxol: heart failure (8% vs 1%), infection (46% vs 27%), chills (42% vs 4%), fever (47% vs 23%), cough (42% vs 22%), rash (39% vs 18%), arthralgia (37% vs 21%), tachycardia (12% vs 4%), diarrhoea (45% vs 30%), hypertonia (11% vs 3%), epistaxis (18% vs 4%), acne (11% vs 3%), herpes simplex (12% vs 3%), accidental injury (13% vs 3%), insomnia (25% vs 13%), rhinitis (22% vs 5%), sinusitis (21% vs 7%), and injection site reaction (7% vs 1%). Some of these frequency differences may be due to the increased number and duration of treatments with Taxol/trastuzumab combination vs single agent Taxol. Severe events were reported at similar rates for Taxol/trastuzumab and single agent Taxol.

When doxorubicin was administered in combination with Taxol in metastatic breast cancer, **cardiac contraction abnormalities** (≥ 20% reduction of left ventricular ejection fraction) were observed in 15% of patients vs. 10% with standard FAC regimen. **Congestive heart failure** was observed in < 1% in both Taxol/doxorubicin and standard FAC arms. Administration of trastuzumab in combination with Taxol in patients previously treated with anthracyclines resulted in an increased frequency and severity of **cardiac dysfunction** in comparison with patients treated with Taxol single agent (NYHA Class I/II 10% vs. 0%; NYHA Class III/IV 2% vs. 1%) and rarely has been associated with death (see trastuzumab Summary of Product Characteristics). In all but these rare cases, patients responded to appropriate medical treatment.

Radiation pneumonitis has been reported in patients receiving concurrent radiotherapy.

AIDS-related Kaposi's sarcoma

Except for haematologic and hepatic undesirable effects (see below), the frequency and severity of undesirable effects are generally similar between KS patients and patients treated with paclitaxel monotherapy for other solid tumours, based on a clinical study including 107 patients.

Blood and the lymphatic system disorders: bone marrow suppression was the major dose-limiting toxicity. Neutropenia is the most important haematological toxicity. During the first course of treatment, severe neutropenia (< 500 cells/mm^3) occurred in 20% of patients. During the entire treatment period, severe neutropenia was observed in 39% of patients. Neutropenia was present for > 7 days in 41% and for 30-35 days in 8% of patients. It resolved within 35 days in all patients who were followed. The incidence of Grade 4 neutropenia lasting ≥ 7 days was 22%.

Neutropenic fever related to paclitaxel was reported in 14% of patients and in 1.3% of treatment cycles. There were 3 septic episodes (2.8%) during paclitaxel administration related to the medicinal product that proved fatal.

Thrombocytopenia was observed in 50% of patients, and was severe (< 50,000 cells/mm^3) in 9%. Only 14% experienced a drop in their platelet count < 75,000 cells/mm^3, at least once while on treatment. Bleeding episodes related to paclitaxel were reported in < 3% of patients, but the haemorrhagic episodes were localised.

Anaemia (Hb < 11 g/dL) was observed in 61% of patients and was severe (Hb < 8 g/dL) in 10%. Red cell transfusions were required in 21% of patients.

Hepato-biliary disorders: Among patients (> 50% on protease inhibitors) with normal baseline liver function, 28%, 43% and 44% had elevations in bilirubin, alkaline phosphatase and AST (SGOT), respectively. For each of these parameters, the increases were severe in 1% of cases.

4.9 Overdose

There is no known antidote for Taxol overdosage. The primary anticipated complications of overdosage would consist of bone marrow suppression, peripheral neurotoxicity and mucositis.

5. PHARMACOLOGICAL PROPERTIES

5.1 Pharmacodynamic properties

Pharmacotherapeutic group / ATC code: cytostatic agent, L01C D01.

Paclitaxel is a novel antimicrotubule agent that promotes the assembly of microtubules from tubulin dimers and stabilises microtubules by preventing depolymerization. This stability results in the inhibition of the normal dynamic reorganisation of the microtubule network that is essential for vital interphase and mitotic cellular functions. In addition, paclitaxel induces abnormal arrays or bundles of microtubules throughout the cell cycle and multiple asters of microtubules during mitosis.

In the first-line chemotherapy of ovarian carcinoma, the safety and efficacy of Taxol were evaluated in two major, randomised, controlled (vs. cyclophosphamide 750 mg/m^2 / cisplatin 75 mg/m^2) trials. In the Intergroup trial (BMS CA139-209), over 650 patients with stage II$_{b-c}$, III or IV primary ovarian cancer received a maximum of 9 treatment courses of Taxol (175 mg/m^2 over 3 hr) followed by cisplatin (75 mg/m^2) or control. The second major trial (GOG-111/ BMS CA139-022) evaluated a maximum of 6 courses of either Taxol (135 mg/m^2 over 24 hrs) followed by cisplatin (75 mg/m^2) or control in over 400 patients with stage III/IV primary ovarian cancer, with a $>$ 1 cm residual disease after staging laparotomy, or with distant metastases. While the two different Taxol posologies were not compared with each other directly, in both trials patients treated with Taxol in combination with cisplatin had a significantly higher response rate, longer time to progression, and longer survival time when compared with standard therapy. Increased neurotoxicity, arthralgia/myalgia but reduced myelosuppression were observed in advanced ovarian cancer patients administered 3-hour infusion Taxol/cisplatin as compared to patients who received cyclophosphamide/cisplatin.

In the adjuvant treatment of breast carcinoma, 3121 patients with node positive breast carcinoma were treated with adjuvant Taxol therapy or no chemotherapy following four courses of doxorubicin and cyclophosphamide (CALGB 9344, BMS CA 139-223). Median follow-up was 69 months. Overall, Taxol patients had a significant reduction of 18% in the risk of disease recurrence relative to patients receiving AC alone (p = 0.0014), and a significant reduction of 19% in the risk of death (p = 0.0044) relative to patients receiving AC alone. Retrospective analyses show benefit in all patient subsets. In patients with hormone receptor negative/ unknown tumours, reduction in risk of disease recurrence was 28% (95%CI: 0.59-0.86). In the patient subgroup with hormone receptor positive tumours, the risk reduction of disease recurrence was 9% (95%CI: 0.78-1.07). However, the design of the study did not investigate the effect of extended AC therapy beyond 4 cycles. It cannot be excluded on the basis of this study alone that the observed effects could be partly due to the difference in duration of chemotherapy between the two arms (AC 4 cycles; AC + Taxol 8 cycles). Therefore, adjuvant treatment with Taxol should be regarded as an alternative to extended AC therapy.

In a second large clinical study in adjuvant node positive breast cancer with a similar design, 3060 patients were randomized to receive or not four courses of Taxol at a higher dose of 225 mg/m^2 following four courses of AC (NSABP B-28, BMS CA139-270). At a median follow-up of 64 months, Taxol patients had a significant reduction of 17% in the risk of disease recurrence relative to patients who received AC alone (p = 0.006); Taxol treatment was associated with a reduction in the risk of death of 7% (95%CI: 0.78-1.12). All subset analyses favored the Taxol arm. In this study patients with hormone receptor positive tumour had a reduction in the risk of disease recurrence of 23% (95%CI: 0.6-0.92); in the patient subgroup with hormone receptor negative tumour the risk reduction of disease recurrence was 10% (95%CI: 0.7-1.11).

In the first-line treatment of metastatic breast cancer, the efficacy and safety of Taxol were evaluated in two pivotal, phase III, randomised, controlled open-label trials.

In the first study (BMS CA139-278), the combination of bolus doxorubicin (50 mg/m^2) followed after 24 hours by Taxol (220 mg/m^2 by 3-hour infusion) (AT), was compared versus standard FAC regimen (5-FU 500 mg/m^2, doxorubicin 50 mg/m^2, cyclophosphamide 500 mg/m^2), both administered every three weeks for eight courses. In this randomised study, 267 patients with metastatic breast cancer, who had either received no prior chemotherapy or only non-anthracycline chemotherapy in the adjuvant setting, were enrolled. Results showed a significant difference in time to progression for patients receiving AT compared to those receiving FAC (8.2 vs. 6.2 months; p= 0.029). The median survival was in favour of Taxol/doxorubicin vs. FAC (23.0 vs. 18.3 months; p= 0.004). In the AT and FAC treatment arm 44% and 48% respectively received follow-up chemotherapy which included taxanes in 7% and 50% respectively. The overall response rate was also significantly higher in the AT arm compared to the FAC arm (68% vs. 55%). Complete responses were seen in 19% of the Taxol/doxorubicin arm patients vs. 8% of the FAC arm patients. All efficacy results have been subsequently confirmed by a blinded independent review.

In the second pivotal study, the efficacy and safety of the Taxol and Herceptin® combination was evaluated in a planned subgroup analysis (metastatic breast cancer patients who formerly received adjuvant anthracyclines) of the study HO648g. The efficacy of Herceptin® in combination with paclitaxel in patients who did not receive prior adjuvant anthracyclines has not been proven. The combination of trastuzumab (4 mg/kg loading dose then 2 mg/kg weekly) and Taxol (175 mg/m^2) 3-hour infusion, every three weeks was compared to single-agent Taxol (175 mg/m^2) 3-hour infusion, every three weeks in 188 patients with metastatic breast cancer overexpressing HER2 (2+ or 3+ as measured by immunohistochemistry), who had previously been treated with anthracyclines. Taxol was administered every three weeks for at least six courses while trastuzumab was given weekly until disease progression. The study showed a significant benefit for the Taxol/trastuzumab combination in terms of time to progression (6.9 vs. 3.0 months), response rate (41% vs. 17%), and duration of response (10.5 vs. 4.5 months) when compared to Taxol alone. The most significant toxicity observed with the Taxol/trastuzumab combination was cardiac dysfunction (see 4.8).

In the treatment of advanced NSCLC, Taxol 175 mg/m^2 followed by cisplatin 80 mg/m^2 has been evaluated in two phase III trials (367 patients on Taxol containing regimens). Both were randomised trials, one compared to treatment with cisplatin 100 mg/m^2, the other used teniposide 100 mg/m^2 followed by cisplatin 80 mg/m^2 as comparator (367 patients on comparator). Results in each trial were similar. For the primary outcome of mortality, there was no significant difference between the Taxol containing regimen and the comparator (median survival times 8.1 and 9.5 months on Taxol containing regimens, 8.6 and 9.9 months on comparators). Similarly, for progression-free survival there was no significant difference between treatments. There was a significant benefit in terms of clinical response rate. Quality of life results are suggestive of a benefit on Taxol containing regimens in terms of appetite loss and provide clear evidence of the inferiority of Taxol containing regimens in terms of peripheral neuropathy ($p < 0.008$).

In the treatment of AIDS-related KS, the efficacy and safety of paclitaxel were investigated in a non-comparative study in patients with advanced KS, previously treated with systemic chemotherapy. The primary end-point was best tumour response. Of the 107 patients, 63 were considered resistant to liposomal anthracyclines. This subgroup is considered to constitute the core efficacy population. The overall success rate (complete/partial response) after 15 cycles of treatment was 57% (CI 44 - 70%) in liposomal anthracycline-resistant patients. Over 50% of the responses were apparent after the first 3 cycles. In liposomal anthracycline-resistant patients, the response rates were comparable for patients who had never received a protease inhibitor (55.6%) and those who received one at least 2 months prior to treatment with paclitaxel (60.9%). The median time to progression in the core population was 468 days (95% CI 257-NE). Median survival could not be computed, but the lower 95% bound was 617 days in core patients.

5.2 Pharmacokinetic properties

Following intravenous administration, paclitaxel exhibits a biphasic decline in plasma concentrations.

The pharmacokinetics of paclitaxel were determined following 3 and 24 hour infusions at doses of 135 and 175 mg/m^2. Mean terminal half-life estimates ranged from 3.0 to 52.7 hours, and mean, non-compartmentally derived, values for total body clearance ranged from 11.6 to 24.0 l/hr/m^2; total body clearance appeared to decrease with higher plasma concentrations of paclitaxel. Mean steady-state volume of distribution ranged from 198 to 688 l/m^2, indicating extensive extravascular distribution and/or tissue binding. With the 3-hour infusion, increasing doses result in non-linear pharmacokinetics. For the 30% increase in dose from 135 mg/m^2 to 175 mg/m^2, the C_{max} and $AUC_{\rightarrow\infty}$ values increased 75% and 81%, respectively.

Following an intravenous dose of 100 mg/ m^2 given as a 3-hour infusion to 19 KS patients, the mean C_{max} was 1,530 ng/ml (range 761 - 2,860 ng/ml) and the mean AUC 5,619 ng.hr/ml (range 2,609 - 9,428 ng.hr/ml). Clearance was 20.6 l/h/ m^2 (range 11-38) and the volume of distribution was 291 l/ m^2 (range 121-638). The terminal elimination half-life averaged 23.7 hours (range 12 - 33).

Intrapatient variability in systemic paclitaxel exposure was minimal. There was no evidence for accumulation of paclitaxel with multiple treatment courses.

In vitro studies of binding to human serum proteins indicate that 89-98% of drug is bound. The presence of cimetidine, ranitidine, dexamethasone or diphenhydramine did not affect protein binding of paclitaxel.

The disposition of paclitaxel has not been fully elucidated in humans. Mean values for cumulative urinary recovery of unchanged drug have ranged from 1.3 to 12.6% of the dose, indicating extensive non-renal clearance. Hepatic metabolism and biliary clearance may be the principal mechanism for disposition of paclitaxel. Paclitaxel appears to be metabolised primarily by cytochrome P450 enzymes. Following administration of a radiolabelled paclitaxel, an average of 26, 2 and 6% of the radioactivity was excreted in the faeces as 6α-hydroxypaclitaxel, 3'-p-hydroxypaclitaxel, and 6α-3'-p-dihydroxy-paclitaxel, respectively. The formation of these hydroxylated metabolites is catalysed by CYP2C8, -3A4, and both -2C8 and -3A4 respectively. The effect of renal or hepatic dysfunction on the disposition of paclitaxel following a 3-hour infusion has not been investigated formally. Pharmacokinetic parameters obtained from one patient undergoing haemodialysis who received a 3-hour infusion of Taxol 135 mg/m^2 were within the range of those defined in non-dialysis patients.

In clinical trials where Taxol and doxorubicin were administered concomitantly, the distribution and elimination of doxorubicin and its metabolites were prolonged. Total plasma exposure to doxorubicin was 30% higher when paclitaxel immediately followed doxorubicin than when there was a 24-hour interval between drugs.

For use of Taxol in combination with other therapies, please consult the Summary of Product Characteristics of cisplatin, doxorubicin or trastuzumab for information on the use of these medicinal products.

5.3 Preclinical safety data

The carcinogenic potential of Taxol has not been studied. However, paclitaxel is a potential carcinogenic and genotoxic agent, based upon its pharmacodynamic mechanism of action. Taxol has been shown to be mutagenic in both *in vitro* and *in vivo* mammalian test systems.

6. PHARMACEUTICAL PARTICULARS

6.1 List of excipients

Ethanol (see 4.4).

Chromatographically purified polyoxyethylated castor oil.

6.2 Incompatibilities

Polyoxyethylated castor oil can result in DEHP (di-(2-ethylhexyl)phthalate) leaching from plasticised polyvinyl chloride (PVC) containers, at levels which increase with time and concentration. Consequently, the preparation, storage and administration of diluted Taxol should be carried out using non-PVC-containing equipment.

6.3 Shelf life

Vial before opening

2 years

After opening before dilution

Chemical and physical in-use stability has been demonstrated for 28 days at 25°C following multiple needle entries and product withdrawal.

From a microbiological point of view, once opened the product may be stored for a maximum of 28 days at 25°C. Other in-use storage times and conditions are the responsibility of the user.

After dilution

Chemical and physical in-use stability of the solution prepared for infusion has been demonstrated at 5°C and at 25°C for 7 days when diluted in 5% Dextrose solution, and for 14 days when diluted in 0.9% Sodium Chloride Injection.

From a microbiological point of view, the product should be used immediately. If not used immediately, in-use storage times and conditions prior to use are the responsibility of the user and would normally not be longer than 24 hours at 2 to 8°C, unless dilution has taken place in controlled and validated aseptic conditions.

6.4 Special precautions for storage

Do not store above 25°C.

Store in original package to protect from light.

Freezing does not adversely affect the product.

Diluted solutions: see 6.3.

6.5 Nature and contents of container

Type 1 glass vials (with butyl rubber stopper) contain 30 mg, 100 mg, 150 mg or 300 mg of paclitaxel in 5 ml, 16.7 ml, 25 ml or 50 ml solution respectively.

The vials are packaged individually in a carton. Boxes containing 10 cartons are also available.

Not all presentations may be marketed in all member states.

6.6 Instructions for use and handling

Handling: as with all antineoplastic agents, caution should be exercised when handling Taxol. Dilution should be carried out under aseptic conditions by trained personnel in a designated area. Adequate protective gloves should be worn. Precautions should be taken to avoid contact with the skin and mucous membranes. In the event of contact with the skin, the area should be washed with soap and water. Following topical exposure, tingling, burning and redness have been observed. In the event of contact with the mucous membranes, these should be flushed thoroughly with water. Upon inhalation, dyspnoea, chest pain, burning throat and nausea have been reported.

If unopened vials are refrigerated, a precipitate may form that redissolves with little or no agitation upon reaching room temperature. Product quality is not affected. If the solution remains cloudy or if an insoluble precipitate is noted, the vial should be discarded.

Following multiple needle entries and product withdrawals, the vials maintain microbial, chemical and physical stability for up to 28 days at 25°C. Other in-use storage times and conditions are the responsibility of the user.

The Chemo-Dispensing Pin device or similar devices with spikes should not be used since they can cause the vial stopper to collapse, resulting in loss of sterile integrity.

Preparation for IV administration: prior to infusion, Taxol must be diluted using aseptic techniques in 0.9% Sodium Chloride Injection, or 5% Dextrose Injection, or 5% Dextrose and 0.9% Sodium Chloride Injection, or 5% Dextrose in Ringer's Injection, to a final concentration of 0.3 to 1.2 mg/ml.

Chemical and physical in-use stability of the solution prepared for infusion has been demonstrated at 5°C and at 25°C for 7 days when diluted in 5% Dextrose solution, and for 14 days when diluted in 0.9% Sodium Chloride Injection. From a microbiological point of view, the product should be used immediately. If not used immediately, in-use storage times and conditions prior to use are the responsibility of the user and would normally not be longer than 24 hours at 2 to 8°C, unless dilution has taken place in controlled and validated aseptic conditions.

After dilution the solution is for single use only.

Upon preparation, solutions may show haziness, which is attributed to the formulation vehicle, and is not removed by filtration. Taxol should be administered through an in-line filter with a microporous membrane $\leqslant 0.22\ \mu m$. No significant losses in potency have been noted following simulated delivery of the solution through IV tubing containing an in-line filter.

There have been rare reports of precipitation during Taxol infusions, usually towards the end of a 24 hour infusion period. Although the cause of this precipitation has not been elucidated, it is probably linked to the supersaturation of the diluted solution. To reduce the precipitation risk, Taxol should be used as soon as possible after dilution, and excessive agitation, vibration or shaking should be avoided. The infusion sets should be flushed thoroughly before use. During infusion, the appearance of the solution should be regularly inspected and the infusion should be stopped if precipitation is present.

To minimise patient exposure to DEHP which may be leached from plasticised PVC infusion bags, sets, or other medical instruments, diluted Taxol solutions should be stored in non-PVC bottles (glass, polypropylene) or plastic bags (polypropylene, polyolefin) and administered through polyethylene-lined administration sets. Use of filter devices (e.g. IVEX-2®) which incorporate short inlet and/or outlet plasticised PVC tubing has not resulted in significant leaching of DEHP.

Disposal: all items used for preparation, administration or otherwise coming into contact with Taxol should undergo disposal according to local guidelines for the handling of cytotoxic compounds.

7. MARKETING AUTHORISATION HOLDER

Bristol-Myers Squibb Pharmaceuticals Limited

Uxbridge Business Park

Sanderson Road

Uxbridge

Middlesex UB8 1DH

United Kingdom

8. MARKETING AUTHORISATION NUMBER(S)

PL 11184/0026

9. DATE OF FIRST AUTHORISATION/RENEWAL OF THE AUTHORISATION

18 November 1993 / 20 September 2003

10. DATE OF REVISION OF THE TEXT

01 August 2005

Taxotere 20mg and 80mg concentrate and solvent for infusion

(sanofi-aventis)

1. NAME OF THE MEDICINAL PRODUCT

TAXOTERE 20 mg concentrate and solvent for solution for infusion

TAXOTERE 80 mg concentrate and solvent for solution for infusion

2. QUALITATIVE AND QUANTITATIVE COMPOSITION

Single-dose vials of TAXOTERE 20 mg concentrate for solution for infusion contain docetaxel which is a trihydrate corresponding to 20 mg of docetaxel (anhydrous). The viscous solution contains 40 mg/ml docetaxel (anhydrous).

Single-dose vials of TAXOTERE 80 mg concentrate for solution for infusion contain docetaxel which is a trihydrate corresponding to 80 mg of docetaxel (anhydrous). The viscous solution contains 40 mg/ml docetaxel (anhydrous).

For excipients, see 6.1.

3. PHARMACEUTICAL FORM

Concentrate and solvent for solution for infusion.

4. CLINICAL PARTICULARS

4.1 Therapeutic indications

Breast cancer

TAXOTERE in combination with doxorubicin and cyclophosphamide is indicated for the adjuvant treatment of patients with operable node- positive breast cancer.

TAXOTERE (docetaxel) in combination with doxorubicin is indicated for the treatment of patients with locally advanced or metastatic breast cancer who have not previously received cytotoxic therapy for this condition.

TAXOTERE (docetaxel) monotherapy is indicated for the treatment of patients with locally advanced or metastatic breast cancer after failure of cytotoxic therapy. Previous chemotherapy should have included an anthracycline or an alkylating agent.

TAXOTERE (docetaxel) in combination with trastuzumab is indicated for the treatment of patients with metastatic breast cancer whose tumors overexpress HER2 and who previously have not received chemotherapy for metastatic disease.

TAXOTERE (docetaxel) in combination with capecitabine is indicated for the treatment of patients with locally advanced or metastatic breast cancer after failure of cytotoxic chemotherapy. Previous therapy should have included an anthracycline.

Non-small cell lung cancer

TAXOTERE (docetaxel) is indicated for the treatment of patients with locally advanced or metastatic non-small cell lung cancer after failure of prior chemotherapy.

TAXOTERE (docetaxel) in combination with cisplatin is indicated for the treatment of patients with unresectable, locally advanced or metastatic non-small cell lung cancer, in patients who have not previously received chemotherapy for this condition.

Prostate cancer

TAXOTERE (docetaxel) in combination with prednisone or prednisolone is indicated for the treatment of patients with hormone refractory metastatic prostate cancer.

The use of docetaxel should be confined to units specialised in the administration of cytotoxic chemotherapy and it should only be administered under the supervision of a physician qualified in the use of anticancer chemotherapy.

4.2 Posology and method of administration

Recommended dosage:

For breast and non-small cell lung cancers, premedication consisting of an oral corticosteroid, such as dexamethasone 16 mg per day (e.g. 8 mg BID) for 3 days starting 1 day prior to docetaxel administration, unless contra-indicated, can be used (see section 4.4). Prophylactic G-CSF may be used to mitigate the risk of hematological toxicities.

For prostate cancer, given the concurrent use of prednisone or prednisolone the recommended premedication regimen is oral dexamethasone 8 mg, 12 hours, 3 hours and 1 hour before the docetaxel infusion (see section 4.4).

Docetaxel is administered as a one-hour infusion every three weeks.

Breast cancer

In the adjuvant treatment of operable node-positive breast cancer, the recommended dose of docetaxel is 75 mg/m^2 administered 1-hour after doxorubicin 50 mg/m^2 and cyclophosphamide 500 mg/m^2 every 3 weeks for 6 cycles (see also Dosage adjustments during treatment).

For the treatment of patients with locally advanced or metastatic breast cancer, the recommended dosage of docetaxel is 100 mg/m^2 in monotherapy. In first-line treatment, docetaxel 75 mg/m^2 is given in combination therapy with doxorubicin (50 mg/m^2). See section 6.6.

In combination with trastuzumab the recommended dose of docetaxel is 100 mg/m^2 every three weeks, with trastuzumab administered weekly. In the pivotal trial the initial docetaxel infusion was started the day following the first dose of trastuzumab. The subsequent docetaxel doses were administered immediately after completion of the trastuzumab infusion, if the preceding dose of trastuzumab was well tolerated. For trastuzumab dosage and administration, see summary of product characteristics.

In combination with capecitabine, the recommended dose of docetaxel is 75 mg/m2 every three weeks, combined with capecitabine at 1250 mg/m2 twice daily (within 30 minutes after a meal) for 2 weeks followed by 1- week rest period. For capecitabine dose calculation according to body surface area, see capecitabine summary of product characteristics.

Non-small cell lung cancer

In chemotherapy naïve patients treated for non-small cell lung cancer, the recommended dose regimen is docetaxel 75 mg/m^2 immediately followed by cisplatin 75 mg/ m^2 over 30-60 minutes. For treatment after failure of prior platinum-based chemotherapy, the recommended dosage is 75 mg/m^2 as a single agent.

Prostate cancer

The recommended dose of docetaxel is 75 mg/m^2. Prednisone or prednisolone 5 mg orally twice daily is administered continuously (see section 5.1).

Dosage adjustments during treatment:

General

Docetaxel should be administered when the neutrophil count is $\geq$ 1,500 cells/mm^3.

In patients who experienced either febrile neutropenia, neutrophil $<$ 500 cells/mm^3 for more than one week, severe or cumulative cutaneous reactions or severe peripheral neuropathy during docetaxel therapy, the dose of docetaxel should be reduced from 100 mg/m^2 to 75 mg/m^2 and/or from 75 to 60 mg/m^2. If the patient continues to experience these reactions at 60 mg/m^2, the treatment should be discontinued.

Adjuvant therapy for breast cancer:

In the pivotal trial in patients who received adjuvant therapy for breast cancer and who experienced complicated neutropenia (including prolonged neutropenia, febrile neutropenia, or infection), it was recommended to use G-CSF to provide prophylactic coverage (eg, day 4 to 11) in all subsequent cycles. Patients who continued to experience this reaction should remain on G-CSF and have their TAXOTERE dose reduced to 60 mg/m^2.

However, in clinical practice neutropenia could occur earlier. Thus the use of G-CSF should be considered function of the neutropenic risk of the patient and current recommendations. Patients who experience Grade 3 or 4 stomatitis should have their dose decreased to 60 mg/m^2.

In combination with cisplatin:

For patients who are dosed initially at docetaxel 75 mg/m^2 in combination with cisplatin and whose nadir of platelet count during the previous course of therapy is $<$25000 cells/mm^3, or in patients who experience febrile neutropenia, or in patients with serious non-hematologic toxicities, the docetaxel dosage in subsequent cycles should be reduced to 65 mg/m^2. For cisplatin dosage adjustments, see manufacturer's summary of product characteristics.

In combination with capecitabine:

- For capecitabine dose modifications, see capecitabine summary of product characteristics.
- For patients developing the first appearance of a Grade 2 toxicity, which persists at the time of the next TAXOTERE/ capecitabine treatment, delay treatment until resolved to Grade 0- 1, and resume at 100% of the original dose.
- For patients developing the second appearance of a Grade 2 toxicity, or the first appearance of a Grade 3 toxicity, at any time during the treatment cycle, delay treatment until resolved to Grade 0- 1, then resume treatment with TAXOTERE 55 mg/m^2.
- For any subsequent appearances of toxicities, or any Grade 4 toxicities, discontinue the TAXOTERE dose.

For trastuzumab dose modifications, see trastuzumab summary of product characteristics

Special populations:

Patients with hepatic impairment: Based on pharmacokinetic data with docetaxel at 100 mg/m^2 as single agent, patients who have both elevations of transaminase (ALT and/or AST) greater than 1.5 times the upper limit of the normal range (ULN) and alkaline phosphatase greater than 2.5 times the ULN, the recommended dose of docetaxel is 75 mg/m^2 (see sections 4.4 and 5.2). For those patients with serum bilirubin $>$ULN and/or ALT and AST$>$3.5 times the ULN associated with alkaline phosphatase $>$6 times the ULN, no dose-reduction can be recommended and docetaxel should not be used unless strictly indicated. No data are available in patients with hepatic impairment treated by docetaxel in combination.

Children: The safety and effectiveness of docetaxel in children have not been established.

Elderly: Based on a population pharmacokinetic analysis, there are no special instructions for use in the elderly.

In combination with capecitabine, for patients 60 years of age or more, a starting dose reduction of capecitabine to 75% is recommended (see capecitabine summary of product characteristics).

4.3 Contraindications

Hypersensitivity reactions to the active substance or to any of the excipients.

Docetaxel should not be used in patients with baseline neutrophil count of $<$1,500 cells/mm^3.

Docetaxel must not be used in pregnant or breast-feeding women.

Docetaxel should not be used in patients with severe liver impairment since there is no data available (see sections 4.4 and 4.2).

Contraindications for other medicinal products also apply, when combined with docetaxel.

4.4 Special warnings and special precautions for use

For breast and non-small cell lung cancers, premedication consisting of an oral corticosteroid, such as dexamethasone 16 mg per day (e.g. 8 mg BID) for 3 days starting 1 day prior to docetaxel administration, unless contraindicated, can reduce the incidence and severity of fluid retention as well as the severity of hypersensitivity reactions. For prostate cancer, the premedication is oral dexamethasone 8 mg, 12 hours, 3 hours and 1 hour before the docetaxel infusion (see section 4.2).

Haematology

Neutropenia is the most frequent adverse reaction of docetaxel. Neutrophil nadirs occurred at a median of 7 days but this interval may be shorter in heavily pre-treated patients. Frequent monitoring of complete blood counts should be conducted on all patients receiving docetaxel. Patients should be retreated with docetaxel when neutrophils recover to a level ≥1,500 cells/mm^3 (See section 4.2).

In the case of severe neutropenia (<500 cells/mm^3 for seven days or more) during a course of docetaxel therapy, a reduction in dose for subsequent courses of therapy or the use of appropriate symptomatic measures are recommended (see section 4.2).

Hypersensitivity reactions

Patients should be observed closely for hypersensitivity reactions especially during the first and second infusions. Hypersensitivity reactions may occur within a few minutes following the initiation of the infusion of docetaxel, thus facilities for the treatment of hypotension and bronchospasm should be available. If hypersensitivity reactions occur, minor symptoms such as flushing or localised cutaneous reactions do not require interruption of therapy. However, severe reactions, such as severe hypotension, bronchospasm or generalised rash/erythema require immediate discontinuation of docetaxel and appropriate therapy. Patients who have developed severe hypersensitivity reactions should not be re-challenged with docetaxel.

Cutaneous reactions

Localised skin erythema of the extremities (palms of the hands and soles of the feet) with oedema followed by desquamation has been observed. Severe symptoms such as eruptions followed by desquamation which lead to interruption or discontinuation of docetaxel treatment were reported (see section 4.2).

Fluid retention

Patients with severe fluid retention such as pleural effusion, pericardial effusion and ascites should be monitored closely.

Patients with liver impairment

In patients treated with docetaxel at 100 mg/m^2 as single agent who have serum transaminase levels (ALT and/or AST) greater than 1.5 times the ULN concurrent with serum alkaline phosphatase levels greater than 2.5 times the ULN, there is a higher risk of developing severe adverse reactions such as toxic deaths including sepsis and gastrointestinal haemorrhage which can be fatal, febrile neutropenia, infections, thrombocytopenia, stomatitis and asthenia. Therefore, the recommended dose of docetaxel in those patients with elevated liver function test (LFTs) is 75 mg/m^2 and LFTs should be measured at baseline and before each cycle (see section 4.2).

For patients with serum bilirubin levels >ULN and/or ALT and AST>3.5 times the ULN concurrent with serum alkaline phosphatase levels >6 times the ULN, no dose-reduction can be recommended and docetaxel should not be used unless strictly indicated.

No data are available in patients with hepatic impairment treated by docetaxel in combination.

Patients with renal impairment

There are no data available in patients with severely impaired renal function treated with docetaxel.

Nervous system

The development of severe peripheral neurotoxicity requires a reduction of dose (see section 4.2).

Cardiac toxicity

Heart failure has been observed in patients receiving TAXOTERE in combination with trastuzumab, particularly following anthracycline (doxorubicin or epirubicin)-containing chemotherapy. This may be moderate to severe and has been associated with death (see section 4.8).

When patients are candidates for treatment with TAXOTERE in combination with trastuzumab, they should undergo baseline cardiac assessment. Cardiac function should be further monitored during treatment (e.g. every three months) to help identify patients who may develop cardiac dysfunction. For more details see Summary of Product Characteristics of trastuzumab.

Others

Contraceptive measures must be taken during and for at least three months after cessation of therapy.

Additional cautions for use in adjuvant treatment of breast cancer

Complicated neutropenia

For patients who experience complicated neutropenia (prolonged neutropenia, febrile neutropenia or infection), G-CSF and dose reduction should be considered (see section 4.2).

Gastrointestinal reactions

Symptoms such as early abdominal pain and tenderness, fever, diarrhea, with or without neutropenia, may be early manifestations of serious gastrointestinal toxicity and should be evaluated and treated promptly.

Congestive heart failure

Patients should be monitored for symptoms of congestive heart failure during therapy and during the follow up period.

Leukemia

In women receiving TAXOTERE, doxorubicin and cyclophosphamide (TAC), the risk of acute myeloid leukemia is comparable to the risk observed for other anthracycline/cyclophosphamide containing regimens.

Patients with 4+ nodes

The benefit/risk ratio for TAC in patients with 4+ nodes was not defined fully at the interim analysis (see section 5.1).

Elderly

There are no data available in patient >70 years of age on TAXOTERE use in combination with doxorubicin and cyclophosphamide.

Of the 333 patients treated with TAXOTERE every three weeks in a prostate cancer study, 209 patients were 65 years of age or greater and 68 patients were older than 75 years. In patients treated with TAXOTERE every three weeks, the incidence of related nail changes occurred at a rate ⩾ 10% higher in patients who were 65 years of age or greater compared to younger patients. The incidence of related fever, diarrhea, anorexia, and peripheral edema occurred at rates ⩾ 10% higher in patients who were 75 years of age or greater versus less than 65 years.

4.5 Interaction with other medicinal products and other forms of Interaction

There have been no formal clinical studies to evaluate the drug interactions of docetaxel.

In vitro studies have shown that the metabolism of docetaxel may be modified by the concomitant administration of compounds which induce, inhibit or are metabolised by (and thus may inhibit the enzyme competitively) cytochrome P450-3A such as ciclosporine, terfenadine, ketoconazole, erythromycin and troleandomycin. As a result, caution should be exercised when treating patients with these drugs as concomitant therapy since there is a potential for a significant interaction.

Docetaxel is highly protein bound >95%). Although the possible *in vivo* interaction of docetaxel with concomitantly administered medication has not been investigated formally, *in vitro* interactions with tightly protein-bound drugs such as erythromycin, diphenhydramine, propranolol, propafenone, phenytoin, salicylate, sulfamethoxazole and sodium valproate did not affect protein binding of docetaxel. In addition, dexamethasone did not affect protein binding of docetaxel. Docetaxel did not influence the binding of digitoxin.

The pharmacokinetics of docetaxel, doxorubicin and cyclophosphamide were not influenced by their coadministration. Limited data from a single uncontrolled study were suggestive of an interaction between docetaxel and carboplatin. When combined to docetaxel, the clearance of carboplatin was about 50% higher than values previously reported for carboplatin monotherapy.

Docetaxel pharmacokinetics in the presence of prednisone was studied in patients with metastatic prostate cancer. Docetaxel is metabolised by CYP3A4 and prednisone is known to induce CYP3A4. No statistically significant effect of prednisone on the pharmacokinetics of docetaxel was observed.

4.6 Pregnancy and lactation

There is no information on the use of docetaxel in pregnant women. Docetaxel has been shown to be both embryotoxic and foetotoxic in rabbits and rats, and to reduce fertility in rats. As with other cytotoxic drugs, docetaxel may cause foetal harm when administered to pregnant women. Therefore, docetaxel must not be used during pregnancy. Women of childbearing age receiving docetaxel should be advised to avoid becoming pregnant, and to inform the treating physician immediately should this occur.

Docetaxel is a lipophilic substance but it is not known whether it is excreted in human milk. Consequently, because of the potential for adverse reactions in nursing infants, breast feeding must be discontinued for the duration of docetaxel therapy.

4.7 Effects on ability to drive and use machines

Docetaxel is unlikely to affect the ability to drive or operate machines.

4.8 Undesirable effects

The adverse reactions considered to be possibly or probably related to the administration of TAXOTERE have been obtained in:.

- 1312 and 121 patients who received 100 mg/m^2 and 75 mg/m^2 of TAXOTEREas a single agent respectively
- 258 patients who received TAXOTERE in combination with doxorubicin
- 406 patients who received TAXOTERE in combination with cisplatin
- 92 patients treated with TAXOTERE in combination with trastuzumab,
- 255 patients who received TAXOTERE in combination with capecitabine,
- 332 patients who received TAXOTERE in combination with prednisone or prednisolone (clinically important treatment related adverse events are presented).
- 744 patients who received TAXOTERE in combination with doxorubicin and cyclophosphamide (clinically important treatment related adverse events are presented).

These reactions were described using the NCI Common Toxicity Criteria (grade 3 = G3; grade 3-4 = G3/4; grade 4 = G4) and the COSTART terms. Frequencies are defined as: very common > 1/10), common >1/100, <1/10); uncommon >1/1,000, <1/100); rare >1/10,000, <1/1,000); very rare (<1/10,000).

The most commonly reported adverse reaction was neutropenia, which was reversible and not cumulative (see sections 4.2 and 4.4). The median day to nadir was 7 days and the median duration of severe neutropenia (<500 cells/mm^3) was 7 days."

For combination with trastuzumab, adverse events (all grades) reported in ⩾10% are displayed. There was an increased incidence of SAEs (40% vs. 31%) and Grade 4 AEs (34% vs. 23%) in the trastuzumab combination arm compared to TAXOTERE monotherapy.

For combination with capecitabine, the most frequent treatment-related undesirable effects (⩾ 5%) reported in a phase III trial in breast cancer patients failing anthracycline treatment are presented (see capecitabine summary of product characteristics).

Neoplasms benign and malignant (including cysts and polyps)

Two patients were diagnosed with leukemia at a median follow-up time of 55 months and one case of leukemia was reported after the follow-up period. No cases of myelodysplastic syndrome occurred.

Blood and the lymphatic system disorders

Bone marrow suppression and other hematologic adverse reactions have been reported.

TAXOTERE 100mg/m^2 single agent:

Very common: Neutropenia (96.6%; G4: 76.4%); Anemia (90.4%; G3/4: 8.9%); Infections (20%; G3/4: 5.7%, including sepsis and pneumonia, fatal in 1.7%); Febrile neutropenia (11.8%).

Common: Thrombocytopenia (7.8%; G4: 0.2%); G3/4 infection associated with neutrophil count <500 cells/mm^3 (4.6%); Bleeding episodes (2.4%).

Rare: Bleeding episodes associated with G3/4 thrombocytopenia.

TAXOTERE 75mg/m^2 single agent:

Very common: Neutropenia (89.8%; G4: 54.2%); Anemia (93.3%; G3/4: 10.8%); Infections (10.7%; G3/4: 5%); Thrombocytopenia (10%; G4: 1.7%).

Common: Febrile neutropenia (8.3%).

TAXOTERE 75mg/m^2 in combination with doxorubicin:

Very common: Neutropenia (99.2%; G4: 91.7%); Anemia (96.1%; G3/4: 9.4%); Infection (35.3%; G3/4: 7.8%); Febrile neutropenia (34.1%); Thrombocytopenia (28.1%; G4: 0.8%).

TAXOTERE 75mg/m^2 in combination with cisplatin:

Very common: Neutropenia (91.1%; G4: 51.5%); Anemia (88.6%; G3/4: 6.9%); Fever in absence of infection (17.2%; G3/4:1.2%); Thrombocytopenia (14.9%; G4: 0.5%); Infections (14.3%; G3/4: 5.7%).

Common: Febrile neutropenia (4.9%).

TAXOTERE 100mg/m^2 in combination with trastuzumab:

Very common: Neutropenia (G3/4: 32%); Febrile neutropenia (includes neutropenia associated with fever and antibiotic use) or neutropenic sepsis (23%)-; Nasopharyngitis (15%).

Haematological toxicity was increased in patients receiving trastuzumab and docetaxel, compared with docetaxel alone (32% grade 3/4 neutropenia versus 22%, using NCI-CTC criteria). The incidence of febrile neutropenia/neutropenic sepsis was also increased in patients treated with Herceptin plus docetaxel (23% versus 17% for patients treated with docetaxel alone).

TAXOTERE 75mg/m^2 in combination with capecitabine:

Very common: Neutropenia (G3/4: 63%), Anemia (G3/4: 10%).

Common: Thrombocytopenia (G3/4: 3%).

TAXOTERE 75mg/m^2 in combination with prednisone or prednisolone:

Very common: Neutropenia (40.9%, G3/4: 32%), Anemia (66.5%, G3/4: 4.9%), Infection (12.0%, G3/4: 3.3%).

Common: Thrombocytopenia (3.4%, G3/4: 0.6%), Febrile neutropenia (2.7%), Epistaxis (3.0%, G3/4: 0%).

TAXOTERE 75mg/m^2 in combination with doxorubicin and cyclophosphamide:

Very common: Anemia (91.5%; G3/4: 4.3%); Neutropenia (71.4%; G3/4: 65.5%); Fever in absence of infection (43.1%; G3/4:1.2%); Thrombocytopenia (39.4%; G3/4: 2.0%); Infection (27.2%; G3/4: 3.2%); Febrile neutropenia (24.7%); Neutropenic infection (12.1%).

There were no septic deaths.

Immune system disorders

Hypersensitivity reactions have generally occurred within a few minutes following the start of the infusion of docetaxel and were usually mild to moderate. The most frequently reported symptoms were flushing, rash with or without pruritus, chest tightness, back pain, dyspnoea and drug fever or chills. Severe reactions, characterised by hypotension and/or bronchospasm or generalized rash/erythema, resolved after discontinuing the infusion and appropriate therapy (see section 4.4).

TAXOTERE 100mg/m² single agent: very common (25.9%; G3/4: 5.3%)

TAXOTERE 75mg/m² single agent: common (2.5%, no severe)

TAXOTERE 75mg/m² in combination with doxorubicin: common (4.7%; G3/4: 1.2%)

TAXOTERE 75mg/m² in combination with cisplatin: very common (10.6%; G3/4: 2.5%)

TAXOTERE 75mg/m² in combination with prednisone or prednisolone: common (6.9%; G3/4: 0.6%)

TAXOTERE 75mg/m² in combination with doxorubicin and cyclophosphamide: very common (10.5%; G3/4: 1.1%)

Skin and subcutaneous tissue disorders

Reversible cutaneous reactions have been observed and were generally considered as mild to moderate. Reactions were characterised by a rash including localised eruptions mainly on the feet and hands, but also on the arms, face or thorax, and frequently associated with pruritus. Eruptions generally occurred within one week after the docetaxel infusion. Less frequently, severe symptoms such as eruptions followed by desquamation which rarely lead to interruption or discontinuation of docetaxel treatment were reported (see sections 4.2 and 4.4). Severe nail disorders are characterised by hypo- or hyperpigmentation and sometimes pain and onycholysis. Very rare cases of bullous eruption such as erythema multiforme or Stevens-Johnson syndrome have been reported with docetaxel and other concomitant factors may have contributed to the development of these effects.

TAXOTERE 100mg/m² single agent:

Very common: Alopecia (79%); Cutaneous reactions (56.6%; G3/4: 5.9%); Nail changes (27.9%; severe 2.6%).

Very rare: one case of alopecia non-reversible at the end of the study.

73% of the cutaneous reactions were reversible within 21 days.

TAXOTERE 75mg/m² single agent:

Very common: Alopecia (38%); Cutaneous reactions (15.7%; G3/4: 0.8%).

Common: Nail changes (9.9%; severe 0.8%).

TAXOTERE 75mg/m² in combination with doxorubicin:

Very common: Alopecia (94.6%); Nail changes (20.2%; severe 0.4%); Cutaneous reactions (13.6%; no severe).

TAXOTERE 75mg/m² in combination with cisplatin:

Very common: Alopecia (73.6%); Nail changes (13.3%; severe 0.7%); Cutaneous reactions (11.1%; G3/4: 0.2%)

TAXOTERE 100mg/m² in combination with trastuzumab:

Very common: Alopecia (67%), Erythema (23%), Rash (24%), Nail disorder (17%).

TAXOTERE 75mg/m² in combination with capecitabine:

Very common: Hand-foot Syndrome (63%; G3/4: 24%); Alopecia (41%; G3/4: 6%); Nail disorder (14%; G3/4: 2%).

Common: Dermatitis (8%); Rash erythematous (8%; G3/4: <1%); Nail discoloration (6%); Onycholysis (5%; G3/4: 1%).

TAXOTERE 75mg/m² in combination with prednisone or prednisolone:

Very common: Alopecia (65.1%); Nail changes (28.3%; no severe);

Common: Rash/Desquamation (3.3%; G3/4: 0.3%).

TAXOTERE 75mg/m² in combination with doxorubicin and cyclophosphamide:

Very common: Alopecia (97.7%); Skin toxicity (18.4%; G3/4: 0.7%); Nail disorders (18.4%; G3/4: 0.4%).

Alopecia was observed to be ongoing at the median follow-up time of 55 months in 22 patients out of the 687 patients with alopecia at the end of the chemotherapy.

Fluid retention

Events such as peripheral oedema and less frequently pleural effusion, pericardial effusion, ascites and weight gain have been reported. The peripheral oedema usually starts at the lower extremities and may become generalised with a weight gain of 3 kg or more. Fluid retention is cumulative in incidence and severity (see section 4.4).

TAXOTERE 100mg/m² single agent: very common (64.1%; severe 6.5%). The median cumulative dose to treatment discontinuation was more than 1,000 mg/m² and the median time to fluid retention reversibility was 16.4 weeks (range 0 to 42 weeks). The onset of moderate and severe retention is delayed (median cumulative dose: 818.9 mg/m²) in patients with premedication compared with patients without premedication (median cumulative dose: 489.7 mg/m²); however, it has been reported in some patients during the early courses of therapy.

TAXOTERE 75mg/m² single agent: very common (24.8%; severe 0.8%)

TAXOTERE 75mg/m² in combination with doxorubicin: very common (35.7%; severe 1.2%)

TAXOTERE 75mg/m² in combination with cisplatin: very common (25.9%; severe 0.7%)

TAXOTERE 100mg/m² in combination with trastuzumab:

Very common: Oedema peripheral (40%), Lymphoedema (11%).

TAXOTERE 75mg/m² in combination with prednisone or prednisolone: very common (24.4%; severe 0.6%)

TAXOTERE 75mg/m² in combination with doxorubicin and cyclophosphamide:

Very common: Peripheral edema (26.7%; G3/4: 0.4%)

Uncommon: Lymphedema (0.3%; G3/4: 0%)

Peripheral edema was observed to be ongoing at the median follow-up time of 55 months in 18 patients out of the 112 patients with peripheral edema at the end of the chemotherapy.

Fluid retention has not been accompanied by acute episodes of oliguria or hypotension. Dehydration and pulmonary oedema have rarely been reported

Gastrointestinal disorders

TAXOTERE 100mg/m² single agent:

Very common: Stomatitis (41.8%; G3/4: 5.3%); Diarrhoea (40.6%; G3/4: 4%); Nausea (40.5%; G3/4: 4%); Vomiting (24.5%; G3/4: 3%).

Common: Taste perversion (10.1%; severe 0.07%); Constipation (9.8%; severe 0.2%); Abdominal pain (7.3%; severe 1%); Gastrointestinal bleeding (1.4%; severe 0.3%).

Uncommon: Esophagitis (1%; severe 0.4%).

TAXOTERE 75mg/m² single agent:

Very common: Nausea (28.9%; G3/4: 3.3%); Stomatitis (24.8%; G3/4: 1.7%); Vomiting (16.5%; G3/4: 0.8%); Diarrhoea (11.6%; G3/4: 1.7%).

Common: Constipation (6.6%).

TAXOTERE 75mg/m² in combination with doxorubicin:

Very common: Nausea (64%; G3/4: 5%); Stomatitis (58.1%; G3/4: 7.8%); Diarrhoea (45.7%; G3/4: 6.2%); Vomiting (45%; G3/4: 5%); Constipation (14.3%).

TAXOTERE 75mg/m² in combination with cisplatin:

Very common: Nausea (69%; G3/4:9.6%); Vomiting (53.4%; G3/4: 7.6%); Diarrhoea (41.1%; G3/4: 6.4%); Stomatitis (23.4%; G3/4: 2%);.

Common: Constipation (9.4%).

TAXOTERE 100mg/m² in combination with trastuzumab:

Very common: Nausea (43%), Diarrhoea (43%), Vomiting (29%), Constipation (27%), Stomatitis (20%), Dyspepsia (14%), Abdominal pain (12%).

TAXOTERE 75mg/m² in combination with capecitabine:

Very common: Stomatitis (67%; G3/4: 18%); Diarrhea (64%; G3/4: 14%); Nausea (43%; G3/4: 6%); Vomiting (33%; G3/4: 4%); Taste disturbance (15%; G3/4: <1%); Constipation (14%; G3/4: 1%); Abdominal pain (14%; G3/4: 2%); Dyspepsia (12%).

Common: Abdominal pain upper (9%); Dry mouth (5%).

TAXOTERE 75mg/m² in combination with prednisone or prednisolone:

Very common: Nausea (35.5%; G3/4: 2.4%); Diarrhoea (24.1%; G3/4: 1.2%); Stomatitis/Pharyngitis (17.8%; G3/4: 0.9%); Taste disturbance (17.5%; G3/4: 0%); Vomiting (13.3%; G3/4: 1.2%).

TAXOTERE 75mg/m² in combination with doxorubicin and cyclophosphamide:

Very common: Nausea (80.4%; G3/4: 5.1%); Stomatitis (69.1%; G3/4: 7.1%); Vomiting (42.6%; G3/4: 4.3%); Diarrhea (30.9%; G3/4: 3.2%); Taste perversion (27.4%; G3/4: 0.7%); Constipation (22.6%; G3/4: 0.4%).

Common: Abdominal pain (7.3%; G3/4: 0.5%).

Uncommon: colitis/enteritis/large intestine perforation (0.5%). Two patients required treatment discontinuation; no deaths due to these events occurred.

Rare occurrences of dehydration as a consequence of gastrointestinal events, gastrointestinal perforation, ischemic colitis, colitis and neutropenic enterocolitis have been reported. Very rare cases of ileus and intestinal obstruction have been reported.

Nervous system disorders

The development of severe peripheral neurotoxicity requires a reduction of dose (see sections 4.2 and 4.4).

Mild to moderate neuro-sensory signs are characterised by paresthesia, dysesthesia or pain including burning. Neuromotor events are mainly characterised by weakness.

TAXOTERE 100mg/m² single agent:

Very common: Neurosensory (50%; G3: 4.1%), Neuromotor (13.8%; G3/4: 4%)

Reversibility data are available among 35.3% of patients who developed neurotoxicity following TAXOTERE treatment at 100 mg/m² as single agent. The events were spontaneously reversible within 3 months.

TAXOTERE 75mg/m² single agent:

Very common: Neurosensory (24%; G3: 0.8%).

Common: Neuromotor (9.9%; G3/4: 2.5%).

TAXOTERE 75mg/m² in combination with doxorubicin:

Very common: Neurosensory (30.2%; G3: 0.4%).

Common: Neuromotor (2.3%; G3/4: 0.4%).

TAXOTERE 75mg/m² in combination with cisplatin:

Very common: Neurosensory (40.4%; G3:3.7%), Neuromotor (12.8%; G3/4: 2%)

TAXOTERE 100mg/m² in combination with trastuzumab:

Very common: Paresthesia (32%), Headache (21%), Dysgeusia (14%), Hypoaesthesia (11%).

TAXOTERE 75mg/m² in combination with capecitabine:

Very common: Paresthesia (11%; G3/4: <1%).

Common: Dizziness (9%); Headache (7%; G3/4: <1%); Peripheral neuropathy (5%).

TAXOTERE 75mg/m² in combination with prednisone or prednisolone:

Very common: Neuropathy Sensory (27.4%; G3/4:1.2%), Common: Neuropathy Motor (3.9%; G3/4: 0%).

TAXOTERE 75mg/m² in combination with doxorubicin and cyclophosphamide:

Very common: Neurosensory (23.8%; G3/4: 0%).

Common: Neuromotor (2.8%; G3/4: 0%); Neurocortical (2.8%; G3/4: 0.3%); Neurocerebellar (1.1%; G3/4: 0.1%).

Uncommon: Syncope (0.5%; G3/4: 0%)

Neurosensory was observed to be ongoing at the median follow-up time of 55 months in 9 patients out of the 73 patients with neurosensory at the end of the chemotherapy.

Rare cases of convulsion or transient loss of consciousness have been observed with docetaxel administration. These reactions sometimes appear during the infusion of the drug.

Cardiac disorders

TAXOTERE 100mg/m² single agent:

Common: Cardiac dysrhythmia (4.1%; G3/4: 0.7%); Hypotension (3.8%); Hypertension (2.4%).

Uncommon: Heart failure (0.5%).

TAXOTERE 75mg/m² single agent:

Common: Cardiac dysrhythmia (2.5%, no severe); Hypotension (1.7%).

TAXOTERE 75mg/m² in combination with doxorubicin:

Common: Heart failure (2.3%); Cardiac dysrhythmia (1.2%; no severe).

Uncommon: Hypotension (0.4%).

TAXOTERE 75mg/m² in combination with cisplatin:

Common: Hypotension (3.7%; G3/4: 0.7%); Cardiac dysrhythmia (2.5%; G3/4: 0.7%).

Uncommon: Heart failure (0.5%)

TAXOTERE 100mg/m² in combination with trastuzumab:

Symptomatic heart failure was reported in 2.2% of the patients who received TAXOTERE plus trastuzumab compared to 0% of patients given TAXOTERE alone. In the TAXOTERE plus trastuzumab arm, 64% had received a prior anthracycline as adjuvant therapy compared with 55% in the docetaxel arm alone.

TAXOTERE 75mg/m² in combination with capecitabine:

Very common: Lower limb oedema (14%; G3/4: 1%).

TAXOTERE 75mg/m² in combination with prednisone or prednisolone:

Common: Cardiac left ventricular function decrease (3.9%; G3/4: 0.3%).

TAXOTERE 75mg/m² in combination with doxorubicin and cyclophosphamide:

Very common: Vasodilatation (20.3%; G3/4: 0.9%).

Common: Cardiac dysrhythmia (3.9%; G3/4: 0.1%); Hypotension (1.5%; G3/4: 0%).

Congestive Heart Failure (CHF) (1.6%) has also been reported. One patient in each treatment arm died due to heart failure.

Rare cases of myocardial infarction have been reported.

Vascular disorders

TAXOTERE 75mg/m² in combination with doxorubicin and cyclophosphamide:

Uncommon: Phlebitis (0.7%; G3/4: 0%).

Venous thromboembolic events have rarely been reported.

Hepato-biliary disorders

TAXOTERE 100mg/m² single agent:

Common: G3/4 bilirubin increase (<5%); G3/4 alkaline phosphatase increase (<4%); G3/4 AST increase (<3%); G3/4 ALT increase (<2%).

TAXOTERE 75mg/m² single agent:

Common: G3/4 bilirubin increase (<2%).

TAXOTERE 75mg/m² in combination with doxorubicin:

Common: G3/4 bilirubin increase (<2.5%); G3/4 alkaline phosphatase increase (<2.5%).

Uncommon: G3/4 AST increase (<1%); G3/4 ALT increase (<1%).

TAXOTERE 75mg/m² in combination with cisplatin:

Common: G3/4 bilirubin increase (2.1%); G3/4 ALT increase (1.3%).

Uncommon: G3/4 AST increase (0.5%); G3/4 alkaline phosphatase increase (0.3%).

TAXOTERE 75mg/m² in combination with capecitabine:

Common: Hyperbilirubinemia (G3/4: 9%)

Very rare cases of hepatitis have been reported.

Metabolism and nutrition disorders

TAXOTERE 100mg/m² single agent: Very common: Anorexia (16.8%).

TAXOTERE 75mg/m² single agent: Very common: Anorexia (19%).

TAXOTERE 75mg/m² in combination with doxorubicin: Common: Anorexia (8.5%).

TAXOTERE 75mg/m² in combination with cisplatin: Very common: Anorexia (28.8%).

TAXOTERE 100mg/m² in combination with trastuzumab: Very common: Anorexia (22%); Weight increased (15%).

TAXOTERE 75mg/m² in combination with capecitabine:

Very common: Anorexia (12%; G3/4: 1%); Appetite decreased (10%).

Common: Dehydration (8%; G3/4: 2%); Weight decreased (6%).

TAXOTERE 75mg/m² in combination with prednisone or prednisolone:

Very common: Anorexia (12.7%, G3/4: 0.6%).

TAXOTERE 75mg/m² in combination with doxorubicin and cyclophosphamide:

Very common: Anorexia (19.9%; G3/4: 2.2%), Weight gain or loss (15.2%; G3/4: 0.3%).

Eye Disorders

Very rare cases of transient visual disturbances (flashes, flashing lights, scotomata) typically occurring during drug infusion and in association with hypersensitivity reactions have been reported. These were reversible upon discontinuation of the infusion.

Cases of lacrimation with or without conjunctivitis, as cases of lacrimal duct obstruction resulting in excessive tearing have been rarely reported.

TAXOTERE 100mg/m² in combination with trastuzumab:

Very common: Lacrimation increased (21%), Conjunctivitis (12%).

TAXOTERE 75mg/m² in combination with capecitabine:

Very common: Lacrimation increased (12%)

TAXOTERE 75mg/m² in combination with prednisone or prednisolone:

Common: Tearing (9.3%, G3/4: 0.6%)

TAXOTERE 75mg/m² in combination with doxorubicin and cyclophosphamide:

Common: Lacrimation disorder (9.8%; G3/4: 0.1%); Conjunctivitis (4.6%; G3/4: 0.3%).

Psychiatric disorders

TAXOTERE 100mg/m² in combination with trastuzumab: Very common: Insomnia 11%).

Musculoskeletal, connective tissue and bone disorders

TAXOTERE 100mg/m² single agent:

Very common: Myalgia (20%; severe 1.4%).

Common: Arthralgia (8.6%).

TAXOTERE 75mg/m² single agent:

Common: Myalgia (5.8%).

TAXOTERE 75mg/m² in combination with doxurubicin:

Common: Myalgia (8.5%).

TAXOTERE 75mg/m² in combination with cisplatin:

Very common: Myalgia (13.8%; severe 0.5%).

TAXOTERE 100mg/m² in combination with trastuzumab:

Very common: Myalgia (27%), Arthralgia (27%), Pain in extremity (16%), Bone pain (14%), Back pain (10%).

TAXOTERE 75mg/m² in combination with capecitabine:

Very common: Myalgia (14%; G3/4: 2%); Arthralgia (11%; G3/4: 1%).

Common: Back pain (7%; G3/4: 1%).

TAXOTERE 75mg/m² in combination with prednisone or prednisolone:

Common: Arthralgia (3.0%, G3/4: 0.3%), Myalgia (6.9%; G3/4: 0.3%).

TAXOTERE 75mg/m² in combination with doxorubicin and cyclophosphamide:

Very common: Myalgia (22.8%; G3/4: 0.8%); Arthralgia (15.1%; G3/4: 0.4%).

Respiratory, thoracic and mediastinal disorders

TAXOTERE 100mg/m² single agent:

Very common: Dyspnea (16.1%; severe 2.7%)

TAXOTERE 100mg/m² in combination with trastuzumab:

Very common: Epistaxis (18%), Pharyngolaryngeal pain (16%), Dyspnoea (14%), Cough (13%), Rhinorrhoea (12%).

TAXOTERE 75mg/m² in combination with capecitabine:

Very common: Sore throat (11%; G3/4: 2%)

Common: Dyspnea (7%; G3/4: 1%); Cough (6%; G3/4: <1%); Epistaxis (5%; G3/4: <1%)

TAXOTERE 75mg/m² in combination with prednisone or prednisolone:

Common: Dyspnea (4.5%; G3/4: 0.6%), Cough (1.2%; G3/4: 0%).

TAXOTERE 75mg/m² in combination with doxorubicin and cyclophosphamide:

Common: Cough (3.1%; G3/4: 0%).

Acute respiratory distress syndrome, interstitial pneumonia and pulmonary fibrosis have rarely been reported.

Reproductive system and breast disorders

TAXOTERE 75mg/m² in combination with doxorubicin and cyclophosphamide:

Very common: Amenorrhea (57.6%).

Amenorrhea was observed to be ongoing at the median follow-up time of 55 months in 133 patients out of the 233 patients with amenorrhea at the end of the chemotherapy.

General disorders and administration site conditions

Infusion site reactions were generally mild and consisted of hyper pigmentation, inflammation, redness or dryness of the skin, phlebitis or extravasation and swelling of the vein.

TAXOTERE 100mg/m² single agent:

Very common: Asthenia (62.6%; severe 11.2%); Pain (16.5%).

Common: Infusion site reactions (5.6%); Chest pain (4.5%; severe 0.4%) without any cardiac or respiratory involvement.

TAXOTERE 75mg/m² single agent:

Very common: Asthenia (48.8%; severe 12.4%); Pain (10.7%).

TAXOTERE 75mg/m² in combination with doxorubicin:

Very common: Asthenia (54.7%; severe 8.1%); Pain (17.1%).

Common: Infusion site reaction (3.1%).

TAXOTERE 75mg/m² in combination with cisplatin:

Very common: Asthenia (51.5%; severe 9.9%).

Common: Infusion site reaction (6.2%); Pain (5.4%).

TAXOTERE 100mg/m² in combination with trastuzumab:

Very common: Asthenia (45%), Pyrexia (29%), Fatigue (24%), Mucosal inflammation (23%), Pain (12%), Influenza like illness (12%), Chest pain (11%), Rigors (11%).

Common: Lethargy (7%).

TAXOTERE 75mg/m² in combination with capecitabine:

Very common: Asthenia (23%; G3/4: 3%); Pyrexia (21%; G3/4: 1%); Fatigue (21%; G3/4: 4%); Weakness (13%; G3/4: 1%).

Common: Pain in limb (9%; G3/4: <1%); Lethargy (6%); Pain (6%); Oral candidiasis (6%; G3/4: < 1%).

TAXOTERE 75mg/m² in combination with prednisone or prednisolone:

Very common: Fatigue (42.8%; G3/4: 3.9%).

TAXOTERE 75mg/m² in combination with doxorubicin and cyclophosphamide:

Very common: Asthenia (79.2%; G3/4: 11%).

Radiation recall phenomena have rarely been reported.

Injury, poisoning and procedural complications

TAXOTERE 100mg/m² in combination with trastuzumab: Very common: Nail toxicity (11%)

4.9 Overdose

There were a few reports of overdose. There is no known antidote for docetaxel overdose. In case of overdose, the patient should be kept in a specialised unit and vital functions closely monitored. The primary anticipated complications of overdose would consist of bone marrow suppression, peripheral neurotoxicity and mucositis. Patients should receive therapeutic G-CSF as soon as possible after discovery of overdose. Other appropriate symptomatic measures should be taken, as needed.

5. PHARMACOLOGICAL PROPERTIES

5.1 Pharmacodynamic properties

Pharmaco-therapeutic group: Antineoplastic agents, ATC Code: L01CD 02

Preclinical data

Docetaxel is an antineoplastic agent which acts by promoting the assembly of tubulin into stable microtubules and inhibits their disassembly which leads to a marked decrease of free tubulin. The binding of docetaxel to microtubules does not alter the number of protofilaments.

Docetaxel has been shown *in vitro* to disrupt the microtubular network in cells which is essential for vital mitotic and interphase cellular functions.

Docetaxel was found to be cytotoxic *in vitro* against various murine and human tumour cell lines and against freshly excised human tumour cells in clonogenic assays. Docetaxel achieves high intracellular concentrations with a long cell residence time. In addition, docetaxel was found to be active on some but not all cell lines over expressing the p-glycoprotein which is encoded by the multidrug resistance gene. *In vivo*, docetaxel is schedule independent and has a broad spectrum of experimental antitumour activity against advanced murine and human grafted tumours.

Clinical data

Breast cancer

TAXOTERE in combination with doxorubicin and cyclophosphamide: adjuvant therapy

Data from a multicenter open label randomized trial support the use of TAXOTERE for the adjuvant treatment of patients with operable node-positive breast cancer and KPS ⩾ 80%, between 18 and 70 years of age. After stratification according to the number of positive lymph nodes (1-3, 4+), 1491 patients were randomized to receive either TAXOTERE 75 mg/m² administered 1-hour after doxorubicin 50 mg/m² and cyclophosphamide 500 mg/m² (TAC arm), or doxorubicin 50 mg/m² followed by fluorouracil 500 mg/m² and cyclosphosphamide 500 mg/m² (FAC arm). Both regimens were administered once every 3 weeks for 6 cycles. TAXOTERE was administered as a 1-hour infusion, all other drugs were given as IV bolus on day one. G-CSF was administered as secondary prophylaxis to patients who experienced complicated neutropenia (febrile neutropenia, prolonged neutropenia, or infection). Patients on the TAC arm received antibiotic prophylaxis with ciprofloxacin 500 mg orally b.i.d. for 10 days starting on day 5 of each cycle, or equivalent. In both arms, after the last cycle of chemotherapy, patients with positive estrogen and/or progesterone receptors received tamoxifen 20 mg daily for up to 5 years. Adjuvant radiation therapy was prescribed according to guidelines in place at participating institutions and was given to 69% of patients who received TAC and 72% of patients who received FAC.

An interim analysis was performed with a median follow up of 55 months. Significantly longer disease-free survival for the TAC arm compared to the FAC arm was demonstrated. Incidence of relapses at 5 years was reduced in patients receiving TAC compared to those who received FAC (25% versus 32%, respectively) i.e. an absolute risk reduction by 7% (p=0.001). Overall survival at 5 years was also significantly increased with TAC compared to FAC (87% versus 81%, respectively) i.e. an absolute reduction of the risk of death by 6% (p=0.008). TAC-treated patient subsets according to prospectively defined major prognostic factors were analyzed:

(see Table 1)

The beneficial effect of TAC was not proven in patients with 4 and more positive nodes (37% of the population) at the interim analysis stage. The effect appears to be less pronounced than in patients with 1-3 positive nodes. The benefit/risk ratio was not defined fully in patients with 4 and more positive nodes at this analysis stage.

TAXOTERE as single agent

Two randomised phase III comparative studies, involving a total of 326 alkylating or 392 anthracycline failure metastatic breast cancer patients, have been performed with docetaxel at the recommended dose and regimen of 100 mg/m² every 3 weeks.

In alkylating-failure patients, docetaxel was compared to doxorubicin (75 mg/m² every 3 weeks). Without affecting overall survival time (docetaxel 15 months vs. doxorubicin 14 months, p=0.38) or time to progression (docetaxel 27 weeks vs. doxorubicin 23 weeks, p=0.54), docetaxel increased response rate (52% vs. 37%, p=0.01) and shortened time to response (12 weeks vs. 23 weeks, p=0.007). Three docetaxel patients (2%) discontinued the treatment due to fluid retention, whereas 15 doxorubicin patients (9%) discontinued due to cardiac toxicity (three cases of fatal congestive heart failure).

In anthracycline-failure patients, docetaxel was compared to the combination of Mitomycin C and Vinblastine (12 mg/m² every 6 weeks and 6 mg/m² every 3 weeks).

Table 1

		Disease Free Survival			Overall Survival		
Patient subset No of positive nodes	**Number of patients**	**Hazard ratio***	**95% CI**	**P=**	**Hazard ratio***	**95% CI**	**P=**
Overall	745	0.72	0.59-0.88	0.001	0.70	0.53-0.91	0.008
1-3	467	0.61	0.46-0.82	0.0009	0.45	0.29-0.70	0.0002
4+	278	0.83	0.63-1.08	0.17	0.94	0.66-1.33	0.72

*a hazard ratio of less than 1 indicates that TAC is associated with a longer disease-free survival and overall survival compared to FAC

Docetaxel increased response rate (33% vs. 12%, p<0.0001), prolonged time to progression (19 weeks vs. 11 weeks, p=0.0004) and prolonged overall survival (11 months vs. 9 months, p=0.01).

During these phase III studies, the safety profile of docetaxel was consistent with the safety profile observed in phase II studies (see section 4.8).

TAXOTERE in combination with doxorubicin

One large randomized phase III study, involving 429 previously untreated patients with metastatic disease, has been performed with doxorubicin (50 mg/m²) in combination with docetaxel (75 mg/m²) (AT arm) versus doxorubicin (60 mg/m²) in combination with cyclophosphamide (600 mg/m²) (AC arm). Both regimens were administered on day 1 every 3 weeks.

- Time to progression (TTP) was significantly longer in the AT arm versus AC arm, p=0.0138. The median TTP was 37.3 weeks (95%CI:33.4 - 42.1) in AT arm and 31.9 weeks (95%CI: 27.4 - 36.0) in AC arm.
- Overall response rate (ORR) was significantly higher in the AT arm versus AC arm, p=0.009. The ORR was 59.3% (95%CI: 52.8 - 65.9) in AT arm versus 46.5% (95%CI: 39.8 - 53.2) in AC arm.

In this trial, AT arm showed a higher incidence of severe neutropenia (90% versus 68.6%), febrile neutropenia (33.3% versus 10%), infection (8% versus 2.4%), diarrhea (7.5% versus 1.4%), asthenia (8.5% versus 2.4%), and pain (2.8% versus 0%) than AC arm. On the other hand, AC arm showed a higher incidence of severe anemia (15.8% versus 8.5%) than AT arm, and, in addition, a higher incidence of severe cardiac toxicity: congestive heart failure (3.8% versus 2.8%), absolute LVEF decrease $\geq$ 20% (13.1 % versus 6.1%), absolute LVEF decrease $\geq$ 30% (6.2% versus 1.1%). Toxic deaths occurred in 1 patient in the AT arm (congestive heart failure) and in 4 patients in the AC arm (1 due to septic shock and 3 due to congestive heart failure).

In both arms, quality of life measured by the EORTC questionnaire was comparable and stable during treatment and follow-up.

TAXOTERE in combination with trastuzumab

TAXOTERE in combination with trastuzumab was studied for the treatment of patients with metastatic breast cancer whose tumors overexpress HER2, and who previously had not received chemotherapy for metastatic disease. One hundred eighty six patients were randomized to receive TAXOTERE (100 mg/m²) with or without trastuzumab; 60% of patients received prior anthracycline-based adjuvant chemotherapy. TAXOTERE plus trastuzumab was efficacious in patients whether or not they had received prior adjuvant anthracyclines. The main test method used to determine HER2 positivity in this pivotal trial was immunohistochemistry (IHC). A minority of patients were tested using fluorescence in-situ hybridization (FISH). In this trial, 87% of patients had disease that was IHC 3+, and 95% of patients entered had disease that was IHC 3+ and/or FISH positive. Efficacy results are summarized in the following table:

Parameter	TAXOTERE plus trastuzumab[1]	TAXOTERE[1]
	n=92	n=94
Response rate (95% CI)	61% (50-71)	34% (25-45)
Median Duration of reponse (95% CI)	11.4 (9.2-15.0)	5.1 (4.4-6.2)
Median TTP (months) (95% CI)	10.6 (7.6-12.9)	5.7 (5.0-6.5)
Median Survival (months) (95% CI)	30.5[2] (26.8-ne)	22.1[2] (17.6-28.9)

TTP=time to progression; "ne" indicates that it could not be estimated or it was not yet reached.

[1]Full analysis set (intent-to-treat)

[2] Estimated median survival

TAXOTERE in combination with capecitabine

Data from one multicenter, randomised, controlled phase III clinical trial support the use of docetaxel in combination with capecitabine for treatment of patients with locally advanced or metastatic breast cancer after failure of cytotoxic chemotherapy, including an anthracycline. In this trial, 255 patients were randomised to treatment with docetaxel (75 mg/m2 as a 1 hour intravenous infusion every 3 weeks) and capecitabine (1250 mg/m2 twice daily for 2 weeks followed by 1-week rest period). 256 patients were randomised to treatment with docetaxel alone (100 mg/ m2 as a 1 hour intravenous infusion every 3 weeks). Survival was superior in the docetaxel +capecitabine combination arm (p=0.0126). Median survival was 442 days (docetaxel + capecitabine) vs. 352 days (docetaxel alone). The overall objective response rates in the all-randomised population (investigator assessment) were 41.6% (docetaxel + capecitabine) vs. 29.7% (docetaxel alone); p = 0.0058. Time to progressive disease was superior in the docetaxel + capecitabine combination arm (p<0.0001). The median time to progression was 186 days (docetaxel + capecitabine) vs. 128 days (docetaxel alone).

Non-Small Cell Lung Cancer

Patients previously treated with chemotherapy with or without radiotherapy

In a phase III study, in previously treated patients, time to progression (12.3 weeks versus 7 weeks) and overall survival were significantly longer for docetaxel at 75 mg/m² compared to Best Supportive Care. The 1-year survival rate was also significantly longer in docetaxel (40%) versus BSC (16%).

There was less use of morphinic analgesic (p<0.01), non-morphinic analgesics (p<0.01), other disease-related medications (p=0.06) and radiotherapy (p<0.01) in patients treated with docetaxel at 75 mg/m² compared to those with BSC.

The overall response rate was 6.8% in the evaluable patients, and the median duration of response was 26.1 weeks.

Taxotere in combination with platinum agents in chemotherapy-naïve patients

In a Phase III trial, 1218 patients with unresectable stage IIIB or IV NSCLC, with KPS of 70% or greater, and who did not receive previous chemotherapy for this condition, were randomised to either Taxotere (T) 75 mg/m² as a 1 hour infusion immediately followed by cisplatin (Cis) 75 mg/ m² over 30-60 minutes every 3 weeks, Taxotere 75 mg/ m² as a 1 hour infusion in combination with carboplatin (AUC 6 mg/ml•min) over 30-60 minutes every 3 weeks, or vinorelbine (V) 25 mg/ m² administered over 6-10 minutes on days 1, 8, 15, 22 followed by cisplatin 100 mg/ m² administered on day 1 of cycles repeated every 4 weeks.

Survival data, median time to progression and response rates for two arms of the study are illustrated in the following table:

(see Table 2)

Secondary end-points included change of pain, global rating of quality of life by EuroQoL-5D, Lung Cancer Symptom Scale, and changes in Karnosfky performance status. Results on these end-points were supportive of the primary end-points results.

For Taxotere/Carboplatin combination, neither equivalent nor non-inferior efficacy could be proven compared to the reference treatment combination VCis.

Prostate Cancer

The safety and efficacy of TAXOTERE in combination with prednisone or prednisolone in patients with hormone refractory metastatic prostate cancer were evaluated in a randomized multicenter Phase III trial. A total of 1006 patients with KPS$\geq$60 were randomized to the following treatment groups:

- TAXOTERE 75 mg/m² every 3 weeks for 10 cycles.
- TAXOTERE 30 mg/m² administered weekly for the first 5 weeks in a 6 week cycle for 5 cycles.
- Mitoxantrone 12 mg/m² every 3 weeks for 10 cycles.

All 3 regimens were administered in combination with prednisone or prednisolone 5 mg twice daily, continuously.

Patients who received docetaxel every three weeks demonstrated significantly longer overall survival compared to those treated with mitoxantrone. The increase in survival seen in the docetaxel weekly arm was not statistically significant compared to the mitoxantrone control arm. Efficacy endpoints for the TAXOTERE arms versus the control arm are summarized in the following table:

(see Table 3 below)

Given the fact that TAXOTERE every week presented a slightly better safety profile than TAXOTERE every 3 weeks, it is possible that certain patients may benefit from TAXOTERE every week.

No statistical differences were observed between treatment groups for Global Quality of Life.

5.2 Pharmacokinetic properties

The pharmacokinetics of docetaxel have been evaluated in cancer patients after administration of 20-115 mg/m² in Phase I studies. The kinetic profile of docetaxel is dose independent and consistent with a three-compartment pharmacokinetic model with half lives for the a, b and g phases of 4 min, 36 min and 11.1 h, respectively. The late phase is due, in part, to a relatively slow efflux of docetaxel from the peripheral compartment. Following

Table 2

	Tcis n=408	Vcis n=404	Statistical Analysis
Overall Survival (Primary end point):			
Median Survival (months)	11.3	10.1	Hazard Ratio: 1.122 [97.2% CI: 0.937, 1.342]*
1-year Survival (%)	46	41	Treatment difference 5.4% [95% CI: -1.1, 12.0]
2-year Survival (%)	21	14	Treatment difference 6.2% [95% CI: 0.2, 12.3]
Median Time to Progression (weeks)	22.0	23.0	Hazard Ratio 1.032 [95% CI: 0.876, 1.216]
Overall Response Rate (%)	31.6	24.5	Treatment difference 7.1% [95% CI: 0.7, 13.5]

*: Corrected for multiple comparisons and adjusted for stratification factors (stage of disease and region of treatment), based on evaluable patient population.

Table 3

Endpoint	*TAXOTERE every 3 weeks*	*TAXOTERE every week*	*Mitoxantrone every 3 weeks*
Number of patients	*335*	*334*	*337*
Median survival (months): (95% CI)	*18.9: (17.0-21.2)*	*17.4: (15.7-19.0)*	*16.5: (14.4-18.6)*
Hazard ratio (95% CI)	*0.761 (0.619-0.936)*	*0.912 (0.747-1.113)*	
p-value	*0.0094*	*0.3624*	–
Number of patients	*291*	*282*	*300*
*PSA** response rate (%): (95% CI)*	*45.4: (39.5-51.3)*	*47.9: (41.9-53.9)*	*31.7: (26.4-37.3)*
*p-value**	*0.0005*	*<0.0001*	–
Number of patients	*153*	*154*	*157*
Pain response rate (%): (95% CI)	*34.6: (27.1-42.7)*	*31.2: (24.0-39.1)*	*21.7: (15.5-28.9)*
*p-value**	*0.0107*	*0.0798*	–
Number of patients	*141*	*134*	*137*
Tumor response rate (%): (95% CI)	*12.1: (7.2-18.6)*	*8.2: (4.2-14.2)*	*6.6: (3.0-12.1)*
*p-value**	*0.1112*	*0.5853*	–

† Stratified log rank test

** Threshold for statistical significance=0.0175*

*** PSA: Prostate-Specific Antigen*

the administration of a 100 mg/m^2 dose given as a one-hour infusion a mean peak plasma level of 3.7 μg/ml was obtained with a corresponding AUC of 4.6 h.μg/ml. Mean values for total body clearance and steady-state volume of distribution were 21 l/h/m^2 and 113 l, respectively. Inter individual variation in total body clearance was approximately 50%. Docetaxel is more than 95% bound to plasma proteins.

A study of ^{14}C-docetaxel has been conducted in three cancer patients. Docetaxel was eliminated in both the urine and faeces following cytochrome P450-mediated oxidative metabolism of the tert-butyl ester group, within seven days, the urinary and faecal excretion accounted for about 6% and 75% of the administered radioactivity, respectively. About 80% of the radioactivity recovered in faeces is excreted during the first 48 hours as one major inactive metabolite and 3 minor inactive metabolites and very low amounts of unchanged drug.

A population pharmacokinetic analysis has been performed with docetaxel in 577 patients. Pharmacokinetic parameters estimated by the model were very close to those estimated from Phase I studies. The pharmacokinetics of docetaxel were not altered by the age or sex of the patient. In a small number of patients (n=23) with clinical chemistry data suggestive of mild to moderate liver function impairment (ALT, AST $\geq$1.5 times the ULN associated with alkaline phosphatase $\geq$2.5 times the ULN), total clearance was lowered by 27% on average (see section 4.2). Docetaxel clearance was not modified in patients with mild to moderate fluid retention and there are no data available in patients with severe fluid retention.

When used in combination, docetaxel does not influence the clearance of doxorubicin and the plasma levels of doxorubicinol (a doxorubicin metabolite). The pharmacokinetics of docetaxel, doxorubicin and cyclophosphamide were not influenced by their coadministration.

Phase I study evaluating the effect of capecitabine on the pharmacokinetics of docetaxel and vice versa showed no effect by capecitabine on the pharmacokinetics of docetaxel (Cmax and AUC) and no effect by docetaxel on the pharmacokinetics of a relevant capecitabine metabolite 5'-DFUR.

Clearance of docetaxel in combination therapy with cisplatin was similar to that observed following monotherapy. The pharmacokinetic profile of cisplatin administered shortly after TAXOTERE infusion is similar to that observed with cisplatin alone

The effect of prednisone on the pharmacokinetics of docetaxel administered with standard dexamethasone premedication has been studied in 42 patients. No effect of prednisone on the pharmacokinetics of docetaxel was observed.

5.3 Preclinical safety data

The carcinogenic potential of docetaxel has not been studied.

Docetaxel has been shown to be mutagenic in the *in vitro* micronucleus and chromosome aberration test in CHO-K1 cells and in the *in vivo* micronucleus test in the mouse. However, it did not induce mutagenicity in the Ames test or the CHO/HGPRT gene mutation assay. These results are consistent with the pharmacological activity of docetaxel.

Adverse effects on the testis observed in rodent toxicity studies suggest that docetaxel may impair male fertility.

6. PHARMACEUTICAL PARTICULARS

6.1 List of excipients

TAXOTERE vial: polysorbate 80.

Solvent vial: ethanol in water for injections.

6.2 Incompatibilities

None known.

6.3 Shelf life

TAXOTERE 20mg vials: 24 months

TAXOTERE 80mg vials: 36 months

Premix solution: The premix solution contains 10 mg/ml docetaxel and should be used immediately after preparation. However the chemical and physical stability of the premix solution has been demonstrated for 8 hours when stored either between 2°C and 8°C or at room temperature.

Infusion solution: the infusion solution should be used within 4 hours at room temperature.

6.4 Special precautions for storage

Vials should be stored between 2°C and 25°C and protected from bright light.

6.5 Nature and contents of container

Each blister carton of TAXOTERE 20 mg or 80 mg concentrate and solvent for solution for infusion contains:

- one single-dose TAXOTERE vial and,
- one single-dose solvent for TAXOTERE vial

TAXOTERE 20 mg concentrate for solution for infusion vial:

The TAXOTERE 20 mg concentrate for solution for infusion vial is a 7 ml clear glass vial with a green flip-off cap.

This vial contains 0.5 ml of a 40 mg/ml solution of docetaxel in polysorbate 80 (fill volume: 24.4mg/0.61 ml). This fill volume has been established during the development of TAXOTERE to compensate for liquid loss during preparation of the premix due to foaming, adhesion to the walls of the vial and "dead-volume". This overfill ensures that after dilution with the entire contents of the accompanying solvent for TAXOTERE vial, there is a minimal extractable premix volume of 2 ml containing 10 mg/ml docetaxel which corresponds to the labelled amount of 20 mg per vial.

Solvent vial:

The solvent vial is a 7 ml clear glass vial with a transparent colourless flip-off cap.

Solvent vial contains 1.5 ml of a 13% w/w solution of ethanol in water for injections (fill volume: 1.98 ml). The addition of the entire contents of the solvent vial to the contents of the TAXOTERE 20 mg concentrate for solution for infusion vial ensures a premix concentration of 10 mg/ml docetaxel.

TAXOTERE 80 mg concentrate for solution for infusion vial:

The TAXOTERE 80 mg concentrate for solution for infusion vial is a 15 ml clear glass vial with a red flip-off cap.

This vial contains 2 ml of a 40 mg/ml solution of docetaxel in polysorbate 80 (fill volume: 94.4 mg/2.36 ml). This fill volume has been established during the development of TAXOTERE to compensate for liquid loss during preparation of the premix due to foaming, adhesion to the walls of the vial and "dead-volume". This overfill ensures that after dilution with the entire contents of the accompanying solvent for TAXOTERE vial, there is a minimal extractable premix volume of 8 ml containing 10 mg/ml docetaxel which corresponds to the labelled amount of 80 mg per vial.

Solvent vial:

The solvent vial is a 15 ml clear glass vial with a transparent colourless flip-off cap.

Solvent vial contains 6 ml of a 13% w/w solution of ethanol in water for injections (fill volume: 7.33 ml). The addition of the entire contents of the solvent vial to the contents of the TAXOTERE 80 mg concentrate for solution for infusion vial ensures a premix concentration of 10 mg/ml docetaxel.

6.6 Instructions for use and handling Recommendations for safe handling

TAXOTERE is an antineoplastic agent and, as with other potentially toxic compounds, caution should be exercised when handling it and preparing TAXOTERE solutions. The use of gloves is recommended.

If TAXOTERE concentrate, premix solution or infusion solution should come into contact with skin, wash immediately and thoroughly with soap and water. If TAXOTERE concentrate, premix solution or infusion solution should come into contact with mucous membranes, wash immediately and thoroughly with water.

Preparation for the intravenous administration

a) Preparation of the TAXOTERE premix solution (10 mg docetaxel/ml)

If the vials are stored under refrigeration, allow the required number of TAXOTERE boxes to stand at room temperature for 5 minutes.

Using a syringe fitted with a needle, aseptically withdraw the entire contents of the solvent for TAXOTERE vial by partially inverting the vial.

Inject the entire contents of the syringe into the corresponding TAXOTERE vial.

Remove the syringe and needle and mix manually by repeated inversions for at least 45 seconds. Do not shake.

Allow the premix vial to stand for 5 minutes at room temperature and then check that the solution is homogenous and clear (foaming is normal even after 5 minutes due to the presence of polysorbate 80 in the formulation).

The premix solution contains 10 mg/ml docetaxel and should be used immediately after preparation. However the chemical and physical stability of the premix solution has been demonstrated for 8 hours when stored either between 2°C and 8°C or at room temperature.

b) Preparation of the infusion solution

More than one premix vial may be necessary to obtain the required dose for the patient. Based on the required dose for the patient expressed in mg, aseptically withdraw the corresponding premix volume containing 10 mg/ml docetaxel from the appropriate number of premix vials using graduated syringes fitted with a needle. For example, a dose of 140 mg docetaxel would require 14 ml docetaxel premix solution.

Inject the required premix volume into a 250 ml infusion bag or bottle containing either 5% glucose solution or 0.9% sodium chloride solution.

If a dose greater than 200 mg of docetaxel is required, use a larger volume of the infusion vehicle so that a concentration of 0.74 mg/ml docetaxel is not exceeded.

Mix the infusion bag or bottle manually using a rocking motion.

The TAXOTERE infusion solution should be used within 4 hours and should be aseptically administered as a 1-hour infusion under room temperature and normal lighting conditions.

As with all parenteral products, TAXOTERE premix solution and infusion solution should be visually inspected prior to use, solutions containing a precipitate should be discarded.

Disposal

All materials that have been utilised for dilution and administration should be disposed of according to standard procedures.

7. MARKETING AUTHORISATION HOLDER

Aventis Pharma S.A., 20 avenue Raymond Aron, 92165 Antony Cedex, France

8. MARKETING AUTHORISATION NUMBER(S)

TAXOTERE 20 mg concentrate and solvent for solution for infusion: EU/1/95/002/001

TAXOTERE 80 mg concentrate and solvent for solution for infusion: EU/1/95/002/002

9. DATE OF FIRST AUTHORISATION/RENEWAL OF THE AUTHORISATION

27 November 1995

10. DATE OF REVISION OF THE TEXT

January 2005

Legal Category: POM

Tazocin

(Wyeth Pharmaceuticals)

1. NAME OF THE MEDICINAL PRODUCT

TAZOCIN 2.25g

TAZOCIN 4.5g

2. QUALITATIVE AND QUANTITATIVE COMPOSITION

Piperacillin sodium/tazobactam sodium (INN)

TAZOCIN 2.25g contains 2 active ingredients; piperacillin 2g and tazobactam 250mg both present as sodium salts.

TAZOCIN 4.5g contains 2 active ingredients; piperacillin 4g and tazobactam 500mg both present as sodium salts.

3. PHARMACEUTICAL FORM

TAZOCIN, an injectable antibacterial combination for intravenous administration is available as a white to off-white sterile, lyophilised powder for solution for injection or infusion packaged in glass vials.

The product contains no excipients or preservatives.

4. CLINICAL PARTICULARS

4.1 Therapeutic indications

TAZOCIN is indicated for treatment of the following systemic and/or local bacterial infections in which susceptible organisms have been detected or are suspected:

Adults and the Elderly

Lower respiratory tract infections

Urinary tract infections (complicated and uncomplicated)

Intra-abdominal infections

Skin and skin structure infections

Bacterial septicaemia

Bacterial infections in neutropenic adults in combination with an aminoglycoside

Children

Appendicitis complicated by rupture with peritonitis and/or abscess formation in children aged 2-12 years.

Bacterial infections in neutropenic children in combination with an aminoglycoside.

TAZOCIN is indicated for the treatment of polymicrobic infections including those where gram-positive and gram-negative aerobic and/or anaerobic organisms are suspected (intra-abdominal, skin and skin structure, lower respiratory tract) see Section 5.1. As such, TAZOCIN is particularly useful in the treatment of polymicrobial infections and in presumptive therapy prior to the availability of the results of sensitivity tests because of its broad spectrum of activity.

4.2 Posology and method of administration

TAZOCIN may be given by slow intravenous injection (over at least 3-5 minutes) or by slow intravenous infusion (over 20-30 minutes).

Neutropenic patients with signs of infection (e.g. fever) should receive immediate empirical antibiotic therapy before laboratory results are available.

Adults and Children Over 12 Years, Each with Normal Renal Function

The usual dosage for adults and children over 12 years is 4.5g TAZOCIN (4g piperacillin / 500mg tazobactam) given every 8 hours.

The total daily dose of TAZOCIN depends on the severity and localisation of the infection and can vary from 2.25g (2g piperacillin / 250mg tazobactam) to 4.5g (4g piperacillin / 500mg tazobactam) administered every 6 or 8 hours.

In neutropenia the recommended dose is 4.5g TAZOCIN (4g piperacillin / 500mg tazobactam) given every 6 hours in combination with an aminoglycoside.

Elderly with Normal Renal Function

TAZOCIN may be used at the same dose levels as adults except in cases of renal impairment (see below):

Renal Insufficiency in Adults, the Elderly and Children Receiving the Adult Dose

In patients with renal insufficiency, the intravenous dose should be adjusted to the degree of actual renal impairment. The suggested daily doses are as follows:

Creatinine Clearance (ml/min)	Recommended Piperacillin/Tazobactam Dosage
20 - 80	12g/1.5g/day Divided Doses 4g/500mg q 8H
< 20	8g/1g/day Divided Doses 4g/500mg q 12H

For patients on haemodialysis, the maximum daily dose is 8g/1g piperacillin/tazobactam. In addition, because haemodialysis removes 30%-50% of piperacillin in 4 hours, one additional dose of 2g/250mg piperacillin/tazobactam should be administered following each dialysis period. For patients with renal failure and hepatic insufficiency, measurement of serum levels of TAZOCIN will provide additional guidance for adjusting dosage.

Children Aged 12 Years and Under with Normal Renal Function

TAZOCIN is only recommended for the treatment of children with neutropenia or complicated appendicitis.

Neutropenia

For children the dose should be adjusted to 90mg/kg (80mg piperacillin / 10mg tazobactam) administered every 6 hours, in combination with an aminoglycoside, not exceeding 4.5g (4g piperacillin / 500mg tazobactam) every 6 hours.

Complicated Appendicitis

For children aged 2–12 years the dose should be adjusted to 112.5mg/kg (100mg piperacillin / 12.5mg tazobactam) administered every 8 hours, not exceeding 4.5g (4g piperacillin / 500mg tazobactam) every 8 hours.

Until further experience is available, TAZOCIN should not be used in children who do not have neutropenia or complicated appendicitis.

Renal Insufficiency in Children Aged 12 Years and Under

In children with renal insufficiency the intravenous dosage should be adjusted to the degree of actual renal impairment as follows:

Creatinine Clearance (ml/min)	Recommended Piperacillin / Tazobactam Dosage
⩾ 40	No adjustment
20-39	90mg (80mg piperacillin / 10mg tazobactam) /kg q 8H, not exceeding 13.5g/day
< 20	90mg (80mg piperacillin / 10mg tazobactam) /kg q 12H, not exceeding 9g/day

For children weighing < 50kg on haemodialysis the recommended dose is 45mg (40mg piperacillin /5mg tazobactam) /kg every 8 hours.

The above dosage modifications are only an approximation. Each patient must be monitored closely for signs of drug toxicity. Drug dose and interval should be adjusted accordingly.

Hepatic Impairment

No dose adjustment is necessary.

Duration of Therapy

The duration of therapy should be guided by the severity of the infection and the patient's clinical and bacteriological progress.

In acute infections, treatment with TAZOCIN should be continued for 48 hours beyond the resolution of clinical symptoms or the fever.

In paediatric complicated appendicitis treatment is recommended for a minimum of 5 days and a maximum of 14 days.

4.3 Contraindications

Hypersensitivity to any of the beta-lactams (including penicillins and cephalosporins) or to beta-lactamase inhibitors.

4.4 Special warnings and special precautions for use

Warnings

Serious and occasionally fatal hypersensitivity (anaphylactic / anaphylactoid [including shock]) reactions have been reported in patients receiving therapy with penicillins including TAZOCIN. These reactions are more likely to occur in persons with a history of sensitivity to multiple allergens.

There have been reports of patients with a history of penicillin hypersensitivity who have experienced severe reactions when treated with a cephalosporin.

If an allergic reaction occurs during therapy with TAZOCIN, the antibiotic should be discontinued. Serious hypersensitivity reactions may require adrenaline and other emergency measures.

Table 1 PROPOSED MINIMUM INHIBITORY CONCENTRATION (MIC) BREAKPOINTS

Pathogens	Susceptible	Intermediate	Resistant
Enterobacteriaceae	⩽ 16 mg/L	32 - 64 mg/L	⩾ 128 mg/L
Pseudomonas	⩽ 64 mg/L	-	⩾ 128 mg/L
Staphylococcus	⩽ 8 mg/L	-	⩾ 16 mg/L
Streptococcus	⩽ 1 mg/L	-	⩾ 2 mg/L
Anaerobes	⩽ 32 mg/L	64 mg/L	⩾ 128 mg/L

Before initiating therapy with TAZOCIN, careful inquiry should be made concerning previous hypersensitivity reactions to penicillins, cephalosporins, and other allergens.

In case of severe, persistent diarrhoea, the possibility of antibiotic-induced, life threatening pseudomembranous colitis must be taken into consideration. The onset of pseudomembranous colitis symptoms may occur during or after antibacterial treatment. Therefore, TAZOCIN must be discontinued immediately in such cases, and suitable therapy be initiated (e.g. oral metronidazole or oral vancomycin). Preparations which inhibit peristalsis are contra-indicated.

Precautions

Leukopenia and neutropenia may occur, especially during prolonged therapy. Therefore, periodic assessment of hematopoietic function should be performed.

Periodic assessment of organ system functions including renal and hepatic during prolonged therapy is advisable.

Bleeding manifestations have occurred in some patients receiving β-lactam antibiotics. These reactions have sometimes been associated with abnormalities of coagulation tests such as clotting time, platelet aggregation and prothrombin time, and are more likely to occur in patients with renal failure. If bleeding manifestations occur, the antibiotic should be discontinued and appropriate therapy instituted.

As with other antibiotics, the possibility of the emergence of resistant organisms which might cause superinfections should be kept in mind, particularly during prolonged treatment. Microbiological follow-up may be required to detect any important superinfection. If this occurs, appropriate measures should be taken.

As with other penicillins, patients may experience neuromuscular excitability or convulsions if higher than recommended doses are given intravenously.

This product contains 2.35mEq (54mg) of sodium per gram of piperacillin which may increase a patient's overall sodium intake. This may be harmful to people on a low sodium diet.

Hypokalaemia may occur in patients with low potassium reserves or who are receiving concomitant medications that may lower potassium levels; periodic electrolyte determinations should be performed in such patients. Modest elevation of indices of liver function may be observed.

Antimicrobials used in high doses for short periods to treat gonorrhoea may mask or delay the symptoms of incubating syphilis. Therefore, prior to treatment, patients with gonorrhoea should also be evaluated for syphilis. Specimens for darkfield examination should be obtained from patients with any suspect primary lesion, and serologic tests should be made for a minimum of 4 months.

4.5 Interaction with other medicinal products and other forms of Interaction

Concurrent administration of probenecid and piperacillin/ tazobactam produced a longer half-life and lower renal clearance for both piperacillin and tazobactam. However, peak plasma concentrations of either drug are unaffected.

Piperacillin either alone or with tazobactam did not cause clinically important alterations to the phamacokinetics of tobramycin in subjects with normal renal function and with mild or moderate renal impairment. The pharmacokinetics of piperacillin, tazobactam, and the M1 metabolite were not significantly altered by tobramycin administration. No clinically important pharmacokinetic interactions have been noted between TAZOCIN and vancomycin in healthy adults with normal renal function.

Whenever TAZOCIN is used concurrently with another antibiotic, especially an aminoglycoside, the drugs must not be mixed in intravenous solutions or administered concurrently due to physical incompatibility. The mixing of TAZOCIN with an aminoglycoside in vitro can result in substantial inactivation of the aminoglycoside.

During simultaneous administration of heparin, oral anticoagulants and other drugs which may affect the blood coagulation system including thrombocyte function, appropriate coagulation tests should be performed more frequently and monitored regularly.

Piperacillin when used concomitantly with vecuronium has been implicated in the prolongation of the neuromuscular blockade of vecuronium. Due to their similar mechanism of action, it is expected that the neuromuscular blockade produced by any of the non-polarizing muscle relaxants could be prolonged in the presence of piperacillin.

Piperacillin may reduce the excretion of methotrexate. Serum levels of methotrexate should be monitored in patients on methotrexate therapy.

As with other penicillins, the administration of TAZOCIN may result in a false-positive reaction for glucose in the urine using a copper-reduction method. It is recommended that glucose tests based on enzymatic glucose oxidase reaction be used.

There have been reports of positive test results using the Bio-Rad Laboratories Platelia *Aspergillus* EIA test in patients receiving piperacillin-tazobactam injection who were subsequently found to be free of *Aspergillus* infection. Cross-reactions with non-*Aspergillus* polysaccharides and polyfuranoses with Bio-Rad Laboratories Platelia *Aspergillus* EIA test have been reported. Therefore, positive test results in patients receiving piperacillin-tazobactam should be interpreted cautiously and confirmed by other diagnostic methods.

4.6 Pregnancy and lactation

Studies in mice and rats have not demonstrated any embryotoxic or teratogenic effects of the piperacillin-tazobactam combination Tazocin. There are no adequate and well-controlled studies with piperacillin-tazobactam combination Tazocin or with piperacillin or tazobactam alone in pregnant women. Piperacillin and tazobactam cross the placenta. Pregnant women should be treated only if the expected benefit outweighs the possible risks to the pregnant woman and foetus.

Piperacillin is excreted in low concentrations in human milk; tazobactam concentrations in human milk have not been studied. Women who are breast-feeding should be treated only if the expected benefit outweighs the possible risks to the nursing woman and child.

4.7 Effects on ability to drive and use machines

TAZOCIN is not known to affect ability to drive or operate machines.

4.8 Undesirable effects

The most commonly reported adverse reactions are diarrhoea, nausea, vomiting, and rash, each having a frequency of ⩾ 1% but ⩽ 10%.

Body System	Adverse Reaction
Infections and infestations	
Uncommon:	Candidal superinfection
Blood and lymphatic system disorders	
Uncommon:	Leucopenia, neutropenia, thrombocytopenia
Rare:	Anaemia, bleeding manifestations (including purpura, epistaxis, bleeding time prolonged), eosinophilia, haemolytic anaemia
Very rare:	Agranulocytosis, Coombs direct test positive, pancytopenia, prolonged partial thromboplastin time, prothrombin time prolonged, thrombocytosis
Immune system disorders	
Uncommon:	Hypersensitivity reaction
Rare:	Anaphylactic/anaphylactoid reaction (including shock)
Metabolism and nutritional disorders	
Very rare:	Hypoalbuminaemia, hypoglycaemia, hypoproteinaemia, hypokalaemia
Nervous system disorders	
Uncommon:	Headache, insomnia
Rare:	Muscular weakness, hallucination, convulsion, dry mouth
Vascular disorders	
Uncommon:	Hypotension, phlebitis, thrombophlebitis
Rare:	Flushing
Gastrointestinal disorders	
Common:	Diarrhoea, nausea, vomiting
Uncommon:	Constipation, dyspepsia, jaundice, stomatitis
Rare:	Abdominal pain, pseudomembranous colitis, hepatitis

Hepatobiliary disorders

Uncommon:	Alanine aminotransferase increased, aspartate aminotransferase increased
Rare:	Bilirubin increased, blood alkaline phosphatase increased, gamma-glutamyltransferase increased, hepatitis

Skin and subcutaneous tissue disorders

Common:	Rash
Uncommon:	Pruritus, urticaria, erythema
Rare:	Bullous dermatitis, erythema multiforme, increased sweating, eczema, exanthema
Very rare:	Stevens-Johnson Syndrome, toxic epidermal necrolysis

Musculoskeletal, connective tissue and bone disorders

Rare:	Arthralgia, myalgia

Renal and urinary disorders

Uncommon:	Blood creatinine increased
Rare:	Interstitial nephritis, renal failure
Very rare:	Blood urea nitrogen increased

General disorders and administration site conditions

Uncommon:	Fever, injection site reaction
Rare:	Rigors, tiredness, oedema

Piperacillin therapy has been associated with an increased incidence of fever and rash in cystic fibrosis patients.

4.9 Overdose

There have been post-marketing reports of overdose with TAZOCIN. The majority of those events experienced including nausea, vomiting, and diarrhoea have also been reported with the usual recommended dosages. Patients may experience neuromuscular excitability or convulsions if higher than recommended doses are given intravenously (particularly in the presence of renal failure).

Treatment of Intoxication

No specific antidote is known.

Treatment should be supportive and symptomatic according to the patient's clinical presentation. In the event of an emergency, all required intensive medical measures are indicated as in the case of piperacillin.

Excessive serum concentrations of either piperacillin or tazobactam may be reduced by haemodialysis.

In case of motor excitability or convulsions, anticonvulsive agents (e.g. diazepam or barbiturates) may be indicated.

In case of severe, anaphylactic reactions, the usual counter-measures are to be initiated.

5. PHARMACOLOGICAL PROPERTIES

5.1 Pharmacodynamic properties

ATC Code: J01CR05

Pharmacotherapeutic group: Beta-lactam antibacterials, penicillins

Piperacillin, a broad spectrum, semisynthetic penicillin active against many gram-positive and gram-negative aerobic and anaerobic bacteria, exerts bactericidal activity by inhibition of both septum and cell wall synthesis. Tazobactam, a triazolylmethyl penicillanic acid sulphone, is a potent inhibitor of many β-lactamases, in particular the plasmid mediated enzymes which commonly cause resistance to penicillins and cephalosporins including third-generation cephalosporins. The presence of tazobactam in the TAZOCIN formulation enhances and extends the antibiotic spectrum of piperacillin to include many β-lactamase producing bacteria normally resistant to it and other β-lactam antibiotics. Thus, TAZOCIN combines the properties of a broad spectrum antibiotic and a β-lactamase inhibitor.

TAZOCIN is highly active against piperacillin-sensitive micro-organisms as well as many β-lactamase producing, piperacillin-resistant micro-organisms. TAZOCIN also acts synergistically with aminoglycosides against certain strains of *Pseudomonas aeruginosa*.

The prevalence of acquired resistance may vary geographically and with time for selected species. Local information of resistance is desirable, particularly when treating severe infections. Please refer to local guidelines for antibiotic sensitivity testing as appropriate.

The minimum inhibitory concentration (MIC) breakpoints separating susceptible from intermediately susceptible and intermediately susceptible from resistant organisms are suggested as follows:

(see Table 1 on previous page)

Resistance has been mainly observed for *Staphylococcus epidermidis*, *Burkholderia cepacia*, *Citrobacter freundii*, *Enterobacter cloacae*, *Pseudomonas* and *Serratia* species, *Enterococcus avium*, *Enterococcus faecium*, *Propionibacterium acnes*, *Acinetobacter* species, *Enterobacter aerogenes*, *Stenotrophomonas maltophilia*, *Corynebacterium jeikeium*, *Staphylococcus aureus* (methicillin resistant), and *Staphylococcus* coagulase negative (methicillin resistant).

Organism susceptibility to TAZOCIN observed in the European clinical studies conducted in adults or children with various infections published from 1997 to 1999 have been summarised in the following table.

It must be noted that this information gives only an approximate guidance on the probability that a micro-organism will be susceptible to TAZOCIN.

ESTIMATED EUROPEAN RANGE OF MICROBIOLOGIC RESISTANCE TO TAZOCIN (PIPERACILLIN/TAZOBACTAM)

Susceptibilty (classification) Pathogen	**Resistance rate**[a]
Susceptible (Gram-Positive Aerobes)	
Brevibacterium species*	
*Corynebacterium xerosis**	
Corynebacterium species	
Enterococcus durans	
*Enterococcus faecalis**	0 - 8 %
Enterococcus species*	0 - 4 %
*Gemella haemolysans**	
*Gemella morbillorum**	
*Lactococcus lactis cremoris**	
*Propionibacterium granulosum**	
Propionibacterium species	
*Staphylococcus aureus, methicillin-susceptible**	0 - 12 %
*Staphylococcus epidermidis**	0 - 25 %
*Staphylococcus haemolyticus**	
*Staphylococcus hominis**	
*Staphylococcus saprophyticus**	
*Staphylococcus sciuri**	
*Staphylococcus xylosus**	
*Staphylococcus species, coagulase negative**	
Streptococcus agalactiae	2 %
*Streptococcus anginosus**	
*Streptococcus beta hemolysans non group A**	
*Streptococcus beta hemolysans group D**	
*Streptococcus constellatus**	
*Streptococcus gordonii**	
*Streptococcus intermedius**	
*Streptococcus milleri**	
*Streptococcus milleri-group**	
*Streptococcus mitis**	
*Streptococcus morbillorum**	
*Streptococcus oralis**	
*Streptococcus pneumoniae**	0 - 2 %
*Streptococcus pyogenes**	0 - 3 %
*Streptococcus sanguis**	
*Streptococcus viridans**	
*Streptococcus viridans group**	0 - 17 %
Streptococcus species*	
Susceptible (Gram-Negative Aerobes)	
Acinetobacter anitratus	0 - 25 %
*Acinetobacter lwoffii**	0 - 4 %
*Aeromonas sobria**	
Alcaligenens species*	
Branhamella catarrhalis	
Burkholderia cepacia	0 - 30 %
Citrobacter diversus	9 %
*Citrobacter farmeri**	
*Citrobacter freundii**	0 - 25 %
Citrobacter koseri	
Citrobacter species*	
*Eikenella corrodens**	
Enterobacter agglomerans	17 %
*Enterobacter cloacae**	0 - 25 %
Enterobacter species	11 - 17 %
*Escherichia coli**	0 - 15 %
*Escherichia hermannii**	0 - 3 %
Escherichia vulneris	
*Haemophilus influenzae**	0 - 3 %
Haemophilus parainfluenzae	0 - 2 %
Haemophilus species	
*Klebsiella ornithinolytica**	
*Klebsiella oxytoca**	3 - 19 %
*Klebsiella pneumoniae**	3 - 17 %
Klebsiella species	0 - 18 %
Morganella morganii	0 - 5 %
*Pasteurella multocida**	
Proteus, indole positive	0 - 4 %
*Proteus mirabilis**	0 - 4 %
*Proteus vulgaris**	0 - 8 %
Proteus species*	
Providencia stuartii	11 %
Providencia species	2 %
*Pseudomonas aeruginosa**	0 - 29 %
Pseudomonas fluorescens	22 %
Pseudomonas putida	20 %
Pseudomonas species	2 - 30 %
Salmonella arizonae	
Salmonella species	0 - 3 %
Serratia liquefaciens	12 - 22 %
*Serratia marcescens**	0 - 38 %
*Serratia odorifera**	
Serratia species*	0 - 48 %
Shigella boydii	
Shigella dysenteriae	
Shigella flexneri	
Shigella sonnei	

Susceptible (Gram-Positive Anaerobes)	
Bifidobacterium species*	
*Clostridium bifermentans**	
*Clostridium butyricum**	
*Clostridium cadaveris**	
*Clostridium clostridiforme**	
*Clostridium difficile**	
*Clostridium hastiforme**	
*Clostridium limosum**	
*Clostridium perfringens**	
*Clostridium ramosum**	
*Clostridium tertium**	
Clostridium species*	
Eubacterium aerofaciens	
*Eubacterium lentum**	
Eubacterium species	
*Peptococcus asaccharolyticus**	
Peptococcus species	
*Peptostreptococcus anaerobius**	
*Peptostreptococcus magnus**	
*Peptostreptococcus micros**	
*Peptostreptococcus prevotii**	
Peptostreptococcus species*	
Susceptible (Gram-Negative Anaerobes)	
*Bacteroides caccae**	0 - 2 %
*Bacteroides capillosus**	
*Bacteroides distasonis**	
*Bacteroides fragilis**	0 - 3 %
Bacteroides fragilis group	
*Bacteroides ovatus**	0 - 15 %
*Bacteroides putredinis**	
*Bacteroides stercoris**	
*Bacteroides thetaiotaomicron**	
*Bacteroides uniformis**	
*Bacteroides ureolyticus**	
*Bacteroides vulgatus**	
Bacteroides species*	0 - 4 %
*Fusobacterium necrophorum**	
*Fusobacterium nucleatum**	
*Fusobacterium varium**	
Fusobacterium species*	
*Porphyromonas asaccharolytica**	
*Porphyromonas gingivalis**	
Porphyromonas species*	
Prevotella bivia	
*Prevotella disiens**	
*Prevotella intermedia**	
*Prevotella melaninogenica**	
*Prevotella oralis**	
Prevotella species*	
Intermediate Susceptible (Gram-Positive Aerobes)	
*Enterococcus avium**	15 - 45 %
*Enterococcus faecium**	15 - 93 %
*Propionibacterium acnes**	50 %
Intermediate Susceptible (Gram-Negative Aerobes)	
*Acinetobacter baumannii**	16 - 63 %
Acinetobacter calcoaceticus	30 - 58 %
Acinetobacter species*	0 - 75 %
Enterobacter aerogenes	7 - 79 %
*Pseudomonas stutzeri**	50 %
Stenotrophomonas maltophilia	1 - 53 %
Resistant (Gram-Positive Aerobes)	
Corynebacterium jeikeium	100 %
Staphylococcus aureus (methicillin resistant)	100 %
Staphylococcus coagulase negative (methicillin resistant)	100 %

[a] When no range is given this indicates that all isolates are susceptible; one percentage number (without any range) means that the organism was cited in one study.

* Clinical efficacy has been demonstrated for susceptible isolates in paediatric appendicitis complicated by rupture with peritonitis and/or abscess formation.

5.2 Pharmacokinetic properties

Distribution

Peak piperacillin and tazobactam plasma concentrations are attained immediately after completion of an intravenous infusion or injection. Piperacillin plasma levels produced when given with tazobactam are similar to those attained when equivalent doses of piperacillin are administered alone.

There is a greater proportional (approximately 28%) increase in plasma levels of piperacillin and tazobactam with increasing dose over the dosage range of 250mg tazobactam/2g piperacillin to 500mg tazobactam/4g piperacillin.

Both piperacillin and tazobactam are 20 to 30% bound to plasma proteins. The protein binding of either piperacillin or tazobactam is unaffected by the presence of the other compound. Protein binding of the tazobactam metabolite is negligible.

TAZOCIN is widely distributed in tissue and body fluids including intestinal mucosa, gallbladder, lung, bile and bone.

Biotransformation

Piperacillin is metabolised to a minor microbiologically active desethyl metabolite. Tazobactam is metabolised to a single metabolite which has been found to be microbiologically inactive.

Elimination

Piperacillin and tazobactam are eliminated by the kidney via glomerular filtration and tubularsecretion.

Piperacillin is excreted rapidly as unchanged drug with 68% of the administered dose appearing in the urine. Tazobactam and its metabolite are eliminated primarily by renal excretion with 80% of the administered dose appearing as unchanged drug and the remainder as the single metabolite. Piperacillin, tazobactam, and desethyl piperacillin are also secreted into the bile.

Following single or multiple doses of TAZOCIN to healthy subjects, the plasma half-life of piperacillin and tazobactam ranged from 0.7 to 1.2 hours and was unaffected by dose or duration of infusion. The elimination half-lives of both piperacillin and tazobactam are increased with decreasing renal clearance.

There are no significant changes in piperacillin pharmacokinetics due to tazobactam. Piperacillin appears to reduce the rate of elimination of tazobactam.

Impaired Renal Function

The half-lives of piperacillin and tazobactam increase with decreasing creatinine clearance. The increase is two-fold and four-fold for piperacillin and tazobactam, respectively, at creatinine clearance of below 20ml/min compared to patients with normal function.

Haemodialysis removes 30% to 50% of TAZOCIN with an additional 5% of the tazobactam dose removed as the tazobactam metabolite. Peritoneal dialysis removes approximately 6% and 21% of the piperacillin and tazobactam doses, respectively, with up to 18% of the tazobactam dose removed as the tazobactam metabolite.

Impaired Liver Function

Plasma concentrations of piperacillin and tazobactam are prolonged in hepatically impaired patients. The half-life of piperacillin and of tazobactam increases by approximately 25% and 18%, respectively, in patients with hepatic cirrhosis compared to healthy subjects. However, dosage adjustments in patients with hepatic impairment are not necessary.

5.3 Preclinical safety data

Preclinical mutagenicity and reproduction studies reveal no special hazards for humans.

Carcinogenicity studies have not been conducted with piperacillin, tazobactam, or the combination.

6. PHARMACEUTICAL PARTICULARS

6.1 List of excipients

TAZOCIN contains no excipients or preservatives.

6.2 Incompatibilities

Whenever TAZOCIN is used concurrently with another antibiotic (e.g. aminoglycosides), the drugs must be administered separately. The mixing of TAZOCIN with an aminoglycoside in vitro can result in substantial inactivation of the aminoglycoside.

TAZOCIN should not be mixed with other drugs in a syringe or infusion bottle since compatibility has not been established.

TAZOCIN should be administered through an infusion set separately from any other drugs unless compatibility is proven.

Because of chemical instability, TAZOCIN should not be used with solutions containing only sodium bicarbonate.

Lactated Ringer's solution is not compatible with TAZOCIN.

TAZOCIN should not be added to blood products or albumin hydrolysates.

6.3 Shelf life

Vials containing sterile powder for injection: 24 months.

6.4 Special precautions for storage

Do not store above 25°C. Store in the original container.

To reduce the risk of microbial contamination TAZOCIN should be used immediately. However, when prepared under aseptic conditions, reconstituted and/or diluted TAZOCIN in vials, syringes or I.V. bags has demonstrated chemical and physical stability for 24 hours when stored in a refrigerator at 2-8 °C.

If not used immediately, in use storage times and conditions prior to administration are the responsibility of the user. Unused solution should be discarded.

6.5 Nature and contents of container

Type I or III glass vial with butyl rubber stopper and aluminium/plastic seal containing TAZOCIN 2.25g or TAZOCIN 4.5g, boxed singly.

Infusion pack containing: One vial made of type I glass with a butyl rubber stopper and violet aluminium/plastic seal containing 4.5g TAZOCIN; a 50ml type III glass bottle with a butyl rubber stopper and blue aluminium plastic seal containing Water For Injections BP; and a transfer needle.

6.6 Instructions for use and handling

Reconstitution Directions

Intravenous Injection

Each vial of TAZOCIN 2.25g should be reconstituted with 10ml of one of the following diluents. Each vial of TAZOCIN 4.5g should be reconstituted with 20ml of one of the following diluents:

- Sterile Water for Injection
- 0.9% Sodium Chloride for Injection

Swirl until dissolved. Intravenous injection should be given over at least 3-5 minutes.

Intravenous Infusion

Each vial of TAZOCIN 2.25g should be reconstituted with 10ml of one of the above diluents. Each vial of TAZOCIN 4.5g should be reconstituted with 20ml of one of the above diluents.

The reconstituted solution should be further diluted to at least 50ml with one of the reconstitution diluents, or with Dextrose 5% in Water.

Displacement Volume

Each gram of TAZOCIN lyophilised powder has a displacement volume of 0.7ml.

2.25g TAZOCIN will displace 1.58ml

4.5g TAZOCIN will displace 3.15ml

7. MARKETING AUTHORISATION HOLDER

John Wyeth & Brother Limited

Trading as:

Wyeth Pharmaceuticals

Huntercombe Lane South

Taplow

Maidenhead

Berkshire SL6 0PH

UK

8. MARKETING AUTHORISATION NUMBER(S)

TAZOCIN 2.25g PL 00011/0292

TAZOCIN 4.5g PL 00011/0293

9. DATE OF FIRST AUTHORISATION/RENEWAL OF THE AUTHORISATION

Tazocin 2.25g: 30 January 2004

Tazocin 4.5g: 30 January 2004

10. DATE OF REVISION OF THE TEXT

2 March 2005

*Trade marks

Tegretol Chewtabs 100mg, 200mg, Tegretol Tablets 100mg, 200mg, 400mg

(Cephalon UK Limited)

1. NAME OF THE MEDICINAL PRODUCT

Tegretol® Tablets 100mg, 200mg and 400mg

Tegretol® Chewtabs 100mg and 200mg

2. QUALITATIVE AND QUANTITATIVE COMPOSITION

The active ingredient is 5-Carbamoyl-5-H-dibenz(b,f)azepine.

Each uncoated tablet contains 100mg, 200mg or 400mg carbamazepine Ph.Eur.

Each chewtab contains 100mg or 200mg carbamazepine Ph.Eur.

3. PHARMACEUTICAL FORM

100mg Tablets: The tablets are white, round, flat, uncoated tablets with bevelled edges, having a breakline on one face and impressed TEGRETOL 100 on the other.

200mg Tablets: The tablets are white, round, flat, uncoated tablets with bevelled edges, having a breakline on one face and impressed TEGRETOL 200 on the other.

400mg Tablets: The tablets are white, flat, rod-shaped tablets with bevelled edges. One side bears the imprint "CG/CG", the other "LR/LR" and both sides are scored.

100mg Chewtabs: The tablets are pale orange, square shaped chewable tablets, with a pronounced orange odour, embossed with "T" on one side and impressed with Tegretol 100 on the other.

200mg Chewtabs: The tablets are pale orange, square shaped chewable tablets, with a pronounced orange odour, embossed with "T" on one side and impressed with Tegretol 200 on the other.

4. CLINICAL PARTICULARS

4.1 Therapeutic indications

Epilepsy - generalised tonic-clonic and partial seizures.

Note: Tegretol is not usually effective in absences (petit mal) and myoclonic seizures. Moreover, anecdotal evidence suggests that seizure exacerbation may occur in patients with atypical absences.

The paroxysmal pain of trigeminal neuralgia.

For the prophylaxis of manic-depressive psychosis in patients unresponsive to lithium therapy.

4.2 Posology and method of administration

Tegretol is given orally, usually in two or three divided doses. Tegretol may be taken during, after or between meals, with a little liquid e.g. a glass of water.

The chewtabs should be chewed before swallowing, preferably with a little liquid to wash down possible remnants of the tablets.

The chewtabs are particularly suitable for children and adults who have difficulty in swallowing tablets.

Epilepsy:

Adults: It is advised that with all formulations of Tegretol, a gradually increasing dosage scheme is used and this should be adjusted to suit the needs of the individual patient. It may be helpful to monitor the plasma concentration of carbamazepine to establish the optimum dose (see Pharmacokinetics, Precautions and Interactions).

Tegretol should be taken in a number of divided doses although initially 100-200mg once or twice daily is recommended. This may be followed by a slow increase until the best response is obtained, often 800-1200mg daily. In some instances, 1600mg or even 2000mg daily may be necessary.

Elderly: Due to the potential for drug interactions, the dosage of Tegretol should be selected with caution in elderly patients.

Children: It is advised that with all formulations of Tegretol, a gradually increasing dosage scheme is used and this should be adjusted to suit the needs of the individual patient. It may be helpful to monitor the plasma concentration of carbamazepine to establish the optimum dose, (see Pharmacokinetics, Precautions and Interactions).

Usual dosage 10-20mg/kg bodyweight daily taken in several divided doses.

Tegretol tablets are not recommended for very young children.

1-5 years: 2-4 × 100mg Chewtabs per day, where appropriate

5-10 years: 2-3 × 200mg tablets per day, to be taken in divided doses.

10-15 years: 3-5 × 200mg tablets per day, to be taken in several divided doses.

Wherever possible, anti-epileptic agents should be prescribed as the sole anti-epileptic agent but if used in polytherapy the same incremental dosage pattern is advised.

When Tegretol is added to existing antiepileptic therapy, this should be done gradually while maintaining or, if necessary, adapting the dosage of the other antiepileptic(s) (see 4.5 **Interaction with other Medicaments and other forms of Interaction**).

Trigeminal neuralgia:

Slowly raise the initial dosage of 200-400mg daily (100mg twice daily in elderly patients) until freedom from pain is achieved (normally at 200mg 3-4 times daily). In the majority of patients a dosage of 200mg 3 or 4 times a day is sufficient to maintain a pain free state. In some instances, doses of 1600mg Tegretol daily may be needed. However, once the pain is in remission, the dosage should be gradually reduced to the lowest possible maintenance level.

For the prophylaxis of manic depressive psychosis in patients unresponsive to lithium therapy:

Initial starting dose of 400mg daily, in divided doses, increasing gradually until symptoms are controlled or a total of 1600mg given in divided doses is reached. The usual dosage range is 400-600mg daily, given in divided doses.

4.3 Contraindications

Known hypersensitivity to carbamazepine or structurally related drugs, (e.g. tricyclic antidepressants) or any other component of the formulation. Patients with atrioventricular block, a history of previous bone marrow depression or a history of acute intermittent porphyria.

Because it is structurally related to tricyclic anti-depressants, the use of Tegretol is not recommended in combination with monoamine oxidase inhibitors (MAOIs); before administering Tegretol, MAOIs should be discontinued for a minimum of 2 weeks, or longer if the clinical situation permits.

4.4 Special warnings and special precautions for use

Warnings

Agranulocytosis and aplastic anaemia have been associated with Tegretol; however, due to the very low incidence of these conditions, meaningful risk estimates for Tegretol are difficult to obtain. The overall risk in the general untreated population has been estimated at 4.7 persons per million per year for agranulocytosis and 2.0 persons per million per year for aplastic anaemia.

Decreased platelet or white blood cell counts occur occasionally to frequently in association with the use of Tegretol. Nonetheless, complete pre-treatment blood counts, including platelets and possibly reticulocytes and serum iron, should be obtained as a baseline, and periodically thereafter.

Patients and their relatives should be made aware of early toxic signs and symptoms indicative of a potential haematological problem, as well as symptoms of dermatological or hepatic reactions. If reactions such as fever, sore throat, rash, ulcers in the mouth, easy bruising, petechial or purpuric haemorrhage appear, the patient should be advised to consult his physician immediately.

If the white blood cell or platelet count is definitely low or decreased during treatment, the patient and the complete blood count should be closely monitored (see Section 4.8 Undesirable Effects). However, treatment with Tegretol should be discontinued if the patient develops leucopenia which is severe, progressive or accompanied by clinical manifestations, e.g. fever or sore throat. Tegretol should also be discontinued if any evidence of significant bone marrow depression appears.

Liver function tests should also be performed before commencing treatment and periodically thereafter, particularly in patients with a history of liver disease and in elderly patients. The drug should be withdrawn immediately in cases of aggravated liver dysfunction or acute liver disease.

Some liver function tests in patients receiving carbamazepine may be found to be abnormal, particularly gamma glutamyl transferase. This is probably due to hepatic enzyme induction. Enzyme induction may also produce modest elevations in alkaline phosphatase. These enhancements of hepatic metabolising capacity are not an indication for the withdrawal of carbamazepine.

Severe hepatic reactions to carbamazepine occur very rarely. The development of signs and symptoms of liver dysfunction or active liver disease should be urgently evaluated and treatment with Tegretol suspended pending the outcome of the evaluation.

Mild skin reactions e.g. isolated macular or maculopapular exanthemata, are mostly transient and not hazardous, and they usually disappear within a few days or weeks, either during the continued course of treatment or following a decrease in dosage; however, the patient should be kept under close surveillance and a worsening rash or accompanying symptoms are an indication for the immediate withdrawal of Tegretol.

If signs and symptoms suggestive of severe skin reactions (e.g. Stevens-Johnson syndrome, Lyell's syndrome (toxic epidermal necrolysis)) appear, Tegretol should be withdrawn at once.

Tegretol should be used with caution in patients with mixed seizures which include absences, either typical or atypical. In all these conditions, Tegretol may exacerbate seizures. In case of exacerbation of seizures, Tegretol should be discontinued.

An increase in seizure frequency may occur during switchover from an oral formulation to suppositories.

Abrupt withdrawal of Tegretol may precipitate seizures:

If treatment with Tegretol has to be withdrawn abruptly, the changeover to another anti-epileptic drug should if necessary be effected under the cover of a suitable drug (e.g. diazepam i.v., rectal; or phenytoin i.v.).

Cross-hypersensitivity can occur between carbamazepine and oxcarbazepine (Trileptal) in approximately 25 – 30% of the patients.

Cross-hypersensitivity can occur between carbamazepine and phenytoin.

Isolated reports of impaired male fertility and/or abnormal spermatogenesis are on file. A causal relationship has not been established.

Tegretol and oestrogen and/or progestogen preparations

Due to hepatic enzyme induction, Tegretol may cause failure of the therapeutic effect of oestrogen and/or progestogen containing products. This may result in failure of contraception, recurrence of symptoms or breakthrough bleeding or spotting.

Patients taking Tegretol and requiring oral contraception should receive a preparation containing not less than 50μg oestrogen or use of some alternative non-hormonal method of contraception should be considered.

Although correlations between dosages and plasma levels of carbamazepine, and between plasma levels and clinical efficacy or tolerability are rather tenuous, monitoring of the plasma levels may be useful in the following conditions: dramatic increase in seizure frequency/verification of patient compliance; during pregnancy; when treating children or adolescents; in suspected absorption disorders; in suspected toxicity when more than one drug is being used (see 4.5 **Interaction with other Medicaments and other forms of Interaction**).

There have been a few cases of neonatal seizures and/or respiratory depression associated with maternal Tegretol and other concomitant anti-epileptic drug use. A few cases of neonatal vomiting, diarrhoea and/or decreased feeding have also been reported in association with maternal Tegretol use. These reactions may represent a neonatal withdrawal syndrome.

Precautions

Tegretol should be prescribed only after a critical benefit-risk appraisal and under close monitoring in patients with a history of cardiac, hepatic or renal damage, adverse haematological reactions to other drugs, or interrupted courses of therapy with Tegretol.

Baseline and periodic complete urinalysis and BUN determinations are recommended.

Tegretol has shown mild anticholinergic activity; patients with increased intraocular pressure should therefore be warned and advised regarding possible hazards.

The possibility of activation of a latent psychosis and, in elderly patients, of confusion or agitation should be borne in mind.

4.5 Interaction with other medicinal products and other forms of Interaction

Cytochrome P450 3A4 (CYP 3A4) is the main enzyme catalysing formation of carbamazepine 10, 11-epoxide. Co-administration of inhibitors of CYP 3A4 may result in increased plasma concentrations which could induce adverse reactions. Co-administration of CYP 3A4 inducers might increase the rate of Tegretol metabolism, thus leading to a potential decrease in carbamazepine serum level and potential decrease in the therapeutic effect.

Similarly, discontinuation of a CYP34A inducer may decrease the rate of metabolism of carbamazepine, leading to an increase in carbamazepine plasma levels.

Agents that may raise Tegretol plasma levels:

Isoniazid, verapamil, diltiazem, ritonavir, dextropropoxyphene, viloxazine, fluoxetine, fluvoxamine, possibly cimetidine, acetazolamide, danazol, nicotinamide (in adults, only in high dosage), nefazodone, macrolide antibiotics (e.g. erythromycin, clarithromycin), azoles (e.g. itraconazole, ketoconazole, fluconazole), terfenadine, loratadine, grapefruit juice, protease inhibitors for HIV treatment (e.g. ritonavir). Since raised plasma carbamazepine levels may result in adverse reactions (e.g. dizziness, drowsiness, ataxia, diplopia), the dosage of Tegretol should be adjusted accordingly and/or the plasma levels monitored.

Agents that may decrease Tegretol plasma levels:

Phenobarbitone, phenytoin, primidone, or theophylline, rifampicin, cisplatin or doxorubicin and, although the data are partly contradictory, possibly also clonazepam or valproic acid, oxcarbazepine. Mefloquine may antagonise the anti-epileptic effect of Tegretol. On the other hand, valproic acid and primidone have been reported to raise the plasma level of the pharmacologically active carbamazepine 10, 11-epoxide metabolite. The dose of Tegretol may consequently have to be adjusted.

Isotretinoin has been reported to alter the bioavailability and/or clearance of carbamazepine and carbamazepine-10, 11-epoxide; carbamazepine plasma concentrations should be monitored.

Serum levels of carbamazepine can be reduced by concomitant use of the herbal remedy St John's wort (*Hypericum perforatum*).

Effect of Tegretol on plasma levels of concomitant agents:

Carbamazepine may lower the plasma level, diminish or even abolish the activity of certain drugs. The dosage of the following drugs may have to be adjusted to clinical requirement: levothyroxine, clobazam, clonazepam, ethosuximide, primidone, valproic acid, alprazolam, corticosteroids, (e.g. prednisolone, dexamethasone); cyclosporin, digoxin, doxycycline; dihydropyridine derivatives, e.g. felodipine and isradipine; indinavir, saquinavir, ritonavir, haloperidol, imipramine, methadone, tramadol, products containing oestrogens and/or progestogens (alternative contraceptive methods should be considered) see Section 4.4 **Special Warnings and Precautions for Use**, gestrinone, tibolone, toremifene, theophylline, oral anticoagulants (warfarin), lamotrigine, tiagabine, topiramate, tricyclic antidepressants (e.g. imipramine, amitriptyline, nortriptyline, clomipramine), clozapine, oxcarbazepine, olanzapine, itraconazole and risperidone.

Plasma phenytoin levels have been reported both to be raised and to be lowered by carbamazepine, and plasma mephenytoin levels have been reported in rare instances to increase.

Combinations to be taken into consideration:

Co-administration of carbamazepine and paracetamol may reduce the bioavailability of paracetamol/acetaminophen.

Concomitant use of carbamazepine and isoniazid has been reported to increase isoniazid-induced hepatotoxicity.

The combination of lithium and carbamazepine may cause enhanced neurotoxicity in spite of lithium plasma concentrations being within the therapeutic range. Combined use of carbamazepine with metoclopramide or major tranquillisers, e.g. haloperidol, thioridazine, may also result in an increase in neurological side-effects.

Because it (carbamazepine) is structurally related to tricyclic anti-depressants, the use of Tegretol is not recommended in combination with monoamine oxidase inhibitors (MAOIs); before administering Tegretol, MAOIs should be discontinued for a minimum of 2 weeks, or longer if the clinical situation permits.

Concomitant medication with Tegretol and some diuretics (hydrochlorothiazide, furosemide) may lead to symptomatic hyponatraemia.

Carbamazepine may antagonise the effects of non-depolarising muscle relaxants (e.g. pancuronium); their dosage should be raised and patients monitored closely for a more rapid recovery from neuromuscular blockade than expected.

Tegretol, like other psychoactive drugs, may reduce alcohol tolerance; it is therefore advisable for the patient to abstain from alcohol.

4.6 Pregnancy and lactation

In animals (mice, rats and rabbits) oral administration of carbamazepine during organogenesis led to increased embryo mortality at a daily doses which caused maternal toxicity (above 200mg/kg b.w. daily i.e. 20 times the usual human dosage). In the rat there was also some evidence of abortion at 300mg/kg body weight daily. Near-term rat foetuses showed growth retardation, again at maternally toxic doses. There was no evidence of teratogenic potential in the three animal species tested but, in one study using mice, carbamazepine (40-240 mg/kg b.w. daily orally) caused defects (mainly dilatation of cerebral ventricles in 4.7% of exposed foetuses as compared with 1.3% in controls).

Pregnant women with epilepsy should be treated with special care.

In women of childbearing age Tegretol should, wherever possible, be prescribed as monotherapy, because the incidence of congenital abnormalities in the offspring of women treated with a combination of anti-epileptic drugs is greater than in those of mothers receiving the individual drugs as monotherapy.

If pregnancy occurs in a woman receiving Tegretol, or if the problem of initiating treatment with Tegretol arises during pregnancy, the drug's potential benefits must be carefully weighed against its possible hazards, particularly in the first three months of pregnancy. Minimum effective doses should be given and monitoring of plasma levels is recommended.

Offspring of epileptic mothers with untreated epilepsy are known to be more prone to developmental disorders, including malformations. The possibility that carbamazepine, like all major anti-epileptic drugs, increases the risk has been reported, although conclusive evidence from controlled studies with carbamazepine monotherapy is lacking. However, there are reports on developmental disorders and malformations, including spina bifida, and also other congenital anomalies e.g. craniofacial defects, cardiovascular malformations and anomalies involving various body systems, have been reported in association with Tegretol. Patients should be counselled regarding the possibility of an increased risk of malformations and given the opportunity of antenatal screening.

Folic acid deficiency is known to occur in pregnancy. Anti-epileptic drugs have been reported to aggravate deficiency. This deficiency may contribute to the increased incidence of birth defects in the offspring of treated epileptic women. Folic acid supplementation has therefore been recommended before and during pregnancy.

Vitamin K_1 to be given to the mother during the last weeks of pregnancy as well as to the new-born to prevent bleeding disorders in the offspring, has also been recommended.

Use during lactation:

Carbamazepine passes into the breast milk (about 25-60% of the plasma concentrations). The benefits of breast-feeding should be weighed against the remote possibility of adverse effects occurring in the infant. Mothers taking Tegretol may breast-feed their infants, provided the infant is observed for possible adverse reactions (e.g. excessive somnolence, allergic skin reaction).

4.7 Effects on ability to drive and use machines

The patient's ability to react may be impaired by dizziness and drowsiness caused by Tegretol, especially at the start of treatment or in connection with dose adjustments; patients should therefore exercise due caution when driving a vehicle or operating machinery.

4.8 Undesirable effects

Particularly at the start of treatment with Tegretol, or if the initial dosage is too high, or when treating elderly patients, certain types of adverse reaction occur very commonly or commonly, e.g. CNS adverse reactions (dizziness, headache, ataxia, drowsiness, fatigue, diplopia); gastrointestinal disturbances (nausea, vomiting), as well as allergic skin reactions.

The dose-related adverse reactions usually abate within a few days, either spontaneously or after a transient dosage reduction. The occurrence of CNS adverse reactions may be a manifestation of relative overdosage or significant fluctuation in plasma levels. In such cases it is advisable to monitor the plasma levels and divide the daily dosage into smaller (i.e. 3-4) fractional doses.

Frequency estimate: very common ≥ 10%, common ≥ 1% to < 10%; uncommon ≥ 0.1% to < 1%; rare ≥ 0.01% to < 0.1%; very rare < 0.01%

Central nervous system:

Neurological:

Very common: Dizziness, ataxia, drowsiness, fatigue.

Common: Headache, diplopia, accommodation disorders (e.g. blurred vision).

Uncommon: Abnormal involuntary movements (e.g. tremor, asterixis, dystonia, tics); nystagmus.

Rare: Orofacial dyskinesia, oculomotor disturbances, speech disorders (e.g. dysarthria or slurred speech), choreoathetotic disorders, peripheral neuritis, paraesthesia, muscle weakness, and paretic symptoms.

Cases of neuroleptic malignant syndrome have been reported. The causative role of carbamazepine in inducing or contributing to the development of a neuromalignant syndrome, especially in conjunction with neuroleptics, is unclear.

Psychiatric:

Rare: Hallucinations (visual or acoustic), depression, loss of appetite, restlessness, aggressive behaviour, agitation, confusion.

Very rare: Activation of psychosis.

Skin and appendages:

Very common: Allergic skin reactions, urticaria, which may be severe.

Uncommon: Exfoliative dermatitis and erythroderma.

Rare: Lupus erythematosus-like syndrome, pruritus.

Very rare: Stevens-Johnson syndrome, toxic epidermal necrolysis, photosensitivity, erythema multiforme and nodosum, alterations in skin pigmentation, purpura, acne, sweating, hair loss.

Very rare cases of hirsutism have been reported, but the causal relationship is not clear.

Blood:

Very common: Leucopenia.

Common: Thrombocytopenia, eosinophilia.

Rare: Leucocytosis, lymphadenopathy, folic acid deficiency.

Very rare: Agranulocytosis, aplastic anaemia, pure red cell aplasia, megaloblastic anaemia, acute intermittent porphyria, reticulocytosis, and possibly haemolytic anaemia.

Liver:

Very common: Elevated gamma-GT (due to hepatic enzyme induction), usually not clinically relevant.

Common: Elevated alkaline phosphatase.

Uncommon: Elevated transaminases.

Rare: Hepatitis of cholestatic, parenchymal (hepatocellular) or mixed type, jaundice.

Very rare: Granulomatous hepatitis. Hepatic failure.

Gastro-intestinal tract:

Very common: Nausea, vomiting.

Common: Dryness of the mouth, with suppositories rectal irritation may occur.

Uncommon: Diarrhoea or constipation.

Rare: Abdominal pain.

Very rare: Glossitis, stomatitis, pancreatitis.

Hypersensitivity reactions:

Rare: A delayed multi-organ hypersensitivity disorder with fever, skin rashes, vasculitis, lymphadenopathy, disorders mimicking lymphoma, arthralgia, leucopenia, eosinophilia, hepato-splenomegaly and abnormal liver function tests, occurring in various combinations. Other organs may also be affected (e.g. liver, lungs, kidneys, pancreas, myocardium, colon).

Very rare: Aseptic meningitis, with myoclonus and peripheral eosinophilia; anaphylactic reaction, angioedema.

Treatment must be discontinued immediately if such hypersensitivity reactions occur.

Cardiovascular system:

Rare: Disturbances of cardiac conduction, hypertension or hypotension.

Very rare: Bradycardia, arrhythmias, AV-block with syncope, collapse, congestive heart failure, aggravation of coronary artery disease, thrombophlebitis, thromboembolism.

Endocrine system and metabolism:

Common: Oedema, fluid retention, weight increase, hyponatraemia and reduced plasma osmolality due to an antidiuretic hormone (ADH)-like effect, leading in rare cases to water intoxication accompanied by lethargy, vomiting, headache, mental confusion, neurological abnormalities.

Very rare: Increase in prolactin with or without clinical symptoms such as galactorrhoea, gynaecomastia, abnormal thyroid function tests; decreased l-thyroxin (FT4, T4, T3) and increased TSH, usually without clinical manifestations, disturbances of bone metabolism (decrease in plasma calcium and 25-OH-cholecalciferol), leading to osteomalacia, elevated levels of cholesterol, including HDL cholesterol and triglycerides.

Urogenital system:

Very rare: Interstitial nephritis, renal failure, renal dysfunction (e.g. albuminuria, haematuria, oliguria and elevated BUN/ azotaemia), urinary frequency, urinary retention, sexual disturbances/impotence.

Sense organs:

Very rare: Taste disturbances; lens opacities, conjunctivitis, hearing disorders, e.g. tinnitus, hyperacusis, hypoacusis, change in pitch perception.

Musculoskeletal system:

Very rare: Arthralgia, muscle pain or cramp.

Respiratory tract:

Very rare: Pulmonary hypersensitivity characterised e.g. by fever, dyspnoea, pneumonitis or pneumonia.

4.9 Overdose

Signs and symptoms

The presenting signs and symptoms of overdosage involve the central nervous, cardiovascular or respiratory systems.

Central nervous system: CNS depression; disorientation, somnolence, agitation, hallucination, coma; blurred vision, slurred speech, dysarthria, nystagmus, ataxia, dyskinesia, initially hyperreflexia, later hyporeflexia; convulsions, psychomotor disturbances, myoclonus, hypothermia, mydriasis.

Respiratory system: Respiratory depression, pulmonary oedema.

Cardiovascular system: Tachycardia, hypotension and at times hypertension, conduction disturbance with widening of QRS complex; syncope in association with cardiac arrest.

Gastro-intestinal system: Vomiting, delayed gastric emptying, reduced bowel motility.

Renal function: Retention of urine, oliguria or anuria; fluid retention, water intoxication due to ADH-like effect of carbamazepine.

Laboratory findings: Hyponatraemia, possibly metabolic acidosis, possibly hyperglycaemia, increased muscle creatinine phosphokinase.

Treatment

There is no specific antidote.

Management should initially be guided by the patient's clinical condition; admission to hospital. Measurement of the plasma level to confirm carbamazepine poisoning and to ascertain the size of the overdose.

Evacuation of the stomach, gastric lavage, and administration of activated charcoal. Delay in evacuating the stomach may result in delayed absorption, leading to relapse during recovery from intoxication. Supportive medical care in an intensive care unit with cardiac monitoring and careful correction of electrolyte imbalance.

Special recommendations:

Hypotension: Administer dopamine or dobutamine i.v.

Disturbances of cardiac rhythm: To be handled on an individual basis.

Convulsions: Administer a benzodiazepine (e.g. diazepam) or another anticonvulsant, e.g. phenobarbitone (with caution because of increased respiratory depression) or paraldehyde.

Hyponatraemia (water intoxication): Fluid restriction and slow and careful NaCl 0.9% infusion i.v. These measures may be useful in preventing brain damage.

Charcoal haemoperfusion has been recommended. Forced diuresis, haemodialysis, and peritoneal dialysis have been reported not to be effective.

Relapse and aggravation of symptomatology on the 2nd and 3rd day after overdose, due to delayed absorption, should be anticipated.

5. PHARMACOLOGICAL PROPERTIES

5.1 Pharmacodynamic properties

Therapeutic class: Anti-epileptic, neurotropic and psychotropic agent; (ATC Code: N03 AX 1). Dibenzazepine derivative.

As an antiepileptic agent its spectrum of activity embraces: partial seizures (simple and complex) with and without secondary generalisation; generalised tonic-clonic seizures, as well as combinations of these types of seizures.

The mechanism of action of carbamazepine, the active substance of Tegretol, has only been partially elucidated. Carbamazepine stabilises hyperexcited nerve membranes, inhibits repetitive neuronal discharges, and reduces synaptic propagation of excitatory impulses. It is conceivable that prevention of repetitive firing of sodium-dependent action potentials in depolarised neurons via use- and voltage-dependent blockade of sodium channels may be its main mechanism of action.

Whereas reduction of glutamate release and stabilisation of neuronal membranes may account for the antiepileptic effects, the depressant effect on dopamine and noradrenaline turnover could be responsible for the antimanic properties of carbamazepine.

5.2 Pharmacokinetic properties

Absorption

Carbamazepine is absorbed almost completely but relatively slowly from the tablets. The conventional tablets yield mean peak plasma concentrations of the unchanged substance within 12 hours (chewable tablets 6 hours; syrup 2 hours) following single oral doses. With respect to the amount of active substance absorbed, there is no clinically relevant difference between the oral dosage forms. After a single oral dose of 400mg carbamazepine (tablets) the mean peak concentration of unchanged carbamazepine in the plasma is approx. 4.5μg/ml.

The bioavailability of Tegretol in various oral formulations has been shown to lie between 85-100%.

Ingestion of food has no significant influence on the rate and extent of absorption, regardless of the dosage form of Tegretol.

Steady-state plasma concentrations of carbamazepine are attained within about 1-2 weeks, depending individually upon auto-induction by carbamazepine and hetero-induction by other enzyme-inducing drugs, as well as on pre-treatment status, dosage, and duration of treatment.

Different preparations of carbamazepine may vary in bioavailability; to avoid reduced effect or risk of breakthrough seizures or excessive side effects, it may be prudent to avoid changing the formulation.

Distribution

Carbamazepine is bound to serum proteins to the extent of 70-80%. The concentration of unchanged substance in cerebrospinal fluid and saliva reflects the non-protein bound portion in plasma (20-30%). Concentrations in breast milk were found to be equivalent to 25-60% of the corresponding plasma levels.

Carbamazepine crosses the placental barrier. Assuming complete absorption of carbamazepine, the apparent volume of distribution ranges from 0.8 to 1.9 L/kg.

Elimination

The elimination half-life of unchanged carbamazepine averages approx. 36 hours following a single oral dose, whereas after repeated administration it averages only 16-24 hours (auto-induction of the hepatic mono-oxygenase system), depending on the duration of the medication. In patients receiving concomitant treatment with other enzyme-inducing drugs (e.g. phenytoin, phenobarbitone), half-life values averaging 9-10 hours have been found.

The mean elimination half-life of the 10, 11-epoxide metabolite in the plasma is about 6 hours following single oral doses of the epoxide itself.

After administration of a single oral dose of 400mg carbamazepine, 72% is excreted in the urine and 28% in the faeces. In the urine, about 2% of the dose is recovered as unchanged drug and about 1% as the pharmacologically active 10, 11-epoxide metabolite. Carbamazepine is metabolised in the liver, where the epoxide pathway of biotransformation is the most important one, yielding the 10, 11-transdiol derivative and its glucuronide as the main metabolites.

Cytochrome P450 3A4 has been identified as the major isoform responsible for the formation of carbamazepine 10, 11-epoxide from carbamazepine. 9-Hydroxy-methyl-10-carbamoyl acridan is a minor metabolite related to this pathway. After a single oral dose of carbamazepine about 30% appears in the urine as end-products of the epoxide pathway.

Other important biotransformation pathways for carbamazepine lead to various monohydroxylated compounds, as well as to the N-glucuronide of carbamazepine.

Characteristics in patients

The steady-state plasma concentrations of carbamazepine considered as "therapeutic range" vary considerably inter-individually; for the majority of patients a range between 4-12μg/ml corresponding to 17-50μmol/l has been reported. Concentrations of carbamazepine 10, 11-epoxide (pharmacologically active metabolite): about 30% of carbamazepine levels.

Owing to enhanced carbamazepine elimination, children may require higher doses of carbamazepine (in mg/kg) than adults to maintain therapeutic concentrations.

There is no indication of altered pharmacokinetics of carbamazepine in elderly patients as compared with young adults.

No data are available on the pharmacokinetics of carbamazepine in patients with impaired hepatic or renal function.

5.3 Preclinical safety data

In rats treated with carbamazepine for two years, the incidence of tumours of the liver was found to be increased. The significance of these findings relative to the use of carbamazepine in humans is, at present, unknown. Bacterial and mammalian mutagenicity studies yielded negative results.

6. PHARMACEUTICAL PARTICULARS

6.1 List of excipients

Tegretol Tablets: Each uncoated tablet contains aerosil 200 standard, avicel PH 102, nymcel ZSB-10 and magnesium stearate.

Tegretol Chewtabs: Each tablet contains crospovidone, red iron oxide (E 172), yellow iron oxide (E 172), magnesium stearate, orange flavour 51,941/AP, sorbitol, stearic acid

6.2 Incompatibilities

None known

6.3 Shelf life

Five years

6.4 Special precautions for storage

Tegretol 400mg tablets are protected from moisture. Medicines should be kept out of reach of children.

Tegretol Chewtabs: Protect from heat. (Store below 30°C).

6.5 Nature and contents of container

Tegretol 100mg come in PVC/PVdC blister packs of 84 tablets, and securitainers of 500 tablets.

Tegretol 200mg come in PVC/PVdC blister packs of 84.

Tegretol 400mg come in PVC blister packs of 56.

Tegretol Chewtabs 100mg come in aluminium blister packs of 56 tablets.

Tegretol Chewtabs 200mg come in aluminium blister packs of 56 tablets.

6.6 Instructions for use and handling

None

7. MARKETING AUTHORISATION HOLDER

Novartis Pharmaceuticals UK Limited

Trading as Geigy Pharmaceuticals

Frimley Business Park

Frimley

Camberley

Surrey

GU16 7SR

England.

8. MARKETING AUTHORISATION NUMBER(S)

Tegretol 100mg Tablets: PL 00101/0461

Tegretol 200mg Tablets: PL 00101/0462

Tegretol 400mg Tablets: PL 00101/0463

Tegretol Chewtabs 100mg: PL 00101/0454

Tegretol Chewtabs 200mg: PL 00101/0455

9. DATE OF FIRST AUTHORISATION/RENEWAL OF THE AUTHORISATION

Tegretol 100mg Tablets: 4 July 1997/ 28 July 1999

Tegretol 200mg Tablets: 4 July 1997 / 28 July 1999

Tegretol 400mg Tablets: 4 July 1997

Tegretol Chewtabs 100mg: 4 July 1997 / 26 March 2001

Tegretol Chewtabs 200mg: 4 July 1997 / 26 March 2001

10. DATE OF REVISION OF THE TEXT

Tegretol Tablets: 31 January 2003

Tegretol Chewtabs: 31 January 2003

Legal category:

POM

Tegretol Liquid 100 mg/5ml

(Cephalon UK Limited)

1. NAME OF THE MEDICINAL PRODUCT

Tegretol® Liquid 100mg/5ml

2. QUALITATIVE AND QUANTITATIVE COMPOSITION

The active ingredient is 5-Carbamoyl-5-H-dibenz(b,f)azepine.

The liquid contains 100mg carbamazepine Ph.Eur. in each 5ml.

3. PHARMACEUTICAL FORM

Tegretol Liquid is a white oral suspension.

4. CLINICAL PARTICULARS

4.1 Therapeutic indications

Epilepsy - generalised tonic-clonic and partial seizures.

Note: Tegretol is not usually effective in absences (petit mal) and myoclonic seizures. Moreover, anecdotal evidence suggests that seizure exacerbation may occur in patients with atypical absences.

The paroxysmal pain of trigeminal neuralgia.

For the prophylaxis of manic-depressive psychosis in patients unresponsive to lithium therapy.

4.2 Posology and method of administration

Tegretol Liquid is given orally, usually in two or three divided doses.

Tegretol Liquid (the liquid should be shaken before use) may be taken during, after or between meals.

Since a given dose of Tegretol Liquid will produce higher peak levels than the same dose in tablet form, it is advisable to start with low doses of the liquid and to increase them slowly so as to avoid adverse effects on the central nervous system such as dizziness and lethargy.

When switching a patient from tablets to liquid the same overall dose may be used but in smaller, more frequent, doses.

Epilepsy:

Adults: It is advised that with all formulations of Tegretol, a gradually increasing dosage scheme is used and this should be adjusted to suit the needs of the individual patient. It may be helpful to monitor the plasma concentration of carbamazepine to establish the optimum dose (see Pharmacokinetics, Precautions and Interactions).

Tegretol should be taken in a number of divided doses although initially 100-200mg once to twice daily is recommended. This may be followed by a slow increase until the best response is obtained, often 800-1200mg daily. In some instances, 1600mg or even 2000mg daily may be necessary.

Elderly: Due to the potential for drug interactions, the dosage of Tegretol should be selected with caution in elderly patients.

Children: It is advised that with all formulations of Tegretol, a gradually increasing dosage scheme is used and this should be adjusted to suit the needs of the individual patient. It may be helpful to monitor the plasma concentration of carbamazepine to establish the optimum dose (see Pharmacokinetics, Precautions and Interactions).

Usual dosage 10-20mg/kg bodyweight daily in several divided doses.

Age up to 1 year: 5-10ml liquid per day

1-5 years: 10-20ml liquid per day

5-10 years: 20-30ml liquid per day to be taken in divided doses

10-15 years: 30-50ml liquid per day to be taken in several divided doses.

Wherever possible anti-epileptic agents should be prescribed as the sole drug anti-epileptic agent but if used in polytherapy, the same incremental dosage pattern is advised.

When Tegretol is added to existing antiepileptic therapy, this should be done gradually while maintaining or, if necessary, adapting the dosage of the other antiepileptic(s) (see 4.5 **Interaction with other Medicaments and other forms of Interaction**).

Trigeminal neuralgia:

Slowly raise the initial dosage of 200-400mg daily (100mg twice daily in elderly patients) until freedom from pain is achieved (normally at 200mg 3-4 times daily). In the majority of patients a dosage of 200mg 3 or 4 times a day is sufficient to maintain a pain free state. In some instances, doses of 1600mg Tegretol daily may be needed. However, once the pain is in remission, the dosage should be gradually reduced to the lowest possible maintenance level.

For the prophylaxis of main depressive psychosis in patients unresponsive to lithium therapy:

Initial starting dose of 100-200mg daily, in divided doses, increasing gradually until symptoms are controlled or a total of 1600mg given in divided doses is reached. The usual dosage range is 400-600mg daily, given in divided doses.

4.3 Contraindications

Known hypersensitivity to carbamazepine or structurally related drugs (e.g. tricyclic antidepressants) or any other component of the formulation.

Patients with atrioventricular block, a history of bone marrow depression or a history of acute intermittent porphyria.

Because it is structurally related to tricyclic anti-depressants, the use of Tegretol is not recommended in combination with monoamine oxidase inhibitors (MAOIs); before administering Tegretol, MAOIs should be discontinued for a minimum of 2 weeks, or longer if the clinical situation permits.

4.4 Special warnings and special precautions for use

Warnings

Agranulocytosis and aplastic anaemia have been associated with Tegretol; however, due to the very low incidence of these conditions, meaningful risk estimates for Tegretol are difficult to obtain. The overall risk in the general untreated population has been estimated at 4.7 persons per million per year for agranulocytosis and 2.0 persons per million per year for aplastic anaemia.

Decreased platelet or white blood cell counts occur occasionally to frequently in association with the use of Tegretol. Nonetheless, complete pre-treatment blood counts, including platelets and possibly reticulocytes and serum iron, should be obtained as a baseline, and periodically thereafter.

Patients and their relatives should be made aware of early toxic signs and symptoms indicative of a potential haematological problem, as well as symptoms of dermatological or hepatic reactions. If reactions such as fever, sore throat, rash, ulcers in the mouth, easy bruising, petechial or purpuric haemorrhage appear, the patient should be advised to consult his physician immediately.

If the white blood cell or platelet count is definitely low or decreased during treatment, the patient and the complete blood count should be closely monitored (see Section 4.8 **Undesirable Effects**). However, treatment with Tegretol should be discontinued if the patient develops leucopenia which is severe, progressive or accompanied by clinical manifestations, e.g. fever or sore throat. Tegretol should also be discontinued if any evidence of significant bone marrow depression appears.

Liver function tests should also be performed before commencing treatment and periodically thereafter, particularly in patients with a history of liver disease and in elderly patients. The drug should be withdrawn immediately in cases of aggravated liver dysfunction or acute liver disease.

Some liver function tests in patients receiving carbamazepine may be found to be abnormal, particularly gamma glutamyl transferase. This is probably due to hepatic enzyme induction. Enzyme induction may also produce modest elevations in alkaline phosphatase. These enhancements of hepatic metabolising capacity are not an indication for the withdrawal of carbamazepine.

Severe hepatic reactions to carbamazepine occur very rarely. The development of signs and symptoms of liver dysfunction or active liver disease should be urgently evaluated and treatment with Tegretol suspended pending the outcome of the evaluation.

Mild skin reactions e.g. isolated macular or maculopapular exanthemata, are mostly transient and not hazardous, and they usually disappear within a few days or weeks, either during the continued course of treatment or following a decrease in dosage; however, the patient should be kept under close surveillance and a worsening rash or accompanying symptoms are an indication for the immediate withdrawal of Tegretol.

If signs and symptoms suggestive of severe skin reactions (e.g. Stevens-Johnson syndrome, Lyell's syndrome (toxic epidermal necrolysis)) appear, Tegretol should be withdrawn at once.

Tegretol should be used with caution in patients with mixed seizures which include absences, either typical or atypical. In all these conditions, Tegretol may exacerbate seizures. In case of exacerbation of seizures, Tegretol should be discontinued.

An increase in seizure frequency may occur during switchover from an oral formulation to suppositories.

Abrupt withdrawal of Tegretol may precipitate seizures:

If treatment with Tegretol has to be withdrawn abruptly, the changeover to another anti-epileptic drug should if necessary be effected under the cover of a suitable drug (e.g. diazepam i.v., rectal; or phenytoin i.v.).

Cross-hypersensitivity can occur between carbamazepine and oxcarbazepine (Trileptal) in approximately 25 – 30% of the patients.

Cross-hypersensitivity can occur between carbamazepine and phenytoin.

Isolated reports of impaired male fertility and/or abnormal spermatogenesis are on file. A causal relationship has not been established.

Tegretol and oestrogen and/or progestogen preparations

Due to hepatic enzyme induction, Tegretol may cause failure of the therapeutic effect of oestrogen and/or progestogen containing products. This may result in failure of contraception, recurrence of symptoms or breakthrough bleeding or spotting.

Patients taking Tegretol and requiring oral contraception should receive a preparation containing not less than 50μg oestrogen or use of some alternative non-hormonal method of contraception should be considered.

Although correlations between dosages and plasma levels of carbamazepine, and between plasma levels and clinical efficacy or tolerability are rather tenuous, monitoring of the plasma levels may be useful in the following conditions: dramatic increase in seizure frequency/verification of patient compliance; during pregnancy; when treating children or adolescents; in suspected absorption disorders; in suspected toxicity when more than one drug is being used (see 4.5 **Interaction with other Medicaments and other forms of Interaction**).

There have been a few cases of neonatal seizures and/or respiratory depression associated with maternal Tegretol and other concomitant anti-epileptic drug use. A few cases of neonatal vomiting, diarrhoea and/or decreased feeding have also been reported in association with maternal Tegretol use. These reactions may represent a neonatal withdrawal syndrome.

Precautions

Tegretol should be prescribed only after a critical benefit-risk appraisal and under close monitoring in patients with a history of cardiac, hepatic or renal damage, adverse haematological reactions to other drugs, or interrupted courses of therapy with Tegretol.

Baseline and periodic complete urinalysis and BUN determinations are recommended.

Tegretol has shown mild anticholinergic activity; patients with increased intraocular pressure should therefore be warned and advised regarding possible hazards.

The possibility of activation of a latent psychosis and, in elderly patients, of confusion or agitation should be borne in mind.

4.5 Interaction with other medicinal products and other forms of Interaction

Cytochrome P450 3A4 (CYP 3A4) is the main enzyme catalysing formation of carbamazepine 10, 11-epoxide. Co-administration of inhibitors of CYP 3A4 may result in increased plasma concentrations which could induce adverse reactions. Co-administration of CYP 3A4 inducers might increase the rate of Tegretol metabolism, thus leading to a potential decrease in carbamazepine serum level and potential decrease in the therapeutic effect.

Similarly, discontinuation of a CYP34A inducer may decrease the rate of metabolism of carbamazepine, leading to an increase in carbamazepine plasma levels.

Agents that may raise Tegretol plasma levels:

Isoniazid, verapamil, diltiazem, ritonavir, dextropropoxyphene, viloxazine, fluoxetine, fluvoxamine, possibly cimetidine, acetazolamide, danazol, nicotinamide (in adults, only in high dosage), nefazodone, macrolide antibiotics (e.g. erythromycin, clarithromycin), azoles (e.g. itraconazole, ketoconazole, fluconazole), terfenadine, loratadine grapefruit juice, protease inhibitors for HIV treatment (e.g. ritonavir). Since raised plasma carbamazepine levels may result in adverse reactions (e.g. dizziness, drowsiness, ataxia, diplopia), the dosage of Tegretol should be adjusted accordingly and/or the plasma levels monitored.

Agents that may decrease Tegretol plasma levels:

Phenobarbitone, phenytoin, primidone, or theophylline, rifampicin, cisplatin or doxorubicin and, although the data are partly contradictory, possibly also clonazepam or valproic acid, oxcarbazepine. Mefloquine may antagonise the anti-epileptic effect of Tegretol. On the other hand, valproic acid and primidone have been reported to raise the plasma level of the pharmacologically active carbamazepine 10, 11-epoxide metabolite. The dose of Tegretol may consequently have to be adjusted.

Isotretinoin has been reported to alter the bioavailability and/or clearance of carbamazepine and carbamazepine-10, 11-epoxide; carbamazepine plasma concentrations should be monitored.

Serum levels of carbamazepine can be reduced by concomitant use of the herbal remedy St John's wort (Hypericum perforatum).

Effect of Tegretol on plasma levels of concomitant agents:

Carbamazepine may lower the plasma level, diminish or even abolish the activity of certain drugs. The dosage of the following drugs may have to be adjusted to clinical requirement: levothyroxine, clobazam, clonazepam, ethosuximide, primidone, valproic acid, alprazolam, corticosteroids, (e.g. prednisolone, dexamethasone); cyclosporin, digoxin, doxycycline; dihydropyridine derivatives, e.g. felodipine and isradipine; indinavir, saquinavir, ritonavir, haloperidol, imipramine, methadone, tramadol, products containing oestrogens and/or progestogens (alternative contraceptive methods should be considered) see Section 4.4 **Special Warnings and Precautions for Use**, gestrinone, tibolone, toremifene, theophylline, oral anticoagulants (warfarin), lamotrigine, tiagabine, topiramate, tricyclic antidepressants (e.g. imipramine, amitriptyline, nortriptyline, clomipramine), clozapine, oxcarbazepine, olanzapine, itraconazole and risperidone.

Plasma phenytoin levels have been reported both to be raised and to be lowered by carbamazepine, and plasma mephenytoin levels have been reported in rare instances to increase.

Combinations to be taken into consideration:

Co-administration of carbamazepine and paracetamol may reduce the bioavailability of paracetamol/acetaminophen.

Concomitant use of carbamazepine and isoniazid has been reported to increase isoniazid-induced hepatotoxicity.

The combination of lithium and carbamazepine may cause enhanced neurotoxicity in spite of lithium plasma concentrations being within the therapeutic range. Combined use of carbamazepine with metoclopramide or major tranquillisers, e.g. haloperidol, thioridazine, may also result in an increase in neurological side-effects.

Because it (carbamazepine) is structurally related to tricyclic anti-depressants, the use of Tegretol is not recommended in combination with monoamine oxidase inhibitors (MAOIs); before administering Tegretol, MAOIs should be discontinued for a minimum of 2 weeks, or longer if the clinical situation permits.

Concomitant medication with Tegretol and some diuretics (hydrochlorothiazide, furosemide) may lead to symptomatic hyponatraemia.

Carbamazepine may antagonise the effects of non-depolarising muscle relaxants (e.g. pancuronium); their dosage should be raised and patients monitored closely for a more rapid recovery from neuromuscular blockade than expected.

Tegretol, like other psychoactive drugs, may reduce alcohol tolerance; it is therefore advisable for the patient to abstain from alcohol.

4.6 Pregnancy and lactation

In animals (mice, rats and rabbits) oral administration of carbamazepine during organogenesis led to increased embryo mortality at a daily doses which caused maternal toxicity (above 200mg/kg b.w. daily i.e. 20 times the usual human dosage). In the rat there was also some evidence of abortion at 300mg/kg body weight daily. Near-term rat foetuses showed growth retardation, again at maternally toxic doses. There was no evidence of teratogenic potential in the three animal species tested but, in one study using mice, carbamazepine (40-240 mg/kg b.w. daily orally) caused defects (mainly dilatation of cerebral ventricles in 4.7% of exposed foetuses as compared with 1.3% in controls).

Pregnant women with epilepsy should be treated with special care.

In women of childbearing age Tegretol should, wherever possible, be prescribed as monotherapy, because the incidence of congenital abnormalities in the offspring of women treated with a combination of anti-epileptic drugs is greater than in those of mothers receiving the individual drugs as monotherapy.

If pregnancy occurs in a woman receiving Tegretol, or if the problem of initiating treatment with Tegretol arises during pregnancy, the drug's potential benefits must be carefully weighed against its possible hazards, particularly in the first three months of pregnancy. Minimum effective doses should be given and monitoring of plasma levels is recommended.

Offspring of epileptic mothers with untreated epilepsy are known to be more prone to developmental disorders, including malformations. The possibility that carbamazepine, like all major anti-epileptic drugs, increases the risk has been reported, although conclusive evidence from controlled studies with carbamazepine monotherapy is lacking. However, there are reports on developmental disorders and malformations, including spina bifida, and also other congenital anomalies e.g. craniofacial defects, cardiovascular malformations and anomalies involving various body systems, have been reported in association with Tegretol. Patients should be counselled regarding the possibility of an increased risk of malformations and given the opportunity of antenatal screening.

Folic acid deficiency is known to occur in pregnancy. Anti-epileptic drugs have been reported to aggravate deficiency. This deficiency may contribute to the increased incidence of birth defects in the offspring of treated epileptic women. Folic acid supplementation has therefore been recommended before and during pregnancy.

Vitamin K_1 to be given to the mother during the last weeks of pregnancy as well as to the new-born to prevent bleeding disorders in the offspring, has also been recommended.

Use during lactation:

Carbamazepine passes into the breast milk (about 25-60% of the plasma concentrations). The benefits of breast-feeding should be weighed against the remote possibility of adverse effects occurring in the infant. Mothers taking Tegretol may breast-feed their infants, provided the infant is observed for possible adverse reactions (e.g. excessive somnolence, allergic skin reaction).

4.7 Effects on ability to drive and use machines

The patient's ability to react may be impaired by dizziness and drowsiness caused by Tegretol, especially at the start of treatment or in connection with dose adjustments;

patients should therefore exercise due caution when driving a vehicle or operating machinery.

4.8 Undesirable effects
Particularly at the start of treatment with Tegretol, or if the initial dosage is too high, or when treating elderly patients, certain types of adverse reaction occur very commonly or commonly, e.g. CNS adverse reactions (dizziness, headache, ataxia, drowsiness, fatigue, diplopia); gastrointestinal disturbances (nausea, vomiting), as well as allergic skin reactions.

The dose-related adverse reactions usually abate within a few days, either spontaneously or after a transient dosage reduction. The occurrence of CNS adverse reactions may be a manifestation of relative overdosage or significant fluctuation in plasma levels. In such cases it is advisable to monitor the plasma levels and divide the daily dosage into smaller (i.e. 3-4) fractional doses.

Frequency estimate: very common $\geqslant$ 10%, common $\geqslant$ 1% to < 10%; uncommon $\geqslant$ 0.1% to < 1%; rare $\geqslant$ 0.01% to < 0.1%; very rare < 0.01%

Central nervous system:

Neurological:

Very common: Dizziness, ataxia, drowsiness, fatigue.

Common: Headache, diplopia, accommodation disorders (e.g. blurred vision).

Uncommon: Abnormal involuntary movements (e.g. tremor, asterixis, dystonia, tics); nystagmus.

Rare: Orofacial dyskinesia, oculomotor disturbances, speech disorders (e.g. dysarthria or slurred speech), choreoathetotic disorders, peripheral neuritis, paraesthesia, muscle weakness, and paretic symptoms.

Cases of neuroleptic malignant syndrome have been reported. The causative role of carbamazepine in inducing or contributing to the development of a neuromalignant syndrome, especially in conjunction with neuroleptics, is unclear.

Psychiatric:

Rare: Hallucinations (visual or acoustic), depression, loss of appetite, restlessness, aggressive behaviour, agitation, confusion.

Very rare: Activation of psychosis.

Skin and appendages:

Very common: Allergic skin reactions, urticaria, which may be severe.

Uncommon: Exfoliative dermatitis and erythroderma.

Rare: Lupus erythematosus-like syndrome, pruritus.

Very rare: Stevens-Johnson syndrome, toxic epidermal necrolysis, photosensitivity, erythema multiforme and nodosum, alterations in skin pigmentation, purpura, acne, sweating, hair loss.

Very rare cases of hirsutism have been reported, but the causal relationship is not clear.

Blood:

Very common: Leucopenia.

Common: Thrombocytopenia, eosinophilia.

Rare: Leucocytosis, lymphadenopathy, folic acid deficiency.

Very rare: Agranulocytosis, aplastic anaemia, pure red cell aplasia, megaloblastic anaemia, acute intermittent porphyria, reticulocytosis, and possibly haemolytic anaemia.

Liver:

Very common: Elevated gamma-GT (due to hepatic enzyme induction), usually not clinically relevant.

Common: Elevated alkaline phosphatase.

Uncommon: Elevated transaminases.

Rare: Hepatitis of cholestatic, parenchymal (hepatocellular) or mixed type, jaundice.

Very rare: Granulomatous hepatitis. Hepatic failure.

Gastro-intestinal tract:

Very common: Nausea, vomiting.

Common: Dryness of the mouth, with suppositories rectal irritation may occur.

Uncommon: Diarrhoea or constipation.

Rare: Abdominal pain.

Very rare: Glossitis, stomatitis, pancreatitis.

Hypersensitivity reactions:

Rare: A delayed multi-organ hypersensitivity disorder with fever, skin rashes, vasculitis, lymphadenopathy, disorders mimicking lymphoma, arthralgia, leucopenia, eosinophilia, hepato-splenomegaly and abnormal liver function tests, occurring in various combinations. Other organs may also be affected (e.g. liver, lungs, kidneys, pancreas, myocardium, colon).

Very rare: Aseptic meningitis, with myoclonus and peripheral eosinophilia; anaphylactic reaction, angioedema.

Treatment must be discontinued immediately if such hypersensitivity reactions occur.

Cardiovascular system:

Rare: Disturbances of cardiac conduction, hypertension or hypotension.

Very rare: Bradycardia, arrhythmias, AV-block with syncope, collapse, congestive heart failure, aggravation of coronary artery disease, thrombophlebitis, thromboembolism.

Endocrine system and metabolism:

Common: Oedema, fluid retention, weight increase, hyponatraemia and reduced plasma osmolality due to an antidiuretic hormone (ADH)-like effect, leading in rare cases to water intoxication accompanied by lethargy, vomiting, headache, mental confusion, neurological abnormalities.

Very rare: Increase in prolactin with or without clinical symptoms such as galactorrhoea, gynaecomastia, abnormal thyroid function tests; decreased I-thyroxin (FT4, T4, T3) and increased TSH, usually without clinical manifestations, disturbances of bone metabolism (decrease in plasma calcium and 25-OH-cholecalciferol), leading to osteomalacia, elevated levels of cholesterol, including HDL cholesterol and triglycerides.

Urogenital system:

Very rare: Interstitial nephritis, renal failure, renal dysfunction (e.g. albuminuria, haematuria, oliguria and elevated BUN/ azotaemia), urinary frequency, urinary retention, sexual disturbances/impotence.

Sense organs:

Very rare: Taste disturbances; lens opacities, conjunctivitis, hearing disorders, e.g. tinnitus, hyperacusis, hypoacusis, change in pitch perception.

Musculoskeletal system:

Very rare: Arthralgia, muscle pain or cramp.

Respiratory tract:

Very rare: Pulmonary hypersensitivity characterised e.g. by fever, dyspnoea, pneumonitis or pneumonia.

4.9 Overdose
Signs and symptoms

The presenting signs and symptoms of overdosage involve the central nervous, cardiovascular or respiratory systems.

Central nervous system: CNS depression; disorientation, somnolence, agitation, hallucination, coma; blurred vision, slurred speech, dysarthria, nystagmus, ataxia, dyskinesia, initially hyperreflexia, later hyporeflexia; convulsions, psychomotor disturbances, myoclonus, hypothermia, mydriasis.

Respiratory system: Respiratory depression, pulmonary oedema.

Cardiovascular system: Tachycardia, hypotension and at times hypertension, conduction disturbance with widening of QRS complex; syncope in association with cardiac arrest.

Gastro-intestinal system: Vomiting, delayed gastric emptying, reduced bowel motility.

Renal function: Retention of urine, oliguria or anuria; fluid retention, water intoxication due to ADH-like effect of carbamazepine.

Laboratory findings: Hyponatraemia, possibly metabolic acidosis, possibly hyperglycaemia, increased muscle creatinine phosphokinase.

Treatment

There is no specific antidote.

Management should initially be guided by the patient's clinical condition; admission to hospital. Measurement of the plasma level to confirm carbamazepine poisoning and to ascertain the size of the overdose.

Evacuation of the stomach, gastric lavage, and administration of activated charcoal. Delay in evacuating the stomach may result in delayed absorption, leading to relapse during recovery from intoxication. Supportive medical care in an intensive care unit with cardiac monitoring and careful correction of electrolyte imbalance.

Special recommendations:

Hypotension: Administer dopamine or dobutamine i.v.

Disturbances of cardiac rhythm: To be handled on an individual basis.

Convulsions: Administer a benzodiazepine (e.g. diazepam) or another anticonvulsant, e.g. phenobarbitone (with caution because of increased respiratory depression) or paraldehyde.

Hyponatraemia (water intoxication): Fluid restriction and slow and careful NaCl 0.9% infusion i.v. These measures may be useful in preventing brain damage.

Charcoal haemoperfusion has been recommended. Forced diuresis, haemodialysis, and peritoneal dialysis have been reported not to be effective.

Relapse and aggravation of symptomatology on the 2nd and 3rd day after overdose, due to delayed absorption, should be anticipated.

5. PHARMACOLOGICAL PROPERTIES
5.1 Pharmacodynamic properties
Therapeutic class: Anti-epileptic, neurotropic and psychotropic agent; (ATC Code: N03 AX 1). Dibenzazepine derivative.

As an antiepileptic agent its spectrum of activity embraces: partial seizures (simple and complex) with and without secondary generalisation; generalised tonic-clonic seizures, as well as combinations of these types of seizures.

The mechanism of action of carbamazepine, the active substance of Tegretol, has only been partially elucidated. Carbamazepine stabilises hyperexcited nerve membranes, inhibits repetitive neuronal discharges, and reduces synaptic propagation of excitatory impulses. It is conceivable that prevention of repetitive firing of sodium-dependent action potentials in depolarised neurons via use- and voltage-dependent blockade of sodium channels may be its main mechanism of action.

Whereas reduction of glutamate release and stabilisation of neuronal membranes may account for the antiepileptic effects, the depressant effect on dopamine and noradrenaline turnover could be responsible for the antimanic properties of carbamazepine.

5.2 Pharmacokinetic properties
Absorption

Carbamazepine is absorbed almost completely but relatively slowly from the tablets. The conventional tablets yield mean peak plasma concentrations of the unchanged substance within 12 hours (liquid 2 hours) following single oral doses. With respect to the amount of active substance absorbed, there is no clinically relevant difference between the oral dosage forms. After a single oral dose of 400mg carbamazepine (tablets) the mean peak concentration of unchanged carbamazepine in the plasma is approx. 4.5μg/ml.

The bioavailability of Tegretol in various oral formulations has been shown to lie between 85-100%.

Ingestion of food has no significant influence on the rate and extent of absorption, regardless of the dosage form of Tegretol.

Steady-state plasma concentrations of carbamazepine are attained within about 1-2 weeks, depending individually upon auto-induction by carbamazepine and hetero-induction by other enzyme-inducing drugs, as well as on pre-treatment status, dosage, and duration of treatment.

Different preparations of carbamazepine may vary in bioavailability; to avoid reduced effect or risk of breakthrough seizures or excessive side effects, it may be prudent to avoid changing the formulation.

Distribution

Carbamazepine is bound to serum proteins to the extent of 70-80%. The concentration of unchanged substance in cerebrospinal fluid and saliva reflects the non-protein bound portion in plasma (20-30%). Concentrations in breast milk were found to be equivalent to 25-60% of the corresponding plasma levels.

Carbamazepine crosses the placental barrier. Assuming complete absorption of carbamazepine, the apparent volume of distribution ranges from 0.8 to 1.9 L/kg.

Elimination

The elimination half-life of unchanged carbamazepine averages approx. 36 hours following a single oral dose, whereas after repeated administration it averages only 16-24 hours (auto-induction of the hepatic mono-oxygenase system), depending on the duration of the medication. In patients receiving concomitant treatment with other enzyme-inducing drugs (e.g. phenytoin, phenobarbitone), half-life values averaging 9-10 hours have been found.

The mean elimination half-life of the 10, 11-epoxide metabolite in the plasma is about 6 hours following single oral doses of the epoxide itself.

After administration of a single oral dose of 400mg carbamazepine, 72% is excreted in the urine and 28% in the faeces. In the urine, about 2% of the dose is recovered as unchanged drug and about 1% as the pharmacologically active 10, 11-epoxide metabolite. Carbamazepine is metabolised in the liver, where the epoxide pathway of biotransformation is the most important one, yielding the 10, 11-transdiol derivative and its glucuronide as the main metabolites.

Cytochrome P450 3A4 has been identified as the major isoform responsible for the formation of carbamazepine 10, 11-epoxide from carbamazepine. 9-Hydroxy-methyl-10-carbamoyl acridan is a minor metabolite related to this pathway. After a single oral dose of carbamazepine about 30% appears in the urine as end-products of the epoxide pathway.

Other important biotransformation pathways for carbamazepine lead to various monohydroxylated compounds, as well as to the N-glucuronide of carbamazepine.

Characteristics in patients

The steady-state plasma concentrations of carbamazepine considered as "therapeutic range" vary considerably inter-individually; for the majority of patients a range between 4-12μg/ml corresponding to 17-50μmol/l has been reported. Concentrations of carbamazepine 10, 11-epoxide (pharmacologically active metabolite): about 30% of carbamazepine levels.

Owing to enhanced carbamazepine elimination, children may require higher doses of carbamazepine (in mg/kg) than adults to maintain therapeutic concentrations.

There is no indication of altered pharmacokinetics of carbamazepine in elderly patients as compared with young adults.

No data are available on the pharmacokinetics of carbamazepine in patients with impaired hepatic or renal function.

5.3 Preclinical safety data

In rats treated with carbamazepine for two years, the incidence of tumours of the liver was found to be increased. The significance of these findings relative to the use of carbamazepine in humans is, at present, unknown. Bacterial and mammalian mutagenicity studies yielded negative results.

6. PHARMACEUTICAL PARTICULARS

6.1 List of excipients

Cremophor S9, Avicel RC581, sorbitol solution 70%, saccharin sodium, Natrosol 250g, methyl hydroxybenzoate, propyl hydroxybenzoate, sorbic acid, propylene glycol, caramel flavour 52.929A (E150), purified water.

6.2 Incompatibilities

None known

6.3 Shelf life

Five years

6.4 Special precautions for storage

Protect from heat (store below 25°C). Keep container tightly closed.

6.5 Nature and contents of container

Tegretol Liquid comes in a 300ml amber glass bottle with a child resistant/tamper evident cap.

6.6 Instructions for use and handling

None

7. MARKETING AUTHORISATION HOLDER

Novartis Pharmaceuticals UK Limited

Trading as Geigy Pharmaceuticals

Frimley Business Park

Frimley

Camberley

Surrey

GU16 7SR

England.

8. MARKETING AUTHORISATION NUMBER(S)

PL 00101/0456

9. DATE OF FIRST AUTHORISATION/RENEWAL OF THE AUTHORISATION

4 July 1997 / 28 June 1999

10. DATE OF REVISION OF THE TEXT

31 January 2003

Legal Category

POM

Tegretol Retard Tablets 200mg, 400mg

(Cephalon UK Limited)

1. NAME OF THE MEDICINAL PRODUCT

Tegretol® Retard Tablets 200mg and 400mg

2. QUALITATIVE AND QUANTITATIVE COMPOSITION

The active ingredient is 5-Carbamoyl-5-H-dibenz(b,f)azepine.

Each coated tablet contains 200mg or 400mg carbamazepine Ph.Eur.

3. PHARMACEUTICAL FORM

The 200mg tablets are beige-orange, oval, slightly biconvex, coated tablets with a score on each side. One side bears the imprint "H/C", the other "C/G".

The 400mg tablets are brownish-orange, oval, slightly biconvex coated tablets with a score on each side. One side bears the imprint "ENE/ENE", the other "C/G".

4. CLINICAL PARTICULARS

4.1 Therapeutic indications

Epilepsy - generalised tonic-clonic and partial seizures. Tegretol Retard is indicated in newly diagnosed patients with epilepsy and in those patients who are uncontrolled or unable to tolerate their current anti-convulsant therapy.

Note: Carbamazepine is not usually effective in absences (petit mal) and myoclonic seizures. Moreover, anecdotal evidence suggests that seizure exacerbation may occur in patients with atypical absences.

The paroxysmal pain of trigeminal neuralgia.

For the prophylaxis of manic-depressive psychoses in patients unresponsive to lithium therapy.

4.2 Posology and method of administration

Tegretol Retard is given orally, generally in the same total daily dose as conventional Tegretol dosage forms but usually in two divided doses. In a few patients when changing from other oral dosage forms of Tegretol to Tegretol Retard the total daily dose may need to be increased, particularly when it is used in polytherapy. When starting treatment with Tegretol Retard in monotherapy, 100-200mg once or twice daily is recommended. This may be followed by a slow increase in dosage until the best response is obtained, often 800-1200mg daily. In some instances, 1600mg or even 2000mg daily may be necessary.

Tegretol Retard (either the whole or half divisible tablet as prescribed), should not be chewed but should be swallowed with a little liquid, before, during or between meals. The divisible tablet presentation enables flexibility of dosing to be achieved.

Epilepsy

Adults

It is advised that with all formulations of Tegretol, a gradually increasing dosage scheme is used and this should be adjusted to suit the needs of the individual patient. It may be helpful to monitor the plasma concentration of carbamazepine to establish the optimum dose (see Pharmacokinetics, Precautions and Interactions).

Elderly

Due to the potential for drug interactions, the dosage of Tegretol should be selected with caution in elderly patients.

Children

It is advised that with all formulations of Tegretol, a gradually increasing dosage scheme is used and this should be adjusted to suit the needs of the individual patient. It may be helpful to monitor the plasma concentration of carbamazepine to establish the optimum dose (see Pharmacokinetics, Precautions and Interactions).

Usual dosage 10-20mg/kg bodyweight daily in several divided doses.

Age

- up to 5 years: Tegretol Retard Tablets are not recommended
- 5-10 years: 400-600mg daily
- 10-15 years: 600-1000mg

Wherever possible, Tegretol Retard should be used as the sole drug anti-epileptic agent but if used in polytherapy, the same incremental dosage pattern is advised.

When Tegretol is added to existing antiepileptic therapy, this should be done gradually while maintaining or, if necessary, adapting the dosage of the other antiepileptic(s) (see 4.5 Interaction with other Medicaments and other forms of Interaction).

Trigeminal neuralgia

Slowly raise the initial dosage of 200-400mg daily (100mg twice daily in elderly patients) until freedom from pain is achieved (normally at 200mg 3-4 times daily). In the majority of patients a dosage of 200mg 3 or 4 times a day is sufficient to maintain a pain free state. In some instances, doses of 1600mg Tegretol daily may be needed. However, once the pain is in remission, the dosage should be gradually reduced to the lowest possible maintenance level.

For the prophylaxis of manic depressive psychosis in patients unresponsive to lithium therapy

Initial starting dose of 400mg daily, in divided doses, increasing gradually until symptoms are controlled or a total of 1600mg given in divided doses is reached. The usual dosage range is 400-600mg daily, given in divided doses.

4.3 Contraindications

Known hypersensitivity to carbamazepine or structurally related drugs e.g. tricyclic antidepressants or any other component of the formulation.

Patients with atrioventricular block, a history of bone marrow depression or a history of acute intermittent porphyria.

Because it is structurally related to tricyclic antidepressants, the use of Tegretol is not recommended in combination with monoamine oxidase inhibitors (MAOIs); before administering Tegretol, MAOIs should be discontinued for a minimum of 2 weeks, or longer if the clinical situation permits.

4.4 Special warnings and special precautions for use

Warnings

Agranulocytosis and aplastic anaemia have been associated with Tegretol; however, due to the very low incidence of these conditions, meaningful risk estimates for Tegretol are difficult to obtain. The overall risk in the general untreated population has been estimated at 4.7 persons per million per year for agranulocytosis and 2.0 persons per million per year for aplastic anaemia.

Decreased platelet or white blood cell counts occur occasionally to frequently in association with the use of Tegretol. Nonetheless, complete pre-treatment blood counts, including platelets and possibly reticulocytes and serum iron, should be obtained as a baseline, and periodically thereafter.

Patients and their relatives should be made aware of early toxic signs and symptoms indicative of a potential haematological problem, as well as symptoms of dermatological or hepatic reactions. If reactions such as fever, sore throat, rash, ulcers in the mouth, easy bruising, petechial or purpuric haemorrhage appear, the patient should be advised to consult his physician immediately.

If the white blood cell or platelet count is definitely low or decreased during treatment, the patient and the complete blood count should be closely monitored (see Section 4.8 Undesirable Effects). However, treatment with Tegretol should be discontinued if the patient develops leucopenia which is severe, progressive or accompanied by clinical manifestations, e.g. fever or sore throat. Tegretol should also be discontinued if any evidence of significant bone marrow depression appears.

Liver function tests should also be performed before commencing treatment and periodically thereafter, particularly in patients with a history of liver disease and in elderly patients. The drug should be withdrawn immediately in cases of aggravated liver dysfunction or acute liver disease.

Some liver function tests in patients receiving carbamazepine may be found to be abnormal, particularly gamma glutamyl transferase. This is probably due to hepatic enzyme induction. Enzyme induction may also produce modest elevations in alkaline phosphatase. These enhancements of hepatic metabolising capacity are not an indication for the withdrawal of carbamazepine.

Severe hepatic reactions to carbamazepine occur very rarely. The development of signs and symptoms of liver dysfunction or active liver disease should be urgently evaluated and treatment with Tegretol suspended pending the outcome of the evaluation.

Mild skin reactions e.g. isolated macular or maculopapular exanthemata, are mostly transient and not hazardous, and they usually disappear within a few days or weeks, either during the continued course of treatment or following a decrease in dosage; however, the patient should be kept under close surveillance and a worsening rash or accompanying symptoms are an indication for the immediate withdrawal of Tegretol.

If signs and symptoms suggestive of severe skin reactions (e.g. Stevens-Johnson syndrome, Lyell's syndrome (toxic epidermal necrolysis)) appear, Tegretol should be withdrawn at once.

Tegretol should be used with caution in patients with mixed seizures which include absences, either typical or atypical. In all these conditions, Tegretol may exacerbate seizures. In case of exacerbation of seizures, Tegretol should be discontinued.

An increase in seizure frequency may occur during switchover from an oral formulation to suppositories.

Abrupt withdrawal of Tegretol may precipitate seizures.

If treatment with Tegretol has to be withdrawn abruptly, the changeover to another anti-epileptic drug should, if necessary, be effected under the cover of a suitable drug (e.g. diazepam i.v., rectal; or phenytoin i.v.).

Cross-hypersensitivity can occur between carbamazepine and oxcarbazepine (Trileptal) in approximately 25 – 30% of the patients.

Cross-hypersensitivity can occur between carbamazepine and phenytoin.

Isolated reports of impaired male fertility and/or abnormal spermatogenesis are on file. A causal relationship has not been established.

Tegretol and oestrogen and/or progestogen preparations

Due to hepatic enzyme induction, Tegretol may cause failure of the therapeutic effect of oestrogen and/or progestogen containing products. This may result in failure of contraception, recurrence of symptoms or breakthrough bleeding or spotting.

Patients taking Tegretol and requiring oral contraception should receive a preparation containing not less than 50μg oestrogen or use of some alternative non-hormonal method of contraception should be considered.

Although correlations between dosages and plasma levels of carbamazepine, and between plasma levels and clinical efficacy or tolerability are rather tenuous, monitoring of the plasma levels may be useful in the following conditions: dramatic increase in seizure frequency/verification of patient compliance; during pregnancy; when treating children or adolescents; in suspected absorption disorders; in suspected toxicity when more than one drug is being used (see 4.5 Interaction with other Medicaments and other forms of Interaction).

There have been a few cases of neonatal seizures and/or respiratory depression associated with maternal Tegretol and other concomitant anti-epileptic drug use. A few cases of neonatal vomiting, diarrhoea and/or decreased feeding have also been reported in association with maternal Tegretol use. These reactions may represent a neonatal withdrawal syndrome.

Precautions

Tegretol should be prescribed only after a critical benefit-risk appraisal and under close monitoring in patients with a history of cardiac, hepatic or renal damage, adverse haematological reactions to other drugs, or interrupted courses of therapy with Tegretol.

Baseline and periodic complete urinalysis and BUN determinations are recommended.

Tegretol has shown mild anticholinergic activity; patients with increased intraocular pressure should therefore be warned and advised regarding possible hazards.

The possibility of activation of a latent psychosis and, in elderly patients, of confusion or agitation should be borne in mind.

4.5 Interaction with other medicinal products and other forms of Interaction

Cytochrome P450 3A4 (CYP 3A4) is the main enzyme catalysing formation of carbamazepine 10, 11-epoxide. Co-administration of inhibitors of CYP 3A4 may result in increased plasma concentrations which could induce adverse reactions. Co-administration of CYP 3A4 inducers might increase the rate of Tegretol metabolism, thus leading to a potential decrease in carbamazepine serum level and potential decrease in the therapeutic effect.

Similarly, discontinuation of a CYP3A4 inducer may decrease the rate of metabolism of carbamazepine, leading to an increase in carbamazepine plasma levels.

Agents that may raise Tegretol plasma levels

- Isoniazid
- Verapamil
- Diltiazem
- Ritonavir
- Dextropropoxyphene
- Viloxazine
- Fluoxetine
- Fluvoxamine
- Possibly cimetidine
- Acetazolamide
- Danazol
- Nicotinamide (in adults, only in high dosage)
- Nefazodone
- Macrolide antibiotics (e.g. erythromycin, clarithromycin)
- Azoles (e.g. itraconazole, ketoconazole, fluconazole)
- Terfenadine
- Loratadine
- Grapefruit juice
- Protease inhibitors for HIV treatment (e.g. ritonavir).

Since raised plasma carbamazepine levels may result in adverse reactions (e.g. dizziness, drowsiness, ataxia, diplopia), the dosage of Tegretol should be adjusted accordingly and/or the plasma levels monitored.

Agents that may decrease Tegretol plasma levels

- Phenobarbitone
- Phenytoin
- Primidone
- Theophylline
- Rifampicin
- Cisplatin
- Doxorubicin

and, although the data are partly contradictory, possibly also

- Clonazepam
- Valproic acid
- Oxcarbazepine.

Mefloquine may antagonise the anti-epileptic effect of Tegretol. On the other hand, valproic acid and primidone have been reported to raise the plasma level of the pharmacologically active carbamazepine 10, 11-epoxide metabolite. The dose of Tegretol may consequently have to be adjusted.

Isotretinoin has been reported to alter the bioavailability and/or clearance of carbamazepine and carbamazepine-10, 11-epoxide; carbamazepine plasma concentrations should be monitored.

Serum levels of carbamazepine can be reduced by concomitant use of the herbal remedy St John's wort (*Hypericum perforatum*).

Effect of Tegretol on plasma levels of concomitant agents

Carbamazepine may lower the plasma level, diminish or even abolish the activity of certain drugs.

The dosage of the following drugs may have to be adjusted to clinical requirement:

- Levothyroxine
- Clobazam
- Clonazepam
- Ethosuximide
- Primidone
- Valproic acid
- Alprazolam
- Corticosteroids, (e.g. prednisolone, dexamethasone)
- Cyclosporine
- Digoxin
- Doxycycline
- Dihydropyridine derivatives, e.g. felodipine and isradipine
- Indinavir
- Saquinavir
- Ritonavir
- Haloperidol
- Imipramine
- Methadone
- Tramadol
- Products containing oestrogens and/or progestogens (alternative contraceptive methods should be considered) see Section 4.4 "Special Warnings and Precautions for Use"
- Gestrinone
- Tibolone
- Toremifene
- Theophylline
- Oral anticoagulants (warfarin)
- Lamotrigine
- Tiagabine
- Topiramate
- Tricyclic antidepressants (e.g. imipramine, amitriptyline, nortriptyline, clomipramine)
- Clozapine
- Oxcarbazepine
- Olanzapine
- Itraconazole
- Risperidone.

Plasma phenytoin levels have been reported both to be raised and to be lowered by carbamazepine, and plasma mephenytoin levels have been reported in rare instances to increase.

Combinations to be taken into consideration

Co-administration of carbamazepine and paracetamol may reduce the bioavailability of paracetamol/acetaminophen.

Concomitant use of carbamazepine and isoniazid has been reported to increase isoniazid-induced hepatotoxicity.

The combination of lithium and carbamazepine may cause enhanced neurotoxicity in spite of lithium plasma concentrations being within the therapeutic range. Combined use of carbamazepine with metoclopramide or major tranquillisers, e.g. haloperidol, thioridazine, may also result in an increase in neurological side-effects.

Because it (carbamazepine) is structurally related to tricyclic anti-depressants, the use of Tegretol is not recommended in combination with monoamine oxidase inhibitors (MAOIs); before administering Tegretol, MAOIs should be discontinued for a minimum of 2 weeks, or longer if the clinical situation permits.

Concomitant medication with Tegretol and some diuretics (hydrochlorothiazide, furosemide) may lead to symptomatic hyponatraemia.

Carbamazepine may antagonise the effects of non-depolarising muscle relaxants (e.g. pancuronium); their dosage should be raised and patients monitored closely for a more rapid recovery from neuromuscular blockade than expected.

Tegretol, like other psychoactive drugs, may reduce alcohol tolerance; it is therefore advisable for the patient to abstain from alcohol.

4.6 Pregnancy and lactation

In animals (mice, rats and rabbits) oral administration of carbamazepine during organogenesis led to increased embryo mortality at a daily doses which caused maternal toxicity (above 200mg/kg b.w. daily i.e. 20 times the usual human dosage). In the rat there was also some evidence of abortion at 300mg/kg body weight daily. Near-term rat foetuses showed growth retardation, again at maternally toxic doses. There was no evidence of teratogenic potential in the three animal species tested but, in one study using mice, carbamazepine (40-240 mg/kg b.w. daily orally) caused defects (mainly dilatation of cerebral ventricles in 4.7% of exposed foetuses as compared with 1.3% in controls).

Pregnant women with epilepsy should be treated with special care.

In women of childbearing age Tegretol should, wherever possible, be prescribed as monotherapy, because the incidence of congenital abnormalities in the offspring of women treated with a combination of anti-epileptic drugs is greater than in those of mothers receiving the individual drugs as monotherapy.

If pregnancy occurs in a woman receiving Tegretol, or if the problem of initiating treatment with Tegretol arises during pregnancy, the drug's potential benefits must be carefully weighed against its possible hazards, particularly in the first three months of pregnancy. Minimum effective doses should be given and monitoring of plasma levels is recommended.

Offspring of epileptic mothers with untreated epilepsy are known to be more prone to developmental disorders, including malformations. The possibility that carbamazepine, like all major anti-epileptic drugs, increases the risk has been reported, although conclusive evidence from controlled studies with carbamazepine monotherapy is lacking. However, there are reports on developmental disorders and malformations, including spina bifida, and also other congenital anomalies e.g. craniofacial defects, cardiovascular malformations and anomalies involving various body systems, have been reported in association with Tegretol. Patients should be counselled regarding the possibility of an increased risk of malformations and given the opportunity of antenatal screening.

Folic acid deficiency is known to occur in pregnancy. Anti-epileptic drugs have been reported to aggravate deficiency. This deficiency may contribute to the increased incidence of birth defects in the offspring of treated epileptic women. Folic acid supplementation has therefore been recommended before and during pregnancy.

Vitamin K_1 to be given to the mother during the last weeks of pregnancy as well as to the new-born to prevent bleeding disorders in the offspring, has also been recommended.

Use during lactation

Carbamazepine passes into the breast milk (about 25-60% of the plasma concentrations). The benefits of breast-feeding should be weighed against the remote possibility of adverse effects occurring in the infant. Mothers taking Tegretol may breast-feed their infants, provided the infant is observed for possible adverse reactions (e.g. excessive somnolence, allergic skin reaction).

4.7 Effects on ability to drive and use machines

The patient's ability to react may be impaired by dizziness and drowsiness caused by Tegretol, especially at the start of treatment or in connection with dose adjustments; patients should therefore exercise due caution when driving a vehicle or operating machinery.

4.8 Undesirable effects

Particularly at the start of treatment with Tegretol, or if the initial dosage is too high, or when treating elderly patients, certain types of adverse reaction occur very commonly or commonly, e.g. CNS adverse reactions (dizziness, headache, ataxia, drowsiness, fatigue, diplopia); gastrointestinal disturbances (nausea, vomiting), as well as allergic skin reactions.

The dose-related adverse reactions usually abate within a few days, either spontaneously or after a transient dosage reduction. The occurrence of CNS adverse reactions may be a manifestation of relative overdosage or significant fluctuation in plasma levels. In such cases it is advisable to monitor the plasma levels and divide the daily dosage into smaller (i.e. 3-4) fractional doses.

Frequency estimate: very common $\geqslant$ 10%, common $\geqslant$ 1% to < 10%; uncommon $\geqslant$ 0.1% to < 1%; rare $\geqslant$ 0.01% to < 0.1%; very rare < 0.01%

Central nervous system:

Neurological:

Very common: Dizziness, ataxia, drowsiness, fatigue.

Common: Headache, diplopia, accommodation disorders (e.g. blurred vision).

Uncommon: Abnormal involuntary movements (e.g. tremor, asterixis, dystonia, tics); nystagmus.

Rare: Orofacial dyskinesia, oculomotor disturbances, speech disorders (e.g. dysarthria or slurred speech), choreoathetotic disorders, peripheral neuritis, paraesthesia, muscle weakness, and paretic symptoms.

Cases of neuroleptic malignant syndrome have been reported. The causative role of carbamazepine in inducing or contributing to the development of a neuromalignant syndrome, especially in conjunction with neuroleptics, is unclear.

Psychiatric:

Rare: Hallucinations (visual or acoustic), depression, loss of appetite, restlessness, aggressive behaviour, agitation, confusion.

Very rare: Activation of psychosis.

Skin and appendages:

Very common: Allergic skin reactions, urticaria, which may be severe.

Uncommon: Exfoliative dermatitis and erythroderma.

Rare: Lupus erythematosus-like syndrome, pruritus.

Very rare: Stevens-Johnson syndrome, toxic epidermal necrolysis, photosensitivity, erythema multiforme and nodosum, alterations in skin pigmentation, purpura, acne, sweating, hair loss.

Very rare cases of hirsutism have been reported, but the causal relationship is not clear.

Blood:

Very common: Leucopenia.

Common: Thrombocytopenia, eosinophilia.

Rare: Leucocytosis, lymphadenopathy, folic acid deficiency.

Very rare: Agranulocytosis, aplastic anaemia, pure red cell aplasia, megaloblastic anaemia, acute intermittent porphyria, reticulocytosis, and possibly haemolytic anaemia.

Liver:

Very common: Elevated gamma-GT (due to hepatic enzyme induction), usually not clinically relevant.

Common: Elevated alkaline phosphatase.

Uncommon: Elevated transaminases.

Rare: Hepatitis of cholestatic, parenchymal (hepatocellular) or mixed type, jaundice.

Very rare: Granulomatous hepatitis. Hepatic failure.

Gastro-intestinal tract:

Very common: Nausea, vomiting.

Common: Dryness of the mouth, with suppositories rectal irritation may occur.

Uncommon: Diarrhoea or constipation.

Rare: Abdominal pain.

Very rare: Glossitis, stomatitis, pancreatitis.

Hypersensitivity reactions:

Rare: A delayed multi-organ hypersensitivity disorder with fever, skin rashes, vasculitis, lymphadenopathy, disorders mimicking lymphoma, arthralgia, leucopenia, eosinophilia, hepato-splenomegaly and abnormal liver function tests, occurring in various combinations. Other organs may also be affected (e.g. liver, lungs, kidneys, pancreas, myocardium, colon).

Very rare: Aseptic meningitis, with myoclonus and peripheral eosinophilia; anaphylactic reaction, angioedema.

Treatment must be discontinued immediately if such hypersensitivity reactions occur.

Cardiovascular system:

Rare: Disturbances of cardiac conduction, hypertension or hypotension.

Very rare: Bradycardia, arrhythmias, AV-block with syncope, collapse, congestive heart failure, aggravation of coronary artery disease, thrombophlebitis, thromboembolism.

Endocrine system and metabolism:

Common: Oedema, fluid retention, weight increase, hyponatraemia and reduced plasma osmolality due to an antidiuretic hormone (ADH)-like effect, leading in rare cases to water intoxication accompanied by lethargy, vomiting, headache, mental confusion, neurological abnormalities.

Very rare: Increase in prolactin with or without clinical symptoms such as galactorrhoea, gynaecomastia, abnormal thyroid function tests; decreased l-thyroxine (FT4, T4, T3) and increased TSH, usually without clinical manifestations, disturbances of bone metabolism (decrease in plasma calcium and 25-OH-cholecalciferol), leading to osteomalacia, elevated levels of cholesterol, including HDL cholesterol and triglycerides.

Urogenital system:

Very rare: Interstitial nephritis, renal failure, renal dysfunction (e.g. albuminuria, haematuria, oliguria and elevated BUN/ azotaemia), urinary frequency, urinary retention, sexual disturbances/impotence.

Sense organs:

Very rare: Taste disturbances; lens opacities, conjunctivitis, hearing disorders, e.g. tinnitus, hyperacusis, hypoacusis, change in pitch perception.

Musculoskeletal system:

Very rare: Arthralgia, muscle pain or cramp.

Respiratory tract:

Very rare: Pulmonary hypersensitivity characterised e.g. by fever, dyspnoea, pneumonitis or pneumonia.

4.9 Overdose

Signs and symptoms

The presenting signs and symptoms of overdosage involve the central nervous, cardiovascular or respiratory systems.

Central nervous system

CNS depression; disorientation, somnolence, agitation, hallucination, coma; blurred vision, slurred speech, dysarthria, nystagmus, ataxia, dyskinesia, initially hyperreflexia, later hyporeflexia; convulsions, psychomotor disturbances, myoclonus, hypothermia, mydriasis.

Respiratory system

Respiratory depression, pulmonary oedema.

Cardiovascular system

Tachycardia, hypotension and at times hypertension, conduction disturbance with widening of QRS complex; syncope in association with cardiac arrest.

Gastro-intestinal system

Vomiting, delayed gastric emptying, reduced bowel motility.

Renal function

Retention of urine, oliguria or anuria; fluid retention, water intoxication due to ADH-like effect of carbamazepine.

Laboratory findings

Hyponatraemia, possibly metabolic acidosis, possibly hyperglycaemia, increased muscle creatinine phosphokinase.

Treatment

There is no specific antidote.

Management should initially be guided by the patient's clinical condition; admission to hospital. Measurement of the plasma level to confirm carbamazepine poisoning and to ascertain the size of the overdose.

Evacuation of the stomach, gastric lavage, and administration of activated charcoal. Delay in evacuating the stomach may result in delayed absorption, leading to relapse during recovery from intoxication. Supportive medical care in an intensive care unit with cardiac monitoring and careful correction of electrolyte imbalance.

Special recommendations

Hypotension

Administer dopamine or dobutamine i.v.

Disturbances of cardiac rhythm

To be handled on an individual basis.

Convulsions

Administer a benzodiazepine (e.g. diazepam) or another anticonvulsant, e.g. phenobarbitone (with caution because of increased respiratory depression) or paraldehyde.

Hyponatraemia (water intoxication)

Fluid restriction and slow and careful NaCl 0.9% infusion i.v. These measures may be useful in preventing brain damage.

Charcoal haemoperfusion has been recommended. Forced diuresis, haemodialysis, and peritoneal dialysis have been reported not to be effective.

Relapse and aggravation of symptomatology on the 2nd and 3rd day after overdose, due to delayed absorption, should be anticipated.

5. PHARMACOLOGICAL PROPERTIES

5.1 Pharmacodynamic properties

Therapeutic class: Anti-epileptic, neurotropic and psychotropic agent; (ATC Code: N03 AX 1). Dibenzazepine derivative.

As an antiepileptic agent its spectrum of activity embraces: partial seizures (simple and complex) with and without secondary generalisation; generalised tonic-clonic seizures, as well as combinations of these types of seizures.

The mechanism of action of carbamazepine, the active substance of Tegretol, has only been partially elucidated. Carbamazepine stabilises hyperexcited nerve membranes, inhibits repetitive neuronal discharges, and reduces synaptic propagation of excitatory impulses. It is conceivable that prevention of repetitive firing of sodium-dependent action potentials in depolarised neurons via use- and voltage-dependent blockade of sodium channels may be its main mechanism of action.

Whereas reduction of glutamate release and stabilisation of neuronal membranes may account for the antiepileptic effects, the depressant effect on dopamine and noradrenaline turnover could be responsible for the antimanic properties of carbamazepine.

5.2 Pharmacokinetic properties

Absorption

Carbamazepine is almost completely absorbed but the rate of absorption from the tablets is slow and may vary amongst the various formulations and between patients. Peak concentrations of active substance in the plasma are attained within 24 hours of administration of single dose of Tegretol Retard tablets.

The retard formulation shows about 15% lower bioavailability than standard preparations due mainly to the considerable reduction in peak plasma levels occasioned by controlled release of the same dosage of carbamazepine. Plasma concentrations show less fluctuation but auto-induction of carbamazepine occurs as with standard carbamazepine preparations.

The bioavailability of Tegretol in various oral formulations has been shown to lie between 85-100%.

Ingestion of food has no significant influence on the rate and extent of absorption, regardless of the dosage form of Tegretol.

Steady-state plasma concentrations of carbamazepine are attained within about 1-2 weeks, depending individually upon auto-induction by carbamazepine and hetero-induction by other enzyme-inducing drugs, as well as on pre-treatment status, dosage, and duration of treatment.

Different preparations of carbamazepine may vary in bioavailability; to avoid reduced effect or risk of breakthrough seizures or excessive side effects, it may be prudent to avoid changing the formulation.

Distribution

Carbamazepine is bound to serum proteins to the extent of 70-80%. The concentration of unchanged substance in cerebrospinal fluid and saliva reflects the non-protein bound portion in plasma (20-30%). Concentrations in breast milk were found to be equivalent to 25-60% of the corresponding plasma levels.

Carbamazepine crosses the placental barrier. Assuming complete absorption of carbamazepine, the apparent volume of distribution ranges from 0.8 to 1.9 L/kg.

Elimination

The elimination half-life of unchanged carbamazepine averages approx. 36 hours following a single oral dose, whereas after repeated administration it averages only 16-24 hours (auto-induction of the hepatic mono-oxygenase system), depending on the duration of the medication. In patients receiving concomitant treatment with other enzyme-inducing drugs (e.g. phenytoin, phenobarbitone), half-life values averaging 9-10 hours have been found.

The mean elimination half-life of the 10, 11-epoxide metabolite in the plasma is about 6 hours following single oral doses of the epoxide itself.

After administration of a single oral dose of 400mg carbamazepine, 72% is excreted in the urine and 28% in the faeces. In the urine, about 2% of the dose is recovered as unchanged drug and about 1% as the pharmacologically active 10, 11-epoxide metabolite. Carbamazepine is metabolised in the liver, where the epoxide pathway of biotransformation is the most important one, yielding the 10, 11-transdiol derivative and its glucuronide as the main metabolites.

Cytochrome P450 3A4 has been identified as the major isoform responsible for the formation of carbamazepine 10, 11-epoxide from carbamazepine. 9-Hydroxy-methyl-10-carbamoyl acridan is a minor metabolite related to this pathway. After a single oral dose of carbamazepine about 30% appears in the urine as end-products of the epoxide pathway.

Other important biotransformation pathways for carbamazepine lead to various monohydroxylated compounds, as well as to the N-glucuronide of carbamazepine.

Characteristics in patients

The steady-state plasma concentrations of carbamazepine considered as "therapeutic range" vary considerably inter-individually; for the majority of patients a range between 4-12μg/ml corresponding to 17-50μmol/l has been reported. Concentrations of carbamazepine 10, 11-epoxide (pharmacologically active metabolite): about 30% of carbamazepine levels.

Owing to enhanced carbamazepine elimination, children may require higher doses of carbamazepine (in mg/kg) than adults to maintain therapeutic concentrations.

There is no indication of altered pharmacokinetics of carbamazepine in elderly patients as compared with young adults.

No data are available on the pharmacokinetics of carbamazepine in patients with impaired hepatic or renal function.

5.3 Preclinical safety data

In rats treated with carbamazepine for two years, the incidence of tumours of the liver was found to be increased. The significance of these findings relative to the use of carbamazepine in humans is, at present, unknown. Bacterial and mammalian mutagenicity studies yielded negative results.

6. PHARMACEUTICAL PARTICULARS

6.1 List of excipients

Each 200mg and 400mg tablet contains

- Colloidal silicon dioxide
- Ethylcellulose aqueous dispersion (30%)
- Microcrystalline cellulose
- Ethyl acrylate/methyl methacrylate copolymer
- Magnesium stearate
- Croscarmellose sodium type A
- Talc
- Hydroxypropylmethylcellulose
- Glyceryl polyoxyethylene glycol stearate
- Red iron oxide (E.172)
- Yellow iron oxide (E.172)
- Titanium dioxide (E.171).

6.2 Incompatibilities

None known

6.3 Shelf life

Three years

6.4 Special precautions for storage

Store below 25°C and protect from moisture.

6.5 Nature and contents of container

Tegretol Retard Tablets 200mg and 400mg come in PVC/PCTFE (PVC 190-270 micron; PCTFE 15-25 micron; aluminium foil 26-34 micron) or PVC/PE/PVdC (PVC 190-270 micron; PE 20-40 micron; PVdC 32-59 micron; aluminium foil 26-34 micron) blister packs of 56 tablets.

6.6 Instructions for use and handling

None

7. MARKETING AUTHORISATION HOLDER

Novartis Pharmaceuticals UK Limited

Trading as Geigy Pharmaceuticals

Frimley Business Park

Frimley

Camberley

Surrey

GU16 7SR

England.

8. MARKETING AUTHORISATION NUMBER(S)

Tegretol Retard Tablets 200mg: PL 00101/0457

Tegretol Retard Tablets 400mg: PL 00101/0458

9. DATE OF FIRST AUTHORISATION/RENEWAL OF THE AUTHORISATION

4 July 1997 / 26 March 2001

10. DATE OF REVISION OF THE TEXT

22 June 2004

Legal Category

POM

Tegretol Suppositories 125mg, 250mg

(Cephalon UK Limited)

1. NAME OF THE MEDICINAL PRODUCT

Tegretol® Suppositories 125mg

Tegretol® Suppositories 250mg

2. QUALITATIVE AND QUANTITATIVE COMPOSITION

The active ingredient is 5-Carbamoyl-5-H-dibenz(b,f)azepine.

Each 125mg suppository contains 125 mg carbamazepine Ph.Eur.

Each 250mg suppository contains 250 mg carbamazepine Ph.Eur.

3. PHARMACEUTICAL FORM

White to practically white, torpedo-shaped suppositories.

4. CLINICAL PARTICULARS

4.1 Therapeutic indications

Epilepsy - generalised tonic-clonic and partial seizures.

Note: Tegretol is not usually effective in absences (petit mal) and myoclonic seizures. Moreover, anecdotal evidence suggests that seizure exacerbation may occur in patients with atypical absences.

No clinical data are available on the use of Tegretol Suppositories in indications other than epilepsy.

4.2 Posology and method of administration

Epilepsy:

Adults, Elderly and Children: 125 mg and 250 mg suppositories are available for short-term use as replacement therapy (maximum period recommended: 7 days) in patients for whom oral treatment is temporarily not possible, for example in post-operative or unconscious subjects.

When switching from oral formulations to suppositories the dosage should be increased by approximately 25% (the 125 and 250mg suppositories correspond to 100 and 200mg tablets respectively). The final dose adjustment should always depend on the clinical response in the individual patient (plasma level monitoring is recommended). Tegretol Suppositories have been shown to provide plasma levels which are well within the therapeutic range (see Pharmacokinetics).

Where Suppositories are used the maximum daily dose is limited to 1000mg (250mg qid at 6 hour intervals, see Pharmacokinetics).

Due to the potential for drug interactions, the dosage of Tegretol should be selected with caution in elderly patients.

When Tegretol is added to existing antiepileptic therapy, this should be done gradually while maintaining or, if necessary, adapting the dosage of the other antiepileptic(s) (see 4.5 **Interaction with other Medicaments and other forms of Interaction**).

Route of administration: Rectal.

4.3 Contraindications

Known hypersensitivity to carbamazepine or structurally related drugs (e.g. tricyclic antidepressants) or any other component of the formulation.

Patients with atrioventricular block, a history of bone marrow depression or a history of acute intermittent porphyria.

Because it is structurally related to tricyclic anti-depressants, the use of Tegretol is not recommended in combination with monoamine oxidase inhibitors (MAOIs); before administering Tegretol, MAOIs should be discontinued for a minimum of 2 weeks, or longer if the clinical situation permits.

4.4 Special warnings and special precautions for use

Warnings

Agranulocytosis and aplastic anaemia have been associated with Tegretol; however, due to the very low incidence of these conditions, meaningful risk estimates for Tegretol are difficult to obtain. The overall risk in the general untreated population has been estimated at 4.7 persons per million per year for agranulocytosis and 2.0 persons per million per year for aplastic anaemia.

Decreased platelet or white blood cell counts occur occasionally to frequently in association with the use of Tegretol. Nonetheless, complete pre-treatment blood counts, including platelets and possibly reticulocytes and serum iron, should be obtained as a baseline, and periodically thereafter.

Patients and their relatives should be made aware of early toxic signs and symptoms indicative of a potential haematological problem, as well as symptoms of dermatological or hepatic reactions. If reactions such as fever, sore throat, rash, ulcers in the mouth, easy bruising, petechial or purpuric haemorrhage appear, the patient should be advised to consult his physician immediately.

If the white blood cell or platelet count is definitely low or decreased during treatment, the patient and the complete blood count should be closely monitored (see Section 4.8 Undesirable Effects). However, treatment with Tegretol should be discontinued if the patient develops leucopenia which is severe, progressive or accompanied by clinical manifestations, e.g. fever or sore throat. Tegretol should also be discontinued if any evidence of significant bone marrow depression appears.

Liver function tests should also be performed before commencing treatment and periodically thereafter, particularly in patients with a history of liver disease and in elderly patients. The drug should be withdrawn immediately in cases of aggravated liver dysfunction or acute liver disease.

Some liver function tests in patients receiving carbamazepine may be found to be abnormal, particularly gamma glutamyl transferase. This is probably due to hepatic enzyme induction. Enzyme induction may also produce modest elevations in alkaline phosphatase. These enhancements of hepatic metabolising capacity are not an indication for the withdrawal of carbamazepine.

Severe hepatic reactions to carbamazepine occur very rarely. The development of signs and symptoms of liver dysfunction or active liver disease should be urgently evaluated and treatment with Tegretol suspended pending the outcome of the evaluation.

Mild skin reactions e.g. isolated macular or maculopapular exanthemata, are mostly transient and not hazardous, and they usually disappear within a few days or weeks, either during the continued course of treatment or following a decrease in dosage; however, the patient should be kept under close surveillance and a worsening rash or accompanying symptoms are an indication for the immediate withdrawal of Tegretol.

If signs and symptoms suggestive of severe skin reactions (e.g. Stevens-Johnson syndrome, Lyell's syndrome (toxic epidermal necrolysis)) appear, Tegretol should be withdrawn at once.

Tegretol should be used with caution in patients with mixed seizures which include absences, either typical or atypical. In all these conditions, Tegretol may exacerbate seizures. In case of exacerbation of seizures, Tegretol should be discontinued.

An increase in seizure frequency may occur during switchover from an oral formulation to suppositories.

Abrupt withdrawal of Tegretol may precipitate seizures:

If treatment with Tegretol has to be withdrawn abruptly, the changeover to another anti-epileptic drug should if necessary be effected under the cover of a suitable drug (e.g. diazepam i.v., rectal; or phenytoin i.v.).

Cross-hypersensitivity can occur between carbamazepine and oxcarbazepine (Trileptal) in approximately 25 – 30% of the patients.

Cross-hypersensitivity can occur between carbamazepine and phenytoin.

Isolated reports of impaired male fertility and/or abnormal spermatogenesis are on file. A causal relationship has not been established.

Tegretol and oestrogen and/or progestogen preparations

Due to hepatic enzyme induction, Tegretol may cause failure of the therapeutic effect of oestrogen and/or progestogen containing products. This may result in failure of contraception, recurrence of symptoms or breakthrough bleeding or spotting.

Patients taking Tegretol and requiring oral contraception should receive a preparation containing not less than 50μg oestrogen or use of some alternative non-hormonal method of contraception should be considered.

Although correlations between dosages and plasma levels of carbamazepine, and between plasma levels and clinical efficacy or tolerability are rather tenuous, monitoring of the plasma levels may be useful in the following conditions: dramatic increase in seizure frequency/verification of patient compliance; during pregnancy; when treating children or adolescents; in suspected absorption disorders; in suspected toxicity when more than one drug is being used (see 4.5 Interaction with other Medicaments and other forms of Interaction).

There have been a few cases of neonatal seizures and/or respiratory depression associated with maternal Tegretol and other concomitant anti-epileptic drug use. A few cases of neonatal vomiting, diarrhoea and/or decreased feeding have also been reported in association with maternal Tegretol use. These reactions may represent a neonatal withdrawal syndrome.

Precautions

Tegretol should be prescribed only after a critical benefit-risk appraisal and under close monitoring in patients with a history of cardiac, hepatic or renal damage, adverse haematological reactions to other drugs, or interrupted courses of therapy with Tegretol.

Baseline and periodic complete urinalysis and BUN determinations are recommended.

Tegretol has shown mild anticholinergic activity; patients with increased intraocular pressure should therefore be warned and advised regarding possible hazards.

The possibility of activation of a latent psychosis and, in elderly patients, of confusion or agitation should be borne in mind.

4.5 Interaction with other medicinal products and other forms of Interaction

Cytochrome P450 3A4 (CYP 3A4) is the main enzyme catalysing formation of carbamazepine 10, 11-epoxide. Co-administration of inhibitors of CYP 3A4 may result in increased plasma concentrations which could induce adverse reactions. Co-administration of CYP 3A4 inducers might increase the rate of Tegretol metabolism, thus leading to a potential decrease in carbamazepine serum level and potential decrease in the therapeutic effect.

Similarly, discontinuation of a CYP34A inducer may decrease the rate of metabolism of carbamazepine, leading to an increase in carbamazepine plasma levels.

Agents that may raise Tegretol plasma levels:

Isoniazid, verapamil, diltiazem, ritonavir, dextropropoxyphene, viloxazine, fluoxetine, fluvoxamine, possibly cimetidine, acetazolamide, danazol, nicotinamide (in adults, only in high dosage), nefazodone, macrolide antibiotics (e.g. erythromycin, clarithromycin), azoles (e.g. itraconazole, ketoconazole, fluconazole), terfenadine, loratadine grapefruit juice, protease inhibitors for HIV treatment (e.g. ritonavir). Since raised plasma carbamazepine levels may result in adverse reactions (e.g. dizziness, drowsiness, ataxia, diplopia), the dosage of Tegretol should be adjusted accordingly and/or the plasma levels monitored.

Agents that may decrease Tegretol plasma levels:

Phenobarbitone, phenytoin, primidone, or theophylline, rifampicin, cisplatin or doxorubicin and, although the data are partly contradictory, possibly also clonazepam or valproic acid, oxcarbazepine. Mefloquine may antagonise the anti-epileptic effect of Tegretol. On the other hand, valproic acid and primidone have been reported to raise the plasma level of the pharmacologically active carbamazepine 10, 11-epoxide metabolite. The dose of Tegretol may consequently have to be adjusted.

Isotretinoin has been reported to alter the bioavailability and/or clearance of carbamazepine and carbamazepine-10, 11-epoxide; carbamazepine plasma concentrations should be monitored.

Serum levels of carbamazepine can be reduced by concomitant use of the herbal remedy St John's wort (Hypericum perforatum).

Effect of Tegretol on plasma levels of concomitant agents:

Carbamazepine may lower the plasma level, diminish or even abolish the activity of certain drugs. The dosage of the following drugs may have to be adjusted to clinical requirement: levothyroxine, clobazam, clonazepam, ethosuximide, primidone, valproic acid, alprazolam, corticosteroids, (e.g. prednisolone, dexamethasone); cyclosporin, digoxin, doxycycline; dihydropyridine derivatives, e.g. felodipine and isradipine; indinavir, saquinavir, ritonavir, haloperidol, imipramine, methadone, tramadol, products containing oestrogens and/or progestogens (alternative contraceptive methods should be considered) see Section 4.4 **Special Warnings and Precautions for Use**, gestrinone, tibolone, toremifene, theophylline, oral anticoagulants (warfarin), lamotrigine, tiagabine, topiramate, tricyclic antidepressants (e.g. imipramine, amitriptyline, nortriptyline, clomipramine), clozapine, oxcarbazapine, olanzapine, itraconazole and risperidone.

Plasma phenytoin levels have been reported both to be raised and to be lowered by carbamazepine, and plasma mephenytoin levels have been reported in rare instances to increase.

Combinations to be taken into consideration:

Co-administration of carbamazepine and paracetamol may reduce the bioavailability of paracetamol/acetaminophen.

Concomitant use of carbamazepine and isoniazid has been reported to increase isoniazid-induced hepatotoxicity.

The combination of lithium and carbamazepine may cause enhanced neurotoxicity in spite of lithium plasma concentrations being within the therapeutic range. Combined use of carbamazepine with metoclopramide or major tranquillisers, e.g. haloperidol, thioridazine, may also result in an increase in neurological side-effects.

Because it (carbamazepine) is structurally related to tricyclic anti-depressants, the use of Tegretol is not recommended in combination with monoamine oxidase inhibitors (MAOIs); before administering Tegretol, MAOIs should be discontinued for a minimum of 2 weeks, or longer if the clinical situation permits.

Concomitant medication with Tegretol and some diuretics (hydrochlorothiazide, furosemide) may lead to symptomatic hyponatraemia.

Carbamazepine may antagonise the effects of non-depolarising muscle relaxants (e.g. pancuronium); their dosage should be raised and patients monitored closely for a more rapid recovery from neuromuscular blockade than expected.

Tegretol, like other psychoactive drugs, may reduce alcohol tolerance; it is therefore advisable for the patient to abstain from alcohol.

4.6 Pregnancy and lactation

In animals (mice, rats and rabbits) oral administration of carbamazepine during organogenesis led to increased embryo mortality at a daily doses which caused maternal toxicity (above 200mg/kg b.w. daily i.e. 20 times the usual human dosage). In the rat there was also some evidence of abortion at 300mg/kg body weight daily. Near-term rat foetuses showed growth retardation, again at maternally toxic doses. There was no evidence of teratogenic potential in the three animal species tested but, in one study using mice, carbamazepine (40-240 mg/kg b.w. daily orally) caused defects (mainly dilatation of cerebral ventricles in 4.7% of exposed foetuses as compared with 1.3% in controls).

Pregnant women with epilepsy should be treated with special care.

In women of childbearing age Tegretol should, wherever possible, be prescribed as monotherapy, because the incidence of congenital abnormalities in the offspring of women treated with a combination of anti-epileptic drugs is greater than in those of mothers receiving the individual drugs as monotherapy.

If pregnancy occurs in a woman receiving Tegretol, or if the problem of initiating treatment with Tegretol arises during pregnancy, the drug's potential benefits must be carefully weighed against its possible hazards, particularly in the first three months of pregnancy. Minimum effective doses should be given and monitoring of plasma levels is recommended.

Offspring of epileptic mothers with untreated epilepsy are known to be more prone to developmental disorders, including malformations. The possibility that carbamazepine, like all major anti-epileptic drugs, increases the risk has been reported, although conclusive evidence from controlled studies with carbamazepine monotherapy is lacking. However, there are reports on developmental disorders and malformations, including spina bifida, and also other congenital anomalies e.g. craniofacial defects, cardiovascular malformations and anomalies involving various body systems, have been reported in association with Tegretol. Patients should be counselled regarding the possibility of an increased risk of malformations and given the opportunity of antenatal screening.

Folic acid deficiency is known to occur in pregnancy. Anti-epileptic drugs have been reported to aggravate deficiency. This deficiency may contribute to the increased incidence of birth defects in the offspring of treated epileptic women. Folic acid supplementation has therefore been recommended before and during pregnancy.

Vitamin K_1 to be given to the mother during the last weeks of pregnancy as well as to the new-born to prevent bleeding disorders in the offspring, has also been recommended.

Use during lactation:

Carbamazepine passes into the breast milk (about 25-60% of the plasma concentrations). The benefits of breast-feeding should be weighed against the remote possibility of adverse effects occurring in the infant. Mothers taking Tegretol may breast-feed their infants, provided the infant is observed for possible adverse reactions (e.g. excessive somnolence, allergic skin reaction).

4.7 Effects on ability to drive and use machines

The patient's ability to react may be impaired by dizziness and drowsiness caused by Tegretol, especially at the start of treatment or in connection with dose adjustments; patients should therefore exercise due caution when driving a vehicle or operating machinery.

4.8 Undesirable effects

Particularly at the start of treatment with Tegretol, or if the initial dosage is too high, or when treating elderly patients, certain types of adverse reaction occur very commonly or commonly, e.g. CNS adverse reactions (dizziness, headache, ataxia, drowsiness, fatigue, diplopia); gastrointestinal disturbances (nausea, vomiting), as well as allergic skin reactions.

The dose-related adverse reactions usually abate within a few days, either spontaneously or after a transient dosage reduction. The occurrence of CNS adverse reactions may be a manifestation of relative overdosage or significant fluctuation in plasma levels. In such cases it is advisable to monitor the plasma levels and divide the daily dosage into smaller (i.e. 3-4) fractional doses.

Frequency estimate: very common ⩾ 10%, common ⩾ 1% to < 10%; uncommon ⩾ 0.1% to < 1%; rare ⩾ 0.01% to < 0.1%; very rare < 0.01%

Central nervous system:

Neurological:

Very common: Dizziness, ataxia, drowsiness, fatigue.

Common: Headache, diplopia, accommodation disorders (e.g. blurred vision).

Uncommon: Abnormal involuntary movements (e.g. tremor, asterixis, dystonia, tics); nystagmus.

Rare: Orofacial dyskinesia, oculomotor disturbances, speech disorders (e.g. dysarthria or slurred speech), choreoathetotic disorders, peripheral neuritis, paraesthesia, muscle weakness, and paretic symptoms.

Cases of neuroleptic malignant syndrome have been reported. The causative role of carbamazepine in inducing or contributing to the development of a neuromalignant syndrome, especially in conjunction with neuroleptics, is unclear.

Psychiatric:

Rare: Hallucinations (visual or acoustic), depression, loss of appetite, restlessness, aggressive behaviour, agitation, confusion.

Very rare: Activation of psychosis.

Skin and appendages:

Very common: Allergic skin reactions, urticaria, which may be severe.

Uncommon: Exfoliative dermatitis and erythroderma.

Rare: Lupus erythematosus-like syndrome, pruritus.

Very rare: Stevens-Johnson syndrome, toxic epidermal necrolysis, photosensitivity, erythema multiforme and nodosum, alterations in skin pigmentation, purpura, acne, sweating, hair loss.

Very rare cases of hirsutism have been reported, but the causal relationship is not clear.

Blood:

Very common: Leucopenia.

Common: Thrombocytopenia, eosinophilia.

Rare: Leucocytosis, lymphadenopathy, folic acid deficiency.

Very rare: Agranulocytosis, aplastic anaemia, pure red cell aplasia, megaloblastic anaemia, acute intermittent porphyria, reticulocytosis, and possibly haemolytic anaemia.

Liver:

Very common: Elevated gamma-GT (due to hepatic enzyme induction), usually not clinically relevant.

Common: Elevated alkaline phosphatase.

Uncommon: Elevated transaminases.

Rare: Hepatitis of cholestatic, parenchymal (hepatocellular) or mixed type, jaundice.

Very rare: Granulomatous hepatitis. Hepatic failure.

Gastro-intestinal tract:

Very common: Nausea, vomiting.

Common: Dryness of the mouth, with suppositories rectal irritation may occur.

Uncommon: Diarrhoea or constipation.

Rare: Abdominal pain.

Very rare: Glossitis, stomatitis, pancreatitis.

Hypersensitivity reactions:

Rare: A delayed multi-organ hypersensitivity disorder with fever, skin rashes, vasculitis, lymphadenopathy, disorders mimicking lymphoma, arthralgia, leucopenia, eosinophilia, hepato-splenomegaly and abnormal liver function tests, occurring in various combinations. Other organs may also be affected (e.g. liver, lungs, kidneys, pancreas, myocardium, colon).

Very rare: Aseptic meningitis, with myoclonus and peripheral eosinophilia; anaphylactic reaction, angioedema.

Treatment must be discontinued immediately if such hypersensitivity reactions occur.

Cardiovascular system:

Rare: Disturbances of cardiac conduction, hypertension or hypotension.

Very rare: Bradycardia, arrhythmias, AV-block with syncope, collapse, congestive heart failure, aggravation of coronary artery disease, thrombophlebitis, thromboembolism.

Endocrine system and metabolism:

Common: Oedema, fluid retention, weight increase, hyponatraemia and reduced plasma osmolality due to an antidiuretic hormone (ADH)-like effect, leading in rare cases to water intoxication accompanied by lethargy, vomiting, headache, mental confusion, neurological abnormalities.

Very rare: Increase in prolactin with or without clinical symptoms such as galactorrhoea, gynaecomastia, abnormal thyroid function tests; decreased l-thyroxin (FT4, T4, T3) and increased TSH, usually without clinical manifestations, disturbances of bone metabolism (decrease in plasma calcium and 25-OH-cholecalciferol), leading to osteomalacia, elevated levels of cholesterol, including HDL cholesterol and triglycerides.

Urogenital system:

Very rare: Interstitial nephritis, renal failure, renal dysfunction (e.g. albuminuria, haematuria, oliguria and elevated BUN/ azotaemia), urinary frequency, urinary retention, sexual disturbances/impotence.

Sense organs:

Very rare: Taste disturbances; lens opacities, conjunctivitis, hearing disorders, e.g. tinnitus, hyperacusis, hypoacusis, change in pitch perception.

Musculoskeletal system:

Very rare: Arthralgia, muscle pain or cramp.

Respiratory tract:

Very rare: Pulmonary hypersensitivity characterised e.g. by fever, dyspnoea, pneumonitis or pneumonia.

4.9 Overdose

Signs and symptoms

The presenting signs and symptoms of overdosage involve the central nervous, cardiovascular or respiratory systems.

Central nervous system: CNS depression; disorientation, somnolence, agitation, hallucination, coma; blurred vision, slurred speech, dysarthria, nystagmus, ataxia, dyskinesia, initially hyperreflexia, later hyporeflexia; convulsions, psychomotor disturbances, myoclonus, hypothermia, mydriasis.

Respiratory system: Respiratory depression, pulmonary oedema.

Cardiovascular system: Tachycardia, hypotension and at times hypertension, conduction disturbance with widening of QRS complex; syncope in association with cardiac arrest.

Gastro-intestinal system: Vomiting, delayed gastric emptying, reduced bowel motility.

Renal function: Retention of urine, oliguria or anuria; fluid retention, water intoxication due to ADH-like effect of carbamazepine.

Laboratory findings: Hyponatraemia, possibly metabolic acidosis, possibly hyperglycaemia, increased muscle creatinine phosphokinase.

Treatment

There is no specific antidote.

Management should initially be guided by the patient's clinical condition; admission to hospital. Measurement of the plasma level to confirm carbamazepine poisoning and to ascertain the size of the overdose.

Evacuation of the stomach, gastric lavage, and administration of activated charcoal. Delay in evacuating the stomach may result in delayed absorption, leading to relapse during recovery from intoxication. Supportive medical care in an intensive care unit with cardiac monitoring and careful correction of electrolyte imbalance, if required.

Special recommendations:

Hypotension: Administer dopamine or dobutamine i.v.

Disturbances of cardiac rhythm: To be handled on an individual basis.

Convulsions: Administer a benzodiazepine (e.g. diazepam) or another anticonvulsant, e.g. phenobarbitone (with caution because of increased respiratory depression) or paraldehyde.

Hyponatraemia (water intoxication): Fluid restriction and slow and careful NaCl 0.9% infusion i.v. These measures may be useful in preventing brain damage.

Charcoal haemoperfusion has been recommended. Forced diuresis, haemodialysis, and peritoneal dialysis have been reported not to be effective.

Relapse and aggravation of symptomatology on the 2nd and 3rd day after overdose, due to delayed absorption, should be anticipated.

5. PHARMACOLOGICAL PROPERTIES

5.1 Pharmacodynamic properties

Therapeutic class: Anti-epileptic, neurotropic and psychotropic agent; (ATC Code: N03 AX 1). Dibenzazepine derivative.

As an antiepileptic agent its spectrum of activity embraces: partial seizures (simple and complex) with and without secondary generalisation; generalised tonic-clonic seizures, as well as combinations of these types of seizures.

The mechanism of action of carbamazepine, the active substance of Tegretol, has only been partially elucidated. Carbamazepine stabilises hyperexcited nerve membranes, inhibits repetitive neuronal discharges, and reduces synaptic propagation of excitatory impulses. It is conceivable that prevention of repetitive firing of sodium-dependent action potentials in depolarised neurons via use- and voltage-dependent blockade of sodium channels may be its main mechanism of action.

Whereas reduction of glutamate release and stabilisation of neuronal membranes may account for the antiepileptic effects, the depressant effect on dopamine and noradrenaline turnover could be responsible for the antimanic properties of carbamazepine.

5.2 Pharmacokinetic properties

Absorption

As measured by AUC calculations the total bioavailability of carbamazepine from Tegretol suppositories is approximately 25% less than from oral formulations. For doses up to 300mg approximately 75% of the total amount absorbed reaches the general circulation within 6 hours of application. For these reasons the maximum recommended daily dose is limited to 250mg qid (1000mg per day), the equivalent to 800mg per day orally. Clinical trials have shown that when Tegretol suppositories are substituted for oral dosage forms plasma levels within the range 5-8μg/ml (19-34μmol/l) are reached. It should be possible, therefore, to maintain therapeutically effective plasma levels in most patients.

Distribution

Carbamazepine is bound to serum proteins to the extent of 70-80%. The concentration of unchanged substance in cerebrospinal fluid and saliva reflects the non-protein bound portion in plasma (20-30%). Concentrations in breast milk were found to be equivalent to 25-60% of the corresponding plasma levels.

Carbamazepine crosses the placental barrier. Assuming complete absorption of carbamazepine, the apparent volume of distribution ranges from 0.8 to 1.9 L/kg.

Elimination

The elimination half-life of unchanged carbamazepine averages approx. 36 hours following a single oral dose, whereas after repeated administration it averages only 16-24 hours (auto-induction of the hepatic mono-oxygenase system), depending on the duration of the medication. In patients receiving concomitant treatment with other enzyme-inducing drugs (e.g. phenytoin, phenobarbitone), half-life values averaging 9-10 hours have been found.

The mean elimination half-life of the 10, 11-epoxide metabolite in the plasma is about 6 hours following single oral doses of the epoxide itself.

After administration of a single oral dose of 400mg carbamazepine, 72% is excreted in the urine and 28% in the faeces. In the urine, about 2% of the dose is recovered as unchanged drug and about 1% as the pharmacologically active 10, 11-epoxide metabolite. Carbamazepine is metabolised in the liver, where the epoxide pathway of biotransformation is the most important one, yielding the 10, 11-transdiol derivative and its glucuronide as the main metabolites.

Cytochrome P450 3A4 has been identified as the major isoform responsible for the formation of carbamazepine 10, 11-epoxide from carbamazepine. 9-Hydroxy-methyl-10-carbamoyl acridan is a minor metabolite related to this pathway. After a single oral dose of carbamazepine about 30% appears in the urine as end-products of the epoxide pathway.

Other important biotransformation pathways for carbamazepine lead to various monohydroxylated compounds, as well as to the N-glucuronide of carbamazepine.

Characteristics in patients

The steady-state plasma concentrations of carbamazepine considered as "therapeutic range" vary considerably inter-individually; for the majority of patients a range between 4-12μg/ml corresponding to 17-50μmol/l has been reported. Concentrations of carbamazepine 10, 11-epoxide (pharmacologically active metabolite): about 30% of carbamazepine levels.

Owing to enhanced carbamazepine elimination, children may require higher doses of carbamazepine (in mg/kg) than adults to maintain therapeutic concentrations.

There is no indication of altered pharmacokinetics of carbamazepine in elderly patients as compared with young adults.

No data are available on the pharmacokinetics of carbamazepine in patients with impaired hepatic or renal function.

5.3 Preclinical safety data

In rats treated with carbamazepine for two years, the incidence of tumours of the liver was found to be increased. The significance of these findings relative to the use of carbamazepine in humans is, at present, unknown. Bacterial and mammalian mutagenicity studies yielded negative results.

6. PHARMACEUTICAL PARTICULARS

6.1 List of excipients

Each suppository contains hydroxypropylmethylcellulose and suppository mass 15.

6.2 Incompatibilities

None known

6.3 Shelf life

Three years

6.4 Special precautions for storage

Protect from heat (store below 30°C).

6.5 Nature and contents of container

Tegretol Suppositories are sealed in polyethylene laminated aluminium foil and come in packs of 5.

6.6 Instructions for use and handling

None

7. MARKETING AUTHORISATION HOLDER

Novartis Pharmaceuticals UK Limited
Trading as Geigy Pharmaceuticals
Frimley Business Park
Frimley
Camberley
Surrey
GU16 7SR
England.

8. MARKETING AUTHORISATION NUMBER(S)

Tegretol Suppositories 125mg: PL 00101/0459
Tegretol Suppositories 250mg: PL 00101/0460

9. DATE OF FIRST AUTHORISATION/RENEWAL OF THE AUTHORISATION

4 July 1997/ 28 November 1998

10. DATE OF REVISION OF THE TEXT

31 January 2003

Legal category

POM

Telfast 120 and 180

(sanofi-aventis)

1. NAME OF THE MEDICINAL PRODUCT

Telfast ™ 120 mg film-coated tablets

Telfast ™ 180 mg film-coated tablets

2. QUALITATIVE AND QUANTITATIVE COMPOSITION

Telfast 120 mg film-coated tablets: Each tablet contains 120 mg of fexofenadine hydrochloride, which is equivalent to 112 mg of fexofenadine.

Telfast 180 mg film-coated tablets: Each tablet contains 180 mg of fexofenadine hydrochloride, which is equivalent to 168 mg of fexofenadine.

For excipients see 6.1.

3. PHARMACEUTICAL FORM

Telfast 120 mg film-coated tablets:

Film coated tablets.

Peach, modified capsule shaped, debossed, film-coated tablet

Telfast 180 mg film-coated tablets:

Film coated tablets.

Peach, capsule shaped, debossed, film-coated tablet

4. CLINICAL PARTICULARS

4.1 Therapeutic indications

Telfast 120 mg film-coated tablets: Relief of symptoms associated with seasonal allergic rhinitis.

Telfast 180 mg film-coated tablets: Relief of symptoms associated with chronic idiopathic urticaria.

4.2 Posology and method of administration

Adults and children aged 12 years and over

Telfast 120 mg film-coated tablets: The recommended dose of fexofenadine hydrochloride for adults and children aged 12 years and over is 120mg once daily taken before a meal.

Telfast 180 mg film-coated tablets: The recommended dose of fexofenadine hydrochloride for adults and children aged 12 years and over is 180mg once daily taken before a meal.

Fexofenadine is a pharmacologically active metabolite of terfenadine.

Children under 12 years of age

The efficacy and safety of fexofenadine hydrochloride has not been studied in children under 12.

Special risk groups

Studies in special risk groups (elderly, renally or hepatically impaired patients) indicate that it is not necessary to adjust the dose of fexofenadine hydrochloride in these patients.

4.3 Contraindications

The product is contraindicated in patients with known hypersensitivity to any of its ingredients.

4.4 Special warnings and special precautions for use

As with most new drugs there is only limited data in the elderly and renally or hepatically impaired adult patients. Fexofenadine hydrochloride should be administered with care in these special groups.

4.5 Interaction with other medicinal products and other forms of Interaction

Fexofenadine does not undergo hepatic biotransformation and therefore will not interact with other drugs through hepatic mechanisms. Coadministration of fexofenadine hydrochloride with erythromycin or ketoconazole has been found to result in a 2-3 times increase in the level of fexofenadine in plasma. The changes were not accompanied by any effects on the QT interval and were not associated with any increase in adverse events compared to the drugs given singly.

Animal studies have shown that the increase in plasma levels of fexofenadine observed after coadministration of erythromycin or ketoconazole, appears to be due to an increase in gastrointestinal absorption and either a decrease in biliary excretion or gastrointestinal secretion, respectively.

No interaction between fexofenadine and omeprazole was observed. However, the administration of an antacid containing aluminium and magnesium hydroxide gels 15 minutes prior to fexofenadine hydrochloride caused a reduction in bioavailability, most likely due to binding in the gastrointestinal tract. It is advisable to leave 2 hours between administration of fexofenadine hydrochloride and aluminium and magnesium hydroxide containing antacids.

4.6 Pregnancy and lactation

Pregnancy

There are no adequate data from the use of fexofenadine hydrochloride in pregnant women. Limited animal studies do not indicate direct or indirect harmful effects with respect to effects on pregnancy, embryonal/foetal development, parturition or postnatal development (see section 5.3). Fexofenadine hydrochloride should not be used during pregnancy unless clearly necessary.

Lactation

There are no data on the content of human milk after administering fexofenadine hydrochloride. However, when terfenadine was administered to nursing mothers, fexofenadine was found to cross into human breast milk. Therefore fexofenadine hydrochloride is not recommended for mothers breast feeding their babies.

4.7 Effects on ability to drive and use machines

On the basis of the pharmacodynamic profile and reported adverse events it is unlikely that fexofenadine hydrochloride tablets will produce an effect on the ability to drive or use machines. In objective tests, Telfast has been shown to have no significant effects on central nervous system function. This means that patients may drive or perform tasks that require concentration. However, in order to identify sensitive people who have an unusual reaction to drugs, it is advisable to check the individual response before driving or performing complicated tasks.

4.8 Undesirable effects

In controlled clinical trials the most commonly reported adverse events were headache (7.3%), drowsiness (2.3%), nausea (1.5%) and dizziness (1.5%) The incidence of these events observed with fexofenadine was similar to that observed with placebo.

Events that have been reported with incidences less than 1% and similar to placebo in controlled trials and have also been reported rarely during postmarketing surveillance include: fatigue, insomnia, nervousness and sleep disorders or paroniria, such as nightmares. In rare cases, rash, urticaria, pruritus, and hypersensitivity reactions with manifestations such as angioedema, chest tightness, dyspnoea, flushing and systemic anaphylaxis have also been reported.

4.9 Overdose

Dizziness, drowsiness, fatigue and dry mouth have been reported with overdose of fexofenadine hydrochloride. Single doses up to 800 mg and doses up to 690 mg twice daily for 1 month or 240 mg once daily for 1 year have been administered to healthy subjects without the development of clinically significant adverse events as compared with placebo. The maximum tolerated dose of fexofenadine hydrochloride has not been established.

Standard measures should be considered to remove any unabsorbed drug. Symptomatic and supportive treatment is recommended. Haemodialysis does not effectively remove fexofenadine hydrochloride from blood.

5. PHARMACOLOGICAL PROPERTIES

5.1 Pharmacodynamic properties

Pharmacotherapeutic Group: Antihistamines for systemic use, ATC code: RO6A X26

Fexofenadine hydrochloride is a non-sedating H_1 antihistamine. Fexofenadine is a pharmacologically active metabolite of terfenadine.

Human histamine wheal and flare studies following single and twice daily doses of fexofenadine hydrochloride demonstrate that the drug exhibits an antihistaminic effect beginning within one hour, achieving maximum at 6 hours and lasting 24 hours. There was no evidence of tolerance to these effects after 28 days of dosing. A positive dose-response relationship between doses of 10mg to 130mg taken orally was found to exist. In this model of antihistaminic activity, it was found that doses of at least 130mg were required to achieve a consistent effect that was maintained over a 24 hour period. Maximum inhibition in skin wheal and flare areas were greater than 80%. Clinical studies conducted in seasonal allergic rhinitis have shown that a dose of 120mg is sufficient for 24 hour efficacy.

No significant differences in QT_c intervals were observed in seasonal allergic rhinitis patients given fexofenadine hydrochloride up to 240 mg twice daily for 2 weeks when compared to placebo. Also, no significant change in QT_c intervals was observed in healthy subjects given fexofenadine hydrochloride up to 60 mg twice daily for 6 months, 400 mg twice daily for 6.5 days and 240 mg once daily for 1 year, when compared to placebo. Fexofenadine at concentrations 32 times greater than the therapeutic concentration in man had no effect on the delayed rectifier K+ channel cloned from human heart.

Fexofenadine hydrochloride (5-10mg/kg po) inhibited antigen induced bronchospasm in sensitised guinea pigs and inhibited histamine release at supratherapeutic concentrations (10-100μM) from peritoneal mast cells.

5.2 Pharmacokinetic properties

Fexofenadine hydrochloride is rapidly absorbed into the body following oral administration, with T_{max} occurring at approximately 1-3 hours post dose. The mean C_{max} value was approximately 427ng/ml following the administration of a 120mg dose once daily and approximately 494ng/ml following the administration of a 180mg dose once daily.

Fexofenadine is 60-70% plasma protein bound. Fexofenadine undergoes negligible metabolism (hepatic or non-hepatic), as it was the only major compound identified in urine and faeces of animals and man. The plasma concentration profiles of fexofenadine follow a bi-exponential decline with a terminal elimination half-life ranging from 11 to 15 hours after multiple dosing. The single and multiple dose pharmacokinetics of fexofenadine are linear for oral doses up to 120mg BID. A dose of 240mg BID produced slightly greater than proportional increase (8.8%) in steady state area under the curve, indicating that fexofenadine pharmacokinetics are practically linear at these doses between 40mg and 240mg taken daily. The major route of elimination is believed to be via biliary excretion while up to 10% of ingested dose is excreted unchanged through the urine.

5.3 Preclinical safety data

Dogs tolerated 450mg/kg administered twice daily for 6 months and showed no toxicity other than occasional emesis. Also, in single dose dog and rodent studies, no treatment-related gross findings were observed following necropsy.

Radiolabelled fexofenadine hydrochloride in tissue distribution studies of the rat indicated that fexofenadine did not cross the blood brain barrier.

Fexofenadine hydrochloride was found to be non-mutagenic in various *in vitro* and *in vivo* mutagenicity tests.

The carcinogenic potential of fexofenadine hydrochloride was assessed using terfenadine studies with supporting pharmacokinetic studies showing fexofenadine hydrochloride exposure (via plasma AUC values). No evidence of carcinogenicity was observed in rats and mice given terfenadine (up to 150mg/kg/day).

In a reproductive toxicity study in mice, fexofenadine hydrochloride did not impair fertility, was not teratogenic and did not impair pre- or postnatal development.

6. PHARMACEUTICAL PARTICULARS

6.1 List of excipients

Tablet core

Microcrystalline Cellulose

Pregelatinised Maize Starch

Croscarmellose Sodium

Magnesium Stearate

Film coat

Hypromellose

Povidone

Titanium Dioxide (E171)

Colloidal Anhydrous Silica

Macrogol 400

Iron oxide (E172)

6.2 Incompatibilities

None.

6.3 Shelf life

3 years.

6.4 Special precautions for storage

No special precautions for storage.

6.5 Nature and contents of container

PVC/PE/PVDC/A1 blisters packaged into cardboard boxes.

Telfast 120 mg film-coated tablets: 30 peach, modified capsule-shaped tablets per package.

Telfast 180 mg film-coated tablets: 30 peach, capsule-shaped tablets per package.

6.6 Instructions for use and handling

No special requirements.

7. MARKETING AUTHORISATION HOLDER

Aventis Pharma Ltd

50 Kings Hill Avenue

Kings Hill

West Malling

Kent ME19 4AH

8. MARKETING AUTHORISATION NUMBER(S)

Telfast 120 mg film-coated tablets: PL 04425/0157

Telfast 180 mg film-coated tablets: PL 04425/0158

9. DATE OF FIRST AUTHORISATION/RENEWAL OF THE AUTHORISATION

Telfast 120 mg & 180 mg film-coated tablets: 4 December 1996/ 29 June 2001

10. DATE OF REVISION OF THE TEXT

September 2004

11. Legal Category

POM

Telfast 30mg tablets

(sanofi-aventis)

1. NAME OF THE MEDICINAL PRODUCT

Telfast TM 30 mg film-coated tablets

2. QUALITATIVE AND QUANTITATIVE COMPOSITION

Each tablet contains 30 mg of fexofenadine hydrochloride, which is equivalent to 28mg of fexofenadine.

For excipients, see 6.1.

3. PHARMACEUTICAL FORM

Film-coated tablet.

Peach round film-coated tablet.

4. CLINICAL PARTICULARS

4.1 Therapeutic indications

Relief of symptoms associated with seasonal allergic rhinitis.

4.2 Posology and method of administration

Children 6 to 11 years of age.

The recommended dose of fexofenadine hydrochloride in children aged 6 to 11 years is 30mg twice daily.

Children under 6 years of age

The efficacy and safety of fexofenadine hydrochloride has not been established in children under 6.

Special risk groups

The safety and efficacy of fexofenadine hydrochloride in renally or hepatically impaired children have not been established (see section 4.4).

Studies conducted in adults in special risk groups (renally or hepatically impaired patients) indicate that it is not necessary to adjust the dose of fexofenadine hydrochloride in adults.

4.3 Contraindications

Hypersensitivity to the active substance or to any of the excipients.

4.4 Special warnings and special precautions for use

The safety and efficacy of fexofenadine hydrochloride in renally or hepatically impaired children have not been established (see section 4.2). Fexofenadine Hydrochloride should be administered with caution in these patients.

4.5 Interaction with other medicinal products and other forms of Interaction

Fexofenadine does not undergo hepatic biotransformation and therefore will not interact with other medicinal products through hepatic mechanisms. Coadministration of fexofenadine hydrochloride with erythromycin or ketoconazole has been found to result in a 2-3 times increase in the level of fexofenadine in plasma. The changes were not accompanied by any effects on the QT interval and were not associated with any increase in adverse events compared to the medicinal products given singly.

Animal studies have shown that the increase in plasma levels of fexofenadine observed after coadministration of erythromycin or ketoconazole, appears to be due to an increase in gastrointestinal absorption and either a decrease in biliary excretion or gastrointestinal secretion, respectively.

No interaction between fexofenadine hydrochloride and omeprazole was observed. However, the administration of an antacid containing aluminium and magnesium hydroxide gels 15 minutes prior to fexofenadine hydrochloride caused a reduction in bioavailability, most likely due to binding in the gastrointestinal tract. It is advisable to leave 2 hours between administration of fexofenadine hydrochloride and aluminium and magnesium hydroxide containing antacids.

4.6 Pregnancy and lactation

Pregnancy

There are no adequate data from the use of fexofenadine hydrochloride in pregnant women. Limited animal studies do not indicate direct or indirect harmful effects with respect to effects on pregnancy, embryonal/foetal development, parturition or postnatal development (see section 5.3). Fexofenadine hydrochloride should not be used during pregnancy unless clearly necessary.

Lactation

There are no data on the content of human milk after administering fexofenadine hydrochloride. However, when terfenadine was administered to nursing mothers, fexofenadine was found to cross into human breast milk. Therefore fexofenadine hydrochloride is not recommended for mothers breast feeding their babies.

4.7 Effects on ability to drive and use machines

On the basis of the pharmacodynamic profile and reported adverse events it is unlikely that fexofenadine hydrochloride tablets will produce an effect on the ability to drive or use machines. In objective tests, Telfast has been shown to have no significant effects on central nervous system function. This means that patients may drive or perform tasks that require concentration. However, in order to identify sensitive people who have an unusual reaction to drugs, it is advisable to check the individual response before driving or performing complicated tasks.

4.8 Undesirable effects

In controlled clinical trials in children aged 6 to 11 years, the most commonly reported adverse reaction considered at least possibly related to fexofenadine hydrochloride by the investigator was headache. The incidence of headache in pooled data from clinical trials was 1.0% for patients taking fexofenadine hydrochloride 30 mg (673 children) and for patients taking placebo (700 children). There are no clinical safety data in children treated with fexofenadine hydrochloride for periods longer than two weeks.

In adults, the following undesirable effects have been reported in clinical trials, with an incidence similar to that observed with placebo:

Nervous system disorders

Common ($\geqslant$1/100, $<$1/10): headache, drowsiness, dizziness.

Gastrointestinal disorders

Common ($\geqslant$1/100, $<$1/10): nausea

General disorder

Uncommon ($\geqslant$1/1000, $<$1/100): fatigue

In adults, the following undesirable effects have been rarely ($\geqslant$1/10 000, $<$1/1 000) reported in post-marketing surveillance:

Psychiatric disorders

insomnia, nervousness, sleep disorders or paroniria, such as nightmares.

Skin and subcutaneous tissue disorders

rash, urticaria, pruritus

Immune system disorders

hypersensitivity reactions with manifestations such as angioedema, chest tightness, dyspnoea, flushing and systemic anaphylaxis

4.9 Overdose

Dizziness, drowsiness, fatigue and dry mouth have been reported with overdose of fexofenadine hydrochloride. Doses up to 60 mg twice daily for two weeks have been administered to children, and single doses up to 800 mg and doses up to 690 mg twice daily for 1 month or 240 mg once daily for 1 year have been administered to healthy subjects without the development of clinically significant adverse events as compared with placebo. The maximum tolerated dose of fexofenadine hydrochloride has not been established.

Standard measures should be considered to remove any unabsorbed drug. Symptomatic and supportive treatment is recommended. Haemodialysis does not effectively remove fexofenadine hydrochloride from blood.

5. PHARMACOLOGICAL PROPERTIES

5.1 Pharmacodynamic properties

Pharmacotherapeutic Group: Antihistamines for systemic use, ATC code: RO6A X26

Fexofenadine hydrochloride is a non-sedating H_1 antihistamine. Fexofenadine is a pharmacologically active metabolite of terfenadine.

In children aged 6 to 11 years, the suppressive effects of fexofenadine hydrochloride on histamine – induced wheal and flare were comparable to that in adults at similar exposure.

Inhibition of histamine-induced wheal and flare was observed at one hour post dose following single doses of 30 and 60 mg fexofenadine hydrochloride. Peak inhibitory effects of fexofenadine generally occurred at 3-6 hours post dose.

In a pooled analysis of three placebo-controlled double-blind phase III studies, involving 1369 children with seasonal allergic rhinitis aged 6 to 11 years, fexofenadine hydrochloride at 30 mg twice daily was significantly better than placebo in reducing total symptom score (p=0.0001). All individual component symptoms including rhinorrhea (p=0.0058), sneezing (p=0.0001), itchy/ watery/red eyes (p=0.0001), itchy nose/ palate and throat (p=0.0001), and nasal congestion (p=0.0334) were significantly improved by fexofenadine hydrochloride.

In children aged 6 to 11 years, no significant differences in QT_c were observed following up to 60 mg fexofenadine hydrochloride twice daily for two weeks compared with placebo. No significant differences in QT_c intervals were observed in adult and adolescent patients with seasonal allergic rhinitis, when given fexofenadine hydrochloride up to 240 mg twice daily for 2 weeks when compared with placebo. Also, no significant change in QT_c intervals was observed in healthy adult subjects given fexofenadine hydrochloride up to 60 mg twice daily for 6 months, 400 mg twice daily for 6.5 days and 240 mg once daily for 1 year, when compared with placebo. Fexofenadine at concentrations 32 times greater than the therapeutic concentration in man had no effect on the delayed rectifier K+ channel cloned from human heart.

5.2 Pharmacokinetic properties

Fexofenadine hydrochloride is rapidly absorbed into the body following oral administration, with T_{max} occurring at approximately 1-3 hours post dose. In children, the mean C_{max} value was approximately 128 ng/ml following a single dose oral administration of 30 mg fexofenadine hydrochloride.

A dose of 30 mg BID was determined to provide plasma levels (AUC) in paediatric patients which are comparable to those achieved in adults with the approved adult regimen of 120 mg once daily.

After oral administration in adults, fexofenadine is 60-70% plasma protein bound. Fexofenadine undergoes negligible metabolism (hepatic or non-hepatic), as it was the only major compound identified in urine and faeces of animals and man. The plasma concentration profiles of fexofenadine follow a bi-exponential decline with a terminal elimination half-life ranging from 11 to 15 hours after multiple dosing. The single and multiple dose pharmacokinetics of fexofenadine are linear for oral doses up to 120mg BID. A dose of 240mg BID produced slightly greater than proportional increase (8.8%) in steady state area under the curve, indicating that fexofenadine pharmacokinetics are practically linear at these doses between 40mg and 240mg taken daily. The major route of elimination is believed to be via biliary excretion while up to 10% of ingested dose is excreted unchanged through the urine.

5.3 Preclinical safety data

Dogs tolerated 450mg/kg administered twice daily for 6 months and showed no toxicity other than occasional emesis. Also, in single dose dog and rodent studies, no treatment-related gross findings were observed following necropsy.

Radiolabelled fexofenadine hydrochloride in tissue distribution studies of the rat indicated that fexofenadine did not cross the blood brain barrier.

Fexofenadine hydrochloride was found to be non-mutagenic in various *in vitro* and *in vivo* mutagenicity tests.

The carcinogenic potential of fexofenadine hydrochloride was assessed using terfenadine studies with supporting pharmacokinetic studies showing fexofenadine hydrochloride exposure (via plasma AUC values). No evidence of carcinogenicity was observed in rats and mice given terfenadine (up to 150mg/kg/day).

In a reproductive toxicity study in mice, fexofenadine hydrochloride did not impair fertility, was not teratogenic and did not impair pre- or postnatal development.

6. PHARMACEUTICAL PARTICULARS

6.1 List of excipients

Tablet core

Microcrystalline Cellulose

Pregelatinised Maize Starch

Croscarmellose Sodium

Magnesium Stearate

Film coat

Hypromellose

Povidone

Titanium Dioxide (E171)

Colloidal Anhydrous Silica

Macrogol

Pink Iron oxide (E172) blend

Yellow Iron oxide (E172) blend

6.2 Incompatibilities

Not applicable.

6.3 Shelf life

3 years.

6.4 Special precautions for storage

This medicinal product does not require any special storage conditions

6.5 Nature and contents of container

PVC/PE/PVDC/A1 blisters packaged into cardboard boxes.

60 tablets per package.

6.6 Instructions for use and handling

No special requirements.

7. MARKETING AUTHORISATION HOLDER

Aventis Pharma Ltd

50 Kings Hill Avenue

Kings Hill

West Malling

Kent ME19 4AH

8. MARKETING AUTHORISATION NUMBER(S)

PL 04425/0162

9. DATE OF FIRST AUTHORISATION/RENEWAL OF THE AUTHORISATION

1st April 2003

10. DATE OF REVISION OF THE TEXT

September 2004

11. Legal Category

POM

Telzir 700 mg film coated-tablets

(GlaxoSmithKline UK)

1. NAME OF THE MEDICINAL PRODUCT

Telzir▼ 700 mg film-coated tablets.

2. QUALITATIVE AND QUANTITATIVE COMPOSITION

Each film-coated tablet contains 700 mg of fosamprenavir as fosamprenavir calcium (equivalent to approximately 600 mg of amprenavir).

For excipients, see section 6.1.

3. PHARMACEUTICAL FORM

Film-coated tablets.

Pink film coated, capsule shaped, biconvex tablets, marked with GXLL7 on one side.

4. CLINICAL PARTICULARS

4.1 Therapeutic indications

Telzir in combination with low dose ritonavir is indicated for the treatment of Human Immunodeficiency Virus Type 1 (HIV-1) infected adults in combination with other antiretroviral medicinal products.

In moderately antiretroviral experienced patients, Telzir in combination with low dose ritonavir has not been shown to be as effective as lopinavir / ritonavir.

In heavily pretreated patients the use of Telzir in combination with low dose ritonavir has not been sufficiently studied.

In protease inhibitor (PI) experienced patients the choice of Telzir should be based on individual viral resistance testing and treatment history (see section 5.1).

4.2 Posology and method of administration

Telzir must only be given with low dose ritonavir as a pharmacokinetic enhancer of amprenavir and in combination with other antiretroviral medicinal products. The Summary of Product Characteristics of ritonavir must therefore be consulted prior to initiation of therapy with Telzir.

Therapy should be initiated by a physician experienced in the management of HIV infection.

Telzir (fosamprenavir) is a pro-drug of amprenavir and must not be administered concomitantly with other medicinal products containing amprenavir.

The importance of complying with the full recommended dosing regimen should be stressed to all patients.

<u>Adults (greater than or equal to 18 years of age)</u>

For antiretroviral naïve and experienced patients the recommended dose is 700 mg fosamprenavir twice daily with 100 mg ritonavir twice daily, in combination with other antiretroviral medicinal products (see section 5.1).

Caution is advised if the recommended doses of fosamprenavir with ritonavir detailed above are exceeded (see section 4.4).

<u>Children (less than 12 years of age) and adolescents (12 to 17 years of age)</u>

The safety and efficacy of Telzir with ritonavir has not yet been established in these patient populations. Therefore, this combination must not be used in this age group until further data becomes available.

<u>Elderly (over 65 years of age)</u>

The pharmacokinetics of fosamprenavir have not been studied in this patient population (see section 5.2).

<u>Renal impairment</u>

No initial dose adjustment is considered necessary in patients with renal impairment (see section 5.2).

<u>Hepatic impairment</u>

There are limited data regarding the use of Telzir with ritonavir when co-administered to patients with hepatic impairment and therefore specific dosage recommendations cannot be made. Consequently, Telzir in combination with ritonavir should be used with caution in patients with mild or moderate hepatic impairment and is contraindicated in those with severe hepatic impairment (see sections 4.3, 4.4 and 5.2).

Telzir is administered orally. Telzir (tablets) with ritonavir can be taken with or without food.

Telzir is also available as an oral suspension for use in adults unable to swallow tablets.

4.3 Contraindications

Hypersensitivity to fosamprenavir, amprenavir or to any of the excipients of Telzir, or to ritonavir.

Patients with severe hepatic impairment (see sections 4.4 and 5.2).

Telzir must not be administered concurrently with medicinal products with narrow therapeutic windows that are substrates of cytochrome P450 3A4 (CYP3A4), e.g. amiodarone, astemizole, bepridil, cisapride, dihydroergotamine, ergotamine, pimozide, quinidine, terfenadine (see section 4.5).

Telzir with ritonavir must not be co-administered with medicinal products with narrow therapeutic windows that are highly dependent on CYP2D6 metabolism, e.g. flecainide and propafenone (see section 4.5).

Rifampicin must not be administered concurrently with Telzir (see section 4.5).

Herbal preparations containing St John's wort (*Hypericum perforatum*) must not be used while taking Telzir due to the risk of decreased plasma concentrations and reduced clinical effects of amprenavir (see section 4.5).

4.4 Special warnings and special precautions for use

Patients should be advised that treatment with Telzir, or any other current antiretroviral therapy, does not cure HIV and that they may still develop opportunistic infections and other complications of HIV infection. Current antiretroviral therapies, including Telzir, have not been proven to prevent the risk of transmission of HIV to others through sexual contact or blood contamination. Appropriate precautions should continue to be taken.

Fosamprenavir contains a sulphonamide moiety. The potential for cross-sensitivity between medicinal products in the sulphonamide class and fosamprenavir is unknown. In the pivotal studies of Telzir, in patients receiving fosamprenavir with ritonavir there was no evidence of an increased risk of rashes in patients with a history of sulphonamide allergy versus those who did not have a sulphonamide allergy. Yet, Telzir should be used with caution in patients with a known sulphonamide allergy.

Co-administration of Telzir 700 mg twice daily with ritonavir in doses greater than 100 mg twice daily has not been clinically evaluated. The use of higher ritonavir doses might alter the safety profile of the combination and therefore is not recommended.

<u>Liver disease</u>

The safety and efficacy of Telzir have not been established in patients with significant underlying liver disease. Telzir should be used with caution in patients with mild or moderate hepatic impairment and is contraindicated in patients with severe hepatic impairment. Patients with chronic hepatitis B or C and treated with combination antiretroviral therapy are at an increased risk of severe and potentially fatal hepatic adverse events. In case of concomitant antiviral therapy for hepatitis B or C, please refer also to the relevant Summary of Product Characteristics for these medicinal products.

Patients with pre-existing liver dysfunction, including chronic active hepatitis, have an increased frequency of liver function abnormalities during combination antiretroviral therapy and should be monitored according to standard practice. If there is evidence of worsening liver disease in such patients, interruption or discontinuation of treatment must be considered.

<u>Medicinal products – interactions</u>

The use of Telzir concomitantly with midazolam or triazolam is not recommended (see section 4.5).

The use of Telzir concomitantly with halofantrine or lidocaine (systemic) is not recommended (see section 4.5).

The use of Telzir concomitantly with PDE5 inhibitors (e.g. sildenafil and vardenafil) is not recommended (see section 4.5).

Concomitant use of Telzir with simvastatin or lovastatin is not recommended due to an increased risk of myopathy, including rhabdomyolysis (see section 4.5).

A reduction in the rifabutin dosage by at least 75 % is recommended when administered with Telzir with ritonavir. Further dose reduction may be necessary (see section 4.5).

Because of the interactions with amprenavir, the efficacy of hormonal contraceptives may be impaired. Therefore, alternative reliable barrier methods of contraception are recommended for women of childbearing potential (see section 4.5).

Anticonvulsants (carbamazepine, phenobarbital, phenytoin) should be used with caution. Telzir may be less effective due to decreased amprenavir plasma concentrations in patients taking these medicinal products concomitantly (see section 4.5).

Therapeutic concentration monitoring is recommended for immunosuppressant medicinal products (cyclosporine, tacrolimus, rapamycin) when co-administered with Telzir (see section 4.5).

Therapeutic concentration monitoring is recommended for tricyclic antidepressants (e.g. desipramine and nortriptyline) when coadministered with Telzir (see section 4.5).

When methadone is coadministered with Telzir, patients should be closely monitored for opiate abstinence syndrome (see section 4.5).

When warfarin or other oral anticoagulants are coadministered with Telzir a reinforced monitoring of INR (International Normalised Ratio) is recommended (see section 4.5).

<u>Rash / cutaneous reactions</u>

Most patients with mild or moderate rash can continue Telzir. Appropriate antihistamines (e.g. cetirizine dihydrochloride) may reduce pruritus and hasten the resolution of rash. Severe and life-threatening skin reactions, including Stevens-Johnson syndrome, were reported in less than 1 % of patients included in the clinical development programme. Telzir should be permanently discontinued in case of severe rash, or in case of rash of moderate intensity with systemic or mucosal symptoms (see section 4.8).

<u>Haemophiliac patients</u>

There have been reports of increased bleeding including spontaneous skin haematomas and haemarthroses in haemophiliac patients type A and B treated with protease inhibitors (PIs). In some patients administration of factor VIII was necessary. In more than half of the reported cases, treatment with protease inhibitors was continued, or reintroduced if treatment had been discontinued. A causal relationship has been evoked, although the mechanism of action has not been elucidated. Haemophiliac patients should therefore be informed of the possibility of increased bleeding.

<u>Hyperglycaemia</u>

New onset of diabetes mellitus, hyperglycaemia or exacerbations of existing diabetes mellitus have been reported in patients receiving antiretroviral therapy, including protease inhibitors. In some of these, the hyperglycaemia was severe and in some cases also associated with ketoacidosis. Many of the patients had confounding medical conditions, some of which required therapy with medicinal products that have been associated with the development of diabetes mellitus or hyperglycaemia.

Lipodystrophy

Combination antiretroviral therapy has been associated with the redistribution of body fat (lipodystrophy) in HIV patients. The long-term consequences of these events are currently unknown. Knowledge about the mechanism is incomplete. A connection between visceral lipomatosis and protease inhibitors and lipoatrophy and nucleoside reverse transcriptase inhibitors has been hypothesised. A higher risk of lipodystrophy has been associated with individual factors such as older age, and with drug related factors such as longer duration of antiretroviral treatment and associated metabolic disturbances. Clinical examination should include evaluation for physical signs of fat redistribution. Consideration should be given to the measurement of fasting serum lipids and blood glucose. Lipid disorders should be managed as clinically appropriate (see section 4.8).

Immune Reactivation Syndrome

In HIV-infected patients with severe immune deficiency at the time of institution of combination antiretroviral therapy (CART), an inflammatory reaction to asymptomatic or residual opportunistic pathogens may arise and cause serious clinical conditions, or aggravation of symptoms. Typically, such reactions have been observed within the first few weeks or months of initiation of CART. Relevant examples are cytomegalovirus retinitis, generalised and/or focal mycobacterium infections, and *Pneumocystis carinii* pneumonia. Any inflammatory symptoms should be evaluated and treatment instituted when necessary.

4.5 Interaction with other medicinal products and other forms of Interaction

When fosamprenavir and ritonavir are co-administered, the ritonavir metabolic drug interaction profile may predominate because ritonavir is a more potent CYP3A4 inhibitor. The full prescribing information for ritonavir must therefore be consulted prior to initiation of therapy with Telzir with ritonavir. Ritonavir also inhibits CYP2D6 but to a lesser extent than CYP3A4. Ritonavir induces CYP3A4, CYP1A2, CYP2C9 and glucuronosyl transferase.

Additionally, both amprenavir, the active metabolite of fosamprenavir, and ritonavir are primarily metabolised in the liver by CYP3A4. Therefore, any medicinal products that either share this metabolic pathway or modify CYP3A4 activity may modify the pharmacokinetics of amprenavir and ritonavir. Similarly administration of fosamprenavir with ritonavir may modify the pharmacokinetics of other active substances that share this metabolic pathway.

• Associations contraindicated (see section 4.3)

CYP3A4 substrates with narrow therapeutic index

Telzir must not be administered concurrently with medicinal products with narrow therapeutic windows containing active substances that are substrates of cytochrome P450 3A4 (CYP3A4). Co-administration may result in competitive inhibition of the metabolism of these active substances thus increasing their plasma level and leading to serious and / or life-threatening adverse reactions such as cardiac arrhythmia (e.g. amiodarone, astemizole, bepridil, cisapride, pimozide, quinidine, terfenadine) or peripheral vasospasm or ischaemia (e.g. ergotamine, dihydroergotamine).

CYP2D6 substrates with narrow therapeutic index

Telzir with ritonavir must not be co-administered with medicinal products containing active substances that are highly dependent on CYP2D6 metabolism and for which elevated plasma concentrations are associated with serious and / or life-threatening adverse reactions. These active substances include flecainide and propafenone.

Rifampicin

Rifampicin reduces the amprenavir plasma AUC by approximately 82 %. Based on information for other protease inhibitors, it is expected that co-administration of Telzir with ritonavir with rifampicin will also result in large decreases in plasma concentrations of amprenavir. Accordingly, Telzir with ritonavir must not be co-administered with rifampicin.

St John's wort (*Hypericum perforatum*)

Serum levels of amprenavir and ritonavir can be reduced by concomitant use of the herbal preparation St John's wort (*Hypericum perforatum*). This is due to induction of drug metabolising enzymes by St John's wort. Herbal preparations containing St John's wort should therefore not be combined with Telzir with ritonavir. If a patient is already taking St John's wort, check amprenavir, ritonavir and if possible viral levels and stop St John's wort. Amprenavir and ritonavir levels may increase on stopping St John's wort. The inducing effect may persist for at least 2 weeks after cessation of treatment with St John's wort.

• Other combinations

Antiretroviral medicinal products

Non-nucleoside reverse transcriptase inhibitors

Efavirenz: there was no clinically relevant interaction when fosamprenavir 700 mg twice daily and ritonavir 100 mg twice daily was used concurrently with efavirenz (600 mg once daily).

Nevirapine: based on the effect of nevirapine on other HIV protease inhibitors, nevirapine may decrease the serum concentration of amprenavir. Appropriate doses of the combination with respect to safety and efficacy have not been established. This combination should be used with caution.

Nucleoside / Nucleotide reverse transcriptase inhibitors

Interaction studies with abacavir, lamivudine and zidovudine have been performed with amprenavir without ritonavir. Based on data derived from these studies and because ritonavir is not expected to have a significant impact on the pharmacokinetics of NRTIs, the co-administration of fosamprenavir and ritonavir with these medicinal products is not expected to significantly alter the exposure of the co-administered active substances.

Didanosine chewable tablet: no pharmacokinetic study has been performed with fosamprenavir in combination with didanosine. Clinically significant interaction resulting from an increase in the stomach pH due to the didanosine antacid component is unlikely and no dose separation or adjustment is considered necessary when fosamprenavir and didanosine are administered concomitantly (see chapter, Antacids). No significant interaction is expected with didanosine gastro-resistant capsule.

Tenofovir: no recommendations can be drawn at this stage on the co-administration of fosamprenavir with ritonavir with tenofovir.

Protease Inhibitors

Lopinavir / ritonavir: no dose recommendation can be given for the co-administration of Telzir with ritonavir and lopinavir / ritonavir, but close monitoring is advised because the safety and efficacy of this combination is unknown. The C_{max}, AUC and C_{min} of lopinavir were increased by 30 %, 37 % and 52 % respectively when lopinavir 400 mg with ritonavir 100 mg twice daily was given with fosamprenavir 700 mg with ritonavir 100 mg twice daily for two weeks. The C_{max}, AUC and C_{min} of amprenavir were decreased by 58 %, 63 % and 65 % respectively.

When lopinavir 533 mg with ritonavir 133 mg was administered in combination with fosamprenavir 1400 mg twice daily for two weeks, the C_{max}, AUC, and C_{min} of lopinavir were unchanged compared to values observed for lopinavir 400 mg with ritonavir 100 mg twice daily. However, the AUC and C_{min} of amprenavir were decreased by 26 % and 42 %, respectively; whereas, C_{max} was not significantly altered compared to values obtained for fosamprenavir 700 mg with ritonavir 100 mg twice daily.

No interaction studies have been undertaken between fosamprenavir with ritonavir and the protease inhibitors: indinavir, saquinavir, nelfinavir and atazanavir.

Antibiotics / Antifungals

Clarithromycin: a reduction in the clarithromycin dose should be considered when co-administered with Telzir with ritonavir in patients with renal impairment as moderate increases in clarithromycin concentrations are expected when co-administered with Telzir with ritonavir.

Erythromycin: no pharmacokinetic study has been performed with fosamprenavir with ritonavir in combination with erythromycin, however, plasma levels of erythromycin may be increased when co-administered.

Ketoconazole / Itraconazole: co-administration of amprenavir with ketoconazole increased ketoconazole AUC by 44 %. When ritonavir is co-administered, a larger increase in ketoconazole concentration may occur. Itraconazole concentrations are expected to increase in the same manner as ketoconazole. In the absence of specific studies of fosamprenavir with ritonavir in combination with ketoconazole or itraconazole, no recommendations can be drawn in terms of dose adjustment.

Rifabutin: co-administration of amprenavir with rifabutin results in a 200 % increase in rifabutin plasma concentrations (AUC) which could potentially lead to an increase of rifabutin related adverse reactions, notably uveitis. When ritonavir is co-administered a larger increase in rifabutin concentrations may occur. A reduction in the rifabutin dosage by at least 75 % is recommended when administered with Telzir with ritonavir. Further dose reduction may be necessary.

Other medicinal products

Medicinal products that may reduce plasma amprenavir concentrations when co-administered with Telzir

Antacids, Histamine H_2 receptor antagonist and Proton-Pump inhibitors: no dose adjustment for any of the respective medicinal products is considered necessary when antacids, proton-pump inhibitors or histamine H_2 receptor antagonists are administered concomitantly with fosamprenavir. The AUC and C_{max} of amprenavir were decreased by 18 % and 35 % respectively, whilst the C_{min} (C12h) was comparable, when a single 1400 mg dose of fosamprenavir was co-administered with a single 30 ml dose of antacid suspension (equivalent to 3.6 grams aluminium hydroxide and 1.8 grams magnesium hydroxide).

Serum levels of amprenavir can be reduced by concomitant use of histamine H_2 receptor antagonists (for example ranitidine and cimetidine). Concurrent administration of ranitidine (300 mg single dose) with fosamprenavir (1400 mg single dose) decreased plasma amprenavir AUC by 30 % and C_{max} by 51 %. There was, however, no change observed in the amprenavir C_{min} (C12h).

Anticonvulsant active substances: concomitant administration of anticonvulsant active substances known as enzymatic inductors (phenytoin, phenobarbital, carbamazepine) with fosamprenavir may lead to a decrease in the plasma concentrations of amprenavir. These combinations should be used with caution.

Medicinal products whose plasma levels may be increased when co-administered with Telzir

Other medicinal products with a narrow therapeutic window: some substances (e.g. lidocaine (by systemic route) and halofantrine) given with Telzir may cause serious adverse reactions. Concomitant use is not recommended.

Benzodiazepines: concomitant use of Telzir with midazolam or triazolam could result in prolonged sedation or respiratory depression and thus is not recommended.

Erectile dysfunction medicinal products: concomitant use is not recommended. Based on data for ritonavir and other protease inhibitors, plasma concentrations of PDE5 inhibitors (e.g. sildenafil and vardenafil) are expected to substantially increase when co-administered with Telzir with ritonavir and may result in an increase in PDE5 inhibitor associated adverse reactions, including hypotension, visual changes and priapism.

HMG-CoA reductase inhibitors: if treatment with a HMG-CoA reductase inhibitor is indicated, pravastatin or fluvastatin is recommended because their metabolism is not dependent on CYP 3A4 and interactions are not expected with protease inhibitors. HMG-CoA reductase inhibitors which are highly dependent on CYP3A4 for metabolism, such as lovastatin and simvastatin, are expected to have markedly increased plasma concentrations when co-administered with Telzir with ritonavir. Since increased concentrations of HMG-CoA reductase inhibitors may cause myopathy, including rhabdomyolysis, the combination of lovastatin or simvastatin with Telzir with ritonavir is not recommended. No adjustment of the fosamprenavir or ritonavir dose is required when co-administered with atorvastatin.

The C_{max} , AUC and C_{min} of atorvastatin were increased by 184 %, 153 % and 73 % respectively when atorvastatin (10 mg once daily for 4 days) was given with fosamprenavir 700 mg twice daily with ritonavir 100 mg twice daily for two weeks. The C_{max}, AUC and C_{min} of amprenavir were unchanged. When used with Telzir with ritonavir, doses of atorvastatin no greater than 20 mg / day should be administered, with careful monitoring for atorvastatin toxicity.

Immunosuppressants: frequent therapeutic concentration monitoring of immunosuppresant levels is recommended until levels have stabilised as plasma concentrations of cyclosporin, rapamycin and tacrolimus may be increased when co-administered with fosamprenavir with ritonavir.

Tricyclic antidepressants: careful monitoring of the therapeutic and adverse reactions of tricyclic antidepressants is recommended when they (for example desipramine and nortriptyline) are concomitantly administered with Telzir.

Medicinal products whose plasma levels may be decreased when co-administered with Telzir

Methadone: no data are available on the co-administration of fosamprenavir with ritonavir and methadone. Amprenavir and ritonavir both decrease plasma concentrations of methadone. When methadone is co-administered with Telzir with ritonavir, patients should be closely monitored for opiate abstinence syndrome, with concomitant monitoring of methadone plasma levels.

Oral anticoagulants: a reinforced monitoring of the International Normalised Ratio is recommended in case of administration of Telzir with ritonavir with warfarin or other oral anticoagulants, due to a possible decrease or increase of their antithrombotic effect.

Oral contraceptives: alternative reliable barrier methods of contraception are recommended for women of childbearing potential. Oestrogens and progestogens may interact with fosamprenavir and ritonavir, thus concomitant use may impair the efficacy of hormonal contraceptives.

4.6 Pregnancy and lactation

Pregnancy

There is no clinical experience with fosamprenavir in pregnant women. In animal studies at systemic plasma exposures (AUC) to amprenavir lower than therapeutic exposure in patients treated with Telzir, some developmental toxicity was observed (see section 5.3). In view of the low exposure in reproductive toxicity studies, the potential developmental toxicity of Telzir has not been fully determined.

Telzir should be used during pregnancy only if the potential benefit justifies the potential risk to the foetus.

Lactation

Amprenavir-related material was found in rat milk, but it is not known whether amprenavir is excreted in human milk. Rat pups exposed pre and post-natally to amprenavir and fosamprenavir showed developmental toxicity (see section 5.3).

It is therefore recommended that mothers treated with Telzir do not breast-feed their infants. As a general rule, it is recommended that HIV-infected women must not breast-feed under any circumstances to avoid transmission of HIV.

4.7 Effects on ability to drive and use machines

No studies on the effects of Telzir in combination with ritonavir on the ability to drive and use machines have been performed. The adverse reaction profile of Telzir should be borne in mind when considering the patient's ability to drive or operate machinery (see section 4.8).

4.8 Undesirable effects

The safety of fosamprenavir has been studied in 755 patients in Phase II and III controlled clinical trials. The safety of the co-administration of fosamprenavir with low dose ritonavir was established in two pivotal Phase III trials: APV30002 (n = 322) in antiretroviral naïve patients, fosamprenavir (1400 mg) given once daily in combination with ritonavir (200 mg) as part of a triple regimen including abacavir and lamivudine. APV30003 in protease inhibitor experienced patients, fosamprenavir given in combination with low dose ritonavir either once daily (1400 mg / 200 mg) (n = 106) or twice daily (700 mg / 100 mg) (n = 106) in combination with two active reverse transcriptase inhibitors (RTIs).

The adverse reaction profile was similar across all the respective studies: antiretroviral naïve (APV30002) and protease inhibitor experienced (twice daily dosing, APV30003) patient populations.

The adverse reactions are listed by body system, organ class and absolute frequency. Frequencies are defined as: Very common (⩾ 1/10), Common (⩾ 1/100, < 1/10), Uncommon (⩾ 1/1,000, < 1/100), Rare (⩾ 1/10,000, < 1/1,000) or Very rare (< 1/10,000), including isolated reports. The frequency of the reactions were calculated using adverse reactions that were of at least moderate intensity (Grade 2 or more) and reported by investigators as being attributable to the medicinal products used in the studies. The most frequent clinical adverse reactions (occurring in at least 1 % of patients) reported in the two large clinical studies in adults with at least a possible casual relationship to Telzir are summarised below.

Body System	Adverse reaction	Frequency
Nervous system disorders	Headache, dizziness	Common
Gastrointestinal disorders	Diarrhoea	Very common
	Loose stools, nausea, vomiting, abdominal pain	Common
Skin and subcutaneous tissue disorders	Rash	Common
General disorders and administration site conditions	Fatigue	Common

Rash / cutaneous reactions: erythematous or maculopapular cutaneous eruptions, with or without pruritus, may occur during therapy. The rash generally will resolve spontaneously without the necessity of discontinuing treatment with the fosamprenavir with ritonavir.

Severe or life-threatening rash, including Stevens-Johnson syndrome is rare, reported in less than 1 % of patients included in the clinical development programme. Fosamprenavir with ritonavir therapy should be definitively stopped in case of severe rash or in case of rash of mild or moderate intensity associated with systemic or mucosal signs (see section 4.4).

Clinical chemistry abnormalities: clinical chemistry abnormalities (Grade 3 or 4) potentially related to treatment with fosamprenavir with ritonavir and reported in greater than or equal to 1 % of patients, included:

increased ALT (*common*), AST (*common*), serum lipase (*common*) and triglycerides (*very common*). Grade 3 or 4 elevations in total cholesterol values were observed in less than 1 % of patients (< 1 % APV30002; 0 % APV 30003).

Lipodystrophy: combination antiretroviral therapy has been associated with redistribution of body fat (lipodystrophy) in HIV patients including the loss of peripheral and facial subcutaneous fat, increased intra-abdominal and visceral fat, breast hypertrophy and dorsocervical fat accumulation (buffalo hump) (see section 4.4).

Metabolic abnormalities: combination antiretroviral therapy has been associated with metabolic abnormalities such as hypertriglyceridaemia, hypercholesterolaemia, insulin resistance, hyperglycaemia and hyperlactataemia (see section 4.4).

Hyperglycaemia: new onset of diabetes mellitus, hyperglycaemia or exacerbations of existing diabetes mellitus have been reported in patients receiving antiretroviral protease inhibitors (see section 4.4).

Rhabdomyolysis: an increase in CPK, myalgia, myositis, and rarely, rhabdomyolysis, have been reported with protease inhibitors, more specifically in association with nucleoside analogues.

Haemophiliac patients: there have been reports of increased spontaneous bleeding in haemophiliac patients receiving antiretroviral protease inhibitors (see section 4.4).

Immune Reactivation Syndrome: in HIV-infected patients with severe immune deficiency at the time of initiation of combination antiretroviral therapy (CART), an inflammatory reaction to asymptomatic or residual opportunistic infections may arise (see section 4.4).

4.9 Overdose

There is no known antidote for Telzir. It is not known whether amprenavir can be removed by peritoneal dialysis or haemodialysis. If overdosage occurs, the patient should be monitored for evidence of toxicity (see section 4.8) and standard supportive treatment applied as necessary.

5. PHARMACOLOGICAL PROPERTIES

5.1 Pharmacodynamic properties

Pharmacotherapeutic group: Antivirals for systemic use, protease inhibitor, ATC Code: J05A (pending)

Mechanism of action

Fosamprenavir is rapidly converted to amprenavir by cellular or serum phosphatases *in vivo*. Amprenavir is a competitive inhibitor of HIV-1 protease. Amprenavir binds to the active site of HIV-1 protease and thereby prevents the processing of viral gag and gag-pol polyprotein precursors, resulting in the formation of immature non-infectious viral particles.

Fosamprenavir has little or no antiviral activity *in vitro*. The *in vitro* antiviral activity observed with fosamprenavir is due to the presence of trace amounts of amprenavir. The *in vitro* antiviral activity of amprenavir was evaluated against HIV-1 IIIB in both acutely and chronically infected lymphoblastic cell lines (MT-4, CEM-CCRF, H9) and in peripheral blood lymphocytes. The 50% inhibitory concentration (IC_{50}) of amprenavir ranged from 0.012 to 0.08 μM in acutely infected cells and was 0.41 μM in chronically infected cells (1 μM = 0.50 μg/ml). *In vitro,* amprenavir exhibited synergistic anti-HIV-1 activity in combination with the nucleoside reverse transcriptase inhibitors (NRTIs) abacavir, didanosine and zidovudine and the protease inhibitor saquinavir, and additive anti-HIV-1 activity in combination with indinavir, nelfinavir and ritonavir. The relationship between *in vitro* anti-HIV-1 activity of amprenavir and the inhibition of HIV-1 replication in humans has not been defined.

Co-administration of ritonavir with fosamprenavir increase plasma amprenavir AUC by approximately 2-fold and plasma $C_{\tau,ss}$ by 4- to 6-fold, compared to values obtained when fosamprenavir is administered alone. Administration of fosamprenavir 700 mg twice daily with ritonavir 100 mg twice daily results in plasma amprenavir trough concentrations (geometric mean plasma C_{min} 1.74 μg/ml, reported in study APV30003 in antiretroviral experienced patients) above the median IC_{50} value reported in this study (0.008 μg/ml [0.001 – 0.144]).

Resistance

HIV-1 isolates with a decreased susceptibility to amprenavir have been selected during *in vitro* serial passage experiments. Reduced susceptibility to amprenavir was associated with virus that had developed I50V or I84V or V32I+I47V or I54M mutations.

No development of genotypic or phenotypic amprenavir resistance was detected in virus from thirty-two anti retroviral therapy naïve patients receiving fosamprenavir 1400 mg with ritonavir 200 mg once daily (Study APV30002) and experiencing virological failure or on-going viral replication. A significantly higher proportion of nelfinavir treated patients acquired primary and / or secondary PRO mutations (nelfinavir 27/54 (50 %)) (p< 0.001).

Development of amprenavir resistance was detected in viral isolates from protease experienced patients receiving fosamprenavir 1400 mg with ritonavir 200 mg once daily or 700 mg fosamprenavir with 100 mg ritonavir twice daily (Study APV30003) and having virological failure or having on-going viral replication. 58% (19/33) versus 25% (7/28) patients acquired primary and / or secondary PRO mutations in the fosamprenavir with ritonavir arm versus the lopinavir / ritonavir arm. The following amprenavir resistance–associated mutations developed either alone or in combination: V32I, M46I/L, I47V, I50V, I54L/M and I84V.

Cross-Resistance

The data are currently too limited to determine a clinically relevant phenotypic cut-off for fosamprenavir with ritonavir.

Cross-resistance between amprenavir and reverse transcriptase inhibitors is unlikely to occur because the enzyme targets are different.

Telzir is not recommended for use as monotherapy, due to the rapid emergence of resistant virus.

Clinical experience

The clinical experience is mainly based on two open label studies performed in comparison to nelfinavir in antiretroviral naïve patients (study APV30002) and in comparison to lopinavir / ritonavir in antiretroviral experienced patients (study APV30003). In both studies fosamprenavir was used boosted with ritonavir.

Antiretroviral Naïve Patients

In antiretroviral naïve patients in APV30002, fosamprenavir (1400 mg) given once daily in combination with low dose ritonavir (200 mg) as part of a triple regimen including abacavir (300 mg twice daily) and lamivudine (150 mg twice daily) showed similar efficacy over 48 weeks compared to nelfinavir (1250 mg) given twice daily in combination with abacavir with lamivudine (300 and 150 mg twice daily).

Non-inferiority was demonstrated between fosamprenavir with ritonavir and nelfinavir based on the proportions of patients achieving plasma HIV-1 RNA levels < 400 copies/ml at 48 weeks (primary endpoint). In the ITT (Rebound or Discontinuation = Failure) analysis, 69 % (221 / 322) of patients receiving fosamprenavir with ritonavir achieved < 400 copies/ml compared to 68 % (221 / 327) of patients receiving nelfinavir.

The median plasma HIV-1 RNA had decreased by 3.1 $\log_{10}$ copies/ml and 3.0 $\log_{10}$ copies/ml at Week 48 in the fosamprenavir with ritonavir and nelfinavir arms respectively.

The median baseline CD4 cell count was low (170 cells/mm^3 overall) in both groups. CD4 + cell counts increased in both the fosamprenavir with ritonavir and nelfinavir groups, with median increases above baseline being similar in magnitude at Week 48 (+ 203 and + 207 cells/mm^3, respectively).

The data presented above demonstrates that the once daily regimen of fosamprenavir with ritonavir (1400 / 200 mg OD) in antiretroviral naïve patients showed similar efficacy compared to nelfinavir given twice daily. However, the demonstration of efficacy in this population is only based on one open label study versus nelfinavir. Another clinical study is planned to reinforce the efficacy demonstration of the medicinal product in this population. Therefore, as a conservative approach, based on enhanced amprenavir C_{trough} levels, the twice daily dosing regimen of fosamprenavir with ritonavir is recommended for optimal therapeutic management of this population (see section 4.2).

Antiretroviral Experienced Patients

In a randomised open-label study (APV30003) in protease inhibitor experienced patients with virological failure (less than or equal to two PIs) the fosamprenavir with ritonavir combination (700 / 100 mg twice daily or 1400 / 200 mg once daily) did not demonstrate non-inferiority to lopinavir / ritonavir with regard to viral suppression as measured by the average area under the curve minus baseline (AAUCMB) for plasma HIV-1 RNA over 48 weeks (the primary end point). Results were in favour of the lopinavir / ritonavir arm as detailed below.

All patients in this study had failed treatment with a previous protease inhibitor regimen (defined as plasma HIV-1 RNA that never went below 1,000 copies/ml after at least 12 consecutive weeks of therapy, or initial suppression of HIV-1 RNA which subsequently rebounded to ⩾ 1,000 copies/ml). However, only 65 % of patients were receiving a PI based regimen at study entry.

The population enrolled mainly consisted of moderately antiretroviral experienced patients. The median durations of prior exposure to NRTIs were 257 weeks for patients receiving fosamprenavir with ritonavir twice daily (79 % had ⩾ 3 prior NRTIs) and 210 weeks for patients receiving lopinavir/ritonavir (64 % had ⩾ 3 prior NRTIs). The median durations of prior exposure to protease inhibitors were 149 weeks for patients receiving fosamprenavir with ritonavir twice daily (49 % received ⩾ 2 prior PIs) and 130 weeks for patients receiving lopinavir/ritonavir (40 % received ⩾ 2 prior PIs).

The mean AAUCMBs ($\log_{10}$ c/ml) in the ITT (E) population (Observed analysis) at 48 weeks are described in the table below:

Plasma HIV-1 RNA Average Area Under the Curve Minus Baseline (AAUCMB) Values ($\log_{10}$ copies/ml) at week 48 by Randomisation Strata in APV30003 ITT (E) Population (Observed Analysis)

(see Table 1 on next page)

When considering the proportion of patients with undetectable viral load in the fosamprenavir with ritonavir twice daily dosing regimens and lopinavir / ritonavir arms respectively, results showed a trend in favour of the lopinavir / ritonavir arms: 58 % versus 61 % (plasma HIV-1 RNA < 400 copies/ml) or 46 % versus 50 % (plasma HIV-1 RNA < 50 copies/ml) at Week 48 (secondary efficacy endpoint) in the intent to treat (RD=F) analysis.

In patients with high viral load at baseline > 100,000 copies/ml) 7/14 (50 %) patients in the lopinavir / ritonavir group and 6/19 (32 %) patients in the fosamprenavir with ritonavir group had plasma HIV-1 RNA < 400 copies/ml.

The fosamprenavir with ritonavir twice daily regimen and the lopinavir / ritonavir twice daily regimen showed similar immunological improvements through 48 weeks of treatment as measured by median change from baseline in CD4 + cell count (fosamprenavir with ritonavir twice daily: 81 cells/mm^3: lopinavir / ritonavir twice daily: 91 cells/mm^3).

There are insufficient data to recommend the use of fosamprenavir with ritonavir in heavily pre-treated patients.

5.2 Pharmacokinetic properties

After oral administration, fosamprenavir is rapidly and almost completely hydrolysed to amprenavir and inorganic phosphate prior to reaching the systemic circulation. The conversion of fosamprenavir to amprenavir appears to primarily occur in the gut epithelium.

Table 1 Plasma HIV-1 RNA Average Area Under the Curve Minus Baseline (AAUCMB) Values (log_{10} copies/ml) at week 48 by Randomisation Strata in APV30003 ITT (E) Population (Observed Analysis)

Plasma HIV-1 RNA stratum	Observed analysis FOS/RTV BID N=107 Mean (n)	Observed analysis LPV/RTV BID N=103 Mean (n)	Observed analysis Mean Diff. (97.5% CI) FOS/RTV BID vs LPV/RTV BID
1000 – 10,000 copies/ml	-1.53 (41)	-1.43 (43)	-0.104 (-0.550, 0.342)
>10,000 – 100,000 copies/ml	-1.59 (45)	-1.81 (46)	0.216 (-0.213, 0.664)
>100,000 copies/ml	-1.38 (19)	-2.61 (14)	1.232 (0.512, 1.952)
Total population	-1.53 (105)	-1.76 (103)	0.244 (-0.047, 0.536)

Key: FOS/RTV BID – Fosamprenavir with ritonavir twice daily, LPV/RTV BID – Lopinavir / ritonavir twice daily

The pharmacokinetic properties of amprenavir following co-administration of Telzir with ritonavir have been evaluated in healthy adult subjects and HIV-infected patients and no substantial differences were observed between these two groups.

Telzir tablet and oral suspension formulations, both given fasted, delivered equivalent plasma amprenavir AUC_∞ values and the Telzir oral suspension formulation delivered a 14 % higher plasma amprenavir C_{max} as compared to the oral tablet formulation.

Absorption

After single dose administration of fosamprenavir, amprenavir peak plasma concentrations are observed approximately 2 hours after administration. Fosamprenavir AUC values are, in general, less than 1 % of those observed for amprenavir. The absolute bioavailability of fosamprenavir in humans has not been established.

After multiple dose oral administration of equivalent fosamprenavir and amprenavir doses, comparable amprenavir AUC values were observed; however, C_{max} values were approximately 30 % lower and C_{min} values were approximately 28 % higher with fosamprenavir.

After multiple dose oral administration of fosamprenavir 700 mg with ritonavir 100 mg twice daily, amprenavir was rapidly absorbed with a geometric mean (95 % CI) steady state peak plasma amprenavir concentration (C_{max}) of 6.08 (5.38-6.86) μg/ml occurring approximately 1.5 (0.75-5.0) hours after dosing (t_{max}). The mean steady state plasma amprenavir trough concentration (C_{min}) was 2.12 (1.77-2.54) μg/ml and $AUC_{0\text{-}tau}$ was 39.6 (34.5–45.3) h*μg/ml.

Administration of the fosamprenavir tablet formulation with a high fat meal did not alter plasma amprenavir pharmacokinetics (C_{max}, t_{max} or $AUC_{0\text{-}\infty}$) compared to the administration of this formulation in the fasted state. Telzir tablets may be taken without regard to food intake.

Co-administration of amprenavir with grapefruit juice was not associated with clinically significant changes in plasma amprenavir pharmacokinetics.

Distribution

The apparent volume of distribution of amprenavir following administration of Telzir is approximately 430 l (6 l/kg assuming a 70 kg body weight), suggesting a large volume of distribution, with penetration of amprenavir freely into tissues beyond the systemic circulation. This value is decreased by approximately 40 % when Telzir is co-administered with ritonavir, most likely due to an increase in amprenavir bioavailability.

In *in vitro* studies, the protein binding of amprenavir is approximately 90 %. It is bound to the alpha-1-acid glycoprotein (AAG) and albumin, but has a higher affinity for AAG. Concentrations of AAG have been shown to decrease during the course of antiretroviral therapy. This change will decrease the total active substance concentration in the plasma, however the amount of unbound amprenavir, which is the active moiety, is likely to be unchanged.

CSF penetration of amprenavir is negligible in humans. Amprenavir appears to penetrate into semen, though semen concentrations are lower than plasma concentrations.

Metabolism

Fosamprenavir is rapidly and almost completely hydrolysed to amprenavir and inorganic phosphate as it is absorbed through the gut epithelium, following oral administration. Amprenavir is primarily metabolised by the liver with less than 1 % excreted unchanged in the urine. The primary route of metabolism is via the cytochrome P450 3A4 enzyme. Amprenavir metabolism is inhibited by ritonavir, via inhibition of CYP3A4, resulting in increased plasma concentrations of amprenavir. Amprenavir in addition is also an inhibitor of the CYP3A4 enzyme, although to a lesser extent than ritonavir. Therefore medicinal products that are inducers, inhibitors or substrates of CYP3A4 must be used with caution when administered concurrently with Telzir with ritonavir (see sections 4.3 and 4.5).

Elimination

Following administration of Telzir, the half-life of amprenavir is 7.7 hours. When Telzir is co-administered with ritonavir, the half-life of amprenavir is increased to 15 – 23 hours.

The primary route of elimination of amprenavir is via hepatic metabolism with less than 1 % excreted unchanged in the urine and no detectable amprenavir in faeces. Metabolites account for approximately 14 % of the administered amprenavir dose in the urine, and approximately 75 % in the faeces.

Special populations

Paediatrics

The pharmacokinetics of fosamprenavir in combination with ritonavir has not been studied in paediatric patients.

Elderly

The pharmacokinetics of fosamprenavir in combination with ritonavir has not been studied in patients over 65 years of age.

Renal impairment

Patients with renal impairment have not been specifically studied. Less than 1 % of the therapeutic dose of amprenavir is excreted unchanged in the urine. Renal clearance of ritonavir is also negligible, therefore the impact of renal impairment on amprenavir and ritonavir elimination should be minimal.

Hepatic impairment

Fosamprenavir is converted in man to amprenavir. The principal route of amprenavir and ritonavir elimination is hepatic metabolism. There are limited data regarding the use of this combination in patients with hepatic impairment and therefore specific dosage recommendations cannot be made (see sections 4.3 and 4.4).

5.3 Preclinical safety data

Toxicity was similar to that of amprenavir and occurred at amprenavir plasma exposure levels below human exposure after treatment with fosamprenavir in combination with ritonavir at the recommended dose.

In repeated dose toxicity studies in adult rats and dogs, fosamprenavir produced evidence of gastrointestinal disturbances (salivation, vomiting and soft to liquid faeces), and hepatic changes (increased liver weights, raised serum liver enzyme activities and microscopic changes, including hepatocyte necrosis).

In reproductive toxicity studies with fosamprenavir in rats, male fertility was not affected, but in females gravid uterine weights, numbers of ovarian corpora lutea and uterine implantation sites were reduced. In pregnant rats and rabbits there were no major effects on embryo-foetal development. However, the number of abortions increased. In rabbits, systemic exposure at the high dose level was only 0.3 times human exposure at the maximum clinical dose and thus the developmental toxicity of fosamprenavir has not been fully determined. In rats exposed pre- and post-natally to fosamprenavir, pups showed impaired physical and functional development and reduced growth. Pup survival was decreased. In addition, decreased number of implantation sites per litter and a prolongation of gestation were seen when pups were mated after reaching maturity.

Fosamprenavir was not mutagenic or genotoxic in a standard battery of *in vitro* and *in vivo* assays. Carcinogenicity studies of fosamprenavir in rats and mice have not yet been completed; however, in long-term carcinogenicity studies with amprenavir in mice and rats, there were benign hepatocellular adenomas in males at exposure levels equivalent to 2.0-fold (mice) or 3.8-fold (rats) those in humans given 1200 mg twice daily of amprenavir alone. In male mice altered hepatocellular foci were seen at doses that were at least 2.0 times human therapeutic exposure.

A higher incidence of hepatocellular carcinoma was seen in all amprenavir male mouse treatment groups. However, this increase was not statistically significantly different from male control mice by appropriate tests. The mechanism for the hepatocellular adenomas and carcinomas found in these studies has not been elucidated and the significance of the observed effects for humans is uncertain. However, there is little evidence from the exposure data in humans, both in clinical trials and from marketed use, to suggest that these findings are of clinical significance.

6. PHARMACEUTICAL PARTICULARS

6.1 List of excipients

Tablet core:

Microcrystalline cellulose

Croscarmellose sodium

Povidone K30

Magnesium stearate

Colloidal anhydrous silica

Tablet film-coat:

Hypromellose

Titanium dioxide (E171)

Glycerol triacetate

Iron oxide red (E172)

6.2 Incompatibilities

Not applicable.

6.3 Shelf life

3 years.

6.4 Special precautions for storage

This medicinal product does not require any special storage conditions.

6.5 Nature and contents of container

HDPE bottles with a child resistant polypropylene closure containing 60 tablets.

6.6 Instructions for use and handling

No special requirements.

Administrative Data

7. MARKETING AUTHORISATION HOLDER

Glaxo Group Ltd

Greenford Road

Greenford

Middlesex UB6 0NN

United Kingdom

8. MARKETING AUTHORISATION NUMBER(S)

EU/1/04/282/001

9. DATE OF FIRST AUTHORISATION/RENEWAL OF THE AUTHORISATION

12 July 2004

10. DATE OF REVISION OF THE TEXT

17 December 2004

Telzir Oral Suspension

(GlaxoSmithKline UK)

1. NAME OF THE MEDICINAL PRODUCT

Telzir▼ 50 mg/ml oral suspension.

2. QUALITATIVE AND QUANTITATIVE COMPOSITION

Each ml of oral suspension contains 50 mg fosamprenavir as fosamprenavir calcium (equivalent to approximately 43 mg amprenavir).

For excipients, see section 6.1.

3. PHARMACEUTICAL FORM

Oral suspension.

The suspension is white to off-white in colour.

4. CLINICAL PARTICULARS

4.1 Therapeutic indications

Telzir in combination with low dose ritonavir is indicated for the treatment of Human Immunodeficiency Virus Type 1 (HIV-1) infected adults in combination with other antiretroviral medicinal products.

In moderately antiretroviral experienced patients, Telzir in combination with low dose ritonavir has not been shown to be as effective as lopinavir / ritonavir.

In heavily pretreated patients the use of Telzir in combination with low dose ritonavir has not been sufficiently studied.

In protease inhibitor (PI) experienced patients, the choice of Telzir should be based on individual viral resistance testing and treatment history (see section 5.1).

4.2 Posology and method of administration

Telzir must only be given with low dose ritonavir as a pharmacokinetic enhancer of amprenavir and in combination with other antiretroviral medicinal products. The Summary of Product Characteristics of ritonavir must therefore be consulted prior to initiation of therapy with Telzir.

Therapy should be initiated by a physician experienced in the management of HIV infection.

Telzir (fosamprenavir) is a pro-drug of amprenavir and must not be administered concomitantly with other medicinal products containing amprenavir.

The importance of complying with the full recommended dosing regimen should be stressed to all patients.

Adults (greater than or equal to 18 years of age)

For antiretroviral naïve and experienced patients the recommended dose is 700 mg fosamprenavir twice daily with 100 mg ritonavir twice daily, in combination with other antiretroviral medicinal products (see section 5.1).

Caution is advised if the recommended doses of fosamprenavir with ritonavir detailed above are exceeded (see section 4.4).

Children (less than 12 years of age) and adolescents (12 to 17 years of age)

The safety and efficacy of Telzir with ritonavir has not yet been established in these patient populations. Therefore, this combination must not be used in this age group until further data becomes available.

Elderly (over 65 years of age)

The pharmacokinetics of fosamprenavir have not been studied in this patient population (see section 5.2).

Renal impairment

No initial dose adjustment is considered necessary in patients with renal impairment (see section 5.2).

Hepatic impairment

There are limited data regarding the use of Telzir with ritonavir when co-administered to patients with hepatic impairment and therefore specific dosage recommendations cannot be made. Consequently, Telzir in combination with ritonavir should be used with caution in patients with mild or moderate hepatic impairment and is contraindicated in those with severe hepatic impairment (see sections 4.3, 4.4 and 5.2).

Telzir is administered orally. Telzir is also available as 700 mg film-coated tablets.

The oral suspension **should** be taken **without** food and on an empty stomach.

Shake the bottle vigorously for 20 seconds before first dose is removed and 5 seconds before each subsequent dose.

4.3 Contraindications

Hypersensitivity to fosamprenavir, amprenavir or to any of the excipients of Telzir, or to ritonavir.

Patients with severe hepatic impairment (see sections 4.4 and 5.2).

Telzir must not be administered concurrently with medicinal products with narrow therapeutic windows that are substrates of cytochrome P450 3A4 (CYP3A4), e.g. amiodarone, astemizole, bepridil, cisapride, dihydroergotamine, ergotamine, pimozide, quinidine, terfenadine (see section 4.5).

Telzir with ritonavir must not be co-administered with medicinal products with narrow therapeutic windows that are highly dependent on CYP2D6 metabolism e.g. flecainide and propafenone (see section 4.5).

Rifampicin must not be administered concurrently with Telzir (see section 4.5).

Herbal preparations containing St John's wort (*Hypericum perforatum*) must not be used while taking Telzir due to the risk of decreased plasma concentrations and reduced clinical effects of amprenavir (see section 4.5).

4.4 Special warnings and special precautions for use

Patients should be advised that treatment with the Telzir, or any other current antiretroviral therapy, does not cure HIV and that they may still develop opportunistic infections and other complications of HIV infection. Current antiretroviral therapies, including Telzir, have not been proven to prevent the risk of transmission of HIV to others through sexual contact or blood contamination. Appropriate precautions should continue to be taken.

Fosamprenavir contains a sulphonamide moiety. The potential for cross-sensitivity between medicinal products in the sulphonamide class and fosamprenavir is unknown. In the pivotal studies of Telzir, in patients receiving fosamprenavir with ritonavir there was no evidence of an increased risk of rashes in patients with a history of sulphonamide allergy versus those who did not have a sulphonamide allergy. Yet, Telzir should be used with caution in patients with a known sulphonamide allergy.

The Telzir oral suspension contains propyl and methyl parahydroxybenzoate. These products may cause an allergic reaction in some individuals. This reaction may be delayed.

Co-administration of Telzir 700 mg twice daily with ritonavir in doses greater than 100 mg twice daily has not been clinically evaluated. The use of higher ritonavir doses might alter the safety profile of the combination and therefore is not recommended.

Liver disease

The safety and efficacy of Telzir have not been established in patients with significant underlying liver disease. Telzir should be used with caution in patients with mild or moderate hepatic impairment and is contraindicated in patients with severe hepatic impairment. Patients with chronic hepatitis B or C and treated with combination antiretroviral therapy are at an increased risk of severe and potentially fatal hepatic adverse events. In case of concomitant antiviral therapy for hepatitis B or C, please refer also to the relevant Summary of Product Characteristics for these medicinal products.

Patients with pre-existing liver dysfunction, including chronic active hepatitis, have an increased frequency of liver function abnormalities during combination antiretroviral therapy and should be monitored according to standard practice. If there is evidence of worsening liver disease in such patients, interruption or discontinuation of treatment must be considered.

Medicinal products – interactions

The use of Telzir concomitantly with midazolam or triazolam is not recommended (see section 4.5).

The use of Telzir concomitantly with halofantrine or lidocaine (systemic) is not recommended.

The use of Telzir concomitantly with PDE5 inhibitors (e.g. sildenafil and vardenafil) is not recommended (see section 4.5).

Concomitant use of Telzir with simvastatin or lovastatin is not recommended due to an increased risk of myopathy, including rhabdomyolysis (see section 4.5).

A reduction in the rifabutin dosage by at least 75 % is recommended when administered with Telzir with ritonavir. Further dose reduction may be necessary (see section 4.5).

Because of the interactions with amprenavir, the efficacy of hormonal contraceptives may be impaired. Therefore, alternative reliable barrier methods of contraception are recommended for women of childbearing potential (see section 4.5).

Anticonvulsants (carbamazepine, phenobarbital, phenytoin) should be used with caution. Telzir may be less effective due to decreased amprenavir plasma concentrations in patients taking these medicinal products concomitantly (see section 4.5).

Therapeutic concentration monitoring is recommended for immunosuppressant medicinal products (cyclosporine, tacrolimus, rapamycin) when co-administered with Telzir (see section 4.5).

Therapeutic concentration monitoring is recommended for tricyclic antidepressants (e.g. desipramine and nortriptyline) when co-administered with Telzir (see section 4.5).

When methadone is co-administered with Telzir, patients should be closely monitored for opiate abstinence syndrome (see section 4.5).

When warfarin or other oral anticoagulants are co-administered with Telzir a reinforced monitoring of INR (International normalised ratio) is recommended (see section 4.5).

Rash / cutaneous reactions

Most patients with mild or moderate rash can continue Telzir. Appropriate antihistamines (e.g. cetirizine dihydrochloride) may reduce pruritus and hasten the resolution of rash. Severe and life-threatening skin reactions, including Stevens-Johnson syndrome, were reported in less than 1 % of patients included in the clinical development programme. Telzir should be permanently discontinued in case of severe rash, or in case of rash of moderate intensity with systemic or mucosal symptoms (see section 4.8).

Haemophiliac patients

There have been reports of increased bleeding including spontaneous skin haematomas and haemarthroses in haemophiliac patients type A and B treated with protease inhibitors (PIs). In some patients administration of factor VIII was necessary. In more than half of the reported cases, treatment with protease inhibitors was continued, or reintroduced if treatment had been discontinued. A causal relationship has been evoked, although the mechanism of action has not been elucidated. Haemophiliac patients should therefore be informed of the possibility of increased bleeding.

Hyperglycaemia

New onset of diabetes mellitus, hyperglycaemia or exacerbations of existing diabetes mellitus have been reported in patients receiving antiretroviral therapy, including protease inhibitors. In some of these, the hyperglycaemia was severe and in some cases also associated with ketoacidosis. Many of the patients had confounding medical conditions, some of which required therapy with medicinal products that have been associated with the development of diabetes mellitus or hyperglycaemia.

Lipodystrophy

Combination antiretroviral therapy has been associated with the redistribution of body fat (lipodystrophy) in HIV patients. The long-term consequences of these events are currently unknown. Knowledge about the mechanism is incomplete. A connection between visceral lipomatosis and protease inhibitors and lipoatrophy and nucleoside reverse transcriptase inhibitors has been hypothesised. A higher risk of lipodystrophy has been associated with individual factors such as older age, and with drug related factors such as longer duration of antiretroviral treatment and associated metabolic disturbances. Clinical examination should include evaluation for physical signs of fat redistribution. Consideration should be given to the measurement of fasting serum lipids and blood glucose. Lipid disorders should be managed as clinically appropriate (see section 4.8).

Immune Reactivation Syndrome

In HIV-infected patients with severe immune deficiency at the time of institution of combination antiretroviral therapy (CART), an inflammatory reaction to asymptomatic or residual opportunistic pathogens may arise and cause serious clinical conditions, or aggravation of symptoms. Typically, such reactions have been observed within the first few weeks or months of initiation of CART. Relevant examples are cytomegalovirus retinitis, generalised and/or focal mycobacterium infections, and *Pneumocystis carinii* pneumonia. Any inflammatory symptoms should be evaluated and treatment instituted when necessary.

4.5 Interaction with other medicinal products and other forms of Interaction

When fosamprenavir and ritonavir are co-administered, the ritonavir metabolic drug interaction profile may predominate because ritonavir is a more potent CYP3A4 inhibitor. The full prescribing information for ritonavir must therefore be consulted prior to initiation of therapy with Telzir with ritonavir. Ritonavir also inhibits CYP2D6 but to a lesser extent than CYP3A4. Ritonavir induces CYP3A4, CYP1A2, CYP2C9 and glucuronosyl transferase.

Additionally, both amprenavir, the active metabolite of fosamprenavir, and ritonavir are primarily metabolised in the liver by CYP3A4. Therefore, any medicinal products that either share this metabolic pathway or modify CYP3A4 activity may modify the pharmacokinetics of amprenavir and ritonavir. Similarily, administration of fosamprenavir with ritonavir may modify the pharmacokinetics of other active substances that share this metabolic pathway.

• Associations contraindicated (see section 4.3)

CYP3A4 substrates with narrow therapeutic index

Telzir must not be administered concurrently with medicinal products with narrow therapeutic windows containing active substances that are substrates of cytochrome P450 3A4 (CYP3A4). Co-administration may result in competitive inhibition of the metabolism of these active substances thus increasing their plasma levels and leading to serious and / or life-threatening adverse reactions such as cardiac arrhythmia (e.g. amiodarone, astemizole, bepridil, cisapride, pimozide, quinidine, terfenadine) or peripheral vasospasm or ischaemia (e.g. ergotamine, dihydroergotamine).

CYP2D6 substrates with narrow therapeutic index

Telzir with ritonavir must not be co-administered with medicinal products containing active substances that are highly dependent on CYP2D6 metabolism and for which elevated plasma concentrations are associated with serious and / or life-threatening adverse reactions. These active substances include flecainide and propafenone.

Rifampicin

Rifampicin reduces the amprenavir plasma AUC by approximately 82 %. Based on information for other protease inhibitors, it is expected that co-administration of Telzir with ritonavir with rifampicin will also result in large decreases in plasma concentrations of amprenavir. Accordingly, Telzir with ritonavir must not be co-administered with rifampicin.

St John's wort (*Hypericum perforatum*)

Serum levels of amprenavir and ritonavir can be reduced by concomitant use of the herbal preparation St John's wort (*Hypericum perforatum*). This is due to induction of drug metabolising enzymes by St John's wort. Herbal preparations containing St John's wort should therefore not be combined with Telzir with ritonavir. If a patient is already taking St John's wort, check amprenavir, ritonavir and if possible viral levels and stop St John's wort. Amprenavir and ritonavir levels may increase on stopping St John's wort. The inducing effect may persist for at least 2 weeks after cessation of treatment with St John's wort.

• Other combinations

Antiretroviral medicinal products

Non-nucleoside reverse transcriptase inhibitors

Efavirenz: there was no clinically relevant interaction when fosamprenavir 700 mg twice daily and ritonavir 100 mg twice daily was used concurrently with efavirenz (600 mg once daily).

Nevirapine: based on the effect of nevirapine on other HIV protease inhibitors, nevirapine may decrease the serum concentration of amprenavir. Appropriate doses of the combination with respect to safety and efficacy have not been established. This combination should be used with caution.

Nucleoside / Nucleotide reverse transcriptase inhibitors

Interaction studies with abacavir, lamivudine and zidovudine have been performed with amprenavir without ritonavir. Based on data derived from these studies and because ritonavir is not expected to have a significant impact on the pharmacokinetics of NRTIs, the co-administration of fosamprenavir and ritonavir with these medicinal products is not expected to significantly alter the exposure of the co-administered active substances.

Didanosine chewable tablet: no pharmacokinetic study has been performed with fosamprenavir in combination with didanosine. Clinically significant interaction resulting from an increase in the stomach pH due to the didanosine antacid component is unlikely and no dose separation or adjustment is considered necessary when fosamprenavir and didanosine are administered concomitantly (see chapter, Antacids). No significant interaction is expected with didanosine gastro-resistent capsule

Tenofovir: no recommendations can be drawn at this stage on the co-administration of fosamprenavir with ritonavir with tenofovir.

Protease Inhibitors

Lopinavir / ritonavir: no dose recommendation can be given for the co-administration of Telzir with ritonavir and lopinavir / ritonavir, but close monitoring is advised because the safety and efficacy of this combination is unknown. The C_{max}, AUC and C_{min} of lopinavir were increased by 30 %, 37 % and 52 % respectively when lopinavir 400 mg with ritonavir 100 mg was given with fosamprenavir 700 mg with ritonavir 100 mg twice daily for two weeks. The C_{max}, AUC and C_{min} of amprenavir were decreased by 58 %, 63 % and 65 % respectively.

When lopinavir 533 mg with ritonavir 133 mg was administered in combination with fosamprenavir 1400 mg twice daily for two weeks, the C_{max}, AUC, and C_{min} of lopinavir were unchanged compared to values observed for lopinavir 400 mg with ritonavir 100 mg twice daily. However, the AUC and C_{min} of amprenavir were decreased by 26 % and 42 %, respectively; whereas, C_{max} was not significantly altered compared to values obtained for fosamprenavir 700 mg with ritonavir 100 mg twice daily.

No interaction studies have been undertaken between fosamprenavir with ritonavir and the following protease inhibitors: indinavir, saquinavir, nelfinavir and atazanavir.

Antibiotics / Antifungals

Clarithromycin: a reduction in the clarithromycin dose should be considered when co-administered with Telzir with ritonavir in patients with renal impairment as moderate increases in clarithromycin concentrations are expected when coadministered with Telzir with ritonavir.

Erythromycin: no pharmacokinetic study has been performed with fosamprenavir with ritonavir in combination with erythromycin, however, plasma levels of erythromycin may be increased when co-administered.

Ketoconazole / Itraconazole: co-administration of amprenavir with ketoconazole increased ketoconazole AUC by 44%. When ritonavir is co-administered, a larger increase in ketoconazole concentration may occur. Itraconazole concentrations are expected to increase in the same manner as ketoconazole. In the absence of specific studies of fosamprenavir with ritonavir in combination with ketoconazole or itraconazole, no recommendations can be drawn in terms of dose adjustment.

Rifabutin: co-administration of amprenavir with rifabutin results in a 200 % increase in rifabutin plasma concentrations (AUC) which could potentially lead to an increase of rifabutin related adverse reactions, notably uveitis. When ritonavir is co-administered a larger increase in rifabutin concentrations may occur. A reduction in the rifabutin dosage by at least 75 % is recommended when administered with Telzir with ritonavir. Further dose reduction may be necessary.

Other medicinal products

Medicinal products that may reduce plasma amprenavir concentrations when co-administered with Telzir

Antacids, Histamine H_2 receptor antagonist and Proton-Pump inhibitors*:* no dose adjustment for any of the respective medicinal products is considered necessary when antacids, proton-pump inhibitors or histamine H_2 receptor antagonists are administered concomitantly with fosamprenavir. The AUC and C_{max} of amprenavir were decreased by 18 % and 35 % respectively, whilst the C_{min} (C12h) was comparable, when a single 1400 mg dose of fosamprenavir was co-administered with a single 30 ml dose of antacid suspension (equivalent to 3.6 grams aluminium hydroxide and 1.8 grams magnesium hydroxide).

Serum levels of amprenavir can be reduced by concomitant use of histamine H_2 receptor antagonists (for example ranitidine and cimetidine). Concurrent administration of ranitidine (300 mg single dose) with fosamprenavir (1400 mg single dose) decreased plasma amprenavir AUC by 30 % and C_{max} by 51 %. There was, however, no change observed in the amprenavir C_{min} (C12h).

Anticonvulsant active substances*:* concomitant administration of anticonvulsant active substances known as enzymatic inductors (phenytoin, phenobarbital, carbamazepine) with fosamprenavir may lead to a decrease in the plasma concentrations of amprenavir. These combinations should be used with caution.

Medicinal products whose plasma levels may be increased when co-administered with Telzir

Other medicinal products with a narrow therapeutic window*:* some substances (e.g. lidocaine (by systemic route) and halofantrine) given with Telzir may cause serious adverse reactions. Concomitant use is not recommended.

Benzodiazepines: concomitant use of Telzir with midazolam or triazolam could result in prolonged sedation or respiratory depression and thus is not recommended.

Erectile dysfunction medicinal products*:* concomitant use is not recommended. Based on data for ritonavir and other protease inhibitors, plasma concentrations of PDE5 inhibitors (e.g. sildenafil and vardenafil) are expected to substantially increase when co-administered with Telzir with ritonavir and may result in an increase in PDE5 inhibitor associated adverse reactions, including hypotension, visual changes and priapism.

HMG-CoA reductase inhibitors*:* if treatment with a HMG-CoA reductase inhibitor is indicated, pravastatin or fluvastatin is recommended because their metabolism is not dependent on CYP3A4 and interactions are not expected with protease inhibitors. HMG-CoA reductase inhibitors which are highly dependent on CYP3A4 for metabolism, such as lovastatin and simvastatin, are expected to have markedly increased plasma concentrations when co-administered with Telzir with ritonavir. Since increased concentrations of HMG-CoA reductase inhibitors may cause myopathy, including rhabdomyolysis, the combination of lovastatin or simvastatin with Telzir with ritonavir is not recommended. No adjustment of the fosamprenavir or ritonavir dose is required when co-administered with atorvastatin.

The C_{max}, AUC and C_{min} of atorvastatin were increased by 184 %, 153 % and 73 % respectively when atorvastatin (10 mg once daily for 4 days) was given with fosamprenavir 700 mg twice daily with ritonavir 100 mg twice daily for two weeks. The C_{max}, AUC and C_{min} of amprenavir were unchanged. When used with Telzir with ritonavir, doses of atorvastatin no greater than 20 mg/day should be administered, with careful monitoring for atorvastatin toxicity.

Immunosuppressants*:* frequent therapeutic concentration monitoring of immunosuppresant levels is recommended until levels have stabilised as plasma concentrations of cyclosporin, rapamycin and tacrolimus may be increased when co-administered with fosamprenavir with ritonavir.

Tricyclic antidepressants: careful monitoring of the therapeutic and adverse reactions of tricyclic antidepressants is recommended when they (for example desipramine and nortriptyline) are concomitantly administered with Telzir.

Medicinal products whose plasma levels may be decreased when co-administered with Telzir

Methadone*:* no data are available on the co-administration of fosamprenavir with ritonavir and methadone. Amprenavir and ritonavir both decrease plasma concentrations of methadone. When methadone is co-administered with Telzir with ritonavir, patients should be closely monitored for opiate abstinence syndrome, with concomitant monitoring of methadone plasma levels.

Oral anticoagulants*:* a reinforced monitoring of the International Normalised Ratio is recommended in case of administration of Telzir with ritonavir with warfarin or other oral anticoagulants, due to a possible decrease or increase of their antithrombotic effect.

Oral contraceptives*:* alternative reliable barrier methods of contraception are recommended for women of childbearing potential. Oestrogens and progestogens may interact with fosamprenavir and ritonavir, thus concomitant use may impair the efficacy of hormonal contraceptives.

4.6 Pregnancy and lactation

Pregnancy

There is no clinical experience with fosamprenavir in pregnant women. In animal studies at systemic plasma exposures (AUC) to amprenavir lower than therapeutic exposure in patients treated with Telzir, some developmental toxicity was observed (see section 5.3). In view of the low exposure in reproductive toxicity studies, the potential developmental toxicity of Telzir has not been fully determined.

Telzir should be used during pregnancy only if the potential benefit justifies the potential risk to the foetus.

Lactation

Amprenavir-related material was found in rat milk, but it is not known whether amprenavir is excreted in human milk. Rat pups exposed pre and post-natally to amprenavir and fosamprenavir showed developmental toxicity (see section 5.3).

It is therefore recommended that mothers treated with Telzir do not breast-feed their infants. As a general rule, it is recommended that HIV-infected women must not breast-feed under any circumstances to avoid transmission of HIV.

4.7 Effects on ability to drive and use machines

No studies on the effects of Telzir in combination with ritonavir on the ability to drive and use machines have been performed. The adverse reaction profile of Telzir should be borne in mind when considering the patient's ability to drive or operate machinery (see section 4.8).

4.8 Undesirable effects

It should be noted that the Telzir oral suspension has not been evaluated clinically and that the adverse reaction profile detailed in this section is based on the experience with the Telzir film coated tablets.

The safety of fosamprenavir has been studied in 755 patients in Phase II and III controlled clinical trials. The safety of the co-administration of fosamprenavir with low dose ritonavir was established in two pivotal Phase III trials: APV30002 (n = 322) in antiretroviral naïve patients, fosamprenavir (1400 mg) given once daily in combination with ritonavir (200 mg) as part of a triple regimen including abacavir and lamivudine. APV30003 in protease inhibitor experienced patients, fosamprenavir given in combination with low dose ritonavir either once daily (1400 mg / 200 mg) (n = 106) or twice daily (700 mg / 100 mg) (n = 106) in combination with two active reverse transcriptase inhibitors (RTIs).

The adverse reaction profile was similar across all the respective studies: antiretroviral naïve (APV30002) and protease inhibitor experienced (twice daily dosing, APV30003) patient populations.

The adverse reactions are listed by body system, organ class and absolute frequency. Frequencies are defined as: Very common (≥ 1/10), Common (≥ 1/100, < 1/10), Uncommon (≥ 1/1,000, < 1/100), Rare (≥ 1/10,000, < 1/1,000) or Very rare (< 1/10,000), including isolated reports. The frequency of the reactions were calculated using adverse reactions that were of at least moderate intensity (Grade 2 or more) and reported by investigators as being attributable to the medicinal products used in the studies. The most frequent clinical adverse reactions (occurring in at least 1 % of patients) reported in the two large clinical studies in adults with at least a possible casual relationship to Telzir are summarised below.

Body System	Adverse reaction	Frequency
Nervous system disorders	Headache, dizziness	Common
Gastrointestinal disorders	Diarrhoea	Very common
	Loose stools, nausea, vomiting, abdominal pain	Common
Skin and subcutaneous tissue disorders	Rash	Common
General disorders and administration site conditions	Fatigue	Common

Rash / cutaneous reactions: erythematous or maculopapular cutaneous eruptions, with or without pruritus, may occur during therapy. The rash generally will resolve spontaneously without the necessity of discontinuing treatment with the fosamprenavir with ritonavir.

Severe or life-threatening rash, including Stevens-Johnson syndrome is rare, reported in less than 1 % of patients included in the clinical development programme. Fosamprenavir with ritonavir therapy should be definitively stopped in case of severe rash or in case of rash of mild or moderate intensity associated with systemic or mucosal signs (see section 4.4).

Clinical chemistry abnormalities: clinical chemistry abnormalities (Grade 3 or 4) potentially related to treatment with fosamprenavir with ritonavir and reported in greater than or equal to 1 % of patients, included:

increased ALT (*common*), AST (*common*), serum lipase (*common*) and triglycerides (*very common*). Grade 3 or 4 elevations in total cholesterol values were observed in less than 1 % of patients (< 1 % APV30002; 0 % APV 30003).

Lipodystrophy: combination antiretroviral therapy has been associated with redistribution of body fat (lipodystrophy) in HIV patients including the loss of peripheral and facial subcutaneous fat, increased intra-abdominal and visceral fat, breast hypertrophy and dorsocervical fat accumulation (buffalo hump) (see section 4.4).

Metabolic abnormalities: combination antiretroviral therapy has been associated with metabolic abnormalities such as hypertriglyceridaemia, hypercholesterolaemia, insulin resistance, hyperglycaemia and hyperlactataemia (see section 4.4).

Hyperglycaemia: new onset of diabetes mellitus, hyperglycaemia or exacerbations of existing diabetes mellitus have been reported in patients receiving antiretroviral protease inhibitors (see section 4.4).

Rhabdomyolysis: an increase in CPK, myalgia, myositis, and rarely, rhabdomyolysis, have been reported with protease inhibitors, more specifically in association with nucleoside analogues.

Haemophiliac patients: there have been reports of increased spontaneous bleeding in haemophiliac patients receiving antiretroviral protease inhibitors (see section 4.4).

Immune Reactivation Syndrome: in HIV-infected patients with severe immune deficiency at the time of initiation of combination antiretroviral therapy (CART), an inflammatory reaction to asymptomatic or residual opportunistic infections may arise (see section 4.4).

4.9 Overdose

There is no known antidote for Telzir. It is not known whether amprenavir can be removed by peritoneal dialysis or haemodialysis. If overdosage occurs, the patient should be monitored for evidence of toxicity (see section 4.8) and standard supportive treatment applied as necessary.

5. PHARMACOLOGICAL PROPERTIES

5.1 Pharmacodynamic properties

Pharmacotherapeutic group: Antivirals for systemic use, protease inhibitor, ATC Code: J05A (pending)

Mechanism of action

Fosamprenavir is rapidly converted to amprenavir by cellular or serum phosphatases *in vivo*. Amprenavir is a competitive inhibitor of HIV-1 protease. Amprenavir binds to the active site of HIV-1 protease and thereby prevents the processing of viral gag and gag-pol polyprotein precursors, resulting in the formation of immature non-infectious viral particles.

Fosamprenavir has little or no antiviral activity *in vitro*. The *in vitro* antiviral activity observed with fosamprenavir is due to the presence of trace amounts of amprenavir. The *in vitro* antiviral activity of amprenavir was evaluated against HIV-1 IIIB in both acutely and chronically infected lymphoblastic cell lines (MT-4, CEM-CCRF, H9) and in peripheral blood lymphocytes. The 50% inhibitory concentration (IC_{50}) of amprenavir ranged from 0.012 to 0.08 μM in acutely infected cells and was 0.41 μM in chronically infected cells (1 μM = 0.50 μg/ml). *In vitro*, amprenavir exhibited synergistic anti-HIV-1 activity in combination with the nucleoside reverse transcriptase inhibitors (NRTIs) abacavir, didanosine and zidovudine and the protease inhibitor saquinavir, and additive anti-HIV-1 activity in combination with indinavir, nelfinavir and ritonavir. The relationship between *in vitro* anti-HIV-1 activity of amprenavir and the inhibition of HIV-1 replication in humans has not been defined.

Co-administration of ritonavir with fosamprenavir increase plasma amprenavir AUC by approximately 2-fold and plasma $C_{\tau,ss}$ by 4- to 6-fold, compared to values obtained when fosamprenavir is administered alone. Administration of fosamprenavir 700 mg twice daily with ritonavir 100 mg twice daily results in plasma amprenavir trough concentrations (geometric mean plasma C_{min} 1.74 μg/ml, reported in study APV30003 in antiretroviral experienced patients) above the median IC_{50} value reported in this study (0.008 μg/ml [0.001 – 0.144]).

Resistance

HIV-1 isolates with a decreased susceptibility to amprenavir have been selected during *in vitro* serial passage experiments. Reduced susceptibility to amprenavir was associated with virus that had developed I50V or I84V or V32I+I47V or I54M mutations.

No development of genotypic or phenotypic amprenavir resistance was detected in virus from thirty-two antiretroviral therapy naïve patients receiving fosamprenavir 1400 mg with ritonavir 200 mg once daily (Study APV30002) and experiencing virological failure or on-going viral replication. A significantly higher proportion of nelfinavir treated patients acquired primary and /or secondary PRO mutations (nelfinavir 27/54 (50 %)) ($p < 0.001$).

Development of amprenavir resistance was detected in viral isolates from protease experienced patients receiving fosamprenavir 1400 mg with ritonavir 200 mg once daily or 700 mg fosamprenavir with 100 mg ritonavir twice daily (Study APV30003) and having virological failure or having on-going viral replication. 58% (19/33) versus 25% (7/28) patients acquired primary and / or secondary PRO mutations in the fosamprenavir with ritonavir arm versus the lopinavir / ritonavir arm. The following amprenavir resistance–associated mutations developed either alone or in combination: V32I, M46I/L, I47V, I50V, I54L/M and I84V.

Cross-Resistance

The data are currently too limited to determine a clinically relevant phenotypic cut-off for fosamprenavir with ritonavir.

Cross-resistance between amprenavir and reverse transcriptase inhibitors is unlikely to occur because the enzyme targets are different.

Telzir is not recommended for use as monotherapy, due to the rapid emergence of resistant virus.

Clinical experience

The clinical experience is mainly based on two open label studies performed in comparison to nelfinavir in antiretroviral naïve patients (study APV30002) and in comparison to lopinavir / ritonavir in antiretroviral experienced patients (study APV30003). In both studies fosamprenavir was used boosted with ritonavir.

Antiretroviral Naïve Patients

In antiretroviral naïve patients in APV30002, fosamprenavir (1400 mg) given once daily in combination with low dose ritonavir (200 mg) as part of a triple regimen including abacavir (300 mg twice daily) and lamivudine (150 mg twice daily) showed similar efficacy over 48 weeks compared to nelfinavir (1250 mg) given twice daily in combination with abacavir plus lamivudine (300 and 150 mg twice daily).

Non-inferiority was demonstrated between fosamprenavir with ritonavir and nelfinavir based on the proportions of patients achieving plasma HIV-1 RNA levels < 400 copies/ml at 48 weeks (primary endpoint). In the ITT (Rebound or Discontinuation = Failure) analysis, 69 % (221 / 322) of patients receiving fosamprenavir with ritonavir achieved < 400 copies/ml compared to 68 % (221 / 327) of patients receiving nelfinavir.

The median plasma HIV-1 RNA had decreased by 3.1 $\log_{10}$ copies/ml and 3.0 $\log_{10}$ copies/ml at Week 48 in the fosamprenavir with ritonavir and nelfinavir arms respectively.

The median baseline CD4 cell count was low (170 cells/mm^3 overall) in both groups. CD4+ cell counts increased in both the fosamprenavir with ritonavir and nelfinavir groups, with median increases above baseline being similar in magnitude at Week 48 (+203 and +207 cells/mm^3, respectively).

The data presented above demonstrates that the once daily regimen of fosamprenavir with ritonavir (1400/200 mg OD) in antiretroviral naïve patients showed similar efficacy compared to nelfinavir given twice daily. However, the demonstration of efficacy in this population is only based on one open label study versus nelfinavir. Another clinical study is planned to reinforce the efficacy demonstration of the medicinal product in this population. Therefore, as a conservative approach, based on enhanced amprenavir C_{trough} levels, the twice daily dosing regimen of fosamprenavir with ritonavir is recommended for optimal therapeutic management of this population (see section 4.2).

Antiretroviral Experienced Patients

In a randomised open-label study (APV30003) in protease inhibitor experienced patients with virological failure (less than or equal to two PIs) the fosamprenavir with ritonavir (700 / 100 mg twice daily or 1400 / 200 mg once daily) did not demonstrate non-inferiority to lopinavir / ritonavir with regard to viral suppression as measured by the average area under the curve minus baseline (AAUCMB) for plasma HIV-1 RNA over 48 weeks (the primary end point). Results were in favour of the lopinavir / ritonavir arm as detailed below.

All patients in this study had failed treatment with a previous protease inhibitor regimen (defined as plasma HIV-1 RNA that never went below 1,000 copies/ml after at least 12 consecutive weeks of therapy, or initial suppression of HIV-1 RNA which subsequently rebounded to $\geqslant$ 1,000 copies/ml). However, only 65 % of patients were receiving a PI based regimen at study entry.

The population enrolled mainly consisted of moderately antiretroviral experienced patients. The median durations of prior exposure to NRTIs were 257 weeks for patients receiving fosamprenavir with ritonavir twice daily (79 % had $\geqslant$ 3 prior NRTIs) and 210 weeks for patients receiving lopinavir/ritonavir (64 % had $\geqslant$ 3 prior NRTIs). The median durations of prior exposure to protease inhibitors were 149 weeks for patients receiving fosamprenavir with ritonavir twice daily (49 % received $\geqslant$ 2 prior PIs) and 130 weeks for patients receiving lopinavir/ritonavir (40 % received $\geqslant$2 prior PIs).

The mean AAUCMBs ($\log_{10}$ c/ml) in the ITT (E) population (Observed analysis) at 48 weeks are described in the table below:

Plasma HIV-1 RNA Average Area Under the Curve Minus Baseline (AAUCMB) Values ($\log_{10}$ copies/ml) at week 48 by Randomisation Strata in APV30003 ITT (E) Population (Observed Analysis)

(see Table 1)

When considering the proportion of patients with undetectable viral load in the fosamprenavir with ritonavir twice daily dosing regimens and lopinavir / ritonavir arms respectively, results showed a trend in favour of the lopinavir / ritonavir arms: 58 % versus 61 % (plasma HIV-1 RNA < 400 copies/ml) or 46 % versus 50 % (plasma HIV-1 RNA < 50 copies/ml) at Week 48 (secondary efficacy endpoint) in the intent to treat (RD=F) analysis.

In patients with high viral load at baseline > 100,000 copies/ml 7/14 (50 %) patients in the lopinavir / ritonavir group and 6/19 (32 %) patients in the fosamprenavir with ritonavir group had plasma HIV-1 RNA < 400 copies/ml.

The fosamprenavir with ritonavir twice daily regimen and the lopinavir / ritonavir twice daily regimen showed similar immunological improvements through 48 weeks of treatment as measured by median change from baseline in CD4+ cell count (fosamprenavir with ritonavir twice daily: 81 cells/mm^3: lopinavir / ritonavir twice daily: 91 cells/mm^3).

There are insufficient data to recommend the use of fosamprenavir with ritonavir in heavily pre-treated patients.

5.2 Pharmacokinetic properties

After oral administration, fosamprenavir is rapidly and almost completely hydrolysed to amprenavir and inorganic phosphate prior to reaching the systemic circulation. The conversion of fosamprenavir to amprenavir appears to primarily occur in the gut epithelium.

The pharmacokinetic properties of amprenavir following co-administration of Telzir with ritonavir have been evaluated in healthy adult subjects and HIV-infected patients and no substantial differences were observed between these two groups.

Telzir tablet and oral suspension formulations, both given fasted, delivered equivalent plasma amprenavir AUC_∞ values and the Telzir oral suspension formulation delivered a 14 % higher plasma amprenavir C_{max} as compared to the oral tablet formulation. However, the bioequivalence could not be demonstrated when the oral suspension was given with food. Therefore the Telzir oral suspension should be taken without food and on an empty stomach (see section 4.2).

Absorption

After single dose administration of fosamprenavir, amprenavir peak plasma concentrations are observed approximately 2 hours after administration. Fosamprenavir AUC values are, in general, less than 1 % of those observed for amprenavir. The absolute bioavailability of fosamprenavir in humans has not been established.

After multiple dose oral administration of equivalent fosamprenavir and amprenavir doses, comparable amprenavir AUC values were observed; however, C_{max} values were approximately 30 % lower and C_{min} values were approximately 28 % higher with fosamprenavir.

After multiple dose oral administration of fosamprenavir 700 mg with ritonavir 100 mg twice daily, amprenavir was rapidly absorbed with a geometric mean (95 % CI) steady state peak plasma amprenavir concentration (C_{max}) of 6.08 (5.38-6.86) μg/ml occurring approximately 1.5 (0.75-5.0) hours after dosing (t_{max}). The mean steady state plasma amprenavir trough concentration (C_{min}) was 2.12 (1.77-2.54) μg/ml and $AUC_{0\text{-}tau}$ was 39.6 (34.5–45.3) h*μg/ml.

Administration of the fosamprenavir oral suspension formulation with a high fat meal reduced plasma amprenavir AUC by approximately 25 % and C_{max} by approximately 40 % as compared to the administration of this formulation in the fasted state.

Co-administration of amprenavir with grapefruit juice was not associated with clinically significant changes in plasma amprenavir pharmacokinetics.

Distribution

The apparent volume of distribution of amprenavir following administration of Telzir is approximately 430 l (6 l/kg assuming a 70 kg body weight), suggesting a large volume of distribution, with penetration of amprenavir freely into tissues beyond the systemic circulation. This value is decreased by approximately 40 % when Telzir is co-administered with ritonavir, most likely due to an increase in amprenavir bioavailability.

In *in vitro* studies, the protein binding of amprenavir is approximately 90 %. It is bound to the alpha-1-acid glycoprotein (AAG) and albumin, but has a higher affinity for AAG. Concentrations of AAG have been shown to decrease during the course of antiretroviral therapy. This change will decrease the total active substance concentration in the plasma, however the amount of unbound amprenavir, which is the active moiety, is likely to be unchanged.

CSF penetration of amprenavir is negligible in humans. Amprenavir appears to penetrate into semen, though semen concentrations are lower than plasma concentrations.

Metabolism

Fosamprenavir is rapidly and almost completely hydrolysed to amprenavir and inorganic phosphate as it is absorbed through the gut epithelium, following oral administration. Amprenavir is primarily metabolised by the liver with less than 1 % excreted unchanged in the urine. The primary route of metabolism is via the cytochrome P450 3A4 enzyme. Amprenavir metabolism is inhibited by ritonavir, via inhibition of CYP3A4, resulting in increased plasma concentrations of amprenavir. Amprenavir in addition is also an inhibitor of the CYP3A4 enzyme, although to a lesser extent than ritonavir. Therefore medicinal products that are inducers, inhibitors or substrates of CYP3A4 must be used with caution when administered concurrently with Telzir with ritonavir (see sections 4.3 and 4.5).

Elimination

Following administration of Telzir, the half-life of amprenavir is 7.7 hours. When Telzir is co-administered with ritonavir, the half-life of amprenavir is increased to 15 – 23 hours.

The primary route of elimination of amprenavir is via hepatic metabolism with less than 1 % excreted unchanged in the urine and no detectable amprenavir in

Table 1 Plasma HIV-1 RNA Average Area Under the Curve Minus Baseline (AAUCMB) Values ($\log_{10}$ copies/ml) at week 48 by Randomisation Strata in APV30003 ITT (E) Population (Observed Analysis)

Plasma HIV-1 RNA stratum	Observed analysis FOS/RTV BID N=107 Mean (n)	Observed analysis LPV/RTV BID N=103 Mean (n)	Observed analysis Mean Diff. (97.5% CI) FOS/RTV BID vs LPV/RTV BID
1000 – 10,000 copies/ml	-1.53 (41)	-1.43 (43)	-0.104 (-0.550, 0.342)
>10.000 – 100,000 copies/ml	-1.59 (45)	-1.81 (46)	0.216 (-0.213, 0.664)
>100,000 copies/ml	-1.38 (19)	-2.61 (14)	1.232 (0.512, 1.952)
Total population	-1.53 (105)	-1.76 (103)	0.244 (-0.047, 0.536)

Key: FOS/RTV BID – Fosamprenavir with ritonavir twice daily, LPV/RTV BID – Lopinavir / ritonavir twice daily

faeces. Metabolites account for approximately 14 % of the administered amprenavir dose in the urine, and approximately 75 % in the faeces.

Special populations

Paediatrics

The pharmacokinetics of fosamprenavir in combination with ritonavir has not been studied in paediatric patients.

Elderly

The pharmacokinetics of fosamprenavir in combination with ritonavir has not been studied in patients over 65 years of age.

Renal impairment

Patients with renal impairment have not been specifically studied. Less than 1 % of the therapeutic dose of amprenavir is excreted unchanged in the urine. Renal clearance of ritonavir is also negligible, therefore the impact of renal impairment on amprenavir and ritonavir elimination should be minimal.

Hepatic impairment

Fosamprenavir is converted in man to amprenavir. The principal route of amprenavir and ritonavir elimination is hepatic metabolism. There are limited data regarding the use of this combination in patients with hepatic impairment and therefore specific dosage recommendations cannot be made (see sections 4.3 and 4.4).

5.3 Preclinical safety data

Toxicity was similar to that of amprenavir and occurred at amprenavir plasma exposure levels below human exposure after treatment with fosamprenavir in combination with ritonavir at the recommended dose.

In repeated dose toxicity studies in adult rats and dogs, fosamprenavir produced evidence of gastrointestinal disturbances (salivation, vomiting and soft to liquid faeces), and hepatic changes (increased liver weights, raised serum liver enzyme activities and microscopic changes, including hepatocyte necrosis).

In reproductive toxicity studies with fosamprenavir in rats, male fertility was not affected, but in females gravid uterine weights, numbers of ovarian corpora lutea and uterine implantation sites were reduced. In pregnant rats and rabbits there were no major effects on embryo-foetal development. However, the number of abortions increased. In rabbits, systemic exposure at the high dose level was only 0.3 times human exposure at the maximum clinical dose and thus the development toxicity of fosamprenavir has not been fully determined. In rats exposed pre- and post-natally to fosamprenavir, pups showed impaired physical and functional development and reduced growth. Pup survival was decreased. In addition, decreased number of implantation sites per litter and a prolongation of gestation were seen when pups were mated after reaching maturity.

Fosamprenavir was not mutagenic or genotoxic in a standard battery of *in vitro* and *in vivo* assays. Carcinogenicity studies of fosamprenavir in rats and mice have not yet been completed; however, in long-term carcinogenicity studies with amprenavir in mice and rats, there were benign hepatocellular adenomas in males at exposure levels equivalent to 2.0-fold (mice) or 3.8-fold (rats) those in humans given 1200 mg twice daily of amprenavir alone. In male mice altered hepatocellular foci were seen at doses that were at least 2.0 times human therapeutic exposure.

A higher incidence of hepatocellular carcinoma was seen in all amprenavir male mouse treatment groups. However, this increase was not statistically significantly different from male control mice by appropriate tests. The mechanism for the hepatocellular adenomas and carcinomas found in these studies has not been elucidated and the significance of the observed effects for humans is uncertain. However, there is little evidence from the exposure data in humans, both in clinical trials and from marketed use, to suggest that these findings are of clinical significance.

6. PHARMACEUTICAL PARTICULARS

6.1 List of excipients

Hypromellose

Sucralose

Propylene glycol

Methyl parahydroxybenzoate (E218)

Propyl parahydroxybenzoate (E216)

Polysorbate 80

Calcium chloride dehydrate

Artificial grape bubblegum flavour

Natural peppermint flavour

Purified water

6.2 Incompatibilities

In the absence of compatibility studies, this medicinal product must not be mixed with other medicinal products.

6.3 Shelf life

2 years.

Discard 28 days after first opening.

6.4 Special precautions for storage

Do not freeze.

6.5 Nature and contents of container

HDPE bottle with a child resistant polypropylene closure containing 225 millilitres oral suspension.

A 10 ml graduated polypropylene dosing syringe and polyethylene adapter are provided in the pack.

6.6 Instructions for use and handling

No special requirements.

Administrative Data

7. MARKETING AUTHORISATION HOLDER

Glaxo Group Ltd
Greenford Road
Greenford
Middlesex UB6 0NN
United Kingdom

8. MARKETING AUTHORISATION NUMBER(S)

EU/1/04/282/002

9. DATE OF FIRST AUTHORISATION/RENEWAL OF THE AUTHORISATION

12 July 2004

10. DATE OF REVISION OF THE TEXT

17 December 2004

Temazepam Elixir

(Pharmacia Limited)

1. NAME OF THE MEDICINAL PRODUCT

Temazepam Elixir

2. QUALITATIVE AND QUANTITATIVE COMPOSITION

A solution containing Temazepam 10 mg/5 ml in a formulation as described in the application.

3. PHARMACEUTICAL FORM

Elixir for human administration

4. CLINICAL PARTICULARS

4.1 Therapeutic indications

Temazepam Elixir is indicated for the short-term treatment of sleep disturbances considered severe or disabling or where insomnia is subjecting the individual to extreme distress. This product is especially useful in those patients for whom the persistence of hypnotic effect after rising would be undesirable.

4.2 Posology and method of administration

Route of administration: Oral

Insomnia: Treatment should be as short as possible. Generally the duration of treatment should vary from a few days to two weeks with a maximum, including the tapering off process, of four weeks, in certain cases extension beyond the maximum treatment period may be necessary; if so, it should not take place without re-evaluation of the patient's status. The product should be taken on retiring or up to 30 minutes before going to bed.

Adults

10-20 mg (5-10 ml). In exceptional circumstances the dose may be increased to 30-40 mg (15-20 ml).

Elderly

10 mg (5 ml). In exceptional circumstances the dose may be increased to 20 mg (10 ml).

Treatment should be started with the lowest recommended dose. The maximum dose should not be exceeded. Patients with impaired liver function should have a reduced dose.

4.3 Contraindications

Hypersensitivity to benzodiazepines, severe respiratory insufficiency, myasthenia gravis, sleep apnoea syndrome, children, severe hepatic insufficiency.

4.4 Special warnings and special precautions for use

Tolerance: Some loss of efficacy to the hypnotic effects of short acting benzodiazepines may develop after repeated use for a few weeks.

Dependence: Use of benzodiazepines may lead to the development of physical and psychic dependence upon these products. The risk of dependence increases with dose and duration of treatment; it is also greater in patients with a history of alcohol and drug abuse. Once physical dependence has developed, abrupt termination of treatment will be accompanied by withdrawal symptoms. These may consist of headaches, muscle pain, extreme anxiety, tension, restlessness, confusion and irritability. In severe cases the following symptoms may occur: derealization, depersonalisation, hyperacusis and tingling of the extremities, hypersensitivity to light, noise and physical contact, hallucinations or epileptic seizures.

Rebound insomnia: A transient syndrome whereby the symptoms that led to treatment with benzodiazepine recur in an enhanced form, may occur on withdrawal of hypnotic treatment. It may be accompanied by other reactions including mood changes, anxiety and restlessness. Since the risk of withdrawal phenomena/rebound phenomena is greater after abrupt discontinuation of treatment it is recommended that the dosage is decreased gradually.

Duration of treatment: The duration of treatment should be as short as possible (see dosage), but should not exceed 4 weeks, including the tapering off process. Extension beyond this period should not take place without re-evaluation of the situation. It may be useful to inform the patient at the start of treatment that it will be of limited duration and to explain precisely how the dosage will be progressively decreased. Moreover, it is important that the patient should be made aware of the possibility of rebound phenomena to minimise anxiety over such symptoms should they occur while the medicinal product is being discontinued. There is some evidence to suggest that for benzodiazepines with a short duration of action, withdrawal phenomena can occur within the dosage interval, especially when the dosage is high.

Amnesia: Benzodiazepines may induce anterograde amnesia. The condition occurs most often several hours after ingesting the product and therefore to reduce the risk, patients should ensure that they will be able to have an uninterrupted sleep of 7-8 hours (see also undesirable effects).

Psychiatric and 'paradoxical' reactions: Reactions like restlessness, agitation, irritability, aggressiveness, delusion, rages, nightmares, hallucinations, psychoses, inappropriate behaviour and other adverse behavioural effects are known to occur when using benzodiazepines. Should this occur, use of the product should be discontinued. These reactions are more likely to occur in children and the elderly.

Specific patient groups: Elderly-see dosage recommendations. A lower dose is also recommended for patients with chronic respiratory insufficiency due to the risk of respiratory depression. Benzodiazepines are contraindicated in patients with severe hepatic insufficiency as their use may precipitate encephalopathy. Benzodiazepines are not recommended for the primary treatment of psychotic illness.

Benzodiazepines should not be used alone to treat depression or anxiety associated with depression (suicide may be precipitated in such patients). Benzodiazepines should be used with extreme caution in patients with a history of alcohol or drug abuse.

4.5 Interaction with other medicinal products and other forms of Interaction

Not recommended: Concomitant intake with alcohol. The sedative effect may be enhanced when the product is used in combination with alcohol. This affects the ability to drive or use machines.

Take into account: Combination with CNS depressants. Enhancement of the central depressive effect may occur during concomitant use with antipsychotics (neuroleptics), hypnotics, anxiolytics/sedatives, antidepressant agents, narcotic analgesic, antiepileptic drugs, anaesthetics and sedative antihistamines. In the case of narcotic analgesics enhancement of the euphoria may also occur leading to an increase in psychotic dependence.

4.6 Pregnancy and lactation

Insufficient data are available on temazepam to assess its safety during pregnancy and lactation.

If the product is prescribed to a woman of childbearing age, she should be warned to contact her physician about stopping the product if she intends to become, or suspects that she is, pregnant. If for compelling medical reasons, temazepam is administered during the late phase of pregnancy, or during labour, effects on the neonate, such as hypothermia, hypotonia and moderate respiratory depression, can be expected due to the pharmacological action of the product. Moreover, infants born to mothers who took benzodiazepines chronically during the later stages of pregnancy may have develops physical dependence and may be at some risk of developing withdrawal symptoms in the postnatal period.

Since benzodiazepines are found in the breast milk, temazepam should not be administered to breast-feeding mothers.

4.7 Effects on ability to drive and use machines

Sedation, amnesia, impaired concentration and impaired muscular function may adversely affect the ability to drive or to use machines. If insufficient sleep duration occurs, the likelihood of impaired alertness may be increased. (See also interactions).

4.8 Undesirable effects

Drowsiness during the day, numbed emotions, reduced alertness, confusion, fatigue, headaches, dizziness, muscle weakness, ataxia, or double vision. These phenomena occur predominantly at the start of therapy and usually disappear thereafter. Other side effects like gastrointestinal disturbances, changes in libido or skin reactions have been reported occasionally.

Amnesia: Anterograde amnesia may occur using therapeutic dosages, the risk increasing at higher dosages. Amnesia may be associated with inappropriate behaviour. (See warnings and precautions.)

Depression: Pre-existing depression may be unmasked during benzodiazepine use.

Psychiatric and 'paradoxical' reactions: Reactions like restlessness, agitation, irritability, aggressiveness, delusion, rages, nightmares, hallucinations, psychoses, inappropriate behaviour and other adverse behavioural effects are known to occur when using benzodiazepines. Should this occur, use of the product should be discontinued. These reactions are more likely to occur in children and the elderly.

Dependence: Use (even at therapeutic doses) may lead to the development of physical dependence: Discontinuation of therapy may result in withdrawal or rebound phenomena (see warnings and precautions). Psychic dependence may occur. Abuse has been reported in polydrug users.

4.9 Overdose

As with other benzodiazepines, overdose should not present a treat to life unless combined with other CNS depressants (including alcohol). In the management of overdose with any medicinal product, it should be borne in mind that multiple agents may have been taken.

Following overdose with oral benzodiazepines, vomiting should be induced (within one hour) if the patient is conscious or gastric lavage undertaken with the airway protected if the patient is unconscious. If there is no advantage in emptying the stomach, activated charcoal should be given to reduce absorption. The value of dialysis has not been determined for temazepam. 3-OH benzodiazepines are, as a rule, not dialysable and their metabolites (glucuronides) only dialysable with difficulty. Special attention should be paid to respiratory and cardiovascular function in intensive care.

Overdose of benzodiazepines is usually manifested by degrees of central nervous system depression ranging from drowsiness to coma.

In mild cases, symptoms include drowsiness, mental confusion and lethargy; in more serious cases, symptoms may include ataxia, hypotonia, hypotension, respiratory depression, rarely coma and very rarely death. Flumazenil may be used as an antidote.

5. PHARMACOLOGICAL PROPERTIES

5.1 Pharmacodynamic properties

Temazepam is a benzodiazepine; it has anxiolytic, sedative and hypnotic characteristics as well as possible muscle relaxant and anticonvulsant characteristics.

5.2 Pharmacokinetic properties

Absorption: Pharmacokinetic studies have shown that temazepam is well absorbed (90-100% and the first pass effect is slight-about 5%). The time to reach peak plasma levels is usually about 50 mins when given orally. Maximum plasma levels observed after doses of 20 mg are 660-1100 ng/ml. With multiple dosing steady state is obtained by the third day and there is little or no accumulation of parent drug or metabolites.

Distribution: The volume of distribution is 1.3 to 1.5 l/kg body weight; for the unbound fraction 43-68 l/kg. Approximately 96% of unchanged drug is bound to plasma proteins.

Metabolism: Temazepam is metabolised principally in the liver where most of the unchanged drug is directly conjugated to the glucuronide and excreted in the urine. Less than 5% of the drug is demethylated to oxazepam and eliminated as the glucuronide. The glucuronides of temazepam have no demonstrable CNS activity.

Elimination: Temazepam is rapidly eliminated, most studies showing an elimination half-life in the range of 7-11 hours (mean 8 hours). Following a single dose, 80% of the dose appears in the urine, mostly as conjugates and 12% of the dose in the faeces. Less than 2% of the dose is excreted unchanged in the urine.

Elimination in reduced renal function: In established renal insufficiency the metabolic clearance of temazepam as well as the plasma level of non-protein bound temazepam remain within the normal range. The elimination half-life for temazepam glucuronide is however increased by which this inactive metabolite accumulates. As stated under 'overdose' it is unlikely that temazepam may be significantly removed by dialysis.

5.3 Preclinical safety data

None stated.

6. PHARMACEUTICAL PARTICULARS

6.1 List of excipients

Povidone 25	BP
Polyethylene glycol 400	BP
Ethanol	BP
Glycerol	BP
Sodium phosphate	BP
Citric acid	BP
Chlorophyll (E141)	HSE
Sorbitol solution (70%)	BP
Peppermint oil	BP
Lemon flavour supara BL2300	HSE

6.2 Incompatibilities

None stated.

6.3 Shelf life

The shelf life for Temazepam Elixir packed in amber glass bottles, opaque plastic bottles or amber pet bottles is 30 months. The shelf life for Temazepam Elixir packed in single dose plastic containers is 24 months.

6.4 Special precautions for storage

Store below 25°C and protect from direct light.

6.5 Nature and contents of container

Temazepam Elixir is packed in amber glass bottles (30, 100, 300 and 2000 ml), opaque plastic bottles (100, 300, 500 and 2000 ml), amber pet bottles (300, 500, 1000 and 2000 ml) or single dose plastic containers (2.5, 5 and 10 ml).

6.6 Instructions for use and handling

None.

7. MARKETING AUTHORISATION HOLDER

Pharmacia Limited

Davy Avenue

Milton Keynes

MK5 8PH

UK

8. MARKETING AUTHORISATION NUMBER(S)

PL 00032/0491

9. DATE OF FIRST AUTHORISATION/RENEWAL OF THE AUTHORISATION

Date of first Authorisation: 13 September 2002

10. DATE OF REVISION OF THE TEXT

Legal Category

POM.

Temgesic 200 microgram Sublingual Tablets

(Schering-Plough Ltd)

1. NAME OF THE MEDICINAL PRODUCT

Temgesic 200 microgram Sublingual Tablets

2. QUALITATIVE AND QUANTITATIVE COMPOSITION

Buprenorphine hydrochloride 216μg/tablet, equivalent to 200μg buprenorphine base.

3. PHARMACEUTICAL FORM

Sublingual tablets

4. CLINICAL PARTICULARS

4.1 Therapeutic indications

As a strong analgesic for the relief of moderate to severe pain.

4.2 Posology and method of administration

Administration by the sublingual route.

<u>Adults and children over 12</u>:

1-2 tablets (200-400 micrograms) to be dissolved under the tongue every 6-8 hours or as required. The recommended starting dose for moderate to severe pain of the type typically presenting in general practice is 1 to 2 tablets, 8 hourly.

<u>Elderly</u>:

There is no evidence that dosage needs to be modified for the elderly.

<u>Children under 12 years:</u>

Temgesic Sublingual is suitable for use in children under 12 as follows:

16 - 25 kg (35 - 55lb) ½ tablet

25 - 37.5 kg (55 - 82.5lb) ½-1 tablet

37.5 - 50 kg (82.5 - 110lb) 1-1½ tablets

The recommended dose should be administered every 6 to 8 hours.

Sublingual administration is not suitable for children under the age of six years.

Temgesic sublingual may be used in balanced anaesthetic techniques at a dose of 400 micrograms.

4.3 Contraindications

Not to be given to patients who are known to be allergic to Temgesic or other opiates. Hypersensitivity to any of the constituents

4.4 Special warnings and special precautions for use

Temgesic occasionally causes significant respiratory depression and, as with other strong centrally acting analgesics, care should be taken when treating patients with impaired respiratory function or patients who are receiving drugs which can cause respiratory depression. Although volunteer studies have indicated that opiate antagonists may not fully reverse the effects of Temgesic, clinical experience has shown that Naloxone may be of benefit in reversing a reduced respiratory rate. Respiratory stimulants such as Doxapram are also effective. The intensity and duration of action may be affected in patients with impaired liver failure.

Controlled human and animal studies indicate that buprenorphine has a substantially lower dependence liability than pure agonist analgesics. In patients abusing opioids in moderate doses substitution with buprenorphine may prevent withdrawal symptoms. In man limited euphorigenic effects have been observed. This has resulted in some abuse of the product and caution should be exercised when prescribing it to patients known to have, or suspected of having, problems with drug abuse.

4.5 Interaction with other medicinal products and other forms of Interaction

There is evidence to indicate that therapeutic doses of buprenorphine do not reduce the analgesic efficacy of standard doses of an opioid agonist and that when buprenorphine is employed within the normal therapeutic range, standard doses of opioid agonist may be administered before the effects of the former have ended without compromising analgesia. However, in individuals on high doses of opioids buprenorphine may precipitate abstinence effects due to its properties as a partial agonist.

Temgesic may cause some drowsiness which may be potentiated by other centrally acting agents, including alcohol, tranquillisers, sedatives and hypnotics. Temgesic should be used with caution in patients receiving monoamine oxidase inhibitors, although animals studies have given no evidence of interactions.

Although interaction studies have not been performed, since this drug is metabolised by CYP3A4 (see section 5.2 pharmacokinetic properties), it is expected that gestodene, troleandomycin, ketoconazole, norfluoxetine, ritonavir, indinavir and saquinavir inhibit its metabolism. Alternatively, inducers of this enzyme such as phenobarbital, carbamazepine, phenytoin and rifampicin may reduce the levels of the drug. Since the magnitude of an inducing or inhibitory effect is unknown, such drug combinations should be avoided.

Temgesic has no known effects on diagnostic laboratory tests.

4.6 Pregnancy and lactation

Temgesic is not recommended for use during pregnancy. Animal studies indicate that the amounts of buprenorphine excreted in milk are very low and in human use are unlikely to be of clinical significance to the baby. There is indirect evidence in animal studies to suggest that Temgesic may cause a reduction in milk flow during lactation. Although this occurred only at doses well in excess of the human dose, it should be borne in mind when treating lactating women.

4.7 Effects on ability to drive and use machines

Ambulant patients should be warned not to drive or operate machinery until they are certain they can tolerate Temgesic.

4.8 Undesirable effects

Nausea, vomiting, dizziness, sweating and drowsiness have been reported and may be more frequent in ambulant patients. Hallucinations and other psychotomimetic effects have occurred although more rarely than with other agonists/antagonists. Elderly patients would be expected to be more susceptible to these effects. Hypotension leading to syncope may occur. Rashes, headache, urinary retention and blurring of vision have occasionally been reported. Rarely, a serious allergic reaction may occur following a single dose. Temgesic occasionally causes significant respiratory depression (see section 4.4, Special Warnings and Precautions for Use).

Cases of bronchospasm, angioneurotic oedema and anaphylactic shock have also been reported.

4.9 Overdose

Supportive measures should be instituted and if appropriate Naloxone or respiratory stimulants can be used. The expected symptoms of overdosage would be drowsiness, nausea and vomiting; marked miosis may occur.

5. PHARMACOLOGICAL PROPERTIES

5.1 Pharmacodynamic properties

Buprenorphine is a μ (mu) opioid partial agonist and κ (kappa) antagonist. It is a strong analgesic of the partial agonist (mixed agonist/antagonist) class.

5.2 Pharmacokinetic properties

Absorption

When taken orally, buprenorphine undergoes first-pass hepatic metabolism with N-dealkylation and glucuroconjugation in the small intestine. The use of this medication by the oral route is therefore inappropriate.

Peak plasma concentrations are achieved 90 minutes after sublingual administration.

Distribution

The absorption of buprenorphine is followed by a rapid distribution phase and a half-life of 2 to 5 hours.

Metabolism and elimination

Buprenorphine is oxidatively metabolised by 14-N-dealkylation to N-desalkyl-buprenorphine (also known as norbuprenorphine) via cytochrome P450 CYP3A4 and by glucuroconjugation of the parent molecule and the dealkylated metabolite. Norbuprenorphine is a μ (mu) agonist with weak intrinsic activity.

Elimination of buprenorphine is bi- or tri- exponential, with a long terminal elimination phase of 20 to 25 hours, due in part to reabsorption of buprenorphine after intestinal hydrolysis of the conjugated derivative, and in part to the highly lipophilic nature of the molecule.

Buprenorphine is essentially eliminated in the faeces by biliary excretion of the glucuroconjugated metabolites (80%), the rest being eliminated in the urine.

5.3 Preclinical safety data

None stated.

6. PHARMACEUTICAL PARTICULARS

6.1 List of excipients

Lactose, mannitol, maize starch, povidone K30, citric acid anhydrous, magnesium stearate, sodium citrate, purified water and alcohol (96%).

6.2 Incompatibilities

None stated.

6.3 Shelf life

36 months.

6.4 Special precautions for storage

Not applicable.

6.5 Nature and contents of container

Cartons of 50 tablets contained in strips packed in units of 10 tablets each.

6.6 Instructions for use and handling

To be dissolved under the tongue and not to be chewed or swallowed.

Administrative Data

7. MARKETING AUTHORISATION HOLDER

Schering-Plough Ltd
Shire Park
Welwyn Garden City
Hertfordshire AL7 1TW
UK

8. MARKETING AUTHORISATION NUMBER(S)

PL 00201/0245

9. DATE OF FIRST AUTHORISATION/RENEWAL OF THE AUTHORISATION

16 March 1992 / 9 November 2000

10. DATE OF REVISION OF THE TEXT

April 2004

Temgesic 400 microgram Sublingual Tablets

(Schering-Plough Ltd)

1. NAME OF THE MEDICINAL PRODUCT

Temgesic 400 microgram Sublingual Tablets

2. QUALITATIVE AND QUANTITATIVE COMPOSITION

Buprenorphine hydrochloride 432μg/tablet, equivalent to 400μg buprenorphine base.

3. PHARMACEUTICAL FORM

Sublingual tablets

4. CLINICAL PARTICULARS

4.1 Therapeutic indications

As a strong analgesic for the relief of moderate to severe pain.

4.2 Posology and method of administration

Administration by the sublingual route.

Adults and children over 12:

200-400 micrograms to be dissolved under the tongue every 6-8 hours or as required. The recommended starting dose for moderate to severe pain of the type typically presenting in general practice is 200-400 micrograms 8 hourly. The tablet should not be chewed or swallowed as this will reduce efficacy.

Elderly:

There is no indication that dosage needs to be modified for the elderly.

Children under 12 years:

Temgesic sublingual is suitable for use in children under 12 as follows:

16 - 25 kg (35 - 55lb) 100 micrograms

25 - 37.5 kg (55 - 82.5lb) 100-200 micrograms

37.5 - 50 kg (82.5 - 110 lb) 200-300 micrograms.

The recommended dose should be administered every 6 to 8 hours.

Sublingual administration is not suitable for children under the age of six years.

Temgesic sublingual may be used in balanced anaesthetic techniques at a dose of 400 micrograms.

4.3 Contraindications

Not to be given to patients who are known to be allergic to Temgesic or other opiates. Hypersensitivity to any of the constituents.

4.4 Special warnings and special precautions for use

Temgesic occasionally causes significant respiratory depression and, as with other strong centrally acting analgesics, care should be taken when treating patients with impaired respiratory function or patients who are receiving drugs which can cause respiratory depression. Although volunteer studies have indicated that opiate antagonists may not fully reverse the effects of Temgesic, clinical experience has shown that Naloxone may be of benefit in reversing a reduced respiratory rate. Respiratory stimulants such as Doxapram are also effective. The intensity and duration of action may be affected in patients with impaired liver failure.

Controlled human and animal studies indicate that buprenorphine has a substantially lower dependence liability than pure agonist analgesics. In patients abusing opioids in moderate doses substitution with buprenorphine may prevent withdrawal symptoms. In man limited euphorigenic effects have been observed. This has resulted in some abuse of the product and caution should be exercised when prescribing it to patients known to have, or suspected of having, problems with drug abuse.

4.5 Interaction with other medicinal products and other forms of Interaction

There is evidence to indicate that therapeutic doses of buprenorphine do not reduce the analgesic efficacy of standard doses of an opioid agonist and that when buprenorphine is employed within the normal therapeutic range, standard doses of opioid agonist may be administered before the effects of the former have ended without compromising analgesia. However, in individuals on high doses of opioids buprenorphine may precipitate abstinence effects due to its properties as a partial agonist.

Temgesic may cause some drowsiness which may be potentiated by other centrally acting agents, including alcohol, tranquillisers, sedatives and hypnotics. Temgesic should be used with caution in patients receiving monoamine oxidase inhibitors, although animals studies have given no evidence of interactions.

Although interaction studies have not been performed, since this drug is metabolised by CYP3A4 (see section 5.2 pharmacokinetic properties), it is expected that gestodene, troleandomycin, ketoconazole, norfluoxetine, ritonavir, indinavir and saquinavir inhibit its metabolism. Alternatiely, inducers of this enzyme such as phenobarbitol, carbamazepine, phenytoin and rifampicin may reduce the levels of the drug. Since the magnitude of an inducing or inhibitory effect is unknown, such drug combinations should be avoided.

Temgesic has no known effects on diagnostic laboratory tests.

4.6 Pregnancy and lactation

Temgesic is not recommended for use during pregnancy. Animal studies indicate that the amounts of buprenorphine excreted in milk are very low and in human use are unlikely to be of clinical significance to the baby. There is indirect evidence in animal studies to suggest that Temgesic may cause a reduction in milk flow during lactation. Although this occurred only at doses well in excess of the human dose, it should be borne in mind when treating lactating women.

4.7 Effects on ability to drive and use machines

Ambulant patients should be warned not to drive or operate machinery until they are certain they can tolerate Temgesic.

4.8 Undesirable effects

Nausea, vomiting, dizziness, sweating and drowsiness have been reported and may be more frequent in ambulant patients. Hallucinations and other psychotomimetic effects have occurred although more rarely than with other agonists/antagonists. Elderly patients would be expected to be more susceptible to these effects. Hypotension leading to syncope may occur. Rashes, headache, urinary retention and blurring of vision have occasionally been reported. Rarely, a serious allergic reaction may occur following a single dose. Temgesic occasionally causes significant respiratory depression (see section 4.4, Special Warnings and Precautions for Use).

Cases of bronchospasm, angioneurotic oedema and anaphylactic shock have also been reported.

4.9 Overdose

Supportive measures should be instituted and if appropriate Naloxone or respiratory stimulants can be used. The expected symptoms of overdosage would be drowsiness, nausea and vomiting; marked miosis may occur.

5. PHARMACOLOGICAL PROPERTIES

5.1 Pharmacodynamic properties

Buprenorphine is a μ (mu) opioid partial agonist and κ (kappa) antagonist. It is a strong analgesic of the partial agonist (mixed agonist/antagonist) class.

5.2 Pharmacokinetic properties

Absorption

When taken orally, buprenorphine undergoes first-pass hepatic metabolism with N-dealkylation and glucuroconjugation in the small intestine. The use of this medication by the oral route is therefore inappropriate.

Peak plasma concentrations are achieved 90 minutes after sublingual administration.

Distribution

The absorption of buprenorphine is followed by a rapid distribution phase and a half-life of 2 to 5 hours.

Metabolism and elimination

Buprenorphine is oxidatively metabolised by 14-N-dealkylation to N-desalkyl-buprenorphine (also known as norbuprenorphine) via cytochrome P450 CYP3A4 and by glucuroconjugation of the parent molecule and the dealkylated metabolite. Norbuprenorphine is a μ (mu) agonist with weak intrinsic activity.

Elimination of buprenorphine is bi- or tri- exponential, with a long terminal elimination phase of 20 to 25 hours, due in part to reabsorption of buprenorphine after intestinal hydrolysis of the conjugated derivative, and in part to the highly lipophilic nature of the molecule.

Buprenorphine is essentially eliminated in the faeces by biliary excretion of the glucuroconjugated metabolites (80%), the rest being eliminated in the urine.

5.3 Preclinical safety data

None stated.

6. PHARMACEUTICAL PARTICULARS

6.1 List of excipients

Lactose, mannitol, maize starch, povidone K30, citric acid anhydrous, magnesium stearate, sodium citrate, purified water and alcohol (96%).

6.2 Incompatibilities

None stated.

6.3 Shelf life

36 months.

6.4 Special precautions for storage

Not applicable.

6.5 Nature and contents of container

Cartons of 50 tablets contained in strips packed in units of 10 tablets each.

6.6 Instructions for use and handling

To be dissolved under the tongue and not to be chewed or swallowed.

Administrative Data

7. MARKETING AUTHORISATION HOLDER

Schering-Plough Ltd
Shire Park
Welwyn Garden City
Hertfordshire AL7 1TW
UK

8. MARKETING AUTHORISATION NUMBER(S)

PL 00201/0244

9. DATE OF FIRST AUTHORISATION/RENEWAL OF THE AUTHORISATION

May 1998

10. DATE OF REVISION OF THE TEXT

April 2004

Temgesic Injection 1ml

(Schering-Plough Ltd)

1. NAME OF THE MEDICINAL PRODUCT

Temgesic Injection 1ml

2. QUALITATIVE AND QUANTITATIVE COMPOSITION

Buprenorphine hydrochloride 324μg/ml, equivalent to 300μg buprenorphine base.

3. PHARMACEUTICAL FORM

Terminally sterilised solution for injection.

4. CLINICAL PARTICULARS

4.1 Therapeutic indications

As a strong analgesic for the relief of moderate to severe pain.

4.2 Posology and method of administration

Administration by i.m. or slow i.v. injection.

Adults and children over 12 years: 1-2 ml (300-600 micrograms of buprenorphine) every 6-8 hours or as required.

Children aged under 12 years: 3-6 micrograms/kg body weight every 6-8 hours. In refractory cases up to 9 micrograms/kg may be administered. There is no clinical experience in infants below the age of 6 months.

There is no evidence that dosage need be modified for the elderly.

Temgesic Injection may be employed in balanced anaesthetic techniques as a pre-medication at a dose of 300 micrograms i.m., or as an analgesic supplement at doses of 300 to 450 micrograms i.v.

4.3 Contraindications

Not to be given to patients who are known to be allergic to Temgesic or other opiates.

Hypersensitivity to any of the constituents.

4.4 Special warnings and special precautions for use

Temgesic occasionally causes significant respiratory depression and, as with other strong centrally acting analgesics, care should be taken when treating patients with impaired respiratory function or patients who are receiving drugs which can cause respiratory depression.

Although volunteer studies have indicated that opiate antagonists may not fully reverse the effects of Temgesic, clinical experience has shown that Naloxone may be of benefit in reversing a reduced respiratory rate. Respiratory stimulants such as Doxapram are also effective. The intensity and duration of action may be affected in patients with impaired liver failure.

Controlled human and animal studies indicate that buprenorphine has a substantially lower dependence liability than pure agonist analgesics. In patients abusing opioids in moderate doses substitution with buprenorphine may prevent withdrawal symptoms. In man limited euphorigenic effects have been observed. This has resulted in some abuse of the product and caution should be exercised when prescribing it to patients known to have, or suspected of having, problems with drug abuse.

4.5 Interaction with other medicinal products and other forms of Interaction

There is evidence to indicate that therapeutic doses of buprenorphine do not reduce the analgesic efficacy of standard doses of an opioid agonist and that when buprenorphine is employed within the normal therapeutic range, standard doses of opioid agonist may be administered before the effects of the former have ended without compromising analgesia. However, in individuals on high doses of opioids buprenorphine may precipitate abstinence effects due to its properties as a partial agonist.

Temgesic may cause some drowsiness which may be potentiated by other centrally acting agents, including alcohol, tranquillisers, sedatives and hypnotics. Temgesic should be used with caution in patients receiving monoamine oxidase inhibitors, although animals studies have given no evidence of interactions.

Although interaction studies have not been performed, since this drug is metabolised by CYP3A4 (see section 5.2 pharmacokinetic properties), it is expected that gestodene, troleandomycin, ketonazole, norfluoxetine, ritonavir, indinavir and saquinavir inhibit its metabolism. Alternatively, inducers of this enzyme such as phenobarbital, carbamazepine, phenytoin and rifampicin may reduce the levels of the drug. Since the magnitude of an inducing or inhibitory effect is unknown, such drug combinations should be avoided.

Temgesic has no known effects on diagnostic laboratory tests.

4.6 Pregnancy and lactation

Temgesic is not recommended for use during pregnancy. Animal studies indicate that the amounts of buprenorphine excreted in milk are very low and in human use are unlikely to be of clinical significance to the baby.

There is indirect evidence in animal studies to suggest that Temgesic may cause a reduction in milk flow during lactation. Although this occurred only at doses well in excess of the human dose, it should be borne in mind when treating lactating women.

4.7 Effects on ability to drive and use machines

Ambulant patients should be warned not to drive or operate machinery until they are certain they can tolerate Temgesic.

4.8 Undesirable effects

Nausea, vomiting, dizziness, sweating and drowsiness have been reported and may be more frequent in ambulant patients. Hallucinations and other psychotomimetic effects have occurred although more rarely than with other agonists/antagonists. Elderly patients would be expected to be more susceptible to these effects. Hypotension leading to syncope may occur. Rashes, headache, urinary retention and blurring of vision have occasionally been reported. Rarely, a serious allergic reaction may occur following a single dose. Temgesic occasionally causes significant respiratory depression (see section 4.4, Special Warnings and Precautions for Use).

Cases of bronchospasm, angioneurotic oedema and anaphylactic shock have also been reported.

4.9 Overdose

Supportive measures should be instituted and if appropriate Naloxone or respiratory stimulants can be used. The expected symptoms of overdosage would be drowsiness, nausea and vomiting; marked miosis may occur.

5. PHARMACOLOGICAL PROPERTIES

5.1 Pharmacodynamic properties

Buprenorphine is a μ (mu) opioid partial agonist and κ (kappa) antagonist. It is a strong analgesic of the partial agonist (mixed agonist (antagonist) class.

5.2 Pharmacokinetic properties

Buprenorphine is readily available by i.v. or i.m. routes; the relative bioavailability i.m. to i.v. was 1.07. Peak plasma levels are achieved within a few minutes of i.m. administration and after 10 minutes are not significantly different from those observed after the same dose given i.v.

Buprenorphine is oxidatively metabolised by 14-N-dealkylation to N-desalkyl-buprenorphine (also known as norbuprenorphine) via cytokine P450 CYP3A4 and by glucuroconjungation of the parent molecule and the dealkylated metabolite. Norbuprenorphine is a μ (mu) agonist with weak intrinsic activity.

Elimination of buprenorphine is bi- or tri- exponential, with a long terminal elimination phase of 20 to 25 hours, due in part to reabsorption of buprenorphine after intestinal hydrolysis of the conjugated derivative, and in part to the highly lipophilic nature of the molecule.

Buprenorphine is essentially eliminated in the faeces by biliary excretion of the glucuroconjugated metabolites (80%), the rest being eliminated in the urine.

5.3 Preclinical safety data

No preclinical findings of relevance to the prescriber have been reported.

6. PHARMACEUTICAL PARTICULARS

6.1 List of excipients

Dextrose anhydrous parenteral

Hydrochloric acid

Water for injections.

6.2 Incompatibilities

None stated.

6.3 Shelf life

Five years

6.4 Special precautions for storage

The product, though stable, should be kept cool and protected from light.

6.5 Nature and contents of container

Sealed Type I glass ampoules. Pack size: five ampoules.

6.6 Instructions for use and handling

Administration by i.m. or slow i.v. injection.

Administrative Data

7. MARKETING AUTHORISATION HOLDER

Schering-Plough Ltd

Shire Park

Welwyn Garden City

Hertfordshire AL7 1TW

UK

8. MARKETING AUTHORISATION NUMBER(S)

PL 00201/0246

9. DATE OF FIRST AUTHORISATION/RENEWAL OF THE AUTHORISATION

April 2004

10. DATE OF REVISION OF THE TEXT

Legal Category

CD (Sch 3), POM

Temodal 5mg, 20mg, 100mg or 250mg hard capsules

(Schering-Plough Ltd)

1. NAME OF THE MEDICINAL PRODUCT

Temodal 5 mg, 20 mg, 100 mg or 250 mg hard capsules.

2. QUALITATIVE AND QUANTITATIVE COMPOSITION

Each Temodal capsule contains 5 mg, 20 mg, 100 mg or 250 mg temozolomide.

For excipients, see 6.1.

3. PHARMACEUTICAL FORM

Hard capsule

The hard capsules are white, opaque and imprinted with a specific colour imprinting ink that is unique for each strength.

4. CLINICAL PARTICULARS

4.1 Therapeutic indications

Temodal capsules are indicated for the treatment of patients with:

- newly diagnosed glioblastoma multiforme concomitantly with radiotherapy and subsequently as monotherapy treatment

- malignant glioma, such as glioblastoma multiforme or anaplastic astrocytoma, showing recurrence or progression after standard therapy.

4.2 Posology and method of administration

Temodal should only be prescribed by physicians experienced in the oncological treatment of brain tumours.

<u>Posology</u>

<u>Adult patients with newly diagnosed glioblastoma multiforme</u>

Temodal is administered in combination with focal radiotherapy (concomitant phase) followed by up to 6 cycles of temozolomide monotherapy.

<u>Concomitant phase</u>

Temodal is administered orally at a dose of 75 mg/m^2 daily for 42 days concomitant with focal radiotherapy (60 Gy administered in 30 fractions). No dose reductions will be made, but delay or discontinuation of temozolomide administration will be decided weekly according to haematological and non-haematological toxicity criteria. The Temodal dose can be continued throughout the 42 day concomitant period (up to 49 days) if all of the following conditions are met: absolute neutrophil count $\geqslant 1.5 \times 10^9$/l, thrombocyte count $\geqslant 100 \times 10^9$/l, Common Toxicity Criteria (CTC) non-haematological toxicity $\leqslant$ Grade 1 (except for alopecia, nausea and vomiting). During treatment a complete blood count should be obtained weekly. Temodal administration should be interrupted or discontinued during concomitant phase according to the haematological and non-haematological toxicity criteria as noted in **Table 1.**

Table 1. Temozolomide dosing interruption or discontinuation during concomitant radiotherapy and temozolomide

Toxicity	TMZ interruption[a]	TMZ discontinuation
Absolute Neutrophil Count	$\geqslant 0.5$ and $< 1.5 \times 10^9$/l	$< 0.5 \times 10^9$/l
Thrombocyte Count	$\geqslant 10$ and $< 100 \times 10^9$/l	$< 10 \times 10^9$/l
CTC Non-haematological toxicity (except for alopecia, nausea, vomiting)	CTC Grade 2	CTC Grade 3 or 4

a: Treatment with concomitant TMZ can be continued when all of the following conditions are met: absolute neutrophil count $\geqslant 1.5 \times 10^9$/l; thrombocyte count $\geqslant 100 \times 10^9$/l; CTC non-haematological toxicity $\leqslant$ Grade 1 (except for alopecia, nausea, vomiting).

TMZ = temozolomide; CTC = Common Toxicity Criteria.

<u>Monotherapy phase</u>

Four weeks after completing the Temodal + Radiotherapy phase, Temodal is administered for up to 6 cycles of monotherapy treatment. Dosage in Cycle 1 (monotherapy) is 150 mg/m^2 once daily for 5 days followed by 23 days without treatment. At the start of Cycle 2, the dose is escalated to 200 mg/m^2 if the CTC non-haematological toxicity for Cycle 1 is Grade $\leqslant$ 2 (except for alopecia, nausea and vomiting), absolute neutrophil count (ANC) is $\geqslant 1.5 \times 10^9$/l, and the thrombocyte count is $\geqslant 100 \times 10^9$/l. If the dose was not escalated at Cycle 2, escalation should not be done in subsequent cycles. Once escalated, the dose remains at 200 mg/m^2 per day for the first 5 days of each subsequent cycle except if toxicity occurs. Dose reductions and discontinuations during the monotherapy phase should be applied according to **Tables 2 and 3.**

During treatment a complete blood count should be obtained on Day 22 (21 days after the first dose of Temodal). The Temodal dose should be reduced or discontinued according to **Table 3**.

Table 2 Temodal dose levels for monotherapy treatment

Dose Level	Dose (mg/m^2/day)	Remarks
–1	100	Reduction for prior toxicity
0	150	Dose during Cycle 1
1	200	Dose during Cycles 2-6 in absence of toxicity

Table 3. Temodal dose reduction or discontinuation during monotherapy treatment

Toxicity	Reduce TMZ by 1 dose level[a]	Discontinue TMZ
Absolute Neutrophil Count	$< 1.0 \times 10^9$/l	See footnote b
Thrombocyte Count	$< 50 \times 10^9$/l	See footnote b
CTC Non-haematological Toxicity (except for alopecia, nausea, vomiting)	CTC Grade 3	CTC Grade 4[b]

a: TMZ dose levels are listed in Table 2.

b: TMZ is to be discontinued if:

• dose level -1 (100 mg/m^2) still results in unacceptable toxicity

• the same Grade 3 non-haematological toxicity (except for alopecia, nausea, vomiting) recurs after dose reduction.

TMZ = temozolomide; CTC = Common Toxicity Criteria.

<u>Recurrent or progressive malignant glioma</u>:

<u>Adult patients</u>

A treatment cycle comprises 28 days. In patients previously untreated with chemotherapy, Temodal is administered orally at a dose of 200 mg/m^2 once daily for the first 5 days followed by a 23 day treatment interruption (total of 28 days). In patients previously treated with chemotherapy, the initial dose is 150 mg/m^2 once daily, to be increased in the second cycle to 200 mg/m^2 once daily, for 5 days if there is no haematological toxicity (see section **4.4**)

Paediatric patients

In patients 3 years of age or older, a treatment cycle comprises 28 days. Temodal is administered orally at a dose of 200 mg/m^2 once daily for the first 5 days followed by a 23 day treatment interruption (total of 28 days). Paediatric patients previously treated with chemotherapy should receive an initial dose of 150 mg/m^2 once daily for 5 days, with escalation to 200 mg/m^2 once daily for 5 days at the next cycle if there is no haematological toxicity (see section **4.4**).

Patients with hepatic or renal dysfunction

The pharmacokinetics of temozolomide were comparable in patients with normal hepatic function and in those with mild or moderate hepatic dysfunction. No data are available on the administration of Temodal in patients with severe hepatic dysfunction (Child's Class III) or with renal dysfunction. Based on the pharmacokinetic properties of temozolomide, it is unlikely that dose reductions are required in patients with severe hepatic or renal dysfunction. However, caution should be exercised when Temodal is administered in these patients.

Elderly patients

Based on pharmacokinetic analysis, clearance of temozolomide is not affected by age. However, special care should be taken when Temodal is administered in elderly patients (see section **4.4**).

Method of administration

Temodal should be administered in the fasting state.

Temodal capsules must be swallowed whole with a glass of water and must not be opened or chewed. The prescribed dose should be administered using the minimum number of capsules possible.

Anti-emetic therapy may be administered prior to or following administration of Temodal (see section **4.4**). If vomiting occurs after the dose is administered, a second dose should not be administered that day.

4.3 Contraindications

Temodal is contraindicated in patients who have a history of hypersensitivity to its components or to dacarbazine (DTIC).

Temodal is contraindicated in patients with severe myelosuppression (see section **4.4**).

Temodal is contraindicated in women who are pregnant or breast-feeding (see section **4.6**).

4.4 Special warnings and special precautions for use

Patients who received concomitant Temodal and radiotherapy in a pilot trial for the prolonged 42 day schedule were shown to be at particular risk for developing *Pneumocystis carinii* pneumonia. Thus, prophylaxis against *Pneumocystis carinii* pneumonia is required for all patients receiving concomitant Temodal and radiotherapy for the 42 day regimen (with a maximum of 49 days) regardless of lymphocyte count. If lymphopenia occurs, they are to continue the prophylaxis until recovery of lymphopenia to grade ⩽ 1.

Anti-emetic therapy: Nausea and vomiting are very commonly associated with Temodal, and guidelines are provided:

Patients with newly diagnosed glioblastoma multiforme:

- anti-emetic prophylaxis is recommended prior to the initial dose of concomitant temozolomide,
- anti-emetic prophylaxis is strongly recommended during the monotherapy phase.

Patients with recurrent or progressive malignant glioma:

Patients who have experienced severe (Grade 3 or 4) vomiting in previous treatment cycles may require anti-emetic therapy.

This medicinal product contains lactose; thus, patients with rare hereditary problems of galactose intolerance, the Lapp lactase deficiency or glucose-galactose malabsorption should not take this medicine.

Laboratory parameters

Prior to dosing, the following laboratory parameters must be met: ANC $\geqslant$ 1.5 $\times$ 10^9/l and platelet count $\geqslant$ 100 $\times$ 10^9/l. A complete blood count should be obtained on Day 22 (21 days after the first dose) or within 48 hours of that day, and weekly until ANC is above 1.5 $\times$ 10^9/l and platelet count exceeds 100 $\times$ 10^9/l. If ANC falls to < 1.0 $\times$ 10^9/l or the platelet count is < 50 $\times$ 10^9/l during any cycle, the next cycle should be reduced one dose level. Dose levels include 100 mg/m^2, 150 mg/m^2, and 200 mg/m^2. The lowest recommended dose is 100 mg/m^2.

Paediatric use

There is no clinical experience with use of Temodal in children under the age of 3 years. Experience in older children is very limited.

Use in elderly patients

Elderly patients (> 70 years of age) appear to be at increased risk of neutropenia and thrombocytopenia, compared with younger patients. Therefore, special care should be taken when Temodal is administered in elderly patients.

Table 4 Temodal (TMZ) and radiotherapy: Treatment-emergent events during concomitant and monotherapy treatment

Very Common (> 1/10); Common (> 1/100, < 1/10); Uncommon (> 1/1,000, < 1/100) CIOMS III		
Body System	**TMZ + concomitant radiotherapy** n=288*	**TMZ monotherapy** n=224
Infections and infestations		
Common:	Candidiasis oral, *herpes simplex*, infection, pharyngitis, wound infection	Candidiasis oral, infection
Uncommon:		*Herpes simplex*, Herpes zoster, influenza-like symptoms
Blood and lymphatic system disorders		
Common:	Leukopenia, lymphopenia, neutropenia, thrombocytopenia	Anaemia, febrile neutropenia, leukopenia, thrombocytopenia
Uncommon:	Anaemia, febrile neutropenia	Lymphopenia, petechiae
Endocrine disorders		
Uncommon:	Cushingoid	Cushingoid
Metabolism and nutrition disorders		
Very Common:	Anorexia	Anorexia
Common:	Hyperglycaemia, weight decreased	Weight decreased
Uncommon:	Hypokalemia, alkaline phosphatase increased, weight increased	Hyperglycaemia, weight increased
Psychiatric disorders		
Common:	Anxiety, emotional lability, insomnia	Anxiety, depression, emotional lability, insomnia
Uncommon:	Agitation, apathy, behaviour disorder, depression, hallucination	Hallucination, amnesia
Nervous system disorders		
Very Common:	Headache	Headache, convulsions
Common:	Dizziness, aphasia, balance impaired, concentration impaired, confusion, consciousness decreased, convulsions, memory impairment, neuropathy, paresthesia, somnolence, speech disorder, tremor	Dizziness, aphasia, balance impaired, concentration impaired, confusion, dysphasia, hemiparesis, memory impairment, neurological disorder (NOS), neuropathy, peripheral neuropathy, paresthesia, somnolence, speech disorder, tremor
Uncommon:	Ataxia, cognition impaired, dysphasia, extrapyramidal disorder, gait abnormal, hemiparesis, hyperesthesia, hypoesthesia, neurological disorder (NOS), peripheral neuropathy, status epilepticus	Ataxia, coordination abnormal, gait abnormal, hemiplegia, hyperesthesia, sensory disturbance
Eye disorders		
Common:	Vision blurred	Vision blurred, diplopia, visual field defect
Uncommon:	Eye pain, hemianopia, vision disorder, visual acuity reduced, visual field defect	Eye pain, eyes dry, visual acuity reduced
Ear and labyrinth disorders		
Common:	Hearing impairment	Hearing impairment, tinnitus
Uncommon:	Earache, hyperacusis, tinnitus, otitis media	Deafness, earache, vertigo
Cardiac disorders		
Uncommon:	Palpitation	
Vascular disorders		
Common:	Oedema, oedema leg, haemorrhage	Oedema leg, haemorrhage, deep venous thrombosis
Uncommon:	Hypertension, cerebral haemorrhage	Oedema, oedema peripheral, embolism pulmonary
Respiratory, thoracic and mediastinal disorders		
Common:	Coughing, dyspnoea	Coughing, dyspnoea
Uncommon:	Pneumonia, upper respiratory infection, nasal congestion	Pneumonia, sinusitis, upper respiratory infection, bronchitis
Gastrointestinal disorders		
Very Common:	Constipation, nausea, vomiting	Constipation, nausea, vomiting

Common:	Abdominal pain, diarrhoea, dyspepsia, dysphagia, stomatitis	Diarrhoea, dyspepsia, dysphagia, mouth dry, stomatitis
Uncommon:		Abdominal distension, fecal incontinence, gastrointestinal disorder (NOS), gastroenteritis, haemorrhoids
Skin and subcutaneous tissue disorders		
Very Common:	Alopecia, rash	Alopecia, rash
Common:	Dermatitis, dry skin, erythema, pruritus	Dry skin, pruritus
Uncommon:	Photosensitivity reaction, pigmentation abnormal, skin exfoliation	Erythema, pigmentation abnormal, sweating increased
Musculoskeletal and connective tissue disorders		
Common:	Arthralgia, muscle weakness	Arthralgia, musculoskeletal pain, myalgia, muscle weakness
Uncommon:	Back pain, musculoskeletal pain, myalgia, myopathy	Back pain, myopathy
Renal and urinary disorders		
Common:	Micturition frequency, urinary incontinence	Urinary incontinence
Uncommon:		Dysuria
Reproductive system and breast disorders		
Uncommon:	Impotence	Amenorrhea, breast pain, menorrhagia, vaginal haemorrhage, vaginitis
General disorders and administration site conditions		
Very Common:	Fatigue	Fatigue
Common:	Fever, pain, allergic reaction, radiation injury, face oedema, taste perversion	Fever, pain, allergic reaction, radiation injury, taste perversion
Uncommon:	Flushing, hot flushes, asthenia, condition aggravated, rigors, tongue discolouration, parosmia, thirst	Asthenia, condition aggravated, pain, rigors, tooth disorder, face oedema, taste perversion
Investigations		
Common:	ALT increased	ALT increased
Uncommon:	Gamma GT increased, hepatic enzymes increased, AST increased	

*A patient who was randomised to the RT arm only, received Temodal + RT.

Table 5 Treatment related undesirable effects: Recurrent or progressive malignant glioma

Very common (> 1/10); Common (> 1/100, < 1/10); Uncommon (> 1/1,000, < 1/100); Rare (> 1/10,000, < 1/1,000); Very rare (< 1/10,000) (CIOMS III)	
Infections and infestations Rare:	 Opportunistic infections, including *pneumocystis carinii* pneumonia (PCP)
Blood and lymphatic system disorders Very common: Uncommon:	 Thrombocytopenia, neutropenia or lymphopenia (grade 3-4), Pancytopenia, leukopenia, anaemia (grade 3-4)
Metabolism and nutrition disorders Very common: Common:	 Anorexia Weight decrease
Nervous system disorders Very common: Common:	 Headache Somnolence, dizziness, paresthesia
Respiratory, thoracic and mediastinal disorders Common:	 Dyspnoea
Gastrointestinal disorders Very common: Common:	 Nausea, vomiting, constipation Diarrhoea, abdominal pain, dyspepsia
Skin and subcutaneous tissue disorders Common: Very rare:	 Rash, alopecia, pruritus Urticaria, exanthema, erythroderma, erythema multiforme
General disorders and administration site conditions Very common: Common: Very rare:	 Fatigue Fever, asthenia, pain, rigors, malaise, taste perversion Allergic reactions, including anaphylaxis, angioedema

Male patients

Temozolomide can have genotoxic effects. Therefore, men being treated with temozolomide are advised not to father a child during up to 6 months after treatment and to seek advice on cryoconservation of sperm prior to treatment because of the possibility of irreversible infertility due to therapy with temozolomide.

4.5 Interaction with other medicinal products and other forms of Interaction

Administration of Temodal with ranitidine did not result in alterations in the extent of absorption of temozolomide or the exposure to monomethyl triazenoimidazole carboxamide (MTIC).

Administration of Temodal with food resulted in a 33 % decrease in C_{max} and a 9 % decrease in area under the curve (AUC).

As it cannot be excluded that the change in C_{max} is clinically significant, Temodal should be administered without food.

Based on an analysis of population pharmacokinetics observed in Phase II trials, co-administration of dexamethasone, prochlorperazine, phenytoin, carbamazepine, ondansetron, H_2 receptor antagonists, or phenobarbital did not alter the clearance of temozolomide. Co-administration with valproic acid was associated with a small but statistically significant decrease in clearance of temozolomide.

No studies have been conducted to determine the effect of temozolomide on the metabolism or elimination of other medicinal products. However, since temozolomide does not require hepatic metabolism and exhibits low protein binding, it is unlikely that it would affect the pharmacokinetics of other medications.

Use of Temodal in combination with other myelosuppressive agents may increase the likelihood of myelosuppression.

4.6 Pregnancy and lactation

Pregnancy

There are no studies in pregnant women. In preclinical studies in rats and rabbits administered 150 mg/m^2, teratogenicity and/or foetal toxicity were demonstrated. Temodal, therefore, should not normally be administered to pregnant women. If use during pregnancy must be considered, the patient should be apprised of the potential risk to the foetus. Women of childbearing potential should be advised to avoid pregnancy while they are receiving Temodal.

Lactation

It is not known whether temozolomide is excreted in human milk; thus, Temodal must not be used by women who are breast-feeding.

4.7 Effects on ability to drive and use machines

The ability to drive and use machines may be impaired in patients treated with Temodal due to fatigue and somnolence.

4.8 Undesirable effects

Newly diagnosed glioblastoma multiforme

Table 4 provides treatment emergent adverse events in patients with newly diagnosed glioblastoma multiforme during the concomitant and monotherapy phases of treatment.

Table 4: Temodal (TMZ) and radiotherapy: Treatment-emergent events during concomitant and monotherapy treatment

(see Table 4 on previous page)

Laboratory results: Myelosuppression (neutropenia and thrombocytopenia), which is known dose limiting toxicity for most cytotoxic agents, including Temodal, was observed. When laboratory abnormalities and adverse events were combined across concomitant and monotherapy treatment phases, Grade 3 or Grade 4 neutrophil abnormalities including neutropenic events were observed in 8 % of the patients. Grade 3 or Grade 4 thrombocyte abnormalities, including thrombocytopenic events were observed in 14 % of the patients who received Temodal.

Recurrent or progressive malignant glioma

In clinical trials, the most frequently occurring treatment-related undesirable effects were gastrointestinal disturbances, specifically nausea (43 %) and vomiting (36 %). These effects were usually Grade 1 or 2 (0 – 5 episodes of vomiting in 24 hours) and were either self-limiting or readily controlled with standard anti-emetic therapy. The incidence of severe nausea and vomiting was 4 %.

Table 5 includes undesirable effects reported during clinical trials for recurrent or progressive malignant glioma and following the marketing of Temodal.

Table 5. Treatment related undesirable effects: Recurrent or progressive malignant glioma

(see Table 5 opposite)

Laboratory results: Grade 3 or 4 thrombocytopenia and neutropenia occurred in 19 % and 17 % respectively, of patients treated for malignant glioma. This led to hospitalisation and/or discontinuation of Temodal in 8 % and 4 %, respectively. Myelosuppression was predictable (usually within the first few cycles, with the nadir between Day 21 and Day 28), and recovery was rapid, usually within 1-2 weeks. No evidence of cumulative myelosuppression was observed. The presence of thrombocytopenia may increase the risk of bleeding, and the presence of neutropenia or leukopenia may increase the risk of infection.

Antineoplastic agents, and notably alkylating agents, have been associated with a potential risk of myelodysplastic syndrome (MDS) and secondary malignancies, including leukemia. Very rare cases of MDS and secondary malignancies, including myeloid leukemia have been reported in patients treated with regimens that included Temodal.

4.9 Overdose

Doses of 500, 750, 1,000, and 1,250 mg/m^2 (total dose per cycle over 5 days) have been evaluated clinically in patients. Dose-limiting toxicity was haematological and was reported with any dose but is expected to be more severe at higher doses. An overdose of 10,000 mg (total dose in a single cycle, over 5 days) was taken by one patient and the adverse events reported were pancytopenia, pyrexia, multi-organ failure and death. There are reports of patients who have taken the recommended dose for more than 5 days of treatment (up to 64 days) with adverse events reported including bone marrow suppression, with or without infection, in some cases severe and prolonged and resulting in death. In the event of an overdose, haematological evaluation is needed. Supportive measures should be provided as necessary.

5. PHARMACOLOGICAL PROPERTIES

5.1 Pharmacodynamic properties

Pharmacotherapeutic group: Antineoplastic agents - Other alkylating agents, ATC code L01A X03

Temozolomide is a triazene, which undergoes rapid chemical conversion at physiologic pH to the active compound MTIC. The cytotoxicity of MTIC is thought to be due primarily to alkylation at the O^6 position of guanine with additional alkylation also occurring at the N^7 position. Cytotoxic lesions that develop subsequently are thought to involve aberrant repair of the methyl adduct.

Newly diagnosed glioblastoma multiforme

Five hundred and seventy-three patients were randomised to receive either temozolomide + Radiotherapy (RT) (n=287) or RT alone (n=286). Patients in the temozolomide + RT arm received concomitant temozolomide (75 mg/m^2) once daily, starting the first day of RT until the last day of RT, for 42 days (with a maximum of 49 days). This was followed by monotherapy temozolomide (150 - 200 mg/m^2) on Days 1 - 5 of every 28-day cycle for up to 6 cycles, starting 4 weeks after the end of RT. Patients in the control arm received RT only. *Pneumocystis carinii* pneumonia (PCP) prophylaxis was required during RT and combined temozolomide therapy.

Temozolomide was administered as salvage therapy in the follow-up phase in 161 patients of the 282 (57 %) in the RT alone arm, and 62 patients of the 277 (22 %) in the temozolomide + RT arm.

The hazard ratio (HR) for overall survival was 1.59 (95 % CI for HR=1.33 -1.91) with a log-rank $p < 0.0001$ in favour of the temozolomide arm. The estimated probability of surviving 2 years or more (26 % vs 10 %) is higher for the RT + temozolomide arm. The addition of concomitant temozolomide to radiotherapy, followed by temozolomide monotherapy in the treatment of patients with newly diagnosed glioblastoma multiforme demonstrated a statistically significant improved overall survival compared with radiotherapy alone (**Figure 1**).

(see Figure 1)

The results from the trial were not consistent in the subgroup of patients with a poor performance status (PS=2, n=70), where overall survival and time to progression were similar in both arms. However, no unacceptable risks appear to be present in this patient group.

Recurrent or progressive malignant glioma

Data on clinical efficacy in patients with glioblastoma multiforme (Karnofsky performance status [KPS] ⩾ 70), progressive or recurrent after surgery and radiotherapy, were based on two clinical trials. One was a non-comparative trial in 138 patients (29 % received prior chemotherapy), and the other was a randomised reference controlled trial of temozolomide and procarbazine in a total of 225 patients (67 % received prior treatment with nitrosourea based chemotherapy.) In both trials, the primary endpoint was progression-free survival (PFS) defined by MRI scans or neurological worsening. In the non-comparative trial, the PFS at 6 months was 19 %, the median progression-free survival was 2.1 months, and the median overall survival 5.4 months. The objective response rate based on MRI scans was 8 %.

In the randomised trial, the 6 month PFS was significantly greater for temozolomide than for procarbazine (21 % vs 8 %, respectively – chi-square p = 0.008) with median PFS of 2.89 and 1.88 months respectively (log rank p = 0.0063). The median survival was 7.34 and 5.66 months for temozolomide and procarbazine, respectively (log rank p = 0.33). At 6 months the fraction of surviving patients was significantly higher in the temozolomide arm (60 %) compared with the procarbazine arm (44 %) (chi-square p = 0.019). In patients with prior chemotherapy a benefit was indicated in those with a KPS of 80 or better.

Data on time to worsening of neurological status favoured temozolomide over procarbazine as did data on time to worsening of performance status (decrease to a KPS of < 70 or a decrease by at least 30 points). The median times to progression in these endpoints ranged from 0.7 to 2.1 months longer for temozolomide than for procarbazine (log rank p = < 0.01 to 0.03).

Anaplastic astrocytoma

In a multicentre, global, prospective phase II trial evaluating the safety and efficacy of oral temozolomide in the treatment of patients with anaplastic astrocytoma at first relapse, the 6 month progression-free survival was 46 %. The median progression-free survival was 5.4 months.

Median overall survival was 14.6 months. Response rate, based on the central reviewer assessment, was 35 % (13 CR and 43 PR) for the intent-to-treat population. In 43 patients stable disease was reported. The 6-month event-free survival for the ITT population was 44 % with a median event-free survival of 4.6 months, which was similar to the results for the progression-free survival. For the eligible histology population, the efficacy results were similar. Achieving a radiological objective response or maintaining progression-free status was strongly associated with maintained or improved quality of life.

5.2 Pharmacokinetic properties

PET studies in humans and preclinical data suggest that temozolomide crosses the blood-brain barrier rapidly and is present in the CSF. CSF penetration was confirmed in one patient; CSF exposure based on AUC of temozolomide was approximately 30 % of that in plasma, which is consistent with animal data. After oral administration to adult patients, temozolomide is absorbed rapidly with peak concentrations reached as early as 20 minutes post-dose (mean times between 0.5 and 1.5 hours). The half-life in plasma is approximately 1.8 hours. Plasma concentrations increase in a dose-related manner. Plasma clearance, volume of distribution and half-life are independent of dose. Temozolomide demonstrates low protein binding (10 % to 20 %), and thus it is not expected to interact with highly protein bound agents. After oral administration of ^{14}C-labelled temozolomide, mean faecal excretion of ^{14}C over 7 days post-dose was 0.8 % indicating complete absorption. The major route of ^{14}C elimination is renal. Following oral administration, approximately 5 % to 10 % of the dose is recovered unchanged in the urine over 24 hours, and the remainder excreted as temozolomide acid, 5-aminoimidazole-4-carboxamide (AIC) or unidentified polar metabolites.

Analysis of population-based pharmacokinetics of temozolomide revealed that plasma temozolomide clearance was independent of age, renal function or tobacco use. In a separate pharmacokinetic study, plasma pharmacokinetic profiles in patients with mild to moderate hepatic dysfunction were similar to those observed in patients with normal hepatic function.

Temozolomide is spontaneously hydrolyzed at physiologic pH primarily to the active species, 3-methyl-(triazen-1-yl)imidazole-4-carboxamide (MTIC). MTIC is spontaneously hydrolyzed to 5-amino-imidazole-4-carboxamide (AIC), a known intermediate in purine and nucleic acid biosynthesis, and to methylhydrazine, which is believed to be the active alkylating species. The cytotoxicity of MTIC is thought to be primarily due to alkylation of DNA mainly at the O^6 and N^7 positions of guanine. Relative to the AUC of temozolomide, the exposure to MTIC and AIC is ~ 2.4 % and 23 %, respectively. *In vivo*, the $t_{1/2}$ of MTIC was similar to that of temozolomide, 1.8 hr.

Paediatric patients had a higher AUC than adult patients; however, the maximum tolerated dose (MTD) was 1,000 mg/m^2 per cycle both in children and in adults.

5.3 Preclinical safety data

Single-cycle (5-day dosing, 23 days non-treatment), three- and six-cycle toxicity studies were conducted in rats and dogs. The primary targets of toxicity included the bone marrow, lymphoreticular system, testes, the gastrointestinal tract and, at higher doses, which were lethal to 60 % to 100 % of rats and dogs tested, degeneration of the retina occurred. Most of the toxicity showed evidence of reversibility, except for adverse events on the male reproductive system and retinal degeneration. However, because the doses implicated in retinal degeneration were in the lethal dose range, and no comparable effect has been observed in clinical studies, this finding was not considered to have clinical relevance.

Temozolomide is an embryotoxic, teratogenic and genotoxic alkylating agent. Temozolomide is more toxic to the rat and dog than to humans, and the clinical dose approximates the minimum lethal dose in rats and dogs. Dose-related reductions in leukocytes and platelets appear to be sensitive indicators of toxicity. A variety of neoplasms, including mammary carcinomas, keratocanthoma of the skin and basal cell adenoma were observed in the six-cycle rat study while no tumours or pre-neoplastic changes were evident in dog studies. Rats appear to be particularly sensitive to oncogenic effects of temozolomide, with the occurrence of first tumours within three months of initiating dosing. This latency period is very short even for an alkylating agent.

Results of the Ames/salmonella and Human Peripheral Blood Lymphocyte (HPBL) chromosome aberration tests showed a positive mutagenicity response.

6. PHARMACEUTICAL PARTICULARS

6.1 List of excipients

The capsule contains anhydrous lactose, colloidal anhydrous silica, sodium starch glycolate, tartaric acid, stearic acid. Capsule shells contain gelatine, titanium dioxide, sodium lauryl sulphate and are imprinted with pharmaceutical ink which contains pharmaceutical grade shellac, propylene glycol, together with:

5mg - green print - ammonium hydroxide, titanium dioxide (E 171), yellow iron oxide (E 172) and indigotin (E 132).

20mg - brown print - ammonium hydroxide, potassium hydroxide, titanium dioxide (E 171), black iron oxide (E 172), yellow iron oxide (E 172), brown iron oxide (E 172) and red iron oxide (E 172).

100mg - blue print - titanium dioxide (E 171) and indigotin (E 132).

250mg - black print - ammonium hydroxide, potassium hydroxide and black iron oxide (E 172).

6.2 Incompatibilities

Not applicable.

6.3 Shelf life

2 years

6.4 Special precautions for storage

Do not store above 30 °C.

6.5 Nature and contents of container

Type I amber glass bottles with child-resistant polypropylene caps containing 5 and 20 capsules.

Not all pack sizes may be marketed.

6.6 Instructions for use and handling

Do not open the capsules. If a capsule becomes damaged, avoid contact of the powder contents with skin or mucous membrane. If contact does occur, wash the affected area.

Keep capsules out of the reach and sight of children, preferably in a locked cupboard. Ingestion can be lethal.

7. MARKETING AUTHORISATION HOLDER

SP Europe
73, rue de Stalle
B-1180 Bruxelles
Belgium

Figure 1 Kaplan-Meier curves for overall survival (ITT population)

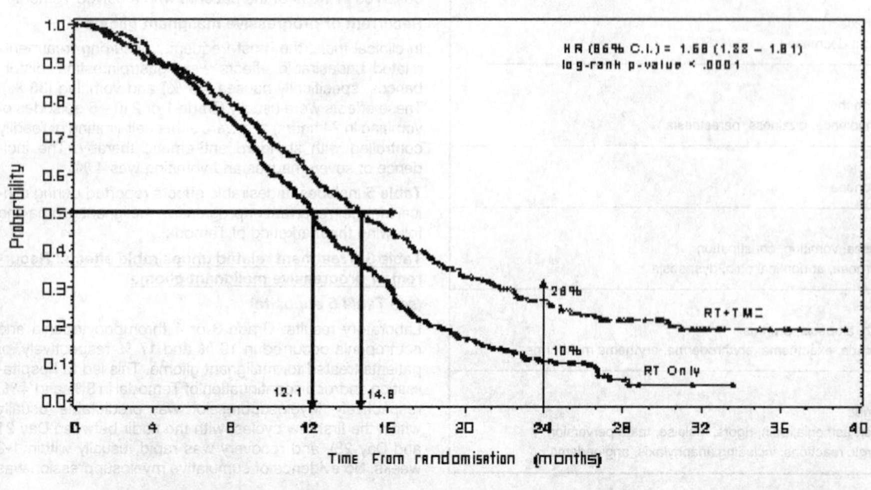

8. MARKETING AUTHORISATION NUMBER(S)

Temodal 5mg Capsules	:	EU/1/98/096/001-2
Temodal 20mg Capsules	:	EU/1/98/096/003-4
Temodal 100mg Capsules	:	EU/1/98/096/005-6
Temodal 250mg Capsules	:	EU/1/98/096/007-8

9. DATE OF FIRST AUTHORISATION/RENEWAL OF THE AUTHORISATION
Date of first authorisation: 26 January 1999

Date of last renewal: 26 January 2004

10. DATE OF REVISION OF THE TEXT
June 3, 2005

Legal Category
Prescription Only Medicine

Temodal/EU/06-05/7

Tenif

(AstraZeneca UK Limited)

1. NAME OF THE MEDICINAL PRODUCT
Tenif

2. QUALITATIVE AND QUANTITATIVE COMPOSITION
Atenolol 50 mg

Nifedipine 20 mg

For excipients, see Section 6.1

3. PHARMACEUTICAL FORM
Capsules

Reddish brown capsules containing atenolol and a slow release formulation of nifedipine.

4. CLINICAL PARTICULARS

4.1 Therapeutic indications
Management of hypertension where therapy with either a calcium channel blocker or a beta-blocking drug proves inadequate.

Management of chronic stable angina pectoris where therapy with a calcium channel blocker or a beta-adrenoceptor blocking drug proves inadequate.

4.2 Posology and method of administration
For administration by the oral route.

Adults

Hypertension: One capsule daily swallowed with water. If necessary, the dosage may be increased to 1 capsule dosed every 12 hours. Patients can be transferred to the combination from other antihypertensive treatments with the *exception of clonidine (see Section 4.4).*

Angina: One capsule every 12 hours swallowed with water. Where additional efficacy is necessary, prophylactic nitrate therapy or additional nifedipine may be of benefit.

Elderly

Dosage should not exceed 1 capsule daily in hypertension or 1 capsule twice daily in angina.

The pharmacokinetics of nifedipine are altered in the elderly so that lower maintenance doses of nifedipine may be required compared to younger patients.

Children

There is no paediatric experience with Tenif and therefore Tenif should not be used in children.

Renal Impairment

Tenif should not be used in patients with marked renal impairment (see Section 4.3)

4.3 Contraindications
Tenif should not be used in patients with any of the following conditions:

- known hypersensitivity to either active component, or any other excipient or other dihydropyridines because of the theoretical risk of cross-reactivity;

- bradycardia;

- cardiogenic shock;

- hypotension;

- metabolic acidosis;

- severe peripheral arterial circulatory disturbances;

- second or third degree heart block;

- sick sinus syndrome;

- untreated phaeochromocytoma;

- uncontrolled heart failure;

- women capable of childbearing or during pregnancy or during lactation;

- patients with clinically significant aortic stenosis;

- patients with marked renal impairment (i.e. creatinine clearance below 15 ml/min/1.73 m^2; serum creatinine greater than 600 micromol/litre);

- patients receiving calcium channel blockers with negative inotropic effects eg.

verapamil and diltiazem;

- unstable angina;

- during or within one month of a myocardial infarction.

Tenif should not be used for the treatment of acute attacks of angina.

The safety of Tenif in malignant hypertension has not been established.

Tenif should not be used for secondary prevention of myocardial infarction.

Due to the nifedipine component, Tenif should not be administered in combination with rifampicin because plasma levels of nifedipine, predictive of efficacy, may not be attained due to enzyme induction. (see Section 4.5).

4.4 Special warnings and special precautions for use
Due to its beta-blocker component, Tenif:

• although contraindicated in uncontrolled heart failure (see Section 4.3), may be substituted with care in patients already treated with a beta-blocking drug, and/or whose signs of heart failure have been controlled. Caution must be exercised in patients with conduction defects or whose cardiac reserve is poor, especially as nifedipine also has negative inotropic effects. However, in patients already treated with a beta-blocker and/or where signs of cardiac failure has been controlled, Tenif may be substituted with care if necessary

• may increase the number and duration of angina attacks in patients with Prinzmetal's angina due to unopposed alpha receptor mediated coronary artery vasoconstriction. Atenolol is a beta$_1$-selective beta-blocking drug; consequently, the use of Tenif may be considered although utmost caution must be exercised.

• although contra-indicated in severe peripheral arterial circulatory disturbances (see Section 4.3), may also aggravate less severe peripheral arterial circulatory disturbances.

• due to its negative effect on conduction time, caution must be exercised if it is given to patients with first degree heart block.

• may modify the tachycardia of hypoglycaemia.

• may mask the signs of thyrotoxicosis.

• will reduce heart rate, as a result of its pharmacological action. In the rare instances when a treated patient develops symptoms, which may be attributable to a slow heart rate, the dose may be reduced.

• should not be discontinued abruptly in patients suffering from ischaemic heart disease.

• may cause a more severe reaction to a variety of allergens, when given to patients with a history of anaphylactic reaction to such allergens. Such patients may be unresponsive to the usual doses of adrenaline used to treat the allergic reactions.

• May cause a hypersensitivity reaction including angioedema and urticaria

Obstructive airways disease:

Tenif contains the cardioselective beta-blocking drug atenolol. Although cardioselective (beta$_1$) beta-blocking drugs may have less effect on lung function than non-selective beta-blocking drugs, as with all beta-blocking drugs, these should be avoided in patients with reversible obstructive airways disease, unless there are compelling clinical reasons for their use. Where such reasons exist, Tenif may be used with caution. Occasionally, some increase in airways resistance may occur in asthmatic patients, however, and this may usually be reversed by commonly used dosage of bronchodilators such as salbutamol or isoprenaline.

The label and patient information leaflet for this product state the following warning: "If you have ever had asthma or wheezing, you should not take this medicine unless you have discussed these symptoms with the prescribing doctor".

Due to its nifedipine component it should be noted that:

• in rare cases, a transient increase in blood glucose has been observed with nifedipine in acute studies. This should be considered in patients suffering from diabetes mellitus. Nifedipine has no diabetogenic effect.

• ischaemic pain occurs in a small proportion of patients following introduction of nifedipine monotherapy. Although a "steal" effect has not been demonstrated, patients experiencing this effect should discontinue nifedipine therapy.

• in single cases of in-vitro fertilisation, calcium antagonists like nifedipine have been associated with reversible biochemical changes in the spermatozoa's head section that may result in impaired sperm function. In those men who are repeatedly unsuccessful in fathering a child by in-vitro fertilisation and where no other explanation can be found, calcium antagonists like nifedipine should be considered as possible causes.

Hypertensive or anginal patients with clinically significant liver disease have not been studied and no dosage adjustment is suggested from the systemic availability of the monocomponents in patients with cirrhosis. However nifedipine is metabolised primarily by the liver and therefore patients with liver dysfunction should be carefully monitored. As a precaution, it is recommended that the dose should not exceed one capsule daily.

4.5 Interaction with other medicinal products and other forms of Interaction
Tenif must not be used in conjunction with calcium channel blockers with negative inotropic effects. eg, verapamil, diltiazem since this can lead to an exaggeration of these effects particularly in patients with impaired ventricular function and/or sino-atrial or atrio-ventricular conduction abnormalities. This may result in severe hypotension, bradycardia and cardiac failure, (see Section 4.3).

Concomitant therapy with additional dihydropyridines eg nifedipine, may increase the risk of hypotension, and cardiac failure may occur in patients with latent cardiac insufficiency.

Atenolol monotherapy:

Digitalis glycosides, in association with beta-blocking drugs, may increase atrio-ventricular conduction time.

beta-blocking drugs may exacerbate the rebound hypertension, which can follow the withdrawal of clonidine. If the two drugs are co-administered, the beta-blocking drug should be withdrawn several days before discontinuing clonidine. If replacing clonidine by beta-blocking drug therapy, the introduction of beta-blocking drugs should be delayed for several days after clonidine administration has stopped.

Caution must be exercised when prescribing a beta-blocking drug with Class I antiarrhythmic agents such as disopyramide.

Concomitant use of sympathomimetic agents, eg adrenaline, may counteract the effect of beta-blocking drugs.

Concomitant use with insulin and oral antidiabetic drugs may lead to the intensification of the blood sugar lowering effects of these drugs.

Concomitant use of prostaglandin synthetase inhibiting drugs, eg ibuprofen or indomethacin, may decrease the hypotensive effects of beta-blocking drugs.

Caution must be exercised when using anaesthetic agents with Tenif. The anaesthetist should be informed and the choice of anaesthetic should be the agent with as little negative inotropic activity as possible. Use of beta-blocking drugs with anaesthetic drugs may result in attenuation of the reflex tachycardia and increase the risk of hypotension. Anaesthetic agents causing myocardial depression are best avoided.

Nifedipine monotherapy:

The antihypertensive effect of nifedipine can be potentiated by simultaneous administration of cimetidine.

The simultaneous administration of nifedipine and quinidine may lead to serum quinidine levels being suppressed regardless of dosage of quinidine.

The simultaneous administration of nifedipine and digoxin may lead to reduced digoxin clearance and hence an increase in the plasma digoxin level. Patients' plasma digoxin levels should be monitored and, if necessary, the digoxin dose reduced.

As with other dihydropyridines, nifedipine should not be taken with grapefruit juice because bioavailability is increased.

Due to enzyme induction, rifampicin has been shown to decrease the nifedipine AUC and C_{max} by 95% (288ng l/ml to 8ng l/ml and 154ng/ml to 7.5ng/ml respectively. This may result in reduced efficacy, therefore ***co-administration of nifedipine is contraindicated.*** (see Section 4.3).

Nifedipine may cause falsely increased spectrophotometric values of urinary vanillylmandellic acid. However, measurement with HPLC is unaffected.

4.6 Pregnancy and lactation
Tenif is contraindicated in women capable of childbearing or during pregnancy or during lactation (see Section 4.3).

4.7 Effects on ability to drive and use machines
The use of Tenif is unlikely to result in any impairment of the ability of patients to drive or operate machinery. However, it should be taken into account that occasionally dizziness or fatigue may occur.

4.8 Undesirable effects
Tenif is well tolerated. In clinical studies, the undesired events reported are usually attributed to the pharmacological actions of its components.

The following undesired events, listed by body system, have been reported:

Tenif

Cardiovascular: flushing, oedema.

CNS: dizziness, headache.

Gastrointestinal: gastrointestinal disturbance.

Haematological: purpura

Reproductive: impotence

Others: fatigue

Atenolol monotherapy

Cardiovascular: bradycardia, heart failure deterioration, postural hypotension which may be associated with syncope, cold extremities. In susceptible patients: precipitation of heart block, intermittent claudication, Raynaud's phenomenon.

CNS: confusion, dizziness, headache, mood changes, nightmares, psychoses and hallucinations, sleep disturbances of the type noted with other beta-blockers.

Gastrointestinal: dry mouth, gastrointestinal disturbances, elevations of transaminase levels have been seen infrequently, rare cases of hepatic toxicity including intrahepatic cholestasis have been reported.

Haematological: purpura, thrombocytopenia.

Integumentary: alopecia, dry eyes, psoriasiform skin reactions, exacerbation of psoriasis, skin rashes.

Neurological: paraesthesia.

Respiratory: bronchospasm may occur in patients with bronchial asthma or a history of asthmatic complaints.

Reproductive: impotence

Special senses: visual disturbances.

Others: hypersensitivity reaction, including angioedema and urticaria, an increase in ANA (antinuclear antibodies) has been observed, however the clinical relevance of this is not clear. Fatigue.

Nifedipine monotherapy

Cardiovascular: palpitations, tachycardia, gravitational oedema, marked reduction in blood pressure in dialysis patients with malignant hypertension and hypovolaemia.

Neurological: paraesthesia.

Respiratory: dyspnoea.

Gastrointestinal: gingival hyperplasia, hypersensitivity type jaundice and disturbances of liver function such as increased transaminase or intra-hepatic cholestasis which regress after discontinuing therapy.

Haematological: agranulocytosis.

Integumentary: skin reactions such as pruritus, urticaria, photosensitive dermatitis, exanthema and exfoliative dermatitis, erythromelalgia and systemic allergic reactions.

Musculoskeletal: myalgia, tremor (both after high doses).

Urogenital: increased frequency of micturition, gynaecomastia (in older men on long term therapy, which usually regresses on withdrawal of therapy).

As with other sustained release dihydropyridines, exacerbation of angina pectoris may occur rarely at the start of treatment with sustained release formulations of nifedipine. The occurrence of myocardial infarction has been described although it is not possible to distinguish such an event from the natural course of ischaemic heart disease.

Discontinuance of Tenif should be considered if, according to clinical judgement, the well-being of the patient is adversely affected by any of the above reactions.

4.9 Overdose

Symptoms

The symptoms of overdosage may include bradycardia, hypotension, acute cardiac insufficiency and bronchospasm.

Treatment

General treatment should include: close supervision, treatment in an intensive care ward, the use of gastric lavage, activated charcoal and a laxative to prevent absorption of any drug still present in the gastrointestinal tract, the use of plasma or plasma substitutes to treat hypotension and shock. The possible use of haemodialysis or haemoperfusion may be considered.

Excessive bradycardia can be countered with atropine 1 to 2 mg intravenously and/or a cardiac pacemaker. If necessary, this may be followed by a bolus dose of glucagon 10 mg intravenously. If required, this may be repeated or followed by an intravenous infusion of glucagon 1 to 10 mg/hour depending on response. Intravenous calcium gluconate combined with metaraminol may be beneficial for hypotension induced by nifedipine. If no response to glucagon occurs or if glucagon is unavailable, a beta-adrenoceptor stimulant such as dobutamine 2.5 to 10 micrograms/kg/minute by intravenous infusion may be given. Dobutamine, because of its positive inotropic effect could also be used to treat hypotension and acute cardiac insufficiency. It is likely that these doses would be inadequate to reverse the cardiac effects of beta-blockade if a large overdose has been taken. The dose of dobutamine should therefore be increased if necessary to achieve the required response according to the clinical condition of the patient. In severe cases of hypotension cardiac pacing with appropriate cardiorespiratory support may be necessary.

Bronchospasm can usually be reversed by bronchodilators.

5. PHARMACOLOGICAL PROPERTIES

5.1 Pharmacodynamic properties

CO7 FB

Beta-blocking agents, selective and other antihypertensives.

Atenolol is a beta-blocking drug which is $beta_1$ selective (i.e. acts preferentially on $beta_1$-adrenergic receptors in the heart). Selectivity decreases with increasing dose.

Atenolol is without intrinsic sympathomimetic and membrane stabilising activities and as with other beta-blocking drugs, atenolol has negative inotropic effects (and is therefore contraindicated in uncontrolled heart failure).

As with other beta-blocking drugs, its mode of action in the treatment of hypertension is unclear.

It is probably the action of atenolol in reducing cardiac rate and contractility which makes it effective in eliminating or reducing the symptoms of patients with angina.

Atenolol is effective and well-tolerated in most ethnic populations although the response may be less in black patients.

It is unlikely that any additional ancillary properties possessed by S(-) atenolol, in comparison with the racemic mixture, will give rise to different therapeutic effects.

Nifedipine is a calcium channel blocker. It is a powerful coronary and peripheral vasodilator which increases myocardial oxygen supply and reduces blood pressure (afterload) and peripheral resistance. Concomitant use of atenolol, therefore, ameliorates the reflex sympathetic response to nifedipine monotherapy by blocking the rise in heart rate, while the tendency of atenolol to increase peripheral resistance is balanced by the vasodilation and increased sympathetic tone induced by the calcium antagonist.

Consequently, greater antihypertensive or antianginal efficacy is achieved by the concomitant use of nifedipine and atenolol than either drug alone. This beneficial pharmacodynamic interaction also results in fewer side effects when lower dosages of the two drugs are used in combination.

5.2 Pharmacokinetic properties

Absorption of atenolol following oral dosing is consistent but incomplete (approximately 40 to 50%) with peak plasma concentrations occurring 2 to 4 hours after dosing. The atenolol blood levels are consistent and subject to little variability. There is no significant hepatic metabolism of atenolol and more than 90% of that absorbed reaches the systemic circulation unaltered. The plasma half-life is about 6 hours but this may rise in severe renal impairment since the kidney is the major route of elimination. Atenolol penetrates tissues poorly due to its low lipid solubility and its concentration in brain tissue is low. Plasma protein binding is low (approximately 3%). Absorption of nifedipine following oral dosing is complete with peak plasma concentrations occurring about 3 hours after dosing. Nifedipine is >90% plasma protein bound. There is significant hepatic metabolism of nifedipine. The plasma half-life is between 6 and 11 hours for the sustained formulation of nifedipine.

Co-administration of atenolol and nifedipine has little effect on the pharmacokinetics of either. In the elderly, the systemic bioavailability and elimination half-life of both components are increased.

Tenif is effective when given either once or twice daily. This simplicity of dosing facilitates compliance by its acceptability to patients.

5.3 Preclinical safety data

Atenolol and nifedipine are drugs on which extensive clinical experience has been obtained. Relevant information for the prescriber is provided elsewhere in the Prescribing Information.

6. PHARMACEUTICAL PARTICULARS

6.1 List of excipients

Gelatin

Iron Oxide Red (E172)

Lactose

Macrogol

Maize starch

Magnesium carbonate

Magnesium stearate

Methylhydroxypropylcellulose

Microcrystalline cellulose

Polysorbate

Sodium Laurilsulfate

Titanium dioxide (E171)

6.2 Incompatibilities

Not applicable

6.3 Shelf life

48 months

6.4 Special precautions for storage

Do not store above 30°C. Protect from light and moisture

Store in original package. Keep the container in the outer carton.

6.5 Nature and contents of container

PVC/PVDC/AL Blister strips of 28 capsules.

6.6 Instructions for use and handling

None

7. MARKETING AUTHORISATION HOLDER

AstraZeneca UK Limited,

600 Capability Green,

Luton, LU1 3LU, UK.

8. MARKETING AUTHORISATION NUMBER(S)

PL 17901/0047

9. DATE OF FIRST AUTHORISATION/RENEWAL OF THE AUTHORISATION

1st June 2000 / 7th December 2004

10. DATE OF REVISION OF THE TEXT

7th December 2004

Tenoret 50

(AstraZeneca UK Limited)

1. NAME OF THE MEDICINAL PRODUCT

Tenoret 50 Film-coated Tablets

2. QUALITATIVE AND QUANTITATIVE COMPOSITION

Atenolol. 50mg

Chlortalidone 12.5 mg

For excipients, see Section 6.1

3. PHARMACEUTICAL FORM

Film-coated tablets.

Brown, biconvex, film-coated tablet imprinted with the name Tenoret 50 on one face, and an 'S' logo on the reverse.

4. CLINICAL PARTICULARS

4.1 Therapeutic indications

The management of hypertension, particularly suited to older patients.

4.2 Posology and method of administration

Tenoret 50 Film-coated Tablets are administered orally.

Adults

One tablet daily.

Elderly

One tablet daily. Older patients with hypertension who do not respond to low dose therapy with a single agent should have a satisfactory response to a single tablet daily of Tenoret 50 Film-coated Tablets. Where hypertensive control is not achieved, addition of a small dose of a third agent e.g. as a vasodilator, may be appropriate.

Children

There is no paediatric experience with Tenoret 50 Film-coated Tablets, therefore this preparation is not recommended for children.

Renal Impairment

In patients with renal impairment a reduction in daily dose or in frequency of administration may be necessary. (See Section 4.4).

4.3 Contraindications

Tenoret 50 Film-coated Tablets should not be used in patients with any of the following:

- known hypersensitivity to either active component or any of the excipients;
- bradycardia;
- cardiogenic shock;
- hypotension;
- metabolic acidosis;
- severe peripheral arterial circulatory disturbances;
- second- or third-degree heart block;
- sick sinus syndrome;
- untreated phaeochromocytoma;
- uncontrolled heart failure.

Tenoret 50 Film-coated Tablets must not be given during pregnancy or lactation.

4.4 Special warnings and special precautions for use

Due to its beta-blocker component Tenoret 50 Film-coated Tablets:

- although contraindicated in uncontrolled heart failure (See Section 4.3),

may be used in patients whose signs of heart failure have been controlled. Caution must be exercised in patients whose cardiac reserve is poor.

- may increase the number and duration of angina attacks in patients with Prinzmetal's angina due to unopposed alpha receptor mediated coronary artery vasoconstriction. Atenolol is a $beta_1$-selective beta-blocker; consequently the use of Tenoret 50 Film-Coated Tablets may be considered although utmost caution must be exercised.
- although contraindicated in severe peripheral arterial circulatory disturbances (See Section 4.3), may also aggravate less severe peripheral arterial circulatory disturbances.
- due to its negative effect on conduction time, caution must be exercised if it is given to patients with first-degree heart block.
- may modify the tachycardia of hypoglycaemia.
- may mask the signs of thyrotoxicosis.
- will reduce heart rate, as a result of its pharmacological action. In the rare instances when a treated patient develops symptoms which may be attributable to a slow heart rate, the dose may be reduced.
- should not be discontinued abruptly in patients suffering from ischaemic heart disease.
- may cause a more severe reaction to a variety of allergens, when given to patients with a history of anaphylactic reactions to such allergens. Such patients may be unresponsive to the usual doses of adrenaline used to treat the allergic reactions.
- may cause a hypersensitivity reaction including angioedema and urticaria.

Tenoret 50 Film-coated Tablets contain the cardioselective beta-blocker atenolol. Although cardioselective (beta$_1$) beta-blockers may have less effect on lung function than non-selective beta-blockers, as with all beta-blockers, these should be avoided in patients with reversible obstructive airways disease, unless there are compelling clinical reasons for their use. Where such reasons exist, Tenoret 50 Film-coated Tablets may be used with caution. Occasionally, some increase in airways resistance may occur in asthmatic patients, however, and this may usually be reversed by commonly used dosage of bronchodilators such as salbutamol or isoprenaline.

The label and patient information leaflet for this product state the following warning: ''If you have ever had asthma or wheezing, you should not take this medicine unless you have discussed these symptoms with the prescribing doctor''.

Due to its chlortalidone component:

- hypokalaemia may occur. Measurement of potassium levels is appropriate, especially in the older patient, those receiving digitalis preparations for cardiac failure, those taking an abnormal (low in potassium) diet or those suffering from gastrointestinal complaints. Hypokalaemia may predispose to arrhythmias in patients receiving digitalis;
- caution must be exercised in patients with severe renal failure (See Section 4.2);
- impaired glucose tolerance may occur and caution must be exercised if chlortalidone is administered to patients with a known pre-disposition to diabetes mellitus;
- hyperuricaemia may occur. Only a minor increase in serum uric acid usually occurs but in cases of prolonged elevation, the concurrent use of a uricosuric agent will reverse the hyperuricaemia.

4.5 Interaction with other medicinal products and other forms of Interaction

Combined use of beta-blockers and calcium channel blockers with negative inotropic effects, e.g. verapamil, diltiazem, can lead to an exaggeration of these effects particularly in patients with impaired ventricular function and/or sino-atrial or atrio-ventricular conduction abnormalities. This may result in severe hypotension, bradycardia and cardiac failure. Neither the beta-blocker nor the calcium channel blocker should be administered intravenously within 48 hours of discontinuing the other.

Concomitant therapy with dihydropyridines e.g. nifedipine, may increase the risk of hypotension, and cardiac failure may occur in patients with latent cardiac insufficiency.

Digitalis glycosides, in association with beta-blockers, may increase atrio-ventricular conduction time.

Beta-blockers may exacerbate the rebound hypertension which can follow the withdrawal of clonidine. If the two drugs are co-administered, the beta-blocker should be withdrawn several days before discontinuing clonidine. If replacing clonidine by beta-blocker therapy, the introduction of -blockers should be delayed for several days after clonidine administration has stopped.

Caution must be exercised when prescribing a beta-blocker with Class 1 antiarrhythmic agents such as disopyramide.

Concomitant use of sympathomimetic agents, e.g. adrenaline, may counteract the effect of beta-blockers.

Concomitant use with insulin and oral antidiabetic drugs may lead to the intensification of the blood sugar lowering effects of these drugs.

Concomitant use of prostaglandin synthetase-inhibiting drugs e.g. ibuprofen and indomethacin, may decrease the hypotensive effects beta-blockers.

Preparations containing lithium should not be given with diuretics because they may reduce its renal clearance.

Caution must be exercised when using anaesthetic agents with Tenoret 50 Film-coated Tablets. The anaesthetist should be informed and the choice of anaesthetic should be an agent with as little negative inotropic activity as possible. Use of beta-blockers with anaesthetic drugs may result in attenuation of the reflex tachycardia and increase the risk of hypotension. Anaesthetic agents causing myocardial depression are best avoided.

4.6 Pregnancy and lactation

Pregnancy:

Tenoret 50 Film-coated Tablets must not be given during pregnancy

Lactation:

Tenoret 50 Film-coated Tablets must not be given during lactation.

4.7 Effects on ability to drive and use machines

Use is unlikely to result in any impairment of the ability of patients to drive or operate machinery. However, it should be taken into account that occasionally dizziness or fatigue may occur.

4.8 Undesirable effects

Tenoret 50 Film-Coated Tablets were well tolerated in clinical studies, the undesired events reported are usually attributable to the pharmacological actions of its components.

The following undesired events, listed by body system, have been reported with Tenoret 50 Film-coated Tablets or either of its components:

Biochemical:

Hyperuricaemia, hypokalaemia, impaired glucose tolerance (See Section 4.4), hyponatraemia related to chlortalidone.

Cardiovascular:

Bradycardia, heart failure deterioration, postural hypotension which may be associated with syncope, cold extremities. In susceptible patients: precipitation of heart block, intermittent claudication, Raynaud's phenomenon.

CNS:

Confusion, dizziness, headache, mood changes, nightmares, psychoses and hallucinations, sleep disturbances of the type noted with other beta-blockers.

Gastrointestinal:

dry mouth, gastrointestinal disturbances, nausea. Elevations of transaminase levels have been seen infrequently, rare cases of hepatic toxicity including intrahepatic cholestasis have been reported. Pancreatitis.

Haematological:

Leucopenia, purpura, thrombocytopenia.

Integumentary:

Alopecia, dry eyes, psoriasiform skin reactions, exacerbation of psoriasis, skin rashes.

Neurological:

paraesthesia.

Respiratory:

bronchospasm may occur in patients with bronchial asthma or a history of asthmatic complaints.

Reproductive:

Impotence

Special senses:

visual disturbances.

Others:

hypersensitivity reactions, including angioedema and urticaria; fatigue, an increase in ANA (Antinuclear Antibodies) has been observed, however the clinical relevance of this is not clear.

Discontinuance of Tenoret 50 Film-coated Tablets should be considered if, according to clinical judgement, the well-being of the patient is adversely affected by any of the above reactions.

4.9 Overdose

The symptoms of overdosage may include bradycardia, hypotension, acute cardiac insufficiency and bronchospasm.

General treatment should include: close supervision, treatment in an intensive care ward, the use of gastric lavage, activated charcoal and a laxative to prevent absorption of any drug still present in the gastrointestinal tract, the use of plasma or plasma substitutes to treat hypotension and shock. The possible use of haemodialysis or haemoperfusion may be considered.

Excessive bradycardia can be countered with atropine 1-2 mg intravenously and/or a cardiac pacemaker. If necessary, this may be followed by a bolus dose of glucagon 10 mg intravenously. If required, this may be repeated or followed by an intravenous infusion of glucagon 1-10 mg/hour depending on response. If no response to glucagon occurs or if glucagon is unavailable, a beta-adrenoceptor stimulant such as dobutamine 2.5 to 10 micrograms/kg/minute by intravenous infusion may be given. Dobutamine, because of its positive inotropic effect, could also be used to treat hypotension and acute cardiac insufficiency. It is likely that these doses would be inadequate to reverse the cardiac effects of beta-blocker blockade if a large overdose has been taken. The dose of dobutamine should therefore be increased if necessary to achieve the required response according to the clinical condition of the patient.

Bronchospasm can usually be reversed by bronchodilators.

Excessive diuresis should be countered by maintaining normal fluid and electrolyte balance.

5. PHARMACOLOGICAL PROPERTIES

Beta-blocking agents, selective, and other diuretics.

C07C B03

5.1 Pharmacodynamic properties

Tenoret 50 Film-coated Tablets combines the antihypertensive activity of two agents, a beta-blocker (atenolol) and a diuretic (chlortalidone).

Atenolol

Atenolol is beta$_1$-selective (i.e. acts preferentially on beta$_1$-adrenergic receptors in the heart). Selectivity decreases with increasing dose.

Atenolol is without intrinsic sympathomimetic and membrane-stabilising activities and, as with other beta-blockers, has negative inotropic effects (and is therefore contraindicated in uncontrolled heart failure).

As with other beta-blockers, the mode of action in the treatment of hypertension is unclear.

It is unlikely that any additional ancillary properties possessed by S (-) atenolol, in comparison with the racemic mixture, will give rise to different therapeutic effects.

Atenolol is effective and well-tolerated in most ethnic populations. Black patients respond better to the combination of atenolol and chlortalidone, than to atenolol alone.

The combination of atenolol with thiazide-like diuretics has been shown to be compatible and generally more effective than either drug used alone.

Chlortalidone

Chlortalidone, a monosulfonamyl diuretic, increases excretion of sodium and chloride. Natriuresis is accompanied by some loss of potassium. The mechanism by which chlortalidone reduces blood pressure is not fully known but may be related to the excretion and redistribution of body sodium.

5.2 Pharmacokinetic properties

Atenolol

Absorption of atenolol following oral dosing is consistent but incomplete (approximately 40-50%) with peak plasma concentrations occurring 2-4 hours after dosing. The atenolol blood levels are consistent and subject to little variability. There is no significant hepatic metabolism of atenolol and more than 90% of that absorbed reaches the systemic circulation unaltered. The plasma half-life is about 6 hours but this may rise in severe renal impairment since the kidney is the major route of elimination. Atenolol penetrates tissues poorly due to its low lipid solubility and its concentration in brain tissue is low. Plasma protein binding is low (approximately 3%).

Chlortalidone

Absorption of chlortalidone following oral dosing is consistent but incomplete (approximately 60%) with peak plasma concentrations occurring about 12 hours after dosing. The chlortalidone blood levels are consistent and subject to little variability. The plasma half-life is about 50 hours and the kidney is the major route of elimination. Plasma protein binding is high (approximately 75%).

Coadministration of chlortalidone and atenolol has little effect on the pharmacokinetics of either.

Tenoret 50 Film-coated Tablets is effective for at least 24 hours after a single oral daily dose. This simplicity of dosing facilitates compliance by its acceptability to patients.

5.3 Preclinical safety data

Atenolol and chlortalidone are drugs on which extensive clinical experience has been obtained. Relevant information for the prescriber is provided elsewhere in the Summary of Product Characteristics.

6. PHARMACEUTICAL PARTICULARS

6.1 List of excipients

Magnesium Carbonate

Maize Starch

Sodium laurilsulfate

Gelatin

Magnesium Stearate

Methylhydroxypropylcellulose

Macrogol 300

Iron Oxide (E172)

6.2 Incompatibilities

Not applicable.

6.3 Shelf life

36 months.

6.4 Special precautions for storage

Do not store above 25°C.

Store in the original package. Keep the container in the outer carton

6.5 Nature and contents of container

Blister packs of 28 tablets contained in a carton.

6.6 Instructions for use and handling

Not applicable.

7. MARKETING AUTHORISATION HOLDER

AstraZeneca UK Limited.,

600 Capability Green,

Luton, LU1 3LU, UK.

8. MARKETING AUTHORISATION NUMBER(S)

PL 17901/0048

9. DATE OF FIRST AUTHORISATION/RENEWAL OF THE AUTHORISATION

01 June 2000/09 February 2005

10. DATE OF REVISION OF THE TEXT

February 2005

Tenoretic

(AstraZeneca UK Limited)

1. NAME OF THE MEDICINAL PRODUCT

Tenoretic Film-coated Tablets

2. QUALITATIVE AND QUANTITATIVE COMPOSITION
Atenolol 100 mg

Chlortalidone 25 mg

For excipients, see Section 6.1

3. PHARMACEUTICAL FORM
Film-coated tablets.

Brown

4. CLINICAL PARTICULARS

4.1 Therapeutic indications
Management of hypertension.

4.2 Posology and method of administration
Tenoretic Film-coated Tablets are administered orally.

Adults

One tablet daily. Most patients with hypertension will give a satisfactory response to a single tablet daily of Tenoretic Film-coated Tablets. There is little or no further fall in blood pressure with increased dosage and, where necessary, another antihypertensive drug, such as a vasodilator, can be added.

Elderly

Dosage requirements are often lower in this age group.

Children

There is no paediatric experience with Tenoretic Film-coated Tablets, therefore this preparation is not recommended for children.

Renal Impairment

In patients with severe renal impairment, a reduction in the daily dose or in frequency of administration may be necessary. (See Section 4.4).

4.3 Contraindications
Tenoretic Film-coated Tablets should not be used in patients with any of the following:
- known hypersensitivity to either active component or any of the excipients;
- bradycardia;
- cardiogenic shock;
- hypotension;
- metabolic acidosis;
- severe peripheral arterial circulatory disturbances;
- second- or third-degree heart block;
- sick sinus syndrome;
- untreated phaeochromocytoma;
- uncontrolled heart failure.

Tenoretic Film-coated Tablets must not be given during pregnancy or lactation.

4.4 Special warnings and special precautions for use
Due to its beta-blocker component Tenoretic Film-coated Tablets:

- although contraindicated in uncontrolled heart failure (See section 4.3) may be used in patients whose signs of heart failure have been controlled. Caution must be exercised in patients whose cardiac reserve is poor.
- may increase the number and duration of angina attacks in patients with Prinzmetal's angina due to unopposed alpha receptor mediated coronary artery vasoconstriction. Atenolol is a $beta_1$-selective beta-blocker; consequently the use of Tenoretic Film-coated Tablets may be considered although utmost caution must be exercised.
- although contraindicated in severe peripheral arterial circulatory disturbances (See section 4.3) may also aggravate less severe peripheral arterial circulatory disturbances.
- due to its negative effect on conduction time, caution must be exercised if it is given to patients with first-degree heart block.
- may modify the tachycardia of hypoglycaemia.
- may mask the signs of thyrotoxicosis.
- will reduce heart rate, as a result of its pharmacological action. In the rare instances when a treated patient develops symptoms which may be attributable to a slow heart rate, the dose may be reduced.
- should not be discontinued abruptly in patients suffering from ischaemic heart disease.
- may cause a more severe reaction to a variety of allergens, when given to patients with a history of anaphylactic reaction to such allergens. Such patients may be unresponsive to the usual doses of adrenaline used to treat the allergic reactions.
- may cause a hypersensitivity reaction including angioedema and urticaria.

Tenoretic Film-coated Tablets contain the cardioselective beta-blocker atenolol. Although cardioselective ($beta_1$) beta-blockers may have less effect on lung function than non-selective beta-blockers, as with all beta-blockers, these should be avoided in patients with reversible obstructive airways disease, unless there are compelling clinical reasons for their use. Where such reasons exist, Tenoretic Film-coated Tablets may be used with caution. Occasionally, some increase in airways resistance may occur in asthmatic patients, however, and this may usually be reversed by commonly used dosage of bronchodilators such as salbutamol or isoprenaline.

The label and patient information leaflet for this product state the following warning:

"If you have ever had asthma or wheezing, you should not take this medicine unless you have discussed these symptoms with the prescribing doctor".

Due to its chlortalidone component:

- hypokalaemia may occur. Measurement of potassium levels is appropriate, especially in the older patient, those receiving digitalis preparations for cardiac failure, those taking an abnormal (low in potassium) diet or those suffering from gastrointestinal complaints. Hypokalaemia may predispose to arrhythmias in patients receiving digitalis;
- caution must be exercised in patients with severe renal failure (See Section 4.2-);
- Impaired glucose tolerance may occur and caution must be exercised if chlortalidone is administered to patients with a known pre-disposition to diabetes mellitus;
- hyperuricaemia may occur. Only a minor increase in serum uric acid usually occurs but in cases of prolonged elevation, the concurrent use of a uricosuric agent will reverse the hyperuricaemia.

4.5 Interaction with other medicinal products and other forms of Interaction
Combined use of beta-blockers and calcium channel blockers with negative inotropic effects e.g. verapamil, diltiazem, can lead to an exaggeration of these effects particularly in patients with impaired ventricular function and/or sino-atrial or atrio-ventricular conduction abnormalities. This may result in severe hypotension, bradycardia and cardiac failure. Neither the beta-blocker nor the calcium channel blocker should be administered intravenously within 48 hours of discontinuing the other.

Concomitant therapy with dihydropyridines e.g. nifedipine, may increase the risk of hypotension, and cardiac failure may occur in patients with latent cardiac insufficiency.

Digitalis glycosides, in association with beta-blockers, may increase atrio-ventricular conduction time.

Beta-blockers may exacerbate the rebound hypertension which can follow the withdrawal of clonidine. If the two drugs are co-administered, the beta-blocker should be withdrawn several days before discontinuing clonidine. If replacing clonidine by beta-blocker therapy, the introduction of beta-blockers should be delayed for several days after clonidine administration has stopped.

Caution must be exercised when prescribing a beta-blockers with Class 1 antiarrhythmic agents such as disopyramide.

Concomitant use of sympathomimetic agents, e.g. adrenaline, may counteract the effect of beta-blockers.

Concomitant use with insulin and oral antidiabetic drugs may lead to the intensification of the blood sugar lowering effects of these drugs.

Concomitant use of prostaglandin synthetase inhibiting drugs (e.g. ibuprofen, indomethacin) may decrease the hypotensive effects of beta-blockers

Preparations containing lithium should not be given with diuretics because they may reduce its renal clearance.

Caution must be exercised when using anaesthetic agents with TenoreticFilm-coated Tablets. The anaesthetist should be informed and the choice of anaesthetic should be an agent with as little negative inotropic activity as possible. Use of beta-blockers with anaesthetic drugs may result in attenuation of the reflex tachycardia and increase the risk of hypotension. Anaesthetic agents causing myocardial depression are best avoided.

4.6 Pregnancy and lactation
Pregnancy:

Tenoretic Film-coated Tablets must not be given during pregnancy.

Lactation:

Tenoretic Film-coated Tablets must not be given during lactation.

4.7 Effects on ability to drive and use machines
Use is unlikely to result in any impairment of the ability of patients to drive or operate machinery. However, it should be taken into account that occasionally dizziness or fatigue may occur.

4.8 Undesirable effects
Tenoretic Film-coated Tablets are well tolerated. In clinical studies, the undesired events reported are usually attributable to the pharmacological actions of its components.

The following undesired events, listed by body system, have been reported with Tenoretic Film-coated Tablets or either of its components:

Biochemical:

hyperuricaemia, hypokalaemia, impaired glucose tolerance (See Section 4.4), hyponatraemia related to chlortalidone.

Cardiovascular:

Bradycardia, heart failure deterioration, postural hypotension which may be associated with syncope, cold extremities. In susceptible patients: precipitation of heart block, intermittent claudication, Raynaud's phenomenon.

CNS:

Confusion, dizziness, headache, mood changes, nightmares, psychoses and hallucinations, sleep disturbances of the type noted with beta-blockers

Gastrointestinal:

dry mouth, gastrointestinal disturbances, nausea. Elevations of transaminase levels have been seen infrequently, rare cases of hepatic toxicity including intrahepatic cholestasis have been reported. Pancreatitis.

Haematological:

Leucopenia, purpura, thrombocytopenia.

Integumentary:

Alopecia, dry eyes, psoriasiform skin reactions, exacerbation of psoriasis, skin rashes.

Neurological:

paraesthesia.

Respiratory:

bronchospasm may occur in patients with bronchial asthma or a history of asthmatic complaints.

Reproductive:

impotence

Special senses:

visual disturbances.

Others:

hypersensitivity reactions, including angioedema and urticaria; fatigue, an increase in ANA (Antinuclear Antibodies) has been observed, however the clinical relevance of this is not clear.

Discontinuance of Tenoretic Film-coated Tablets should be considered if, according to clinical judgement, the well-being of the patient is adversely affected by any of the above reactions.

4.9 Overdose
The symptoms of overdosage may include bradycardia, hypotension, acute cardiac insufficiency and bronchospasm.

General treatment should include: close supervision, treatment in an intensive care ward, the use of gastric lavage, activated charcoal and a laxative to prevent absorption of any drug still present in the gastrointestinal tract, the use of plasma or plasma substitutes to treat hypotension and shock. The possible use of haemodialysis or haemoperfusion may be considered.

Excessive bradycardia may be countered with atropine 1-2 mg intravenously and/or a cardiac pacemaker. If necessary, this may be followed by a bolus dose of glucagon 10 mg intravenously. If required, this may be repeated or followed by an intravenous infusion of glucagon 1-10 mg/hour depending on response. If no response to glucagon occurs or if glucagon is unavailable, a beta-adrenoceptor stimulant such as dobutamine 2.5 to 10 micrograms/kg/minute by intravenous infusion may be given. Dobutamine, because of its positive inotropic effects could be used to treat hypotension and acute cardiac insufficiency. It is likely that these doses would be inadequate to reverse the cardiac effects of beta-blocker blockade if a large overdose has been taken. The dose of dobutamine should therefore be increased if necessary to achieve the required response according to the clinical condition of the patient.

Bronchospasm can usually be reversed by bronchodilators.

Excessive diuresis should be countered by maintaining normal fluid and electrolyte balance.

5. PHARMACOLOGICAL PROPERTIES
Beta-blocking agents, selective, and other diuretics.

C07C B03

5.1 Pharmacodynamic properties
Tenoretic Film-coated Tablets combines the antihypertensive activity of two agents, a beta-blocker (atenolol) and a diuretic (chlortalidone).

Atenolol

Atenolol is $beta_1$-selective (i.e. acts preferentially on $beta_1$-adrenergic receptors in the heart). Selectivity decreases with increasing dose.

Atenolol is without intrinsic sympathomimetic and membrane-stabilising activities and, as with other beta-adrenoceptor blocking drugs, has negative inotropic effects (and is therefore contraindicated in uncontrolled heart failure).

As with other beta-blockers, the mode of action in the treatment of hypertension is unclear.

It is unlikely that any additional ancillary properties possessed by S (-) atenolol, in comparison with the racemic mixture, will give rise to different therapeutic effects.

Atenolol is effective and well-tolerated in most ethnic populations. Black patients respond better to the combination of atenolol and chlortalidone, than to atenolol alone.

The combination of atenolol with thiazide-like diuretics has been shown to be compatible and generally more effective than either drug used alone.

Chlortalidone

Chlortalidone, a monosulfonamyl diuretic, increases excretion of sodium and chloride. Natriuresis is accompanied by some loss of potassium. The mechanism by which chlortalidone reduces blood pressure is not fully known but may be related to the excretion and redistribution of body sodium.

5.2 Pharmacokinetic properties

Atenolol

Absorption of atenolol following oral dosing is consistent but incomplete (approximately 40-50%) with peak plasma concentrations occurring 2-4 hours after dosing. The atenolol blood levels are consistent and subject to little variability. There is no significant hepatic metabolism of atenolol and more than 90% of that absorbed reaches the systemic circulation unaltered. The plasma half-life is about 6 hours but this may rise in severe renal impairment since the kidney is the major route of elimination. Atenolol penetrates tissues poorly due to its low lipid solubility and its concentration in brain tissue is low. Plasma protein binding is low (approximately 3%).

Chlortalidone

Absorption of chlortalidone following oral dosing is consistent but incomplete (approximately 60%) with peak plasma concentrations occurring about 12 hours after dosing. The chlortalidone blood levels are consistent and subject to little variability. The plasma half-life is about 50 hours and the kidney is the major route of elimination. Plasma protein binding is high (approximately 75%).

Coadministration of chlortalidone and atenolol has little effect on the pharmacokinetics of either.

Tenoretic Film-coated Tablets is effective for at least 24 hours after a single oral daily dose. This simplicity of dosing facilitates compliance by its acceptability to patients.

5.3 Preclinical safety data

Atenolol and chlortalidone are drugs on which extensive clinical experience has been obtained. Relevant information for the prescriber is provided elsewhere in the Summary of Product Characteristics.

6. PHARMACEUTICAL PARTICULARS

6.1 List of excipients

Heavy Magnesium Carbonate

Maize Starch.

Sodium laurilsulfate

Gelatin

Magnesium Stearate

Methylhydroxypropylcellulose.

Macrogol 300 BP

Iron Oxide yellow (E172)

Iron Oxide red (E172)

Magnesium Carbonate.

6.2 Incompatibilities

Not applicable.

6.3 Shelf life

4 years.

6.4 Special precautions for storage

Do not store above 25°C.

Store in the original package. Keep the container in the outer carton

6.5 Nature and contents of container

Blister packs of 28 tablets contained in a carton.

6.6 Instructions for use and handling

Not applicable.

7. MARKETING AUTHORISATION HOLDER

AstraZeneca UK Limited
600 Capability Green,
Luton, LU1 3LU, UK.

8. MARKETING AUTHORISATION NUMBER(S)

17901/0049

9. DATE OF FIRST AUTHORISATION/RENEWAL OF THE AUTHORISATION

01.06.00/09.02.05

10. DATE OF REVISION OF THE TEXT

9th February 2005

Tenormin 100mg Tablets

(AstraZeneca UK Limited)

1. NAME OF THE MEDICINAL PRODUCT

'Tenormin' 100mg Tablets

2. QUALITATIVE AND QUANTITATIVE COMPOSITION

Atenolol. 100 mg.

For excipients, see Section 6.1

3. PHARMACEUTICAL FORM

Film coated tablet

orange, film coated tablets

4. CLINICAL PARTICULARS

4.1 Therapeutic indications

i. Management of hypertension

ii. Management of angina pectoris

iii. Management of cardiac arrhythmias

iv. Management of myocardial infarction. Early intervention in the acute phase.

4.2 Posology and method of administration

Oral Administration.

The dose must always be adjusted to individual requirements of the patients, with the lowest possible starting dosage. The following are guidelines.

Adults

Hypertension

One tablet daily. Most patients respond to 100 mg daily given orally as a single dose. Some patients, however, will respond to 50 mg given as a single daily dose. The effect will be fully established after one to two weeks. A further reduction in blood pressure may be achieved by combining Tenormin with other antihypertensive agents. For example co-administration of Tenormin with a diuretic, as in Tenoretic, provides a highly effective and convenient antihypertensive therapy.

Angina

Most patients with angina pectoris will respond to 100 mg given orally once daily or 50 mg given twice daily. It is unlikely that additional benefit will be gained by increasing the dose.

Cardiac Arrhythmias

A suitable initial dose of Tenormin is 2.5 mg (5 ml) injected intravenously over a 2.5 minute period (i.e. 1 mg/minute). (See also prescribing information for Tenormin Injection). This may be repeated at 5 minute intervals, until a response is observed up to a maximum dosage of 10 mg. If Tenormin is given by infusion, 0.15 mg/kg bodyweight may be administered over a 20 minute period. If required, the injection or infusion may be repeated every 12 hours. Having controlled the arrhythmias with intravenous Tenormin, a suitable oral maintenance dosage is 50-100 mg daily, given as a single dose.

Myocardial Infarction

For patients suitable for treatment with intravenous beta-blockade and presenting within 12 hours of the onset of chest pain, Tenormin 5-10 mg should be given by slow intravenous injection (1 mg/minute) followed by Tenormin 50 mg orally about 15 minutes later, provided no untoward effects have occurred from the intravenous dose. This should be followed by a further 50 mg orally 12 hours after the intravenous dose and then 12 hours later by 100 mg orally, once daily. If bradycardia and/or hypotension requiring treatment, or any other untoward effects occur, Tenormin should be discontinued.

Elderly

Dosage requirements may be reduced especially in patients with impaired renal function.

Children

There is no paediatric experience with Tenormin and for this reason it is not recommended for use in children.

Renal Failure

Since Tenormin is excreted via the kidneys, the dosage should be adjusted in cases of severe impairment of renal function.

No significant accumulation of Tenormin occurs in patients who have a creatinine clearance greater than 35 ml/min/1.73 m^2 (normal range is 100-150 ml/min/1.73m^2).

For patients with a creatinine clearance of 15-35 ml/min/1.73m^2 (equivalent to serum creatinine of 300-600 micromol/litre) the oral dose should be 50 mg daily and the intravenous dose should be 10 mg once every two days.

For patients with a creatinine clearance of <15 ml/min/1.73m^2 (equivalent to serum creatinine of >600 micromol/litre) the oral dose should be 25 mg daily or 50 mg on alternate days and the intravenous dose should be 10 mg once every four days.

Patients on haemodialysis should be given 50 mg orally after each dialysis; this should be done under hospital supervision as marked falls in blood pressure can occur.

4.3 Contraindications

Tenormin, as with other beta-blockers, should not be used in patients with any of the following:

cardiogenic shock;

uncontrolled heart failure;

sick sinus syndrome;

second or third degree heart block;

untreated phaeochromocytoma;

metabolic acidosis;

bradycardia ($<$45bpm);

hypotension;

known hypersensitivity to the active substance, or any of the excipients;

severe peripheral arterial circulatory disturbances.

4.4 Special warnings and special precautions for use

Tenormin as with other beta-blockers:

• should not be withdrawn abruptly. The dosage should be withdrawn gradually over a period of 7-14 days, to facilitate a reduction in beta-blocker dosage. Patients should be followed during withdrawal, especially those with ischaemic heart disease.

• when a patient is scheduled for surgery, and a decision is made to discontinue beta-blocker therapy, this should be done at least 24 hours prior to the procedure. The risk-benefit assessment of stopping beta-blockade should be made for each patient. If treatment is continued, an anaesthetic with little negative inotropic activity should be selected to minimise the risk of myocardial depression. The patient may be protected against vagal reactions by intravenous administration of atropine.

• although contraindicated in uncontrolled heart failure (see Section 4.3), may be used in patients whose signs of heart failure have been controlled. Caution must be exercised in patients whose cardiac reserve is poor.

• may increase the number and duration of angina attacks in patients with Prinzmetal's angina due to unopposed alpha-receptor mediated coronary artery vasoconstriction. Tenormin is a $beta_1$ -selective beta-blocker; consequently, its use may be considered although utmost caution must be exercised.

• although contraindicated in severe peripheral arterial circulatory disturbances (see Section 4.3), may also aggravate less severe peripheral arterial circulatory disturbances.

• due to its negative effect on conduction time, caution must be exercised if it is given to patients with first degree heart block.

• may mask the symptoms of hypoglycaemia, in particular, tachycardia.

• may mask the signs of thyrotoxicosis

• will reduce heart rate, as a result of its pharmacological action. In the rare instances when a treated patient develops symptoms which may be attributable to a slow heart rate and the pulse rate drops to less than 50-55bpm at rest, the dose should be reduced.

• may cause a more severe reaction to a variety of allergens, when given to patients with a history of anaphylactic reaction to such allergens. Such patients may be unresponsive to the usual doses of adrenaline used to treat the allergic reactions.

• may cause a hypersensitivity reaction including angioedema and urticaria

• should be used with caution in the elderly, starting with a lesser dose (See Section 4.2).

Since Tenormin is excreted via the kidneys, dosage should be reduced in patients with a creatinine clearance of below 35ml/min/1.7m^2.

Although cardioselective ($beta_1$) beta-blockers may have less effect on lung function than non-selective beta-blockers, as with all, beta-blockers, these should be avoided in patients with reversible obstructive airways disease, unless there are compelling clinical reasons for their use. Where such reasons exist, Tenormin may be used with caution. Occasionally, some increase in airways resistance may occur in asthmatic patients, however, and this may usually be reversed by commonly used dosage of bronchodilators such as salbutamol or isoprenaline. The label and patient information leaflet for this product state the following warning: "If you have ever had asthma or wheezing, you should not take this medicine unless you have discussed these symptoms with the prescribing doctor".

As with other beta-blockers, in patients with a phaeochromocytoma, an alpha-blocker should be given concomitantly.

4.5 Interaction with other medicinal products and other forms of Interaction

Combined use of beta-blockers and calcium channel blockers with negative inotropic effects e.g. verapamil and diltiazem can lead to an exaggeration of these effects particularly in patients with impaired ventricular function and/or sino-atrial or atrio-ventricular conduction abnormalities. This may result in severe hypotension, bradycardia and cardiac failure. Neither the beta-blocker nor the calcium channel blocker should be administered intravenously within 48 hours of discontinuing the other.

Concomitant therapy with dihydropyridines e.g. nifedipine, may increase the risk of hypotension, and cardiac failure may occur in patients with latent cardiac insufficiency.

Digitalis glycosides, in association with beta-blockers, may increase atrio-ventricular conduction time.

Beta-blockers may exacerbate the rebound hypertension which can follow the withdrawal of clonidine. If the two drugs are co-administered, the beta-blocker should be withdrawn several days before discontinuing clonidine. If replacing clonidine by beta-blocker therapy, the introduction of beta-blockers should be delayed for several days after clonidine administration has stopped. (See also prescribing information for clonidine).

Caution must be exercised when prescribing a beta-blocker with Class I antiarrhythmic agents such as disopyramide and quinidine.

Concomitant use of sympathomimetic agents, e.g. adrenaline, may counteract the effect of beta-blockers.

Concomitant use with insulin and oral antidiabetic drugs may lead to the intensification of the blood sugar lowering effects of these drugs. Symptoms of hypoglycaemia, particularly tachycardia, may be masked (See Section 4.4).

Concomitant use of prostaglandin synthetase inhibiting drugs (e.g. ibuprofen and indomethacin), may decrease the hypotensive effects of beta-blockers.

Caution must be exercised when using anaesthetic agents with Tenormin. The anaesthetist should be informed and the choice of anaesthetic should be an agent with as little negative inotropic activity as possible. Use of beta-blockers with anaesthetic drugs may result in attenuation of the reflex tachycardia and increase the risk of hypotension. Anaesthetic agents causing myocardial depression are best avoided.

4.6 Pregnancy and lactation

Tenormin crosses the placental barrier and appears in the cord blood. No studies have been performed on the use of Tenormin in the first trimester and the possibility of foetal injury cannot be excluded. Tenormin has been used under close supervision for the treatment of hypertension in the third trimester. Administration of Tenormin to pregnant women in the management of mild to moderate hypertension has been associated with intra-uterine growth retardation.

The use of Tenormin in women who are, or may become, pregnant requires that the anticipated benefit be weighed against the possible risks, particularly in the first and second trimesters, since beta-blockers, in general, have been associated with a decrease in placental perfusion which may result in intra-uterine deaths, immature and premature deliveries.

There is significant accumulation of Tenormin in breast milk.

Neonates born to mothers who are receiving Tenormin at parturition or breast-feeding may be at risk of hypoglycaemia and bradycardia.

Caution should be exercised when Tenormin is administered during pregnancy or to a woman who is breast-feeding.

4.7 Effects on ability to drive and use machines

Use is unlikely to result in any impairment of the ability of patients to drive or operate machinery. However it should be taken into account that occasionally dizziness or fatigue may occur.

4.8 Undesirable effects

Tenormin is well tolerated. In clinical studies, the undesired events reported are usually attributable to the pharmacological actions of atenolol.

The following undesired events, listed by body system, have been reported.

Cardiovascular: bradycardia; heart failure deterioration; postural hypotension which may be associated with syncope; cold extremities. In susceptible patients: precipitation of heart block; intermittent claudication; Raynaud's phenomenon.

CNS: confusion; dizziness; headache; mood changes; nightmares; psychoses and hallucinations; sleep disturbances of the type noted with other beta-blockers.

Gastrointestinal: dry mouth; gastrointestinal disturbances. Elevations of transaminase levels have been seen infrequently, rare cases of hepatic toxicity, including intrahepatic cholestasis have been reported.

Haematological: purpura; thrombocytopenia.

Integumentary: alopecia; dry eyes; psoriasiform skin reactions; exacerbation of psoriasis; skin rashes.

Neurological: paraesthesia.

Reproductive: impotence

Respiratory: bronchospasm may occur in patients with bronchial asthma or a history of asthmatic complaints.

Special senses: visual disturbances.

Others: hypersensitivity reactions, including angioedema and urticaria; fatigue; an increase in ANA (Antinuclear Antibodies) has been observed, however, the clinical relevance of this is not clear.

Discontinuance of the drug should be considered if, according to clinical judgement, the well-being of the patient is adversely affected by any of the above reactions.

4.9 Overdose

The symptoms of overdosage may include bradycardia, hypotension, acute cardiac insufficiency and bronchospasm.

General treatment should include: close supervision, treatment in an intensive care ward, the use of gastric lavage, activated charcoal and a laxative to prevent absorption of any drug still present in the gastrointestinal tract, the use of plasma or plasma substitutes to treat hypotension and shock. The use of haemodialysis or haemoperfusion may be considered.

Excessive bradycardia can be countered with atropine 1-2 mg intravenously and/or a cardiac pacemaker. If necessary, this may be followed by a bolus dose of glucagon 10 mg intravenously. If required, this may be repeated or followed by an intravenous infusion of glucagon 1-10 mg/hour depending on response. If no response to glucagon occurs or if glucagon is unavailable, a beta-adrenoceptor stimulant such as dobutamine 2.5 to 10 micrograms/kg/minute by intravenous infusion may be given. Dobutamine, because of its positive inotropic effect could also be used to treat hypotension and acute cardiac insufficiency. It is likely that these doses would be inadequate to reverse the cardiac effects of beta-blocker blockade if a large overdose has been taken. The dose of dobutamine should therefore be increased if necessary to achieve the required response according to the clinical condition of the patient.

Bronchospasm can usually be reversed by bronchodilators.

5. PHARMACOLOGICAL PROPERTIES

5.1 Pharmacodynamic properties

Beta Blocking Agents, Plain, Selective

CO7A B03

Atenolol is a beta-blocker which is $beta_1$-selective, (i.e. acts preferentially on $beta_1$-adrenergic receptors in the heart). Selectivity decreases with increasing dose.

Atenolol is without intrinsic sympathomimetic and membrane stabilising activities and as with other beta-blockers, has negative inotropic effects (and is therefore contraindicated in uncontrolled heart failure).

As with other beta-blockers, the mode of action of atenolol in the treatment of hypertension is unclear.

It is probably the action of atenolol in reducing cardiac rate and contractility which makes it effective in eliminating or reducing the symptoms of patients with angina.

It is unlikely that any additional ancillary properties possessed by S (-) atenolol, in comparison with the racemic mixture, will give rise to different therapeutic effects.

Tenormin is effective and well-tolerated in most ethnic populations although the response may be less in black patients.

Tenormin is effective for at least 24 hours after a single oral dose. The drug facilitates compliance by its acceptability to patients and simplicity of dosing. The narrow dose range and early patient response ensure that the effect of the drug in individual patients is quickly demonstrated. Tenormin is compatible with diuretics, other hypotensive agents and antianginals (see Section 4.5). Since it acts preferentially on beta-receptors in the heart, Tenormin may, with care, be used successfully in the treatment of patients with respiratory disease, who cannot tolerate non-selective beta-blockers.

Early intervention with Tenormin in acute myocardial infarction reduces infarct size and decreases morbidity and mortality. Fewer patients with a threatened infarction progress to frank infarction; the incidence of ventricular arrhythmias is decreased and marked pain relief may result in reduced need of opiate analgesics. Early mortality is decreased. Tenormin is an additional treatment to standard coronary care.

5.2 Pharmacokinetic properties

Absorption of atenolol following oral dosing is consistent but incomplete (approximately 40-50%) with peak plasma concentrations occurring 2-4 hours after dosing. The atenolol blood levels are consistent and subject to little variability. There is no significant hepatic metabolism of atenolol and more than 90% of that absorbed reaches the systemic circulation unaltered. The plasma half-life is about 6 hours but this may rise in severe renal impairment since the kidney is the major route of elimination. Atenolol penetrates tissues poorly due to its low lipid solubility and its concentration in brain tissue is low. Plasma protein binding is low (approximately 3%).

5.3 Preclinical safety data

Atenolol is a drug on which extensive clinical experience has been obtained. Relevant information for the prescriber is provided elsewhere in the Prescribing Information.

6. PHARMACEUTICAL PARTICULARS

6.1 List of excipients

Gelatin

Magnesium Carbonate

Macrogol

Magnesium Stearate

Maize Starch.

Methylhydroxypropylcellulose.

Sodium Laurilsulfate.

Sunset yellow lake (E110)

Talc.

Titanium Dioxide (E171)

6.2 Incompatibilities

Not applicable.

6.3 Shelf life

60 months

6.4 Special precautions for storage

Do not store above 25°C

Store in the original package. Keep the container in the outer carton.

6.5 Nature and contents of container

Aluminium PVC/PVDC Blister strips of 14 tablets in cartons: 28 Tablets

Aluminium PVC/PVDC blister strips of 7 tablets: 504 Tablets (for Hospital Use)

(pack is subdivided into 6 cartons each containing 12 blister strips i.e. 84 tablets)

6.6 Instructions for use and handling

Not applicable.

7. MARKETING AUTHORISATION HOLDER

AstraZeneca UK Limited,

600 Capability Green,

Luton, LU1 3LU, UK.

8. MARKETING AUTHORISATION NUMBER(S)

PL 17901/0054

9. DATE OF FIRST AUTHORISATION/RENEWAL OF THE AUTHORISATION

01st June 2000 / 5th November 2003

10. DATE OF REVISION OF THE TEXT

5th November 2003

Tenormin 25mg Tablets

(AstraZeneca UK Limited)

1. NAME OF THE MEDICINAL PRODUCT

'Tenormin' 25mg Tablets

2. QUALITATIVE AND QUANTITATIVE COMPOSITION

Atenolol. 25 mg

For excipients, see Section 6.1

3. PHARMACEUTICAL FORM

Film coated tablet

White film coated tablets

4. CLINICAL PARTICULARS

4.1 Therapeutic indications

i. Management of hypertension

ii. Management of angina pectoris

iii. Management of cardiac arrhythmias

iv. Management of myocardial infarction. Early intervention in the acute phase.

4.2 Posology and method of administration

Oral administration

The dose must always be adjusted to individual requirements of the patients, with the lowest possible starting dosage. The following are guidelines.

Adults

Hypertension

One tablet daily. Most patients respond to 100 mg daily given orally as a single dose. Some patients, however, will respond to 50 mg given as a single daily dose. The effect will be fully established after one to two weeks. A further reduction in blood pressure may be achieved by combining Tenormin with other antihypertensive agents. For example, co-administration of Tenormin with a diuretic, as in Tenoretic provides a highly effective and convenient antihypertensive therapy.

Angina

Most patients with angina pectoris will respond to 100 mg given orally once daily or 50 mg given twice daily. It is unlikely that additional benefit will be gained by increasing the dose.

Cardiac Arrhythmias

A suitable initial dose of Tenormin is 2.5 mg (5 ml) injected intravenously over a 2.5 minute period (i.e. 1 mg/minute). (See also prescribing information for Tenormin Injection). This may be repeated at 5 minute intervals until a response is observed up to a maximum dosage of 10 mg. If Tenormin is given by infusion, 0.15 mg/kg bodyweight may be administered over a 20 minute period. If required, the injection or infusion may be repeated every 12 hours. Having controlled the arrhythmias with intravenous Tenormin, a suitable oral maintenance dosage is 50-100 mg daily, given as a single dose.

Myocardial Infarction

For patients suitable for treatment with intravenous beta-blockade and presenting within 12 hours of the onset of chest pain, Tenormin 5-10 mg should be given by slow intravenous injection (1 mg/minute) followed by Tenormin 50 mg orally about 15 minutes later, provided no untoward effects have occurred from the intravenous dose. This should be followed by a further 50 mg orally 12 hours after the intravenous dose and then 12 hours later by 100 mg orally, once daily. If bradycardia and/or hypotension requiring treatment, or any other untoward effects occur, Tenormin should be discontinued.

Elderly

Dosage requirements may be reduced, especially in patients with impaired renal function.

Children

There is no paediatric experience with Tenormin and for this reason it is not recommended for use in children.

Renal Failure

Since Tenormin is excreted via the kidneys the dosage should be adjusted in cases of severe impairment of renal function.

No significant accumulation of Tenormin occurs in patients who have a creatinine clearance greater than 35 ml/min/1.73 m^2 (normal range is 100-150 ml/min/1.73m^2).

For patients with a creatinine clearance of 15-35 ml/min/1.73m^2 (equivalent to serum creatinine of 300-600 micromol/litre) the oral dose should be 50 mg daily and the intravenous dose should be 10 mg once every two days.

For patients with a creatinine clearance of <15 ml/min/1.73m^2 (equivalent to serum creatinine of >600 micromol/litre) the oral dose should be 25 mg daily or 50 mg on alternate days and the intravenous dose should be 10 mg once every four days.

Patients on haemodialysis should be given 50 mg orally after each dialysis; this should be done under hospital supervision as marked falls in blood pressure can occur.

4.3 Contraindications

Tenormin, as with other beta-blockers, should not be used in patients with any of the following:

cardiogenic shock;

uncontrolled heart failure;

sick sinus syndrome;

second or third degree heart block;

untreated phaeochromocytoma;

metabolic acidosis;

bradycardia (<45bpm);

hypotension;

known hypersensitivity to the active substance, or any of the excipients;

severe peripheral arterial circulatory disturbances.

4.4 Special warnings and special precautions for use

Tenormin as with other beta-blockers:

• should not be withdrawn abruptly. The dosage should be withdrawn gradually over a period of 7-14 days, to facilitate a reduction in beta-blocker dosage. Patients should be followed during withdrawal, especially those with ischaemic heart disease.

• when a patient is scheduled for surgery, and a decision is made to discontinue beta-blocker therapy, this should be done at least 24 hours prior to the procedure. The risk-benefit assessment of stopping beta-blockade should be made for each patient. If treatment is continued, an anaesthetic with little negative inotropic activity should be selected to minimise the risk of myocardial depression. The patient may be protected against vagal reactions by intravenous administration of atropine.

• although contraindicated in uncontrolled heart failure (see Section 4.3), may be used in patients whose signs of heart failure have been controlled. Caution must be exercised in patients whose cardiac reserve is poor.

• may increase the number and duration of angina attacks in patients with Prinzmetal's angina due to unopposed alpha-receptor mediated coronary artery vasoconstriction. Tenormin is a beta$_1$ -selective beta-blocker; consequently, its use may be considered although utmost caution must be exercised.

• although contraindicated in severe peripheral arterial circulatory disturbances (see Section 4.3), may also aggravate less severe peripheral arterial circulatory disturbances.

• due to its negative effect on conduction time, caution must be exercised if it is given to patients with first degree heart block.

• may mask the symptoms of hypoglycaemia, in particular, tachycardia.

• may mask the signs of thyrotoxicosis.

• will reduce heart rate, as a result of its pharmacological action. In the rare instances when a treated patient develops symptoms which may be attributable to a slow heart rate and the pulse rate drops to less than 50-55bpm at rest, the dose should be reduced.

• may cause a more severe reaction to a variety of allergens, when given to patients with a history of anaphylactic reaction to such allergens. Such patients may be unresponsive to the usual doses of adrenaline used to treat the allergic reactions.

• may cause a hypersensitivity reaction including angioedema and urticaria

• should be used with caution in the elderly, starting with a lesser dose (See Section 4.2).

Since Tenormin is excreted via the kidneys, dosage should be reduced in patients with a creatinine clearance of below 35ml/min/1.7m^2.

Although cardioselective (beta$_1$) beta-blockers may have less effect on lung function than non-selective beta-blockers, as with all, beta-blockers, these should be avoided in patients with reversible obstructive airways disease, unless there are compelling clinical reasons for their use. Where such reasons exist, Tenormin may be used with caution. Occasionally, some increase in airways resistance may occur in asthmatic patients, however, and this may usually be reversed by commonly used dosage of bronchodilators such as salbutamol or isoprenaline. The label and patient information leaflet for this product state the following warning: "If you have ever had asthma or wheezing, you should not take this medicine unless you have discussed these symptoms with the prescribing doctor".

As with other beta-blockers, in patients with a phaeochromocytoma, an alpha-blocker should be given concomitantly.

4.5 Interaction with other medicinal products and other forms of Interaction

Combined use of beta-blockers and calcium channel blockers with negative inotropic effects e.g. verapamil and diltiazem can lead to an exaggeration of these effects particularly in patients with impaired ventricular function and/or sino-atrial or atrio-ventricular conduction abnormalities. This may result in severe hypotension, bradycardia and cardiac failure. Neither the beta-blocker nor the calcium channel blocker should be administered intravenously within 48 hours of discontinuing the other.

Concomitant therapy with dihydropyridines e.g. nifedipine, may increase the risk of hypotension, and cardiac failure may occur in patients with latent cardiac insufficiency.

Digitalis glycosides, in association with beta-blockers, may increase atrio-ventricular conduction time.

Beta-blockers may exacerbate the rebound hypertension which can follow the withdrawal of clonidine. If the two drugs are co-administered, the beta-blocker should be withdrawn several days before discontinuing clonidine. If replacing clonidine by beta-blocker therapy, the introduction of beta-blockers should be delayed for several days after clonidine administration has stopped. (See also prescribing information for clonidine).

Caution must be exercised when prescribing a beta-blocker with Class I antiarrhythmic agents such as disopyramide and quinidine.

Concomitant use of sympathomimetic agents, e.g. adrenaline, may counteract the effect of beta-blockers.

Concomitant use with insulin and oral antidiabetic drugs may lead to the intensification of the blood sugar lowering effects of these drugs. Symptoms of hypoglycaemia, particularly tachycardia, may be masked (See Section 4.4).

Concomitant use of prostaglandin synthetase inhibiting drugs (e.g. ibuprofen and indomethacin), may decrease the hypotensive effects of beta-blockers.

Caution must be exercised when using anaesthetic agents with Tenormin. The anaesthetist should be informed and the choice of anaesthetic should be an agent with as little negative inotropic activity as possible. Use of beta-blockers with anaesthetic drugs may result in attenuation of the reflex tachycardia and increase the risk of hypotension. Anaesthetic agents causing myocardial depression are best avoided.

4.6 Pregnancy and lactation

Tenormin crosses the placental barrier and appears in the cord blood. No studies have been performed on the use of Tenormin in the first trimester and the possibility of foetal injury cannot be excluded. Tenormin has been used under close supervision for the treatment of hypertension in the third trimester. Administration of Tenormin to pregnant women in the management of mild to moderate hypertension has been associated with intra-uterine growth retardation.

The use of Tenormin in women who are, or may become, pregnant requires that the anticipated benefit be weighed against the possible risks, particularly in the first and second trimesters, since beta-blockers, in general, have been associated with a decrease in placental perfusion which may result in intra-uterine deaths, immature and premature deliveries.

There is significant accumulation of Tenormin in breast milk.

Neonates born to mothers who are receiving Tenormin at parturition or breast-feeding may be at risk of hypoglycaemia and bradycardia.

Caution should be exercised when Tenormin is administered during pregnancy or to a woman who is breast-feeding.

4.7 Effects on ability to drive and use machines

Use is unlikely to result in any impairment of the ability of patients to drive or operate machinery. However, it should be taken into account that occasionally dizziness or fatigue may occur.

4.8 Undesirable effects

Tenormin is well tolerated. In clinical studies, the undesired events reported are usually attributable to the pharmacological actions of atenolol.

The following undesired events, listed by body system, have been reported.

Cardiovascular: bradycardia; heart failure deterioration; postural hypotension which may be associated with syncope; cold extremities. In susceptible patients: precipitation of heart block; intermittent claudication; Raynaud's phenomenon.

CNS: confusion; dizziness; headache; mood changes; nightmares; psychoses and hallucinations; sleep disturbances of the type noted with other beta-blockers.

Gastrointestinal: dry mouth; gastrointestinal disturbances. Elevations of transaminase levels have been seen infrequently, rare cases of hepatic toxicity, including intrahepatic cholestasis have been reported.

Haematological: purpura; thrombocytopenia.

Integumentary: alopecia; dry eyes; psoriasiform skin reactions; exacerbation of psoriasis; skin rashes.

Neurological: paraesthesia.

Reproductive: impotence

Respiratory: bronchospasm may occur in patients with bronchial asthma or a history of asthmatic complaints.

Special senses: visual disturbances.

Others: hypersensitivity reactions, including angioedema and urticaria; fatigue; an increase in ANA (Antinuclear Antibodies) has been observed, however, the clinical relevance of this is not clear.

Discontinuance of the drug should be considered if, according to clinical judgement, the well-being of the patient is adversely affected by any of the above reactions.

4.9 Overdose

The symptoms of overdosage may include bradycardia, hypotension, acute cardiac insufficiency and bronchospasm.

General treatment should include: close supervision, treatment in an intensive care ward, the use of gastric lavage, activated charcoal and a laxative to prevent absorption of any drug still present in the gastrointestinal tract, the use of plasma or plasma substitutes to treat hypotension and shock. The use of haemodialysis or haemoperfusion may be considered.

Excessive bradycardia can be countered with atropine 1-2 mg intravenously and/or a cardiac pacemaker. If necessary, this may be followed by a bolus dose of glucagon 10 mg intravenously. If required, this may be repeated or followed by an intravenous infusion of glucagon 1-10 mg/hour depending on response. If no response to glucagon occurs or if glucagon is unavailable, a beta-adrenoceptor stimulant such as dobutamine 2.5 to 10 micrograms/kg/minute by intravenous infusion may be given. Dobutamine, because of its positive inotropic effect could also be used to treat hypotension and acute cardiac insufficiency. It is likely that these doses would be inadequate to reverse the cardiac effects of beta-blocker blockade if a large overdose has been taken. The dose of dobutamine should therefore be increased if necessary to achieve the required response according to the clinical condition of the patient.

Bronchospasm can usually be reversed by bronchodilators.

5. PHARMACOLOGICAL PROPERTIES

5.1 Pharmacodynamic properties

Beta blocking agents, plain, selective

CO7A B03

Atenolol is a beta-blocker which is beta$_1$-selective, (i.e. acts preferentially on beta$_1$-adrenergic receptors in the heart). Selectivity decreases with increasing dose.

Atenolol is without intrinsic sympathomimetic and membrane stabilising activities and as with other beta-blockers, has negative inotropic effects (and is therefore contraindicated in uncontrolled heart failure).

As with other beta-blockers, the mode of action of atenolol in the treatment of hypertension is unclear.

It is probably the action of atenolol in reducing cardiac rate and contractility which makes it effective in eliminating or reducing the symptoms of patients with angina.

It is unlikely that any additional ancillary properties possessed by S (-) atenolol, in comparison with the racemic mixture, will give rise to different therapeutic effects.

Tenormin is effective and well-tolerated in most ethnic populations although the response may be less in black patients.

Tenormin is effective for at least 24 hours after a single oral dose. The drug facilitates compliance by its acceptability to patients and simplicity of dosing. The narrow dose range and early patient response ensure that the effect of the drug in individual patients is quickly demonstrated. Tenormin is compatible with diuretics, other hypotensive agents and antianginals (but see Section 4.5). Since it acts preferentially on beta-receptors in the heart, Tenormin may, with care, be used successfully in the treatment of patients with respiratory disease, who cannot tolerate non-selective beta-blockers.

Early intervention with Tenormin in acute myocardial infarction reduces infarct size and decreases morbidity and mortality. Fewer patients with a threatened infarction progress to frank infarction; the incidence of ventricular arrhythmias is decreased and marked pain relief may result in reduced need of opiate analgesics. Early mortality is decreased. Tenormin is an additional treatment to standard coronary care.

5.2 Pharmacokinetic properties

Absorption of atenolol following oral dosing is consistent but incomplete (approximately 40-50%) with peak plasma concentrations occurring 2-4 hours after dosing. The atenolol blood levels are consistent and subject to little variability. There is no significant hepatic metabolism of atenolol and more than 90% of that absorbed reaches the systemic circulation unaltered. The plasma half-life is about 6 hours but this may rise in severe renal impairment since the kidney is the major route of elimination. Atenolol penetrates tissues poorly due to its low lipid solubility and its concentration in brain tissue is low. Plasma protein binding is low (approximately 3%).

5.3 Preclinical safety data

Atenolol is a drug on which extensive clinical experience has been obtained. Relevant information for the prescriber is provided elsewhere in the prescribing information.

6. PHARMACEUTICAL PARTICULARS

6.1 List of excipients

Gelatin.

Glycerol.

Magnesium Carbonate.

Magnesium Stearate.

Maize Starch.

Methylhydroxypropylcellulose.

Sodium Laurilsulfate

Titanium Dioxide (E171).

6.2 Incompatibilities

Not applicable.

6.3 Shelf life

60 months.

6.4 Special precautions for storage

Do not store above 25°C.

Store in the original package. Keep the container in the outer carton.

6.5 Nature and contents of container

Aluminium PVC/PVDC blister strips: 28 tablets

6.6 Instructions for use and handling

Not applicable.

7. MARKETING AUTHORISATION HOLDER

AstraZeneca UK Limited,

600 Capability Green,

Luton, LU1 3LU, UK.

8. MARKETING AUTHORISATION NUMBER(S)

PL 17901/0052

9. DATE OF FIRST AUTHORISATION/RENEWAL OF THE AUTHORISATION

1st June 2000 / 5th November 2003

10. DATE OF REVISION OF THE TEXT

5th November 2003

Tenormin Injection 0.5mg/ml

(AstraZeneca UK Limited)

1. NAME OF THE MEDICINAL PRODUCT

'Tenormin' Injection 0.5mg/ml

2. QUALITATIVE AND QUANTITATIVE COMPOSITION

Atenolol 0.5 mg/ml (5mg in 10ml)

For excipients, see Section 6.1

3. PHARMACEUTICAL FORM

Solution for injection or infusion.

Type I clear glass ampoules containing a clear, colourless, sterile solution

4. CLINICAL PARTICULARS

4.1 Therapeutic indications

Management of arrhythmias and for the early intervention treatment of acute myocardial infarction.

4.2 Posology and method of administration

Administered by the intravenous route.

The dose must always be adjusted to individual requirements of the patients, with the lowest possible starting dosage. The following are guidelines.

Adults

Cardiac Arrhythmias

A suitable initial dose of Tenormin is 2.5mg (5ml) injected intravenously over a 2.5 minute period (i.e.1mg/minute). This may be repeated at 5 minute intervals until a response is observed up to a maximum dosage of 10 mg. If Tenormin is given by infusion, 0.15-mg/kg bodyweight may be administered over a 20 minute period. If required, the injection or infusion may be repeated every 12 hours. Having controlled the arrhythmias with intravenous Tenormin, a suitable oral maintenance dosage is 50 to 100 mg daily (see prescribing information for Tenormin and Tenormin LS tablets).

Myocardial Infarction

For patients suitable for treatment with intravenous beta-blockade and presenting within 12 hours of the onset of chest pain, Tenormin 5-10 mg should be given by slow intravenous injection (1 mg/minute) followed by Tenormin 50 mg orally about 15 minutes later, provided no untoward effects have occurred from the intravenous dose. This should be followed by a further 50 mg orally 12 hours after the intravenous dose and then 12 hours later by 100 mg orally, once daily. If bradycardia and/or hypotension requiring treatment, or any other untoward effects occur, Tenormin should be discontinued

Elderly

Dosage requirements may be reduced especially in patients with impaired renal function.

Children

There is no paediatric experience with Tenormin and for this reason it is not recommended for use in children.

Renal Failure

Since Tenormin is excreted via the kidneys, dosage should be adjusted in cases of severe impairment of renal function.

No significant accumulation of Tenormin occurs in patients who have a creatinine clearance greater than 35 ml/min/ $1.73m^2$ (normal range is 100 to 150 ml/min/$1.73m^2$).

For patients with a creatinine clearance of 15 to 35 ml/min/ $1.73m^2$ (equivalent to serum creatinine of 300 to 600 micromol/litre) the oral dose should be 50 mg daily and intravenous dose should be 10 mg once every two days.

For patients with a creatinine clearance of <15 ml/min/ $1.73m^2$ (equivalent to serum creatinine of >600 micromol/ litre) the oral dose should be 25 mg daily or 50 mg on alternate days and the intravenous dose should be 10 mg once every four days.

Patients on haemodialysis should be given 50 mg orally after each dialysis; this should be done under hospital supervision as marked falls in blood pressure can occur.

4.3 Contraindications

Tenormin, as with other beta-blockers, should not be used in patients with any of the following:

cardiogenic shock

uncontrolled heart failure

sick sinus syndrome

second or third degree heart block

untreated phaeochromocytoma

metabolic acidosis

bradycardia ($<$45bpm)

hypotension

known hypersensitivity to the active substance, or any of the excipients severe peripheral arterial circulatory disturbances.

4.4 Special warnings and special precautions for use

Tenormin as with other beta-blockers:

- should not be withdrawn abruptly. The dosage should be withdrawn gradually over a period of 7-14 days, to facilitate a reduction in beta-blocker dosage. Patients should be followed during withdrawal, especially those with ischaemic heart disease.
- when a patient is scheduled for surgery, and a decision is made to discontinue beta-blocker therapy, this should be done at least 24 hours prior to the procedure. The risk-benefit assessment of stopping beta-blockade should be made for each patient. If treatment is continued, an anaesthetic with little negative inotropic activity should be selected to minimise the risk of myocardial depression. The patient may be protected against vagal reactions by intravenous administration of atropine.
- although contraindicated in uncontrolled heart failure (see Section 4.3), may be used in patients whose signs of heart failure have been controlled. Caution must be exercised in patients whose cardiac reserve is poor.
- may increase the number and duration of angina attacks in patients with Prinzmetal's angina due to unopposed alpha-receptor mediated coronary artery vasoconstriction. Tenormin is a beta$_1$ -selective beta-blocker; consequently, its use may be considered although utmost caution must be exercised.
- although contraindicated in severe peripheral arterial circulatory disturbances (see Section 4.3), may also aggravate less severe peripheral arterial circulatory disturbances.
- due to its negative effect on conduction time, caution must be exercised if it is given to patients with first degree heart block.
- may mask the symptoms of hypoglycaemia, in particular, tachycardia.
- may mask the signs of thyrotoxicosis.
- will reduce heart rate, as a result of its pharmacological action. In the rare instances when a treated patient develops symptoms which may be attributable to a slow heart rate and the pulse rate drops to less than 50-55bpm at rest, the dose should be reduced.
- may cause a more severe reaction to a variety of allergens, when given to patients with a history of anaphylactic reaction to such allergens. Such patients may be unresponsive to the usual doses of adrenaline used to treat the allergic reactions.
- may cause a hypersensitivity reaction including angioedema and urticaria
- should be used with caution in the elderly, starting with a lesser dose (See Section 4.2).

Since Tenormin is excreted via the kidneys, dosage should be reduced in patients with a creatinine clearance of below 35ml/min/$1.7m^2$.

Although cardioselective (beta$_1$) beta-blockers may have less effect on lung function than non-selective beta-blockers, as with all, beta-blockers, these should be avoided in patients with reversible obstructive airways disease, unless there are compelling clinical reasons for their use. Where such reasons exist, Tenormin may be used with caution. Occasionally, some increase in airways resistance may occur in asthmatic patients, however, and this may usually be reversed by commonly used dosage of bronchodilators such as salbutamol or isoprenaline. The label and patient information leaflet for this product state the following warning: "If you have ever had asthma or wheezing, you should not take this medicine unless you have discussed these symptoms with the prescribing doctor".

As with other beta-blockers, in patients with a phaeochromocytoma, an alpha-blocker should be given concomitantly.

4.5 Interaction with other medicinal products and other forms of Interaction

Combined use of beta-blockers and calcium channel blockers with negative inotropic effects e.g. verapamil, and diltiazem can lead to an exaggeration of these effects particularly in patients with impaired ventricular function and/or sino-atrial or atrio-ventricular conduction abnormalities. This may result in severe hypotension, bradycardia and cardiac failure. Neither the beta-blocker nor the calcium channel blocker should be administered intravenously within 48 hours of discontinuing the other.

Concomitant therapy with dihydropyridines e.g. nifedipine, may increase the risk of hypotension, and cardiac failure may occur in patients with latent cardiac insufficiency.

Digitalis glycosides, in association with beta-blockers, may increase atrio-ventricular conduction time.

Beta-blockers may exacerbate the rebound hypertension which can follow the withdrawal of clonidine. If the two drugs are co-administered, the beta-blocker should be withdrawn several days before discontinuing clonidine. If replacing clonidine by beta-blocker therapy, the introduction of beta-blockers should be delayed for several days after clonidine administration has stopped. (See also prescribing information for clonidine).

Caution must be exercised when prescribing a beta-blocker with Class I antiarrhythmic agents such as disopyramide and quinidine.

Concomitant use of sympathomimetic agents, e.g. adrenaline, may counteract the effect of beta-blockers.

Concomitant use with insulin and oral antidiabetic drugs may lead to the intensification of the blood sugar lowering effects of these drugs. Symptoms of hypoglycaemia, particularly tachycardia, may be masked (see Section 4.4).

Concomitant use of prostaglandin synthetase inhibiting drugs (e.g. ibuprofen and indomethacin) may decrease the hypotensive effects of beta-blockers.

Caution must be exercised when using anaesthetic agents with Tenormin. The anaesthetist should be informed and the choice of anaesthetic should be an agent with as little negative inotropic activity as possible. Use of beta-blockers with anaesthetic drugs may result in attenuation of the reflex tachycardia and increase the risk of hypotension. Anaesthetic agents causing myocardial depression are best avoided.

4.6 Pregnancy and lactation

Tenormin crosses the placental barrier and appears in the cord blood. No studies have been performed on the use of Tenormin in the first trimester and the possibility of foetal injury cannot be excluded. Tenormin has been used under close supervision for the treatment of hypertension in the third trimester. Administration of Tenormin to pregnant women in the management of mild to moderate hypertension has been associated with intra-uterine growth retardation.

The use of Tenormin in women who are, or may become, pregnant requires that the anticipated benefit be weighed against the possible risks, particularly in the first and second trimesters, since beta-blockers, in general, have been associated with a decrease in placental perfusion which may result in intra-uterine deaths, immature and premature deliveries.

There is significant accumulation of Tenormin in breast milk.

Neonates born to mothers who are receiving Tenormin at parturition or breast-feeding may be at risk of hypoglycaemia and bradycardia.

Caution should be exercised when Tenormin is administered during pregnancy or to a woman who is breast-feeding.

4.7 Effects on ability to drive and use machines

The use of Tenormin is unlikely to result in any impairment of the ability of patients to drive or operate machinery. However, it should be taken into account that occasionally dizziness or fatigue may occur.

4.8 Undesirable effects

Tenormin is well tolerated. In clinical studies, the undesired events reported are usually attributable to the pharmacological actions of atenolol.

The following undesired events, listed by body system, have been reported.

Cardiovascular: bradycardia; heart failure deterioration; postural hypotension which may be associated with syncope; cold extremities. In susceptible patients: precipitation of heart block; intermittent claudication; Raynaud's phenomenon.

CNS: confusion; dizziness; headache; mood changes; nightmares; psychoses and hallucinations; sleep disturbances of the type noted with other beta-blockers.

Gastrointestinal: dry mouth; gastrointestinal disturbances. Elevations of transaminase levels have been seen infrequently, rare cases of hepatic toxicity, including intrahepatic cholestasis have been reported.

Haematological: purpura; thrombocytopenia.

Integumentary: alopecia; dry eyes; psoriasiform skin reactions; exacerbation of psoriasis; skin rashes.

Neurological: paraesthesia.

Reproductive: impotence

Respiratory: bronchospasm may occur in patients with bronchial asthma or a history of asthmatic complaints.

Special senses: visual disturbances.

Others: hypersensitivity reactions, including angioedema and urticaria; fatigue; an increase in ANA (Antinuclear Antibodies) has been observed, however, the clinical relevance of this is not clear.

Discontinuance of the drug should be considered if, according to clinical judgement, the well-being of the patient is adversely affected by any of the above reactions.

4.9 Overdose

The symptoms of overdosage may include bradycardia, hypotension, acute cardiac insufficiency and bronchospasm.

General treatment should include: close supervision, treatment in an intensive care ward, the use of gastric lavage, activated charcoal and a laxative to prevent absorption of any drug still present in the gastrointestinal tract, the use of plasma or plasma substitutes to treat hypotension and shock. The use of haemodialysis or haemoperfusion may be considered.

Excessive bradycardia can be countered with atropine 1-2 mg intravenously and/or a cardiac pacemaker. If necessary, this may be followed by a bolus dose of glucagon 10 mg intravenously. If required, this may be repeated or followed by an intravenous infusion of glucagon 1-10 mg/hour depending on response. If no response to glucagon occurs or if glucagon is unavailable, a beta-adrenoceptor stimulant such as dobutamine 2.5 to 10 micrograms/kg/minute by intravenous infusion may be given. Dobutamine, because of its positive inotropic effect could also be used to treat hypotension and acute cardiac insufficiency. It is likely that these doses would be inadequate to reverse the cardiac effects of beta-blocker blockade if a large overdose has been taken. The dose of dobutamine should therefore be increased if necessary to achieve the required response according to the clinical condition of the patient.

Bronchospasm can usually be reversed by bronchodilators.

5. PHARMACOLOGICAL PROPERTIES

5.1 Pharmacodynamic properties

Beta blocking agents, plain, selective

CO7A B03

Atenolol is a beta-blocker which is $beta_1$-selective, (i.e. acts preferentially on $beta_1$-adrenergic receptors in the heart). Selectivity decreases with increasing dose.

Atenolol is without intrinsic sympathomimetic and membrane stabilising activities and as with other beta-blockers, has negative inotropic effects (and is therefore contraindicated in uncontrolled heart failure).

As with other beta-blockers, the mode of action of atenolol in the treatment of hypertension is unclear.

It is probably the action of atenolol in reducing cardiac rate and contractility which makes it effective in eliminating or reducing the symptoms of patients with angina.

It is unlikely that any additional ancillary properties possessed by S (-) atenolol, in comparison with the racemic mixture, will give rise to different therapeutic effects.

Tenormin is effective and well-tolerated in most ethnic populations although the response may be less in black patients.

The narrow dose range and early patient response to Tenormin ensure that the effect of the drug in individual patients is quickly demonstrated. Tenormin is compatible with diuretics, other hypotensive agents and antianginals (see Section 4.5). Since it acts preferentially on beta-adrenergic receptors in the heart, Tenormin may, with care be used successfully in the treatment of patients with respiratory disease who cannot tolerate non-selective beta-adrenoceptor blocking drugs.

Early intervention with Tenormin in acute myocardial infarction reduces infarct size and decreases morbidity and mortality. Fewer patients with a threatened infarction progress to frank infarction; the incidence of ventricular arrhythmias is decreased and marked pain relief may result in reduced need of opiate analgesics. Early mortality is decreased. Tenormin is an additional treatment to standard coronary care.

5.2 Pharmacokinetic properties

Following intravenous administration, the blood levels of atenolol decay tri-exponentially with an elimination half-life of about 6 hours. Throughout the intravenous dose range of 5 to 10 mg the blood level profile obeys linear pharmacokinetics and beta-adrenoceptor blockade is still measurable 24 hours after a 10 mg intravenous dose.

Absorption of atenolol following oral dosing is consistent but incomplete (approximately 40 to 50%) with peak plasma concentrations occurring 2 to 4 hours after dosing. The atenolol blood levels are consistent and subject to little variability. There is no significant hepatic metabolism of atenolol and more than 90% of that absorbed reaches the systemic circulation unaltered. The plasma half-life is about 6 hours but this may rise in severe renal impairment since the kidney is the major route of elimination. Atenolol penetrates tissues poorly due to its low lipid solubility and its concentration in brain tissue is low. Plasma protein binding is low (approximately 3%).

5.3 Preclinical safety data

Atenolol is a drug on which extensive clinical experience has been obtained. Relevant information for the prescriber is provided elsewhere in the Prescribing Information.

6. PHARMACEUTICAL PARTICULARS

6.1 List of excipients

Citric acid

Sodium chloride

Sodium hydroxide

Water for Injection

6.2 Incompatibilities

None known

6.3 Shelf life

36 months.

6.4 Special precautions for storage

Do not store above 25°C. Keep the container in the outer carton.

6.5 Nature and contents of container

Glass ampoules.

10 ml ampoules are packed in boxes of 10.

6.6 Instructions for use and handling

Use as instructed by the prescriber.

Tenormin Injection is compatible with sodium chloride intravenous\infusion (0.9%w/v) and Glucose Intravenous Infusion BP (5% w/v).

7. MARKETING AUTHORISATION HOLDER

AstraZeneca UK Limited,

600 Capability Green,

Luton, LU1 3LU, UK.

8. MARKETING AUTHORISATION NUMBER(S)

17901/0050

9. DATE OF FIRST AUTHORISATION/RENEWAL OF THE AUTHORISATION

01 June 2000/18th February 2004

10. DATE OF REVISION OF THE TEXT

18th February 2004

Tenormin LS 50mg Tablets

(AstraZeneca UK Limited)

1. NAME OF THE MEDICINAL PRODUCT

'Tenormin' LS 50mg tablets

2. QUALITATIVE AND QUANTITATIVE COMPOSITION

Atenolol 50 mg

For excipients, see Section 6.1

3. PHARMACEUTICAL FORM

Film coated tablet

White film coated tablets

4. CLINICAL PARTICULARS

4.1 Therapeutic indications

i. Management of hypertension

ii. Management of angina pectoris

iii. Management of cardiac arrhythmias

iv. Management of myocardial infarction. Early intervention in the acute phase.

4.2 Posology and method of administration

Oral administration

The dose must always be adjusted to individual requirements of the patients, with the lowest possible starting dosage. The following are guidelines.

Adults

Hypertension

One tablet daily. Most patients respond to 100 mg daily given orally as a single dose. Some patients, however, will respond to 50 mg given as a single daily dose. The effect will be fully established after one to two weeks. A further reduction in blood pressure may be achieved by combining Tenormin with other antihypertensive agents. For example, co-administration of Tenormin with a diuretic, as in Tenoretic provides a highly effective and convenient antihypertensive therapy.

Angina

Most patients with angina pectoris will respond to 100 mg given orally once daily or 50 mg given twice daily. It is unlikely that additional benefit will be gained by increasing the dose.

Cardiac Arrhythmias

A suitable initial dose of Tenormin is 2.5 mg (5 ml) injected intravenously over a 2.5 minute period. (i.e. 1 mg/minute). (See also prescribing information for Tenormin Injection). This may be repeated at 5 minute intervals until a response is observed up to a maximum dosage of 10 mg. If Tenormin is given by infusion, 0.15 mg/kg bodyweight may be administered over a 20 minute period. If required, the injection or infusion may be repeated every 12 hours. Having controlled the arrhythmias with intravenous Tenormin, a suitable oral maintenance dosage is 50-100 mg daily, given as a single dose.

Myocardial Infarction

For patients suitable for treatment with intravenous beta-blockade and presenting within 12 hours of the onset of chest pain, Tenormin 5-10 mg should be given by slow intravenous injection (1 mg/minute) followed by Tenormin 50 mg orally about 15 minutes later, provided no untoward effects have occurred from the intravenous dose. This should be followed by a further 50 mg orally 12 hours after the intravenous dose and then 12 hours later by 100 mg orally, once daily. If bradycardia and/or hypotension requiring treatment, or any other untoward effects occur, Tenormin should be discontinued.

Elderly

Dosage requirements may be reduced, especially in patients with impaired renal function.

Children

There is no paediatric experience with Tenormin and for this reason it is not recommended for use in children.

Renal Failure

Since Tenormin is excreted via the kidneys the dosage should be adjusted in cases of severe impairment of renal function.

No significant accumulation of Tenormin occurs in patients who have a creatinine clearance greater than 35 ml/min/1.73 m^2 (normal range is 100-150 ml/min/1.73m^2).

For patients with a creatinine clearance of 15-35 ml/min/1.73m^2 (equivalent to serum creatinine of 300-600 micromol/litre) the oral dose should be 50 mg daily and the intravenous dose should be 10 mg once every two days.

For patients with a creatinine clearance of <15 ml/min/1.73m^2 (equivalent to serum creatinine of >600 micromol/litre) the oral dose should be 25 mg daily or 50 mg on alternate days and the intravenous dose should be 10 mg once every four days.

Patients on haemodialysis should be given 50 mg orally after each dialysis; this should be done under hospital supervision as marked falls in blood pressure can occur.

4.3 Contraindications

Tenormin, as with other beta-blockers, should not be used in patients with any of the following:

cardiogenic shock;

uncontrolled heart failure;

sick sinus syndrome;

second or third degree heart block;

untreated phaeochromocytoma;

metabolic acidosis;

bradycardia (<45bpm);

hypotension;

known hypersensitivity to the active substance, or any of the excipients;

severe peripheral arterial circulatory disturbances.

4.4 Special warnings and special precautions for use

Tenormin as with other beta-blockers:

- should not be withdrawn abruptly. The dosage should be withdrawn gradually over a period of 7-14 days, to facilitate a reduction in beta-blocker dosage. Patients should be followed during withdrawal, especially those with ischaemic heart disease.
- when a patient is scheduled for surgery, and a decision is made to discontinue beta-blocker therapy, this should be done at least 24 hours prior to the procedure. The risk-benefit assessment of stopping beta-blockade should be made for each patient. If treatment is continued, an anaesthetic with little negative inotropic activity should be selected to minimise the risk of myocardial depression. The patient may be protected against vagal reactions by intravenous administration of atropine.
- although contraindicated in uncontrolled heart failure (see Section 4.3), may be used in patients whose signs of heart failure have been controlled. Caution must be exercised in patients whose cardiac reserve is poor.
- may increase the number and duration of angina attacks in patients with Prinzmetal's angina due to unopposed alpha-receptor mediated coronary artery vasoconstriction. Tenormin is a $beta_1$ -selective beta-blocker; consequently, its use may be considered although utmost caution must be exercised.
- although contraindicated in severe peripheral arterial circulatory disturbances (see Section 4.3), may also aggravate less severe peripheral arterial circulatory disturbances.
- due to its negative effect on conduction time, caution must be exercised if it is given to patients with first degree heart block.

• may mask the symptoms of hypoglycaemia, in particular, tachycardia.

• may mask the signs of thyrotoxicosis.

• will reduce heart rate, as a result of its pharmacological action. In the rare instances when a treated patient develops symptoms which may be attributable to a slow heart rate and the pulse rate drops to less than 50-55bpm at rest, the dose should be reduced.

• may cause a more severe reaction to a variety of allergens, when given to patients with a history of anaphylactic reaction to such allergens. Such patients may be unresponsive to the usual doses of adrenaline used to treat the allergic reactions.

• may cause a hypersensitivity reaction including angioedema and urticaria

• should be used with caution in the elderly, starting with a lesser dose (See Section 4.2).

Since Tenormin is excreted via the kidneys, dosage should be reduced in patients with a creatinine clearance of below 35ml/min/1.7m^2.

Although cardioselective (beta$_1$) beta-blockers may have less effect on lung function than non-selective beta-blockers, as with all, beta-blockers, these should be avoided in patients with reversible obstructive airways disease, unless there are compelling clinical reasons for their use. Where such reasons exist, Tenormin may be used with caution. Occasionally, some increase in airways resistance may occur in asthmatic patients, however, and this may usually be reversed by commonly used dosage of bronchodilators such as salbutamol or isoprenaline. The label and patient information leaflet for this product state the following warning: "If you have ever had asthma or wheezing, you should not take this medicine unless you have discussed these symptoms with the prescribing doctor".

As with other beta-blockers, in patients with a phaeochromocytoma, an alpha-blocker should be given concomitantly.

4.5 Interaction with other medicinal products and other forms of Interaction

Combined use of beta-blockers and calcium channel blockers with negative inotropic effects e.g. verapamil and diltiazem can lead to an exaggeration of these effects particularly in patients with impaired ventricular function and/or sino-atrial or atrio-ventricular conduction abnormalities. This may result in severe hypotension, bradycardia and cardiac failure. Neither the beta-blocker nor the calcium channel blocker should be administered intravenously within 48 hours of discontinuing the other.

Concomitant therapy with dihydropyridines e.g. nifedipine, may increase the risk of hypotension, and cardiac failure may occur in patients with latent cardiac insufficiency.

Digitalis glycosides, in association with beta-blockers, may increase atrio-ventricular conduction time.

Beta-blockers may exacerbate the rebound hypertension which can follow the withdrawal of clonidine. If the two drugs are co-administered, the beta-blocker should be withdrawn several days before discontinuing clonidine. If replacing clonidine by beta-blocker therapy, the introduction of beta-blockers should be delayed for several days after clonidine administration has stopped. (See also prescribing information for clonidine).

Caution must be exercised when prescribing a beta-blocker with Class I antiarrhythmic agents such as disopyramide and quinidine.

Concomitant use of sympathomimetic agents, e.g. adrenaline, may counteract the effect of beta-blockers.

Concomitant use with insulin and oral antidiabetic drugs may lead to the intensification of the blood sugar lowering effects of these drugs. Symptoms of hypoglycaemia, particularly tachycardia, may be masked (See Section 4.4).

Concomitant use of prostaglandin synthetase inhibiting drugs (e.g. ibuprofen and indomethacin), may decrease the hypotensive effects of beta-blockers.

Caution must be exercised when using anaesthetic agents with Tenormin. The anaesthetist should be informed and the choice of anaesthetic should be an agent with as little negative inotropic activity as possible. Use of beta-blockers with anaesthetic drugs may result in attenuation of the reflex tachycardia and increase the risk of hypotension. Anaesthetic agents causing myocardial depression are best avoided.

4.6 Pregnancy and lactation

Tenormin crosses the placental barrier and appears in the cord blood. No studies have been performed on the use of Tenormin in the first trimester and the possibility of foetal injury cannot be excluded. Tenormin has been used under close supervision for the treatment of hypertension in the third trimester. Administration of Tenormin to pregnant women in the management of mild to moderate hypertension has been associated with intra-uterine growth retardation.

The use of Tenormin in women who are, or may become, pregnant requires that the anticipated benefit be weighed against the possible risks, particularly in the first and second trimesters, since beta-blockers, in general, have been associated with a decrease in placental perfusion which may result in intra-uterine deaths, immature and premature deliveries.

There is significant accumulation of Tenormin in breast milk.

Neonates born to mothers who are receiving Tenormin at parturition or breast-feeding may be at risk of hypoglycaemia and bradycardia.

Caution should be exercised when Tenormin is administered during pregnancy or to a woman who is breast-feeding.

4.7 Effects on ability to drive and use machines

Use is unlikely to result in any impairment of the ability of patients to drive or operate machinery. However, it should be taken into account that occasionally dizziness or fatigue may occur.

4.8 Undesirable effects

Tenormin is well tolerated. In clinical studies, the undesired events reported are usually attributable to the pharmacological actions of atenolol.

The following undesired events, listed by body system, have been reported.

Cardiovascular: bradycardia; heart failure deterioration; postural hypotension which may be associated with syncope; cold extremities. In susceptible patients: precipitation of heart block; intermittent claudication; Raynaud's phenomenon.

CNS: confusion; dizziness; headache; mood changes; nightmares; psychoses and hallucinations; sleep disturbances of the type noted with other beta-blockers.

Gastrointestinal: dry mouth; gastrointestinal disturbances. Elevations of transaminase levels have been seen infrequently, rare cases of hepatic toxicity, including intrahepatic cholestasis have been reported.

Haematological: purpura; thrombocytopenia.

Integumentary: alopecia; dry eyes; psoriasiform skin reactions; exacerbation of psoriasis; skin rashes.

Neurological: paraesthesia.

Reproductive: impotence

Respiratory: bronchospasm may occur in patients with bronchial asthma or a history of asthmatic complaints.

Special senses: visual disturbances.

Others: hypersensitivity reactions, including angioedema and urticaria; fatigue; an increase in ANA (Antinuclear Antibodies) has been observed, however, the clinical relevance of this is not clear.

Discontinuance of the drug should be considered if, according to clinical judgement, the well-being of the patient is adversely affected by any of the above reactions.

4.9 Overdose

The symptoms of overdosage may include bradycardia, hypotension, acute cardiac insufficiency and bronchospasm.

General treatment should include: close supervision, treatment in an intensive care ward, the use of gastric lavage, activated charcoal and a laxative to prevent absorption of any drug still present in the gastrointestinal tract, the use of plasma or plasma substitutes to treat hypotension and shock. The use of haemodialysis or haemoperfusion may be considered.

Excessive bradycardia can be countered with atropine 1-2 mg intravenously and/or a cardiac pacemaker. If necessary, this may be followed by a bolus dose of glucagon 10 mg intravenously. If required, this may be repeated or followed by an intravenous infusion of glucagon 1-10 mg/hour depending on response. If no response to glucagon occurs or if glucagon is unavailable, a beta-adrenoceptor stimulant such as dobutamine 2.5 to 10 micrograms/kg/minute by intravenous infusion may be given. Dobutamine, because of its positive inotropic effect could also be used to treat hypotension and acute cardiac insufficiency. It is likely that these doses would be inadequate to reverse the cardiac effects of beta-blocker blockade if a large overdose has been taken. The dose of dobutamine should therefore be increased if necessary to achieve the required response according to the clinical condition of the patient.

Bronchospasm can usually be reversed by bronchodilators.

5. PHARMACOLOGICAL PROPERTIES

5.1 Pharmacodynamic properties

Beta blocking agents, plain, selective

CO7A B03

Atenolol is a beta-blocker which is beta$_1$-selective, (i.e. acts preferentially on beta$_1$-adrenergic receptors in the heart). Selectivity decreases with increasing dose.

Atenolol is without intrinsic sympathomimetic and membrane stabilising activities and as with other beta-blockers, has negative inotropic effects (and is therefore contraindicated in uncontrolled heart failure).

As with other beta-blockers, the mode of action of atenolol in the treatment of hypertension is unclear.

It is probably the action of atenolol in reducing cardiac rate and contractility which makes it effective in eliminating or reducing the symptoms of patients with angina.

It is unlikely that any additional ancillary properties possessed by S (-) atenolol, in comparison with the racemic mixture, will give rise to different therapeutic effects.

Tenormin is effective and well-tolerated in most ethnic populations although the response may be less in black patients.

Tenormin is effective for at least 24 hours after a single oral dose. The drug facilitates compliance by its acceptability to patients and simplicity of dosing. The narrow dose range and early patient response ensure that the effect of the drug in individual patients is quickly demonstrated. Tenormin is compatible with diuretics, other hypotensive agents and antianginals (see section 4.5). Since it acts preferentially on beta-receptors in the heart, Tenormin may, with care, be used successfully in the treatment of patients with respiratory disease, who cannot tolerate non-selective beta-blockers.

Early intervention with Tenormin in acute myocardial infarction reduces infarct size and decreases morbidity and mortality. Fewer patients with a threatened infarction progress to frank infarction; the incidence of ventricular arrhythmias is decreased and marked pain relief may result in reduced need of opiate analgesics. Early mortality is decreased. Tenormin is an additional treatment to standard coronary care.

5.2 Pharmacokinetic properties

Absorption of atenolol following oral dosing is consistent but incomplete (approximately 40-50%) with peak plasma concentrations occurring 2-4 hours after dosing. The atenolol blood levels are consistent and subject to little variability. There is no significant hepatic metabolism of atenolol and more than 90% of that absorbed reaches the systemic circulation unaltered. The plasma half-life is about 6 hours but this may rise in severe renal impairment since the kidney is the major route of elimination. Atenolol penetrates tissues poorly due to its low lipid solubility and its concentration in brain tissue is low. Plasma protein binding is low (approximately 3%).

5.3 Preclinical safety data

Atenolol is a drug on which extensive clinical experience has been obtained. Relevant information for the prescriber is provided elsewhere in the prescribing information.

6. PHARMACEUTICAL PARTICULARS

6.1 List of excipients

Gelatin

Macrogol 300

Magnesium Carbonate

Magnesium Stearate

Maize Starch

Methylhydoxypropylcellulose

Sodium Lauryl Sulphate Sodium Laurilsulfate

Sunset Yellow Lake (E110).

Talc

Titanium Dioxide. (E171)

6.2 Incompatibilities

Not applicable.

6.3 Shelf life

60 months.

6.4 Special precautions for storage

Do not store above 25°C.

Store in the original package. Keep the container in the outer carton.

6.5 Nature and contents of container

Aluminium PVC/PVDC Blister strips of 14 tablets: 28 Tablets

Aluminium PVC/PVDC blister strips of 7 tablets: 504 Tablets (for Hospital Use)

(pack is subdivided into 6 cartons each containing 12 blister strips i.e. 84 tablets)

6.6 Instructions for use and handling

Not applicable.

7. MARKETING AUTHORISATION HOLDER

AstraZeneca UK Limited,

600 Capability Green,

Luton, LU1 3LU, UK.

8. MARKETING AUTHORISATION NUMBER(S)

PL 17901/0053.

9. DATE OF FIRST AUTHORISATION/RENEWAL OF THE AUTHORISATION

1st June 2000 / 5th November 2003

10. DATE OF REVISION OF THE TEXT

5th November 2003

Tenormin Syrup

(AstraZeneca UK Limited)

1. NAME OF THE MEDICINAL PRODUCT

'Tenormin' Syrup.

2. QUALITATIVE AND QUANTITATIVE COMPOSITION

Atenolol 0.5% w/v.

For excipients, see Section 6.1

3. PHARMACEUTICAL FORM

Syrup.

4. CLINICAL PARTICULARS

4.1 Therapeutic indications

i. Management of hypertension

ii. Management of angina

iii. Management of cardiac arrhythmias

iv. Myocardial infarction. Early intervention in the acute phase.

4.2 Posology and method of administration

Oral administration.

Tenormin syrup is intended for patients unable to swallow Tenormin tablets.

The dose must always be adjusted to individual requirements of the patients, with the lowest possible starting dosage. The following are guidelines.

Adults

Hypertension

Two or four 5 ml spoonfuls daily i.e. 50 mg or 100 mg in patients unable to take 50 mg or 100 mg tablets.

Most patients respond to 100 mg once daily. Some patients, however, will respond to 50 mg given as a single daily dose. The effect will be fully established after one to two weeks. A further reduction in blood pressure may be achieved by combining Tenormin with other antihypertensive agents.

Angina

Most patients with angina pectoris will respond to 100 mg (four 5 ml spoonfuls) given orally once a day, or 50 mg (two 5 ml spoonfuls) given twice daily. It is unlikely that additional benefit will be gained by increasing the dose.

Cardiac Arrhythmias

A suitable initial dose of Tenormin Injection is 2.5 mg (5 ml) given intravenously over a 2.5 minute period (i.e. 1 mg/minute). (See prescribing information for Tenormin Injection). This may be repeated at 5 minute intervals until a response is observed up to a maximum dosage of 10 mg. If Tenormin Injection is given by infusion, 0.15 mg/kg body weight may be administered over a 20 minute period. If required, the injection or infusion may be repeated every 12 hours. Having controlled the arrhythmias, a suitable oral maintenance dosage is 50 - 100 mg (two to four 5 ml spoonfuls of Tenormin Syrup) daily, given as a single dose.

Myocardial Infarction

For patients suitable for treatment with intravenous beta-blockade and presenting within 12 hours of the onset of chest pain, Tenormin 5-10 mg should be given by slow intravenous injection (1 mg/minute) followed by Tenormin 50 mg orally about 15 minutes later, provided no untoward effects have occurred from the intravenous dose. This should be followed by a further 50 mg orally 12 hours after the intravenous dose and then 12 hours later by 100 mg orally, once daily. If bradycardia and/or hypotension requiring treatment, or any other untoward effects occur, Tenormin should be discontinued.

Elderly

Dosage requirements may be reduced, especially in patients with impaired renal function.

Children

There is no paediatric experience with Tenormin and for this reason it is not recommended for use in children.

Renal Failure

Since Tenormin is excreted via the kidneys, dosage should be adjusted in cases of severe impairment of renal function.

No significant accumulation of Tenormin occurs in patients who have a creatinine clearance greater than 35 ml/min/1.73 m^2 (Normal range is 100-150 ml/min/1.73 m^2).

For patients with a creatinine clearance of 15-35 ml/min/1.73 m^2 (equivalent to serum creatinine of 300-600 micromol/litre) the oral dose should be 50 mg daily and the intravenous dose should be 10 mg once every two days.

For patients with a creatinine clearance of $<$15 ml/min/1.73 m^2 (equivalent to serum creatinine of $>$600 micromol/litre) the oral dose should be 25 mg daily or 50 mg on alternate days and the intravenous dose should be 10 mg once every four days.

Patients on haemodialysis should be given 50 mg orally after each dialysis: this should be done under hospital supervision as marked falls in blood pressure can occur.

4.3 Contraindications

Tenormin, as with other beta-blockers, should not be used in patients with any of the following:

cardiogenic shock;

uncontrolled heart failure;

sick sinus syndrome;

second or third degree heart block;

untreated phaeochromocytoma;

metabolic acidosis;

bradycardia ($<$45bpm);

hypotension;

known hypersensitivity to the active substance, or any of the excipients;

severe peripheral arterial circulatory disturbances.

4.4 Special warnings and special precautions for use

Tenormin as with other beta-blockers:

- should not be withdrawn abruptly. The dosage should be withdrawn gradually over a period of 7-14 days, to facilitate a reduction in beta-blocker dosage. Patients should be followed during withdrawal, especially those with ischaemic heart disease.

- when a patient is scheduled for surgery, and a decision is made to discontinue beta-blocker therapy, this should be done at least 24 hours prior to the procedure. The risk-benefit assessment of stopping beta-blockade should be made for each patient. If treatment is continued, an anaesthetic with little negative inotropic activity should be selected to minimise the risk of myocardial depression. The patient may be protected against vagal reactions by intravenous administration of atropine.

- although contraindicated in uncontrolled heart failure (see Section 4.3), may be used in patients whose signs of heart failure have been controlled. Caution must be exercised in patients whose cardiac reserve is poor.

- may increase the number and duration of angina attacks in patients with Prinzmetal's angina due to unopposed alpha-receptor mediated coronary artery vasoconstriction. Tenormin is a $beta_1$ -selective beta-blocker; consequently, its use may be considered although utmost caution must be exercised.

- although contraindicated in severe peripheral arterial circulatory disturbances (see Section 4.3), may also aggravate less severe peripheral arterial circulatory disturbances.

- due to its negative effect on conduction time, caution must be exercised if it is given to patients with first degree heart block.

- may mask the symptoms of hypoglycaemia, in particular, tachycardia.

- may mask the signs of thyrotoxicosis.

- will reduce heart rate, as a result of its pharmacological action. In the rare instances when a treated patient develops symptoms which may be attributable to a slow heart rate and the pulse rate drops to less than 50-55bpm at rest, the dose should be reduced.

- may cause a more severe reaction to a variety of allergens, when given to patients with a history of anaphylactic reaction to such allergens. Such patients may be unresponsive to the usual doses of adrenaline used to treat the allergic reactions.

- may cause a hypersensitivity reaction including angioedema and urticaria

- should be used with caution in the elderly, starting with a lesser dose (See Section 4.2).

Since Tenormin is excreted via the kidneys, dosage should be reduced in patients with a creatinine clearance of below 35ml/min/1.7m^2.

Although cardioselective ($beta_1$) beta-blockers may have less effect on lung function than non-selective beta-blockers, as with all, beta-blockers, these should be avoided in patients with reversible obstructive airways disease, unless there are compelling clinical reasons for their use. Where such reasons exist, Tenormin may be used with caution. Occasionally, some increase in airways resistance may occur in asthmatic patients, however, and this may usually be reversed by commonly used dosage of bronchodilators such as salbutamol or isoprenaline. The label and patient information leaflet for this product state the following warning: "If you have ever had asthma or wheezing, you should not take this medicine unless you have discussed these symptoms with the prescribing doctor".

As with other beta-blockers, in patients with a phaeochromocytoma, an alpha-blocker should be given concomitantly.

4.5 Interaction with other medicinal products and other forms of Interaction

Combined use of beta-blockers and calcium channel blockers with negative inotropic effects e.g. verapamil, and diltiazem can lead to an exaggeration of these effects particularly in patients with impaired ventricular function and/or sino-atrial or atrio-ventricular conduction abnormalities. This may result in severe hypotension, bradycardia and cardiac failure. Neither the beta-blocker nor the calcium channel blocker should be administered intravenously within 48 hours of discontinuing the other.

Concomitant therapy with dihydropyridines e.g. nifedipine, may increase the risk of hypotension, and cardiac failure may occur in patients with latent cardiac insufficiency.

Digitalis glycosides, in association with beta-blockers, may increase atrio-ventricular conduction time.

Beta-blockers may exacerbate the rebound hypertension which can follow the withdrawal of clonidine. If the two drugs are co-administered, the beta-blocker should be withdrawn several days before discontinuing clonidine. If replacing clonidine by beta-blocker therapy, the introduction of beta-blockers should be delayed for several days after clonidine administration has stopped. (See also prescribing information for clonidine).

Caution must be exercised when prescribing a beta-blocker with Class I antiarrhythmic agents such as disopyramide and quinidine.

Concomitant use of sympathomimetic agents, e.g. adrenaline, may counteract the effect of beta-blockers.

Concomitant use with insulin and oral antidiabetic drugs may lead to the intensification of the blood sugar lowering effects of these drugs. Symptoms of hypoglycaemia, particularly tachycardia, may be masked (See Section 4.4).

Concomitant use of prostaglandin synthetase inhibiting drugs (e.g. ibuprofen and indomethacin), may decrease the hypotensive effects of beta-blockers.

Caution must be exercised when using anaesthetic agents with Tenormin. The anaesthetist should be informed and the choice of anaesthetic should be an agent with as little negative inotropic activity as possible. Use of beta-blockers with anaesthetic drugs may result in attenuation of the reflex tachycardia and increase the risk of hypotension. Anaesthetic agents causing myocardial depression are best avoided.

4.6 Pregnancy and lactation

Tenormin crosses the placental barrier and appears in the cord blood. No studies have been performed on the use of Tenormin in the first trimester and the possibility of foetal injury cannot be excluded. Tenormin has been used under close supervision for the treatment of hypertension in the third trimester. Administration of Tenormin to pregnant women in the management of mild to moderate hypertension has been associated with intra-uterine growth retardation.

The use of Tenormin in women who are, or may become, pregnant requires that the anticipated benefit be weighed against the possible risks, particularly in the first and second trimesters, since beta-blockers, in general, have been associated with a decrease in placental perfusion which may result in intra-uterine deaths, immature and premature deliveries.

There is significant accumulation of Tenormin in breast milk.

Neonates born to mothers who are receiving Tenormin at parturition or breast-feeding may be at risk of hypoglycaemia and bradycardia.

Caution should be exercised when Tenormin is administered during pregnancy or to a woman who is breast-feeding.

4.7 Effects on ability to drive and use machines

Use is unlikely to result in any impairment of the ability of patients to drive or operate machinery. However, it should be taken into account that occasionally dizziness or fatigue may occur.

4.8 Undesirable effects

Tenormin is well tolerated. In clinical studies, the undesired events reported are usually attributable to the pharmacological actions of atenolol.

The following undesired events, listed by body system, have been reported.

Cardiovascular: bradycardia; heart failure deterioration; postural hypotension which may be associated with syncope; cold extremities. In susceptible patients: precipitation of heart block; intermittent claudication; Raynaud's phenomenon.

CNS: confusion; dizziness; headache; mood changes; nightmares; psychoses and hallucinations; sleep disturbances of the type noted with other beta-blockers.

Gastrointestinal: dry mouth; gastrointestinal disturbances. Elevations of transaminase levels have been seen infrequently, rare cases of hepatic toxicity, including intrahepatic cholestasis have been reported.

Haematological: purpura; thrombocytopenia.

Integumentary: alopecia; dry eyes; psoriasiform skin reactions; exacerbation of psoriasis; skin rashes.

Neurological: paraesthesia.

Reproductive: impotence

Respiratory: bronchospasm may occur in patients with bronchial asthma or a history of asthmatic complaints.

Special senses: visual disturbances.

Others: hypersensitivity reactions, including angioedema and urticaria; fatigue; an increase in ANA (Antinuclear Antibodies) has been observed, however, the clinical relevance of this is not clear.

Discontinuance of the drug should be considered if, according to clinical judgement, the well-being of the patient is adversely affected by any of the above reactions.

4.9 Overdose

The symptoms of overdosage may include bradycardia, hypotension, acute cardiac insufficiency and bronchospasm.

General treatment should include: close supervision, treatment in an intensive care ward, the use of gastric lavage, activated charcoal and a laxative to prevent absorption of any drug still present in the gastrointestinal tract, the use of plasma or plasma substitutes to treat hypotension and shock. The use of haemodialysis or haemoperfusion may be considered.

Excessive bradycardia can be countered with atropine 1-2 mg intravenously and/or a cardiac pacemaker. If necessary, this may be followed by a bolus dose of glucagon 10 mg intravenously. If required, this may be repeated or followed by an intravenous infusion of glucagon 1-10 mg/hour depending on response. If no response to glucagon occurs or if glucagon is unavailable, a beta-adrenoceptor stimulant such as dobutamine 2.5 to 10 micrograms/kg/minute by intravenous infusion may be given. Dobutamine, because of its positive inotropic effect could also be used to treat hypotension and acute cardiac insufficiency. It is likely that these doses would be inadequate to reverse the cardiac effects of beta-blocker blockade if a large overdose has been taken. The dose of dobutamine should therefore be increased if necessary to achieve the required response according to the clinical condition of the patient.

Bronchospasm can usually be reversed by bronchodilators.

5. PHARMACOLOGICAL PROPERTIES

5.1 Pharmacodynamic properties

Beta blocking agents, plain, selective

CO7 B03

Atenolol is a beta-blocker which is $beta_1$-selective, (i.e. acts preferentially on $beta_1$-adrenergic receptors in the heart). Selectivity decreases with increasing dose.

Atenolol is without intrinsic sympathomimetic and membrane stabilising activities and as with other beta-blockers, has negative inotropic effects (and is therefore contraindicated in uncontrolled heart failure).

As with other beta-blockers, the mode of action of atenolol in the treatment of hypertension is unclear.

It is probably the action of atenolol in reducing cardiac rate and contractility which makes it effective in eliminating or reducing the symptoms of patients with angina.

It is unlikely that any additional ancillary properties possessed by S (-) atenolol, in comparison with the racemic mixture, will give rise to different therapeutic effects.

Tenormin is effective and well-tolerated in most ethnic populations although the response may be less in black patients.

Tenormin is effective for at least 24 hours after once daily dosing with 10 ml or 20 ml Tenormin syrup. Tenormin syrup facilitates compliance by its acceptability to patients and the once daily dosing regimen. The narrow dose range and early patient response ensure that the effect of the drug in individual patients is quickly demonstrated. Tenormin is compatible with diuretics, other hypotensive agents and antianginals (see Section 4.5). Since it acts preferentially on beta-adrenergic receptors in the heart, Tenormin may, with care, be used successfully in the treatment of patients with respiratory disease, who cannot tolerate non-selective beta-blockers.

Early intervention with Tenormin in acute myocardial infarction reduces infarct size and decreases morbidity and mortality. Fewer patients with a threatened infarction progress to frank infarction; the incidence of ventricular arrhythmias is decreased and marked pain relief may result in reduced need of opiate analgesics. Early mortality is decreased. Tenormin is an additional treatment to standard coronary care.

5.2 Pharmacokinetic properties

Absorption of atenolol following oral dosing is consistent but incomplete (approximately 40-50%) with peak plasma concentrations occurring 2-4 hours after dosing. The atenolol blood levels are consistent and subject to little variability. There is no significant hepatic metabolism of atenolol and more than 90% of that absorbed reaches the systemic circulation unaltered. The plasma half-life is about 6 hours but this may rise in severe renal impairment since the kidney is the major route of elimination. Atenolol penetrates tissues poorly due to its low lipid solubility and its concentration in brain tissue is low. Plasma protein binding is low (approximately 3%).

5.3 Preclinical safety data

Atenolol is a drug on which extensive clinical experience has been obtained. Relevant information for the prescriber is provided elsewhere in the Summary of Product Characteristics.

6. PHARMACEUTICAL PARTICULARS

6.1 List of excipients

Citric acid

Lemon and lime flavour

Methyl hydroxybenzoate

Propyl hydroxybenzoate

Purified water

Saccharin sodium

Sodium citrate

Sorbitol solution

6.2 Incompatibilities

Not applicable.

6.3 Shelf life

36 months

6.4 Special precautions for storage

Do not store above 25°C.

Store in the original container.

6.5 Nature and contents of container

Amber coloured PET bottles with white polypropylene screw caps containing 300 ml.

6.6 Instructions for use and handling

Not applicable.

7. MARKETING AUTHORISATION HOLDER

AstraZeneca UK Limited,

600 Capability Green,

Luton, LU1 3LU, UK.

8. MARKETING AUTHORISATION NUMBER(S)

PL.17901/0051

9. DATE OF FIRST AUTHORISATION/RENEWAL OF THE AUTHORISATION

01 June 2000 / 31 October 2003

10. DATE OF REVISION OF THE TEXT

31 October 2003

Tensipine MR 10

(Genus Pharmaceuticals)

1. NAME OF THE MEDICINAL PRODUCT

Tensipine MR 10

2. QUALITATIVE AND QUANTITATIVE COMPOSITION

Tensipine MR 10 tablets: Pink-grey lacquered modified release tablets each containing 10mg nifedipine, one side marked TMR and the reverse side marked 10.

3. PHARMACEUTICAL FORM

Modified release tablets for oral administration.

4. CLINICAL PARTICULARS

4.1 Therapeutic indications

For the prophylaxis of chronic stable angina pectoris and the treatment of hypertension.

4.2 Posology and method of administration

Adults

The recommended starting dose of Tensipine MR is 10mg every 12 hours swallowed with water with subsequent titration of dosage according to response. The dose may be adjusted to 40mg every 12 hours.

Tensipine MR 10 permits titration of initial dosage. The recommended dose is one Tensipine MR 10 tablet (10mg) every 12 hours.

Nifedipine is metabolised primarily by the liver and therefore patients with liver dysfunction should be carefully monitored.

Patients with renal impairment should not require adjustment of dosage.

Elderly patients

The pharmacokinetics of nifedipine are altered in the elderly so that lower maintenance doses of nifedipine may be required compared to younger patients.

Children

Nifedipine is not recommended for use in children.

Treatment may be continued indefinitely.

4.3 Contraindications

Tensipine MR should not be administered to patients with known hypersensitivity to nifedipine or other dihydropyridines because of the theoretical risk of cross-reaction, to women capable of child-bearing or to nursing mothers.

Tensipine MR should not be used in cardiogenic shock, clinically significant aortic stenosis, unstable angina, or during or within one month of a myocardial infarction.

Tensipine MR should not be used for the treatment of acute attacks of angina.

The safety of Tensipine MR in malignant hypertension has not been established.

Tensipine MR should not be used for secondary prevention of myocardial infarction.

Tensipine MR should not be administered concomitantly with rifampicin since effective plasma levels of nifedipine may not be achieved owing to enzyme induction.

4.4 Special warnings and special precautions for use

Tensipine MR is not a beta-blocker and therefore gives no protection against the dangers of abrupt beta-blocker withdrawal; any such withdrawal should be by gradual reduction of the dose of beta-blocker preferably over 8 - 10 days.

Tensipine MR may be used in combination with beta-blocking drugs and other antihypertensive agents but the possibility of an additive effect resulting in postural hypotension should be borne in mind. Tensipine MR will not prevent possible rebound effects after cessation of other antihypertensive therapy.

Tensipine MR should be used with caution in patients whose cardiac reserve is poor. Deterioration of heart failure has occasionally been observed with nifedipine.

Caution should be exercised in patients with severe hypotension.

Diabetic patients taking Tensipine MR may require adjustment of their control.

In dialysis patients with malignant hypertension and hypovolaemia, a marked decrease in blood pressure can occur.

4.5 Interaction with other medicinal products and other forms of Interaction

The antihypertensive effect of Tensipine MR may be potentiated by simultaneous administration of cimetidine.

When used in combination with nifedipine, serum quinidine levels have been shown to be suppressed regardless of dosage of quinidine.

The simultaneous administration of nifedipine and digoxin may lead to reduced digoxin clearance and hence an increase in the plasma digoxin level. Plasma digoxin levels should be monitored and, if necessary, the digoxin dose reduced.

Diltiazem decreases the clearance of nifedipine and hence increases plasma nifedipine levels. Therefore, caution should be taken when both drugs are used in combination and a reduction of the nifedipine dose may be necessary.

Nifedipine may increase the spectrophotometric values of urinary vanillylmandelic acid falsely. However, HPLC measurements are unaffected.

Rifampicin interacts with nifedipine (see Contra-indications).

As with other dihydropyridines, nifedipine should not be taken with grapefruit juice because bioavailability is increased.

4.6 Pregnancy and lactation

Tensipine MR is contra-indicated in women capable of child-bearing and nursing mothers.

4.7 Effects on ability to drive and use machines

None known.

4.8 Undesirable effects

Ischaemic pain has been reported in a small proportion of patients within one to four hours of the introduction of Tensipine MR therapy. Although a "steal" effect has not been demonstrated, patients experiencing this effect should discontinue Tensipine MR.

Most side-effects are consequences of the vasodilatory effects of nifedipine. Headache, flushing, tachycardia and palpitations may occur, most commonly in the early stages of treatment with nifedipine. Gravitational oedema not associated with heart failure or weight gain may also occur.

Paraesthesia, dizziness, lethargy and gastro-intestinal symptoms such as nausea and altered bowel habit occur occasionally.

There are reports of skin reactions such as rash, pruritus and urticaria.

Other less frequently reported side-effects include myalgia, tremor and visual disturbances.

Impotence may occur rarely.

Increased frequency of micturition may occur.

There are reports of gingival hyperplasia and, in older men on long-term therapy, gynaecomastia, which usually regress upon withdrawal of therapy.

Mood changes may occur rarely.

Side-effects which may occur in isolated cases are photosensitivity, exfoliative dermatitis, systemic allergic reactions and purpura. Usually, these regress after discontinuation of the drug.

Rare cases of hypersensitivity-type jaundice have been reported. In addition, disturbances of liver function such as intra-hepatic cholestasis may occur. These regress after discontinuation of therapy.

As with other sustained release dihydropyridines, exacerbation of angina pectoris may occur rarely at the start of treatment. The occurrence of myocardial infarction has been described although it is not possible to distinguish such an event from the natural course of ischaemic heart disease.

4.9 Overdose

Clinical effects

Reports of nifedipine overdosage are limited and symptoms are not necessarily dose-related. Severe hypotension due to vasodilatation, and tachycardia or bradycardia are the most likely manifestations of overdose.

Metabolic disturbances include hyperglycaemia, metabolic acidosis and hypo- or hyperkalaemia.

Cardiac effects may include heart block, AV dissociation and asystole, and cardiogenic shock with pulmonary oedema.

Other toxic effects include nausea, vomiting, drowsiness, dizziness, confusion, lethargy, flushing, hypoxia and unconsciousness to the point of coma.

Treatment

As far as treatment is concerned, elimination of nifedipine and the restoration of stable cardiovascular conditions have priority.

After oral ingestion, gastric lavage is indicated, if necessary in combination with irrigation of the small intestine. Ipecacuanha should be given to children.

Elimination must be as complete as possible, including the small intestine, to prevent the otherwise inevitable subsequent absorption of the active substance. Activated charcoal should be given in 4-hourly doses of 25g for adults, 10g for children.

Blood pressure, ECG, central arterial pressure, pulmonary wedge pressure, urea and electrolytes should be monitored.

Hypotension as a result of cardiogenic shock and arterial vasodilatation should be treated with elevation of the feet and plasma expanders. If these measures are ineffective, hypotension may be treated with 10% calcium gluconate 10 - 20ml intravenously over 5 - 10 minutes. If the effects are inadequate, the treatment can be continued, with ECG monitoring. In addition, beta-sympathomimetics may be given, e.g. isoprenaline 0.2mg slowly i.v. or as a continuous infusion of 5μg/min. If an insufficient increase in blood pressure is achieved with calcium and isoprenaline, vasoconstricting sympathomimetics such as dopamine or noradrenaline should be administered. The dosage of these drugs should be determined by the patient's response.

Bradycardia may be treated with atropine, beta-sympathomimetics or a temporary cardiac pacemaker, as required.

Additional fluids should be administered with caution to avoid cardiac overload.

5. PHARMACOLOGICAL PROPERTIES

5.1 Pharmacodynamic properties

Mode of action

Nifedipine is a specific and potent calcium antagonist. In hypertension, the main action of Tensipine MR is to cause peripheral vasodilatation and thus reduce peripheral resistance.

In angina, Tensipine MR reduces peripheral and coronary vascular resistance, leading to an increase in coronary blood flow, cardiac output and stroke volume, whilst decreasing after-load.

Additionally, nifedipine dilates submaximally both clear and atherosclerotic coronary arteries, thus protecting the heart against coronary artery spasm and improving perfusion to the ischaemic myocardium.

Nifedipine reduces the frequency of painful attacks and the ischaemic ECG changes irrespective of the relative contribution from coronary artery spasm or atherosclerosis.

Tensipine MR administered twice-daily provides 24-hour control of raised blood pressure. Tensipine MR causes reduction in blood pressure such that the percentage lowering is directly related to its initial level. In normotensive individuals, Tensipine MR has little or no effect on blood pressure.

5.2 Pharmacokinetic properties

Nifedipine is absorbed almost completely from the gastro-intestinal tract regardless of the oral formulation used and undergoes extensive metabolism in the liver to inactive metabolites, with less than 1% of the parent drug appearing unchanged in the urine. The rate of absorption determines the drug's apparent elimination. The terminal elimination half-life of the modified release formulation is 6 - 11 hours.

After enteral or intravenous doses, 70 - 80% of activity is eliminated (primarily as metabolites) via the urine. Remaining excretion is via the faeces.

After 24 hours, 90% of the administered dose is eliminated.

Protein binding of nifedipine exceeds 90% in human serum.

5.3 Preclinical safety data

Reproduction toxicology

Nifedipine administration has been associated with a variety of embryotoxic, placentotoxic and fetotoxic effects in rats, mice and rabbits. All of the doses associated with the teratogenic, embryotoxic or fetotoxic effects in animals were maternally toxic and several times the recommended maximum dose for humans.

6. PHARMACEUTICAL PARTICULARS

6.1 List of excipients

Tensipine MR tablets contain the following excipients:

Microcrystalline cellulose, maize starch, lactose, polysorbate 80, magnesium stearate, hydroxypropyl methylcellulose, polyethylene glycol 4000, iron oxide red and titanium dioxide.

6.2 Incompatibilities

Not applicable.

6.3 Shelf life

PVC blister strips: 48 months

PP blister strips: 30 months

6.4 Special precautions for storage

The tablets should be protected from strong light and stored in the manufacturer's original container.

6.5 Nature and contents of container

Tensipine MR 10 tablets: blister strips of 14 tablets in a cardboard outer container, packs of 56 tablets.

Blister strips are composed of red polypropylene foil (0.3mm) with aluminium backing foil (0.02mm) or red PVC foil (0.3mm) with aluminium backing foil (0.02mm).

6.6 Instructions for use and handling

No additional information.

7. MARKETING AUTHORISATION HOLDER

Genus Pharmaceuticals Limited

T/A Genus Pharmaceuticals

Benham Valence

Newbury

Berkshire RG20 8LU

8. MARKETING AUTHORISATION NUMBER(S)

PL 06831/0048

9. DATE OF FIRST AUTHORISATION/RENEWAL OF THE AUTHORISATION

22 April 1996

10. DATE OF REVISION OF THE TEXT

24 November 2004

POM

Tensipine MR 20

(Genus Pharmaceuticals)

1. NAME OF THE MEDICINAL PRODUCT

Tensipine MR 20

2. QUALITATIVE AND QUANTITATIVE COMPOSITION

Tensipine MR 20 tablets: Pink-grey lacquered modified release tablets each containing 20mg nifedipine, one side marked TMR and the reverse side marked 20.

3. PHARMACEUTICAL FORM

Modified release tablets for oral administration.

4. CLINICAL PARTICULARS

4.1 Therapeutic indications

For the prophylaxis of chronic stable angina pectoris and the treatment of hypertension.

4.2 Posology and method of administration

Adults

The recommended starting dose of Tensipine MR is 10mg every 12 hours swallowed with water with subsequent titration of dosage according to response. The dose may be adjusted to 40mg every 12 hours.

Tensipine MR 10 permits titration of initial dosage. The recommended dose is one Tensipine MR 10 tablet (10mg) every 12 hours.

Nifedipine is metabolised primarily by the liver and therefore patients with liver dysfunction should be carefully monitored.

Patients with renal impairment should not require adjustment of dosage.

Elderly patients

The pharmacokinetics of nifedipine are altered in the elderly so that lower maintenance doses of nifedipine may be required compared to younger patients.

Children

Nifedipine is not recommended for use in children.

Treatment may be continued indefinitely.

4.3 Contraindications

Tensipine MR should not be administered to patients with known hypersensitivity to nifedipine or other dihydropyridines because of the theoretical risk of cross-reaction, to women capable of child-bearing or to nursing mothers.

Tensipine MR should not be used in cardiogenic shock, clinically significant aortic stenosis, unstable angina, or during or within one month of a myocardial infarction.

Tensipine MR should not be used for the treatment of acute attacks of angina.

The safety of Tensipine MR in malignant hypertension has not been established.

Tensipine MR should not be used for secondary prevention of myocardial infarction.

Tensipine MR should not be administered concomitantly with rifampicin since effective plasma levels of nifedipine may not be achieved owing to enzyme induction.

4.4 Special warnings and special precautions for use

Tensipine MR is not a beta-blocker and therefore gives no protection against the dangers of abrupt beta-blocker withdrawal; any such withdrawal should be by gradual reduction of the dose of beta-blocker preferably over 8 - 10 days.

Tensipine MR may be used in combination with beta-blocking drugs and other antihypertensive agents but the possibility of an additive effect resulting in postural hypotension should be borne in mind. Tensipine MR will not prevent possible rebound effects after cessation of other antihypertensive therapy.

Tensipine MR should be used with caution in patients whose cardiac reserve is poor. Deterioration of heart failure has occasionally been observed with nifedipine.

Caution should be exercised in patients with severe hypotension.

Diabetic patients taking Tensipine MR may require adjustment of their control.

In dialysis patients with malignant hypertension and hypovolaemia, a marked decrease in blood pressure can occur.

4.5 Interaction with other medicinal products and other forms of Interaction

The antihypertensive effect of Tensipine MR may be potentiated by simultaneous administration of cimetidine.

When used in combination with nifedipine, serum quinidine levels have been shown to be suppressed regardless of dosage of quinidine.

The simultaneous administration of nifedipine and digoxin may lead to reduced digoxin clearance and hence an increase in the plasma digoxin level. Plasma digoxin levels should be monitored and, if necessary, the digoxin dose reduced.

Diltiazem decreases the clearance of nifedipine and hence increases plasma nifedipine levels. Therefore, caution should be taken when both drugs are used in combination and a reduction of the nifedipine dose may be necessary.

Nifedipine may increase the spectrophotometric values of urinary vanillylmandelic acid falsely. However, HPLC measurements are unaffected.

Rifampicin interacts with nifedipine (see Contra-indications).

As with other dihydropyridines, nifedipine should not be taken with grapefruit juice because bioavailability is increased.

4.6 Pregnancy and lactation

Tensipine MR is contra-indicated in women capable of child-bearing and nursing mothers.

4.7 Effects on ability to drive and use machines

None known.

4.8 Undesirable effects

Ischaemic pain has been reported in a small proportion of patients within one to four hours of the introduction of Tensipine MR therapy. Although a "steal" effect has not been demonstrated, patients experiencing this effect should discontinue Tensipine MR.

Most side-effects are consequences of the vasodilatory effects of nifedipine. Headache, flushing, tachycardia and palpitations may occur, most commonly in the early stages of treatment with nifedipine. Gravitational oedema not associated with heart failure or weight gain may also occur.

Paraesthesia, dizziness, lethargy and gastro-intestinal symptoms such as nausea and altered bowel habit occur occasionally.

There are reports of skin reactions such as rash, pruritus and urticaria.

Other less frequently reported side-effects include myalgia, tremor and visual disturbances.

Impotence may occur rarely.

Increased frequency of micturition may occur.

There are reports of gingival hyperplasia and, in older men on long-term therapy, gynaecomastia, which usually regress upon withdrawal of therapy.

Mood changes may occur rarely.

Side-effects which may occur in isolated cases are photosensitivity, exfoliative dermatitis, systemic allergic reactions and purpura. Usually, these regress after discontinuation of the drug.

Rare cases of hypersensitivity-type jaundice have been reported. In addition, disturbances of liver function such as intra-hepatic cholestasis may occur. These regress after discontinuation of therapy.

As with other sustained release dihydropyridines, exacerbation of angina pectoris may occur rarely at the start of treatment. The occurrence of myocardial infarction has been described although it is not possible to distinguish such an event from the natural course of ischaemic heart disease.

4.9 Overdose

Clinical effects

Reports of nifedipine overdosage are limited and symptoms are not necessarily dose-related. Severe hypotension due to vasodilatation, and tachycardia or bradycardia are the most likely manifestations of overdose.

Metabolic disturbances include hyperglycaemia, metabolic acidosis and hypo- or hyperkalaemia.

Cardiac effects may include heart block, AV dissociation and asystole, and cardiogenic shock with pulmonary oedema.

Other toxic effects include nausea, vomiting, drowsiness, dizziness, confusion, lethargy, flushing, hypoxia and unconsciousness to the point of coma.

Treatment

As far as treatment is concerned, elimination of nifedipine and the restoration of stable cardiovascular conditions have priority.

After oral ingestion, gastric lavage is indicated, if necessary in combination with irrigation of the small intestine. Ipecacuanha should be given to children.

Elimination must be as complete as possible, including the small intestine, to prevent the otherwise inevitable subsequent absorption of the active substance. Activated charcoal should be given in 4-hourly doses of 25g for adults, 10g for children.

Blood pressure, ECG, central arterial pressure, pulmonary wedge pressure, urea and electrolytes should be monitored.

Hypotension as a result of cardiogenic shock and arterial vasodilatation should be treated with elevation of the feet and plasma expanders. If these measures are ineffective, hypotension may be treated with 10% calcium gluconate 10 - 20ml intravenously over 5 - 10 minutes. If the effects are inadequate, the treatment can be continued, with ECG monitoring. In addition, beta-sympathomimetics may be given, e.g. isoprenaline 0.2mg slowly i.v. or as a continuous infusion of 5μg/min. If an insufficient increase in blood pressure is achieved with calcium and isoprenaline, vasoconstricting sympathomimetics such as dopamine or noradrenaline should be administered. The dosage of these drugs should be determined by the patient's response.

Bradycardia may be treated with atropine, beta-sympathomimetics or a temporary cardiac pacemaker, as required.

Additional fluids should be administered with caution to avoid cardiac overload.

5. PHARMACOLOGICAL PROPERTIES

5.1 Pharmacodynamic properties

Mode of action

Nifedipine is a specific and potent calcium antagonist. In hypertension, the main action of Tensipine MR is to cause peripheral vasodilatation and thus reduce peripheral resistance.

In angina, Tensipine MR reduces peripheral and coronary vascular resistance, leading to an increase in coronary blood flow, cardiac output and stroke volume, whilst decreasing after-load.

Additionally, nifedipine dilates submaximally both clear and atherosclerotic coronary arteries, thus protecting the heart against coronary artery spasm and improving perfusion to the ischaemic myocardium.

Nifedipine reduces the frequency of painful attacks and the ischaemic ECG changes irrespective of the relative contribution from coronary artery spasm or atherosclerosis.

Tensipine MR administered twice-daily provides 24-hour control of raised blood pressure. Tensipine MR causes reduction in blood pressure such that the percentage lowering is directly related to its initial level. In normotensive individuals, Tensipine MR has little or no effect on blood pressure.

5.2 Pharmacokinetic properties

Nifedipine is absorbed almost completely from the gastro-intestinal tract regardless of the oral formulation used and undergoes extensive metabolism in the liver to inactive metabolites, with less than 1% of the parent drug appearing unchanged in the urine. The rate of absorption determines the drug's apparent elimination. The terminal elimination half-life of the modified release formulation is 6 - 11 hours.

After enteral or intravenous doses, 70 - 80% of activity is eliminated (primarily as metabolites) via the urine. Remaining excretion is via the faeces.

After 24 hours, 90% of the administered dose is eliminated.

Protein binding of nifedipine exceeds 90% in human serum.

5.3 Preclinical safety data

Reproduction toxicology

Nifedipine administration has been associated with a variety of embryotoxic, placentotoxic and fetotoxic effects in rats, mice and rabbits. All of the doses associated with the teratogenic, embryotoxic or fetotoxic effects in animals were maternally toxic and several times the recommended maximum dose for humans.

6. PHARMACEUTICAL PARTICULARS

6.1 List of excipients

Tensipine MR tablets contain the following excipients:

Microcrystalline cellulose, maize starch, lactose, polysorbate 80, magnesium stearate, hydroxypropyl methylcellulose, polyethylene glycol 4000, iron oxide red and titanium dioxide.

6.2 Incompatibilities

Not applicable.

6.3 Shelf life

PVC blister strips: 48 months

PP blister strips: 30 months

6.4 Special precautions for storage

The tablets should be protected from strong light and stored in the manufacturer's original container.

6.5 Nature and contents of container

Tensipine MR 20 tablets: blister strips of 14 tablets in a cardboard outer container, packs of 56 tablets.

Blister strips are composed of red polypropylene foil (0.3mm) with aluminium backing foil (0.02mm) or red PVC foil (0.3mm) with aluminium backing foil (0.02mm).

6.6 Instructions for use and handling

No additional information.

7. MARKETING AUTHORISATION HOLDER

Genus Pharmaceuticals Limited

T/A Genus Pharmaceuticals

Benham Valence

Newbury

Berkshire RG20 8LU

8. MARKETING AUTHORISATION NUMBER(S)

PL 06831/0049

9. DATE OF FIRST AUTHORISATION/RENEWAL OF THE AUTHORISATION

22 April 1996

10. DATE OF REVISION OF THE TEXT

24 November 2004

POM

Teoptic 1% Eye Drops, Teoptic 2% Eye Drops

(Novartis Pharmaceuticals UK Ltd)

1. NAME OF THE MEDICINAL PRODUCT

Teoptic® 1% Eye Drops

Teoptic® 2% Eye Drops

2. QUALITATIVE AND QUANTITATIVE COMPOSITION

Carteolol hydrochloride 1%

Carteolol hydrochloride 2%.

3. PHARMACEUTICAL FORM

Eye Drops

4. CLINICAL PARTICULARS

4.1 Therapeutic indications

For the reduction of intraocular pressure e.g. in ocular hypertension, chronic open angle glaucoma, some secondary glaucomas.

4.2 Posology and method of administration

Adults including the elderly:

Initially one drop of 1% eye drops instilled twice daily in each affected eye. If the clinical response is not adequate the dosage may be altered to one drop of 2% eye drops twice daily in each affected eye.

Children:

Not recommended for use in children.

4.3 Contraindications

- Unsatisfactorily controlled cardiac insufficiency
- Bronchospasm including bronchial asthma or chronic obstructive pulmonary disease
- Hypersensitivity to any of the components of the formulation.

As with all ophthalmic preparations containing benzalkonium chloride, soft contact lenses (hydrophilic lenses) should not be worn during treatment with Teoptic Eye Drops.

4.4 Special warnings and special precautions for use

Unlike miotics, Teoptic Eye Drops reduce intraocular pressure without altering accommodation or pupil diameter. A slight increase in pupil diameter may be noted, however, if patients are transferred from miotic therapy to Teoptic Eye Drops.

4.5 Interaction with other medicinal products and other forms of Interaction

As with other topically applied ophthalmic preparations Teoptic Eye Drops may be absorbed systemically. Teoptic Eye Drops should, therefore, be used with caution in patients receiving systemic beta-adrenergic-receptor blocking therapy and in patients with known contra-indications to systemic beta-blockers, e.g. sinus bradycardia, second and third degree atrio-ventricular block, cardiogenic shock, right ventricular insufficiency due to pulmonary hypertension and congestive heart failure, unsatisfactorily controlled diabetes mellitus.

Teoptic Eye Drops may, if necessary be used in association with pilocarpine, adrenaline, carbachol and carbonic anhydrase inhibitors.

4.6 Pregnancy and lactation

Teoptic Eye Drops have not been studied in human pregnancy and lactation. Use during pregnancy is therefore contraindicated. In animal studies, orally administered carteolol has been shown to penetrate the breast milk and the use of Teoptic Eye Drops in lactating mothers should, therefore, be at the discretion of the physician.

4.7 Effects on ability to drive and use machines

None known.

4.8 Undesirable effects

Local ocular reactions such as irritation, burning, itching and pain, blurred vision, photophobia, xerosis, conjunctival hyperaemia, conjunctival discharge and corneal disorders such as diffuse superficial keratitis may occasionally develop. As with all beta-blocking agents, bradycardia, bronchospasm, rashes, dyspnoea, headache, lassitude and vertigo have occasionally been reported.

4.9 Overdose

There is no experience of overdosage with Teoptic Eye Drops. However, potential symptoms (typical of beta-blocking agents) which may occur after accidental oral ingestion include bradycardia, severe hypotension, acute cardiac failure, bronchospasm, hypoglycaemia, delirium and unconsciousness. Initially treatment should be by removal of any unabsorbed drug (e.g. gastric lavage) and general supportive measures, i.e. marked bradycardia should be treated in the first instance by intravenous atropine sulphate at a dose of 0.5 - 2.0 mg depending on severity; intravenous glucagon and cardiac pacemakers may be required in more severe cases; bronchospasm should be treated with appropriate bronchodilators, including beta$_2$-agonists and aminophylline where necessary. Patients should be monitored for several days as the beta-blocking effects of Teoptic may exceed its plasma half-life.

5. PHARMACOLOGICAL PROPERTIES

5.1 Pharmacodynamic properties

Carteolol hydrochloride is a beta-adrenergic receptor blocking agent with intrinsic sympathomimetic activity. It has no local anaesthetic effect.

5.2 Pharmacokinetic properties

The distribution of radioactivity was studied in New Zealand white rabbits after the instillation in one eye of ^{14}C carteolol hydrochloride. The maximum levels of radioactivity were recorded on the ocular tissues and in the plasma 30 minutes to 1 hour after instillation and then declined rapidly. The highest concentrations were found in the cornea, iris, anterior sclera, ciliary body, conjunctiva, nictitating membrane and extraocular muscle. Moderate concentrations were found in the aqueous humor, posterior sclera, retina, choroid and optic nerve. Low concentrations in the lens, vitreous humor and plasma. The concentrations of radioactivity varied dose-dependently and the elimination rate from each tissue was similar. 8 hours after instillation the levels in all tissues had fallen to 5-10% of the maximum tissue concentrations.

In the tissues of the untreated eyes, the concentrations of radioactivity were generally less than 10% of those in the treated eyes. Most of the radioactivity in the aqueous humor of the treated eyes was due to unchanged carteolol, whereas that in the aqueous humor of the untreated eyes and in the plasma was due predominantly to its metabolites.

6. PHARMACEUTICAL PARTICULARS

6.1 List of excipients

Teoptic 1%:

benzalkonium chloride 0.005 %

sodium chloride 0.7 %

sodium phosphate dibasic 0.1 %

sodium phosphate monobasic 0.04 %

water for injection to 100 %

Teoptic 2%:

benzalkonium chloride 0.005 %

sodium chloride 0.54 %

sodium phosphate dibasic 0.1 %

sodium phosphate monobasic 0.04 %

water for injection to 100 %

6.2 Incompatibilities

None known

6.3 Shelf life

Unopened: 36 months

Opened: 28 days

6.4 Special precautions for storage

Do not store above 25°C.

Do not use later than one month after first breaking the seal.

6.5 Nature and contents of container

1 X 5ml polyethylene dropper bottle

3 X 5ml polyethylene dropper bottle

6.6 Instructions for use and handling

None stated

7. MARKETING AUTHORISATION HOLDER

Novartis Pharmaceuticals UK Ltd

Frimley Business Park

Frimley

Camberley

Surrey

GU16 7SR

United Kingdom

8. MARKETING AUTHORISATION NUMBER(S)

Teoptic 1% - PL 00101/0603

Teoptic 2% - PL 00101/0604

9. DATE OF FIRST AUTHORISATION/RENEWAL OF THE AUTHORISATION

6 December 2001

10. DATE OF REVISION OF THE TEXT

14 January 2002

LEGAL CATEGORY

POM

Terra-Cortril Topical Ointment

(Pfizer Limited)

1. NAME OF THE MEDICINAL PRODUCT
TERRA-CORTRIL®

2. QUALITATIVE AND QUANTITATIVE COMPOSITION
Each gram of Terra-Cortril Ointment contains 30mg oxytetracycline as oxytetracycline hydrochloride Ph Eur and 10mg hydrocortisone Ph. Eur.

3. PHARMACEUTICAL FORM
Ointment for topical administration.

4. CLINICAL PARTICULARS
4.1 Therapeutic indications
Terra-Cortril Ointment is indicated in the following disorders: exudative and secondarily infected eczema including atopic eczema, primary irritant dermatitis, allergic and seborrhoeic dermatitis. Secondarily infected insect bite reactions.

In exudative flexural intertrigo Terra-Cortril Ointment can be used for up to seven days.

Like other tetracyclines, oxytetracycline is generally ineffective against Pseudomonas and Proteus species. Because these are recognised secondary infecting organisms in exudative dermatoses, preliminary identification of the organism and determination of antibiotic sensitivity is important.

4.2 Posology and method of administration
After thorough cleansing of the affected skin areas, a small amount of the ointment should be applied gently. Applications should be made two to four times daily.

Terra-Cortril Ointment is for topical administration only.

Use in the elderly No special precautions.

Use in children Not recommended. (See 'Contra-indications').

Use in renal or hepatic impairment No special precautions.

4.3 Contraindications
Hypersensitivity to one of the components of the preparation.

Primary bacterial infections eg impetigo, pyoderma, furunculosis.

Pregnancy, lactation and in infants and small children because of the theoretical risk of damage to permanent dentition.

4.4 Special warnings and special precautions for use
Terra-Cortril Ointment should not be continued for more than seven days in the absence of any clinical improvement, since in this situation occult extension of infection may occur due to the masking effect of the steroid.

Extended or recurrent application may increase the risk of contact sensitization and should be avoided.

The use of oxytetracycline and other antibiotics may result in an overgrowth of resistant organisms - particularly Candida and staphylococci. Careful observation of the patient for this possibility is essential. If new infections due to nonsusceptible bacteria of fungi appear during therapy, Ointment should be discontinued. If extensive areas are treated or if the occlusive technique is used, there may by increased systemic absorption of the corticosteroid and suitable precautions should be taken.

If irritation develops, the product should be discontinued.

Terra-Cortril Ointment is not recommended for ophthalmic use.

4.5 Interaction with other medicinal products and other forms of Interaction
None established.

4.6 Pregnancy and lactation
Terra-Cortril Ointment is contra-indicated during pregnancy and in nursing mothers, because of the theoretical risk of damage to permanent dentition.

4.7 Effects on ability to drive and use machines
Terra-Cortril Ointment is not expected to have an influence on the ability to drive or operate machinery.

4.8 Undesirable effects
Hydrocortisone and oxytetracycline are well tolerated by the epithelial tissues and may be used topically with minimal untoward effects. Allergic reactions, including contact dermatitis may occur occasionally, but are rare.

Reactions occurring most often from the presence of the anti-infective ingredients are allergic sensitisations.

The following local side effects have been reported with topical corticosteroids, especially under occlusive dressings; burning, itching, irritation, dryness, folliculitis, hypertrichosis, acneiform eruptions, hypopigmentation, perioral dermatitis, allergic contact dermatitis, maceration of the skin, secondary infection, skin atrophy, striae, miliaria.

The use of Terra-Cortril Ointment should be discontinued if such reactions occur.

Secondary infection The development of secondary bacterial or fungal infection has occurred after use of combinations containing steroids and antimicrobials.

4.9 Overdose
There is no specific antidote available. In case of overdosage, discontinue medication, treat symptomatically and institute supportive measures.

5. PHARMACOLOGICAL PROPERTIES
5.1 Pharmacodynamic properties
Terra-Cortril Ointment possesses both the anti-inflammatory activity of hydrocortisone and the broad spectrum antibacterial activity of oxytetracycline, which is active against a wide variety of Gram-positive and Gram-negative organisms.

5.2 Pharmacokinetic properties
Oxytetracycline There is no published information on the systemic absorption of oxytetracycline following dermal application.

Hydrocortisone Following topical steroid application, variable absorption has been reported especially when applied to large surfaces, under occlusive dressing or for prolonged periods of time.

5.3 Preclinical safety data

6. PHARMACEUTICAL PARTICULARS
6.1 List of excipients
Liquid paraffin Ph. Eur., white soft paraffin B.P.

6.2 Incompatibilities
None documented.

6.3 Shelf life
5 Years.

6.4 Special precautions for storage
Store below 25 °C

6.5 Nature and contents of container
Aluminium Tube with screw cap containing 15g ointment.

Aluminium Tube with screw cap containing 30g ointment.

6.6 Instructions for use and handling
None

7. MARKETING AUTHORISATION HOLDER
Pfizer Limited

Ramsgate Road

Sandwich

CT13 9NJ

United Kingdom

8. MARKETING AUTHORISATION NUMBER(S)
PL0057/5076R

9. DATE OF FIRST AUTHORISATION/RENEWAL OF THE AUTHORISATION
26 February 1997

10. DATE OF REVISION OF THE TEXT
February 1997

11. LEGAL CATEGORY
POM

Testim 50mg Gel

(Ipsen Ltd)

1. NAME OF THE MEDICINAL PRODUCT
▼Testim 50mg Gel

2. QUALITATIVE AND QUANTITATIVE COMPOSITION
One tube of 5g contains 50mg testosterone.

For excipients, see section 6.1

3. PHARMACEUTICAL FORM
Gel

A clear to translucent gel

4. CLINICAL PARTICULARS
4.1 Therapeutic indications
Testosterone replacement therapy for male hypogonadism when testosterone deficiency has been confirmed by clinical features and biochemical tests (see 4.4 Special warnings and precautions for use).

4.2 Posology and method of administration
Adults and the Elderly: The recommended starting dose of Testim is testosterone 50mg (1 tube).

Dose titration should be based on serum testosterone levels or the persistence of clinical signs and symptoms related to testosterone deficiency. To ensure proper serum testosterone levels are achieved, early morning serum testosterone should be measured before applying the next dose, approximately 7-14 days after initiation of therapy. Currently there is no consensus about age specific testosterone levels. The normal serum testosterone level for young eugonadal men is generally accepted to be approximately 300 – 1000 ng/dL (10.4 – 34.6 nmol/L). However, it should be taken into account that physiologically testosterone levels are lower with increasing age. If serum testosterone concentrations are below the normal range, the daily testosterone dose may be increased from 50mg (one tube) to 100mg (two tubes) once a day. The duration of treatment and frequency of subsequent testosterone measurements should be determined by the physician. Non-virilised patients may require treatment with one tube for a longer period of time before the dose is increased, as needed. At any time during treatment, after initial titration, the dose may need to be reduced if serum testosterone levels are raised above the upper limit of the normal range. If morning serum testosterone levels are above the normal range while applying 50mg (1 tube) of Testim, the use of Testim should be discontinued. If serum testosterone levels are below the normal limit, the dose may be increased, not exceeding 100mg per day.

Because of the variability in analytical values amongst diagnostic laboratories, all testosterone measurements should be performed at the same laboratory.

The gel should be applied once a day, at about the same time each day, to clean, dry, intact, skin of the shoulders and/or upper arms. It is preferable that the gel is applied in the morning. For patients who wash in the morning, Testim should be applied after washing, bathing or showering.

To apply the gel, patients should open one tube and squeeze the entire contents into the palm of one hand. They should then apply the gel immediately to their shoulders and/or upper arms. The gel should be spread on the skin gently as a thin layer. The gel should then be rubbed until no gel is left on the skin. This process should then be repeated with a second tube of Testim by patients who have been prescribed a daily dose of testosterone 100mg. It is suggested that patients who require two tubes of gel each day use both shoulders (one tube per shoulder) and/or upper arms as application sites. Patients should thoroughly wash their hands immediately with soap and water after Testim has been applied. After application of the gel, patients should allow the application sites to dry for a few minutes and then dress with clothing that covers the application sites.

Patients should be advised not to apply Testim to the genitals.

Children and women:
Testim is not indicated in children and has not been clinically evaluated in males under 18 years of age. For use in women, see Section 4.4 Special Warnings and Precautions for Use.

4.3 Contraindications
Androgens are contraindicated in men with carcinoma of the breast or known or suspected carcinoma of the prostate.

Testim should not be used in patients with known hypersensitivity to the active substance or to any of the excipients.

4.4 Special warnings and special precautions for use
Prior to testosterone initiation, all patients must undergo a detailed examination in order to exclude the risk of preexisting prostate cancer. Careful and regular monitoring of the breast and prostate gland must be performed in accordance with recommended methods (digital rectal examination and estimation of serum PSA) in patients receiving testosterone therapy at least once yearly and twice yearly in elderly patients and at risk patients (those with clinical or familial factors).

Androgens may accelerate the progression of sub-clinical prostate cancer and benign prostatic hyperplasia.

Care should be taken in patients with skeletal metastases due to the risk of hypercalcaemia/hypercalciuria developing from androgen therapy. In these patients, serum calcium levels should be determined regularly.

Testosterone may cause an increase in blood pressure and Testim should be used with caution in patients with hypertension.

In patients suffering from severe cardiac, hepatic or renal insufficiency, treatment with testosterone may cause severe complications characterised by oedema with or without congestive cardiac failure. In this case, treatment must be stopped immediately. In addition diuretic therapy may be required.

Testosterone should be used with caution in patients with ischaemic heart disease.

Testosterone should be used with caution in patients with epilepsy and migraine as these conditions may be aggravated.

There are published reports of increased risk of sleep apnoea in hypogonadal subjects treated with testosterone esters, especially in those with risk factors such as obesity or chronic respiratory disease.

Improved insulin sensitivity may occur in patients treated with androgens who achieve normal testosterone plasma concentrations following replacement therapy.

Certain clinical signs: irritability, nervousness, weight gain, prolonged or frequent erections may indicate excessive androgen exposure requiring dosage adjustment.

If the patient develops a severe application site reaction, treatment should be reviewed and discontinued if necessary.

The following checks should be carried out periodically; Full blood count, lipid profile and liver function tests.

To ensure proper dosing, serum testosterone concentrations should be measured (see section 4.2: Posology and method of administration).

Testim should not be used to treat non-specific symptoms suggestive of hypogonadism if testosterone deficiency has not been demonstrated and if other aetiologies responsible for the symptoms have not been excluded. Testosterone deficiency should be clearly demonstrated by clinical features and confirmed by 2 separate blood testosterone measurements before initiating therapy with any testosterone replacement, including Testim treatment.

Testim is not a treatment for male infertility or sexual dysfunction/impotence in patients without demonstrated testosterone deficiency. For the restoration of fertility in patients with hypogonadotrophic hypogonadism, therapeutic measures in addition to treatment with Testim are required.

Athletes treated for testosterone replacement in primary and secondary male hypogonadism should be advised that the product contains an active substance which may produce a positive reaction in anti-doping tests. Androgens are not suitable for enhancing muscular development in healthy individuals or for increasing physical ability.

Testim should not be used in women due to possible virilising effects.

As washing after Testim administration reduces testosterone levels, patients are advised not to wash or shower for at least 6 hours after applying Testim. When washing occurs up to six hours after the gel application, the absorption of testosterone may be reduced.

Testim contains propylene glycol, which may cause skin irritation.

The contents of each tube are flammable.

Potential for Transfer

If no precaution is taken, testosterone gel can be transferred to other persons by close skin to skin contact, resulting in increased testosterone serum levels and possibly adverse effects (e.g. growth of facial and/or body hair, deepening of the voice, irregularities of the menstrual cycle) in case of repeat contact (inadvertent androgenisation).

The physician should inform the patient carefully about the risk of testosterone transfer and about safety instructions (see below). Testim should not be prescribed in patients with a major risk of non-compliance with safety instructions (e.g. severe alcoholism, drug abuse, severe psychiatric disorders).

This transfer is avoided by wearing clothes covering the application area or showering prior to contact.

As a result, the following precautions are recommended:

For the patient:

- wash hands thoroughly with soap and water after applying the gel
- cover the application area with clothing once the gel has dried
- shower before any situation in which this type of contact is foreseen

For people not being treated with Testim

- in the event of contact with an application area which has not been washed or is not covered with clothing, wash the area of skin onto which testosterone may have been transferred as soon as possible, using soap and water.
- Report the development of signs of excessive androgen exposure such as acne or hair modification.

To guarantee partner safety, the patient should be advised for example to observe a long interval between Testim application and sexual intercourse, to wear a T-shirt covering the application site during contact period, or to shower before sexual intercourse.

Furthermore, it is recommended to wear a T-shirt covering the application site during contact periods with children in order to avoid a contamination risk of children's skin.

Pregnant women must avoid any contact with Testim application sites. In case of pregnancy of the partner, the patient must reinforce his attention to the precautions for use (see section 4.6).

4.5 Interaction with other medicinal products and other forms of Interaction

When androgens are used simultaneously with anti-coagulants, the anti-coagulant effects may be increased. Patients receiving oral anticoagulants require close monitoring, especially when androgen therapy is started or stopped.

In a published pharmacokinetic study of an injectable testosterone product, administration of testosterone cypionate led to an increased clearance of propranolol in the majority of men tested.

The concurrent administration of testosterone with ACTH or corticosteroids may enhance oedema formation; thus these drugs should be administered cautiously, particularly in patients with cardiac or hepatic disease.

Laboratory Test Interactions: Androgens may decrease levels of thyroxine-binding globulin resulting in decreased total T4 serum levels and increased resin uptake of T3 and T4. Free thyroid hormone levels remain unchanged, however, and there is no clinical evidence of thyroid dysfunction.

4.6 Pregnancy and lactation

Testim is not indicated for women and must not be used in pregnant or breastfeeding women.

Testosterone may induce virilising effects on the female foetus.

Pregnant women should avoid skin contact with Testim application sites.

In the event that unwashed or unclothed skin to which Testim has been applied does come into direct contact with the skin of a pregnant woman, the general area of contact on the woman should be washed with soap and water immediately.

4.7 Effects on ability to drive and use machines

No studies on the effects on the ability to drive and use machines have been performed.

4.8 Undesirable effects

The most frequently observed adverse drug reactions were application site erythema and increased PSA, both occurring in approximately 4% of patients.

The most commonly reported adverse events that were possibly or probably related to study drug and reported with an incidence of ⩾ 1% and ⩽ 10% in Testim treated patients in clinical trials are listed in the following table:

Organ System Class	Adverse Reaction
Vascular disorders	Worsening hypertension
Skin and subcutaneous tissue disorders	Acne
General disorders and administration site disorders	Erythema, rash, application site reaction
Investigations	PSA increased, haematocrit increased, haemoglobin increased, red blood cell count increased

Uncommonly, gynaecomastia may develop and persist in patients being treated for hypogonadism with Testim.

Other known adverse drug reactions that may be associated with testosterone treatments include prostate abnormalities and prostate cancer, pruritus, vasodilation, emotional lability, nausea, alopecia, cholestatic jaundice, generalised paresthesia, hirsutism, seborrhoea, decreased libido, anxiety, altered blood lipid levels including a reduction in HDL cholesterol, alteration in liver functions tests, and in prolonged or excessive doses, electrolyte disturbances (such as retention of sodium, chloride, potassium, calcium, inorganic phosphates and water), oligospermia and frequent and/or prolonged erections.

Patients should be instructed to report any of the following to a physician; too frequent or persistent erections of the penis; any changes in skin colour, ankle swelling or unexplained nausea or vomiting; any breathing disturbances including those associated with sleep.

4.9 Overdose

There is a single case of acute testosterone over-dosage reported in the literature. In this case, a cerebrovascular event was associated with testosterone levels of up to 395 nmol/l (11,400ng/dL). It is unlikely that such serum testosterone levels could be achieved using the transdermal route of administration.

5. PHARMACOLOGICAL PROPERTIES

5.1 Pharmacodynamic properties

Pharmacotherapeutic group: Androgens. ATC code: G03B A03.

Testosterone and dihydrotestosterone (DHT), endogenous androgens, are responsible for the normal growth and development of the male sex organs and for the maintenance of secondary sex characteristics. These effects include the growth and maturation of the prostate, seminal vesicles, penis and scrotum; the development of male hair distribution on the face, chest, axillae and pubis; laryngeal enlargement, vocal chord thickening, alterations in body musculature and fat distribution.

Insufficient secretion of testosterone due to testicular failure, pituitary pathology or gonadotropin or luteinising hormone-releasing hormone deficiency results in male hypogonadism and low serum testosterone concentration. Symptoms associated with low testosterone include decreased sexual desire with or without impotence, fatigue, loss of muscle mass, mood depression and regression of secondary sexual characteristics. Restoring testosterone levels to within the normal range can result in improvements over time in muscle mass, mood, sexual desire, libido and sexual function including sexual performance and number of spontaneous erections.

During exogenous administration of testosterone to normal males, endogenous testosterone release may be decreased through feedback inhibition of pituitary luteinising hormone (LH). With large doses of exogenous androgens, spermatogenesis may also be suppressed through inhibition of pituitary follicle stimulating hormone (FSH).

Androgen administration causes retention of sodium, nitrogen, potassium, phosphorus and decreased urinary excretion of calcium. Androgens have been reported to increase protein anabolism and decrease protein catabolism. Nitrogen balance is improved only when there is sufficient intake of calories and protein. Androgens have been reported to stimulate production of red blood cells by enhancing the production of erythropoietin.

5.2 Pharmacokinetic properties

Testim dries very quickly when applied to the skin surface. The skin acts as a reservoir for the sustained release of testosterone into the systemic circulation.

With once daily application of Testim 50mg or 100mg to adult males with early morning serum testosterone levels ⩽ 300 ng/dL, follow up measurements at 30, 60 and 90 days after starting treatment have confirmed that serum testosterone concentrations are generally maintained within the normal range.

Following 50 mg Testim daily in hypogonadal men, the C_{avg} was shown to be 365±187 ng/dL (12.7±6.5 nmol/L), C_{max} was 538±371 ng/dL (18.7±12.9 nmol/L) and C_{min} was 223±126 ng/dl (7.7± 4.4 nmol/L), measured at steady-state. The corresponding concentrations following 100 mg Testim daily were C_{avg} = 612±286 ng/dL (21.3±9.9 nmol/L), C_{max} = 897±566 ng/dL (31.1±19.6 nmol/L) and C_{min} = 394±189 ng/dL (13.7±6.6 nmol/L).

In the young eugonadal man, normal levels of serum testosterone are in the range of 300 – 1000 ng/dL (10.4 – 34.6 nmol/L).

The measurement of serum testosterone levels can be variable depending on the laboratory and method of assay used (see 4.2 Posology and method of administration).

Distribution:

Circulating testosterone is chiefly bound in the serum to sex hormone-binding globulin (SHBG) and albumin. The albumin-bound fraction of testosterone easily dissociates from albumin and is presumed to be bioactive. The portion of testosterone bound to SHBG is not considered biologically active. Approximately 40% of testosterone in plasma is bound to SHBG, 2% remains unbound (free) and the rest is bound to albumin and other proteins.

Metabolism:

There is considerable variation in the half-life of testosterone as reported in the literature, ranging from ten to 100 minutes.

Testosterone is metabolised to various 17-keto steroids through two different pathways. The major active metabolites of testosterone are oestradiol and dihydrotestosterone (DHT). Testosterone is metabolised to DHT by steroid 5α reductase located in the skin, liver and the urogenital tract of the male. DHT binds with greater affinity to SHBG than does testosterone. In many tissues, the activity of testosterone depends on its reduction to DHT, which binds to cytosol receptor proteins. The steroid-receptor complex is transported to the nucleus where it initiates transcription and cellular changes related to androgen action. In reproductive tissues, DHT is further metabolised to 3-$\alpha$and 3-β androstanediol.

Inactivation of testosterone occurs primarily in the liver.

DHT concentrations increased during Testim treatment. After 90 days of treatment, mean DHT concentrations remained within the normal range for Testim treated subjects.

Excretion:

About 90% of testosterone given intramuscularly is excreted in the urine as glucuronic and sulphuric acid conjugates of testosterone and its metabolites; about 6% of a dose is excreted in the faeces, mostly in the unconjugated form.

Special Patient groups:

In patients treated with Testim no differences in the average daily serum testosterone concentration at steady state were observed based on age or cause of hypogonadism.

5.3 Preclinical safety data

Toxicological studies have not revealed effects other than those which can be explained based on the hormonal profile of Testim.

6. PHARMACEUTICAL PARTICULARS

6.1 List of excipients

Purified water

Pentadecalactone

Carbomer 980

Carbomer 1342

Propylene glycol

Glycerol

Macrogol 1000

Ethanol

Trometamol

6.2 Incompatibilities

Not applicable

6.3 Shelf life

2 years

6.4 Special precautions for storage

Do not store above 25°C

6.5 Nature and contents of container

Testim is supplied in unit dose aluminium tubes with epoxy phenolic liners and screw caps, each containing 5g gel.

The tubes are packed in cartons containing 7, 14 or 30 tubes.

Not all pack sizes may be marketed.

6.6 Instructions for use and handling
No special requirements.

7. MARKETING AUTHORISATION HOLDER
Ipsen Limited,
190 Bath Road,
Slough,
Berks SL1 3XE
UK

8. MARKETING AUTHORISATION NUMBER(S)
PL 06958/0027

9. DATE OF FIRST AUTHORISATION/RENEWAL OF THE AUTHORISATION
20 August 2004

10. DATE OF REVISION OF THE TEXT
19 October 2004

Testogel

(Schering Health Care Limited)

1. NAME OF THE MEDICINAL PRODUCT
TESTOGEL® 50 mg, gel in sachet

2. QUALITATIVE AND QUANTITATIVE COMPOSITION
One sachet of 5 g contains 50 mg of testosterone.

For excipients, see 6.1.

3. PHARMACEUTICAL FORM
Gel in sachet.

Testogel is a transparent or slightly opalescent, colourless gel in sachet.

4. CLINICAL PARTICULARS

4.1 Therapeutic indications
Testosterone replacement therapy for male hypogonadism when testosterone deficiency has been confirmed by clinical features and biochemical tests (see 4.4 Special warnings and precautions for use).

4.2 Posology and method of administration
Cutaneous use.

Adult and Elderly men

The recommended dose is 5 g of gel (i.e. 50 mg of testosterone) applied once daily at about the same time, preferably in the morning. The daily dose should be adjusted by the doctor depending on the clinical or laboratory response in individual patients, not exceeding 10 g of gel per day. The adjustment of posology should be achieved by 2.5 g of gel steps.

The application should be administered by the patient himself, onto clean, dry, healthy skin over both shoulders, or both arms or abdomen.

After opening the sachets, the total contents must be extracted from the sachet and applied immediately onto the skin. The gel has just to be simply spread on the skin gently as a thin layer. It is not necessary to rub it on the skin. Allow drying for at least 3-5 minutes before dressing. Wash hands with soap and water after applications.

Do not apply to the genital areas as the high alcohol content may cause local irritation.

Steady state plasma testosterone concentrations are reached approximately on the 2nd day of treatment by Testogel. In order to adjust the testosterone dose, serum testosterone concentrations must be measured in the morning before application from the 3rd day on after starting treatment (one week seems reasonable). The dose may be reduced if the plasma testosterone concentrations are raised above the desired level. If the concentrations are low, the dosage may be increased, not exceeding 10 g of gel per day.

Children

Testogel is not indicated for use in children and has not been evaluated clinically in males under 18 years of age.

4.3 Contraindications
Testogel is contraindicated:

- in cases of known or suspected prostatic cancer or breast carcinoma,

- in cases of known hypersensitivity to testosterone or to any other constituent of the gel.

4.4 Special warnings and special precautions for use
Testogel should be used only if hypogonadism (hyper- and hypogonadotrophic) has been demonstrated and if other etiology, responsible for the symptoms, has been excluded before treatment is started. Testosterone insufficiency should be clearly demonstrated by clinical features (regression of secondary sexual characteristics, change in body composition, asthenia, reduced libido, erectile dysfunction etc.) and confirmed by 2 separate blood testosterone measurements. Currently, there is no consensus about age specific testosterone reference values. However, it should be taken into account that physiologically testosterone serum levels are lower with increasing age.

Due to variability in laboratory values, all measures of testosterone should be carried out in the same laboratory.

Testogel is not a treatment for male sterility or impotence.

Prior to testosterone initiation, all patients must undergo a detailed examination in order to exclude a risk of pre-existing prostatic cancer. Careful and regular monitoring of the prostate gland and breast must be performed in accordance with recommended methods (digital rectal examination and estimation of serum PSA) in patients receiving testosterone therapy at least once yearly and twice yearly in elderly patients and at risk patients (those with clinical or familial factors).

Androgens may accelerate the progression of sub-clinical prostatic cancer and benign prostatic hyperplasia.

Testogel should be used with caution in cancer patients at risk of hypercalcaemia (and associated hypercalciuria), due to bone metastases. Regular monitoring of serum calcium concentrations is recommended in these patients.

In patients suffering from severe cardiac, hepatic or renal insufficiency, treatment with Testogel may cause severe complications characterised by oedema with or without congestive cardiac failure. In this case, treatment must be stopped immediately. In addition, diuretic therapy may be required.

Testogel should be used with caution in patients with ischemic heart disease.

Testosterone may cause a rise in blood pressure and Testogel should be used with caution in patients with hypertension.

Beside laboratory tests of the testosterone concentrations in patients on long-term androgen therapy the following laboratory parameters should be checked periodically: haemoglobin, haematocrit (to detect polycythaemia), liver function tests.

Testogel should be used with caution in patients with epilepsy and migraine as these conditions may be aggravated.

There are published reports of increased risk of sleep apnoea in hypogonadal subjects treated with testosterone esters, especially in those with risk factors such as obesity and chronic respiratory disease.

Improved insulin sensitivity may occur in patients treated with androgens who achieve normal testosterone plasma concentrations following replacement therapy.

Certain clinical signs: irritability, nervousness, weight gain, prolonged or frequent erections may indicate excessive androgen exposure requiring dosage adjustment.

If the patient develops a severe application site reaction, treatment should be reviewed and discontinued if necessary.

The attention of athletes is drawn to the fact that this proprietary medicinal product contains an active substance (testosterone) which may produce a positive reaction in anti-doping tests.

Testogel should not be used by women, due to possibly virilizing effects.

Potential testosterone transfer

If no precaution is taken, testosterone gel can be transferred to other persons by close skin to skin contact, resulting in increased testosterone serum levels and possibly adverse effects (e.g. growth of facial and/or body hair, deepening of the voice, irregularities of the menstrual cycle) in case of repeat contact (inadvertent androgenization).

The physician should inform the patient carefully about the risk of testosterone transfer and about safety instructions (see below). Testogel should not be prescribed in patients with a major risk of non-compliance with safety instructions (e.g. severe alcoholism, drug abuse, severe psychiatric disorders).

This transfer is avoided by wearing clothes covering the application area or showering prior to contact.

As a result, the following precautions are recommended:

* for the patient:

- wash hands with soap and water after applying the gel,

- cover the application area with clothing once the gel has dried,

- shower before any situation in which this type of contact is foreseen.

* for people not being treated with Testogel:

- in the event of contact with an application area which has not been washed or is not covered with clothing, wash the area of skin onto which testosterone may have been transferred as soon as possible, using soap and water,

- report the development of signs of excessive androgen exposure such as acne or hair modification.

According to in vitro absorption studies on testosterone conducted with Testogel, it seems preferable for patients to observe at least 6 hours between gel application and bathing or showering. Occasional baths or showers taken between 1 and 6 hours after application of the gel should not significantly influence the treatment outcome.

To guarantee partner safety the patient should be advised for example to observe a long interval between Testogel application and sexual intercourse, to wear a T-shirt covering the application site, during contact period or to shower before sexual intercourse.

Furthermore, it is recommended to wear a T-shirt, covering the application site, during contact period with children, in order to avoid a contamination risk of children's skin.

Pregnant women must avoid any contact with Testogel application sites. In case of pregnancy of the partner, the patient must reinforce his attention to the precautions for use (see section 4.6).

4.5 Interaction with other medicinal products and other forms of Interaction
+ Oral anticoagulants

Changes in anticoagulant activity (the increased effect of the oral anticoagulant by modification of coagulation factor hepatic synthesis and competitive inhibition of plasma protein binding):

Increased monitoring of the prothrombin time, and INR determinations, are recommended. Patients receiving oral anticoagulants require close monitoring especially when androgens are started or stopped.

Concomitant administration of testosterone and ACTH or corticosteroids may increase the risk of developing oedema. As a result, these medicinal products should be administered cautiously, particularly in patients suffering from cardiac, renal or hepatic disease.

Interaction with laboratory tests: androgens may decrease levels of thyroxin binding globulin, resulting in decreased T_4 serum concentrations and in increased resin uptake of T_3 and T_4. Free thyroid hormone levels, however, remain unchanged and there is no clinical evidence of thyroid insufficiency.

4.6 Pregnancy and lactation
Testogel is intended for use by men only.

Testogel is not indicated in pregnant or breast feeding women. No clinical trials have been conducted with this treatment in women.

Pregnant women must avoid any contact with Testogel application sites (see section 4.4). This product may have adverse virilizing effects on the fœtus. In the event of contact, wash with soap and water as soon as possible.

4.7 Effects on ability to drive and use machines
Testogel has no influence on the ability to drive or use machines.

4.8 Undesirable effects
The most frequently observed adverse drug reactions at the recommended dosage of 5 g of gel per day were skin reactions (10%): reaction at the application site, erythema, acne, dry skin.

Adverse drug reactions reported in 1 - <10% of patients treated with Testogel in the controlled clinical trials are listed in the following table:

Organ system class	Adverse reactions
Body as a whole-general	Changes in laboratory tests (polycythaemia, lipids), headache
Urogenital system	Prostatic disorders, gynaecomastia, mastodynia
Central and peripheral nervous system	Dizziness, paraesthesia amnesia, hyperaesthesia, mood disorders
Cardiovascular system	Hypertension
Gastro-intestinal system	Diarrhoea
Skin and appendages	Alopecia

Gynaecomastia, which may be persistent, is a common finding in patients treated for hypogonadism.

The other known adverse drug reactions of oral or injectable treatments containing testosterone are: prostatic changes and progression of sub-clinical prostatic cancer, urinary obstruction, pruritus, arterial vasodilatation, nausea, cholestatic jaundice, changes in liver function tests, increased libido, depression, nervousness, myalgia and, during high dose prolonged treatment, electrolyte changes (sodium, potassium, calcium, inorganic phosphate and water retention), oligospermia and priapism (frequent or prolonged erections).

Because of the alcohol contained in the product, frequent applications to the skin may cause irritation and dry skin.

4.9 Overdose
Only one case of acute testosterone overdose following an injection has been reported in the literature. This was a case of a cerebrovascular accident in a patient with a high plasma testosterone concentration of 114 ng/ml (395 nmol/l). It would be most unlikely that such plasma testosterone concentrations be achieved using the transdermal route.

5. PHARMACOLOGICAL PROPERTIES

5.1 Pharmacodynamic properties

Pharmacotherapeutic group: Androgens. ATC code: G03B A03.

Endogenous androgens, principally testosterone, secreted by the testes and its major metabolite DHT, are responsible for the development of the external and internal genital organs and for maintaining the secondary sexual characteristics (stimulating hair growth, deepening of the voice, development of the libido); for a general effect on protein anabolism; for development of skeletal muscle and body fat distribution; for a reduction in urinary nitrogen, sodium, potassium, chloride, phosphate and water excretion.

Testosterone does not produce testicular development: it reduces the pituitary secretion of gonadotropins.

The effects of testosterone in some target organs arise after peripheral conversion of testosterone to estradiol, which than binds to oestrogen receptors in the target cell nucleus e.g. the pituitary, fat, brain, bone and testicular Leydig cells.

5.2 Pharmacokinetic properties

The percutaneous absorption of testosterone ranges from approximately 9% to 14% of the applied dose.

Following percutaneous absorption, testosterone diffuses into the systemic circulation at relatively constant concentrations during the 24 hour cycle.

Serum testosterone concentrations increase from the first hour after an application, reaching steady state from day two. Daily changes in testosterone concentrations are then of similar amplitude to those observed during the circadian rhythm of endogenous testosterone. The percutaneous route therefore avoids the blood distribution peaks produced by injections. It does not produce supra-physiological hepatic concentrations of the steroid in contrast to oral androgen therapy.

Administration of 5 g of Testogel produces an average testosterone concentration increase of approximately 2.5 ng/ml (8.7 nmol/l) in plasma.

When treatment is stopped, testosterone concentrations start decreasing approximately 24 hours after the last dose. Concentrations return to baseline approximately 72 to 96 hours after the final dose.

The major active metabolites of testosterone are dihydrotestosterone and estradiol.

Testosterone is excreted, mostly in urine, and in faeces as conjugated testosterone metabolites.

5.3 Preclinical safety data

Testosterone has been found to be non-mutagenic in vitro using the reverse mutation model (Ames test) or hamster ovary cells. A relationship between androgen treatment and certain cancers has been found in studies on laboratory animals. Experimental data in rats have shown increased incidences of prostate cancer after treatment with testosterone.

Sex hormones are known to facilitate the development of certain tumours induced by known carcinogenic agents. No correlation between these findings and the actual risk in human beings has been established.

6. PHARMACEUTICAL PARTICULARS

6.1 List of excipients

Carbomer 980

Isopropyl myristate

Ethanol 96%

Sodium hydroxide

Purified water

6.2 Incompatibilities

Not applicable.

6.3 Shelf life

3 years.

6.4 Special precautions for storage

No special precautions for storage.

6.5 Nature and contents of container

5 g in sachet (PET/Aluminium/PE).

Boxes of 1, 2, 7, 10, 14, 28, 30, 50, 60, 90 or 100 sachets.

Not all the pack sizes may be marketed.

6.6 Instructions for use and handling

No special requirements.

7. MARKETING AUTHORISATION HOLDER

Laboratoires BESINS INTERNATIONAL

5, rue du Bourg l'Abbé

75003 PARIS

France

8. MARKETING AUTHORISATION NUMBER(S)

PL 16468/0005

9. DATE OF FIRST AUTHORISATION/RENEWAL OF THE AUTHORISATION

3 March 2003

10. DATE OF REVISION OF THE TEXT

5 February 2004

LEGAL CATEGORY

POM

Testosterone Enanthate Ampoules

(Cambridge Laboratories)

1. NAME OF THE MEDICINAL PRODUCT

Testosterone Enanthate Ampoules

2. QUALITATIVE AND QUANTITATIVE COMPOSITION

Each ampoule contains 250mg Testosterone Enanthate Ph.Eur in oily solution.

3. PHARMACEUTICAL FORM

Solution for injection.

4. CLINICAL PARTICULARS

4.1 Therapeutic indications

Mammary carcinoma in the female.

Androgen deficiency in the male.

4.2 Posology and method of administration

Females - mammary carcinoma: 250mg every two weeks by intramuscular injection.

Males - Hypogonadism: To stimulate development of underdeveloped androgen-dependent organs and for initial treatment of deficiency symptoms, 250mg Testosterone Enanthate intramuscularly every two to three weeks.

For maintenance treatment: 250mg Testosterone Enanthate intramuscularly every three to six weeks, according to individual requirement.

4.3 Contraindications

Prostatic carcinoma, mammary carcinoma in males and pregnancy. Previous or existing liver tumours (in advanced mammary carcinoma in the female only) if these are not due to metastases.

4.4 Special warnings and special precautions for use

Androgens should not be used for enhancing muscular development in healthy individuals or for increasing physical ability.

High dose or long term administration of testosterone occasionally increases the tendency to water retention and oedema. Caution should therefore be exercised in patients predisposed to oedema.

In rare cases benign and in even rarer cases malignant liver tumours leading in isolated cases to life-threatening intra-abdominal haemorrhage have been observed after the use of hormonal substances such as Testosterone Enanthate. If severe upper abdominal complaints, liver enlargement or signs of intra-abdominal haemorrhage occur, a liver tumour should be included in the differential diagnosis and, if necessary, the preparation should be withdrawn. Regular examination of the prostate is advisable for men receiving androgen therapy.

If, in individual cases, frequent or persistent erections occur, the dose should be reduced or the treatment discontinued in order to avoid injury to the penis.

In women: If hypercalcaemia develops, therapy must be discontinued.

4.5 Interaction with other medicinal products and other forms of Interaction

Phenobarbitone increases the break-down of steroid hormones in the liver (possible impairment of efficacy).

The clotting status should be monitored particularly closely when Testosterone Enanthate is administered together with coumarin derivatives.

4.6 Pregnancy and lactation

Contra-indicated in pregnancy.

4.7 Effects on ability to drive and use machines

None known.

4.8 Undesirable effects

Women treated with Testosterone Enanthate may develop signs of virilization, (e.g. acne, hirsutism, voice changes). Particular care is therefore necessary in women whose occupations involve singing or speaking.

Spermatogenesis is inhibited by long-term and high-dose treatment with Testosterone Enanthate.

In rare cases, coughing, dyspnoea and circulatory irregularities may occur during or immediately after the injection. Experience has shown that these reactions can be avoided by injecting very slowly.

4.9 Overdose

Acute toxicity data show that Testosterone Enanthate can be classified as non-toxic following a single intake. Even in the case of an inadvertent administration of a multiple of the dose required for therapy, no acute toxicity risk is expected.

5. PHARMACOLOGICAL PROPERTIES

5.1 Pharmacodynamic properties

Testosterone Enanthate is an ester of the natural male sex hormone testosterone and exhibits all the pharmacological effects of the natural hormone. It differs in that it has a depot effect, due to the fact that Testosterone Enanthate is only slowly degraded to testosterone in the body.

5.2 Pharmacokinetic properties

Following intramuscular administration of 200mg of Testosterone Enanthate to 6 hypogonadal males:-

- Peak serum testosterone levels of 1233 ± 484 ng/dl were achieved at 24 hours.
- Physiological levels of testosterone (approx. 500 ng/dl) were maintained for 11 days.

Half-life in blood was 2-3 days (healthy male volunteers).

5.3 Preclinical safety data

Studies in animals showed that the formulation has minimal potential for causing sensitisation or local irritation following intramuscular injection. Long-term systemic studies showed no evidence of testicular toxicity although a temporary inhibition of spermatogenesis may occur. No fertility studies with Testosterone Enanthate have been carried out. Administration of Testosterone Enanthate is contra-indicated during pregnancy due to the possibility of virilisation of the female foetus. However, investigations into embryotoxic, in particular teratogenic, effects gave no indication that further impairment of organ development may occur.

In vitro investigations of mutagenicity gave negative results.

6. PHARMACEUTICAL PARTICULARS

6.1 List of excipients

Benzyl benzoate

Castor oil for injection

6.2 Incompatibilities

None so far known.

6.3 Shelf life

5 years.

6.4 Special precautions for storage

Protect from light.

6.5 Nature and contents of container

Clear glass ampoules of 1 ml in packs of 3.

6.6 Instructions for use and handling

Not applicable.

7. MARKETING AUTHORISATION HOLDER

Cambridge Laboratories Limited

Deltic House

Kingfisher Way

Silverlink Business Park

Wallsend

Tyne & Wear

NE28 9NX

8. MARKETING AUTHORISATION NUMBER(S)

PL 12070/0015

9. DATE OF FIRST AUTHORISATION/RENEWAL OF THE AUTHORISATION

19 September 1996

10. DATE OF REVISION OF THE TEXT

September 2003

Tetralysal 300

(Galderma (U.K.) Ltd)

1. NAME OF THE MEDICINAL PRODUCT

Tetralysal 300

2. QUALITATIVE AND QUANTITATIVE COMPOSITION

Lymecycline 408mg equivalent to 300mg tetracycline base

3. PHARMACEUTICAL FORM

Hard gelatin capsule, red cap and yellow body

4. CLINICAL PARTICULARS

4.1 Therapeutic indications

Tetralysal 300 is for the treatment of acne

As Tetralysal 300 contains a broad spectrum antibiotic, it is also recommended for the treatment of infections caused by tetracycline-sensitive organisms and may be utilised in all conditions where tetracycline is indicated, including use in penicillin-sensitive patients for the treatment of staphylococcal infections. Typical indications include: ear, nose and throat infections; acute and chronic bronchitis (including prophylaxis); infections of the gastro-intestinal and urinary tracts; non-gonococcal urethritis of chlamydial origin and other chlamydial infections such as trachoma; rickettsial fevers; soft tissue infections.

4.2 Posology and method of administration

Adults:

The usual dosage for the chronic treatment of acne is 1 capsule daily: treatment should be continued for at least 8 weeks.

For other infections, the usual dosage is 1 capsule b.d. If higher doses are required, 3-4 capsules may be given over 24 hours. Lower doses may be given for prophylaxis.

In the management of sexually transmitted disease both partners should be treated.

Elderly:

As for other tetracyclines, no specific dose adjustment is required.

Children:

Not recommended for children under the age of 12 years. For children over the age of 12 years the adult dosage may be given.

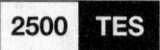

4.3 Contraindications
As lymecycline is mainly excreted by the kidneys, Tetralysal 300 should not be administered to patients with overt renal insufficiency. Its use is also contra-indicated in patients hypersensitive to tetracyclines.

Children under 12 years

Pregnancy and lactation (see section 4.6)

4.4 Special warnings and special precautions for use
Prolonged use of broad spectrum antibiotics may result in the appearance of resistant organisms and superinfection.

Care should be exercised in administering tetracyclines to patients with hepatic impairment. Tetracyclines may cause photosensitivity reactions; however, very rare cases have been reported with lymecycline.

May cause exacerbation of systemic lupus erythematosus. Can cause weak neuromuscular blockade so should be used with caution in Myasthenia Gravis.

4.5 Interaction with other medicinal products and other forms of Interaction
The absorption of tetracyclines may be affected by the simultaneous administration of calcium, aluminium, magnesium, bismuth and zinc salts, antacids, Bismuth containing ulcer-healing drugs, iron preparations and quinapril. These products should not be taken within two hours before or after taking Tetralysal 300.

Unlike earlier tetracyclines, absorption of Tetralysal 300 is not significantly impaired by moderate amounts of milk.

Concomitant use of oral retinoids should be avoided as this may increase the risk of benign intracranial hypertension. An increase in the effects of anticoagulants may occur with tetracyclines. Concomitant use of diuretics should be avoided.

Although not reported for Tetralysal 300, a few cases of pregnancy or breakthrough bleeding have been attributed to the concurrent use of tetracycline or oxytetracycline with oral contraceptives.

4.6 Pregnancy and lactation
Tetracyclines are selectively absorbed by developing bones and teeth and may cause dental staining and enamel hypoplasia. In addition these compounds readily cross the placental barrier and therefore Tetralysal 300 should not be given to pregnant or lactating women.

4.7 Effects on ability to drive and use machines
None known

4.8 Undesirable effects
- Rarely anaphylaxis
- Nausea, vomiting, diarrhoea
- Rarely dysphagia
- A few cases of oesophagitis and oesophageal ulceration have been reported, usually when taken before bed or with inadequate fluids.
- A few cases of pancreatitis have been reported.
- As with all antibiotics overgrowth of nonsusceptible organisms may cause candidiasis, pseudomembranous colitis (Clostridium difficile overgrowth), glossitis, stomatitis, vaginitis, or staphylococcal enterocolitis.
- Transient increases in liver function tests, hepatitis, jaundice and hepatic failure have been reported rarely.
- Bulging fontanelles in infants and benign intracranial hypertension in juveniles and adults have been reported. Presenting features were headache and visual disturbances including blurring of vision, scotomata and diplopia. Permanent visual loss has been reported.
- Skin rashes, photosensitivity, erythematous, and maculopapular rashes, pruritis, bullous dermatoses, exfoliative dermatitis.
- Teeth discoloration – usually only obvious after repeated doses.

4.9 Overdose
There is no specific treatment, but gastric lavage should be performed as soon as possible. Supportive measure should be instituted as required and a high fluid intake maintained.

5. PHARMACOLOGICAL PROPERTIES
5.1 Pharmacodynamic properties
Lymecycline has antimicrobial activity and uses similar to those of tetracycline hydrochloride. It acts by interfering with bacterial protein synthesis and is active against a large number of Gram-positive and Gram-negative pathogenic bacteria including some which are resistant to penicillin.

5.2 Pharmacokinetic properties
Lymecycline is more readily absorbed from the gastrointestinal tract than tetracycline, with a peak serum concentration of approximately 2mg/L after 3 hours following a 300 mg dose. In addition, similar blood concentrations are achieved with small doses. When the dose is doubled an almost correspondingly higher blood concentration has been reported to occur.

The serum half-life of lymecycline is approximately 10 hours.

5.3 Preclinical safety data
No specific information is presented given the vast experience gained with the use of tetracyclines in humans over the last forty years.

6. PHARMACEUTICAL PARTICULARS
6.1 List of excipients
Magnesium stearate

Colloidal hydrated silica

The capsule shells contain

gelatin

titanium dioxide (E171)

erythrosine (E127)

quinoline yellow (E104)

indigotine (E132)

6.2 Incompatibilities
None known

6.3 Shelf life
Thirty-six (36) months (unopened)

6.4 Special precautions for storage

Aluminium and polyethylene strips:	Do not store above 25°C.
	Store in the original container.
Aluminium-PVC/PVDC calendar blister strips:	Do not store above 25°C.
	Keep container in the outer carton.

As with all medicines, Tetralysal 300 should be kept out of the sight and reach of children.

6.5 Nature and contents of container
Aluminium-PVC/PVDC calendar blister strips of 14 capsules; two strips per carton, pack size = 28 capsules or Aluminium and polyethylene strips 28 or 56 capsule pack size.

6.6 Instructions for use and handling
No special instructions

7. MARKETING AUTHORISATION HOLDER
Galderma (UK) Limited

Galderma House

Church Lane

Kings Langley

Herts. WD4 8JP

England

8. MARKETING AUTHORISATION NUMBER(S)
PL 10590/0019

9. DATE OF FIRST AUTHORISATION/RENEWAL OF THE AUTHORISATION
29th September 1995

10. DATE OF REVISION OF THE TEXT
October 2003

10 Legal category
POM

Teveten 300mg, 400mg & 600mg Film-coated Tablets

(Solvay Healthcare Limited)

1. NAME OF THE MEDICINAL PRODUCT
Teveten 300mg Film-coated Tablet

Teveten 400 mg Film-coated Tablet

Teveten 600mg Film-coated Tablet

2. QUALITATIVE AND QUANTITATIVE COMPOSITION
Eprosartan mesylate equivalent to 300mg, 400mg or 600mg eprosartan free base.

For excipients, see section 6.1.

3. PHARMACEUTICAL FORM
300 mg: Oval, biconvex, white film-coated tablets with inscriptions 'SOLVAY' and '5043'.

400 mg: Oval, biconvex, pink film-coated tablets with inscriptions 'SOLVAY' and '5044'.

600 mg: Capsule-shaped, biconvex, white film-coated tablet with the inscription 5046'.

4. CLINICAL PARTICULARS
4.1 Therapeutic indications
Eprosartan is indicated for the treatment of essential hypertension.

4.2 Posology and method of administration
The recommended dose is 600 mg eprosartan once daily.

The dose may be increased to 800 mg eprosartan once daily if further response is required. Achievement of maximal blood pressure reduction in most patients may take 2 to 3 weeks of treatment.

Eprosartan may be used alone or in combination with other anti-hypertensives, e.g. thiazide-type diuretics, calcium channel blockers, if a greater blood pressure lowering effect is required.

Eprosartan should be taken with food.

Elderly >75 years): As clinical experience is limited in patients over 75 years, a starting dose of 300 mg once daily is recommended.

Dosage in hepatically impaired patients: There is limited experience in patients with hepatic impairment (see section 4.3 Contra-indications and section 5.2 Pharmacokinetic properties). In patients with mild to moderate hepatic impairment, a starting dose of 300 mg once daily is recommended.

Dosage in renally impaired patients: No dose adjustment is required in patients with creatinine clearance 60-80 ml/min. As clinical experience is limited in patients with creatinine clearance <60 ml/min, a starting dose of 300mg once daily is recommended (see section 4.4 Special Warnings and Precautions).

Children: As safety and efficacy in children have not been established, treatment of children is not recommended.

4.3 Contraindications
Known hypersensitivity to components of the product.

Pregnancy and lactation.

Severe hepatic impairment.

4.4 Special warnings and special precautions for use
Risk of renal impairment
As a consequence of inhibiting the renin-angiotensin-aldosterone system, changes in renal function including renal failure have been reported with angiotensin converting enzyme (ACE) inhibitors and angiotensin receptor antagonists in susceptible individuals. Such changes in renal function may be reversible upon discontinuation of therapy.

As clinical experience is limited in patients with creatinine clearance <60 ml/min and in patients undergoing dialysis, caution is recommended.

As with other angiotensin II antagonists, pre-treatment and periodic monitoring of serum potassium and creatinine levels is recommended in patients with impaired renal function.

Sodium and/or volume depletion
At the start of therapy, symptomatic hypotension may occur in patients with severe sodium depletion and/or volume depletion (e.g. high dose diuretic therapy). Sodium and/or volume depletion should be corrected before commencing therapy or existing diuretic therapy should be reduced.

Hyperkalaemia
Although eprosartan has no significant effect on serum potassium there is no experience of concomitant administration with K-sparing diuretics or K-supplements. Consequently, as with other angiotensin II antagonists, the risk of hyperkalaemia when taken with K-sparing diuretics or K-supplements cannot be excluded. Regular monitoring for serum potassium levels is recommended when drugs that may increase potassium are administered with eprosartan in patients with renal impairment.

4.5 Interaction with other medicinal products and other forms of Interaction
No clinically significant drug interactions have been observed. No effect on the pharmacokinetics of digoxin and the pharmacodynamics of warfarin or glyburide (glibenclamide) has been shown with eprosartan. Similarly no effect on eprosartan pharmacokinetics has been shown with ranitidine, ketoconazole or fluconazole.

Eprosartan has been safely used concomitantly with thiazide diuretics (e.g. hydrochlorothiazide) and calcium channel blockers (e.g. sustained-release nifedipine) without evidence of clinically significant adverse interactions. It has been safely co-administered with hypolipidaemic agents (e.g. lovastatin, simvastatin, pravastatin, fenofibrate, gemfibrozil, niacin).

Reversible increases in serum lithium concentrations and toxicity have been reported during concomitant administration of lithium with ACE inhibitors. While this is not documented with eprosartan, the possibility of a similar effect can not be excluded and careful monitoring of serum lithium levels is recommended during concomitant use.

Eprosartan has been shown not to inhibit human cytochrome P450 enzymes CYP1A, 2A6, 2C9/8, 2C19, 2D6, 2E and 3A *in vitro*.

4.6 Pregnancy and lactation
Pregnancy: There is little experience with the use of eprosartan during pregnancy. Drugs that act directly on the renin-angiotensin-aldosterone system can cause foetal and neonatal morbidity and death when administered to pregnant women during the second and third trimester. As with other drugs affecting the renin- angiotensin-aldosterone system, eprosartan should not be used in pregnancy, and if pregnancy is detected, eprosartan should be discontinued as soon as possible.

Lactation: Breast feeding women should not be treated with eprosartan (see Contraindications).

4.7 Effects on ability to drive and use machines
The effect of eprosartan on the ability to drive and use machines has not been studied, but based on its pharmacodynamic properties, eprosartan is unlikely to affect this ability. When driving vehicles or operating machines, it should be taken into account, that occasionally dizziness or weariness may occur during treatment of hypertension.

4.8 Undesirable effects

Clinical Trials

In placebo-controlled clinical trials, the overall incidence of adverse experiences reported with eprosartan was comparable to placebo. Adverse experiences have usually been mild and transient in nature and have only required discontinuation of therapy in 4.1% of patients treated with eprosartan in placebo-controlled studies (6.5% for placebo).

The following table shows the adverse experiences, regardless of causality, reported by patients with hypertension in placebo controlled studies of up to 13 weeks duration. It includes all adverse experiences occurring on eprosartan 600 - 800 mg once daily with an incidence at least 1% higher than placebo.

	Eprosartan 600/800mg O.D.	Placebo
Total Number of Patients	326	280
	%	%
Dizziness	4.6	2.9
Arthralgia	1.8	0.7
Rhinitis	1.5	0.4
Flatulence	1.5	0
Hypertriglyceridaemia	1.2	0

Angioedema has been infrequently reported.

Market Experience

The following adverse reactions have been reported during post-marketing experience with the following frequencies (very common >1/10); common >1/100, <1/10); uncommon >1/1000, <1/100); rare >1/10,000, <1/1000); very rare (<1/10,000)

Body as a whole:

Rare: Headache, asthenia

Nervous disorders:

Rare: Dizziness

Cardiovascular disorders:

Very rare: Hypotension (including postural hypotension)

Gastrointestinal disorders:

Very rare: Nausea

Skin disorders:

Rare: Rash, pruritus, urticaria

Very rare: Facial swelling, angioedema

Laboratory Findings

In placebo-controlled clinical studies, significantly elevated serum potassium concentrations were observed in 0.9% of patients treated with eprosartan and 0.3% of patients who received placebo.

Significantly low values of haemoglobin were observed in 0.1% and 0% patients treated with eprosartan and placebo respectively.

In rare cases elevations of BUN values were reported in patients treated with eprosartan. In rare cases increases in liver function values were also observed but were not considered to be causally related to eprosartan treatment.

4.9 Overdose

Limited data are available with regard to overdosage in humans. Eprosartan was well tolerated after oral dosing (maximum unit dose taken to date in humans 1200 mg) with no mortality in rats and mice up to 3000 mg/kg and in dogs up to 1000 mg/kg. The most likely manifestation of overdosage would be hypotension. If symptomatic hypotension occurs, supportive treatment should be instituted.

5. PHARMACOLOGICAL PROPERTIES

5.1 Pharmacodynamic properties

Eprosartan is a potent, synthetic, orally active non-biphenyl non-tetrazole angiotensin II receptor antagonist, which binds selectively to the AT_1 receptor. Angiotensin II is a potent vasoconstrictor and the primary active hormone of the renin-angiotensin-aldosterone system, playing a major part in the pathophysiology of hypertension. Angiotensin II binds to the AT_1 receptor in many tissues (e.g. smooth vascular musculature, suprarenals, kidney, heart) and produces important biological effects such as vasoconstriction, sodium retention and release of aldosterone. More recently, angiotensin II has been implicated in the genesis of cardiac and vascular hypertrophy through its effect on cardiac and smooth muscle cell growth.

Eprosartan antagonised the effect of angiotensin II on blood pressure, renal blood flow and aldosterone secretion in normal volunteers. In hypertensive patients, comparable blood pressure control is achieved when eprosartan is administered as a single dose or in two divided doses. In placebo-controlled studies, in 299 patients treated receiving 600-800 mg once daily, there was no evidence of first dose postural hypotension. Discontinuation of treatment with eprosartan does not lead to a rapid rebound increase in blood pressure.

Eprosartan was evaluated in mild to moderate hypertensive patients (sitting DBP ⩾95 mmHg and <115 mmHg) and severe hypertensive patients (sitting DBP ⩾115 mmHg and ⩽125 mmHg).

A dose of 1200 mg once daily, for 8 weeks, has been shown in 72 patients in clinical trials to be effective. In placebo-controlled studies using doses up to 1200 mg once daily, there is no apparent dose relationship in the incidence of adverse experiences reported.

In patients with hypertension, blood pressure reduction did not produce a change in heart rate.

In hypertensive patients eprosartan does not affect fasting triglycerides, total cholesterol, or LDL (low density lipoprotein) cholesterol levels. In addition, eprosartan has no effect on fasting blood sugar levels.

Eprosartan does not compromise renal autoregulatory mechanisms. In normal adult males eprosartan has been shown to increase mean effective renal plasma flow. Effective renal plasma flow is not altered in patients with essential hypertension and patients with renal insufficiency treated with eprosartan. Eprosartan does not reduce glomerular filtration rate in normal males, in patients with hypertension or in patients with varying degrees of renal insufficiency. Eprosartan has a natriuretic effect in normal subjects on a salt restricted diet.

Eprosartan does not significantly affect the excretion of urinary uric acid.

Eprosartan does not potentiate effects relating to bradykinin (ACE-mediated), e.g. cough. In a study specifically designed to compare the incidence of cough in patients treated with eprosartan and an angiotensin converting enzyme inhibitor, the incidence of dry persistent cough in patients treated with eprosartan (1.5%) was significantly lower ($p<0.05$) than that observed in patients treated with an angiotensin converting enzyme inhibitor (5.4%). In a further study investigating the incidence of cough in patients who had previously coughed while taking an angiotensin converting enzyme inhibitor, the incidence of dry, persistent cough was 2.6% on eprosartan, 2.7% on placebo, and 25.0% on an angiotensin converting enzyme inhibitor ($p<0.01$, eprosartan versus angiotensin converting enzyme inhibitor).

5.2 Pharmacokinetic properties

Absolute bioavailability following a single 300 mg oral dose of eprosartan is about 13%, due to limited oral absorption. Eprosartan plasma concentrations peak at one to two hours after an oral dose in the fasted state. Plasma concentrations are dose proportional from 100 to 200 mg, but less than proportional for 400 and 800 mg doses. The terminal elimination half-life of eprosartan following oral administration is typically five to nine hours. A slight accumulation (14%) is seen with chronic use of eprosartan. Administration of eprosartan with food delays absorption with minor increases (<25%) observed in C_{max} and AUC.

Plasma protein binding of eprosartan is high (approximately 98%) and constant over the concentration range achieved with therapeutic doses. The extent of plasma protein binding is not influenced by gender, age, hepatic dysfunction or mild-moderate renal impairment but has shown to be decreased in a small number of patients with severe renal impairment.

Following oral and intravenous dosing with [^{14}C]eprosartan in human subjects, eprosartan was the only drug-related compound found in the plasma and faeces. In the urine, approximately 20% of the radioactivity excreted was an acyl glucuronide of eprosartan with the remaining 80% being unchanged eprosartan.

The volume of distribution of eprosartan is about 13 litres. Total plasma clearance is about 130 ml/min. Biliary and renal excretion contribute to the elimination of eprosartan. Following intravenous [^{14}C]eprosartan, about 61% of radioactivity is recovered in the faeces and about 37% in the urine. Following an oral dose of [^{14}C]eprosartan, about 90% of radioactivity is recovered in the faeces and about 7% in the urine.

Both AUC and C_{max} values of eprosartan are increased in the elderly (on average, approximately two-fold).

Following administration of a single 100 mg dose of eprosartan, AUC values of eprosartan (but not C_{max}) are increased, on average, by approximately 40% in patients with hepatic impairment. Since an intravenous dose of eprosartan was not administered to patients with hepatic impairment, the plasma clearance of eprosartan could not be measured.

Compared to subjects with normal renal function (n=7), mean AUC and Cmax values were approximately 30% higher in patients with creatinine clearance 30-59 ml/min (n=11) and approximately 50% higher in patients with creatinine clearance 5-29 ml/min (n=3).

In a separate investigation, mean AUC was approximately 60% higher in patients undergoing dialysis (n=9) compared to subjects with normal renal function (n=10).

There is no difference in the pharmacokinetics of eprosartan between males and females.

5.3 Preclinical safety data

General toxicology

Eprosartan given orally at dosages up to 1000 mg/kg per day for up to six months in rat and up to one year in dogs did not result in any significant drug-related toxicity.

Reprotoxicity

In pregnant rabbits, eprosartan has been shown to produce maternal and foetal mortality at 10 mg/kg per day during late pregnancy only. This is most likely due to effects on the renin angiotensin aldosterone system. Maternal toxicity but no foetal effects were observed at 3 mg/kg per day.

Genotoxicity

Genotoxicity was not observed in a battery of *in vitro* and *in vivo* tests.

Carcinogenicity

Carcinogenicity was not observed in rats and mice given up to 600 or 2000 mg/kg per day respectively for two years.

6. PHARMACEUTICAL PARTICULARS

6.1 List of excipients

Tablet cores

Lactose

Microcrystalline cellulose

Pregelatinised starch

Magnesium stearate

Croscarmellose sodium (300 mg and 400 mg tablets only)

Crospovidone (600 mg tablets only)

Film-coat

Hypromellose

Titanium dioxide (E171)

Macrogol 400

Polysorbate 80

Red and yellow iron oxides (E172) (400 mg tablets only)

6.2 Incompatibilities

None known.

6.3 Shelf life

PVC/Aclar blister packs: 36 months

HDPE bottles: 36 months

6.4 Special precautions for storage

Do not store above 25°C.

Keep container in the outer carton.

6.5 Nature and contents of container

Opaque PVC/Aclar blister packs containing 28 tablets or 56 tablets.

HDPE bottles containing 100 tablets.

6.6 Instructions for use and handling

No special instructions.

7. MARKETING AUTHORISATION HOLDER

Solvay Healthcare Limited

Mansbridge Road

West End

Southampton

SO18 3JD

8. MARKETING AUTHORISATION NUMBER(S)

PL 00512/0163-5

9. DATE OF FIRST AUTHORISATION/RENEWAL OF THE AUTHORISATION

300, 400mg: 23 August 1999/17 April 2003

600mg: 29 November 1999/17 April 2003

10. DATE OF REVISION OF THE TEXT

21 April 2005

LEGAL CATEGORY

POM

Thiopental injection

(Link Pharmaceuticals Ltd)

1. NAME OF THE MEDICINAL PRODUCT

Thiopental Injection BP

2. QUALITATIVE AND QUANTITATIVE COMPOSITION

Thiopental Sodium BP 500mg

3. PHARMACEUTICAL FORM

Freeze-dried powder for solution for injection in a vial.

4. CLINICAL PARTICULARS

4.1 Therapeutic indications

1. Thiopental is used for the induction of general anaesthesia and is also used as an adjunct to provide hypnosis during balanced anaesthesia with other anaesthetic agents, including analgesics and muscle relaxants.

2. Thiopental is also used as an adjunct for control of convulsive disorders of various aetiology, including those caused by local anaesthetics.

3. Thiopental has now been used to reduce the intracranial pressure in patients with increased intracranial pressure, if controlled ventilation is provided.

4.2 Posology and method of administration
Intravenous injection.

Thiopental Injection BP is administered intravenously normally as a 2.5% w/v (500mg in 20ml) solution. On occasions it may be administered as a 5% w/v solution (500mg in 10ml).

The intravenous injection preparation should be used after reconstitution of the sterile powder with Water for Injections, usually to produce a 2.5% w/v solution and this should be discarded after seven hours.

Use in anaesthesia
Normal dosage for the induction of anaesthesia is 100mg to 150mg injected over 10 to 15 seconds. If necessary a repeat dose of 100mg to 150mg may be given after one minute. No fixed dosage recommendations for the intravenous injection can be given, since the dosage will need to be carefully adjusted according to the patient's response. Factors such as age, sex, and weight of the patient should be taken into consideration. Thiopental sodium reaches effective concentrations in the brain within 30 seconds and anaesthesia is normally produced within one minute of an intravenous dose.

Adult
100mg to 150mg intravenously over 10 to 15 seconds, normally as a 2.5% w/v solution.

A repeat dose of 100mg to 150mg may be given after one minute.

The intravenous injection should be given slowly and the amounts given titrated against the patient's response to minimise the risk of respiratory depression or the possibility of overdosage. The average dose for an adult of 70kg is roughly 200mg to 300mg (8mls to 12mls of a 2.5% w/v solution) with a maximum of 500mg.

Children
2 to 7mg/kg bodyweight, intravenously over 10 to 15 seconds, normally as a 2.5% w/v solution. A repeat dose of 2 to 7mg/kg may be given after one minute. The dose is 2 to 7mg/kg based on the patient's response. The dose for children should not exceed 7mg/kg.

Elderly
Smaller adult doses are advisable.

Use in convulsive states
75mg to 125mg (3mls to 5mls of a 2.5% w/v solution) should be given as soon as possible after the convulsion begins. Further doses may be required to control convulsions following the use of a local anaesthetic. Other regimens, such as the use of intravenous or rectal diazepam, may be used to control convulsive states.

Use in neurological patients with raised intracranial pressure
Intermittent bolus injections of 1.5 to 3mg/kg of bodyweight may be given to reduce elevations of intracranial pressure if controlled ventilation is provided.

4.3 Contraindications
Thiopental is contraindicated in respiratory obstruction, acute asthma, severe shock and dystrophia myotonica. Administration of any barbiturate is contraindicated in porphyria.

Care should also be exercised with severe cardiovascular diseases, severe respiratory diseases and hypertension of various aetiology.

Patients with hypersensitivity reactions to barbiturates.

4.4 Special warnings and special precautions for use
Special care is needed in administering thiopental to patients with the following conditions:- hypovolaemia, severe haemorrhage, burns, dehydration, severe anaemia, cardiovascular disease, status asthmaticus, severe liver disease, myasthenia gravis and muscular dystrophies, adrenocortical insufficiency (even when controlled by cortisone), cachexia and severe toxaemia, raised intracranial pressure, raised blood urea, raised plasma potassium, metabolic disorders e.g. thyrotoxicosis, myxoedema, diabetes.

Thiopental may precipitate acute circulatory failure in patients with cardiovascular disease, particularly constrictive pericarditis.

Thiopental can cause respiratory depression and a reduction in cardiac output.

Headache is also reported with the use of barbiturate anaesthetics.

Reduced doses are recommended in shock, dehydration, severe anaemia, hyperkalaemia, toxaemia, myxoedema or other metabolic disorders. Thiopental sodium is metabolised primarily by the liver so doses should be reduced in patients with hepatic impairment. Reduced doses are also indicated in the elderly and in patients who have been premedicated with narcotic analgesics.

Thiopental has been shown to interact with sulphafurazole. Reduced initial doses may be required to achieve adequate anaesthesia, but repeat doses may also be necessary to maintain anaesthesia.

Increased doses may be necessary in patients who have either an habituation or addiction to alcohol or drugs of abuse. Under these circumstances it is recommended that supplementary analgesic agents are used.

Accidental intra-arterial injection of thiopental causes severe arterial spasm and an intense burning pain around the injection site. In the case of accidental intra-arterial injection of thiopental the needle should be left in-situ so that an injection of an antispasmodic, such as papaverine or prilocaine hydrochloride may be given. Anticoagulant therapy may also be started to reduce the risk of thrombosis.

Thiopental injection should be used with caution in patients with adrenocortical insufficiency or with raised intracranial pressure.

4.5 Interaction with other medicinal products and other forms of Interaction
Thiopental has been shown to interact with sulphafurazole.

It should be noted that thiopental will interact with beta-blockers and calcium antagonists causing a fall in blood pressure.

The sedative properties of antipsychotics and anxiolytics may be potentiated by thiopental.

4.6 Pregnancy and lactation
Thiopental readily crosses the placental barrier and also appears in breast milk. Therefore, breast-feeding should be temporarily suspended or breast milk expressed before the induction of anaesthesia. It has been shown that thiopental can be used without adverse effects during pregnancy although the total dose should not exceed 250mg. However, when considering use of thiopental the clinician should only use the drug when the expected benefits outweigh any potential risks.

4.7 Effects on ability to drive and use machines
Post-operative vertigo, disorientation and sedation may be prolonged and out-patients given thiopental should therefore be advised not to drive or use machinery, especially within the first 24 to 36 hours.

4.8 Undesirable effects
Laryngeal spasm may occur, together with coughing or sneezing, during the induction procedure. For this reason it is not advised to use thiopental alone for peroral endoscopy.

Extravasation causes local tissue necrosis and severe pain. This can be relieved by application of an ice pack and local injection of hydrocortisone. The 5% w/v solution is hypertonic and may cause pain on injection and thrombophlebitis.

Allergic reactions, skin reactions and hypersensitivity have been rarely reported.

Bronchospasm, respiratory depression and myocardial depression or cardiac arrhythmias may occur.

4.9 Overdose
Overdosage produces acute respiratory depression, hypotension, circulatory failure and apnoea. Treatment must be artificial ventilation, lowering of the patient's head and infusion of plasma volume expanders.

5. PHARMACOLOGICAL PROPERTIES

5.1 Pharmacodynamic properties
Thiopental is a short-acting substituted barbiturate that is more lipid soluble than other groups of barbiturates. The drug reversibly depresses the activity of all excitable tissues. The CNS is particularly sensitive and normally a general anaesthesia can be achieved with thiopental without significant effects on peripheral tissues.

Thiopental acts through the CNS with particular activity in the mesencephalic reticular activating system. The barbiturates exert different effects on synaptic transmission, mostly those dependent on GABA. Autonomic ganglia of the peripheral nervous system are also depressed.

5.2 Pharmacokinetic properties
Following intravenous administration, unconsciousness occurs within 30 seconds and will be continued for 20 to 30 minutes after a single dose. Rapid uptake occurs to most vascular areas of the brain followed by redistribution into other tissues.

Thiopental is strongly bound to plasma protein, which impairs excretion through the kidney. The metabolites are usually inactive and are then excreted. Thiopental, therefore, whilst having a short duration of action, may have a long elimination phase.

5.3 Preclinical safety data
There are no pre-clinical data of relevance to the prescriber which are additional to that already included in other sections of the Summary of Product Characteristics.

6. PHARMACEUTICAL PARTICULARS

6.1 List of excipients
None

6.2 Incompatibilities
Solutions of thiopental injection have a pH of 10 to 11 and are strongly alkaline in order to maintain stability. Solutions are incompatible with acid, acidic salts and solutions such as pethidine, morphine and promethazine.

6.3 Shelf life
48 months.

6.4 Special precautions for storage
Do not store above 25°C. Store reconstituted solution between 2°C to 8°C in an upright position and use within 7 hours. Use once following reconstitution and discard any residue.

6.5 Nature and contents of container
20ml Type III clear glass vials with 20mm bromylbutyl caoutchouc siliconised rubber closures.

Pack size: 25 vials per pack.

6.6 Instructions for use and handling
Not applicable.

7. MARKETING AUTHORISATION HOLDER
Link Pharmaceuticals Limited, Bishops Weald House, Albion Way, Horsham, West Sussex RH12 1AH, UK

8. MARKETING AUTHORISATION NUMBER(S)
PL 12406/0014

9. DATE OF FIRST AUTHORISATION/RENEWAL OF THE AUTHORISATION
5 April 1999

10. DATE OF REVISION OF THE TEXT
January 2003

11. Legal Category
POM

Thiotepa Injection
(Wyeth Pharmaceuticals)

1. NAME OF THE MEDICINAL PRODUCT
Thiotepa Injection

2. QUALITATIVE AND QUANTITATIVE COMPOSITION
Thiotepa 15mg

3. PHARMACEUTICAL FORM
Sterile powder for solution for injection

4. CLINICAL PARTICULARS

4.1 Therapeutic indications
Thiotepa (N,N',N" triethylenethiophosphoramide) is a polyfunctional alkylating agent used alone or in combination with other cytotoxic drugs, or with surgery in the treatment of neoplastic diseases. It is believed to exert its cytotoxic effects by the alkylation of DNA.

4.2 Posology and method of administration
Thiotepa (15mg) should be reconstituted with 1.5ml Water for Injection immediately prior to use. Please refer to specific sections on particular disease types for further reconstitution instructions. Reconstituted solutions should be clear to slightly opaque. Solutions that are grossly opaque or precipitated should be discarded.

Use Luer-Lock fittings on all syringes and sets. Large bore needles are recommended to minimise pressure and possible formation of aerosols. The latter may also be reduced by the use of a venting needle.

Thiotepa may be given by intravenous, intramuscular and intrathecal routes of injection; it may be given directly into pleural, pericardial or peritoneal cavities and as a bladder instillation.

Since absorption from the gastrointestinal tract is variable, Thiotepa should not be administered orally.

Dosage must be carefully individualised. A slow response to Thiotepa does not necessarily indicate a lack of effect. Therefore, increasing the frequency of dosing may only increase toxicity.

For intramuscular injection, bladder and intracavitary instillations:

Dosage: Adults, adolescents over 12 years and the elderly

Up to 60mg in single or divided doses. Doses should be reduced in cases of leucopenia as indicated in Table 1. Single-dose administration of 90mg Thiotepa as a bladder instillation is described under "Bladder Cancer".

Table 1

WBC Count Cells/mm^3	Dose of Thiotepa Adults and Adolescents over 12 years
6000	60mg
5000 - 6000	45mg
4500 - 5000	30mg
4000 - 4500	20mg
3500 - 4000	10mg
3000 - 3500	5mg
below 3000	omit dose

Children: Use in children is not recommended.

Intrathecal injection: Up to a maximum of 10mg.

It is essential that a complete blood count should be performed 12-24 hours before each dose of Thiotepa.

Thrombocytopenia in the absence of leucopenia has been noted.

Dosage schedules of Thiotepa vary widely according to the route of administration and the indication.

Examples of dosage schedules used according to specific tumour types are given below:

Breast Cancer:

Patients with advanced breast cancer have been treated with Thiotepa as part of a combination regime, given intramuscularly in divided doses of 15-30mg three times weekly for two weeks; this representing one course of treatment. An interval of six to eight weeks is recommended between courses to allow bone-marrow recovery.

An alternative schedule employs Thiotepa as part of a combination regime, given as an initial priming dose of 15mg intramuscularly or intravenously each day for four days. This may be followed in three weeks by maintenance doses of 15mg I.M. every 14-21 days.

Bladder Cancer:

Instillations of Thiotepa have been used to treat multiple superficial tumours of the bladder, resulting in a complete clinical response in about one third of patients. Patients are dehydrated for 8-12 hours prior to treatment. Up to 60mg Thiotepa dissolved in 60ml sterile water is instilled into the bladder by catheter once a week for four weeks. During removal of the catheter following instillation, Thiotepa injection is continued to ensure bathing of the prostatic and pendulous urethra. The solution should be retained for up to two hours and the patient should be frequently repositioned to ensure maximum contact with the urothelium.

Patients are generally cystoscoped two weeks after a course of four instillations. If a response is observed a second course of four Thiotepa instillations may be given, generally at a reduced dosage, e.g. 15-60mg with intervals of one to two weeks between instillations.

Second and third courses must be given with caution since bone-marrow depression may be increased. Deaths have occurred after intravesical administration, caused by bone-marrow depression from systemically absorbed drug.

Instillations of Thiotepa have been used prophylactically as an adjunct to surgical resection of superficial tumours of the bladder, resulting in a marked decrease in the recurrence rate. It is recommended that there should be a minimum interval of one week between tumour resection and the commencement of prophylactic instillation of Thiotepa. 30-60mg Thiotepa dissolved in 60ml sterile water is instilled into the bladder for two hours and repeated at intervals of one to two weeks for a total of 4-8 instillations. This initial course may be followed by instillations of Thiotepa, 30-60mg every four to six weeks for one year or longer.

Single-dose Thiotepa instillations have been used prophylactically as an adjunct of surgical resection in the treatment of superficial tumours of the bladder. 90mg Thiotepa dissolved in 100mg sterile water is instilled into the bladder with the patient in the left lateral position. After 15 minutes the patient is transferred to the right lateral position and after a further 15 minutes the bladder is emptied. It is felt that such single-dose administration may decrease the incidence of systemic toxicity by decreasing the extent of systemic absorption of the drug.

Note: Patients who have had previous radiotherapy to the bladder are at increased risk of drug toxicity.

Malignant meningeal disease:

Intrathecal injections of Thiotepa have been found to be useful for the palliative treatment of cases of meningeal infiltration by leukaemia and lymphoma. Clinical experience has shown Thiotepa to be effective in carcinomatous involvement of the meninges, but published data is limited. Thiotepa, at a concentration of 1mg/ml in sterile water, is administered by injection through a lumbar theca, in doses of up to 10mg on alternate days until there is clearance of malignant cells from the cerebrospinal fluid (CSF). It is recommended that if no improvement occurs in the CSF after three injections, then treatment should be changed. Not more than four injections should be given on alternative days. Routine blood counts should be performed prior to each dose of Thiotepa.

Ovarian cancer:

Ovarian cancer has been treated with Thiotepa as a single agent or as part of a combination regime in a variety of schedules. For example, 15mg Thiotepa I.V. or I.M. may be given daily for four days initially and then continued with single doses administered once a week or once every two weeks.

Intracavitary instillation of Thiotepa:

Instillations of Thiotepa have been used to treat malignant pleural effusions and abdominal ascites. The procedure recommended, is first to aspirate as much fluid as possible and then to instil the dose of Thiotepa, 10-60mg in 20-60ml sterile water. This may be repeated once a week or once every two weeks.

Prevention of recurrences of Pterygium:

A 1:2,000 solution of Thiotepa in sterile Ringer's solution (i.e. 15mg powder in 30ml Ringer's), applied topically as eye drops, every three hours daily for up to six weeks after surgical removal of the pterygium, is effective in reducing the recurrence rate following surgery.

Condyloma Acuminata:

Thiotepa applied topically or instilled intraurethrally in a gel, has been successfully used to eradicate condyloma acuminata. The drug may be administered by first reconstituting 60mg Thiotepa with 5ml sterile water. This is diluted to 15ml, using a sterile mixture of water and lubricating jelly made to a consistency viscous enough to remain in the urethra and fluid enough to allow easy injection. This therapy may be repeated at weekly intervals.

4.3 Contraindications

Thiotepa administration is contraindicated in patients with a WBC count below 3,000 and/or a platelet count below 100,000 and in patients with known hypersensitivity to ingredients of this preparation.

4.4 Special warnings and special precautions for use

Death from septicaemia and haemorrhage has occurred as a direct result of haematopoietic depression by Thiotepa. Death has also occurred after intravesical administration, caused by bone-marrow depression from systemically absorbed drug.

Thiotepa is highly toxic to the haematopoietic system. WBC and platelet counts are recommended 12-24 hours before each dose of Thiotepa, at weekly intervals during therapy, and for at least three weeks after therapy has been discontinued, regardless of route of administration, except when used topically as eye drops or in the treatment of condyloma acuminata. Bone marrow depression may be delayed; the nadir in blood cell and platelet counts may occur up to 30 days after treatment is stopped. Myelosuppression has occasionally been prolonged.

Dosage should be adjusted according to WBC count (see table 1, Section 4.2, Posology and Method of Administration). Thiotepa administration is contraindicated in patients with WBC count below 3,000 and/or a platelet count below 100,000 (see Section 4.3 Contraindications). Treatment should be discontinued if the white cell or platelet count falls rapidly.

Thiotepa should in general not be used in patients with existing hepatic, renal or bone- marrow damage and only if the need outweighs the risk in such patients. The lowest effective dosage should be used with hepatic, renal and haematopoietic function tests.

In general, dose selection for an elderly patient should be cautious, usually starting at the low end of the dosing range, reflecting the greater frequency of decreasing hepatic, renal or cardiac function, and of concomitant disease or other drug therapy.

Safe use in children has not been established.

Effective contraception should be used during Thiotepa therapy if either the patient or the partner is of childbearing potential.

Thiotepa should only be used by clinicians who are familiar with the various characteristics of cytotoxic drugs and their clinical toxicity.

Thiotepa must be stored in a refrigerator (2-8°C). The occurrence of a precipitate on reconstitution (with 1.5ml of Water for Injection) indicates that polymerisation has occurred with the formation of less active constituents and the injection must be discarded.

Reconstituted solutions may be stored in a refrigerator (2-8°C) for 24 hours. However, if a precipitate forms, the solution must be discarded.

Thiotepa may be mixed in the same syringe with procaine hydrochloride 2% or with adrenaline 1 in 1,000 or with both.

Trained personnel should reconstitute Thiotepa in a designated area. Caution should be exercised in the handling and preparation of Thiotepa. Adequate protective gloves and goggles should be worn and the work surface should be covered with plastic-backed absorbent paper. Thiotepa is not a vesicant and should not cause harm if it comes in contact with the skin. It should, of course, be washed off with water immediately. If Thiotepa contacts mucous membranes, the membranes should be flushed thoroughly with water. Any transient stinging may be treated with bland cream. The cytotoxic preparation should not be handled by pregnant staff.

Any spillage or waste material may be disposed of by incineration. We do not make any specific recommendations with regard to the temperature of the incinerator.

Thiotepa has been reported to possess mutagenic activity on the basis of bacterial, plant and mammalian mutagenicity tests. It has also been reported to be carcinogenic in mice and rats. These effects are consistent with its activity as an alkylating agent. There is some evidence of carcinogenicity in man. In patients treated with Thiotepa, cases of myelodysplastic syndromes and acute non-lymphocytic leukaemia have been reported.

4.5 Interaction with other medicinal products and other forms of Interaction

It is not advisable to combine, simultaneously or sequentially, cancer chemotherapeutic agents or a cancer chemotherapeutic agent and a therapeutic modality having the same mechanism of action. Therefore, Thiotepa combined with other alkylating agents such as nitrogen mustard or cyclophosphamide or Thiotepa combined with irradiation would serve to intensify toxicity rather than to enhance therapeutic response. If these agents must follow each other, it is important that recovery from the first agent, as indicated by white blood cell count, be complete before therapy with the second agent is instituted.

Other drugs which are known to produce bone-marrow depression should be avoided.

Prolonged apnoea has been reported when succinylcholine was administered prior to surgery, following combined use of Thiotepa and other anticancer agents. It was theorised that this was caused by a decrease of pseudocholinesterase activity caused by the anticancer drugs.

4.6 Pregnancy and lactation

Thiotepa can cause foetal harm when administered to a pregnant woman.

Thiotepa is teratogenic and embryotoxic in mice and rats following intraperitoneal administration. In addition, it has been reported to interfere with spermatogenesis and ovarian function in rodent species.

There are no adequate and well-controlled studies in pregnant women. Patients of childbearing potential should be advised to avoid pregnancy. The drug therefore, should not normally be administered to patients who are pregnant or to mothers who are breast feeding unless the benefit outweighs the risk to foetus or child.

If Thiotepa is used during pregnancy, or if pregnancy occurs during Thiotepa therapy, the patient and partner should be apprised of the potential hazard to the foetus.

There are no data on the excretion of Thiotepa in human breast milk. Breast feeding should be discontinued during and for three months following the use of Thiotepa.

4.7 Effects on ability to drive and use machines

None.

4.8 Undesirable effects

The most serious side-effect is upon the blood-forming elements and is a direct consequence of the cytotoxic effect of the drug. Death from septicaemia and haemorrhage has occurred as a direct consequence of haematopoietic suppression.

Infections and Infestations

Increased susceptibility to infections.

Neoplasms benign and malignant (including cysts and polyps)

Myelodysplastic syndrome, acute non-lymphocytic leukemia.

Blood and lymphatic system disorders

Bone-marrow depression, thrombocytopenia, haematopoietic suppression.

Immune system disorders

Allergic reactions.

Metabolism and nutrition disorders

Anorexia.

Nervous system disorders

Headache, dizziness.

Eye disorders

Depigmentation of periorbital skin after using Thiotepa eye drops, blurred vision, conjunctivitis.

Gastrointestinal disorders

Nausea, vomiting, diarrhoea, abdominal pain.

Skin and subcutaneous tissue disorders

Rash, contact dermatitis, alopecia.

Renal and urinary disorders

Haemorrhagic cystitis after intravesical or intravenous administration, dysuria, urinary retention.

Reproductive system and breast disorders

Impairment of fertility, amenorrhoea, interference with spermatogenesis.

General disorders and administration site conditions

Fatigue, weakness, febrile reaction, pain at injection site, skin discolouration following topical use or exposure, local irritation comparable to mild radiation cystitis following bladder instillations.

4.9 Overdose

Manifestations of overdose are primarily reflections of the decreased blood cell and platelet counts due to haematopoietic toxicity, which may become life-threatening. Bleeding due to low platelet counts may occur, and the patient is more vulnerable to, and less able to, combat infections.

There is no specific antidote. General supportive measures are recommended. Thiotepa may be removed using dialysis. Blood counts should be carried out to estimate damage to the haematopoietic system. Whole blood, platelet or leucocyte transfusions have proven beneficial.

5. PHARMACOLOGICAL PROPERTIES

5.1 Pharmacodynamic properties

Thiotepa is an ethyleneimine compound whose antineoplastic effect is related to its alkylating action. It is not a vesicant and may be given by all parenteral routes, as well as directly into tumour masses.

5.2 Pharmacokinetic properties

Variable absorption occurs from intramuscular injection sites. Absorption through serous membranes such as the bladder and pleura occurs to some extent. Only traces of unchanged Thiotepa and triethylene phosphoramide are excreted in the urine, together with a large proportion of metabolites.

5.3 Preclinical safety data
Thiotepa has been shown to be mutagenic in various *in vitro* assays, and carcinogenic in animal studies.

Studies in animals have shown Thiotepa to impair spermatogenesis and ovarian function.

6. PHARMACEUTICAL PARTICULARS

6.1 List of excipients
Water for Injection

6.2 Incompatibilities
None

6.3 Shelf life
18 months

6.4 Special precautions for storage
Thiotepa must be stored in a refrigerator (2-8°C). Reconstituted solutions may be stored in a refrigerator (2-8°C) for up to 24 hours.

6.5 Nature and contents of container
Flint glass vial with butyl rubber stopper.

Pack Size: 15mg

6.6 Instructions for use and handling
See " Special Warnings and Precautions".

7. MARKETING AUTHORISATION HOLDER
Cyanamid of Great Britain Ltd

Fareham Road

Gosport

Hampshire

PO13 OAS

8. MARKETING AUTHORISATION NUMBER(S)
PL 0095/0234

9. DATE OF FIRST AUTHORISATION/RENEWAL OF THE AUTHORISATION
22 August 1991/ 16 April 2002

10. DATE OF REVISION OF THE TEXT
06 August 2004

Tilade Inhaler and Syncroner

(sanofi-aventis)

1. NAME OF THE MEDICINAL PRODUCT
Tilade Inhaler

Tilade Syncroner

2. QUALITATIVE AND QUANTITATIVE COMPOSITION
The active component per actuation of Tilade is nedocromil sodium 2mg

3. PHARMACEUTICAL FORM
Tilade is presented as a metered dose pressurised aerosol containing nedocromil sodium as a suspension in chlorofluorocarbon propellants, for inhalation.

4. CLINICAL PARTICULARS

4.1 Therapeutic indications
Tilade is recommended for the treatment of bronchial asthma where regular preventative anti-inflammatory therapy is indicated and in particular in patients whose asthma is not adequately controlled by bronchodilators alone. Tilade may be given in addition to all existing therapies and in many cases will provide added therapeutic benefit.

4.2 Posology and method of administration
Adults (including the Elderly) and Children over the age of 6 years:

Initially two actuations (4mg of nedocromil sodium) four times daily. Once symptomatic control has been achieved, the usual maintenance dose is two actuations twice daily.

Tilade is intended for regular daily usage and should not be used for the relief of symptoms in an acute attack.

4.3 Contraindications
Tilade is contraindicated in patients with known hypersensitivity to any constituent of the formulation.

4.4 Special warnings and special precautions for use
Tilade should not be used for the relief of an acute attack of bronchospasm.

4.5 Interaction with other medicinal products and other forms of Interaction
None known.

4.6 Pregnancy and lactation
Studies in pregnant and lactating animals have failed to reveal a hazard. However, as with all medications caution should be exercised especially during the first trimester of pregnancy.

On the basis of animal studies and its physiochemical properties it is considered that only negligible amounts of nedocromil sodium may pass into human breast milk. There is no information to suggest that the use of nedocromil sodium by nursing mothers has any undesirable effects on the baby.

4.7 Effects on ability to drive and use machines
Tilade has no known effect on the ability to drive or operate machinery.

4.8 Undesirable effects
The principal side effects reported are headache and upper gastro-intestinal tract symptoms (nausea, vomiting, dyspepsia and abdominal pain). These are usually mild and transient. In common with other inhaled medications Tilade may produce cough or bronchospasm.

4.9 Overdose
Animal studies have not shown evidence of toxic effects of nedocromil sodium even at high dosage, nor have extended human studies revealed any safety hazard with the drug. Overdosage is unlikely therefore to cause problems.

However, if overdosage is suspected, treatment should be supportive and directed to the control of the relevant symptoms.

5. PHARMACOLOGICAL PROPERTIES

5.1 Pharmacodynamic properties
Tilade contains nedocromil sodium, a non-steroid agent, which has anti-inflammatory properties when administered topically in the lung. In-vivo, ex-vivo and in-vitro studies have shown that nedocromil sodium has beneficial effects on cellular, humoral and neuronal mechanisms thought to be involved in the inflammation of bronchial asthma. In the treatment of bronchial asthma, nedocromil sodium reduces bronchospasm, cough and bronchial hyperreactivity and improves objective measurements of lung function.

5.2 Pharmacokinetic properties
Nedocromil can be detected in the plasma for several hours after administration of a dose of 4mg by inhalation. Approximately 5% of the inhaled dose was found to be absorbed with a rate constant which was lower than the elimination rate constant; this means that absorption from the lungs is rate limiting. After oral administration, the extent of absorption was lower (0.7 to 1.7%) and was shown to occur over a period of at least 72 hours. Following multiple dosing by inhalation there was no accumulation, although the slow oral absorption contributed to the small carry-over that occurred from day to day.

Intravenous administration was used to study the elimination process from the body. The results demonstrated nedocromil to have a high clearance (10ml min^{-1} kg^{-1}) due largely to excretion. The major route was via the urine (70%), the remainder via the alimentary tract.

Plasma protein binding was moderate and readily reversible.

No metabolism of the compound was detected.

5.3 Preclinical safety data
Animal studies have failed to reveal toxic effects with nedocromil sodium even at high doses.

6. PHARMACEUTICAL PARTICULARS

6.1 List of excipients
Dentomint

Saccharin sodium

Sorbitan trioleate

Propellant mixture 12:114 (dichlorodifluoromethane and dichlorotetrafluoroethane)

6.2 Incompatibilities
None known.

6.3 Shelf life
36 months.

6.4 Special precautions for storage
Store below 30°C, away from direct sunlight, but do not freeze.

The canister is pressurised and must not be punctured or burnt even when empty.

6.5 Nature and contents of container
An aluminium aerosol can fitted with a metering valve.

Tilade Inhaler: The pack consists of two cans each delivering 56 actuations. Each can is fitted with a plastic adaptor and dust cap.

Tilade Syncroner: The pack consists of two cans each delivering 112 actuations. Each can is fitted with a spacer device and dust cap.

6.6 Instructions for use and handling
Please refer to enclosed package insert.

7. MARKETING AUTHORISATION HOLDER
Concord Pharmaceuticals Limited

Bishops Weald House

Albion Way

Horsham

West Sussex

RH12 1AH

8. MARKETING AUTHORISATION NUMBER(S)
PL 15638/0012

9. DATE OF FIRST AUTHORISATION/RENEWAL OF THE AUTHORISATION
August 1998

10. DATE OF REVISION OF THE TEXT
June 2004

Legal Category: POM

Tildiem LA 200, Tildiem LA 300

(sanofi-aventis)

1. NAME OF THE MEDICINAL PRODUCT
Tildiem LA 200

Tildiem LA 300

2. QUALITATIVE AND QUANTITATIVE COMPOSITION
Each capsule contains a combination of immediate-release and coated sustained-release pellets with 200mg or 300mg diltiazem hydrochloride as the active ingredient.

For excipients see 6.1

3. PHARMACEUTICAL FORM
Tildiem LA 200: Sustained-release oral capsules (grey body, pink cap).

Tildiem LA 300: Opaque capsules with a white body and yellow cap.

4. CLINICAL PARTICULARS

4.1 Therapeutic indications
Mild to moderate hypertension and angina pectoris.

4.2 Posology and method of administration
Tildiem LA 200 and Tildiem LA 300 are sustained release products for once daily dosing. The capsules should not be chewed but swallowed whole with water, ideally before or during a meal. The dosage requirements may differ in patients with angina or hypertension.

Tildiem (diltiazem hydrochloride) is available in a range of presentations to enable dosage to be adjusted to meet the individual requirements of the patient. Careful titration of the dose should be considered where appropriate, as individual patient response may vary. When changing from one type of Tildiem formulation to another it may be necessary to adjust the dosage until a satisfactory response is obtained. To ensure consistency of response once established, particularly in the sustained release formulations, Tildiem LA 200 and 300 should continue to be prescribed by brand name.

Adults:

Angina and hypertension: The usual starting dose is Tildiem LA 200 once daily. This dose may be increased to Tildiem LA 300 once daily, or 2 capsules of Tildiem LA 200 daily (400 mg), and if clinically indicated a higher dose of one Tildiem LA 300 plus one Tildiem LA 200 capsule (total 500 mg) may be considered.

Elderly and patients with impaired hepatic or renal function:

Heart rate should be monitored and if it falls below 50 beats per minute the dose should not be increased. Plasma levels of diltiazem can be increased in this group of patients.

Angina and hypertension: the initial dose should be one Tildiem LA 200 capsule daily. This dose may be increased to one capsule of Tildiem LA 300 daily if clinically indicated.

Children:

Safety and efficacy in children have not been established. Therefore diltiazem is not recommended for use in children.

4.3 Contraindications
Sick sinus syndrome, 2nd or 3rd degree AV block in patients without a functioning pacemaker.

Severe bradycardia (less than 50 beats per minute).

Left ventricular failure with pulmonary stasis.

Pregnancy, women of child-bearing potential and lactation *(see section 4.6 Pregnancy and lactation)*.

Concurrent use with dantrolene infusion *(see section 4.5 Interactions with other medicinal products and other forms of interaction)*.

Hypersensitivity to diltiazem or to any of the excipients

4.4 Special warnings and special precautions for use
Close observation is necessary in patients with reduced left ventricular function, bradycardia (risk of exacerbation) or with a 1st degree AV block or prolonged PR interval detected on the electrocardiogram (risk of exacerbation and rarely, of complete block).

Plasma diltiazem concentrations can be increased in the elderly and patients with renal or hepatic insufficiency. The contraindications and precautions should be carefully observed and close monitoring, particularly of heart rate, should be carried out at the beginning of treatment.

In the case of general anaesthesia, the anaesthetist must be informed that the patient is taking diltiazem. The depression of cardiac contractility, conductivity and automaticity as well as the vascular dilatation associated with anaesthetics may be potentiated by calcium channel blockers.

4.5 Interaction with other medicinal products and other forms of Interaction

COMBINATION CONTRA-INDICATED FOR SAFETY REASONS:

Dantrolene (infusion)

Lethal ventricular fibrillation is regularly observed in animals when intravenous verapamil and dantrolene are administered concomitantly.

The combination of a calcium antagonist and dantrolene is therefore potentially dangerous *(see section 4.3 Contra-indications)*.

COMBINATIONS REQUIRING CAUTION:

Alpha$_1$-antagonists:

Increased anti-hypertensive effect.

Concomitant treatment with alpha-antagonists may produce or aggravate hypotension. The combination of diltiazem with an alpha antagonist should be considered only with strict monitoring of blood pressure.

Beta-blockers:

Possibility of rhythm disturbances (pronounced bradycardia, sinus arrest), sino-atrial and atrio-ventricular conduction disturbances and heart failure (synergistic effect).

Such a combination must only be used under close clinical and ECG monitoring, particularly at the beginning of treatment.

Amiodarone, Digoxin:

Increased risk of bradycardia; caution is required when these are combined with diltiazem, particularly in elderly subjects and when high doses are used.

Antiarrhythmic agents:

Since diltiazem has antiarrhythmic properties, its concomitant prescription with other antiarrhythmic agents is not recommended due to the risk of increased cardiac adverse effects due to an additive effect. This combination should only be used under close clinical and ECG monitoring.

Nitrate derivatives:

Increased hypotensive effects and faintness (additive vasodilating effects).

In all patients treated with calcium antagonists, the prescription of nitrate derivatives should only be carried out at gradually increasing doses.

Cyclosporin:

Increase in circulating cyclosporin levels. It is recommended that the cyclosporin dose be reduced, renal function be monitored, circulating cyclosporin levels be assayed and that the dose should be adjusted during combined therapy and after its discontinuation.

Carbamazepine:

Increase in circulating carbamazepine levels. It is recommended that the plasma carbamazepine concentrations be assayed and that the dose should be adjusted if necessary.

Theophylline:

Increase in circulating theophylline levels.

Anti-H_2 agents (cimetidine and ranitidine):

Increase in plasma diltiazem concentrations.

Patients currently receiving diltiazem therapy should be carefully monitored when initiating or discontinuing therapy with anti-H_2 agents. An adjustment in diltiazem daily dose may be necessary.

Rifampicin

Risk of decrease of diltiazem plasma levels after initiating therapy with rifampicin. The patient should be carefully monitored when initiating or discontinuing rifampicin treatment.

Lithium

Risk of increase in lithium-induced neurotoxicity.

COMBINATIONS TO BE TAKEN INTO ACCOUNT:

Oral administration of diltiazem can raise the plasma concentration of drugs exclusively metabolised by CYP3A4. The concomitant therapy of diltiazem and such drugs may increase the risk of adverse reactions (e.g. muscular disorders with statins).

4.6 Pregnancy and lactation

Pregnancy: this drug has been shown to be teratogenic in certain animal species and is therefore contraindicated in pregnancy and in women of child-bearing potential.

Breast feeding: as this drug is excreted in breast milk, breast feeding whilst taking diltiazem is contraindicated.

4.7 Effects on ability to drive and use machines

No effect reported to date

4.8 Undesirable effects

Cardiovascular disorders:

The manifestations of vasodilation (orthostatic hypotension, headache, flushing and in particular oedema of the lower limbs) are dose-dependent and appear more frequently in elderly subjects and are related to the pharmacological activity of the product.

Occasional cases of vasculitis.

Rare cases of symptomatic bradycardia and sino-atrial block and atrioventricular block, palpitations.

Development or aggravation of congestive heart failure.

Gastro-intestinal system disorders:

Digestive disturbances such as dyspepsia, gastric pain, nausea, constipation, dry mouth.

Gingival hyperplasia

Skin and appendage disorders:

Muco-cutaneous reactions such as simple erythema, urticaria, or occasionally desquamative erythema, with or without fever and photosensitivity have been reported, recovering when the treatment is discontinued.

Erythema multiforme and/or exfoliative dermatitis and acute generalised exanthematous pustular dermatitis have been reported.

Liver and other biliary system disorders:

Isolated cases of moderate and transient elevation of liver transaminases have been observed at the start of treatment. Isolated cases of clinical hepatitis have been reported which resolved on cessation of diltiazem therapy.

Others:

Malaise, dizziness, asthenia/fatigue.

As with some other calcium channel blockers, exceptional cases of extrapyramidal symptoms and gynaecomastia have been reported, reversible after discontinuation of calcium antagonists.

4.9 Overdose

The clinical effects of acute overdose can involve pronounced hypotension leading to collapse, sinus bradycardia with or without isorhythmic dissociation, and atrioventricular conduction disturbances.

Treatment, under hospital supervision, will include gastric lavage, osmotic diuresis. Conduction disturbances may be managed by temporary cardiac pacing.

Proposed corrective treatments: atropine, vasopressors, inotropic agents, glucagon and calcium gluconate infusion.

5. PHARMACOLOGICAL PROPERTIES

5.1 Pharmacodynamic properties

Calcium antagonist, antihypertensive agent.

Pharmacotherapeutic group: Calcium Channel Blocker, ATC Code: C08D B01

Diltiazem restricts calcium entry into the slow calcium channel of vascular smooth muscle and myocardial muscle fibres in a voltage-dependent manner. By this mechanism, diltiazem reduces the concentration of intracellular calcium in contractile protein.

In animals: diltiazem increases coronary blood flow without inducing any coronary steal phenomena. It acts both on small, large and collateral arteries. This vasodilator effect, which is moderate on peripheral systemic arterial territories, can be seen at doses that are not negatively inotropic.

The two major active circulating metabolites, i.e. desacetyl diltiazem and N-monodesmethyl diltiazem, possess pharmacological activity in angina corresponding to 10 and 20% respectively of that of the parent compound.

In humans: diltiazem increases coronary blood flow by reducing coronary resistance.

Due to its moderate bradycardia-inducing activity and the reduction in systemic arterial resistance, diltiazem reduces cardiac workload.

Tildiem LA does not have a significant myocardial depressant action in man.

5.2 Pharmacokinetic properties

Diltiazem is well absorbed (90%) in healthy volunteers following oral administration.

The sustained release capsule provides prolonged absorption of the active constituent, producing steady state plasma concentrations between 2 and 14 hours post-dose, during which time peak plasma levels occur.

Bioavailability of Tildiem LA relative to the Tildiem 60mg formulation is approximately 80%. The mean apparent plasma half-life is 8 hours.

Diltiazem in plasma is 80 to 85% protein bound and is poorly dialysed. It is extensively metabolised by the liver.

The major circulating metabolite, N-monodesmethyl diltiazem accounts for approximately 35% of the circulating diltiazem.

Less than 5% of diltiazem is excreted unchanged in the urine.

Twenty four hours after intake, plasma concentrations remain, even after the 200 mg dose administration, at the level of 50 ng/ml, in patients. During long term administration in any one patient, plasma concentrations of diltiazem remained constant.

Mean plasma concentrations in the elderly and patients with renal and hepatic insufficiency are higher than in young subjects.

Food intake does not significantly affect the kinetics of Tildiem LA, however, when administered with food, absorption was observed to be higher in the first few hours post-dose.

Diltiazem and its metabolites are poorly dialysed.

Once daily formulations of diltiazem have been shown to have different pharmacokinetic profiles and therefore it is not advised to substitute different brands for one another.

5.3 Preclinical safety data

No data of therapeutic relevance.

6. PHARMACEUTICAL PARTICULARS

6.1 List of excipients

Tildiem LA 200: Microcrystalline cellulose, acrylic and methacrylic esters co-polymer, ethylcellulose, sodium carboxymethylcellulose, diacetylated monoglycerides, magnesium stearate. *In the capsule:* gelatin, black iron oxide (E172), titanium dioxide (E171), red iron oxide (E172).

Tildiem LA 300: Microcrystalline cellulose, acrylic and methacrylic esters copolymer, ethylcellulose, carmellose sodium, diacetylated monoglycerides, magnesium stearate.

In the capsule: gelatin, titanium dioxide (E171), yellow iron oxide (E172).

6.2 Incompatibilities

Not applicable

6.3 Shelf life

Tildiem LA 200: Three years

Tildiem LA 300: Two years

6.4 Special precautions for storage

Tildiem LA 200: To be stored below 25°C.

Tildiem LA 300: Do not store above 25°C.

6.5 Nature and contents of container

28 capsules, in a PVC/foil blister strip.

6.6 Instructions for use and handling

Please consult the package insert before use. Do not use after the stated expiry date on the carton and blister strip.

Keep out of the reach of children.

7. MARKETING AUTHORISATION HOLDER

Sanofi-Synthelabo

PO Box 597

Guildford

Surrey

8. MARKETING AUTHORISATION NUMBER(S)

Tildiem LA 200: PL 11723/0338

Tildiem LA 300: PL 11723/0337

9. DATE OF FIRST AUTHORISATION/RENEWAL OF THE AUTHORISATION

Tildiem LA 200: 12th December 2000

Tildiem LA 300: 12th December 2000 / 27 August 2003

10. DATE OF REVISION OF THE TEXT

Tildiem LA 200: July 2002

Tildiem LA 300: August 2003

Legal Category POM

Tildiem Retard 90mg, Tildiem Retard 120mg

(sanofi-aventis)

1. NAME OF THE MEDICINAL PRODUCT

Tildiem Retard 90mg.

Tildiem Retard 120mg

2. QUALITATIVE AND QUANTITATIVE COMPOSITION

Each 90mg tablet contains 90mg diltiazem hydrochloride as the active ingredient.

Each 120mg tablet contains 120mg diltiazem hydrochloride as the active ingredient.

For excipients see 6.1

3. PHARMACEUTICAL FORM

Sustained release tablet.

Off-white biconvex tablet.

4. CLINICAL PARTICULARS

4.1 Therapeutic indications

Mild to moderate hypertension and angina pectoris.

4.2 Posology and method of administration

Tildiem Retard tablets should be swallowed whole with a little water and not crushed or chewed.

Patients should be advised that the tablet membrane may pass through the gastro-intestinal tract unchanged.

Tildiem (diltiazem hydrochloride) is available in a range of presentations to enable dosage to be adjusted to meet the individual requirements of the patient. Careful titration of the dose should be considered where appropriate, as individual patient response may vary. When changing from one type of Tildiem formulation to another it may be necessary to adjust the dosage until a satisfactory response is obtained. To ensure consistency of response once established, particularly in the sustained release formulations, Tildiem Retard 90mg and 120mg should continue to be prescribed by brand name.

Adults:

Angina and hypertension:

The usual starting dose is one tablet (90mg or 120mg) twice daily. Patient responses may vary and dosage requirements can differ significantly between individual patients. Higher divided doses up to 480mg/day have been used with benefit in some angina patients especially in unstable angina. Doses of 360mg/day may be required to provide adequate BP control in hypertensive patients.

Elderly and patients with impaired hepatic or renal function:

Heart rate should be monitored in these patients and if it falls below 50 beats per minute the dose should not be increased.

Angina:

The recommended starting dose is one Tildiem 60mg tablet twice daily. This dose may be increased to one 90mg or 120mg Tildiem Retard tablet twice daily.

Hypertension:

The starting dose should be one 120mg Tildiem Retard tablet daily. Dose adjustment to one 90mg or one 120mg Tildiem Retard tablet twice daily may be required.

Children:

Safety and efficacy in children have not been established. Therefore diltiazem is not recommended for use in children.

4.3 Contraindications

Sick sinus syndrome, 2nd or 3rd degree AV block in patients without a functioning pacemaker.

Severe bradycardia (less than 50 beats per minute).

Left ventricular failure with pulmonary stasis.

Pregnancy, women of child-bearing potential and lactation *(see section 4.6 Pregnancy and lactation)*.

Concurrent use with dantrolene infusion *(see section 4.5 Interactions with other medicinal products and other forms of interaction)*.

Hypersensitivity to diltiazem or to any of the excipients.

4.4 Special warnings and special precautions for use

Close observation is necessary in patients with reduced left ventricular function, bradycardia (risk of exacerbation) or with a 1st degree AV block detected on the electrocardiogram (risk of exacerbation and rarely of complete block) or prolonged PR interval.

Plasma diltiazem concentrations can be increased in the elderly and patients with renal or hepatic insufficiency. The contraindications and precautions should be carefully observed and close monitoring, particularly of heart rate, should be carried out at the beginning of treatment.

In the case of general anaesthesia, the anaesthetist must be informed that the patient is taking diltiazem. The depression of cardiac contractility, conductivity and automaticity as well as the vascular dilatation associated with anaesthetics may be potentiated by calcium channel blockers.

Diltiazem does not affect the glucose or endogenous insulin responses to hypoglycaemia.

4.5 Interaction with other medicinal products and other forms of Interaction

COMBINATION CONTRAINDICATED FOR SAFETY REASONS:

Dantrolene (infusion)

Lethal ventricular fibrillation is regularly observed in animals when intravenous verapamil and dantrolene are administered concomitantly.

The combination of a calcium antagonist and dantrolene is therefore potentially dangerous *(see section 4.3 Contraindications)*.

COMBINATIONS REQUIRING CAUTION:

Alpha-antagonists:

Increased anti-hypertensive effects.

Concomitant treatment with alpha-antagonists may produce or aggravate hypotension. The combination of diltiazem with an alpha antagonist should be considered only with strict monitoring of blood pressure.

Beta-blockers:

Possibility of rhythm disturbances (pronounced bradycardia, sinus arrest), sino-atrial and atrio-ventricular conduction disturbances and heart failure (synergistic effect).

Such a combination must only be used under close clinical and ECG monitoring, particularly at the beginning of treatment.

Amiodarone, Digoxin:

Increased risk of bradycardia; caution is required when these are combined with diltiazem, particularly in elderly subjects and when high doses are used.

Antiarrhythmic agents:

Since diltiazem has antiarrhythmic properties, its concomitant prescription with other antiarrhythmic agents is not recommended due to the risk of increased cardiac adverse effects due to an additive effect. This combination should only be used under close clinical and ECG monitoring.

Nitrate derivatives:

Increased hypotensive effects and faintness (additive vasodilating effects).

In all patients treated with calcium antagonists, the prescription of nitrate derivatives should only be carried out at gradually increasing doses.

Cyclosporin:

Increase in circulating cyclosporin levels. It is recommended that the cyclosporin dose be reduced, renal function be monitored, circulating cyclosporin levels be assayed and that the dose should be adjusted during combined therapy and after its discontinuation.

Carbamazepine:

Increase in circulating carbamazepine levels.

It is recommended that the plasma carbamazepine concentrations be assayed and that the dose should be adjusted if necessary.

Theophylline:

Increase in circulating theophylline levels.

Anti-H_2 agents (cimetidine and ranitidine):

Increase in plasma diltiazem concentrations.

Patients currently receiving diltiazem therapy should be carefully monitored when initiating or discontinuing therapy with anti-H_2 agents. An adjustment in diltiazem daily dose may be necessary.

Rifampicin

Risk of decrease of diltiazem plasma levels after initiating therapy with rifampicin. The patient should be carefully monitored when initiating or discontinuing rifampicin treatment.

Lithium

Risk of increase in lithium-induced neurotoxicity.

COMBINATIONS TO BE TAKEN INTO ACCOUNT:

Oral administration of diltiazem can raise the plasma concentration of drugs exclusively metabolised by CYP3A4. The concomitant therapy of diltiazem and such drugs may increase the risk of adverse reactions (e.g. muscular disorders with statins).

4.6 Pregnancy and lactation

Pregnancy: this drug has been shown to be teratogenic in certain animal species and is therefore contraindicated in pregnancy and in women of child-bearing potential.

Breast feeding: as this drug is excreted in breast milk, breast feeding whilst taking diltiazem is contraindicated.

4.7 Effects on ability to drive and use machines

No effect reported to date.

4.8 Undesirable effects

Cardiovascular disorders:

The manifestations of vasodilation (orthostatic hypotension, headache, flushing and in particular oedema of the lower limbs) are dose-dependent and appear more frequently in elderly subjects and are related to the pharmacological activity of the product.

Occasional cases of vasculitis.

Rare cases of symptomatic bradycardia and sino-atrial block and atrioventricular block, palpitations.

Development or aggravation of congestive heart failure.

Gastro-intestinal system disorders:

Digestive disturbances such as dyspepsia, gastric pain, nausea, constipation, dry mouth.

Gingival hyperplasia

Skin and appendage disorders:

Muco-cutaneous reactions such as simple erythema, urticaria, or occasionally desquamative erythema, with or without fever and photosensitivity have been reported, recovering when the treatment is discontinued.

Erythema multiforme and/or exfoliative dermatitis and acute generalised exanthematous pustular dermatitis have been reported.

Liver and other biliary system disorders:

Isolated cases of moderate and transient elevation of liver transaminases have been observed at the start of treatment. Isolated cases of clinical hepatitis have been reported which resolved on cessation of diltiazem therapy.

Others:

Malaise, dizziness, asthenia/fatigue.

As with some other calcium channel blockers, exceptional cases of extrapyramidal symptoms and gynaecomastia have been reported, reversible after discontinuation of calcium antagonists.

4.9 Overdose

The clinical effects of acute overdose can involve pronounced hypotension leading to collapse, sinus bradycardia with or without isorhythmic dissociation, and atrioventricular conduction disturbances.

Treatment, under hospital supervision, will include gastric lavage, osmotic diuresis. Conduction disturbances may be managed by temporary cardiac pacing.

Proposed corrective treatments: atropine, vasopressors, inotropic agents, glucagon and calcium gluconate infusion.

5. PHARMACOLOGICAL PROPERTIES

5.1 Pharmacodynamic properties

Pharmacotherapeutic group: Calcium Channel Blocker, ATC code: C08D B01

Tildiem is a calcium antagonist. It restricts the slow channel entry of calcium into the cell and so reduces the liberation of calcium from stores in the sarcoplasmic reticulum. This results in a reduction of the amount of available intracellular calcium reducing myocardial oxygen consumption. It increases exercise capacity and improves all indices of myocardial ischaemia in the angina patient. Tildiem relaxes large and small coronary arteries and relieves the spasm of vasospastic (Prinzmetal's) angina and the response to catecholamines but has little effect on the peripheral vasculature. There is therefore no possibility of reflex tachycardia. A small reduction in heart rate occurs which is accompanied by an increase in cardiac output, improved myocardial perfusion and reduction of ventricular work. In animal studies, Tildiem protects the myocardium against the effects of ischaemia and reduces the damage produced by excessive entry of calcium into the myocardial cell during reperfusion.

5.2 Pharmacokinetic properties

Diltiazem is well absorbed (90%) in healthy volunteers following oral administration.

These formulations of diltiazem hydrochloride provide prolonged absorption of the active ingredient. Peak plasma concentrations occur between 4 and 8 hours post-dose.

Bioavailability of this formulation of diltiazem is approximately 90% of that of the conventional tablet. The mean apparent plasma half-life is 7 - 8 hours.

Diltiazem is 80 to 85% bound to plasma proteins. It is extensively metabolised by the liver.

The major circulating metabolite, N-monodesmethyl diltiazem accounts for approximately 35% of the circulating diltiazem.

Less than 5% of diltiazem is excreted unchanged in the urine.

During long term administration to any one patient, plasma concentrations of diltiazem remain constant.

Mean plasma concentrations in elderly subjects and patients with renal and hepatic insufficiency are higher than in young subjects.

Diltiazem and its metabolites are poorly dialysed.

Twice daily formulations of diltiazem have been shown to have different pharmacokinetic profiles and therefore it is not advised to substitute different brands for one another.

5.3 Preclinical safety data

No data of therapeutic relevance.

6. PHARMACEUTICAL PARTICULARS

6.1 List of excipients

Tablet core: Sodium dihydrogen citrate, sucrose, povidone, magnesium stearate, macrogol 6000.

Coating: Sucrose, coating polymer, acetyl tributyl citrate, castor oil polymerised, sodium hydrogen carbonate, ethyl vanillin, titanium dioxide (E171).

6.2 Incompatibilities

Not applicable

6.3 Shelf life

Two years.

6.4 Special precautions for storage

Do not store above 30°C. Store in the original package.

Tildiem Retard tablets are coated with a porous polymer membrane which enables the diltiazem to diffuse out of the tablet at a gradual rate. This membrane may pass through the gastro-intestinal tract unchanged. This has no bearing on the efficacy of the product.

6.5 Nature and contents of container

56 tablets in PVC/foil strips

6.6 Instructions for use and handling

No special requirements.

7. MARKETING AUTHORISATION HOLDER

Sanofi-Synthelabo,

PO Box 597,

Guildford,

Surrey

8. MARKETING AUTHORISATION NUMBER(S)

Tildiem Retard 90mg 11723/0335

Tildiem Retard 120mg 11723/0336

9. DATE OF FIRST AUTHORISATION/RENEWAL OF THE AUTHORISATION

12 December 2000 / 27 August 2003

10. DATE OF REVISION OF THE TEXT

April 2004

Legal Category: POM

Tildiem Tablets 60mg

(sanofi-aventis)

1. NAME OF THE MEDICINAL PRODUCT

Tildiem tablets 60mg

2. QUALITATIVE AND QUANTITATIVE COMPOSITION

Each modified release tablet contains diltiazem hydrochloride 60mg

3. PHARMACEUTICAL FORM

Modified release tablet

4. CLINICAL PARTICULARS

4.1 Therapeutic indications

Prophylaxis and treatment of Angina Pectoris

4.2 Posology and method of administration

Adults: The usual dose is one tablet (60mg) three times daily. However, patient responses may vary and dosage requirements can differ significantly between individual patients. If necessary the divided dose may be increased to 360mg/day. Higher doses up to 480mg/day have been used with benefit in some patients especially in unstable angina. There is no evidence of any decrease in efficacy at these high doses.

Elderly and patients with impaired hepatic or renal function: The recommended starting dose is one tablet (60mg) twice daily. The heart rate should be measured regularly in these groups of patients and the dose should not be increased if the heart rate falls below 50 beats per minute.

Children: Safety and efficacy in children have not been established.

4.3 Contraindications

Sick sinus syndrome, 2nd or 3rd degree AV block in patients without a functioning pacemaker.

Severe bradycardia (less than 50 beats per minute).

Left ventricular failure with pulmonary stasis.

Pregnancy, women of child-bearing potential and lactation *(see section 4.6 Pregnancy and lactation).*

Concurrent use with dantrolene infusion *(see section 4.5 Interactions with other medicinal products and other forms of interactions).*

Hypersensitivity to diltiazem or to any of the excipients.

4.4 Special warnings and special precautions for use

Close observation is necessary in patients with reduced left ventricular function, bradycardia (risk of exacerbation) or with a 1st degree AV block detected on the electrocardiogram (risk of exacerbation and rarely of complete block) or prolonged PR interval.

Plasma diltiazem concentrations can be increased in the elderly and patients with renal or hepatic insufficiency. The contraindications and precautions should be carefully observed and close monitoring, particularly of heart rate, should be carried out at the beginning of treatment.

In the case of general anaesthesia, the anaesthetist must be informed that the patient is taking diltiazem. The depression of cardiac contractility, conductivity and automaticity as well as the vascular dilatation associated with anaesthetics may be potentiated by calcium channel blockers.

4.5 Interaction with other medicinal products and other forms of Interaction

Combination contraindicated for safety reasons:

Dantrolene (infusion)

Lethal ventricular fibrillation is regularly observed in animals when intravenous verapamil and dantrolene are administered concomitantly.

The combination of a calcium antagonist and dantrolene is therefore potentially dangerous *(see section 4.3 Contra-indications).*

Combinations requiring caution:

Alpha-antagonists: Increased anti-hypertensive effects.

Concomitant treatment with alpha-antagonists may produce or aggravate hypotension. The combination of diltiazem with an alpha antagonist should be considered only with strict monitoring of blood pressure.

Beta-blockers: Possibility of rhythm disturbances (pronounced bradycardia, sinus arrest), sino-atrial and atrioventricular conduction disturbances and heart failure (synergistic effect).

Such a combination must only be used under close clinical and ECG monitoring, particularly at the beginning of treatment.

Amiodarone, Digoxin: Increased risk of bradycardia; caution is required when these are combined with diltiazem, particularly in elderly subjects and when high doses are used.

Antiarrhythmic agents: Since diltiazem has antiarrhythmic properties, its concomitant prescription with other antiarrhythmic agents is not recommended due to the risk of increased cardiac adverse effects due to an additive effect. This combination should only be used under close clinical and ECG monitoring.

Nitrate derivatives: Increased hypotensive effects and faintness (additive vasodilating effects).

In all patients treated with calcium antagonists, the prescription of nitrate derivatives should only be carried out at gradually increasing doses.

Cyclosporin: Increase in circulating cyclosporin levels. It is recommended that the cyclosporin dose be reduced, renal function be monitored, circulating cyclosporin levels be assayed and that the dose should be adjusted during combined therapy and after its discontinuation.

Carbamazepine: Increase in circulating carbamazepine levels.

It is recommended that the plasma carbamazepine concentrations be assayed and that the dose should be adjusted if necessary.

Theophylline: Increase in circulating theophylline levels.

Anti-H_2 agents (cimetidine and ranitidine): Increase in plasma diltiazem concentrations. Patients currently receiving diltiazem therapy should be carefully monitored when initiating or discontinuing therapy with anti-H_2 agents. An adjustment in diltiazem daily dose may be necessary.

Rifampicin: Risk of decrease of diltiazem plasma levels after initiating therapy with rifampicin. The patient should be carefully monitored when initiating or discontinuing rifampicin treatment.

Lithium: Risk of increase in lithium-induced neurotoxicity.

COMBINATIONS TO BE TAKEN INTO ACCOUNT:

Oral administration of diltiazem can raise the plasma concentration of drugs exclusively metabolised by CYP3A4. The concomitant therapy of diltiazem and such drugs may increase the risk of adverse reactions (e.g. muscular disorders with statins).

4.6 Pregnancy and lactation

Pregnancy: this drug has been shown to be teratogenic in certain animal species and is therefore contraindicated in pregnancy and in women of child-bearing potential.

Breast feeding: as this drug is excreted in breast milk, breast feeding whilst taking diltiazem is contraindicated.

4.7 Effects on ability to drive and use machines

Not applicable.

4.8 Undesirable effects

Cardiovascular disorders:

The manifestations of vasodilation (orthostatic hypotension, headache, flushing and in particular oedema of the lower limbs) are dose-dependent and appear more frequently in elderly subjects and are related to the pharmacological activity of the product.

Occasional cases of vasculitis.

Rare cases of symptomatic bradycardia and sino-atrial block and atrioventricular block, palpitations.

Development or aggravation of congestive heart failure.

Gastro-intestinal system disorders:

Digestive disturbances such as dyspepsia, gastric pain, nausea, constipation, dry mouth.

Gingival hyperplasia

Skin and appendage disorders:

Muco-cutaneous reactions such as simple erythema, urticaria, or occasionally desquamative erythema, with or without fever and photosensitivity have been reported, recovering when the treatment is discontinued.

Erythema multiforme and/or exfoliative dermatitis and acute generalised exanthematous pustular dermatitis have been reported.

Liver and other biliary system disorders:

Isolated cases of moderate and transient elevation of liver transaminases have been observed at the start of treatment. Isolated cases of clinical hepatitis have been reported which resolved on cessation of diltiazem therapy.

Others:

Malaise, dizziness, asthenia/fatigue.

As with some other calcium channel blockers, exceptional cases of extrapyramidal symptoms and gynaecomastia have been reported, reversible after discontinuation of calcium antagonists.

4.9 Overdose

The clinical effects of acute overdose can involve pronounced hypotension leading to collapse, sinus bradycardia with or without isorhythmic dissociation, and atrioventricular conduction disturbances.

Treatment, under hospital supervision, will include gastric lavage, osmotic diuresis. Conduction disturbances may be managed by temporary cardiac pacing.

Proposed corrective treatments: atropine, vasopressors, inotropic agents, glucagon and calcium gluconate infusion.

5. PHARMACOLOGICAL PROPERTIES

5.1 Pharmacodynamic properties

Tildiem is a calcium antagonist. It restricts the slow channel entry of calcium into the cell and so reduces the liberation of calcium from stores in the sarcoplasmic reticulum. This results in a reduction of the amount of available intracellular calcium reducing myocardial oxygen consumption. It increases exercise capacity and improves all indices of myocardial ischaemia in the angina patient. Tildiem relaxes large and small coronary arteries and relieves the spasm of vasospastic (prinzmetals) angina and the response to catecholamines but has little effect on the peripheral vasculature. There is therefore no possibility of reflex tachycardia. A small reduction in heart rate occurs which is accompanied by an increase in cardiac output, improved myocardial perfusion and reduction of ventricular work. In animal studies, Tildiem protects the myocardium against the effects of ischaemia and reduces the damage produced by excessive entry of calcium into the myocardial cell during reperfusion.

5.2 Pharmacokinetic properties

Diltiazem hydrochloride is effective in angina, protecting the heart against ischaemia, vasodilating coronary arteries and reducing myocardial oxygen requirements. It is well tolerated and does not generally give rise to side effects associated with peripheral vasodilators, nor cause significant myocardial depression.

Diltiazem is well absorbed (90%) in healthy volunteers following oral administration.

Peak plasma concentrations occur 3 to 4 hours after dosing.

Due to a first pass effect, the bioavailability of the 60 mg tablet is about 40 %.

The mean apparent plasma half-life is 4 - 8 hours.

Diltiazem is 80 to 85% bound to plasma proteins. It is extensively metabolised by the liver.

The major circulating metabolite, N-monodesmethyl diltiazem accounts for approximately 35% of the circulating diltiazem.

Less than 5% of diltiazem is excreted unchanged in the urine.

There is a linear relationship between dose and plasma concentration. During long term administration to any one patient, plasma concentrations of diltiazem remain constant.

Mean plasma concentrations in elderly subjects and patients with renal and hepatic insufficiency are higher than in young subjects.

Diltiazem and its metabolites are poorly dialysed.

5.3 Preclinical safety data

Not applicable

6. PHARMACEUTICAL PARTICULARS

6.1 List of excipients

Lactose, macrogol 6000, hydrogenated caster oil, magnesium stearate

6.2 Incompatibilities

None known

6.3 Shelf life

36 months

6.4 Special precautions for storage

Store below 25°C. Protect from moisture.

6.5 Nature and contents of container

PVC/ foil blister packs of 90 tablets.

6.6 Instructions for use and handling

None stated

Administrative Data

7. MARKETING AUTHORISATION HOLDER

Sanofi-Synthelabo
PO Box 597
Guildford
Surrey

8. MARKETING AUTHORISATION NUMBER(S)

PL 11723/0334

9. DATE OF FIRST AUTHORISATION/RENEWAL OF THE AUTHORISATION

12th December 2000

10. DATE OF REVISION OF THE TEXT

July 2002

Legal Category POM

Timentin 0.8 G, 1.6 G, 3.2 G

(GlaxoSmithKline UK)

1. NAME OF THE MEDICINAL PRODUCT

Timentin® 0.8 G, 1.6 G, 3.2 G

2. QUALITATIVE AND QUANTITATIVE COMPOSITION

Timentin 0.8 g: Contains 50 mg clavulanic acid with 750 mg ticarcillin.

Timentin 1.6 g: Contains 100 mg clavulanic acid with 1.5 g ticarcillin.

Timentin 3.2 g: Contains 200 mg clavulanic acid with 3.0 g ticarcillin.

The clavulanic acid is present as Potassium Clavulanate BP and the ticarcillin as ticarcillin sodium.

3. PHARMACEUTICAL FORM

Powder for solution for infusion.

Vials containing sterile powder for reconstitution.

4. CLINICAL PARTICULARS

4.1 Therapeutic indications

Timentin is an injectable antibiotic agent with a broad spectrum of bactericidal activity against a wide range of Gram-positive and Gram-negative aerobic and anaerobic bacteria. The presence of clavulanate in the formulation extends the spectrum of activity of ticarcillin to include many b-lactamase-producing bacteria normally resistant to ticarcillin and other b-lactam antibiotics.

Timentin is indicated for the treatment of infections in which susceptible organisms have been detected or are suspected.

Typical indications include:

Severe infections in hospitalised patients and proven or suspected infections in patients with impaired or suppressed host defences including: septicaemia, bacteraemia, peritonitis, intra-abdominal sepsis, post-surgical infections, bone and joint infections, skin and soft tissue infections, respiratory tract infections, serious or complicated renal infections (e.g. pyelonephritis), ear, nose and throat infections.

A comprehensive list of sensitive and resistant organisms is provided in Section 5.1. Consideration should be given to official guidance regarding bacterial resistance and the appropriate use of antibacterial agents.

4.2 Posology and method of administration

Adult dosage (including elderly patients):

The usual dosage is 3.2 g Timentin given six to eight hourly. The maximum recommended dosage is 3.2 g four hourly.

Children's dosage:

The usual dosage for children is 80 mg Timentin/kg body weight given every six to eight hours.

For premature infants and full-term infants during the peri-natal period, the dosage is 80 mg Timentin/kg body weight every 12 hours, increasing to every eight hours thereafter.

Dosage in renal impairment:

Mild impairment	Moderate impairment	Severe impairment
(Creatinine Clearance >30 ml/min)	(Creatinine Clearance 10-30 ml/min)	(Creatinine Clearance <10 ml/min)
3.2 g 8 hourly	1.6 g 8 hourly	1.6 g 12 hourly

Similar reductions in dosage should be made for children.

Administration:

Intravenous infusion

4.3 Contraindications

Timentin contains ticarcillin which is a penicillin, and should not be given to patients with a history of hypersensitivity to beta-lactam antibiotics (e.g. penicillins and cephalosporins).

4.4 Special warnings and special precautions for use

Before initiating therapy with Timentin, careful inquiry should be made concerning previous hypersensitivity reactions to beta-lactams (e.g. penicillins and cephalosporins). Serious and occasionally fatal hypersensitivity reactions (anaphylaxis) have been reported in patients receiving beta-lactam antibiotics. These reactions are more likely to occur in individuals with a history of beta-lactam hypersensitivity.

Changes in liver function tests have been observed in some patients receiving Timentin. The clinical significance of these changes is uncertain but Timentin should be used with care in patients with evidence of severe hepatic dysfunction.

In patients with renal impairment, dosage should be adjusted according to the degree of impairment (see Section 4.2). It should be noted that each gram of ticarcillin contains 5.3 mmol of sodium (approx.). This should be included in the daily allowance of patients on sodium restricted diets. Timentin has only rarely been reported to cause hypokalemia; however, the possibility of this occurring should be kept in mind particularly when treating patients with fluid and electrolyte imbalance. Periodic monitoring of serum potassium may be advisable in patients receiving prolonged therapy.

Bleeding manifestations have occurred in some patients receiving beta-lactam antibiotics. These reactions have been associated with abnormalities of coagulation tests such as clotting time, platelet aggregation and prothrombin time and are more likely to occur in patients with renal impairment. If bleeding manifestations appear, Timentin treatment should be discontinued and appropriate therapy instituted.

Prolonged use may occasionally result in overgrowth of non-susceptible organisms.

4.5 Interaction with other medicinal products and other forms of Interaction

Timentin acts synergistically with aminoglycosides against a number of organisms including *Pseudomonas*. Timentin prescribed concurrently with an aminoglycoside, may therefore be preferred in the treatment of life-threatening infections, particularly in patients with impaired host defences. In such instances the two products should be administered separately, at the recommended dosages.

Co-administration of probenecid cannot be recommended. Probenecid decreases the renal tubular secretion of ticarcillin. Concurrent administration of probenecid delays ticarcillin renal excretion but does not delay the excretion of clavulanic acid.

4.6 Pregnancy and lactation

Pregnancy:

Animal studies with Timentin have shown no teratogenic effects. Penicillins are generally considered safe for use in pregnancy. Limited information is available concerning the results of the use of Timentin in human pregnancy. The decision to administer any drug during pregnancy should be taken with the utmost care. Therefore Timentin should only be used in pregnancy when the potential benefits outweigh the potential risks associated with treatment.

Lactation:

Trace quantities of Timentin are excreted in breast milk.

Timentin may be administered during the period of lactation. With the exception of the risk of sensitization, there are no detrimental effects for the breast-fed infant.

4.7 Effects on ability to drive and use machines

Adverse effects on the ability to drive or operate machinery have not been observed.

4.8 Undesirable effects

Hypersensitivity reactions:

Hypersensitivity effects, including skin rashes:

Skin rashes, pruritus, urticaria, and anaphylactic reactions. Bullous reactions (including erythema multiforme, Stevens-Johnson syndrome and toxic epidermal necrolysis) have been reported very rarely.

Gastrointestinal effects:

Nausea, vomiting and diarrhea have been reported. Pseudomembranous colitis has been reported rarely.

Hepatic effects:

A moderate rise in AST and/or ALT has been noted in patients receiving ampicillin class antibiotics. Hepatitis and cholestatic jaundice have been reported very rarely. These events have been noted with other penicillins and cephalosporins.

Renal effects:

Hypokalaemia has been reported rarely.

Central Nervous System effects:

Convulsions may occur rarely, particularly in patients with impaired renal function or in those receiving high doses.

Haematological effects:

Thrombocytopenia, leukopenia, eosinophilia and reduction of haemoglobin have been reported rarely. Haemolytic anaemia has been reported very rarely. Prolongation of prothrombin time and bleeding time. Bleeding manifestations have occurred.

Local effects:

Pain, burning, swelling and induration at the injection site and thrombophlebitis with intravenous administration.

4.9 Overdose

Gastrointestinal effects such as nausea, vomiting and diarrhoea may be evident and should be treated symptomatically.

Disturbances of the fluid and electrolyte balances may be evident and may be treated symptomatically.

Ticarcillin and clavulanic acid may be removed from circulation by haemodialysis.

As with other penicillins, Timentin overdosage has the potential to cause neuromuscular hyperirritability or convulsive seizures.

5. PHARMACOLOGICAL PROPERTIES

5.1 Pharmacodynamic properties

Timentin is an injectable antibiotic, active against a wide range of both Gram-positive and Gram-negative bacteria, including b-lactamase-producing strains.

Resistance to many antibiotics is caused by bacterial enzymes which destroy the antibiotic before it can act on the pathogen. The clavulanate in Timentin anticipates this defence mechanism by blocking the b-lactamase enzymes, thus rendering the organisms sensitive to ticarcillin's rapid bactericidal effect at concentrations readily attainable in the body.

Clavulanate, by itself, has little antibacterial effect; however, in association with ticarcillin, as Timentin it produces an antibiotic agent with a breadth of spectrum suitable for empiric use in a wide range of infections treated parenterally in hospital.

Gram-Positive

Aerobes: *Staphylococcus* species including *Staphylococcus aureus* and *Staphylococcus epidermidis, Streptococcus* species including *Enterococcus faecalis.*

Anaerobes: *Peptococcus* species, *Peptostreptococcus* species, *Clostridium* species, *Eubacterium* species.

Gram-Negative

Aerobes: *Escherichia coli, Haemophilus* species including *Haemophilus influenzae, Moraxella catarrhalis, Klebsiella* species including *Klebsiella pneumoniae, Enterobacter* species, *Proteus* species including indole-positive strains, *Providentia stuartii, Pseudomonas* species including *Pseudomonas aeruginosa, Serratia* species including *Serratia marcescens, Citrobacter* species, *Acinetobacter* species, *Yersinia enterocolitica*

Anaerobes: *Bacteroides* species including *Bacteroides fragilis, Fusobacterium* species, *Veillonella* species.

Breakpoints

The breakpoints listed below have been obtained from the National Committee for Clinical Laboratory Standards (NCCLS) (Performance Standards for Antimicrobial Disk Susceptibility Tests; Approved Standard - Seventh Edition).

Enterobacteriaceae	S ⩽16/2 μg/mL	R ⩾ 128/2 μg/mL
Pseudomonas aeruginosa	S ⩽64/2 μg/mL	R ⩾ 128/2 μg/mL
Other non-Enterobacteriaceae	S ⩽16/2 μg/mL	R ⩾ 128/2 μg/mL
Staphylococcus spp.	S ⩽8/2 μg/mL	R ⩾ 16/2 μg/mL

S = susceptible, R = resistant

There are no NCCLS breakpoints for other organisms listed in this document.

Table 1

Susceptible
Aerobic Gram-positive micro-organisms
Staphylococcus aureus
Aerobic Gram-negative micro-organisms
Acinetobacter species
Escherichia coli
Haemophilus influenzae
Klebsiella pneumoniae
Proteus species
Serratia species
Anaerobic micro-organisms
Bacteroides fragilis
Intermediate
Aerobic Gram-negative micro-organisms
Serratia marcescens
Insusceptible
Aerobic Gram-positive micro-organisms
Enterococcus
Aerobic Gram-negative micro-organisms
Citrobacter species
Enterobacter species
Pseudomonas aeruginosa

The prevalence of resistance may vary geographically and with time for selected species. Where possible, local information on resistance is included. This information gives only an approximate guidance on probabilities whether micro-organisms will be susceptible to ticarcillin disodium clavulanate potassium (commonly known as Timentin) or not.

5.2 Pharmacokinetic properties

The pharmacokinetics of the two components are closely matched and both components are well distributed in body fluids and tissues. Both clavulanate and ticarcillin have low levels of serum binding; about 20% and 45% respectively.

As with other penicillins the major route of elimination for ticarcillin is via the kidney; clavulanate is also excreted by this route.

5.3 Preclinical safety data

Not applicable.

6. PHARMACEUTICAL PARTICULARS

6.1 List of excipients

None

6.2 Incompatibilities

Timentin is not compatible with the following:

Proteinaceous fluids (e.g. protein hydrolysates); blood and plasma; intravenous lipids.

If Timentin is prescribed concurrently with an aminoglycoside the antibiotics should not be mixed in the syringe, intravenous fluid container or giving set because loss of activity of the aminoglycoside can occur under these conditions.

6.3 Shelf life

24 months.

6.4 Special precautions for storage

Timentin should be stored in a dry place at temperatures below 25°C.

6.5 Nature and contents of container

Clear Type I glass vials fitted with a chlorobutyl rubber bung and an aluminium seal. Supplied in packs of four vials.

6.6 Instructions for use and handling

The sterile powder should be dissolved in approximately 5 ml/10 ml (1.6 g/3.2 g vial) prior to dilution into the infusion container (e.g. mini-bag) or in-line burette.

The following approximate infusion volumes are suggested:

	Water for Injections BP	Glucose Intravenous Infusion BP (5% w/v)
3.2 g	100 ml	100-150 ml
1.6 g	50 ml	100 ml

Detailed instructions are given in the Package Enclosure Leaflet.

Each dose of Timentin should be infused intravenously over a period of 30-40 minutes; avoid continuous infusion over longer periods as this may result in subtherapeutic concentrations.

800 mg Timentin has a displacement value of 0.55 ml.

Heat is generated when Timentin dissolves. Reconstituted solutions are normally a pale straw colour.

Timentin presentations are not for multi-dose use or for direct IV or IM injection. Any residual antibiotic solution should be discarded if less than the fully made up vial is used.

Administrative Data

7. MARKETING AUTHORISATION HOLDER

Beecham Group plc, Great West Road

Brentford, Middlesex TW8 9GS

Trading as:

GlaxoSmithKline UK,

Stockley Park West,

Uxbridge,

Middlesex UB11 1BT

8. MARKETING AUTHORISATION NUMBER(S)

00038/0329

9. DATE OF FIRST AUTHORISATION/RENEWAL OF THE AUTHORISATION

15 April 2003

10. DATE OF REVISION OF THE TEXT

01st October 2004

11. Legal Status

POM

Timoptol

(Merck Sharp & Dohme Limited)

1. NAME OF THE MEDICINAL PRODUCT

TIMOPTOL® Ophthalmic Solution 0.25%

TIMOPTOL® Ophthalmic Solution 0.5%

2. QUALITATIVE AND QUANTITATIVE COMPOSITION

'Timoptol' Ophthalmic Solution 0.25% contains timolol maleate Ph Eur equivalent to 0.25% w/v solution of timolol with preservative.

'Timoptol' Ophthalmic Solution 0.5% contains timolol maleate Ph Eur equivalent to 0.5% w/v solution of timolol with preservative.

3. PHARMACEUTICAL FORM

Eye drops solution.

Clear, colourless to light yellow, sterile eye drops solution.

4. CLINICAL PARTICULARS

4.1 Therapeutic indications

'Timoptol' Ophthalmic Solution is a beta-adrenoreceptor blocking agent used topically in the reduction of elevated intra-ocular pressure in various conditions including the following: patients with ocular hypertension; patients with chronic open-angle glaucoma including aphakic patients; some patients with secondary glaucoma.

4.2 Posology and method of administration

Recommended therapy is one drop 0.25% solution in the affected eye twice a day.

If clinical response is not adequate, dosage may be changed to one drop 0.5% solution in each affected eye twice a day. If needed, 'Timoptol' may be used with other agent(s) for lowering intra-ocular pressure. The use of two topical beta-adrenergic blocking agents is not recommended (see 4.4 'Special warnings and special precautions for use').

Intra-ocular pressure should be reassessed approximately four weeks after starting treatment because response to 'Timoptol' may take a few weeks to stabilise.

Provided that the intra-ocular pressure is maintained at satisfactory levels, many patients can than be placed on once-a-day therapy.

Transfer from other agents

When another topical beta-blocking agent is being used, discontinue its use after a full day of therapy and start treatment with 'Timoptol' the next day with one drop of 0.25% 'Timoptol' in each affected eye twice a day. The dosage may be increased to one drop of 0.5% solution in each affected eye twice a day, if the response is not adequate.

When transferring a patient from a single anti-glaucoma agent other than a topical beta-blocking agent, continue the agent and add one drop of 0.25% 'Timoptol' in each affected eye twice a day. On the following day, discontinue the previous agent completely, and continue with 'Timoptol'. If a higher dosage of 'Timoptol' is required, substitute one drop of 0.5% solution in each affected eye twice a day.

'Timoptol' Ophthalmic Solution is also available as 'Timoptol' Unit dose: The Unit-dose Dispenser of 'Timoptol' is free from preservative and should be used for patients who may be sensitive to the preservative benzalkonium chloride, or when use of a preservative-free topical medication is advisable.

Paediatric use: is not currently recommended.

Use in the elderly: there has been wide experience with the use of timolol maleate in elderly patients. The dosage recommendations given above reflect the clinical data derived from this experience.

4.3 Contraindications

Bronchial asthma, history of bronchial asthma or severe chronic obstructive pulmonary disease; sinus bradycardia, second- and third-degree AV block, overt cardiac failure, cardiogenic shock; and hypersensitivity to this product or other beta-blocking agents.

4.4 Special warnings and special precautions for use

Like other topically applied ophthalmic drugs, 'Timoptol' may be absorbed systemically and adverse reactions seen with oral beta-blockers may occur.

Cardiac failure should be adequately controlled before beginning therapy with 'Timoptol'. Patients with a history of severe cardiac disease should be watched for signs of cardiac failure and have their pulse rates checked.

Respiratory and cardiac reactions, including death due to bronchospasm in patients with asthma and, rarely, death associated with cardiac failure have been reported.

The effect on intra-ocular pressure or the known effects of systemic beta-blockade may be exaggerated when 'Timoptol' is given to the patients already receiving a systemic beta-blocking agent. The response of these patients should be closely observed. The use of two topical beta-adrenergic blocking agents is not recommended.

There have been reports of skin rashes and/or dry eyes associated with the use of beta-adrenoreceptor blocking drugs. The reported incidence is small and in most cases the symptoms have cleared when treatment was withdrawn. Discontinuation of the drug should be considered if any such reaction is not otherwise explicable. Cessation of therapy involving beta-blockade should be gradual.

Choroidal detachment has been reported with administration of aqueous suppressant therapy (e.g. timolol, acetazolamide) after filtration procedures.

'Timoptol' has been generally well tolerated in glaucoma patients wearing conventional hard contact lenses. 'Timoptol' has not been studied in patients wearing lenses made with material other than polymethylmethacrylate (PMMA), which is used to make hard contact lenses.

The Ocumeter® Dispenser of 'Timoptol' contains benzalkonium chloride as a preservative which may be deposited in soft contact lenses; therefore 'Timoptol' should not be used while wearing these lenses. The lenses should be removed before application of the drops and not reinserted earlier than 15 minutes after use.

In patients with angle-closure glaucoma, the immediate objective of treatment is to reopen the angle. This requires constricting the pupil with a miotic. 'Timoptol' has little or no effect on the pupil. When 'Timoptol' is used to reduce elevated intra-ocular pressure in angle-closure glaucoma it should be used with a miotic and not alone.

Patients should be advised that if they develop an intercurrent ocular condition (e.g. trauma, ocular surgery or infection), they should immediately seek their physician's advice concerning the continued use of the present multidose container (see 6.6 'Instructions for use and handling').

There have been reports of bacterial keratitis associated with the use of multiple dose containers of topical ophthalmic products. These containers had been inadvertently contaminated by patients who, in most cases, had a concurrent corneal disease or a disruption of the ocular epithelial surface.

Risk from anaphylactic reaction: While taking beta-blockers, patients with a history of atopy or a history of severe anaphylactic reaction to a variety of allergens may be more reactive to repeated challenge with such allergens, either accidental, diagnostic, or therapeutic. Such patients may be unresponsive to the usual doses of epinephrine (adrenaline) used to treat anaphylactic reactions.

4.5 Interaction with other medicinal products and other forms of Interaction

Although 'Timoptol' alone has little or no effect on pupil size, mydriasis has occasionally been reported when 'Timoptol' is given with epinephrine (adrenaline).

Potentiated systemic beta-blockade (e.g. decreased heart rate) has been reported during combined treatment with quinidine and timolol, possibly because quinidine inhibits the metabolism of timolol via the P-450 enzyme, CYP2D6.

Oral β-adrenergic blocking agents may exacerbate the rebound hypertension which can follow the withdrawal of clonidine.

'Timoptol' may potentially add to the effects of oral calcium antagonists, rauwolfia alkaloids or beta-blockers, to induce hypotension and/or marked bradycardia.

Close observation of the patient is recommended when a beta-blocker is administered to patients receiving catecholamine-depleting drugs such as reserpine, because of possible additive effects and the production of hypotension and/or marked bradycardia, which may produce vertigo, syncope, or postural hypotension.

Oral calcium antagonists may be used in combination with beta-adrenergic blocking agents when heart function is normal, but should be avoided in patients with impaired cardiac function.

The potential exists for hypotension, AV conduction disturbances and left ventricular failure to occur in patients receiving a beta-blocking agent when an oral calcium entry blocker is added to the treatment regimen. The nature of any cardiovascular adverse effect tends to depend on the type of calcium blocker used. Dihydropyridine derivatives, such as nifedipine, may lead to hypotension, whereas verapamil or diltiazem have a greater propensity to lead to AV conduction disturbances or left ventricular failure when used with a beta-blocker.

Intravenous calcium channel blockers should be used with caution in patients receiving beta-adrenergic blocking agents.

The concomitant use of beta-adrenergic blocking agents and digitalis with either diltiazem or verapamil may have additive effects in prolonging AV conduction time.

4.6 Pregnancy and lactation

Use in pregnancy: 'Timoptol' has not been studied in human pregnancy. The use of 'Timoptol' requires that the anticipated benefit be weighed against possible hazards.

Breast-feeding mothers: Timolol is detectable in human milk. A decision for breast-feeding mothers, either to stop taking 'Timoptol' or stop nursing, should be based on the importance of the drug to the mother.

4.7 Effects on ability to drive and use machines

Possible side effects such as dizziness and visual disturbances may affect some patients' ability to drive or operate machinery.

4.8 Undesirable effects

Side effects

'Timoptol' is usually well tolerated. The following adverse reactions have been reported with *ocular* administration of this or other timolol maleate formulations, either in clinical trials or since the drug has been marketed. Additional side effects have been reported in clinical experiences with *systemic* timolol maleate, and may be considered potential effects of ophthalmic timolol maleate:

Special senses:

ocular: signs and symptoms of ocular irritation, including burning and stinging, conjunctivitis, blepharitis, keratitis, dry eyes and decreased corneal sensitivity. Tinnitus, visual disturbances, including refractive changes (due to withdrawal of miotic therapy in some cases), diplopia, ptosis and choroidal detachment following filtration surgery (see 4.4 'Special warnings and special precautions for use').

Cardiovascular:

ocular: bradycardia, arrhythmia, hypotension, syncope, heart block, cerebrovascular accident, cerebral ischaemia, congestive heart failure, palpitation, cardiac arrest, oedema, claudication, Raynaud's phenomenon, cold hands and feet.

systemic: AV block (second- or third-degree), sino-atrial block, pulmonary oedema, worsening of arterial insufficiency, worsening of angina pectoris, vasodilation.

Respiratory:

ocular: bronchospasm (predominantly in patients with pre-existing bronchospastic disease), respiratory failure, dyspnoea, cough.

systemic: rales

Body as a whole:

ocular: headache, asthenia, fatigue, chest pain.

systemic: extremity pain, decreased exercise tolerance.

Integumentary:

ocular: alopecia, psoriasiform rash or exacerbation of psoriasis.

systemic: pruritus, sweating, exfoliative dermatitis.

Hypersensitivity:

ocular: signs and symptoms of allergic reactions including anaphylaxis, angioedema, urticaria, localised and generalised rash.

Nervous system/psychiatric:

ocular: dizziness, depression, insomnia, nightmares, memory loss, increase in signs and symptoms of myasthenia gravis, paresthesia.

systemic: vertigo, local weakness, diminished concentration, increased dreaming.

Digestive:

ocular: nausea, diarrhoea, dyspepsia, dry mouth.

systemic: vomiting

Urogenital:

ocular: decreased libido, Peyronie's disease.

systemic: impotence, micturition difficulties.

Immunologic:

ocular: systemic lupus erythematosus

Endocrine:

systemic: hyperglycaemia, hypoglycaemia.

Musculoskeletal:

systemic: arthralgia.

Haematologic:

systemic: non-thrombocytopenic purpura.

4.9 Overdose

There have been reports of inadvertent overdosage with 'Timoptol' resulting in systemic effects similar to those seen with systemic beta-adrenergic blocking agents such as dizziness, headache, shortness of breath, bradycardia, bronchospasm, and cardiac arrest (see 'Side effects').

If overdosage occurs, the following measures should be considered:

1. Gastric lavage, if ingested. Studies have shown that timolol does not dialyse readily.

2. Symptomatic bradycardia: atropine sulphate, 0.25 to 2 mg intravenously, should be used to induce vagal blockade. If bradycardia persists, intravenous isoprenaline hydrochloride should be administered cautiously. In refractory cases, the use of a cardiac pacemaker may be considered.

3. Hypotension: a sympathomimetic pressor agent such as dopamine, dobutamine or noradrenaline should be used. In refractory cases, the use of glucagon has been reported to be useful.

4. Bronchospasm: isoprenaline hydrochloride should be used. Additional therapy with aminophylline may be considered.

5. Acute cardiac failure: conventional therapy with digitalis, diuretics, and oxygen should be instituted immediately. In refractory cases, the use of intravenous aminophylline is suggested. This may be followed, if necessary, by glucagon, which has been reported useful.

6. Heart block (second- or third-degree): isoprenaline hydrochloride or a pacemaker should be used.

5. PHARMACOLOGICAL PROPERTIES

5.1 Pharmacodynamic properties

Timolol maleate is a non-selective beta-adrenergic receptor blocking agent that does not have significant intrinsic sympathomimetic, direct myocardial depressant, or local anaesthetic activity. Timolol maleate combines reversibly with the beta-adrenergic receptor, and this inhibits the usual biologic response that would occur with stimulation of that receptor. This specific competitive antagonism blocks stimulation of the beta-adrenergic stimulating (agonist) activity, whether these originate from an endogenous or exogenous source. Reversal of this blockade can be accomplished by increasing the concentration of the agonist which will restore the usual biological response.

Unlike miotics, 'Timoptol' reduces IOP with little or no effect on accommodation or pupil size. In patients with cataracts, the inability to see around lenticular opacities when the pupil is constricted is avoided. When changing patients from miotics to 'Timoptol' a refraction might be necessary when the effects of the miotic have passed.

Diminished response after prolonged therapy with 'Timoptol' has been reported in some patients.

5.2 Pharmacokinetic properties

The onset of reduction in intra-ocular pressure can be detected within one-half hour after a single dose. The maximum effect occurs in one or two hours; significant lowering of IOP can be maintained for as long as 24 hours with a single dose.

5.3 Preclinical safety data

No adverse ocular effects were observed in rabbits and dogs administered 'Timoptol' topically in studies lasting one and two years, respectively. The oral LD_{50} of the drug is 1,190 and 900 mg/kg in female mice and female rats, respectively.

Carcinogenesis, mutagenesis, impairment of fertility

In a two-year oral study of timolol maleate in rats there was a statistically significant ($p \leq 0.05$) increase in the incidence of adrenal phaeochromocytomas in male rats administered 300 mg/kg/day (300 times the maximum recommended human oral dose). Similar differences were not observed in rats administered oral doses equivalent to 25 or 100 times the maximum recommended human oral dose.

In a lifetime oral study in mice, there were statistically significant ($p \leq 0.05$) increases in the incidence of benign and malignant pulmonary tumours, benign uterine polyps and mammary adenocarcinoma in female mice at 500 mg/kg/day (500 times the maximum recommended human dose), but not at 5 or 50 mg/kg/day. In a subsequent study in female mice, in which post-mortem examinations were limited to uterus and lungs, a statistically significant increase in the incidence of pulmonary tumours was again observed at 500 mg/kg/day.

The increased occurrence of mammary adenocarcinoma was associated with elevations in serum prolactin which occurred in female mice administered timolol at 500 mg/kg/day, but not at doses of 5 or 50 mg/kg/day. An increased incidence of mammary adenocarcinomas in rodents has been associated with administration of several other therapeutic agents which elevate serum prolactin, but no correlation between serum prolactin levels and mammary tumours has been established in man. Furthermore, in adult human female subjects who received oral dosages of up to 60 mg of timolol maleate, the maximum recommended human oral dosage, there were no clinically meaningful changes in serum prolactin.

Timolol maleate was devoid of mutagenic potential when evaluated *in vivo* (mouse) in the micronucleus test and cytogenetic assay (doses up to 800 mg/kg) and *in vitro* in a neoplastic cell transformation assay (up to 100 mcg/ml). In Ames tests the highest concentrations of timolol employed, 5,000 or 10,000 mcg/plate, were associated with statistically significant ($p \leq 0.05$) elevations of revertants observed with tester strain TA100 (in seven replicate assays) but not in the remaining three strains. In the assays with tester strain TA100, no consistent dose-response relationship was observed, nor did the ratio of test to control revertants reach 2. A ratio of 2 is usually considered the criterion for a positive Ames test.

Reproduction and fertility studies in rats showed no adverse effect on male or female fertility at doses up to 150 times the maximum recommended human oral dose.

6. PHARMACEUTICAL PARTICULARS

6.1 List of excipients

Disodium phosphate dodecahydrate (may be replaced by equivalent amounts of the dihydrate or anhydrous)

Sodium dihydrogen phosphate dihydrate (may be replaced by equivalent amounts of monohydrate)

Sodium hydroxide

Benzalkonium chloride

Water for injection

6.2 Incompatibilities

None known.

6.3 Shelf life

ALP bottle: 36 months.

Ocumeter bottle: 24 months

Discard 'Timoptol' Ophthalmic Solution 28 days after opening the bottle.

6.4 Special precautions for storage

Do not store above 25°C. Store the bottle in the outer carton.

6.5 Nature and contents of container

Both the 0.25% and the 0.5% w/v solutions are presented in:

ALP container:

The ALP (Automated Liquid packaging) vial consists of an oval, translucent, low-density polyethylene container with a metered-drop tip and polypropylene cap. The tip and cap are covered with a transparent, tamper-evident, disposable over-cap. The ALP vial contains 5 ml of solution.

OCUMETER Plus ophthalmic dispenser:

The OCUMETER Plus ophthalmic dispenser consists of a translucent high-density polyethylene container with a sealed dropper tip, a flexible fluted side area, which is depressed to dispense the drops, and a two-piece cap assembly. The two-piece cap mechanism punctures the sealed dropper tip upon initial use, then locks together to provide a single cap during the usage period. Tamper evidence is provided by two perforated tabs on the container label extending on to the cap. The OCUMETER Plus ophthalmic dispenser contains 5 ml of solution.

6.6 Instructions for use and handling

Patients should be instructed to avoid allowing the tip of the dispensing container to contact the eye or surrounding structures.

Patients should also be instructed that ocular solutions, if handled improperly, can become contaminated by common bacteria known to cause ocular infections. Serious damage to the eye and subsequent loss of vision may result from using contaminated solutions.

7. MARKETING AUTHORISATION HOLDER

Merck Sharp & Dohme Limited

Hertford Road, Hoddesdon, Hertfordshire EN11 9BU, UK

8. MARKETING AUTHORISATION NUMBER(S)

0.25% Ophthalmic Solution 0025/0134

0.5% Ophthalmic Solution 0025/0135

9. DATE OF FIRST AUTHORISATION/RENEWAL OF THE AUTHORISATION

Granted: 5 January 1979

Last renewed: 12 February 2002

10. DATE OF REVISION OF THE TEXT

May 2002.

LEGAL CATEGORY:

POM

® denotes registered trademark of Merck & Co., Inc., Whitehouse Station, NJ, USA.

MSD (logo)

Merck Sharp & Dohme Limited

Hertford Road, Hoddesdon, Hertfordshire EN11 9BU, UK

SPC.TOTOS.01.UK.0712

May 2002

Timoptol Unit Dose Ophthalmic Solution

(Merck Sharp & Dohme Limited)

1. NAME OF THE MEDICINAL PRODUCT

TIMOPTOL® Unit Dose Ophthalmic Solution

2. QUALITATIVE AND QUANTITATIVE COMPOSITION

'Timoptol' Unit Dose Ophthalmic Solution 0.25% contains timolol maleate Ph Eur equivalent to 0.25% w/v solution of timolol without preservative.

'Timoptol' Unit Dose Ophthalmic Solution 0.5% contains timolol maleate Ph Eur equivalent to 0.5% w/v solution of timolol without preservative.

3. PHARMACEUTICAL FORM

Clear, colourless to light yellow, sterile eye drops.

4. CLINICAL PARTICULARS

4.1 Therapeutic indications

'Timoptol' Ophthalmic Solution is a beta-adrenoreceptor blocking agent used topically in the reduction of elevated intra-ocular pressure in various conditions including the following: patients with ocular hypertension; patients with chronic open-angle glaucoma including aphakic patients; some patients with secondary glaucoma.

4.2 Posology and method of administration

Recommended therapy is one drop 0.25% solution in the affected eye twice a day.

If clinical response is not adequate, dosage may be changed to one drop 0.5% solution in each affected eye twice a day. If needed, 'Timoptol' may be used with other agent(s) for lowering intra-ocular pressure. The use of two topical beta-adrenergic blocking agents is not recommended (see 4.4 'Special warnings and special precautions for use').

Intra-ocular pressure should be reassessed approximately four weeks after starting treatment because response to 'Timoptol' may take a few weeks to stabilise.

Provided that the intra-ocular pressure is maintained at satisfactory levels, many patients can than be placed on once-a-day therapy.

Transfer from other agents

When another topical beta-blocking agent is being used, discontinue its use after a full day of therapy and start treatment with 'Timoptol' the next day with one drop of 0.25% 'Timoptol' in each affected eye twice a day. The dosage may be increased to one drop of 0.5% solution in each affected eye twice a day if the response is not adequate.

When transferring a patient from a single anti-glaucoma agent other than a topical beta-blocking agent, continue the agent and add one drop of 0.25% 'Timoptol' in each affected eye twice a day. On the following day, discontinue the previous agent completely, and continue with 'Timoptol'. If a higher dosage of 'Timoptol' is required, substitute one drop of 0.5% solution in each affected eye twice a day.

'Timoptol' Unit dose: The Unit-dose Dispenser of 'Timoptol' is free from preservative and should be used for patients who may be sensitive to the preservative benzalkonium chloride, or when use of a preservative-free topical medication is advisable.

'Timoptol' Unit-dose is a sterile solution. The solution from one individual unit is to be used immediately after opening for administration to one or both eyes. Since sterility cannot be maintained after the individual unit is opened, the remaining contents should be discarded immediately after administration.

Paediatric use: is not currently recommended.

Use in the elderly: there has been wide experience with the use of timolol maleate in elderly patients. The dosage recommendations given above reflect the clinical data derived from this experience.

4.3 Contraindications

Bronchial asthma, history of bronchial asthma or severe chronic obstructive pulmonary disease; sinus bradycardia, second- and third-degree AV block, overt cardiac failure, cardiogenic shock; and hypersensitivity to this product or other beta-blocking agents.

4.4 Special warnings and special precautions for use

Like other topically applied ophthalmic drugs, 'Timoptol' may be absorbed systemically and adverse reactions seen with oral beta-blockers may occur.

Cardiac failure should be adequately controlled before beginning therapy with 'Timoptol'. Patients with a history of severe cardiac disease should be watched for signs of cardiac failure and have their pulse rates checked.

Respiratory and cardiac reactions, including death due to bronchospasm in patients with asthma and, rarely, death associated with cardiac failure have been reported.

The effect on intra-ocular pressure or the known effects of systemic beta-blockade may be exaggerated when 'Timoptol' is given to patients already receiving a systemic beta-blocking agent. The response of these patients should be closely observed. The use of two topical beta-adrenergic blocking agents is not recommended.

There have been reports of skin rashes and/or dry eyes associated with the use of beta-adrenoreceptor blocking drugs. The reported incidence is small and in most cases the symptoms have cleared when treatment was withdrawn. Discontinuation of the drug should be considered if any such reaction is not otherwise explicable. Cessation of therapy involving beta-blockade should be gradual.

Choroidal detachment has been reported with administration of aqueous suppressant therapy (e.g. timolol, acetazolamide) after filtration procedures.

'Timoptol' has been generally well tolerated in glaucoma patients wearing conventional hard contact lenses. 'Timoptol' has not been studied in patients wearing lenses made with material other than polymethylmethacrylate (PMMA), which is used to make hard contact lenses.

The Unit-dose Dispenser of 'Timoptol' is free from preservative and should, therefore, be discarded after single use to one or both eyes.

In patients with angle-closure glaucoma, the immediate objective of treatment is to reopen the angle. This requires constricting the pupil with a miotic. 'Timoptol' has little or no effect on the pupil. When 'Timoptol' is used to reduce elevated intra-ocular pressure in angle-closure glaucoma it should be used with a miotic and not alone.

Patients should be advised that if they develop an intercurrent ocular condition (e.g. trauma, ocular surgery or infection), they should immediately seek their physician's advice concerning the continued use of the present multidose container (see 6.6 'Instructions for use/handling').

There have been reports of bacterial keratitis associated with the use of multiple dose containers of topical ophthalmic products. These containers had been inadvertently contaminated by patients who, in most cases, had a concurrent corneal disease or a disruption of the ocular epithelial surface.

Risk from anaphylactic reaction: While taking beta-blockers, patients with a history of atopy or a history of severe anaphylactic reaction to a variety of allergens may be more reactive to repeated challenge with such allergens, either accidental, diagnostic, or therapeutic. Such patients may be unresponsive to the usual doses of epinephrine (adrenaline) used to treat anaphylactic reactions.

4.5 Interaction with other medicinal products and other forms of Interaction

Although 'Timoptol' alone has little or no effect on pupil size, mydriasis has occasionally been reported when 'Timoptol' is given with epinephrine (adrenaline).

Potentiated systemic beta-blockade (e.g. decreased heart rate) has been reported during combined treatment with quinidine and timolol, possibly because quinidine inhibits the metabolism of timolol via the P-450 enzyme, CYP2D6.

Oral β-adrenergic blocking agents may exacerbate the rebound hypertension which can follow the withdrawal of clonidine.

'Timoptol' may potentially add to the effects of oral calcium antagonists, rauwolfia alkaloids or beta-blockers, to induce hypotension and/or marked bradycardia.

Close observation of the patient is recommended when a beta-blocker is administered to patients receiving catecholamine-depleting drugs such as reserpine, because of possible additive effects and the production of hypotension and/or marked bradycardia, which may produce vertigo, syncope, or postural hypotension.

Oral calcium antagonists may be used in combination with beta-adrenergic blocking agents when heart function is normal, but should be avoided in patients with impaired cardiac function.

The potential exists for hypotension, AV conduction disturbances and left ventricular failure to occur in patients receiving a beta-blocking agent when an oral calcium entry blocker is added to the treatment regimen. The nature of any cardiovascular adverse effect tends to depend on the type of calcium blocker used. Dihydropyridine derivatives, such as nifedipine, may lead to hypotension, whereas verapamil or diltiazem have a greater propensity to lead to AV conduction disturbances or left ventricular failure when used with a beta-blocker.

Intravenous calcium channel blockers should be used with caution in patients receiving beta-adrenergic blocking agents.

The concomitant use of beta-adrenergic blocking agents and digitalis with either diltiazem or verapamil may have additive effects in prolonging AV conduction time.

4.6 Pregnancy and lactation

Use in pregnancy: 'Timoptol' has not been studied in human pregnancy. The use of 'Timoptol' requires that the anticipated benefit be weighed against possible hazards.

Breast-feeding mothers: Timolol is detectable in human milk. A decision for breast-feeding mothers, either to stop taking 'Timoptol' or stop nursing, should be based on the importance of the drug to the mother.

4.7 Effects on ability to drive and use machines

Possible side effects such as dizziness and visual disturbances may affect some patients' ability to drive or operate machinery.

4.8 Undesirable effects

Side effects

'Timoptol' is usually well tolerated. The following adverse reactions have been reported with *ocular* administration of this or other timolol maleate formulations, either in clinical trials or since the drug has been marketed. Additional side effects have been reported in clinical experiences with *systemic* timolol maleate, and may be considered potential effects of ophthalmic timolol maleate:

Special senses:

ocular: signs and symptoms of ocular irritation, including burning and stinging, conjunctivitis, blepharitis, keratitis, dry eyes, and decreased corneal sensitivity. Tinnitus, visual disturbances, including refractive changes (due to withdrawal of miotic therapy in some cases), diplopia, ptosis and choroidal detachment following filtration surgery (see 4.4 'Special warnings and special precautions for use').

Cardiovascular:

ocular: bradycardia, arrhythmia, hypotension, syncope, heart block, cerebrovascular accident, cerebral ischaemia, congestive heart failure, palpitation, cardiac arrest, oedema, claudication, Raynaud's phenomenon, cold hands and feet.

systemic: AV block (second- or third-degree), sino-atrial block, pulmonary oedema, worsening of arterial insufficiency, worsening of angina pectoris, vasodilation.

Respiratory:

ocular: bronchospasm (predominantly in patients with pre-existing bronchospastic disease), respiratory failure, dyspnoea, cough.

systemic: rales

Body as a whole:

ocular: headache, asthenia, fatigue, chest pain.

systemic: extremity pain, decreased exercise tolerance.

Integumentary:

ocular: alopecia, psoriasiform rash or exacerbation of psoriasis.

systemic: pruritus, sweating, exfoliative dermatitis.

Hypersensitivity:

ocular: signs and symptoms of allergic reactions including anaphylaxis, angioedema, urticaria, localised and generalised rash.

Nervous system/psychiatric:

ocular: dizziness, depression, insomnia, nightmares, memory loss, increase in signs and symptoms of myasthenia gravis, paraesthesia.

systemic: vertigo, local weakness, diminished concentration, increased dreaming.

Digestive:

ocular: nausea, diarrhoea, dyspepsia, dry mouth.

systemic: vomiting.

Urogenital:

ocular: decreased libido, Peyronie's disease.

systemic: impotence, micturition difficulties.

Immunologic:

ocular: systemic lupus erythematosus.

Endocrine:

systemic: hyperglycaemia, hypoglycaemia.

Musculoskeletal:

systemic: arthralgia.

Haematologic:

systemic: non-thrombocytopenic purpura.

4.9 Overdose

There have been reports of inadvertent overdosage with 'Timoptol' resulting in systemic effects similar to those seen with systemic beta-adrenergic blocking agents such as dizziness, headache, shortness of breath, bradycardia, bronchospasm, and cardiac arrest (see 4.8 'Undesirable effects').

If overdosage occurs, the following measures should be considered:

1. Gastric lavage, if ingested. Studies have shown that timolol does not dialyse readily.

2. Symptomatic bradycardia: atropine sulphate, 0.25 to 2 mg intravenously, should be used to induce vagal blockade. If bradycardia persists, intravenous isoprenaline hydrochloride should be administered cautiously. In refractory cases, the use of a cardiac pacemaker may be considered.

3. Hypotension: a sympathomimetic pressor agent such as dopamine, dobutamine or noradrenaline should be used. In refractory cases, the use of glucagon has been reported to be useful.

4. Bronchospasm: isoprenaline hydrochloride should be used. Additional therapy with aminophylline may be considered.

5. Acute cardiac failure: conventional therapy with digitalis, diuretics, and oxygen should be instituted immediately. In refractory cases, the use of intravenous aminophylline is suggested. This may be followed, if necessary, by glucagon, which has been reported useful.

6. Heart block (second- or third-degree): isoprenaline hydrochloride or a pacemaker should be used.

5. PHARMACOLOGICAL PROPERTIES

5.1 Pharmacodynamic properties

Timolol maleate is a non-selective beta-adrenergic receptor blocking agent that does not have significant intrinsic sympathomimetic, direct myocardial depressant, or local anaesthetic activity. Timolol maleate combines reversibly with the beta-adrenergic receptor, and this inhibits the usual biologic response that would occur with stimulation of that receptor. This specific competitive antagonism blocks stimulation of the beta-adrenergic stimulating (agonist) activity, whether these originate from an endogenous or exogenous source. Reversal of this blockade can be accomplished by increasing the concentration of the agonist which will restore the usual biological response.

Unlike miotics, 'Timoptol' reduces IOP with little or no effect on accommodation or pupil size. In patients with cataracts, the inability to see around lenticular opacities when the pupil is constricted is avoided. When changing patients from miotics to 'Timoptol' a refraction might be necessary when the effects of the miotic have passed.

Diminished response after prolonged therapy with 'Timoptol' has been reported in some patients.

5.2 Pharmacokinetic properties

The onset of reduction in intra-ocular pressure can be detected within one-half hour after a single dose. The maximum effect occurs in one or two hours; significant lowering of IOP can be maintained for as long as 24 hours with a single dose.

5.3 Preclinical safety data

No adverse ocular effects were observed in rabbits and dogs administered 'Timoptol' topically in studies lasting one and two years, respectively. The oral LD_{50} of the drug is 1,190 and 900 mg/kg in female mice and female rats, respectively.

Carcinogenesis, mutagenesis, impairment of fertility

In a two-year oral study of timolol maleate in rats there was a statistically significant ($p \leqslant 0.05$) increase in the incidence of adrenal phaeochromocytomas in male rats administered 300 mg/kg/day (300 times the maximum recommended human oral dose). Similar differences were not observed in rats administered oral doses equivalent to 25 or 100 times the maximum recommended human oral dose.

In a lifetime oral study in mice, there were statistically significant ($p \leqslant 0.05$) increases in the incidence of benign and malignant pulmonary tumours, benign uterine polyps and mammary adenocarcinoma in female mice at 500 mg/kg/day (500 times the maximum recommended human dose), but not at 5 or 50 mg/kg/day. In a subsequent study in female mice, in which post-mortem examinations were limited to uterus and lungs, a statistically significant increase in the incidence of pulmonary tumours was again observed at 500 mg/kg/day.

The increased occurrence of mammary adenocarcinoma was associated with elevations in serum prolactin which occurred in female mice administered timolol at 500 mg/kg/day, but not at doses of 5 or 50 mg/kg/day. An increased incidence of mammary adenocarcinomas in rodents has been associated with administration of several other therapeutic agents which elevate serum prolactin, but no correlation between serum prolactin levels and mammary tumors has been established in man. Furthermore, in adult human female subjects who received oral dosages of up to 60 mg of timolol maleate, the maximum recommended human oral dosage, there were no clinically meaningful changes in serum prolactin.

Timolol maleate was devoid of mutagenic potential when evaluated *in vivo* (mouse) in the micronucleus test and cytogenetic assay (doses up to 800 mg/kg) and *in vitro* in a neoplastic cell transformation assay (up to 100 mcg/ml). In Ames tests the highest concentrations of timolol employed, 5,000 or 10,000 mcg/plate, were associated with statistically significant ($p \leqslant 0.05$) elevations of revertants observed with tester strain TA100 (in seven replicate assays) but not in the remaining three strains. In the assays with tester strain TA100, no consistent dose-response relationship was observed, nor did the ratio of test to control revertants reach 2. A ratio of 2 is usually considered the criterion for a positive Ames test.

Reproduction and fertility studies in rats showed no adverse effect on male or female fertility at doses up to 150 times the maximum recommended human oral dose.

6. PHARMACEUTICAL PARTICULARS

6.1 List of excipients

'Timoptol' Unit Dose Ophthalmic Solution contains the following inactive ingredients:

Disodium phosphate dodecahydrate

(may be replaced by equivalent amounts of the dihydrate or anhydrous form)

Sodium dihydrogen phosphate dihydrate

(may be replaced by equivalent amounts of the monohydrate)

Sodium hydroxide

Water for injection

6.2 Incompatibilities

None known.

6.3 Shelf life

36 months.

'Timoptol' Unit Dose Ophthalmic Solution should be used immediately after opening and any remaining contents should be discarded immediately after administration.

6.4 Special precautions for storage

Do not store above 25°C and keep in outer carton.

6.5 Nature and contents of container

Both the 0.25% and the 0.5% w/v solutions are presented in:

Unit-dose Dispensers, available in cartons of 30 unit doses.

6.6 Instructions for use and handling

Patients should be instructed to avoid allowing the tip of the dispensing container to contact the eye or surrounding structures.

Patients should also be instructed that ocular solutions, if handled improperly, can become contaminated by common bacteria known to cause ocular infections. Serious damage to the eye and subsequent loss of vision may result from using contaminated solutions.

7. MARKETING AUTHORISATION HOLDER

Merck Sharp & Dohme Limited

Hertford Road, Hoddesdon, Hertfordshire EN11 9BU, UK

8. MARKETING AUTHORISATION NUMBER(S)

0.25% Ophthalmic Solution, 0.20 ml Unit Dose, 0025/0210

0.5% Ophthalmic Solution, 0.20 ml Unit Dose, 0025/0211

9. DATE OF FIRST AUTHORISATION/RENEWAL OF THE AUTHORISATION

Granted: 17 March 1992

Last renewed: 21 March 2002

10. DATE OF REVISION OF THE TEXT

May 2002.

LEGAL CATEGORY

POM.

SPC.TOTUD.01.UK.0713

May 2002

Timoptol-LA

(Merck Sharp & Dohme Limited)

1. NAME OF THE MEDICINAL PRODUCT

TIMOPTOL®-LA Ophthalmic Gel-Forming Solution 0.25%

TIMOPTOL®-LA Ophthalmic Gel-Forming Solution 0.5%

2. QUALITATIVE AND QUANTITATIVE COMPOSITION

Each millilitre of 0.25% w/v solution contains an amount of timolol maleate equivalent to 2.5 mg/ml timolol.

Each millilitre of 0.5% w/v solution contains an amount of timolol maleate equivalent to 5 mg/ml timolol.

3. PHARMACEUTICAL FORM

Sterile ophthalmic gel-forming solution.

4. CLINICAL PARTICULARS

4.1 Therapeutic indications

A beta-adrenoreceptor blocker used topically in the reduction of elevated intra-ocular pressure in various conditions including the following: patients with ocular hypertension; patients with chronic open-angle glaucoma including aphakic patients; some patients with secondary glaucoma.

4.2 Posology and method of administration

Invert the closed container and shake once before each use. It is not necessary to shake the container more than once.

Recommended therapy is one drop 0.25% solution in each affected eye once a day.

If clinical response is not adequate, dosage may be changed to one drop 0.5% solution in each affected eye once a day.

If needed, 'Timoptol'-LA may be used with other agent(s) for lowering intra-ocular pressure. Other topically applied medication should be administered not less than 10 minutes before 'Timoptol'-LA. The use of two topical beta-adrenergic blocking agents is not recommended (see section 4.4 'Special warnings and special precautions for use').

Intra-ocular pressure should be reassessed approximately four weeks after starting treatment because response to 'Timoptol'-LA may take a few weeks to stabilise.

Transfer from other agents: When transferring a patient from 'Timoptol' to 'Timoptol'-LA, discontinue 'Timoptol' after a full day of therapy, starting treatment with the same concentration of 'Timoptol'-LA on the following day.

When another topical beta-blocking agent is being used, discontinue its use after a full day of therapy and start treatment with 'Timoptol'-LA the next day with one drop of 0.25% 'Timoptol'-LA in each affected eye once a day. The dosage may be increased to one drop of 0.5% solution in each affected eye once a day if the response is not adequate.

When transferring a patient from a single anti-glaucoma agent other than a topical beta-blocking agent, continue the agent and add one drop of 0.25% 'Timoptol'-LA in each affected eye once a day. On the following day, discontinue the previous agent completely, and continue with 'Timoptol'-LA. If a higher dosage of 'Timoptol'-LA is required, substitute one drop of 0.5% solution in each affected eye once a day (see section 5.1 'Pharmacodynamic properties').

Paediatric use: is not currently indicated.

Use in the elderly: there has been wide-experience with the use of timolol maleate in elderly patients. The dosage recommendations given above reflect the clinical data derived from this experience.

4.3 Contraindications

Bronchial asthma, history of bronchial asthma or severe chronic obstructive pulmonary disease; sinus bradycardia, second- or third-degree AV block, overt cardiac failure, cardiogenic shock; and hypersensitivity to any component of this product or other beta-blocking agents. 'Timoptol'-LA should not be used in patients wearing contact lenses as it has not been studied in these patients.

4.4 Special warnings and special precautions for use

Like other topically applied ophthalmic drugs, this drug may be absorbed systemically and adverse reactions seen with oral beta-blockers may occur.

Cardiac failure should be adequately controlled before beginning therapy with 'Timoptol'-LA. Patients with a history of severe cardiac disease should be watched for signs of cardiac failure and have their pulse rates monitored.

Respiratory and cardiac reactions, including death due to bronchospasm in patients with asthma and, rarely, death associated with cardiac failure, are potential complications of therapy with 'Timoptol'-LA.

The effect on intra-ocular pressure or the known effects of systemic beta-blockade may be exaggerated when 'Timoptol'-LA is given to patients already receiving a systemic beta-blocking agent. The response of these patients should be closely observed. The use of two topical beta-adrenergic blocking agents is not recommended.

There have been reports of skin rashes and/or dry eyes associated with the use of beta-adrenoreceptor blocking drugs. The reported incidence is small and in most cases the symptoms have cleared when treatment was withdrawn. Discontinuation of the drug should be considered if any such reaction is not otherwise explicable. Cessation of therapy involving beta-blockade should be gradual.

The dispenser of 'Timoptol'-LA contains benzododecinium bromide as a preservative. In a clinical study, the time required to eliminate 50% of the gellan solution from the eye was up to 30 minutes.

In patients with angle-closure glaucoma, the immediate objective of treatment is to reopen the angle. This requires constricting the pupil with a miotic. 'Timoptol'-LA has little or no effect on the pupil. When 'Timoptol'-LA is used to reduce elevated intra-ocular pressure in angle-closure glaucoma it should be used with a miotic and not alone.

Choroidal detachment has been reported with administration of aqueous suppressant therapy (e.g. timolol, acetazolamide) after filtration procedures.

Transient blurred vision following instillation may occur, generally lasting from 30 seconds to 5 minutes, and in rare cases up to 30 minutes or longer. Blurred vision and potential visual disturbances may impair the ability to perform hazardous tasks such as operating machinery or driving a motor vehicle.

Patients should be advised that if they develop an intercurrent ocular condition (e.g. trauma, ocular surgery or infection), they should immediately seek their physician's advice concerning the continued use of the present multi-dose container (see section 6.6 'Instructions for use/handling').

There have been reports of bacterial keratitis associated with the use of multiple dose containers of topical ophthalmic products. These containers had been inadvertently contaminated by patients who, in most cases, had a concurrent corneal disease or a disruption of the ocular epithelial surface.

Risk from anaphylactic reactions: While taking beta-blockers, patients with a history of atopy or a history of severe anaphylactic reaction to a variety of allergens may be more reactive to repeated challenge with such allergens, either accidental, diagnostic, or therapeutic. Such patients may be unresponsive to the usual doses of epinephrine (adrenaline) used to treat anaphylactic reactions.

4.5 Interaction with other medicinal products and other forms of Interaction

Although 'Timoptol' alone has little or no effect on pupil size, mydriasis has occasionally been reported when 'Timoptol' is given with epinephrine (adrenaline). The potential for mydriasis exists from concomitant therapy with 'Timoptol'-LA and epinephrine.

Close observation of the patient is recommended when a beta-blocker is administered to patients receiving catecholamine-depleting drugs such as reserpine, because of possible additive effects and the production of hypotension and/or marked bradycardia, which may produce vertigo, syncope, or postural hypotension.

The potential exists for hypotension, atrioventricular (AV) conduction disturbances and left ventricular failure to occur in patients receiving a beta-blocking agent when an oral calcium-channel blocker is added to the treatment regimen. The nature of any cardiovascular adverse effect tends to depend on the type of calcium-channel blocker used. Dihydropyridine derivatives, such as nifedipine, may lead to hypotension, whereas verapamil or diltiazem have a greater propensity to lead to AV conduction disturbances or left ventricular failure when used with a beta-blocker.

The concomitant use of beta-adrenergic blocking agents and digitalis with either diltiazem or verapamil may have additive effects in prolonging AV conduction time.

Oral calcium-channel antagonists may be used in combination with beta-adrenergic blocking agents when heart function is normal, but should be avoided in patients with impaired cardiac function.

Intravenous calcium-channel blockers should be used with caution in patients receiving beta-adrenergic blocking agents.

Potentiated systemic beta-blockade (e.g. decreased heart rate) has been reported during combined treatment with quinidine and timolol, possibly because quinidine inhibits the metabolism of timolol via the P-450 enzyme, CYP2D6.

Oral-β-adrenergic blocking agents may exacerbate the rebound hypertension which can follow the withdrawal of clonidine.

4.6 Pregnancy and lactation

Use in pregnancy: 'Timoptol'-LA has not been studied in human pregnancy. The use of 'Timoptol'-LA requires that the anticipated benefit be weighed against possible hazards.

Breast-feeding mothers: Timolol is detectable in human milk. Because of the potential for adverse reactions to 'Timoptol'-LA in infants, a decision should be made whether to discontinue nursing or to discontinue the drug, taking into account the importance of the drug to the mother.

4.7 Effects on ability to drive and use machines

Transient blurred vision following instillation may occur, generally lasting from 30 seconds to 5 minutes, and in rare cases, up to 30 minutes or longer. Blurred vision and potential visual disturbances may impair the ability to perform hazardous tasks such as operating machinery or driving a motor vehicle.

4.8 Undesirable effects

Side effects

'Timoptol'-LA is usually well tolerated. The most frequent drug-related complaint in clinical studies was transient blurred vision (6.0%), lasting from 30 seconds to 5 minutes following instillation.

The following possibly, probably, or definitely drug-related adverse reactions occurred with frequency of at least 1% in parallel active treatment controlled clinical trials:

Ocular: burning and stinging, discharge, foreign body sensation, itching.

The following side effects reported with 'Timoptol', either in clinical trials or since the drug has been marketed, are potential side effects of 'Timoptol'-LA. Additional side effects have been reported in clinical experiences with *systemic* timolol maleate, and may be considered potential effects of ophthalmic timolol maleate

Special senses:

ocular: signs and symptoms of ocular irritation, including conjunctivitis, blepharitis, keratitis, decreased corneal sensitivity and dry eyes. Tinnitus, visual disturbances, including refractive changes (due to withdrawal of miotic therapy in some cases), diplopia, and ptosis. Choroidal detachment following filtration surgery (see section 4.4 'Special warnings and precautions for use').

Cardiovascular:

ocular: bradycardia, arrhythmia, hypotension, syncope, heart block, cerebrovascular accident, cerebral ischaemia, congestive heart failure, palpitation, cardiac arrest, oedema, claudication, Raynaud's phenomenon, cold hands and feet.

systemic: AV block (second- or third-degree), sino-atrial block, pulmonary oedema, worsening of arterial insufficiency, worsening of angina pectoris, vasodilation.

Respiratory:

ocular: bronchospasm (predominantly in patients with pre-existing bronchospastic disease), respiratory failure, dyspnoea, cough.

systemic: rales

Body as a whole:

ocular: headache, asthenia, fatigue, chest pain.

systemic: extremity pain, decreased exercise tolerance.

Integumentary:

ocular: alopecia, psoriasiform rash or exacerbation of psoriasis.

systemic: pruritis, sweating, exfoliative dermatitis.

Hypersensitivity:

ocular: signs and symptoms of allergic reactions including anaphylaxis, angioedema, urticaria, localised and generalised rash.

Nervous system/psychiatric:

ocular: dizziness, depression, insomnia, nightmares, memory loss, paraesthesia.

systemic: vertigo, local weakness, diminished concentration, increased dreaming.

Neuromuscular:

ocular: increase in signs and symptoms of myasthenia gravis.

Digestive:

ocular: nausea, diarrhoea, dyspepsia, dry mouth.

systemic: vomiting.

Urogenital:

ocular: decreased libido, Peyronie's disease.

systemic: impotence, micturition difficulties.

Immunologic:

ocular: systemic lupus erythematosus.

Endocrine:

systemic: hyperglycaemia, hypoglycaemia.

Musculoskeletal:

systemic: arthralgia.

Haematological:

systemic: non-thrombocytopenic purpura.

4.9 Overdose

There have been reports of inadvertent overdosage with 'Timoptol' resulting in systemic effects similar to those seen with systemic beta-adrenergic blocking agents such as dizziness, headache, shortness of breath, bradycardia, bronchospasm, and cardiac arrest (see section 4.8 'Undesirable effects' - Side effects).

If overdosage occurs, the following measures should be considered:

1. Symptomatic bradycardia: atropine sulphate, 0.25 to 2 mg intravenously, should be used to induce vagal blockade. If bradycardia persists, intravenous isoprenaline hydrochloride should be administered cautiously. In refractory cases, the use of a cardiac pacemaker may be considered.

2. Hypotension: a sympathomimetic pressor agent such as dopamine, dobutamine or norepinephrine (noradrenaline) should be used. In refractory cases, the use of glucagon has been reported to be useful.

3. Bronchospasm: isoprenaline hydrochloride should be used. Additional therapy with aminophylline may be considered.

4. Acute cardiac failure: conventional therapy with digitalis, diuretics, and oxygen should be instituted immediately. In refractory cases, the use of intravenous aminophylline is suggested. This may be followed, if necessary, by glucagon, which has been reported useful.

5. Heart block (second- or third-degree): isoprenaline hydrochloride or a pacemaker should be used.

Timolol does not dialyse readily.

5. PHARMACOLOGICAL PROPERTIES

5.1 Pharmacodynamic properties

Pharmacotherapeutic group

Beta-adrenergic receptor blocking agent.

Mechanism of action

The precise mechanism of action of timolol maleate in lowering intra-ocular pressure is not clearly established. A fluorescein study and tonography studies indicate that the predominant action may be related to reduced aqueous formation. However, in some studies a slight increase in outflow facility was also observed.

'Timoptol'-LA is an ophthalmic formulation comprising timolol maleate, which reduces intra-ocular pressure, whether or not associated with glaucoma, and a new delivery vehicle. Gellan solution contains a highly purified anionic heteropolysaccharide derived from gellan gum. Aqueous solutions of gellan gum form a clear transparent gel at low polymer concentrations in the presence of cations. When 'Timoptol'-LA contacts the precorneal tear film, it becomes a gel. Gellan gum increases the contact time of the drug with the eye.

Pharmacodynamics

In parallel active treatment controlled, double-masked, multiclinic studies in patients with untreated elevated intra-ocular pressure of greater than 22 mmHg in one or both eyes, 0.25% and 0.5% 'Timoptol'-LA administered once daily had an intra-ocular pressure-lowering effect equivalent to the same concentration of 'Timoptol' administered twice daily (see table below).

For the five independent comparative studies listed in the table below, the entrance criterion was an intra-ocular pressure of greater than 22 mmHg in one or both eyes after a washout period of one week for most antiglaucoma medications and up to three weeks for ophthalmic beta-adrenergic antagonists. The dosage used was one drop of 'Timoptol'-LA in each affected eye once daily versus one drop of 'Timoptol' in each affected eye twice daily.

Mean change in intra-ocular pressure (mmHg) from baseline at trough (immediately before the morning dose) for the final week of the double-masked study

(see Table 1)

Table 1

Concentration	'Timoptol'-LA (n)	'Timoptol' (n)	Week
0.25%	-5.8 (94)	-5.9 (96)	12
0.25%	-6.0 (74)	-5.9 (73)	12
0.50%	-8.3 (110)*	-8.2 (111)*	12
0.50%	-5.6 (189)	-6.3 (94)	24
0.50%	-6.4 (212)	-6.1 (109)	24

*The baseline intra-ocular pressure was elevated in comparison to the other studies due to the higher intra-ocular pressure of patients with pseudoexfoliative glaucoma.

Onset of action of timolol maleate is usually rapid, occurring approximately 20 minutes after topical application to the eye.

Maximum reduction of intra-ocular pressure occurs in two to four hours with 'Timoptol'-LA. Significant lowering of intra-ocular pressure has been maintained for 24 hours with both 0.25% and 0.5% 'Timoptol'-LA.

As compared with 0.5% 'Timoptol' administered twice daily, in three clinical studies 0.5% 'Timoptol'-LA administered once daily reduced mean heart rate less and produced bradycardia less frequently (see section 4.4 'Special warnings and special precautions for use'). At trough (24 hours post-dose 'Timoptol'-LA, 12 hours post-dose 'Timoptol'), the mean reduction in heart rate was 0.8 beats/minute for 'Timoptol'-LA and 3.6 beats/minute for 'Timoptol'; whereas at two hours post-dose, the mean reduction was comparable (3.8 beats/minute for 'Timoptol'-LA and 5 beats/minute for 'Timoptol').

Timolol maleate is a non-selective beta-adrenergic receptor blocking agent that does not have significant intrinsic sympathomimetic, direct myocardial depressant, or local anaesthetic (membrane-stabilising) activity.

Unlike miotics, timolol maleate reduces intra-ocular pressure with little or no effect on accommodation or pupil size. Thus, changes in visual acuity due to increased accommodation are uncommon, and the dim or blurred vision and night blindness produced by miotics are not evident. In addition, in patients with cataracts the inability to see around lenticular opacities when the pupil is constricted by miotics is avoided. When changing patients from miotics to 'Timoptol'-LA, refraction may be necessary after the effects of the miotic have passed.

As with other antiglaucoma drugs, diminished responsiveness to timolol maleate after prolonged therapy has been reported in some patients. However, in clinical studies of 'Timoptol' in which 164 patients were followed for at least three years, no significant difference in mean intra-ocular pressure was observed after initial stabilisation. This indicates that the intra-ocular pressure-lowering effects of timolol maleate is well maintained.

5.2 Pharmacokinetic properties

Onset of action of timolol maleate is usually rapid, occurring approximately 20 minutes after topical application to the eye.

Maximum reduction of intra-ocular pressure occurs in two to four hours with 'Timoptol'-LA. Significant lowering of intra-ocular pressure has been maintained for 24 hours with both 0.25% and 0.5% 'Timoptol'-LA. In a study of plasma timolol concentrations, the systemic exposure to timolol was less when normal healthy volunteers received 0.5% 'Timoptol'-LA once daily than when they received 0.5% 'Timoptol' twice daily.

5.3 Preclinical safety data

No adverse ocular effects were observed in monkeys and rabbits administered 'Timoptol'-LA topically in studies lasting 12 months and one month, respectively. The oral LD_{50} of timolol is 1,190 and 900 mg/kg in female mice and female rats, respectively. The oral LD_{50} of gellan gum is greater than 5,000 mg/kg in rats.

In a two-year oral study of timolol maleate in rats there was a statistically significant ($p \leqslant 0.05$) increase in the incidence of adrenal phaeochromocytomas in male rats administered 300 mg/kg/day (300 times the maximum recommended human oral dose*). Similar differences were not observed in rats administered oral doses equivalent to 25 or 100 times the maximum recommended human oral dose.

In a lifetime oral study in mice, there were statistically significant ($p \leqslant 0.05$) increases in the incidence of benign and malignant pulmonary tumours, benign uterine polyps and mammary adenocarcinoma in female mice at 500 mg/kg/day (500 times the maximum recommended human dose), but not at 5 or 50 mg/kg/day. In a subsequent study in female mice, in which post-mortem examinations were limited to uterus and lungs, a statistically significant increase in the incidence of pulmonary tumours was again observed at 500 mg/kg/day.

The increased occurrence of mammary adenocarcinoma was associated with elevations in serum prolactin which occurred in female mice administered timolol at 500 mg/kg/day, but not at doses of 5 or 50 mg/kg/day. An increased incidence of mammary adenocarcinomas in rodents has been associated with administration of several other therapeutic agents which elevate serum prolactin, but no correlation between serum prolactin levels and mammary tumours has been established in man. Furthermore, in adult human female subjects who received oral dosages of up to 60 mg of timolol maleate, the maximum recommended human oral dosage, there were no clinically meaningful changes in serum prolactin.

In oral studies of gellan gum administered to rats for up to 105 weeks at concentrations up to 5% of their diet and to mice for 96-98 weeks at concentrations up to 3% of their diet, no overt signs of toxicity and no increase in the incidence of tumours was observed.

Timolol maleate was devoid of mutagenic potential when evaluated *in vivo* (mouse) in the micronucleus test and cytogenetic assay (doses up to 800 mg/kg) and *in vitro* in a neoplastic cell-transformation assay (up to 100 mcg/ml). In Ames tests the highest concentrations of timolol employed, 5,000 or 10,000 mcg/plate, were associated with statistically significant ($p \leqslant 0.05$) elevations of revertants observed with tester strain TA100 (in seven replicate assays), but not in the remaining three strains. In the assays with tester strain TA100, no consistent dose-response relationship was observed, nor did the ratio of test to control revertants reach 2. A ratio of 2 is usually considered the criterion for a positive Ames test.

Gellan gum was devoid of mutagenic potential when evaluated *in vivo* (mouse) in micronucleus assay using doses up to 450 mg/kg. In addition, gellan gum in concentrations up to 20 mg/ml was not detectably mutagenic in the following *in-vitro* assays:

(1) unscheduled DNA synthesis in rat hepatocytes assay, (2) V-79 mammalian cell mutagenesis assay, and (3) chromosomal aberrations in Chinese hamster ovary cells assay.

In Ames tests, gellan gum (in concentrations up to 1,000 mcg/plate, which is its limit of solubility) did not induce a twofold or greater increase in revertants relative to the solvent control. It is therefore not detectably mutagenic.

*The maximum recommended daily oral dose of timolol is 60 mg. One drop of 0.5% 'Timoptol'-LA contains about 1/300 of this dose, which is about 0.2 mg.

6. PHARMACEUTICAL PARTICULARS

6.1 List of excipients

Gellan gum, trometamol, mannitol E421, and water for injection. Benzododecinium bromide (0.012%) is added as preservative.

6.2 Incompatibilities

None known.

6.3 Shelf life

The shelf life is 24 months. After opening the shelf life is 28 days.

6.4 Special precautions for storage

Do not store above 25°C. Do not freeze. Store bottle in the outer carton.

6.5 Nature and contents of container

ALP Container:

The 5 ml ALP container consists of an oval translucent, low-density polyethylene bottle with a controlled-drop tip, and a blue coloured (light-blue 0.25% or dark-blue 0.5%) polypropylene cap. The tip and cap are covered with a translucent, tamper-evident, disposable over cap. The ALP vial contains 2.5 ml of solution.

Ocumeter Plus Ophthalmic Dispenser:

The OCUMETER Plus ophthalmic dispenser consists of a translucent high-density polyethylene container with a sealed dropper tip, a flexible fluted side area, which is depressed to dispense the drops, and a two-piece assembly. The two-piece cap mechanism punctures the sealed dropper tip upon initial use, then locks together to provide a single cap during the usage period. Tamper evidence is provided by a safety strip on the container label. The OCUMETER Plus ophthalmic dispenser contains 2.5 ml of solution.

'Timoptol'-LA Ophthalmic Gel-Forming solution is available in single bottles containing 2.5 ml of solution.

6.6 Instructions for use and handling

Invert the container and shake once before each use. It is not necessary to shake the container more than once.

Discard 28 days after opening.

Patients should be instructed to avoid allowing the tip of the dispensing container to contact the eye or surrounding structures.

Patients should also be instructed that ocular solutions, if handled improperly, can become contaminated by common bacteria known to cause ocular infections. Serious damage to the eye and subsequent loss of vision may result from using contaminated solutions.

7. MARKETING AUTHORISATION HOLDER

Merck Sharp & Dohme Limited

Hertford Road, Hoddesdon, Hertfordshire EN11 9BU, UK.

8. MARKETING AUTHORISATION NUMBER(S)

0.25% PL 0025/0310

0.5% PL 0025/0311

9. DATE OF FIRST AUTHORISATION/RENEWAL OF THE AUTHORISATION

Granted: 2 April 1996/Renewed: 2 April 2001

10. DATE OF REVISION OF THE TEXT

May 2002.

LEGAL CATEGORY
POM.

MSD (logo)

Merck Sharp & Dohme Limited

Hertford Road, Hoddesdon, Hertfordshire EN11 9BU, UK

SPC.TOTX.01.UK.0711

TOBI 300 mg/5 ml Nebuliser Solution

(Chiron Corporation Limted)

1. NAME OF THE MEDICINAL PRODUCT
TOBI®

300 mg/5 mL Nebuliser Solution

2. QUALITATIVE AND QUANTITATIVE COMPOSITION
One ampoule of 5mL contains tobramycin 300mg as a single dose.

For excipients, see 6.1.

3. PHARMACEUTICAL FORM
Nebuliser solution.

Clear, slightly yellow solution.

4. CLINICAL PARTICULARS
4.1 Therapeutic indications
Long-term management of chronic pulmonary infection due to *Pseudomonas aeruginosa* in cystic fibrosis (CF) patients aged 6 years and older.

Consideration should be given to official guidance on the appropriate use of antibacterial agents.

4.2 Posology and method of administration
TOBI® is supplied for use via inhalation and is not for parenteral use.

Posology
The recommended dose for adults and children is one ampoule twice-daily for 28 days. The dose interval should be as close as possible to 12 hours and not less than 6 hours. After 28 days of therapy, patients should stop TOBI therapy for the next 28 days. A cycle of 28 days of active therapy and 28 days of rest from treatment should be maintained.

Dosage is not adjusted for weight. All patients should receive one ampoule of TOBI (300 mg of tobramycin) twice daily.

Controlled clinical studies, conducted for a period of 6 months using the following TOBI dosage regimen, have shown that improvement in lung function was maintained above baseline during the 28 day rest periods.

TOBI Dosing Regimen in Controlled Clinical Studies

(see Table 1)

Safety and efficacy have been assessed in controlled and open label studies for up to 96 weeks (12 cycles), but have not been studied in patients under the age of 6 years, patients with forced expiratory volume in 1 second (FEV_1) <25% or >75% predicted, or patients colonised with *Burkholderia cepacia*.

Therapy should be initiated by a physician experienced in the management of cystic fibrosis. Treatment with TOBI should be continued on a cyclical basis for as long as the physician considers the patient is gaining clinical benefit from the inclusion of TOBI in their treatment regimen. If clinical deterioration of pulmonary status is evident, additional anti-pseudomonal therapy should be considered. Clinical studies have shown that a microbiological report indicating *in vitro* drug resistance does not necessarily preclude a clinical benefit for the patient.

Method of administration
The contents of one ampoule should be emptied into the nebuliser and administered by inhalation over approximately a 15-minute period using a hand-held PARI LC PLUS reusable nebuliser with a suitable compressor. Suitable compressors are those which, when attached to a PARI LC Plus nebuliser, deliver a flow rate of 4-6 L/min and/or a back pressure of 110-217 kPa. The manufacturers' instructions for the care and use of the nebuliser and compressor should be followed.

TOBI is inhaled whilst the patient is sitting or standing upright and breathing normally through the mouthpiece of the nebuliser. Nose clips may help the patient breathe through the mouth. The patient should continue their standard regimen of chest physiotherapy. The use of appropriate bronchodilators should continue as thought clinically necessary. Where patients are receiving several different respiratory therapies it is recommended that they are taken in the following order: bronchodilator, chest physiotherapy, other inhaled medicinal products, and finally TOBI.

Maximum tolerated daily dose
The maximum tolerated daily dose of TOBI® has not been established.

4.3 Contraindications
Administration of TOBI® is contraindicated in any patient with known hypersensitivity to any aminoglycoside.

4.4 Special warnings and special precautions for use
General Warnings
For information on pregnancy and lactation see 4.6.

TOBI should be used with caution in patients with known or suspected renal, auditory, vestibular or neuromuscular dysfunction, or with severe, active haemoptysis.

The Serum concentration of tobramycin should only be monitored through venipuncture and not finger prick blood sampling, which is a non validated dosing method. It has been observed that contamination of the skin of the fingers from the preparation and nebulisation of TOBI may lead to falsely increased serum levels of the drug. This contamination cannot be completely avoided by hand washing before testing.

Bronchospasm
Bronchospasm can occur with inhalation of medicinal products and has been reported with nebulised tobramycin. The first dose of TOBI should be given under supervision, using a pre-nebulisation bronchodilator if this is part of the current regimen for the patient. FEV_1 should be measured before and after nebulisation. If there is evidence of therapy-induced bronchospasm in a patient not receiving a bronchodilator the test should be repeated, on a separate occasion, using a bronchodilator. Evidence of bronchospasm in the presence of bronchodilator therapy may indicate an allergic response. If an allergic response is suspected TOBI should be discontinued. Bronchospasm should be treated as medically appropriate.

Neuromuscular disorders
TOBI should be used with great caution in patients with neuromuscular disorders such as parkinsonism or other conditions characterised by myasthenia, including myasthenia gravis, as aminoglycosides may aggravate muscle weakness due to a potential curare-like effect on neuromuscular function.

Nephrotoxicity
Although nephrotoxicity has been associated with parenteral aminoglycoside therapy, there was no evidence of nephrotoxicity during clinical trials with TOBI.

The product should be used with caution in patients with known or suspected renal dysfunction and serum concentrations of tobramycin should be monitored. Patients with severe renal impairment, i.e., serum creatinine >2 mg/dL (176.8 μmol/L), were not included in the clinical studies.

Current clinical practice suggests baseline renal function should be assessed. Urea and creatinine levels should be reassessed after every 6 complete cycles of TOBI therapy (180 days of nebulised aminoglycoside therapy). If there is evidence of nephrotoxicity, all tobramycin therapy should be discontinued until trough serum concentrations fall below 2 μg/mL. TOBI® therapy may then be resumed at the physician's discretion. Patients receiving concomitant parenteral aminoglycoside therapy should be monitored as clinically appropriate taking into account the risk of cumulative toxicity.

Ototoxicity
Ototoxicity, manifested as both auditory and vestibular toxicity, has been reported with parenteral aminoglycosides. Vestibular toxicity may be manifested by vertigo, ataxia or dizziness. Auditory toxicity, as measured by complaints of hearing loss or by audiometric evaluations, did not occur with TOBI therapy during controlled clinical studies. In open label studies and post-marketing experience, some patients with a history of prolonged previous or concomitant use of intravenous aminoglycosides have experienced hearing loss. Physicians should consider the potential for aminoglycosides to cause vestibular and cochlear toxicity and carry out appropriate assessments of auditory function during TOBI therapy. In patients with a predisposing risk due to previous prolonged, systemic aminoglycoside therapy it may be necessary to consider audiological assessment before initiating TOBI therapy. The onset of tinnitus warrants caution as it is a sentinel symptom of ototoxicity. If a patient reports tinnitus or hearing loss during aminoglycoside therapy the physician should consider referring them for audiological assessment. Patients receiving concomitant parenteral aminoglycoside therapy should be monitored as clinically appropriate taking into account the risk of cumulative toxicity.

Haemoptysis
Inhalation of nebulised solutions may induce a cough reflex. The use of TOBI in patients with active, severe haemoptysis should be undertaken only if the benefits of treatment are considered to outweigh the risks of inducing further haemorrhage.

Microbial Resistance
In clinical studies, some patients on TOBI therapy showed an increase in aminoglycoside Minimum Inhibitory Concentrations for *P. aeruginosa* isolates tested. There is a theoretical risk that patients being treated with nebulised tobramycin may develop *P. aeruginosa* isolates resistant to intravenous tobramycin (see 5.1).

4.5 Interaction with other medicinal products and other forms of Interaction
In clinical studies, patients taking TOBI concomitantly with dornase alfa, β-agonists, inhaled corticosteroids, and other oral or parenteral anti-pseudomonal antibiotics, demonstrated adverse experience profiles which were similar to those of the control group.

Concurrent and/or sequential use of TOBI with other medicinal products with nephrotoxic or ototoxic potential should be avoided. Some diuretics can enhance aminoglycoside toxicity by altering antibiotic concentrations in serum and tissue. TOBI should not be administered concomitantly with furosemide, urea or mannitol.

Other medicinal products that have been reported to increase the potential toxicity of parenterally administered aminoglycosides include:

Amphotericin B, cefalotin, ciclosporin, tacrolimus, polymyxins (risk of increased nephrotoxicity);

Platinum compounds (risk of increased nephrotoxicity and ototoxicity);

Anticholinesterases, botulinum toxin (neuromuscular effects).

4.6 Pregnancy and lactation
TOBI should not be used during pregnancy or lactation unless the benefits to the mother outweigh the risks to the foetus or baby.

Pregnancy
There are no adequate data from the use of tobramycin administered by inhalation in pregnant women. Animal studies do not indicate a teratogenic effect of tobramycin (see 5.3 Preclinical data). However, aminoglycosides can cause foetal harm (e.g., congenital deafness) when high systemic concentrations are achieved in a pregnant woman. If TOBI is used during pregnancy, or if the patient becomes pregnant while taking TOBI, she should be informed of the potential hazard to the foetus.

Lactation
Systemic tobramycin is excreted in breast milk. It is not known if administration of TOBI will result in serum concentrations high enough for tobramycin to be detected in breast milk. Because of the potential for ototoxicity and nephrotoxicity with tobramycin in infants, a decision should be made whether to terminate nursing or discontinue TOBI therapy.

4.7 Effects on ability to drive and use machines
On the basis of reported adverse drug reactions, TOBI is presumed to be unlikely to produce an effect on the ability to drive and use machinery.

4.8 Undesirable effects
In controlled clinical trials, voice alteration and tinnitus were the only undesirable effects reported in significantly more patients treated with TOBI; (13% TOBI vs 7% control) and (3% TOBI vs 0% control) respectively. These episodes of tinnitus were transient and resolved without discontinuation of TOBI therapy, and were not associated with permanent loss of hearing on audiogram testing. The risk of tinnitus did not increase with repeated cycles of exposure to TOBI.

Additional undesirable effects, some of which are common sequelae of the underlying disease, but where a causal relationship to TOBI could not be excluded were: sputum discolouration, respiratory tract infection, myalgia, nasal polyp and otitis media.

(see Table 2 on next page)

In open label studies and post-marketing experience, some patients with a history of prolonged previous or concomitant use of intravenous aminoglycosides have experienced hearing loss (see 4.4). Parenteral aminoglycosides have been associated with hypersensitivity, ototoxicity and nephrotoxicity (see 4.3, 4.4).

4.9 Overdose
Administration by inhalation results in low systemic bioavailability of tobramycin. Symptoms of aerosol overdose may include severe hoarseness.

In the event of accidental ingestion of TOBI, toxicity is unlikely as tobramycin is poorly absorbed from an intact gastrointestinal tract.

In the event of inadvertent administration of TOBI by the intravenous route, signs and symptoms of parenteral tobramycin overdose may occur that include dizziness, tinnitus, vertigo, loss of hearing acuity, respiratory distress and/or neuromuscular blockade and renal impairment.

Table 1

Cycle 1		Cycle 2		Cycle 3	
28 Days	28 Days	28 Days	28 Days	28 Days	28 Days
TOBI 300 mg twice daily plus standard care	standard care	TOBI 300 mg twice daily plus standard care	standard care	TOBI 300 mg twice daily plus standard care	standard care

Table 2

In the POSTMARKETING phase, undesirable effects have been reported at the following frequencies:

Body as a Whole	
Rare:	Chest pain, Asthenia, Fever, Headache, Pain,
Very Rare:	Abdominal pain, Fungal infection, Malaise, Back pain, Allergic reactions including urticaria and pruritus
Digestive System	
Rare:	Nausea, Anorexia, Mouth ulceration, Vomiting
Very Rare:	Diarrhoea, Oral moniliasis
Haemic and Lymphatic System	
Very Rare:	Lymphadenopathy
Nervous System	
Rare:	Dizziness
Very Rare:	Somnolence
Respiratory System	
Uncommon:	Voice alteration (including hoarseness), Dyspnoea, Cough increased, Pharyngitis
Rare:	Bronchospasm, chest tightness, cough, shortness of breath, Lung disorder, Sputum Increased, Haemoptysis, Lung function decreased, Laryngitis, Epistaxis, Rhinitis, Asthma
Very Rare:	Hyperventilation, Hypoxia, Sinusitis
Special Senses	
Rare:	Tinnitus, Taste perversion, Hearing loss, Aphonia
Very Rare:	Ear disorder, Ear pain
Skin and Appendages	
Rare:	Rash

Acute toxicity should be treated with immediate withdrawal of TOBI, and baseline tests of renal function should be undertaken. Tobramycin serum concentrations may be helpful in monitoring overdose. In the case of any overdosage, the possibility of drug interactions with alterations in the elimination of TOBI or other medicinal products should be considered.

5. PHARMACOLOGICAL PROPERTIES

5.1 Pharmacodynamic properties

Pharmacotherapeutic group (ATC code) Aminoglycoside Antibacterials J01GB01General properties

Tobramycin is an aminoglycoside antibiotic produced by *Streptomyces tenebrarius*. It acts primarily by disrupting protein synthesis leading to altered cell membrane permeability, progressive disruption of the cell envelope and eventual cell death. It is bactericidal at concentrations equal to or slightly greater than inhibitory concentrations.

Breakpoints

Established susceptibility breakpoints for parenteral administration of tobramycin are inappropriate in the aerosolised administration of the medicinal product. Cystic fibrosis (CF) sputum exhibits an inhibitory action on the local biological activity of nebulised aminoglycosides. This necessitates sputum concentrations of aerosolised tobramycin to be some ten and twenty–five fold above the Minimum Inhibitory Concentration (MIC) for, respectively, *P. aeruginosa* growth suppression and bactericidal activity. In controlled clinical trials, 97% of patients receiving TOBI achieved sputum concentrations 10 fold the highest *P. aeruginosa* MIC cultured from the patient, and 95% of patients receiving TOBI achieved 25 fold the highest MIC. Clinical benefit is still achieved in a majority of patients who culture strains with MIC values above the parenteral breakpoint.

Susceptibility

In the absence of conventional susceptibility breakpoints for the nebulised route of administration, caution must be exercised in defining organisms as susceptible or insusceptible to nebulised tobramycin.

In clinical studies with TOBI, most patients with *P. aeruginosa* isolates with tobramycin MICs <128 μg/mL at baseline showed improved lung function following treatment with TOBI. Patients with a *P. aeruginosa* isolate with a MIC ⩾ 128 μg/mL at baseline are less likely to show a clinical response. However, seven of 13 patients (54%) in the placebo-controlled trials who acquired isolates with MICs of ⩾ 128 μg/mL while using TOBI had improvement in pulmonary function.

Based upon *in vitro* data and/or clinical trial experience, the organisms associated with pulmonary infections in CF may be expected to respond to TOBI therapy as follows:

Susceptible	*Pseudomonas aeruginosa* *Haemophilus influenzae* *Staphylococcus aureus*
Insusceptible	*Burkholderia cepacia* *Stenotrophomonas maltophilia* *Alcaligenes xylosoxidans*

Treatment with the TOBI regimen in clinical studies showed a small but clear increase in tobramycin, amikacin and gentamicin Minimum Inhibitory Concentrations for *P. aeruginosa* isolates tested. Each additional 6 months of treatment resulted in incremental increases similar in magnitude to that observed in the 6 months of controlled studies. The most prevalent aminoglycoside resistance mechanism seen in *P. aeruginosa* isolated from chronically infected CF patients is impermeability, defined by a general lack of susceptibility to all aminoglycosides. *P. aeruginosa* isolated from CF patients has also been shown to exhibit adaptive aminoglycoside resistance that is characterised by a reversion to susceptibility when the antibiotic is removed.

Other Information

There is no evidence that patients treated with up to 18 months of TOBI were at a greater risk for acquiring *B. cepacia, S. maltophilia or A. xylosoxidans,* than would be expected in patients not treated with TOBI. *Aspergillus* species were more frequently recovered from the sputum of patients who received TOBI; however, clinical sequelae such as Allergic Bronchopulmonary Aspergillosis (ABPA) were reported rarely and with similar frequency as in the control group.

5.2 Pharmacokinetic properties

Absorption and distribution

Sputum concentrations: Ten minutes after inhalation of the first 300 mg dose of TOBI, the average sputum concentration of tobramycin was 1,237 μg/g (range: 35 to 7,414 μg/g). Tobramycin does not accumulate in sputum; after 20 weeks of therapy with the TOBI regimen, the average sputum concentration of tobramycin 10 minutes after inhalation was 1,154 μg/g (range: 39 to 8,085 μg/g). High variability of sputum tobramycin concentrations was observed. Two hours after inhalation, sputum concentrations declined to approximately 14% of tobramycin levels measured at 10 minutes after inhalation.

Serum concentrations: The median serum concentration of tobramycin 1 hour after inhalation of a single 300 mg dose of TOBI by CF patients was 0.95 μg/mL (range: below limit of quantitation [BLQ] – 3.62μg/mL). After 20 weeks of therapy on the TOBI regimen, the median serum tobramycin concentration 1 hour after dosing was 1.05 μg/mL (range: BLQ- 3.41μg/mL).

Elimination

The elimination of tobramycin administered by the inhalation route has not been studied.

Following intravenous administration, systemically absorbed tobramycin is eliminated principally by glomerular filtration. The elimination half-life of tobramycin from serum is approximately 2 hours. Less than 10% of tobramycin is bound to plasma proteins.

Unabsorbed tobramycin following TOBI administration is probably eliminated primarily in expectorated sputum.

5.3 Preclinical safety data

Preclinical data reveal that the main hazard for humans, based on studies of safety pharmacology, repeated dose toxicity, genotoxicity, or toxicity to reproduction, consists of renal toxicity and ototoxicity. In repeated dose toxicity studies, target organs of toxicity are the kidneys and vestibular/cochlear functions. In general, toxicity is seen at higher systemic tobramycin levels than are achievable by inhalation at the recommended clinical dose.

No reproduction toxicology studies have been conducted with tobramycin administered by inhalation, but subcutaneous administration at doses of 100 mg/kg/day in rats and the maximum tolerated dose of 20 mg/kg/day in rabbits, during organogenesis, was not teratogenic. Teratogenicity could not be assessed at higher parenteral doses in rabbits as they induced maternal toxicity and abortion. Based on available data from animals a risk of toxicity (e.g. ototoxicity) at prenatal exposure levels cannot be excluded.

6. PHARMACEUTICAL PARTICULARS

6.1 List of excipients

Sodium chloride

Water for injections

Sulphuric acid and sodium hydroxide for pH adjustment

6.2 Incompatibilities

TOBI should not be diluted or mixed with any other medicinal product in the nebuliser.

6.3 Shelf life

3 years.

The contents of the whole ampoule should be used immediately after opening (see 6.6).

6.4 Special precautions for storage

Store at 2-8°C. Store in the original package in order to protect from light.

After removal from the refrigerator, or if refrigeration is unavailable, TOBI pouches (intact or opened) may be stored at up to 25°C for up to 28 days.

TOBI solution is normally slightly yellow, but some variability in colour may be observed, which does not indicate loss of activity if the product has been stored as recommended.

6.5 Nature and contents of container

TOBI is supplied in 5 mL single-use low density polyethylene ampoules. One outer carton contains a total of 56 ampoules comprising 4 sealed foil pouches, each containing 14 ampoules packed in a plastic tray.

6.6 Instructions for use and handling

TOBI is a sterile, non-pyrogenic, aqueous preparation for single use only. As it is preservative-free, the contents of the whole ampoule should be used immediately after opening and any unused solution discarded. Opened ampoules should never be stored for re-use.

7. MARKETING AUTHORISATION HOLDER

Chiron Corporation Limited

Symphony House

Cowley Business Park

The High Street

Uxbridge

UB8 2AD

UK

8. MARKETING AUTHORISATION NUMBER(S)

PL 17092/0002

9. DATE OF FIRST AUTHORISATION/RENEWAL OF THE AUTHORISATION

10 December 1999

Date of Last Renewal

10 December 2004

10. DATE OF REVISION OF THE TEXT

December 2004

Legal Category: POM

Tomudex

(AstraZeneca UK Limited)

1. NAME OF THE MEDICINAL PRODUCT

'Tomudex'

2. QUALITATIVE AND QUANTITATIVE COMPOSITION

'Tomudex' contains 2 mg raltitrexed (INN applied for) in each vial.

3. PHARMACEUTICAL FORM

Powder for solution for injection.

4. CLINICAL PARTICULARS

4.1 Therapeutic indications

The palliative treatment of advanced colorectal cancer where 5-Fluorouracil and folinic acid based regimens are either not tolerated or inappropriate.

4.2 Posology and method of administration

Adults: - The dose of 'Tomudex' is calculated on the basis of the body surface area. The recommended dose is 3 mg/m^2 given intravenously, as a single short, intravenous infusion in 50 to 250 ml of either 0.9% sodium chloride solution or 5% dextrose (glucose) solution. It is recommended that the infusion is given over a 15 minute period. Other drugs should not be mixed with 'Tomudex' in the same infusion container. In the absence of toxicity, treatment may be repeated every 3 weeks.

Dose escalation above 3 mg/m^2 is not recommended, since higher doses have been associated with an increased incidence of life-threatening or fatal toxicity.

Prior to the initiation of treatment and before each subsequent treatment a full blood count (including a differential count and platelets), liver transaminases, serum bilirubin and serum creatinine measurements should be performed. The total white cell count should be greater than 4,000/mm^3, the neutrophil count greater than 2,000/mm^3 and the platelet count greater than 100,000/mm^3 prior to treatment. In the event of toxicity the next scheduled dose should be withheld until signs of toxic effects regress. In particular, signs of gastrointestinal toxicity (diarrhoea or mucositis) and haematological toxicity (neutropenia or thrombocytopenia) should have completely resolved before subsequent treatment is allowed. Patients who develop signs of gastrointestinal toxicity should have their full blood counts monitored at least weekly for signs of haematological toxicity.

Based on the worst grade of gastrointestinal and haematological toxicity observed on the previous treatment and provided that such toxicity has completely resolved, the following dose reductions are recommended for subsequent treatment:

* 25% dose reduction: in patients with WHO grade 3 haematological toxicity (neutropenia or thrombocytopenia) or WHO grade 2 gastrointestinal toxicity (diarrhoea or mucositis).

* 50% dose reduction: in patients with WHO grade 4 haematological toxicity (neutropenia or thrombocytopenia) or WHO grade 3 gastrointestinal toxicity (diarrhoea or mucositis).

Once a dose reduction has been made, all subsequent doses should be given at the reduced dose.

Treatment should be discontinued in the event of any WHO grade 4 gastrointestinal toxicity (diarrhoea or mucositis) or in the event of a WHO grade 3 gastrointestinal toxicity associated with WHO grade 4 haematological toxicity. Patients with such toxicity should be managed promptly with standard supportive care measures including i.v. hydration and bone marrow support. In addition pre-clinical data suggest that consideration should be given to the administration of folinic acid. From clinical experience with other antifolates folinic acid may be given at a dose of 25mg/m^2 i.v. every 6 hours until the resolution of symptoms. Further use of 'Tomudex' in such patients is not recommended.

It is essential that the dose reduction scheme should be adhered to since the potential for life threatening and fatal toxicity increases if the dose is not reduced or treatment not stopped as appropriate.

Elderly: - Dosage and administration as for adults. However, as with other cytotoxics, 'Tomudex' should be used with caution in elderly patients (see Warnings/Precautions).

Children: - 'Tomudex' is not recommended for use in children as safety and efficacy have not been established in this group of patients.

Renal impairment:- For patients with abnormal serum creatinine, before the first or any subsequent treatment, a creatinine clearance should be performed or calculated. For patients with a normal serum creatinine when the serum creatinine may not correlate well with the creatinine clearance due to factors such as age or weight loss, the same procedure should be followed. If creatinine clearance is < 65 ml/min, the following dose modifications are recommended:

Dose modification in the presence of renal impairment

Creatinine Clearance	Dose as % of 3.0 mg/m^2	Dosing Interval
> 65 ml/min	Full dose	3-weekly
55 to 65 ml/min	75%	4-weekly
25 to 54 ml/min	50%	4-weekly
< 25 ml/min	No therapy	Not applicable

See Contraindications for use in patients with severe renal impairment

Hepatic Impairment:- No dosage adjustment is recommended for patients with mild to moderate hepatic impairment. However, given that a proportion of the drug is excreted via the faecal route, (see Section 5.2 Pharmacokinetic Properties) and that these patients usually form a poor prognosis group, patients with mild to moderate hepatic impairment need to be treated with caution. (See Section 4.4 Warnings and Precautions for Use). 'Tomudex' has not been studied in patients with severe hepatic impairment, clinical jaundice or decompensated liver disease and its use in such patients is not recommended.

4.3 Contraindications

'Tomudex' should not be used in pregnant women, in women who may become pregnant during treatment or women who are breast feeding. Pregnancy should be excluded before treatment with 'Tomudex' is commenced. (see Pregnancy section).

'Tomudex' is contraindicated in patients with severe renal impairment.

4.4 Special warnings and special precautions for use

It is recommended that 'Tomudex' is only given by or under the supervision of a physician who is experienced in cancer chemotherapy, and in the management of chemotherapy-related toxicity. Patients undergoing therapy should be subject to appropriate supervision so that signs of possible toxic effects or adverse reactions (particularly diarrhoea) may be detected and treated promptly (see Posology and Method of Administration).

In common with other cytotoxic agents of this type, caution is necessary in patients with depressed bone marrow function, poor general condition, or prior radiotherapy.

Patients whose disease progressed on previous treatment for advanced disease with 5-Fluorouracil based regimens may also be resistant to the effects of 'Tomudex'.

Elderly patients are more vulnerable to the toxic effects of 'Tomudex'. Extreme care should be taken to ensure adequate monitoring of adverse reactions especially signs of gastrointestinal toxicity (diarrhoea or mucositis).

A proportion of the 'Tomudex' is excreted via the faecal route, (see section 5.2 Pharmacokinetic properties) therefore, patients with mild to moderate hepatic impairment should be treated with caution.

Treatment with 'Tomudex' in patients with severe hepatic impairment is not recommended.

It is recommended that pregnancy should be avoided during treatment and for at least 6 months after cessation of treatment if either partner is receiving 'Tomudex' (see also Pregnancy and Lactation).

There is no clinical experience with extravasation. However, perivascular tolerance studies in animals did not reveal any significant irritant reaction.

'Tomudex' is a cytotoxic agent and should be handled according to normal procedures adopted for such agents (see Instructions for use/handling).

4.5 Interaction with other medicinal products and other forms of Interaction

No specific interaction studies have been conducted in man.

Folinic acid, folic acid or vitamin preparations containing these agents must not be given immediately prior to or during administration of 'Tomudex', since they may interfere with its action.

Clinical trials evaluating the use of Tomudex in combination with other antitumour therapies are currently ongoing.

'Tomudex' is 93% protein bound and while it has the potential to interact with similarly highly protein bound drugs, no displacement interaction with warfarin has been observed in vitro. Data suggest that active tubular secretion may contribute to the renal excretion of raltitrexed, indicating a potential interaction with other actively secreted drugs such as non-steroidal anti-inflammatory drugs (NSAIDS). However, a review of the clinical trial safety database did not reveal evidence of clinically significant interaction in patients treated with 'Tomudex' who also received concomitant NSAIDS, warfarin and other commonly prescribed drugs.

4.6 Pregnancy and lactation

Pregnancy should be avoided if either partner is receiving 'Tomudex'. It is also recommended that conception should be avoided for at least 6 months after cessation of treatment.

'Tomudex' should not be used during pregnancy or in women who may become pregnant during treatment (see the Pre-clinical Safety Data). Pregnancy should be excluded before treatment with 'Tomudex' is started. 'Tomudex' should not be given to women who are breast feeding.

Fertility studies in the rat indicate that 'Tomudex' can cause impairment of male fertility. Fertility returned to normal three months after dosing ceased. 'Tomudex' caused embryolethality and foetal abnormalities in pregnant rats.

4.7 Effects on ability to drive and use machines

'Tomudex' may cause malaise or asthenia following infusion and the ability to drive/use machinery could be impaired whilst such symptoms continue.

4.8 Undesirable effects

As with other cytotoxic drugs, 'Tomudex' may be associated with certain adverse drug reactions. These mainly include reversible effects on the haemopoietic system, liver enzymes and gastrointestinal tract.

The following effects were reported as possible adverse drug reactions. The incidences represent those that were reported in the colorectal cancer clinical trials irrespective of the clinician's assessment of causality.

Gastrointestinal System

The most frequent effects were nausea in 57% of patients, diarrhoea (36%), vomiting (35%) and anorexia (26%). The incidence of severe (WHO Grade 3 and 4) gastrointestinal adverse events were 12% for nausea and vomiting, 12% for diarrhoea and 2% for mucositis. Other effects include mouth ulceration, dyspepsia and constipation. Gastrointestinal bleeding which may be associated with mucositis and/or thrombocytopenia has been reported rarely.

Diarrhoea is usually mild or moderate (WHO grade 1 and 2) and can occur at any time following the administration of 'Tomudex'. However severe diarrhoea may be associated with concurrent haematological suppression, especially leucopenia. Subsequent treatment may need to be discontinued or the dose reduced according to the grade of toxicity (see Posology and Method of Administration).

Nausea and vomiting are usually mild (WHO grade 1 and 2), occur usually in the first week following the administration of 'Tomudex', and are usually responsive to antiemetics.

Haemopoietic system

Leucopenia (neutropenia in particular)(21%), anaemia (16%) and thrombocytopenia (5%), alone or in combination, have been reported in clinical trials. They are usually mild to moderate, and occur in the first and second week after treatment and recover by the third week. Severe (WHO grade 3 and 4) leucopenia (neutropenia in particular) and thrombocytopenia of WHO grade 4 can occur. The incidence of severe (WHO Grade 4) leucopenia or thrombocytopenia was 5% and 1% respectively. These may be potentially life-threatening or fatal especially if associated with signs of gastrointestinal toxicity (see Posology and Method of Administration).

Metabolic and Nutritional

Reversible increases of 14% each in both AST and ALT have been commonly reported in clinical trials. Such changes have usually been asymptomatic and self-limiting when not associated with progression of the underlying malignancy. Other effects were weight loss, dehydration, peripheral oedema, hyperbilirubinaemia and increases in alkaline phosphatase.

Musculoskeletal and Nervous System

Arthralgia and hypertonia (usually muscular cramps) have each been reported in less than 2% of patients.

Skin, Appendages and Special Senses

Rash was commonly reported in clinical trials (13% of patients) sometimes associated with pruritus. Other effects were desquamation, alopecia, sweating, taste perversion and conjunctivitis each in less than 5% of patients.

Whole Body

The most frequent effects were asthenia (46%) and fever (20%) which were usually mild to moderate following the first week of administration of 'Tomudex' and reversible. Severe asthenia can occur and may be associated with malaise and a flu-like syndrome. Other effects were abdominal pain (23%), pain (8%) headache (7%) and infections (5%). Cellulitis and sepsis were also reported each in less than 5% of patients.

4.9 Overdose

There is no clinically proven antidote available. In the case of inadvertent or accidental administration of an overdose, preclinical data suggest that consideration should be given to the administration of folinic acid. From clinical experience with other antifolates folinic acid may be given at a dose of 25mg/m^2 i.v. every 6 hours. As the time interval between 'Tomudex' administration and folinic acid rescue increases, its effectiveness in counteracting toxicity may diminish.

The expected manifestations of overdose are likely to be an exaggerated form of the adverse drug reactions anticipated with the administration of the drug. Patients should, therefore, be carefully monitored for signs of gastrointestinal and haematological toxicity. Symptomatic treatment and standard supportive care measures for the management of this toxicity should be applied.

5. PHARMACOLOGICAL PROPERTIES

5.1 Pharmacodynamic properties

Raltitrexed is a folate analogue belonging to the family of anti-metabolites and has potent inhibitory activity against the enzyme thymidylate synthase (TS). Compared to other antimetabolites such as 5-Fluorouracil or methotrexate, raltitrexed acts as a direct and specific TS inhibitor. TS is a key enzyme in the de novo synthesis of thymidine triphosphate (TTP), a nucleotide required exclusively for deoxyribonucleic acid (DNA) synthesis. Inhibition of TS leads to DNA fragmentation and cell death. Raltitrexed is transported into cells via a reduced folate carrier (RFC) and is then extensively polyglutamated by the enzyme folyl polyglutamate synthetase (FPGS) to polyglutamate forms that are retained in cells and are even more potent inhibitors of TS. Raltitrexed polyglutamation enhances TS inhibitory potency and increases the duration of TS inhibition in cells which may improve antitumour activity. Polyglutamation could also contribute to increased toxicity due to drug retention in normal tissues.

In clinical trials, 'Tomudex' at the dose of 3mg/m^2 i.v. every 3 weeks has demonstrated clinical antitumour activity with an acceptable toxicity profile in patients with advanced colorectal cancer.

Four large clinical trials have been conducted with 'Tomudex' in advanced colorectal cancer. Of the three comparative trials, two showed no statistical difference between 'Tomudex' and the combination of 5-fluorouracil plus folinic acid for survival while one trial showed a statistically significant difference in favour of the combination of 5-fluorouracil plus folinic acid. 'Tomudex' as a single agent was as effective as the combination of 5-fluorouracil and folinic acid in terms of objective response rate in all trials.

5.2 Pharmacokinetic properties

Following intravenous administration at 3.0 mg/m^2, the concentration-time profile in patients was triphasic: Peak concentrations, found at the end of the infusion, were followed by a rapid initial decline in concentration. This was followed by a slow elimination phase. The key pharmacokinetic parameters are presented below:

Table 1 Summary of mean pharmacokinetic parameters in patients administered 3.0 mg/m² Raltitrexed by intravenous infusion

C_{max} (ng/ml)	$AUC_{0-\infty}$ (ng.h/ml)	CL (ml/min)	CL_r (ml/min)	V_{ss} (l)	$t_{1/2}\beta$ (h)	$t_{1/2}\gamma$ (h)
656	1856	51.6	25.1	548	1.79	198

Key: **C_{max}**: Peak plasma concentration. **AUC**: Area under plasma concentration- time curve.
CL: Clearance. **CLr**: Renal clearance
Vss: Volume of distribution at steady state. **$t_{1/2}\beta$**: Half life of the second (β) phase.
$t_{1/2}\gamma$: Terminal half life.

Summary of mean pharmacokinetic parameters in patients administered 3.0 mg/m² Raltitrexed by intravenous infusion

(see Table 1 above)

The maximum concentrations of raltitrexed increased linearly with dose over the clinical dose range tested.

During repeated administration at three week intervals, there was no clinically significant plasma accumulation of raltitrexed in patients with normal renal function.

Apart from the expected intracellular polyglutamation, raltitrexed was not metabolised and was excreted unchanged, mainly in the urine, 40 - 50%. Raltitrexed was also excreted in the faeces with approximately 15% of the radioactive dose being eliminated over a 10 day period. In the [14C] - raltitrexed trial approximately half of the radiolabel was not recovered during the study period. This suggests that a proportion of the raltitrexed dose is retained within tissues, perhaps as raltitrexed polyglutamates, beyond the end of the measurement period (29 days). Trace levels of radiolabel were detected in red blood cells on Day 29.

Raltitrexed pharmacokinetics are independent of age and gender. Pharmacokinetics have not been evaluated in children.

Mild to moderate hepatic impairment led to a small reduction in plasma clearance of less than 25%.

Mild to moderate renal impairment (creatinine clearance of 25 to 65 ml/min) led to a significant reduction (approximately 50%) in raltitrexed plasma clearance.

5.3 Preclinical safety data

Perivascular tolerance in studies in animals did not reveal any significant irritant reaction.

Acute toxicity

The approximate LD_{50} values for the mouse and rat are 875-1249 mg/kg and >500 mg/kg respectively. In the mouse, levels of 750 mg/kg and above caused death by general intoxication.

Chronic toxicity

In one month continuous and six month intermittent dosing studies in the rat, toxicity was related entirely to the cytotoxic nature of the drug. Principal target organs were the gastrointestinal tract, bone marrow and the testes. In similar studies in the dog, cumulative dose levels similar to that used clinically, elicited only pharmacologically-related changes to proliferating tissue. Target organs in the dog were therefore similar to the rat.

Mutagenicity

'Tomudex' was not mutagenic in the Ames test or in supplementary tests using E. coli or chinese hamster ovary cells. 'Tomudex' caused increased levels of chromosome damage in an in vitro assay of human lymphocytes. This effect was ameliorated by the addition of thymidine, thus confirming it to be due to the anti-metabolic nature of the drug. An in vivo micronucleus study in the rat indicated that at cytotoxic dose levels, 'Tomudex' is capable of causing chromosome damage in the bone marrow.

Reproductive toxicology

Fertility studies in the rat indicate that 'Tomudex' can cause impairment of male fertility. Fertility returned to normal three months after dosing ceased. 'Tomudex' caused embryolethality and foetal abnormalities in pregnant rats.

Carcinogenicity

The carcinogenic potential of 'Tomudex' has not been evaluated.

6. PHARMACEUTICAL PARTICULARS

6.1 List of excipients

Mannitol Ph Eur, USP

Dibasic sodium phosphate heptahydrate USP

Sodium hydroxide Ph Eur, USNF

6.2 Incompatibilities

There is no information on incompatibilities at present and therefore 'Tomudex' should not be mixed with any other drug.

6.3 Shelf life

The expiry life of 'Tomudex' is 36 months when stored below 25°C, protected from light.

Once reconstituted, 'Tomudex' is chemically stable for 24 hours at 25°C exposed to ambient light. For storage recommendation, see Instructions for Use/Handling.

6.4 Special precautions for storage

Unopened vial - Do not store above 25°C. Keep container in the outer carton.

Reconstituted vial - Refrigerate at 2-8°C.

6.5 Nature and contents of container

'Tomudex' is packed in 5ml clear neutral type I glass vials, with a bromobutyl rubber closure and an aluminium crimp seal with a plastic flip-off cover.

The vials are packed in individual cartons to protect the product from light.

6.6 Instructions for use and handling

Each vial, containing 2mg of raltitrexed, should be reconstituted with 4ml of sterile water for injections to produce a 0.5 mg/ml solution.

The appropriate dose of solution is diluted in 50 - 250 ml of either 0.9% sodium chloride or 5% glucose (dextrose) injection and administered by a short intravenous infusion over a period of 15 minutes.

There is no preservative or bacteriostatic agent present in 'Tomudex' or the materials specified for reconstitution or dilution. 'Tomudex' must therefore be reconstituted and diluted under aseptic conditions and it is recommended that solutions of 'Tomudex' should be used as soon as possible. Reconstituted 'Tomudex' solution may be stored refrigerated (2 - 8°C) for up to 24 hours.

In accordance with established guidelines, when diluted in 0.9% sodium chloride or 5% glucose (dextrose) solution, it is recommended that administration of the admixed solution should commence as soon as possible after admixing. The admixed solution must be completely used or discarded within 24 hours of reconstitution of 'Tomudex' intravenous injection.

Reconstituted and diluted solutions do not need to be protected from light.

Do not store partially used vials or admixed solutions for future patient use.

Any unused injection or reconstituted solution should be discarded in a suitable manner for cytotoxics.

'Tomudex' should be reconstituted for injection by trained personnel in a designated area for the reconstitution of cytotoxic agents. Cytotoxic preparations such as 'Tomudex' should not be handled by pregnant women.

Reconstitution should normally be carried out in a partial containment facility with extraction e.g. a laminar air flow cabinet, and work surfaces should be covered with disposable plastic-backed absorbent paper.

Appropriate protective clothing, including normal surgical disposable gloves and goggles, should be worn. In case of contact with skin, immediately wash thoroughly with water. For splashes in the eyes irrigate with clean water, holding the eyelids apart, for at least 10 minutes. Seek medical attention.

Any spillages should be cleared up using standard procedures.

Waste material should be disposed of by incineration in a manner consistent with the handling of cytotoxic agents.

7. MARKETING AUTHORISATION HOLDER

AstraZeneca UK Limited,

600 Capability Green,

Luton, LU1 3LU, UK.

8. MARKETING AUTHORISATION NUMBER(S)

PL 17901/0056

9. DATE OF FIRST AUTHORISATION/RENEWAL OF THE AUTHORISATION

25th June 2000

10. DATE OF REVISION OF THE TEXT

25th October 2001

Topal

(Pierre Fabre Limited)

1. NAME OF THE MEDICINAL PRODUCT

TOPAL, chewable tablets.

2. QUALITATIVE AND QUANTITATIVE COMPOSITION

Dried aluminium hydroxide gel 30 mg

Magnesium carbonate (light) 40 mg

Alginic acid 200 mg

3. PHARMACEUTICAL FORM

Chewable tablets.

4. CLINICAL PARTICULARS

4.1 Therapeutic indications

Relief of discomfort due to gastric reflux or mucosal irritation in conditions such as:

- Heartburn
- Reflux oesophagitis
- Hiatus hernia
- Gastritis
- Acid dyspepsia.

4.2 Posology and method of administration

Oral route.

Adults including the elderly: 1 to 3 tablets 4 times a day.

Children: half the adult dose.

4.3 Contraindications

No specific contraindications.

4.4 Special warnings and special precautions for use

- Care should be observed if used by diabetics because of the sugar content: sucrose 880 mg, lactose 220 mg.
- Each tablet contains 40 mg sodium bicarbonate.
- TOPAL is not recommended in patients who are severely debilitated or on low phosphorus diets and in patients with severe renal insufficiency alkalosis or hypermagnesaemia.

4.5 Interaction with other medicinal products and other forms of Interaction

Antiacids may interfere with the absorption of some drugs especially tetracyclines.

4.6 Pregnancy and lactation

There are no adequate data from the use of TOPAL tablets in pregnant women. Animal studies are insufficient with respect to effects on pregnancy, embryonal and foetal development, parturition and post-natal development (see section 5.3).

The potential risk for humans is unknown. TOPAL tablets should not be used during pregnancy unless clearly necessary.

4.7 Effects on ability to drive and use machines

None stated

4.8 Undesirable effects

TOPAL is well tolerated and any side effects which occur are likely to be mild and transient.

4.9 Overdose

Treatment should be symptomatic.

5. PHARMACOLOGICAL PROPERTIES

5.1 Pharmacodynamic properties

Formation of a supernatant gel on the surface of the gastric fluid (lighter than water). This coats the cardio-tuberosity zone (shown by fiberoptic endoscopy) and rises up into the oesophagus if reflux occurs.

Able to coat the mucosa.

5.2 Pharmacokinetic properties

Rapid (within 6 to 14 minutes) and persistent (lasting 2 to 4 hours) action confirmed by a double-blind, crossover placebo-controlled study.

5.3 Preclinical safety data

6. PHARMACEUTICAL PARTICULARS

6.1 List of excipients

Sucrose, lactose monohydrate, silica gel, povidone, citric acid monohydrate, sodium hydrogen carbonate, caramel flavour, vanillin, strawberry flavour and magnesium stearate.

6.2 Incompatibilities

None stated.

6.3 Shelf life

3 years.

6.4 Special precautions for storage

Do not store above 30°C unopened and protect from moisture.

6.5 Nature and contents of container

Aluminium PVC/ blisters cards strips containing 14 tablets in a carton of 42 (3 strips of 14).

6.6 Instructions for use and handling

No special instructions.

7. MARKETING AUTHORISATION HOLDER

Pierre Fabre Limited

Hyde Abbey house

23 Hyde street

Winchester

Hampshire

SO23 7DR

United Kingdom

8. MARKETING AUTHORISATION NUMBER(S)

PL 0603/0021

9. DATE OF FIRST AUTHORISATION/RENEWAL OF THE AUTHORISATION

2 August 1979 / 15 March 1995

10. DATE OF REVISION OF THE TEXT

October 2003.

Topamax 25 mg, 50mg, 100mg, 200mg Tablets and Sprinkle Capsules 15, 25 or 50 mg.

(Janssen-Cilag Ltd)

1. NAME OF THE MEDICINAL PRODUCT

TOPAMAX® 25 mg Tablets

TOPAMAX® 50 mg Tablets

TOPAMAX® 100 mg Tablets

TOPAMAX® 200 mg Tablets

TOPAMAX® Sprinkle Capsules 15, 25 or 50 mg.

2. QUALITATIVE AND QUANTITATIVE COMPOSITION

Each tablet contains 25, 50, 100 and 200 mg of topiramate.

Topamax Sprinkle Capsules contain topiramate 15, 25 or 50 mg.

For excipients see Section 6.1.

3. PHARMACEUTICAL FORM

Topamax Tablets are available as engraved, round, film-coated tablets in the following strengths and colours: 25 mg - white, 50 mg – light - yellow, 100 mg - yellow, 200 mg - salmon. The tablets are engraved as follows:

25 mg "TOP" on one side; "25" on the other

50 mg "TOP" on one side; "50" on the other

100 mg "TOP" on one side; "100" on the other

200 mg "TOP" on one side; "200" on the other

Topamax Sprinkle Capsules are available as hard gelatin capsules containing topiramate in coated beads.

4. CLINICAL PARTICULARS

4.1 Therapeutic indications

Epilepsy

Topamax is indicated as monotherapy in adults and children aged 6 years and above with newly diagnosed epilepsy who have generalised tonic-clonic seizures or partial seizures with or without secondarily generalised seizures.

Topamax is indicated as adjunctive therapy for adults and children over 2 years of age who are inadequately controlled on conventional first line antiepileptic drugs for: partial seizures with or without secondarily generalised seizures; seizures associated with Lennox Gastaut Syndrome and primary generalised tonic-clonic seizures.

The efficacy and safety of conversion from adjunctive therapy to Topamax monotherapy has not been demonstrated.

Migraine

Topamax is indicated in adults for the prophylaxis of migraine headache. Initiation of treatment with topiramate should be restricted to specialist care and treatment should be managed under specialist supervision or shared care arrangements.

Prophylactic treatment of migraine may be considered in situations such as: Adults experiencing three or more migraine attacks per month; frequent migraine attacks that significantly interfere with the patient's daily routine.

Continuing therapy should be reviewed every six months.

The usefulness of Topamax in the acute treatment of migraine has not been studied.

4.2 Posology and method of administration

4.2.1 General

For optimal seizure control in both adults and children, it is recommended that therapy be initiated at a low dose followed by titration to an effective dose.

Tablets should not be broken. Topamax can be taken without regard to meals.

Topamax Sprinkle Capsules may be swallowed whole or may be administered by carefully opening the capsule and sprinkling the entire contents on a small amount (teaspoon) of soft food e.g. apple sauce, mashed banana, ice cream or yoghurts. This drug/food mixture should be swallowed immediately and not chewed. It should not be stored for future use.

It is not necessary to monitor topiramate plasma concentrations to optimise Topamax therapy.

The dosing recommendations apply to children and to all adults, including the elderly, in the absence of underlying renal disease. (See 4.4 Special warnings and special precautions for use.)

Since Topamax is removed from plasma by haemodialysis, a supplemental dose of Topamax equal to approximately one-half the daily dose should be administered on haemodialysis days. The supplemental dose should be administered in divided doses at the beginning and completion of the haemodialysis procedure. The supplemental dose may differ based on the characteristics of the dialysis equipment being used.

4.2.2 Epilepsy

a) Monotherapy

Adults and children over 16 years

Titration should begin at 25 mg nightly for 1 week. The dosage should then be increased at 1- or 2-week intervals by increments of 25 or 50 mg/day, administered in two divided doses. If the patient is unable to tolerate the titration regimen, smaller increments or longer intervals between increments can be used. Dose and titration rate should be guided by clinical outcome.

The recommended initial target dose for topiramate monotherapy in adults with newly diagnosed epilepsy is 100 mg/day and the maximum recommended daily dose is 400 mg. These dosing recommendations apply to all adults including the elderly in the absence of underlying renal disease.

Children aged 6-16 years

Treatment of children aged 6 years and above should begin at 0.5 to 1 mg/kg nightly for the first week. The dosage should then be increased at 1- or 2-week intervals by increments of 0.5 to 1 mg/kg/day, administered in two divided doses. If the child is unable to tolerate the titration regimen, smaller increments or longer intervals between dose increments can be used. Dose and dose titration rate should be guided by clinical outcome.

The recommended initial target dose range for topiramate monotherapy in children with newly diagnosed epilepsy aged 6 years and above is 3 to 6 mg/kg/day. Higher doses have been tolerated and rarely doses up to 16 mg/kg/day have been given.

The tablet formulations are not appropriate for children requiring doses of less than 25 mg/day. A suitable formulation (eg Topamax Sprinkle Capsules) should be prescribed.

b) Adjunctive Therapy

Adults and children over 16 years

The minimal effective dose as adjunctive therapy is 200 mg per day. The usual total daily dose is 200 mg to 400 mg in two divided doses. Some patients may require doses up to 800 mg per day, which is the maximum recommended dose. It is recommended that therapy be initiated at a low dose, followed by titration to an effective dose.

Titration should begin at 25 mg daily for one week. The total daily dose should then be increased by 25-50 mg increments at one to two weekly intervals and should be taken in two divided doses. If the patient is unable to tolerate the titration regimen then lower increments or longer intervals between increments may be used. Dose titration should be guided by clinical outcome.

Children aged 2 - 16 years

The recommended total daily dose of Topamax (topiramate) as adjunctive therapy is approximately 5 to 9 mg/kg/day in two divided doses. Titration should begin at 25 mg nightly for the first week. The dosage should then be increased at 1- or 2-week intervals by increments of 1 to 3 mg/kg/day (administered in two divided doses), to achieve optimal clinical response. Dose titration should be guided by clinical outcome.

Daily doses up to 30 mg/kg/day have been studied and were generally well tolerated.

4.2.3 Migraine

Adults and children over 16 years

Titration should begin at 25 mg nightly for 1 week. The dosage should then be increased in increments of 25 mg/day administered at 1-week intervals. If the patient is unable to tolerate the titration regimen, longer intervals between dose adjustments can be used.

The recommended total daily dose of topiramate as treatment for the prophylaxis of migraine headache is 100 mg/day administered in two divided doses. Some patients may experience a benefit at a total daily dose of 50 mg/day. No extra benefit has been demonstrated from the administration of doses higher than 100 mg/day. Dose and titration rate should be guided by clinical outcome.

Children

Topamax in migraine prophylaxis has not been studied in children under 16 years.

4.3 Contraindications

Hypersensitivity to any component of this product.

4.4 Special warnings and special precautions for use

4.4.1 General

Antiepileptic drugs, including Topamax, should be withdrawn gradually to minimise the potential of increased seizure frequency. In clinical trials, dosages were decreased by 100 mg/day at weekly intervals. In some patients, withdrawal was accelerated without complications.

The major route of elimination of unchanged topiramate and its metabolites is via the kidney. Renal elimination is dependent on renal function and is independent of age. Patients with moderate or severe renal impairment may take 10 to 15 days to reach steady-state plasma concentrations as compared to 4 to 8 days in patients with normal renal function.

As with all patients, the titration schedule should be guided by clinical outcome (e.g. seizure control, avoidance of side effects, prophylaxis of migraine headache) with the knowledge that subjects with known renal impairment may require a longer time to reach steady state at each dose.

Some patients, especially those with a predisposition to nephrolithiasis, may be at increased risk for renal stone formation and associated signs and symptoms such as renal colic, renal pain or flank pain. Adequate hydration whilst using topiramate is very important as it can reduce the risk of developing renal stones. In addition, it may reduce the risk of heat-related adverse events during exercise and exposure to particularly warm environments (see section 4.8).

Risk factors for nephrolithiasis include prior stone formation, a family history of nephrolithiasis and hypercalciuria. None of these risk factors can reliably predict stone formation during topiramate treatment. In addition, patients taking other medication associated with nephrolithiasis may be at increased risk.

In hepatically impaired patients, topiramate should be administered with caution as the clearance of topiramate may be decreased.

Depression and mood alterations have been reported in patients treated with topiramate. In double blind clinical trials, suicide related events (SREs) (suicidal ideation, suicide attempts and suicide) occurred at a frequency of 0.5% in topiramate treated patients (43 out of 7,999 patients treated) and at a 3 fold higher incidence than in those treated with placebo (0.15%; 5 out of 3,150 patients treated).

Patients should be monitored for signs of depression and referred for appropriate treatment if necessary. Patients (and caregivers of patients) should be advised to seek medical advice immediately should suicidal thoughts emerge.

In accordance with good clinical practice, patients with a history of depression and/or suicidal behaviour, adolescents and young adults may be at a greater risk of suicidal thoughts or suicide attempts, and should receive careful monitoring during treatment.

Acute myopia with secondary angle-closure glaucoma has been reported rarely in both children and adults receiving Topamax. Symptoms typically occur within 1 month of the start of treatment and include decreased visual acuity and/or ocular pain. Ophthalmological findings include bilateral myopia, anterior chamber shallowing, hyperaemia and increased intra-ocular pressure with or without mydriasis. There may be supraciliary effusion resulting in anterior displacement of the lens and iris. Treatment includes discontinuation of Topamax as rapidly as is clinically feasible and appropriate measures to reduce intraocular pressure. These measures generally result in a decrease in intraocular pressure. If increased intraocular pressure is suspected, immediate specialist advice should be sought.

Metabolic Acidosis: Hyperchloraemic, non-anion gap, metabolic acidosis (ie decreased serum bicarbonate below the normal reference range in the absence of respiratory alkalosis) is associated with topiramate treatment. This decrease in serum bicarbonate is due to the inhibitory effect of topiramate on renal carbonic anhydrase. Generally, the decrease in bicarbonate occurs early in treatment although it can occur at any time during treatment. These decreases are usually mild to moderate (average decrease of 4 mmol/L at doses of 100 mg/day or above in adults and at approximately 6 mg/kg/day in paediatric patients). Rarely, patients have experienced decreases to values below 10 mmol/L. Conditions or therapies that predispose to acidosis (such as renal disease, severe respiratory disorders, status epilepticus, diarrhoea, surgery, ketogenic diet, or certain drugs) may be additive to the bicarbonate lowering effects of topiramate.

Chronic metabolic acidosis in paediatric patients can reduce growth rates. The effect of topiramate on growth and bone-related sequelae has not been systematically investigated in paediatric or adult populations.

Depending on underlying conditions, appropriate evaluation including serum bicarbonate levels is recommended with topiramate therapy. If metabolic acidosis develops and persists, consideration should be given to reducing the dose or discontinuing topiramate (using dose tapering).

A dietary supplement or increased food intake may be considered if the patient is losing weight or has inadequate weight gain while on this medication.

Patients with rare hereditary problems of galactose intolerance, the Lapp lactase deficiency or glucose-galactose malabsorption should not take this medicine.

4.4.2 Migraine Prophylaxis

In migraine prophylaxis, before discontinuation of treatment, dosage should be gradually reduced over at least 2 weeks to minimise the possibility of rebound migraine headaches.

Weight loss

During the double-blind treatment with topiramate 100 mg/day, the mean change from baseline to the final visit in body weight was -2.5 kg, compared to -0.1 kg in the placebo group. Overall, 68% of patients treated with topiramate 100 mg/day lost weight during the trials, compared to 33% of patients receiving placebo. Weight decrease was reported as an adverse event in 1% of all placebo-treated patients and in 9% of all patients receiving topiramate 100 mg/day.

Significant weight loss may occur during long-term topiramate treatment for migraine prophylaxis. In clinical studies of topiramate 100 mg in migraine prophylaxis, a continuing weight decrease was observed with a mean weight decrease of 5.5 kg over 20 months. Twenty-five per cent of patients treated with topiramate for migraine prophylaxis had a weight loss of ⩾ 10% of their body weight.

It is recommended that patients on long term topiramate for migraine prophylaxis should be regularly weighed and monitored for continuing weight loss.

4.5 Interaction with other medicinal products and other forms of Interaction

For purposes of this section, a no effect dose is defined as a ⩽ 15% change.

Effects of Topamax on Other Antiepileptic Drugs

The addition of Topamax to other antiepileptic drugs (phenytoin, carbamazepine, valproic acid, phenobarbital, primidone) has no clinically significant effect on their steady-state plasma concentrations, except in some patients where the addition of Topamax to phenytoin may result in an increase of plasma concentrations of phenytoin. Consequently, it is advised that any patient on phenytoin should have phenytoin levels monitored.

A pharmacokinetic interaction study of patients with epilepsy indicated the addition of topiramate to lamotrigine had no effect on steady state plasma concentration of lamotrigine at topiramate doses of 100 to 400 mg/day. In addition, there was no change in steady state plasma concentration of topiramate during or after removal of lamotrigine treatment (mean dose of 327 mg/day).

Effects of Other Antiepileptic Drugs on Topamax

Phenytoin and carbamazepine decrease the plasma concentration of topiramate. The addition or withdrawal of phenytoin or carbamazepine to Topamax therapy may require an adjustment in dosage of the latter. This should be done by titrating to clinical effect.

The addition or withdrawal of valproic acid does not produce clinically significant changes in plasma concentrations of topiramate and, therefore, does not warrant dosage adjustment of Topamax.

The results of these interactions are summarised in the following table:

(see Table 1 below)

Other Drug Interactions

Digoxin: In a single-dose study, serum digoxin area under plasma concentration curve (AUC) decreased 12% due to concomitant administration of Topamax. The clinical relevance of this observation has not been established. When Topamax is added or withdrawn in patients on digoxin therapy, careful attention should be given to the routine monitoring of serum digoxin.

CNS Depressants: Concomitant administration of Topamax and alcohol or other CNS depressant drugs has not been evaluated in clinical studies. Because of the potential of topiramate to cause CNS depression, as well as other cognitive and/or neuropsychiatric adverse events, topiramate should be used with caution if used in combination with alcohol and other CNS depressants.

Oral Contraceptives: In an interaction study with a combined oral contraceptive, Topamax increased plasma clearance of the oestrogenic component significantly. Consequently, and bearing in mind the potential risk of teratogenicity, patients should receive a preparation containing not less than 50 μg of oestrogen or use some alternative non-hormonal method of contraception. Patients taking oral contraceptives should be asked to report any change in their bleeding patterns.

Hydrochlorothiazide (HCTZ): A drug-drug interaction study conducted in healthy volunteers evaluated the steady-state pharmacokinetics of HCTZ (25 mg q24h) and topiramate (96 mg q12h) when administered alone and concomitantly. The results of this study indicate that topiramate Cmax increased by 27% and AUC increased by 29% when HCTZ was added to topiramate. The clinical significance of this change is unknown. The addition of HCTZ to topiramate therapy may require an adjustment of the topiramate dose. The steady-state pharmacokinetics of HCTZ were not significantly influenced by the concomitant administration of topiramate. Clinical laboratory results indicated decreases in serum potassium after topiramate or HCTZ administration, which were greater when HCTZ and topiramate were administered in combination.

Metformin: A drug-drug interaction study conducted in healthy volunteers evaluated the steady-state pharmacokinetics of metformin 500mg bd and topiramate 100mg bd in plasma when metformin was given alone and when metformin and topiramate were given simultaneously. The results of this study indicated that metformin mean C_{max} and mean AUC_{0-12h} increased by 18% and 25%, respectively, while mean CL/F decreased 20% when metformin was co-administered with topiramate. Topiramate did not affect metformin t_{max}. The clinical significance of the effect of topiramate on metformin pharmacokinetics is unclear. Oral plasma clearance of topiramate appears to be reduced when administered with metformin. The extent of change in the clearance is unknown. The clinical significance of the effect of metformin on topiramate pharmacokinetics is unclear. When Topamax is added or withdrawn in patients on metformin therapy, careful attention should be given to the routine monitoring for adequate control of their diabetic disease state.

Pioglitazone: A drug-drug interaction study conducted in healthy volunteers evaluated the steady-state pharmacokinetics of topiramate and pioglitazone when administered alone and concomitantly. A 15% decrease in the AUCτ,ss of pioglitazone with no alteration in Cmax,ss was observed. This finding was not statistically significant. In addition, a 13% and 16% decrease in Cmax,ss and AUCτ,ss respectively, of the active hydroxy-metabolite was noted as well as a 60% decrease in Cmax,ss and AUCτ,ss of the active keto-metabolite. The clinical significance of these findings is not known. When Topamax is added to pioglitazone therapy or pioglitazone is added to Topamax therapy, careful attention should be given to the routine monitoring of patients for adequate control of their diabetic disease state.

Others: Topamax, when used concomitantly with other agents predisposing to nephrolithiasis, may increase the risk of nephrolithiasis. While using Topamax, agents like these should be avoided since they may create a physiological environment that increases the risk of renal stone formation. The interaction with benzodiazepines has not been studied.

Additional Pharmacokinetic Drug Interaction Studies: Clinical studies have been conducted to assess the potential pharmacokinetic drug interaction between topiramate and other agents. The changes in Cmax or AUC as a result of the interactions are summarized below. The second column (concomitant drug concentration) describes what happens to the concentration of the concomitant drug listed in the first column when topiramate is added. The third column (topiramate concentration) describes how the coadministration of a drug listed in the first column modifies the concentration of topiramate.

Summary of Results from Additional Clinical Pharmacokinetic Drug Interaction Studies

Concomitant Drug	Concomitant Drug Concentration[a]	Topiramate Concentration[a]
Amitriptyline	↔ 20% increase in C_{max} and AUC of nortriptyline metabolite	NS
Dihydroergotamine (Oral and Subcutaneous)	↔	↔
Haloperidol	↔ 31% increase in AUC of the reduced metabolite	NS
Propranolol	↔ 17% increase in C_{max} for 4-OH propranolol (TPM 50 mg q12h)	16% increase in C_{max}, 17% increase in AUC (80 mg propranolol q12h)
Sumatriptan (Oral and Subcutaneous)	↔	NS
Pizotifen	↔	↔

[a] % values are the changes in treatment mean C_{max} or AUC with respect to monotherapy

↔ = No effect on C_{max} and AUC (⩽ 15% change) of the parent compound

NS = Not studied

Interaction studies showed that Topamax did not significantly alter the serum levels of amitriptyline, propranolol or dihydroergotamine mesylate. The combination of Topamax with each of these drugs was well tolerated and no dose adjustments were necessary.

Laboratory Tests:

Clinical trial data indicates that topiramate has been associated with an average decrease of 4 mmol/L in the serum bicarbonate level (see Section 4.4 Special warnings and special precautions for use Metabolic Acidosis).

4.6 Pregnancy and lactation

Topiramate was teratogenic in mice, rats and rabbits. In rats, topiramate crosses the placental barrier.

There are no studies using Topamax in pregnant women. However, Topamax should not be used during pregnancy unless, in the opinion of the physician, the potential benefit outweighs the potential risk to the foetus.

Before starting Topamax, women of childbearing potential should be fully informed of the possible effects of Topamax on the unborn foetus and the risks should be discussed with the patient in relation to the benefits of Topamax treatment in migraine prophylaxis.

In post-marketing experience, hypospadias has been reported in male infants exposed in-utero to topiramate, with or without other anticonvulsants; however, a causal relationship with topiramate has not been established.

It is recommended that women of child bearing potential use adequate contraception.

Topiramate is excreted in the milk of lactating rats. The excretion of topiramate in human milk has not been evaluated in controlled studies. Limited observations in patients suggests an extensive excretion of topiramate into breast milk. Topamax should not be used during breast feeding.

4.7 Effects on ability to drive and use machines

As with all antiepileptic drugs, Topamax may produce central nervous system related adverse events. Drowsiness is likely and Topamax may be more sedating than other antiepileptic drugs. These adverse events could potentially be dangerous in patients driving a vehicle or operating machinery, particularly until such time as the individual patient's experience with the drug is established.

4.8 Undesirable effects

4.8.1 Epilepsy

a) Monotherapy

Qualitatively, the types of adverse events observed in monotherapy trials were generally similar to those observed during adjunctive therapy trials (see below). With the exception of paraesthesia and fatigue in adults, these adverse events were reported at similar or lower incidence rates in monotherapy trials.

Adults:

In double-blind monotherapy clinical trials, the most common adverse events, i.e., those occurring in 10% or more of the topiramate-treated adult patients were paraesthesia, headache, fatigue, dizziness, somnolence, weight decrease, nausea and anorexia.

Adverse events occurring at 5% or more but less than 10% included: insomnia, difficulty with memory, depression, difficulty with concentration/attention, abdominal pain, nervousness, hypoaesthesia, mood problems and anxiety.

Children:

In double-blind monotherapy clinical trials, the most common adverse events, i.e., those occurring in 10% or more of the topiramate-treated children were headache, anorexia and somnolence.

Adverse events occurring at 5% or more but less than 10% included: difficulty with concentration/attention, fatigue, weight decrease, dizziness, paraesthesia, insomnia and nervousness.

b) Adjunctive Therapy

Adults:

Since Topamax has most frequently been co-administered with other antiepileptic agents, it is not possible to determine which agents, if any, are associated with adverse effects. In double blind clinical trials, some of which included a rapid titration period, adverse events which occurred with a frequency greater than or equal to 5% and with a higher incidence in the topiramate-treated adult patients than in placebo included: abdominal pain, ataxia, anorexia, asthenia, confusion, difficulty with concentration/attention, difficulty with memory, diplopia, dizziness, fatigue, language problems, nausea, nystagmus, paraesthesia, psychomotor slowing, somnolence, speech disorders/related speech problems, abnormal vision and weight decrease. Topamax may cause agitation and emotional lability (which may manifest mood problems and nervousness) and depression. Other less common adverse effects include, gait abnormal, aggressive reaction, apathy, cognitive problems, co-ordination problems, leucopenia, psychotic symptoms (such as hallucinations) and taste perversion.

Isolated cases of venous thromboembolic events have been reported. A causal association with the drug has not been established.

Reports of increases in liver enzymes in patients taking Topamax with and without other medications have been received. Isolated reports have been received of hepatitis and hepatic failure occurring in patients taking multiple medications while being treated with Topamax.

Table 1

AED Coadministered	AED Concentration	Topiramate Concentration
Phenytoin	↔**	↓
Carbamazepine (CBZ)	↔	↓
Valproic Acid	↔	↔
Lamotrigine	↔	↔
Phenobarbital	↔	NS
Primidone	↔	NS

↔ = No effect on plasma concentration (⩽ 15% change)

** = Plasma concentrations increase in some patients

↓ = Plasma concentrations decrease

NS = Not studied

AED = antiepileptic drug

Children

In double blind clinical trials, some of which included a rapid titration period, adverse events which occurred with a frequency greater than or equal to 5% and with a higher incidence in the topiramate-treated children than in placebo included: somnolence, anorexia, fatigue, insomnia, nervousness, personality disorder (behaviour problems), difficulty with concentration/attention, aggressive reaction, weight decrease, gait abnormal, mood problems, ataxia, saliva increased, nausea, difficulty with memory, hyperkinesia, dizziness, speech disorders/related speech problems and paraesthesia.

Adverse events that occurred less frequently but were considered potentially medically relevant included: emotional lability, agitation, apathy, cognitive problems, psychomotor slowing, confusion, hallucination, depression and leucopenia.

4.8.2 Migraine prophylaxis

In double-blind clinical trials, clinically relevant adverse events which occurred at a frequency of 5% or more and seen at a higher incidence in topiramate-treated patients than placebo-treated patients included: fatigue, paraesthesia, dizziness, hypoaesthesia, language problems, nausea, diarrhoea, dyspepsia, dry mouth, weight decrease, anorexia, somnolence, difficulty with memory, difficulty with concentration/attention, insomnia, anxiety, mood problems, depression, taste perversion, abnormal vision. Fifty per cent of patients in these trials experienced paraesthesia.

During 6-month double-blind treatment with topiramate 100 mg/day for migraine prophylaxis, weight decrease was reported as an adverse event in 1% of all placebo-treated patients and in 9% of all patients receiving topiramate 100 mg/day. Weight loss continued with long-term topiramate treatment (see Section 4.4 Special warnings and special precautions for use).

Children

The effect of Topamax in children less than 16 years old with migraine has not been studied.

4.8.3 General

Topamax increases the risk of nephrolithiasis especially in those with a predisposition (see 4.4 Special warnings and special precautions for use). In the initial clinical trials none of the calculi required open surgery and three-quarters were passed spontaneously. Most of the patients opted to continue treatment despite nephrolithiasis.

Reduced sweating has been rarely reported. The majority of cases have been in children and some have been associated with flushing and raised temperature.

Acute myopia associated with secondary acute angle closure glaucoma has been reported rarely. (See section 4.4)

Metabolic acidosis has been reported rarely (see Section 4.4 Special warnings and special precautions for use).

Suicidal ideation or attempts have been reported uncommonly (see Section 4.4. special warnings and special precautions for use).

Very rarely, reports have been received for bullous skin and mucosal reactions (including erythema multiforme, pemphigus, Stevens-Johnson syndrome and toxic epidermal necrolysis). The majority of these reports have occurred in patients taking other medications also associated with bullous skin and mucosal reactions.

4.9 Overdose

Signs and Symptoms

Overdoses of topiramate have been reported. Signs and symptoms included convulsions, drowsiness, speech disturbances, blurred vision, diplopia, mentation impaired, lethargy, abnormal co-ordination, stupor, hypotension, abdominal pain, agitation, dizziness and depression. The clinical consequences were not severe in most cases, but deaths have been reported after polydrug overdoses involving topiramate.

Topiramate overdose can result in severe metabolic acidosis.

A patient who ingested a dose calculated to be between 96 and 110 g topiramate was admitted to hospital with coma lasting 20-24 hours followed by full recovery after 3 to 4 days.

Treatment

In acute topiramate overdose, if the ingestion is recent, the stomach should be emptied immediately by lavage or by induction of emesis. Activated charcoal has been shown to adsorb topiramate *in vitro*. Treatment should be appropriately supportive. Haemodialysis has been shown to be an effective means of removing topiramate from the body. The patient should be well hydrated.

5. PHARMACOLOGICAL PROPERTIES

5.1 Pharmacodynamic properties

Topiramate is classified as a sulphamate-substituted monosaccharide. Three pharmacological properties of topiramate have been identified that may contribute to its anticonvulsant activity:

Topiramate reduces the frequency at which action potentials are generated when neurones are subjected to a sustained depolarisation indicative of a state-dependent blockade of voltage-sensitive sodium channels.

Topiramate markedly enhances the activity of GABA at some types of GABA receptors but has no apparent effect on the activity of N-methyl-D-aspartate (NMDA) at the NMDA receptor subtype.

Topiramate weakly antagonises the excitatory activity of kainate/AMPA subtype of glutamate receptor.

In addition, topiramate inhibits some isoenzymes of carbonic anhydrase. This pharmacologic effect is much weaker than that of acetazolamide, a known carbonic anhydrase inhibitor, and is not thought to be a major component of topiramate's antiepileptic activity.

5.2 Pharmacokinetic properties

Topiramate is rapidly and well absorbed. Based on recovery of radioactivity from the urine, the mean extent of absorption of a 100 mg dose of ^{14}C topiramate was at least 81%. There is no clinically significant effect of food on topiramate. Generally 13-17% of topiramate is bound to plasma proteins. The mean apparent volume of distribution has been measured as 0.55-0.8 L/kg for single doses up to 1200 mg. There is an effect of gender on the volume of distribution. Values for females are circa 50% of those for males.

Topiramate is not extensively metabolised (≈20%) in healthy volunteers. Topiramate is metabolised up to 50% in patients receiving concomitant antiepileptic therapy with known inducers of drug metabolising enzymes. Six metabolites have been isolated, characterised and identified from plasma, urine and faeces of humans. Two metabolites, which retained most of the structure of topiramate, were tested and found to have little or no anticonvulsant activity.

In humans, the major route of elimination of unchanged topiramate and its metabolites is via the kidney. Overall, plasma clearance is approximately 20 to 30 mL/min in humans following oral administration.

Topiramate exhibits low intersubject variability in plasma concentrations and, therefore, has predictable pharmacokinetics. The pharmacokinetics of topiramate are linear with plasma clearance remaining constant and area under the plasma concentration curve increasing in a dose-proportional manner over a 100 to 400 mg single oral dose range in healthy subjects. Patients with normal renal function may take 4 to 8 days to reach steady-state plasma concentrations. The mean C_{max} following multiple, twice a day oral doses of 100 mg to healthy subjects was 6.76 μg/mL. Following administration of multiple doses of 50 mg and 100 mg of topiramate twice a day, the mean plasma elimination half-life was approximately 21 hours.

The plasma and renal clearance of topiramate are decreased in patients with impaired renal function (CLCR $\leqslant$ 60 mL/min), and the plasma clearance is decreased in patients with end-stage renal disease.

Plasma clearance of topiramate is unchanged in elderly subjects in the absence of underlying renal disease.

Plasma clearance of topiramate is decreased in patients with moderate to severe hepatic impairment.

The pharmacokinetics of topiramate in children, as in adults receiving add-on therapy, are linear, with clearance independent of dose and steady-state plasma concentrations increasing in proportion to dose. Children, however, have a higher clearance and shorter elimination half-life. Consequently, the plasma concentrations of topiramate for the same mg/kg dose may be lower in children compared to adults. As in adults, hepatic enzyme inducing anti-epileptic drugs decrease the steady-state plasma concentrations.

5.3 Preclinical safety data

Preclinical data reveal no special hazard for humans based on conventional studies of repeated dose toxicity and genotoxicity.

As with other antiepileptic drugs, topiramate was teratogenic in mice, rats and rabbits. Overall numbers of foetal malformations in mice were increased for all drug-treated groups, but no significant differences or dosage-response relationships were observed for overall or specific malformations, suggesting that other factors such as maternal toxicity may be involved.

6. PHARMACEUTICAL PARTICULARS

6.1 List of excipients

Topamax contains the following inactive ingredients:

Lactose monohydrate

Pregelatinized starch

Carnauba wax

Microcrystalline cellulose

Sodium starch glycolate

Magnesium stearate

OPADRY White, Yellow, Pink, Red (depending on the colour, contains hydroxypropyl methylcellulose, titanium dioxide (E171), polyethylene glycol, synthetic iron oxide and polysorbate 80).

Topamax Sprinkle Capsules contain the following inactive ingredients:

Sugar spheres

Povidone

Cellulose Acetate

Capsule Composition

Gelatin

Titanium dioxide (E171)

Silicon dioxide

Sodium lauryl sulphate

Ink Composition

OPACODE contains synthetic iron oxide, pharmaceutical glaze, n-butyl alcohol, alcohol, hydroxypropyl methyl cellulose, propylene glycol, ammonium hydroxide, simethicone and distilled water.

6.2 Incompatibilities

None known

6.3 Shelf life

Topamax Tablets: 36 months.

Topamax Sprinkle Capsules: 24 months.

6.4 Special precautions for storage

Topamax Tablets: Do not store above 25°C. Keep container tightly closed.

Topamax Sprinkle Capsules: Do not store above 25°C. Keep container tightly closed.

6.5 Nature and contents of container

Topamax Tablets: Available in high density polyethylene (HDPE) bottles with low density polyethylene (LDPE) tamper-evident closures containing 60 tablets. Each bottle contains a desiccant sachet.

Topamax Sprinkle Capsules: Available in opaque HDPE containers with tamper evident closures containing 60 capsules. The closures consist of either an HDPE outer shell and polypropylene inner shell or polypropylene outer shell and LDPE inner shell.

6.6 Instructions for use and handling

Not applicable.

7. MARKETING AUTHORISATION HOLDER

Janssen-Cilag Limited

Saunderton

High Wycombe

Buckinghamshire

HP14 4HJ

UK

8. MARKETING AUTHORISATION NUMBER(S)

Topamax 25 mg Tablets PL 00242/0301

Topamax 50 mg Tablets PL 00242/0302

Topamax 100 mg Tablets PL 00242/0303

Topamax 200 mg Tablets PL 00242/0304

Topamax Sprinkle Capsules 15 mg PL 00242/0348

Topamax Sprinkle Capsules 25 mg PL 00242/0349

Topamax Sprinkle Capsules 50 mg PL 00242/0350

9. DATE OF FIRST AUTHORISATION/RENEWAL OF THE AUTHORISATION

Topamax Tablets: 18 July 1995 / 30 March 2005

Topamax Sprinkle Capsules: 17 February 1999 / 30 March 2005

10. DATE OF REVISION OF THE TEXT

29 July 2005

Legal Category: POM

Topicycline

(Shire Pharmaceuticals Limited)

1. NAME OF THE MEDICINAL PRODUCT

Topicycline Powder and Solvent for Topicycline Powder

2. QUALITATIVE AND QUANTITATIVE COMPOSITION

One bottle of powder containing 154 mg of Tetracycline Hydrochloride.

One bottle containing 70 ml of solvent for use only with Topicycline Powder PL 10536/0025. Once reconstituted, Topicycline contains tetracycline hydrochloride 2.2 mg per ml.

For excipients, see section 6.1.

3. PHARMACEUTICAL FORM

Powder and Solvent for Cutaneous Solution.

Topicycline is presented in two separate bottles as a yellow powder and as a solvent which must be combined prior to topical application.

4. CLINICAL PARTICULARS

4.1 Therapeutic indications

For the treatment of acne vulgaris.

4.2 Posology and method of administration

Topicycline is first prepared by the Pharmacist according to the manufacturer's instructions.

Once reconstituted, Topicycline is applied topically, twice daily. It should be applied generously to the entire affected area, not just to the individual lesions, until the skin is thoroughly wet.

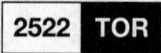

The average amount of Topicycline delivered to the skin by application to the face and neck twice a day is approximately 1.3 ml/day. This quantity of the medication contains approximately 2.9 mg of tetracycline hydrochloride. Twice-daily use of Topicycline on other acne-involved areas, in addition to the face and neck, has resulted in an average application of about 2.2 ml/day, or 4.8 mg of tetracycline hydrochloride.

4.3 Contraindications
In patients who have shown hypersensitivity to any of its ingredients or to any of the other tetracyclines.

4.4 Special warnings and special precautions for use
Cross resistance between tetracyclines in micro-organisms and cross sensitisation in patients may develop.

Prolonged use of an anti-infective agent may result in the development of infection due to micro-organisms resistant to the agent.

Topicycline is for external use only, and care should be taken to keep it out of eyes, nose and other mucosal surfaces. Liver damage from Topicycline is highly unlikely because of the low levels of systemic absorption, however the warnings and precautions associated with the use of oral tetracyclines should be considered before prescribing to patients with renal impairment.

Photosensitisation may occur in patients exposed to sunlight during use of tetracycline. Appropriate precautions should be taken. This is particularly important in fair skinned individuals.

4.5 Interaction with other medicinal products and other forms of Interaction
None.

4.6 Pregnancy and lactation
Reproduction studies in rats and rabbits have revealed no evidence of impaired fertility or harm to the foetus from Topicycline. There are no data on the use of this product in pregnant women. It is not known whether tetracycline or any other component of Topicycline, administered in this topical form, is secreted in human milk. Because many drugs are secreted in human milk, caution should be exercised if Topicycline is administered to nursing mothers.

4.7 Effects on ability to drive and use machines
None.

4.8 Undesirable effects
Some patients may experience stinging or tingling sensations, skin rashes and skin discolouration at the site of application. The stinging or tingling reaction normally occurs for no more than a few minutes, does not occur on every application and often diminishes with continued use.

Topicycline may leave a faint yellow colour on the skin which could result in the staining of clothing and bed linen. This can be avoided by advising the patient to wash lightly the affected area one hour after applying Topicycline.

4.9 Overdose
Not applicable.

5. PHARMACOLOGICAL PROPERTIES

5.1 Pharmacodynamic properties
Topicycline is a topical antibiotic preparation containing the active ingredient tetracycline hydrochloride. It has a broad spectrum of antimicrobial activity against both gram positive and gram negative pathogenic bacteria and it is mainly bacteriostatic.

In this topical preparation, Topicycline delivers tetracycline hydrochloride to the pilosebaceous apparatus and the adjacent tissues. Topicycline reduces the inflammatory acne lesions but its mode of action is not fully understood.

5.2 Pharmacokinetic properties
Very small amounts of tetracycline hydrochloride are absorbed systemically after application of Topicycline to the skin, compared with oral dosing. The serum level of tetracycline resulting from the use of Topicycline is less than 0.1 ug/ml which is less than 7% of the level associated with an oral therapeutic dose of 500 mg/day.

5.3 Preclinical safety data
Not applicable.

6. PHARMACEUTICAL PARTICULARS

6.1 List of excipients
The powder also contains 4-epitetracycline hydrochloride and sodium bisulphite (E222). The solvent contains n-decyl methyl sulphoxide and citric acid (E330) in 70 ml of a 40% ethanol solution.

6.2 Incompatibilities
None.

6.3 Shelf life
Shelf life of unreconstituted product is 24 months.

Shelf life of solvent is 24 months.

Shelf life of reconstituted product is 8 weeks.

6.4 Special precautions for storage
Do not store above 25°C.

6.5 Nature and contents of container
A single carton containing a plastic bottle and cap for the powder with an applicator and overcap supplied for the reconstituted product. The carton also contains a plastic bottle and cap for the solvent. On reconstitution of active powder (PL 10536/0025) and solvent (PL 10536/0026), the pack size is 70 ml.

6.6 Instructions for use and handling
At the time of dispensing the entire contents of the solvent-containing bottle are poured into the bottle containing the powder. The resultant mixture is then shaken well. Any unused material should be discarded.

7. MARKETING AUTHORISATION HOLDER
Monmouth Pharmaceuticals Limited
Hampshire International Business Park
Chineham
Basingstoke
Hampshire
RG24 8EP
United Kingdom

8. MARKETING AUTHORISATION NUMBER(S)

Topicycline Powder	PL 10536/0025
Solvent for Topicycline Powder	PL 10536/0026

9. DATE OF FIRST AUTHORISATION/RENEWAL OF THE AUTHORISATION
23 October 1995

10. DATE OF REVISION OF THE TEXT
June 2004.

Toradol Injection

(Roche Products Limited)

1. NAME OF THE MEDICINAL PRODUCT
Toradol

2. QUALITATIVE AND QUANTITATIVE COMPOSITION
Toradol contains ketorolac trometamol 10mg or 30mg in ampoules of 1ml. It also contains ethanol, sodium chloride and water.

3. PHARMACEUTICAL FORM
Toradol is a clear, slightly yellow solution for intramuscular or bolus intravenous injection.

4. CLINICAL PARTICULARS

4.1 Therapeutic indications
Toradol is indicated for the short-term management of moderate to severe acute post-operative pain.

4.2 Posology and method of administration
Toradol is for administration by intramuscular or bolus intravenous injection. Bolus intravenous doses should be given over no less than 15 seconds. Toradol should not be used for epidural or spinal administration.

The time to onset of analgesic effect following both IV and IM administration is similar and is approximately 30 minutes, with maximum analgesia occurring within one to two hours. The median duration of analgesia is generally four to six hours.

Dosage should be adjusted according to the severity of the pain and the patient response.

The administration of continuous multiple daily doses of ketorolac intramuscularly or intravenously should not exceed two days because adverse events may increase with prolonged usage. There has been limited experience with dosing for longer periods since the vast majority of patients have transferred to oral medication, or no longer require analgesic therapy after this time.

Adults

The recommended initial dose of Toradol is 10mg, followed by 10 to 30mg every four to six hours as required. In the initial post-operative period, Toradol may be given as often as every two hours if needed. The lowest effective dose should be given. A total daily dose of 90mg for non-elderly and 60mg for the elderly, renally-impaired patients and patients less than 50kg should not be exceeded. The maximum duration of treatment should not exceed two days.

Reduce dosage in patients under 50kg.

Opioid analgesics (e.g. morphine, pethidine) may be used concomitantly, and may be required for optimal analgesic effect in the early post-operative period when pain is most severe. Ketorolac does not interfere with opioid binding and does not exacerbate opioid-related respiratory depression or sedation. When used in association with Toradol IM/IV, the daily dose of opioid is usually less than that normally required. However, opioid side-effects should still be considered, especially in day-case surgery.

For patients receiving parenteral Toradol, and who are converted to Toradol oral tablets, the total combined daily dose should not exceed 90mg (60mg for the elderly, renally-impaired patients and patients less than 50kg) and the oral component should not exceed 40mg on the day the change of formulation is made. Patients should be converted to oral treatment as soon as possible.

Elderly

For patients over 65 years, the lower end of the dosage range is recommended; a total daily dose of 60mg should not be exceeded (see section *4.4 Special warnings and special precautions for use*).

Children

Safety and efficacy in children have not been established. Therefore, Toradol is not recommended for use in children under 16 years of age.

Renal impairment

Contra-indicated in moderate to severe renal impairment; reduce dosage in lesser impairment (not exceeding 60mg/day IV or IM) (see section *4.3 Contra-indications*).

4.3 Contraindications
– a history of, or active, peptic ulceration or gastro-intestinal bleeding

– suspected or confirmed cerebrovascular bleeding

– haemorrhagic diatheses, including coagulation disorders

– hypersensitivity to ketorolac trometamol or any of its ingredients, or other NSAIDs and those patients in whom aspirin or other prostaglandin synthesis inhibitors induce allergic reactions (severe anaphylactic-like reactions have been observed in such patients)

– the complete or partial syndrome of nasal polyps, angioedema or bronchospasm

– concurrent treatment with other NSAIDs, oxpentifylline, probenecid or lithium salts

– hypovolaemia from any cause or dehydration

– moderate or severe renal impairment (serum creatinine > 160 micromol/l)

– a history of asthma

– patients who have had operations with a high risk of haemorrhage or incomplete haemostasis

– patients on anti-coagulants including low dose heparin (2500 - 5000 units twelve hourly)

– during pregnancy, labour, delivery or lactation

– children under 16 years of age

– Toradol is contra-indicated as prophylactic analgesia before surgery due to inhibition of platelet aggregation and is contra-indicated intra-operatively because of the increased risk of bleeding

– Toradol is contra-indicated in patients currently receiving aspirin.

4.4 Special warnings and special precautions for use
Physicians should be aware that in some patients pain relief may not occur until upwards of 30 minutes after IV or IM administration.

Use in the elderly: Patients over the age of 65 years may be at a greater risk of experiencing adverse events than younger patients. This age-related risk is common to all NSAIDs. Compared to young adults, the elderly have an increased plasma half-life and reduced plasma clearance of ketorolac. With Toradol IM/IV, a total daily dose greater than 60mg is not recommended. With Toradol tablets, a longer dosing interval is advisable (see section *4.2 Posology and method of administration*).

Effects on fertility: The use of Toradol, as with any drug known to inhibit cyclo-oxygenase/prostaglandin synthesis may impair fertility and is not recommended in women attempting to conceive. In women who have difficulty conceiving or are undergoing investigation for fertility, withdrawal of Toradol should be considered.

Gastro-intestinal effects: Toradol can cause gastro-intestinal irritation, ulcers or bleeding in patients with or without a history of previous symptoms. Elderly and debilitated patients are more prone to develop these reactions. The incidence increases with dose and duration of treatment.

In a non-randomised, in-hospital post-marketing surveillance study, increased rates of clinically serious GI bleeding were seen in patients < 65 years of age who received an average daily dose of > 90mg ketorolac IM as compared to those patients receiving parenteral opioids.

Respiratory effects: Bronchospasm may be precipitated in patients with a history of asthma.

Renal effects: Drugs that inhibit prostaglandin biosynthesis (including non-steroidal anti-inflammatory drugs) have been reported to cause nephrotoxicity, including but not limited to glomerular nephritis, interstitial nephritis, renal papillary necrosis, nephrotic syndrome and acute renal failure. In patients with renal, cardiac or hepatic impairment, caution is required since the use of NSAIDs may result in deterioration of renal function.

As with other drugs that inhibit prostaglandin synthesis, elevations of serum urea, creatinine and potassium have been reported with ketorolac trometamol and may occur after one dose.

Patients with impaired renal function: Since ketorolac trometamol and its metabolites are excreted primarily by the kidney, patients with moderate to severe impairment of renal function (serum creatinine greater than 160 micromol/l) should not receive Toradol. Patients with lesser renal impairment should receive a reduced dose of ketorolac (not exceeding 60mg/day IM or IV) and their renal status should be closely monitored.

Caution should be observed in patients with conditions leading to a reduction in blood volume and/or renal blood flow, where renal prostaglandins have a supportive role in the maintenance of renal perfusion. In these patients, administration of an NSAID may cause a dose-dependent reduction in renal prostaglandin formation and may precipitate overt renal failure. Patients at greatest risk of this reaction are those who are volume depleted because of blood loss or severe dehydration, patients with impaired renal function, heart failure, liver dysfunction, the elderly and those taking diuretics. Discontinuation of NSAID therapy is typically followed by recovery to the pre-treatment state. Inadequate fluid/blood replacement during surgery, leading to hypovolaemia, may lead to renal dysfunction which could be exacerbated when Toradol is administered. Therefore, volume depletion should be corrected and close monitoring of serum urea and creatinine and urine output is recommended until the patient is normovolaemic. In patients on renal dialysis, ketorolac clearance was reduced to approximately half the normal rate and terminal half-life increased approximately three-fold.

Fluid retention and oedema: Fluid retention and oedema have been reported with the use of Toradol and it should therefore be used with caution in patients with cardiac decompensation, hypertension or similar conditions.

Use in patients with impaired liver function: Patients with impaired hepatic function from cirrhosis do not have any clinically important changes in ketorolac clearance or terminal half-life.

Borderline elevations of one or more liver function tests may occur. These abnormalities may be transient, may remain unchanged, or may progress with continued therapy. Meaningful elevations (greater than three times normal) of serum glutamate pyruvate transaminase (SGPT/ALT) or serum glutamate oxaloacetate transaminase (SGOT/AST) occurred in controlled clinical trials in less than 1% of patients. If clinical signs and symptoms consistent with liver disease develop, or if systemic manifestations occur, Toradol should be discontinued.

Haematological effects: Patients with coagulation disorders should not receive Toradol. Patients on anti-coagulation therapy may be at increased risk of bleeding if given Toradol concurrently. The concomitant use of ketorolac and prophylactic low-dose heparin (2500 - 5000 units twelve hourly) has not been studied extensively and may also be associated with an increased risk of bleeding. Patients already on anti-coagulants or who require low-dose heparin should not receive ketorolac. Patients who are receiving other drug therapy that interferes with haemostasis should be carefully observed if Toradol is administered. In controlled clinical studies, the incidence of clinically significant post-operative bleeding was less than 1%.

Ketorolac inhibits platelet aggregation and prolongs bleeding time. In patients with normal bleeding function, bleeding times were raised, but not outside the normal range of two to eleven minutes. Unlike the prolonged effects from aspirin, platelet function returns to normal within 24 to 48 hours after ketorolac is discontinued.

In post-marketing experience, post-operative wound haemorrhage has been reported in association with the immediate peri-operative use of Toradol IM/IV. Therefore, ketorolac should not be used in patients who have had operations with a high risk of haemorrhage or incomplete haemostasis. Caution should be used where strict haemostasis is critical, e.g. in cosmetic or day-case surgery. Haematomata and other signs of wound haemorrhage and epistaxis have been reported with the use of Toradol. Physicians should be aware of the pharmacological similarity of ketorolac to other non-steroidal anti-inflammatory drugs that inhibit cyclo-oxygenase and the risk of bleeding, particularly in the elderly.

Toradol is not an anaesthetic agent and possesses no sedative or anxiolytic properties; therefore it is not recommended as a pre-operative medication for the support of anaesthesia when these effects are required.

The risk of clinically serious gastro-intestinal bleeding is dose-dependent. This is particularly true in elderly patients who receive an average daily dose greater than 60mg/day of Toradol.

4.5 Interaction with other medicinal products and other forms of Interaction

Toradol should not be used with other NSAIDs or in patients receiving aspirin because of the potential for additive side-effects.

Ketorolac is highly bound to human plasma protein (mean 99.2%) and binding is concentration-independent.

Ketorolac did not alter digoxin protein binding. *In vitro* studies indicated that at therapeutic concentrations of salicylate (300μg/ml) and above, the binding of ketorolac was reduced from approximately 99.2% to 97.5%. Therapeutic concentrations of digoxin, warfarin, paracetamol, phenytoin and tolbutamide did not alter ketorolac protein binding. Because ketorolac is a highly potent drug and present in low concentrations in plasma, it would not be expected to displace other protein-bound drugs significantly.

Care should be taken when administering Toradol with anti-coagulants since co-administration may cause an enhanced anti-coagulant effect.

There is no evidence in animal or human studies that ketorolac trometamol induces or inhibits the hepatic enzymes capable of metabolising itself or other drugs. Hence Toradol would not be expected to alter the pharmacokinetics of other drugs due to enzyme induction or inhibition mechanisms.

In normovolaemic healthy subjects, ketorolac reduces the diuretic response to frusemide by approximately 20%, so particular care should be taken in patients with cardiac decompensation.

Toradol and other non-steroidal anti-inflammatory drugs can reduce the anti-hypertensive effect of beta-blockers and may increase the risk of renal impairment when administered concurrently with ACE inhibitors, particularly in volume depleted patients.

NSAIDs may exacerbate cardiac failure, reduce GFR and increase plasma cardiac glycoside levels when co-administered with cardiac glycosides.

Caution is advised when methotrexate is administered concurrently, since some prostaglandin synthesis inhibiting drugs have been reported to reduce the clearance of methotrexate, and thus possibly enhance its toxicity.

Probenecid should not be administered concurrently with ketorolac because of increases in ketorolac plasma level and half-life.

As with all NSAIDs caution is advised when cyclosporin is co-administered because of the increased risk of nephrotoxicity.

NSAIDs should not be used for eight to twelve days after mifepristone administration as NSAIDs can reduce the effects of mifepristone.

As with all NSAIDs, caution should be taken when co-administering with cortico-steroids because of the increased risk of gastro-intestinal bleeding.

Patients taking quinolones may have an increased risk of developing convulsions.

Co-administration with diuretics can lead to a reduced diuretic effect, and increase the risk of nephrotoxicity of NSAIDs.

Because of an increased tendency to bleeding when oxpentifylline is administered concurrently, this combination should be avoided.

In patients receiving lithium, there is a possible inhibition of renal lithium clearance, increased plasma lithium concentration, and potential lithium toxicity. (See section *4.3 Contra-indications*).

4.6 Pregnancy and lactation

There was no evidence of teratogenicity in rats or rabbits studied at maternally-toxic doses of ketorolac. Prolongation of the gestation period and/or delayed parturition were seen in the rat. Ketorolac and its metabolites have been shown to pass into the foetus and milk of animals. Ketorolac has been detected in human milk at low levels. Safety in human pregnancy has not been established. Congenital abnormalities have been reported in association with NSAID administration in man, however these are low in frequency and do not follow any discernible pattern. Ketorolac is therefore contra-indicated during pregnancy, labour or delivery, or in mothers who are breast-feeding.

4.7 Effects on ability to drive and use machines

Some patients may experience dizziness, drowsiness, visual disturbances, headaches, vertigo, insomnia or depression with the use of Toradol. If patients experience these, or other similar undesirable effects, patients should not drive or operate machinery.

4.8 Undesirable effects

The following side-effects have been reported with Toradol.

Gastro-intestinal: Nausea, dyspepsia, gastro-intestinal pain, gastro-intestinal bleeding, abdominal discomfort, haematemesis, gastritis, oesophagitis, diarrhoea, eructation, constipation, flatulence, fullness, melaena, peptic ulcer, non-peptic gastro-intestinal ulceration, rectal bleeding, ulcerative stomatitis, vomiting, haemorrhage, perforation, pancreatitis.

Central nervous/musculoskeletal systems: Anxiety, drowsiness, dizziness, headache, sweating, dry mouth, nervousness, paraesthesia, functional disorders, abnormal thinking, depression, euphoria, convulsions, excessive thirst, inability to concentrate, insomnia, malaise, fatigue, stimulation, vertigo, abnormal taste and vision, optic neuritis, myalgia, abnormal dreams, hallucinations, hyperkinesia, hearing loss, tinnitus, aseptic meningitis, psychotic reactions.

Renal: Nephrotoxicity including increased urinary frequency, oliguria, acute renal failure, hyponatraemia, hyperkalaemia, haemolytic uraemic syndrome, flank pain (with or without haematuria), raised serum urea and creatinine, interstitial nephritis, urinary retention, nephrotic syndrome.

Cardiovascular/haematological: Flushing, bradycardia, pallor, purpura, thrombocytopenia, neutropenia, agranulocytosis, aplastic anaemia, haemolytic anaemia, hypertension, palpitations, chest pain.

Reproductive, female: Infertility.

Respiratory: Dyspnoea, asthma, pulmonary oedema.

Dermatological: Pruritus, urticaria, skin photosensitivity, Lyell's syndrome, Stevens-Johnson syndrome, exfoliative dermatitis, maculopapular rash.

Hypersensitivity reactions: Anaphylaxis, bronchospasm, laryngeal oedema, hypotension, flushing and rash. Such reactions may occur in patients with or without known sensitivity to Toradol or other non-steroidal anti-inflammatory drugs.

These may also occur in individuals with a history of angioedema, bronchospastic reactivity (e.g. asthma and nasal polyps). Anaphylactoid reactions, like anaphylaxis, may have a fatal outcome (see section *4.3 Contra-indications*).

Bleeding: Post-operative wound haemorrhage, haematomata, epistaxis, increased bleeding time.

Other: Asthenia, oedema, weight gain, abnormalities of liver function tests, hepatitis, liver failure, jaundice, fever. Injection site pain has been reported in some patients.

4.9 Overdose

Doses of 360mg given intramuscularly over an eight hour interval for five consecutive days have caused abdominal pain and peptic ulcers which have healed after discontinuation of dosing. Two patients recovered from unsuccessful suicide attempts. One patient experienced nausea after 210mg ketorolac, and the other hyperventilation after 300mg ketorolac.

5. PHARMACOLOGICAL PROPERTIES

5.1 Pharmacodynamic properties

Toradol is a potent analgesic agent of the non-steroidal, anti-inflammatory class (NSAID). It is not an opioid and has no known effects on opioid receptors. Its mode of action is to inhibit the cyclo-oxygenase enzyme system and hence prostaglandin synthesis, and it demonstrates a minimal anti-inflammatory effect at its analgesic dose.

5.2 Pharmacokinetic properties

IM: Following intramuscular administration, ketorolac trometamol was rapidly and completely absorbed, a mean peak plasma concentration of 2.2μg/ml occurring an average of 50 minutes after a single 30mg dose. The influences of age, kidney and liver function on terminal plasma half-life and mean total clearance are outlined in the table below (estimated from a single 30mg IM dose of ketorolac).

Type of subjects	Total clearance (l/hr/kg) mean (range)	Terminal half-life (hrs) mean (range)
Normal subjects (n = 54)	0.023 (0.010 - 0.046)	5.3 (3.5 - 9.2)
Patients with hepatic dysfunction (n = 7)	0.029 (0.013 - 0.066)	5.4 (2.2 - 6.9)
Patients with renal impairment (n = 25) (serum creatinine 160 - 430 micromol/l)	0.016 (0.005 - 0.043)	10.3 (5.9 - 19.2)
Renal dialysis patients (n = 9)	0.016 (0.003 - 0.036)	13.6 (8.0 - 39.1)
Healthy elderly subjects (n = 13) (mean age 72)	0.019 (0.013 - 0.034)	7.0 (4.7 - 8.6)

IV: Intravenous administration of a single 10mg dose of ketorolac trometamol resulted in a mean peak plasma concentration of 2.4μg/ml occurring an average of 5.4 minutes after dosing, with a terminal plasma elimination half-life of 5.1 hours, an average volume of distribution of 0.15 l/kg, and a total plasma clearance of 0.35ml/min/kg.

The pharmacokinetics of ketorolac in man following single or multiple doses are linear. Steady-state plasma levels are achieved after dosing every six hours for one day. No changes in clearance occurred with chronic dosing. The primary route of excretion of ketorolac and its metabolites is renal: 91.4% (mean) of a given dose being found in the urine and 6.1% (mean) in the faeces.

More than 99% of the ketorolac in plasma is protein-bound over a wide concentration range.

5.3 Preclinical safety data

An 18-month study in mice with oral doses of ketorolac trometamol at 2mg/kg/day (0.9 times human systemic exposure at the recommended IM or IV dose of 30mg qid, based on area-under-the-plasma-concentration curve [AUC]), and a 24-month study in rats at 5mg/kg/day (0.5 times the human AUC), showed no evidence of tumourigenicity.

Ketorolac trometamol was not mutagenic in the Ames test, unscheduled DNA synthesis and repair, and in forward mutation assays. Ketorolac trometamol did not cause chromosome breakage in the *in vivo* mouse micronucleus assay. At 1590μg/ml and at higher concentrations, ketorolac trometamol increased the incidence of chromosomal aberrations in Chinese hamster ovarian cells.

Impairment of fertility did not occur in male or female rats at oral doses of 9mg/kg (0.9 times the human AUC) and 16mg/kg (1.6 times the human AUC) of ketorolac trometamol, respectively.

6. PHARMACEUTICAL PARTICULARS

6.1 List of excipients

Ethanol

Sodium Chloride

Water

6.2 Incompatibilities

Toradol should not be mixed in a small volume (e.g. in a syringe) with morphine sulphate, pethidine hydrochloride, promethazine hydrochloride or hydroxyzine hydrochloride as precipitation of ketorolac will occur.

It is compatible with normal saline, 5% dextrose, Ringer's, lactated Ringer's or Plasmacyte solutions. Compatibility of Toradol with other drugs is unknown.

6.3 Shelf life

24 months.

6.4 Special precautions for storage

Store at controlled room temperature (15 - 30°C) and protect from light. Do not use if particulate matter is present.

6.5 Nature and contents of container

Toradol 10mg and 30mg is available in single-dose ampoules containing 1ml of solution in cartons of 1, 5 or 10.

6.6 Instructions for use and handling

No special instructions applicable.

7. MARKETING AUTHORISATION HOLDER

Roche Products Limited, 40 Broadwater Road, Welwyn Garden City, Hertfordshire, AL7 3AY.

8. MARKETING AUTHORISATION NUMBER(S)

PL 0031/0480 (ampoules 10mg/ml)

PL 0031/0481 (ampoules 30mg/ml)

9. DATE OF FIRST AUTHORISATION/RENEWAL OF THE AUTHORISATION

31 May 1996/30 October 2000

10. DATE OF REVISION OF THE TEXT

October 2002

Toradol is a registered trade mark

P927009/903

Toradol Tablets

(Roche Products Limited)

1. NAME OF THE MEDICINAL PRODUCT

Toradol

2. QUALITATIVE AND QUANTITATIVE COMPOSITION

Ketorolac Trometamol 10mg.

3. PHARMACEUTICAL FORM

White to creamy white film coated, round tablet, marked "KET 10" on one face, the other face blank.

4. CLINICAL PARTICULARS

4.1 Therapeutic indications

Toradol tablets are indicated for the short-term management of moderate postoperative pain.

4.2 Posology and method of administration

Toradol tablets are recommended for short-term use only (up to 7 days) and are not recommended for chronic use.

Adults

10mg every 4 to 6 hours as required. Doses exceeding 40mg per day are not recommended.

Opioid analgesics (e.g. morphine, pethidine) may be used concomitantly, and may be required for optimal analgesic effect in the early postoperative period when pain is most severe. Ketorolac does not interfere with opioid binding and does not exacerbate opioid-related respiratory depression or sedation.

For patients receiving parenteral Toradol, and who are converted to Toradol oral tablets, the total combined daily dose should not exceed 90mg (60mg for the elderly, renally-impaired patients and patients less than 50kg) and the oral component should not exceed 40mg on the day the change of formulation is made. Patients should be converted to oral treatment as soon as possible.

Elderly

A longer dosing interval, e.g. 6 - 8 hourly, is advisable in the elderly. The lower end of the dosage range is recommended for patients over 65 years of age.

Children

Toradol is not recommended for use in children under 16 years of age.

4.3 Contraindications

– a history of peptic ulcer or gastro-intestinal bleeding

– suspected or confirmed cerebrovascular bleeding

– haemorrhagic diatheses, including coagulation disorders

– hypersensitivity to ketorolac trometamol or other NSAIDs and those patients in whom aspirin or other prostaglandin synthesis inhibitors induce allergic reactions (severe anaphylactic-like reactions have been observed in such patients)

– the complete or partial syndrome of nasal polyps, angioedema or bronchospasm

– concurrent treatment with other NSAIDs, oxpentifylline, probenecid or lithium salts

– hypovolaemia from any cause or dehydration

– moderate or severe renal impairment (serum creatinine > 160 micromol/l)

– a history of asthma

– patients who have had operations with a high risk of haemorrhage or incomplete haemostasis

– patients on anticoagulants including low dose heparin (2500 - 5000 units 12-hourly)

– during pregnancy, labour, delivery or lactation

– children under 16 years of age

– Toradol is contra-indicated as prophylactic analgesia before surgery due to inhibition of platelet aggregation and is contra-indicated intraoperatively because of the increased risk of bleeding

– Toradol is contra-indicated in patients currently receiving aspirin.

4.4 Special warnings and special precautions for use

Use in the elderly: Patients over the age of 65 years may be at a greater risk of experiencing adverse events than younger patients. This age-related risk is common to all NSAIDs. Compared to young adults, the elderly have an increased plasma half-life and reduced plasma clearance of ketorolac. A longer dosing interval is advisable (see *Posology and method of administration*).

Effects on fertility: The use of Toradol, as with any drug known to inhibit cyclo-oxygenase/prostaglandin synthesis, may impair fertility and is not recommended in women attempting to conceive. In women who have difficulty conceiving or are undergoing investigation of fertility, withdrawal of Toradol should be considered.

Gastro-intestinal effects: Toradol can cause gastro-intestinal irritation, ulcers or bleeding in patients with or without a history of previous symptoms. Elderly and debilitated patients are more prone to develop these reactions. The incidence increases with dose and duration of treatment.

In a non-randomised, in-hospital post-marketing surveillance study, increased rates of clinically serious GI bleeding were seen in patients ⩽ 65 years of age who received an average daily dose of > 90mg ketorolac IM as compared to those patients receiving parenteral opioids.

Respiratory effects: Bronchospasm may be precipitated in patients with a history of asthma.

Renal effects: Drugs that inhibit prostaglandin biosynthesis (including non-steroidal anti-inflammatory drugs) have been reported to cause nephrotoxicity, including but not limited to glomerular nephritis, interstitial nephritis, renal papillary necrosis, nephrotic syndrome and acute renal failure. In patients with renal, cardiac or hepatic impairment, caution is required since the use of NSAIDs may result in deterioration of renal function.

As with other drugs that inhibit prostaglandin synthesis, elevations of serum urea, creatinine and potassium have been reported with ketorolac trometamol and may occur after one dose.

Patients with impaired renal function: Since ketorolac trometamol and its metabolites are excreted primarily by the kidney, patients with moderate to severe impairment of renal function (serum creatinine greater than 160 micromol/l) should not receive Toradol. Patients with lesser renal impairment should receive a reduced dose of ketorolac (not exceeding 60mg/day IM or IV) and their renal status should be closely monitored.

Caution should be observed in patients with conditions leading to a reduction in blood volume and/or renal blood flow, where renal prostaglandins have a supportive role in the maintenance of renal perfusion. In these patients, administration of an NSAID may cause a dose-dependent reduction in renal prostaglandin formation and may precipitate overt renal failure. Patients at greatest risk of this reaction are those who are volume depleted because of blood loss or severe dehydration, patients with impaired renal function, heart failure, liver dysfunction, the elderly and those taking diuretics. Discontinuation of NSAID therapy is typically followed by recovery to the pre-treatment state. Inadequate fluid/blood replacement during surgery, leading to hypovolaemia, may lead to renal dysfunction which could be exacerbated when Toradol is administered. Therefore, volume depletion should be corrected and close monitoring of serum urea and creatinine and urine output is recommended until the patient is normovolaemic. In patients on renal dialysis, ketorolac clearance was reduced to approximately half the normal rate and terminal half-life increased approximately three-fold.

Fluid retention and oedema: Fluid retention and oedema have been reported with the use of Toradol and it should therefore be used with caution in patients with cardiac decompensation, hypertension or similar conditions.

Use in patients with impaired liver function: Patients with impaired hepatic function from cirrhosis do not have any clinically important changes in ketorolac clearance or terminal half-life.

Borderline elevations of one or more liver function tests may occur. These abnormalities may be transient, may remain unchanged, or may progress with continued therapy. Meaningful elevations (greater than 3 times normal) of serum glutamate pyruvate transaminase (SGPT/ALT) or serum glutamate oxaloacetate transaminase (SGOT/AST) occurred in controlled clinical trials in less than 1% of patients. If clinical signs and symptoms consistent with liver disease develop, or if systemic manifestations occur, Toradol should be discontinued.

Haematological effects: Patients with coagulation disorders should not receive Toradol. Patients on anticoagulation therapy may be at increased risk of bleeding if given Toradol concurrently. The concomitant use of ketorolac and prophylactic low-dose heparin (2500 - 5000 units 12-hourly) has not been studied extensively and may also be associated with an increased risk of bleeding. Patients already on anticoagulants or who require low-dose heparin should not receive ketorolac. Patients who are receiving other drug therapy that interferes with haemostasis should be carefully observed if Toradol is administered. In controlled clinical studies, the incidence of clinically significant postoperative bleeding was less than 1%.

Ketorolac inhibits platelet aggregation and prolongs bleeding time. In patients with normal bleeding function, bleeding times were raised, but not outside the normal range of 2 - 11 minutes. Unlike the prolonged effects from aspirin, platelet function returns to normal within 24 to 48 hours after ketorolac is discontinued.

In post-marketing experience, postoperative wound haemorrhage has been reported in association with the immediate peri-operative use of Toradol IM/IV. Therefore, ketorolac should not be used in patients who have had operations with a high risk of haemorrhage or incomplete haemostasis. Caution should be used where strict haemostasis is critical, e.g. in cosmetic or day-case surgery. Haematomata and other signs of wound haemorrhage and epistaxis have been reported with the use of Toradol. Physicians should be aware of the pharmacological similarity of ketorolac to other non-steroidal anti-inflammatory drugs that inhibit cyclo-oxygenase and the risk of bleeding, particularly in the elderly.

Toradol is not an anaesthetic agent and possesses no sedative or anxiolytic properties; therefore it is not recommended as a pre-operative medication for the support of anaesthesia when these effects are required.

The risk of clinically serious gastro-intestinal bleeding is dose-dependent. This is particularly true in elderly patients who receive an average daily dose greater than 60mg/day of Toradol.

4.5 Interaction with other medicinal products and other forms of Interaction

Toradol should not be used with other NSAIDs or in patients receiving aspirin because of the potential for additive side-effects.

Ketorolac is highly bound to human plasma protein (mean 99.2%) and binding is concentration-independent.

Ketorolac did not alter digoxin protein binding. *In vitro* studies indicated that at therapeutic concentrations of salicylate (300mcg/ml) and above, the binding of ketorolac was reduced from approximately 99.2% to 97.5%. Therapeutic concentrations of digoxin, warfarin, paracetamol, phenytoin and tolbutamide did not alter ketorolac protein binding. Because ketorolac is a highly potent drug and present in low concentrations in plasma, it would not be expected to displace other protein-bound drugs significantly.

There is no evidence in animal or human studies that ketorolac trometamol induces or inhibits the hepatic enzymes capable of metabolising itself or other drugs. Hence Toradol would not be expected to alter the pharmacokinetics of other drugs due to enzyme induction or inhibition mechanisms.

In normovolaemic healthy subjects, ketorolac reduces the diuretic response to frusemide by approximately 20%, so particular care should be taken in patients with cardiac decompensation.

There is an increased risk of renal impairment when ketorolac is administered concurrently with ACE inhibitors, particularly in volume depleted patients.

Caution is advised when methotrexate is administered concurrently, since some prostaglandin synthesis inhibiting drugs have been reported to reduce the clearance of methotrexate, and thus possibly enhance its toxicity.

Probenecid should not be administered concurrently with ketorolac because of increases in ketorolac plasma level and half-life.

Because of an increased tendency to bleeding when oxpentifylline is administered concurrently, this combination should be avoided.

In patients receiving lithium, there is a possible inhibition of renal lithium clearance, increased plasma lithium concentration, and potential lithium toxicity. (See *Contra-indications*).

4.6 Pregnancy and lactation

There was no evidence of teratogenicity in rats or rabbits studied at maternally-toxic doses of ketorolac. Prolongation of the gestation period and/or delayed parturition were seen in the rat. Ketorolac and its metabolites have been shown to pass into the foetus and milk of animals. Ketorolac has been detected in human milk at low levels. Safety in human pregnancy has not been established. Ketorolac is therefore contra-indicated during pregnancy, labour or delivery, or in mothers who are breast-feeding.

4.7 Effects on ability to drive and use machines
Some patients may experience drowsiness, dizziness, vertigo, insomnia or depression with the use of Toradol. If patients experience these, or other similar undesirable effects, they should exercise caution in carrying out activities that require alertness.

4.8 Undesirable effects
The following side-effects have been reported with Toradol.

Gastro-intestinal: Nausea, dyspepsia, gastro-intestinal pain, gastro-intestinal bleeding, abdominal discomfort, haematemesis, gastritis, oesophagitis, diarrhoea, eructation, constipation, flatulence, fullness, melaena, peptic ulcer, rectal bleeding, stomatitis, vomiting, haemorrhage, perforation, pancreatitis.

Central nervous/musculoskeletal systems: Anxiety, drowsiness, dizziness, headache, sweating, dry mouth, nervousness, paraesthesia, functional disorders, abnormal thinking, depression, euphoria, convulsions, excessive thirst, inability to concentrate, insomnia, stimulation, vertigo, abnormal taste and vision, myalgia, abnormal dreams, hallucinations, hyperkinesia, hearing loss, tinnitus, aseptic meningitis, psychotic reactions.

Renal: increased urinary frequency, oliguria, acute renal failure, hyponatraemia, hyperkalaemia, haemolytic uraemic syndrome, flank pain (with or without haematuria), raised serum urea and creatinine, interstitial nephritis, urinary retention, nephrotic syndrome.

Cardiovascular/haematological: Flushing, bradycardia, pallor, purpura, thrombocytopenia, hypertension, palpitations, chest pain.

Reproductive, female: Infertility.

Respiratory: Dyspnoea, asthma, pulmonary oedema.

Dermatological: Pruritus, urticaria, Lyell's syndrome, Stevens-Johnson syndrome, exfoliative dermatitis, maculopapular rash.

Hypersensitivity reactions: Anaphylaxis, bronchospasm, laryngeal oedema, hypotension, flushing and rash. Such reactions may occur in patients with or without known sensitivity to Toradol or other non-steroidal anti-inflammatory drugs.

These may also occur in individuals with a history of angioedema, bronchospastic reactivity (e.g. asthma and nasal polyps). Anaphylactoid reactions, like anaphylaxis, may have a fatal outcome (see *Contra-indications*).

Bleeding: Postoperative wound haemorrhage, haematomata, epistaxis, increased bleeding time.

Other: Asthenia, oedema, weight gain, abnormalities of liver function tests, hepatitis, liver failure, fever.

4.9 Overdose
Doses of 360mg given intramuscularly over an 8-hour interval for five consecutive days have caused abdominal pain and peptic ulcers which have healed after discontinuation of dosing. Two patients recovered from unsuccessful suicide attempts. One patient experienced nausea after 210mg ketorolac, and the other hyperventilation after 300mg ketorolac.

5. PHARMACOLOGICAL PROPERTIES
5.1 Pharmacodynamic properties
Ketorolac trometamol is a non-narcotic analgesic. It is a non-steroidal anti-inflammatory agent that exhibits anti-inflammatory and weak antipyretic activity.

Ketorolac trometamol inhibits the synthesis of prostaglandins and is considered a peripherally acting analgesic. It does not have known effects on opiate receptors.

No evidence of respiratory depression has been observed after administration of ketorolac trometamol in controlled clinical trials. Ketorolac trometamol does not cause pupil constriction.

5.2 Pharmacokinetic properties
Ketorolac trometamol is rapidly and completely absorbed following oral administration with a peak plasma concentration of 0.87mcg/ml occurring 50 minutes after a single 10mg dose. The terminal plasma elimination half-life averages 5.4 hours (S.D. = 1.0) in healthy subjects. In elderly subjects (mean age 72) it is 6.2 hours (S.D. = 1.0). More than 99% of the ketorolac in plasma is protein bound.

The pharmacokinetics of ketorolac in man following single or multiple doses are linear. Steady state plasma levels are achieved after 1 day of Q.I.D. dosing. No changes occurred with chronic dosing. Following a single intravenous dose, the volume of distribution is 0.25 l/kg, the half-life is 5 hours and the clearance 0.55ml/min/kg. The primary route of excretion of ketorolac and its metabolites (conjugates and the p-hydroxymetabolite) is in the urine (91.4%) and the remainder is excreted in the faeces.

A high fat diet decreased the rate, but not the extent of absorption, while antacid had no effect on ketorolac absorption.

5.3 Preclinical safety data
None stated.

6. PHARMACEUTICAL PARTICULARS
6.1 List of excipients
Microcrystalline cellulose EP
Spray dried lactose EP
Magnesium stearate EP
Coating suspension:
Opadry white YS-1-7002
Purified water

6.2 Incompatibilities
None known.

6.3 Shelf life
3 years.

6.4 Special precautions for storage
Protect from moisture.

6.5 Nature and contents of container
White HDPE bottles with polypropylene screw containers containing 50, 56, 100, 250 or 500 tablets.

Polypropylene securitainers containing 50, 56, 100, 250 or 500 tablets.

Amber or white PVC/aluminium foil blister packs in outer cardboard carton containing 4, 20, 28, 50, 56, 100, 250 or 500 tablets.

6.6 Instructions for use and handling
None stated.

7. MARKETING AUTHORISATION HOLDER
Roche Products Limited, 40 Broadwater Road, Welwyn Garden City, Hertfordshire, AL7 3AY.

8. MARKETING AUTHORISATION NUMBER(S)
PL 0031/0482

9. DATE OF FIRST AUTHORISATION/RENEWAL OF THE AUTHORISATION
31 May 1996

10. DATE OF REVISION OF THE TEXT
October 2002

Toradol is a registered trade mark

P927008/903

Torem

(Roche Products Limited)

1. NAME OF THE MEDICINAL PRODUCT
Torem 2.5mg Tablets
Torem 5mg Tablets
Torem 10mg Tablets

2. QUALITATIVE AND QUANTITATIVE COMPOSITION
Torem 2.5mg Tablets: Each tablet contains 2.5mg torasemide.

Torem 5mg Tablets: Each tablet contains 5.0mg torasemide.

Torem 10mg Tablets: Each tablet contains 10.0mg torasemide.

For excipients, see 6.1

3. PHARMACEUTICAL FORM
Tablets.

Torem 2.5mg Tablets: White to off-white, round tablet marked BM/B4 on one side.

Torem 5mg Tablets: White to off-white, round tablet marked BM/C9 on one side.

Torem 10mg Tablets: White to off-white, round tablet marked BM/D7 on one side.

4. CLINICAL PARTICULARS
4.1 Therapeutic indications
Torem 2.5mg Tablets:
Essential hypertension.

Torem 5mg Tablets:
Essential hypertension; oedema due to congestive heart failure; hepatic, pulmonary or renaloedema.

Torem 10mg Tablets:
Oedema due to congestive heart failure; hepatic, pulmonary or renal oedema.

4.2 Posology and method of administration
Adults
Essential hypertension: A dose of 2.5mg torasemide p.o. once daily is recommended. If necessary, the dose may be increased to 5mg once daily. Studies suggest that doses above 5mg daily will not lead to further reduction in blood pressure. The maximum effect is exhibited after approximately twelve weeks of continuous treatment.

Oedema: The usual dose is 5mg p.o. once daily. If necessary, the dose can be increased stepwise up to 20mg once daily. In individual cases, as much as 40mg torasemide/day has been administered.

Elderly
No special dosage adjustments are necessary.

Children
There is no experience of torasemide in children.

4.3 Contraindications
Renal failure with anuria; hepatic coma and pre-coma; hypotension; pregnancy and lactation; hypersensitivity to torasemide and sulphonylureas; cardiac arrhythmias, simultaneous therapy with aminoglycosides or cephalosporins, or renal dysfunction due to drugs which cause renal damage.

4.4 Special warnings and special precautions for use
Hypokalaemia, hyponatraemia, hypovolaemia and disorders of micturition must be corrected before treatment.

On long-term treatment with torasemide, regular monitoring of the electrolyte balance, glucose, uric acid, creatinine and lipids in the blood, is recommended.

Careful monitoring of patients with a tendency to hyperuricaemia and gout is recommended. Carbohydrate metabolism in latent or manifest diabetes mellitus should be monitored.

As for other drugs which produce changes in blood pressure, patients taking torasemide should be warned not to drive or operate machinery if they experience dizziness or related symptoms.

Patients with rare hereditary problems of glucose intolerance, the Lapp lactase deficiency of glucose-galactose malabsorption should not take this medication.

4.5 Interaction with other medicinal products and other forms of Interaction
When used simultaneously with cardiac glycosides, a potassium and/or magnesium deficiency may increase sensitivity of the cardiac muscle to such drugs. The kaliuretic effect of mineralo-and glucocorticoids and laxatives may be increased.

As with other diuretics, the effect of antihypertensive drugs given concomitantly may be potentiated.

Torasemide, especially at high doses, may potentiate the toxicity of aminoglycoside antibiotics, cisplatin preparations, the nephrotoxic effects of cephalosporins, and the cardio-and neurotoxic effect of lithium. The action of curare-containing muscle relaxants and of theophylline can be potentiated. In patients receiving high doses of salicylates, salicylate toxicity may be increased. The action of antidiabetic drugs may be reduced.

Sequential or combined treatment, or starting a new comedication with an ACE inhibitor may result in transient hypotension. This may be minimised by lowering the starting dose of the ACE inhibitor and/or reducing or stopping temporarily the dose of torasemide. Torasemide may decrease arterial responsiveness to pressor agents e.g. adrenaline, noradrenaline.

Non-steroidal anti-inflammatory drugs (eg. Indometacin) and probenecid may reduce the diuretic and hypotensive effect of torasemide.

Concomitant use of torasemide and colestyramine has not been studied in humans, but in an animal study co-administration of colestyramine decreased absorption of oral torasemide.

4.6 Pregnancy and lactation
There are no data from experience in humans of the effect of torasemide on the embryo and foetus. Whilst studies in the rat have shown no teratogenic effect, malformed foetuses have been observed after high doses in pregnant rabbits. No studies have been conducted on excretion in breast milk. Consequently, torasemide is contra-indicated in pregnancy and lactation.

4.7 Effects on ability to drive and use machines
As for other drugs which produce changes in blood pressure, patients taking torasemide should be warned not to drive or operate machinery if they experience dizziness or related symptoms.

4.8 Undesirable effects
Blood chemistry/volume:
As with other diuretics, depending on the dosage and duration of treatment, there may be disturbances of water and electrolyte balance, especially with markedly limited salt intake.

Hypokalaemia may occur (especially if a low potassium diet is being taken, or if vomiting, diarrhoea, or excessive use of laxatives takes place, or in cases of hepatic failure).

Symptoms and signs of electrolyte and volume depletion, such as headache, dizziness, hypotension, weakness, drowsiness, confusional states, loss of appetite and cramps, can occur if diuresis is marked, especially at the start of treatment and in elderly patients. Dose adjustment may be necessary.

Raised serum uric acid, glucose and lipids can occur.

There may be aggravation of metabolic alkalosis.

Cardiovascular system:
In isolated cases, thromboembolic complications and circulatory disturbances due to haemoconcentration may occur.

Gastro-intestinal system:
Patients may experience gastro-intestinal symptoms.

Pancreatitis has been reported in isolated cases.

Renal and Urinary system:
In patients with urinary outflow obstruction, retention of urine may be precipitated.

Raised serum urea and creatinine may occur.

Liver:

Increases in certain liver enzymes, eg. gamma-GT.

Haematology:

Isolated cases of decreases in red and white blood cells and platelets have been reported.

Skin/allergy:

In isolated cases, there may be allergic reactions, such as pruritis, rash and photosensitivity.

Nervous system:

Isolated reports of visual disturbance.

Tinnitus and hearing loss have occurred in isolated cases.

Rarely, limb paraesthesia has been reported.

Others:

Dry mouth.

4.9 Overdose

Symptoms and signs

No typical picture of intoxication is known. If overdosage occurs, then there may be marked diuresis with the danger of loss of fluid and electrolytes which may lead to somnolence and confusion, hypotension, circulatory collapse. Gastrointestinal disturbances may occur.

Treatment

No specific antidote is known. Symptoms and signs of overdosage require the reduction of the dose or withdrawal of torasemide, and simultaneous replacement of fluid and electrolytes.

5. PHARMACOLOGICAL PROPERTIES

5.1 Pharmacodynamic properties

Torasemide is a loop diuretic. However, at low doses its pharmacodynamic profile resembles that of the thiazide class regarding the level and duration of diuresis. At higher doses, torasemide induces a brisk diuresis in a dose dependant manner with a high ceiling of effect.

5.2 Pharmacokinetic properties

Absorption

Torasemide is absorbed rapidly and almost completely after oral administration, and peak serum levels are reached after one to two hours.

Serum protein binding

More than 99% of torasemide is bound to plasma proteins.

Distribution

The apparent distribution volume is 16 litres.

Metabolism

Torasemide is metabolised to three metabolites, M1, M3 and M5 by stepwise oxidation, hydroxylation or ring hydroxylation.

Elimination

The terminal half-life of torasemide and its metabolites is three to four hours in healthy subjects. Total clearance of torasemide is 40ml/min and renal clearance about 10ml/min. About 80% of the dose administered is excreted as torasemide and metabolites into the renal tubule - torasemide 24%, M1 12%, M3 3%, M5 41%.

In the presence of renal failure, elimination half-life of torasemide is unchanged.

5.3 Preclinical safety data

Acute toxicity

Very low toxicity.

Chronic toxicity

The changes observed in toxicity studies in dogs and rats at high doses are attributable to an excess pharmacodynamic action (diuresis). Changes observed were weight reduction, increases in creatinine and urea and renal alterations such as tubular dilatation and interstitial nephritis. All drug induced changes were shown to be reversible.

Teratogenicity

Reproduction toxicology studies in the rat have shown no teratogenic effect, but malformed foetuses have been observed after high doses in pregnant rabbits. No effects on fertility have been seen.

Torasemide showed no mutagenic potential. Carcinogenicity studies in rats and mice showed no tumourigenic potential.

6. PHARMACEUTICAL PARTICULARS

6.1 List of excipients

Lactose monohydrate,

Maize starch,

Colloidal silicon dioxide,

Magnesium stearate

6.2 Incompatibilities

Not applicable.

6.3 Shelf life

Torem 2.5mg Tablets: 5 years

Torem 5mg Tablets: 5 years

Torem 10mg Tablets: 4 years

6.4 Special precautions for storage

No special precautions for storage.

6.5 Nature and contents of container

Blister packs, PVC/aluminium, containing 14, 28, 100 or 112 tablets.

6.6 Instructions for use and handling

Not applicable.

7. MARKETING AUTHORISATION HOLDER

Roche Products Limited, 40 Broadwater Road, Welwyn Garden City, Hertfordshire, AL7 3AY.

8. MARKETING AUTHORISATION NUMBER(S)

Torem 2.5mg Tablets: PL 00031/0539

Torem 5mg Tablets: PL 00031/0540

Torem 10mg Tablets: PL 00031/0541

9. DATE OF FIRST AUTHORISATION/RENEWAL OF THE AUTHORISATION

26 February 2005

10. DATE OF REVISION OF THE TEXT

February 2005

Torem is a registered trade mark

P905014/201

TRACLEER

(Actelion Pharmaceuticals UK)

1. NAME OF THE MEDICINAL PRODUCT

Tracleer ▼ 62.5 mg film-coated tablets

Tracleer ▼ 125 mg film-coated tablets

2. QUALITATIVE AND QUANTITATIVE COMPOSITION

Each film-coated tablet contains 62.5 mg bosentan (as bosentan monohydrate)

or 125 mg bosentan (as bosentan monohydrate).

For excipients, see 6.1.

3. PHARMACEUTICAL FORM

Film-coated tablet:

Orange-white, round, biconvex, film-coated tablets, embossed with "62,5" on one side.

Orange-white, oval, biconvex, film-coated tablets, embossed with "125" on one side.

4. CLINICAL PARTICULARS

4.1 Therapeutic indications

Treatment of pulmonary arterial hypertension (PAH) to improve exercise capacity and symptoms in patients with grade III functional status. Efficacy has been shown in:

- Primary PAH
- PAH secondary to scleroderma without significant interstitial pulmonary disease

4.2 Posology and method of administration

Treatment should only be initiated and monitored by a physician experienced in the treatment of pulmonary arterial hypertension. Tracleer treatment should be initiated at a dose of 62.5 mg twice daily for 4 weeks and then increased to the maintenance dose of 125 mg twice daily. Tablets are to be taken orally morning and evening, with or without food.

In the case of clinical deterioration (e.g., decrease in 6-minute walk test distance by at least 10% compared with pre-treatment measurement) despite Tracleer treatment for at least 8 weeks (target dose for at least 4 weeks), alternative therapies should be considered. However, some patients who show no response after 8 weeks of treatment with Tracleer may respond favourably after an additional 4 to 8 weeks of treatment. If the decision to withdraw Tracleer is taken, it should be done gradually while an alternative therapy is introduced.

In the case of late clinical deterioration despite treatment with Tracleer (i.e., after several months of treatment), the treatment should be re-assessed. Some patients not responding well to 125 mg twice daily of Tracleer may slightly improve their exercise capacity when the dose is increased to 250 mg twice daily. A careful risk/benefit assessment should be made, taking into consideration that the liver toxicity is dose dependent (see sections 4.4 and 5.1).

Discontinuation of treatment

There is limited experience with abrupt discontinuation of Tracleer. No evidence for acute rebound has been observed. However, to avoid the possible occurrence of harmful clinical deterioration due to potential rebound effect, gradual dose reduction (halving the dose for 3 to 7 days) should be considered. Intensified monitoring is recommended during the discontinuation period.

Dosage in hepatic impairment

No dose adjustment is needed in patients with mild hepatic impairment (i.e., Child-Pugh class A) (see section 5.2). Tracleer is contraindicated in patients with moderate to severe liver dysfunction (see sections 4.3, 4.4 and 5.2).

Dosage in renal impairment

No dose adjustment is required in patients with renal impairment. No dose adjustment is required in patients undergoing dialysis (see section 5.2).

Dosage in elderly patients

No dose adjustment is required in patients over the age of 65 years.

Children

Safety and efficacy in patients under the age of 12 years have not been substantially documented.

The following dosing regimen was used in study AC-052-356 (BREATHE-3):

Body Weight (kg)	Initiation Dose (4 weeks)	Maintenance Dose
$10 \leqslant x \leqslant 20$	31.25 mg once daily	31.25 mg twice daily
$20 < x \leqslant 40$	31.25 mg twice daily	62.5 mg twice daily
> 40 kg	62.5 mg twice daily	125 mg twice daily

This study was primarily designed to assess pharmacokinetics in children. The number of patients studied in each dose group was insufficient to establish the optimal dosing regimen in patients under the age of 12 years (see also section 5.1). The pharmacokinetic findings showed that systemic exposure was lower than in adults with pulmonary hypertension (see section 5.2) which may provide sub-optimal effect on pulmonary vasculature. However the safety of higher doses has not been established in children.

No data are available in children under 3 years.

Patients with low body weight

There is limited experience in patients with a body weight below 40 kg.

4.3 Contraindications

- Hypersensitivity to bosentan or any of the excipients
- Child-Pugh Class B or C, i.e., moderate to severe hepatic impairment (see section 5.2)
- Baseline values of liver aminotransferases, i.e., aspartate aminotransferases (AST) and/or alanine aminotransferases (ALT), greater than 3 times the upper limit of normal (see section 4.4)
- Concomitant use of cyclosporine A (see section 4.5)
- Pregnancy
- Women of childbearing potential who are not using a reliable method of contraception (see sections 4.4, 4.5 and 4.6)

4.4 Special warnings and special precautions for use

The efficacy of Tracleer has not been established in patients with severe pulmonary arterial hypertension. Transfer to a therapy that is recommended at the severe stage of the disease (e.g., epoprostenol) should be considered if the clinical condition deteriorates (see section 4.2).

The benefit/risk balance of bosentan has not been established in patients with WHO class I or II functional status of pulmonary arterial hypertension. No studies have been performed in secondary pulmonary arterial hypertension other than related to connective tissue diseases (primarly scleroderma).

Tracleer should only be initiated if the systemic systolic blood pressure is higher than 85 mmHg.

Liver function

Elevations in liver aminotransferases, i.e., aspartate and alanine aminotransferases (AST and/or ALT), associated with bosentan are dose dependent. Liver enzyme changes typically occur within the first 16 weeks of treatment (see section 4.8). These increases may be partly due to competitive inhibition of the elimination of bile salts from hepatocytes but other mechanisms, which have not been clearly established, are probably also involved in the occurrence of liver dysfunction. The accumulation of bosentan in hepatocytes leading to cytolysis with potentially severe damage of the liver, or an immunological mechanism, are not excluded. Liver dysfunction risk may also be increased when medicinal products that are inhibitors of the bile salt export pump (BSEP), e.g., rifampicin, glibenclamide and cyclosporine A (see sections 4.3 and 4.5), are co-administered with bosentan, but limited data are available.

Liver aminotransferase levels must be measured prior to initiation of treatment and subsequently at monthly intervals. In addition, liver aminotransferase levels must be measured 2 weeks after any dose increase.

Recommendations in case of ALT/AST elevations

ALT/AST levels	Treatment and monitoring recommendations
> 3 and ⩽ 5 × ULN	Confirm by another liver test; if confirmed, reduce the daily dose or stop treatment (see section 4.2), monitor aminotransferase levels at least every 2 weeks. If the aminotransferase levels return to pre-treatment values consider continuing or re-introducing Tracleer according to the conditions described below.

> 5 and ⩽ 8 × ULN	Confirm by another liver test; if confirmed, stop treatment (see section 4.2) and monitor aminotransferase levels at least every 2 weeks. If the aminotransferase levels return to pre-treatment values consider re-introducing Tracleer according to the conditions described below.
> 8 × ULN	Treatment must be stopped and re-introduction of Tracleer is not to be considered

In case of associated clinical symptoms of liver injury, i.e., nausea, vomiting, fever, abdominal pain, jaundice, unusual lethargy or fatigue, flu-like syndrome (arthralgia, myalgia, fever), **treatment must be stopped and re-introduction of Tracleer is not to be considered.**

Re-introduction of treatment

Re-introduction of treatment with Tracleer should only be considered if the potential benefits of treatment with Tracleer outweigh the potential risks and when liver aminotransferase levels are within pre-treatment values. The advice of a hepatologist is recommended. Re-introduction must follow the guidelines detailed in section 4.2. **Aminotransferase levels must then be checked within 3 days after re-introduction, then again after a further 2 weeks, and thereafter according to the recommendations above.**

ULN= Upper Limit of Normal

Haemoglobin concentration

Treatment with bosentan was associated with a dose-related, modest decrease in haemoglobin concentration (see section 4.8). Bosentan-related decreases in haemoglobin concentration are not progressive, and stabilise after the first 4–12 weeks of treatment. It is recommended that haemoglobin concentrations be checked prior to initiation of treatment, every month during the first 4 months, and quarterly thereafter. If a clinically relevant decrease in haemoglobin concentration occurs, further evaluation and investigation should be undertaken to determine the cause and need for specific treatment.

Use in women of child-bearing potential

Tracleer treatment must not be initiated in women of child-bearing potential unless they practise reliable contraception (see section 4.5) and the result of the pre-treatment pregnancy test is negative (see section 4.6). Monthly pregnancy tests during treatment with Tracleer are recommended.

Pulmonary veno-occlusive disease

No data are available with bosentan in patients with pulmonary hypertension associated with pulmonary veno-occlusive disease. However, cases of life threatening pulmonary oedema have been reported with vasodilators (mainly prostacyclin) when used in those patients. Consequently, should signs of pulmonary oedema occur when bosentan is administered in patients with pulmonary hypertension, the possibility of associated veno-occlusive disease should be considered.

Pulmonary arterial hypertension patients with concomitant left ventricular failure

No specific study has been performed in patients with pulmonary hypertension and concomitant left ventricular dysfunction. However, 1,611 patients (804 Tracleer- and 807 placebo-treated patients) with severe chronic heart failure (CHF) were treated for a mean duration of 1.5 years in a placebo-controlled study (study AC-052-301/302 [ENABLE 1 and 2]). In this study there was an increased incidence of hospitalisation due to CHF during the first 4–8 weeks of treatment with Tracleer, which could have been the result of fluid retention. In this study, fluid retention was manifested by early weight gain, decreased haemoglobin concentration and increased incidence of leg oedema. At the end of this study, there was no difference in overall hospitalisations for heart failure nor in mortality between Tracleer- and placebo-treated patients. Consequently, it is recommended that patients be monitored for signs of fluid retention (e.g., weight gain), especially if they concomitantly suffer from severe systolic dysfunction. Should this occur, starting treatment with diuretics is recommended, or the dose of existing diuretics should be increased. Treatment with diuretics should be considered in patients with evidence of fluid retention before the start of treatment with Tracleer.

Concomitant use with other medicinal products

Glibenclamide: Tracleer should not be used concomitantly with glibenclamide, due to an increased risk of elevated liver aminotransferases (see section 4.5). An alternative antidiabetic medicinal product should be used in patients in whom an antidiabetic treatment is indicated.

Fluconazole: concomitant use of Tracleer with fluconazole is not recommended (see section 4.5). Although not studied, this combination may lead to large increases in plasma concentrations of bosentan.

Concomitant administration of both a CYP3A4 inhibitor and a CYP2C9 inhibitor should be avoided (see section 4.5).

4.5 Interaction with other medicinal products and other forms of Interaction

Bosentan is an inducer of the cytochrome P450 (CYP) isoenzymes CYP2C9 and CYP3A4. *In vitro* data also suggest an induction of CYP2C19. Consequently, plasma concentrations of substances metabolised by these isoenzymes will be decreased when Tracleer is co-administered. The possibility of altered efficacy of medicinal products metabolised by these isoenzymes should be considered. The dosage of these products may need to be adjusted after initiation, dose change or discontinuation of concomitant Tracleer treatment.

Bosentan is metabolised by CYP2C9 and CYP3A4. Inhibition of these isoenzymes may increase the plasma concentration of bosentan (see ketoconazole). The influence of CYP2C9 inhibitors on bosentan concentration has not been studied. The combination should be used with caution. Concomitant administration with fluconazole, which inhibits mainly CYP2C9, but to some extent also CYP3A4, could lead to large increases in plasma concentrations of bosentan. The combination is not recommended (see section 4.4). For the same reason, concomitant administration of both a potent CYP3A4 inhibitor (such as ketoconazole, itraconazole and ritonavir) and a CYP2C9 inhibitor (such as voriconazole) with Tracleer is not recommended (see section 4.4).

Hormonal contraceptives: no specific interaction studies have been performed with hormonal contraceptives (including oral, injectable, implantable and transdermal contraceptives). Because oestrogens and progestogens are partially metabolised by CYP450, there is a possibility of failure of contraception when Tracleer is co-administered. Therefore, women of childbearing potential must use an additional or an alternative reliable method of contraception when taking Tracleer (see sections 4.3 and 4.6).

Specific interaction studies have demonstrated the following:

Cyclosporine A: co-administration of Tracleer and cyclosporine A (a calcineurin inhibitor) is contraindicated (see section 4.3). Indeed, when co-administered, initial trough concentrations of bosentan were approximately 30-fold higher than those measured after bosentan alone. At steady state, bosentan plasma concentrations were 3- to 4-fold higher than with bosentan alone. The mechanism of this interaction is unknown. The blood concentrations of cyclosporine A (a CYP3A4 substrate) decreased by approximately 50%.

Tacrolimus, sirolimus: co-administration of tacrolimus or sirolimus and Tracleer has not been studied in man but co-administration of tacrolimus or sirolimus and Tracleer may result in increased plasma concentrations of bosentan in analogy to co-administration with cyclosporine A. Concomitant Tracleer may reduce the plasma concentrations of tacrolimus and sirolimus. Therefore, concomitant use of Tracleer and tacrolimus or sirolimus is not advisable. Patients in need of the combination should be closely monitored for adverse events related to Tracleer and for tacrolimus and sirolimus blood concentrations.

Glibenclamide: co-administration of Tracleer 125 mg twice daily for 5 days decreased the plasma concentrations of glibenclamide (a CYP3A4 substrate) by 40%, with potential significant decrease of the hypoglycaemic effect. The plasma concentrations of bosentan were also decreased by 29%. In addition, an increased incidence of elevated aminotransferases was observed in patients receiving concomitant therapy. Both glibenclamide and bosentan inhibit the bile salt export pump, which could explain the elevated aminotransferases. In this context, this combination should not be used (see section 4.4). No drug-drug interaction data are available with the other sulfonylureas.

Warfarin: co-administration of bosentan 500 mg twice daily for 6 days decreased the plasma concentrations of both S-warfarin (a CYP2C9 substrate) and R-warfarin (a CYP3A4 substrate) by 29% and 38%, respectively. Clinical experience of concomitant administration of bosentan with warfarin in patients with pulmonary arterial hypertension did not result in clinically relevant changes in International Normalized Ratio (INR) or warfarin dose (baseline versus end of the clinical studies). In addition, the frequency of changes in warfarin dose during the trials due to changes in INR or due to adverse events was similar among bosentan- and placebo-treated patients. No dose adjustment is needed for warfarin and similar oral anticoagulant agents when bosentan is initiated but intensified monitoring of INR is recommended, especially during bosentan initiation and the up-titration period.

Simvastatin: co-administration of Tracleer 125 mg twice daily for 5 days decreased the plasma concentrations of simvastatin (a CYP3A4 substrate), and its active β-hydroxy acid metabolite by 34% and 46%, respectively. The plasma concentrations of bosentan were not affected by concomitant simvastatin. Monitoring of cholesterol levels and subsequent dosage adjustment should be considered.

Ketoconazole: co-administration of Tracleer 62.5 mg twice daily for 6 days and ketoconazole, a potent CYP3A4 inhibitor, increased the plasma concentrations of bosentan approximately 2-fold. No dose adjustment of Tracleer is considered necessary. Although not demonstrated through *in vivo* studies, similar increases in bosentan plasma concentrations are expected with the other potent CYP3A4 inhibitors (such as itraconazole and ritonavir). However, when combined with a CYP3A4 inhibitor, patients who are poor metabolisers of CYP2C9 are at risk of increases in bosentan plasma concentrations that may be of higher magnitude, thus leading to potential harmful adverse events.

Digoxin: co-administration of bosentan 500 mg twice daily for 7 days decreased the AUC, C_{max} and C_{min} of digoxin by 12%, 9% and 23%, respectively. The mechanism for this interaction may be induction of P-glycoprotein. This interaction is unlikely to be of clinical relevance.

Epoprostenol: limited data obtained from a study (AC-052-356, BREATHE-3) in which 10 paediatric patients received the combination of Tracleer and epoprostenol indicate that after both single- and multiple-dose administration, the C_{max} and AUC values of bosentan were similar in patients with or without continuous infusion of epoprostenol (see section 5.1).

4.6 Pregnancy and lactation

Pregnancy

Studies in animals have shown reproductive toxicity (teratogenicity, embryotoxicity, see section 5.3). There are minimal data on the use of Tracleer in pregnant women from very few cases received in the post-marketing period. The potential risk for humans is still unknown, but Tracleer must be considered a human teratogen and must not be used during pregnancy. Women must not become pregnant for at least 3 months after stopping treatment with Tracleer. Tracleer is contraindicated in pregnancy (see section 4.3).

Women of childbearing potential must use reliable contraception during treatment with Tracleer and for at least 3 months after cessation of treatment. Tracleer may render hormonal contraceptives ineffective (see section 4.5). Therefore, women of childbearing potential must not use hormonal contraceptives as the sole method of contraception but must use an additional or an alternative reliable method of contraception. Monthly pregnancy tests during treatment with Tracleer are recommended.

Women who become pregnant while receiving Tracleer must be informed of the potential hazard to the foetus.

Use during lactation

It is not known whether bosentan is excreted into human milk. Nursing women taking Tracleer should be advised to discontinue breast-feeding.

4.7 Effects on ability to drive and use machines

No studies on the effect of Tracleer on the ability to drive and use machines have been performed. Tracleer may cause dizziness, which could influence the ability to drive or use machines.

4.8 Undesirable effects

Adverse events

All placebo-controlled trials

In eight placebo-controlled studies, six of which were for indications other than pulmonary arterial hypertension, a total of 677 patients were treated with bosentan at daily doses ranging from 100 mg to 2000 mg and 288 patients were treated with placebo. The foreseen duration of treatment ranged from 2 weeks to 6 months. The adverse drug reactions that occurred more frequently on bosentan than on placebo (⩾ 3% of bosentan-treated patients, with ⩾ 2% difference) were headache (15.8% vs 12.8%), flushing (6.6% vs 1.7%), abnormal hepatic function (5.9% vs 2.1%), leg oedema (4.7% vs 1.4%), and anaemia (3.4% vs 1.0%), all of which were dose related.

Placebo-controlled trials in pulmonary arterial hypertension

The table below shows the adverse drug reactions that occurred in ⩾ 3% of patients treated with Tracleer (125 and 250 mg twice daily) in placebo-controlled trials in pulmonary arterial hypertension, and which were more frequent in these patients:

Adverse drug reactions occurring in ⩾ 3% of patients, and more frequently in patients on Tracleer (125 and 250 mg twice daily), in placebo-controlled trials in pulmonary arterial hypertension

Body system / Adverse event	Placebo		Tracleer (all)	
	N = 80		N = 165	
	No.	%	No.	%
Respiratory, thoracic and mediastinal disorders				
Upper respiratory tract infection	9	11%	20	12%
Nasopharyngitis	6	8%	18	11%
Pneumonia	1	1%	5	3%
Cardiac disorders				
Oedema lower limb	4	5%	13	8%
Palpitations	1	1%	8	5%

Oedema	2	3%	7	4%
Gastrointestinal disorders				
Dyspepsia	-		7	4%
Dry mouth	1	1%	5	3%
Nervous system disorders				
Headache	16	20%	36	22%
Vascular disorders				
Flushing	4	5%	15	9%
Hypotension	3	4%	11	7%
Skin & subcutaneous tissue disorders				
Pruritus	-		6	4%
General disorders and administration site conditions				
Fatigue	1	1%	6	4%
Hepato-biliary disorders				
Hepatic function abnormal	2	3%	14	8%

Note: only AEs with onset from start of treatment to 1 calendar day after end of treatment are included. One patient could have had more than one AE.

At the recommended maintenance dose or double the dose (i.e., 125 or 250 mg twice daily) the adverse drug reactions that occurred more frequently with Tracleer than with placebo (in ⩾ 3% of Tracleer-treated patients, with ⩾ 2% difference) were nasopharyngitis, flushing, abnormal hepatic function, leg oedema, hypotension, palpitations, dyspepsia, fatigue and pruritus. Adverse drug reactions that occurred in ⩾ 1% and < 3% of these patients and more frequently on Tracleer than on placebo (⩾ 2% difference) were anaemia, gastro-oesophageal reflux disease and rectal haemorrhage, all 2.4% on Tracleer versus 0% on placebo.

Treatment discontinuations due to adverse events, during the clinical trials in patients with pulmonary arterial hypertension, at doses of 125 and 250 mg twice daily, were less frequent in Tracleer- than in placebo-treated patients (5.5% vs 10%, respectively).

Laboratory abnormalities

<u>Liver test abnormalities</u>

Bosentan has been associated with dose-related elevations in liver aminotransferases, i.e., aspartate and alanine aminotransferases. Liver enzyme changes generally occurred within the first 16 weeks of treatment, usually developed gradually, and were mainly asymptomatic. They returned, in all cases during the clinical programme, to pre-treatment levels, without sequelae, within a few days to 9 weeks either spontaneously or after dose reduction or discontinuation.

The mechanism of this adverse effect is unclear. These elevations in aminotransferases may reverse spontaneously while continuing treatment with the maintenance dose of Tracleer or after dose reduction, but interruption or cessation may be necessary (see section 4.4).

In eight placebo-controlled studies, six of which were for indications other than pulmonary arterial hypertension, elevations in liver aminotransferases by greater than 3 times the upper limit of normal (ULN) were observed in 11.2% of the bosentan-treated patients as compared to 1.8% of the placebo-treated patients. Bilirubin increases to > 3 × ULN were associated with aminotransferase increases > 3 × ULN) in 2 of 658 (0.3%) of patients treated with bosentan. Nine of the 74 bosentan-treated patients who had elevated liver aminotransferases > 3 × ULN) also had symptoms such as abdominal pain, nausea/vomiting, and fever.

In studies in patients with pulmonary arterial hypertension, the incidence of elevated liver aminotransferases > 3 × ULN) was 12.7% in bosentan-treated patients (N = 165), 11.6% in patients treated with 125 mg twice daily and 14.3% in patients treated with 250 mg twice daily. Eight-fold increases were seen in 2.1% of pulmonary arterial hypertension patients on 125 mg twice daily and 7.1% of pulmonary arterial hypertension patients on 250 mg twice daily.

<u>Haemoglobin</u>

The mean decrease in haemoglobin concentration from baseline to trial completion for the bosentan-treated patients was 0.9 g/dl and for the placebo-treated patients was 0.1 g/dl.

In eight placebo-controlled studies, clinically relevant decreases in haemoglobin > 15% decrease from baseline resulting in values < 11 g/dl) were observed in 5.6% of bosentan-treated patients as compared with 2.6% of placebo-treated patients. In patients with pulmonary arterial hypertension treated with doses of 125 and 250 mg twice daily, clinically relevant decreases in haemoglobin occurred in 3.0% and 1.3% of the bosentan- and placebo-treated patients, respectively.

<u>Post-Marketing Experience</u>

Based on an exposure of about 13,000 patients to Tracleer in the post-marketing period, the majority of adverse events have been similar to those reported in clinical trials.

Undesirable effects are ranked under headings of frequency using the following convention; very common (⩾1/10); common >1/100, <1/10); uncommon >1/1,000, ⩽1/100); rare >1/10,000, ⩽1/1,000); very rare (⩽1/10,000).

Gastrointestinal disorders:

Common: nausea.

Uncommon: vomiting, abdominal pain, diarrhoea.

Hepato-biliary disorders:

Uncommon: aminotransferase elevations associated with hepatitis and/or jaundice.

Skin and subcutaneous tissue disorders:

Uncommon: hypersensitivity reactions including dermatitis, pruritus and rash.

Immune system:

Rare: anaphylaxis and/or angioedema

4.9 Overdose

Bosentan has been administered as a single dose of up to 2400 mg to healthy subjects and up to 2000 mg/day for 2 months in patients with a disease other than pulmonary hypertension. The most common adverse event was headache of mild to moderate intensity.

There is no specific experience of overdose with Tracleer beyond the doses described above. Massive overdose may result in pronounced hypotension requiring active cardiovascular support.

5. PHARMACOLOGICAL PROPERTIES

5.1 Pharmacodynamic properties

Pharmacotherapeutic group: other antihypertensives, ATC code: C02KX01

<u>Mechanism of action</u>

Bosentan is a dual endothelin receptor antagonist (ERA) with affinity for both endothelin A and B (ET_A and ET_B) receptors. Bosentan decreases both pulmonary and systemic vascular resistance resulting in increased cardiac output without increasing heart rate.

The neurohormone endothelin-1 (ET-1) is one of the most potent vasoconstrictors known and can also promote fibrosis, cell proliferation, cardiac hypertrophy, and remodeling and is pro-inflammatory. These effects are mediated by endothelin binding to ET_A and ET_B receptors located in the endothelium and vascular smooth muscle cells. ET-1 concentrations in tissues and plasma are increased in several cardiovascular disorders and connective tissue diseases, including pulmonary arterial hypertension, scleroderma, acute and chronic heart failure, myocardial ischaemia, systemic hypertension and atherosclerosis, suggesting a pathogenic role of ET-1 in these diseases. In pulmonary arterial hypertension and heart failure, in the absence of endothelin receptor antagonism, elevated ET-1 concentrations are strongly correlated with the severity and prognosis of these diseases.

Bosentan competes with the binding of ET-1 and other ET peptides to both ET_A and ET_B receptors, with a slightly higher affinity for ET_A receptors (K_i = 4.1–43 nM) than for ET_B receptors (K_i = 38-730 nM). Bosentan specifically antagonises ET receptors and does not bind to other receptors.

<u>Efficacy</u>

Animal models

In animal models of pulmonary hypertension, chronic oral administration of bosentan reduced pulmonary vascular resistance and reversed pulmonary vascular and right ventricular hypertrophy. In an animal model of pulmonary fibrosis, bosentan reduced collagen deposition in the lungs.

Efficacy in adult patients with pulmonary arterial hypertension

Two randomised, double-blind, multi-centre, placebo-controlled trials have been conducted in 32 (Study AC-052-351) and 213 (Study AC-052-352, BREATHE-1) adult patients with WHO functional class III–IV pulmonary arterial hypertension (primary pulmonary hypertension or pulmonary hypertension secondary mainly to scleroderma). After 4 weeks of Tracleer 62.5 mg twice daily, the maintenance doses studied in these trials were 125 mg twice daily in AC-052-351 and 125 mg twice daily and 250 mg twice daily in AC-052-352.

Tracleer was added to patients' current therapy, which could include a combination of anticoagulants, vasodilators (e.g., calcium channel blockers), diuretics, oxygen, and digoxin, but not epoprostenol. Control was placebo plus current therapy.

The primary endpoint for each study was change in 6-minute walk distance at 12 weeks for the first study and 16 weeks for the second study. In both trials, treatment with Tracleer resulted in significant increases in exercise capacity. The placebo-corrected increases in walk distance compared to baseline were 76 metres (p = 0.02; t-test) and 44 metres (p = 0.0002; Mann-Whitney U test) at the primary endpoint of each trial, respectively. The differences between the two groups 125 mg twice daily and 250 mg twice daily were not statistically significant but there was a trend towards improved exercise capacity in the group treated with 250 mg twice daily.

The improvement in walk distance was apparent after 4 weeks of treatment, was clearly evident after 8 weeks of treatment and was maintained for up to 28 weeks of double-blind treatment in a subset of the patient population.

In a retrospective responder analysis based on change in walking distance, WHO functional class and dyspnoea of the 95 patients randomised to Tracleer 125 mg twice daily in the placebo-controlled trials, it was found that at week 8, 66 patients had improved, 22 were stable and 7 had deteriorated. Of the 22 patients stable at week 8, 6 improved at week 12/16 and 4 deteriorated compared with baseline. Of the 7 patients that deteriorated at week 8, 3 improved at week 12/16 and 4 deteriorated compared with baseline.

Invasive haemodynamic parameters were assessed in the first study only. Treatment with Tracleer led to a significant increase in cardiac index associated with a significant reduction in pulmonary artery pressure, pulmonary vascular resistance and mean right atrial pressure.

A reduction in symptoms of pulmonary arterial hypertension was observed with Tracleer treatment. Dyspnoea measurement during walk tests showed an improvement in Tracleer-treated patients. In the AC-052-352 trial, 92% of the 213 patients were classified at baseline as WHO functional class III and 8% as class IV. Treatment with Tracleer led to a WHO functional class improvement in 42.4% of patients (placebo 30.4%). The overall change in WHO functional class during both trials was significantly better among Tracleer-treated patients as compared with placebo-treated patients. Treatment with Tracleer was associated with a significant reduction in the rate of clinical worsening compared with placebo at 28 weeks (10.7% vs 37.1%, respectively; p = 0.0015).

Study performed in children with pulmonary arterial hypertension

One study has been conducted in children with pulmonary hypertension. Tracleer has been evaluated in an open-label non-controlled study in 19 paediatric patients with pulmonary arterial hypertension (AC-052-356, BREATHE-3: primary pulmonary hypertension 10 patients, and pulmonary arterial hypertension related to congenital heart diseases 9 patients). This study was primarily designed as a pharmacokinetic study (see section 5.2). Patients were divided into and dosed according to three body-weight groups (see section 4.2) for 12 weeks. Half of the patients in each group were already being treated with intravenous epoprostenol and the dose of epoprostenol remained constant for the duration of the trial. The age range was 3–15 years. Patients were in WHO functional class II (N = 15 patients, 79%) or class III (N = 4 patients, 21%) at baseline.

Haemodynamics were measured in 17 patients. The mean increase from baseline in cardiac index was 0.5 l/min/m^2, the mean decrease in mean pulmonary arterial pressure was 8 mmHg, and the mean decrease in pulmonary vascular resistance was 389 dyn·sec·cm^{-5}. These haemodynamic improvements from baseline were similar with or without co-administration of epoprostenol. Changes in exercise test parameters at week 12 from baseline were highly variable and none were significant.

Combination with epoprostenol

The combination of Tracleer and epoprostenol has been investigated in two studies: AC-052-355 (BREATHE-2) and AC-052-356 (BREATHE-3). AC-052-355 was a multi-centre, randomised, double-blind, parallel-group trial of Tracleer versus placebo in 33 patients with severe pulmonary arterial hypertension who were receiving concomitant epoprostenol therapy. AC-052-356 was an open-label, non-controlled trial; 10 of the 19 paediatric patients were on concomitant Tracleer and epoprostenol therapy during the 12-week trial. The safety profile of the combination was not different from the one expected with each component and the combination therapy was well tolerated in children and adults. The clinical benefit of the combination has not been demonstrated.

5.2 Pharmacokinetic properties

The pharmacokinetics of bosentan have mainly been documented in healthy subjects. Limited data in patients show that the exposure to bosentan in adult pulmonary arterial hypertension patients is approximately 2-fold greater than in healthy adult subjects.

In healthy subjects, bosentan displays dose- and time-dependent pharmacokinetics. Clearance and volume of distribution decrease with increased intravenous doses and increase with time. After oral administration, the systemic exposure is proportional to dose up to 500 mg. At higher oral doses C_{max} and AUC increase less than proportionally to the dose.

<u>Absorption</u>

In healthy subjects the absolute bioavailability of bosentan is approximately 50% and is not affected by food. The maximum plasma concentrations are attained within 3–5 hours.

Distribution

Bosentan is highly bound > 98%) to plasma proteins, mainly albumin. Bosentan does not penetrate into erythrocytes.

A volume of distribution (V_{ss}) of about 18 litres was determined after an intravenous dose of 250 mg.

Biotransformation and elimination

After a single intravenous dose of 250 mg, the clearance was 8.2 l/h. The terminal elimination half-life ($t_{1/2}$) is 5.4 hours.

Upon multiple dosing, plasma concentrations of bosentan decrease gradually to 50%–65% of those seen after single dose administration. This decrease is probably due to auto-induction of metabolising liver enzymes. Steady-state conditions are reached within 3–5 days.

Bosentan is eliminated by biliary excretion following metabolism in the liver by the cytochrome P450 isoenzymes, CYP2C9 and CYP3A4. Less than 3% of an administered oral dose is recovered in urine.

Bosentan forms three metabolites and only one of these is pharmacologically active. This metabolite is mainly excreted unchanged via the bile. In adult patients, the exposure to the active metabolite is greater than in healthy subjects. In patients with evidence of the presence of cholestasis, the exposure to the active metabolite may be increased.

Bosentan is an inducer of CYP2C9 and CYP3A4 and possibly also of CYP2C19 and the P-glycoprotein. *In vitro*, bosentan inhibits the bile salt export pump in hepatocyte cultures.

In vitro data demonstrated that bosentan had no relevant inhibitory effect on the CYP isoenzymes tested (CYP1A2, 2A6, 2B6, 2C8, 2C9, 2D6, 2E1, 3A4). Consequently, bosentan is not expected to increase the plasma concentrations of medicinal products metabolised by these isoenzymes.

Pharmacokinetics in special populations

Based on the investigated range of each variable, it is not expected that the pharmacokinetics of bosentan will be influenced by gender, body weight, race, or age in the adult population to any relevant extent. No kinetic data are available in children under 3 years.

Children

The pharmacokinetics of single and multiple oral doses were studied in paediatric patients with pulmonary arterial hypertension who were dosed on the basis of body weight (see sections 4.2 and 5.1). The exposure to bosentan decreased with time in a manner consistent with the known auto-induction properties of bosentan. The mean AUC (CV%) values of bosentan in paediatric patients treated with 31.25, 62.5 or 125 mg b.i.d. were 3496 (49), 5428 (79), and 6124 (27) ng·h/ml, respectively, and were lower than the value of 8149 (47) ng·h/ml observed in adult patients with pulmonary arterial hypertension receiving 125 mg b.i.d. At steady state the systemic exposure in paediatric patients weighing 10–20 kg, 20–40 kg and > 40kg were 43%, 67% and 75%, respectively, of the adult systemic exposure. The reason for this difference is unclear and possibly related to an increased hepatic metabolism and excretion. The consequences of these findings regarding hepatotoxicity are unknown. Gender and the concomitant use of intravenous epoprostenol had no significant effect on the pharmacokinetics of bosentan.

Hepatic impairment

In patients with mildly impaired liver function (Child-Pugh class A) no relevant changes in the pharmacokinetics have been observed. The steady state AUC of bosentan was 9% higher and the AUC of the active metabolite, Ro 48-5033, was 33% higher in patients with mild hepatic impairment than in healthy volunteers. The pharmacokinetics of bosentan have not been studied in patients with Child-Pugh class B or C hepatic impairment and Tracleer is contra-indicated in this patient population (see section 4.3).

Renal impairment

In patients with severe renal impairment (creatinine clearance 15–30 ml/min), plasma concentrations of bosentan decreased by approximately 10%. Plasma concentrations of bosentan metabolites increased about 2-fold in these patients as compared to subjects with normal renal function. No dose adjustment is required in patients with renal impairment. There is no specific clinical experience in patients undergoing dialysis. Based on physicochemical properties and the high degree of protein binding, bosentan is not expected to be removed from the circulation by dialysis to any significant extent (see section 4.2).

5.3 Preclinical safety data

A 2-year carcinogenicity study in mice showed an increased combined incidence of hepatocellular adenomas and carcinomas in males, but not in females, at plasma concentrations about 2 to 4 times the plasma concentrations achieved at the therapeutic dose in humans. In rats, oral administration of bosentan for 2 years produced a small, significant increase in the combined incidence of thyroid follicular cell adenomas and carcinomas in males, but not in females, at plasma concentrations about 9 to 14 times the plasma concentrations achieved at the therapeutic dose in humans. Bosentan was negative in tests for genotoxicity. There was evidence for a mild thyroid hormonal imbalance induced by bosentan in rats. However, there was no evidence of bosentan affecting thyroid function (thyroxine, TSH) in humans.

The effect of bosentan on mitochondrial function is unknown.

Bosentan has been shown to be teratogenic in rats at plasma levels higher than 1.5 times the plasma concentrations achieved at the therapeutic dose in humans. Teratogenic effects, including malformations of the head and face and of the major vessels, were dose dependent. The similarities of the pattern of malformations observed with other ET receptor antagonists and in ET knock-out mice indicate a class effect. Appropriate precautions must be taken for women of child-bearing potential (see sections 4.3, 4.4, 4.6).

In fertility studies in male and female rats at plasma concentrations 21 and 43 times, respectively, the expected therapeutic level in humans, no effects on sperm count, motility and viability, or on mating performance or fertility were observed, nor was there any adverse effect on the development of the pre-implantation embryo or on implantation.

6. PHARMACEUTICAL PARTICULARS

6.1 List of excipients

Tablet core:

Maize starch

Pregelatinised starch

Sodium starch glycollate

Povidone

Glycerol dibehenate

Magnesium stearate

Film coat:

Hypromellose

Glycerol triacetate

Talc

Titanium dioxide (E171)

Iron oxide yellow (E172)

Iron oxide red (E172)

Ethylcelluiose

6.2 Incompatibilities

Not applicable.

6.3 Shelf life

3 years

6.4 Special precautions for storage

Do not store above 30°C.

6.5 Nature and contents of container

PVC/PE/PVDC/aluminium-blisters containing 14 film-coated tablets.

62.5 mg: Cartons contain 14, 56 or 112 film-coated tablets.

PVC/PE/PVDC/aluminium-blisters containing 14 film-coated tablets.

125 mg: Cartons contain 56 or 112 film-coated tablets.

Not all pack sizes may be marketed.

6.6 Instructions for use and handling

No special requirements.

7. MARKETING AUTHORISATION HOLDER

Actelion Registration Ltd

BSI Building 13th Floor

389 Chiswick High Road

London W4 4AL

United Kingdom

8. MARKETING AUTHORISATION NUMBER(S)

EU/1/02/220/001

EU/1/02/220/002

EU/1/02/220/003

EU/1/02/220/004

EU/1/02/220/005

9. DATE OF FIRST AUTHORISATION/RENEWAL OF THE AUTHORISATION

15 May 2002

10. DATE OF REVISION OF THE TEXT

September 2004

Tracrium Injection

(GlaxoSmithKline UK)

1. NAME OF THE MEDICINAL PRODUCT

Tracrium Injection

2. QUALITATIVE AND QUANTITATIVE COMPOSITION

Atracurium Besilate HSE 10mg/ml

3. PHARMACEUTICAL FORM

Injection

4. CLINICAL PARTICULARS

4.1 Therapeutic indications

Tracrium is a highly selective, competitive or non-depolarising neuromuscular blocking agent. It is used as an adjunct to general anaesthesia or sedation in the intensive care unit (ICU), to relax skeletal muscles, and to facilitate tracheal intubation and mechanical ventilation.

4.2 Posology and method of administration

Route of administration: Intravenous injection or continuous infusion.

Used by injection in adults: Tracrium is administered by intravenous injection.

The dosage range recommended for adults is 0.3 to 0.6 mg/kg (depending on the duration of full block required) and will provide adequate relaxation for about 15 to 35 minutes.

Endotracheal intubation can usually be accomplished within 90 seconds from the intravenous injection of 0.5 to 0.6 mg/kg.

Full block can be prolonged with supplementary doses of 0.1 to 0.2 mg/kg as required. Successive supplementary dosing does not give rise to accumulation of neuromuscular blocking effect.

Spontaneous recovery from the end of full block occurs in about 35 minutes as measured by the restoration of the tetanic response to 95% of normal neuromuscular function.

The neuromuscular block produced by Tracrium can be rapidly reversed by standard doss of anticholinesterase agents, such as neostigmine and edrophonium, accompanied or preceded by atropine, with no evidence of recurarisation.

Use as an infusion in adults: After an initial bolus dose of 0.2 to 0.6mg/kg, Tracrium can be used to maintain neuromuscular block during long surgical procedures by administration as a continuous infusion at rates of 0.3 to 0.6mg/kg/hour.

Tracrium can be administered by infusion during cardiopulmonary bypass surgery at the recommended infusion rates. Induced hypothermia to a body temperature of 25°C to 26°C reduces the rate of inactivation of atracurium, therefore full neuromuscular block may be maintained by approximately half the original infusion rate at these low temperatures.

Tracrium is compatible with the following infusion solutions for the times stated below:

Infusion solution stability	*Period of*
Sodium Chloride Intravenous Infusion BP (0.9% w/v)	24 hours
Glucose Intravenous Infusion BP (5% w/v)	8 hours
Ringer's Injection USP	8 hours
Sodium Chloride (0.18%w/v) and Glucose (4% w/v) Intravenous Infusion BP	8 hours
Compound Sodium Lactate Intravenous Infusion BP (Hartmann's Solution for Injection)	4 hours

When diluted in these solutions to give atracurium besilate concentrations of 0.5 mg/ml and above, the resultant solutions will be stable in daylight for the stated periods at temperatures of up to 30°C.

Use in Children: The dosage in children over the age of one month is similar to that in adults on a bodyweight basis.

Use in Neonates: The use of Tracrium is not recommended in neonates since there are insufficient data available.

Use in the elderly: Tracrium may be used at standard dosage in elderly patients. It is recommended, however, that the initial dose be at the lower end of the range and that it be administered slowly.

Use in patients with reduced renal and/or hepatic function: Tracrium may be used at standard dosage at all levels of renal or hepatic function, including end stage failure.

Use in patients with cardiovascular disease: In patients with clinically significant cardiovascular disease, the initial dose of Tracrium should be administered over a period of 60 seconds.

Use in intensive care unit (ICU) patients: After an optional initial bolus dose of Tracrium of 0.3 to 0.6 mg/kg, Tracrium can be used to maintain neuromuscular block by administering a continuous infusion at rates of between 11 and 13 microgram/kg/min (0.65 to 0.78 mg/kg/hr). There may be wide inter-patient variability in dosage requirements and these may increase or decrease with time. Infusion rates as low as 4.5 microgram/kg/min (0.27 mg/kg/hr) or as high as 29.5 microgram/kg/min (1.77 mg/kg/hr) are required in some patients.

The rate of spontaneous recovery from neuromuscular block after infusion of Tracrium in ICU patients is independent of the duration of administration.

Spontaneous recovery to a train-of-four rati >0.75 (the ratio of the height of the fourth to the first twitch in a train-of-four) can be expected to occur in approximately 60 minutes. A range of 32 to 108 minutes has been observed in clinical trials.

Monitoring: In common with all neuromuscular blocking agents, monitoring of neuromuscular function is recommended during the use of Tracrium in order to individualise dosage requirements.

4.3 Contraindications

Tracrium should not be administered to patients known to have an allergic hypersensitivity to the drug.

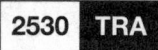

4.4 Special warnings and special precautions for use

Precautions: In common with all the other neuromuscular blocking agents, Tracrium paralyses the respiratory muscles as well as other skeletal muscles but has no effect on consciousness. Tracrium should be administered only with adequate general anaesthesia and only by or under the close supervision of an experienced anaesthetist with adequate facilities for endotracheal intubation and artificial ventilation.

In common with other neuromuscular blocking agents, the potential for histamine release exists in susceptible patients during Tracrium administration. Caution should be exercised in administering Tracrium to patients with a history suggestive of an increased sensitivity to the effects of histamine.

Monitoring of serial creatinine phosphate (cpk) values should be considered in asthmatic patients receiving high dose corticosteroids and neuromuscular blocking agents in ICU.

Tracrium does not have significant vagal or ganglionic blocking properties in the recommended dosage range. Consequently, Tracrium has no clinically significant effects on heart rate in the recommended dosage range and it will not counteract the bradycardia produced by many anaesthetic agents or by vagal stimulation during surgery.

In common with other non-depolarising neuromuscular blocking agents, increased sensitivity to atracurium may be expected in patients with myasthenia gravis and other forms of neuromuscular disease.

As with other neuromuscular blocking agents severe acid-base and/or serum electrolyte abnormalities may increase or decrease the sensitivity of patients to atracurium.

As with other non-depolarising neuromuscular blockers hypophosphataemia may prolong recovery. Recovery may be hastened by correcting this condition.

Tracrium should be administered over a period of 60 seconds to patients who may be unusually sensitive to falls in arterial blood pressure, for example those who are hypovolaemic.

Tracrium is inactivated by high pH and so must not be mixed in the same syringe with thiopental or any alkaline agent.

When a small vein is selected as the injection site, Tracrium should be flushed through the vein with physiological saline after injection. When other anaesthetic drugs are administered through the same in-dwelling needle or cannula as Tracrium it is important that each drug is flushed through with an adequate volume of physiological saline. Atracurium besilate is hypotonic and must not be administered into the infusion line of a blood transfusion.

Studies in malignant hyperthermia in susceptible animals (swine), and clinical studies in patients susceptible to malignant hypothermia indicate that Tracrium does not trigger this syndrome.

In common with other non-depolarising neuromuscular blocking agents, resistance may develop in patients suffering from burns. Such patients may require increased doses, dependent on the time elapsed since the burn injury and the extent of the burn.

Intensive Care Unit (ICU) patients: When administered to laboratory animals in high doses, Laudanosine, a metabolite of atracrium has been associated with transient hypotension and, in some species, cerebral excitatory effects. Although seizures have been seen in ICU patients receiving atracurium, a causal relationship to laudanosine has not been established (see Undesirable Effects).

Carcinogenicity: Carcinogenicity studies have not been performed.

Teratogenicity: Animal studies have indicated that Tracrium has no significant effects on foetal development.

Fertility: Fertility studies have not been performed.

4.5 Interaction with other medicinal products and other forms of Interaction

The neuromuscular block produced by Tracrium may be increased by the concomitant use of inhalational anaesthetics such as halothane, isoflurane and enflurane.

In common with all non-depolarising neuromuscular blocking agents the magnitude and/or duration of a non-depolarising neuromuscular block may be increased as a result of interaction with: antibiotics, including the aminoglycosides, polymyxins, spectinomycin, tetracyclines, lincomycin and clindamycin; antiarrhythmic drugs, propranolol, calcium channel blockers, lidocaine, procainamide and quinidine; diuretics: furosemide and possibly mannitol, thiazide diuretics and acetazolamide; magnesium sulphate, ketamine, lithium salts, ganglion blocking agents, trimetaphan, hexamethonium.

Rarely certain drugs may aggravate or unmask latent myasthenia gravis or actually induce a myasthenic syndrome; increased sensitivity to Tracrium would be consequent on such a development. Such drugs include various antibiotics, β-blockers (propranolol, oxprenolol), antiarrhythmic drugs (procainamide, quinidine), antirheumatic drugs (chloroquine, D-penicillamine), trimetaphan, chlorpromazine, steroids, phenytoin and lithium.

The onset of non-depolarising neuromuscular block is likely to be lengthened and the duration of block shortened in patients receiving chronic anticonvulsant therapy.

The administration of combinations of non-depolarising neuromuscular blocking agents in conjunction with Tracrium may produce a degree of neuromuscular blockage in excess of that which might be expected were an equipotent total dose of Tracrium administered. Any synergistic effect may vary between different drug combinations.

A depolarising muscle relaxant such as suxamethonium chloride should not be administered to prolong the neuromuscular blocking effects of non-depolarising blocking agents such as atracurium, as this may result in a prolonged and complex block which can be difficult to reverse with anticholinesterase drugs.

4.6 Pregnancy and lactation

In common with all neuromuscular blocking agents, Tracrium should be used during pregnancy only if the potential benefit to the mother outweighs any potential risk to the foetus.

Tracrium is suitable for maintenance of muscle relaxation during Caesarean section as it does not cross the placenta in clinically significant amounts following recommended doses. It is not known whether Tracrium is excreted in human milk.

4.7 Effects on ability to drive and use machines

None known.

4.8 Undesirable effects

Associated with the use of Tracrium there have been reports of skin flushing and mild transient hypotension or bronchospasm, which have been attributed to histamine release. Very rarely, severe anaphylactoid reactions have been reported in patients receiving Tracrium in conjunction with one or more anaesthetic agents.

There have been rare reports of seizures in ICU patients who have been receiving atracurium concurrently with several other agents. These patients usually had one or more medical conditions predisposing to seizures (e.g. cranial trauma, cerebral oedema, viral encephalitis, hypoxic encephalopathy, uraemia). A causal relationship to laudanosine has not been established. In clinical trials, there appears to be no correlation between plasma laudanosine concentration and the occurrence of seizures.

There have been some reports of muscle weakness and/or myopathy following prolonged use of muscle relaxants in severely ill patients in the ICU. Most patients were receiving concomitant corticosteroids. These events have been seen infrequently in association with Tracrium. A causal relationship has not been established.

4.9 Overdose

Prolonged muscle paralysis and its consequences are the main signs of overdosage.

Treatment: It is essential to maintain a patient airway together with assisted positive pressure ventilation until spontaneous respiration is adequate. Full sedation will be required since consciousness is not impaired. Recovery may be hastened by the administration of anticholinesterase agents accompanied by atropine or glycopyrrolate, once evidence of spontaneous recovery is present.

5. PHARMACOLOGICAL PROPERTIES

5.1 Pharmacodynamic properties

Atracurium is a highly selective competitive (non-depolarising) neuromuscular blocking agent with an intermediate duration of action. Non-depolarising agents antagonise the neurotransmitter action of acetylcholine by binding with receptor sites on the motor-end-plate. Atracurium can be used in a wide range of surgical procedures and to facilitate controlled ventilation.

5.2 Pharmacokinetic properties

The pharmacokinetics of Atracurium in man are essentially linear with the 0.3-0.6 mg/kg dose range. The elimination half-life is approximately 20 minutes.

Atracurium is degraded spontaneously mainly by a non-enzymatic decomposition process (Hofmann elimination) which occurs at plasma pH and at body temperature and produces breakdown products which are inactive. Degradation also occurs by ester hydrolysis catalysed by non-specific esterases. Elimination of atracurium is not dependent on kidney or liver function.

The main breakdown products are laudanosine and a monoquaternary alcohol which have no neuromuscular blocking activity. The monoquaternary alcohol is degraded spontaneously by hofmann elimination and excreted by the kidney. Laudanosine is excreted by the kidney and metabolised by the liver. The half-life of laudanosine ranges from 3-6h in patients with normal kidney and liver function. It is about 15h in renal failure and is about 40h in renal and hepatic failure. Peak plasma levels of laudanosine are highest in patients without kidney or liver function and average 4 μg/ml with wide variation.

Concentration of metabolites are higher in ICU patients with abnormal renal and/or hepatic function (see Special Warnings and Special Precautions for Use). These metabolites do not contribute to neuromuscular block.

5.3 Preclinical safety data

There are no pre-clinical data of relevance to the prescriber which are additional to that already included in other sections of the SMPC.

6. PHARMACEUTICAL PARTICULARS

6.1 List of excipients

Benzene Sulphonic acid

Water for Injections

6.2 Incompatibilities

None

6.3 Shelf life

24 months

6.4 Special precautions for storage

Store between 2 and 8°C. Do not freeze. Keep container in the outer carton.

Any unused Tracrium from opened ampoules or vials should be discarded.

6.5 Nature and contents of container

Neutral glass ampoules or vials. Vials are closed with a rubber stopper, sealed with an aluminium collar and fitted with a plastic flip-off top. Pack sizes: Boxes of 5 × 2.5ml ampoules, 5 × 5ml ampoules and 2 × 25ml vials.

6.6 Instructions for use and handling

None

Administrative Data

7. MARKETING AUTHORISATION HOLDER

The Wellcome Foundation Ltd trading as:

GlaxoSmithKline UK

Stockley Park West

Uxbridge

Middlesex UB11 1BT

Glaxo Wellcome House

Berkeley Avenue

Greenford

Middlesex UB6 ONN

8. MARKETING AUTHORISATION NUMBER(S)

PL0003/0166

9. DATE OF FIRST AUTHORISATION/RENEWAL OF THE AUTHORISATION

12th January 1999

10. DATE OF REVISION OF THE TEXT

January 2005

11. Legal Status

POM

Tractocile 7.5 mg/ml Concentrate for Solution for Infusion

(Ferring Pharmaceuticals Ltd)

1. NAME OF THE MEDICINAL PRODUCT

TRACTOCILE 7.5 mg/ml concentrate for solution for infusion

2. QUALITATIVE AND QUANTITATIVE COMPOSITION

One ml solution contains 7.5 mg atosiban free-base in the form of atosiban acetate.

After dilution, the concentration of atosiban is 0.75 mg/ml.

For excipients, see section 6.1.

3. PHARMACEUTICAL FORM

Concentrate for solution for infusion

Visual appearance: clear, colourless solution without particles.

4. CLINICAL PARTICULARS

4.1 Therapeutic indications

TRACTOCILE is indicated to delay imminent pre-term birth in pregnant women with:

– regular uterine contractions of at least 30 seconds duration at a rate of ⩾ 4 per 30 minutes

– a cervical dilation of 1 to 3 cm (0-3 for nulliparas) and effacement of ⩾ 50%

– age ⩾ 18 years

– a gestational age from 24 until 33 completed weeks

– a normal fetal heart rate

4.2 Posology and method of administration

Treatment with TRACTOCILE should be initiated and maintained by a physician experienced in the treatment of pre-term labour.

TRACTOCILE is administered intravenously in three successive stages: an initial bolus dose (6.75 mg), performed with TRACTOCILE 7.5 mg/ml solution for injection, immediately followed by a continuous high dose infusion (loading infusion 300 micrograms/min) of TRACTOCILE 7.5 mg/ml concentrate for solution for infusion during three hours, followed by a lower dose of TRACTOCILE 7.5 mg/ml concentrate for solution for infusion (subsequent infusion 100 micrograms/min) up to 45 hours. The duration of the treatment should not exceed 48 hours. The total dose given during a full course of TRACTOCILE therapy should preferably not exceed 330 mg of the active substance.

Intravenous therapy using the initial bolus injection of TRACTOCILE 7.5 mg/ml, solution for injection (see Summary of Product Characteristics of this product) should be started as soon as possible after diagnosis of pre-term labour. Once the bolus has been injected, proceed with the infusion. In the case of persistence of uterine contractions during treatment with TRACTOCILE, alternative therapy should be considered.

There is no data available regarding the need for dose adjustments in patients with renal or liver insufficiency.

The following table shows the full posology of the bolus injection followed by the infusion:

(see Table 1 below)

Re-treatment

In case a re-treatment with atosiban is needed, it should also commence with a bolus injection of TRACTOCILE 7.5 mg/ml, solution for injection followed by infusion with TRACTOCILE 7.5 mg/ml, concentrate for solution for infusion.

4.3 Contraindications

TRACTOCILE should not be used in the following conditions:

– Gestational age below 24 or over 33 completed weeks
– Premature rupture of the membranes >30 weeks of gestation
– Intrauterine growth retardation and abnormal fetal heart rate
– Antepartum uterine haemorrhage requiring immediate delivery
– Eclampsia and severe pre-eclampsia requiring delivery
– Intrauterine fetal death
– Suspected intrauterine infection
– Placenta praevia
– Abruptio placenta
– Any other conditions of the mother or fetus, in which continuation of pregnancy is hazardous
– Known hypersensitivity to the active substance or any of the excipients.

4.4 Special warnings and special precautions for use

When atosiban is used in patients in whom premature rupture of membranes cannot be excluded, the benefits of delaying delivery should be balanced against the potential risk of chorioamnionitis.

There is no experience with atosiban treatment in patients with impaired function of the liver or kidneys (see sections 4.2 and 5.2).

Atosiban has not been used in patients with an abnormal placental site.

There is only limited clinical experience in the use of atosiban in multiple pregnancies or the gestational age group between 24 and 27 weeks, because of the small number of patients treated. The benefit of atosiban in these subgroups is therefore uncertain.

Re-treatment with TRACTOCILE is possible, but there is only limited clinical experience available with multiple re-treatments, up to 3 re-treatments (see section 4.2).

In case of intrauterine growth retardation, the decision to continue or reinitiate the administration of TRACTOCILE depends on the assessment of fetal maturity.

Monitoring of uterine contractions and fetal heart rate during administration of atosiban and in case of persistent uterine contractions should be considered.

As an antagonist of oxytocin, atosiban may theoretically facilitate uterine relaxation and postpartum bleeding therefore blood loss after delivery should be monitored. However, inadequate uterus contraction postpartum was not observed during the clinical trials.

4.5 Interaction with other medicinal products and other forms of Interaction

It is unlikely that atosiban is involved in cytochrome P450 mediated drug-drug interactions as *in vitro* investigations have shown that atosiban is not a substrate for the cytochrome P450 system, and does not inhibit the drug metabolising cytochrome P450 enzymes.

Interaction studies were performed in healthy, female volunteers with betamethasone and labetalol. No clinically relevant interaction was observed between atosiban and betamethasone. When atosiban and labetalol were co-administrated, C_{max} of labetalol was decreased by 36% and T_{max} increased by 45 minutes. However, the extent of labetalol bioavailability in terms of AUC did not change. The interaction observed has no clinical relevance. Labetalol had no effect on atosiban pharmacokinetics.

No interaction study has been performed with antibiotics, ergot alkaloids, and anti-hypertensive agents other than labetalol.

4.6 Pregnancy and lactation

Atosiban should only be used when pre-term labour has been diagnosed between 24 and 33 completed weeks of gestation.

In atosiban clinical trials no effects were observed on lactation. Small amounts of atosiban have been shown to pass from plasma into the breast milk of lactating women.

Embryo-fetal toxicity studies have not shown toxic effects of atosiban. No studies were performed that covered fertility and early embryonic development (see section 5.3).

4.7 Effects on ability to drive and use machines

Not applicable.

4.8 Undesirable effects

Possible undesirable effects of atosiban were described for the mother during the use of atosiban in clinical trials. The observed undesirable effects were generally of a mild severity. In total 48% of the patients treated with atosiban experienced undesirable effects.

For the newborn, the clinical trials did not reveal any specific undesirable effects of atosiban. The infant adverse events were in the range of normal variation and were comparable with both placebo and beta-mimetic group incidences.

The undesirable effects in the women were the following:

Very common (>1/10)	*Gastrointestinal disorders:* nausea.
Common (>1/100, <1/10)	*Metabolism and nutrition disorders:* hyperglycaemia *Nervous system disorders:* headache, dizziness *Cardiac disorders:* tachycardia *Vascular disorders:* hot flush, hypotension *Gastrointestinal disorders:* vomiting *General disorders and administration site conditions:* injection site reaction
Uncommon (>1/1,000, <1/100)	*Psychiatric disorders:* insomnia *Skin and subcutaneous tissue disorders:* pruritis, rash *General disorders and administration site conditions:* pyrexia
Rare (>1/10,000, <1/1,000)	Incidental cases of uterine haemorrhage/uterine atony were reported. The frequency did not exceed that of the control groups in clinical trials. One case of allergic reaction was reported, which was considered to be probably related to atosiban.

4.9 Overdose

Few cases of atosiban overdosing were reported, they occurred without any specific signs or symptoms. There is no known specific treatment in case of an overdose.

5. PHARMACOLOGICAL PROPERTIES

5.1 Pharmacodynamic properties

Pharmacotherapeutic group: Other gynecologicals, ATC code: G02CX01

TRACTOCILE contains atosiban (INN), a synthetic peptide ([Mpa^1,D-Tyr(Et)^2,Thr^4,Orn^8]-oxytocin) which is a competitive antagonist of human oxytocin at receptor level. In rats and guinea pigs, atosiban was shown to bind to oxytocin receptors, to decrease the frequency of contractions and the tone of the uterine musculature, resulting in a suppression of uterine contractions. Atosiban was also shown to bind to the vasopressin receptor, thus inhibiting the effect of vasopressin. In animals atosiban did not exhibit cardiovascular effects.

In human pre-term labour, atosiban at the recommended dosage antagonises uterine contractions and induces uterine quiescence. The onset of uterus relaxation following atosiban is rapid, uterine contractions being significantly reduced within 10 minutes to achieve stable uterine quiescence ($\leqslant$ 4 contractions/hour) for 12 hours.

Phase III clinical trials (CAP-001 studies) include data from 742 women who were diagnosed with pre-term labour at 23–33 weeks of gestation and were randomised to receive either atosiban (according to this labelling) or β-agonist (dose-titrated).

Primary endpoint: the primary efficacy outcome was the proportion of women remaining undelivered and not requiring alternative tocolysis within 7 days of treatment initiation. The data show that 59.6% (n=201) and 47.7% (n=163) of atosiban- and β-agonist-treated women (p=0.0004), respectively, were undelivered and did not require alternative tocolysis within 7 days of starting treatment. Most of the treatment failures in CAP-001 were caused by poor tolerability. Treatment failures caused by insufficient efficacy were significantly (p=0.0003) more frequent in atosiban (n=48, 14.2%) than in the β-agonist-treated women (n=20, 5.8%).

In the CAP-001 studies the probability of remaining undelivered and not requiring alternative tocolytics within 7 days of treatment initiation was similar for atosiban and beta-mimetics treated women at gestational age of 24-28 weeks. However, this finding is based on a very small sample (n=129 patients).

Secondary endpoints: secondary efficacy parameters included the proportion of women remaining undelivered within 48 h of treatment initiation. There was no difference between the atosiban and beta-mimetic groups with regard to this parameter.

Mean (SD) gestational age at delivery was the same in the two groups: 35.6 (3.9) and 35.3 (4.2) weeks for the atosiban and β-agonist groups, respectively (p=0.37). Admission to a neonatal intensive care unit (NICU) was similar for both treatment groups (approximately 30%), as was length of stay and ventilation therapy. Mean (SD) birth weight was 2491 (813) grams in the atosiban group and 2461 (831) grams in the β-agonist group (p=0.58).

Fetal and maternal outcome did apparently not differ between the atosiban and the β-agonist group, but the clinical studies were not powered enough to rule out a possible difference.

Of the 361 women who received atosiban treatment in the phase III studies, 73 received at least one re-treatment, 8 received at least 2 re-treatments and 2 received 3 re-treatments (see section 4.4).

As the safety and efficacy of atosiban in women with a gestational age of less than 24 completed weeks has not been established in controlled randomised studies, the treatment of this patient group with atosiban is not recommended (see section 4.3).

In a placebo-controlled study, fetal/infant deaths were 5/295 (1.7%) in the placebo group and 15/288 (5.2%) in the atosiban group, of which two occurred at five and eight months of age. Eleven out of the 15 deaths in the atosiban group occurred in pregnancies with a gestational age of 20 to 24 weeks, although in this subgroup patient distribution was unequal (19 women on atosiban, 4 on placebo). For women with a gestational age greater than 24 weeks there was no difference in mortality rate (1.7% in the placebo group and 1.5% in the atosiban group).

5.2 Pharmacokinetic properties

In healthy non-pregnant subjects receiving atosiban infusions (10 to 300 micrograms/min over 12 hours), the steady state plasma concentrations increased proportionally to the dose.

The clearance, volume of distribution and half-life were found to be independent of the dose.

In women in pre-term labour receiving atosiban by infusion (300 micrograms/min for 6 to 12 hours), steady state plasma concentrations were reached within one hour following the start of the infusion (mean 442 ± 73 ng/ml, range 298 to 533 ng/ml).

Following completion of the infusion, plasma concentration rapidly declined with an initial (t_α) and terminal (t_β) half-life of 0.21 ± 0.01 and 1.7 ± 0.3 hours, respectively. Mean value for clearance was 41.8 ± 8.2 litres/h. Mean value of volume of distribution was 18.3 ± 6.8 litres.

Plasma protein binding of atosiban is 46 to 48% in pregnant women. It is not known whether the free fraction in the maternal and fetal compartments differs substantially. Atosiban does not partition into red blood cells.

Atosiban passes the placenta. Following an infusion of 300 micrograms/min in healthy pregnant women at term, the fetal/maternal atosiban concentration ratio was 0.12.

Two metabolites were identified in the plasma and urine from human subjects. The ratios of the main metabolite M1 (des-(Orn^8, Gly-NH$_2$^{9})-[Mpa^1, D-Tyr(Et)^2, Thr^4]-oxytocin) to atosiban concentrations in plasma were 1.4 and 2.8 at the second hour and at the end of the infusion respectively. It is not known whether M1 accumulates in tissues. Atosiban is found in only small quantities in urine, its urinary concentration is about 50 times lower than that of M1. The proportion of atosiban eliminated in faeces is not known. Main metabolite M1 is apparently as potent as the parent compound in inhibiting oxytocin-induced uterine contractions *in vitro*. Metabolite M1 is excreted in milk (see section 4.6).

There is no experience with atosiban treatment in patients with impaired function of the liver or kidneys (see sections 4.2 and 4.4).

It is unlikely that atosiban inhibits hepatic cytochrome P450 isoforms in humans (see section 4.5).

5.3 Preclinical safety data

No systemic toxic effects were observed during the two-week intravenous toxicity studies (in rats and dogs) at doses which are approximately 10 times higher than the human therapeutic dose, and during the three-months toxicity studies in rats and dogs (up to 20 mg/kg/day s.c.). The highest atosiban subcutaneous dose not producing any adverse effects was approximately two times the therapeutic human dose.

No studies were performed that covered fertility and early embryonic development. Reproduction toxicity studies,

Table 1

Step	Regimen	Injection/infusion rate	Atosiban dose
1	0.9 ml intravenous bolus	over 1 minute	6.75 mg
2	3 hours intravenous loading infusion	24 ml/hour	18 mg/hour
3	subsequent intravenous infusion	8 ml/hour	6 mg/hour

with dosing from implantation up to late stage pregnancy, showed no effects on mothers and fetuses. The exposure of the rat fetus was approximately four times that received by the human fetus during intravenous infusions in women. Animal studies have shown inhibition of lactation as expected from the inhibition of action of oxytocin.

Atosiban was neither oncogenic nor mutagenic in *in vitro* and *in vivo* tests.

6. PHARMACEUTICAL PARTICULARS

6.1 List of excipients

Mannitol

Hydrochloric acid 1M

Water for injections

6.2 Incompatibilities

In the absence of compatibility studies, this medicinal product must not be mixed with other medicinal products except those mentioned in section 6.6.

6.3 Shelf life

2 years.

Once the vial has been opened, the dilution must be performed immediately.

Diluted solution for intravenous administration should be used within 24 hours after preparation.

6.4 Special precautions for storage

Store in a refrigerator (2°C - 8°C).

Store in the original package.

6.5 Nature and contents of container

One vial of concentrate for solution for infusion contains 5 ml solution, corresponding to 37.5 mg atosiban.

Colourless glass vials, clear borosilicated (type I) sealed with grey siliconised bromo-butyl rubber stopper, type I, and flip-off cap of polypropylene and aluminium.

6.6 Instructions for use and handling

The vials should be inspected visually for particulate matter and discoloration prior to administration.

Preparation of the intravenous infusion solution:

For intravenous infusion, following the bolus dose, TRACTOCILE 7.5 mg/ml, concentrate for solution for infusion should be diluted in one of the following solutions:

- 0.9% w/v NaCl
- Ringer's lactate solution
- 5% w/v glucose solution.

Withdraw 10 ml solution from a 100 ml infusion bag and discard. Replace it by 10 ml TRACTOCILE 7.5 mg/ml concentrate for solution for infusion from two 5 ml vials to obtain a concentration of 75 mg atosiban in 100 ml.

The reconstituted product is a clear, colourless solution without particles.

The loading infusion is given by infusing 24 ml/hour (i.e. 18 mg/h) of the above prepared solution over the 3 hour period under adequate medical supervision in an obstetric unit. After three hours the infusion rate is reduced to 8 ml/hour.

Prepare new 100 ml bags in the same way as described to allow the infusion to be continued.

If an infusion bag with a different volume is used, a proportional calculation should be made for the preparation.

To achieve accurate dosing, a controlled infusion device is recommended to adjust the rate of flow in drops/min. An intravenous microdrip chamber can provide a convenient range of infusion rates within the recommended dose levels for TRACTOCILE.

In the absence of compatibility studies, this medicinal product must not be mixed with other medicinal products (see section 6.2). If other medicinal products need to be given intravenously at the same time, the intravenous cannula can be shared or another site of intravenous administration can be used. This permits the continued independent control of the rate of infusion.

7. MARKETING AUTHORISATION HOLDER

Ferring AB

Soldattorpsvägen 5

Box 30 047

SE - 20061 - Limhamn

Sweden.

8. MARKETING AUTHORISATION NUMBER(S)

EU/1/99/124/002.

9. DATE OF FIRST AUTHORISATION/RENEWAL OF THE AUTHORISATION

20 January 2005.

10. DATE OF REVISION OF THE TEXT

January 2005.

11. LEGAL CATEGORY

POM.

Tractocile 7.5 mg/ml Solution for Injection

(Ferring Pharmaceuticals Ltd)

1. NAME OF THE MEDICINAL PRODUCT

TRACTOCILE 7.5 mg/ml solution for injection

2. QUALITATIVE AND QUANTITATIVE COMPOSITION

One ml solution contains 7.5 mg atosiban free-base in the form of atosiban acetate.

For excipients, see section 6.1.

3. PHARMACEUTICAL FORM

Solution for injection

Visual appearance: clear, colourless solution without particles.

4. CLINICAL PARTICULARS

4.1 Therapeutic indications

TRACTOCILE is indicated to delay imminent pre-term birth in pregnant women with:

- regular uterine contractions of at least 30 seconds duration at a rate of ⩾ 4 per 30 minutes
- a cervical dilation of 1 to 3 cm (0-3 for nulliparas) and effacement of ⩾ 50%
- age ⩾ 18 years
- a gestational age from 24 until 33 completed weeks
- a normal fetal heart rate

4.2 Posology and method of administration

Treatment with TRACTOCILE should be initiated and maintained by a physician experienced in the treatment of pre-term labour.

TRACTOCILE is administered intravenously in three successive stages: an initial bolus dose (6.75 mg), performed with TRACTOCILE 7.5 mg/ml solution for injection, immediately followed by a continuous high dose infusion (loading infusion 300 micrograms/min) of TRACTOCILE 7.5 mg/ml concentrate for solution for infusion during three hours, followed by a lower dose of TRACTOCILE 7.5 mg/ml concentrate for solution for infusion (subsequent infusion 100 micrograms/min) up to 45 hours. The duration of the treatment should not exceed 48 hours. The total dose given during a full course of TRACTOCILE therapy should preferably not exceed 330 mg of the active substance.

Intravenous therapy using the initial bolus injection should be started as soon as possible after diagnosis of pre-term labour. Once the bolus has been injected, proceed with the infusion (See Summary of Product Characteristics of TRACTOCILE 7.5 mg/ml, concentrate for solution for infusion). In the case of persistence of uterine contractions during treatment with TRACTOCILE, alternative therapy should be considered.

There is no data available regarding the need for dose adjustments in patients with renal or liver insufficiency.

The following table shows the full posology of the bolus injection followed by the infusion:

(see Table 1 on next page)

Re-treatment

In case a re-treatment with atosiban is needed, it should also commence with a bolus injection of TRACTOCILE 7.5 mg/ml, solution for injection followed by infusion with TRACTOCILE 7.5 mg/ml, concentrate for solution for infusion.

4.3 Contraindications

TRACTOCILE should not be used in the following conditions:

- Gestational age below 24 or over 33 completed weeks
- Premature rupture of the membranes >30 weeks of gestation
- Intrauterine growth retardation and abnormal fetal heart rate
- Antepartum uterine haemorrhage requiring immediate delivery
- Eclampsia and severe pre-eclampsia requiring delivery
- Intrauterine fetal death
- Suspected intrauterine infection
- Placenta praevia
- Abruptio placenta
- Any other conditions of the mother or fetus, in which continuation of pregnancy is hazardous
- Known hypersensitivity to the active substance or any of the excipients.

4.4 Special warnings and special precautions for use

When atosiban is used in patients in whom premature rupture of membranes cannot be excluded, the benefits of delaying delivery should be balanced against the potential risk of chorioamnionitis.

There is no experience with atosiban treatment in patients with impaired function of the liver or kidneys (see sections 4.2 and 5.2).

Atosiban has not been used in patients with an abnormal placental site.

There is only limited clinical experience in the use of atosiban in multiple pregnancies or the gestational age group between 24 and 27 weeks, because of the small number of patients treated. The benefit of atosiban in these subgroups is therefore uncertain.

Re-treatment with TRACTOCILE is possible, but there is only limited clinical experience available with multiple re-treatments, up to 3 re-treatments (see section 4.2).

In case of intrauterine growth retardation, the decision to continue or reinitiate the administration of TRACTOCILE depends on the assessment of fetal maturity.

Monitoring of uterine contractions and fetal heart rate during administration of atosiban and in case of persistent uterine contractions should be considered.

As an antagonist of oxytocin, atosiban may theoretically facilitate uterine relaxation and postpartum bleeding therefore blood loss after delivery should be monitored. However, inadequate uterus contraction postpartum was not observed during the clinical trials.

4.5 Interaction with other medicinal products and other forms of Interaction

It is unlikely that atosiban is involved in cytochrome P450 mediated drug-drug interactions as *in vitro* investigations have shown that atosiban is not a substrate for the cytochrome P450 system, and does not inhibit the drug metabolising cytochrome P450 enzymes.

Interaction studies were performed in healthy, female volunteers with betamethasone and labetalol. No clinically relevant interaction was observed between atosiban and betamethasone. When atosiban and labetalol were co-administrated, C_{max} of labetalol was decreased by 36% and T_{max} increased by 45 minutes. However, the extent of labetalol bioavailability in terms of AUC did not change. The interaction observed has no clinical relevance. Labetalol had no effect on atosiban pharmacokinetics.

No interaction study has been performed with antibiotics, ergot alkaloids, and anti-hypertensive agents other than labetalol.

4.6 Pregnancy and lactation

Atosiban should only be used when pre-term labour has been diagnosed between 24 and 33 completed weeks of gestation.

In atosiban clinical trials no effects were observed on lactation. Small amounts of atosiban have been shown to pass from plasma into the breast milk of lactating women.

Embryo-fetal toxicity studies have not shown toxic effects of atosiban. No studies were performed that covered fertility and early embryonic development (see section 5.3).

4.7 Effects on ability to drive and use machines

Not applicable.

4.8 Undesirable effects

Possible undesirable effects of atosiban were described for the mother during the use of atosiban in clinical trials. The observed undesirable effects were generally of a mild severity. In total 48% of the patients treated with atosiban experienced undesirable effects.

For the newborn, the clinical trials did not reveal any specific undesirable effects of atosiban. The infant adverse events were in the range of normal variation and were comparable with both placebo and beta-mimetic group incidences.

The undesirable effects in the women were the following:

Very common (>1/10)	*Gastrointestinal disorders:* nausea.
Common (>1/100, <1/10)	*Metabolism and nutrition disorders:* hyperglycaemia *Nervous system disorders:* headache, dizziness *Cardiac disorders:* tachycardia *Vascular disorders:* hot flush, hypotension *Gastrointestinal disorders:* vomiting *General disorders and administration site conditions:* injection site reaction
Uncommon (>1/1,000, <1/100)	*Psychiatric disorders:* insomnia *Skin and subcutaneous tissue disorders:* pruritis, rash *General disorders and administration site conditions:* pyrexia
Rare (>1/10,000, <1/1,000)	Incidental cases of uterine haemorrhage/uterine atony were reported. The frequency did not exceed that of the control groups in clinical trials. One case of allergic reaction was reported, which was considered to be probably related to atosiban.

4.9 Overdose

Few cases of atosiban overdosing were reported, they occurred without any specific signs or symptoms. There is no known specific treatment in case of an overdose.

5. PHARMACOLOGICAL PROPERTIES

5.1 Pharmacodynamic properties

Pharmacotherapeutic group: Other gynecologicals, ATC code: G02CX01

TRACTOCILE contains atosiban (INN), a synthetic peptide ([Mpa^1,D-Tyr(Et)^2,Thr^4,Orn^8]-oxytocin) which is a competitive antagonist of human oxytocin at receptor level. In rats and guinea pigs, atosiban was shown to bind to oxytocin receptors, to decrease the frequency of contractions and

Table 1

Step	Regimen	Injection/infusion rate	Atosiban dose
1	0.9 ml intravenous bolus	over 1 minute	6.75 mg
2	3 hours intravenous loading infusion	24 ml/hour	18 mg/hour
3	subsequent intravenous infusion	8 ml/hour	6 mg/hour

the tone of the uterine musculature, resulting in a suppression of uterine contractions. Atosiban was also shown to bind to the vasopressin receptor, thus inhibiting the effect of vasopressin. In animals atosiban did not exhibit cardiovascular effects.

In human pre-term labour, atosiban at the recommended dosage antagonises uterine contractions and induces uterine quiescence. The onset of uterus relaxation following atosiban is rapid, uterine contractions being significantly reduced within 10 minutes to achieve stable uterine quiescence (≤ 4 contractions/hour) for 12 hours.

Phase III clinical trials (CAP-001 studies) include data from 742 women who were diagnosed with pre-term labour at 23–33 weeks of gestation and were randomised to receive either atosiban (according to this labelling) or β-agonist (dose-titrated).

Primary endpoint: the primary efficacy outcome was the proportion of women remaining undelivered and not requiring alternative tocolysis within 7 days of treatment initiation. The data show that 59.6% (n=201) and 47.7% (n=163) of atosiban- and β-agonist-treated women (p=0.0004), respectively, were undelivered and did not require alternative tocolysis within 7 days of starting treatment. Most of the treatment failures in CAP-001 were caused by poor tolerability. Treatment failures caused by insufficient efficacy were significantly (p=0.0003) more frequent in atosiban (n=48, 14.2%) than in the β-agonist-treated women (n=20, 5.8%).

In the CAP-001 studies the probability of remaining undelivered and not requiring alternative tocolytics within 7 days of treatment initiation was similar for atosiban and beta-mimetics treated women at gestational age of 24-28 weeks. However, this finding is based on a very small sample (n=129 patients).

Secondary endpoints: secondary efficacy parameters included the proportion of women remaining undelivered within 48 h of treatment initiation. There was no difference between the atosiban and beta-mimetic groups with regard to this parameter.

Mean (SD) gestational age at delivery was the same in the two groups: 35.6 (3.9) and 35.3 (4.2) weeks for the atosiban and β-agonist groups, respectively (p=0.37). Admission to a neonatal intensive care unit (NICU) was similar for both treatment groups (approximately 30%), as was length of stay and ventilation therapy. Mean (SD) birth weight was 2491 (813) grams in the atosiban group and 2461 (831) grams in the β-agonist group (p=0.58).

Fetal and maternal outcome did apparently not differ between the atosiban and the β-agonist group, but the clinical studies were not powered enough to rule out a possible difference.

Of the 361 women who received atosiban treatment in the phase III studies, 73 received at least one re-treatment, 8 received at least 2 re-treatments and 2 received 3 re-treatments (see section 4.4).

As the safety and efficacy of atosiban in women with a gestational age of less than 24 completed weeks has not been established in controlled randomised studies, the treatment of this patient group with atosiban is not recommended (see section 4.3).

In a placebo-controlled study, fetal/infant deaths were 5/295 (1.7%) in the placebo group and 15/288 (5.2%) in the atosiban group, of which two occurred at five and eight months of age. Eleven out of the 15 deaths in the atosiban group occurred in pregnancies with a gestational age of 20 to 24 weeks, although in this subgroup patient distribution was unequal (19 women on atosiban, 4 on placebo). For women with a gestational age greater than 24 weeks there was no difference in mortality rate (1.7% in the placebo group and 1.5% in the atosiban group).

5.2 Pharmacokinetic properties

In healthy non-pregnant subjects receiving atosiban infusions (10 to 300 micrograms/min over 12 hours), the steady state plasma concentrations increased proportionally to the dose.

The clearance, volume of distribution and half-life were found to be independent of the dose.

In women in pre-term labour receiving atosiban by infusion (300 micrograms/min for 6 to 12 hours), steady state plasma concentrations were reached within one hour following the start of the infusion (mean 442 ± 73 ng/ml, range 298 to 533 ng/ml).

Following completion of the infusion, plasma concentration rapidly declined with an initial (t_α) and terminal (t_β) half-life of 0.21 ± 0.01 and 1.7 ± 0.3 hours, respectively. Mean value for clearance was 41.8 ± 8.2 litres/h. Mean value of volume of distribution was 18.3 ± 6.8 litres.

Plasma protein binding of atosiban is 46 to 48% in pregnant women. It is not known whether the free fraction in the maternal and fetal compartments differs substantially. Atosiban does not partition into red blood cells.

Atosiban passes the placenta. Following an infusion of 300 micrograms/min in healthy pregnant women at term, the fetal/maternal atosiban concentration ratio was 0.12.

Two metabolites were identified in the plasma and urine from human subjects. The ratios of the main metabolite M1 (des-(Orn^8, Gly-NH$_2^9$)-[Mpa^1, D-Tyr(Et)^2, Thr^4]-oxytocin) to atosiban concentrations in plasma were 1.4 and 2.8 at the second hour and at the end of the infusion respectively. It is not known whether M1 accumulates in tissues. Atosiban is found in only small quantities in urine, its urinary concentration is about 50 times lower than that of M1. The proportion of atosiban eliminated in faeces is not known. Main metabolite M1 is apparently as potent as the parent compound in inhibiting oxytocin-induced uterine contractions *in vitro*. Metabolite M1 is excreted in milk (see section 4.6).

There is no experience with atosiban treatment in patients with impaired function of the liver or kidneys (see sections 4.2 and 4.4).

It is unlikely that atosiban inhibits hepatic cytochrome P450 isoforms in humans (see section 4.5).

5.3 Preclinical safety data

No systemic toxic effects were observed during the two-week intravenous toxicity studies (in rats and dogs) at doses which are approximately 10 times higher than the human therapeutic dose, and during the three-months toxicity studies in rats and dogs (up to 20 mg/kg/day s.c.). The highest atosiban subcutaneous dose not producing any adverse effects was approximately two times the therapeutic human dose.

No studies were performed that covered fertility and early embryonic development. Reproduction toxicity studies, with dosing from implantation up to late stage pregnancy, showed no effects on mothers and fetuses. The exposure of the rat fetus was approximately four times that received by the human fetus during intravenous infusions in women. Animal studies have shown inhibition of lactation as expected from the inhibition of action of oxytocin.

Atosiban was neither oncogenic nor mutagenic in *in vitro* and *in vivo* tests.

6. PHARMACEUTICAL PARTICULARS

6.1 List of excipients

Mannitol

Hydrochloric acid 1M

Water for injections

6.2 Incompatibilities

In the absence of compatibility studies, this medicinal product must not be mixed with other medicinal products.

6.3 Shelf life

2 years.

Once the vial has been opened, the product must be used immediately.

6.4 Special precautions for storage

Store in a refrigerator (2°C - 8°C).

Store in the original package.

6.5 Nature and contents of container

One vial of solution for injection contains 0.9 ml solution, corresponding to 6.75 mg atosiban.

Colourless glass vials, clear borosilicated (type I) sealed with grey siliconised bromo-butyl rubber stopper, type I, and flip-off cap of polypropylene and aluminium.

6.6 Instructions for use and handling

The vials should be inspected visually for particulate matter and discoloration prior to administration.

Preparation of the initial intravenous injection:

Withdraw 0.9 ml of a 0.9 ml labelled vial of TRACTOCILE 7.5 mg/ml, solution for injection and administer slowly as an intravenous bolus dose over one minute, under adequate medical supervision in an obstetric unit. The TRACTOCILE 7.5 mg/ml, solution for injection should be used immediately.

In the absence of compatibility studies, this medicinal product must not be mixed with other medicinal products (see section 6.2).

7. MARKETING AUTHORISATION HOLDER

Ferring AB

Soldattorpsvägen 5

Box 30 047

SE - 20061 - Limhamn

Sweden.

8. MARKETING AUTHORISATION NUMBER(S)

EU/1/99/124/001.

9. DATE OF FIRST AUTHORISATION/RENEWAL OF THE AUTHORISATION

20 January 2005.

10. DATE OF REVISION OF THE TEXT

January 2005.

11. LEGAL CATEGORY

POM.

Tramacet 37.5 mg/325 mg film-coated tablets

(Janssen-Cilag Ltd)

1. NAME OF THE MEDICINAL PRODUCT

TRAMACET® ▼37.5 mg/325 mg, film-coated tablets

2. QUALITATIVE AND QUANTITATIVE COMPOSITION

One film-coated tablet contains 37.5 mg tramadol hydrochloride and 325 mg paracetamol

For excipients, see 6.1.

3. PHARMACEUTICAL FORM

Film-coated tablet

Pale yellow film-coated tablet.

4. CLINICAL PARTICULARS

4.1 Therapeutic indications

Tramacet tablets are indicated for the symptomatic treatment of moderate to severe pain.

The use of Tramacet should be restricted to patients whose moderate to severe pain is considered to require a combination of tramadol and paracetamol (see also Section 5.1).

4.2 Posology and method of administration

Posology

ADULTS AND ADOLESCENTS (12 years and older)

The use of Tramacet should be restricted to patients whose moderate to severe pain is considered to require a combination of tramadol and paracetamol.

The dose should be individually adjusted according to intensity of pain and response of the patient.

An initial dose of two tablets of Tramacet is recommended. Additional doses can be taken as needed, not exceeding 8 tablets (equivalent to 300 mg tramadol and 2600 mg paracetamol) per day.

The dosing interval should not be less than six hours.

Tramacet should under no circumstances be administered for longer than is strictly necessary (see also section 4.4 - Special warnings and precautions for use). If repeated use or long term treatment with Tramacet is required as a result of the nature and severity of the illness, then careful, regular monitoring should take place (with breaks in the treatment, where possible), to assess whether continuation of the treatment is necessary.

Children

The effective and safe use of Tramacet has not been established in children below the age of 12 years. Treatment is therefore not recommended in this population.

Elderly patients

The usual dosages may be used although it should be noted that in volunteers aged over 75 years the elimination half life of tramadol was increased by 17% following oral administration. In patients over 75 years old, it is recommended that the minimum interval between doses should be not less than 6 hours, due to the presence of tramadol.

Renal insufficiency

Because of the presence of tramadol, the use of Tramacet is not recommended in patients with severe renal insufficiency (creatinine clearance <10 ml/min). In cases of moderate renal insufficiency (creatinine clearance between 10 and 30 ml/min), the dosing should be increased to 12-hourly intervals. As tramadol is removed only very slowly by haemodialysis or by haemofiltration, post dialysis administration to maintain analgesia is not usually required.

Hepatic insufficiency

In patients with severe hepatic impairment Tramacet should not be used (see Section 4.3). In moderate cases prolongation of the dosage interval should be carefully considered (see Section 4.4).

Method of administration

Oral use.

Tablets must be swallowed whole, with a sufficient quantity of liquid. They must not be broken or chewed.

4.3 Contraindications

- Hypersensitivity to tramadol, paracetamol or to any of the excipients (see 6.1. List of excipients) of the medicinal product,

- acute intoxication with alcohol, hypnotic drugs, centrally-acting analgesics, opioids or psychotropic drugs,

- Tramacet should not be administered to patients who are receiving monoamine oxidase inhibitors or within two weeks of their withdrawal (see 4.5. Interactions with other medicinal products and other forms of interaction),

- severe hepatic impairment,
- epilepsy not controlled by treatment (see. 4.4. Special Warnings).

4.4 Special warnings and special precautions for use

-Warnings:

- In adults and adolescents 12 years and older. The maximum dose of 8 tablets of Tramacet should not be exceeded. In order to avoid inadvertent overdose, patients should be advised not to exceed the recommended dose and not to use any other paracetamol (including over the counter) or tramadol hydrochloride containing products concurrently without the advice of a physician.
- In severe renal insufficiency (creatinine clearance <10 ml/mm), Tramacet is not recommended.
- In patients with severe hepatic impairment Tramacet should not be used (See Section 4.3). The hazards of paracetamol overdose are greater in patients with non-cirrhotic alcoholic liver disease. In moderate cases prolongation of dosage interval should be carefully considered.
- In severe respiratory insufficiency, Tramacet is not recommended.
- Tramadol is not suitable as a substitute in opioid-dependent patients. Although it is an opioid agonist, tramadol cannot suppress morphine withdrawal symptoms.
- Convulsions have been reported in tramadol-treated patients susceptible to seizures or taking other medications that lower the seizure threshold, especially selective serotonin re-uptake inhibitors, tricyclic antidepressants, antipsychotics, centrally acting analgesics or local anaesthesia. Epileptic patients controlled by a treatment or patients susceptible to seizures should be treated with Tramacet only if there are compelling circumstances. Convulsions have been reported in patients receiving tramadol at the recommended dose levels. The risk may be increased when doses of tramadol exceed the recommended upper dose limit.
- Concomitant use of opioid agonists-antagonists (nalbuphine, buprenorphine, pentazocine) is not recommended (see 4.5 Interactions with other medicinal products and other forms of interaction).

Precautions for use

Tramacet should be used with caution in opioid dependent patients, or in patients with cranial trauma, in patients prone to convulsive disorder, biliary tract disorders, in a state of shock, in an altered state of consciousness for unknown reasons, with problems affecting the respiratory centre or the respiratory function, or with an increased intracranial pressure.

Paracetamol in overdosage may cause hepatic toxicity in some patients.

At therapeutic doses, tramadol has the potential to cause withdrawal symptoms. Rarely, cases of dependence and abuse have been reported.

Symptoms of withdrawal reactions, similar to those occurring during opiate withdrawal may occur as follows: agitation, anxiety, nervousness, insomnia, hyperkinesia, tremor and gastrointestinal symptoms.

In one study, use of tramadol during general anaesthesia with enflurane and nitrous oxide was reported to enhance intra-operative recall. Until further information is available, use of tramadol during light planes of anaesthesia should be avoided.

4.5 Interaction with other medicinal products and other forms of Interaction

Concomitant use is contraindicated with:

• Non-selective MAO Inhibitors

Risk of serotoninergic syndrome: diarrhoea, tachycardia, sweating, trembling, confusion, even coma.

• Selective-A MAO Inhibitors

Extrapolation from non-selective MAO inhibitors

Risk of serotoninergic syndrome: diarrhoea, tachycardia, sweating, trembling, confusion, even coma.

• Selective-B MAO Inhibitors

Central excitation symptoms evocative of a serotoninergic syndrome: diarrhoea, tachycardia, sweating, trembling, confusion, even coma.

In case of recent treatment MAO inhibitors, a delay of two weeks should occur before treatment with tramadol

Concomitant use is not recommended with:

• Alcohol

Alcohol increases the sedative effect of opioid analgesics.

The effect on alertness can make driving of vehicles and the use of machines dangerous.

Avoid intake of alcoholic drinks and of medicinal products containing alcohol.

• Carbamazepine and other enzyme inducers

Risk of reduced efficacy and shorter duration due to decreased plasma concentrations of tramadol.

• Opioid agonists-antagonists (buprenorphine, nalbuphine, pentazocine)

Decrease of the analgesic effect by competitive blocking effect at the receptors, with the risk of occurrence of withdrawal syndrome.

Concomitant use which needs to be taken into consideration:

• In isolated cases there have been reports of Serotonin Syndrome in a temporal connection with the therapeutic use of tramadol in combination with other serotoninergic medicines such as selective serotonin re-uptake inhibitors (SSRIs) and triptans. Signs of Serotonin Syndrome may be for example, confusion, agitation, fever, sweating, ataxia, hyperreflexia, myoclonus and diarrhoea.

• Other opioid derivatives (including antitussive drugs and substitutive treatments), benzodiazepines and barbiturates.

Increased risk of respiratory depression which can be fatal in cases of overdose.

• Other central nervous system depressants, such as other opioid derivatives (including antitussive drugs and substitutive treatments), barbiturates, benzodiazepines, other anxiolytics, hypnotics, sedative antidepressants, sedative antihistamines, neuroleptics, centrally-acting antihypertensive drugs, thalidomide and baclofen.

These drugs can cause increased central depression. The effect on alertness can make driving of vehicles and the use of machines dangerous.

• As medically appropriate, periodic evaluation of prothrombin time should be performed when Tramacet and warfarin like compounds are administered concurrently due to reports of increased INR.

• Other drugs known to inhibit CYP3A4, such as ketoconazole and erythromycin, might inhibit the metabolism of tramadol (N-demethylation) probably also the metabolism of the active O-demethylated metabolite. The clinical importance of such an interaction has not been studied.

Medicinal products reducing the seizure threshold, such as bupropion, serotonin reuptake inhibitor antidepressants, tricyclic antidepressants and neuroleptics. Concomitant use of tramadol with these drugs can increase the risk of convulsions. The speed of absorption of paracetamol may be increased by metoclopramide or domperidone and absorption reduced by cholestyramine.

4.6 Pregnancy and lactation

Pregnancy:

Since Tramacet is a fixed combination of active ingredients including tramadol, it should not be used during pregnancy.

• Data regarding paracetamol:

Epidemiological studies in human pregnancy have shown no ill effects due to paracetamol used in the recommended dosages.

• Data regarding tramadol:

Tramadol should not be used during pregnancy as there is inadequate evidence available to assess the safety of tramadol in pregnant women. Tramadol administered before or during birth does not affect uterine contractility. In neonates it may induce changes in the respiratory rate which are usually not clinically relevant.

Lactation:

Since Tramacet is a fixed combination of active ingredients including tramadol, it should not be ingested during breast feeding.

• Data regarding paracetamol:

Paracetamol is excreted in breast milk but not in a clinically significant amount. Available published data do not contraindicate breast feeding by women using single ingredient medicinal products containing only paracetamol.

• Data regarding tramadol:

Tramadol and its metabolites are found in small amounts in human breast milk. An infant could ingest about 0.1% of the dose given to the mother. Tramadol should not be ingested during breast feeding.

4.7 Effects on ability to drive and use machines

Tramadol may cause drowsiness or dizziness, which may be enhanced by alcohol or other CNS depressants. If affected, the patient should not drive or operate machinery.

4.8 Undesirable effects

The most commonly reported undesirable effects during the clinical trials performed with the paracetamol/tramadol combination were nausea, dizziness and somnolence, observed in more than 10% of the patients.

-Cardiovascular system disorders:

- Uncommon (0.1%-1%): hypertension, palpitations, tachycardia, arrhythmia.

Central and peripheral nervous system disorders:

• Very common >10%): dizziness, somnolence

• Common (1%-10%): headache, trembling

• Uncommon (0.1%-1%): involuntary muscular contractions, paraesthesia, tinnitus

• Rare (<0.1%): ataxia, convulsions.

Psychiatric disorders:

• Common (1%-10%): confusion, mood changes (anxiety, nervousness, euphoria), sleep disorders

• Uncommon (0.1%-1%): depression, hallucinations, nightmares, amnesia

• Rare (<0.1%): drug dependence.

Vision disorders:

• Rare (<0.1%): blurred vision

Respiratory system disorders:

• Uncommon (0.1%-1%): dyspnoea

Gastro-intestinal disorders:

• Very common >10%): nausea

• Common (1%-10%): vomiting, constipation, dry mouth, diarrhoea, abdominal pain, dyspepsia, flatulence

• Uncommon (0.1%-1%): dysphagia, melaena.

Liver and biliary system disorders:

• Uncommon (0.1%-1%): hepatic transaminases increase.

Skin and appendages disorders:

• Common (1%-10%): sweating, pruritus

• Uncommon (0.1%-1%): dermal reactions (e.g. rash, urticaria).

Urinary system disorders:

• Uncommon (0.1%-1%): albuminuria, micturition disorders (dysuria and urinary retention).

Body as a whole:

• Uncommon (0.1%-1%): shivers, hot flushes, thoracic pain.

* Although not observed during clinical trials, the occurrence of the following undesirable effects known to be related to the administration of tramadol or paracetamol cannot be excluded:

Tramadol

• Postural hypotension, bradycardia, collapse (tramadol).

• Post-marketing surveillance of tramadol has revealed rare alterations of warfarin effect, including elevation of prothrombin times.

• Rare cases (< 0.1%): allergic reactions with respiratory symptoms (e.g. dyspnoea, bronchospasm, wheezing, angioneurotic oedema) and anaphylaxis.

• Rare cases (<0.1%): changes in appetite, motor weakness, and respiratory depression.

• Psychic side-effects may occur following administration of tramadol which vary individually in intensity and nature (depending on personality and duration of medication). These include changes in mood (usually elation, occasionally dysphoria), changes in activity (usually suppression, occasionally increase) and changes in cognitive and sensorial capacity (e.g. decision behaviour perception disorders).

• Worsening of asthma has been reported though a causal relationship has not been established.

• Symptoms of withdrawal reactions, similar to those occurring during opiate withdrawal may occur as follows: agitation, anxiety, nervousness, insomnia, hyperkinesia, tremor and gastrointestinal symptoms.

Paracetamol

• Adverse effects of paracetamol are rare but hypersensitivity including skin rash may occur. There have been reports of blood dyscrasias including thrombocytopenia and agranulocytosis, but these were not necessarily causally related to paracetamol.

• There have been several reports that suggest that paracetamol may produce hypoprothrombinaemia when administered with warfarin-like compounds. In other studies, prothrombin time did not change.

4.9 Overdose

Tramacet is a fixed combination of active ingredients. In case of overdose, the symptoms may include the signs and symptoms of toxicity of tramadol or paracetamol or of both these active ingredients.

- Symptoms of overdose from tramadol:

In principle, on intoxication with tramadol, symptoms similar to those of other centrally acting analgesics (opioids) are to be expected. These include in particular, miosis, vomiting, cardiovascular collapse, consciousness disorders up to coma, convulsions and respiratory depression up to respiratory arrest.

Miosis, vomiting, cardiovascular collapse, drowsiness including coma, convulsions and respiratory depression which could result in respiratory arrest.

- Symptoms of overdose from paracetamol:

An overdose is of particular concern in young children. Symptoms of paracetamol overdosage in the first 24 hours are pallor, nausea, vomiting, anorexia and abdominal pain. Liver damage may become apparent 12 to 48 hours after ingestion. Abnormalities of glucose metabolism and metabolic acidosis may occur. In severe poisoning, hepatic failure may progress to encephalophathy, coma and death. Acute renal failure with acute tubular necrosis may develop even in the absence of severe liver damage. Cardiac arrhythmias and pancreatitis have been reported.

Liver damage is possible in adults who have taken 7.5-10 g or more of paracetamol. It is considered that excess quantities of a toxic metabolite (usually adequately detoxified by glutathione when normal doses of paracetamol are ingested), become irreversibly bound to liver tissue.

<u>- Emergency treatment:</u>

- Transfer immediately to a specialised unit.
- Maintain respiratory and circulatory functions.

- Prior to starting treatment, a blood sample should be taken as soon as possible after overdose in order to measure the plasma concentration of paracetamol and tramadol and in order to perform hepatic tests.

- Perform hepatic tests at the start (of overdose) and repeat every 24 hours. An increase in hepatic enzymes (ASAT, ALAT) is usually observed, which normalizes after one or two weeks.

- Empty the stomach by causing the patient to vomit (when the patient is conscious) by irritation or gastric lavage.

- Supportive measures such as maintaining the patency of the airway and maintaining cardiovascular function should be instituted; naloxone should be used to reverse respiratory depression; fits can be controlled with diazepam.

- Tramadol is minimally eliminated from the serum by haemodialysis or haemofiltration. Therefore treatment of acute intoxication with Tramacet with haemodialysis or haemofiltration alone is not suitable for detoxification.

Immediate treatment is essential in the management of paracetamol overdose. Despite a lack of significant early symptoms, patients should be referred to hospital urgently for immediate medical attention and any adult or adolescent who had ingested around 7.5 g or more of paracetamol in the preceding 4 hours or any child who has ingested ⩾150 mg/kg of paracetamol in the preceding 4 hours should undergo gastric lavage. Paracetamol concentrations in blood should be measured later than 4 hours after overdose in order to be able to assess the risk of developing liver damage (via the paracetamol overdose nomogram). Administration of oral methionine or intravenous N-acetylcysteine (NAC) which may have a beneficial effect up to at least 48 hours after the overdose, may be required. Administration of intravenous NAC is most beneficial when initiated within 8 hours of overdose ingestion. However, NAC should still be given if the time to presentation is greater than 8 hours after overdose and continued for a full course of therapy. NAC treatment should be started immediately when massive overdose is suspected. General supportive measures must be available.

Irrespective of the reported quantity of paracetamol ingested, the antidote for paracetamol, NAC, should be administered orally or intravenously, as quickly as possible. If possible, within 8 hours following the overdose.

5. PHARMACOLOGICAL PROPERTIES

5.1 Pharmacodynamic properties

Pharmacotherapeutic group: Tramadol, combinations

ATC code: No 2A X 52

ANALGESICS

Tramadol is an opioid analgesic that acts on the central nervous system. Tramadol is a pure non selective agonist of the μ, δ, and κ opioid receptors with a higher affinity for the μ receptors. Other mechanisms which contribute to its analgesic effect are inhibition of neuronal reuptake of noradrenaline and enhancement of serotonin release. Tramadol has an antitussive effect. Unlike morphine, a broad range of analgesic doses of tramadol has no respiratory depressant effect. Similarly, the gastro-intestinal motility is not modified. The cardiovascular effects are generally slight. The potency of tramadol is considered to be one-tenth to one-sixth that of morphine.

The precise mechanism of the analgesic properties of paracetamol is unknown and may involve central and peripheral effects.

Tramacet is positioned as a step II analgesic in the WHO pain ladder and should be utilised accordingly by the physician.

5.2 Pharmacokinetic properties

Tramadol is administered in racemic form and the [-] and [+] forms of tramadol and its metabolite M1, are detected in the blood. Although tramadol is rapidly absorbed after administration, its absorption is slower (and its half-life longer) than that of paracetamol.

After a single oral administration of a tramadol/paracetamol (37.5 mg/325 mg) tablet, peak plasma concentrations of 64.3/55.5 ng/ml [(+)-tramadol/(-)-tramadol] and 4.2 μg/ml (paracetamol) are reached after 1.8 h [(+)-tramadol/(-)-tramadol] and 0.9 h (paracetamol) respectively. The mean elimination half-lives $t_{1/2}$ are 5.1/4.7 h [(+)-tramadol/(-)-tramadol] and 2.5 h (paracetamol).

During pharmacokinetic studies in healthy volunteers after single and repeated oral administration of Tramacet, no clinical significant change was observed in the kinetic parameters of each active ingredient compared to the parameters of the active ingredients used alone.

Absorption:

Racemic tramadol is rapidly and almost completely absorbed after oral administration. The mean absolute bioavailability of a single 100 mg dose is approximately 75%. After repeated administration, the bioavailability is increased and reaches approximately 90%.

After administration of Tramacet, the oral absorption of paracetamol is rapid and nearly complete and takes place mainly in the small intestine. Peak plasma concentrations of paracetamol are reached in one hour and are not modified by concomitant administration of tramadol.

The oral administration of Tramacet with food has no significant effect on the peak plasma concentration or extent of absorption of either tramadol or paracetamol so that Tramacet can be taken independently of meal times.

Distribution:

Tramadol has a high tissue affinity ($V_{d,\beta}$=203 ± 40 l). It has a plasma protein binding of about 20%.

Paracetamol appears to be widely distributed throughout most body tissues except fat. Its apparent volume of distribution is about 0.9 L/kg. A relative small portion (~20%) of paracetamol is bound to plasma proteins.

Metabolism:

Tramadol is extensively metabolised after oral administration. About 30% of the dose is excreted in urine as unchanged drug, whereas 60% of the dose is excreted as metabolites.

Tramadol is metabolised through *O*-demethylation (catalysed by the enzyme CYP2D6) to the metabolite M1, and through *N*-demethylation (catalysed by CYP3A) to the metabolite M2. M1 is further metabolised through N-demethylation and by conjugation with glucuronic acid. The plasma elimination half-life of M1 is 7 hours. The metabolite M1 has analgesic properties and is more potent than the parent drug. The plasma concentrations of M1 are several-fold lower than those of tramadol and the contribution to the clinical effect is unlikely to change on multiple dosing.

Paracetamol is principally metabolised in the liver through two major hepatic routes: glucuronidation and sulphation. The latter route can be rapidly saturated at doses above the therapeutic doses. A small fraction (less than 4%) is metabolised by cytochrome P 450 to an active intermediate (the N-acetyl benzoquinoneimine) which, under normal conditions of use, is rapidly detoxified by reduced glutathione and excreted in urine after conjugation to cysteine and mercapturic acid. However, during massive overdose, the quantity of this metabolite is increased.

Elimination:

Tramadol and its metabolites are eliminated mainly by the kidneys. The half-life of paracetamol is approximately 2 to 3 hours in adults. It is shorter in children and slightly longer in the newborn and in cirrhotic patients. Paracetamol is mainly eliminated by dose-dependent formation of gluco- and sulfo-conjugate derivatives. Less than 9% of paracetamol is excreted unchanged in urine. In renal insufficiency, the half-life of both compounds is prolonged.

5.3 Preclinical safety data

No preclinical study has been performed with the fixed combination (tramadol and paracetamol) to evaluate its carcinogenic or mutagenic effects or its effects on fertility.

No teratogenic effect that can be attributed to the medicine has been observed in the progeny of rats treated orally with the combination tramadol/paracetamol.

The combination tramadol/paracetamol has proven to be embryotoxic and foetotoxic in the rat at materno-toxic dose (50/434 mg/kg tramadol/paracetamol), i.e., 8.3 times the maximum therapeutic dose in man. No teratogenic effect has been observed at this dose. The toxicity to the embryo and the foetus results in a decreased foetal weight and an increase in supernumerary ribs. Lower doses, causing less severe materno-toxic effect (10/87 and 25/217 mg/kg tramadol/paracetamol) did not result in toxic effects in the embryo or the foetus.

Results of standard mutagenicity tests did not reveal a potential genotoxic risk for tramadol in man.

Results of carcinogenicity tests do not suggest a potential risk of tramadol for man.

Animal studies with tramadol revealed, at very high doses, effects on organ development, ossification and neonatal mortality, associated with maternotoxicity. Fertility reproductive performance and development of offspring were unaffected. Tramadol crosses the placenta. No effect on fertility has been observed after oral administration of tramadol up to doses of 50 mg/kg in the male rat and 75 mg/kg in the female rat.

Extensive investigations showed no evidence of a relevant genotoxic risk of paracetamol at therapeutic (i.e. non-toxic) doses.

Long-term studies in rats and mice yielded no evidence of relevant tumorigenic effects at non-hepatotoxic dosages of paracetamol.

Animal studies and extensive human experience to date yield no evidence of reproductive toxicity.

6. PHARMACEUTICAL PARTICULARS

6.1 List of excipients

Tablet core:

powdered cellulose

pregelatinised starch

sodium starch glycolate (Type A)

maize starch

magnesium stearate

Film-coating:

OPADRY yellow YS-1-6382 G (hypromellose, titanium dioxide (E171),

macrogol 400, yellow iron oxide (E172), polysorbate 80),

carnauba wax

6.2 Incompatibilities

Not applicable.

6.3 Shelf life

3 years in thermoformed blister packs of (polypropylene/aluminium) and of (polypropylene/polypropylene)

3 years in thermoformed blister packs of (PVC/aluminium)

6.4 Special precautions for storage

No special precautions for storage.

6.5 Nature and contents of container

Tramacet tablets are packed in transparent or white opaque PVC/PVDC/aluminium foil, white opaque polypropylene/aluminium foil or white opaque polypropylene/white opaque polypropylene blisters. Box of 2 tablets, or 10, 20, 30, 40, 50, 60, 70, 80, 90 and 100 tablets.

Not all packaging sizes may be marketed.

6.6 Instructions for use and handling

No special requirements.

7. MARKETING AUTHORISATION HOLDER

Janssen-Cilag Ltd

Saunderton

High Wycombe

Buckinghamshire

HP14 4HJ

UK

8. MARKETING AUTHORISATION NUMBER(S)

PL 0242/0384

9. DATE OF FIRST AUTHORISATION/RENEWAL OF THE AUTHORISATION

25 September 2003

10. DATE OF REVISION OF THE TEXT

24 September 2004

Trandate Injection

(UCB Pharma Limited)

1. NAME OF THE MEDICINAL PRODUCT

Trandate Injection

2. QUALITATIVE AND QUANTITATIVE COMPOSITION

Labetalol hydrochloride 5mg/ml.

3. PHARMACEUTICAL FORM

Solution for Injection

4. CLINICAL PARTICULARS

4.1 Therapeutic indications

Trandate Injection is indicated for the treatment of:-

1. Severe hypertension, including severe hypertension of pregnancy, when rapid control of blood pressure is essential.

2. Anaesthesia when a hypotensive technique is indicated.

3. Hypertensive episodes following acute myocardial infarction.

4.2 Posology and method of administration

Adults:

Trandate Injection is intended for intravenous use in hospitalised patients. The plasma concentrations achieved after intravenous dose of Trandate in severe hypertension are substantially greater than those following oral administration of the drug and provide a greater degree of blockade of alpha-adrenoceptors necessary to control the more severe disease. Patients should, therefore, always receive the drug whilst in the supine or left lateral position. Raising the patient into the upright position, within three hours of intravenous Trandate administration, should be avoided since excessive postural hypotension may occur.

Bolus injection

If it is essential to reduce blood pressure quickly, as for example, in hypertensive encephalopathy, a dose of 50mg of Trandate should be given by intravenous injection over a period of at least one minute. If necessary, doses of 50mg may be repeated at five minute intervals until a satisfactory response occurs. The total dose should not exceed 200mg. After bolus injection, the maximum effect usually occurs within five minutes and the effective duration of action is usually about six hours but may be as long as eighteen hours.

Intravenous infusion

An alternative method of administering Trandate is intravenous infusion of a solution made by diluting the contents of two ampoules (200mg) to 200ml with Sodium Chloride and Dextrose Injection BP or 5% Dextrose Intravenous Infusion BP. The resultant infusion solution contains 1mg/ml of Trandate. It should be administered using a paediatric giving set fitted with a 50ml graduated burette to facilitate dosage.

In the hypertension of pregnancy: The infusion can be started at the rate of 20mg per hour and this dose may be doubled every thirty minutes until a satisfactory reduction in blood pressure has been obtained or a dosage of 160mg per hour is reached. Occasionally, higher doses may be necessary.

In hypertensive episodes following acute myocardial infarction: The infusion should be commenced at 15mg per hour and gradually increased to a maximum of 120mg per hour depending on the control of blood pressure.

In hypertension due to other causes: The rate of infusion of Trandate should be about 2mg (2ml of infusion solution) per minute, until a satisfactory response is obtained; the infusion should then be stopped. The effective dose is usually in the range of 50-200mg depending on the severity of the hypertension. For most patients it is unnecessary to administer more than 200mg but larger doses may be required especially in patients with phaeochromocytoma. The rate of infusion may be adjusted according to the response, at the discretion of the physician. The blood pressure and pulse rate should be monitored throughout the infusion.

It is desirable to monitor the heart rate after injection and during infusion. In most patients, there is a small decrease in the heart rate; severe bradycardia is unusual but may be controlled by injecting atropine 1-2 mg intravenously. Respiratory function should be observed particularly in patients with any known impairment.

Once the blood pressure has been adequately reduced, maintenance therapy with Trandate tablets should be instituted with a starting dose of one 100mg tablet twice daily (see Trandate tablets SmPC for further details). Trandate Injection has been administered to patients with uncontrolled hypertension already receiving other hypotensive agents, including beta-blocking drugs, without adverse effects.

In hypotensive anaesthesia: Induction should be with standard agents (e.g. sodium thiopentone) and anaesthesia maintained with nitrous oxide and oxygen with or without halothane. The recommended starting dose of Trandate Injection is 10-20mg intravenously depending on the age and condition of the patient. Patients for whom halothane is contra-indicated usually require a higher initial dose of Trandate (25-30mg). If satisfactory hypotension is not achieved after five minutes, increments of 5-10mg should be given until the desired level of blood pressure is attained.

Halothane and Trandate act synergistically therefore the halothane concentration should not exceed 1-1.5% as profound falls in blood pressure may be precipitated.

Following Trandate Injection the blood pressure can be quickly and easily adjusted by altering the halothane concentration and / or adjusting table tilt. The mean duration of hypotension following 20-25mg of Trandate is fifty minutes.

Hypotension induced by Trandate Injection is readily reversed by atropine 0.6mg and discontinuation of halothane.

Tubocurarine and pancuronium may be used when assisted or controlled ventilation is required. Intermittent Positive Pressure Ventilation (IPPV) may further increase the hypotension resulting from Trandate Injection and / or halothane.

Children:

Safety and efficacy have not been established.

4.3 Contraindications

- Cardiogenic shock.
- Uncontrolled, incipient or digitalis refractory heart failure.
- Sick sinus syndrome (including sino-atrial block).
- Second or third degree heart block.
- Prinzmetal's angina.
- History of wheezing or asthma.
- Untreated phaeochromocytoma.
- Metabolic acidosis.
- Bradycardia (<45-50 bpm).
- Hypotension.
- Hypersensitivity to labetalol.
- Severe peripheral circulatory disturbances.
- Where peripheral vasoconstriction suggests low cardiac output, the use of Trandate Injection to control hypertensive episodes following acute myocardial infarction is contra-indicated.

4.4 Special warnings and special precautions for use

There have been reports of skin rashes and/ or dry eyes associated with the use of beta-adrenoceptor blocking drugs. The reported incidence is small and in most cases the symptoms have cleared when the treatment was withdrawn. Gradual discontinuance of the drug should be considered if any such reaction is not otherwise explicable.

There have been rare reports of severe hepatocellular injury with labetalol therapy. The hepatic injury is usually reversible and has occurred after both short and long term treatment. Appropriate laboratory testing should be done at the first sign or symptom of liver dysfunction. If there is laboratory evidence of liver injury or the patient is jaundiced, labetalol therapy should be stopped and not restarted.

Due to negative inotropic effects, special care should be taken with patients whose cardiac reserve is poor and heart failure should be controlled before starting Trandate therapy.

Patients particularly those with ischemic heart disease, should not interrupt/ discontinue abruptly Trandate therapy. The dosage should gradually be reduced, ie. over 1-2 weeks, if necessary at the same time initiating replacement therapy, to prevent exacerbation of angina pectoris. In addition, hypertension and arrhythmias may develop.

It is not necessary to discontinue Trandate therapy in patients requiring anaesthesia, but the anaesthetist must be informed and the patient should be given intravenous atropine prior to induction. During anaesthesia Trandate may mask the compensatory physiological responses to sudden haemorrhage (tachycardia and vasoconstriction). Close attention must therefore be paid to blood loss and the blood volume maintained. If beta-blockade is interrupted in preparation for surgery, therapy should be discontinued for at least 24 hours. Anaesthetic agents causing myocardial depression (eg. cyclopropane, trichloroethylene) should be avoided. Trandate may enhance the hypotensive effects of halothane.

In patients with peripheral circulatory disorders (Raynaud's disease or syndrome, intermittent claudication), beta-blockers should be used with great caution as aggravation of these disorders may occur.

Beta-blockers may induce bradycardia. If the pulse rate decreases to less than 50-55 beats per minute at rest and the patient experiences symptoms related to the bradycardia, the dosage should be reduced.

Beta-blockers, even those with apparent cardioselectivity, should not be used in patients with asthma or a history of obstructive airways disease unless no alternative treatment is available. In such cases the risk of inducing bronchospasm should be appreciated and appropriate precautions taken. If bronchospasm should occur after the use of Trandate it can be treated with a $beta_2$-agonist by inhalation, e.g. salbutamol (the dose of which may need to be greater than the usual in asthma) and, if necessary, intravenous atropine 1mg

Due to a negative effect on conduction time, beta-blockers should only be given with caution to patients with first degree heart block. Patients with liver or kidney insufficiency may need a lower dosage, depending on the pharmacokinetic profile of the compound. The elderly should be treated with caution, starting with a lower dosage but tolerance is usually good in the elderly.

Patients with a history of psoriasis should take beta-blockers only after careful consideration.

Risk of anaphylactic reaction: While taking beta-blockers, patients with a history of severe anaphylactic reaction to a variety of allergens may be more reactive to repeated challenge, either accidental, diagnostic or therapeutic. Such patients may be unresponsive to the usual doses of epinephrine use to treat allergic reaction.

The label will state "Do not take Trandate if you have a history of wheezing or asthma as it can make your breathing worse."

4.5 Interaction with other medicinal products and other forms of Interaction

Concomitant use not recommended:

- Calcium antagonists such as verapamil and to a lesser extent diltiazem have a negative influence on contractility and atrio-ventricular conduction.
- Digitalis glycosides used in association with beta-blockers may increase atrio-ventricular conduction time.
- Clonidine: Beta-blockers increase the risk of rebound hypertension. When clonidine is used in conjunction with non-selective beta-blockers, such as propranolol, treatment with clonidine should be continued for some time after treatment with the beta-blocker has been discontinued.
- Monoamineoxidase inhibitors (except MOA-B inhibitors).

Use with caution:

- Class I antiarrhythmic agents (eg. disopyramide, quinidine) and amiodarone may have potentiating effects on atrial conduction time and induce negative inotropic effect.
- Insulin and oral antidiabetic drugs may intensify the blood sugar lowering effect, especially of non-selective beta-blockers. Beta- blockade may prevent the appearance of signs of hypoglycaemia (tachycardia).
- Anaesthetic drugs may cause attenuation of reflex tachycardia and increase the risk of hypotension. Continuation of beta-blockade reduces the risk of arrhythmia during induction and intubation. The anaesthesiologist should be informed when the patient is receiving a beta-blocking agent. Anaesthetic agents causing myocardial depression, such as cyclopropane and trichlorethylene, are best avoided.
- Cimetidine, hydralazine and alcohol may increase the bioavailability of labetalol.

Take into account:

- Calcium antagonists: dihydropyridine derivates such as nifedipine. The risk of hypotension may be increased. In patients with latent cardiac insufficiency, treatment with beta-blockers may lead to cardiac failure.
- Prostaglandin synthetase inhibiting drugs may decrease the hypotensive effect of beta-blockers.
- Sympathicomimetic agents may counteract the effect of beta-adrenergic blocking agents.
- Concomitant use of tricyclic antidepressants, barbiturates, phenothiazines or other antihypertensive agents may increase the blood pressure lowering effect of labetalol. Concomitant use of tricyclic antidepressants may increase the incidence of tremor.
- Labetalol has been shown to reduce the uptake of radioisotopes of metaiodobenzylguanidine (MIBG), and may increase the likelihood of a false negative study. Care should therefore be taken in interpreting results from MIBG scintigraphy. Consideration should be given to withdrawing labetalol for several days at least before MIBG scintigraphy, and substituting other beta or alpha-blocking drugs.

4.6 Pregnancy and lactation

Although no teratogenic effects have been demonstrated in animals, Trandate should only be used during the first trimester of pregnancy if the potential benefit outweighs the potential risk.

Trandate crosses the placental barrier and the possibility of the consequences of alpha- and beta- adrenoceptor blockade in the foetus and neonate should be borne in mind. Perinatal and neonatal distress (bradycardia, hypotension, respiratory depression, hypoglycaemia, hypothermia) has been rarely reported. Sometimes these symptoms have developed a day or two after birth. Response to supportive measures (e.g. intravenous fluids and glucose) is usually prompt but with severe pre-eclampsia, particularly after prolonged intravenous labetalol, recovery may be slower. This may be related to diminished liver metabolism in premature babies.

Beta-blockers reduce placental perfusion, which may result in intrauterine foetal death, immature and premature deliveries. There is an increased risk of cardiac and pulmonary complications in the neonate in the post-natal period. Intra-uterine and neonatal deaths have been reported with Trandate but other drugs (e.g. vasodilators, respiratory depressants) and the effects of pre-eclampsia, intra-uterine growth retardation and prematurity were implicated. Such clinical experience warns against unduly prolonging high dose labetalol and delaying delivery and against co-administration of hydralazine.

Trandate is excreted in breast milk. Breast-feeding is therefore not recommended.

4.7 Effects on ability to drive and use machines

There are no studies on the effect of this medicine on the ability to drive. When driving vehicles or operating machines it should be taken into account that occasionally dizziness or fatigue may occur.

4.8 Undesirable effects

Trandate Injection is usually well tolerated. Excessive postural hypotension may occur if patients are allowed to assume an upright position within three hours of receiving Trandate Injection.

Most side-effects are transient and occur during the first few weeks of treatment with Trandate. They include headache, tiredness, dizziness, depressed mood and lethargy, nasal congestion, sweating, and rarely, ankle oedema. A tingling sensation in the scalp, usually transient, also may occur in a few patients early in treatment. Tremor has been reported in the treatment of hypertension of pregnancy. Acute retention of urine, difficulty in micturition, ejaculatory failure, epigastric pain, nausea and vomiting have been reported.

There have been rare reports of positive anti-nuclear antibodies unassociated with disease, cases of systemic lupus erythematosus, drug fever, toxic myopathy, hypersensitivity (rash, pruritus, angioedema and dyspnoea), reversible lichenoid rash, impaired vision, dry eyes, cramps, raised liver function tests, jaundice (both hepatocellular and cholestatic), hepatitis and hepatic necrosis, bradycardia and heart block.

Other possible side effects of beta-blockers are: heart failure, cold or cyanotic extremities, Raynaud's phenomenon, paraesthesia of the extremities, increase of an existing intermittent claudication, hallucinations, psychoses, confusion, sleep disturbances, nightmares, diarrhoea, bronchospasm (in patients with asthma or a history of asthma), masking of the symptoms of thyrotoxicosis or hypoglycaemia.

4.9 Overdose

Symptoms of overdosage are bradycardia, hypotension, bronchospasm and acute cardiac insufficiency.

After an overdose or in case of hypersensitivity, the patient should be kept under close supervision and be treated in an intensive-care ward. Artificial respiration may be required. Bradycardia or extensive vagal reactions should be treated by administering atropine or methylatropine. Hypotension and shock should be treated with plasma/ plasma substitutes and, if necessary, catecholamines. The beta-blocking effect can be counteracted by slow intravenous administration of isoprenaline hydrochloride, starting with a dose of approximately 5mcg/min, or dobutamine, starting with a dose of approximately 2.5mcg/min, until the required effect has been obtained. If this does not produce the desired effect, intravenous administration of 8-10 mg glucagon may be considered. If required the injection should be repeated within one hour, to be followed, if necessary, by an iv infusion of glucagon at 1-3mg/hour. Administration of calcium ions, or the use of a cardiac pacemaker, may also be considered.

Oliguric renal failure has been reported after massive overdosage of labetalol orally. In one case, the use of dopamine to increase the blood pressure may have aggravated the renal failure.

Labetalol does have membrane stabilising activity which may have clinical significance in overdosage.

Haemodialysis removes less than 1% labetalol hydrochloride from the circulation.

5. PHARMACOLOGICAL PROPERTIES

5.1 Pharmacodynamic properties

Labetalol lowers the blood pressure primarily by blocking peripheral arteriolar alpha-adrenoceptors thus reducing peripheral resistance and, by concurrent beta-blockade, protects the heart from reflex sympathetic drive that would otherwise occur. Cardiac output is not significantly reduced at rest or after moderate exercise. Increases in systolic blood pressure during exercise are reduced but corresponding changes in diastolic pressure are essentially normal.

In patients with angina pectoris co-existing with hypertension, the reduced peripheral resistance decreases myocardial afterload and oxygen demand. All these effects would be expected to benefit hypertensive patients and those with co-existing angina.

5.2 Pharmacokinetic properties

The plasma half-life of labetalol is about 4 hours. About 50% of labetalol in the blood is protein bound. Labetalol is metabolised mainly through conjugation to inactive glucuronide metabolites. These are excreted both in urine and via the bile into the faeces.

Only negligible amounts of the drug cross the blood brain barrier in animal studies.

5.3 Preclinical safety data

Not applicable since Trandate Injection has been used in clinical practice for many years and its effects in man are well known.

6. PHARMACEUTICAL PARTICULARS

6.1 List of excipients

Hydrochloric acid dilute

Sodium hydroxide

Water for Injection

6.2 Incompatibilities

Trandate injection has been shown to be incompatible with sodium bicarbonate injection BP 4.2% w/v

6.3 Shelf life

24 months

6.4 Special precautions for storage

Protect from light. Store below 30°C

6.5 Nature and contents of container

Type I Glass ampoules: 5 ampoules per pack. Pack size 20.

6.6 Instructions for use and handling

None

7. MARKETING AUTHORISATION HOLDER

UCB Pharma Limited

208 Bath Road

Slough

Berkshire

SL1 3WE

UK

8. MARKETING AUTHORISATION NUMBER(S)

PL 0039/0492

9. DATE OF FIRST AUTHORISATION/RENEWAL OF THE AUTHORISATION

1 November 1996/ 3 October 1999

10. DATE OF REVISION OF THE TEXT

June 2005

POM

Trandate Tablets 50mg, 100mg, 200mg or 400mg

(UCB Pharma Limited)

1. NAME OF THE MEDICINAL PRODUCT

Trandate Tablets 50mg, 100mg, 200mg or 400mg

2. QUALITATIVE AND QUANTITATIVE COMPOSITION

Each tablet contains 50mg, 100mg, 200mg or 400mg Labetalol hydrochloride

3. PHARMACEUTICAL FORM

Orange coloured, circular, biconvex film-coated tablets engraved Trandate 50, 100, 200 or 400 on one face

4. CLINICAL PARTICULARS

4.1 Therapeutic indications

Trandate Tablets are indicated for the treatment of:-

1. Mild, moderate or severe hypertension
2. Hypertension in pregnancy
3. Angina pectoris with existing hypertension

4.2 Posology and method of administration

Trandate tablets should be taken orally with food.

Adults:

Hypertension

Treatment should start with 100mg twice daily. In patients already being treated with antihypertensives and in those of low body weight this may be sufficient to control blood pressure. In others, increases in dose of 100mg twice daily should be made at fortnightly intervals. Many patients' blood pressure is controlled by 200mg twice daily and up to 800mg daily may be given as a twice daily regimen. In severe, refractory hypertension, daily doses up to 2400mg have been given. Such doses should be divided into a three or four times a day regimen.

Elderly

In elderly patients, an initial dose of 50mg twice daily is recommended. This has provided satisfactory control in some cases.

In the hypertension of pregnancy

The initial dose of 100mg twice daily may be increased, if necessary, at weekly intervals by 100mg twice daily. During the second and third trimester, the severity of the hypertension may require further dose titration to a three times daily regimen, ranging from 100mg tds to 400mg tds. A total daily dose of 2400mg should not be exceeded.

Hospital in-patients with severe hypertension, particularly of pregnancy, may have daily increases in dosage.

General

If rapid reduction of blood pressure is necessary, see the SPC for Trandate Injection. If long-term control of hypertension following the use of Trandate Injection is required, oral therapy with Trandate tablets should start with 100mg twice daily.

Additive hypotensive effects may be expected if Trandate tablets are administered together with other antihypertensives e.g. diuretics, methyldopa etc. When transferring patients from such agents, Trandate tablets should be introduced with a dosage of 100mg twice daily and the previous therapy gradually decreased. Abrupt withdrawal of clonidine or beta-blocking agents is undesirable.

Angina co-existing with hypertension

In patients with angina pectoris co-existing with hypertension, the dose of Trandate will be that required to control the hypertension.

Children:

Safety and efficacy in children have not been established.

4.3 Contraindications

- Cardiogenic shock.
- Uncontrolled, incipient or digitalis-refractory heart failure.
- Sick sinus syndrome (including sino-atrial block).
- Second or third degree heart block.
- Prinzmetal's angina.
- History of wheezing or asthma.
- Untreated phaeochromocytoma.
- Metabolic acidosis.
- Bradycardia (<45-50 bpm).
- Hypotension.
- Hypersensitivity to labetalol.
- Severe peripheral circulatory disturbances.

4.4 Special warnings and special precautions for use

There have been reports of skin rashes and/ or dry eyes associated with the use of beta-adrenoceptor blocking drugs. The reported incidence is small and in most cases the symptoms have cleared when the treatment was withdrawn. Gradual discontinuance of the drug should be considered if any such reaction is not otherwise explicable.

There have been rare reports of severe hepatocellular injury with labetalol therapy. The hepatic injury is usually reversible and has occurred after both short and long term treatment. Appropriate laboratory testing should be done at the first sign or symptom of liver dysfunction. If there is laboratory evidence of liver injury or the patient is jaundiced, labetalol therapy should be stopped and not restarted.

Due to negative inotropic effects, special care should be taken with patients whose cardiac reserve is poor and heart failure should be controlled before starting Trandate therapy.

Patients particularly those with ischemic heart disease, should not interrupt/ discontinue abruptly Trandate therapy. The dosage should gradually be reduced, ie. over 1-2 weeks, if necessary at the same time initiating replacement therapy, to prevent exacerbation of angina pectoris. In addition, hypertension and arrhythmias may develop.

It is not necessary to discontinue Trandate therapy in patients requiring anaesthesia but the anaesthetist must be informed and the patient should be given intravenous atropine prior to induction. If beta-blockade is interrupted in preparation for surgery, therapy should be discontinued for at least 24 hours. Anaesthetic agents causing myocardial depression (eg. cyclopropane, trichloroethylene) should be avoided. Trandate may enhance the hypotensive effects of halothane.

In patients with peripheral circulatory disorders (Raynaud's disease or syndrome, intermittent claudication), beta-blockers should be used with great caution as aggravation of these disorders may occur.

Beta-blockers may induce bradycardia. If the pulse rate decreases to less than 50-55 beats per minute at rest and the patient experiences symptoms related to the bradycardia, the dosage should be reduced.

Beta-blockers, even those with apparent cardioselectivity, should not be used in patients with asthma or a history of obstructive airways disease unless no alternative treatment is available. In such cases the risk of inducing bronchospasm should be appreciated and appropriate precautions taken. If bronchospasm should occur after the use of Trandate it can be treated with a $beta_2$-agonist by inhalation, e.g. salbutamol (the dose of which may need to be greater than the usual in asthma) and, if necessary, intravenous atropine 1mg.

Due to a negative effect on conduction time, beta-blockers should only be given with caution to patients with first degree heart block. Patients with liver or kidney insufficiency may need a lower dosage, depending on the pharmacokinetic profile of the compound. The elderly should be treated with caution, starting with a lower dosage but tolerance is usually good in the elderly.

Patients with a history of psoriasis should take beta-blockers only after careful consideration.

Risk of anaphylactic reaction: While taking beta-blockers, patients with a history of severe anaphylactic reaction to a variety of allergens may be more reactive to repeated challenge, either accidental, diagnostic or therapeutic. Such patients may be unresponsive to the usual doses of epinephrine used to treat allergic reaction.

The label will state "Do not take Trandate if you have a history of wheezing or asthma as it can make your breathing worse."

Trandate Tablets contain sodium benzoate which is a mild irritant to the eyes, nose and mucous membranes. It may increase the risk of jaundice in newborn babies.

4.5 Interaction with other medicinal products and other forms of Interaction

Concomitant use not recommended:

- Calcium antagonists such as verapamil and to a lesser extent diltiazem have a negative influence on contractility and atrio-ventricular conduction.
- Digitalis glycosides used in association with beta-blockers may increase atrio-ventricular conduction time.
- Clonidine: Beta-blockers increase the risk of rebound hypertension. When clonidine is used in conjunction with non-selective beta-blockers, such as propranolol, treatment with clonidine should be continued for some time after treatment with the beta-blocker has been discontinued.
- Monoamineoxidase inhibitors (except MOA-B inhibitors).

Use with caution:

- Class I antiarrhythmic agents (eg. disopyramide, quinidine) and amiodarone may have potentiating effects on atrial conduction time and induce negative inotropic effect.
- Insulin and oral antidiabetic drugs may intensify the blood sugar lowering effect, especially of non-selective beta-blockers. Beta- blockade may prevent the appearance of signs of hypoglycaemia (tachycardia).
- Anaesthetic drugs may cause attenuation of reflex tachycardia and increase the risk of hypotension. Continuation of beta-blockade reduces the risk of arrhythmia during induction and intubation. The anaesthesiologist should be informed when the patient is receiving a beta-blocking agent. Anaesthetic agents causing myocardial depression, such as cyclopropane and trichlorethylene, are best avoided.
- Cimetidine, hydralazine and alcohol may increase the bioavailability of labetalol.

Take into account:

- Calcium antagonists: dihydropyridine derivates such as nifedipine. The risk of hypotension may be increased. In patients with latent cardiac insufficiency, treatment with beta-blockers may lead to cardiac failure.
- Prostaglandin synthetase inhibiting drugs may decrease the hypotensive effect of beta-blockers.
- Sympathicomimetic agents may counteract the effect of beta-adrenergic blocking agents.
- Concomitant use of tricyclic antidepressants, barbiturates, phenothiazines or other antihypertensive agents may increase the blood pressure lowering effect of labetalol. Concomitant use of tricyclic antidepressants may increase the incidence of tremor.
- Labetalol has been shown to reduce the uptake of radioisotopes of metaiodobenzylguanidine (MIBG), and may increase the likelihood of a false negative study. Care should therefore be taken in interpreting results from MIBG scintigraphy. Consideration should be given to withdrawing labetalol for several days at least before MIBG scintigraphy, and substituting other beta or alpha-blocking drugs.

4.6 Pregnancy and lactation

Although no teratogenic effects have been demonstrated in animals, Trandate should only be used during the first trimester of pregnancy if the potential benefit outweighs the potential risk.

Trandate crosses the placental barrier and the possible consequences of alpha- and beta-adrenoceptor blockade in the foetus and neonate should be borne in mind. Perinatal and neonatal distress (bradycardia, hypotension, respiratory depression, hypoglycaemia, hypothermia) has been rarely reported. Sometimes these symptoms have developed a day or two after birth. Response to supportive measures (e.g. intravenous fluids and glucose) is usually prompt but with severe pre-eclampsia, particularly after prolonged intravenous labetalol, recovery may be slower. This may be related to diminished liver metabolism in premature babies.

Beta-blockers reduce placental perfusion, which may result in intrauterine foetal death, immature and premature deliveries. There is an increased risk of cardiac and pulmonary complications in the neonate in the post-natal period. Intra-uterine and neonatal deaths have been reported with Trandate but other drugs (e.g. vasodilators, respiratory depressants) and the effects of pre-eclampsia, intra-uterine growth retardation and prematurity were implicated. Such clinical experience warns against unduly prolonging high dose labetalol and delaying delivery and against co-administration of hydralazine.

Trandate is excreted in breast milk. Breast-feeding is therefore not recommended.

4.7 Effects on ability to drive and use machines

There are no studies on the effect of this medicine on the ability to drive. When driving vehicles or operating machines it should be taken into account that occasionally dizziness or fatigue may occur.

4.8 Undesirable effects

Most side-effects are transient and occur during the first few weeks of treatment with Trandate. They include headache, tiredness, dizziness, depressed mood and lethargy, nasal congestion, sweating, and rarely, ankle oedema. Postural hypotension is uncommon except at very high doses or if the initial dose is too high or doses are increased too rapidly. A tingling sensation in the scalp, usually transient, also may occur in a few patients early in treatment. Tremor has been reported in the treatment of hypertension of pregnancy. Acute retention of urine, difficulty in micturition, ejaculatory failure, epigastric pain, nausea and vomiting have been reported.

There have been rare reports of positive anti-nuclear antibodies unassociated with disease, cases of systemic lupus erythematosus, drug fever, toxic myopathy, hypersensitivity (rash, pruritus, angioedema and dyspnoea), reversible lichenoid rash, impaired vision, dry eyes, cramps, raised liver function tests, jaundice (both hepatocellular and cholestatic), hepatitis and hepatic necrosis, bradycardia and heart block.

Other possible side effects of beta-blockers are: heart failure, cold or cyanotic extremities, Raynaud's phenomenon, paraesthesia of the extremities, increase of an existing intermittent claudication, hallucinations, psychoses, confusion, sleep disturbances, nightmares, diarrhoea, bronchospasm (in patients with asthma or a history of asthma), masking of the symptoms of thyrotoxicosis or hypoglycaemia.

4.9 Overdose

Symptoms of overdosage are bradycardia, hypotension, bronchopasm and acute cardiac insufficency.

After ingestion of an overdose or in case of hypersensitivity, the patient should be kept under close supervision and be treated in an intensive-care ward. Absorption of any drug material still present in the gastro-intestinal tract can be prevented by gastric lavage, administration of activated charcoal and a laxative. Artificial respiration may be required. Bradycardia or extensive vagal reactions should be treated by administering atropine or methylatropine. Hypotension and shock should be treated with plasma/plasma substitutes and, if necessary, catecholamines. The beta-blocking effect can be counteracted by slow intravenous administration of isoprenaline hydrochloride, starting with a dose of approximately 5mcg/min, or dobutamine, starting with a dose of approximately 2.5mcg/min, until the required effect has been obtained. If this does not produce the desired effect, intravenous administration of 8-10 mg glucagon may be considered. If required the injection should be repeated within one hour, to be followed, if necessary, by an iv infusion of glucagon at 1-3mg/hour. Administration of calcium ions, or the use of a cardiac pacemaker, may also be considered.

Oliguric renal failure has been reported after massive overdosage of labetalol orally. In one case, the use of dopamine to increase the blood pressure may have aggravated the renal failure.

Labetalol does have membrane stabilising activity which may have clinical significance in overdosage.

Haemodialysis removes less than 1% labetalol hydrochloride from the circulation.

5. PHARMACOLOGICAL PROPERTIES

5.1 Pharmacodynamic properties

Labetalol lowers the blood pressure by blocking peripheral arteriolar alpha-adrenoceptors thus reducing peripheral resistance, and by concurrent beta-blockade, protects the heart from reflex sympathetic drive that would otherwise occur. Cardiac output is not significantly reduced at rest or after moderate exercise. Increases in systolic blood pressure during exercise are reduced but corresponding changes in diastolic pressure are essentially normal.

In patients with angina pectoris co-existing with hypertension, the reduced peripheral resistance decreases myocardial afterload and oxygen demand. All these effects would be expected to benefit hypertensive patients and those with co-existing angina.

5.2 Pharmacokinetic properties

The plasma half-life of labetalol is about 4 hours. About 50% of labetalol in the blood is protein bound. Labetalol is metabolised mainly through conjugation to inactive glucuronide metabolites. These are excreted both in urine and via the bile into the faeces.

Only negligible amounts of the drug cross the blood brain barrier in animal studies.

5.3 Preclinical safety data

Not applicable since Trandate Tablets have been used in clinical practice for many years and its effects in man are well known.

6. PHARMACEUTICAL PARTICULARS

6.1 List of excipients

Tablet Core:

Lactose

Magnesium stearate

Starch maize special

Starch maize pregelatinised

Film coating suspension:

Hydroxypropylmethylcellulose

Sodium benzoate

Titanium dioxide

Sunset yellow

Methyl hydroxybenzoate

Propyl hydroxybenzoate

IMS 740P

Purified Water

6.2 Incompatibilities

None stated

6.3 Shelf life

60 months

6.4 Special precautions for storage

No special storage conditions are necessary

6.5 Nature and contents of container

50 mg, 100mg, 200mg:

Calendar blister pack containing 56 tablets; composed of hard tempered aluminium foil and opaque PVC blister.

100 mg, 200mg:

Polypropylene container with tamper-evident polyethylene lid containing 250mg tablets.

400 mg:

Propylene container with tamper-evident polyethylene lids containing 56 or 250 tablets.

6.6 Instructions for use and handling

None

7. MARKETING AUTHORISATION HOLDER

UCB Pharma Ltd

208 Bath Road

Slough

Berkshire

SL1 3WE

UK

8. MARKETING AUTHORISATION NUMBER(S)

50 mg:

PL 00039/0493

100 mg:

PL 00039/0494

200 mg:

PL 00039/0495

400 mg:

PI 00039/0496

9. DATE OF FIRST AUTHORISATION/RENEWAL OF THE AUTHORISATION

1 November 1996/ 17 February 1999

10. DATE OF REVISION OF THE TEXT

June 2005.

11. Legal Category

POM

Tranexamic Acid 500 mg Film Coated Tablets

(Pharmacia Limited)

1. NAME OF THE MEDICINAL PRODUCT

Tranexamic Acid 500 mg film coated tablets

2. QUALITATIVE AND QUANTITATIVE COMPOSITION

Each tablet contains 500 mg tranexamic acid.

For excipients see section 6.1.

3. PHARMACEUTICAL FORM

Film-coated tablets

White, oblong tablets, 8x18 mm, engraved TX with an arc above and below the lettering, for oral use.

4. CLINICAL PARTICULARS

4.1 Therapeutic indications

Short-term use for haemorrhage or risk of haemorrhage in increased fibrinolysis or fibrinogenolysis. Local fibrinolysis as occurs in the following conditions:

Prostatectomy and bladder surgery

Menorrhagia

Epistaxis

Conisation of the cervix

Traumatic hyphaema

Hereditary angioneurotic oedema

Management of dental extraction in haemophiliacs

4.2 Posology and method of administration

Route of administration: Oral.

Local fibrinolysis: The recommended standard dosage is 15-25mg/kg bodyweight (i.e. 2-3 tablets) two to three times daily. For the indications listed below the following doses may be used:

1a. Prostatectomy: Prophylaxis and treatment of haemorrhage in high risk patients should commence per- or post-operatively with tranexamic acid injection; thereafter 2 tablets three to four times daily until macroscopic haematuria is no longer present.

1b. Menorrhagia: 2 tablets three times daily as long as needed for up to 4 days. If very heavy bleeding, dosage may be increased. A total dose of 4g daily (8 tablets) should not be exceeded. Tranexamic acid therapy is initiated only after heavy bleeding has started.

1c. Epistaxis: Where recurrent bleeding is anticipated oral therapy (2 tablets three times daily) should be administered for 7 days.

1d. Conisation of the cervix: 3 tablets three times daily.

1e. Traumatic hyphaema: 2-3 tablets three times daily. The dose is based on 25 mg/kg three times a day.

2. Haemophilia: In the management of dental extractions 2-3 tablets every eight hours. The dose is based on 25 mg/kg.

3. Hereditary angioneurotic oedema: Some patients are aware of the onset of the illness; suitable treatment for these patients is intermittently 2-3 tablets two to three times daily for some days. Other patients are treated continuously at this dosage.

Children's dosage: This should be calculated according to body weight at 25 mg/kg per dose.

Elderly patients: No reduction in dosage is necessary unless there is evidence of renal failure (see guidelines below).

Renal insufficiency: By extrapolation from clearance data relating to the intravenous dosage form, the following reduction in the oral dosage is recommended for patients with mild to moderate renal insufficiency.

Serum Creatinine (μmol/L)	Dose tranexamic acid
120-249	15mg/kg bodyweight twice daily
250-500	15mg/kg bodyweight/day

4.3 Contraindications

Severe renal failure because of risk of accumulation.

Hypersensitivity to tranexamic acid or any of the other ingredients.

Active thromboembolic disease.

4.4 Special warnings and special precautions for use

Patients with irregular menstrual bleeding should not use tranexamic acid until the cause of irregular bleeding has been established. If menstrual bleeding is not adequately reduced by tranexamic acid, an alternative treatment should be considered.

Patients with a previous thromboembolic event and a family history of thromboembolic disease (patients with thrombophilia) should use tranexamic acid only if there is a strong medical indication and under strict medical supervision.

The blood levels are increased in patients with increased renal insufficiency, therefore a dose reduction is recommended (see section 4.2).

In massive haematuria from the upper urinary tract (especially in haemophilia) since, in a few cases, ureteric obstruction has been reported.

When disseminated intravascular coagulation is in progress.

In the long-term treatment of patients with hereditary angioneurotic oedema, regular eye examinations (e.g. visual acuity, slit lamp, intraocular pressure, visual fields) and liver function tests should be performed.

The use of tranexamic acid in cases of increased fibrinolysis due to disseminated intravascular coagulation is not recommended.

Clinical experience with tranexamic acid in menorrhagic children under 15 years of age is not available.

4.5 Interaction with other medicinal products and other forms of Interaction

Tranexamic acid will counteract the thrombolytic effect of fibrinolytic preparations.

4.6 Pregnancy and lactation
Pregnancy
Although there is no evidence from animal studies of a teratogenic effect, the usual caution with the use of drugs in pregnancy should be observed. Tranexamic acid crosses the placenta.

Lactation
Tranexamic acid passes into breast milk to a concentration of approximately one hundredth of the concentration in the maternal blood. An antifibrinolytic effect in the infant is unlikely.

4.7 Effects on ability to drive and use machines
No effects on the ability to drive or use machines have been observed.

4.8 Undesirable effects
Gastrointestinal disorders (nausea, vomiting, diarrhoea) may occur but disappear when the dosage is reduced. Rare instances of colour vision disturbances have been reported. Patients who experience disturbance of colour vision should be withdrawn from treatment. Rare cases of thromboembolic events have been reported. Rare cases of allergic skin reactions have also been reported.

4.9 Overdose
Symptoms may be nausea, vomiting, orthostatic symptoms and/or hypotension. Initiate vomiting, then stomach lavage, and charcoal therapy. Maintain a high fluid intake to promote renal excretion. There is a risk of thrombosis in predisposed individuals. Anticoagulant treatment should be considered.

5. PHARMACOLOGICAL PROPERTIES
5.1 Pharmacodynamic properties
Tranexamic acid tablets contain tranexamic acid, an antifibrinolytic that is an inhibitor of the activation of plasminogen to plasmin in the fibrinolytic system. The treatment of menorrhagia is symptomatic since it does not affect the underlying pathogenesis of the increased menstrual flow.

5.2 Pharmacokinetic properties
The bioavailability is approximately 35% in the dose range of 0.5 – 2 gram and is not affected by simultaneous food intake. Following a single oral dose, C_{max} and urinary excretion increased linearly with doses between 0.5 and 2 gram. Following a single oral dose of 0.5 g, C_{max} is approximately 5 μg/ml and after a dose of 2 g, C_{max} is 15μg/ml.

Therapeutic concentration is maintained in plasma up to 6 hours after an oral single dose of 2 gram. Binding to plasma proteins (plasminogen) is approximately 3% at therapeutic plasma levels. Plasma clearance is approximately 7 l/hour. Prevailing plasma half-life is approximately 2 hours following a single intravenous dose. After repeated oral administration the half-life is longer. The terminal half-life is about 3 hours. Approximately 95% of the absorbed dose is excreted unchanged in the urine. Two metabolites have been identified: an N-acetylated and a deaminated derivative.

Impaired kidney function constitutes a risk for accumulation of tranexamic acid.

5.3 Preclinical safety data
Preclinical data reveal no special hazard for humans in addition to those included in other sections of the SPC. These data have been based on conventional studies of safety pharmacology, repeated dose toxicity, reproductive toxicity, genotoxicity or carcinogenicity.

Retinal abnormalities were found in long term toxicity studies in dog and cat: increased reflectivity, photoreceptor segment atrophy, peripheral retinal atrophy, atrophy of rods and cones. These ocular changes were dose related and occurred in high doses.

6. PHARMACEUTICAL PARTICULARS
6.1 List of excipients
Core
Microcrystalline cellulose, hydroxypropyl cellulose, talc, magnesium stearate, colloidal anhydrous silica, Povidone

Coating
Methacrylate polymers, titanium dioxide (E171), talc, magnesium stearate, Macrogol 8000, vanillin

6.2 Incompatibilities
None known.

6.3 Shelf life
Three years.

6.4 Special precautions for storage
Do not store above 25°C

6.5 Nature and contents of container
Blister packs of PVC/PVDC with aluminium foil backing containing 1 or 5 blister strips of 12 tablets each

6.6 Instructions for use and handling
None

7. MARKETING AUTHORISATION HOLDER
Pharmacia Limited
Davy Avenue
Milton Keynes
MK5 8PH
United Kingdom

8. MARKETING AUTHORISATION NUMBER(S)
PL 00032/0257

9. DATE OF FIRST AUTHORISATION/RENEWAL OF THE AUTHORISATION
8 November 2000

10. DATE OF REVISION OF THE TEXT
December 2003

11. LEGAL CATEGORY
POM
Ref: CKC 1_0 UK

Tranexamic Acid 500mg tablets
(Link Pharmaceuticals Ltd)

1. NAME OF THE MEDICINAL PRODUCT
Tranexamic acid 500mg tablets.

2. QUALITATIVE AND QUANTITATIVE COMPOSITION
Each tablet contains 500mg tranexamic acid. For excipients see 6.1.

3. PHARMACEUTICAL FORM
Tablet.

Tranexamic acid tablets are white caplet shaped tablets marked LINK on one face and blank on the reverse.

4. CLINICAL PARTICULARS
4.1 Therapeutic indications
Short-term use for haemorrhage or risk of haemorrhage in increased fibrinolysis or fibrinogenolysis.

Local fibrinolysis may occur in the following conditions: prostatectomy, menorrhagia, epistaxis, conisation of the cervix, traumatic hyphaema.

Management of dental extraction in haemophiliacs.

Hereditary angioneurotic oedema.

4.2 Posology and method of administration
Local fibrinolysis: The recommended standard dose is 15mg/kg to 25mg/kg body weight i.e. 2 to 3 tablets two to three times daily. For the indications listed below the following doses may be used:

Prostatectomy: Prophylaxis and treatment of haemorrhage in high risk patients should commence pre- or post-operatively with tranexamic acid intravenously; thereafter 2 tablets, three or four times daily until macroscopic haematuria is no longer present.

Menorrhagia: 2 to 3 tablets three to four times daily for three to four days. Therapy is indicated only after heavy bleeding has started.

Epistaxis: Where recurrent bleeding is anticipated, oral therapy (2 tablets three times daily) should be administered for seven days.

Conisation of the cervix: 3 tablets three times daily.

Traumatic hyphaema: 2 to 3 tablets three times daily. The dose is based on 25mg/kg three times a day.

Haemophilia: In the management of dental extractions 2 to 3 tablets every eight hours. The dose is based on 25mg/kg.

Hereditary angioneurotic oedema: Some patients are aware of the onset of the illness; suitable treatment for these patients is intermittently 2 to 3 tablets two to three times daily for some days. Other patients are treated continuously at this dosage.

Children: The dose should be calculated according to body weight, at 25mg/kg per dose.

The Elderly: No reduction in dosage is necessary unless there is evidence of renal failure (see 4.4).

4.3 Contraindications
Known allergy to tranexamic acid or any of the excipients.

A history of thromboembolic disease.

4.4 Special warnings and special precautions for use
In patients with renal insufficiency, because of the risk of accumulation. By extrapolation from clearance data relating to an intravenous dosage form, the following reduction in the oral dosage is recommended.

Serum creatinine	*Oral dose*	*Dose frequency*
120 to 250 micromol/l	25mg/kg	twice daily
250 to 500 micromol/l	25mg/kg	every 24 hours
>500 micromol/l	12.5mg/kg	every 24 hours

In massive haematuria from the upper urinary tract (especially in haemophilia) since, in a few cases, ureteric obstruction has been reported.

When disseminated intravascular coagulation is in progress it should not be treated with any antifibrinolytic agent unless both bleeding tendency and systemic fibrinogenolysis are present. Such cases would require careful surveillance and anticoagulant cover.

In the long-term treatment of patients with hereditary angioneurotic oedema regular eye examination (e.g. visual acuity, slit lamp, intra-ocular pressure, visual fields) and liver function tests should be performed (see 4.8).

4.5 Interaction with other medicinal products and other forms of Interaction
Drugs which also have effects on haemostasis should be given with caution to patients receiving tranexamic acid. There is a theoretical risk of increased potential for thrombus formation e.g. with oestrogens. Alternatively the action of the antifibrinolytic could be antagonised by thrombolytics.

4.6 Pregnancy and lactation
Pregnancy: Although there is no evidence from animal studies of a teratogenic effect, the usual caution with use of drugs in pregnancy should be observed.

Lactation: Tranexamic acid passes into breast milk to a concentration of approximately one hundredth of the concentration in the maternal blood. An antifibrinolytic effect in the infant is unlikely but caution is recommended.

4.7 Effects on ability to drive and use machines
Tranexamic acid is not expected to affect a patient's ability to drive and/or operate machines.

4.8 Undesirable effects
Gastro-intestinal disorders (nausea, vomiting, diarrhoea) may occur but disappear when the dosage is reduced. Rare instances of transient colour vision disturbances have been reported. Patients who experience disturbance of colour vision should be withdrawn from treatment. Rare cases of thromboembolic events have been reported.

4.9 Overdose
No cases of overdosage have been reported. Symptoms may be nausea, vomiting, orthostatic symptoms and/or hypotension. Initiate vomiting, then stomach lavage and charcoal therapy. Maintain a high fluid intake to promote renal excretion.

5. PHARMACOLOGICAL PROPERTIES
5.1 Pharmacodynamic properties
ATC Code: B02A A02.

Tranexamic acid is an antifibrinolytic agent that competitively inhibits the activation of plasminogen to plasmin.

5.2 Pharmacokinetic properties
Absorption of tranexamic acid from the gastro-intestinal tract is 30% to 50% and is not influenced by food. Peak concentrations occur in about 3 hours.

The apparent elimination half-life is about 2 hours.

At therapeutic concentrations, (5mg/l to 10mg/l) tranexamic acid is very weakly protein bound, about 3%. This is explained by its binding to plasminogen which is saturated at very low concentrations. Its volume of distribution is about 1 l/kg.

Tranexamic acid is distributed into a number of tissues, including the large intestine, kidneys and prostate. The drug also passes into seminal fluid, inhibiting its fibrinolytic activity but has no effect on sperm migration. Tranexamic acid also crosses the blood-aqueous barrier in the eye and the damaged blood-brain barrier and diffuses rapidly to the joint fluid and synovial membrane.

Tranexamic acid crosses the placenta and its concentration in cord blood may reach that of the maternal blood. The concentration of tranexamic acid in breast milk of lactating women 1 hour after the last dose of a 2 day treatment was about one hundredth of the peak serum concentration.

Approximately 90% of a (intravenous) dose of tranexamic acid is recovered in the urine by 24 hours post dose (30% at 1 hour; 45% at 3 hours). This suggests that very little metabolism of the drug occurs.

Renal failure

The drug is excreted, unmetabolised, by the kidney, and so in renal impairment the dose should be reduced to avoid accumulation (see 4.4).

5.3 Preclinical safety data
There are no pre-clinical data of relevance to the prescriber which are additional to that already included in other sections of the Summary of Product Characteristics.

6. PHARMACEUTICAL PARTICULARS
6.1 List of excipients
Calcium hydrogen phosphate (anhydrous), croscarmellose sodium, povidone, talc and magnesium stearate.

6.2 Incompatibilities
Not applicable.

6.3 Shelf life
3 years.

6.4 Special precautions for storage
Do not store above 25°C.

6.5 Nature and contents of container
Blister packs of white PVC coated with PVdC and hard-tempered aluminium foil on the reverse, in cardboard boxes of 60 tablets.

6.6 Instructions for use and handling
Not applicable.

7. MARKETING AUTHORISATION HOLDER
Link Pharmaceuticals Limited, Bishops Weald House, Albion Way, Horsham, West Sussex, RH12 1AH.

8. MARKETING AUTHORISATION NUMBER(S)
PL 12406/0022

9. DATE OF FIRST AUTHORISATION/RENEWAL OF THE AUTHORISATION
December 2001

10. DATE OF REVISION OF THE TEXT
June 2002

11. Legal Category
POM

Trangina XL

(Alpharma Limited)

1. NAME OF THE MEDICINAL PRODUCT
TRANGINA XL 60mg TABLETS.

2. QUALITATIVE AND QUANTITATIVE COMPOSITION
Each tablet contains 60mg isosorbide-5-mononitrate.

3. PHARMACEUTICAL FORM
Prolonged-release tablets.

White, oval-shaped tablets impressed "C" on one face and the identifying letters "CY" on either side of a central division line on the reverse.

4. CLINICAL PARTICULARS

4.1 Therapeutic indications
Prophylatic treatment of angina pectoris.

4.2 Posology and method of administration
Posology

Adults: Isosorbide mononitrate (one tablet) once daily to be taken in the morning. The dose of 60mg may be increased to 120mg (two tablets) daily, both to be taken once daily in the morning. The dose can be titrated to minimise the possibility of headache, by initiating treatment with 30mg (half a tablet) for the first 2-4 days.

Isosorbide mononitrate tablets must not be chewed or crushed. They should be swallowed whole with half a glass of water.

Children: The safety and efficacy of isosorbide mononitrate in children has not been established.

Elderly: No evidence of a need for routine dosage adjustment in the elderly has been found, but special care may be needed in those with increased susceptibility to hypotension or marked hepatic or renal insufficiency.

The core of the tablet is insoluble in the digestive juices but disintegrates into small particles when all active substance has been released. Very occasionally the matrix may pass through the gastrointestinal tract without disintegrating and be found visible in the stool, but all active substance has been released.

Method of Administration

For oral use.

4.3 Contraindications
Hypersensitivity to nitrates or any ingredients in the tablet.

Severe cerebrovascular insufficiency or hypotension are relative contraindications to the use of isosorbide mononitrate.

4.4 Special warnings and special precautions for use
Isosorbide mononitrate is not indicated for relief of acute angina attacks; in the event of an acute attack, sublingual or buccal glyceryl trinitrate tablets should be used.

4.5 Interaction with other medicinal products and other forms of Interaction
Alcohol: enhanced hypotensive effect.

4.6 Pregnancy and lactation
For isosorbide-5-mononitrate no clinical data on exposed pregnancies is available. Studies in animals have shown reproductive toxicity (see section 5.3). The relevance of these data for humans is unknown. Trangina XL 60mg Tablets should not be used during pregnancy unless clearly necessary.

4.7 Effects on ability to drive and use machines
Isosorbide-5-mononitrate has a moderate influence on the ability of an individual to drive and use machines. Isosorbide mononitrate may cause dizziness. Patients should make sure they are not affected before driving or operating machinery.

4.8 Undesirable effects
Most of the adverse reactions are pharmacodynamic mediated and dose dependent. Headache may occur when treatment is initiated but usually disappears after continued treatment. Hypotension with symptoms such as dizziness and nausea has occasionally been reported. These symptoms generally disappear during long-term treatment.

4.9 Overdose
Symptoms: Pulsing headache. More serious symptoms are excitation, flushing, cold perspiration, nausea, vomiting, vertigo, syncope, tachycardia and a fall in blood pressure.

Treatment: Induction of emesis, activated charcoal. In case of pronounced hypotension the patient should first be placed in the supine position with legs raised. If necessary intravenous administration of fluid.

5. PHARMACOLOGICAL PROPERTIES

5.1 Pharmacodynamic properties
Isosorbide mononitrate is an active metabolite of the vasodilator isosorbide dinitrate.

Isosorbide-5-mononitrate is a potent venodilator and to a lesser extent an arterial dilator. Both intravenous and oral formulations reduce systemic arterial pressure and venous return, thereby lowering cardiac volume, dimensions and work. While the precise mechanism of action remains unclear, it is probably due to nitric oxide (NO) release which activates guanylate cyclase and increases the synthesis of cyclic GMP. It is possible that NO combines with sulphydryl groups in the endothelium and produces S-nitrosothiols that stimulate guanylate cyclase production. This is enhanced by N-acetylcysteine, which provides a source of sulphydryl groups. How cyclic GMP produces vascular relaxation is not exactly known.

5.2 Pharmacokinetic properties
Isosorbide mononitrate is readily absorbed from the gastro-intestinal tract. Following oral administration of conventional tablets, peak plasma levels are reached in about 1 hour. Unlike isosorbide dinitrate, isosorbide mononitrate does not undergo first-pass hepatic metabolism and bioavailability is nearly 100%. Isosorbide mononitrate is widely distributed with a large apparent volume of distribution. It is taken up by smooth muscle cells of blood vessels and the nitrate group is cleaved to inorganic nitrite and then to nitric oxide. Isosorbide mononitrate is metabolised to inactive metabolites, including isosorbide and isosorbide glucuronide. Only 2% of isosorbide mononitrate is excreted unchanged in the urine. An elimination half-life of about 4 to 5 hours has been reported.

5.3 Preclinical safety data
High concentrations of isosorbide-5-mononitrate in rats are associated with prolonged gestation and parturition, stillbirths and neonatal death.

6. PHARMACEUTICAL PARTICULARS

6.1 List of excipients
The tablets also contain: lactose, hypromellose (E464), glyceryl palmitostearate, maize starch, magnesium stearate.

6.2 Incompatibilities
Not applicable.

6.3 Shelf life
Shelf-life

Two years from date of manufacture.

Shelf-life after dilution/reconstitution

Not applicable.

Shelf-life after first opening

Not applicable.

6.4 Special precautions for storage
Do not store above 25°C.

Keep container in the outer carton.

6.5 Nature and contents of container
Aluminium (25μm)/PVC (250μm) strips in a carton box.

Pack sizes: 28, 56 (Al/PVC)

6.6 Instructions for use and handling
Not applicable.

Administrative Data

7. MARKETING AUTHORISATION HOLDER
Alpharma Limited

(Trading styles: Alpharma, Cox Pharmaceuticals)

Whiddon Valley

BARNSTAPLE

N Devon EX32 8NS

8. MARKETING AUTHORISATION NUMBER(S)
PL 0142/0462.

9. DATE OF FIRST AUTHORISATION/RENEWAL OF THE AUTHORISATION
Not applicable.

10. DATE OF REVISION OF THE TEXT
April 2001

Transiderm Nitro 10

(Novartis Pharmaceuticals UK Ltd)

1. NAME OF THE MEDICINAL PRODUCT
TRANSIDERM NITRO 10.

2. QUALITATIVE AND QUANTITATIVE COMPOSITION
Nitroglycerin on lactose 500mg equivalent to nitroglycerin 50mg.

3. PHARMACEUTICAL FORM
Transdermal patch.

4. CLINICAL PARTICULARS

4.1 Therapeutic indications
Prophylactic treatment of attacks of angina pectoris, as monotherapy or in combination with other anti-anginal agents.

4.2 Posology and method of administration
For dermal administration.

Adults:

Angina: Treatment should be initiated with one TRANSIDERM-NITRO 5 patch daily. If a higher dosage is required a TRANSIDERM-NITRO 10 patch may be substituted. The dosage may be increased to a maximum of two TRANSIDERM-NITRO 10 patches daily in resistant cases. TRANSIDERM-NITRO may be given either continuously, or intermittently with a patch off period of 8-12 hours, usually at night, during each 24 hour period. Development of tolerance or attenuation of therapeutic effect commonly occurs with prolonged or frequent administration of all long-acting nitrates. Recent evidence suggests that intermittent therapy with TRANSIDERM-NITRO may reduce the incidence of tolerance.

Prior to the use of intermittent therapy, the clinical benefits to the patients should be weighed against the risks of angina in the patch-free interval. In patients considered to be at risk, concomitant anti-anginal therapy should be implemented (see "Precautions").

It is recommended that the patch is applied to the lateral chest wall. The replacement patch should be applied to a new area of skin. Allow several days to elapse before applying a fresh patch to the same area of skin. If acute attacks of angina pectoris occur, rapidly acting nitrates may be required.

Use in the elderly

No specific information on use in the elderly is available; however no evidence exists to suggest that an alteration in dosage is required.

Use in children

There is insufficient knowledge of the effects of TRANSIDERM-NITRO in children and, therefore, recommendations for its use cannot be made.

4.3 Contraindications
TRANSIDERM-NITRO should not be prescribed to patients hypersensitive to nitrates.

Severe hypotension.

Increased intracranial pressure.

Myocardial insufficiency due to obstruction (e.g. in the presence of aortic or mitral stenosis or of constrictive pericarditis).

Sildenafil has been shown to potentiate the hypotensive effects of nitrates and its co-administration with nitrates or nitric oxide donors is therefore contraindicated.

4.4 Special warnings and special precautions for use
In recent myocardial infarction or acute heart failure, TRANSIDERM-NITRO should be employed only under careful surveillance.

As with all anti-anginal nitrate preparations, withdrawal of long-term treatment should be gradual, by replacement with decreasing doses of long-acting oral nitrates.

The system should be removed before cardioversion or DC defibrillation is attempted. This is to avoid the possibility of arcing between the patch and the electrodes. Also the system should be removed before diathermy treatment.

Caution should be exercised in patients with arterial hypoxaemia due to severe anaemia because, in such patients the biotransformation of nitroglycerin is reduced. Similarly, caution is called for in patients with hypoxaemia and a ventilation/perfusion imbalance due to lung disease or ischaemic heart failure.

Nitrate therapy may aggravate the angina caused by hypertrophic cardiotherapy.

The possibility of increased frequency of angina during patch-off periods should be considered. In such cases, the use of concomitant anti-anginal therapy is desirable.

If tolerance to nitroglycerin patches develops, the effects of sublingual nitroglycerin on exercise tolerance may be partially diminished.

4.5 Interaction with other medicinal products and other forms of Interaction
Concomitant treatment with other vasodilators, calcium antagonists, ACE inhibitors, beta-blockers, diuretics, antihypertensives, tricyclic antidepressants and major tranquillisers, as well as the consumption of alcohol, may potentiate the blood pressure lowering effects of TRANSIDERM-NITRO.

Concurrent administration of TRANSIDERM-NITRO with dihydroergotamine may increase the bioavailability of dihydroergotamine and lead to coronary vasoconstriction.

The possibility that the ingestion of acetylsalicylic acid and non-steroidal anti-inflammatory drugs might diminish the therapeutic response to TRANSIDERM-NITRO cannot be excluded.

The hypotensive effects of nitrates are potentiated by concurrent administration of sildenafil

4.6 Pregnancy and lactation
As with all drugs, TRANSIDERM-NITRO should not be prescribed during pregnancy, particularly during the first trimester, unless there are compelling reasons for doing so.

It is not known whether the active substance passes into the breast milk. The benefits for the mother must be weighed against the risks for the child.

4.7 Effects on ability to drive and use machines
Postural hypotension has been reported rarely following initiation of treatment with TRANSIDERM-NITRO and care is advised when driving or operating machinery.

4.8 Undesirable effects
Central nervous system:
Like other preparations, TRANSIDERM-NITRO may give rise to headache, which is due to cerebral vasodilation and is dose-dependent. Such headaches, however, may regress after a few days despite continuation of the therapy. If they do not disappear, they should be treated with mild analgesics. In cases where headaches are unresponsive to treatment, the dosage of nitroglycerin should be reduced or use of the product discontinued.

Skin:
Reddening of the skin, with or without local itching or burning sensation, as well as allergic contact dermatitis may occasionally occur. Upon removal of the patch, any slight reddening of the skin will usually disappear within a few hours. The application site should be changed on patch replacement to prevent local irritation.

Cardiovascular:
Facial flushing, faintness, dizziness or lightheadedness, and postural hypotension, which may be associated with reflex-induced tachycardia, have been reported rarely. Reflex tachycardia can be controlled by concomitant treatment with a beta-blocker.

Gastro-intestinal:
Rarely nausea, vomiting.

4.9 Overdose
Signs:
High doses of glyceryl trinitrate are known to cause pronounced systemic side effects, e.g. a marked fall in blood pressure and reflex tachycardia resulting in collapse and syncope. Methemoglobinaemia has also been reported following accidental overdosage of nitroglycerin. However, with TRANSIDERM-NITRO, the release membrane will reduce the likelihood of overdosage occurring.

Management:
In contrast to long acting oral nitrate preparations, the effect of TRANSIDERM-NITRO can be rapidly terminated simply by removing the system. Any fall in blood pressure or signs of collapse that may occur, may be managed by general resuscitative measures.

5. PHARMACOLOGICAL PROPERTIES

5.1 Pharmacodynamic properties
Nitroglycerin relaxes smooth muscle. It acts chiefly on systemic veins and large coronary arteries, with more predominant effects on the former. In angina pectoris the fundamental mechanism of action of nitroglycerin is based on an increase in venous capacitance leading to a decreased return of blood to the heart. Owing to this, preload and hence filling volume diminshes, resulting in a decreased myocardial oxygen requirement at rest and especially during exercise.

In the coronary arterial circulation nitroglycerin dilates extramural conductance and small resistance vessels. It appears to cause redistribution of coronary blood flow to the ischaemic subendocardium by selectively dilating large epicardial vessels and also relaxes vasospasm.

Nitroglycerin dilates the arteriolar vascular bed, as a result of which afterload and left ventricular systolic wall tension decrease, leading to a reduction in myocardial oxygen consumption.

5.2 Pharmacokinetic properties
Following single application, plasma concentrations of nitroglycerin reach a plateau within 2 hours, which is maintained throughout the day until patch removal. The height of this plateau is directly proportional to the size of the system's drug-releasing area.

The same plasma levels are attained regardless of whether the system is applied to the skin of the upper arm, pelvis or chest. Upon removal of TRANSIDERM-NITRO the plasma level falls rapidly. After repeated application of TRANSIDERM-NITRO no cumulation occurs.

5.3 Preclinical safety data
None stated.

6. PHARMACEUTICAL PARTICULARS

6.1 List of excipients
Lactose, silicone oil, silica dioxide, ethylene-vinyl acetate copolymer, silicone-based adhesive (medical adhesive CH15).

6.2 Incompatibilities
None.

6.3 Shelf life
36 months.

6.4 Special precautions for storage
Store below 25°C.

6.5 Nature and contents of container
Individual patches in a sealed pouch (made of paper/PE/AL/surlyn*). 28 sealed patches in each cardboard container.

* Aluminium $12\mu m$ ±10%, polyethylene 16g/m^2 ± 20%, surlyn 20g/m^2 ±15%.

6.6 Instructions for use and handling
None stated.

7. MARKETING AUTHORISATION HOLDER
Novartis Pharmaceuticals UK Limited

Trading as Ciba Laboratories

Frimley Business Park

Frimley

Camberley

Surrey

GU16 7SR

8. MARKETING AUTHORISATION NUMBER(S)
00101/0465.

9. DATE OF FIRST AUTHORISATION/RENEWAL OF THE AUTHORISATION
21 July 1997.

10. DATE OF REVISION OF THE TEXT
July 2000.

Transiderm Nitro 5

(Novartis Pharmaceuticals UK Ltd)

1. NAME OF THE MEDICINAL PRODUCT
TRANSIDERM NITRO 5.

2. QUALITATIVE AND QUANTITATIVE COMPOSITION
Nitroglycerin on lactose 250mg equivalent to nitroglycerin 25mg.

3. PHARMACEUTICAL FORM
Transdermal patch.

4. CLINICAL PARTICULARS

4.1 Therapeutic indications
Prophylactic treatment of attacks of angina pectoris, as monotherapy or in combination with other anti-anginal agents.

Prophylactic treatment of phlebitis and extravasation secondary to venous cannulation for intravenous fluid and drug administration when the duration of treatment is expected to last for 2 days or longer.

4.2 Posology and method of administration
For dermal administration

Adults:
Angina:
Treatment should be initiated with one TRANSIDERM-NITRO 5 patch daily. If a higher dosage is required a TRANSIDERM-NITRO 10 patch may be substituted. The dosage may be increased to a maximum of two TRANSIDERM-NITRO 10 patches daily in resistant cases. TRANSIDERM-NITRO may be given either continuously, or intermittently with a patch off period of 8-12 hours, usually at night, during each 24 hour period. Development of tolerance or attenuation of therapeutic effect commonly occurs with prolonged or frequent administration of all long-acting nitrates. Recent evidence suggests that intermittent therapy with TRANSIDERM-NITRO may reduce the incidence of tolerance.

Prior to the use of intermittent therapy, the clinical benefits to the patients should be weighed against the risks of angina in the patch-free interval. In patients considered to be at risk, concomitant anti-anginal therapy should be implemented (see "Precautions").

It is recommended that the patch is applied to the lateral chest wall. The replacement patch should be applied to a new area of skin. Allow several days to elapse before applying a fresh patch to the same area of skin. If acute attacks of angina pectoris occur, rapidly acting nitrates may be required.

Phlebitis and extravasation:
One TRANSIDERM-NITRO 5 patch is to be applied distal to the site of intravenous cannulation at the time of venepuncture. The patch should be removed after 3-4 days and a new replacement patch applied to a different area of skin. Treatment with TRANSIDERM-NITRO should be discontinued once intravenous therapy has stopped.

Use in the elderly
No specific information on use in the elderly is available; however no evidence exists to suggest that an alteration in dosage is required.

Use in children
There is insufficient knowledge of the effects of TRANSIDERM-NITRO in children and, therefore, recommendations for its use cannot be made.

4.3 Contraindications
TRANSIDERM-NITRO should not be prescribed to patients hypersensitive to nitrates.

Severe hypotension.

Increased intracranial pressure.

Myocardial insufficiency due to obstruction (e.g. in the presence of aortic or mitral stenosis or of constrictive pericarditis).

Sildenafil has been shown to potentiate the hypotensive effects of nitrates and its co-administration with nitrates or nitric oxide donors is, therefore, contraindicated

4.4 Special warnings and special precautions for use
In recent myocardial infarction or acute heart failure, TRANSIDERM-NITRO should be employed only under careful surveillance.

As with all anti-anginal nitrate preparations, withdrawal of long-term treatment should be gradual, by replacement with decreasing doses of long-acting oral nitrates.

The system should be removed before cardioversion or DC defibrillation is attempted. This is to avoid the possibility of arcing between the patch and the electrodes. Also the system should be removed before diathermy treatment.

Caution should be exercised in patients with arterial hypoxaemia due to severe anaemia because, in such patients the biotransformation of nitroglycerin is reduced. Similarly, caution is called for in patients with hypoxaemia and a ventilation/perfusion imbalance due to lung disease or ischaemic heart failure.

Nitrate therapy may aggravate the angina caused by hypertrophic cardiotherapy.

The possibility of increased frequency of angina during patch-off periods should be considered. In such cases, the use of concomitant anti-anginal therapy is desirable.

If tolerance to nitroglycerin patches develops, the effects of sublingual nitroglycerin on exercise tolerance may be partially diminished.

4.5 Interaction with other medicinal products and other forms of Interaction
Concomitant treatment with other vasodilators, calcium antagonists, ACE inhibitors, beta-blockers, diuretics, antihypertensives, tricyclic antidepressants and major tranquillisers, as well as the consumption of alcohol, may potentiate the blood pressure lowering effects of TRANSIDERM-NITRO.

Concurrent administration of TRANSIDERM-NITRO with dihydroergotamine may increase the bioavailability of dihydroergotamine and lead to coronary vasoconstriction.

The possibility that the ingestion of acetylsalicylic acid and non-steroidal anti-inflammatory drugs might diminish the therapeutic response to TRANSIDERM-NITRO cannot be excluded.

The hypotensive effects of nitrates are potentiated by concurrent administration of sildenafil

4.6 Pregnancy and lactation
As with all drugs, TRANSIDERM-NITRO should not be prescribed during pregnancy, particularly during the first trimester, unless there are compelling reasons for doing so.

It is not known whether the active substance passes into the breast milk. The benefits for the mother must be weighed against the risks for the child.

4.7 Effects on ability to drive and use machines
Postural hypotension has been reported rarely following initiation of treatment with TRANSIDERM-NITRO and care is advised when driving or operating machinery.

4.8 Undesirable effects
Central nervous system:
Like other preparations, TRANSIDERM-NITRO may give rise to headache, which is due to cerebral vasodilation and is dose-dependent. Such headaches, however, may regress after a few days despite continuation of the therapy. If they do not disappear, they should be treated with mild analgesics. In cases where headaches are unresponsive to treatment, the dosage of nitroglycerin should be reduced or use of the product discontinued.

Skin:
Reddening of the skin, with or without local itching or burning sensation, as well as allergic contact dermatitis may occasionally occur. Upon removal of the patch, any slight reddening of the skin will usually disappear within a few hours. The application site should be changed on patch replacement to prevent local irritation.

Cardiovascular:
Facial flushing, faintness, dizziness or lightheadedness, and postural hypotension, which may be associated with reflex-induced tachycardia, have been reported rarely. Reflex tachycardia can be controlled by concomitant treatment with a beta-blocker.

Gastro-intestinal:
Rarely nausea, vomiting.

4.9 Overdose
Signs:
High doses of glyceryl trinitrate are known to cause pronounced systemic side effects, e.g. a marked fall in blood pressure and reflex tachycardia resulting in collapse and syncope. Methemoglobinaemia has also been reported following accidental overdosage of nitroglycerin. However, with TRANSIDERM-NITRO, the release membrane will reduce the likelihood of overdosage occurring.

Management:

In contrast to long acting oral nitrate preparations, the effect of TRANSIDERM-NITRO can be rapidly terminated simply by removing the system. Any fall in blood pressure or signs of collapse that may occur, may be managed by general resuscitative measures.

5. PHARMACOLOGICAL PROPERTIES

5.1 Pharmacodynamic properties

Nitroglycerin relaxes smooth muscle. It acts chiefly on systemic veins and large coronary arteries, with more predominant effects on the former. In angina pectoris the fundamental mechanism of action of nitroglycerin is based on an increase in venous capacitance leading to a decreased return of blood to the heart. Owing to this, preload and hence filling volume diminshes, resulting in a decreased myocardial oxygen requirement at rest and especially during exercise.

In the coronary arterial circulation nitroglycerin dilates extramural conductance and small resistance vessels. It appears to cause redistribution of coronary blood flow to the ischaemic subendocardium by selectively dilating large epicardial vessels and also relaxes vasospasm.

Nitroglycerin dilates the arteriolar vascular bed, as a result of which afterload and left ventricular systolic wall tension decrease, leading to a reduction in myocardial oxygen consumption.

5.2 Pharmacokinetic properties

Following single application, plasma concentrations of nitroglycerin reach a plateau within 2 hours, which is maintained throughout the day until patch removal. The height of this plateau is directly proportional to the size of the system's drug-releasing area.

The same plasma levels are attained regardless of whether the system is applied to the skin of the upper arm, pelvis or chest. Upon removal of TRANSIDERM-NITRO the plasma level falls rapidly. After repeated application of TRANSIDERM-NITRO no cumulation occurs.

5.3 Preclinical safety data

None stated.

6. PHARMACEUTICAL PARTICULARS

6.1 List of excipients

Lactose, silicone oil, silica dioxide, ethylene-vinyl acetate, silicone-based adhesive (medical adhesive CH15).

6.2 Incompatibilities

None.

6.3 Shelf life

36 months.

6.4 Special precautions for storage

Store below 25°C.

6.5 Nature and contents of container

Individual patches in a sealed pouch (made of paper/PE/AL/surlyn*). 28 sealed patches in each cardboard container.

* Aluminium 12μm ± 10%, polyethylene 16g/m² ± 20%, surlyn 20g/m² ± 15%.

6.6 Instructions for use and handling

None stated.

7. MARKETING AUTHORISATION HOLDER

Novartis Pharmaceuticals UK Limited

Trading as Ciba Laboratories

Frimley Business Park

Frimley

Camberley

Surrey

GU16 7SR

8. MARKETING AUTHORISATION NUMBER(S)

00101/0464.

9. DATE OF FIRST AUTHORISATION/RENEWAL OF THE AUTHORISATION

21 July 1997.

10. DATE OF REVISION OF THE TEXT

July 2000.

TRANSTEC transdermal patch

(Napp Pharmaceuticals Limited)

1. NAME OF THE MEDICINAL PRODUCT

TRANSTEC® 35 μg/h transdermal patch

TRANSTEC® 52.5 μg/h transdermal patch

TRANSTEC® 70 μg/h transdermal patch

2. QUALITATIVE AND QUANTITATIVE COMPOSITION

TRANSTEC 35 μg/h:

One transdermal patch contains 20 mg buprenorphine.

Area containing the active substance: 25 cm²

Nominal release rate: 35 μg buprenorphine per hour (over a period of 72 hours).

TRANSTEC 52.5 μg/h:

One transdermal patch contains 30 mg buprenorphine.

Area containing the active substance: 37.5 cm²

Nominal release rate: 52.5 μg buprenorphine per hour (over a period of 72 hours).

TRANSTEC 70 μg/h:

One transdermal patch contains 40 mg buprenorphine.

Area containing the active substance: 50 cm²

Nominal release rate: 70 μg buprenorphine per hour (over a period of 72 hours).

(For excipients see section 6.1)

3. PHARMACEUTICAL FORM

Transdermal patch

Skin coloured patch with rounded corners marked:

TRANSTEC 35 μg/h, buprenorphinum 20 mg

TRANSTEC 52.5 μg/h, buprenorphinum 30 mg

TRANSTEC 70 μg/h, buprenorphinum 40 mg

4. CLINICAL PARTICULARS

4.1 Therapeutic indications

Moderate to severe cancer pain and severe pain which does not respond to non-opioid analgesics.

TRANSTEC is not suitable for the treatment of acute pain.

4.2 Posology and method of administration

Posology

Patients over 18 years of age

The TRANSTEC dosage should be adapted to the condition of the individual patient (pain intensity, suffering, individual reaction). The lowest possible dosage providing adequate pain relief should be given. Three patch strengths are available to provide such adaptive treatment: TRANSTEC 35 μg/h, TRANSTEC 52.5 μg/h and TRANSTEC 70 μg/h.

Initial dose selection: patients who have previously not received any analgesics should start with the lowest patch strength (TRANSTEC 35 μg/h). Patients previously given a WHO step-I analgesic (non-opioid) should also begin with TRANSTEC 35 μg/h. According to the WHO recommendations, the administration of a non-opioid analgesic can be continued, depending on the patient's overall medical condition.

When switching from an opioid analgesic to TRANSTEC and choosing the initial patch strength, the nature of the previous medication, administration and the mean daily dose should be taken into account in order to avoid the recurrence of pain. The details in the following table serve as a guideline.

(see Table 1)

The data in the table are naturally only a rough guideline. The necessary strength of TRANSTEC must be adapted to the requirements of the individual patient and checked at regular intervals.

After application of the first TRANSTEC patch the buprenorphine serum concentrations rise slowly both in patients who have been treated previously with analgesics and in those who have not. Therefore initially, there is unlikely to be a rapid onset of effect. Consequently, a first evaluation of the analgesic effect should only be made after 24 hours.

Dose titration and maintenance therapy

The TRANSTEC patch should be replaced every 72 hours. The dose should be titrated individually until analgesic efficacy is attained. If analgesia is insufficient at the end of the initial application period (72 hours), the dose may be increased, either by applying more than one TRANSTEC patch of the same strength or by switching to the next patch strength. At the same time no more than two patches regardless of the patch strength should be applied.

Before application of the next TRANSTEC patch strength the amount of buprenorphine sublingual tablets administered in addition to the previous TRANSTEC patch should be taken into consideration, i.e. the total amount of buprenorphine required, and the dosage adjusted accordingly. Patients requiring a supplementary analgesic (e.g. for breakthrough pain) may take one to two 0.2 mg buprenorphine sublingual tablets every 24 hours in addition to the patch. If the regular addition of 0.4 – 0.6 mg sublingual buprenorphine is necessary, the next patch strength should be used.

Patients under 18 years of age

As TRANSTEC has not been studied in patients under 18 years of age, the use of the medicinal product in patients below this age is not recommended.

Elderly patients

No dosage adjustment of TRANSTEC is required for elderly patients.

Patients with renal insufficiency

Since the pharmacokinetics of buprenorphine is not altered during the course of renal failure, its use in patients with renal insufficiency is possible.

Patients with hepatic insufficiency

Buprenorphine is metabolised in the liver. The intensity and duration of its action may be affected in patients with impaired liver function. Therefore patients with liver insufficiency should be carefully monitored during treatment with TRANSTEC.

Method of application

TRANSTEC should be applied to non-irritated skin on a non-hairy flat surface, but not to any parts of the skin with large scars. Preferable sites on the upper body are: upper back or below the collar-bone on the chest. Any remaining hairs should be cut off with a pair of scissors (not shaved). If the site of application requires cleansing, this should be done with water. Soap or any other cleansing agents should not be used. Skin preparations that might affect adhesion of the patch to the area selected for application of TRANSTEC should be avoided.

The skin must be completely dry before application. TRANSTEC is to be applied immediately after removal from the sachet. Following removal of the release liner, the patch should be pressed firmly in place with the palm of the hand for approximately 30 seconds. The patch will not be affected when bathing, showering or swimming. However, it should not be exposed to excessive heat (e.g. sauna, infrared-radiation).

Each TRANSTEC patch should be worn continuously for 72 hours. After removal of the previous patch a new TRANSTEC patch should be applied to a different skin site. At least 6 days should elapse before a new patch is applied to the same area of skin.

Duration of administration

TRANSTEC should under no circumstances be administered for longer than absolutely necessary. If long-term pain treatment with TRANSTEC is necessary in view of the nature and severity of the illness, then careful and regular monitoring should be carried out (if necessary with breaks in treatment) to establish whether and to what extent further treatment is necessary.

Experience regarding application for more than two months is so far limited.

Discontinuation of the TRANSTEC patch

After removal of the TRANSTEC patch buprenorphine serum concentrations decrease gradually and thus the analgesic effect is maintained for a certain amount of time. This should be considered when therapy with TRANSTEC is to be followed by other opioids. As a general rule, a subsequent opioid should not be administered within 24

Table 1

Pretreatment with opioids (mg/24 h)				
Weak opioids				
dihydrocodeine, oral	120-240 mg	-360 mg		
tramadol, parenteral	100-200 mg	-300 mg	-400 mg	
tramadol, oral	150-300 mg	-450 mg	-600 mg	
Strong opioids				
buprenorphine,parenteral	0.3-0.6 mg	-0.9 mg	-1.2 mg	-2.4 mg
buprenorphine, sublingual	0.4-0.8 mg	-1.2 mg	-1.6 mg	-3.2 mg
morphine, parenteral	10-20 mg	-30 mg	-40 mg	-80 mg
morphine, oral	30-60 mg	-90 mg	-120 mg	-240 mg
Initial patch strength				
TRANSTEC	**35 μ g/h**	**52.5 μ g/h**	**70 μ g/h**	**2 × 70 μ g/h**

hours after removal of the TRANSTEC patch. For the time being only limited information is available on the starting dose of other opioids administered after discontinuation of the TRANSTEC patch.

4.3 Contraindications

TRANSTEC is contraindicated in:

- known hypersensitivity towards the active substance buprenorphine or to any of the excipients (for the excipients see section 6.1)
- in opioid-dependent patients and for narcotic withdrawal treatment
- conditions in which the respiratory centre and function are severely impaired or may become so
- patients who are receiving MAO inhibitors or have taken them within the last two weeks (see 4.5 Interactions)
- patients suffering from myasthenia gravis
- patients suffering from delirium tremens.

4.4 Special warnings and special precautions for use

TRANSTEC must only be used with particular caution in acute alcohol intoxication, convulsive disorders, in patients with head injury, shock, a reduced level of consciousness of uncertain origin, increased intracranial pressure without the possibility of ventilation.

Buprenorphine occasionally causes respiratory depression. Therefore care should be taken when treating patients with impaired respiratory function or patients receiving medication which can cause respiratory depression.

Buprenorphine has a substantially lower dependence liability than pure opioid agonists. In healthy volunteer and patient studies with TRANSTEC, withdrawal reactions have not been observed. However, after long-term use of TRANSTEC withdrawal symptoms, similar to those occurring during opiate withdrawal, cannot be entirely excluded (see also 4.8 Undesirable effects). These symptoms are: agitation, anxiety, nervousness, insomnia, hyperkinesia, tremor and gastrointestinal disorders.

In patients abusing opioids, substitution with buprenorphine may prevent withdrawal symptoms. This has resulted in some abuse of buprenorphine and caution should be exercised when prescribing it to patients suspected of having drug abuse problems.

Buprenorphine is metabolised in the liver. The intensity and duration of effect may be altered in patients with liver function disorders. Therefore such patients should be carefully monitored during TRANSTEC treatment.

As TRANSTEC has not been studied in patients under 18 years of age, the use of the medicinal product in patients below this age is not recommended.

Patients with fever / external heat

Fever and the presence of heat may increase the permeability of the skin. Theoretically in such situations buprenorphine serum concentrations may be raised during TRANSTEC treatment. Therefore on treatment with TRANSTEC, attention should be paid to the increased possibility of opioid reactions in febrile patients or those with increased skin temperature due to other causes.

4.5 Interaction with other medicinal products and other forms of Interaction

On administration of MAO inhibitors in the last 14 days prior to the administration of the opioid pethidine life-threatening interactions have been observed affecting the central nervous system and respiratory and cardiovascular function. The same interactions between MAO inhibitors and TRANSTEC cannot be ruled out (see also 4.3 Contraindications).

When TRANSTEC is applied together with other opioids, anaesthetics, hypnotics, sedatives, antidepressants, neuroleptics, and in general, drugs that depress respiration and the central nervous system, the CNS effects may be intensified. This applies also to alcohol.

Administered together with inhibitors or inducers of CYP 3A4 the efficacy of TRANSTEC may be intensified (inhibitors) or weakened (inducers).

4.6 Pregnancy and lactation

Pregnancy

There are no adequate data from the use of TRANSTEC in pregnant women. Studies in animals have shown reproductive toxicity (see Section 5.3). The potential risk for humans is unknown.

Towards the end of pregnancy high doses of buprenorphine may induce respiratory depression in the neonate even after a short period of administration. Long-term administration of buprenorphine during the last three months of pregnancy may cause a withdrawal syndrome in the neonate.

Therefore TRANSTEC is contraindicated during pregnancy.

Lactation

Studies in rats have shown that buprenorphine may inhibit lactation. Excretion of buprenorphine into the milk in rats has been observed. Data on excretion into human milk are not available.

Therefore the use of TRANSTEC during lactation should be avoided.

4.7 Effects on ability to drive and use machines

Even when used according to instructions, TRANSTEC may affect the patient's reactions to such an extent that road safety and the ability to operate machinery may be impaired. This applies particularly in conjunction with other centrally acting substances including alcohol, tranquillisers, sedatives and hypnotics.

Patients wearing a TRANSTEC patch should not drive or use machines, nor for at least 24 hours after the patch has been removed.

4.8 Undesirable effects

Any undesirable effects occurring in the double-blind (phase III) clinical studies with all three patch strengths are presented in the following table:

SYSTEM ORGAN CLASS	**TRANSTEC patch** (n=323) % of patients
CENTRAL NERVOUS SYSTEM DISORDERS	
Nausea	16.7
Dizziness	6.8
Tiredness	5.6
Headache	1.5
Drowsiness	0.9
Sedation	0.6
GASTRO-INTESTINAL SYSTEM DISORDERS	
Vomiting	9.3
Constipation	5.3
BODY AS A WHOLE - GENERAL DISORDERS	
Diaphoresis	3.7
Oedema	1.5
RESPIRATORY SYSTEM DISORDERS	
Dyspnoea	2.2
URINARY SYSTEm disorders	
Micturition disorders	0.9
Urinary retention	0.6
SKIN AND SUBCUTANEOUS DISORDERS	
Erythema	17
Pruritus	14.7

Following TRANSTEC patch removal the most frequent local skin reactions were erythema and pruritus. Both symptoms were mainly mild and subsided within 24 hours of patch removal. On repeated patch application for a mean of five months up to two years exanthema developed in 7.5% of the patients. In isolated cases delayed local allergic reactions occurred with marked signs of inflammation. In such cases treatment with TRANSTEC should be terminated.

During pharmacokinetic studies (phase I) in healthy volunteers (n = 86) the tolerability of the TRANSTEC application was also tested. In addition to the above listed undesirable effects in patients, the following symptoms were observed in pain-free healthy volunteers:

<u>Systemic effects</u>

In several cases: concentration impaired, visual disturbance, muscle fasciculation, sleep disorder, hiccups, dry mouth, hot flushes and thoracic pain.

In individual cases: numbness, appetite lost, retching, dysequilibrium, parageusia, speech disorder, pyrosis, weariness, mood swings, decreased libido, ear pain, hyperventilation and eyelid oedema.

<u>Local effects</u>

In several cases: itching and pustules

In individual cases: vesicles, rash and prickling skin sensation.

In common with other strong analgesics, other side effects with buprenorphine have been reported, such as respiratory depression, miosis, rashes, blurring of vision, serious allergic reactions, hallucinations and other psychotomimetic effects.

Buprenorphine has a low risk of dependence. After discontinuation of TRANSTEC, withdrawal symptoms are unlikely. This is due to the gradual decrease of buprenorphine serum concentrations (usually over a period of 30 hours after removal of the last patch). However, after long-term use of the TRANSTEC patch withdrawal symptoms, similar to those occurring during opiate withdrawal, cannot be entirely excluded. These symptoms include: agitation, anxiety, nervousness, insomnia, hyperkinesia, tremor and gastrointestinal disorders.

4.9 Overdose

Buprenorphine has a wide safety margin. Due to the rate-controlled delivery of small amounts of buprenorphine into the blood circulation high or toxic buprenorphine concentrations in the blood are unlikely. The maximum serum concentration of buprenorphine after the application of the TRANSTEC 70 μg/h patch is ten times less than after the intravenous administration of the therapeutic dose of 0.3 mg buprenorphine.

Symptoms

In principal, on overdosage with buprenorphine, symptoms similar to those of other centrally acting analgesics (opioids) are to be expected. These are: respiratory depression, sedation, drowsiness, nausea, vomiting, cardiovascular collapse, and marked miosis.

Treatment

General emergency measures apply. Keep the airway open (aspiration!), maintain respiration and circulation depending on the symptoms. Naloxone is of limited usefulness in antagonising respiratory depression, and then only in high doses. Therefore, adequate ventilation should be established.

5. PHARMACOLOGICAL PROPERTIES

5.1 Pharmacodynamic properties

Buprenorphine is an opioid analgesic, ATC code: N02AE. Buprenorphine acts as a partial agonist at μ opioid receptors and as an antagonist at κ receptors.

Adverse effects are similar to those of other strong opioid analgesics. Buprenorphine appears to have a lower dependence liability than morphine.

5.2 Pharmacokinetic properties

a) General characteristics of the active substance

Buprenorphine has a plasma protein binding of about 96%.

Buprenorphine is metabolised in the liver to *N*-dealkylbuprenorphine (norbuprenorphine) and to glucuronide conjugated metabolites. $^2/_3$ of the drug is eliminated unchanged in the faeces and $^1/_3$ eliminated unchanged or dealkylated via the urinary system. There is evidence of enterohepatic recirculation.

Studies in non-pregnant and pregnant rats have shown that buprenorphine passes the blood-brain and placental barriers. Concentrations in the brain (which contained only unchanged buprenorphine) after parenteral administration were 2-3 times higher than after oral administration. After i.m. or oral administration buprenorphine apparently accumulates in the foetal gastrointestinal lumen – presumably due to biliary excretion, as enterohepatic circulation has not fully developed.

b) Characteristics of TRANSTEC in healthy volunteers

After the application of TRANSTEC, buprenorphine is absorbed through the skin. The continuous delivery of buprenorphine into the systemic circulation is by controlled release from the adhesive polymer-based matrix system.

After the initial application of TRANSTEC the plasma concentrations of buprenorphine gradually increase, and after 12-24 h the plasma concentrations reach the minimum effective concentration of 100 pg/ml. The plasma concentrations increase to a maximum of Cmax = 305 pg/ml (TRANSTEC 35 μg/h) and Cmax = 624 pg/ml (TRANSTEC 70 μg/h) at tmax = 57 h (TRANSTEC 35 μg/h) and tmax = 59 h (TRANSTEC 70 μg/h).

After removal of the TRANSTEC patch the plasma concentrations of buprenorphine steadily decrease and are eliminated with a half-life of approx. 30 hours (range 25 - 36). Due to the continuous absorption of buprenorphine from the depot in the skin elimination is slower than after intravenous administration.

5.3 Preclinical safety data

Standard toxicological studies have not shown evidence of any particular potential risks for humans. In tests with repeated doses of buprenorphine in rats the increase in body weight was reduced.

Studies on fertility and general reproductive capacity of rats showed no detrimental effects. Studies in rats and rabbits revealed signs of fetotoxicity and increased post-implantation loss.

Studies in rats showed diminished intra-uterine growth, delays in the development of certain neurological functions and high peri/post natal mortality in the neonates after treatment of the dams during gestation or lactation. There is evidence that complicated delivery and reduced lactation contributed to these effects. There was no evidence of embryotoxicity including teratogenicity in rats or rabbits.

In-vitro and in-vivo examinations on the mutagenic potential of buprenorphine did not indicate any clinically relevant effects.

In long-term studies in rats and mice there was no evidence of any carcinogenic potential relevant for humans.

Toxicological data available did not indicate a sensitising potential of the additives of the transdermal patches.

6. PHARMACEUTICAL PARTICULARS

6.1 List of excipients

Adhesive matrix (containing buprenorphine): [(Z)-octadec-9-en-1-yl] oleate, povidone K90, 4-oxopentanic acid, poly[acrylic acid-co-butylacrylate-co-(2-ethylhexyl)acrylate-co-vinylacetate] (5:15:75:5), cross-linked

Adhesive matrix (without buprenorphine): poly[acrylic acid-co-butylacrylate-co-(2-ethylhexyl)acrylate-co-vinylacetate] (5:15:75:5), cross-linked

Separating foil between the adhesive matrices with and without buprenorphine: poly(ethyleneterephthalate) - foil

Backing layer: poly(ethyleneterephthalate) – tissue

Release liner (on the front covering the adhesive matrix containing buprenorphine) (to be removed before applying the patch): poly(ethyleneterephthalate) – foil, siliconised, coated on one side with aluminium

6.2 Incompatibilities
Not applicable.

6.3 Shelf life
The shelf life of the medicinal product in the intact container (sealed sachet): 36 months.

6.4 Special precautions for storage
No special precautions.

6.5 Nature and contents of container
Type of container:

Sealed sachet, composed of identical top and bottom layers of heat-sealable laminate, comprising (from outside to inside) paper, low density polyethylene, aluminum and poly(acrylic acid-co-ethylene) (= surlyn).

Pack sizes:

Packs containing 5 individually sealed patches.

6.6 Instructions for use and handling
No special requirements

7. MARKETING AUTHORISATION HOLDER
Grünenthal GmbH,

Zieglerstrasse 6,

52078 Aachen,

Germany

8. MARKETING AUTHORISATION NUMBER(S)
PL 04539/0014

PL 04539/0015

PL 04539/0016

9. DATE OF FIRST AUTHORISATION/RENEWAL OF THE AUTHORISATION
27 February 2002

10. DATE OF REVISION OF THE TEXT
11 July 2005

11. LEGAL CATEGORY
POM CD (Sch 3)

TRASICOR Tablets 20mg, 40mg & 80mg

(Amdipharm)

1. NAME OF THE MEDICINAL PRODUCT
TRASICOR Tablets 20mg, 40mg & 80mg.

2. QUALITATIVE AND QUANTITATIVE COMPOSITION
Oxprenolol hydrochloride EP 20mg, 40mg & 80mg.

3. PHARMACEUTICAL FORM
Tablets.

4. CLINICAL PARTICULARS

4.1 Therapeutic indications
Angina Pectoris: For long-term prophylactic use (if necessary nitrates should be employed for alleviating acute attacks).

Hypertension: As monotherapy or for use in combination with other antihypertensives, e.g. with a diuretic, peripheral vasodilator, calcium channel blocker or ACE inhibitor.

Disturbances of cardiac rhythm: Especially supraventricular tachycardia, atrial fibrillation and digitalis-induced arrhythmias, ventricular tachycardia.

Short-term relief of functional cardiovascular disorders due to adrenergic hyperactivity: Such as cardiac neurosis, hyperkinetic heart syndrome and anxiety-induced cardiovascular disorders.

4.2 Posology and method of administration
The dosage should be individualised. Before raising the dosage, the heart rate at rest should always be checked. If it is 50-55 beats/min, the dosage should not be increased, see contraindications. The tablets should be swallowed with liquid.

If the maximum recommended dose is insufficient to produce the desired response appropriate combined therapy should be considered.

When discontinuing prolonged treatment with a beta-blocker, the medication should not be interrupted abruptly, but withdrawn gradually.

Higher doses using conventional Trasicor Tablets may be administered in two or more divided doses.

<u>Elderly</u>

No special dosage regime is necessary but concurrent hepatic insufficiency should be taken into account.

<u>Children</u>

No adequate experience has been acquired on the use of Trasicor in children.

Hypertension: 80 – 160mg total daily dose, given in 2 to 3 doses. If necessary, the dosage can be raised to 320mg.

Angina pectoris: 80 – 160mg total daily dose, given in 2 to 3 doses. If necessary, the dosage can be raised to 320mg.

Distribution of cardiac rhythm: 40 – 240mg total daily dose given in 2 – 3 doses. The maximum recommended dose is 240mg/day.

Short-term relief of functional cardiovascular disorders due to adrenergic hyperactivity e.g. short-term relief of sympathomimetic symptoms of anxiety: 40 – 80mg daily, given in 1 or 2 doses, is usually sufficient.

4.3 Contraindications
Trasicor is contraindicated in patients with

Hypersensitivity to oxprenolol and related derivatives, cross-sensitivity to other beta-blockers or to any of the excipients.

Cardiogenic shock.

Second or third degree atrioventricular block.

Uncontrolled heart failure.

Sick-sinus syndrome.

Bradycardia (< 45 – 50bpm).

Hypotension.

Untreated phaeochromocytoma.

Severe peripheral arterial circulatory disturbances.

History of bronchospasm and bronchial asthma. (A warning stating "Do not take this medicine if you have a history of wheezing or asthma" will appear on the label)

Prinzmetal's angina (variant angina pectoris).

Use of anaesthetics which are known to have a negative inotropic effect.

Metabolic acidosis.

4.4 Special warnings and special precautions for use
Owing to the risk of bronchoconstriction, non-selective beta-blockers such as Trasicor/Slow Trasicor should be used with particular caution in patients with chronic obstructive lung disease. (see "Contra-indications").

As beta-blockers increase the AV conduction time, beta-blockers should only be given with caution to patients with first degree AV block.

Beta-blockers should not be used in patients with untreated congestive heart failure. This condition should first be stabilised.

If the patient develops increasing bradycardia less than 50-55 beats per minute at rest and the patient experiences symptoms related to bradycardia, the dosage should be reduced or gradually withdrawn (see "Contra-indications").

Beta-blockers are liable to affect carbohydrate metabolism. Diabetic patients, especially those dependent on insulin, should be warned that beta-blockers can mask symptoms of hypoglycaemia (e.g. tachycardia) (see "Interactions with other medicaments and other forms of interaction"). Hypoglycaemia, producing loss of consciousness in some cases, may occur in non-diabetic individuals who are taking beta-blockers, particularly those who undergo prolonged fasting or severe exercise. The concurrent use of beta-blockers and anti-diabetic medication should always be monitored to confirm that diabetic control is well maintained.

Beta-blockers may mask certain clinical signs (e.g. tachycardia) of hyperthyroidism and the patient should be carefully monitored.

Beta-blockers may reduce liver function and thus affect the metabolism of other drugs. Like many beta-blockers oxprenolol undergoes substantial first-pass hepatic metabolism. In the presence of liver cirrhosis the bioavailability of oxprenolol may be increased leading to higher plasma concentrations (see "Pharmacokinetic properties"). Patients with severe renal failure might be more susceptible to the effects of anthihypertensive drugs due to haemodynamic effects. Careful monitoring is advisable (see "Pharmacokinetic properties").

In patients with peripheral circulatory disorders (e.g. Reynaud's disease or syndrome, intermittent claudication), beta-blockers should be used with great caution as aggravation of these disorders may occur (see "Contra-indications").

In patients with phaeochromocytoma a beta-blocker should only be given together with an alpha-blocker, (see "Contra-indications").

Owing to the danger of cardiac arrest, a calcium antagonist of the verapamil type must not be administered intravenously to the patient already receiving treatment with a beta-blocker. Furthermore, since beta-blockers may potentiate the negative-inotropic and dromotropic effects of calcium antagonists, like verapamil or diltiazem, any oral co-medication (e.g. in angina pectoris) requires close clinical control (see also "Interactions with other medicaments and other forms of interaction").

Anaphylactic reactions precipitated by other agents may be particularly severe in patients taking beta-blockers, especially non-selective drugs, and may require higher than normal doses of adrenaline for treatment. Whenever possible, beta-blockers should be discontinued in patients who are at increased risk for anaphylaxis.

Especially in patients with ischaemic heart disease, treatment should not be discontinued suddenly. The dosage should gradually be reduced, i.e. over 1-3 weeks, if necessary, at the same time initiating alternative therapy, to prevent exacerbation of angina pectoris.

If a patient receiving oxprenolol requires anaesthesia, the anaesthetist should be informed of the use of the medication prior to the use of general anaesthetic to permit him to take the necessary precautions. The anaesthetic selected should be one exhibiting as little inotropic activity as possible, e.g. halothane/nitrous oxide. If on the other hand, inhibition of sympathetic tone during the operation is regarded as undesirable, the beta-blocker should be withdrawn gradually at least 48 hours prior to surgery.

The full development of the "oculomucocutaneous syndrome", as previously described with practolol has not been reported with oxprenolol. However some features of this syndrome have been noted such as dry eyes alone or occasionally associated with skin rash. In most cases the symptoms cleared after withdrawal of the treatment. Discontinuation of oxprenolol should be considered, and a switch to another antihypertensive drug might be advisable, see advice on discontinuation above.

4.5 Interaction with other medicinal products and other forms of Interaction
Calcium channel blockers: e.g. verapamil, diltiazem: Potentiation of bradycardia, myocardial depression and hypotension; particularly after intravenous administration of verapamil in patients taking oral beta-blockers, the possibility of hypotension and cardiac arrhythmias cannot be excluded (see "Special Warnings and Precautions").

Class I anti-arrhythmic drugs and amiodarone: Drugs like disopyramide, quinidine and amiodarone may increase atrial-conduction time and induce negative inotropic effect when administered concomitantly with beta-blockers.

Sympathomimetic drugs: Non-cardioselective beta-blockers such as oxprenolol enhance the pressor response to sympathomimetic drugs such as adrenaline, noradrenaline, isoprenaline, ephedrine and phenylephrine (e.g. local anaesthetics in dentistry, nasal and ocular drops), resulting in hypertension and bradycardia.

Clonidine: When clonidine is used in conjunction with non-selective beta-blockers, such as oxprenolol, treatment with clonidine should be continued for some time after beta-blocker has been discontinued to reduce the danger of rebound hypertension.

Catecholamine-depleting drugs: e.g. guanethidine, reserpine, may have an additive effect when administered concomitantly with beta-blockers. Patients should be closely observed for hypotension.

Beta-blockers may modify blood glucose concentrations in patients being treated with insulin and oral antidiabetic drugs and may alter the response to hypoglycaemia by prolonging the recovery (blood glucose rise) from hypoglycaemia, causing hypotension and blocking tachycardia. In diabetic patients receiving beta-blockers hypoglycaemic episodes may not result in the expected tachycardia but hypoglycaemia-induced sweating will occur and may even be intensified and prolonged. (see "Special Warnings and Precautions).

Non-steroidal anti-inflammatory drugs (NSAIDs): Non-steroidal anti-inflammatory drugs (NSAIDs) can reduce the hypotensive effect of beta-blockade.

Cimetidine: Hepatic metabolism of beta-blockers may be reduced resulting in increased plasma levels of beta-blocker and prolonged serum half-life. Marked bradycardia may occur.

Ergot alkaloids: Concomitant administration with beta-blockers may enhance the vasoconstrictive action of ergot alkaloids.

Anaesthetic drugs: Beta-blockers and certain anaesthetics (e.g. halothane) are additive in their cardiodepressant effect. However, continuation of beta-blockers reduces the risk of arrhythmia during anaesthesia (see "Special Warnings and Precautions").

Digitalis glycosides: Beta-blockers and digitalis glycosides may be additive in their depressant effect on myocardial conduction, particularly through the atrioventricular node, resulting in bradycardia or heart block.

Lidocaine: Concomitant administration with beta-blockers may increase lidocaine blood concentrations and potential toxicity; patients should be closely monitored for increased lidocaine effects.

Alcohol and beta-blocker effects on the central nervous system have been observed to be additive and it is possible that symptoms such as dizziness may be exaggerated if alcohol and Trasicor are taken together (see also "Special Warnings and Precautions").

4.6 Pregnancy and lactation
As in the case of any form of drug therapy, oxprenolol should be employed with caution during pregnancy, especially in the first 3 months.

Beta-blockers may reduce placental perfusion, which may result in intrauterine foetal death, immature and premature deliveries. Use the lowest possible dose. If possible, discontinue beta-blocker therapy at least 2 to 3 days prior to delivery to avoid the effects on uterine contractility and possible adverse effects, especially bradycardia and hypoglycaemia, in the foetus and neonate.

Oxprenolol is excreted into breast milk (see "Pharmacokinetic properties"). However, although the estimated daily infant dose derived from breast-feeding is likely to be very low, breast feeding is not recommended.

4.7 Effects on ability to drive and use machines

Patients receiving oxprenolol should be warned that dizziness, fatigue or visual disturbances (see "Undesirable Effects") may occur, in which case they should not drive, operate machinery or do anything else requiring alertness, particularly if they also consume alcohol.

4.8 Undesirable effects

Side-Effects: Frequency estimate: very common > 10%, common > 1% - < 10%, uncommon > 0.1% - < 1%, rare > 0.01% - < 0.1%, very rare < 0.01%.

Central nervous system:

Common: Fatigue, dizziness, headache, mental depression.

Uncommon: Sleep disturbances, nightmares.

Rare: Hallucinations, exertional tiredness.

Cardiovascular system:

Common: Hypotension, heart failure, peripheral vascular disorders (e.g. cold extremities, paraesthesia).

Uncommon: Bradycardia, disturbance of cardiac conduction.

Rare: Raynaud-like symptoms.

Gastro-intestinal tract:

Very common: Dry mouth, constipation.

Common: Nausea.

Uncommon: Diarrhoea, vomiting, flatulence.

Skin and appendages:

Uncommon: Allergic skin rash (e.g. urticarial, psoriasiform, eczematous, lichenoid).

Rare: Worsening of psoriasis.

Respiratory system:

Common: Dyspnoea, bronchoconstriction (see "Special Warnings and Precautions" and "Contra-indications").

Sense organs:

Uncommon: Visual disturbances ("blurred vision", "vision abnormal").

Rare: Dry eyes, keratoconjuctivitis.

Others:

Common: Disturbances of libido and potency.

Very rare: Thrombocytopenia.

4.9 Overdose

Signs and symptoms:

Poisoning due to an overdosage of beta-blocker may lead to pronounced hypotension, bradycardia, hypoglycaemia, heart failure, cardiogenic shock, conduction abnormalities (first or second degree block, complete heart block, asystole), or even cardiac arrest. In addition, dyspnoea, bronchospasm, vomiting, impairment of consciousness, and also generalised convulsions may occur.

The manifestations of poisoning with beta-blocker are dependent on the pharmacological properties of the ingested drug. Although the onset of action is rapid, effects of massive overdose may persist for several days despite declining plasma levels. Watch carefully for cardiovascular or respiratory deterioration in an intensive care setting, particularly in the early hours. Observe mild overdose cases for at least 4 hours for the development of signs of poisoning.

Treatment:

Patients who are seen soon after potentially life-threatening overdosage (within 4 hours) should be treated by gastric lavage and activated charcoal.

Treatment of symptoms is based on modern methods of intensive care, with continuous monitoring of cardiac function, blood gases, and electrolytes, and if necessary, emergency measures such as artificial respiration, resuscitation or cardiac pacemaker.

Significant bradycardia should be treated initially with atropine. Large doses of isoprenaline may be necessary for control of heart rate and hypotension. Glucagon has positive chronotropic and inotropic effects on the heart that are independent of interactions with beta-adrenergic receptors and it represents a useful alternative treatment for hypotension and heart failure.

For seizures, diazepam has been effective and is the drug of choice.

For bronchospasm, aminophylline, salbutamol or terbutaline (beta$_2$-agonist) are effective bronchodilator drugs. Monitor the patient for dysrhythmias during and after administration.

Patients who recover should be observed for signs of beta-blocker withdrawal phenomenon (see "Special Warnings and Precautions").

5. PHARMACOLOGICAL PROPERTIES

5.1 Pharmacodynamic properties

Oxprenolol, the active substance of Trasicor, is a non-selective, lipophilic beta-blocker exerting a sympatholytic effect and displaying mild to modest partial agonistic activity (PAA), also known as intrinsic sympathomimetic activity (ISA).

Drugs like oxprenolol with PAA cause comparatively less slowing of the resting heart rate and a less marked negative-inotropic effect than those without PAA. The risk of substantial bradycardia at rest and heart failure is lessened.

The antiarrhythmic effect of oxprenolol is primarily due to suppression of the arrhythmogenic sympathetic influence of catecholamines. Evidence that increased sympathetic stimulation predisposes to many arrhythmias is strong. This is supported by the increased incidence of arrhythmias in man in situations associated with high sympathetic drive or myocardial sensitisation to catecholamines e.g. exercise, emotional stress, phaeochromocytoma, trauma, myocardial ischaemia, anaesthesia, hyperthyroidism.

Oxprenolol decreases cardiac impulse formation in the sinus node with resultant slowing of the sinus rate; it slightly prolongs the sino-atrial conduction time; both the atrioventricular (AV) conduction time and the AV node refractory periods are lengthened.

Some beta-blockers such as oxprenolol possess a membrane stabilising activity (MSA) on the cardiac action potential, also known as "quinidine-like" or "local anaesthetic" action, a property that tends to result in greater cardiac depression than is seen with beta-blockers which do not have this pharmacological characteristic. However, at normal therapeutic doses, this property is probably clinically irrelevant and it only becomes manifest after overdose.

In coronary artery disease, oxprenolol is beneficial in increasing exercise tolerance and decreasing the frequency and severity of anginal attacks.

Emotional stress and anxiety states, the symptoms of which are largely caused by increased sympathetic drive, are alleviated by the sympatholytic effect of oxprenolol.

The exact way in which beta-blockers exert their antihypertensive action is still not fully understood. Various modes of action have been postulated. During chronic therapy the antihypertensive effect of beta-blockers is associated with a decline in peripheral resistance.

Oxprenolol is effective in lowering elevated supine, standing and exercise blood pressure; postural hypotension is unlikely to occur.

5.2 Pharmacokinetic properties

Absorption:

Oral oxprenolol is rapidly and completely absorbed. Food has no significant effect on absorption. Peak plasma concentrations are achieved approximately 1 hour after drug administration.

Biotransformation:

Oxprenolol is subject to first-pass metabolism. Its systemic bioavailability is 20 – 70%.

Distribution:

Oxprenolol has a plasma-protein binding rate of approx. 80% and a calculated distribution volume of 1.2 l/kg.

Oxprenolol crosses the placental barrier. The concentration in the breast milk is equivalent to approx. 30% of that in the plasma.

Elimination:

Oxprenolol has an elimination half-life of 1 – 2 hours. Oxprenolol is extensively metabolised, direct O-glucuronidation being the major metabolic pathway and oxidative reactions minor ones. Oxprenolol is excreted chiefly in the urine (almost exclusively in the form of inactive metabolites). The drug is not likely to accumulate.

Characteristics in patients:

Age has no effect on the pharmacokinetics of oxprenolol.

In patients with acute or chronic inflammatory diseases an increase in the plasma levels of oxprenolol has been observed. The plasma levels may also increase in the presence of severe hepatic insufficiency associated with a reduced metabolism.

Impaired renal function generally leads to an increase in the blood levels of oxprenolol, but the concentrations measured remain within – although at the upper limit of – the concentration range recorded in subjects with healthy kidneys. In addition, in patients with renal failure the apparent elimination half-life for unchanged, i.e. active, oxprenolol is comparable with the corresponding half-life values determined in subjects with no renal disease. Hence, there is no need to readjust the dosage in the presence of impaired renal function.

5.3 Preclinical safety data

None stated.

6. PHARMACEUTICAL PARTICULARS

6.1 List of excipients

20 mg and 40mg Tablets:

Calcium phosphate tribasic, magnesium stearate, polyvinylpyrollidone K25, sucrose, purified talc special, wheat starch, cellulose-HP-M-603, Kollidon VA64, titanium dioxide E171.

80 mg Tablets:

Calcium phosphate, maize starch, Povidone K25, Aerosil 200V, sodium starch glycollate, purified talc special, magnesium stearate, hydroxypropylmethylcellulose 3 CPS, polysorbate 80, titanium dioxide E171, yellow iron oxide 17268 E172.

6.2 Incompatibilities

None known.

6.3 Shelf life

60 months.

6.4 Special precautions for storage

Protect from moisture.

6.5 Nature and contents of container

PVC* Blister packs of 56 (20 mg, 40 mg and 80 mg tablets) and 100 (20 mg and 40 mg tablets only) tablets.

*PVC 250 micron, aluminium foil 20 micron.

6.6 Instructions for use and handling

None.

7. MARKETING AUTHORISATION HOLDER

Amdipharm plc

Regency House

Miles Gray Road

Basildon

Essex

SS14 3AF

UK

8. MARKETING AUTHORISATION NUMBER(S)

Trasicor Tablets 20 mg – PL 20072/0018

Trasicor Tablets 40 mg – PL 20072/0019

Trasicor Tablets 80 mg – PL 20072/0020

9. DATE OF FIRST AUTHORISATION/RENEWAL OF THE AUTHORISATION

Trasicor Tablets 20 mg – 1st January 2005

Trasicor Tablets 40 mg – 1st January 2005

Trasicor Tablets 80 mg – 1st January 2005

10. DATE OF REVISION OF THE TEXT

Trasylol

(Bayer plc)

1. NAME OF THE MEDICINAL PRODUCT

TRASYLOL

2. QUALITATIVE AND QUANTITATIVE COMPOSITION

Each 50 ml vial contains aprotinin solution corresponding to 70 mg aprotinin (= 500,000 Kallikrein Inactivator Units, KIU = 277.8 European Pharmacopoeia Units, E.P. units) in 0.9 % sodium chloride solution.

For excipients see Section 6.1.

3. PHARMACEUTICAL FORM

Solution for infusion.

4. CLINICAL PARTICULARS

4.1 Therapeutic indications

Trasylol is indicated for the treatment of patients at high risk of major blood loss during and following open heart surgery with extracorporeal circulation. These include:

Patients requiring re-operation through a previous median sternotomy.

Patients with septic endocarditis.

Patients with known blood dyscrasias and coagulopathy, e.g. haemophiliacs, patients with von Willebrand's disease, patients receiving treatment with aspirin.

Trasylol is also indicated for the treatment of patients in whom optimal blood conservation during open heart surgery is an absolute priority. These include:

Jehovah's Witnesses who are to undergo open heart surgery with extracorporeal circulation.

Patients who require open heart surgery and are known carriers of a highly infectious virus, e.g. Hepatitis B, HIV.

Patients with rare blood groups who require open heart surgery.

Since Trasylol can contribute to the re-establishment of haemostasis by inactivating free plasmin, it is indicated for the treatment of life-threatening haemorrhage due to hyperplasminaemia. Such haemorrhage has occasionally been observed during the mobilisation and dissection of malignant tumours, in acute promyelocytic leukaemia, and following thrombolytic therapy.

4.2 Posology and method of administration

A 1 ml (10,000 KIU) initial dose should always be administered at least 10 minutes prior to the remainder of the dose due to the risk of allergic/anaphylactic reactions (see Section 4.8). This is especially important in patients with documented previous exposure to aprotinin and in those patients for whom a previous exposure is uncertain.

After the uneventful administration of the initial 1 ml dose, the therapeutic dose may be given.

Trasylol must be given only to patients in the supine position and must be given slowly (maximum 5-10 ml/min) as an intravenous injection or a short infusion.

Open heart surgery

Adults

The recommended regimen involves a loading dose, maintenance dose and a pump prime dose, administered as follows:

(i) *Loading dose*

A loading dose of 200 ml (2 million KIU) is administered as a slow intravenous injection or infusion over 20 minutes after induction of anaesthesia and prior to sternotomy.

(ii) *Maintenance dose*

The loading dose should be followed by the administration of a continuous infusion of 50 ml (500,000 KIU) per hour until the end of the operation except in patients with septic endocarditis where it may be continued into the early post-operative period.

(iii) *Pump prime dose*

An additional 200 ml (2 million KIU) should be added to the priming volume of the extracorporeal circuit. In patients with septic endocarditis 300 ml (3 million KIU) should be added to the pump prime.

In general, the total amount of aprotinin administered per treatment course should not exceed 7 million KIU.

Elderly

No dosage adjustment in the elderly is necessary.

Children

The dosage has not been established.

Hyperplasminaemia

Adults

Initially 50 ml (500,000 KIU) to 100 ml (1 million KIU) should be given by slow intravenous injection or infusion (maximum rate 10 ml/min). If necessary, this should be followed by 20 ml (200,000 KIU) hourly until bleeding stops.

Children

The dose should be calculated in proportion to the adult dose on the basis of body weight.

4.3 Contraindications

Known hypersensitivity to aprotinin.

For use in pregnancy see Section 4.6.

4.4 Special warnings and special precautions for use

If an allergic/anaphylactic reaction occurs during the injection, administration should be stopped immediately and the appropriate therapeutic measures instituted, e.g. adrenaline, antihistamines and intravenous corticosteroids. Intravenous fluids, bronchodilators and respiratory support may also be needed.

The addition of Trasylol to heparinised blood will prolong the activated clotting time (ACT). Thus, the ACT should not be taken as a reliable indicator of the need to administer additional heparin during a prolonged period of cardiopulmonary bypass. Furthermore, a prolonged ACT in the presence of Trasylol does not necessarily signify excess heparin requiring additional protamine. It is therefore not necessary to adjust the usual heparin/protamine regimen during treatment with Trasylol.

An increase in renal failure and mortality compared to age-matched historical controls has been reported for aprotinin-treated patients undergoing cardiopulmonary bypass with deep hypothermic circulatory arrest during operation on the thoracic aorta. Trasylol should therefore be used with extreme caution under these circumstances. Adequate anti-coagulation with heparin must be assured (see also additional note below).

Additional note on use with extracorporeal circulation

In patients undergoing cardiopulmonary bypass with Trasylol therapy, one of the following methods is recommended to maintain adequate anticoagulation:

1. ACT – An ACT is not a standardised coagulation test, and different formulations of the assay are affected differently by the presence of aprotinin. The test is further influenced by variable dilution effects and the temperature experienced during cardiopulmonary bypass. It has been observed that kaolin-based ACTs are not increased to the same degree by aprotinin as are diatomaceous earth-based (celite) ACTs. While protocols vary, a minimal celite-ACT of 750 seconds or kaolin-ACT of 480 seconds, independent of the effects of haemodilution and hypothermia, is recommended in the presence of aprotinin. Consult the manufacturer of the ACT test regarding the interpretation of the assay in the presence of Trasylol.

2. Fixed Heparin Dosing - A standard loading dose of heparin, administered prior to cannulation of the heart, plus the quantity of heparin added to the prime volume of the cardiopulmonary bypass circuit, should total at least 350 IU/kg. Additional heparin should be administered in a fixed-dose regimen based on patient weight and duration of cardiopulmonary bypass.

3. Heparin Titration – Protamine titration, a method that is not affected by aprotinin, can be used to measure heparin levels. A heparin dose response, assessed by protamine titration, should be performed prior to administration of aprotinin to determine the heparin loading dose. Additional heparin should be administered on the basis of heparin levels measured by protamine titration. Heparin levels during bypass should not be allowed to drop below 2.7 U/ml (2.0 mg/kg) or below the level indicated by heparin dose-response testing performed prior to administration of aprotinin.

In Trasylol treated patients the neutralisation of heparin by protamine after discontinuation of cardiopulmonary bypass should either be based on a fixed ratio to the amount of heparin applied or be controlled by a protamine titration method.

Trasylol is not a heparin-sparing agent.

4.5 Interaction with other medicinal products and other forms of interaction

Trasylol has a dose-dependent inhibitory effect on the action of thrombolytic agents, e.g. streptokinase, urokinase, alteplase (r-tPA).

4.6 Pregnancy and lactation

No evidence of teratogenic or embryotoxic effects has been seen in animals. Experience in human pregnancy and lactation is limited and inadequate to assess safety. Hence, Trasylol should only be used during pregnancy after a careful risk/benefit assessment.

No studies are available on the use of Trasylol during lactation. However, since aprotinin is not bioavailable after oral administration, any drug contained in the milk would be very unlikely to have any effect on the baby.

4.7 Effects on ability to drive and use machines

None known.

4.8 Undesirable effects

Spontaneous reports

The following undesirable effects have been noted in spontaneous reports with aprotinin:

Body as a whole

Allergic/anaphylactic reactions are rare in patients with no prior exposure to aprotinin. A retrospective review showed that the incidence of an allergic/anaphylactic reaction following re-exposure is increased when the re-exposure occurs within 6 months of the initial administration (5% for re-exposure within 6 months and 0.9% for re-exposures greater than 6 months). The incidence of severe anaphylactic reactions to aprotinin may further increase when patients are re-exposed more than twice within 6 months. Even when a second exposure to aprotinin has been tolerated without symptoms, a subsequent administration may result in severe allergic reactions or anaphylactic shock with, in rare cases, a fatal outcome.

The symptoms of allergic/anaphylactic shock may include:

Cardiovascular:	bradycardia, hypotension, tachycardia, vasodilatation
Digestive:	nausea
Respiratory:	asthma (bronchospasm), dyspnoea
Skin:	cyanosis, pallor, pruritis, urticaria

If allergic reactions occur during injection or infusion, administration should be stopped immediately. Standard emergency treatment may be required (see section 4.4).

Cardiovascular system

As with all venepunctures, local thrombophlebitic reactions may occur after Trasylol injections or infusions.

Urogenital system

Abnormal kidney function has been observed in clinical studies. During post-marketing surveillance single cases of reversible kidney failure have been reported.

Clinical trials

During placebo-controlled clinical studies (aprotinin, n = 3107; placebo, n = 2228), the following adverse drug reactions were reported (placebo subtracted incidence):

Uncommon ($\geqslant$ *0.1%* $<$ *1%*)

Cardiovascular:	coronary thrombosis, cardiac arrest, heart failure, myocardial infarction, pericardial effusion, thrombosis, ventricular fibrillation
Urogenital:	abnormal kidney function

Rare ($\geqslant$ *0.01%* $<$ *0.1%*)

Cardiovascular:	arterial thrombosis, myocardial ischaemia

For all clinical trials with aprotinin including those with no placebo group (n = 3797), the cardiovascular adverse drug reaction of haemorrhage was uncommonly reported ($\geqslant$ 0.1% $<$ 1%) in addition to those reported for the placebo-controlled clinical studies.

Cardiovascular system additional notes

In two clinical studies, where patients underwent a second coronary bypass surgery, an increased incidence of peri-operative fatal/non-fatal myocardial infarction was observed in the aprotinin group compared with the placebo group. It has been suggested that the increased risk in this patient-population and/or inadequate heparinisation contributed to this result (ACT-determination with celite activated system; see note on heparinisation in Section 4.4). These findings have not been confirmed in another study of basically identical design.

In a multicentre study in patients undergoing primary coronary artery bypass graft surgery there was an increased risk of graft occlusion for aprotinin treated patients compared with patients who received placebo. Two centres mainly negatively influenced this result. Subanalyses clearly demonstrated that for one centre inadequate heparinisation was the primary issue while the other centre used a non-standard graft conservation technique. In addition to the note on heparinisation (see section 4.4) the practice of using blood from the aprotinin central infusion line is strongly discouraged. No differences between the treatment groups were observed for the incidence of myocardial infarctions or deaths in the study.

4.9 Overdose

Symptoms of overdosage are not known and there is no specific antidote.

5. PHARMACOLOGICAL PROPERTIES

5.1 Pharmacodynamic properties

ATC code: B 02 AB 01

Trasylol is a protease inhibitor which contributes to the re-establishment of haemostasis by inactivating free plasmin, thus supplementing the natural plasmin inhibitors, like alpha-2-antiplasmin, which are depleted in the hyperplasminaemic state. Trasylol also inhibits the fibrinolytic activity of the plasmin streptokinase complex formed following thrombolytic therapy with streptokinase.

5.2 Pharmacokinetic properties

Following intravenous injection of aprotinin, an initial rapid clearance is followed by a slower exponential decrease ($T_{½}$'s of approximately two and seven hours respectively).

A constant infusion of 250,000 KIU/hour provides a steady-state plasma concentration of 40-50 KIU/ml. This is equivalent to about 1μmol/L which is of the same order of magnitude as the concentration of alpha-2-antiplasmin in normal plasma. Normally aprotinin does not cross the blood-brain barrier.

Aprotinin is degraded by lysosomal activity in the kidney. The resulting products are excreted renally. Aprotinin is not excreted unchanged in the urine.

5.3 Preclinical safety data

In rat intravenous studies, daily doses of up to 80,000 KIU/kg produced no maternal toxicity, embryotoxicity, or foetotoxicity.

6. PHARMACEUTICAL PARTICULARS

6.1 List of excipients

0.9 % sodium chloride solution.

6.2 Incompatibilities

Trasylol has been shown to be incompatible with corticosteroids, heparin and nutrient solutions containing amino acids or fat emulsions and tetracyclines. Administration of Trasylol in mixed infusions (particularly with beta-lactam antibiotics) should be avoided. Trasylol is compatible with electrolyte and sugar solutions.

6.3 Shelf life

The shelf-life of Trasylol is 48 months.

Any unused solution should be discarded immediately. Do not use the contents of the vials after the expiry date shown on the label.

6.4 Special precautions for storage

Do not store above 25 °C.

6.5 Nature and contents of container

Type II glass infusion bottles, colourless: vials of 500,000 KIU/50 ml.

Sealed with chlorobutyl stoppers.

6.6 Instructions for use and handling

If the contents are cloudy, the product must not be used.

7. MARKETING AUTHORISATION HOLDER

Bayer plc

Bayer House

Strawberry Hill

Newbury, Berkshire

RG14 1JA

Trading as Bayer plc, Pharmaceutical Division.

8. MARKETING AUTHORISATION NUMBER(S)

PL 0010/5900R

9. DATE OF FIRST AUTHORISATION/RENEWAL OF THE AUTHORISATION

Date of first authorisation: 5 July 1990

Date of last renewal: 13 November 2000

10. DATE OF REVISION OF THE TEXT

August 2002

LEGAL CATEGORY

POM

Trental 400

(sanofi-aventis)

1. NAME OF THE MEDICINAL PRODUCT

TRENTAL 400.

2. QUALITATIVE AND QUANTITATIVE COMPOSITION

Pentoxifylline 400MG.

3. PHARMACEUTICAL FORM
Modified release tablet.

4. CLINICAL PARTICULARS

4.1 Therapeutic indications
Trental 400 is indicated in the treatment of peripheral vascular disease, including intermittent claudication and rest pain.

4.2 Posology and method of administration
The recommended initial dose is 1 tablet (400 mg) three times daily; two tablets daily may prove sufficient in some patients, particularly for maintenance therapy. Tablets should be taken with or immediately after meals, and swallowed whole with plenty of water.

Elderly: No special dosage requirements.

Children: Trental 400 is not suitable for use in children.

Special Cases: In patients with impairment of renal function (creatinine clearance below 30ml/min) a dose reduction by approximately 30% to 50% may be necessary guided by individual tolerance.

4.3 Contraindications
Trental 400 is contra-indicated in cases where there is known hypersensitivity to the active constituent, pentoxifylline other methyl xanthines or any of the excipients. Also in patients with cerebral haemorrhage, extensive retinal haemorrhage, acute myocardial infarction and severe cardiac arrhythmias.

4.4 Special warnings and special precautions for use
In patients with hypotension or severe coronary artery disease, Trental 400 should be used with caution, as a transient hypotensive effect is possible and, in isolated cases, might result in a reduction in coronary artery perfusion.

Particularly careful monitoring is required in patients with impaired renal function. In patients with a creatinine clearance of less than 30 ml/min it may be necessary to reduce the daily dose of Trental 400 to one or two tablets to avoid accumulation. In patients with severely impaired liver function the dosage may need to be reduced.

4.5 Interaction with other medicinal products and other forms of Interaction
High doses of Trental injection have been shown, in rare cases, to intensify the hypoglycaemic action of insulin and oral hypoglycaemic agents. However, no effect on insulin release has been observed with Trental following oral administration.

Trental 400 may potentiate the effect of anti-hypertensive agents and the dosage of the latter may need to be reduced.

Trental 400 should not be given concomitantly with ketorolac as there is increased risk of bleeding and/or prolongation of prothrombin time.

Concomitant administration of pentoxifylline and theophylline may increase theophylline levels in some patients. Therefore there may be an increase in and intensification of adverse effects of theophylline.

4.6 Pregnancy and lactation
There is no information on the use of Trental in pregnancy but no untoward effects have been found in animal studies. Trental 400 should not be administered during pregnancy.

Pentoxifylline passes into breast milk in minute quantities. Because insufficient experience has been gained, the possible risks and benefits must be weighed before administration of Trental 400 to breast feeding mothers.

4.7 Effects on ability to drive and use machines
No effect known.

4.8 Undesirable effects
Gastrointestinal side-effects (e.g. nausea, vomiting, diarrhoea), may occur which, in individual cases, could necessitate discontinuation of treatment. Headache, dizziness, agitation and sleep disorders may occasionally occur as well as, in isolated cases intrahepatic cholestasis and transaminase elevation.

There have been reports of flushing, occasionally tachycardia and rarely angina pectoris and hypotension, particularly if using high doses of pentoxifylline. In such cases a discontinuation of the medication or a reduction of the daily dosage is required.

Hypersensitivity reactions such as pruritus, rash, urticaria, anaphylactic or anaphylactoid reactions with angioneurotic edema or bronchospasm may occur in isolated cases and usually disappear rapidly after discontinuation of the drug treatment.

A few very rare events of bleeding (e.g. skin, mucosa) have been reported in patients treated with Trental with and without anticoagulants or platelet aggregation inhibitors. The serious cases are predominantly concentrated in the gastrointestinal, genitourinary, multiple site and surgical wound areas and are associated with bleeding risk factors. A causal relationship between Trental therapy and bleeding has not been established. Thrombocytopenia has occurred in isolated cases.

4.9 Overdose
The treatment of overdosage should be symptomatic with particular attention to supporting the cardiovascular system.

5. PHARMACOLOGICAL PROPERTIES

5.1 Pharmacodynamic properties
Leukocyte properties of haemorrheologic importance have been modified in animal and in vitro human studies. Pentoxifylline has been shown to increase leukocyte deformability and to inhibit neutrophil adhesion and activation.

5.2 Pharmacokinetic properties
The half life of absorption of Trental 400 is 4-6 hours. Pentoxifylline is extensively metabolised, mainly in the liver. Sixty percent of a single dose of Trental 400 is eliminated via the kidney over 24 hours.

5.3 Preclinical safety data
Nothing of clinical relevance.

6. PHARMACEUTICAL PARTICULARS

6.1 List of excipients
Hydroxyethyl cellulose, povidone, talc, magnesium stearate, hypromellose, macrogol 8000, erythrosine (E127). titanium dioxide (E171).

6.2 Incompatibilities
None known.

6.3 Shelf life
5 years.

6.4 Special precautions for storage
Do not store above 25°C. Store in the original package.

6.5 Nature and contents of container
Blister Pack (Alu/PVC): 90 tablets.

6.6 Instructions for use and handling
None.

7. MARKETING AUTHORISATION HOLDER
Aventis Pharma Ltd.
50 Kings Hill Avenue
Kings Hill
West Malling
Kent
ME19 4AH
UK

8. MARKETING AUTHORISATION NUMBER(S)
PL 04425/0213

9. DATE OF FIRST AUTHORISATION/RENEWAL OF THE AUTHORISATION
15th April 2002

10. DATE OF REVISION OF THE TEXT
September 2004
Legal category: POM

Treosulfan Capsules 250 mg

(medac GmbH)

1. NAME OF THE MEDICINAL PRODUCT
Treosulfan Capsules 250 mg

2. QUALITATIVE AND QUANTITATIVE COMPOSITION
White opaque capsules each containing 250 mg treosulfan.

3. PHARMACEUTICAL FORM
Capsules

4. CLINICAL PARTICULARS

4.1 Therapeutic indications
For the treatment of all types of ovarian cancer, either supplementary to surgery or palliatively. Some uncontrolled studies have suggested activity in a wider range of neoplasms.

Because of a lack of cross-resistance reported between Treosulfan and other cytotoxic agents Treosulfan may be useful in any neoplasm refractive to conventional therapy.

Treosulfan has been used in combination regimens in conjunction with vincristine, methotrexate, 5-FU and procarbazine.

4.2 Posology and method of administration
The following dosage regimens have been indicated. All regimens indicate that a total dose of 21-28 g of treosulfan should be given in the initial 8 weeks of treatment.

Regimen A: 1 g daily, given in four divided doses for four weeks, followed by four weeks off therapy.

Regimen B: 1 g daily, given in four divided doses for two weeks, followed by two weeks off therapy.

Regimen C: 1.5 g daily, given in three divided doses for one week only, followed by three weeks off therapy. If no evidence of haematological toxicity at this dose in Regimen C, increase to 2 g daily in four divided doses for one week for the second and subsequent courses.

These cycles should be repeated with the dose being adjusted if necessary, as outlined below, according to the effect on the peripheral blood counts. The capsules should be swallowed whole and not allowed to disintegrate within the mouth.

Dose modification (all regimens): For excessive haematological toxicity (white blood cell count less than 3.000/microlitre or thrombocyte count less than 100.000/microlitre, a repeat blood count should be made after 1-2 weeks interval and treatment restarted if haematological parameters are satisfactory, reducing dose as follows:

Regimen A: 1 g daily × 28 to 0.75 g daily × 28 (and to 0.5 g daily × 28 if necessary).

Regimen B: 1 g daily × 14 to 0.75 g daily × 14 (and to 0.5 g daily × 14 if necessary).

Regimen C: 2 g daily × 7 to 1.5 g daily × 7 (and to 1 g daily × 7 if necessary).

Present evidence, whilst not definitive, suggests that Regimens B and C are less myelosuppressive than Regimen A, whilst retaining maximum cytotoxic efficacy.

Dosage in the elderly
Treosulfan is renally excreted. Blood counts should be carefully monitored in the elderly and the dosage adjusted accordingly.

Children
Not recommended

4.3 Contraindications
Severe and lasting bone marrow depression.

4.4 Special warnings and special precautions for use
None

4.5 Interaction with other medicinal products and other forms of Interaction
In one patient the effect of ibuprofen/chloroquine was reduced with concomitant administration of treosulfan.

4.6 Pregnancy and lactation
Warning: This product should not normally be administered to patients who are pregnant or to mothers who are breast feeding.

Woman of childbearing age should take adequate contraceptive precautions.

4.7 Effects on ability to drive and use machines
Because of nausea and vomiting the ability to drive or operate machines may be influenced.

4.8 Undesirable effects
The dose-limiting side effect of treosulfan is a myelosuppression, which is usually reversible. It is manifested by a reduction in leukocytes and platelets and a decrease in haemoglobin.

The leukocytes and platelets usually reach their baseline level after 28 days.

Because the inhibition of bone marrow function is cumulative, the blood count should be monitored at shorter intervals starting with the third course of treatment.

This is especially important if combined with other forms of therapy that suppress bone marrow function such as radiotherapy.

During long-term therapy with oral treosulfan doses eight patients (1.4 % of 553 patients) developed an acute non-lymphatic leukaemia.

Skin
Mild alopecia is observed in 16 % of the patients and a skin pigmentation in the form of a bronze discoloration in up to 30 % of the cases.

The occurrence of urticaria, erythemas, a scleroderma and triggering of a psoriasis have been reported.

Respiratory
In rare cases allergic alveolitis, pneumonia and pulmonary fibrosis have developed.

Gastrointestinal
Nausea with or without vomiting is observed in approx. 50 % of the patients.

Stomatitis may occur if the patients chew the capsule.

Other adverse reactions
In rare cases flu-like complaints, a paraesthesia, haemorrhagic cystitis, Addison's disease and hypoglycaemia have been observed. It cannot be totally ruled out that one case of cardiomyopathy was related to treosulfan.

Because of the possible development of a haemorrhagic cystitis patients are advised to drink more fluids for up to 24 hours after infusion.

4.9 Overdose
Although there is no experience of acute overdosage with treosulfan, nausea, vomiting and gastritis may occur. Prolonged or excessive therapeutic doses may result in bone marrow depression which has occasionally been irreversible. The drug should be withdrawn, a blood transfusion given and general supportive measures given.

5. PHARMACOLOGICAL PROPERTIES

5.1 Pharmacodynamic properties
Treosulfan is a bifunctional alkylating agent which has been shown to possess antineoplastic activity in the animal tumor screen and in clinical trials. The activity of treosulfan is due to the formation of epoxide compounds in vivo.

Treosulfan is converted in vitro under physiological conditions (pH 7.4; 37 °C) non-enzymatically via a monoepoxide to the diepoxide (diepoxybutane) with a half-life of 2.2 hours.

The epoxides formed react with nucleophilic centres of the DNA and are responsible via secondary biological mechanisms for the antineoplastic effect. It is important that in vivo the monoepoxide first formed can already alkylate a nucleophilic centre of the DNA. This fixes the compound to this centre by chemical reaction before the second epoxide ring is formed.

5.2 Pharmacokinetic properties

Oral absorption from treosulfan is excellent with the bioavailability approaching 100 %.

5.3 Preclinical safety data

Acute toxicity

In mice the oral LD_{50} is 3360 mg treosulfan/kg body weight and the intravenous $LD_{50}>2500$ mg treosulfan/kg body weight.

In rats the oral LD_{50} is 2575 mg treosulfan/kg body weight and the intraperitoneal $LD_{50}>$ 2860 mg treosulfan/kg body weight.

Subacute toxicity

In monkeys receiving a subacute dose (56-111 mg/kg/day) the haematopoietic system was damaged. At higher doses (222-445 mg/kg/day) diarrhoea, anorexia and marked weight loss were also noted.

Chronic toxicity

Administration of treosulfan to rats for seven months led to a reduction in spermiogenesis in males and cycle disturbances in females. All other organs were unchanged.

Tumorogenic and mutagenic potential

In long-term therapy with oral treosulfan doses an acute non-lymphatic leukaemia was observed in 1.4 % of the patients.

Treosulfan, like other cytostatic agents with alkylating properties, has a mutagenic potential. Therefore, patients of child-bearing age should practice contraception while receiving treosulfan.

Reproductive toxicity

Treosulfan has not been tested for reproductive toxicity in animal experiments. However, during chronic toxicity testing in rats, a delayed spermiogenesis and the absence of corpora lutea and follicles was determined.

6. PHARMACEUTICAL PARTICULARS

6.1 List of excipients

Capsule content: maize starch, hydroxypropyl methylcellulose, magnesium stearate

Capsule shell: titanium dioxide E171, gelatine

6.2 Incompatibilities

None known

6.3 Shelf life

Treosulfan capsules have a shelf-life of 5 years.

6.4 Special precautions for storage

None

6.5 Nature and contents of container

Amber glass bottles of 100 capsules.

6.6 Instructions for use and handling

The capsules should be swallowed whole and not allowed to disintegrate within the mouth.

7. MARKETING AUTHORISATION HOLDER

medac
Gesellschaft fuer klinische Spezialpraeparate
Fehlandtstrasse 3 · D-20354 Hamburg
Germany

Full information is available on request from

medac
Gesellschaft für klinische Spezialpräparate
Scion House
Stirling University Innovation Park
Stirling FK9 4NF
Tel.: 01786/ 458 086
Fax: 01786/ 458 032

8. MARKETING AUTHORISATION NUMBER(S)

11587/0001

9. DATE OF FIRST AUTHORISATION/RENEWAL OF THE AUTHORISATION

20/01/1992

10. DATE OF REVISION OF THE TEXT

September 2005

Treosulfan Injection

(medac GmbH)

1. NAME OF THE MEDICINAL PRODUCT

Treosulfan Injection

2. QUALITATIVE AND QUANTITATIVE COMPOSITION

Infusion bottles containing 1 g or 5 g treosulfan, a white crystalline powder.

3. PHARMACEUTICAL FORM

Powder for reconstitution and parenteral administration by injection or infusion

4. CLINICAL PARTICULARS

4.1 Therapeutic indications

For the treatment of all types of ovarian cancer, either supplementary to surgery or palliatively. Some uncontrolled studies have suggested activity in a wider range of neoplasms.

Because of a lack of cross-resistance reported between treosulfan and other cytotoxic agents treosulfan may be useful in any neoplasm refractive to conventional therapy.

Treosulfan has been used in combination regimens in conjunction with vincristine, methotrexate, 5-FU and procarbazine.

4.2 Posology and method of administration

3 - 8 g/m2 i.v. every 1-3 weeks depending on blood count and concurrent chemotherapy. Single injections of up to 8 g/m2 have been given with no serious adverse effects. Doses up to 1.5 g/m2 have been given intraperitoneally. Doses up to 3 g/m2 treosulfan may be given as a bolus injection. Larger doses should be administered as an i.v. infusion at a rate of 3 g/m2 every 5-10 minutes (8 g/m2 as a 30 minutes infusion).

Treatment should not be given if the white blood cell count is less than 3.000/microlitre or the thrombocyte count less than 100.000/microlitre. A repeat blood count should be made after a weeks interval, when treatment may be restarted if haematological parameters are satisfactory. Lower doses of treosulfan should be used if other cytotoxic drugs or radiotherapy are being given concurrently. Treatment is initiated as soon as possible after diagnosis.

Care should be taken in administration of the injection to avoid extravasation into tissues since this will cause local pain and tissue damage. If extravasation occurs, the injection should be discontinued immediately and any remaining portion of the dose should be introduced into another vein.

Dosage in the elderly

Treosulfan is renally excreted. Blood counts should be carefully monitored in the elderly and the dosage adjusted accordingly.

Children

Not recommended

4.3 Contraindications

Severe and lasting bone marrow depression.

4.4 Special warnings and special precautions for use

None

4.5 Interaction with other medicinal products and other forms of Interaction

In one patient the effect of ibuprofen/chloroquine was reduced with concomitant administration of treosulfan.

4.6 Pregnancy and lactation

Warning: This product should not normally be administered to patients who are pregnant or to mothers who are breast feeding.

Woman of childbearing age should take adequate contraceptive precautions.

4.7 Effects on ability to drive and use machines

Because of nausea and vomiting the ability to drive or operate machines may be influenced.

4.8 Undesirable effects

The dose-limiting side effect of treosulfan is a myelosuppression, which is usually reversible. It is manifested by a reduction in leukocytes and platelets and a decrease in haemoglobin.

The leukocytes and platelets usually reach their baseline level after 28 days.

Because the inhibition of bone marrow function is cumulative, the blood count should be monitored at shorter intervals starting with the third course of treatment.

This is especially important if combined with other forms of therapy that suppress bone marrow function such as radiotherapy.

During long-term therapy with oral treosulfan doses eight patients (1.4 % of 553 patients) developed an acute non-lymphatic leukaemia.

Skin

Mild alopecia is observed in 16 % of the patients and a skin pigmentation in the form of a bronze discoloration in up to 30 % of the cases.

The occurrence of urticaria, erythemas, a scleroderma and triggering of a psoriasis have been reported.

Respiratory

In rare cases allergic alveolitis, pneumonia and pulmonary fibrosis have developed.

Gastrointestinal

Nausea with or without vomiting is observed in approx. 50 % of the patients.

Other adverse reactions

In rare cases flu-like complaints, a paraesthesia, haemorrhagic cystitis, Addison's disease and hypoglycaemia have been observed. It cannot be totally ruled out that one case of cardiomyopathy was related to treosulfan.

Because of the possible development of a haemorrhagic cystitis patients are advised to drink more fluids for up to 24 hours after infusion.

During infusion, care must be taken to use a flawless technique, since painful inflammatory reactions may occur as a result of extravasation of treosulfan solution into surrounding tissue.

4.9 Overdose

Although there is no experience of acute overdosage with treosulfan, nausea, vomiting and gastritis may occur. Prolonged or excessive therapeutic doses may result in bone marrow depression which has occasionally been irreversible. The drug should be withdrawn, a blood transfusion given and general supportive measures given.

5. PHARMACOLOGICAL PROPERTIES

5.1 Pharmacodynamic properties

Treosulfan is a bifunctional alkylating agent which has been shown to possess antineoplastic activity in the animal tumor screen and in clinical trials. The activity of treosulfan is due to the formation of epoxide compounds in vivo.

Treosulfan is converted in vitro under physiological conditions (pH 7.4; 37 °C) non-enzymatically via a monoepoxide to the diepoxide (diepoxybutane) with a half-life of 2.2 hours.

The epoxides formed react with nucleophilic centres of the DNA and are responsible via secondary biological mechanisms for the antineoplastic effect. It is important that in vivo the monoepoxide first formed can already alkylate a nucleophilic centre of the DNA. This fixes the compound to this centre by chemical reaction before the second epoxide ring is formed.

5.2 Pharmacokinetic properties

After intravenous administration treosulfan is rapidly distributed in the body.

Elimination follows a 1st order kinetics with a half-life of 1.6 h. Approximately 30 % of the substance are excreted unchanged with the urine within 24 hours, nearly 90 % of which within the first 6 hours after administration.

5.3 Preclinical safety data

Acute toxicity

In mice the oral LD_{50} is 3360 mg treosulfan/kg body weight and the intravenous $LD_{50}>2500$ mg treosulfan/kg body weight.

In rats the oral LD_{50} is 2575 mg treosulfan/kg body weight and the intraperitoneal $LD_{50}>$ 2860 mg treosulfan/kg body weight.

Subacute toxicity

In monkeys receiving a subacute dose (56-111 mg/kg/day) the haematopoietic system was damaged. At higher doses (222-445 mg/kg/day) diarrhoea, anorexia and marked weight loss were also noted.

Chronic toxicity

Administration of treosulfan to rats for seven months led to a reduction in sper-miogenesis in males and cycle disturbances in females. All other organs were unchanged.

Tumorogenic and mutagenic potential

In long-term therapy with oral treosulfan doses an acute non-lymphatic leukaemia was observed in 1.4 % of the patients.

Treosulfan, like other cytostatic agents with alkylating properties, has a mutagenic potential. Therefore, patients of child-bearing age should practice contraception while receiving treosulfan.

Reproductive toxicity

Treosulfan has not been tested for reproductive toxicity in animal experiments. However, during chronic toxicity testing in rats, a delayed spermiogenesis and the absence of corpora lutea and follicles was determined.

6. PHARMACEUTICAL PARTICULARS

6.1 List of excipients

None

6.2 Incompatibilities

No incompatibilities are as yet known.

6.3 Shelf life

Treosulfan Injection has a shelf-life of 5 years when stored at room temperature.

The drug product should not be used after the expiration date.

Once brought into solution the injection should be used immediately.

6.4 Special precautions for storage

None

6.5 Nature and contents of container

100 ml colourless glass vial with butyl rubber stopper and cap of aluminium completed with plastic bottle holder.

Each vial contains 1 g or 5 g treosulfan.

The vials are packed in boxes of 5.

6.6 Instructions for use and handling

Route of administration

Treosulfan Injection 1 g or 5 g is used for intravenous infusion after being dissolved in 20 or 100 ml of water for injection.

As with all cytotoxic substances, appropriate precautions should be taken when handling treosulfan.

Guidelines for the safe handling of antineoplastic agents:

1. Trained personnel should reconstitute the drug.
2. This should be performed in a designated area.
3. Adequate protective gloves, masks and clothing should be worn.
4. Precautions should be taken to avoid the drug accidentally coming into contact with the eyes.
5. Cytotoxic preparations should not be handled by staff who may be pregnant.
6. Adequate care and precautions should be taken in the disposal of items (syringes, needles, etc.) used to reconstitute cytotoxic drugs.
7. The work surface should be covered with disposable plastic-backed absorbent paper.
8. Use Luer-lock fittings on all syringes and sets. Large bore needles are recommended to minimise pressure and the possible formation of aerosols. The latter may also be reduced by the use of a venting needle.

Instructions for reconstitution of Treosulfan Injection

To avoid solubility problems during reconstitution the following aspects should be regarded.

1. The solvent, water for injection, is warmed to 25 - 30 °C (not higher !) by using a water bath.
2. The treosulfan is carefully removed from the inner surface of the infusion bottle by shaking.

This procedure is very important, because moistening of powder that sticks to the surface results in caking. In case caking occurs the bottle has to be shaken long and vigorously.

3. One side of the double sided cannula is put into the rubber stopper of the water bottle. The treosulfan bottle is then put on the other end of the cannula with the bottom on top. The whole construction is converted and the water let run into the lower bottle while the bottle is shaken gently.

If followed these instructions, the whole reconstitution procedure should take not longer than 2 minutes.

7. MARKETING AUTHORISATION HOLDER

medac

Gesellschaft fuer klinische Spezialpraeparate

Fehlandtstrasse 3 · D-20354 Hamburg

Germany

8. MARKETING AUTHORISATION NUMBER(S)

11587/0002

9. DATE OF FIRST AUTHORISATION/RENEWAL OF THE AUTHORISATION

20/01/1992

10. DATE OF REVISION OF THE TEXT

September 2005

Full information is available on request from

medac

Gesellschaft für klinische Spezialpräparate

Scion House

Stirling University Innovation Park

Stirling FK9 4NF

Tel.: 01786/ 458 086

Fax: 01786/ 458 032

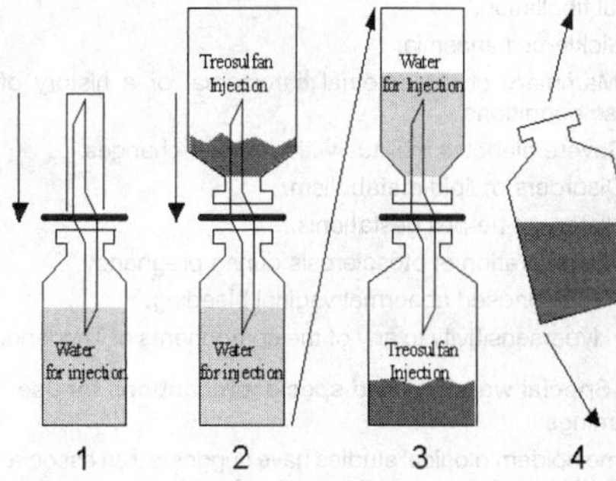

1

Tri-Adcortyl Cream, Ointment

(E. R. Squibb & Sons Limited)

1. NAME OF THE MEDICINAL PRODUCT

TRI-ADCORTYL CREAM

TRI-ADCORTYL OINTMENT

2. QUALITATIVE AND QUANTITATIVE COMPOSITION

Containing in each gram the following: Triamcinolone acetonide 0.1%, Neomycin (as sulphate) 0.25%, Gramicidin 0.025%, Nystatin 100,000 units.

3. PHARMACEUTICAL FORM

Topical Cream.

Topical Ointment

4. CLINICAL PARTICULARS

4.1 Therapeutic indications

In the treatment of corticosteroid sensitive dermatoses complicated by infections due to micro-organisms sensitive to the anti-infectives.

4.2 Posology and method of administration

Adults and children:

Apply to the affected area two or occasionally three times daily.

Elderly:

Corticosteroids should be used sparingly and for short periods of time, as natural thinning of the skin occurs in the elderly.

If, after about 7 days application, little or no improvement has occurred, cultural isolation of the offending organism should be followed by appropriate local or systemic antimicrobial therapy.

This product is not recommended for children under one year of age.

4.3 Contraindications

In tuberculous and most viral lesions of the skin, particularly herpes simplex and varicella. Also in fungal lesions not susceptible to nystatin.

In patients with hypersensitivity to any of the components.

Should not be used for facial rosacea, acne vulgaris or perioral dermatitis.

Should not be applied to the external auditory canal in patients with perforated eardrums.

The products should not be used for extensive areas because of possible risk of systemic absorption and neomycin-induced ototoxicity.

Should not be used in children under one year of age.

4.4 Special warnings and special precautions for use

Adrenal suppression can occur, even without occlusion. The use of occlusive dressings should be avoided because of the increased risk of sensitivity reactions and increased percutaneous absorption. The possibility of sensitivity to neomycin should be taken into consideration especially in the treatment of patients suffering from leg ulcers.

Steroid-antibiotic combinations should not be continued for more than 7 days in the absence of any clinical improvement, since in this situation occult extension of infection may occur due to the masking effect of the steroid.

Extended or recurrent application may increase the risk of contact sensitisation and should be avoided.

If used on the face, courses should be limited to 5 days and occlusion should not be used.

Contact with the eyes or mucous membranes should be avoided.

Children Older Than 1 Year

In infants, long-term continuous topical steroid therapy should be avoided. Courses should be limited to 5 days and occlusion should not be used.

4.5 Interaction with other medicinal products and other forms of Interaction

Not applicable

4.6 Pregnancy and lactation

There is inadequate evidence of safety in human pregnancy. Topical administration of corticosteroids to pregnant animals can cause abnormalities of foetal development including cleft palate and intra-uterine growth retardation. There may, therefore, be a very small risk of such effects in the human foetus. There are theoretical risks of neomycin-induced foetal ototoxicity; therefore the product should be used with caution only when the benefit outweighs the potential risk.

4.7 Effects on ability to drive and use machines

Not applicable.

4.8 Undesirable effects

Triamcinolone Acetonide:

The following side effects have been reported. Usually with prolonged usage: dermatologic - impaired wound healing, thinning of the skin, petechiae and ecchymoses, facial erythema and telangiectasia, increased sweating, purpura, striae, hirsutism, acneiform eruptions, lupus erythematosus-like lesions and suppressed reactions to skin tests. These effects may be enhanced with occlusive dressings.

The possibility of the systemic effects which are associated with all steroid therapy should be considered. These include reversible hypothalamic-pituitary-adrenal (HPA) axis suppression, manifestations of Cushings syndrome, hyperglycaemia and glucosuria in some patients. Following discontinuation, recovery of HPA axis function is generally prompt and complete.

Neomycin:

Sensitivity reactions may occur especially with prolonged use. Ototoxicity and nephrotoxicity have been reported. The product should be used with caution and in small amounts in the treatment of skin infections following extensive burns, trophic ulceration and other conditions where absorption of neomycin is possible. The product should be used with care in patients with established hearing loss.

Gramicidin:

Sensitivity has occasionally been reported.

Nystatin:

There have been no substantiated reports of sensitivity associated with topical nystatin.

4.9 Overdose

Topically applied corticosteroids can be absorbed in sufficient amounts to produce systemic effects (see side effects).

In the event of accidental ingestion, the patient should be observed and treated symptomatically.

5. PHARMACOLOGICAL PROPERTIES

5.1 Pharmacodynamic properties

Triamcinolone acetonide is a potent fluorinated corticosteroid with rapid anti- inflammatory, antipruritic and anti-allergic actions.

The combined action of the antibiotics neomycin and gramicidin provides comprehensive antibacterial therapy against a wide range of gram-positive and gram-negative bacteria, including those micro-organisms responsible for most bacterial skin infections.

Nystatin is an antifungal antibiotic, active against a wide range of yeasts and yeast-like fungi, including candida albicans.

5.2 Pharmacokinetic properties

Not applicable.

5.3 Preclinical safety data

No further relevant data

6. PHARMACEUTICAL PARTICULARS

6.1 List of excipients

Cream:	Aluminium hydroxide, antifoam emulsion, benzyl alcohol, ethanol, ethylenediamine, hydrochloric acid, macrogol ether, perfume, polysorbate 60, propylene glycol, sorbitol, titanium dioxide, white soft paraffin, water.
Ointment:	Polyethylene resin, liquid paraffin.

6.2 Incompatibilities

None known.

6.3 Shelf life

Cream:	24 months.
Ointment:	48 months

6.4 Special precautions for storage

Cream:	Do not store above 25°C. Avoid freezing.
Ointment:	Do not store above 25°C

6.5 Nature and contents of container

Aluminium tubes of 30g.

6.6 Instructions for use and handling

None.

7. MARKETING AUTHORISATION HOLDER

E.R. Squibb & Sons Limited,

Uxbridge Business Park,

Sanderson Road,

Uxbridge,

Middlesex UB8 1DH

8. MARKETING AUTHORISATION NUMBER(S)

Cream:	PL 0034/5093R
Ointment:	PL 0034/5094R

9. DATE OF FIRST AUTHORISATION/RENEWAL OF THE AUTHORISATION

Cream:	31st January 1991 / 1st July 2002
Ointment:	25th February 1991 / 1st July 2002

10. DATE OF REVISION OF THE TEXT

24th June 2005

Tri-Adcortyl Otic Ointment

(E. R. Squibb & Sons Limited)

1. NAME OF THE MEDICINAL PRODUCT

TRI-ADCORTYL OTIC OINTMENT

2. QUALITATIVE AND QUANTITATIVE COMPOSITION

Containing in each gram the following:Triamcinolone acetonide 0.1%, Neomycin (as sulphate) 0.25%, Gramicidin 0.025%, Nystatin 100,000 units.

3. PHARMACEUTICAL FORM

Aural Ointment.

4. CLINICAL PARTICULARS

4.1 Therapeutic indications

For the topical treatment of otitis externa, known to respond to topical steroid therapy, complicated by infections due to micro-organisms sensitive to the anti-infectives.

4.2 Posology and method of administration

Adults and children:

Apply a small amount directly from the tube into the aural canal two or occasionally three times daily.

Elderly:

Corticosteroids should be used sparingly and for short periods of time, as natural thinning of the skin occurs in the elderly.

If, after about 7 days application, little or no improvement has occurred, cultural isolation of the offending organism should be followed by appropriate local or systemic antimicrobial therapy.

This product is not recommended for children under one year of age.

4.3 Contraindications

In tuberculous and most viral lesions of the skin, particularly herpes simplex and varicella. Also in fungal lesions not susceptible to nystatin.

In patients with hypersensitivity to any of the components.

Should not be used for facial rosacea, acne vulgaris or perioral dermatitis.

Should not be applied to the external auditory canal in patients with perforated eardrums.

The product should not be used for extensive areas because of possible risk of systemic absorption and neomycin-induced ototoxicity.

Should not be used in children under one year of age.

4.4 Special warnings and special precautions for use

Adrenal suppression can occur, even without occlusion. The use of occlusive dressings should be avoided because of the increased risk of sensitivity reactions and increased percutaneous absorption. The possibility of sensitivity to neomycin should be taken into consideration especially in the treatment of patients suffering from leg ulcers.

Steroid-antibiotic combinations should not be continued for more than 7 days in the absence of any clinical improvement, since in this situation occult extension of infection may occur due to the masking effect of the steroid.

Extended or recurrent application may increase the risk of contact sensitisation and should be avoided.

If used in childhood, or on the face, courses should be limited to 5 days and occlusion should not be used.

Not for ophthalmic use. Contact with the eyes or mucous membranes should be avoided.

Children Older Than 1 Year

In infants, long-term continuous topical steroid therapy should be avoided. Courses should be limited to 5 days and occlusion should not be used.

4.5 Interaction with other medicinal products and other forms of Interaction

Not applicable

4.6 Pregnancy and lactation

There is inadequate evidence of safety in human pregnancy. Topical administration of corticosteroids to pregnant animals can cause abnormalities of foetal development including cleft palate and intra-uterine growth retardation. There may, therefore, be a very small risk of such effects in the human foetus. There are theoretical risks of neomycin-induced foetal ototoxicity; therefore the product should be used with caution only when the benefit outweighs the potential risk.

4.7 Effects on ability to drive and use machines

Not applicable.

4.8 Undesirable effects

Triamcinolone Acetonide:

Triamcinolone acetonide is well tolerated. Where adverse reactions occur they are usually reversible on cessation of therapy. However the following side effects have been reported usually with prolonged usage:

Dermatologic - impaired wound healing, thinning of the skin, petechiae and ecchymoses, facial erythema and telangiectasia, increased sweating, purpura, striae, hirsutism, acneiform eruptions, lupus erythematosus-like lesions and suppressed reactions to skin tests.

These effects may be enhanced with occlusive dressings.

Signs of systemic toxicity such as oedema and electrolyte imbalance have not been observed even when high topical dosage has been used. The possibility of the systemic effects which are associated with all steroid therapy should be considered. These include reversible hypothalamic-pituitary-adrenal (HPA) axis suppression, manifestations of Cushings syndrome, hyperglycaemia and glucosuria in some patients. Following discontinuation, recovery of HPA axis function is generally prompt and complete.

Neomycin:

Sensitivity reactions may occur especially with prolonged use. Ototoxicity and nephrotoxicity have been reported. The product should be used with caution and in small amounts in the treatment of skin infections following extensive burns, trophic ulceration and other conditions where absorption of neomycin is possible. The product should be used with care in patients with established hearing loss.

Gramicidin:

Sensitivity has occasionally been reported.

Nystatin:

There have been no substantiated reports of sensitivity associated with topical nystatin.

4.9 Overdose

Topically applied corticosteroids can be absorbed in sufficient amounts to produce systemic effects (see side effects).

In the event of accidental ingestion, the patient should be observed and treated symptomatically.

5. PHARMACOLOGICAL PROPERTIES

5.1 Pharmacodynamic properties

Triamcinolone acetonide is a potent fluorinated corticosteroid with rapid anti- inflammatory, antipruritic and anti-allergic actions.

The combined action of the antibiotics neomycin and gramicidin provides comprehensive antibacterial therapy against a wide range of gram-positive and gram-negative bacteria, including those micro-organisms responsible for most bacterial skin infections.

Nystatin is an antifungal antibiotic, active against a wide range of yeasts and yeast-like fungi, including *candida albicans*.

5.2 Pharmacokinetic properties

Not applicable.

5.3 Preclinical safety data

No further relevant data

6. PHARMACEUTICAL PARTICULARS

6.1 List of excipients

Polylethylene resin and liquid paraffin

6.2 Incompatibilities

None known.

6.3 Shelf life

48 months.

6.4 Special precautions for storage

Do not store above 25°C.

6.5 Nature and contents of container

Aluminium tubes of 10g.

6.6 Instructions for use and handling

None.

7. MARKETING AUTHORISATION HOLDER

E.R. Squibb & Sons Limited
Uxbridge Business Park,
Sanderson Road,
Uxbridge,
Middlesex UB8 1DH

8. MARKETING AUTHORISATION NUMBER(S)

PL 0034/5095R

9. DATE OF FIRST AUTHORISATION/RENEWAL OF THE AUTHORISATION

25th February 1991 / 1st July 2002

10. DATE OF REVISION OF THE TEXT

24th June 2005

Triadene

(Schering Health Care Limited)

1. NAME OF THE MEDICINAL PRODUCT

TRIADENE®

2. QUALITATIVE AND QUANTITATIVE COMPOSITION

The memo pack holds six beige tablets containing 30 micrograms ethinylestradiol and 50 micrograms gestodene, five dark brown tablets containing 40 micrograms ethinylestradiol and 70 micrograms gestodene, and ten white tablets containing 30 micrograms ethinylestradiol and 100 micrograms gestodene.

3. PHARMACEUTICAL FORM

Sugar-coated tablets

4. CLINICAL PARTICULARS

4.1 Therapeutic indications

Oral contraception and the recognised gynaecological indications for such oestrogen-progestogen combinations.

4.2 Posology and method of administration

First treatment cycle: 1 tablet daily for 21 days, starting on the first day of the menstrual cycle. Contraceptive protection begins immediately.

Subsequent cycles: Tablet taking from the next pack of Triadene is continued after a 7-day interval, beginning on the same day of the week as the first pack.

Changing from 21-day combined oral contraceptives: The first tablet of Triadene should be taken on the first day immediately after the end of the previous oral contraceptive course. Additional contraceptive precautions are not required.

Changing from a combined Every Day pill (28 day tablets): Triadene should be started after taking the last active tablet from the Every Day Pill pack. The first Triadene tablet is taken the next day. Additional contraceptive precautions are not then required.

Changing from a progestogen-only pill (POP): The first tablet of Triadene should be taken on the first day of bleeding, even if a POP has already been taken on that day. Additional contraceptive precautions are not then required. The remaining progestogen-only pills should be discarded.

Post-partum and post-abortum use: After pregnancy, oral contraception can be started 21 days after a vaginal delivery, provided that the patient is fully ambulant and there are no puerperal complications. Additional contraceptive precautions will be required for the first 7 days of tablet taking. Since the first post-partum ovulation may precede the first bleeding, another method of contraception should be used in the interval between childbirth and the first course of tablets. After a first-trimester abortion, oral contraception may be started immediately in which case no additional contraceptive precautions are required.

Special circumstances requiring additional contraception

Incorrect administration: A single delayed tablet should be taken as soon as possible, and if this can be done within 12 hours of the correct time, contraceptive protection is maintained. With longer delays, additional contraception is needed. Only the most recently delayed tablet should be taken, earlier missed tablets being omitted, and additional non-hormonal methods of contraception (except the rhythm or temperature methods) should be used for the next 7 days, while the next 7 tablets are being taken. Additionally, therefore, if tablet(s) have been missed during the last 7 days of a pack, there should be no break before the next pack is started. In this situation, a withdrawal bleed should not be expected until the end of the second pack. Some breakthrough bleeding may occur on tablet taking days but this is not clinically significant. If the patient does not have a withdrawal bleed during the tablet-free interval following the end of the second pack, the possibility of pregnancy must be ruled out before starting the next pack.

Gastro-intestinal upset: Vomiting or diarrhoea may reduce the efficacy of oral contraceptives by preventing full absorption. Tablet-taking from the current pack should be continued. Additional non-hormonal methods of contraception (except the rhythm or temperature methods) should be used during the gastro-intestinal upset and for 7 days following the upset. If these 7 days overrun the end of a pack, the next pack should be started without a break. In this situation, a withdrawal bleed should not be expected until the end of the second pack. If the patient does not have a withdrawal bleed during the tablet-free interval following the end of the second pack, the possibility of pregnancy must be ruled out before starting the next pack. Other methods of contraception should be considered if the gastro-intestinal disorder is likely to be prolonged.

4.3 Contraindications

1. Pregnancy.

2. Severe disturbances of liver function, jaundice or persistent itching during a previous pregnancy, Dubin-Johnson syndrome, Rotor syndrome, previous or existing liver tumours.

3. History of confirmed venous thromboembolism (VTE). Family history of idiopathic VTE. Other known risk factors for VTE.

4. Existing or previous arterial thrombotic or embolic processes, conditions which predispose to them e.g. disorders of the clotting processes, valvular heart disease and atrial fibrillation.

5. Sickle-cell anaemia.

6. Mammary or endometrial carcinoma, or a history of these conditions.

7. Severe diabetes mellitus with vascular changes.

8. Disorders of lipid metabolism.

9. History of herpes gestationis.

10. Deterioration of otosclerosis during pregnancy.

11. Undiagnosed abnormal vaginal bleeding.

12. Hypersensitivity to any of the components of Triadene.

4.4 Special warnings and special precautions for use

Warnings:

Some epidemiological studies have suggested an association between the use of combined oral contraceptives (COCs) and an increased risk of arterial and venous thrombotic and thromboembolic diseases such as myocardial infarction, stroke, deep venous thrombosis and pulmonary embolism. These events occur rarely. Full recovery from such disorders does not always occur, and it should be realised that in a few cases they are fatal.

The use of any combined oral contraceptive carries an increased risk of venous thromboembolism (VTE) compared with no use. The excess risk of VTE is highest during the first year a woman ever uses a combined oral contraceptive. This increased risk is less than the risk of VTE associated with pregnancy which is estimated as 60 cases per 100 000 pregnancies. Some epidemiological studies have reported a greater risk of VTE for women using combined oral contraceptives containing desogestrel or gestodene (the so-called third generation pills) than for women using pills containing levonorgestrel (the so-called second generation pills).

The spontaneous incidence of VTE in healthy non-pregnant women (not taking any oral contraceptive) is about 5 cases per 100,000 women per year. The incidence in users of second generation pills is about 15 per 100,000 women per year of use. The incidence in users of third generation pills is about 25 cases per 100,000 women per year of use; this excess incidence has not been satisfactorily explained by bias or confounding. The level of all of these risks of VTE increases with age and is likely to be further increased in women with other known risk factors for VTE such as obesity.

The risk of venous and/or arterial thrombosis associated with combined oral contraceptives increases with:

- age;
- smoking (with heavier smoking and increasing age the risk further increases, especially in women over 35 years of age);
- a positive family history (i.e. venous or arterial thromboembolism ever in a sibling or parent at a relatively early age). If a hereditary predisposition is suspected, the woman should be referred to a specialist for advice before deciding about any COC use;
- obesity (body mass index over 30 kg/m^2);
- dyslipoproteinaemia;
- hypertension;
- valvular heart disease;
- atrial fibrillation;
- prolonged immobilisation, major surgery, any surgery to the legs, or major trauma. In these situations it is advisable to discontinue COC use (in the case of elective surgery at least six weeks in advance) and not to resume until two weeks after complete remobilisation.
- There is no consensus about the possible role of varicose veins and superficial thrombophlebitis in venous thromboembolism.
- The increased risk of thromboembolism in the puerperium must be considered (for information on "Pregnancy and Lactation" see Section 4.6).
- Other medical conditions which have been associated with adverse circulatory events include diabetes mellitus, systemic lupus erythematosus, haemolytic uraemic syndrome, chronic inflammatory bowel disease (Crohn's disease or ulcerative colitis), sickle cell disease and subarachnoid haemorrhage.
- An increase in frequency or severity of migraine during COC use (which may be prodromal of a cerebrovascular event) may be a reason for immediate discontinuation of the COC.
- Biochemical factors that may be indicative of hereditary or acquired predisposition for venous or arterial thrombosis include Activated Protein C (APC) resistance, hyperhomocysteinaemia, antithrombin-III deficiency, protein C deficiency, protein S deficiency, antiphospholipid antibodies (anticardiolipin antibodies, lupus anticoagulant).

When considering risk/benefit, the physician should take into account that adequate treatment of a condition may reduce the associated risk of thrombosis and that the risk associated with pregnancy is higher than that associated with COC use.

Numerous epidemiological studies have been reported on the risks of ovarian, endometrial, cervical and breast cancer in women using combined oral contraceptives. The evidence is clear that combined oral contraceptives offer substantial protection against both ovarian and endometrial cancer.

An increased risk of cervical cancer in long-term users of combined oral contraceptives has been reported in some studies, but there continues to be controversy about the extent to which this is attributable to the confounding effects of sexual behaviour and other factors.

A meta-analysis from 54 epidemiological studies reported that there is a slightly increased relative risk (RR = 1.24) of having breast cancer diagnosed in women who are currently using combined oral contraceptives (COCs). The observed pattern of increased risk may be due to an earlier diagnosis of breast cancer in COC users, the biological effects of COCs or a combination of both. The additional breast cancers diagnosed in current users of COCs or in women who have used COCs in the last ten years are more likely to be localised to the breast than those in women who never used COCs.

Breast cancer is rare among women under 40 years of age whether or not they take COCs. Whilst this background risk increases with age, the excess number of breast cancer diagnoses in current and recent COC users is small in relation to the overall risk of breast cancer (see bar chart).

The most important risk factor for breast cancer in COC users is the age women discontinue the COC; the older the age at stopping, the more breast cancers are diagnosed. Duration of use is less important and the excess risk gradually disappears during the course of the 10 years after stopping COC use such that by 10 years there appears to be no excess.

The possible increase in risk of breast cancer should be discussed with the user and weighed against the benefits of COCs taking into account the evidence that they offer substantial protection against the risk of developing certain other cancers (e.g. ovarian and endometrial cancer).

Estimated cumulative numbers of breast cancers per 10,000 women diagnosed in 5 years of use and up to 10 years after stopping COCs, compared with numbers of breast cancers diagnosed in 10,000 women who had never used COCs.

(see Figure 1)

The possibility cannot be ruled out that certain chronic diseases may occasionally deteriorate during the use of combined oral contraceptives (see '*Precautions*').

The combination of ethinylestradiol and gestodene, like other contraceptive steroids, is associated with an increased incidence of neoplastic nodules in the rat liver, the relevance of which to man is unknown. Malignant liver tumours have been reported on rare occasions in long-term users of oral contraceptives.

In rare cases benign and, in even rarer cases, malignant liver tumours leading in isolated cases to life-threatening intra-abdominal haemorrhage have been observed after the use of hormonal substances such as those contained in Triadene. If severe upper abdominal complaints, liver enlargement or signs of intra-abdominal haemorrhage occur, the possibility of a liver tumour should be included in the differential diagnosis.

Reasons for stopping oral contraception immediately:

1. Occurrence for the first time, or exacerbation, of migrainous headaches or unusually frequent or unusually severe headaches.
2. Sudden disturbances of vision, of hearing or other perceptual disorders.
3. First signs of thrombophlebitis or thromboembolic symptoms (e.g. unusual pains in or swelling of the leg(s), stabbing pains on breathing or coughing for no apparent reason). Feeling of pain and tightness in the chest.
4. Six weeks before an elective major operation (e.g. abdominal, orthopaedic), any surgery to the legs, medical treatment for varicose veins or prolonged immobilisation, e.g. after accidents or surgery. Do not restart until 2 weeks after full ambulation. In case of emergency surgery, thrombotic prophylaxis is usually indicated e.g. subcutaneous heparin.
5. Onset of jaundice, hepatitis, itching of the whole body.
6. Increase in epileptic seizures.
7. Significant rise in blood pressure.
8. Onset of severe depression.
9. Severe upper abdominal pain or liver enlargement.
10. Clear exacerbation of conditions known to be capable of deteriorating during oral contraception or pregnancy.
11. Pregnancy is a reason for stopping immediately because it has been suggested by some investigations that oral contraceptives taken in early pregnancy may slightly increase the risk of foetal malformations. Other investigations have failed to support these findings. The possibility therefore cannot be excluded, but it is certain that if a risk exists at all, it is very small.

Precautions:

Assessment of women prior to starting oral contraceptives (and at regular intervals thereafter) should include a personal and family medical history of each woman. Physical examination should be guided by this and by the contraindications (section 4.3) and warnings (section 4.4) for this product. The frequency and nature of these assessments should be based upon relevant guidelines and should be adapted to the individual woman, but should include measurement of blood pressure and, if judged appropriate by the clinician, breast, abdominal and pelvic examination including cervical cytology.

The following conditions require strict medical supervision during medication with oral contraceptives. Deterioration or first appearance of any of these conditions may indicate that use of the oral contraceptive should be discontinued:

Diabetes mellitus, or a tendency towards diabetes mellitus (e.g. unexplained glycosuria), hypertension, varicose veins, a history of phlebitis, otosclerosis, multiple sclerosis, epilepsy, porphyria, tetany, disturbed liver function, Sydenham's chorea, renal dysfunction, family history of clotting disorders (see also contraindications), obesity, family history of breast cancer and patient history of benign breast disease, history of clinical depression, systemic lupus erythematosus, uterine fibroids and migraine, gallstones, cardiovascular diseases, chloasma, asthma, an intolerance to contact lenses, or any disease that is prone to worsen during pregnancy.

Some women may experience amenorrhoea or oligomenorrhoea after discontinuation of oral contraceptives, especially when these conditions existed prior to use. Women should be informed of this possibility.

4.5 Interaction with other medicinal products and other forms of Interaction

Hepatic enzyme inducers such as barbiturates, primidone, phenobarbitone, phenytoin, phenylbutazone, rifampicin, carbamazepine and griseofulvin can impair the efficacy of Triadene. For women receiving long-term therapy with hepatic enzyme inducers, another method of contraception should be used. The use of antibiotics may also reduce the efficacy of Triadene, possibly by altering the intestinal flora.

Women receiving short courses of enzyme inducers or broad spectrum antibiotics should take additional, non-hormonal (except rhythm or temperature method) contraceptive precautions during the time of concurrent medication and for 7 days afterwards. If these 7 days overrun the end of a pack, the next pack should be started without a break. In this situation, a withdrawal bleed should not be expected until the end of the second pack. If the patient does not have a withdrawal bleed during the tablet-free interval following the end of the second pack, the possibility of pregnancy must be ruled out before resuming with the next pack. With rifampicin, additional contraceptive precautions should be continued for 4 weeks after treatment stops, even if only a short course was administered.

The requirement for oral antidiabetics or insulin can change as a result of the effect on glucose tolerance.

The herbal remedy St John's wort (Hypericum perforatum) should not be taken concomitantly with Triadene as this could potentially lead to a loss of contraceptive effect.

4.6 Pregnancy and lactation

If pregnancy occurs during medication with oral contraceptives, the preparation should be withdrawn immediately (see Section 4.4. 'Reasons for stopping oral contraception immediately').

The use of Triadene during lactation may lead to a reduction in the volume of milk produced and to a change in its composition. Minute amounts of the active substances are excreted with the milk. Mothers who are breast-feeding may be advised instead to use a progestogen-only pill.

4.7 Effects on ability to drive and use machines

None known.

4.8 Undesirable effects

In rare cases, headaches, gastric upsets, nausea, vomiting, breast tenderness, changes in body weight, changes in libido, depressive moods can occur.

In predisposed women, use of Triadene can sometimes cause chloasma which is exacerbated by exposure to sunlight. Such women should avoid prolonged exposure to sunlight.

Estimated cumulative numbers of breast cancers per 10,000 women diagnosed in 5 years of use and up to 10 years after stopping COCs, compared with numbers of breast cancers diagnosed in 10,000 women who had never used COCs.

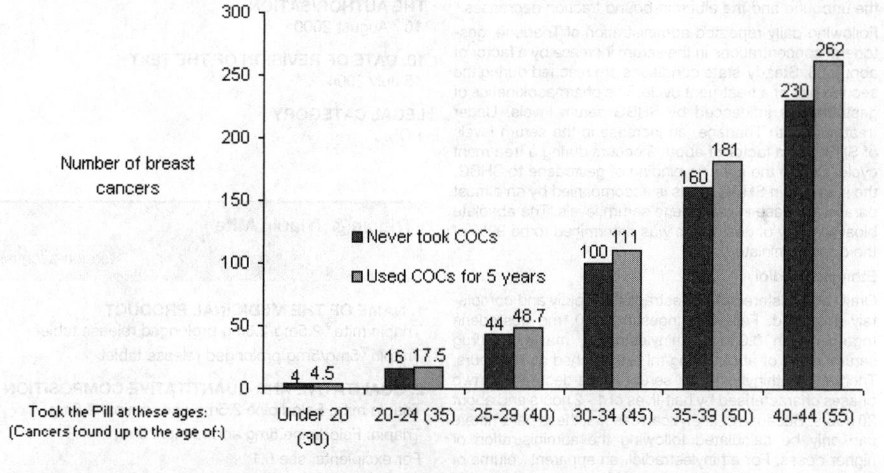

Individual cases of poor tolerance of contact lenses have been reported with use of oral contraceptives. Contact lens wearers who develop changes in lens tolerance should be assessed by an ophthalmologist.

Menstrual changes:

1. Reduction of menstrual flow:

This is not abnormal and it is to be expected in some patients. Indeed, it may be beneficial where heavy periods were previously experienced.

2. Missed menstruation:

Occasionally, withdrawal bleeding may not occur at all. If the tablets have been taken correctly, pregnancy is very unlikely. If withdrawal bleeding fails to occur at the end of a second pack, the possibility of pregnancy must be ruled out before resuming with the next pack.

3. Intermenstrual bleeding:

'Spotting' or heavier 'breakthrough bleeding' sometimes occur during tablet taking, especially in the first few cycles, and normally cease spontaneously. Triadene should therefore, be continued even if irregular bleeding occurs. If irregular bleeding is persistent, appropriate diagnostic measures to exclude an organic cause are indicated and may include curettage. This also applies in the case of spotting which occurs at irregular intervals in several consecutive cycles or which occurs for the first time after long use of Triadene.

4. Effect on blood chemistry:

The use of oral contraceptives may influence the results of certain laboratory tests including biochemical parameters of liver, thyroid, adrenal and renal function, plasma levels of carrier proteins and lipid/lipoprotein fractions, parameters of carbohydrate metabolism and parameters of coagulation and fibrinolysis. Laboratory staff should therefore be informed about oral contraceptive use when laboratory tests are requested.

Refer to Section 4.4. 'Special warnings and precautions for use' for additional information.

4.9 Overdose

Overdosage may cause nausea, vomiting and, in females, withdrawal bleeding.

There are no specific antidotes and treatment should be symptomatic.

5. PHARMACOLOGICAL PROPERTIES

5.1 Pharmacodynamic properties

This oestrogen-progestogen combination acts by inhibiting ovulation by suppression of the mid-cycle surge of luteinising hormone, the inspissation of cervical mucus so as to constitute a barrier to sperm, and the rendering of the endometrium unreceptive to implantation.

5.2 Pharmacokinetic properties

Gestodene

Orally administered gestodene is rapidly and completely absorbed. Following ingestion of 0.1mg gestodene together with 0.03mg ethinylestradiol (which represents the combination with the highest gestodene content of the tri-step formulation), maximum drug serum levels of about 5.6ng/ml are reached at 0.5 hour. Thereafter, gestodene serum levels decrease in two phases, characterised by half-lives of 0.1 hours and about 18 hours. For gestodene, an apparent volume of distribution of 0.7 l/kg and a metabolic clearance rate from serum of about 0.8ml/min/kg were determined. Gestodene is not excreted in unchanged form but as metabolites, which are eliminated with a half-life of about 1 day. Gestodene metabolites are excreted at an urinary to biliary ratio of about 6: 4. The biotransformation follows the known pathways of steroid metabolism. No pharmacologically active metabolites are known.

Gestodene is bound to serum albumin and to SHBG (sex hormone binding globulin). Only 1.3% of the total serum drug levels are present as free steroid, but 68.5% are specifically bound to SHBG. The relative distribution (free, albumin-bound, SHBG-bound) depends on the SHBG concentrations in the serum. Following induction of the binding protein, the SHBG bound fraction increases while the unbound and the albumin-bound fraction decreases.

Following daily repeated administration of Triadene, gestodene concentrations in the serum increase by a factor of about 2.8. Steady-state conditions are reached during the second half of a treatment cycle. The pharmacokinetics of gestodene is influenced by SHBG serum levels. Under treatment with Triadene, an increase in the serum levels of SHBG by a factor of about 3 occurs during a treatment cycle. Due to the specific binding of gestodene to SHBG, the increase in SHBG levels is accompanied by an almost parallel increase in gestodene serum levels. The absolute bioavailability of gestodene was determined to be 99% of the dose administered.

Ethinylestradiol

Orally administered ethinylestradiol is rapidly and completely absorbed. Following ingestion of 0.1mg gestodene together with 0.03mg ethinylestradiol, maximum drug serum levels of about 90pg/ml are reached at 1.3 hours. Thereafter, ethinylestradiol serum levels decrease in two phases characterised by half-lives of 1 - 2 hours and about 20 hours. Because of analytical reasons, these parameters can only be calculated following the administration of higher doses. For ethinylestradiol, an apparent volume of distribution of about 5 l/kg and a metabolic clearance rate from serum of about 5ml/min/kg were determined. Ethinylestradiol is highly but non-specifically bound to serum albumin. About 2% of drug levels are present unbound. During absorption and first liver passage, ethinylestradiol is metabolised resulting in a reduced absolute and variable oral bioavailability. Unchanged drug is not excreted. Ethinylestradiol metabolites are excreted at an urinary to biliary ratio of 4: 6 with a half-life of about 1 day.

According to the half-life of the terminal disposition phase from serum and the daily ingestion, steady-state serum levels are reached after 3 - 4 days and are higher by 30 - 40% as compared to a single dose.

During established lactation, 0.02% of the daily maternal dose could be transferred to the newborn via the milk.

The systemic availability of ethinylestradiol might be influenced in both directions by other drugs. There is, however, no interaction with high doses of vitamin C. Ethinylestradiol induces the hepatic synthesis of SHBG of CBG (corticoid binding globulin) during continuous use. The extent of SHBG induction, however, depends on the chemical structure and the dose of the co-administered progestogen. During treatment with Triadene, SHBG concentrations in the serum increased from about 74nmol/l to 187nmol/l and the serum concentration of CBG were increased from about 42μg/ml to 87μg/ml.

5.3 Preclinical safety data

There are no preclinical safety data which could be of relevance to the prescriber and which are not already included in other relevant sections of the SPC.

6. PHARMACEUTICAL PARTICULARS

6.1 List of excipients

lactose

maize starch

povidone 700 000

calcium disodium edetate

magnesium stearate (E 572)

sucrose

polyethylene glycol 6000

calcium carbonate (E 170)

talc

montan glycol wax

titanium dioxide (E 171)

ferric oxide pigment (brown and yellow) (E 172)

glycerol (E 422)

6.2 Incompatibilities

None known.

6.3 Shelf life

5 years.

6.4 Special precautions for storage

Not applicable.

6.5 Nature and contents of container

Deep drawn circular strips made of polyvinyl chloride film with counter-sealing foil made of aluminium with heat sealable coating.

Presentation

Each carton contains 3 blister memo-packs. Each blister memo-pack contains 21 active tablets.

6.6 Instructions for use and handling

Keep out of the reach of children.

7. MARKETING AUTHORISATION HOLDER

Schering Health Care Limited

The Brow

Burgess Hill

West Sussex RH15 9NE

8. MARKETING AUTHORISATION NUMBER(S)

0053/0205

9. DATE OF FIRST AUTHORISATION/RENEWAL OF THE AUTHORISATION

10th August 2000

10. DATE OF REVISION OF THE TEXT

15 July 2004

LEGAL CATEGORY

POM

Triapin & Triapin Mite

(sanofi-aventis)

1. NAME OF THE MEDICINAL PRODUCT

Triapin mite▼2.5mg/2.5mg prolonged release tablet

Triapin▼5mg/5mg prolonged release tablet

2. QUALITATIVE AND QUANTITATIVE COMPOSITION

Triapin mite: Felodipine 2.5mg and ramipril 2.5mg

Triapin: Felodipine 5mg and ramipril 5mg

For excipients, see 6.1

3. PHARMACEUTICAL FORM

Prolonged release tablet

Triapin Mite: An apricot coloured, circular, biconvex, prolonged release tablet engraved $\frac{\mathrm{H}}{\mathrm{OD}}$ on one side and 2.5 on the other side, with a diameter of approximately 9 mm.

Triapin: A reddish-brown, circular, biconvex, prolonged release tablet engraved $\frac{\mathrm{H}}{\mathrm{OE}}$ on one side and 5 on the other side, with a diameter of approximately 9 mm.

4. CLINICAL PARTICULARS

4.1 Therapeutic indications

Treatment of essential hypertension. Triapin mite and Triapin fixed dose combinations are indicated in patients whose blood pressure is not adequately controlled on felodipine or ramipril alone.

4.2 Posology and method of administration

Adults, including elderly: One tablet Triapin mite or Triapin daily. The maximum dose is two tablets Triapin mite once daily, or one tablet Triapin daily.

Patients with impaired liver function: See sections 4.3 Contraindications and 4.4, Special warnings and special precautions for use.

Patients with impaired renal function or patients already on diuretic treatment: See sections 4.3. Contraindications and 4.4. Special warnings and special precautions for use.

Individual dose titration with the components can be recommended and when clinically appropriate, direct change from monotherapy to the fixed combination may be considered

Children: No experience is available. Triapin mite or Triapin should not be given to children.

The tablets should be swallowed whole with a sufficient amount of liquid. The tablets must not be divided, crushed or chewed.

The tablet can be administered without food or following a light meal not rich in fat or carbohydrate.

4.3 Contraindications

Triapin Mite or Triapin must not be used:

- in patients with hypersensitivity to felodipine (or other dihydropyridines), ramipril, orother angiotensin converting enzyme (ACE) inhibitors or any of the excipients of Triapin mite or Triapin.
- in patients with a history of angioneurotic oedema.
- in unstable haemodynamic conditions: cardiovascular shock, untreated heart failure, acute myocardial infarction, unstable angina pectoris, stroke.
- in patients with AV block II or III.
- in patients with severely impaired hepatic function.
- in patients with severely impaired renal function (creatinine clearance less than 20 ml/min) and in patients on dialysis.
- during pregnancy.
- during lactation.

4.4 Special warnings and special precautions for use

Angio-oedema occurring during treatment with an ACE inhibitor necessitates immediate discontinuation of the drug. Angio-oedema may involve the tongue, glottis or larynx and, if so, may necessitate emergency measures.

Angio-oedema involving the tongue, glottis or larynx may be fatal. Emergency therapy should be given including, but not necessarily limited to, immediate subcutaneous adrenaline solution 1:1000 (0.3 to 0.5ml) or slow intravenous adrenaline 1 mg/ml (observe dilution instructions) with control of ECG and blood pressure. The patient should be hospitalised and observed for at least 12 to 24 hours and should not be discharged until complete resolution of symptoms has occurred.

Compared with non-black patients, a higher incidence of angio-oedema has been reported in black patients treated with ACE inhibitors.

Renal function should be monitored, particularly in the initial weeks of treatment with ACE inhibitors. Caution should be observed in patients with an activated renin-angiotensin system.

Patients with mild to moderately impaired renal function (creatinine clearance 20-60 ml/min) and patients already on diuretic treatment. For dosage see the respective monoproducts

Proteinuria: It may occur particularly in patients with existing renal function impairment or on relatively high doses of ACE inhibitors.

Renovascular hypertension/renal artery stenosis: There is an increased risk of severe hypotension and renal insufficiency when patients with renovascular hypertension and pre-existing bilateral renal artery stenosis or stenosis of the artery to a solitary kidney are treated with ACE inhibitors. Loss of renal function may occur with only mild changes in serum creatinine even in patients with unilateral renal artery stenosis.

There is no experience regarding the administration of Triapin or Triapin mite in patients with a recent kidney transplantation.

Hepatic failure: Rarely, ACE inhibitors have been associated with a syndrome that starts with cholestatic jaundice and progress to fulminant hepatic necrosis and (sometimes) death. The mechanism of this syndrome is not understood. Patients receiving ACE inhibitors who develop jaundice or marked elevations of hepatic enzymes should discontinue the ACE inhibitor and receive appropriate medical follow up.

Patients with mild to moderately impaired liver funcion: For dosage see respective monoproducts

Surgery/Anaesthesia: Hypotension may occur in patients undergoing major surgery or during treatment with anaesthetic agents that are known to lower blood pressure. If hypotension occurs, it may be corrected by volume expansion.

Aoritic stenosis/Hypertrophic cardiomyopathy: ACE inhibitors should be used with caution in patients with haemodynamically relevant left-ventricular inflow or outflow impediment (e.g. stenosis of the aortic or mitral valve, obstructive cardiomyopathy).

Symptomathic hypotension: In some patients, symptomatic hypotension may be observed after the initial dose, mainly in patients with heart failure (with or without renal insufficiency) treated with high doses of loop diuretics, in hyponatraemia or in reduced renal function. Therefore, Triapin mite or Triapin should only be given to such patients after special consideration and after the doses of the individual components have been carefully titrated. Triapin mite or Triapin should only be given if the patient is in a stable circulatory condition (see 4.3 Contra-indications). In hypertensive patients without cardiac and renal insufficiency, hypotension may occur especially in patients with decreased blood volume due to diuretic therapy, salt restriction, diarrhoea or vomiting.

Patients who would be at particular risk from an undesirably pronounced reduction in blood pressure (e.g. patients with coronory or cerebrovascular insufficiency) should be treated with ramipril and felodipine in a free combination. If satisfactory and stable blood pressure control is achieved with the doses of ramipril and felodipine included in Triapin mite or Triapin, the patient can be switched to this combination. In some cases, felodipine may cause hypotension with tachycardia, which may aggravate angina pectoris.

Neutropenia/Agranulocytosis: Triapin mite or Triapin may cause agranulocytosis and neutropenia. These undesirable effects have also been shown with other ACE inhibitors, rarely in uncomplicated patients but more frequently in patients with some degree of renal impairment, especially when it is associated with collagen vascular disease (e.g. systemic lupus erythematodes, scleroderma) and therapy with immunosuppressive agents. Monitoring of white blood cell counts should be considered for patients who have collagen vascular disease, especially if the disease is associated with impaired renal function. Neutropenia and agranulocytosis are reversible after discontinuation of the ACE inhibitor. Should symptoms such as fever, swelling of the lymph nodes, and/or inflammation of the throat occur in the course of therapy with Triapin mite or Triapin, the treating physician must be consulted and the white blood picture investigated immediately.

Cough: During treatment with an ACE inhibitor a dry cough may occur which disapperars after discontinuation.

Concomitant treatment with ACE inhibitors and antidiabetics (insulin and oral antidiabetics) may lead to an enhanced hypoglycaemic effect with the risk of hypoglycaemia. This effect may me most pronounced at the beginning of treatment and in patients with impaired renal function.

Felodipine is metabolised by CYP3A4. Therefore, combination with medicinal products which are potent CYP3A4 inhibitors or inducers should be avoided. For the same reason, the concomitant intake of grapefruit juice should be avoided (see 4.5 Interaction with other medicinal products and other forms of interaction).

Potassium-sparing diuretics and potassium supplements increase the risk of hyperkalaemia and should, therefore, generally not be given together with Triapin mite or Triapin.

The combination of lithium and ACE inhibitor is not recommended.

LDL-apheresis: Concomitant use of ACE inhibitors and extracorporeal treatments leading to contact of blood with negatively charged surfaces should be avoided since it may lead to severe anaphylactoid reactions. Such extracorporeal treatments include dialysis or haemofiltration with certain high-flux (e.g. polyacrylonitrile) membranes and low-density lipoprotein apheresis with dextran sulphate.

Desensitisation therapy: Increased likelihood and greater severity of anaphylactic and anaphylactoid reactions to insect venom (e.g. bee and wasp) as for other ACE inhibitors.

Ethnic differences: As with other angiotensin converting enzyme inhibitors, ramipril is apparently less effective in lowering blood pressure in black people than in non-blacks, possibly because of a higher prevalence of low-renin states in the black hypertensive population.

Children, patients with creatinine clearance under 20 ml/min and dialysis-treated patients: No experience is available. Triapin mite or Triapin should not be given to these patient groups.

4.5 Interaction with other medicinal products and other forms of Interaction

Not recommended associations.

Potassium salts, potassium-relating diuretics: Rise in serum potassium concentration is to be anticipated. Concomitant treatment with potassium-retaining diuretics (e.g. spironolactone, triamterene, or amiloride) or with potassium salts requires close monitoring of serum potassium.

Felodipine is a CYP3A4 substrate. Drugs that induce or inhibit CYP3A4 will have large influence on felodipine plasma concentrations.

Drugs that increase the metabolism of felodipine through induction of cytochrome P450 3A4 include carbamazepine, phenytoin, phenobarbital and rifampin as well as St John's wort (Hypericum perforatum). During concomitant administration of felodipine with carbamazepine, phenytoin, phenobarbital, AUC decreased by 93% and C_{max} by 82%. A similar effect is expected with St John's wort. Combination with CYP3A4 inducers should be avoided.

Potent inhibitors of cytochrome P450 3A4 include azole antifungals, macrolide antibiotics, telithomycin and HIV protease inhibitors. During concomitant administration of felodipine with itraconazole, C_{max} increased 8-fold and AUC 6-fold. During concomitant administration of felodipine with erythromycin, C_{max} and AUC increased approximately 2.5-fold. Combination with potent CYP3A4 inhibitors should be avoided.

Grapefruit juice inhibits cytochrome P450 3A4. Concomitant administration of felodipine with grapefruit juice increased felodipine C_{max} and AUC approximately 2-fold. The combination should be avoided.

Caution is recommended with concomitant use

Lithium: Excretion of lithium may be reduced by ACE inhibitors, leading to lithium toxicity. Lithium levels must, therefore, be monitored.

Antihypertensive agents and other substances with blood pressure lowering potential (e.g. nitrates, antipsychotics, narcotics, anaesthetics): Potentiation of the antihypertensive effect of Triapin mite or Triapin is to be anticipated.

Allopurinol, immunosuppressants, corticosteroids, procainamide, cytostatics and other substances that may change the blood picture: Increased likelihood of haematological reactions.

Nonsteroidal anti-inflammatory drugs (NSAIDS): Attenuation of the effect of ramipril is to be expected. Furthermore, concomitant treatment with ACE inhibitors and such drugs may lead to an increased risk of worsening of the renal function and an increase in serum potassium.

Vasopressor sympathomimetics: These may reduce the antihypertensive effect of Triapin mite or Triapin. Particularly close blood pressure monitoring is recommended.

Insulin, metformin, sulphonylureas: Concomitant treatment with ACE inhibitors and antidiabetic agents may cause a pronounced hypoglycaemic effect with the risk of hypoglycaemia. This effect is most pronounced at the beginning of treatment.

Theophylline: Concomitant administration of felodipine and oral theophylline reduces theophylline absorption by approximately 20%. This is probably of minor clinical importance.

Tacrolimus: Felodipine may increase the concentration of tacrolimus. When used together, the tacrolimus serum concentration should be followed and the tacrolimus dose may need to be adjusted.

Heparin: Rise in serum potassium concentration possible.

Salt: Increased dietary salt intake may attenuate the antihypertensive effect of Triapin mite or Triapin.

Alcohol: Increased vasodilatation. The antihypertensive effect of Triapin mite or Triapin may increase.

4.6 Pregnancy and lactation

Pregnancy

Triapin mite or Triapin must not be given during pregnancy (see 4.3 Contra-indications).

Calcium antagonists may inhibit contractions of the uterus during labour. Definite evidence that labour is prolonged in full-term pregnancy is lacking. Risk of foetal hypoxia may occur if the mother is hypotensive and perfusion of the uterus is reduced due to redistribution of the blood-flow through peripheral vasodilatation. In animal experiments, calcium antagonists have caused embryotoxic and/or teratogenic effects, especially in the form of distal skeletal malformations in several species.

Appropriate and well-controlled studies with ramipril have not been done in humans. ACE inhibitors cross the placenta and can cause foetal and neonatal morbidity and mortality when administered to pregnant women.

Foetal exposure to ACE inhibitors during the second and third trimesters has been associated with neonatal hypotension, renal failure, face or skull deformities and/or death. Maternal oligohydramnios have also been reported reflecting decreasing renal function in the foetus. Limb contractures, craniofacial deformities, hypoplastic lung development and intrauterine growth retardation have been reported in association with oligohydramnios. Intrauterine growth retardation, prematurity, persistent ductus arteriosus and foetal death have also been reported, but it is not clear whether they are related to the ACE inhibitor or to the underlying maternal disease. Whether exposure limited to the first trimester can adversely effect foetal outcome is not known.

Lactation

In animals, ramipril is excreted in milk. No information is available on whether or not ramipril is excreted in human breast-milk. Felodipine is excreted in human breast-milk.

Women must not breast-feed during treatment with Triapin mite or Triapin (see 4.3. Contra-indications).

4.7 Effects on ability to drive and use machines

Some undesirable effects (e.g. some symptoms of reduction in blood pressure such as dizziness) may be accompanied by an impairment of the ability to concentrate and react. This may constitute a risk in situations where these

Table 1

Frequencies/ Organ System	Common (⩾ 1/100)	Uncommon (> 1/1000, < 1/100)	Rare (> 1/10 000, < 1/1000)	Very rare (< 1/10 000)
Nervous System Disorders	Headache	Dizziness, paraesthesiae	Syncope	
Vascular Disorders	Flush, peripheral oedema			Leucocytoclastic vasculitis
Cardiac Disorders		Tachycardia, palpitations		
Gastrointestinal Disorders		Nausea, abdominal pain	Vomiting	Gingival hyperplasia, gingivitis
Metabolism and nutrition disorders				Hyperglycaemia
Skin and Subcutaneous Tissue Disorders		Rash, pruritus	Urticaria	Photosensitivity reactions, angio-oedema
General Disorders and Administration Site conditions		Fatigue		Fever
Musculoskeletal and Connective Tissue Disorders			Arthralgia, myalgia	
Psychiatric Disorders			Impotence/ sexual dysfunction	
Hepatobiliary Disorders				Increased liver enzymes
Renal and Urinary Disorders				Pollakisuria
Immune System Disorder				Hypersensitivity reactions

abilities are of special importance, e.g., when driving a car or operating machinery.

4.8 Undesirable effects

The following undesirable effects may occur in connection with felodipine treatment

(see Table 1 on previous page)

The following undesirable effects may occur in connection with ramipril treatment

(see Table 2 opposite)

4.9 Overdose

Symptoms

Overdosage may cause excessive peripheral vasodilatation with marked hypotension, bradycardia, shock, electrolyte disturbances and renal failure.

Management

Primary detoxification by, for example, gastric lavage, administration of adsorbents and/or sodium sulphate (if possible during the first 30 minutes). In case of hypotension, administration of α_1-adrenergic sympathomimetics and angiotensin II must be considered in addition to volume and salt substitution. Bradycardia or extensive vagal reactions should be treated by administering atropine.

No experience is available concerning the efficacy of forced diuresis, alteration in urine pH, haemofiltration, or dialysis in speeding up the elimination of ramipril or ramiprilat. If dialysis or haemofiltration is nevertheless considered, see also under 4.4 Special Warnings and Special Precautions for use.

5. PHARMACOLOGICAL PROPERTIES

5.1 Pharmacodynamic properties

Pharmacotherapeutic group: Antihypertensive drugs. ATC code: C09B B05

Both the calcium antagonist felodipine and the ACE inhibitor ramipril reduce blood pressure by dilation of the peripheral blood vessels. Calcium antagonists dilate the arterial beds while ACE inhibitors dilate both arterial and venous beds. Vasodilatation and thereby reduction of blood pressure may lead to activation of the sympathetic nervous system and the renin-angiotensin system. Inhibition of ACE results in decreased plasma angiotensin II.

The onset of the antihypertensive effect of a single dose of Triapin mite or Triapin is 1 to 2 hours. The maximum antihypertensive effect is achieved within 2 to 4 weeks and is maintained during long-term therapy. The blood pressure reduction is maintained throughout the 24-hour dosage interval. Morbidity and mortality data are not available.

Felodipineis a vascular selective calcium antagonist, which lowers arterial blood pressure by decreasing peripheral vascular resistance via a direct relaxant action on vascular smooth muscles. Due to its selectivity for smooth muscle in the arterioles, felodipine, in therapeutic doses, has no direct effect on cardiac contractility or conduction. The renal vascular resistance is decreased by felodipine. The normal glomerular filtration rate is not influenced. In patients with impaired renal function, the glomerular filtration rate may increase. Felodipine possesses a mild natriuretic/diuretic effect and fluid retention does not occur.

Ramiprilis a prodrug which hydrolyses to the active metabolite ramiprilat, a potent and long-acting ACE (angiotensin converting enzyme) inhibitor. In plasma and tissue, ACE catalyses the conversion of angiotensin I to the vasoconstrictor angiotensin II and also the breakdown of the vasodilator bradykinin. The vasodilatation induced by the ACE inhibitor reduces blood pressure pre-load and after-load. Since angiotensin II also stimulates the release of aldosterone, ramiprilat reduces secretion of aldosterone. Ramipril reduces peripheral arterial resistance without major changes in renal plasma flow or glomerular filtration rate. In hypertensive patients, ramipril leads to a reduction in supine and standing blood pressure without a compensatory rise in heart rate.

5.2 Pharmacokinetic properties

General characteristics of the active substances

Felodipine ER (extended-release formulation): The bioavailability is approximately 15% and is not influenced by concomitant intake of food. The peak plasma concentration is reached after 3 to 5 hours. Binding to plasma proteins is more than 99%. The distribution volume at steady state is 10 l/kg. The half-life for felodipine in the elimination phase is approximately 25 hours and steady state is reached after 5 days. There is no risk of accumulation during long-term treatment. Mean clearance is 1200 ml/min. Decreased clearance in elderly patients leads to higher plasma concentrations of felodipine. Age only partly explains the inter-individual variation in plasma concentration, however. Felodipine is metabolised in the liver and all identified metabolites are devoid of vasodilating properties. Approximately 70% of a given dose is excreted as metabolites in the urine and about 10% with the faeces. Less than 0.5% of the dose is excreted unchanged in the urine. Impaired renal function does not influence the plasma concentration of felodipine.

Ramipril: The pharmacokinetic parameters of ramiprilat are calculated after intravenous administration of ramipril. Ramipril is metabolised in the liver, and aside from the

Table 2

Frequencies/ Organ System	**Common ($\geq$ 1/100)**	**Uncommon (> 1/1000, < 1/100)**	**Rare (> 1/10 000, < 1/1000)**	**Very rare (< 1/10 000)**
Respiratory, Thoracic and Mediastinal Disorders	Dry tickling cough			
Nervous System Disorders		Headache, disorders of balance, impaired reactions	Dizziness, syncope, tremor, smell and taste disturbances, loss of taste	Paraesthesia
Vascular Disorders		Tachycardia	Peripheral oedema, flushing	Exacerbation of perfusion disturbances due to vascular stenosis, precipitation or intensification of Raynauds phenomenon, vasculitis, transient ischemic attack, ischemic stroke, cerebral ischemia
Gastrointestinal Disorders		Nausea	Dryness of the mouth, glossitis, inflammatory reactions of the oral cavity and gastrointestinal tract, abdominal discomfort, gastric pain, digestive disturbances, constipation, diarrhoea, vomiting	Ileus
Investigation and Electrolyte Balance		Increase in serum urea and serum creatinine	Increase in serum potassium, increased levels of pancreatic enzymes	Decrease in serum sodium, raised titers of antinuclear antibodies
General Disorders and Administration Site conditions		Weakness, drowsiness, lightheadedness	Fatigue, sweating	Fever
Eye Disorders		Conjunctivitis	Visual disturbances	
Skin and Subcutaneous Tissue Disorders		Angioneurotic oedema, pruritus, rash, urticaria		Maculopapular rash, pemphigus, exacerbation of psoriasis, psoriasiform, pemphigoid or lichenoid exanthema, enanthema, erythema multiforme, Steven-Johnson syndrome, toxic epidermal necrolysis, alopecia, onycholysis, photosensitivity, serositis
Hepatobiliary Disorders		Increases in serum levels of hepatic enzymes and/or bilirubin, cholestatic jaundice		Pancreatitis, liver failure, hepatocellular or cholestatic hepatitis
Cardiac Disorders			Severe hypotension, palpitations, disturbed orthostatic regulation, angina pectoris, cardiac arrhythmias	Myocardial ischemia, myocardial infarction, cardiovascular shock, coronary insufficiency
Musculoskeletal and Connective Tissue Disorders			Muscle cramps	Myalgia, arthralgia, myositis
Blood and Lymphatic System Disorders			Reduction in the red blood cell count and haemoglobin content, white blood cell or blood platelet	Agranulocytosis, pancytopenia, bone marrow depression, haemolytical anaemia, eosinophilia, SR-elevation, leucocytosis
Immune System Disorders			Anaphylactic or anaphylactoid reactions	
Respiratory, Thoracic and Mediastinal Disorders			Sinusitis, bronchitis, bronchospasm, dyspnoea, aggravation of asthma, rhinitis	
Psychiatric Disorders			Nervousness, depressed mood, restlessness, confusion, sleep disturbances, feeling of anxiety, somnolence, reduced libido	
Metabolism and Nutrition Disorders			Loss of appetite	
Ear and Labyrinth Disorders			Tinnitus, disturbed hearing	
Reproductive System and Breast Disorders			Transient erectile impotence	
Endocrine Disorders				Gynaecomastia

active metabolite ramiprilat, pharmacologically inactive metabolites have been identified. The formation of active ramiprilat may be decreased in patients with impaired liver function. The metabolites are excreted mainly via the kidneys. The bioavailability of ramiprilat is approximately 28% after oral administration of ramipril. After intravenous administration of 2.5 mg ramipril, approximately 53% of the dose is converted to ramiprilat. A maximum serum concentration of ramiprilat is achieved after 2 to 4 hours. Absorption and bioavailability are not influenced by concomitant intake of food. The protein binding of ramiprilat is approximately 55%. The distribution volume is approximately 500 litres. The effective half-life, after repeated daily dosage of 5 to 10 mg, is 13 to 17 hours. Steady-state is achieved after approximately 4 days. Renal clearance is 70 to 100 ml/min and total clearance is approximately 380 ml/min. Impaired renal function delays the elimination of ramiprilat and excretion in the urine is reduced.

Characteristics of the combination product

In Triapin mite or Triapin the pharmacokinetics of ramipril, ramiprilat and felodipine are essentially unaltered compared to the monoproducts, felodipine ER tablets and ramipril tablets. Felodipine does not influence the ACE inhibition caused by ramiprilat. The fixed combination tablets are thus regarded as bioequivalent to the free combination.

5.3 Preclinical safety data

Repeated-dose toxicity studies performed with the combination in rats and monkeys did not demonstrate any synergistic effects.

Pre-clinical data for felodipine and ramipril reveal no special hazard for humans based on conventional studies of genotoxicity and carcinogenic potential.

Reproduction toxicity

Felodipine: In investigations on fertility and general reproductive performance in rats, a prolongation of parturition resulting in difficult labour/increased foetal deaths and early postnatal deaths was observed. Reproduction toxicity studies in rabbits have shown a dose-related reversible enlargement of the mammary glands of the parent animals and dose-related digital anomalies in the foetuses.

Ramipril: Studies in rats, rabbits and monkeys did not disclose any teratogenic properties. Daily doses during pregnancy and lactation in rats produced irreversible renal pelvis dilatation in the offspring.

6. PHARMACEUTICAL PARTICULARS

6.1 List of excipients

Cellulose microcrystalline

Hyprolose

Hypromellose

Iron oxides E172

Lactose anhydrous

Macrogol 6000

Macrogolglycerol hydroxystearate

Maize starch

Paraffin

Propyl gallate

Sodium aluminium silicate

Sodium stearyl fumarate

Titanium dioxide E 171

6.2 Incompatibilities

Not applicable.

6.3 Shelf life

Triapin mite: 24 months

Triapin: 30 months

6.4 Special precautions for storage

Do not store above 30 °C.

6.5 Nature and contents of container

PVC/PVDC blisters: 28 tablets

6.6 Instructions for use and handling

No special requirements.

Administrative Data

7. MARKETING AUTHORISATION HOLDER

Aventis Pharma Ltd.

50 Kings Hill Avenue

Kings Hill

West Malling

Kent

ME19 4AH

UK

8. MARKETING AUTHORISATION NUMBER(S)

Triapin Mite: PL 04425/0321

Triapin: PL 04425/0320

9. DATE OF FIRST AUTHORISATION/RENEWAL OF THE AUTHORISATION

15th April 2002

10. DATE OF REVISION OF THE TEXT

19th December 2003

Legal category:

POM

Triclofos Elixir BP

(Celltech Manufacturing Services Limited)

1. NAME OF THE MEDICINAL PRODUCT

Triclofos Elixir BP

2. QUALITATIVE AND QUANTITATIVE COMPOSITION

Triclofos Sodium BP 10%w/v

3. PHARMACEUTICAL FORM

An elixir for oral administration

4. CLINICAL PARTICULARS

4.1 Therapeutic indications

For the short-term treatment of insomnia

4.2 Posology and method of administration

As directed by a medical practitioner.

The following doses of Triclofos Elixir should be administered 15 to 30 minutes before bedtime:

Adults and Children over 12 years

1-2g (10-20ml)

Children

up to 1 year: 25-30mg/kg body weight

1-5 years: 250-500mg (2.5-5ml)

6-12 years: 500mg-1g (5-10ml)

Elderly

No specific dosage recommendations (but see Special Warnings and Precautions for Use)

4.3 Contraindications

The use of Triclofos Elixir is contraindicated in:

cardiac disease, hepatic impairment, hypersensitivity (or previous idiosyncrasy) to Triclofos (or chloral hydrate), nursing mothers, pregnancy, renal impairment.

The use of Triclofos Elixir is not recommended in patients with gastritis, or in those with a history of acute attacks of porphyria.

4.4 Special warnings and special precautions for use

There is a danger of misuse with Triclofos and habituation may develop. Tolerance to Triclofos may develop with high or prolonged dosage and dependence may occur. Sudden withdrawal after long term use may result in delirium. Other withdrawal symptoms which may occur include: apprehension, weakness, anxiety, headache, dizziness, irritability, tremors, nausea, vomiting, abdominal cramps, insomnia, visual distortions, muscle twitches, convulsions and hallucinations. Potential sequelae of such misuse are gastritis and parenchymatous renal injury. Delirium may occur, especially in the elderly, and particularly when Triclofos is used in conjunction with psychotropic or anticholinergic agents

4.5 Interaction with other medicinal products and other forms of Interaction

Patients established on anticoagulant therapy should be monitored for changes in prothrombin time when Triclofos is added or removed from the treatment regimen. Triclofos is known to potentiate the effects of alcohol. Administration of intravenous frusemide following administration of Triclofos may provoke a hypermetabolic state characterised by sweating, hot flushes, and variable blood pressure.

Coadministration of barbiturates and other sedatives may potentiate the drowsiness that can be caused by Triclofos

4.6 Pregnancy and lactation

Contra-indicated

4.7 Effects on ability to drive and use machines

Patients should be warned that their ability to drive or use machines may be impaired by drowsiness.

4.8 Undesirable effects

Abdominal distension and flatulence; malaise; gastric irritation (gastro-intestinal upset, nausea and vomiting); eosinophilia, ketonuria, reduction in total white cell count; CNS type reactions (ataxia, drowsiness, headache, light-headedness, staggering gait, vertigo, confusion, sometimes with paranoia, excitement, hangover, nightmares); hypersensitivity reactions including skin reactions (angioedema, purpura, bullous lesions (erythema multiforme, Stevens Johnson syndrome)) and urticaria, have all been reported in patients following administration of Triclofos.

4.9 Overdose

Symptoms of overdose may include respiratory depression, arrhythmias, hypothermia, pin-point pupils, hypotension, coma, gastric irritation, areflexia, muscle flaccidity, oesophageal stricture, gastric perforation, gastro-intestinal haemorrhage and vomiting. Gastric necrosis, icterus, hepatic damage, albuminuria and renal damage may also occur. Serious problems have arisen in adults with doses as little as 4g and 10g can be fatal in adults.

Treatment: provided that the patient is conscious and a patient airway can be maintained, it may be appropriate to empty the stomach contents by gastric lavage. Activated charcoal should then be administered. General supportive measures, including ECG monitoring, should be employed. It may be necessary to consider haemodialysis or haemoperfusion in patients who deteriorate despite general supportive measures.

5. PHARMACOLOGICAL PROPERTIES

5.1 Pharmacodynamic properties

Triclofos sodium has hypnotic and sedative actions similar to those of chloral hydrate. It is hydrolysed in the body to trichloroethanol which is probably the active metabolite.

5.2 Pharmacokinetic properties

Following oral administration, triclofos is rapidly and completely hydrolysed in the gastro-intestinal tract to trichloroethanol. Peak serum levels of trichloroethanol are achieved within about one hour. Trichloroethanol is subject to conjugation with glucuronic acid and further metabolism to trichloroacetic acid. Trichloroethanol and trichloroacetic acid are approximately 35% and 95% protein bound respectively. Their half lives are estimated as between 8 and 11 hours and between 67 and 75 hours respectively. Approximately 12% of a dose is excreted in the urine within 24 hours. In infants the half lives are longer. The value for trichloroethanol is 35 hours, whilst for trichloroacetic acid the half life exceeds six days, with significant plasma concentrations present at 14 days.

5.3 Preclinical safety data

Triclofos Sodium has the same major metabolites as chloral hydrate, which has been shown to induce liver tumours in male mice, with no tumourigenic effects in rats. The mechanism of tumour induction is not known, but in the absence of clear evidence of mutagenic and clastogenic potential it is unlikely to be relevant to man. No data are available on the genotoxic or carcinogenic potential of triclofos sodium.

6. PHARMACEUTICAL PARTICULARS

6.1 List of excipients

Sugar Granulated

Vanillin

Nipastat GL75 containing: methyl-, ethyl-, propyl- and butyl-4- hydroxybenzoates

Disodium Edetate

Sodium Bicarbonate Powder

Sunset Yellow Ariavit 311831

Flavour IFF 1211

Purified Water

Activated Charcoal

6.2 Incompatibilities

None

6.3 Shelf life

24 months unopened - all bottles.

6 months once opened - 100ml and 300ml bottles.

6.4 Special precautions for storage

Store below 25°C. Keep well closed.

6.5 Nature and contents of container

Amber glass bottles (100ml) with screw on white pigmented polypropylene closure with saran faced expanded polyethylene wad.

Amber glass bottles (300ml) with screw on white pigmented polypropylene child resistant closure with natural expanded polyethylene wad

2 litre amber glass bottles with screw on white pigmented polypropylene closure with natural expanded polyethylene wad.

6.6 Instructions for use and handling

Discard elixir 6 months after first opening.

7. MARKETING AUTHORISATION HOLDER

Celltech Manufacturing Services Limited

Vale of Bardsley

Ashton-under-Lyne

Lancashire

OL7 9RR

United Kingdom

8. MARKETING AUTHORISATION NUMBER(S)

PL 18816/0018

9. DATE OF FIRST AUTHORISATION/RENEWAL OF THE AUTHORISATION

18 July 2001

10. DATE OF REVISION OF THE TEXT

September 2002

Tridestra

(Orion Pharma (UK) Limited)

1. NAME OF THE MEDICINAL PRODUCT

Tridestra

2. QUALITATIVE AND QUANTITATIVE COMPOSITION

Tridestra tablet (white):

Estradiol valerate 2 mg

Tridestra tablet (blue):

Estradiol valerate 2 mg

Medroxyprogesterone acetate 20 mg

Tridestra tablet (yellow):

Placebo

For excipients, see 6.1

3. PHARMACEUTICAL FORM

Tablets, oral.

4. CLINICAL PARTICULARS

4.1 Therapeutic indications

i) Hormone replacement therapy (HRT) for oestrogen deficiency symptoms in peri-and post-menopausal women.

ii) Prevention of osteoporosis in postmenopausal women at high risk of future fractures who are intolerant of, or contra-indicated for, other medicinal products approved for the prevention of osteoporosis.

Please also refer to section 4.4

The experience of treating women older than 65 years is limited.

4.2 Posology and method of administration

Tridestra is a cyclic HRT, that produces a vaginal bleed every 3 months. The bleeding occurs during treatment when the yellow (placebo) tablets are taken and is similar to the monthly bleed experienced during the normal menstrual cycle.

Tridestra consists of 91 tablets in a blister pack bearing calendar markings. Dosage is according to the calendar pack. One tablet should be taken daily without a break between packs.

The dosage during days 1 to 70 (inclusive) of the cycle is 2 mg oestradiol valerate (white tablets). From day 71 to day 84 (inclusive) it is 2 mg of oestradiol valerate and 20 mg of medroxyprogesterone acetate (blue tablets). From day 85 to day 91 (inclusive) a placebo preparation (yellow tablets) is taken when a menstrual like bleed occurs.

For initiation and continuation of treatment of postmenopausal symptoms, the lowest effective dose for the shortest duration (see also Section 4.4) should be used.

Women with amenorrhoea who are not taking HRT or who are switching to Tridestra from continuous combined HRT product, may start treatment on any day.

Women who are still having periods may start treatment 5 days after the start of the period.

Women who are switching from a cyclic or sequential HRT product to Tridestra treatment may start one week after completion of the cycle (28 days) ie at the end of a withdrawal bleed.

If the patient has forgotten to take one tablet, it should be taken within 12 hours otherwise the forgotten tablet should be discarded and the usual tablet taken the following day. Missing a dose may increase the likelihood of breakthrough bleeding and spotting.

4.3 Contraindications

- Known, past or suspected breast cancer
- Known or suspected oestrogen-dependent malignant tumours (e.g. endometrial cancer)
- Undiagnosed genital bleeding
- Untreated endometrial hyperplasia
- Previous idiopathic or current venous thromboembolism [deep venous thrombosis (DVT), pulmonary embolism]
- Active or recent arterial thromboembolic disease (e.g. angina, myocardial infarction)
- Acute liver disease or a history of liver disease as long as liver function tests have failed to return to normal
- Known hypersensitivity to the active substances or to any of the excipients
- Porphyria

4.4 Special warnings and special precautions for use

For the treatment of postmenopausal symptoms, HRT should only be initiated for symptoms that adversely affect quality of life. In all cases, a careful appraisal of the risks and benefits should be undertaken at least annually and HRT should only be continued as long as the benefit outweighs the risk.

Medical examination/follow-up

Before initiating or reinstituting HRT, a complete personal and family medical history should be taken. Physical (including pelvic and breast) examination should be guided by this and by the contraindications and warnings for use. During treatment, periodic check-ups are recommended of a frequency and nature adapted to the individual woman. Women should be advised what changes in their breasts should be reported to their doctor or nurse (see 'Breast Cancer' below). Investigations, including mammography, should be carried out in accordance with currently accepted screening practices, modified to the clinical needs of the individual.

Conditions which need supervision

If any of the following conditions are present, have occurred previously and/or have been aggravated during pregnancy or previous hormone treatment, the patient should be closely supervised. It should be taken into account that these conditions may recur or be aggravated during treatment with Tridestra, in particular:

- Leiomyoma (uterine fibroids) or endometriosis
- A history of or risk factors for thromboembolic disorders (see below)
- Risk factors for oestrogen dependent tumours, e.g. 1st degree heredity for breast cancer
- Hypertension
- Liver disorders (e.g. liver adenoma)
- Diabetes mellitus with or without vascular involvement
- Cholelithiasis
- Migraine or (severe) headache
- Systemic lupus erythematosus
- A history of endometrial hyperplasia (see below)
- Epilepsy
- Asthma
- Otosclerosis

Reasons for immediate withdrawal of therapy

Therapy should be discontinued in case a contra-indication is discovered and in the following situations:

- Jaundice or deterioration of liver function
- Significant increase in blood pressure
- New onset of migraine-type headache
- Pregnancy

Endometrial hyperplasia

- The risk of endometrial hyperplasia and carcinoma is increased when oestrogens are administered alone for prolonged periods (see Section 4.8). The addition of a progestagen for at least 12 days per cycle in non-hysterectomised women greatly reduces this risk.
- Breakthrough bleeding and spotting may occur during the first months of treatment. If breakthrough bleeding or spotting appears after some time of therapy, or continues after treatment has been discontinued, the reason should be investigated, which may include endometrial biopsy to excluded endometrial malignancy.

Breast cancer

A randomised placebo-controlled trial, the Women's Health Initiative study (WHI) and epidemiological studies including the Million Women Study (MWS), have reported an increased risk of breast cancer in women taking oestrogens, oestrogen-progestagen combinations or tibolone for HRT for several years (see Section 4.8). For all HRT, an excess risk becomes apparent within a few years of use and increase with duration of intake but returns to baseline within a few (at most 5 years) after stopping treatment.

In the MWS, the relative risk of breast cancer with conjugated equine oestrogens (CEE) or oestrodial (E2) was greater when a progestagen was added, either sequentially or continuously, and regardless of type of progestagen. There was no evidence of a difference in risk between the different routes of administration.

In the WHI study, the continuous combined conjugated equine oestrogen and medroxyprogesterone acetate (CEE + MPA) product used was associated with breast cancers that were slightly larger in size and more frequently had local lymph node metastases compared to placebo.

HRT, especially oestrogen-progestagen combined treatment, increases the density of mammographic images which may adversely affect the radiological detection of breast cancer.

Venous thromboembolism

- HRT is associated with a higher relative risk of developing venous thromboembolism (VTE), i.e. deep vein thrombosis or pulmonary embolism. One randomised controlled trial and epidemiological studies found a two-to threefold higher risk for users compared with non-users. For non-users it is estimated that the number of cases of VTE that will occur over a 5 year period is about 3 per 1000 women aged 50-59 years and 8 per 1000 women aged between 60-69 years. It is estimated that in healthy women who use HRT for 5 years, the number of additional cases of VTE over a 5 year period will be between 2 and 6 (best estimate = 4) per 1000 women aged 50-59 years and between 5 and 15 (best estimate = 9) per 1000 women aged 60-69 years. The occurrence of such an event is more likely in the first year of HRT than later.
- Generally recognised risk factors for VTE include a personal history or family history, severe obesity (BMI > 30 kg/m^2) and systemic lupus erythematosus (SLE). There is no consensus about the possible role of varicose veins in VTE.
- Patients with a history of VTE or known thrombophilic states have an increased risk of VTE. HRT may add to this risk. Personal or strong family history of thromboembolism or recurrent spontaneous abortion should be investigated in order to exclude a thrombophilic predisposition. Until a thorough evaluation of thrombophilic factors has been made or anticoagulant treatment initiated, use of HRT in such patients should be viewed as contraindicated. Those women already on anticoagulant treatment require careful consideration of the benefit-risk of use of HRT.
- The risk of VTE may be temporarily increased with prolonged immobilisation, major trauma or major surgery. As in all postoperative patients, scrupulous attention should be given to prophylactic measures to prevent VTE following surgery. Where prolonged immobilisation is liable to follow elective surgery, particularly abdominal or orthopaedic surgery to the lower limbs, consideration should be given to temporarily stopping HRT 4 to 6 weeks earlier, if possible. Treatment should not be restarted until the woman is completely mobilised.
- If VTE develops after initiating therapy, the drug should be discontinued. Patients should be told to contact their doctors immediately when they are aware of a potential thromboembolic symptom (eg, painful swelling of a leg, sudden pain in the chest, dyspnea).

Coronary artery disease (CAD)

- There is no evidence from randomised controlled trials of cardiovascular benefit with continuous combined conjugated oestrogens and medroxyprogesterone acetate (MPA). Two large clinical trials (WHI and HERS i.e. Heart and Estrogen/progestin Replacement Study) showed a possible increased risk of cardiovascular morbidity in the first year of use and no overall benefit. For other HRT products there are only limited data from randomised controlled trials examining effects in cardiovascular morbidity and mortality. Therefore, it is uncertain whether these findings also extend to other HRT products.

Stroke

- One large randomised clinical trial (WHI-trial) found, as a secondary outcome, an increased risk of ischaemic stroke in healthy women during treatment with continuous combined conjugated oestrogens and MPA. For women who do not use HRT, it is estimated that the number of cases of stroke that will occur over a 5 year period is about 3 per 1000 women aged 50-59 years and 11 per 1000 women aged 60-69 years. It is estimated that for women who use conjugated estrogens and MPA for 5 years, the number of additional cases will be between 0 and 3 (best estimate = 1) per 1000 users aged 50-59 years and between 1 and 9 (best estimate = 4) per 1000 users aged 60-69 years. It is unknown whether the increased risk also extends to other HRT products.

Ovarian cancer

- Long-term (at least 5-10 years) use of oestrogen-only HRT products in hysterectomised women has been associated with an increased risk of ovarian cancer in some epidemiological studies. It is uncertain whether long-term use of combined HRT confers a different risk than oestrogen-only products.

Other conditions

- Oestrogens may cause fluid retention and, therefore, patients with cardiac or renal dysfunction should be carefully observed. Patients with terminal renal insufficiency should be closely observed, since it is expected that the level of circulating active ingredients of Tridestra is increased.
- Women with pre-existing hypertriglyceridaemia should be followed closely during oestrogen replacement or HRT, since rare cases of large increases of plasma triglycerides leading to pancreatitis have been reported with oestrogen therapy in this condition.
- Oestrogens increase thyroid binding globulin (TBG), leading to increased circulating total thyroid hormone, as measured by protein-bound iodine (PBI), T4 levels (by column or by radio-immunoassay) or T3 levels (by radio-immunoassay). T3 resin uptake is decreased, reflecting the elevated TBG. Free T4 and free T3 concentrations are unaltered. Other binding proteins may be elevated in serum, i.e. corticoid binding globulin (CBG), sex-hormone-binding globulin (SHBG) leading to increased circulating corticosteroids and sex steroids, respectively. Free or biological active hormone concentrations are unchanged. Other plasma proteins may be increased (angiotensinogen/renin substrate, alpha-1-antitrypsin, ceruloplasmin).
- There is no conclusive evidence for improvement of cognitive function. There is some evidence from the WHI trial of increased risk of probable dementia in women who start using continuous combined CEE and MPA after the age of 65. It is unknown whether the findings apply to younger post-menopausal women or other HRT products.

4.5 Interaction with other medicinal products and other forms of Interaction

The metabolism of oestrogens and progestogens may be increased by concomitant use of substances known to induce drug-metabolising enzymes, specifically cytochrome P450 enzymes, such as anticonvulsants (e.g. phenobarbital, phenytoin, carbamazepine) and anti-infectives (e.g. rifampicin, rifabutin, nevirapine, efavirenz).

Ritonavir and nelfinavir, although known as strong inhibitors, by contrast exhibit inducing properties when used concomitantly with steroid hormones. Herbal preparations containing St John's wort (Hypericum perforatum) may induce the metabolism of oestrogens and progestogens.

Clinically, an increased metabolism of oestrogens and progestogens may lead to decreased effect and changes in the uterine bleeding profile.

4.6 Pregnancy and lactation

Tridestra is not indicated during pregnancy. If pregnancy occurs during medication with Tridestra treatment should be withdrawn immediately.

Clinically, data on a limited number of exposed pregnancies indicate no adverse effects of medroxyprogesterone acetate on the foetus.

The results of most epidemiological studies to date relevant to inadvertent foetal exposure to combinations of oestrogens and progestogen indicate no teratogenic or foetotoxic effect.

Lactation

Tridestra is not indicated during lactation.

Table 1

Organ group	Common (> 1/100)	Uncommon >1/1,000, < 1/100	Rare > 1/10,000; < 1/1,000
Gastrointestinal disorders	Nausea, abdominal pain	vomiting	
Skin and subcutaneous tissue disorders			
Nervous System disorders	Headache, migraine		
Vision disorders	Visual disturbances		
Cardiac and vascular disorders			
Reproductive disorders and breast disorders	Dysmenorrhoea, breast tenderness, breast enlargement, breakthrough bleeding.	Uterine fibroids	Endometrial hyperplasia, menorrhagia
Miscellaneous	Oedema, tiredness, weigth increase, changes in mood, Changes in libido		

4.7 Effects on ability to drive and use machines

No effects on ability to drive and use machines have been observed

4.8 Undesirable effects

Adverse drug reactions occur most commonly in the first months of the treatment. The most common adverse effect is breakthrough bleeding and spotting appearing in 22% of patients. The overall percentage of treated patients experiencing at least 1 adverse reaction is 47%.

(see Table 1 above)

Breast Cancer

According to evidence from a large number of epidemiological studies and one randomised placebo-controlled trial, the Women's Health Initiative (WHI), the overall risk of breast cancer increases with increasing duration of HRT use in current or recent HRT users.

For oestrogen only HRT, estimates of relative risk (RR) from a reanalysis of original data from 51 epidemiological studies (in which > 80% of HRT use was oestrogen only HRT) and from the epidemiological Million Women Study (MWS) are similar at 1.35 (95% CI 1.21-1.49) and 1.30 (95% CI 1.21-1.40), respectively.

For oestrogen plus progestagen combined HRT, several epidemiological studies have reported an overall higher risk for breast cancer than with oestrogens alone.

The MWS reported that, compared to never users, the use of various types of oestrogen-progestagen combined HRT was associated with a higher risk of breast cancer (RR = 2.00, 95%CI: 1.88-2.12) than use of oestrogens alone (RR = 1.30, 95%CI: 1.21 – 1.40) or use of tibolone (RR=1.45; 95%CI 1.25-1.68).

The WHI trial reported a risk estimate of 1.24 (95% CI: 1.01-1.54) after 5.6 years of use of oestrogen-progestagen combined HRT (CEE + MPA) in all users compared with placebo.

The absolute risks calculated from the MWS and the WHI trials are presented below:

The MWS has estimated, from the known average incidence of breast cancer in developed countries, that:

- For women not using HRT, about 32 in every 1000 are expected to have breast cancer diagnosed between the ages of 50 and 64 years.
- For 1000 current or recent users of HRT, the number of additional cases during the corresponding period will be
- For users of oestrogen only replacement therapy,
  - between 0 and 3 (best estimate = 1.5) for 5 years' use
  - between 3 and 7 (best estimate = 5) for 10 years' use.
- For users of oestrogen plus progestagen combined HRT,
  - between 5 and 7 (best estimate = 6) for 5 years' use
  - between 18 and 20 (best estimate = 19) for 10 years' use.

The WHI trial estimated that after 5.6 years of follow-up of women between the ages of 50 and 79 years, an additional 8 cases of invasive breast cancer would be due to oestrogen-progestagen combined HRT (CEE + MPA) per 10,000 women years.

According to calculations from the trial data, it is estimated that:

- For 1000 women in the placebo group,
  - about 16 cases of invasive breast cancer would be diagnosed in 5 years.
- For 1000 women who used oestrogen + progestagen combined HRT (CEE + MPA), the number of additional cases would be
  - between 0 and 9 (best estimate = 4) for 5 years' use.

The number of additional cases of breast cancer in women who use HRT is broadly similar for women who start HRT irrespective of age at start of use (between the ages of 45-65) (see section 4.4).

Endometrial cancer

In women with an intact uterus, the risk of endometrial hyperplasia and endometrial cancer increases with increasing duration of use of unopposed oestrogens. According to data from epidemiological studies, the best estimate of the risk is that for women not using HRT, about 5 in every 1000 are expected to have endometrial cancer diagnosed between the ages of 50 and 65. Depending on the duration of treatment and oestrogen dose, the reported increase in endometrial cancer risk among unopposed oestrogen users varies from 2-to 12-fold greater compared with non-users. Adding a progestagen to oestrogen-only therapy greatly reduces this increased risk.

Other adverse reactions have been reported in association with oestrogen/progestagen treatment:

- Oestrogen-dependent neoplasms benign and malignant, e.g. endometrial cancer.
- Venous thromboembolism, i.e. deep leg or pelvic venous thrombosis and pulmonary embolism, is more frequent among HRT users than among non-users. For further information see sections 4.3. Contraindications and 4.4. Special warnings and precautions for use.
- Myocardial infarction and stroke.
- Gall bladder disease.
- Skin and subcutaneous disorders: chloasma, erythema multiforme, erythema nodosum, vascular purpura.
- Probable dementia (see section 4.4)

4.9 Overdose

Overdosage of oestrogen may cause nausea, headache and withdrawal bleeding. Serious ill effects have not been reported following acute ingestion of large doses of oestrogens and progestogens in contraceptive formulations by young children. When needed, therapy is symptomatic.

5. PHARMACOLOGICAL PROPERTIES

5.1 Pharmacodynamic properties

Pharmacotherapeutic group: Progestogens and Oestrogens in Combination

ATC code: G03FB 06

- **Oestradiol / Oestradiol valerate**: the active ingredient, synthetic 17β-oestradiol, is chemically and biologically identical to endogenous human oestradiol. It substitutes for the loss of oestrogen production in menopausal women, and alleviates menopausal symptoms. Oestrogens prevent bone loss following menopause or ovariectomy.

Progestagen: Medroxyprogesterone acetate (MPA) is a synthetic derivative of natural progesterone, a 17-α-hydroxy-6-methylprogesterone acetate. It has a similar effect to progesterone with slight androgenic activity. As oestrogens promote the growth of the endometrium, unopposed oestrogens increase the risk of endometrial hyperplasia and cancer. The addition of a progestagen greatly reduces the oestrogen-induced risk of endometrial hyperplasia in non-hysterectomised women.

- **Relief of oestrogen-deficiency symptoms and bleeding patterns**

- Relief of menopausal symptoms was achieved during the first few weeks of treatment.

- Tridestra causes a withdrawal bleed at the end of a 3 monthly cycle

- Regular withdrawal bleeding occurred in 77% of women with a mean duration of 5 days. Withdrawal bleeding usually started 2-3 days after the last tablet is taken of the 14 days of the oestrogen/progestagen phase (2 mg E_2 V + 20 mg MPA). Break through bleeding and/or spotting appeared in 15% of the women during the first three months of therapy and in 27% during months 10-12 of treatment. Amenorrhoea (no bleeding or spotting) occurred in 0% of the cycles during the first year of treatment (for cyclic or sequential products).

- **Prevention of osteoporosis**

- Oestrogen deficiency at menopause is associated with an increasing bone turnover and decline in bone mass. The effect of oestrogens on bone mineral density (BMD) is dose dependent. Protection appears to be effective for as long as treatment is continued. After discontinuation of HRT, bone mass is lost at a rate similar to that in untreated women.

- Evidence from the WHI trial and meta-analysed trials shows that current use of HRT, alone or in combination with a progestagen – given to predominantly healthy women – reduces the risk of hip, vertebral and other osteoporotic fractures. HRT may also prevent fractures in women with low bone density and/or established osteoporosis, but evidence for that is limited.

- After 1 year of treatment with Tridestra, the increase in lumbar spine bone mineral density (BMD) was 3.3±3.6 % (mean±SD). The percentage of women who maintained or gained BMD in lumbar zone during treatment was 72.7%. After 2 years of treatment with Tridestra, the increase in BMD was 5.9±3.0 % (mean±SD). The percentage of women who maintained or gained BMD in lumber zone during treatment was 95.2%.

- Tridestra also had an effect on hip BMD. The increase after 1 year was 2.3%±3.4% (mean±SD) at the femoral neck. The percentage of women who maintained or gained BMD in the hip zone during treatment was 72.7%. The increase after 2 years was 0.6%±3.6% (mean±SD) at femoral neck. The percentage of women who maintained or gained BMD in the hip zone during treatment was 52.4%.

5.2 Pharmacokinetic properties

Maximum plasma levels (C_{max}) of oestradiol (about 250 pmol/l) are reached in about 5-7 hours. The trough concentration (C_{min}) of oestradiol was about 142 pmol/l and the average concentration ($C_{average}$) about 185 pmol/l. In circulation, natural oestrogens are bound to sex hormone binding globulin and albumin. Free oestradiol is metabolised in the liver and partly converted to less active oestrogens like oestrone.

Maximum plasma levels (C_{max}) of oestrone (about 1790 pmol/l) are reached in 5–7 hours after intake of the tablet. C_{min} of oestrone was about 864 pmol/l, $C_{average}$ about 1160 pmol/l. Oestrone is subjected to an enterohepatic cycle and its half-life is 15–20 hours. The majority of oestrogens are excreted via kidneys as conjugates (sulphates or glucuronides).

MPA is well absorbed from the gastrointestinal tract and rapidly distributed from circulation to extravascular tissues. After the intake of the Tridestra combination tablet, the maximum plasma level (C_{max}) of MPA (about 5 μg/L) is reached in about 2 hours. $C_{average}$ (after a single dose) was about 1.3 μg/L. The elimination half-life is 40-50 hours. MPA is metabolised in the liver and excreted as glucuronides both in urine and bile. The extent of absorption from the combination tablet is comparable to MPA given alone.

5.3 Preclinical safety data

Data from animal toxicity studies with oestrodial and medroxyprogesterone acetate have shown expected oestrogenic and gestagenic effects, and do not reveal any particular risk for humans in the therapeutic dose-range.

6. PHARMACEUTICAL PARTICULARS

6.1 List of excipients

Tridestra tablet (white):

Lactose

Maize starch

Gelatine

Purified water

Magnesium stearate

Talc

Tridestra tablet (blue):

Lactose

Maize starch

Gelatine

Purified water

Magnesium stearate

Indigo carmine (E132)

Tridestra tablet (yellow):

Lactose

Maize starch

Gelatine

Purified water

Magnesium stearate

Yellow iron oxide (E172)

6.2 Incompatibilities

None

6.3 Shelf life
3 years

6.4 Special precautions for storage
Do not store above 25 °C
Store in a dry place

6.5 Nature and contents of container
A PVC/PVDC/AL thermofoiled blister pack.
Quantity: 91

6.6 Instructions for use and handling
No special requirements

7. MARKETING AUTHORISATION HOLDER
Orion Corporation
P.O. Box 65,
FIN-02101 Espoo
Finland

8. MARKETING AUTHORISATION NUMBER(S)
PL 13911/0007

9. DATE OF FIRST AUTHORISATION/RENEWAL OF THE AUTHORISATION
1 February 2000

10. DATE OF REVISION OF THE TEXT
24th May 2004

Trileptal 150 mg, 300 mg, 600 mg Film-coated tablets

(Novartis Pharmaceuticals UK Ltd)

1. NAME OF THE MEDICINAL PRODUCT
Trileptal® 150 mg Film-coated Tablets
Trileptal® 300 mg Film-coated Tablets
Trileptal® 600 mg Film-coated Tablets

2. QUALITATIVE AND QUANTITATIVE COMPOSITION
Each film-coated tablet contains 150 mg, 300 mg or 600 mg oxcarbazepine.

For excipients, see 6.1.

3. PHARMACEUTICAL FORM
Film-coated tablets.

150 mg: pale grey green, ovaloid tablets, scored on both sides. Embossed with T/D on one side and C/G on the other side.

300 mg: yellow, ovaloid tablets, scored on both sides. Embossed with TE/TE on one side and CG/CG on the other side.

600 mg: light pink, ovaloid tablets scored on both sides. Embossed with TF/TF on one side and CG/CG on the other side.

4. CLINICAL PARTICULARS
4.1 Therapeutic indications
Trileptal is indicated for the treatment of partial seizures with or without secondarily generalised tonic-clonic seizures.

Trileptal is indicated for use as monotherapy or adjunctive therapy in adults and in children of 6 years of age and above.

4.2 Posology and method of administration
In mono- and adjunctive therapy, treatment with Trileptal is initiated with a clinically effective dose given in two divided doses. The dose may be increased depending on the clinical response of the patient. When other antiepileptic medicinal products are replaced by Trileptal, the dose of the concomitant antiepileptic medicinal product(s) should be reduced gradually on initiation of Trileptal therapy. In adjunctive therapy, as the total antiepileptic medicinal product load of the patient is increased, the dose of concomitant antiepileptic medicinal product(s) may need to be reduced and/or the Trileptal dose increased more slowly (see Section 4.5 "Interaction with other medicinal products and other forms of interaction").

Trileptal can be taken with or without food.

The following dosing recommendations apply to all patients, in the absence of impaired renal function (see Section 5.2 "Pharmacokinetic properties"). Drug plasma level monitoring is not necessary to optimise Trileptal therapy.

The tablets are scored and can be broken in two halves in order to make it easier for the patient to swallow the tablet.

Adults

Monotherapy

Trileptal should be initiated with a dose of 600 mg/day (8-10 mg/kg/day) given in 2 divided doses. If clinically indicated, the dose may be increased by a maximum of 600 mg/day increments at approximately weekly intervals from the starting dose to achieve the desired clinical response. Therapeutic effects are seen at doses between 600 mg/day and 2400 mg/day.

Controlled monotherapy trials in patients not currently being treated with antiepileptic medicinal products showed 1200 mg/day to be an effective dose; however, a dose of 2400 mg/day has been shown to be effective in more refractory patients converted from other antiepileptic medicinal products to Trileptal monotherapy.

In a controlled hospital setting, dose increases up to 2400 mg/day have been achieved over 48 hours.

Adjunctive therapy

Trileptal should be initiated with a dose of 600 mg/day (8-10 mg/kg/day) given in 2 divided doses. If clinically indicated, the dose may be increased by a maximum of 600 mg/day increments at approximately weekly intervals from the starting dose to achieve the desired clinical response. Therapeutic responses are seen at doses between 600 mg/day and 2400 mg/day.

Daily doses from 600 to 2400 mg/day have been shown to be effective in a controlled adjunctive therapy trial, although most patients were not able to tolerate the 2400 mg/day dose without reduction of concomitant antiepileptic medicinal products, mainly because of CNS-related adverse events. Daily doses above 2400 mg/day have not been studied systematically in clinical trials.

Elderly

Adjustment of the dose is recommended in the elderly with compromised renal function (see 'Patients with renal impairment'). For patients at risk of hyponatraemia see Section 4.4 'Special warnings and special precautions for use'.

Children

In mono- and adjunctive therapy, Trileptal should be initiated with a dose of 8-10 mg/kg/day given in 2 divided doses. In adjunctive therapy, therapeutic effects were seen at a median maintenance dose of approximately 30 mg/kg/day. If clinically indicated, the dose may be increased by a maximum of 10 mg/kg/day increments at approximately weekly intervals from the starting dose, to a maximum dose of 46 mg/kg/day, to achieve the desired clinical response (see Section 5.2 "Pharmacokinetic properties").

Trileptal is recommended for use in children of 6 years of age and above. Safety has been evaluated in children from 2 years of age.

All the above dosing recommendations are based on the doses studied in clinical trials for all age groups. However, lower initiation doses may be considered where appropriate.

Patients with hepatic impairment

No dosage adjustment is required for patients with mild to moderate hepatic impairment. Trileptal has not been studied in patients with severe hepatic impairment, therefore, caution should be exercised when dosing severely impaired patients (see Section 5.2 "Pharmacokinetics properties").

Patients with renal impairment

In patients with impaired renal function (creatinine clearance less than 30 ml/min) Trileptal therapy should be initiated at half the usual starting dose (300 mg/day) and increased, in at least weekly intervals, to achieve the desired clinical response (see Section 5.2 "Pharmacokinetic properties").

Dose escalation in renally impaired patients may require more careful observation.

4.3 Contraindications
Hypersensitivity to the active substance or to any of the excipients.

4.4 Special warnings and special precautions for use
Patients who have exhibited hypersensitivity reactions to carbamazepine should be informed that approximately 25-30 % of these patients may experience hypersensitivity reactions (e.g. severe skin reactions) with Trileptal (see Section 4.8 "Undesirable effects").

Hypersensitivity reactions may also occur in patients without history of hypersensitivity to carbamazepine. In general, if signs and symptoms suggestive of hypersensitivity reactions occur (see Section 4.8 "Undesirable effects"), Trileptal should be withdrawn immediately.

Serious dermatological reactions, including Stevens-Johnson syndrome, toxic epidermal necrolysis (Lyell's syndrome) and erythema multiforme, have been reported very rarely in association with Trileptal use. Patients with serious dermatological reactions may require hospitalization, as these conditions may be life-threatening and very rarely be fatal. Trileptal associated cases occurred in both children and adults. The median time to onset was 19 days. Several isolated cases of recurrence of the serious skin reaction when rechallenged with Trileptal were reported. Patients who develop a skin reaction with Trileptal should be promptly evaluated and Trileptal withdrawn immediately unless the rash is clearly not drug related. In case of treatment withdrawal, consideration should be given to replacing Trileptal with other antiepileptic drug therapy to avoid withdrawal seizures. Trileptal should not be restarted in patients who discontinued treatment due to a hypersensitivity reaction (see section 4.3 Contraindications).

Serum sodium levels below 125 mmol/l, usually asymptomatic and not requiring adjustment of therapy, have been observed in up to 2.7 % of Trileptal treated patients. Experience from clinical trials shows that serum sodium levels returned towards normal when the Trileptal dosage was reduced, discontinued or the patient was treated conservatively (e.g. restricted fluid intake). In patients with pre-existing renal conditions associated with low sodium or in patients treated concomitantly with sodium-lowering medicinal products (e.g. diuretics, desmopressin) as well as NSAIDs (e.g. indomethacin), serum sodium levels should be measured prior to initiating therapy. Thereafter, serum sodium levels should be measured after approximately two weeks and then at monthly intervals for the first three months during therapy, or according to clinical need. These risk factors may apply especially to elderly patients. For patients on Trileptal therapy when starting on sodium-lowering medicinal products, the same approach for sodium checks should be followed. In general, if clinical symptoms suggestive of hyponatraemia occur on Trileptal therapy (see Section 4.8 "Undesirable effects"), serum sodium measurement may be considered. Other patients may have serum sodium assessed as part of their routine laboratory studies.

All patients with cardiac insufficiency and secondary heart failure should have regular weight measurements to determine occurrence of fluid retention. In case of fluid retention or worsening of the cardiac condition, serum sodium should be checked. If hyponatraemia is observed, water restriction is an important counter-measurement. As oxcarbazepine may, very rarely, lead to impairment of cardiac conduction, patients with pre-existing conduction disturbances (e.g. atrioventricular-block, arrhythmia) should be followed carefully.

Very rare cases of hepatitis have been reported, which in most of the cases resolved favourably. When a hepatic event is suspected, liver function should be evaluated and discontinuation of Trileptal should be considered.

Female patients of childbearing age should be warned that the concurrent use of Trileptal with hormonal contraceptives may render this type of contraceptive ineffective (see Section 4.5 "Interaction with other medicinal products and other forms of interaction"). Additional non-hormonal forms of contraception are recommended when using Trileptal.

Caution should be exercised if alcohol is taken in combination with Trileptal therapy, due to a possible additive sedative effect.

As with all antiepileptic medicinal products, Trileptal should be withdrawn gradually to minimise the potential of increased seizure frequency.

4.5 Interaction with other medicinal products and other forms of Interaction
Enzyme induction

Oxcarbazepine and its pharmacologically active metabolite (the monohydroxy derivative, MHD) are weak inducers *in vitro* and *in vivo* of the cytochrome P450 enzymes CYP3A4 and CYP3A5 responsible for the metabolism of a very large number of drugs, for example, immunosuppressants (e.g. cyclosporine, tacrolimus), oral contraceptives (see below), and some other antiepileptic medicinal products (e.g. carbamazepine) resulting in a lower plasma concentration of these medicinal products (see table below summarizing results with other antiepileptic medicinal products).

In vitro, oxcarbazepine and MHD are weak inducers of UDP-glucuronyl transferases (effects on specific enzymes in this family are not known). Therefore, *in vivo* oxcarbazepine and MHD may have a small inducing effect on the metabolism of medicinal products which are mainly eliminated by conjugation through the UDP-glucuronyl transferases. When initiating treatment with Trileptal or changing the dose, it may take 2 to 3 weeks to reach the new level of induction.

In case of discontinuation of Trileptal therapy, a dose reduction of the concomitant medications may be necessary and should be decided upon by clinical and/or plasma level monitoring. The induction is likely to gradually decrease over 2 to 3 weeks after discontinuation.

Hormonal contraceptives: Trileptal was shown to have an influence on the two components, ethinylestradiol (EE) and levonorgestrel (LNG), of an oral contraceptive. The mean AUC values of EE and LNG were decreased by 48-52 % and 32-52% respectively. Therefore, concurrent use of Trileptal with hormonal contraceptives may render these contraceptives ineffective (see Section 4.4 "Special warnings and special precautions for use"). Another reliable contraceptive method should be used.

Enzyme inhibition

Oxcarbazepine and MHD inhibit CYP2C19. Therefore, interactions could arise when co-administering high doses of Trileptal with medicinal products that are mainly metabolised by CYP2C19 (e.g. phenytoin). Phenytoin plasma levels increased by up to 40 % when Trileptal was given at doses above 1200 mg/day (see table below summarizing results with other anticonvulsants). In this case, a reduction of co-administered phenytoin may be required (see section 4.2 "Posology and method of administration").

Antiepileptic medicinal products

Potential interactions between Trileptal and other antiepileptic medicinal products were assessed in clinical studies. The effect of these interactions on mean AUCs and C_{min} are summarised in the following table.

Summary of antiepileptic medicinal product interactions with Trileptal

Antiepileptic medicinal product	Influence of Trileptal on antiepileptic medicinal product	Influence of antiepileptic medicinal product on MHD
Co-administered	Concentration	Concentration
Carbamazepine	0 - 22 % decrease (30 % increase of carbamazepine-epoxide)	40 % decrease
Clobazam	Not studied	No influence
Felbamate	Not studied	No influence
Lamotrigine	Slight decrease*	No influence
Phenobarbitone	14 - 15 % increase	30 - 31 % decrease
Phenytoin	0 - 40 % increase	29 - 35 % decrease
Valproic acid	No influence	0 – 18 % decrease

* Preliminary results indicate that oxcarbazepine may result in lower lamotrigine concentrations, possibly of importance in children, but the interaction potential of oxcarbazepine appears lower than seen with concomitant enzyme inducing drugs (carbamazepine, phenobarbitone, and phenytoin).

Strong inducers of cytochrome P450 enzymes (i.e. carbamazepine, phenytoin and phenobarbitone) have been shown to decrease the plasma levels of MHD (29-40 %). Concomitant therapy of Trileptal and lamotrigine has been associated with an increased risk of adverse events (nausea, somnolence, dizziness and headache). When one or several antiepileptic medicinal products are concurrently administered with Trileptal, a careful dose adjustment and/or plasma level monitoring may be considered on a case by case basis, notably in paediatric patients treated concomitantly with lamotrigine.

No autoinduction has been observed with Trileptal.

Other medicinal product interactions

Cimetidine, erythromycin, viloxazine, warfarin and dextropropoxyphene had no effect on the pharmacokinetics of MHD.

The interaction between oxcarbazepine and MAOIs is theoretically possible based on a structural relationship of oxcarbazepine to tricyclic antidepressants.

Patients on tricyclic antidepressant therapy were included in clinical trials and no clinically relevant interactions have been observed.

The combination of lithium and oxcarbazepine might cause enhanced neurotoxicity.

4.6 Pregnancy and lactation

Pregnancy

Risk related to epilepsy and antiepileptic medicinal products in general:

It has been shown that in the offspring of women with epilepsy, the prevalence of malformations is two to three times greater than the rate of approximately 3% in the general population. In the treated population, an increase in malformations has been noted with polytherapy, however, the extent to which the treatment and/or the illness is responsible has not been elucidated.

Moreover, effective anti-epileptic therapy must not be interrupted, since the aggravation of the illness is detrimental to both the mother and the foetus.

Risk related to oxcarbazepine:

Clinical data on exposure during pregnancy are still insufficient to assess the teratogenic potential of oxcarbazepine. In animal studies, increased embryo mortality, delayed growth and malformations were observed at maternally toxic dose levels (see section 5.3 "Preclinical safety data").

Taking these data into consideration:

- If women receiving Trileptal become pregnant or plan to become pregnant, the use of this product should be carefully re-evaluated. Minimum effective doses should be given, and monotherapy whenever possible should be preferred at least during the first three months of pregnancy.

- Patients should be counselled regarding the possibility of an increased risk of malformations and given the opportunity of antenatal screening.

- During pregnancy, an effective antiepileptic oxcarbazepine treatment must not be interrupted, since the aggravation of the illness is detrimental to both the mother and the foetus.

Monitoring and prevention:

Antiepileptic medicinal products may contribute to folic acid deficiency, a possible contributory cause of foetal abnormality. Folic acid supplementation is recommended before and during pregnancy. As the efficacy of this supplementation is not proved, a specific antenatal diagnosis can be offered even for women with a supplementary treatment of folic acid.

In the newborn child:

Bleeding disorders in the newborn caused by antiepileptic agents have been reported. As a precaution, vitamin K_1 should be administered as a preventive measure in the last few weeks of pregnancy and to the newborn.

Lactation

Oxcarbazepine and its active metabolite (MHD) are excreted in human breast milk. A milk-to-plasma concentration ratio of 0.5 was found for both. The effects on the infant exposed to Trileptal by this route are unknown. Therefore, Trileptal should not be used during breast-feeding.

4.7 Effects on ability to drive and use machines

The use of Trileptal has been associated with adverse reactions such as dizziness or somnolence (see Section 4.8 "Undesirable effects"). Therefore, patients should be advised that their physical and/ or mental abilities required for operating machinery or driving a car might be impaired.

4.8 Undesirable effects

The most commonly reported adverse reactions are somnolence, headache, dizziness, diplopia, nausea, vomiting and fatigue occurring in more than 10% of patients.

The undesirable effect profile by body system is based on AEs from clinical trials assessed as related to Trileptal. In addition, clinically meaningful reports on adverse experiences from named patient programs and postmarketing experience were taken into account.

Frequency estimate:- very common: $\geqslant$ 1/10; common: $\geqslant$ 1/100 - < 1/10; uncommon: $\geqslant$ 1/1,000 - < 1 /100; rare: $\geqslant$ 1/10,000 - < 1/1,000; very rare: < 1/10,000*

Blood and lymphatic system disorders	
Uncommon	leucopenia.
Very rare	thrombocytopenia.
Immune system disorders	
Very rare	hypersensitivity (characterised by features such as abnormal liver function tests, rash, fever, lymphadenopathy, eosinophilia, arthralgia).
Metabolism and nutrition disorders	
Common	hyponatraemia
Very rare	hyponatraemia associated with signs and symptoms such as seizures, confusion, depressed level of consciousness, encephalopathy (see also Nervous system disorders for further undesirable effects), vision disorders (e.g. blurred vision), vomiting, nausea†.
Psychiatric disorders	
Common	confusional state, depression, apathy, agitation (e.g. nervousness), affect lability.
Nervous system disorders	
Very common	somnolence, headache, dizziness.
Common	ataxia, tremor, nystagmus, disturbance in attention, amnesia.
Eye disorders	
Very common	diplopia.
Common	vision blurred, visual disturbance.
Ear and labyrinth disorders	
Common	vertigo.
Cardiac disorders	
Very rare	arrhythmia, atrioventricular block.
Gastrointestinal disorders	
Very common	nausea, vomiting.
Common	diarrhoea, constipation, abdominal pain.
Very rare	pancreatitis and/or lipase and/or amylase increase.
Hepato-biliary disorders	
Very rare	hepatitis.
Skin and subcutaneous tissue disorders	
Common	rash, alopecia, acne.
Uncommon	urticaria.
Very rare	angioedema, Stevens-Johnson syndrome, toxic epidermal necrolysis (Lyell's syndrome), erythema multiforme (see section 4.4 Special warnings and special precautions for use).
Musculoskeletal, connective tissue and bone disorders	
Very rare	systemic lupus erythematosus.
General disorders and administration site conditions	
Very common	fatigue.
Common	asthenia.
Investigations	
Uncommon	hepatic enzymes increased, blood alkaline phosphatase increased.

* according to CIOMS III frequency classification

† Very rarely clinically significant hyponatraemia (sodium <125 mmol/l) can develop during Trileptal use. It generally occurred during the first 3 months of treatment with Trileptal, although there were patients who first developed a serum sodium <125 mmol/l more than 1 year after initiation of therapy (see Section 4.4 "Special warnings and special precautions for use").

4.9 Overdose

Isolated cases of overdose have been reported. The maximum dose taken was approximately 24,000 mg. All patients recovered with symptomatic treatment. Symptoms of overdose include somnolence, dizziness, nausea, vomiting, hyperkinesia, hyponatraemia, ataxia and nystagmus. There is no specific antidote. Symptomatic and supportive treatment should be administered as appropriate. Removal of the medicinal product by gastric lavage and/or inactivation by administering activated charcoal should be considered.

5. PHARMACOLOGICAL PROPERTIES

5.1 Pharmacodynamic properties

Pharmacotherapeutic group: Antiepileptics

ATC code: N03A F 02

Pharmacodynamic effects

The pharmacological activity of oxcarbazepine is primarily exerted through the metabolite (MHD) (see Section 5.2 "Pharmacokinetic properties"- Biotransformation). The mechanism of action of oxcarbazepine and MHD is thought to be mainly based on blockade of voltage-sensitive sodium channels, thus resulting in stabilisation of hyperexcited neural membranes, inhibition of repetitive neuronal firing, and diminishment of propagation of synaptic impulses. In addition, increased potassium conductance and modulation of high-voltage activated calcium channels may also contribute to the anticonvulsant effects. No significant interactions with brain neurotransmitter or modulator receptor sites were found.

Oxcarbazepine and its active metabolite (MHD), are potent and efficacious anticonvulsants in animals. They protected rodents against generalised tonic-clonic and, to a lesser degree, clonic seizures, and abolished or reduced the frequency of chronically recurring partial seizures in Rhesus monkeys with aluminum implants. No tolerance (i.e. attenuation of anticonvulsive activity) against tonic-clonic seizures was observed when mice and rats were treated daily for 5 days or 4 weeks, respectively, with oxcarbazepine or MHD.

5.2 Pharmacokinetic properties

Absorption

Following oral administration of Trileptal, oxcarbazepine is completely absorbed and extensively metabolised to its pharmacologically active metabolite (MHD).

After single dose administration of 600 mg Trileptal to healthy male volunteers under fasted conditions, the mean C_{max} value of MHD was 34 μmol/l, with a corresponding median t_{max} of 4.5 hours.

In a mass balance study in man, only 2 % of total radioactivity in plasma was due to unchanged oxcarbazepine, approximately 70 % was due to MHD, and the remainder attributable to minor secondary metabolites which were rapidly eliminated.

Food has no effect on the rate and extent of absorption of oxcarbazepine, therefore, Trileptal can be taken with or without food.

Distribution

The apparent volume of distribution of MHD is 49 litres.

Approximately 40 % of MHD, is bound to serum proteins, predominantly to albumin. Binding was independent of the serum concentration within the therapeutically relevant range. Oxcarbazepine and MHD do not bind to alpha-1-acid glycoprotein.

Oxcarbazepine and MHD cross the placenta. Neonatal and maternal plasma MHD concentrations were similar in one case.

Biotransformation

Oxcarbazepine is rapidly reduced by cytosolic enzymes in the liver to MHD, which is primarily responsible for the pharmacological effect of Trileptal. MHD is metabolised further by conjugation with glucuronic acid. Minor amounts (4 % of the dose) are oxidised to the pharmacologically inactive metabolite (10, 11-dihydroxy derivative, DHD).

Elimination

Oxcarbazepine is cleared from the body mostly in the form of metabolites which are predominantly excreted by the kidneys. More than 95 % of the dose appears in the urine, with less than 1 % as unchanged oxcarbazepine. Faecal excretion accounts for less than 4 % of the administered dose. Approximately 80 % of the dose is excreted in the urine either as glucuronides of MHD (49 %) or as unchanged MHD (27 %), whereas the inactive DHD accounts for approximately 3 % and conjugates of oxcarbazepine account for 13 % of the dose.

Oxcarbazepine is rapidly eliminated from the plasma with apparent half-life values between 1.3 and 2.3 hours. In contrast, the apparent plasma half-life of MHD averaged 9.3 ± 1.8 h.

Dose proportionality

Steady-state plasma concentrations of MHD are reached within 2 - 3 days in patients when Trileptal is given twice a day. At steady-state, the pharmacokinetics of MHD are linear and show dose proportionality across the dose range of 300 to 2400 mg/day.

Special populations

Patients with hepatic impairment

The pharmacokinetics and metabolism of oxcarbazepine and MHD were evaluated in healthy volunteers and hepatically-impaired subjects after a single 900 mg oral dose. Mild to moderate hepatic impairment did not affect the pharmacokinetics of oxcarbazepine and MHD. Trileptal has not been studied in patients with severe hepatic impairment.

Patients with renal impairment

There is a linear correlation between creatinine clearance and the renal clearance of MHD. When Trileptal is administered as a single 300 mg dose, in renally impaired patients (creatinine clearance < 30 mL/min) the elimination half-life of MHD is prolonged by 60-90 % (16 to 19 hours) with a two fold increase in AUC compared to adults with normal renal function (10 hours).

Children

After a single dose administration of 5 or 15 mg/kg of Trileptal, the dose-adjusted AUC values of MHD were 30 % lower in children aged 2 - 5 years than in older children aged 6 - 12 years. In general, in children with normal renal function, renal clearance of MHD normalised for bodyweight is higher than in adults. In children, 10 to 50 % reduction of MHD elimination half-life (5 to 9 hours) was observed compared to adults (10 hours).

Elderly

Following administration of single (300 mg) and multiple doses (600 mg/day) of Trileptal in elderly volunteers (60 - 82 years of age), the maximum plasma concentrations and AUC values of MHD were 30 % - 60 % higher than in younger volunteers (18 - 32 years of age). Comparisons of creatinine clearances in young and elderly volunteers indicate that the difference was due to age-related reductions in creatinine clearance. No special dose recommendations are necessary because therapeutic doses are individually adjusted.

Gender

No gender related pharmacokinetic differences have been observed in children, adults, or the elderly.

5.3 Preclinical safety data

Preclinical data indicated no special hazard for humans based on repeated dose toxicity, safety pharmacology and genotoxicity studies with oxcarbazepine and the pharmacologically active metabolite, monohydroxy derivative (MHD).

Evidence of nephrotoxicity was noted in repeated dose toxicity rat studies but not in dog or mice studies. As there are no reports of such changes in patients, the clinical relevance of this finding in rats remains unknown.

Immunostimulatory tests in mice showed that MHD (and to a lesser extent oxcarbazepine) can induce delayed hypersensitivity.

Animal studies revealed effects such as increases in the incidence of embryo mortality and some delay in antenatal and/or postnatal growth at maternally toxic dose levels. There was an increase in rat foetal malformations in one of the eight embryo toxicity studies, which were conducted with either oxcarbazepine or the pharmacologically active metabolite (MHD), at a dose which also showed maternal toxicity (see Section 4.6 "Pregnancy and lactation").

In the carcinogenicity studies, liver (rats and mice), testicular and female genital tract granular cell (rats) tumours were induced in treated animals. The occurrence of liver tumours was most likely a consequence of the induction of hepatic microsomal enzymes; an inductive effect which, although it cannot be excluded, is weak or absent in patients treated with Trileptal. Testicular tumours may have been induced by elevated luteinizing hormone concentrations. Due to the absence of such an increase in humans, these tumours are considered to be of no clinical relevance. A dose-related increase in the incidence of granular cell tumours of the female genital tract (cervix and vagina) was noted in the rat carcinogenicity study with MHD. These effects occurred at exposure levels comparable with the anticipated clinical exposure. The mechanism for the development of these tumours has not been elucidated. Thus, the clinical relevance of these tumours is unknown.

6. PHARMACEUTICAL PARTICULARS

6.1 List of excipients

Tablet core:

silica, colloidal anhydrous

cellulose, microcrystalline

hypromellose

crospovidone

magnesium stearate.

Tablet coating:

hypromellose

talc

titanium dioxide (E 171).

150 mg coating only:

macrogol 4000

iron oxide, yellow (E 172)

iron oxide red (E 172)

iron oxide black (E 172).

300 mg tablet coating only:

macrogol 8000

iron oxide, yellow (E 172).

600 mg coating only:

macrogol 4000

iron oxide red (E 172)

iron oxide black (E 172).

6.2 Incompatibilities

Not applicable.

6.3 Shelf life

3 years.

6.4 Special precautions for storage

This medicinal product does not require any special storage conditions.

6.5 Nature and contents of container

Blister containing 10 tablets. Blister material: PVC/PE/PVDC with aluminium foil backing.

Tablets 150 mg: blister pack of 30, 50, 100, 200 and/or 500 tablets.

Tablets 300 mg: blister pack of 30, 50, 100, 200 and/or 500 tablets.

Tablets 600 mg: blister pack of 30, 50, 100, 200 and/or 500 tablets.

Not all pack sizes may be marketed.

6.6 Instructions for use and handling

No special requirements.

7. MARKETING AUTHORISATION HOLDER

Novartis Pharmaceuticals UK Limited

Frimley Business Park

Frimley

Camberley

Surrey

GU16 7SR

Unite Kingdom

8. MARKETING AUTHORISATION NUMBER(S)

Trileptal Tablets 150mg PL 00101/0581

Trileptal Tablets 300mg PL 00101/0582

Trileptal Tablets 600mg PL 00101/0583

9. DATE OF FIRST AUTHORISATION/RENEWAL OF THE AUTHORISATION

7 January 2000

10. DATE OF REVISION OF THE TEXT

06 July 2005

Legal Category

POM

Trileptal 60 mg/ml Oral Suspension

(Novartis Pharmaceuticals UK Ltd)

1. NAME OF THE MEDICINAL PRODUCT

Trileptal® 60 mg/ml Oral Suspension.

2. QUALITATIVE AND QUANTITATIVE COMPOSITION

1 ml of the oral suspension contains 60 mg oxcarbazepine.

For excipients, see 6.1.

3. PHARMACEUTICAL FORM

Oral suspension.

Off-white to slightly reddish brown oral suspension.

4. CLINICAL PARTICULARS

4.1 Therapeutic indications

Trileptal is indicated for the treatment of partial seizures with or without secondarily generalised tonic-clonic seizures.

Trileptal is indicated for use as monotherapy or adjunctive therapy in adults and in children of 6 years of age and above.

4.2 Posology and method of administration

In mono- and adjunctive therapy, treatment with Trileptal is initiated with a clinically effective dose given in two divided doses. The dose may be increased depending on the clinical response of the patient. When other antiepileptic medicinal products are replaced by Trileptal, the dose of the concomitant antiepileptic medicinal product(s) should be reduced gradually on initiation of Trileptal therapy. In adjunctive therapy, as the total antiepileptic medicinal product load of the patient is increased, the dose of concomitant antiepileptic medicinal product(s) may need to be reduced and/or the Trileptal dose increased more slowly (see Section 4.5 "Interaction with other medicinal products and other forms of interaction").

Trileptal can be taken with or without food.

The prescription for Trileptal oral suspension should be given in millilitres (see conversion table below which gives the milligram dose in millilitres). The prescribed dose in millilitres is rounded to the nearest 0.5 ml.

The doses given in the table below are only applicable to patients aged 6 years and above. These doses are to be administered twice a day.

Dose in milligrams (to be given b.i.d)	Dose in millilitres (to be given b.i.d)
45 - 75 mg	1.0 ml
76 - 105 mg	1.5 ml
106 - 135 mg	2.0 ml
136 - 165 mg	2.5 ml
166 - 195 mg	3.0 ml
196 - 225 mg	3.5 ml
226 - 255 mg	4.0 ml
256 - 285 mg	4.5 ml
286 - 315 mg	5.0 ml
316 - 345 mg	5.5 ml
346 – 375 mg	6.0 ml
376 – 405 mg	6.5 ml
406 – 435 mg	7.0 ml
436 – 465 mg	7.5 ml
466 – 495 mg	8.0 ml
496 – 525 mg	8.5 ml
526 – 555 mg	9.0 ml

556 – 585 mg	9.5 ml
586 – 616 mg	10.0 ml
616 – 645 mg	10.5 ml
646 – 675 mg	11.0 ml
676 – 705 mg	11.5 ml
706 – 735 mg	12.0 ml
736 – 765 mg	12.5 ml
766 – 795 mg	13.0 ml
796 – 825 mg	13.5 ml
826 – 855 mg	14.0 ml
856 – 885 mg	14.5 ml
886 – 915 mg	15.0 ml
916 – 945 mg	15.5 ml
946 – 975 mg	16.0 ml
976 – 1005 mg	16.5 ml
1006 – 1035 mg	17.0 ml
1036 – 1065 mg	17.5 ml
1066 – 1095 mg	18.0 ml
1096 – 1125 mg	18.5 ml
1126 – 1155 mg	19.0 ml
1156 – 1185 mg	19.5 ml
1186 – 1215 mg	20.0 ml

Before taking Trileptal oral suspension, the bottle should be shaken well and the dose prepared immediately afterwards. The prescribed amount of oral suspension should be withdrawn from the bottle using the oral syringe supplied. Trileptal oral suspension may be swallowed directly from the syringe or can be mixed in a small glass of water just prior to administration. After each use, the bottle should be closed and the outside of the syringe wiped with a dry, clean tissue.

Trileptal oral suspension and Trileptal film-coated tablets may be interchanged at equal doses.

The following dosing recommendations apply to all patients, in the absence of impaired renal function (see Section 5.2 "Pharmacokinetic properties"). Drug plasma level monitoring is not necessary to optimise Trileptal therapy.

Adults

Monotherapy

Trileptal should be initiated with a dose of 600 mg/day (8-10 mg/kg/day) given in 2 divided doses. If clinically indicated, the dose may be increased by a maximum of 600 mg/day increments at approximately weekly intervals from the starting dose to achieve the desired clinical response. Therapeutic effects are seen at doses between 600 mg/day and 2400 mg/day.

Controlled monotherapy trials in patients not currently being treated with antiepileptic medicinal products showed 1200 mg/day to be an effective dose; however, a dose of 2400 mg/day has been shown to be effective in more refractory patients converted from other antiepileptic medicinal products to Trileptal monotherapy.

In a controlled hospital setting, dose increases up to 2400 mg/day have been achieved over 48 hours.

Adjunctive therapy

Trileptal should be initiated with a dose of 600 mg/day (8-10 mg/kg/day) given in 2 divided doses. If clinically indicated, the dose may be increased by a maximum of 600 mg/day increments at approximately weekly intervals from the starting dose to achieve the desired clinical response. Therapeutic responses are seen at doses between 600 mg/day and 2400 mg/day.

Daily doses from 600 to 2400 mg/day have been shown to be effective in a controlled adjunctive therapy trial, although most patients were not able to tolerate the 2400 mg/day dose without reduction of concomitant antiepileptic medicinal products, mainly because of CNS-related adverse events. Daily doses above 2400 mg/day have not been studied systematically in clinical trials.

Elderly

Adjustment of the dose is recommended in the elderly with compromised renal function (see 'Patients with renal impairment'). For patients at risk of hyponatraemia see Section 4.4 'Special warnings and special precautions for use'.

Children

In mono- and adjunctive therapy, Trileptal should be initiated with a dose of 8-10 mg/kg/day given in 2 divided doses. In adjunctive therapy, therapeutic effects were seen at a median maintenance dose of approximately 30 mg/kg/day. If clinically indicated, the dose may be increased by a maximum of 10 mg/kg/day increments at approximately weekly intervals from the starting dose, to a maximum dose of 46 mg/kg/day, to achieve the desired clinical response (see Section 5.2 "Pharmacokinetic properties").

Trileptal is recommended for use in children of 6 years of age and above. Safety has been evaluated in children from 2 years of age.

All the above dosing recommendations are based on the doses studied in clinical trials for all age groups. However, lower initiation doses may be considered where appropriate.

Patients with hepatic impairment

No dosage adjustment is required for patients with mild to moderate hepatic impairment. Trileptal has not been studied in patients with severe hepatic impairment, therefore, caution should be exercised when dosing severely impaired patients (see Section 5.2 "Pharmacokinetics properties").

Patients with renal impairment

In patients with impaired renal function (creatinine clearance less than 30 ml/min) Trileptal therapy should be initiated at half the usual starting dose (300 mg/day) and increased, in at least weekly intervals, to achieve the desired clinical response (see Section 5.2 "Pharmacokinetic properties").

Dose escalation in renally impaired patients may require more careful observation.

4.3 Contraindications

Hypersensitivity to the active substance or to any of the excipients.

4.4 Special warnings and special precautions for use

Patients who have exhibited hypersensitivity reactions to carbamazepine should be informed that approximately 25-30 % of these patients may experience hypersensitivity reactions (e.g. severe skin reactions) with Trileptal (see Section 4.8 "Undesirable effects").

Hypersensitivity reactions may also occur in patients without history of hypersensitivity to carbamazepine. In general, if signs and symptoms suggestive of hypersensitivity reactions occur (see Section 4.8 "Undesirable effects"), Trileptal should be withdrawn immediately.

Serious dermatological reactions, including Stevens-Johnson syndrome, toxic epidermal necrolysis (Lyell's syndrome) and erythema multiforme, have been reported very rarely in association with Trileptal use. Patients with serious dermatological reactions may require hospitalization, as these conditions may be life-threatening and very rarely be fatal. Trileptal associated cases occurred in both children and adults. The median time to onset was 19 days. Several isolated cases of recurrence of the serious skin reaction when rechallenged with Trileptal were reported. Patients who develop a skin reaction with Trileptal should be promptly evaluated and Trileptal withdrawn immediately unless the rash is clearly not drug related. In case of treatment withdrawal, consideration should be given to replacing Trileptal with other antiepileptic drug therapy to avoid withdrawal seizures. Trileptal should not be restarted in patients who discontinued treatment due to a hypersensitivity reaction (see section 4.3 Contraindications).

Serum sodium levels below 125 mmol/l, usually asymptomatic and not requiring adjustment of therapy, have been observed in up to 2.7 % of Trileptal treated patients. Experience from clinical trials shows that serum sodium levels returned towards normal when the Trileptal dosage was reduced, discontinued or the patient was treated conservatively (e.g. restricted fluid intake). In patients with pre-existing renal conditions associated with low sodium or in patients treated concomitantly with sodium-lowering medicinal products (e.g. diuretics, desmopressin) as well as NSAIDs (e.g. indomethacin), serum sodium levels should be measured prior to initiating therapy. Thereafter, serum sodium levels should be measured after approximately two weeks and then at monthly intervals for the first three months during therapy, or according to clinical need. These risk factors may apply especially to elderly patients. For patients on Trileptal therapy when starting on sodium-lowering medicinal products, the same approach for sodium checks should be followed. In general, if clinical symptoms suggestive of hyponatraemia occur on Trileptal therapy (see Section 4.8 "Undesirable effects"), serum sodium measurement may be considered. Other patients may have serum sodium assessed as part of their routine laboratory studies.

All patients with cardiac insufficiency and secondary heart failure should have regular weight measurements to determine occurrence of fluid retention. In case of fluid retention or worsening of the cardiac condition, serum sodium should be checked. If hyponatraemia is observed, water restriction is an important counter-measurement. As oxcarbazepine may, very rarely, lead to impairment of cardiac conduction, patients with pre-existing conduction disturbances (e.g. atrioventricular-block, arrhythmia) should be followed carefully.

Very rare cases of hepatitis have been reported, which in most of the cases resolved favourably. When a hepatic event is suspected, liver function should be evaluated and discontinuation of Trileptal should be considered.

Female patients of childbearing age should be warned that the concurrent use of Trileptal with hormonal contraceptives may render this type of contraceptive ineffective (see Section 4.5 "Interaction with other medicinal products and other forms of interaction"). Additional non-hormonal forms of contraception are recommended when using Trileptal.

Caution should be exercised if alcohol is taken in combination with Trileptal therapy, due to a possible additive sedative effect.

As with all antiepileptic medicinal products, Trileptal should be withdrawn gradually to minimise the potential of increased seizure frequency.

Trileptal oral suspension contains ethanol, less than 100 mg per dose. It contains parabenes which may cause allergic reactions (possibly delayed). It contains sorbitol and, therefore, should not be administered to patients with rare hereditary problems of fructose intolerance.

4.5 Interaction with other medicinal products and other forms of Interaction

Enzyme induction

Oxcarbazepine and its pharmacologically active metabolite (the monohydroxy derivative, MHD) are weak inducers *in vitro* and *in vivo* of the cytochrome 450 enzymes CYP3A4 and CYP3A5 responsible for the metabolism of a very large number of drugs, for example, immunosuppressants (e.g. cyclosporine, tacrolimus), oral contraceptives (see below), and some other antiepileptic medicinal products (e.g. carbamazepine) resulting in a lower plasma concentration of these medicinal products (see table below summarizing results with other antiepileptic medicinal products).

In vitro, oxcarbazepine and MHD are weak inducers of UDP-glucuronyl transferases (effects on specific enzymes in this family are not known). Therefore, *in vivo* oxcarbazepine and MHD may have a small inducing effect on the metabolism of medicinal products which are mainly eliminated by conjugation through the UDP-glucuronyl transferases. When initiating treatment with Trileptal or changing the dose, it may take 2 to 3 weeks to reach the new level of induction.

In case of discontinuation of Trileptal therapy, a dose reduction of the concomitant medications may be necessary and should be decided upon by clinical and/or plasma level monitoring. The induction is likely to gradually decrease over 2 to 3 weeks after discontinuation.

Hormonal contraceptives: Trileptal was shown to have an influence on the two components, ethinylestradiol (EE) and levonorgestrel (LNG), of an oral contraceptive. The mean AUC values of EE and LNG were decreased by 48-52 % and 32-52% respectively. Therefore, concurrent use of Trileptal with hormonal contraceptives may render these contraceptives ineffective (see Section 4.4 "Special warnings and special precautions for use"). Another reliable contraceptive method should be used.

Enzyme inhibition

Oxcarbazepine and MHD inhibit CYP2C19. Therefore, interactions could arise when co-administering high doses of Trileptal with medicinal products that are metabolised by CYP2C19 (e.g. phenytoin). Phenytoin plasma levels increased by up to 40 % when Trileptal was given at doses above 1200 mg/day (see table below summarizing results with other anticonvulsants). In this case, a reduction of co-administered phenytoin may be required (see Section 4.2 "Posology and method of administration").

Antiepileptic medicinal products

Potential interactions between Trileptal and other antiepileptic medicinal products were assessed in clinical studies. The effect of these interactions on mean AUCs and C_{min} are summarised in the following table.

Summary of antiepileptic medicinal product interactions with Trileptal

Antiepileptic medicinal product	Influence of Trileptal on antiepileptic medicinal product	Influence of antiepileptic medicinal product on MHD
Co-administered Carbamazepine	Concentration 0 - 22 % decrease (30 % increase of carbamazepine-epoxide)	Concentration 40 % decrease
Clobazam	Not studied	No influence
Felbamate	Not studied	No influence
Lamotrigine	Slight decrease*	No influence
Phenobarbitone	14 - 15 % increase	30 - 31 % decrease

Phenytoin	0 - 40 % increase	29 - 35 % decrease
Valproic acid	No influence	0 - 18 % decrease

* Preliminary results indicate that oxcarbazepine may result in lower lamotrigine concentrations, possibly of importance in children, but the interaction potential of oxcarbazepine appears lower than seen with concomitant enzyme inducing drugs (carbamazepine, phenobarbitone, and phenytoin).

Strong inducers of cytochrome P450 enzymes (i.e. carbamazepine, phenytoin and phenobarbitone) have been shown to decrease the plasma levels of MHD (29-40 %). Concomitant therapy of Trileptal and lamotrigine has been associated with an increased risk of adverse events (nausea, somnolence, dizziness and headache). When one or several antiepileptic medicinal products are concurrently administered with Trileptal, a careful dose adjustment and/or plasma level monitoring may be considered on a case by case basis, notably in paediatric patients treated concomitantly with lamotrigine.

No autoinduction has been observed with Trileptal.

Other medicinal product interactions

Cimetidine, erythromycin, viloxazine, warfarin and dextropropoxyphene had no effect on the pharmacokinetics of MHD.

The interaction between oxcarbazepine and MAOIs is theoretically possible based on a structural relationship of oxcarbazepine to tricyclic antidepressants.

Patients on tricyclic antidepressant therapy were included in clinical trials and no clinically relevant interactions have been observed.

The combination of lithium and oxcarbazepine might cause enhanced neurotoxicity.

4.6 Pregnancy and lactation

Pregnancy

Risk related to epilepsy and antiepileptic medicinal products in general:

It has been shown that in the offspring of women with epilepsy, the prevalence of malformations is two to three times greater than the rate of approximately 3% in the general population. In the treated population, an increase in malformations has been noted with polytherapy, however, the extent to which the treatment and/or the illness is responsible has not been elucidated.

Moreover, effective anti-epileptic therapy must not be interrupted, since the aggravation of the illness is detrimental to both the mother and the foetus.

Risk related to oxcarbazepine:

Clinical data on exposure during pregnancy are still insufficient to assess the teratogenic potential of oxcarbazepine. In animal studies, increased embryo mortality, delayed growth and malformations were observed at maternally toxic dose levels (see section 5.3 "Preclinical safety data").

Taking these data into consideration:

- If women receiving Trileptal become pregnant or plan to become pregnant, the use of this product should be carefully re-evaluated. Minimum effective doses should be given, and monotherapy whenever possible should be preferred at least during the first three months of pregnancy.

- Patients should be counselled regarding the possibility of an increased risk of malformations and given the opportunity of antenatal screening.

- During pregnancy, an effective antiepileptic oxcarbazepine treatment must not be interrupted, since the aggravation of the illness is detrimental to both the mother and the foetus.

Monitoring and prevention:

Antiepileptic medicinal products may contribute to folic acid deficiency, a possible contributory cause of foetal abnormality. Folic acid supplementation is recommended before and during pregnancy. As the efficacy of this supplementation is not proved, a specific antenatal diagnosis can be offered even for women with a supplementary treatment of folic acid.

In the newborn child:

Bleeding disorders in the newborn caused by antiepileptic agents have been reported. As a precaution, vitamin K_1 should be administered as a preventive measure in the last few weeks of pregnancy and to the newborn.

Lactation

Oxcarbazepine and its active metabolite (MHD) are excreted in human breast milk. A milk-to-plasma concentration ratio of 0.5 was found for both. The effects on the infant exposed to Trileptal by this route are unknown. Therefore, Trileptal should not be used during breast-feeding.

4.7 Effects on ability to drive and use machines

The use of Trileptal has been associated with adverse reactions such as dizziness or somnolence (see Section 4.8 "Undesirable effects"). Therefore, patients should be advised that their physical and/ or mental abilities required for operating machinery or driving a car might be impaired.

4.8 Undesirable effects

The most commonly reported adverse reactions are somnolence, headache, dizziness, diplopia, nausea, vomiting and fatigue occurring in more than 10% of patients.

The undesirable effect profile by body system is based on AEs from clinical trials assessed as related to Trileptal. In addition, clinically meaningful reports on adverse experiences from named patient programs and post-marketing experience were taken into account.

Frequency estimate:- very common: ⩾ 1/10; common: ⩾ 1/100 - < 1/10; uncommon: ⩾ 1/1,000 - < 1/100; rare: ⩾ 1/10,000 - < 1/1,000; very rare: < 1/10,000*

Blood and lymphatic system disorders	
Uncommon	leucopenia.
Very rare	thrombocytopenia.
Immune system disorders	
Very rare	hypersensitivity (characterised by features such as abnormal liver function tests, rash, fever, lymphadenopathy, eosinophilia, arthralgia).
Metabolism and nutrition disorders	
Common	hyponatraemia.
Very rare	hyponatraemia associated with signs and symptoms such as seizures, confusion, depressed level of consciousness, encephalopathy (see also Nervous system disorders for further undesirable effects), vision disorders (e.g. blurred vision), vomiting, nausea[†].
Psychiatric disorders	
Common	confusional state, depression, apathy, agitation (e.g. nervousness), affect lability.
Nervous system disorders	
Very common	somnolence, headache, dizziness.
Common	ataxia, tremor, nystagmus, disturbance in attention, amnesia.
Eye disorders	
Very common	diplopia.
Common	vision blurred, visual disturbance.
Ear and labyrinth disorders	
Common	vertigo.
Cardiac disorders	
Very rare	arrhythmia, atrioventricular block.
Gastrointestinal disorders	
Very common	nausea, vomiting.
Common	diarrhoea, constipation, abdominal pain.
Very rare	pancreatitis and/or lipase and/or amylase increase.
Hepato-biliary disorders	
Very rare	hepatitis.
Skin and subcutaneous tissue disorders	
Common	rash, alopecia, acne.
Uncommon	urticaria.
Very rare	angioedema, Stevens-Johnson syndrome, toxic epidermal necrolysis (Lyell's syndrome), erythema multiforme (see section 4.4 Special warnings and special precautions for use).
Musculoskeletal, connective tissue and bone disorders	
Very rare	systemic lupus erythematosus.
General disorders and administration site conditions	
Very common	fatigue.
Common	asthenia.
Investigations	
Uncommon	hepatic enzymes increased, blood alkaline phosphatase increased.

* according to CIOMS III frequency classification

† Very rarely clinically significant hyponatraemia (sodium <125 mmol/l) can develop during Trileptal use. It generally occurred during the first 3 months of treatment with Trileptal, although there were patients who first developed a serum sodium <125 mmol/l more than 1 year after initiation of therapy (see Section 4.4 "Special warnings and special precautions for use").

4.9 Overdose

Isolated cases of overdose have been reported. The maximum dose taken was approximately 24,000 mg. All patients recovered with symptomatic treatment. Symptoms of overdose include somnolence, dizziness, nausea, vomiting, hyperkinesia, hyponatraemia, ataxia and nystagmus. There is no specific antidote. Symptomatic and supportive treatment should be administered as appropriate. Removal of the medicinal product by gastric lavage and/or inactivation by administering activated charcoal should be considered.

5. PHARMACOLOGICAL PROPERTIES

5.1 Pharmacodynamic properties

Pharmacotherapeutic group: Antiepileptics

ATC code: N03A F 02

Pharmacodynamic effects

The pharmacological activity of oxcarbazepine is primarily exerted through the metabolite (MHD) (see Section 5.2 "Pharmacokinetic properties"- Biotransformation). The mechanism of action of oxcarbazepine and MHD is thought to be mainly based on blockade of voltage-sensitive sodium channels, thus resulting in stabilisation of hyperexcited neural membranes, inhibition of repetitive neuronal firing, and diminishment of propagation of synaptic impulses. In addition, increased potassium conductance and modulation of high-voltage activated calcium channels may also contribute to the anticonvulsant effects. No significant interactions with brain neurotransmitter or modulator receptor sites were found.

Oxcarbazepine and its active metabolite (MHD), are potent and efficacious anticonvulsants in animals. They protected rodents against generalised tonic-clonic and, to a lesser degree, clonic seizures, and abolished or reduced the frequency of chronically recurring partial seizures in Rhesus monkeys with aluminum implants. No tolerance (i.e. attenuation of anticonvulsive activity) against tonic-clonic seizures was observed when mice and rats were treated daily for 5 days or 4 weeks, respectively, with oxcarbazepine or MHD.

5.2 Pharmacokinetic properties

Absorption

Following oral administration of Trileptal tablets, oxcarbazepine is completely absorbed and extensively metabolised to its pharmacologically active metabolite (MHD).

After single dose administration of 600 mg Trileptal oral suspension to healthy male volunteers under fasted conditions, the mean C_{max} value of MHD was 24.9 μmol/l, with a corresponding median t_{max} of 6 hours.

In a mass balance study in man, only 2 % of total radioactivity in plasma was due to unchanged oxcarbazepine, approximately 70 % was due to MHD, and the remainder attributable to minor secondary metabolites which were rapidly eliminated.

Food has no effect on the rate and extent of absorption of oxcarbazepine, therefore, Trileptal can be taken with or without food.

Distribution

The apparent volume of distribution of MHD is 49 litres.

Approximately 40 % of MHD, is bound to serum proteins, predominantly to albumin. Binding was independent of the serum concentration within the therapeutically relevant range. Oxcarbazepine and MHD do not bind to alpha-1-acid glycoprotein.

Oxcarbazepine and MHD cross the placenta. Neonatal and maternal plasma MHD concentrations were similar in one case.

Biotransformation

Oxcarbazepine is rapidly reduced by cytosolic enzymes in the liver to MHD, which is primarily responsible for the pharmacological effect of Trileptal. MHD is metabolised further by conjugation with glucuronic acid. Minor amounts (4 % of the dose) are oxidised to the pharmacologically inactive metabolite (10, 11-dihydroxy derivative, DHD).

Elimination

Oxcarbazepine is cleared from the body mostly in the form of metabolites which are predominantly excreted by the kidneys. More than 95 % of the dose appears in the urine, with less than 1 % as unchanged oxcarbazepine. Faecal excretion accounts for less than 4 % of the administered dose. Approximately 80 % of the dose is excreted in the urine either as glucuronides of MHD (49 %) or as unchanged MHD (27 %), whereas the inactive DHD accounts for approximately 3 % and conjugates of oxcarbazepine account for 13 % of the dose.

Oxcarbazepine is rapidly eliminated from the plasma with apparent half-life values between 1.3 and 2.3 hours. In contrast, the apparent plasma half-life of MHD averaged 9.3 ± 1.8 h.

Dose proportionality

Steady-state plasma concentrations of MHD are reached within 2 - 3 days in patients when Trileptal is given twice a day. At steady-state, the pharmacokinetics of MHD are linear and show dose proportionality across the dose range of 300 to 2400 mg/day.

Special populations

Patients with hepatic impairment

The pharmacokinetics and metabolism of oxcarbazepine and MHD were evaluated in healthy volunteers and hepatically-impaired subjects after a single 900 mg oral dose. Mild to moderate hepatic impairment did not affect the pharmacokinetics of oxcarbazepine and MHD. Trileptal has not been studied in patients with severe hepatic impairment.

Patients with renal impairment

There is a linear correlation between creatinine clearance and the renal clearance of MHD. When Trileptal is administered as a single 300 mg dose, in renally impaired patients (creatinine clearance < 30 ml/min) the elimination half-life of MHD is prolonged by 60-90 % (16 to 19 hours) with a two fold increase in AUC compared to adults with normal renal function (10 hours).

Children

After a single dose administration of 5 or 15 mg/kg of Trileptal, the dose-adjusted AUC values of MHD were 30 % lower in children aged 2 - 5 years than in older children aged 6 - 12 years. In general, in children with normal renal function, renal clearance of MHD normalised for bodyweight is higher than in adults. In children, 10 to 50 % reduction of MHD elimination half-life (5 to 9 hours) was observed compared to adults (10 hours).

Elderly

Following administration of single (300 mg) and multiple doses (600 mg/day) of Trileptal in elderly volunteers (60 - 82 years of age), the maximum plasma concentrations and AUC values of MHD were 30 % - 60 % higher than in younger volunteers (18 - 32 years of age). Comparisons of creatinine clearances in young and elderly volunteers indicate that the difference was due to age-related reductions in creatinine clearance. No special dose recommendations are necessary because therapeutic doses are individually adjusted.

Gender

No gender related pharmacokinetic differences have been observed in children, adults, or the elderly.

5.3 Preclinical safety data

Preclinical data indicated no special hazard for humans based on repeated dose toxicity, safety pharmacology and genotoxicity studies with oxcarbazepine and the pharmacologically active metabolite, monohydroxy derivative (MHD).

Evidence of nephrotoxicity was noted in repeated dose toxicity rat studies but not in dog or mice studies. As there are no reports of such changes in patients, the clinical relevance of this finding in rats remains unknown.

Immunostimulatory tests in mice showed that MHD (and to a lesser extent oxcarbazepine) can induce delayed hypersensitivity.

Animal studies revealed effects such as increases in the incidence of embryo mortality and some delay in antenatal and/or postnatal growth at maternally toxic dose levels. There was an increase in rat foetal malformations in one of the eight embryo toxicity studies, which were conducted with either oxcarbazepine or the pharmacologically active metabolite (MHD), at a dose which also showed maternal toxicity (see Section 4.6 "Pregnancy and lactation").

In the carcinogenicity studies, liver (rats and mice), testicular and female genital tract granular cell (rats) tumours were induced in treated animals. The occurrence of liver tumours was most likely a consequence of the induction of hepatic microsomal enzymes; an inductive effect which, although it cannot be excluded, is weak or absent in patients treated with Trileptal. Testicular tumours may have been induced by elevated luteinizing hormone concentrations. Due to the absence of such an increase in humans, these tumours are considered to be of no clinical relevance. A dose-related increase in the incidence of granular cell tumours of the female genital tract (cervix and vagina) was noted in the rat carcinogenicity study with MHD. These effects occurred at exposure levels comparable with the anticipated clinical exposure. The mechanism for the development of these tumours has not been elucidated. Thus, the clinical relevance of these tumours is unknown.

6. PHARMACEUTICAL PARTICULARS

6.1 List of excipients

Propyl parahydroxybenzoate (E 216)

saccharin sodium

sorbic acid (E 200)

macrogol stearate 400

methyl parahydroxybenzoate (E 218)

yellow-plum-lemon flavour

ascorbic acid (E 300)

dispersible cellulose

propylene glycol

sorbitol 70% (non-crystallising)

water purified.

Ethanol is a component of the flavour.

6.2 Incompatibilities

Not applicable.

6.3 Shelf life

3 years.

Use within 7 weeks after first opening the bottle.

6.4 Special precautions for storage

This medicinal product does not require any special storage conditions.

6.5 Nature and contents of container

Brown (amber) type III glass bottles containing 250 ml of oral suspension. The bottles have a child-resistant cap and are packed in a cardboard box together with a 10 ml polypropylene oral syringe and press-in bottle adaptor.

Pack size: 1 bottle

6.6 Instructions for use and handling

No special requirements.

7. MARKETING AUTHORISATION HOLDER

Novartis Pharmaceuticals UK Limited

Frimley Business Park

Frimley

Camberley

Surrey

GU16 7SR

United Kingdom

8. MARKETING AUTHORISATION NUMBER(S)

PL 00101/0631

9. DATE OF FIRST AUTHORISATION/RENEWAL OF THE AUTHORISATION

13 November 2001

10. DATE OF REVISION OF THE TEXT

06 July 2005

Legal Category

POM

TRI-MINULET

(Wyeth Pharmaceuticals)

Presentation:

The memo pack holds six beige tablets containing 30 micrograms ethinyloestradiol and 50 micrograms gestodene, five dark brown tablets containing 40 micrograms ethinyloestradiol and 70 micrograms gestodene, and ten white tablets containing 30 micrograms ethinyloestradiol and 100 micrograms gestodene.

All tablets have a lustrous, sugar-coating.

Uses:

Oral contraception and the recognised gynaecological indications for such oestrogen-progestogen combinations. The mode of action includes the inhibition of ovulation by suppression of the mid-cycle surge of luteinising hormone, the inspissation of cervical mucus so as to constitute a barrier to sperm, and the rendering of the endometrium unreceptive to implantation.

Dosage and Administration

First treatment cycle: 1 tablet daily for 21 days, starting with the tablet marked number 1, on the first day of the menstrual cycle. Additional contraception (barriers and spermicide) is not required.

Subsequent cycles: Each subsequent course is started when seven tablet-free days have followed the preceding course. A withdrawal bleed should occur during the 7 tablet-free days.

Changing from another 21 day combined oral contraceptive: The first tablet of Tri-Minulet should be taken on the first day immediately after the end of the previous oral contraceptive course. Additional contraception is not required. A withdrawal bleed should not be expected until the end of the first pack of Tri-Minulet.

Changing from an Every Day (ED) 28 day combined oral contraceptive: The first tablet of Tri-Minulet should be taken on the day immediately after the day on which the last active pill in the ED pack has been taken. The remaining tablets in the ED pack should be discarded. Additional contraception is not required. A withdrawal bleed should not be expected until the end of the first pack of Tri-Minulet.

Changing from a Progestogen-only-Pill (POP): The first tablet of Tri-Minulet should be taken on the first day of menstruation even if the POP for that day has already been taken. The remaining tablets in the POP pack should be discarded. Additional contraception is not required.

Post-partum and post-abortum use: After pregnancy combined oral contraception can be started in non-lactating women 21 days after a vaginal delivery, provided that the patient is fully ambulant and there are no puerperal complications.

If the pill is started later than 21 days after delivery, then alternative contraception (barriers and spermicides) should be used until oral contraception is started and for the first 7 days of pill-taking. If unprotected intercourse has taken place after 21 days post partum, then oral contraception should not be started until the first menstrual bleed after childbirth.

After a miscarriage or abortion oral contraception may be started immediately.

Special Circumstances Requiring Additional Contraception

Missed Pills:

If a tablet is delayed it should be taken as soon as possible and if it is taken within 12 hours of the correct time, additional contraception is not needed. Further tablets should then be taken at the usual time. If the delay exceeds 12 hours, the last missed pill should be taken when remembered, the earlier missed pills left in the pack and normal pill-taking resumed. If one or more tablets are omitted from the 21 days of pill-taking, additional contraception (barriers and spermicides) should be used for the next 7 days of pill-taking. In addition, if one or more pills are missed during the last 7 days of pill-taking, the subsequent pill-free interval should be disregarded and the next pack started the day after taking the last tablet from the previous pack. In this case, a withdrawal bleed should not be expected until the end of the second pack. If the patient does not have a withdrawal bleed at the end of the second pack she must return to her doctor to exclude the possibility of pregnancy.

Gastro-Intestinal Upset:

Vomiting or diarrhoea may reduce the efficacy by preventing full absorption. Additional contraception (barriers and spermicides) should be used during the stomach upset and for the 7 days following the upset. If these 7 days overrun the end of a pack, the next pack should be started without a break. In this case, a withdrawal bleed should not be expected until the end of the second pack. If the patient does not have a withdrawal bleed at the end of the second pack she must return to her doctor to exclude the possibility of pregnancy.

Mild laxatives do not impair contraceptive action.

Interaction with other drugs: Some drugs accelerate the metabolism of oral contraceptives when taken concurrently and these include barbiturates, phenytoin, phenylbutazone and rifampicin. Other drugs suspected of having the capacity to reduce the efficacy of oral contraceptives include ampicillin and other antibiotics. It is, therefore, advisable to use non-hormonal methods of contraception (barriers and spermicides) in addition to the oral contraceptive as long as an extremely high degree of protection is required during treatment with such drugs. The additional contraception should be used while the concurrent medication continues and for 7 days afterwards. If these extra precautions overrun the end of the pack, the next pack should be started without a break. In this case, a withdrawal bleed should not be expected until the end of the second pack. If the patient does not have a withdrawal bleed at the end of the second pack she must return to her doctor to exclude the possibility of pregnancy.

The herbal remedy St John's wort (*Hypericum perforatum*) should not be taken concomitantly with this medicine as it could potentially lead to a loss of contraceptive effect.

Contra-indications, warnings etc.

Contra-indications:

1. Suspected pregnancy.

2. History of confirmed venous thromboembolism (VTE). Family history of idiopathic VTE. Other known risk factors for VTE. Thrombotic disorders and a history of these conditions, sickle-cell anaemia, disorders of lipid metabolism and other conditions in which, in individual cases, there is known or suspected to be a much increased risk of thrombosis.

3. Acute or severe chronic liver diseases. Dubin-Johnson syndrome. Rotor syndrome. History, during pregnancy, of idiopathic jaundice or severe pruritus.

4. History of herpes gestationis.

5. Mammary or endometrial carcinoma, or a history of these conditions.

6. Abnormal vaginal bleeding of unknown cause.

7. Deterioration of otosclerosis during pregnancy.

Warnings:

1. Venous and Arterial Thrombosis and Thromboembolism

Use of COCs is associated with an increased risk of venous and arterial thrombotic and thromboembolic events.

Minimising exposure to oestrogens and progestogens is in keeping with good principles of therapeutics. For any particular oestrogen/progestogen combination, the dosage regimen prescribed should be one that contains the least amount of oestrogen and progestogen that is compatible with a low failure rate and the needs of the patient.

Unless clinically indicated otherwise, new users of COCs should be started on preparations containing less than 50µg of oestrogen.

Venous Thrombosis and Thromboembolism

Use of COCs increases the risk of venous thrombotic and thromboembolic events. Reported events include deep venous thrombosis and pulmonary embolism.

The use of any COC carries an increased risk of venous thrombotic and thromboembolic events compared with no use. The excess risk is highest during the first year a woman ever uses a combined oral contraceptive. This increased risk is less than the risk of venous thrombotic and thromboembolic events associated with pregnancy which is estimated as 60 cases per 100,000 woman-years. Venous thromboembolism is fatal in 1-2% of cases.

Some epidemiological studies have reported a greater risk of VTE for women using combined oral contraceptives containing desogestrel or gestodene (the so-called third generation pills) than for women using pills containing levonorgestrel (the so-called second generation pills).

The spontaneous incidence of VTE in healthy non-pregnant women (not taking any oral contraceptive) is about 5 cases per 100,000 women per year. The incidence in users of the second generation pills is about 15 per 100,000 women per year of use. The incidence in users of third generation pills (such as Tri-Minulet) is about 25 cases per 100,000 women per year of use; this excess incidence has not been satisfactorily explained by bias or confounding. The level of all these risks of VTE increases with age and is likely to be further increased in women with other known risk factors of VTE.

All this information should be taken into account when prescribing this COC. When counselling on the choice of contraceptive method(s) all of the above information should be considered.

The risk of venous thrombotic and thromboembolic events is further increased in women with conditions predisposing for venous thrombosis and thromboembolism. Caution must be exercised when prescribing COCs for such women.

Examples of predisposing conditions for venous thrombosis are:

- Certain inherited or acquired thrombophilias (the presence of an inherited thrombophilia may be indicated by a family history of venous thrombotic/thromboembolic events
- Obesity (body mass index of 30kg/m^2 or over)
- Surgery or trauma with increased risk of thrombosis (see reasons for discontinuation)
- Recent delivery or second-trimester abortion
- Prolonged immobilisation
- Increasing age
- Systemic Lupus Erythematosus (SLE)

The relative risk of post-operative thromboembolic complications has been reported to be increased two- or four-fold with the use of COCs (see reasons for discontinuation).

Since the immediate post-partum period is associated with an increased risk of thromboembolism, COCs should be started no earlier than day 28 after delivery or second-trimester abortion.

Arterial Thrombosis and Thromboembolism

The use of COCs increases the risk or arterial thrombotic and thromboembolic events. Reported events include myocardial infarction and cerebrovascular events (ischaemic and haemorrhagic stroke).

The risk of arterial thrombotic and thromboembolic events is further increased in women with underlying risk factors.

Caution must be exercised when prescribing COCs for women with risk factors for arterial thrombotic and thromboembolic events.

Examples of risk factors for arterial thrombotic and thromboembolic event are:

- Smoking, especially over the age of 35
- Certain inherited and acquired thrombophilias
- Hypertension
- Dyslipoproteinaemias
- Thrombogenic valvular heart disease, atrial fibrillation
- Obesity (body mass index of 30kg/m^2)
- Increasing age
- Diabetes
- Systemic Lupus Erythematosus (SLE)

COC users with migraine (particularly migraine with aura) may be at increased risk of stroke.

There is no consensus about the possible role of varicose veins and superficial thrombophlebitis in venous thromboembolism.

The suitability of a combined oral contraceptive should be judged according to the severity of such conditions in the individual case, and should be discussed with the patient before she decides to take it.

2. The risk of arterial thrombosis associated with combined oral contraceptives increases with age, and this risk is aggravated by cigarette smoking. The use of combined oral contraceptives by women in the older age group, especially those who are cigarette smokers, should therefore be discouraged and alternative methods used.

3. The possibility cannot be ruled out that certain chronic diseases may occasionally deteriorate during the use of combined oral contraceptives. (See 'Precautions').

4. The combination of ethinyloestradiol and gestodene, like other contraceptive steroids, is associated with an increased incidence of neoplastic nodules in the rat liver, the relevance of which to man is unknown.

5. Malignant liver tumours have been reported on rare occasions in long-term users of oral contraceptives. Benign hepatic tumours have also been associated with oral contraceptive usage. A hepatic tumour should be considered in the differential diagnosis when upper abdominal pain, enlarged liver or signs of intra-abdominal haemorrhage occur.

6. Numerous epidemiological studies have been reported on the risks of ovarian, endometrial, cervical and breast cancer in women using combined oral contraceptives. The evidence is clear that combined oral contraceptives offer substantial protection against both ovarian and endometrial cancer.

An increased risk of cervical cancer in long-term users of combined oral contraceptives has been reported in some studies, but there continues to be controversy about the extent to which this is attributable to the confounding effects of sexual behaviour and other factors.

A meta-analysis from 54 epidemiological studies reported that there is a slightly increased relative risk (RR = 1.24) of having breast cancer diagnosed in women who are currently using combined oral contraceptives (COCs). The observed pattern of increased risk may be due to an earlier diagnosis of breast cancer in COC users, the biological effects of COCs or a combination of both. The additional breast cancers diagnosed in current users of COCs or in women who have used COCs in the last ten years are more likely to be localised to the breast than those in women who never used COCs.

Breast cancer is rare among women under 40 years of age whether or not they take COCs. Whilst this background risk increases with age, the excess number of breast cancer diagnoses in current and recent COC users is small in relation to the overall risk of breast cancer (see bar chart).

(see Figure 1 below)

The most important risk factor for breast cancer in COC users is the age women discontinue the COC; the older the age at stopping, the more breast cancers are diagnosed. Duration of use is less important and the excess risk gradually disappears during the course of the 10 years after stopping COC use such that by 10 years there appears to be no excess.

The possible increase in risk of breast cancer should be discussed with the user and weighed against the benefits of COCs taking into account the evidence that they offer substantial protection against the risk of developing certain other cancers (e.g. ovarian and endometrial cancer).

Reasons for stopping oral contraception immediately:

1. Occurrence of migraine in patients who have never previously suffered from it. Exacerbation of pre-existing migraine. Any unusually frequent or unusually severe headaches.

2. Any kind of acute disturbance of vision.

3. Suspicion of thrombosis or infarction including symptoms such as unusual pains in or swelling of the legs, stabbing pains on breathing, persistent cough or coughing blood, pain or tightness in the chest.

4. Six weeks before elective operations and during immobilisation, e.g. after accidents, etc.

5. Significant rise in blood pressure.

6. Jaundice.

7. Clear exacerbation of conditions known to be capable of deteriorating during oral contraception or pregnancy.

8. Pregnancy is a reason for stopping immediately because it has been suggested by some investigations that oral contraceptives taken in early pregnancy may slightly increase the risk of foetal malformations. Other investigations have failed to support these findings. The possibility therefore cannot be excluded, but it is certain that if a risk exists at all, it is very small.

If oral contraception is stopped for any reason and pregnancy is not desired, it is recommended that alternative non-hormonal methods of contraception (such as barriers or spermicides) are used to ensure contraceptive protection is maintained.

Precautions:

1. Assessment of women prior to starting oral contraceptives (and at regular intervals thereafter) should include a personal and family medical history of each woman. Physical examination should be guided by this and by the contraindications (section 4.3) and warnings (section 4.4) for this product. The frequency and nature of these assessments should be based upon relevant guidelines and should be adapted to the individual woman, but should include measurement of blood pressure and, if judged appropriate by the clinician, breast, abdominal and pelvic examination including cervical cytology.

2. Before starting treatment, pregnancy must be excluded.

3. The following conditions require careful observation during medication: a history of severe depressive states, varicose veins, diabetes, hypertension, epilepsy, migraine, otosclerosis, multiple sclerosis, porphyria, tetany, disturbed liver function, gall-stones, cardiovascular diseases, renal diseases, chloasma, uterine fibroids, asthma, the

Figure 1 Breast cancer is rare among women under 40 years of age whether or not they take COCs. Whilst this background risk increases with age, the excess number of breast cancer diagnoses in current and recent COC users is small in relation to the overall risk of breast cancer (see bar chart).

Estimated cumulative numbers of breast cancers per 10,000 women diagnosed in 5 years of use and up to 10 years after stopping COCs, compared with numbers of breast cancers diagnosed in 10,000 women who had never used COCs

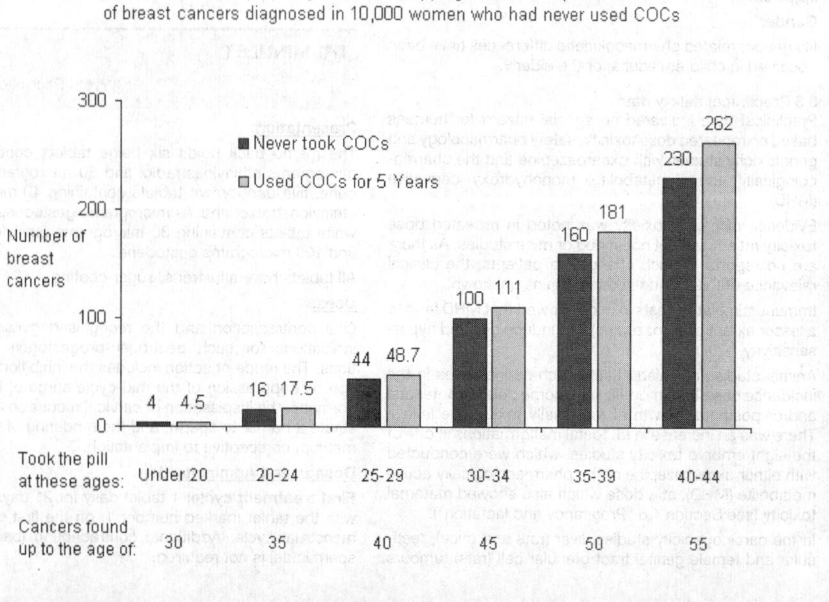

wearing of contact lenses, or any disease that is prone to worsen during pregnancy. The first appearance or deterioration of any of these conditions may indicate that the oral contraceptive should be stopped.

4. The risk of the deterioration of chloasma, which is often not fully reversible, is reduced by the avoidance of excessive exposure to sunlight.

Side-effects:

See "Warnings and Precautions"

There is an increased risk of venous thromboembolism for all women using a combined oral contraceptive. For information on differences in risk between oral contraceptives, see "Warnings".

Occasional side-effects may include nausea, vomiting, headaches, breast tenderness, changed body weight or libido, depressive moods and chloasma.

Menstrual changes:

1. Reduction of menstrual flow: This is not abnormal and it is to be expected in some patients. Indeed, it may be beneficial where heavy periods were previously experienced.

2. Missed menstruation: Occasionally, withdrawal bleeding may not occur at all. If the tablets have been taken correctly, pregnancy is very unlikely, but should be ruled out before a new course of tablets is started.

Intermenstrual bleeding: Very light 'spotting' or heavier 'breakthrough bleeding' may occur during tablet-taking, especially in the first few cycles. It appears to be generally of no significance, except where it indicates errors of tablet-taking, or where the possibility of interaction with other drugs exists (q.v.). However, if irregular bleeding is persistent, an organic cause should be considered.

Effect on adrenal and thyroid glands: Oral contraceptives have no significant influence on adrenocortical function. The ACTH function test for the adrenal cortex remains unchanged. The reduction in corticosteroid excretion and the elevation of plasma corticosteroids are due to an increased cortisol-binding capacity of the plasma proteins.

The response to metyrapone is less pronounced than in untreated women and is thus similar to that during pregnancy.

The radio-iodine uptake shows that thyroid function is unchanged. There is a rise in serum protein-bound iodine, similar to that in pregnancy and during the administration of oestrogens. This is due to the increased capacity of the plasma proteins for binding thyroid hormones, rather than to any change in glandular function. In women taking oral contraceptives, the content of protein-bound iodine in blood serum should therefore, not be used for evaluation of thyroid function.

Effect on blood chemistry: Oral contraceptives may accelerate erythrocyte sedimentation in the absence of any disease. This effect is due to a change in the proportion of the plasma protein fractions. Increases in plasma copper, iron and alkaline phosphatase have also been recorded.

Overdosage:

There have been no reports of serious ill-effects from overdosage, even when a considerable number of tablets have been taken by a small child. In general, it is, therefore, unnecessary to treat overdosage. However, if overdosage is discovered within two or three hours and is so large that treatment seems desirable, gastric lavage can be safely used.

There are no specific antidotes and further treatment should be symptomatic.

Pharmaceutical precautions:	Store in cool, dry conditions. Shelf-life five years
Legal category:	POM
Package quantities:	Individual packs containing 3 months' supply.
Further information:	NIL
Product Licence Number:	PL 0011/0140
Date of Last Revision:	3rd March 2003

Wyeth Pharmaceuticals,
Huntercombe Lane South,
Taplow,
Maidenhead,
Berkshire SL6 0PH
UK

Trimovate

(GlaxoSmithKline UK)

1. NAME OF THE MEDICINAL PRODUCT

Trimovate Cream

Trimovate

Clobetasone Butyrate

2. QUALITATIVE AND QUANTITATIVE COMPOSITION

Trimovate Cream is a yellow water-miscible cream containing clobetasone butyrate 0.05% w/w, oxytetracycline 3.0% w/w as calcium oxytetracycline and nystatin 100,000 units per gram.

3. PHARMACEUTICAL FORM

Cream for topical administration.

4. CLINICAL PARTICULARS

4.1 Therapeutic indications

Clobetasone butyrate is a topically active corticosteroid which provides an exceptional combination of activity and safety. Topical formulations have been shown to be more effective in the treatment of eczemas than 1% hydrocortisone, yet to have little effect on hypothalamic-pituitary-adrenal function.

The combination of the topically active antibiotics, nystatin and oxytetracycline, provides a broad spectrum of antibacterial and anticandidal activity against many of the organisms associated with infected dermatoses. Trimovate is indicated for the treatment and management of steroid responsive dermatoses where candidal or bacterial infection is present, suspected or likely to occur and the use of a more potent topical corticosteroid is not required. These include infected eczemas, intertrigo, napkin rash, anogenital pruritus and seborrhoeic dermatitis.

4.2 Posology and method of administration

Apply to the affected area up to four times a day.

Suitable for treating infants, children and adults.

4.3 Contraindications

Primary cutaneous infections caused by viruses (e.g. herpes simplex, chickenpox) fungi and bacteria. Secondary infections due to dermatophytes, Pseudomonas or Proteus species.

Hypersensitivity to the preparation.

4.4 Special warnings and special precautions for use

Although generally regarded as safe, even for long term administration in adults, there is a potential for overdosage, and in children this may result in adrenal suppression. Extreme caution is required in dermatoses in such patients and treatment should not normally exceed seven days. In infants, the napkin may act as an occlusive dressing, and increase absorption.

If infection persists, systemic chemotherapy is likely to be required: Any spread of infection requires withdrawal of topical corticosteroid therapy. Bacterial infection is encouraged by the warm, moist conditions induced by occlusive dressings, and the skin should be cleansed before a fresh dressing is applied. Do not continue for more than seven days in the absence of clinical improvement, since occult extension of infection may occur due to the masking effect of the steroid.

As with all corticosteroids, prolonged application to the face is undesirable. If applied to the eyelids, care is needed to ensure that the preparation does not enter the eye, as glaucoma might result.

Trimovate may cause slight staining of hair, skin or fabric, but this can be removed by washing. The application may be covered with a non-occlusive dressing to protect clothing.

Extended or recurrent application may increase the risk of contact sensitisation.

Products which contain antimicrobial agents should not be diluted.

4.5 Interaction with other medicinal products and other forms of Interaction

None reported.

4.6 Pregnancy and lactation

There is inadequate evidence of safety in human pregnancy. Topical administration of corticosteroids to pregnant animals can cause abnormalities of fetal development including cleft palate and intra-uterine growth retardation. There may therefore be a very small risk of such effects in the human fetus.

4.7 Effects on ability to drive and use machines

None stated.

4.8 Undesirable effects

In the unlikely event of signs of hypersensitivity appearing, application should be stopped immediately.

If large areas of the body were to be treated with Trimovate, it is possible that some patients would absorb sufficient steroid to cause transient adrenal suppression despite the low degree of systemic activity associated with clobetasone butyrate.

Local atrophic changes could possibly occur in situations where moisture increases absorption of clobetasone butyrate, but only after prolonged use.

There are reports of pigmentation changes and hypertrichosis with topical steroids. Exacerbation of symptoms may occur with extensive use.

4.9 Overdose

Acute overdosage is very unlikely to occur, however, in the case of chronic overdosage or misuse the features of hypercorticism may appear and in this situation topical steroids should be discontinued.

5. PHARMACOLOGICAL PROPERTIES

5.1 Pharmacodynamic properties

Clobetasone butyrate is a topically active corticosteroid.

Clobetasone butyrate is less potent than other available corticosteroid preparations and has been shown not to suppress the hypothalamo-pituitary-adrenal axis in patients treated for psoriasis or eczema. Pharmacological studies in man and animals have shown that clobetasone butyrate has a relatively high level of topical activity accompanied by a low level of systemic activity.

The use of nystatin in the local treatment of candidal infections of the skin and of the tetracyclines in localised bacterial infections is well known. Nystatin is included in Trimovate at the standard concentration recommended by the British Pharmaceutical codex for the topical preparation nystatin ointment (100,000 units/g) and oxytetracycline calcium is included at a concentration to give approximately the same level of activity as recommended for Oxytetracycline Ointment BPC (3.0% w/w).

The principle action of the preparation is based on the anti-inflammatory activity of the corticosteroid. The broad spectrum antibacterial and anti-candidal activity provided by the combination of oxytecycline and nystatin allow this effect to be utilised in the treatment of conditions which are or are likely to become infected.

5.2 Pharmacokinetic properties

Trimovate has been shown to have a satisfactory pharmacokinetic profile by many years of successful clinical experience.

5.3 Preclinical safety data

No additional data of relevance.

6. PHARMACEUTICAL PARTICULARS

6.1 List of excipients

Titanium dioxide, glyceryl monostearate, cetostearyl alcohol, soft paraffin white, polyoxyl 40 stearate, dimethicone 20, glycerol, chlorocresol, sodium metabisulphite, sodium acid phosphate, disodium hydrogen phosphate anhydrous, purified water.

6.2 Incompatibilities

None reported.

6.3 Shelf life

18 months.

6.4 Special precautions for storage

Store below 25°C.

6.5 Nature and contents of container

Collapsible latex banded aluminium tube, internally coated with epoxy resin based lacquer with polypropylene cap.

6.6 Instructions for use and handling

None stated.

Administrative Data

7. MARKETING AUTHORISATION HOLDER

Glaxo Wellcome UK Ltd trading as GlaxoSmithKline UK,

Stockley Park West,

Uxbridge, Middlesex.

UB11 1BT.

8. MARKETING AUTHORISATION NUMBER(S)

PL 10949/0040

9. DATE OF FIRST AUTHORISATION/RENEWAL OF THE AUTHORISATION

29 May 2002

10. DATE OF REVISION OF THE TEXT

29 January 2002

11. Legal Category

POM.

Trinordiol

(Wyeth Pharmaceuticals)

1. NAME OF THE MEDICINAL PRODUCT

Trinordiol

2. QUALITATIVE AND QUANTITATIVE COMPOSITION

Each light brown tablet contains 50 micrograms Levonorgestrel Ph. Eur. and 30 micrograms Ethinylestradiol Ph. Eur.

Each white tablet contains 75 micrograms Levonorgestrel Ph. Eur and 40 micrograms Ethinylestradiol Ph. Eur.

Each ochre tablet contains 125 micrograms Levonorgestrel Ph. Eur and 30 micrograms Ethinylestradiol Ph. Eur.

For excipients see 6.1.

3. PHARMACEUTICAL FORM

White or ochre or light brown lustrous sugar coated tablets.

4. CLINICAL PARTICULARS

4.1 Therapeutic indications

Oral contraception.

4.2 Posology and method of administration

First treatment cycle: 1 tablet daily for 21 days, starting with the tablet marked number 1, on the first day of the menstrual cycle. Additional contraception (barriers and spermicide) is not required.

Subsequent cycles: Each subsequent course is started when seven tablet-free days have followed the preceding course. A withdrawal bleed should occur during the 7 tablet-free days.

Changing from another 21 day combined oral contraceptive: The first tablet of Trinordiol should be taken on the first day immediately after the end of the previous oral contraceptive course. Additional contraception is not required. A withdrawal bleed should not be expected until the end of the first pack of Trinordiol.

Changing from an Every Day (ED) 28 day combined oral contraceptive: The first tablet of Trinordiol should be taken on the day immediately after the day on which the last active pill in the ED pack has been taken. The remaining tablets in the ED pack should be discarded. Additional contraception is not required. A withdrawal bleed should not be expected until the end of the first pack of Trinordiol.

Changing from a Progestogen-only-Pill (POP): The first tablet of Trinordiol should be taken on the first day of menstruation even if the POP for that day has already been taken. The remaining tablets in the POP pack should be discarded. Additional contraception is not required.

Post-partum and post-abortum use: After pregnancy combined oral contraception can be started in non-lactating women 21 days after a vaginal delivery, provided that the patient is fully ambulant and there are no puerperal complications.

If the pill is started later than 21 days after delivery, then alternative contraception (barriers and spermicides) should be used until oral contraception is started and for the first 7 days of pill-taking. If unprotected intercourse has taken place after 21 days post partum, then oral contraception should not be started until the first menstrual bleed after childbirth.

After a miscarriage or abortion oral contraception may be started immediately.

Elderly: Not applicable

Children: Not applicable

Special Circumstances Requiring Additional Contraception

Missed Pills:

If a tablet is delayed it should be taken as soon as possible and if it is taken within 12 hours of the correct time, additional contraception is not needed. Further tablets should then be taken at the usual time. If the delay exceeds 12 hours, the last missed pill should be taken when remembered, the earlier missed pills left in the pack and normal pill-taking resumed. If one or more tablets are omitted from the 21 days of pill-taking, additional contraception (barriers and spermicides) should be used for the next 7 days of pill-taking. In addition, if one or more pills are missed during the last 7 days of pill-taking, the subsequent pill-free interval should be disregarded and the next pack started the day after taking the last tablet from the previous pack. In this case, a withdrawal bleed should not be expected until the end of the second pack. If the patient does not have a withdrawal bleed at the end of the second pack she must return to her doctor to exclude the possibility of pregnancy.

Gastro-Intestinal Upset:

Vomiting or diarrhoea may reduce the efficacy by preventing full absorption. Additional contraception (barriers and spermicides) should be used during the stomach upset and for the 7 days following the upset. If these 7 days overrun the end of a pack, the next pack should be started without a break. In this case, a withdrawal bleed should not be expected until the end of the second pack. If the patient does not have a withdrawal bleed at the end of the second pack she must return to her doctor to exclude the possibility of pregnancy.

Mild laxatives do not impair contraceptive action.

Interaction with other drugs:

Some drugs may reduce the efficacy of oral contraceptives (refer to "4.5. Interaction with other medicaments and other forms of interaction."). It is therefore, advisable to use non-hormonal methods of contraception (barriers and spermicides) in addition to the oral contraceptive as long as an extremely high degree of protection is required during treatment with such drugs. The additional contraception should be used while the concurrent medication continues and for 7 days afterwards. If these extra precautions overrun the end of the pack, the next pack should be started without a break. In this case, a withdrawal bleed should not be expected until the end of the second pack. If the patient does not have a withdrawal bleed at the end of the second pack she must return to her doctor to exclude the possibility of pregnancy.

4.3 Contraindications

Suspected pregnancy.

1. History of confirmed venous thromboembolism (VTE). Family history of idiopathic VTE. Other known risk factors for VTE.

2. Arterial thrombotic disorders and a history of these conditions, sickle-cell anaemia, disorders of lipid metabolism and other conditions in which, in individual cases, there is known or suspected to be a much increased risk of thrombosis.

3. Sickle-cell anaemia.

4. Acute or severe chronic liver diseases. Dubin-Johnson syndrome. Rotor syndrome. History, during pregnancy, of idiopathic jaundice or severe pruritus.

5. History of herpes gestationis.

6. Mammary or endometrial carcinoma, or a history of these conditions.

7. Abnormal vaginal bleeding of unknown cause.

8. Deterioration of otosclerosis during pregnancy.

4.4 Special warnings and special precautions for use
Warnings:

1. Venous and Arterial Thrombosis and Thromboembolism

Use of COCs is associated with an increased risk of venous and arterial thrombotic and thromboembolic events.

Minimising exposure to oestrogens and progestogens is in keeping with good principles of therapeutics. For any particular oestrogen/progestogen combination, the dosage regimen prescribed should be one that contains the least amount of oestrogen and progestogen that is compatible with a low failure rate and the needs of the patient.

Unless clinically indicated otherwise, new users of COCs should be started on preparations containing less than 50μg of oestrogen.

Venous Thrombosis and Thromboembolism

Use of COCs increases the risk of venous thrombotic and thromboembolic events. Reported events include deep venous thrombosis and pulmonary embolism.

The use of any COC carries an increased risk of venous thrombotic and thromboembolic events compared with no use. The excess risk is highest during the first year a woman ever uses a combined oral contraceptive. This increased risk is less than the risk of venous thrombotic and thromboembolic events associated with pregnancy which is estimated as 60 cases per 100,000 woman-years. Venous thromboembolism is fatal in 1-2% of cases.

Some epidemiological studies have reported a greater risk of VTE for women using combined oral contraceptives containing desogestrel or gestodene (the so-called third generation pills) than for women using pills containing levonorgestrel (the so-called second generation pills).

The spontaneous incidence of VTE in healthy non-pregnant women (not taking any oral contraceptive) is about 5 cases per 100,000 women per year. The incidence in users of the second generation pills (such as Trinordiol) is about 15 per 100,000 women per year of use. The incidence in users of third generation pills is about 25 cases per 100,000 women per year of use; this excess incidence has not been satisfactorily explained by bias or confounding. The level of all these risks of VTE increases with age and is likely to be further increased in women with other known risk factors of VTE.

All this information should be taken into account when prescribing this COC. When counselling on the choice of contraceptive method(s) all of the above information should be considered.

The risk of venous thrombotic and thromboembolic events is further increased in women with conditions predisposing for venous thrombosis and thromboembolism. Caution must be exercised when prescribing COCs for such women.

Examples of predisposing conditions for venous thrombosis are:

- Certain inherited or acquired thrombophilias (the presence of an inherited thrombophilia may be indicated by a family history of venous thrombotic/thromboembolic events)
- Obesity (body mass index of 30kg/m^2 or over)
- Surgery or trauma with increased risk of thrombosis (see reasons for discontinuation)
- Recent delivery or second-trimester abortion
- Prolonged immobilisation
- Increasing age
- Systemic Lupus Erythematosus (SLE)

The relative risk of post-operative thromboembolic complications has been reported to be increased two- or four-fold with the use of COCs (see reasons for discontinuation).

Since the immediate post-partum period is associated with an increased risk of thromboembolism, COCs should be started no earlier than day 28 after delivery or second-trimester abortion.

Arterial Thrombosis and Thromboembolism

The use of COCs increases the risk or arterial thrombotic and thromboembolic events. Reported events include myocardial infarction and cerebrovascular events (ischaemic and haemorrhagic stroke).

The risk of arterial thrombotic and thromboembolic events is further increased in women with underlying risk factors.

Caution must be exercised when prescribing COCs for women with risk factors for arterial thrombotic and thromboembolic events.

Examples of risk factors for arterial thrombotic and thromboembolic events are:

- Smoking, especially over the age of 35
- Certain inherited and acquired thrombophilias
- Hypertension
- Dyslipoproteinaemias
- Thrombogenic valvular heart disease, atrial fibillation
- Obesity (body mass index of 30kg/m^2)
- Increasing age
- Diabetes
- Systemic Lupus Erythematosus (SLE)

COC users with migraine (particularly migraine with aura) may be at increased risk of stroke.

There is no consensus about the possible role of varicose veins and superficial thrombophlebitis in venous thromboembolism

The suitability of a combined oral contraceptive should be judged according to the severity of such conditions in the individual case, and should be discussed with the patient before she decides to take it.

2. The risk of arterial thrombosis associated with combined oral contraceptives increases with age, and this risk is aggravated by cigarette smoking. The use of combined oral contraceptives by women in the older age group, especially those who are cigarette smokers, should therefore be discouraged and alternative methods used.

3. The possibility cannot be ruled out that certain chronic diseases may occasionally deteriorate during the use of combined oral contraceptives. (See 'Precautions').

4. Malignant liver tumours have been reported on rare occasions in long-term users of oral contraceptives. Benign hepatic tumours have also been associated with oral contraceptive usage. A hepatic tumour should be considered in the differential diagnosis when upper abdominal pain, enlarged liver or signs of intra-abdominal haemorrhage occur.

5. Numerous epidemiological studies have been reported on the risks of ovarian, endometrial, cervical and breast cancer in women using combined oral contraceptives. The evidence is clear that combined oral contraceptives offer substantial protection against both ovarian and endometrial cancer.

An increased risk of cervical cancer in long term users of combined oral contraceptives has been reported in some studies, but there continues to be controversy about the extent to which this is attributable to the confounding effects of sexual behaviour and other factors.

A meta-analysis from 54 epidemiological studies reported that there is a slightly increased relative risk (RR = 1.24) of having breast cancer diagnosed in women who are currently using combined oral contraceptives (COCs). The observed pattern of increased risk may be due to an earlier diagnosis of breast cancer in COC users, the biological effects of COCs or a combination of both. The additional breast cancers diagnosed in current users of COCs or in women who have used COCs in the last ten years are more likely to be localised to the breast than those in women who never used COCs.

Breast cancer is rare among women under 40 years of age whether or not they take COCs. Whilst this background risk increases with age, the excess number of breast cancer diagnoses in current and recent COC users is small in relation to the overall risk of breast cancer (see bar chart).

(see Figure 1 on next page)

The most important risk factor for breast cancer in COC users is the age women discontinue the COC; the older the age at stopping, the more breast cancers are diagnosed. Duration of use is less important and the excess risk gradually disappears during the course of the 10 years after stopping COC use such that by 10 years there appears to be no excess.

The possible increase in risk of breast cancer should be discussed with the user and weighed against the benefits of COCs taking into account the evidence that they offer substantial protection against the risk of developing certain other cancers (e.g. ovarian and endometrial cancer).

Reasons for stopping oral contraception immediately:

1. Occurrence of migraine in patients who have never previously suffered from it. Exacerbation of pre-existing migraine. Any unusually frequent or unusually severe headaches.

2. Any kind of acute disturbance of vision.

3. Suspicion of thrombosis or infarction including symptoms such as unusual pains in or swelling of the legs, stabbing pains on breathing, persistent cough or coughing blood, pain or tightness in the chest.

4. Six weeks before elective operations or treatment of varicose veins by sclerotherapy and during immobilisation, e.g. after accidents, etc.

5. Significant rise in blood-pressure.

6. Jaundice.

7. Clear exacerbation of conditions known to be capable of deteriorating during oral contraception or pregnancy.

8. Pregnancy is a reason for stopping immediately because it has been suggested by some investigations that oral contraceptives taken in early pregnancy may slightly increase the risk of foetal malformations. Other investigations have failed to support these findings. The possibility

Figure 1

Estimated cumulative numbers of breast cancers per 10,000 women diagnosed in 5 years of use and up to 10 years after stopping COCs, compared with numbers of breast cancers diagnosed in 10,000 women who had never used COCs

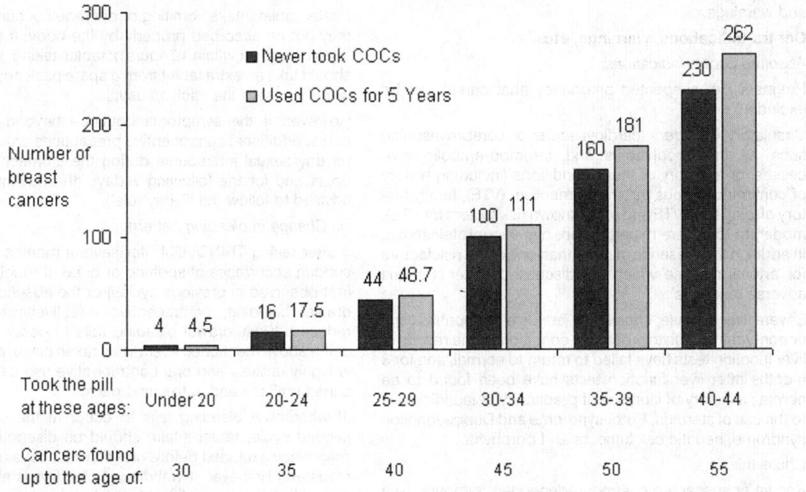

therefore cannot be excluded, but it is certain that if a risk exists at all, it is very small.

If oral contraception is stopped for any reason and pregnancy is not desired, it is recommended that alternative non-hormonal methods of contraception (such as barriers or spermicides) are used to ensure contraceptive protection is maintained.

Precautions:

1. Assessment of women prior to starting oral contraceptives (and at regular intervals thereafter) should include a personal and family medical history of each woman. Physical examination should be guided by this and by the contraindications (section 4.3) and warnings (section 4.4) for this product. The frequency and nature of these assessments should be based upon relevant guidelines and should be adapted to the individual woman, but should include measurement of blood pressure and, if judged appropriate by the clinician, breast, abdominal and pelvic examination including cervical cytology.

2. Before starting treatment, pregnancy must be excluded.

3. The following conditions require careful observation during medication: a history of severe depressive states, varicose veins, diabetes, hypertension, epilepsy, otosclerosis, multiple sclerosis, porphyria, tetany, disturbed liver function, gall-stones, cardiovascular diseases, renal diseases, chloasma, uterine fibroids, asthma, the wearing of contact lenses, or any disease that is prone to worsen during pregnancy. The first appearance or deterioration of any of these conditions may indicate that the oral contraceptive should be stopped.

4. The risk of the deterioration of chloasma, which is often not fully reversible, is reduced by the avoidance of excessive exposure to sunlight.

Menstrual changes:

1. Reduction of menstrual flow: This is not abnormal and it is to be expected in some patients.

2. Missed menstruation: Occasionally withdrawal bleeding may not occur at all. If the tablets have been taken correctly, pregnancy is very unlikely but should be ruled out before a new course of tablets is started.

Intermenstrual bleeding:

Very light "spotting" or heavier "break through bleeding" may occur during tablet-taking, especially in the first few cycles. It appears to be generally of no significance, except where it indicates errors of tablet-taking, or where the possibility of interaction with other drugs exists. However, if irregular bleeding is persistent an organic cause should be considered.

4.5 Interaction with other medicinal products and other forms of Interaction

Some drugs accelerate the metabolism of oral contraceptives when taken concurrently and these include barbiturates, phenytoin, phenylbutazone and rifampicin. Other drugs suspected of having the capacity to reduce the efficacy of oral contraceptives include ampicillin and other antibiotics. It is therefore, advisable to use non-hormonal methods of contraception (barriers and spermicides). Please refer to "4.2 Posology and Method of Administration, Interaction with other drugs.".

The response to metyrapone is less pronounced than in untreated women and is thus similar to that during pregnancy.

ACTH function test remains unchanged. Reduction in corticosteroid excretion and elevation of plasma corticosteroids are due to increased cortisol-binding capacity of the plasma proteins.

Serum protein-bound iodine levels should not be used for evaluation of thyroid function as levels may rise due to increased thyroid hormone binding capacity of plasma proteins.

Erythrocyte sedimentation may be accelerated in absence of any disease due to a change in the proportion of plasma protein fractions. Increases in plasma copper, iron and alkaline phosphatase have been recorded.

The herbal remedy St John's Wort *(Hypericum perforatum)* should not be taken concomitantly with this medicine as it could potentially lead to a loss of contraceptive effect.

4.6 Pregnancy and lactation

Pregnancy is a reason for stopping administration immediately because it has been suggested by some investigations that oral contraceptives taken in early pregnancy may slightly increase the risk of foetal malformations. Other investigations have failed to support these findings. The possibility, therefore, can not be excluded, but it is certain that if a risk exists at all, it is very small. After pregnancy combined oral contraception can be started in non-lactating women 21 days after a vaginal delivery, provided that the patient is fully ambulant and there are no puerperal complications. Please refer to "4.2 Posology and Method of Administration, Post-partum and Post-abortum use".

Administration of oestrogens to lactating women may decrease the quantity or quality of the milk.

4.7 Effects on ability to drive and use machines

None known.

4.8 Undesirable effects

See "4.4 Special Warnings and Special Precautions for Use".

There is an increased risk of venous thromboembolism for all women using a combined oral contraceptive. For information on differences in risk between oral contraceptives, see Section 4.4.

Occasional side-effects may include nausea, vomiting, headaches, breast tenderness, irregular bleeding or missed bleeds, changed body weight or libido, depressive moods, chloasma and altered serum lipid profile.

4.9 Overdose

There have been no reports of serious ill-effects from overdosage, even when a considerable number of tablets have been taken by a small child. In general, it is therefore unnecessary to treat overdosage. However, if overdosage is discovered within two or three hours and is so large that treatment seems desirable, gastric lavage can be safely used.

There are no specific antidotes and further treatment should be symptomatic.

5. PHARMACOLOGICAL PROPERTIES

5.1 Pharmacodynamic properties

Ethinylestradiol is a synthetic oestrogen which has actions and uses similar to those of oestradiol, but is more potent.

Norgestrel is a progestational agent with actions similar to those of progesterone. It is much more potent as an inhibitor of ovulation than norethisterone and has androgenic activity.

5.2 Pharmacokinetic properties

Ethinylestradiol is absorbed by the gastro-intestinal tract. It is only slowly metabolised and excreted in the urine.

Norgestrel is absorbed from the gastro-intestinal tract. Metabolites are excreted in the urine and faeces as glucuronide and sulphate conjugates.

5.3 Preclinical safety data

No pre-clinical safety data other than those described elsewhere in this document are considered relevant to the prescriber.

6. PHARMACEUTICAL PARTICULARS

6.1 List of excipients

Lactose

Maize starch

Povidone (E1201)

Magnesium stearate (E572)

Sucrose

Polyethylene glycol 6000

Calcium carbonate (E170)

Talc (E553b)

Glycerol (E442)

Titanium dioxide (E171)

Wax E

Iron oxide pigment (E172) red brown (light brown tablets)

Iron oxide pigment (E172) yellow (light brown and ochre tablets)

6.2 Incompatibilities

None known.

6.3 Shelf life

5 years

6.4 Special precautions for storage

Store at or below room temperature

6.5 Nature and contents of container

Primary container: Polyvinylchloride (PVC) / aluminium foil blister pack.

Secondary container: Cardboard carton.

Presentation: Memo pack containing 21 tablets -

6 light brown tablets: 50 micrograms Levonorgestrel / 30 micrograms Ethinylestradiol

5 white tablets: 75 micrograms Levonorgestrel / 40 micrograms Ethinylestradiol

10 ochre tablets: 125 micrograms Levonorgestrel / 30 micrograms Ethinylestradiol

6.6 Instructions for use and handling

Not applicable.

7. MARKETING AUTHORISATION HOLDER

John Wyeth and Brother Limited

Trading as Wyeth Laboratories

Huntercombe Lane South

Taplow

Maidenhead

Berkshire SL6 0PH

UK

8. MARKETING AUTHORISATION NUMBER(S)

PL 0011/0066

9. DATE OF FIRST AUTHORISATION/RENEWAL OF THE AUTHORISATION

Last renewal: 18th December 1995

10. DATE OF REVISION OF THE TEXT

3rd March 2003

TRINOVUM®

(Janssen-Cilag Ltd)

Presentation

TRINOVUM® oral contraceptive tablets are 1/4 inch diameter, circular tablets with flat faces and bevelled edges. The 7 white tablets contain 500 µg norethisterone and 35 µg ethinyloestradiol and are engraved C over 535 on each face. The 7 light peach coloured tablets contain 750 µg norethisterone and 35 µg ethinyloestradiol and are engraved C over 735 on each face. The 7 peach coloured tablets contain 1.0 mg norethisterone and 35 µg ethinyloestradiol and are engraved C over 135 on each face.

Uses

Contraception and the recognised indications for such oestrogen/progestogen combinations.

Action

Through the mechanism of gonadotrophin suppression by the oestrogenic and progestational actions of the ingredients.

Although the primary mechanism of action is inhibition of ovulation, alterations to the cervical mucus and to the endometrium may also contribute to the efficacy of the product.

Dosage and administration

It is preferable that tablet intake from the first pack is started on the first day of menstruation in which case no extra contraceptive precautions are necessary.

If menstruation has already begun (that is 2, 3 or 4 days previously), tablet taking should commence on day 5 of the menstrual period. In this case additional contraceptive precautions must be taken for the first 7 days of tablet taking. (See further information for additional contraceptive precautions.)

If menstruation began more than 5 days previously then the patient should be advised to wait until her next menstrual period before starting to take TRINOVUM®.

How to take TRINOVUM®:

One tablet is taken daily at the same time (preferably in the evening) without interruption for 21 days, followed by a break of 7 tablet-free days (a white tablet is taken every day for 7 days, then a pale peach coloured tablet every day for 7 days, then a peach coloured tablet every day for 7 days, then 7 tablet-free days). Each subsequent pack is started after the 7 tablet-free days have elapsed. Additional contraceptive precautions are not then required.

Use during pregnancy:

TRINOVUM® is contra-indicated for use during pregnancy or suspected pregnancy, since it has been suggested that combined oral contraceptives, in common with many other substances, might be capable of affecting the normal development of the child in the early stages of pregnancy. It can be definitely concluded, however, that, if a risk of abnormality exists at all, it must be very small.

Post-partum administration:

Following a vaginal delivery, oral contraceptive administration to non-breast feeding mothers can be started 21 days post-partum, provided the patient is fully ambulant and there are no puerperal complications. No additional contraceptive precautions are required. If post-partum administration begins more than 21 days after delivery, additional contraceptive precautions are required for the first 7 days of pill-taking. If intercourse has taken place post-partum, oral contraceptive use should be delayed until the first day of the first menstrual period.

N.B. Mothers who are breast feeding should be advised not to use the combined pill since this may reduce the amount of breast-milk, but may be advised instead to use a progestogen-only pill (POP).

After miscarriage or abortion administration should start immediately in which case no additional contraceptive precautions are required.

Changing from a 21 day pill or 22 day pill to TRINOVUM®:

All tablets in the old pack should be finished. The first TRINOVUM® tablet is taken the next day i.e. no gap is left between taking tablets nor does the patient need to wait for her period to begin. Tablets should be taken as instructed in 'How to take TRINOVUM®'. Additional contraceptive precautions are not required. The patient will not have a period until the end of the first TRINOVUM® pack, but this is not harmful, nor does it matter if she experiences some bleeding on tablet-taking days.

Changing from a combined Every Day Pill (28 day tablets) to TRINOVUM®:

TRINOVUM® should be started after taking the last active tablet from the 'Every Day Pill' pack (i.e. after taking 21 or 22 tablets). The first TRINOVUM® tablet is taken the next day i.e. no gap is left between taking tablets nor does the patient need to wait for her period to begin. Tablets should be taken as instructed in 'How to take TRINOVUM®'. Additional contraceptive precautions are not required. Remaining tablets from the Every Day (ED) pack should be discarded. The patient will not have a period until the end of the first TRINOVUM® pack, but this is not harmful, nor does it matter if she experiences some bleeding on tablet-taking days.

Changing from a Progestogen-only Pill (POP or Mini Pill) to TRINOVUM®:

The first TRINOVUM® tablet should be taken on the first day of the period, even if the patient has already taken a mini pill on that day. Tablets should be taken as instructed in 'How to take TRINOVUM®'. Additional contraceptive precautions are not required. All the remaining progestogen-only pills in the mini pill pack should be discarded.

If the patient is taking a (mini) pill, then she may not always have a period, especially when she is breast feeding. The first TRINOVUM® tablet should be taken on the day after stopping the mini pill. All remaining pills in the mini pill packet must be discarded. Additional contraceptive precautions must be taken for the first 7 days.

To skip a period:

To skip a period, a new pack of TRINOVUM® should be started on the day after finishing the current pack (the patient skips the tablet-free days). Tablet-taking should be continued in the usual way. During the use of the second pack she may experience slight spotting or break-through bleeding but contraceptive protection will not be diminished provided there are no tablet omissions.

The next pack of TRINOVUM® is started after the usual 7 tablet-free days, regardless of whether the period has completely finished or not.

Reduced reliability:

The reliability of TRINOVUM® may be reduced under the following circumstances.

Forgotten tablets:

For further advice on the above please see precautions and warnings.

Vomiting or diarrhoea:

For further advice on the above, please see precautions and warnings.

Interactions:

For further advice on the above, please see precautions and warnings.

Contra-indications, warnings, etc

Absolute contra-indications:

Pregnancy or suspected pregnancy (that cannot yet be excluded).

Circulatory disorders (cardiovascular or cerebrovascular) such as thrombophlebitis and thrombo-embolic processes, or a history of these conditions (including history of confirmed venous thrombo-embolism (VTE), family history of idiopathic VTE and other known risk factors for VTE), moderate to severe hypertension, hyperlipoproteinaemia. In addition the presence of more than one of the risk factors for arterial disease which are discussed under 'Serious adverse reactions'.

Severe liver disease, cholestatic jaundice or hepatitis (viral or non-viral) or a history of these conditions if the results of liver function tests have failed to return to normal, and for 3 months after liver function tests have been found to be normal; a history of jaundice of pregnancy or jaundice due to the use of steroids, Rotor syndrome and Dubin-Johnson syndrome, hepatic cell tumours and porphyria.

Cholelithiasis.

Known or suspected oestrogen-dependent tumours, (see 'Serious Adverse Reactions'); endometrial hyperplasia; undiagnosed vaginal bleeding.

Systemic lupus erythematosus or a history of this condition.

A history during pregnancy or previous use of steroids of: severe pruritus; herpes gestationis; a manifestation or deterioration of otosclerosis.

Relative contra-indications:

If any relative contra-indication listed below is present, the benefits of oestrogen/progestogen-containing preparations must be weighed against the possible risk for each individual case and the patient kept under close supervision. In case of aggravation or appearance of any of these conditions whilst the patient is taking the pill, its use should be discontinued.

- Conditions implicating an increasing risk of developing venous thrombo-embolic complications, e.g. severe varicose veins or prolonged immobilisation or major surgery (see Precautions and Warnings).
- Disorders of coagulation.
- Presence of any risk factor for arterial disease e.g. smoking, hyperlipidaemia or hypertension (see 'Serious Adverse Reactions').
- Other conditions associated with an increased risk of circulatory disease such as latent or overt cardiac failure, renal dysfunction, or a history of these conditions.
- Epilepsy or a history of this condition.
- Migraine or a history of this condition.
- A history of cholelithiasis.
- Presence of any risk factor for oestrogen-dependent tumours; oestrogen-sensitive gynaecological disorders such as uterine fibromyomata and endometriosis (see also under 'Serious Adverse Reactions').
- Diabetes mellitus.
- Severe depression or a history of this condition. If this is accompanied by a disturbance in tryptophan metabolism, administration of vitamin B6 might be of therapeutic value.
- Sickle cell haemoglobinopathy, since under certain circumstances, e.g. during infections or anoxia, oestrogen-containing preparations may induce thrombo-embolic process in patients with this condition.
- If the results of liver function tests become abnormal, use should be discontinued.

Precautions and Warnings

Reduced reliability:

When TRINOVUM® is taken according to the directions for use the occurrence of pregnancy is highly unlikely. However, the reliability of oral contraceptives may be reduced under the following circumstances:

(i) Forgotten tablets:

If the patient forgets to take a tablet, she should take it as soon as she remembers and take the next one at the normal time. This may mean that two tablets are taken in one day. Provided she is less than 12 hours late in taking her tablet, TRINOVUM® will still give contraceptive protection during this cycle and the rest of the pack should be taken as usual.

If she is more than 12 hours late in taking one or more tablets then she should take the last missed pill as soon as she remembers but leave the other missed pills in the pack. She should continue to take the rest of the pack as usual but must use extra precautions (e.g. sheath, diaphragm plus spermicide) and follow the '7-day rule' (see further information for '7-day rule'). If there are 7 or more pills left in the pack after the missed and delayed pills then the usual 7-day break can be left before starting the next pack. If there are less than 7 pills left in the pack after the missed and delayed pills then when the pack is finished the next pack should be started the next day. If withdrawal bleeding does not occur at the end of the second pack then a pregnancy test should be performed.

(ii) Vomiting or diarrhoea:

If after tablet intake vomiting or diarrhoea occurs, a tablet may not be absorbed properly by the body. If the symptoms disappear within 12 hours of tablet-taking, the patient should take an extra tablet from a spare pack and continue with the rest of the pack as usual.

However, if the symptoms continue beyond those 12 hours, additional contraceptive precautions are necessary for any sexual intercourse during the stomach or bowel upset and for the following 7 days (the patient must be advised to follow the '7-day rule').

(iii) Change in bleeding pattern:

If after taking TRINOVUM® for several months there is a sudden occurrence of spotting or break-through bleeding (not observed in previous cycles) or the absence of withdrawal bleeding, contraceptive effectiveness may be reduced. If withdrawal bleeding fails to occur and none of the above mentioned events has taken place, pregnancy is highly unlikely and oral contraceptive use can be continued until the end of the next pack.

(If withdrawal bleeding fails to occur at the end of the second cycle, tablet intake should be discontinued and pregnancy excluded before oral contraceptive use can be resumed.) However, if withdrawal bleeding is absent and any of the above mentioned events has occurred, tablet intake should be discontinued and pregnancy excluded before oral contraceptive use can be resumed.

Interactions

Irregular cycles and reduced reliability of oral contraceptives may occur when these preparations are used concomitantly with drugs such as anticonvulsants, barbiturates, antibiotics, (e.g. tetracyclines, ampicillin, rifampicin, etc.), griseofulvin, activated charcoal and certain laxatives. Special consideration should be given to patients being treated with antibiotics for acne. They should be advised to use a non-hormonal method of contraception, or to use an oral contraceptive containing a progestogen showing minimal androgenicity, which have been reported as helping to improve acne without using an antibiotic. Oral contraceptives may diminish glucose tolerance and increase the need for insulin or other antidiabetic drugs in diabetics.

The herbal remedy St John's Wort *(Hypericum perforatum)* should not be taken concomitantly with this medicine as this could potentially lead to a loss of contraceptive effect.

Medical examination/consultation:

Assessment of women prior to starting oral contraceptives (and at regular intervals thereafter) should include a personal and family medical history of each woman. Physical examination should be guided by this and by the contra-indications (Section 4.3) and warnings (Section 4.4) for this product. The frequency and nature of these assessments should be based upon relevant guidelines and should be adapted to the individual woman, but should include measurement of blood pressure and, if judged appropriate by the clinician, breast, abdominal and pelvic examination including cervical cytology.

Caution should be observed when prescribing oral contraceptives to young women whose cycles are not yet stabilised.

Venous thrombo-embolic disease

An increased risk of venous thrombo-embolic disease (VTE) associated with the use of oral contraceptives is well established but is smaller than that associated with pregnancy, which has been estimated at 60 cases per 100,000 pregnancies. Some epidemiological studies have reported a greater risk of VTE for women using combined oral contraceptives containing desogestrel or gestodene (the so-called 'third generation' pills) than for women using pills containing levonorgestrel or norethisterone (the so-called 'second generation' pills).

The spontaneous incidence of VTE in healthy non-pregnant women (not taking any oral contraceptive) is about 5 cases per 100,000 per year. The incidence in users of second generation pills is about 15 per 100,000 women per year of use. The incidence in users of third generation pills is about 25 cases per 100,000 women per year of use; this excess incidence has not been satisfactorily explained by bias or confounding. The level of all of these risks of VTE increases with age and is likely to be further increased in women with other known risk factors for VTE such as obesity. The excess risk of VTE is highest during the first year a woman ever uses a combined oral contraceptive.

Surgery, varicose veins or immobilisation

In patients using oestrogen-containing preparations the risk of deep vein thrombosis may be temporarily increased when undergoing a major operation (e.g. abdominal, orthopaedic), any surgery to the legs, medical treatment for varicose veins or prolonged immobilisation. Therefore, it is advisable to discontinue oral contraceptive use at least 4 to 6 weeks prior to these procedures if performed electively and to (re)start not less than 2 weeks after full ambulation. The latter is also valid with regard to immobilisation after an accident or emergency surgery. In case of emergency surgery, thrombotic prophylaxis is usually indicated e.g. with subcutaneous heparin.

Chloasma

Chloasma may occasionally occur, especially in women with a history of chloasma gravidarum. Women with a tendency to chloasma should avoid exposure to the sun or ultraviolet radiation whilst taking this preparation. Chloasma is often not fully reversible.

Laboratory tests

The use of steroids may influence the results of certain laboratory tests. In the literature, at least a hundred different parameters have been reported to possibly be influenced by oral contraceptive use, predominantly by the oestrogenic component. Among these are: biochemical parameters of the liver, thyroid, adrenal and renal function, plasma levels of (carrier) proteins and lipid/lipoprotein fractions and parameters of coagulation and fibrinolysis.

Adverse reactions

Various adverse reactions have been associated with oral contraceptive use. The serious reactions are dealt with in more detail. The first appearance of symptoms indicative of any one of these reactions necessitates immediate cessation of oral contraceptive use while appropriate diagnostic and therapeutic measures are undertaken.

Serious adverse reactions

There is a general opinion, based on statistical evidence that users of combined oral contraceptives experience more often than non-users various disorders of the circulation. How often these disorders occur in users of modern low-oestrogen oral contraceptives is unknown, but there are reasons for suggesting that they may occur less often than with the older types of pill which contain more oestrogen.

Various reports have associated oral contraceptive use with the occurrence of deep venous thrombosis, pulmonary embolism and other embolisms. Other investigations of these oral contraceptives have suggested an increased risk or oestrogen and /or progestogen dose-dependent coronary and cerebrovascular accidents, predominantly in heavy smokers. Thrombosis has very rarely been reported to occur in other veins or arteries, e.g. hepatic, mesenteric, renal or retinal.

It should be noted that there is no consensus about the often contradictory findings obtained in early studies. The physician should bear in mind the possibility of vascular accidents occurring and that there may not be full recovery from such disorders and they may be fatal. The physician should take into account the presence of risk factors for arterial disease and deep venous thrombosis when prescribing oral contraceptives. Risk factors for arterial disease include smoking, the presence of hyperlipidaemia, hypertension or diabetes.

Signs and symptoms of a thrombotic event may include: sudden severe pain in the chest, whether or not reaching to the left arm; sudden breathlessness; any unusual severe, prolonged headache, especially if it occurs for the first time or gets progressively worse, or is associated with any of the following symptoms: sudden partial or complete loss of vision or diplopia, aphasia, vertigo, a bad fainting attack or collapse with or without focal epilepsy, weakness or very marked numbness suddenly affecting one side or one part of the body, motor disturbances; severe pain in the calf of one leg; acute abdomen.

Cigarette smoking increases the risk of serious cardiovascular adverse reactions to oral contraceptive use. The risk increases with age and with heavy smoking and is more marked in women over 35 years of age. Women who use oral contraceptives should be strongly advised not to smoke.

The use of oestrogen-containing oral contraceptives may promote growth of existing sex steroid dependent tumours. For this reason, the use of these oral contraceptives in patients with such tumours is contra-indicated.

Numerous epidemiological studies have been reported of the risk or ovarian, endometrial, cervical and breast cancer in women using combined oral contraceptives.

The evidence is clear that combined oral contraceptives offer substantial protection against both ovarian and endometrial cancer. An increased risk of cervical cancer in long term users of combined oral contraceptives has been reported in some studies, but there continues to be controversy about the extent to which this is attributable to the confounding effects of sexual behaviour and other factors.

A meta-analysis from 54 epidemiological studies reported that there is a slightly increased relative risk (RR = 1.24) of having breast cancer diagnosed in women who are currently using combined oral contraceptives (COCs). The observed pattern of increased risk may be due to an earlier diagnosis of breast cancer in COC users, the biological effects of COCs or a combination of both. The additional breast cancers diagnosed in current users of COCs or in women who have used COCs in the last 10 years are more likely to be localised to the breast than those in women who never used COCs.

Breast cancer is rare among women under 40 years of age whether or not they take COCs. Whilst this background risk increases with age, the excess number of breast cancer diagnoses in current and recent COC users is small in relation to the overall risk of breast cancer (see bar chart).

Figure 1

Estimated number of breast cancers found in 10,000 women who took the Pill for 5 years then stopped, or who never took the Pill

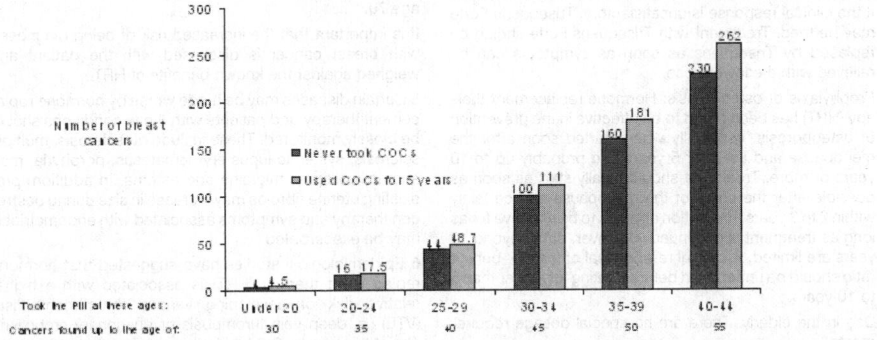

The most important risk factor for breast cancer in COC users is the age women discontinue the COC; the older the age at stopping, the more breast cancers are diagnosed. Duration of use is less important and the excess risk gradually disappears during the course of the 10 years after stopping COC use such that by 10 years there appears to be no excess.

The possible increase in risk of breast cancer should be discussed with the user and weighed against the benefits of COCs taking into account the evidence that they offer substantial protection against the risk of developing certain other cancers (eg ovarian and endometrial cancer).

(see Figure 1 above)

Malignant hepatic tumours have been reported on rare occasions in long-term users of oral contraceptives. Benign hepatic tumours have also been associated with oral contraceptive usage. A hepatic tumour should be considered in the differential diagnosis when upper abdominal pain, enlarged liver or signs of intra-abdominal haemorrhage occur.

The use of oral contraceptives may sometimes lead to the development of cholestatic jaundice or cholelithiasis.

On rare occasions the use of oral contraceptives may trigger or reactivate systemic lupus erythematosus.

A further rare complication of oral contraceptive use is the occurrence of chorea which can be reversed by discontinuing the pill. The majority of cases of oral-contraceptive-induced chorea show a pre-existing predisposition which often relates to acute rheumatism.

Other adverse reactions:

Cardiovascular System

Rise of blood pressure. If hypertension develops, treatment should be discontinued.

Genital Tract

Intermenstrual bleeding, post-medication amenorrhoea, changes in cervical secretion, increase in size of uterine fibromyomata, aggravation of endometriosis, certain vaginal infections, e.g. candidiasis.

Breast

Tenderness, pain, enlargement, secretion.

Gastro Intestinal Tract

Nausea, vomiting, cholelithiasis, cholestatic jaundice.

Skin

Erythema nodosum, rash, chloasma, erythema multiforme, hirsutism, loss of scalp hair.

Eyes

Discomfort of the cornea if contact lenses are used.

CNS

Headache, migraine, mood changes, depression.

Metabolic

Fluid retention, change in body weight, reduced glucose tolerance.

Other

Changes in libido, leg cramps, premenstrual -like syndrome.

Overdosage

There have been no reports of serious ill-health from overdosage even when a considerable number of tablets have been taken by a small child. In general, it is therefore unnecessary to treat overdosage. However, if overdosage is discovered within 2 or 3 hours and is large, then gastric lavage can be safely used. There are no antidotes and further treatment should be symptomatic.

Further Information

Additional contraceptive precautions

When additional contraceptive precautions are required the patient should be advised either not to have sex, or to use a cap plus spermicide or for her partner to use a condom. Rhythm methods should not be advised as the pill disrupts the usual cyclical changes associated with the natural menstrual cycle e.g. changes in temperature and cervical mucus.

The 7-day rule

If any one tablet is forgotten for more than 12 hours.

If the patient has vomiting or diarrhoea for more than 12 hours.

If the patient is taking any of the drugs listed under 'Interactions':

The patient should continue to take her tablets as usual

• and additional contraceptive precautions must be taken for the next 7 days.

BUT - if these 7 days run beyond the end of the current pack, the next pack must be started as soon as the current one is finished, i.e. no gap should be left between packs. (This prevents an extended break in tablet taking which may increase the risk of the ovaries releasing an egg and thus reducing contraceptive protection.) The patient will not have a period until the end of 2 packs but this is not harmful nor does it matter if she experiences some bleeding on tablet taking days.

Pharmaceutical precautions

Store at room temperature (below 25°C).

Protect from light.

Legal Category

POM

Package quantities

Carton containing 3 push packs of 21 tablets - sufficient for 3 cycles.

Product Licence Number

0242/0279

Product Licence Holder

Janssen-Cilag Limited
Saunderton
High Wycombe
Buckinghamshire
HP14 4HJ
UK

Date of preparation

18 December 2001

Trisequens

(Novo Nordisk Limited)

1. NAME OF THE MEDICINAL PRODUCT

Trisequens®

2. QUALITATIVE AND QUANTITATIVE COMPOSITION

28 sequential tablets: 12 blue, 10 white, 6 red.

Active ingredients:

Blue tablets - Estradiol hemihydrate EP corresponding to estradiol 2mg

White tablets - Estradiol hemihydrate EP corresponding to estradiol 2mg

Norethisterone acetate EP 1mg

Red tablets - Estradiol hemihydrate EP corresponding to estradiol 1mg

3. PHARMACEUTICAL FORM

Film-coated tablets for oral administration.

4. CLINICAL PARTICULARS

4.1 Therapeutic indications

a) The treatment of symptoms due to oestrogen deficiency.

b) Second line therapy for prevention of osteoporosis in postmenopausal women at high risk of future fractures who are intolerant of, or contraindicated for, other medicinal products approved for the prevention of osteoporosis.

4.2 Posology and method of administration

4.2.1 **Dosage**: Adults: Menopausal symptoms and prophylaxis of osteoporosis.

Trisequens is administered orally, without chewing, one tablet daily without interruption, starting with the blue tablets. Treatment should be instituted with Trisequens. If the clinical response is unsatisfactory, Trisequens Forte may be tried. Treatment with Trisequens Forte should be replaced by Trisequens as soon as symptoms can be relieved with the lower dose.

Prophylaxis of osteoporosis: Hormone replacement therapy (HRT) has been found to be effective in the prevention of osteoporosis, especially when started soon after the menopause and used for 5 years and probably up to 10 years or more. Treatment should ideally start as soon as possible after the onset of the menopause and certainly within 2 to 3 years. Protection appears to be effective for as long as treatment is continued. However, data beyond 10 years are limited. A careful re-appraisal of the risk-benefit ratio should be undertaken before treating for longer than 5 to 10 years.

Use in the elderly: There are no special dosage requirements.

Not intended for children or males.

4.2.2 Administration: In menstruating women the first tablet should be taken on the fifth day of menstrual bleeding. If menstruation has stopped altogether or is infrequent and sporadic (2-4 monthly intervals) the first tablet can be taken at any time.

A regular shedding of the endometrium is usually induced during the red tablet phase or at the end of the white tablet phase.

Before initiation of therapy it is recommended that the patient is fully informed of all likely benefits and potential risks.

Since progestogens are only administered to protect against hyperplastic changes of the endometrium, patients without a uterus should be treated with an oestrogen-only preparation.

4.3 Contraindications

1 Known, suspected or past history of cancer of the breast.

2 Known or suspected oestrogen-dependent neoplasia.

3 Undiagnosed irregular vaginal bleeding.

4 Known or suspected pregnancy.

5 Active deep venous thrombosis, thromboembolic disorders or a history of confirmed venous thromboembolism.

6 Active or chronic liver disease or history of liver disease where the liver function tests have failed to return to normal.

7 Rotor's syndrome or Dubin-Johnson syndrome.

8 Severe cardiac or renal disease.

9 Hypersensitivity to one or more of the constituents.

4.4 Special warnings and special precautions for use

1 Assessment of each woman prior to taking hormone replacement therapy (and at regular intervals thereafter) should include a personal and family medical history. Physical examination should be guided by this and by the contraindications (section 4.3) and warnings (section 4.4) for this product. During assessment of each individual woman clinical examination of the breasts and pelvic examination should be performed where clinically indicated rather than as a routine procedure. Women should be encouraged to participate in the national breast cancer screening programme (mammography) and the national cervical cancer screening programme (cervical cytology) as appropriate for their age. Breast awareness should also be encouraged and women advised to report any changes in their breasts to their doctor or nurse.

2 Endometrial assessment should be carried out if indicated; this may be particularly relevant in patients who are, or who have been, treated with oestrogen unopposed by a progestogen.

In the female there is an increased risk of endometrial hyperplasia and carcinoma associated with unopposed oestrogen administered long term (for more than one year). However, the appropriate addition of a progestogen to an oestrogen regimen lowers this additional risk.

3 If abnormal or irregular vaginal bleeding occurs during or shortly after therapy, diagnostic measures, including endometrial sampling when indicated, should be undertaken to rule out the possibility of uterine malignancy.

4 A reanalysis of original data from 51 epidemiological studies reported a small or moderate increase in the probability of having breast cancer *diagnosed* in women currently or recently using HRT. The findings may be due to biological effects of HRT, earlier diagnosis, or a combination of both. The relative risk increased with duration of treatment (by 2.3% per year of use) and returned to normal in the course of five years after cessation of HRT use. This is comparable to the increase in relative risk when natural menopause is delayed in the absence of HRT. Breast cancers diagnosed in current or recent users of HRT are more likely to be localised to the breast than those found in non-users. HRT use may not be associated with increased mortality from breast cancer.

Between the ages of 50 and 70, about 45 women in every 1000 not using HRT will have breast cancer diagnosed. It is estimated that among those who use HRT for 5 years starting at age 50, 2 extra cases of breast cancer will be detected by age 70 in every 1000 women. For those who use HRT for 10 years there will be 6 extra cases of breast cancer, and for 15 years use, 12 extra cases of breast cancer in every 1000 women during the 20 year period until age 70.

It is important that the increased risk of being diagnosed with breast cancer is discussed with the patient and weighed against the known benefits of HRT.

5 Certain diseases may be made worse by hormone replacement therapy and patients with these conditions should be closely monitored. These include otosclerosis, multiple sclerosis, systemic lupus erythematosus, porphyria, melanoma, epilepsy, migraine and asthma. In addition, pre-existing uterine fibroids may increase in size during oestrogen therapy and symptoms associated with endometriosis may be exacerbated.

6 Epidemiological studies have suggested that hormone replacement therapy (HRT) is associated with a higher relative risk of developing venous thromboembolism (VTE) i.e. deep vein thrombosis or pulmonary embolism. The studies find a 2-3 fold higher risk for users compared with non-users which for healthy women amounts to one extra case of VTE each year for every 5000 patients taking HRT.

Generally recognised risk factors for VTE include a personal history or family history and severe obesity (Body Mass Index >30 kg/m^2). In women with these factors the benefits of treatment with HRT need to be carefully weighed against the risks. There is no consensus about the possible role of varicose veins in VTE.

The risk of VTE may be temporarily increased with prolonged immobilisation, major trauma or major surgery. In women on HRT scrupulous attention should be given to prophylactic measures to prevent VTE following surgery. Where prolonged immobilisation is likely to follow elective surgery, particularly abdominal or orthopaedic surgery to the lower limbs, consideration should be given to temporarily stopping HRT 4 weeks earlier, if possible.

If venous thromboembolism develops after initiating therapy the drug should be discontinued.

7 Oestrogens may cause fluid retention and, therefore, patients with cardiac or renal dysfunction should be carefully observed.

8 If jaundice, migraine-like headaches, visual disturbance or a significant increase in blood pressure develop after initiating therapy, the medication should be discontinued while the cause is investigated.

9 Trisequens is not a contraceptive, neither will it restore fertility.

10 Most studies indicate that oestrogen replacement therapy has little effect on blood pressure and some indicate that oestrogen use may be associated with a small decrease in B.P. In addition, most studies on combined therapy, including Trisequens, indicate that the addition of a progestogen also has little effect on blood pressure. Rarely, idiosyncratic hypertension may occur.

However, when oestrogens are administered to hypertensive women, supervision is necessary and blood pressure should be monitored at regular intervals.

11 Diabetic patients should be carefully observed when initiating hormone replacement therapy, as worsening glucose tolerance may occur.

12 Changed oestrogen levels may affect certain endocrine and liver function tests.

13 It has been reported that there is an increase in the risk of surgically confirmed gall bladder disease in women receiving postmenopausal oestrogens.

4.5 Interaction with other medicinal products and other forms of Interaction

May potentiate side effects of phenothiazines. Drugs such as barbiturates, phenytoin and rifampicin, which induce the activity of hepatic microsomal drug metabolising enzymes, may decrease the effectiveness of Trisequens. Mineral oil may decrease the intestinal absorption of Trisequens.

4.6 Pregnancy and lactation

Trisequens is contra-indicated during pregnancy and lactation.

4.7 Effects on ability to drive and use machines

No effects known.

4.8 Undesirable effects

The following side effects have been reported with oestrogen/progestogen therapy:

1 Genitourinary system: irregular vaginal bleeding, premenstrual-like syndrome, increase in size of uterine fibromyomata.

2 Breasts - tenderness, enlargement, secretion.

3 Gastrointestinal - nausea, vomiting, abdominal cramps, bloating, cholestatic jaundice.

4 Skin - chloasma or melasma which may persist when drug is discontinued, erythema multiforme, erythema nodosum, haemorrhagic eruption, loss of scalp hair, hirsutism.

5 Eyes - steepening of corneal curvature, intolerance to contact lenses.

6 CNS - headaches, migraine, dizziness, mental depression, chorea.

7 Miscellaneous - increase or decrease in weight, reduced carbohydrate tolerance, aggravation of porphyria, oedema, change in libido, leg cramps.

4.9 Overdose

Overdosage may be manifested by nausea and vomiting. There is no specific antidote and treatment should be symptomatic.

5. PHARMACOLOGICAL PROPERTIES

5.1 Pharmacodynamic properties

The oestrogen component of Trisequens substitutes for the loss of endogenous oestrogen production which occurs in women around the time of the menopause, whilst the progestogen component counteracts hyperstimulation of the endometrium. A regular shedding of the endometrium is usually induced during the red tablet phase or at the end of the white tablet phase. Studies based on measurement of bone mineral content have shown that Trisequens is effective in the prevention of progressive bone loss following the menopause.

During treatment with Trisequens total cholesterol and LDL-C are lowered significantly whereas HDL-C and triglycerides are unchanged.

5.2 Pharmacokinetic properties

The micronised 17β-estradiol in Trisequens is absorbed rapidly and efficiently from the gastrointestinal tract, reaching a peak plasma concentration in 2-4 hours. Following administration of Trisequens, the steady state plasma level of estradiol ranges from between 70-100 pg/ml. Estradiol has a half life of approximately 14-16 hours. In the blood stream more than 90% of estradiol is bound to plasma proteins. Estradiol is oxidized to oestrone, which is converted to oestriol. Both transformations take place mainly in the liver. Oestrogens are excreted into the bile and then undergo reabsorption from the intestine. During this enterohepatic circulation, degradation occurs. Estradiol and its metabolites are excreted either in the urine (90-95%) as biologically inactive glucuronide and sulphate conjugates or in the faeces (5-10%) mostly unconjugated.

Norethisterone acetate is rapidly absorbed and transformed to norethisterone, then metabolised and excreted as glucuronide and sulphate conjugates. About half the dose is recovered in the urine within 24 hours, the remainder being reduced to less than 1% of the dose within 5-6 days. The mean plasma half life is 3-6 hours.

6. PHARMACEUTICAL PARTICULARS

6.1 List of excipients

Lactose monohydrate

Maize starch

Gelatin

Talc

Magnesium stearate

Methyl hydroxypropyl cellulose

Purified water

Blue tablets: Indigo carmine (E132)

Titanium dioxide (E171)

Polyethylene glycol

White tablets: Triacetin

Red tablets: Iron oxide (E172)

Titanium dioxide (E171)

Propylene glycol

6.2 Incompatibilities

None known.

6.3 Shelf life

48 months.

6.4 Special precautions for storage

Store in a dry place, protected from light. Store below 25°C. Do not refrigerate.

6.5 Nature and contents of container

Polypropylene/polystyrene calendar dial pack containing 28 tablets. Calendar dial packs (3 × 28 tablets) are contained within outer carton.

6.6 Instructions for use and handling

Each carton contains a patient information leaflet with instructions for use of the calendar dial pack.

7. MARKETING AUTHORISATION HOLDER

Novo Nordisk Limited

Broadfield Park, Brighton Road

Crawley, West Sussex, RH11 9RT

8. MARKETING AUTHORISATION NUMBER(S)

PL 3132/0122.

9. DATE OF FIRST AUTHORISATION/RENEWAL OF THE AUTHORISATION

29 January 1998.

10. DATE OF REVISION OF THE TEXT

February 1998, April 1999, April 2001, April 2002, December 2003

LEGAL CATEGORY

Prescription-only medicine (POM).

Tritace Tablets

(sanofi-aventis)

1. NAME OF THE MEDICINAL PRODUCT

Tritace 1.25 mg Tablets

Tritace 2.5 mg Tablets

Tritace 5 mg Tablets

Tritace 10 mg Tablets

2. QUALITATIVE AND QUANTITATIVE COMPOSITION

1.25 mg ramipril.

2.5 mg ramipril.

5 mg ramipril

10 mg ramipril.

For excipients, see 6.1.

3. PHARMACEUTICAL FORM

Tablet

1.25mg: White to almost white oblong tablets with score-line.

Upper stamp: 1.25 & logo ( )

Lower stamp: HMN & 1.25

2.5mg: Yellowish to yellow oblong tablets with score-line.

Upper stamp: 2.5 & logo ( )

Lower stamp: HMR & 2.5

5mg: Pale red oblong tablets with score-line.

Upper stamp: 5 & logo ( )

Lower stamp: HMP & 5.

10mg: White to almost white, oblong tablets with a score-line

Upper stamp: HMO/HMO

Lower stamp: anonymous

4. CLINICAL PARTICULARS

4.1 Therapeutic indications

For reducing the risk of myocardial infarction, stroke, cardiovascular death or need for revascularisation procedures in patients of 55 years or more who have clinical evidence of cardiovascular disease (previous MI, unstable angina or multivessel CABG or multivessel PTCA), stroke or peripheral vascular disease.

Also for reducing the risk of myocardial infarction, stroke, cardiovascular death or need for revascularisation procedures in diabetic patients of 55 years or more who have one or more of the following clinical findings: hypertension (systolic blood pressure > 160mmHg or diastolic blood pressure > 90mmHg); high total cholesterol > 5.2 mmol/L); low HDL (< 0.9 mmol/L); current smoker; known microalbuminuria; clinical evidence of previous vascular disease.

Tritace is indicated for the treatment of mild to moderate hypertension.

Congestive heart failure as adjunctive therapy to diuretics with or without cardiac glycosides.

Tritace has been shown to reduce mortality when given to patients surviving acute myocardial infarction with clinical evidence of heart failure.

4.2 Posology and method of administration

Oral administration.

Dosage and Administration:

Reducing the risk of myocardial infarction, stroke or cardiovascular death and/or the need for revascularisation procedures: The recommended initial dose is 2.5mg Tritace once a day. Depending on the tolerability, the dose should be gradually increased. It is therefore recommended that this dose is doubled after about one week of treatment then, after a further 3 weeks, it should be finally increased to 10mg. The usual maintenance dose is 10mg Tritace once a day. Patients already stabilised on lower doses of Tritace for other indications where possible should be titrated to 10mg Tritace once daily.

Hypertension: ([a-z])he recommended initial dosage in patients not on diuretics and without congestive heart failure is 1.25 mg Tritace once a day. Dosage should be increased incrementally at intervals of 1 – 2 weeks, based on patient response, up to a maximum of 10 mg once a day.

A 1.25 mg dose will only achieve a therapeutic response in a minority of patients. The usual maintenance dose is 2.5 -—5 mg as a single daily dose. If the patient response is still unsatisfactory at a dose of 10 mg Tritace, combination treatment is recommended.

In hypertensive patients who also have congestive heart failure, with or without associated renal insufficiency, symptomatic hypotension has been observed after treatment with ACE inhibitors. In these patients therapy should be started at a dose of 1.25 mg under close medical supervision in hospital.

Congestive heart failure: Recommended initial dose: In patients stabilised on diuretic therapy the initial dose is 1.25 mg once daily. Depending on the patient's response, the dose may be increased. It is recommended that the dose, if increased, be doubled at intervals of 1 to 2 weeks. If a daily dose of 2.5 mg or more is required, this may be taken as a single dose or as two divided doses. Maximum permitted daily dose: 10 mg.

Post myocardial infarction: Initiation of therapy: Treatment must be started in hospital between day 3 and day 10 following AMI. The starting dose is 2.5 mg twice a day which is increased to 5 mg twice a day after 2 days. If the initial 2.5 mg dose is not tolerated a dose of 1.25 mg twice a day should be given for two days before increasing to 2.5 mg and 5.0 mg twice a day. If the dose cannot be increased to 2.5 mg twice a day treatment should be withdrawn.

Sufficient experience is still lacking in the treatment of patients with severe (NYHA IV) heart failure immediately after myocardial infarction. Should the decision be taken to treat these patients, it is recommended that therapy be started at 1.25mg once daily and that particular caution be exercised in any dose increase.

Maintenance dose: 2.5 to 5.0 mg twice a day.

Maximum daily dose: 10mg.

Patients on diuretics/Patients with salt depletion: In diuretic treated patients, the diuretic should be discontinued for 2-3 days (or longer depending on the duration of action of the diuretic), or at least the dose reduced, to reduce the likelihood of symptomatic hypotension. It may be resumed later if required. The initial daily dose in patients previously treated with a diuretic is generally 1.25mg Tritace.

In patients with incompletely corrected fluid or salt depletion, in patients with severe hypertension, as well as in patients in whom a hypotensive reaction would constitute a particular risk, (e.g., with relevant stenoses of the coronary or cerebral vessels), a reduced initial dose of 1.25mg Tritace should be considered.

Dosage adjustment in renal impairment: The usual dose of Tritace is recommended for patients with a creatinine clearance > 30 ml/min (serum creatinine < 165 μmol/l). For patients with a creatinine clearance < 30 ml/min (serum creatinine >165 μmol/l) the initial dose is 1.25 mg Tritace once daily and the maximum dose 5 mg Tritace once daily.

In patients with severe renal impairment (creatinine clearance < 10 ml/min and serum creatinine of 400-650 μmol/l), the recommended initial dose is also 1.25 mg Tritace once a day, but the maintenance dose should not exceed 2.5 mg Tritace once a day.

Dosage in hepatic impairment: In patients with impaired liver function the metabolism of the parent compound ramipril, and therefore the formation of the bioactive metabolite ramiprilat, is delayed due to a diminished activity of esterases in the liver, resulting in elevated plasma ramipril levels. Treatment with ramipril should therefore be initiated at a dose of 1.25 mg under close medical supervision in patients with impaired liver function. Higher doses should be used with caution.

Elderly: Caution in all elderly patients especially those with concomitant use of diuretics, congestive heart failure or renal or hepatic insufficiency. A reduced initial dose of 1.25mg Tritace should be considered. The dose should then be titrated accordingly

Children: Tritace has not been studied in children, and therefore use in this age group is not recommended.

Tritace should be taken with a glass of water. The absorption of ramipril is not affected by food.

4.3 Contraindications

Hypersensitivity to ramipril, any of the excipients of Tritace, or to any other ACE inhibitor.

History of angioneurotic oedema.

Haemodynamically relevant renal artery stenosis.

Hypotensive or haemodynamically unstable patients.

Pregnancy.

Lactation.

4.4 Special warnings and special precautions for use

Warnings:

Angioneurotic oedema occurring during treatment with an ACE inhibitor necessitates immediate discontinuation of the drug. Angioneurotic oedema may involve the tongue, glottis or larynx and hospitalisation of the patient is advisable.

Tritace should not be used in patients with aortic or mitral valve stenosis or outflow obstruction (see Precautions section below).

Precautions:

Assessment of renal function: Evaluation of the patient should include assessment of renal function prior to initiation of therapy and during treatment.

Impaired renal function: Patients with renal insufficiency may require reduced or less frequent doses of Tritace; their renal function should be closely monitored. In the majority, renal function will not alter. There is a risk of impairment of renal function, particularly in patients with congestive heart failure or after a renal transplant, renal insufficiency, bilateral renal artery stenosis and unilateral renal artery stenosis in the single kidney. In the latter patient group, even a small increase in serum creatinine may be indicative of unilateral loss of renal function. If recognised early, such impairment of renal function is reversible upon discontinuation of therapy.

Patients haemodialysed using high flux polyacrylonitrile ('AN69') membranes are highly likely to experience anaphylactoid reactions if they are treated with ACE inhibitors. This combination should therefore be avoided, either by use of alternative antihypertensive drugs or alternative membranes for dialysis.

Similar reactions have been observed during low-density lipoprotein apheresis with dextran sulphate. This method should, therefore, not be used in patients treated with ACE inhibitors.

Some hypertensive patients with no apparent pre-existing renal disease may develop minor and usually transient increases in blood urea nitrogen and serum creatinine when Tritace is given, in particular concomitantly with a diuretic. Dosage reduction of Tritace and/or discontinuation of the diuretic may be required.

Impaired liver function: As ramipril is a prodrug metabolised to its active moiety in the liver, particular caution and close monitoring should be applied to patients with impaired liver function. The metabolism of the parent compound, and therefore the formation of the bioactive metabolite ramiprilat, may be diminished resulting in markedly elevated plasma levels of the parent compound (due to the reduced activity of esterases in the liver).

In patients in whom severe liver cirrhosis with oedema and/or ascites is present, the renin angiotensin system may be significantly activated; therefore, particular caution must be exercised in treating these patients (see also above and under "4.2 Posology and Method of Administration").

Symptomatic hypotension: In patients with uncomplicated hypertension, symptomatic hypotension has been observed rarely after the initial dose of Tritace as well as after increasing the dose of Tritace. It is more likely to occur in patients who have been volume- and salt-depleted by prolonged diuretic therapy, dietary salt restriction, dialysis, diarrhoea, vomiting or patients with severe heart failure. Therefore, in these patients, diuretic therapy should be discontinued and volume and/or salt depletion should be corrected before initiating therapy with Tritace.

Agranulocytosis and bone marrow depression: In patients on angiotensin converting enzyme inhibitors agranulocytosis and bone marrow depression have been seen rarely, as well as a reduction in red cell count, haemoglobin content and platelet count. These are more frequent in patients with renal impairment, especially if they have a collagen vascular disease. Regular monitoring of white blood cell counts (to permit detection of a possible leucopenia) and protein levels in urine should be considered in patients with collagen vascular disease (e.g. lupus erythematosus and scleroderma), especially associated with impaired renal function and concomitant therapy particularly with corticosteroids and anti metabolites. Patients on allopurinol, immunosuppressants and other substances that may change the blood picture also have increased likelihood of other blood picture changes.

Hyperkalaemia: Elevated serum potassium has been observed very rarely in hypertensive patients. Risk factors for the development of hyperkalaemia include renal insufficiency, potassium sparing diuretics and the concomitant use of agents to treat hypokalaemia. It is recommended that serum potassium be monitored regularly. More frequent monitoring of serum potassium is necessary in patients with impaired renal function.

Patients with hyper-stimulated renin angiotensin system: In the treatment of patients with a hyper-stimulated renin angiotensin system, particular caution must be exercised (see also under "4.2 Posology and Method of Administration"). Such patients are at risk of an acute pronounced fall in blood pressure and deterioration of renal function due to ACE inhibition, especially when an ACE inhibitor or a concomitant diuretic is given for the first time or for the first time at an increased dose. Initial doses or initial dose increases must be accompanied by close blood pressure monitoring until such time as no further acute reduction in blood pressure is to be anticipated.

Significant activation of the renin angiotensin system is to be anticipated, for example:

- in patients with severe and/or malignant hypertension.
- in patients with heart failure, particularly if severe or if treated with other substances having antihypertensive potential.
- in patients with haemodynamically relevant left-ventricular inflow or outflow obstruction (e.g., aortic or mitral valve stenosis).
- in patients pre-treated with diuretics.
- in patients with fluid or salt depletion, or in those whom it may develop (as a result of insufficient fluid or salt intake, or as a result of, e.g., dialysis, diarrhoea, vomiting or excessive sweating in cases where salt and fluid replacement is inadequate).

Generally, it is recommended that dehydration, hypovolaemia or salt depletion be corrected before initiating treatment (in patients with heart failure, however, such corrective action must be carefully weighed against other risks of volume overload). When these conditions have become clinically relevant, treatment with Tritace must only be started or continued if appropriate steps are taken concurrently to prevent an excessive fall in blood pressure and deterioration of renal function.

For all of the above, the initial phase of treatment requires close medical supervision.

Patients at particular risk from a pronounced reduction in blood pressure: If symptomatic hypotension occurs, the patient should be placed in a supine position and, if necessary, receive an intravenous infusion of physiological saline. Intravenous atropine may be necessary if there is associated bradycardia. Treatment with Tritace may usually be continued following restoration of effective blood volume and blood pressure.

Surgery/anaesthesia: In patients undergoing surgery or during anaesthesia with agents producing hypotension, Tritace may block angiotensin II formation secondary to compensatory renin release. If hypotension occurs and is considered to be due to this mechanism, it can be corrected by appropriate treatment.

4.5 Interaction with other medicinal products and other forms of Interaction

Vasopressor sympathomimetics: These may reduce the antihypertensive effect of Tritace. Particularly close blood pressure monitoring is recommended.

Allopurinol, immunosuppressants, corticosteroids, procainamide, cytostatics and other substances that may change the blood picture: Increased likelihood of haematological reactions (see also under "4.4 Special Warnings and Special Precautions for use").

Lithium Salts: Excretion of lithium may be reduced by ACE inhibitors. Such reduction may lead to increased serum lithium levels and increased lithium toxicity. Lithium levels must, therefore, be monitored.

Diuretics and other antihypertensive agents: Combination with diuretics or other antihypertensive agents may potentiate the antihypertensive response to Tritace. Potassium sparing diuretics (spironolactone, amiloride, triamterene) or potassium supplements may increase the risk of hyperkalaemia. Tritace may attenuate the potassium loss caused by thiazide-type diuretics. Regular monitoring of serum sodium and potassium is recommended in patients undergoing concurrent diuretic therapy. Adrenergic-blocking drugs should only be combined with ramipril under careful supervision.

Combination with antidiabetics: When antidiabetic agents (insulin and sulphonylurea derivatives) are used concurrently, the possibility of increased blood-sugar reduction must be considered. Particularly close blood glucose monitoring is therefore recommended in the initial phase of co-administration.

Combination with NSAIDS: When ACE inhibitors are administered simultaneously with non-steroidal anti-inflammatory drugs (e.g. acetylsalicylic acid and indomethacin), attenuation of the antihypertensive effect may occur. Furthermore, concomitant use of ACE inhibitors and NSAIDs may lead to an increased risk of worsening of renal function and an increase in serum potassium.

Heparin: Rise in serum potassium concentration possible.

Desensitisation therapy: The likelihood and severity of anaphylactic and anaphylactoid reactions to insect venoma is increased under ACE inhibition. It is assumed that this effect may also occur in connection with other allergens.

The protein binding of ramipril is about 73% and of ramiprilat about 56%.

4.6 Pregnancy and lactation

Tritace must not be taken during pregnancy. Therefore, pregnancy must be excluded before starting treatment. If the patient intends to become or becomes pregnant, treatment with ACE inhibitors must be discontinued, i.e. replaced by another form of treatment. Pregnancy must be avoided in cases where treatment with ACE inhibitors is indispensable.

It is not known if exposure limited to the first trimester only can harm the fetus. Exposure of the mother to ACE inhibitors in mid or late pregnancy has been associated with oligohydramnios and neonatal hypotension with anuria or renal failure.

From animal experiments it is known that use of ramipril may cause a decreased utero-placental perfusion. There is also a potential risk of fetal or post-natal effect as ACE inhibitors also influence the local renin-angiotensin system. In peri-post natal studies increased renal pelvic dilation was observed in the first generation offspring. However, ramipril was not fetotoxic in our studies although ACE inhibitors have shown fetotoxicity in some species.

If treatment with Tritace is necessary during lactation, the patient must not breast feed in order to prevent the infant from ingesting small quantities of ramipril with breast milk.

4.7 Effects on ability to drive and use machines

In individual cases, as a result of a reduction in blood pressure, treatment with Tritace may affect the ability to drive and operate machinery. This occurs especially at the start of treatment, when changing over from other preparations and during concomitant use of alcohol. After the first dose or subsequent increases in dose it is not advisable to drive or operate machinery for several hours.

4.8 Undesirable effects

Generally, adverse reactions have been mild and transient, and do not require discontinuation of therapy. The most frequently reported adverse reactions are nausea, dizziness and headache. Uncommonly drowsiness, light-headedness or impaired reactions may occur.

Reactions such as peripheral oedema, tinnitus, fatigue, visual disturbances, sweating, disturbed hearing, disturbed orthostatic regulation are rare.

Cardiovascular: Symptomatic hypotension accompanied by dizziness, weakness and nausea may occur after the initial dose of Tritace and after an increase in the dose of Tritace. It has been rarely observed, but may occur in severely salt/volume-depleted patients such as those treated with diuretics, patients on dialysis and in patients with severe congestive heart failure. Syncope has also been observed rarely.

Myocardial infarction or cerebrovascular accident possibly secondary to severe hypotension in high risk patients, chest pain, palpitations, rhythm disturbances, angina pectoris may occur.

Renal: Treatment with Tritace may impair renal function and in isolated cases progression to acute renal failure may occur.

Gastrointestinal: Treatment with Tritace may be associated with symptoms in the digestive tract, e.g. rarely dryness of the mouth, glossitis, irritation or inflammation of the oral mucosa, digestive disturbances, constipation, diarrhoea, nausea, and vomiting, (gastritis-like) stomach pain, abdominal discomfort (sometimes with increased levels of pancreatic enzymes). Uncommonly increases in hepatic enzymes and/or serum bilirubin, jaundice due to impaired excretion of bile pigment (cholestatic jaundice), acute hepatitis, potentially leading to liver failure.

Pancreatitis has been reported rarely in patients treated with ACE inhibitors; in some cases this has proved fatal.

Allergic: Hypersensitivity reactions accompanied by pruritus, rash, shortness of breath and sometimes fever may occur, but usually resolve spontaneously after withdrawal of Tritace.

In addition, the following cutaneous and mucosal reactions may occur: reddening of skin areas with accompanying heat sensation, conjunctivitis, itching, urticaria, other skin or mucosal eruptions (maculo-papular and lichenoid exanthema and enanthema, erythema multiforme), sometimes pronounced hair loss, exacerbation of perfusion disturbances due to vascular stenoses and precipitation or intensification of Raynaud's phenomenon. In isolated cases, pemphigus, exacerbation of psoriasis, psoriasiform and pemphigoid exanthema and enanthema, Stevens-Johnson syndrome, toxic epidermal necrolysis, hypersensitivity of the skin to light, and onycholysis have been observed.

See Section 4.5 (Interactions) for advice on reactions to insect venoma.

Haematological reactions: Rarely, a mild - in isolated cases severe – reduction in the red blood cell count and haemoglobin content, white blood cell or blood platelet count may develop. In isolated cases, agranulocytosis, pancytopenia and bone marrow depression may occur.

In isolated cases haemolytic anaemia may develop.

Vasculitis, muscle and joint pains, fever, or eosinophilia may occur. Raised titres of antinuclear antibodies have been seen with other ACE inhibitors.

Angioneurotic oedema: See Section 4.4 (Special Warnings and Special Precautions for use). Serious reactions of this type and other, non-pharmacologically mediated anaphylactic or anaphylactoid reactions to ramipril or any of the other ingredients are rare

Respiratory tract: A dry tickling cough may occur. This is possibly due to the desired ACE inhibition as are the following adverse effects: rhinitis, sinusitis, bronchitis and, especially in patients with tickling cough, bronchospasm.

Other adverse reactions: Disturbances of balance, headache, nervousness, restlessness, tremor, sleep disorders, confusion, loss of appetite, depressed mood, feeling of anxiety, paraesthesiae, uncommonly, disturbances of smell and taste or partial, sometimes complete loss of taste, muscle cramps, erectile impotence and reduced sexual desire may occur.

Laboratory test findings: Increases in blood urea nitrogen and serum creatinine may occur, in particular with renal insufficiency or in patients pre-treated with a diuretic. Pre-existing proteinuria may deteriorate (though ACE inhibitors usually reduce proteinuria), or there may be an increase in urinary output.

Sodium/Potassium serum levels – See Section 4.5 (Special warnings and special precautions for use).

4.9 Overdose

Symptoms

Overdosage may cause excessive peripheral vasodilation (with marked hypotension, shock), bradycardia, electrolyte disturbances, and renal failure.

Management

In the event of prolonged hypotension, administration of α_1-adrenergic agonists (e.g. norepinephrine, dopamine) and angiotensin II (angiotensinamide) must be considered in addition to volume and salt substitution.

5. PHARMACOLOGICAL PROPERTIES

5.1 Pharmacodynamic properties

Pharmacotherapeutic group: Converting Enzyme Blockers, ATC code CO2E A05.

Ramipril is a prodrug, which after absorption from the gastrointestinal tract, is hydrolysed in the liver to form the active angiotensin converting enzyme (ACE) inhibitor, ramiprilat, which is a potent and long acting ACE inhibitor. Administration of ramipril causes an increase in plasma renin activity and a decrease in plasma concentrations of angiotensin II and aldosterone. The beneficial haemodynamic effects resulting from ACE inhibition are a consequence of the reduction in angiotensin II causing dilation of peripheral vessels and reduction in vascular resistance. There is evidence suggesting that tissue ACE particularly in the vasculature, rather than circulating ACE, is the primary factor determining the haemodynamic effects.

Angiotensin converting enzyme is identical with kininase II, one of the enzymes responsible for the degradation of bradykinin. There is evidence that ACE inhibition by ramiprilat appears to have some effects on the kallikrein-kinin-prostaglandin systems. It is assumed that effects on these systems contribute to the hypotensive action of ramipril.

Administration of Tritace to hypertensive patients results in reduction of both supine and standing blood pressure. The antihypertensive effect is evident within one to two hours after the drug intake; peak effect occurs 3 - 6 hours after drug intake and has been shown to be maintained for at least 24 hours after usual therapeutic doses.

In a large endpoint study – HOPE - ramipril significantly reduced the incidence of stroke, myocardial infarction and/or cardiovascular death when compared with placebo. These benefits occurred largely in normotensive patients and were shown, using standard regression analysis techniques, to be only partially due to the relatively modest reductions in blood pressure demonstrated in the study. The 10mg dose, currently the highest safe dose level approved, was selected by the HOPE investigators from previous dose-ranging studies (SECURE, HEART) and was considered to be the most likely dose to effect full blockade of the renin-angiotensin-aldosterone system. This and other studies suggest that ACE inhibitors like ramipril are likely to have other direct effects on the cardiovascular system. These may include the antagonism of angiotensin II mediated vasoconstriction, the inhibition of proliferating vascular smooth muscle and plaque rupture, the enhancement of endothelial function, the reduction of LV hypertrophy and positive effects on fibrinolysis. Additional effects in diabetic patients may also contribute e.g. effects on insulin clearance and pancreatic blood flow.

5.2 Pharmacokinetic properties

Following oral administration ramipril is rapidly absorbed from the gastrointestinal tract; peak plasma concentrations of ramipril are reached within one hour. Peak plasma concentrations of the active metabolite, ramiprilat, are reached within 2 – 4 hours.

Plasma concentrations of ramiprilat decline in a polyphasic manner. The effective half-life of ramiprilat after multiple once daily administration of ramipril is 13 – 17 hours for 5 – 10 mg ramipril and markedly longer for lower doses, 1.25 – 2.5 mg ramipril. This difference is related to the long terminal phase of the ramiprilat concentration time curve observed at very low plasma concentrations. This terminal phase is independent of the dose, indicating a saturable capacity of the enzyme to bind ramiprilat. Steady-state plasma concentrations of ramiprilat after once daily dosing with the usual doses of ramipril are reached by about the fourth day of treatment.

Ramipril is almost completely metabolised and the metabolites are excreted mainly via the kidneys. In addition to the bioactive metabolite, ramiprilat, other, inactive metabolites have been identified, including diketopiperazine ester, diketopiperazine acid and conjugates.

5.3 Preclinical safety data

Reproduction toxicology studies in the rat, rabbit and monkey did not disclose any teratogenic properties. Fertility was not impaired either in male or in female rats. The administration of ramipril to female rats during the fetal period and lactation produced irreversible renal damage (dilation of the renal pelvis) in the offspring at daily doses of 50 mg/kg body weight and higher.

6. PHARMACEUTICAL PARTICULARS

6.1 List of excipients

1.25mg and 10mg: Methylhydroxypropylcellulose, pregelatinised starch, microcrystalline cellulose, sodium stearyl fumarate.

2.5mg: Methylhydroxypropylcellulose, pregelatinised starch, microcrystalline cellulose, sodium stearyl fumarate, yellow ferric oxide.

5mg: Methylhydroxypropylcellulose, pregelatinised starch, microcrystalline cellulose, sodium stearyl fumarate, red ferric oxide.

6.2 Incompatibilities

None known.

6.3 Shelf life

5 years (1.25mg, 2.5mg and 5mg tablets)

4 years (10mg tablets)

6.4 Special precautions for storage

Store below 25°C

6.5 Nature and contents of container

PVC aluminium blisters containing tablets. Available in packs of 28 tablets

6.6 Instructions for use and handling

None

7. MARKETING AUTHORISATION HOLDER

Aventis Pharma Ltd.
50 Kings Hill Avenue
Kings Hill
West Malling
Kent ME19 4AH

8. MARKETING AUTHORISATION NUMBER(S)

1.25mg: PL 04425/0356
2.5mg: PL 04425/0357
5mg: PL 04425/0358
10mg: PL 04425/0359

9. DATE OF FIRST AUTHORISATION/RENEWAL OF THE AUTHORISATION

30th September 2003

10. DATE OF REVISION OF THE TEXT

February 2004

Legal category: POM

Tritace Titration Pack

(sanofi-aventis)

1. NAME OF THE MEDICINAL PRODUCT

Tritace™ Titration Pack

2. QUALITATIVE AND QUANTITATIVE COMPOSITION

2.5 mg, 5.0 mg or 10 mg ramipril.

3. PHARMACEUTICAL FORM

2.5 mg: Orange opaque/white opaque hard gelatin capsules.

5.0 mg: Scarlet opaque/white opaque hard gelatin capsules.

10 mg: Blue opaque/white opaque hard gelatin capsules.

4. CLINICAL PARTICULARS

4.1 Therapeutic indications

For reducing the risk of myocardial infarction, stroke, cardiovascular death or need for revascularisation procedures in patients of 55 years or more who have clinical evidence of cardiovascular disease (previous MI, unstable angina or multivessel CABG or multivessel PTCA), stroke or peripheral vascular disease.

Also for reducing the risk of myocardial infarction, stroke, cardiovascular death or need for revascularisation procedures in diabetic patients of 55 years or more who have one or more of the following clinical findings: hypertension (systolic blood pressure > 160mmHg or diastolic blood pressure > 90mmHg); high total cholesterol >5.2 mmol/L); low HDL (<0.9 mmol/L); current smoker; known microalbuminuria; clinical evidence of previous vascular disease.

Oral administration.

4.2 Posology and method of administration

Dosage and Administration:

Tritace Titration Pack is a multi-strength pack containing a total of 35 capsules. The dose regimen is based on the fixed titration process to titrate the patient up to a maintenance dose of 10mg Tritace once a day, as shown below.

- Tritace 2.5mg once a day for 7 days
- Tritace 5mg once a day for 21 days
- Tritace 10mg once a day for 7 days

The patient opens the pack from the top to access the first week's treatment of Tritace 2.5mg. When this is finished the patient tears away the dividing cardboard layer to reach the next 3 weeks treatment of Tritace 5mg. The patient repeats this process to get to the final weeks worth of treatment of Tritace 10mg.

Tritace Titration Pack should only be used in patients for whom this titration schedule is thought to be suitable.

Caution is required in patients with concomitant use of diuretics, congestive heart failure, renal or hepatic insufficiency, incompletely corrected fluid or salt depletion, severe hypertension, or in patients in whom a hypotensive reaction would constitute a particular risk, (e.g., with relevant stenoses of the coronary or cerebral vessels). In these cases the fixed titration regimen may not be suitable and an individual titration schedule should be considered.

Elderly: Caution in all elderly patients.

Children: Tritace has not been studied in children, and therefore use in this age group is not recommended.

Tritace capsules should be taken with a glass of water. The absorption of ramipril is not affected by food.

4.3 Contraindications

Hypersensitivity to ramipril, any of the excipients of Tritace, or to any other ACE inhibitor.

History of angioneurotic oedema.

Haemodynamically relevant renal artery stenosis.

Hypotensive or haemodynamically unstable patients.

Pregnancy.

Lactation.

4.4 Special warnings and special precautions for use

Warnings:

Tritace Titration Pack should only be used in patients for whom this fixed dosage regimen is suitable. Those patients needing a lower starting dose or longer periods of time on the lower strengths of capsules should not be prescribed Tritace Titration Pack.

Angioneurotic oedema occurring during treatment with an ACE inhibitor necessitates immediate discontinuation of the drug. Angioneurotic oedema may involve the tongue, glottis or larynx and hospitalisation of the patient is advisable.

Tritace should not be used in patients with aortic or mitral valve stenosis or outflow obstruction (see Precautions section below).

Precautions:

Assessment of renal function: Evaluation of the patient should include assessment of renal function prior to initiation of therapy and during treatment.

Impaired renal function: Patients with renal insufficiency may require reduced or less frequent doses of Tritace; their renal function should be closely monitored. In the majority, renal function will not alter. There is a risk of impairment of renal function, particularly in patients with congestive heart failure or after a renal transplant, renal insufficiency, bilateral renal artery stenosis and unilateral renal artery stenosis in the single kidney. In the latter patient group, even a small increase in serum creatinine may be indicative of unilateral loss of renal function. If recognised early, such impairment of renal function is reversible upon discontinuation of therapy.

Patients haemodialysed using high flux polyacrylonitrile ('AN69') membranes are highly likely to experience anaphylactoid reactions if they are treated with ACE inhibitors. This combination should therefore be avoided, either by use of alternative antihypertensive drugs or alternative membranes for dialysis.

Similar reactions have been observed during low-density lipoprotein apheresis with dextran sulphate. This method should, therefore, not be used in patients treated with ACE inhibitors.

Some hypertensive patients with no apparent pre-existing renal disease may develop minor and usually transient increases in blood urea nitrogen and serum creatinine when Tritace is given, in particular concomitantly with a diuretic. Dosage reduction of Tritace and/or discontinuation of the diuretic may be required.

Impaired liver function: As ramipril is a prodrug metabolised to its active moiety in the liver, particular caution and close monitoring should be applied to patients with impaired liver function. The metabolism of the parent compound, and therefore the formation of the bioactive metabolite ramiprilat, may be diminished resulting in markedly elevated plasma levels of the parent compound (due to the reduced activity of esterases in the liver).

In patients in whom severe liver cirrhosis with oedema and/or ascites is present, the renin angiotensin system may be significantly activated; therefore, particular caution must be exercised in treating these patients (see also above and under "4.2 Posology and Method of Administration").

Agranulocytosis and bone marrow depression: In patients on angiotensin converting enzyme inhibitors agranulocytosis and bone marrow depression have been seen rarely, as well as a reduction in red cell count, haemoglobin content and platelet count. These are more frequent in patients with renal impairment, especially if they have a collagen vascular disease. Regular monitoring of white blood cell counts (to permit detection of a possible leucopenia) and protein levels in urine should be considered in patients with collagen vascular disease (e.g. lupus erythematosus and scleroderma), especially associated with impaired renal function and concomitant therapy particularly with corticosteroids and anti metabolites. Patients on allopurinol, immunosuppressants and other substances that may change the blood picture also have increased likelihood of other blood picture changes.

Hyperkalaemia: Elevated serum potassium has been observed very rarely in hypertensive patients. Risk factors for the development of hyperkalaemia include renal insufficiency, potassium sparing diuretics and the concomitant use of agents to treat hypokalaemia. It is recommended that serum potassium be monitored regularly. More frequent monitoring of serum potassium is necessary in patients with impaired renal function.

Patients with hyper-stimulated renin angiotensin system: In the treatment of patients with a hyper-stimulated renin angiotensin system, particular caution must be exercised (see also under "4.2 Posology and Method of Administration"). Such patients are at risk of an acute pronounced fall in blood pressure and deterioration of renal function due to ACE inhibition, especially when an ACE inhibitor or a concomitant diuretic is given for the first time or for the first time at an increased dose. Initial doses or initial dose increases must be accompanied by close blood pressure monitoring until such time as no further acute reduction in blood pressure is to be anticipated.

Significant activation of the renin angiotensin system is to be anticipated, for example:

- in patients with severe and/or with malignant hypertension.
- in patients with heart failure, particularly if severe or if treated with other substances having antihypertensive potential.
- in patients with haemodynamically relevant left-ventricular inflow or outflow obstruction (e.g., aortic or mitral valve stenosis).
- in patients pre-treated with diuretics.
- in patients with fluid or salt depletion, or in those in whom it may develop (as a result of insufficient fluid or salt intake, or as a result of, e.g., dialysis, diarrhoea, vomiting or excessive sweating in cases where salt and fluid replacement is inadequate).

Generally, it is recommended that dehydration, hypovolaemia or salt depletion be corrected before initiating treatment (in patients with heart failure, however, such corrective action must be carefully weighed against other risks of volume overload). When these conditions have become clinically relevant, treatment with Tritace must only be started or continued if appropriate steps are taken concurrently to prevent an excessive fall in blood pressure and deterioration of renal function.

For all of the above, the initial phase of treatment requires close medical supervision.

Patients at particular risk from a pronounced reduction in blood pressure: If symptomatic hypotension occurs, the patient should be placed in a supine position and, if necessary, receive an intravenous infusion of physiological saline. Intravenous atropine may be necessary if there is associated bradycardia. Treatment with Tritace may usually be continued following restoration of effective blood volume and blood pressure.

Surgery/anaesthesia: In patients undergoing surgery or during anaesthesia with agents producing hypotension, Tritace may block angiotensin II formation secondary to compensatory renin release. If hypotension occurs and is considered to be due to this mechanism, it can be corrected by appropriate treatment.

4.5 Interaction with other medicinal products and other forms of Interaction

Vasopressor sympathomimetics: These may reduce the antihypertensive effect of Tritace. Particularly close blood pressure monitoring is recommended.

Allopurinol, immunosuppressants, corticosteroids, procainamide, cytostatics and other substances that may change the blood picture: Increased likelihood of haematological reactions (see also under "4.4 Special Warnings and Special Precautions for use").

Lithium Salts: Excretion of lithium may be reduced by ACE inhibitors. Such reduction may lead to increased serum lithium levels and increased lithium toxicity. Lithium levels must, therefore, be monitored.

Diuretics and other antihypertensive agents: Combination with diuretics or other antihypertensive agents may potentiate the antihypertensive response to Tritace. Potassium sparing diuretics (spironolactone, amiloride, triamterene) or potassium supplements may increase the risk of hyperkalaemia. Tritace may attenuate the potassium loss caused by thiazide-type diuretics. Regular monitoring of serum sodium and potassium is recommended in patients undergoing concurrent diuretic therapy. Adrenergic-blocking drugs should only be combined with ramipril under careful supervision.

Combination with antidiabetics: When antidiabetic agents (insulin and sulphonylurea derivatives) are used concurrently, the possibility of increased blood-sugar reduction must be considered. Particularly close blood glucose monitoring is therefore recommended in the initial phase of co-administration.

Combination with NSAIDs: When ACE inhibitors are administered simultaneously with non-steroidal anti-inflammatory drugs (e.g. acetylsalicylic acid and indomethacin), attenuation of the antihypertensive effect may occur. Furthermore, concomitant use of ACE inhibitors and NSAIDs may lead to an increased risk of worsening of renal function and an increase in serum potassium.

Heparin: Rise in serum potassium concentration possible.

Desensitisation therapy: The likelihood and severity of anaphylactic and anaphylactoid reactions to insect venoma is increased under ACE inhibition. It is assumed that this effect may also occur in connection with other allergens.

The protein binding of ramipril is about 73% and of ramiprilat about 56%.

4.6 Pregnancy and lactation

Tritace must not be taken during pregnancy. Therefore, pregnancy must be excluded before starting treatment. If the patient intends to become or becomes pregnant, treatment with ACE inhibitors must be discontinued, i.e. replaced by another form of treatment. Pregnancy must be avoided in cases where treatment with ACE inhibitors is indispensable.

It is not known if exposure limited to the first trimester only can harm the fetus. Exposure of the mother to ACE inhibitors in mid or late pregnancy has been associated with oligohydramnios and neonatal hypotension with anuria or renal failure.

From animal experiments it is known that use of ramipril may cause a decreased utero-placental perfusion. There is also a potential risk of fetal or post-natal effect as ACE inhibitors also influence the local renin-angiotensin system. In peri-post natal studies increased renal pelvic dilatation was observed in the first generation offspring. However, ramipril was not fetotoxic in our studies although ACE inhibitors have shown fetotoxicity in some species.

If treatment with Tritace is necessary during lactation, the patient must not breast feed in order to prevent the infant from ingesting small quantities of ramipril with breast milk.

4.7 Effects on ability to drive and use machines

In individual cases, as a result of a reduction in blood pressure, treatment with Tritace may affect the ability to drive and operate machinery. This occurs especially at the start of treatment, when changing over from other preparations and during concomitant use of alcohol. After the first dose or subsequent increases in dose it is not advisable to drive or operate machinery for several hours.

4.8 Undesirable effects

Generally, adverse reactions have been mild and transient, and do not require discontinuation of therapy. The most frequently reported adverse reactions are nausea, dizziness and headache. Uncommonly drowsiness, light-headedness or impaired reactions may occur.

Reactions such as peripheral oedema, tinnitus, fatigue, visual disturbances, sweating, disturbed hearing, disturbed orthostatic regulation are rare.

Cardiovascular: Symptomatic hypotension accompanied by dizziness, weakness and nausea may occur after the initial dose of Tritace and after an increase in the dose of Tritace. It has been rarely observed, but may occur in severely salt/volume-depleted patients such as those treated with diuretics, patients on dialysis and in patients with severe congestive heart failure. Syncope has also been observed rarely.

Myocardial infarction or cerebrovascular accident possibly secondary to severe hypotension in high risk patients, chest pain, palpitations, rhythm disturbances, angina pectoris may occur.

Renal: Treatment with Tritace may impair renal function and in isolated cases progression to acute renal failure may occur.

Gastrointestinal: Treatment with Tritace may be associated with symptoms in the digestive tract, e.g. rarely dryness of the mouth, glossitis, irritation or inflammation of the oral mucosa, digestive disturbances, constipation, diarrhoea, nausea, and vomiting, (gastritis-like) stomach pain, abdominal discomfort (sometimes with increased levels of pancreatic enzymes). Uncommonly, increases in hepatic enzymes and/or serum bilirubin, jaundice due to impaired excretion of bile pigment (cholestatic jaundice), acute hepatitis, potentially leading to liver failure.

Pancreatitis has been reported rarely in patients treated with ACE inhibitors; in some cases this has proved fatal.

Allergic: Hypersensitivity reactions accompanied by pruritus, rash, shortness of breath and sometimes fever may occur, but usually resolve spontaneously after withdrawal of Tritace.

In addition, the following cutaneous and mucosal reactions may occur: reddening of skin areas with accompanying heat sensation, conjunctivitis, itching, urticaria, other skin or mucosal eruptions (maculo-papular and lichenoid exanthema and enanthema, erythema multiforme), sometimes pronounced hair loss, exacerbation of disturbances due to vascular stenoses and precipitation or intensification of Raynaud's phenomenon. In isolated cases, pemphigus, exacerbation of psoriasis, psoriasiform and pemphigoid exanthema and enanthema, Stevens-Johnson syndrome, toxic epidermal necrolysis, hypersensitivity of the skin to light and onycholysis have been observed.

See Section 4.5 (Interactions) for advice on reactions to insect venoma

Haematological reactions: Rarely, a mild - in isolated cases severe – reduction in the red blood cell count and haemoglobin content, white blood cell or blood platelet count may develop. In isolated cases, agranulocytosis, pancytopenia and bone marrow depression may occur.

In isolated cases haemolytic anaemia may develop.

Vasculitis, muscle and joint pains, fever, or eosinophilia may occur. Raised titres of antinuclear antibodies have been seen with other ACE inhibitors.

Angioneurotic oedema: See Section 4.4 (Special Warnings and Special Precautions for Use). Serious reactions of this type and other, non-pharmacologically mediated anaphylactic or anaphylactoid reactions to ramipril or any of the other ingredients are rare.

Respiratory tract: A dry tickling cough may occur. This is possibly due to the desired ACE inhibition as are the following adverse effects: rhinitis, sinusitis, bronchitis and, especially in patients with tickling cough, bronchospasm.

Other adverse reactions: Disturbances of balance, headache, nervousness, restlessness, tremor, sleep disorders, confusion, loss of appetite, depressed mood, feeling of anxiety, paraesthesiae, uncommonly disturbances of smell and taste or partial, sometimes complete, loss of taste, muscle cramps, erectile impotence and reduced sexual desire may occur.

Laboratory test findings: Increases in blood urea nitrogen and serum creatinine may occur, in particular with renal insufficiency or in patients pretreated with a diuretic. Pre-existing proteinuria may deteriorate (though ACE inhibitors usually reduce proteinuria), or there may be an increase in urinary output.

Sodium/Potassium serum levels – See Section 4.5 (Special warnings and special precautions for use).

4.9 Overdose

Symptoms

Overdosage may cause excessive peripheral vasodilatation (with marked hypotension, shock), bradycardia, electrolyte disturbances, and renal failure.

Management

In the event of prolonged hypotension, administration of α_1-adrenergic agonists (e.g. norepinephrine, dopamine) and angiotensin II (angiotensinamide) must be considered in addition to volume and salt substitution.

*

5. PHARMACOLOGICAL PROPERTIES

5.1 Pharmacodynamic properties

Ramipril is a prodrug which, after absorption from the gastrointestinal tract, is hydrolysed in the liver to form the active angiotensin converting enzyme (ACE) inhibitor, ramiprilat which is a potent and long acting ACE inhibitor. Administration of ramipril causes an increase in plasma renin activity and a decrease in plasma concentrations of angiotensin II and aldosterone. The beneficial haemodynamic effects resulting from ACE inhibition are a consequence of the reduction in angiotensin II causing dilation of peripheral vessels and reduction in vascular resistance. There is evidence suggesting that tissue ACE particularly in the vasculature, rather than circulating ACE, is the primary factor determining the haemodynamic effects.

Angiotensin converting enzyme is identical with kininase II, one of the enzymes responsible for the degradation of bradykinin. There is evidence that ACE inhibition by ramiprilat appears to have some effects on the kallikrein-kinin-prostaglandin systems. It is assumed that effects on these systems contribute to the hypotensive and metabolic activity of ramipril.

In a large endpoint study – HOPE - ramipril significantly reduced the incidence of stroke, myocardial infarction and/or cardiovascular death when compared with placebo. These benefits occurred largely in normotensive patients and were shown, using standard regression analysis techniques, to be only partially due to the relatively modest reductions in blood pressure demonstrated in the study. The 10mg dose, currently the highest safe dose level approved, was selected by the HOPE investigators from previous dose-ranging studies (SECURE, HEART) and was considered to be the most likely dose to effect full blockade of the renin-angiotensin-aldosterone system. This and other studies suggest that ACE inhibitors like ramipril are likely to have other direct effects on the cardiovascular system. These may include the antagonism of angiotensin II mediated vasoconstriction, the inhibition of proliferating vascular smooth muscle and plaque rupture, the enhancement of endothelial function, the reduction of LV hypertrophy and positive effects on fibrinolysis. Additional effects in diabetic patients may also contribute e.g. effects on insulin clearance and pancreatic blood flow.

5.2 Pharmacokinetic properties

Following oral administration ramipril is rapidly absorbed from the gastrointestinal tract; peak plasma concentrations of ramipril are reached within one hour. Peak plasma concentrations of the active metabolite, ramiprilat, are reached within 2 – 4 hours.

Plasma concentrations of ramiprilat decline in a polyphasic manner. The effective half-life of ramiprilat after multiple once daily administration of ramipril is 13 – 17 hours for 5 – 10 mg ramipril and markedly longer for lower doses, 1.25 – 2.5 mg ramipril. This difference is related to the long terminal phase of the ramiprilat concentration time curve observed at very low plasma concentrations. This terminal phase is independent of the dose, indicating a saturable capacity of the enzyme to bind ramiprilat. Steady-state plasma concentrations of ramiprilat after once daily dosing with the usual doses of ramipril are reached by about the fourth day of treatment.

Ramipril is almost completely metabolised and the metabolites are excreted mainly via the kidneys. In addition to the bioactive metabolite, ramiprilat, other, inactive metabolites have been identified, including diketopiperazine ester, diketopiperazine acid and conjugates.

5.3 Preclinical safety data

Reproduction toxicology studies in the rat, rabbit and monkey did not disclose any teratogenic properties. Fertility was not impaired either in male or in female rats. The administration of ramipril to female rats during the fetal period and lactation produced irreversible renal damage (dilation of the renal pelvis) in the offspring at daily doses of 50 mg/kg body weight and higher.

6. PHARMACEUTICAL PARTICULARS

6.1 List of excipients

Pregelatinised starch. Gelatin in the capsule shell, together with colours: E127, E171, E172 (2.5 mg); E127, E131, E171 (5.0 mg); E127, E132, E171, E172 (10 mg).

6.2 Incompatibilities

None known.

6.3 Shelf life

Maximum of 36 months

6.4 Special precautions for storage

Do not store above 25°C

6.5 Nature and contents of container

PVC/Aluminium Blister packs of 35 capsules. 7 × 2.5mg, 21 × 5mg and 7 × 10mg capsules

6.6 Instructions for use and handling

None.

7. MARKETING AUTHORISATION HOLDER

Aventis Pharma Ltd
50 Kings Hill Avenue
Kings Hill
West Malling
Kent
ME19 4AH
UK

8. MARKETING AUTHORISATION NUMBER(S)

PL 04425/0298

9. DATE OF FIRST AUTHORISATION/RENEWAL OF THE AUTHORISATION

21/12/01

10. DATE OF REVISION OF THE TEXT

August 2003

11. LEGAL STATUS

POM

Trizivir film-coated tablets

(GlaxoSmithKline UK)

1. NAME OF THE MEDICINAL PRODUCT

TRIZIVIR film-coated tablets

2. QUALITATIVE AND QUANTITATIVE COMPOSITION

Each film-coated tablet contains 300 mg of abacavir as abacavir sulfate, 150 mg lamivudine and 300 mg zidovudine.

For excipients see section 6.1.

3. PHARMACEUTICAL FORM

Film-coated tablet.

Blue-green capsule-shaped film-coated tablets engraved with "GX LL1" on one side.

4. CLINICAL PARTICULARS

4.1 Therapeutic indications

Trizivir is indicated for the treatment of Human Immunodeficiency Virus (HIV) infection in adults. This fixed combination replaces the three components (abacavir, lamivudine and zidovudine) used separately in similar dosages. It is recommended that treatment is started with abacavir, lamivudine, and zidovudine separately for the first 6-8 weeks (see section 4.4). The choice of this fixed combination should be based not only on potential adherence criteria, but mainly on expected efficacy and risk related to the three nucleoside analogues.

The demonstration of the benefit of Trizivir is mainly based on results of studies performed in treatment naive patients or moderately antiretroviral experienced patients with non-advanced disease. In patients with high viral load > 100,000 copies/ml) choice of therapy needs special consideration (see section 5.1).

4.2 Posology and method of administration

Therapy should be prescribed by a physician experienced in the management of HIV infection.

The recommended dose of Trizivir in adults (18 years and over) is one tablet twice daily.

Trizivir can be taken with or without food.

Where discontinuation of therapy with one of the active substances of Trizivir is indicated, or where dose reduction is necessary separate preparations of abacavir, lamivudine and zidovudine are available.

Renal impairment: Whilst no dosage adjustment of abacavir is necessary in patients with renal dysfunction, lamivudine and zidovudine concentrations are increased in patients with renal impairment due to decreased clearance. Therefore, as dosage adjustments of these may be necessary, it is recommended that separate preparations of abacavir, lamivudine and zidovudine be administered to patients with reduced renal function (creatinine clearance ≤ 50 ml/min). Physicians should refer to the individual summary of product characteristics of these medicinal products. Trizivir should not be administered to patients with end-stage renal disease (see sections 4.3 and 5.2).

Hepatic impairment: Trizivir is contra-indicated in patients with hepatic impairment (see sections 4.3 and 5.2).

Elderly: No pharmacokinetic data are currently available in patients over 65 years of age. Special care is advised in this age group due to age associated changes such as the decrease in renal function and alteration of haematological parameters.

Dosage adjustments in patients with haematological adverse reactions: Dosage adjustment of zidovudine may be necessary if the haemoglobin level falls below 9 g/dl or 5.59 mmol/l or the neutrophil count falls below 1.0×10^9/l (see sections 4.3 and 4.4). As dosage adjustment of Trizivir is not possible, separate preparations of abacavir, lamivudine and zidovudine should be used. Physicians should refer to the individual summary of product characteristics of these medicinal products.

4.3 Contraindications

Trizivir is contraindicated in patients with known hypersensitivity to abacavir, lamivudine or zidovudine, or to any of the excipients. See BOXED INFORMATION ON HYPERSENSITIVITY REACTIONS in section 4.4 and section 4.8.

Trizivir is contraindicated in patients with end-stage renal disease.

Trizivir is contraindicated in patients with hepatic impairment.

Due to the active substance zidovudine, Trizivir is contraindicated in patients with abnormally low neutrophil counts ($< 0.75 \times 10^9$/l), or abnormally low haemoglobin levels (< 7.5 g/dl or 4.65 mmol/l) (see section 4.4).

4.4 Special warnings and special precautions for use

The special warnings and precautions relevant to abacavir, lamivudine and zidovudine are included in this section. There are no additional precautions or warnings relevant to the combination Trizivir.

(see Table 1)

Table 1

Hypersensitivity Reaction (see also section 4.8):
In clinical studies approximately 5 % of subjects receiving abacavir (which is also the active substance of Ziagen) develop a hypersensitivity reaction. Some of these cases were life-threatening and resulted in a fatal outcome despite taking precautions.

• Description
Hypersensitivity reactions are characterised by the appearance of symptoms indicating multi-organ system involvement. Almost all hypersensitivity reactions will have fever and/or rash as part of the syndrome.
Other signs and symptoms may include respiratory signs and symptoms such as dyspnoea, sore throat, cough, and abnormal chest x-ray findings (predominantly infiltrates, which can be localised), gastrointestinal symptoms, such as nausea, vomiting, diarrhoea, or abdominal pain, **and may lead to misdiagnosis of hypersensitivity as respiratory disease (pneumonia, bronchitis, pharyngitis), or gastroenteritis.**
Other frequently observed signs or symptoms of the hypersensitivity reaction may include lethargy or malaise and musculoskeletal symptoms (myalgia, rarely myolysis, arthralgia).
The symptoms related to this hypersensitivity reaction worsen with continued therapy and can be life-threatening. These symptoms usually resolve upon discontinuation of abacavir.

• Management
Hypersensitivity reaction symptoms usually appear within the first six weeks of initiation of treatment with abacavir, although these reactions **may occur at any time during therapy**. Patients should be monitored closely, especially during the first two months of treatment with Trizivir, with consultation every two weeks.
Patients who are diagnosed with a hypersensitivity reaction whilst on therapy **MUST discontinue Trizivir immediately. Trizivir, or any other medicinal product containing abacavir (i.e. Kivexa, Ziagen), MUST NEVER be restarted in patients who have stopped therapy due to a hypersensitivity reaction.**
Restarting abacavir following a hypersensitivity reaction results in a prompt return of symptoms within hours. This recurrence is usually more severe than on initial presentation, and may include life-threatening hypotension and death.
To avoid a delay in diagnosis and minimise the risk of a life-threatening hypersensitivity reaction, Trizivir must be permanently discontinued if hypersensitivity cannot be ruled out, even when other diagnoses are possible (respiratory diseases, flu-like illness, gastroenteritis or reactions to other medications).
Special care is needed for those patients simultaneously starting treatment with Trizivir and other medicinal products known to induce skin toxicity (such as non-nucleoside reverse transcriptase inhibitors - NNRTIs). This is because it is currently difficult to differentiate between rashes induced by these products and abacavir related hypersensitivity reactions.

• Management after an interruption of Trizivir therapy
If therapy with Trizivir has been discontinued for any reason and restarting therapy is under consideration, the reason for discontinuation must be established to assess whether the patient had any symptoms of a hypersensitivity reaction. **If a hypersensitivity reaction cannot be ruled out, Trizivir or any other medicinal product containing abacavir (i.e. Kivexa, Ziagen) must not be restarted.**
Hypersensitivity reactions with rapid onset, including life-threatening reactions have occurred after restarting abacavir in patients who had only one of the key symptoms of hypersensitivity (skin rash, fever, gastrointestinal, respiratory or constitutional symptoms such as lethargy and malaise) prior to stopping abacavir. The most common isolated symptom of a hypersensitivity reaction was a skin rash. Moreover, on very rare occasions hypersensitivity reactions have been reported in patients who have restarted therapy, and who had no preceding symptoms of a hypersensitivity reaction.
In both cases if a decision is made to restart Trizivir this must be done in a setting where medical assistance is readily available.

• Essential patient information
***Prescribers* must ensure that patients are fully informed regarding the following information on the hypersensitivity reaction:**
- Patients must be made aware of the possibility of a hypersensitivity reaction to abacavir that may result in a life-threatening reaction or death.
- Patients developing signs or symptoms possibly linked with a hypersensitivity reaction
MUST CONTACT their doctor IMMEDIATELY.
- Patients who are hypersensitive to abacavir should be reminded that they must never take Trizivir or any other medicinal product containing abacavir (i.e. Kivexa, Ziagen) again.
- In order to avoid restarting Trizivir, patients who have experienced a hypersensitivity reaction should dispose of their remaining Trizivir tablets in their possession in accordance with the local requirements, and ask their doctor or pharmacist for advice.
- Patients who have stopped Trizivir for any reason, and particularly due to possible adverse reactions or illness, must be advised to contact their doctor before restarting.
- Patients should be advised of the importance of taking Trizivir regularly.
- Each patient should be reminded to read the Package Leaflet included in the Trizivir pack.
They should be reminded of the importance of removing the Alert Card included in the pack, and keeping it with them at all times.

Lactic acidosis: lactic acidosis, usually associated with hepatomegaly and hepatic steatosis, has been reported with the use of nucleoside analogues. Early symptoms (symptomatic hyperlactatemia) include benign digestive symptoms (nausea, vomiting and abdominal pain), non-specific malaise, loss of appetite, weight loss, respiratory symptoms (rapid and/or deep breathing) or neurological symptoms (including motor weakness).

Lactic acidosis has a high mortality and may be associated with pancreatitis, liver failure, or renal failure.

Lactic acidosis generally occurred after a few or several months of treatment.

Treatment with nucleoside analogues should be discontinued in the setting of symptomatic hyperlactatemia and metabolic/lactic acidosis, progressive hepatomegaly, or rapidly elevating aminotransferase levels.

Caution should be exercised when administering nucleoside analogues to any patient (particularly obese women) with hepatomegaly, hepatitis or other known risk factors for liver disease and hepatic steatosis (including certain medicinal products and alcohol). Patients co-infected with hepatitis C and treated with alpha interferon and ribavirin may constitute a special risk.

Patients at increased risk should be followed closely.

Mitochondrial dysfunction: nucleoside and nucleotide analogues have been demonstrated *in vitro* and *in vivo* to cause a variable degree of mitochondrial damage. There have been reports of mitochondrial dysfunction in HIV-negative infants exposed *in utero* and/or post-natally to nucleoside analogues. The main adverse events reported are haematological disorders (anaemia, neutropenia), metabolic disorders (hyperlactatemia, hyperlipasemia). These events are often transitory. Some late-onset neurological disorders have been reported (hypertonia, convulsion, abnormal behaviour). Whether the neurological disorders are transient or permanent is currently unknown. Any child exposed *in utero* to nucleoside and nucleotide analogues, even HIV-negative children, should have clinical and laboratory follow-up and should be fully investigated for possible mitochondrial dysfunction in case of relevant signs or symptoms. These findings do not affect current national recommendations to use antiretroviral therapy in pregnant women to prevent vertical transmission of HIV.

Lipodystrophy: combination antiretroviral therapy has been associated with the redistribution of body fat (lipodystrophy) in HIV patients. The long-term consequences of these events are currently unknown. Knowledge about the mechanism is incomplete. A connection between visceral lipomatosis and protease inhibitors (PIs) and lipoatrophy and nucleoside reverse transcriptase inhibitors (NRTIs) has been hypothesised. A higher risk of lipodystrophy has been associated with individual factors such as older age, and with drug related factors such as longer duration of antiretroviral treatment and associated metabolic disturbances. Clinical examination should include evaluation for physical signs of fat redistribution. Consideration should be given to the measurement of fasting serum lipids and blood glucose. Lipid disorders should be managed as clinically appropriate (see section 4.8).

Haematological adverse reactions: anaemia, neutropenia and leucopenia (usually secondary to neutropenia) can be expected to occur in patients receiving zidovudine. These occurred more frequently at higher zidovudine dosages (1200-1500 mg/day) and in patients with poor bone marrow reserve prior to treatment, particularly with advanced HIV disease. Haematological parameters should therefore be carefully monitored (see section 4.3) in patients receiving Trizivir. These haematological effects are not usually observed before four to six week's therapy. For patients with advanced symptomatic HIV disease, it is generally recommended that blood tests are performed at least every two weeks for the first three months of therapy and at least monthly thereafter.

In patients with early HIV disease haematological adverse reactions are infrequent. Depending on the overall condition of the patient, blood tests may be performed less often, for example every one to three months. Additionally dosage adjustment of zidovudine may be required if severe anaemia or myelosuppression occurs during treatment with Trizivir, or in patients with pre-existing bone marrow compromise e.g. haemoglobin < 9 g/dl (5.59 mmol/l) or neutrophil count $< 1.0 \times 10^9$/l (see section 4.2). As dosage adjustment of Trizivir is not possible separate preparations of zidovudine, abacavir and lamivudine should be used. Physicians should refer to the individual prescribing information for these medicinal products.

Pancreatitis: cases of pancreatitis have occurred rarely in patients treated with abacavir, lamivudine and zidovudine. However it is not clear whether these cases were due to treatment with these medicinal products or to the underlying HIV disease. Treatment with Trizivir should be stopped immediately if clinical signs, symptoms or laboratory abnormalities suggestive of pancreatitis occur.

Liver disease: if lamivudine is being used concomitantly for the treatment of HIV and HBV, additional information relating to the use of lamivudine in the treatment of hepatitis B infection is available in the Zeffix SPC.

The safety and efficacy of Trizivir has not been established in patients with significant underlying liver disorders. Trizivir is contraindicated in patients with hepatic impairment (see section 4.3).

Patients with chronic hepatitis B or C and treated with combination antiretroviral therapy are at an increased risk of severe and potentially fatal hepatic adverse events. In case of concomitant antiviral therapy for hepatitis B or C, please refer also to the relevant product information for these medicinal products.

If Trizivir is discontinued in patients co-infected with hepatitis B virus, periodic monitoring of both liver function tests and markers of HBV replication is recommended, as withdrawal of lamivudine may result in an acute exacerbation of hepatitis (see Zeffix SPC).

Patients with pre-existing liver dysfunction including chronic active hepatitis have an increased frequency of liver function abnormalities during combination antiretroviral therapy and should be monitored according to standard practice. If there is evidence of worsening liver disease in such patients, interruption or discontinuation of treatment must be considered.

Children and adolescents: because insufficient data are available, the use of Trizivir in children or adolescents is not recommended. In this patient population, hypersensitivity reactions are particularly difficult to identify.

Immune Reactivation Syndrome: in HIV-infected patients with severe immune deficiency at the time of institution of combination antiretroviral therapy (CART), an inflammatory reaction to asymptomatic or residual opportunistic pathogens may arise and cause serious clinical conditions, or aggravation of symptoms. Typically, such reactions have been observed within the first few weeks or months of initiation of CART. Relevant examples are cytomegalovirus retinitis, generalised and/or focal mycobacterial infections, and *Pneumocystis carinii* pneumonia. Any inflammatory symptoms should be evaluated and treatment instituted when necessary.

Opportunistic infections: patients should be advised that Trizivir or any other antiretroviral therapy does not cure HIV infection and that they may still develop opportunistic infections and other complications of HIV infection. Therefore patients should remain under close clinical observation by physicians experienced in the treatment of these associated HIV diseases.

Miscellaneous: patients should be advised that current antiretroviral therapy, including Trizivir, has not been proven to prevent the risk of transmission of HIV to others through sexual contact or blood contamination. Appropriate precautions should continue to be taken.

To date there are insufficient data on the efficacy and safety of Trizivir given concomitantly with NNRTIs or PIs (see section 5.1).

4.5 Interaction with other medicinal products and other forms of Interaction

As Trizivir contains abacavir, lamivudine and zidovudine, any interactions that have been identified with these agents individually may occur with Trizivir.

The likelihood of metabolic interactions with lamivudine is low due to limited metabolism and plasma protein binding, and almost complete renal clearance. Zidovudine is primarily eliminated by hepatic conjugation to an inactive glucuronidated metabolite. Medicinal products that are primarily eliminated by hepatic metabolism especially via glucuronidation may have the potential to inhibit metabolism of zidovudine. Based on the results of *in vitro* experiments and the known major metabolic pathways of abacavir, the potential for P450 mediated interactions with other medicinal products involving abacavir are low. Clinical studies have shown that there are no clinically significant interactions between abacavir, lamivudine and zidovudine.

The interactions listed below should not be considered exhaustive but are representative of the classes of medicinal products where caution should be exercised.

Interactions relevant to abacavir

Based on the results of *in vitro* experiments and the known major metabolic pathways of abacavir, the potential for P450 mediated interactions with other medicinal products involving abacavir is low. P450 does not play a major role in the metabolism of abacavir, and abacavir does not inhibit metabolism mediated by CYP 3A4. Abacavir has also been shown *in vitro* not to inhibit CYP 3A4, CYP 2C9 or CYP 2D6 enzymes at clinically relevant concentrations. Therefore, there is little potential for interactions with antiretroviral PIs and other medicinal products metabolised by major P450 enzymes.

Potent enzymatic inducers such as rifampicin, phenobarbital and phenytoin may via their action on UDP-glucuronyltransferases slightly decrease the plasma concentrations of abacavir.

The metabolism of abacavir is altered by concomitant ethanol resulting in an increase in AUC of abacavir of about 41 %. These findings are not considered clinically significant. Abacavir has no effect on the metabolism of ethanol.

Retinoid compounds are eliminated via alcohol dehydrogenase. Interaction with abacavir is possible but has not been studied.

In a pharmacokinetic study, coadministration of 600 mg abacavir twice daily with methadone showed a 35 % reduction in abacavir C_{max} and a 1 hour delay in t_{max}, but the AUC was unchanged. The changes in abacavir pharmacokinetics are not considered clinically relevant. In this study, abacavir increased the mean methadone systemic clearance by 22 %. The induction of drug metabolizing enzymes cannot therefore be excluded. Patients being treated with methadone and abacavir should be monitored for evidence of withdrawal symptoms indicating under dosing, as occasionally methadone re-titration may be required.

Interactions relevant to lamivudine

The possibility of interactions with other medicinal products administered concurrently with Trizivir should be considered, particularly when the main route of elimination is active renal secretion especially via the cationic transport system e.g. trimethoprim. Nucleoside analogues (e.g. zidovudine, didanosine and zalcitabine) and other medicinal products (e.g. ranitidine, cimetidine) are eliminated only in part by this mechanism and were shown not to interact with lamivudine.

Administration of trimethoprim/sulfamethoxazole 160 mg/800 mg results in a 40 % increase in lamivudine exposure, because of the trimethoprim component; the sulfamethoxazole component does not interact. However, unless the patient has renal impairment, no dosage adjustment of lamivudine is necessary (see section 4.2). Lamivudine has no effect on the pharmacokinetics of trimethoprim or sulfamethoxazole. When concomitant administration with co-trimoxazole is warranted, patients should be monitored clinically. Co-administration of Trizivir with high doses of co-trimoxazole for the treatment of *Pneumocystis carinii* pneumonia (PCP) and toxoplasmosis should be avoided.

Co-administration of lamivudine with intravenous ganciclovir or foscarnet is not recommended until further information is available.

Lamivudine may inhibit the intracellular phosphorylation of zalcitabine when the two medicinal products are used concurrently. Trizivir is therefore not recommended to be used in combination with zalcitabine.

Lamivudine metabolism does not involve CYP 3A, making interactions with medicinal products metabolised by this system (e.g. PIs and non-nucleosides) unlikely.

Interactions relevant to zidovudine

Limited data suggests that co-administration of zidovudine and rifampicin decreases the AUC of zidovudine by 48 % ± 34 %. However the clinical significance of this is unknown.

Limited data suggest that probenecid increases the mean half-life and area under the plasma concentration curve of zidovudine by decreasing glucuronidation. Renal excretion of the glucuronide (and possibly zidovudine itself) is reduced in the presence of probenecid.

Phenytoin blood levels have been reported to be low in some patients receiving zidovudine, while in one patient a high level was noted. These observations suggest that phenytoin concentrations should be carefully monitored in patients receiving Trizivir and phenytoin.

In a pharmacokinetic study co-administration of zidovudine and atovaquone showed a decrease in zidovudine oral clearance leading to a 35 % ± 23 % increase in plasma zidovudine AUC. Given the limited data available the clinical significance of this is unknown.

Valproic acid or methadone when co-administered with zidovudine have been shown to increase the AUC, with a corresponding decrease in its clearance. As only limited data are available the clinical significance of this is not known.

Other medicinal products, including but not limited to, acetyl salicylic acid, codeine, morphine, indomethacin, ketoprofen, naproxen, oxazepam, lorazepam, cimetidine, clofibrate, dapsone and isoprinosine, may alter the metabolism of zidovudine by competitively inhibiting glucuronidation or directly inhibiting hepatic microsomal metabolism. Careful thought should be given to the possibilities of interactions before using such medicinal products, particularly for chronic therapy, in combination with Trizivir.

Zidovudine in combination with either ribavirin or stavudine are antagonistic *in vitro*. The concomitant use of either ribavirin or stavudine with Trizivir should be avoided.

Concomitant treatment, especially acute therapy, with potentially nephrotoxic or myelosuppressive medicinal products (e.g. systemic pentamidine, dapsone, pyrimethamine, co-trimoxazole, amphotericin, flucytosine, ganciclovir, interferon, vincristine, vinblastine and doxorubicin) may also increase the risk of adverse reactions to zidovudine. If concomitant therapy with Trizivir and any of these medicinal products is necessary then extra care should be taken in monitoring renal function and haematological parameters and, if required, the dosage of one or more agents should be reduced.

Limited data from clinical trials do not indicate a significantly increased risk of adverse reactions to zidovudine with co-trimoxazole (see interaction information above relating to lamivudine and cotrimoxazole) aerosolised pentamidine, pyrimethamine and acyclovir.

Co-administration of Trizivir with high doses of co-trimoxazole for the treatment of *Pneumocystis carinii* pneumonia (PCP) and toxoplasmosis should be avoided.

4.6 Pregnancy and lactation

Pregnancy

Trizivir is not recommended during pregnancy. There are no data on the use of Trizivir in pregnancy. Placental transfer of lamivudine and zidovudine occurs in humans, and for abacavir has been confirmed in animals. Studies with abacavir, lamivudine and zidovudine in animals have shown reproductive toxicity (see section 5.3). As the active substances of Trizivir may inhibit DNA replication any use, especially during the first trimester, presents a potential risk to the foetus.

Lactation

Both lamivudine and zidovudine are excreted in human milk at similar concentrations to those found in serum. It is expected that abacavir will also be secreted into human milk, although this has not been confirmed. It is therefore recommended that mothers do not breast-feed their babies while receiving treatment with Trizivir. Additionally, it is recommended that HIV infected women do not breast-feed their infants under any circumstances in order to avoid transmission of HIV.

4.7 Effects on ability to drive and use machines

No studies on the effects on ability to drive and use machines have been performed. The clinical status of the patient and the adverse event profile of Trizivir should be borne in mind when considering the patient's ability to drive or operate machinery.

4.8 Undesirable effects

Overview

Adverse events have been reported with abacavir, lamivudine and zidovudine used separately or in combination for therapy of HIV disease. Because Trizivir contains abacavir, lamivudine and zidovudine, the adverse events associated with these compounds may be expected. The assessment of the safety profile of Trizivir in clinical studies is not yet available.

The adverse events reported with abacavir, lamivudine and zidovudine are presented in Table 3 below. For many of these, it is unclear whether they are related to the active substance, the wide range of other medicinal products used in the management of HIV infection, or whether they are a result of the underlying disease process.

Hypersensitivity to abacavir (see also section 4.4):

In clinical studies, approximately 5 % of subjects receiving abacavir developed a hypersensitivity reaction; some of these were life-threatening and resulted in fatal outcome despite taking precautions. This reaction is characterised by the appearance of symptoms indicating multi-organ/body-system involvement.

Almost all patients developing hypersensitivity reactions will have fever and/or rash (usually maculopapular or urticarial) as part of the syndrome, however hypersensitivity reactions have occurred without rash or fever.

The signs and symptoms associated with hypersensitivity to abacavir are summarised in Table 2. These have been identified either from clinical studies or post marketing surveillance.

Some patients with hypersensitivity reactions were initially thought to have gastroenteritis, respiratory disease (pneumonia, bronchitis, pharyngitis) or a flu-like illness. This delay in diagnosis of hypersensitivity has resulted in abacavir being continued or re-introduced, leading to more severe hypersensitivity reactions or death. Therefore, the diagnosis of hypersensitivity reaction should be carefully considered for patients presenting with symptoms of these diseases.

Symptoms usually appeared within the first six weeks (median time to onset 11 days) of initiation of treatment with abacavir, although these reactions may occur at any time during therapy. Close medical supervision is necessary during the first two months, with consultations every two weeks.

Risk factors that may predict the occurrence or severity of hypersensitivity to abacavir have not been identified. However, it is likely that intermittent therapy may increase the risk of developing sensitisation and therefore occurrence of clinically significant hypersensitivity reactions. Consequently, patients should be advised of the importance of taking Trizivir regularly.

Restarting Trizivir, or any other medicinal product containing abacavir, following a hypersensitivity reaction would result in a prompt return of symptoms within hours. This recurrence of the hypersensitivity reaction was usually more severe than on initial presentation and may include life-threatening hypotension and death. **Patients who develop this hypersensitivity reaction must discontinue Trizivir and must never be rechallenged with Trizivir, or any other medicinal product containing abacavir (i.e. Kivexa, Ziagen).**

To avoid a delay in diagnosis and minimise the risk of a life-threatening hypersensitivity reaction, Trizivir must be permanently discontinued if hypersensitivity cannot be ruled out, even when other diagnoses are possible (respiratory disease, flu-like illness, gastroenteritis or reactions to other medications).

Hypersensitivity reactions with rapid onset, including life-threatening reactions have occurred after restarting abacavir in patients who had only one of the key symptoms of hypersensitivity (skin rash, fever, gastrointestinal, respiratory or constitutional symptoms such as lethargy and malaise) prior to stopping abacavir. The most common isolated symptom of a hypersensitivity reaction was a skin rash. Moreover, on very rare occasions hypersensitivity reactions have been reported in patients who have restarted therapy and who had no preceding symptoms of a hypersensitivity reaction. In both cases if a decision is made to restart Trizivir this must be done in a setting where medical assistance is readily available.

Each patient must be warned about this hypersensitivity reaction to abacavir.

Table 2: Summary of signs and symptoms associated with hypersensitivity to abacavir

(Signs and symptoms reported in at least 10 % of patients with a hypersensitivity reaction to abacavir are in **bold text**).

Body system	Adverse event
Gastrointestinal tract	**Nausea, vomiting, diarrhoea, abdominal pain**, mouth ulceration
Neurological/ psychiatry	**Headache**, paraesthesia
Haematological	Lymphopenia
Liver/pancreas	**Elevated liver function tests**, hepatitis, hepatic failure

Musculoskeletal	**Myalgia,** rarely myolysis, arthralgia, elevated creatine phosphokinase
Respiratory tract	**Dyspnoea,** sore throat, **cough,** adult respiratory distress syndrome, respiratory failure
Skin	**Rash** (usually maculopapular or urticarial)
Urology	Elevated creatinine, renal failure
Miscellaneous	**Fever, lethargy, malaise,** oedema, lymphadenopathy, hypotension, conjunctivitis, anaphylaxis

Undesirable effects reported with the individual substances

The adverse events reported with the individual components of Trizivir are presented in table 3. Care however must be taken to eliminate the possibility of a hypersensitivity reaction if any of these symptoms occur.

Table 3: Adverse events reported with the individual components of Trizivir

(Adverse events occurring in at least 5 % of patients are **in bold text**).

(see Table 3 opposite)

Adverse events associated with abacavir:

Many of the adverse events listed above occur commonly (nausea, vomiting, diarrhoea, fever, lethargy, rash) in patients with abacavir hypersensitivity. Therefore, patients with any of these symptoms should be carefully evaluated for the presence of this hypersensitivity reaction. If Trizivir has been discontinued in patients due to experiencing any one of these symptoms and a decision is made to restart a medicinal product containing abacavir, this must be done in a setting where medical assistance is readily available (see Section 4.4). Very rarely cases of erythema multiforme, Stevens Johnson syndrome or toxic epidermal necrolysis have been reported where abacavir hypersensitivity could not be ruled out. In such cases medicinal products containing abacavir should be permanently discontinued.

Haematological adverse events with zidovudine

Anaemia, neutropenia and leucopenia occurred more frequently at higher dosages (1200-1500 mg/day) and in patients with advanced HIV disease (especially when there is poor bone marrow reserve prior to treatment) and particularly in patients with CD4 cell counts less than 100/mm^3. Dosage reduction or cessation of therapy may become necessary (see section 4.4). The anaemia may necessitate transfusions.

The incidence of neutropenia was also increased in those patients whose neutrophil counts, haemoglobin levels and serum vitamin B_{12} levels were low at the start of zidovudine therapy.

Lactic acidosis

Treatment with nucleoside analogues has been associated with cases of lactic acidosis, sometimes fatal, usually associated with severe hepatomegaly and hepatic steatosis, (see section 4.4).

Lipodystrophy/metabolic abnormalities

Combination antiretroviral therapy has been associated with redistribution of body fat (lipodystrophy) in HIV patients including the loss of peripheral and facial subcutaneous fat, increased intra-abdominal and visceral fat, breast hypertrophy and dorsocervical fat accumulation (buffalo hump).

Combination antiretroviral therapy has been associated with metabolic abnormalities such as hypertriglyceridaemia, hypercholesterolaemia, insulin resistance, hyperglycaemia and hyperlactataemia (see section 4.4).

Immune Reactivation Syndrome

In HIV-infected patients with severe immune deficiency at the time of initiation of combination antiretroviral therapy (CART) an inflammatory reaction to asymptomatic or residual opportunistic infections may arise (see section 4.4).

4.9 Overdose

There is no experience of overdose with Trizivir. No specific symptoms or signs have been identified following acute overdose with zidovudine or lamivudine apart from those listed as undesirable effects. No fatalities occurred, and all patients recovered. Single doses up to 1200 mg and daily doses up to 1800 mg of abacavir have been administered to patients in clinical studies. No unexpected adverse reactions were reported. The effects of higher doses are not known.

If overdose occurs the patient should be monitored for evidence of toxicity (see section 4.8), and standard supportive treatment applied as necessary. Since lamivudine is dialysable, continuous haemodialysis could be used in the treatment of overdose, although this has not been studied. Haemodialysis and peritoneal dialysis appear to have a limited effect on elimination of zidovudine, but enhance the elimination of the glucuronide metabolite. It is not known whether abacavir can be removed by peritoneal dialysis or haemodialysis.

Table 3 Adverse events reported with the individual components of Trizivir

	Abacavir	Lamivudine	Zidovudine
IMPORTANT: for information on abacavir hypersensitivity, see the description above in the boxed information and Table 2			
Cardiovascular			Cardiomyopathy.
Gastrointestinal tract	**Nausea, vomiting, diarrhoea.**	**Nausea, vomiting, diarrhoea, abdominal pain or cramps.**	**Nausea, vomiting, anorexia,** diarrhoea, abdominal pain, oral mucosa pigmentation, dyspepsia and flatulence.
Neurological/ psychiatry	**Headache**.	**Headache, insomnia,** peripheral neuropathy (or paraesthesia).	**Headache, insomnia,** paraesthesia, dizziness, somnolence, loss of mental acuity, convulsions, anxiety, depression.
Haematological		Neutropenia and anaemia (both occasionally severe) have occurred in combination with zidovudine, thrombocytopenia, very rarely pure red cell aplasia.	Anaemia, neutropenia and leucopenia (see below for further details), thrombocytopenia, and pancytopenia with marrow hypoplasia, very rarely pure red cell aplasia, very rarely aplastic anaemia.
Liver/pancreas	Pancreatitis.	Transient rises in liver enzymes (AST, ALT), rarely hepatitis, rises in serum amylase and pancreatitis.	Liver disorders such as severe hepatomegaly with steatosis, rises in blood levels of liver enzymes and bilirubin, pancreatitis.
Musculoskeletal		**Muscle disorders,** arthralgia, rhabdomyolysis.	**Myalgia,** myopathy.
Respiratory tract		**Cough, nasal symptoms.**	Cough, dyspnoea.
Skin	rash (without systemic symptoms). Very rare reports of erythema multiforme, Stevens-Johnson syndrome and toxic epidermal necrolysis.	**Rash, alopecia.**	Rash, nail and skin pigmentation, urticaria, pruritus, sweating.
Metabolic/endocrine	Lactic acidosis.	Lactic acidosis.	Lactic acidosis.
Miscellaneous	**Fever, lethargy, fatigue,** anorexia.	**Fever, malaise, fatigue.**	**Malaise,** fever, urinary frequency, taste perversion, generalised pain, chills, chest pain, influenza-like syndrome, gynaecomastia, asthenia.

5. PHARMACOLOGICAL PROPERTIES

5.1 Pharmacodynamic properties

Pharmacotherapeutic group, nucleoside reverse transcriptase inhibitors, ATC Code: J05A F30.

Mechanism of action and resistance

Abacavir, lamivudine and zidovudine are all NRTIs, and are potent selective inhibitors of HIV-1 and HIV-2.

All three medicinal products are metabolised sequentially by intracellular kinases to the respective 5′-triphosphate (TP). Lamivudine-TP, carbovir-TP (the active triphosphate form of abacavir) and zidovudine-TP are substrates for and competitive inhibitors of HIV reverse transcriptase. However, their main antiviral activity is through incorporation of the monophosphate form into the viral DNA chain, resulting in chain termination. Abacavir, lamivudine and zidovudine triphosphates show significantly less affinity for host cell DNA polymerases.

Lamivudine has been shown to be highly synergistic with zidovudine, inhibiting the replication of HIV in cell culture. Abacavir shows synergy *in vitro* in combination with nevirapine and zidovudine. It has been shown to be additive in combination with didanosine, zalcitabine, stavudine and lamivudine.

Abacavir-resistant isolates of HIV-1 have been selected *in vitro* and are associated with specific genotypic changes in the reverse transcriptase (RT) codon region (codons M184V, K65R, L74V and Y115F). Viral resistance to abacavir develops relatively slowly *in vitro* and *in vivo*, requiring multiple mutations to reach an eight-fold increase in IC_{50} over wild-type virus, which may be a clinically relevant level. Isolates resistant to abacavir may also show reduced sensitivity to lamivudine, zalcitabine and/or didanosine, but remain sensitive to zidovudine and stavudine.

Cross-resistance between abacavir, lamivudine or zidovudine and PIs or NNRTIs is unlikely. Reduced susceptibility to abacavir has been demonstrated in clinical isolates of patients with uncontrolled viral replication, who have been pre-treated with and are resistant to other nucleoside inhibitors. Clinical isolates with three or more mutations associated with NRTIs are unlikely to be susceptible to abacavir.

Clinical experience

One randomised, double blind, placebo controlled clinical study has compared the combination of abacavir, lamivudine and zidovudine to the combination of indinavir, lamivudine and zidovudine in treatment naive patients. Due to the high proportion of premature discontinuation (42 % of patients discontinued randomised treatment by week 48), no definitive conclusion can be drawn regarding the equivalence between the treatment regimens at week 48. Although a similar antiviral effect was observed between the abacavir and indinavir containing regimens in terms of proportion of patients with undetectable viral load (≤ 400 copies/ml; intention to treat analysis (ITT), 47 % versus 49 %; as treated analysis (AT), 86 % versus 94 % for abacavir and indinavir combinations respectively), results favoured the indinavir combination, particularly in the subset of patients with high viral load > 100,000 copies/ml at baseline; ITT, 46 % versus 55 %; AT, 84 % versus 93 % for abacavir and indinavir respectively).

In an ongoing clinical study over 16 weeks in treatment-naive patients, the combination of abacavir, lamivudine and zidovudine showed a similar antiviral effect to the combination with nelfinavir, lamivudine and zidovudine.

In antiretroviral-naïve patients the triple combination of abacavir, lamivudine and zidovudine was superior in terms of durability of viral load response over 48 weeks to lamivudine and zidovudine. In a similar patient population durability of antiviral response over 120 weeks was demonstrated in approximately 70 % of subjects.

In antiretroviral-naive patients treated with a combination of abacavir, lamivudine, zidovudine and efavirenz in a small, ongoing, open label pilot study, the proportion of patients with undetectable viral load (< 400 copies/ml) was approximately 90 % with 80 % having < 50 copies/ml after 24 weeks of treatment.

In patients with a low baseline viral load (< 5,000 copies/ml) and moderate exposure to antiretroviral therapy, addition of abacavir to previous treatment including lamivudine and zidovudine, produced a moderate impact on viral load at 48 weeks.

Currently there are no data on the use of Trizivir in heavily pre-treated patients, patients failing on other therapies or patients with advanced disease (CD4 cells < 50 cells/mm^3).

The degree of benefit of this nucleoside combination in heavily pre-treated patients will depend on the nature and duration of prior therapy that may have selected for HIV-1 variants with cross-resistance to abacavir, lamivudine or zidovudine.

To date there are insufficient data on the efficacy and safety of Trizivir given concomitantly with NNRTIs or PIs.

5.2 Pharmacokinetic properties

Absorption

Abacavir, lamivudine and zidovudine are rapidly and well absorbed from the gastro-intestinal tract following oral administration. The absolute bioavailability of oral abacavir, lamivudine and zidovudine in adults is about 83 %, 80 - 85 % and 60 - 70 % respectively.

In a pharmacokinetic study in HIV-1 infected patients, the steady state pharmacokinetic parameters of abacavir, lamivudine and zidovudine were similar when either Trizivir alone or the combination tablet lamivudine/zidovudine and abacavir in combination were administered, and also similar to the values obtained in the bioequivalence study of Trizivir in healthy volunteers.

A bioequivalence study compared Trizivir with abacavir 300 mg, lamivudine 150 mg and zidovudine 300 mg taken together. The effect of food on the rate and extent of absorption was also studied. Trizivir was shown to be bioequivalent to abacavir 300 mg, lamivudine 150 mg and zidovudine 300 mg given as separate tablets for AUC_∞ and C_{max}. Food decreased the rate of absorption of Trizivir (slight decrease C_{max} (mean 18 - 32 %) and increase t_{max} (approximately 1 hour), but not the extent of absorption (AUC_∞). These changes are not considered clinically relevant and no food restrictions are recommended for administration of Trizivir.

At a therapeutic dosage (one Trizivir tablet twice daily) in patients, the mean (CV) steady-state C_{max} of abacavir, lamivudine and zidovudine in plasma are 3.49 μg/ml (45 %), 1.33 μg/ml (33 %) and 1.56 μg/ml (83 %), respectively. Corresponding values for C_{min} could not be established for abacavir and are 0.14 μg/ml (70 %) for lamivudine and 0.01 μg/ml (64 %) for zidovudine. The mean (CV) AUCs for abacavir, lamivudine and zidovudine over a dosing interval of 12 hours are 6.39 μg.h/ml (31 %), 5.73 μg.h/ml (31 %) and 1.50 μg.h/ml (47 %), respectively.

A modest increase in C_{max} (28 %) was observed for zidovudine when administered with lamivudine, however overall exposure (AUC) was not significantly altered. Zidovudine has no effect on the pharmacokinetics of lamivudine. An effect of abacavir is observed on zidovudine (C_{max} reduced with 20 %) and on lamivudine (C_{max} reduced with 35 %).

Distribution

Intravenous studies with abacavir, lamivudine and zidovudine showed that the mean apparent volume of distribution is 0.8, 1.3 and 1.6 l/kg respectively. Lamivudine exhibits linear pharmacokinetics over the therapeutic dose range and displays limited binding to the major plasma protein albumin (< 36 % serum albumin in vitro). Zidovudine plasma protein binding is 34 % to 38 %. Plasma protein binding studies in vitro indicate that abacavir binds only low to moderately (~ 49 %) to human plasma proteins at therapeutic concentrations. This indicates a low likelihood for interactions with other medicinal products through plasma protein binding displacement.

Interactions involving binding site displacement are not anticipated with Trizivir.

Data show that abacavir, lamivudine and zidovudine penetrate the central nervous system (CNS) and reach the cerebrospinal fluid (CSF). The mean ratios of CSF/serum lamivudine and zidovudine concentrations 2 - 4 hours after oral administration were approximately 0.12 and 0.5 respectively. The true extent of CNS penetration of lamivudine and its relationship with any clinical efficacy is unknown.

Studies with abacavir demonstrate a CSF to plasma AUC ratio of between 30 to 44 %. The observed values of the peak concentrations are 9 fold greater than the IC_{50} of abacavir of 0.08 μg/ml or 0.26 μM when abacavir is given at 600 mg twice daily.

Metabolism

Metabolism of lamivudine is a minor route of elimination. Lamivudine is predominately cleared by renal excretion of unchanged lamivudine. The likelihood of metabolic drug interactions with lamivudine is low due to the small extent of hepatic metabolism (5 - 10 %) and low plasma binding.

The 5'-glucuronide of zidovudine is the major metabolite in both plasma and urine, accounting for approximately 50 - 80 % of the administered dose eliminated by renal excretion. 3'-amino-3'-deoxythymidine (AMT) has been identified as a metabolite of zidovudine following intravenous dosing.

Abacavir is primarily metabolised by the liver with approximately 2 % of the administered dose being renally excreted, as unchanged compound. The primary pathways of metabolism in man are by alcohol dehydrogenase and by glucuronidation to produce the 5'-carboxylic acid and 5'-glucuronide which account for about 66 % of the dose excreted in the urine.

Elimination

The observed lamivudine half-life of elimination is 5 to 7 hours. The mean systemic clearance of lamivudine is approximately 0.32 l/h/kg, with predominantly renal clearance > 70 %) via the organic cationic transport system. Studies in patients with renal impairment show lamivudine elimination is affected by renal dysfunction. Dose reduction is required for patients with creatinine clearance ⩽ 50 ml/min (see section 4.2).

From studies with intravenous zidovudine, the mean terminal plasma half-life was 1.1 hours and the mean systemic clearance was 1.6 l/h/kg. Renal clearance of zidovudine is estimated to be 0.34 l/h/kg, indicating glomerular filtration and active tubular secretion by the kidneys. Zidovudine concentrations are increased in patients with advanced renal failure.

The mean half-life of abacavir is about 1.5 hours. Following multiple oral doses of abacavir 300 mg twice a day there is no significant accumulation of abacavir. Elimination of abacavir is via hepatic metabolism with subsequent excretion of metabolites primarily in the urine. The metabolites and unchanged abacavir account for about 83 % of the administered abacavir dose in the urine the remainder is eliminated in the faeces.

Special populations

Hepatically impaired: There are no data available on the use of Trizivir in hepatically impaired patients. Limited data in patients with cirrhosis suggest that accumulation of zidovudine may occur in patients with hepatic impairment because of decreased glucuronidation. Data obtained in patients with moderate to severe hepatic impairment show that lamivudine pharmacokinetics are not significantly affected by hepatic dysfunction.

Abacavir is metabolised primarily by the liver. The pharmacokinetics of abacavir have been studied in patients with mild hepatic impairment (Child-Pugh score 5-6) receiving a single 600 mg dose. The results showed that there was a mean increase of 1.89 fold [1.32; 2.70] in the abacavir AUC, and 1.58 [1.22; 2.04] fold in the elimination half-life. No recommendation on dosage reduction is possible in patients with mild hepatic impairment due to substantial variability of abacavir exposure in this patient population. The pharmacokinetics of abacavir have not been studied in patients with moderate or severe hepatic impairment. Plasma concentrations of abacavir are expected to be variable and substantially increased in these patients (see section 4.3).

Renally impaired: The observed lamivudine half-life of elimination is 5 to 7 hours. The mean systemic clearance of lamivudine is approximately 0.32 l/h/kg, with predominantly renal clearance > 70 %) via the organic cationic transport system. Studies in patients with renal impairment show lamivudine elimination is affected by renal dysfunction.

From studies with intravenous zidovudine, the mean terminal plasma half-life was 1.1 hours and the mean systemic clearance was 1.6 l/h/kg. Renal clearance of zidovudine is estimated to be 0.34 l/h/kg, indicating glomerular filtration and active tubular secretion by the kidneys. Zidovudine concentrations are increased in patients with advanced renal failure.

Abacavir is primarily metabolised by the liver with approximately 2 % of abacavir excreted unchanged in the urine. The pharmacokinetics of abacavir in patients with end-stage renal disease is similar to patients with normal renal function, and, therefore, no dose reduction is required in patients with renal impairment.

As dosage adjustments of lamivudine and zidovudine may be necessary it is recommended that separate preparations of abacavir, lamivudine and zidovudine be administered to patients with reduced renal function (creatinine clearance ⩽ 50 ml/min). Trizivir is contraindicated in patients with end-stage renal disease (see section 4.3).

Elderly: No pharmacokinetic data are available in patients over 65 years of age.

5.3 Preclinical safety data

There are no data available on treatment with the combination of abacavir, lamivudine and zidovudine in animals. The clinically relevant toxicological effects of these three medicinal products are anaemia, neutropenia and leucopenia.

Mutagenicity and carcinogenicity

Neither abacavir, lamivudine nor zidovudine is mutagenic in bacterial tests, but like many nucleoside analogues they show activity in the *in vitro* mammalian tests such as the mouse lymphoma assay. This is consistent with the known activity of other nucleoside analogues.

Lamivudine has not shown any genotoxic activity in the *in vivo* studies at doses that gave plasma concentrations up to 40 - 50 times higher than clinical plasma levels. Zidovudine showed clastogenic effects in oral repeated dose micronucleus tests in mice and rats. Peripheral blood lymphocytes from AIDS patients receiving zidovudine treatment have also been observed to contain higher numbers of chromosome breakages.

A pilot study has demonstrated that zidovudine is incorporated into leukocyte nuclear DNA of adults, including pregnant women, taking zidovudine as treatment for HIV-1 infection, or for the prevention of mother to child viral transmission. Zidovudine was also incorporated into DNA from cord blood leukocytes of infants from zidovudine-treated mothers. A transplacental genotoxicity study conducted in monkeys compared zidovudine alone with the combination of zidovudine and lamivudine at human-equivalent exposures. The study demonstrated that foetuses exposed *in utero* to the combination sustained a higher level of nucleoside analogue-DNA incorporation into multiple foetal organs, and showed evidence of more telomere shortening than in those exposed to zidovudine alone. The clinical significance of these findings is unknown.

Abacavir has a weak potential to cause chromosomal damage both *in vitro* and *in vivo* at high test concentrations and therefore any potential risk to man must be balanced against the expected benefits of treatment.

The carcinogenic potential of a combination of abacavir, lamivudine and zidovudine has not been tested. In long-term oral carcinogenicity studies in rats and mice, lamivudine did not show any carcinogenic potential. In oral carcinogenicity studies with zidovudine in mice and rats, late appearing vaginal epithelial tumours were observed. A subsequent intravaginal carcinogenicity study confirmed the hypothesis that the vaginal tumours were the result of long term local exposure of the rodent vaginal epithelium to high concentrations of unmetabolised zidovudine in urine. There were no other zidovudine-related tumours observed in either sex of either species.

In addition, two transplacental carcinogenicity studies have been conducted in mice. In one study, by the US National Cancer Institute, zidovudine was administered at maximum tolerated doses to pregnant mice from day 12 to 18 of gestation. One year postnatally, there was an increase in the incidence of tumours in the lung, liver and female reproductive tract of offspring exposed to the highest dose level (420 mg/kg term body weight).

In a second study, mice were administered zidovudine at doses up to 40 mg/kg for 24 months, with exposure beginning prenatally on gestation day 10. Treatment related findings were limited to late-occurring vaginal epithelial tumours, which were seen with a similar incidence and time of onset as in the standard oral carcinogenicity study. The second study thus provided no evidence that zidovudine acts as a transplacental carcinogen.

It is concluded that as the increase in incidence of tumours in the first transplacental carcinogenicity study represents a hypothetical risk, this should be balanced against the proven therapeutic benefit.

Carcinogenicity studies with orally administered abacavir in mice and rats showed an increase in the incidence of malignant and non-malignant tumours. Malignant tumours occurred in the preputial gland of males and the clitoral gland of females of both species, and in rats in the thyroid gland of males and and in the liver, urinary bladder, lymph nodes and the subcutis of females.

The majority of these tumours occurred at the highest abacavir dose of 330 mg/kg/day in mice and 600 mg/kg/day in rats. The exception was the preputial gland tumour which occurred at a dose of 110 mg/kg in mice. The systemic exposure at the no effect level in mice and rats was equivalent to 3 and 7 times the human systemic exposure during therapy. While the carcinogenic potential in humans is unknown, these data suggest that a carcinogenic risk to humans is outweighed by the potential clinical benefit.

Repeat-dose toxicity:

In toxicology studies abacavir was shown to increase liver weights in rats and monkeys. The clinical relevance of this is unknown. There is no evidence from clinical studies that abacavir is hepatotoxic. Additionally, autoinduction of abacavir metabolism or induction of the metabolism of other medicinal products hepatically metabolised has not been observed in man.

Mild myocardial degeneration in the heart of mice and rats was observed following administration of abacavir for two years. The systemic exposures were equivalent to 7 to 24 times the expected systemic exposure in humans. The clinical relevance of this finding has not been determined.

Reproductive toxicology

Lamivudine was not teratogenic in animal studies but there were indications of an increase in early embryonic deaths in the rabbit at relatively low systemic exposures, comparable to those achieved in humans. A similar effect was not seen in rats even at very high systemic exposure.

Zidovudine had a similar effect in both species, but only at very high systemic exposures. At maternally toxic doses, zidovudine given to rats during organogenesis resulted in an increased incidence of malformations, but no evidence of foetal abnormalities was observed at lower doses.

Abacavir demonstrated toxicity to the developing embryo and foetus in rats, but not in rabbits. These findings included decreased foetal body weight, foetal oedema, and an increase in skeletal variations/malformations, early intra-uterine deaths and still births. No conclusion can be drawn with regard to the teratogenic potential of abacavir because of this embryo-foetal toxicity.

A fertility study in the rat has shown that abacavir had no effect on male or female fertility. Likewise, neither lamivudine nor zidovudine had any effect on fertility. Zidovudine has not been shown to affect the number of sperm, sperm morphology and motility in man.

6. PHARMACEUTICAL PARTICULARS

6.1 List of excipients

Core: microcrystalline cellulose, sodium starch glycollate (type A), magnesium stearate.

Coating: Opadry Green 03B11434 containing: hypromellose, titanium dioxide, polyethylene glycol, indigo carmine aluminium lake, iron oxide yellow.

6.2 Incompatibilities

Not applicable

6.3 Shelf life

2 years

6.4 Special precautions for storage

Do not store above 30°C

6.5 Nature and contents of container

Trizivir tablets are available in opaque PVC/Aclar blister packs containing 40 or 60 tablets or child-resistant HDPE bottles containing 60 tablets.

6.6 Instructions for use and handling

No special requirements

Administrative Data

7. MARKETING AUTHORISATION HOLDER

Glaxo Group Ltd

Greenford

Middlesex UB6 0NN

United Kingdom

8. MARKETING AUTHORISATION NUMBER(S)

EU/1/00/156/001 - Blister pack (40 Tablets)

EU/1/00/156/002 - Blister pack (60 Tablets)

EU/1/00/156/003 -Bottle pack (60 Tablets)

9. DATE OF FIRST AUTHORISATION/RENEWAL OF THE AUTHORISATION

28 December 2000

10. DATE OF REVISION OF THE TEXT

5 January 2005

Trosyl Nail Solution

(Pfizer Limited)

1. NAME OF THE MEDICINAL PRODUCT

TROSYL NAIL SOLUTION

2. QUALITATIVE AND QUANTITATIVE COMPOSITION

Tioconazole 283 mg/ml.

For excipients, see 6.1.

3. PHARMACEUTICAL FORM

Cutaneous solution. Clear pale yellow solution for topical application.

4. CLINICAL PARTICULARS

4.1 Therapeutic indications

Tioconazole is a broad spectrum imidazole antifungal agent. Trosyl Nail Solution is indicated for the topical treatment of nail infections due to susceptible fungi (dermatophytes and yeasts) and bacteria.

4.2 Posology and method of administration

Route of administration: Topical.

Adults The solution should be applied to the affected nails and immediately surrounding skin every twelve hours using the applicator brush supplied.

The duration of treatment is up to six months but may be extended to twelve months.

Use in the elderly No special precautions are required. Use the adult dose.

Use in children No special precautions are required. Use the adult dose.

4.3 Contraindications

Trosyl Nail Solution is contra-indicated in individuals who have been shown to be hypersensitive to imidazole antifungal agents, or to any of the components of the solution.

Use is contraindicated during pregnancy.

4.4 Special warnings and special precautions for use

Trosyl Nail Solution is not for ophthalmic use.

4.5 Interaction with other medicinal products and other forms of Interaction

None known.

4.6 Pregnancy and lactation

Use DuringPregnancy: In animal studies tioconazole was not teratogenic. At high doses it increased the incidence of renal abnormalities in rat embryos, but this effect was minor and transient and was not evident in weaned animals.

There is insufficient evidence as to the drug's safety in human pregnancy although absorption after topical administration is negligible. Because of the extensive duration of treatment required for nail infections, the use of Trosyl Nail Solution is contra-indicated throughout pregnancy.

Use During Lactation: It is unknown whether this drug is excreted in human milk. Because many drugs are excreted in human milk, nursing should be temporarily discontinued while Trosyl is administered.

4.7 Effects on ability to drive and use machines

None known.

4.8 Undesirable effects

Trosyl Nail Solution is well tolerated upon local application. Symptoms of local irritation have been reported by some patients, but are usually seen during the first week of treatment and are transient and mild.

However, if a sensitivity reaction develops with the use of Trosyl Nail Solution, treatment should be discontinued and appropriate therapy instituted.

Skin and subcutaneous tissue disorders (at the application site): Bullous eruption, dermatitis, pruritis, pain, oedema, tingling/burning sensation, contact dermatitis, dry skin, nail disorder (including nail discoloration, periungual inflammation and nail pain), rash, skin exfoliation, skin irritation.

Immune system disorders: Allergic Reaction (including peripheral oedema, periorbital oedema and urticaria).

4.9 Overdose

No cases of overdosage with Trosyl Nail Solution have been reported. In the event of excessive oral ingestion, gastrointestinal symptoms may occur. Appropriate means of gastric lavage should be considered.

5. PHARMACOLOGICAL PROPERTIES

5.1 Pharmacodynamic properties

Pharmacotherapeutic group: Imidazole and triazole derivatives; ATC-code: D01AC07.

Tioconazole is an imidazole which is active against commonly occurring dermatophyte and yeast-like fungal species. It is fungicidal in murine models vs. Candida spp., *T. rubrum* and *T. mentacrophytes*. *In vitro* it is fungicidal to pathenogenic dermatophytes, yeasts and other fungi. All dermatophytes and Candida spp. were inhibited by 6.25 or 12.5 mg/l respectively. It is also inhibitory vs. Staph. spp. and Strep. spp. at 100 mg/l or less.

Oral doses (200 mg/kg) did not affect behaviour in rats but 25 mg/kg i.v. produced dose-related respiratory distress, gasping, tremors and prostration. Slight but dose-related impairment of performance of mice on the rotating rod occurred from 25 mg/kg. Slight anti-cholinergic and antihistamine (H_1) activity was recorded *in vitro* but no effect on mice pupil size *in vivo*. Oral tioconazole prolonged alcohol and pentobarbitone sleeping time at 150 and 37.5 mg/kg respectively.

In the anaesthetised cat i.v. tioconazole 2.5 - 10 mg/kg produced brief falls in blood pressure and increased heart rate, haematuria, tremors and twitches.

5.2 Pharmacokinetic properties

Absorption is rapid and extensive on oral administration to rats, monkeys and man, the major metabolite being a glucuronide conjugate of tioconazole. Tissue uptake in rat and monkey was highest in liver, kidney and intestinal tract with excretion in all species mainly in faeces.

Rat studies using oral, dermal and vaginal administration of C^{14} labelled tioconazole confirm significantly lower absorption via the topical route.

In man, oral formulations of tioconazole (500mg) gave plasma concentrations of 1300ng/ml. Topical administration of dermal cream 1% (20mg/day) for 28 days, or vaginal cream 2% (100mg/day) for 30 days gave negligible mean peak plasma levels, i.e. 10.1 and 11.5ng/ml respectively.

After single dose administration of tioconazole vaginal ointment 6.5% w/w (tioconazole 300mg) the mean peak plasma concentration was 18ng/ml in humans, achieved approximately 8 hours post dose.

5.3 Preclinical safety data

None relevant to the prescriber.

6. PHARMACEUTICAL PARTICULARS

6.1 List of excipients

Undecylenic acid, ethyl acetate.

6.2 Incompatibilities

Not applicable.

6.3 Shelf life

24 months.

6.4 Special precautions for storage

Do not store above 25°C. Avoid flame and heat. Do not refrigerate.

6.5 Nature and contents of container

Trosyl Nail Solution is contained in an amber glass bottle with a screw cap fitted with an applicator containing 12 ml.

6.6 Instructions for use and handling

No special instructions are required.

7. MARKETING AUTHORISATION HOLDER

Pfizer Limited

Ramsgate Road

Sandwich

Kent

CT13 9NJ

United Kingdom

8. MARKETING AUTHORISATION NUMBER(S)

PL 00057/0236

9. DATE OF FIRST AUTHORISATION/RENEWAL OF THE AUTHORISATION

21 July 1999

10. DATE OF REVISION OF THE TEXT

May 2004

LEGAL CATEGORY

POM

TY4_0

Trusopt

(Merck Sharp & Dohme Limited)

1. NAME OF THE MEDICINAL PRODUCT

TRUSOPT® 2% Eye drops, solution

2. QUALITATIVE AND QUANTITATIVE COMPOSITION

Each ml contains 20 mg dorzolamide (as 22.3 mg of dorzolamide hydrochloride).

3. PHARMACEUTICAL FORM

Eye drops, solution.

Isotonic, buffered, slightly viscous, aqueous solution of dorzolamide hydrochloride.

4. CLINICAL PARTICULARS

4.1 Therapeutic indications

'Trusopt' is indicated:

- as adjunctive therapy to beta-blockers,
- as monotherapy in patients unresponsive to beta-blockers or in whom beta-blockers are contra-indicated, in the treatment of elevated intra-ocular pressure in:
- ocular hypertension,
- open-angle glaucoma,
- pseudo-exfoliative glaucoma.

4.2 Posology and method of administration

When used as monotherapy, the dose is one drop of dorzolamide in the conjunctival sac of the affected eye(s), three times daily.

When used as adjunctive therapy with an ophthalmic beta-blocker, the dose is one drop of dorzolamide in the conjunctival sac of the affected eye(s), two times daily.

When substituting dorzolamide for another ophthalmic antiglaucoma agent, discontinue the other agent after proper dosing on one day, and start dorzolamide on the next day.

If more than one topical ophthalmic drug is being used, the drugs should be administered at least ten minutes apart.

Please see section 6.6 'Instructions for use and handling.'

Paediatric use:

Safety and effectiveness in children have not been established.

4.3 Contraindications

Dorzolamide is contra-indicated in patients who are hypersensitive to any component of this product.

Dorzolamide has not been studied in patients with severe renal impairment (CrCl <30 ml/min) or with hyperchloraemic acidosis. Because dorzolamide and its metabolites are excreted predominantly by the kidney, dorzolamide is therefore contra-indicated in such patients.

4.4 Special warnings and special precautions for use

Dorzolamide has not been studied in patients with hepatic impairment and should therefore be used with caution in such patients.

The management of patients with acute angle-closure glaucoma requires therapeutic interventions in addition to ocular hypotensive agents. Dorzolamide has not been studied in patients with acute angle-closure glaucoma.

Dorzolamide is a sulphonamide and although administered topically, is absorbed systemically. Therefore, the same types of adverse reactions that are attributable to sulphonamides may occur with topical administration. If signs of serious reactions of hypersensitivity occur, discontinue the use of this preparation.

Therapy with oral carbonic anhydrase inhibitors has been associated with urolithiasis as a result of acid-base disturbances, especially in patients with a prior history of renal calculi. Although no acid-base disturbances have been observed with dorzolamide, urolithiasis has been reported infrequently. Because dorzolamide is a topical carbonic anhydrase inhibitor that is absorbed systemically, patients with a prior history of renal calculi may be at increased risk of urolithiasis while using dorzolamide.

In clinical studies, local ocular adverse effects, primarily conjunctivitis and lid reactions, were reported with chronic administration of dorzolamide. Some of these reactions had the clinical appearance and course of an allergic-type reaction that resolved upon discontinuation of drug therapy. If such reactions are observed, discontinuation of treatment should be considered.

There is a potential for an additive effect on the known systemic effects of carbonic anhydrase inhibition in patients receiving an oral carbonic anhydrase inhibitor and dorzolamide. The concomitant administration of dorzolamide and oral carbonic anhydrase inhibitors is not recommended.

Corneal oedemas and irreversible corneal decompensations have been reported in patients with pre-existing chronic corneal defects and/or a history of intra-ocular surgery while using 'Trusopt'. Topical dorzolamide should be used with caution in such patients.

Choroidal detachment concomitant with ocular hypotony have been reported after filtration procedures with administration of aqueous suppressant therapies.

Dorzolamide has not been studied in patients wearing contact lenses. However, 'Trusopt' contains the preservative benzalkonium chloride, which may be absorbed by soft contact lenses. Therefore dorzolamide should not be administered while wearing soft contact lenses. Contact lenses should be removed before application of the drops and not be re-inserted earlier than 15 minutes after use.

4.5 Interaction with other medicinal products and other forms of Interaction

Specific drug interaction studies have not been performed with dorzolamide.

In clinical studies, dorzolamide was used concomitantly with the following medications without evidence of adverse interactions: timolol ophthalmic solution, betaxolol ophthalmic solution and systemic medications, including ACE-inhibitors, calcium-channel blockers, diuretics, non-steroidal anti-inflammatory drugs including aspirin, and hormones (e.g. oestrogen, insulin, thyroxine).

Association between dorzolamide and miotics and adrenergic agonists has not been fully evaluated during glaucoma therapy.

Dorzolamide is a carbonic anhydrase inhibitor and, although administered topically, is absorbed systemically. In clinical studies, dorzolamide was not associated with acid-base disturbances. However, these disturbances have been reported with oral carbonic anhydrase inhibitors and have, in some instances, resulted in drug interactions (e.g. toxicity associated with high-dose salicylate therapy). Therefore, the potential for such drug interactions should be considered in patients receiving dorzolamide.

4.6 Pregnancy and lactation

Pregnancy: No studies were performed on pregnant women. Dorzolamide should not be used during pregnancy. In rabbits given maternotoxic doses associated with metabolic acidosis, malformations of the vertebral bodies were observed.

Lactation: There are no data showing whether the drug is excreted in human milk. Dorzolamide should not be used during lactation. In lactating rats, decreases in the body-weight gain of offspring were observed.

4.7 Effects on ability to drive and use machines

Possible side effects such as dizziness and visual disturbances may affect the ability to drive and use machines (see also 4.8 'Undesirable effects').

4.8 Undesirable effects

The following adverse reactions have been reported either during clinical trials or during post-marketing experience:

Eye disorders: burning and stinging, blurred vision, eye itching, tearing, conjunctivitis, eyelid inflammation, eyelid irritation, eyelid crusting, irritation including redness, pain, superficial punctate keratitis, corneal oedema, iridocyclitis, transient myopia (which resolved upon discontinuation of therapy), ocular hypotony and choroidal detachment following filtration surgery (see also 4.4);

General disorders: Hypersensitivity: signs and symptoms of local reactions (palpebral reactions) and systemic allergic reactions including angioedema, urticaria and pruritus, rash, shortness of breath, rarely bronchospasm;

Gastro-intestinal disorders: bitter taste, nausea, dry mouth, throat irritation;

Respiratory disorders: epistaxis;

Skin disorders: contact dermatitis;

Nervous system disorders: headache, asthenia/fatigue, dizziness, paraesthesia;

Renal and urinary disorders: urolithiasis;

Laboratory findings: Dorzolamide was not associated with clinically meaningful electrolyte disturbances.

4.9 Overdose

Only limited information is available with regard to human overdosage by accidental or deliberate ingestion of dorzolamide hydrochloride. The following have been reported with oral ingestion: somnolence; topical application: nausea, dizziness, headache, fatigue, abnormal dreams, and dysphagia.

Treatment should be symptomatic and supportive. Electrolyte imbalance, development of an acidotic state, and possible central nervous system effects may occur. Serum electrolyte levels (particularly potassium) and blood pH levels should be monitored.

5. PHARMACOLOGICAL PROPERTIES

5.1 Pharmacodynamic properties

ATC code: S01 EC 03

Topical anti-glaucomatous agent.

Carbonic anhydrase inhibitor.

Mechanism of action

Carbonic anhydrase (CA) is an enzyme found in many tissues of the body, including the eye. In humans, carbonic anhydrase exists as a number of isoenzymes, the most active being carbonic anhydrase II (CA-II) found primarily in red blood cells (RBCs) but also in other tissues. Inhibition of carbonic anhydrase in the ciliary processes of the eye decreases aqueous-humor secretion. The result is a reduction in intra-ocular pressure (IOP).

'Trusopt' contains dorzolamide hydrochloride, a potent inhibitor of human carbonic anhydrase II. Following topical ocular administration, dorzolamide reduces elevated intra-ocular pressure, whether or not associated with glaucoma. Elevated intra-ocular pressure is a major risk factor in the pathogenesis of optic nerve damage and visual-field loss. Dorzolamide does not cause pupillary constriction and reduces intra-ocular pressure without side effects such as night blindness, accommodative spasm. Dorzolamide has minimal or no effect on pulse rate or blood pressure.

Topically applied beta-adrenergic blocking agents also reduce IOP by decreasing aqueous humor secretion but by a different mechanism of action. Studies have shown that when dorzolamide is added to a topical beta-blocker, additional reduction in IOP is observed; this finding is consistent with the reported additive effects of beta-blockers and oral carbonic anhydrase inhibitors.

Pharmacodynamic effects

Clinical effects: In patients with glaucoma or ocular hypertension, the efficacy of dorzolamide given t.d.s. as monotherapy (baseline IOP $\geq$23 mmHg) or given b.d. as adjunctive therapy while receiving ophthalmic beta-blockers (baseline IOP $\geq$22 mmHg) was demonstrated in large-scale clinical studies of up to one- year duration. The IOP-lowering effect of dorzolamide as monotherapy and as adjunctive therapy was demonstrated throughout the day and this effect was maintained during long-term administration. Efficacy during long-term monotherapy was similar to betaxolol and slightly less than timolol. When used as adjunctive therapy to ophthalmic beta-blockers, dorzolamide demonstrated additional IOP lowering similar to pilocarpine 2% q.d.s.

5.2 Pharmacokinetic properties

Unlike oral carbonic anhydrase inhibitors, topical administration of dorzolamide hydrochloride allows for the drug to exert its effects directly in the eye at substantially lower doses and therefore with less systemic exposure. In clinical trials, this resulted in a reduction in IOP without the acid-base disturbances or alterations in electrolytes characteristic of oral carbonic anhydrase inhibitors.

When topically applied, dorzolamide reaches the systemic circulation. To assess the potential for systemic carbonic anhydrase inhibition following topical administration, drug and metabolite concentrations in RBCs and plasma and carbonic anhydrase inhibition in RBCs were measured. Dorzolamide accumulates in RBCs during chronic dosing as a result of selective binding to CA-II while extremely low concentrations of free drug in plasma are maintained. The parent drug forms a single N-desethyl metabolite that inhibits CA-II less potently than the parent drug but also inhibits a less active isoenzyme (CA-I). The metabolite also accumulates in RBCs where it binds primarily to CA-I. Dorzolamide binds moderately to plasma proteins (approximately 33%). Dorzolamide is primarily excreted unchanged in the urine; the metabolite is also excreted in urine. After dosing ends, dorzolamide washes out of RBCs non-linearly, resulting in a rapid decline of drug concentration initially, followed by a slower elimination phase with a half-life of about four months.

When dorzolamide was given orally to simulate the maximum systemic exposure after long-term topical ocular administration, steady state was reached within 13 weeks. At steady state, there was virtually no free drug or metabolite in plasma; CA inhibition in RBCs was less than that anticipated to be necessary for a pharmacological effect on renal function or respiration. Similar pharmacokinetic results were observed after chronic, topical administration of dorzolamide.

However, some elderly patients with renal impairment (estimated CrCl 30-60 ml/min) had higher metabolite concentrations in RBCs, but no meaningful differences in carbonic anhydrase inhibition, and no clinically significant systemic side effects were directly attributable to this finding.

5.3 Preclinical safety data

The main findings in animal studies with dorzolamide hydrochloride administered orally were related to the pharmacological effects of systemic carbonic anhydrase inhibition. Some of these findings were species-specific and/ or were a result of metabolic acidosis.

In clinical studies, patients did not develop signs of metabolic acidosis or serum electrolyte changes that are indicative of systemic CA inhibition. Therefore, it is not expected that the effects noted in animal studies would be observed in patients receiving therapeutic doses of dorzolamide.

6. PHARMACEUTICAL PARTICULARS

6.1 List of excipients

Hydroxyethyl cellulose, mannitol, sodium citrate, sodium hydroxide (to adjust q.s. pH = 5.65), benzalkonium chloride, water for injections.

6.2 Incompatibilities

None known.

6.3 Shelf life

The shelf-life is 2 years.

'Trusopt' should be used no longer than 28 days after first opening of the container.

6.4 Special precautions for storage

Store bottle in outer carton.

6.5 Nature and contents of container

The OCUMETER Plus ophthalmic dispenser consists of a translucent, high-density polyethylene container with a sealed dropper tip, a flexible fluted side area which is depressed to dispense the drops, and a two-piece cap assembly. The two-piece cap mechanism punctures the sealed dropper tip upon initial use, then locks together to provide a single cap during the usage period. Tamper evidence is provided by a safety strip on the container label. The OCUMETER Plus ophthalmic dispenser contains 5 ml of solution.

'Trusopt' is available in the following packaging configurations:

1 × 5 ml (single 5-ml container)

3 × 5 ml (three 5-ml containers)

6 × 5 ml (six 5-ml containers)

6.6 Instructions for use and handling

Patients should be instructed to avoid allowing the tip of the dispensing container to contact the eye or surrounding structures.

Patients should also be instructed that ocular solutions, if handled improperly, can become contaminated by common bacteria known to cause ocular infections. Serious damage to the eye and subsequent loss of vision may result from using contaminated solutions.

Patients should be informed of the correct handling of the OCUMETER Plus bottles.

Usage instructions:

1. Before using the medication for the first time, be sure the safety strip on the front of the bottle is unbroken. A gap between the bottle and the cap is normal for an unopened bottle.

2. Tear off the safety strip to break the seal.

3. To open the bottle, unscrew the cap by turning as indicated by the arrows.

4. Tilt your head back and pull your lower eyelid down slightly to form a pocket between your eyelid and your eye.

5. Invert the bottle, and press lightly with the thumb or index finger over the "Finger Push Area" until a single drop is dispensed into the eye as directed by your doctor. DO NOT TOUCH YOUR EYE OR EYELID WITH THE DROPPER TIP.

6. Repeat steps 4 & 5 with the other eye if instructed to do so by your doctor.

7. Replace the cap by turning until it is firmly touching the bottle. Do not over-tighten the cap.

8 The dispenser tip is designed to provide a pre-measured drop; therefore, do NOT enlarge the hole of the dispenser tip.

9 After you have used all doses, there will be some 'Trusopt' left in the bottle. You should not be concerned since an extra amount of 'Trusopt' has been added and you will get the full amount of 'Trusopt' that your doctor prescribed. Do not attempt to remove the excess medicine from the bottle.

7. MARKETING AUTHORISATION HOLDER

Merck Sharp & Dohme Limited

Hertford Road, Hoddesdon, Hertfordshire EN11 9BU, UK

8. MARKETING AUTHORISATION NUMBER(S)

2% Eye drops, solution: PL 0025/0323.

9. DATE OF FIRST AUTHORISATION/RENEWAL OF THE AUTHORISATION

9 January 1995/ 11 November 1999.

10. DATE OF REVISION OF THE TEXT

Revision approved: April 2002.

LEGAL CATEGORY

P.O.M.

® denotes registered trademark of Merck & Co., Inc., Whitehouse Station, NJ, USA.

MSD (logo)

Merck Sharp & Dohme Limited

Hertford Road, Hoddesdon, Hertfordshire EN11 9BU, UK.

SPC.DZH.01.UK/IRL.0732(W21)

Truvada film-coated tablets

(Gilead Sciences International Limited)

1. NAME OF THE MEDICINAL PRODUCT
Truvada film-coated tablets. ▼

2. QUALITATIVE AND QUANTITATIVE COMPOSITION
Each film-coated tablet contains 200 mg of emtricitabine and 245 mg of tenofovir disoproxil (equivalent to 300 mg of tenofovir disoproxil fumarate or 136 mg of tenofovir).

For excipients, see section 6.1.

3. PHARMACEUTICAL FORM
Film-coated tablet.

Blue, capsule-shaped, film-coated tablet, debossed on one side with "GILEAD" and on the other side with "701".

4. CLINICAL PARTICULARS

4.1 Therapeutic indications
Truvada is a fixed dose combination of emtricitabine and tenofovir disoproxil fumarate. It is indicated in antiretroviral combination therapy for the treatment of HIV-1 infected adults.

The demonstration of the benefit of the combination emtricitabine and tenofovir disoproxil fumarate in antiretroviral therapy is based solely on studies performed in treatment-naïve patients (see section 5.1).

4.2 Posology and method of administration
Therapy should be initiated by a physician experienced in the management of HIV infection.

Posology

Adults: The recommended dose of Truvada is one tablet, taken orally, once daily. In order to optimise the absorption of tenofovir, it is recommended that Truvada should be taken with food. Even a light meal improves absorption of tenofovir from the combination tablet (see section 5.2).

Where discontinuation of therapy with one of the components of Truvada is indicated or where dose modification is necessary, separate preparations of emtricitabine and tenofovir disoproxil fumarate are available. Please refer to the Summary of Product Characteristics for these medicinal products.

Children and adolescents: The safety and efficacy of Truvada have not been established in patients under the age of 18 years. Consequently, Truvada should not be administered to children or adolescents.

Elderly: No data are available on which to make a dose recommendation for patients over the age of 65 years. However, no adjustment in the recommended daily dose for adults should be required unless there is evidence of renal insufficiency.

Renal insufficiency: Exposure to emtricitabine and tenofovir may be significantly increased when Truvada is administered to patients with moderate to severe renal impairment as emtricitabine and tenofovir are principally eliminated by renal excretion. Dosing interval adjustment of Truvada is required in patients with moderate renal impairment (creatinine clearance between 30 and 49 ml/min), as detailed below.

	Creatinine Clearance (ml/min)*	
	≥ 50	30-49
Recommended Dosing Interval	Every 24 hours	Every 48 hours

* Calculated using ideal (lean) body weight

The safety and efficacy of these dosing interval adjustment guidelines have not been clinically evaluated. Therefore, clinical response to treatment and renal function should be closely monitored in these patients (see sections 4.4 and 5.2).

Truvada is not recommended for patients with severe renal impairment (creatinine clearance < 30 ml/min) and in patients who require haemodialysis since appropriate dose reductions cannot be achieved with the combination tablet.

Hepatic impairment: The pharmacokinetics of Truvada and emtricitabine have not been studied in patients with hepatic impairment. The pharmacokinetics of tenofovir have been studied in patients with hepatic impairment and no dose adjustment is required for tenofovir disoproxil fumarate in these patients. Based on minimal hepatic metabolism and the renal route of elimination for emtricitabine, it is unlikely that a dose adjustment would be required for Truvada in patients with hepatic impairment (see sections 4.4 and 5.2).

Method of administration

If patients have difficulty in swallowing, Truvada can be disintegrated in approximately 100 ml of water, orange juice or grape juice and taken immediately.

4.3 Contraindications
Hypersensitivity to emtricitabine, tenofovir, tenofovir disoproxil fumarate or to any of the excipients.

4.4 Special warnings and special precautions for use
Truvada should not be administered concomitantly with other medicinal products containing emtricitabine, tenofovir disoproxil (as fumarate) or other cytidine analogues, such as lamivudine and zalcitabine (see section 4.5).

Triple nucleoside therapy: There have been reports of a high rate of virological failure and of emergence of resistance at an early stage when tenofovir disoproxil fumarate was combined with lamivudine and abacavir as well as with lamivudine and didanosine as a once daily regimen. There is close structural similarity between lamivudine and emtricitabine and similarities in the pharmacokinetics and pharmacodynamics of these two agents. Therefore, the same problems may be seen if Truvada is administered with a third nucleoside analogue.

Patients receiving Truvada or any other antiretroviral therapy may continue to develop opportunistic infections and other complications of HIV infection, and therefore should remain under close clinical observation by physicians experienced in the treatment of patients with HIV associated diseases.

Patients must be advised that antiretroviral therapies, including Truvada, have not been proven to prevent the risk of transmission of HIV to others through sexual contact or blood contamination. Appropriate precautions must continue to be used.

Truvada contains lactose monohydrate. Consequently, patients with rare hereditary problems of galactose intolerance, the Lapp lactase deficiency, or glucose-galactose malabsorption should not take this medicine.

Renal impairment: Emtricitabine and tenofovir are primarily excreted by the kidneys by a combination of glomerular filtration and active tubular secretion. Emtricitabine and tenofovir exposure may be markedly increased in patients with moderate or severe renal impairment. Consequently, a dose interval adjustment is required in patients with creatinine clearance between 30 and 49 ml/min (see section 5.2). The safety and efficacy of Truvada in patients with renal impairment have not been established. Careful monitoring for signs of toxicity, such as deterioration of renal function, and for changes in viral load is required in patients with pre-existing renal impairment once Truvada has been started at prolonged dosing intervals. Truvada is not recommended for patients with creatinine clearance < 30 ml/min or patients who require haemodialysis, as the required dose modifications for emtricitabine and tenofovir disoproxil fumarate cannot be achieved with Truvada (see section 4.2).

Renal events, which may include hypophosphataemia, have been reported with the use of tenofovir disoproxil fumarate in clinical practice (see section 4.8).

Careful monitoring of renal function (serum creatinine and serum phosphate) is recommended before taking Truvada, every four weeks during the first year, and then every three months. In patients with a history of renal dysfunction or in patients who are at risk for renal dysfunction, consideration should be given to more frequent monitoring of renal function.

Use of Truvada should be avoided with concurrent or recent use of a nephrotoxic medicinal product (see section 4.5).

Truvada should be avoided in antiretroviral-experienced patients with HIV-1 harbouring the K65R mutation (see section 5.1).

In a 144-week controlled clinical study that compared tenofovir disoproxil fumarate with stavudine in combination with lamivudine and efavirenz in antiretroviral-naïve patients, small decreases in bone mineral density of the hip and spine were observed in both treatment groups. Decreases in bone mineral density of spine and changes in bone biomarkers from baseline were significantly greater in the tenofovir disoproxil fumarate treatment group at 144 weeks. Decreases in bone mineral density of hip were significantly greater in this group until 96 weeks. However, there was no increased risk of fractures or evidence for clinically relevant bone abnormalities over 144 weeks. If bone abnormalities are suspected then appropriate consultation should be obtained.

Patients with HIV and hepatitis B or C virus co-infection: Patients with chronic hepatitis B or C treated with antiretroviral therapy are at an increased risk for severe and potentially fatal hepatic adverse reactions.

Physicians should refer to current HIV treatment guidelines for the optimal management of HIV infection in patients co-infected with hepatitis B virus (HBV).

In case of concomitant antiviral therapy for hepatitis B or C, please refer also to the relevant Summary of Product Characteristics for these medicinal products.

The safety and efficacy of Truvada have not been established for the treatment of chronic HBV infection. Emtricitabine and tenofovir individually and in combination have shown activity against HBV in pharmacodynamic studies (see section 5.1). Limited clinical experience suggests that emtricitabine and tenofovir disoproxil fumarate have anti-HBV activity when used in antiretroviral combination therapy to control HIV infection.

Exacerbations of hepatitis have been reported in patients after the discontinuation of emtricitabine or tenofovir disoproxil fumarate. Patients co-infected with HIV and HBV should be closely monitored with both clinical and laboratory follow-up for at least several months after stopping treatment with Truvada.

Liver disease: The safety and efficacy of Truvada have not been established in patients with significant underlying liver disorders. The pharmacokinetics of Truvada and emtricitabine have not been studied in patients with hepatic impairment. The pharmacokinetics of tenofovir have been studied in patients with hepatic impairment and no dose adjustment is required in these patients. Based on minimal hepatic metabolism and the renal route of elimination for emtricitabine, it is unlikely that a dose adjustment would be required for Truvada in patients with hepatic impairment (see section 5.2).

Patients with pre-existing liver dysfunction, including chronic active hepatitis, have an increased frequency of liver function abnormalities during combination antiretroviral therapy and should be monitored according to standard practice. If there is evidence of worsening liver disease in such patients, interruption or discontinuation of treatment must be considered.

Lactic acidosis: Lactic acidosis, usually associated with hepatic steatosis, has been reported with the use of nucleoside analogues. Early symptoms (symptomatic hyperlactataemia) include benign digestive symptoms (nausea, vomiting and abdominal pain), non-specific malaise, loss of appetite, weight loss, respiratory symptoms (rapid and/or deep breathing) or neurological symptoms (including motor weakness). Lactic acidosis has a high mortality and may be associated with pancreatitis, liver failure or renal failure. Lactic acidosis generally occurred after a few or several months of treatment.

Treatment with nucleoside analogues should be discontinued in the setting of symptomatic hyperlactataemia and metabolic/lactic acidosis, progressive hepatomegaly, or rapidly elevating aminotransferase levels.

Caution should be exercised when administering nucleoside analogues to any patient (particularly obese women) with hepatomegaly, hepatitis or other known risk factors for liver disease and hepatic steatosis (including certain medicinal products and alcohol). Patients co-infected with hepatitis C and treated with alpha interferon and ribavirin may constitute a special risk.

Patients at increased risk should be followed closely.

Lipodystrophy: Combination antiretroviral therapy has been associated with the redistribution of body fat (lipodystrophy) in HIV patients. The long-term consequences of these events are currently unknown. Knowledge about the mechanism is incomplete. A connection between visceral lipomatosis and protease inhibitors and lipoatrophy and nucleoside reverse transcriptase inhibitors has been hypothesised. A higher risk of lipodystrophy has been associated with individual factors such as older age, and with drug related factors such as longer duration of antiretroviral treatment and associated metabolic disturbances. Clinical examination should include evaluation for physical signs of fat redistribution. Consideration should be given to the measurement of fasting serum lipids and blood glucose. Lipid disorders should be managed as clinically appropriate (see section 4.8).

Tenofovir is structurally related to nucleoside analogues hence the risk of lipodystrophy cannot be excluded. However, 144-week clinical data from antiretroviral-naïve patients indicate that the risk of lipodystrophy was lower with tenofovir disoproxil fumarate than with stavudine when administered with lamivudine and efavirenz.

Mitochondrial dysfunction: Nucleoside and nucleotide analogues have been demonstrated *in vitro* and *in vivo* to cause a variable degree of mitochondrial damage. There have been reports of mitochondrial dysfunction in HIV negative infants exposed *in utero* and/or postnatally to nucleoside analogues. The main adverse events reported are haematological disorders (anaemia, neutropenia), metabolic disorders (hyperlactataemia, hyperlipasaemia). These events are often transitory. Some late-onset neurological disorders have been reported (hypertonia, convulsion, abnormal behaviour). Whether the neurological disorders are transient or permanent is currently unknown. Any child exposed *in utero* to nucleoside and nucleotide analogues, even HIV negative children, should have clinical and laboratory follow-up and should be fully investigated for possible mitochondrial dysfunction in case of relevant signs or symptoms. These findings do not affect current national recommendations to use antiretroviral therapy in pregnant women to prevent vertical transmission of HIV.

Immune Reactivation Syndrome: In HIV infected patients with severe immune deficiency at the time of institution of combination antiretroviral therapy (CART), an inflammatory reaction to asymptomatic or residual opportunistic pathogens may arise and cause serious clinical conditions, or aggravation of symptoms. Typically, such reactions have been observed within the first few weeks or months of initiation of CART. Relevant examples are cytomegalovirus retinitis, generalised and/or focal mycobacterial infections, and *Pneumocystis carinii* pneumonia. Any inflammatory symptoms should be evaluated and treatment instituted when necessary.

Co-administration of tenofovir disoproxil fumarate and didanosine resulted in increased systemic exposure to didanosine. Patients receiving tenofovir disoproxil fumarate and didanosine should be carefully monitored for didanosine-related adverse events including, but not limited to, pancreatitis and peripheral neuropathy (see section 4.5).

4.5 Interaction with other medicinal products and other forms of Interaction
The steady-state pharmacokinetics of emtricitabine and tenofovir were unaffected when emtricitabine and tenofovir disoproxil fumarate were administered together *versus* each medicinal product dosed alone.

In vitro and clinical pharmacokinetic interaction studies have shown the potential for CYP450 mediated interactions involving emtricitabine and tenofovir disoproxil fumarate with other medicinal products is low.

Interactions relevant to emtricitabine:

In vitro, emtricitabine did not inhibit metabolism mediated by any of the following human CYP450 isoforms: 1A2, 2A6, 2B6, 2C9, 2C19, 2D6 and 3A4. Emtricitabine did not inhibit the enzyme responsible for glucuronidation.

There are no clinically significant interactions when emtricitabine is co-administered with indinavir, zidovudine, stavudine or famciclovir.

Emtricitabine is primarily excreted via glomerular filtration and active tubular secretion. With the exception of famciclovir and tenofovir disoproxil fumarate, the effect of co-administration of emtricitabine with medicinal products that are excreted by the renal route, or other medicinal products known to affect renal function, has not been evaluated. Co-administration of Truvada with medicinal products that are eliminated by active tubular secretion may lead to an increase in serum concentrations of either emtricitabine or a co-administered medicinal product due to competition for this elimination pathway.

There is no clinical experience with the co-administration of emtricitabine and cytidine analogues. Consequently, Truvada should not be administered in combination with lamivudine or zalcitabine for the treatment of HIV infection (see section 4.4).

Interactions relevant to tenofovir:

Co-administration of lamivudine, indinavir or efavirenz with tenofovir disoproxil fumarate did not result in any interaction.

When tenofovir disoproxil fumarate was administered with lopinavir/ritonavir, no changes were observed in the pharmacokinetics of lopinavir and ritonavir. Tenofovir AUC was increased by approximately 30% when tenofovir disoproxil fumarate was administered with lopinavir/ritonavir.

When didanosine gastro-resistant capsules were administered 2 hours prior to or concurrently with tenofovir disoproxil fumarate, the AUC for didanosine was on average increased by 48% and 60% respectively. The mean increase in the AUC of didanosine was 44% when the buffered tablets were administered 1 hour prior to tenofovir. In both cases the pharmacokinetic parameters for tenofovir administered with a light meal were unchanged. No recommendation could be drawn at this stage with regard to a specific dosage adjustment when these medicinal products are co-administered (see section 4.4).

When tenofovir disoproxil fumarate was administered with atazanavir, a decrease in concentrations of atazanavir was observed (decrease of 25% and 40% of AUC and C_{min} respectively compared to atazanavir 400 mg). When ritonavir was added to atazanavir, the negative impact of tenofovir on atazanavir C_{min} was significantly reduced, whereas the decrease of AUC was of the same magnitude (decrease of 25% and 26% of AUC and C_{min} respectively compared to atazanavir/ritonavir 300/100 mg).

Tenofovir is excreted renally, both by filtration and active secretion via the human organic anion transporter 1 (hOAT1). Co-administration of tenofovir disoproxil fumarate with other medicinal products that are also actively secreted via the anion transporter (e.g. cidofovir) may result in increased concentrations of tenofovir or of the co-administered medicinal product.

Tenofovir disoproxil fumarate has not been evaluated in patients receiving nephrotoxic medicinal products (e.g. aminoglycosides, amphotericin B, foscarnet, ganciclovir, pentamidine, vancomycin, cidofovir or interleukin-2). Use of tenofovir disoproxil fumarate should be avoided with concurrent or recent use of a nephrotoxic medicinal product. If concomitant use of Truvada and nephrotoxic agents is unavoidable, renal function should be monitored weekly (see section 4.4).

Co-administration of tenofovir disoproxil fumarate and methadone, ribavirin, adefovir dipivoxil or the hormonal contraceptive norgestimate/ethinyl oestradiol did not result in any pharmacokinetic interaction.

4.6 Pregnancy and lactation
Pregnancy:

For emtricitabine and tenofovir disoproxil fumarate, insufficient data on exposed pregnancies are available.

Animal studies do not indicate direct or indirect harmful effects of emtricitabine or tenofovir disoproxil fumarate with respect to pregnancy, embryonal/foetal development, parturition or postnatal development (see section 5.3).

However, Truvada should not be used during pregnancy unless no other alternative is available.

The use of Truvada must be accompanied by the use of effective contraception.

Lactation:

It is not known whether emtricitabine or tenofovir are excreted in human milk.

It is recommended that HIV infected women do not breast-feed their infants under any circumstances in order to avoid transmission of HIV to the infant.

4.7 Effects on ability to drive and use machines
No studies on the effects of Truvada on the ability to drive and use machines have been performed. However, patients should be informed that dizziness has been reported during treatment with both emtricitabine and tenofovir disoproxil fumarate.

4.8 Undesirable effects
As Truvada contains emtricitabine and tenofovir disoproxil fumarate, the type and severity of adverse reactions associated with these antiretrovirals may be expected to occur with the combination tablet. Data from two clinical studies in which emtricitabine and tenofovir disoproxil fumarate were co-administered did not show new patterns of adverse reactions compared to previous experience with each agent.

The adverse reactions considered at least possibly related to treatment with the components of Truvada from clinical trial and post-marketing experience are listed below by body system organ class and absolute frequency. Frequencies are defined as very common (⩾ 1/10), common (⩾ 1/100, < 1/10), uncommon (⩾ 1/1,000, < 1/100), rare (⩾ 1/10,000, < 1/1,000) or very rare (< 1/10,000) including isolated reports.

Blood and lymphatic system disorders:

Common: neutropenia

Immune system disorders:

Common: allergic reaction

Metabolism and nutrition disorders:

Very common: hypophosphataemia

Common: hypertriglyceridaemia, hyperglycaemia

Rare: lactic acidosis

Lactic acidosis, usually associated with hepatic steatosis, has been reported with the use of nucleoside analogues (see section 4.4).

Psychiatric disorders:

Common: insomnia

Nervous system disorders:

Very common: dizziness, headache

Common: abnormal dreams

Respiratory, thoracic and mediastinal disorders:

Very rare: dyspnoea

Gastrointestinal disorders:

Very common: diarrhoea, nausea, vomiting

Common: flatulence, dyspepsia, abdominal pain, elevated serum lipase, elevated amylase including elevated pancreatic amylase

Rare: pancreatitis

Hepatobiliary disorders:

Common: hyperbilirubinaemia, increased liver enzymes including serum aspartate aminotransferase (AST) and/or elevated serum alanine aminotransferase (ALT) and gamma-glutamyl transferase (gamma GT)

Very rare: hepatitis

Skin and subcutaneous tissue disorders:

Common: rash, pruritus, maculopapular rash, urticaria, vesiculobullous rash, pustular rash and skin discolouration (increased pigmentation)

Musculoskeletal and connective tissue disorders:

Very common: elevated creatine kinase

Renal and urinary disorders:

Rare: renal failure (acute and chronic), acute tubular necrosis, proximal tubulopathy including Fanconi syndrome, proteinuria, increased creatinine

Very rare: polyuria

General disorders and administration site conditions:

Common: pain

Very rare: asthenia

The adverse reaction profile in patients co-infected with HBV is similar to that observed in patients infected with HIV without co-infection with HBV. However, as would be expected in this patient population, elevations in AST and ALT occurred more frequently than in the general HIV infected population.

Combination antiretroviral therapy has been associated with metabolic abnormalities such as hypertriglyceridaemia, hypercholesterolaemia, insulin resistance, hyperglycaemia and hyperlactataemia (see section 4.4).

Combination antiretroviral therapy has been associated with redistribution of body fat (lipodystrophy) in HIV patients including the loss of peripheral and facial subcutaneous fat, increased intra-abdominal and visceral fat, breast hypertrophy and dorsocervical fat accumulation (buffalo hump) (see section 4.4).

In a 144-week controlled clinical study in antiretroviral-naïve patients that compared tenofovir disoproxil fumarate with stavudine in combination with lamivudine and efavirenz, patients who received tenofovir disoproxil had a significantly lower incidence of lipodystrophy compared with patients who received stavudine. The tenofovir disoproxil fumarate arm also had significantly smaller mean increases in fasting triglycerides and total cholesterol than the comparator arm.

In HIV infected patients with severe immune deficiency at the time of initiation of combination antiretroviral therapy (CART), an inflammatory reaction to asymptomatic or residual opportunistic infections may arise (see section 4.4).

4.9 Overdose
If overdose occurs the patient must be monitored for evidence of toxicity (see section 4.8), and standard supportive treatment applied as necessary.

Up to 30% of the emtricitabine dose and approximately 10% of the tenofovir dose can be removed by haemodialysis. It is not known whether emtricitabine or tenofovir can be removed by peritoneal dialysis.

5. PHARMACOLOGICAL PROPERTIES

5.1 Pharmacodynamic properties
Pharmacotherapeutic group: Antiviral for systemic use: Nucleoside and nucleotide reverse transcriptase inhibitors, ATC code: J05AF30

Mechanism of action and pharmacodynamic effects: Emtricitabine is a nucleoside analogue of cytidine. Tenofovir disoproxil fumarate is converted *in vivo* to tenofovir, a nucleoside monophosphate (nucleotide) analogue of adenosine monophosphate. Both emtricitabine and tenofovir have activity that is specific to human immunodeficiency virus (HIV-1 and HIV-2) and hepatitis B virus.

Emtricitabine and tenofovir are phosphorylated by cellular enzymes to form emtricitabine triphosphate and tenofovir diphosphate, respectively. *In vitro* studies have shown that both emtricitabine and tenofovir can be fully phosphorylated when combined together in cells. Emtricitabine triphosphate and tenofovir diphosphate competitively inhibit HIV-1 reverse transcriptase, resulting in DNA chain termination.

Both emtricitabine triphosphate and tenofovir diphosphate are weak inhibitors of mammalian DNA polymerases and there was no evidence of toxicity to mitochondria *in vitro* and *in vivo*.

Antiviral activity in vitro: Synergistic antiviral activity was observed with the combination of emtricitabine and tenofovir *in vitro*. Additive to synergistic effects were observed in combination studies with protease inhibitors, and with nucleoside and non-nucleoside analogue inhibitors of HIV reverse transcriptase.

Resistance: Resistance has been seen *in vitro* and in some HIV-1 infected patients due to the development of the M184V/I mutation with emtricitabine and the K65R mutation with tenofovir. No other pathways of resistance to emtricitabine or tenofovir have been identified. Emtricitabine-resistant viruses with the M184V/I mutation were cross-resistant to lamivudine, but retained sensitivity to didanosine, stavudine, tenofovir, zalcitabine and zidovudine. The K65R mutation can also be selected by abacavir, didanosine or zalcitabine and results in reduced susceptibility to these agents plus lamivudine, emtricitabine and tenofovir. Tenofovir disoproxil fumarate should be avoided in patients with HIV-1 harbouring the K65R mutation.

Patients with HIV-1 expressing three or more thymidine analogue associated mutations (TAMs) that included either the M41L or L210W reverse transcriptase mutation showed reduced susceptibility to tenofovir disoproxil fumarate.

Clinical experience: There are no clinical data specific to the administration of Truvada. The clinical experience of the combined use of the two agents is from studies with the separate presentations of emtricitabine and tenofovir disoproxil fumarate within antiretroviral combination therapy.

Preliminary 24-week data from an ongoing clinical study in antiretroviral-naïve patients treated with the once daily combination of emtricitabine, tenofovir disoproxil fumarate and efavirenz showed a similar antiviral effect to the combination of zidovudine and lamivudine twice daily with efavirenz once daily. The percentage of patients who achieved and maintained a viral load < 400 copies/ml was 88% in the emtricitabine/tenofovir disoproxil fumarate group and 80% in the zidovudine/lamivudine group (p-value = 0.019); the corresponding percentages for a viral load < 50 copies/ml were 74% in the emtricitabine/tenofovir disoproxil fumarate group and 66% in the zidovudine/lamivudine group (p-value = 0.075). Mean changes in CD4 cell count from baseline to week 24 were +129 and +111 cells/mm^3 for the emtricitabine/tenofovir disoproxil fumarate and zidovudine/lamivudine groups, respectively.

Antiretroviral-naïve adults were also treated once daily with emtricitabine and tenofovir disoproxil fumarate in combination with lopinavir/ritonavir given once or twice daily. At 48 weeks, 70% and 64% of patients demonstrated HIV RNA < 50 copies/ml with the once and twice daily regimens of lopinavir/ritonavir, respectively. The mean changes in CD4 cell count from baseline were +185 cells/mm^3 and +196 cells/mm^3 with the once and twice daily regimens of lopinavir/ritonavir, respectively.

Limited clinical experience in patients co-infected with HIV and HBV suggests that treatment with emtricitabine or tenofovir disoproxil fumarate in antiretroviral combination therapy to control HIV infection also results in a reduction in HBV DNA (4 to 5 log_{10} reduction or 3 log_{10} reduction, respectively) (see section 4.4).

5.2 Pharmacokinetic properties

Absorption: The bioequivalence of one Truvada film-coated tablet with one emtricitabine 200 mg hard capsule and one tenofovir disoproxil fumarate 245 mg film-coated tablet was established following single dose administration to fasting healthy subjects. Following oral administration of Truvada to healthy subjects, emtricitabine and tenofovir disoproxil fumarate are rapidly absorbed and tenofovir disoproxil fumarate is converted to tenofovir. Maximum emtricitabine and tenofovir concentrations are observed in serum within 0.5 to 3.0 h of dosing in the fasted state. Administration of Truvada with food resulted in a delay of approximately three quarters of an hour in reaching maximum tenofovir concentrations and increases in tenofovir AUC and C_{max} of approximately 35% and 15%, respectively, when administered with a high fat or light meal, compared to administration in the fasted state. In order to optimise the absorption of tenofovir, it is recommended that Truvada should be taken with food.

Distribution: Following intravenous administration the volume of distribution of emtricitabine and tenofovir was approximately 1.4 l/kg and 800 ml/kg, respectively. After oral administration of emtricitabine or tenofovir disoproxil fumarate, emtricitabine and tenofovir are widely distributed throughout the body. *In vitro* binding of emtricitabine to human plasma proteins was < 4% and independent of concentration over the range of 0.02 to 200 μg/ml. *In vitro* protein binding of tenofovir to plasma or serum protein was less than 0.7 and 7.2%, respectively, over the tenofovir concentration range 0.01 to 25 μg/ml.

Biotransformation: There is limited metabolism of emtricitabine. The biotransformation of emtricitabine includes oxidation of the thiol moiety to form the 3'-sulphoxide diastereomers (approximately 9% of dose) and conjugation with glucuronic acid to form 2'-O-glucuronide (approximately 4% of dose). *In vitro* studies have determined that neither tenofovir disoproxil fumarate nor tenofovir are substrates for the CYP450 enzymes. Neither emtricitabine nor tenofovir inhibited *in vitro* drug metabolism mediated by any of the major human CYP450 isoforms involved in drug biotransformation. Also, emtricitabine did not inhibit uridine-5'-diphosphoglucuronyl transferase, the enzyme responsible for glucuronidation.

Elimination: Emtricitabine is primarily excreted by the kidneys with complete recovery of the dose achieved in urine (approximately 86%) and faeces (approximately 14%). Thirteen percent of the emtricitabine dose was recovered in urine as three metabolites. The systemic clearance of emtricitabine averaged 307 ml/min. Following oral administration, the elimination half-life of emtricitabine is approximately 10 hours.

Tenofovir is primarily excreted by the kidney by both filtration and an active tubular transport system with approximately 70-80% of the dose excreted unchanged in urine following intravenous administration. The apparent clearance of tenofovir averaged approximately 307 ml/min. Renal clearance has been estimated to be approximately 210 ml/min, which is in excess of the glomerular filtration rate. This indicates that active tubular secretion is an important part of the elimination of tenofovir. Following oral administration, the elimination half-life of tenofovir is approximately 12 to 18 hours.

Age, gender and ethnicity: Emtricitabine and tenofovir pharmacokinetics are similar in male and female patients. In general, the pharmacokinetics of emtricitabine in infants, children and adolescents (aged 4 months up to 18 years) are similar to those seen in adults. Pharmacokinetic studies have not been performed with tenofovir in children and adolescents (under 18 years). Pharmacokinetic studies have not been performed with emtricitabine or tenofovir in the elderly (over 65 years).

Renal impairment: The pharmacokinetics of emtricitabine and tenofovir after co-administration of separate preparations or as Truvada have not been studied in patients with renal impairment. Pharmacokinetic parameters were determined following administration of single doses of emtricitabine 200 mg or tenofovir disoproxil 245 mg to non-HIV infected patients with varying degrees of renal impairment. The degree of renal impairment was defined according to baseline creatinine clearance (CrCl) (normal renal function when CrCl > 80 ml/min; mild impairment with CrCl = 50-79 ml/min; moderate impairment with CrCl = 30-49 ml/min and severe impairment with CrCl = 10-29 ml/min).

The mean (%CV) emtricitabine drug exposure increased from 12 (25%) μg•h/ml in subjects with normal renal function, to 20 (6%) μg•h/ml, 25 (23%) μg•h/ml and 34 (6%) μg•h/ml, in patients with mild, moderate and severe renal impairment, respectively.

The mean (%CV) tenofovir drug exposure increased from 2,185 (12%) ng•h/ml in patients with normal renal function, to 3,064 (30%) ng•h/ml, 6,009 (42%) ng•h/ml and 15,985 (45%) ng•h/ml, in patients with mild, moderate and severe renal impairment, respectively.

The increased dose interval for Truvada in patients with moderate renal impairment is expected to result in higher peak plasma concentrations and lower C_{min} levels as compared to patients with normal renal function. The clinical implications of this are unknown.

In patients with end-stage renal disease (ESRD) requiring haemodialysis, between dialysis drug exposures substantially increased over 72 hours to 53 (19%) μg•h/ml of emtricitabine, and over 48 hours to 42,857 (29%) ng•h/ml of tenofovir.

It is recommended that the dosing interval for Truvada is modified in patients with creatinine clearance between 30 and 49 ml/min. Truvada is not suitable for patients with CrCl < 30 ml/min or for those on haemodialysis (see section 4.2).

Hepatic impairment: The pharmacokinetics of Truvada have not been studied in patients with hepatic impairment. However, it is unlikely that a dose adjustment would be required for Truvada in patients with hepatic impairment.

The pharmacokinetics of emtricitabine have not been studied in non-HBV infected subjects with varying degrees of hepatic insufficiency. In general, emtricitabine pharmacokinetics in HBV infected subjects were similar to those in healthy subjects and in HIV infected subjects.

A single 245 mg dose of tenofovir disoproxil was administered to non-HIV infected patients with varying degrees of hepatic impairment defined according to Child-Pugh-Turcotte (CPT) classification. Tenofovir pharmacokinetics were not substantially altered in subjects with hepatic impairment suggesting that no dose adjustment is required in these subjects. The mean (%CV) tenofovir C_{max} and $AUC_{0-\infty}$ values were 223 (34.8%) ng/ml and 2,050 (50.8%) ng•h/ml, respectively, in normal subjects compared with 289 (46.0%) ng/ml and 2,310 (43.5%) ng•h/ml in subjects with moderate hepatic impairment, and 305 (24.8%) ng/ml and 2,740 (44.0%) ng•h/ml in subjects with severe hepatic impairment.

5.3 Preclinical safety data

Non-clinical data on emtricitabine reveal no special hazard for humans based on conventional studies of safety pharmacology, repeated dose toxicity, genotoxicity and reproductive/developmental toxicity. Emtricitabine did not show any carcinogenic potential in long-term oral carcinogenicity studies in mice and rats.

Preclinical studies of tenofovir disoproxil fumarate conducted in rats, dogs and monkeys revealed target organ effects in gastrointestinal tract, kidney, bone and a decrease in serum phosphate concentration. Bone toxicity was diagnosed as osteomalacia (monkeys) and reduced bone mineral density (rats and dogs). Findings in the rat and monkey studies indicated that there was a substance-related decrease in intestinal absorption of phosphate with potential secondary reduction in bone mineral density. The mechanisms of these toxicities are not completely understood.

Conventional reproductive/developmental toxicity studies reveal no special hazard for humans.

Tenofovir disoproxil fumarate was positive in two out of three *in vitro* genotoxicity studies but negative in the *in vivo* micronucleus assay.

Tenofovir disoproxil fumarate did not show any carcinogenic potential in a long-term oral carcinogenicity study in rats. A long-term oral carcinogenicity study in mice showed a low incidence of duodenal tumours, considered likely related to high local concentrations in the gastrointestinal tract at a dose of 600 mg/kg/day. While the mechanism of tumour formation is uncertain, the findings are unlikely to be of relevance to humans.

6. PHARMACEUTICAL PARTICULARS

6.1 List of excipients

Tablet core:

Croscarmellose sodium

Lactose monohydrate

Magnesium stearate (E572)

Microcrystalline cellulose (E460)

Pregelatinised starch (gluten free)

Film-coating:

Glycerol triacetate (E1518)

Hypromellose (E464)

Indigo carmine aluminium lake (E132)

Lactose monohydrate

Titanium dioxide (E171)

6.2 Incompatibilities

Not applicable.

6.3 Shelf life

2 years.

6.4 Special precautions for storage

Store in the original container. Keep the container tightly closed.

6.5 Nature and contents of container

HDPE bottle with a child-resistant closure containing 30 film-coated tablets and a silica gel desiccant.

6.6 Instructions for use and handling

No special requirements.

7. MARKETING AUTHORISATION HOLDER

Gilead Sciences International Limited

Cambridge

CB1 6GT

United Kingdom

8. MARKETING AUTHORISATION NUMBER(S)

EU/1/04/305/001

9. DATE OF FIRST AUTHORISATION/RENEWAL OF THE AUTHORISATION

21 February 2005

10. DATE OF REVISION OF THE TEXT

21 February 2005

Tuinal

(Flynn Pharma Ltd)

1. NAME OF THE MEDICINAL PRODUCT

TUINAL

2. QUALITATIVE AND QUANTITATIVE COMPOSITION

Capsules (orange and blue, coded F65) containing 100mg Tuinal (50mg Secobarbitone Sodium PhEur and 50mg Amylobarbitone Sodium PhEur). (The British Approved Name for Secobarbitone is quinalbarbitone.)

3. PHARMACEUTICAL FORM

Capsule

4. CLINICAL PARTICULARS

4.1 Therapeutic indications

For the short-term treatment of severe, intractable insomnia in patients already taking barbiturates. New patients should not be started on this preparation. Attempts should be made to wean patients off this preparation by gradual reduction of the dose over a period of days or weeks *(see drug abuse and dependence)*. Abrupt discontinuation should be avoided as this may precipitate withdrawal effects *(see warnings)*.

4.2 Posology and method of administration

For adults only: 100 - 200 mg at bedtime.

THE ELDERLY

Tuinal should not be administered to elderly or debilitated patients.

CHILDREN

Tuinal should not be administered to children or young adults.

Attempts should be made to wean patients off this preparation, but this should be done gradually (see 'Warnings' and 'Undesirable Effects').

In studies, secobarbital sodium has been found to lose most of its effectiveness for both inducing and maintaining sleep by the end of 2 weeks of continued drug administration, even with the use of multiple doses.

4.3 Contraindications

Hypersensitivity to barbiturates, a history of manifest or latent porphyria, marked impairment of liver function or respiratory disease in which dyspnoea or obstruction is evident.

Barbiturates should not be administered to children, young adults, patients with a history of drug or alcohol addiction or abuse, the elderly and the debilitated.

4.4 Special warnings and special precautions for use

Addiction potential: Barbiturates have a high addiction potential. Long-term use, or use of high dosage for short periods, may lead to tolerance and subsequently to physical and psychological dependence. Patients who have psychological dependence on barbiturates may increase the dosage or decrease the dosage interval without consulting a doctor, and subsequently may develop a physical dependence on barbiturates.

Signs of acute intoxication with barbiturates include unsteady gait, slurred speech and sustained nystagmus. Symptoms of dependence or chronic intoxication include confusion, defective judgement, loss of emotional control, insomnia and somatic complaints.

To minimise the possibility of overdosage or development of dependence, the amount prescribed should be limited to that required for the interval until the next appointment.

Withdrawal symptoms occur after long-term normal use (and particularly after abuse) on rapid cessation of barbiturate treatment. Symptoms include nightmares, irritability and insomnia, and in severe cases, tremors, delirium, convulsions and death.

Barbiturates should be withdrawn gradually from any patient known to be taking excessive doses over long periods.

Information for patients: The following information should be given to patients receiving Tuinal:

1. The use of Tuinal carries with it an associated risk of psychological and/or physical dependence. The patient should be warned against increasing the dose of the drug without consulting a physician.

2. Tuinal may impair the mental and/or physical abilities required for the performance of potentially hazardous

tasks, such as driving a car or operating machinery. The patient should be cautioned accordingly.

3. Alcohol should not be consumed while taking Tuinal. The concurrent use of Tuinal with other CNS depressants (e.g. alcohol, narcotics, tranquillisers and antihistamines) may result in additional CNS depressant effects.

Drug abuse and dependence: Barbiturates may be habit forming; tolerance, psychological and physical dependence may occur especially following prolonged use of high doses. Daily administration in excess of 400 mg secobarbitone, for approximately 90 days, is likely to produce some degree of physical dependence.

A dosage of 600 - 800 mg, for at least 35 days, is sufficient to produce withdrawal seizures. The average daily dose for the barbiturate addict is usually about 1.5g.

As tolerance to barbiturates develops, the amount needed to maintain the same level of intoxication increases; tolerance to a fatal dosage, however, does not increase more than twofold. As this occurs, the margin between intoxicating dosage and fatal dosage becomes smaller. The lethal dose of a barbiturate is far less if alcohol is also ingested.

Symptoms of acute intoxication include unsteady gait, slurred speech and sustained nystagmus. Mental signs of chronic intoxication include confusion, poor judgement, irritability, insomnia and somatic complaints.

The symptoms of barbiturate withdrawal can be severe and may cause death. Minor withdrawal symptoms may appear 8 to 12 hours after the last dose of a barbiturate. These symptoms usually appear in the following order: anxiety, muscle twitching, tremor of hands and fingers, progressive weakness, dizziness, distortion in visual perception, nausea, vomiting, insomnia and orthostatic hypotension. Major withdrawal symptoms (convulsions and delirium) may occur within 16 hours and last up to five days after abrupt cessation of barbiturates. Intensity of withdrawal symptoms gradually declines over a period of approximately 15 days. Individuals susceptible to barbiturate abuse and dependence include alcoholics and opiate abusers, as well as other sedative-hypnotic and amphetamine abusers.

Dependence on barbiturates arises from repeated administration on a continuous basis, generally in amounts exceeding therapeutic dose levels. Treatment of dependence consists of cautious and gradual withdrawal of the drug. Barbiturate-dependent patients can be withdrawn by using a number of withdrawal regimens. In all cases, withdrawal takes an extended period. One method involves substituting a 30 mg dose of phenobarbitone for each 100 - 200 mg dose of barbiturate that the patient has been taking. The total daily amount of phenobarbitone is then administered in three or four divided doses, not to exceed 600 mg daily. Should signs of withdrawal occur on the first day of treatment, a loading dose of 100 to 200 mg of phenobarbitone may be administered intramuscularly in addition to the oral dose. After stabilisation on phenobarbitone, the total daily dose is decreased by 30 mg a day as long as withdrawal is proceeding smoothly. A modification of this regimen involves initiating treatment at the patient's regular dosage level and decreasing the daily dosage by 10% as tolerated by the patient.

Infants that are physically dependent on barbiturates may be given phenobarbitone, 3 to 10 mg/kg/day. After withdrawal symptoms (hyperactivity, disturbed sleep, tremors and hyperreflexia) are relieved, the dosage of phenobarbitone should be gradually decreased and completely withdrawn over a two week period.

Carcinogenesis: Animal data show that phenobarbitone can be carcinogenic after lifetime administration.

Human data: In a 29 year epidemiological study of 9136 patients who were treated on an anticonvulsant protocol that included phenobarbitone, results indicated a higher than normal incidence of hepatic carcinoma. Previously some of these patients had been treated with thorotrast, a drug that is known to produce hepatic carcinomas. Thus, this study did not provide sufficient evidence that phenobarbitone is carcinogenic in humans.

A retrospective study of 84 children with brain tumours, matched to 73 normal controls and 78 cancer controls (malignant disease other than brain tumours), suggested an association between exposure to barbiturates prenatally and an increased incidence of brain tumours.

Barbiturates should be administered with caution, if at all, to patients who are mentally depressed or have suicidal tendencies. They should also be used with great caution and at reduced dosage in those with hepatic disease, marked renal dysfunction, shock or respiratory depression.

Elderly or debilitated patients may react to barbiturates with marked excitement, depression or confusion (see 'Contra-indications'). In some persons, barbiturates repeatedly produce excitement rather than depression.

Barbiturates should not be administered to patients showing the premonitory signs of hepatic coma(see 'Contra-indications').

A cumulative effect may occur with the barbiturates leading to features of chronic poisoning including headache, depression and slurred speech.

Automatism may follow the use of a hypnotic dose of barbiturate.

The systemic affects of exogenous and endogenous corticosteroids may be diminished by amylobarbitone. This product should therefore be administered with caution to patients with borderline hypoadrenal function, regardless of whether it is of pituitary or of primary adrenal origin.

Laboratory tests: Prolonged therapy with barbiturates should be accompanied by periodic evaluation of, for example, the haematopoietic, renal and hepatic systems (but see 'Uses).

4.5 Interaction with other medicinal products and other forms of Interaction

Toxic effects and fatalities have occurred following overdoses of Tuinal alone and in combination with other CNS depressants. Caution should be exercised in prescribing unnecessarily large amounts of Tuinal for patients who have a history of emotional disturbances or suicidal ideation or who have misused alcohol or other CNS drugs.

Anticoagulants: Barbiturates cause induction of the liver microsomal enzymes responsible for metabolising many other drugs. In particular they may result in increased metabolism and decreased anticoagulant response of oral anticoagulants (eg warfarin). Patients stabilised on anticoagulant therapy may require dosage adjustments if barbiturates are added to or withdrawn from their regimen.

Corticosteroids: Barbiturates appear to enhance the metabolism of exogenous corticosteroids and steroid dosage may also need adjustment.

Griseofulvin: Barbiturates may interfere with the absorption of oral griseofulvin, thus decreasing its blood level. Concomitant administration should be avoided if possible.

Doxycycline: Barbiturates may shorten the half-life of doxycycline for as long as two weeks after the barbiturate is discontinued. If administered concomitantly the clinical response to doxycycline should be monitored closely.

Phenytoin, Sodium Valproate, Valproic Acid: The effect of barbiturates on phenytoin metabolism is variable. Phenytoin and barbiturate blood levels should be monitored more frequently if administered concomitantly. Sodium valproate and valproic acid decrease barbiturate metabolism. Therefore, barbiturate blood levels should be monitored and dosage adjustments made as clinically indicated.

CNS Depressants: Concomitant use of other CNS depressants, including other sedatives or hypnotics, antihistamines, tranquillisers or alcohol, may produce additive depressant effects.

Monoamine Oxidase Inhibitors (MAOIS): Prolong the effects of barbiturates.

Oestradiol, oestrone, progesterone and other steroidal hormones: There have been reports of patients treated with antiepileptic drugs (eg phenobarbitone) who became pregnant while taking oral contraceptives. Barbiturates may decrease the effect of oestradiol. An alternative contraceptive method might be suggested to women taking barbiturates.

4.6 Pregnancy and lactation

Usage in Pregnancy: Barbiturates are contraindicated during pregnancy since they can cause foetal harm. A higher than expected incidence of foetal abnormalities may be connected with maternal consumption of barbiturates. Barbiturates readily cross the placental barrier and are distributed throughout foetal tissues with highest concentrations in placenta, foetal liver and brain. Withdrawal symptoms occur in infants born to women who receive barbiturates during the last trimester of pregnancy. If a patient becomes pregnant whilst taking this drug, she should be told of the potential hazard to the foetus.

Reports of infants suffering from long term barbiturate exposure *in utero* included the acute withdrawal syndrome of seizures and hyper-irritability from birth to a delayed onset of up to 14 days.

Labour and Delivery: Respiratory depression has been noted in infants born following the use of barbiturates during labour. Premature infants are particularly susceptible. Resuscitation equipment should be available.

Nursing Mothers: Small amounts of barbiturates are excreted in the milk and they are therefore contraindicated for the nursing mother.

4.7 Effects on ability to drive and use machines

Tuinal may impair the mental and/or physical abilities required for the performance of potentially hazardous tasks such as driving a car or operating machinery. The patient should be cautioned accordingly

4.8 Undesirable effects

The following adverse reactions and their incidences were compiled from surveillance of thousands of hospitalised patients who received barbiturates. As such patients may be less aware of certain of the milder adverse effects of barbiturates, the incidence of these reactions may be somewhat higher in fully ambulatory patients.

More than 1 in 100 patients: The most common adverse reaction, estimated to occur at a rate of 1 to 3 patients per 100, is the following:

NERVOUS SYSTEM: Somnolence

LESS THAN 1 IN 100 PATIENTS: Adverse reactions estimated to occur at a rate of less than 1 in 100 patients are listed below grouped by organ system and by decreasing frequency:

NEUROLOGICAL: Agitation, confusion, hyperkinesia, ataxia, CNS depression, nightmares, nervousness, psychiatric disturbance, hallucinations, insomnia, anxiety, dizziness, abnormal thinking.

RESPIRATORY: Hypoventilation, apnoea.

CARDIOVASCULAR: Bradycardia, hypotension, syncope.

DIGESTIVE: Nausea, vomiting, constipation

OTHER: Headache, hypersensitivity reactions (angioneurotic oedema, rashes, exfoliative dermatitis), fever, liver damage. Hypersensitivity is more likely to occur in patients with asthma, urticaria or angioneurotic oedema. Megaloblastic anaemia has followed chronic phenobarbitone use.

4.9 Overdose

The toxic dose of barbiturates varies considerably. In general, an oral dose of 1g of most barbiturates produces serious poisoning in an adult. Death commonly occurs after 2 to 10g of ingested barbiturate. The sedated, therapeutic blood levels of amylobarbitone and secobarbitone range between 2 and 10 mg/1 and 0.5 and 5 mg/l, respectively; the usual lethal blood levels range from 40 to 80 mg/l with amylobarbitone and 15 to 40 mg/l with secobarbitone. Barbiturate intoxication may be confused with alcoholism, bromide intoxication, and various neurological disorders. Potential tolerance must be considered when evaluating significance of dose and plasma concentration.

SIGNS AND SYMPTOMS: Symptoms of oral overdose may occur within 15 minutes and begin with CNS depression, absent or sluggish reflexes, underventilation, hypotension and hypothermia, which may progress to pulmonary oedema and death. Haemorrhagic blisters may develop, especially at pressure points.

Complications such as pneumonia, pulmonary oedema, cardiac arrhythmias, congestive heart failure and renal failure may occur. Uraemia may increase CNS sensitivity to barbiturates if renal function is impaired. Differential diagnosis should include hypoglycaemia, head trauma, cerebrovascular accidents, convulsive states and diabetic coma.

TREATMENT OF OVERDOSAGE

General management should consist of symptomatic and supportive therapy. Activated charcoal may be more effective than emesis or lavage. Diuresis and peritoneal dialysis are of little value. Haemodialysis and haemoperfusion enhance drug clearance and should be considered in serious poisoning. If the patient has chronically abused sedatives, withdrawal reactions may be manifest following acute overdose.

5. PHARMACOLOGICAL PROPERTIES

5.1 Pharmacodynamic properties

Amylobarbitone sodium and secobarbitone sodium are non-selective central nervous system depressents that are primarily used as sedative-hypnotics.

Barbiturates are capable of producing all levels of CNS mood alteration, from excitation to mild sedation, hypnosis and deep coma. Overdosage can product death. Barbiturates depress the sensory cortex, decrease motor activity, alter cerebellar function and produce drowsiness, sedation and hypnosis.

Tuinal is a combination of equal parts of amylobarbitone sodium (50mg per capsule) and secobarbitone sodium (50mg per capsule). It is a moderately long-acting barbiturate which in ordinary doses acts as a hypnotic. Its onset of action occurs in 15 to 30 minutes and the duration of action ranges from 3 to 11 hours.

Barbiturate-induced sleep differs from physiologic sleep. Sleep laboratory studies have demonstrated that barbiturates reduce the amount of time spent in the rapid eye movement (REM) phase of sleep, or dreaming stage. Also stages III and IV sleep are decreased. Following abrupt cessation of barbiturates used regularly, patients may experience markedly increased dreaming, nightmares and/or insomnia. Therefore, withdrawal of a single therapeutic dose over five or six days has been recommended to lessen the REM rebound and disturbed sleep which contribute to drug withdrawal syndrome (for example, decrease the dose from 3 to 2 doses a day for 1 week).

5.2 Pharmacokinetic properties

Barbiturates are weak acids that are absorbed and rapidly distributed to all tissues and fluids, with high concentrations in the brain, liver and kidneys. Lipid solubility of the barbiturates is the dominant factor in their distribution within the body. Barbiturates are bound to plasma and tissue proteins; the degree of binding increases as a function of lipid solubility.

Amylobarbitone sodium and secobarbitone sodium are weak acids that are absorbed and rapidly distributed to all tissues and fluids with high concentrations in the brain, liver and kidneys. They are bound to plasma and tissue proteins to a varying degree. The barbiturates are metabolised by the liver and the metabolites excreted in the urine and less commonly in the faeces.

5.3 Preclinical safety data

Carcinogenesis: Animal data show that phenobarbitone can be carcinogenic after lifetime administration.

6. PHARMACEUTICAL PARTICULARS

6.1 List of excipients
Starch, Silicone, Erythrosine, Patent blue V, Quinoline yellow, Gelatin

6.2 Incompatibilities
Not applicable

6.3 Shelf life
60 months

6.4 Special precautions for storage
Store below 25°C. Keep lid tightly closed.

6.5 Nature and contents of container
High density polyethylene bottles with screw caps containing 100 capsules.

6.6 Instructions for use and handling
Not applicable

7. MARKETING AUTHORISATION HOLDER
Flynn Pharma Ltd.

Alton House

4 Herbert Street

Dublin 2

Republic of Ireland

8. MARKETING AUTHORISATION NUMBER(S)
PL 13621/0004

9. DATE OF FIRST AUTHORISATION/RENEWAL OF THE AUTHORISATION
1995

10. DATE OF REVISION OF THE TEXT
December 1995

Legal Category
CD (Sch 2), POM

Twinrix Adult Vaccine

(GlaxoSmithKline UK)

1. NAME OF THE MEDICINAL PRODUCT
Twinrix Adult, suspension for injection in prefilled syringe

Inactivated hepatitis A and hepatitis B recombinant, adsorbed vaccine.

2. QUALITATIVE AND QUANTITATIVE COMPOSITION
1 dose (1 ml) contains:

Inactivated hepatitis A virus* 720 ELISA Units

Hepatitis B virus surface antigen recombinant (S protein)** 20 micrograms

*adsorbed on aluminium oxide hydrated Total: 0.05 milligrams Al^{3+}

**adsorbed on aluminium phosphate Total: 0.4 milligrams Al^{3+}

and produced on genetically-engineered yeast cells (*Saccharomyces Cerevisiae*)

For excipients, see 6.1.

3. PHARMACEUTICAL FORM
Suspension for injection in prefilled syringe

4. CLINICAL PARTICULARS

4.1 Therapeutic indications
Twinrix Adult is indicated for use in non immune adults and adolescents 16 years of age and above who are at risk of both hepatitis A and hepatitis B infection.

4.2 Posology and method of administration
- Posology

- Dosage

A dose of 1.0 ml is recommended for adults and adolescents 16 years of age and above.

- Primary vaccination schedule

The standard primary course of vaccination with Twinrix Adult consists of three doses, the first administered at the elected date, the second one month later and the third six months after the first dose.

In exceptional circumstances in adults, when travel is anticipated within one month or more after initiating the vaccination course, but where insufficient time is available to allow the standard 0, 1, 6 month schedule to be completed, a schedule of three intramuscular injections given at 0, 7 and 21 days may be used. When this schedule is applied, a fourth dose is recommended 12 months after the first dose.

The recommended schedule should be adhered to. Once initiated, the primary course of vaccination should be completed with the same vaccine.

- Booster dose

Long-term antibody persistence data following vaccination with TWINRIX Adult are available up to 60 months after vaccination. The anti-HBs and anti-HAV antibody titres observed following a primary vaccination course with the combined vaccine are in the range of what is seen following vaccination with the monovalent vaccines. The kinetics of antibody decline are also similar. General guidelines for booster vaccination can therefore be drawn from experience with the monovalent vaccines.

Hepatitis B

The need for a booster dose of hepatitis B vaccine in healthy individuals who have received a full primary vaccination course has not been established; however some official vaccination programmes currently include a recommendation for a booster dose of hepatitis B vaccine and these should be respected.

For some categories of subjects or patients exposed to HBV (e.g. haemodialysis or immunocompromised patients) a precautionary attitude should be considered to ensure a protective antibody level ⩾ 10IU/l.

Hepatitis A

It is not yet fully established whether immunocompetent individuals who have responded to hepatitis A vaccination will require booster doses as protection in the absence of detectable antibodies may be ensured by immunological memory. Guidelines for boosting are based on the assumption that antibodies are required for protection; anti-HAV antibodies have been predicted to persist for at least 10 years.

In situations where a booster dose of both hepatitis A and hepatitis B are desired, Twinrix Adult can be given. Alternatively, subjects primed with Twinrix Adult may be administered a booster dose of either of the monovalent vaccines.

Method of Administration

Twinrix Adult is for intramuscular injection, preferably in the deltoid region.

Exceptionally the vaccine may be administered subcutaneously in patients with thrombocytopenia or bleeding disorders. However, this route of administration may result in suboptimal immune response to the vaccine. (see 4.4).

4.3 Contraindications
Twinrix Adult should not be administered to subjects with known hypersensitivity to any constituent of the vaccine, or to subjects having shown signs of hypersensitivity after previous administration of Twinrix Adult or the monovalent hepatitis A or hepatitis B vaccine.

As with other vaccines, the administration of Twinrix Adult should be postponed in subjects suffering from acute severe febrile illness.

4.4 Special warnings and special precautions for use
It is possible that subjects may be in the incubation period of a hepatitis A or hepatitis B infection at the time of vaccination. It is not known whether Twinrix Adult will prevent hepatitis A and hepatitis B in such cases.

The vaccine will not prevent infection caused by other agents such as hepatitis C and hepatitis E and other pathogens known to infect the liver.

Twinrix Adult is not recommended for postexposure prophylaxis (e.g. needle stick injury).

The vaccine has not been tested in patients with impaired immunity. In haemodialysis patients and persons with an impaired immune system, adequate anti-HAV and anti-HBs antibody titers may not be obtained after the primary immunisation course and such patients may therefore require administration of additional doses of vaccine.

A number of factors have been observed to reduce the immune response to hepatitis B vaccines. These factors include older age, male gender, obesity, smoking, route of administration, and some chronic underlying diseases. Consideration should be given to serological testing of those subjects who may be at risk of not achieving seroprotection following a complete course of Twinrix Adult. Additional doses may need to be considered for persons who do not respond or have a sub-optimal response to a course of vaccinations.

As with all injectable vaccines, appropriate medical treatment and supervision should always be readily available in case of a rare anaphylactic event following the administration of the vaccine.

Since intradermal injection or intramuscular administration into the gluteal muscle could lead to a suboptimal response to the vaccine, these routes should be avoided. However, exceptionally Twinrix Adult can be administered subcutaneously to subjects with thrombocytopenia or bleeding disorders since bleeding may occur following an intramuscular administration to these subjects (see 4.2.).

TWINRIX ADULT SHOULD UNDER NO CIRCUMSTANCES BE ADMINISTERED INTRAVASCULARLY.

Thiomersal (an organomercuric compound) has been used in the manufacturing process of this medicinal product and residues of it are present in the final product. Therefore, sensitisation reactions may occur.

4.5 Interaction with other medicinal products and other forms of Interaction
No data on concomitant administration of Twinrix Adult with specific hepatitis A immunoglobulin or hepatitis B immunoglobulin have been generated. However, when the monovalent hepatitis A and hepatitis B vaccines were administered concomitantly with specific immunoglobulins, no influence on seroconversion was observed although it may result in lower antibody titres.

Although the concomitant administration of Twinrix Adult and other vaccines has not specifically been studied, it is anticipated that, if different syringes and other injection sites are used, no interaction will be observed.

It may be expected that in patients receiving immunosuppressive treatment or patients with immunodeficiency, an adequate response may not be achieved.

4.6 Pregnancy and lactation
Pregnancy

The effect of Twinrix Adult on foetal development has not been assessed.

However, as with all inactivated vaccines, one does not expect harm to the foetus. Twinrix Adult should be used during pregnancy only when there is a clear risk of hepatitis A and hepatitis B.

Lactation

The effect on breastfed infants of the administration of Twinrix Adult to their mothers has not been evaluated in clinical studies. Twinrix Adult should therefore be used with caution in breastfeeding women.

4.7 Effects on ability to drive and use machines
Twinrix Adult has no or negligible influence on the ability to drive and use machines.

4.8 Undesirable effects
In controlled clinical studies performed with Twinrix Adult, the most commonly reported adverse events were reactions at the injection site, including pain, redness and swelling.

In a comparative study it was noted that the frequency of solicited adverse events following the administration of Twinrix Adult is not different from the frequency of solicited adverse events following the administration of the monovalent vaccines.

Frequencies are reported as:

Very common: (⩾ 10%)

Common: (⩾ 1% and < 10%)

Uncommon: (⩾ 0.1% and < 1%)

Rare: (⩾ 0.01% and < 0.1%)

Very rare: (< 0.01%)

General reactions that may occur in temporal association with Twinrix Adult vaccination include:

Body as a whole:

very common: fatigue

common: headache, malaise

uncommon: fever

Gastro-intestinal system:

common: nausea

uncommon: vomiting

In a clinical trial where Twinrix Adult was administered at 0, 7, 21 days, solicited general symptoms were reported with the same categories of frequency as defined above, except for headache which was very commonly reported. After a fourth dose given at month 12, the incidence of systemic adverse reactions was comparable to that seen after vaccination at 0, 7, 21 days.

During postmarketing surveillance, the following undesirable events have been reported in temporal association with vaccination.

Body as a whole:

very rare: flu-like symptoms (fever, chills, headache, myalgia, arthralgia), fatigue, allergic reactions including anaphylactic and anaphylactoid reactions and serum sickness like disease

Cardiovascular general:

very rare: syncope, hypotension

Central and peripheral nervous system:

very rare: dizziness, paresthesia

Gastro-intestinal system:

very rare: nausea, vomiting, decreased appetite, diarrhoea, abdominal pain

Liver and biliary system:

very rare: abnormal liver function tests

Neurological disorders:

very rare: convulsions

Platelet, bleeding and clotting:

very rare: thrombocytopenia, thrombocytopenic purpura

Skin and appendages:

very rare: rash, pruritis, urticaria

White cell and reticuloendothelial system:

very rare: lymphadenopathy

Following widespread use of the monovalent hepatitis A and/or hepatitis B vaccines, the following undesirable events have additionally been reported in temporal association with vaccination.

Central and peripheral nervous system:

very rare: cases of peripheral and/or central neurological disorders, and may include multiple sclerosis, optic neuritis, myelitis, Bell's palsy, polyneuritis such as Guillain-Barré syndrome (with ascending paralysis), meningitis, encephalitis, encephalopathy

Skin and appendages:

very rare: erythema exsudativum multiforme

Vascular extracardiac:

very rare: vasculitis

4.9 Overdose
No case of overdose has been reported.

5. PHARMACOLOGICAL PROPERTIES

5.1 Pharmacodynamic properties
Pharmaco-therapeutic group: Hepatitis vaccines, ATC code JO7BC.

Twinrix Adult is a combined vaccine formulated by pooling bulk preparations of the purified, inactivated hepatitis A (HA) virus and purified hepatitis B surface antigen (HBsAg), separately adsorbed onto aluminium hydroxide and aluminium phosphate. The HA virus is propagated in MRC_5 human diploid cells. HBsAg is produced by culture, in a selective medium, of genetically engineered yeast cells.

Twinrix Adult confers immunity against HAV and HBV infection by inducing specific anti-HAV and anti-HBs antibodies.

Protection against hepatitis A and hepatitis B develops within 2-4 weeks. In the clinical studies, specific humoral antibodies against hepatitis A were observed in approximately 94% of the adults one month after the first dose and in 100% one month after the third dose (i.e. month 7). Specific humoral antibodies against hepatitis B were observed in 70% of the adults after the first dose and approximately 99% after the third dose.

The 0, 7 and 21 day primary schedule plus a fourth dose at month 12 is for use in exceptional circumstances in adults. In a clinical trial where Twinrix Adult was administered according to this schedule, 82% and 85% of vaccinees had seroprotective levels of anti-HBV antibodies at 1 and 5 weeks respectively following the third dose (i.e. at months 1 and 2 after the initial dose). The seroprotection rate against hepatitis B increased to 95.1% by three months after the first dose.

Seropositivity rates for anti-HAV antibodies were 100%, 99.5% and 100% at months 1, 2 and 3 after the initial dose. One month after the fourth dose, all vaccinees demonstrated seroprotective levels of anti-HBs antibodies and were seropositive for anti-HAV antibodies.

In two long term clinical studies conducted in adults, persistence of anti-HAV and anti-HBs antibodies has been proven up to 60 months following the initiation of a primary vaccination course of Twinrix Adult in the majority of vaccinees. The kinetics of decline of anti-HAV and anti-HBs antibodies were shown to be similar to those of the monovalent vaccines.

5.2 Pharmacokinetic properties
Evaluation of pharmacokinetic properties is not required for vaccines.

5.3 Preclinical safety data
Preclinical data reveal no special hazard for humans based on general safety studies.

6. PHARMACEUTICAL PARTICULARS

6.1 List of excipients
Aluminium oxide hydrated

Aluminium phosphate

Formaldehyde

Neomycin sulphate

Phenoxyethanol

Soldium chloride

Water for injections

6.2 Incompatibilities
In the absence of compatibility studies, this medicinal product must not be mixed with other medicinal products.

6.3 Shelf life
3 years.

6.4 Special precautions for storage
Store at 2°C-8°C (in a refrigerator).

Do not freeze.

Store in the original package, in order to protect from light.

6.5 Nature and contents of container
1 ml of suspension in prefilled syringe (type I glass) with a plunger stopper (rubber butyl) with or without needles – pack size of 1, 10 or 25.

Not all pack sizes may be marketed.

6.6 Instructions for use and handling
Upon storage, a fine white deposit with a clear colourless supernatant can be observed.

The vaccine should be well shaken to obtain a slightly opaque, white suspension and visually inspected for any foreign particulate matter and/or variation of physical aspect prior to administration. In the event of either being observed, discard the vaccine.

Administrative Data

7. MARKETING AUTHORISATION HOLDER
GlaxoSmithKline Biologicals s.a.

rue de l'Institut 89

1330 Rixensart, Belgium

Telephone: +32 (0)2 656 8111

Fax: +32 (0)2 656 8000

Telex: 63251 SB BIO B

8. MARKETING AUTHORISATION NUMBER(S)
EU/1/96/020/007 pack of 1 prefilled syringe with non-fixed needle EU/1/96/020/008 pack of 10 prefilled syringes with non-fixed needles

9. DATE OF FIRST AUTHORISATION/RENEWAL OF THE AUTHORISATION
20 September 1996

10. DATE OF REVISION OF THE TEXT
12th February 2004

11. Legal Category
POM

Twinrix Paediatric Vaccine

(GlaxoSmithKline UK)

1. NAME OF THE MEDICINAL PRODUCT
Twinrix Paediatric, suspension for injection in prefilled syringe

Inactivated hepatitis A and hepatitis B recombinant, adsorbed vaccine.

2. QUALITATIVE AND QUANTITATIVE COMPOSITION
1 dose (0.5 ml) contains:

Inactivated hepatitis A virus* 360 ELISA Units

Hepatitis B virus surface antigen recombinant (S protein)** 10 micrograms

* adsorbed on aluminium oxide hydrated Total: 0.025 milligrams Al^{3+}

** adsorbed on aluminium phosphate Total: 0.2 milligrams Al^{3+}

and produced on genetically-engineered yeast cells (*Saccharomyces Cerevisiae*)

For excipients, see 6.1.

3. PHARMACEUTICAL FORM
Suspension for injection in prefilled syringe

4. CLINICAL PARTICULARS

4.1 Therapeutic indications
Twinrix Paediatric is indicated for use in non immune infants, children and adolescents from 1 year up to and including 15 years who are at risk of both hepatitis A and hepatitis B infection.

4.2 Posology and method of administration
- Posology

- Dosage

The dose of 0.5 ml (360 ELISA Units HA/10 μg HBsAg) is recommended for infants, children and adolescents from 1 year up to and including 15 years of age.

- Primary vaccination schedule

The standard primary course of vaccination with Twinrix Paediatric consists of three doses, the first administered at the elected date, the second one month later and the third six months after the first dose. The recommended schedule should be adhered to. Once initiated, the primary course of vaccination should be completed with the same vaccine.

- Booster dose.

Long-term antibody persistence data following vaccination with Twinrix Paediatric are available up to 48 months after vaccination. The anti-HBs and anti-HAV antibody titres observed following a primary vaccination course with the combined vaccine are in the range of what is seen following vaccination with the monovalent vaccines. The kinetics of antibody decline are also similar. General guidelines for booster vaccination can therefore be drawn from experience with the monovalent vaccines.

Hepatitis B

The need for a booster dose of hepatitis B vaccine in healthy individuals who have received a full primary vaccination course has not been established; however some official vaccination programmes currently include a recommendation for a booster dose of hepatitis B vaccine and these should be respected.

For some categories of subjects or patients exposed to HBV (e.g. haemodialysis or immunocompromised patients) a precautionary attitude should be considered to ensure a protective antibody level ⩾ 10IU/l.

Hepatitis A

It is not yet fully established whether immunocompetent individuals who have responded to hepatitis A vaccination will require booster doses as protection in the absence of detectable antibodies may be insured by immunological memory. Guidelines for boosting are based on the assumption that antibodies are required for protection; anti-HAV antibodies have been predicted to persist for at least 10 years.

In situations where a booster dose of both hepatitis A and hepatitis B are desired, Twinrix Paediatric can be given. Alternatively, subjects primed with Twinrix Paediatric may be administered a booster dose of either of the monovalent vaccines.

Method of administration

Twinrix Paediatric is for intramuscular injection, preferably in the deltoid region in adolescents and children or in the anterolateral thigh in infants.

Exceptionally, the vaccine may be administered subcutaneously in patients with thrombocytopenia or bleeding disorders. However, this route of administration may result in suboptimal immune response to the vaccine. (see 4.4)

4.3 Contraindications
Twinrix Paediatric should not be administered to subjects with known hypersensitivity to any constituent of the vaccine, or to subjects having shown signs of hypersensitivity after previous administration of Twinrix Paediatric or the monovalent HA or HB vaccine.

As with other vaccines, the administration of Twinrix Paediatric should be postponed in subjects suffering from acute severe febrile illness.

4.4 Special warnings and special precautions for use
It is possible that subjects may be in the incubation period of a HA or HB infection at the time of vaccination. It is not known whether Twinrix Paediatric will prevent HA and HB in such cases.

The vaccine will not prevent infection caused by other agents such as hepatitis C and hepatitis E and other pathogens known to infect the liver.

Twinrix Paediatric is not recommended for postexposure prophylaxis (e.g. needle stick injury).

The vaccine has not been tested in patients with impaired immunity. In haemodialysis patients, patients receiving immunosuppressive treatment or patients with an impaired immune system, the anticipated immune response may not be achieved after the primary immunisation course. Such patients may require additional doses of vaccine; nevertheless immunocompromised patients may fail to demonstrate an adequate response.

As with all injectable vaccines, appropriate medical treatment and supervision should always be readily available in case of a rare anaphylactic event following the administration of the vaccine.

Since intradermal injection or intramuscular administration into the gluteal muscle could lead to a suboptimal response to the vaccine, these routes should be avoided. However, exceptionally Twinrix Paediatric can be administered subcutaneously to subjects with thrombocytopenia or bleeding disorders since bleeding may occur following an intramuscular administration to these subjects. (see 4.2)

TWINRIX PAEDIATRIC SHOULD UNDER NO CIRCUMSTANCES BE ADMINISTERED INTRAVASCULARLY.

Thiomersal (an organomercuric compound) has been used in the manufacturing process of this medicinal product and residues of it are present in the final product. Therefore, sensitisation reactions may occur.

4.5 Interaction with other medicinal products and other forms of Interaction
No data on concomitant administration of Twinrix Paediatric with specific hepatitis A immunoglobulin or hepatitis B immunoglobulin have been generated. However, when the monovalent hepatitis A and hepatitis B vaccines were administered concomitantly with specific immunoglobulins, no influence on seroconversion was observed although it may result in lower antibody titers.

See also 4.4.

As the concomitant administration of Twinrix Paediatric and other vaccines has not specifically been studied it is advised that the vaccine should not be administered at the same time as other vaccines.

4.6 Pregnancy and lactation
Pregnancy

The effect of Twinrix Paediatric on foetal development has not been assessed.

However, as with all inactivated vaccines, one does not expect harm to the foetus. Twinrix Paediatric should be used during pregnancy only when there is a clear risk of hepatitis A and hepatitis B.

Lactation

The effect on breastfed infants of the administration of Twinrix Paediatric to their mothers has not been evaluated in clinical studies. Twinrix Paediatric should therefore be used with caution in breastfeeding women.

4.7 Effects on ability to drive and use machines
Twinrix Paediatric has no or negligible influence on the ability to drive and use machines.

4.8 Undesirable effects
During clinical studies performed with Twinrix Paediatric, the most commonly reported adverse events were reactions at the injection site, including pain, redness and swelling.

During postmarketing surveillance, the following undesirable events have been reported in temporal association with vaccination.

Frequencies are reported as:

very rare: < 0.01%

Body as a whole:

very rare: flu-like symptoms (fever, chills, headache, myalgia, arthralgia), fatigue, allergic reactions including anaphylactic and anaphylactoid reactions and serum sickness like disease, malaise

Cardiovascular general:

very rare: syncope, hypotension

Central and peripheral nervous system:

very rare: dizziness, paresthesia

Gastro-intestinal system:

very rare: nausea, vomiting, decreased appetite, diarrhoea, abdominal pain

Liver and biliary system:

very rare: abnormal liver function tests

Neurological disorders:

very rare: convulsions

Platelet, bleeding and clotting:

very rare: thrombocytopenia, thrombocytopenic purpura

Skin and appendages:

rare: rash, pruritis, urticaria

White cell and reticuloendothelial system:

very rare: lymphadenopathy

Following widespread use of the monovalent hepatitis A and/or hepatitis B vaccines, the following undesirable events have additionally been reported in temporal association with vaccination.

Central and peripheral nervous system:

very rare: cases of peripheral and/or central neurological disorders, and may include multiple sclerosis, optic neuritis, myelitis, Bell's palsy, polyneuritis such as Guillain-Barré syndrome (with ascending paralysis), meningitis, encephalitis, encephalopathy

Skin and appendages:

very rare: erythema exsudativum multiforme

Vascular extracardiac:

very rare: vasculitis

4.9 Overdose

No case of overdose has been reported.

5. PHARMACOLOGICAL PROPERTIES

5.1 Pharmacodynamic properties

Pharmaco-therapeutic group: Hepatitis vaccines, ATC code JO7BC.

Twinrix Paediatric is a combined vaccine formulated by pooling bulk preparations of the purified, inactivated hepatitis A (HA) virus and purified hepatitis B surface antigen (HBsAg), separately adsorbed onto aluminium hydroxide and aluminium phosphate.

The HA virus is propagated in MRC_5 human diploid cells. HBsAg is produced by culture, in a selective medium, of genetically engineered yeast cells.

Twinrix Paediatric confers immunity against HAV and HBV infection by inducing specific anti-HA and anti-HBs antibodies.

Protection against hepatitis A and hepatitis B develops within 2-4 weeks. In the clinical studies, specific humoral antibodies against hepatitis A were observed in approximately 89% of the subjects one month after the first dose and in 100% one month after the third dose (i.e. month 7). Specific humoral antibodies against hepatitis B were observed in approximately 67% of the subjects after the first dose and 100% after the third dose.

In a long term clinical trial, persistence of anti-HAV and anti-HBs antibodies has been demonstrated up to 48 months following the initiation of a primary vaccination course of Twinrix Paediatric in the majority of vaccines (see 4.2). The kinetics of decline of anti-HAV and anti-HBs antibodies were shown to be similar to those of the monovalent vaccines.

5.2 Pharmacokinetic properties

Evaluation of pharmacokinetic properties is not required for vaccines.

5.3 Preclinical safety data

Preclinical data reveal no special hazard for humans based on general safety studies.

6. PHARMACEUTICAL PARTICULARS

6.1 List of excipients

Aluminium oxide hydrated

Aluminium phosphate

Formaldehyde

Neomycin sulphate

Phenoxyethanol

Sodium chloride

Water for injections

6.2 Incompatibilities

In the absence of compatibility studies, this medicinal product must not be mixed with other medicinal products.

6.3 Shelf life

3 years.

6.4 Special precautions for storage

Store at 2°C-8°C (in a refrigerator).

Do not freeze.

Store in the original package, in order to protect from light.

6.5 Nature and contents of container

0.5 ml of suspension in prefilled syringe (type I glass) with a plunger stopper (rubber butyl) with or without needles – pack size of 1 or 10.

Not all pack sizes may be marketed.

6.6 Instructions for use and handling

Upon storage, a fine white deposit with a clear colourless supernatant can be observed.

The vaccine should be well shaken to obtain a slightly opaque, white suspension and visually inspected for any foreign particulate matter and/or variation of physical aspect prior to administration. In the event of either being observed, discard the vaccine.

Administrative Data

7. MARKETING AUTHORISATION HOLDER

GlaxoSmithKline Biologicals s.a.

rue de l'Institut 89

1330 Rixensart, Belgium

Telephone: +32 (0)2 656 8111

Fax: +32 (0)2 656 8000

Telex: 63251 SB BIO B

8. MARKETING AUTHORISATION NUMBER(S)

EU/1/97/029/006 pack of 1 prefilled syringe

9. DATE OF FIRST AUTHORISATION/RENEWAL OF THE AUTHORISATION

10 February 1997

10. DATE OF REVISION OF THE TEXT

11 April 2002

11. Legal Category

POM

Tylex Capsules

(SCHWARZ PHARMA Limited)

1. NAME OF THE MEDICINAL PRODUCT

TYLEX CAPSULES

2. QUALITATIVE AND QUANTITATIVE COMPOSITION

Each capsule contains 30mg of codeine phosphate hemihydrate and 500mg of paracetamol.

3. PHARMACEUTICAL FORM

Capsules

4. CLINICAL PARTICULARS

4.1 Therapeutic indications

For the relief of severe pain.

4.2 Posology and method of administration

Adults: The capsules are given orally. The usual dose is one or two capsules every four hours as required. The total daily dose should not exceed 240mg of codeine phosphate hemihydrate (i.e. not more than four doses (8 capsules) per 24 hours should be taken).

Elderly: A reduced dose may be required.

Children: Use in children under 12 years of age is not recommended.

Dosage should be adjusted according to the severity of the pain and the response of the patient. However, it should be kept in mind that tolerance to codeine can develop with continued use and that the incidence of untoward effects is dose related. Doses of codeine higher than 60mg fail to give commensurate relief of pain but merely prolong analgesia and are associated with an appreciably increased incidence of undesirable side effects.

4.3 Contraindications

These capsules should not to be administered to patients who have previously exhibited hypersensitivity to either paracetamol or codeine, or to any of its excipients.

These capsules are not recommended for children under the age of 12 years.

4.4 Special warnings and special precautions for use

Because safety and effectiveness in the administration of paracetamol with codeine in children under 12 years of age have not been established, such use is not recommended.

These capsules contain sodium metabisulphite, a sulphite that may cause allergic reactions including anaphylactic symptoms and life threatening or less severe asthmatic episodes in certain susceptible people. The overall prevalence of sulphite sensitivity in the general population is unknown and probably low. Sulphite sensitivity is seen more frequently in asthmatic than non-asthmatic people.

These capsules should be used with caution in patients with head injuries, increased intracranial pressure, acute abdominal conditions, the elderly and debilitated, and those with severe impairment of hepatic or renal function, hypothyroidism, Addison's disease and prostatic hypertrophy or urethral stricture.

The hazard of overdose is greater in those with non-cirrhotic alcoholic liver disease.

Chronic heavy alcohol abusers may be at increased risk of liver toxicity from excessive paracetamol use, although reports of this event are rare. Reports almost invariably involve cases of severe chronic alcoholics and the dosages of paracetamol most often exceed recommended doses and often involve substantial overdose. Professionals should alert their patients who regularly consume large amounts of alcohol not to exceed recommended doses of paracetamol.

At high doses codeine has most of the disadvantages of morphine, including respiratory depression. Codeine can produce drug dependence of the morphine type, and therefore has the potential for being abused. Codeine may impair the mental and/or physical abilities required for the performance of potentially hazardous tasks.

Patients should be advised that immediate medical advice should be sought in the event of an overdose, because of the risk of delayed, serious liver damage. They should be advised not to exceed the recommended dose, not to take other paracetamol-containing products concurrently, to consult their doctor if symptoms persist and to keep the product out of the reach of children.

4.5 Interaction with other medicinal products and other forms of Interaction

Patients receiving other central nervous system depressants (including other opioid analgesics, tranquillisers, sedative hypnotics and alcohol) concomitantly with these capsules may exhibit an additive depressant effect. When such therapy is contemplated, the dose of one or both agents should be reduced.

Concurrent use of MAO inhibitors or tricyclic antidepressants with codeine may increase the effect of either the antidepressant or codeine. Concurrent use of anticholinergics and codeine may produce paralytic ileus.

The speed of absorption of paracetamol may be increased by metoclopramide or domperidone and absorption reduced by cholestyramine.

The anti-coagulant effect of warfarin and other coumarins may be enhanced by prolonged regular daily use of paracetamol with increased risk of bleeding; occasional doses have no significant effect.

4.6 Pregnancy and lactation

These capsules are not recommended during pregnancy or lactation since safety in pregnant women or nursing mothers has not been established.

4.7 Effects on ability to drive and use machines

Patients should be advised not to drive or operate machinery if affected by dizziness or sedation.

4.8 Undesirable effects

The most frequently observed reactions include light headedness, dizziness, sedation, shortness of breath, nausea and vomiting. These effects seem more prominent in ambulatory than non-ambulatory patients and some of these adverse reactions may be alleviated if the patient lies down. Other adverse reactions include allergic reactions, (including skin rash), euphoria, dysphoria, constipation, abdominal pain and pruritus.

In clinical use of paracetamol-containing products, there have been a few reports of blood dyscrasias including thrombocytopenia and agranulocytosis but these were not necessarily causally related to paracetamol.

4.9 Overdose

Symptoms of paracetamol overdosage in the first 24 hours are pallor, nausea, vomiting, anorexia and abdominal pain. Liver damage may become apparent 12 to 48 hours after ingestion. Abnormalities of glucose metabolism and metabolic acidosis may occur. In severe poisoning, hepatic failure may progress to encephalopathy, coma and death. Acute renal failure with acute tubular necrosis may develop even in the absence of severe liver damage. Cardiac arrhythmias and pancreatitis have been reported. Liver damage is possible in adults who have taken 10g or more of paracetamol. It is considered that excess quantities of a toxic metabolite (usually adequately detoxified by glutathione when normal doses of paracetamol are ingested), become irreversibly bound to liver tissue.

Immediate treatment is essential in the management of paracetamol overdose. Despite a lack of significant early symptoms, patients should be referred to hospital urgently for immediate medical attention and any patient who has ingested around 7.5g or more of paracetamol in the preceding 4 hours should undergo gastric lavage. Administration of oral methionine or intravenous N-acetylcysteine which may have a beneficial effect up to at least 48 hours after the overdose, may be required. General supportive measures must be available.

Serious overdose with codeine is characterised by respiratory depression, extreme somnolence progressing to stupor or coma, skeletal muscle flaccidity, cold and clammy skin and sometimes bradycardia and hypotension. In severe overdose with codeine, apnoea, circulatory collapse, cardiac arrest and death may occur. Primary attention should be given to the re-establishment of adequate respiratory exchange through the provision of a patient airway and the institution of controlled ventilation. Oxygen, intravenous fluids, vasopressors and other supportive measures should be employed as indicated. Opioid antagonists may be employed. Gastric lavage should be considered.

5. PHARMACOLOGICAL PROPERTIES

5.1 Pharmacodynamic properties

Paracetamol has analgesic and antipyretic actions similar to those of aspirin with weak anti-inflammatory effects. Paracetamol is only a weak inhibitor of prostaglandin biosynthesis, although there is some evidence to suggest that it may be more effective against enzymes in the CNS than those in the periphery. This fact may partly account for its well documented ability to reduce fever and to induce analgesia, effects that involve actions on neural tissues. Single or repeated therapeutic doses of paracetamol have no effect on the cardiovascular and respiratory systems. Acid-based changes do not occur and gastric irritation, erosion or bleeding is not produced as may occur after salicylates. There is only a weak effect upon platelets and no effect on bleeding time or the excretion of uric acid.

Codeine is an analgesic with uses similar to those of morphine but has only mild sedative effects. The major effect is on the CNS and the bowel. The effects are remarkably diverse and include analgesia, drowsiness, changes in mood, respiratory depression, decreased gastrointestinal motility, nausea, vomiting and alterations of the endocrine and autonomic nervous systems. The relief of pain is relatively selective, in that other sensory modalities, (touch, vibration, vision, hearing etc.) are not obtunded.

5.2 Pharmacokinetic properties

Paracetamol is readily absorbed from the gastro-intestinal tract with peak plasma concentration occurring about 30 minutes to 2 hours after ingestion. It is metabolised in the liver and excreted in the urine mainly as the glucuronide and sulphate conjugates. Less than 5% is excreted as unchanged paracetamol. The elimination half-life varies from about 1 to 4 hours. Plasma-protein binding is negligible at usual therapeutic concentrations but increases with increasing concentrations.

A minor hydroxylated metabolite which is usually produced in very small amounts by mixed-function oxidases in the liver and which is usually detoxified by conjugation with liver glutathione may accumulate following paracetamol overdosage and cause liver damage.

Codeine and its salts are absorbed from the gastro intestinal tract. Ingestion of codeine phosphate hemihydrate produces peak plasma codeine concentrations in about one hour. Codeine is metabolised by O- & N-demethylation in the liver to morphine and norcodeine. Codeine and its metabolites are excreted almost entirely by the kidney, mainly as conjugates with glucuronic acid.

The plasma half-life has been reported to be between 3 and 4 hours after administration by mouth or intravascular injection.

5.3 Preclinical safety data

None stated.

6. PHARMACEUTICAL PARTICULARS

6.1 List of excipients

Pregelatinised starch

Calcium stearate

Aerosol OT-B (dioctyl sodium sulfosuccinate, sodium benzoate (E211))

Sodium metabisulphite

Gelatin capsule:

Titanium dioxide (E171)

Erythrosine (E127)

Indigo carmine (E132)

Printing ink:

Shellac

Soya lecithin

2-ethyoxyethanol

Dimethylpolysiloxane

Iron oxide E172

6.2 Incompatibilities

None pertinent

6.3 Shelf life

36 months –HPDE bottles and PVC/aluminium foil blisters

36 months –PP securitainers

6.4 Special precautions for storage

Do not store above 25°C. Keep container in the outer carton.

6.5 Nature and contents of container

Tamper-evident high density polyethylene bottles fitted with low density polyethylene caps containing 24, 100 or 500 capsules.

PVC/aluminium foil blister strips containing 1x7, 2x7, 4x7, 1x8, 3x8, 50x6, 100x6, 5x20 capsules.

Polypropylene securitainers containing 8, 16, 24, 32, 56 or 64 capsules.

Not all pack sizes may be marketed.

6.6 Instructions for use and handling

None

7. MARKETING AUTHORISATION HOLDER

Schwarz Pharma Ltd

Schwarz House

East Street

Chesham

Buckinghamshire

HP5 1DG

England

8. MARKETING AUTHORISATION NUMBER(S)

PL 04438/0046

9. DATE OF FIRST AUTHORISATION/RENEWAL OF THE AUTHORISATION

29 March 1996

10. DATE OF REVISION OF THE TEXT

August 2001

Tylex Effervescent

(SCHWARZ PHARMA Limited)

1. NAME OF THE MEDICINAL PRODUCT

Tylex Effervescent

2. QUALITATIVE AND QUANTITATIVE COMPOSITION

Each effervescent tablet contains 500 mg of paracetamol Ph.Eur. and 30 mg of codeine phosphate hemihydrate Ph. Eur.

3. PHARMACEUTICAL FORM

Effervescent tablets

4. CLINICAL PARTICULARS

4.1 Therapeutic indications

For the relief of severe pain.

4.2 Posology and method of administration

Adults: The tablets are given orally and should be dissolved in at least half a tumbler-full of water before taking. The usual dose is one or two tablets every four hours as required. The total daily dose should not exceed 240 mg of codeine phosphate hemihydrate (i.e. not more than eight tablets per 24 hours should be taken).

Elderly: A reduced dose may be required.

Children: Use in children under 12 years of age is not recommended.

Dosage should be adjusted according to the severity of the pain and the response of the patient. However, it should be kept in mind that tolerance to codeine can develop with continued use and that the incidence of untoward effects is dose related. Doses of codeine higher than 60 mg fail to give commensurate relief of pain but merely prolong analgesia and are associated with an appreciably increased incidence of undesirable side effects.

4.3 Contraindications

Tylex Effervescent should not to be administered to patients who have previously exhibited hypersensitivity to either paracetamol or codeine, or to any of its excipients.

Tylex Effervescent is not recommended for children under the age of 12 years.

4.4 Special warnings and special precautions for use

Because safety and effectiveness in the administration of paracetamol with codeine in children under 12 years of age have not been established, such use is not recommended.

Tylex Effervescent should be used with caution in patients with head injuries, increased intracranial pressure, acute abdominal conditions, the elderly and debilitated, and those with severe impairment of hepatic or renal function, hypothyroidism, Addison's disease and prostatic hypertrophy or urethral stricture.

The hazard of overdose is greater in those with non-cirrhotic alcoholic liver disease.

Chronic heavy alcohol abusers may be at increased risk of liver toxicity from excessive paracetamol use, although reports of this event are rare. Reports almost invariably involve cases of severe chronic alcoholics and the dosages of paracetamol most often exceed recommended doses and often involve substantial overdose. Professionals should alert their patients who regularly consume large amounts of alcohol not to exceed recommended doses of paracetamol.

Tylex Effervescent contains 312.9 mg sodium/tablet and this should be taken into account when prescribing for patients for whom sodium restriction is indicated. The product also contains 25 mg aspartame/tablet and therefore care should be taken in phenylketonuria.

At high doses codeine has most of the disadvantages of morphine, including respiratory depression. Codeine can produce drug dependence of the morphine type, and therefore has the potential for being abused. Codeine may impair the mental/or physical abilities required for the performance of potentially hazardous tasks.

Patients should be advised that immediate medical advice should be sought in the event of an overdose, because of the risk of delayed, serious liver damage. They should be advised not to exceed the recommended dose, not to take other paracetamol-containing products concurrently, to consult their doctor if symptoms persist and to keep the product out of the reach of children.

4.5 Interaction with other medicinal products and other forms of Interaction

Patients receiving other central nervous system depressants (including other opioid analgesics, tranquillisers, sedative hypnotics and alcohol) concomitantly with Tylex Effervescent may exhibit an additive depressant effect. When such therapy is contemplated, the dose of one or both agents should be reduced.

Concurrent use of MAO inhibitors or tricyclic antidepressants with codeine may increase the effect of either the antidepressant or codeine. Concurrent use of anticholinergics and codeine may produce paralytic ileus.

The speed of absorption of paracetamol may be increased by metoclopramide or domperidone and absorption reduced by cholestyramine.

The anti-coagulant effect of warfarin and other coumarins may be enhanced by prolonged regular daily use of paracetamol with increased risk of bleeding; occasional doses have no significant effect.

4.6 Pregnancy and lactation

The use of Tylex Effervescent is not recommended during pregnancy or lactation since safety in pregnant women or nursing mothers has not been established.

4.7 Effects on ability to drive and use machines

Patients should be advised not to drive or operate machinery if affected by dizziness or sedation.

4.8 Undesirable effects

The most frequently observed reactions include light headedness, dizziness, sedation, shortness of breath, nausea and vomiting. These effects seem more prominent in ambulatory than non-ambulatory patients and some of these adverse reactions may be alleviated if the patient lies down. Other adverse reactions include allergic reactions(including skin rash), euphoria, dysphoria, constipation, abdominal pain and pruritus.

In clinical use of paracetamol-containing products, there have been a few reports of blood dyscrasias including thrombocytopenia and agranulocytosis but these were not necessarily causally related to paracetamol.

4.9 Overdose

Symptoms of paracetamol overdosage in the first 24 hours are pallor, nausea, vomiting, anorexia and abdominal pain. Liver damage may become apparent 12 to 48 hours after ingestion. Abnormalities of glucose metabolism and metabolic acidosis may occur. In severe poisoning, hepatic failure may progress to encephalopathy, coma and death. Acute renal failure with acute tubular necrosis may develop even in the absence of severe liver damage. Cardiac arrhythmias and pancreatitis have been reported. Liver damage is possible in adults who have taken 10 g or more of paracetamol. It is considered that excess quantities of a toxic metabolite (usually adequately detoxified by glutathione when normal doses of paracetamol are ingested), become irreversibly bound to liver tissue.

Immediate treatment is essential in the management of paracetamol overdose. Despite a lack of significant early symptoms, patients should be referred to hospital urgently for immediate medical attention and any patient who has ingested around 7.5 g or more of paracetamol in the preceding 4 hours should undergo gastric lavage. Administration of oral methionine or intravenous N-acetylcysteine which may have a beneficial effect up to at least 48 hours after the overdose, may be required. General supportive measures must be available.

Serious overdose with codeine is characterised by respiratory depression, extreme somnolence progressing to stupor or coma, skeletal muscle flaccidity, cold and clammy skin and sometimes bradycardia and hypotension. In severe overdose with codeine, apnoea, circulatory collapse, cardiac arrest and death may occur. Primary attention should be given to the re-establishment of adequate respiratory exchange through the provision of a patient airway and the institution of controlled ventilation. Oxygen, intravenous fluids, vasopressors and other supportive measures should be employed as indicated. Opioid antagonists may be employed. Gastric lavage should be considered.

5. PHARMACOLOGICAL PROPERTIES

5.1 Pharmacodynamic properties

Paracetamol has analgesic and antipyretic actions similar to those of aspirin with weak anti-inflammatory effects. Paracetamol is only a weak inhibitor of prostaglandin biosynthesis, although there is some evidence to suggest that it may be more effective against enzymes in the CNS than those in the periphery. This fact may partly account for its well documented ability to reduce fever and to induce analgesia, effects that involve actions on neural tissues. Single or repeated therapeutic doses of paracetamol have no effect on the cardiovascular and respiratory systems. Acid-based changes do not occur and gastric irritation, erosion or bleeding is not produced as may occur after salicylates. There is only a weak effect upon platelets and no effect on bleeding time or the excretion of uric acid.

Codeine is an analgesic with uses similar to those of morphine but has only mild sedative effects. The major effect is on the CNS and the bowel. The effects are remarkably diverse and include analgesia, drowsiness, changes in mood, respiratory depression, decreased gastrointestinal motility, nausea, vomiting and alterations of the endocrine and autonomic nervous systems. The relief of pain is relatively selective, in that other sensory modalities, (touch, vibration, vision, hearing etc.) are not obtunded.

5.2 Pharmacokinetic properties
Paracetamol is readily absorbed from the gastro-intestinal tract with peak plasma concentration occurring about 30 minutes to 2 hours after ingestion. It is metabolised in the liver and excreted in the urine mainly as the glucuronide and sulphate conjugates. Less than 5% is excreted as unchanged paracetamol. The elimination half-life varies from about 1 to 4 hours. Plasma-protein binding is negligible at usual therapeutic concentrations but increases with increasing concentrations.

A minor hydroxylated metabolite which is usually produced in very small amounts by mixed-function oxidases in the liver and which is usually detoxified by conjugation with liver glutathione may accumulate following paracetamol overdosage and cause liver damage.

Codeine and its salts are absorbed from the gastro intestinal tract. Ingestion of codeine phosphate hemihydrate produces peak plasma codeine concentrations in about one hour. Codeine is metabolised by O- & N-demethylation in the liver to morphine and norcodeine. Codeine and its metabolites are excreted almost entirely by the kidney, mainly as conjugates with glucuronic acid.

The plasma half-life has been reported to be between 3 and 4 hours after administration by mouth or intravascular injection.

5.3 Preclinical safety data
None stated.

6. PHARMACEUTICAL PARTICULARS

6.1 List of excipients
Citric acid anhydrous

Sodium bicarbonate

Sodium carbonate anhydrous

Aspartame

Blackcurrant flavour no. 78004-31

Polyethylene glycol 6000

Magnesium stearate

Ethanol 96% (not detected in the finished product)

6.2 Incompatibilities
None pertinent

6.3 Shelf life
36 months

6.4 Special precautions for storage
Store at room temperature (at or below 25°C) in a dry place. Protect from light.

6.5 Nature and contents of container
Paper/aluminium laminate blister strips packed in cardboard cartons.

Pack sizes: 1x1, 1x6, 4x2, 4x6, 5x6, 6x6, 7x6 and 15x6.

6.6 Instructions for use and handling
None

7. MARKETING AUTHORISATION HOLDER
SCHWARZ PHARMA Ltd

Schwarz House

East Street

Chesham

Buckinghamshire

HP5 1DG

England

8. MARKETING AUTHORISATION NUMBER(S)
PL 04438/0045

9. DATE OF FIRST AUTHORISATION/RENEWAL OF THE AUTHORISATION
29 March 1996

10. DATE OF REVISION OF THE TEXT
February 2005

Typherix

(GlaxoSmithKline UK)

1. NAME OF THE MEDICINAL PRODUCT
'Typherix' 25 micrograms/0.5ml

Vi-polysaccharide typhoid vaccine.

Solution for injection

2. QUALITATIVE AND QUANTITATIVE COMPOSITION
Each 0.5 ml dose of vaccine contains

Vi polysaccharide of Salmonella typhi. 25 micrograms

For excipients, see 6.1.

3. PHARMACEUTICAL FORM
Solution for injection.

'Typherix' is a clear isotonic colourless solution.

4. CLINICAL PARTICULARS

4.1 Therapeutic indications
Active immunisation against typhoid fever for both adults and children two years of age and older.

4.2 Posology and method of administration
Posology

A single dose of 0.5 ml is recommended for both adults and children two years of age and older.

The vaccine should be administered at least two weeks prior to risk of exposure to typhoid fever.

Subjects who remain at risk of typhoid fever should be revaccinated using a single dose of vaccine with an interval of not more than 3 years.

Method of administration

'Typherix' is for intramuscular injection.

'Typherix' should under no circumstances be administered intravascularly.

4.3 Contraindications
'Typherix' should not be administered to subjects with known hypersensitivity to any component of the vaccine or to subjects having shown signs of hypersensitivity after previous administration.

4.4 Special warnings and special precautions for use
The vaccine protects against typhoid fever caused by *Salmonella typhi.* Protection is not conferred against *Salmonella paratyphi* and other non-typhoidal Salmonellae.

'Typherix' has not been evaluated in children under 2 years of age. Polysaccharide vaccines in general have lower immunogenicity under this age.

Different injectable vaccines should always be administered at different injection sites.

The administration of 'Typherix' should be postponed in subjects suffering from acute severe febrile illness.

'Typherix' should be administered with caution to subjects with thrombocytopenia or bleeding disorders since bleeding may occur following an intramuscular administration to these subjects: following injection, firm pressure should be applied to the site (without rubbing) for at least two minutes.

It may be expected that in patients receiving immunosuppressive treatment or patients with immunodeficiency, an adequate response may not be achieved.

Appropriate medical treatment and supervision should always be readily available in case of a rare anaphylactic reaction following administration of the vaccine.

4.5 Interaction with other medicinal products and other forms of Interaction
In clinical studies in adults aged over 18 years, 'Typherix' has been administered concomitantly in opposite arms with 'Havrix' Monodose (1440), SmithKline Beecharns' inactivated hepatitis A vaccine.

There was no adverse impact on either the reactogenicity or immunogenicity of the vaccines when they were administered simultaneously in opposite arms.

No interaction studies with other vaccines have been performed.

4.6 Pregnancy and lactation
Pregnancy

The effect of 'Typherix' on fetal development has not been assessed.

'Typherix' should only be used during pregnancy when there is a high risk of infection.

Lactation

The effect on breastfed infants of the administration of 'Typherix' to their mothers has not been evaluated.

'Typherix' should therefore only be used in breastfeeding women when there is a high risk of infection.

4.7 Effects on ability to drive and use machines
Some of the effects mentioned under section 4.8 "Undesirable Effects" may affect the ability to drive or operate machinery.

4.8 Undesirable effects
During clinical studies, the most commonly reported adverse events after the first dose, were reactions at the injection site, including soreness redness and swelling.

General reactions that may occur in temporal association with Typherix vaccination include:

Body as a whole:

Common: fever, headache, general aches, malaise

Gastro-intestinal system:

Common: nausea

Skin appendages:

Common: itching

Following a second dose, there was an increased incidence of redness and soreness >10%).

Local reactions were usually reported during the first 48 hours and systemic reactions were also transient.

The following reactions have been reported in post-marketing experience:

Body as a whole:

Very rare: anaphylaxis, allergic reactions, including anaphylactoid reactions

Skin appendages:

Very rare: urticaria

4.9 Overdose
Occasional reports of overdose have been received. The symptoms reported in these cases are not different from those reported following normal dosage.

5. PHARMACOLOGICAL PROPERTIES
Pharmaco-therapeutic group: Bacterial vaccine, ATC code: J07AP

5.1 Pharmacodynamic properties
In comparative clinical studies, the immune response to Typherix was shown to be equivalent to a licensed comparator Vi polysaccharide vaccine. Seroconversion was observed in >95% of Typherix recipients when measured at two weeks after administration. Two years after vaccination 61% were seropositive, and at three years 46%.

The protective efficacy of Typherix has not been investigated in clinical trials.

For individuals who remain at - or who may be re-exposed to - risk of typhoid fever, it is recommended that they be revaccinated using a single dose of vaccine with an interval of not more than 3 years.

5.2 Pharmacokinetic properties
Evaluation of pharmacokinetic properties is not required for vaccines and formal pharmacokinetic studies have not been performed.

5.3 Preclinical safety data
No preclinical safety testing with the vaccine has been conducted.

6. PHARMACEUTICAL PARTICULARS

6.1 List of excipients
Sodium dihydrogen phosphate dihydrate

Disodium phosphate dihydrate

Sodium chloride

Phenol (1.1 mg/dose)

Water for injection

6.2 Incompatibilities
In the absence of compatibility studies, this medicinal product must not be mixed with other medicinal products.

6.3 Shelf life
2 years.

6.4 Special precautions for storage
Store at 2 C - 8 C (in a refrigerator)

Do not freeze.

Store in the original package, in order to protect from light.

6.5 Nature and contents of container
Solution in prefilled syringe (Type I glass) (0.5 ml) with an elastomer plunger stopper (butyl)- pack sizes of 1, 10, 50 or 100.

Not all pack sizes may be marketed.

6.6 Instructions for use and handling
Vaccines should be inspected for any foreign particulate matter and/or variation of physical aspect. In the event of either being observed, discard the vaccine.

Shake before use.

Administrative Data

7. MARKETING AUTHORISATION HOLDER
SmithKline Beecham plc

980 Great West Road

Brentford

Middlesex TW8 9BD

Trading as:

GlaxoSmithKline UK

Stockley Park West

Uxbridge

Middlesex, UB11 1BT

8. MARKETING AUTHORISATION NUMBER(S)
PL 10592/0126

9. DATE OF FIRST AUTHORISATION/RENEWAL OF THE AUTHORISATION
5 April 2003

10. DATE OF REVISION OF THE TEXT
17 September 2002

11. Legal Status
POM

TYPHIM Vi

(Sanofi Pasteur MSD)

1. NAME OF THE MEDICINAL PRODUCT
TYPHIM Vi®

Vi Capsular Polysaccharide Typhoid Vaccine.

2. QUALITATIVE AND QUANTITATIVE COMPOSITION
Each dose of 0.5 millilitre contains:

Purified Vi capsular polysaccharide of Salmonella typhi - 25 micrograms

3. PHARMACEUTICAL FORM
Sterile solution.

4. CLINICAL PARTICULARS

4.1 Therapeutic indications
Active immunisation against typhoid fever.

4.2 Posology and method of administration
Adults and Children over 18 months of age: A single dose of 0.5 millilitre administered by deep subcutaneous or intramuscular injection.

Children under 18 months of age: Since the response to the vaccine may be sub-optimal, the use of the product should be based upon the risk of exposure to the disease.

Elderly: As for adults and children over 18 months of age.

Revaccination: A single dose at 3 yearly intervals in subjects who remain at risk from typhoid fever.

4.3 Contraindications
Acute infectious illness.

Hypersensitivity to the vaccine or its components.

4.4 Special warnings and special precautions for use
The vaccine does not protect against paratyphoid fever. As with all vaccines, facilities for the management of anaphylaxis should always be available during vaccination.

4.5 Interaction with other medicinal products and other forms of Interaction
None known

4.6 Pregnancy and lactation
No reproductive studies have been conducted in animals. There are no data on the use of this vaccine in pregnancy and lactation. The vaccine should not normally be used in pregnancy or during lactation unless the benefit outweighs the risk.

4.7 Effects on ability to drive and use machines
Not applicable.

4.8 Undesirable effects
The effects reported after vaccination are usually mild and short lasting. They consist mainly of local reactions at the site of injection (pain, oedema, redness).

Systemic reactions have also been reported rarely: fever, headache, malaise, fatigue, joint pain, myalgia, nausea, vomiting, diarrhoea and abdominal pain.

Very rarely, cases of pruritis, rash, urticaria and exceptionally asthma, serum sickness and anaphylactoid reactions have been reported.

4.9 Overdose
Not applicable.

5. PHARMACOLOGICAL PROPERTIES

5.1 Pharmacodynamic properties
Not applicable.

5.2 Pharmacokinetic properties
Not applicable.

5.3 Preclinical safety data
Not applicable.

6. PHARMACEUTICAL PARTICULARS

6.1 List of excipients

Phenol (preservative)	⩽1.250 milligrams
Isotonic buffer solution*	q.s. 0.5 millilitre

*Composition of the isotonic buffer solution:

Sodium Chloride	4.150 milligrams
Disodium phosphate	0.065 milligram
Monosodium phosphate	0.023 milligram
Water for Injections	q.s. 0.5 millilitre

6.2 Incompatibilities
Not applicable.

6.3 Shelf life
36 months.

6.4 Special precautions for storage
Store between +2°C and +8°C. Do not freeze.

6.5 Nature and contents of container
The vaccine is supplied in:

single dose (0.5 millilitre) prefilled syringes (with or without attached needle); in single syringe packs and packs of 10 syringes.

6.6 Instructions for use and handling
Shake well immediately before use.

7. MARKETING AUTHORISATION HOLDER
Sanofi Pasteur MSD Ltd

Mallards Reach

Bridge Avenue

Maidenhead

Berkshire

SL6 1QP

8. MARKETING AUTHORISATION NUMBER(S)
PL 6745/0039

9. DATE OF FIRST AUTHORISATION/RENEWAL OF THE AUTHORISATION
5 May 1992

10. DATE OF REVISION OF THE TEXT
May 2005

Ubretid

(sanofi-aventis)

1. NAME OF THE MEDICINAL PRODUCT
Ubretid™.

2. QUALITATIVE AND QUANTITATIVE COMPOSITION
Active ingredient Distigmine bromide 5mg.

3. PHARMACEUTICAL FORM
Tablets.

4. CLINICAL PARTICULARS

4.1 Therapeutic indications
Anticholinesterase. Post-operative urinary retention. Post operative ileus and intestinal atony. To assist emptying of the neurogenic bladder. As an adjunct in the treatment of myasthenia gravis.

4.2 Posology and method of administration
ADULTS
In prevention of urinary retention, ileus or intestinal atony following surgery:
One Ubretid tablet daily, half an hour before breakfast.
In neurogenic bladder:
One Ubretid tablet daily or on alternate days, half an hour before breakfast, on an empty stomach.
In myasthenia gravis:
Dosage to be individualised for each patient, dependent upon the severity of the condition, the degree and duration of response and the side effects encountered. The tablets should always be taken on an empty stomach half an hour before breakfast. Dosage should commence at 1 tablet daily and may be adjusted at intervals of three to four days to a total not exceeding 4 tablets daily.
CHILDREN
Up to 2 tablets daily according to age.
ELDERLY
No dosage adjustment is necessary for elderly patients.
Ubretid tablets are for oral administration.

4.3 Contraindications
Ubretid is contraindicated in cases of severe post operative shock, serious circulatory insufficiency, severe constipation, serious spastic and mechanical ileus, asthma and mechanical urinary obstruction.

4.4 Special warnings and special precautions for use
Caution should be taken in conditions where the potentiation of the effects of acetylcholine is undesirable, eg cardiac dysfunction, bronchospasm, peptic ulcer, oesophagitis, epilepsy and Parkinsonism. The patient should be supervised in the early stages of dosage titration to guard against the possibility of myasthenic crisis or cholinergic crisis.

4.5 Interaction with other medicinal products and other forms of Interaction
Use with caution in patients receiving concomitantly drugs acting on the cardiovascular system, e.g. beta blockers, drugs with local anaesthetic properties and muscle relaxants. In myasthenia gravis, where short acting cholinergic drugs are taken concurrently, their dosage should be reduced to the minimum required to control symptoms.

4.6 Pregnancy and lactation
Ubretid should be avoided during pregnancy. No information is available on lactation.

4.7 Effects on ability to drive and use machines
None stated.

4.8 Undesirable effects
The following side effects may occur infrequently: bradycardia, AV block, hypotension, bronchospasm, dyspnoea, increased bronchial secretions, sweating, salivation and lacrimation, muscle twitching, abdominal cramps, diarrhoea, urinary frequency and miosis. These effects of Ubretid may be controlled with atropine, giving 2mg intramuscularly; atropinisation should be maintained for at least 24 hours.

4.9 Overdose
Overdosage of Ubretid may also produce skeletal muscle fatigue, weakness and eventually paralysis. The muscarinic effects of overdosage may be controlled with atropine 2mg intramuscularly repeated at intervals indicated by the clinical response until signs of mild atropinisation (dry mouth, mydriasis) appear. The patient should be kept fully atropinised for at least 24 hours.

5. PHARMACOLOGICAL PROPERTIES

5.1 Pharmacodynamic properties
Distigmine is an inhibitor of cholinesterase by the formation of complexes with the enzyme. This process is reversible. Specific cholinesterase or acetylcholinesterase is inhibited more strongly than pseudo or plasma cholinesterase.

5.2 Pharmacokinetic properties
Maximum inhibition of plasma cholinesterase occurs 9 hours after a single intramuscular dose and persists for about 24 hours.

Tritium labelled Ubretid was used to determine the urinary and biliary excretion of the drug in the rat. Activity in the urine was demonstrated quickly, amounting to 43% after 8 hours. Biliary excretion was shown to be insignificant. In man, results suggested that about 50% of a 0.5mg 1ml dose was excreted in 24 hours.

5.3 Preclinical safety data
There are no preclinical data of relevance to the prescriber which are additional to that already included in other sections of the SPC.

6. PHARMACEUTICAL PARTICULARS

6.1 List of excipients
Lactose BP, Maize starch BP, Purified talc BP and Magnesium stearate BP.

6.2 Incompatibilities
None stated.

6.3 Shelf life
36 months.

6.4 Special precautions for storage
Store in a dry place below 25°C.

6.5 Nature and contents of container
Blisters of 20μm aluminium foil and 250μm UPVC/PVdC opaque white film containing 30 tablets.

6.6 Instructions for use and handling
None.

7. MARKETING AUTHORISATION HOLDER
Rhone-Poulenc Rorer

RPR House

50 Kings Hill Avenue

Kings Hill

West Malling

Kent

ME19 4AH

8. MARKETING AUTHORISATION NUMBER(S)
PL 05272/0029

9. DATE OF FIRST AUTHORISATION/RENEWAL OF THE AUTHORISATION
26 November 1996

10. DATE OF REVISION OF THE TEXT
August 1997

11. Legal Category
POM

Ucerax Tablets 25 mg

(UCB Pharma Limited)

1. NAME OF THE MEDICINAL PRODUCT
UCERAX TABLETS 25 mg.

2. QUALITATIVE AND QUANTITATIVE COMPOSITION
Hydroxyzine hydrochloride 25 mg.

For excipients, see 6.1.

3. PHARMACEUTICAL FORM
Film-coated tablets.

4. CLINICAL PARTICULARS

4.1 Therapeutic indications
UCERAX is indicated to assist in the management of anxiety.

UCERAX is indicated to assist in the management of pruritus associated with acute and chronic urticaria, including cholinergic and physical types, and in atopic and contact dermatosis in adults and children.

4.2 Posology and method of administration
Adults:

Anxiety.

50 mg/day in 3 separate administrations of 12.5-12.5-25mg. In more severe cases, doses up to 300mg/day can be used.

Pruritus.

Starting dose of 25 mg at night, increasing as necessary to 25 mg three or four times daily.

The maximum single dose in adults should not exceed 200mg whereas the maximum daily doses should not exceed 300mg.

Children:

Children aged from 12 months to 6 years: 1mg/kg/day up to 2.5mg/kg/day in divided doses.

Children aged over 6 years:1mg/kg/day up to 2mg/kg/day in divided doses.

The dosage should be adjusted according to the patient's response to therapy.

In the elderly, it is advised to start with half the recommended dose due to the prolonged action.

In patients with hepatic dysfunction, it is recommended to reduce the daily dose by 33%.

Dosage should be reduced in patients with moderate or severe renal impairment due to decreased excretion of its metabolite cetirizine.

4.3 Contraindications
UCERAX is contra-indicated in patients with a history of hypersensitivity to any of its constituents, to cetirizine, to other piperazine derivatives, to aminophylline, or to ethylenediamine.

UCERAX is contra-indicated during pregnancy and lactation.

UCERAX is contra-indicated in patients with porphyria.

4.4 Special warnings and special precautions for use
UCERAX should be administered cautiously in patients with increased potential for convulsions.

Young children are more susceptible to develop adverse events related to the central nervous system (see section 4.8). In children, convulsions have been more frequently reported than in adults.

Because of its potential anticholinergic effects, UCERAX should be used cautiously in patients suffering from glaucoma, bladder outflow obstruction, decreased gastrointestinal motility, myasthenia gravis, or dementia.

Dosage adjustments may be required if UCERAX is used simultaneously with other central nervous system depressant drugs or with drugs having anticholinergic properties (see section 4.5).

The concomitant use of alcohol and UCERAX should be avoided (see section 4.5).

Caution is needed in patients who have a known predisposing factor to cardiac arrhythmia, or who are concomitantly treated with a potentially arrhythmogenic drug.

In the elderly, it is advised to start with half the recommended dose due to a prolonged action.

UCERAX dosage should be reduced in patients with hepatic dysfunction and in patients with moderate or severe renal impairment (see section 4.2).

The treatment should be stopped at least 5 days before allergy testing or methacholine bronchial challenge, to avoid effects on the test results.

Due to the presence of lactose, patients with rare hereditary problems of galactose intolerance, the Lapp lactase deficiency or glucose-galactose malabsorption should not take this medicine.

4.5 Interaction with other medicinal products and other forms of Interaction
Patients should be informed that UCERAX may potentiate the effects of barbiturates, other CNS depressants or drugs having anticholinergic properties.

Alcohol also potentiates the effects of UCERAX.

UCERAX antagonizes the effects of betahistine, and of anticholinesterase drugs.

The treatment should be stopped at least 5 days before allergy testing or methacholine bronchial challenge, to avoid effects on the test results.

Simultaneous administration of UCERAX with monoamine oxidase inhibitors should be avoided.

UCERAX counteracts the epinephrine pressor action.

In rats, hydroxyzine antagonised the anticonvulsant action of phenytoin.

Cimetidine 600 mg bid has been shown to increase the serum concentrations of hydroxyzine by 36% and to decrease peak concentrations of the metabolite cetirizine by 20%.

UCERAX is an inhibitor of cytochrome P450 2D6 (Ki: 3.9 μM; 1.7 μg/ml) and may cause at high doses drug-drug interactions with CYP2D6 substrates.

UCERAX has no inhibitory effect at 100 μM on UDP-glucuronyl transferase isoforms 1A1 and 1A6 in human liver microsomes. It inhibits cytochrome P_{450} 2C9/C10, 2C19 and 3A4 isoforms at concentrations (IC_{50} : 19 to 140 μM; 7 to 52 μg/ml) well above peak plasma concentrations. The metabolite cetirizine at 100 μM has no inhibitory effect on human liver cytochrome P_{450} (1A2, 2A6, 2C9/C10, 2C19, 2D6, 2E1 and 3A4) and UDP-glucuronyl transferase isoforms. Therefore, UCERAX is unlikely to impair the metabolism of drugs which are substrates for these enzymes.

As hydroxyzine is metabolized in the liver, an increase in hydroxyzine blood concentrations may be expected when hydroxyzine is co-administered with other drugs known to be potent inhibitors of liver enzymes.

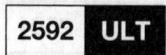

4.6 Pregnancy and lactation
Animal studies have shown reproductive toxicity.

Hydroxyzine crosses the placental barrier leading to higher fetal than maternal concentrations.

To date, no relevant epidemiological data are available relating to exposure to UCERAX during pregnancy.

In neonates whose mothers received UCERAX during late pregnancy and/or labour, the following events were observed immediately or only a few hours after birth: hypotonia, movement disorders including extrapyramidal disorders, clonic movements, CNS depression, neonatal hypoxic conditions, or urinary retention.

Therefore, UCERAX should not be used during pregnancy.

UCERAX is contra-indicated during lactation. Breast-feeding should be stopped if UCERAX therapy is needed.

4.7 Effects on ability to drive and use machines
Alertness or reaction time may be impaired by UCERAX therefore patients' driving capacity or ability to use machines may be reduced. Concomitant use of UCERAX with alcohol or other sedative drugs should be avoided as it aggravates these effects.

4.8 Undesirable effects
Undesirable effects are mainly related to CNS depressant or paradoxical CNS stimulation effects, to anticholinergic activity, or to hypersensitivity reactions. The following adverse reactions, in MedDRA terms, have been spontaneously reported:

Cardiac disorders:

Tachycardia NOS

Eye disorders:

Accommodation disorder, vision blurred

Gastrointestinal disorders:

Constipation, dry mouth, nausea, vomiting NOS

General disorders and administration site conditions:
Fatigue, malaise, pyrexia

Immune system disorders:
Anaphylactic shock, hypersensitivity NOS

Investigations:

Liver function tests NOS abnormal

Nervous system disorders:

Convulsions NOS, dizziness, dyskinesia NEC, headache NOS, insomnia NEC, sedation, somnolence, tremor NEC

Psychiatric disorders:

Agitation, confusion, disorientation, hallucination NOS

Renal and urinary disorders:

Urinary retention

Respiratory, thoracic and mediastinal disorders:

Bronchospasm NOS

Skin and subcutaneous tissue disorders:

Angioneurotic oedema, dermatitis NOS, pruritus NOS, rash erythematous, rash maculo-papular, sweating increased, urticaria NOS

Vascular disorders:

Hypotension NOS

4.9 Overdose
Symptoms observed after an important overdose are mainly associated with excessive anticholinergic load, CNS depression or CNS paradoxical stimulation. They include nausea, vomiting, tachycardia, pyrexia, somnolence, impaired pupillary reflex, tremor, confusion, or hallucination. This may be followed by depressed level of consciousness, respiratory depression, convulsions, hypotension, or cardiac arrhythmia. Deepening coma and cardiorespiratory collapse may ensue.

Airway, breathing and circulatory status must be closely monitored with continuous ECG recording and an adequate oxygen supply should be available. Cardiac and blood pressure monitoring should be maintained until the patient is free of symptoms for 24 hours. Patients with altered mental status should be checked for simultaneous intake of other drugs or alcohol and should be given oxygen, naloxone, glucose, and thiamine if deemed necessary.

Norepinephrine or metaraminol should be used if vasopressor is needed. Epinephrine should not be used.

Syrup of ipecac should not be administered in symptomatic patients or those who could rapidly become obtunded, comatose or convulsing, as this could lead to aspiration pneumonitis. Gastric lavage with prior endotracheal intubation may be performed if a clinically significant ingestion has occurred. Activated charcoal may be left in the stomach but there are scant data to support its efficacy.

It is doubtful that hemodialysis or hemoperfusion would be of any value.

There is no specific antidote.

Literature data indicate that, in the presence of severe, life-threatening, intractable anticholinergic effects unresponsive to other agents, a therapeutic trial dose of physostigmine may be useful. Physostigmine should not be used just to keep the patient awake. If cyclic antidepressants have been coingested, use of physostigmine may precipitate seizures and intractable cardiac arrest. Also avoid physostigmine in patients with cardiac conduction defects.

5. PHARMACOLOGICAL PROPERTIES

5.1 Pharmacodynamic properties
Hydroxyzine is an anxiolytic compound with a rapid onset of action and a wide margin of safety. It is unrelated chemically to the phenothiazines, reserpine, meprobamate or benzodiazepines.

Its action may be due to a suppression of activity in certain key regions of the subcortical area of the CNS.

Hydroxyzine also has potent antihistaminic properties.

5.2 Pharmacokinetic properties
In man a mean maximum hydroxyzine plasma concentration of about 30 to 80 ng/ml occurs about 2 to 5 hours after single oral doses of 25 to 100 mg. The drug and its metabolites are widely distributed in the tissues. Hydroxyzine crosses the blood - brain barrier and the placental barrier. Elimination is biphasic with a terminal half-life of about 20 hours.

5.3 Preclinical safety data
There is no pre-clinical data of relevance to the subscriber additional to that noted in other sections of this SPC.

6. PHARMACEUTICAL PARTICULARS

6.1 List of excipients
Lactose monohydrate.

Microcrystalline cellulose

Magnesium stearate

Anhydrous colloidal silica

Purified water

Opadry® Y-1-7000 containing:

Titanium dioxide

Hydroxypropylmethylcellulose 2910 5cP

Macrogol 400.

6.2 Incompatibilities
None.

6.3 Shelf life
5 years.

6.4 Special precautions for storage
Keep container in the outer pack.

6.5 Nature and contents of container
Aluminium foil / PVC blister packs containing 25, 30, 50 or 60 tablets.

6.6 Instructions for use and handling
Not applicable.

7. MARKETING AUTHORISATION HOLDER
UCB Pharma Limited

UCB House

3, George Street

Watford

Herts WD18 0UH

8. MARKETING AUTHORISATION NUMBER(S)
PL / 8972 / 0001.

9. DATE OF FIRST AUTHORISATION/RENEWAL OF THE AUTHORISATION
16.08.2001

10. DATE OF REVISION OF THE TEXT
February 2002

Ultiva Injection

(GlaxoSmithKline UK)

1. NAME OF THE MEDICINAL PRODUCT
Ultiva (remifentanil hydrochloride) for Injection 1 mg

Ultiva (remifentanil hydrochloride) for Injection 2 mg

Ultiva (remifentanil hydrochloride) for Injection 5 mg

2. QUALITATIVE AND QUANTITATIVE COMPOSITION
Ultiva is a sterile, endotoxin-free, preservative-free, white to off white, lyophilized powder, to be reconstituted before use.

When reconstituted as directed, solutions of Ultiva are clear and colourless and contain 1mg/ml of remifentanil base as remifentanil hydrochloride.

Ultiva for injection is available in glass vials containing 1 mg, 2 mg or 5 mg of remifentanil base.

3. PHARMACEUTICAL FORM
Lyophilized powder for reconstitution for intravenous administration.

4. CLINICAL PARTICULARS

4.1 Therapeutic indications
Ultiva is indicated as an analgesic agent for use during induction and/or maintenance of general anaesthesia under close supervision.

Ultiva is indicated for provision of analgesia and sedation in mechanically ventilated intensive care patients 18 years of age and over.

4.2 Posology and method of administration
Ultiva should be administered only in a setting fully equipped for the monitoring and support of respiratory and cardiovascular function and by persons specifically trained in the use of anaesthetic drugs and the recognition and management of the expected adverse effects of potent opioids, including respiratory and cardiac resuscitation. Such training must include the establishment and maintenance of a patent airway and assisted ventilation.

Ultiva is for intravenous use only and must not be administered by epidural or intrathecal injection (see Section 4.3 Contra-indications).

There is a potential for the development of tolerance during administration of μ-opioid agonists.

Ultiva may be given by target controlled infusion (TCI) with an approved infusion device incorporating the Minto pharmacokinetic model with covariates for age and lean body mass (LBM) (Anesthesiology 1997;86;10-23)

Ultiva is stable for 24 hours at room temperature after reconstitution and further dilution with one of the following IV fluids listed below:

Sterilised Water for Injections

5% Dextrose Injection

5% Dextrose and 0.9% Sodium Chloride Injection

0.9% Sodium Chloride Injection0.45% Sodium Chloride Injection

For manually-controlled infusion Ultiva can be diluted to concentrations of 20 to 250 micrograms/ml (50 micrograms/ml is the recommended dilution for adults and 20 to 25 micrograms/ml for paediatric patients aged 1 year and over).

For TCI the recommended dilution of Ultiva is 20 to 50 micrograms/ml.

(See Section 6.6 Instructions for use/handling for additional information, including tables to help titrate Ultiva to the patient's anaesthetic needs).

General Anaesthesia - Adults

Administration by Manually-Controlled Infusion

The administration of Ultiva must be individualised based on the patient's response. Specific dosing guidelines for patients undergoing cardiac surgery are provided in the section headed 'Cardiac Surgery' below.

The following table summarises the starting infusion rates and dose range:

DOSING GUIDELINES FOR ADULTS

(see Table 1 on next page)

When given by bolus injection at induction Ultiva should be administered over not less than 30 seconds.

At the doses recommended above, remifentanil significantly reduces the amount of hypnotic agent required to maintain anaesthesia. Therefore, isoflurane and propofol should be administered as recommended above to avoid excessive depth of anaesthesia (see Concomitant medication below).

Induction of anaesthesia: Ultiva should be administered with an hypnotic agent, such as propofol, thiopentone, or isoflurane, for the induction of anaesthesia. Administering Ultiva after an hypnotic agent will reduce the incidence of muscle rigidity. Ultiva can be administered at an infusion rate of 0.5 to 1 microgram/kg/min, with or without an initial bolus injection of 1 microgram/kg given over not less than 30 seconds. If endotracheal intubation is to occur more than 8 to 10 minutes after the start of the infusion of Ultiva, then a bolus injection is not necessary.

Maintenance of anaesthesia in ventilated patients: After endotracheal intubation, the infusion rate of Ultiva should be decreased, according to anaesthetic technique, as indicated in the above table. Due to the fast onset and short duration of action of Ultiva, the rate of administration during anaesthesia can be titrated upward in 25% to 100% increments or downward in 25% to 50% decrements, every 2 to 5 minutes to attain the desired level of μ-opioid response. In response to light anaesthesia, supplemental bolus injections may be administered every 2 to 5 minutes.

Spontaneous ventilation anaesthesia: In spontaneous ventilation anaesthesia respiratory depression is likely to occur. Special care is needed to adjust the dose to the patient and ventilatory support may be required. The recommended starting dose is 0.04 microgram/kg/min with titration to effect. A range of infusion rates from 0.025 to 0.1 microgram/kg/min has been studied. Bolus doses are not recommended.

Concomitant medication: Ultiva decreases the amounts or doses of inhaled anaesthetics, hypnotics and benzodiazepines required for anaesthesia (see Section 4.5 Interaction with other medicaments and other forms of interaction).

Doses of the following agents used in anaesthesia: isoflurane, thiopentone, propofol and temazepam have been reduced by up to 75% when used concurrently with remifentanil.

Guidelines for discontinuation: Due to the very rapid offset of action of Ultiva no residual opioid activity will be present within 5 to 10 minutes after discontinuation. For those patients undergoing surgical procedures where post-operative pain is anticipated, analgesics should be administered prior to discontinuation of Ultiva. Sufficient

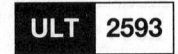

Table 1 DOSING GUIDELINES FOR ADULTS

INDICATION	BOLUS INJECTION (microgram/kg)	CONTINUOUS INFUSION (microgram/kg/min)	
		Starting Rate	Range
Induction of anaesthesia	1(give over not less than 30 seconds)	0.5 to 1	–
Maintenance of anaesthesia in ventilated patients			
• Nitrous oxide (66%)	0.5 to 1	0.4	0.1 to 2
• Isoflurane (starting dose 0.5MAC)	0.5 to 1	0.25	0.05 to 2
• Propofol (Starting dose 100 microgram/kg/min)	0.5 to 1	0.25	0.05 to 2

time must be allowed to reach the maximum effect of the longer acting analgesic. The choice of analgesic should be appropriate for the patient's surgical procedure and the level of post-operative care.

Care should be taken to avoid inadvertent administration of Ultiva remaining in IV lines and cannulae (see Section 4.4 Special warnings and precautions for use).

Guidance on provision of analgesia and sedation in mechanically ventilated intensive care patients is provided below (see Intensive Care).

Administration by Target-Controlled Infusion

Induction and maintenance of anaesthesia in ventilated patients: Ultiva TCI should be used in association with an intravenous or inhalational hypnotic agent during the induction and maintenance of anaesthesia in ventilated adult patients (see the table in *Dosing Guidelines For Adults* under *4.2 Posology and method of administration – General Anaesthesia – Adults - Administration by Manually-Controlled Infusion*). In association with these agents, adequate analgesia for induction of anaesthesia and surgery can generally be achieved with target blood remifentanil concentrations ranging from 3 to 8 nanograms/ml. Ultiva should be titrated to individual patient response. For particularly stimulating surgical procedures target blood concentrations up to 15 nanograms/ml may be required.

At the doses recommended above, remifentanil significantly reduces the amount of hypnotic agent required to maintain anaesthesia. Therefore, isoflurane and propofol should be administered as recommended above to avoid excessive depth of anaesthesia (see *Dosing Guidelines for Adults* and *Concomitant Medication* under *4.2 Posology and method of administration – General Anaesthesia – Adults - Administration by Manually-Controlled Infusion).*

For information on blood remifentanil concentrations achieved with manually-controlled infusion see Table 8.

There are insufficient data to make recommendations on the use of TCI for spontaneous ventilation anaesthesia.

Guidelines for discontinuation/continuation into the immediate post-operative period: At the end of surgery when the TCI infusion is stopped or the target concentration reduced, spontaneous respiration is likely to return at calculated remifentanil concentrations in the region of 1 to 2 nanograms/ml. As with manually-controlled infusion, post-operative analgesia should be established before the end of surgery with longer acting analgesics (see *Guidelines for discontinuation* under *4.2 Posology and method of administration – General Anaesthesia – Adults - Administration by Manually-Controlled Infusion*)

As there are insufficient data, the administration of Ultiva by TCI for the management of post-operative analgesia is not recommended.

General Anaesthesia - Paediatric patients (1 to12 years of age)

Co-administration of Ultiva with induction agents has not been studied. Ultiva TCI has not been studied in paediatric patients.

When given by bolus injection Ultiva should be administered over not less than 30 seconds. Surgery should not commence until at least 5 minutes after the start of the Ultiva infusion, if a simultaneous bolus dose has not been given. Paediatric patients should be monitored and the dose titrated to the depth of analgesia appropriate for the surgical procedure.

Induction of anaesthesia: The use of remifentanil for induction of anaesthesia in patients aged 1 to12 years is not recommended as there are no data available in this patient population.

Maintenance of anaesthesia: The following doses of Ultiva are recommended for maintenance of anaesthesia:

DOSING GUIDELINES FOR PAEDIATRIC PATIENTS (1 to12 years of age)

(see Table 2 below)

Concomitant medication: At the doses recommended above, remifentanil significantly reduces the amount of hypnotic agent required to maintain anaesthesia. Therefore, isoflurane, halothane and sevoflurane should be administered as recommended above to avoid excessive depth of anaesthesia. No data are available for dosage recommendations for simultaneous use of other hypnotics with remifentanil (see section 4.2. Posology and method of administration, General Anaesthesia – Adults, Concomitant medication).

Guidelines for patient management in the immediate post-operative period/ Establishment of alternative analgesia prior to discontinuation of Ultiva: Due to the very rapid offset of action of Ultiva, no residual activity will be present within 5 to 10 minutes after discontinuation. For those patients undergoing surgical procedures where post-operative pain is anticipated, analgesics should be administered prior to discontinuation of Ultiva. Sufficient time must be allowed to reach the therapeutic effect of the longer acting analgesic. The choice of agent(s), the dose and the time of administration should be planned in advance and individually tailored to be appropriate for the patient's surgical procedure and the level of post-operative care anticipated (see Section 4.4. Special warnings and precautions for use).

Neonates/infants (aged less than 1 year):

The pharmacokinetic profile of remifentanil in neonates/infants (aged less than 1 year) is comparable to that seen in adults after correction for body weight differences. However, there are insufficient clinical data to make dosage recommendations for this age group.

Elderly (over 65 years of age):

General anaesthesia: Caution should be exercised in the administration of Ultiva in this population. The initial starting dose of Ultiva administered to patients over 65 should be half the recommended adult dose and then titrated to individual patient need as an increased sensitivity to the pharmacodynamic effects of remifentanil has been seen in this patient population.

Because of the increased sensitivity of elderly patients to Ultiva, when administering Ultiva by TCI in this population the initial target concentration should be 1.5 to 4 nanograms/ml with subsequent titration to response.

Cardiac anaesthesia: No initial dose reduction is required (See Cardiac Surgery below).

Intensive Care: No initial dose reduction is required (see Intensive Care).

Cardiac Surgery

Administration by Manually-Controlled Infusion

DOSING GUIDELINES FOR CARDIAC ANAESTHESIA

(see Table 3)

Ultiva is not recommended for use in patients with poor left ventricular function (left ventricular ejection fraction less than 0.35), since the safe use of the product in this patient group has not been established. There are no data available on use in patients under 18 years of age undergoing cardiac surgery.

Induction period of anaesthesia: After administration of hypnotic to achieve loss of consciousness, Ultiva should be administered at an initial infusion rate of 1 microgram/kg/min. The use of bolus injections of Ultiva during induction in cardiac surgical patients is not recommended. Endotracheal intubation should not occur until at least 5 minutes after the start of the infusion.

Maintenance period of anaesthesia: After endotracheal intubation the infusion rate of Ultiva can be titrated upward in 25% to 100% increments, or downward in 25% to 50% decrements, every 2 to 5 minutes according to patient need. Supplemental bolus doses, administered over not less than 30 seconds, may also be given every 2 to 5 minutes as required. High risk cardiac patients, such as those undergoing valve surgery, should be administered a maximum bolus dose of 0.5 microgram/kg. These dosing recommendations also apply during hypothermic cardiopulmonary bypass (see Section 5.2 Pharmacokinetic properties - Cardiac anaesthesia).

Concomitant medication: At the doses recommended above, remifentanil significantly reduces the amount of hypnotic agent required to maintain anaesthesia. Therefore, isoflurane and propofol should be administered as recommended above to avoid excessive depth of anaesthesia. No data are available for dosage recommendations for simultaneous use of other hypnotics with remifentanil (see above under General Anaesthesia - Adults - Concomitant medication).

Continuation of Ultiva post-operatively to provide analgesia prior to weaning for extubation: It is recommended that the infusion of Ultiva should be maintained at the final intra-operative rate during transfer of patients to the post-operative care area. Upon arrival into this area, the patient's level of analgesia and sedation should be closely monitored and the Ultiva infusion rate adjusted to meet the individual patient's requirements (see Intensive care, below, for further information on management of intensive care patients.

Establishment of alternative analgesia prior to discontinuation of Ultiva: Due to the very rapid offset of action of Ultiva, no residual opioid activity will be present within 5 to 10 minutes after discontinuation. Prior to discontinuation of Ultiva, patients must be given alternative analgesic and sedative agents at a sufficient time in advance to allow the therapeutic effects of these agents to become established. It is therefore recommended that the choice of agent(s), the dose and the time of administration are planned, before weaning the patient from the ventilator. When other opioid agents are administered as part of the regimen for transition to alternative analgesia, the patient must be carefully monitored. The benefit of providing adequate post-operative analgesia must always be balanced against the potential risk of respiratory depression with these agents.

Guidelines for discontinuation of Ultiva: Due to the very rapid offset of action of Ultiva, hypertension, shivering and aches have been reported in cardiac patients immediately following discontinuation of Ultiva (see section 4.8 Undesirable effects). To minimise the risk of these occurring, adequate alternative analgesia must be established (as described above), before the Ultiva infusion is

Table 2 DOSING GUIDELINES FOR PAEDIATRIC PATIENTS (1 to12 years of age)

*CONCOMITANT ANAESTHETIC AGENT	BOLUS INJECTION (microgram/kg)	CONTINUOUS INFUSION (microgram/kg/min)	
		Starting Rate	Range
Halothane (starting dose 0.3MAC)	1	0.25	0.05 to 1.3
Sevoflurane (starting dose 0.3MAC)	1	0.25	0.05 to 0.9
Isoflurane (starting dose 0.5MAC)	1	0.25	0.06 to 0.9

*co-administered with nitrous oxide/oxygen in a ratio of 2:1

Table 3 DOSING GUIDELINES FOR CARDIAC ANAESTHESIA

INDICATION	BOLUS INJECTION (microgram/kg)	CONTINUOUS INFUSION (microgram/kg/min)	
		Starting Rate	Range
Induction of anaesthesia	Not recommended	1	–
Maintenance of anaesthesia in ventilated patients:			
• Isoflurane (starting dose 0.4MAC)	0.5 to 1	1	0.003 to 4
• Propofol (Starting dose 50 microgram/kg/min)	0.5 to 1	1	0.01 to 4.3
Continuation of post-operative analgesia, prior to extubation	Not recommended	1	0 to 1

discontinued. The infusion rate should be reduced by 25% decrements in at least 10-minute intervals until the infusion is discontinued. During weaning from the ventilator the Ultiva infusion should not be increased and only down titration should occur, supplemented as required with alternative analgesics. Haemodynamic changes such as hypertension and tachycardia should be treated with alternative agents as appropriate.

Administration by Target-Controlled Infusion

Induction and maintenance of anaesthesia: Ultiva TCI should be used in association with an intravenous or inhalational hypnotic agent during the induction and maintenance of anaesthesia in ventilated adult patients (see the table in *Dosing Guidelines for Cardiac Anaesthesia* under *4.2 Posology and method of administration – Cardiac Surgery - Administration by Manually-Controlled Infusion*). In association with these agents, adequate analgesia for cardiac surgery is generally achieved at the higher end of the range of target blood remifentanil concentrations used for general surgical procedures. Following titration of remifentanil to individual patient response, blood concentrations as high as 20 nanograms/ml have been used in clinical studies. At the doses recommended above, remifentanil significantly reduces the amount of hypnotic agent required to maintain anaesthesia. Therefore, isoflurane and propofol should be administered as recommended above to avoid excessive depth of anaesthesia (see table in *Dosing Guidelines for Cardiac Anaesthesia* and *Concomitant medication* paragraph under *4.2 Posology and method of administration - Cardiac Surgery -Administration by Manually-Controlled Infusion*).

For information on blood remifentanil concentrations achieved with manually-controlled infusion see Table 8.

Guidelines for discontinuation/continuation into the immediate post-operative period: At the end of surgery when the TCI infusion is stopped or the target concentration reduced, spontaneous respiration is likely to return at calculated remifentanil concentrations in the region of 1 to 2 nanograms/ml. As with manually-controlled infusion, post-operative analgesia should be established before the end of surgery with longer acting analgesics (see *Guidelines for discontinuation* under *4.2 Posology and method of administration – Cardiac Surgery - Administration by Manually-Controlled Infusion*)

As there are insufficient data, the administration of Ultiva by TCI for the management of post-operative analgesia is not recommended.

Intensive Care - Adults

Ultiva can be initially used alone for the provision of analgesia and sedation in mechanically ventilated intensive care patients.

It is recommended that Ultiva is initiated at an infusion rate of 0.1 microgram/kg/min (6 microgram/kg/h) to 0.15 microgram/kg/min (9 microgram/kg/h). The infusion rate should be titrated in increments of 0.025 microgram/kg/min (1.5 microgram/kg/h) to achieve the desired level of sedation and analgesia. A period of at least 5 minutes should be allowed between dose adjustments. The level of sedation and analgesia should be carefully monitored, regularly reassessed and the Ultiva infusion rate adjusted accordingly. If an infusion rate of 0.2 microgram/kg/min (12 microgram/kg/h) is reached and the desired level of sedation is not achieved, it is recommended that dosing with an appropriate sedative agent is initiated (see below). The dose of sedative agent should be titrated to obtain the desired level of sedation. Further increases to the Ultiva infusion rate in increments of 0.025 microgram/kg/min (1.5 microgram/kg/h) may be made if additional analgesia is required.

Ultiva has been studied in intensive care patients in well controlled clinical trials for up to three days. As patients were not studied beyond three days, no evidence of safety and efficacy for longer treatment has been established.

The following table summarises the starting infusion rates and typical dose range for provision of analgesia and sedation in individual patients:

DOSING GUIDELINES FOR USE OF ULTIVA WITHIN THE INTENSIVE CARE SETTING

CONTINUOUS INFUSION microgram/kg/min (microgram/kg/h)	
Starting Rate	Range
0.1 (6) to 0.15 (9)	0.006 (0.36) to 0.74 (44.4)

Bolus doses of Ultiva are not recommended in the intensive care setting.

The use of Ultiva will reduce the dosage requirement of any concomitant sedative agents. Typical starting doses for sedative agents, if required, are given below:

RECOMMENDED STARTING DOSE OF SEDATIVE AGENTS, IF REQUIRED

Sedative Agent	Bolus (mg/kg)	Infusion (mg/kg/h)
Propofol	Up to 0.5	0.5
Midazolam	Up to 0.03	0.03

To allow separate titration of the respective agents sedative agents should not be administered as an admixture.

Additional analgesia for ventilated patients undergoing stimulating procedures: An increase in the existing Ultiva infusion rate may be required to provide additional analgesic cover for ventilated patients undergoing stimulating and/or painful procedures such as endotracheal suctioning, wound dressing and physiotherapy. It is recommended that an Ultiva infusion rate of at least 0.1 microgram/kg/min (6 microgram/kg/h) should be maintained for at least 5 minutes prior to the start of the stimulating procedure. Further dose adjustments may be made every 2 to 5 minutes in increments of 25%-50% in anticipation of, or in response to, additional requirement for analgesia. A mean infusion rate of 0.25 microgram/kg/min (15 microgram/kg/h), maximum 0.75 microgram/kg/min (45 microgram/kg/h), has been administered for provision of additional analgesia during stimulating procedures.

Establishment of alternative analgesia prior to discontinuation of Ultiva: Due to the very rapid offset of action of Ultiva, no residual opioid activity will be present within 5 to 10 minutes after discontinuation regardless of the duration of infusion. Prior to discontinuation of Ultiva, patients must be given alternative analgesic and sedative agents at a sufficient time in advance to allow the therapeutic effects of these agents to become established. It is therefore recommended that the choice of agent(s), the dose and the time of administration are planned prior to discontinuation of Ultiva.

Guidelines for extubation and discontinuation of Ultiva: In order to ensure a smooth emergence from an Ultiva-based regimen it is recommended that the infusion rate of Ultiva is titrated in stages to 0.1 microgram/kg/min (6 microgram/kg/h) over a period up to 1 hour prior to extubation.

Following extubation, the infusion rate should be reduced by 25% decrements in at least 10-minute intervals until the infusion is discontinued. During weaning from the ventilator the Ultiva infusion should not be increased and only down titration should occur, supplemented as required with alternative analgesics.

Upon discontinuation of Ultiva, the IV cannula should be cleared or removed to prevent subsequent inadvertent administration.

When other opioid agents are administered as part of the regimen for transition to alternative analgesia, the patient must be carefully monitored. The benefit of providing adequate analgesia must always be balanced against the potential risk of respiratory depression.

Ultiva TCI has not been studied in intensive care patients

Intensive Care - Paediatric patients

The use of remifentanil in intensive care patients under the age of 18 years is not recommended as there are no data available in this patient population.

Renally-impaired intensive care patients

No adjustments to the doses recommended above are necessary in renally-impaired patients, including those undergoing renal replacement therapy (see Section 5.2 Pharmacokinetic properties).

Neurosurgery

Limited clinical experience in patients undergoing neurosurgery has shown that no special dosage recommendations are required.

ASA III/IV patients

General anaesthesia: As the haemodynamic effects of potent opioids can be expected to be more pronounced in ASA III/IV patients, caution should be exercised in the administration of Ultiva in this population. Initial dosage reduction and subsequent titration to effect is therefore recommended.

For TCI, a lower initial target of 1.5 to 4 nanograms/ml should be used in ASA III or IV patients and subsequently titrated to response.

Cardiac anaesthesia: No initial dose reduction is required.

Obese patients

For manually-controlled infusion it is recommended that for obese patients the dosage of Ultiva should be reduced and based upon ideal body weight as the clearance and volume of distribution of remifentanil are better correlated with ideal body weight than actual body weight.

With the calculation of lean body mass (LBM) used in the Minto model, LBM is likely to be underestimated in female patients with a body mass index (BMI) greater than 35 kg/m^2 and in male patients with BMI greater than 40 kg/m^2. To avoid underdosing in these patients, remifentanil TCI should be titrated carefully to individual response.

Renal impairment

On the basis of investigations carried out to date, a dose adjustment in patients with impaired renal function, including intensive care patients, is not necessary.

Hepatic impairment

No adjustment of the initial dose, relative to that used in healthy adults, is necessary as the pharmacokinetic profile of remifentanil is unchanged in this patient population. However, patients with severe hepatic impairment may be slightly more sensitive to the respiratory depressant effects of remifentanil. These patients should be closely monitored and the dose of Ultiva titrated to individual patient need.

4.3 Contraindications

As glycine is present in the formulation Ultiva is contra-indicated for epidural and intrathecal use.

Ultiva is contra-indicated in patients with known hypersensitivity to any component of the preparation and other fentanyl analogues.

Ultiva is contra-indicated for use as the sole agent for induction of anaesthesia.

4.4 Special warnings and special precautions for use

Ultiva should be administered only in a setting fully equipped for the monitoring and support of respiratory and cardiovascular function, and by persons specifically trained in the use of anaesthetic drugs and the recognition and management of the expected adverse effects of potent opioids, including respiratory and cardiac resuscitation. Such training must include the establishment and maintenance of a patent airway and assisted ventilation.

Rapid offset of action

Due to the very rapid offset of action of Ultiva, patients may emerge rapidly from anaesthesia and no residual opioid activity will be present within 5-10 minutes after the discontinuation of Ultiva. For those patients undergoing surgical procedures where post-operative pain is anticipated, analgesics should be administered prior to discontinuation of Ultiva. Sufficient time must be allowed to reach the maximum effect of the longer acting analgesic. The choice of analgesic should be appropriate for the patient's surgical procedure and the level of post-operative care. When other opioid agents are administered as part of the regimen for transition to alternative analgesia, the benefit of providing adequate post-operative analgesia must always be balanced against the potential risk of respiratory depression with these agents. Common post-operative events associated with the emergence from general anaesthesia, such as shivering, agitation, tachycardia, hypertension, may occur earlier following discontinuation of Ultiva.

Inadvertent administration

A sufficient amount of Ultiva may be present in the dead space of the IV line and/or cannula to cause respiratory depression, apnoea and/or muscle rigidity if the line is flushed with IV fluids or other drugs. This may be avoided by administering Ultiva into a fast flowing IV line or via a dedicated IV line which is removed when Ultiva is discontinued.

Muscle rigidity - prevention and management

At the doses recommended muscle rigidity may occur. As with other opioids, the incidence of muscle rigidity is related to the dose and rate of administration. Therefore, bolus injections should be administered over not less than 30 seconds.

Muscle rigidity induced by remifentanil must be treated in the context of the patient's clinical condition with appropriate supporting measures including ventilatory support. Excessive muscle rigidity occurring during the induction of anaesthesia should be treated by the administration of a neuromuscular blocking agent and/or additional hypnotic agents. Muscle rigidity seen during the use of remifentanil as an analgesic may be treated by stopping or decreasing the rate of administration of remifentanil. Resolution of muscle rigidity after discontinuing the infusion of remifentanil occurs within minutes. Alternatively an opioid antagonist may be administered, however this may reverse or attenuate the analgesic effect of remifentanil.

Respiratory depression - management

As with all potent opioids, profound analgesia is accompanied by marked respiratory depression. Therefore, remifentanil should only be used in areas where facilities for monitoring and dealing with respiratory depression are available. The appearance of respiratory depression should be managed appropriately, including decreasing the rate of infusion by 50%, or by a temporary discontinuation of the infusion. Unlike other fentanyl analogues, remifentanil has not been shown to cause recurrent respiratory depression even after prolonged administration. However, as many factors may affect post-operative recovery it is important to ensure that full consciousness and adequate spontaneous ventilation are achieved before the patient is discharged from the recovery area.

Cardiovascular effects

Hypotension and bradycardia (see Section 4.8 Undesirable Effects) may be managed by reducing the rate of infusion of Ultiva or the dose of concurrent anaesthetics or by using IV fluids, vasopressor or anticholinergic agents as appropriate.

Debilitated, hypovolaemic, and elderly patients may be more sensitive to the cardiovascular effects of remifentanil.

Drug abuse

As with other opioids remifentanil may produce dependency.

4.5 Interaction with other medicinal products and other forms of Interaction

Remifentanil is not metabolised by plasmacholinesterase, therefore, interactions with drugs metabolised by this enzyme are not anticipated.

As with other opioids remifentanil, whether given by manually-controlled infusion or TCI, decreases the amounts or doses of inhaled and IV anaesthetics, and benzodiazepines required for anaesthesia (See Section 4.2 Posology and method of administration, General Anaesthesia – Adults, Paediatric Patients, and Cardiac Surgery). If doses of concomitantly administered CNS depressant drugs are not reduced patients may experience an increased incidence of adverse effects associated with these agents.

The cardiovascular effects of Ultiva (hypotension and bradycardia), may be exacerbated in patients receiving concomitant cardiac depressant drugs, such as beta-blockers and calcium channel blocking agents.

4.6 Pregnancy and lactation

There are no adequate and well-controlled studies in pregnant women. Ultiva should be used during pregnancy only if the potential benefit justifies the potential risk to the foetus.

It is not known whether remifentanil is excreted in human milk. However, because fentanyl analogues are excreted in human milk and remifentanil-related material was found in rat milk after dosing with remifentanil, caution should be exercised when remifentanil is administered to a nursing mother.

For a summary of the reproductive toxicity study findings please refer to Section 5.3 Preclinical safety data.

Labour and delivery

The safety profile of remifentanil during labour or delivery has not been demonstrated. There are insufficient data to recommend remifentanil for use during labour and Caesarean section. Remifentanil crosses the placental barrier and fentanyl analogues can cause respiratory depression in the child.

4.7 Effects on ability to drive and use machines

If an early discharge is envisaged, following treatment using anaesthetic agents, patients should be advised not to drive or operate machinery.

4.8 Undesirable effects

The most common adverse events associated with remifentanil are direct extensions of μ-opioid agonist pharmacology. These are acute respiratory depression, bradycardia, hypotension and/or skeletal muscle rigidity. These adverse events resolve within minutes of discontinuing or decreasing the rate of remifentanil administration.

Post-operative shivering, apnoea, hypertension, hypoxia, pruritis, constipation, aches, sedation, nausea and vomiting have also been reported.

Very rarely, allergic reactions including anaphylaxis have been reported in patients receiving remifentanil in conjunction with one or more anaesthetic agents.

In common with other opioids, very rare cases of asystole, usually preceded by severe bradycardia, have been reported in patients receiving remifentanil in conjunction with other anaesthetic agents.

4.9 Overdose

As with all potent opioid analgesics, overdose would be manifested by an extension of the pharmacologically predictable actions of remifentanil. Due to the very short duration of action of Ultiva, the potential for deleterious effects due to overdose is limited to the immediate time period following drug administration. Response to discontinuation of the drug is rapid, with return to baseline within ten minutes.

In the event of overdose, or suspected overdose, take the following actions: discontinue administration of Ultiva, maintain a patent airway, initiate assisted or controlled ventilation with oxygen, and maintain adequate cardiovascular function. If depressed respiration is associated with muscle rigidity, a neuromuscular blocking agent may be required to facilitate assisted or controlled respiration. Intravenous fluids and vasopressor agents for the treatment of hypotension and other supportive measures may be employed.

Intravenous administration of an opioid antagonist such as naloxone may be given as a specific antidote in addition to ventilatory support to manage severe respiratory depression. The duration of respiratory depression following overdose with Ultiva is unlikely to exceed the duration of action of the opioid antagonist.

5. PHARMACOLOGICAL PROPERTIES

5.1 Pharmacodynamic properties

Remifentanil is a selective μ-opioid agonist with a rapid onset and very short duration of action. The μ-opioid activity, of remifentanil, is antagonised by narcotic antagonists, such as naloxone.

Assays of histamine in patients and normal volunteers have shown no elevation in histamine levels after administration of remifentanil in bolus doses up to 30 microgram/kg.

5.2 Pharmacokinetic properties

Following administration of the recommended doses of remifentanil, the effective biological half-life is 3-10 minutes. The average clearance of remifentanil in young healthy adults is 40ml/min/kg, the central volume of distribution is 100ml/kg and the steady-state volume of distribution is 350ml/kg. In children aged 1 to 12 years, remifentanil clearance and volume of distribution decreases with increasing age; the values of these parameters in neonates are approximately twice those of healthy young adults.

Table 4 Ultiva for Injection Infusion Rates (ml/kg/h)

Drug Delivery Rate	Infusion Delivery Rate (ml/kg/h) for Solution Concentrations of		
(microgram/kg/min)	25 microgram/ml 1mg/40ml	50 microgram/ml 1mg/20ml	250 microgram/ml 10mg/40ml
0.0125	0.03	0.015	Not recommended
0.025	0.06	0.03	Not recommended
0.05	0.12	0.06	0.012
0.075	0.18	0.09	0.018
0.1	0.24	0.12	0.024
0.15	0.36	0.18	0.036
0.2	0.48	0.24	0.048
0.25	0.6	0.3	0.06
0.5	1.2	0.6	0.12
0.75	1.8	0.9	0.18
1.0	2.4	1.2	0.24
1.25	3.0	1.5	0.3
1.5	3.6	1.8	0.36
1.75	4.2	2.1	0.42
2.0	4.8	2.4	0.48

Table 5 Ultiva for Injection Infusion Rates (ml/h) for a 25 microgram/ml Solution

Infusion Rate	Patient Weight (kg)									
(microgram/kg/min)	10	20	30	40	50	60	70	80	90	100
0.0125	0.3	0.6	0.9	1.2	1.5	1.8	2.1	2.4	2.7	3.0
0.025	0.6	1.2	1.8	2.4	3.0	3.6	4.2	4.8	5.4	6.0
0.05	1.2	2.4	3.6	4.8	6.0	7.2	8.4	9.6	10.8	12.0
0.075	1.8	3.6	5.4	7.2	9.0	10.8	12.6	14.4	16.2	18.0
0.1	2.4	4.8	7.2	9.6	12.0	14.4	16.8	19.2	21.6	24.0
0.15	3.6	7.2	10.8	14.4	18.0	21.6	25.2	28.8	32.4	36.0
0.2	4.8	9.6	14.4	19.2	24.0	28.8	33.6	38.4	43.2	48.0

Blood concentrations of remifentanil are proportional to the dose administered throughout the recommended dose range. For every 0.1 microgram/kg/min increase in infusion rate, the blood concentration of remifentanil will rise 2.5nanograms/ml. Remifentanil is approximately 70% bound to plasma proteins.

Metabolism

Remifentanil is an esterase metabolised opioid that is susceptible to metabolism by non-specific blood and tissue esterases. The metabolism of remifentanil results in the formation of an essentially inactive carboxylic acid metabolite (1/4600th as potent as remifentanil). The half life of the metabolite in healthy adults is 2 hours. Approximately 95% of remifentanil is recovered in the urine as the carboxylic acid metabolite. Remifentanil is not a substrate for plasma cholinesterase.

Cardiac anaesthesia

The clearance of remifentanil is reduced by approximately 20% during hypothermic (28°C) cardiopulmonary bypass. A decrease in body temperature lowers elimination clearance by 3% per degree centigrade.

Renal impairment

The rapid recovery from remifentanil-based sedation and analgesia is unaffected by renal status.

The pharmacokinetics of remifentanil are not significantly changed in patients with varying degrees of renal impairment even after administration for up to 3 days in the intensive care setting.

The clearance of the carboxylic acid metabolite is reduced in patients with renal impairment. In intensive care patients with moderate/severe renal impairment, the concentration of the carboxylic acid metabolite is expected to reach approximately 100-fold the level of remifentanil at steady-state. Clinical data demonstrate that the accumulation of the metabolite does not result in clinically relevant μ-opioid effects even after administration of remifentanil infusions for up to 3 days in these patients.

There is no evidence that remifentanil is extracted during renal replacement therapy.

The carboxylic acid metabolite is extracted during haemodialysis by 25 - 35 %.

Hepatic impairment

The pharmacokinetics of remifentanil are not changed in patients with severe hepatic impairment awaiting liver transplant, or during the anhepatic phase of liver transplant surgery. Patients with severe hepatic impairment may be slightly more sensitive to the respiratory depressant effects of remifentanil. These patients should be closely monitored and the dose of remifentanil should be titrated to the individual patient need.

Paediatric patients

The average clearance and steady state volume of distribution of remifentanil are increased in younger children and decline to young healthy adult values by age 17. The elimination half-life of remifentanil in neonates is not significantly different from that of young healthy adults. Changes in analgesic effect after changes in infusion rate of remifentanil should be rapid and similar to those seen in young healthy adults. The pharmacokinetics of the carboxylic acid metabolite in paediatric patients 2-17 years of age are similar to those seen in adults after correcting for differences in body weight.

Elderly

The clearance of remifentanil is slightly reduced (approximately 25%) in elderly patients >65 years) compared to young patients. The pharmacodynamic activity of remifentanil increases with increasing age. Elderly patients have a remifentanil EC50 for formation of delta waves on the electroencephalogram (EEG) that is 50% lower than young patients; therefore, the initial dose of remifentanil should be reduced by 50% in elderly patients and then carefully titrated to meet the individual patient need.

Table 6 Ultiva for Injection Infusion Rates (ml/h) for a 50 microgram/ml Solution

Infusion Rate	Patient Weight (kg)							
(microgram/kg/min)	30	40	50	60	70	80	90	100
0.025	0.9	1.2	1.5	1.8	2.1	2.4	2.7	3.0
0.05	1.8	2.4	3.0	3.6	4.2	4.8	5.4	6.0
0.075	2.7	3.6	4.5	5.4	6.3	7.2	8.1	9.0
0.1	3.6	4.8	6.0	7.2	8.4	9.6	10.8	12.0
0.15	5.4	7.2	9.0	10.8	12.6	14.4	16.2	18.0
0.2	7.2	9.6	12.0	14.4	16.8	19.2	21.6	24.0
0.25	9.0	12.0	15.0	18.0	21.0	24.0	27.0	30.0
0.5	18.0	24.0	30.0	36.0	42.0	48.0	54.0	60.0
0.75	27.0	36.0	45.0	54.0	63.0	72.0	81.0	90.0
1.0	36.0	48.0	60.0	72.0	84.0	96.0	108.0	120.0
1.25	45.0	60.0	75.0	90.0	105.0	120.0	135.0	150.0
1.5	54.0	72.0	90.0	108.0	126.0	144.0	162.0	180.0
1.75	63.0	84.0	105.0	126.0	147.0	168.0	189.0	210.0
2.0	72.0	96.0	120.0	144.0	168.0	192.0	216.0	240.0

Table 7 Ultiva for Injection Infusion Rates (ml/h) for a 250 microgram/ml Solution

Infusion Rate	Patient Weight (kg)							
(microgram/kg/min)	30	40	50	60	70	80	90	100
0.1	0.72	0.96	1.20	1.44	1.68	1.92	2.16	2.40
0.15	1.08	1.44	1.80	2.16	2.52	2.88	3.24	3.60
0.2	1.44	1.92	2.40	2.88	3.36	3.84	4.32	4.80
0.25	1.80	2.40	3.00	3.60	4.20	4.80	5.40	6.00
0.5	3.60	4.80	6.00	7.20	8.40	9.60	10.80	12.00
0.75	5.40	7.20	9.00	10.80	12.60	14.40	16.20	18.00
1.0	7.20	9.60	12.00	14.40	16.80	19.20	21.60	24.00
1.25	9.00	12.00	15.00	18.00	21.00	24.00	27.00	30.00
1.5	10.80	14.40	18.00	21.60	25.20	28.80	32.40	36.00
1.75	12.60	16.80	21.00	25.20	29.40	33.60	37.80	42.00
2.0	14.40	19.20	24.00	28.80	33.60	38.40	43.20	48.00

5.3 Preclinical safety data

Intrathecal administration of the glycine formulation without remifentanil to dogs caused agitation, pain and hind limb dysfunction and incoordination. These effects are believed to be secondary to the glycine excipient. Glycine is a commonly used excipient in intravenous products and this finding has no relevance for intravenous administration of Ultiva.

Reproductive toxicity studies

Remifentanil has been shown to reduce fertility in male rats when administered daily by intravenous injection for at least 70 days at a dose of 0.5mg/kg, or approximately 250 times the maximum recommended human bolus dose of 2 microgram/kg. The fertility of female rats was not affected at doses up to 1mg/kg when administered for at least 15 days prior to mating. No teratogenic effects have been observed with remifentanil at doses up to 5mg/kg in rats and 0.8mg/kg in rabbits. Administration of remifentanil to rats throughout late gestation and lactation at doses up to 5mg/kg IV had no significant effect on the survival, development, or reproductive performance of the F1 generation.

Genotoxicity

Remifentanil was devoid of genotoxic activity in bacteria and in rat liver or mouse bone marrow cells in vivo. However, a positive response was seen in vitro in different mammalian cell systems in the presence of a metabolic activation system. This activity was seen only at concentrations more than three orders of magnitude higher than therapeutic blood levels.

6. PHARMACEUTICAL PARTICULARS

6.1 List of excipients

Glycine Ph. Eur.

Hydrochloric acid Ph. Eur.

6.2 Incompatibilities

Ultiva should only be admixed with those infusion solutions recommended (See Section 6.6 Instructions for use/handling).

It should not be admixed with Lactated Ringer's Injection or Lactated Ringer's and 5% Dextrose Injection.

Ultiva should not be mixed with propofol in the same intravenous admixture solution.

Administration of Ultiva into the same intravenous line with blood/serum/plasma is not recommended. Non-specific esterases in blood products may lead to the hydrolysis of remifentanil to its inactive metabolite.

Ultiva should not be mixed with other therapeutic agents prior to administration.

6.3 Shelf life

Ultiva for Injection 1mg: 18 months

Ultiva for Injection 2mg: 2 years

Ultiva for Injection 5mg: 3 years

6.4 Special precautions for storage

Store at or below 25°C.

The reconstituted solution of Ultiva is chemically and physically stable for 24 hours at room temperature. However, Ultiva does not contain an antimicrobial preservative and thus care must be taken to assure the sterility of prepared solutions, reconstituted product should be used promptly, and any unused material discarded.

6.5 Nature and contents of container

Ultiva for Injection 1mg for intravenous use is available as 1mg of Remifentanil lyophilised powder in 3ml vials, in cartons of 5.

Ultiva for Injection 2mg for intravenous use is available as 2mg of Remifentanil lyophilised powder in 5ml vials, in cartons of 5.

Ultiva for Injection 5mg for intravenous use is available as 5mg of Remifentanil lyophilised powder in 10ml vials, in cartons of 5.

6.6 Instructions for use and handling

Ultiva is stable for 24 hours at room temperature after reconstitution and further dilution with one of the following IV fluids listed below:

Sterilised Water for Injections

5% Dextrose Injection

5% Dextrose and 0.9% Sodium Chloride Injection

0.9% Sodium Chloride Injection

0.45% Sodium Chloride Injection

For manually-controlled infusion Ultiva can be diluted to concentrations of 20 to 250 micrograms/ml (50 microgram/ml is the recommended dilution for adults and 20 to 25 micrograms/ml for paediatric patents aged 1 year and over).

For TCI the recommended dilution of Ultiva is 20 to 50 micrograms/ml.

Ultiva has been shown to be compatible with the following intravenous fluids when administered into a running IV catheter:

Lactated Ringer's Injection

Lactated Ringer's and 5% Dextrose Injection

Ultiva has been shown to be compatible with propofol when administered into a running IV catheter.

The following tables give guidelines for infusion rates of Ultiva for manually-controlled infusion:

Table 4 Ultiva for Injection Infusion Rates (ml/kg/h)

(see Table 4 on previous page)

Table 5 Ultiva for Injection Infusion Rates (ml/h) for a 25 microgram/ml Solution

(see Table 5 on previous page)

Table 6. Ultiva for Injection Infusion Rates (ml/h) for a 50 microgram/ml Solution

(see Table 6)

Table 7. Ultiva for Injection Infusion Rates (ml/h) for a 250 microgram/ml Solution

(see Table 7)

The following table provides the equivalent blood remifentanil concentration using a TCI approach for various manually-controlled infusion rates at steady state:

Table 8. Remifentanil Blood Concentrations (nanograms/ml) estimated using the Minto (1997) Pharmacokinetic Model in a 70 kg, 170 cm, 40 Year Old Male Patient for Various Manually-Controlled Infusion rates (micrograms /kg/min) at Steady State.

Ultiva Infusion Rate (micrograms /kg/min)	Remifentanil Blood Concentration (nanograms/ml)
0.05	1.3
0.10	2.6
0.25	6.3
0.40	10.4
0.50	12.6
1.0	25.2
2.0	50.5

Administrative Data

7. MARKETING AUTHORISATION HOLDER

GlaxoSmithKline UK Ltd

980 Great West Rd

Brentford

Middlesex

TW8 9GS

8. MARKETING AUTHORISATION NUMBER(S)

19494/0026 < Ultiva for Injection 1mg >

19494/0027 <Ultiva for Injection 2mg >

19494/0028 < Ultiva for Injection 5m >

9. DATE OF FIRST AUTHORISATION/RENEWAL OF THE AUTHORISATION

01 May 2004

10. DATE OF REVISION OF THE TEXT

27 May 2005

Uniflu Tablets

(Alliance Pharmaceuticals)

1. NAME OF THE MEDICINAL PRODUCT
Uniflu Tablets

2. QUALITATIVE AND QUANTITATIVE COMPOSITION
Caffeine BP 30.0 mg

Codeine Phosphate BP 10.0 mg

Diphenhydramine Hydrochloride BP 15.0 mg

Paracetamol BP 500.0 mg

Phenylephrine Hydrochloride BP 10.0 mg

3. PHARMACEUTICAL FORM
Lilac, oblong, sugar coated tablet.

4. CLINICAL PARTICULARS
4.1 Therapeutic indications
For the symptomatic relief from the discomforts associated with influenza and colds *i.e.* nasal and sinus congestion, headache, fever, aching limbs, coughing and runny nose; and for the symptomatic relief of nasal congestion in allergic conditions such as hay fever.

4.2 Posology and method of administration
Adults: One Uniflu tablet to be swallowed whole with water, followed by one tablet every six hours until the symptoms disappear.

Not more than four tablets of Uniflu to be taken in 24 hours.

Elderly: As adult dose.

Children: Under 12 years - Not recommended.

Over 12 years - One tablet every eight hours until symptoms disappear.

Not more than three tablets of Uniflu to be taken in 24 hours.

4.3 Contraindications
Hypersensitivity to paracetamol or any of the other constituents. The phenylephrine content of Uniflu tablets contra-indicates their use in hyperthyroidism and hypertension, cardiovascular and coronary disease and should not be given to patients being treated with monoamine oxidase inhibitors or within fourteen days of stopping such treatment. Uniflu tablets are contra-indicated in chronic obstructive airways disease.

4.4 Special warnings and special precautions for use
Regarding paracetamol, Uniflu should be administered with care to patients with severe renal or severe hepatic impairment. The hazard of overdose is greater in those with non-cirrhotic alcoholic liver disease. Caution is required in patients with epilepsy, prostatic hypertrophy and glaucoma.

Do not exceed the stated dose. Keep out of the reach of children.

If symptoms persist consult your doctor. Patients receiving other regular medication should be warned to consult their physician before using this product. Patients should be advised not to take other paracetamol-containing products concurrently.

4.5 Interaction with other medicinal products and other forms of Interaction
Alcohol and other central nervous system depressants can potentiate the sedative effect of Uniflu tablets. Patients are warned to avoid alcoholic drink whilst using the product. Phenylephrine may antagonise the effects of concurrent antihypertensive therapy. The speed of absorption of paracetamol may be increased by metoclopramide or domperidone and absorption reduced by cholestyramine.

Paracetamol may cause a marginal increase in blood levels of chloramphenicol.

The anticoagulant effect of warfarin and other coumarins may be enhanced by prolonged regular daily use of paracetamol with increased risk of bleeding; occasional doses have no significant effect.

4.6 Pregnancy and lactation
The safe use of Uniflu tablets in pregnancy has not been established. They should not, therefore, be used in pregnancy except under close medical supervision. Epidemiological studies in human pregnancy have shown no ill effects due to paracetamol used in the recommended dosage, but patients should follow the advice of their doctor regarding its use.

Paracetamol is excreted in breast milk but not in a clinically significant amount. Available published data do not contra-indicate breast feeding. Uniflu tablets should also be avoided in nursing mothers.

4.7 Effects on ability to drive and use machines
Drowsiness may be experienced during treatment with Uniflu tablets and patients are advised not to drive or operate machinery if affected.

4.8 Undesirable effects
Headache, dry mouth, blurred vision, gastro-intestinal disturbance, urinary retention and occasional rashes have been reported. Hypertension may occur due to phenylephrine. Adverse effects of paracetamol are rare but hypersensitivity including skin rash may occur. There have been a few reports of blood dyscrasias including thrombocytopenia and agranulocytosis but these were not necessarily causally related to paracetamol.

4.9 Overdose
Overdosage may lead to tachycardia, hypertension, nausea, vomiting, delayed onset hepatic failure due to paracetamol and respiratory depression due to codeine.

Immediate medical advice should be sought in the event of an overdose, even if you feel well, because of the risk of delayed, serious liver damage.

Treatment consists of supportive measures, gastric lavage, as well as correction of any fluid or electrolyte imbalance. Intravenous N-acetylcysteine and naloxone may be needed as antidotes in severe cases. In cases of severe hypertension, intravenous phentolamine may be required.

Symptoms of paracetamol overdosage in the first 24 hours are pallor, nausea, vomiting, anorexia and abdominal pain. Liver damage may become apparent 12 to 48 hours after ingestion. Abnormalities of glucose metabolism and metabolic acidosis may occur. In severe poisoning, hepatic failure may progress to encephalopathy, coma and death. Acute renal failure with acute tubular necrosis may develop even in the absence of severe liver damage. Cardiac arrhythmias and pancreatitis have been reported. Liver damage is possible in adults who have taken 10 g or more of paracetamol. It is considered that excess quantities of a toxic metabolite (usually adequately detoxified by glutathione when normal doses of paracetamol are ingested), become irreversibly bound to liver tissue.

Immediate treatment is essential in the management of paracetamol overdose. Despite a lack of significant early symptoms, patients should be referred to hospital urgently for immediate medical attention and any patient who has ingested around 7.5 g or more of paracetamol in the preceding 4 hours should undergo gastric lavage. Administration of oral methionine or intravenous N-acetylcysteine which may have a beneficial effect up to at least 48 hours after the overdose, may be required. General supportive measures must be available.

5. PHARMACOLOGICAL PROPERTIES
5.1 Pharmacodynamic properties
Caffeine

Caffeine, like other xanthines, stimulates the central nervous system, increases respiration, affects smooth muscle and exerts a diuretic effect. These effects are all thought to be mediated by the inhibition of phosphodiesterase resulting in a raised cyclic AMP concentration. Of the xanthines, caffeine is the most active in stimulating the central nervous system and is principally used for this purpose and has the least diuretic effect. Its action on the central nervous system is mainly on the higher centres producing a condition of wakefulness and increased mental activity. Caffeine may stimulate the respiratory centre and increase the rate and depth of respiration.

Codeine Phosphate

Codeine phosphate has analgesic, antidiarrhoeal and antitussive actions. Codeine is the antitussive agent against which all other antitussives are evaluated. It acts by depressing the central pathways of the cough reflex in the medulla. The dosage of codeine phosphate employed in Uniflu tablets is that which is necessary to produce antitussive action.

Diphenhydramine Hydrochloride

Diphenhydramine hydrochloride is an ethanolamine derivative with the properties and use of antihistamine. It is less potent than promethazine hydrochloride but has a shorter duration of action. It has sedative, anti-emetic, anticholinergic and local anaesthetic properties.

Diphenhydramine hydrochloride is a histamine H_1-receptor antagonist. It has action on the contraction of smooth muscle and the dilatation and increased permeability of the capillaries. It also has anticholinergic activity.

Paracetamol

Paracetamol has both antipyretic and analgesic activities but no useful anti-inflammatory properties. Its mechanism of analgesic effect is not yet defined. Prostaglandin synthetase from the central nervous system is sensitive to paracetamol, explaining its antipyretic effect. It does not, however, have an anti-inflammatory effect as the peripheral tissue prostaglandin synthetase is not affected.

Phenylephrine Hydrochloride

Phenylephrine hydrochloride is a sympathomimetic agent with mainly direct effects on adrenergic receptors. It has predominantly α-adrenergic activity and is without stimulator effects on the central nervous system. It is used for its bronchodilator effects and to elicit sympathetic responses (vasoconstriction) where there is congestion and inflammation of the nasal mucosa.

5.2 Pharmacokinetic properties
Caffeine

Caffeine is absorbed erratically from the gastro-intestinal tract and does not appear to accumulate in any particular tissue. It passes readily into the central nervous system and saliva.

Caffeine is almost completely metabolised and is excreted in the urine as 1-methyluric acid, 1-methylxanthine and other metabolites. Only about 1% remains unchanged.

Codeine Phosphate

Codeine phosphate is absorbed from the gastro-intestinal tract with peak plasma codeine concentrations produced in about one hour. Codeine is metabolised by O and N-demethylation in the liver to morphine and norcodeine. About 10% of an oral dose is demethylated to morphine. The plasma half life of Codeine in healthy volunteers has been found to be about 3.5 hours. Codeine and its metabolites are excreted almost entirely by the kidneys, mainly as conjugates with glucuronic acid.

Diphenhydramine Hydrochloride

Diphenhydramine hydrochloride is absorbed from the gastro-intestinal tract, metabolised by the liver and excreted mainly as metabolites in the urine. Any unchanged diphenhydramine is eliminated more rapidly than its metabolites. It has been reported to be 98% bound to plasma proteins with a normal half-life of 4 to 7 hours.

Paracetamol

Paracetamol is a weak acid which is readily absorbed from the gastro-intestinal tract with peak plasma concentration occurring about 30 minutes to 2 hours after ingestion. Following absorption it is mainly biotransformed by conjugation to the sulphate and glucuronide. Plasma-protein binding is negligible at the usual therapeutic concentrations.

The elimination of paracetamol does not appear to follow saturation kinetics. The half-life of paracetamol ranges from 2-4 hours in healthy adults. In adults, the sulphate and glucuronide account for about 90% of the urinary recovery of paracetamol, each metabolite contributing to half this amount. Less than 5% is excreted as unchanged paracetamol.

In the overdose situation (10g paracetamol or above), the defence mechanisms of the liver which lead to non-toxic glucuronide and sulphate formation are overwhelmed. Normally minor metabolic pathways therefore participate actively in the overall biotransformation of the drug and these produce hepatoxic metabolites.

Phenylephrine Hydrochloride

The bioavailability of phenylephrine is reduced due to first pass metabolism by monoamine oxidase in the gut and liver.

5.3 Preclinical safety data
There are no pre-clinical data of relevance to the prescriber which are additional to that already included in other sections of the SPC.

6. PHARMACEUTICAL PARTICULARS
6.1 List of excipients
Acacia

Acacia Powder

Protein S (Byco C) (Hydrolysed Gelatin)

Alginic Acid (E400)

Magnesium Stearate

Stearic Acid

Sodium Starch Glycollate (Type A)

Opaglos Regular

(includes Shellac, Polyvinylpyrollidone)

Refined Sugar (Sucrose)

Calcium Sulphate Dihydrate

Sodium Carboxymethylcellulose (E466)

Opalux (Lavender) AS 1117

(includes Sucrose, Erythrosine (E127), Indigo Carmine (E132),

Titanium Dioxide (E171), Sodium Benzoate (E211)

Carnauba Wax

IMS 99

Purified Water

6.2 Incompatibilities
No major incompatibilities have been reported.

6.3 Shelf life
24 months, as packaged for sale.

6.4 Special precautions for storage
Uniflu Tablets should be stored in cool, dry place not exceeding 25°C.

6.5 Nature and contents of container
The product is presented in press through blisters containing six Uniflu tablets with six Gregovite 'C' tablets. The blister pack is made from PVC/PVDC with a printed aluminium foil lidding. The foil is printed (red on gold) with the name and PL number of both products, together with the company name.

The product is available in two pack sizes:

i. 12 tablet box containing 1 blister strip

ii. 24 tablet box containing 2 blister strips

6.6 Instructions for use and handling
Not applicable.

7. MARKETING AUTHORISATION HOLDER

Alliance Pharmaceuticals Ltd

Avonbridge House

Bath Road

Chippenham

Wiltshire

SN15 2BB

United Kingdom

8. MARKETING AUTHORISATION NUMBER(S)

PL 16853/0086

9. DATE OF FIRST AUTHORISATION/RENEWAL OF THE AUTHORISATION

18th April 2005

10. DATE OF REVISION OF THE TEXT

April 2005

Uniphyllin Continus tablets

(Napp Pharmaceuticals Limited)

1. NAME OF THE MEDICINAL PRODUCT

UNIPHYLLIN® CONTINUS® tablets 200, 300 and 400 mg.

2. QUALITATIVE AND QUANTITATIVE COMPOSITION

Tablets containing 200, 300 or 400 mg of Theophylline PhEur.

For excipients, see 6.1

3. PHARMACEUTICAL FORM

Prolonged release tablets

200 mg	Capsule shaped, white tablet with a scoreline on one side and U200 on the other.
300 mg	Capsule shaped, white tablet with a scoreline on one side and U300 on the other.
400 mg	Capsule shaped, white tablet with UNIPHYLLIN on one side and the Napp logo and U400 on either side of a scoreline on the reverse.

4. CLINICAL PARTICULARS

4.1 Therapeutic indications

For the treatment and prophylaxis of bronchospasm associated with asthma, chronic obstructive pulmonary disease and chronic bronchitis. Also indicated for the treatment of left ventricular and congestive cardiac failure.

4.2 Posology and method of administration

Route of Administration

Oral

The tablets should be swallowed whole and not chewed. Patients vary in their response to xanthines and it may be necessary to titrate the dose on an individual basis.

The usual maintenance dose for adults and elderly patients is 200 mg 12 hourly. This may be titrated to either 300 mg or 400 mg dependent on the therapeutic response. Plasma theophylline concentrations should ideally be maintained between 5 and 15 mg/l. A plasma level of 5 mg/l probably represents the lower level of clinical effectiveness. Significant adverse reactions are usually seen at plasma theophylline levels greater than 20 mg/l. Patients may require monitoring of plasma theophylline levels when higher dosages are prescribed or when co-administered with medication that reduces theophylline clearance.

Children: The maintenance dose is 9 mg/kg twice daily. Some children with chronic asthma require and tolerate much higher doses (10-16 mg/kg twice daily). Lower dosages (based on usual adult dose) may be required for adolescents.

It may be appropriate to administer a larger evening or morning dose in some patients, in order to achieve optimum therapeutic effect when symptoms are most severe e.g. at the time of the 'morning dip' in lung function.

In patients whose night time or day time symptoms persist despite other therapy and who are not currently receiving theophylline, then the total daily requirement of UNIPHYLLIN CONTINUS tablets (as specified above) may be added to their treatment regimen as either a single evening or morning dose.

4.3 Contraindications

Porphyria; hypersensitivity to xanthines or any of the tablet constituents; concomitant administration with ephedrine in children.

4.4 Special warnings and special precautions for use

The patient's response to therapy should be carefully monitored – worsening of asthma symptoms requires medical attention.

Use with caution in patients with cardiac arrhythmias, peptic ulcer, hyperthyroidism, severe hypertension, hepatic dysfunction, chronic alcoholism or acute febrile illness.

The half-life of theophylline may be prolonged in the elderly and in patients with heart failure, hepatic impairment or viral infections. Toxic accumulation may occur (see Section 4.9 Overdose). A reduction of dosage may be necessary in the elderly patient.

Avoid concomitant use with other xanthine-containing products.

The hypokalaemia resulting from beta agonist therapy, steroids, diuretics and hypoxia may be potentiated by xanthines. Particular care is advised in patients suffering from severe asthma who require hospitalisation. It is recommended that serum potassium levels are monitored in such situations.

Alternative treatment is advised for patients with a history of seizure activity.

4.5 Interaction with other medicinal products and other forms of Interaction

The following increase clearance and it may therefore be necessary to increase dosage to ensure a therapeutic effect: aminoglutethimide, carbamazepine, isoprenaline, moracizine, phenytoin, rifampicin, ritonavir, sulphinpyrazone, barbiturates and hypericum perforatum. Plasma concentrations of theophylline can be reduced by concomitant use of the herbal remedy St John's Wort (hypericum perforatum). Smoking and alcohol consumption can also increase clearance of theophylline.

The following reduce clearance and a reduced dosage may therefore be necessary to avoid side-effects: allopurinol, carbimazole, cimetidine, ciprofloxacin, clarithromycin, diltiazem, disulfiram, erythromycin, fluconazole, interferon, isoniazid, methotrexate, mexiletine, nizatidine, norfloxacin, oxpentifylline, propafenone, propranolol, ofloxacin, thiabendazole, verapamil, viloxazine hydrochloride and oral contraceptives (see Section 4.9 Overdose). The concomitant use of theophylline and fluvoxamine should usually be avoided. Where this is not possible, patients should have their theophylline dose halved and plasma theophylline should be monitored closely.

Factors such as viral infections, liver disease and heart failure also reduce theophylline clearance (see Section 4.9 Overdose). There are conflicting reports concerning the potentiation of theophylline by influenza vaccine and physicians should be aware that interaction may occur. A reduction in dosage may be necessary in elderly patients. Thyroid disease or associated treatment may alter theophylline plasma levels. There is also a pharmacological interaction with adenosine, benzodiazepines, halothane, lomustine and lithium and these drugs should be used with caution.

Theophylline may decrease steady state phenytoin levels.

Co-administration with β-blockers may cause antagonism of bronchodilation; with ketamine may cause reduced convulsive threshold; with doxapram may cause increased CNS stimulation.

4.6 Pregnancy and lactation

There are no adequate data from well controlled studies of the use of theophylline in pregnant women. Theophylline has been reported to give rise to teratogenic effects in mice, rats and rabbits (See section 5.3). The potential risk for humans is unknown. Theophylline should not be administered during pregnancy unless clearly necessary. Theophylline is secreted in breast milk, and may be associated with irritability in the infant, therefore it should only be given to breast feeding women when the anticipated benefits outweigh the risk to the child.

4.7 Effects on ability to drive and use machines

No known effects.

4.8 Undesirable effects

The risk of side-effects usually associated with theophylline and xanthine derivatives such as nausea, gastric irritation, headache, CNS stimulation, tachycardia, palpitations, arrhythmias and convulsions is significantly reduced when UNIPHYLLIN CONTINUS tablet preparations are given (see Section 4.9 Overdose).

4.9 Overdose

Over 3 g could be serious in an adult (40 mg/kg in a child). The fatal dose may be as little as 4.5 g in an adult (60 mg/kg in a child), but is generally higher.

Symptoms

Warning: Serious features may develop as long as 12 hours after overdosage with prolonged release formulations.

Alimentary features: Nausea, vomiting (which is often severe), epigastric pain and haematemesis. Consider pancreatitis if abdominal pain persists.

Neurological features: Restlessness, hypertonia, exaggerated limb reflexes and convulsions. Coma may develop in very severe cases.

Cardiovascular features: Sinus tachycardia is common. Ectopic beats and supraventricular and ventricular tachycardia may follow.

Metabolic features: Hypokalaemia due to shift of potassium from plasma into cells is common, can develop rapidly and may be severe. Hyperglycaemia, hypomagnesaemia and metabolic acidosis may also occur. Rhabdomyolysis may also occur.

Management

Activated charcoal or gastric lavage should be considered if a significant overdose has been ingested within 1-2 hours. Repeated doses of activated charcoal given by mouth can enhance theophylline elimination. Measure the plasma potassium concentration urgently, repeat frequently and correct hypokalaemia. BEWARE! If large amounts of potassium have been given, serious hyperkalaemia may develop during recovery. If plasma potassium is low, then the plasma magnesium concentration should be measured as soon as possible.

In the treatment of ventricular arrhythmias, proconvulsant antiarrhythmic agents such as lignocaine (lidocaine) should be avoided because of the risk of causing or exacerbating seizures.

Measure the plasma theophylline concentration regularly when severe poisoning is suspected, until concentrations are falling. Vomiting should be treated with an antiemetic such as metoclopramide or ondansetron.

Tachycardia with an adequate cardiac output is best left untreated. Beta-blockers may be given in extreme cases but not if the patient is asthmatic. Control isolated convulsions with intravenous diazepam. Exclude hypokalaemia as a cause.

5. PHARMACOLOGICAL PROPERTIES

5.1 Pharmacodynamic properties

Theophylline is a bronchodilator. In addition it affects the function of a number of cells involved in the inflammatory processes associated with asthma and chronic obstructive airways disease. Of most importance may be enhanced suppressor, T-lymphocyte activity and reduction of eosinophil and neutrophil function. These actions may contribute to an anti-inflammatory prophylactic activity in asthma and chronic obstructive airways disease. Theophylline stimulates the myocardium and produces a diminution of venous pressure in congestive heart failure leading to marked increase in cardiac output.

5.2 Pharmacokinetic properties

Theophylline is well absorbed from UNIPHYLLIN CONTINUS tablets and at least 60% may be bound to plasma proteins. The main urinary metabolites are 1,3-dimethyl uric acid and 3-methylxanthine. About 10% is excreted unchanged.

5.3 Preclinical safety data

In studies in which mice, rats and rabbits were dosed during the period of organogenesis, theophylline produced teratogenic effects.

6. PHARMACEUTICAL PARTICULARS

6.1 List of excipients

Hydroxyethylcellulose

Povidone (K25)

Cetostearyl Alcohol

Macrogol 6000

Talc

Magnesium Stearate

6.2 Incompatibilities

Not applicable.

6.3 Shelf life

Three years.

6.4 Special precautions for storage

Do not store above 25°C.

6.5 Nature and contents of container

Blister packs consisting of aluminium foil sealed to 250 μm PVC with a PVdC coating of at least 40 gsm thickness, containing 56 tablets.

6.6 Instructions for use and handling

None.

Administrative Data

7. MARKETING AUTHORISATION HOLDER

Napp Pharmaceuticals Ltd

Cambridge Science Park

Milton Road

Cambridge CB4 0GW

8. MARKETING AUTHORISATION NUMBER(S)

PL 16950/0066-0068

9. DATE OF FIRST AUTHORISATION/RENEWAL OF THE AUTHORISATION

200 mg - 23 August 1979/15 May 2003

300 mg – 22 February 1988/15 May 2003

400 mg – 29 October 1982/15 May 2003

10. DATE OF REVISION OF THE TEXT

July 2004

11. Legal Category

P

®UNIPHYLLIN, CONTINUS and the Napp Device are Registered Trade Marks.

Uniroid-HC Ointment

(Chemidex Pharma Ltd.)

1. NAME OF THE MEDICINAL PRODUCT

Uniroid-HC™ Ointment

2. QUALITATIVE AND QUANTITATIVE COMPOSITION

Each gram of ointment contains:

Hydrocortisone Ph.Eur. 5.0mg

Cinchocaine Hydrochloride B.P. 5.0mg

3. PHARMACEUTICAL FORM

An off-white, odourless, smooth, translucent ointment.

4. CLINICAL PARTICULARS

4.1 Therapeutic indications

Uniroid-HC Ointment is indicated primarily for the treatment of external haemorrhoids for the short term relief of pain, irritation and associated pruritus ani. Uniroid-HC Ointment can also be used for internal haemorrhoids.

4.2 Posology and method of administration

Adults

Treatment with Uniroid-HC Ointment should be limited to seven days. Patients should be advised to return to their doctor if the condition persists beyond this time.

Directions for use and dosage schedule:

First wash the anal area gently with water and pat dry with cotton wool. With the finger, spread a small quantity of the ointment on the painful area without rubbing. Do not use toilet paper.

Apply the ointment twice a day (morning and evening) and after each bowel movement, or as prescribed by the doctor.

The ointment can be used internally by means of the nozzle applicator which is supplied. Insert the nozzle applicator to full extent and squeeze the tube gently from the lower end whilst withdrawing.

The nozzle applicator must be cleaned thoroughly in warm, soapy water before and after each use.

The ointment may be used separately or concurrently with the suppositories.

The Elderly

Dosage modifications are not required in the elderly.

Children

Uniroid-HC Ointment is not recommended for use in children under 12 years of age unless directed by a doctor.

4.3 Contraindications

Known hypersensitivity to any of the constituents and to local anaesthetics. This product is contra-indicated in tuberculosis, anal thrush and most viral lesions of the skin including herpes simplex, vaccinia and varicella.

4.4 Special warnings and special precautions for use

Since the use of occlusive dressings may increase the risk of sensitivity, such dressings should be avoided. Uniroid-HC Ointment is not recommended for use in children unless recommended by a doctor.

4.5 Interaction with other medicinal products and other forms of Interaction

No interactions have been reported.

4.6 Pregnancy and lactation

There is inadequate evidence of safety in human pregnancy. Topical administration of corticosteroids to pregnant animals can cause abnormalities of foetal development including cleft palate and intra-uterine growth retardation. There may, therefore, be a very small risk of such effects in the human foetus. Uniroid-HC Ointment can be used post-partum, provided the mother is not breast-feeding.

4.7 Effects on ability to drive and use machines

Not applicable.

4.8 Undesirable effects

Recurrent or prolonged application may increase the risk of contact sensitisation particularly to cinchocaine. The possibility of systemic absorption should be borne in mind when prescribing preparations containing corticosteroids which can cause adrenal suppression in large doses.

4.9 Overdose

Not applicable to a product with this route of administration.

5. PHARMACOLOGICAL PROPERTIES

5.1 Pharmacodynamic properties

Hydrocortisone

The principle pharmacological actions of hydrocortisone are on gluconeogensis, glycogen deposition, protein and calcium metabolism and inhibition of corticotrophin secretion and anti-inflammatory activity (glucocorticoid actions). When applied topically hydrocortisone causes reduction of inflammation, pruritus and exudation in disorders of the skin and perianal region.

Cinchocaine hydrochloride

Cinchocaine hydrochloride is a local anaesthetic agent and is suitable for surface or spinal anaesthesia and for relaxing sphincteric spasms. It is an anaesthetic of the amide type. It is more toxic than cocaine by local application but its local anaesthetic action is greater so it can be used in lower concentrations. Its action is more prolonged than lignocaine.

Surface or topical anaesthetics such as cinchocaine block the sensory nerve endings in the skin preventing transmissions of impulses along the nerve fibres and inhibiting depolarisation and ion-exchange. These effects are reversible. Before this blocking action can occur the lipid soluble anaesthetic base must penetrate the lipoprotein nerve sheath and the effectiveness of the anaesthetic depends on the concentration attained in the nerve fibre. The onset of action varies depending on the anaesthetic used. Cinchocaine has a rapid onset of action and is also long lasting.

5.2 Pharmacokinetic properties

Hydrocortisone

Hydrocortisone is passed through the skin, particularly in denuded areas. About 90% of plasma hydrocortisone is bound to plasma proteins, mainly to globulin, less so to albumin. In the liver and most body tissues it is metabolised to hydrogenated and degraded forms such as tetrahydrocortisone and tetrahydrocortisol. These degraded forms are excreted in the urine. They are mainly conjugated as glucuronides. A very small proportion of unchanged hydrocortisone is excreted in the urine.

Cinchocaine hydrochloride

Most local anaesthetics such as cinchocaine hydrochloride are absorbed through damaged skin. Cinchocaine hydrochloride is an ester-type local anaesthetic. Following absorption it is hydrolysed by esterases in the plasma and liver.

5.3 Preclinical safety data

There are no pre-clinical data of relevance to the prescriber which are additional to that already included in other sections of the SPC.

6. PHARMACEUTICAL PARTICULARS

6.1 List of excipients

Cetostearyl alcohol BP, white soft paraffin BP

6.2 Incompatibilities

None reported

6.3 Shelf life

36 months, as packaged for sale.

6.4 Special precautions for storage

Uniroid-HC Ointment should be stored in a cool, dry place at a temperature not exceeding 25°C (77°F).

6.5 Nature and contents of container

Externally white enamelled and printed; internally lacquered aluminium tube with medium density polyethylene nozzle applicator and white plug seal cap.

The product is available in tubes of 30g and 15g.

6.6 Instructions for use and handling

Not applicable.

Administrative Data

7. MARKETING AUTHORISATION HOLDER

Chemidex Pharma Limited,

Chemidex House,

Egham Business Village,

Crabtree Road,

Egham,

Surrey TW20 8RB.

United Kingdom.

8. MARKETING AUTHORISATION NUMBER(S)

PL 17736 / 0001

9. DATE OF FIRST AUTHORISATION/RENEWAL OF THE AUTHORISATION

3 November 2000 / 25 April 2003

10. DATE OF REVISION OF THE TEXT

April 2003

Uniroid-HC Suppositories

(Chemidex Pharma Ltd.)

1. NAME OF THE MEDICINAL PRODUCT

Uniroid-HC® Suppositories

2. QUALITATIVE AND QUANTITATIVE COMPOSITION

Each suppository contains:

Hydrocortisone Ph. Eur. 5.0 mg

Cinchocaine Hydrochloride B.P. 5.0 mg

3. PHARMACEUTICAL FORM

An off-white, odourless, smooth, suppository.

4. CLINICAL PARTICULARS

4.1 Therapeutic indications

Uniroid-HC Suppositories are indicated for use in the treatment of internal haemorrhoids for the short term relief of pain, irritation and associated pruritus ani.

4.2 Posology and method of administration

Adults

Treatment with Uniroid-HC Suppositories should be limited to seven days. Patients should be advised to return to their doctor if the condition persists beyond this time.

Directions for use and dosage schedule:

Remove the plastic protective shell and insert a suppository as far as possible into the anus.

One suppository to be inserted twice a day (morning and evening) and after each bowel movement, or as prescribed by the doctor.

The suppositories may be used separately or concurrently with the ointment.

The Elderly

Dosage modifications are not required in the elderly.

Children

Uniroid-HC Suppositories are not recommended for use in children under 12 years of age unless directed by a doctor.

4.3 Contraindications

Known hypersensitivity to any of the constituents and to local anaesthetics. This product is contra-indicated in tuberculosis, anal thrush and most viral lesions of the skin including herpes simplex, vaccinia and varicella.

4.4 Special warnings and special precautions for use

Uniroid-HC Suppositories are not recommended for use in children unless recommended by a doctor.

4.5 Interaction with other medicinal products and other forms of Interaction

No interactions have been reported.

4.6 Pregnancy and lactation

There is inadequate evidence of safety in human pregnancy. Topical administration of corticosteroids to pregnant animals can cause abnormalities of foetal development including cleft palate and intra-uterine growth retardation. There may, therefore, be a very small risk of such effects in the human foetus. Uniroid-HC Suppositories can be used post-partum, provided the mother is not breast-feeding.

4.7 Effects on ability to drive and use machines

Not applicable.

4.8 Undesirable effects

Recurrent or prolonged application may increase the risk of contact sensitisation particularly to cinchocaine. The possibility of systemic absorption should be borne in mind when prescribing preparations containing corticosteroids which can cause adrenal suppression in large doses.

4.9 Overdose

Not applicable to a product with this route of administration.

5. PHARMACOLOGICAL PROPERTIES

5.1 Pharmacodynamic properties

Hydrocortisone

The principle pharmacological actions of hydrocortisone are on gluconeogensis, glycogen deposition, protein and calcium metabolism and inhibition of corticotrophin secretion and anti-inflammatory activity (glucocorticoid actions). When applied topically hydrocortisone causes reduction of inflammation, pruritus and exudation in disorders of the skin and perianal region.

Cinchocaine hydrochloride

Cinchocaine hydrochloride is a local anaesthetic agent and is suitable for surface or spinal anaesthesia and for relaxing sphincteric spasms. It is an anaesthetic of the amide type. It is more toxic than cocaine by local application but its local anaesthetic action is greater so it can be used in lower concentrations. Its action is more prolonged than lignocaine.

Surface or topical anaesthetics such as cinchocaine block the sensory nerve endings in the skin preventing transmissions of impulses along the nerve fibres and inhibiting depolarisation and ion- exchange. These effects are reversible. Before this blocking action can occur the lipid soluble anaesthetic base must penetrate the lipoprotein nerve sheath and the effectiveness of the anaesthetic depends on the concentration attained in the nerve fibre. The onset of action varies depending on the anaesthetic used. Cinchocaine has a rapid onset of action and is also long lasting.

5.2 Pharmacokinetic properties

Hydrocortisone

Hydrocortisone is passed through the skin, particularly in denuded areas. About 90% of plasma hydrocortisone is bound to plasma proteins, mainly to globulin, less so to albumin. In the liver and most body tissues it is metabolised to hydrogenated and degraded forms such as tetrahydrocortisone and tetrahydrocortisol. These degraded forms are excreted in the urine. They are mainly conjugated as glucuronides. A very small proportion of unchanged hydrocortisone is excreted in the urine.

Cinchocaine hydrochloride

Most local anaesthetics such as cinchocaine hydrochloride are absorbed through damaged skin. Cinchocaine hydrochloride is an ester-type local anaesthetic. Following absorption it is hydrolysed by esterases in the plasma and liver.

5.3 Preclinical safety data

There are no pre-clinical data of relevance to the prescriber which are additional to that already included in other sections of the SPC.

6. PHARMACEUTICAL PARTICULARS

6.1 List of excipients

Adeps Solidus (Witepsol H15) Ph. Eur.

6.2 Incompatibilities

None reported.

6.3 Shelf life

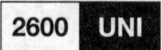

36 months, as packaged for sale.

6.4 Special precautions for storage

Uniroid-HC Suppositories should be stored in a cool, dry place at a temperature not exceeding 25°C (77°F).

6.5 Nature and contents of container

Printed PVC laminate; white thermoplastic film of laminated polyvinyl chloride 95 microns thick and polythene 27-30 microns thick.

The product is available in packs of 12. It may also be marketed in packs of 10.

6.6 Instructions for use and handling

Not applicable.

7. MARKETING AUTHORISATION HOLDER

Chemidex Pharma Limited
Chemidex House
Egham Business Village
Crabtree Road
Egham
Surrey TW20 8RB
United Kingdom

8. MARKETING AUTHORISATION NUMBER(S)

PL 17736/0002

9. DATE OF FIRST AUTHORISATION/RENEWAL OF THE AUTHORISATION

3 November 2000

10. DATE OF REVISION OF THE TEXT

February 2001

Univer Capsules

(Zeneus Pharma Ltd)

1. NAME OF THE MEDICINAL PRODUCT

Univer Capsules

2. QUALITATIVE AND QUANTITATIVE COMPOSITION

Verapamil hydrochloride 120mg, 180mg and 240mg.

For excipients, see 6.1.

3. PHARMACEUTICAL FORM

Prolonged-release capsule, hard.

Capsules are blue and yellow and printed with V120, V180 or V240.

4. CLINICAL PARTICULARS

4.1 Therapeutic indications

Mild to moderate hypertension. Angina pectoris.

4.2 Posology and method of administration

For oral administration only. The capsules should be swallowed whole and not chewed.

The bioequivalence of Univer to other prolonged release verapamil formulations may not have been evaluated. As such, this product should not be directly substituted for other non-identical formulations of verapamil and vice-versa.

Adults: Mild to moderate hypertension: Initial dose in adult patients new to verapamil therapy should be 120 mg once daily. This can be increased to 240 mg once daily which is the normal maintenance dosage. The dose may be further increased to a maximum of 480 mg once daily if required.

Angina: The usual adult dose is 360 mg once daily. Dosage may be increased to a maximum of 480 mg daily if required.

Elderly: Elderly patients show enhanced bioavailability of verapamil and therapeutic control may be achieved with lower doses in this patient population.

Children: Not recommended in children and adolescents under the age of 18 years.

Hepatic impairment: Verapamil is extensively metabolised in the liver and for those patients with impaired liver function, the dose should be reduced and carefully titrated.

Renal impairment: About 70% of an administered dose of verapamil is excreted as metabolites in the urine. Verapamil should be prescribed cautiously when renal function is impaired. Careful patient monitoring is recommended.

4.3 Contraindications

Acute myocardial infarction with complications such as bradycardia, hypotension, left ventricular decompensation or congestive heart failure.

Second or third degree atrioventricular block without pacemaker.

Sick sinus syndrome, sino-atrial block, or severe sinus bradycardia (except in patients with functioning artificial ventricular pacemaker).

Uncompensated cardiac failure.

Atrial flutter or atrial fibrillation associated with an accessory pathway (e.g. Wolff-Parkinson-White, Lown-Ganong-Levine syndrome).

Porphyria.

Hypotension (systolic pressure <90 mm Hg) or cardiogenic shock.

Intravenous dantrolene (see section 4.5).

Known hypersensitivity to any of the ingredients.

Concomitant ingestion of grapefruit juice.

4.4 Special warnings and special precautions for use

Special care should be taken in hypotension (see section 4.3), especially in acute myocardial infarction as this is a condition where atrioventricular conduction defects may develop and contractility may be impaired.

Use with caution in patients with first degree atrioventricular block.

Left ventricular contractility may be affected and although the effect is small, cardiac failure may be precipitated or aggravated. Hence incipient cardiac failure should be controlled using appropriate therapy before verapamil is given.

Verapamil is extensively metabolised in the liver and special care should be taken in cases where liver damage exists, as plasma levels of verapamil may be increased (see section 4.2).

4.5 Interaction with other medicinal products and other forms of Interaction

Dantrolene: the association of this muscle relaxant given intravenously and verapamil is potentially dangerous (can cause fatal ventricular fibrillation in animals) and is contraindicated.

The combination of verapamil and beta-blockers, antiarrhythmic agents or inhaled anaesthetics may lead to additive cardiovascular effects (e.g. AV block, bradycardia, hypotension, heart failure). A period between stopping beta-blocking therapy and starting therapy with this product may be advisable. Concomitant use of verapamil and beta-blockers or antiarrhythmics, if necessary, should only be administered to patients in a closely monitored clinical setting. Intravenous beta-blockers should not be given to patients under treatment with verapamil. The effects of verapamil may be additive to other hypotensive agents.

Caution is required when verapamil is given with digoxin, theophylline, midazolam, ciclosporin and carbamazepine as plasma levels of these drugs may rise. With rifampicin, phenytoin and phenobarbital, plasma levels of verapamil may be reduced, whilst with alcohol and cimetidine, plasma verapamil levels may be increased.

Lithium toxicity may be enhanced.

Lithium can enhance neuromuscular block during anaesthesia and hence verapamil with lithium may potentiate the neuromuscular blocking effect.

Grapefruit juice – an increase in verapamil serum level has been reported.

4.6 Pregnancy and lactation

Animal studies have shown no teratogenic effects and data on a limited number of exposed pregnancies showed no adverse effects on the health of the foetus or newborn child.

Caution should be exercised, however, when prescribing to pregnant women and verapamil should be avoided in the first trimester unless the benefits clearly outweigh the risks.

Verapamil is excreted in breast milk and rare hypersensitivity reactions have been reported. Verapamil should only be used during lactation if, in the clinicians judgement, it is essential for the welfare of the patient.

4.7 Effects on ability to drive and use machines

It is possible that a patient's ability to drive a vehicle or operate machinery may be impaired, particularly when starting treatment.

4.8 Undesirable effects

Occasionally, particularly in high doses or with prior myocardial damage, cardiovascular effects may be larger than desired giving rise to bradycardic arrhythmias, such as sinus bradycardia, second and third degree atrioventricular block, bradyarrhythmia in atrial fibrillation, transient asystole, hypotension, heart failure.

Constipation may occur. Headaches, dizziness, fatigue and ankle oedema are uncommon. Very infrequently nausea, vomiting, flushing and allergic reactions have been observed. Reversible impairment of liver function has been rarely reported and is most likely a hypersensitivity reaction.

There have been rare reports of gynaecomastia, gingival hyperplasia, erythromelalgia, paraesthesia and elevated prolactin levels.

4.9 Overdose

Normal resuscitation procedures should be initiated in the event of cardiovascular collapse, i.e. if atrioventricular conduction defects such as second or third degree block develop these should be treated in the usual way using atropine, isoprenaline or the temporary insertion of a pacemaker, as required. Hypotension may be observed and, if persistent, and in the absence of a conduction defect, treatment with systemic dopaminergic agents, e.g. dopamine, dobutamine or noradrenaline should be started. Specific antidote may be given, e.g. slow intravenous injection, or an infusion, of 10-20 ml calcium gluconate 10% solution. Overdose with modified-release preparations may result in prolonged toxicity of delayed onset.

5. PHARMACOLOGICAL PROPERTIES

5.1 Pharmacodynamic properties

Verapamil is a phenylalkylamine calcium antagonist with effects upon arterial smooth muscle, myocardial cells and cells of the cardiac conduction system. It lowers heart rate, increases myocardial perfusion and reduces coronary spasm. It decreases vascular peripheral resistance and lowers blood pressure by vasodilation without reflex tachycardia. The effects are more pronounced on high blood pressure than on normal pressure because of its use-dependent action on the voltage-operated calcium channel.

5.2 Pharmacokinetic properties

Approximately 90% of verapamil is absorbed following oral administration and is subject to extensive first pass metabolism in the liver. There is considerable interindividual variation in plasma concentrations. About 70% of the oral dose is excreted by the kidneys and 16% with the faeces.

Where liver damage exists plasma levels of verapamil may be increased. Renal failure does not significantly alter the kinetics of the drug. Elderly subjects show enhanced bioavailability of verapamil.

Univer provides prolonged release of verapamil in the gastrointestinal tract and a pharmacokinetic profile consistent with a prolonged release formulation. A study in healthy volunteers compared the pharmacokinetics of Univer 240 mg administered once daily and immediate-release verapamil 80 mg administered three times daily. The comparative steady state kinetic data are shown below:

Steady State	Univer, dose 240 mg	Verapamil immediate release, dose 80 mg
C_{max} (ng/ml)	117.60	172.23
T_{max} (hr)	7.68	1.16
AUC_{0-8hr} (ng × hr/ml)	—	694.15
AUC_{0-24hr} (ng × hr/ml)	1572.98	—
Half-life (hr)	9.01	6.38
Elimination Rate (hr^{-1})	0.08	0.12

5.3 Preclinical safety data

There is no evidence of teratogenicity or carcinogenicity with verapamil. There are no additional preclinical safety data of relevance to the prescriber.

6. PHARMACEUTICAL PARTICULARS

6.1 List of excipients

Capsule contents:

Fumaric acid
Sugar spheres (containing sucrose and maize starch)
Talc
Povidone
Shellac

Capsule shell:

Gelatin
Titanium dioxide (E171)
Erythrosine (E127)
Indigotine (E132)
Yellow iron oxide (E172)

Printing ink:

Titanium dioxide (E171)
Black iron oxide (E172)
Shellac
Soya lecithin
Antifoam DC 1510

6.2 Incompatibilities

None stated

6.3 Shelf life

2 years

6.4 Special precautions for storage

Do not store above 25°C. Store in the original package.

6.5 Nature and contents of container

PVC/aluminium blister packs of 4, 8, 28 or 56 capsules.

Containers of 100 or 500.

6.6 Instructions for use and handling

None

7. MARKETING AUTHORISATION HOLDER

Elan Pharma Ltd
Monksland
Athlone
Co Westmeath
Ireland

Trading as:
Elan Pharma
Abel Smith House
Gunnels Wood Road
Stevenage
Hertfordshire
SG1 2FG
UK

8. MARKETING AUTHORISATION NUMBER(S)
Univer Capsules 120 mg: PL 10038/0033
Univer Capsules 180 mg: PL 10038/0034
Univer Capsules 240 mg: PL 10038/0035

9. DATE OF FIRST AUTHORISATION/RENEWAL OF THE AUTHORISATION
14 May 2001

10. DATE OF REVISION OF THE TEXT
August 2003

Legal Category

POM

Univer Capsules 120mg

(Zeneus Pharma Ltd)

1. NAME OF THE MEDICINAL PRODUCT
Univer 120 mg Capsules

2. QUALITATIVE AND QUANTITATIVE COMPOSITION
Verapamil hydrochloride 120 mg.

For excipients, see 6.1.

3. PHARMACEUTICAL FORM
Prolonged-release capsule, hard.

Capsules are blue and yellow and printed with V120.

4. CLINICAL PARTICULARS
4.1 Therapeutic indications
Mild to moderate hypertension. Angina pectoris.

4.2 Posology and method of administration
For oral administration only. The capsules should be swallowed whole and not chewed.

The bioequivalence of Univer to other prolonged release verapamil formulations may not have been evaluated. As such, this product should not be directly substituted for other non-identical formulations of verapamil and vice-versa.

Adults: Mild to moderate hypertension: Initial dose in adult patients new to verapamil therapy should be 120 mg once daily. This can be increased to 240 mg once daily which is the normal maintenance dosage. The dose may be further increased to a maximum of 480 mg once daily if required.

Angina: The usual adult dose is 360 mg once daily. Dosage may be increased to a maximum of 480 mg daily if required.

Elderly: Elderly patients show enhanced bioavailability of verapamil and therapeutic control may be achieved with lower doses in this patient population.

Children: Not recommended in children and adolescents under the age of 18 years.
Hepatic impairment: Verapamil is extensively metabolised in the liver and for those patients with impaired liver function, the dose should be reduced and carefully titrated.

Renal impairment: About 70% of an administered dose of verapamil is excreted as metabolites in the urine. Verapamil should be prescribed cautiously when renal function is impaired. Careful patient monitoring is recommended.

4.3 Contraindications
• Acute myocardial infarction with complications such as bradycardia, hypotension, left ventricular decompensation or congestive heart failure.

• Second or third degree atrioventricular block without pacemaker.

• Sick sinus syndrome, sino-atrial block, or severe sinus bradycardia (except in patients with functioning artificial ventricular pacemaker).

• Uncompensated cardiac failure.

• Atrial flutter or atrial fibrillation associated with an accessory pathway (e.g. Wolff-Parkinson-White, Lown-Ganong-Levine syndrome).

• Porphyria.

• Hypotension (systolic pressure <90 mm Hg) or cardiogenic shock.

• Intravenous dantrolene (see section 4.5).

• Known hypersensitivity to any of the ingredients.

• Concomitant ingestion of grapefruit juice.

4.4 Special warnings and special precautions for use
Special care should be taken in hypotension (see section 4.3), especially in acute myocardial infarction as this is a condition where atrioventricular conduction defects may develop and contractility may be impaired.

Use with caution in patients with first degree atrioventricular block.

Left ventricular contractility may be affected and although the effect is small, cardiac failure may be precipitated or aggravated. Hence incipient cardiac failure should be controlled using appropriate therapy before verapamil is given.

Verapamil is extensively metabolised in the liver and special care should be taken in cases where liver damage exists, as plasma levels of verapamil may be increased (see section 4.2).

4.5 Interaction with other medicinal products and other forms of Interaction
Dantrolene: the association of this muscle relaxant given intravenously and verapamil is potentially dangerous (can cause fatal ventricular fibrillation in animals) and is contra-indicated.

The combination of verapamil and beta-blockers, antiarrhythmic agents or inhaled anaesthetics may lead to additive cardiovascular effects (e.g. AV block, bradycardia, hypotension, heart failure). A period between stopping beta-blocking therapy and starting therapy with this product may be advisable. Concomitant use of verapamil and beta-blockers or antiarrhythmics, if necessary, should only be administered to patients in a closely monitored clinical setting. Intravenous beta-blockers should not be given to patients under treatment with verapamil. The effects of verapamil may be additive to other hypotensive agents.

Caution is required when verapamil is given with digoxin, theophylline, midazolam, ciclosporin and carbamazepine as plasma levels of these drugs may rise. With rifampicin, phenytoin and phenobarbital, plasma levels of verapamil may be reduced, whilst with alcohol and cimetidine, plasma verapamil levels may be increased.

Lithium toxicity may be enhanced.

Lithium can enhance neuromuscular block during anaesthesia and hence verapamil with lithium may potentiate the neuromuscular blocking effect.

Grapefruit juice – an increase in verapamil serum level has been reported.

4.6 Pregnancy and lactation
Animal studies have shown no teratogenic effects and data on a limited number of exposed pregnancies showed no adverse effects on the health of the foetus or newborn child.

Caution should be exercised, however, when prescribing to pregnant women and verapamil should be avoided in the first trimester unless the benefits clearly outweigh the risks.

Verapamil is excreted in breast milk and rare hypersensitivity reactions have been reported. Verapamil should only be used during lactation if, in the clinicians judgement, it is essential for the welfare of the patient.

4.7 Effects on ability to drive and use machines
It is possible that a patient's ability to drive a vehicle or operate machinery may be impaired, particularly when starting treatment.

4.8 Undesirable effects
Occasionally, particularly in high doses or with prior myocardial damage, cardiovascular effects may be larger than desired giving rise to bradycardic arrhythmias, such as sinus bradycardia, second and third degree atrioventricular block, bradyarrhythmia in atrial fibrillation, transient asystole, hypotension, heart failure.

Constipation may occur. Headaches, dizziness, fatigue and ankle oedema are uncommon. Very infrequently nausea, vomiting, flushing and allergic reactions have been observed. Reversible impairment of liver function has been rarely reported and is most likely a hypersensitivity reaction.

There have been rare reports of gynaecomastia, gingival hyperplasia, erythromelalgia, paraesthesia and elevated prolactin levels.

4.9 Overdose
Normal resuscitation procedures should be initiated in the event of cardiovascular collapse, i.e. if atrioventricular conduction defects such as second or third degree block develop these should be treated in the usual way using atropine, isoprenaline or the temporary insertion of a pacemaker, as required. Hypotension may be observed and, if persistent, and in the absence of a conduction defect, treatment with systemic dopaminergic agents, e.g. dopamine, dobutamine or noradrenaline should be started. Specific antidote may be given, e.g. slow intravenous injection, or an infusion, of 10-20 ml calcium gluconate 10% solution. Overdose with modified-release preparations may result in prolonged toxicity of delayed onset.

5. PHARMACOLOGICAL PROPERTIES
5.1 Pharmacodynamic properties
Verapamil is a phenylalkylamine calcium antagonist with effects upon arterial smooth muscle, myocardial cells and cells of the cardiac conduction system. It lowers heart rate, increases myocardial perfusion and reduces coronary spasm. It decreases vascular peripheral resistance and lowers blood pressure by vasodilation without reflex tachycardia. The effects are more pronounced on high blood pressure than on normal pressure because of its use-dependent action on the voltage-operated calcium channel.

5.2 Pharmacokinetic properties
Approximately 90% of verapamil is absorbed following oral administration and is subject to extensive first pass metabolism in the liver. There is considerable interindividual variation in plasma concentrations. About 70% of the oral dose is excreted by the kidneys and 16% with the faeces.

Where liver damage exists plasma levels of verapamil may be increased. Renal failure does not significantly alter the kinetics of the drug. Elderly subjects show enhanced bioavailability of verapamil.

Univer provides prolonged release of verapamil in the gastrointestinal tract and a pharmacokinetic profile consistent with a prolonged release formulation. A study in healthy volunteers compared the pharmacokinetics of Univer 240 mg administered once daily and immediate-release verapamil 80 mg administered three times daily. The comparative steady state kinetic data are shown below:

Steady State	Univer, dose 240 mg	Verapamil immediate release, dose 80 mg
C_{max} (ng/ml)	117.60	172.23
T_{max} (hr)	7.68	1.16
AUC_{0-8hr} (ng × hr/ml)	—	694.15
AUC_{0-24hr} (ng × hr/ml)	1572.98	—
Half-life (hr)	9.01	6.38
Elimination Rate (hr^{-1})	0.08	0.12

5.3 Preclinical safety data
There is no evidence of teratogenicity or carcinogenicity with verapamil. There are no additional preclinical safety data of relevance to the prescriber.

6. PHARMACEUTICAL PARTICULARS
6.1 List of excipients
Capsule contents:
Fumaric acid
Sugar spheres (containing sucrose and maize starch)
Talc
Povidone
Shellac
Capsule shell:
Gelatin
Titanium dioxide (E171)
Erythrosine (E127)
Indigotine (E132)
Yellow iron oxide (E172)
Printing ink:
Titanium dioxide (E171)
Black iron oxide (E172)
Shellac
Soya lecithin
Antifoam DC 1510

6.2 Incompatibilities
None stated.

6.3 Shelf life
2 years.

6.4 Special precautions for storage
Do not store above 25°C. Store in the original package.

6.5 Nature and contents of container
PVC/aluminium blister packs of 4, 8, 28 or 56 capsules.

Containers of 100 or 500.

6.6 Instructions for use and handling
None

7. MARKETING AUTHORISATION HOLDER
Elan Pharma Ltd
Monksland
Athlone
Co. Westmeath
Ireland
Trading as:
Elan Pharma
Abel Smith House
Gunnels Wood Road
Stevenage
Hertfordshire
SG1 2FG

8. MARKETING AUTHORISATION NUMBER(S)
PL 10038/0033

9. DATE OF FIRST AUTHORISATION/RENEWAL OF THE AUTHORISATION
14 May 2001

10. DATE OF REVISION OF THE TEXT
August 2003

11. LEGAL CATEGORY
POM

Univer Capsules 180mg

(Zeneus Pharma Ltd)

1. NAME OF THE MEDICINAL PRODUCT
Univer 180 mg Capsules

2. QUALITATIVE AND QUANTITATIVE COMPOSITION
Verapamil hydrochloride 180 mg.

For excipients, see 6.1.

3. PHARMACEUTICAL FORM
Prolonged-release capsule, hard.

Capsules are yellow and printed with V180.

4. CLINICAL PARTICULARS

4.1 Therapeutic indications
Mild to moderate hypertension. Angina pectoris.

4.2 Posology and method of administration
For oral administration only. The capsules should be swallowed whole and not chewed.

The bioequivalence of Univer to other prolonged release verapamil formulations may not have been evaluated. As such, this product should not be directly substituted for other non-identical formulations of verapamil and vice-versa.

Adults: Mild to moderate hypertension: Initial dose in adult patients new to verapamil therapy should be 120 mg once daily. This can be increased to 240 mg once daily which is the normal maintenance dosage. The dose may be further increased to a maximum of 480 mg once daily if required.

Angina: The usual adult dose is 360 mg once daily. Dosage may be increased to a maximum of 480 mg daily if required.

Elderly: Elderly patients show enhanced bioavailability of verapamil and therapeutic control may be achieved with lower doses in this patient population.

Children: Not recommended in children and adolescents under the age of 18 years.

Hepatic impairment: Verapamil is extensively metabolised in the liver and for those patients with impaired liver function, the dose should be reduced and carefully titrated.

Renal impairment: About 70% of an administered dose of verapamil is excreted as metabolites in the urine. Verapamil should be prescribed cautiously when renal function is impaired. Careful patient monitoring is recommended.

4.3 Contraindications

• Acute myocardial infarction with complications such as bradycardia, hypotension, left ventricular decompensation or congestive heart failure.

• Second or third degree atrioventricular block without pacemaker.

• Sick sinus syndrome, sino-atrial block, or severe sinus bradycardia (except in patients with functioning artificial ventricular pacemaker).

• Uncompensated cardiac failure.

• Atrial flutter or atrial fibrillation associated with an accessory pathway (e.g. Wolff-Parkinson-White, Lown-Ganong-Levine syndrome).

• Porphyria.

• Hypotension (systolic pressure <90 mm Hg) or cardiogenic shock.

• Intravenous dantrolene (see section 4.5).

• Known hypersensitivity to any of the ingredients.

• Concomitant ingestion of grapefruit juice.

4.4 Special warnings and special precautions for use
Special care should be taken in hypotension (see section 4.3), especially in acute myocardial infarction as this is a condition where atrioventricular conduction defects may develop and contractility may be impaired.

Use with caution in patients with first degree atrioventricular block.

Left ventricular contractility may be affected and although the effect is small, cardiac failure may be precipitated or aggravated. Hence incipient cardiac failure should be controlled using appropriate therapy before verapamil is given.

Verapamil is extensively metabolised in the liver and special care should be taken in cases where liver damage exists, as plasma levels of verapamil may be increased (see section 4.2).

4.5 Interaction with other medicinal products and other forms of Interaction
Dantrolene: the association of this muscle relaxant given intravenously and verapamil is potentially dangerous (can cause fatal ventricular fibrillation in animals) and is contra-indicated.

The combination of verapamil and beta-blockers, antiarrhythmic agents or inhaled anaesthetics may lead to additive cardiovascular effects (e.g. AV block, bradycardia, hypotension, heart failure). A period between stopping beta-blocking therapy and starting therapy with this product may be advisable. Concomitant use of verapamil and beta-blockers or antiarrhythmics, if necessary, should only be administered to patients in a closely monitored clinical setting. Intravenous beta-blockers should not be given to patients under treatment with verapamil. The effects of verapamil may be additive to other hypotensive agents.

Caution is required when verapamil is given with digoxin, theophylline, midazolam, ciclosporin and carbamazepine as plasma levels of these drugs may rise. With rifampicin, phenytoin and phenobarbital, plasma levels of verapamil may be reduced, whilst with alcohol and cimetidine, plasma verapamil levels may be increased.

Lithium toxicity may be enhanced.

Lithium can enhance neuromuscular block during anaesthesia and hence verapamil with lithium may potentiate the neuromuscular blocking effect.

Grapefruit juice – an increase in verapamil serum level has been reported.

4.6 Pregnancy and lactation
Animal studies have shown no teratogenic effects and data on a limited number of exposed pregnancies showed no adverse effects on the health of the foetus or newborn child.

Caution should be exercised, however, when prescribing to pregnant women and verapamil should be avoided in the first trimester unless the benefits clearly outweigh the risks.

Verapamil is excreted in breast milk and rare hypersensitivity reactions have been reported. Verapamil should only be used during lactation if, in the clinicians judgement, it is essential for the welfare of the patient.

4.7 Effects on ability to drive and use machines
It is possible that a patient's ability to drive a vehicle or operate machinery may be impaired, particularly when starting treatment.

4.8 Undesirable effects
Occasionally, particularly in high doses or with prior myocardial damage, cardiovascular effects may be larger than desired giving rise to bradycardic arrhythmias, such as sinus bradycardia, second and third degree atrioventricular block, bradyarrhythmia in atrial fibrillation, transient asystole, hypotension, heart failure.

Constipation may occur. Headaches, dizziness, fatigue and ankle oedema are uncommon. Very infrequently nausea, vomiting, flushing and allergic reactions have been observed. Reversible impairment of liver function has been rarely reported and is most likely a hypersensitivity reaction.

There have been rare reports of gynaecomastia, gingival hyperplasia, erythromelalgia, paraesthesia and elevated prolactin levels.

4.9 Overdose
Normal resuscitation procedures should be initiated in the event of cardiovascular collapse, i.e. if atrioventricular conduction defects such as second or third degree block develop these should be treated in the usual way using atropine, isoprenaline or the temporary insertion of a pacemaker, as required. Hypotension may be observed and, if persistent, and in the absence of a conduction defect, treatment with systemic dopaminergic agents, e.g. dopamine, dobutamine or noradrenaline should be started. Specific antidote may be given, e.g. slow intravenous injection, or an infusion, of 10-20 ml calcium gluconate 10% solution. Overdose with modified-release preparations may result in prolonged toxicity of delayed onset.

5. PHARMACOLOGICAL PROPERTIES

5.1 Pharmacodynamic properties
Verapamil is a phenylalkylamine calcium antagonist with effects upon arterial smooth muscle, myocardial cells and cells of the cardiac conduction system. It lowers heart rate, increases myocardial perfusion and reduces coronary spasm. It decreases vascular peripheral resistance and lowers blood pressure by vasodilation without reflex tachycardia. The effects are more pronounced on high blood pressure than on normal pressure because of its use-dependent action on the voltage-operated calcium channel.

5.2 Pharmacokinetic properties
Approximately 90% of verapamil is absorbed following oral administration and is subject to extensive first pass metabolism in the liver. There is considerable interindividual variation in plasma concentrations. About 70% of the oral dose is excreted by the kidneys and 16% with the faeces.

Where liver damage exists plasma levels of verapamil may be increased. Renal failure does not significantly alter the kinetics of the drug. Elderly subjects show enhanced bioavailability of verapamil.

Univer provides prolonged release of verapamil in the gastrointestinal tract and a pharmacokinetic profile consistent with a prolonged release formulation. A study in healthy volunteers compared the pharmacokinetics of Univer 240 mg administered once daily and immediate-release verapamil 80 mg administered three times daily.

The comparative steady state kinetic data are shown below:

Steady State	Univer, dose 240 mg	Verapamil immediate release, dose 80 mg
C_{max} (ng/ml)	117.60	172.23
T_{max} (hr)	7.68	1.16
AUC_{0-8hr} (ng × hr/ml)	—	694.15
AUC_{0-24hr} (ng × hr/ml)	1572.98	—
Half-life (hr)	9.01	6.38
Elimination Rate (hr^{-1})	0.08	0.12

5.3 Preclinical safety data
There is no evidence of teratogenicity or carcinogenicity with verapamil. There are no additional preclinical safety data of relevance to the prescriber.

6. PHARMACEUTICAL PARTICULARS

6.1 List of excipients
Capsule contents:

Fumaric acid

Sugar spheres (containing sucrose and maize starch)

Talc

Povidone

Shellac

Capsule shell:

Gelatin

Titanium dioxide (E171)

Erythrosine (E127)

Yellow iron oxide (E172)

Printing ink:

Titanium dioxide (E171)

Black iron oxide (E172)

Shellac

Soya lecithin

Antifoam DC 1510

6.2 Incompatibilities
None stated.

6.3 Shelf life
2 years.

6.4 Special precautions for storage
Do not store above 25°C. Store in the original package.

6.5 Nature and contents of container
PVC/aluminium blister packs of 4, 8, 28 or 56 capsules.

Containers of 100 or 500.

6.6 Instructions for use and handling
None

7. MARKETING AUTHORISATION HOLDER
Elan Pharma Ltd
Monksland
Athlone
Co. Westmeath
Ireland
Trading as:
Elan Pharma
Abel Smith House
Gunnels Wood Road
Stevenage
Hertfordshire
SG1 2FG

8. MARKETING AUTHORISATION NUMBER(S)
PL 10038/0034

9. DATE OF FIRST AUTHORISATION/RENEWAL OF THE AUTHORISATION
14 May 2001

10. DATE OF REVISION OF THE TEXT
August 2003

11. LEGAL CATEGORY
POM

Univer Capsules 240mg

(Zeneus Pharma Ltd)

1. NAME OF THE MEDICINAL PRODUCT
Univer 240 mg Capsules

2. QUALITATIVE AND QUANTITATIVE COMPOSITION
Verapamil hydrochloride 240 mg.

For excipients, see 6.1.

3. PHARMACEUTICAL FORM
Prolonged-release capsule, hard.

Capsules are blue and yellow and printed with V240.

4. CLINICAL PARTICULARS

4.1 Therapeutic indications
Mild to moderate hypertension. Angina pectoris.

4.2 Posology and method of administration
For oral administration only. The capsules should be swallowed whole and not chewed.

The bioequivalence of Univer to other prolonged release verapamil formulations may not have been evaluated. As such, this product should not be directly substituted for other non-identical formulations of verapamil and vice-versa.

Adults: Mild to moderate hypertension: Initial dose in adult patients new to verapamil therapy should be 120 mg once daily. This can be increased to 240 mg once daily which is the normal maintenance dosage. The dose may be further increased to a maximum of 480 mg once daily if required.

Angina: The usual adult dose is 360 mg once daily. Dosage may be increased to a maximum of 480 mg daily if required.

Elderly: Elderly patients show enhanced bioavailability of verapamil and therapeutic control may be achieved with lower doses in this patient population.

Children: Not recommended in children and adolescents under the age of 18 years.

Hepatic impairment: Verapamil is extensively metabolised in the liver and for those patients with impaired liver function, the dose should be reduced and carefully titrated.

Renal impairment: About 70% of an administered dose of verapamil is excreted as metabolites in the urine. Verapamil should be prescribed cautiously when renal function is impaired. Careful patient monitoring is recommended.

4.3 Contraindications

- Acute myocardial infarction with complications such as bradycardia, hypotension, left ventricular decompensation or congestive heart failure.
- Second or third degree atrioventricular block without pacemaker.
- Sick sinus syndrome, sino-atrial block, or severe sinus bradycardia (except in patients with functioning artificial ventricular pacemaker).
- Uncompensated cardiac failure.
- Atrial flutter or atrial fibrillation associated with an accessory pathway (e.g. Wolff-Parkinson-White, Lown-Ganong-Levine syndrome).
- Porphyria.
- Hypotension (systolic pressure <90 mm Hg) or cardiogenic shock.
- Intravenous dantrolene (see section 4.5).
- Known hypersensitivity to any of the ingredients.
- Concomitant ingestion of grapefruit juice.

4.4 Special warnings and special precautions for use
Special care should be taken in hypotension (see section 4.3), especially in acute myocardial infarction as this is a condition where atrioventricular conduction defects may develop and contractility may be impaired.

Use with caution in patients with first degree atrioventricular block.

Left ventricular contractility may be affected and although the effect is small, cardiac failure may be precipitated or aggravated. Hence incipient cardiac failure should be controlled using appropriate therapy before verapamil is given.

Verapamil is extensively metabolised in the liver and special care should be taken in cases where liver damage exists, as plasma levels of verapamil may be increased (see section 4.2).

4.5 Interaction with other medicinal products and other forms of Interaction
Dantrolene: the association of this muscle relaxant given intravenously and verapamil is potentially dangerous (can cause fatal ventricular fibrillation in animals) and is contra-indicated.

The combination of verapamil and beta-blockers, antiarrhythmic agents or inhaled anaesthetics may lead to additive cardiovascular effects (e.g. AV block, bradycardia, hypotension, heart failure). A period between stopping beta-blocking therapy and starting therapy with this product may be advisable. Concomitant use of verapamil and beta-blockers or antiarrhythmics, if necessary, should only be administered to patients in a closely monitored clinical setting. Intravenous beta-blockers should not be given to patients under treatment with verapamil. The effects of verapamil may be additive to other hypotensive agents.

Caution is required when verapamil is given with digoxin, theophylline, midazolam, ciclosporin and carbamazepine as plasma levels of these drugs may rise. With rifampicin, phenytoin and phenobarbital, plasma levels of verapamil may be reduced, whilst with alcohol and cimetidine, plasma verapamil levels may be increased.

Lithium toxicity may be enhanced.

Lithium can enhance neuromuscular block during anaesthesia and hence verapamil with lithium may potentiate the neuromuscular blocking effect.

Grapefruit juice – an increase in verapamil serum level has been reported.

4.6 Pregnancy and lactation
Animal studies have shown no teratogenic effects and data on a limited number of exposed pregnancies showed no adverse effects on the health of the foetus or newborn child.

Caution should be exercised, however, when prescribing to pregnant women and verapamil should be avoided in the first trimester unless the benefits clearly outweigh the risks.

Verapamil is excreted in breast milk and rare hypersensitivity reactions have been reported. Verapamil should only be used during lactation if, in the clinicians judgement, it is essential for the welfare of the patient.

4.7 Effects on ability to drive and use machines
It is possible that a patient's ability to drive a vehicle or operate machinery may be impaired, particularly when starting treatment.

4.8 Undesirable effects
Occasionally, particularly in high doses or with prior myocardial damage, cardiovascular effects may be larger than desired giving rise to bradycardic arrhythmias, such as sinus bradycardia, second and third degree atrioventricular block, bradyarrhythmia in atrial fibrillation, transient asystole, hypotension, heart failure.

Constipation may occur. Headaches, dizziness, fatigue and ankle oedema are uncommon. Very infrequently nausea, vomiting, flushing and allergic reactions have been observed. Reversible impairment of liver function has been rarely reported and is most likely a hypersensitivity reaction.

There have been rare reports of gynaecomastia, gingival hyperplasia, erythromelalgia, paraesthesia and elevated prolactin levels.

4.9 Overdose
Normal resuscitation procedures should be initiated in the event of cardiovascular collapse, i.e. if atrioventricular conduction defects such as second or third degree block develop these should be treated in the usual way using atropine, isoprenaline or the temporary insertion of a pacemaker, as required. Hypotension may be observed and, if persistent, and in the absence of a conduction defect, treatment with systemic dopaminergic agents, e.g. dopamine, dobutamine or noradrenaline should be started. Specific antidote may be given, e.g. slow intravenous injection, or an infusion, of 10-20 ml calcium gluconate 10% solution. Overdose with modified-release preparations may result in prolonged toxicity of delayed onset.

5. PHARMACOLOGICAL PROPERTIES

5.1 Pharmacodynamic properties
Verapamil is a phenylalkylamine calcium antagonist with effects upon arterial smooth muscle, myocardial cells and cells of the cardiac conduction system. It lowers heart rate, increases myocardial perfusion and reduces coronary spasm. It decreases vascular peripheral resistance and lowers blood pressure by vasodilation without reflex tachycardia. The effects are more pronounced on high blood pressure than on normal pressure because of its use-dependent action on the voltage-operated calcium channel.

5.2 Pharmacokinetic properties
Approximately 90% of verapamil is absorbed following oral administration and is subject to extensive first pass metabolism in the liver. There is considerable interindividual variation in plasma concentrations. About 70% of the oral dose is excreted by the kidneys and 16% with the faeces.

Where liver damage exists plasma levels of verapamil may be increased. Renal failure does not significantly alter the kinetics of the drug. Elderly subjects show enhanced bioavailability of verapamil.

Univer provides prolonged release of verapamil in the gastrointestinal tract and a pharmacokinetic profile consistent with a prolonged release formulation. A study in healthy volunteers compared the pharmacokinetics of Univer 240 mg administered once daily and immediate-release verapamil 80 mg administered three times daily. The comparative steady state kinetic data are shown below:

Steady State	Univer, dose 240 mg	Verapamil immediate release, dose 80 mg
C_{max} (ng/ml)	117.60	172.23
T_{max} (hr)	7.68	1.16
$AUC_{0\text{-}8hr}$ (ng × hr/ml)	—	694.15
$AUC_{0\text{-}24hr}$ (ng × hr/ml)	1572.98	—
Half-life (hr)	9.01	6.38
Elimination Rate (hr^{-1})	0.08	0.12

5.3 Preclinical safety data
There is no evidence of teratogenicity or carcinogenicity with verapamil. There are no additional preclinical safety data of relevance to the prescriber.

6. PHARMACEUTICAL PARTICULARS

6.1 List of excipients
Capsule contents:
Fumaric acid
Sugar spheres (containing sucrose and maize starch)
Talc
Povidone
Shellac
Capsule shell:
Gelatin
Titanium dioxide (E171)
Erythrosine (E127)
Indigotine (E132)
Yellow iron oxide (E172)
Printing ink:
Titanium dioxide (E171)
Black iron oxide (E172)
Shellac
Soya lecithin
Antifoam DC 1510

6.2 Incompatibilities
None stated.

6.3 Shelf life
2 years.

6.4 Special precautions for storage
Do not store above 25°C. Store in the original package.

6.5 Nature and contents of container
PVC/aluminium blister packs of 4, 8, 28 or 56 capsules.

Containers of 100 or 500.

6.6 Instructions for use and handling
None

7. MARKETING AUTHORISATION HOLDER
Elan Pharma Ltd
Monksland
Athlone
Co. Westmeath
Ireland
Trading as:
Elan Pharma
Abel Smith House
Gunnels Wood Road
Stevenage
Hertfordshire
SG1 2FG

8. MARKETING AUTHORISATION NUMBER(S)
PL 10038/0035

9. DATE OF FIRST AUTHORISATION/RENEWAL OF THE AUTHORISATION
14 May 2001

10. DATE OF REVISION OF THE TEXT
August 2003

11. LEGAL CATEGORY
POM

URDOX (Ursodeoxycholic) Acid Tablets 300mg

(Wockhardt UK Ltd)

1. NAME OF THE MEDICINAL PRODUCT
Urdox Tablets 300mg.

2. QUALITATIVE AND QUANTITATIVE COMPOSITION
Ursodeoxycholic acid 300mg.

For excipients, see 6.1

3. PHARMACEUTICAL FORM
Film coated tablets

Urdox tablets are white. film coated, convex tablets with "URDOX" on one side.

4. CLINICAL PARTICULARS

4.1 Therapeutic indications
Urdox tablets are indicated for the dissolution of small to medium sized radiolucent, cholesterol-rich gall-stones in functioning gall bladders.

Cholesterol stones coated with calcium or stones composed of bile pigments are not dissolved by ursodeoxycholic acid. Urdox has a particular place in the treatment of patients in whom surgery is contraindicated or who are anxious to avoid surgery.

4.2 Posology and method of administration
Urdox tablets are for oral administration

To be taken with a drink of water.

Adults and Elderly:

The usual dose is 6 - 12mg/kg/day either as a single night time dose or in divided doses. This may be increased to 15mg/kg/day in obese patients, if necessary.

The duration of treatment may be up to two years, depending on the size of the stone(s), and should be continued for three months after the apparent dissolution of the stone(s).

Children:

Not recommended.

4.3 Contraindications
1. Use in patients with radio-opaque calcified gall-stones, or in those with non-functioning gall bladders.

2. Use in women who may become pregnant.

3. Use in patients with chronic liver disease, peptic ulcers or in those with inflammatory diseases of the small intestine and colon.

4.4 Special warnings and special precautions for use
None known

4.5 Interaction with other medicinal products and other forms of Interaction
Urdox tablets should not be administered with oral contraceptives, oestrogenic hormones and other drugs which reduce the blood cholesterol level and increase the bile cholesterol level. Antacids bind bile acids in the gut. Drugs such as charcoal, colestipol and cholestyramine bind bile acids *in vitro*. All the above should be avoided during bile acid therapy as they may limit the effectiveness of therapy. Ursodeoxycholic acid may increase the absorption and serum levels of ciclosporin in some patients.

4.6 Pregnancy and lactation
This product should not be used during pregnancy or lactation. Measures should be taken to prevent pregnancy if given to women of childbearing age. A non-hormonal contraceptive should be used. Treatment should be discontinued immediately if pregnancy occurs and medical advice sought.

4.7 Effects on ability to drive and use machines
None known.

4.8 Undesirable effects
Urdox may give rise to nausea, vomiting, diarrhoea and pruritus. A calcified layer may develop on the surface of the stone making it unable to be dissolved by bile acid therapy, resulting in surgery for some patients.

4.9 Overdose
Bile acids are removed in the faeces either unchanged or as bacterial metabolites. It is unlikely therefore that serious toxicity would occur following overdose. The most likely result is diarrhoea which should be treated symptomatically and supportively.

5. PHARMACOLOGICAL PROPERTIES

5.1 Pharmacodynamic properties
When given by mouth, ursodeoxycholic acid reduces the ratio of cholesterol to bile salts plus phospholipids in bile, causing desaturation of cholesterol saturated bile. The exact mechanism of action has not been fully elucidated.

5.2 Pharmacokinetic properties
Ursodeoxycholic acid is absorbed from the gastro-intestinal tract and undergoes first pass metabolism and enterohepatic recycling. It is partially conjugated in the liver before being excreted into bile and undergoing 7-α-dehydroxylation to lithocholic acid, some of which is excreted directly in the faeces. The rest is absorbed and mainly conjugated and sulphated by the liver before excretion in the faeces.

5.3 Preclinical safety data
There are no pre-clinical data of relevance to the prescriber which are additional to those already included in other sections.

6. PHARMACEUTICAL PARTICULARS

6.1 List of excipients
Lactose

Maize starch

Povidone

Sodium starch glycollate

Magnesium stearate

Purified water

Tablet Coating

Hydroxypropylmethylcellulose (E464)

Titanium dioxide (E171)

Polyethylene glycol

6.2 Incompatibilities
None known.

6.3 Shelf life
Three years.

6.4 Special precautions for storage
Do not store above 25°C.

Store in the original container.

6.5 Nature and contents of container
Polypropylene or polyethylene tablet container with tamper evident closure of 60, 100 or 500 tablets.

Strips of 60 tablets in white opaque 250 micron UPVC with 20 micron hard tempered foil.

6.6 Instructions for use and handling
None.

Administrative Data

7. MARKETING AUTHORISATION HOLDER
CP Pharmaceuticals Ltd

Ash Road North

Wrexham

LL13 9UF

United Kingdom

8. MARKETING AUTHORISATION NUMBER(S)
PL 4543/0318

9. DATE OF FIRST AUTHORISATION/RENEWAL OF THE AUTHORISATION

Date of first authorisation	24 February 1992
Date of last renewal	21 May 2002

10. DATE OF REVISION OF THE TEXT
January 2002

Urispas 200

(Shire Pharmaceuticals Limited)

1. NAME OF THE MEDICINAL PRODUCT
Urispas 200

2. QUALITATIVE AND QUANTITATIVE COMPOSITION
Each Urispas tablet contains flavoxate hydrochloride 200 mg.

For excipients, see 6.1.

3. PHARMACEUTICAL FORM
Film-coated tablet.

White, film-coated tablets embossed with 'F 200'.

4. CLINICAL PARTICULARS

4.1 Therapeutic indications
Urispas is indicated for the symptomatic relief of dysuria, urgency, nocturia, vesical supra-pubic pain, frequency and incontinence as may occur in cystitis, prostatitis, urethritis, urethro-cystitis and urethrotrigonitis.

In addition, the preparation is indicated for the relief of vesico-urethral spasms due to catheterisation, cystoscopy or indwelling catheters; prior to cystoscopy or catheterisation; sequelae of surgical intervention of the lower urinary tract.

4.2 Posology and method of administration
For oral administration.

Adults (including the elderly):

The recommended adult dosage is one tablet three times a day for as long as required.

Children:

Urispas tablets are not recommended for children under 12 years of age.

4.3 Contraindications
The following obstructive conditions: pyloric or duodenal obstruction, obstructive intestinal lesions or ileus, achalasia, gastro-intestinal haemorrhage and obstructive uropathies of the lower urinary tract.

Hypersensitivity to flavoxate hydrochloride or to any of the excipients of Urispas 200.

4.4 Special warnings and special precautions for use
Urispas should be used with caution in patients with suspected glaucoma.

Where evidence of urinary infection is present, appropriate anti-infective therapy should be instituted concomitantly.

Patients with rare hereditary problems of galactose intolerance, the Lapp lactose deficiency or glucose-galactose malabsorption should not take this medicine.

4.5 Interaction with other medicinal products and other forms of Interaction
None known.

4.6 Pregnancy and lactation
Since there is no evidence of the drug's safety in human pregnancy, nor any evidence from animal work that it is free from hazard, Urispas should be avoided in pregnancy unless there is no safer alternative. It is not known whether flavoxate is excreted in human milk. Because many drugs are excreted in human milk, caution should be exercised when Urispas is administered during breast-feeding.

4.7 Effects on ability to drive and use machines
In the event of drowsiness and blurred vision, the patient should not operate a motor vehicle or machinery.

4.8 Undesirable effects
In clinical trials comparing Urispas with other antispasmodic agents, the incidence of side-effects was low. The following adverse reactions have been observed:

Blood and lymphatic disorders: Eosinophilia, leukopenia.

Immune system disorders: Angioedema.

Nervous system disorders: Drowsiness, dizziness, headache, mental confusion (especially in the elderly), nervousness, vertigo.

Eye disorders: Blurred vision, disturbances in eye accommodation, increased ocular tension.

Cardiac disorders: Palpitations, tachycardia.

Gastrointestinal disorders: Diarrhoea, dry mouth, dyspepsia, dysphagia, nausea, vomiting.

Skin and subcutaneous tissue disorders: Urticaria and other dermatoses.

Renal and urinary disorders: Dysuria.

General disorders: Fatigue, hyperpyrexia.

4.9 Overdose
Patients who have taken an overdosage of Urispas should have gastric lavage performed within four hours of the overdosage occurring. If overdosage is extreme, or there is a delay in removing the drug from the stomach, administration of a parasympathomimetic drug should be considered.

5. PHARMACOLOGICAL PROPERTIES

5.1 Pharmacodynamic properties

Pharmacotherapeutic Group:	Urinary antispasmodics – Flavoxate
ATC code:	G04BD02

Flavoxate hydrochloride (and its main metabolite methyl flavone carboxylic acid, MFCA) is an antispasmodic selective to the urinary tract. In animal and human studies, flavoxate hydrochloride has been shown to have a direct antispasmodic action on smooth muscle fibres.

The mechanism of action involves intracellular cyclic AMP accumulation and calcium blocking activity. It inhibits bladder contractions induced by various agonists or by electrical stimulation and inhibits the frequency of bladder voiding contractions. It increases bladder volume capacity, reduces the threshold and micturition pressure.

In addition, animal studies have shown flavoxate hydrochloride to have analgesic and local anaesthetic properties.

Flavoxate does not significantly affect cardiac or respiratory functions.

5.2 Pharmacokinetic properties
Oral studies in man have indicated that flavoxate is readily absorbed from the intestine and converted, to a large extent, almost immediately to MFCA.

Following an IV dose (equimolar to 100 mg), the following parameters were calculated for flavoxate: $T_{½}$ 83.3 mins: apparent volume of distribution 2.89 l/kg. The apparent distribution of MFCA was 0.20 l/kg. No free flavoxate was found in urine (24 hours). However, 47% of the dose was excreted as MFCA.

Following single oral dosing to volunteers of 200 mg and 400 mg flavoxate, almost no free flavoxate was detected in the plasma. The peak level of MFCA was attained at 30-60 mins after the 200 mg dose and at around two hours following the 400 mg dose. The AUC for the 400 mg dose was approximately twice as large as the AUC for the 200 mg dose. About 50% of the dose was excreted as MFCA within 12 hours; most being excreted within the first 6 hours.

After repeated oral dosing (200 mg, TDS, 7 days) the cumulative excretion of metabolites stabilised at 60% of the dose on the third day remaining almost unchanged after one week.

5.3 Preclinical safety data
None stated.

6. PHARMACEUTICAL PARTICULARS

6.1 List of excipients
Tablet Core:

Lactose

Sodium starch glycollate

Povidone

Talc

Magnesium stearate

Cellulose microcrystalline

Tablet Coating:

Hypromellose

Cellulose microcrystalline

Macrogol 6000

Macrogol stearate

Magnesium stearate

Titanium dioxide (E171)

6.2 Incompatibilities
None known.

6.3 Shelf life

3 years.

6.4 Special precautions for storage

Do not store above 30°C. Keep blister strips in the outer carton.

6.5 Nature and contents of container

PVC / aluminium blister strips in a pack size of 90 tablets.

6.6 Instructions for use and handling

Not applicable.

7. MARKETING AUTHORISATION HOLDER

Shire Pharmaceuticals Limited

Hampshire International Business Park

Chineham

Basingstoke

Hampshire RG24 8EP

United Kingdom

8. MARKETING AUTHORISATION NUMBER(S)

PL 08557/0034

9. DATE OF FIRST AUTHORISATION/RENEWAL OF THE AUTHORISATION

30 May 1997/16 March 2003

10. DATE OF REVISION OF THE TEXT

July 2004

LEGAL CATEGORY

POM

Ursofalk Capsules

(Dr Falk Pharma UK Limited)

1. NAME OF THE MEDICINAL PRODUCT

Ursofalk

2. QUALITATIVE AND QUANTITATIVE COMPOSITION

Each capsule of Ursofalk contains the following active ingredient:

Ursodeoxycholic Acid 250mg

3. PHARMACEUTICAL FORM

White, opaque, hard gelatine capsule

4. CLINICAL PARTICULARS

4.1 Therapeutic indications

Ursofalk is indicated in the treatment of primary biliary cirrhosis (PBC) and for the dissolution of radiolucent gallstones in patients with a functioning gall bladder.

4.2 Posology and method of administration

Method of administration: Oral

Primary Biliary Cirrhosis

Adults and the Elderly: 10-15mg ursodeoxycholic acid (UDCA) per kg per day in two to four divided doses. The following dosage regimen is recommended:

Body Weight (kg)	Capsules Daily (in 2-4 divided doses)	1 Mg (UDCA)/kg/day
50 - 62	2 - 4	10.0 - 16.1
63 - 85	3 - 5	11.9 - 14.7
86 - 120	4 - 7	11.6 - 14.6

Children: Dosage should be related to bodyweight.

Dissolution of gallstones

Adults: 8-12mg ursodeoxycholic acid (UDCA) per kg per day in two divided doses. The following dosage regimen is recommended:

Body Weight (kg)	Capsules Daily (in 2 divided doses)	1 Mg (UDCA)/kg/day
50 - 62	2	8.1 - 10
63 - 85	3	8.8 - 11.9
86 - 120	4	8.3 - 11.6

If doses are unequal the larger dose should be taken in late evening to counteract the rise in biliary cholesterol saturation which occurs in the early morning. The late evening dose may usefully be taken with food to help maintain bile flow overnight.

The time required for dissolution of gallstones is likely to range from 6 to 24 months depending on stone size and composition. Follow-up cholecystograms or ultrasound investigation may be useful at 6 month intervals until the gallstones have disappeared.

Treatment should be continued until 2 successive cholecystograms and/or ultrasound investigations 4-12 weeks apart have failed to demonstrate gallstones. This is because these techniques do not permit reliable visualisation of stones less than 2mm in diameter.

The likelihood of recurrence of gallstones after dissolution by bile acid treatment has been estimated as up to 50% at 5 years.

The efficiency of Ursofalk in treating radio-opaque or partially radio opaque gallstones has not been tested but these are generally thought to be less soluble than radiolucent stones.

Non-cholesterol stones account for 10-15% radiolucent stones and may not be dissolved by bile acids.

Elderly: There is no evidence to suggest that any alteration in the adult dose is needed but the relevant precautions should be taken into account.

Children: Cholesterol rich gallstones are rare in children but when they occur, dosage should be related to bodyweight.

4.3 Contraindications

Ursofalk is not suitable for the dissolution of radio-opaque gallstones and should not be used in patients with a non-functioning gall bladder.

4.4 Special warnings and special precautions for use

A product of this class has been found to be carcinogenic in animals. The relevance of these findings to the clinical use of Ursofalk has not been established.

4.5 Interaction with other medicinal products and other forms of Interaction

Some drugs, such as cholestyramine, charcoal, colestipol and certain antacids (e.g. aluminium hydroxide) bind bile acids *in vitro*. They could therefore have a similar effect *in vivo* and may interfere with the absorption of Ursofalk.

Drugs which increase cholesterol elimination in bile, such as oestrogenic hormones, oestrogen-rich contraceptive agents and certain blood cholesterol lowering agents, such as Clofibrate, should not be taken with Ursofalk.

UDCA may increase the absorption of cyclosporin in transplantation patients.

4.6 Pregnancy and lactation

Ursofalk should not be used in pregnancy. When treating women of childbearing potential, non-hormonal or low oestrogen oral contraceptive measures are recommended.

4.7 Effects on ability to drive and use machines

Ursofalk is not expected to affect ability to drive and use machines.

4.8 Undesirable effects

Diarrhoea may occur rarely.

4.9 Overdose

Serious adverse effects are unlikely to occur in overdosage. However, liver function should be monitored. If necessary, ion-exchange resins may be used to bind bile acids in the intestines.

5. PHARMACOLOGICAL PROPERTIES

5.1 Pharmacodynamic properties

UDCA is a bile acid which effects a reduction in cholesterol in biliary fluid primarily by dispersing the cholesterol and forming a liquid-crystal phase.

5.2 Pharmacokinetic properties

Ursodeoxycholic acid occurs naturally in the body. When given orally it is rapidly and completely absorbed. It is 96-98% bound to plasma proteins and efficiently extracted by the liver and excreted in the bile as glycine and taurine conjugates. In the intestine some of the conjugates are deconjugated and reabsorbed. The conjugates may also be dehydroxylated to lithocholic acid, part of which is absorbed, sulphated by the liver and excreted via the biliary tract.

5.3 Preclinical safety data

Not applicable.

6. PHARMACEUTICAL PARTICULARS

6.1 List of excipients

Ursofalk contains the following excipients:

Maize starch, colloidal anhydrous silica, magnesium stearate, gelatin, titanium dioxide.

6.2 Incompatibilities

None known.

6.3 Shelf life

36 months.

6.4 Special precautions for storage

None.

6.5 Nature and contents of container

Clear PVC blister strips with aluminium foil backing packed in cardboard cartons. Available in cartons containing 60 capsules packaged in six blister strips of 10 capsules or 100 capsules packaged in 4 blister strips of 25 capsules.

6.6 Instructions for use and handling

None.

7. MARKETING AUTHORISATION HOLDER

Dr Falk Pharma UK Ltd

Unit K

Bourne End Business Park

Cores End Road

Bourne End

Bucks

SL8 5AS

United Kingdom

8. MARKETING AUTHORISATION NUMBER(S)

PL 10341/0006

9. DATE OF FIRST AUTHORISATION/RENEWAL OF THE AUTHORISATION

31st December 2004

10. DATE OF REVISION OF THE TEXT

Ursofalk Suspension

(Dr Falk Pharma UK Limited)

1. NAME OF THE MEDICINAL PRODUCT

Ursofalk Suspension.

2. QUALITATIVE AND QUANTITATIVE COMPOSITION

5ml (=1 measuring spoon) of Ursofalk Suspension contains the following active ingredient:

Ursodeoxycholic acid 250mg.

3. PHARMACEUTICAL FORM

Suspension for oral administration.

4. CLINICAL PARTICULARS

4.1 Therapeutic indications

Ursofalk Suspension is indicated in the treatment of primary biliary cirrhosis (PBC) and for the dissolution of radiolucent gallstones in patients with a functioning gall bladder.

4.2 Posology and method of administration

Method of administration: Oral.

Primary Biliary Cirrhosis

Adults and the elderly: 10-15mg ursodeoxycholic acid (UDCA) per kg per day in two to four divided doses. The following dosage regimen is recommended:

Body Weight (kg)	Spoonfuls (5ml) (in 2-4 divided doses)	mg (UDCA)/kg/day
50 - 62	2 - 4	10.0 - 16.1
63 - 85	3 - 5	11.9 - 14.7
86 - 120	4 - 7	11.6 - 14.6

Children: Dosage should be related to bodyweight.

Dissolution of Gallstones

Adults: 8-12mg ursodeoxycholic acid (UDCA) per kg per day in two divided doses. The following dosage regimen is recommended:

Body Weight (kg)	Spoonfuls (5ml) (in 2 divided doses)	mg (UDCA)/kg/day
50 - 62	2	8.1 - 10.0
63 - 85	3	8.8 - 11.9
86 - 120	4	8.3 - 11.6

If doses are unequal the larger dose should be taken in late evening to counteract the rise in biliary cholesterol saturation which occurs in the early morning. The late evening dose may usefully be taken with food to help maintain bile flow overnight.

The time required for dissolution of gallstones is likely to range from 6 to 24 months depending on stone size and composition.

Follow-up cholecystograms or ultrasound investigation may be useful at 6 month intervals until the gallstones have disappeared.

Treatment should be continued until 2 successive cholecystograms and/or ultrasound investigations 4-12 weeks apart have failed to demonstrate gallstones. This is because these techniques do not permit reliable visualisation of stones less then 2mm in diameter.

The likelihood of recurrence of gallstones after dissolution by bile acid treatment has been estimated as up to 50% at 5 years.

The efficiency of Ursofalk Suspension in treating radio-opaque or partially radio-opaque gallstones has not been tested but these are generally thought to be less soluble than radiolucent stones.

Non-cholesterol stones account for 10-15% of radiolucent stones and may not be dissolved by bile acids.

Elderly: There is no evidence to suggest that any alteration in the adult dose is needed but the relevant precautions should be taken into account.

Children: Cholesterol rich gallstones are rare in children but when they occur, dosage should be related to bodyweight.

4.3 Contraindications
Ursofalk Suspension is not suitable for the dissolution of radio-opaque gallstones and should not be used in patients with a non-functioning gall bladder.

4.4 Special warnings and special precautions for use
A product of this class has been found to be carcinogenic in animals.

The relevance of these findings to the clinical use of Ursofalk Suspension has not been established.

4.5 Interaction with other medicinal products and other forms of Interaction
Some drugs, such as cholestyramine, charcoal, colestipol and certain antacids (e.g.aluminium hydroxide) bind bile acids in vitro. They could therefore have a similar effect in vivo and may interfere with the absorption of Ursofalk Suspension.

Drugs which increase cholesterol elimination in bile, such as oestrogenic hormones, oestrogen-rich contraceptive agents and certain blood cholesterol lowering agents, such as clofibrate, should not be taken with Ursofalk Suspension.

UDCA may increase the absorption of cyclosporin in transplantation patients.

4.6 Pregnancy and lactation
Ursofalk Suspension should not be used in pregnancy. When treating women of childbearing potential, non-hormonal or low oestrogen oral contraceptive measures are recommended.

4.7 Effects on ability to drive and use machines
Ursofalk Suspension is not expected to affect ability to drive and use machines.

4.8 Undesirable effects
Diarrhoea may occur rarely.

4.9 Overdose
Serious adverse effects are unlikely to occur in overdosage. However liver function should be monitored. If necessary, ion-exchange resins may be used to bind bile acids in the intestines.

5. PHARMACOLOGICAL PROPERTIES

5.1 Pharmacodynamic properties
UDCA is a bile acid which effects a reduction in cholesterol biliary fluid primarily by dispersing the cholesterol and forming a liquid-crystal phase. UDCA affects the enterohepatic circulation of bile salts by reducing the ileal reabsorption of endogenous more hydrophobic and potentially toxic salts such as cholic and chenedeoxycholic acids.

In-vitro studies show that UDCA has a direct hepatoprotective effect and reduces the hepatotoxicity of hydrophobic bile salts. Immunological effects have also been demonstrated with a reduction in abnormal expression of HLS Class I antigens on hepatocytes as well as suppression of cytokine and interleukin production.

5.2 Pharmacokinetic properties
Ursodeoxycholic acid occurs naturally in the body. When given orally it is rapidly and completely absorbed. It is 96-98% bound to plasma proteins and efficiently extracted by the liver and excreted in the bile as glycine and taurine conjugates. In the intestine some of the conjugates are deconjugated and reabsorbed. The conjugates may also be dehyroxylated to lithocholic acid, part of which is absorbed, sulphated by the liver and excreted bia the biliary tract.

5.3 Preclinical safety data
None Stated.

6. PHARMACEUTICAL PARTICULARS

6.1 List of excipients
Ursofalk Suspension contains the following excipients:

Benzoic acid (E210), microcrystalline cellulose and carboxymethyl-cellulose sodium, sodium chloride, sodium citrate, citric acid anhydrous, glycerol, propylene glycol, xylitol, sodium cyclamate, lemon flavouring (Givaudan 87017) and purified water.

6.2 Incompatibilities
None known other than the interactions identified in Section 4.5.

6.3 Shelf life
48 months.

6.4 Special precautions for storage
Do not refrigerate or freeze.

6.5 Nature and contents of container
Amber glass bottle closed with a plastic screw cap, containing 100ml or 250ml of suspension.

6.6 Instructions for use and handling
Shake well before use. After opening bottle, do not use after 4 months.

7. MARKETING AUTHORISATION HOLDER
Dr Falk Pharma UK Ltd
Unit K
Bourne End Business Park
Cores End Road
Bourne End
Bucks
SL8 5AS
United Kingdom

8. MARKETING AUTHORISATION NUMBER(S)
PL 10341/0007

9. DATE OF FIRST AUTHORISATION/RENEWAL OF THE AUTHORISATION
31st December 2004

10. DATE OF REVISION OF THE TEXT

Utinor Tablets 400mg

(Merck Sharp & Dohme Limited)

1. NAME OF THE MEDICINAL PRODUCT
UTINOR® 400 mg Tablets

2. QUALITATIVE AND QUANTITATIVE COMPOSITION
'Utinor' contains 400 mg of the active ingredient, norfloxacin.

For excipients, see 6.1

3. PHARMACEUTICAL FORM
'Utinor' is supplied as off-white oval tablets marked 'MSD 705'.

4. CLINICAL PARTICULARS

4.1 Therapeutic indications
Norfloxacin is a broad-spectrum, quinolone bactericidal agent indicated for the treatment of:

Upper and lower, complicated and uncomplicated, acute and chronic urinary tract infections. These infections include cystitis, pyelitis, pyelonephritis, chronic prostatitis and those urinary infections associated with urological surgery, neurogenic bladder or nephrolithiasis caused by bacteria susceptible to 'Utinor'.

Consideration should be given to official local guidance (e.g. national recommendations) on the appropriate use of bacterial agents.

Susceptibility of the causative organism to the treatment should be tested (if possible), although therapy may be initiated before the results are available.

4.2 Posology and method of administration
'Utinor' should be taken with a glass of water at least one hour before or two hours after a meal or milk ingestion. Multivitamins, products containing iron or zinc, antacids containing magnesium and aluminium, sucralfate or products containing didanosine should not be taken within 2 hours of administration of norfloxacin.

Susceptibility of the causative organism to 'Utinor' should be tested. However, therapy may be initiated before obtaining the results of these tests.

Diagnosis	Dosage	Therapy duration
Uncomplicated lower urinary tract infections (e.g. cystitis)*	400 mg twice daily	3 days
Urinary tract infections	400 mg twice daily	7-10 days
Chronic relapsing urinary tract infection**	400 mg twice daily	Up to 12 weeks

* Trials in over 600 patients have demonstrated the efficacy and tolerability of 'Utinor' in the three-day treatment of uncomplicated urinary tract infections.

** If adequate suppression is obtained within the first four weeks of therapy, the dose of 'Utinor' may be reduced to 400 mg daily.

Patients with renal impairment

'Utinor' is suitable for the treatment of patients with renal impairment. In studies involving patients whose creatinine clearance was less than 30 ml/min/1.73m^2, but who did not require haemodialysis, the plasma half-life of norfloxacin was approximately eight hours. Clinical studies showed there was no difference in the mean half-life of norfloxacin in patients with a creatinine clearance of less than 10 ml/min/1.73m^2, compared to patients with creatinine clearance of 10-30 ml/min/1.73m^2. Hence, for these patients, the recommended dose is one 400 mg tablet once daily. At this dosage, concentrations in appropriate body tissues or fluids exceed the MICs for most pathogens sensitive to norfloxacin.

Use in the elderly

Pharmacokinetic studies have shown no appreciable changes when compared to younger patients, apart from a slight prolongation of half-life. In the absence of renal impairment, no adjustment of dosage is necessary. Limited clinical studies have shown 'Utinor' to be well tolerated.

4.3 Contraindications
Hypersensitivity to any component of this product or any chemically related quinolone antibacterials.

'Utinor' is contra-indicated in prepubertal children and growing adolescents.

4.4 Special warnings and special precautions for use
As with other drugs in this class, 'Utinor' should not be used in patients with a history of convulsions or known factors that predispose to seizures unless there is an overwhelming clinical need. Convulsions have been reported rarely with norfloxacin.

Tendinitis and/or tendon rupture, particularly affecting the Achilles tendon, may occur with quinolone antibiotics. Such reactions have been observed, particularly in older patients and in those treated concurrently with corticosteroids. At the first sign of pain or inflammation, patients should discontinue 'Utinor' and rest the affected limbs.

Photosensitivity reactions have been observed in patients who are exposed to excessive sunlight while receiving some members of this drug class. Excessive sunlight should be avoided. Therapy should be discontinued if photosensitivity occurs.

Quinolones, including norfloxacin, may exacerbate the signs of myasthenia gravis and lead to life threatening weakness of the respiratory muscles. Caution should be exercised when using quinolones, including 'Utinor', in patients with myasthenia gravis (see section 4.8 'Undesirable effects').

Rarely, haemolytic reactions have been reported in patients with latent or actual defects in glucose-6-phosphate dehydrogenase activity who take quinolone antibacterial agents, including norfloxacin (see 4.8 'Undesirable effects').

Very rarely, some quinolones have been associated with prolongation of the QTc interval on the electrocardiogram and infrequent cases of arrhythmia (including extremely rare cases of torsade de pointes) have been observed. As with other agents associated with prolongation of the QTc interval, caution should be exercised when using 'Utinor' in patients with hypokalaemia, significant bradycardia or undergoing concurrent treatment with class Ia or class III antiarrhythmics.

Some quinolones including 'Utinor' should be used with caution in patients using cisapride, erythromycin, antipsychotics, tricyclic antidepressants or who have any personal or family history of QTc prolongation.

Use in children

As with other quinolones, 'Utinor' has been shown to cause arthropathy in immature animals. The safety of 'Utinor' in children has not been adequately explored and therefore the use of 'Utinor' in prepubertal children or growing adolescents is contra-indicated.

4.5 Interaction with other medicinal products and other forms of Interaction
Co-administration of probenecid does not affect serum concentrations of norfloxacin, but urinary excretion of the drug diminishes.

As with other organic acid antibacterials, antagonism has been demonstrated *in vitro* between 'Utinor' and nitrofurantoin.

Elevated plasma levels of theophylline have been reported with concomitant quinolone use. There have been rare reports of theophylline-related side effects in patients on concomitant therapy with norfloxacin and theophylline. Therefore, monitoring of theophylline plasma levels should be considered and dosage of theophylline adjusted as required.

Elevated serum levels of cyclosporin have been reported with concomitant use of norfloxacin. Cyclosporin serum levels should be monitored and appropriate cyclosporin dosage adjustments made when these drugs are used concomitantly.

Quinolones, including norfloxacin, may enhance the effects of the anticoagulant warfarin, or its derivatives, by displacing significant amounts from serum albumin-binding sites. When concomitant administration of these products cannot be avoided, measurements of prothrombin time or other suitable coagulation tests should be carried out.

The concomitant administration of quinolones including norfloxacin with glibenclamide (a sulfonylurea agent) has, on occasions, resulted in severe hypoglycaemia. Therefore monitoring of blood glucose is recommended when these agents are co-administered.

Multivitamins, products containing iron or zinc, antacids or sucralfate should not be administered concomitantly with, or within two hours of, the administration of norfloxacin because they may interfere with absorption, resulting in lower serum and urine levels of norfloxacin.

Products containing didanosine should not be administered concomitantly with, or within 2 hours of the administration of norfloxacin, because the products may interfere with absorption resulting in lower serum and urine levels of norfloxacin.

Some quinolones, including norfloxacin, have also been shown to interfere with the metabolism of caffeine. This may lead to reduced clearance of caffeine and a prolongation of its plasma half-life.

Animal data have shown that quinolones in combination with fenbufen can lead to convulsions. Therefore, concomitant administration of quinolones and fenbufen should be avoided.

4.6 Pregnancy and lactation
There is no evidence from animal studies that norfloxacin has any teratogenic or mutagenic effects. Embryotoxicity secondary to maternotoxicity was observed after large doses in rabbits. Embryonic losses were observed in cynomolgus monkeys without any teratogenic effects. The relevance of these findings for humans is uncertain.

The safe use of 'Utinor' in pregnant women has not been established; however, as with other quinolones, norfloxacin has been shown to cause arthropathy in immature animals and therefore its use during pregnancy is not recommended.

It is not known whether 'Utinor' is excreted in human milk; administration to breast-feeding mothers is thus not recommended.

4.7 Effects on ability to drive and use machines
There are side-effects associated with this product that may affect some patients' ability to drive or operate machinery (see 4.8 'Undesirable effects').

4.8 Undesirable effects
The overall incidence of drug-related side effects reported during clinical trials was approximately 3%.

The most common side effects have been gastro-intestinal, neuropsychiatric and skin reactions, and include nausea, headache, dizziness, rash, heartburn, abdominal pain/cramps, and diarrhoea.

Less commonly, other side effects such as anorexia, sleep disturbances, depression, anxiety/nervousness, irritability, euphoria, disorientation, hallucination, tinnitus, and epiphora have been reported.

Abnormal laboratory side effects observed during clinical trials included:

leucopenia, elevation of ALAT (SGPT), ASAT (SGOT), eosinophilia, neutropenia, thrombocytopenia.

With more widespread use the following additional side effects have been reported:

Hypersensitivity reactions

Hypersensitivity reactions including anaphylaxis, angioedema, dyspnoea, vasculitis, urticaria, arthritis, myalgia, arthralgia and interstitial nephritis.

Skin

Photosensitivity, Stevens-Johnson syndrome, toxic epidermal necrolysis, exfoliative dermatitis, erythema multiforme, pruritus.

Gastro-intestinal

Pseudomembranous colitis, pancreatitis (rare), hepatitis, jaundice including cholestatic jaundice and elevated liver-function tests.

Musculoskeletal

Tendinitis, tendon rupture, exacerbation of myasthenia gravis, elevated creatinine kinase (CK).

Nervous system/psychiatric

Polyneuropathy including Guillaine-Barré syndrome, confusion, paraesthesia, psychic disturbances including psychotic reactions, convulsions, tremors, myoclonus.

Haematological

Haemolytic anaemia, sometimes associated with glucose-6-phosphate dehydrogenase deficiency.

Genito-urinary

Vaginal candidiasis.

Renal function

Renal failure.

Special senses

Dysgeusia, visual disturbances.

Cardiovascular

Very rarely: prolonged QTc interval and ventricular arrhythmia (including torsade de pointes) may occur with some quinolones including norfloxacin.

4.9 Overdose
No information is available at present.

In the event of recent acute overdosage, the stomach should be emptied by induced vomiting or by gastric lavage and the patient carefully observed and given symptomatic and supportive treatment. Adequate hydration must be maintained.

5. PHARMACOLOGICAL PROPERTIES
Pharmacotherapeutic group: Fluoroquinolones

ATC code: J01 MA06

5.1 Pharmacodynamic properties
Mechanism of Action

Norfloxacin inhibits bacterial deoxyribonucleic acid synthesis and is bactericidal. At the molecular level, three specific events were attributed to norfloxacin in *Escherichia coli* cells:

(1) Inhibition of the ATP-dependent DNA supercoiling reaction catalysed by DNA gyrase

(2) Inhibition of the relaxation of supercoiled DNA

(3) Promotion of double-stranded DNA breakage.

'Utinor' has a broad spectrum of antibacterial activity against Gram-positive and Gram-negative aerobic pathogens. The fluorine atom at the 6 position provides increased potency against Gram-negative organisms and the piperazine moiety at the 7 position is responsible for the anti-pseudomonal activity.

Break points (NCCLS)

The general MIC susceptibility test breakpoints to separate susceptible (S) pathogens from resistant (R) pathogens are:

S ⩽ 4 mcg/mL, R ⩾ 16 mcg/mL.

For *Neisseria gonorrhoeae* MIC breakpoint not defined.

Susceptibility

The prevalence of resistance may vary geographically and with time for selected species and local information on resistance is desirable, particularly when treating severe infections. The information below gives only approximate guidance on the probability as to whether the microorganism will be susceptible to norfloxacin or not.

Organism	Prevalence of Resistance (Range) [European Union]
SUSCEPTIBLE	
Gram-positive aerobes:	
Bacillus cereus	
Enterococcus faecalis	13 to 64%
Group G streptococci	
Staphylococcus coag. Negative	0 to 80%
Staphylococcus aureus (Methicillin-sensitive strains only)	0 to 20%
Staphylococcus epidermidis (Methicillin-sensitive strains only)	7 to 22%
Staphylococcus saprophyticus (Methicillin-sensitive strains only)	0 to 17%
Streptococcus agalactiae	0 to 67%
Viridans group streptococci	
Gram-negative aerobes:	
Aeromonas hydrophilia	0 to 33%
Campylobacter fetus subsp. Jejuni	
Citrobacter koseri (formerly *Citrobacter diversus*)	0%
Citrobacter freundii	0 to 33%
Edwardsiella tarda	
Enterobacter aerogenes	0 to 67%
Enterobacter agglomerans	
Enterobacter cloacae	0 to 36%
Enterotoxigenic *Escherichia coli*	
Escherichia coli	0 to 75%
Hafnia alvei	0%
Haemophilus ducreyi	
Haemophilus influenzae	
Klebsiella oxytoca	0 to 27%
Klebsiella pneumoniae	0 to 13%
Morganella morganii	0 to 53%
*Neisseria gonorrhoeae**	
Plesiomonas shigelloides	
Proteus mirabilis	0 to 33%
Proteus vulgaris	0 to 7%
Providencia rettgeri	0 to 33%
Providencia stuartii	0 to 100%
Pseudomonas aeruginosa	0 to 47%
Pseudomonas cepacia	
Pseudomonas fluorescens	
Pseudomonas stutzeri	
Salmonella spp.	0 to 8%
Salmonella typhi	
Serratia marcescens	0 to 27%
Shigella spp.	0 to 17%
Shigella boydii	
Shigella dysenteriae	
Shigella flexneri	
Shigella sonnei	
Vibrio cholerae	
Vibrio parahaemolyticus	
Yersinia enterocolitica	
Other:	
Flavobacterium spp.	
Ureaplasma urealyticum	
RESISTANT	
Gram-positive aerobes:	
Enterococcus spp. (other than *E. faecalis*)	
Methicillin-resistant *Staphylococcus aureus*	
Methicillin-resistant *Staphylococcus epidermidis*	
Gram-negative aerobes:	
Acinetobacter spp.	
Acinetobacter baumannii	0 to 93%
Gram-positive anaerobes:	
Actinomyces spp.	
Clostridium spp (other than *C. perfringens*)	
Gram-negative anaerobes:	
Bacteroides spp.	
Fusobacterium spp.	

* Breakpoint not defined.

Mechanism/s of Resistance

The major mechanism of resistance to the quinolones, including norfloxacin, is through mutations in the genes that encode for DNA gyrase and topoisomerase IV, the targets of quinolone action. Additional mechanisms of resistance include mutations in the cell membrane proteins, which alter membrane permeability and the development of efflux pumps.

There is no cross-resistance between norfloxacin and structurally unrelated antibacterial agents such as penicillins, cephalosporins, tetracyclines, macrolides, aminocyclitols and sulfonamides, 2, 4 diaminopyrimidines, or combinations thereof (e.g. co-trimoxazole).

5.2 Pharmacokinetic properties
Norfloxacin is rapidly absorbed following oral administration. In healthy volunteers, at least 30-40% of an oral dose of norfloxacin is absorbed. This results in a serum concentration of 1.5 mcg/ml being attained approximately 1 hour after administration of a 400 mg dose. Mean serum half-life is 3 to 4 hours, and is independent of dose.

The following are mean concentrations of norfloxacin in various fluids and tissues measured 1 to 4 hours post-dose after the two 400 mg doses, unless otherwise indicated:

Renal parenchyma	7.3 mcg/g
Prostate	2.5 mcg/g
Seminal fluid	2.7 mcg/ml
Testicle	1.6 mcg/g

Uterus/cervix	3.0 mcg/g
Vagina	4.3 mcg/g
Fallopian tube	1.9 mcg/g
Bile	6.9 mcg/ml (after 2 × 200 mg doses).

Norfloxacin is eliminated through metabolism, biliary excretion and renal excretion. After a single 400 mg dose of norfloxacin, mean antimicrobial activities equivalent to 278, 773 and 82 mcg of norfloxacin/g of faeces were obtained at 12, 24 and 48 hours, respectively.

Renal excretion occurs by both glomerular filtration and net tubular secretion, as evidenced by the high rate of renal clearance (approximately 275 ml/min). After a single 400 mg dose, urinary concentrations reach a value of 200 or more mcg/ml in healthy volunteers and remain above 30 mcg/ml for at least 12 hours. In the first 24 hours, 33-48% of the drug is recovered in the urine.

Norfloxacin exists in the urine as norfloxacin and six active metabolites of lesser antimicrobial potency. The parent compound accounts for over 70% of total excretion. The bactericidal potency of norfloxacin is not affected by the pH of urine.

Protein binding is less than 15%.

5.3 Preclinical safety data

Norfloxacin, when administered to 3- to 5-month-old dogs at doses four or more times the usual human dose, produced blister formation and eventual erosion of the articular cartilage of the weight-bearing joints. Similar changes have been produced by other structurally related drugs. Dogs six months or older were not susceptible to these changes.

Teratology studies in mice and rats and fertility studies in mice at oral doses of 30 to 50 times the usual dose for humans did not reveal teratogenic or foetal toxic effects. Embryotoxicity was observed in rabbits at doses of 100 mg/kg/day. This was secondary to maternal toxicity and it is a non-specific antimicrobial effect in the rabbit due to an unusual sensitivity to antibiotic-induced changes in the gut microflora.

Although the drug was not teratogenic in cynomolgus monkeys at several times the therapeutic human dosage, an increased percentage of embryonic losses was observed.

6. PHARMACEUTICAL PARTICULARS

6.1 List of excipients

'Utinor' contains the following inactive ingredients:

Croscarmellose sodium USNF

Magnesium stearate Ph Eur

Microcrystalline cellulose Ph Eur

Hydroxypropylcellulose Ph Eur

Hypromellose Ph Eur

Titanium dioxide Ph Eur

Carnauba wax Ph Eur

6.2 Incompatibilities

None

6.3 Shelf life

36 months shelf-life for blister packs.

6.4 Special precautions for storage

Store below 25°C, in a dry place protected from light.

6.5 Nature and contents of container

'Utinor' is available as blister packs of 6 and 14 tablets.

6.6 Instructions for use and handling

None.

7. MARKETING AUTHORISATION HOLDER

Merck Sharp & Dohme Limited

Hertford Road, Hoddesdon, Hertfordshire EN11 9BU, UK

8. MARKETING AUTHORISATION NUMBER(S)

PL 0025/0254

9. DATE OF FIRST AUTHORISATION/RENEWAL OF THE AUTHORISATION

Authorisation first granted 3 August 1990. Licence last renewed 4 December 2001.

10. DATE OF REVISION OF THE TEXT

July 2004

® denotes registered trademark of Merck & Co., Inc., Whitehouse Station, NJ, USA.

SPC.NRX.02.UK.0850

Utovlan Tablets

(Pharmacia Limited)

1. NAME OF THE MEDICINAL PRODUCT

Utovlan.

2. QUALITATIVE AND QUANTITATIVE COMPOSITION OF THE FINISHED PRODUCT

Each tablet contains 5mg norethisterone Ph Eur.

For excipients see Section 6.1.

3. PHARMACEUTICAL FORM

White, flat, circular, bevel-edged tablet inscribed 'SEARLE' on one side and 'U' on the other.

4. CLINICAL PARTICULARS

4.1 Therapeutic indications

At low dose: Dysfunctional uterine bleeding, endometriosis, polymenorrhoea, menorrhagia, metropathia, haemorrhagia, postponement of menstruation and premenstrual syndrome.

At high dose: Disseminated carcinoma of the breast.

4.2 Posology and method of administration

Oral Administration

Low dose

Dysfunctional uterine bleeding, polymenorrhoea, menorrhagia, dysmenorrhoea and metropathia haemorrhagia: 1 tablet three times daily for 10 days; bleeding usually stops within 48 hours. Withdrawal bleeding resembling true menstruation occurs a few days after the end of treatment. One tablet twice daily, from days 19 to 26 of the two subsequent cycles, should be given to prevent recurrence of the condition.

Endometriosis: 1 tablet three times daily for a minimum treatment period of six months. The dosage should be increased to 4 or 5 tablets a day if spotting occurs. The initial dosage should be resumed when bleeding or spotting stops.

Postponement of menstruation: 1 tablet three times daily, starting three days before the expected onset of menstruation. Menstruation usually follows within three days of finishing the treatment.

Pre-menstrual syndrome: 1 tablet daily from days 16 to 25 of the menstrual cycle.

High dose

For disseminated breast carcinoma the starting dose is 8 tablets (40mg) per day increasing to 12 tablets (60mg) if no regression is noted.

4.3 Contraindications

Pregnancy

Previous idiopathic or current venous thromboembolism (deep vein thrombosis, pulmonary embolism)

Active or recent arterial thromboembolic disease (e.g. angina, myocardial infarction)

Disturbance of liver function

History during pregnancy of idiopathic jaundice

Severe pruritus or pemphigoid gestationis

Undiagnosed irregular vaginal bleeding

Porphyria

Known hypersensitivity to norethisterone or any of the excipients

4.4 Special warnings and special precautions for use

If menstrual bleeding should fail to follow a course of Utovlan, the possibility of pregnancy must be excluded before a further course is given.

Therapy should be discontinued if the following occur:

- Jaundice or deterioration in liver function
- Significant increase in blood pressure
- New onset of migraine-type headache

Progestogens may cause fluid retention. Special care should be taken when prescribing norethisterone in patients with conditions which might be aggravated by this factor:

- Epilepsy
- Migraine
- Asthma
- Cardiac dysfunction
- Renal dysfunction

Risk of venous thromboembolism (VTE)

Long term use of low dose progestogens as part of combined oral contraception or combined hormone replacement therapy has been associated with an increased risk of venous thromboembolism, although the role of progestogens in this aetiology is uncertain. A patient who develops symptoms suggestive of thromboembolic complications should have her status and need for treatment carefully assessed before continuing therapy.

Any patient who develops an acute impairment of vision, proptosis, diplopia or migraine headache should be carefully evaluated ophthalmologically to exclude papilloedema or retinal vascular lesions before continuing medication.

Generally recognised risk factors for VTE include a personal history or family history, severe obesity (BMI > 30 kg/m^2) and systemic lupus erythematosus (SLE). There is no consensus about the possible role of varicose veins in VTE.

Treatment with steroid hormones may add to these risk factors. Personal or strong family history of thromboembolism or recurrent spontaneous abortion should be investigated in order to exclude a thrombophillic predisposition. Until a thorough evaluation of thrombophillic factors has been made or anticoagulant treatment initiated, use of progestogens in these patients should be viewed as contraindicated. Where a patient is already taking anticoagulants, the risks and benefits of progestogen therapy should be carefully considered.

The risk of VTE may be temporarily increased with prolonged immobilisation, major trauma or major surgery. As in all post-operative patients, scrupulous attention should be given to prophylactic measures to prevent VTE. Where prolonged immobilisation is likely to follow elective surgery, particularly abdominal or orthopaedic surgery to the lower limbs, consideration should be given to stopping progestogen therapy 4-6 weeks pre-operatively. Treatment should not be restarted until the patient is fully remobilised.

If VTE develops after initiating therapy the drug should be withdrawn. Patients should be advised to contact their doctor immediately if they become aware of a potential thromboembolic symptom (e.g., painful swelling in the leg, sudden pain in the chest, dyspnoea).

4.5 Interaction with other medicinal products and other forms of Interaction

Interaction with other medicines

The metabolism of progestogens may be increased by concommitant administration of compounds known to induce drug-metabolising enzymes, specifically cytochrome P450 enzymes. These compopunds include anticonvulsants (e.g., phenobarbital, phenytoin, carbamezapin) and anti-infectives (e.g., rifampicin, rifabutin, nevirapine, efavirenz, tetracyclines, ampicillin, oxacillin and cotrimoxazole)

Ritonavir and nelfinavir, although known as strong inhibitors, by contrast exhibit inducing properties when used concomitantly with steroid hormones. Herbal preparations containing St John's Wort (Hypericum Perforatum) may induce the metabolism of progestogens. Progestogen levels may therefore be reduced.

Aminoglutethimide has been reported to decrease plasma levels of some progestogens.

Concurrent administration of cyclosporin and norethisterone has been reported to lead to increased plasma cyclosporin levels and/or decreased plamsa norethisterone levels.

When used in combination with cytotoxic drugs, it is possible that progestogens may reduce the haematological toxicity of chemotherapy.

Special care should be taken when progestogens are administered with other drugs which also cause fluid retention, such as NSAIDs and vasodilators.

Other forms of interaction

Progestogens can influence certain laboratory tests (e.g., tests for hepatic function, thyroid function and coagulation).

4.6 Pregnancy and lactation

Contra-indicated in pregnancy.

4.7 Effects on ability to drive and use machines

None.

4.8 Undesirable effects

Progestogens given alone at low doses have been associated with the following undesirable effects:

Genitourinary	breakthrough bleeding, spotting, amenorrhoea, abnormal uterine bleeding, (irregular, increase, decrease), alterations of cervical secretions, cervical erosions, prolonged anovulation
Breast	Galactorrhoea, mastodynia, tenderness
Central Nervous System	depression, headache, dizziness, fatigue, insomnia, nervousness, somnolence, confusion, euphoria, loss of concentration, vision disorders
Gastrointestinal/ Hepatobiliary	nausea, vomiting, cholestatic icterus/ jaundice, constipation, diarrhoea, dry mouth, disturbed liver function
Metabolic & Nutritional	altered serum lipid and lipoprotein profiles, increased fasting glucose levels, increased fasting insulin levels, decreased glucose tolerance, adrenergic-like effects (e.g., fine hand tremors, sweating, cramps in calves at night), corticoid-like effects (e.g., Cushingoid syndrome), diabetic cataract, exacerbation of diabetes mellitus, glycosuria
Cardiovascular	thrombo-embolic disorders, cerebral and myocardial infarction, congestive heart failure, increased blood pressure, palpitations, pulmonary embolism, retinal thrombosis, tachycardia, thrombophlebitis

Skin & Mucous Membranes	acne, hirsutism, alopecia, pruritis, rash, urticaria
Allergy	hypersensitivity reactions (e.g., anaphylaxis & anaphylactoid reactions, angioedema)
Miscellaneous	oedema/fluid retention, bloating, weight gain, pyrexia, change in appetite, change in libido, hypercalcaemia, malaise

4.9 Overdose
Overdosage may be manifested by nausea, vomiting, breast enlargement and later vaginal bleeding. There is no specific antidote and treatment should be symptomatic.

Gastric lavage may be employed if the overdosage is large and the patient is seen sufficiently early (within four hours).

5. PHARMACOLOGICAL PROPERTIES
Pharmotherapeutic group (ATC code) L02A B.

5.1 Pharmacodynamic properties
Norethisterone given at intermediate doses (5-10mg) suppresses ovulation via its effect on the pituitary. The endogenous production of oestrogens and progesterones are also suppressed, and the ectopic endometrium is converted to a decidua resembling that of pregnancy. In carcinoma norethisterone may act by pituitary inhibition or by direct action on tumour deposits.

5.2 Pharmacokinetic properties
Norethisterone is rapidly and completely absorbed after oral administration, peak plasma concentration occurring in the majority of subjects between 1 and 3 hours. Due to first-pass metabolism, blood levels after oral administration are 60% of those after i.v. administration. The half life of elimination varies from 5 to 12 hours, with a mean of 7.6 hours. Norethisterone is metabolised mainly in the liver. Approximately 60% of the administered dose is excreted as metabolites in urine and faeces.

5.3 Preclinical safety data
The toxicity of norethisterone is very low. Reports of teratogenic effects in animals are uncommon. No carcinogenic effects have been found even in long-term studies.

6. PHARMACEUTICAL PARTICULARS

6.1 List of excipients
maize starch

polyvidone

magnesium stearate

lactose

6.2 Incompatibilities
None stated.

6.3 Shelf life
The shelf life of Utovlan tablets is 3 years.

6.4 Special precautions for storage
Store in a dry place, below 25°C, away from direct sunlight.

6.5 Nature and contents of container
Utovlan tablets are supplied in pvc/foil blister packs of 30 and 90 tablets.

6.6 Instructions for use and handling
None.

7. MARKETING AUTHORISATION HOLDER
Pharmacia Limited

Davy Avenue, Milton Keynes

MK5 8PH, UK

8. MARKETING AUTHORISATION NUMBER(S)
PL 00032/0423

9. DATE OF FIRST AUTHORISATION/RENEWAL OF THE AUTHORISATION
15th July 2002/15th February 2003

10. DATE OF REVISION OF THE TEXT
June 2003

Vagifem

(Novo Nordisk Limited)

1. NAME OF THE MEDICINAL PRODUCT

Vagifem

2. QUALITATIVE AND QUANTITATIVE COMPOSITION

Active ingredient: Estradiol 25 micrograms

3. PHARMACEUTICAL FORM

Film-coated vaginal tablet inset in disposable applicator.

4. CLINICAL PARTICULARS

4.1 Therapeutic indications

The treatment of atrophic vaginitis due to oestrogen deficiency.

4.2 Posology and method of administration

4.2.1 Dosage

Vagifem is administered intravaginally using the applicator. An initial dose of one tablet daily for two weeks will usually improve vaginal atrophy and associated symptoms; a maintenance dose of two tablets per week may then be instituted. Treatment should be discontinued after about three months to assess whether further therapy is necessary.

Not intended for children or males.

Use in the elderly: there are no special dosage requirements.

4.2.2 Administration

The applicator is inserted into the vagina up to the end of the smooth part of the applicator (approximately 9 cms). The tablet is released by pressing the plunger. The applicator is then withdrawn and disposed of.

4.3 Contraindications

1 Known, suspected or past history of carcinoma of the breast.

2 Known or suspected oestrogen-dependent neoplasia, eg endometrial carcinoma or other hormone-dependent tumours.

3 Abnormal genital bleeding of unknown aetiology.

4 Active deep venous thrombosis, thromboembolic disorders or a history of confirmed venous thromboembolism. See Warnings and Precautions number 6.

4.4 Special warnings and special precautions for use

1. Assessment of each woman prior to taking hormone replacement therapy (and at regular intervals thereafter) should include a personal and family medical history. Physical examination should be guided by this and by the contraindications (section 4.3) and warnings (section 4.4) for this product. During assessment of each individual woman clinical examination of the breasts and pelvic examination should be performed where clinically indicated rather than as a routine procedure. Women should be encouraged to participate in the national breast cancer screening programme (mammography) and the national cervical cancer screening programme (cervical cytology) as appropriate for their age. Breast awareness should also be encouraged and women advised to report any changes in their breasts to their doctor or nurse.

2. Vaginal infections should be treated before initiation of Vagifem therapy.

3. Although the dose of oestradiol is low and the treatment is local, a minor degree of systemic absorption may occur. Because of this, the increased risk of endometrial cancer after treatment with unopposed oestrogens should be kept in mind. Endometrial hyperplasia (atypical or adenomatous) often precedes endometrial cancer.

4. Persistent or recurring vaginal bleeding should be investigated.

5. A reanalysis of original data from 51 epidemiological studies reported a small or moderate increase in the probability of having breast cancer *diagnosed* in women currently or recently using HRT. The findings may be due to biological effects of HRT, earlier diagnosis, or a combination of both. The relative risk increased with duration of treatment (by 2.3% per year of use) and returned to normal in the course of five years after cessation of HRT use. This is comparable to the increase in relative risk when natural menopause is delayed in the absence of HRT. Breast cancers diagnosed in current or recent users of HRT are more likely to be localised to the breast than those found in non-users. HRT use may not be associated with increased mortality from breast cancer.

Between the ages of 50 and 70, about 45 women in every 1000 not using HRT will have breast cancer diagnosed. It is estimated that among those who use HRT for 5 years starting at age 50, 2 extra cases of breast cancer will be detected by age 70 in every 1000 women. For those who use HRT for 10 years there will be 6 extra cases of breast cancer, and for 15 years use, 12 extra cases of breast cancer in every 1000 women during the 20 year period until age 70.

It is important that the increased risk of being diagnosed with breast cancer is discussed with the patient and weighed against the known benefits of HRT.

6. Epidemiological studies have suggested that hormone replacement therapy (HRT) is associated with a higher relative risk of developing venous thromboembolism (VTE), i.e. deep vein thrombosis or pulmonary embolism. The studies find a 2-3 fold higher risk for users compared with non-users which for healthy women amounts to one extra case of VTE each year for every 5000 patients taking HRT.

Generally recognised risk factors for VTE include a personal or family history and severe obesity (Body Mass Index > 30 kg/m^2). In women with these factors the benefits of treatment with HRT need to be carefully weighed against risks. There is no consensus about the possible role of varicose veins in VTE.

The risk of VTE may be temporarily increased with prolonged immobilisation, major trauma or major surgery. In women on HRT scrupulous attention should be given to prophylactic measures to prevent VTE following surgery. Where prolonged immobilisation is liable to follow elective surgery, particularly abdominal or orthopaedic surgery to the lower limbs, consideration should be given to temporarily stopping HRT four weeks earlier, if possible.

If venous thromboembolism develops after initiating therapy the drug should be discontinued.

7. Patients with the following conditions who are treated with Vagifem should be monitored more frequently and if any of the conditions worsen Vagifem treatment should be withdrawn:

- Acute or chronic liver disease or history of liver disease where the liver function tests have failed to return to normal.
- Thrombophlebitis, thromboembolic disorders, or cerebro vascular accident, or a past history of these disorders.
- Haemoglobinopathies or sickle cell anaemia.
- Porphyria.
- Epilepsy.
- Migraine.
- Diabetes.
- Asthma
- Cardiac dysfunction
- Hypertension requiring treatment.

4.5 Interaction with other medicinal products and other forms of Interaction

Not applicable due to the low systemic absorption.

4.6 Pregnancy and lactation

Vagifem is contra-indicated in pregnant women.

4.7 Effects on ability to drive and use machines

No effects known.

4.8 Undesirable effects

Few side effects have been observed. Slight vaginal bleeding, vaginal discharge and skin rash have rarely been reported.

4.9 Overdose

Vagifem is intended for intravaginal use. The dose of oestradiol is so low that a considerable number of tablets would have to be ingested to approach a significant dose.

5. PHARMACOLOGICAL PROPERTIES

5.1 Pharmacodynamic properties

17-β oestradiol is the principal and most active of the naturally occurring human oestrogens. It has pharmacological actions in common with all oestrogenic compounds. The action on the vagina is to increase maturation of vaginal epithelial cells and increase cervical secretory activity.

5.2 Pharmacokinetic properties

Oestrogens are well absorbed from the vagina. After treatment with Vagifem, marginal elevations of plasma oestradiol and conjugated oestrogens as well as suppression of pituitary gonadotrophins have been observed. This indicates that there is an absorption of the oestradiol. This absorption is, however, low and no other systemic oestrogen effect could be determined.

6. PHARMACEUTICAL PARTICULARS

6.1 List of excipients

Methyl hydroxypropyl cellulose (E464)

Lactose

Maize starch

Magnesium stearate

Polyethylene glycol 6000

Purified water

6.2 Incompatibilities

None known

6.3 Shelf life

36 months

6.4 Special precautions for storage

Store in a dry place, protect from light. Store below 25°C. Do not refrigerate.

6.5 Nature and contents of container

Laminated bubble strips containing 5 applicators with inset tablet. Packed in cartons containing 3 strips (15 tablets and applicators).

6.6 Instructions for use and handling

Each carton contains a patient information leaflet with instructions for use.

7. MARKETING AUTHORISATION HOLDER

Novo Nordisk A/S

Novo Alle

DK-2880 Bagsvaerd

Denmark

The registered office in the UK is:-

Novo Nordisk Limited

Broadfield Park

Crawley

West Sussex

RH11 9RT

Tel: (01293) 613555

8. MARKETING AUTHORISATION NUMBER(S)

PL 4668/0026

9. DATE OF FIRST AUTHORISATION/RENEWAL OF THE AUTHORISATION

First authorised August 1990.

Authorisation renewed August 1995.

10. DATE OF REVISION OF THE TEXT

August 1995, April 2001

LEGAL CATEGORY

Prescription only medicine (POM)

Valcyte

(Roche Products Limited)

1. NAME OF THE MEDICINAL PRODUCT

Valcyte® ▼ 450mg film-coated tablets.

2. QUALITATIVE AND QUANTITATIVE COMPOSITION

Each tablet contains 496.3mg of valganciclovir hydrochloride equivalent to 450mg of valganciclovir (as free base).

For excipients, see section *6.1*.

3. PHARMACEUTICAL FORM

Film-coated tablet.

Pink, convex oval film-coated tablet, with "VGC" embossed on one side and "450" on the other side.

4. CLINICAL PARTICULARS

4.1 Therapeutic indications

Valcyte is indicated for the induction and maintenance treatment of cytomegalovirus (CMV) retinitis in patients with acquired immunodeficiency syndrome (AIDS).

Valcyte is indicated for the prevention of CMV disease in CMV-negative patients who have received a solid organ transplant from a CMV-positive donor.

4.2 Posology and method of administration

Caution – Strict adherence to dosage recommendations is essential to avoid overdose; see section *4.4 Special warnings and precautions for use* and section *4.9 Overdose*.

Valganciclovir is rapidly and extensively metabolised to ganciclovir after oral dosing. Oral valganciclovir 900mg b.i.d. is therapeutically equivalent to intravenous ganciclovir 5mg/kg b.i.d.

Standard dosage in adults

Induction treatment of CMV retinitis:

For patients with active CMV retinitis, the recommended dose is 900mg valganciclovir (two Valcyte 450mg tablets) twice a day for 21 days and, whenever possible, taken with food. Prolonged induction treatment may increase the risk of bone marrow toxicity (see section *4.4 Special warnings and precautions for use*).

Maintenance treatment of CMV retinitis:

Following induction treatment, or in patients with inactive CMV retinitis, the recommended dose is 900mg valganciclovir (two Valcyte 450mg tablets) once daily and, whenever possible, taken with food. Patients whose retinitis worsens may repeat induction treatment; however, consideration should be given to the possibility of viral drug resistance.

Prevention of CMV disease in solid organ transplantation:

For patients who have received a transplant, the recommended dose is 900mg (two Valcyte 450mg tablets) once daily, starting within 10 days of transplantation and continuing until 100 days post-transplantation. Whenever possible, the tablets should be taken with food.

Special dosage instructions

Patients with renal impairment:

Serum creatinine levels or creatinine clearance should be monitored carefully. Dosage adjustment is required according to creatinine clearance, as shown in the table below (see section *4.4 Special warnings and precautions for use* and section *5.2 Pharmacokinetic properties*).

An estimated creatinine clearance (mL/min) can be related to serum creatinine by the following formulae:

$$\text{For males} = \frac{(140 - \text{age[years]}) \times (\text{body weight [kg]})}{(72) \times (0.011 \times \text{serum creatinine [micromol/ L]})}$$

$$\text{For females} = 0.85 \times \text{male value}$$

CrCl (mL/min)	Induction dose of valganciclovir	Maintenance/ Prevention dose of valganciclovir
⩾ 60	900mg (2 tablets) twice daily	900mg (2 tablets) once daily
40 – 59	450mg (1 tablet) twice daily	450mg (1 tablet) once daily
25 – 39	450mg (1 tablet) once daily	450mg (1 tablet) every 2 days
10 – 24	450mg (1 tablet) every 2 days	450mg (1 tablet) twice weekly

Patients undergoing haemodialysis:

For patients on haemodialysis (CrCl < 10mL/min) a dose recommendation cannot be given. Thus Valcyte should not be used in these patients (see section *4.4 Special warnings and precautions for use* and section *5.2 Pharmacokinetic properties*).

Patients with hepatic impairment:

Safety and efficacy of Valcyte tablets have not been studied in patients with hepatic impairment (see section *5.2 Pharmacokinetic properties*).

Paediatric patients:

Safety and efficacy have not been established in this patient population (see section *4.4 Special warnings and precautions for use* and section *5.3 Preclinical safety data*).

Elderly patients:

Safety and efficacy have not been established in this patient population.

Patients with severe leucopenia, neutropenia, anaemia, thrombocytopenia and pancytopenia: see section *4.4 Special warnings and precautions for use* before initiation of therapy.

If there is a significant deterioration of blood cell counts during therapy with Valcyte, treatment with haematopoietic growth factors and/or dose interruption should be considered (see section *4.4 Special warnings and precautions for use* and section *4.8 Undesirable effects*).

Method of administration

Valcyte is administered orally, and whenever possible, should be taken with food (see section *5.2 Pharmacokinetic properties, Absorption*).

The tablets should not be broken or crushed. Since Valcyte is considered a potential teratogen and carcinogen in humans, caution should be observed in handling broken tablets (see section *4.4 Special warnings and precautions for use*). Avoid direct contact of broken or crushed tablets with skin or mucous membranes. If such contact occurs, wash thoroughly with soap and water, rinse eyes thoroughly with sterile water, or plain water if sterile water is unavailable.

4.3 Contraindications

Valcyte is contra-indicated in patients with hypersensitivity to valganciclovir, ganciclovir or to any of the excipients.

Due to the similarity of the chemical structure of Valcyte and that of aciclovir and valaciclovir, a cross-hypersensitivity reaction between these drugs is possible. Therefore, Valcyte is contra-indicated in patients with hypersensitivity to aciclovir and valaciclovir.

Valcyte is contra-indicated during lactation, refer to section *4.6 Pregnancy and lactation*.

4.4 Special warnings and special precautions for use

Prior to the initiation of valganciclovir treatment, patients should be advised of the potential risks to the foetus. In animal studies, ganciclovir was found to be mutagenic, teratogenic, aspermatogenic and carcinogenic, and a suppressor of female fertility. Valcyte should, therefore, be considered a potential teratogen and carcinogen in humans with the potential to cause birth defects and cancers (see section *5.3 Preclinical safety data*). It is also considered likely that Valcyte causes temporary or permanent inhibition of spermatogenesis. Women of child bearing potential must be advised to use effective contraception during treatment. Men must be advised to practise barrier contraception during treatment, and for at least 90 days thereafter, unless it is certain that the female partner is not at risk of pregnancy (see section *4.6 Pregnancy and lactation*, section *4.8 Undesirable effects* and section *5.3 Preclinical safety data*).

The use of Valcyte in children and adolescents is not recommended because the pharmacokinetic characteristics of Valcyte have not been established in these patient populations (see section *4.2 Posology and method of administration*). Furthermore, valganciclovir has the potential to cause carcinogenicity and reproductive toxicity in the long term.

Severe leucopenia, neutropenia, anaemia, thrombocytopenia, pancytopenia, bone marrow depression and aplastic anaemia have been observed in patients treated with Valcyte (and ganciclovir). Therapy should not be initiated if the absolute neutrophil count is less than 500 cells/μL, or the platelet count is less than 25000/μL, or the haemoglobin level is less than 8g/dL (see section *4.2 Posology and method of administration* and section *4.8 Undesirable effects*).

Valcyte should be used with caution in patients with pre-existing haematological cytopenia or a history of drug-related haematological cytopenia and in patients receiving radiotherapy.

It is recommended that complete blood counts and platelet counts be monitored during therapy. Increased haematological monitoring may be warranted in patients with renal impairment. In patients developing severe leucopenia, neutropenia, anaemia and/or thrombocytopenia, it is recommended that treatment with haematopoietic growth factors and/or dose interruption be considered (see section *4.2 Posology and method of administration, Special dosage instructions* and section *4.8 Undesirable effects*).

The bioavailability of ganciclovir after a single dose of 900mg valganciclovir is approximately 60%, compared with approximately 6% after administration of 1000mg oral ganciclovir (as capsules). Excessive exposure to ganciclovir may be associated with life-threatening adverse reactions. Therefore, careful adherence to the dose recommendations is advised when instituting therapy, when switching from induction to maintenance therapy, and in patients who may switch from oral ganciclovir to valganciclovir as Valcyte cannot be substituted for ganciclovir capsules on a one-to-one basis. Patients switching from ganciclovir capsules should be advised of the risk of overdosage if they take more than the prescribed number of Valcyte tablets (see section *4.2 Posology and method of administration* and section *4.9 Overdose*).

In patients with impaired renal function, dosage adjustments based on creatinine clearance are required (see section *4.2 Posology and method of administration, Special dosage instructions* and section *5.2 Pharmacokinetic properties, Pharmacokinetics in special populations*).

Valcyte should not be used in patients on haemodialysis (see section 4.2 *Posology and method of administration, Special dosage instructions* and section 5.2 *Pharmacokinetic properties, Pharmacokinetics in special populations*).

Convulsions have been reported in patients taking imipenem-cilastatin and ganciclovir. Valcyte should not be used concomitantly with imipenem-cilastatin unless the potential benefits outweigh the potential risks (see section *4.5 Interaction with other medicinal products and other forms of interaction*).

Patients treated with Valcyte and (a) didanosine, (b) drugs that are known to be myelosuppressive (e.g. zidovudine), or (c) substances affecting renal function, should be closely monitored for signs of added toxicity (see section *4.5 Interaction with other medicinal products and other forms of interaction*).

The controlled clinical study using valganciclovir for the prophylactic treatment of CMV disease in transplantation, as detailed in section 5.1 *Pharmacodynamic properties, Clinical efficacy*, did not include lung and intestinal transplant patients. Therefore, experience in these transplant patients is limited.

4.5 Interaction with other medicinal products and other forms of Interaction

Drug interactions with valganciclovir

In-vivo drug interaction studies with Valcyte have not been performed. Since valganciclovir is extensively and rapidly metabolised to ganciclovir; drug interactions associated with ganciclovir will be expected for valganciclovir.

Drug interactions with ganciclovir

Imipenem-cilastatin

Convulsions have been reported in patients taking ganciclovir and imipenem-cilastatin concomitantly. These drugs should not be used concomitantly unless the potential benefits outweigh the potential risks (see section *4.4 Special warnings and precautions for use*).

Probenecid

Probenecid given with oral ganciclovir resulted in statistically significantly decreased renal clearance of ganciclovir (20%) leading to statistically significantly increased exposure (40%). These changes were consistent with a mechanism of interaction involving competition for renal tubular secretion. Therefore, patients taking probenecid and Valcyte should be closely monitored for ganciclovir toxicity.

Zidovudine

When zidovudine was given in the presence of oral ganciclovir there was a small (17%), but statistically significant increase in the AUC of zidovudine. There was also a trend towards lower ganciclovir concentrations when administered with zidovudine, although this was not statistically significant. However, since both zidovudine and ganciclovir have the potential to cause neutropenia and anaemia, some patients may not tolerate concomitant therapy at full dosage (see section *4.4 Special warnings and precautions for use*).

Didanosine

Didanosine plasma concentrations were found to be consistently raised when given with ganciclovir (both intravenous and oral). At ganciclovir oral doses of 3 and 6g/day, an increase in the AUC of didanosine ranging from 84 to 124% has been observed, and likewise at intravenous doses of 5 and 10mg/kg/day, an increase in the AUC of didanosine ranging from 38 to 67% has been observed. There was no clinically significant effect on ganciclovir concentrations. Patients should be closely monitored for didanosine toxicity (see section *4.4 Special warnings and precautions for use*).

Mycophenolate Mofetil

Based on the results of a single dose administration study of recommended doses of oral mycophenolate mofetil (MMF) and intravenous ganciclovir and the known effects of renal impairment on the pharmacokinetics of MMF and ganciclovir, it is anticipated that co-administration of these agents (which have the potential to compete for renal tubular secretion) will result in increases in phenolic glucuronide of mycophenolic acid (MPAG) and ganciclovir concentration. No substantial alteration of mycophenolic acid (MPA) pharmacokinetics is anticipated and MMF dose adjustment is not required. In patients with renal impairment to whom MMF and ganciclovir are co-administered, the dose recommendation of ganciclovir should be observed and the patients monitored carefully. Since both MMF and ganciclovir have the potential to cause neutropenia and leucopenia, patients should be monitored for additive toxicity.

Zalcitabine

No clinically significant pharmacokinetic changes were observed after concomitant administration of ganciclovir and zalcitabine. Both valganciclovir and zalcitabine have the potential to cause peripheral neuropathy and patients should be monitored for such events.

Stavudine

No clinically significant interactions were observed when stavudine and oral ganciclovir were given in combination.

Trimethoprim

No clinically significant pharmacokinetic interaction was observed when trimethoprim and oral ganciclovir were given in combination. However, there is a potential for toxicity to be enhanced since both drugs are known to be myelosuppressive and therefore both drugs should be used concomitantly only if the potential benefits outweigh the risks.

Other antiretrovirals

At clinically relevant concentrations, there is unlikely to be either a synergistic or antagonistic effect on the inhibition of either HIV in the presence of ganciclovir or CMV in the presence of a variety of antiretroviral drugs. Metabolic interactions with, for example, protease inhibitors and non-nucleoside reverse transcriptase inhibitors (NNRTIs) are unlikely due to the lack of P450 involvement in the metabolism of either valganciclovir or ganciclovir.

Other potential drug interactions

Toxicity may be enhanced when valganciclovir is co-administered with, or is given immediately before or after, other drugs that inhibit replication of rapidly dividing cell populations such as occur in the bone marrow, testes and germinal layers of the skin and gastrointestinal mucosa. Examples of these types of drugs are dapsone, pentamidine, flucytosine, vincristine, vinblastine, adriamycin, amphotericin B, trimethoprim/sulpha combinations, nucleoside analogues and hydroxyurea.

Since ganciclovir is excreted through the kidney (section 5.2), toxicity may also be enhanced during co-administration of valganciclovir with drugs that might reduce the renal clearance of ganciclovir and hence increase its exposure. The renal clearance of ganciclovir might be inhibited by two mechanisms: (a) nephrotoxicity, caused by drugs such as cidofovir and foscarnet, and (b) competitive inhibition of active tubular secretion in the kidney by, for example, other nucleoside analogues.

Therefore, all of these drugs should be considered for concomitant use with valganciclovir only if the potential benefits outweigh the potential risks (see section *4.4 Special warnings and precautions for use*).

4.6 Pregnancy and lactation

There are no data from the use of Valcyte in pregnant women. Its active metabolite, ganciclovir, readily diffuses across the human placenta. Based on its pharmacological mechanism of action and reproductive toxicity observed in animal studies with ganciclovir (see section 5.3 *Preclinical* safety data) there is a theoretical risk of teratogenicity in humans.

Valcyte should not be used in pregnancy unless the therapeutic benefit for the mother outweighs the potential risk of teratogenic damage to the child.

Women of child-bearing potential must be advised to use effective contraception during treatment. Male patients must be advised to practise barrier contraception during, and for at least 90 days following treatment with Valcyte unless it is certain that the female partner is not at risk of pregnancy (see section *5.3 Preclinical safety data*).

It is unknown if ganciclovir is excreted in breast milk, but the possibility of ganciclovir being excreted in the breast milk and causing serious adverse reactions in the nursing infant cannot be discounted. Therefore, breast-feeding must be discontinued.

4.7 Effects on ability to drive and use machines

No studies on the effects on ability to drive and use machines have been performed.

Convulsions, sedation, dizziness, ataxia, and/or confusion have been reported with the use of Valcyte and/or ganciclovir. If they occur, such effects may affect tasks requiring alertness, including the patient's ability to drive and operate machinery.

4.8 Undesirable effects

Valganciclovir is a prodrug of ganciclovir, which is rapidly and extensively metabolised to ganciclovir after oral administration. The undesirable effects known to be associated with ganciclovir usage can be expected to occur with valganciclovir. All of the undesirable effects observed in valganciclovir clinical studies have been previously observed with ganciclovir. The most commonly reported adverse drug reactions following administration of valganciclovir are neutropenia, anaemia and diarrhoea.

The oral formulations, valganciclovir and ganciclovir, are associated with a higher risk of diarrhoea compared to intravenous ganciclovir. In addition, valganciclovir is associated with a higher risk of neutropenia and leucopenia compared to oral ganciclovir.

Severe neutropenia (< 500 ANC/μL) is seen more frequently in CMV retinitis patients undergoing treatment with valganciclovir than in solid organ transplant patients receiving valganciclovir or oral ganciclovir.

The frequency of adverse reactions reported in clinical trials with either valganciclovir, oral ganciclovir, or intravenous ganciclovir is presented in the table below. The adverse reactions listed were reported in clinical trials in patients with AIDS for the induction or maintenance treatment of CMV retinitis, or in liver, kidney or heart transplant patients for the prophylaxis of CMV disease. The term (severe) in parenthesis in the table indicates that the adverse reaction has been reported in patients at both mild/moderate intensity and severe/life-threatening intensity at that specific frequency.

Infections and infestations:	
Common (≥ 1/100, <1/10):	oral candidiasis, sepsis (bacteraemia, viraemia), cellulitis, urinary tract infection.
Blood and lymphatic system disorders:	
Very common (≥ 1/10):	(severe) neutropenia, anaemia.
Common (≥ 1/100, <1/10):	severe anaemia, (severe) thrombocytopenia, (severe) leucopenia, (severe) pancytopenia.
Uncommon (≥ 1/1000, <1/100):	bone marrow depression.
Immune system disorders:	
Uncommon (≥ 1/1000, <1/100):	anaphylactic reaction.
Metabolic and nutrition disorders:	
Common (≥ 1/100, <1/10)	appetite decreased, anorexia.
Psychiatric disorders:	
Common (≥ 1/100, <1/10):	depression, anxiety, confusion, abnormal thinking.
Uncommon (≥ 1/1000, <1/100):	agitation, psychotic disorder.
Nervous system disorders:	
Common (≥ 1/100, <1/10):	headache, insomnia, dysgeusia (taste disturbance), hypoaesthesia, paraesthesia, peripheral neuropathy, dizziness (excluding vertigo), convulsions.
Uncommon (≥ 1/1000, <1/100):	tremor.
Eye disorders:	
Common (≥ 1/100, <1/10):	macular oedema, retinal detachment, vitreous floaters, eye pain.
Uncommon (≥ 1/1000, <1/100):	vision abnormal, conjunctivitis.
Ear and labyrinth disorders:	
Common (≥ 1/100, <1/10):	ear pain.
Uncommon (≥ 1/1000, <1/100):	deafness.
Cardiac disorders:	
Uncommon (≥ 1/1000, <1/100):	arrhythmias.
Vascular disorders:	
Uncommon (≥ 1/1000, <1/100):	hypotension.
Respiratory, thoracic and mediastinal disorders:	
Very common (≥ 1/10):	dyspnoea.
Common (≥ 1/100, <1/10):	cough.
Gastrointestinal disorders:	
Very common (≥ 1/10):	diarrhoea.
Common (≥ 1/100, <1/10):	nausea, vomiting, abdominal pain, abdominal pain upper, dyspepsia, constipation, flatulence, dysphagia.
Uncommon (≥ 1/1000, <1/100):	abdominal distention, mouth ulcerations, pancreatitis.
Hepato-biliary disorders:	
Common (≥ 1/100, <1/10):	(severe) hepatic function abnormal, blood alkaline phosphatase increased, aspartate aminotransferase increased.
Uncommon (≥ 1/1000, <1/100):	alanine aminotransferase increased.
Skin and subcutaneous disorders:	
Common (≥ 1/100, <1/10):	dermatitis, night sweats, pruritus.
Uncommon (≥ 1/1000, <1/100):	alopecia, urticaria, dry skin.
Musculoskeletal, connective tissue and bone disorders:	
Common (≥ 1/100, <1/10):	back pain, myalgia, arthralgia, muscle cramps.
Renal and urinary disorders:	
Common (≥ 1/100, <1/10):	creatinine clearance renal decreased, renal impairment.
Uncommon (≥ 1/1000, <1/100):	haematuria, renal failure.
Reproductive system and breast disorders:	
Uncommon (≥ 1/1000, <1/100):	male infertility.
General disorders and administration site conditions:	
Common (≥ 1/100, <1/10):	fatigue, pyrexia, rigors, pain, chest pain, malaise, asthenia.
Investigations:	
Common (≥ 1/100, <1/10):	weight decreased, blood creatinine increased.

4.9 Overdose

Overdose experience with Valganciclovir

One adult developed fatal bone marrow depression (medullary aplasia) after several days of dosing that was at least 10-fold greater than recommended for the patient's degree of renal impairment (decreased creatinine clearance).

It is expected that an overdose of valganciclovir could also possibly result in increased renal toxicity (see section *4.2 Posology and method of administration* and section *4.4 Special warnings and precautions for use*).

Haemodialysis and hydration may be of benefit in reducing blood plasma levels in patients who receive an overdose of valganciclovir (see section *5.2 Pharmacokinetic properties, Patients undergoing haemodialysis*).

Overdose experience with intravenous ganciclovir

Reports of overdoses with intravenous ganciclovir have been received from clinical trials and during post-marketing experience. In some of these cases no adverse events were reported. The majority of patients experienced one or more of the following adverse events:

- *Haematological toxicity*: pancytopenia, bone marrow depression, medullary aplasia, leucopenia, neutropenia, granulocytopenia.
- *Hepatotoxicity*: hepatitis, liver function disorder.
- *Renal toxicity*: worsening of haematuria in a patient with pre-existing renal impairment, acute renal failure, elevated creatinine.
- *Gastrointestinal toxicity*: abdominal pain, diarrhoea, vomiting.
- *Neurotoxicity*: generalised tremor, convulsion.

5. PHARMACOLOGICAL PROPERTIES

5.1 Pharmacodynamic properties

Pharmacotherapeutic group: ATC code: J05A B14 (anti-infectives for systemic use, antivirals for systemic use, direct acting antivirals).

Mechanism of action:

Valganciclovir is an L-valyl ester (prodrug) of ganciclovir. After oral administration, valganciclovir is rapidly and extensively metabolised to ganciclovir by intestinal and hepatic esterases. Ganciclovir is a synthetic analogue of 2'-deoxyguanosine and inhibits replication of herpes viruses *in vitro* and *in vivo*. Sensitive human viruses include human cytomegalovirus (HCMV), herpes simplex virus-1 and -2 (HSV-1 and HSV-2), human herpes virus -6, -7 and -8 (HHV-6, HHV-7, HHV8), Epstein-Barr virus (EBV), varicella-zoster virus (VZV) and hepatitis B virus (HBV).

In CMV-infected cells, ganciclovir is initially phosphorylated to ganciclovir monophosphate by the viral protein kinase, pUL97. Further phosphorylation occurs by cellular kinases to produce ganciclovir triphosphate, which is then slowly metabolised intracellularly. Triphosphate metabolism has been shown to occur in HSV- and HCMV- infected cells with half-lives of 18 and between 6 and 24 hours respectively, after the removal of extracellular ganciclovir. As the phosphorylation is largely dependent on the viral kinase, phosphorylation of ganciclovir occurs preferentially in virus-infected cells.

The virustatic activity of ganciclovir is due to inhibition of viral DNA synthesis by: (a) competitive inhibition of incorporation of deoxyguanosine-triphosphate into DNA by viral DNA polymerase, and (b) incorporation of ganciclovir triphosphate into viral DNA causing termination of, or very limited, further viral DNA elongation.

Antiviral Activity

The in-vitro anti-viral activity, measured as IC_{50} of ganciclovir against CMV, is in the range of 0.08μM (0.02μg/mL) to 14μM (3.5μg/mL).

The clinical antiviral effect of Valcyte has been demonstrated in the treatment of AIDS patients with newly diagnosed CMV retinitis (Clinical trial WV15376). CMV shedding was decreased in urine from 46% (32/69) of patients at study entry to 7% (4/55) of patients following four weeks of Valcyte treatment.

Clinical efficacy

Treatment of CMV retinitis:

Patients with newly diagnosed CMV retinitis were randomised in one study to induction therapy with either Valcyte 900mg b.i.d or intravenous ganciclovir 5mg/kg b.i.d. The proportion of patients with photographic progression of CMV retinitis at week 4 was comparable in both treatment groups, 7/70 and 7/71 patients progressing in the intravenous ganciclovir and valganciclovir arms respectively.

Following induction treatment dosing, all patients in this study received maintenance treatment with Valcyte given at the dose of 900mg daily. The mean (median) time from randomisation to progression of CMV retinitis in the group receiving induction and maintenance treatment with Valcyte was 226 (160) days and in the group receiving induction treatment with intravenous ganciclovir and maintenance treatment with Valcyte was 219 (125) days.

Prevention of CMV disease in transplantation:

A double-blind, double-dummy clinical active comparator study has been conducted in heart, liver and kidney transplant patients (lung and gastro-intestinal transplant patients were not included in the study) at high-risk of CMV disease (D+/R-) who received either Valcyte (900mg od) or oral ganciclovir (1000mg tid) starting within 10 days of transplantation until Day 100 post-transplant. The incidence of CMV disease (CMV syndrome + tissue invasive disease) during the first 6 months post-transplant was 12.1% in the Valcyte arm (n=239) compared with 15.2% in the oral ganciclovir arm (n=125). The large majority of cases occurred following cessation of prophylaxis (post-Day 100) with cases in the valganciclovir arm occurring on average later than those in the oral ganciclovir arm. The incidence of acute rejection in the first 6 months was 29.7% in patients randomised to valganciclovir compared with 36.0% in the oral ganciclovir arm, with the incidence of graft loss being equivalent, occurring in 0.8% of patients, in each arm.

Viral Resistance

Virus resistant to ganciclovir can arise after chronic dosing with valganciclovir by selection of mutations in the viral kinase gene (UL97) responsible for ganciclovir monophosphorylation and/or the viral polymerase gene (UL54). Viruses containing mutations in the UL97 gene are resistant to ganciclovir alone, whereas viruses with mutations in the UL54 gene are resistant to ganciclovir but may show cross-resistance to other antivirals that also target the viral polymerase.

Treatment of CMV retinitis:

Genotypic analysis of CMV in polymorphonuclear leucocytes (PMNL) isolates from 148 patients with CMV retinitis enrolled in one clinical study has shown that 2.2%, 6.5%, 12.8%, and 15.3% contain UL97 mutations after 3, 6, 12 and 18 months, respectively, of valganciclovir treatment.

Prevention of CMV disease in transplantation:

Resistance was studied by genotypic analysis of CMV in PMNL samples collected i) on Day 100 (end of study drug prophylaxis) and ii) in cases of suspected CMV disease up to 6 months after transplantation. From the 245 patients randomised to receive valganciclovir, 198 Day 100 samples were available for testing and no ganciclovir resistance mutations were observed. This compares with 2 ganciclovir resistance mutations detected in the 103 samples tested (1.9%) for patients in the oral ganciclovir comparator arm.

Of the 245 patients randomised to receive valganciclovir, samples from 50 patients with suspected CMV disease were tested and no resistance mutations were observed. Of the 127 patients randomised on the ganciclovir comparator arm, samples from 29 patients with suspected CMV disease were tested, from which two resistance

Table 1

Parameter	Ganciclovir (5mg/kg, i.v.) n = 18	Valganciclovir (900mg, p.o.) n = 25	
		Ganciclovir	Valganciclovir
AUC(0 - 12 h) (μg.h/ml)	28.6 ± 9.0	32.8 ± 10.1	0.37 ± 0.22
C_{max} (μg/ml)	10.4 ± 4.9	6.7 ± 2.1	0.18 ± 0.06

mutations were observed, giving an incidence of resistance of 6.9%.

5.2 Pharmacokinetic properties

The pharmacokinetic properties of valganciclovir have been evaluated in HIV- and CMV-seropositive patients, patients with AIDS and CMV retinitis and in solid organ transplant patients.

Absorption

Valganciclovir is a prodrug of ganciclovir. It is well absorbed from the gastrointestinal tract and rapidly and extensively metabolised in the intestinal wall and liver to ganciclovir. Systemic exposure to valganciclovir is transient and low. The absolute bioavailability of ganciclovir from valganciclovir is approximately 60% across all the patient populations studied and the resultant exposure to ganciclovir is similar to that after its intravenous administration (please see below). For comparison, the bioavailability of ganciclovir after administration of 1000mg oral ganciclovir (as capsules) is 6 - 8%.

Valganciclovir in HIV+, CMV+ patients:

Systemic exposure of HIV+, CMV+ patients after twice daily administration of ganciclovir and valganciclovir for one week is:

(see Table 1 above)

The efficacy of ganciclovir in increasing the time-to-progression of CMV retinitis has been shown to correlate with systemic exposure (AUC).

Valganciclovir in solid organ transplant patients:

Steady state systemic exposure of solid organ transplant patients to ganciclovir after daily oral administration of ganciclovir and valganciclovir is:

Parameter	Ganciclovir (1000mg tid.) n = 82	Valganciclovir (900mg, od) n = 161
		Ganciclovir
AUC(0 - 24 h) (μg.h/ml)	28.0 ± 10.9	46.3 ± 15.2
C_{max} (μg/ml)	1.4 ± 0.5	5.3 ± 1.5

The systemic exposure of ganciclovir to heart, kidney and liver transplant recipients was similar after oral administration of valganciclovir according to the renal function dosing algorithm.

Food effect:

Dose proportionality with respect to ganciclovir AUC following administration of valganciclovir in the dose range 450 to 2625mg was demonstrated only under fed conditions. When valganciclovir was given with food at the recommended dose of 900mg, higher values were seen in both mean ganciclovir AUC (approximately 30%) and mean ganciclovir C_{max} values (approximately 14%) than in the fasting state. Also, the inter-individual variation in exposure of ganciclovir decreases when taking Valcyte with food. Valcyte has only been administered with food in clinical studies. Therefore, it is recommended that Valcyte be administered with food (see section *4.2 Posology and method of administration*).

Distribution:

Because of rapid conversion of valganciclovir to ganciclovir, protein binding of valganciclovir was not determined. Plasma protein binding of ganciclovir was 1 - 2% over concentrations of 0.5 and 51μg/mL. The steady state volume of distribution of ganciclovir after intravenous administration was 0.680 ± 0.161 L/kg (n=114).

Metabolism

Valganciclovir is rapidly and extensively metabolised to ganciclovir; no other metabolites have been detected. No metabolite of orally administered radiolabelled ganciclovir (1000mg single dose) accounted for more than 1 - 2% of the radioactivity recovered in the faeces or urine.

Elimination

Following dosing with Valcyte, renal excretion, as ganciclovir, by glomerular filtration and active tubular secretion is the major route of elimination of valganciclovir. Renal clearance accounts for 81.5% ± 22% (n=70) of the systemic clearance of ganciclovir. The half-life of ganciclovir from valganciclovir is 4.1 ± 0.9 hours in HIV- and CMV-seropositive patients.

Pharmacokinetics in special clinical situations

Patients with renal impairment

Decreasing renal function resulted in decreased clearance of ganciclovir from valganciclovir with a corresponding increase in terminal half-life. Therefore, dosage adjustment is required for renally impaired patients (see section *4.2 Posology and method of administration* and section *4.4 Special warnings and precautions for use*).

Patients undergoing haemodialysis

For patients receiving haemodialysis dose recommendations for Valcyte 450mg film-coated tablets cannot be given. This is because an individual dose of Valcyte required for these patients is less than the 450mg tablet strength. Thus, Valcyte should not be used in these patients (see section *4.2 Posology and method of administration* and section *4.4 Special warnings and precautions for use*).

Patients with hepatic impairment

The safety and efficacy of Valcyte tablets have not been studied in patients with hepatic impairment. Hepatic impairment should not affect the pharmacokinetics of ganciclovir since it is excreted renally and, therefore, no specific dose recommendation is made.

5.3 Preclinical safety data

Valganciclovir is a pro-drug of ganciclovir and therefore effects observed with ganciclovir apply equally to valganciclovir. Toxicity of valganciclovir in pre-clinical safety studies was the same as that seen with ganciclovir and was induced at ganciclovir exposure levels comparable to, or lower than, those in humans given the induction dose.

These findings were gonadotoxicity (testicular cell loss) and nephrotoxicity (uraemia, cell degeneration), which were irreversible; myelotoxicity (anaemia, neutropenia, lymphocytopenia) and gastrointestinal toxicity (mucosal cell necrosis), which were reversible.

Further studies have shown ganciclovir to be mutagenic, carcinogenic, teratogenic, embryotoxic, aspermatogenic (i.e. impairs male fertility) and to suppress female fertility.

6. PHARMACEUTICAL PARTICULARS

6.1 List of excipients

Tablet core	Tablet film-coat
Povidone K30	Opadry Pink YS-1-14519A containing:
Crospovidone	Hypromellose
Microcrystalline cellulose	Titanium dioxide (E171)
Stearic acid	Macrogol 400
	Red iron oxide (E172)
	Polysorbate 80

6.2 Incompatibilities

Not applicable.

6.3 Shelf life

3 years.

6.4 Special precautions for storage

No special precautions for storage.

6.5 Nature and contents of container

High density polyethylene (HDPE) bottle, with child-resistant polypropylene closure, and cotton pad enclosed.

60 tablets.

6.6 Instructions for use and handling

Any unused product or waste material should be disposed of in accordance with local requirements.

7. MARKETING AUTHORISATION HOLDER

Roche Products Limited, 40 Broadwater Road, Welwyn Garden City, Hertfordshire, AL7 3AY, UK.

8. MARKETING AUTHORISATION NUMBER(S)

PL 00031/0599

9. DATE OF FIRST AUTHORISATION/RENEWAL OF THE AUTHORISATION

April 2002

10. DATE OF REVISION OF THE TEXT

June 2003

P232029/603

Vallergan Tablets, Syrup, Forte Syrup

(sanofi-aventis)

1. NAME OF THE MEDICINAL PRODUCT

Vallergan tablets 10mg

Vallergan Forte Syrup

Vallergan Syrup

2. QUALITATIVE AND QUANTITATIVE COMPOSITION

Vallergan tablets 10mg: Alimemazine tartrate 10mg

Vallergan Forte Syrup: Alimemazine tartrate 30mg per 5ml

Vallergân Syrup: Alimemazine tartrate 7.5mg per 5ml

For a full list of excipients, see section 6.1

3. PHARMACEUTICAL FORM

Vallergan tablets 10mg: Circular, film coated biconvex tablet with bevelled edge, dark blue in colour, one face impressed V/10. The reverse side is plain

Vallergan Forte Syrup: Syrup

Vallergan Syrup: Syrup

4. CLINICAL PARTICULARS

4.1 Therapeutic indications

Vallergan has a central sedative effect comparable to that of chlorpromazine but largely devoid of the latter's anti adrenaline action. It has powerful antihistamine and anti-emetic actions. In the management of urticaria and pruritus.

In pre-medication as a sedative before anaesthesia in children aged between 2 to 7 years.

4.2 Posology and method of administration

The product is administered orally

Not recommended for infants less than 2 years old.

Urticaria and pruritus

Adults: 10mg two or three times daily; up to 100mg per day have been used in intractable cases.

Elderly: Dosage should be reduced to 10mg once or twice daily.

Children over

2 years of age: The use of Vallergan Syrup is recommended. 2.5-5 mg (approx. 1.7 – 3.3ml) three or four times daily

As a sedative before anaesthesia

The dosage for children is best achieved by use of Vallergan Syrup. Children aged 2-7 years: the maximum dosage recommended is 2mg (approx. 1.3ml) per kg bodyweight 1-2 hours before the operation.

4.3 Contraindications

Vallergan should be avoided in patients with hepatic or renal dysfunction, epilepsy, Parkinson's disease, hypothyroidism, phaeochromocytoma, myasthenia gravis, prostatic hypertrophy. It should be avoided in patients known to be hypersensitive to phenothiazines or to any of the excipients or with history of narrow angle glaucoma.

4.4 Special warnings and special precautions for use

Vallergan should be used with caution in:

- elderly or volume depleted patients who are more susceptible to orthostatic hypotension (see section 4.8)
- Elderly patients presenting chronic constipation (risk of paralytic ileus),
- Elderly patients with possible prostatic hypertrophy (see section 4.3);
- Elderly patients in hot and cold weather (risk of hyper/hypothermia) (see section 4.8)
- patients with certain cardiovascular diseases, due to the tachycardia-inducing and hypotensive effects of phenothiazines (see section 4.8)

Patients are strongly advised not to consume alcoholic beverages or medicines containing alcohol throughout treatment (see section 4.5 Interactions).

Exposure to sunlight should be avoided during treatment. (see section 4.8)

There is a risk of post-operative restlessness especially if the child is in pain.

4.5 Interaction with other medicinal products and other forms of Interaction

The sedative effects of phenothiazines may be intensified (additively) by alcohol (see section 4.4), anxiolytics & hypnotics, opiates, barbiturates and other sedatives. There may be increased antimuscarinic and sedative effects of phenothiazines with tricyclic antidepressants & MAOI's (including moclobemide). Respiratory depression may occur.

The hypotensive effect of most antihypertensive drugs especially alpha adrenoreceptor blocking agents may be exaggerated by phenothiazines. The use of antimuscarinics will increase the risk of antimuscarinic side effects when in conjunction with antihistamines.

The mild anticholinergic effect of phenothiazines may be enhanced by other anticholinergic drugs possibly leading to constipation, heat stroke, etc

The action of some drugs may be opposed by phenothiazines; these include amfetamine, levodopa, clonidine, guanethidine, adrenaline.

Anticholinergic agents may reduce the antipsychotic effect of phenothiazines.

Some drugs interfere with absorption of phenothiazines: antacids, anti-Parkinson, lithium. Increases or decreases in the plasma concentrations of a number of drugs, eg propranolol, phenobarbital have been observed but were not of clinical significance.

High doses of phenothiazines reduce the response to hypoglycaemic agents, the dosage of which may have to be raised. Adrenaline must not be used in patients overdosed with phenothiazines.

4.6 Pregnancy and lactation
There is inadequate evidence of the safety of Vallergan in human pregnancy, but it has been widely used for many years without apparent ill consequence. Some phenothiazines have shown evidence of harmful effects in animals. Vallergan, like other drugs, should be avoided in pregnancy unless the physician considers it essential. Neuroleptics may occasionally prolong labour and at such a time should be withheld until the cervix is dilated 3-4cm. Possible adverse effects on the neonate include lethargy or paradoxical hyperexcitability, tremor and low Apgar score. Phenothiazines may be excreted in milk: breast feeding should be suspended during treatment.

4.7 Effects on ability to drive and use machines
Patients should be warned about drowsiness during the early days of treatment, and advised not to drive or operate machinery.

4.8 Undesirable effects
Minor side-effects are nasal stuffiness, dry mouth, insomnia, agitation.

Liver function: Jaundice, usually transient, occurs in a very small percentage of patients. A premonitory sign may be a sudden onset of fever after one to three weeks of treatment followed by the development of jaundice. Neuroleptic jaundice has the biochemical and other characteristics of obstructive jaundice and is associated with obstructions of the canaliculi by bile thrombi; the frequent presence of an accompanying eosinophilia indicates the allergic nature of this phenomenon. Treatment should be withheld on the development of jaundice.

Cardiorespiratory: hypotension, or pallor may occur in children. Elderly or volume depleted subjects are particularly susceptible to postural hypotension (see section 4.4).

Cardiac arrhythmias, including atrial arrhythmia. A-V block, ventricular tachycardia and fibrillation have been reported during therapy, possibly related to dosage. Pre-existing cardiac disease, old age, hypokalaemia and concurrent tricyclic antidepressants may predispose. ECG changes, usually benign, include widened QT interval, ST depression, U-waves and T-wave changes.

Respiratory depression is possible in susceptible patients.

Blood picture: A mild leukopaenia occurs in up to 30% of patients on prolonged high dosage. Agranulocytosis may occur rarely; it is not dose related. The occurrence of unexplained infections or fever requires immediate haematological investigation.

Extrapyramidal: Acute dystonias or dyskinesias, usually transitory are commoner in children and young adults and usually occur within the first 4 days of treatment or after dosage increases.

- akathisia characteristically occurs after large doses.

- Parkinsonism is commoner in adults and the elderly. It usually develops after weeks or months of treatment. One or more of the following may be seen: tremor, rigidity, akinesia or other features of Parkinsonism. Commonly just tremor.

- tardive dyskinesia: If this occurs it is usually, but not necessarily, after prolonged or high dosage. It can even occur after treatment has been stopped. Dosage should therefore be kept low whenever possible.

Skin and eyes: contact skin sensitisation is a serious but rare complication in those frequently handling preparations of phenothiazines: Care must be taken to avoid contact of the drug with the skin. Skin rashes of various kinds may also be seen in patients treated with the drug. Patients on high dosage may develop photosensitivity in sunny weather and should avoid exposure to direct sunlight (see section 4.4). Ocular changes and the development of a metallic greyish-mauve colouration of exposed skin have been noted in some individuals, mainly females, who have received chlorpromazine continuously for long periods (four to eight years).

Endocrine: hyperprolactinaemia which may result in galactorrhoea, gynaecomastia, amenorrhoea: impotence.

Neuroleptic malignant syndrome (hyperthermia, rigidity, autonomic dysfunction and altered consciousness) may occur.

Paradoxical excitement has been noted.

4.9 Overdose
Symptoms of phenothiazine overdosage include drowsiness or loss of consciousness, hypotension, tachycardia, ECG changes, ventricular arrhythmias and hypothermia. Severe extra-pyramidal dyskinesias may occur.

If the patient is seen sufficiently soon (up to 6 hours) after ingestion of a toxic dose, gastric lavage may be attempted. Pharmacological induction of emesis is unlikely to be of any use. Activated charcoal should be given. There is no specific antidote. Treatment is supportive.

Generalised vasodilatation may result in circulatory collapse; Raising the patient's legs may suffice, in severe cases, volume expansion by intravenous fluids may be needed; infusion fluids should be warmed before administration in order not to aggravate hypothermia.

Positive inotropic agents such as dopamine may be tried if fluid replacement is insufficient to correct the circulatory collapse. Peripheral vasoconstrictor agents are not generally recommended; avoid the use of adrenaline.

Ventricular or supraventricular tachy-arrhythmias usually respond to restoration of normal body temperature and correction of circulatory or metabolic disturbances. If persistent or life-threatening, appropriate anti-arrhythmic therapy may be considered. Avoid lidocaine and, as far as possible, long acting anti-arrhythmic drugs.

Pronounced central nervous system depression requires airway maintenance or, in extreme circumstances, assisted respiration. Severe dystonic reactions, usually respond to procyclidine (5-10mg) or orphenadrine (20-40mg) administered intramuscularly or intravenously. Convulsions should be treated with intravenous diazepam.

Neuroleptic malignant syndrome should be treated with cooling. Dantrolene sodium may be tried.

5. PHARMACOLOGICAL PROPERTIES
5.1 Pharmacodynamic properties
Antihistamines for Systemic Use, Phenothiazine derivatives (R06AD01)

Alimemazine has a central sedative effect, comparable to that of chlorpromazine, but largely devoid of the latter's anti-adrenaline action. It has powerful antihistamine and anti-emetic actions.

5.2 Pharmacokinetic properties
There is little information about blood levels, distribution and excretion in humans. The rate of metabolism and excretion of phenothiazines decreases in old age.

5.3 Preclinical safety data
There are no pre-clinical data of relevance to the prescriber which are additional to that already included in other sections of the SPC

6. PHARMACEUTICAL PARTICULARS
6.1 List of excipients
Vallergan tablets 10mg: Microcrystalline cellulose, Lactose spray dried, Colloidal Silicone Dioxide, Magnesium stearate, Sodium starch glycollate, Hydroxypropyl Methylcellulose, Polyethylene glycol 200, Blue opaspray M-1-4229 (purified water, Indigo Carmine, Titanium Dioxide, Industrial Methylated Spirits 74 OP, Hydroxypropyl methylcellulose), Demineralised water

Vallergan Forte Syrup: Sucrose, Apricot Flavour no. 1 NS, Ethanol 96% v/v, Citric acid anhydrous, Sodium citrate gran., Sodium benzoate, Sodium sulphite anhydrous, Sodium metabisulphite powder, L(+) Ascorbic acid, Demineralised water

Vallergan Syrup: Sucrose, Apricot Flavour no. 1 NS, Ethanol 96% v/v, Caramel HT, Citric acid anhydrous, Sodium citrate gran, Sodium benzoate, Sodium sulphite anhydrous, Sodium metabisulphite powder, L(+) Ascorbic acid, Demineralised water

6.2 Incompatibilities
None stated

6.3 Shelf life
Vallergan Tablets: 36 months

Vallergan Syrup and Forte Syrup: 36 months unopened

1 month after first opening.

Diluted product shelf life 28 days.

6.4 Special precautions for storage
Protect from light.

Vallergan Tablets: Store below 30 °C

Vallergan Syrup and Forte Syrup: Store below 25 °C.

6.5 Nature and contents of container
Vallergan tablets 10mg: PVDC coated uPVC/Al foil blister pack containing 28 tablets

Vallergan Forte Syrup: Glass bottle 100ml

Vallergan Syrup: Glass bottle 100ml

6.6 Instructions for use and handling
Not applicable

7. MARKETING AUTHORISATION HOLDER
Castlemead Healthcare Limited

20 Clanwilliam Terrace

Dublin 2

Ireland

8. MARKETING AUTHORISATION NUMBER(S)
Vallergan tablets 10mg: PL 16946/0009

Vallergan Forte Syrup: PL 16946/0011

Vallergan Syrup: PL16946/0010

9. DATE OF FIRST AUTHORISATION/RENEWAL OF THE AUTHORISATION
September 1998

10. DATE OF REVISION OF THE TEXT
July 2005

Legal category: POM

Valoid Injection

(Amdipharm)

1. NAME OF THE MEDICINAL PRODUCT
Valoid Injection

2. QUALITATIVE AND QUANTITATIVE COMPOSITION
Cyclizine Base B.P. 3.735 w/v

3. PHARMACEUTICAL FORM
Injection

4. CLINICAL PARTICULARS
4.1 Therapeutic indications
Valoid is indicated for the prevention and treatment of nausea and vomiting including motion sickness, nausea and vomiting caused by narcotic analgesics and by general anaesthetics in the post-operative period and radiotherapy, especially for breast cancer since cyclizine does not elevate prolactin levels.

Valoid may be of value in relieving vomiting and attacks of vertigo associated with Meniere's disease and other forms of vestibular disturbance when the oral route cannot be used.

Valoid injection, by the intravenous route, is also indicated pre-operatively in patients undergoing emergency surgery in order to reduce the hazard of regurgitation and aspiration of gastric contents during induction of general anaesthesia.

4.2 Posology and method of administration
Adults
50mg intramuscularly or intravenously up to three times daily.

When used intravenously, Valoid should be injected slowly into the bloodstream, with only minimal withdrawal of blood into the syringe.

For the prevention of postoperative nausea and vomiting, administer the first dose by slow intravenous injection 20 minutes before the anticipated end of surgery.

Cyclizine given intravenously, in half the recommended dose, increases the lower oesophageal sphincter tone and thereby reduces the hazard of regurgitation and aspiration of gastric contents if given to patients, undergoing emergency surgery, before induction of general anaesthesia.

Use in the Elderly
There have been no specific studies of Valoid in the elderly. Experience has indicated that normal adult dosage is appropriate.

4.3 Contraindications
Valoid should not be given to individuals with known hypersensitivity to cyclizine.

4.4 Special warnings and special precautions for use
As with other anticholinergic agents, Valoid should be used with caution and appropriate monitoring in patients with glaucoma, obstructive disease of the gastrointestinal tract and in males with possible prostatic hypertrophy. Valoid injection, may have a hypotensive effect.

Cyclizine should be used with caution in patients with severe heart failure. In such patients, cyclizine may cause a fall in cardiac output associated with increases in heart rate, mean arterial pressure and pulmonary wedge pressure.

There have been no specific studies in hepatic and/or renal dysfunction.

4.5 Interaction with other medicinal products and other forms of Interaction
Valoid may have additive effects with alcohol and other central nervous system depressants e.g. hypnotics, tranquillisers. Valoid enhances the soporific effect of pethidine. Because of its anticholinergic activity, cyclizine may enhance the side-effects of other anticholinergic drugs.

4.6 Pregnancy and lactation
Some animal studies are interpreted as indicating that cyclizine may be teratogenic.

In the absence of any definitive human data, the use of Valoid in pregnancy is not advised.

It is not known whether cyclizine or its metabolite are excreted in human milk.

4.7 Effects on ability to drive and use machines
Although studies designed to detect drowsiness did not reveal sedation in healthy adults who took a single oral therapeutic dose (50mg) of cyclizine, sedation of short duration was reported by subjects receiving intravenous cyclizine. Patients should not drive or operate machinery until they have determined their own response.

Although there are no data available, patients should be cautioned that Valoid may have additive effects with alcohol and other central nervous system depressants, e.g. hypnotics and tranquillisers.

4.8 Undesirable effects

Urticaria, drug rash, drowsiness, dryness of the mouth, nose and throat, blurred vision, tachycardia, urinary retention, constipation, restlessness, nervousness, insomnia and auditory and visual hallucinations have been reported, particularly when dosage recommendations have been exceeded. Other Central Nervous System effects which have been reported rarely include dystonia, dyskinesia, extrapyramidal motor disturbances, tremor, twitching, muscle spasms, convulsions, disorientation, dizziness, decreased consciousness and transient speech disorders. Cholestatic jaundice has occurred in association with cyclizine.

Injection site reactions including vein tracking, erythema, pain and thrombophlebitis have been reported rarely.

Single case reports have been documented of fixed drug eruption, generalised chorea, hypersensitivity, hepatitis and agranulocytosis.

A single case of anaphylaxis has been recorded following intravenous administration of cyclizine co-administered with propanidid in the same syringe.

4.9 Overdose

Symptoms

Symptoms of acute toxicity from cyclizine arise from peripheral anticholinergic effects and effects on the central nervous system.

Peripheral anticholinergic symptoms include, dry mouth, nose and throat, blurred vision, tachycardia and urinary retention. Central nervous system effects include drowsiness, dizziness, incoordination, ataxia, weakness, hyperexcitability, disorientation, impaired judgement, hallucinations, hyperkinesia, extrapyramidal motor disturbances, convulsions, hyperpyrexia and respiratory depression.

An oral dose of 5mg/kg is likely to be associated with at least one of the clinical symptoms stated above. Younger children are more susceptible to convulsions. The incidence of convulsions, in children less than 5 years, is about 60% when the oral dose ingested exceeds 40mg/kg.

Treatment

In the management of acute overdosage with Valoid, gastric lavage and supportive measures for respiration and circulation should be performed if necessary. Convulsions should be controlled in the usual way with parenteral anticonvulsant therapy.

5. PHARMACOLOGICAL PROPERTIES

5.1 Pharmacodynamic properties

Cyclizine is a histamine H_1 receptor antagonist of the piperazine class which is characterised by a low incidence of drowsiness. It possesses anticholingergic and antiemetic properties. The exact mechanism by which cyclizine can prevent or suppress both nausea and vomiting from various causes is unknown. Cyclizine increases lower oesophageal sphincter tone and reduces the sensitivity of the labyrinthine apparatus. It may inhibit the part of the midbrain known collectively as the emetic centre.

5.2 Pharmacokinetic properties

In healthy adult volunteers the administration of a single oral dose of 50mg cyclizine resulted in a peak plasma concentration of approximately 70ng/ml occurring at about 2 hours after drug administration. The plasma elimination half life was approximately 20 hours.

Cyclizine produces its antiemetic effect within 2 hours and lasts approximately 4 hours.

The N-demethylated derivative, norcyclizine, has been identified as a metabolite of cyclizine. Norcyclizine has little antihistaminic (H_1) activity compared to cyclizine and has a plasma elimination half life of approximately 20 hours. After a single dose of 50mg cyclizine given to a single adult male volunteer, urine collected over the following 24 hours contained less than 1% of the total dose administered.

5.3 Preclinical safety data

A. Mutagenicity

Cyclizine was not mutagenic in a full Ames test, including use of S9-microsomes.

B. Carcinogencity

No long term studies have been conducted in animals to determine whether cyclizine has a potential for carcinogenesis.

C. Teratogenicity

Some animal studies are interpreted as indicating that cyclizine may be teratogenic.

D. Fertility

In a study involving prolonged administration of cyclizine to male and female rats there was no evidence of impaired fertility after continuous treatment for 90-100 days. There is no experience of the effect of Valoid on human fertility.

6. PHARMACEUTICAL PARTICULARS

6.1 List of excipients

Lactic Acid

Water for Injections

6.2 Incompatibilities

None stated.

6.3 Shelf life

48 months

6.4 Special precautions for storage

Store below 25°C

Protect from Light

6.5 Nature and contents of container

1ml neutral glass ampoules. 5 ampoules in a carton.

6.6 Instructions for use and handling

No special instructions.

7. MARKETING AUTHORISATION HOLDER

Amdipharm PLC

Trading as Amdipharm

Regency House

Miles Gray Road

Basildon

Essex

SS14 3AF

United Kingdom

8. MARKETING AUTHORISATION NUMBER(S)

PL 20072/0010

9. DATE OF FIRST AUTHORISATION/RENEWAL OF THE AUTHORISATION

1 December 2003

10. DATE OF REVISION OF THE TEXT

October 2004

Valoid Tablets

(Amdipharm)

1. NAME OF THE MEDICINAL PRODUCT

Valoid Tablets

2. QUALITATIVE AND QUANTITATIVE COMPOSITION

Cyclizine hydrochloride BP 50.0 mg per tablet.

3. PHARMACEUTICAL FORM

Tablet

4. CLINICAL PARTICULARS

4.1 Therapeutic indications

Valoid is indicated for the prevention and treatment of nausea and vomiting including motion sickness, nausea and vomiting caused by narcotic analgesics and by general anaesthetics in the post-operative period and radiotherapy, especially for breast cancer since cyclizine does not elevate prolactin levels.

Valoid may be of value in relieving vomiting and attacks of vertigo associated with Meniere's disease and other forms of vestibular disturbance.

4.2 Posology and method of administration

Route of administration: oral

Adults and Children over 12 Years:

One tablet up to three times daily.

Children 6 – 12 Years:

Half a tablet up to three times daily.

Under 6 Years:

Formulation not applicable.

Use in the Elderly:

There have been no specific studies of Valoid in the elderly. Experience has indicated that normal adult dosage is appropriate.

4.3 Contraindications

Valoid should not be given to individuals with known hypersensitivity to cyclizine.

4.4 Special warnings and special precautions for use

As with other anticholinergic agents, Valoid should be used with caution and appropriate monitoring in patients with glaucoma, obstructive disease of the gastrointestinal tract and in males with possible prostatic hypertrophy.

Cyclizine should be used with caution in patients with severe heart failure. In such patients, cyclizine may cause a fall in cardiac output associated with increases in heart rate, mean arterial pressure and pulmonary wedge pressure.

There have been no specific studies in hepatic and/or renal dysfunction.

Cyclizine was not mutagenic in a full Ames test, including use of S9-microsomes.

No long-term studies have been conducted in animals to determine whether cyclizine has a potential for carcinogenesis.

4.5 Interaction with other medicinal products and other forms of Interaction

Valoid may have additive effects with alcohol and other central nervous system depressants e.g. hypnotics, tranquillisers. Valoid enhances the soporific effect of pethidine. Because of its anticholinergic activity cyclizine may enhance the side-effects of other anticholinergic drugs.

4.6 Pregnancy and lactation

Some animal studies are interpreted as indicating that cyclizine may be teratogenic.

In a study involving prolonged administration of cyclizine to male and female rats there was no evidence of impaired fertility after continuous treatment for 90 to 100 days. There is no experience of the effect of Valoid on human fertility.

In the absence of any definitive human data, the use of Valoid in pregnancy is not advised.

It is not known whether cyclizine or its metabolite are excreted in human milk.

4.7 Effects on ability to drive and use machines

Studies designed to detect drowsiness did not reveal sedation in healthy adults who took a single oral therapeutic dose (50 mg) of cyclizine.

Patients should not drive or operate machinery until they have determined their own response.

Although there are no data available, patients should be cautioned that Valoid may have additive effects with alcohol and other central nervous system depressants, e.g. hypnotics and tranquillisers.

4.8 Undesirable effects

Urticaria, drug rash, drowsiness, dryness of the mouth, nose and throat, blurred vision, tachycardia, urinary retention, constipation, restlessness, nervousness, insomnia and auditory and visual hallucinations have been reported, particularly when dosage recommendations have been exceeded. Other Central Nervous System effects which have been recorded rarely include dystonia, dyskinesia, extrapyramidal motor disturbances, tremor, twitching, muscle spasms, convulsions, disorientation, dizziness, decreased consciousness and transient speech disorders. Cholestatic jaundice has occurred in association with cyclizine. Single case reports have been documented of fixed drug eruption, generalised chorea, hypersensitivity hepatitis and agranulocytosis.

4.9 Overdose

Symptoms: Symptoms of acute toxicity from cyclizine arise from peripheral anticholinergic effects and effects on the central nervous system.

Peripheral anticholinergic symptoms include, dry mouth, nose and throat, blurred vision, tachycardia and urinary retention. Central nervous system effects include drowsiness, dizziness, inco-ordination, ataxia, weakness, hyperexcitability, disorientation, impaired judgement, hallucinations, hyperkinesia, extrapyramidal motor disturbances, convulsions, hyperpyrexia and respiratory depression.

An oral dose of 5 mg/kg is likely to be associated with at least one of the clinical symptoms stated above. Younger children are more susceptible to convulsions. The incidence of convulsions, in children less than 5 years, is about 60% when the oral dose ingested exceeds 40 mg/kg.

Treatment: In the management of acute overdosage with Valoid, gastric lavage and supportive measures for respiration and circulation should be performed if necessary. Convulsions should be controlled in the usual way with parenteral anticonvulsant therapy.

5. PHARMACOLOGICAL PROPERTIES

5.1 Pharmacodynamic properties

Cyclizine is a piperazine derivative with the general properties of H_1-blocking drugs but is used as an anti-emetic in a variety of clinical situations including drug-induced and motion sickness, vertigo, post-operative vomiting and radiation sickness. The mechanism of the anti-emetic effect is unclear. Cyclizine also possesses anticholinergic activity but does not have marked sedative effects.

5.2 Pharmacokinetic properties

H_1-blockers are well absorbed from the GI tract. Following oral administration effects develop within 30 minutes, are maximal within 1-2 hours and last, for cyclizine, for 4-6 hours. Cyclizine is extensively N-demethylated to norcyclizine which is widely distributed throughout the tissues and has a plasma half-life of less than 1 day.

5.3 Preclinical safety data

There are no preclinical data of relevance to the prescriber which are additional to that in other sections of the SmPC.

6. PHARMACEUTICAL PARTICULARS

6.1 List of excipients

Lactose

Potato starch

Acacia

Magnesium stearate

Purified water

6.2 Incompatibilities

None known.

6.3 Shelf life

60 months.

6.4 Special precautions for storage

Store below 25°C.

6.5 Nature and contents of container

Amber glass bottle with low density polyethylene snap fit closure.

Pack size: 100 tablets

6.6 Instructions for use and handling
No special instructions.

7. MARKETING AUTHORISATION HOLDER
Amdipharm PLC
Trading as Amdipharm
Regency House
Miles Gray Road
Basildon
Essex SS14 3AF
United Kingdom

8. MARKETING AUTHORISATION NUMBER(S)
PL 20072/0011

9. DATE OF FIRST AUTHORISATION/RENEWAL OF THE AUTHORISATION
1 December 2003

10. DATE OF REVISION OF THE TEXT

Valtrex Tablets 500mg

(GlaxoSmithKline UK)

1. NAME OF THE MEDICINAL PRODUCT
Valtrex™ Tablets 500mg

2. QUALITATIVE AND QUANTITATIVE COMPOSITION
500mg of valaciclovir

3. PHARMACEUTICAL FORM
Film coated tablets

4. CLINICAL PARTICULARS
4.1 Therapeutic indications
Valtrex is indicated for the treatment of herpes zoster (shingles).

Valtrex is indicated for the treatment of herpes simplex infections of the skin and mucous membranes, including initial and recurrent genital herpes.

Valtrex is indicated for the suppression (prevention) of recurrent herpes simplex infections of the skin and mucous membranes, including genital herpes.

Valtrex can reduce transmission of genital herpes when taken as suppressive therapy and combined with safer sex practices (particularly the use of condoms).

Valtrex is indicated for the prophylaxis of cytomegalovirus (CMV) infection and disease, following renal transplantation.

4.2 Posology and method of administration
Route of administration: oral

Dosage in adults:

Treatment of herpes zoster:

1000 mg of Valtrex to be taken 3 times daily for 7 days.

Treatment of herpes simplex:

Valtrex can prevent lesion development when taken at the first signs and symptoms of an HSV recurrence.

500 mg of Valtrex to be taken twice daily. For recurrent episodes, treatment should be for 5 days. For initial episodes, which can be more severe, treatment may have to be extended to 10 days. Dosing should begin as early as possible. For recurrent episodes of herpes simplex, this should ideally be during the prodromal period or immediately the first signs or symptoms appear.

Suppression (prevention) of herpes simplex infection:

For immunocompetent patients the total daily dose is 500mg. This can be taken as 250mg twice daily. A dose of 500mg once daily is also effective, especially in patients with fewer than 10 recurrences per year.

For immunocompromised patients the dose is 500mg twice daily.

Reduction of transmission of genital herpes:

In immunocompetent heterosexual adult patients with 9 or fewer recurrences per year, 500 mg of Valtrex to be taken once daily by the infected partner in order to reduce transmission to a sexual partner negative for HSV-2 antibodies. Safer sex practices (particularly condom use) should be maintained, and sexual contact avoided if lesions are present.

There are no data on the reduction of transmission beyond 8 months in other patient populations.

Prophylaxis of cytomegalovirus infection (CMV) and disease

Dosage in adults and adolescents (from 12 years of age):

The dosage of Valtrex is 2g four times a day, to be initiated within 72 hours post-transplant, or as soon as oral medication can be tolerated. This dose should be reduced according to creatinine clearance (see Dosage in renal impairment below).

The duration of treatment will usually be 90 days.

Dosage in children:

There are no data available on the use of Valtrex in children.

Dosage in the elderly:

Dosage modification is not required unless renal function is significantly impaired (see Dosage in renal impairment, below). Adequate hydration should be maintained.

Dosage in renal impairment:

Herpes zoster treatment and herpes simplex treatment, suppression and reduction of transmission:

The dosage of Valtrex should be reduced in patients with significantly impaired renal function as shown in the table below:

Therapeutic indication	Creatinine clearance ml/min	Valtrex dosage
Herpes zoster	15-30	1 g twice a day
	less than 15	1 g once a day
Herpes simplex (treatment)	less than 15	500 mg once a day
Herpes simplex prevention (suppression):		
- immunocompetent patients	less than 15	250 mg once a day
- immunocompromised patients	less than 15	500 mg once a day
Reduction of transmission of genital herpes:	less than 15	250 mg once a day

In patients on haemodialysis, the Valtrex dosage recommended for patients with a creatinine clearance of less than 15 ml/min should be used, but this should be administered after the haemodialysis has been performed.

CMV prophylaxis: The dosage of Valtrex should be reduced in patients with impaired renal function as shown in the table below:

Creatinine clearance ml/min	Valtrex dosage
75 or greater	*2 g four times a day*
50 to less than75	*1.5 g four times a day*
25 to less than50	*1.5 g three times a day*
10 to less than25	*1.5 g twice a day*
less than 10 or dialysis	*1.5 g once a day*

In patients on haemodialysis, the Valtrex dosage should be administered after the haemodialysis has been performed.

The creatinine clearance should be monitored frequently, and the Valtrex dosage adjusted accordingly. It is recommended that creatinine clearance is monitored daily for optimum dose adjustments, especially during the first 10 days post-transplant, and at least twice weekly during hospitalisation, and as considered necessary thereafter.

Dosage in hepatic impairment:

Studies with a 1g unit dose of Valtrex show that dose modification is not required in patients with mild or moderate cirrhosis (hepatic synthetic function maintained). Pharmacokinetic data in patients with advanced cirrhosis (impaired hepatic synthetic function and evidence of portal-systemic shunting) do not indicate the need for dosage adjustment. However, clinical experience is limited.

There are no data available on the use of higher doses of Valtrex (for CMV prophylaxis) in patients with liver disease. However, following a 1g unit dose of Valtrex, aciclovir AUCs were elevated in patients with moderate or severe cirrhosis. Therefore, caution should be exercised when administering higher doses of Valtrex to patients with hepatic impairment.

4.3 Contraindications
Valtrex is contra-indicated in patients known to be hypersensitive to valaciclovir, aciclovir or any components of formulations of Valtrex.

4.4 Special warnings and special precautions for use
Hydration status:

Care should be taken to ensure adequate fluid intake in patients who are at risk of dehydration, particularly the elderly.

Use in renal impairment:

The Valtrex dose should be reduced in patients with renal impairment (see 4.2 Posology and Method of Administration).

Patients with a history of renal impairment are also at increased risk of developing reversible psychiatric reactions (see 4.8 Undesirable Effects).

Use of high dose Valtrex in hepatic impairment:

There are no data available on the use of higher doses of Valtrex (for CMV prophylaxis) in patients with liver disease. However, following a 1g unit dose of Valtrex, aciclovir AUCs were elevated in patients with moderate or severe cirrhosis. Therefore, caution should be exercised when administering higher doses of Valtrex to patients with hepatic impairment.

Use in genital herpes: Suppressive therapy with Valtrex reduces the risk of transmitting genital herpes. It does not cure genital herpes or completely eliminate the risk of transmission. In addition to therapy with Valtrex, it is recommended that patients use safer sex practices (particularly the use of condoms).

4.5 Interaction with other medicinal products and other forms of Interaction
No clinically significant interactions have been identified.

Aciclovir is eliminated primarily unchanged in the urine via active tubular secretion. Any drugs administered concurrently that compete with this mechanism for elimination may increase aciclovir plasma concentrations following Valtrex administration.

In patients receiving high dose Valtrex (8g/day) for CMV prophylaxis, caution is required during concurrent administration with drugs which compete with aciclovir elimination, because of the potential for increased plasma levels of one or both drugs or their metabolites. Following 1g Valtrex, cimetidine and probenecid increase the AUC of aciclovir by this mechanism, and reduce aciclovir renal clearance. However, no dosage adjustment is necessary at this dose of 1g because of the wide therapeutic index of aciclovir. Alternative agents, which do not interact with other agents excreted primarily via the kidney, may be considered for the management of excess gastric acid production and urate-lowering therapy when administering high dose valaciclovir.

Increases in plasma AUCs of aciclovir and of the inactive metabolite of mycophenolate mofetil, an immunosuppressant agent used in transplant patients, have been shown when the drugs are coadministered; there is limited clinical experience with the use of this combination.

Care is also required, with monitoring for changes in renal function (see 4.2, Posology and Method of Administration), if administering high-dose Valtrex with drugs which affect other aspects of renal physiology (e.g. cyclosporin, tacrolimus).

4.6 Pregnancy and lactation
Teratogenicity:

Valaciclovir was not teratogenic in rats or rabbits. Valaciclovir is almost completely metabolised to aciclovir. Subcutaneous administration of aciclovir in internationally accepted tests did not produce teratogenic effects in rats or rabbits. In additional studies in rats, foetal abnormalities were observed at subcutaneous doses that produced plasma levels of 100 μg/ml and maternal toxicity.

Fertility:

Valaciclovir did not affect fertility in male or female rats dosed by the oral route.

Pregnancy:

There are limited data on the use of Valtrex in pregnancy. Valtrex should only be used in pregnancy if the potential benefits of treatment outweigh the potential risk.

In prospective aciclovir studies, there has not been an increased incidence of birth defects in approximately 550 women exposed to systemic aciclovir (most at oral doses up to 1000mg per day) during the first trimester of pregnancy, as compared with the incidence in the general population. The reported defects show no uniqueness or pattern to suggest a common aetiology.

The daily aciclovir AUC (area under plasma concentration-time curve) following Valtrex 1000 mg and 8000 mg would be approximately 2 and 9 times greater than that expected with oral aciclovir 1000 mg daily, respectively.

Lactation:

The principle metabolite of valaciclovir is aciclovir which is excreted in breast milk. Aciclovir has been detected in breast milk at concentrations ranging from 0.6 to 4.1 times the corresponding aciclovir plasma concentrations. Following oral administration of 200 mg aciclovir five times a day, the mean steady state peak plasma concentration (C^{ss} max) is 3.1 microM (0.7 mcg/ml). These levels would potentially expose nursing infants to aciclovir dosages of up to 0.3 mg/kg/day. The elimination half-life of aciclovir from breast milk has been reported to be 2.8 hours, similar to that in plasma.

Caution is therefore advised if Valtrex is to be administered to a nursing woman. However, aciclovir is used to treat neonatal herpes simplex at intravenous doses of 30 mg/kg /day.

4.7 Effects on ability to drive and use machines
No special precautions necessary.

4.8 Undesirable effects
Adverse reactions are listed below by MedDRA body system organ class and by frequency.

The frequency categories used are:

Very common ⩾ 1 in 10,

Common ⩾ 1 in 100 and < 1 in 10,

Uncommon ⩾ 1 in 1,000 and < 1 in 100,

Rare ⩾ 1 in 10,000 and < 1 in 1,000,

Very rare < 1 in 10,000.

Blood and lymphatic system disorders

Very rare: Thrombocytopenia.

Immune system disorders

Very rare: Anaphylaxis.

Psychiatric and nervous system disorders

Common: *Headache

Rare: Dizziness, confusion, hallucinations, decreased consciousness.

Very rare: Tremor, ataxia, dysarthria, convulsions, encephalopathy, coma.

The above events are reversible and usually seen in patients with renal impairment or with other predisposing factors. In renal transplant patients receiving high doses (8 g daily) of Valtrex for CMV prophylaxis, psychiatric reactions (confusion, hallucinations and thinking disorders) occurred more frequently compared with lower doses for other indications. They were mainly mild to moderate in nature, reversible upon dose adjustment, and occurred mainly in the immediate post-transplant period. Therefore, it is important to monitor creatinine clearance frequently in these patients, and to adjust the dose accordingly (see 4.2 Posology and Method of Administration). The cause of these events appears to be multi-factorial, including over-exposure to aciclovir, renal impairment, dialysis, administration of psychotropic agents, and other underlying medical conditions.

Respiratory, thoracic and mediastinal disorders

Uncommon: Dyspnoea.

Gastrointestinal disorders

Common: *Nausea

Rare: Abdominal discomfort, vomiting, diarrhoea.

Hepato-biliary disorders

Very rare: Reversible increases in liver function tests.

These are occasionally described as hepatitis.

Skin and subcutaneous tissue disorders

Uncommon: Rashes including photosensitivity.

Rare: Pruritus.

Very rare: Urticaria, angioedema.

Renal and urinary disorders

Rare: Renal impairment.

Very rare: Acute renal failure.

Other: There have been reports of renal insufficiency, microangiopathic haemolytic anaemia and thrombocytopenia (sometimes in combination) in severely immunocompromised patients, particularly those with advanced HIV disease, receiving high doses (8 g daily) of valaciclovir for prolonged periods in clinical trials. These findings have been observed in patients not treated with valaciclovir who have the same underlying or concurrent conditions.

* Clinical trial data have been used to assign frequency categories to these adverse reactions. For all other adverse events, spontaneous post-marketing data has been used as a basis for allocating frequency.

4.9 Overdose

Symptoms and signs:

There are at present limited data available on overdosage with Valtrex. However patients have ingested single overdoses of up to 20g of aciclovir, which is only partially absorbed in the gastrointestinal tract, usually without toxic effects. Accidental, repeated overdoses of oral aciclovir over several days have been associated with gastrointestinal effects (such as nausea and vomiting) and neurological effects (headache and confusion). Overdosage of intravenous aciclovir has resulted in elevations of serum creatinine and subsequent renal failure. Neurological effects including confusion, hallucinations, agitation, seizures and coma have been described in association with intravenous overdosage.

Management:-

Patients should be observed closely for signs of toxicity. Haemodialysis significantly enhances the removal of aciclovir from the blood and may, therefore, be considered a management option in the event of symptomatic overdose.

5. PHARMACOLOGICAL PROPERTIES

5.1 Pharmacodynamic properties

Pharmacotherapeutic group:

Valaciclovir, an antiviral, is the L-valine ester of aciclovir. Aciclovir is a purine (guanine) nucleoside analogue.

Mode of action:

Valaciclovir is rapidly and almost completely converted in man to aciclovir and valine, probably by the enzyme referred to as valaciclovir hydrolase.

Aciclovir is a specific inhibitor of the herpes viruses with in vitro activity against herpes simplex viruses (HSV) type 1 and type 2, varicella zoster virus (VZV), cytomegalovirus (CMV), Epstein-Barr Virus (EBV), and human herpes virus 6 (HHV-6). Aciclovir inhibits herpes virus DNA synthesis once it has been phosphorylated to the active triphosphate form.

The first stage of phosphorylation requires the activity of a virus-specific enzyme. In the case of HSV, VZV and EBV this enzyme is the viral thymidine kinase (TK), which is only present in virus infected cells. Selectivity is maintained in CMV with phosphorylation, at least in part, being mediated through the phosphotransferase gene product of UL97. This requirement for activation of aciclovir by a virus specific enzyme largely explains its selectivity.

The phosphorylation process is completed (conversion from mono- to triphosphate) by cellular kinases. Aciclovir triphosphate competitively inhibits the virus DNA polymerase and incorporation of this nucleoside analogue results in obligate chain termination, halting virus DNA synthesis and thus blocking virus replication.

CMV prophylaxis with Valtrex significantly reduces HSV disease in renal transplant patients.

Extensive monitoring of clinical HSV and VZV isolates from patients receiving aciclovir therapy or prophylaxis has revealed that virus with reduced sensitivity to aciclovir is extremely rare in the immunocompetent and is only found infrequently in severely immunocompromised individuals e.g. solid organ or bone marrow transplant recipients, patients receiving chemotherapy for malignant disease and people infected with the human immunodeficiency virus (HIV).

Resistance is normally due to a thymidine kinase deficient phenotype, which results in a virus that is profoundly disadvantaged in the natural host. Infrequently, reduced sensitivity to aciclovir has been described as a result of subtle alterations in either the virus thymidine kinase or DNA polymerase. The virulence of these variants resembles that of the wild-type virus.

5.2 Pharmacokinetic properties

General characteristics:

After oral administration valaciclovir is well absorbed and rapidly and almost completely converted to aciclovir and valine. This conversion is probably mediated by an enzyme isolated from human liver referred to as valaciclovir hydrolase.

The bioavailability of aciclovir from 1000 mg valaciclovir is 54%, and is not reduced by food. Mean peak aciclovir concentrations are 10-37 μM (2.2-8.3μg/ml) following single doses of 250-2000 mg valaciclovir to healthy subjects with normal renal function, and occur at a median time of l.00 –2.00 hours post dose.

Peak plasma concentrations of valaciclovir are only 4% of aciclovir levels, occur at a median time of 30 to 100 minutes post dose, and are at or below the limit of quantification 3 hours after dosing. The valaciclovir and aciclovir pharmacokinetic profiles are similar after single and repeat dosing. Binding of valaciclovir to plasma proteins is very low (15%).

In patients with normal renal function, the elimination plasma half-life of aciclovir after both single and multiple dosing with valaciclovir is approximately 3 hours. In patients with end-stage renal disease, the average elimination half-life of aciclovir after valaciclovir administration is approximately 14 hours. Less than 1% of the administered dose of valaciclovir is recovered in the urine as unchanged drug. Valaciclovir is eliminated principally as aciclovir (greater than 80% of the recovered dose) and the known aciclovir metabolite, 9-carboxymethoxymethylguanine (CMMG), in the urine.

Characteristics in patients:

Herpes zoster and herpes simplex do not significantly alter the pharmacokinetics of valaciclovir and aciclovir after oral administration of Valtrex.

In patients with HIV infection, the disposition and pharmacokinetic characteristics of aciclovir after oral administration of single or multiple doses of 1000 mg or 2000 mg Valtrex are unaltered compared with healthy subjects.

In renal transplant recipients receiving valaciclovir 2g 4 times daily, aciclovir peak concentrations are similar to or greater than those in healthy volunteers with comparable doses and renal function. However, the estimated daily AUCs are appreciably greater.

5.3 Preclinical safety data

Mutagenicity:

The results of mutagenicity tests in vitro and in vivo indicate that valaciclovir is unlikely to pose a genetic risk to humans.

Carcinogenicity:

Valaciclovir was not carcinogenic in bio-assays performed in mice and rats.

6. PHARMACEUTICAL PARTICULARS

6.1 List of excipients

Tablet core:

Microcrystalline cellulose

Crospovidone

Povidone K90

Magnesium stearate

Colloidal silicon dioxide

Purified water

Film coat:

White Colour Concentrate YS-1-18043 containing;

Hydroxypropylmethylcellulose

Titanium dioxide

Polyethylene glycol 400

Polysorbate 80

Purified water

Printing ink:

Brilliant Blue Printing Ink FT203 containing Brilliant Blue, E133

Polish:

Carnauba wax

6.2 Incompatibilities

No data.

6.3 Shelf life

Three years

6.4 Special precautions for storage

Store below 30°C

6.5 Nature and contents of container

Tablets are packed into blister packs prepared from unplasticised polyvinyl chloride and aluminium foil.

Pack sizes	4 × 500mg
	10 × 500mg
	42 × 500mg

Tablets are packed into polypropylene containers with polyethylene snap-fitting caps Pack size: 500 × 500mg

6.6 Instructions for use and handling

No special instructions for use.

Administrative Data

7. MARKETING AUTHORISATION HOLDER

The Wellcome Foundation Ltd

Glaxo Wellcome House

Berkeley Avenue

Greenford

Middlesex

UB6 0NN

8. MARKETING AUTHORISATION NUMBER(S)

PL 00003/0352

9. DATE OF FIRST AUTHORISATION/RENEWAL OF THE AUTHORISATION

20 January 1995

10. DATE OF REVISION OF THE TEXT

18 November 2004

11. Legal Status

POM

Vancocin CP Injection

(Flynn Pharma Ltd)

1. NAME OF THE MEDICINAL PRODUCT

'Vancocin' CP.

2. QUALITATIVE AND QUANTITATIVE COMPOSITION

Vial Size	Quantity of Vancomycin
10ml	500mg
20ml	1g

3. PHARMACEUTICAL FORM

Injection of vancomycin hydrochloride.

4. CLINICAL PARTICULARS

4.1 Therapeutic indications

Vancomycin is indicated in potentially life-threatening infections which cannot be treated with other effective, less toxic antimicrobial drugs, including the penicillins and cephalosporins.

Vancomycin is useful in the therapy of severe staphylococcal infections in patients who cannot receive or who have failed to respond to the penicillins and cephalosporins, or who have infections with staphylococci resistant to other antibiotics.

Vancomycin is used in the treatment of endocarditis and as prophylaxis against endocarditis in patients at risk from dental or surgical procedures.

Its effectiveness has been documented in other infections due to staphylococci, including osteomyelitis, pneumonia, septicaemia and soft tissue infections.

Vancomycin may be used orally for the treatment of staphylococcal enterocolitis and pseudomembranous colitis due to *Clostridium difficile*. Parenteral administration of vancomycin is not effective for these indications. Intravenous administration may be used concomitantly if required.

4.2 Posology and method of administration

For intravenous infusion and oral use only and not for intramuscular administration.

Figure 1

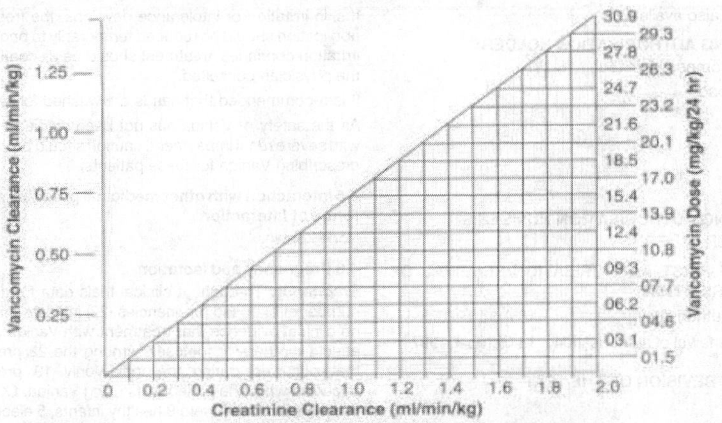

Dosage nomogram for vancomycin in patients with impaired renal function

Infusion-related adverse events are related to both concentration and rate of administration of vancomycin.

Concentrations of no more than 5mg/ml are recommended. In selected patients in need of fluid restriction, a concentration up to 10mg/ml may be used; use of such higher concentrations may increase the risk of infusion-related events. Infusions should be given over at least 60 minutes. In adults, if doses exceeding 500mg are used, a rate of infusion of no more than 10mg/min is recommended. Infusion-related events may occur, however, at any rate or concentration.

Intravenous infusion in patients with normal renal function

Adults: The usual intravenous dose is 500mg every six hours or 1g every 12 hours, in Sodium Chloride Intravenous Infusion BP or 5% Dextrose Intravenous Infusion BP. Each dose should be administered at no more than 10mg/min. Other patient factors, such as age, obesity or pregnancy, may call for modification of the usual daily dose. The majority of patients with infections caused by organisms sensitive to the antibiotic show a therapeutic response within 48-72 hours. The total duration of therapy is determined by the type and severity of the infection and the clinical response of the patient. In staphylococcal endocarditis, treatment for three weeks or longer is recommended.

Pregnancy: It has been reported that significantly increased doses may be required to achieve therapeutic serum concentrations in pregnant patients, but see 'Warnings'.

The elderly: Dosage reduction may be necessary to a greater extent than expected because of decreasing renal function (see below). Monitor auditory function - see 'Warnings' and 'Precautions'.

Children: The usual intravenous dosage is 10mg/kg per dose given every 6 hours (total daily dosage 40mg/kg of body weight). Each dose should be administered over a period of at least 60 minutes.

In neonates and young infants, the total daily dosage may be lower. An initial dose of 15mg/kg is suggested, followed by 10mg/kg every 12 hours in the first week of life and every 8 hours thereafter until one month of age. Each dose should be administered over 60 minutes. Close monitoring of serum vancomycin concentrations may be warranted in these patients.

Patients with impaired renal function

Dosage adjustments must be made to avoid toxic serum levels. In premature infants and the elderly, greater dosage reductions than expected may be necessary because of decreased renal function. Regular monitoring of serum levels is advised in such patients, as accumulation has been reported, especially after prolonged therapy. Vancomycin serum concentrations may be determined by use of a microbiological assay, radioimmunoassay, fluorescence polarisation immunoassay, fluorescence immunoassay or high-pressure liquid chromatography. The following nomogram, based on creatinine clearance values, is provided:

(see Figure 1 above)

The nomogram is not valid for functionally anephric patients on dialysis. For such patients, a loading dose of 15mg/kg body weight should be given to achieve therapeutic serum levels promptly, and the dose required to maintain stable levels is 1.9mg/kg/24 hours. Since individual maintenance doses of 250mg to 1g are convenient, in patients with marked renal impairment a dose may be given every several days rather than on a daily basis. In anuria a dose of 1g every 7 to 10 days has been recommended.

Preparation of solutions: See 'Instructions for use/handling'.

Measurement of serum concentrations

Following multiple intravenous doses, peak serum concentrations, measured 2 hours after infusion is complete, range from 18-26mg/l. Trough levels measured immediately prior to the next dose should be 5-10mg/l. Ototoxicity has been associated with serum drug levels of 80-100mg/l, but this is rarely seen when serum levels are kept at or below 30mg/l.

Oral administration

The contents of vials for parenteral administration may be used.

Adults and the elderly: The usual daily dose given is 500mg in divided doses for 7 to 10 days, although up to 2g/day have been used in severe cases. The total daily dosage should not exceed 2g. Each dose may be reconstituted in 30ml water and either given to the patient to drink, or administered by nasogastric tube.

Children: The usual daily dose is 40mg/kg in three or four divided doses for 7 to 10 days. The total daily dosage should not exceed 2g.

Common flavouring syrups may be added to the solution at the time of administration to improve the taste.

Capsules are also available.

4.3 Contraindications

Hypersensitivity to vancomycin.

4.4 Special warnings and special precautions for use

Warnings

Rapid bolus administration (eg, over several minutes) may be associated with exaggerated hypotension, including shock, and, rarely, cardiac arrest. Vancomycin should be infused in a dilute solution over a period of not less than 60 minutes to avoid rapid infusion-related reactions. Stopping the infusion usually results in a prompt cessation of these reactions (see 'Posology and method of administration' and 'Undesirable effects' sections).

Some patients with inflammatory disorders of the intestinal mucosa may have significant systemic absorption of oral vancomycin and, therefore, may be at risk for the development of adverse reactions associated with the parenteral administration of vancomycin. The risk is greater in patients with renal impairment. It should be noted that the total systemic and renal clearances of vancomycin are reduced in the elderly.

Due to its potential ototoxicity and nephrotoxicity, vancomycin should be used with care in patients with renal insufficiency and the dose should be reduced according to the degree of renal impairment. The risk of toxicity is appreciably increased by high blood concentrations or prolonged therapy. Blood levels should be monitored and renal function tests should be performed regularly.

Vancomycin should also be avoided in patients with previous hearing loss. If it is used in such patients, the dose should be regulated, if possible, by periodic determination of the drug level in the blood. Deafness may be preceded by tinnitus. The elderly are more susceptible to auditory damage. Experience with other antibiotics suggests that deafness may be progressive despite cessation of treatment.

Usage in paediatrics: In premature neonates and young infants, it may be appropriate to confirm desired vancomycin serum concentrations. Concomitant administration of vancomycin and anaesthetic agents has been associated with erythema and histamine-like flushing in children.

Usage in the elderly: The natural decrement of glomerular filtration with increasing age may lead to elevated vancomycin serum concentrations if dosage is not adjusted (see 'Posology and method of administration').

Precautions

Clinically significant serum concentrations have been reported in some patients being treated for active *C. difficile*-induced pseudomembranous colitis after multiple oral doses of vancomycin. Therefore, monitoring of serum concentrations may be appropriate in these patients.

Patients with borderline renal function and individuals over the age of 60 should be given serial tests of auditory function and of vancomycin blood levels. All patients receiving the drug should have periodic haematological studies, urine analysis and renal function tests.

Vancomycin is very irritating to tissue, and causes injection site necrosis when injected intramuscularly; it must be infused intravenously. Injection site pain and thrombophlebitis occur in many patients receiving vancomycin and are occasionally severe.

The frequency and severity of thrombophlebitis can be minimised by administering the drug slowly as a dilute solution (2.5 to 5.0g/l) and by rotating the sites of infusion.

Prolonged use of vancomycin may result in the overgrowth of non-susceptible organisms. Careful observation of the patient is essential. If superinfection occurs during therapy, appropriate measures should be taken. In rare instances, there have been reports of pseudomembranous colitis, due to *C. difficile*, developing in patients who received intravenous vancomycin.

4.5 Interaction with other medicinal products and other forms of Interaction

Concomitant administration of vancomycin and anaesthetic agents has been associated with erythema, histamine-like flushing and anaphylactoid reactions.

There have been reports that the frequency of infusion-related events increases with the concomitant administration of anaesthetic agents. Infusion-related events may be minimised by the administration of vancomycin as a 60-minute infusion prior to anaesthetic induction.

Concurrent or sequential systemic or topical use of other potentially neurotoxic or nephrotoxic drugs, such as amphotericin B, aminoglycosides, bacitracin, polymixin B, colistin, viomycin or cisplatin, when indicated, requires careful monitoring.

4.6 Pregnancy and lactation

Usage in pregnancy: Teratology studies have been performed at 5 times the human dose in rats and 3 times the human dose in rabbits, and have revealed no evidence of harm to the foetus due to vancomycin. In a controlled clinical study, the potential ototoxic and nephrotoxic effects of vancomycin hydrochloride on infants were evaluated when the drug was administered to pregnant women for serious staphylococcal infections complicating intravenous drug abuse. Vancomycin hydrochloride was found in cord blood. No sensorineural hearing loss or nephrotoxicity attributable to vancomycin was noted. One infant, whose mother received vancomycin in the third trimester, experienced conductive hearing loss that was not attributable to vancomycin. Because vancomycin was administered only in the second and third trimesters, it is not known whether it causes foetal harm. Vancomycin should be given in pregnancy only if clearly needed and blood levels should be monitored carefully to minimise the risk of foetal toxicity. It has been reported, however, that pregnant patients may require significantly increased doses of vancomycin to achieve therapeutic serum concentrations.

Usage in nursing mothers: Vancomycin hydrochloride is excreted in human milk. Caution should be exercised when vancomycin is administered to a nursing woman. It is unlikely that a nursing infant can absorb a significant amount of vancomycin from its gastro-intestinal tract.

4.7 Effects on ability to drive and use machines

Not applicable

4.8 Undesirable effects

Infusion-related events: During or soon after rapid infusion of vancomycin, patients may develop anaphylactoid reactions including hypotension, wheezing, dyspnoea, urticaria or pruritus. Rapid infusion may also cause flushing of the upper-body ('red-neck syndrome') or pain and muscle spasm of the chest and back. These reactions usually resolve within 20 minutes but may persist for several hours. In animal studies, hypotension and bradycardia occurred in animals given large doses of vancomycin at high concentrations and rates. Such events are infrequent if vancomycin is given by slow infusion over 60 minutes. In studies of normal volunteers, infusion-related events did not occur when vancomycin was administered at a rate of 10mg/min or less.

Nephrotoxicity: Rarely, renal failure, principally manifested by increased serum creatinine or blood urea concentrations, have been observed, especially in patients given large doses of intravenously administered vancomycin. Rare cases of interstitial nephritis have been reported. Most occurred in patients who were given aminoglycosides concomitantly or who had pre-existing kidney dysfunction. When vancomycin was discontinued, azotaemia resolved in most patients.

Ototoxicity: Hearing loss associated with intravenously administered vancomycin has been reported. Most of these patients had kidney dysfunction, pre-existing hearing loss, or concomitant treatment with an ototoxic drug. Vertigo, dizziness and tinnitus have been reported rarely.

Haematological: Reversible neutropenia, usually starting one week or more after onset of intravenous therapy or after a total dose of more than 25g. Neutropenia appears to be promptly reversible when vancomycin is discontinued. Thrombocytopenia has rarely been reported. Reversible agranulocytosis (less than 500 granulocytes per mm^3) has been reported rarely, although causality has not been established.

Miscellaneous: Phlebitis, hypersensitivity reactions, anaphylaxis, nausea, chills, drug fever, eosinophilia, rashes (including exfoliative dermatitis) and rare cases of vasculitis. Vancomycin has been associated with the bullous eruption disorders Stevens-Johnson syndrome, toxic epidermal necrolysis and linear IgA bullous dermatosis. If a bullous disorder is suspected, the drug should be discontinued and specialist dermatological assessment should be carried out.

4.9 Overdose

Supportive care is advised, with maintenance of glomerular filtration. Vancomycin is poorly removed from the blood by haemodialysis or peritoneal dialysis. Haemoperfusion with Amberlite resin XAD-4 has been reported to be of limited benefit.

5. PHARMACOLOGICAL PROPERTIES

5.1 Pharmacodynamic properties

Vancomycin is a glycopeptide antibiotic derived from *Nocardia orientalis* (formerly *Streptomyces orientalis*), and is active against many Gram-positive bacteria, including *Staphylococcus aureus*, *Staph. epidermidis*, alpha and beta haemolytic streptococci, group D streptococci, corynebacteria and clostridia.

5.2 Pharmacokinetic properties

Vancomycin is not significantly absorbed from the normal gastro-intestinal tract and is therefore not effective by the oral route for infections other than staphylococcal enterocolitis and pseudomembranous colitis due to *Clostridium difficile*.

5.3 Preclinical safety data

Although no long-term studies in animals have been performed to evaluate carcinogenic potential, no mutagenic potential of vancomycin was found in standard laboratory tests. No definitive fertility studies have been performed.

6. PHARMACEUTICAL PARTICULARS

6.1 List of excipients

Vials of Vancocin contain only the active ingredient, vancomycin hydrochloride.

6.2 Incompatibilities

Vancomycin solution has a low pH that may cause chemical or physical instability when it is mixed with other compounds.

6.3 Shelf life

500mg vial: 2 years.

1g vial: 2 years.

6.4 Special precautions for storage

Store below 25°C.

After reconstitution: May be stored in a refrigerator (2°-8°C) for 24 hours.

Prior to administration, parenteral drug products should be inspected visually for particulate matter and discolouration whenever solution or container permits.

Solutions of the parenteral powder intended for oral administration may be stored in a refrigerator (2°-8°C) for 96 hours.

6.5 Nature and contents of container

Rubber-stoppered 10ml vials each containing chromatographically purified vancomycin hydrochloride, 500,000iu, equivalent to 500mg vancomycin, as an off-white lyophilised plug.

Rubber-stoppered 20ml vials containing chromatographically purified vancomycin hydrochloride, 1,000,000iu, equivalent to 1g vancomycin, as an off-white lyophilised plug.

6.6 Instructions for use and handling

Preparation of solution: At the time of use, add 10ml of Water for Injections PhEur to the 500mg vial, or 20ml Water for Injections PhEur to the 1g vial. Vials reconstituted in this manner will give a solution of 50mg/ml.

FURTHER DILUTION IS REQUIRED. Read instructions which follow:

1. *Intermittent infusion* is the preferred method of administration. Reconstituted solutions containing 500mg vancomycin must be diluted with at least 100ml diluent. Reconstituted solutions containing 1g vancomycin must be diluted with at least 200ml diluent. Sodium Chloride Intravenous Infusion BP or 5% Dextrose Intravenous Infusion BP are suitable diluents. The desired dose should be given by intravenous infusion over a period of at least 60 minutes. If administered over a shorter period of time or in higher concentrations, there is the possibility of inducing marked hypotension in addition to thrombophlebitis. Rapid administration may also produce flushing and a transient rash over the neck and shoulders.

2. *Continuous infusion* (should be used only when intermittent infusion is not feasible). 1-2g can be added to a sufficiently large volume of Sodium Chloride Intravenous Infusion BP or 5% Dextrose Intravenous Infusion BP to permit the desired daily dose to be administered slowly by intravenous drip over a 24 hour period.

3. *Oral administration*

The contents of vials for parenteral administration may be used.

Common flavouring syrups may be added to the solution at the time of administration to improve the taste.

Capsules are also available.

7. MARKETING AUTHORISATION HOLDER

Eli Lilly and Company Limited
Kingsclere Road
Basingstoke
Hampshire
RG21 6XA
England

8. MARKETING AUTHORISATION NUMBER(S)

PL 0006/5076R

9. DATE OF FIRST AUTHORISATION/RENEWAL OF THE AUTHORISATION

Date of first authorisation: 18 April 1990

Date of last renewal of authorisation: 13 October 1997

10. DATE OF REVISION OF THE TEXT

May 2000

LEGAL CATEGORY

POM

PACKAGE QUANTITIES

Vials 500mg (500,000iu vancomycin). Single vials.

Vials 1g (1,000,000iu vancomycin). Single vials.

'VANCOCIN' is an Eli Lilly and Company Limited trademark VA.21M

Vaniqa 11.5% Cream

(Shire Pharmaceuticals Limited)

1. NAME OF THE MEDICINAL PRODUCT

Vaniqa ▼ 11.5% cream

2. QUALITATIVE AND QUANTITATIVE COMPOSITION

Each gram of Vaniqa 11.5% w/w cream contains 115 mg eflornithine (as monohydrate chloride).

For excipients, see 6.1.

3. PHARMACEUTICAL FORM

Cream.

4. CLINICAL PARTICULARS

4.1 Therapeutic indications

Treatment of facial hirsutism in women.

4.2 Posology and method of administration

Apply a thin layer of the cream to clean and dry affected areas twice daily, at least eight hours apart. Rub in thoroughly. For maximal efficacy, the treated area should not be cleansed within four hours of application. Cosmetics (including sunscreens) can be applied over the treated areas, but no sooner than five minutes after application.

Efficacy has only been demonstrated for affected areas of the face and under the chin. Application should be limited to these areas. The product should be applied such that no visual residual product remains on the treated areas after rub-in. Maximal applied doses used safely in clinical trials were up to 30 grams per month.

Improvement in the condition may be noticed within eight weeks of starting treatment.

Continued treatment may result in further improvement and is necessary to maintain beneficial effects. The condition may return to pre-treatment levels within eight weeks following discontinuation of treatment.

Use should be discontinued if no beneficial effects are noticed within four months of commencing therapy.

Patients may need to continue to use a hair removal method (e.g. shaving or plucking) in conjunction with Vaniqa. In that case, the cream should be applied no sooner than five minutes after shaving or use of other hair removal methods, as increased stinging or burning may otherwise occur.

Elderly: (> 65 years) no dosage adjustment is necessary.

Children and Adolescents: (< 12 years) safety and efficacy of Vaniqa have not been established.

Hepatic/renal impairment: the safety and efficacy of Vaniqa in women with hepatic or renal impairment have not been established.

4.3 Contraindications

Hypersensitivity to eflornithine or to any of the excipients (see 6.1).

4.4 Special warnings and special precautions for use

Excessive hair growth can result from serious underlying disorders (e.g. polycystic ovary syndrome, androgen secreting neoplasm) or certain medications (e.g. cyclosporin, glucocorticoids, minoxidil, phenobarbitone, phenytoin, combined oestrogen-androgen hormone replacement therapy). These factors should be considered in the overall medical treatment of patients who might be prescribed Vaniqa.

Vaniqa is for cutaneous use only. Contact with eyes or mucous membranes (e.g. nose or mouth) should be avoided. Transient stinging or burning may occur when the cream is applied to abraded or broken skin.

If skin irritation or intolerance develops, the frequency of application should be reduced temporarily to once a day. If irritation continues, treatment should be discontinued and the physician consulted.

It is recommended that hands are washed following use.

As the safety of Vaniqa has not been studied in patients with severe renal impairment, caution should be used when prescribing Vaniqa for these patients.

4.5 Interaction with other medicinal products and other forms of Interaction

None known.

4.6 Pregnancy and lactation

Pregnancy: Throughout clinical trials data from a limited number of exposed pregnancies (22) indicate that there is no clinical evidence that treatment with Vaniqa adversely affects mothers or foetuses. Among the 22 pregnancies that occurred during the trials, only 19 pregnancies occurred while the patient was using Vaniqa. Of these 19 pregnancies, there were 9 healthy infants, 5 elective abortions, 4 spontaneous abortions and 1 birth defect (Down's Syndrome to a 35 year old). To date, no other relevant epidemiological data are available. Animal studies have shown reproductive toxicity (see 5.3). The potential risk to humans is unknown. Therefore, women who are pregnant or planning pregnancy should use an alternative means to manage facial hair.

Lactation: it is not known if eflornithine is excreted in human milk. Women should not use Vaniqa whilst breast-feeding.

4.7 Effects on ability to drive and use machines

Vaniqa has not been studied for its possible effects on the ability to drive or use machinery. No effect is expected.

4.8 Undesirable effects

The mostly skin related adverse reactions reported were primarily mild in intensity and resolved without discontinuation of Vaniqa or initiation of medical treatment. The most frequently reported undesirable effect was acne, which was generally mild. In the vehicle controlled trials (n= 594), acne was observed in 41% of patients at baseline; 7% of patients treated with Vaniqa and 8% treated with vehicle experienced a worsening of their condition. Of those with no acne at baseline, similar percentages (14%) reported acne following treatment with Vaniqa or vehicle.

The following listing notes the frequency of adverse skin reactions seen in clinical trials, according to MedDRA convention. MedDRA conventions for frequency are very common (> 10%), common (> 1% to < 10%), uncommon (> 0.1% to < 1%), rare (> 0.01% to < 0.1%), or very rare (< 0.01%), including isolated reports. Note that over 1350 patients were treated with Vaniqa in these trials for 6 months to one year, while only slightly more than 200 patients were treated with vehicle for 6 months. Most events were reported at similar rates between Vaniqa and vehicle. The skin effects of burning, stinging, tingling, rash and erythema were reported at higher levels in Vaniqa treated patients compared to vehicle, as indicated by the asterisk (*).

Frequency of adverse skin reactions seen in Vaniqa clinical trials, (according to MedDRA frequency convention).

Skin and subcutaneous tissue disorders

Very common (> 10%)	Acne
Common (> 1% to < 10%)	Pseudofolliculitis barbae, alopecia, stinging skin*, burning skin*, dry skin, pruritis, erythema*, tingling skin*, irritated skin, rash*, folliculitis
Uncommon (> 0.1% to < 1%)	Ingrown hair, oedema face, dermatitis, oedema mouth, papular rash, bleeding skin, herpes simplex, eczema, cheilitis, furunculosis, contact dermatitis, hair disorder, hypopigmentation, flushing skin, lip numbness, skin soreness
Rare (> 0.01% to < 0.1%)	Rosacea, seborrheic dermatitis, skin neoplasm, maculopapular rash, skin cysts, vesiculobullous rash, skin disorder, hirsutism, skin tightness

4.9 Overdose

Given the minimal cutaneous penetration of eflornithine (see 5.2), overdose is highly unlikely. However, should very high dose cutaneous administration or accidental oral ingestion occur, attention should be paid to the effects seen with therapeutic doses of intravenous eflornithine (400 mg/kg/day or approximately 24 g/day) used in the treatment of *Trypanosoma brucei gambiense* infection (African sleeping sickness): hair loss, facial swelling, seizures, hearing impairment, gastrointestinal disturbance, loss of appetite, headache, weakness, dizziness, anaemia, thrombocytopenia and leucopenia.

5. PHARMACOLOGICAL PROPERTIES

5.1 Pharmacodynamic properties

Pharmacotherapeutic group: other dermatologicals, ATC code: D11A X.

Eflornithine irreversibly inhibits ornithine decarboxylase, an enzyme involved in the production of the hair shaft by the hair follicle. Vaniqa has been shown to reduce the rate of hair growth.

The safety and efficacy of Vaniqa was evaluated in two double-blind, randomised, vehicle-controlled clinical trials involving 594 women of skin types I-VI (393 on Vaniqa, 201 on vehicle) treated for up to 24 weeks. Physicians assessed the change from baseline on a 4-point scale, 48 hours after women had shaved the treated areas of the affected areas of the face and under the chin, considering parameters such as hair length and density, and darkening of the skin associated with the presence of terminal hair. Improvement was seen as early as 8 weeks after initiation of treatment.

The combined results of these two trials are presented below:

Outcome*	Vaniqa 11.5% cream	Vehicle
Clear / almost clear	6%	0%
Marked improvement	29%	9%
Improved	35%	33%
No improvement / worse	30%	58%

* At end of therapy (Week 24). For patients who discontinued therapy during the trial last observations were carried forward to Week 24.

Statistically significant ($p \leqslant 0.001$) improvement for Vaniqa versus vehicle was seen in each of these studies for women with marked improvement and clear/almost clear responses. These improvements resulted in a corresponding reduction in the darkening appearance of the facial skin associated with the presence of terminal hair. Subgroup analysis revealed a difference in treatment success where 27% of non-white women and 39% of white women showed a marked or better improvement. Subgroup analysis also showed that 29% of obese women (BMI $\geqslant$ 30) and 43% of normal weight women (BMI < 30) showed a marked or better improvement. About 12% of women in the clinical trials were postmenopausal. Significant improvement ($p < 0.001$) versus vehicle was seen in postmenopausal women.

Patient self-assessments demonstrated a significantly reduced psychological discomfort with the condition, as measured by responses to 6 questions on a visual analogue scale. Vaniqa significantly reduced how bothered patients felt by their facial hair and by the time spent removing, treating, or concealing facial hair. Patient comfort in various social and work settings was also improved. Patient self-assessments were found to correlate with physician observations of efficacy. These patient-observable differences were seen 8 weeks after initiating treatment.

The condition returned to pre-treatment levels within eight weeks after discontinuation of treatment.

5.2 Pharmacokinetic properties

Steady state cutaneous penetration of eflornithine in women from Vaniqa on facial skin of shaving women was 0.8%.

The steady state plasma half-life of eflornithine was approximately 8 hours. Steady state was reached within four days. The steady state peak and trough plasma concentrations of eflornithine were approximately 10 ng/ml and 5 ng/ml, respectively. The steady state 12-hour area under the plasma concentration versus time curve was 92.5 ng.hr/ml.

Eflornithine is not known to be metabolised and is eliminated primarily in the urine.

5.3 Preclinical safety data

Preclinical data reveal no special hazard for humans based on conventional studies of repeat dose toxicity, genotoxicity and carcinogenic potential, including one photocarcinogenicity study in mice.

In a dermal fertility study in rats, no adverse effects on fertility were observed at up to 180 times the human dose. In dermal teratology studies, no teratogenic effects were observed in rats and rabbits at doses up to 180 and 36 times the human dose, respectively. Higher doses resulted in maternal and foetal toxicity without evidence of teratogenicity.

6. PHARMACEUTICAL PARTICULARS

6.1 List of excipients

Cetostearyl alcohol;

Macrogol 20 cetostearyl ether;

Dimeticone;

Glyceryl stearate;

Macrogol 100 stearate;

Methyl parahydroxybenzoate (E218);

Mineral oil;

Phenoxyethanol;

Propyl parahydroxybenzoate (E216);

Purified water and

Stearyl alcohol.

6.2 Incompatibilities

Not applicable.

6.3 Shelf life

3 years.

6.4 Special precautions for storage

Do not store above 25°C.

6.5 Nature and contents of container

High density polyethylene tube with a polypropylene screw cap containing 15 g, 30 g or 60 g of cream. Not all pack sizes may be marketed.

6.6 Instructions for use and handling

Wash hands after applying this medicine.

7. MARKETING AUTHORISATION HOLDER

Shire Pharmaceutical Contracts Ltd

Hampshire International Business Park

Chineham

Basingstoke

Hampshire RG24 8EP

United Kingdom

8. MARKETING AUTHORISATION NUMBER(S)

EU/1/01/173/001-003

9. DATE OF FIRST AUTHORISATION/RENEWAL OF THE AUTHORISATION

March 2001

10. DATE OF REVISION OF THE TEXT

October 2004

VAQTA Paediatric

(Sanofi Pasteur MSD)

1. NAME OF THE MEDICINAL PRODUCT

VAQTA® Paediatric

Hepatitis A Vaccine, Purified Inactivated, for Paediatrics and Adolescents

2. QUALITATIVE AND QUANTITATIVE COMPOSITION

Each 0.5ml dose contains:

Strain CR 326F Hepatitis A virus, inactivated.............25U

Adsorbed onto approximately 0.225 mg of aluminium provided as amorphous aluminium hydroxyphosphate sulphate

For excipients, see section 6.1

3. PHARMACEUTICAL FORM

VAQTA® Paediatric is a sterile suspension for intramuscular use.

4. CLINICAL PARTICULARS

4.1 Therapeutic indications

VAQTA® Paediatric is indicated for active pre-exposure prophylaxis of children and adolescents 12 months of age up to and including 17 years of age, against disease caused by hepatitis A virus.

4.2 Posology and method of administration

Posology

Children and adolescents aged 12 months to 17 years of age should receive a single 0.5 millilitre (25U) dose of vaccine at an elected date and a second (booster) dose of 0.5 millilitre (25U) 6 to 18 months later.

The vaccine should not be used in children under 12 months old since safety and immunogenicity have not been evaluated in this age group.

A single dose of VAQTA® Paediatric may also be given at 6 to 12 months following the administration of a single (first) dose of another inactivated hepatitis A vaccine in order to complete the vaccination series.

Healthy children ($\geqslant$ 2 years of age) and adolescents who received two doses of VAQTA® Paediatric with a 6-month interval have been shown to remain seropositive for up to 9 years (see section 5.1).

Studies are ongoing to evaluate the need, if any, for additional booster doses.

Method of administration

VAQTA® Paediatric should be injected INTRAMUSCULARLY in the deltoid region. The vaccine should not be administered subcutaneously or intradermally since administration by these routes may result in a less than optimal antibody response.

VAQTA® Paediatric must not be administered intravenously.

4.3 Contraindications

VAQTA® Paediatric should not be administered to subjects with known hypersensitivity to any component of the vaccine, to subjects who showed signs of hypersensitivity after a previous dose of the vaccine or to subjects who are hypersensitive to neomycin or formaldehyde.

As with other vaccines, administration of VAQTA® Paediatric should be postponed in subjects suffering from an acute severe febrile illness. The presence of a minor infection, however, is not a contra-indication for vaccination.

4.4 Special warnings and special precautions for use

As with all injectable vaccines, appropriate medical treatment and supervision should always be readily available in case of a rare anaphylactic event following the administration of the vaccine.

Testing for antibodies to hepatitis A prior to a decision on immunisation should be performed in patients born in areas of high endemicity and/or with a history of jaundice.

VAQTA® Paediatric does not cause immediate protection against hepatitis A, and there may be a period of 2 to 4 weeks before antibody induction occurs.

Because of the long incubation period (approximately 20 to 50 days) for hepatitis A, it is possible for unrecognised hepatitis A infection to be present at the time the vaccine is given. The vaccine may not prevent hepatitis A in such individuals.

VAQTA® Paediatric will not prevent hepatitis caused by infectious agents other than hepatitis A virus.

In subjects with an impaired immune system, adequate anti-HAV antibody titres may not be obtained. If the immunosuppression is due to medical treatment, vaccination should be delayed if possible until the completion of therapy and immune system recovery.

The vaccine has been evaluated in human immunodeficiency virus (HIV) infected adults. There are no data on the use of VAQTA Paediatric in HIV infected subjects.

As with any vaccine, vaccination with VAQTA® Paediatric may not result in a protective response in all susceptible vaccines.

As no studies have been performed with VAQTA® Paediatric in subjects with liver disease, caution is advised if administering the vaccine in these subjects.

4.5 Interaction with other medicinal products and other forms of Interaction

VAQTA® Paediatric must not be mixed with other vaccines or medicinal products in the same syringe.

VAQTA® Paediatric may be given concomitantly with MMR®II [Measles, Mumps and Rubella Virus Vaccine Live] and oral or inactivated polio vaccines. (see Section 5.1 Pharmacodynamic properties).

VAQTA® Paediatric may be administered comcomitantly with immunoglobulin using separate syringes and separate limbs for the injections when combined intermediate and longer-term protection is desirable.

In a clinical study conducted in healthy adults seropositivity rates for hepatitis A when VAQTA®, yellow fever and polysaccharide typhoid vaccines were administered concomitantly were generally similar to when VAQTA® was given alone. Also antibody response rates for yellow fever and typhoid vaccines were equivalent when administered with and without VAQTA®.

Immunogenicity data are insufficient to support concomitant administration of VAQTA with VARIVAX or VAQTA with DTaP.

Other interaction studies have not been performed. However, interactions with other vaccines are not anticipated when vaccines are administered at different injection sites.

4.6 Pregnancy and lactation

Animal reproduction studies have not been conducted with VAQTA® Paediatric. It is not known whether VAQTA® Paediatric can cause foetal harm when administered to a pregnant woman or can affect reproduction capacity. VAQTA® Paediatric is not recommended in pregnancy unless there is a high risk of hepatitis A infection, and the attending physician judges that the possible benefits of vaccination outweigh the risks to the foetus.

It is not known whether VAQTA® Paediatric is excreted in human milk, and the effect on breastfed infants following administration of VAQTA® Paediatric to mothers has not been studied. Hence, VAQTA® Paediatric should be used with caution in women who are breastfeeding.

4.7 Effects on ability to drive and use machines

There are no specific data. However, asthenia/fatigue and headache have been reported following administration of VAQTA® Paediatric.

4.8 Undesirable effects

Children and adolescents from 12 months to 17 years of age

In combined clinical trials involving 706 healthy children 12 months to 23 months of age and 2595 healthy children ($\geqslant$2 years of age) and adolescents who received one or more 25U doses of hepatitis A vaccine with or without other paediatric vaccines, subjects were followed for elevated temperature and local reactions during a 5-day period post vaccination and systemic adverse experiences including fever during a 14 day period post vaccination. Of the 706 children, 241 received VAQTA without other paediatric vaccines for one of the two doses. Fever and injection-site reactions, generally mild and transient were the most frequently reported adverse experiences. Adverse experiences reported as vaccine related for the two age groups (12 months to 23 months and 2 to 17 years of age) are listed below in decreasing order of frequency within each system organ classification.

[Very common: ($\geqslant$1/10), Common: ($\geqslant$1/100, <1/10), Uncommon: ($\geqslant$1/1000, <1/100 and Rare: ($\geqslant$1/10,000, <1/1000)]

Children aged 12 months up to and including 23 months of age

Metabolism and nutrition disorders:

Uncommon:anorexia

Psychiatric disorders:

Common: irritability

Uncommon: crying, nervousness; insomnia; agitation

Nervous system disorders:

Uncommon: somnolence;dizziness; hypersomnia; loss of balance.

Respiratory, thoracic and mediastinal disorders:

Uncommon: rhinorrhea; cough; respiratory congestion;

Gastrointestinal disorders:

Uncommon: diarrhea; vomiting; eructation; flatulence; abdominal distension;

Skin and subcutaneous tissue disorders:

Common: rash

Uncommon: miliaria rubra; sweating; clammy skin; eczema;

General disorders and administrative site conditions:

Common: fever, injection-site pain/tenderness/soreness, swelling, erythema, and warmth

Uncommon: gait abnormality; injection-site ecchymosis; malaise.

Children/Adolescents (2 years up to and including 17 years of age)

Metabolism and nutrition disorders:

Rare: anorexia

Psychiatric disorders:

Uncommon: irritability

Rare: nervousness

Nervous system disorders:

Common: headache

Uncommon: dizziness

Rare: somnolence; paraesthesia

Ear and labyrinth disorders:

Rare: ear pain

Vascular disorders:

Rare: flushing

Respiratory, thoracic and mediastinal disorders:

Rare: nasal congestion; cough; rhinorrhea

Gastrointestinal disorders:

Uncommon: abdominal pain; vomiting; diarrhoea; nausea

Skin and subcutaneous tissue disorders:

Uncommon: rash; pruritus

Rare: urticaria; sweating

Musculoskeletal, connective tissue and bone disorders:

Uncommon: arm pain (in the injected limb); arthralgia; myalgia

Rare: stiffness

General disorders and administrative site conditions:

Very common: injection-site pain and tenderness

Common: injection-site warmth, erythema and swelling; fever; injection-site ecchymosis

Uncommon: asthenia/fatigue; injection-site pruritus and pain/soreness

Rare: injection-site induration; flu-like illness; chest pain; pain; warm sensation; injection-site scab; stiffness/tightness and stinging

Additional complaints not reported in infants, children and adolescents have been reported in clinical trials involving adult subjects.

Should anaphylactic reactions occur see section 4.4 Special Warnings and Precautions for Use.

Marketed experience

As with other vaccines, single cases of central or peripheral affections of the nervous system including Guillain-Barré Syndrome and haematologic autoimmune diseases like thrombocytopenia have been reported.

Post-marketing Safety Study

In a post-marketing safety study, a total of 42,110 individuals > 2 years of age received 1 or 2 doses of VAQTA. There were no vaccine related serious adverse reactions in the 30 days after vaccination.

4.9 Overdose

There are no data with regard to overdose, however overdose is unlikely given the presentation of the product in single dose vials or syringes.

5. PHARMACOLOGICAL PROPERTIES

5.1 Pharmacodynamic properties

VAQTA® Paediatric is derived from hepatitis A virus that has been cultured in human MRC-5 diploid fibroblasts. It contains inactivated virus of a strain which was originally derived by further serial passage of a proven attenuated strain.

The onset of seroconversion following a single dose of VAQTA® Paediatric was shown to parallel the onset of protection against clinical hepatitis A disease. A very high degree of protection has been demonstrated after a single dose of VAQTA® Paediatric in 1037 children and adolescents 2 to 16 years of age in a US community with recurrent outbreaks of hepatitis A (The Monroe Efficacy Study). Seroconversion was achieved in more than 99% of vaccine recipients within 4 weeks of the vaccination. The protective efficacy of a single dose of VAQTA® Paediatric was observed to be 100%. A booster dose was administered to most vaccinees 6, 12 or 18 months after the primary dose. The effectiveness of VAQTA® Paediatric for use in this community has been demonstrated by the fact that after 9 years, no cases of hepatitis A disease ⩾16 days after vaccination have occurred in the vaccinees.

Clinical studies showed seropositivity rates of more than 96% in children and adolescents within 4-6 weeks after the recommended primary dose. In children (⩾2 years of age) and adolescents seropositivity has been shown to persist up to 18 months after a single 25U dose. Persistence of immunologic memory has been demonstrated by eliciting an anamnestic antibody response to a second (booster) of 25U given 6 to 18 months after the primary dose to children (⩾ 2 years of age) and adolescents.

In studies of healthy children and adolescents who received two doses (25U) of VAQTA® Paediatric at 0 and 6 to 18 months, the hepatitis A antibody response has been shown to persist for up to 9 years. The geometric mean antibody titres (GMTs) tend to decline over time. A mathematical model predicts duration of protection lasting for many years after the booster.

Use With Other Vaccines

A concomitant use study was conducted among 617 healthy children who were randomized to receive VAQTA (~25U) with or without M-M-R II and VARIVAX* [Varicella Virus Vaccine Live (Oka/Merck)] at ~12 months of age, and VAQTA (~25U) with or without DTaP (Diphtheria, Tetanus, and acellular Pertussis) vaccine (and an optional dose of polio vaccine) at ~18 months of age. In this study, the concomitant administration of VAQTA with other vaccines at separate injection sites was generally well tolerated. The safety profile of VAQTA administered alone at ~12 months and ~18 months of age was comparable to the safety profile of VAQTA administered alone to children 2 to 16 years of age. The safety profile of the concomitant administration of VAQTA with other vaccines at ~12 months and ~18 months of age was comparable to the safety profile of VAQTA administered alone at ~12 months and ~18 months of age.

The hepatitis A response rates after each dose of VAQTA when VAQTA was given alone or concomitantly with M-M-R II and VARIVAX or DTaP and an optional dose of polio vaccine were similar. The hepatitis A response rates also were similar to predefined historical rates seen in 2- to 3-year-old children administered VAQTA alone. When VAQTA was administered concomitantly with M-M-R II and VARIVAX, the measles, mumps, and rubella response rates were similar to the historical rates for M-M-R II. VAQTA may be given concomitantly at separate injection sites with M-M-R II. Data suggest that VAQTA may be administered concomitantly with oral or inactivated polio vaccine. Immunogenicity data are insufficient to support concomitant administration of VAQTA with VARIVAX or VAQTA with DTaP.

Use in Children With Maternal Antibody to Hepatitis A

In a concomitant use study, children received VAQTA (~25U) at ~12 months and ~18 months of age with or without other pediatric vaccines. After each dose of VAQTA (~25U), the hepatitis A antibody titers were comparable between children who were initially seropositive to hepatitis A and children who were initially seronegative to hepatitis A. These data suggest that maternal antibody to hepatitis A in children ~12 months of age does not affect the immune response to VAQTA.

5.2 Pharmacokinetic properties

Not applicable

5.3 Preclinical safety data

None stated.

6. PHARMACEUTICAL PARTICULARS

6.1 List of excipients

Sodium borate

Sodium chloride

Water for injections

For adjuvant see section 2.0 Qualitative and Quantitative Composition

Neomycin and formaldehyde are used in the manufacturing process

6.2 Incompatibilities

Do not mix in the same syringe with other vaccines/drugs.

6.3 Shelf life

36 months when stored between +2°C and +8°C.

Expiry date has been printed on the package (month followed by year) and is applicable only if the vaccine has been stored between +2°C and +8°C. Potency of this vaccine is not significantly affected after exposure to temperatures up to 28°C for up to 3 months. However this is NOT a storage recommendation and if kept longer than three months at this temperature it should not be used.

6.4 Special precautions for storage

Store vaccine between +2°C and +8°C (+36°F and +46°F). DO NOT FREEZE since freezing destroys potency.

6.5 Nature and contents of container

Single dose (0.5ml, approx 25U) vial and prefilled syringe.

6.6 Instructions for use and handling

The vaccine should be used as supplied; no reconstitution is necessary.

Shake well immediately before withdrawal and use. Thorough agitation is necessary to maintain suspension of the vaccine.

Parenteral drug products should be inspected visually for extraneous particulate matter and discoloration prior to administration. After thorough agitation, VAQTA® Paediatric is a slightly opaque white suspension.

It is important to use a separate sterile syringe and needle for each individual to prevent transmission of infections from one person to another.

7. MARKETING AUTHORISATION HOLDER

Sanofi Pasteur MSD Limited
Mallards Reach
Bridge Avenue
Maidenhead
Berkshire
SL6 1QP

8. MARKETING AUTHORISATION NUMBER(S)

PL 6745/0064

9. DATE OF FIRST AUTHORISATION/RENEWAL OF THE AUTHORISATION

15 August 1996

10. DATE OF REVISION OF THE TEXT

July 2005

® Registered trademark

Varidase Topical 125,000 Units Per Vial

(Wyeth Pharmaceuticals)

1. NAME OF THE MEDICINAL PRODUCT

Varidase Topical 125,000 units per vial.

2. QUALITATIVE AND QUANTITATIVE COMPOSITION

Varidase Topical contains streptokinase 100,000 IU and streptodornase 25,000 IU.

3. PHARMACEUTICAL FORM

Powder and solvent for solution for cutaneous use or powder for solution for cutaneous use.

4. CLINICAL PARTICULARS

4.1 Therapeutic indications

Varidase Topical is indicated wherever removal of clotted blood, fibrinous or purulent accumulations is required.

It is indicated in the treatment of suppurative surface lesions such as ulcers, pressure sores, amputation sites, diabetic gangrene, radiation necrosis, infected wounds and surgical incisions, until the wound is thoroughly cleansed of clots, fibrinous exudates and pus.

It is also indicated in the treatment of burns and may be used prior to skin grafting.

Varidase Topical can be used to dissolve clots in the bladder or in urinary catheters.

4.2 Posology and method of administration

Adults, children and the elderly:

Directions for use in the cleansing of necrotic infected and sloughy wounds.

Refer to Section 6.6 for instructions on reconstitution.

Standard methods of application:

Pre-soak gauze with Varidase Topical solution then apply to the wound. Following application, a semi-occlusive dressing is necessary to prevent drying out of the wound, e.g. a polyethylene film taped on two sides. Alternatively the wound may be packed with dry gauze which is then soaked with Varidase Topical solution and dressed with a semi-occlusive dressing.

Alternative method of application:

Where wounds are covered by a thick dry eschar it is usually necessary to cross hatch the eschar into approximately 3-5mm squares and to a sufficient depth to allow the access of the enzymes to the underlying fibrinous purulent material.

Alternatively, Varidase Topical may be introduced under the eschar, taking care that the solution enters only the cavity beneath and that the volume is not sufficient to cause pain through increased pressure. Introducing Varidase Topical in this way often results in the eschar becoming partly detached thus facilitating its mechanical removal.

Special technique of application:

Varidase Topical may be applied in jelly form. This can be prepared by dissolving the contents of one vial in 5ml of sterile water and mixing the resulting solution thoroughly, but gently, with 15ml of inert jelly, such as K-Y or carboxymethylcellulose (CMC) jelly. This method can be particularly useful in cases of burns where dressings are not employed.

Frequency of application:

Varidase Topical treatment should be repeated once or twice a day. Care should be taken to irrigate the lesion thoroughly with physiological saline to remove loosened material prior to the next application.

Duration of treatment:

Treatment should be continued until healthy granulations are present and re-epithelialisation has begun, usually within one to two weeks. In mixed wounds, where granulation has started in some areas, Varidase use can continue until the entire wound is clean and granulating without any harmful effects to the healthy tissues.

4.3 Contraindications

Active haemorrhage.

Hypersensitivity to any component of the medicinal product.

Severe uncontrolled hypertension.

Intravenous or intramusucular use.

4.4 Special warnings and special precautions for use

Varidase Topical is intended for local use only. This product contains streptokinase, which when used systemically is known to be antigenic.

There have been reports of hypersensitivity and anaphylactic/anaphylactoid reactions (including shock, dyspnoea, and urticaria) associated with the use of streptodornase-streptokinase.

Streptokinase and streptodornase are antigenic, and antibodies may develop in patients. As a result, decreased efficacy may occur after repeated use. Topical administration of streptokinase causes a significant humoral response by one month, then declines. It may be preferable to avoid intravenous strepokinase in patients who have been treated with topical streptokinase in the preceding six months.

Use with caution in patients with a history of decreased hepatic function. Hepatic dysfunction may be caused by the high activities of the proteolytic enzymes plasminogen activator and plasmin, which are generated by the action of streptokinase. This has been reported with I.V. use.

The beneficial action of the enzymes causes an accumulation of tissue fluid. However, drainage and aspiration, particularly of closed spaces, such as the bladder, may be required because of the accumulation of tissue fluid.

In order to avoid cross-infection, a new vial of Varidase Topical and a separate sterile syringe and needle should be used for each individual patient.

Varidase Topical has been shown to be a sensitiser when administered at relatively low intradermal doses to guinea pigs. The potential may exist to induce allergic reactions as described under "Undesirable Effects".

4.5 Interaction with other medicinal products and other forms of Interaction

The preparation is buffered to physiological pH. The enzymes of Varidase Topical can be inactivated by the concomitant use of other preparations of an acidic or alkaline pH. Aluminium reacts with Varidase Topical. If the reconstituting fluid has a high calcium content, the solution becomes opalescent, but this does not affect the potency of the enzymes.

4.6 Pregnancy and lactation

Safe use of Varidase Topical during pregnancy and lactation has not been established. While only minimal amounts of streptokinase cross the placenta, streptokinase-specific antibodies are found in foetal blood. Use in these circumstances should be avoided unless considered essential by the physician.

4.7 Effects on ability to drive and use machines

None known.

4.8 Undesirable effects

Allergic reactions to the application of Varidase Topical may be minimised by careful and frequent removal of exudate followed by thorough irrigation using physiological saline prior to retreatment with Varidase Topical.

System Organ Class	Adverse Reaction
Blood and lymphatic system disorders	
Frequency undetermined	Haemorrhage
Immune system disorders	
Frequency undetermined	Hypersensitivity and anaphylactic/anaphylactoid reactions (including shock, dyspnoea and urticaria)
Skin and subcutaneous tissue disorders	
Frequency undetermined	Rash erythematous, dermatitis contact, dermatitis, injection site reaction, pruritus
Renal and urinary disorders	
Frequency undetermined	Haematuria following bladder instillation
General disorders and administration site conditions	
Frequency undetermined	Fever/pyrexia, burning sensation, pain.

4.9 Overdose

There is no specific antidote. Removal of the preparation by careful washing or by irrigation/suction drainage is recommended.

5. PHARMACOLOGICAL PROPERTIES

5.1 Pharmacodynamic properties

Streptokinase acts indirectly upon a substrate of fibrin or fibrinogen by activating a fibrinolytic enzyme in human serum. Upon application of streptokinase in situ, the activation of this fibrinolytic system brings about rapid dissolution of blood clots and the fibrinous portion of exudates. Streptodornase liquefies the viscous nucleoprotein of dead cells or pus. Thus the action of the enzymes results in the liquefaction of the two main viscous substances resulting from inflammatory or infectious processes thereby facilitating cleansing and de-sloughing of wounds.

Varidase Topical has no effect on collagen, living cells or healthy tissue.

5.2 Pharmacokinetic properties

There are no published reports concerning the pharmacokinetics of Varidase.

5.3 Preclinical safety data

Not applicable.

6. PHARMACEUTICAL PARTICULARS

6.1 List of excipients

Powder for solution for cutaneous use

Sodium phosphate monobasic, sodium phosphate dibasic.

Diluent for powder for solution for cutaneous use

Sodium chloride

Purified water

6.2 Incompatibilities

None known.

6.3 Shelf life

18 months (unopened).

1 day (reconstituted solution stored in a refrigerator at 2-8°C).

6.4 Special precautions for storage

The unreconstituted and reconstituted product should be stored in a refrigerator (2-8°C). Do not freeze.

6.5 Nature and contents of container

25ml borosilicate Type 1 glass vial with butyl rubber stopper and metal seal with pull-tab.

The product is available in:

1. Boxes containing a single vial of Varidase Topical sterile powder.

2. Combi-packs containing 1 vial of Varidase Topical sterile powder, 1 vial of Diluent (20ml of sterile sodium chloride 0.9% solution BP) and 1 sterile transfer needle.

6.6 Instructions for use and handling

Reconstitution:

Single vial: The contents should be gently mixed with 20ml of sterile physiological saline or, if unavailable, 20ml of Water for Injection until the powder is completely dissolved. The resulting clear solution can then be withdrawn into a syringe.

Combi-Pack: Insert one end of the sterile transfer needle into the diluent vial and push the Varidase vial down onto the outer end of the needle.

(Ensure that the transfer needle goes centrally through the upraised circle on the stoppers).

Invert the vials so that the Varidase vial is under the diluent vial and allow the full 20ml of diluent to run into the Varidase vial to dissolve the powder. Remove the empty diluent vial and discard. If necessary, gently agitate the Varidase vial until the powder is completely dissolved. The resulting clear solution can then be poured from the transfer needle.

As Varidase Topical is packed under vacuum, care should be taken when inserting a needle into the vial.

Excess agitation of the vial should be avoided to prevent frothing and denaturing of the enzymes.

As Varidase Topical does not contain a preservative, multi-dose use is not recommended.

7. MARKETING AUTHORISATION HOLDER

Cyanamid of Great Britain Ltd

Fareham Road

Gosport

Hants

PO13 0AS

8. MARKETING AUTHORISATION NUMBER(S)

Varidase Topical 125,000 units per vial - PL 0095/5038R.

Diluent for Varidase Topical (Combi-Pack) - PL 1502/0006R.

9. DATE OF FIRST AUTHORISATION/RENEWAL OF THE AUTHORISATION

17th September 1996.

10. DATE OF REVISION OF THE TEXT

17th May 2004

Varilrix

(GlaxoSmithKline UK)

1. NAME OF THE MEDICINAL PRODUCT

Varilrix® ▼, $10^{3.3}$ PFU/0.5ml, powder and solvent for solution for injection.

2. QUALITATIVE AND QUANTITATIVE COMPOSITION

One dose (0.5 ml) contains:

Live attenuated varicella-zoster (Oka strain) virus* $10^{3.3}$ plaque forming units (PFU)

*propagated in MRC5 human diploid cells

For excipients, see 6.1.

3. PHARMACEUTICAL FORM

Powder and solvent for solution for injection.

Pink to red solution.

4. CLINICAL PARTICULARS

4.1 Therapeutic indications

Varilrix is indicated for active immunisation against varicella in healthy adults and adolescents (⩾ 13 years) who have been found to be seronegative with respect to the varicella-zoster virus and are, therefore, at risk of developing chickenpox.

Varilrix is not indicated for routine use in children. However, it may be administered to seronegative healthy children of 1-12 years of age who are close contacts (e.g. household) of persons considered to be at high risk of severe varicella infections.

4.2 Posology and method of administration

Posology

Adolescents (⩾ 13 years) and Adults

Two doses (each of 0.5 ml of reconstituted vaccine) should be given, with an interval between doses of approximately eight weeks (minimum interval of six weeks).

There are insufficient data to determine the long-term protective efficacy of the vaccine. However, there is currently no evidence that further doses are routinely required following completion of a two-dose regimen in healthy adolescents and adults (see section 5.1).

If Varilrix is to be administered to seronegative subjects before a period of planned or possible future immunosuppression (such as those awaiting organ transplantation and those in remission from malignant disease), the timing of the vaccinations should take into account the delay after the second dose before maximal protection might be expected (see also sections 4.3, 4.4 and 5.1).

Children 1-12 years

Varilrix is not indicated for routine use in children. However, under the circumstances described in section 4.1, a single dose of 0.5 ml of reconstituted vaccine should be given.

Varilrix should not be administered to children aged less than one year.

Elderly

There are no data on immune responses to Varilrix in the elderly.

Method of administration

Varilrix is for subcutaneous administration only. The upper arm (deltoid region) is the preferred site of injection.

Varilrix should not be administered intradermally.

Varilrix must under no circumstances be administered intravascularly.

There are no data on the immune responses when different varicella-zoster vaccines are used for the first and second doses. Therefore, it is recommended that the same vaccine should be used for both doses.

Varilrix must not be mixed with any other medicinal product in the same syringe (see also sections 4.5 and 6.2).

4.3 Contraindications

Varilrix is contra-indicated in subjects who have a history of hypersensitivity to neomycin, or to any of the excipients in the vaccine, or to any other varicella vaccine.

A second dose of Varilrix is contra-indicated in subjects who have had a hypersensitivity reaction following the first dose.

Varilrix is contra-indicated during pregnancy and breast-feeding (see also sections 4.4 and 4.6).

Varilrix must not be administered to subjects with primary or acquired immunodeficiency states, such as subjects with leukaemias, lymphomas, blood dyscrasias, clinically manifest HIV infection, or patients receiving immunosuppressive therapy (including high dose corticosteroids).

Administration of Varilrix must be postponed in subjects suffering from acute, severe febrile illness.

4.4 Special warnings and special precautions for use

As with all injectable vaccines, appropriate medical treatment and supervision should always be readily available in case of a rare anaphylactic reaction following the administration of the vaccine.

Varilrix contains a live attenuated varicella-zoster virus and administration is contra-indicated during pregnancy (see sections 4.3 and 4.6). Due to an unknown degree of risk to the mother and to the fetus, female candidates for vaccination must be advised to take adequate precautions to prevent pregnancy occurring between the two doses and for three months after the second dose.

Serological studies of efficacy and post-marketing experience indicate that the vaccine does not completely protect all individuals from naturally-acquired varicella and cannot be expected to provide maximal protection against infection with varicella-zoster virus until about six weeks after the second dose (see section 5.1).

Administration of Varilrix to subjects who are in the incubation period of the infection cannot be expected to protect against clinically manifest varicella or to modify the course of the disease.

The rash produced during naturally-acquired primary infection with varicella-zoster may be more severe in those with existing severe skin damage, including severe eczematous conditions. It is not known if there is an increased risk of vaccine-associated skin lesions in such persons, but this possibility should be taken into consideration before vaccination.

Transmission of the vaccine viral strain

Transmission of vaccine viral strain has been shown to occur from healthy vaccinees to healthy contacts, to pregnant contacts and to immunosuppressed contacts. However, transmission to any of these groups occurs rarely or very rarely and has not been confirmed to occur in the absence of vaccine-associated cutaneous lesions in the vaccinee (see section 4.8).

In healthy contacts of vaccinees, seroconversion has sometimes occurred in the absence of any clinical manifestations of infection. Clinically apparent infections due to transmission of the vaccine viral strain have been associated with few skin lesions and minimal systemic upset.

However, contact with the following groups must be avoided if the vaccinee develops a cutaneous rash thought likely to be vaccine-related (especially vesicular or papulovesicular) within four to six weeks of the first or second dose and until this rash has completely disappeared (see also sections 4.6 and 5.1).

- varicella-susceptible pregnant women and
- individuals at high risk of severe varicella, such as those with primary and acquired immunodeficiency states. These include individuals with leukaemias, lymphomas, blood dyscrasias, clinically manifest HIV infections, and patients who are receiving immunosuppressive therapy, including high dose corticosteroids.

In the absence of a rash in the vaccinee, the risk of transmission of the vaccine viral strain to contacts in the above groups appears to be extremely small. Nevertheless, vaccinees (*e.g.* healthcare workers) who are very likely to come into contact with persons in the above groups should preferably avoid any such contact during the period between vaccinations and for 4-6 weeks after the second dose. If this is not feasible, then vaccinees should be vigilant regarding the reporting of any skin rash during this period, and should take steps as above if a rash is discovered.

Healthy seronegative children may be vaccinated if they are close contacts of persons who are at high risk of severe varicella infection (see sections 4.1 and 4.2). In these circumstances, continued contact between the vaccinee and the person at risk may be unavoidable. Therefore, the risk of transmission of the attenuated vaccine viral strain from the vaccinee should be weighed against the potential for acquisition of wild-type varicella-zoster by the at-risk person.

The Oka vaccine viral strain has recently been shown to be sensitive to acyclovir.

4.5 Interaction with other medicinal products and other forms of Interaction

In subjects who have received immune globulins or a blood transfusion, vaccination should be delayed for at least three months because of the likelihood of vaccine failure due to passively acquired antibody to the varicella-zoster virus.

Aspirin and systemic salicylates should not be given to children under the age of 16, except under medical supervision, because of the risk of Reye's syndrome. Reye's syndrome has been reported in children treated with aspirin during natural varicella infection. However, there is no evidence to suggest that vaccination with Varilrix should be contrainidicated for older age-groups who need to take aspirin.

In a study in which Varilrix was administered to toddlers at the same time as, but at a different site to, a combined measles, mumps and rubella vaccine, there was no evidence of significant immune interference between the live viral antigens.

If it is considered necessary to administer another live vaccine at the same time as Varilrix, the vaccines must be given as separate injections and at different body sites.

4.6 Pregnancy and lactation

Pregnancy

Varicella-zoster virus may cause severe clinical disease in pregnant individuals and may adversely affect the fetus and/or result in perinatal varicella, depending on the gestational stage when the infection occurs. Because the possible effects of infection with the vaccine viral strain on the mother and on the fetus are unknown, Varilrix must not be administered to pregnant women.

Furthermore, female candidates for vaccination must be advised to take adequate precautions to avoid pregnancy occurring between the two vaccine doses and for three months following the second dose.

Lactation

The infants of seronegative women would not have acquired transplacental antibody to varicella-zoster virus. Therefore, due to the theoretical risk of transmission of the vaccine viral strain from mother to infant, women should not be vaccinated while breastfeeding.

4.7 Effects on ability to drive and use machines

It would not be expected that vaccination would affect the ability to drive or operate machinery.

4.8 Undesirable effects

Clinical studies

Undesirable effects that occurred during the 4-6 week period after vaccination were monitored using symptom checklists. The adverse events listed below were reported in temporal relationship with vaccination.

Frequencies, based on a total of 1141 doses administered to adolescents and adults, are reported as follows:

Very common: (≥ 10%)

Common: (≥ 1% and < 10%)

Uncommon: (≥ 0.1% and < 1%)

In adolescents and adults, the incidence of adverse reactions was not higher after the second dose with respect to the first.

The adverse events listed below were reported with similar frequencies following vaccination of 2624 children.

Injection site reactions:

very common: pain, redness, swelling

uncommon: inflammation, mass

Body as a whole:

common: fatigue, fever

uncommon: chest pain, malaise, pain

Central and peripheral nervous system:

common: headache

uncommon: dizziness, migraine

Gastrointestinal system:

uncommon: gastroenteritis, nausea

Musculoskeletal system:

uncommon: arthralgia, back pain, myalgia

Psychiatric:

uncommon: somnolence

Respiratory system:

uncommon: coughing, pharyngitis, rhinitis

Skin and appendages:

common: papulovesicular rash

uncommon: pruritis

White cell and reticuloendothelial system:

uncommon: lymphadenopathy

Post-marketing surveillance

Transmission of the vaccine virus from healthy vaccinees to healthy contacts has been shown to occur very rarely.

The following adverse events have been reported following vaccination of children, adolescents and adults with a frequency of less than 0.01%.

Injection site reactions

pain, redness, swelling

Body as a whole

fever

urticaria

anaphylactoid reaction

Skin and appendages

papulovesicular rash

There have been isolated reports of ataxia, myelitis and thrombocytopenia in temporal association with, but with an indeterminate relationship to, Varilrix.

4.9 Overdose

There is no experience of administration of an overdose of Varilrix. Accidental administration of an excessive dose is very unlikely because the vaccine is presented in single dose vials.

5. PHARMACOLOGICAL PROPERTIES

5.1 Pharmacodynamic properties

ATC code J07B K01

The Oka strain virus contained in Varilrix was initially obtained from a child with natural varicella; the virus was then attenuated through sequential passage in tissue culture.

Natural infection induces a cellular and humoral immune response to the varicella-zoster virus, which can be rapidly detected following infection. IgG, IgM and IgA directed against viral proteins usually appear at the same time that a cellular immune response can be demonstrated, making the relative contribution of humoral and cellular immunity to disease progression difficult to ascertain. Vaccination has been shown to induce both humoral and cell-mediated types of immunity.

In clinical trials, the immune response to vaccination was routinely measured using an immunofluorescence assay. Antibody titres of ≥ 1:4 (the detection level of the test) were considered as positive.

In clinical trials that enrolled 211 adolescents and 213adults, all vaccinees had detectable levels of antibodies in blood samples taken six weeks after the second vaccine dose. Virtually all (98.7%) of the 1637 children tested had detectable antibodies six weeks after immunisation with one dose of vaccine.

In a follow-up study over 2 years in 159 vaccinated adult health care workers, 2 out of 72 (3%) vaccinees reporting contacts with wild-type chickenpox experienced mild breakthrough disease. Approximately one-third of the vaccinees showed an increase in antibody titre over the follow-up period, indicative of contact with the virus, without clinical evidence of varicella infection.

The percentage of vaccinees who will later experience herpes-zoster due to reactivation of the Oka strain virus is currently unknown. However, the risk of zoster after vaccination is currently thought to be much lower than would be expected after wild-type virus infection, due to attenuation of the vaccine strain.

5.2 Pharmacokinetic properties

Evaluation of pharmacokinetic properties is not required for vaccines.

5.3 Preclinical safety data

There is no other relevant information that has not already been stated above.

6. PHARMACEUTICAL PARTICULARS

6.1 List of excipients

Amino acids, human albumin, lactose, neomycin sulphate, mannitol, sorbitol

6.2 Incompatibilities

Varilrix should not be mixed with other vaccines in the same syringe.

6.3 Shelf life

2 years.

The vaccine should be used immediately after reconstitution. If not used immediately, in-use storage times and conditions prior to use are the responsibility of the user and should normally not be longer than 1 hour at +2°C to +8°C (in a refrigerator). Do not freeze.

6.4 Special precautions for storage

Store at +2°C to +8°C (in a refrigerator).

The lyophilised vaccine is not affected by freezing.

6.5 Nature and contents of container

Powder for reconstitution

Slightly pink-coloured pellet in 3 ml vials (Type I glass) with stopper (bromobutyl rubber) and flip-off cap (aluminium).

Solvent for reconstitution

Water for Injections in 1 ml ampoule (Type I glass).

Packs of one.

6.6 Instructions for use and handling

Due to minor variations of its pH, the colour of the reconstituted vaccine may vary from pink to red. The diluent and the reconstituted vaccine should be inspected visually for any foreign particulate matter and/or variation of physical appearance prior to administration. In the event of either being observed, discard the diluent or the reconstituted vaccine.

Varilrix must be reconstituted by adding the contents of the supplied container of water for injections diluent to the vial containing the pellet. After the addition of the diluent to the pellet, the mixture should be well shaken until the pellet is completely dissolved in the diluent.

Alcohol and other disinfecting agents must be allowed to evaporate from the skin before injection of the vaccine since they may inactivate the virus.

Any unused product or waste material should be disposed of in accordance with local requirements.

Administrative Data

7. MARKETING AUTHORISATION HOLDER

SmithKline Beecham plc
980, Great West Road
Brentford
Middlesex TW8 9GS
United Kingdom

Trading as:

GlaxoSmithKline UK
Stockley Park West
Uxbridge
Middlesex UB11 1BT
United Kingdom

8. MARKETING AUTHORISATION NUMBER(S)

Vaccine: PL 10592/0121
Diluent: PL 10592/0021

9. DATE OF FIRST AUTHORISATION/RENEWAL OF THE AUTHORISATION
25 June 2002

10. DATE OF REVISION OF THE TEXT
30 September 2004

11. Legal Status
POM

VARIVAX

(Sanofi Pasteur MSD)

1. NAME OF THE MEDICINAL PRODUCT
VARIVAX® ▼powder and solvent for suspension for injection

[Varicella Vaccine (live)]

2. QUALITATIVE AND QUANTITATIVE COMPOSITION
The vaccine is a lyophilised preparation of a live attenuated varicella virus (Oka/Merck strain).

After reconstitution, one dose (0,5 mL) contains:

Varicella virus** (Oka/Merck strain) ⩾1350 PFU***

** Produced on human diploid cells (MRC-5)

***PFU = Plaque-forming units

For excipients, see section 6.1.

3. PHARMACEUTICAL FORM
Powder and solvent for suspension for injection.

White to off-white powder and solvent.

When reconstituted, VARIVAX is a clear, colourless to pale yellow liquid.

4. CLINICAL PARTICULARS

4.1 Therapeutic indications
Active immunisation for the primary prevention of varicella in individuals 12 months of age and older.

VARIVAX may also be administered to susceptible individuals who have been exposed to varicella. Vaccination within 3 days of exposure may prevent a clinically apparent infection or modify the course of the infection. In addition, there are limited data that indicate that vaccination up to 5 days after exposure may modify the course of the infection (see section 5.1).

VARIVAX is to be used on the basis of applicable official recommendations.

4.2 Posology and method of administration
Posology

Individuals 12 months to 12 years of age should receive a single 0,5 mL dose. VARIVAX should not be administered to individuals less than 1 year of age.

Individuals 12 months to 12 years of age with asymptomatic HIV infection [CDC Class 1] with an age-specific CD4+ T-lymphocyte percentage ⩾25% should receive two doses of 0,5 mL given 12 weeks apart.

Individuals 13 years of age and older should receive two doses of 0,5 mL given 4-8 weeks apart. If the interval between doses exceeds 8 weeks, the second dose should be given as soon as possible. Some individuals may not be protected until after the second dose has been administered.

There are data available on protective efficacy for up to 9 years post-vaccination (see section 5.1). However, the need for booster doses has not been determined as yet.

If VARIVAX is to be administered to seronegative subjects before a period of planned or possible future immunosuppression (such as those awaiting organ transplantation and those in remission from a malignant disease), the timing of the vaccinations should take into account the interval after the second dose before maximal protection might be expected (see sections 4.3, 4.4, and 5.1).

Elderly

There are no data on protective efficacy or immune responses to VARIVAX in seronegative persons over 65 years of age.

Method of administration

The vaccine is to be injected by the SUBCUTANEOUS ROUTE in the deltoid region or in the higher anterolateral region of the thigh.

DO NOT INJECT INTRAVASCULARLY.

4.3 Contraindications
• History of hypersensitivity to any varicella vaccine, to any of the excipients or to gelatin or neomycin (which may be present as trace residues, see sections 4.4 and 6.1).

• Blood dyscrasias, leukaemia, lymphomas of any type, or other malignant neoplasms affecting the hemic and lymphatic systems.

• Individuals receiving immunosuppressive therapy (including high doses of corticosteroids).

• Individuals with humoral or cellular (primary or acquired) immunodeficiency, including hypogammaglobulinemia and individuals with AIDS, or symptomatic HIV infection or a CDC Class 2 or higher or an age-specific CD4+ T-lymphocyte percentage <25% (see section 4.4).

• Individuals with a family history of congenital or hereditary immunodeficiency, unless the immune competence of the potential vaccine recipient is demonstrated.

• Active untreated tuberculosis.

• Any illness with fever >38,5°C; however, low-grade fever itself is not a contraindication to vaccination.

• Pregnancy (see also sections 4.4 and 4.6).

4.4 Special warnings and special precautions for use
As with all injectable vaccines, appropriate medical treatment and supervision should always be readily available in case of a rare anaphylactic reaction following the administration of the vaccine.

Before vaccination of women of child-bearing potential, pregnancy must be excluded and effective contraception must be used for 3 months following vaccination (see sections 4.3 and 4.6). In addition, VARIVAX is not generally recommended for breastfeeding mothers (see section 4.6).

As with other vaccines, VARIVAX does not completely protect all individuals from naturally acquired varicella. Clinical trials have only assessed efficacy beginning 6 weeks after a single dose in healthy individuals up to 12 years of age or 6 weeks after the second dose in older subjects (see section 5.1).

As for other vaccines, there is the possibility of hypersensitivity reactions, not only to the active principle, but also to the following excipients and trace residuals present in the vaccine: gelatin and neomycin; residual components of MRC-5 cells, including DNA and proteins; and trace quantities of bovine calf serum from MRC-5 culture medium.

There are limited data on the safety and efficacy of the vaccine in individuals 12 months of age and older who are known to be infected with human immunodeficiency virus with and without evidence of immunosuppression. However, VARIVAX may be given to individuals 12 months to 12 years of age with asymptomatic HIV infection [CDC Class 1] with an age-specific CD4+ T-lymphocytes percentage ⩾25% (see section 4.3).

Vaccine recipients should avoid use of salicylates for 6 weeks after vaccination (see section 4.5).

Transmission

Transmission of vaccine virus may rarely occur between healthy vaccinees who develop a varicella-like rash and healthy susceptible contacts, pregnant contacts and immunosuppressed contacts (see section 4.8).

Therefore, vaccine recipients should attempt to avoid, whenever possible, close association with susceptible high-risk individuals for up to 6 weeks following vaccination.

In circumstances where contact with high-risk individuals is unavoidable, before vaccination, the potential risk of transmission of the vaccine virus should be weighed against the risk of acquiring and transmitting the wild-type varicella virus.

Susceptible high-risk individuals include:

• Immunocompromised individuals (see section 4.3);

• Pregnant women without documented positive history of chickenpox or laboratory evidence of prior infection;

• Newborns of mothers without documented positive history of chickenpox or laboratory evidence of prior infection.

4.5 Interaction with other medicinal products and other forms of Interaction
VARIVAX must not be mixed with any other vaccine or other medicinal product in the same syringe. Other injectable vaccines or other medicinal products must be given as separate injections and at different body sites.

Concomitant administration with other vaccines

VARIVAX has been administered to toddlers at the same time as, but at a different injection site from, a combined measles, mumps, and rubella vaccine, *Haemophilus influenzae* type b conjugate vaccine, hepatitis B vaccine, diphtheria/tetanus/whole-cell pertussis vaccine, and oral polio virus vaccine. There was no evidence of a clinically relevant difference in the immune responses to any of the antigens when co-administered with VARIVAX. If varicella vaccine (live) (Oka/Merck strain) is not given concomitantly with measles, mumps, and rubella virus vaccine live, a 1-month interval between the 2 live virus vaccines should be observed.

Concurrent administration of VARIVAX and tetravalent, pentavalent or hexavalent (diphtheria, tetanus, and acelular pertussis [DTaP])-based vaccines has not been evaluated.

Vaccination should be deferred for at least 5 months following blood or plasma transfusions, or administration of normal human immune globulin or varicella zoster immune globulin (VZIG).

Administration of varicella zoster virus antibody-containing blood products, including VZIG or other immune globulin preparations, within 1 month following a dose of VARIVAX may reduce the immune response to the vaccine and hence reduce its protective efficacy. Therefore, administration of any of these products should be avoided within 1 month after a dose of VARIVAX unless considered to be essential.

Vaccine recipients should avoid use of salicylates for 6 weeks after vaccination with VARIVAX as Reye's syndrome has been reported following use of salicylates during wild-type varicella infection (see section 4.4).

4.6 Pregnancy and lactation
Studies with the vaccine have not been conducted in pregnant women. It is not known whether the vaccine can cause foetal harm when administered to a pregnant woman or can affect reproduction capacity. However, wild-type varicella is known to cause foetal harm, and is associated with an increased risk of herpes zoster in the first year of life and severe chickenpox in the newborn infant. **Therefore, VARIVAX must not be administered to pregnant women** (see section 4.3). Before vaccination of women of child-bearing potential, pregnancy must be excluded and effective contraception must be used for 3 months following vaccination.

Lactation

Due to the theoretical risk of transmission of the vaccine viral strain from mother to infant, VARIVAX is not generally recommended for breastfeeding mothers (see also section 4.4). Vaccination of exposed women with negative history of varicella or known to be seronegative to varicella should be assessed on an individual basis.

4.7 Effects on ability to drive and use machines
It would not be expected that vaccination with VARIVAX would affect the ability to drive or operate machinery.

4.8 Undesirable effects
Clinical Studies

Overall safety profile of varicella vaccine (live) (Oka/Merck strain)

In clinical trials, frozen and refrigerator-stable formulations of varicella vaccine (live) (Oka/Merck strain) were administered to approximately 17.000 healthy individuals ⩾12 months of age who were monitored for up to 42 days after each dose. There appeared to be no increased risk for adverse events with the use of VARIVAX in seropositive individuals. The safety profile of refrigerator-stable varicella vaccine (live) (Oka/Merck strain) was generally similar to the safety profile for earlier formulations of the vaccine.

In a double-blind, placebo-controlled study among 956 healthy individuals 12 months to 14 years of age, 914 of whom were serologically confirmed to be susceptible to varicella, the only adverse events that occurred at a significantly greater rate in vaccine recipients than in placebo recipients were pain (26,7% versus 18,1%) and redness (5,7% versus 2,4%) at the injection site and non-injection-site varicella-like rash (2,2% versus 0,2%).

Across clinical studies in which causality was assessed (5129 subjects), the following adverse events were reported in temporal association with vaccination:

Very common (⩾ 1/10), Common (⩾ 1/100, <1/10), Uncommon (⩾ 1/1000, <1/100), Rare (⩾ 1/10,000, <1/1000)

Healthy individuals 12 months to 12 years of age (1-dose)

Infections and infestations

Common: upper respiratory infection

Uncommon: influenza, gastroenteritis, otitis, otitis media, pharyngitis, varicella, viral exanthema, viral infection

Rare: infection, candidiasis, flu-like illness, non-venomous bite/sting

Blood and lymphatic system disorders

Rare: lymphadenopathy, lymphadenitis, thrombocytopenia

Metabolism and nutrition disorders

Uncommon: anorexia

Psychiatric disorders

Common: irritability

Uncommon: crying, insomnia, sleep disorder

Nervous system disorders

Uncommon: headache, somnolence

Rare: apathy, nervousness, agitation, hypersomnia, dream abnormality, emotional changes, gait abnormality, febrile seizure, tremor

Eye disorders

Uncommon: conjunctivitis

Rare: acute conjunctivitis, tearing, edema of the eyelid, irritation

Ear and labyrinth disorders

Rare: ear pain

Vascular disorders

Rare: extravasation

Respiratory, thoracic and mediastinal disorders

Uncommon: cough, nasal congestion, respiratory congestion, rhinorrhoea

Rare: sinusitis, sneezing, pulmonary congestion, epistaxis, rhinitis, wheezing, bronchitis, respiratory infection, pneumonia

Gastrointestinal disorders

Uncommon: diarrhoea, vomiting

Rare: abdominal pain, nausea, flatulence, hematochezia, mouth ulcer

Skin and subcutaneous tissue disorders

Common: rash, measles/rubella-like rash, varicella-like rash

Uncommon: contact dermatitis, diaper rash, erythema, miliaria rubra, pruritus, urticaria

Rare: flushing, vesicle, atopic dermatitis, eczema, acne, herpes simplex, hive-like rash, contusion, dermatitis, drug eruption, impetigo, skin infection, measles, sunburn

Musculoskeletal and connective site conditions

Rare: musculoskeletal pain, myalgia, pain of the hip, leg or neck, stiffness

General disorders and administration site conditions

Very common: fever

Common: injection site erythema, rash, pain/tenderness/soreness, swelling, and varicella-like rash

Uncommon: asthenia/fatigue; injection site ecchymosis, hematoma, induration, rash; malaise

Rare: injection site eczema, lump, warmth, hive-like rash, discoloration, inflammation, stiffness, trauma, roughness/dryness, edema/swelling, pain/tenderness/soreness; warm sensation; warm to touch; venipuncture site hemorrhage; lip abnormality.

The following serious adverse events temporally associated with the vaccination were reported in individuals 12 months to 12 years of age given varicella vaccine (live) (Oka/Merck strain): diarrhoea, febrile seizure, fever, post-infectious arthritis, vomiting.

Healthy individuals 13 years of age and older (majority received 2 doses 4 to 8 weeks apart)

Causality was not assessed in individuals 13 years of age and older with the exception of serious adverse events. However, across clinical studies (1648 subjects) the following events were temporally associated with vaccination:

Skin and subcutaneous tissue disorders

Common: varicella-like rash, generalized

General disorders and administration site conditions

Very common: fever ⩾37,7°C oral; injection site erythema, soreness and swelling

Common: injection site rash, pruritus and varicella-like rash

Uncommon: injection site ecchymosis, hematoma, induration, numbness and warmth

Rare: heaviness, hyperpigmentation, stiffness.

Elderly

Clinical trial experience has not identified differences in the safety profile between the elderly (individuals ⩾65 years of age) and younger subjects.

Cases of herpes zoster in clinical studies

In clinical trials, 12 cases of herpes zoster have been reported in 9543 vaccinated individuals 12 months to 12 years of age during 84.414 person-years of follow-up. This resulted in a calculated incidence of at least 14 cases per 100.000 person-years, compared with 77 cases per 100.000 person-years following wild-type varicella infection. In 1652 vaccinated individuals 13 years of age and older, 2 cases of herpes zoster were reported. All 14 cases were mild and no sequelae were reported. The long-term effect of varicella vaccine (live) (Oka/Merck strain) on the incidence of herpes zoster, particularly in those vaccinees exposed to wild-type varicella, is unknown at present.

Concomitant use of varicella vaccine (live) (Oka/Merck strain) with other pediatric vaccines

When varicella vaccine (live) (Oka/Merck strain) was given concurrently with measles, mumps, rubella vaccine (M-M-R II) to 12- to 23-month-old individuals, fever (⩾38,9°C; oral equivalent, Days 0 to 42 postvaccination) was reported at a rate of 26-40%.

Post-Marketing Clinical Studies

In a post-marketing study with varicella vaccine (live) (Oka/Merck strain), conducted to evaluate short-term safety (follow-up of 30 or 60 days) in approximately 86.000 children, 12 months to 12 years of age, and in 3600 individuals, 13 years of age and older, no vaccine-related serious adverse events were reported.

Post-Marketing Surveillance

After marketing authorisation, other undesirable effects have been reported very rarely (<1/10.000) in temporal relation to vaccination.

Infections and infestations

Encephalitis*; pharyngitis; pneumonia*; herpes zoster*

Blood and the lymphatic system disorders

Thrombocytopenia

Immune system disorders

Anaphylaxis in individuals with or without an allergic history

Nervous system disorders

Cerebrovascular accident; febrile and non-febrile convulsions; Guillain-Barré syndrome; transverse myelitis; Bell's palsy; ataxia*; vertigo/dizziness; paresthesia

Respiratory, thoracic and mediastinal disorders

Pharyngitis; pneumonitis

Skin and subcutaneous tissue disorders

Stevens-Johnson syndrome; erythema multiforme; Henoch-Schönlein purpura; secondary bacterial infections of skin and soft tissues, including impetigo and cellulitis.

* These selected adverse events reported with varicella vaccine (live) (Oka/Merck strain) are also a consequence of wild-type varicella infection. There is no indication of an increased risk of these adverse events following vaccination compared with wild-type disease from active post-marketing surveillance studies or passive post-marketing surveillance reporting (see section 5.1 and *Post-Marketing Clinical Studies*).

Postvaccination rashes in which the Oka/Merck strain was isolated were generally mild (see section 5.1).

Transmission

The vaccine virus may rarely be transmitted to contacts of vaccinees who develop a varicella-like rash (see section 4.4). In particular, this kind of transmission has been documented 3 times as of May 2003, since the product was first marketed (1995). During this time more than 40 million doses have been distributed. Transmission of vaccine virus from vaccinees without a varicella-like rash has been reported but has not been confirmed.

4.9 Overdose

Accidental administration of more than the recommended dose of varicella vaccine (live) (Oka/Merck strain) has been reported (either a larger dose than recommended was injected, more than one injection was given, or the interval between injections was shorter than that recommended). Of these cases, the following adverse events were reported: injection-site redness, soreness, inflammation; irritability; gastrointestinal complaints (i.e., hematemesis, fecal emesis, gastroenteritis with vomiting and diarrhea); cough and viral infection. None of the cases had long-term sequelae.

5. PHARMACOLOGICAL PROPERTIES

5.1 Pharmacodynamic properties

Pharmacotherapeutic group: virus vaccines - varicella viruses

ATC code: JO7BK

Evaluation of clinical efficacy

Healthy individuals 12 months to 12 years of age

In combined clinical trials using earlier formulations of the varicella vaccine (live) (Oka/Merck strain) at doses ranging from approximately 1000 to 17.000 PFU, the majority of subjects who received the varicella vaccine (live) (Oka/Merck strain) and were exposed to wild-type virus were either completely protected from chickenpox or developed a milder form of the disease.

In particular, the protective efficacy of varicella vaccine (live) (Oka/Merck strain) beginning 42 days postvaccination was evaluated in three different ways:

1) by a double-blind, placebo-controlled trial over 2 years (N=956; efficacy 95 to 100%; formulation containing 17.430 PFU);

2) by assessment of protection from disease following household exposure over 7 to 9 years of observation (N=259; efficacy 81 to 88%; formulation containing 1000-9000 PFU); and

3) by comparing chickenpox rates over 7 to 9 years in vaccinees versus historical control data from 1972 through 1978 (N=5404; efficacy 83 to 94%; formulation containing 1000-9000 PFU).

In a group of 9202 individuals 12 months to 12 years of age who had received a dose of the varicella vaccine (live) (Oka/Merck strain), 1149 cases of infection (occurring more than 6 weeks postvaccination) were observed over a follow-up period of up to 13 years. Out of these 1149 cases, 20 (1,7%) were classified as severe (number of lesions ⩾300, oral body temperature ⩾37,8°C). The above-mentioned data, compared with the 36% proportion of severe cases observed following the wild-type virus infection in the unvaccinated historical controls, corresponds to a 95% relative decrease in the proportion of severe cases observed in the vaccinees who acquired infection after vaccination.

Protective efficacy following two doses given 4 or 8 weeks apart in individuals 13 years of age or older was evaluated based on household exposure over 6 to 7 years after vaccination. The clinical efficacy rate ranged from approximately 80 to 100%.

Prophylaxis of varicella by vaccination up to 3 days following exposure has been investigated in two small controlled trials. The first study demonstrated that none of 17 children developed varicella following household exposure compared with 19 of 19 unvaccinated contacts. In a second placebo-controlled trial of post-exposure prophylaxis, one of 10 children in the vaccine group versus 12 of 13 in the placebo group developed varicella. In an uncontrolled trial in a hospital setting, 148 patients, of whom 35 were immunocompromised, received a dose of varicella vaccine 1 to 3 days post-exposure and none developed varicella.

Published data on prevention of varicella at 4 to 5 days post-exposure are limited. In a double-blind trial, 26 susceptible siblings of children with active varicella were randomized to placebo or varicella vaccine. In the varicella vaccine group, 4 of 13 children (30,8%) developed varicella, of whom 3 children were vaccinated on Days 4 to 5. However, the disease was mild (1, 2, and 50 lesions). In contrast, 12 of 13 children (92,3%) in the placebo group developed typical varicella (60 to 600 lesions). Thus, vaccination 4 to 5 days after exposure to varicella may modify the course of any secondary cases of varicella.

Immunogenicity of varicella vaccine (live) (Oka/Merck strain)

Clinical studies have established that the immunogenicity of the refrigerator-stable formulation is similar to the immunogenicity of earlier formulations that were evaluated for efficacy.

A titer ⩾5 gpELISA units (gpELISA is a highly sensitive assay that is not commercially available) at 6 weeks post-vaccination has been shown to be an approximate correlate of clinical protection. However, it is not known whether a titer of ⩾0,6 gpELISA units correlates with long-term protection.

Humoral immune response in individuals 12 months to 12 years of age

Seroconversion (based on assay cutoff that generally corresponds to ⩾0,6 gpELISA units) was observed in 98% of 9610 susceptible individuals 12 months to 12 years of age who received doses ranging from 1000 to 50.000 PFU. Varicella antibody titers ⩾5 gpELISA units were induced in approximately 83% of these individuals.

In individuals 12 to 23 months of age, the administration of VARIVAX refrigerated (8000 PFU/dose or 25.000 PFU/dose) induced varicella antibody titers ⩾5 gpELISA units at 6 weeks postvaccination, in 93% of individuals vaccinated.

Humoral immune response in individuals 13 years of age and older

In 934 individuals 13 years of age and older, several clinical trials with varicella vaccine (live) (Oka/Merck strain) at doses ranging from approximately 900 to 17.000 PFU, have shown a seroconversion rate (varicella antibody titer ⩾0,6 gpELISA units) after 1 dose of vaccine ranging from 73 to 100%. The proportion of subjects with antibody titers ⩾5 gpELISA units ranged from 22 to 80%.

After 2 doses of vaccine (601 subjects) at doses ranging from approximately 900 to 9000 PFU, the seroconversion rate ranged from 97 to 100% and the proportion of subjects with antibody titers ⩾5 gpELISA units ranged from 76 to 98%.

There are no data on immune responses to VARIVAX in VZV-seronegative persons ⩾65 years of age.

Onset of immune response

In a clinical study in individuals 12 months to 12 years of age given a single dose of varicella vaccine (live) (Oka/Merck strain) (872 to 8715 PFU), the kinetics of the antibody response were evaluated by immune adherence hemagglutination assay. At 2 weeks, 91% (32/35) seroconverted; at 4 weeks 100% (31/31) seroconverted.

Duration of immune response

Individuals 12 months to 12 years of age

In those clinical studies involving healthy individuals 12 months to 12 years of age who have been followed long-term after single-dose vaccination, detectable varicella antibodies (gpELISA ⩾0,6 units) were present in 99,1% (3092/3120) at 1 year, 99,4% (1382/1391) at 2 years, 98,7% (1032/1046) at 3 years, 99,3% (997/1004) at 4 years, 99,2% (727/733) at 5 years, and 100% (432/432) at 6 years postvaccination.

Individuals 13 years of age and older

In clinical studies involving healthy individuals 13 years of age and older who received 2 doses of vaccine, detectable varicella antibodies (gpELISA ⩾0,6 units) were present in 97,9% (568/580) at 1 year, 97,1% (34/35) at 2 years, 100% (144/144) at 3 years, 97,0% (98/101) at 4 years, 97,5% (78/80) at 5 years, and 100% (45/45) at 6 years postvaccination.

A boost in antibody levels has been observed in vaccinees following exposure to wild-type varicella, which could account for the apparent long-term persistence of antibody levels after vaccination in these studies. The duration of immune response following administration of varicella vaccine (live) (Oka/Merck strain) in the absence of wild-type boosting is unknown (see section 4.2).

Immune memory was demonstrated by administering a booster dose of varicella vaccine (live) (Oka/Merck strain) 4 to 6 years after the first vaccination in 419 individuals who were 1 to 17 years of age at the time of the first injection. The GMT prior to the booster dose was 25,7 gpELISA units/mL and increased to 143,6 gpELISA units/mL approximately 7-10 days after the booster dose.

5.2 Pharmacokinetic properties

Evaluation of pharmacokinetic properties is not required for vaccines.

5.3 Preclinical safety data

Traditional preclinical safety studies were not performed, but there are no preclinical concerns considered relevant to clinical safety beyond data included in other sections of the SPC.

6. PHARMACEUTICAL PARTICULARS

6.1 List of excipients

Powder:

Sucrose

Hydrolysed gelatin

Urea

Sodium chloride

Monosodium L-glutamate

Anhydrous disodium phosphate

Potassium dihydrogen phosphate

Potassium chloride

For information regarding residual components in trace quantities, see sections 4.3 and 4.4.

Solvent:

Water for Injections

6.2 Incompatibilities

The vaccine should not be mixed with other medicinal products.

6.3 Shelf life

18 months.

After reconstitution, the vaccine should be used immediately. However, the in-use stability has been demonstrated for 30 minutes between +20°C and +25°C.

Discard the vaccine if it is not used within 30 minutes after its preparation.

6.4 Special precautions for storage

Store at +2°C to +8 °C (in a refrigerator). Keep vial in the outer carton to protect from light.

In-use storage times and conditions prior to use should not be longer than 30 minutes at +20°C to +25 °C.

Do not freeze.

6.5 Nature and contents of container

Vial

3 mL vial (Type I glass) with stopper (butyl rubber) and flip-off cap (aluminum).

Pre-filled syringe

1 mL pre-filled syringe (Type 1 glass) with plunger stopper (chlorobutyl rubber) and tip cap (chlorobutyl rubber), without needle, 1 mL pre-filled syringe (Type 1 glass) with plunger stopper (chlorobutyl rubber) and tip cap (chlorobutyl rubber), with 2 separate needles in the blister or 1 mL pre-filled syringe (Type 1 glass) with plunger stopper (chlorobutyl rubber) with needle.

Pack of one and ten doses.

Not all pack sizes may be marketed.

6.6 Instructions for use and handling

Directions for the vaccine preparation

Avoid contact with disinfectants.

To reconstitute the vaccine, use only water for injections provided in the prefilled syringe.

2 separate needles may be available in the secondary packaging of the presentations containing prefilled syringes without attached needle.

The needle should be pushed into the extremity of the syringe by operating a rotation of a quarter of a tour (90°).

Inject the entire content of the pre-filled syringe into the vial containing the powder. Gently agitate to mix thoroughly. Withdraw the entire content in the same provided syringe and inject the vaccine by subcutaneous route.

Reconstituted vaccine not used within 30 minutes should be discarded.

The reconstituted vaccine should be inspected visually for any foreign particulate matter and/or variation in physical appearance. The vaccine must not be used if any particulate matter is noted or if the appearance of the vaccine differs from that described in section 3.

It is important to use a separate sterile syringe and needle for each patient to prevent transmission of infectious agents from one individual to another.

Any unused product or waste material should be disposed of in accordance with local requirements.

7. MARKETING AUTHORISATION HOLDER

Sanofi Pasteur MSD Ltd

Mallards Reach

Bridge Avenue

Maidenhead

Berkshire SL6 1QP, United Kingdom

8. MARKETING AUTHORISATION NUMBER(S)

PL06745/0124

9. DATE OF FIRST AUTHORISATION/RENEWAL OF THE AUTHORISATION

27 January 2004

10. DATE OF REVISION OF THE TEXT

March 2005

11. LEGAL CATEGORY

POM

Vascace

(Roche Products Limited)

1. NAME OF THE MEDICINAL PRODUCT

Vascace®

2. QUALITATIVE AND QUANTITATIVE COMPOSITION

One film coated tablet 0.5mg contains:

Cilazapril, anhydrous 0.5mg, in the form of the monohydrate (cilazapril 0.522mg).

One film coated tablet 1.0mg contains:

Cilazapril, anhydrous 1.0mg, in the form of the monohydrate (cilazapril 1.044mg).

One film coated tablet 2.5mg contains:

Cilazapril, anhydrous 2.5mg, in the form of the monohydrate (cilazapril 2.61mg).

One film coated tablet 5.0mg contains:

Cilazapril, anhydrous 5mg, in the form of the monohydrate (cilazapril 5.22mg).

3. PHARMACEUTICAL FORM

Tablets.

4. CLINICAL PARTICULARS

4.1 Therapeutic indications

Vascace is indicated in treatment of all grades of essential hypertension. Vascace is also indicated in the treatment of chronic heart failure, usually as an adjunctive therapy with digitalis and/or diuretics.

4.2 Posology and method of administration

Vascace should be administered once-daily. As food intake has no clinically significant influence on absorption, Vascace can be administered before or after a meal. The dose should always be taken at about the same time of day.

Special Dosage Instructions:

Essential hypertension

The recommended initial dosage is 1mg once a day. Dosage should be adjusted individually in accordance with the blood pressure response until control is achieved. Most patients can be maintained on between 2.5 and 5.0mg/day. If the blood pressure is not adequately controlled with 5mg Vascace once daily, a low dose of a non-potassium-sparing diuretic may be administered concomitantly to enhance the anti-hypertensive effect.

Hypertensive patients receiving diuretics

The diuretic should be discontinued two to three days before beginning therapy with Vascace to reduce the likelihood of symptomatic hypotension. It may be resumed later if required. The recommended starting dose in these patients is 0.5mg once daily.

Chronic heart failure

Vascace can be used as adjunctive therapy with digitalis and/or diuretics in patients with chronic heart failure. Therapy with Vascace should be initiated with a recommended starting dose of 0.5mg once daily under close medical supervision. The dose should be increased to the lowest maintenance dose of 1mg daily according to tolerability and clinical status. Further titration within the usual maintenance dose of 1mg to 2.5mg daily should be carried out based on patients response, clinical status and tolerability. The usual maximum dose is 5mg once daily.

Results from clinical trials showed that clearance of cilazaprilat in patients with chronic heart failure is correlated with creatinine clearance. Thus in patients with chronic heart failure and impaired renal function special dosage recommendation as given under "Impaired Renal Function" should be followed.

Impaired renal function

Reduced dosages may be required for patients with renal impairment, depending on their creatinine clearance.

The following dose schedules are recommended:

Creatinine clearance	Initial dose of Vascace	Maximal dose of Vascace
> 40ml/min	1mg once daily	5mg once daily
10 - 40ml/min	0.5mg once daily	2.5mg once daily
< 10ml/min	Not recommended	Not recommended

In patients requiring haemodialysis, Vascace should be administered on days when dialysis is not performed and the dosage should be adjusted according to blood pressure response.

Elderly

In the treatment of hypertension, Vascace should be initiated with between 0.5mg and 1mg once daily. Thereafter, the maintenance dose must be adapted to individual response.

In the treatment of chronic heart failure, Vascace should be initiated with a dose of 0.5mg daily. The maintenance dose of 1mg to 2.5mg must be adapted to individual tolerability, response and clinical status.

In elderly patients with chronic heart failure on high diuretic dosage the recommended starting dose of Vascace 0.5mg must be strictly followed.

Children

Safety and efficacy in children have not been established therefore there is no recommendation for administration of cilazapril to children.

4.3 Contraindications

Vascace is contra-indicated in patients who are hypersensitive to cilazapril, other ACE-inhibitors or any of the product exipients, in patients with ascites and in pregnancy and lactation.

Vascace is also contra-indicated in patients with a history of angioedema after treatment with other ACE-inhibitors.

4.4 Special warnings and special precautions for use

(See also *Special Dosage Instructions* under section *4.2 Posology and method of administration*)

Vascace should be used with caution in patients with aortic stenosis, hypertrophic cardiomyopathy or outflow obstruction.

In elderly patients with chronic heart failure on high diuretic dosage the recommended starting dose of Vascace 0.5mg must be strictly followed.

Although the mechanism involved has not been definitely established, there is clinical evidence that haemodialysis with polyacrylonitrile methallyl sulphate high-flux membranes (e.g. AN69), haemofiltration or LDL-apheresis, if performed in patients being treated with ACE-inhibitors, including cilazapril, can lead to the provocation of anaphylaxis/anaphylactoid reactions including life-threatening shock. The above-mentioned procedures must therefore be avoided in such patients.

Symptomatic hypotension

Occasionally, symptomatic hypotension has been reported with ACE-inhibitor therapy, particularly in patients with sodium or volume depletion in connection with conditions such as vomiting, diarrhoea, pre-treatment with diuretics, low sodium diet or after dialysis. In patients with angina pectoris or cerebrovascular disease, treatment with ACE-inhibitors should be started under close medical supervision, as excessive hypotension could result in myocardial infarction or cerebrovascular accident.

Patients with chronic heart failure, especially those taking high doses of loop diuretics, may experience a pronounced blood pressure decrease in response to ACE-inhibitors. This should be treated by having the patient rest in the supine position and may require infusion of normal saline or volume expanders. After volume repletion, Vascace therapy may be continued. However, if symptoms persist, the dosage should be reduced or the drug discontinued.

Renal impairment

Reduced dosages may be required for patients with renal impairment, depending on their creatinine clearance (see section *4.2 Special dosage instructions*). In patients whose renal function depends primarily on the activity of the renin-angiotensin-aldosterone system, such as patients with severe heart failure or with unilateral or bilateral renal artery stenosis, treatment with ACE-inhibitors including Vascace may produce increases in blood urea nitrogen and/or serum creatinine. Although these alterations are usually reversible upon discontinuation of Vascace and/or diuretic therapy, cases of severe renal dysfunction and, rarely, acute renal failure have been reported.

In this patient population, renal function should be monitored during the first weeks of therapy.

For haemodialysis using high-flux polyacrylonitrile (AN69) membranes please see above statement under the heading of *Special warnings and special precautions for use*.

Hepatic impairment

In patients with severe liver function impairment, hypotension may occur.

Hepatic failure

Rarely, ACE-inhibitors have been associated with hepatotoxicity including cholestatic and hepatocellular hepatitis. More severe reactions such as fulminant hepatic necrosis have also been reported. Patients receiving ACE-inhibitors who develop jaundice or elevations of hepatic enzymes should discontinue the ACE-inhibitor and receive appropriate medical follow-up.

Serum potassium

Concomitant administration of potassium-sparing diuretics, potassium supplements or potassium containing salt substitutes may lead to increases in serum potassium, particularly in patients with renal impairment. Therefore, if concomitant use for such agents is indicated, their dosage should be reduced when Vascace is initiated and serum potassium and renal function should be monitored carefully.

Surgery anaesthesia

The use of ACE-inhibitors in combination with anaesthetic drugs in surgery that also have blood-pressure-lowering effects, can produce arterial hypotension. If this occurs, volume expansion by means of intravenous infusion or - if resistant to these measures - angiotensin II infusion is indicated.

4.5 Interaction with other medicinal products and other forms of Interaction

There was no increase in plasma digoxin concentrations when Vascace was administered concomitantly with digoxin. No clinically significant drug interactions were observed when Vascace was administered concomitantly with nitrates, oral antidiabetics, H2-receptor blockers and coumarin anticoagulants. No significant pharmacokinetic drug interactions between Vascace and furosemide or thiazides were noted. An additive effect may be observed when Vascace is administered in combination with other blood-pressure-lowering agents.

Potassium-sparing diuretics, potassium supplements or potassium containing salt substitutes administered together with Vascace can lead to increases in serum potassium, particularly in patients with renal impairment (see section *4.4 Special warnings and special precautions for use*).

As with other ACE-inhibitors, use of Vascace concomitantly with a non-steroidal anti-inflammatory drug (NSAID) may diminish the anti-hypertensive effect of Vascace.

Anaphylactic reactions can occur in patients undergoing desensitisation therapy with wasp or bee venom while receiving an ACE-inhibitor. Cilazapril must therefore be interrupted before the start of desensitisation therapy. Additionally, in this situation, cilazapril must not be replaced by a beta blocker.

Concomitant administration of ACE-inhibitors and antidiabetic medicines (insulin, oral hypoglycaemic agents) may cause an increased blood glucose lowering effect with the risk of hypoglycaemia. This phenomenon may be more likely to occur during the first weeks of combined treatment and in patients with renal impairment.

The concomitant administration of ACE-inhibitors with lithium may reduce the excretion of lithium. Serum lithium levels should be monitored frequently.

Concomitant administration of allopurinol, cytostatic or immunosuppressive agents, systemic corticosteroids or procainamide with ACE-inhibitors may lead to an increased risk of leucopenia.

4.6 Pregnancy and lactation

Vascace is contra-indicated in pregnancy since foetotoxicity has been observed for ACE-inhibitors in animals. Although there is no experience with Vascace, other ACE-inhibitors in human pregnancy have been associated with oligohydramnios and neonatal hypotension and/or anuria. It is not known whether cilazapril passes into human breast milk, but since animal data show the presence of cilazaprilat in rat milk, Vascace should not be administered to nursing mothers.

4.7 Effects on ability to drive and use machines

As with other ACE-inhibitors, impairment of performance in activities requiring complete mental alertness (e.g. driving a motor vehicle) is not to be expected with Vascace. However, it should be noted that dizziness may occasionally occur in some people.

4.8 Undesirable effects

Headache, dizziness and coughing are the most frequently reported events in patients taking Vascace. Undesirable effects occurring in < 2% of the patients include fatigue, hypotension, dyspepsia, nausea, and rash. In most cases undesirable effects were transient, mild or moderate in degree, and did not require discontinuation of therapy.

Hepatic disorders

Single cases of liver function disorders, such as increased liver function tests (transaminases, bilirubin, alkaline phosphatase, gamma GT) and cholestatic hepatitis with or without necrosis, have been reported.

Idiosyncratic

ACE-inhibitors have been documented to induce cough in a substantial number of patients. Rarely dyspnoea, sinusitis, rhinitis, glossitis, bronchitis and bronchospasm have been reported.

As with other ACE-inhibitors, angioneurotic oedema has been reported, although rarely, in patients receiving Vascace. Angioedema involving the tongue, glottis or larynx may be **fatal**. If involvement of the face, lips, tongue, glottis and/or larynx occurs Vascace should be discontinued, replaced by an agent belonging to another class of drugs and appropriate therapy instituted without delay. Emergency therapy should be given including, but not necessarily limited to, immediate intramuscular adrenaline (epinephrine) solution 1:1000 (0.3 to 0.5ml) or slow intravenous adrenaline 1mg/ml (observing dilution instructions) with control of ECG and blood pressure. The patient should be hospitalised and observed for at least 12 to 24 hours and should not be discharged until complete resolution of symptoms has occurred.

Pancreatitis has been reported rarely in patients treated with ACE-inhibitors (including Vascace); in some cases this has proved fatal.

Laboratory test findings

Clinically relevant changes in laboratory test values possibly or probably related to Vascace treatment have been observed only rarely.

Minor, mostly reversible increases in serum creatinine/urea have been observed in patients treated with Vascace. Such changes are likely to occur in patients with renal artery stenosis or with renal impairment (see section *4.4 Special warnings and special precautions for use*), but they have also occasionally been observed in patients with normal renal function, particularly in those receiving concomitant diuretics. Isolated cases of acute renal failure have been reported in patients with severe heart failure, renal artery stenosis or renal disorders (see section *4.4 Special warnings and special precautions for use*).

In some patients decreases in haemoglobin, haematocrit and/or white blood cell count have been reported, but in no case has a definite causal relationship to Vascace been established.

4.9 Overdose

While single doses of up to 160mg Vascace have been administered to normal healthy volunteers without untoward effects on blood pressure, only a few data on overdose are available in patients.

The most likely symptoms of overdosage are severe hypotension, shock, stupor, bradycardia, electrolyte disturbances and renal failure.

After ingestion of an overdose, the patient should be kept under close supervision, preferably in an intensive care unit. Serum electrolytes and creatinine should be monitored frequently. Therapeutic measures depend on the nature and severity of the symptoms. Measurements to prevent absorption such as gastric lavage, administration of adsorbents and sodium sulphate within 30 minutes after intake, and to hasten elimination should be applied if ingestion is recent. If hypotension occurs, the patient should be placed in the shock position and salt and volume supplementation should be given, rapidly. Treatment with angiotensin II should be considered. Bradycardia or extensive vagal reactions should be treated by administering atropine. The use of a pacemaker may be considered. ACE-inhibitors may be removed from the circulation by haemodialysis. The use of high-flux polyacrylonitrile membranes should be avoided.

5. PHARMACOLOGICAL PROPERTIES

5.1 Pharmacodynamic properties

Vascace (cilazapril) is a specific, long-acting angiotensin-converting enzyme (ACE) inhibitor which suppresses the renin-angiotensin-aldosterone system and thereby the conversion of the inactive angiotensin I to angiotensin II which is a potent vasoconstrictor. At recommended doses, the effect of Vascace in hypertensive patients and in patients with chronic heart failure is maintained for up to 24 hours.

In patients with normal renal function, serum potassium usually remains within the normal range during Vascace treatment. In patients concomitantly taking potassium-sparing diuretics, potassium levels may rise.

Hypertension

Vascace induces a reduction of both supine and standing systolic and diastolic blood pressure, usually with no orthostatic component. It is effective in all degrees of essential hypertension as well as in renal hypertension. The anti-hypertensive effect of Vascace is usually apparent within the first hour after administration, with maximum effect observed between three and seven hours after dosing. In general the heart rate remains unchanged. Reflex tachycardia is not induced, although small, clinically insignificant alterations of heart rate may occur. In some patients blood pressure reduction may diminish toward the end of the dosage interval.

The initial dosage seldom achieves the desired therapeutic response. Blood pressure should be assessed and dosage adjusted as required. Should the effect of Vascace at the top of the recommended dose be insufficient it can be combined with non-potassium-sparing diuretics.

The anti-hypertensive effect of Vascace is maintained during long-term therapy. No rapid increase in blood pressure has been observed after abrupt withdrawal of Vascace.

In hypertensive patients with moderate to severe renal impairment, the glomerular filtration rate and renal blood flow remained in general unchanged with Vascace despite a clinically significant blood pressure reduction.

As with other ACE-inhibitors, the blood pressure-lowering effect of Vascace in black patients may be less pronounced than in non-blacks. However, racial differences in response are no longer evident when Vascace is administered in combination with hydrochlorothiazide.

Chronic heart failure

In patients with chronic heart failure the renin-angiotensin-aldosterone and the sympathetic nervous systems are generally activated leading to enhanced systemic vasoconstriction and to the promotion of sodium and water retention. By suppressing the renin-angiotensin-aldosterone system, Vascace improves loading conditions in the failing heart by reducing systemic vascular resistance (afterload) and pulmonary capillary wedge pressure (preload) in patients on diuretics and/or digitalis. Furthermore, the exercise tolerance of these patients increases significantly showing an improvement in quality of life. The haemodynamic and clinical effects occur promptly and persist.

5.2 Pharmacokinetic properties

Cilazapril is efficiently absorbed and rapidly converted to the active form, cilazaprilat. Ingestion of food immediately prior to Vascace administration, delays and reduces the absorption to a minor extent which, however, is therapeutically irrelevant. The bioavailability of cilazaprilat from oral cilazapril approximates 60% based on urinary recovery data. Maximum plasma concentrations are reached within two hours after administration and are directly related to dosage.

Cilazaprilat is eliminated unchanged by the kidneys, with an effective half-life of nine hours after once-daily dosing with Vascace. In patients with renal impairment, higher plasma concentrations of cilazaprilat are observed than in patients with normal renal function, since drug clearance is reduced when creatinine clearance is lower. There is no elimination in patients with complete renal failure, but haemodialysis reduces concentrations of both cilazapril and cilazaprilat to a limited extent.

In elderly patients whose renal function is normal for age, plasma concentrations of cilazaprilat may be up to 40% higher, and the clearance 20% lower than in younger patients. Similar changes in the pharmacokinetics occur in patients with moderate to severe liver cirrhosis.

In patients with chronic heart failure the clearance of cilazaprilat is correlated with the creatinine clearance. Thus, dosage adjustments beyond those recommended for patients with impaired renal functions (see section *4.2 Special Dosage Instructions*) should not be necessary.

5.3 Preclinical safety data

Please refer to section *4.6 Pregnancy and lactation.*

6. PHARMACEUTICAL PARTICULARS

6.1 List of excipients

In the tablet core:

Lactose

Maize starch

Hypromellose 3cp

Talc

Sodium stearyl fumarate

In the film coat:

Hypromellose 6cp

Talc

Titanium dioxide E171

Red iron oxide E172 (2.5mg and 5.0mg only)

Yellow iron oxide E172 (1.0mg and 2.5mg only)

6.2 Incompatibilities

Not applicable.

6.3 Shelf life

3 years.

6.4 Special precautions for storage

Do not store above 25°C.

6.5 Nature and contents of container

Glass Bottles and Aluminium Blisters* in the following quantities:

0.5mg: 2, 28*, 30 or 100 tablets

1.0mg: 2, 28*, 30 or 100 tablets

2.5mg: 4, 28*, 30, 98 or 100 tablets

5.0mg: 28*, 30, 98 or 100 tablets

*Marketed packs

6.6 Instructions for use and handling

None stated.

7. MARKETING AUTHORISATION HOLDER

Roche Products Limited, 40 Broadwater Road, Welwyn Garden City, Hertfordshire AL7 3AY.

8. MARKETING AUTHORISATION NUMBER(S)

PL 0031/0244 0.5mg Tablets

PL 0031/0245 1.0mg Tablets

PL 0031/0246 2.5mg Tablets

PL 0031/0247 5.0mg Tablets

9. DATE OF FIRST AUTHORISATION/RENEWAL OF THE AUTHORISATION

26 October 1990/7 December 2001

10. DATE OF REVISION OF THE TEXT

November 2002

11. LEGAL STATUS

POM.

Vascace is a registered trade mark P999683/1202

Vascalpha 10mg Prolonged Release Tablet

(Alpharma Limited)

1. NAME OF THE MEDICINAL PRODUCT

VASCALPHA 10 mg PROLONGED RELEASE TABLETS (FELODIPINE)

2. QUALITATIVE AND QUANTITATIVE COMPOSITION

Each prolonged release tablet contains 10mg of felodipine.

For excipients, see 6.1.

3. PHARMACEUTICAL FORM

Prolonged release tablet.

Reddish brown, round, biconvex, film coated prolonged release tablets with imprint 10.

4. CLINICAL PARTICULARS

4.1 Therapeutic indications

Essential hypertension

4.2 Posology and method of administration

Vascalpha (felodipine) prolonged release tablets should usually be administered as follows:

The recommended starting dose is 5 mg felodipine once daily.

If necessary, the dose may be increased to 10 mg felodipine once daily or another antihypertensive agent added. Dose increases should occur at intervals of at least 2 weeks. The usual maintenance dose is 5-10mg once daily.

The maximum daily dose is 10 mg felodipine.

The dose should be adjusted to the individual requirements of the patient.

Elderly

The recommended starting dose should be adapted in the elderly.

Subsequent dose increases should be undertaken with particular caution.

Impaired hepatic function

In patients with mild to moderate hepatic impairment, the recommended starting dose should be lowered to the minimal therapeutic effective dose of felodipine.

The dose should only be increased after carefully balancing the benefits against the risks (see 5.2 Pharmacokinetic properties). It is contraindicated in patients with severe hepatic impairment.

Impaired renal function

The pharmacokinetics are not significantly affected in patients with mild to moderate impaired renal function. Caution should be taken in patients with severe renal impairment (see section 4.4 Special warnings and precautions for use and section 5.2. Pharmacokinetic properties).

Children

Felodipine should not be used in children, as its safety and efficacy in this population have not been established.

Administration

The prolonged release tablets should be taken in the morning with a sufficient amount of fluid (e.g. a glass of water, but it should NOT be taken with grapefruit juice!) (see 4.5 Interaction with other medicinal products and other forms of interaction).

The prolonged release tablets should be swallowed whole and not chewed or crushed. The tablets may be taken on an empty stomach or with a light meal, however a high fat meal should be avoided (see 5.2 Pharmacokinetic properties).

4.3 Contraindications

Felodipine is contra-indicated in patients with:

- hypersensitivity to felodipine (or other dihydropyridines) or to any of the excipients
- cardiogenic shock
- severe aortic and mitral stenosis
- obstructive hyperthrophic cardiomyopathy
- unstable angina pectoris
- acute myocardial infarction (within 4-8 weeks of a myocardial infarction)
- decompensated heart failure
- severe hepatic impairment
- pregnancy

4.4 Special warnings and special precautions for use

Felodipine should be used with caution in patients with:

- conduction disorders, compensated heart failure, tachycardia and aortic or mitral valve stenosis.
- mild to moderate hepatic impairment, as the anti-hypertensive effect may be enhanced. Adjustment of the dosage should be considered.
- severe renal impairment (GFR <30ml/min, creatinine >1.8mg/dl)
- AV block of the second or third degree

If treatment with felodipine is discontinued abruptly, a hypertensive crisis may occur in individual cases.

Felodipine could cause significant hypotension (vasodilation effect) with consecutive tachycardia, leading to myocardial ischaemia in sensitive patients, therefore predisposed patients may suffer from myocardial infarction (see section 5.1 Pharmacodynamic properties).

Dihydropyridines may cause acute hypotension. In some cases there is a risk of hypoperfusion accompanied by reflex tachycardia (paradoxical angor) (see section 5.1 Pharmacodynamic properties).

Felodipine is metabolised by CYP3A4 enzymes. Therefore, combination with medicinal products which are potent CYP3A4 inhibitors or inducers should be avoided (see section 4.5 Interaction with other medicinal products and other forms of interaction). Due to the same reason the concomitant intake of grapefruit juice should be avoided (see section 4.5 Interaction with other medicinal products and other forms of interaction).

4.5 Interaction with other medicinal products and other forms of Interaction

Felodipine is a CYP3A4 substrate. Drugs that induce or inhibit CYP3A4 will have large influence on felodipine concentrations.

The anti-hypertensive effect of felodipine may be enhanced by other anti-hypertensives and tricyclic antidepressants.

The concomitant intake of felodipine and drugs which inhibit the cytochrome P450 isoenzyme 3A4 of the liver (such as cimetidine, azole antifungals [itraconazole or ketoconazole], macrolide antibiotics [erythromycin] or HIV protease inhibitors leads to increased felodipine plasma levels (see section 4.4 Special warnings and precautions for use). Grapefruit juice results in increased peak plasma levels and bioavailability possibly due to interaction with flavanoids in the fruit juice. Therefore grapefruit juice should not be taken together with felodipine.

Cocomitant treatment with drugs such as carbamazepine, phenytoin and barbiturates (e.g. phenobarbital) and rifampicin reduces the plasma levels of felodipine via enzyme induction in the liver (cytochrome P450 System). Therefore a dose increase of felodipine may be necessary.

Hydrochlorothiazide may enhance the antihypertensive effect of felodipine.

Felodipine can induce an increase of Cmax of ciclosporin. Additionally, ciclosporin may inhibit felodipine metabolism, which may create a potential risk of felodipine toxicity.

Blood levels of digoxin increase during concomitant administration of felodipine. Therefore, decreasing of digoxin dosage should be taken into account when the two drugs are administered concurrently.

4.6 Pregnancy and lactation

Pregnancy

Felodipine is contra-indicated during the entire duration of pregnancy, as animal experiments have demonstrated foetal damage (see 5.3 Preclinical safety data). Pregnancy must be excluded before starting treatment with felodipine.

Lactation

Felodipine is excreted in breast milk. If the breast-feeding mother is taking therapeutic doses of felodipine, a fully breast-fed infant absorbs only a very low dose of the active substance with the breast milk. There is no experience of the risk this may pose to the newborn, therefore as a precaution breast-feeding should be discontinued during treatment.

4.7 Effects on ability to drive and use machines

Treatment with felodipine requires regular medical supervision. Felodipine can influence individual reactions to such an extent that the ability to take an active part in road traffic or to operate machines (or work without suitable safeguards) may be impaired. This is particularly the case at start of therapy, or when the dose is increased, or medication is changed as well as after concomitant ingestion of alcohol.

4.8 Undesirable effects

Very commonly (> 10%) flushing, headache or tinnitus may occur, particularly at the beginning of treatment, when the dose is increased or when high doses are administered. Generally, these effects subside on continued treatment.

Commonly (> 1% - < 10%), peripheral oedema occurs (The degree of ankle swelling is dose related.). Commonly, particularly at the beginning of treatment, angina pectoris attacks may occur, or in patients with pre-existing angina pectoris there may be an increase in the frequency, duration and severity of the attacks.

Uncommonly (> 0.1% - < 1%) dizziness, fatigue, hypotension, syncope, palpitations, tachycardia and dyspnoea, restlessness, paraesthesia, tremors, myalgia, arthralgia, gastro-intestinal complaints (e.g. nausea, vomiting, diarrhoea, constipation), weight gain, sweating, pollakisuria, skin and hypersensitivity reactions such as pruritus, urticaria, exanthema, and photosensitisation have been observed. Uncommonly felodipine treatment may lead to gingival hyperplasia and gingivitis.

Rarely (> 0.01% - < 0.1%) leucocytoclastic vasculitis has been observed.

Very rarely including isolated reports (> 0.01%) hepatic function disorders (elevated transaminase levels), exfoliative dermatitis, angiooedema and fever, as well as erection disorders and gynecomastia, myocardial infarction and menorrhagia have been reported.

4.9 Overdose

Symptoms of intoxication

Overdose may lead to excessive peripheral vasodilatation with marked hypotension and in rare cases bradycardia.

Management of intoxication

The therapeutic measures should focus on elimination of the active ingredient and monitoring of the vital signs. If severe hypotension occurs, symptomatic treatment should be provided, the patient should be placed supine with the legs elevated. In case of accompanying bradycardia, atropine (0.5 – 1.0 mg) should be given intravenously. Additional intravenous fluids should be cautiously administered under haemodynamic supervision to prevent cardiac overloading. Sympathomimetic drugs with predominant effect on the α_1-adrenoreceptor (such as dobutamine, dopamine, norepinephrine or adrenaline) may also be given. Dosage depends on the efficacy obtained.

Felodipine is only dialysable to a minimal extent (approx. 9%).

5. PHARMACOLOGICAL PROPERTIES

5.1 Pharmacodynamic properties

Pharmacotheraputic group: 1,4-didydropyridine derivative/calcium antagonist

ATC code: C08C A02

Felodipine is a calcium antagonist of the dihydropyridine class of calcium channel blockers. Calcium antagonists interfere with the voltage-dependent L-type (slow) calcium channels in the plasma membranes of smooth muscle cells and reduce the inflow of calcium ions. This results in vasodilatation.

Felodipine has a greater selectivity for vascular smooth muscle than myocardial muscle. Felodipine selectively dilates arterioles with no effects on venous vessels. Felodipine leads to a dose-related lowering of blood pressure via vasodilatation and consequently a reduction of peripheral vascular resistance. It reduces both systolic and diastolic blood pressure. The haemodynamic effect of felodipine is accompanied by reflex (baroreceptor-mediated) tachycardia. In therapeutic doses, felodipine has no direct effect on either cardiac contractility or cardiac conduction. Felodipine reduces renal vascular resistance. The glomerular filtration rate remains unchanged.

Felodipine has a weak natriuretic/diuretic effect and does not provoke fluid retention.

Felodipine can be used as a monotherapy but also concomitantly with beta-blockers, diuretics and ACE inhibitors.

5.2 Pharmacokinetic properties

Absorption

Felodipine is completely absorbed following oral administration. Peak plasma levels are reached with the prolonged release formulation after 3 – 5 hours and result in even felodipine plasma concentrations within the therapeutic range for 24 hours. Steady state is reached approx. 3 days after starting treatment. Due to an extensive first-pass effect, only approx. 15 % of the administered dose is systemically available.

Distribution

The plasma protein binding of felodipine is > 99 %. The volume of distribution is approximately 10 l/kg at steady state, so that felodipine is indicating large tissue distribution. There is no significant accumulation during long-term treatment.

Metabolism

Felodipine is extensively metabolised in the liver by CYP3A4. All identified metabolites are inactive.

Elimination

No unchanged parent substance is detectable in the urine. The average half-life of felodipine in the terminal phase is 25 hours. The inactive hydrophilic metabolites formed by hepatic biotransformation are mainly eliminated renally (to approx. 70 %), and the remainder is excreted in the faeces. The mean plasma clearance is 1100 ml/l and depends on the hepatic blood flow.

Elderly

Increased plasma concentrations have been measured in elderly patients.

Impaired hepatic function

Increased plasma concentrations of up to 100% have been measured in patients with impaired hepatic function.

Impaired renal function

Renal impairment does not affect the pharmacokinetics of felodipine, although accumulation of inactive metabolites occurs in renal failure.

Effect of food

The rate, but not the extent of absorption is affected by the simultaneous ingestion of fatty food. Cmax was 2 to 2.5 times higher following intake of a high-fat meal compared to a fasting state.

5.3 Preclinical safety data

Preclinical data reveal no special hazard for humans based on conventional studies of safety pharmacology, repeated dose toxicity, genotoxicity and carcinogenic potential. In animal studies with respect to the reproduction, adverse effects were found. Effects in rats (prolonged duration of pregnancy and difficult labour) and rabbits (impaired development of distal phalanges, presumably due to decreased uteroplacental perfusion) revealed no evidence of a direct teratogenic effect, but indicate secondary consequences of the pharmacodynamic effect. In monkeys, an abnormal position of the distal phalanges was found. The significance of these observations for humans is unknown.

6. PHARMACEUTICAL PARTICULARS

6.1 List of excipients

Tablet core:

Lactose monohydrate, microcrystalline cellulose, hypromellose, povidone, propyl gallate, colloidal anhydrous silica, magnesium stearate

Tablet coat:

Hypromellose, talcum, propylene glycol, titanium dioxide (E171), iron oxide red (E172), iron oxide yellow (E172).

6.2 Incompatibilities
Not applicable.

6.3 Shelf life
48 months

6.4 Special precautions for storage
Do not store above 25°C.

6.5 Nature and contents of container
PVC/PE/PVDC aluminium blister.

Pack sizes: 10, 14, 20, 28, 30, 50, 56, 60, 90, 98, 100, 250, 500 and 1000 prolonged release tablets.

Not all pack sizes may be marketed.

6.6 Instructions for use and handling
Not applicable.

7. MARKETING AUTHORISATION HOLDER
Alpharma Limited (Trading styles: Alpharma and Cox Pharmaceuticals)

Whiddon Valley

Barnstaple

North Devon

EX32 8NS

8. MARKETING AUTHORISATION NUMBER(S)
PL 00142/0542

9. DATE OF FIRST AUTHORISATION/RENEWAL OF THE AUTHORISATION
21 July 2003

10. DATE OF REVISION OF THE TEXT
August 2003

Vascalpha 5mg Prolonged Release Tablet

(Alpharma Limited)

1. NAME OF THE MEDICINAL PRODUCT
VASCALPHA 5 mg PROLONGED RELEASE TABLETS (FELODIPINE)

2. QUALITATIVE AND QUANTITATIVE COMPOSITION
Each prolonged release tablet contains 5mg of felodipine.

For excipients, see 6.1

3. PHARMACEUTICAL FORM
Prolonged release tablet.

Light pink, round, biconvex, film-coated prolonged release tablets with imprint 5.

4. CLINICAL PARTICULARS

4.1 Therapeutic indications
Essential hypertension

4.2 Posology and method of administration
Vascalpha (felodipine) prolonged release tablets should usually be administered as follows:

The recommended starting dose is 5 mg felodipine once daily.

If necessary, the dose may be increased to 10 mg felodipine once daily or another antihypertensive agent added. Dose increases should occur at intervals of at least 2 weeks. The usual maintenance dose is 5-10mg once daily.

The maximum daily dose is 10 mg felodipine.

The dose should be adjusted to the individual requirements of the patient.

Elderly

The recommended starting dose should be adapted in the elderly.

Subsequent dose increases should be undertaken with particular caution.

Impaired hepatic function

In patients with mild to moderate hepatic impairment, the recommended starting dose should be lowered to the minimal therapeutic effective dose of felodipine.

The dose should only be increased after carefully balancing the benefits against the risks (see 5.2 Pharmacokinetic properties). It is contraindicated in patients with severe hepatic impairment.

Impaired renal function

The pharmacokinetics are not significantly affected in patients with mild to moderate impaired renal function. Caution should be taken in patients with severe renal impairment (see section 4.4 Special warnings and precautions for use and section 5.2. Pharmacokinetic properties).

Children

Felodipine should not be used in children, as its safety and efficacy in this population have not been established.

Administration

The prolonged release tablets should be taken in the morning with a sufficient amount of fluid (e.g. a glass of water, but it should NOT be taken with grapefruit juice!) (see 4.5 Interaction with other medicinal products and other forms of interaction).

The prolonged release tablets should be swallowed whole and not chewed or crushed. The tablets may be taken on an empty stomach or with a light meal, however a high fat meal should be avoided (see 5.2 Pharmacokinetic properties).

4.3 Contraindications
Felodipine is contra-indicated in patients with:

- hypersensitivity to felodipine (or other dihydropyridines) or to any of the excipients
- cardiogenic shock
- severe aortic and mitral stenosis
- obstructive hyperthrophic cardiomyopathy
- unstable angina pectoris
- acute myocardial infarction (within 4-8 weeks of a myocardial infarction)
- decompensated heart failure
- severe hepatic impairment
- pregnancy

4.4 Special warnings and special precautions for use
Felodipine should be used with caution in patients with:

- conduction disorders, compensated heart failure, tachycardia and aortic or mitral valve stenosis.

- mild to moderate hepatic impairment, as the anti-hypertensive effect may be enhanced. Adjustment of the dosage should be considered.

- severe renal impairment (GFR <30ml/min, creatinine >1.8mg/dl)

- AV block of the second or third degree

If treatment with felodipine is discontinued abruptly, a hypertensive crisis may occur in individual cases.

Felodipine could cause significant hypotension (vasodilation effect) with consecutive tachycardia, leading to myocardial ischaemia in sensitive patients, therefore predisposed patients may suffer from myocardial infarction (see section 5.1 Pharmacodynamic properties).

Dihydropyridines may cause acute hypotension. In some cases there is a risk of hypoperfusion accompanied by reflex tachycardia (paradoxical angor) (see section 5.1 Pharmacodynamic properties).

Felodipine is metabolised by CYP3A4 enzymes. Therefore, combination with medicinal products which are potent CYP3A4 inhibitors or inducers should be avoided (see section 4.5 Interaction with other medicinal products and other forms of interaction). Due to the same reason the concomitant intake of grapefruit juice should be avoided (see section 4.5 Interaction with other medicinal products and other forms of interaction).

4.5 Interaction with other medicinal products and other forms of Interaction
Felodipine is a CYP3A4 substrate. Drugs that induce or inhibit CYP3A4 will have large influence on felodipine concentrations.

The anti-hypertensive effect of felodipine may be enhanced by other anti-hypertensives and tricyclic antidepressants.

The concomitant intake of felodipine and drugs which inhibit the cytochrome P450 isoenzyme 3A4 of the liver (such as cimetidine, azole antifungals [itraconazole or ketoconazole], macrolide antibiotics [erythromycin] or HIV protease inhibitors) leads to increased felodipine plasma levels (see section 4.4 Special warnings and precautions for use). Grapefruit juice results in increased peak plasma levels and bioavailability possibly due to interaction with flavanoids in the fruit juice. Therefore grapefruit juice should not be taken together with felodipine.

Concomitant treatment with drugs such as carbamazepine, phenytoin and barbiturates (e.g. phenobarbital) and rifampicin reduces the plasma levels of felodipine via enzyme induction in the liver (cytochrome P450 System). Therefore a dose increase of felodipine may be necessary.

Hydrochlorothiazide may enhance the antihypertensive effect of felodipine.

Felodipine can induce an increase of Cmax of ciclosporin. Additionally, ciclosporin may inhibit felodipine metabolism, which may create a potential risk of felodipine toxicity.

Blood levels of digoxin increase during concomitant administration of felodipine. Therefore, decreasing of digoxin dosage should be taken into account when the two drugs are administered concurrently.

4.6 Pregnancy and lactation

Pregnancy

Felodipine is contra-indicated during the entire duration of pregnancy, as animal experiments have demonstrated foetal damage (see 5.3 Preclinical safety data). Pregnancy must be excluded before starting treatment with felodipine.

Lactation

Felodipine is excreted in breast milk. If the breast-feeding mother is taking therapeutic doses of felodipine, a fully breast-fed infant absorbs only a very low dose of the active substance with the breast milk. There is no experience of the risk this may pose to the newborn, therefore as a precaution breast-feeding should be discontinued during treatment.

4.7 Effects on ability to drive and use machines
Treatment with felodipine requires regular medical supervision. Felodipine can influence individual reactions to such an extent that the ability to take an active part in road traffic or to operate machines (or work without suitable safeguards) may be impaired. This is particularly the case at start of therapy, or when the dose is increased, or medication is changed as well as after concomitant ingestion of alcohol.

4.8 Undesirable effects
Very commonly > 10%) flushing, headache or tinnitus may occur, particularly at the beginning of treatment, when the dose is increased or when high doses are administered. Generally, these effects subside on continued treatment.

Commonly > 1% - < 10%), peripheral oedema occurs (The degree of ankle swelling is dose related.). Commonly, particularly at the beginning of treatment, angina pectoris attacks may occur, or in patients with pre-existing angina pectoris there may be an increase in the frequency, duration and severity of the attacks.

Uncommonly > 0.1% - < 1%) dizziness, fatigue, hypotension, syncope, palpitations, tachycardia and dyspnoea, restlessness, paraesthesia, tremors, myalgia, arthralgia, gastro-intestinal complaints (e.g. nausea, vomiting, diarrhoea, constipation), weight gain, sweating, pollakisuria, skin and hypersensitivity reactions such as pruritus, urticaria, exanthema, and photosensitisation have been observed. Uncommonly felodipine treatment may lead to gingival hyperplasia and gingivitis.

Rarely > 0.01% - < 0.1%) leucocytoclastic vasculitis has been observed.

Very rarely including isolated reports (< 0.01%) hepatic function disorders (elevated transaminase levels), exfoliative dermatitis, angioedema and fever, as well as erection disorders and gynecomastia, myocardial infarction and menorrhagia have been reported.

4.9 Overdose
Symptoms of intoxication

Overdose may lead to excessive peripheral vasodilatation with marked hypotension and in rare cases bradycardia.

Management of intoxication

The therapeutic measures should focus on elimination of the active ingredient and monitoring of the vital signs. If severe hypotension occurs, symptomatic treatment should be provided, the patient should be placed supine with the legs elevated. In case of accompanying bradycardia, atropine (0.5 – 1.0 mg) should be given intravenously. Additional intravenous fluids should be cautiously administered under haemodynamic supervision to prevent cardiac overloading. Sympathomimetic drugs with predominant effect on the α_1-adrenoreceptor (such as dobutamine, dopamine, norepinephrine or adrenaline) may also be given. Dosage depends on the efficacy obtained.

Felodipine is only dialysable to a minimal extent (approx. 9%).

5. PHARMACOLOGICAL PROPERTIES

5.1 Pharmacodynamic properties
Pharmacotheraputic group: 1,4-didydropyridine derivative/calcium antagonist

ATC code: C08C A02

Felodipine is a calcium antagonist of the dihydropyridine class of calcium channel blockers. Calcium antagonists interfere with the voltage-dependent L-type (slow) calcium channels in the plasma membranes of smooth muscle cells and reduce the inflow of calcium ions. This results in vasodilatation.

Felodipine has a greater selectivity for vascular smooth muscle than myocardial muscle. Felodipine selectively dilates arterioles with no effects on venous vessels. Felodipine leads to a dose-related lowering of blood pressure via vasodilatation and consequently a reduction of peripheral vascular resistance. It reduces both systolic and diastolic blood pressure. The haemodynamic effect of felodipine is accompanied by reflex (baroreceptor-mediated) tachycardia. In therapeutic doses, felodipine has no direct effect on either cardiac contractility or cardiac conduction. Felodipine reduces renal vascular resistance. The glomerular filtration rate remains unchanged.

Felodipine has a weak natriuretic/diuretic effect and does not provoke fluid retention.

Felodipine can be used as a monotherapy but also concomitantly with beta-blockers, diuretics and ACE inhibitors.

5.2 Pharmacokinetic properties
Absorption

Felodipine is completely absorbed following oral administration. Peak plasma levels are reached with the prolonged release formulation after 3 – 5 hours and result in even felodipine plasma concentrations within the therapeutic range for 24 hours. Steady state is reached approximately 3 days after starting treatment. Due to an extensive first-pass effect, only approx. 15 % of the administered dose is systemically available.

Distribution

The plasma protein binding of felodipine is > 99 %. The volume of distribution is approximately 10 l/kg at steady state, so that felodipine is indicating large tissue distribution. There is no significant accumulation during long-term treatment.

Metabolism

Felodipine is extensively metabolised in the liver by CYP3A4. All identified metabolites are inactive.

Elimination

No unchanged parent substance is detectable in the urine. The average half-life of felodipine in the terminal phase is 25 hours. The inactive hydrophilic metabolites formed by hepatic biotransformation are mainly eliminated renally (to approximately 70 %), and the remainder is excreted in the faeces. The mean plasma clearance is 1100 ml/l and depends on the hepatic blood flow.

Elderly

Increased plasma concentrations have been measured in elderly patients.

Impaired hepatic function

Increased plasma concentrations of up to 100% have been measured in patients with impaired hepatic function.

Impaired renal function

Renal impairment does not affect the pharmacokinetics of felodipine, although accumulation of inactive metabolites occurs in renal failure.

Effect of food

The rate, but not the extent of absorption is affected by the simultaneous ingestion of fatty food. Cmax was 2 to 2.5 times higher following intake of a high-fat meal compared to a fasting state.

5.3 Preclinical safety data

Preclinical data reveal no special hazard for humans based on conventional studies of safety pharmacology, repeated dose toxicity, genotoxicity and carcinogenic potential. In animal studies with respect to the reproduction, adverse effects were found. Effects in rats (prolonged duration of pregnancy and difficult labour) and rabbits (impaired development of distal phalanges, presumably due to decreased uteroplacental perfusion) revealed no evidence of a direct teratogenic effect, but indicate secondary consequences of the pharmacodynamic effect. In monkeys, an abnormal position of the distal phalanges was found. The significance of these observations for humans is unknown.

6. PHARMACEUTICAL PARTICULARS

6.1 List of excipients

Tablet core:

Lactose monohydrate, microcrystalline cellulose, hypromellose, povidone, propyl gallate, colloidal anhydrous silica, magnesium stearate

Tablet coat:

Hypromellose, talcum, propylene glycol, titanium dioxide (E171), iron oxide red (E172), iron oxide yellow (E172).

6.2 Incompatibilities

Not applicable.

6.3 Shelf life

48 months

6.4 Special precautions for storage

Do not store above 25°C.

6.5 Nature and contents of container

PVC/PE/PVDC aluminium blister.

Pack sizes: 10, 14, 20, 28, 30, 50, 56, 60, 90, 98, 100, 250, 500 and 1000 prolonged release tablets.

Not all pack sizes may be marketed.

6.6 Instructions for use and handling

Not applicable.

7. MARKETING AUTHORISATION HOLDER

Alpharma Limited (Trading styles: Alpharma and Cox Pharmaceuticals)

Whiddon Valley

Barnstaple

North Devon

EX32 8NS

8. MARKETING AUTHORISATION NUMBER(S)

PL 00142/0541

9. DATE OF FIRST AUTHORISATION/RENEWAL OF THE AUTHORISATION

21 July 2003

10. DATE OF REVISION OF THE TEXT

August 2003

Vasogen Cream

(Forest Laboratories UK Limited)

1. NAME OF THE MEDICINAL PRODUCT

VASOGEN CREAM

2. QUALITATIVE AND QUANTITATIVE COMPOSITION

Dimethicone (as silicone fluid 200) BP 20.0% w/w

Zinc oxide Ph.Eur. 7.5% w/w

Calamine BP 1.5% w/w

3. PHARMACEUTICAL FORM

Cream

4. CLINICAL PARTICULARS

4.1 Therapeutic indications

The prevention and treatment of nappy rash and bedsores. Local protection of skin around the stoma after ileostomy and colostomy.

4.2 Posology and method of administration

Vasogen is applied topically to the skin and may be either rubbed in gently or applied thinly and left to dry. Further application can be made as required.

4.3 Contraindications

Use in patients with known hypersensitivity to the product or any of its ingredients, e.g. lanolin or phenonip. Vasogen should not be applied when it is considered that free drainage is necessary, e.g. weeping dermatitis.

4.4 Special warnings and special precautions for use

None

4.5 Interaction with other medicinal products and other forms of Interaction

None known

4.6 Pregnancy and lactation

No restrictions

4.7 Effects on ability to drive and use machines

Not applicable

4.8 Undesirable effects

Side-effects such as local sensitivity reactions are extremely rare.

4.9 Overdose

Not applicable

5. PHARMACOLOGICAL PROPERTIES

5.1 Pharmacodynamic properties

Dimethicone is an inert polymer which has a low surface tension and is a water repellent. It is widely used in barrier creams. Zinc oxide is a mild astringent and antiseptic. Calamine has a mild astringent activity and is widely used in various dermatological conditions.

5.2 Pharmacokinetic properties

Not applicable

5.3 Preclinical safety data

There are no preclinical data of relevance to the prescriber which are additional to that already included in other sections of the SPC.

6. PHARMACEUTICAL PARTICULARS

6.1 List of excipients

Aluminium Hydroxide (wet gel)

Lanolin (anhydrous)

Methylcellulose

Phenonip

Purified Water

6.2 Incompatibilities

None known.

6.3 Shelf life

3 years

6.4 Special precautions for storage

Do not store above 25°C.

6.5 Nature and contents of container

White low-density polyethylene tube with white polypropylene cap.

Pack sizes 14, 50 and 100g.

6.6 Instructions for use and handling

None

7. MARKETING AUTHORISATION HOLDER

Forest Laboratories UK Limited

Bourne Road

Bexley

Kent DA5 1NX

8. MARKETING AUTHORISATION NUMBER(S)

PL 0108/5033R

9. DATE OF FIRST AUTHORISATION/RENEWAL OF THE AUTHORISATION

29 August 1989/26 March 1996

10. DATE OF REVISION OF THE TEXT

January 2001

11. Legal Category

GSL

VELCADE 3.5 mg powder for solution for injection.

(Janssen-Cilag Ltd)

1. NAME OF THE MEDICINAL PRODUCT

VELCADE ▼ 3.5 mg powder for solution for injection.

2. QUALITATIVE AND QUANTITATIVE COMPOSITION

Each vial contains 3.5 mg bortezomib (as a mannitol boronic ester).

After reconstitution, 1 ml of solution for injection contains 1 mg bortezomib.

For excipients, see section 6.1.

3. PHARMACEUTICAL FORM

Powder for solution for injection.

White to off-white cake or powder.

4. CLINICAL PARTICULARS

4.1 Therapeutic indications

VELCADE is indicated as mono-therapy for the treatment of progressive multiple myeloma in patients who have received at least 1 prior therapy and who have already undergone or are unsuitable for bone marrow transplantation.

4.2 Posology and method of administration

Treatment must be initiated and administered under the supervision of a physician qualified and experienced in the use of chemotherapeutic agents.

Recommended dosage

The recommended starting dose of bortezomib is 1.3 mg/m^2 body surface area twice weekly for two weeks (days 1, 4, 8, and 11) followed by a 10-day rest period (days 12-21). This 3-week period is considered a treatment cycle. At least 72 hours should elapse between consecutive doses of VELCADE.

It is recommended that patients with a confirmed complete response receive 2 additional cycles of VELCADE beyond a confirmation. It is also recommended that responding patients who do not achieve a complete remission receive a total of 8 cycles of VELCADE therapy.

Currently there are limited data concerning retreatment with VELCADE.

Recommended dosage adjustments during treatment and re-initiation of treatment

VELCADE treatment must be withheld at the onset of any Grade 3 non-haematological or any Grade 4 haematological toxicities, excluding neuropathy as discussed below (see also section 4.4). Once the symptoms of the toxicity have resolved, VELCADE treatment may be re-initiated at a 25% reduced dose (1.3 mg/m^2 reduced to 1.0 mg/m^2; 1.0 mg/m^2 reduced to 0.7 mg/m^2). If the toxicity is not resolved or if it recurs at the lowest dose, discontinuation of VELCADE must be considered unless the benefit of treatment clearly outweighs the risk.

Patients who experience VELCADE related neuropathic pain and/or peripheral neuropathy are to be managed as presented in Table 1. Patients with pre-existing severe neuropathy may be treated with VELCADE only after careful risk/benefit assessment.

Table 1: Recommended* dose modifications for VELCADE related neuropathic pain and/or peripheral sensory neuropathy.

Severity of peripheral neuropathy	Modification of dose and regimen
Grade 1 (paraesthesia and/or loss of reflexes) with no pain or loss of function	No action
Grade 1 with pain or Grade 2 (interfering with function but no activities of daily living)	Reduce to 1.0 mg/m^2
Grade 2 with pain or Grade 3 (interfering with activities of daily living)	Withhold VELCADE treatment until symptoms of toxicity have resolved. When toxicity resolves re-initiate VELCADE treatment and reduce dose to 0.7 mg/m^2 and change treatment schedule to once per week.
Grade 4 (permanent sensory loss that interferes with function)	Discontinue VELCADE

*Based on dose modifications in phase II & III multiple myeloma studies

Administration

The reconstituted solution is administered as a 3-5 second bolus intravenous injection through a peripheral or central intravenous catheter followed by a flush with 9 mg/ml (0.9%) sodium chloride solution for injection.

Paediatric patients

VELCADE has not been studied in children and adolescents. Therefore, it should not be used in the paediatric age group until further data become available.

Elderly patients

There is no evidence to suggest that dose adjustments are necessary in the elderly (see section 4.8).

Use in patients with impaired renal function

VELCADE has not been formally studied in patients with impaired renal function. Patients with compromised renal function should be monitored carefully, especially if creatinine clearance is ≤30 ml/min and a dose reduction should be considered (see section 4.4 and 4.8).

Use in patients with impaired hepatic function

VELCADE has not been studied in patients with impaired hepatic function. Significant hepatic impairment may have an impact on the elimination of bortezomib and may increase the likelihood of drug-drug interactions. Patients with impaired liver function should be treated with extreme caution and a dose reduction should be considered (see section 4.3 and 4.4).

4.3 Contraindications

Hypersensitivity to bortezomib, boron or to any of the excipients.

Severe hepatic impairment.

4.4 Special warnings and special precautions for use

Gastrointestinal

Gastrointestinal toxicity, including nausea, diarrhoea, vomiting and constipation are very common with VELCADE treatment. Cases of ileus have been reported, therefore patients who experience constipation should be closely monitored.

Haematological

VELCADE treatment is very commonly associated with haematological toxicities (thrombocytopenia, neutropenia and anaemia). The most common haematologic toxicity is transient thrombocytopenia. Platelets were lowest at Day 11 of each cycle of VELCADE treatment. There was no evidence of cumulative thrombocytopenia, including in the phase II extension study. The mean platelet count nadir measured was approximately 40% of baseline. In patients with advanced myeloma the severity of thrombocytopenia was related to pre-treatment platelet count: for baseline platelet counts <75,000/μl, 90% of 21 patients had a count ≤25,000/μl during the study, including 14% <10,000/μl; in contrast, with a baseline platelet count >75,000/μl, only 14% of 309 patients had a count $\leqslant 25 \times 10^9$/L during the study. Platelet counts should be monitored prior to each dose of VELCADE. Therapy should be held when the platelet count is <25,000/μl and re-initiated at a reduced dose after resolution (see section 4.2). Potential benefit of the treatment should be carefully weighed against the risks, particularly in case of moderate to severe thrombocytopenia and risk factors for bleeding.

Therefore, complete blood counts (CBC) including platelet counts should be frequently monitored throughout treatment with VELCADE.

Peripheral Neuropathy

Treatment with VELCADE is very commonly associated with peripheral neuropathy, which is predominantly sensory, although cases of motor neuropathy have been reported. The incidence of peripheral neuropathy increases early in the treatment and has been observed to peak during cycle 5.

It is recommended that patients be carefully monitored for symptoms of neuropathy such as a burning sensation, hyperesthesia, hypoesthesia, paraesthesia, discomfort or neuropathic pain. Patients experiencing new or worsening peripheral neuropathy may require the dose and schedule of VELCADE to be modified (see section 4.2). Neuropathy has been managed with supportive care and other therapies. Improvement in, or resolution of, peripheral neuropathy was reported in 51% of patients with ≥ Grade 2 peripheral neuropathy in phase III and 71% of patients with grade 3 or 4 peripheral neuropathy or peripheral neuropathy leading to discontinuation of treatment in phase II studies, respectively.

In addition to peripheral neuropathy, there may be a contribution of autonomic neuropathy to some adverse reactions such as postural hypotension and severe constipation with ileus. Information on autonomic neuropathy and its contribution to these undesirable effects is limited.

Seizures

Seizures have been uncommonly reported in patients without previous history of seizures or epilepsy. Special care is required when treating patients with any risk factors for seizures.

Hypotension

VELCADE treatment is commonly associated with orthostatic/postural hypotension. Most undesirable effects are mild to moderate in nature and are observed throughout treatment. Patients developing orthostatic hypotension on VELCADE did not have evidence of orthostatic hypotension prior to treatment with VELCADE. Most patients required treatment for their orthostatic hypotension. A minority of patients with orthostatic hypotension experienced syncopal events. Orthostatic/postural hypotension was not acutely related to bolus infusion of VELCADE. The mechanism of this event is unknown although a component may be due to autonomic neuropathy. Autonomic neuropathy may be related to bortezomib or bortezomib may aggravate an underlying condition such as diabetic neuropathy. Caution is advised when treating patients with a history of syncope receiving medicinal products known to be associated with hypotension; or who are dehydrated due to recurrent diarrhoea or vomiting. Management of orthostatic/postural hypotension may include adjustment of antihypertensive medicinal products, rehydration or administration of mineralocorticosteroids and/or sympathomimetics. Patients should be instructed to seek medical advice if they experience symptoms of dizziness, lightheadedness or fainting spells.

Heart failure

Development or exacerbation of congestive heart failure has been reported during bortezomib treatment. In a phase III randomized, comparative study the incidence of heart failure in the VELCADE group was similar to that in the dexamethasone group. Fluid retention may be a predisposing factor for signs and symptoms of heart failure.

ECG Investigations

There have been isolated cases of QT-interval prolongation in clinical studies, causality has not been established.

Renal Impairment

The incidence of serious undesirable effects has been shown to increase in patients with mild to moderate renal impairment compared to patients with normal renal function (see section 4.8). Renal complications are frequent in patients with multiple myeloma. Such patients should be monitored closely and dose reduction considered.

Hepatic Impairment

Patients with hepatic impairment should be treated with extreme caution and a dose reduction should be considered (see sections 4.2 and 4.3).

Tumour lysis syndrome

Because bortezomib is a cytotoxic agent and can rapidly kill malignant plasma cells, the complications of tumour lysis syndrome may occur. The patients at risk of tumour lysis syndrome are those with high tumour burden prior to treatment. These patients should be monitored closely and appropriate precautions taken.

Amyloidosis

The impact of proteasome inhibition by bortezomib on disorders associated with protein accumulation such as amyloidosis is unknown. Caution is advised in these patients.

Precautions with certain concomitant medicinal products

Patients should be monitored closely when given bortezomib in combination with potent CYP3A4-inhibitors. Caution should be exercised when bortezomib is combined with CYP3A4- or CYP2C19 substrates (see section 4.5).

Normal liver function should be confirmed and caution should be exercised in patients receiving oral hypoglycemics (see section 4.5).

Potentially immunocomplex-mediated reactions

Potentially immunocomplex-mediated reactions, such as serum-sickness –type reaction, polyarthritis with rash and proliferative glomerulonephritis have been reported uncommonly. Bortezomib should be discontinued if serious reactions occur.

4.5 Interaction with other medicinal products and other forms of Interaction

No formal drug-drug interaction studies have been conducted with bortezomib. *In vitro* studies indicate that bortezomib is a weak inhibitor of the cytochrome P450 (CYP) isozymes 1A2, 2C9, 2C19, 2D6 and 3A4. Based on the limited contribution (7%) of CYP2D6 to the metabolism of bortezomib, the CYP2D6 poor metabolizer phenotype is not expected to affect the overall disposition of bortezomib.

Patients should be monitored closely when given bortezomib in combination with potent CYP3A4-inhibitors (e.g. ketoconazole, ritonavir), CYP2C19-inhibitors (fluoxetine) or CYP3A4-inducers (e.g. rifampicin). Caution should be exercised when bortezomib is combined with CYP3A4- or CYP2C19 substrates (see section 4.4).

During clinical trials, hypoglycemia and hyperglycemia were reported in diabetic patients receiving oral hypoglycemics. Patients on oral antidiabetic agents receiving VELCADE treatment may require close monitoring of their blood glucose levels and adjustment of the dose of their antidiabetics.

4.6 Pregnancy and lactation

For VELCADE no clinical data on exposed pregnancies are available. The teratogenic potential of bortezomib has not been fully investigated.

In non-clinical studies, bortezomib had no effects on embryonal foetal development in rats and rabbits at the highest maternally tolerated dosages. Animal studies were not conducted to determine the parturition and post-natal development (see section 5.3)

Males and females of childbearing capacity should use effective contraceptive measures during treatment and for 3 months following VELCADE therapy. If VELCADE is used during pregnancy, or if the patient becomes pregnant while receiving this medicinal product, the patient needs to be informed of potential for hazards to the foetus.

It is not known whether VELCADE is excreted in human milk. Because of the potential for serious undesirable effects in breast-fed infants from VELCADE, women are advised against breast feeding while receiving VELCADE.

4.7 Effects on ability to drive and use machines

VELCADE may have a moderate influence on the ability to drive and use machines. VELCADE may be associated with fatigue, dizziness, syncope, orthostatic/postural hypotension or blurred vision. Therefore, patients must be cautious when operating machinery, or when driving (see section 4.8).

4.8 Undesirable effects

The following undesirable effects were considered to have at least a possible or probable causal relationship to VELCADE by the investigators during the conduct of 5 non-comparative Phase II studies and 1 comparative phase III trial VELCADE vs dexamethasone in 663 patients with relapsed or refractory multiple myeloma, of whom 331 received VELCADE as single agent. The safety database comprises data from patients with multiple myeloma or B-cell lymphocytic leukemia (CLL). Patients were treated with VELCADE as a single agent, or in combination with dexamethasone.

ADRs are listed below by system organ class and frequency. Frequencies are defined as: Very common >1/10); common >1/100, <1/10); uncommon >1/1,000, <1/100); rare >1/10,000, <1/1,000); very rare (<1/10,000), including isolated reports.

Infections and infestations

Common: herpes zoster, pneumonia, bronchitis, sinusitis, nasopharyngitis, herpes simplex.

Uncommon: candidal infection, gastroenteritis, upper and lower respiratory tract infection, infection, influenza, fungal infection, sepsis, urinary tract infection, catheter related infection, haemophilus infection, pneumonia pneumococcal, post herpetic neuralgia, bacteraemia, blepharitis, bronchopneumonia, cytomegalovirus infection, infectious mononucleosis, varicella, oral candidiasis, pleural infection.

Neoplasms benign, malignant and unspecified (including cysts and polyps)

Uncommon: tumour lysis syndrome (see section 4.4).

Blood and lymphatic system disorders (see section 4.4)

Very Common: thrombocytopenia, anaemia, neutropenia.

Common: leukopenia, lymphopenia.

Uncommon: lymphadenopathy, febrile neutropenia, pancytopenia, haemolytic anaemia, thrombocytopenic purpura.

Immune system disorders

Uncommon: hypersensitivity, immunocomplex mediated hypersensitivity.

Metabolism and nutrition disorders

Very Common: appetite decreased.

Common: dehydration, hyperglycaemia, hypokalaemia.

Uncommon: hypercalcaemia, hyperkalaemia, hyperuricaemia, hyponatraemia, hypernatraemia, hypocalcaemia, hypomagnesaemia, hypophosphataemia, hypoglycaemia, appetite increased, cachexia, vitamin B12 deficiency.

Endocrine disorders

Uncommon: Inappropriate antidiuretic hormone (ADH) secretion.

Psychiatric disorders

Common: insomnia, anxiety, confusion, depression.

Uncommon: agitation, delirium, restlessness, mood swings, mental status changes, sleep disorder, irritability, hallucinations, abnormal dreams.

Nervous system disorders(see sections 4.4 and 4.7)

Very Common: peripheral neuropathy, peripheral sensory neuropathy (see section 4.4), headache, paraesthesia.

Common: dizziness (excluding vertigo), dysgeusia, peripheral neuropathy aggravated, polyneuropathy, dysaesthesia, hypoaesthesia, tremor.

Uncommon: convulsions (see section 4.4), syncope, disturbance in attention, increased activity, ageusia, somnolence, migraine, peripheral motor neuropathy, jerky movements, dizziness postural, sciatica, cognitive disorder, mononeuropathy, paresis, restless leg syndrome, speech disorder, intracranial haemorrhage, paraplegia, subarachnoid haemorrhage.

Eye disorders

Common: vision blurred (see section 4.7), eye pain.

Uncommon: dry eye, conjunctivitis, eye discharge, vision abnormal, eye haemorrhage, photophobia, eye irritation, lacrimation increased, conjunctival hyperaemia, eye swelling.

Ear and labyrinth disorders

Common: vertigo.

Uncommon: tinnitus, deafness, hypoacusis, hearing impaired.

Cardiac disorders

Uncommon: Development or exacerbation of congestive heart failure (see section 4.4), cardiac failure, ventricular hypokinesia, pulmonary oedema and acute pulmonary oedema, cardiac arrest, cardiogenic shock, tachycardia, sinus tachycardia, supraventricular tachycardia, arrhythmia, atrial fibrillation, palpitations, sinus arrest, atrioventricular block complete, angina pectoris, angina unstable, myocardial infarction.

Vascular disorders

Common: hypotension, orthostatic and postural hypotension (see sections 4.4 and 4.7), phlebitis, haematoma, hypertension.

Uncommon: flushing, petechiae, hot flushes, ecchymosis, purpura, cerebral hemorrhage, vasculitis, vein discolouration, vein distended, wound hemorrhage, pulmonary hypertension, cerebrovascular accident.

Respiratory, thoracic and mediastinal disorders

Very Common: dyspnoea.

Common: epistaxis, dyspnoea exertional, cough, rhinorrhoea.

Uncommon: nasal congestion, wheezing, pleural effusion, hoarseness, chest wall pain, hypoxia, pulmonary congestion, rhinitis, asthma, hyperventilation, orthopnoea, sinus pain, throat tightness, productive cough, respiratory alkalosis, respiratory arrest, tachypnoea.

Gastrointestinal disorders (see section 4.4)

Very Common: nausea, diarrhoea, vomiting, constipation.

Common: abdominal pain, dyspepsia, loose stools, abdominal pain upper, flatulence, abdominal distension, hiccups, mouth ulceration, pharyngolaryngeal pain, stomatitis, dry mouth.

Uncommon: ileus paralytic, abdominal discomfort, eructation, gastrointestinal motility disorder, oral pain, retching, antibiotic associated colitis, change in bowel habit, diarrhoea haemorrhagic, gastrointestinal haemorrhage, spleen pain, colitis, dysphagia, oesophagitis, gastritis, gastro-oesophageal reflux disease, gastrointestinal pain, gingival bleeding, gingival pain, haematemesis, hiatus hernia, irritable bowel syndrome, oral mucosal petechiae, rectal haemorrhage, salivary hypersecretion, tongue coated, tongue discolouration, enteritis, faecal impaction, acute pancreatitis.

Hepatobiliary disorders (see section 4.4)

Uncommon: hepatitis, hepatic haemorrhage, hypoproteinaemia.

Skin and subcutaneous tissue disorders

Very Common: rash.

Common: pruritus, erythema, periorbital oedema, urticaria, rash pruritic, sweating increased, dry skin, eczema.

Uncommon: night sweats, rash erythematous, alopecia, contusion, pruritus generalised, rash macular, rash papular, skin nodule, rash generalized, dermatitis, eyelid oedema, nail disorder, photosensitivity reaction, skin discolouration, dermatitis atopic, hair texture abnormal, heat rash, psoriasis, vasculitic rash, face oedema, pressure sore, ichthyosis.

Musculoskeletal and connective tissue disorders

Very Common: myalgia.

Common: pain in limb, muscle cramps, arthralgia, bone pain, peripheral swelling, muscle weakness, back pain, musculoskeletal pain.

Uncommon: joint stiffness, buttock pain, joint swelling, muscle spasms, muscle twitching or sensation of heaviness, muscle stiffness, swelling, pain in jaw.

Renal and urinary disorders

Common: renal impairment, dysuria.

Uncommon: renal failure acute, renal colic, haematuria, proteinuria, urinary frequency, difficulty in micturition, renal failure, oliguria, urinary retention, loin pain, urinary incontinence, micturition urgency.

General disorders and administration site conditions

Very Common: fatigue (see section 4.7), pyrexia.

Common: weakness, rigors, malaise, influenza like illness, oedema peripheral, pain, lethargy, oedema, chest pain, asthenia.

Uncommon: fall, mucosal inflammation, feeling cold, chest pressure sensation, injection site phlebitis, mucosal haemorrhage, tenderness, injection site erythema, neuralgia, chest discomfort, groin pain, chest tightness, extravasation inflammation.

Investigations

Common: weight decreased, blood lactate dehydrogenase increased.

Uncommon: alanine aminotransferase increased, aspartate aminotransferase increased, blood alkaline phosphatase increased, blood creatinine increased, blood urea increased, gamma-glutamyltransferase increased, blood amylase increased, blood bilirubin increased, blood phosphate decreased, liver function tests abnormal, red blood cell count decreased, weight increased, white blood cell count decreased, blood bicarbonate decreased, heart rate irregular, C-reactive protein increased.

Injury, poisoning and procedural complications

Uncommon: catheter related complications, post procedural pain, post procedural haemorrhage, burns.

Reproductive system and breast disorders

Uncommon: testicular pain, erectile dysfunction.

Table 2 Dosing regimens in Phase II and Phase III studies

Phase/arm	Drug Schedule	Dose	Regimen
II	VELCADE: Day 1,4,8,11, (rest Day 12-21)	1.3 mg/m^2 (IV bolus)	Q3 weeks × 8cycles (extension**)
III	VELCADE* a) Days 1,4,8,11, (Rest Day 12-21) b) Days 1,8,15,22	1.3 mg/m^2 (IV bolus)	a) Q3weeks × 8, then b) Q5 weeks × 3
III	DEXAMETHASONE a) Days 1–4, 9–12, 17–20 b) Days 1–4	40 mg (PO)	a) Q5 week × 4 b) Q4 week × 5
II	Add DEXAMETHASONE***	20 mg (PO) (Days 1,2,4,5,8,9, 11,12)	Q3 weeks

* a) is the initial treatment, a) and b) represent a full course of treatment

**An extension study authorised patients benefiting from treatment to continue receiving VELCADE

*** If after 2 or 4 cycles of VELCADE, the patients had progressive disease or stable disease, respectively, they could receive dexamethasone

Table 3 Patient characteristics in Phase II and Phase III studies

	Phase II VELCADE	Phase III VELCADE	Phase III Dex
Pt Number, ITT analysis	202	333	336
Male %	60	56	60
Median age, yrs (range)	59 (34-84)	61 (33-84)	61 (27-86)
Caucasian	81	90 %	88 %
Karnofsky PS > 80%	80	87%	84 %
Platelets < 75'000/μl	21 %	6 %	4 %
Hemoglobin < 100g/l	44 %	32 %	28 %
Median Creatinine Clearance, ml/min (range)	74 (14-221)	73.3 (15.6-170.7)	73.3 (15.3-261.1)
Myeloma IgG	60 %	60 %	59%
Myeloma IgA	24 %	23 %	24%
Myeloma light chain	14 %	12 %	13 %
Median duration since diagnosis (yrs)	4.0	3.5	3.1
Chromosome 13 abnormalities	15%	25.7%	25.0%
Med. $\beta 2$ μglobulin (mg/L)	3.5	3.7	3.6
Median number prior treatment lines* (range)	6 (2-15)	2 (1-7)	2 (1-8)
1 prior line > 1 prior line	0	N=132(40%) N= 186 (60%)	N= 119 (35%) N= 194 (65%)

*Including steroids, alkylating agents, anthracyclines, thalidomide and stem cell transplants

Potentially immunocomplex-mediated reactions (see section 4.4)

Potentially immunocomplex-mediated reactions, such as serum-sickness –type reaction, polyarthritis with rash and proliferative glomerulonephritis have been reported uncommonly.

Post Marketing Experience

Clinically significant adverse reactions are listed if they have been reported during post approval use of VELCADE and have not been reported in clinical trials:

Uncommon: cardiac tamponade, ischemic colitis, encephalopathy.

4.9 Overdose

In patients, overdosage more than twice the recommended dose has been associated with the acute onset of symptomatic hypotension and thrombocytopenia with fatal outcomes. (Refer to section 5.3 for preclinical cardiovascular safety pharmacology studies).

There is no known specific antidote for VELCADE overdosage. In the event of an overdosage, the patient's vital signs should be monitored and appropriate supportive care given to maintain blood pressure (such as fluids, pressors, and/or inotropic agents) and body temperature (See Sections 4.2 and 4.4).

5. PHARMACOLOGICAL PROPERTIES

5.1 Pharmacodynamic properties

Pharmacotherapeutic group: Antineoplastic agent

ATC code: LO1XX32

Bortezomib is a proteasome inhibitor. It is specifically designed to inhibit the chymotrypsin-like activity of the 26S proteasome in mammalian cells. The 26S proteasome is a large protein complex that degrades ubiquitinated proteins. The ubiquitin-proteasome pathway plays an essential role in orchestrating the turnover of specific proteins, thereby maintaining homeostasis within cells. Inhibition of the 26S proteasome prevents this targeted proteolysis and affects multiple signalling cascades within the cell, ultimately resulting in cancer cell death.

Bortezomib is highly selective for the proteasome. At 10 μM concentrations, bortezomib does not inhibit any of a wide variety of receptors and proteases screened and is more than 1500-fold more selective for the proteasome than for its next preferable enzyme. The kinetics of proteasome inhibition were evaluated *in vitro*, and bortezomib was shown to dissociate from the proteasome with a $t_{½}$ of 20 minutes, thus demonstrating that proteasome inhibition by bortezomib is reversible.

Bortezomib mediated proteasome inhibition affects cancer cells in a number of ways, including, but not limited to, altering regulatory proteins, which control cell cycle progression and Nuclear Factor kappa B (NF-kB) activation. Inhibition of the proteasome results in cell cycle arrest and apoptosis. NF-kB is a transcription factor whose activation is required for many aspects of tumourogenesis, including cell growth and survival, angiogenesis, cell:cell interactions, and metastasis. In myeloma, bortezomib affects the ability of myeloma cells to interact with the bone marrow microenvironment.

Experiments have demonstrated that bortezomib is cytotoxic to a variety of cancer cell types and that cancer cells are more sensitive to the proapoptotic effects of proteasome inhibition than normal cells. Bortezomib causes reduction of tumour growth *in vivo* in many preclinical tumour models, including multiple myeloma.

Table 4 Patient exposure to treatment with VELCADE during phase 2 and 3 studies

	Phase II VELCADE	Phase III VELCADE	Phase III Dex
Received at least 1 dose	N= 202	N=331	N= 332
Completed 4 cycles a) all initial cycles (number) b) full course (number) c) extension *	62% 27% (8 cycles) NA N= 63 pts (median 7 cycles) or total median 14 cycles (range 7-32)	69% 29 % (8 cycles) 9% (11 cycles) NA	 36 % (4 cycles) 5 % (9 cycles) NA

*Patients could continue on treatment after completing 8 cycles, in case of benefit

NA = not applicable

<u>Clinical Trials</u>

The safety and efficacy of VELCADE were evaluated in 2 studies at the recommended dose of 1.3 mg/m^2: a phase III randomized, comparative study, versus Dexamethasone (Dex), of 669 patients with relapsed or refractory multiple myeloma who had received 1-3 prior lines of therapy, and a phase II single-arm study of 202 patients with relapsed and refractory multiple myeloma, who had received at least 2 prior lines of treatment and who were progressing on their most recent treatment. (See Tables 2, 3 and 4).

Table 2: Dosing regimens in Phase II and Phase III studies (see Table 2 on previous page)

Table 3: Patient characteristics in Phase II and Phase III studies (see Table 3 on previous page)

Table 4: Patient exposure to treatment with VELCADE during phase 2 and 3 studies (see Table 4 above)

In the phase III study, treatment with VELCADE led to a significantly longer time to progression, a significantly prolonged survival and a significantly higher response rate, compared to treatment with dexamethasone (see Table 5), in all patients as well as in patients who have received 1 prior line of therapy. As a result of a preplanned interim analysis, the Dexamethasone arm was halted at the recommendation of the data monitoring committee and all patients randomised to dexamethasone were then offered VELCADE, regardless of disease status. Due to this early crossover, the median duration of follow-up for surviving patients is 8.3 months. Both in patients who were refractory to their last prior therapy and those who were not refractory, overall survival was significantly longer and response rate was significantly higher on the VELCADE arm.

Of the 669 patients enrolled, 245 (37%) were 65 years of age or older. Response parameters as well as TTP remained significantly better for VELCADE independently of age. Regardless of $\beta 2$- microglobulin levels at baseline, all efficacy parameters (time to progression and overall survival, as well as response rate) were significantly improved on the VELCADE arm.

In the refractory population of the Phase II study, responses were determined by an independent review committee and the response criteria were those of the European Bone Marrow Transplant Group. The median survival of all patients enrolled was 17 months (range <1 to 36+ months). This survival was greater than the six-to-nine month median survival anticipated by consultant clinical investigators for a similar patient population. By multivariate analysis, the response rate was independent of myeloma type, performance status, chromosome 13 deletion status, or the number, or type of previous therapies; patients who had received 2 to 3 prior therapeutic regimens had a response rate of 32% (10/32) and patients who received greater than 7 prior therapeutic regimens had a response rate of 31% (21/67).

Table 5: Summary of Disease Outcomes from the Phase III and Phase II studies

(see Table 5 below)

In the phase II study, patients who did not obtain an optimal response to therapy with VELCADE alone were able to receive high-dose dexamethasone in conjunction with VELCADE (see Table 2). The protocol allowed patients to receive dexamethasone if they had had a less than optimal response to VELCADE alone. A total of 74 evaluable patients were administered dexamethasone in combination with VELCADE. Eighteen percent of patients achieved, or had an improved response (MR (11%) or PR (7%)) with combination treatment.

5.2 Pharmacokinetic properties

After single intravenous dose administration, plasma concentrations of bortezomib decline in a biphasic manner characterized by a rapid distribution phase followed by a longer terminal elimination phase. The rapid distribution period has a half-life of less than 10 minutes. In humans, the terminal elimination of bortezomib has an estimated half-life ranging from 5 to 15 hours. Exposure to bortezomib appears to be dose-dependent over the dose range of 1.45 to 2.0 mg/m^2, with dose-proportional increases observed from 1.0 to 1.3 mg/m^2.

In a group of patients with solid tumours (n=17), treated with both bortezomib and gemcitabine, the mean terminal elimination of bortezomib after the first dose (1.0 mg/m^2) was 5.45 hours and the mean $AUC_{0\text{-}24}$ was 30.1 hr × ng/ml.

Following multiple doses of bortezomib, a decrease in clearance is observed resulting in a corresponding increase in terminal elimination half-life and AUC. Repeated dosing does not have an effect on the initial distribution kinetics of bortezomib, so no changes in estimated C_{max} or the distribution half-life are observed. In the patients with solid tumours, the mean terminal elimination half-life increased from 5.45 to 19.7 hours, and the $AUC_{0\text{-}24}$ increased from 30.1 hr*ng/mL to 54.0 hr*ng/mL after the first and third doses of the first cycle, respectively. Similar findings have also been observed in nonclinical studies in rats and cynomolgus monkeys.

Over a bortezomib concentration range of 0.01 to 1.0 μg/ml, the in vitro protein binding averaged 82.9% in human plasma. The percent of bortezomib bound to plasma proteins was not concentration dependent.

The elimination pathways of bortezomib have not been evaluated in vivo. In vitro, CYP3A4 and CYP2C19 are quantitatively the major enzymes responsible for the metabolism of bortezomib. Only a small amount of parent compound has been recovered in urine while no intact bortezomib has been recovered in bile or faeces.

Formal studies in patients with severely impaired renal and hepatic functions have not been conducted to date; consequently caution is recommended when administering bortezomib to these classes of patients (see 4.4). In the absence of data VELCADE is contraindicated in patients with severe liver impairment (see 4.3).

5.3 Preclinical safety data

Bortezomib was positive for clastogenic activity (structural chromosomal aberrations) in the *in vitro* chromosomal aberration assay using Chinese hamster ovary cells at concentrations as low as 3.125 μg/ml, which was the lowest concentration evaluated. Bortezomib was not genotoxic when tested in the *in vitro* mutagenicity assay (Ames assay) and *in vivo* micronucleus assay in mice.

Developmental toxicity studies in the rat and rabbit have shown embryo-fetal lethality at maternally toxic dosages, but no direct embryo-foetal toxicity below maternally toxic dosages. Fertility studies were not performed but evaluation of reproductive tissues has been performed in the general toxicity studies. In the 6-month rat study, degenerative effects in both the testes and the ovary have been observed. It is, therefore, likely that bortezomib could have a potential effect on either male or female fertility. Peri- and postnatal development studies were not conducted.

In multi-cycle general toxicity studies conducted in the rat and monkey the principal target organs included the gastrointestinal tract resulting in vomiting and/or diarrhea, hematopoietic and lymphatic tissues resulting in peripheral blood cytopenias and lymphoid tissue atrophy and hematopoietic bone marrow hypocellularity, peripheral neuropathy (observed in monkeys, mice and dogs) involving sensory nerve axons, and mild changes in the kidneys. All these target organs have shown partial to full recovery following discontinuation of treatment.

Based on animal studies, the penetration of bortezomib through the blood-brain barrier appears to be limited, if any and the relevance to humans is unknown.

Cardiovascular safety pharmacology studies in monkeys and dogs show that IV doses approximately two to three times the recommended clinical dose on a mg/m^2 basis are associated with increases in heart rate, decreases in contractility, hypotension and death. In dogs the decreased cardiac contractility and hypotension responded to acute intervention with positive inotropic or pressor agents. Moreover, in dog studies, a slight increase in the corrected QT interval was observed.

6. PHARMACEUTICAL PARTICULARS

6.1 List of excipients

Mannitol (E 421).

Nitrogen.

6.2 Incompatibilities

This medicinal product must not be mixed with other medicinal products except those mentioned in 6.6.

6.3 Shelf life

2 years

Reconstituted solution: 8 hours

6.4 Special precautions for storage

Do not store above 30°C. Keep the container in the outer carton in order to protect from light.

The reconstituted solution should be used immediately after preparation. If the reconstituted solution is not used immediately, in-use storage times and conditions prior to use are the responsibility of the user. However, the chemical and physical in-use stability of the reconstituted solution has been demonstrated for 8 hours at 25 °C stored

Table 5 Summary of Disease Outcomes from the Phase III and Phase II studies

	Phase III		Phase III		Phase III		Phase II
	All Patients		1 Prior Line of Therapy		>1 Prior Line of Therapy		⩾ 2 prior lines
<u>Time related events</u>	**VELCADE N=333[a]**	**Dex N=336[a]**	**VELCADE N=132[a]**	**Dex N=119[a]**	**VELCADE N=200[a]**	**Dex N=217[a]**	**VELCADE N=202[a]**
TTP, days [95% CI]	189[b] [148, 211]	106[b] [86, 128]	212[d] [188, 267]	169[d] [105, 191]	148[b] [129, 192]	87[b] [84, 107]	210 [154, 281]
1 year survival, % [95% CI]	80[d] [74,85]	66[d] [59,72]	89[d] [82,95]	72[d] [62,83]	73 [64,82]	62 [53,71]	60
<u>Best Response (%)</u>	**VELCADE N=315[c]**	**Dex N=312[c]**	**VELCADE N=128**	**Dex N=110**	**VELCADE N=187**	**Dex N=202**	**VELCADE N=193**
CR	20 (6) [b]	2 (<1) [b]	8 (6)	2 (2)	12 (6)	0 (0)	(4)**
CR + nCR	41 (13) [b]	5 (2) [b]	16 (13)	4 (4)	25 (13)	1 (<1)	(10)**
CR+ nCR + PR	121 (38) [b]	56 (18) [b]	57 (45) [d]	29 (26) [d]	64 (34) [b]	27 (13) [b]	(27)**
CR + nCR+ PR+MR	146 (46)	108 (35)	66 (52)	45 (41)	80 (43)	63 (31)	(35)**
Median duration Days (months)	242 (8.0)	169 (5.6)	246 (8.1)	189 (6.2)	238 (7.8)	126 (4.1)	385*
Time To Response CR + PR (days)	43	43	44	46	41	27	38*

[a] Intent to Treat (ITT) population

[b] p-value from the stratified log-rank test; analysis by line of therapy excludes stratification for therapeutic history; $p < 0.0001$

[c] Response population includes patients who had measurable disease at baseline and received at least 1 dose of study drug.

[d] p-value from the Cochran-Mantel-Haenszel chi-square test adjusted for the stratification factors; analysis by line of therapy excludes stratification for therapeutic history

*CR+PR+MR **CR=CR, (IF-); nCR=CR (IF+)

NA = not applicable, NE = not estimated

in the original vial and/or a syringe prior to administration, with a maximum of 8 hours in the syringe.

6.5 Nature and contents of container

10 ml, type 1, glass vial with a grey bromobutyl stopper and an aluminium seal.

The vial is contained in a transparent blister pack consisting of a tray with a lid.

1 vial contains 38.5 mg powder for solution for injection.

VELCADE is available in cartons containing 1 single-use vial.

6.6 Instructions for use and handling

For single use only.

VELCADE is a cytotoxic agent. Therefore, as with other potentially toxic compounds, caution should be used during handling and preparation. Use of gloves and other protective clothing to prevent skin contact is recommended.

ASEPTIC TECHNIQUE MUST BE STRICTLY OBSERVED THROUGHOUT HANDLING OF VELCADE SINCE NO PRESERVATIVE IS PRESENT.

VELCADE is provided as a lyophilised powder in the form of a mannitol boronic ester. When reconstituted, the mannitol ester is in equilibrium with its hydrolysis product, the monomeric boronic acid.

When reconstituted, each vial of VELCADE 3.5 mg yields a solution with a concentration of 1 mg/ml. Each vial must be reconstituted with 3.5 ml of 9 mg/ml (0.9%) sodium chloride for injection. Dissolution is completed in less than 2 minutes. The reconstituted solution is clear and colourless, with a final pH of 4 to 7. The reconstituted solution must be inspected visually for particulate matter and discolouration prior to administration. If any discolouration or particulate matter is observed, the reconstituted product must be discarded.

Procedure for proper disposal

Any unused product or waste material should be disposed of in accordance with local requirements.

7. MARKETING AUTHORISATION HOLDER

JANSSEN-CILAG INTERNATIONAL NV

Turnhoutseweg, 30, B-2340 Beerse

Belgium

8. MARKETING AUTHORISATION NUMBER(S)

EU/1/04/274/001

9. DATE OF FIRST AUTHORISATION/RENEWAL OF THE AUTHORISATION

26/04/2004

10. DATE OF REVISION OF THE TEXT

27/07/2005

Velosef Capsules 250mg, 500mg, Syrup 250mg/5ml

(E. R. Squibb & Sons Limited)

1. NAME OF THE MEDICINAL PRODUCT

VELOSEF CAPSULES 250MG & 500MG

VELOSEF SYRUP 250MG/5ML

2. QUALITATIVE AND QUANTITATIVE COMPOSITION

Capsules 250mg: Opaque, orange body with opaque blue cap printed Squibb and 113 in white on each half. Each capsule contains 250mg cefradine.

Capsules 500mg: Opaque blue printed in white with Squibb and 114 on each half. Each capsule contains 500mg cefradine.

Syrup 250mg/5ml: When reconstituted contains 250mg cefradine per 5 ml.

3. PHARMACEUTICAL FORM

Oral Capsules.

Oral powder for reconstitution.

4. CLINICAL PARTICULARS

4.1 Therapeutic indications

In the treatment of infections of the urinary and respiratory tracts and of the skin and soft tissues. These include:

Upper respiratory infections - pharyngitis, sinusitis, otitis media, tonsillitis, laryngo-tracheo bronchitis.

Lower respiratory infections - acute and chronic bronchitis, lobar and bronchopneumonia.

Urinary tract infections - cystitis, urethritis, pyelonephritis.

Skin and soft tissue infections - abscess, cellulitis, furunculosis, impetigo.

Cefradine has been shown to be effective in reducing the incidence of postoperative infections in patients undergoing surgical procedures associated with a high risk of infection. It is also of value where postoperative infections would be disastrous and where patients have a reduced host resistance to bacterial infection. Protection is best ensured by achieving adequate local tissue concentrations at the time contamination is likely to occur. Thus, cefradine should be administered immediately prior to surgery and continued during the postoperative period.

Bacteriology studies to determine the causative organisms and their sensitivity to cefradine should be performed. Therapy may be instituted prior to receiving the results of the sensitivity test.

4.2 Posology and method of administration

Cefradine may be given without regard to meals.

Adults:

For urinary tract infections the usual dose is 500mg four times daily or 1g twice daily; severe or chronic infections may require larger doses. Prolonged intensive therapy is needed for complications such as prostatitis and epididymitis. For respiratory tract infections and skin and soft tissue infections the usual dose is 250mg or 500mg four times daily or 500mg or 1g twice daily depending on the severity and site of infections.

Children:

The usual dose is from 25 to 50mg/kg/day total, given in two or four equally divided doses.

For otitis media daily doses from 75 to 100mg/kg in divided doses every 6 to 12 hours are recommended. Maximum dose 4g per day.

Elderly:

There are no specific dosage recommendations or precautions for use in the elderly except, as with other drugs, to monitor those patients with impaired renal or hepatic function.

All patients, irrespective of age and weight

Larger doses (up to 1g four times daily) may be given for severe or chronic infections. Therapy should be continued for a minimum of 48-72 hours after the patient becomes asymptomatic or evidence of bacterial eradication has been obtained. In infections caused by haemolytic strains of streptococci, a minimum of 10 days' treatment is recommended to guard against the risk of rheumatic fever or glomerulonephritis. In the treatment of chronic urinary tract infections, frequent bacteriological and clinical appraisal is necessary during therapy and may be necessary for several months afterwards. Persistent infections may require treatment for several weeks. Smaller doses than those indicated above should not be used. Doses for children should not exceed doses recommended for adults. As cefradine is available in both injectable and oral form, patients may be changed from the cefradine injectable to cefradine oral at the same dosage level.

Renal Impairment Dosage:

Patients not on dialysis:

The following dosage schedule is suggested as a guideline based on a dosage of 500mg Q6H and on creatinine clearance. Further modification in the dosage schedule may be required because of the dosage selected and individual variation.

Creatinine Clearance	Dose	Time Interval
More than 20 ml/min	500 mg	6 hours
5 - 20 ml/min	250 mg	6 hours
Less than 5 ml/min	250 mg	12 hours

Patients on chronic, intermittent haemodialysis:

250 mg	At start of haemodialysis
250 mg	6 - 12 hours after start
250 mg	36 - 48 hours after start
250 mg	At start of next haemodialysis if >30 hours after previous dose.

Further modification of the dosage schedule may be necessary in children.

4.3 Contraindications

Patients with known hypersensitivity to the cephalosporin antibiotics or to any component of the formulation.

4.4 Special warnings and special precautions for use

There is evidence of partial cross-allergenicity between the penicillins and the cephalosporins. Therefore cefradine should be used with caution in those patients with known hypersensitivity to penicillins. There have been instances of patients who have had reactions to both drug classes (including anaphylaxis).

Dosage should be reduced in renal failure (see Section 4.2.).

After treatment with cefradine, a false positive reaction for glucose in the urine may occur with Benedict's or Fehling's solution or with reagent tablets such as Clinitest*, but not with enzyme-based tests such as Clinistix* or Diastix*.

As with all antibiotics, prolonged use may result in overgrowth of non-susceptible organisms.

4.5 Interaction with other medicinal products and other forms of Interaction

Loop diuretics may increase nephrotoxicity of cephalosporins.

Probenecid has been seen to raise serum concentrations of cefradine, by reducing renal clearance of the cephalosporins.

4.6 Pregnancy and lactation

Although animal studies have not demonstrated any teratogenicity, safety in pregnancy has not been established.

Cefradine is excreted in breast milk and should be used with caution in lactating mothers.

4.7 Effects on ability to drive and use machines

Since this medicine may cause dizziness, patients should be cautioned about operating hazardous machinery, including automobiles.

4.8 Undesirable effects

Limited essentially to gastro-intestinal disturbances and on occasion to hypersensitivity phenomena. The latter are more likely to occur in individuals who have previously demonstrated hypersensitivity and those with a history of allergy, asthma, hay fever or urticaria. The majority of reported side-effects have been mild and are rare, and include glossitis, heartburn, dizziness, tightness in the chest, headache, nausea, vomiting, diarrhoea, abdominal pain, vaginitis, candidal overgrowth. Skin and hypersensitivity reactions include urticaria, pruritus, skin rashes, fever, athralgia and oedema.

As with other cephalosporins, there have been rare reports of erythema multiforme, Stevens Johnson Syndrome, anaphylaxis and toxic epidermal necrolysis. Also, mild transient eosinophilia, leucopenia and neutropenia, rarely positive direct Coombs tests and pseudomembraneous colitis have been reported.

Elevations of BUN and serum creatinine and reversible interstitial nephritis have been reported. Transient hepatitis and cholestatic jaundice have been reported very rarely. Elevations of ALT, AST, total bilirubin and alkaline phosphatase have been observed.

4.9 Overdose

None known.

5. PHARMACOLOGICAL PROPERTIES

5.1 Pharmacodynamic properties

Actions:

Cefradine is a broad-spectrum, bactericidal antibiotic active against both Gram-positive and Gram-negative bacteria. It is also highly active against most strains of penicillinase-producing Staphylococci.

Microbiology:

The following organisms have shown in vitro sensitivity to cefradine.

Gram-positive - Staphylococci (both penicillin sensitive and resistant strains), Streptococci, *Streptococcus pyogenes* (beta-haemolytic) and *Streptococcus pneumoniae.*

Gram-negative - *Escherichia coli, Klebsiella* spp, *Proteus mirabilis, Haemophilus influenzae, Shigella* spp., *Salmonella* spp. (including *Salmonella typhi*) and *Neisseria* spp.

Because cefradine is unaffected by penicillinase, many strains of *Escherichia coli* and *Staphylococcus aureus* which produce this enzyme are susceptible to cefradine but resistant to ampicillin.

5.2 Pharmacokinetic properties

Cefradine has a high degree of stability to many beta-lactamases. It has a low degree of protein-binding and a large volume of distribution. Therefore, tissue levels are generally found to be high. Oral cefradine can be given twice or four times daily, and is well absorbed.

Human Pharmacology: Cefradine is acid stable and is rapidly absorbed following oral administration in the fasting state. Following doses of 250mg, 500mg and 1000mg average peak serum levels of approximately 9, 16.5, and 24.2 micrograms/ml, respectively, were obtained at one hour. The presence of food in the gastrointestinal tract delays the absorption but does not affect the total amount of cefradine absorbed. Measurable serum levels are present six hours after administration. Over 90% of the drug is excreted unchanged in the urine within 6 hours. Peak urine concentrations are approximately 1600 micrograms/ml following a 250mg dose, 3200 micrograms/ml following a 500mg dose, and 4000 micrograms/ml following a 1000mg dose. After 48 hours' administration of 100mg/kg/day of cefradine for the treatment of otitis media, cefradine has been measured in the middle ear exudate at an average level of 3.6 microgram/ml.

5.3 Preclinical safety data

No relevant further data available.

6. PHARMACEUTICAL PARTICULARS

6.1 List of excipients

Capsules 250mg: Erythrosine, gelatin capsules, indigo carmine, iron oxide, lactose, magnesium stearate, titanium dioxide.

Capsules 500mg: Gelatin capsules, indigo carmine, lactose, magnesium stearate, titanium dioxide.

Syrup: Citric acid, blood orange flavour, cinnamon flavour and tutti frutti flavour, guar gum, methylcellulose, sodium citrate, sucrose.

6.2 Incompatibilities

None known

6.3 Shelf life

Capsules:	36 months
Syrup:	48 months

6.4 Special precautions for storage

Capsules: Store below 25°C.

Syrup: Store in a cool place in dry form.
After reconstitution: discard unused syrup after 14 days if stored in a refrigerator, or 7 days at below 25°C.

6.5 Nature and contents of container

Capsules: Blister packs of 20 or 100 capsules.

Syrup: Bottles of 100 ml.

6.6 Instructions for use and handling

Not applicable

7. MARKETING AUTHORISATION HOLDER

E. R. Squibb & Sons Limited
Uxbridge Business Park
Sanderson Road
Uxbridge
Middlesex
UB8 1DH

8. MARKETING AUTHORISATION NUMBER(S)

Velosef Capsules 250mg: PL 0034/0133R
Velosef Capsules 500mg: PL 0034/0134R
Velosef Syrup 250mg/5ml: PL 0034/0136R

9. DATE OF FIRST AUTHORISATION/RENEWAL OF THE AUTHORISATION

Capsules: 25.01 91 / 25.09.01
Syrup: 30.01.91 / 25.09.01

10. DATE OF REVISION OF THE TEXT

June 2005

Velosef for Injection 500 mg and 1g

(E. R. Squibb & Sons Limited)

1. NAME OF THE MEDICINAL PRODUCT

VELOSEF FOR INJECTION 500MG
VELOSEF FOR INJECTION 1G

2. QUALITATIVE AND QUANTITATIVE COMPOSITION

Velosef for Injection is a sterile powder blend of cefradine and L-arginine. After reconstitution, Velosef for Injection 500mg provides 500mg of cefradine activity and Velosef for Injection 1g provides 1g of cefradine activity.

3. PHARMACEUTICAL FORM

Powder for solution for injection; intramuscular or intravenous injection and intravenous infusion.

4. CLINICAL PARTICULARS

4.1 Therapeutic indications

The treatment of infections of the urinary and respiratory tracts, and of the skin and soft tissues, bones and joints; also septicaemia and endocarditis. These include:

Upper respiratory infections - pharyngitis, sinusitis, otitis media, tonsillitis, laryngo-tracheo-bronchitis.

Lower respiratory infections - acute and chronic bronchitis, lobar and bronchopneumonia.

Urinary tract infections - cystitis, urethritis, pyelonephritis.

Skin and soft tissue infections - abscess, cellulitis, furunculosis, impetigo.

Cefradine has been shown to be effective in reducing the incidence of postoperative infections in patients undergoing surgical procedures associated with a high risk of infection. It is also of value where post-operative infection would be disastrous and where patients have a reduced host resistance to bacterial infection. Protection is best ensured by achieving adequate local tissue concentrations at the time contamination is likely to occur. Thus, cefradine should be administered immediately prior to surgery and continued during the postoperative period.

Bacteriological studies to determine the causative organisms and their sensitivity to cefradine should be performed. Therapy may be instituted prior to receiving the results of the sensitivity test.

4.2 Posology and method of administration

Sterile cefradine for injection is indicated primarily as an intramuscular injection for those patients unable to tolerate oral medication. It is also indicated for intravenous use either by direct injection or by intravenous infusion for the treatment of serious and life-threatening infections.

Instructions for reconstitution for intramuscular or intravenous injection and intravenous infusion are given in section 6.6.

Adults:

Treatment:

The usual dose range of cefradine for injection is 2-4g daily in four equally divided doses. This may be increased up to 8g a day for severe infections, e.g. septicaemia and endocarditis. For the majority of infections, the usual dose is 500mg q.i.d. in equally spaced doses; severe or chronic infections may require larger doses. Prolonged intensive therapy is needed for complications such as prostatitis and epididymitis. Patients who are severely ill and who require high serum levels of cefradine for treating their infections should be started on intravenous therapy.

Limited experience indicates that intraperitoneal administration of cefradine may be effective after surgery in cases of peritonitis where a surgical drainage system has been established.

Prophylaxis:

The recommended dose for surgical prophylaxis is a single, pre-operative 1-2g IM or IV dose. Subsequent parenteral or oral doses can be administered as appropriate.

Children:

The usual dose is 50-100mg/kg/day total given in four equally divided doses. More serious illnesses may require 200-300mg/kg/day.

Elderly:

There are no specific dosage recommendations or precautions for use in the elderly except, as with other drugs, to monitor those patients with impaired renal or hepatic function.

All patients, regardless of age and weight:

Therapy should be continued for a minimum of 48-72 hours after the patient becomes asymptomatic or evidence of bacterial eradication has been obtained. In infections caused by haemolytic strains of streptococci, a minimum of 10 days of treatment is recommended to guard against the risk of rheumatic fever or glomerulonephritis. In the treatment of chronic urinary tract infections, frequent bacteriological and clinical appraisal is necessary during therapy and may be necessary for several months afterwards. Persistent infections may require treatment for several weeks. Smaller doses than those indicated above should not be used. Doses for children should not exceed doses recommended for adults. As cefradine is available in both injectable and oral form, patients may be changed from the cefradine injectable to cefradine oral at the same dosage level.

Renal Impairment Dosage:

Patients not on dialysis:

The following dosage schedule is suggested as a guideline based on a dosage of 500mg Q6H and on creatinine clearance. Further modification in the dosage schedule may be required because of the dosage selected and individual variation.

Creatinine Clearance	Dose	Time Interval
More than 20 ml/min	500 mg	6 hours
5 - 20 ml/min	250 mg	6 hours
Less than 5 ml/min	250 mg	12 hours

Patients on chronic, intermittent haemodialysis:

250 mg	At start of haemodialysis
250 mg	6 - 12 hours after start
250 mg	36 - 48 hours after start
250 mg	At start of next haemodialysis if >30 hours after previous dose.

Further modification of the dosage schedule may be necessary in children.

4.3 Contraindications

Patients with known hypersensitivity to the cephalosporin antibiotics or to any component of the formulation.

4.4 Special warnings and special precautions for use

There is evidence of partial cross-allergenicity between the penicillins and the cephalosporins. Therefore cefradine should be used with caution in those patients with known hypersensitivity to penicillins. There have been instances of patients who have had reactions to both drug classes (including anaphylaxis).

Dosage should be reduced in renal failure (see Section 4.2)

After treatment with cefradine a false positive reaction for glucose in the urine may occur with Benedict's solution or Fehling's solution or with reagent tablets such as Clinitest*, but not with enzyme-based tests such as Clinistix* or Diastix*.

As with all antibiotics, prolonged use may result in overgrowth of non-susceptible organisms.

4.5 Interaction with other medicinal products and other forms of Interaction

Loop diuretics may increase nephrotoxicity of cephalosporins.

Probenecid has been seen to raise serum concentrations of cefradine, by reducing renal clearance of the cephalosporins.

4.6 Pregnancy and lactation

Although animal studies have not demonstrated any teratogenicity, safety in pregnancy has not been established. Cefradine is excreted in breast milk and should be used with caution in lactating mothers.

4.7 Effects on ability to drive and use machines

Since this medicine may cause dizziness, patients should be cautioned about operating hazardous machinery, including automobiles.

4.8 Undesirable effects

Limited essentially to gastro-intestinal disturbances and on occasion to hypersensitivity phenomena. The latter are more likely to occur in individuals who have previously demonstrated hypersensitivity and those with a history of allergy, asthma, hay fever or urticaria. The majority of reported side-effects have been mild and are rare, and include glossitis, heartburn, headache, dizziness, dyspnoea, paraesthesia, nausea, vomiting, diarrhoea, abdominal pain, candidal overgrowth, vaginitis. Skin and hypersensitivity reactions include urticaria, pruritus, skin rashes, fever, arthralgia and oedema.

As with other cephalosporins, there have been rare reports of erythema multiforme, Stevens Johnson Syndrome, anaphylaxis and toxic epidermal necrolysis. Also, mild transient eosinophilia, leucopenia and neutropenia, rarely positive direct Coombs tests and pseudomembranous colitis have been reported.

Elevations of BUN, serum creatinine and reversible interstitial nephritis have been reported. Transient hepatitis and cholestatic jaundice have been reported very rarely. Elevations of ALT, AST, total bilirubin and alkaline phosphatase have been observed.

Injection:

As with other parenterally administered antibiotics, transient pain may be experienced at the injection site, but is seldom the cause for discontinuing treatment. Thrombophlebitis has been reported following intravenous injection.

Since sterile abscesses have been reported following accidental subcutaneous injection, the preparation should be administered by deep intramuscular injection.

4.9 Overdose

None known

5. PHARMACOLOGICAL PROPERTIES

5.1 Pharmacodynamic properties

Actions:

Cefradine is a broad-spectrum bactericidal antibiotic active against both Gram-positive and Gram-negative bacteria. It is also highly active against most strains of penicillinase-producing Staphylococci.

Microbiology:

The following organisms have shown *in vitro* sensitivity to cefradine:

Gram-positive - *Staphylococci* (both penicillin sensitive and resistant strains), *Streptococci*, *Streptococcus pyogenes* (beta haemolytic) and *Streptococcus pneumoniae*.

Gram-negative - *E. coli*, *Klebsiella*, *spp*, *P. mirabilis*, *Haemophilus influenzae*, *Salmonella spp.* (including *Salmonella typhi*) and *Neisseria spp.*

Because cefradine is unaffected by penicillinase, many strains of *E. coli* and *Staphylococcus aureus* which produce this enzyme are susceptible to cefradine but resistant to ampicillin.

Cefradine has a high degree of stability to beta-lactamases. It has a low degree of protein binding and a large volume of distribution. Therefore, tissue levels are generally found to be high.

5.2 Pharmacokinetic properties

Following intramuscular administration of a single 0.5g dose of cefradine to normal volunteers, the average peak serum concentration was 8.41 microgram/ml with the time to peak concentration being 0.93 hours. The serum half-life averaged 1.25 hours. A single 1g intravenous dose resulted in serum concentrations of 86 micrograms/ml at 5 minutes and 12 micrograms/ml at 1 hour; these concentrations declined to 1 microgram/ml at 4 hours. Continuous infusion of 500mg per hour into a 70kg man maintained a concentration of about 21.4 microgram/ml cefradine activity; this study showed that a serum concentration of approximately 3 microgram/ml can be obtained for each milligram of cefradine administered per kg of body weight per hour of infusion.

Cefradine is excreted unchanged in the urine. The kidneys excrete 57% to 80% of an intramuscular dose in the first six hours; this results in a high urine concentration, e.g. 880 micrograms/ml of urine after a 500mg intramuscular dose. Probenecid slows tubular secretion and almost doubles peak serum concentration.

Assays of bone obtained at surgery have shown that cefradine penetrates bone tissue.

5.3 Preclinical safety data

No further information is available for this established product.

6. PHARMACEUTICAL PARTICULARS

6.1 List of excipients

L-Arginine sterile.

6.2 Incompatibilities

None known.

6.3 Shelf life

36 months.

6.4 Special precautions for storage

Storage before reconstitution: Do not store above 25°C.

Storage after reconstitution: Solutions for IM or IV Injection should be used immediately (see also section 6.6 below).

6.5 Nature and contents of container

500mg or 1g Type III Ph Eur clear glass vial with siliconed, butyl rubber stopper and aluminium seal.

500mg: packs of 5 vials

1g: single vial pack.

6.6 Instructions for use and handling

Reconstitution:

For intramuscular use: Aseptically add sterile water for injections or 0.9% sodium chloride injection according to following table:

Single dose* Vial Size	Volume of Diluent to be Added
500 mg	2.0 ml
1 g	4.0 ml

* The preparation contains no bactericide and is intended for single use only and not multiple dose.

Shake to effect solution and withdraw the entire contents

For intravenous use: Cefradine for injection may be administered by direct intravenous injection or by infusion. A 3 microgram/ml serum concentration can be maintained for each milligram of cefradine per kg body weight per hour of infusion.

For direct intravenous administration: Suitable reconstitution solutions for intravenous injection solutions are:

Sterile Water for Injections;

5% Dextrose Injection;

0.9% Sodium Chloride Injection.

Aseptically add 5ml of the reconstitution solution to the 500mg vial or 10ml of the reconstituted solution to the 1g vial. Shake to effect solution and withdraw the entire contents. The solution may be slowly injected directly into a vein over a 3 to 5 minute period.

For continuous or intermittent intravenous infusion:

Suitable reconstitution solutions for intravenous infusion solutions are:

Sterile Water for Injections (50mg/ml cefradine solutions are approximately isotonic);

5% or 10% Dextrose Injection;

0.9% Sodium Chloride Injection;

Sodium Lactate Injection (M/6 sodium lactate);

Dextrose and Sodium Chloride Injection;

Lactated Ringer's Injection; Ringer's Injection;

5% Dextrose in Lactated Ringer's Injection;

5% Dextrose in Ringer's Injection.

Aseptically add 5ml of the reconstitution solution to the 500mg vial or 10ml of the reconstituted solution to the 1g vial and shake to effect solution. Aseptically transfer the entire contents to the IV infusion diluent.

Reconstituted solutions may vary in colour from light to straw yellow; however, this does not affect the potency.

Protect solutions of cefradine from concentrated light or direct sunlight.

Stability

From a microbial point of view, all strengths of reconstituted product should be used immediately, unless reconstitution has taken place in controlled and validated aseptic conditions.

If the reconstituted product is not used immediately, in-use storage times and conditions prior to use are the responsibility of the user.

For solutions for intramuscular and direct intravenous injection, chemical and physical in-use stability has been demonstrated for 2 hours at room temperature (25°C) and 12 hours when stored in a refrigerator at 2°-8°C.

For solutions for intravenous infusion, using Water for Injection, Glucose 5% or Sodium Chloride 0.9%, for concentrations up to 10mg/ml (1%), chemical and physical in-use stability has been demonstrated for 12 hours at room temperature (25°C) and 1 week when stored in a refrigerator at 2°-8°C and, for concentrations up to 50mg/ml (5%), chemical and physical in-use stability has been demonstrated for 10 hours at room temperature (25°C) or 48 hours at 2°-8°C.

In the case of prolonged infusion, replace 5% infusions every 10 hours and 1% infusions every 12 hours with freshly-prepared solutions.

7. MARKETING AUTHORISATION HOLDER

E. R. Squibb & Sons Limited

Uxbridge Business Park
Sanderson Road
Uxbridge
Middlesex
UB8 1DH

8. MARKETING AUTHORISATION NUMBER(S)

Velosef Injection 500 mg:	PL 0034/0198
Velosef Injection 1 g:	PL 0034/0199

9. DATE OF FIRST AUTHORISATION/RENEWAL OF THE AUTHORISATION

Velosef Injection 500 mg:	22 July 1981 / 24 February 1999 / 23 February 2004
Velosef Injection 1 g:	22 July 1981 / 5 July 1999 / 5 July 2004

10. DATE OF REVISION OF THE TEXT

June 2005

Velosulin 100 IU/ml in a vial.

(Novo Nordisk Limited)

1. NAME OF THE MEDICINAL PRODUCT

Velosulin 100 IU/ml in a vial

Solution for injection or infusion.

2. QUALITATIVE AND QUANTITATIVE COMPOSITION

Insulin human, rDNA (produced by recombinant DNA technology in *Saccharomyces cerevisiae*).

Each vial contains 10 ml of solution equivalent to 1000 IU of insulin human (100 IU per ml).

One IU (International Unit) corresponds to 0.035 mg of anhydrous human insulin.

For excipients, see Section 6.1. List of excipients.

3. PHARMACEUTICAL FORM

Solution for injection or infusion in a vial.

Velosulin is a clear, colourless, aqueous solution.

4. CLINICAL PARTICULARS

4.1 Therapeutic indications

Treatment of diabetes mellitus.

4.2 Posology and method of administration

This phosphate-buffered soluble insulin is intended for continuous subcutaneous insulin infusion (CSII) in external insulin infusion pumps.

Velosulin is a fast-acting insulin and may be used in combination with certain longer-acting insulin products. For incompatibilities see section 6.2.

Dosage

Dosage is individual and determined by the physician in accordance with the needs of the patient.

Usually, 40-60% of the total daily dose is given as a continuous basal rate and the remaining 40-60% as boluses divided between the three main meals.

In general, when patients are transferred from injection to infusion therapy, it may be advisable to reduce the dosage by initiating the patient at 90% of the previous total daily dosage, with 40% as basal rate and 50% as boluses divided between the three main meals.

The individual insulin requirement is usually between 0.3 and 1.0 IU/kg/day. The daily insulin requirement may be higher in patients with insulin resistance (e.g. during puberty or due to obesity) and lower in patients with residual, endogenous insulin production.

In patients with diabetes mellitus optimised glycaemic control delays the onset and slows the progression of late diabetic complications. Close blood glucose monitoring is recommended.

Meal time insulin injections or infusions should be followed within 30 minutes by a meal or snack containing carbohydrates.

Dosage adjustment

Concomitant illness, especially infections and feverish conditions, usually increases the patient's insulin requirement.

Renal or hepatic impairment may reduce insulin requirement.

Adjustment of dosage may also be necessary if patients change physical activity or their usual diet.

Dosage adjustment may be necessary when transferring patients from one insulin preparation to another (see section 4.4 Special warnings and special precautions for use).

Administration

For subcutaneous and intravenous use.

Insulin infusion (CSII):

Continuous subcutaneous insulin infusion (CSII) in external insulin infusion pumps is usually administered in the abdominal wall. Velosulin should never be mixed with any other insulin products when used in a pump.

Patients started on CSII must receive comprehensive instruction in the use of the pump, and the necessary actions in case of illness, hypoglycaemia, hyperglycaemia or pump failure.

The patient should read and follow the instructions that accompany the infusion pump and use the correct reservoir and catheter for the pump (see section 6.6).

The infusion set should be changed every 48 hours using aseptic technique when inserting the infusion set.

When filling a new syringe, no large air bubbles should be left in either the syringe or the catheter.

The patient should follow the instructions from the doctor about the basal infusion rate and the mealtime insulin boluses to be taken.

To get the benefit of insulin infusion, and to detect possible malfunction of the pump, the patient should measure his blood glucose level regularly.

In the event of a hypoglycaemic episode, the infusion should be stopped until the episode is resolved. If repeated or severe low blood glucose levels occur, the patient should notify the health care professional and the need to reduce or stop the insulin administration should be considered. A pump malfunction or obstruction of the infusion set can result in a rapid rise in glucose levels. If the patient suspects an interruption to insulin flow the patient should notify the health care professional.

Patients administering Velosulin by CSII must have injection syringes and alternative insulin readily available in case of emergency or pump interruption or failure, in order that insulin can be administered by subcutaneous injection.

Insulin injection:

Administration of Velosulin is also possible by subcutaneous or intravenous injection.

Subcutaneous injection is usually done in the abdominal wall, although the thigh, the gluteal region or the deltoid region may also be used. Subcutaneous injection into the abdominal wall ensures a faster absorption than from other injection sites.

Injection into a lifted skin fold minimises the risk of unintended intramuscular injection.

Keep the needle under the skin for at least 6 seconds to make sure the entire dose is injected.

Injection sites should be rotated within an anatomic region in order to avoid lipodystrophy.

Velosulin may also be administered intravenously, which should only be carried out by health care professionals.

Velosulin is accompanied by a package leaflet with detailed instruction for use to be followed.

Velosulin vials may be used with insulin syringes with a corresponding unit scale. When two types of insulin are mixed, draw the amount of fast-acting insulin first, followed by the amount of long-acting insulin.

4.3 Contraindications

Hypoglycaemia

Hypersensitivity to human insulin or to any of the excipients (see section 6.1 List of excipients).

4.4 Special warnings and special precautions for use

Inadequate dosage or discontinuation of treatment, especially in type 1 diabetes, may lead to **hyperglycaemia**.

Usually the first symptoms of hyperglycaemia set in gradually, over a period of hours or days. They include thirst, increased frequency of urination, nausea, vomiting, drowsiness, flushed dry skin, dry mouth, loss of appetite as well as acetone odour of breath.

In type 1 diabetes, untreated hyperglycaemic events eventually lead to diabetic ketoacidosis which is potentially lethal.

Due to the lack of long-acting insulin, patients receiving continuous subcutaneous insulin infusion via an insulin pump are at risk of fast development of ketoacidosis in case of prolonged interruption of continuous subcutaneous insulin infusion.

Hypoglycaemia may occur if the insulin dose is too high in relation to the insulin requirement (see section 4.8 and 4.9).

Omission of a meal or unplanned, strenuous physical exercise may lead to hypoglycaemia.

Patients whose blood glucose control is greatly improved e.g. by intensified insulin therapy, may experience a change in their usual warning symptoms of hypoglycaemia and should be advised accordingly.

Usual warning symptoms may disappear in patients with long-standing diabetes.

Transferring a patient to another type or brand of insulin should be done under strict medical supervision. Changes in strength, brand (manufacturer), type (fast-, dual-, long-acting insulin etc.), origin (animal, human or analogue insulin) and/or method of manufacture (recombinant DNA versus animal source insulin) may result in a need for a change in dosage. If an adjustment is needed when switching the patients to Velosulin, it may occur with the first dose or during the first several weeks or months.

A few patients who have experienced hypoglycaemic reactions after transfer from animal source insulin have reported that early warning symptoms of hypoglycaemia were less pronounced or different from those experienced with their previous insulin.

Before travelling between different time zones, the patient should be advised to consult the doctor, since this may mean that the patient has to take insulin and meals at different times.

Patients using CSII may be more prone to infection at the site of infusion. Infections can be minimised by careful attention to personal hygiene of the hands and infusion site and by frequent changes of catheter (maximum usage 2 days).

Velosulin contains metacresol, which may cause allergic reactions.

4.5 Interaction with other medicinal products and other forms of Interaction

A number of medicinal products are known to interact with glucose metabolism. The physician must therefore take possible interactions into account and should always ask their patients about any medicinal products they take.

The following substances may reduce insulin requirement:

Oral hypoglycaemic agents (OHA), monoamine oxidase inhibitors (MAOI), non-selective beta-blocking agents, angiotensin converting enzyme (ACE) inhibitors, salicylates and alcohol.

The following substances may increase insulin requirement:

Thiazides, glucocorticoids, thyroid hormones and beta-sympathomimetics, growth hormone and danazol.

Beta-blocking agents may mask the symptoms of hypoglycaemia and delay recovery from hypoglycaemia.

Octreotide/lanreotide may both decrease and increase insulin requirement.

Alcohol may intensify and prolong the hypoglycaemic effect of insulin.

4.6 Pregnancy and lactation

There are no restrictions on treatment of diabetes with insulin during pregnancy, as insulin does not pass the placental barrier.

Both hypoglycaemia and hyperglycaemia, which can occur in inadequately controlled diabetes therapy, increase the risk of malformations and death *in utero*. Intensified control in the treatment of pregnant women with diabetes is therefore recommended throughout pregnancy and when contemplating pregnancy.

Insulin requirements usually fall in the first trimester and increase subsequently during the second and third trimesters.

After delivery, insulin requirements return rapidly to pre-pregnancy values.

Insulin treatment of the nursing mother presents no risk to the baby. However, the Velosulin dosage may need to be adjusted.

4.7 Effects on ability to drive and use machines

The patient's ability to concentrate and react may be impaired as a result of hypoglycaemia. This may constitute a risk in situations where these abilities are of special importance (e.g. driving a car or operating machinery).

Patients should be advised to take precautions to avoid hypoglycaemia whilst driving. This is particularly important in those who have reduced or absent awareness of the warning signs of hypoglycaemia or have frequent episodes of hypoglycaemia. The advisability of driving should be considered in these circumstances.

4.8 Undesirable effects

As for other insulin products, hypoglycaemia, in general is the most frequently occurring undesirable effect. It may occur if the insulin dose is too high in relation to the insulin requirement. In clinical trials and during marketed use the frequency varies with patient population and dose regimens. Therefore, no specific frequency can be presented. Severe hypoglycaemia may lead to unconsciousness and/or convulsions and may result in temporary or permanent impairment of brain function or even death.

Frequencies of adverse drug reactions from clinical trials, that are considered related to fast-acting human insulin (Actrapid) are listed below. The frequencies are defined as: Uncommon >1/1000, < 1/100). Isolated spontaneous cases are presented as very rare defined as < 1/10,000.

Immune system disorders

Uncommon – Urticaria, rash

Very rare – Anaphylactic reactions

Symptoms of generalized hypersensitivity may include generalized skin rash, itching, sweating, gastrointestinal upset, angioneurotic oedema, difficulties in breathing, palpitation, reduction in blood pressure and fainting/loss of consciousness. Generalised hypersensitivity reactions are potentially life threatening.

Nervous system disorders

Uncommon – Peripheral neuropathy

Fast improvement in blood glucose control may be associated with a condition termed "acute painful neuropathy", which is usually reversible.

Eye disorders

Uncommon – Refraction disorders

Refraction anomalies may occur upon initiation of insulin therapy. These symptoms are usually of transitory nature.

Very rare – Diabetic retinopathy

Long-term improved glycaemic control decreases the risk of progression of diabetic retinopathy. However, intensification of insulin therapy with abrupt improvement in glycaemic control may be associated with temporary worsening of diabetic retinopathy.

Skin and subcutaneous tissue disorders

Uncommon – Lipodystrophy

Lipodystrophy may occur at the injection site as a consequence of failure to rotate injection sites within an area.

General disorders and administration site conditions

Uncommon – Injection site reactions

Injection site reactions (redness, swelling, itching, pain and haematoma at the injection site) may occur during treatment with insulin. Most reactions are transitory and disappear during continued treatment.

Very rare – Oedema

Oedema may occur upon initiation of insulin therapy. These symptoms are usually of transitory nature.

4.9 Overdose

A specific overdose of insulin cannot be defined. However, hypoglycaemia may develop over sequential stages:

- Mild hypoglycaemic episodes can be treated by oral administration of glucose or sugary products. It is therefore recommended that the diabetic patient carry some sugar lumps, sweets, biscuits or sugary fruit juice.
- Severe hypoglycaemic episodes, where the patient has become unconscious, can be treated by glucagon (0.5 to 1 mg) given intramuscularly or subcutaneously by a person who has received appropriate instruction, or by glucose given intravenously by a medical professional. Glucose must also be given intravenously, if the patient does not respond to glucagon within 10 to 15 minutes.

Upon regaining consciousness, administration of oral carbohydrate is recommended for the patient in order to prevent relapse.

5. PHARMACOLOGICAL PROPERTIES

5.1 Pharmacodynamic properties

Pharmacotherapeutic group: insulins and analogues, fast-acting, insulin (human). ATC code: A10A B01.

The blood glucose lowering effect of insulin is due to the facilitated uptake of glucose following binding of insulin to receptors on muscle and fat cells and to the simultaneous inhibition of glucose output from the liver.

A clinical trial in a single intensive care unit treating hyperglycaemia (blood glucose above 10 mmol/L) in 204 diabetic and 1344 non-diabetic patients undergoing major surgery showed that normoglycaemia (blood glucose 4.4 – 6.1 mmol/L) induced by intravenous treatment with another fast-acting human insulin (Actrapid) reduced mortality by 42% (8% versus 4.6%).

Velosulin is a fast-acting insulin.

When Velosulin is administered as a bolus injection onset of action is within ½ hour, reaches a maximum effect within 1.5-3.5 hours and the entire time of duration is approximately 7-8 hours.

5.2 Pharmacokinetic properties

Insulin in the blood stream has a half-life of a few minutes. Consequently, the time-action profile of an insulin preparation is determined solely by its absorption characteristics.

This process is influenced by several factors (e.g. insulin dosage, injection route and site, thickness of subcutaneous fat, type of diabetes). The pharmacokinetics of insulins is therefore affected by significant intra- and inter-individual variation.

Continuous subcutaneous infusion eliminates some of the variations/fluctuations inherent to injection therapy.

The relatively fast absorption of soluble insulin ensures a constant supply of insulin to the blood from a relatively small pool under the skin.

Absorption

The maximum plasma concentration is reached within 1.5-2.5 hours after subcutaneous administration.

Distribution

No profound binding to plasma proteins, except circulating insulin antibodies (if present) has been observed.

Metabolism

Human insulin is reported to be degraded by insulin protease or insulin-degrading enzymes and possibly protein disulfide isomerase. A number of cleavage (hydrolysis) sites on the human insulin molecule have been proposed; none of the metabolites formed following the cleavage are active.

Elimination

The terminal half-life is determined by the rate of absorption from the subcutaneous tissue. The terminal half-life ($t_{½}$) is therefore a measure of the absorption rather than of the elimination *per se* of insulin from plasma (insulin in the blood stream has a $t_{½}$ of a few minutes). Trials have indicated a $t_{½}$ of about 2-5 hours.

The pharmacokinetic profile has been studied in a small number (n=18) of diabetic children (aged 6-12 years) and adolescents (aged 13-17 years) using another fast-acting human insulin (Actrapid). The data are limited but suggest that the pharmacokinetic profile in children and adolescents may be similar to that in adults. However, there were differences between age groups in C_{max}, stressing the importance of individual titration of human insulin.

5.3 Preclinical safety data

Preclinical data reveal no special hazard for humans based on conventional studies of safety pharmacology, repeated dose toxicity, genotoxicity, carcinogenic potential, toxicity to reproduction.

6. PHARMACEUTICAL PARTICULARS

6.1 List of excipients

Zinc chloride

Glycerol

Metacresol

Disodium phosphate dihydrate

Sodium hydroxide or/and hydrochloric acid (for pH adjustment)

Water for injections

6.2 Incompatibilities

Medicinal products added to the insulin solution may cause degradation of the insulin, e.g. if the medicinal products contain thiols or sulphites. Upon mixing Velosulin with infusion fluids an unpredictable amount of insulin will be adsorbed to the infusion material. Monitoring of the patient's blood glucose during infusion is therefore recommended.

When administered by CSII no other medicinal products or other insulins should be mixed in the reservoir of the infusion pump with Velosulin.

When combination with long-acting insulin is necessary it is only possible to mix Velosulin with isophane or premixed insulins. Velosulin should not be mixed with insulin zinc suspensions since the phosphate buffer may interact with the zinc in the suspension and alter the timing of action of the insulin in an unpredictable way.

Concerning compatibility with insulin infusion pumps, reservoirs, catheters and needles, see section 6.6 Instructions for use and handling.

6.3 Shelf life

30 months.

After first opening: 6 weeks.

After first use as infusion, the insulin solution may be stored in the pump reservoir for six days.

6.4 Special precautions for storage

Store in a refrigerator (2°C - 8°C).

Do not freeze.

Keep the vial in the outer carton in order to protect from light.

During use: do not refrigerate. Do not store above 25°C.

After first use as infusion: the insulin solution may be stored in the pump reservoir at up to 37°C (close to the body).

Protect from excessive heat and sunlight.

6.5 Nature and contents of container

Glass vial (type 1) closed with a bromobutyl/polyisoprene rubber stopper and a protective tamper-proof cap.

Pack size: 1 vial × 10 ml.

6.6 Instructions for use and handling

Insulin preparations, which have been frozen, must not be used.

Insulin solutions should not be used if they do not appear water clear and colourless.

Insulin infusion (CSII):

Use only syringes made of polyethylene, polypropylene or glass.

Use only catheters where the material in contact with the insulin is made of polyethylene or polypropylene.

Use only teflon-coated or stainless steel needles.

7. MARKETING AUTHORISATION HOLDER

Novo Nordisk A/S

Novo Allé

DK-2880 Bagsværd

Denmark

8. MARKETING AUTHORISATION NUMBER(S)

EU/1/02/232/001

9. DATE OF FIRST AUTHORISATION/RENEWAL OF THE AUTHORISATION

October 2002

10. DATE OF REVISION OF THE TEXT

2 August 2004

Legal Status

POM

Ventavis

(Schering Health Care Limited)

1. NAME OF THE MEDICINAL PRODUCT

▼Ventavis 10 microgram/ml nebuliser solution.

2. QUALITATIVE AND QUANTITATIVE COMPOSITION

1 ml solution contains 10 micrograms iloprost (as iloprost trometamol). Each 2-ml ampoule contains 20 micrograms iloprost (as iloprost trometamol).

For excipients, see 6.1.

3. PHARMACEUTICAL FORM

Nebuliser solution.

Clear, colourless solution.

4. CLINICAL PARTICULARS

4.1 Therapeutic indications

Treatment of patients with primary pulmonary hypertension, classified as NYHA functional class III, to improve exercise capacity and symptoms.

4.2 Posology and method of administration

Ventavis should only be initiated and monitored by a physician experienced in the treatment of pulmonary hypertension.

Ventavis is intended for inhalation use by nebulisation.

Adults

Dose per inhalation session:

The recommended dose is 2.5 micrograms or 5.0 micrograms of inhaled iloprost (as delivered at the mouthpiece of the nebuliser) according to the individual need and tolerability.

Two compressed air nebuliser systems, HaloLite and Prodose, have been shown to be suitable nebulisers for the administration of Ventavis. With both systems the mass median aerodynamic diameter of the aerosol droplet (MMAD) with iloprost was between 2.6 and 2.7 μm. For each inhalation session the content of one 2-ml ampoule of Ventavis will be transferred into the nebuliser medication chamber immediately before use. HaloLite and Prodose are dosimetric systems. They stop automatically after the pre-set dose has been delivered. The inhalation time depends on the patient's breathing pattern.

Device	Dose of iloprost at mouthpiece	Estimated Inhalation time (frequency of 15 breaths per minute)
HaloLite	2.5 μg 5 μg	4 to 5 min 8 to 10 min
Prodose	2.5 μg 5 μg	4 to 5 min 8 to 10 min

For a dose of 5 μg iloprost at mouthpiece it is recommended to complete two inhalation cycles with 2.5 μg pre-set dose program with a filling of one 2-ml ampoule.

In addition Venta-Neb, a portable ultrasonic battery-powered nebuliser, has been shown to be suitable for the administration of Ventavis. The measured MMAD of the aerosol droplets was 2.6 μm. For each inhalation session, the content of one 2-ml ampoule of Ventavis will be transferred into the nebuliser medication chamber immediately before use.

Two programs can be operated:

PI Program 1: 5,0 μg active substance on the mouth piece 25 inhalation cycles.

P2 Program 2: 2,5 μg active substance on the mouth piece 10 inhalation cycles.

The selection of the pre set program is made by the physician.

Venta-Neb prompts the patient to inhale by an optical and an acoustic signal. It stops after the pre-set dose has been administered. To obtain the optimal droplet size for the administration of Ventavis the green baffle plate should be used. For details refer to the instruction manual of the Venta-Neb nebuliser.

Device	Dose of iloprost at mouthpiece	Estimated Inhalation time
Venta-Neb	2.5 μg 5 μg	4 min 8 min

The efficacy and tolerability of inhaled iloprost when administered with other nebulising systems, which provide different nebulisation characteristics of iloprost solution, have not been established.

Daily dose:

The dose per inhalation session should be administered 6 to 9 times per day according to the individual need and tolerability.

Duration of treatment:

The duration of treatment depends on clinical status and is left to the physician's discretion. Should patients deteriorate on this treatment intravenous prostacyclin treatment should be considered.

Patients with hepatic impairment

Iloprost elimination is reduced in patients with hepatic dysfunction (see section 5.2).

To avoid undesired accumulation over the day, special caution has to be exercised with these patients during initial dose titration. Initially, doses of 2.5 μg should be administered with dosing intervals of at least 3 hours (corresponds to administration of max. 6 times per day). Thereafter, dosing intervals may be shortened cautiously based on individual tolerability. If a further increase in the dose up to 5.0 μg is indicated, again dosing intervals of at least 3 hours should be chosen initially and shortened according to individual tolerability. A further undesired accumulation of the medicinal product following treatment over several days is not likely due to the overnight break in administration of the medicinal product.

Patients with renal impairment

There is no need for dose adaptation in patients with a creatinine clearance > 30 ml/min (as determined from serum creatinine using the Cockroft and Gault formula). Patients with a creatinine clearance of ⩽ 30 ml/min were not investigated in the clinical trials.

Children and adolescents (below 18 years of age)

Currently no experience in children and adolescents is available.

4.3 Contraindications

Hypersensitivity to iloprost or to any of the excipients.

Conditions where the effects of Ventavis on platelets might increase the risk of haemorrhage (e.g. active peptic ulcers, trauma, intracranial haemorrhage).

Severe coronary heart disease or unstable angina; myocardial infarction within the last six months; decompensated cardiac failure if not under close medical supervision; severe arrhythmias; cerebrovascular events (e.g. transient ischaemic attack, stroke) within the last 3 months.

Pulmonary hypertension due to venous occlusive disease.

Congenital or acquired valvular defects with clinically relevant myocardial function disorders not related to pulmonary hypertension.

Pregnancy, lactation.

4.4 Special warnings and special precautions for use

The use of Ventavis is not recommended in patients with unstable pulmonary hypertension, with advanced right heart failure. In case of deterioration or worsening of right heart failure transfer to other medicinal products should be considered.

The pulmonary vasodilatory effect of inhaled iloprost is of short duration (one to two hours). Patients who experience syncope in association with pulmonary hypertension should avoid any exceptional straining, for example during physical exertion. Before physical exertion it might be useful to inhale. The occurrence of a nocturnal or exertional syncope reflects therapeutic gaps and/or insufficient efficiency, and the need to adapt and/or change the therapy should be considered (see section 4.8).

The benefit of Ventavis has not been established in patients with chronic pulmonary bronchitis and severe asthma. Patients with acute pulmonary infections should be carefully monitored.

In patients with low systemic blood pressure, care should be taken to avoid further hypotension. Ventavis should not be initiated in patients with systolic arterial hypotension less than 85 mmHg.

Should signs of pulmonary oedema occur when inhaled iloprost is administered in patients with pulmonary hypertension, the possibility of associated pulmonary veno-occlusive disease should be considered. The treatment should be stopped.

In case of interruption of Ventavis therapy, the risk of rebound effect is not formally excluded. Careful monitoring of the patient should be performed, when inhaled iloprost therapy is stopped and an alternative treatment should be considered in critically ill patients.

Iloprost elimination is reduced in patients with hepatic dysfunction and in patients with renal failure requiring dialysis (see section 5.2). A cautious initial dose titration using dosing intervals of at least 3 hours is recommended (see section 4.2).

Prolonged oral treatment with iloprost clathrate in dogs up to one year was associated with slightly increased fasted serum glucose levels. It cannot be excluded that this is also relevant to man on prolonged Ventavis therapy.

To minimise accidental exposure, it is recommended to use Ventavis with nebulisers with inhalation-triggered systems (HaloLite/Prodose), and to keep the room well ventilated.

Ventavis nebuliser solution should not come into contact with skin and eyes; oral ingestion of Ventavis solution should be avoided. During nebulisation sessions a facial mask must be avoided and only a mouthpiece should be used.

4.5 Interaction with other medicinal products and other forms of Interaction

Iloprost may increase the effect of vasodilatators and antihypertensive agents.

Iloprost can inhibit platelet function and its use with anticoagulants (such as heparin, coumarin-type anticoagulants) or other inhibitors of platelet aggregation (such as acetylsalicylic acid, non-steroidal anti-inflammatory drugs, ticlopidine, clopidogrel and glycoprotein IIb/IIIa antagonists: abciximab, eptifibatide and tirofiban) may increase the risk of bleeding. A careful monitoring of the patients taking anticoagulants according to common medical practice is recommended. The concomitant use of other platelet inhibitors should be avoided in patients taking anticoagulants.

Intravenous infusion of iloprost has no effect either on the pharmacokinetics of multiple oral doses of digoxin or on the pharmacokinetics of co-administered tissue plasminogen activator (t-PA) in patients.

Although, clinical studies have not been conducted, *in vitro* studies investigating the inhibitory potential of iloprost on the activity of cytochrome P450 enzymes revealed that no relevant inhibition of drug metabolism via these enzymes by iloprost have to be expected.

4.6 Pregnancy and lactation

• Pregnancy

There are no adequate data from the use of Ventavis in pregnant women. Animal studies have shown reproductive toxicity (see section 5.3). The potential risk for humans is unknown. Ventavis is contra-indicated during pregnancy. Women of child-bearing potential should use effective contraceptive measures during treatment.

• Lactation

It is not known whether Ventavis enters the breast milk. The medicinal product must not be administered to breast feeding mothers (see section 4.3).

4.7 Effects on ability to drive and use machines

Care should be exercised during initiation of therapy until any effects on the individual have been determined. In patients experiencing hypotensive symptoms such as dizziness, the ability to drive or operate machines may be affected.

4.8 Undesirable effects

In addition to local effects resulting from administration of iloprost by inhalation such as increased cough, adverse reactions with iloprost are related to the pharmacological properties of prostacyclins.

The frequencies of the adverse reactions reported below (very common >10%, common >1 - 10%) are based on clinical trial data.

Cardiovascular disorders

Very common: vasodilatation, hypotension

Common: syncope

Syncope is a common symptom of the disease itself, but can also occur under therapy. The increased occurrence of syncopes can be related to the deterioration of the disease or insufficient effectiveness of the product (see section 4.4).

Respiratory, thoracic and mediastinal disorders

Very common: increased cough

Nervous system disorders

Common: headache

Musculoskeletal disorders

Common: trismus

Bleeding events (mostly haematoma) were common as expected in this patient population with a high proportion of patients taking anticoagulant co-medication. The frequency of bleeding events did not differ between iloprost and placebo-treated patients.

4.9 Overdose

• Symptoms

No case of overdose has been reported. Hypotensive/vasovagal reaction might be anticipated as well as headache, flushing, nausea, vomiting, and diarrhoea.

• Therapy

A specific antidote is not known. Interruption of the inhalation session, monitoring and symptomatic measures are recommended.

5. PHARMACOLOGICAL PROPERTIES

5.1 Pharmacodynamic properties

Pharmacotherapeutic group: Platelet aggregation inhibitors excluding heparin, ATC code: B01A C

Iloprost, the active substance of Ventavis, is a synthetic prostacyclin analogue. The following pharmacological effects have been observed *in vitro*:

• Inhibition of platelet aggregation, platelet adhesion and release reaction

• Dilatation of arterioles and venules

• Increase of capillary density and reduction of increased vascular permeability caused by mediators such as serotonin or histamine in the microcirculation

• Stimulation of endogenous fibrinolytic potential

The pharmacological effects after inhalation of Ventavis are:

Direct vasodilatation of the pulmonary arterial bed occur with consecutive significant improvement of pulmonary artery pressure, pulmonary vascular resistance and cardiac output as well as mixed venous oxygen saturation.

No clinical trial data are available comparing directly in intra-patient observations the acute haemodynamic response after intravenous to that after inhaled iloprost. The haemodynamics observed suggest an acute response with preferential effect of inhaled treatment on the pulmonary vessels. The pulmonary vasodilatory effect of each single inhalation levels off within one to two hours.

However, the predictive value of these acute haemodynamic data are considered to be of limited value as acute response does not in all cases correlate with long-term benefit of treatment with inhaled iloprost.

Efficacy in adult patients with pulmonary hypertension

A randomised, double-blind, multi-centre, placebo-controlled phase III trial (study RRA02997) has been conducted in 203 adult patients (inhaled iloprost: N=101; placebo n=102) with stable pulmonary hypertension. Inhaled iloprost (or placebo) was added to patients' current therapy, which could include a combination of anticoagulants, vasodilators (e.g. calcium channel blockers), diuretics, oxygen, and digitalis, but not PGI2 (prostacyclin or its analogues). 108 of the patients included were diagnosed with primary pulmonary hypertension, 95 were diagnosed with secondary pulmonary hypertension of which 56 were associated with chronic thromboembolic disease, 34 with connective tissue disease (including CREST and scleroderma) and 4 were considered appetite suppressant drug related. The baseline 6-minute walk test values reflected a moderate exercise limitation: in the iloprost group the mean was 332 meters (median value: 340 meters) and in the placebo group the mean was 315 meters (median value: 321 meters). In the iloprost group, the median daily inhaled dose was 30 μg (range 12.5 to 45 μg/day). The primary efficacy endpoint defined for this study, was a combined response criterion consisting of improvement in exercise capacity (6 minute walk test) at 12 weeks by at least 10% versus baseline, and improvement by at least one NYHA class at 12 weeks versus baseline, and no deterioration of pulmonary hypertension or death at any time before 12 weeks. The rate of responders to iloprost was 16.8% (17/101) and the rate of responders in the placebo group was 4.9% (5/102) (p=0.007).

In the iloprost group, the mean change from baseline after 12 weeks of treatment in the 6 minute walking distance was an increase of 22 meters (-3.3 meters in the placebo group, no data imputation for death or missing values).

In the iloprost group the NYHA class was improved in 26% of patients (placebo: 15%) (p = 0.032), unchanged in 67.7% of patients (placebo: 76%) and deteriorated in 6.3% of patients (placebo: 9%). Invasive haemodynamic parameters were assessed at baseline and after 12 weeks treatment.

A subgroup analysis showed that no treatment effect was observed as compared to placebo on the

6-minute walk test in the subgroup of patients with secondary pulmonary hypertension.

A mean increase in the 6-minute walk test of 44.7 meters from a baseline mean value of 329 meters vs. a change of -7.4 meters from a baseline mean value of 324 meters in the placebo group (no data imputation for death or missing values) was observed in the subgroup of 49 patients with primary pulmonary hypertension receiving treatment of inhaled iloprost for 12 weeks (46 patients in the placebo group).

No study has been performed with Ventavis in children with pulmonary hypertension.

5.2 Pharmacokinetic properties

• Absorption

When iloprost is administered via inhalation in patients with pulmonary hypertension (iloprost dose at the mouthpiece: 5 micrograms), peak serum levels of 100 to 200 picograms/ml were observed at the end of inhalation session. These levels decline with half-lives between approximately 5 and 25 minutes. Within 30 minutes to 1 hour after the end of inhalation, iloprost is not detectable in the central compartment (limit of quantification 25 picograms/ml).

• Distribution

No studies performed following inhalation.

Following intravenous infusion, the apparent steady-state volume of distribution was 0.6 to 0.8 l/kg in healthy subjects. Total plasma protein binding of iloprost is concentration-independent in the range of 30 to 3000 picograms/ml and amounts to approximately 60 %, of which 75 % is due to albumin binding.

• Metabolism

No studies performed following inhalation.

Iloprost is extensively metabolised principally via β-oxidation of the carboxyl side chain. No unchanged substance is eliminated. The main metabolite is tetranor-iloprost, which is found in the urine in free and conjugated form in 4 diastereoisomers. Tetranor-iloprost is pharmacologically inactive as shown in animal experiments. Results of *in vitro* studies reveal that CYP 450-dependent metabolism plays only a minor role in the biotransformation of iloprost. Further in vitro studies suggest that metabolism of iloprost in the lungs is similar after intravenous administration or inhalation.

• Elimination

No studies performed following inhalation.

In subjects with normal renal and hepatic function, the disposition of iloprost following intravenous infusion is characterised in most cases by a two-phase profile with mean half-lives of 3 to 5 minutes and 15 to 30 minutes.

A mass-balance study was done using ^{3}H-iloprost in healthy subjects. Following intravenous infusion, the recovery of total radioactivity is 81 %, and the respective recoveries in urine and faeces are 68 % and 12 %. The metabolites are eliminated from plasma and urine in 2 phases, for which half-lives of about 2 and 5 hours (plasma) and 2 and 18 hours (urine) have been calculated.

• Characteristics in patients

Renal dysfunction:

In a study with intravenous infusion of iloprost, patients with end-stage renal failure undergoing intermittent dialysis treatment are shown to have a significantly lower clearance (mean CL = 5 ± 2 ml/minute/kg) than that observed in patients with renal failure not undergoing intermittent dialysis treatment (mean CL = 18 ± 2 ml/minute/kg).

Hepatic dysfunction:

Because iloprost is extensively metabolised by the liver, the plasma levels of the active substance are influenced by changes in hepatic function. In an intravenous study, results were obtained involving 8 patients suffering from liver cirrhosis. The mean clearance of iloprost is estimated to be 10 ml/minute/kg.

Age and gender:

Age and gender are not of clinical relevance to the pharmacokinetics of iloprost.

5.3 Preclinical safety data

• Systemic toxicity

In acute toxicity studies, single intravenous and oral doses of iloprost caused severe symptoms of intoxication or death (IV) at doses about two orders of magnitude above the intravenous therapeutic dose. Considering the high pharmacological potency of iloprost and the absolute doses required for therapeutic purposes the results obtained in acute toxicity studies do not indicate a risk of acute adverse effects in humans. As expected for a prostacyclin, iloprost produced haemodynamic effects (vasodilatation, reddening of skin, hypotension, inhibition of platelet function, respiratory distress) and general signs of intoxication such as apathy, gait disturbances, and postural changes.

Continuous IV/SC infusion of iloprost up to 26 weeks in rodents and non-rodents did not cause any organ toxicity at dose levels which exceeded the human therapeutic systemic exposure between 14 and 47 times (based on plasma levels). Only expected pharmacological effects like hypotension, reddening of skin, dyspnoea, increased intestinal motility were observed.

Based on Cmax values in rats the systemic exposure in these parenteral studies was approximately 3.5 times higher than the maximum achievable exposure after inhalation. This highest achievable dose of 48.7 micrograms/kg/day was also the "no observed adverse effect level" (NOAEL) as evaluated in inhalation toxicity studies in rats up to 26 weeks. Following inhalation the systemic exposure based on AUC values in rats exceeded the corresponding therapeutic exposure in human patients by approximately 13 times.

• Genotoxic potential, tumorigenicity

Iloprost is not a gene mutagen in bacterial and mammalian cells *in vitro* and is not clastogenic in human lymphocytes up to cytotoxic concentrations and in the micronucleus test *in vivo*.

No tumorigenic potential of iloprost could be demonstrated in tumorigenicity studies in rats and mice.

• Reproduction toxicology

In embryo- and foetotoxicity studies in rats continuous intravenous administration of iloprost led to anomalies of single phalanges of the forepaws in a few foetuses/pups without dose dependence.

These alterations are not considered as true teratogenic effects, but are most likely related to iloprost induced growth retardation in late organogenesis due to haemodynamic alterations in the foetoplacental unit. In comparable embryotoxicity studies in rabbits and monkeys no such digit anomalies or other gross-structural abnormalities were observed in the foetuses/pups up to the highest tested dose.

In rats, passage of extremely low levels of iloprost into the milk was observed.

• Local tolerance, contact sensitising and antigenicity potential

In inhalation studies in rats, the administration of an iloprost formulation with a concentration of 20 micrograms/ml up to 26 weeks did not cause any local irritation of the upper and lower respiratory tract.

A dermal sensitisation (maximisation test) and an antigenicity study in guinea pigs showed no sensitising potential.

6. PHARMACEUTICAL PARTICULARS

6.1 List of excipients

trometamol

ethanol 96 %

sodium chloride

hydrochloric acid for pH adjustment

water for injections

6.2 Incompatibilities

In the absence of compatibility studies, this medicinal product must not be mixed with other medicinal products.

6.3 Shelf life

2 years

6.4 Special precautions for storage

No special precautions for storage.

6.5 Nature and contents of container

Ampoules of 3 ml, colourless, glass type I, containing 2 ml nebuliser solution.

Packages containing 30, 100 and 300 ampoules.

6.6 Instructions for use and handling

For each inhalation session the contents of one opened ampoule of Ventavis has to be transferred into the nebuliser medication chamber immediately before use. After each inhalation session, any solution remaining in the nebuliser should be discarded.

7. MARKETING AUTHORISATION HOLDER

Schering AG, D-13342 Berlin, Germany

8. MARKETING AUTHORISATION NUMBER(S)

EU/1/03/255/001

EU/1/03/255/002

EU/1/03/255/003

9. DATE OF FIRST AUTHORISATION/RENEWAL OF THE AUTHORISATION

16 September 2003

10. DATE OF REVISION OF THE TEXT

5 September 2005

LEGAL CATEGORY

POM

Ventodisks

(Allen & Hanburys)

1. NAME OF THE MEDICINAL PRODUCT

Ventodisks 200mcg

Ventodisks 400mcg

2. QUALITATIVE AND QUANTITATIVE COMPOSITION

200mcg or 400mcg Salbutamol (as Sulphate) per blister.

3. PHARMACEUTICAL FORM

Unit dose of powder in multidose presentation pack for inhalation use.

4. CLINICAL PARTICULARS

4.1 Therapeutic indications

Salbutamol is a selective β_2 adrenoceptor agonist. At therapeutic doses it acts on the β_2 adrenoceptors of bronchial muscle. With its fast onset of action, it is particularly suitable for the relief of acute asthma symptoms and the prevention of exercise induced asthma.

Salbutamol provides short-acting (4-6 hour) bronchodilation with fast onset (within 5 minutes) in reversible airways obstruction.

Ventodisks should be used to relieve symptoms when they occur and to prevent them in those circumstances recognised by the patient to precipitate an asthma attack (e.g. before exercise or unavoidable allergen exposure).

Ventodisks are particularly valuable as relief medication in mild, moderate or severe asthma, provided that reliance on it does not delay the introduction and use of regular inhaled corticosteroid therapy.

4.2 Posology and method of administration

Route of Administration

Ventodisks are for administration by the inhaled route only using a ventolin diskhaler.

Adults

For the relief of acute asthma symptoms 200 micrograms or 400 micrograms may be taken administered as a single dose.

The maximum dose is 400 micrograms four times daily.

To prevent allergen- or exercise-induced symptoms, 400 micrograms should be taken 10-15 minutes before exertion.

Children

The recommended dose for relief of acute bronchospasm or before allergen exposure or exercise is 200 micrograms. The maximum daily dose is 200 micrograms four times a day.

Elderly patients

The normal adult dose is applicable.

On-demand use of Ventodisks should not exceed four times daily. Reliance on such frequent supplementary use, or a sudden increase in dose, indicates deteriorating or poorly controlled asthma (see precautions).

4.3 Contraindications

Although intravenous salbutamol, and occasionally salbutamol tablets, are used in the management of premature labour, uncomplicated by conditions such as placenta praevia, ante-partum haemorrhage, or toxaemia of pregnancy, salbutamol preparations are not appropriate for managing premature labour. Salbutamol preparations should not be used for threatened abortion.

Ventodisks are contra-indicated in patients with a history of hypersensitivity to any of the components. (See Pharmaceutical Particulars – List of Excipients)

4.4 Special warnings and special precautions for use

Bronchodilators should not be the only or main treatment in patients with severe or unstable asthma. Severe asthma requires regular medical assessment, including lung-function testing, as patients are at risk of severe attacks and even death. Physicians should consider using oral corticosteroid therapy and/or the maximum recommended dose of inhaled corticosteroid in these patients.

Increasing use of bronchodilators in particular β_2-agonists to relieve symptoms indicates deterioration of asthma control. If patients find that short acting relief bronchodilator treatment with ventodisks becomes less effective or they need more inhalations than usual, medical attention must be sought.

In this situation patient should be reassessed and consideration given to the need for increased anti-inflammatory therapy (e.g. higher doses of inhaled corticosteroids or a course of oral corticosteroids). Severe exacerbations of asthma must be treated in the normal way.

In the event of a previously effective dose of inhaled salbutamol failing to give relief lasting at least three hours, the patient should be advised to seek medical advice in order that any necessary additional treatment may be instituted.

As there may be adverse effects associated with excessive dosing, the dosage or frequency of administration should only be increased on medical advice.

Salbutamol should be administered cautiously to patients suffering from thyrotoxicosis.

Salbutamol oral preparations and non-selective β-blocking drugs such as propranolol, should not usually be prescribed together.

Potentially serious hypokalaemia may result from β_2 agonist therapy, mainly from parenteral and nebulised administration. Particular caution is advised in acute severe asthma as this effect may be potentiated by hypoxia and by concomitant treatment with xanthine derivatives, steroids and diuretics. Serum potassium levels should be monitored in such situations.

4.5 Interaction with other medicinal products and other forms of Interaction

None known.

4.6 Pregnancy and lactation

Administration of drugs during pregnancy should only be considered if the expected benefit to the mother is greater than any possible risk to the fetus.

As with the majority of drugs, there is little published evidence of the safety of salbutamol in the early stages of human pregnancy, but in animal studies there was evidence of some harmful effects on the fetus at very high dose levels.

As salbutamol is probably secreted in breast milk, its use in nursing mothers requires careful consideration. It is not known whether salbutamol has a harmful effect on the neonate, and so its use should be restricted to situations where it is felt that the expected benefit to the mother is likely to outweigh any potential risk to the neonate.

4.7 Effects on ability to drive and use machines

None known

4.8 Undesirable effects

Ventodisks may cause a fine tremor of skeletal muscle, usually the hands are most obviously affected. This effect is dose-related and is common to all β-adrenergic stimulants.

Occasionally headaches have been reported.

Tachycardia, with or without peripheral vasodilatation, may rarely occur. In common with other β_2 agonists, cardiac arrhythmias (including atrial fibrillation, supraventricular tachycardia and extrasystoles) have been reported in association with the use of salbutamol, usually in susceptible patients.

There have been very rare reports of muscle cramps.

Hypersensitivity reactions including angioedema, urticaria, bronchospasm, hypotension and collapse have been reported very rarely.

Potentially serious hypokalaemia may result from β_2 agonist therapy.

As with other inhalation therapy, paradoxical bronchospasm may occur with an immediate increase in wheezing after dosing. This should be treated immediately with an alternative presentation or a different fast-acting inhaled bronchodilator. The preparation should be discontinued immediately, the patient assessed and, if necessary, alternative therapy instituted.

As with other β_2 agonists hyperactivity in children has been reported rarely.

Mouth and throat irritation may occur with inhaled salbutamol.

4.9 Overdose

The preferred antidote for overdosage with salbutamol is a cardioselective β-blocking agent, but β-blocking drugs should be used with caution in patients with a history of bronchospasm.

Hypokalaemia may occur following overdose with salbutamol. Serum potassium levels should be monitored.

5. PHARMACOLOGICAL PROPERTIES

5.1 Pharmacodynamic properties

Salbutamol is a selective β_2 adrenoceptor agonist. At therapeutic doses it acts on the β_2 adrenoceptors of bronchial muscle, with little or no action on the β_1 adrenoceptors of cardiac muscle.

5.2 Pharmacokinetic properties

Salbutamol administered intravenously has a half-life of 4 to 6 hours and is cleared partly renally and partly by metabolism to the inactive 4'-O-Sulphate (Phenolic Sulphate) which is also excreted primarily in the urine. The faeces are a minor route of excretion. The majority of a dose of Salbutamol given intravenously, orally or by inhalation is excreted within 72 hours. Salbutamol is bound to plasma proteins to the extent of 10%.

After administration by the inhaled route between 10 and 20% of the dose reaches the lower airways. The remainder is retained in the delivery system or is deposited in the oropharynx from where it is swallowed. The fraction deposited in the airways is absorbed into the pulmonary tissues and circulated but is not metabolised by the lung. On reaching the systemic circulation it becomes accessible to hepatic metabolism and is excreted, primarily in the urine, as unchanged drug and as phenolic sulphate.

The swallowed portion of an inhaled dose is absorbed from the gastrointestinal tract and undergoes considerable first-pass metabolism to the phenolic sulphate. Both unchanged drug and conjugate are excreted primarily in the urine.

5.3 Preclinical safety data

None stated.

6. PHARMACEUTICAL PARTICULARS

6.1 List of excipients

Lactose BP (which contains milk protein)

6.2 Incompatibilities

None reported.

6.3 Shelf life

36 months

6.4 Special precautions for storage

Store below 30°C

6.5 Nature and contents of container

Circular double aluminium foil blister pack. 8 unit doses per Ventodisk. Ventodisks are supplied as follows:

1) Carton containing 14 disks plus a diskhaler

2) Carton containing 5 disks plus a diskhaler (Hospital pack)

3) Refill pack of 14 disks

4) A starter/sample pack consisting of a diskhaler preloaded with one disk

Carton containing 15 disks plus a diskhaler

Refill pack of 15 disks

Note: Not all packs sizes may be marketed.

6.6 Instructions for use and handling

None.

7. MARKETING AUTHORISATION HOLDER

Glaxo Wellcome UK Ltd, trading as Allen & Hanburys,

Stockley Park West,

Middlesex, UB11 1BT

8. MARKETING AUTHORISATION NUMBER(S)

Ventodisks 200mcg PL 10949/0079

Ventodisks 400mcg PL10949/0080

9. DATE OF FIRST AUTHORISATION/RENEWAL OF THE AUTHORISATION

3 December 1998

10. DATE OF REVISION OF THE TEXT

15th June 2003

11. Legal Status

POM

Ventolin Accuhaler

(Allen & Hanburys)

1. NAME OF THE MEDICINAL PRODUCT

Ventolin™ Accuhaler™

2. QUALITATIVE AND QUANTITATIVE COMPOSITION

Ventolin Accuhaler is a plastic inhaler device containing a foil strip with 60 regularly spaced blisters each containing a mixture of 200 micrograms of microfine salbutamol (as sulphate) and larger particle lactose.

3. PHARMACEUTICAL FORM

Multi-dose dry powder inhalation device.

4. CLINICAL PARTICULARS

4.1 Therapeutic indications

Ventolin Accuhaler can be used in the management of asthma, bronchospasm and/or reversible airways obstruction.

Ventolin Accuhaler is particularly suitable for the relief of asthma symptoms. It should be used to relieve symptoms when they occur, and to prevent them in those circumstances recognised by the patient to precipitate an asthma attack (e.g. before exercise or unavoidable allergen exposure).

Ventolin Accuhaler is particularly valuable as relief medication in mild, moderate or severe asthma, provided that reliance on it does not delay the introduction and use of regular inhaled corticosteroid therapy.

4.2 Posology and method of administration

Ventolin Accuhaler is for inhalation use only. Ventolin Accuhaler is suitable for many patients including those who cannot use a metered-dose inhaler successfully.

Adults (including the elderly): For the relief of acute bronchospasm, 200 micrograms as a single dose. The maximum daily dose is 200 micrograms four times a day.

To prevent allergen- or exercise-induced symptoms, 200 micrograms should be taken 10-15 minutes before challenge.

Children: The recommended dose for relief of acute bronchospasm or before allergen exposure or exercise is 200 micrograms. The maximum daily dose is 200 micrograms four times a day.

On-demand use of Ventolin Accuhaler should not exceed four times daily. Reliance on such frequent supplementary use, or a sudden increase in dose, indicates poorly controlled or deteriorating asthma (see *Precautions*).

4.3 Contraindications

Although intravenous salbutamol, and occasionally salbutamol tablets, are used in the management of premature labour uncomplicated by conditions such as placenta praevia, ante-partum haemorrhage, or toxaemia of pregnancy, inhaled salbutamol preparations are not appropriate for managing premature labour. Salbutamol preparations should not be used for threatened abortion.

Ventolin Accuhaler is contra-indicated in patients with a history of hypersensitivity to any of the components. (See Pharmaceutical Particulars – List of Excipients).

4.4 Special warnings and special precautions for use

Bronchodilators should not be the only or main treatment in patients with severe or unstable asthma. Severe asthma requires regular medical assessment, including lung-function testing, as patients are at risk of severe attacks and even death. Physicians should consider using the maximum recommended dose of inhaled corticosteroid and/or oral corticosteroid therapy in these patients.

The dosage or frequency of administration should only be increased on medical advice.

Increasing use of bronchodilators, in particular short-acting inhaled β_2-agonists to relieve symptoms, indicates deterioration of asthma control. The patient should be instructed to seek medical advice if short-acting relief bronchodilator treatment becomes less effective, or more inhalations than usual are required. In this situation the patient should be assessed and consideration given to the need for increased anti-inflammatory therapy (e.g. higher doses of inhaled corticosteroid or a course of oral corticosteroid).

Severe exacerbations of asthma must be treated in the normal way.

Salbutamol should be administered cautiously to patients suffering from thyrotoxicosis.

Potentially serious hypokalaemia may result from β_2-agonist therapy, mainly from parenteral and nebulised administration. Particular caution is advised in acute severe asthma as this effect may be potentiated by hypoxia and by concomitant treatment with xanthine derivatives, steroids and diuretics. Serum potassium levels should be monitored in such situations.

4.5 Interaction with other medicinal products and other forms of Interaction

Salbutamol and non-selective β-blocking drugs such as propranolol, should not usually be prescribed together.

4.6 Pregnancy and lactation

Pregnancy: Administration of drugs during pregnancy should only be considered if the expected benefit to the mother is greater than any possible risk to the fetus. As with the majority of drugs, there is little published evidence of the safety of salbutamol in the early stages of human pregnancy, but in animal studies there was evidence of some harmful effects on the fetus at very high dose levels.

Lactation: As salbutamol is probably secreted in breast milk, its use in nursing mothers requires careful consideration. It is not known whether salbutamol has a harmful effect on the neonate, and so its use should be restricted to situations where it is felt that the expected benefit to the mother is likely to outweigh any potential risk to the neonate.

4.7 Effects on ability to drive and use machines

None reported.

4.8 Undesirable effects

As with other inhalation therapy, paradoxical bronchospasm may occur with an immediate increase in wheezing after dosing. This should be treated immediately with an alternative presentation or a different fast-acting inhaled bronchodilator. The preparation should be discontinued immediately, the patient assessed, and, if necessary, alternative therapy instituted.

Hypersensitivity reactions including angioedema, urticaria, bronchospasm, hypotension and collapse have been reported very rarely.

Potentially serious hypokalaemia may result from β_2-agonist therapy.

Ventolin Accuhaler may cause a fine tremor of skeletal muscle, usually the hands are most obviously affected. This effect is dose-related and is common to all -adrenergic stimulants.

Tachycardia, with or without peripheral vasodilatation, may rarely occur. In common with other β_2 agonists, cardiac arrhythmias (including atrial fibrillation, supraventricular tachycardia and extrasystoles) have been reported in association with the use of salbutamol, usually in susceptible patients.

Headaches have occasionally been reported.

Mouth and throat irritation may occur with inhaled salbutamol.

As with other β_2-agonists hyperactivity in children has been reported rarely.

There have been very rare reports of muscle cramps.

4.9 Overdose

The preferred antidote for overdosage with salbutamol is a cardioselective β-blocking agent, but β-blocking drugs should be used with caution in patients with a history of bronchospasm.

Hypokalaemia may occur following overdose with salbutamol. Serum potassium levels should be monitored.

5. PHARMACOLOGICAL PROPERTIES

5.1 Pharmacodynamic properties

Salbutamol is a selective β_2-adrenoceptor agonist. At therapeutic doses it acts on the β_2-adrenoceptors of bronchial muscle, with little or no action on the β_1-adrenoceptors of cardiac muscle.

Salbutamol provides short-acting (4-6 hour) bronchodilatation with a fast onset (within 5 minutes) in reversible airways obstruction.

5.2 Pharmacokinetic properties

Salbutamol administered intravenously has a half-life of 4 to 6 hours and is cleared partly renally, and partly by metabolism to the inactive 4'-O-sulphate (phenolic sulphate) which is also excreted primarily in the urine. The faeces are a minor route of excretion. After administration by the inhaled route between 10 and 20% of the dose reaches the lower airways. The remainder is retained in the delivery system or is deposited in the oropharynx from where it is swallowed. The fraction deposited in the airways is absorbed into the pulmonary tissues and circulation, but is not metabolised by the lung. On reaching the systemic circulation it becomes accessible to hepatic metabolism and is excreted, primarily in the urine, as unchanged drug and as the phenolic sulphate. The swallowed portion of an inhaled dose is absorbed from the gastrointestinal tract and undergoes considerable first-pass metabolism to the phenolic sulphate. Both unchanged drug and conjugate are excreted primarily in the urine. Almost all of a dose of salbutamol given intravenously, orally or by inhalation is excreted within 72 hours. Salbutamol is bound to plasma proteins to the extent of 10%.

5.3 Preclinical safety data

In common with other potent selective β_2-receptor agonists, salbutamol has been shown to be teratogenic in mice when given subcutaneously. In a reproductive study, 9.3% of fetuses were found to have cleft palate at 2.5mg/kg, 4 times the maximum human oral dose. In rats, treatment at the levels of 0.5, 2.32, 10.75 and 50mg/kg/day orally throughout pregnancy resulted in no significant fetal abnormalities. The only toxic effect was an increase in neonatal mortality at the highest dose level as the result of lack of maternal care. A reproductive study in rabbits revealed cranial malformations in 37% of fetuses at 50mg/kg/day, 78 times the maximum human oral dose.

6. PHARMACEUTICAL PARTICULARS

6.1 List of excipients

Lactose (which contains milk protein)

6.2 Incompatibilities

None reported.

6.3 Shelf life

24 months.

6.4 Special precautions for storage

Do not store above 30°C. Keep in the original container

6.5 Nature and contents of container

The powder mix of salbutamol (as sulphate) and lactose is filled into a blister strip consisting of a formed base foil with a peelable foil laminate lid. The foil strip is contained within the Accuhaler device.

6.6 Instructions for use and handling

The powdered medicine is inhaled through the mouth into the lungs.

The Accuhaler device contains the medicine in individual blisters which areopened as the device is manipulated.

For detailed instructions for use refer to the Patient Information Leaflet in every pack.

Adminstrative Details

7. MARKETING AUTHORISATION HOLDER

Glaxo Wellcome UK Ltd,

trading as Allen & Hanburys,

Stockley Park West,

Uxbridge, Middlesex,

UB11 1BT.

8. MARKETING AUTHORISATION NUMBER(S)

10949/0252

9. DATE OF FIRST AUTHORISATION/RENEWAL OF THE AUTHORISATION

December 1995

10. DATE OF REVISION OF THE TEXT

15th Sep 03

11. Legal Status

POM.

Ventolin Evohaler

(Allen & Hanburys)

1. NAME OF THE MEDICINAL PRODUCT

Ventolin$_{TM}$ Evohaler$_{TM}$.

2. QUALITATIVE AND QUANTITATIVE COMPOSITION

Ventolin Evohaler is a pressurised metered-dose inhaler delivering 100 micrograms of salbutamol (as Salbutamol Sulphate BP) per actuation. Ventolin Evohaler contains a new propellant (HFA 134a) and does not contain any chlorofluorocarbons.

3. PHARMACEUTICAL FORM

Aerosol.

4. CLINICAL PARTICULARS

4.1 Therapeutic indications

Ventolin Evohaler provides short-acting (4 to 6 hour) bronchodilatation with fast onset (within 5 minutes) in reversible airways obstruction.

It is particularly suitable for the relief and prevention of asthma symptoms. It should be used to relieve symptoms when they occur, and to prevent them in those circumstances recognised by the patient to precipitate an asthma attack (e.g. before exercise or unavoidable allergen exposure).

Ventolin Evohaler is particularly valuable as relief medication in mild, moderate or severe asthma, provided that reliance on it does not delay the introduction and use of regular inhaled corticosteroid therapy.

4.2 Posology and method of administration

Ventolin Evohaler is for oral inhalation use only. A spacer device may be used in patients who find it difficult to synchronise aerosol actuation with inspiration of breath.

Adults (including the elderly): For the relief of acute asthma symptoms including bronchospasm, one inhalation (100 micrograms) may be administered as a single minimum starting dose. This may be increased to two inhalations if necessary. To prevent allergen- or exercise-induced symptoms, two inhalations should be taken 10-15 minutes before challenge.

For chronic therapy, two inhalations up to four times a day.

Children: For the relief of acute asthma symptoms including bronchospasm, or before allergen exposure or exercise, one inhalation, or two if necessary.

For chronic therapy, two inhalations up to four times a day.

The Babyhaler$_{TM}$ spacer device may be used to facilitate administration to children under 5 years of age.

On-demand use of Ventolin Evohaler should not exceed 8 inhalations in any 24 hours. Reliance on such frequent supplementary use, or a sudden increase in dose, indicates poorly controlled or deteriorating asthma (see *Special warnings and precautions for use*).

4.3 Contraindications

Although intravenous salbutamol, and occasionally salbutamol tablets, are used in the management of premature labour uncomplicated by conditions such as placenta praevia, ante-partum haemorrhage or toxaemia of pregnancy, inhaled salbutamol preparations are not appropriate for managing premature labour. Salbutamol preparations should not be used for threatened abortion.

Ventolin Evohaler is contra-indicated in patients with a history of hypersensitivity to any of the components.

4.4 Special warnings and special precautions for use

Patients inhaler technique should be checked to make sure that aerosol actuation is synchronised with inspiration of breath for optimum delivery of drug to the lungs. Patients should be warned that they may experience a different taste upon inhalation compared to their previous inhaler.

Bronchodilators should not be the only or main treatment in patients with severe or unstable asthma. Severe asthma requires regular medical assessment, including lung-function testing, as patients are at risk of severe attacks and even death. Physicians should consider using the maximum recommended dose of inhaled corticosteroid and/or oral corticosteroid therapy in these patients.

The dosage or frequency of administration should only be increased on medical advice. If a previously effective dose of inhaled salbutamol fails to give relief lasting at least three hours, the patient should be advised to seek medical advice.

Increasing use of bronchodilators, in particular short-acting inhaled β_2-agonists, to relieve symptoms, indicates deterioration of asthma control. The patient should be instructed to seek medical advice if short-acting relief bronchodilator treatment becomes less effective, or more inhalations than usual are required. In this situation the patient should be assessed and consideration given to the need for increased anti-inflammatory therapy (e.g. higher doses of inhaled corticosteroid or a course of oral corticosteroid).

Severe exacerbations of asthma must be treated in the normal way.

Salbutamol should be administered cautiously to patients with thyrotoxicosis.

Potentially serious hypokalaemia may result from β_2-agonist therapy, mainly from parenteral and nebulised administration. Particular caution is advised in acute severe asthma as this effect may be potentiated by hypoxia and by concomitant treatment with xanthine derivatives, steroids and diuretics. Serum potassium levels should be monitored in such situations.

4.5 Interaction with other medicinal products and other forms of Interaction

Salbutamol and non-selective β-blocking drugs such as propranolol, should not usually be prescribed together.

4.6 Pregnancy and lactation

Administration of drugs during pregnancy should only be considered if the expected benefit to the mother is greater than any possible risk to the fetus. As with the majority of drugs, there is little published evidence of the safety of salbutamol in the early stages of human pregnancy, but in animal studies there was evidence of some harmful effects on the fetus at very high dose levels. A full range of reproductive studies with the non-chlorofluorocarbon propellant HFA 134a, have shown no effect on fetal development in animals.

Specific teratology studies with Ventolin Evohaler have shown no effects over and above those consistent with the known effects of high doses of beta-agonists. However, there is no experience on use in pregnancy and lactation in humans.

As salbutamol is probably secreted in breast milk, its use in nursing mothers requires careful consideration. It is not known whether salbutamol has a harmful effect on the neonate, and so its use should be restricted to situations where it is felt that the expected benefit to the mother is likely to outweigh any potential risk to the neonate.

4.7 Effects on ability to drive and use machines

None reported.

4.8 Undesirable effects

Adverse events are listed below by system organ class and frequency. Frequencies are defined as: very common (≥1/10), common (≥1/100 and <1/10), uncommon (≥1/1000 and <1/100), rare (≥1/10,000 and <1/1000) and very rare (<1/10,000) including isolated reports. Very common and common events were generally determined from clinical trial data. Rare and very rare events were generally determined from spontaneous data.

Immune system disorders

Very rare:Hypersensitivity reactions including angioedema, urticaria, bronchospasm, hypotension and collapse.

Metabolism and nutrition disorders

Rare: Hypokalaemia.

Potentially serious hypokalaemia may result from *beta*$_2$ agonist therapy.

Nervous system disorders

Common: Tremor, headache.

Very rare: Hyperactivity.

Cardiac disorders

Common: Tachycardia.

Very rare: Cardiac arrhythmias (including atrial fibrillation, supraventricular tachycardia and extrasystoles).

Vascular disorders

Rare: Peripheral vasodilatation.

Respiratory, thoracic and mediastinal disorders

Very rare: Paradoxical bronchospasm.

As with other inhalation therapy, paradoxical bronchospasm may occur with an immediate increase in wheezing after dosing. This should be treated immediately with an alternative presentation or a different fast-acting inhaled bronchodilator. EVOHALER should be discontinued immediately, the patient assessed, and, if necessary, alternative therapy instituted.

Gastrointestinal disorders

Uncommon: Mouth and throat irritation.

Musculoskeletal and connective tissue disorders

Uncommon: Muscle cramps.

4.9 Overdose

The preferred antidote for overdosage with salbutamol is a cardioselective β-blocking agent, but β-blocking drugs should be used with caution in patients with a history of bronchospasm.

Hypokalaemia may occur following overdose with salbutamol. Serum potassium levels should be monitored.

5. PHARMACOLOGICAL PROPERTIES

5.1 Pharmacodynamic properties

Salbutamol is a selective β_2-adrenoceptor agonist. At therapeutic doses it acts on the β_2-adrenoceptors of bronchial muscle providing short acting (4-6 hour) bronchodilatation with a fast onset (within 5 minutes) in reversible airways obstruction.

5.2 Pharmacokinetic properties

Salbutamol administered intravenously has a half life of 4 to 6 hours and is cleared partly renally and partly by metabolism to the inactive 4'-O-sulphate (phenolic sulphate) which is also excreted primarily in the urine. The faeces are a minor route of excretion.

After administration by the inhaled route between 10 and 20% of the dose reaches the lower airways. The remainder is retained in the delivery system or is deposited in the oropharynx from where it is swallowed. The fraction deposited in the airways is absorbed into the pulmonary tissues and circulation, but is not metabolised by the lung. On reaching the systemic circulation it becomes accessible to hepatic metabolism and is excreted, primarily in the urine, as unchanged drug and as the phenolic sulphate.

The swallowed portion of an inhaled dose is absorbed from the gastrointestinal tract and undergoes considerable first-pass metabolism to the phenolic sulphate. Both unchanged drug and conjugate are excreted primarily in the urine. Most of a dose of salbutamol given intravenously, orally or by inhalation is excreted within 72 hours. Salbutamol is bound to plasma proteins to the extent of 10%.

5.3 Preclinical safety data

In common with other potent selective β_2-agonists, salbutamol has been shown to be teratogenic in mice when given subcutaneously. In a reproductive study, 9.3% of fetuses were found to have cleft palate at 2.5mg/kg dose. In rats, treatment at the levels of 0.5, 2.32, 10.75 and 50mg/kg/day orally throughout pregnancy resulted in no significant fetal abnormalities. The only toxic effect was an increase in neonatal mortality at the highest dose level as the result of lack of maternal care. Reproductive studies in the rabbit at doses of 50mg/kg/day orally (i.e. much higher than the normal human dose) have shown fetuses with treatment related changes; these included open eyelids (ablepharia), secondary palate clefts (palatoschisis), changes in ossification of the frontal bones of the cranium (cranioschisis) and limb flexure. Reformulation of the Ventolin Evohaler has not altered the known toxicological profile of salbutamol.

The non-CFC propellant, HFA 134a, has been shown to have no toxic effect at very high vapour concentrations, far in excess of those likely to be experienced by patients, in a wide range of animal species exposed daily for periods of two years.

6. PHARMACEUTICAL PARTICULARS

6.1 List of excipients

HFA 134a.

6.2 Incompatibilities

None reported.

6.3 Shelf life

24 months when stored below 30°C.

6.4 Special precautions for storage

Store below 30°C (86°F).

Protect from frost and direct sunlight.

As with most inhaled medications in aerosol canisters, the therapeutic effect of this medication may decrease when the canister is cold.

The canister should not be broken, punctured or burnt, even when apparently empty.

6.5 Nature and contents of container

An inhaler comprising an aluminium alloy can sealed with a metering valve, actuator and dust cap. Each canister contains 200 metered actuations providing 100 micrograms of salbutamol (as Salbutamol Sulphate BP).

6.6 Instructions for use and handling

The aerosol spray is inhaled through the mouth into the lungs. After shaking the inhaler, the mouthpiece is placed in the mouth and the lips closed around it. The actuator is depressed to release a spray, which must coincide with inspiration of breath.

For detailed instructions for use refer to the Patient Information Leaflet in every pack.

7. MARKETING AUTHORISATION HOLDER

Glaxo Wellcome UK Ltd trading as Allen & Hanburys

Stockley Park West

Uxbridge

Middlesex, UB11 1BT

8. MARKETING AUTHORISATION NUMBER(S)

PL 10949/0274.

9. DATE OF FIRST AUTHORISATION/RENEWAL OF THE AUTHORISATION

28 June 2003

10. DATE OF REVISION OF THE TEXT

12 April 2005

11. Legal Status

POM.

Babyhaler, Evohaler and Ventolin are trade marks of the GlaxoSmithKline group of companies.

Ventolin Injection 500mcg

(Allen & Hanburys)

1. NAME OF THE MEDICINAL PRODUCT

Ventolin Injection 500 micrograms (0.5mg) in 1ml

2. QUALITATIVE AND QUANTITATIVE COMPOSITION

Ventolin Injection 500 micrograms (0.5mg) in 1ml (500 micrograms/ml) is presented as ampoules of 1ml, each containing 500 micrograms salbutamol as salbutamol sulphate BP in a sterile isotonic solution.

3. PHARMACEUTICAL FORM

A colourless or faintly straw coloured solution for injection.

4. CLINICAL PARTICULARS

4.1 Therapeutic indications

Ventolin Injection provides short-acting (4-6 hour) bronchodilatation with a fast onset (within 5 minutes) in reversible airways obstruction. It is indicated for the relief of severe bronchospasm.

4.2 Posology and method of administration

Ventolin Injection may be administered by the subcutaneous, intramuscular or intravenous route, under the direction of a physician.

Adults:

Subcutaneous route: 500 micrograms (8 micrograms/kg body weight) and repeated every four hours as required.

Intramuscular route: 500 micrograms (8 micrograms/kg body weight) and repeated every four hours as required.

Slow intravenous injection:

250 micrograms (4 micrograms/kg bodyweight) injected slowly. If necessary the dose may be repeated.

The use of Ventolin Injection 500 micrograms in 1ml (500 micrograms/ml, for intravenenous administration may be facilitated by dilution to 10ml with Water for Injection BP (final concentration of 50 micrograms/ml) and 5mls of the diluted preparation (250 micrograms/5ml) administered by slow intravenous injection.

Children:

At present there are insufficient data to recommend a dosage regimen for routine use.

Instructions to open the ampoule

Ampoules are equipped with the OPC (One Point Cut) opening system and must be opened using the following instructions:

hold with the hand the bottom part of the ampoule as indicated in picture 1

put the other hand on the top of the ampoule positioning the thumb above the coloured point and press as indicated in picture 2

Picture 1

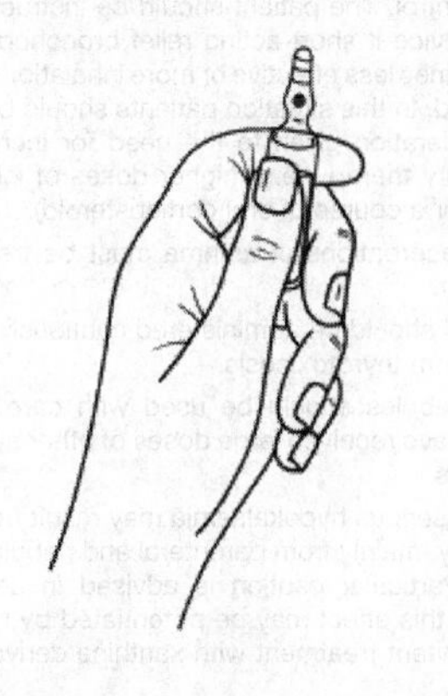

Picture 2

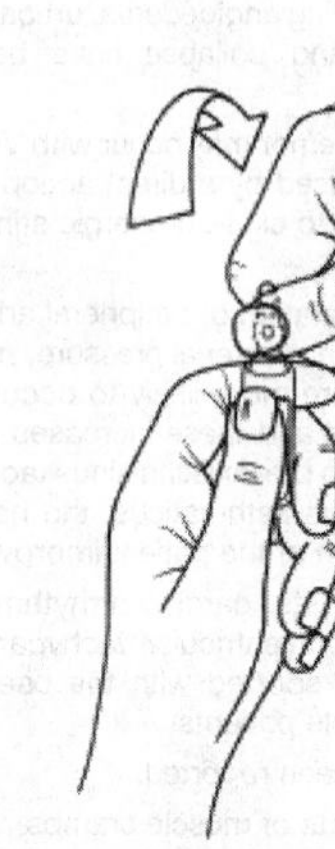

4.3 Contraindications

Although intravenous salbutamol, and occasionally salbutamol tablets, are used in the management of premature labour uncomplicated by conditions such as placenta praevia, ante-partum haemorrhage or toxaemia of pregnancy, salbutamol preparations should not be used for threatened abortion.

Ventolin Injection is contra-indicated in patients with a history of hypersensitivity to any of the components.

4.4 Special warnings and special precautions for use

Bronchodilators should not be the only or main treatment in patients with severe or unstable asthma. Severe asthma requires regular medical assessment, including lung-function testing, as patients are at risk of severe attacks and even death. Physicians should consider using the maximum recommended dose of inhaled corticosteroid and/or oral corticosteroid therapy in these patients.

The dosage or frequency of administration should only be increased on medical advice.

Patients being treated with Ventolin Injection may also be receiving short-acting inhaled bronchodilators to relieve symptoms. Increasing use of bronchodilators, in particular short-acting inhaled $_2$-agonists to relieve symptoms, indicates deterioration of asthma control.

The patient should be instructed to seek medical advice if short-acting relief bronchodilator treatment becomes less effective, or more inhalations than usual are required. In this situation the patient should be assessed and consideration given to the need for increased anti-inflammatory therapy (e.g. higher doses of inhaled corticosteroid or a course of oral corticosteroid).

Salbutamol should be administered cautiously to patients suffering from thyrotoxicosis.

Potentially serious hypokalaemia may result from β_2-agonist therapy, mainly from parenteral and nebulised administration. Particular caution is advised in acute severe asthma as this effect may be potentiated by hypoxia and by concomitant treatment with xanthine derivatives, steroids and diuretics. Serum potassium levels should be monitored in such situations.

Severe exacerbations of asthma must be treated in the normal way.

The use of Ventolin Injection in the treatment of severe bronchospasm does not obviate the requirement for corticosteroid therapy as appropriate. When practicable, administration of oxygen concurrently with Ventolin Injection is recommended. In common with other β-adrenoceptor agonists, salbutamol can induce reversible metabolic changes such as hypokalaemia and increased blood glucose levels. Diabetic patients may be unable to compensate for the increase in blood glucose and the development of ketoacidosis has been reported. Concurrent administration of corticosteroids can exaggerate this effect.

4.5 Interaction with other medicinal products and other forms of Interaction

Salbutamol and non-selective beta-blocking drugs such as propranolol, should not usually be prescribed together.

4.6 Pregnancy and lactation

Administration of drugs during pregnancy should only be considered if the expected benefit to the mother is greater than any possible risk to the foetus.

As with the majority of drugs, there is little published evidence of the safety of salbutamol in the early stages of human pregnancy, but in animal studies there was evidence of some harmful effects on the foetus at very high dose levels.

As salbutamol is probably secreted in breast milk its use in nursing mothers is not recommended unless the expected benefits outweigh any potential risk. In such situations the use of the inhaled route may be preferable although it is not known whether salbutamol has a harmful effect on the neonate.

4.7 Effects on ability to drive and use machines

Not applicable.

4.8 Undesirable effects

Hypersensitivity reactions including angioedema, urticaria, bronchospasm, hypotension and collapse have been reported very rarely.

Enhancement of physiological tremor may occur with Ventolin Injection. This effect is caused by a direct action on skeletal muscle and is common to all β-adrenergic stimulants.

Tachycardia, with or without dilatation of peripheral arterioles leading to a small reduction in arterial pressure, may occur. Increases in heart rate are more likely to occur in patients with normal heart rates and these increases are dose-dependent. In patients with pre-existing sinus tachycardia, especially those in status asthmaticus, the heart rate tends to fall as the condition of the patient improves.

In common with other β_2-agonists, cardiac arrhythmias (including atrial fibrillation, supraventricular tachycardia and extrasystoles) have been reported with the use of salbutamol, usually in susceptible patients.

Headaches have occasionally been reported.

There have been very rare reports of muscle cramps.

Potentially serious hypokalaemia may result from β_2-agonist therapy.

Intramuscular use of the undiluted injection may produce slight pain or stinging.

4.9 Overdose

The preferred antidote for overdosage with salbutamol is a cardioselective beta-blocking agent, but β-blocking drugs should be used with caution in patients with a history of bronchospasm.

Hypokalaemia may occur following overdose with salbutamol. Serum potassium levels should be monitored.

5. PHARMACOLOGICAL PROPERTIES

5.1 Pharmacodynamic properties

Salbutamol is a selective β_2-adrenoceptor agonist. At therapeutic doses it acts on β_2-adrenoceptors of bronchial muscle providing short-acting (4-6 hour) bronchodilation with a fast onset (within 5 minutes) in reversible airways obstruction.

5.2 Pharmacokinetic properties

Salbutamol administered intravenously has a half-life of 4 to 6 hours and is cleared partly renally and partly by metabolism to the inactive 4'-O-sulphate (phenolic sulphate) which is also excreted primarily in the urine. The faeces are a minor route of excretion. The majority of a dose of salbutamol given intravenously, orally or by inhalation is excreted within 72 hours. Salbutamol is bound to plasma proteins to the extent of 10%.

5.3 Preclinical safety data

There are no additional preclinical safety data other than are provided in the other sections of the Summary of Product Characteristics.

6. PHARMACEUTICAL PARTICULARS

6.1 List of excipients

Sodium chloride

Sodium hydroxide pellets

Dilute sulphuric acid

Water for injections

Nitrogen (oxygen free)

6.2 Incompatibilities

None stated

6.3 Shelf life

36 months

24 hours – shelf life of admixtures with infusion fluids.

6.4 Special precautions for storage

Store below 30°C and keep the ampoule in the outer container.

6.5 Nature and contents of container

Clear, neutral glass ampoules, packed in plastic trays with a cardboard sleeve over the trays.

Pack size: 1ml ampoules in plastic trays of 5.

6.6 Instructions for use and handling

The only recommended diluents for Ventolin Injection are water for injections BP, sodium chloride injection BP, sodium chloride and dextrose injection BP or dextrose injection BP.

All unused admixtures of Ventolin Injection should be discarded 24 hours after preparation.

Ventolin Injection should not be administered in the same syringe as any other medication.

Administrative Data

7. MARKETING AUTHORISATION HOLDER

Glaxo Wellcome UK Ltd
Stockley Park West
Uxbridge
Middlesex
UB11 1BT

8. MARKETING AUTHORISATION NUMBER(S)

PL 10949/0084

9. DATE OF FIRST AUTHORISATION/RENEWAL OF THE AUTHORISATION

6 September 2000

10. DATE OF REVISION OF THE TEXT

May 2004

11. Legal Status

POM

Ventolin Nebules 2.5mg, 5mg

(Allen & Hanburys)

1. NAME OF THE MEDICINAL PRODUCT

Ventolin Nebules 2.5mg.

Ventolin Nebules 5 mg.

2. QUALITATIVE AND QUANTITATIVE COMPOSITION

Plastic ampoule containing 2.5ml of a sterile 0.1% or 0.2% w/v solution of salbutamol (as Salbutamol Sulphate BP) in normal saline.

3. PHARMACEUTICAL FORM

Solution for inhalation via a nebuliser.

4. CLINICAL PARTICULARS

4.1 Therapeutic indications

Salbutamol is a selective $\beta 2$-agonist providing short-acting (4-6 hour) bronchodilatation with a fast onset (within 5 minutes) in reversible airways obstruction.

Ventolin Nebules are indicated for use in the routine management of chronic bronchospasm unresponsive to conventional therapy, and in the treatment of acute severe asthma.

4.2 Posology and method of administration

Ventolin Nebules are for inhalation use only under the direction of a physician, using a suitable nebuliser.

The solution should not be injected or administered orally.

Adults (including the elderly): 2.5mg to 5mg salbutamol up to four times a day. Up to 40mg per day can be given under strict medical supervision in hospital.

Children: 2.5mg to 5mg up to four times a day.

In infants under 18 months old the clinical efficacy of nebulised salbutamol is uncertain. As transient hypoxia may occur supplemental oxygen therapy should be considered.

Ventolin Nebules are intended to be used undiluted. However, if prolonged delivery time (more than 10 minutes) is required, the solution may be diluted with sterile normal saline.

4.3 Contraindications

Although intravenous salbutamol, and occasionally salbutamol tablets, are used in the management of premature labour uncomplicated by conditions such as placenta praevia, ante-partum haemorrhage or toxaemia of pregnancy, inhaled salbutamol preparations are not appropriate for managing premature labour. Salbutamol preparations should not be used for threatened abortion.

Ventolin Nebules are contra-indicated in patients with a history of hypersensitivity to any of the components.

4.4 Special warnings and special precautions for use

Bronchodilators should not be the only or main treatment in patients with severe or unstable asthma. Severe asthma requires regular medical assessment, including lung-function testing, as patients are at risk of severe attacks and even death. Physicians should consider using the maximum recommended dose of inhaled corticosteroid and/or oral corticosteroid therapy in these patients.

Patients receiving treatment at home should seek medical advice if treatment with Ventolin Nebules becomes less effective. The dosage or frequency of administration should only be increased on medical advice.

Patients being treated with Ventolin Nebules may also be receiving other dosage forms of short-acting inhaled bronchodilators to relieve symptoms. Increasing use of bronchodilators, in particular short-acting inhaled $\beta 2$-agonists to relieve symptoms, indicates deterioration of asthma control. The patient should be instructed to seek medical advice if short-acting relief bronchodilator treatment becomes less effective or more inhalations than usual are required. In this situation patients should be assessed and consideration given to the need for increased anti-inflammatory therapy (e.g. higher doses of inhaled corticosteroid or a course of oral corticosteroid).

Severe exacerbations of asthma must be treated in the normal way.

Salbutamol should be administered cautiously to patients suffering from thyrotoxicosis.

Ventolin Nebules should be used with care in patients known to have received large doses of other sympathomimetic drugs.

Potentially serious hypokalaemia may result from $\beta 2$-agonist therapy, mainly from parenteral and nebulised administration. Particular caution is advised in acute severe asthma as this effect may be potentiated by hypoxia and by concomitant treatment with xanthine derivatives, steroids and diuretics. Serum potassium levels should be monitored in such situations.

In common with other β-adrenoceptor agonists, salbutamol can induce reversible metabolic changes such as increased blood glucose levels. Diabetic patients may be unable to compensate for the increase in blood glucose and the development of ketoacidosis has been reported. Concurrent administration of corticosteroids can exaggerate this effect.

A small number of cases of acute angle-closure glaucoma have been reported in patients treated with a combination of nebulised salbutamol and ipratropium bromide. A combination of nebulised salbutamol with nebulised anticholinergics should therefore be used cautiously. Patients should receive adequate instruction in correct administration and be warned not to let the solution or mist enter the eye.

4.5 Interaction with other medicinal products and other forms of Interaction

Salbutamol and non-selective β-blocking drugs such as propranolol, should not usually be prescribed together.

4.6 Pregnancy and lactation

Administration of drugs during pregnancy should only be considered if the expected benefit to the mother is greater than any possible risk to the fetus. As with the majority of drugs, there is little published evidence of the safety of salbutamol in the early stages of human pregnancy, but in animal studies there was evidence of some harmful effects on the fetus at very high dose levels.

As salbutamol is probably secreted in breast milk, its use in nursing mothers requires careful consideration. It is not known whether salbutamol has a harmful effect on the neonate, and so its use should be restricted to situations where it is felt that the expected benefit to the mother is likely to outweigh any potential risk to the neonate.

4.7 Effects on ability to drive and use machines

None reported.

4.8 Undesirable effects

As with other inhalation therapy, paradoxical bronchospasm may occur with an immediate increase in wheezing after dosing. This should be treated immediately with an alternative presentation or a different fast-acting inhaled bronchodilator. The preparation should be discontinued immediately, the patient assessed, and, if necessary, alternative therapy instituted.

Solutions which are not of neutral pH may rarely cause bronchospasm.

Hypersensitivity reactions including angioedema, urticaria, bronchospasm, hypotension and collapse have been reported very rarely.

Potentially serious hypokalaemia may result from $\beta 2$-agonist therapy.

Ventolin Nebules may cause a fine tremor of skeletal muscle, usually the hands are most obviously affected. This effect is dose-related and is common to all β-adrenergic stimulants.

Tachycardia, with or without peripheral vasodilatation, may rarely occur. In common with other $\beta 2$ agonists, cardiac arrhythmias (including atrial fibrillation, supraventricular tachycardia and extrasystoles) have been reported in association with the use of salbutamol, usually in susceptible patients.

Headaches have occasionally been reported.

Mouth and throat irritation may occur with inhaled salbutamol.

As with other $\beta 2$-agonists hyperactivity in children has been reported rarely.

There have been very rare reports of muscle cramps.

4.9 Overdose

The preferred antidote to overdosage with salbutamol is a cardioselective β-blocking agent, but β-blocking drugs should be used with caution in patients with a history of bronchospasm.

Hypokalaemia may occur following overdose with salbutamol. Serum potassium levels should be monitored.

5. PHARMACOLOGICAL PROPERTIES

5.1 Pharmacodynamic properties

Salbutamol is a selective $\beta 2$-agonist providing short-acting (4-6 hour) bronchodilatation with a fast onset (within 5 minutes) in reversible airways obstruction. At therapeutic doses it acts on the $\beta 2$-adrenoceptors of bronchial muscle. With its fast onset of action, it is particularly suitable for the management and prevention of attack in asthma.

5.2 Pharmacokinetic properties

Salbutamol administered intravenously has a half-life of 4 to 6 hours and is cleared partly renally, and partly by metabolism to the inactive 4'-O-sulphate (phenolic sulphate) which is also excreted primarily in the urine. The faeces are a minor route of excretion. Most of a dose of salbutamol given intravenously, orally or by inhalation is excreted within 72 hours. Salbutamol is bound to plasma proteins to the extent of 10%.

After administration by the inhaled route between 10 and 20% of the dose reaches the lower airways. The remainder is retained in the delivery system or is deposited in the oropharynx from where it is swallowed. The fraction deposited in the airways is absorbed into the pulmonary tissues and circulation, but is not metabolised by the lung. On reaching the systemic circulation it becomes accessible to hepatic metabolism and is excreted, primarily in the urine, as unchanged drug and as the phenolic sulphate.

The swallowed portion of an inhaled dose is absorbed from the gastrointestinal tract and undergoes considerable first-pass metabolism to the phenolic sulphate. Both unchanged drug and conjugate are excreted primarily in the urine.

5.3 Preclinical safety data
No additional preclinical safety data are included here.

6. PHARMACEUTICAL PARTICULARS
6.1 List of excipients
Sodium chloride

Sulphuric acid if required to adjust pH

Purified water

6.2 Incompatibilities
None known.

6.3 Shelf life
3 years if unopened.

3 months after removal from the foil overwrap, (see below).

6.4 Special precautions for storage
Ventolin Nebules should be stored below 30°C. The Nebules should be protected from light after removal from the foil tray.

6.5 Nature and contents of container
Low density polyethylene ampoules available in boxes of 20 or 40 in strips of 5 or 10. Sample pack of 5.

6.6 Instructions for use and handling
The nebulised solution may be inhaled through a face mask, T-piece or via an endotracheal tube. Intermittent positive pressure ventilation (IPPV) may be used but is rarely necessary. When there is a risk of anoxia through hypoventilation, oxygen should be added to the inspired air.

As many nebulisers operate on a continuous flow basis, it is likely that some nebulised drug will be released into the local environment. Ventolin Nebules should therefore be administered in a well-ventilated room, particularly in hospitals when several patients may be using nebulisers at the same time.

Dilution: Ventolin Nebules may be diluted with Sodium Chloride Injection BP, (normal saline). Solutions in nebulisers should be replaced daily.

Administrative Data
7. MARKETING AUTHORISATION HOLDER
Allen & Hanburys

Stockley Park West

Uxbridge

Middlesex UB11 1BT

8. MARKETING AUTHORISATION NUMBER(S)
Ventolin Nebules 2.5mgPL10949/0085

Ventolin Nebules 5 mg. PL10949/0086

9. DATE OF FIRST AUTHORISATION/RENEWAL OF THE AUTHORISATION
10th July 2002

10. DATE OF REVISION OF THE TEXT
June 1998

11. Legal Status
POM.

Ventolin Respirator Solution

(Allen & Hanburys)

1. NAME OF THE MEDICINAL PRODUCT
Ventolin™ Respirator Solution.

2. QUALITATIVE AND QUANTITATIVE COMPOSITION
Aqueous, colourless to light yellow solution, pH 3.5, providing 5mg/ml of salbutamol (as Salbutamol Sulphate BP).

3. PHARMACEUTICAL FORM
Solution for nebulisation.

4. CLINICAL PARTICULARS
4.1 Therapeutic indications
Ventolin Respirator Solution is indicated for use in the routine management of chronic bronchospasm unresponsive to conventional therapy, and in the treatment of acute severe asthma.

4.2 Posology and method of administration
Ventolin Respirator Solution is for inhalation use only under the direction of a physician, using a suitable nebuliser. The solution should not be injected or administered orally. Ventolin Respirator Solution may be administered intermittently or continuously. Salbutamol has a duration of action of 4 to 6 hours in most patients.

Intermittent administration
Adults: Ventolin Respirator solution 0.5ml (2.5mg of salbutamol) should be diluted to a final volume of 2ml with normal saline for injection. This may be increased to 1ml (5mg of salbutamol) diluted to a final volume of 2.5ml. The resulting solution is inhaled from a suitably driven nebuliser until aerosol generation ceases. Using a correctly matched nebuliser and driving source this should take about ten minutes.

Ventolin Respirator Solution may be used undiluted for intermittent administration. For this, 2ml of Ventolin Respirator Solution (10mg of salbutamol) is placed in the nebuliser and the patient allowed to inhale the nebulised solution until bronchodilatation is achieved. This usually takes 3 - 5 minutes. Some adult patients may require higher doses of salbutamol up to 10mg, in which case nebulisation of the undiluted solution may continue until aerosol generation ceases.

Children: The same mode of administration for intermittent administration is also applicable to children. The minimum starting dosage for children under the age of twelve years is 0.5ml (2.5mg of salbutamol) diluted to 2 to 2.5ml with normal saline for injection. Some children may, however, require higher doses of salbutamol up to 5mg. Intermittent treatment may be repeated up to four times daily.

Continuous administration
Ventolin Respirator Solution is diluted with normal saline for injection to contain 50-100 micrograms of salbutamol per ml, (1-2ml solution made up to 100ml with diluent). The diluted solution is administered as an aerosol by a suitably driven nebuliser. The usual rate of administration is 1-2mg per hour.

In infants under 18 months the clinical efficacy of nebulised salbutamol is uncertain. As transient hypoxaemia may occur supplemental oxygen therapy should be considered.

4.3 Contraindications
Hypersensitivity.

Threatened abortion.

4.4 Special warnings and special precautions for use
Bronchodilators should not be the only or main treatment in patients with severe or unstable asthma. Severe asthma requires regular medical assessment, including lung-function testing, as patients are at risk of severe attacks and even death. Physicians should consider using the maximum recommended dose of inhaled corticosteroid and/or oral corticosteroid therapy in these patients.

Patients receiving treatment at home should be warned to seek medical advice if treatment with Ventolin Respirator Solution becomes less effective. As there may be adverse effects associated with excessive dosing the dosage or frequency of administration should only be increased on medical advice.

Patients being treated with Ventolin Respirator Solution may also be receiving other dosage forms of short-acting inhaled bronchodilators to relieve symptoms.

Increasing use of bronchodilators, in particular short-acting inhaled $\beta 2$-agonists, to relieve symptoms, indicates deterioration of asthma control. The patient should be instructed to seek medical advice if short-acting relief bronchodilator treatment becomes less effective, or more inhalations than usual are required. In this situation the patient should be assessed and consideration given to the need for increased anti-inflammatory therapy (e.g. higher doses of inhaled corticosteroid or a course of oral corticosteroid).

Severe exacerbations of asthma must be treated in the normal way.

Ventolin Respirator Solution should be used with care in patients known to have received large doses of other sympathomimetic drugs.

Potentially serious hypokalaemia may result from β_2-agonist therapy, mainly from parenteral and nebulised administration. Particular caution is advised in acute severe asthma as this effect may be potentiated by hypoxia and by concomitant treatment with xanthine derivatives, steroids and diuretics. Serum potassium levels should be monitored in such situations.

In common with other β-adrenoceptor agonists, salbutamol can induce reversible metabolic changes such as increased blood glucose levels. Diabetic patients may be unable to compensate for the increase in blood glucose and the development of ketoacidosis has been reported. Concurrent administration of corticosteroids can exaggerate this effect.

A small number of cases of acute angle-closure glaucoma have been reported in patients treated with a combination of nebulised salbutamol and ipratropium bromide. A combination of nebulised salbutamol with nebulised anticholinergics should therefore be used cautiously. Patients should receive adequate instruction in correct administration and be warned not to let the solution or mist enter the eye.

Salbutamol should be administered cautiously to patients suffering from thyrotoxicosis.

4.5 Interaction with other medicinal products and other forms of Interaction
Should not normally be prescribed with non-selective β-blocking drugs such as propranolol.

4.6 Pregnancy and lactation
Administration of drugs during pregnancy should only be considered if the expected benefit to the mother is greater than any possible risk to the foetus. As with the majority of drugs, there is little published evidence of the safety of salbutamol in the early stages of human pregnancy, but in animal studies there was evidence of some harmful effects on the foetus at very high dose levels.

As salbutamol is probably secreted in breast milk, its use in nursing mothers requires careful consideration. It is not known whether salbutamol has a harmful effect on the neonate, and so its use should be restricted to situations where it is felt that the expected benefit to the mother is likely to outweigh any potential risk to the neonate.

4.7 Effects on ability to drive and use machines
None reported.

4.8 Undesirable effects
As with other inhalation therapy, paradoxical bronchospasm may occur with an immediate increase in wheezing after dosing. This should be treated immediately with an alternative presentation or a different fast-acting inhaled bronchodilator. The preparation should be discontinued immediately, the patient assessed and, if necessary, alternative therapy instituted.

Non-isotonic solutions, or solutions which are not of neutral pH, or which contain benzalkonium chloride, may rarely cause paradoxical bronchospasm.

Hypersensitivity reactions including angioedema, urticaria, bronchospasm, hypotension and collapse have been reported very rarely.

Potentially serious hypokalaemia may result from β_2-agonist therapy.

Ventolin Respirator Solution may cause a fine tremor of skeletal muscle, usually the hands are most obviously affected. This effect is dose-related and is common to all β-adrenergic stimulants.

Tachycardia, with or without peripheral vasodilatation, may rarely occur. In common with other β_2 agonists, cardiac arrhythmias (including atrial fibrillation, supraventricular tachycardia and extrasystoles) have been reported in association with the use of salbutamol, usually in susceptible patients.

Headaches have occasionally been reported.

Mouth and throat irritation may occur with inhaled salbutamol.

As with other β_2-agonists hyperactivity in children has been reported rarely.

There have been very rare reports of muscle cramps.

4.9 Overdose
Discontinue administration of Ventolin Respirator Solution if there are any signs of overdosage. The preferred antidote for overdosage with salbutamol is a cardioselective -blocking agent, but β-blocking drugs should be used with caution in patients with a history of bronchospasm. Hypokalaemia may occur following overdose with salbutamol. Serum potassium levels should be monitored.

5. PHARMACOLOGICAL PROPERTIES
5.1 Pharmacodynamic properties
Salbutamol is a selective $\beta 2$-agonist providing short-acting (4-6 hour) bronchodilatation with a fast onset (within 5 minutes) in reversible airways obstruction. At therapeutic doses it acts on the β_2-adrenoceptors of bronchial muscle. With its fast onset of action, it is particularly suitable for the management and prevention of attack in asthma.

5.2 Pharmacokinetic properties
Salbutamol administered intravenously has a half-life of 4 to 6 hours and is cleared partly renally and partly by metabolism to the inactive 4'-0-sulphate (phenolic sulphate) which is also excreted primarily in the urine. The faeces are a minor route of excretion. Most of a dose of salbutamol given intravenously, orally or by inhalation is excreted within 72 hours. Salbutamol is bound to plasma proteins to the extent of 10%.

After administration by the inhaled route between 10 and 20% of the dose reaches the lower airways. The remainder is retained in the delivery system or is deposited in the oropharynx from where it is swallowed. The fraction deposited in the airways is absorbed into the pulmonary tissues and circulation, but is not metabolised by the lung. On reaching the systemic circulation it becomes accessible to hepatic metabolism and is excreted, primarily in the urine, as unchanged drug and as the phenolic sulphate.

The swallowed portion of an inhaled dose is absorbed from the gastrointestinal tract and undergoes considerable first-pass metabolism to the phenolic sulphate. Both unchanged drug and conjugate are excreted primarily in the urine.

5.3 Preclinical safety data
No additional preclinical safety data are included here.

6. PHARMACEUTICAL PARTICULARS
6.1 List of excipients
Preservative: Benzalkonium chloride. Sulphuric acid if required to adjust to pH 3.5.

Purified water.

6.2 Incompatibilities
None known.

6.3 Shelf life
Unopened: 3 years. Following opening for the first time: 28 days.

6.4 Special precautions for storage
Store below 25°C. Protect from light. Discard any contents remaining one month after opening the bottle.

6.5 Nature and contents of container
Screw-capped 10ml amber glass bottle.

Screw-capped 20ml amber glass bottle.

6.6 Instructions for use and handling
Inhalation use only, using a suitable nebuliser.

The nebulised solution may be inhaled through a face mask, "T" piece or via an endotracheal tube. Intermittent positive pressure ventilation (IPPV) may be used, but is rarely necessary. When there is a risk of anoxia through hypoventilation, oxygen should be added to the inspired air.

As many nebulisers operate on a continuous flow basis, it is likely that nebulised drug will be released into the local environment. Ventolin Respirator Solution should therefore be administered in a well ventilated room, particularly in hospitals when several patients may be using nebulisers at the same time.

Administrative Data
7. MARKETING AUTHORISATION HOLDER
Glaxo Wellcome UK Ltd

trading as Allen & Hanburys

Stockley Park West

Uxbridge

Middlesex UB11 1BT.

8. MARKETING AUTHORISATION NUMBER(S)
PL 10949/0244

9. DATE OF FIRST AUTHORISATION/RENEWAL OF THE AUTHORISATION
02 September 2005

10. DATE OF REVISION OF THE TEXT
02 September 2005

11. Legal Category
POM.

Ventolin Rotacaps 200mcg, 400mcg

(Allen & Hanburys)

1. NAME OF THE MEDICINAL PRODUCT
Ventolin TM RotacapsTM 200mcg

Ventolin TM RotacapsTM 400mcg

2. QUALITATIVE AND QUANTITATIVE COMPOSITION
200mcg microfine salbutamol (as sulphate) in each light blue capsule, marked Ventolin 200 or

400mcg microfine salbutamol (as sulphate) in each dark blue capsule, marked Ventolin 400.

3. PHARMACEUTICAL FORM
Hard gelatin capsule containing powder for inhalation.

4. CLINICAL PARTICULARS
4.1 Therapeutic indications
Salbutamol is a selective β_2-agonist providing short-acting (4-6 hour) bronchodilatation with a fast onset (within 5 minutes) in reversible airways obstruction.

Ventolin Rotacaps can be used in the management of asthma, bronchospasm and/or reversible airways obstruction.

Ventolin Rotacaps are particularly suitable for the relief of asthma symptoms. They should be used to relieve symptoms when they occur, and to prevent them in those circumstances recognised by the patient to precipitate an asthma attack (e.g. before exercise or unavoidable allergen exposure).

Ventolin Rotacaps are particularly valuable as relief medication in mild, moderate or severe asthma, provided that reliance on them does not delay the introduction and use of regular inhaled corticosteroid therapy.

4.2 Posology and method of administration
Ventolin Rotacaps are for oral inhalation use only, using a Ventolin RotahalerTM. Ventolin Rotacaps are suitable for many patients including those who cannot use a metered-dose inhaler successfully.

Adults (including the elderly): For the relief of acute bronchospasm: 200 micrograms or 400 micrograms as a single dose. The maximum daily dose is 400 micrograms four times a day.

To prevent allergen- or exercise-induced symptoms: 400 micrograms 10-15 minutes before challenge.

Children: The recommended dose for the relief of acute bronchospasm or before allergen exposure or exercise is 200 micrograms. The maximum daily dose is 200 micrograms four times a day.

On-demand use of Ventolin Rotacaps should not exceed four times daily. Reliance on such frequent supplementary use, or a sudden increase in dose, indicates poorly controlled or deteriorating asthma (see *Special warning and precautions for use*).

4.3 Contraindications
Although intravenous salbutamol, and occasionally salbutamol tablets, are used in the management of premature labour uncomplicated by conditions such as placenta praevia, ante-partum haemorrhage or toxaemia of pregnancy, inhaled salbutamol preparations are not appropriate for managing premature labour. Salbutamol preparations should not be used for threatened abortion.

Ventolin Rotacaps are contra-indicated in patients with a history of hypersensitivity to any of the components. (See Pharmaceutical Particulars – List of Exceipients).

4.4 Special warnings and special precautions for use
Patients should be instructed in the proper use of the Rotahaler device to ensure that the drug reaches the target area within the lungs.

Bronchodilators should not be the only or main treatment in patients with severe or unstable asthma. Severe asthma requires regular medical assessment, including lung-function testing, as patients are at risk of severe attacks and even death. Physicians should consider using the maximum recommended dose of inhaled corticosteroid and/or oral corticosteroid therapy in these patients.

The dosage or frequency of administration should only be increased on medical advice.

Increasing use of bronchodilators, in particular short-acting inhaled β_2-agonists to relieve symptoms, indicates deterioration of asthma control. The patient should be instructed to seek medical advice if short-acting relief bronchodilator treatment becomes less effective, or more inhalations than usual are required. In this situation the patient should be assessed, and consideration given to the need for increased anti-inflammatory therapy (e.g. higher doses of inhaled corticosteroid or a course of oral corticosteroid).

Severe exacerbations of asthma must be treated in the normal way.

Salbutamol should be administered cautiously to patients suffering from thyrotoxicosis.

Potentially serious hypokalaemia may result from β_2-agonist therapy, mainly from parenteral and nebulised administration. Particular caution is advised in acute severe asthma as this effect may be potentiated by hypoxia and by concomitant treatment with xanthine derivatives, steroids and diuretics. Serum potassium levels should be monitored in such situations.

4.5 Interaction with other medicinal products and other forms of Interaction
Salbutamol and non-selective β-blocking drugs such as propranolol, should not usually be prescribed together.

4.6 Pregnancy and lactation
Administration of drugs during pregnancy should only be considered if the expected benefit to the mother is greater then any possible risk to the fetus. As with the majority of drugs, there is little published evidence of the safety of salbutamol in the early stages of human pregnancy, but in animals studies there was evidence of some harmful effects on the fetus at very high dose levels.

As salbutamol is probably secreted in breast milk, its use in nursing mothers requires careful consideration. It is not known whether salbutamol has a harmful effect on the neonate, and so its use should be restricted to situations where it is felt that the expected benefit to the mother is likely to outweigh any potential risk to the neonate.

4.7 Effects on ability to drive and use machines
None reported.

4.8 Undesirable effects
As with other inhalation therapy, paradoxical bronchospasm may occur with an immediate increase in wheezing after dosing. This should be treated immediately with an alternative presentation or a different fast-acting inhaled bronchodilator. The preparation should be discontinued immediately, the patient assessed and, if necessary, alternative therapy instituted.

Hypersensitivity reactions including angioedema, urticaria, bronchospasm, hypotension and collapse have been reported very rarely.

Potentially serious hypokalaemia may result from β_2-agonist therapy.

Ventolin Rotacaps may cause a fine tremor of skeletal muscle, usually the hands are most obviously affected. This effect is dose-related and is common to all β-adrenergic stimulants.

Tachycardia, with or without peripheral vasodilatation, may rarely occur. In common with other β_2-agonists, cardiac arrhythmias (including atrial fibrillation, supraventricular tachycardia and extrasystoles) have been reported in association with the use of salbutamol, usually in susceptible patients.

Headaches have occasionally been reported.

Mouth and throat irritation may occur with inhaled salbutamol.

As with other β_2-agonists hyperactivity in children has been reported rarely.

There have been very rare reports of muscle cramps.

4.9 Overdose
The preferred antidote for overdosage with salbutamol is a cardioselective β-blocking agent, but β-blocking drugs should be used with caution in patients with a history of bronchospasm.

Hypokalaemia may occur following overdose with salbutamol. Serum potassium levels should be monitored.

5. PHARMACOLOGICAL PROPERTIES
5.1 Pharmacodynamic properties
Salbutamol is a selective β_2-adrenoceptor agonist. At therapeutic doses it acts on the β_2-adrenoceptors of bronchial muscle providing short acting (4-6 hour) bronchodilatation with a fast onset (within 5 minutes) in reversible airways obstruction.

5.2 Pharmacokinetic properties
Salbutamol administered intravenously has a half life of 4 to 6 hours and is cleared partly renally and partly by metabolism to the inactive 4'-O-sulphate (phenolic sulphate) which is also excreted primarily in the urine. The faeces are a minor route of excretion.

After administration by the inhaled route between 10 and 20% of the dose reaches the lower airways. The remainder is retained in the delivery system or is deposited in the oropharynx from where it is swallowed. The fraction deposited in the airways is absorbed into the pulmonary tissues and circulation, but is not metabolised by the lung. On reaching the systemic circulation it becomes accessible to hepatic metabolism and is excreted, primarily in the urine, as unchanged drug and as the phenolic sulphate.

The swallowed portion of an inhaled dose is absorbed from the gastrointestinal tract and undergoes considerable first-pass metabolism to the phenolic sulphate. Both unchanged drug and conjugate are excreted primarily in the urine. Most of a dose of salbutamol given intravenously, orally or by inhalation is excreted within 72 hours. Salbutamol is bound to plasma proteins to the extent of 10%.

5.3 Preclinical safety data
There are no pre-clinical data of relevance to the prescriber which are additional to that already included in other sections of the SPC.

6. PHARMACEUTICAL PARTICULARS
6.1 List of excipients
Lactose (which contains milk protein).

6.2 Incompatibilities
None reported.

6.3 Shelf life
3 years.

6.4 Special precautions for storage
Store in a dry place below 30°C.

6.5 Nature and contents of container
Ventolin Rotacaps are supplied in polypropylene containers with snap-on tamper-evident polyethylene caps containing 112 capsules.

6.6 Instructions for use and handling
The contents of the Rotacaps capsule are inhaled through the mouth into the lungs. The capsule is inserted into a Rotahaler device which separates the two halves. The drug is released as the patient inhales through the mouth.

A capsule should only be inserted into the Rotahaler device when required for use.

For detailed instructions for use refer to the Patient Information Leaflet in every pack.

Administrative Data
7. MARKETING AUTHORISATION HOLDER
Glaxo Wellcome UK Limited

trading as Allen & Hanburys,

Stockley Park West,

Uxbridge,

Middlesex, UB11 1BT.

8. MARKETING AUTHORISATION NUMBER(S)
Ventolin TM RotacapsTM 200mcg PL10949/0072

Ventolin TM RotacapsTM 400mcg PL10949/0073

9. DATE OF FIRST AUTHORISATION/RENEWAL OF THE AUTHORISATION
19/03/2003

10. DATE OF REVISION OF THE TEXT
15th September 2003

11. Legal Status
POM.

Rotacaps, Rotahaler and Ventolin are trade marks of the Glaxo Wellcome Group of Companies.

Ventolin Solution for IV Infusion

(Allen & Hanburys)

1. NAME OF THE MEDICINAL PRODUCT
VentolinTM Solution for Intravenous Infusion 5mg in 5ml (1mg/ml).

2. QUALITATIVE AND QUANTITATIVE COMPOSITION
Ventolin Solution for Intravenous Infusion 5mg in 5ml (1mg/ml) is presented as ampoules of 5ml, each containing 5mg salbutamol as Salbutamol Sulphate BP in a sterile isotonic solution.

3. PHARMACEUTICAL FORM
Clear, colourless or pale straw-coloured solution for intravenous infusion.

4. CLINICAL PARTICULARS

4.1 Therapeutic indications
Ventolin Solution for Intravenous Infusion should be administered under the direction of a physician. It is indicated for two distinct clinical situations:

a) For the relief of severe bronchospasm.

b) In the management of premature labour; to arrest uncomplicated labour between 24 and 33 weeks of gestation in patients with no medical or obstetric contra-indication to tocolytic therapy. Data suggest that the main effect of tocolytic therapy is a delay in delivery of up to 48 hours. This delay may be used to administer glucocorticoids or to implement other measures known to improve perinatal health.

4.2 Posology and method of administration
Ventolin Solution for Intravenous Infusion is used to prepare an infusion solution. It should not be injected undiluted. Ventolin Solution for Intravenous Infusion should not be administered in the same syringe or infusion as any other medication.

1) In severe bronchospasm.

Adults: A suitable solution for infusion providing 10 micrograms salbutamol/ml is prepared by diluting 5ml Ventolin Solution for Intravenous Infusion to 500ml with an infusion solution such as Sodium Chloride and Dextrose Injection BP. Other suitable diluents are Water for Injections BP, Sodium Chloride Injection BP or Dextrose Injection BP.

Infusion rates providing 3 to 20 micrograms salbutamol/minute (0.3 to 2ml/minute of the above infusion solution) are usually adequate. Higher doses have been used with success in patients with respiratory failure. Children: There are insufficient data to recommend a dosage regime for routine use.

2. In the management of premature labour.

The infusion, prepared as described below, should be administered as early as possible after the diagnosis of premature labour, and after evaluation of the patient to eliminate any contra-indications to the use of salbutamol (see Contra-indications).

During infusion the maternal pulse rate should be monitored and the infusion rate djusted to avoid excessive maternal heart rate (above 140 beats/minute).

It is essential that the volume of infusion fluid is kept to a minimum to control the level of hydration and so avoid the risk of maternal pulmonary oedema (see Undesirable effects). A controlled infusion device, preferably a syringe pump, should be used.

Infusion rates providing 10 to 45 micrograms salbutamol/minute are generally adequate to control uterine contractions. A starting rate of 10 micrograms/minute is recommended, increasing the rate at 10-minute intervals until there is evidence of patient response shown by diminution in strength, frequency or duration of contractions. Thereafter, the infusion rate may be increased slowly until contractions cease. Once uterine contractions have ceased the infusion rate should be maintained at the same level for one hour and then reduced by 50% decrements at six hourly intervals. If labour progresses despite treatment the infusion should be stopped. If contractions have been successfully inhibited by the infusion, treatment may be continued orally with Ventolin Tablets 4mg given three or four times daily.

Dilution: The recommended diluent is 5% Dextrose (see precautions for use in diabetic patients).

For use in a syringe pump*:* Prepare a solution providing 200 micrograms salbutamol/ml by diluting 10ml Ventolin Solution for Intravenous Infusion with 40ml diluent. An infusion rate of 10 to 45 micrograms/minute is equivalent to 0.05 to 0.225ml/minute of this solution.

Other infusion methods*:* Prepare a solution providing 20 micrograms salbutamol/ml by diluting 10ml Ventolin Solution for Intravenous Infusion with 490ml diluent. An infusion rate of 10 to 45 micrograms/minute is equivalent to 0.5 to 2.25ml/minute of this solution.

<u>Instructions to open the ampoule</u>

Ampoules are equipped with the OPC (One Point Cut) opening system and must be opened using the following instructions:

- hold with the hand the bottom part of the ampoule as indicated in picture 1
- put the other hand on the top of the ampoule positioning the thumb above the coloured point and press as indicated in picture 2

Picture 1

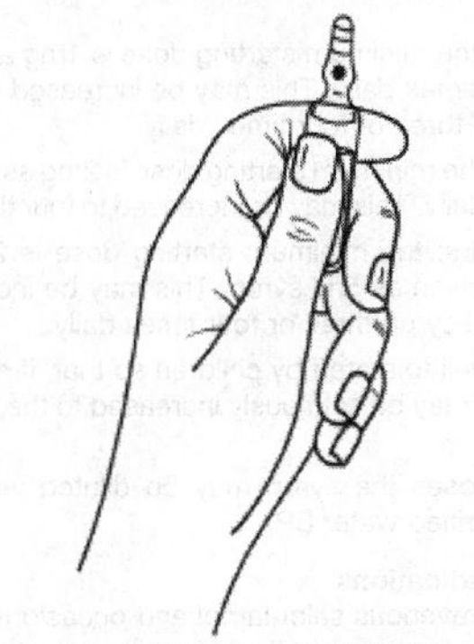

Picture 2

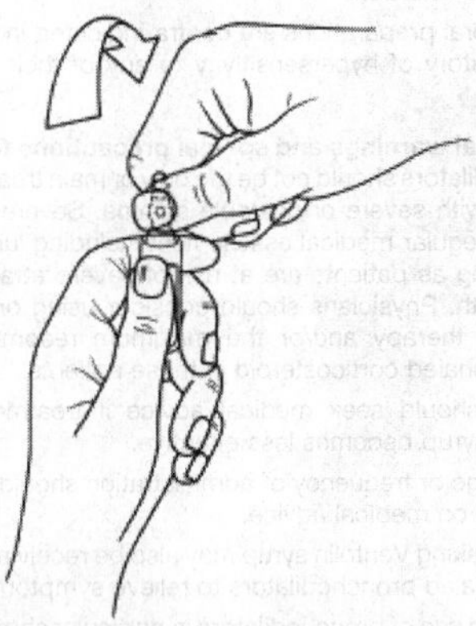

4.3 Contraindications
Although Ventolin Solution for Intravenous Infusion and occasionally salbutamol tablets, are used in the management of premature labour uncomplicated by conditions such as placenta praevia, ante-partum haemorrhage or toxaemia of pregnancy, salbutamol preparations should not be used for threatened abortion.

Ventolin Solution for Intravenous Infusion is contra-indicated in patients with a history of hypersensitivity to any of the components.

4.4 Special warnings and special precautions for use
Bronchodilators should not be the only or main treatment in patients with severe or unstable asthma. Severe asthma requires regular medical assessment, including lung-function testing, as patients are at risk of severe attacks and even death. Physicians should consider using the maximum recommended dose of inhaled corticosteroid and/or oral corticosteroid therapy in these patients.

The dosage or frequency of administration should only be increased on medical advice.

Patients being treated with Ventolin Solution for Intravenous Infusion may also be receiving short-acting inhaled bronchodilators to relieve symptoms. Increasing use of bronchodilators, in particular short-acting inhaled β_2-agonists to relieve symptoms, indicates deterioration of asthma control. The patient should be instructed to seek medical advice if short-acting relief bronchodilator treatment becomes less effective, or more inhalations than usual are required. In this situation the patient should be assessed and consideration given to the need for increased anti-inflammatory therapy (e.g. higher doses of inhaled corticosteroid or a course of oral corticosteroid). Severe exacerbations of asthma must be treated in the normal way. The use of Ventolin Solution for Intravenous Infusion in the treatment of severe bronchospasm does not obviate the requirement for corticosteroid therapy as appropriate. When practicable, administration of oxygen concurrently with parenteral Ventolin is recommended, particularly when it is given by intravenous infusion to hypoxic patients. In common with other β-adrenoceptor agonists, salbutamol can induce reversible metabolic changes such as hypokalaemia and increased blood glucose levels. Diabetic patients may be unable to compensate for the increase in blood glucose and the development of ketoacidosis has been reported. Concurrent administration of corticosteroids can exaggerate this effect.

Therefore, diabetic patients and those concurrently receiving corticosteroids should be monitored frequently during intravenous infusion of Ventolin so that remedial steps (e.g. an increase in insulin dosage) can be taken to counter any metabolic change occurring. For these patients it may be preferable to dilute Ventolin Solution for Intravenous Infusion in Sodium Chloride Injection BP rather than in diluents containing dextrose.

Salbutamol should be administered cautiously to patients suffering from thyrotoxicosis.

Potentially serious hypokalaemia may result from β_2-agonist therapy, mainly from parenteral and nebulised administration. Particular caution is advised in acute severe asthma as this effect may be potentiated by hypoxia and by concomitant treatment with xanthine derivatives, steroids and diuretics. Serum potassium levels should be monitored in such situations.

As maternal pulmonary oedema has been reported during or following treatment of premature labour with β_2-agonists, careful attention should be given to fluid balance and cardio-respiratory function monitored. In patients being treated for premature labour by intravenous infusion of salbutamol, increases in maternal heart rate of the order of 20 to 50 beats per minute usually accompany the infusion. The maternal pulse rate should be monitored and not normally allowed to exceed a steady rate of 140 beats per minute. Maternal blood pressure may fall slightly during the infusion; the effect being greater on diastolic than on systolic pressure. Falls in diastolic pressure are usually within the range of 10 to 20mmHg. The effect of infusion on fetal heart rate is less marked, but increases of up to 20 beats per minute may occur. In the treatment of premature labour, before Ventolin Solution for Intravenous Infusion is given to any patient with known heart disease, an adequate assessment of the patient's cardiovascular status should be made by a physician experienced in cardiology. In order to minimise the risk of hypotension associated with tocolytic therapy, special care should be taken to avoid caval compression by keeping the patient in the left or right lateral positions throughout the infusion.

4.5 Interaction with other medicinal products and other forms of Interaction
Ventolin Solution for Intravenous Infusion should not be administered in the same syringe or infusion as any other medication.

Salbutamol and non-selective β-blocking drugs such as propranolol, should not usually be prescribed together.

4.6 Pregnancy and lactation
Administration of drugs during pregnancy should only be considered if the expected benefit to the mother is greater than any possible risk to the fetus. As with the majority of drugs, there is little published evidence of the safety of salbutamol in the early stages of human pregnancy, but in animal studies there was evidence of some harmful effects on the fetus at very high dose levels. As salbutamol is probably secreted in breast milk, its use in nursing mothers requires careful consideration. It is not known whether salbutamol has a harmful effect on the neonate, and so its use should be restricted to situations where it is felt that the expected benefit to the mother is likely to outweigh any potential risk to the neonate.

4.7 Effects on ability to drive and use machines
None reported.

4.8 Undesirable effects
Hypersensitivity reactions including angioedema, urticaria, bronchospasm, hypotension and collapse have been reported very rarely. Enhancement of physiological tremor may occur with Ventolin Solution for Intravenous Infusion. This effect is caused by a direct action on skeletal muscle and is common to all β-adrenergic stimulants.

Tachycardia, with or without dilatation of peripheral arterioles leading to a small reduction in arterial pressure, may occur. Increases in heart rate are more likely to occur in patients with normal heart rates and these increases are dose-dependent. In patients with pre-existing sinus tachycardia, especially those in status asthmaticus, the heart rate tends to fall as the condition of the patient improves. In common with other β2-agonists, cardiac arrhythmias (including atrial fibrillation, Supraventricular tachycardia and extrasystoles) have been reported in association with the use of salbutamol, usually in susceptible patients.

Maternal pulmonary oedema has been reported in association with use of β-agonists, including salbutamol, for the management of premature labour; in some cases this has proved fatal. Predisposing factors include fluid overload, multiple pregnancy, pre-existing cardiac disease and maternal infection. Close monitoring of the patient's state of hydration is essential. If signs of pulmonary oedema develop (e.g. cough, shortness of breath), treatment should be discontinued immediately and diuretic therapy instituted.

Headaches have occasionally been reported.

There have been very rare reports of muscle cramps.

Potentially serious hypokalaemia may result from β_2-agonist therapy.

In the management of premature labour, intravenous infusion of Ventolin has occasionally been associated with nausea, vomiting and headaches.

4.9 Overdose
The preferred antidote for overdosage with salbutamol is a cardioselective β-blocking agent, but β-blocking drugs should be used with caution in patients with a history of bronchospasm.

Hypokalaemia may occur following overdose with salbutamol. Serum potassium levels should be monitored.

5. PHARMACOLOGICAL PROPERTIES

5.1 Pharmacodynamic properties

Salbutamol is a selective β_2-agonist which acts on the β_2-adrenoceptors of the bronchi and uterus.

5.2 Pharmacokinetic properties

Salbutamol administered intravenously has a half-life of 4 to 6 hours and is cleared partly renally and partly by metabolism to the inactive 4'-0-sulphate (phenolic sulphate) which is also excreted primarily in the urine. The faeces are a minor route of excretion. Most of a dose of salbutamol given intravenously, orally or by inhalation is excreted within 72 hours. Salbutamol is bound to plasma proteins to the extent of 10%.

5.3 Preclinical safety data

No additional preclinical safety data are included here.

6. PHARMACEUTICAL PARTICULARS

6.1 List of excipients

Sodium chloride, sodium hydroxide, sulphuric acid and Water for Injections.

6.2 Incompatibilities

None stated.

6.3 Shelf life

36 months.

24 hours after mixing with infusion fluids.

6.4 Special precautions for storage

Store below 30°C and keep container in the outer carton.

6.5 Nature and contents of container

Clear, neutral glass ampoules, available in boxes of 10 ampoules or 5 ampoules.

6.6 Instructions for use and handling

Ventolin Solution for Intravenous Infusion must be diluted before use. The recommended diluents are Water for Injections BP, Sodium Chloride Injection BP, Sodium Chloride and Dextrose Injection BP and Dextrose Injection BP. (See Posology and method of administration.)

All unused admixtures of Ventolin Solution for Intravenous Infusion with infusion fluids should be discarded twenty-four hours after preparation.

Administrative Data

7. MARKETING AUTHORISATION HOLDER

Glaxo Wellcome UK Ltd,

trading as Allen & Hanburys,

Stockley Park West,

Uxbridge,

Middlesex,

UB11 1BT.

8. MARKETING AUTHORISATION NUMBER(S)

PL 10949/0087

9. DATE OF FIRST AUTHORISATION/RENEWAL OF THE AUTHORISATION

11 September 2000

10. DATE OF REVISION OF THE TEXT

21st October 2003

11. Legal Status

POM.

Ventolin is a trade mark of the Glaxo Wellcome Group of Companies

Ventolin Syrup

(Allen & Hanburys)

1. NAME OF THE MEDICINAL PRODUCT

Ventolin Syrup

2. QUALITATIVE AND QUANTITATIVE COMPOSITION

Each 5 ml contains 2 mg Salbutamol (as Salbutamol Sulphate BP).

3. PHARMACEUTICAL FORM

Syrup

4. CLINICAL PARTICULARS

4.1 Therapeutic indications

Salbutamol is a selective beta-2 adrenoceptor agonist providing short-acting (4-6 hour) bronchodilatation in reversible airways obstruction. Ventolin syrup can be used in the management of asthma, bronchospasm and/or reversible airways obstruction.

Relief of bronchospasm in bronchial asthma of all types.

Ventolin syrup is suitable oral therapy for children and adults who are unable to use an inhaler device.

4.2 Posology and method of administration

Route of administration: oral

Adults

The minimum starting dose is 2mg three times a day given as 5ml syrup. The usual effective dose is 4mg (10ml syrup) three or four times a day, which may be increased to a maximum of 8mg (20ml syrup) three or four times a day if adequate bronchodilatation is not obtained.

Elderly

In elderly patients or in those known to be unusually sensitive to beta-adrenergic stimulant drugs, it is advisable to initiate treatment with the minimum starting dose.

Children

2 - 6 years: the minimum starting dose is 1mg as 2.5ml of syrup three times daily. This may be increased to 2mg as 5ml of syrup three or four times daily.

6-12 years: the minimum starting dose is 2mg as 5ml syrup three times daily. This may be increased to four times daily.

Over 12 years: the minimum starting dose is 2mg three times daily given as 5ml syrup. This may be increased to 4mg as 10ml syrup three or four times daily.

Ventolin is well tolerated by children so that, if necessary, these doses may be cautiously increased to the maximum dose.

For lower doses the syrup may be diluted with freshly prepared purified water BP.

4.3 Contraindications

Although intravenous salbutamol and occasionally salbutamol tablets are used in the management of premature labour, uncomplicated by conditions such as placenta praevia, ante-partum haemorrhage, or toxaemia of pregnancy, salbutamol presentations should not be used for threatened abortion.

Ventolin oral preparations are contra-indicated in patients with a history of hypersensitivity to any of their components.

4.4 Special warnings and special precautions for use

Bronchodilators should not be the only or main treatment in patients with severe or unstable asthma. Severe asthma requires regular medical assessment including lung function testing as patients are at risk of severe attacks and even death. Physicians should consider using oral corticosteroid therapy and/or the maximum recommended dose of inhaled corticosteroid in those patients.

Patients should seek medical advice if treatment with Ventolin syrup becomes less effective.

The dosage or frequency of administration should only be increased on medical advice.

Patients taking Ventolin syrup may also be receiving short-acting inhaled bronchodilators to relieve symptoms.

Increasing use of bronchodilators in particular short-acting inhaled beta$_2$-agonists to relieve symptoms indicates deterioration of asthma control. The patient should be instructed to seek medical advice if short-acting relief bronchodilator treatment becomes less effective or they need more inhalations than usual.

In this situation patients should be reassessed and consideration given to the need for increased anti-inflammatory therapy (eg. Higher doses of inhaled corticosteroids or a course of oral corticosteroid). Severe exacerbations of asthma must be treated in the normal way.

Patients should be warned that if either the usual relief with Ventolin oral preparations is diminished or the usual duration of action reduced, they should not increase the dose or its frequency of administration, but should seek medical advice.

Ventolin syrup and non-selective beta-blocking drugs, such as propranolol, should not usually be prescribed together.

Salbutamol should be administered cautiously to patients suffering from thyrotoxicosis.

Potentially serious hypokalaemia may result from beta-2 agonist therapy mainly from parenteral and nebulised administration. Particular caution is advised in acute severe asthma as this effect may be potentiated by hypoxia and by concomitant treatment with xanthine derivatives, steroids. It is recommended that serum potassium levels are monitored is such situations.

In common with other β-adrenoceptor agonists, salbutamol can induce reversible metabolic changes such as increased blood glucose levels. Diabetic patients may be unable to compensate for the increase in blood glucose and the development of ketoacidosis has been reported. Concurrent administration of corticosteroids can exaggerate this effect.

4.5 Interaction with other medicinal products and other forms of Interaction

None known.

4.6 Pregnancy and lactation

Administration of drugs during pregnancy should only be considered if the expected benefit to the mother is greater than any possible risk to the foetus.

As with the majority of drugs, there is little published evidence of its safety in the early stages of human pregnancy, but in animal studies there was evidence of some harmful effects on the foetus at very high dose levels.

As salbutamol is probably secreted in breast milk its use in nursing mothers requires careful consideration. It is not known whether salbutamol has a harmful effect on the neonate, and so its use should be restricted to situations where it is felt that the expected benefit to the mother is likely to outweigh any potential risk to the neonate.

4.7 Effects on ability to drive and use machines

None known.

4.8 Undesirable effects

Adverse events are listed below by system organ class and frequency. Frequencies are defined as: very common (≥1/10), common (≥1/100 and <1/10), uncommon (≥1/1000 and <1/100), rare (≥1/10,000 and <1/1000) and very rare (<1/10,000) including isolated reports. Very common and common events were generally determined from clinical trial data. Rare and very rare events were generally determined from spontaneous data.

Immune system disorders

Very rare: Hypersensitivity reactions including angioedema, urticaria, bronchospasm, hypotension and collapse.

Metabolism and nutrition disorders

Rare: Hypokalaemia.

Potentially serious hypokalaemia may result from beta agonist therapy.

Nervous system disorders

Very common: Tremor.

Common: Headache.

Very rare: Hyperactivity.

Cardiac disorders

Common: Tachycardia.

Rare: Cardiac arrhythmias including atrial fibrillation, supraventricular tachycardia and extrasystoles

Vascular disorders

Rare: Peripheral vasodilatation.

Musculoskeletal and connective tissue disorders

Common: Muscle cramps.

Very rare: Feeling of muscle tension.

4.9 Overdose

The preferred antidote for overdosage with Ventolin is a cardio-selective beta-blocking agent but beta-blocking drugs should be used with caution in patients with a history of bronchospasm.

Hypokalaemia may occur following overdose with salbutamol. Serum potassium levels should be monitored.

5. PHARMACOLOGICAL PROPERTIES

5.1 Pharmacodynamic properties

Salbutamol is a selective beta-2 adrenoceptor agonist. At therapeutic doses it acts on the beta-2 adrenoceptors of bronchial muscle.

5.2 Pharmacokinetic properties

Salbutamol administered intravenously has a half life of 4 to 6 hours and is cleared partly renally and partly by metabolism to the inactive 4' -O-sulphate (phenolic sulphate) which is also excreted primarily in the urine. The faeces are a minor route of excretion. The majority of a dose of salbutamol given intravenously, orally or by inhalation is excreted within 72 hours. Salbutamol is bound to plasma proteins to the extent of 10%.

After oral administration, salbutamol is absorbed from the gastrointestinal tract and undergoes considerable first-pass metabolism to the phenolic sulphate. Both unchanged drug and conjugate are excreted primarily in the urine. The bioavailability of orally administered salbutamol is about 50%.

5.3 Preclinical safety data

There are no preclinical data of relevance to the prescriber which are additional to that in other sections of the SmPC.

6. PHARMACEUTICAL PARTICULARS

6.1 List of excipients

Sodium citrate

Citric acid monohydrate

Hydroxypropyl methylcellulose

Sodium benzoate

Saccharin sodium

Sodium chloride

Orange flavour IFF 17.42.8187

Purified water

6.2 Incompatibilities

None known.

Ventolin syrup is sugar free. If dilution is required freshly prepared Purified Water BP should be used. The diluted mixture must be protected from light and stored below 25°C.

6.3 Shelf life

36 months.

6.4 Special precautions for storage

Store at a temperature not exceeding 30°C.

Protect from light.

Ventolin syrup may be diluted with freshly Purified Water BP. The diluted mixture must be protected from light and stored below 25°C. Discard after 28 days.

6.5 Nature and contents of container

Amber glass bottle.

Closure (150ml): plastic tamper evident, child resistant or plastic child resistant or ROPP aluminium (lacquered internally and externally) with either PVdC faced EPE or

LDPE faced PVdC/EPE OR LLDPE/PVdC-PVC/LLDPE/EPE (single or double faced) wad.

Closure (2000ml): polypropylene cap with wadding as for 150ml.

Pack size: 150ml, 2000ml.

6.6 Instructions for use and handling
No special instructions.

Administrative Data

7. MARKETING AUTHORISATION HOLDER
Glaxo Wellcome UK Ltd
trading as Allen & Hanburys
Stockley Park West
Uxbridge
Middlesex, UB11 1BT

8. MARKETING AUTHORISATION NUMBER(S)
PL 10949/0088

9. DATE OF FIRST AUTHORISATION/RENEWAL OF THE AUTHORISATION
27 April 2000

10. DATE OF REVISION OF THE TEXT
12 April 2005

Babyhaler, Evohaler, Ventolin and Volumatic are trade marks of the Glaxo Wellcome Group of Companies.

Vepesid Capsules 50 mg and 100 mg

(Bristol-Myers Pharmaceuticals)

1. NAME OF THE MEDICINAL PRODUCT
Vepesid Capsules 50 mg and 100 mg

2. QUALITATIVE AND QUANTITATIVE COMPOSITION
Pale pink, soft gelatin capsules containing 50 mg or 100 mg etoposide.

3. PHARMACEUTICAL FORM
Oral capsules

4. CLINICAL PARTICULARS

4.1 Therapeutic indications
Vepesid is an anti-neoplastic drug for intravenous or oral use, which can be used alone or in combination with other oncolytic drugs.

Present data indicate that Vepesid is applicable in the therapy of: small cell lung cancer, resistant non-seminomatous testicular carcinoma.

4.2 Posology and method of administration
The recommended course of Vepesid capsules is 120-240 mg/m^2 orally daily, for five consecutive days. The dose of Vepesid capsules is based on the recommended i.v. dose with consideration given to the bioavailability of Vepesid capsules appearing to be dependent upon the dose administered. The bioavailability also varies from patient to patient following any oral dose. This should be taken into consideration when prescribing this medication. In view of significant intra-patient variability, dose adjustments may be required in order to achieve the desired therapeutic effect. As Vepesid produces myelosuppression, courses may not be repeated more frequently than at 21 day intervals. In any case, a repeat course of Vepesid should not be given until the blood picture has been checked for evidence of myelosuppression and found to be satisfactory.

The capsules should be taken on an empty stomach.

Elderly:

No dosage adjustment is necessary.

Paediatric use:

Safety and effectiveness in children have not been established.

4.3 Contraindications
Vepesid is contra-indicated in patients with severe hepatic dysfunction or in those patients who have demonstrated hypersensitivity to the drug.

4.4 Special warnings and special precautions for use
Vepesid should be administered by individuals experienced in the use of anti-neoplastic therapy.

When Vepesid is administered intravenously care should be taken to avoid extravasation.

If radiotherapy and/or chemotherapy has been given prior to starting Vepesid treatment, an adequate interval should be allowed to enable the bone marrow to recover. If the leucocyte count falls below 2,000mm^3, treatment should be suspended until the circulating blood elements have returned to acceptable levels (platelets above 100,000 mm^3, leucocytes above 4,000/mm^3), this is usually within 10 days.

Peripheral blood counts and liver function should be monitored. (See Undesirable Effects.)

Bacterial infections should be brought under control before treatment with Vepesid commences.

The occurrence of acute leukaemia, which can occur with or without a preleukaemic phase has been reported rarely in patients treated with etoposide in association with other anti-neoplastic drugs.

Neither the cumulative risk, nor the predisposing factors related to the development of secondary leukaemia are known. The roles of both administration schedules and cumulative doses of etoposide have been suggested, but have not been clearly defined.

An 11q23 chromosome abnormality has been observed in some cases of secondary leukaemia in patients who have received epipodophyllotoxins. This abnormality has also been seen in patients developing secondary leukaemia after being treated with chemotherapy regimens not containing epipodophyllotoxins and in leukaemia occurring *de novo*. Another characteristic that has been associated with secondary leukaemia in patients who have received epipodophyllotoxins appears to be a short latency period, with average median time to development of leukaemia being approximately 32 months.

Tumour lysis syndrome (sometimes fatal) has been reported following the use of etoposide in association with other chemotherapeutic drugs. Close monitoring of patients is needed to detect early signs of tumour lysis syndrome, especially in patients with risk factors such as bulky treatment-sensitive tumours, and renal insufficiency. Appropriate preventive measures should also be considered in patients at risk of this complication of therapy.

4.5 Interaction with other medicinal products and other forms of Interaction
Co-administration of oral etoposide with high doses of cyclosporin (resulting in concentrations above 2000 ng/ml) has led to an 80% increase in etoposide exposure (AUC). Total body clearance of etoposide decreased by 38% compared to etoposide alone.

4.6 Pregnancy and lactation
Vepesid is teratogenic in rats and mice at dose levels equivalent to those employed clinically. There are no adequate and well-controlled studies in pregnant women.

Vepesid should not normally be administered to patients who are pregnant or to mothers who are breast feeding. Women of childbearing potential should be advised to avoid becoming pregnant.

The influence of Vepesid on human reproduction has not been determined.

In-vitro tests indicate that Vepesid is mutagenic.

4.7 Effects on ability to drive and use machines
None stated.

4.8 Undesirable effects
Haematological:

The dose limiting toxicity of Vepesid is myelosuppression, predominantly leucopenia and thrombocytopenia. Anaemia occurs infrequently.

The leucocyte count nadir occurs approximately 21 days after treatment.

Alopecia:

Alopecia occurs in approximately two-thirds of patients and is reversible on cessation of therapy.

Gastrointestinal:

Nausea and vomiting are the major gastrointestinal toxicities and occur in over one-third of patients. Anti-emetics are useful in controlling these side effects. Abdominal pain, anorexia, diarrhoea, oesophagitis and stomatitis occur infrequently.

Other Toxicities:

Hypotension may occur following an excessively rapid infusion and may be reversed by slowing the infusion rate.

Anaphylactoid reactions have been reported following administration of Vepesid. Higher rates of anaphylactoid reactions have been reported in children who received infusions at concentrations higher than those recommended. The role that concentration of infusion (or rate of infusion) plays in the development of anaphylactoid reactions is uncertain. These reactions have usually responded to cessation of therapy and administration of pressor agents, corticosteroids, antihistamines or volume expanders as appropriate.

Apnoea with spontaneous resumption of breathing following discontinuation of etoposide injection has been reported. Sudden fatal reactions associated with bronchospasm have been reported. Hypertension and/or flushing have also been reported. Blood pressure usually returns to normal within a few hours after cessation of the infusion.

The use of etoposide has been reported infrequently to cause peripheral neuropathy.

Vepesid has been shown to reach high concentrations in the liver and kidney, thus presenting a potential for accumulation in cases of functional impairment.

Somnolence, fatigue, aftertaste, fever, rash, pigmentation, pruritus, urticaria, dysphagia, transient cortical blindness and a single case of radiation recall dermatitis have also been reported following the administration of Vepesid.

Neoplasms benign, malignant and unspecified:

Tumour lysis syndrome (sometimes fatal) has been reported very rarely (see Section 4.4 Special Warnings and Precautions for Use).

4.9 Overdose
No proven antidotes have been established for Vepesid overdosage. Treatment should be symptomatic and supportive.

Total doses of 2.4 to 3.5 g/m^2 administered i.v. over three days have resulted in severe mucositis and myelotoxicity. Metabolic acidosis and cases of severe hepatic toxicity have been reported in patients receiving higher than recommended doses of etoposide.

5. PHARMACOLOGICAL PROPERTIES

5.1 Pharmacodynamic properties
Etoposide is a semi-synthetic derivative of podophyllotoxin.

Experimental data indicate that etoposide arrests the cell cycle in the G^2 phase. Etoposide differs from the vinca alkaloids in that it does not cause an accumulation of cells in metaphase, but prevents cells from entering mitosis or destroys cells in the G^2 phase. The incorporation of thymidine into DNA is inhibited *in vitro* by etoposide. Etoposide does not interfere with microtubule assembly.

5.2 Pharmacokinetic properties
Etoposide is approximately 94% protein-bound in human serum. Plasma decay kinetics follow a bi-exponential curve and correspond to a two compartmental model. The mean volume of distribution is approximately 32% of body weight. Etoposide demonstrates relatively poor penetration into the cerebrospinal fluid. Urinary excretion is approximately 45% of an administered dose, 29% being excreted unchanged in 72 hours.

5.3 Preclinical safety data
No further relevant data.

6. PHARMACEUTICAL PARTICULARS

6.1 List of excipients
Other ingredients: Citric acid, glycerol, polyethylene glycol 400, water. Gelatin capsules containing glycerol, iron oxide, sodium hydroxybenzoic acid ethyl ester, sodium propylhydroxybenzoate, titanium dioxide, water.

6.2 Incompatibilities
None stated.

6.3 Shelf life
36 months

6.4 Special precautions for storage
Do not store above 25°C. Do not open any blister in which there is evidence of capsule leakage.

6.5 Nature and contents of container
Vepesid 50 mg capsules are packed in blister packs of 20 capsules, each capsule containing 50 mg etoposide.

Vepesid 100 mg capsules are packed in blister packs of 10 capsules, each capsule containing 100 mg etoposide.

6.6 Instructions for use and handling
Vepesid should be administered by individuals experienced in the use of anti-neoplastic therapy.

7. MARKETING AUTHORISATION HOLDER
Bristol-Myers Squibb Holdings Limited
t/a Bristol-Myers Pharmaceuticals
Uxbridge Business Park
Sanderson Road
Uxbridge
Middlesex
UB8 1DH

8. MARKETING AUTHORISATION NUMBER(S)

Vepesid Capsules 50 mg	PL 0125/0153
Vepesid Capsules 100mg	PL 0125/0124

9. DATE OF FIRST AUTHORISATION/RENEWAL OF THE AUTHORISATION

Vepesid Capsules 50 mg	29 April 1983 / 18 September 2002
Vepesid Capsules 100mg	03 July 1981 / 26 November 2003

10. DATE OF REVISION OF THE TEXT
July 2005

Vepesid Injection for Infusion 20mg/ml (5.0 ml Vial)

(Bristol-Myers Pharmaceuticals)

1. NAME OF THE MEDICINAL PRODUCT
VEPESID INJECTION FOR INFUSION 20MG/ML (5.0 ML VIAL)

2. QUALITATIVE AND QUANTITATIVE COMPOSITION
Etoposide 20mg/ml. The 5ml vials contains 100mg etoposide.

3. PHARMACEUTICAL FORM
Concentrate for solution for infusion.

4. CLINICAL PARTICULARS

4.1 Therapeutic indications

Vepesid is an anti-neoplastic drug for intravenous or oral use, which can be used alone or in combination with other oncolytic drugs.

Present data indicate that Vepesid is applicable in the therapy of: small cell lung cancer, resistant non-seminomatous testicular carcinoma.

4.2 Posology and method of administration

Adults:

The recommended course of Vepesid Injection is 60-120mg/m^2, i.v. daily for five consecutive days. As Vepesid produces myelosuppression, courses may not be repeated more frequently than at 21 day intervals. In any case, repeat courses of Vepesid should not be given until the blood picture has been checked for evidence for myelosuppression and found to be satisfactory.

Immediately before administration, the required dose of Vepesid Injection must be diluted with 0.9% saline solution for injection to give a solution concentration of not more than 0.25mg/ml of etoposide; it should then be given by intravenous infusion over a period of not less than 30 minutes.

Care should be taken to avoid extravasation.

Children:

Safety and effectiveness in children have not been established.

Elderly:

No dosage adjustment is necessary.

4.3 Contraindications

Vepesid is contra-indicated in patients with severe hepatic dysfunction or in those patients who have demonstrated hypersensitivity to the drug.

Vepesid must not be given by intra-cavitary injection

4.4 Special warnings and special precautions for use

Vepesid should be administered by individuals experienced in the use of anti-neoplastic therapy.

When Vepesid is administered intravenously care should be taken to avoid extravasation.

If radiotherapy and/or chemotherapy has been given prior to starting Vepesid treatment, an adequate interval should be allowed to enable the bone marrow to recover. If the leucocyte count falls below 2000/mm^3, treatment should be suspended until the circulating blood elements have returned to acceptable levels (platelets above 100,000/mm^3, leucocytes above 4000/mm^3), this is usually within 10 days.

Peripheral blood counts and liver function should be monitored. (See Undesirable effects.)

Bacterial infections should be brought under control before treatment with Vepesid commences.

The occurrence of acute leukaemia, which can occur with or without a preleukaemic phase has been reported rarely in patients treated with etoposide in association with other anti-neoplastic drugs.

Tumour lysis syndrome (sometimes fatal) has been reported following the use of etoposide in association with other chemotherapeutic drugs. Close monitoring of patients is needed to detect early signs of tumour lysis syndrome, especially in patients with risk factors such as bulky treatment-sensitive tumours, and renal insufficiency. Appropriate preventive measures should also be considered in patients at risk of this complication of therapy.

4.5 Interaction with other medicinal products and other forms of Interaction

None known.

4.6 Pregnancy and lactation

Vepesid is teratogenic in rats and mice at dose levels equivalent to those employed clinically. There are no adequate and well-controlled studies in pregnant women.

Vepesid should not normally be administered to patients who are pregnant or to mothers who are breast feeding. Women of childbearing potential should be advised to avoid becoming pregnant.

The influence of Vepesid on human reproduction has not been determined. *In-vitro* tests indicate that Vepesid is mutagenic.

4.7 Effects on ability to drive and use machines

None known.

4.8 Undesirable effects

Haematological: The dose limiting toxicity of Vepesid is myelosuppression, predominantly leucopenia and thrombocytopenia. Anaemia occurs infrequently. The leucocyte count nadir occurs approximately 21 days after treatment.

Alopecia: Alopecia occurs in approximately two-thirds of patients and is reversible on cessation of therapy.

Gastrointestinal: Nausea and vomiting are the major gastrointestinal toxicities and occur in over one-third of patients. Anti-emetics are useful in controlling these side-effects. Abdominal pain, anorexia, diarrhoea, oesophagitis and stomatitis occur infrequently.

Other Toxicities: Hypotension may occur following an excessively rapid infusion and may be reversed by slowing the infusion rate.

Anaphylactoid reactions have been reported following administration of Vepesid. Higher rates of anaphylactoid reactions have been reported in children who received infusions at concentrations higher than those recommended. The role that concentration of infusion (or rate of infusion) plays in the development of anaphylactoid reactions is uncertain. These reactions have usually responded to cessation of therapy and administration of pressor agents, corticosteroids, antihistamines or volume expanders as appropriate.

Apnoea with spontaneous resumption of breathing following discontinuation of etoposide injection has been reported. Sudden fatal reactions associated with bronchospasm have been reported. Hypertension and/or flushing have also been reported. Blood pressure usually returns to normal within a few hours after cessation of the infusion.

The use of etoposide has been reported infrequently to cause peripheral neuropathy.

Vepesid has been shown to reach high concentrations in the liver and kidney, thus presenting a potential for accumulation in cases of functional impairment.

Somnolence, fatigue, aftertaste, fever, rash, pigmentation, pruritus, urticaria, dysphagia, transient cortical blindness and a single case of radiation recall dermatitis have also been reported following the administration of Vepesid.

Neoplasms benign, malignant and unspecified:

Tumour lysis syndrome (sometimes fatal) has been reported very rarely (see Section 4.4 Special Warnings and Precautions for Use).

4.9 Overdose

No proven antidotes have been established for Vepesid overdosage. Treatment should be symptomatic and supportive.

Total doses of 2.4 to 3.5 g/m^2 administered i.v. over three days have resulted in severe mucositis and myelotoxicity. Metabolic acidosis and cases of severe hepatic toxicity have been reported in patients receiving higher than recommended doses of etoposide.

5. PHARMACOLOGICAL PROPERTIES

5.1 Pharmacodynamic properties

Etoposide is a semisynthetic derivative of podophyllotoxin.

Experimental data indicate that etoposide arrests the cell cycle in the G_2 phase. Etoposide differs from the vinca alkaloids in that it does not cause an accumulation of cells in the metaphase, but prevents cells from entering mitosis or destroys cells in the G_2 phase. The incorporation of the thymidine into DNA is inhibited *in-vitro* by etoposide. Etoposide does not interfere with microtubule assembly.

5.2 Pharmacokinetic properties

Etoposide is approximately 94% protein-bound in human serum. Plasma decay kinetics follow a bi-exponential curve and correspond to a two compartmental model. The mean volume of distribution is approximately 32% of body weight. Etoposide demonstrates relatively poor penetration into the cerebrospinal fluid. Urinary excretion is approximately 45% of an administered dose, 29% being excreted unchanged in 72 hours.

5.3 Preclinical safety data

No further relevant data.

6. PHARMACEUTICAL PARTICULARS

6.1 List of excipients

Benzyl alcohol, citric acid anhydrous, dehydrated ethanol, polyethylene glycol 300, polysorbate 80.

6.2 Incompatibilities

None known

6.3 Shelf life

3 Years.

6.4 Special precautions for storage

Unopened vials:	Do not store above 25°C. Protect from light.
Diluted infusion solution:	After dilution as recommended to a concentration of 0.2 or 0.4 mg/ml, the infusion solution has been demonstrated to be physically and chemically stable at 25°C for 96 and 24 hours respectively.

From a microbiological point of view, the product should be used immediately after dilution.

Other in-use storage times and conditions prior to use are the responsibility of the user.

6.5 Nature and contents of container

Type I flint glass vial with grey butyl rubber parenteral stopper and sealed with flip-off plastic/aluminium cap. Vepesid Injection is packed in cartons containing '10 × 5ml' vials.

6.6 Instructions for use and handling

Preparation of Intravenous Solution:

Immediately before administration the required dose of Vepesid Injection must be diluted with 0.9% saline solution for injection to give a solution concentration of not more than 0.25mg/ml of etoposide; it should then be given by intravenous infusion over a period of not less than 30 minutes. The infusion solution should be used immediately after dilution. Solutions of concentration greater than 0.25mg/ml may show signs of precipitation, and are therefore not recommended. Any solutions showing signs of precipitation should be discarded.

The intravenous solution is suitable for infusion in glass or PVC containers.

Hard plastic devices made of acrylic or ABS (a polymer composed of acrylonitrile, butadiene and styrene) have been reported to crack and leak when used with undiluted Vepesid Injection. This effect has not been reported with diluted Vepesid Injection.

Vepesid should not be physically mixed with any other drug.

Guidelines for the Safe Handling of Antineoplastic Agents:

1. Trained personnel should reconstitute the drug.
2. This should be performed in a designated area.
3. Adequate protective gloves should be worn.
4. Precautions should be taken to avoid the drug accidentally coming into contact with the eyes. In the event of contact with the eyes, irrigate with large amounts of water and/or saline.
5. The cytotoxic preparation should not be handled by pregnant staff.
6. Adequate care and precautions should be taken in the disposal of items (syringes, needles etc) used to reconstitute cytotoxic drugs. Excess material and body waste may be disposed of by placing in double sealed polythene bags and incinerating at a temperature of 1,000°C. Liquid waste may be flushed with copious amounts of water.
7. The work surface should be covered with disposable plastic-backed absorbent paper.
8. Use Luer-lock fittings on all syringes and sets. Large bore needles are recommended to minimise pressure and the possible formation of aerosols. The latter may also be reduced by the use of a venting needle.

7. MARKETING AUTHORISATION HOLDER

Bristol-Myers Squibb Holdings Limited

t/a Bristol-Myers Pharmaceuticals

Uxbridge Business Park

Sanderson Road

Uxbridge

Middlesex

UB8 1DH

8. MARKETING AUTHORISATION NUMBER(S)

PL 0125/0184

9. DATE OF FIRST AUTHORISATION/RENEWAL OF THE AUTHORISATION

03 March 1988 / 26 November 2003

10. DATE OF REVISION OF THE TEXT

July 2005

Vermox Suspension

(Janssen-Cilag Ltd)

1. NAME OF THE MEDICINAL PRODUCT

Vermox™ Suspension.

2. QUALITATIVE AND QUANTITATIVE COMPOSITION

Each 5 ml of suspension contains mebendazole PhEur 100 mg.

3. PHARMACEUTICAL FORM

White homogeneous oral suspension.

4. CLINICAL PARTICULARS

4.1 Therapeutic indications

Broad spectrum gastrointestinal anthelmintic indicated for the treatment of:

Enterobius vermicularis (threadworm/pinworm)

Oxyuris vermicularis

Trichuris trichuria (whipworm)

Ascaris lumbricoides (large roundworm)

Ancylostoma duodenale (common hookworm)

Necator americanus (American hookworm)

There is no evidence that Vermox Suspension is effective in the treatment of cysticercosis.

4.2 Posology and method of administration

Method of administration.

Oral Use

Adults and children over 2 years:

Enterobiasis:

1 × 5 ml (1 dosing cup).

It is highly recommended that a second dose is taken after two weeks, if reinfection is suspected.

Ascariasis, trichuriasis, ancylostomiasis, necatoriasis and mixed infections:

1 × 5 ml (1 dosing cup) bd for three days.

4.3 Contraindications
Vermox is contra-indicated in pregnancy and in patients who have shown hypersensitivity to the product or any components.

4.4 Special warnings and special precautions for use
Not recommended in the treatment of children under 2 years.

A case-control study of a single outbreak of Stevens-Johnson syndrome /toxic epidermal necrolysis (SJS/TEN) suggested a possible association with the concomitant use of metronidazole with mebendazole. Although there are no additional data on this potential interaction, concomitant use of mebendazole and metronidazole should be avoided.

4.5 Interaction with other medicinal products and other forms of Interaction
Concomitant treatment with cimetidine may inhibit the metabolism of mebendazole in the liver, resulting in increased plasma concentrations of the drug.

Concomitant use of mebendazole and metronidazole should be avoided (see section 4.4).

4.6 Pregnancy and lactation
Since Vermox is contra-indicated in pregnancy, patients who think they are or may be pregnant should not take this preparation.

As it is not known whether mebendazole is excreted in human milk, it is not advisable to breast feed following administration of Vermox.

4.7 Effects on ability to drive and use machines
None known.

4.8 Undesirable effects
At the recommended dose, Vermox is generally well tolerated. However, patients with high parasitic burdens when treated with Vermox have manifested diarrhoea and abdominal pain.

Post-marketing experience

Within each system organ class, the adverse drug reactions are ranked under the headings of reporting frequency, using the following convention:

Very common >1/10) Common >1/100, < 1/10) Uncommon >1/1000, < 1/100) Rare >1/10000, < 1/1000) Very rare (< 1/10000) including isolated reports.

Immune system disorders

Very rare: hypersensitivity reactions such as anaphylactic and anaphylactoid reactions

Nervous system disorders

Very rare: convulsions in infants

Gastrointestinal disorders

Very rare: abdominal pain, diarrhoea (these symptoms can also be the result of the worm infestation itself)

Skin and subcutaneous tissue disorders

Very rare: toxic epidermal necrolysis, Stevens-Johnson syndrome (see also section 4.4), exanthema, angioedema, urticaria, rash

Adverse drug reactions reported with prolonged use at dosages substantially above those recommended

Liver function disturbances, hepatitis, glomerulonephritis and neutropenia.

4.9 Overdose
Symptoms

In the event of accidental overdosage, abdominal cramps, nausea, vomiting and diarrhoea may occur.

See also section 4.8. subheading 'Adverse drug reactions reported with prolonged use at dosages substantially above those recommended'.

Treatment

There is no specific antidote. Within the first hour after ingestion, gastric lavage may be performed. Activated charcoal may be given if considered appropriate.

5. PHARMACOLOGICAL PROPERTIES

5.1 Pharmacodynamic properties
In vitro and *in vivo* work suggests that mebendazole blocks the uptake of glucose by adult and larval forms of helminths, in a selective and irreversible manner. Inhibition of glucose uptake appears to lead to endogenous depletion of glycogen stores within the helminth. Lack of glycogen leads to decreased formation of ATP and ultrastructural changes in the cells.

There is no evidence that Vermox is effective in the treatment of cysticercosis.

5.2 Pharmacokinetic properties
Using a tracer dose of ^{3}H-mebendazole, the pharmacokinetics and bioavailability of a solution and IV drug have been examined. After oral administration, the half life was 0.93 hours. Absorption of this tracer dose was almost complete but low availability indicated a high first pass effect. At normal therapeutic doses, it is very hard to measure levels in the plasma.

5.3 Preclinical safety data
No relevant information additional to that contained elsewhere in the Summary of Product Characteristics.

6. PHARMACEUTICAL PARTICULARS

6.1 List of excipients
Sucrose

Microcrystalline cellulose and sodium carboxymethyl cellulose

Methylcellulose 15 mPa.s

Methylparaben

Propylparaben

Sodium lauryl sulphate

Banana 1

Citric acid, monohydrate

Purified water

6.2 Incompatibilities
None known.

6.3 Shelf life
5 years.

6.4 Special precautions for storage
Shake well before use.

Keep out of reach and sight of children.

6.5 Nature and contents of container
Amber glass flask containing 30 ml suspension, with either:

• Pilfer-proof screw cap. Cork insert in cap is coated on both sides with polyvinylchloride

or

• Child-resistant polypropylene screw cap, lined inside with a LDPE insert.

A 5ml natural polypropylene (food-grade) dosing cup is also provided, graduated for 2.5 ml and 5 ml.

6.6 Instructions for use and handling
Not applicable.

7. MARKETING AUTHORISATION HOLDER
Janssen-Cilag Ltd
Saunderton
High Wycombe
Buckinghamshire
HP14 4HJ
UK

8. MARKETING AUTHORISATION NUMBER(S)
PL 0242/0050

9. DATE OF FIRST AUTHORISATION/RENEWAL OF THE AUTHORISATION
Date of First Authorisation: 17 November 1977

Date of Renewal of Authorisation: 15 December 2002

10. DATE OF REVISION OF THE TEXT
June 2005

Legal category POM

(TM) trademark

Vermox Tablets

(Janssen-Cilag Ltd)

1. NAME OF THE MEDICINAL PRODUCT
Vermox tablets.

2. QUALITATIVE AND QUANTITATIVE COMPOSITION
Each tablet contains mebendazole 100 mg.

3. PHARMACEUTICAL FORM
Tablet.

4. CLINICAL PARTICULARS

4.1 Therapeutic indications
For the treatment of *Trichuris trichuria* (whipworm), *Enterobius vermicularis* (pinworm or threadworm), *Ascaris lumbricoides* (roundworm), *Ancylostoma duodenale* (common hookworm), *Necator americanus* (American hookworm) in single or mixed gastrointestinal infestations.

There is no evidence that Vermox Tablets are effective in the treatment of cysticercosis.

4.2 Posology and method of administration
Adults and children over 2 years:

For the control of trichuriasis, ascariasis and hookworm infections, one tablet twice a day for three consecutive days.

For the control of enterobiasis a single tablet is administered. It is highly recommended that a second tablet is taken after two weeks, if re-infection is suspected.

Tablets may be chewed or swallowed whole. Crush the tablet before giving it to a young child. Always supervise a child while they are taking this medicine.

Method of Administration

Oral use.

4.3 Contraindications
Vermox is contra-indicated in pregnancy and in patients who have shown hypersensitivity to the product or any components.

4.4 Special warnings and special precautions for use
Not recommended in the treatment of children under 2 years.

A case-control study of a single outbreak of Stevens-Johnson syndrome /toxic epidermal necrolysis (SJS/TEN) suggested a possible association with the concomitant use of metronidazole with mebendazole. Although there are no additional data on this potential interaction, concomitant use of mebendazole and metronidazole should be avoided.

4.5 Interaction with other medicinal products and other forms of Interaction
Concomitant treatment with cimetidine may inhibit the metabolism of mebendazole in the liver, resulting in increased plasma concentrations of the drug.

Concomitant use of mebendazole and metronidazole should be avoided (see section 4.4).

4.6 Pregnancy and lactation
Since Vermox is contra-indicated in pregnancy, patients who think they are, or may be, pregnant should not take this preparation.

Lactation

As it is not known whether mebendazole is excreted in human milk, it is not advisable to breast feed following administration of Vermox.

4.7 Effects on ability to drive and use machines
None stated.

4.8 Undesirable effects
At the recommended dose, Vermox is generally well tolerated. However, patients with high parasitic burdens when treated with Vermox have manifested diarrhoea and abdominal pain.

Post-marketing experience

Within each system organ class, the adverse drug reactions are ranked under the headings of reporting frequency, using the following convention:

Very common >1/10) Common >1/100, < 1/10) Uncommon >1/1000, < 1/100) Rare >1/10000, < 1/1000) Very rare (< 1/10000) including isolated reports.

Immune system disorders

Very rare: hypersensitivity reactions such as anaphylactic and anaphylactoid reactions

Nervous system disorders

Very rare: convulsions in infants

Gastrointestinal disorders

Very rare: abdominal pain, diarrhoea (these symptoms can also be the result of the worm infestation itself)

Skin and subcutaneous tissue disorders

Very rare: toxic epidermal necrolysis, Stevens-Johnson syndrome (see also section 4.4), exanthema, angioedema, urticaria, rash

Adverse drug reactions reported with prolonged use at dosages substantially above those recommended

Liver function disturbances, hepatitis, glomerulonephritis and neutropenia.

4.9 Overdose
Symptoms

In the event of accidental overdosage, abdominal cramps, nausea, vomiting and diarrhoea may occur.

See also section 4.8. subheading 'Adverse drug reactions reported with prolonged use at dosages substantially above those recommended'.

Treatment

There is no specific antidote. Within the first hour after ingestion, gastric lavage may be performed. activated charcoal may be given if considered appropriate.

5. PHARMACOLOGICAL PROPERTIES

5.1 Pharmacodynamic properties
In vitro and *in vivo* work suggests that mebendazole blocks the uptake of glucose by adult and larval forms of helminths, in a selective and irreversible manner. Inhibition of glucose uptake appears to lead to endogenous depletion of glycogen stores within the helminth. Lack of glycogen leads to decreased formation of ATP and ultrastructural changes in the cells.

There is no evidence that Vermox is effective in the treatment of cysticercosis.

5.2 Pharmacokinetic properties
Using a tracer dose of ^{3}H-mebendazole, the pharmacokinetics and bioavailability of a solution and IV drug have been examined. After oral administration, the half life was 0.93 hours. Absorption of this tracer dose was almost complete but low availability indicated a high first pass effect. At normal therapeutic doses, it is very hard to measure levels in the plasma.

5.3 Preclinical safety data
No relevant information additional to that contained elsewhere in the Summary of Product Characteristics.

6. PHARMACEUTICAL PARTICULARS

6.1 List of excipients

Microcrystalline cellulose

Sodium starch glycolate

Talc

Maize starch

Sodium saccharin

Magnesium stearate

Hydrogenated vegetable oil

Orange flavour

Colloidal anhydrous silica

Sodium lauryl sulphate

Orange yellow S

Purified water*

2-propanol*

* Not present in the final product.

6.2 Incompatibilities

Not applicable.

6.3 Shelf life

60 months.

6.4 Special precautions for storage

None.

6.5 Nature and contents of container

Blister strips of PVC genotherm glass clear aluminium foil coated on the inside with a heat seal lacquer.

Pack sizes: 1 and 6 tablet packs.

6.6 Instructions for use and handling

Not applicable

7. MARKETING AUTHORISATION HOLDER

Janssen-Cilag Ltd

Saunderton

High Wycombe

Buckinghamshire

HP14 4HJ

UK

8. MARKETING AUTHORISATION NUMBER(S)

PL 0242/0011

9. DATE OF FIRST AUTHORISATION/RENEWAL OF THE AUTHORISATION

Date of First Authorisation: 9 April 1975

Date of Renewal of Authorisation: 30 September 2003

10. DATE OF REVISION OF THE TEXT

June 2005

LEGAL CATEGORY POM.

Vesanoid

(Roche Products Limited)

1. NAME OF THE MEDICINAL PRODUCT

Vesanoid® 10mg capsules.

2. QUALITATIVE AND QUANTITATIVE COMPOSITION

1 capsule contains 10mg of tretinoin (all-trans retinoic acid)

For excipients, see section *6.1*.

3. PHARMACEUTICAL FORM

Capsule, soft.

Bi-coloured orange-yellow / reddish-brown capsules marked "ROCHE" on one side.

4. CLINICAL PARTICULARS

4.1 Therapeutic indications

Vesanoid (tretinoin) is indicated for induction of remission in acute promyelocytic leukaemia (APL; FAB classification AML-M3).

This treatment is intended for previously untreated patients as well as patients who relapse after a standard chemotherapy (anthracycline and cytosine arabinoside or equivalent therapies) or patients who are refractory to chemotherapy.

The association of tretinoin with chemotherapy increases the duration of survival and reduces the risk of relapse compared to chemotherapy alone.

4.2 Posology and method of administration

A total daily dose of 45mg/m^2 body surface divided in two equal doses is recommended for oral administration. This is approximately 8 capsules per adult dose.

It is recommended to take the capsules with a meal or shortly thereafter.

There is limited safety and efficacy information on the use of tretinoin in children.

Paediatric patients can be treated with 45mg/m^2 unless severe toxicity becomes apparent. Dose reduction should be particularly considered for children with intractable headache.

Treatment should be continued until complete remission has been achieved or up to a maximum of 90 days.

Due to limited information on patients with hepatic and/or renal insufficiency, the dose will be decreased to 25mg/m^2 as a precautionary measure.

Full-dose anthracycline-based chemotherapy should be added to the tretinoin regimen as follows (see section *4.4 Special warnings and special precautions for use*):

• When the leukocyte count at start of therapy is greater than 5 × 10^9/L, chemotherapy should be started together with tretinoin on day one.

• When the leukocyte count at start of therapy is less than 5 × 10^9/L but rapidly increases during tretinoin therapy, chemotherapy should be **immediately** added to the tretinoin regimen if the leukocyte count reaches greater than 6 × 10^9/L by day five, or greater than 10 × 10^9/L by day ten, or greater than 15 × 10^9/L by day 28.

• All other patients should receive chemotherapy immediately after complete remission is attained.

If chemotherapy is added to tretinoin because of hyperleukocytosis, it is not necessary to modify the dose of tretinoin.

After completion of tretinoin therapy and the first chemotherapy course, consolidation anthracycline-based chemotherapy should be given, for example, a further two courses at 4 to 6 week intervals.

In some patients the plasma levels of tretinoin may fall significantly in spite of continued administration.

4.3 Contraindications

Known allergy to a product in the class of retinoids or to any of the excipients.

Pregnancy (see section *4.6 Pregnancy and lactation*).

Lactation (see section *4.6 Pregnancy and lactation*).

Tetracyclines (see section *4.5 Interactions with other medicinal products and other forms of interactions*).

Vitamin A (see section *4.5 Interactions with other medicinal products and other forms of interactions*).

4.4 Special warnings and special precautions for use

Tretinoin should be administered to patients with acute promyelocytic leukaemia only under the strict supervision of a physician who is experienced in the treatment of haematological/oncological diseases.

Supportive care appropriate for patients with acute promyelocytic leukaemia, for example prophylaxis for bleeding and prompt therapy for infection, should be maintained during therapy with tretinoin. The patient's haematologic profile, coagulation profile, liver function test results, and triglyceride and cholesterol levels should be monitored frequently.

During clinical trials hyperleukocytosis has been frequently observed (in 75% of the cases), sometimes associated with the "Retinoic Acid Syndrome". Retinoic acid syndrome has been reported in many acute promyelocytic leukaemia patients (up to 25% in some centres) treated with tretinoin.

Retinoic acid syndrome is characterised by fever, dyspnoea, acute respiratory distress, pulmonary infiltrates, pleural and pericardial effusions, hypotension, oedema, weight gain, hepatic, renal and multi-organ failure.

Retinoic acid syndrome is frequently associated with hyperleukocytosis and may be fatal.

The incidence of the retinoic acid syndrome is diminished when full dose chemotherapy is added to the tretinoin regimen based on the white blood cell count. The current therapeutic treatment recommendations and method of administration are detailed in section *4.2 Posology and method of administration*.

Immediate treatment with dexamethasone (10mg every 12 hours for up to maximum 3 days or until resolution of the symptoms) should be given, if the patient presents any symptom(s) or sign(s) of this syndrome.

In cases of moderate and severe retinoic acid syndrome, temporary interruption of Vesanoid therapy should be considered.

Vesanoid may cause pseudotumor cerebri. This condition should be treated according to standard medical practice. Temporary discontinuation of Vesanoid should be considered in patients not responding to treatment.

Sweet's syndrome or acute febrile neutrophilic dermatitis responded dramatically to corticosteroid treatment.

There is a risk of thrombosis (both venous and arterial) which may involve any organ system, during the first month of treatment (see section *4.8 Undesirable effects*). Therefore, caution should be exercised when treating patients with the combination of Vesanoid and anti-fibrinolytic agents, such as tranexamic acid, aminocaproic acid or aprotinin (see section *4.5 Interactions with other medicinal products and other forms of interactions*).

Because hypercalcaemia may occur during therapy, serum calcium levels should be monitored.

Micro-dosed progesterone preparations ("minipill") are an inadequate method of contraception during treatment with tretinoin (see section *4.6 Pregnancy and lactation*).

4.5 Interaction with other medicinal products and other forms of Interaction

Tetracyclines: systemic treatment with retinoids may cause elevation of the intracranial pressure. As tetracyclines may also cause elevation of the intracranial pressure, patients must not be treated with tretinoin and tetracyclines at the same time (see section *4.3 Contra-indications*).

Vitamin A: As with other retinoids, tretinoin must not be administered in combination with vitamin A because symptoms of hypervitaminosis A could be aggravated (see section *4.3 Contraindications*).

The effect of food on the bioavailability of tretinoin has not been characterised. Since the bioavailability of retinoids, as a class, is known to increase in the presence of food, it is recommended that tretinoin be administered with a meal or shortly thereafter.

As tretinoin is metabolised by the hepatic P450 system, there is the potential for alteration of pharmacokinetics parameters in patients administered concomitant medications that are also inducers or inhibitors of this system. Medications that generally induce hepatic P450 enzymes include rifampicin, glucocorticoids, phenobarbital and pentobarbital. Medications that generally inhibit hepatic P450 enzymes include ketoconazole, cimetidine, erythromycin, verapamil, diltiazem and cyclosporine. There are no data to suggest that co-use with these medications increases or decreases either efficacy or toxicity of tretinoin.

Cases of fatal thrombotic complications have been reported rarely in patients concomitantly treated with all-trans retinoic acid and anti-fibrinolytic agents such as tranexamic acid, aminocaproic acid and aprotinin (see section *4.4 Special warnings and special precautions for use*). Therefore, caution should be exercised when administering all-trans retinoic acid concomitantly with these agents.

There are no data on a possible pharmacokinetic interaction between tretinoin and daunorubicin or AraC.

4.6 Pregnancy and lactation

All the measures listed below should be considered in relationship to the severity of the disease and the urgency of the treatment.

Pregnancy: Tretinoin is teratogenic. Its use is contraindicated in pregnant women and women who might become pregnant during the treatment with tretinoin and within one month after cessation of treatment, unless the benefit of tretinoin treatment outweighs the risk of foetal abnormalities due to the severity of the patient's condition and the urgency of treatment.

There is a very high risk for any exposed foetus that a deformed infant will result if pregnancy occurs while taking tretinoin, irrespective of the dose or duration of the treatment.

Therapy with tretinoin should only be started in female patients of child-bearing age if each of the following conditions is met:

• She is informed by her physician of the hazards of becoming pregnant during and one month after treatment with tretinoin.

• She is willing to comply with the mandatory effective contraception measures: to use a reliable contraception method without interruption during therapy and for one month after discontinuation of treatment with tretinoin (see section *4.4 Special warnings and special precautions for use*).

• Pregnancy tests must be performed at monthly intervals during therapy.

In spite of these precautions, should pregnancy occur during treatment with tretinoin or up to one month after its discontinuation, there is a high risk of severe malformation of the foetus, particularly when tretinoin is given during the first trimester of pregnancy.

Lactation: Nursing must be discontinued if therapy with tretinoin is initiated.

4.7 Effects on ability to drive and use machines

The ability to drive or operate machinery might be impaired in patients treated with tretinoin, particularly if they are experiencing dizziness or severe headache.

4.8 Undesirable effects

In patients treated with the recommended daily doses of tretinoin the most frequent undesirable effects are consistent with the signs and symptoms of the hypervitaminosis A syndrome (as for other retinoids).

Retinoic acid syndrome has been reported in many acute promyelocytic leukaemia patients (up to 25% in some centres) treated with tretinoin. Retinoic acid syndrome is characterised by fever, dyspnoea, acute respiratory distress, pulmonary infiltrates, pleural and pericardial effusions, hypotension, oedema, weight gain, hepatic, renal and multi-organ failure. Retinoic acid syndrome is frequently associated with hyperleukocytosis and may be fatal. For prevention and treatment of retinoic acid syndrome see section *4.4 Special warnings and special precautions for use*.

Skin: (> 75% of patients) dryness, erythema, rash, pruritus, hair loss, sweating.

Genital ulcerations, including Fournier's gangrene, Sweet's syndrome and erythema nodosum have been reported rarely.

Mucous membranes: (> 75% of patients) cheilitis, dryness of mouth, nose, conjunctiva and other mucous membranes, with or without inflammatory symptoms.

Central nervous system: (> 75% of patients) headache, intra-cranial hypertension, pseudotumor cerebri syndrome (mainly in children) (see also section *4.4 Special warnings and special precautions for use*), fever, shivering, dizziness, confusion, anxiety, depression, paraesthesias, insomnia, malaise.

Neuro-sensory system: (25% - 50% of patients) vision and hearing disorders.

Musculo-skeletal system: (50% - 75% of patients) bone pain, chest pain. Myositis has been reported rarely.

Gastrointestinal tract: (> 75% of patients) nausea, vomiting, abdominal pain, diarrhoea, constipation, diminished appetite, pancreatitis.

Metabolic, hepatic and renal dysfunctions: (50% - 75% of patients) elevation in serum triglycerides, cholesterol, transaminases (ALAT, ASAT), creatinine. Rare cases of hypercalcaemia have been reported (see also section *4.4 Special warnings and special precautions for use*).

Respiratory system: (50% - 75% of patients) dyspnoea, respiratory insufficiency, pleural effusion, asthma-like syndrome.

Cardiovascular system: (50% - 75% of patients) arrhythmias, flushing, oedema. Cases of thrombosis (both venous and arterial) involving various sites (e.g. cerebrovascular accident, myocardial infarction, renal infarct) have been reported uncommonly (see section *4.4 Special warnings and special precautions for use*).

Haematologic: Marked basophilia with or without symptomatic hyperhistaminaemia has been reported rarely, mainly in patients with the rare APL variant associated with basophilic differentiation. Thrombocytosis has been reported rarely.

Others: Vasculitis, predominantly involving the skin, has been reported rarely.

The decision to interrupt or continue therapy should be based on an evaluation of the benefit of the treatment versus the severity of the side-effects.

Teratogenicity: See section *4.6 Pregnancy and lactation*.

There is limited safety information on the use of tretinoin in children. There have been some reports of increased toxicity in children treated with tretinoin, particularly increased pseudotumor cerebri.

4.9 Overdose

No cases of acute overdosage with tretinoin have been reported.

In the event of accidental overdosage of tretinoin, reversible signs of hyper-vitaminosis A (headache, nausea, vomiting) can appear.

The recommended dose in acute promyelocytic leukaemia is one-quarter of the maximum tolerated dose in solid tumour patients and below the maximum tolerated dose in children.

There is no specific treatment in the case of an overdose, however it is important that the patient be treated in a special haematological unit.

5. PHARMACOLOGICAL PROPERTIES

5.1 Pharmacodynamic properties

Cytostatic-differentiating agent.

Tretinoin is a natural metabolite of retinol and belongs to the class of retinoids, comprising natural and synthetic analogues.

In vitro studies with tretinoin have demonstrated induction of differentiation and inhibition of cell proliferation in transformed haemopoietic cell lines, including human myeloid leukaemia cell lines.

The mechanism of action in acute promyelocytic leukaemia is not known but it may be due to a modification in binding of tretinoin to a nuclear retinoic acid receptor (RAR) given that the α-receptor of retinoic acid is altered by fusion with a protein called PML.

5.2 Pharmacokinetic properties

Tretinoin is an endogenous metabolite of vitamin A which is normally present in plasma.

After oral administration, tretinoin is absorbed by the digestive tract and maximum plasma concentrations in healthy volunteers are attained after 3 hours.

There is a large inter-patient and intra-patient variation in plasma levels of tretinoin.

Tretinoin is extensively bound to plasma proteins. Following peak levels, plasma concentrations decline with a mean elimination half life of 0.7 hours. Plasma concentrations return to endogenous levels after 7 to 12 hours following a single 40mg dose. No accumulation is seen after multiple doses and tretinoin is not retained in body tissues.

After an oral dose of radiolabelled tretinoin, about 60% of the radioactivity was excreted in urine and about 30% in faeces. The metabolites found in urine were formed by oxidation and glucuronidation.

During continuous administration a marked decrease in plasma concentration can occur, possibly due to cytochrome P-450 enzyme induction which increases clearance and decreases bioavailability after oral doses.

At present there are no data on a possible interaction between tretinoin and daunorubicin.

The requirement for dosage adjustment in patients with renal or hepatic insufficiency has not been investigated. As a precautionary measure, the dose will be decreased (see section *4.2 Posology and method of administration*).

5.3 Preclinical safety data

Oral administration of tretinoin to animals indicated that the compound had very low acute toxicity in all species investigated.

In animal experimental tests it was shown that in all investigated species the acute toxicity of tretinoin administered orally is low. After a longer period of administration rats exhibit a dose- and time-dependent bone matrix dissolution, a decrease in erythrocyte count and toxic alterations in kidney and testes.

Dogs mainly exhibited disorders concerning spermatogenesis and hyperplasia of the bone marrow.

The major metabolites of tretinoin (4-oxo-tretinoin, isotretinoin and 4-oxo-isotretinoin) are less effective than tretinoin in inducing differentiation of human leukaemic cells (HL-60)

Subchronic and chronic toxicity studies in rats indicated that the no effect oral dose was at or below 1mg/kg/day; in dogs, 30mg/kg/day was associated with toxic effects including weight loss, dermatological and testicular changes.

Reproduction studies in animals have demonstrated the teratogenic activity of tretinoin.

No evidence of mutagenicity has been found.

6. PHARMACEUTICAL PARTICULARS

6.1 List of excipients

Yellow beeswax, Hydrogenated soybean oil, Partially hydrogenated soybean oil, Soybean oil.

Gelatin, Glycerol, Karion (Sorbitol, Mannitol, Starch), Titanium dioxide (E 171), Iron oxide yellow (E 172), Iron oxide red (E 172)

6.2 Incompatibilities

Not applicable.

6.3 Shelf life

3 years.

6.4 Special precautions for storage

Bottles:

Keep the bottle tightly closed.

Protect from light. Store between 5°C and 30°C.

Blister packs:

Protect from light. Store between 5°C and 30°C.

6.5 Nature and contents of container

Amber glass-bottles of 100 capsules.

PVC/PE/PVDC/Aluminium- blister packs of 100 capsules.

6.6 Instructions for use and handling

None.

7. MARKETING AUTHORISATION HOLDER

Roche Products Limited, 40, Broadwater Road, Welwyn Garden City, Hertfordshire, AL7 3AY, UK.

8. MARKETING AUTHORISATION NUMBER(S)

PL 00031/0618

PA 50/154/1

9. DATE OF FIRST AUTHORISATION/RENEWAL OF THE AUTHORISATION

July 2001 (UK)

August 2001 (Ireland)

10. DATE OF REVISION OF THE TEXT

August 2004 (UK)

July 2004 (Ireland)

Vesanoid is a registered trade mark

Vesicare 5mg & 10mg film-coated tablets

(Astellas Pharma Limited)

1. NAME OF THE MEDICINAL PRODUCT

Vesicare®▼5 mg, film-coated tablet

Vesicare®▼10 mg, film-coated tablet

2. QUALITATIVE AND QUANTITATIVE COMPOSITION

Vesicare 5 mg film-coated tablet: Each tablet contains 5 mg solifenacin succinate, corresponding to 3.8 mg solifenacin.

Vesicare 10 mg film-coated tablet: Each tablet contains 10 mg solifenacin succinate, corresponding to 7.5 mg solifenacin.

For excipients, see Section 6.1.

3. PHARMACEUTICAL FORM

Film-coated tablets

Vesicare 5 mg film-coated tablet: Each 5 mg tablet is a round, light-yellow tablet marked with the Yamanouchi logo and "150" on the same side.

Vesicare 10 mg film-coated tablet: Each 10 mg tablet is a round, light-pink tablet marked with the Yamanouchi logo and "151"on the same side.

4. CLINICAL PARTICULARS

4.1 Therapeutic indications

Symptomatic treatment of urge incontinence and/or increased urinary frequency and urgency as may occur in patients with overactive bladder syndrome.

4.2 Posology and method of administration

Posology

Adults, including the elderly

The recommended dose is 5 mg solifenacin succinate once daily. If needed, the dose may be increased to 10 mg solifenacin succinate once daily.

Children and adolescents

Safety and effectiveness in children have not yet been established. Therefore, Vesicare should not be used in children.

Special Populations

Patients with renal impairment

No dose adjustment is necessary for patients with mild to moderate renal impairment (creatinine clearance > 30 ml/min). Patients with severe renal impairment (creatinine clearance ⩽ 30 ml/min) should be treated with caution and receive no more than 5 mg once daily (see Section 5.2).

Patients with hepatic impairment

No dose adjustment is necessary for patients with mild hepatic impairment. Patients with moderate hepatic impairment (Child-Pugh score of 7 to 9) should be treated with caution and receive no more than 5 mg once daily (see Section 5.2).

Potent inhibitors of cytochrome P450 3A4

The maximum dose of Vesicare should be limited to 5 mg when treated simultaneously with ketoconazole or therapeutic doses of other potent CYP3A4 inhibitors e.g. ritonavir, nelfinavir, itraconazole (see Section 4.5).

Method of administration

Vesicare should be taken orally and should be swallowed whole with liquids. It can be taken with or without food.

4.3 Contraindications

- Solifenacin is contraindicated in patients with urinary retention, severe gastrointestinal condition (including toxic megacolon), myasthenia gravis or narrow-angle glaucoma and in patients at risk for these conditions.
- Patients hypersensitive to the active substance or to any of the excipients.
- Patients undergoing haemodialysis (see Section 5.2).
- Patients with severe hepatic impairment (see Section 5.2).
- Patients with severe renal impairment or moderate hepatic impairment and who are on treatment with a potent CYP3A4 inhibitor, e.g. ketoconazole (see Section 4.5).

4.4 Special warnings and special precautions for use

Other causes of frequent urination (heart failure or renal disease) should be assessed before treatment with Vesicare. If urinary tract infection is present, an appropriate antibacterial therapy should be started.

Vesicare should be used with caution in patients with:

- clinically significant bladder outflow obstruction at risk of urinary retention.
- gastrointestinal obstructive disorders.
- risk of decreased gastrointestinal motility.
- severe renal impairment (creatinine clearance ⩽ 30 ml/min; see Section 4.2 and 5.2) and doses should not exceed 5 mg for these patients.
- moderate hepatic impairment (Child-Pugh score of 7 to 9; see Section 4.2 and 5.2) and doses should not exceed 5 mg for these patients.
- concomitant use of a potent CYP3A4 inhibitor, e.g. ketoconazole (see 4.2 and 4.5).
- hiatus hernia/gastroesophageal reflux and/or who are concurrently taking medicinal products (such as bisphosphonates) that can cause or exacerbate oesophagitis.
- autonomic neuropathy.

Safety and efficacy have not yet been established in patients with a neurogenic cause for detrusor overactivity.

Patients with rare hereditary problems of galactose intolerance, the Lapp lactase deficiency or glucose-galactose malabsorption should not take this medicinal product.

The maximum effect of Vesicare can be determined after 4 weeks at the earliest.

4.5 Interaction with other medicinal products and other forms of Interaction

Pharmacological interactions

Concomitant medication with other medicinal products with anticholinergic properties may result in more pronounced therapeutic effects and undesirable effects. An interval of approximately one week should be allowed after stopping treatment with Vesicare before commencing other anticholinergic therapy. The therapeutic effect of solifenacin may be reduced by concomitant administration of cholinergic receptor agonists.

Solifenacin can reduce the effect of medicinal products that stimulate the motility of the gastrointestinal tract, such as metoclopramide and cisapride.

Pharmacokinetic interactions

In vitro studies have demonstrated that at therapeutic concentrations, solifenacin does not inhibit CYP1A1/2, 2C9, 2C19, 2D6, or 3A4 derived from human liver microsomes. Therefore, solifenacin is unlikely to alter the clearance of drugs metabolised by these CYP enzymes.

Effect of other medicinal products on the pharmacokinetics of solifenacin

Solifenacin is metabolised by CYP3A4. Simultaneous administration of ketoconazole (200 mg/day), a potent CYP3A4 inhibitor, resulted in a two-fold increase of the AUC of solifenacin, while ketoconazole at a dose of 400 mg/day resulted in a three-fold increase of the AUC of solifenacin. Therefore, the maximum dose of Vesicare should be restricted to 5 mg when used simultaneously with ketoconazole or therapeutic doses of other potent CYP3A4 inhibitors (e.g. ritonavir, nelfinavir, itraconazole) (see Section 4.2). Simultaneous treatment of solifenacin and a potent CYP3A4 inhibitor is contraindicated in patients with severe renal impairment or moderate hepatic impairment.

The effects of enzyme induction on the pharmacokinetics of solifenacin and its metabolites have not been studied as well as the effect of higher affinity CYP3A4 substrates on solifenacin exposure. Since solifenacin is metabolised by CYP3A4, pharmacokinetic interactions are possible with other CYP3A4 substrates with higher affinity (e.g. verapamil, diltiazem) and CYP3A4 inducers (e.g. rifampicin, phenytoin, carbamazepine).

Effect of solifenacin on the pharmacokinetics of other medicinal products

Oral Contraceptives

Intake of Vesicare showed no pharmacokinetic interaction of solifenacin on combined oral contraceptives (ethinyl - estradiol/levonorgestrel).

Warfarin

Intake of Vesicare did not alter the pharmacokinetics of *R*-warfarin or *S*-warfarin or their effect on prothrombin time.

Digoxin

Intake of Vesicare showed no effect on the pharmacokinetics of digoxin.

4.6 Pregnancy and lactation

Pregnancy

No clinical data are available from women who became pregnant while taking solifenacin. Animal studies do not indicate direct harmful effects on fertility, embryonal / foetal development or parturition (see Section 5.3). The potential risk for humans is unknown. Caution should be exercised when prescribing to pregnant women.

Lactation

No data on the excretion of solifenacin in human milk are available. In mice, solifenacin and/or its metabolites was excreted in milk, and caused a dose dependent failure to thrive in neonatal mice (see Section 5.3). The use of Vesicare should therefore be avoided during breast-feeding.

4.7 Effects on ability to drive and use machines

Since solifenacin, like other anticholinergics may cause blurred vision, and, uncommonly, somnolence and fatigue (see section 4.8. Undesirable effects), the ability to drive and use machines may be negatively affected.

4.8 Undesirable effects

Due to the pharmacological effect of solifenacin, Vesicare may cause anticholinergic undesirable effects of (in general) mild or moderate severity. The frequency of anticholinergic undesirable effects is dose related. The most commonly reported adverse reaction with Vesicare was dry mouth. It occurred in 11% of patients treated with 5 mg once daily, in 22% of patients treated with 10 mg once daily and in 4% of placebo-treated patients. The severity of dry mouth was generally mild and only occasionally led to discontinuation of treatment. In general, medicinal product compliance was very high (approximately 99%) and approximately 90% of the patients treated with Vesicare completed the full study period of 12 weeks treatment.

The table below reflects the data obtained with Vesicare in clinical trials.

(see Table 1 below)

Allergic reactions were not observed during the clinical development. However, the occurrence of allergic reactions can never be excluded.

4.9 Overdose

The highest dose of solifenacin succinate given to human volunteers was 100 mg as a single dose. At this dose, the most frequent adverse events were headache (mild), dry mouth (moderate), dizziness (moderate), drowsiness (mild) and blurred vision (moderate).

No cases of acute overdose have been reported. In the event of overdose with solifenacin succinate, the patient should be treated with activated charcoal. Gastric lavage may be performed, but vomiting should not be induced.

As for other anticholinergics, symptoms can be treated as follows:

- Severe central anticholinergic effects such as hallucinations or pronounced excitation: treat with physostigmine or carbachol.
- Convulsions or pronounced excitation: treat with benzodiazepines.
- Respiratory insufficiency: treat with artificial respiration.
- Tachycardia: treat with beta-blockers.
- Urinary retention: treat with catheterisation.
- Mydriasis: treat with pilocarpine eye drops and/or place patient in a dark room.

As with other antimuscarinics, in case of overdosing, specific attention should be paid to patients with known risk for QT-prolongation (i.e. hypokalaemia, bradycardia and concurrent administration of medicinal products known to prolong QT-interval) and relevant pre-existing cardiac diseases (i.e. myocardial ischaemia, arrhythmia, congestive heart failure).

5. PHARMACOLOGICAL PROPERTIES

5.1 Pharmacodynamic properties

Pharmacotherapeutic group: Urinary antispasmodics, ATC code: G04B D08.

Mechanism of action:

Solifenacin is a competitive, specific cholinergic-receptor antagonist.

The urinary bladder is innervated by parasympathetic cholinergic nerves. Acetylcholine contracts the detrusor smooth muscle through muscarinic receptors of which the M_3 subtype is predominantly involved. *In vitro* and *in vivo* pharmacological studies indicate that solifenacin is a competitive inhibitor of the muscarinic M_3 subtype receptor. In addition, solifenacin showed to be a specific antagonist for muscarinic receptors by displaying low or no affinity for various other receptors and ion channels tested.

Pharmacodynamic effects:

Treatment with Vesicare in doses of 5 mg and 10 mg daily was studied in several double-blind, randomised, controlled clinical trials in men and women with overactive bladder.

As shown in the table below, both the 5 mg and 10 mg doses of Vesicare produced statistically significant improvements in the primary and secondary endpoints compared with placebo. Efficacy was observed within one week of starting treatment and stabilised over a period of 12 weeks. A long-term open- label study demonstrated that efficacy was maintained for at least 12 months. After 12 weeks of treatment, approximately 50% of patients suffering from incontinence before treatment were free of incontinence episodes, and in addition 35% of patients achieved a micturition frequency of less than 8 micturitions per day. Treatment of the symptoms of overactive bladder also results in a benefit on a number of Quality of Life measures, such as general health perception, incontinence impact, role limitations, physical limitations, social limitations, emotions, symptom severity, severity measures and sleep/energy.

Results (pooled data) of four controlled Phase 3 studies with a treatment duration of 12 weeks

(see Table 2 on next page)

5.2 Pharmacokinetic properties

General characteristics

Absorption

After intake of Vesicare tablets, maximum solifenacin plasma concentrations (C_{max}) are reached after 3 to 8 hours. The t_{max} is independent of the dose. The C_{max} and area under the curve (AUC) increase in proportion to the dose between 5 to 40 mg. Absolute bioavailability is approximately 90%. Food intake does not affect the C_{max} and AUC of solifenacin.

Distribution

The apparent volume of distribution of solifenacin following intravenous administration is about 600 L. Solifenacin is to a great extent (approximately 98%) bound to plasma proteins, primarily α_1-acid glycoprotein.

Metabolism

Solifenacin is extensively metabolised by the liver, primarily by cytochrome P450 3A4 (CYP3A4). However, alternative metabolic pathways exist, that can contribute to the metabolism of solifenacin. The systemic clearance of solifenacin is about 9.5 L/h and the terminal half life of solifenacin is 45 - 68 hours. After oral dosing, one pharmacologically active (4*R*-hydroxy solifenacin) and three inactive metabolites (*N*-glucuronide, *N*-oxide and 4*R*- hydroxy-*N*-oxide of solifenacin) have been identified in plasma in addition to solifenacin.

Excretion

After a single administration of 10 mg [^{14}C-labelled]-solifenacin, about 70% of the radioactivity was detected in urine and 23% in faeces over 26 days. In urine, approximately 11% of the radioactivity is recovered as unchanged active substance; about 18% as the *N*-oxide metabolite, 9% as the 4*R*-hydroxy- *N*-oxide metabolite and 8% as the 4*R*-hydroxy metabolite (active metabolite).

Dose Proportionality

Pharmacokinetics are linear in the therapeutic dose range.

Characteristics in patients

Age

No dosage adjustment based on patient age is required. Studies in the elderly have shown that the exposure to solifenacin, expressed as the AUC, after administration of solifenacin succinate (5 mg and 10 mg once daily) was similar in healthy elderly subjects (aged 65 - 80 years) and healthy young subjects (aged less than 55 years). The mean rate of absorption expressed as t_{max} was slightly slower in the elderly and the terminal half-life was approximately 20% longer in elderly subjects. These modest differences were considered not clinically significant.

The pharmacokinetics of solifenacin have not been established in children and adolescents.

Gender

The pharmacokinetics of solifenacin are not influenced by gender.

Race

The pharmacokinetics of solifenacin are not influenced by race.

Renal impairment

The AUC and C_{max} of solifenacin in mild and moderate renally impaired patients was not significantly different from that found in healthy volunteers. In patients with severe renal impairment (creatinine clearance $\leqslant$ 30 ml/min), exposure to solifenacin was significantly greater than in the controls, with increases in C_{max} of about 30%, AUC of more than 100% and $t_{½}$ of more than 60%. A statistically significant relationship was observed between creatinine clearance and solifenacin clearance.

Pharmacokinetics in patients undergoing haemodialysis has not been studied.

Table 1

MedDRA system organ class	Common >1/100, <1/10	Uncommon >1/1000, <1/100	Rare >1/10000, <1/1000
Gastrointestinal disorders	Constipation Nausea Dyspepsia Abdominal pain	Gastroesophageal reflux diseases Dry throat	Colonic obstruction Faecal impaction
Infections and infestations		Urinary tract infection Cystitis	
Nervous system disorders		Somnolence Dysgeusia	
Eye disorders	Blurred vision	Dry eyes	
General disorders and administration site conditions		Fatigue Oedema lower limb	
Respiratory, thoracic and mediastinal disorders		Nasal dryness	
Skin and subcutaneous tissue disorders		Dry skin	
Renal and urinary disorders		Difficulty in micturition	Urinary retention

Table 2 Results (pooled data) of four controlled Phase 3 studies with a treatment duration of 12 weeks

	Placebo	Vesicare 5 mg o.d.	Vesicare 10 mg o.d.	Tolterodin 2 mg b.i.d.
No. of micturitions/24 h				
Mean baseline	11.9	12.1	11.9	12.1
Mean reduction from baseline	1.4	2.3	2.7	1.9
% change from baseline	(12%)	(19%)	(23%)	(16%)
n	1138	552	1158	250
p-value*		<0.001	<0.001	0.004
No. of urgency episodes/24 h				
Mean baseline	6.3	5.9	6.2	5.4
Mean reduction from baseline	2.0	2.9	3.4	2.1
% change from baseline	(32%)	(49%)	(55%)	(39%)
n	1124	548	1151	250
p-value*		<0.001	<0.001	0.031
No. of incontinence episodes/24 h				
Mean baseline	2.9	2.6	2.9	2.3
Mean reduction from baseline	1.1	1.5	1.8	1.1
% change from baseline	(38%)	(58%)	(62%)	(48%)
n	781	314	778	157
p-value*		<0.001	<0.001	0.009
No. of nocturia episodes/24 h				
Mean baseline	1.8	2.0	1.8	1.9
Mean reduction from baseline	0.4	0.6	0.6	0.5
% change from baseline	(22%)	(30%)	(33%)	(26%)
n	1005	494	1035	232
p-value*		0.025	<0.001	0.199
Volume voided/micturition				
Mean baseline	166 ml	146 ml	163 ml	147 ml
Mean increase from baseline	9 ml	32 ml	43 ml	24 ml
% change from baseline	(5%)	(21%)	(26%)	(16%)
n	1135	552	1156	250
p-value*		<0.001	<0.001	<0.001
No. of pads/24 h				
Mean baseline	3.0	2.8	2.7	2.7
Mean reduction from baseline	0.8	1.3	1.3	1.0
% change from baseline	(27%)	(46%)	(48%)	(37%)
n	238	236	242	250
p-value*		<0.001	<0.001	0.010

Note: In 4 of the pivotal studies, Vesicare 10 mg and placebo were used. In 2 out of the 4 studies also Vesicare 5 mg was used and one of the studies included tolterodine 2 mg bid.

Not all parameters and treatment groups were evaluated in each individual study. Therefore, the numbers of patients listed may deviate per parameter and treatment group.

* P-value for the pair-wise comparison to placebo

Hepatic impairment

In patients with moderate hepatic impairment (Child-Pugh score of 7 to 9) the C_{max} is not affected, AUC increased by 60% and $t_{½}$ doubled. Pharmacokinetics of solifenacin in patients with severe hepatic impairment has not been studied.

5.3 Preclinical safety data

Preclinical data reveal no special hazard for humans based on conventional studies of safety pharmacology, repeated dose toxicity, fertility, embryofetal development, genotoxicity, and carcinogenic potential. In the pre- and postnatal development study in mice, solifenacin treatment of the mother during lactation caused dose-dependent lower postpartum survival rate, decreased pup weight and slower physical development at clinically relevant levels.

6. PHARMACEUTICAL PARTICULARS

6.1 List of excipients

Core tablet:

Maize starch

Lactose monohydrate

Hypromellose

Magnesium stearate

Film Coating:

Macrogol 8000

Talc

Hypromellose

Titanium dioxide (E171)

Yellow ferric oxide (E172) - Vesicare 5 mg

Red ferric oxide (E172) - Vesicare 10 mg

6.2 Incompatibilities

Not applicable.

6.3 Shelf life

3 years.

6.4 Special precautions for storage

This medicinal product does not require any special storage conditions.

6.5 Nature and contents of container

Container:

The tablets are packed in PVC/Aluminium blisters.

Pack sizes:

3, 5, 10, 20, 30, 50, 60, 90 or 100 tablets (not all pack sizes may be marketed).

6.6 Instructions for use and handling

No special requirements.

7. MARKETING AUTHORISATION HOLDER

Yamanouchi Pharma Ltd.

Yamanouchi House,

Pyrford Road,

West Byfleet,

Surrey.

KT14 6RA

8. MARKETING AUTHORISATION NUMBER(S)

PL 00166/0197 Vesicare 5 mg

PL 00166/0198 Vesicare 10 mg

9. DATE OF FIRST AUTHORISATION/RENEWAL OF THE AUTHORISATION

16 August 2004

10. DATE OF REVISION OF THE TEXT

8 June 2005

11. LEGAL CATEGORY

POM

VFEND 50 mg and 200 mg film-coated tablets, VFEND 200 mg powder for solution for infusion, VFEND 40 mg/ml powder for oral suspension

(Pfizer Limited)

1. NAME OF THE MEDICINAL PRODUCT

VFEND 50 mg and 200 mg film-coated tablets.

VFEND 200 mg powder for solution for infusion.

VFEND 40 mg/ml powder for oral suspension.

2. QUALITATIVE AND QUANTITATIVE COMPOSITION

Film-coated tablets:

Each tablet contains 50 mg or 200 mg voriconazole.

For excipients, see section 6.1.

Powder for solution for infusion:

Vials contain 200 mg voriconazole, equivalent to a 10 mg/ml solution following reconstitution (see section 6.6).

For excipients, see section 6.1.

Powder for oral suspension:

Each bottle contains 45 g powder for oral suspension providing 40 mg/ml voriconazole when constituted with water.

For excipients, see section 6.1.

3. PHARMACEUTICAL FORM

Film-coated tablets:

White, round tablets, debossed "Pfizer" on one side and "VOR50" on the reverse.

White, capsule-shaped tablets, debossed "Pfizer" on one side and "VOR200" on the reverse.

Powder for solution for infusion:

VFEND powder for solution for infusion is a white lyophilised powder containing nominally 200 mg voriconazole presented in a 30 ml clear glass vial.

Powder for oral suspension:

White to off-white powder for oral suspension providing a white to off-white, orange flavoured suspension when constituted.

4. CLINICAL PARTICULARS

4.1 Therapeutic indications

VFEND, voriconazole, is a broad spectrum, triazole antifungal agent and is indicated as follows:

Treatment of invasive aspergillosis.

Treatment of candidemia in non-neutropenic patients

Treatment of fluconazole-resistant serious invasive *Candida* infections (including *C. krusei*).

Treatment of serious fungal infections caused by *Scedosporium* spp. and *Fusarium* spp.

VFEND should be administered primarily to patients with progressive, possibly life-threatening infections.

4.2 Posology and method of administration

Film-coated tablets:

VFEND film-coated tablets are to be taken at least one hour before, or one hour following, a meal.

Powder for solution for infusion:

VFEND requires reconstitution and dilution (see section 6.6) prior to administration as an intravenous infusion. Not for bolus injection.

It is recommended that VFEND is administered at a maximum rate of 3 mg/kg per hour over 1 to 2 hours.

Electrolyte disturbances such as hypokalaemia, hypomagnesaemia and hypocalcaemia should be monitored and corrected, if necessary, prior to initiation and during voriconazole therapy (see section 4.4).

Use in adults

Therapy must be initiated with the specified loading dose regimen of either intravenous or oral VFEND to achieve plasma concentrations on Day 1 that are close to steady state. On the basis of the high oral bioavailability (96 %; see section 5.2), switching between intravenous and oral administration is appropriate when clinically indicated.

Detailed information on dosage recommendations is provided in the following table:

(see Table 1 on next page)

Powder for oral suspension:

VFEND oral suspension is to be taken at least one hour before, or two hours following, a meal.

Electrolyte disturbances such as hypokalaemia, hypomagnesaemia and hypocalcaemia should be monitored and corrected, if necessary, prior to initiation and during voriconazole therapy (see section 4.4).

VFEND is also available for oral use as 50 mg and 200 mg film-coated tablets.

Use in adults

Therapy must be initiated with the specified loading dose regimen of either intravenous or oral VFEND to achieve plasma concentrations on Day 1 that are close to steady state. On the basis of the high oral bioavailability (96 %; see section 5.2), switching between intravenous and oral administration is appropriate when clinically indicated.

Table 1

	Intravenous	Oral	
		Patients 40 kg and above	Patients less than 40 kg
Loading Dose Regimen(first 24 hours)	6 mg/kg every 12 hours (for the first 24 hours)	400 mg every 12 hours (for the first 24 hours)	200 mg every 12 hours (for the first 24 hours)
Maintenance Dose (after first 24 hours)	4 mg/kg twice daily	200 mg twice daily	100 mg twice daily

Table 2

	Intravenous	Oral Suspension	
		Patients 40 kg and above	Patients less than 40 kg
Loading Dose Regimen(first 24 hours)	6 mg/kg every 12 hours (for the first 24 hours)	400 mg (10 ml) every 12 hours (for the first 24 hours)	200 mg (5 ml) every 12 hours (for the first 24 hours)
Maintenance Dose (after first 24 hours)	4 mg/kg twice daily	200 mg (5 ml) twice daily	100 mg (2.5 ml) twice daily

Detailed information on dosage recommendations is provided in the following table:

(see Table 2 above)

Dosage adjustment

Film-coated tablets:

If patient response is inadequate, the maintenance dose may be increased to 300 mg twice daily for oral administration. For patients less than 40 kg the oral dose may be increased to 150 mg twice daily.

If patients are unable to tolerate treatment at these higher doses reduce the oral dose by 50 mg steps to the 200 mg twice daily (or 100 mg twice daily for patients less than 40 kg) maintenance dose.

Phenytoin may be co-administered with voriconazole if the maintenance dose of voriconazole is increased from 200 mg to 400 mg orally, twice daily (100 mg to 200 mg orally, twice daily in patients less than 40 kg), see sections 4.4 and 4.5.

Rifabutin may be co-administered with voriconazole if the maintenance dose of voriconazole is increased from 200 mg to 350 mg orally, twice daily (100 mg to 200 mg orally, twice daily in patients less than 40 kg), see sections 4.4 and 4.5.

Treatment duration depends upon patients' clinical and mycological response.

Powder for solution for infusion:

If patients are unable to tolerate treatment at 4 mg/kg twice daily, reduce the intravenous dose to 3 mg/kg twice daily.

Rifabutin or phenytoin may be co-administered with voriconazole if the maintenance dose of voriconazole is increased to 5 mg/kg intravenously twice daily, see sections 4.4 and 4.5.

Treatment duration depends upon patients' clinical and mycological response. The duration of treatment with the intravenous formulation should be no longer than 6 months (see section 5.3).

Use in the elderly

No dose adjustment is necessary for elderly patients (see section 5.2).

Use in patients with renal impairment

Film-coated tablets:

The pharmacokinetics of orally administered voriconazole are not affected by renal impairment. Therefore, no adjustment is necessary for oral dosing for patients with mild to severe renal impairment (see section 5.2).

Voriconazole is haemodialysed with a clearance of 121 ml/min. A four hour haemodialysis session does not remove a sufficient amount of voriconazole to warrant dose adjustment.

Powder for solution for infusion:

In patients with moderate to severe renal dysfunction (creatinine clearance < 50 ml/min), accumulation of the intravenous vehicle, SBECD, occurs. Oral voriconazole should be administered to these patients, unless an assessment of the risk benefit to the patient justifies the use of intravenous voriconazole. Serum creatinine levels should be closely monitored in these patients and, if increases occur, consideration should be given to changing to oral voriconazole therapy.

Voriconazole is haemodialysed with a clearance of 121 ml/min. A 4 hour haemodialysis session does not remove a sufficient amount of voriconazole to warrant dose adjustment.

The intravenous vehicle, SBECD, is haemodialysed with a clearance of 55 ml/min.

Use in patients with hepatic impairment

No dose adjustment is necessary in patients with acute hepatic injury, manifested by elevated liver function tests (ALAT, ASAT) (but continued monitoring of liver function tests for further elevations is recommended).

It is recommended that the standard loading dose regimens be used but that the maintenance dose be halved in patients with mild to moderate hepatic cirrhosis (Child-Pugh A and B) receiving VFEND (see section 5.2).

VFEND has not been studied in patients with severe chronic hepatic cirrhosis (Child-Pugh C).

VFEND has been associated with elevations in liver function tests and clinical signs of liver damage, such as jaundice, and must only be used in patients with severe hepatic impairment if the benefit outweighs the potential risk. Patients with hepatic impairment must be carefully monitored for drug toxicity (see also section 4.8).

Use in children

Safety and effectiveness in paediatric subjects below the age of 2 years has not been established (see also section 5.1 -). Therefore voriconazole is not recommended for children less than 2 years of age. Limited data are currently available to determine the optimal posology. However, the following regimen has been used in paediatric studies.

Children aged 2 to < 12 years:

	Intravenous	Oral
Loading Dose Regimen (first 24 hours)	6 mg/kg every 12 hours (for the first 24 hours)	6 mg/kg every 12 hours (for the first 24 hours)
Maintenance Dose (after first 24 hours)	4 mg/kg twice daily	4 mg/kg twice daily

If a child is able to swallow tablets, the dose should be administered to the nearest mg/kg dose possible using whole 50 mg tablets.

The pharmacokinetics and tolerability of higher doses have not been characterised in paediatric populations.

Adolescents (12 to 16 years of age): should be dosed as adults.

Powder for oral suspension:

If patient response is inadequate, the maintenance dose may be increased to 300 mg twice daily for oral administration. For patients less than 40kg the oral dose may be increased to 150 mg twice daily.

If patients are unable to tolerate treatment at these higher doses reduce the oral dose by 50 mg steps to the 200 mg twice daily (or 100 mg twice daily for patients less than 40 kg) maintenance dose.

Phenytoin may be coadministered with voriconazole if the maintenance dose of voriconazole is increased from 200 mg to 400 mg orally, twice daily (100 mg to 200 mg orally, twice daily in patients less than 40 kg), see sections 4.4 and 4.5.

Rifabutin may be coadministered with voriconazole if the maintenance dose of voriconazole is increased from 200 mg to 350 mg orally, twice daily (100 mg to 200 mg orally, twice daily in patients less than 40 kg), see sections 4.4 and 4.5.

Treatment duration depends upon patients' clinical and mycological response.

Use in the elderly

No dose adjustment is necessary for elderly patients (see section 5.2).

Use in patients with renal impairment

The pharmacokinetics of orally administered voriconazole are not affected by renal impairment. Therefore, no adjustment is necessary for oral dosing for patients with mild to severe renal impairment (see section 5.2).

Voriconazole is haemodialysed with a clearance of 121 ml/min. A 4 hour haemodialysis session does not remove a sufficient amount of voriconazole to warrant dose adjustment.

Use in patients with hepatic impairment

No dose adjustment is necessary in patients with acute hepatic injury, manifested by elevated liver function tests (ALAT, ASAT) (but continued monitoring of liver function tests for further elevations is recommended).

It is recommended that the standard loading dose regimens be used but that the maintenance dose be halved in patients with mild to moderate hepatic cirrhosis (Child-Pugh A and B) receiving VFEND (see section 5.2).

VFEND has not been studied in patients with severe chronic hepatic cirrhosis (Child-Pugh C).

VFEND has been associated with elevations in liver function tests and clinical signs of liver damage, such as jaundice, and must only be used in patients with severe hepatic impairment if the benefit outweighs the potential risk. Patients with hepatic impairment must be carefully monitored for drug toxicity (see also section 4.8).

Use in children

Safety and effectiveness in paediatric subjects below the age of 2 years has not been established (see also 5.1). Therefore voriconazole is not recommended for children less than 2 years of age.

Limited data are currently available to determine the optimal posology (see section 5.2). However, the following regimen has been used in paediatric studies.

Children aged 2 to < 12 years:

	Intravenous	Oral Suspension
Loading Dose Regimen (first 24 hours)	6 mg/kg every 12 hours (for the first 24 hours)	6 mg/kg every 12 hours (for the first 24 hours)
Maintenance Dose (after first 24 hours)	4 mg/kg twice daily	4 mg/kg twice daily

The dose should be administered to the nearest 20 mg (0.5 ml) as the oral syringe is graduated in increments of 0.5 ml.

The pharmacokinetics and tolerability of higher doses have not been characterised in paediatric populations.

Adolescents (12 to 16 years of age): should be dosed as adults.

4.3 Contraindications

VFEND is contraindicated in patients with known hypersensitivity to voriconazole or to any of the excipients.

Co-administration of the CYP3A4 substrates, terfenadine, astemizole, cisapride, pimozide or quinidine with VFEND is contraindicated since increased plasma concentrations of these medicinal products can lead to QTc prolongation and rare occurrences of *torsades de pointes* (see section 4.5).

Co-administration of VFEND with rifampicin, carbamazepine and phenobarbital is contraindicated since these medicinal products are likely to decrease plasma voriconazole concentrations significantly (see section 4.5).

Coadministration of VFEND with efavirenz is contraindicated because efavirenz significantly decreases voriconazole plasma concentrations while VFEND also significantly increases efavirenz plasma concentrations (see section 4.5).

Co-administration of VFEND with ritonavir (400 mg and above twice daily) is contraindicated because ritonavir significantly decreases plasma voriconazole concentrations in healthy subjects (see section 4.5).

Co-administration of ergot alkaloids (ergotamine, dihydroergotamine), which are CYP3A4 substrates, is contraindicated since increased plasma concentrations of these medicinal products can lead to ergotism (see section 4.5).

Co-administration of voriconazole and sirolimus is contraindicated, since voriconazole is likely to increase plasma concentrations of sirolimus significantly (see section 4.5).

4.4 Special warnings and special precautions for use

Hypersensitivity: Caution should be used in prescribing VFEND to patients with hypersensitivity to other azoles (see also section 4.8).

Cardiovascular:

Some azoles, including voriconazole have been associated with QT interval prolongation. There have been rare cases of torsade de pointes in patients taking voriconazole who had risk factors, such as history of cardiotoxic chemotherapy, cardiomyopathy, hypokalaemia and concomitant medications that may have been contributory. Voriconazole should be administered with caution to patients with potentially proarrhythmic conditions, such as

- Congenital or acquired QT-prolongation
- Cardiomyopathy, in particular when heart failure is present
- Sinus bradycardia
- Existing symptomatic arrhythmias
- Concomitant medication that is known to prolong QT interval.

Electrolyte disturbances such as hypokalaemia, hypomagnesaemia and hypocalcaemia should be monitored and corrected, if necessary, prior to initiation and during voriconazole therapy (see section 4.2). A study has been conducted in healthy volunteers which examined the effect on QT interval of single doses of voriconazole up to 4 times the usual daily dose. No subject experienced an interval exceeding the potentially clinically relevant threshold of 500 msec (see section 5.1).

Infusion-related reactions: Infusion-related reactions, predominantly flushing and nausea, have been observed during administration of the intravenous formulation of voriconazole. Depending on the severity of symptoms, consideration should be given to stopping treatment (see section 4.8).

Hepatic toxicity: In clinical trials, there have been uncommon cases of serious hepatic reactions during treatment with VFEND (including clinical hepatitis, cholestasis and fulminant hepatic failure, including fatalities). Instances of hepatic reactions were noted to occur primarily in patients with serious underlying medical conditions (predominantly haematological malignancy). Transient hepatic reactions, including hepatitis and jaundice, have occurred among patients with no other identifiable risk factors. Liver dysfunction has usually been reversible on discontinuation of therapy (see section 4.8).

Monitoring of hepatic function: Patients at the beginning of therapy with voriconazole and patients who develop abnormal liver function tests during VFEND therapy must be routinely monitored for the development of more severe hepatic injury. Patient management should include laboratory evaluation of hepatic function (particularly liver function tests and bilirubin). Discontinuation of VFEND should be considered if clinical signs and symptoms are consistent with liver disease development.

Renal adverse events: Acute renal failure has been observed in severely ill patients undergoing treatment with VFEND. Patients being treated with voriconazole are likely to be treated concomitantly with nephrotoxic medications and have concurrent conditions that may result in decreased renal function (see section 4.8).

Monitoring of renal function: Patients should be monitored for the development of abnormal renal function. This should include laboratory evaluation, particularly serum creatinine.

Dermatological reactions: Patients have rarely developed exfoliative cutaneous reactions, such as Stevens-Johnson syndrome, during treatment with VFEND. If patients develop a rash they should be monitored closely and VFEND discontinued if lesions progress.

In addition VFEND has been associated with photosensitivity skin reaction especially during long term therapy. It is recommended that patients should be informed to avoid sunlight during the treatment.

Paediatric use: Safety and effectiveness in paediatric subjects below the age of two years has not been established (see also section 5.1).

Phenytoin (CYP2C9 substrate and potent CYP450 inducer): Careful monitoring of phenytoin levels is recommended when phenytoin is co-administered with voriconazole. Concomitant use of voriconazole and phenytoin should be avoided unless the benefit outweighs the risk (see section 4.5).

Rifabutin (CYP450 inducer): Careful monitoring of full blood counts and adverse reactions to rifabutin (e.g. uveitis) is recommended when rifabutin is co-administered with voriconazole. Concomitant use of voriconazole and rifabutin should be avoided unless the benefit outweighs the risk (see section 4.5).

Methadone (CYP3A4 substrate). Frequent monitoring for adverse events and toxicity related to methadone, including QTc prolongation, is recommended when coadministered with voriconazole since methadone levels increased following co-administration of voriconazole. Dose reduction of methadone may be needed (see section 4.5).

VFEND tablets contain lactose and should not be given to patients with rare hereditary problems of galactose intolerance, Lapp lactase deficiency or glucose-galactose malabsorption.

VFEND oral suspension contains sucrose and should not be given to patients with rare hereditary problems of fructose intolerance, sucrase-isomaltase deficiency or glucose-galactose malabsorption.

4.5 Interaction with other medicinal products and other forms of Interaction

Unless otherwise specified, drug interaction studies have been performed in healthy male subjects using multiple dosing to steady state with oral voriconazole at 200 mg twice daily. These results are relevant to other populations and routes of administration.

This section addresses the effects of other medicinal products on voriconazole, the effects of voriconazole on other medicinal products and two-way interactions. The interactions for the first two sections are presented in the following order: contraindications, those requiring dosage adjustment and careful clinical and/or biological monitoring and finally those that have no significant pharmacokinetic interaction but may be of clinical interest in this therapeutic field.

Effects of other medicinal products on voriconazole

Voriconazole is metabolised by cytochrome P450 isoenzymes, CYP2C19, CYP2C9 and CYP3A4. Inhibitors or inducers of these isoenzymes may increase or decrease voriconazole plasma concentrations respectively.

Rifampicin(CYP450 inducer): Rifampicin (600 mg once daily) decreased the C_{max} (maximum plasma concentration) and AUC_τ (area under the plasma concentration time curve within a dose interval) of voriconazole by 93 % and 96 %, respectively. Co-administration of voriconazole and rifampicin is contraindicated (see section 4.3).

Ritonavir (potent CYP450 inducer; CYP3A4 inhibitor and substrate): Ritonavir (400 mg twice daily) decreased the steady state C_{max} and AUC_τ of oral voriconazole by an average of 66% and 82%, respectively, in healthy subjects with the exception of one subject in whom a 2.5 fold increases in AUC_τ was observed. No extrapolation can be made for ritonavir doses lower than 400 mg. Repeat oral administration of voriconazole did not have a significant effect on steady state C_{max} and AUC_τ of ritonavir following repeat dose administration in healthy subjects. Coadministration of voriconazole and ritonavir (400 mg and above twice daily) is contraindicated (see section 4.3).

Carbamazepine and phenobarbital(potent CYP450 inducers): Although not studied, carbamazepine or phenobarbital are likely to significantly decrease plasma voriconazole concentrations. Co-administration of voriconazole with carbamazepine and phenobarbital is contraindicated (see section 4.3).

Cimetidine(non-specific CYP450 inhibitor and increases gastric pH): Cimetidine (400 mg twice daily) increased voriconazole C_{max} and AUC_τ by 18 % and 23 %, respectively. No dosage adjustment of voriconazole is recommended.

Ranitidine(increases gastric pH): Ranitidine (150 mg twice daily) had no significant effect on voriconazole C_{max} and AUC_τ.

Macrolide antibiotics: Erythromycin (CYP3A4 inhibitor; 1g twice daily) and azithromycin (500 mg once daily) had no significant effect on voriconazole C_{max} and AUC_τ.

Effects of voriconazole on other medicinal products

Voriconazole inhibits the activity of cytochrome P450 isoenzymes, CYP2C19, CYP2C9 and CYP3A4. Therefore there is potential for voriconazole to increase the plasma levels of substances metabolised by these CYP450 isoenzymes.

Terfenadine, astemizole, cisapride, pimozide and quinidine(CYP3A4 substrates): Although not studied, coadministration of voriconazole with terfenadine, astemizole, cisapride, pimozide, or quinidine is contraindicated, since increased plasma concentrations of these medicinal products can lead to QTc prolongation and rare occurrences of *torsades de pointes* (see section 4.3).

Sirolimus (CYP3A4 substrate): Voriconazole increased sirolimus (2 mg single dose) C_{max} and AUC_τ by 556 % and 1014 %, respectively. Co-administration of voriconazole and sirolimus is contraindicated (see section 4.3).

Ergot alkaloids (CYP3A4 substrates): Although not studied, voriconazole may increase the plasma concentrations of ergot alkaloids (ergotamine and dihydroergotamine) and lead to ergotism. Co-administration of voriconazole with ergot alkaloids is contraindicated (see section 4.3).

Cyclosporin(CYP3A4 substrate): In stable, renal transplant recipients, voriconazole increased cyclosporin C_{max} and AUC_τ by at least 13 % and 70 %, respectively. When initiating voriconazole in patients already receiving cyclosporin it is recommended that the cyclosporin dose be halved and cyclosporin level carefully monitored. Increased cyclosporin levels have been associated with nephrotoxicity. When voriconazole is discontinued, cyclosporin levels must be carefully monitored and the dose increased as necessary.

Methadone (CYP3A4 substrate): In subjects receiving a methadone maintenance dose (32-100 mg once daily) coadministration of oral voriconazole (400 mg twice daily for 1 day, then 200 mg twice daily for four days) increased the C_{max} and AUC_τ of pharmacologically active R-methadone by 31 % and 47 %, respectively, whereas the C_{max} and AUC_τ of the S-enantiomer increased by approximately 65 % and 103 %, respectively. Voriconazole plasma concentrations during coadministration of methadone were comparable to voriconazole levels (historical data) in healthy subjects without any comedication. Frequent monitoring for adverse events and toxicity related to increased plasma concentrations of methadone, including QT prolongation, is recommended during coadministration. Dose reduction of methadone may be needed.

Tacrolimus(CYP3A4 substrate): Voriconazole increased tacrolimus (0.1 mg/kg single dose) C_{max} and AUC_t (area under the plasma concentration time curve to the last quantifiable measurement) by 117 % and 221 %, respectively. When initiating voriconazole in patients already receiving tacrolimus, it is recommended that the tacrolimus dose be reduced to a third of the original dose and tacrolimus level carefully monitored. Increased tacrolimus levels have been associated with nephrotoxicity. When voriconazole is discontinued, tacrolimus levels must be carefully monitored and the dose increased as necessary.

Oral anticoagulants:

Warfarin (CYP2C9 substrate): Co-administration of voriconazole (300 mg twice daily) with warfarin (30 mg single dose) increased maximum prothrombin time by 93 %. Close monitoring of prothrombin time is recommended if warfarin and voriconazole are co-administered.

Other oral anticoagulants e.g. phenprocoumon, acenocoumarol (CYP2C9, CYP3A4 substrates): Although not studied, voriconazole may increase the plasma concentrations of coumarins and therefore may cause an increase in prothrombin time. If patients receiving coumarin preparations are treated simultaneously with voriconazole, the prothrombin time should be monitored at close intervals and the dosage of anticoagulants adjusted accordingly.

Sulphonylureas(CYP2C9 substrates): Although not studied, voriconazole may increase the plasma levels of sulphonylureas, (e.g. tolbutamide, glipizide, and glyburide) and therefore cause hypoglycaemia. Careful monitoring of blood glucose is recommended during co-administration.

Statins(CYP3A4 substrates): Although not studied clinically, voriconazole has been shown to inhibit lovastatin metabolism *in vitro* (human liver microsomes). Therefore, voriconazole is likely to increase plasma levels of statins that are metabolised by CYP3A4. It is recommended that dose adjustment of the statin be considered during co-administration. Increased statin levels have been associated with rhabdomyolysis.

Benzodiazepines(CYP3A4 substrates): Although not studied clinically, voriconazole has been shown to inhibit midazolam metabolism *in vitro* (human liver microsomes). Therefore, voriconazole is likely to increase the plasma levels of benzodiazepines that are metabolised by CYP3A4 (e.g. midazolam and triazolam) and lead to a prolonged sedative effect. It is recommended that dose adjustment of the benzodiazepine be considered during co-administration.

Vinca Alkaloids (CYP3A4 substrates): Although not studied, voriconazole may increase the plasma levels of the vinca alkaloids (e.g. vincristine and vinblastine) and lead to neurotoxicity.

Prednisolone(CYP3A4 substrate): Voriconazole increased C_{max} and AUC_τ of prednisolone (60 mg single dose) by 11 % and 34 %, respectively. No dosage adjustment is recommended.

Digoxin(P-glycoprotein mediated transport): Voriconazole had no significant effect on C_{max} and AUC_τ of digoxin (0.25 mg once daily).

Mycophenolic acid (UDP-glucuronyl transferase substrate): Voriconazole had no effect on the C_{max} and AUC_t of mycophenolic acid (1 g single dose).

Two-way interactions

Phenytoin (CYP2C9 substrate and potent CYP450 inducer): Concomitant use of voriconazole and phenytoin should be avoided unless the benefit outweighs the risk.

Phenytoin (300 mg once daily) decreased the C_{max} and AUC_τ of voriconazole by 49 % and 69 %, respectively. Voriconazole (400 mg twice daily, see section 4.2) increased C_{max} and AUC_τ of phenytoin (300 mg once daily) by 67 % and 81 %, respectively. Careful monitoring of phenytoin plasma levels is recommended when phenytoin is co-administered with voriconazole.

Phenytoin may be co-administered with voriconazole if the maintenance dose of voriconazole is increased to 5 mg /kg intravenously twice daily or from 200 mg to 400 mg orally, twice daily (100 mg to 200 mg orally, twice daily in patients less than 40 kg), see section 4.2.

Rifabutin(CYP450 inducer): Concomitant use of voriconazole and rifabutin should be avoided unless the benefit outweighs the risk.

Rifabutin (300 mg once daily) decreased the C_{max} and AUC_τ of voriconazole at 200 mg twice daily by 69 % and 78 %, respectively. During co-administration with rifabutin, the C_{max} and AUC_τ of voriconazole at 350 mg twice daily were 96 % and 68 % of the levels when administered alone at 200 mg twice daily. At a voriconazole dose of 400 mg twice daily C_{max} and AUC_τ were 104 % and 87 % higher, respectively, compared with voriconazole alone at 200 mg twice daily. Voriconazole at 400 mg twice daily increased C_{max} and AUC_τ of rifabutin by 195 % and 331 %, respectively.

If rifabutin co-administration with voriconazole is justified then the maintenance dose of voriconazole may be increased to 5 mg/kg intravenously twice daily or from 200 mg to 350 mg orally, twice daily (100 mg to 200 mg orally, twice daily in patients less than 40 kg) (see section 4.2). Careful monitoring of full blood counts and adverse reactions to rifabutin (e.g. uveitis) is recommended when rifabutin is co-administered with voriconazole.

Omeprazole(CYP2C19 inhibitor; CYP2C19 and CYP3A4 substrate): Omeprazole (40 mg once daily) increased voriconazole C_{max} and AUC_τ by 15 % and 41 %, respectively. No dosage adjustment of voriconazole is recommended. Voriconazole increased omeprazole C_{max} and AUC_τ by 116 % and 280 %, respectively. When initiating voriconazole in patients already receiving omeprazole, it is recommended that the omeprazole dose be halved. The metabolism of other proton pump inhibitors which are CYP2C19 substrates may also be inhibited by voriconazole.

Indinavir(CYP3A4 inhibitor and substrate): Indinavir (800 mg three times daily) had no significant effect on voriconazole C_{max}, C_{min} and AUC_τ. Voriconazole did not have a significant effect on C_{max} and AUC_τ of indinavir (800 mg three times daily).

Efavirenz (a non-nucleoside reverse transcriptase inhibitor (CYP450 inducer; CYP3A4 inhibitor and substrate): Steady-state efavirenz (400mg orally once daily) decreased the steady state C_{max} and AUC_τ of voriconazole by an average of 61% and 77%, respectively, in healthy subjects. In the same study voriconazole at steady state increased the steady state C_{max} and AUC_τ of efavirenz by an average of 38% and 44% respectively, in healthy subjects. Coadministration of voriconazole and efavirenz is contraindicated (see section 4.3).

Other HIV protease inhibitors (CYP3A4 inhibitors): *In vitro* studies suggest that voriconazole may inhibit the metabolism of HIV protease inhibitors (e.g. saquinavir, amprenavir and nelfinavir). *In vitro* studies also show that the metabolism of voriconazole may be inhibited by HIV protease inhibitors. However results of the combination of voriconazole with other HIV protease inhibitors cannot be predicted in humans only from *in vitro* studies. Patients should be carefully monitored for any occurrence of drug toxicity and/or loss of efficacy during the co-administration of voriconazole and HIV protease inhibitors.

Non-nucleoside reverse transcriptase inhibitors (NNRTI)(CYP3A4 substrates, inhibitors or CYP450 inducers): *In vitro* studies show that the metabolism of voriconazole may be inhibited by delavirdine. Although not studied, the metabolism of voriconazole may be induced by nevirapine. An in-vivo study showed that voriconazole inhibited the metabolism of efavirenz. Voriconazole may also inhibit the metabolism of NNRTIs besides efavirenz. Patients should be carefully monitored for any occurrence of drug toxicity and/or lack of efficacy during the co-administration of voriconazole and NNRTIs. Coadministration of voriconazole with efavirenz is contraindicated (see section 4.3)

Voriconazole should be administered with caution in patients with concomitant medication that is known to prolong QT interval. When there is also a potential for voriconazole to increase the plasma levels of substances metabolised by CYP3A4 isoenzymes (certain antihistamines, quinidine, cisapride, pimozide) co-administration is contraindicated (see section 4.3).

4.6 Pregnancy and lactation

Pregnancy

No adequate information on the use of VFEND in pregnant women is available.

Studies in animals have shown reproductive toxicity (see section 5.3). The potential risk to humans is unknown.

VFEND must not be used during pregnancy unless the benefit to the mother clearly outweighs the potential risk to the foetus.

Women of child-bearing potential

Women of child-bearing potential must always use effective contraception during treatment.

Lactation

The excretion of voriconazole into breast milk has not been investigated. Breast-feeding must be stopped on initiation of treatment with VFEND.

4.7 Effects on ability to drive and use machines

Voriconazole may cause transient and reversible changes to vision, including blurring, altered/enhanced visual perception and/or photophobia. Patients must avoid potentially hazardous tasks, such as driving or operating machinery while experiencing these symptoms.

4.8 Undesirable effects

The safety profile of voriconazole is based on an integrated safety database of more than 2000 subjects (1655 patients in therapeutic trials). This represents a heterogeneous population, containing patients with haematological malignancy, HIV infected patients with oesophageal candidiasis and refractory fungal infections, non-neutropenic patients with candidaemia or aspergillosis and healthy volunteers. Five hundred and sixty one patients had a duration of voriconazole therapy of greater than 12 weeks, with 136 patients receiving voriconazole for over 6 months.

In the table below, since the majority of the studies were of an open nature, all causality adverse events, by system organ class and frequency (very common $>1/10$, common $>1/100$ and $<1/10$, uncommon $>1/1000$ and $<1/100$ and rare, $<1/1000$) if possibly causally related are listed. The most commonly reported adverse reactions were visual disturbances, fever, rash, vomiting, nausea, diarrhoea, headache, peripheral oedema and abdominal pain.

The severity of the adverse reactions was generally mild to moderate. No clinically significant differences were seen when the safety data were analysed by age, race, or gender.

Undesirable effects reported in subjects receiving voriconazole

Body System	Adverse Drug Reactions
Body as a whole	
Very common	Fever, headache, abdominal pain
Common	Chills, asthenia, back pain, chest pain, injection site reaction/ inflammation, face oedema, flu syndrome
Uncommon	Allergic reaction, anaphylactoid reaction, angioedema, peritonitis
Cardiovascular	
Common	Hypotension, thrombophlebitis, phlebitis
Uncommon	Atrial arrhythmia, bradycardia, syncope, tachycardia, ventricular arrhythmia, ventricular fibrillation, supraventricular tachycardia, QT interval prolongation
Rare	AV complete block, bundle branch block, nodal arrhytmia, ventricular tachycardia, torsade de pointes,
Digestive	
Very common	Nausea, vomiting, diarrhoea
Common	Elevated liver function tests (including ASAT, ALAT, alkaline phosphatase, GGT, LDH, bilirubin), jaundice, cheilitis, cholestatic jaundice, gastroenteritis
Uncommon	Cholecystitis, cholelithiasis, constipation, duodenitis, dyspepsia, enlarged liver, gingivitis, glossitis, hepatitis, hepatic failure, pancreatitis, tongue oedema
Rare	Pseudomembranous colitis, hepatic coma
Endocrine	
Uncommon	Adrenal cortex insufficiency
Haemic and lymphatic	
Common	Thrombocytopenia, anaemia (including macrocytic, microcytic, normocytic, megaloblastic, aplastic), leukopenia, pancytopenia, purpura
Uncommon	Lymphadenopathy, agranulocytosis, eosinophilia, disseminated intravascular coagulation, marrow depression
Rare	Lymphangitis
Metabolic and nutritional	
Very common	Peripheral oedema
Common	Hypokalaemia, creatinine increased, hypoglycaemia
Uncommon	BUN increased, albuminuria, hypercholesterolaemia
Rare	Hyperthyroidism, hypothyroidism
Musculoskeletal	
Uncommon	Arthritis
Nervous	
Common	Dizziness, hallucinations, confusion, depression, anxiety, tremor, agitation, paraesthesia
Uncommon	Ataxia, brain oedema, diplopia, hypoaesthesia, nystagmus, vertigo
Rare	Guillain-Barre syndrome, oculogyric crisis, hypertonia, Extrapyramidal syndrome, insomnia, encephalopathy, somnolence during infusion
Respiratory	
Common	Respiratory distress syndrome, lung oedema, sinusitis
Skin and appendages	
Very common	Rash
Common	Pruritus, maculopapular rash, photosensitivity skin reaction, alopecia, exfoliative dermatitis
Uncommon	Fixed drug eruption, eczema, psoriasis, Stevens-Johnson syndrome, urticaria
Rare	Discoid lupus erythematosis, erythema multiforme, toxic epidermal necrolysis
Special senses	
Very common	Visual disturbances (including altered/enhanced visual perception, blurred vision, colour vision change, photophobia)
Uncommon	Blepharitis, optic neuritis, papilloedema, scleritis, altered taste perception
Rare	Retinal haemorrhage, corneal opacity, optic atrophy, hypoacusis, tinnitus
Urogenital	
Common	Acute kidney failure, haematuria
Uncommon	Nephritis
Rare	Kidney tubular necrosis

Altered taste perception

In the combined data from three bioequivalence studies using the powder for oral suspension formulation, treatment related taste perversion was recorded in 12 (14%) of subjects.

Visual disturbances

Voriconazole treatment-related visual disturbances were very common. In clinical trials, short-term as well as long-term treatment, approximately 30 % of subjects experienced altered/enhanced visual perception, blurred vision, colour vision change or photophobia. The visual disturbances are transient and fully reversible, with the majority spontaneously resolving within 60 minutes and no clinically significant long-term visual effects were observed. There is evidence of attenuation with repeated doses of voriconazole. The visual disturbance is generally mild, rarely results in discontinuation and has not been associated with long-term sequelae. Visual disturbances may be associated with higher plasma concentrations and/or doses.

The mechanism of action is unknown, although the site of action is most likely to be within the retina.

In a study in healthy volunteers investigating the impact of voriconazole on retinal function, voriconazole caused a decrease in the electroretinogram (ERG) waveform amplitude. The ERG measures electrical currents in the retina. The ERG changes did not progress over 29 days of treatment and were fully reversible on withdrawal of voriconazole.

Dermatological reactions

Dermatological reactions were common in patients treated with voriconazole in clinical trials, but these patients had serious underlying diseases and were receiving multiple concomitant medications. The majority of rashes were of mild to moderate severity. Patients have rarely developed serious cutaneous reactions, including Stevens-Johnson syndrome, toxic epidermal necrolysis and erythema multiforme during treatment with VFEND.

If patients develop a rash they should be monitored closely and VFEND discontinued if lesions progress.

Photosensitivity reactions have been reported, especially during long-term therapy (see also section 4.4).

Liver function tests

The overall incidence of clinically significant transaminase abnormalities in the voriconazole clinical programme was 13.4 % (200/1493) of subjects treated with voriconazole. Liver function test abnormalities may be associated with higher plasma concentrations and/or doses. The majority of abnormal liver function tests either resolved during treatment without dose adjustment or following dose adjustment, including discontinuation of therapy.

Voriconazole has been infrequently associated with cases of serious hepatic toxicity in patients with other serious underlying conditions. This includes cases of jaundice, and rare cases of hepatitis and hepatic failure leading to death (see section 4.4).

Infusion-related reactions

During infusion of the intravenous formulation of voriconazole in healthy subjects, anaphylactoid-type reactions, including flushing, fever, sweating, tachycardia, chest tightness, dyspnoea, faintness, nausea, pruritus and rash have occurred. Symptoms appeared immediately upon initiating the infusion (see also section 4.4).

4.9 Overdose

In clinical trials there were 3 cases of accidental overdose. All occurred in paediatric patients, who received up to five times the recommended intravenous dose of voriconazole. A single adverse reaction of photophobia of 10 minutes duration was reported.

There is no known antidote to voriconazole.

Voriconazole is haemodialysed with a clearance of 121 ml/min. The intravenous vehicle, SBECD, is haemodialysed with a clearance of 55 ml/min. In an overdose, haemodialysis may assist in the removal of voriconazole and SBECD from the body.

5. PHARMACOLOGICAL PROPERTIES

5.1 Pharmacodynamic properties

Pharmacotherapeutic group: ATC code: J02A C03

Antimycotics for Systemic Use – Triazole derivatives

Mechanism of action

In vitro, voriconazole displays broad-spectrum antifungal activity with antifungal potency against *Candida* species (including fluconazole resistant *C. krusei* and resistant strains of *C. glabrata* and *C. albicans*) and fungicidal activity against all *Aspergillus* species tested. In addition voriconazole shows *in vitro* fungicidal activity against emerging fungal pathogens, including those such as *Scedosporium* or *Fusarium* which have limited susceptibility to existing antifungal agents. Its mode of action is inhibition of fungal cytochrome P450-mediated 14α-sterol demethylation, an essential step in ergosterol biosynthesis.

In animal studies there is a correlation between minimum inhibitory concentration values and efficacy against experimental mycoses. By contrast, in clinical studies, there appears to be no correlation between minimum inhibitory concentration values and clinical outcome. Furthermore, there does not appear to be a correlation between plasma levels and clinical outcome. This is typical of azole antimycotics.

Microbiology

Clinical efficacy (with partial or complete response, see below under Clinical Experience) has been demonstrated for *Aspergillus* spp. including *A. flavus, A. fumigatus, A. terreus, A. niger, A. nidulans, Candida* spp., including *C. albicans, C. glabrata, C. krusei, C. parapsilosis* and *C. tropicalis* and limited numbers of *C. dubliniensis, C. inconspicuaa*nd *C. guilliermondii, Scedosporium* spp., including *S. apiospermum, S. prolificans* and *Fusarium* spp.

Other treated fungal infections (with often partial or complete response, see below under Clinical Experience) included isolated cases of *Alternaria* spp., *Blastomyces dermatitidis, Blastoschizomyces capitatus, Cladosporium* spp., *Coccidioides immitis, Conidiobolus coronatus, Cryptococcus neoformans, Exserohilum rostratum, Exophiala spinifera, Fonsecaea pedrosoi, Madurella mycetomatis, Paecilomyces lilacinus, Penicillium* spp. including *P. marneffei, Phialophora richardsiae, Scopulariopsis brevicaulis* and *Trichosporon* spp. including *T. beigelii* infections.

In vitro activity against clinical isolates has been observed for *Acremonium* spp., *Alternaria* spp., *Bipolaris* spp., *Cladophialophora* spp., *Histoplasma capsulatum,* with most strains being inhibited by concentrations of voriconazole in the range 0.05 to 2 μg/ml.

In vitro activity against the following pathogens has been shown, but the clinical significance is unknown: *Curvularia* spp. and *Sporothrix* spp.

Specimens for fungal culture and other relevant laboratory studies (serology, histopathology) should be obtained prior to therapy to isolate and identify causative organisms. Therapy may be instituted before the results of the cultures and other laboratory studies are known; however, once these results become available, anti-infective therapy should be adjusted accordingly.

Clinical isolates with decreased susceptibility to voriconazole have been identified. However, elevated minimum inhibitory concentrations did not always correlate with clinical failure and clinical success has been observed in patients infected with organisms resistant to other azoles. Correlation of *in vitro* activity with clinical outcome is difficult owing to the complexity of the patients studied in clinical trials; breakpoints for voriconazole remain to be established.

Clinical Experience

Successful outcome in this section is defined as complete or partial response.

Aspergillus **infections** – efficacy in aspergillosis patients with poor prognosis

Voriconazole has *in vitro* fungicidal activity against *Aspergillus* spp. The efficacy and survival benefit of voriconazole versus conventional amphotericin B in the primary treatment of acute invasive aspergillosis was demonstrated in an open, randomised, multicentre study in 277 immunocompromised patients treated for 12 weeks. A satisfactory global response (complete or partial resolution of all attributable symptoms signs, radiographic/bronchoscopic abnormalities present at baseline) was seen in 53 % of voriconazole-treated patients compared to 31 % of patients treated with comparator. The 84-day survival rate for voriconazole was statistically significantly higher than that for the comparator and a clinically and statistically significant benefit was shown in favour of voriconazole for both time to death and time to discontinuation due to toxicity.

This study confirmed findings from an earlier, prospectively designed study where there was a positive outcome in subjects with risk factors for a poor prognosis, including graft versus host disease, and, in particular, cerebral infections (normally associated with almost 100 % mortality).

The studies included cerebral, sinus, pulmonary and disseminated aspergillosis in patients with bone marrow and solid organ transplants, haematological malignancies, cancer and AIDS.

Candidaemiain non-neutropenic patients.

The efficacy of voriconazole compared to the regimen of amphotericin B followed by fluconazole in the primary treatment of candidaemia was demonstrated in an open, comparative study. Three hundred and seventy non-neutropenic patients (above 12 years of age) with documented candidaemia were included in the study, of whom 248 were treated with voriconazole. Nine subjects in the voriconazole group and five in the amphotericin B followed by fluconazole group also had mycologically proven infection in deep tissue. Patients with renal failure were excluded from this study. The median treatment duration was 15 days in both treatment arms. In the primary analysis, successful response as assessed by a Data Review Committee (DRC) blinded to study medication was defined as resolution/improvement in all clinical signs and symptoms of infection with eradication of *Candida* from blood and infected deep tissue sites at 12 weeks after the end of therapy (EOT). Patients who did not have an assessment 12 weeks after EOT were counted as failures. In this analysis a successful response was seen in 41% of patients in both treatment arms.

In a secondary analysis, which utilised *DRC* assessments at the latest evaluable time point (EOT, or 2, 6, or 12 weeks after EOT) voriconazole and the regimen of amphotericin B followed by fluconazole had successful response rates of 65% and 71%, respectively. The Investigator's assessment of successful outcome at each of these time points is shown in the following table.

Timepoint	*Voriconazole (N=248)*	*Amphotericin B → fluconazole (N=122)*
EOT	*178 (72%)*	*88 (72%)*
2 weeks after EOT	*125 (50%)*	*62 (51%)*
6 weeks after EOT	*104 (42%)*	*55 (45%)*
12 weeks after EOT	*104 (42%)*	*51 (42%)*

There are no data in children below the age of 12 years for this indication.

Serious refractory *Candida* infections

The study comprised 55 patients with serious refractory systemic *Candida* infections (including candidaemia, disseminated and other invasive candidiasis) where prior antifungal treatment, particularly with fluconazole, had been ineffective. Successful response was seen in 24 patients (15 complete, 9 partial responses). In fluconazole-resistant non *albicans* species, a successful outcome was seen in 3/3 *C. krusei* (complete responses) and 6/8 *C. glabrata* (5 complete, 1 partial response) infections. The clinical efficacy data were supported by limited susceptibility data.

Scedosporium **and *Fusarium* infections**

Voriconazole was shown to be effective against the following rare fungal pathogens:

Scedosporium spp.: Successful response to voriconazole therapy was seen in 16 (6 complete, 10 partial responses) of 28 patients with *S. apiospermum* and in 2 (both partial responses) of 7 patients with *S. prolificans* infection. In addition, a successful response was seen in 1 of 3 patients with infections caused by more than one organism including *Scedosporium* spp.

Fusarium spp.: Seven (3 complete, 4 partial responses) of 17 patients were successfully treated with voriconazole. Of these 7 patients, 3 had eye, 1 had sinus, and 3 had disseminated infection. Four additional patients with fusariosis had an infection caused by several organisms; two of them had a successful outcome.

The majority of patients receiving voriconazole treatment of the above mentioned rare infections were intolerant of, or refractory to, prior antifungal therapy.

Duration of treatment

In clinical trials, 561 patients received voriconazole therapy for greater than 12 weeks, with 136 patients receiving voriconazole for over 6 months.

Experience in paediatric patients

Sixty one paediatric patients aged 9 months up to 15 years who had definite or probable invasive fungal infections, were treated with voriconazole. This population included 34 patients 2 to < 12 years old and 20 patients 12-15 years of age.

The majority (57/61) had failed previous antifungal therapies. Therapeutic studies included 5 patients aged 12-15 years, the remaining patients received voriconazole in the compassionate use programmes. Underlying diseases in these patients included haematological malignancies and aplastic anaemia (27 patients) and chronic granulomatous disease (14 patients). The most commonly treated fungal infection was aspergillosis (43/61; 70 %).

Clinical Studies Examining QT Interval

A placebo-controlled, randomized, single-dose, crossover study to evaluate the effect on the QT interval of healthy volunteers was conducted with three oral doses of voriconazole and ketoconazole. The placebo-adjusted mean maximum increases in QTc from baseline after 800, 1200 and 1600 mg of voriconazole were 5.1, 4.8, and 8.2 msec, respectively and 7.0 msec for ketoconazole 800 mg. No subject in any group had an increase in QTc of $\geqslant$60 msec from baseline. No subject experienced an interval exceeding the potentially clinically relevant threshold of 500 msec.

5.2 Pharmacokinetic properties

General pharmacokinetic characteristics

The pharmacokinetics of voriconazole have been characterised in healthy subjects, special populations and patients. During oral administration of 200 mg or 300 mg twice daily for 14 days in patients at risk of aspergillosis (mainly patients with malignant neoplasms of lymphatic or haematopoietic tissue), the observed pharmacokinetic characteristics of rapid and consistent absorption, accumulation and non-linear pharmacokinetics were in agreement with those observed in healthy subjects.

The pharmacokinetics of voriconazole are non-linear due to saturation of its metabolism. Greater than proportional increase in exposure is observed with increasing dose. It is estimated that, on average, increasing the oral dose from 200 mg twice daily to 300 mg twice daily leads to a 2.5-fold increase in exposure (AUC_τ). When the recommended intravenous or oral loading dose regimens are administered, plasma concentrations close to steady state are achieved within the first 24 hours of dosing. Without the loading dose, accumulation occurs during twice daily multiple dosing with steady-state plasma voriconazole concentrations being achieved by day 6 in the majority of subjects.

Absorption

Voriconazole is rapidly and almost completely absorbed following oral administration, with maximum plasma concentrations (C_{max}) achieved 1-2 hours after dosing. The absolute bioavailability of voriconazole after oral administration is estimated to be 96 %. When multiple doses of voriconazole are administered with high fat meals, C_{max} and AUC_τ are reduced by 34 % and 24 %, respectively. The absorption of voriconazole is not affected by changes in gastric pH.

Distribution

The volume of distribution at steady state for voriconazole is estimated to be 4.6 l/kg, suggesting extensive distribution into tissues. Plasma protein binding is estimated to be 58 %. Cerebrospinal fluid samples from eight patients in a compassionate programme showed detectable voriconazole concentrations in all patients.

Metabolism

In vitro studies showed that voriconazole is metabolised by the hepatic cytochrome P450 isoenzymes, CYP2C19, CYP2C9 and CYP3A4.

The inter-individual variability of voriconazole pharmacokinetics is high.

In vivo studies indicated that CYP2C19 is significantly involved in the metabolism of voriconazole. This enzyme exhibits genetic polymorphism. For example, 15-20 % of Asian populations may be expected to be poor metabolisers. For Caucasians and Blacks the prevalence of poor metabolisers is 3-5 %. Studies conducted in Caucasian and Japanese healthy subjects have shown that poor metabolisers have, on average, 4-fold higher voriconazole exposure (AUC_τ) than their homozygous extensive metaboliser counterparts. Subjects who are heterozygous extensive metabolisers have on average 2-fold higher voriconazole exposure than their homozygous extensive metaboliser counterparts.

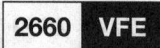

The major metabolite of voriconazole is the N-oxide, which accounts for 72 % of the circulating radiolabelled metabolites in plasma. This metabolite has minimal antifungal activity and does not contribute to the overall efficacy of voriconazole

Excretion

Voriconazole is eliminated via hepatic metabolism with less than 2 % of the dose excreted unchanged in the urine.

After administration of a radiolabelled dose of voriconazole, approximately 80 % of the radioactivity is recovered in the urine after multiple intravenous dosing and 83 % in the urine after multiple oral dosing. The majority > 94 %) of the total radioactivity is excreted in the first 96 hours after both oral and intravenous dosing.

The terminal half-life of voriconazole depends on dose and is approximately 6 hours at 200 mg (orally). Because of non-linear pharmacokinetics, the terminal half-life is not useful in the prediction of the accumulation or elimination of voriconazole.

Pharmacokinetic-Pharmacodynamic relationships

In 10 therapeutic studies, the median for the average and maximum plasma concentrations in individual subjects across the studies was 2425 ng/ml (inter-quartile range 1193 to 4380 ng/ml) and 3742 ng/ml (inter-quartile range 2027 to 6302 ng/ml), respectively. A positive association between mean, maximum or minimum plasma voriconazole concentration and efficacy in therapeutic studies was not found.

Pharmacokinetic-Pharmacodynamic analyses of clinical trial data identified positive associations between plasma voriconazole concentrations and both liver function test abnormalities and visual disturbances.

Pharmacokinetics in special patient groups

Gender

In an oral multiple dose study, C_{max} and AUC_{τ} for healthy young females were 83 % and 113 % higher, respectively, than in healthy young males (18-45 years). In the same study, no significant differences in C_{max} and AUC_{τ} were observed between healthy elderly males and healthy elderly females (⩾ 65 years).

In the clinical programme, no dosage adjustment was made on the basis of gender. The safety profile and plasma concentrations observed in male and female patients were similar. Therefore, no dosage adjustment based on gender is necessary.

Elderly

In an oral multiple dose study C_{max} and AUC_{τ} in healthy elderly males (⩾ 65 years) were 61 % and 86 % higher, respectively, than in healthy young males (18-45 years). No significant differences in C_{max} and AUC_{τ} were observed between healthy elderly females (⩾ 65 years) and healthy young females (18- 45 years).

In the therapeutic studies no dosage adjustment was made on the basis of age. A relationship between plasma concentrations and age was observed. The safety profile of voriconazole in young and elderly patients was similar and, therefore, no dosage adjustment is necessary for the elderly (see section 4.2).

Paediatrics *(For 200mg powder for solution for infusion only)*

A population pharmacokinetic analysis was conducted on data from 35 immunocompromised subjects aged 2 to < 12 years old who were included in the intravenous single or multiple dose pharmacokinetic studies. Twenty four of these subjects received multiple doses of voriconazole. Average steady state plasma concentrations in children receiving a maintenance dose of 4 mg/kg every 12 hours were similar to those in adults receiving 3 mg/kg every 12 hours, with medians of 1186 ng/ml in children and 1155 ng/ml in adults. Therefore a maintenance dose of 4 mg/kg every 12 hours is recommended for children aged between 2 to < 12 years of age (see Ssection 4.2).

Renal impairment

Film-coated tablets:

In an oral single dose (200 mg) study in subjects with normal renal function and mild (creatinine clearance 41-60 ml/min) to severe (creatinine clearance < 20 ml/min) renal impairment, the pharmacokinetics of voriconazole were not significantly affected by renal impairment. The plasma protein binding of voriconazole was similar in subjects with different degrees of renal impairment. See dosing and monitoring recommendations under sections 4.2 and 4.4.

Powder for solution for infusion:

In patients with moderate to severe renal dysfunction (serum creatinine levels >2.5 mg /dl), accumulation of the intravenous vehicle, SBECD, occurs. See dosing and monitoring recommendations under sections 4.2 and 4.4.

Hepatic impairment

After an oral single dose (200 mg), AUC was 233 % higher in subjects with mild to moderate hepatic cirrhosis (Child-Pugh A and B) compared with subjects with normal hepatic function. Protein binding of voriconazole was not affected by impaired hepatic function.

In an oral multiple dose study, AUC_{τ} was similar in subjects with moderate hepatic cirrhosis (Child-Pugh B) given a maintenance dose of 100 mg twice daily and subjects with normal hepatic function given 200 mg twice daily. No pharmacokinetic data are available for patients with severe hepatic cirrhosis (Child-Pugh C). See dosing and monitoring recommendations under sections 4.2 and 4.4.

5.3 Preclinical safety data

Repeated-dose toxicity studies with voriconazole indicated the liver to be the target organ. Hepatotoxicity occurred at plasma exposures similar to those obtained at therapeutic doses in humans, in common with other antifungal agents. In rats, mice and dogs, voriconazole also induced minimal adrenal changes. Conventional studies of safety pharmacology, genotoxicity or carcinogenic potential did not reveal a special hazard for humans.

In reproduction studies, voriconazole was shown to be teratogenic in rats and embryotoxic in rabbits at systemic exposures equal to those obtained in humans with therapeutic doses. In the pre and postnatal development study in rats at exposures lower than those obtained in humans with therapeutic doses, voriconazole prolonged the duration of gestation and labour and produced dystocia with consequent maternal mortality and reduced perinatal survival of pups. The effects on parturition are probably mediated by species-specific mechanisms, involving reduction of oestradiol levels, and are consistent with those observed with other azole antifungal agents.

Preclinical data on the intravenous vehicle, SBECD indicated that the main effects were vacuolation of urinary tract epithelium and activation of macrophages in the liver and lungs in the repeated-dose toxicity studies. As GPMT (guinea pig maximisation test) result was positive, prescribers should be aware of the hypersensitivity potential of the intravenous formulation. Standard genotoxicity and reproduction studies with the excipient SBECD reveal no special hazard for humans. Carcinogenicity studies were not performed with SBECD. An impurity, present in SBECD, has been shown to be an alkylating mutagenic agent with evidence for carcinogenicity in rodents. This impurity should be considered a substance with carcinogenic potential in humans. In the light of these data the duration of treatment of the intravenous formulation should be no longer than 6 months.

6. PHARMACEUTICAL PARTICULARS

6.1 List of excipients

Film-coated tablets:

Tablet core:

Lactose Monohydrate

Pregelatinised Starch

Croscarmellose Sodium

Povidone

Magnesium Stearate

Film-coat:

Hypromellose

Titanium Dioxide (E171)

Lactose Monohydrate

Glycerol Triacetate

Powder for solution for infusion:

Sulphobutylether beta cyclodextrin sodium (SBECD)

Powder for oral suspension:

Sucrose (0.54 g per ml of suspension)

Silica, Colloidal

Titanium Dioxide (E171)

Xanthan Gum

Sodium Citrate

Sodium Benzoate (E211)

Citric Acid

Natural Orange Flavour (containing orange oil, maltodextrin and tocopherol)

6.2 Incompatibilities

Film-coated tablets:

Not applicable

Powder for solution for infusion:

VFEND must not be infused into the same line or cannula concomitantly with infusions of other medicinal products including parenteral nutrition (e.g. Aminofusin 10 % Plus). 4.2 % Sodium Bicarbonate Intravenous Infusion is not compatible with VFEND and is not recommended for use as a diluent. Compatibility with other concentrations is unknown.

This medicinal product must not be mixed with other medicinal products except those mentioned in section 6.6.

Infusions of blood products must not occur simultaneously with voriconazole.

Infusion of total parenteral nutrition can occur simultaneously with voriconazole but not in the same line or cannula.

Powder for oral suspension:

This medicinal product must not be mixed with other medicinal products except those mentioned in 6.6. It is not intended that the suspension be further diluted with water or other vehicles.

6.3 Shelf life

VFEND film-coated tablets: 3 years.

VFEND powder for solution for infusion: 3 years.

VFEND is a single dose unpreserved sterile lyophile. Therefore, from a microbiological point of view, once reconstituted, the product must be used immediately. If not used immediately, in-use storage times and conditions prior to use are the responsibility of the user and would normally not be longer than 24 hours at 2°C to 8°C, unless reconstitution has taken place in controlled and validated aseptic conditions.

Chemical and physical in-use stability has been demonstrated for 24 hours at 2°C to 8°C.

Powder for oral suspension:

The shelf-life of the powder for oral suspension is 2 years.

The shelf-life of the constituted suspension is 14 days.

6.4 Special precautions for storage

Film-coated tablets:

No special precautions for storage.

Powder for solution for infusion:

Reconstituted concentrate: Store at 2°C-8°C for up to 24 hours (in a refrigerator).

Powder for oral suspension:

Powder for oral suspension: Store at 2°C - 8°C (in a refrigerator) before constitution.

Constituted suspension: Do not store above 30°C, do not refrigerate or freeze.

Keep the container tightly closed.

Any remaining suspension should be discarded 14 days after constitution.

6.5 Nature and contents of container

Film-coated tablets:

HDPE tablet containers of 2, 30 and 100. Not all bottle sizes may be marketed.

PVC / Aluminium blister in cartons of 2, 10, 14, 20, 28, 30, 50, 56 and 100.

Not all pack sizes may be marketed.

Powder for solution for infusion:

Packs of 1 single use 30 ml clear Type I glass vials with rubber stoppers and aluminium caps with plastic seals.

Powder for oral suspension:

One 100 ml high-density polyethylene (HDPE) bottle (with a polypropylene child resistant closure) contains 45 g of powder for oral suspension. Following constitution, the volume of the suspension is 75 ml, providing a usable volume of 70 ml.

A measuring cup (graduated to indicate 23 mL), 5 ml oral syringe and a press-in bottle adaptor are also provided.

Pack size: 1 bottle

6.6 Instructions for use and handling

Film-coated tablets:

Not applicable.

Powder for solution for infusion:

The powder is reconstituted with 19 ml of Water for Injections to obtain an extractable volume of 20 ml of clear concentrate containing 10 mg/ml of voriconazole. Discard the VFEND vial if vacuum does not pull the diluent into the vial. It is recommended that a standard 20 ml (non-automated) syringe be used to ensure that the exact amount (19.0 ml) of Water for Injections is dispensed. This medicinal product is for single use only and any unused solution should be discarded and only clear solutions without particles should be used.

For administration, the required volume of the reconstituted concentrate is added to a recommended compatible infusion solution (detailed below) to obtain a final voriconazole solution containing 0.5-5 mg/ml.

Required Volumes of 10 mg/ml VFEND Concentrate

(see Table 3 on next page)

Voriconazole is a single dose unpreserved sterile lyophile. Therefore, from a microbiological point of view, the reconstituted solution must be used immediately. If not used immediately, in-use storage times and conditions prior to use are the responsibility of the user and would normally not be longer than 24 hours at 2 to 8°C, unless reconstitution has taken place in controlled and validated aseptic conditions.

The reconstituted solution can be diluted with:

9 mg/ml (0.9 %) Sodium Chloride for Infusion

Lactated Ringer's Intravenous Infusion

5 % Glucose and Lactated Ringer's Intravenous Infusion

5 % Glucose and 0.45 % Sodium Chloride Intravenous Infusion

5 % Glucose Intravenous Infusion

5 % Glucose in 20 mEq Potassium Chloride Intravenous Infusion

0.45 % Sodium Chloride Intravenous Infusion

5 % Glucose and 0.9 % Sodium Chloride Intravenous Infusion

The compatibility of voriconazole with diluents other than described above or in section 6.2 is unknown.

Table 3 Required Volumes of 10 mg/ml VFEND Concentrate

Body Weight(kg)	Volume of VFEND Concentrate (10 mg/ml) required for:		
	3 mg/kg dose(number of vials)	4 mg/kg dose(number of vials)	6 mg/kg dose(number of vials)
30	9.0 ml (1)	12 ml (1)	18 ml(1)
35	10.5 ml (1)	14 ml (1)	21 ml (2)
40	12.0 ml (1)	16 ml (1)	24 ml (2)
45	13.5 ml (1)	18 ml (1)	27 ml (2)
50	15.0 ml (1)	20 ml (1)	30 ml (2)
55	16.5 ml (1)	22 ml (2)	33 ml (2)
60	18.0 ml (1)	24 ml (2)	36 ml (2)
65	19.5 ml (1)	26 ml (2)	39 ml (2)
70	21.0 ml (2)	28 ml (2)	42 ml (3)
75	22.5 ml (2)	30 ml (2)	45 ml (3)
80	24.0 ml (2)	32 ml (2)	48 ml (3)
85	25.5 ml (2)	34 ml (2)	51 ml (3)
90	27.0 ml (2)	36 ml (2)	54 ml (3)
95	28.5 ml (2)	38 ml (2)	57 ml (3)
100	30.0 ml (2)	40 ml (2)	60 ml (3)

Powder for oral suspension:

Constitution instructions:

1. Tap the bottle to release the powder.
2. Measure 23 ml of water by filling the measuring cup to the top of the marked line. Add the water to the bottle. Using the cup measure another 23 ml of water and add this to the bottle.
3. Shake the closed bottle vigorously for about 1 minute.
4. Remove child-resistant cap. Press bottle adaptor into the neck of the bottle.
5. Replace the cap.
6. Write the date of expiration of the constituted suspension on the bottle label (the shelf-life of the constituted suspension is 14 days).

Instructions for use:

Shake the closed bottle of constituted suspension for approximately 10 seconds before each use.

Once constituted, VFEND oral suspension should only be administered using the oral syringe supplied with each pack. Refer to the patient leaflet for more detailed instructions for use.

7. MARKETING AUTHORISATION HOLDER

Pfizer Limited, Ramsgate Road, Sandwich, Kent CT13 9NJ, United Kingdom

8. MARKETING AUTHORISATION NUMBER(S)

EU/1/02/212/001 VFEND 50 mg Film-coated tablets; Pack size 2 tablets; Blister

EU/1/02/212/002 VFEND 50 mg Film-coated tablets; Pack size 10 tablets; Blister

EU/1/02/212/003 VFEND 50 mg Film-coated tablets; Pack size 14 tablets; Blister

EU/1/02/212/004 VFEND 50 mg Film-coated tablets; Pack size 20 tablets; Blister

EU/1/02/212/005 VFEND 50 mg Film-coated tablets; Pack size 28 tablets; Blister

EU/1/02/212/006 VFEND 50 mg Film-coated tablets; Pack size 30 tablets; Blister

EU/1/02/212/007 VFEND 50 mg Film-coated tablets; Pack size 50 tablets; Blister

EU/1/02/212/008 VFEND 50 mg Film-coated tablets; Pack size 56 tablets; Blister

EU/1/02/212/009 VFEND 50 mg Film-coated tablets; Pack size 100 tablets; Blister

EU/1/02/212/010 VFEND 50 mg Film-coated tablets; Pack size 2 tablets; Bottle

EU/1/02/212/011 VFEND 50 mg Film-coated tablets; Pack size 30 tablets; Bottle

EU/1/02/212/012 VFEND 50 mg Film-coated tablets; Pack size 100 tablets; Bottle

EU/1/02/212/013 VFEND 200 mg Film-coated tablets; Pack size 2 tablets; Blister

EU/1/02/212/014 VFEND 200 mg Film-coated tablets; Pack size 10 tablets; Blister

EU/1/02/212/015 VFEND 200 mg Film-coated tablets; Pack size 14 tablets; Blister

EU/1/02/212/016 VFEND 200 mg Film-coated tablets; Pack size 20 tablets; Blister

EU/1/02/212/017 VFEND 200 mg Film-coated tablets; Pack size 28 tablets; Blister

EU/1/02/212/018 VFEND 200 mg Film-coated tablets; Pack size 30 tablets; Blister

EU/1/02/212/019 VFEND 200 mg Film-coated tablets; Pack size 50 tablets; Blister

EU/1/02/212/020 VFEND 200 mg Film-coated tablets; Pack size 56 tablets; Blister

EU/1/02/212/021 VFEND 200 mg Film-coated tablets; Pack size 100 tablets; Blister

EU/1/02/212/022 VFEND 200 mg Film-coated tablets; Pack size 2 tablets; Bottle

EU/1/02/212/023 VFEND 200 mg Film-coated tablets; Pack size 30 tablets; Bottle

EU/1/02/212/024 VFEND 200 mg Film-coated tablets; Pack size 100 tablets; Bottle

EU/1/02/212/025 VFEND 200 mg Powder for solution for infusion; Vial

EU/1/02/212/026 VFEND 40 mg/ml Powder for oral suspension; Bottle

9. DATE OF FIRST AUTHORISATION/RENEWAL OF THE AUTHORISATION

19 March 2002

10. DATE OF REVISION OF THE TEXT

29 March 2005

LEGAL CATEGORY

POM

Ref: VF 8_0

Viagra 25mg, 50mg, 100mg

(Pfizer Limited)

1. NAME OF THE MEDICINAL PRODUCT

VIAGRA® 25 mg film-coated tablets.

VIAGRA® 50 mg film-coated tablets.

VIAGRA® 100 mg film-coated tablets.

2. QUALITATIVE AND QUANTITATIVE COMPOSITION

Each tablet contains 25mg, 50mg or 100mg of sildenafil, as the citrate.

For excipients, see Section 6.1.

3. PHARMACEUTICAL FORM

Film-coated tablet.

The 25 mg tablets are blue film-coated, rounded diamond-shaped tablets, marked "PFIZER" on one side and "VGR 25" on the other.

The 50 mg tablets are blue film-coated, rounded diamond-shaped tablets, marked "PFIZER" on one side and "VGR 50" on the other.

The 100 mg tablets are blue film-coated, rounded diamond-shaped tablets, marked "PFIZER" on one side and "VGR 100" on the other.

4. CLINICAL PARTICULARS

4.1 Therapeutic indications

Treatment of men with erectile dysfunction, which is the inability to achieve or maintain a penile erection sufficient for satisfactory sexual performance.

In order for VIAGRA to be effective, sexual stimulation is required.

4.2 Posology and method of administration

For oral use.

Use in adults

The recommended dose is 50mg taken as needed approximately one hour before sexual activity. Based on efficacy and toleration, the dose may be increased to 100mg or decreased to 25mg. The maximum recommended dose is 100 mg. The maximum recommended dosing frequency is once per day. If VIAGRA is taken with food, the onset of activity may be delayed compared to the fasted state (see Section 5.2).

Use in the elderly

Dosage adjustments are not required in elderly patients.

Use in patients with impaired renal function

The dosing recommendations described in "Use in adults" apply to patients with mild to moderate renal impairment (creatinine clearance = 30-80 ml/min).

Since sildenafil clearance is reduced in patients with severe renal impairment (creatinine clearance < 30 ml/min) a 25mg dose should be considered. Based on efficacy and toleration, the dose may be increased to 50mg and 100mg.

Use in patients with impaired hepatic function

Since sildenafil clearance is reduced in patients with hepatic impairment (e.g. cirrhosis) a 25mg dose should be considered. Based on efficacy and toleration, the dose may be increased to 50mg and 100mg.

Use in children

VIAGRA is not indicated for individuals below 18 years of age.

Use in patients using other medicines

With the exception of ritonavir for which co-administration with sildenafil is not advised (see Section 4.4) a starting dose of 25mg should be considered in patients receiving concomitant treatment with CYP3A4 inhibitors (see Section 4.5).

In order to minimize the potential for developing postural hypotension, patients should be stable on alpha-blocker therapy prior to initiating sildenafil treatment. In addition, initiation of sildenafil at a dose of 25 mg should be considered (see Sections 4.4 and 4.5).

4.3 Contraindications

Hypersensitivity to the active substance or to any of the excipients.

Consistent with its known effects on the nitric oxide/cyclic guanosine monophosphate (cGMP) pathway (see Section 5.1), sildenafil was shown to potentiate the hypotensive effects of nitrates, and its co-administration with nitric oxide donors (such as amyl nitrite) or nitrates in any form is therefore contraindicated.

Agents for the treatment of erectile dysfunction, including sildenafil, should not be used in men for whom sexual activity is inadvisable (e.g. patients with severe cardiovascular disorders such as unstable angina or severe cardiac failure).

The safety of sildenafil has not been studied in the following sub-groups of patients and its use is therefore contraindicated: severe hepatic impairment, hypotension (blood pressure < 90/50 mmHg), recent history of stroke or myocardial infarction and known hereditary degenerative retinal disorders such as retinitis pigmentosa (a minority of these patients have genetic disorders of retinal phosphodiesterases).

4.4 Special warnings and special precautions for use

A medical history and physical examination should be undertaken to diagnose erectile dysfunction and determine potential underlying causes, before pharmacological treatment is considered.

Prior to initiating any treatment for erectile dysfunction, physicians should consider the cardiovascular status of their patients, since there is a degree of cardiac risk associated with sexual activity. Sildenafil has vasodilator properties, resulting in mild and transient decreases in blood pressure (see Section 5.1). Prior to prescribing sildenafil, physicians should carefully consider whether their patients with certain underlying conditions could be adversely affected by such vasodilatory effects, especially in combination with sexual activity. Patients with increased susceptibility to vasodilators include those with left ventricular outflow obstruction (e.g., aortic stenosis, hypertrophic obstructive cardiomyopathy), or those with the rare syndrome of multiple system atrophy manifesting as severely impaired autonomic control of blood pressure.

VIAGRA potentiates the hypotensive effect of nitrates (see Section 4.3).

Serious cardiovascular events, including myocardial infarction, unstable angina, sudden cardiac death, ventricular arrhythmia, cerebrovascular haemorrhage, transient ischaemic attack, hypertension and hypotension have been reported post-marketing in temporal association with the use of VIAGRA. Most, but not all, of these patients had pre-existing cardiovascular risk factors. Many events were reported to occur during or shortly after sexual intercourse and a few were reported to occur shortly after the use of VIAGRA without sexual activity. It is not possible to determine whether these events are related directly to these factors or to other factors.

Agents for the treatment of erectile dysfunction, including sildenafil, should be used with caution in patients with anatomical deformation of the penis (such as angulation, cavernosal fibrosis or Peyronie's disease), or in patients who have conditions which may predispose them to priapism (such as sickle cell anaemia, multiple myeloma or leukaemia).

The safety and efficacy of combinations of sildenafil with other treatments for erectile dysfunction have not been studied. Therefore the use of such combinations is not recommended.

Co-administration of sildenafil with ritonavir is not advised (see Section 4.5).

Caution is advised when sildenafil is administered to patients taking an alpha-blocker, as the coadministration may lead to symptomatic hypotension in a few susceptible individuals (see Section 4.5). This is most likely to occur within 4 hours post sildenafil dosing. In order to minimise the potential for developing postural hypotension, patients should be hemodynamically stable on alpha-blocker therapy prior to initiating sildenafil treatment. Initiation of sildenafil at a dose of 25 mg should be considered (see Section 4.2). In addition, physicians should advise patients what to do in the event of postural hypotensive symptoms.

Studies with human platelets indicate that sildenafil potentiates the antiaggregatory effect of sodium nitroprusside *in vitro*. There is no safety information on the administration of sildenafil to patients with bleeding disorders or active peptic ulceration. Therefore sildenafil should be administered to these patients only after careful benefit-risk assessment.

VIAGRA is not indicated for use by women.

4.5 Interaction with other medicinal products and other forms of Interaction

Effects of other medicinal products on sildenafil

In vitro studies:

Sildenafil metabolism is principally mediated by the cytochrome P450 (CYP) isoforms 3A4 (major route) and 2C9 (minor route). Therefore, inhibitors of these isoenzymes may reduce sildenafil clearance.

In vivo studies:

Population pharmacokinetic analysis of clinical trial data indicated a reduction in sildenafil clearance when co-administered with CYP3A4 inhibitors (such as ketoconazole, erythromycin, cimetidine). Although no increased incidence of adverse events was observed in these patients, when sildenafil is administered concomitantly with CYP3A4 inhibitors, a starting dose of 25mg should be considered.

Co-administration of the HIV protease inhibitor ritonavir, which is a highly potent P450 inhibitor, at steady state (500mg b.i.d.) with sildenafil (100mg single dose) resulted in a 300% (4-fold) increase in sildenafil C_{max} and a 1,000% (11-fold) increase in sildenafil plasma AUC. At 24 hours, the plasma levels of sildenafil were still approximately 200ng/ml, compared to approximately 5ng/ml when sildenafil was dosed alone. This is consistent with ritonavir's marked effects on a broad range of P450 substrates. Sildenafil had no effect on ritonavir pharmacokinetics. Based on these pharmacokinetic results co-administration of sildenafil with ritonavir is not advised (see Section 4.4) and in any event the maximum dose of sildenafil should under no circumstances exceed 25mg within 48 hours.

Co-administration of the HIV protease inhibitor saquinavir, a CYP3A4 inhibitor, at steady state (1200mg t.i.d.) with sildenafil (100mg single dose) resulted in a 140% increase in sildenafil C_{max} and a 210% increase in sildenafil AUC. Sildenafil had no effect on saquinavir pharmacokinetics (see Section 4.2). Stronger CYP3A4 inhibitors such as ketoconazole and itraconazole would be expected to have greater effects.

When a single 100mg dose of sildenafil was administered with erythromycin, a specific CYP3A4 inhibitor, at steady state (500mg twice daily for 5 days), there was a 182% increase in sildenafil systemic exposure (AUC). In normal healthy male volunteers, there was no evidence of an effect of azithromycin (500mg daily for 3 days) on the AUC, C_{max}, T_{max}, elimination rate constant, or subsequent half-life of sildenafil or its principal circulating metabolite. Cimetidine (800mg), a cytochrome P450 inhibitor and non-specific CYP3A4 inhibitor, caused a 56% increase in plasma sildenafil concentrations when co-administered with sildenafil (50mg) to healthy volunteers.

Grapefruit juice is a weak inhibitor of CYP3A4 gut wall metabolism and may give rise to modest increases in plasma levels of sildenafil.

Table 1

MedDRA System Organ Class	Adverse Reaction	Sildenafil (%) N=3350	Placebo (%) N=2995
Nervous system disorders *Very common*	Headache	10.8	2.8
Common	Dizziness	2.9	1.0
Eye disorders *Common*	Altered vision (increased perception of light, blurred vision)	2.5	0.4
Common	Chromatopsia (mild and transient, predominantly colour tinge to vision)	1.1	0.03
Cardiac disorders *Common*	Palpitation	1.0	0.2
Vascular disorders *Very common*	Flushing	10.9	1.4
Respiratory, thoracic and mediastinal disorders *Common*	Nasal congestion	2.1	0.3
Gastrointestinal disorders *Common*	Dyspepsia	3.0	0.4

Single doses of antacid (magnesium hydroxide/aluminium hydroxide) did not affect the bioavailability of sildenafil.

Although specific interaction studies were not conducted for all medicinal products, population pharmacokinetic analysis showed no effect of concomitant medication on sildenafil pharmacokinetics when grouped as CYP2C9 inhibitors (such as tolbutamide, warfarin, phenytoin), CYP2D6 inhibitors (such as selective serotonin reuptake inhibitors, tricyclic antidepressants), thiazide and related diuretics, loop and potassium sparing diuretics, angiotensin converting enzyme inhibitors, calcium channel blockers, beta-adrenoreceptor antagonists or inducers of CYP450 metabolism (such as rifampicin, barbiturates).

Nicorandil is a hybrid of potassium channel opener and nitrate. Due to the nitrate component it has the potential to have serious interaction with sildenafil.

Effects of sildenafil on other medicinal products

In vitro studies:

Sildenafil is a weak inhibitor of the cytochrome P450 isoforms 1A2, 2C9, 2C19, 2D6, 2E1 and 3A4 (IC_{50} >150 microM). Given sildenafil peak plasma concentrations of approximately 1 microM after recommended doses, it is unlikely that VIAGRA will alter the clearance of substrates of these isoenzymes.

There are no data on the interaction of sildenafil and non-specific phosphodiesterase inhibitors such as theophylline or dipyridamole.

In vivo studies:

Consistent with its known effects on the nitric oxide/cGMP pathway (see Section 5.1), sildenafil was shown to potentiate the hypotensive effects of nitrates, and its co-administration with nitric oxide donors or nitrates in any form is therefore contraindicated (see Section 4.3).

Concomitant administration of sildenafil to patients taking alpha-blocker therapy may lead to symptomatic hypotension in a few susceptible individuals. This is most likely to occur within 4 hours post sildenafil dosing (see Sections 4.2 and 4.4). In three specific drug-drug interaction studies, the alpha-blocker doxazosin (4 mg and 8 mg) and sildenafil (25 mg, 50 mg, or 100 mg) were administered simultaneously to patients with benign prostatic hyperplasia (BPH) stabilized on doxazosin therapy. In these study populations, mean additional reductions of supine blood pressure of 7/7 mmHg, 9/5 mmHg, and 8/4 mmHg, and mean additional reductions of standing blood pressure of 6/6 mmHg, 11/4 mmHg, and 4/5 mmHg, respectively, were observed. When sildenafil and doxazosin were administered simultaneously to patients stabilized on doxazosin therapy, there were infrequent reports of patients who experienced symptomatic postural hypotension. These reports included dizziness and light-headedness, but not syncope.

No significant interactions were shown when sildenafil (50mg) was co-administered with tolbutamide (250mg) or warfarin (40mg), both of which are metabolised by CYP2C9.

Sildenafil (50mg) did not potentiate the increase in bleeding time caused by acetyl salicylic acid (150mg).

Sildenafil (50mg) did not potentiate the hypotensive effects of alcohol in healthy volunteers with mean maximum blood alcohol levels of 80 mg/dl.

Pooling of the following classes of antihypertensive medication; diuretics, beta-blockers, ACE inhibitors, angiotensin II antagonists, antihypertensive medicinal products (vasodilator and centrally-acting), adrenergic neurone blockers, calcium channel blockers and alpha-adrenoceptor blockers, showed no difference in the side effect profile in patients taking sildenafil compared to placebo treatment. In a specific interaction study, where sildenafil (100mg) was co-administered with amlodipine in hypertensive patients, there was an additional reduction on supine systolic blood pressure of 8 mmHg. The corresponding additional reduction in supine diastolic blood pressure was 7 mmHg. These additional blood pressure reductions were of a similar magnitude to those seen when sildenafil was administered alone to healthy volunteers (see Section 5.1).

Sildenafil (100mg) did not affect the steady state pharmacokinetics of the HIV protease inhibitors, saquinavir and ritonavir, both of which are CYP3A4 substrates.

4.6 Pregnancy and lactation

VIAGRA is not indicated for use by women.

No relevant adverse effects were found in reproduction studies in rats and rabbits following oral administration of sildenafil.

4.7 Effects on ability to drive and use machines

As dizziness and altered vision were reported in clinical trials with sildenafil, patients should be aware of how they react to VIAGRA, before driving or operating machinery.

4.8 Undesirable effects

Adverse reactions (with incidence of ⩾1%) were reported in patients treated with the recommended dosing regimen in placebo-controlled clinical trials. Adverse reactions were mild to moderate in nature and the incidence and severity increased with dose. In fixed dose studies, dyspepsia (12%) and altered vision (11%) were more common at 100 mg than at lower doses. The most commonly reported adverse reactions were headache and flushing, see Table 1.

Very common: ⩾ 1/10

Common: ⩾ 1/100 and < 1/10

Uncommon: ⩾ 1/1000 and < 1/100

Rare: ⩾ 1/10,000 and < 1/1000

Very Rare: < 1/10,000

(see Table 1 above)

There were reports of muscle aches when sildenafil was administered more frequently than the recommended dosing regimen.

In postmarketing surveillance the following adverse events have been uncommonly or rarely reported (Table 2):

Table 2	
Immune system disorders	Hypersensitivity reactions
Eye disorders	Eye pain Red eyes/ bloodshot eyes
Cardiac disorders	Tachycardia, ventricular arrhythmia, myocardial infarction, unstable angina, sudden cardiac death (Section 4.4).
Vascular disorders	Hypotension, (see Sections 4.4 and 4.5), hypertension, epistaxis, syncope, cerebrovascular haemorrhage, transient ischemic attack (see Section 4.4)
Gastrointestinal disorders	Vomiting

Skin and subcutaneous tissue disorders	Skin rash
Reproductive system and breast disorders	Prolonged erection, priapism

4.9 Overdose

In single dose volunteer studies of doses up to 800mg, adverse reactions were similar to those seen at lower doses, but the incidence rates and severities were increased. Doses of 200mg did not result in increased efficacy but the incidence of adverse reactions (headache, flushing, dizziness, dyspepsia, nasal congestion, altered vision) was increased.

In cases of overdose, standard supportive measures should be adopted as required. Renal dialysis is not expected to accelerate clearance as sildenafil is highly bound to plasma proteins and not eliminated in the urine.

5. PHARMACOLOGICAL PROPERTIES

5.1 Pharmacodynamic properties

Pharmacotherapeutic group: Drugs used in erectile dysfunction. ATC Code: G04B E03.

Sildenafil is an oral therapy for erectile dysfunction. In the natural setting, i.e. with sexual stimulation, it restores impaired erectile function by increasing blood flow to the penis.

The physiological mechanism responsible for erection of the penis involves the release of nitric oxide (NO) in the corpus cavernosum during sexual stimulation. Nitric oxide then activates the enzyme guanylate cyclase, which results in increased levels of cyclic guanosine monophosphate (cGMP), producing smooth muscle relaxation in the corpus cavernosum and allowing inflow of blood.

Sildenafil is a potent and selective inhibitor of cGMP specific phosphodiesterase type 5 (PDE5) in the corpus cavernosum, where PDE5 is responsible for degradation of cGMP. Sildenafil has a peripheral site of action on erections. Sildenafil has no direct relaxant effect on isolated human corpus cavernosum but potently enhances the relaxant effect of NO on this tissue. When the NO/cGMP pathway is activated, as occurs with sexual stimulation, inhibition of PDE5 by sildenafil results in increased corpus cavernosum levels of cGMP. Therefore sexual stimulation is required in order for sildenafil to produce its intended beneficial pharmacological effects.

Studies *in vitro* have shown that sildenafil is selective for PDE5, which is involved in the erection process. Its effect is more potent on PDE5 than on other known phosphodiesterases. There is a 10-fold selectivity over PDE6 which is involved in the phototransduction pathway in the retina. At maximum recommended doses, there is an 80-fold selectivity over PDE1, and over 700-fold over PDE 2, 3, 4, 7, 8, 9, 10 and 11. In particular, sildenafil has greater than 4,000-fold selectivity for PDE5 over PDE3, the cAMP-specific phosphodiesterase isoform involved in the control of cardiac contractility.

Two clinical studies were specifically designed to assess the time window after dosing during which sildenafil could produce an erection in response to sexual stimulation. In a penile plethysmography (RigiScan) study of fasted patients, the median time to onset for those who obtained erections of 60% rigidity (sufficient for sexual intercourse) was 25 minutes (range 12-37 minutes) on sildenafil. In a separate RigiScan study, sildenafil was still able to produce an erection in response to sexual stimulation 4-5 hours post-dose.

Sildenafil causes mild and transient decreases in blood pressure which, in the majority of cases, do not translate into clinical effects. The mean maximum decreases in supine systolic blood pressure following 100mg oral dosing of sildenafil was 8.4 mmHg. The corresponding change in supine diastolic blood pressure was 5.5 mmHg. These decreases in blood pressure are consistent with the vasodilatory effects of sildenafil, probably due to increased cGMP levels in vascular smooth muscle. Single oral doses of sildenafil up to 100mg in healthy volunteers produced no clinically relevant effects on ECG.

In a study of the hemodynamic effects of a single oral 100mg dose of sildenafil in 14 patients with severe coronary artery disease (CAD) (>70% stenosis of at least one coronary artery), the mean resting systolic and diastolic blood pressures decreased by 7% and 6% respectively compared to baseline. Mean pulmonary systolic blood pressure decreased by 9%. Sildenafil showed no effect on cardiac output, and did not impair blood flow through the stenosed coronary arteries.

No clinical relevant differences were demonstrated in time to limiting angina for sildenafil when compared with placebo in a double blind, placebo controlled exercise stress trial in 144 patients with erectile dysfunction and chronic stable angina, who were taking on a regular basis anti-anginal medications (except nitrates).

Mild and transient differences in colour discrimination (blue/green) were detected in some subjects using the Farnsworth-Munsell 100 hue test at 1 hour following a 100mg dose, with no effects evident after 2 hours post-dose. The postulated mechanism for this change in colour discrimination is related to inhibition of PDE6, which is involved in the phototransduction cascade of the retina. Sildenafil has no effect on visual acuity or contrast sensitivity. In a small size placebo-controlled study of patients with documented early age-related macular degeneration (n=9), sildenafil (single dose, 100mg) demonstrated no significant changes in visual tests conducted (visual acuity, Amsler grid, colour discrimination simulated traffic light, Humphrey perimeter and photostress).

There was no effect on sperm motility or morphology after single 100mg oral doses of sildenafil in healthy volunteers.

Further information on clinical trials

In clinical trials sildenafil was administered to more than 3000 patients aged 19-87. The following patient groups were represented: elderly (21%), patients with hypertension (24%), diabetes mellitus (16%), ischaemic heart disease and other cardiovascular diseases (14%), hyperlipidaemia (14%), spinal cord injury (6%), depression (5%), transurethral resection of the prostate (5%), radical prostatectomy (4%). The following groups were not well represented or excluded from clinical trials: patients with pelvic surgery, patients post-radiotherapy, patients with severe renal or hepatic impairment and patients with certain cardiovascular conditions (see Section 4.3).

In fixed dose studies, the proportions of patients reporting that treatment improved their erections were 62% (25mg), 74% (50mg) and 82% (100mg) compared to 25% on placebo. In controlled clinical trials, the discontinuation rate due to sildenafil was low and similar to placebo.

Across all trials, the proportion of patients reporting improvement on sildenafil were as follows: psychogenic erectile dysfunction (84%), mixed erectile dysfunction (77%), organic erectile dysfunction (68%), elderly (67%), diabetes mellitus (59%), ischaemic heart disease (69%), hypertension (68%), TURP (61%), radical prostatectomy (43%), spinal cord injury (83%), depression (75%). The safety and efficacy of sildenafil was maintained in long term studies.

5.2 Pharmacokinetic properties

Absorption

Sildenafil is rapidly absorbed. Maximum observed plasma concentrations are reached within 30 to 120 minutes (median 60 minutes) of oral dosing in the fasted state. The mean absolute oral bioavailability is 41% (range 25-63%). After oral dosing of sildenafil AUC and C_{max} increase in proportion with dose over the recommended dose range (25-100mg).

When sildenafil is taken with food, the rate of absorption is reduced with a mean delay in T_{max} of 60 minutes and a mean reduction in C_{max} of 29%.

Distribution

The mean steady state volume of distribution (V_d) for sildenafil is 105 l, indicating distribution into the tissues. After a single oral dose of 100 mg, the mean maximum total plasma concentration of sildenafil is approximately 440 ng/ml (CV 40%). Since sildenafil (and its major circulating N-desmethyl metabolite) is 96% bound to plasma proteins, this results in the mean maximum free plasma concentration for sildenafil of 18 ng/ml (38 nM). Protein binding is independent of total drug concentrations.

In healthy volunteers receiving sildenafil (100mg single dose), less than 0.0002% (average 188ng) of the administered dose was present in ejaculate 90 minutes after dosing.

Metabolism

Sildenafil is cleared predominantly by the CYP3A4 (major route) and CYP2C9 (minor route) hepatic microsomal isoenzymes. The major circulating metabolite results from N-demethylation of sildenafil. This metabolite has a phosphodiesterase selectivity profile similar to sildenafil and an *in vitro* potency for PDE5 approximately 50% that of the parent drug. Plasma concentrations of this metabolite are approximately 40% of those seen for sildenafil. The N-desmethyl metabolite is further metabolised, with a terminal half life of approximately 4 h.

Elimination

The total body clearance of sildenafil is 41 l/h with a resultant terminal phase half life of 3-5 h. After either oral or intravenous administration, sildenafil is excreted as metabolites predominantly in the faeces (approximately 80% of administered oral dose) and to a lesser extent in the urine (approximately 13% of administered oral dose).

Pharmacokinetics in special patient groups

Elderly

Healthy elderly volunteers (65 years or over) had a reduced clearance of sildenafil, resulting in approximately 90% higher plasma concentrations of sildenafil and the active N-desmethyl metabolite compared to those seen in healthy younger volunteers (18-45 years). Due to age-differences in plasma protein binding, the corresponding increase in free sildenafil plasma concentration was approximately 40%.

Renal insufficiency

In volunteers with mild to moderate renal impairment (creatinine clearance = 30-80 ml/min), the pharmacokinetics of sildenafil were not altered after receiving a 50mg single oral dose. The mean AUC and C_{max} of the N-desmethyl metabolite increased 126% and 73% respectively, compared to age-matched volunteers with no renal impairment. However, due to high inter-subject variability, these differences were not statistically significant. In volunteers with severe renal impairment (creatinine clearance < 30 ml/min), sildenafil clearance was reduced, resulting in mean increases in AUC and C_{max} of 100% and 88% respectively compared to age-matched volunteers with no renal impairment. In addition, N-desmethyl metabolite AUC and C_{max} values were significantly increased 79% and 200% respectively.

Hepatic insufficiency

In volunteers with mild to moderate hepatic cirrhosis (Child-Pugh A and B) sildenafil clearance was reduced, resulting in increases in AUC (84%) and C_{max} (47%) compared to age-matched volunteers with no hepatic impairment. The pharmacokinetics of sildenafil in patients with severely impaired hepatic function have not been studied.

5.3 Preclinical safety data

Preclinical data revealed no special hazard for humans based on conventional studies of safety pharmacology, repeated dose toxicity, genotoxicity, carcinogenicity potential, and toxicity to reproduction.

6. PHARMACEUTICAL PARTICULARS

6.1 List of excipients

Tablet core: microcrystalline cellulose, calcium hydrogen phosphate (anhydrous), croscarmellose sodium, magnesium stearate.

Film coat: hypromellose, titanium dioxide (E171), lactose, triacetin, indigo carmine aluminium lake (E132).

6.2 Incompatibilities

Not applicable.

6.3 Shelf life

5 years.

6.4 Special precautions for storage

Do not store above 30°C.

Store in the original package, in order to protect from moisture.

6.5 Nature and contents of container

PVC/Aluminium foil blisters in cartons of 1, 4, 8 or 12 tablets. Not all pack sizes may be marketed.

6.6 Instructions for use and handling

No special requirements.

7. MARKETING AUTHORISATION HOLDER

Pfizer Limited, Sandwich, Kent, CT13 9NJ, United Kingdom.

8. MARKETING AUTHORISATION NUMBER(S)

EU/1/98/077/001 - Viagra tablets 25 mg; pack size 1 tablet

EU/1/98/077/002 - Viagra tablets 25 mg; pack size 4 tablets

EU/1/98/077/003 - Viagra tablets 25 mg; pack size 8 tablets

EU/1/98/077/004 - Viagra tablets 25 mg; pack size 12 tablets

EU/1/98/077/005 - Viagra tablets 50 mg; pack size 1 tablet

EU/1/98/077/006 - Viagra tablets 50 mg; pack size 4 tablets

EU/1/98/077/007 - Viagra tablets 50 mg; pack size 8 tablets

EU/1/98/077/008 - Viagra tablets 50 mg; pack size 12 tablets

EU/1/98/077/009 - Viagra tablets 100 mg; pack size 1 tablet

EU/1/98/077/010 - Viagra tablets 100 mg; pack size 4 tablets

EU/1/98/077/011 - Viagra tablets 100 mg; pack size 8 tablets

EU/1/98/077/012 - Viagra tablets 100 mg; pack size 12 tablets

9. DATE OF FIRST AUTHORISATION/RENEWAL OF THE AUTHORISATION

14 September 1998/14 September 2003

10. DATE OF REVISION OF THE TEXT

27 April 2005

LEGAL CATEGORY

POM

Ref: VI 11_1

ViATIM

(Sanofi Pasteur MSD)

1. NAME OF THE MEDICINAL PRODUCT

ViATIM®, Suspension and solution for injection in a pre-filled dual chamber syringe

Hepatitis A (inactivated, adsorbed) and Typhoid polysaccharide vaccine.

2. QUALITATIVE AND QUANTITATIVE COMPOSITION

The dual chamber syringe contains 0.5 millilitre of purified Vi polysaccharide typhoid vaccine and 0.5 millilitre of inactivated hepatitis A vaccine which are mixed prior to administration.

After reconstitution, 1 dose (1ml) contains:

Originally contained in the suspension:

Hepatitis A virus, GBM strain (inactivated)[1,2] ....160 U[3]

1 produced in human diploid (MRC-5) cells

2 adsorbed on aluminium hydroxide, hydrated (0.3 milligrams Al)

3 In the absence of an international standardised reference, the antigen content is expressed using an in-house reference

Originally contained in the solution:

Salmonella typhi (Ty 2 strain) capsular Vi polysaccharide25 micrograms

For excipients, see section 6.1.

3. PHARMACEUTICAL FORM

Suspension and solution for suspension for injection in a pre-filled dual chamber syringe

The vaccine is presented in a dual-chamber syringe.

The purified Vi polysaccharide typhoid vaccine (solution for injection) is contained in the chamber of the syringe closest to the needle, and the inactivated hepatitis A vaccine (suspension for injection) in the chamber closest to the plunger.

The component Hepatitis A (inactivated, adsorbed) is a cloudy and white suspension and the component Typhoid polysaccharide is a clear and colourless solution.

4. CLINICAL PARTICULARS

4.1 Therapeutic indications

ViATIM® is indicated for simultaneous active immunisation against typhoid fever and hepatitis A virus infection in subjects from 16 years of age.

ViATIM® should be given in accordance with official recommendations.

4.2 Posology and method of administration

Posology

The recommended dosage for subjects of at least 16 years of age is 1 millilitre of the mixed vaccine.

Initial protection is achieved with one single dose of ViATIM®. Protective levels of antibody may not be reached until 14 days after administration of the vaccine.

There are serological data to show that there should be continuing protection against hepatitis A for up to 36 months after a first dose in subjects who responded to the initial vaccination.

In order to provide long-term protection against infection caused by the hepatitis A virus, a second dose (booster) of an inactivated hepatitis A vaccine should be given. The second dose is preferably given between 6 to 12 months after the primary immunisation but may be given up to 36 months after the primary immunisation (see Section 5.1).

It is predicted that HAV antibodies persist for many years (at least 10 years) after the second (booster) dose.

The combined vaccine may be used to provide the second (booster) dose of hepatitis A vaccine if protection against typhoid fever is also desirable. In these instances, the combined vaccine should preferably be given between 6 and 12 months after the first dose of hepatitis A vaccine (monovalent) but may be given up to 36 months later.

However if the initial dose of hepatitis A vaccine was given as a combined typhoid and hepatitis A vaccine, then the second dose of combined vaccine should usually be given approximately 36 months after the first dose.

In subjects who remain at risk of typhoid fever, revaccination against typhoid fever should be carried out with a single dose of a purified Vi polysaccharide typhoid vaccine every 3 years, unless it is also appropriate to administer a booster of hepatitis A vaccine in which case ViATIM may be used (see Section 5.1).

Method of administration

ViATIM® should be administered by slow intramuscular injection in the deltoid region. ViATIM® must not be administered intravascularly.

ViATIM® should not be administered into the buttocks due to the varying amount of fatty tissue in this region, nor by the intradermal route, since these methods of administration may induce a weaker immune response. ViATIM® may be administered by the subcutaneous route in patients with thrombocytopenia or in those at risk of haemorrhage.

4.3 Contraindications

Known hypersensitivity to any constituent of ViATIM®.

Known hypersensitivity to neomycin (present in trace amounts as a residual of the manufacturing process).

Vaccination should be delayed in subjects with an acute severe febrile illness.

4.4 Special warnings and special precautions for use

As with all vaccines, appropriate facilities and medication such as epinephrine (adrenaline) should be readily available for immediate use in case of anaphylaxis or hypersensitivity following injection.

Immunogenicity of ViATIM® could be impaired by immunosuppressive treatment or in immunodeficient subjects. It is recommended to delay vaccination until the completion of any immunosuppressive treatment. Subjects with chronic immunodeficiency such as HIV infection may be vaccinated if the underlying immunodeficiency allows the induction of an antibody response, even if limited.

Because of the incubation period of hepatitis A disease, infection may be present but not clinically apparent at the time of vaccination. It is not known whether ViATIM® will prevent hepatitis A in this case.

ViATIM® does not protect against infection caused by other known liver pathogens including hepatitis B, hepatitis C and hepatitis E viruses.

ViATIM® does not protect against infection by Salmonella enterica other than serotype typhi.

As with any vaccine, a protective immune response may not be elicited in all vaccinees.

4.5 Interaction with other medicinal products and other forms of Interaction

ViATIM® must not be mixed with any other vaccine in the same syringe.

ViATIM® is a combination of purified Vi polysaccharide typhoid vaccine and inactivated hepatitis A vaccine. Although concomitant administration with other inactivated vaccines using different syringes and at different injection sites has not been specifically studied, it is anticipated that no interaction will be observed.

Concomitant administration of yellow fever vaccine with ViATIM® has not been specifically assessed. However, based on data obtained from the concomitant administration of the monovalent vaccines (purified Vi polysaccharide typhoid vaccine and inactivated hepatitis A vaccine) with yellow fever vaccine, no interference with the immune responses to any of these antigens would be expected.

The effect of concomitant administration of immunoglobulins on the immunogenicity of ViATIM® has not been assessed. Therefore, interference with the immune response of ViATIM® cannot be ruled out. Data obtained from concomitant administration of immunoglobulins with the monovalent inactivated hepatitis A vaccine showed that anti-HAV seroconversion rates were not modified whereas anti-HAV antibody titres could be lower than after vaccination with the monovalent vaccine alone.

4.6 Pregnancy and lactation

Pregnancy

Data regarding exposure during pregnancy are available for more than 150 cases with monovalent Vi polysaccharide typhoid vaccine, more than 40 cases with monovalent inactivated hepatitis A vaccine, and more than 10 cases with ViATIM® or the two components given simultaneously. These data indicated no adverse effects on pregnancy or on the health of foetus/newborn child.

Animal studies performed with the monovalent Vi polysaccharide typhoid vaccine do not indicate direct or indirect harmful effects with respect to pregnancy, embryonal/foetal development, parturition or postnatal development.

Nevertheless, ViATIM® should only be used during pregnancy after careful consideration of the risk-benefit relationship. When the patient is considered to be at risk of only one of hepatitis A or typhoid fever, the monovalent vaccine should be used.

Lactation

There are no data on the effect of administration of ViATIM® during lactation.

ViATIM® should only be used during breastfeeding after careful consideration of the risk-benefit relationship.

4.7 Effects on ability to drive and use machines

Dizziness has been observed as an uncommon reaction following administration of this vaccine.

4.8 Undesirable effects

The safety profile of ViATIM® was evaluated in nearly 1100 subjects included in 5 clinical studies. The most commonly reported reactions were those occurring at the injection site.

The adverse reactions observed with ViATIM® were as follows:

Nervous system disorders

Uncommon (0.1 - 1%): dizziness.

Gastrointestinal disorders

Common (1-10%): nausea; diarrhoea.

Skin and subcutaneous tissue disorders

Uncommon (0.1 - 1%): pruritus; rash.

Musculoskeletal, connective tissue and bone disorders

Common (1 - 10%): arthralgia.

Very Common (> 10%): myalgia.

General disorders

Very common (> 10%): asthenia; headache, malaise.

Common (1 - 10%): fever.

Administration site conditions

Very common (> 10%): pain, induration/oedema, and erythema at the injection site.

Pain at the ViATIM® injection site was reported in 89.9% of subjects (severe in 4.5%). For subjects who received the two monovalent vaccines concomitantly at separate injection sites, pain was reported in 83.2% of subjects (severe in 5.0%) for both vaccine sites combined. Pain was reported by 79.3% of subjects (severe in 5.0%) at the Vi vaccine site and by 50.3% of subjects (severe in 0.6%) at the hepatitis A vaccine site.

Pain at the injection site lasting more than 3 days was reported by 17.4% of subjects after ViATIM®, by 2.8% of subjects for the monovalent Vi vaccine site and by 0.6% of subjects for the monovalent hepatitis A vaccine site.

Severe oedema/induration (> 5 cm) was reported in 7.9% of subjects at the ViATIM® site. For subjects who received the two monovalent vaccines concomitantly at separate injection sites, severe oedema/induration was reported in 1.7% of subjects for both vaccine sites combined (in 1.1% of subjects at the Vi vaccine site and in 0.6% of subjects at the hepatitis A vaccine site).

The overall incidence of systemic reactions was similar between subjects who were vaccinated with ViATIM® and subjects who received the two monovalent vaccines concomitantly at separate injection sites.

All reactions resolved without any sequelae.

Undesirable effects reported following use of the monovalent purified Vi polysaccharide vaccine (and not listed above for ViATIM®) include:

Vomiting, abdominal pain have been reported rarely. Very rarely, cases of allergic reactions such as urticaria, serum sickness and anaphylactoid reactions have been reported. Very rarely, aggravation of asthma has been reported. Paraesthesia has been reported very rarely.

Undesirable effects reported following use of the monovalent inactivated hepatitis A vaccine (and not listed above for ViATIM®) include:

The appearance of a nodule at the injection site was observed in very rare cases. Mild reversible elevation of serum transaminase has been observed on rare occasions. In post marketing surveillance, skin reactions such as urticaria were very rarely observed.

4.9 Overdose

There are no data on overdose of ViATIM®.

5. PHARMACOLOGICAL PROPERTIES

5.1 Pharmacodynamic properties

Pharmacotherapeutic group: Bacterial and viral vaccines combined, ATC code J07C (combined)/P03 (typhoid)/C02 (hepatitis A).

Four clinical studies provided useful data on immune responses to ViATIM®. A total of 1090 subjects were included, with 179, 610, 243 and 58 subjects vaccinated in each study.

After the primary vaccination the seroprotection rate for HAV (⩾ 20mIU/mL) ranged between 95.6% and 99.4% after 14 days and between 98.7% and 100% after 28 days.

The seroprotection rate for Vi (⩾ 1μg/mL) ranged between 83% and 89% after 14 days and between 69.8% and 91% after 28 days

In one study that evaluated anti-Vi antigen seroprotection rates at years 1, 2 and 3 after the first dose of ViATIM and after re-vaccination with ViATIM at year 3, results were as follows:

(see Table 1 below)

Anti-HAV antigen seroprotection rates at years 1, 2 and 3 after the first dose of ViATIM and after re-vaccination with ViATIM at year 3 were as follows:

(see Table 2 on next page)

Similar results were seen at all timepoints in the control group who received concomitant monovalent purified Vi polysaccharide and inactivated hepatitis A vaccines.

5.2 Pharmacokinetic properties

Not relevant for vaccines.

Table 1

	Viatim			
	Year 1	Year 2	Year 3	28 days after Re-vaccination at Year 3
Number of vaccinees	139	124	112	46
% of vaccinees seroprotected (95% CI)	44.6 (36.2-53.3)	40.3 (31.6-49.5)	32.1 (23.6-41.6)	69.6 (54.2-82.3)

Table 2

	Viatim			
	Year 1	Year 2	Year 3	28 days after Re-vaccination at Year 3
Number of vaccinees	140	124	12	46
% ⩾ 20 mIU/ml	99.3	98.4	99.1	100
(95% CI)	(96.1-100)	(94.3-99.8)	(95.1-100)	(92.3-100)

5.3 Preclinical safety data
Preclinical safety data obtained with the monovalent vaccines contained in this combined vaccine reveal no special hazard to humans.

6. PHARMACEUTICAL PARTICULARS

6.1 List of excipients
Purified Vi polysaccharide typhoid vaccine component:

- Phosphate buffer solution:
- Sodium chloride
- Disodium phosphate dihydrate
- Sodium dihydrogen phosphate dihydrate
- Water for Injections

Inactivated hepatitis A vaccine component:

- 2-Phenoxyethanol solution
- Formaldehyde
- Medium 199 Hanks (without phenol red)* supplemented with polysorbate 80

*Medium 199 Hanks (without phenol red) is a complex mixture of amino acids (including phenylalanine), mineral salts, vitamins and other components (including glucose), diluted in water for injections and pH adjusted with hydrochloric acid or sodium hydroxide

6.2 Incompatibilities
In the absence of compatibility studies, this vaccine must not be mixed with other medicinal products in the same syringe.

6.3 Shelf life
3 years.

6.4 Special precautions for storage
Store at 2°C – 8°C (in a refrigerator).

Do not freeze. If frozen, the vaccine should be discarded.

6.5 Nature and contents of container
A prefilled syringe (type I glass) with a dual-chamber (0.5 millilitre of vaccine in each chamber) with elastomer (chlorobutyl and bromobutyl rubber blend) plunger-stopper, elastomer tip cap and elastomer by-pass stopper.

Pack of 1 or 10 prefilled syringes supplied with or without needle.

6.6 Instructions for use and handling
The two vaccine components should only be mixed immediately prior to injection.

Shake before mixing and again prior to injection to obtain a homogeneous suspension. The contents of the two compartments are mixed by slowly advancing the plunger. The final volume to be injected is 1 millilitre.

The vaccine should be visually inspected before administration for any foreign particulate matter. The mixed vaccine is a cloudy, whitish suspension.

Any unused product or waste material should be disposed of in accordance with local requirements.

7. MARKETING AUTHORISATION HOLDER
Sanofi Pasteur MSD Ltd
Mallards Reach
Bridge Avenue
Maidenhead
Berkshire
SL6 1QP

8. MARKETING AUTHORISATION NUMBER(S)
PL 06745/0114

9. DATE OF FIRST AUTHORISATION/RENEWAL OF THE AUTHORISATION
3rd September 2001

10. DATE OF REVISION OF THE TEXT
May 2005

Viazem XL 120mg

(Genus Pharmaceuticals)

1. NAME OF THE MEDICINAL PRODUCT
VIAZEM® XL 120mg

2. QUALITATIVE AND QUANTITATIVE COMPOSITION
Diltiazem hydrochloride: 120 mg capsule.

For excipients, see section 6.1

3. PHARMACEUTICAL FORM
Prolonged release capsule, hard.

Lavender opaque capsule. Each capsule is printed on the caps and body, in white ink Viazem XL 120

4. CLINICAL PARTICULARS

4.1 Therapeutic indications
VIAZEM XL is indicated for the management of stable angina pectoris and the treatment of mild to moderate hypertension.

4.2 Posology and method of administration
Dosage requirements may differ between patients with angina and patients with hypertension. In addition individual patients response may vary, necessitating careful titration. The range of strengths facilitates titration to the optimal dose.

One capsule of VIAZEM XL is to be taken before or during a meal. The dose should be taken at approximately the same time each day.

The capsule should not be chewed but swallowed whole, with a glass of water.

Due to the variability of release profile in individual patients, when changing from one type of sustained release diltiazem preparation to another, it may be necessary to adjust the dose.

Adults:

Hypertension: The usual starting dose is 180 mg once daily. The dose may be increased after 2-4 weeks according to the patient's response and the usual maintenance dose is 240mg-360mg once daily. The maximum daily dose is 360 mg. However, the single daily doses of 300 mg and 360 mg should only be administered to patients when no satisfactory therapeutic effect has been effected with lower doses and after the benefit risk-ratio has been carefully assessed by the doctor.

Angina: Care should be taken when titrating patients with stable angina in order to establish the optimal dose. The usual starting dose is 180 mg once daily. The dose may be increased after 2-4 weeks according to the patient's response. The maximum daily dose is 360 mg. However, the single daily doses of 300 mg and 360 mg should only be administered to patients when no satisfactory therapeutic effect has been effected with lower doses and after the benefit risk-ratio has been carefully assessed by the doctor.

Elderly and patients with impaired hepatic or renal function:
Plasma levels of diltiazem can be increased in the elderly, and in patients with impaired hepatic renal or hepatic function. In these cases, the starting dose should be one 120mg VIAZEM XL capsule once daily. Heart rate should be monitored and if it falls below 50 beats per minute, the dose should not be increased. Dose adjustment may be required to obtain a satisfactory clinical response.

Children:
Safety and efficacy in children have not been established.

4.3 Contraindications
Diltiazem depresses atrioventricular node conduction and is therefore contraindicated in patients with severe bradycardia (less than 50 bpm), sick sinus syndrome, congestive heart failure, and left ventricular failure with second or third degree AV or sino-atrial block, except in the presence of a functioning pacemaker. Diltiazem is also contraindicated in left ventricular failure with pulmonary stasis as diltiazem may have mild negative effects on contractility.

Diltiazem is contraindicated in acute complicated myocardial infarction (e.g. bradycardia hypotension, congestive heart failure/reduced LV function), pulmonary congestion, hypotension (<90 mmHg systolic) cerebrovascular accident, cardiac shock and unstable angina pectoris.

Diltiazem is contraindicated in pre-excitation syndrome (e.g. WPW) accompanied with atrial flutter, fibrillation and in digitalis intoxication, as diltiazem may precipitate ventricular tachycardia.

Diltiazem should not be used in patients with known hypersensitivity to diltiazem.

Diltiazem should not be used during pregnancy, by women of child-bearing potential, or by women who are breast-feeding.

4.4 Special warnings and special precautions for use
Patients treated with beta-adrenoreceptor blocking drugs and patients with conduction disturbances (bradycardia, bundle branch block, first degree AV block, prolonged PR interval) should only be treated with VIAZEM XL after special consideration due to the risk of serious bradyarrhythmias.

This product should be used with caution in patients with hepatic dysfunction. Abnormalities of liver function may appear during therapy. The higher single daily doses of VIAZEM XL capsules 300mg and 360mg should not be administered to patients with impaired renal and/or hepatic function and to elderly patients (prolonged half life of elimination) because there is no experience on the use of such high dosages in these patient categories.

In patients undergoing long-term therapy with cyclosporin, plasma levels of cyclosporin should be monitored when concurrent administration of diltiazem is initiated, or discontinued or if the dose of diltiazem is changed.

Abnormally short transit time through the gastrointestinal tract could lead to incomplete release of contents of the capsule e.g. in chronic conditions with associated diarrhoea such as Crohns disease or ulcerative colitis.

4.5 Interaction with other medicinal products and other forms of Interaction
Combinations contraindicated as a safety measure:

In animals, fatal ventricular fibrillations are constantly seen during administration of verapamil and dantrolene via the i.v. route. The combination of a calcium antagonist and dantrolene is therefore potentially dangerous. The concurrent iv administration of beta-adrenergic blocking agents with diltiazem should be avoided because an additive effect on SA and AV conduction and ventricular function will occur. The use of such a combination requires ECG monitoring especially at the beginning of treatment.

Combinations requiring safety precautions:

In common with other calcium antagonists, when diltiazem is used with drugs which may induce bradycardia or with antiarrhythmic drugs (e.g. amiodarone) or other antihypertensive drugs, the possibility of an additive effect should be borne in mind. Inhalation anaesthetics should be used with caution during diltiazem therapy. Tri/tetracyclic antidepressants and neuroleptics may increase the antihypertensive effects of diltiazem whilst the concomitant use of lithium with diltiazem may lead to neurotoxicity (extrapyramidal effects). Rifampin and other hepatic enzyme inducers may reduce the bioavailability of diltiazem and high doses of Vitamin D and/or high intake of calcium salts leading to elevated serum calcium levels may reduce the response to diltiazem.

Diltiazem is metabolised by CYP3A4 and could, by competitive inhibition of CYP3A4, affect the pharmacokinetics of other drugs metabolised by this enzyme. In addition inhibitors and inducers of CYP3A4 may affect the pharmacokinetics of diltiazem.

Diltiazem prolongs the sedative effect of medazolam and triazolam via metabolic interaction and decreases nifedipine clearance by 50%. Diltiazem may cause increases in the levels of digitoxin. Diltiazem has been shown to increase the bioavailability of imipramine by 30% probably due to inhibition of its first pass metabolism.

Diltiazem has been used safely in combination with diuretics, ACE-inhibitors and other anti-hypertensive agents. It is recommended that patients receiving these combinations should be regularly monitored. Concomitant use of diltiazem with alpha-blockers such as prazosin should be strictly monitored because of the possible synergistic hypotensive effect of the combination.

Case reports have suggested that blood levels of carbamazepine, cyclosporin, theophylline and phenytoin may be increased when given concurrently with diltiazem. Care should be exercised in patients taking these drugs. In common with other calcium antagonists diltiazem may cause small increases in plasma levels of digoxin. In patients taking H_2-antagonists concurrently with diltiazem there may be increased levels of diltiazem.

Magnification of the hypotensive and lipothymic effects (summation of vasodilator properties) of nitrate derivatives can occur. In patients on calcium inhibitors, prescriptions of nitrate derivatives should be made at progressively increasing doses. Diltiazem treatment has been continued without problem during anaesthesia, but diltiazem may potentiate the activity of curare-like and depolarising neuromuscular blocking agents, therefore the anaesthetist should be informed that the patient is receiving a calcium antagonist.

4.6 Pregnancy and lactation
Pregnancy:

Diltiazem should not be taken during pregnancy. Women of child bearing-potential should exclude the possibility of pregnancy before commencing treatment by taking suitable contraceptive measures if necessary. In animal tests, Diltiazem was found to have a tetratogenic effects in some species of animal.

Diltiazem may suppress the contractility of the uterus. Definite evidence that this will prolong partus in full-term pregnancy is lacking. A risk of hypoxia in the foetus may arise in the event of hypotension in the mother and reduced perfusion of the uterus due to redistribution of blood flow due to peripheral vasodilatation. In animal experiments diltiazem has exhibited teratogenic effects in some animal species. In the absence of adequate evidence of safety in human pregnancy, VIAZEM XL should not be used in pregnancy or in women of childbearing potential.

Lactation:

Diltiazem is excreted in breast milk in concentrations similar to those in serum. If the use of diltiazem is considered essential, an alternative method of infant feeding should be instituted.

4.7 Effects on ability to drive and use machines

There are no studies on the effect of diltiazem when driving vehicles or operating machines. It should be taken into account that occasionally asthenia/fatigue and dizziness may occur. Treatment of hypertension with this medicinal product requires regular monitoring. Individual different reactions may affect the ability to drive. This risk should be considered especially at the beginning of treatment, when changing the drug, or in combination with alcohol.

4.8 Undesirable effects

Certain undesirable effects may lead to suspension of treatment: sinus bradycardia, sino-atrial heart block, 2nd and 3rd degree atrioventricular heart block, skin rash, oedema of the lower limbs.

In hypertensive patients, adverse effects are generally mild and transient and are most commonly vasodilatory related events.

The following have been described in decreasing order of frequency: lower limb oedema, headache, hot flushes/flushing, asthenia/fatigue, palpitations, malaise, minor gastro-intestinal disorders (dyspepsia, abdominal pain, dry mouth, nausea, vomiting, diarrhoea, constipation) and skin rash. Erythema multiforme and Stevens Johnson syndrome have been reported infrequently in patients receiving diltiazem hydrochloride. Vasodilatory related events (in particular, oedema) are dose-dependent and appear to be more frequent in elderly subjects.

Rare cases of symptomatic bradycardia and exceptionally sino-atrial block and atrioventricular block, hypotension, syncope, reduced left ventricular function have also been recorded. Isolated cases of hallucinations, depression, insomnia, hyperglycaemia and impotence have been reported.

Experience with use in other indications and with other formulations has shown that skin rashes are usually localised and are limited to cases of erythema, urticaria or occasionally desquamative erthema, with or without fever, which regress when treatment is discontinued.

Isolated cases of moderate and transient elevations of liver transaminases have been observed at the start of treatment. Isolated cases of clinical hepatitis have been reported which resolved with cessation of therapy.

Dizziness, pruritis, nervousness, paraesthesia, articular/muscular pain, photo sensitisation, hypotension, gingival hyperplasia, and gynaecomastia, have also been observed.

4.9 Overdose

The clinical consequences of overdose can be severe hypotension leading to collapse, and sinus bradycardia which may be accompanied by isorhythmic dissociation and atrioventricular conduction disturbances. Observation in a coronary care unit is advisable. Vasopressors such as adrenaline may be indicated in patients exhibiting profound hypotension. Calcium gluconate may help reverse the effects of calcium entry blockade. Atropine administration and temporary cardiac pacing may be required to manage bradycardia and/or conduction disturbances.

Glucagon can be used in cases of established hypoglycaemia.

Diltiazem and its metabolites are very poorly dialysable.

5. PHARMACOLOGICAL PROPERTIES

5.1 Pharmacodynamic properties

Diltiazem is classified as a calcium channel blocker, benziothiazepine derivative, C08DB01, under the ATC classification. It selectively reduces calcium entry through voltage-dependent calcium-n channels into vascular smooth muscle cells and myocardial cells. This lowers the concentration of intracellular calcium which is available to activate contractile proteins. This action of diltiazem results in dilation of coronary arteries causing an increase in myocardial oxygen supply. It reduces cardiac work by moderating the heart rate and by reducing systemic vascular resistance thus reducing oxygen demand. Diltiazem also prolongs AV conduction and has mild effects on contractility. Clinical data on morbidity and mortality are not available.

5.2 Pharmacokinetic properties

Multiple dose pharmacokinetic studies have shown that the kinetics of VIAZEM XL are non-linear within the 120mg-360mg dosage range. Diltiazem is well absorbed, but has a highly saturable first pass effect leading to a variable absolute bioavailability, which is on average 35%. The saturable first pass effect results in higher than expected systemic exposure with increasing doses.

The protein binding is 80 to 85% and the volume of distribution is 5.0 l/kg.

Diltiazem is metabolised by CYP3A4 in the liver and 70% of the dose is excreted in urine, mainly as metabolites. The plasma levels of the two main metabolites, N-monodesmethyldiltiazem and desacetyldiltiazem, represent 35% and 15% of diltiazem levels respectively. The metabolites contribute around 50% of the clinical effect. Plasma clearance of diltiazem is approximately 0.5 l/h/kg. Plasma half-life of diltiazem is approximately 5-7 hours.

VIAZEM XL capsules allow a prolonged absorption of diltiazem and maximum levels are reached within 6 to 12 hours. Concomitant food intake with VIAZEM XL does not influence the pharmacokinetics of diltiazem. For most patients, chronic administration of VIAZEM XL 300mg once daily, results in therapeutic diltiazem levels (50-200ng/ml) over 24 hours. However, the inter-individual variability is high and individual dose adjustment based on therapeutic response is therefore necessary.

5.3 Preclinical safety data

Tests on reproductive functions in animals show that diltiazem decreases fertility in rats and that it is teratogenic in mice, rats and rabbits. Exposure during late pregnancy induces dystocia and a decrease in the number of live newborns in rats.

Detailed mutagenicity and carcinnogenicity tests performed negative.

6. PHARMACEUTICAL PARTICULARS

6.1 List of excipients

Sucrose Stearate

Microcrystalline cellulose

Povidone

Magnesium Stearate

Talc

Titanium dioxide

Hypromellose

Polysorbate 80

Polyacrylate dispersion 30% (dry)

Simethicone emulsion

Gelatine capsule

Gelatin capsule colours

120 mg	Capsule body	Capsule cap
	Lavender opaque[1]	Lavender opaque[1]

1 = Colour is composed of	Azorubine E122 Indigotine E132 Titanium Dioxide E171

Gelatin capsule markings:

120 mg	Capsule body Viazem XL 120	Capsule cap Viazem XL 120
(Capsule Size 3)	(white ink EEC approved)	(white ink EEC approved)

White printing ink contains:

Shellac, Ethyl Alcohol, Isopropyl Alcohol, n-Butyl, Propylene Glycol, Sodium Hydroxide, Polyvinylpyrrolidone, Titanium Dioxide

6.2 Incompatibilities

Not applicable.

6.3 Shelf life

3 years

6.4 Special precautions for storage

Do not store above 25°C. Store in original package in a dry place away from any heat source, e.g. direct sunlight, heaters, steam, etc.

6.5 Nature and contents of container

The capsules are packed in PVC/aluminium blisters. Pack sizes are 28 capsules per blister.

6.6 Instructions for use and handling

Swallow capsules whole, with a glass of water do not chew.

7. MARKETING AUTHORISATION HOLDER

Stada Arzneimittel AG

Stadastrasse 2-18

61118 Bad Vilbel

Germany

8. MARKETING AUTHORISATION NUMBER(S)

PL 11204/0090

9. DATE OF FIRST AUTHORISATION/RENEWAL OF THE AUTHORISATION

2nd April 1997

10. DATE OF REVISION OF THE TEXT

20 November 2001

Viazem XL 180mg

(Genus Pharmaceuticals)

1. NAME OF THE MEDICINAL PRODUCT

VIAZEM® XL 180mg

2. QUALITATIVE AND QUANTITATIVE COMPOSITION

Diltiazem hydrochloride: 180 mg capsule.

For excipients, see section 6.1

3. PHARMACEUTICAL FORM

Prolonged release capsule, hard.

White and blue-green opaque capsules. Each capsule is printed on the cap and body, in black ink, with Viazem XL 180.

4. CLINICAL PARTICULARS

4.1 Therapeutic indications

VIAZEM XL is indicated for the management of stable angina pectoris and the treatment of mild to moderate hypertension.

4.2 Posology and method of administration

Dosage requirements may differ between patients with angina and patients with hypertension. In addition individual patients response may vary, necessitating careful titration. The range of strengths facilitates titration to the optimal dose.

One capsule of VIAZEM XL is to be taken before or during a meal. The dose should be taken at approximately the same time each day.

The capsule should not be chewed but swallowed whole, with a glass of water.

Due to the variability of release profile in individual patients, when changing from one type of sustained release diltiazem preparation to another, it may be necessary to adjust the dose.

Adults:

Hypertension: The usual starting dose is 180 mg once daily. The dose may be increased after 2-4 weeks according to the patient's response and the usual maintenance dose is 240mg-360mg once daily. The maximum daily dose is 360 mg. However, the single daily doses of 300 mg and 360 mg should only be administered to patients when no satisfactory therapeutic effect has been effected with lower doses and after the benefit risk-ratio has been carefully assessed by the doctor.

Angina: Care should be taken when titrating patients with stable angina in order to establish the optimal dose. The usual starting dose is 180 mg once daily. The dose may be increased after 2-4 weeks according to the patient's response. The maximum daily dose is 360 mg. However, the single daily doses of 300 mg and 360 mg should only be administered to patients when no satisfactory therapeutic effect has been effected with lower doses and after the benefit risk-ratio has been carefully assessed by the doctor.

Elderly and patients with impaired hepatic or renal function:

Plasma levels of diltiazem can be increased in the elderly, and in patients with impaired hepatic renal or hepatic function. In these cases, the starting dose should be one 120mg VIAZEM XL capsule once daily. Heart rate should be monitored and if it falls below 50 beats per minute, the dose should not be increased. Dose adjustment may be required to obtain a satisfactory clinical response.

Children:

Safety and efficacy in children have not been established.

4.3 Contraindications

Diltiazem depresses atrioventricular node conduction and is therefore contraindicated in patients with severe bradycardia (less than 50 bpm), sick sinus syndrome, congestive heart failure, and left ventricular failure with second or third degree AV or sino-atrial block, except in the presence of a functioning pacemaker. Diltiazem is also contraindicated in left ventricular failure with pulmonary stasis as diltiazem may have mild negative effects on contractility.

Diltiazem is contraindicated in acute complicated myocardial infarction (e.g. bradycardia hypotension, congestive heart failure/reduced LV function), pulmonary congestion, hypotension (<90 mmHg systolic) cerebrovascular accident, cardiac shock and unstable angina pectoris.

Diltiazem is contraindicated in pre-excitation syndrome (e.g. WPW) accompanied with atrial flutter, fibrillation and in digitalis intoxication, as diltiazem may precipitate ventricular tachycardia.

Diltiazem should not be used in patients with known hypersensitivity to diltiazem.

Diltiazem should not be used during pregnancy, by women of child-bearing potential, or by women who are breast-feeding.

4.4 Special warnings and special precautions for use

Patients treated with beta-adrenoreceptor blocking drugs and patients with conduction disturbances (bradycardia, bundle branch block, first degree AV block, prolonged PR interval) should only be treated with VIAZEM XL after special consideration due to the risk of serious bradyarrhythmias.

This product should be used with caution in patients with hepatic dysfunction. Abnormalities of liver function may appear during therapy. The higher single daily doses of VIAZEM XL capsules 300mg and 360mg should not be administered to patients with impaired renal and/or hepatic function and to elderly patients (prolonged half life of elimination) because there is no experience on the use of such high dosages in these patient categories.

In patients undergoing long-term therapy with cyclosporin, plasma levels of cyclosporin should be monitored when concurrent administration of diltiazem is initiated, or discontinued or if the dose of diltiazem is changed.

Abnormally short transit time through the gastrointestinal tract could lead to incomplete release of contents of the capsule e.g. in chronic conditions with associated diarrhoea such as Crohns disease or ulcerative colitis.

4.5 Interaction with other medicinal products and other forms of Interaction

Combinations contraindicated as a safety measure:

In animals, fatal ventricular fibrillations are constantly seen during administration of verapamil and dantrolene via the i.v. route. The combination of a calcium antagonist and dantrolene is therefore potentially dangerous. The concurrent iv administration of beta-adrenergic blocking agents with diltiazem should be avoided because an additive effect on SA and AV conduction and ventricular function will occur. The use of such a combination requires ECG monitoring especially at the beginning of treatment.

Combinations requiring safety precautions:

In common with other calcium antagonists, when diltiazem is used with drugs which may induce bradycardia or with antiarrhythmic drugs (e.g. amiodarone) or other antihypertensive drugs, the possibility of an additive effect should be borne in mind. Inhalation anaesthetics should be used with caution during diltiazem therapy. Tri/tetracyclic antidepressants and neuroleptics may increase the antihypertensive effects of diltiazem whilst the concomitant use of lithium with diltiazem may lead to neurotoxicity (extrapyramidal effects). Rifampin and other hepatic enzyme inducers may reduce the bioavailability of diltiazem and high doses of Vitamin D and/or high intake of calcium salts leading to elevated serum calcium levels may reduce the response to diltiazem.

Diltiazem is metabolised by CYP3A4 and could, by competitive inhibition of CYP3A4, affect the pharmacokinetics of other drugs metabolised by this enzyme. In addition inhibitors and inducers of CYP3A4 may affect the pharmacokinetics of diltiazem.

Diltiazem prolongs the sedative effect of medazolam and triazolam via metabolic interaction and decreases nifedipine clearance by 50%. Diltiazem may cause increases in the levels of digitoxin. Diltiazem has been shown to increase the bioavailability of imipramine by 30% probably due to inhibition of its first pass metabolism.

Diltiazem has been used safely in combination with diuretics, ACE-inhibitors and other anti-hypertensive agents. It is recommended that patients receiving these combinations should be regularly monitored. Concomitant use of diltiazem with alpha-blockers such as prazosin should be strictly monitored because of the possible synergistic hypotensive effect of the combination.

Case reports have suggested that blood levels of carbamazepine, cyclosporin, theophylline and phenytoin may be increased when given concurrently with diltiazem. Care should be exercised in patients taking these drugs. In common with other calcium antagonists diltiazem may cause small increases in plasma levels of digoxin. In patients taking H_2-antagonists concurrently with diltiazem there may be increased levels of diltiazem.

Magnification of the hypotensive and lipothymic effects (summation of vasodilator properties) of nitrate derivatives can occur. In patients on calcium inhibitors, prescriptions of nitrate derivatives should be made at progressively increasing doses. Diltiazem treatment has been continued without problem during anaesthesia, but diltiazem may potentiate the activity of curare-like and depolarising neuromuscular blocking agents, therefore the anaesthetist should be informed that the patient is receiving a calcium antagonist.

4.6 Pregnancy and lactation

Pregnancy:

Diltiazem should not be taken during pregnancy. Women of child bearing-potential should exclude the possibility of pregnancy before commencing treatment by taking suitable contraceptive measures if necessary. In animal tests, Diltiazem was found to have a tetratogenic effects in some species of animal.

Diltiazem may suppress the contractility of the uterus. Definite evidence that this will prolong partus in full-term pregnancy is lacking. A risk of hypoxia in the foetus may arise in the event of hypotension in the mother and reduced perfusion of the uterus due to redistribution of blood flow due to peripheral vasodilatation. In animal experiments diltiazem has exhibited teratogenic effects in some animal species. In the absence of adequate evidence of safety in human pregnancy, VIAZEM XL should not be used in pregnancy or in women of childbearing potential.

Lactation:

Diltiazem is excreted in breast milk in concentrations similar to those in serum. If the use of diltiazem is considered essential, an alternative method of infant feeding should be instituted.

4.7 Effects on ability to drive and use machines

There are no studies on the effect of diltiazem when driving vehicles or operating machines. It should be taken into account that occasionally asthenia/fatigue and dizziness may occur. Treatment of hypertension with this medicinal product requires regular monitoring. Individual different reactions may affect the ability to drive. This risk should be considered especially at the beginning of treatment, when changing the drug, or in combination with alcohol.

4.8 Undesirable effects

Certain undesirable effects may lead to suspension of treatment: sinus bradycardia, sino-atrial heart block, 2nd and 3rd degree atrioventricular heart block, skin rash, oedema of the lower limbs.

In hypertensive patients, adverse effects are generally mild and transient and are most commonly vasodilatory related events.

The following have been described in decreasing order of frequency: lower limb oedema, headache, hot flushes/flushing, asthenia/fatigue, palpitations, malaise, minor gastro-intestinal disorders (dyspepsia, abdominal pain, dry mouth, nausea, vomiting, diarrhoea, constipation) and skin rash. Erythema multiform and Stevens Johnson syndrome have been reported infrequently in patients receiving diltiazem hydrochloride. Vasodilatory related events (in particular, oedema) are dose-dependent and appear to be more frequent in elderly subjects.

Rare cases of symptomatic bradycardia and exceptionally sino-atrial block and atrioventricular block, hypotension, syncope, reduced left ventricular function have also been recorded. Isolated cases of hallucinations, depression, insomnia, hyperglycaemia and impotence have been reported.

Experience with use in other indications and with other formulations has shown that skin rashes are usually localised and are limited to cases of erythemia, urticaria or occasionally desquamative erthema, with or without fever, which regress when treatment is discontinued.

Isolated cases of moderate and transient elevations of liver transaminases have been observed at the start of treatment. Isolated cases of clinical hepatitis have been reported which resolved with cessation of therapy.

Dizziness, pruritis, nervousness, paraesthesia, articular/muscular pain, photo sensitisation, hypotension, gingival hyperplasia, and gynaecomastia, have also been observed.

4.9 Overdose

The clinical consequences of overdose can be severe hypotension leading to collapse, and sinus bradycardia which may be accompanied by isorhythmic dissociation and atrioventricular conduction disturbances. Observation in a coronary care unit is advisable. Vasopressors such as adrenaline may be indicated in patients exhibiting profound hypotension. Calcium gluconate may help reverse the effects of calcium entry blockade. Atropine administration and temporary cardiac pacing may be required to manage bradycardia and/or conduction disturbances.

Glucagon can be used in cases of established hypoglycaemia.

Diltiazem and its metabolites are very poorly dialysable.

5. PHARMACOLOGICAL PROPERTIES

5.1 Pharmacodynamic properties

Diltiazem is classified as a calcium channel blocker, benziothiazepine derivative, C08DB01, under the ATC classification. It selectively reduces calcium entry through voltage-dependent calcium-n channels into vascular smooth muscle cells and myocardial cells. This lowers the concentration of intracellular calcium which is available to activate contractile proteins. This action of diltiazem results in dilation of coronary arteries causing an increase in myocardial oxygen supply. It reduces cardiac work by moderating the heart rate and by reducing systemic vascular resistance thus reducing oxygen demand. Diltiazem also prolongs AV conduction and has mild effects on contractility. Clinical data on morbidity and mortality are not available.

5.2 Pharmacokinetic properties

Multiple dose pharmacokinetic studies have shown that the kinetics of VIAZEM XL are non-linear within the 120mg-360mg dosage range. Diltiazem is well absorbed, but has a highly saturable first pass effect leading to a variable absolute bioavailability, which is on average 35%. The saturable first pass effect results in higher than expected systemic exposure with increasing doses.

The protein binding is 80 to 85% and the volume of distribution is 5.0 l/kg.

Diltiazem is metabolised by CYP3A4 in the liver and 70% of the dose is excreted in urine, mainly as metabolites. The plasma levels of the two main metabolites, N-monodesmethyldiltiazem and desacetyldiltiazem, represent 35% and 15% of diltiazem levels respectively. The metabolites contribute around 50% of the clinical effect. Plasma clearance of diltiazem is approximately 0.5 l/h/kg. Plasma half-life of diltiazem is approximately 5-7 hours.

VIAZEM XL capsules allow a prolonged absorption of diltiazem and maximum levels are reached within 6 to 12 hours. Concomitant food intake with VIAZEM XL does not influence the pharmacokinetics of diltiazem. For most patients, chronic administration of VIAZEM XL 300mg once daily, results in therapeutic diltiazem levels (50-200ng/ml) over 24 hours. However, the inter-individual variability is high and individual dose adjustment based on therapeutic response is therefore necessary.

5.3 Preclinical safety data

Tests on reproductive functions in animals show that diltiazem decreases fertility in rats and that it is teratogenic in mice, rats and rabbits. Exposure during late pregnancy induces dystocia and a decrease in the number of live newborns in rats.

Detailed mutagenicity and carcinogenicity tests proved negative.

6. PHARMACEUTICAL PARTICULARS

6.1 List of excipients

Sucrose Stearate

Microcrystalline cellulose

Povidone

Magnesium Stearate

Talc

Titanium dioxide

Hypromellose

Polysorbate 80

Polyacrylate dispersion 30% (dry)

Simethicone emulsion

Gelatine capsule

Gelatin capsule colours

180 mg	Capsule body	Capsule cap
	White opaque[1]	Blue Green opaque[2]

1 = Colour is composed of	Titanium Dioxide E171
2 = Colour is composed of	Quinoline Yellow E104 Indigotine E132 Titanium Dioxide E171

Gelatin capsule markings:

180 mg	Capsule body	Capsule cap
	Viazem XL 180	Viazem XL 180
(Capsule Size 2)	(Black ink EEC approved)	(Black ink EEC approved)

Black printing ink contains:

Shellac, Ethyl Alcohol, Isopropyl Alcohol, n-Butyl, Propylene Glycol, Water (Purified) Ammonium Hydroxide, Potassium Hydroxide, Black Iron Oxide

6.2 Incompatibilities

Not applicable.

6.3 Shelf life

3 years

6.4 Special precautions for storage

Do not store above 25°C. Store in original package in a dry place away from any heat source, e.g. direct sunlight, heaters, steam, etc.

6.5 Nature and contents of container

The capsules are packed in PVC/aluminium blisters. Pack sizes are 28 capsules per blister.

6.6 Instructions for use and handling

Swallow capsules whole, with a glass of water do not chew.

7. MARKETING AUTHORISATION HOLDER

Stada Arzneimittel AG

Stadastrasse 2-18

61118 Bad Vilbel

Germany

8. MARKETING AUTHORISATION NUMBER(S)

PL 11201/0091

9. DATE OF FIRST AUTHORISATION/RENEWAL OF THE AUTHORISATION

2nd April 1997

10. DATE OF REVISION OF THE TEXT

20 November 2001

Viazem XL 240mg

(Genus Pharmaceuticals)

1. NAME OF THE MEDICINAL PRODUCT

VIAZEM® XL 240mg

2. QUALITATIVE AND QUANTITATIVE COMPOSITION

Diltiazem hydrochloride: 240 mg capsule.

For excipients, see section 6.1

3. PHARMACEUTICAL FORM

Prolonged release capsule, hard.

Blue-green and lavender opaque colourless. Each capsule is printed on the cap and body, in white ink, with Viazem XL 240.

4. CLINICAL PARTICULARS

4.1 Therapeutic indications

VIAZEM XL is indicated for the management of stable angina pectoris and the treatment of mild to moderate hypertension.

4.2 Posology and method of administration

Dosage requirements may differ between patients with angina and patients with hypertension. In addition individual patients response may vary, necessitating careful titration. The range of strengths facilitates titration to the optimal dose.

One capsule of VIAZEM XL is to be taken before or during a meal. The dose should be taken at approximately the same time each day.

The capsule should not be chewed but swallowed whole, with a glass of water.

Due to the variability of release profile in individual patients, when changing from one type of sustained release diltiazem preparation to another, it may be necessary to adjust the dose.

Adults:

Hypertension: The usual starting dose is 180 mg once daily. The dose may be increased after 2-4 weeks according to the patient's response and the usual maintenance dose is 240mg-360mg once daily. The maximum daily dose is 360 mg. However, the single daily doses of 300 mg and 360 mg should only be administered to patients when no satisfactory therapeutic effect has been effected with lower doses and after the benefit risk-ratio has been carefully assessed by the doctor.

Angina: Care should be taken when titrating patients with stable angina in order to establish the optimal dose. The usual starting dose is 180 mg once daily. The dose may be increased after 2-4 weeks according to the patient's response. The maximum daily dose is 360 mg. However, the single daily doses of 300 mg and 360 mg should only be administered to patients when no satisfactory therapeutic effect has been effected with lower doses and after the benefit risk-ratio has been carefully assessed by the doctor.

Elderly and patients with impaired hepatic or renal function:

Plasma levels of diltiazem can be increased in the elderly, and in patients with impaired hepatic renal or hepatic function. In these cases, the starting dose should be one 120mg VIAZEM XL capsule once daily. Heart rate should be monitored and if it falls below 50 beats per minute, the dose should not be increased. Dose adjustment may be required to obtain a satisfactory clinical response.

Children:

Safety and efficacy in children have not been established.

4.3 Contraindications

Diltiazem depresses atrioventricular node conduction and is therefore contraindicated in patients with severe bradycardia (less than 50 bpm), sick sinus syndrome, congestive heart failure, and left ventricular failure with second or third degree AV or sino-atrial block, except in the presence of a functioning pacemaker. Diltiazem is also contraindicated in left ventricular failure with pulmonary stasis as diltiazem may have mild negative effects on contractility.

Diltiazem is contraindicated in acute complicated myocardial infarction (e.g. bradycardia hypotension, congestive heart failure/reduced LV function), pulmonary congestion, hypotension (<90 mmHg systolic) cerebrovascular accident, cardiac shock and unstable angina pectoris.

Diltiazem is contraindicated in pre-excitation syndrome (e.g. WPW) accompanied with atrial flutter, fibrillation and in digitalis intoxication, as diltiazem may precipitate ventricular tachycardia.

Diltiazem should not be used in patients with known hypersensitivity to diltiazem.

Diltiazem should not be used during pregnancy, by women of child-bearing potential, or by women who are breast-feeding.

4.4 Special warnings and special precautions for use

Patients treated with beta-adrenoreceptor blocking drugs and patients with conduction disturbances (bradycardia, bundle branch block, first degree AV block, prolonged PR interval) should only be treated with VIAZEM XL after special consideration due to the risk of serious bradyarrhythmias.

This product should be used with caution in patients with hepatic dysfunction. Abnormalities of liver function may appear during therapy. The higher single daily doses of VIAZEM XL capsules 300mg and 360mg should not be administered to patients with impaired renal and/or hepatic function and to elderly patients (prolonged half life of elimination) because there is no experience on the use of such high dosages in these patient categories.

In patients undergoing long-term therapy with cyclosporin, plasma levels of cyclosporin should be monitored when concurrent administration of diltiazem is initiated, or discontinued or if the dose of diltiazem is changed.

Abnormally short transit time through the gastrointestinal tract could lead to incomplete release of contents of the capsule e.g. in chronic conditions with associated diarrhoea such as Crohns disease or ulcerative colitis.

4.5 Interaction with other medicinal products and other forms of Interaction

Combinations contraindicated as a safety measure:

In animals, fatal ventricular fibrillations are constantly seen during administration of verapamil and dantrolene via the i.v. route. The combination of a calcium antagonist and dantrolene is therefore potentially dangerous. The concurrent iv administration of beta-adrenergic blocking agents with diltiazem should be avoided because an additive effect on SA and AV conduction and ventricular function will occur. The use of such a combination requires ECG monitoring especially at the beginning of treatment.

Combinations requiring safety precautions:

In common with other calcium antagonists, when diltiazem is used with drugs which may induce bradycardia or with antiarrhythmic drugs (e.g. amiodarone) or other antihypertensive drugs, the possibility of an additive effect should be borne in mind. Inhalation anaesthetics should be used with caution during diltiazem therapy. Tri/tetracyclic antidepressants and neuroleptics may increase the antihypertensive effects of diltiazem whilst the concomitant use of lithium with diltiazem may lead to neurotoxicity (extrapyramidal effects). Rifampin and other hepatic enzyme inducers may reduce the bioavailability of diltiazem and high doses of Vitamin D and/or high intake of calcium salts leading to elevated serum calcium levels may reduce the response to diltiazem.

Diltiazem is metabolised by CYP3A4 and could, by competitive inhibition of CYP3A4, affect the pharmacokinetics of other drugs metabolised by this enzyme. In addition inhibitors and inducers of CYP3A4 may affect the pharmacokinetics of diltiazem.

Diltiazem prolongs the sedative effect of medazolam and triazolam via metabolic interaction and decreases nifedipine clearance by 50%. Diltiazem may cause increases in the levels of digitoxin. Diltiazem has been shown to increase the bioavailability of imipramine by 30% probably due to inhibition of its first pass metabolism.

Diltiazem has been used safely in combination with diuretics, ACE-inhibitors and other anti-hypertensive agents. It is recommended that patients receiving these combinations should be regularly monitored. Concomitant use of diltiazem with alpha-blockers such as prazosin should be strictly monitored because of the possible synergistic hypotensive effect of the combination.

Case reports have suggested that blood levels of carbamazepine, cyclosporin, theophylline and phenytoin may be increased when given concurrently with diltiazem. Care should be exercised in patients taking these drugs. In common with other calcium antagonists diltiazem may cause small increases in plasma levels of digoxin. In patients taking H_2-antagonists concurrently with diltiazem there may be increased levels of diltiazem.

Magnification of the hypotensive and lipothymic effects (summation of vasodilator properties) of nitrate derivatives can occur. In patients on calcium inhibitors, prescriptions of nitrate derivatives should be made at progressively increasing doses. Diltiazem treatment has been continued without problem during anaesthesia, but diltiazem may potentiate the activity of curare-like and depolarising neuromuscular blocking agents, therefore the anaesthetist should be informed that the patient is receiving a calcium antagonist.

4.6 Pregnancy and lactation

Pregnancy:

Diltiazem should not be taken during pregnancy. Women of child bearing-potential should exclude the possibility of pregnancy before commencing treatment by taking suitable contraceptive measures if necessary. In animal tests, Diltiazem was found to have a tetratogenic effects in some species of animal.

Diltiazem may suppress the contractility of the uterus. Definite evidence that this will prolong partus in full-term pregnancy is lacking. A risk of hypoxia in the foetus may arise in the event of hypotension in the mother and reduced perfusion of the uterus due to redistribution of blood flow due to peripheral vasodilatation. In animal experiments diltiazem has exhibited teratogenic effects in some animal species. In the absence of adequate evidence of safety in human pregnancy, VIAZEM XL should not be used in pregnancy or in women of childbearing potential.

Lactation:

Diltiazem is excreted in breast milk in concentrations similar to those in serum. If the use of diltiazem is considered essential, an alternative method of infant feeding should be instituted.

4.7 Effects on ability to drive and use machines

There are no studies on the effect of diltiazem when driving vehicles or operating machines. It should be taken into account that occasionally asthenia/fatigue and dizziness may occur. Treatment of hypertension with this medicinal product requires regular monitoring. Individual different reactions may affect the ability to drive. This risk should be considered especially at the beginning of treatment, when changing the drug, or in combination with alcohol.

4.8 Undesirable effects

Certain undesirable effects may lead to suspension of treatment: sinus bradycardia, sino-atrial heart block, 2nd and 3rd degree atrioventricular heart block, skin rash, oedema of the lower limbs.

In hypertensive patients, adverse effects are generally mild and transient and are most commonly vasodilatory related events.

The following have been described in decreasing order of frequency: lower limb oedema, headache, hot flushes/flushing, asthenia/fatigue, palpitations, malaise, minor gastro-intestinal disorders (dyspepsia, abdominal pain, dry mouth, nausea, vomiting, diarrhoea, constipation) and skin rash. Erythema multiform and Stevens Johnson syndrome have been reported infrequently in patients receiving diltiazem hydrochloride. Vasodilatory related events (in particular, oedema) are dose-dependent and appear to be more frequent in elderly subjects.

Rare cases of symptomatic bradycardia and exceptionally sino-atrial block and atrioventricular block, hypotension, syncope, reduced left ventricular function have also been recorded. Isolated cases of hallucinations, depression, insomnia, hyperglycaemia and impotence have been reported.

Experience with use in other indications and with other formulations has shown that skin rashes are usually localised and are limited to cases of erythemia, urticaria or occasionally desquamative erthema, with or without fever, which regress when treatment is discontinued.

Isolated cases of moderate and transient elevations of liver transaminases have been observed at the start of treatment. Isolated cases of clinical hepatitis have been reported which resolved with cessation of therapy.

Dizziness, pruritis, nervousness, paraesthesia, articular/muscular pain, photo sensitisation, hypotension, gingival hyperplasia, and gynaecomastia, have also been observed.

4.9 Overdose

The clinical consequences of overdose can be severe hypotension leading to collapse, and sinus bradycardia which may be accompanied by isorhythmic dissociation and atrioventricular conduction disturbances. Observation in a coronary care unit is advisable. Vasopressors such as adrenaline may be indicated in patients exhibiting profound hypotension. Calcium gluconate may help reverse the effects of calcium entry blockade. Atropine administration and temporary cardiac pacing may be required to manage bradycardia and/or conduction disturbances.

Glucagon can be used in cases of established hypoglycaemia.

Diltiazem and its metabolites are very poorly dialysable.

5. PHARMACOLOGICAL PROPERTIES

5.1 Pharmacodynamic properties

Diltiazem is classified as a calcium channel blocker, benziothiazepine derivative, C08DB01, under the ATC classification. It selectively reduces calcium entry through voltage-dependent calcium-n channels into vascular smooth muscle cells and myocardial cells. This lowers the concentration of intracellular calcium which is available to activate contractile proteins. This action of diltiazem results in dilation of coronary arteries causing an increase in myocardial oxygen supply. It reduces cardiac work by moderating the heart rate and by reducing systemic vascular resistance thus reducing oxygen demand. Diltiazem also prolongs AV conduction and has mild effects on contractility. Clinical data on morbidity and mortality are not available.

5.2 Pharmacokinetic properties

Multiple dose pharmacokinetic studies have shown that the kinetics of VIAZEM XL are non-linear within the 120mg-360mg dosage range. Diltiazem is well absorbed, but has a highly saturable first pass effect leading to a variable absolute bioavailability, which is on average 35%. The saturable first pass effect results in higher than expected systemic exposure with increasing doses.

The protein binding is 80 to 85% and the volume of distribution is 5.0 l/kg.

Diltiazem is metabolised by CYP3A4 in the liver and 70% of the dose is excreted in urine, mainly as metabolites. The plasma levels of the two main metabolites, N-monodesmethyldiltiazem and desacetyldiltiazem, represent 35% and 15% of diltiazem levels respectively. The metabolites contribute around 50% of the clinical effect. Plasma clearance of diltiazem is approximately 0.5 l/h/kg. Plasma half-life of diltiazem is approximately 5-7 hours.

VIAZEM XL capsules allow a prolonged absorption of diltiazem and maximum levels are reached within 6 to 12 hours. Concomitant food intake with VIAZEM XL does not influence the pharmacokinetics of diltiazem. For most patients, chronic administration of VIAZEM XL 300mg once daily, results in therapeutic diltiazem levels (50-200ng/ml) over 24 hours. However, the inter-individual variability is high and individual dose adjustment based on therapeutic response is therefore necessary.

5.3 Preclinical safety data

Tests on reproductive functions in animals show that diltiazem decreases fertility in rats and that it is teratogenic in mice, rats and rabbits. Exposure during late pregnancy induces dystocia and a decrease in the number of live newborns in rats.

Detailed mutagenicity and carcinogenicity tests proved negative.

6. PHARMACEUTICAL PARTICULARS

6.1 List of excipients

Sucrose Stearate

Microcrystalline cellulose

Povidone

Magnesium Stearate

Talc

Titanium dioxide

Hypromellose

Polysorbate 80

Polyacrylate dispersion 30% (dry)

Simethicone emulsion

Gelatine capsule

Gelatin capsule colours

	Capsule body	Capsule cap
240 mg	Blue Green opaque[1]	Lavender opaque[2]

1 = Colour is composed of	Quinoline Yellow E104 Indigotine E132 Titanium Dioxide E171
2 = Colour is composed of	Azorubine E122 Indigotine E132 Titanium Dioxide E171

Gelatin capsule markings:

	Capsule body	Capsule cap
240 mg	Viazem XL 240	Viazem XL 240
(Capsule Size 1)	(White ink EEC approved)	(White ink EEC approved)

White printing ink contains:

Shellac, Ethyl Alcohol, Isopropyl Alcohol, n-Butyl, Propylene Glycol, Sodium Hydroxide, Polyvinylpyrrolidone, Titanium Dioxide

6.2 Incompatibilities

Not applicable.

6.3 Shelf life

3 years

6.4 Special precautions for storage

Do not store above 25°C. Store in original package in a dry place away from any heat source, e.g. direct sunlight, heaters, steam, etc.

6.5 Nature and contents of container

The capsules are packed in PVC/aluminium blisters. Pack sizes are 28 capsules per blister.

6.6 Instructions for use and handling

Swallow capsules whole, with a glass of water do not chew.

7. MARKETING AUTHORISATION HOLDER

Stada Arzneimittel AG

Stadastrasse 2-18

61118 Bad Vilbel

Germany

8. MARKETING AUTHORISATION NUMBER(S)

PL 11204/0092

9. DATE OF FIRST AUTHORISATION/RENEWAL OF THE AUTHORISATION

2nd April 1997

10. DATE OF REVISION OF THE TEXT

20 November 2001

Viazem XL 300mg

(Genus Pharmaceuticals)

1. NAME OF THE MEDICINAL PRODUCT

VIAZEM® XL 300mg

2. QUALITATIVE AND QUANTITATIVE COMPOSITION

Diltiazem hydrochloride: 300 mg capsule.

For excipients, see section 6.1

3. PHARMACEUTICAL FORM

Prolonged release capsule, hard.

White and lavender opaque capsules. Each capsule is printed on the cap and body, in black ink, with Viazem XL 300.

4. CLINICAL PARTICULARS

4.1 Therapeutic indications

VIAZEM XL is indicated for the management of stable angina pectoris and the treatment of mild to moderate hypertension.

4.2 Posology and method of administration

Dosage requirements may differ between patients with angina and patients with hypertension. In addition individual patients response may vary, necessitating careful titration. The range of strengths facilitates titration to the optimal dose.

One capsule of VIAZEM XL is to be taken before or during a meal. The dose should be taken at approximately the same time each day.

The capsule should not be chewed but swallowed whole, with a glass of water.

Due to the variability of release profile in individual patients, when changing from one type of sustained release diltiazem preparation to another, it may be necessary to adjust the dose.

Adults:

Hypertension: The usual starting dose is 180 mg once daily. The dose may be increased after 2-4 weeks according to the patient's response and the usual maintenance dose is 240mg-360mg once daily. The maximum daily dose is 360 mg. However, the single daily doses of 300 mg and 360 mg should only be administered to patients when no satisfactory therapeutic effect has been effected with lower doses and after the benefit risk-ratio has been carefully assessed by the doctor.

Angina: Care should be taken when titrating patients with stable angina in order to establish the optimal dose. The usual starting dose is 180 mg once daily. The dose may be increased after 2-4 weeks according to the patient's response. The maximum daily dose is 360 mg. However, the single daily doses of 300 mg and 360 mg should only be administered to patients when no satisfactory therapeutic effect has been effected with lower doses and after the benefit risk-ratio has been carefully assessed by the doctor.

Elderly and patients with impaired hepatic or renal function:

Plasma levels of diltiazem can be increased in the elderly, and in patients with impaired hepatic renal or hepatic function. In these cases, the starting dose should be one 120mg VIAZEM XL capsule once daily. Heart rate should be monitored and if it falls below 50 beats per minute, the dose should not be increased. Dose adjustment may be required to obtain a satisfactory clinical response.

Children:

Safety and efficacy in children have not been established.

4.3 Contraindications

Diltiazem depresses atrioventricular node conduction and is therefore contraindicated in patients with severe bradycardia (less than 50 bpm), sick sinus syndrome, congestive heart failure, and left ventricular failure with second or third degree AV or sino-atrial block, except in the presence of a functioning pacemaker. Diltiazem is also contraindicated in left ventricular failure with pulmonary stasis as diltiazem may have mild negative effects on contractility.

Diltiazem is contraindicated in acute complicated myocardial infarction (e.g. bradycardia hypotension, congestive heart failure/reduced LV function), pulmonary congestion, hypotension (<90 mmHg systolic) cerebrovascular accident, cardiac shock and unstable angina pectoris.

Diltiazem is contraindicated in pre-excitation syndrome (e.g. WPW) accompanied with atrial flutter, fibrillation and in digitalis intoxication, as diltiazem may precipitate ventricular tachycardia.

Diltiazem should not be used in patients with known hypersensitivity to diltiazem.

Diltiazem should not be used during pregnancy, by women of child-bearing potential, or by women who are breastfeeding.

4.4 Special warnings and special precautions for use

Patients treated with beta-adrenoreceptor blocking drugs and patients with conduction disturbances (bradycardia, bundle branch block, first degree AV block, prolonged PR interval) should only be treated with VIAZEM XL after special consideration due to the risk of serious bradyarrhythmias.

This product should be used with caution in patients with hepatic dysfunction. Abnormalities of liver function may appear during therapy. The higher single daily doses of VIAZEM XL capsules 300mg and 360mg should not be administered to patients with impaired renal and/or hepatic function and to elderly patients (prolonged half life of elimination) because there is no experience on the use of such high dosages in these patient categories.

In patients undergoing long-term therapy with cyclosporin, plasma levels of cyclosporin should be monitored when concurrent administration of diltiazem is initiated, or discontinued or if the dose of diltiazem is changed.

Abnormally short transit time through the gastrointestinal tract could lead to incomplete release of contents of the capsule e.g. in chronic conditions with associated diarrhoea such as Crohns disease or ulcerative colitis.

4.5 Interaction with other medicinal products and other forms of Interaction

Combinations contraindicated as a safety measure:

In animals, fatal ventricular fibrillations are constantly seen during administration of verapamil and dantrolene via the i.v. route. The combination of a calcium antagonist and dantrolene is therefore potentially dangerous. The concurrent iv administration of beta-adrenergic blocking agents with diltiazem should be avoided because an additive effect on SA and AV conduction and ventricular function will occur. The use of such a combination requires ECG monitoring especially at the beginning of treatment.

Combinations requiring safety precautions:

In common with other calcium antagonists, when diltiazem is used with drugs which may induce bradycardia or with antiarrhythmic drugs (e.g. amiodarone) or other antihypertensive drugs, the possibility of an additive effect should be borne in mind. Inhalation anaesthetics should be used with caution during diltiazem therapy. Tri/tetracyclic antidepressants and neuroleptics may increase the antihypertensive effects of diltiazem whilst the concomitant use of lithium with diltiazem may lead to neurotoxicity (extrapyramidal effects). Rifampin and other hepatic enzyme inducers may reduce the bioavailability of diltiazem and high doses of Vitamin D and/or high intake of calcium salts leading to elevated serum calcium levels may reduce the response to diltiazem.

Diltiazem is metabolised by CYP3A4 and could, by competitive inhibition of CYP3A4, affect the pharmacokinetics of other drugs metabolised by this enzyme. In addition inhibitors and inducers of CYP3A4 may affect the pharmacokinetics of diltiazem.

Diltiazem prolongs the sedative effect of medazolam and triazolam via metabolic interaction and decreases nifedipine clearance by 50%. Diltiazem may cause increases in the levels of digitoxin. Diltiazem has been shown to increase the bioavailability of imipramine by 30% probably due to inhibition of its first pass metabolism.

Diltiazem has been used safely in combination with diuretics, ACE-inhibitors and other anti-hypertensive agents. It is recommended that patients receiving these combinations should be regularly monitored. Concomitant use of diltiazem with alpha-blockers such as prazosin should be strictly monitored because of the possible synergistic hypotensive effect of the combination.

Case reports have suggested that blood levels of carbamazepine, cyclosporin, theophylline and phenytoin may be increased when given concurrently with diltiazem. Care should be exercised in patients taking these drugs. In common with other calcium antagonists diltiazem may cause small increases in plasma levels of digoxin. In patients taking H_2-antagonists concurrently with diltiazem there may be increased levels of diltiazem.

Magnification of the hypotensive and lipothymic effects (summation of vasodilator properties) of nitrate derivatives can occur. In patients on calcium inhibitors, prescriptions of nitrate derivatives should be made at progressively increasing doses. Diltiazem treatment has been continued without problem during anaesthesia, but diltiazem may potentiate the activity of curare-like and depolarising neuromuscular blocking agents, therefore the anaesthetist should be informed that the patient is receiving a calcium antagonist.

4.6 Pregnancy and lactation

Pregnancy:

Diltiazem should not be taken during pregnancy. Women of child bearing-potential should exclude the possibility of pregnancy before commencing treatment by taking suitable contraceptive measures if necessary. In animal tests, Diltiazem was found to have a tetratogenic effects in some species of animal.

Diltiazem may suppress the contractility of the uterus. Definite evidence that this will prolong partus in full-term pregnancy is lacking. A risk of hypoxia in the foetus may arise in the event of hypotension in the mother and reduced perfusion of the uterus due to redistribution of blood flow due to peripheral vasodilatation. In animal experiments diltiazem has exhibited teratogenic effects in some animal species. In the absence of adequate evidence of safety in human pregnancy, VIAZEM XL should not be used in pregnancy or in women of childbearing potential.

Lactation:

Diltiazem is excreted in breast milk in concentrations similar to those in serum. If the use of diltiazem is considered essential, an alternative method of infant feeding should be instituted.

4.7 Effects on ability to drive and use machines

There are no studies on the effect of diltiazem when driving vehicles or operating machines. It should be taken into account that occasionally asthenia/fatigue and dizziness may occur. Treatment of hypertension with this medicinal product requires regular monitoring. Individual different reactions may affect the ability to drive. This risk should be considered especially at the beginning of treatment, when changing the drug, or in combination with alcohol.

4.8 Undesirable effects

Certain undesirable effects may lead to suspension of treatment: sinus bradycardia, sino-atrial heart block, 2nd and 3rd degree atrioventricular heart block, skin rash, oedema of the lower limbs.

In hypertensive patients, adverse effects are generally mild and transient and are most commonly vasodilatory related events.

The following have been described in decreasing order of frequency: lower limb oedema, headache, hot flushes/flushing, asthenia/fatigue, palpitations, malaise, minor gastro-intestinal disorders (dyspepsia, abdominal pain, dry mouth, nausea, vomiting, diarrhoea, constipation) and skin rash. Erythema multiform and Stevens Johnson syndrome have been reported infrequently in patients receiving diltiazem hydrochloride. Vasodilatory related events (in particular, oedema) are dose-dependent and appear to be more frequent in elderly subjects.

Rare cases of symptomatic bradycardia and exceptionally sino-atrial block and atrioventricular block, hypotension, syncope, reduced left ventricular function have also been recorded. Isolated cases of hallucinations, depression, insomnia, hyperglycaemia and impotence have been reported.

Experience with use in other indications and with other formulations has shown that skin rashes are usually localised and are limited to cases of erythemia, urticaria or occasionally desquamative erthema, with or without fever, which regress when treatment is discontinued.

Isolated cases of moderate and transient elevations of liver transaminases have been observed at the start of treatment. Isolated cases of clinical hepatitis have been reported which resolved with cessation of therapy.

Dizziness, pruritis, nervousness, paraesthesia, articular/muscular pain, photo sensitisation, hypotension, gingival hyperplasia, and gynaecomastia, have also been observed.

4.9 Overdose

The clinical consequences of overdose can be severe hypotension leading to collapse, and sinus bradycardia which may be accompanied by isorhythmic dissociation and atrioventricular conduction disturbances. Observation in a coronary care unit is advisable. Vasopressors such as adrenaline may be indicated in patients exhibiting profound hypotension. Calcium gluconate may help reverse the effects of calcium entry blockade. Atropine administration and temporary cardiac pacing may be required to manage bradycardia and/or conduction disturbances.

Glucagon can be used in cases of established hypoglycaemia.

Diltiazem and its metabolites are very poorly dialysable.

5. PHARMACOLOGICAL PROPERTIES

5.1 Pharmacodynamic properties

Diltiazem is classified as a calcium channel blocker, benziothiazepine derivative, C08DB01, under the ATC classification. It selectively reduces calcium entry through voltage-dependent calcium-n channels into vascular smooth muscle cells and myocardial cells. This lowers the concentration of intracellular calcium which is available to activate contractile proteins. This action of diltiazem results in dilation of coronary arteries causing an increase in myocardial oxygen supply. It reduces cardiac work by moderating the heart rate and by reducing systemic vascular resistance thus reducing oxygen demand. Diltiazem also prolongs AV conduction and has mild effects on contractility. Clinical data on morbidity and mortality are not available.

5.2 Pharmacokinetic properties

Multiple dose pharmacokinetic studies have shown that the kinetics of VIAZEM XL are non-linear within the 120mg-360mg dosage range. Diltiazem is well absorbed, but has a highly saturable first pass effect leading to a variable absolute bioavailability, which is on average 35%. The saturable first pass effect results in higher than expected systemic exposure with increasing doses.

The protein binding is 80 to 85% and the volume of distribution is 5.0 l/kg.

Diltiazem is metabolised by CYP3A4 in the liver and 70% of the dose is excreted in urine, mainly as metabolites. The plasma levels of the two main metabolites, N-monodesmethyldiltiazem and desacetyldiltiazem, represent 35% and 15% of diltiazem levels respectively. The metabolites contribute around 50% of the clinical effect. Plasma clearance of diltiazem is approximately 0.5 l/h/kg. Plasma half-life of diltiazem is approximately 5-7 hours.

VIAZEM XL capsules allow a prolonged absorption of diltiazem and maximum levels are reached within 6 to 12 hours. Concomitant food intake with VIAZEM XL does not influence the pharmacokinetics of diltiazem. For most patients, chronic administration of VIAZEM XL 300mg once daily, results in therapeutic diltiazem levels (50-200ng/ml) over 24 hours. However, the inter-individual variability is high and individual dose adjustment based on therapeutic response is therefore necessary.

5.3 Preclinical safety data

Tests on reproductive functions in animals show that diltiazem decreases fertility in rats and that it is teratogenic in mice, rats and rabbits. Exposure during late pregnancy induces dystocia and a decrease in the number of live newborns in rats.

Detailed mutagenicity and carcinogenicity tests proved negative.

6. PHARMACEUTICAL PARTICULARS

6.1 List of excipients

Sucrose Stearate

Microcrystalline cellulose

Povidone

Magnesium Stearate

Talc

Titanium dioxide

Hypromellose

Polysorbate 80

Polyacrylate dispersion 30% (dry)

Simethicone emulsion

Gelatine capsule

Gelatin capsule colours

	Capsule body	Capsule cap
300 mg	White opaque[1]	Lavender opaque[2]

1 = Colour is composed of Titanium Dioxide E171

2 = Colour is composed of Azorubine E122 Indigotine E132 Titanium Dioxide E171

Gelatin capsule markings:

	Capsule body	Capsule cap
300 mg	Viazem XL 300	Viazem XL 300
(Capsule Size 0)	(Black ink EEC approved)	(Black ink EEC approved)

Black printing ink contains:

Shellac, Ethyl Alcohol, Isopropyl Alcohol, n-Butyl, Propylene Glycol, Water (Purified) Ammonium Hydroxide, Potassium Hydroxide, Black Iron Oxide

6.2 Incompatibilities

Not applicable.

6.3 Shelf life

3 years

6.4 Special precautions for storage

Do not store above 25°C. Store in original package in a dry place away from any heat source, e.g. direct sunlight, heaters, steam, etc.

6.5 Nature and contents of container

The capsules are packed in PVC/aluminium blisters. Pack sizes are 28 capsules per blister.

6.6 Instructions for use and handling

Swallow capsules whole, with a glass of water do not chew.

7. MARKETING AUTHORISATION HOLDER

Stada Arzneimittel AG

Stadastrasse 2-18

61118 Bad Vilbel

Germany

8. MARKETING AUTHORISATION NUMBER(S)

PL 11204/0093

9. DATE OF FIRST AUTHORISATION/RENEWAL OF THE AUTHORISATION

2nd April 1997

10. DATE OF REVISION OF THE TEXT

20 November 2001

Viazem XL 360mg

(Genus Pharmaceuticals)

1. NAME OF THE MEDICINAL PRODUCT

VIAZEM® XL 360mg

2. QUALITATIVE AND QUANTITATIVE COMPOSITION

Diltiazem hydrochloride: 360 mg capsule.

For excipients see section 6.1

3. PHARMACEUTICAL FORM

Prolonged release capsule, hard.

Blue-green opaque capsules. Each capsule is printed on the cap and body, in white ink, with Viazem XL 360.

4. CLINICAL PARTICULARS

4.1 Therapeutic indications

VIAZEM XL is indicated for the management of stable angina pectoris and the treatment of mild to moderate hypertension.

4.2 Posology and method of administration

Dosage requirements may differ between patients with angina and patients with hypertension. In addition individual patients response may vary, necessitating careful titration. The range of strengths facilitates titration to the optimal dose.

One capsule of VIAZEM XL is to be taken before or during a meal. The dose should be taken at approximately the same time each day.

The capsule should not be chewed but swallowed whole, with a glass of water.

Due to the variability of release profile in individual patients, when changing from one type of sustained release diltiazem preparation to another, it may be necessary to adjust the dose.

Adults:

Hypertension: The usual starting dose is 180 mg once daily. The dose may be increased after 2-4 weeks according to the patient's response and the usual maintenance dose is 240mg-360mg once daily. The maximum daily dose is 360 mg. However, the single daily doses of 300 mg and 360 mg should only be administered to patients when no satisfactory therapeutic effect has been effected with lower doses and after the benefit risk-ratio has been carefully assessed by the doctor.

Angina: Care should be taken when titrating patients with stable angina in order to establish the optimal dose. The usual starting dose is 180 mg once daily. The dose may be increased after 2-4 weeks according to the patient's response. The maximum daily dose is 360 mg. However, the single daily doses of 300 mg and 360 mg should only be administered to patients when no satisfactory therapeutic effect has been effected with lower doses and after the benefit risk-ratio has been carefully assessed by the doctor.

Elderly and patients with impaired hepatic or renal function:

Plasma levels of diltiazem can be increased in the elderly, and in patients with impaired hepatic renal or hepatic function. In these cases, the starting dose should be one 120mg VIAZEM XL capsule once daily. Heart rate should be monitored and if it falls below 50 beats per minute, the dose should not be increased. Dose adjustment may be required to obtain a satisfactory clinical response.

Children:

Safety and efficacy in children have not been established.

4.3 Contraindications

Diltiazem depresses atrioventricular node conduction and is therefore contraindicated in patients with severe bradycardia (less than 50 bpm), sick sinus syndrome, congestive heart failure, and left ventricular failure with second or third degree AV or sino-atrial block, except in the presence of a functioning pacemaker. Diltiazem is also contraindicated in left ventricular failure with pulmonary stasis as diltiazem may have mild negative effects on contractility.

Diltiazem is contraindicated in acute complicated myocardial infarction (e.g. bradycardia hypotension, congestive heart failure/reduced LV function), pulmonary congestion, hypotension (<90 mmHg systolic) cerebrovascular accident, cardiac shock and unstable angina pectoris.

Diltiazem is contraindicated in pre-excitation syndrome (e.g. WPW) accompanied with atrial flutter, fibrillation and in digitalis intoxication, as diltiazem may precipitate ventricular tachycardia.

Diltiazem should not be used in patients with known hypersensitivity to diltiazem.

Diltiazem should not be used during pregnancy, by women of child-bearing potential, or by women who are breast-feeding.

4.4 Special warnings and special precautions for use

Patients treated with beta-adrenoreceptor blocking drugs and patients with conduction disturbances (bradycardia, bundle branch block, first degree AV block, prolonged PR interval) should only be treated with VIAZEM XL after special consideration due to the risk of serious bradyarrhythmias.

This product should be used with caution in patients with hepatic dysfunction. Abnormalities of liver function may appear during therapy. The higher single daily doses of VIAZEM XL capsules 300mg and 360mg should not be administered to patients with impaired renal and/or hepatic function and to elderly patients (prolonged half life of elimination) because there is no experience on the use of such high dosages in these patient categories.

In patients undergoing long-term therapy with cyclosporin, plasma levels of cyclosporin should be monitored when concurrent administration of diltiazem is initiated, or discontinued or if the dose of diltiazem is changed.

Abnormally short transit time through the gastrointestinal tract could lead to incomplete release of contents of the capsule e.g. in chronic conditions with associated diarrhoea such as Crohns disease or ulcerative colitis.

4.5 Interaction with other medicinal products and other forms of Interaction

Combinations contraindicated as a safety measure:

In animals, fatal ventricular fibrillations are constantly seen during administration of verapamil and dantrolene via the i.v. route. The combination of a calcium antagonist and dantrolene is therefore potentially dangerous. The concurrent iv administration of beta-adrenergic blocking agents with diltiazem should be avoided because an additive effect on SA and AV conduction and ventricular function will occur. The use of such a combination requires ECG monitoring especially at the beginning of treatment.

Combinations requiring safety precautions:

In common with other calcium antagonists, when diltiazem is used with drugs which may induce bradycardia or with antiarrhythmic drugs (e.g. amiodarone) or other antihypertensive drugs, the possibility of an additive effect should be borne in mind. Inhalation anaesthetics should be used with caution during diltiazem therapy. Tri/tetracyclic antidepressants and neuroleptics may increase the antihypertensive effects of diltiazem whilst the concomitant use of lithium with diltiazem may lead to neurotoxicity (extrapyramidal effects). Rifampin and other hepatic enzyme inducers may reduce the bioavailability of diltiazem and high doses of Vitamin D and/or high intake of calcium salts leading to elevated serum calcium levels may reduce the response to diltiazem.

Diltiazem is metabolised by CYP3A4 and could, by competitive inhibition of CYP3A4, affect the pharmacokinetics of other drugs metabolised by this enzyme. In addition inhibitors and inducers of CYP3A4 may affect the pharmacokinetics of diltiazem.

Diltiazem prolongs the sedative effect of medazolam and triazolam via metabolic interaction and decreases nifedipine clearance by 50%. Diltiazem may cause increases in the levels of digitoxin. Diltiazem has been shown to increase the bioavailability of imipramine by 30% probably due to inhibition of its first pass metabolism.

Diltiazem has been used safely in combination with diuretics, ACE-inhibitors and other anti-hypertensive agents. It is recommended that patients receiving these combinations should be regularly monitored. Concomitant use of diltiazem with alpha-blockers such as prazosin should be strictly monitored because of the possible synergistic hypotensive effect of the combination.

Case reports have suggested that blood levels of carbamazepine, cyclosporin, theophylline and phenytoin may be increased when given concurrently with diltiazem. Care should be exercised in patients taking these drugs. In common with other calcium antagonists diltiazem may cause small increases in plasma levels of digoxin. In patients taking H_2-antagonists concurrently with diltiazem there may be increased levels of diltiazem.

Magnification of the hypotensive and lipothymic effects (summation of vasodilator properties) of nitrate derivatives can occur. In patients on calcium inhibitors, prescriptions of nitrate derivatives should be made at progressively increasing doses. Diltiazem treatment has been continued without problem during anaesthesia, but diltiazem may potentiate the activity of curare-like and depolarising neuromuscular blocking agents, therefore the anaesthetist should be informed that the patient is receiving a calcium antagonist.

4.6 Pregnancy and lactation

Pregnancy:

Diltiazem should not be taken during pregnancy. Women of child bearing-potential should exclude the possibility of pregnancy before commencing treatment by taking suitable contraceptive measures if necessary. In animal tests, Diltiazem was found to have a tetratogenic effects in some species of animal.

Diltiazem may suppress the contractility of the uterus. Definite evidence that this will prolong partus in full-term pregnancy is lacking. A risk of hypoxia in the foetus may arise in the event of hypotension in the mother and reduced perfusion of the uterus due to redistribution of blood flow due to peripheral vasodilatation. In animal experiments diltiazem has exhibited teratogenic effects in some animal species. In the absence of adequate evidence of safety in human pregnancy, VIAZEM XL should not be used in pregnancy or in women of childbearing potential.

Lactation:

Diltiazem is excreted in breast milk in concentrations similar to those in serum. If the use of diltiazem is considered essential, an alternative method of infant feeding should be instituted.

4.7 Effects on ability to drive and use machines

There are no studies on the effect of diltiazem when driving vehicles or operating machines. It should be taken into account that occasionally asthenia/fatigue and dizziness may occur. Treatment of hypertension with this medicinal product requires regular monitoring. Individual different reactions may affect the ability to drive. This risk should be considered especially at the beginning of treatment, when changing the drug, or in combination with alcohol.

4.8 Undesirable effects

Certain undesirable effects may lead to suspension of treatment: sinus bradycardia, sino-atrial heart block, 2nd and 3rd degree atrioventricular heart block, skin rash, oedema of the lower limbs.

In hypertensive patients, adverse effects are generally mild and transient and are most commonly vasodilatory related events.

The following have been described in decreasing order of frequency: lower limb oedema, headache, hot flushes/flushing, asthenia/fatigue, palpitations, malaise, minor gastro-intestinal disorders (dyspepsia, abdominal pain, dry mouth, nausea, vomiting, diarrhoea, constipation) and skin rash. Erythema multiforme and Stevens Johnson syndrome have been reported infrequently in patients receiving diltiazem hydrochloride. Vasodilatory related events (in particular, oedema) are dose-dependent and appear to be more frequent in elderly subjects.

Rare cases of symptomatic bradycardia and exceptionally sino-atrial block and atrioventricular block, hypotension, syncope, reduced left ventricular function have also been recorded. Isolated cases of hallucinations, depression, insomnia, hyperglycaemia and impotence have been reported.

Experience with use in other indications and with other formulations has shown that skin rashes are usually localised and are limited to cases of erythemia, urticaria or occasionally desquamative erthema, with or without fever, which regress when treatment is discontinued.

Isolated cases of moderate and transient elevations of liver transaminases have been observed at the start of treatment. Isolated cases of clinical hepatitis have been reported which resolved with cessation of therapy.

Dizziness, pruritis, nervousness, paraesthesia, articular/muscular pain, photo sensitisation, hypotension, gingival hyperplasia, and gynaecomastia, have also been observed.

4.9 Overdose

The clinical consequences of overdose can be severe hypotension leading to collapse, and sinus bradycardia which may be accompanied by isorhythmic dissociation and atrioventricular conduction disturbances. Observation in a coronary care unit is advisable. Vasopressors such as adrenaline may be indicated in patients exhibiting profound hypotension. Calcium gluconate may help reverse the effects of calcium entry blockade. Atropine administration and temporary cardiac pacing may be required to manage bradycardia and/or conduction disturbances.

Glucagon can be used in cases of established hypoglycaemia.

Diltiazem and its metabolites are very poorly dialysable.

5. PHARMACOLOGICAL PROPERTIES

5.1 Pharmacodynamic properties

Diltiazem is classified as a calcium channel blocker, benziothiazepine derivative, C08DB01, under the ATC classification. It selectively reduces calcium entry through voltage-dependent calcium-n channels into vascular smooth muscle cells and myocardial cells. This lowers the concentration of intracellular calcium which is available to activate contractile proteins. This action of diltiazem results in dilation of coronary arteries causing an increase in myocardial oxygen supply. It reduces cardiac work by moderating the heart rate and by reducing systemic vascular resistance thus reducing oxygen demand. Diltiazem also prolongs AV conduction and has mild effects on contractility. Clinical data on morbidity and mortality are not available.

5.2 Pharmacokinetic properties

Multiple dose pharmacokinetic studies have shown that the kinetics of VIAZEM XL are non-linear within the 120mg-360mg dosage range. Diltiazem is well absorbed, but has a highly saturable first pass effect leading to a variable absolute bioavailability, which is on average 35%. The saturable first pass effect results in higher than expected systemic exposure with increasing doses.

The protein binding is 80 to 85% and the volume of distribution is 5.0 l/kg.

Diltiazem is metabolised by CYP3A4 in the liver and 70% of the dose is excreted in urine, mainly as metabolites. The plasma levels of the two main metabolites, N-monodesmethyldiltiazem and desacetyldiltiazem, represent 35% and 15% of diltiazem levels respectively. The metabolites contribute around 50% of the clinical effect. Plasma clearance of diltiazem is approximately 0.5 l/h/kg. Plasma half-life of diltiazem is approximately 5-7 hours.

VIAZEM XL capsules allow a prolonged absorption of diltiazem and maximum levels are reached within 6 to 12 hours. Concomitant food intake with VIAZEM XL does not influence the pharmacokinetics of diltiazem. For most patients, chronic administration of VIAZEM XL 300mg once daily, results in therapeutic diltiazem levels (50-200ng/ml) over 24 hours. However, the inter-individual variability is high and individual dose adjustment based on therapeutic response is therefore necessary.

5.3 Preclinical safety data

Tests on reproductive functions in animals show that diltiazem decreases fertility in rats and that it is teratogenic in mice, rats and rabbits. Exposure during late pregnancy induces dystocia and a decrease in the number of live newborns in rats.

Detailed mutagenicity and carcinogenicity tests proved negative.

6. PHARMACEUTICAL PARTICULARS

6.1 List of excipients

Sucrose Stearate

Microcrystalline cellulose

Povidone

Magnesium Stearate

Talc

Titanium dioxide

Hypromellose

Polysorbate 80

Polyacrylate dispersion 30% (dry)

Simethicone emulsion

Gelatine capsule

Gelatin capsule colours

	Capsule body	Capsule cap
360 mg	Blue Green opaque[1]	Blue Green opaque[1]

1 = Colour is composed of Quinoline Yellow E104
Indigotine E132
Titanium Dioxide E171

Gelatin capsule markings (printed radially):

	Capsule body	Capsule cap
360 mg	Viazem XL 360	Viazem XL 360
(Capsule Size 0)	(White ink EEC approved)	(White ink EEC approved)

White printing ink contains:

Shellac, Ethyl Alcohol, Isopropyl Alcohol, n-Butyl, Propylene Glycol, Sodium Hydroxide, Polyvinylpyrrolidone, Titanium Dioxide

6.2 Incompatibilities

Not applicable.

6.3 Shelf life

3 years

6.4 Special precautions for storage

Do not store above 25°C. Store in original package in a dry place away from any heat source, e.g. direct sunlight, heaters, steam, etc.

6.5 Nature and contents of container

The capsules are packed in PVC/aluminium blisters. Pack sizes are 28 capsules per blister.

6.6 Instructions for use and handling

Swallow capsules whole, with a glass of water do not chew.

7. MARKETING AUTHORISATION HOLDER

Stada Arzneimittel AG

Stadastrasse 2-18

61118 Bad Vilbel

Germany

8. MARKETING AUTHORISATION NUMBER(S)

PL 11204/0094

9. DATE OF FIRST AUTHORISATION/RENEWAL OF THE AUTHORISATION

2nd April 1997

10. DATE OF REVISION OF THE TEXT

20 November 2001

Vibramycin Acne Pack

(Pfizer Limited)

1. NAME OF THE MEDICINAL PRODUCT

VIBRAMYCIN™ ACNE PACK

2. QUALITATIVE AND QUANTITATIVE COMPOSITION

Doxycycline base 50mg (as doxycycline hyclate Ph. Eur.).

3. PHARMACEUTICAL FORM

Capsules.

Hard gelatin capsules coloured pale green and white and marked "VBM C50", containing spherical yellow to yellowish coated microgranules, intended for oral administration to human beings.

4. CLINICAL PARTICULARS

4.1 Therapeutic indications

As a bacteriostatic antibiotic, doxycycline is clinically effective in the treatment of a variety of infections caused by a wide range of gram-negative and gram-positive bacteria, as well as certain other micro-organisms.

Dermatological infections: *Acne vulgaris*.

4.2 Posology and method of administration

Use in adults Acne vulgaris: In the treatment of *acne vulgaris* the recommended dose is 50mg daily with food or fluid. Duration of treatment will vary from 6 to 12 weeks.

Conventional capsule forms of the tetracycline class of drugs are liable to cause oesophageal irritation and ulceration. Administration of adequate amounts of fluid is therefore recommended to combat this problem. If, however, gastric irritation does occur, doxycycline capsules can be given with food or milk. The absorption of doxycycline is not markedly influenced by simultaneous ingestion of food or milk.

If the recommended dose is exceeded, an increase in the incidence of side-effects may ensue.

Use in children Vibramycin is contra-indicated in children under 12 years of age. For children over 12 years of age, the usual adult dose should be used.

Use in patients with renal/hepatic impairment (See section 4.4 'Special warnings and precautions for use'.)

4.3 Contraindications

Persons who have shown hypersensitivity to doxycycline, any of its inert ingredients or to any of the tetracyclines.

The use of drugs of the tetracycline class during tooth development (pregnancy, infancy and childhood to the age of 12 years) may cause permanent discolouration of the teeth (yellow-grey-brown). This adverse reaction is more common during long-term use of the drugs but has been observed following repeated short-term courses. Enamel hypoplasia has also been reported. Vibramycin is therefore contra-indicated in these groups of patients.

Pregnancy Vibramycin is contra-indicated in pregnancy. It appears that the risks associated with the use of tetracyclines during pregnancy are predominantly due to effects on teeth and skeletal development. (See above about use during tooth development).

Nursing mothers Tetracyclines are excreted into milk and are therefore contra-indicated in nursing mothers. (See above about use during tooth development).

Children Vibramycin is contra-indicated in children under the age of 12 years. As with other tetracyclines, Vibramycin forms a stable calcium complex in any bone-forming tissue. A decrease in the fibula growth rate has been observed in prematures given oral tetracyclines in doses of 25mg/kg every 6 hours. This reaction was shown to be reversible when the drug was discontinued. (See above about use during tooth development).

4.4 Special warnings and special precautions for use

Photosensitivity Photosensitivity manifested by an exaggerated sunburn reaction has been observed in some individuals taking tetracyclines, including doxycycline. Patients likely to be exposed to direct sunlight or ultraviolet light should be advised that this reaction can occur with tetracycline drugs and treatment should be discontinued at the first evidence of skin erythema.

Microbiological overgrowth The use of antibiotics may occasionally result in the overgrowth of nonsusceptible organisms including *Candida*. If a resistant organism appears, the antibiotic should be discontinued and appropriate therapy instituted.

Pseudomembranous colitis has been reported with nearly all antibacterial agents, including doxycycline, and has ranged in severity from mild to life-threatening. It is important to consider this diagnosis in patients who present with diarrhoea subsequent to the administration of antibacterial agents.

Oesophagitis Instances of oesophagitis and oesophageal ulcerations have been reported in patients receiving capsule and tablet forms of drugs in the tetracycline class, including doxycycline. Most of these patients took medications immediately before going to bed or with inadequate amounts of fluid.

Achlorhydria Patients known to have, or suspected to have, achlorhydria should not be prescribed Vibramycin Acne Pack.

Bulging fontanelles in infants and benign intracranial hypertension in juveniles and adults have been reported in individuals receiving full therapeutic dosages. Treatment should be withdrawn if evidence of raised intracranial pressure develops. These conditions disappeared rapidly when the drug was discontinued.

Porphyria There have been rare reports of porphyria in patients receiving tetracyclines.

Myasthenia gravis Due to a potential for weak neuromuscular blockade, care should be taken in administering tetracyclines to patients with myasthenia gravis.

Systemic lupus erythematosus Tetracyclines can cause exacerbation of SLE.

Methoxyflurane Caution is advised in administering tetracyclines with methoxyflurane. See section 4.5.

Use in patients with renal impairment No dosage adjustment is necessary in the presence of renal impairment.

Excretion of doxycycline by the kidney is about 40%/72 hours in individuals with normal renal function. This percentage excretion may fall to a range as low as 1-5%/72 hours in individuals with severe renal insufficiency (creatinine clearance below 10ml/min). Studies have shown no significant difference in the serum half-life of doxycycline in individuals with normal and severely impaired renal function. Haemodialysis does not alter the serum half-life of doxycycline. The anti-anabolic action of the tetracyclines may cause an increase in blood urea. Studies to date indicate that this anti-anabolic effect does not occur with the use of Vibramycin in patients with impaired renal function.

Use in patients with impaired hepatic function Vibramycin should be administered with caution to patients with hepatic impairment or those receiving potentially hepatotoxic drugs.

Abnormal hepatic function has been reported rarely and has been caused by both the oral and parenteral administration of tetracyclines, including doxycycline.

4.5 Interaction with other medicinal products and other forms of Interaction

The absorption of doxycycline may be impaired by concurrently administered antacids containing aluminium, calcium, magnesium or other drugs containing these cations; oral zinc, iron salts or bismuth preparations. Dosages should be maximally separated.

There have been reports of prolonged prothrombin time in patients taking warfarin and doxycycline. Tetracyclines depress plasma prothrombin activity and reduced doses of concomitant anticoagulants may be necessary.

The serum half-life of doxycycline may be shortened when patients are concurrently receiving barbiturates, carbamazepine or phenytoin.

A few cases of pregnancy or breakthrough bleeding have been attributed to the concurrent use of tetracycline antibiotics with oral contraceptives.

Since bacteriostatic drugs may interfere with the bactericidal action of penicillin, it is advisable to avoid giving Vibramycin in conjunction with penicillin.

Alcohol may decrease the half-life of doxycycline.

Doxycycline may increase the plasma concentration of cyclosporin. Co-administration should only be undertaken with appropriate monitoring.

The concurrent use of tetracyclines and methoxyflurane has been reported to result in fatal renal toxicity. See section 4.4.

Laboratory test interactions

False elevations of urinary catecholamine levels may occur due to interference with the fluorescence test.

4.6 Pregnancy and lactation

See "Contra-indications".

4.7 Effects on ability to drive and use machines

The effect of doxycycline on the ability to drive or operate heavy machinery has not been studied. There is no evidence to suggest that doxycycline may affect these abilities.

4.8 Undesirable effects

The following adverse reactions have been observed in patients receiving tetracyclines including doxycycline:

Autonomic nervous system Flushing.

Body as a whole Hypersensitivity reactions, including anaphylactic shock, anaphylaxis, anaphylactoid reaction, anaphylactoid purpura, hypotension, pericarditis, angioneurotic oedema, exacerbation of systemic lupus erythematosus, dyspnoea, serum sickness, peripheral oedema, tachycardia and urticaria.

Central and Peripheral nervous system Headache. Bulging fontanelles in infants and benign intracranial hypertension in juveniles and adults have been reported in individuals receiving full therapeutic dosages of tetracyclines. In relation to benign intracranial hypertension, symptoms included blurring of vision, scotomata and diplopia. Permanent visual loss has been reported.

Gastro-intestinalGastro-intestinal symptoms are usually mild and seldom necessitate discontinuation of treatment. Abdominal pain, anorexia, nausea, vomiting, diarrhoea, dyspepsia and rarely dysphagia. Oesophagitis and oesophageal ulceration have been reported in patients receiving Vibramycin. A significant proportion of these occurred with the hyclate salt in the capsule form. (See 'Special warnings and precautions for use' section).

Hearing/Vestibular Tinnitus.

Haemopoietic Haemolytic anaemia, thrombocytopenia, neutropenia, porphyria, and eosinophilia have been reported with tetracyclines.

Liver/Biliary Transient increases in liver function tests, hepatitis, jaundice, hepatic failure and pancreatitis have been reported rarely.

Musculo-Skeletal Arthralgia and myalgia.

Skin Rashes including maculopapular and erythematous rashes, exfoliative dermatitis, erythema multiforme, Steven-Johnson syndrome and toxic epidermal necrolysis. Photosensitivity skin reactions (see 'Special warnings and precautions for use' section).

Superinfection As with all antibiotics, overgrowth of non-susceptible organisms may cause candidiasis, glossitis, staphylococcal enterocolitis, pseudomembranous colitis (with *Clostridium difficile* overgrowth) and inflammatory lesions (with candidal overgrowth) in the anogenital region. Similarly there have been reports for products in the tetracycline class of stomatitis and vaginitis.

Urinary system Increased blood urea. (See 'Special warnings and precautions for use' section.)

Other When given over prolonged periods, tetracyclines have been reported to produce brown-black microscopic discolouration of thyroid tissue. No abnormalities of thyroid function are known to occur.

Tetracyclines may cause discoloration of teeth and enamel hypoplasia, but usually only after long-term use.

4.9 Overdose

Acute overdosage with antibiotics is rare. In the event of overdosage discontinue medication. Gastric lavage plus appropriate supportive treatment is indicated.

Dialysis does not alter the serum half-life and thus would not be of benefit in treating cases of overdosage.

5. PHARMACOLOGICAL PROPERTIES

5.1 Pharmacodynamic properties

As an antibiotic, doxycycline exerts its antimicrobial effect by the inhibition of protein synthesis and is considered to be primarily bacteriostatic. Doxycycline is clinically effective in the treatment of a variety of infections caused by a wide range of gram-negative and gram-positive bacteria, as well as certain other micro-organisms.

5.2 Pharmacokinetic properties

Absorption Absorption is rapid (effective concentrations are attained as from the first hour), and the peak serum concentration occurs after 2 to 4 hours.

Almost all of the product is absorbed in the upper part of digestive tract.

Absorption is not notably modified by administration with meals, milk has little effect.

Distribution In adults, an oral dose of 200mg results in:

- a peak serum concentration of more than 3μg/ml
- a residual concentration of more than 1μg/ml after 24 hours
- a serum half-life of 16 - 22 hours
- protein binding varying between 82 and 93% (labile binding).

Intra- and extracellular diffusion is good. With usual doses, effective concentrations are found in the skin, ovaries, uterine tubes, uterus, placenta, testicles, prostate, bladder, kidneys, lung tissue, muscles, lymph glands, sinus secretions, maxillary sinus, nasal polyps, tonsils, liver, hepatic and gallbladder bile, gall bladder, stomach, intestine, appendix, omentum, saliva and gingival fluid. Only small amounts are diffused into the cerebrospinal fluid.

Excretion The antibiotic is concentrated in the bile. About 40% of the administered dose is eliminated in 3 days in active form in the urine and about 32% in the faeces. Urinary concentrations are roughly 10 times higher than plasma concentrations at the same time. In the presence of impaired renal function, urinary elimination decreases, faecal elimination increases and the half-life remains unchanged. The half-life is not affected by haemodialysis.

5.3 Preclinical safety data

Not applicable.

6. PHARMACEUTICAL PARTICULARS

6.1 List of excipients

Sucrose and maize starch microgranules, Crospovidone, Polymethacrylate, Talc, Gelatin (capsule shell).

Colourants - capsule shell: Titanium dioxide (E 171), Indigo Carmine (E 132), Quinoline Yellow (E 104), Iron Oxide (E 172)

6.2 Incompatibilities

Nil.

6.3 Shelf life

4 years.

6.4 Special precautions for storage

Store below 25°C.

6.5 Nature and contents of container

Doxycycline Capsules are packed in blister packs (200 micron rigid, opaque white polyvinylchloride and 20 micron aluminium).

Doxycycline Capsules 50 mg are supplied in packs of 56 capsules.

6.6 Instructions for use and handling

See Section 4.2 'Posology and method and administration'.

7. MARKETING AUTHORISATION HOLDER

Pfizer Limited
Ramsgate Road
Sandwich
Kent CT13 9NJ
United Kingdom

8. MARKETING AUTHORISATION NUMBER(S)

PL 00057/0410

9. DATE OF FIRST AUTHORISATION/RENEWAL OF THE AUTHORISATION

29 May 1997

10. DATE OF REVISION OF THE TEXT

26 February 2002

11. Legal Category

POM

Ref: VM3_1

Vibramycin, Vibramycin 50, Vibramycin -D

(Pfizer Limited)

1. NAME OF THE MEDICINAL PRODUCT

VIBRAMYCIN®, VIBRAMYCIN 50, VIBRAMYCIN-D.

2. QUALITATIVE AND QUANTITATIVE COMPOSITION

Active Ingredient: doxycycline.

Vibramycin 50 Capsules contain 50mg doxycycline as doxycycline hyclate Ph. Eur.

Vibramycin Capsules contain 100mg doxycycline as doxycycline hyclate Ph. Eur.

Vibramycin-D Dispersible Tablets contain l00mg doxycycline as doxycycline monohydrate.

3. PHARMACEUTICAL FORM

Vibramycin 50 capsules are green and ivory, coded 'Pfizer' and 'VBM 50'.

Vibramycin capsules 100mg are green, coded 'Pfizer' and 'VBM 100'.

Vibramycin-D Dispersible Tablets are light yellow, round tablets scored on one face and coded 'VN' on the other.

4. CLINICAL PARTICULARS

4.1 Therapeutic indications

Vibramycin has been found clinically effective in the treatment of a variety of infections caused by susceptible strains of Gram-positive and Gram-negative bacteria and certain other micro-organisms.

Respiratory tract infections Pneumonia and other lower respiratory tract infections due to susceptible strains of *Streptococcus pneumoniae*, *Haemophilus influenzae*,

Klebsiella pneumoniae and other organisms. *Mycoplasma pneumoniae* pneumonia. Treatment of chronic bronchitis, sinusitis.

Urinary tract infections caused by susceptible strains of Klebsiella species, Enterobacter species, *Escherichia coli, Streptococcus faecalis* and other organisms.

Sexually transmitted diseases Infections due to *Chlamydia trachomatis* including uncomplicated urethral, endocervical or rectal infections. Non-gonococcal urethritis caused by *Ureaplasma urealyticum* (T-mycoplasma). Vibramycin is also indicated in chancroid, granuloma inguinale and lymphogranuloma venereum. Vibramycin is an alternative drug in the treatment of gonorrhoea and syphilis.

Skin infections Acne vulgaris, when antibiotic therapy is considered necessary.

Since Vibramycin is a member of the tetracycline series of antibiotics, it may be expected to be useful in the treatment of infections which respond to other tetracyclines, such as:

Ophthalmic infections Due to susceptible strains of gonococci, staphylococci and *Haemophilus influenzae*. Trachoma, although the infectious agent, as judged by immunofluorescence, is not always eliminated. Inclusion conjunctivitis may be treated with oral Vibramycin alone or in combination with topical agents.

Rickettsial infections Rocky Mountain spotted fever, typhus group, Q fever, Coxiella endocarditis and tick fevers.

Other infections Psittacosis, brucellosis (in combination with streptomycin), cholera, bubonic plague, louse and tick-borne relapsing fever, tularaemia glanders, melioidosis, chloroquine-resistant falciparum malaria and acute intestinal amoebiasis (as an adjunct to amoebicides).

Vibramycin is an alternative drug in the treatment of leptospirosis, gas gangrene and tetanus.

Vibramycin is indicated for prophylaxis in the following conditions: Scrub typhus, travellers' diarrhoea (enterotoxigenic *Escherichia coli),* leptospirosis and malaria. Prophylaxis of malaria should be used in accordance to current guidelines, as resistance is an ever changing problem.

4.2 Posology and method of administration

Adults

The usual dosage of Vibramycin for the treatment of acute infections in adults is 200mg on the first day (as a single dose or in divided doses) followed by a maintenance dose of 100mg/day. In the management of more severe infections, 200mg daily should be given throughout treatment.

Capsules and Dispersible Tablets are for oral administration only.

Vibramycin-D tablets are administered by drinking a suspension of the tablets in a small amount of water.

Vibramycin capsules should be administered with adequate amounts of fluid. This should be done in the sitting or standing position and well before retiring at night to reduce the risk of oesophageal irritation and ulceration. If gastric irritation occurs, it is recommended that Vibramycin be given with food or milk. Studies indicate that the absorption of Vibramycin is not notably influenced by simultaneous ingestion of food or milk.

Exceeding the recommended dosage may result in an increased incidence of side effects. Therapy should be continued for at least 24 to 48 hours after symptoms and fever have subsided.

When used in streptococcal infections, therapy should be continued for 10 days to prevent the development of rheumatic fever or glomerulonephritis.

Dosage recommendations in specific infections:

Acne vulgaris 50mg daily with food or fluid for 6 to 12 weeks.

Sexually transmitted diseases 100mg twice daily for 7 days is recommended in the following infections: uncomplicated gonococcal infections (except anorectal infections in men); uncomplicated urethral, endocervical or rectal infection caused by *Chlamydia trachomatis*; non-gonococcal urethritis caused by *Ureaplasma urealyticum*. Acute epididymo-orchitis caused by *Chlamydia trachomatis* or *Neisseria gonorrhoea* 100mg twice daily for 10 days. Primary and secondary syphilis: Non-pregnant penicillin-allergic patients who have primary or secondary syphilis can be treated with the following regimen: doxycycline 200mg orally twice daily for two weeks, as an alternative to penicillin therapy.

Louse and tick-borne relapsing fevers A single dose of 100 or 200mg according to severity.

Treatment of chloroquine-resistant falciparum malaria 200mg daily for at least 7 days. Due to the potential severity of the infection, a rapid-acting schizonticide such as quinine should always be given in conjunction with Vibramycin; quinine dosage recommendations vary in different areas.

Prophylaxis of malaria100mg daily in adults and children over the age of 12 years. Prophylaxis can begin 1-2 days before travel to malarial areas. It should be continued daily during travel in the malarial areas and for 4 weeks after the traveller leaves the malarial area. For current advice on geographical resistance patterns and appropriate chemoprophylaxis, current guidelines or the Malaria Reference Laboratory should be consulted, details of which can be found in the British National Formulary (BNF).

For the prevention of scrub typhus 200mg as a single dose.

For the prevention of travellers' diarrhoea in adults 200mg on the first day of travel (administered as a single dose or as 100mg every 12 hours) followed by 100mg daily throughout the stay in the area. Data on the use of the drug prophylactically are not available beyond 21 days.

For the prevention of leptospirosis 200mg once each week throughout the stay in the area and 200mg at the completion of the trip. Data on the use of the drug prophylactically are not available beyond 21 days.

Use for childrenSee under "Contra-indications".

Use in the elderlyVibramycin may be prescribed in the elderly in the usual dosages with no special precautions. No dosage adjustment is necessary in the presence of renal impairment. The Vibramycin-D dispersible tablet may be preferred for the elderly since it is less likely to be associated with oesophageal irritation and ulceration.

Use in patients with impaired hepatic functionSee under "Special warnings and precautions for use".

Use in patients with renal impairmentStudies to date have indicated that administration of Vibramycin at the usual recommended doses does not lead to accumulation of the antibiotic in patients with renal impairment see under "Special warnings and precautions for use".

4.3 Contraindications

Persons who have shown hypersensitivity to doxycycline, any of its inert ingredients or to any of the tetracyclines.

The use of drugs of the tetracycline class during tooth development (pregnancy, infancy and childhood to the age of 12 years) may cause permanent discolouration of the teeth (yellow-grey-brown). This adverse reaction is more common during long-term use of the drugs but has been observed following repeated short-term courses. Enamel hypoplasia has also been reported. Vibramycin is therefore contra-indicated in these groups of patients.

Pregnancy Vibramycin is contra-indicated in pregnancy. It appears that the risks associated with the use of tetracyclines during pregnancy are predominantly due to effects on teeth and skeletal development. (See above about use during tooth development).

Nursing mothers Tetracyclines are excreted into milk and are therefore contra-indicated in nursing mothers. (See above about use during tooth development).

Children Vibramycin is contra-indicated in children under the age of 12 years. As with other tetracyclines, Vibramycin forms a stable calcium complex in any bone-forming tissue. A decrease in the fibula growth rate has been observed in prematures given oral tetracyclines in doses of 25mg/kg every 6 hours. This reaction was shown to be reversible when the drug was discontinued. (See above about use during tooth development).

4.4 Special warnings and special precautions for use

Use in patients with impaired hepatic function Vibramycin should be administered with caution to patients with hepatic impairment or those receiving potentially hepatotoxic drugs.

Abnormal hepatic function has been reported rarely and has been caused by both the oral and parenteral administration of tetracyclines, including doxycycline.

Use in patients with renal impairmentExcretion of doxycycline by the kidney is about 40%/72 hours in individuals with normal renal function. This percentage excretion may fall to a range as low as 1-5%/72 hours in individuals with severe renal insufficiency (creatinine clearance below 10ml/min). Studies have shown no significant difference in the serum half-life of doxycycline in individuals with normal and severely impaired renal function. Haemodialysis does not alter the serum half-life of doxycycline. The anti-anabolic action of the tetracyclines may cause an increase in blood urea. Studies to date indicate that this anti-anabolic effect does not occur with the use of Vibramycin in patients with impaired renal function.

Photosensitivity Photosensitivity manifested by an exaggerated sunburn reaction has been observed in some individuals taking tetracyclines, including doxycycline. Patients likely to be exposed to direct sunlight or ultraviolet light should be advised that this reaction can occur with tetracycline drugs and treatment should be discontinued at the first evidence of skin erythema.

Microbiological overgrowth The use of antibiotics may occasionally result in the overgrowth of non-susceptible organisms including Candida. If a resistant organism appears, the antibiotic should be discontinued and appropriate therapy instituted.

Pseudomembranous colitis has been reported with nearly all antibacterial agents, including doxycycline, and has ranged in severity from mild to life-threatening. It is important to consider this diagnosis in patients who present with diarrhoea subsequent to the administration of antibacterial agents.

Oesophagitis Instances of oesophagitis and oesophageal ulcerations have been reported in patients receiving capsule and tablet forms of drugs in the tetracycline class, including doxycycline. Most of these patients took medications immediately before going to bed or with inadequate amounts of fluid.

Bulging fontanelles in infants and benign intracranial hypertension in juveniles and adults have been reported in individuals receiving full therapeutic dosages. These conditions disappeared rapidly when the drug was discontinued.

Porphyria There have been rare reports of porphyria in patients receiving tetracyclines.

Venereal disease When treating venereal disease, where co-existent syphilis is suspected, proper diagnostic procedures including dark-field examinations should be utilised. In all such cases monthly serological tests should be made for at least four months.

Beta-haemolytic streptococci infections Infections due to group A beta-haemolytic streptococci should be treated for at least 10 days.

Myasthenia gravis Due to a potential for weak neuromuscular blockade, care should be taken in administering tetracyclines to patients with myasthenia gravis.

Systemic lupus erythematosus Tetracyclines can cause exacerbation of SLE.

Methoxyflurane Caution is advised in administering tetracyclines with methoxyflurane. See section 4.5.

4.5 Interaction with other medicinal products and other forms of Interaction

The absorption of doxycycline may be impaired by concurrently administered antacids containing aluminium, calcium, magnesium or other drugs containing these cations; oral zinc, iron salts or bismuth preparations. Dosages should be maximally separated.

Since bacteriostatic drugs may interfere with the bactericidal action of penicillin, it is advisable to avoid giving Vibramycin in conjunction with penicillin.

There have been reports of prolonged prothrombin time in patients taking warfarin and doxycycline. Tetracyclines depress plasma prothrombin activity and reduced doses of concomitant anticoagulants may be necessary.

The serum half-life of doxycycline may be shortened when patients are concurrently receiving barbiturates, carbamazepine or phenytoin. An increase in the daily dosage of Vibramycin should be considered.

Alcohol may decrease the half-life of doxycycline.

A few cases of pregnancy or breakthrough bleeding have been attributed to the concurrent use of tetracycline antibiotics with oral contraceptives.

Doxycycline may increase the plasma concentration of cyclosporin. Co-administration should only be undertaken with appropriate monitoring.

The concurrent use of tetracyclines and methoxyflurane has been reported to result in fatal renal toxicity. See section 4.4

Laboratory test interactions

False elevations of urinary catecholamine levels may occur due to interference with the fluorescence test.

4.6 Pregnancy and lactation

See "Contra-indications".

4.7 Effects on ability to drive and use machines

The effect of doxycycline on the ability to drive or operate heavy machinery has not been studied. There is no evidence to suggest that doxycycline may affect these abilities.

4.8 Undesirable effects

The following adverse reactions have been observed in patients receiving tetracyclines, including doxycycline.

Autonomic nervous system Flushing.

Body as a whole Hypersensitivity reactions, including anaphylactic shock, anaphylaxis, anaphylactoid reaction, anaphylactoid purpura, hypotension, pericarditis, angioneurotic oedema, exacerbation of systemic lupus erythematosus, dyspnoea, serum sickness, peripheral oedema, tachycardia and urticaria.

Central and Peripheral nervous systemHeadache. Bulging fontanelles in infants and benign intracranial hypertension in juveniles and adults have been reported in individuals receiving full therapeutic dosages of tetracyclines. In relation to benign intracranial hypertension, symptoms included blurring of vision, scotomata and diplopia. Permanent visual loss has been reported.

Gastro-intestinalGastro-intestinal symptoms are usually mild and seldom necessitate discontinuation of treatment. Abdominal pain, anorexia, nausea, vomiting, diarrhoea, dyspepsia and rarely dysphagia. Oesophagitis and oesophageal ulceration have been reported in patients receiving Vibramycin. A significant proportion of these occurred with the hyclate salt in the capsule form. (See 'Special warnings and precautions for use' section).

Hearing/Vestibular Tinnitus.

HaemopoieticHaemolytic anaemia, thrombocytopenia, neutropenia, porphyria, and eosinophilia have been reported with tetracyclines.

Liver/Biliary Transient increases in liver function tests, hepatitis, jaundice, hepatic failure and pancreatitis have been reported rarely.

Musculo-Skeletal Arthralgia and myalgia.

Skin Rashes including maculopapular and erythematous rashes, exfoliative dermatitis, erythema multiforme, Steven-Johnson syndrome and toxic epidermal necrolysis. Photosensitivity skin reactions (see 'Special warnings and precautions for use' section).

Superinfection As with all antibiotics, overgrowth of non-susceptible organisms may cause candidiasis, glossitis, staphylococcal enterocolitis, pseudomembranous colitis (with *Clostridium difficile* overgrowth) and inflammatory lesions (with candidal overgrowth) in the anogenital region. Similarly there have been reports for products in the tetracycline class of stomatitis and vaginitis.

Urinary system Increased blood urea. (See 'Special warnings and precautions for use' section.)

Other When given over prolonged periods, tetracyclines have been reported to produce brown-black microscopic discolouration of thyroid tissue. No abnormalities of thyroid function are known to occur.

Tetracyclines may cause discoloration of teeth and enamel hypoplasia, but usually only after long-term use.

4.9 Overdose

Acute overdosage with antibiotics is rare. In the event of overdosage discontinue medication. Gastric lavage plus appropriate supportive treatment is indicated.

Dialysis does not alter serum half-life and thus would not be of benefit in treating cases of overdosage.

5. PHARMACOLOGICAL PROPERTIES

5.1 Pharmacodynamic properties

Vibramycin is primarily bacteriostatic and is believed to exert its antimicrobial effect by the inhibition of protein synthesis. Vibramycin is active against a wide range of Gram-positive and Gram-negative bacteria and certain other micro-organisms.

5.2 Pharmacokinetic properties

Tetracyclines are readily absorbed and are bound to plasma proteins in varying degrees. They are concentrated by the liver in the bile and excreted in the urine and faeces at high concentrations and in a biologically active form. Doxycycline is virtually completely absorbed after oral administration. Studies reported to date indicate that the absorption of doxycycline, unlike certain other tetracyclines, is not notably influenced by the ingestion of food or milk. Following a 200mg dose, normal adult volunteers averaged peak serum levels of 2.6 micrograms/ml of doxycycline at 2 hours decreasing to 1.45 micrograms/ml at 24 hours. Doxycycline has a high degree of lipid solubility and a low affinity for calcium. It is highly stable in normal human serum. Doxycycline will not degrade into an epianhydro form.

6. PHARMACEUTICAL PARTICULARS

6.1 List of excipients

Vibramycin 100mg capsules: Maize Starch Ph. Eur., Lactose Ph.Eur., alginic acid, Magnesium Stearate NF, Sodium Lauryl Sulphate Ph.Eur. The capsule shell contains: Gelatin BP, titanium dioxide (E171), patent blue V (E131) and quinoline yellow (E104).

Vibramycin 50mg capsules: Maize Starch Ph.Eur., Lactose Ph.Eur., alginic acid, Magnesium Stearate NF, Sodium Lauryl Sulphate Ph Eur. In addition the capsule shell cap contains: Gelatin BP, titanium dioxide (E171), patent blue V (E131) and quinoline yellow (E104) and the body contains yellow iron oxide (E172), indigotine (E132) and titanium dioxide (E171).

Vibramycin D Dispersible tablets: Anhydrous Colloidal Silica Ph.Eur., Microcrystalline Cellulose Ph.Eur. and Magnesium Stearate Ph.Eur.

6.2 Incompatibilities

None stated.

6.3 Shelf life

Vibramycin 50 and 100mg capsules 48 months.

Vibramycin D Dispersible tablets 48 months.

6.4 Special precautions for storage

Store below 25°C.

6.5 Nature and contents of container

Vibramycin Capsules 100mg are available as:

Packs of 8 Capsules. Aluminium/PVC blister strips, a single strip of 8 capsules in a carton box.

Vibramycin 50 Capsules 50mg are available as:

Calendar Packs of 28 Capsules. Aluminium/PVC blister strips, 14 capsules per strip, 2 strips in a carton box.

Vibramycin-D Dispersible Tablets 100mg are available as:

Packs of 8 Tablets. Aluminium/PVC blister strips, a single strip of 8 tablets in a carton box.

6.6 Instructions for use and handling

No special requirements.

7. MARKETING AUTHORISATION HOLDER

Pfizer Limited

Ramsgate Road

Sandwich

Kent CT13 9NJ

United Kingdom

8. MARKETING AUTHORISATION NUMBER(S)

Vibramycin Capsules 100mg 0057/5059R

Vibramycin Capsules 50mg 0057/0238

Vibramycin-D Dispersible Tablets l00mg 0057/0188

9. DATE OF FIRST AUTHORISATION/RENEWAL OF THE AUTHORISATION

Vibramycin Capsules 100mg 29/10/00

Vibramycin Capsules 50mg 29/10/00

Vibramycin-D Dispersible Tablets l00mg 29/10/00

10. DATE OF REVISION OF THE TEXT

July 2004

Legal Category

POM

Ref: VM6_1

Videx 25mg Chewable or Dispersible Tablet

(Bristol-Myers Squibb Pharmaceuticals Ltd)

1. NAME OF THE MEDICINAL PRODUCT

Videx 25 mg chewable or dispersible tablet

2. QUALITATIVE AND QUANTITATIVE COMPOSITION

Each chewable or dispersible tablet contains 25 mg of didanosine.

For excipients, see 6.1

3. PHARMACEUTICAL FORM

Chewable or dispersible tablet

White tablet, imprinted with "25" on one side and "VIDEX" on the other side.

4. CLINICAL PARTICULARS

4.1 Therapeutic indications

Videx is indicated in combination with other antiretroviral drugs for the treatment of HIV infected patients.

4.2 Posology and method of administration

Oral use.

Because didanosine absorption is reduced in the presence of food, Videx should be administered at least 30 minutes before a meal (see 5.2).

Posology

Different tablet strengths of Videx may be administered on a once-daily or a twice daily (BID) regimen (see 5.1). To ensure that patients receive a sufficient amount of antacid, and to avoid degradation of didanosine at an acidic pH, each dose must be given minimally as 2 tablets.

Adults: The recommended daily dose is dependent on patient weight:

ADULT DOSING GUIDELINES

Patient Weight	BID(*) (dose, mg)	once-daily (**) (dose, mg)
≥ 60 kg	200	400
< 60 kg	125	250

(*) To ensure that patients receive a sufficient amount of antacid, each dose must be given as 2 tablets (e.g. the 200 mg BID dose should be given as 2 doses of 2 × 100 mg tablets with approximately 12 hours between each dose).

(**) To ensure that patients receive a sufficient amount of antacid, each dose must be given as minimally 2 tablets (e.g. the 400 mg once-daily dose should be given as one dose of (2 × 150 mg + 1 × 100 mg tablets); the 250 mg once-daily dose as (1 × 100 mg + 1 × 150 mg tablets) (see 5.1)

Children: The recommended daily dose, based on body surface area, is 240 mg/m²/day (180 mg/m²/day in combination with zidovudine) on a BID or once-daily schedule.

PAEDIATRIC DOSING GUIDELINES

(see Table 1 below)

Infants younger than 3 months: Insufficient clinical experience exists to recommend a dosing regimen.

Dose adjustment

Pancreatitis: Significant elevations of serum amylase should prompt discontinuation of therapy and careful evaluation of the possibility of pancreatitis, even in the absence of symptoms of pancreatitis. Fractionation of amylase may help distinguish amylase of salivary origin. Only after pancreatitis has been ruled out or after clinical and biological parameters have returned to normal, should dosing be resumed, and then only if treatment is considered essential. Treatment should be re-initiated with low doses and increased slowly, if appropriate.

Renal impairment: The following dose adjustments are recommended:

Patient Weight	≥ 60 kg (dose, mg*)		< 60 kg (dose, mg*)	
Creatinine Clearance (ml/min)	BID	once-daily	BID	once-daily
≥ 60	200	400	125	250
30-59	100	200	75	150
10-29	(**)	150	(**)	100
< 10	(**)	100	(**)	75

(*) To ensure that patients receive a sufficient amount of antacid, each dose must be given as minimally 2 tablets (e.g. the 400 mg once-daily dose should be given as one dose of (2 × 150 mg + 1 × 100 mg tablets); the 200 mg BID dose as 2 doses of 2 × 100 mg tablets, with approximately 12 hours between each dose).

(**) These patients should only receive a once-daily regimen.

The dose should preferably be administered after dialysis (see 4.). However, it is not necessary to administer a supplemental dose of Videx following haemodialysis.

Children: Since urinary excretion is also a major route of elimination of didanosine in children, the clearance of didanosine may be altered in children with renal impairment. Although there are insufficient data to recommend a specific dosage adjustment of Videx in this patient population, a reduction in the dose and/or an increase in the interval between doses should be considered.

Neuropathy: Many patients who present with symptoms of neuropathy and who experience resolution of symptoms upon drug discontinuation will tolerate a reduced dose of Videx (see 4.4).

Hepatic impairment: No specific dose adjustment can be recommended in patients with hepatic impairment. These patients should be monitored closely for clinical evidence of didanosine toxicity. Plasma level monitoring of didanosine may help to identify outliers, but currently available data do not allow specific recommendations with regard to target plasma levels (see 5.2).

Method of administration

Adults: Patients should take minimally two tablets in each dose, to provide sufficient antacid against acid degradation of didanosine. The tablets should be thoroughly chewed or dispersed in at least 30 ml of water prior to consumption. To disperse tablets, stir until a uniform dispersion forms, and drink the entire dispersion immediately. If additional flavouring is desired, the dispersion may be diluted with 30 ml of clear apple juice. Stir the further dispersion just prior to consumption.

Children: Children older than 1 year of age should receive a 2-tablet dose, children under

1 year should receive a 1-tablet dose. Tablets should be chewed or dispersed in water prior to consumption, as described above. When a one tablet dose is required, the volume of water for dispersion should be 15 ml. Fifteen ml of clear apple juice may be added to the dispersion as a flavouring. Stir the further dispersion just prior to consumption.

4.3 Contraindications

Hypersensitivity to didanosine or to any of the excipients.

4.4 Special warnings and special precautions for use

Pancreatitis is a known serious complication among HIV infected patients. It has also been associated with didanosine therapy and has been fatal in some cases. Didanosine should be used only with extreme caution in patients with a history of pancreatitis. Positive relationships have been found between the risk of pancreatitis and daily dose of didanosine.

Whenever warranted by clinical conditions, didanosine should be suspended until the diagnosis of pancreatitis is excluded by appropriate laboratory and imaging techniques. Similarly, when treatment with other medicinal products known to cause pancreatic toxicity is required (e.g. pentamidine), didanosine should be suspended during

Table 1 PAEDIATRIC DOSING GUIDELINES

	Body Surface Area (m²)	Total Daily Dose (mg/day)	BID (tablets, mg)	once-daily (tablets, mg)
240 mg/m²/day	0.5	120	50 + 25	100 + 25
	1.0	240	100 + 25	100 + 150
	1.5	360	150 + 25	150 + 150 + 50
180 mg/m²/day	0.5	90	25 + 25	50 + 50
	1.0	180	50 + 50	150 + 25
	1.5	270	100 + 50	150 + 100 + 25

therapy whenever possible. If concomitant therapy is unavoidable, there should be close observation. Dose interruption should be considered when biochemical markers of pancreatitis have significantly increased, even in the absence of symptoms. Significant elevations of triglycerides are a known cause of pancreatitis and warrant close observation.

Peripheral neuropathy: Patients on didanosine may develop toxic peripheral neuropathy, usually characterised by bilateral symmetrical distal numbness, tingling, and pain in feet and, less frequently, hands. Whenever warranted by clinical conditions, didanosine therapy should be suspended until resolution of symptoms. Many patients tolerate a reduced dose after resolution of symptoms.

Retinal or optic nerve changes: Children on didanosine have demonstrated retinal or optic nerve changes on rare occasions, particularly at doses above those recommended. There have been reports of retinal depigmentation in adult patients. Especially for children, periodic dilated retinal examinations (every 6 months), or if a change in vision occurs, should be considered.

Lactic acidosis: lactic acidosis, usually associated with hepatomegaly and hepatic steatosis, has been reported with the use of nucleoside analogues. Early symptoms (symptomatic hyperlactatemia) include benign digestive symptoms (nausea, vomiting and abdominal pain), non-specific malaise, loss of appetite, weight loss, respiratory symptoms (rapid and/or deep breathing) or neurological symptoms (including motor weakness). Lactic acidosis has a high mortality and may be associated with pancreatitis, liver failure, or renal failure.

Lactic acidosis generally occurred after a few or several months of treatment.

Treatment with nucleoside analogues should be discontinued in the setting of symptomatic hyperlactatemia and metabolic/lactic acidosis, progressive hepatomegaly, or rapidly elevating aminotransferase levels. Caution should be exercised when administering nucleoside analogues to any patient (particularly obese women) with hepatomegaly, hepatitis or other known risk factors for liver disease and hepatic steatosis (including certain medicinal products and alcohol). Patients co-infected with hepatitis C and treated with alpha interferon and ribavirin may constitute a special risk.

Patients at increased risk should be followed closely. (See also 4.6).

Renal impairment: The half-life of didanosine after oral administration increased from an average of 1.4 hours in subjects with normal renal function to 4.1 hours in subjects with severe renal impairment requiring dialysis. After an oral dose, didanosine was not detectable in peritoneal dialysis fluid; recovery in haemodialysate ranged from 0.6% to 7.4% of the dose over a 3-4 hour dialysis period. Patients with a creatinine clearance < 60 ml/min may be at greater risk of didanosine toxicity due to decreased drug clearance. A dose reduction is recommended for these patients (see 4.2).

Further, the magnesium content of each Videx tablet is 8.6 mEq, which may represent an excessive load of magnesium to patients with significant renal impairment.

Liver disease: Liver failure of unknown aetiology has occurred rarely in patients on didanosine. Patients should be observed for liver enzyme elevations and didanosine should be suspended if enzymes rise to >5 times the upper limit of normal. Rechallenge should be considered only if the potential benefits clearly outweigh the potential risks.

The safety and efficacy of Videx has not been established in patients with significant underlying liver disorders. Patients with chronic hepatitis B or C and treated with combination antiretroviral therapy are at an increased risk for severe and potentially fatal hepatic adverse events. In case of concomitant antiviral therapy for hepatitis B or C, please refer also to the relevant product information for these medicinal products.

Patients with pre-existing liver dysfunction including chronic active hepatitis have an increased frequency of liver function abnormalities during combination antiretroviral therapy and should be monitored according to standard practice. If there is evidence of worsening liver disease in such patients, interruption or discontinuation of treatment must be considered.

Immune Reactivation Syndrome: In HIV-infected patients with severe immune deficiency at the time of institution of combination antiretroviral therapy (CART), an inflammatory reaction to asymptomatic or residual opportunistic pathogens may arise and cause serious clinical conditions, or aggravation of symptoms. Typically, such reactions have been observed within the first few weeks or months of initiation of CART. Relevant examples are cytomegalovirus retinitis, generalised and/or focal mycobacterial infections, and Pneumocystis carinii pneumonia. Any inflammatory symptoms should be evaluated and treatment instituted when necessary.

Lipodystrophy and metabolic abnormalities: Combination antiretroviral therapy has been associated with the redistribution of body fat (lipodystrophy) in HIV patients. The long-term consequences of these events are currently unknown. Knowledge about the mechanism is incomplete. A connection between visceral lipomatosis and PIs and lipoatrophy and NRTIs has been hypothesised. A higher risk of lipodystrophy has been associated with individual factors such as older age, and with drug related factors such as longer duration of antiretroviral treatment and associated metabolic disturbances. Clinical examination should include evaluation for physical signs of fat redistribution. Consideration should be given to the measurement of fasting serum lipids and blood glucose. Lipid disorders should be managed as clinically appropriate (see 4.8).

Infants younger than 3 months: Insufficient clinical experience exists to recommend a dosing regimen.

Mitochondrial dysfunction: Nucleoside and nucleotide analogues have been demonstrated *in vitro* and *in vivo* to cause a variable degree of mitochondrial damage. There have been reports of mitochondrial dysfunction in HIV-negative infants exposed *in utero* and/or post-natally to nucleoside analogues. The main adverse events reported are haematological disorders (anemia, neutropenia), metabolic disorders (hyperlactatemia, hyperlipasemia). These events are often transitory. Some late-onset neurological disorders have been reported (hypertonia, convulsion, abnormal behaviour). Whether the neurological disorders are transient or permanent is currently unknown. Any child exposed *in utero* to nucleoside and nucleotide analogues, even HIV-negative children, should have clinical and laboratory follow-up and should be fully investigated for possible mitochondrial dysfunction in case of relevant signs or symptoms. These findings do not affect current national recommendations to use antiretroviral therapy in pregnant women to prevent vertical transmission of HIV.

Opportunistic infections: Patients receiving didanosine or any antiretroviral therapy may continue to develop opportunistic infections and other complications of HIV infection or therapy. They therefore should remain under close clinical observation by physicians experienced in the treatment of patients with HIV associated diseases.

Interaction with other medicinal products: Co-administration of didanosine and tenofovir disoproxil fumarate results in a 40-60% increase in systemic exposure to didanosine that may increase the risk for didanosine-related adverse events (see 4.5). Rare cases of pancreatitis and lactic acidosis, sometimes fatal, have been reported.

A reduced didanosine dose (250 mg) has been tested to avoid over-exposure to didanosine in case of co-administration with tenofovir disoproxil fumarate, but this has been associated with reports of high rate of virological failure and of emergence of resistance at early stage within several tested combinations.

Co-administration of didanosine and tenofovir disoproxil fumarate is therefore not recommended, especially in patients with high viral load and low CD4 cell count. If this combination is judged strictly necessary, patients should be carefully monitored for efficacy and didanosine related adverse events.

Triple nucleoside therapy: There have been reports of a high rate of virological failure and of emergence of resistance at an early stage when didanosine was combined with tenofovir disoproxil fumarate and lamivudine as a once daily regimen.

Phenylketonurics: Videx tablets contain 36.5 mg phenylalanine (from the aspartame). Therefore, the use of Videx in phenylketonuria patients should be considered only if clearly indicated.

Sorbitol: Videx tablets contain sorbitol (342 mg, 333 mg, 316 mg and 300 mg for the 25 mg, 50 mg, 100 mg and 150 mg tablets respectively). Therefore the use of Videx tablets in patients with fructose intolerance should be considered only if clearly indicated.

4.5 Interaction with other medicinal products and other forms of Interaction

Specific drug interaction studies have been conducted with zidovudine, stavudine, ranitidine, loperamide, metoclopramide, foscarnet, trimethoprim, sulfamethoxazole, dapsone, and rifabutin without evidence of interaction. Based upon the results from a study with ketoconazole, it is recommended that medicines which can be affected by stomach acidity (e.g. oral azoles such as ketoconazole and itraconazole), be given at least 2 hours prior to dosing with didanosine.

Administration of didanosine 2 hours prior to, or concurrent with, ganciclovir was associated with a mean increase of 111% in the steady state AUC for didanosine. A minor decrease (21%) in the steady state AUC of ganciclovir was seen when didanosine was given 2 hours prior to ganciclovir, but not when both medicines were given simultaneously. There were no changes in renal clearance for either drug. It is not known whether these changes are associated with alterations in either the safety of didanosine or the efficacy of ganciclovir. There is no evidence that Videx potentiates the myelosuppressive effects of ganciclovir or zidovudine.

Co-administration of didanosine with medicines that are known to cause peripheral neuropathy or pancreatitis may increase the risk of these toxicities. Patients who receive these medicines should be carefully observed.

Based on *in vitro* data, ribavirin may increase the intracellular triphosphate levels of didanosine and potentially increase the risk of adverse reactions (see 4. and 4.8); therefore, unless further clinical data are available, caution should be used, if these drugs need to be co-administered.

As with other products containing magnesium and / or aluminium antacid components, Videx tablets should not be taken with any tetracycline antibiotic. Likewise, plasma concentrations of some quinolone antibiotics (e.g. ciprofloxacin) are decreased by administration with antacids contained in or administered with Videx. It is recommended that medicines that may interact with antacids should not be administered within 2 hours of taking Videx tablets.

When didanosine gastro-resistant capsules were administered 2 hours prior to or concurrently with tenofovir disoproxil fumarate, the AUC for didanosine was on average increased by 48% and 60% respectively. The mean increase in the AUC of didanosine was 44% when the buffered tablets were administered 1 hour prior to tenofovir. In both cases the pharmacokinetic parameters for tenofovir administered with a light meal were unchanged. The co-administration of didanosine and tenofovir disoproxil fumarate is not recommended (see 4.4).

Xanthine oxidase is an enzyme involved in the metabolism of didanosine. Inhibitors of xanthine oxidase, such as allopurinol, may increase exposure to didanosine when administered together and thus increase the potential for didanosine associated undesirable effects. Patients should be closely monitored for didanosine related undesirable effects (see 4.8).

Ingestion of Videx with food alters the pharmacokinetics of didanosine (see 5.2).

4.6 Pregnancy and lactation

Pregnancy: There are no adequate and well-controlled studies in pregnant women and it is not known whether didanosine can cause foetal harm or affect reproductive capacity when administered during pregnancy. Lactic acidosis (see 4.4), sometimes fatal, has been reported in pregnant women who received the combination of didanosine and stavudine with or without other antiretroviral treatment. Therefore, the use of didanosine during pregnancy should be considered only if clearly indicated, and only when the potential benefit outweighs the possible risk.

Teratology studies in rats and rabbits did not produce evidence of embryotoxic, foetotoxic, or teratogenic effects. A study in rats showed that didanosine and/or its metabolites are transferred to the foetus through the placenta.

Lactation: It is not known whether didanosine is excreted in human milk. It is recommended that women taking didanosine do not breast-feed because of the potential for serious adverse reactions in nursing infants.

At the 1000 mg/kg/day dose levels in rats, didanosine was slightly toxic to females and pups during mid and late lactation (reduced food intake and body weight gains), but the physical and functional development of the subsequent offsprings were not impaired. A further study showed that, following oral administration, didanosine and/or its metabolites were excreted into the milk of lactating rats.

4.7 Effects on ability to drive and use machines

No effects on the ability to drive and use machines have been observed.

4.8 Undesirable effects

Adults: Most of the serious adverse events observed have generally reflected the recognised clinical course of HIV infection.

In data collected earlier involving monotherapy regimens, no different safety concerns were seen compared to the triple regimen data presented below. In comparative studies between Videx once-daily and BID, no significant difference in terms of incidence of pancreatitis and peripheral neuropathy has been shown.

Pancreatitis, which may be fatal in some cases, was reported in <1% of the patients receiving Videx gastro-resistant capsule; patients with advanced HIV disease or a history of pancreatitis may be at increased risk of developing pancreatitis.

Peripheral neurologic symptoms (8%) have been associated with Videx.

In HIV-infected patients with severe immune deficiency at the time of initiation of combination antiretroviral therapy (CART), an inflammatory reaction to asymptomatic or residual opportunistic infections may arise (see 4.4).

Lipodystrophy and metabolic abnormalities: Combination antiretroviral therapy has been associated with redistribution of body fat (lipodystrophy) in HIV patients including the loss of peripheral and facial subcutaneous fat, increased intra-abdominal and visceral fat, breast hypertrophy and dorsocervical fat accumulation (buffalo hump).

Combination antiretroviral therapy has been associated with metabolic abnormalities such as hypertriglyceridaemia, hypercholesterolaemia, insulin resistance, hyperglycaemia and hyperlactataemia (see 4.4).

In an open label clinical study (study-148), involving 482 patients treated with Videx tablet plus stavudine and nelfinavir, and in a clinical study (study-152) evaluating Videx gastro-resistant capsules as part of a triple regimen in 255 treatment naive HIV infected adults, the following undesirable effects (moderate to severe), which occured at a frequency of ≥2%, and which are considered possibly related to study regimen based on the investigators' attribution, were reported:

Nervous system disorders:

common: peripheral neurologic symptoms (including neuropathy), headache

Gastrointestinal disorders:

very common: diarrhoea

common: nausea, vomiting, abdominal pain

Skin and subcutaneous tissue disorders:

common: rash

General disorders:

common: fatigue

Laboratory abnormalities:

Laboratory abnormalities (grade 3-4) reported in studies -148 (tablets) and -152 (gastro-resistant capsules) included increase of lipase in 7% and 5% respectively, increase of ALT in 3% and 6% respectively, increase of AST in 3% and 5%, respectively, increase in uric acid in 2% in both studies, and increase of bilirubin in 1% and <1% respectively, of the patients. Neutropenia (grade 3-4) was reported in 2% in both studies 148 and 152, anemia in <1% and 1% in study 148 and in study 152 respectively, and thrombocytopenia in 1% and <1%, respectively, of the patients.

Children: Safety data for children were generally similar to those seen in adults. A higher haematotoxicity has been reported with the combination with zidovudine compared to didanosine monotherapy. Retinal or optic nerve changes have been reported in a small number of children usually at doses above those recommended. It is recommended that children on didanosine treatment undergo dilated retinal examination every 6 months or if a change in vision occurs.

Postmarketing:

Cases of lactic acidosis, sometimes fatal, usually associated with severe hepatomegaly and hepatic steatosis have been reported with the use of nucleoside analogues (see 4.4).

The following events (frequency rare to very rare) have been identified during post approval use of Videx:

General disorders and administration site conditions: asthenia, chills and fever, pain **Gastrointestinal disorders**: flatulence, parotid gland enlargement, dry mouth

Metabolism and nutrition disorders: lactic acidosis, anorexia, diabetes mellitus, hypoglycaemia, hyperglycaemia

Skin and subcutaneous tissue disorders: alopecia

Hepatobiliary disorders: hepatic steatosis, hepatitis, liver failure

Infections and infestations: sialoadenitis

Blood and lymphatic system disorders: anaemia, leukopenia, thrombocytopenia

Immune system disorders: anaphylactic reaction

Eye disorders: dry eyes, retinal depigmentation, optic neuritis

Musculoskeletal, connective tissue and bone disorders: myalgia (with or without increases in creatine phosphokinase), rhabdomyolysis including acute renal failure and hemodialysis, arthralgia, myopathy

Investigations: increased/abnormal serum amylase, alkaline phosphatase and creatine phosphokinase

4.9 Overdose

There is no known antidote for didanosine overdosage. Experience in early studies, in which didanosine was initially administered at doses ten times the recommended doses, indicates that the anticipated complications of overdosage could include pancreatitis, peripheral neuropathy, hyperuricemia and hepatic dysfunction.

Didanosine is not dialyzable by peritoneal dialysis, although there is some clearance by haemodialysis. (The fractional removal of didanosine during an average haemodialysis session of 3 to 4 hours was approximately 20-35% of the dose present in the body at the start of dialysis.)

5. PHARMACOLOGICAL PROPERTIES

5.1 Pharmacodynamic properties

Nucleoside reverse transcriptase inhibitor: ATC Code: J05AF02

Didanosine (2',3'-dideoxyinosine) is an inhibitor of the *in vitro* replication of HIV in cultured human cells and cell lines. After didanosine enters the cell, it is enzymatically converted to dideoxyadenosine-triphosphate (ddATP), its active metabolite. In viral nucleic acid replication, incorporation of this 2',3'-dideoxynucleoside prevents chain extension, and thereby inhibits viral replication.

In addition, ddATP inhibits HIV-reverse transcriptase by competing with dATP for binding to the enzyme's active site, preventing proviral DNA synthesis.

The relationship between *in vitro* susceptibility of HIV to didanosine and clinical response to therapy has not been established. Likewise, *in vitro* sensitivity results vary greatly and methods to establish virologic responses have not been proven.

Using the Videx tablet formulation, the effect of Videx BID administration, alone or in combination with zidovudine, was evaluated in several major randomised, controlled clinical trials (ACTG 175, ACTG 152, DELTA, CPCRA 007). These trials confirmed the reduced risk of HIV disease progression or death with Videx tablets therapy, alone or in combination with zidovudine, as compared with zidovudine monotherapy in HIV infected individuals, including symptomatic and asymptomatic adults with CD4 counts < 500 cells/mm^3 and children with evidence of immunosuppression. The primary demonstration of clinical benefits of didanosine has been made through the ACTG 175 trial with the buffered tablet formulation of Videx administered twice daily (BID). This study showed that eight weeks of treatment with zidovudine, Videx tablets BID, or Videx tablets BID plus zidovudine decreased mean plasma HIV RNA by 0.26, 0.65 and 0.93 log_{10} copies/ml, respectively. In the tritherapy setting, the combination of Videx (200 mg) BID plus stavudine and indinavir has been compared to zidovudine plus lamivudine and indinavir in a randomised open label study (START II, n= 205): through 48 weeks of treatment, results were in favour of the Videx arm. However, no formal conclusion can be drawn on the equivalence of the 2 regimens.

Since didanosine exhibits a very long intracellular half-life (> 24 hours), permitting the accumulation of its pharmacologically active ddATP-moiety for extended time periods, administration of the total daily dose of Videx in a once-daily dosing regimen has been explored through clinical studies.

Several clinical studies have been performed with Videx (tablet) administered once daily (once-daily), including the following:

In the tritherapy setting, the randomised open label study -147 indicates that, in mostly asymptomatic patients (n= 123) that were stable on their first combination therapy containing Videx BID, the shift to a similar combination therapy with Videx once-daily did not impact at short term (24 weeks) on the existing antiviral efficacy.

The randomised open label study -148 (n= 756) compared Videx once-daily plus stavudine and nelfinavir to zidovudine plus lamivudine and nelfinavir. After 48 weeks of treatment, results were in favour of the zidovudine (BID), lamivudine and nelfinavir arm compared to Videx (once-daily), stavudine and nelfinavir arm in term of proportion of patients with undetectable viral load (the proportion of patients with HIV RNA copies < 400 copies/ml was 53% for the Videx-containing arm and 62% for the comparator). However, no formal conclusions can be drawn on this study due to methodological issues.

Current evidence indicates that the incidence of resistance to didanosine is an infrequent event and the resistance generated is modest in degree. Didanosine-resistant isolates have been selected in vivo and are associated with specific genotype changes in the reverse transcriptase codon region (codons L74V (most prevalent), K65R, M184V and T69S/G/D/N). Clinical isolates that exhibited a decrease in didanosine susceptibility harbored one or more didanosine-associated mutations. Mutant viruses containing the L74V substitution show a decline in viral fitness and these mutants quickly revert to wild type in the absence of didanosine. Cross-resistance between didanosine and protease inhibitors or non nucleoside reverse transcriptase inhibitor is unlikely. Cross-resistance between didanosine and nucleoside reverse transcriptase inhibitor is observed in isolates containing multi-resistant mutations such as Q151M and T69S-XX (an amino acid substitution with a 2-amino acid insertion) and multiple nucleoside analogue associated mutations (NAMs).

5.2 Pharmacokinetic properties

Adults

Absorption: Didanosine is rapidly degraded at an acidic pH. Therefore, the tablets contain buffering agents designed to increase gastric pH. The administration of didanosine with a meal results in a significant decrease (about 50%) in bioavailability. Videx tablets should be administered at least 30 minutes before a meal. A study in 10 asymptomatic HIV seropositive patients demonstrated that administration of Videx tablets 30 min to 1 hour before a meal did not result in any significant changes in the bioavailability of didanosine compared to administration under fasting conditions. Administration of the tablets 1 to 2 hours after a meal was associated with a 55% decrease in C_{max} and AUC values, which was comparable to the decrease observed when the formulation was given immediately after a meal.

In 30 patients receiving didanosine 400 mg once daily in the fasted state as Videx buffered tablets, single dose AUC was 2516 ± 847 ng·h/ml (34%) (mean ± SD [%CV]) and C_{max} was 1475 ± 673 ng/ml (46%).

Distribution: The volume of distribution at steady state averages 54 l, suggesting that there is some uptake of didanosine by body tissues. The level of didanosine in the cerebrospinal fluid (CSF), one hour after infusion, averages 21% of that of the simultaneous plasma level.

Biotransformation: The metabolism of didanosine in man has not been evaluated. However, based on animal studies, it is presumed that it follows the same pathways responsible for the elimination of endogenous purines.

Elimination: The average elimination half-life after IV administration of didanosine is approximately 1.4 hours. Renal clearance represents 50% of total body clearance (800 ml/min), indicating that active tubular secretion, in addition to glomerular filtration, is responsible for the renal elimination of didanosine. Urinary recovery of didanosine is approximately 20% of the dose after oral treatment. There is no evidence of didanosine accumulation after the administration of oral doses for 4 weeks.

Hepatic impairment: No significant changes in the pharmacokinetics of didanosine were observed among haemophiliac patients with chronic, persistent elevations in liver function enzymes (n=5), which may be indicative of impaired hepatic function; haemophiliac patients with normal or less severe increases in liver function enzymes (n=8); and non-haemophiliac patients with normal enzyme levels (n=8) following a single IV or oral dose. No conclusion can be drawn regarding the metabolism of didanosine, which may be altered in patients with severe hepatic impairment (see 4.2).

Children

Absorption: Variability in the amount of didanosine absorbed in children is greater than in adults. The absolute bioavailability of didanosine administered orally was approximately 36% after the first dose and 47% at steady state.

Distribution: The CSF didanosine level averages 46% of that of the simultaneous plasma level after IV administration of doses of 60 or 90 mg/m^2 and equivalent oral doses of 120 or 180 mg/m^2. Measurable concentrations of didanosine in the CSF were detectable for up to 3.5 hours after dosing.

Elimination: The average elimination half-life after IV didanosine administration is approximately 0.8 hours. Renal clearance represents approximately 59% of the total body clearance (315 ml/min/m^2), indicating that both renal and nonrenal pathways are involved in the elimination. Urinary recovery of didanosine is approximately 17% of dose after oral treatment. There is no evidence of didanosine accumulation after oral administration for an average of 26 days.

5.3 Preclinical safety data

The lowest dose to cause death in acute toxicity studies in the mouse, rat and dog was greater than 2000 mg/kg which is equivalent to approximately 300 times the maximum recommended human dose.

Repeated dose toxicity: Repeat-dose oral toxicity studies revealed evidence of a dose-limiting skeletal muscle toxicity in rodents (but not in dogs) following long-term (> 90 days) dosing with didanosine at doses that were approximately 1.2 - 12 times the estimated human dose. Additionally, in repeat dose studies, leukopenia was observed in dogs and rats, and gastrointestinal disturbances (soft stool, diarrhoea) were seen in dogs at doses approximately 5 - 14 times the maximum human dose.

Carcinogenicity: In the carcinogenicity studies, non-neoplastic alterations have been observed including skeletal muscle myopathy, hepatic alterations and an exacerbation of spontaneous age-related cardiomyopathy. Lifetime dietary carcinogenicity studies were conducted in mice and rats for 22 or 24 months, respectively. No drug-related neoplasms were observed in any didanosine-treated groups of mice during, or at the end of, the dosing period. In rats, statistically significant increased incidences of granulosa cell tumours in females receiving the high dose, of subcutaneous fibrosarcomas and histiocytic sarcomas in males receiving the high dose and of haemangiomas in males receiving the high and intermediate dose of didanosine were noted. The drug-relationship and clinical relevance of these statistical findings were not clear.

Genotoxicity: Results from the genotoxicity studies suggest that didanosine is not mutagenic at biologically and pharmacologically relevant doses. At significantly elevated concentrations *in vitro*, the genotoxic effects of didanosine are similar in magnitude to those seen with natural DNA nucleosides.

Reproduction: In rats, didanosine did not impair the reproduction ability of male or female parents following treatment prior to and during mating, gestation and lactation at daily didanosine doses up to 1000 mg/kg/day. In a perinatal and postnatal reproduction study in rats, didanosine did not induce toxic effects.

6. PHARMACEUTICAL PARTICULARS

6.1 List of excipients

Calcium carbonate, magnesium hydroxide, aspartame, sorbitol, microcrystalline cellulose, crospovidone, mandarin orange flavour (tangerine oil, mandarin oil, gum arabic, alpha tocopherol, colloidal silica) and magnesium stearate.

6.2 Incompatibilities

Not applicable

6.3 Shelf life

2 years.

After dispersion in water, the dispersion is physically and chemically stable for 1 hour.

6.4 Special precautions for storage

Do not store above 30°C. Keep the container tightly closed in order to protect from moisture.

6.5 Nature and contents of container

High-density polyethylene bottle with child-resistant cap.

Package size: 60 tablets per bottle.

6.6 Instructions for use and handling

No special requirements.

7. MARKETING AUTHORISATION HOLDER

Bristol-Myers Squibb Pharmaceuticals Limited
Bristol-Myers Squibb House,
141-149 Staines Road,
Hounslow,
Middlesex TW3 3JA

8. MARKETING AUTHORISATION NUMBER(S)

25 mg: PL 11184/0008

9. DATE OF FIRST AUTHORISATION/RENEWAL OF THE AUTHORISATION

17th February 1994

10. DATE OF REVISION OF THE TEXT

3 March 2005

Videx 200 mg Chewable or Dispersible Tablet

(Bristol-Myers Squibb Pharmaceuticals Ltd)

1. NAME OF THE MEDICINAL PRODUCT

Videx® 200 mg chewable or dispersible tablet

2. QUALITATIVE AND QUANTITATIVE COMPOSITION

Each chewable or dispersible tablet contains 200 mg of didanosine.

For excipients, see 6.1

3. PHARMACEUTICAL FORM

Chewable or dispersible tablet

White tablet, imprinted with "200" on one side and "VIDEX" on the other side.

4. CLINICAL PARTICULARS

4.1 Therapeutic indications

Videx is indicated in combination with other antiretroviral drugs for the treatment of HIV infected patients.

4.2 Posology and method of administration

Oral use.

Because didanosine absorption is reduced in the presence of food, Videx should be administered at least 30 minutes before a meal (see 5.2).

Posology

Different tablet strengths of Videx may be administered on a once-daily or a twice-daily (BID) regimen (see 5.1). The 200 mg tablet can only be used in once-daily regimens.

To ensure that patients receive a sufficient amount of antacid, and to avoid degradation of didanosine at an acidic pH, each dose must be given minimally as 2 tablets.

Adults: The recommended daily dose is dependent on patient weight:

ADULT DOSING GUIDELINES

Patient Weight	Total Daily Dose	Number of tablets (every 24 hours)
⩾ 60 kg	400 mg	2 × 200 mg once-daily
< 60 kg	250 mg	1 × 200 mg + 1 × 50 mg once-daily

Children: The recommended daily dose, based on body surface area, is 240 mg/m^2/day (180 mg/m^2/day in combination with zidovudine). The 200 mg tablet can only be used in once-daily regimens and for body surface areas ⩾ 1.5 m^2. For other body surface areas, one should refer to the other tablet strengths or to the non-buffered powder for oral solution.

PAEDIATRIC DOSING GUIDELINES

(see Table 1 below)

Infants younger than 3 months: Insufficient clinical experience exists to recommend a dosing regimen.

Dose adjustment

Pancreatitis: Significant elevations of serum amylase should prompt discontinuation of therapy and careful evaluation of the possibility of pancreatitis, even in the absence of symptoms of pancreatitis. Fractionation of amylase may help distinguish amylase of salivary origin. Only after pancreatitis has been ruled out or after clinical and biological parameters have returned to normal, should dosing be resumed, and then only if treatment is considered essential. Treatment should be re-initiated with low doses and increased slowly, if appropriate.

Renal impairment: Specific dose adjustment is recommended in patients with a creatinine clearance < 60 ml/min which is not possible with the 200 mg tablet. In this case one should refer to the other tablet strengths (see 4.4).

Neuropathy: Many patients who present with symptoms of neuropathy and who experience resolution of symptoms upon drug discontinuation will tolerate a reduced dose of Videx (see 4.4).

Hepatic impairment: No specific dose adjustment can be recommended in patients with hepatic impairment. These patients should be monitored closely for clinical evidence of didanosine toxicity. Plasma level monitoring of didanosine may help to identify outliers, but currently available data do not allow specific recommendations with regard to target plasma levels (see 5.2).

Method of administration

The tablets should be thoroughly chewed or dispersed in at least 30 ml of water prior to ingestion. To disperse tablets, stir until a uniform dispersion forms, and drink the entire dispersion immediately. If additional flavouring is desired, the dispersion may be diluted with 30 ml of clear apple juice. Stir the further dispersion just prior to consumption.

4.3 Contraindications

Hypersensitivity to didanosine or to any of the excipients.

4.4 Special warnings and special precautions for use

Pancreatitis is a known serious complication among HIV infected patients. It has also been associated with didanosine therapy and has been fatal in some cases. Didanosine should be used only with extreme caution in patients with a history of pancreatitis. Positive relationships have been found between the risk of pancreatitis and daily dose of didanosine.

Whenever warranted by clinical conditions, didanosine should be suspended until the diagnosis of pancreatitis is excluded by appropriate laboratory and imaging techniques. Similarly, when treatment with other medicinal products known to cause pancreatic toxicity is required (e.g. pentamidine), didanosine should be suspended whenever possible. If concomitant therapy is unavoidable, there should be close observation. Dose interruption should be considered when biochemical markers of pancreatitis have significantly increased, even in the absence of symptoms. Significant elevations of triglycerides are a known cause of pancreatitis and warrant close observation.

Peripheral neuropathy: Patients on didanosine may develop toxic peripheral neuropathy, usually characterised by bilateral symmetrical distal numbness, tingling, and pain in feet and, less frequently, hands. Whenever warranted by clinical conditions, didanosine therapy should be suspended until resolution of symptoms. Many patients tolerate a reduced dose after resolution of symptoms.

Retinal or optic nerve changes: Children on didanosine have demonstrated retinal or optic nerve changes on rare occasions, particularly at doses above those recommended. There have been reports of retinal depigmentation in adult patients. Especially for children, periodic dilated retinal examinations (every 6 months), or if a change in vision occurs, should be considered.

Lactic acidosis:
lactic acidosis, usually associated with hepatomegaly and hepatic steatosis, has been reported with the use of nucleoside analogues. Early symptoms (symptomatic hyperlactatemia) include benign digestive symptoms (nausea, vomiting and abdominal pain), non-specific malaise, loss of appetite, weight loss, respiratory symptoms (rapid and/or deep breathing) or neurological symptoms (including motor weakness). Lactic acidosis has a high mortality and may be associated with pancreatitis, liver failure, or renal failure.
Lactic acidosis generally occurred after a few or several months of treatment.
Treatment with nucleoside analogues should be discontinued in the setting of symptomatic hyperlactatemia and metabolic/lactic acidosis, progressive hepatomegaly, or rapidly elevating aminotransferase levels. Caution should be exercised when administering nucleoside analogues to any patient (particularly obese women) with hepatomegaly, hepatitis or other known risk factors for liver disease and hepatic steatosis (including certain medicinal products and alcohol). Patients co-infected with hepatitis C and treated with alpha interferon and ribavirin may constitute a special risk.
Patients at increased risk should be followed closely. (See also 4.6).

Renal impairment: The half-life of didanosine after oral administration increased from an average of 1.4 hours in subjects with normal renal function to 4.1 hours in subjects with severe renal impairment requiring dialysis. After an oral dose, didanosine was not detectable in peritoneal dialysis fluid; recovery in haemodialysate ranged from 0.6% to 7.4% of the dose over a 3-4 hour dialysis period. Patients with a creatinine clearance < 60 ml/min may be at greater risk of didanosine toxicity due to decreased drug clearance. A dose reduction is recommended for these patients (see 4.2).

Further, the magnesium content of each Videx tablet is 8.6 mEq, which may represent an excessive load of magnesium to patients with significant renal impairment.

Liver disease: Liver failure of unknown aetiology has occurred rarely in patients on didanosine. Patients should be observed for liver enzyme elevations and didanosine should be suspended if enzymes rise to >5 times the upper limit of normal. Rechallenge should be considered only if the potential benefits clearly outweigh the potential risks.

The safety and efficacy of Videx has not been established in patients with significant underlying liver disorders. Patients with chronic hepatitis B or C and treated with combination antiretroviral therapy are at an increased risk for severe and potentially fatal hepatic adverse events. In case of concomitant antiviral therapy for hepatitis B or C, please refer also to the relevant product information for these medicinal products.

Patients with pre-existing liver dysfunction including chronic active hepatitis have an increased frequency of liver function abnormalities during combination antiretroviral therapy and should be monitored according to standard practice. If there is evidence of worsening liver disease in such patients, interruption or discontinuation of treatment must be considered.

Immune Reactivation Syndrome: In HIV-infected patients with severe immune deficiency at the time of institution of combination antiretroviral therapy (CART), an inflammatory reaction to asymptomatic or residual opportunistic pathogens may arise and cause serious clinical conditions, or aggravation of symptoms. Typically, such reactions have been observed within the first few weeks or months of initiation of CART. Relevant examples are cytomegalovirus retinitis, generalised and/or focal mycobacterial infections, and Pneumocystis carinii pneumonia. Any inflammatory symptoms should be evaluated and treatment instituted when necessary.

Lipodystrophy and metabolic abnormalities: Combination antiretroviral therapy has been associated with the redistribution of body fat (lipodystrophy) in HIV patients. The long-term consequences of these events are currently unknown. Knowledge about the mechanism is incomplete. A connection between visceral lipomatosis and PIs and lipoatrophy and NRTIs has been hypothesised. A higher risk of lipodystrophy has been associated with individual factors such as older age, and with drug related factors such as longer duration of antiretroviral treatment and associated metabolic disturbances. Clinical examination should include evaluation for physical signs of fat redistribution. Consideration should be given to the measurement of fasting serum lipids and blood glucose. Lipid disorders should be managed as clinically appropriate (see 4.8).

Infants younger than 3 months of age: Insufficient clinical experience exists to recommend a dosing regimen.

Mitochondrial dysfunction: Nucleoside and nucleotide analogues have been demonstrated *in vitro* and *in vivo* to cause a variable degree of mitochondrial damage. There have been reports of mitochondrial dysfunction in HIV-negative infants exposed *in utero* and/or post-natally to nucleoside analogues. The main adverse events reported are haematological disorders (anaemia, neutropenia), metabolic disorders (hyperlactataemia, hyperlipasemia). These events are often transitory. Some late-onset neurological disorders have been reported (hypertonia, convulsion, abnormal behaviour). Whether the neurological disorders are transient or permanent is currently unknown. Any child exposed *in utero* to nucleoside and nucleotide analogues, even HIV-negative children, should have clinical and laboratory follow-up and should be fully investigated for possible mitochondrial dysfunction in case of relevant signs or symptoms. These findings do not affect current national recommendations to use antiretroviral therapy in pregnant women to prevent vertical transmission of HIV.

Opportunistic infections: Patients receiving didanosine or any antiretroviral therapy may continue to develop opportunistic infections and other complications of HIV infection or therapy. They therefore should remain under close clinical observation by physicians experienced in the treatment of patients with HIV associated diseases.

Interaction with other medicinal products: Co-administration of didanosine and tenofovir disoproxil fumarate results in a 40-60% increase in systemic exposure to didanosine that may increase the risk for didanosine-related adverse events (see 4.5). Rare cases of pancreatitis and lactic acidosis, sometimes fatal, have been reported.

A reduced didanosine dose (250 mg) has been tested to avoid over-exposure to didanosine in case of co-administration with tenofovir disoproxil fumarate, but this has been

Table 1 PAEDIATRIC DOSING GUIDELINES

	Body Surface Area (m^2)	Total Daily Dose (mg/day)	Number of tablets (every 24 hours)
240 mg/m^2/day	1.5	360	1 × 200 mg + 1 × 150 mg once-daily
180 mg/m^2/day	1.5	270	1 × 200 mg + 1 × 50 mg + 1 × 25 mg once-daily

associated with reports of high rate of virological failure and of emergence of resistance at early stage within several tested combinations.

Co-administration of didanosine and tenofovir disoproxil fumarate is therefore not recommended, especially in patients with high viral load and low CD4 cell count. If this combination is judged strictly necessary, patients should be carefully monitored for efficacy and didanosine related adverse events.

Triple nucleoside therapy: There have been reports of a high rate of virological failure and of emergence of resistance at an early stage when didanosine was combined with tenofovir disoproxil fumarate and lamivudine as a once daily regimen.

Phenylketonurics: Videx tablets contain 36.5 mg phenylalanine (from the aspartame). Therefore, the use of Videx in phenylketonuria patients should be considered only if clearly indicated.

Sorbitol: Videx tablets contain 280 mg sorbitol. Therefore the use of Videx tablets in patients with fructose intolerance should be considered only if clearly indicated.

4.5 Interaction with other medicinal products and other forms of Interaction

Specific drug interaction studies have been conducted with zidovudine, stavudine, ranitidine, loperamide, metoclopramide, foscarnet, trimethoprim, sulfamethoxazole, dapsone, and rifabutin without evidence of interaction.

Based upon the results from a study with ketoconazole, it is recommended that medicines which can be affected by stomach acidity (e.g. oral azoles such as ketoconazole and itraconazole), be given at least 2 hours prior to dosing with didanosine.

Administration of didanosine 2 hours prior to, or concurrent with, ganciclovir was associated with a mean increase of 111% in the steady state AUC for didanosine. A minor decrease (21%) in the steady state AUC of ganciclovir was seen when didanosine was given 2 hours prior to ganciclovir, but not when both medicines were given simultaneously. There were no changes in renal clearance for either drug. It is not known whether these changes are associated with alterations in either the safety of didanosine or the efficacy of ganciclovir. There is no evidence that Videx potentiates the myelosuppressive effects of ganciclovir or zidovudine.

Co-administration of didanosine with medicines that are known to cause peripheral neuropathy or pancreatitis may increase the risk of these toxicities. Patients who receive these medicines should be carefully observed.

Based on *in vitro* data, ribavirin may increase the intracellular triphosphate levels of didanosine and potentially increase the risk of adverse reactions (see 4.4 and 4.8); therefore, unless further clinical data are available, caution should be used, if these drugs need to be co-administered.

As with other products containing magnesium and /or aluminium antacid components, Videx tablets should not be taken with any tetracycline antibiotic. Likewise, plasma concentrations of some quinolone antibiotics (e.g. ciprofloxacin) are decreased by administration with antacids contained in or administered with Videx. It is recommended that medicines that may interact with antacids should not be administered within 2 hours of taking Videx tablets.

When didanosine gastro-resistant capsules were administered 2 hours prior to or concurrently with tenofovir disoproxil fumarate, the AUC for didanosine was on average increased by 48% and 60% respectively. The mean increase in the AUC of didanosine was 44% when the buffered tablets were administered 1 hour prior to tenofovir. In both cases the pharmacokinetic parameters for tenofovir administered with a light meal were unchanged. The co-administration of didanosine and tenofovir disoproxil fumarate is not recommended (see 4.4).

Xanthine oxidase is an enzyme involved in the metabolism of didanosine. Inhibitors of xanthine oxidase, such as allopurinol, may increase exposure to didanosine when administered together and thus increase the potential for didanosine associated undesirable effects. Patients should be closely monitored for didanosine related undesirable effects (see 4.8).

Ingestion of Videx with food alters the pharmacokinetics of didanosine (see 5.2).

4.6 Pregnancy and lactation

Pregnancy: There are no adequate and well-controlled studies in pregnant women and it is not known whether didanosine can cause foetal harm or affect reproductive capacity when administered during pregnancy. Lactic acidosis (see 4.4), sometimes fatal, has been reported in pregnant women who received the combination of didanosine and stavudine with or without other antiretroviral treatment. Therefore, the use of didanosine during pregnancy should be considered only if clearly indicated, and only when the potential benefit outweighs the possible risk.

Teratology studies in rats and rabbits did not produce evidence of embryotoxic, foetotoxic, or teratogenic effects. A study in rats showed that didanosine and/or its metabolites are transferred to the foetus through the placenta.

Lactation: It is not known whether didanosine is excreted in human milk. It is recommended that women taking didanosine do not breast-feed because of the potential for serious adverse reactions in nursing infants.

At the 1000 mg/kg/day dose levels in rats, didanosine was slightly toxic to females and pups during mid and late lactation (reduced food intake and body weight gains), but the physical and functional development of the subsequent offsprings were not impaired. A further study showed that, following oral administration, didanosine and/or its metabolites were excreted into the milk of lactating rats.

4.7 Effects on ability to drive and use machines

No effects on the ability to drive and use machines have been observed.

4.8 Undesirable effects

Adults: Most of the serious adverse events observed have generally reflected the recognised clinical course of HIV infection.

In data collected earlier involving monotherapy regimens, no different safety concerns were seen compared to the triple regimen data presented below. In comparative studies between Videx once-daily and BID, no significant difference in terms of incidence of pancreatitis and peripheral neuropathy has been shown.

Pancreatitis, which may be fatal in some cases, was reported in <1% of the patients receiving Videx gastro-resistant capsule; patients with advanced HIV disease or a history of pancreatitis may be at increased risk of developing pancreatitis.

Peripheral neurologic symptoms (8%) have been associated with Videx.

In HIV-infected patients with severe immune deficiency at the time of initiation of combination antiretroviral therapy (CART), an inflammatory reaction to asymptomatic or residual opportunistic infections may arise (see 4.4).

Lipodystrophy and metabolic abnormalities: Combination antiretroviral therapy has been associated with redistribution of body fat (lipodystrophy) in HIV patients including the loss of peripheral and facial subcutaneous fat, increased intra-abdominal and visceral fat, breast hypertrophy and dorsocervical fat accumulation (buffalo hump).

Combination antiretroviral therapy has been associated with metabolic abnormalities such as hypertriglyceridaemia, hypercholesterolaemia, insulin resistance, hyperglycaemia and hyperlactataemia (see 4.4).

In an open label clinical study (study-148), involving 482 patients treated with Videx tablet plus stavudine and nelfinavir, and in a clinical study (study-152) evaluating Videx gastro-resistant capsules as part of a triple regimen in 255 treatment naive HIV infected adults, the following undesirable effects (moderate to severe), which occurred at a frequency of ⩾2%, and which are considered possibly related to study regimen based on the investigators' attribution, were reported:

Nervous system disorders:

common: peripheral neurologic symptoms (including neuropathy), headache

Gastrointestinal disorders:

very common: diarrhoea

common: nausea, vomiting, abdominal pain

Skin and subcutaneous tissue disorders:

common: rash

General disorders:

common: fatigue

Laboratory abnormalities:

Laboratory abnormalities (grade 3-4) reported in studies -148 (tablets) and -152 (gastro-resistant capsules) included increase of lipase in 7% and 5% respectively, increase of ALT in 3% and 6% respectively, increase of AST in 3% and 5%, respectively, increase in uric acid in 2% in both studies, and increase of bilirubin in 1% and <1% respectively, of the patients. Neutropenia (grade 3-4) was reported in 2% in both studies 148 and 152, anaemia in <1% and 1% in study 148 and in study 152 respectively, and thrombocytopenia in 1% and <1%, respectively, of the patients.

Children: Safety data for children were generally similar to those seen in adults. A higher haematotoxicity has been reported with the combination with zidovudine compared to didanosine monotherapy. Retinal or optic nerve changes have been reported in a small number of children usually at doses above those recommended. It is recommended that children on didanosine treatment undergo dilated retinal examination every 6 months or if a change in vision occurs.

Postmarketing:

Cases of lactic acidosis, sometimes fatal, usually associated with severe hepatomegaly and hepatic steatosis have been reported with the use of nucleoside analogues (see 4.4).

The following events (frequency rare to very rare) have been identified during post approval use of Videx:

General disorders and administration site conditions: asthenia, chills and fever, pain

Gastrointestinal disorders: flatulence, parotid gland enlargement, dry mouth

Metabolism and nutrition disorders: lactic acidosis, anorexia, diabetes mellitus, hypoglycaemia, hyperglycaemia

Skin and subcutaneous tissue disorders: alopecia

Hepatobiliary disorders: hepatic steatosis, hepatitis, liver failure

Infections and infestations: sialoadenitis

Blood and lymphatic system disorders: anaemia, leukopenia, thrombocytopenia

Immune system disorders: anaphylactic reaction

Eye disorders: dry eyes, retinal depigmentation, optic neuritis

Musculoskeletal, connective tissue and bone disorders: myalgia (with or without increases in creatine phosphokinase), rhabdomyolysis including acute renal failure and hemodialysis, arthralgia, myopathy

Investigations: increased/abnormal serum amylase, alkaline phosphatase and creatine phosphokinase

4.9 Overdose

There is no known antidote for didanosine overdosage. Experience in early studies, in which didanosine was initially administered at doses ten times the recommended doses, indicates that the anticipated complications of overdosage could include pancreatitis, peripheral neuropathy, hyperuricemia and hepatic dysfunction.

Didanosine is not dialyzable by peritoneal dialysis, although there is some clearance by haemodialysis. (The fractional removal of didanosine during an average haemodialysis session of 3 to 4 hours was approximately 20-35% of the dose present in the body at the start of dialysis.)

5. PHARMACOLOGICAL PROPERTIES

5.1 Pharmacodynamic properties

Nucleoside reverse transcriptase inhibitor: ATC Code: J05AF02

Didanosine (2',3'-dideoxyinosine) is an inhibitor of the *in vitro* replication of HIV in cultured human cells and cell lines. After didanosine enters the cell, it is enzymatically converted to dideoxyadenosine-triphosphate (ddATP), its active metabolite. In viral nucleic acid replication, incorporation of this 2',3'-dideoxynucleoside prevents chain extension, and thereby inhibits viral replication.

In addition, ddATP inhibits HIV-reverse transcriptase by competing with dATP for binding to the enzyme's active site, preventing proviral DNA synthesis.

The relationship between *in vitro* susceptibility of HIV to didanosine and clinical response to therapy has not been established. Likewise, *in vitro* sensitivity results vary greatly and methods to establish virologic responses have not been proven.

Using the Videx tablet formulation, the effect of Videx BID administration, alone or in combination with zidovudine, was evaluated in several major randomised, controlled clinical trials (ACTG 175, ACTG 152, DELTA, CPCRA 007). These trials confirmed the reduced risk of HIV disease progression or death with Videx tablets therapy, alone or in combination with zidovudine, as compared with zidovudine monotherapy in HIV infected individuals, including symptomatic and asymptomatic adults with CD4 counts < 500 cells/mm^3 and children with evidence of immunosuppression. The primary demonstration of clinical benefits of didanosine has been made through the ACTG 175 trial with the buffered tablet formulation of Videx administered twice daily (BID). This study showed that eight weeks of treatment with zidovudine, Videx tablets BID, or Videx tablets BID plus zidovudine decreased mean plasma HIV RNA by 0.26, 0.65 and 0.93 log_{10} copies/ml, respectively. In the tritherapy setting, the combination of Videx (200 mg) BID plus stavudine and indinavir has been compared to zidovudine plus lamivudine and indinavir in a randomised open label study (START II, n= 205): through 48 weeks of treatment, results were in favour of the Videx arm. However, no formal conclusion can be drawn on the equivalence of the 2 regimens.

Since didanosine exhibits a very long intracellular half-life (> 24 hours), permitting the accumulation of its pharmacologically active ddATP-moiety for extended time periods, administration of the total daily dose of Videx in a once-daily dosing regimen has been explored through clinical studies.

Several clinical studies have been performed with Videx (tablet) administered once daily, including the following:

In the tritherapy setting, the randomised open label study -147 demonstrated that, in mostly asymptomatic patients (n= 123) that were stable on their first combination therapy containing Videx BID, the shift to a similar combination therapy with Videx once-daily did not impact at short term (24 weeks) on the existing antiviral efficacy.

The randomised open label study -148 (n= 756) compared Videx once-daily plus stavudine and nelfinavir to zidovudine plus lamivudine and nelfinavir. After 48 weeks of treatment, results were in favour of the zidovudine (BID), lamivudine and nelfinavir arm compared to Videx (once-daily), stavudine and nelfinavir arm in term of proportion of patients with undetectable viral load (the proportion of patients with HIV RNA copies < 400 copies/ml was 53% for the Videx-containing arm and 62% for the comparator). However, no formal conclusions can be drawn on this study due to methodological issues.

Current evidence indicates that the incidence of resistance to didanosine is an infrequent event and the resistance generated is modest in degree. Didanosine-resistant isolates have been selected in vivo and are associated with specific genotype changes in the reverse transcriptase codon region (codons L74V (most prevalent), K65R, M184V and T69S/G/D/N). Clinical isolates that exhibited a decrease in didanosine susceptibility harboured one or more didanosine-associated mutations. Mutant viruses containing the L74V substitution show a decline in viral fitness and these mutants quickly revert to wild type in the absence of didanosine. Cross-resistance between didanosine and protease inhibitors or non nucleoside reverse transcriptase inhibitor is unlikely. Cross-resistance between didanosine and nucleoside reverse transcriptase inhibitor is observed in isolates containing multi-resistant mutations such as Q151M and T69S-XX (an amino acid substitution with a 2-amino acid insertion) and multiple nucleoside analogue associated mutations (NAMs).

5.2 Pharmacokinetic properties

Adults

Absorption: Didanosine is rapidly degraded at an acidic pH. Therefore, the tablets contain buffering agents designed to increase gastric pH. The administration of didanosine with a meal results in a significant decrease (about 50%) in bioavailability. Videx tablets should be administered at least 30 minutes before a meal. A study in 10 asymptomatic HIV seropositive patients demonstrated that administration of Videx tablets 30 min to 1 hour before a meal did not result in any significant changes in the bioavailability of didanosine compared to administration under fasting conditions. Administration of the tablets 1 to 2 hours after a meal was associated with a 55% decrease in C_{max} and AUC values, which was comparable to the decrease observed when the formulation was given immediately after a meal.

In 30 patients receiving didanosine 400 mg once daily in the fasted state as Videx buffered tablets, single dose AUC was 2516 ± 847 ng•h/ml (34%) (mean ± SD [%CV]) and C_{max} was 1475 ± 673 ng/ml (46%).

Distribution: The volume of distribution at steady state averages 54 l, suggesting that there is some uptake of didanosine by body tissues. The level of didanosine in the cerebrospinal fluid (CSF), one hour after infusion, averages 21% of that of the simultaneous plasma level.

Biotransformation: The metabolism of didanosine in man has not been evaluated. However, based on animal studies, it is presumed that it follows the same pathways responsible for the elimination of endogenous purines.

Elimination: The average elimination half-life after IV administration of didanosine is approximately 1.4 hours. Renal clearance represents 50% of total body clearance (800 ml/min), indicating that active tubular secretion, in addition to glomerular filtration, is responsible for the renal elimination of didanosine. Urinary recovery of didanosine is approximately 20% of the dose after oral treatment. There is no evidence of didanosine accumulation after the administration of oral doses for 4 weeks.

Hepatic impairment: No significant changes in the pharmacokinetics of didanosine were observed among haemophiliac patients with chronic, persistent elevations in liver function enzymes (n=5), which may be indicative of impaired hepatic function; haemophiliac patients with normal or less severe increases in liver function enzymes (n=8); and non-haemophiliac patients with normal enzyme levels (n=8) following a single IV or oral dose. No conclusion can be drawn regarding the metabolism of didanosine, which may be altered in patients with severe hepatic impairment (see 4.2).

Children

Absorption: Variability in the amount of didanosine absorbed in children is greater than in adults. The absolute bioavailability of didanosine administered orally was approximately 36% after the first dose and 47% at steady state.

Distribution: The CSF didanosine level averages 46% of that of the simultaneous plasma level after IV administration of doses of 60 or 90 mg/m^2 and equivalent oral doses of 120 or 180 mg/m^2. Measurable concentrations of didanosine in the CSF were detectable for up to 3.5 hours after dosing.

Elimination: The average elimination half-life after IV didanosine administration is approximately 0.8 hours. Renal clearance represents approximately 59% of the total body clearance (315 ml/min/m^2), indicating that both renal and nonrenal pathways are involved in the elimination. Urinary recovery of didanosine is approximately 17% of dose after oral treatment. There is no evidence of didanosine accumulation after oral administration for an average of 26 days.

5.3 Preclinical safety data

The lowest dose to cause death in acute toxicity studies in the mouse, rat and dog was greater than 2000 mg/kg which is equivalent to approximately 300 times the maximum recommended human dose.

Repeated dose toxicity: Repeat-dose oral toxicity studies revealed evidence of a dose-limiting skeletal muscle toxicity in rodents (but not in dogs) following long-term (> 90 days) dosing with didanosine at doses that were approximately 1.2 - 12 times the estimated human dose. Additionally, in repeat dose studies, leukopenia was observed in dogs and rats, and gastrointestinal disturbances (soft stool, diarrhoea) were seen in dogs at doses approximately 5 - 14 times the maximum human dose.

Carcinogenicity: In the carcinogenicity studies, non-neoplastic alterations have been observed including skeletal muscle myopathy, hepatic alterations and an exacerbation of spontaneous age-related cardiomyopathy.

Lifetime dietary carcinogenicity studies were conducted in mice and rats for 22 or 24 months, respectively. No drug-related neoplasms were observed in any didanosine-treated groups of mice during, or at the end of, the dosing period. In rats, statistically significant increased incidences of granulosa cell tumours in females receiving the high dose, of subcutaneous fibrosarcomas and histiocytic sarcomas in males receiving the high dose and of haemangiomas in males receiving the high and intermediate dose of didanosine were noted. The drug-relationship and clinical relevance of these statistical findings were not clear.

Genotoxicity: Results from the genotoxicity studies suggest that didanosine is not mutagenic at biologically and pharmacologically relevant doses. At significantly elevated concentrations *in vitro*, the genotoxic effects of didanosine are similar in magnitude to those seen with natural DNA nucleosides.

Reproduction: In rats, didanosine did not impair the reproduction ability of male or female parents following treatment prior to and during mating, gestation and lactation at daily didanosine doses up to 1000 mg/kg/day. In a perinatal and postnatal reproduction study in rats, didanosine did not induce toxic effects.

6. PHARMACEUTICAL PARTICULARS

6.1 List of excipients

Calcium carbonate, magnesium hydroxide, aspartame, sorbitol, microcrystalline cellulose, crospovidone, mandarin orange flavour (tangerine oil, mandarin oil, gum arabic, alpha tocopherol, colloidal silica) and magnesium stearate.

6.2 Incompatibilities

Not applicable

6.3 Shelf life

2 years.

After dispersion in water, the dispersion is physically and chemically stable for 1 hour.

6.4 Special precautions for storage

Do not store above 30°C. Keep the container tightly closed in order to protect from moisture.

6.5 Nature and contents of container

High-density polyethylene bottle with child-resistant cap.

Package size: 60 tablets per bottle.

6.6 Instructions for use and handling

No special requirements.

7. MARKETING AUTHORISATION HOLDER

Bristol-Myers Squibb Pharmaceuticals Limited

Uxbridge Business Park,

Sanderson Road,

Uxbridge,

Middlesex UB8 1DH

8. MARKETING AUTHORISATION NUMBER(S)

PL 11184/0076

9. DATE OF FIRST AUTHORISATION/RENEWAL OF THE AUTHORISATION

10 December 1999

10. DATE OF REVISION OF THE TEXT

25 August 2005

Videx EC 125mg, 200mg, 250mg and 400mg Gastro-resistant Capsules

(Bristol-Myers Squibb Pharmaceuticals Ltd)

1. NAME OF THE MEDICINAL PRODUCT

Videx® EC 125 mg gastro-resistant capsule

Videx® EC 200 mg gastro-resistant capsule

Videx® EC 250 mg gastro-resistant capsule

Videx® EC 400 mg gastro-resistant capsule

2. QUALITATIVE AND QUANTITATIVE COMPOSITION

Each gastro-resistant capsule, hard contains 125 mg, 200 mg, 250 mg or 400 mg of didanosine.

For excipients, see 6.1

3. PHARMACEUTICAL FORM

Gastro-resistant capsule, hard

Videx® EC 125 mg: Gastro-resistant capsules are opaque white and embossed in tan with "6671" on one half, and "BMS 125 mg" on the other half.

Videx® EC 200 mg: Gastro-resistant capsules are opaque white and embossed in green with "6672" on one half, and "BMS 200 mg" on the other half.

Videx® EC 250 mg: Gastro-resistant capsules are opaque white and embossed in blue with "6673" on one half, and "BMS 250 mg" on the other half.

Videx® EC 400 mg: Gastro-resistant capsules are opaque white and embossed in red with "6674" on one half, and "BMS 400 mg" on the other half.

4. CLINICAL PARTICULARS

4.1 Therapeutic indications

Videx is indicated in combination with other antiretroviral drugs for the treatment of HIV infected patients.

4.2 Posology and method of administration

Oral use.

Because didanosine absorption is reduced in the presence of food, Videx gastro-resistant capsules should be administered on an empty stomach (at least 2 hours before or after a meal) (see 5.2).

Posology

Videx gastro-resistant capsules may be administered on a once-daily (QD) or a twice-daily (BID) regimen (see 5.1).

Adults: The recommended daily dose is dependent on patient weight:

§ for patients ⩾ 60 kg: 400 mg per day

§ for patients < 60 kg: 250 mg per day

The following table defines the administration schedule for all strengths of the gastro-resistant capsules:

Patient Weight	Total Daily Dose	Corresponding Regimen
⩾ 60 kg	400 mg	1 capsule of 400 mg (once-daily) or 1 capsule of 200 mg (twice-daily)
< 60 kg	250 mg	1 capsule of 250 mg (once-daily) or 1 capsule of 125 mg (twice-daily)

Children older than 6 years: The use of Videx gastro-resistant capsules has not been specifically studied in children. The recommended daily dose (based on body surface area) is 240 mg/m^2 (180 mg/m^2 in combination with zidovudine).

Children younger than 6 years: The gastro-resistant capsules should not be opened as there is a potential for inadvertent aspiration. Therefore, this medicine is contra-indicated in this age group. Other more appropriate Videx formulations are available.

Dose adjustment

Pancreatitis: Significant elevations of serum amylase should prompt discontinuation of therapy and careful evaluation of the possibility of pancreatitis, even in the absence of symptoms of pancreatitis. Fractionation of amylase may help distinguish amylase of salivary origin. Only after pancreatitis has been ruled out or after clinical and biological parameters have returned to normal, should dosing be resumed, and then only if treatment is considered essential. Treatment should be re-initiated with low doses and increased slowly, if appropriate.

Renal impairment: The following dose adjustments are recommended:

Creatinine Clearance (ml/min)	Patient Weight ⩾ 60 kg Total Daily Dose	Patient Weight < 60 kg Total Daily Dose
⩾ 60	400 mg	250 mg
30 – 59	200 mg	150 mg*
10 – 29	150 mg*	100 mg*
< 10	100 mg*	75 mg*

* These strengths of Videx gastro-resistant capsules are not available. An alternative Videx formulation should be used.

The dose should preferably be administered after dialysis (see 4.). However, it is not necessary to administer a supplemental dose of Videx following haemodialysis.

Neuropathy: Many patients who present with symptoms of neuropathy and who experience resolution of symptoms upon drug discontinuation will tolerate a reduced dose of didanosine (see 4.4).

Hepatic impairment: No specific dose adjustment can be recommended in patients with hepatic impairment. These patients should be monitored closely for clinical evidence of didanosine toxicity. Plasma level monitoring of didanosine may help to identify outliers, but currently available data do not allow specific recommendations with regard to target plasma levels (see 5.2).

Method of administration

To optimise absorption, the gastro-resistant capsule should be taken intact with at least 100 ml of water. Patients should be instructed not to open the capsule to facilitate administration, since this could reduce absorption (see 5.2).

4.3 Contraindications

Hypersensitivity to didanosine or to any of the excipients.

Children younger than 6 years (risk of inadvertent aspiration).

4.4 Special warnings and special precautions for use

Pancreatitis is a known serious complication among HIV infected patients. It has also been associated with didanosine therapy and has been fatal in some cases. Didanosine should be used only with extreme caution in patients with a history of pancreatitis. Positive relationships have been found between the risk of pancreatitis and daily dose of didanosine.

Whenever warranted by clinical conditions, didanosine should be suspended until the diagnosis of pancreatitis is excluded by appropriate laboratory and imaging techniques. Similarly, when treatment with other medicinal products known to cause pancreatic toxicity is required (e.g. pentamidine), didanosine should be suspended whenever possible. If concomitant therapy is unavoidable, close observation is warranted. Dose interruption should be considered when biochemical markers of pancreatitis have significantly increased, even in the absence of symptoms. Significant elevations of triglycerides are a known cause of pancreatitis and warrant close observation.

Peripheral neuropathy: Patients on didanosine may develop toxic peripheral neuropathy, usually characterised by bilateral symmetrical distal numbness, tingling, and pain in feet and, less frequently, hands. Whenever warranted by clinical conditions, didanosine therapy should be suspended until resolution of symptoms. Many patients tolerate a reduced dose after resolution of symptoms.

Retinal or optic nerve changes: Children on didanosine have demonstrated retinal or optic nerve changes on rare occasions, particularly at doses above those recommended. There have been reports of retinal depigmentation in adults. Especially for children, periodic dilated retinal examinations (every 6 months), or if a change in vision occurs, should be considered.

Lactic acidosis:
lactic acidosis, usually associated with hepatomegaly and hepatic steatosis, has been reported with the use of nucleoside analogues. Early symptoms (symptomatic hyperlactatemia) include benign digestive symptoms (nausea, vomiting and abdominal pain), non-specific malaise, loss of appetite, weight loss, respiratory symptoms (rapid and/or deep breathing) or neurological symptoms (including motor weakness). Lactic acidosis has a high mortality and may be associated with pancreatitis, liver failure, or renal failure.
Lactic acidosis generally occurred after a few or several months of treatment.
Treatment with nucleoside analogues should be discontinued in the setting of symptomatic hyperlactatemia and metabolic/lactic acidosis, progressive hepatomegaly, or rapidly elevating aminotransferase levels. Caution should be exercised when administering nucleoside analogues to any patient (particularly obese women) with hepatomegaly, hepatitis or other known risk factors for liver disease and hepatic steatosis (including certain medicinal products and alcohol). Patients co-infected with hepatitis C and treated with alpha interferon and ribavirin may constitute a special risk.
Patients at increased risk should be followed closely. (See also 4.6).

Renal impairment: The half-life of didanosine after oral administration increased from an average of 1.4 hours in subjects with normal renal function to 4.1 hours in subjects with severe renal impairment requiring dialysis. After an oral dose, didanosine was not detectable in peritoneal dialysis fluid; recovery in haemodialysate ranged from 0.6% to 7.4% of the dose over a 3-4 hour dialysis period. Patients with a creatinine clearance < 60 ml/min may be at greater risk of didanosine toxicity due to decreased drug clearance. A dose reduction is recommended for these patients (see 4.2).

Liver disease: Liver failure of unknown aetiology has occurred rarely in patients on didanosine. Patients should be observed for liver enzyme elevations and didanosine should be suspended if enzymes rise to >5 times the upper limit of normal. Rechallenge should be considered only if the potential benefits clearly outweigh the potential risks.

The safety and efficacy of Videx has not been established in patients with significant underlying liver disorders. Patients with chronic hepatitis B or C and treated with combination antiretroviral therapy are at an increased risk for severe and potentially fatal hepatic adverse events. In case of concomitant antiviral therapy for hepatitis B or C, please refer also to the relevant product information for these medicinal products.

Patients with pre-existing liver dysfunction including chronic active hepatitis have an increased frequency of liver function abnormalities during combination antiretroviral therapy and should be monitored according to standard practice. If there is evidence of worsening liver disease in such patients, interruption or discontinuation of treatment must be considered.

Immune Reactivation Syndrome: In HIV-infected patients with severe immune deficiency at the time of institution of combination antiretroviral therapy (CART), an inflammatory reaction to asymptomatic or residual opportunistic pathogens may arise and cause serious clinical conditions, or aggravation of symptoms. Typically, such reactions have been observed within the first few weeks or months of initiation of CART. Relevant examples are cytomegalovirus retinitis, generalised and/or focal mycobacterial infections, and Pneumocystis carinii pneumonia. Any inflammatory symptoms should be evaluated and treatment instituted when necessary.

Lipodystrophy and metabolic abnormalities: Combination antiretroviral therapy has been associated with the redistribution of body fat (lipodystrophy) in HIV patients. The long-term consequences of these events are currently unknown. Knowledge about the mechanism is incomplete. A connection between visceral lipomatosis and PIs and lipoatrophy and NRTIs has been hypothesised. A higher risk of lipodystrophy has been associated with individual factors such as older age, and with drug related factors such as longer duration of antiretroviral treatment and associated metabolic disturbances. Clinical examination should include evaluation for physical signs of fat redistribution. Consideration should be given to the measurement of fasting serum lipids and blood glucose. Lipid disorders should be managed as clinically appropriate (see 4.8).

Mitochondrial dysfunction: Nucleoside and nucleotide analogues have been demonstrated *in vitro* and *in vivo* to cause a variable degree of mitochondrial damage. There have been reports of mitochondrial dysfunction in HIV-negative infants exposed *in utero* and/or post-natally to nucleoside analogues. The main adverse events reported are haematological disorders (anemia, neutropenia), metabolic disorders (hyperlactatemia, hyperlipasemia). These events are often transitory. Some late-onset neurological disorders have been reported (hypertonia, convulsion, abnormal behaviour). Whether the neurological disorders are transient or permanent is currently unknown. Any child exposed *in utero* to nucleoside and nucleotide analogues, even HIV-negative children, should have clinical and laboratory follow-up and should be fully investigated for possible mitochondrial dysfunction in case of relevant signs or symptoms. These findings do not affect current national recommendations to use antiretroviral therapy in pregnant women to prevent vertical transmission of HIV.

Opportunistic infections: Patients receiving didanosine or any antiretroviral therapy may continue to develop opportunistic infections and other complications of HIV infection or therapy. They therefore should remain under close observation by physicians experienced in the treatment of HIV associated diseases.

Interaction with other medicinal products: Co-administration of didanosine and tenofovir disoproxil fumarate results in a 40-60% increase in systemic exposure to didanosine that may increase the risk for didanosine-related adverse events (see 4.5). Rare cases of pancreatitis and lactic acidosis, sometimes fatal, have been reported.

A reduced didanosine dose (250 mg) has been tested to avoid over-exposure to didanosine in case of co-administration with tenofovir disoproxil fumarate, but this has been associated with reports of high rate of virological failure and of emergence of resistance at early stage within several tested combinations.

Co-administration of didanosine and tenofovir disoproxil fumarate is therefore not recommended, especially in patients with high viral load and low CD4 cell count. If this combination is judged strictly necessary, patients should be carefully monitored for efficacy and didanosine related adverse events.

Triple nucleoside therapy: There have been reports of a high rate of virological failure and of emergence of resistance at an early stage when didanosine was combined with tenofovir disoproxil fumarate and lamivudine as a once daily regimen.

Patients on sodium restricted diet:

Each Videx® 125 mg gastro-resistant capsule contains 0.53 mg sodium.

Each Videx® 200 mg gastro-resistant capsule contains 0.85 mg sodium.

Each Videx® 250 mg gastro-resistant capsule contains 1.0 mg sodium.

Each Videx® 400 mg gastro-resistant capsule contains 1.7 mg sodium.

4.5 Interaction with other medicinal products and other forms of Interaction

Specific interaction studies have been conducted with zidovudine, stavudine, ranitidine, loperamide, metoclopramide, foscarnet, trimethoprim, sulfamethoxazole, dapsone and rifabutin, without evidence of interaction.

Administration of didanosine 2 hours prior to, or concurrent with, ganciclovir was associated with a mean increase of 111% in the steady state AUC for didanosine. A minor decrease (21%) in the steady state AUC of ganciclovir was seen when didanosine was given 2 hours prior to ganciclovir, but not when both medicines were given simultaneously. There were no changes in renal clearance for either drug. It is not known whether these changes are associated with alterations in either the safety of didanosine or the efficacy of ganciclovir. There is no evidence that didanosine potentiates the myelosuppressive effects of ganciclovir or zidovudine.

Co-administration of didanosine with medicines that are known to cause peripheral neuropathy or pancreatitis may increase the risk of these toxicities. Patients who receive these medicines should be carefully observed.

Based on *in vitro* data, ribavirin may increase the intracellular triphosphate levels of didanosine and potentially increase the risk of adverse reactions (see 4. and 4.8); therefore, unless further clinical data are available, caution should be used, if these drugs need to be co-administered.

Unlike the Videx chewable/dispersible tablets, Videx gastro-resistant capsules do not contain antacids and therefore drug interactions mediated by altered gastric pH are not anticipated when Videx gastro-resistant capsules are co-administered with medicinal products where absorption is influenced by gastric acidity. Specific interaction studies with ciprofloxacin, indinavir, and fluconazole showed no evidence of significant interaction. Studies with ketoconazole and itraconazole showed statistically significant interactions, which seem unlikely to be clinically relevant. Thus, even if the interaction cannot be formally excluded, Videx gastro-resistant capsules can be prescribed concomitantly with these medicines.

When didanosine gastro-resistant capsules were administered 2 hours prior to or concurrently with tenofovir disoproxil fumarate, the AUC for didanosine was on average increased by 48% and 60% respectively. The mean increase in the AUC of didanosine was 44% when the buffered tablets were administered 1 hour prior to tenofovir. In both cases the pharmacokinetic parameters for tenofovir administered with a light meal were unchanged. The co-administration of didanosine and tenofovir disoproxil fumarate is not recommended (see 4.4).

Xanthine oxidase is an enzyme involved in the metabolism of didanosine. Inhibitors of xanthine oxidase, such as allopurinol, may increase exposure to didanosine when administered together and thus increase the potential for didanosine associated undesirable effects. Patients should be closely monitored for didanosine related undesirable effects (see 4.8).

Ingestion of Videx with food alters the pharmacokinetics of didanosine (see 5.2).

4.6 Pregnancy and lactation

Pregnancy: There are no adequate and well-controlled studies in pregnant women and it is not known whether didanosine can cause foetal harm or affect reproductive capacity when administered during pregnancy. Lactic acidosis (see 4.4), sometimes fatal, has been reported in pregnant women who received the combination of didanosine and stavudine with or without other antiretroviral treatment. Therefore, the use of didanosine during pregnancy should be considered only if clearly indicated, and only when the potential benefit outweighs the possible risk.

Teratology studies in rats and rabbits did not produce evidence of embryotoxic, foetotoxic, or teratogenic effects. A study in rats showed that didanosine and/or its metabolites are transferred to the foetus through the placenta.

Lactation: It is not known whether didanosine is excreted in human milk. It is recommended that women taking didanosine do not breast-feed because of the potential for serious adverse reactions in nursing infants.

At the 1000 mg/kg/day dose levels in rats, didanosine was slightly toxic to females and pups during mid and late lactation (reduced food intake and body weight gains), but the physical and functional development of the subsequent offspring were not impaired. A further study showed that, following oral administration, didanosine and/or its metabolites were excreted in the milk of lactating rats.

4.7 Effects on ability to drive and use machines

No effects on the ability to drive and use machines have been observed.

4.8 Undesirable effects

Adults: Most of the serious adverse events observed have generally reflected the recognised clinical course of HIV infection.

In data collected earlier involving monotherapy regimens, no different safety concerns were seen compared to the triple regimen data presented below. In comparative studies between Videx QD and BID (tablets), no significant difference in terms of incidence of pancreatitis and peripheral neuropathy has been shown.

Pancreatitis, which may be fatal in some cases, was reported in <1% of the patients receiving Videx gastro-resistant capsule; patients with advanced HIV disease or a history of pancreatitis may be at increased risk of developing pancreatitis.

Peripheral neurologic symptoms (8%) have been associated with Videx.

In HIV-infected patients with severe immune deficiency at the time of initiation of combination antiretroviral therapy (CART), an inflammatory reaction to asymptomatic or residual opportunistic infections may arise (see 4.4).

Lipodystrophy and metabolic abnormalities: Combination antiretroviral therapy has been associated with redistribution of body fat (lipodystrophy) in HIV patients including the loss of peripheral and facial subcutaneous fat, increased intra-abdominal and visceral fat, breast hypertrophy and dorsocervical fat accumulation (buffalo hump).

Combination antiretroviral therapy has been associated with metabolic abnormalities such as hypertriglyceridaemia, hypercholesterolaemia, insulin resistance, hyperglycaemia and hyperlactataemia (see 4.4).

In an open label clinical study (study-148), involving 482 patients treated with Videx tablet plus stavudine and nelfinavir, and in a clinical study (study-152) evaluating Videx gastro-resistant capsules as part of a triple regimen in 255 treatment naive HIV infected adults, the following undesirable effects (moderate to severe), which occured at a frequency of ⩾2%, and which are considered possibly related to study regimen based on the investigators' attribution, were reported:

Nervous system disorders:

common: peripheral neurologic symptoms (including neuropathy), headache

Gastrointestinal disorders:

very common: diarrhoea

common: nausea, vomiting, abdominal pain

Skin and subcutaneous tissue disorders:

common: rash

General disorders:

common: fatigue

Laboratory abnormalities:

Laboratory abnormalities (grade 3-4) reported in studies -148 (tablets) and -152 (gastro-resistant capsules) included increase of lipase in 7% and 5% respectively, increase of ALT in 3% and 6% respectively, increase of AST in 3% and 5%, respectively, increase in uric acid in 2% in both studies, and increase of bilirubin in 1% and <1% respectively, of the patients. Neutropenia (grade 3-4) was reported in 2% in both studies 148 and 152, anemia in <1% and 1% in study 148 and in study 152 respectively, and thrombocytopenia in 1% and <1%, respectively, of the patients.

Children: Safety data for children were generally similar to those seen in adults. A higher haematotoxicity has been reported with the combination with zidovudine compared to didanosine monotherapy. Retinal or optic nerve changes have been reported in a small number of children usually at doses above those recommended. It is recommended that children on didanosine treatment undergo dilated retinal examination every 6 months or if a change in vision occurs.

Postmarketing:

Cases of lactic acidosis, sometimes fatal, usually associated with severe hepatomegaly and hepatic steatosis have been reported with the use of nucleoside analogues (see 4.4).

The following events (frequency rare to very rare) have been identified during post approval use of Videx:

General disorders and administration site conditions: asthenia, chills and fever, pain **Gastrointestinal disorders**: flatulence, parotid gland enlargement, dry mouth

Metabolism and nutrition disorders: lactic acidosis, anorexia, diabetes mellitus, hypoglycaemia, hyperglycaemia

Skin and subcutaneous tissue disorders: alopecia

Hepatobiliary disorders: hepatic steatosis, hepatitis, liver failure

Infections and infestations: sialoadenitis

Blood and lymphatic system disorders: anaemia, leukopenia, thrombocytopenia

Immune system disorders: anaphylactic reaction

Eye disorders: dry eyes, retinal depigmentation, optic neuritis

Musculoskeletal, connective tissue and bone disorders: myalgia (with or without increases in creatine phosphokinase), rhabdomyolysis including acute renal failure and hemodialysis, arthralgia, myopathy

Investigations: increased/abnormal serum amylase, alkaline phosphatase and creatine phosphokinase

4.9 Overdose

There is no known antidote for didanosine overdosage. Experience in early studies, in which didanosine was initially administered at doses ten times the recommended doses, indicates that the anticipated complications of overdosage could include pancreatitis, peripheral neuropathy, hyperuricemia and hepatic dysfunction.

Didanosine is not dialyzable by peritoneal dialysis, although there is some clearance by haemodialysis. (The fractional removal of didanosine during an average haemodialysis session of 3 to 4 hours was approximately 20-35% of the dose present in the body at the start of dialysis.)

5. PHARMACOLOGICAL PROPERTIES

5.1 Pharmacodynamic properties

Nucleoside reverse transcriptase inhibitor: ATC Code: J05AF02

Didanosine (2', 3'-dideoxyinosine) is an inhibitor of the *in vitro* replication of HIV in cultured human cells and cell lines. After didanosine enters the cell, it is enzymatically converted to dideoxyadenosine-triphosphate (ddATP), its active metabolite. In viral nucleic acid replication, incorporation of this 2', 3'-dideoxynucleoside prevents chain extension, and thereby inhibits viral replication.

In addition, ddATP inhibits HIV-reverse transcriptase by competing with dATP for binding to the enzyme's active site, preventing proviral DNA synthesis.

The relationship between *in vitro* susceptibility of HIV to didanosine and clinical response to therapy has not been established. Likewise, *in vitro* sensitivity results vary greatly and methods to establish virologic responses have not been proven.

Using the Videx tablet formulation, the effect of Videx BID administration, alone or in combination with zidovudine, was evaluated in several major randomised, controlled clinical trials (ACTG 175, ACTG 152, DELTA, CPCRA 007). These trials confirmed the reduced risk of HIV disease progression or death with Videx tablets therapy, alone or in combination with zidovudine, as compared with zidovudine monotherapy in HIV infected individuals, including symptomatic and asymptomatic adults with CD4 counts < 500 cells/mm^3 and children with evidence of immunosuppression. The primary demonstration of clinical benefits of didanosine has been made through the ACTG 175 trial with the buffered tablet formulation of Videx administered twice daily (BID). This study showed that eight weeks of treatment with zidovudine, Videx tablets BID, or Videx tablets BID plus zidovudine decreased mean plasma HIV RNA by 0.26, 0.65 and 0.93 log_{10} copies/ml, respectively. In the tritherapy setting, the combination of Videx (200 mg) BID plus stavudine and indinavir has been compared to zidovudine plus lamivudine and indinavir in a randomised open label study (START II, n = 205): through 48 weeks of treatment, results were in favour of the Videx arm. However, no formal conclusion can be drawn on the equivalence of the two regimens.

Since didanosine exhibits a very long intracellular half-life (> 24 hours), permitting the accumulation of its pharmacologically active ddATP-moiety for extended time periods, administration of the total daily dose of Videx in a QD dosing regimen has been explored through clinical studies.

Several clinical studies have been performed with Videx (tablet) administered once daily (QD), including the following:

In the tritherapy setting, the randomised open label study – 147 indicates that, in mostly asymptomatic patients (n= 123) that were stable on their first combination therapy containing Videx BID, the shift to a similar combination therapy with Videx QD did not impact at short term (24 weeks) on the existing antiviral efficacy.

The randomised open label study –148 (n= 756) compared Videx QD plus stavudine and nelfinavir to zidovudine plus lamivudine and nelfinavir. After 48 weeks of treatment, results were in favour of the zidovudine (BID), lamivudine and nelfinavir arm compared to Videx QD, stavudine and nelfinavir arm in terms of proportion of patients with undetectable viral load (the proportion of patients with HIV RNA copies < 400 copies/ml was 53% for the Videx-containing arm and 62% for the comparator). However, no formal conclusions can be drawn on this study due to methodological issues.

The efficacy of Videx gastro-resistant capsules was evaluated in treatment-naive HIV infected adults as part of a triple regimen in two (48-week) randomised open label clinical trials. Study –152 (n= 466) compared Videx gastro-resistant capsules (QD) plus stavudine and nelfinavir to zidovudine plus lamivudine and nelfinavir. The protocol-defined analysis showed the proportion of patients with HIV RNA levels < 400 copies/ml at week 48 to be similar for the Videx gastro-resistant arm and for the comparator. Similar log_{10} plasma HIV RNA decreases from baseline (Time Averaged Difference) were observed between treatment arms.

In study -158 (n= 138) the antiviral activity and tolerability of Videx gastro-resistant capsules were compared to tablets, each given QD in combination with stavudine and nelfinavir. At 24 weeks of follow-up, there were similar log_{10} plasma HIV RNA decreases from baseline (Time Averaged Difference) between treatment arms. The percentages of patients with undetectable viral load (limit of detection < 400 copies/ml) were of the same magnitude between the two Videx arms. Due to the high drop-out rate (> 50%) in this study, no definitive conclusion could be drawn on the long-term data. The efficacy of Videx gastro-resistant capsules has not been established in advanced disease or in highly antiretroviral experienced patients.

Current evidence indicates that the incidence of resistance to didanosine is an infrequent event and the resistance generated is modest in degree. Didanosine-resistant isolates have been selected in vivo and are associated with specific genotype changes in the reverse transcriptase codon region (codons L74V (most prevalent), K65R, M184V and T69S/G/D/N). Clinical isolates that exhibited a decrease in didanosine susceptibility harbored one or more didanosine-associated mutations. Mutant viruses containing the L74V substitution show a decline in viral fitness and these mutants quickly revert to wild type in the absence of didanosine. Cross-resistance between didanosine and protease inhibitors or non nucleoside reverse transcriptase inhibitor is unlikely. Cross-resistance between didanosine and nucleoside reverse transcriptase inhibitor is observed in isolates containing multi-resistant mutations such as Q151M and T69S-XX (an amino acid substitution with a 2-amino acid insertion) and multiple nucleoside analogue associated mutations (NAMs).

5.2 Pharmacokinetic properties

Adults

Absorption: Didanosine is rapidly degraded at an acidic pH. Therefore, the granules in the Videx gastro-resistant capsules release didanosine into the higher pH of the small intestine.

Compared to the fasting condition, the administration of Videx gastro-resistant capsules with a high fat meal significantly decreases the didanosine AUC (19%) and C_{max}(46%). Co-administering Videx gastro-resistant capsules with a light meal, 1 hour before or 2 hours after a light meal, results in a significant decrease in both AUC (27%, 24% and 10% respectively) and C_{max} of didanosine (22%, 15% and 15% respectively) compared to the fasting condition.

In another study, administration of Videx gastro-resistant capsules 1.5, 2 and 3 hours prior to a light meal results in equivalent C_{max} and AUC values compared to those obtained under fasting conditions.

To minimise the impact of food on the didanosine pharmacokinetics, Videx gastro-resistant capsules should be administered on an empty stomach at least 2 hours before or 2 hours after a meal (see 4.2).

Relative to administration of intact Videx gastro-resistant capsule on empty stomach, co-administration of didanosine enteric coated beadlets sprinkled on yoghurt and applesauce resulted in a significant decrease in the AUC (20% and 18%, respectively) and C_{max} (30% and 24%, respectively).

Equivalent values for AUC are observed for the tablet and capsule formulations of Videx in healthy volunteers and subjects infected with HIV. The rate of absorption from Videx capsules is slower compared to the tablet; the value for C_{max} for the gastro-resistant capsule is 60% of the value for the tablet. The time to reach C_{max} is approximately 2 hours for the Videx gastro-resistant capsule and 0.67 hour for the Videx tablet.

In 30 patients receiving didanosine 400 mg once daily in the fasted state as Videx gastro-resistant capsules, single dose AUC was 2432 ± 919 ng·h/ml (38%) (mean ± SD [%CV]) and C_{max} was 933 ± 434 ng/ml (47%).

Distribution: The volume of distribution at steady state averages 54 l, suggesting that there is some uptake of didanosine by body tissues. The level of didanosine in the cerebrospinal fluid, one hour after infusion, averages 21% of that of the simultaneous plasma level.

Biotransformation: The metabolism of didanosine in man has not been evaluated. However, based on animal studies, it is presumed that it follows the same pathways responsible for the elimination of endogenous purines.

Elimination: The average elimination half-life after IV administration of didanosine is approximately 1.4 hours. Renal clearance represents 50% of total body clearance (800 ml/min), indicating that active tubular secretion, in addition to glomerular filtration, is responsible for the renal elimination of didanosine. Urinary recovery of didanosine is approximately 20% of the dose after oral treatment. There is no evidence of didanosine accumulation after the administration of oral doses for 4 weeks.

Hepatic impairment: No significant changes in the pharmacokinetics of didanosine were observed among haemophiliac patients with chronic, persistent elevations in liver function enzymes (n=5), which may be indicative of impaired hepatic function; haemophiliac patients with normal or less severe increases in liver function enzymes (n=8); and non-haemophiliac patients with normal enzyme levels (n=8) following a single IV or oral dose. No conclusion can be drawn regarding the metabolism of didanosine, which may be altered in patients with severe hepatic impairment (see 4.2).

Children

There are no specific pharmacokinetic data from children treated with Videx gastro-resistant capsules.

5.3 Preclinical safety data

The lowest dose to cause death in acute toxicity studies in the mouse, rat and dog was greater than 2000 mg/kg which is equivalent to approximately 300 times the maximum recommended human dose (tablet).

Repeated dose toxicity: Repeat-dose oral toxicity studies revealed evidence of a dose-limiting skeletal muscle toxicity in rodents (but not in dogs) following long-term (> 90 days) dosing with didanosine at doses that were approximately 1.2 - 12 times the estimated human dose. Additionally, in repeat dose studies, leukopenia was observed in dogs and rats, and gastrointestinal disturbances (soft stool, diarrhoea) were seen in dogs at doses approximately 5 - 14 times the maximum human dose.

Carcinogenicity: In the carcinogenicity studies, non-neoplastic alterations have been observed including skeletal muscle myopathy, hepatic alterations and an exacerbation of spontaneous age-related cardiomyopathy.

Lifetime dietary carcinogenicity studies were conducted in mice and rats for 22 or 24 months, respectively. No drug-related neoplasms were observed in any didanosine-treated groups of mice during, or at the end of, the dosing period. In rats, statistically significant increased incidences of granulosa cell tumours in females receiving the high dose, of subcutaneous fibrosarcomas and histiocytic sarcomas in males receiving the high dose and of haemangiomas in males receiving the high and intermediate dose of didanosine were noted. The drug-relationship and clinical relevance of these statistical findings were not clear.

Genotoxicity: Results from the genotoxicity studies suggest that didanosine is not mutagenic at biologically and pharmacologically relevant doses. At significantly elevated concentrations *in vitro*, the genotoxic effects of didanosine are similar in magnitude to those seen with natural DNA nucleosides.

Reproduction: In rats, didanosine did not impair the reproduction ability of male or female parents following treatment prior to and during mating, gestation and lactation at daily didanosine doses up to 1000 mg/kg/day. In a perinatal and postnatal reproduction study in rats, didanosine did not induce toxic effects.

6. PHARMACEUTICAL PARTICULARS

6.1 List of excipients

Videx EC 125 mg, 200 mg, 250 mg and 400mg

Sodium carmellose, diethyl phthalate, 30% methacrylic acid copolymer dispersion (EUDRAGIT L30D-55), sodium starch glycolate and talc.

Capsule shell - gelatin, sodium laurilsulfate, colloidal anhydrous silica and titanium dioxide (E171).

Capsule shell imprints (edible ink)

Videx EC 125 mg: shellac, propylene glycol, potassium hydroxide, titanium dioxide (E171), yellow and red iron oxide (E172).

Videx EC 200 mg: shellac, propylene glycol, FD&C Blue #2 Aluminum Lake (E132), titanium dioxide (E171) and yellow iron oxide (E172).

Videx EC 250 mg: shellac, propylene glycol, FD&C Blue #2 Aluminum Lake (E132).

Videx EC 400 mg: shellac, ammonium hydroxide, propylene glycol, simethicone and red iron oxide (E172).

6.2 Incompatibilities

Not applicable

6.3 Shelf life

2 years

6.4 Special precautions for storage

Do not store above 25°C.

6.5 Nature and contents of container

Polyvinyl Chloride/Polyethylene/ACLAR/Aluminium foil blisters with 10 hard capsules per blister card and 3 cards (30 capsules) per carton or with 10 hard capsules per blister card and 6 cards (60 capsules) per carton. Not all pack sizes may be marketed.

6.6 Instructions for use and handling

No special requirements.

7. MARKETING AUTHORISATION HOLDER

Bristol-Myers Squibb Pharmaceuticals Limited,

Uxbridge Business Park,

Sanderson Road,

Uxbridge,

Middlesex UB8 1DH

8. MARKETING AUTHORISATION NUMBER(S)

Videx EC 125 mg:	PL 11184/0083
Videx EC 200 mg:	PL 11184/0084
Videx EC 250 mg:	PL 11184/0085
Videx EC 400 mg:	PL 11184/0086

9. DATE OF FIRST AUTHORISATION/RENEWAL OF THE AUTHORISATION

19 September 2000

10. DATE OF REVISION OF THE TEXT

25 August 2005

Vioform Hydrocortisone Cream, Hydrocortisone Ointment

(Novartis Consumer Health)

1. NAME OF THE MEDICINAL PRODUCT

Vioform Hydrocortisone Cream

Vioform Hydrocortisone Ointment

2. QUALITATIVE AND QUANTITATIVE COMPOSITION

Both pharmaceutical forms contain: Clioquinol BP 3% w/w

Hydrocortisone Ph Eur 1% w/w

3. PHARMACEUTICAL FORM

Cream and ointment

4. CLINICAL PARTICULARS

4.1 Therapeutic indications

Exudative and secondarily infected eczema and dermatitis, including atopic eczema, primary irritant dermatitis, allergic and seborrhoeic dermatitis, infected insect bites reactions, genital or perianal intertrigo.

4.2 Posology and method of administration

Vioform-Hydrocortisone is indicated for external application only.

The preparation should be applied sparingly to the affected area, 1-3 times daily. Treatment should be limited to 7 days. Occlusive dressings should not be used.

If there is little improvement after 7 days treatment with Vioform-Hydrocortisone, the appropriate microbiological investigations should be carried out and local or systemic antibiotic treatment given.

Use in the elderly

There is no evidence to suggest that dosage should be different in the elderly.

Use in children

Vioform-Hydrocortisone is contra-indicated in children below the age of 2 years.

4.3 Contraindications

Hypersensitivity to any component of the formulation or iodine. Primary bacterial viral or fungal infections of the skin. Secondary infections due to yeasts. Application to ulcerated areas. Use in children below the age of 2 years

4.4 Special warnings and special precautions for use

Long-term continuous topical therapy should be avoided since this can lead to adrenal suppression even without occlusion.

Application to relatively large and/or eroded areas of skin, use of occlusive dressings, and treatment for longer than one week should be avoided, because this may lead to a marked increase in protein-bound iodine (PBI). Thyroid function tests such as PBI, radioactive iodine and butanol extractable iodine may be affected, consequently it is advisable that such tests are not performed within one month of discontinuing treatment. However, other thyroid function tests, such as the T3 resin sponge test or T4 determination are unaffected.

The ferric chloride test for phenylketonuria may yield a false-positive result when clioquinol is present in the urine.

Vioform-Hydrocortisone should be used with caution in patients suffering from hepatic and/or renal failure.

Vioform-Hydrocortisone should not be allowed to come into contact with the conjunctiva.

4.5 Interaction with other medicinal products and other forms of Interaction

None known via this topical route.

4.6 Pregnancy and lactation

There is inadequate evidence of safety in human pregnancy. Topical administration of corticosteroids to pregnant animals can cause abnormalities of foetal development, including cleft palate, and intra-uterine growth retardation. There may be, therefore, a very small risk of such effects in the human foetus.

It is not known whether the active substances of Vioform-Hydrocortisone and/or their metabolite(s) pass into the breast milk after topical administration. Use in lactating mothers should only be at the doctor's discretion.

4.7 Effects on ability to drive and use machines

None known.

4.8 Undesirable effects

Vioform-Hydrocortisone is usually well tolerated but occasionally, at the site of application, there may be signs of irritation, such as a burning sensation, itching or skin rash. Hypersensitivity reactions may also occasionally occur. Treatment should be discontinued if patients experience severe irritation or sensitisation.

Vioform-Hydrocortisone may cause hair discoloration.

4.9 Overdose

Vioform-Hydrocortisone is for topical (external) use only. If accidental ingestion of large quantities occurs, there is no specific antidote and general measures to eliminate the drug and reduce its absorption should be undertaken. Symptomatic treatment should be administered as appropriate.

5. PHARMACOLOGICAL PROPERTIES

5.1 Pharmacodynamic properties

Vioform-Hydrocortisone combines the anti-fungal, and anti-bacterial properties of clioquinol with the anti-inflammatory, anti-allergic and anti-pruritic effects of hydrocortisone.

5.2 Pharmacokinetic properties

Following topical application of Vioform-Hydrocortisone, clioquinol has been shown to be absorbed to an extent of about 2% to 3%, as judged by the urinary excretion. Clioquinol is excreted in the urine mainly in glucuronide form and to a smaller extent as sulphate, whereas unchanged clioquinol is found in traces only.

There are no pharmacokinetic data available on hydrocortisone for the combination of Vioform Hydrocortisone.

5.3 Preclinical safety data

Not applicable.

6. PHARMACEUTICAL PARTICULARS

6.1 List of excipients

Cream: Glycerol

Sodium lauryl sulphate

2-Phenoxyethanol

Cetostearyl alcohol

Cetyl palmitate

White soft paraffin

Purified water

Ointment: Light liquid paraffin

Soft white paraffin

6.2 Incompatibilities

None

6.3 Shelf life

60 months.

6.4 Special precautions for storage

Protect from heat.

6.5 Nature and contents of container

Collapsible aluminium tube.

Pack size: 30g.

6.6 Instructions for use and handling

Medicines should be kept out of the reach of children.

7. MARKETING AUTHORISATION HOLDER

Novartis Consumer Health UK Ltd

Trading as Novartis Consumer Health

Wimblehurst Road

Horsham

West Sussex, RH12 5AB

Trading style: Novartis Consumer Health

8. MARKETING AUTHORISATION NUMBER(S)

Vioform Hydrocortisone Cream PL 0030/0050

Vioform Hydrocortisone Ointment PL 0030/0051

9. DATE OF FIRST AUTHORISATION/RENEWAL OF THE AUTHORISATION

PL 0030/0050 Granted: 14 January 1991; Date of renewal: 14 January 1996

PL 0030/0051 Granted: 14 January 1991; Date of renewal: 21 November 1995

10. DATE OF REVISION OF THE TEXT

18 March 1997

Additional information

Legal category:

Prescription only

Viracept Film-coated Tablets

(Roche Products Limited)

1. NAME OF THE MEDICINAL PRODUCT

VIRACEPT 250 mg film-coated tablets.

2. QUALITATIVE AND QUANTITATIVE COMPOSITION

VIRACEPT 250 mg film-coated tablets contain 292.25 mg of nelfinavir mesilate corresponding to 250 mg of nelfinavir (as free base). For excipients, see section 6.1.

3. PHARMACEUTICAL FORM

Film-coated tablets.

4. CLINICAL PARTICULARS

4.1 Therapeutic indications

VIRACEPT is indicated in antiretroviral combination treatment of human immunodeficiency virus (HIV-1) infected adults, adolescents and children of 3 years of age and older.

In protease inhibitor (PI) experienced patients the choice of nelfinavir should be based on individual viral resistance testing and treatment history.

See section 5.1.

4.2 Posology and method of administration

Therapy with VIRACEPT should be initiated by a physician experienced in the management of HIV infection.

VIRACEPT film-coated tablets are administered orally and should always be ingested with food (see section 5.2).

Patients older than 13 years: the recommended dosage of VIRACEPT film-coated tablets is 1250 mg (five 250 mg tablets) twice a day (BID) or 750 mg (three 250 mg tablets) three times a day (TID) by mouth.

The efficacy of the BID regimen has been evaluated versus the TID regimen primarily in patients naïve to PIs (see section 5.1, pharmacodynamic properties).

Patients aged 3 to 13 years: for children, the recommended starting dose is 50-55 mg/kg BID or, if using a TID regimen, 25 – 30 mg/kg body weight per dose. For children unable to take tablets, VIRACEPT oral powder may be administered (see Summary of Product Characteristics for VIRACEPT oral powder).

The recommended dose of VIRACEPT film-coated tablets to be administered **BID to children aged 3 to 13 years** is as follows:

Body Weight kg	Number of VIRACEPT 250 mg film-coated tablets per dose*
18 to < 22	4
⩾ 22	5

The recommended dose of VIRACEPT film-coated tablets to be administered **TID to children aged 3 to 13 years** is as follows:

Body Weight kg	Number of VIRACEPT 250 mg film-coated tablets per dose*
18 to < 23	2
⩾ 23	3

*see Summary of Product Characteristics for VIRACEPT oral powder for patients with less than 18 kg body weight.

Renal and hepatic impairment: there are no data specific for patients with renal impairment and therefore specific dosage recommendations cannot be made. Nelfinavir is principally metabolised and eliminated by the liver. There are not sufficient data from patients with liver impairment and therefore specific dose recommendations cannot be made (see section 5.2). Caution should be used when administering VIRACEPT to patients with impaired renal or hepatic function.

4.3 Contraindications

Hypersensitivity to the active substance or to any of the excipients.

Co-administration with medicinal products with narrow therapeutic windows and which are substrates of CYP3A4 (e.g., terfenadine, astemizole, cisapride, amiodarone, quinidine, pimozide, triazolam, midazolam, ergot derivatives; see section 4.5).

Co-administration with rifampicin (see section 4.5).

Herbal preparations containing St. John's wort *(Hypericum perforatum)* must not be used while taking nelfinavir due to the risk of decreased plasma concentrations and reduced clinical effects of nelfinavir (see section 4.5).

4.4 Special warnings and special precautions for use

Patients should be instructed that VIRACEPT is not a cure for HIV infection, that they may continue to develop infections or other illnesses associated with HIV disease, and that VIRACEPT has not been shown to reduce the risk of transmission of HIV disease through sexual contact or blood contamination.

For use during pregnancy and lactation, see section 4.6.

Immune Reactivation Syndrome:

In HIV-infected patients with severe immune deficiency at the time of institution of combination antiretroviral therapy (CART), an inflammatory reaction to asymptomatic or residual opportunistic pathogens may arise and cause serious clinical conditions, or aggravation of symptoms. Typically, such reactions have been observed within the first few weeks or months of initiation of CART. Relevant examples are cytomegalovirus retinitis, generalised and/or focal mycobacterium infections, and *Pneumocystis carinii* pneumonia. Any inflammatory symptoms should be evaluated and treatment instituted when necessary.

Liver Disease:

The safety and efficacy of nelfinavir has not been established in patients with significant underlying liver disorders. Patients with chronic hepatitis B or C and treated with combination antiretroviral therapy are at an increased risk for severe and potentially fatal hepatic adverse events. In case of concomitant antiviral therapy for hepatitis B or C, please refer also to the relevant product information for these medicinal products.

Patients with pre-existing liver dysfunction including chronic active hepatitis have an increased frequency of liver function abnormalities during combination antiretroviral therapy and should be monitored according to standard practice. If there is evidence of worsening liver disease in such patients, interruption or discontinuation of treatment must be considered.

Renal Impairment:

Caution should be used when administering VIRACEPT to patients with impaired renal function (see section 4.2).

The safety and activity of nelfinavir in children below the age of 3 years have not been established.

Caution is advised whenever VIRACEPT is co-administered with medicinal products which are inducers or inhibitors and/or substrates of CYP3A4; such combinations may require dose adjustment (see also sections 4.3, 4.5 and 4.8).

The HMG-CoA reductase inhibitors simvastatin and lovastatin are highly dependent on CYP3A4 for metabolism, thus concomitant use of VIRACEPT with simvastatin or lovastatin is not recommended due to an increased risk of myopathy including rhabdomyolysis. Caution must also be exercised if VIRACEPT is used concurrently with atorvastatin, which is metabolised to a lesser extent by CYP3A4. In this situation a reduced dose of atorvastatin should be considered. If treatment with a HMG-CoA reductase inhibitor is indicated, pravastatin or fluvastatin is recommended (see section 4.5).

Particular caution should be used when prescribing sildenafil in patients receiving PIs, including nelfinavir. Co-administration of a PI with sildenafil is expected to substantially increase sildenafil concentration and may result in an increase in sildenafil associated adverse events, including hypotension, visual changes, and priapism (see section 4.5).

Potent inducers of CYP3A (e.g., phenobarbital and carbamazepine) may reduce nelfinavir plasma concentrations. Physicians should consider using alternatives when a patient is taking VIRACEPT (see sections 4.3 and 4.5).

VIRACEPT may lead to a decreased AUC of phenytoin; therefore phenytoin concentrations should be monitored during concomitant use with VIRACEPT (see section 4.5).

Methadone AUC may be decreased when co-administered with VIRACEPT; therefore upward adjustment of methadone dose may be required during concomitant use with VIRACEPT (see section 4.5).

Co-administration of the combination oral contraceptive containing norethindrone and 17 α-ethinylestradiol with VIRACEPT resulted in a decrease in AUC of the contraceptive drug; therefore alternative contraceptive measure should also be considered (see section 4.5).

New onset diabetes mellitus, hyperglycaemia or exacerbation of existing diabetes mellitus has been reported in patients receiving PIs. In some of these the hyperglycaemia was severe and in some cases also associated with ketoacidosis. Many patients had confounding medical conditions, some of which required therapy with agents that have been associated with the development of diabetes or hyperglycaemia.

There have been reports of increased bleeding, including spontaneous skin haematomas and haemarthroses, in haemophiliac patients type A and B treated with PIs. In some patients additional factor VIII was given. In more than half of the reported cases, treatment with PIs was continued or reintroduced if treatment had been discontinued. A causal relationship has been evoked, although the mechanism of action has not been elucidated. Haemophiliac patients should therefore be made aware of the possibility of increased bleeding.

Combination antiretroviral therapy has been associated with the redistribution of body fat (lipodystrophy) in HIV patients. The long-term consequences of these events are currently unknown. Knowledge about the mechanism is incomplete. A connection between visceral lipomatosis and PIs and lipoatrophy and nucleoside analogue reverse transcriptase inhibitors (NRTIs) has been hypothesised. A higher risk of lipodystrophy has been associated with individual factors such as older age, and with drug related factors such as longer duration of antiretroviral treatment and associated metabolic disturbances. Clinical examination should include evaluation for physical signs of fat redistribution. Consideration should be given to the measurement of fasting serum lipids and blood glucose. Lipid disorders should be managed as clinically appropriate (see section 4.8).

4.5 Interaction with other medicinal products and other forms of Interaction

Nelfinavir is primarily metabolised via the cytochrome P450 isoenzymes CYP3A and CYP2C19 (see section 5.2). Co-administration with medicinal products that are substrates for CYP3A4 and which have narrow therapeutic windows (e.g., terfenadine, astemizole, cisapride, amiodarone, quinidine, pimozide, triazolam, midazolam, ergot derivatives) is contraindicated (see section 4.3 and below).

Caution should be used when co-administering medicinal products that induce CYP3A or potentially toxic medicinal products which are themselves metabolised by CYP3A (see section 4.3 and below). Based on *in vitro* data, nelfinavir is unlikely to inhibit other cytochrome P450 isoforms at concentrations in the therapeutic range.

Other antiretrovirals:

Nucleoside Analogue Reverse Transcriptase Inhibitors (NRTIs):

Clinically significant interactions have not been observed between nelfinavir and nucleoside analogues (specifically zidovudine plus lamivudine, stavudine, and stavudine plus didanosine). At present, there is no evidence of inadequate efficacy of zidovudine in the CNS that could be associated with the modest reduction in plasma levels of zidovudine when coadministered with nelfinavir. Since it is recommended that didanosine be administered on an empty stomach, VIRACEPT should be administered (with food) one hour after or more than 2 hours before didanosine.

Other Protease Inhibitors (PIs)

Ritonavir: administration of a single 750 mg dose of nelfinavir following 3 doses of ritonavir 500 mg BID resulted in a 152 % increase in AUC and a 156 % increase in the elimination half-life of nelfinavir. Administration of a single 500 mg dose of ritonavir following six doses of nelfinavir 750 mg TID resulted in minimal increase (8 %) in ritonavir plasma AUC.

Addition of low dose ritonavir (either 100 or 200 mg BID) to nelfinavir 1250 mg BID resulted in a 20 % increase in nelfinavir plasma AUC after morning administration and a 39 % increase after evening administration at steady state. The AUC of the nelfinavir metabolite M8 increased by 74 % and 86 % after morning and evening administrations, respectively (see section 5.2 regarding the formation and further metabolism of M8). There were no significant differences between low doses of ritonavir (either 100 or 200 mg BID) for effects on AUCs of nelfinavir and M8. The clinical relevance of these findings has not been established.

Indinavir: administration of a single 750 mg dose of nelfinavir following indinavir 800 mg every 8 hours for 7 days resulted in an 83 % increase in nelfinavir plasma AUC and a 22 % increase in the elimination half-life of nelfinavir. Administration of a single 800 mg dose of indinavir following nelfinavir 750 mg TID for 7 days resulted in a 51 % increase in indinavir plasma AUC concentrations, with a 5-fold increase in trough concentrations measured at 8 hours, but no increase in peak concentrations. The safety of this combination has not been established.

Saquinavir soft gelatin capsule: administration of a single 750 mg dose of nelfinavir following 4 days of saquinavir soft gelatin capsule 1200 mg TID resulted in a 30 % increase in nelfinavir plasma AUC. Administration of a single 1200 mg dose of saquinavir soft gelatin capsule following 4 days of nelfinavir 750 mg TID resulted in a 392 % increase in saquinavir plasma AUC.

Amprenavir: Co-administration of amprenavir 800 mg TID with nelfinavir 750 mg TID resulted in a small increase in nelfinavir and amprenavir plasma AUC and a 189 % increase in amprenavir C_{min}. No dose adjustment is necessary for either medicinal product when nelfinavir is administered in combination with amprenavir.

Non-nucleoside Analogue Reverse Transcriptase Inhibitors (NNRTIs):

Efavirenz: Co-administration of efavirenz 600 mg once daily (qd) with nelfinavir 750 mg TID increased nelfinavir AUC by 20 % with no change in efavirenz AUC. A dose adjustment is not needed when efavirenz is administered with VIRACEPT.

Delavirdine: Co-administration of nelfinavir 750 mg TID with delavirdine 400 mg TID resulted in a 107 % increase in nelfinavir AUC and a 31 % decrease in delavirdine AUC. The safety of this drug combination has not been established and this combination is not recommended.

Nevirapine: Current evidence suggests that there is unlikely to be a clinically relevant interaction when nelfinavir 750 mg TID and nevirapine 200 mg BID are co-administered. A dose adjustment is not needed when nevirapine is administered with VIRACEPT.

Metabolic enzyme inducers: rifampicin decreases nelfinavir plasma AUC by 82 % and its concomitant use with nelfinavir is contraindicated (see section 4.3). Other potent inducers of CYP3A (e.g., phenobarbital, carbamazepine) may also reduce nelfinavir plasma concentrations. If therapy with such medicinal products is warranted, physicians should consider using alternatives when a patient is taking VIRACEPT.

Rifabutin: Co-administration of nelfinavir 750 mg TID and rifabutin 300 mg once a day results in a 32 % decrease in nelfinavir plasma AUC and a 207 % increase in rifabutin plasma AUC (see also section 4.4). Co-administration of nelfinavir 750 mg TID with half the standard dose of rifabutin 150 mg once a day resulted in a 23 % decrease in nelfinavir plasma AUC and an 83 % increase in rifabutin plasma AUC. In contrast co-administration of VIRACEPT 1250 mg BID with half the standard dose of rifabutin 150 mg qd resulted in no change in nelfinavir plasma AUC. Dosage reduction of rifabutin to 150 mg once a day is necessary when nelfinavir 750 mg TID or 1250 mg BID and rifabutin are co-administered.

Phenytoin: Co-administration of nelfinavir 1250 mg BID with phenytoin 300 mg once a day did not change the concentration of nelfinavir. However, AUC values of phenytoin and free phenytoin were reduced by 29 % and 28 % by co-administration of nelfinavir, respectively. No dose adjustment for nelfinavir is recommended. Phenytoin concentrations should be monitored during co-administration with nelfinavir.

St. John's wort *(Hypericum perforatum)*: Plasma levels of nelfinavir can be reduced by concomitant use of the herbal preparation St. John's wort *(Hypericum perforatum)*. This is due to induction of drug metabolising enzymes and/or transport proteins by St. John's wort. Herbal preparations containing St. John's wort must not be used concomitantly with VIRACEPT. If a patient is already taking St. John's wort, stop St. John's wort, check viral levels and if possible nelfinavir levels. Nelfinavir levels may increase on stopping St. John's wort, and the dose of VIRACEPT may need adjusting. The inducing effect of St. John's wort may persist for at least 2 weeks after cessation of treatment (see section 4.3).

Metabolic enzyme inhibitors: co-administration of nelfinavir and a strong inhibitor of CYP3A, ketoconazole, resulted in a 35 % increase in nelfinavir plasma AUC. This change is not considered clinically significant and no dose adjustment is needed when ketoconazole and VIRACEPT are co-administered. Based on the metabolic profiles, a clinically relevant drug interaction would not be expected with other specific inhibitors of CYP3A (e.g., fluconazole, itraconazole, clarithromycin, erythromycin); however, the possibility cannot be excluded.

Co-administration of nelfinavir with inhibitors of CYP2C19 (e.g., fluconazole, fluoxetine, paroxetine, omeprazole, lansoprazole, imipramine, amitriptyline and diazepam) may be expected to reduce the conversion of nelfinavir to its major active metabolite M8 (*tert-butyl* hydroxy nelfinavir) with a concomitant increase in plasma nelfinavir levels (see section 5.2). Limited clinical trial data from patients receiving one or more of these medicinal products with nelfinavir indicated that a clinically significant effect on safety and efficacy is not expected. However, such an effect cannot be ruled out.

HMG-CoA reductase inhibitors which are highly dependent on CYP3A4 metabolism, such as lovastatin and simvastatin, are expected to have markedly increased plasma concentrations when co-administered with VIRACEPT. Co-administration of nelfinavir 1250 mg BID and simvastatin 20 mg once a day increased the plasma AUC of simvastatin by 506 %. Since increased concentrations of HMG-CoA reductase inhibitors may cause myopathy, including rhabdomyolysis, the combination of these medicinal products with VIRACEPT is not recommended. Atorvastatin is less dependent on CYP3A4 for metabolism. Co-administration of nelfinavir 1250 mg BID and atorvastatin 10 mg once a day increased the AUC of atorvastatin by 74 %. When used with VIRACEPT, the lowest possible dose of atorvastatin should be administered. The metabolism of pravastatin and fluvastatin is not dependent on CYP3A4, and interactions are not expected with PIs. If treatment with a HMG-CoA reductase inhibitor is indicated, pravastatin or fluvastatin is recommended.

Methadone: Co-administration of nelfinavir 1250 mg BID with methadone 80 +/- 21 mg once a day in HIV negative methadone maintenance patients resulted in a 47 % decrease in methadone AUC. None of the subjects experienced withdrawal symptoms in this study; however, due to the pharmacokinetic changes, it should be expected that some patients who received this drug combination may experience withdrawal symptoms and require an upward adjustment of the methadone dose.

Other potential interactions (see also section 4.3): Nelfinavir increases terfenadine plasma concentrations; therefore, VIRACEPT must not be administered concurrently with terfenadine because of the potential for serious and/or life-threatening cardiac arrhythmias. Because similar interactions are likely with astemizole and cisapride, VIRACEPT must not be administered concurrently with these drugs. Although specific studies have not been done, potent sedatives metabolised by CYP3A, such as triazolam or midazolam, must not be co-administered with VIRACEPT due to the potential for prolonged sedation or respiratory depression resulting from competitive inhibition of the metabolism of these medicinal products when they are co-administered.

Similarly, concomitant administration of nelfinavir with any of amiodarone, quinidine, pimozide and ergot derivatives is contraindicated. For other compounds that are substrates for CYP3A (e.g. calcium channel blockers including bepridil, immunosuppressants including tacrolimus and ciclosporin and sildenafil) plasma concentrations may be elevated when co-administered with VIRACEPT; therefore, patients should be monitored for toxicities associated with such medicinal products.

Oral contraceptives: administration of nelfinavir 750 mg TID and a combination oral contraceptive which included 0.4 mg of norethindrone and 35 μg of 17 α-ethinylestradiol for 7 days resulted in a 47 % decrease in ethinylestradiol and an 18 % decrease in norethindrone plasma AUC. Alternative contraceptive measures should be considered.

4.6 Pregnancy and lactation

No treatment-related adverse effects were seen in animal reproductive toxicity studies in rats at doses providing systemic exposure comparable to that observed with the clinical dose. Clinical experience in pregnant women is limited. VIRACEPT should be given during pregnancy only if the expected benefit justifies the possible risk to the foetus.

It is recommended that HIV-infected women must not breast-feed their infants under any circumstances in order to avoid transmission of HIV. Studies in lactating rats showed that nelfinavir is excreted in breast milk. There is no data available on nelfinavir excretion into human breast milk. Mothers must be instructed to discontinue breast-feeding if they are receiving VIRACEPT.

4.7 Effects on ability to drive and use machines

VIRACEPT has no or negligible influence on the ability to drive and use machines.

4.8 Undesirable effects

Experience from clinical trials with the VIRACEPT 250 mg tablet

The safety of the VIRACEPT 250 mg tablet was studied in controlled clinical trials with over 1300 patients.

The majority of patients in these studies received either 750 mg TID either alone or in combination with nucleoside analogues or 1250 mg BID in combination with nucleoside analogues.

The most frequently reported adverse drug reaction among patients (n=514) receiving VIRACEPT in two phase III, double-blind studies was diarrhoea (70.6 %, n=350). Diarrhoea was of mild or moderate intensity in 97.7 % of these 350 patients. Although formal analyses of the time to onset of diarrhoea were not performed, onset of diarrhoea generally occurs shortly after beginning treatment with VIRACEPT; onset of diarrhoea is less likely to occur in patients who have been receiving VIRACEPT for longer periods of time. In addition, over 4000 patients ⩾ 13 years in the expanded access programmes received VIRACEPT at a dose of 750 mg TID. The majority of adverse events were of mild intensity.

Across the two phase III, double-blind studies adverse reactions of moderate to severe intensity reported by investigators as at least possibly related to VIRACEPT or of unknown relationship in ≥ 2 % of patients treated with the 750 mg TID dose of VIRACEPT (n = 200) in combination with nucleoside analogues (for 24 weeks) included the following undesirable effects:

Gastrointestinal disorders: diarrhoea (25.9 %), flatulence (2.5 %), nausea (4.5 %),

Skin and subcutaneous tissue disorders: rash (3.0 %).

Safety data up to 48 weeks is available from 554 patients in the study comparing 1250 mg VIRACEPT BID (n=344) versus 750 mg VIRACEPT TID (n=210), each in combination with lamivudine and stavudine. The incidence of adverse reactions of moderate to severe intensity reported by investigators as at least possibly related to VIRACEPT or of unknown relationship in ⩾ 2 % of patients treated was similar for the BID and TID arms: diarrhoea (21.2 % versus 18.2 %), nausea (2.9 % versus 3.3 %) and rash (1.7 % versus 1.4 %).

Marked clinical laboratory abnormalities (change from grade 0 to grade 3 or 4, or change from grade 1 to grade 4) reported in ⩾ 2 % of patients treated with 750 mg TID of VIRACEPT (for 24 weeks) across the same studies included increased creatine kinase (3.9 %), and decreased neutrophils (4.5 %). Marked increases in transaminases occurred in less than 2 % of patients receiving VIRACEPT 750 mg TID and were sometimes accompanied by clinical signs and symptoms of acute hepatitis. Some of these patients were known to be chronic carriers of hepatitis B and/or C viruses. With the exception of diarrhoea, there were no significant differences in the adverse experiences reported by patients treated with VIRACEPT versus the control arms containing zidovudine plus lamivudine or stavudine alone.

In the study comparing VIRACEPT 1250 mg BID with VIRACEPT 750 mg TID each in combination with lamivudine and stavudine, the incidence of marked clinical laboratory abnormalities (change from grade 0 to grade 3 or 4, or change from grade 1 to grade 4) reported in ⩾ 2 % of patients was: AST (2 % versus 1 %), ALT (3 % versus 0 %), neutropenia (2 % versus 1 %).

Post marketing experience

The following additional adverse reactions have been reported in the post-marketing experience:

Infections and infestations:

Rare (⩾0.01 % - ⩽ 0.1%): hepatitis, abnormal liver enzymes and jaundice when nelfinavir is used in combination with other antiretroviral agents.

Immune system disorders:

Uncommon (⩾ 0.1 % - ⩽ 0.1 %): hypersensitivity reactions including bronchospasm, fever, pruritus, facial oedema and rash (maculopapular or bullous).

Metabolism and nutrition disorders:

Rare (⩾ 0.01 % - ⩽ 0.1 %): new onset diabetes mellitus, or exacerbation of existing diabetes mellitus.

Vascular disorders:

Rare (⩾ 0.01 % - ⩽ 0.1 %): increased spontaneous bleeding in patients with haemophilia.

Gastrointestinal disorders:

Rare (⩾ 0.01 % - ⩽ 0.1 %): abdominal distension,

Uncommon (⩾ 0.1 % - ⩽ 1 %): vomiting, pancreatitis/increased amylase.

Skin and subcutaneous tissue disorders:

Uncommon - rare (⩾ 0.01 % - ⩽ 1 %): Combination antiretroviral therapy has been associated with redistribution of body fat (lipodystrophy) in HIV patients including the loss of peripheral and facial subcutaneous fat, increased intra-abdominal and visceral fat, breast hypertrophy and dorsocervical fat accumulation (buffalo hump).

Very rare (⩽ 0.01 %), including isolated reports: Erythema multiforme.

Musculoskeletal and connective tissue disorders:

Rare (⩾ 0.01 % - ⩽ 0.1 %): Increased CPK, myalgia, myositis and rhabdomyolysis have been reported with PIs, particularly in combination with nucleoside analogues.

Combination antiretroviral therapy has been associated with metabolic abnormalities such as hypertriglyceridaemia, hypercholesterolaemia, insulin resistance, hyperglycaemia and hyperlactaemia (see section 4.4).

In HIV-infected patients with severe immune deficiency at the time of initiation of combination antiretroviral therapy (CART), an inflammatory reaction to asymptomatic or residual opportunistic infections may arise (see section 4.4).

4.9 Overdose

Human experience of acute overdose with VIRACEPT is limited. There is no specific antidote for overdose with nelfinavir. If indicated, elimination of unabsorbed nelfinavir should be achieved by emesis or gastric lavage. Administration of activated charcoal may also be used to aid removal of unabsorbed nelfinavir. Since nelfinavir is highly protein bound, dialysis is unlikely to significantly remove it from blood.

Overdoses of nelfinavir could theoretically be associated with prolongation of the QT-interval of the ECG (see also section 5.3). Monitoring of overdosed patients is warranted.

5. PHARMACOLOGICAL PROPERTIES

5.1 Pharmacodynamic properties

Pharmacotherapeutic group: antiviral agent, ATC code: J05A E04

Mechanism of action: HIV protease is an enzyme required for the proteolytic cleavage of the viral polyprotein precursors to the individual proteins found in infectious HIV. The cleavage of these viral polyproteins is essential for the maturation of infectious virus. Nelfinavir reversibly binds to the active site of HIV protease and prevents cleavage of the polyproteins resulting in the formation of immature non-infectious viral particles.

Antiviral activity *in vitro*: the antiviral activity of nelfinavir *in vitro* has been demonstrated in both HIV acute and chronic infections in lymphoblastoid cell lines, peripheral blood lymphocytes and monocytes/macrophages. Nelfinavir was found to be active against a broad range of laboratory strains and clinical isolates of HIV-1 and the HIV-2 strain ROD. The EC_{95} (95 % effective concentration) of nelfinavir ranged from 7 to 111 nM (mean of 58 nM). Nelfinavir demonstrated additive to synergistic effects against HIV in combination with reverse transcriptase inhibitors zidovudine (ZDV), lamivudine (3TC), didanosine (ddI), zalcitabine (ddC) and stavudine (d4T) without enhanced cytotoxicity.

Drug Resistance: HIV isolates with reduced susceptibility to nelfinavir have been selected *in vitro*. HIV isolates from selected patients treated with nelfinavir alone or in combination with reverse transcriptase inhibitors were monitored for phenotypic (n=19) and genotypic (n=195, 157 of which were assessable) changes in clinical trials over a period of 2 to 82 weeks. One or more viral protease mutations at amino acid positions 30, 35, 36, 46, 71, 77 and 88 were detected in > 10 % of patients with assessable isolates. Of 19 patients for whom both phenotypic and genotypic analyses were performed on clinical isolates, 9 patients isolates showed reduced susceptibility (5- to 93-fold) to nelfinavir *in vitro*. Isolates from all 9 patients possessed one or more mutations in the viral protease gene. Amino acid position 30 appeared to be the most frequent mutation site.

The overall incidence of the D30N mutation in the viral protease of assessable isolates (n=157) from patients receiving nelfinavir monotherapy or nelfinavir in combination with zidovudine and lamivudine or stavudine was 54.8 %. The overall incidence of other mutations associated with primary PI resistance was 9.6 % for the L90M substitution where as substitutions at 48, 82 and 84 were not observed.

Cross resistance: HIV isolates obtained from 5 patients during nelfinavir therapy showed a 5- to 93-fold decrease in nelfinavir susceptibility *in vitro* when compared to matched baseline isolates but did not demonstrate a concordant decrease in susceptibility to indinavir, ritonavir, saquinavir or amprenavir *in vitro*. Conversely, following ritonavir therapy, 6 of 7 clinical isolates with decreased ritonavir susceptibility (8- to 113-fold) *in vitro* compared to baseline also exhibited decreased susceptibility to nelfinavir *in vitro* (5- to 40 fold). An HIV isolate obtained from a patient receiving saquinavir therapy showed decreased susceptibility to saquinavir (7- fold) but did not demonstrate a concordant decrease in susceptibility to nelfinavir. Cross-resistance between nelfinavir and reverse transcriptase inhibitors is unlikely because different enzyme targets are involved. Clinical isolates (n=5) with decreased susceptibility to zidovudine, lamivudine, or nevirapine remain fully susceptible to nelfinavir *in vitro*.

Clinical pharmacodynamic data: treatment with nelfinavir alone or in combination with other antiretroviral agents has been documented to reduce viral load and increase CD4 cell counts in HIV-1 seropositive patients. Decreases in HIV RNA observed with nelfinavir monotherapy were less pronounced and of shorter duration. The effects of nelfinavir (alone or combined with other antiretroviral agents) on biological markers of disease activity, CD4 cell count and viral RNA, were evaluated in several studies involving HIV-1 infected patients.

The efficacy of the BID regimen has been evaluated versus the TID regimen with VIRACEPT 250 mg tablets primarily in patients naïve to PIs. A randomised open-label study compared the HIV RNA suppression of nelfinavir 1250 mg BID versus nelfinavir 750 mg TID in PI naïve patients also receiving stavudine (30-40 mg BID) and lamivudine (150 mg BID).

(see Table 1 on next page)

The BID regimen produced statistically significantly higher peak nelfinavir plasma levels versus the TID regimen. Small, non-statistically significant differences were observed in other pharmacokinetic parameters with no trend favouring one regimen over the other. Although study 542 showed no statistically significant differences between

Table 3

Proportion of patients with HIV RNA below LOQ (sensitive and ultrasensitive assays) at Week 48				
Assay	**Analysis**	**Viracept BID (%)**	**Viracept TID (%)**	**95% CI**
Sensitive	Observed data	135/164 (82%)	146/169 (86%)	(-12, +4)
	LOCF	145/200 (73%)	161/206 (78%)	(-14, +3)
	ITT (NC = F)	135/200 (68%)	146/206 (71%)	(-12, +6)
Ultrasensitive	Observed data	114/164 (70%)	125/169 (74%)	(-14, +5)
	LOCF	121/200 (61%)	136/206 (66%)	(-15, +4)
	ITT (NC = F)	114/200 (57%)	125/206 (61%)	(-13, +6)

LOCF= Last observation carried forward
ITT = Intention to Treat
NC = F: non-completers = failures

the two regimens in efficacy in a predominantly antiretroviral naïve patient population, the significance of these findings for antiretroviral experienced patients is unknown.

In a study of 297 HIV-1 seropositive patients receiving zidovudine and lamivudine plus nelfinavir (2 different doses) or zidovudine and lamivudine alone, the mean baseline CD4 cell count was 288 cells/mm^3 and the mean baseline plasma HIV RNA was 5.21 log_{10} copies/ml (160,394 copies/ml). The mean decrease in plasma HIV RNA using a PCR assay (< 400 copies/ml) at 24 weeks was 2.33 log_{10} in patients receiving combination therapy with nelfinavir 750 mg TID, compared to 1.34 log_{10} in patients receiving zidovudine and lamivudine alone. At 24 weeks, the percentage of patients whose plasma HIV RNA levels had decreased to below the limit of detection of the assay (< 400 copies/ml) were 81 % and 8 % for the groups treated with nelfinavir 750 mg TID plus zidovudine and lamivudine or zidovudine and lamivudine, respectively. Mean CD4 cell counts at 24 weeks were increased by 150 and 95 cells/mm^3 for the groups treated with nelfinavir 750 mg TID plus zidovudine and lamivudine or zidovudine and lamivudine, respectively. At 48 weeks, approximately 75 % of the patients treated with nelfinavir 750 mg TID plus zidovudine and lamivudine remained below the level of detection of the assay (< 400 copies/ml); mean increase in CD4 cell counts was 198 cells/mm^3 at 48 weeks in this group.

No important differences in safety or tolerability were observed between the BID and TID dosing groups, with the same proportion of patients in each arm experiencing adverse events of any intensity, irrespective of relationship to trial medication.

5.2 Pharmacokinetic properties

The pharmacokinetic properties of nelfinavir have been evaluated in healthy volunteers and HIV-infected patients. No substantial differences have been observed between healthy volunteers and HIV-infected patients.

Absorption: after single or multiple oral doses of 500 to 750 mg (two to three 250 mg tablets) with food, peak nelfinavir plasma concentrations were typically achieved in 2 to 4 hours. After multiple dosing with 750 mg every 8 hours for 28 days (steady-state), peak plasma concentrations (C_{max}) averaged 3-4 μg/ml and plasma concentrations prior to the next dose (trough) were 1-3 μg/ml. A greater than dose-proportional increase in nelfinavir plasma concentrations was observed after single doses; however, this was not observed after multiple dosing.

A pharmacokinetic study in HIV-positive patients compared multiple doses of 1250 mg twice daily (BID) with multiple doses of 750 mg three times daily (TID) for 28 days. Patients receiving VIRACEPT BID (n=10) achieved nelfinavir C_{max} of 4.0 ± 0.8 μg/ml and morning and evening trough concentrations of 2.2 ± 1.3 μg/ml and 0.7 ± 0.4 μg/ml, respectively. Patients receiving VIRACEPT TID (n=11) achieved nelfinavir peak plasma concentrations (C_{max}) of 3.0 ± 1.6 μg/ml and morning and evening trough concentrations of 1.4 ± 0.6 μg/ml and 1.0 ± 0.5 μg/ml, respectively. The difference between morning and afternoon or evening trough concentrations for the TID and BID regimens was also observed in healthy volunteers who were dosed at precise 8- or 12-hour intervals.

The pharmacokinetics of nelfinavir are similar during BID and TID administration. In patients, the nelfinavir AUC_{0-24} with 1250 mg BID administration was 52.8 ± 15.7 μg>/>h/ml (n=10) and with 750 mg TID administration was 43.6 ± 17.8 μg>/>h/ml (n=11). Trough drug exposures remain at least twenty fold greater than the mean IC95 throughout the dosing interval for both regimens. The clinical relevance of relating *in vitro* measures to drug potency and clinical outcome has not been established. A greater than dose-proportional increase in nelfinavir plasma concentrations was observed after single doses; however, this was not observed after multiple dosing.

The absolute bioavailability of VIRACEPT has not been determined.

Effect of food on gastrointestinal absorption: maximum plasma concentrations and area under the plasma concentration-time curve were consistently 2 to 3-fold higher under fed conditions compared to fasting. The increased plasma concentrations with food were independent of fat content of the meals. The effect of meal content on nelfinavir exposure was investigated in a study using the 250 mg film-coated tablets formulation. Steady state nelfinavir AUC and C_{max} were respectively 15 % and 20 % higher when doses followed a 800 kcal/50 % fat meal compared to those following a light meal (350 kcal/33 % fat), suggesting that meal content has less effect on nelfinavir exposures during multiple dosing than would be anticipated based on data from single dose studies.

Distribution: in both animals and humans, the estimated volumes of distribution (2-7 l/kg) exceeded total body water, suggesting extensive penetration of nelfinavir into tissues. Although no studies have been conducted in humans, studies with a single 50 mg/kg dose of ^{14}C-nelfinavir in rats showed that concentrations in the brain were lower than in other tissues, but exceeded the *in vitro* EC_{95} for antiviral activity. Nelfinavir in serum is extensively protein-bound ⩾(98 %).

Metabolism: unchanged nelfinavir comprised 82-86 % of the total plasma radioactivity after a single oral 750 mg dose of ^{14}C-nelfinavir. *In vitro*, multiple cytochrome P-450 isoforms including CYP3A, CYP2C19/C9 and CYP2D6 are responsible for metabolism of nelfinavir. One major and several minor oxidative metabolites were found in plasma.

The major oxidative metabolite, M8 (*tert-butyl* hydroxy nelfinavir), has *in vitro* antiviral activity equal to the parent drug and its formation is catalysed by the polymorphic cytochrome CYP2C19. The further degradation of M8 appears to be catalysed by CYP3A4. In subjects with normal CYP2C19 activity, plasma levels of this metabolite are approximately 25 % of the total plasma nelfinavir-related concentration. It is expected that in CYP2C19 poor metabolisers or in patients receiving concomitantly strong CYP2C19 inhibitors (see section 4.5), nelfinavir plasma levels would be elevated whereas levels of *tert-butyl* hydroxy nelfinavir would be negligible or non-measurable. Limited clinical data suggest that patients with very low or non-measurable plasma concentrations of the metabolite and elevated concentrations of nelfinavir do not show a reduced virological response or a different safety profile when compared with the whole study population.

Elimination: oral clearance estimates after single doses (24-33 l/h) and multiple doses (26-61 l/h) indicate that nelfinavir exhibits medium to high hepatic bioavailability. The terminal half-life in plasma was typically 3.5 to 5 hours. The majority (87 %) of an oral 750 mg dose containing ^{14}C-nelfinavir was recovered in the faeces; total faecal radioactivity consisted of nelfinavir (22 %) and numerous oxidative metabolites (78 %). Only 1-2 % of the dose was recovered in urine, of which unchanged nelfinavir was the major component.

Pharmacokinetics in special clinical situations:

Pharmacokinetics in children and the elderly: in children between the ages of 2 and 13 years, the clearance of orally administered nelfinavir is approximately 2 to 3 times higher than in adults, with large intersubject variability. Administration of VIRACEPT oral powder or film-coated tablets with food at a dose of approximately 25-30 mg/kg TID achieves steady-state plasma concentrations similar to adult patients receiving 750 mg TID.

In an open prospective study, the pharmacokinetics of BID and TID VIRACEPT regimens in 18 HIV infected children aged 2-14 years were investigated. Children weighing less than 25 kg received 30-37 mg/kg nelfinavir TID or 45-55 mg/kg nelfinavir BID. Children over 25 kg received 750 mg TID or 1250 mg BID.

The C_{min}, C_{max} and AUC_{0-24} were all significantly higher with the BID regimen compared with the TID regimen. In addition, in twice daily application, 14 out of 18 (78 %) and 11 out of 18 (61 %) reached C_{min} values of 1-3 μg/ml and C_{max} values of 3-4 μg/ml, whereas in TID application only 4 out of 18 (22 %) and 7 out of 18 (39 %) reached these values.

There are no data available in the elderly.

Pharmacokinetics in patients with liver impairment:

Pharmacokinetics of nelfinavir after a single dose of 750 mg was studied in patients with liver impairment and healthy volunteers. A 49 %-69 % increase was observed in AUC of nelfinavir in the hepatically impaired groups with impairment (Child-Turcotte Classes A to C) compared to the healthy group. Specific dose recommendations for nelfinavir cannot be made based on the results of this study.

5.3 Preclinical safety data

During *in vitro* studies, cloned human cardiac potassium channels (hERG) were inhibited by high concentrations of nelfinavir and its active metabolite M8. hERG potassium channels were inhibited by 20 % at nelfinavir and M8 concentrations that are about four- to five-fold and seventy-fold, respectively, above the average free therapeutic levels in humans. By contrast, no effects suggesting prolongation of the QT-interval of the ECG were observed at similar doses in dogs or in isolated cardiac tissue. The clinical relevance of these *in vitro* data is unknown. However, based on data from products known to prolong the QT-interval, a block of hERG potassium channels of > 20 % may be clinically relevant. Therefore the potential for QT prolongation should be considered in cases of overdose (see section 4.9).

Acute and chronic toxicity: oral acute and chronic toxicity studies were conducted in the mouse (500 mg/kg/day), rat (up to 1,000 mg/kg/day) and monkey (up to 800 mg/kg/day). There were increased liver weights and dose-related thyroid follicular cell hypertrophy in rats. Weight loss and general physical decline was observed in monkeys together with general evidence of gastrointestinal toxicity.

Mutagenicity: *in vitro* and *in vivo* studies with and without metabolic activation have shown that nelfinavir has no mutagenic or genotoxic activity.

Carcinogenicity: Two year oral carcinogenicity studies with nelfinavir mesilate were conducted in mice and rats. In mice, administration of up to 1000 mg/kg/day did not result in any evidence for an oncogenic effect. In rats administration of 1000 mg/kg/day resulted in increased incidences of thyroid follicular cell adenoma and carcinoma, relative to those for controls. Systemic exposures were 3 to 4 times those for humans given therapeutic doses. Administration of 300 mg/kg/day resulted in an increased incidence of thyroid follicular cell adenoma. Chronic nelfinavir treatment of rats has been demonstrated to produce effects consistent with enzyme induction, which predisposed rats, but not humans, to thyroid neoplasms. The weight of evidence indicates that nelfinavir is unlikely to be a carcinogen in humans.

6. PHARMACEUTICAL PARTICULARS

6.1 List of excipients

Each tablet contains the following excipients:

Tablet core:

Calcium silicate,

Crospovidone,

Magnesium stearate,

Indigo carmine (E132) as powder.

Tablet coat:

Hypromellose,

Glycerol triacetate.

6.2 Incompatibilities

Not applicable.

6.3 Shelf life

3 years.

6.4 Special precautions for storage

Store in the original container. Do not store above 30°C.

6.5 Nature and contents of container

VIRACEPT film-coated tablets are provided in HDPE plastic bottles containing either 270 or 300 tablets, fitted with HDPE child resistant closures with polyethylene liners. A cotton wad is included in the 270 tablet presentation. Not all pack sizes may be marketed.

6.6 Instructions for use and handling

No special requirements.

7. MARKETING AUTHORISATION HOLDER

Roche Registration Limited

40 Broadwater Road

Welwyn Garden City

Hertfordshire, AL7 3AY

United Kingdom

8. MARKETING AUTHORISATION NUMBER(S)

EU/1/97/054/004 - EU/1/97/054/005

9. DATE OF FIRST AUTHORISATION/RENEWAL OF THE AUTHORISATION

5.3.2001- 19.7.2001 / 3.2.2003

10. DATE OF REVISION OF THE TEXT

10 June 2005

Viracept Oral Powder

(Roche Products Limited)

1. NAME OF THE MEDICINAL PRODUCT

VIRACEPT 50 mg/g oral powder.

2. QUALITATIVE AND QUANTITATIVE COMPOSITION

VIRACEPT 50 mg/g oral powder contains 58.45 mg of nelfinavir mesilate corresponding to 50 mg of nelfinavir (as free base) per gram of powder. For excipients, see section 6.1.

3. PHARMACEUTICAL FORM

Oral powder.

4. CLINICAL PARTICULARS

4.1 Therapeutic indications

VIRACEPT is indicated in antiretroviral combination treatment of human immunodeficiency virus (HIV-1) infected adults, adolescents and children of 3 years of age and older.

In protease inhibitor (PI) experienced patients the choice of nelfinavir should be based on individual viral resistance testing and treatment history.

See section 5.1.

4.2 Posology and method of administration

Therapy with VIRACEPT should be initiated by a physician experienced in the management of HIV infection.

VIRACEPT 50 mg/g oral powder should always be ingested with food (see section 5.2).

Patients older than 13 years: VIRACEPT 250 mg tablets are recommended for adults and older children (see Summary of Product Characteristics for VIRACEPT 250 mg tablets). The recommended dose of VIRACEPT 50 mg/g oral powder is 1250 mg twice a day (BID) or 750 mg three times a day (TID), for patients unable to take tablets. All patients older than 13 years should take either 5 level scoops of the 5 gram spoon twice daily or 3 level scoops of the 5 gram spoon three times daily.

The efficacy of the BID regimen has been evaluated versus the TID regimen primarily in patients naïve to PIs (see section 5.1, pharmacodynamic properties).

Patients aged 3 to 13 years: for children, the recommended starting dose is 50-55 mg/kg BID or if using a TID regimen, 25 – 30 mg/kg body weight per dose. For children able to take tablets, VIRACEPT tablets may be administered instead of the oral powder (see Summary of Product Characteristics for VIRACEPT tablets).

The recommended dose of VIRACEPT oral powder to be administered **BID to children aged 3 to 13 years, using a combination of both the 1 gram and 5 gram scoop** is shown in the following table. The prescriber should advise the patient to use the handle of the second scoop to scrape off extra powder and obtain a level scoop.

(see Table 1)

The recommended dose of VIRACEPT oral powder to be administered **TID to children aged 3 to 13 years, using a combination of both the 1 gram and 5 gram scoop** is shown in the following table. The prescriber should advise the patient to use the handle of the second scoop to scrape off extra powder and obtain a level scoop.

(see Table 2)

The oral powder may be mixed with water, milk, formula, soy formula, soy milk, dietary supplements, or pudding. It is recommended that VIRACEPT 50 mg/g oral powder mixed in these media be used within 6 hours. Dosing media not recommended, due to taste, includes any acidic food or juice (e.g., orange juice, apple juice or apple sauce). Do not add water to bottles of VIRACEPT 50 mg/g oral powder.

Renal and hepatic impairment: there are no data specific for patients with renal impairment and therefore specific dosage recommendations cannot be made. Nelfinavir is principally metabolised and eliminated by the liver. There are not sufficient data from patients with liver impairment and therefore specific dose recommendations cannot be made (see section 5.2). Caution should be used when administering VIRACEPT to patients with impaired renal or hepatic function.

4.3 Contraindications

Hypersensitivity to the active substance or to any of the excipients.

Co-administration with medicinal products with narrow therapeutic windows and which are substrates of CYP3A4 (e.g., terfenadine, astemizole, cisapride, amiodarone, quinidine, pimozide, triazolam, midazolam, ergot derivatives; see section 4.5).

Co-administration with rifampicin (see section 4.5).

Herbal preparations containing St. John's wort *(Hypericum perforatum)* must not be used while taking nelfinavir due to the risk of decreased plasma concentrations and reduced clinical effects of nelfinavir (see section 4.5).

4.4 Special warnings and special precautions for use

Patients should be instructed that VIRACEPT is not a cure for HIV infection, that they may continue to develop infections or other illnesses associated with HIV disease, and that VIRACEPT has not been shown to reduce the risk of transmission of HIV disease through sexual contact or blood contamination.

For use during pregnancy and lactation, see section 4.6.

Immune Reactivation Syndrome:

In HIV-infected patients with severe immune deficiency at the time of institution of combination antiretroviral therapy (CART), an inflammatory reaction to asymptomatic or residual opportunistic pathogens may arise and cause serious clinical conditions, or aggravation of symptoms. Typically, such reactions have been observed within the first few weeks or months of initiation of CART. Relevant examples are cytomegalovirus retinitis, generalised and/or focal mycobacterium infections, and *Pneumocystis carinii* pneumonia. Any inflammatory symptoms should be evaluated and treatment instituted when necessary.

Liver Disease:

The safety and efficacy of nelfinavir has not been established in patients with significant underlying liver disorders. Patients with chronic hepatitis B or C and treated with combination antiretroviral therapy are at an increased risk for severe and potentially fatal hepatic adverse events. In case of concomitant antiviral therapy for hepatitis B or C, please refer also to the relevant product information for these medicinal products.

Patients with pre-existing liver dysfunction including chronic active hepatitis have an increased frequency of liver function abnormalities during combination antiretroviral therapy and should be monitored according to standard practice. If there is evidence of worsening liver disease in such patients, interruption or discontinuation of treatment must be considered.

Renal Impairment:

Caution should be used when administering VIRACEPT to patients with impaired renal function (see section 4.2).

The safety and activity of nelfinavir in children below the age of 3 years have not been established.

Caution is advised whenever VIRACEPT is co-administered with medicinal products which are inducers or inhibitors and/or substrates of CYP3A4; such combinations may require dose adjustment (see also sections 4.3, 4.5 and 4.8).

The HMG-CoA reductase inhibitors simvastatin and lovastatin are highly dependent on CYP3A4 for metabolism, thus concomitant use of VIRACEPT with simvastatin or lovastatin is not recommended due to an increased risk of myopathy including rhabdomyolysis. Caution must also be exercised if VIRACEPT is used concurrently with atorvastatin, which is metabolised to a lesser extent by CYP3A4. In this situation a reduced dose of atorvastatin should be considered. If treatment with a HMG-CoA reductase inhibitor is indicated, pravastatin or fluvastatin is recommended (see section 4.5).

Particular caution should be used when prescribing sildenafil in patients receiving PIs, including nelfinavir. Co-administration of a PI with sildenafil is expected to substantially increase sildenafil concentration and may result in an increase in sildenafil associated adverse events, including hypotension, visual changes, and priapism (see section 4.5).

Potent inducers of CYP3A (e.g., phenobarbital and carbamazepine) may reduce nelfinavir plasma concentrations. Physicians should consider using alternatives when a patient is taking VIRACEPT (see sections 4.3 and 4.5).

VIRACEPT may lead to a decreased AUC of phenytoin; therefore phenytoin concentrations should be monitored during concomitant use with VIRACEPT (see section 4.5).

Methadone AUC may be decreased when co-administered with VIRACEPT; therefore upward adjustment of methadone dose may be required during concomitant use with VIRACEPT (see section 4.5).

Co-administration of the combination oral contraceptive containing norethindrone and 17 α-ethinylestradiol with VIRACEPT resulted in a decrease in AUC of the contraceptive drug; therefore alternative contraceptive measure should also be considered (see section 4.5).

VIRACEPT 50 mg/g oral powder contains aspartame as a sweetening agent. Aspartame provides a source of phenylalanine and, therefore, may not be suitable for persons with phenylketonuria.

New onset diabetes mellitus, hyperglycaemia or exacerbation of existing diabetes mellitus has been reported in patients receiving PIs. In some of these the hyperglycaemia was severe and in some cases also associated with ketoacidosis. Many patients had confounding medical conditions, some of which required therapy with agents that have been associated with the development of diabetes or hyperglycaemia.

There have been reports of increased bleeding, including spontaneous skin haematomas and haemarthroses, in haemophiliac patients type A and B treated with PIs. In some patients additional factor VIII was given. In more than half of the reported cases, treatment with PIs was continued or reintroduced if treatment had been discontinued. A causal relationship has been evoked, although the mechanism of action has not been elucidated. Haemophiliac patients should therefore be made aware of the possibility of increased bleeding.

Combination antiretroviral therapy has been associated with the redistribution of body fat (lipodystrophy) in HIV patients. The long-term consequences of these events are currently unknown. Knowledge about the mechanism is incomplete. A connection between visceral lipomatosis and PIs and lipoatrophy and nucleoside analogue reverse transcriptase inhibitors (NRTIs) has been hypothesised. A higher risk of lipodystrophy has been associated with individual factors such as older age, and with drug related

Table 1

Body Weight of the patient kg	Total grams of Powder per dose	White Scoop 1 gram		Blue Scoop 5 gram
7.5 to ⩽ 8.5	8	3	plus	1
> 8.5 to ⩽ 10.5	10	0	plus	2
> 10.5 to ⩽ 12	12	2	plus	2
> 12 to ⩽ 14	14	4	plus	2
> 14 to ⩽ 16	16	1	plus	3
> 16 to ⩽ 18	18	3	plus	3
> 18 to ⩽ 22	21	1	plus	4
> 22	25	0	plus	5

Table 2

Body Weight of the patient kg	Total grams of Powder per dose	White Scoop 1 gram		Blue Scoop 5 gram
7.5 to < 8.5	4	4	plus	0
8.5 to < 10.5	5	0	plus	1
10.5 to < 12	6	1	plus	1
12 to < 14	7	2	plus	1
14 to < 16	8	3	plus	1
16 to < 18	9	4	plus	1
18 to < 23	10	0	plus	2
⩾ 23	15	0	plus	3

factors such as longer duration of antiretroviral treatment and associated metabolic disturbances. Clinical examination should include evaluation for physical signs of fat redistribution. Consideration should be given to the measurement of fasting serum lipids and blood glucose. Lipid disorders should be managed as clinically appropriate (see section 4.8).

4.5 Interaction with other medicinal products and other forms of Interaction

Nelfinavir is primarily metabolised via the cytochrome P450 isoenzymes CYP3A and CYP2C19 (see section 5.2). Co-administration with medicinal products that are substrates for CYP3A4 and which have narrow therapeutic windows (e.g., terfenadine, astemizole, cisapride, amiodarone, quinidine, pimozide, triazolam, midazolam, ergot derivatives) is contraindicated (see section 4.3 and below).

Caution should be used when co-administering medicinal products that induce CYP3A or potentially toxic medicinal products which are themselves metabolised by CYP3A (see section 4.3 and below). Based on *in vitro* data, nelfinavir is unlikely to inhibit other cytochrome P450 isoforms at concentrations in the therapeutic range.

Other antiretrovirals:

Nucleoside Analogue Reverse Transcriptase Inhibitors (NRTIs):

Clinically significant interactions have not been observed between nelfinavir and nucleoside analogues (specifically zidovudine plus lamivudine, stavudine, and stavudine plus didanosine). At present, there is no evidence of inadequate efficacy of zidovudine in the CNS that could be associated with the modest reduction in plasma levels of zidovudine when co-administered with nelfinavir. Since it is recommended that didanosine be administered on an empty stomach, VIRACEPT should be administered (with food) one hour after or more than 2 hours before didanosine.

Other Protease Inhibitors (PIs):

Ritonavir: administration of a single 750 mg dose of nelfinavir following 3 doses of ritonavir 500 mg BID resulted in a 152 % increase in AUC and a 156 % increase in the elimination half-life of nelfinavir. Administration of a single 500 mg dose of ritonavir following six doses of nelfinavir 750 mg TID resulted in minimal increase (8 %) in ritonavir plasma AUC.

Addition of low dose ritonavir (either 100 or 200 mg BID) to nelfinavir 1250 mg BID resulted in a 20 % increase in nelfinavir plasma AUC after morning administration and a 39 % increase after evening administration at steady state. The AUC of the nelfinavir metabolite M8 increased by 74 % and 86 % after morning and evening administrations, respectively (see section 5.2 regarding the formation and further metabolism of M8). There were no significant differences between low doses of ritonavir (either 100 or 200 mg BID) for effects on AUCs of nelfinavir and M8. The clinical relevance of these findings has not been established.

Indinavir: administration of a single 750 mg dose of nelfinavir following indinavir 800 mg every 8 hours for 7 days resulted in an 83 % increase in nelfinavir plasma AUC and a 22 % increase in the elimination half-life of nelfinavir. Administration of a single 800 mg dose of indinavir following nelfinavir 750 mg TID for 7 days resulted in a 51 % increase in indinavir plasma AUC concentrations, with a 5-fold increase in trough concentrations measured at 8 hours, but no increase in peak concentrations. The safety of this combination has not been established.

Saquinavir soft gelatin capsule: administration of a single 750 mg dose of nelfinavir following 4 days of saquinavir soft gelatin capsule 1200 mg TID resulted in a 30 % increase in nelfinavir plasma AUC. Administration of a single 1200 mg dose of saquinavir soft gelatin capsule following 4 days of nelfinavir 750 mg TID resulted in a 392 % increase in saquinavir plasma AUC.

Amprenavir: Co-administration of amprenavir 800 mg TID with nelfinavir 750 mg TID resulted in a small increase in nelfinavir and amprenavir plasma AUC and a 189 % increase in amprenavir C_{min}. No dose adjustment is necessary for either medicinal product when nelfinavir is administered in combination with amprenavir.

Non-nucleoside Analogue Reverse Transcriptase Inhibitors (NNRTIs):

Efavirenz: Co-administration of efavirenz 600 mg once daily (qd) with nelfinavir 750 mg TID increased nelfinavir AUC by 20 % with no change in efavirenz AUC. A dose adjustment is not needed when efavirenz is administered with VIRACEPT.

Delavirdine: Co-administration of nelfinavir 750 mg TID with delavirdine 400 mg TID resulted in a 107 % increase in nelfinavir AUC and a 31 % decrease in delavirdine AUC. The safety of this drug combination has not been established and this combination is not recommended.

Nevirapine: Current evidence suggests that there is unlikely to be a clinically relevant interaction when nelfinavir 750 mg TID and nevirapine 200 mg BID are co-administered. A dose adjustment is not needed when nevirapine is administered with VIRACEPT.

Metabolic enzyme inducers: rifampicin decreases nelfinavir plasma AUC by 82 % and its concomitant use with nelfinavir is contraindicated (see section 4.3). Other potent inducers of CYP3A (e.g., phenobarbital, carbamazepine) may also reduce nelfinavir plasma concentrations. If therapy with such medicinal products is warranted, physicians should consider using alternatives when a patient is taking VIRACEPT.

Rifabutin: Co-administration of nelfinavir 750 mg TID and rifabutin 300 mg once a day results in a 32 % decrease in nelfinavir plasma AUC and a 207 % increase in rifabutin plasma AUC (see also section 4.4). Co-administration of nelfinavir 750 mg TID with half the standard dose of rifabutin 150 mg once a day resulted in a 23 % decrease in nelfinavir plasma AUC and an 83 % increase in rifabutin plasma AUC. In contrast co-administration of VIRACEPT 1250 mg BID with half the standard dose of rifabutin 150 mg qd resulted in no change in nelfinavir plasma AUC. Dosage reduction of rifabutin to 150 mg once a day is necessary when nelfinavir 750 mg TID or 1250 mg BID and rifabutin are co-administered.

Phenytoin: Co-administration of nelfinavir 1250 mg BID with phenytoin 300 mg once a day did not change the concentration of nelfinavir. However, AUC values of phenytoin and free phenytoin were reduced by 29 % and 28 % by co-administration of nelfinavir, respectively. No dose adjustment for nelfinavir is recommended. Phenytoin concentrations should be monitored during co-administration with nelfinavir.

St. John's wort *(Hypericum perforatum)*: Plasma levels of nelfinavir can be reduced by concomitant use of the herbal preparation St. John's wort *(Hypericum perforatum)*. This is due to induction of drug metabolising enzymes and/or transport proteins by St. John's wort. Herbal preparations containing St. John's wort must not be used concomitantly with VIRACEPT. If a patient is already taking St. John's wort, stop St. John's wort, check viral levels and if possible nelfinavir levels. Nelfinavir levels may increase on stopping St. John's wort, and the dose of VIRACEPT may need adjusting. The inducing effect of St. John's wort may persist for at least 2 weeks after cessation of treatment (see section 4.3).

Metabolic enzyme inhibitors: co-administration of nelfinavir and a strong inhibitor of CYP3A, ketoconazole, resulted in a 35 % increase in nelfinavir plasma AUC. This change is not considered clinically significant and no dose adjustment is needed when ketoconazole and VIRACEPT are co-administered. Based on the metabolic profiles, a clinically relevant drug interaction would not be expected with other specific inhibitors of CYP3A (e.g., fluconazole, itraconazole, clarithromycin, erythromycin); however, the possibility cannot be excluded.

Co-administration of nelfinavir with inhibitors of CYP2C19 (e.g., fluconazole, fluoxetine, paroxetine, omeprazole, lansoprazole, imipramine, amitriptyline and diazepam) may be expected to reduce the conversion of nelfinavir to its major active metabolite M8 (*tert-butyl* hydroxy nelfinavir) with a concomitant increase in plasma nelfinavir levels (see section 5.2). Limited clinical trial data from patients receiving one or more of these medicinal products with nelfinavir indicated that a clinically significant effect on safety and efficacy is not expected. However, such an effect cannot be ruled out.

HMG-CoA reductase inhibitors which are highly dependent on CYP3A4 metabolism, such as lovastatin and simvastatin, are expected to have markedly increased plasma concentrations when co-administered with VIRACEPT. Co-administration of nelfinavir 1250 mg BID and simvastatin 20 mg once a day increased the plasma AUC of simvastatin by 506 %. Since increased concentrations of HMG-CoA reductase inhibitors may cause myopathy, including rhabdomyolysis, the combination of these medicinal products with VIRACEPT is not recommended. Atorvastatin is less dependent on CYP3A4 for metabolism. Co-administration of nelfinavir 1250 mg BID and atorvastatin 10 mg once a day increased the AUC of atorvastatin by 74 %. When used with VIRACEPT, the lowest possible dose of atorvastatin should be administered. The metabolism of pravastatin and fluvastatin is not dependent on CYP3A4, and interactions are not expected with PIs. If treatment with a HMG-CoA reductase inhibitor is indicated, pravastatin or fluvastatin is recommended.

Methadone: Co-administration of nelfinavir 1250 mg BID with methadone 80 +/- 21 mg once a day in HIV negative methadone maintenance patients resulted in a 47 % decrease in methadone AUC. None of the subjects experienced withdrawal symptoms in this study; however, due to the pharmacokinetic changes, it should be expected that some patients who received this drug combination may experience withdrawal symptoms and require an upward adjustment of the methadone dose.

Other potential interactions (see also section 4.3): Nelfinavir increases terfenadine plasma concentrations; therefore, VIRACEPT must not be administered concurrently with terfenadine because of the potential for serious and/or life-threatening cardiac arrhythmias. Because similar interactions are likely with astemizole and cisapride, VIRACEPT must not be administered concurrently with these drugs. Although specific studies have not been done, potent sedatives metabolised by CYP3A, such as triazolam or midazolam, must not be co-administered with VIRACEPT due to the potential for prolonged sedation or respiratory depression resulting from competitive inhibition of the metabolism of these medicinal products when they are co-administered.

Similarly, concomitant administration of nelfinavir with any of amiodarone, quinidine, pimozide and ergot derivatives is contraindicated. For other compounds that are substrates for CYP3A (e.g., calcium channel blockers including bepridil, immunosuppressants including tacrolimus and ciclosporin, and sildenafil) plasma concentrations may be elevated when co-administered with VIRACEPT; therefore, patients should be monitored for toxicities associated with such medicinal products.

Oral contraceptives: administration of nelfinavir 750 mg TID and a combination oral contraceptive which included 0.4 mg of norethindrone and 35 μg of 17 α-ethinylestradiol for 7 days resulted in a 47 % decrease in ethinylestradiol and an 18 % decrease in norethindrone plasma AUC. Alternative contraceptive measures should be considered.

4.6 Pregnancy and lactation

No treatment-related adverse effects were seen in animal reproductive toxicity studies in rats at doses providing systemic exposure comparable to that observed with the clinical dose. Clinical experience in pregnant women is limited. VIRACEPT should be given during pregnancy only if the expected benefit justifies the possible risk to the foetus.

It is recommended that HIV-infected women must not breast-feed their infants under any circumstances in order to avoid transmission of HIV. Studies in lactating rats showed that nelfinavir is excreted in breast milk. There is no data available on nelfinavir excretion into human breast milk. Mothers must be instructed to discontinue breast-feeding if they are receiving VIRACEPT.

4.7 Effects on ability to drive and use machines

VIRACEPT has no or negligible influence on the ability to drive and use machines.

4.8 Undesirable effects

Experience from clinical trials with the VIRACEPT 250 mg tablet

The safety of the VIRACEPT 250 mg tablet was studied in controlled clinical trials with over 1300 patients.

The majority of patients in these studies received either 750 mg TID either alone or in combination with nucleoside analogues or 1250 mg BID in combination with nucleoside analogues.

The most frequently reported adverse drug reaction among patients (n=514) receiving VIRACEPT in two phase III, double-blind studies was diarrhoea (70.6 %, n=350). Diarrhoea was of mild or moderate intensity in 97.7 % of these 350 patients. Although formal analyses of the time to onset of diarrhoea were not performed, onset of diarrhoea generally occurs shortly after beginning treatment with VIRACEPT; onset of diarrhoea is less likely to occur in patients who have been receiving VIRACEPT for longer periods of time. In addition, over 4000 patients $\geqslant$ 13 years in the expanded access programmes received VIRACEPT at a dose of 750 mg TID. The majority of adverse events were of mild intensity.

Across the two phase III, double-blind studies adverse reactions of moderate to severe intensity reported by investigators as at least possibly related to VIRACEPT or of unknown relationship in $\geq$ 2 % of patients treated with the 750 mg TID dose of VIRACEPT (n = 200) in combination with nucleoside analogues (for 24 weeks) included the following undesirable effects:

Gastrointestinal disorders: diarrhoea (25.9 %), flatulence (2.5 %), nausea (4.5 %),

Skin and subcutaneous tissue disorders: rash (3.0 %).

Safety data up to 48 weeks is available from 554 patients in the study comparing 1250 mg VIRACEPT BID (n=344) versus 750 mg VIRACEPT TID (n=210), each in combination with lamivudine and stavudine. The incidence of adverse reactions of moderate to severe intensity reported by investigators as at least possibly related to VIRACEPT or of unknown relationship in $\geqslant$ 2 % of patients treated was similar for the BID and TID arms: diarrhoea (21.2 % versus 18.2 %), nausea (2.9 % versus 3.3 %) and rash (1.7 % versus 1.4 %).

Marked clinical laboratory abnormalities (change from grade 0 to grade 3 or 4, or change from grade 1 to grade 4) reported in $\geqslant$ 2 % of patients treated with 750 mg TID of VIRACEPT (for 24 weeks) across the same studies included increased creatine kinase (3.9 %), and decreased neutrophils (4.5 %). Marked increases in transaminases occurred in less than 2 % of patients receiving VIRACEPT 750 mg TID and were sometimes accompanied by clinical signs and symptoms of acute hepatitis. Some of these patients were known to be chronic carriers of hepatitis B and/or C viruses. With the exception of diarrhoea, there were no significant differences in the adverse experiences reported by patients treated with VIRACEPT versus the control arms containing zidovudine plus lamivudine or stavudine alone.

In the study comparing VIRACEPT 1250 mg BID with VIRACEPT 750 mg TID each in combination with lamivudine and stavudine, the incidence of marked clinical laboratory abnormalities (change from grade 0 to grade 3 or 4, or change from grade 1 to grade 4) reported in $\geqslant$ 2 % of patients was: AST (2 % versus 1 %), ALT (3 % versus 0 %), neutropenia (2 % versus 1 %).

Post marketing experience

The following additional adverse reactions have been reported in the post-marketing experience:

Infections and infestations:

Rare (≥ 0.01 % - ≤ 0.1 %): hepatitis, abnormal liver enzymes and jaundice when nelfinavir is used in combination with other antiretroviral agents.

Immune system disorders:

Uncommon (≥ 0.1 % - ≤ 1 %): hypersensitivity reactions including bronchospasm, fever, pruritus, facial oedema and rash (maculopapular or bullous).

Metabolism and nutrition disorders:

Rare (≥ 0.01 % - ≤ 0.1 %): new onset diabetes mellitus, or exacerbation of existing diabetes mellitus.

Vascular disorders:

Rare (≥ 0.01 % - ≤ 0.1 %): increased spontaneous bleeding in patients with haemophilia.

Gastrointestinal disorders:

Rare (≥ 0.01 % - ≤ 0.1 %): abdominal distension,

Uncommon (≥ 0.1 % - ≤ 1 %): vomiting, pancreatitis/increased amylase.

Skin and subcutaneous tissue disorders:

Uncommon - rare (≥ 0.01 % - ≤ 1 %): Combination antiretroviral therapy has been associated with redistribution of body fat (lipodystrophy) in HIV patients including the loss of peripheral and facial subcutaneous fat, increased intra-abdominal and visceral fat, breast hypertrophy and dorsocervical fat accumulation (buffalo hump).

Very rare (≤ 0.01 %), including isolated reports: Erythema multiforme.

Musculoskeletal and connective tissue disorders:

Rare (≥ 0.01 % - ≤ 0.1 %): Increased CPK, myalgia, myositis and rhabdomyolysis have been reported with PIs, particularly in combination with nucleoside analogues.

Combination antiretroviral therapy has been associated with metabolic abnormalities such as hypertriglyceridaemia, hypercholesterolaemia, insulin resistance, hyperglycaemia and hyperlactaemia (see section 4.4).

In HIV-infected patients with severe immune deficiency at the time of initiation of combination antiretroviral therapy (CART), an inflammatory reaction to asymptomatic or residual opportunistic infections may arise (see section 4.4).

4.9 Overdose

Human experience of acute overdose with VIRACEPT is limited. There is no specific antidote for overdose with nelfinavir. If indicated, elimination of unabsorbed nelfinavir should be achieved by emesis or gastric lavage. Administration of activated charcoal may also be used to aid removal of unabsorbed nelfinavir. Since nelfinavir is highly protein bound, dialysis is unlikely to significantly remove it from blood.

Overdoses of nelfinavir could theoretically be associated with prolongation of the QT-interval of the ECG (see also section 5.3). Monitoring of overdosed patients is warranted.

5. PHARMACOLOGICAL PROPERTIES

5.1 Pharmacodynamic properties

Pharmacotherapeutic group: antiviral agent, ATC code: J05A E04.

Mechanism of action: HIV protease is an enzyme required for the proteolytic cleavage of the viral polyprotein precursors to the individual proteins found in infectious HIV. The cleavage of these viral polyproteins is essential for the maturation of infectious virus. Nelfinavir reversibly binds to the active site of HIV protease and prevents cleavage of the polyproteins resulting in the formation of immature non-infectious viral particles.

Antiviral activity *in vitro*: the antiviral activity of nelfinavir *in vitro* has been demonstrated in both HIV acute and chronic infections in lymphoblastoid cell lines, peripheral blood lymphocytes and monocytes/macrophages. Nelfinavir was found to be active against a broad range of laboratory strains and clinical isolates of HIV-1 and the HIV-2 strain ROD. The EC_{95} (95 % effective concentration) of nelfinavir ranged from 7 to 111 nM (mean of 58 nM). Nelfinavir demonstrated additive to synergistic effects against HIV in combination with reverse transcriptase inhibitors zidovudine (ZDV), lamivudine (3TC), didanosine (ddI), zalcitabine (ddC) and stavudine (d4T) without enhanced cytotoxicity.

Drug Resistance: HIV isolates with reduced susceptibility to nelfinavir have been selected *in vitro*. HIV isolates from selected patients treated with nelfinavir alone or in combination with reverse transcriptase inhibitors were monitored for phenotypic (n=19) and genotypic (n=195, 157 of which were assessable) changes in clinical trials over a period of 2 to 82 weeks. One or more viral protease mutations at amino acid positions 30, 35, 36, 46, 71, 77 and 88 were detected in > 10 % of patients with assessable isolates. Of 19 patients for whom both phenotypic and genotypic analyses were performed on clinical isolates, 9 patients isolates showed reduced susceptibility (5- to 93-fold) to nelfinavir *in vitro*. Isolates from all 9 patients possessed one or more mutations in the viral protease gene. Amino acid position 30 appeared to be the most frequent mutation site.

The overall incidence of the D30N mutation in the viral protease of assessable isolates (n=157) from patients receiving nelfinavir monotherapy or nelfinavir in combination with zidovudine and lamivudine or stavudine was 54.8 %. The overall incidence of other mutations associated with primary PI resistance was 9.6 % for the L90M substitution where as substitutions at 48, 82 and 84 were not observed.

Cross resistance: HIV isolates obtained from 5 patients during nelfinavir therapy showed a 5- to 93-fold decrease in nelfinavir susceptibility *in vitro* when compared to matched baseline isolates but did not demonstrate a concordant decrease in susceptibility to indinavir, ritonavir, saquinavir or amprenavir *in vitro*. Conversely, following ritonavir therapy, 6 of 7 clinical isolates with decreased ritonavir susceptibility (8- to 113-fold) *in vitro* compared to baseline also exhibited decreased susceptibility to nelfinavir *in vitro* (5- to 40 fold). An HIV isolate obtained from a patient receiving saquinavir therapy showed decreased susceptibility to saquinavir (7- fold) but did not demonstrate a concordant decrease in susceptibility to nelfinavir. Cross-resistance between nelfinavir and reverse transcriptase inhibitors is unlikely because different enzyme targets are involved. Clinical isolates (n=5) with decreased susceptibility to zidovudine, lamivudine, or nevirapine remain fully susceptible to nelfinavir *in vitro*.

Clinical pharmacodynamic data: treatment with nelfinavir alone or in combination with other antiretroviral agents has been documented to reduce viral load and increase CD4 cell counts in HIV-1 seropositive patients. Decreases in HIV RNA observed with nelfinavir monotherapy were less pronounced and of shorter duration. The effects of nelfinavir (alone or combined with other antiretroviral agents) on biological markers of disease activity, CD4 cell count and viral RNA, were evaluated in several studies involving HIV-1 infected patients.

The efficacy of the BID regimen has been evaluated versus the TID regimen with VIRACEPT 250 mg tablets primarily in patients naïve to PIs. A randomised open-label study compared the HIV RNA suppression of nelfinavir 1250 mg BID versus nelfinavir 750 mg TID in PI naïve patients also receiving stavudine (30-40 mg BID) and lamivudine (150 mg BID).

(see Table 3)

Table 3 Proportion of patients with HIV RNA below LOQ (sensitive and ultrasensitive assays) at Week 48

Assay	Analysis	Viracept BID (%)	Viracept TID (%)	95% CI
Sensitive	Observed data	135/164 (82%)	146/169 (86%)	(-12, +4)
	LOCF	145/200 (73%)	161/206 (78%)	(-14, +3)
	ITT (NC = F)	135/200 (68%)	146/206 (71%)	(-12, +6)
Ultrasensitive	Observed data	114/164 (70%)	125/169 (74%)	(-14, +5)
	LOCF	121/200 (61%)	136/206 (66%)	(-15, +4)
	ITT (NC = F)	114/200 (57%)	125/206 (61%)	(-13, +6)

LOCF= Last observation carried forward

ITT = Intention to Treat

NC = F: non-completers = failures

The BID regimen produced statistically significantly higher peak nelfinavir plasma levels versus the TID regimen. Small, non-statistically significant differences were observed in other pharmacokinetic parameters with no trend favouring one regimen over the other. Although study 542 showed no statistically significant differences between the two regimens in efficacy in a predominantly antiretroviral naïve patient population, the significance of these findings for antiretroviral experienced patients is unknown.

In a study of 297 HIV-1 seropositive patients receiving zidovudine and lamivudine plus nelfinavir (2 different doses) or zidovudine and lamivudine alone, the mean baseline CD4 cell count was 288 cells/mm^3 and the mean baseline plasma HIV RNA was 5.21 $\log_{10}$ copies/ml (160,394 copies/ml). The mean decrease in plasma HIV RNA using a PCR assay (< 400 copies/ml) at 24 weeks was 2.33 $\log_{10}$ in patients receiving combination therapy with nelfinavir 750 mg TID, compared to 1.34 $\log_{10}$ in patients receiving zidovudine and lamivudine alone. At 24 weeks, the percentage of patients whose plasma HIV RNA levels had decreased to below the limit of detection of the assay (< 400 copies/ml) were 81 % and 8 % for the groups treated with nelfinavir 750 mg TID plus zidovudine and lamivudine or zidovudine and lamivudine, respectively. Mean CD4 cell counts at 24 weeks were increased by 150 and 95 cells/mm^3 for the groups treated with nelfinavir 750 mg TID plus zidovudine and lamivudine or zidovudine and lamivudine, respectively. At 48 weeks, approximately 75 % of the patients treated with nelfinavir 750 mg TID plus zidovudine and lamivudine remained below the level of detection of the assay (< 400 copies/ml); mean increase in CD4 cell counts was 198 cells/mm^3 at 48 weeks in this group.

No important differences in safety or tolerability were observed between the BID and TID dosing groups, with the same proportion of patients in each arm experiencing adverse events of any intensity, irrespective of relationship to trial medication.

5.2 Pharmacokinetic properties

The pharmacokinetic properties of nelfinavir have been evaluated in healthy volunteers and HIV-infected patients. No substantial differences have been observed between healthy volunteers and HIV-infected patients.

Absorption: after single or multiple oral doses of 500 to 750 mg (two to three 250 mg tablets) with food, peak nelfinavir plasma concentrations were typically achieved in 2 to 4 hours.

After multiple dosing with 750 mg every 8 hours for 28 days (steady-state), peak plasma concentrations (C_{max}) averaged 3-4 μg/ml and plasma concentrations prior to the next dose (trough) were 1-3 μg/ml. A greater than dose-proportional increase in nelfinavir plasma concentrations was observed after single doses; however, this was not observed after multiple dosing.

A pharmacokinetic study in HIV-positive patients compared multiple doses of 1250 mg twice daily (BID) with multiple doses of 750 mg three times daily (TID) for 28 days. Patients receiving VIRACEPT BID (n=10) achieved nelfinavir C_{max} of 4.0 ± 0.8 μg/ml and morning and evening trough concentrations of 2.2 ± 1.3 μg/ml and 0.7 ± 0.4 μg/ml, respectively. Patients receiving VIRACEPT TID (n=11) achieved nelfinavir peak plasma concentrations (C_{max}) of 3.0 ± 1.6 μg/ml and morning and evening trough concentrations of 1.4 ± 0.6 μg/ml and 1.0 ± 0.5 μg/ml, respectively. The difference between morning and afternoon or evening trough concentrations for the TID and BID regimens was also observed in healthy volunteers who were dosed at precise 8- or 12-hour intervals.

The pharmacokinetics of nelfinavir are similar during BID and TID administration. In patients, the nelfinavir AUC_{0-24} with 1250 mg BID administration was 52.8 ± 15.7 μg>/>h/ml (n=10) and with 750 mg TID administration was 43.6 ± 17.8 μg>/>h/ml (n=11). Trough drug exposures remain at least twenty fold greater than the mean IC95 throughout the dosing interval for both regimens. The clinical relevance of relating *in vitro* measures to drug potency and clinical outcome has not been established. A greater than dose-proportional increase in nelfinavir plasma concentrations was observed after single doses; however, this was not observed after multiple dosing.

The absolute bioavailability of VIRACEPT has not been determined.

Effect of food on gastrointestinal absorption: maximum plasma concentrations and area under the plasma concentration-time curve were consistently 2 to 3-fold higher under fed conditions compared to fasting. The increased plasma concentrations with food were independent of fat content of the meals. The effect of meal content on nelfinavir exposure was investigated in a study using the 250 mg film-coated tablets formulation. Steady state nelfinavir AUC and C_{max} were respectively 15 % and 20 % higher when doses followed a 800 kcal/50 % fat meal compared to those following a light meal (350 kcal/33 % fat), suggesting that meal content has less effect on nelfinavir exposures during multiple dosing than would be anticipated based on data from single dose studies.

Distribution: in both animals and humans, the estimated volumes of distribution (2-7 l/kg) exceeded total body water, suggesting extensive penetration of nelfinavir into tissues. Although no studies have been conducted in humans, studies with a single 50 mg/kg dose of ^{14}C-nelfinavir in rats showed that concentrations in the brain were lower than in other tissues, but exceeded the *in vitro* EC_{95} for antiviral activity. Nelfinavir in serum is extensively protein-bound (≥ 98 %).

Metabolism: unchanged nelfinavir comprised 82-86 % of the total plasma radioactivity after a single oral 750 mg dose of ^{14}C-nelfinavir. *In vitro*, multiple cytochrome P-450 isoforms including CYP3A, CYP2C19/C9 and CYP2D6 are responsible for metabolism of nelfinavir. One major and several minor oxidative metabolites were found in plasma.

The major oxidative metabolite, M8 (*tert-butyl* hydroxy nelfinavir), has *in vitro* antiviral activity equal to the parent drug and its formation is catalysed by the polymorphic cytochrome CYP2C19. The further degradation of M8 appears to be catalysed by CYP3A4. In subjects with normal CYP2C19 activity, plasma levels of this metabolite are approximately 25 % of the total plasma nelfinavir-related concentration. It is expected that in CYP2C19 poor metabolisers or in patients receiving concomitantly strong CYP2C19 inhibitors (see section 4.5), nelfinavir plasma levels would be elevated whereas levels of *tert-butyl* hydroxy nelfinavir would be negligible or non-measurable. Limited clinical data suggest that patients with very low or non-measurable plasma concentrations of the metabolite and elevated concentrations of nelfinavir do not show a reduced virological response or a different safety profile when compared with the whole study population.

Elimination: oral clearance estimates after single doses (24-33 l/h) and multiple doses (26-61 l/h) indicate that nelfinavir exhibits medium to high hepatic bioavailability. The terminal half-life in plasma was typically 3.5 to 5 hours. The majority (87 %) of an oral 750 mg dose containing ^{14}C-nelfinavir was recovered in the faeces; total faecal radioactivity consisted of nelfinavir (22 %) and numerous oxidative metabolites (78 %). Only 1-2 % of the dose was recovered in urine, of which unchanged nelfinavir was the major component.

Pharmacokinetics in special clinical situations:

Pharmacokinetics in children and the elderly: in children between the ages of 2 and 13 years, the clearance of orally administered nelfinavir is approximately 2 to 3 times higher than in adults, with large intersubject variability. Administration of VIRACEPT oral powder or tablets with food at a dose of approximately 25-30 mg/kg TID achieves steady-state plasma concentrations similar to adult patients receiving 750 mg TID.

In an open prospective study, the pharmacokinetics of BID and TID VIRACEPT regimens in 18 HIV infected children aged 2-14 years were investigated. Children weighing less than 25 kg received 30-37 mg/kg nelfinavir TID or 45-55 mg/kg nelfinavir BID. Children over 25 kg received 750 mg TID or 1250 mg BID. The C_{min}, C_{max} and AUC_{0-24} were all significantly higher with the BID regimen compared with the TID regimen. In addition, in twice daily application, 14 out of 18 (78 %) and 11 out of 18 (61 %) reached C_{min} values of 1-3 μg/ml and C_{max} values of 3-4 μg/ml, whereas in TID application only 4 out of 18 (22 %) and 7 out of 18 (39 %) reached these values.

There are no data available in the elderly.

Pharmacokinetics in patients with liver impairment:

Pharmacokinetics of nelfinavir after a single dose of 750 mg was studied in patients with liver impairment and healthy volunteers. A 49 %-69 % increase was observed in AUC of nelfinavir in the hepatically impaired groups with impairment (Child-Turcotte Classes A to C) compared to the healthy group. Specific dose recommendations for nelfinavir cannot be made based on the results of this study.

5.3 Preclinical safety data

During *in vitro* studies, cloned human cardiac potassium channels (hERG) were inhibited by high concentrations of nelfinavir and its active metabolite M8. hERG potassium channels were inhibited by 20 % at nelfinavir and M8 concentrations that are about four- to five-fold and seventy-fold, respectively, above the average free therapeutic levels in humans. By contrast, no effects suggesting prolongation of the QT-interval of the ECG were observed at similar doses in dogs or in isolated cardiac tissue. The clinical relevance of these *in vitro* data is unknown. However, based on data from products known to prolong the QT-interval, a block of hERG potassium channels of > 20 % may be clinically relevant. Therefore the potential for QT prolongation should be considered in cases of overdose (see section 4.9).

Acute and chronic toxicity: oral acute and chronic toxicity studies were conducted in the mouse (500 mg/kg/day), rat (up to 1,000 mg/kg/day) and monkey (up to 800 mg/kg/day). There were increased liver weights and dose-related thyroid follicular cell hypertrophy in rats. Weight loss and general physical decline was observed in monkeys together with general evidence of gastrointestinal toxicity.

Mutagenicity: *in vitro* and *in vivo* studies with and without metabolic activation have shown that nelfinavir has no mutagenic or genotoxic activity.

Carcinogenicity: Two year oral carcinogenicity studies with nelfinavir mesilate were conducted in mice and rats. In mice, administration of up to 1000 mg/kg/day did not result in any evidence for an oncogenic effect. In rats administration of 1000 mg/kg/day resulted in increased incidences of thyroid follicular cell adenoma and carcinoma, relative to those for controls. Systemic exposures were 3 to 4 times those for humans given therapeutic doses. Administration of 300 mg/kg/day resulted in an increased incidence of thyroid follicular cell adenoma. Chronic nelfinavir treatment of rats has been demonstrated to produce effects consistent with enzyme induction, which predisposed rats, but not humans, to thyroid neoplasms. The weight of evidence indicates that nelfinavir is unlikely to be a carcinogen in humans.

6. PHARMACEUTICAL PARTICULARS

6.1 List of excipients

The oral powder contains microcrystalline cellulose, maltodextrin, dibasic potassium phosphate, crospovidone, hydroxypropyl methylcellulose, aspartame (E951), sucrose palmitate, and natural and artificial flavour.

6.2 Incompatibilities

VIRACEPT oral powder should not be mixed with acidic substances due to taste (see section 4.2).

6.3 Shelf life

2 years.

6.4 Special precautions for storage

Store in the original container. Do not store above 30°C.

6.5 Nature and contents of container

VIRACEPT 50 mg/g oral powder is provided in HDPE plastic bottles fitted with polypropylene child resistant closures with a polyethylene liner. Each bottle contains 144 grams of oral powder and is supplied with a 1 gram (white) and a 5 gram (blue) polypropylene scoop.

6.6 Instructions for use and handling

No special requirements.

7. MARKETING AUTHORISATION HOLDER

Roche Registration Limited
40 Broadwater Road
Welwyn Garden City
Hertfordshire, AL7 3AY
United Kingdom

8. MARKETING AUTHORISATION NUMBER(S)

EU/1/97/054/001

9. DATE OF FIRST AUTHORISATION/RENEWAL OF THE AUTHORISATION

22.1.1998 / 3.2.2003

10. DATE OF REVISION OF THE TEXT

10 June 2005

Viraferon 18 million IU, solution for injection, multidose pen

(Schering-Plough Ltd)

1. NAME OF THE MEDICINAL PRODUCT

Viraferon 18 million IU solution for injection, multidose pen

2. QUALITATIVE AND QUANTITATIVE COMPOSITION

One cartridge contains 18 million IU of recombinant interferon alfa-2b* in 1.2 ml.

*produced in *E.coli* by recombinant DNA technology.

One ml contains 15 million IU of interferon alfa-2b.

The pen is designed to deliver its contents of 18 million IU in doses ranging from 1.5 to 6 million IU. The pen will deliver a maximum of 12 doses of 1.5 million IU over a period not to exceed 4 weeks.

For excipients, see section 6.1.

3. PHARMACEUTICAL FORM

Solution for injection

Solution is clear and colourless.

4. CLINICAL PARTICULARS

4.1 Therapeutic indications

Chronic Hepatitis B: Treatment of adult patients with chronic hepatitis B associated with evidence of hepatitis B viral replication (presence of HBV-DNA and HBeAg), elevated ALT and histologically proven active liver inflammation and/or fibrosis.

Chronic Hepatitis C:

Adult patients:

Viraferon is indicated for the treatment of adult patients with chronic hepatitis C who have elevated transaminases without liver decompensation and who are positive for serum HCV-RNA or anti-HCV (see section **4.4**).

The best way to use Viraferon in this indication is in combination with ribavirin.

Chidren and adolescents:

Viraferon is intended for use, in a combination regimen with ribavirin, for the treatment of children and adolescents 3 years of age and older, who have chronic hepatitis C, not previously treated, without liver decompensation, and who are positive for serum HCV-RNA. The decision to treat should be made on a case by case basis, taking into account any evidence of disease progression such as hepatic inflammation and fibrosis, as well as prognostic factors for response, HCV genotype and viral load. The expected benefit of treatment should be weighed against the safety findings observed for paediatric subjects in the clinical trials (see sections **4.4**, **4.8** and **5.1**).

4.2 Posology and method of administration

Viraferon may be administered using either glass or plastic disposable injection syringes.

Not all dosage forms and strengths are appropriate for some indications. Please make sure to select an appropriate dosage form and strength.

Treatment must be initiated by a physician experienced in the management of the disease.

If adverse events develop during the course of treatment with Viraferon for any indication, modify the dosage or discontinue therapy temporarily until the adverse events abate. If persistent or recurrent intolerance develops following adequate dosage adjustment, or disease progresses, discontinue treatment with Viraferon. At the discretion of the physician, the patient may self-administer the dose for maintenance dosage regimens administered subcutaneously.

Chronic Hepatitis B: The recommended dosage is in the range 5 to 10 million IU administered subcutaneously three times a week (every other day) for a period of 4 to 6 months.

The administered dose should be reduced by 50 % in case of occurrence of haematological disorders (white blood cells < 1,500/mm^3, granulocytes < 1,000/mm^3, thrombocytes < 100,000/mm^3). Treatment should be discontinued in case of severe leukopaenia (< 1,200/mm^3), severe neutropaenia (< 750/mm^3) or severe thrombocytopaenia (< 70,000/mm^3).

For all patients, if no improvement on serum HBV-DNA is observed after 3 to 4 months of treatment (at the maximum tolerated dose), discontinue Viraferon therapy.

Chronic Hepatitis C: Viraferon is administered subcutaneously at a dose of 3 million IU three times a week (every other day) to adult patients, whether administered as monotherapy or in combination with ribavirin.

Children 3 years of age or older and adolescents: Interferon alfa-2b 3 MIU/m^2 is administered subcutaneously 3 times a week (every other day) in combination with ribavirin capsules or oral solution administered orally in two divided doses daily with food (morning and evening).

(See ribavirin capsule SPC for dose of ribavirin capsules and dosage modification guidelines for combination therapy. For paediatric patients who weigh < 47 kg or cannot swallow capsules, see ribavirin oral solution SPC).

Relapse patients (adults):

Viraferon is given in combination with ribavirin.

Based on the results of clinical trials, in which data are available for 6 months of treatment, it is recommended that patients be treated with Viraferon in combination with ribavirin for 6 months.

Naïve patients:

Adults: The efficacy of Viraferon is enhanced when given in combination with ribavirin. Viraferon should be given alone mainly in case of intolerance or contraindication to ribavirin.

Viraferon in combination with ribavirin:

Based on the results of clinical trials, in which data are available for 12 months of treatment, it is recommended that patients be treated with Viraferon in combination with ribavirin for at least 6 months.

Treatment should be continued for another 6-month period (i.e., a total of 12 months) in patients who exhibit negative HCV-RNA at month 6, and with viral genotype 1 (as determined in a pre-treatment sample) and high pre-treatment viral load.

Other negative prognostic factors (age > 40 years, male gender, bridging fibrosis) should be taken into account in order to extend therapy to 12 months.

During clinical trials, patients who failed to show a virologic response after 6 months of treatment (HCV-RNA below lower limit of detection) did not become sustained virologic responders (HCV-RNA below lower limit of detection six months after withdrawal of treatment).

Viraferon alone:

The optimal duration of therapy with Viraferon alone is not yet fully established, but a therapy of between 12 and 18 months is advised.

It is recommended that patients be treated with Viraferon alone for at least 3 to 4 months, at which point HCV-RNA status should be determined. Treatment should be continued in patients who exhibit negative HCV-RNA.

Children and adolescents: The efficacy and safety of Viraferon in combination with ribavirin has been studied in children and adolescents who have not been previously treated for chronic hepatitis C.

Genotype 1: The recommended duration of treatment is one year. Patients who fail to achieve virological response at 12 weeks are highly unlikely to become sustained virological responders (negative predictive value 96 %). Virological response is defined as absence of detectable HCV-RNA at Week 12. Treatment should be discontinued in these patients.

Genotype 2/3: The recommended duration of treatment is 24 weeks.

Virological responses after 1 year of treatment and 6 months of follow-up were 36 % for genotype 1 and 81 % for genotype 2/3/4.

4.3 Contraindications

- Hypersensitivity to the active substance or to any of the excipients
- A history of severe pre-existing cardiac disease, e.g., uncontrolled congestive heart failure, recent myocardial infarction, severe arrhythmic disorders
- Severe renal or hepatic dysfunction; including that caused by metastases
- Epilepsy and/or compromised central nervous system (CNS) function (see section **4.4**)
- Chronic hepatitis with decompensated cirrhosis of the liver
- Chronic hepatitis in patients who are being or have been treated recently with immunosuppressive agents excluding short term corticosteroid withdrawal
- Autoimmune hepatitis; or history of autoimmune disease; immunosuppressed transplant recipients

- Pre-existing thyroid disease unless it can be controlled with conventional treatment

Children and adolescents:

- Existence of, or history of severe psychiatric condition, particularly severe depression, suicidal ideation or suicide attempt.

Combination therapy with ribavirin: Also see ribavirin labelling if interferon alfa-2b is to be administered in combination with ribavirin in patients with chronic hepatitis C.

4.4 Special warnings and special precautions for use

For all patients:

Acute hypersensitivity reactions (e.g., urticaria, angioedema, bronchoconstriction, anaphylaxis) to interferon alfa-2b have been observed rarely during Viraferon therapy. If such a reaction develops, discontinue the medication and institute appropriate medical therapy. Transient rashes do not necessitate interruption of treatment.

Moderate to severe adverse experiences may require modification of the patient's dosage regimen, or in some cases, termination of Viraferon therapy. Any patient developing liver function abnormalities during treatment with Viraferon must be monitored closely and treatment discontinued if signs and symptoms progress.

Hypotension may occur during Viraferon therapy or up to two days post-therapy and may require supportive treatment.

Adequate hydration must be maintained in patients undergoing Viraferon therapy since hypotension related to fluid depletion has been seen in some patients. Fluid replacement may be necessary.

While fever may be associated with the flu-like syndrome reported commonly during interferon therapy, other causes of persistent fever must be ruled out.

Viraferon must be used cautiously in patients with debilitating medical conditions, such as those with a history of pulmonary disease (e.g., chronic obstructive pulmonary disease) or diabetes mellitus prone to ketoacidosis. Caution must be observed also in patients with coagulation disorders (e.g., thrombophlebitis, pulmonary embolism) or severe myelosuppression.

Pulmonary infiltrates, pneumonitis, and pneumonia, occasionally resulting in fatality, have been observed rarely in interferon alpha treated patients, including those treated with Viraferon. The aetiology has not been defined. These symptoms have been reported more frequently when shosaikoto, a Chinese herbal medicine, is administered concomitantly with interferon alpha (see section **4.5**). Any patient developing fever, cough, dyspnea or other respiratory symptoms must have a chest X-ray taken. If the chest X-ray shows pulmonary infiltrates or there is evidence of pulmonary function impairment, the patient is to be monitored closely, and, if appropriate, discontinue interferon alpha. While this has been reported more often in patients with chronic hepatitis C treated with interferon alpha, it has also been reported in patients with oncologic diseases treated with interferon alpha. Prompt discontinuation of interferon alpha administration and treatment with corticosteroids appear to be associated with resolution of pulmonary adverse events.

Ocular adverse events (see section **4.8**) including retinal haemorrhages, cotton wool spots, and retinal artery or vein obstruction have been reported in rare instance after treatment with alpha interferons. All patients should have a baseline eye examination. Any patient complaining of changes in visual acuity or visual fields, or reporting other ophthalmologic symptoms during treatment with Viraferon, must have a prompt and complete eye examination. Periodic visual examinations during Viraferon therapy are recommended particularly in patients with disorders that may be associated with retinopathy, such as diabetes mellitus or hypertension. Discontinuation of Viraferon should be considered in patients who develop new or worsening ophthalmological disorders.

Psychiatric and central nervous system (CNS): Severe CNS effects, particularly depression, suicidal ideation and attempted suicide have been observed in some patients during Viraferon therapy, and in the follow-up period. Among children and adolescents treated with Viraferon in combination with ribavirin, suicidal ideation or attempts were reported more frequently compared to adult patients (2.4 % vs 1 %) during treatment and during the 6-month follow-up after treatment. As in adult patients, children and adolescents experienced other psychiatric adverse events (e.g., depression, emotional lability, and somnolence). Other CNS effects including aggressive behaviour (sometimes directed against others), confusion and alterations of mental status have been observed with alpha interferons. If patients develop psychiatric or CNS problems, including clinical depression, it is recommended that the patient be carefully monitored by the prescribing physicians during treatment and in the follow-up period. If such symptoms appear, the potential seriousness of these undesirable effects must be borne in mind by the prescribing physician. If psychiatric symptoms persist or worsen, or suicidal ideation is identified, it is recommended that treatment with Viraferon be discontinued, and the patient followed, with psychiatric intervention, as appropriate.

Patients with existence of or history of severe psychiatric conditions:

If a treatment with interferon alfa-2b is judged necessary in adult patients with existence or history of severe psychiatric conditions, this should only be initiated after having ensured appropriate individualised diagnostic and therapeutic management of the psychiatric condition. The use of interferon alfa-2b in children and adolescents with existence of or history of severe psychiatric conditions is contraindicated (see section **4.3**).

More significant obtundation and coma, including cases of encephalopathy, have been observed in some patients, usually elderly, treated at higher doses. While these effects are generally reversible, in a few patients full resolution took up to three weeks. Very rarely, seizures have occurred with high doses of Viraferon.

Adult patients with a history of congestive heart failure, myocardial infarction and/or previous or current arrhythmic disorders, who require Viraferon therapy, must be closely monitored. It is recommended that those patients who have pre-existing cardiac abnormalities and/or are in advanced stages of cancer have electrocardiograms taken prior to and during the course of treatment. Cardiac arrhythmias (primarily supraventricular) usually respond to conventional therapy but may require discontinuation of Viraferon therapy. There are no data in children or adolescents with a history of cardiac disease.

Hypertriglyceridemia and aggravation of hypertriglyceridemia, sometimes severe, have been observed. Monitoring of lipid levels is, therefore, recommended.

Due to reports of interferon alpha exacerbating pre-existing psoriatic disease and sarcoidosis, use of Viraferon in patients with psoriasis or sarcoidosis is recommended only if the potential benefit justifies the potential risk.

Preliminary data indicates that interferon alpha therapy may be associated with an increased rate of kidney graft rejection. Liver graft rejection has also been reported.

The development of auto-antibodies and autoimmune disorders has been reported during treatment with alpha interferons. Patients predisposed to the development of autoimmune disorders may be at increased risk. Patients with signs or symptoms compatible with autoimmune disorders should be evaluated carefully, and the benefit-risk of continued interferon therapy should be reassessed (see also section **4.4Chronic hepatitis C, Monotherapy** (thyroid abnormalities) and section **4.8**).

Discontinue treatment with Viraferon in patients with chronic hepatitis who develop prolongation of coagulation markers which might indicate liver decompensation.

Appropriate vaccination (hepatitis A and B) should be considered for patients in regular/repeated receipt of human plasma-derived albumin.

Standard measures to prevent infections resulting from the use of medicinal products prepared from human blood or plasma include selection of donors, screening of individual donations and plasma pools for specific markers of infection and the inclusion of effective manufacturing steps for the inactivation/removal of viruses. Despite this, when medicinal products prepared from human blood or plasma are administered, the possibility of transmitting infective agents cannot be totally excluded. This also applies to unknown or emerging viruses and other pathogens.

There are no reports of virus transmissions with albumin manufactured to European Pharmacopoeia specifications by established processes.

It is strongly recommended that every time that Viraferon is administered to a patient, the name and batch number of the product are recorded in order to maintain a link between the patient and the batch of the product.

Chronic Hepatitis C:

Combination therapy with ribavirin: Also see ribavirin labelling if Viraferon is to be administered in combination with ribavirin in patients with chronic hepatitis C.

All patients in the chronic hepatitis C studies had a liver biopsy before inclusion, but in certain cases (i.e. patients with genotype 2 and 3), treatment may be possible without histological confirmation. Current treatment guidelines should be consulted as to whether a liver biopsy is needed prior to commencing treatment.

Monotherapy: Infrequently, adult patients treated for chronic hepatitis C with Viraferon developed thyroid abnormalities, either hypothyroidism or hyperthyroidism. In clinical trials using Viraferon therapy, 2.8 % patients overall developed thyroid abnormalities. The abnormalities were controlled by conventional therapy for thyroid dysfunction. The mechanism by which Viraferon may alter thyroid status is unknown. Prior to initiation of Viraferon therapy for the treatment of chronic hepatitis C, evaluate serum thyroid-stimulating hormone (TSH) levels. Any thyroid abnormality detected at that time must be treated with conventional therapy. Viraferon treatment may be initiated if TSH levels can be maintained in the normal range by medication. Determine TSH levels if, during the course of Viraferon therapy, a patient develops symptoms consistent with possible thyroid dysfunction. In the presence of thyroid dysfunction, Viraferon treatment may be continued if TSH levels can be maintained in the normal range by medication. Discontinuation of Viraferon therapy has not reversed thyroid dysfunction occurring during treatment (also see Children and adolescents, Thyroid monitoring).

Supplemental monitoring specific for children and adolescents

Thyroid Monitoring: Approximately 12 % of children treated with interferon alfa-2b and ribavirin developed increase in TSH. Another 4 % had a transient decrease below the lower limit of normal. Prior to initiation of Viraferon therapy, TSH levels must be evaluated and any thyroid abnormality detected at that time must be treated with conventional therapy. Viraferon therapy may be initiated if TSH levels can be maintained in the normal range by medication. Thyroid dysfunction during treatment with interferon alfa-2b and ribavirin has been observed. If thyroid abnormalities are detected, the patient's thyroid status should be evaluated and treated as clinically appropriate. Children and adolescents should be monitored every 3 months for evidence of thyroid dysfunction (e.g. TSH).

Growth and Development: During a 1-year course of therapy there was a decrease in the rate of linear growth (mean percentile decrease of 9 %) and a decrease in the rate of weight gain (mean percentile decrease of 13 %). A general reversal of these trends was noted during the 6 months follow-up post treatment. However, based on interim data from a long-term follow-up study, 12 (14 %) of 84 children had a > 15 percentile decrease in rate of linear growth, of whom 5 (6 %) children had a > 30 percentile decrease despite being off treatment for more than 1 year. There are no data on long term effects on growth and development and on sexual maturation.

HCV/HIV Coinfection: Patients co-infected with HIV and receiving Highly Active Anti-Retroviral Therapy (HAART) may be at increased risk of developing lactic acidosis. Caution should be used when adding Viraferon and ribavirin to HAART therapy (see ribavirin SPC).

Co-infected patients with advanced cirrhosis receiving HAART may be at increased risk of hepatic decompensation and death. Adding treatment with alfa interferons alone or in combination with ribavirin may increase the risk in this patient subset.

Laboratory Tests:

Standard haematological tests and blood chemistries (complete blood count and differential, platelet count, electrolytes, liver enzymes, serum protein, serum bilirubin and serum creatinine) are to be conducted in all patients prior to and periodically during systemic treatment with Viraferon.

During treatment for hepatitis B or C the recommended testing schedule is at weeks 1, 2, 4, 8, 12, 16, and every other month, thereafter, throughout treatment. If ALT flares during Viraferon therapy to greater than or equal to 2 times baseline, Viraferon therapy may be continued unless signs and symptoms of liver failure are observed. During ALT flare, liver function tests: ALT, prothrombin time, alkaline phosphatase, albumin and bilirubin must be monitored at two-week intervals.

Effect on fertility: Interferon may impair fertility (see section **4.6** and section **5.3**).

4.5 Interaction with other medicinal products and other forms of Interaction

Narcotics, hypnotics or sedatives must be administered with caution when used concomitantly with Viraferon.

Interactions between Viraferon and other medicinal products have not been fully evaluated. Caution must be exercised when administering Viraferon in combination with other potentially myelosuppressive agents.

Interferons may affect the oxidative metabolic process. This must be considered during concomitant therapy with medicinal products metabolised by this route, such as the xanthine derivatives theophylline or aminophylline. During concomitant therapy with xanthine agents, serum theophylline levels must be monitored and dosage adjusted if necessary.

Pulmonary infiltrates, pneumonitis, and pneumonia, occasionally resulting in fatality, have been observed rarely in interferon alpha treated patients, including those treated with Viraferon. The aetiology has not been defined. These symptoms have been reported more frequently when shosaikoto, a Chinese herbal medicine, is administered concomitantly with interferon alpha (see section **4.4**).

(Also see ribavirin labelling if Viraferon is to be administered in combination with ribavirin in patients with chronic hepatitis C).

4.6 Pregnancy and lactation

Women of childbearing potential have to use effective contraception during treatment. Viraferon must be used with caution in fertile men. Decreased serum estradiol and progesterone concentrations have been reported in women treated with human leukocyte interferon.

There are no adequate data from the use of interferon alfa-2b in pregnant women. Studies in animals have shown reproductive toxicity (see section **5.3**). The potential risk for humans is unknown. Viraferon is to be used during pregnancy only if the potential benefit justifies the potential risk to the foetus.

It is not known whether the components of this medicinal product are excreted in human milk. Because of the potential for adverse events from Viraferon in nursing infants, a decision must be made whether to discontinue nursing or to discontinue the medicinal product, taking into account the importance of the treatment to the mother.

Combination therapy with ribavirin: Ribavirin causes serious birth defects when administered during pregnancy. Viraferon in combination with ribavirin is contraindicated (see ribavirin SPC). Females of childbearing potential have to use effective contraception during treatment and for 4 months after treatment.

4.7 Effects on ability to drive and use machines

Patients are to be advised that they may develop fatigue, somnolence, or confusion during treatment with Viraferon, and therefore it is recommended that they avoid driving or operating machinery.

4.8 Undesirable effects

See ribavirin labelling for ribavirin-related undesirable effects if Viraferon is to be administered in combination with ribavirin in patients with chronic hepatitis C.

In clinical trials conducted in a broad range of indications and at a wide range of doses (from 6 MIU/m^2/week in hairy cell leukaemia up to 100 MIU/m^2/week in melanoma), the most commonly reported undesirable effects were fever, fatigue, headache and myalgia. Fever and fatigue were often reversible within 72 hours of interruption or cessation of treatment.

The safety profile shown here was determined from 4 clinical trials in hepatitis C in which patients were treated with Viraferon alone or in combination with ribavirin for one year. All patients in these trials received 3 MIU of Viraferon three times a week. The percentage of patients reporting (treatment related) undesirable effects ⩾ 10 % is presented in **Table 1** as a range to capture the incidences reported in individual treatment groups among these clinical trials in naïve patients treated for one year. Severity was generally mild to moderate.

Table 1. Undesirable effects reported very commonly in any of the clinical trials in naïve patients treated for one year with monotherapy or combination therapy,
Very common (> 1/10) (CIOMS III)

Body System	Viraferon n=806	Viraferon + Rebetol n=1,010
Infections and infestations		
Infection viral	0-7 %	3-10 %
Metabolism and nutrition disorders		
Weight decrease	6-11 %	9-19 %
Psychiatric disorders		
Depression	16-36 %	25-34 %
Irritability	13-27 %	18-34 %
Insomnia	21-28 %	33-41 %
Anxiety	8-12 %	8-16 %
Concentration impaired	8-14 %	9-21 %
Emotional lability	5-8 %	5-11 %
Nervous system disorders		
Headache	51-64 %	48-64 %
Respiratory, thoracic and mediastinal disorders		
Pharyngitis	3-7 %	7-13 %
Coughing	3-7 %	8-11 %
Dyspnoea	2-9 %	10-22 %
Gastrointestinal disorders		
Nausea/Vomiting	18-31 %/ 3-10 %	25-44 %/ 6-10 %
Anorexia	14-19 %	19-26 %
Diarrhoea	12-22 %	13-18 %
Abdominal pain	9-17 %	9-14 %
Skin and subcutaneous tissue disorders		
Alopecia	22-31 %	26-32 %
Pruritus	6-9 %	18-27 %
Skin dry	5-8 %	10-21 %
Rash	5-7 %	15-24 %
Musculoskeletal and connective tissue disorders		
Myalgia	41-61 %	30-62 %
Arthralgia	25-31 %	21-29 %
Musculoskeletal pain	15-20 %	11-20 %
General disorders and administration site conditions		
Injection site inflammation	9-16 %	6-17 %
Injection site reaction	5-8 %	3-36 %
Fatigue	42-70 %	43-68 %
Rigors	15-39 %	19-41 %
Fever	29-39 %	29-41 %
Flu-like symptoms	19-37 %	18-29 %
Asthenia	9-30 %	9-30 %
Dizziness	8-18 %	10-22 %

Table 2. Undesirable effects reported commonly in clinical trials of 483 patients treated with Viraferon + Ribavirin
(Viraferon 3 MIU 3 times a week, ribavirin > 10.6 mg/kg for one year)
Common (> 1/100, < 1/10)
(CIOMS III)

Body System	Viraferon + Rebetol
Infections and infestations 1-5 %	Herpes simplex (resistance)
Blood and lymphatic system disorders 5-10 %: 1-5 %:	Leukopaenia Thrombocytopaenia, lymphadenopathy, lymphopenia
Endocrine disorders 1-5 %:	Hyperthyroidism, hypothyroidism
Metabolism and nutrition disorders 1-5 %:	Hyperuricemia, hypocalcemia, thirst
Psychiatric disorders 5-10 %: 1-5 %:	Agitation, nervousness Sleep disorder, somnolence, libido decreased
Nervous system disorders 5-10 %: 1-5 %:	Mouth dry, sweating increased Hypoesthesia, vertigo, confusion, parasthesia, tremor, migraine, flushing, lacrimal gland disorder
Eye disorders 5-10 %: 1-5 %:	Vision blurred Conjunctivitis, eye pain, vision abnormal
Ear and labyrinth disorders 1-5 %:	Tinnitus
Cardiac disorders 1-5 %:	Palpitation, tachycardia
Vascular disorders 1-5 %:	Hypertension
Respiratory, thoracic and mediastinal disorders 1-5 %:	Bronchitis, cough nonproductive, epistaxis, nasal congestion, respiratory disorder, rhinitis, rhinorrhea, sinusitis
Gastrointestinal disorders 5-10 %: 1-5 %:	Dyspepsia, stomatitis Constipation, dehydration, gingivitis, glossitis, loose stools, stomatitis ulcerative, taste perversion
Hepatobiliary disorders 1-5 %:	Hepatomegaly
Skin and subcutaneous tissue disorders 1-5 %:	Eczema, psoriasis (new or aggravated), rash erythematous, rash maculopapular, skin disorder, erythema
Musculoskeletal and connective tissue disorders 1-5 %:	Arthritis
Renal and urinary disorders 1-5 %:	Micturition frequency
Reproductive system and breast disorders 1-5 %:	Amenorrhea, breast pain, dysmenorrhea, menorrhagia, menstrual disorder, vaginal disorder
General disorders and administration site conditions 5-10 %: 1-5 %:	Malaise, chest pain Injection site pain, right upper quadrant pain

These undesirable effects have also been reported with Viraferon alone.

Additional adverse events were reported rarely (> 1/10,000, < 1/1,000) or very rarely (< 1/10,000) during clinical trials in other indications or following the marketing of interferon alfa-2b:

Immune system disorders:

very rarely: sarcoidosis or exacerbation of sarcoidosis

Endocrine disorders:

very rarely: diabetes, aggravated diabetes

Metabolism and nutrition disorders:

very rarely: hyperglycaemia, hypertriglyceridaemia

Psychiatric disorders:

rarely: suicide ideation

very rarely: aggressive behaviour (sometimes directed against others), suicide attempts, suicide, psychosis, including hallucinations

Nervous system disorders:

very rarely: impaired consciousness, neuropathy, polyneuropathy, seizure, encephalopathy, cerebrovascular ischaemia, cerebrovascular haemorrhage

Eye disorders:

rarely: retinal haemorrhages, retinopathies (including macular oedema), cotton-wool spots, retinal artery or vein obstruction, loss of visual acuity or visual field, optic neuritis and papilloedema

Ear and labyrinth disorders:

very rarely: hearing disorder, hearing loss

Cardiac disorders:

very rarely: cardiac ischaemia and myocardial infarction

Vascular disorders:

very rarely: hypotension; peripheral ischaemia

Respiratory, thoracic and mediastinal disorders:

rarely: pneumonia

very rarely: pulmonary infiltrates, pneumonitis

Gastrointestinal:

very rarely: pancreatitis; increased appetite; gingival bleeding; colitis, mainly ulcerative and ischemic

Hepatobiliary disorders:

very rarely: hepatotoxicity, including fatality

Skin and subcutaneous tissue disorders:

very rarely: face oedema, erythema multiforme, Stevens Johnson syndrome, toxic epidermal necrolysis, injection site necrosis

Musculoskeletal and connective tissue disorders:

very rarely: rhabdomyolysis, sometimes serious; leg cramps; back pain; myositis

Renal and urinary disorders:

very rarely: nephrotic syndrome, renal insufficiency, renal failure

Very rarely Viraferon used alone or in combination with ribavirin may be associated with aplastic anaemia.

Cardiovascular (CVS) adverse events, particularly arrhythmia, appeared to be correlated mostly with pre-existing CVS disease and prior therapy with cardiotoxic agents (see section **4.4**). Cardiomyopathy, that may be reversible upon discontinuation of interferon alpha, has been reported rarely in patients without prior evidence of cardiac disease.

A wide variety of autoimmune and immune-mediated disorders have been reported with alpha interferons including thyroid disorders, systemic lupus erythematosus, rheumatoid arthritis (new or aggravated), idiopathic and thrombotic thrombocytopenic purpura, vasculitis, neuropathies including mononeuropathies (see also section **4.4**).

Clinically significant laboratory abnormalities, most frequently occurring at doses greater than 10 million IU daily, include reduction in granulocyte and white blood cell counts; decreases in haemoglobin level and platelet count; increases in alkaline phosphatase, LDH, serum creatinine and serum urea nitrogen levels. Increase in serum ALT/AST (SGPT/SGOT) levels have been noted as an abnormality in some non-hepatitis subjects and also in some patients with chronic hepatitis B coincident with clearance of viral DNAp.

For safety with respect to transmissible agents, see section **4.4**.

Children and adolescents – Chronic Hepatitis C

In clinical trials of 118 children or adolescents 3 to 16 years of age, 6 % discontinued therapy due to adverse events. In general, the adverse event profile in the limited paediatric population studied was similar to that observed in adults, although there is a paediatric specific concern regarding growth inhibition as decrease in height (mean percentile decrease of growth velocity of 9 %) and weight (mean percentile decrease of 13 %) percentile were observed during treatment (see section **4.4**). Furthermore, suicidal ideation or attempts were reported more frequently compared to adult patients (2.4 % vs 1 %) during treatment and during the 6 month follow-up after treatment. As in adult patients, children and adolescents also experienced other psychiatric adverse events (e.g., depression, emotional lability, and somnolence) (see section **4.4**). In addition, injection site disorders, fever, anorexia, vomiting, and emotional lability occurred more frequently in children and adolescents compared to adult patients. Dose modifications were required in 30 % of patients, most commonly for anaemia and neutropaenia.

Undesirable effects reported in paediatric clinical trials, and not previously reported at an incidence ⩾ 1 % in adults, are shown in **Table 3**. All effects reported at a ⩾ 10 % incidence in paediatric trials were previously reported in adults (**Table 2**) and are not repeated in the paediatric table.

(see Table 3 opposite)

4.9 Overdose

No case of overdose has been reported that has led to acute clinical manifestations. However, as for any pharmacologically active compound, symptomatic treatment with frequent monitoring of vital signs and close observation of the patient is indicated.

5. PHARMACOLOGICAL PROPERTIES

5.1 Pharmacodynamic properties

Pharmacotherapeutic group: Immunostimulants, cytokines and immunomodulators, interferons, interferon alfa-2b, ATC code: L03A B05

Viraferon is a sterile, stable, formulation of highly purified interferon alfa-2b produced by recombinant DNA techniques. Recombinant interferon alfa-2b is a water-soluble protein with a molecular weight of approximately 19,300 daltons. It is obtained from a clone of E. coli, which harbours a genetically engineered plasmid hybrid encompassing an interferon alfa-2b gene from human leukocytes.

The activity of Viraferon is expressed in terms of IU, with 1 mg of recombinant interferon alfa-2b protein corresponding to 2.6×10^8 IU. International Units are determined by comparison of the activity of the recombinant interferon alfa-2b with the activity of the international reference preparation of human leukocyte interferon established by the World Health Organisation.

The interferons are a family of small protein molecules with molecular weights of approximately 15,000 to 21,000 daltons. They are produced and secreted by cells in response to viral infections or various synthetic and biological inducers. Three major classes of interferons have been identified: alpha, beta and gamma. These three main classes are themselves not homogeneous and may contain several different molecular species of interferon. More than 14 genetically distinct human alpha interferons have been identified. Viraferon has been classified as recombinant interferon alfa-2b.

Interferons exert their cellular activities by binding to specific membrane receptors on the cell surface. Human interferon receptors, as isolated from human lymphoblastoid (Daudi) cells, appear to be highly asymmetric proteins. They exhibit selectivity for human but not murine interferons, suggesting species specificity. Studies with other interferons have demonstrated species specificity. However, certain monkey species, eg, rhesus monkeys, are susceptible to pharmacodynamic stimulation upon exposure to human type 1 interferons.

The results of several studies suggest that, once bound to the cell membrane, interferon initiates a complex sequence of intracellular events that include the induction of certain enzymes. It is thought that this process, at least in part, is responsible for the various cellular responses to interferon, including inhibition of virus replication in virus-infected cells, suppression of cell proliferation and such immunomodulating activities as enhancement of the phagocytic activity of macrophages and augmentation of the specific cytotoxicity of lymphocytes for target cells. Any or all of these activities may contribute to interferon's therapeutic effects.

Recombinant interferon alfa-2b has exhibited antiproliferative effects in studies employing both animal and human cell culture systems as well as human tumour xenografts in animals. It has demonstrated significant immunomodulatory activity *in vitro*.

Recombinant interferon alfa-2b also inhibits viral replication *in vitro* and *in vivo*. Although the exact antiviral mode of action of recombinant interferon alfa-2b is unknown, it appears to alter the host cell metabolism. This action inhibits viral replication or if replication occurs, the progeny virions are unable to leave the cell.

<u>Chronic hepatitis B:</u>

Current clinical experience in patients who remain on interferon alfa-2b for 4 to 6 months indicates that therapy can produce clearance of serum HBV-DNA. An improvement in liver histology has been observed. In adult patients with loss of HBeAg and HBV-DNA, a significant reduction in morbidity and mortality has been observed.

Interferon alfa-2b (6 MIU/m^2 3 times a week for 6 months) has been given to children with chronic active hepatitis B. Because of a methodological flaw, efficacy could not be demonstrated. Moreover children treated with interferon alfa-2b experienced a reduced rate of growth and some cases of depression were observed.

<u>Chronic hepatitis C:</u>

In adult patients receiving interferon in combination with ribavirin, the achieved sustained response rate is 47 %. Superior efficacy has been demonstrated with the combination of pegylated interferon with ribavirin (sustained response rate of 61 % achieved in a study performed in naïve patients with a ribavirin dose > 10.6 mg/kg, $p < 0.01$).

Table 3 Undesirable effects very commonly and commonly reported in paediatric clinical trials (⩾ 1 % of patients treated with Viraferon + ribavirin) Very common (> 1/10) - Common (> 1/100, < 1/10)

Body system	⩾ 10%	5 % - < 10 %	1 % - < 5 %
Infection and infestations	Viral infection		Tooth abscess, bacterial infection, fungal infection, herpes simplex, otitis media
Neoplasms benign, malignant and unspecified (including cysts and polyps)			Neoplasm (unspecified),
Blood and lymphatic system disorders	Anaemia, neutropenia		Bruise, thrombocytopaenia, lymphadenopathy
Endocrine disorders	Hypothyroidism		Hyperthyroidism, virilism,
Metabolism and nutrition disorders			Hypertriglyceridemia, hyperuricemia
Psychiatric disorders	Depression, emotional lability, insomnia, irritability	Agitation, somnolence	Aggressive reaction, anxiety, apathy, increased appetite, behavior disorder, concentration impaired, abnormal dreaming, nervousness, sleep disorder, somnambulism, suicidal ideation
Nervous system disorders	Headache, dizziness	Tremor	Confusion, hyperkinesia, dysphonia, paresthaesia, hyperaesthesia, hypoaesthesia
Eye disorders			Conjunctivitis, eye pain, abnormal vision,, lacrimal gland disorder
Vascular disorders		Pallor	Raynaud's disease
Respiratory, thoracic and mediastinal disorders	Pharyngitis	Epistaxis	Coughing, dyspnoea, nasal congestion, nasal irritation, pulmonary infection, rhinorrhea, sneezing, tachypnea
Gastrointestinal disorders	Abdominal pain, anorexia, diarrhoea, nausea, vomiting		Constipation, dyspepsia, gastroenteritis, gastroesophogeal reflux, gastrointestinal disorder, glossitis, loose stools, mouth ulceration, rectal disorder, stomatitis, stomatitis ulcerative, toothache, tooth disorder
Hepatobiliary disorders			Hepatic function abnormal
Skin and subcutaneous tissue disorders	Alopecia, rash	Pruritus	Acne, eczema, skin laceration, nail disorder, dry skin, photosensitivity reaction, maculopapular rash, skin discolouration, skin disorder, erythema, sweating increased
Musculoskeletal and connective tissue disorders	Arthralgia, musculoskeletal pain, myalgia		
Renal and urinary disorders			Enuresis, micturition disorder, urinary tract infection, urinary incontinence
Reproductive system and breast disorders			<u>Female</u>: amenorrhea, menorrhagia, menstrual disorder, vaginal disorder, vaginitis <u>Male</u>: testicular pain
General disorders and administration site conditions	Injection site reaction, injection site inflammation, fatigue, fever, rigors, influenza-like symptoms, malaise, growth rate decrease (height and/or weight decrease for age)	Injection site pain	Asthenia, flushing, oedema, chest pain, right upper quadrant pain

Adult patients: Viraferon alone or in combination with ribavirin has been studied in 4 randomised Phase III clinical trials in 2,552 interferon-naïve patients with chronic hepatitis C. The trials compared the efficacy of Viraferon used alone or in combination with ribavirin. Efficacy was defined as sustained virologic response, 6 months after the end of treatment. Eligible patients for these trials had chronic hepatitis C confirmed by a positive HCV-RNA polymerase chain reaction assay (PCR) (> 100 copies/ml), a liver

Table 4 Sustained virologic response rates with Viraferon + ribavirin (one year of treatment) by genotype and viral load

HCV Genotype	I N=503 C95-132/I95-143	I/R N=505 C95-132/I95-143	I/R N=505 C/I98-580
All Genotypes	**16 %**	**41 %**	**47 %**
Genotype 1	9 %	29 %	33 %
Genotype 1 ⩽ 2 million copies/ml	25 %	33 %	45 %
Genotype 1 > 2 million copies/ml	3 %	27 %	29 %
Genotype 2/3	31 %	65 %	79 %

I   Viraferon (3 MIU 3 times a week)

I/R   Viraferon (3 MIU 3 times a week) + ribavirin (1,000/1,200 mg/day)

biopsy consistent with a histologic diagnosis of chronic hepatitis with no other cause for the chronic hepatitis, and abnormal serum ALT.

Viraferon was administered at a dose of 3 MIU 3 times a week as monotherapy or in combination with ribavirin. The majority of patients in these clinical trials were treated for one year. All patients were followed for an additional 6 months after the end of treatment for the determination of sustained virologic response. Sustained virologic response rates for treatment groups treated for one year with Viraferon alone or in combination with ribavirin (from two studies) are shown in **Table 4**.

Co-administration of Viraferon with ribavirin increased the efficacy of Viraferon by at least two fold for the treatment of chronic heptatitis C in naïve patients. HCV genotype and baseline virus load are prognostic factors which are known to affect response rates. The increased response rate to the combination of Viraferon + ribavirin, compared with Viraferon alone, is maintained across all subgroups. The relative benefit of combination therapy with Viraferon + ribavirin is particularly significant in the most difficult to treat subgroup of patients (genotype 1 and high virus load) (**Table 4**).

Response rates in these trials were increased with compliance. Regardless of genotype, patients who received Viraferon in combination with ribavirin and received ⩾ 80 % of their treatment had a higher sustained response 6 months after 1 year of treatment than those who took < 80 % of their treatment (56 % vs. 32 % in trial C/I98-580).

(see Table 4 above)

Relapse patients: A total of 345 interferon alpha relapse patients were treated in two clinical trials with Viraferon monotherapy or in combination with ribavirin. In these patients, the addition of ribavirin to Viraferon increased by as much as 10-fold the efficacy of Viraferon used alone in the treatment of chronic hepatitis C (48.6 % vs. 4.7 %). This enhancement in efficacy included loss of serum HCV (< 100 copies/ml by PCR), improvement in hepatic inflammation, and normalisation of ALT, and was sustained when measured 6 months after the end of treatment.

Clinical trials in paediatric patients with chronic hepatitis C:

Children and adolescents 3 to 16 years of age with compensated chronic hepatitis C and detectable HCV-RNA (assessed by a central laboratory using a research-based RT-PCR assay) were enrolled in two multicentre trials and received Viraferon 3 MIU/m² 3 times a week plus ribavirin 15 mg/kg per day for 1 year followed by 6 months follow-up after-treatment. A total of 118 patients were enrolled: 57 % male, 80 % Caucasian, and 78 % genotype 1, 64 % ⩽ 12 years of age. The population enrolled mainly consisted in children with mild to moderate hepatitis C. Sustained virological response rates in children and adolescents were similar to those in adults. Due to the lack of data in children with severe progression of the disease, and the potential for undesirable effects, the benefit/risk of the combination of ribavirin and interferon alfa-2b needs to be carefully considered in this population (see sections **4.1**, **4.4** and **4.8**).

Study results are summarized in **Table 5**.

Table 5. Virological response in previously untreated paediatric patients

	Viraferon 3 MIU/m² 3 times a week + **ribavirin 15 mg/kg/day**
Overall Response[1] (n=118)	54 (46 %)*
Genotype 1 (n=92)	33 (36 %)*
Genotype 2/3/4 (n=26)	21 (81 %)*

*Number (%) of patients

1. Defined as HCV-RNA below limit of detection using a research based RT-PCR assay at end of treatment and during follow-up period

5.2 Pharmacokinetic properties

The pharmacokinetics of Viraferon were studied in healthy volunteers following single 5 million IU/m² and 10 million IU doses administered subcutaneously, at 5 million IU/m² administered intramuscularly and as a 30-minute intravenous infusion. The mean serum interferon concentrations following subcutaneous and intramuscular injections were comparable. C_{max} occurred three to 12 hours after the lower dose and six to eight hours after the higher dose. The elimination half-lives of interferon injections were approximately two to three hours, and six to seven hours, respectively. Serum levels were below the detection limit 16 and 24 hours, respectively, post-injection. Both subcutaneous and intramuscular administration resulted in bioavailabilities greater than 100 %.

After intravenous administration, serum interferon levels peaked (135 to 273 IU/ml) by the end of the infusion, then declined at a slightly more rapid rate than after subcutaneous or intramuscular administration of medicinal product, becoming undetectable four hours after the infusion. The elimination half-life was approximately two hours.

Urine levels of interferon were below the detection limit following each of the three routes of administration.

Children and adolescents: Multiple-dose pharmacokinetic properties for Viraferon injection and ribavirin capsules in children and adolescents with chronic hepatitis C, between 5 and 16 years of age, are summarized in **Table 6**. The pharmacokinetics of Viraferon and ribavirin (dose-normalized) are similar in adults and children or adolescents.

Table 6. Mean (% CV) multiple-dose pharmacokinetic parameters for Viraferon and ribavirin capsules when administered to children or adolescents with chronic hepatitis C

Parameter	**Ribavirin** 15 mg/kg/day as 2 divided doses (n = 17)	**Viraferon** 3 MIU/m² 3 times a week (n = 54)
T_{max} (hr)	1.9 (83)	5.9 (36)
C_{max} (ng/ml)	3,275 (25)	51 (48)
AUC*	29,774 (26)	622 (48)
Apparent clearance l/hr/kg	0.27 (27)	Not done

*AUC_{12} (ng.hr/ml) for ribavirin; AUC_{0-24} (IU.hr/ml) for Viraferon

Interferon neutralising factor assays were performed on serum samples of patients who received Viraferon in Schering-Plough monitored clinical trials. Interferon neutralising factors are antibodies which neutralise the antiviral activity of interferon. The clinical incidence of neutralising factors developing in cancer patients treated systemically is 2.9 % and in chronic hepatitis patients is 6.2 %. The detectable titres are low in almost all cases and have not been regularly associated with loss of response or any other autoimmune phenomenon. In patients with hepatitis, no loss of response was observed apparently due to the low titres.

5.3 Preclinical safety data

Although interferon is generally recognised as being species specific, toxicity studies in animals were conducted. Injections of human recombinant interferon alfa-2b for up to three months have shown no evidence of toxicity in mice, rats, and rabbits. Daily dosing of cynomolgus monkeys with 20 × 10^6 IU/kg/day for 3 months caused no remarkable toxicity. Toxicity was demonstrated in monkeys given 100 × 10^6 IU/kg/day for 3 months.

In studies of interferon use in non-human primates, abnormalities of the menstrual cycle have been observed (see section **4.4**).

Results of animal reproduction studies indicate that recombinant interferon alfa-2b was not teratogenic in rats or rabbits, nor did it adversely affect pregnancy, foetal development or reproductive capacity in offspring of treated rats. Interferon alfa-2b has been shown to have abortifacient effects in *Macaca mulatta* (rhesus monkeys) at 90 and 180 times the recommended intramuscular or subcutaneous dose of 2 million IU/m². Abortion was observed in all dose groups (7.5 million, 15 million and 30 million IU/kg), and was statistically significant versus control at the mid- and high-dose groups (corresponding to 90 and 180 times the recommended intramuscular or subcutaneous dose of 2 million IU/m²). High doses of other forms of interferons alpha and beta are known to produce dose-related anovulatory and abortifacient effects in rhesus monkeys.

Mutagenicity studies with interferon alfa-2b revealed no adverse events.

No studies have been conducted in juvenile animals to examine the effects of treatment on growth, development, sexual maturation, and behaviour.

6. PHARMACEUTICAL PARTICULARS

6.1 List of excipients

Sodium phosphate dibasic, sodium phosphate monobasic, edetate disodium, sodium chloride, m-cresol, polysorbate 80, water for injections q.s. Deliverable volume from pen = 1.2 ml (an overfill is included for proper dispensing from the pen delivery system).

6.2 Incompatibilities

This medicinal product must not be mixed with other medicinal products except those mentioned in section 6.6.

6.3 Shelf life

15 months

Chemical and physical in-use stability has been demonstrated for 27 days at 2°C – 8°C.

From a microbiological point of view, once opened, the product may be stored for a maximum of 27 days at 2°C – 8°C. Other in-use storage times and conditions are the responsibility of the user.

6.4 Special precautions for storage

Store in a refrigerator (2°C – 8°C). Do not freeze.

6.5 Nature and contents of container

The solution is contained in a 1.5 ml cartridge, type I flint glass. The cartridge is sealed at one end with an aluminium cap containing a bromobutyl rubber liner and at the other end by a bromobutyl rubber plunger.

The pen is designed to deliver its contents of 18 million IU in doses ranging from 1.5 to 6 million IU. The pen will deliver a maximum of 12 doses of 1.5 million IU over a period not to exceed 4 weeks.

- 1 pen, 12 injection needles and 12 cleansing swabs
- 2 pens, 24 injection needles and 24 cleansing swabs
- 8 pens, 96 injection needles and 96 cleansing swabs

Not all pack sizes may be marketed.

6.6 Instructions for use and handling

Not all dosage forms and strengths are appropriate for some indications. Please make sure to select an appropriate dosage form and strength (see section **4.2**).

Viraferon, solution for injection, multidose pen is injected subcutaneously after attaching an injection needle and dialing the prescribed dose.

Remove the pen from the refrigerator approximately 30 minutes before administration to allow the injectable solution to reach room temperature (not more than 25°C).

Detailed instructions for the subcutaneous use of the product are provided with the package leaflet.

Each pen is intended for a maximum four-week use period and must then be discarded. A new injection needle must be used for each dose. After each use, the injection needle must be discarded safely and the pen must be returned immediately to the refrigerator. A maximum of 48 hours (two days) of exposure to 25°C is permitted over the four-week use period to cover accidental delays in returning the pen to the refrigerator.

Sufficient needles and swabs are provided to use the Viraferon pen for administering the smallest measurable doses. Instruct the patient that any extra needles and swabs that remain after the final dose has been taken from the pen, must be discarded appropriately and safely.

As with all parenteral medicinal products, prior to administration inspect Viraferon, solution for injection, visually for particulate matter and discolouration. The solution should be clear and colourless.

7. MARKETING AUTHORISATION HOLDER

SP Europe

73, rue de Stalle

B-1180 Bruxelles

Belgium

8. MARKETING AUTHORISATION NUMBER(S)
EU/1/99/128/029

EU/1/99/128/030

EU/1/99/128/031

9. DATE OF FIRST AUTHORISATION/RENEWAL OF THE AUTHORISATION
Date of first authorisation: 9 March 2000

Date of last renewal: 23 May 2005

10. DATE OF REVISION OF THE TEXT
23 May 2005

Legal Category
Prescription Only Medicine

ViraPen/05-05/7

Viraferon 18 million IU solution for injection

(Schering-Plough Ltd)

1. NAME OF THE MEDICINAL PRODUCT
Viraferon 18 million IU solution for injection

2. QUALITATIVE AND QUANTITATIVE COMPOSITION
Each vial of Viraferon solution for injection, multiple dose vial, contains 18 million IU of recombinant interferon alfa-2b in 3 ml of solution.

For excipients, see section 6.1.

3. PHARMACEUTICAL FORM
Solution for injection

Solution is clear and colourless.

4. CLINICAL PARTICULARS
4.1 Therapeutic indications
Chronic Hepatitis B: Treatment of adult patients with chronic hepatitis B associated with evidence of hepatitis B viral replication (presence of HBV-DNA and HBeAg), elevated ALT and histologically proven active liver inflammation and/or fibrosis.

Chronic Hepatitis C:

Adult patients:

Viraferon is indicated for the treatment of adult patients with chronic hepatitis C who have elevated transaminases without liver decompensation and who are positive for serum HCV-RNA or anti-HCV (see section **4.4**).

The best way to use Viraferon in this indication is in combination with ribavirin.

Children and adolescents:

Viraferon is intended for use, in a combination regimen with ribavirin, for the treatment of children and adolescents 3 years of age and older, who have chronic hepatitis C, not previously treated, without liver decompensation, and who are positive for serum HCV-RNA. The decision to treat should be made on a case by case basis, taking into account any evidence of disease progression such as hepatic inflammation and fibrosis, as well as prognostic factors for response, HCV genotype and viral load. The expected benefit of treatment should be weighed against the safety findings observed for paediatric subjects in the clinical trials (see sections **4.4**, **4.8** and **5.1**).

4.2 Posology and method of administration
Viraferon may be administered using either glass or plastic disposable injection syringes.

Treatment must be initiated by a physician experienced in the management of the disease.

If adverse events develop during the course of treatment with Viraferon for any indication, modify the dosage or discontinue therapy temporarily until the adverse events abate. If persistent or recurrent intolerance develops following adequate dosage adjustment, or disease progresses, discontinue treatment with Viraferon. At the discretion of the physician, the patient may self-administer the dose for maintenance dosage regimens administered subcutaneously.

Chronic Hepatitis B: The recommended dosage is in the range 5 to 10 million IU administered subcutaneously three times a week (every other day) for a period of 4 to 6 months.

The administered dose should be reduced by 50 % in case of occurrence of haematological disorders (white blood cells < 1,500/mm^3, granulocytes < 1,000/mm^3, thrombocytes < 100,000/mm^3). Treatment should be discontinued in case of severe leukopaenia (< 1,200/mm^3), severe neutropaenia (< 750/mm^3) or severe thrombocytopaenia (< 70,000/mm^3).

For all patients, if no improvement on serum HBV-DNA is observed after 3 to 4 months of treatment (at the maximum tolerated dose), discontinue Viraferon therapy.

Chronic Hepatitis C: Viraferon is administered subcutaneously at a dose of 3 million IU three times a week (every other day) to adult patients, whether administered as monotherapy or in combination with ribavirin.

Children 3 years of age or older and adolescents: Interferon alfa-2b 3 MIU/m^2 is administered subcutaneously 3 times a week (every other day) in combination with ribavirin capsules or oral solution administered orally in two divided doses daily with food (morning and evening).

(See ribavirin capsule SPC for dose of ribavirin capsules and dosage modification guidelines for combination therapy. For paediatric patients who weigh < 47 kg or cannot swallow capsules, see ribavirin oral solution SPC).

Relapse patients (adults):

Viraferon is given in combination with ribavirin.

Based on the results of clinical trials, in which data are available for 6 months of treatment, it is recommended that patients be treated with Viraferon in combination with ribavirin for 6 months.

Naïve patients:

Adults: The efficacy of Viraferon is enhanced when given in combination with ribavirin. Viraferon should be given alone mainly in case of intolerance or contraindication to ribavirin.

Viraferon in combination with ribavirin:

Based on the results of clinical trials, in which data are available for 12 months of treatment, it is recommended that patients be treated with Viraferon in combination with ribavirin for at least 6 months.

Treatment should be continued for another 6-month period (i.e., a total of 12 months) in patients who exhibit negative HCV-RNA at month 6, and with viral genotype 1 (as determined in a pre-treatment sample) and high pre-treatment viral load.

Other negative prognostic factors (age > 40 years, male gender, bridging fibrosis) should be taken into account in order to extend therapy to 12 months.

During clinical trials, patients who failed to show a virologic response after 6 months of treatment (HCV-RNA below lower limit of detection) did not become sustained virologic responders (HCV-RNA below lower limit of detection six months after withdrawal of treatment).

Viraferon alone:

The optimal duration of therapy with Viraferon alone is not yet fully established, but a therapy of between 12 and 18 months is advised.

It is recommended that patients be treated with Viraferon alone for at least 3 to 4 months, at which point HCV-RNA status should be determined. Treatment should be continued in patients who exhibit negative HCV-RNA.

Children and adolescents: The efficacy and safety of Viraferon in combination with ribavirin has been studied in children and adolescents who have not been previously treated for chronic hepatitis C.

Genotype 1: The recommended duration of treatment is one year. Patients who fail to achieve virological response at 12 weeks are highly unlikely to become sustained virological responders (negative predictive value 96 %). Virological response is defined as absence of detectable HCV-RNA at Week 12. Treatment should be discontinued in these patients.

Genotype 2/3: The recommended duration of treatment is 24 weeks.

Virological responses after 1 year of treatment and 6 months of follow-up were 36 % for genotype 1 and 81 % for genotype 2/3/4.

4.3 Contraindications
- Hypersensitivity to the active substance or to any of the excipients

- A history of severe pre-existing cardiac disease, e.g., uncontrolled congestive heart failure, recent myocardial infarction, severe arrhythmic disorders

- Severe renal or hepatic dysfunction; including that caused by metastases

- Epilepsy and/or compromised central nervous system (CNS) function (see section **4.4**)

- Chronic hepatitis with decompensated cirrhosis of the liver

- Chronic hepatitis in patients who are being or have been treated recently with immunosuppressive agents excluding short term corticosteroid withdrawal

- Autoimmune hepatitis; or history of autoimmune disease; immunosuppressed transplant recipients

- Pre-existing thyroid disease unless it can be controlled with conventional treatment

Children and adolescents:

- Existence of, or history of severe psychiatric condition, particularly severe depression, suicidal ideation or suicide attempt.

Combination therapy with ribavirin: Also see ribavirin labelling if interferon alfa-2b is to be administered in combination with ribavirin in patients with chronic hepatitis C.

4.4 Special warnings and special precautions for use
For all patients:

Acute hypersensitivity reactions (e.g., urticaria, angioedema, bronchoconstriction, anaphylaxis) to interferon alfa-2b have been observed rarely during Viraferon therapy. If such a reaction develops, discontinue the medication and institute appropriate medical therapy. Transient rashes do not necessitate interruption of treatment.

Moderate to severe adverse experiences may require modification of the patient's dosage regimen, or in some cases, termination of Viraferon therapy. Any patient developing liver function abnormalities during treatment with Viraferon must be monitored closely and treatment discontinued if signs and symptoms progress.

Hypotension may occur during Viraferon therapy or up to two days post-therapy and may require supportive treatment.

Adequate hydration must be maintained in patients undergoing Viraferon therapy since hypotension related to fluid depletion has been seen in some patients. Fluid replacement may be necessary.

While fever may be associated with the flu-like syndrome reported commonly during interferon therapy, other causes of persistent fever must be ruled out.

Viraferon must be used cautiously in patients with debilitating medical conditions, such as those with a history of pulmonary disease (e.g., chronic obstructive pulmonary disease) or diabetes mellitus prone to ketoacidosis. Caution must be observed also in patients with coagulation disorders (e.g., thrombophlebitis, pulmonary embolism) or severe myelosuppression.

Pulmonary infiltrates, pneumonitis, and pneumonia, occasionally resulting in fatality, have been observed rarely in interferon alpha treated patients, including those treated with Viraferon. The aetiology has not been defined. These symptoms have been reported more frequently when shosaikoto, a Chinese herbal medicine, is administered concomitantly with interferon alpha (see section **4.5**). Any patient developing fever, cough, dyspnea or other respiratory symptoms must have a chest X-ray taken. If the chest X-ray shows pulmonary infiltrates or there is evidence of pulmonary function impairment, the patient is to be monitored closely, and, if appropriate, discontinue interferon alpha. While this has been reported more often in patients with chronic hepatitis C treated with interferon alpha, it has also been reported in patients with oncologic diseases treated with interferon alpha. Prompt discontinuation of interferon alpha administration and treatment with corticosteroids appear to be associated with resolution of pulmonary adverse events.

Ocular adverse events (see section **4.8**) including retinal haemorrhages, cotton wool spots, and retinal artery or vein obstruction have been reported in rare instance after treatment with alpha interferons. All patients should have a baseline eye examination. Any patient complaining of changes in visual acuity or visual fields, or reporting other ophthalmologic symptoms during treatment with Viraferon, must have a prompt and complete eye examination. Periodic visual examinations during Viraferon therapy are recommended particularly in patients with disorders that may be associated with retinopathy, such as diabetes mellitus or hypertension. Discontinuation of Viraferon should be considered in patients who develop new or worsening ophthalmological disorders.

Psychiatric and central nervous system (CNS): Severe CNS effects, particularly depression, suicidal ideation and attempted suicide have been observed in some patients during Viraferon therapy, and in the follow-up period. Among children and adolescents treated with Viraferon in combination with ribavirin, suicidal ideation or attempts were reported more frequently compared to adult patients (2.4 % vs 1 %) during treatment and during the 6-month follow-up after treatment. As in adult patients, children and adolescents experienced other psychiatric adverse events (e.g., depression, emotional lability, and somnolence). Other CNS effects including aggressive behaviour, confusion and alterations of mental status have been observed with alpha interferons. If patients develop psychiatric or CNS problems, including clinical depression, it is recommended that the patient be carefully monitored by the prescribing physicians during treatment and in the follow-up period. If such symptoms appear, the potential seriousness of these undesirable effects must be borne in mind by the prescribing physician. If psychiatric symptoms persist or worsen, or suicidal ideation is identified, it is recommended that treatment with Viraferon be discontinued, and the patient followed, with psychiatric intervention, as appropriate.

Patients with existence of or history of severe psychiatric conditions:

If a treatment with interferon alfa-2b is judged necessary in adult patients with existence or history of severe psychiatric conditions, this should only be initiated after having ensured appropriate individualised diagnostic and therapeutic management of the psychiatric condition. The use of interferon alfa-2b in children and adolescents with existence of or history of severe psychiatric conditions is contraindicated (see section **4.3**).

More significant obtundation and coma, including cases of encephalopathy, have been observed in some patients, usually elderly, treated at higher doses. While these effects are generally reversible, in a few patients full resolution took up to three weeks. Very rarely, seizures have occurred with high doses of Viraferon.

Adult patients with a history of congestive heart failure, myocardial infarction and/or previous or current arrhythmic disorders, who require Viraferon therapy, must be closely monitored. It is recommended that those patients who have pre-existing cardiac abnormalities and/or are in advanced stages of cancer have electrocardiograms taken prior to and during the course of treatment. Cardiac arrhythmias (primarily supraventricular) usually respond to conventional therapy but may require discontinuation of Viraferon therapy. There are no data in children or adolescents with a history of cardiac disease.

Hypertriglyceridemia and aggravation of hypertriglyceridemia, sometimes severe, have been observed. Monitoring of lipid levels is, therefore, recommended.

Due to reports of interferon alpha exacerbating pre-existing psoriatic disease and sarcoidosis, use of Viraferon in patients with psoriasis or sarcoidosis is recommended only if the potential benefit justifies the potential risk.

Preliminary data indicates that interferon alpha therapy may be associated with an increased rate of kidney graft rejection. Liver graft rejection has also been reported.

The development of auto-antibodies and autoimmune disorders has been reported during treatment with alpha interferons. Patients predisposed to the development of autoimmune disorders may be at increased risk. Patients with signs or symptoms compatible with autoimmune disorders should be evaluated carefully, and the benefit-risk of continued interferon therapy should be reassessed (see also section **4.4 Chronic hepatitis C, Monotherapy** (thyroid abnormalities) and section **4.8**).

Discontinue treatment with Viraferon in patients with chronic hepatitis who develop prolongation of coagulation markers which might indicate liver decompensation.

Chronic Hepatitis C:

Combination therapy with ribavirin: Also see ribavirin labelling if Viraferon is to be administered in combination with ribavirin in patients with chronic hepatitis C.

All patients in the chronic hepatitis C studies had a liver biopsy before inclusion, but in certain cases (i.e. patients with genotype 2 and 3), treatment may be possible without histological confirmation. Current treatment guidelines should be consulted as to whether a liver biopsy is needed prior to commencing treatment.

Monotherapy: Infrequently, adult patients treated for chronic hepatitis C with Viraferon developed thyroid abnormalities, either hypothyroidism or hyperthyroidism. In clinical trials using Viraferon therapy, 2.8 % patients overall developed thyroid abnormalities. The abnormalities were controlled by conventional therapy for thyroid dysfunction. The mechanism by which Viraferon may alter thyroid status is unknown. Prior to initiation of Viraferon therapy for the treatment of chronic hepatitis C, evaluate serum thyroid-stimulating hormone (TSH) levels. Any thyroid abnormality detected at that time must be treated with conventional therapy. Viraferon treatment may be initiated if TSH levels can be maintained in the normal range by medication.

Determine TSH levels if, during the course of Viraferon therapy, a patient develops symptoms consistent with possible thyroid dysfunction. In the presence of thyroid dysfunction, Viraferon treatment may be continued if TSH levels can be maintained in the normal range by medication. Discontinuation of Viraferon therapy has not reversed thyroid dysfunction occurring during treatment (also see Children and adolescents, Thyroid monitoring).

Supplemental monitoring specific for children and adolescents

Thyroid Monitoring: Approximately 12 % of children treated with interferon alfa-2b and ribavirin developed increase in TSH. Another 4 % had a transient decrease below the lower limit of normal. Prior to initiation of IntronA therapy, TSH levels must be evaluated and any thyroid abnormality detected at that time must be treated with conventional therapy. Viraferon therapy may be initiated if TSH levels can be maintained in the normal range by medication. Thyroid dysfunction during treatment with interferon alfa-2b and ribavirin has been observed. If thyroid abnormalities are detected, the patient's thyroid status should be evaluated and treated as clinically appropriate. Children and adolescents should be monitored every 3 months for evidence of thyroid dysfunction (e.g. TSH).

Growth and Development: During a 1-year course of therapy there was a decrease in the rate of linear growth (mean percentile decrease of 9 %) and a decrease in the rate of weight gain (mean percentile decrease of 13 %). A general reversal of these trends was noted during the 6 months follow-up post treatment. However, based on interim data from a long-term follow-up study, 12 (14 %) of 84 children had a > 15 percentile decrease in rate of linear growth, of whom 5 (6 %) children had a > 30 percentile decrease despite being off treatment for more than 1 year. There are no data on long term effects on growth and development and on sexual maturation.

HCV/HIV Coinfection: Patients co-infected with HIV and receiving Highly Active Anti-Retroviral Therapy (HAART) may be at increased risk of developing lactic acidosis. Caution should be used when adding Viraferon and ribavirin to HAART therapy (see ribavirin SPC).

Co-infected patients with advanced cirrhosis receiving HAART may be at increased risk of hepatic decompensation and death. Adding treatment with alfa interferons alone or in combination with ribavirin may increase the risk in this patient subset.

Laboratory Tests:

Standard haematological tests and blood chemistries (complete blood count and differential, platelet count, electrolytes, liver enzymes, serum protein, serum bilirubin and serum creatinine) are to be conducted in all patients prior to and periodically during systemic treatment with Viraferon.

During treatment for hepatitis B or C the recommended testing schedule is at weeks 1, 2, 4, 8, 12, 16, and every other month, thereafter, throughout treatment. If ALT flares during Viraferon therapy to greater than or equal to 2 times baseline, Viraferon therapy may be continued unless signs and symptoms of liver failure are observed. During ALT flare, liver function tests: ALT, prothrombin time, alkaline phosphatase, albumin and bilirubin must be monitored at two-week intervals.

Effect on fertility: Interferon may impair fertility (see section **4.6** and section **5.3**).

4.5 Interaction with other medicinal products and other forms of Interaction

Narcotics, hypnotics or sedatives must be administered with caution when used concomitantly with Viraferon.

Interactions between Viraferon and other medicinal products have not been fully evaluated. Caution must be exercised when administering Viraferon in combination with other potentially myelosuppressive agents.

Interferons may affect the oxidative metabolic process. This must be considered during concomitant therapy with medicinal products metabolised by this route, such as the xanthine derivatives theophylline or aminophylline. During concomitant therapy with xanthine agents, serum theophylline levels must be monitored and dosage adjusted if necessary.

Pulmonary infiltrates, pneumonitis, and pneumonia, occasionally resulting in fatality, have been observed rarely in interferon alpha treated patients, including those treated with Viraferon. The aetiology has not been defined. These symptoms have been reported more frequently when shosaikoto, a Chinese herbal medicine, is administered concomitantly with interferon alpha (see section **4.4**).

(Also see ribavirin labelling if Viraferon is to be administered in combination with ribavirin in patients with chronic hepatitis C).

4.6 Pregnancy and lactation

Decreased serum estradiol and progesterone concentrations have been reported in women treated with human leukocyte interferon. Women of childbearing potential must use effective contraception during treatment. Viraferon must be used with caution in fertile men.

For interferon alfa-2b, no clinical data are available on exposed pregnancies.

Studies in animals have shown reproductive toxicity (see section **5.3**). The relevance of these data for humans is unknown. Viraferon is to be used during pregnancy only if the potential benefit justifies the potential risk to the foetus.

It is not known whether the components of this medicinal product are excreted in human milk. Because of the potential for adverse events from Viraferon in nursing infants, a decision must be made whether to discontinue nursing or to discontinue the medicinal product, taking into account the importance of the treatment to the mother.

Combination therapy with ribavirin: Ribavirin causes serious birth defects when administered during pregnancy. Viraferon in combination with ribavirin is contraindicated (see ribavirin SPC). Females of childbearing potential have to use effective contraception during treatment and for 4 months after treatment.

4.7 Effects on ability to drive and use machines

Patients are to be advised that they may develop fatigue, somnolence, or confusion during treatment with Viraferon, and therefore it is recommended that they avoid driving or operating machinery.

4.8 Undesirable effects

See ribavirin labelling for ribavirin-related undesirable effects if Viraferon is to be administered in combination with ribavirin in patients with chronic hepatitis C.

In clinical trials conducted in a broad range of indications and at a wide range of doses (from 6 MIU/m^2/week in hairy cell leukaemia up to 100 MIU/m^2/week in melanoma), the most commonly reported undesirable effects were fever, fatigue, headache and myalgia. Fever and fatigue were often reversible within 72 hours of interruption or cessation of treatment.

The safety profile shown here was determined from 4 clinical trials in hepatitis C in which patients were treated with Viraferon alone or in combination with ribavirin for one year. All patients in these trials received 3 MIU of Viraferon three times a week. The percentage of patients reporting (treatment related) undesirable effects ≥ 10 % is presented in **Table 1** as a range to capture the incidences reported in individual treatment groups among these clinical trials in naïve patients treated for one year. Severity was generally mild to moderate.

Table 1: Undesirable effects reported in clinical trials in naïve patients treated for one year (≥ 10 % of patients)

	Viraferon (n = 806)	**Viraferon + ribavirin (n = 1,010)**
Application site disorder		
Injection site inflammation		
Injection site	9-16 %	6-17 %
reaction	5-8 %	3-36 %
Body as a whole		
Headache	51-64 %	48-64 %
Fatigue	42-70 %	43-68 %
Rigors	15-39 %	19-41 %
Fever	29-39 %	29-41 %
Flu-like symptoms	19-37 %	18-29 %
Asthenia	9-30 %	9-30 %
Weight decrease	6-11 %	9-19 %
Gastrointestinal		
Nausea	18-31 %	25-44 %
Anorexia	14-19 %	19-26 %
Diarrhoea	12-22 %	13-18 %
Abdominal pain	9-17 %	9-14 %
Vomiting	3-10 %	6-10 %
Musculoskeletal		
Myalgia	41-61 %	30-62 %
Arthralgia	25-31 %	21-29 %
Musculoskeletal pain	15-20 %	11-20 %
Psychiatric		
Depression	16-36 %	25-34 %
Irritability	13-27 %	18-34 %
Insomnia	21-28 %	33-41 %
Anxiety	8-12 %	8-16 %
Concentration impaired	8-14 %	9-21 %
Emotional lability	5-8 %	5-11 %
Skin and appendages		
Alopecia	22-31 %	26-32 %
Pruritus	6-9 %	18-27 %
Skin dry	5-8 %	10-21 %
Rash	5-7 %	15-24 %
Respiratory system		
Pharyngitis	3-7 %	7-13 %
Coughing	3-7 %	8-11 %
Dyspnoea	2-9 %	10-22 %
Other		
Dizziness	8-18 %	10-22 %
Infection viral	0-7 %	3-10 %

Table 2: Undesirable effects (< 10%) reported in clinical trial of 483 patients treated with Viraferon + ribavirin (Viraferon 3 MIU 3 times a week, ribavirin > 10.6 mg/kg for one year)

Body system	**5 < 10%**	**1 < 5%**
Application Site		injection site pain
Autonomic Nervous	mouth dry, sweating increased	flushing, lacrimal gland disorder
Body as a Whole	malaise, chest pain	right upper quadrant pain
Cardiovascular		hypertension
Central and Peripheral Nervous		hypoesthesia, vertigo, confusion, paraesthesia, tremor, migraine
Endocrine		hyperthyroidism, hypothyroidism
Gastrointestinal	dyspepsia, stomatitis	constipation, dehydration, gingivitis, glossitis, loose stools, stomatitis ulcerative
Hearing and Vestibular		tinnitus
Heart Rate and Rhythm		palpitation, tachycardia
Liver and Biliary		hepatomegaly
Metabolic and Nutritional		hyperuricemia, hypocalcemia, thirst
Musculoskeletal		arthritis

Platelet, bleeding and clotting		thrombocytopaenia
Psychiatric	agitation, nervousness	sleep disorder, somnolence, libido decreased
Reproductive, female		amenorrhea, breast pain, dysmenorrhea, menorrhagia, menstrual disorder, vaginal disorder
Resistance Mechanism		herpes simplex
Respiratory		bronchitis, cough nonproductive, epistaxis, nasal congestion, respiratory disorder, rhinitis, rhinorrhea, sinusitis
Skin and Appendages		eczema, psoriasis (new or aggravated), rash erythematous, rash maculopapular, skin disorder, erythema
Special Senses		taste perversion
Urinary		micturition frequency
Vision	vision blurred	conjunctivitis, eye pain, vision abnormal
White Cell and Resistance	leukopaenia	lymphadenopathy, lymphopenia

These undesirable effects have also been reported with Viraferon alone.

Additional adverse events were reported rarely (> 1/10,000, < 1/1,000) or very rarely (< 1/10,000) during clinical trials in other indications or following the marketing of interferon alfa-2b:

Body as a whole:

very rarely: face oedema

Cardiovascular:

very rarely: hypotension; cardiac ischaemia and myocardial infarction

Central and peripheral nervous system:

very rarely: impaired consciousness, neuropathy, polyneuropathy, seizure, encephalopathy, cerebrovascular ischaemia, cerebrovascular haemorrhage

Ear and labyrinth:

very rarely: hearing disorder, hearing loss

Endocrine disorders:

very rarely: diabetes, aggravated diabetes

Gastrointestinal:

very rarely: pancreatitis; increased appetite; gingival bleeding; colitis, mainly ulcerative and ischemic

Immune system disorders:

very rarely: sarcoidosis or exacerbation of sarcoidosis

Liver and biliary system:

very rarely: hepatotoxicity, including fatality

Metabolic and nutritional disorders:

very rarely: hyperglycaemia, hypertriglyceridaemia

Musculoskeletal:

very rarely: rhabdomyolysis, sometimes serious; leg cramps; back pain; myositis

Psychiatric:

rarely: suicide ideation

very rarely: aggressive behaviour, suicide attempts, suicide, psychosis, including hallucinations

Respiratory system:

rarely: pneumonia

very rarely: pulmonary infiltrates, pneumonitis

Skin and appendages:

very rarely: erythema multiforme, Stevens Johnson syndrome, toxic epidermal necrolysis, injection site necrosis

Urinary system:

very rarely: nephrotic syndrome, renal insufficiency, renal failure

Vascular (extracardiac disorders):

very rarely: peripheral ischaemia

Visual disorders:

rarely: retinal haemorrhages, retinopathies (including macular oedema), cotton-wool spots, retinal artery or vein obstruction, loss of visual acuity or visual field, optic neuritis and papilloedema

Table 3 Undesirable effects in paediatric clinical trials (≥ 1% of patients treated with Rebetol + interferon alfa-2b injection)

Body system	≥ 10%	5 % - < 10%	1 % - < 5%
Application site disorder	Injection site reaction, injection site inflammation	Injection site pain	
Autonomic nervous system			Flushing, lacrimal gland disorder, sweating increased
Body as a whole	Fatigue, fever, headache, influenza-like symptoms, malaise, rigors, growth rate decrease (height and/or weight decrease for age)		Asthenia, chest pain, erythema, neoplasm (unspecified), oedema, right upper quadrant pain
Central and peripheral nervous	Dizziness	Tremor	Confusion, dysphonia, hyperkinesia, hyperaesthesia, hypoaesthesia, paresthaesia, urinary incontinence
Endocrine	Hypothyroidism		Hyperthyroidism, virilism
Gastrointestinal	Abdominal pain, anorexia, diarrhoea, nausea, vomiting		Constipation, dyspepsia, gastroenteritis, gastroesophogeal reflux, gastrointestinal disorder, glossitis, loose stools, mouth ulceration, rectal disorder, stomatitis, stomatitis ulcerative, toothache, tooth disorder
Infection and infestations			Tooth abscess
Liver and biliary			Hepatic function abnormal
Metabolic and nutritional			Hypertriglyceridemia, hyperuricemia
Musculoskeletal	Arthralgia, musculoskeletal pain, myalgia		
Platelet, bleeding and clotting			Bruise, thrombocytopaenia
Psychiatric	Depression, emotional lability, insomnia, irritability	Agitation, somnolence	Aggressive reaction, anxiety, apathy, increased appetite, behavior disorder, concentration impaired, abnormal dreaming, nervousness, sleep disorder, somnambulism, suicidal ideation
Red blood cell	Anaemia		
Renal and urinary			Enuresis, micturition disorder, urinary tract infection
Reproductive disorder, female and male			Female: amenorrhea, menorrhagia, menstrual disorder, vaginal disorder, vaginitis Male: testicular pain
Resistance mechanism disorder	Viral infection		Bacterial infection, fungal infection, herpes simplex, otitis media
Respiratory system	Pharyngitis	Epistaxis	Coughing, dyspnoea, nasal congestion, nasal irritation, pulmonary infection, rhinorrhea, sneezing, tachypnea
Skin and appendages	Alopecia, rash	Pruritus	Acne, eczema, skin laceration, nail disorder, dry skin, photosensitivity reaction, maculopapular rash, skin discolouration, skin disorder
Vascular (extracardiac)		Pallor	Raynaud's disease
Vision			Conjunctivitis, eye pain, abnormal vision
White cell and resistance	Neutropenia		Lymphadenopathy

Very rarely Viraferon used alone or in combination with ribavirin may be associated with aplastic anaemia.

Cardiovascular (CVS) adverse events, particularly arrhythmia, appeared to be correlated mostly with pre-existing CVS disease and prior therapy with cardiotoxic agents (see section **4.4**). Cardiomyopathy, that may be reversible upon discontinuation of interferon alpha, has been reported rarely in patients without prior evidence of cardiac disease.

A wide variety of autoimmune and immune-mediated disorders have been reported with alpha interferons including thyroid disorders, idiopathic and thrombotic thrombocytopenic purpura, vasculitis, neuropathies including mononeuropathies (see also section **4.4**).

Clinically significant laboratory abnormalities, most frequently occurring at doses greater than 10 million IU daily, include reduction in granulocyte and white blood cell counts; decreases in haemoglobin level and platelet count; increases in alkaline phosphatase, LDH, serum creatinine and serum urea nitrogen levels. Increase in serum ALT/AST (SGPT/SGOT) levels have been noted as an abnormality in some non-hepatitis subjects and also in some patients with chronic hepatitis B coincident with clearance of viral DNAp.

Children and adolescents – Chronic Hepatitis C

In clinical trials of 118 children or adolescents 3 to 16 years of age, 6 % discontinued therapy due to adverse events. In general, the adverse event profile in the limited paediatric population studied was similar to that observed in adults, although there is a paediatric specific concern regarding growth inhibition as decrease in height (mean percentile decrease of growth velocity of 9 %) and weight (mean percentile decrease of 13 %) percentile were observed during treatment (see section **4.4**). Furthermore, suicidal ideation or attempts were reported more frequently compared to adult patients (2.4 % vs 1 %) during treatment and during the 6 month follow-up after treatment. As in adult patients, children and adolescents also experienced other psychiatric adverse events (e.g., depression, emotional lability, and somnolence) (see section **4.4**). In addition, injection site disorders, fever, anorexia, vomiting, and emotional lability occurred more frequently in children and adolescents compared to adult patients. Dose modifications were required in 30 % of patients, most commonly for anaemia and neutropaenia.

Undesirable effects reported in paediatric clinical trials, and not previously reported at an incidence ⩾ 1 % in adults, are shown in **Table 3**. All effects reported at a ⩾ 10 % incidence in paediatric trials were previously reported in adults (**Table 2**) and are not repeated in the paediatric table.

(see Table 3 on previous page)

4.9 Overdose

No case of overdose has been reported that has led to acute clinical manifestations. However, as for any pharmacologically active compound, symptomatic treatment with frequent monitoring of vital signs and close observation of the patient is indicated.

5. PHARMACOLOGICAL PROPERTIES

5.1 Pharmacodynamic properties

Pharmacotherapeutic group: Immunostimulants, cytokines and immunomodulators, interferons, interferon alfa-2b, ATC code: L03A B05

Viraferon is a sterile, stable, formulation of highly purified interferon alfa-2b produced by recombinant DNA techniques. Recombinant interferon alfa-2b is a water-soluble protein with a molecular weight of approximately 19,300 daltons. It is obtained from a clone of E. coli, which harbours a genetically engineered plasmid hybrid encompassing an interferon alfa-2b gene from human leukocytes.

The activity of Viraferon is expressed in terms of IU, with 1 mg of recombinant interferon alfa-2b protein corresponding to 2.6 $\times$ 10^8 IU. International Units are determined by comparison of the activity of the recombinant interferon alfa-2b with the activity of the international reference preparation of human leukocyte interferon established by the World Health Organisation.

The interferons are a family of small protein molecules with molecular weights of approximately 15,000 to 21,000 daltons. They are produced and secreted by cells in response to viral infections or various synthetic and biological inducers. Three major classes of interferons have been identified: alpha, beta and gamma. These three main classes are themselves not homogeneous and may contain several different molecular species of interferon. More than 14 genetically distinct human alpha interferons have been identified. Viraferon has been classified as recombinant interferon alfa-2b.

Interferons exert their cellular activities by binding to specific membrane receptors on the cell surface. Human interferon receptors, as isolated from human lymphoblastoid (Daudi) cells, appear to be highly asymmetric proteins. They exhibit selectivity for human but not murine interferons, suggesting species specificity. Studies with other interferons have demonstrated species specificity. However, certain monkey species, eg, rhesus monkeys, are susceptible to pharmacodynamic stimulation upon exposure to human type 1 interferons.

The results of several studies suggest that, once bound to the cell membrane, interferon initiates a complex sequence of intracellular events that include the induction of certain enzymes. It is thought that this process, at least in part, is responsible for the various cellular responses to interferon, including inhibition of virus replication in virus-infected cells, suppression of cell proliferation and such immunomodulating activities as enhancement of the phagocytic activity of macrophages and augmentation of the specific cytotoxicity of lymphocytes for target cells. Any or all of these activities may contribute to interferon's therapeutic effects.

Recombinant interferon alfa-2b has exhibited antiproliferative effects in studies employing both animal and human cell culture systems as well as human tumour xenografts in animals. It has demonstrated significant immunomodulatory activity *in vitro*.

Recombinant interferon alfa-2b also inhibits viral replication *in vitro* and *in vivo*. Although the exact antiviral mode of action of recombinant interferon alfa-2b is unknown, it appears to alter the host cell metabolism. This action inhibits viral replication or if replication occurs, the progeny virions are unable to leave the cell.

<u>Chronic hepatitis B:</u>

Current clinical experience in patients who remain on interferon alfa-2b for 4 to 6 months indicates that therapy can produce clearance of serum HBV-DNA. An improvement in liver histology has been observed. In adult patients with loss of HBeAg and HBV-DNA, a significant reduction in morbidity and mortality has been observed.

Interferon alfa-2b (6 MIU/m² 3 times a week for 6 months) has been given to children with chronic active hepatitis B. Because of a methodological flaw, efficacy could not be demonstrated. Moreover children treated with interferon alfa-2b experienced a reduced rate of growth and some cases of depression were observed.

<u>Chronic hepatitis C:</u>

Adult patients: Viraferon alone or in combination with ribavirin has been studied in 4 randomised Phase III clinical trials in 2,552 interferon-naïve patients with chronic hepatitis C. The trials compared the efficacy of Viraferon used alone or in combination with ribavirin. Efficacy was defined as sustained virologic response, 6 months after the end of treatment. Eligible patients for these trials had chronic hepatitis C confirmed by a positive HCV-RNA polymerase chain reaction assay (PCR) (> 100 copies/ml), a liver biopsy consistent with a histologic diagnosis of chronic hepatitis with no other cause for the chronic hepatitis, and abnormal serum ALT.

Viraferon was administered at a dose of 3 MIU 3 times a week as monotherapy or in combination with ribavirin. The majority of patients in these clinical trials were treated for one year. All patients were followed for an additional 6 months after the end of treatment for the determination of sustained virologic response. Sustained virologic response rates for treatment groups treated for one year with Viraferon alone or in combination with ribavirin (from two studies) are shown in **Table 3**.

Co-administration of Viraferon with ribavirin increased the efficacy of Viraferon by at least two fold for the treatment of chronic heptatitis C in naïve patients. HCV genotype and baseline virus load are prognostic factors which are known to affect response rates. The increased response rate to the combination of Viraferon + ribavirin, compared with Viraferon alone, is maintained across all subgroups. The relative benefit of combination therapy with Viraferon + ribavirin is particularly significant in the most difficult to treat subgroup of patients (genotype 1 and high virus load) (**Table 4**).

Response rates in these trials were increased with compliance. Regardless of genotype, patients who received Viraferon in combination with ribavirin and received ⩾ 80 % of their treatment had a higher sustained response 6 months after 1 year of treatment than those who took < 80 % of their treatment (56 % vs. 32 % in trial C/I98-580).

(see Table 4 below)

Relapse patients: A total of 345 interferon alpha relapse patients were treated in two clinical trials with Viraferon monotherapy or in combination with ribavirin. In these patients, the addition of ribavirin to Viraferon increased by as much as 10-fold the efficacy of Viraferon used alone in the treatment of chronic hepatitis C (48.6 % vs. 4.7 %). This enhancement in efficacy included loss of serum HCV (< 100 copies/ml by PCR), improvement in hepatic inflammation, and normalisation of ALT, and was sustained when measured 6 months after the end of treatment.

Clinical trials in paediatric patients with chronic hepatitis C:

Children and adolescents 3 to 16 years of age with compensated chronic hepatitis C and detectable HCV-RNA (assessed by a central laboratory using a research-based RT-PCR assay) were enrolled in two multicentre trials and received Viraferon 3 MIU/m² 3 times a week plus ribavirin 15 mg/kg per day for 1 year followed by 6 months follow-up after-treatment. A total of 118 patients were enrolled: 57 % male, 80 % Caucasian, and 78 % genotype 1, 64 % ⩽ 12 years of age. The population enrolled mainly consisted in children with mild to moderate hepatitis C. Sustained virological response rates in children and adolescents were similar to those in adults. Due to the lack of data in children with severe progression of the disease, and the potential for undesirable effects, the benefit/risk of the combination of ribavirin and interferon alfa-2b needs to be carefully considered in this population (see sections **4.1**, **4.4** and **4.8**).

Study results are summarized in **Table 5**.

Table 5. Virological response in previously untreated paediatric patients

	Viraferon 3 MIU/m² 3 times a week **+ ribavirin 15 mg/kg/day**
Overall Response[1] (n=118)	54 (46 %)*
Genotype 1 (n=92)	33 (36 %)*
Genotype 2/3/4 (n=26)	21 (81 %)*

*Number (%) of patients

1. Defined as HCV-RNA below limit of detection using a research based RT-PCR assay at end of treatment and during follow-up period

5.2 Pharmacokinetic properties

The pharmacokinetics of Viraferon were studied in healthy volunteers following single 5 million IU/m² and 10 million IU doses administered subcutaneously, at 5 million IU/m² administered intramuscularly and as a 30-minute intravenous infusion. The mean serum interferon concentrations following subcutaneous and intramuscular injections were comparable. C_{max} occurred three to 12 hours after the lower dose and six to eight hours after the higher dose. The elimination half-lives of interferon injections were approximately two to three hours, and six to seven hours, respectively. Serum levels were below the detection limit 16 and 24 hours, respectively, post-injection. Both subcutaneous and intramuscular administration resulted in bioavailabilities greater than 100 %.

After intravenous administration, serum interferon levels peaked (135 to 273 IU/ml) by the end of the infusion, then declined at a slightly more rapid rate than after subcutaneous or intramuscular administration of medicinal product, becoming undetectable four hours after the infusion. The elimination half-life was approximately two hours.

Urine levels of interferon were below the detection limit following each of the three routes of administration.

Children and adolescents: Multiple-dose pharmacokinetic properties for Viraferon injection and ribavirin capsules in children and adolescents with chronic hepatitis C, between 5 and 16 years of age, are summarized in **Table 6**. The pharmacokinetics of Viraferon and ribavirin (dose-normalized) are similar in adults and children or adolescents.

Table 6. Mean (% CV) multiple-dose pharmacokinetic parameters for Viraferon and ribavirin capsules when administered to children or adolescents with chronic hepatitis C

Parameter	**Ribavirin** 15 mg/kg/day as 2 divided doses (n = 17)	**Viraferon** 3 MIU/m² 3 times a week (n = 54)
T_{max} (hr)	1.9 (83)	5.9 (36)
C_{max} (ng/ml)	3,275 (25)	51 (48)
AUC*	29,774 (26)	622 (48)
Apparent clearance l/hr/kg	0.27 (27)	Not done

*AUC_{12} (ng.hr/ml) for ribavirin; AUC_{0-24} (IU.hr/ml) for Viraferon

Interferon neutralising factor assays were performed on serum samples of patients who received Viraferon in Schering-Plough monitored clinical trials. Interferon neutralising factors are antibodies which neutralise the antiviral activity of interferon. The clinical incidence of neutralising

Table 4 Sustained virologic response rates with Viraferon + ribavirin (one year of treatment) by genotype and viral load

HCV Genotype	**I** **N=503** **C95-132/I95-143**	**I/R** **N=505** **C95-132/I95-143**	**I/R** **N=505** **C/I98-580**
All Genotypes	**16 %**	**41 %**	**47 %**
Genotype 1	9 %	29 %	33 %
Genotype 1 ⩽ 2 million copies/ml	25 %	33 %	45 %
Genotype 1 > 2 million copies/ml	3 %	27 %	29 %
Genotype 2/3	31 %	65 %	79 %

I Viraferon (3 MIU 3 times a week)

I/R Viraferon (3 MIU 3 times a week) + ribavirin (1,000/1,200 mg/day)

factors developing in cancer patients treated systemically is 2.9 % and in chronic hepatitis patients is 6.2 %. The detectable titres are low in almost all cases and have not been regularly associated with loss of response or any other autoimmune phenomenon. In patients with hepatitis, no loss of response was observed apparently due to the low titres.

5.3 Preclinical safety data

Although interferon is generally recognised as being species specific, toxicity studies in animals were conducted. Injections of human recombinant interferon alfa-2b for up to three months have shown no evidence of toxicity in mice, rats, and rabbits. Daily dosing of cynomolgus monkeys with 20 × 10^6 IU/kg/day for 3 months caused no remarkable toxicity. Toxicity was demonstrated in monkeys given 100 × 10^6 IU/kg/day for 3 months.

In studies of interferon use in non-human primates, abnormalities of the menstrual cycle have been observed (see section **4.4**).

Results of animal reproduction studies indicate that recombinant interferon alfa-2b was not teratogenic in rats or rabbits, nor did it adversely affect pregnancy, foetal development or reproductive capacity in offspring of treated rats. Interferon alfa-2b has been shown to have abortifacient effects in *Macaca mulatta* (rhesus monkeys) at 90 and 180 times the recommended intramuscular or subcutaneous dose of 2 million IU/m^2. Abortion was observed in all dose groups (7.5 million, 15 million and 30 million IU/kg), and was statistically significant versus control at the mid- and high-dose groups (corresponding to 90 and 180 times the recommended intramuscular or subcutaneous dose of 2 million IU/m^2). High doses of other forms of interferons alpha and beta are known to produce dose-related anovulatory and abortifacient effects in rhesus monkeys.

Mutagenicity studies with interferon alfa-2b revealed no adverse events.

No studies have been conducted in juvenile animals to examine the effects of treatment on growth, development, sexual maturation, and behaviour.

6. PHARMACEUTICAL PARTICULARS

6.1 List of excipients

Sodium phosphate dibasic, sodium phosphate monobasic, edetate disodium, sodium chloride, m-cresol, polysorbate 80 and water for injections.

6.2 Incompatibilities

This medicinal product must not be mixed with other medicinal products except those mentioned in section 6.6.

6.3 Shelf life

2 years

After first opening the container: Chemical and physical in-use stability has been demonstrated for 28 days at 2°C – 8°C.

From a microbiological point of view, once opened, the product may be stored for a maximum of 28 days at 2°C – 8°C. Other in-use storage times and conditions are the responsibility of the user.

6.4 Special precautions for storage

Store in a refrigerator (2°C – 8°C). Do not freeze. For the purpose of transport, the solution can be kept at or below 25°C for a period up to seven days before use. Viraferon can be put back in the refrigerator at any time during this seven-day period. If the product is not used during the seven-day period, it cannot be put back in the refrigerator for a new storage period and is to be discarded.

6.5 Nature and contents of container

The solution is contained in a 5 ml vial, type I flint glass, with a halobutyl rubber stopper in an aluminium flip-off seal with a polypropylene bonnet.

- 1 vial

- 1 vial, 6 injection syringes, 6 injection needles and 12 cleansing swabs

- 2 vials,

- 12 vials

Not all pack sizes may be marketed.

6.6 Instructions for use and handling

Viraferon solution for injection, may be injected directly after withdrawal of the appropriate doses from the vial with a sterile injection syringe.

As with all parenteral medicinal products, prior to administration inspect Viraferon, solution for injection, visually for particulate matter and discolouration. The solution should be clear and colourless.

7. MARKETING AUTHORISATION HOLDER

SP Europe

73, rue de Stalle

B-1180 Bruxelles

Belgium

8. MARKETING AUTHORISATION NUMBER(S)

EU/1/99/128/021

EU/1/99/128/022

EU/1/99/128/023

EU/1/99/128/024

9. DATE OF FIRST AUTHORISATION/RENEWAL OF THE AUTHORISATION

9 March 2000

10. DATE OF REVISION OF THE TEXT

25 January 2005

Legal Category

Prescription Only Medicine

Viraferon/01-05/6

ViraferonPeg 50, 80, 100, 120 or 150 micrograms powder and solvent for solution for injection

(Schering-Plough Ltd)

1. NAME OF THE MEDICINAL PRODUCT

ViraferonPeg 50 micrograms, 80 micrograms, 100 micrograms, 120 micrograms and 150 micrograms powder and solvent for solution for injection

2. QUALITATIVE AND QUANTITATIVE COMPOSITION

Each vial of ViraferonPeg, powder for solution for injection contains 50, 80, 100, 120 or 150 micrograms of peginterferon alfa-2b as measured on a protein basis.

Each vial provides 50 micrograms/0.5 ml of peginterferon alfa-2b when reconstituted as recommended.

The active substance is a covalent conjugate of recombinant interferon alfa-2b* with monomethoxy polyethylene glycol. The potency of this product should not be compared to that of another pegylated or non-pegylated protein of the same therapeutic class. For more information, see section **5.1.**

*produced by rDNA technology in *E.coli* cells harbouring a genetically engineered plasmid hybrid encompassing an interferon alfa-2b gene from human leukocytes

For excipients, see section 6.1.

3. PHARMACEUTICAL FORM

Powder and solvent for solution for injection

White powder.

Clear and colourless solvent.

4. CLINICAL PARTICULARS

4.1 Therapeutic indications

ViraferonPeg is indicated for the treatment of adult patients with chronic hepatitis C who have elevated transaminases without liver decompensation and who are positive for serum HCV-RNA or anti-HCV (see section **4.4**).

The best way to use ViraferonPeg in this indication is in combination with ribavirin.

This combination is indicated in naïve patients as well as in patients who have previously responded (with normalisation of ALT at the end of treatment) to interferon alpha monotherapy but who have subsequently relapsed.

Interferon monotherapy, including ViraferonPeg, is indicated mainly in case of intolerance or contraindication to ribavirin.

Please refer also to the ribavirin Summary of Product Characteristics (SPC) when ViraferonPeg is to be used in combination with ribavirin.

4.2 Posology and method of administration

Treatment should be initiated and monitored only by a physician experienced in the management of patients with hepatitis C.

Dose to be administered

ViraferonPeg should be administered as a once weekly subcutaneous injection. The dose administered depends on whether it is used in combination with ribavirin or as monotherapy.

Combination therapy

ViraferonPeg 1.5 micrograms/kg/week in combination with ribavirin capsules.

The intended dose of 1.5 μg/kg of ViraferonPeg to be used in combination with ribavirin may be delivered in weight categories with the pen/vial strengths according to **Table 1.** Ribavirin capsules are to be administered orally each day in two divided doses with food (morning and evening).

Table 1 - Dosing for Combination Therapy

(see Table 1 below)

Duration of treatment

Predictability of sustained virological response: Patients infected with virus genotype 1 who fail to achieve virological response at Week 12 are highly unlikely to become sustained virological responders (see also section **5.1**).

Genotype 1: For patients who exhibit virological response at week 12, treatment should be continued for another nine month period (i.e., a total of 48 weeks).

In the subset of patients with genotype 1 infection and low viral load (< 600,000 IU/ml) who become HCV-RNA negative at treatment week 4 and remain HCV-RNA negative at week 24, the treatment could either be stopped after this 24 week treatment course or pursued for an additional 24 weeks (i.e. overall 48 weeks treatment duration). However, an overall 24 weeks treatment duration may be associated with a higher risk of relapse than a 48 weeks treatment duration (see section **5.1**).

• **Genotypes 2 or 3**: It is recommended that all patients be treated for 24 weeks.

• **Genotype 4:** In general, patients infected with genotype 4 are considered harder to treat and limited study data (n=66) indicate they are compatible with a posology as for genotype 1.

ViraferonPeg monotherapy

As monotherapy the ViraferonPeg regimen is 0.5 or 1.0 microgram/kg/week. The lowest vial or pen strength available is 50 μg/0.5 ml; therefore for patients prescribed 0.5 μg/kg/week, doses must be adjusted by volume as shown in **Table 2.** For the 1.0 μg/kg dose, similar volume adjustments can be made or alternate vial strengths can be used as shown in **Table 2.**

Table 2 - Monotherapy Dosing

(see Table 2 on next page)

Duration of treatment

For patients who exhibit virological response at Week 12, treatment should be continued for at least another three-month period (i.e., a total of six months). The decision to extend therapy to one year of treatment should be based on prognostic factors (e.g., genotype, age > 40 years, male gender, bridging fibrosis).

Dose modification for all patients

If severe adverse reactions or laboratory abnormalities develop during treatment with ViraferonPeg monotherapy or ViraferonPeg in combination with ribavirin, modify the dosages of each product as appropriate, until the adverse reactions abate. As adherence might be of importance for outcome of therapy, the dose should be kept as close as possible to the recommended standard dose. Guidelines were developed in clinical trials for dose modification.

Combination Therapy Dose Reduction Guidelines

(see Table 2a on next page)

Dose reduction of ViraferonPeg may be accomplished by either reducing the prescribed volume by one-half or by utilizing a lower dose strength as shown in **Table 2b.**

(see Table 2b on next page)

ViraferonPeg Monotherapy Dose Reduction Guidelines

Dose modification guidelines for patients who use ViraferonPeg monotherapy are shown in **Table 3a.**

(see Table 3a on next page)

Table 1 Dosing for Combination Therapy

Body Weight (kg)	ViraferonPeg		Ribavirin Capsules	
	Vial/Pen Strength (μg/0.5ml)	Administer Once Weekly (ml)	Total Daily Dose (mg)	Number of Capsules (200 mg)
< 40	50	0.5	800	4^a
40-50	80	0.4	800	4^a
51-64	80	0.5	800	4^a
65-75	100	0.5	1,000	5^b
76-85	120	0.5	1,000	5^b
> 85	150	0.5	1,200	6^c

a: 2 morning, 2 evening

b: 2 morning, 3 evening

c: 3 morning, 3 evening

Table 2 Monotherapy Dosing

	0.5 μg/kg		1.0 μg/kg	
Body Weight (kg)	**Vial/Pen Strength (μg/0.5ml)**	**Administer Once Weekly (ml)**	**Vial/Pen Strength (μg/0.5ml)**	**Administer Once Weekly (ml)**
30-35	50*	0.15	50	0.3
36-45	50*	0.2	50	0.4
46-56	50*	0.25	50	0.5
57-72	50	0.3	80	0.4
73-88	50	0.4	80	0.5
89-106	50	0.5	100	0.5
> 106**	80	0.4	120	0.5

* Must use vial. Minimum delivery for pen is 0.3 ml.

** For patients > 120 kg, use 80 μg/0.5 ml vial

Table 2a Dose modification guidelines for combination therapy (with ribavirin)

Laboratory values	Reduce only ribavirin dose to 600 mg/day* if:	Reduce only ViraferonPeg dose to one-half dose if:	Discontinue combination therapy if:
Haemoglobin	< 10 g/dl	-	< 8.5 g/dl
Haemoglobin in: Patients with history of stable cardiac disease	⩾ 2 g/dl decrease in haemoglobin during any four week period during treatment (permanent dose reduction)		< 12 g/dl after four weeks of dose reduction
White blood cells	-	< 1.5 × 10^9/l	< 1.0 × 10^9/l
Neutrophils	-	< 0.75 × 10^9/l	< 0.5 × 10^9/l
Platelets	-	< 50 × 10^9/l	< 25 × 10^9/l
Bilirubin – direct	-		2.5 × ULN**
Bilirubin - indirect	> 5 mg/dl		> 4 mg/dl (for > 4 weeks)
Creatinine	-	-	> 2.0 mg/dl
ALT/AST	-		2 × baseline and > 10 × ULN**

* Patients whose dose of ribavirin is reduced to 600 mg daily receive one 200 mg capsule in the morning and two 200 mg capsules in the evening.

** Upper limit of normal

Table 2b Reduced ViraferonPeg Dosing for Combination Therapy

Body Weight (kg)	Target Reduced Dose (μg)	Vial/Pen Strength (μg/0.5 ml)	Administer Once Weekly (ml)	Amount Delivered (μg)
< 40	25	50*	0.25	25
40-50	32	50	0.3	30
51-64	40	50	0.4	40
65-75	50	50	0.5	50
76-85	60	80	0.4	64
> 85	75	100	0.4	80

*Must use vial. Minimum delivery for pen is 0.3 ml.

Table 3a Dose modification guidelines for ViraferonPeg monotherapy

Laboratory values	Reduce ViraferonPeg to one-half dose if:	Discontinue ViraferonPeg if:
Neutrophils	< 0.75 × 10^9/l	< 0.5 × 10^9/l
Platelets	< 50 × 10^9/l	< 25 × 10^9/l

Dose reduction for patients who use 0.5 μg/kg ViraferonPeg monotherapy must be accomplished by reducing the prescribed volume by one-half. The 50 μg/0.5 ml vial must be used if necessary since the pen can only deliver a minimum volume of 0.3 ml.

For patients who use 1.0 μg/kg ViraferonPeg monotherapy, dose reduction may be accomplished by reducing the prescribed volume by one-half or by utilizing a lower dose strength as shown in **Table 3b**.

(see Table 3b on next page)

Special populations

Use in renal impairment: The clearance of ViraferonPeg is reduced in patients with significant renal impairment. Patients with creatinine clearance ⩽ 50 ml/minute must not be treated with ViraferonPeg (see section **5.2**). It is recommended that patients with moderate renal impairment be closely monitored and that their weekly dose of ViraferonPeg be reduced if medically appropriate.

Use in hepatic impairment: The safety and efficacy of ViraferonPeg therapy has not been evaluated in patients with severe hepatic dysfunction, therefore ViraferonPeg must not be used for these patients.

Use in the elderly (⩾ 65 years of age): There are no apparent age-related effects on the pharmacokinetics of ViraferonPeg. Data from elderly patients treated with a single dose of ViraferonPeg suggest no alteration in ViraferonPeg dose is necessary based on age (see section **5.2**).

Use in patients under the age of 18 years: ViraferonPeg is not recommended for use in children or adolescents under the age of 18, as there is no experience in this group.

4.3 Contraindications

- Hypersensitivity to the active substance or to any interferon or to any of the excipients;
- Use in pregnant women;
- Use in women who are breast-feeding;
- A history of severe pre-existing cardiac disease, including unstable or uncontrolled cardiac disease in the previous six months (see section **4.4**);
- Severe, debilitating medical conditions, including patients with chronic renal failure or creatinine clearance < 50 ml/minute;
- Autoimmune hepatitis or a history of autoimmune disease;
- Severe hepatic dysfunction or decompensated cirrhosis of the liver;
- Pre-existing thyroid disease unless it can be controlled with conventional treatment;
- Epilepsy and/or compromised central nervous system (CNS) function.

4.4 Special warnings and special precautions for use

There is no experience with ViraferonPeg in combination with ribavirin in patients who have relapsed after interferon alpha + ribavirin therapy.

All patients in the chronic hepatitis C studies had a liver biopsy before inclusion, but in certain cases (i.e. patients with genotype 2 and 3), treatment may be possible without histological confirmation. Current treatment guidelines should be consulted as to whether a liver biopsy is needed prior to commencing treatment.

Acute hypersensitivity: Acute hypersensitivity reactions (e.g., urticaria, angioedema, bronchoconstriction, anaphylaxis) have been observed rarely during interferon alfa-2b therapy. If such a reaction develops during treatment with ViraferonPeg, discontinue treatment and institute appropriate medical therapy immediately. Transient rashes do not necessitate interruption of treatment.

Cardiovascular system: As with interferon alfa-2b, patients with a history of congestive heart failure, myocardial infarction and/or previous or current arrhythmic disorders, receiving ViraferonPeg therapy require close monitoring. It is recommended that patients who have pre-existing cardiac abnormalities have electrocardiograms taken prior to and during the course of treatment. Cardiac arrhythmias (primarily supraventricular) usually respond to conventional therapy but may require discontinuation of ViraferonPeg therapy.

Psychiatric and Central Nervous System (CNS): If treatment with peginterferon alfa-2b is judged necessary in patients with existence or history of severe psychiatric conditions, this should only be initiated after having ensured appropriate individualised diagnostic and therapeutic management of the psychiatric condition.

Severe CNS effects, particularly depression, suicidal ideation and attempted suicide have been observed in some patients during ViraferonPeg therapy. Other CNS effects including aggressive behaviour (sometimes directed against others), confusion and alterations of mental status have been observed with alpha interferon. If patients develop psychiatric or CNS problems, including clinical depression, it is recommended that the patient be carefully monitored due to the potential seriousness of these undesirable effects. If symptoms persist or worsen, discontinue ViraferonPeg therapy.

More significant obtundation and coma, including cases of encephalopathy, have been observed in some patients, usually elderly, treated at higher doses for oncology indications. While these effects are generally reversible, in a few patients full resolution took up to three weeks. Very rarely, seizures have occurred with high doses of interferon alpha.

Liver function: As with all interferons, discontinue treatment with ViraferonPeg in patients who develop prolongation of coagulation markers which might indicate liver decompensation.

Fever: While fever may be associated with the flu-like syndrome reported commonly during interferon therapy, other causes of persistent fever must be ruled out.

Hydration: Adequate hydration must be maintained in patients undergoing ViraferonPeg therapy since hypotension related to fluid depletion has been seen in some patients treated with alpha interferons. Fluid replacement may be necessary.

Pulmonary changes: Pulmonary infiltrates, pneumonitis, and pneumonia, occasionally resulting in fatality, have been observed rarely in interferon alpha treated patients. Any patient developing fever, cough, dyspnea or other respiratory symptoms must have a chest X-ray taken. If the chest X-ray shows pulmonary infiltrates or there is evidence of pulmonary function impairment, the patient

Table 3b Reduced ViraferonPeg Dose for the 1.0 μg/kg Monotherapy Regimen

Body Weight (kg)	Target Reduced Dose (μg)	Vial/Pen Strength (μg/0.5ml)	Administer Once Weekly (ml)	Amount Delivered (μg)
30-35	15	50*	0.15	15
36-45	20	50*	0.20	20
46-56	25	50*	0.25	25
57-72	32	50	0.3	30
73-89	40	50	0.4	40
90-106	50	50	0.5	50
> 106	60	80	0.4	64

*Must use vial. Minimum delivery for pen is 0.3 ml.

is to be monitored closely, and, if appropriate, discontinue interferon alpha. Prompt discontinuation of interferon alpha administration and treatment with corticosteroids appear to be associated with resolution of pulmonary adverse events.

Autoimmune disease: The development of auto-antibodies and autoimmune disorders has been reported during treatment with alpha interferons. Patients predisposed to the development of autoimmune disorders may be at increased risk. Patients with signs or symptoms compatible with autoimmune disorders should be evaluated carefully, and the benefit-risk of continued interferon therapy should be reassessed (see also section **4.4 Thyroid changes** and **4.8**).

Ocular changes: Ophthalmologic disorders, including retinal haemorrhages, cotton wool spots, and retinal artery or vein obstruction have been reported in rare instances after treatment with alpha interferons (see section **4.8**). All patients should have a baseline eye examination. Any patient complaining of ocular symptoms, including loss of visual acuity or visual field must have a prompt and complete eye examination. Periodic visual examinations are recommended during ViraferonPeg therapy, particularly in patients with disorders that may be associated with retinopathy, such as diabetes mellitus or hypertension. Discontinuation of ViraferonPeg should be considered in patients who develop new or worsening ophthalmological disorders.

Thyroid changes: Infrequently, patients treated for chronic hepatitis C with interferon alpha have developed thyroid abnormalities, either hypothyroidism or hyperthyroidism. Determine thyroid stimulating hormone (TSH) levels if, during the course of therapy, a patient develops symptoms consistent with possible thyroid dysfunction. In the presence of thyroid dysfunction, ViraferonPeg treatment may be continued if TSH levels can be maintained in the normal range by medication.

Metabolic disturbances: Hypertriglyceridemia and aggravation of hypertriglyceridemia, sometimes severe, have been observed. Monitoring of lipid levels is, therefore, recommended.

HCV/HIV Coinfection

Patients co-infected with HIV and receiving Highly Active Anti-Retroviral Therapy (HAART) may be at increased risk of developing lactic acidosis. Caution should be used when adding ViraferonPeg and ribavirin to HAART therapy (see ribavirin SPC).

Co-infected patients with advanced cirrhosis receiving HAART may be at increased risk of hepatic decompensation and death. Adding treatment with alfa interferons alone or in combination with ribavirin may increase the risk in this patient subset.

Organ transplant recipients: The safety and efficacy of ViraferonPeg alone or in combination with ribavirin for the treatment of hepatitis C in liver or other organ transplant recipients have not been studied. Preliminary data indicates that interferon alpha therapy may be associated with an increased rate of kidney graft rejection. Liver graft rejection has also been reported.

Other: Due to reports of interferon alpha exacerbating pre-existing psoriatic disease and sarcoidosis, use of ViraferonPeg in patients with psoriasis or sarcoidosis is recommended only if the potential benefit justifies the potential risk.

Laboratory tests: Standard haematologic tests, blood chemistry and a test of thyroid function must be conducted in all patients prior to initiating therapy. Acceptable baseline values that may be considered as a guideline prior to initiation of ViraferonPeg therapy are:

- Platelets ⩾ 100,000/mm^3
- Neutrophil count ⩾ 1,500/mm^3
- TSH level must be within normal limits

Laboratory evaluations are to be conducted at weeks 2 and 4 of therapy, and periodically thereafter as clinically appropriate.

Important information about some of the ingredients of ViraferonPeg:

This medicinal product contains less than 1 mmol sodium (23 mg) per 0.7 ml, i.e., essentially "sodium-free".

4.5 Interaction with other medicinal products and other forms of Interaction

Results from a multiple-dose probe study assessing P450 substrates in chronic hepatitis C patients receiving once weekly ViraferonPeg (1.5 μg/kg) for 4 weeks demonstrated an increase in activity of CYP2D6 and CYP2C8/9. No change in activity of CYP1A2, CYP3A4, or N-acetyltransferase was observed.

Caution should be used when administering peginterferon alfa-2b with medications metabolised by CYP2D6 and CYP2C8/9, especially those with narrow therapeutic window, such as warfarin and phenytoin (CYP2C9) and flecainide (CYP2D6).

These findings may partly relate to improved metabolic capacity due to reduced hepatic inflammation in patients undergoing treatment with ViraferonPeg. Caution is therefore advised when ViraferonPeg treatment is initiated for chronic hepatitis in patients treated with medication with a narrow therapeutic window and sensitive to mild metabolic impairment of the liver.

No pharmacokinetic interactions were noted between ViraferonPeg and ribavirin in a multiple-dose pharmacokinetic study.

4.6 Pregnancy and lactation

There are no adequate data from the use of interferon alfa-2b in pregnant women. Interferon alfa-2b has been shown to be abortifacient in primates. ViraferonPeg is likely to also cause this effect. ViraferonPeg is contraindicated in pregnancy (see sections **4.3** and **5.3**).

ViraferonPeg is recommended for use in fertile women only when they are using effective contraception during the treatment period.

Lactation: It is not known whether the components of this medicinal product are excreted in human milk. Because of the potential for adverse reactions in nursing infants, nursing must be discontinued prior to initiation of treatment.

Combination therapy with ribavirin:

Ribavirin causes serious birth defects when administered during pregnancy. Women of childbearing potential have to use effective contraception during and up to for 4 months after treatment (see section **5.3** and the respective informing texts of ribavirin containing medicinal products).

4.7 Effects on ability to drive and use machines

Patients who develop fatigue, somnolence or confusion during treatment with ViraferonPeg are cautioned to avoid driving or operating machinery.

4.8 Undesirable effects

The safety of ViraferonPeg is evaluated from data from two clinical trials: one with ViraferonPeg monotherapy, one with ViraferonPeg in combination with ribavirin. In both cases, patients were treated for one year.

Table 4 describes the regimens and patient exposure for one year of treatment in patients with no previous exposure to interferon (interferon-naïve patients). Because of a significant overlap in the pattern of undesirable effects with ViraferonPeg monotherapy, groups of patients have been brought together in **Table 5** to show the pattern of reported effects for all monotherapy groups.

Table 4 Regimens and patient exposure

Treatment	Regimen	Number of patients treated for one year
ViraferonPeg + ribavirin	ViraferonPeg (1.5 micrograms/kg/ week) + ribavirin (> 10.6 mg/kg/day)	188
Interferon alfa-2b + ribavirin	Interferon alfa-2b (3 MIU three times a week) + ribavirin (1,000/1,200 mg/ day)	505
ViraferonPeg monotherapy	ViraferonPeg (0.5 microgram/kg/ week)	315
	ViraferonPeg (1.0 microgram/kg/ week)	297
	ViraferonPeg (1.5 micrograms/kg/ week)	304

(see Table 5 on next page - right hand column)

Table 6 Undesirable effects commonly reported in clinical trials in patients treated with ViraferonPeg + ribavirin or ViraferonPeg monotherapy
Common (> 1/100, < 1/10)

Body system	5-10%	1- <5%
Infections and infestations		otitis media, fungal infection, bacterial infection, herpes simplex
Blood and lymphatic system disorders	anaemia, leukopaenia	thrombocytopenia, lymphadenopathy
Endocrine disorders	Hypothyroidism	hyperthyroidism
Metabolism and nutrition disorders		hyperuricemia, hypocalcemia, thirst
Psychiatric disorders	agitation, nervousness	aggressive behaviour, somnolence, behavior disorder, apathy, appetite increased, sleep disorder, dreaming abnormal, decreased libido
Nervous system disorders	paresthesia, increased sweating	hypoaesthesia, hyperaesthesia, hypertonia, confusion, tremor, vertigo, migraine, ataxia, neuralgia
Eye disorders		blurred vision, conjunctivitis, lacrimal gland disorder, eye pain
Cardiac disorders		tachycardia, palpitation
Vascular disorders		hypotension, hypertension, syncope, flushing
Ear and labyrinth disorders		tinnitus, hearing impairment/loss
Respiratory, thoracic and mediastinal disorders		nonproductive cough, rhinitis, sinusitis, bronchitis, respiratory disorder, nasal congestion, rhinorrhea, dysphonia, epistaxis
Gastrointestinal disorders	dyspepsia	constipation, taste perversion, loose stools, stomatitis, ulcerative stomatitis, gingival bleeding, glossitis, flatulence, hemorrhoids, gastroesophageal reflux, gingivitis, dehydration

Hepatobiliary disorders		hepatomegaly, hyperbilirubinemia
Skin and subcutaneous tissue disorders		erythematous rash, eczema, photosensitivity reaction, maculopapular rash, abnormal hair texture, acne, dermatitis, furunculosis, nail disorder, psoriasis, urticaria, erythema, face or peripheral oedema
Musculoskeletal and connective tissue disorders		arthritis
Renal and urinary disorders		micturition frequency, urine abnormal
Reproductive system and breast disorders	menstrual disorder, menorrhagia	ovarian disorder, vaginal disorder, sexual dysfunction (not specified), impotence, breast pain, amenorrhoea, prostatitis
General disorders and administration site conditions	RUQ pain, malaise, chest pain	injection site pain

Most cases of neutropaenia and thrombocytopaenia were mild (WHO grades 1 or 2). There were some cases of more severe neutropenia in patients treated with the recommended doses of ViraferonPeg in combination with ribavirin (WHO grade 3: 39 of 186 [21 %]; and WHO grade 4: 13 of 186 [7 %]).

In a clinical trial, approximately 1.2 % of patients treated with ViraferonPeg or interferon alfa-2b in combination with ribavirin reported life-threatening psychiatric events during treatment. These events included suicidal ideation and attempted suicide (see section **4.4**). Following marketing, psychosis and hallucination have been reported rarely.

Rarely (> 1/10,000, < 1/1,000) or very rarely (< 1/10,000) reported events with interferon alfa-2b, including ViraferonPeg, include:

Immune system disorders:

very rarely: sarcoidosis or exacerbation of sarcoidosis

Endocrine disorders:

rarely: diabetes

Nervous system disorders:

rarely: seizure, peripheral neuropathy

very rarely: cerebrovascular ischaemia, cerebrovascular haemorrhage, encephalopathy

Cardiac disorders:

rarely: arrhythmia

very rarely: cardiac ischaemia, myocardial infarction

Respiratory, thoracic and mediastinal disorders:

very rarely: interstitial lung disease

Gastrointestinal disorders:

rarely: pancreatitis

very rarely: ulcerative and ischaemic colitis

Skin and subcutaneous tissue disorders:

very rarely: erythema multiforme, Stevens Johnson syndrome, toxic epidermal necrolysis, injection site necrosis

Musculoskeletal and connective tissue disorders:

rarely: rhabdomyolysis, myositis

Renal and urinary disorders:

rarely: renal insufficiency and renal failure

Cardiovascular (CVS) adverse events, particularly arrhythmia, appeared to be correlated mostly with pre-existing CVS disease and prior therapy with cardiotoxic agents (see section **4.4**). Cardiomyopathy, that may be reversible upon discontinuation of interferon alpha, has been reported rarely in patients without prior evidence of cardiac disease.

Very rarely, interferon alfa-2b or ViraferonPeg used alone or in combination with ribavirin may be associated with aplastic anaemia.

Ophthalmological disorders that have been reported rarely with alpha interferons include retinopathies (including macular oedema), retinal haemorrhages, retinal artery or vein obstruction, cotton wool spots, loss of visual acuity or visual field, optic neuritis, and papilloedema (see section **4.4**).

A wide variety of autoimmune and immune-mediated disorders have been reported with alpha interferons including thyroid disorders, systemic lupus erythematosus, rheumatoid arthritis (new or aggravated), idiopathic and thrombotic thrombocytopenic purpura, vasculitis, neuropathies

Table 5 Undesirable effects very commonly reported in clinical trials > 10 % of patients in ViraferonPeg + ribavirin group Very common (> 1/10)

	ViraferonPeg + ribavirin	Interferon alfa-2b + ribavirin	ViraferonPeg monotherapy
Infections and infestations			
Infection viral	10 %	5 %	4-5 %
Metabolism and nutrition disorders			
Weight decrease	30 %	19 %	8-18 %
Psychiatric disorders			
Depression	34 %	32 %	26 %
Irritability	32 %	34 %	19 %
Insomnia	37 %	41 %	16-19 %
Anxiety	14 %	14 %	8 %
Concentration impaired	18 %	21 %	9-10 %
Emotional lability	11 %	10 %	5 %
Nervous system disorders			
Headache	58 %	57 %	57-63 %
Mouth dry	10 %	8 %	4-8 %
Respiratory, thoracic and mediastinal disorders			
Pharyngitis	10 %	7 %	3 %
Coughing	14 %	11 %	4 %
Dyspnea	26 %	22 %	5 %
Gastrointestinal disorders			
Nausea	43 %	31 %	20-23 %
Anorexia	35 %	26 %	10-25 %
Diarrhoea	20 %	13 %	14-17 %
Abdominal pain	12 %	9 %	11 %
Vomiting	16 %	10 %	4-7 %
Skin and subcutaneous tissue disorders			
Alopecia	45 %	32 %	20-34 %
Pruritus	27 %	27 %	7-9 %
Skin dry	23 %	21 %	6-9 %
Rash	21 %	21 %	5-7 %
Musculoskeletal and connective tissue disorders			
Myalgia	49 %	49 %	46-60 %
Arthralgia	31 %	26 %	23-28 %
Musculoskeletal pain	15 %	11 %	11-13 %
General disorders and administration site conditions			
Injection site inflammation	20 %	17 %	39-44 %
Injection site reaction	54 %	36 %	7-9 %
Fatigue	56 %	59 %	43 %
Rigors	42 %	40 %	33-43 %
Fever	39 %	32 %	29-43 %
Flu-like symptoms	21 %	23 %	18-25 %
Asthenia	28 %	17 %	12-14 %
Dizziness	17 %	16 %	7-12 %

Table 7 Sustained virological response (% patients HCV negative)

	ViraferonPeg monotherapy				ViraferonPeg + ribavirin		
Treatment regimen	**P 1.5**	**P 1.0**	**P 0.5**	**I**	**P 1.5/R**	**P 0.5/R**	**I/R**
Number of Patients	304	297	315	303	511	514	505
Response at end of treatment	49%	41%	33%	24%	65%	56%	54%
Sustained response	**23%**	**25%**	**18%**	**12%**	**54%**	**47%**	**47%**

P 1.5 ViraferonPeg 1.5 micrograms/kg
P 1.0 ViraferonPeg 1.0 microgram/kg
P 0.5 ViraferonPeg 0.5 microgram/kg
I Interferon alfa-2b 3 MIU
P 1.5/R ViraferonPeg (1.5 micrograms/kg) + ribavirin (800 mg)
P 0.5/R ViraferonPeg (1.5 to 0.5 microgram/kg) + ribavirin (1,000/1,200 mg)
I/R Interferon alfa-2b (3 MIU) + ribavirin (1,000/1,200 mg)
* $p < 0.001$ P 1.5 vs. I
** $p = 0.0143$ P 1.5/R vs. I/R

including mononeuropathies (see also section **4.4, Autoimmune disorders**).

4.9 Overdose

In clinical trials, cases of accidental overdose, at never more than twice the prescribed dose, were reported. There were no serious reactions. Undesirable effects resolved during continued administration of ViraferonPeg.

5. PHARMACOLOGICAL PROPERTIES

5.1 Pharmacodynamic properties

Pharmacotherapeutic group: Immunostimulants, Cytokines and immunomodulators, Interferons, Peginterferon alfa-2b, ATC code: L03A B10.

Recombinant interferon alfa-2b is covalently conjugated with monomethoxy polyethylene glycol at an average degree of substitution of 1 mole of polymer/mole of protein. The average molecular mass is approximately 31,300 daltons of which the protein moiety constitutes approximately 19,300.

Interferon alfa-2b

In vitro and *in vivo* studies suggest that the biological activity of ViraferonPeg is derived from its interferon alfa-2b moiety.

Interferons exert their cellular activities by binding to specific membrane receptors on the cell surface. Studies with other interferons have demonstrated species specificity. However, certain monkey species, e.g., Rhesus monkeys, are susceptible to pharmacodynamic stimulation upon exposure to human type 1 interferons.

Once bound to the cell membrane, interferon initiates a complex sequence of intracellular events that include the induction of certain enzymes. It is thought that this process, at least in part, is responsible for the various cellular responses to interferon, including inhibition of virus replication in virus-infected cells, suppression of cell proliferation and such immunomodulating activities as enhancement of the phagocytic activity of macrophages and augmentation of the specific cytotoxicity of lymphocytes for target cells. Any or all of these activities may contribute to interferon's therapeutic effects.

Recombinant interferon alfa-2b also inhibits viral replication *in vitro* and *in vivo*. Although the exact antiviral mode of action of recombinant interferon alfa-2b is unknown, it appears to alter the host cell metabolism. This action inhibits viral replication or if replication occurs, the progeny virions are unable to leave the cell.

ViraferonPeg

ViraferonPeg pharmacodynamics were assessed in a rising single-dose trial in healthy subjects by examining changes in oral temperature, concentrations of effector proteins such as serum neopterin and 2'5'-oligoadenylate synthetase (2'5'-OAS), as well as white cell and neutrophil counts. Subjects treated with ViraferonPeg showed mild dose-related elevations in body temperature. Following single doses of ViraferonPeg between 0.25 and 2.0 micrograms/kg/week, serum neopterin concentration was increased in a dose-related manner. Neutrophil and white cell count reductions at the end of week 4 correlated with the dose of ViraferonPeg.

ViraferonPeg clinical trials

Two pivotal trials have been conducted, one (C/I97-010) with ViraferonPeg monotherapy; the other (C/I98-580) with ViraferonPeg in combination with ribavirin. Eligible patients for these trials had chronic hepatitis C confirmed by a positive HCV-RNA polymerase chain reaction (PCR) assay (> 30 IU/ml), a liver biopsy consistent with a histological diagnosis of chronic hepatitis with no other cause for the chronic hepatitis, and abnormal serum ALT.

In the ViraferonPeg monotherapy trial, a total of 916 naïve chronic hepatitis C patients were treated with ViraferonPeg (0.5, 1.0 or 1.5 micrograms/kg/week) for one year with a follow-up period of six months. In addition, 303 patients received interferon alfa-2b (3 million International Units [MIU] three times a week as a comparator. This study showed that ViraferonPeg was superior to interferon alfa-2b (**Table 7**).

In the ViraferonPeg combination trial, 1,530 naïve patients were treated for one year with one of the following combination regimens:

- ViraferonPeg (1.5 micrograms/kg/week) + ribavirin (800 mg/day), (n = 511).
- ViraferonPeg (1.5 micrograms/kg/week for one month followed by 0.5 microgram/kg/week for 11 months) + ribavirin (1,000/1,200 mg/day), (n = 514).
- Interferon alfa-2b (3 MIU three times a week) + ribavirin (1,000/1,200 mg/day) (n = 505).

In this trial, the combination of ViraferonPeg (1.5 micrograms/kg/week) and ribavirin was significantly more effective than the combination of interferon alfa-2b and ribavirin (**Table 7**), particularly in patients infected with Genotype 1 (**Table 8**). Sustained response was assessed by the response rate six months after the cessation of treatment.

HCV genotype and baseline virus load are prognostic factors which are known to affect response rates. However, response rates in this trial were shown to be dependent also on the dose of ribavirin administered in combination with ViraferonPeg or interferon alfa-2b. In those patients that received > 10.6 mg/kg ribavirin (800 mg dose in typical 75 kg patient), regardless of genotype or viral load, response rates were significantly higher than in those patients that received ⩽ 10.6 mg/kg ribavirin (**Table 8**), while response rates in patients that received > 13.2 mg/kg ribavirin were even higher.

(see Table 7 above)

(see Table 8 below)

In the ViraferonPeg monotherapy study, the Quality of Life was generally less affected by 0.5 microgram/kg of ViraferonPeg than by either 1.0 microgram/kg of ViraferonPeg once weekly or 3 MIU of interferon alfa-2b three times a week.

In a separate trial, 224 patients with genotype 2 or 3 received ViraferonPeg, 1.5 microgram/kg subcutaneously, once weekly, in combination with ribavirin 800 mg – 1,400 mg p.o. for 6 months (based on body weight, only three patients weighing > 105 kg, received the 1,400 mg dose, which has not yet been validated) (**Table 9**). Twenty-four % had bridging fibrosis or cirrhosis (Knodell 3/4).

Table 9. Virologic Response at End of Treatment, Sustained Virologic Response and Relapse by HCV Genotype and Viral Load*

(see Table 9 on next page)

The 6 month treatment duration in this trial was better tolerated than one year of treatment in the pivotal combination trial; for discontinuation 5 % vs. 14 %, for dose modification 18 % vs. 49 %.

In a non-comparative trial, 235 patients with genotype 1 and low viral load (< 600,000 IU/ml) received ViraferonPeg, 1.5 microgram/kg subcutaneously, once weekly, in combination with weight adjusted ribavirin. The overall sustained response rate after a 24-week treatment duration was 50 %. Forty-one percent of subjects (97/235) had nondetectable plasma HCV-RNA levels at Week 4 and Week 24 of therapy. In this subgroup, there was a 92 % (89/97) sustained virological response rate. The high sustained response rate in this subgroup of patients was identified in an interim analysis (n=49) and prospectively confirmed (n=48).

Limited historical data indicate that treatment for 48 weeks might be associated with a higher sustained response rate (11/11) and with a lower risk of relapse (0/11 as compared to 7/96 following 24 weeks of treatment).

Predictability of sustained virological response

Virological reponse by week 12, defined as a 2-log viral load decrease or undetectable levels of HCV RNA has been shown to be predictive for sustained response (**Table 10**).

(see Table 10 on next page)

The negative predictive value for sustained response in patients treated with ViraferonPeg in monotherapy was 98 %.

5.2 Pharmacokinetic properties

ViraferonPeg is a well characterized polyethylene glycol-modified ("pegylated") derivative of interferon alfa-2b and is predominantly composed of monopegylated species. The plasma half-life of ViraferonPeg is prolonged compared with non-pegylated interferon alfa-2b. ViraferonPeg has a potential to depegylate to free interferon alfa-2b. The biologic activity of the pegylated isomers is qualitatively similar, but weaker than free interferon alfa-2b.

Table 8 Sustained response rates with ViraferonPeg + ribavirin (by ribavirin dose, genotype and viral load)

HCV Genotype	**Rebetol dose (mg/kg)**	**P 1.5/R**	**P 0.5/R**	**I/R**
All Genotypes	**All**	**54 %**	**47 %**	**47 %**
	⩽ 10.6	50 %	41 %	27 %
	> 10.6	61 %	48 %	47 %
Genotype 1	**All**	**42 %**	**34 %**	**33 %**
	⩽ 10.6	38 %	25 %	20 %
	> 10.6	48 %	34 %	34 %
Genotype 1 ⩽ 600,000 IU/ml	All	73 %	51 %	45 %
	⩽ 10.6	74 %	25 %	33 %
	> 10.6	71 %	52 %	45 %
Genotype 1 > 600,000 IU/ml	All	30 %	27 %	29 %
	⩽ 10.6	27 %	25 %	17 %
	> 10.6	37 %	27 %	29 %
Genotype 2/3	**All**	**82 %**	**80 %**	**79 %**
	⩽ 10.6	79 %	73 %	50 %
	> 10.6	88 %	80 %	80 %

P 1.5/R ViraferonPeg (1.5 micrograms/kg) + ribavirin (800 mg)
P 0.5/R ViraferonPeg (1.5 to 0.5 microgram/kg) + ribavirin (1,000/1,200 mg)
I/R Interferon alfa-2b (3 MIU) + ribavirin (1,000/1,200 mg)

Table 9 Virologic Response at End of Treatment, Sustained Virologic Response and Relapse by HCV Genotype and Viral Load*

	ViraferonPeg 1.5 μg/kg Once Weekly Plus Rebetol 800-1400 mg/day		
	End of Treatment Response	Sustained Virologic Response	Relapse
All Subjects	94 % (211/224)	81 % (182/224)	12 % (27/224)
HCV 2	100 % (42/42)	93 % (39/42)	7 % (3/42)
⩽ 600,000 IU/ml	100 % (20/20)	95 % (19/20)	5 % (1/20)
> 600,000 IU/mL	100 % (22/22)	91 % (20/22)	9 % (2/22)
HCV 3	93 % (169/182)	79 % (143/182)	14 % (24/166)
⩽ 600,000 IU/ml	93 % (92/99)	86 % (85/99)	8 % (7/91)
> 600,000 IU/ml	93 % (77/83)	70 % (58/83)	23 % (17/75)

* Any subject with an undetectable HCV-RNA level at the Follow-Up Week 12 visit and missing data at the Follow-Up Week 24 visit was considered a sustained responder. Any subject with missing data in and after the Follow-Up Week 12 window was considered to be a non-responder at Week 24 of follow-up.

Table 10 Predictability of sustained response by viral response at week 12 and genotype*

Treatment	Genotype	Viral response at week 12	Sustained response	Negative predictive value
ViraferonPeg 1.5 + ribavirin (> 10.6 mg/kg) 48-week treatment	1	Yes 75 % (82/110)	71 % (58/82)	—
		No 25 % (28/110)	0 % (0/28)	100 %
ViraferonPeg 1.5 + ribavirin 800-1,400 mg 24-week treatment	2 and 3	Yes 99 % (213/215)	83 % (177/213)	—
		No 1 % (2/215)	50 % (1/2)	50 %

* reflects patients with 12 week data available

Following subcutaneous administration, maximal serum concentrations occur between 15-44 hours post-dose, and are sustained for up to 48-72 hours post-dose.

ViraferonPeg C_{max} and AUC measurements increase in a dose-related manner. Mean apparent volume of distribution is 0.99 l/kg.

Upon multiple dosing, there is an accumulation of immunoreactive interferons. There is, however, only a modest increase in biologic activity as measured by a bioassay.

Mean (SD) ViraferonPeg elimination half-life is approximately 40 hours (13.3 hours), with apparent clearance of 22.0 ml/hr•kg. The mechanisms involved in clearance of interferons in man have not yet been fully elucidated. However, renal elimination may account for a minority (approximately 30 %) of ViraferonPeg apparent clearance.

Renal function: Renal clearance appears to account for 30 % of total clearance of ViraferonPeg. In a single dose study (1.0 microgram/kg) in patients with impaired renal function, C_{max}, AUC, and half-life increased in relation to the degree of renal impairment.

Based on these data, no dose modification is recommended based on creatinine clearance. However, because of marked intra-subject variability in interferon pharmacokinetics, it is recommended that patients be monitored closely during treatment with ViraferonPeg (see section **4.2**). Patients with severe renal dysfunction or creatinine clearance < 50 ml/min must not be treated with ViraferonPeg.

Hepatic function: The pharmacokinetics of ViraferonPeg have not been evaluated in patients with severe hepatic dysfunction.

Elderly patients ⩾ 65 years of age: The pharmacokinetics of ViraferonPeg following a single subcutaneous dose of 1.0 microgram/kg were not affected by age. The data suggest that no alteration in ViraferonPeg dosage is necessary based on advancing age.

Patients under the age of 18 years: Specific pharmacokinetic evaluations have not been performed on these patients. ViraferonPeg is indicated for the treatment of chronic hepatitis C only in patients 18 years of age or older.

Interferon neutralising factors: Interferon neutralising factor assays were performed on serum samples of patients who received ViraferonPeg in the clinical trial. Interferon neutralising factors are antibodies which neutralise the antiviral activity of interferon. The clinical incidence of neutralising factors in patients who received ViraferonPeg 0.5 micrograms/kg is 1.1 %.

5.3 Preclinical safety data

ViraferonPeg: Adverse events not observed in clinical trials were not seen in toxicity studies in monkeys. These studies were limited to four weeks due to the appearance of anti-interferon antibodies in most monkeys.

Reproduction studies of ViraferonPeg have not been performed. Interferon alfa-2b has been shown to be an abortifacient in primates. ViraferonPeg is likely to also cause this effect. Effects on fertility have not been determined. It is not known whether the components of this medicinal product are excreted into experimental animal or human milk (see section **4.6** for relevant human data on pregnancy and lactation). ViraferonPeg showed no genotoxic potential.

The relative non-toxicity of monomethoxy-polyethylene glycol (mPEG), which is liberated from ViraferonPeg by metabolism *in vivo* has been demonstrated in preclinical acute and subchronic toxicity studies in rodents and monkeys, standard embryo-foetal development studies and in *in vitro* mutagenicity assays.

ViraferonPeg plus ribavirin: When used in combination with ribavirin, ViraferonPeg did not cause any effects not previously seen with either active substance alone. The major treatment-related change was a reversible, mild to moderate anaemia, the severity of which was greater than that produced by either active substance alone.

6. PHARMACEUTICAL PARTICULARS

6.1 List of excipients

Powder for solution for injection:

Disodium phosphate, anhydrous,

Sodium dihydrogen phosphate dihydrate,

Sucrose,

Polysorbate 80.

Solvent for parenteral use:

Water for injections.

6.2 Incompatibilities

This medicinal product should only be reconstituted with the solvent provided (see section **6.6**). In the absence of compatibility studies, this medicinal product must not be mixed with other medicinal products.

6.3 Shelf life

3 years

After reconstitution:

- Chemical and physical in-use stability has been demonstrated for 24 hours at 2°C - 8°C.

- From a microbiological point of view, the product is to be used immediately. If not used immediately, in-use storage times and conditions prior to use are the responsibility of the user and would normally not be longer than 24 hours at 2°C - 8°C.

6.4 Special precautions for storage

Store in a refrigerator (2°C - 8°C).

6.5 Nature and contents of container

The powder is contained in a 2 ml vial, Type I flint glass, with a butyl rubber stopper in an aluminium flip-off seal with a polypropylene bonnet. The solvent is presented in a 2 ml ampoule, Type I flint glass.

ViraferonPeg 50, 80, 100, 120, or 150 micrograms is supplied as:

- 1 vial of powder for solution for injection and 1 ampoule of solvent for parenteral use;

- 1 vial of powder for solution for injection, 1 ampoule of solvent for parenteral use, 1 injection syringe, 2 injection needles and 1 cleansing swab;

- 4 vials of powder for solution for injection and 4 ampoules of solvent for parenteral use;

- 4 vials of powder for solution for injection, 4 ampoules of solvent for parenteral use, 4 injection syringes, 8 injection needles and 4 cleansing swabs;

- 6 vials of powder for solution for injection and 6 ampoules of solvent for parenteral use.

- 12 vials of powder for solution for injection, 12 ampoules of solvent for parenteral use, 12 injection syringes, 24 injection needles and 12 cleansing swabs.

Not all pack sizes may be marketed

6.6 Instructions for use and handling

ViraferonPeg is supplied as a powder of peginterferon alfa-2b at a strength of 50, 80, 100, 120, or 150 micrograms for single use. Each vial must be reconstituted with 0.7 ml of water for injections for administration of up to 0.5 ml of solution. A small volume is lost during preparation of ViraferonPeg for injection when the dose is measured and injected. Therefore, each vial contains an excess amount of solvent and ViraferonPeg powder to ensure delivery of the labelled dose in 0.5 ml of ViraferonPeg, solution for injection. The reconstituted solution has a concentration of 50 micrograms/0.5 ml, 80 micrograms/0.5 ml, 100 micrograms/0.5 ml, 120 micrograms/0.5 ml or 150 micrograms/0.5 ml.

Using a sterilised injection syringe and injection needle, inject 0.7 ml of water for injections into the vial of ViraferonPeg. Agitate gently to complete dissolution of powder. The appropriate dose can then be withdrawn with a sterilised injection syringe and injected. A complete set of instructions is provided in the Annex to the Package Leaflet.

As for all parenteral medicinal products, inspect visually the reconstituted solution prior to administration. The reconstituted solution should be clear and colourless. Do not use if discolouration or particulate matter is present. Discard any unused material.

7. MARKETING AUTHORISATION HOLDER

SP Europe

73, rue de Stalle

B-1180 Bruxelles

Belgium

8. MARKETING AUTHORISATION NUMBER(S)

ViraferonPeg 50 micrograms: EU/1/00/132/001-005; 026

ViraferonPeg 80 micrograms: EU/1/00/132/006-010; 027

ViraferonPeg 100 micrograms: EU/1/00/132/011-015; 028

ViraferonPeg 120 micrograms: EU/1/00/132/016-020; 029

ViraferonPeg 150 micrograms: EU/1/00/132/021-025; 030

9. DATE OF FIRST AUTHORISATION/RENEWAL OF THE AUTHORISATION

Date of first authorisation: 29 May 2000

Date of last renewal: 23 May 2005

10. DATE OF REVISION OF THE TEXT

8 September 2005

11. Legal Category

Prescription Only Medicine

ViraferonPegP&S/09-05/12

ViraferonPeg Pen 50, 80, 100, 120 or 150 micrograms powder and solvent for solution for injection in pre-filled pen

(Schering-Plough Ltd)

1. NAME OF THE MEDICINAL PRODUCT

ViraferonPeg 50, 80, 100, 120 and 150 micrograms, powder and solvent for solution for injection in pre-filled pen

2. QUALITATIVE AND QUANTITATIVE COMPOSITION

Each pre-filled pen of ViraferonPeg 50, 80, 100, 120 or 150 micrograms contains a sufficient amount of peginterferon alfa-2b as measured on a protein basis in a powder for solution for injection, and the corresponding amount of solvent, to provide 50, 80, 100, 120 or 150 micrograms in 0.5 ml of peginterferon alfa-2b when reconstituted as recommended.

The active substance is a covalent conjugate of recombinant interferon alfa-2b* with monomethoxy polyethylene glycol. The potency of this product should not be compared to that of another pegylated or non-pegylated protein of the same therapeutic class. For more information, see section **5.1.**

*produced by rDNA technology in *E.coli* cells harbouring a genetically engineered plasmid hybrid encompassing an interferon alfa-2b gene from human leukocytes

For excipients, see section 6.1.

3. PHARMACEUTICAL FORM

Powder and solvent for solution for injection in pre-filled pen

Table 1 Dosing for Combination Therapy

Body Weight (kg)	ViraferonPeg		Ribavirin Capsules	
	Vial/Pen Strength (µ g/0.5ml)	Administer Once Weekly (ml)	Total Daily Dose (mg)	Number of Capsules (200 mg)
< 40	50	0.5	800	4[a]
40-50	80	0.4	800	4[a]
51-64	80	0.5	800	4[a]
65-75	100	0.5	1,000	5[b]
76-85	120	0.5	1,000	5[b]
> 85	150	0.5	1,200	6[c]

a: 2 morning, 2 evening
b: 2 morning, 3 evening
c: 3 morning, 3 evening

White powder.

Clear and colourless solvent.

4. CLINICAL PARTICULARS

4.1 Therapeutic indications

ViraferonPeg is indicated for the treatment of adult patients with chronic hepatitis C who have elevated transaminases without liver decompensation and who are positive for serum HCV-RNA or anti-HCV (see section **4.4**).

The best way to use ViraferonPeg in this indication is in combination with ribavirin.

This combination is indicated in naïve patients as well as in patients who have previously responded (with normalisation of ALT at the end of treatment) to interferon alpha monotherapy but who have subsequently relapsed.

Interferon monotherapy, including ViraferonPeg, is indicated mainly in case of intolerance or contraindication to ribavirin.

Please refer also to the ribavirin Summary of Product Characteristics (SPC) when ViraferonPeg is to be used in combination with ribavirin.

4.2 Posology and method of administration

Treatment should be initiated and monitored only by a physician experienced in the management of patients with hepatitis C.

Dose to be administered

ViraferonPeg should be administered as a once weekly subcutaneous injection. The dose administered depends on whether it is used in combination with ribavirin or as monotherapy.

Combination therapy

ViraferonPeg 1.5 micrograms/kg/week in combination with ribavirin capsules.

The intended dose of 1.5 µg/kg of ViraferonPeg to be used in combination with ribavirin may be delivered in weight categories with the pen/vial strengths according to **Table 1**. Ribavirin capsules are to be administered orally each day in two divided doses with food (morning and evening).

Table 1 - Dosing for Combination Therapy

(see Table 1 above)

Duration of treatment

Predictability of sustained virological response: Patients infected with virus genotype 1 who fail to achieve virological response at Week 12 are highly unlikely to become sustained virological responders (see also section **5.1**).

• **Genotype 1**: For patients who exhibit virological response at week 12, treatment should be continued for another nine month period (i.e., a total of 48 weeks).

In the subset of patients with genotype 1 infection and low viral load (< 600,000 IU/ml) who become HCV-RNA negative at treatment week 4 and remain HCV-RNA negative at week 24, the treatment could either be stopped after this 24 week treatment course or pursued for an additional 24 weeks (i.e. overall 48 weeks treatment duration). However, an overall 24 weeks treatment duration may be associated with a higher risk of relapse than a 48 weeks treatment duration (see section **5.1**).

• **Genotypes 2 or 3**: It is recommended that all patients be treated for 24 weeks.

• **Genotype 4:** In general, patients infected with genotype 4 are considered harder to treat and limited study data (n=66) indicate they are compatible with a posology as for genotype 1.

ViraferonPeg monotherapy

As monotherapy the ViraferonPeg regimen is 0.5 or 1.0 microgram/kg/week. The lowest vial or pen strength available is 50 µg/0.5 ml; therefore for patients prescribed 0.5 µg/kg/week, doses must be adjusted by volume as shown in **Table 2**. For the 1.0 µg/kg dose, similar volume adjustments can be made or alternate vial strengths can be used as shown in **Table 2**.

Table 2 - Monotherapy Dosing

(see Table 2 below)

Duration of treatment

For patients who exhibit virological response at Week 12, treatment should be continued for at least another three-month period (i.e., a total of six months). The decision to extend therapy to one year of treatment should be based on prognostic factors (e.g., genotype, age > 40 years, male gender, bridging fibrosis).

Dose modification for all patients

If severe adverse reactions or laboratory abnormalities develop during treatment with ViraferonPeg monotherapy or ViraferonPeg in combination with ribavirin, modify the dosages of each product as appropriate, until the adverse reactions abate. As adherence might be of importance for outcome of therapy, the dose should be kept as close as possible to the recommended standard dose. Guidelines were developed in clinical trials for dose modification.

Combination Therapy Dose Reduction Guidelines

(see Table 2a below)

Dose reduction of ViraferonPeg may be accomplished by either reducing the prescribed volume by one-half or by utilizing a lower dose strength as shown in **Table 2b**.

(see Table 2b on next page)

ViraferonPeg Monotherapy Dose Reduction Guidelines

Dose modification guidelines for patients who use ViraferonPeg monotherapy are shown in **Table 3a**.

Table 3a Dose modification guidelines for ViraferonPeg monotherapy

Laboratory values	Reduce ViraferonPeg <u>to one-half dose</u> if:	Discontinue ViraferonPeg if:
Neutrophils	< 0.75 × 109/l	< 0.5 × 109/l
Platelets	< 50 × 109/l	< 25 × 109/l

Dose reduction for patients who use 0.5 µg/kg ViraferonPeg monotherapy must be accomplished by reducing the prescribed volume by one-half. The 50 µg/0.5 ml vial must be used if necessary since the pen can only deliver a minimum volume of 0.3 ml.

For patients who use 1.0 µg/kg ViraferonPeg monotherapy, dose reduction may be accomplished by reducing the prescribed volume by one-half or by utilizing a lower dose strength as shown in **Table 3b**.

(see Table 3b on next page)

Table 2 Monotherapy Dosing

	0.5 µ g/kg		1.0 µ g/kg	
Body Weight (kg)	Vial/Pen Strength (µ g/0.5ml)	Administer Once Weekly (ml)	Vial/Pen Strength (µ g/0.5ml)	Administer Once Weekly(ml)
30-35	50*	0.15	50	0.3
36-45	50*	0.2	50	0.4
46-56	50*	0.25	50	0.5
57-72	50	0.3	80	0.4
73-88	50	0.4	80	0.5
89-106	50	0.5	100	0.5
> 106**	80	0.4	120	0.5

* Must use vial. Minimum delivery for pen is 0.3 ml.
** For patients > 120 kg, use 80 µg/0.5 ml vial

Table 2a Dose modification guidelines for combination therapy (with ribavirin)

Laboratory values	Reduce only ribavirin dose <u>to 600 mg/day</u>* if:	Reduce only ViraferonPeg <u>dose to one-half dose</u> if:	Discontinue combination therapy if:
Haemoglobin	< 10 g/dl	-	< 8.5 g/dl
Haemoglobin in: Patients with history of stable cardiac disease	⩾ 2 g/dl decrease in haemoglobin during any four week period during treatment (permanent dose reduction)		< 12 g/dl after four weeks of dose reduction
White blood cells	-	< 1.5 × 10^9/l	< 1.0 × 10^9/l
Neutrophils	-	< 0.75 × 10^9/l	< 0.5 × 10^9/l
Platelets	-	< 50 × 10^9/l	< 25 × 10^9/l
Bilirubin – direct	-	-	2.5 × ULN**
Bilirubin - indirect	> 5 mg/dl	-	> 4 mg/dl (for > 4 weeks)
Creatinine	-	-	> 2.0 mg/dl
ALT/AST	-	-	2 × baseline and > 10 × ULN**

* Patients whose dose of ribavirin is reduced to 600 mg daily receive one 200 mg capsule in the morning and two 200 mg capsules in the evening.
** Upper limit of normal

Table 2b Reduced ViraferonPeg Dosing for Combination Therapy

Body Weight (kg)	Target Reduced Dose (μ g)	Vial/Pen Strength (μ g/0.5 ml)	Administer Once Weekly(ml)	Amount Delivered (μ g)
< 40	25	50*	0.25	25
40-50	32	50	0.3	30
51-64	40	50	0.4	40
65-75	50	50	0.5	50
76-85	60	80	0.4	64
> 85	75	100	0.4	80

*Must use vial. Minimum delivery for pen is 0.3 ml.

Table 3b Reduced ViraferonPeg Dose for the 1.0 μg/kg Monotherapy Regimen

Body Weight (kg)	Target Reduced Dose (μ g)	Vial/Pen Strength (μ g/0.5ml)	Administer Once Weekly(ml)	Amount Delivered (μ g)
30-35	15	50*	0.15	15
36-45	20	50*	0.20	20
46-56	25	50*	0.25	25
57-72	32	50	0.3	30
73-89	40	50	0.4	40
90-106	50	50	0.5	50
> 106	60	80	0.4	64

*Must use vial. Minimum delivery for pen is 0.3 ml.

Special populations

Use in renal impairment: The clearance of ViraferonPeg is reduced in patients with significant renal impairment. Patients with creatinine clearance ⩽ 50 ml/minute must not be treated with ViraferonPeg (see section **5.2**). It is recommended that patients with moderate renal impairment be closely monitored and that their weekly dose of ViraferonPeg be reduced if medically appropriate.

Use in hepatic impairment: The safety and efficacy of ViraferonPeg therapy has not been evaluated in patients with severe hepatic dysfunction, therefore ViraferonPeg must not be used for these patients.

Use in the elderly (⩾ 65 years of age): There are no apparent age-related effects on the pharmacokinetics of ViraferonPeg. Data from elderly patients treated with a single dose of ViraferonPeg suggest no alteration in ViraferonPeg dose is necessary based on age (see section **5.2**).

Use in patients under the age of 18 years: ViraferonPeg is not recommended for use in children or adolescents under the age of 18, as there is no experience in this group.

4.3 Contraindications

- Hypersensitivity to the active substance or to any interferon or to any of the excipients;
- Use in pregnant women;
- Use in women who are breast-feeding;
- A history of severe pre-existing cardiac disease, including unstable or uncontrolled cardiac disease in the previous six months (see section **4.4**);
- Severe, debilitating medical conditions, including patients with chronic renal failure or creatinine clearance < 50 ml/minute;
- Autoimmune hepatitis or a history of autoimmune disease;
- Severe hepatic dysfunction or decompensated cirrhosis of the liver;
- Pre-existing thyroid disease unless it can be controlled with conventional treatment;
- Epilepsy and/or compromised central nervous system (CNS) function.

4.4 Special warnings and special precautions for use

There is no experience with ViraferonPeg in combination with ribavirin in patients who have relapsed after interferon alpha + ribavirin therapy.

All patients in the chronic hepatitis C studies had a liver biopsy before inclusion, but in certain cases (i.e. patients with genotype 2 and 3), treatment may be possible without histological confirmation. Current treatment guidelines should be consulted as to whether a liver biopsy is needed prior to commencing treatment.

Acute hypersensitivity: Acute hypersensitivity reactions (e.g., urticaria, angioedema, bronchoconstriction, anaphylaxis) have been observed rarely during interferon alfa-2b therapy. If such a reaction develops during treatment with ViraferonPeg, discontinue treatment and institute appropriate medical therapy immediately. Transient rashes do not necessitate interruption of treatment.

Cardiovascular system: As with interferon alfa-2b, patients with a history of congestive heart failure, myocardial infarction and/or previous or current arrhythmic disorders, receiving ViraferonPeg therapy require close monitoring. It is recommended that patients who have pre-existing cardiac abnormalities have electrocardiograms taken prior to and during the course of treatment. Cardiac arrhythmias (primarily supraventricular) usually respond to conventional therapy but may require discontinuation of ViraferonPeg therapy.

Psychiatric and Central Nervous System (CNS): If treatment with peginterferon alfa-2b is judged necessary in patients with existence or history of severe psychiatric conditions, this should only be initiated after having ensured appropriate individualised diagnostic and therapeutic management of the psychiatric condition.

Severe CNS effects, particularly depression, suicidal ideation and attempted suicide have been observed in some patients during ViraferonPeg therapy. Other CNS effects including aggressive behaviour (sometimes directed against others), confusion and alterations of mental status have been observed with alpha interferon. If patients develop psychiatric or CNS problems, including clinical depression, it is recommended that the patient be carefully monitored due to the potential seriousness of these undesirable effects. If symptoms persist or worsen, discontinue ViraferonPeg therapy.

More significant obtundation and coma, including cases of encephalopathy, have been observed in some patients, usually elderly, treated at higher doses for oncology indications. While these effects are generally reversible, in a few patients full resolution took up to three weeks. Very rarely, seizures have occurred with high doses of interferon alpha.

Liver function: As with all interferons, discontinue treatment with ViraferonPeg in patients who develop prolongation of coagulation markers which might indicate liver decompensation.

Fever: While fever may be associated with the flu-like syndrome reported commonly during interferon therapy, other causes of persistent fever must be ruled out.

Hydration: Adequate hydration must be maintained in patients undergoing ViraferonPeg therapy since hypotension related to fluid depletion has been seen in some patients treated with alpha interferons. Fluid replacement may be necessary.

Pulmonary changes: Pulmonary infiltrates, pneumonitis, and pneumonia, occasionally resulting in fatality, have been observed rarely in interferon alpha treated patients. Any patient developing fever, cough, dyspnea or other respiratory symptoms must have a chest X-ray taken. If the chest X-ray shows pulmonary infiltrates or there is evidence of pulmonary function impairment, the patient is to be monitored closely, and, if appropriate, discontinue interferon alpha. Prompt discontinuation of interferon alpha administration and treatment with corticosteroids appear to be associated with resolution of pulmonary adverse events.

Autoimmune disease: The development of auto-antibodies and autoimmune disorders has been reported during treatment with alpha interferons. Patients predisposed to the development of autoimmune disorders may be at increased risk. Patients with signs or symptoms compatible with autoimmune disorders should be evaluated carefully, and the benefit-risk of continued interferon therapy should be reassessed (see also section **4.4 Thyroid changes** and **4.8**).

Ocular changes: Ophthalmologic disorders, including retinal haemorrhages, cotton wool spots, and retinal artery or vein obstruction have been reported in rare instances after treatment with alpha interferons (see section **4.8**). All patients should have a baseline eye examination. Any patient complaining of ocular symptoms, including loss of visual acuity or visual field must have a prompt and complete eye examination. Periodic visual examinations are recommended during ViraferonPeg therapy, particularly in patients with disorders that may be associated with retinopathy, such as diabetes mellitus or hypertension. Discontinuation of ViraferonPeg should be considered in patients who develop new or worsening ophthalmological disorders.

Thyroid changes: Infrequently, patients treated for chronic hepatitis C with interferon alpha have developed thyroid abnormalities, either hypothyroidism or hyperthyroidism. Determine thyroid stimulating hormone (TSH) levels if, during the course of therapy, a patient develops symptoms consistent with possible thyroid dysfunction. In the presence of thyroid dysfunction, ViraferonPeg treatment may be continued if TSH levels can be maintained in the normal range by medication.

Metabolic disturbances: Hypertriglyceridemia and aggravation of hypertriglyceridemia, sometimes severe, have been observed. Monitoring of lipid levels is, therefore, recommended.

HCV/HIV Coinfection

Patients co-infected with HIV and receiving Highly Active Anti-Retroviral Therapy (HAART) may be at increased risk of developing lactic acidosis. Caution should be used when adding ViraferonPeg and ribavirin to HAART therapy (see ribavirin SPC).

Co-infected patients with advanced cirrhosis receiving HAART may be at increased risk of hepatic decompensation and death. Adding treatment with alfa interferons alone or in combination with ribavirin may increase the risk in this patient subset.

Organ transplant recipients: The safety and efficacy of ViraferonPeg alone or in combination with ribavirin for the treatment of hepatitis C in liver or other organ transplant recipients have not been studied. Preliminary data indicates that interferon alpha therapy may be associated with an increased rate of kidney graft rejection. Liver graft rejection has also been reported.

Other: Due to reports of interferon alpha exacerbating pre-existing psoriatic disease and sarcoidosis, use of ViraferonPeg in patients with psoriasis or sarcoidosis is recommended only if the potential benefit justifies the potential risk.

Laboratory tests: Standard haematologic tests, blood chemistry and a test of thyroid function must be conducted in all patients prior to initiating therapy. Acceptable baseline values that may be considered as a guideline prior to initiation of ViraferonPeg therapy are:

- Platelets ⩾ 100,000/mm^3
- Neutrophil count ⩾ 1,500/mm^3
- TSH level must be within normal limits

Laboratory evaluations are to be conducted at weeks 2 and 4 of therapy, and periodically thereafter as clinically appropriate.

Important information about some of the ingredients of ViraferonPeg:

This medicinal product contains less than 1 mmol sodium (23 mg) per 0.7 ml, i.e., essentially "sodium-free".

4.5 Interaction with other medicinal products and other forms of Interaction

Results from a multiple-dose probe study assessing P450 substrates in chronic hepatitis C patients receiving once weekly ViraferonPeg (1.5 μg/kg) for 4 weeks demonstrated an increase in activity of CYP2D6 and CYP2C8/9. No change in activity of CYP1A2, CYP3A4, or N-acetyltransferase was observed.

Caution should be used when administering peginterferon alfa-2b with medications metabolised by CYP2D6 and CYP2C8/9, especially those with narrow therapeutic window, such as warfarin and phenytoin (CYP2C9) and flecainide (CYP2D6).

These findings may partly relate to improved metabolic capacity due to reduced hepatic inflammation in patients undergoing treatment with ViraferonPeg. Caution is therefore advised when ViraferonPeg treatment is initiated for chronic hepatitis in patients treated with medication with a narrow therapeutic window and sensitive to mild metabolic impairment of the liver.

No pharmacokinetic interactions were noted between ViraferonPeg and ribavirin in a multiple-dose pharmacokinetic study.

4.6 Pregnancy and lactation

There are no adequate data from the use of interferon alfa-2b in pregnant women. Interferon alfa-2b has been shown to be abortifacient in primates. ViraferonPeg is likely to also cause this effect. ViraferonPeg is contraindicated in pregnancy (see sections **4.3** and **5.3**).

ViraferonPeg is recommended for use in fertile women only when they are using effective contraception during the treatment period.

Lactation: It is not known whether the components of this medicinal product are excreted in human milk. Because of the potential for adverse reactions in nursing infants, nursing must be discontinued prior to initiation of treatment.

Combination therapy with ribavirin:

Ribavirin causes serious birth defects when administered during pregnancy. Women of childbearing potential have to use effective contraception during and up to for 4 months after treatment (see section **5.3** and the respective informing texts of ribavirin containing medicinal products).

4.7 Effects on ability to drive and use machines

Patients who develop fatigue, somnolence or confusion during treatment with ViraferonPeg are cautioned to avoid driving or operating machinery.

4.8 Undesirable effects

The safety of ViraferonPeg is evaluated from data from two clinical trials: one with ViraferonPeg monotherapy, one with ViraferonPeg in combination with ribavirin. In both cases, patients were treated for one year.

Table 4 describes the regimens and patient exposure for one year of treatment in patients with no previous exposure to interferon (interferon-naïve patients). Because of a significant overlap in the pattern of undesirable effects with ViraferonPeg monotherapy, groups of patients have been brought together in **Table 5** to show the pattern of reported effects for all monotherapy groups.

Table 4 Regimens and patient exposure

Treatment	Regimen	Number of patients treated for one year
ViraferonPeg + ribavirin	ViraferonPeg (1.5 micrograms/kg/week) + ribavirin > 10.6 mg/kg/day)	188
Interferon alfa-2b + ribavirin	Interferon alfa-2b (3 MIU three times a week) + ribavirin (1,000/1,200 mg/day)	505
ViraferonPeg monotherapy	ViraferonPeg (0.5 microgram/kg/week)	315
	ViraferonPeg (1.0 microgram/kg/week)	297
	ViraferonPeg (1.5 micrograms/kg/week)	304

(see Table 5 on next page)

Table 6 Undesirable effects commonly reported in clinical trials in patients treated with ViraferonPeg + ribavirin or ViraferonPeg monotherapy Common > 1/100, < 1/10)

Body system	5-10%	1-<5%
Infections and infestations		otitis media, fungal infection, bacterial infection, herpes simplex
Blood and lymphatic system disorders	anaemia, leukopaenia	thrombocytopenia, lymphadenopathy
Endocrine disorders	hypothyroidism	hyperthyroidism
Metabolism and nutrition disorders		hyperuricemia, hypocalcemia, thirst
Psychiatric disorders	agitation, nervousness	aggressive behaviour, somnolence, behavior disorder, apathy, appetite increased, sleep disorder, dreaming abnormal, decreased libido
Nervous system disorders	paresthesia, increased sweating	hypoaesthesia, hyperaesthesia, hypertonia, confusion, tremor, vertigo, migraine, ataxia, neuralgia
Eye disorders		blurred vision, conjunctivitis, lacrimal gland disorder, eye pain
Cardiac disorders		tachycardia, palpitation
Vascular disorders		hypotension, hypertension, syncope, flushing
Ear and labyrinth disorders		tinnitus, hearing impairment/loss
Respiratory, thoracic and mediastinal disorders		nonproductive cough, rhinitis, sinusitis, bronchitis, respiratory disorder, nasal congestion, rhinorrhea, dysphonia, epistaxis
Gastrointestinal disorders	dyspepsia	constipation, taste perversion, loose stools, stomatitis, ulcerative stomatitis, gingival bleeding, glossitis, flatulence, hemorrhoids, gastroesophageal reflux, gingivitis, dehydration
Hepatobiliary disorders		hepatomegaly, hyperbilirubinemia
Skin and subcutaneous tissue disorders		erythematous rash, eczema, photosensitivity reaction, maculopapular rash, abnormal hair texture, acne, dermatitis, furunculosis, nail disorder, psoriasis, urticaria, erythema, face or peripheral oedema
Musculoskeletal and connective tissue disorders		arthritis
Renal and urinary disorders		micturition frequency, urine abnormal
Reproductive system and breast disorders	menstrual disorder, menorrhagia	ovarian disorder, vaginal disorder, sexual dysfunction (not specified), impotence, breast pain, amenorrhoea, prostatitis
General disorders and administration site conditions	RUQ pain, malaise, chest pain	injection site pain

Most cases of neutropaenia and thrombocytopaenia were mild (WHO grades 1 or 2). There were some cases of more severe neutropenia in patients treated with the recommended doses of ViraferonPeg in combination with ribavirin (WHO grade 3: 39 of 186 [21 %]; and WHO grade 4: 13 of 186 [7 %]).

In a clinical trial, approximately 1.2 % of patients treated with ViraferonPeg or interferon alfa-2b in combination with ribavirin reported life-threatening psychiatric events during treatment. These events included suicidal ideation and attempted suicide (see section **4.4**). Following marketing, psychosis and hallucination have been reported rarely.

Rarely > 1/10,000, < 1/1,000) or very rarely (< 1/10,000) reported events with interferon alfa-2b, including ViraferonPeg, include:

Immune system disorders:

very rarely: sarcoidosis or exacerbation of sarcoidosis

Endocrine disorders:

rarely: diabetes

Nervous system disorders:

rarely: seizure, peripheral neuropathy

very rarely: cerebrovascular ischaemia, cerebrovascular haemorrhage, encephalopathy

Cardiac disorders:

rarely: arrhythmia

very rarely: cardiac ischaemia, myocardial infarction

Respiratory, thoracic and mediastinal disorders:

very rarely: interstitial lung disease

Gastrointestinal disorders:

rarely: pancreatitis

very rarely: ulcerative and ischaemic colitis

Skin and subcutaneous tissue disorders:

very rarely: erythema multiforme, Stevens Johnson syndrome, toxic epidermal necrolysis, injection site necrosis

Musculoskeletal and connective tissue disorders:

rarely: rhabdomyolysis, myositis

Renal and urinary disorders:

rarely: renal insufficiency and renal failure

Cardiovascular (CVS) adverse events, particularly arrhythmia, appeared to be correlated mostly with pre-existing CVS disease and prior therapy with cardiotoxic agents (see section **4.4**). Cardiomyopathy, that may be reversible upon discontinuation of interferon alpha, has been reported rarely in patients without prior evidence of cardiac disease.

Very rarely, interferon alfa-2b or ViraferonPeg used alone or in combination with ribavirin may be associated with aplastic anaemia.

Ophthalmological disorders that have been reported rarely with alpha interferons include retinopathies (including macular oedema), retinal haemorrhages, retinal artery or vein obstruction, cotton wool spots, loss of visual acuity or visual field, optic neuritis, and papilloedema (see section **4.4**).

A wide variety of autoimmune and immune-mediated disorders have been reported with alpha interferons including thyroid disorders, systemic lupus erythematosus, rheumatoid arthritis (new or aggravated), idiopathic and thrombotic thrombocytopenic purpura, vasculitis, neuropathies including mononeuropathies (see also section **4.4, Autoimmune disorders**).

4.9 Overdose

In clinical trials, cases of accidental overdose, at never more than twice the prescribed dose, were reported. There were no serious reactions. Undesirable effects resolved during continued administration of ViraferonPeg.

5. PHARMACOLOGICAL PROPERTIES

5.1 Pharmacodynamic properties

Pharmacotherapeutic group: Immunostimulants, Cytokines and immunomodulators, Interferons, Peginterferon alfa-2b, ATC code: L03A B10.

Recombinant interferon alfa-2b is covalently conjugated with monomethoxy polyethylene glycol at an average degree of substitution of 1 mole of polymer/mole of protein. The average molecular mass is approximately 31,300 daltons of which the protein moiety constitutes approximately 19,300.

Interferon alfa-2b

In vitro and *in vivo* studies suggest that the biological activity of ViraferonPeg is derived from its interferon alfa-2b moiety.

Interferons exert their cellular activities by binding to specific membrane receptors on the cell surface. Studies with other interferons have demonstrated species specificity. However, certain monkey species, e.g., Rhesus monkeys, are susceptible to pharmacodynamic stimulation upon exposure to human type 1 interferons.

Once bound to the cell membrane, interferon initiates a complex sequence of intracellular events that include the induction of certain enzymes. It is thought that this process, at least in part, is responsible for the various cellular responses to interferon, including inhibition of virus replication in virus-infected cells, suppression of cell proliferation and such immunomodulating activities as enhancement of the phagocytic activity of macrophages and augmentation of the specific cytotoxicity of lymphocytes for target cells. Any or all of these activities may contribute to interferon's therapeutic effects.

Recombinant interferon alfa-2b also inhibits viral replication *in vitro* and *in vivo*. Although the exact antiviral mode of action of recombinant interferon alfa-2b is unknown, it appears to alter the host cell metabolism. This action inhibits viral replication or if replication occurs, the progeny virions are unable to leave the cell.

ViraferonPeg

ViraferonPeg pharmacodynamics were assessed in a rising single-dose trial in healthy subjects by examining changes in oral temperature, concentrations of effector proteins such as serum neopterin and 2'5'-oligoadenylate synthetase (2'5'-OAS), as well as white cell and neutrophil

Table 5 Undesirable effects very commonly reported in clinical trials > 10 % of patients in ViraferonPeg + ribavirin group Very common > 1/10)

	ViraferonPeg + ribavirin	Interferon alfa-2b + ribavirin	ViraferonPeg monotherapy
Infections and infestations			
Infection viral	10 %	5 %	4-5 %
Metabolism and nutrition disorders			
Weight decrease	30 %	19 %	8-18 %
Psychiatric disorders			
Depression	34 %	32 %	26 %
Irritability	32 %	34 %	19 %
Insomnia	37 %	41 %	16-19 %
Anxiety	14 %	14 %	8 %
Concentration impaired	18 %	21 %	9-10 %
Emotional lability	11 %	10 %	5 %
Nervous system disorders			
Headache	58 %	57 %	57-63 %
Mouth dry	10 %	8 %	4-8 %
Respiratory, thoracic and mediastinal disorders			
Pharyngitis	10 %	7 %	3 %
Coughing	14 %	11 %	4 %
Dyspnea	26 %	22 %	5 %
Gastrointestinal disorders			
Nausea	43 %	31 %	20-23 %
Anorexia	35 %	26 %	10-25 %
Diarrhoea	20 %	13 %	14-17 %
Abdominal pain	12 %	9 %	11 %
Vomiting	16 %	10 %	4-7 %
Skin and subcutaneous tissue disorder s			
Alopecia	45 %	32 %	20-34 %
Pruritus	27 %	27 %	7-9 %
Skin dry	23 %	21 %	6-9 %
Rash	21 %	21 %	5-7 %
Musculoskeletal and connective tissue disorders			
Myalgia	49 %	49 %	46-60 %
Arthralgia	31 %	26 %	23-28 %
Musculoskeletal pain	15 %	11 %	11-13 %
General disorders and administration site conditions			
Injection site inflammation	20 %	17 %	39-44 %
Injection site reaction	54 %	36 %	7-9 %
Fatigue	56 %	59 %	43 %
Rigors	42 %	40 %	33-43 %
Fever	39 %	32 %	29-43 %
Flu-like symptoms	21 %	23 %	18-25
Asthenia	28 %	17 %	12-14 %
Dizziness	17 %	16 %	7-12 %

counts. Subjects treated with ViraferonPeg showed mild dose-related elevations in body temperature. Following single doses of ViraferonPeg between 0.25 and 2.0 micrograms/kg/week, serum neopterin concentration was increased in a dose-related manner. Neutrophil and white cell count reductions at the end of week 4 correlated with the dose of ViraferonPeg.

ViraferonPeg clinical trials

Two pivotal trials have been conducted, one (C/I97-010) with ViraferonPeg monotherapy; the other (C/I98-580) with ViraferonPeg in combination with ribavirin. Eligible patients for these trials had chronic hepatitis C confirmed by a positive HCV-RNA polymerase chain reaction (PCR) assay > 30 IU/ml), a liver biopsy consistent with a histological diagnosis of chronic hepatitis with no other cause for the chronic hepatitis, and abnormal serum ALT.

In the ViraferonPeg monotherapy trial, a total of 916 naïve chronic hepatitis C patients were treated with ViraferonPeg (0.5, 1.0 or 1.5 micrograms/kg/week) for one year with a follow-up period of six months. In addition, 303 patients received interferon alfa-2b (3 million International Units [MIU] three times a week as a comparator. This study showed that ViraferonPeg was superior to interferon alfa-2b (**Table 7**).

In the ViraferonPeg combination trial, 1,530 naïve patients were treated for one year with one of the following combination regimens:

- ViraferonPeg (1.5 micrograms/kg/week) + ribavirin (800 mg/day), (n = 511).
- ViraferonPeg (1.5 micrograms/kg/week for one month followed by 0.5 microgram/kg/week for 11 months) + ribavirin (1,000/1,200 mg/day), (n = 514).
- Interferon alfa-2b (3 MIU three times a week) + ribavirin (1,000/1,200 mg/day) (n = 505).

In this trial, the combination of ViraferonPeg (1.5 micrograms/kg/week) and ribavirin was significantly more effective than the combination of interferon alfa-2b and ribavirin (**Table 7**), particularly in patients infected with Genotype 1 (**Table 8**). Sustained response was assessed by the response rate six months after the cessation of treatment.

HCV genotype and baseline virus load are prognostic factors which are known to affect response rates. However, response rates in this trial were shown to be dependent also on the dose of ribavirin administered in combination with ViraferonPeg or interferon alfa-2b. In those patients that received > 10.6 mg/kg ribavirin (800 mg dose in typical 75 kg patient), regardless of genotype or viral load, response rates were significantly higher than in those patients that received ≤ 10.6 mg/kg ribavirin (**Table 8**), while response rates in patients that received > 13.2 mg/kg ribavirin were even higher.

(see Table 7 on next page)

(see Table 8 on next page)

In the ViraferonPeg monotherapy study, the Quality of Life was generally less affected by 0.5 microgram/kg of ViraferonPeg than by either 1.0 microgram/kg of ViraferonPeg once weekly or 3 MIU of interferon alfa-2b three times a week.

In a separate trial, 224 patients with genotype 2 or 3 received ViraferonPeg, 1.5 microgram/kg subcutaneously, once weekly, in combination with ribavirin 800 mg – 1,400 mg p.o. for 6 months (based on body weight, only three patients weighing > 105 kg, received the 1,400 mg dose, which has not yet been validated) (**Table 9**). Twenty-four % had bridging fibrosis or cirrhosis (Knodell 3/4).

Table 9. Virologic Response at End of Treatment, Sustained Virologic Response and Relapse by HCV Genotype and Viral Load*

(see Table 9 on next page)

The 6 month treatment duration in this trial was better tolerated than one year of treatment in the pivotal combination trial; for discontinuation 5 % vs. 14 %, for dose modification 18 % vs. 49 %.

In a non-comparative trial, 235 patients with genotype 1 and low viral load (< 600,000 IU/ml) received ViraferonPeg, 1.5 microgram/kg subcutaneously, once weekly, in combination with weight adjusted ribavirin. The overall sustained response rate after a 24-week treatment duration was 50 %. Forty-one percent of subjects (97/235) had nondetectable plasma HCV-RNA levels at Week 4 and Week 24 of therapy. In this subgroup, there was a 92 % (89/97) sustained virological response rate. The high sustained response rate in this subgroup of patients was identified in an interim analysis (n=49) and prospectively confirmed (n=48).

Limited historical data indicate that treatment for 48 weeks might be associated with a higher sustained response rate (11/11) and with a lower risk of relapse (0/11 as compared to 7/96 following 24 weeks of treatment).

Predictability of sustained virological response

Virological reponse by week 12, defined as a 2-log viral load decrease or undetectable levels of HCV RNA has been shown to be predictive for sustained response (**Table 10**).

(see Table 10 on page 2709)

The negative predictive value for sustained response in patients treated with ViraferonPeg in monotherapy was 98 %.

5.2 Pharmacokinetic properties

ViraferonPeg is a well characterized polyethylene glycol-modified ("pegylated") derivative of interferon alfa-2b and is predominantly composed of monopegylated species. The plasma half-life of ViraferonPeg is prolonged compared with non-pegylated interferon alfa-2b. ViraferonPeg has a potential to depegylate to free interferon alfa-2b. The biologic activity of the pegylated isomers is qualitatively similar, but weaker than free interferon alfa-2b.

Following subcutaneous administration, maximal serum concentrations occur between 15-44 hours post-dose, and are sustained for up to 48-72 hours post-dose.

Table 7 Sustained virological response (% patients HCV negative)

	ViraferonPeg monotherapy				ViraferonPeg + ribavirin		
Treatment regimen	**P 1.5**	**P 1.0**	**P 0.5**	**I**	**P 1.5/R**	**P 0.5/R**	**I/R**
Number of patients	304	297	315	303	511	514	505
Response at end of treatment	49 %	41 %	33 %	24 %	65 %	56 %	54 %
Sustained response	23 %*	25 %	18 %	12 %	54 %**	47 %	47 %

P 1.5 ViraferonPeg 1.5 micrograms/kg
P 1.0 ViraferonPeg 1.0 microgram/kg
P 0.5 ViraferonPeg 0.5 microgram/kg
I Interferon alfa-2b 3 MIU
P 1.5/R ViraferonPeg (1.5 micrograms/kg) + ribavirin (800 mg)
P 0.5/R ViraferonPeg (1.5 to 0.5 microgram/kg) + ribavirin (1,000/1,200 mg)
I/R Interferon alfa-2b (3 MIU) + ribavirin (1,000/1,200 mg)
* $p < 0.001$ P 1.5 vs. I
** $p = 0.0143$ P 1.5/R vs. I/R

Table 8 Sustained response rates with ViraferonPeg + ribavirin(by ribavirin dose, genotype and viral load)

HCV Genotype	**Rebetol dose (mg/kg)**	**P 1.5/R**	**P 0.5/R**	I/R
All Genotypes	**All**	**54 %**	**47 %**	**47 %**
	≤ 10.6	50 %	41 %	27 %
	> 10.6	61 %	48 %	47 %
Genotype 1	**All**	**42 %**	**34 %**	**33 %**
	≤ 10.6	38 %	25 %	20 %
	> 10.6	48 %	34 %	34 %
Genotype 1 ≤ 600,000 IU/ml	All	73 %	51 %	45 %
	≤ 10.6	74 %	25 %	33 %
	> 10.6	71 %	52 %	45 %
Genotype 1 > 600,000 IU/ml	All	30 %	27 %	29 %
	≤ 10.6	27 %	25 %	17 %
	> 10.6	37 %	27 %	29 %
Genotype 2/3	**All**	**82 %**	**80 %**	**79 %**
	≤ 10.6	79 %	73 %	50 %
	> 10.6	88 %	80 %	80 %

P 1.5/R ViraferonPeg (1.5 micrograms/kg) + ribavirin (800 mg)
P 0.5/R ViraferonPeg (1.5 to 0.5 microgram/kg) + ribavirin (1,000/1,200 mg)
I/R Interferon alfa-2b (3 MIU) + ribavirin (1,000/1,200 mg)

Table 9 Virologic Response at End of Treatment, Sustained Virologic Response and Relapse by HCV Genotype and Viral Load*

	ViraferonPeg 1.5 μg/kg Once Weekly Plus Rebetol 800-1400 mg/day		
	End of Treatment Response	Sustained Virologic Response	Relapse
All Subjects	94 % (211/224)	81 % (182/224)	12 % (27/224)
HCV 2	100 % (42/42)	93 % (39/42)	7 % (3/42)
≤ 600,000 IU/ml	100 % (20/20)	95 % (19/20)	5 % (1/20)
> 600,000 IU/mL	100 % (22/22)	91 % (20/22)	9 % (2/22)
HCV 3	93 % (169/182)	79 % (143/182)	14 % (24/166)
≤ 600,000 IU/ml	93 % (92/99)	86 % (85/99)	8 % (7/91)
> 600,000 IU/ml	93 % (77/83)	70 % (58/83)	23 % (17/75)

* Any subject with an undetectable HCV-RNA level at the Follow-Up Week 12 visit and missing data at the Follow-Up Week 24 visit was considered a sustained responder. Any subject with missing data in and after the Follow-Up Week 12 window was considered to be a non-responder at Week 24 of follow-up.

ViraferonPeg C_{max} and AUC measurements increase in a dose-related manner. Mean apparent volume of distribution is 0.99 l/kg.

Upon multiple dosing, there is an accumulation of immunoreactive interferons. There is, however, only a modest increase in biologic activity as measured by a bioassay.

Mean (SD) ViraferonPeg elimination half-life is approximately 40 hours (13.3 hours), with apparent clearance of 22.0 ml/hr•kg. The mechanisms involved in clearance of interferons in man have not yet been fully elucidated. However, renal elimination may account for a minority (approximately 30 %) of ViraferonPeg apparent clearance.

Renal function: Renal clearance appears to account for 30 % of total clearance of ViraferonPeg. In a single dose study (1.0 microgram/kg) in patients with impaired renal function, C_{max}, AUC, and half-life increased in relation to the degree of renal impairment.

Based on these data, no dose modification is recommended based on creatinine clearance. However, because of marked intra-subject variability in interferon pharmacokinetics, it is recommended that patients be monitored closely during treatment with ViraferonPeg (see section **4.2**). Patients with severe renal dysfunction or creatinine clearance < 50 ml/min must not be treated with ViraferonPeg.

Hepatic function: The pharmacokinetics of ViraferonPeg have not been evaluated in patients with severe hepatic dysfunction.

Elderly patients ≥ 65 years of age: The pharmacokinetics of ViraferonPeg following a single subcutaneous dose of 1.0 microgram/kg were not affected by age. The data suggest that no alteration in ViraferonPeg dosage is necessary based on advancing age.

Patients under the age of 18 years: Specific pharmacokinetic evaluations have not been performed on these patients. ViraferonPeg is indicated for the treatment of chronic hepatitis C only in patients 18 years of age or older.

Interferon neutralising factors: Interferon neutralising factor assays were performed on serum samples of patients who received ViraferonPeg in the clinical trial. Interferon neutralising factors are antibodies which neutralise the antiviral activity of interferon. The clinical incidence of neutralising factors in patients who received ViraferonPeg 0.5 micrograms/kg is 1.1 %.

5.3 Preclinical safety data

ViraferonPeg: Adverse events not observed in clinical trials were not seen in toxicity studies in monkeys. These studies were limited to four weeks due to the appearance of anti-interferon antibodies in most monkeys.

Reproduction studies of ViraferonPeg have not been performed. Interferon alfa-2b has been shown to be an abortifacient in primates. ViraferonPeg is likely to also cause this effect. Effects on fertility have not been determined. It is not known whether the components of this medicinal product are excreted into experimental animal or human milk (see section **4.6** for relevant human data on pregnancy and lactation). ViraferonPeg showed no genotoxic potential.

The relative non-toxicity of monomethoxy-polyethylene glycol (mPEG), which is liberated from ViraferonPeg by metabolism *in vivo* has been demonstrated in preclinical acute and subchronic toxicity studies in rodents and monkeys, standard embryo-foetal development studies and in *in vitro* mutagenicity assays.

ViraferonPeg plus ribavirin: When used in combination with ribavirin, ViraferonPeg did not cause any effects not previously seen with either active substance alone. The major treatment-related change was a reversible, mild to moderate anaemia, the severity of which was greater than that produced by either active substance alone.

6. PHARMACEUTICAL PARTICULARS

6.1 List of excipients

Powder for solution for injection:

Disodium phosphate, anhydrous,

Sodium dihydrogen phosphate dihydrate,

Sucrose,

Polysorbate 80.

Solvent for parenteral use:

Water for injections.

Deliverable volume from pen = 0.5 ml.

6.2 Incompatibilities

This medicinal product should only be reconstituted with the solvent provided (see section **6.6**). In the absence of compatibility studies, this medicinal product must not be mixed with other medicinal products.

6.3 Shelf life

3 years

After reconstitution:

- Chemical and physical in-use stability has been demonstrated for 24 hours at 2°C - 8°C.

- From a microbiological point of view, the product is to be used immediately. If not used immediately, in-use storage times and conditions prior to use are the responsibility of the user and would normally not be longer than 24 hours at 2°C - 8°C.

6.4 Special precautions for storage

Store in a refrigerator (2°C - 8°C).

6.5 Nature and contents of container

The powder and solvent are both contained in a two-chamber cartridge, Type I flint glass, separated by a bromobutyl rubber plunger. The cartridge is sealed at one end with a polypropylene cap containing a bromobutyl rubber liner and at the other end by a bromobutyl rubber plunger.

ViraferonPeg 50, 80, 100, 120 or 150 micrograms is supplied as:

- 1 pen containing powder and solvent for solution for injection, 1 injection needle and 2 cleansing swabs;

Table 10 Predictability of sustained response by viral response at week 12 and genotype*

Treatment	Genotype	Viral response at week 12	Sustained response	Negative predictive value
ViraferonPeg 1.5 + ribavirin > 10.6 mg/kg) 48-week treatment	1	Yes 75 % (82/110)	71 % (58/82)	
		No 25 % (28/110)	0 % (0/28)	100 %
ViraferonPeg 1.5 + ribavirin 800-1,400 mg 24-week treatment	2 and 3	Yes 99 % (213/215)	83 % (177/213)	——
		No 1 % (2/215)	50 % (1/2)	50 %

* reflects patients with 12 week data available

- 4 pens containing powder and solvent for solution for injection, 4 injection needles and 8 cleansing swabs;
- 6 pens containing powder and solvent for solution for injection, 6 injection needles and 12 cleansing swabs;
- 12 pens containing powder and solvent for solution for injection, 12 injection needles and 24 cleansing swabs.

Not all pack sizes may be marketed

6.6 Instructions for use and handling

ViraferonPeg pre-filled pen contains a powder of peginterferon alfa-2b and a solvent for solution at a strength of 50 micrograms for single use. Each pen is reconstituted with the solvent provided in the two-chamber cartridge (water for injections) for administration of up to 0.5 ml of solution. A small volume is lost during preparation of ViraferonPeg for injection when the dose is measured and injected. Therefore, each pen contains an excess amount of solvent and ViraferonPeg powder to ensure delivery of the labelled dose in 0.5 ml of ViraferonPeg, solution for injection. The reconstituted solution has a concentration of 50 micrograms in 0.5 ml.

ViraferonPeg is injected subcutaneously after reconstituting the powder as instructed, attaching an injection needle and setting the prescribed dose. A complete set of instructions is provided in the Annex to the Package Leaflet.

As for all parenteral medicinal products, inspect visually the reconstituted solution prior to administration. The reconstituted solution should be clear and colourless. Do not use if discolouration or particulate matter is present. After administering the dose, discard the ViraferonPeg pre-filled pen and any unused solution contained in it.

7. MARKETING AUTHORISATION HOLDER

SP Europe
73, rue de Stalle
B-1180 Bruxelles
Belgium

8. MARKETING AUTHORISATION NUMBER(S)

ViraferonPeg 50 micrograms: EU/1/00/132/031-034
ViraferonPeg 80 micrograms: EU/1/00/132/035-038
ViraferonPeg 100 micrograms: EU/1/00/132/039-042
ViraferonPeg 120 micrograms: EU/1/00/132/043-046
ViraferonPeg 150 micrograms: EU/1/00/132/047-050

9. DATE OF FIRST AUTHORISATION/RENEWAL OF THE AUTHORISATION

Date of first authorisation: 6 February 2002
Date of last renewal: 23 May 2005

10. DATE OF REVISION OF THE TEXT

8 September 2005

11. LEGAL CATEGORY

Prescription Only Medicine

ViraferonPeg Pen/09-05/10

Viramune Tablets

(Boehringer Ingelheim Limited)

1. NAME OF THE MEDICINAL PRODUCT

VIRAMUNE 200 mg tablets

2. QUALITATIVE AND QUANTITATIVE COMPOSITION

Tablets each containing 200 mg of nevirapine anhydrate (active substance).

For excipients, see 6.1.

3. PHARMACEUTICAL FORM

Tablet

VIRAMUNE 200 mg tablets are white, oval, biconvex tablets. One side is embossed with the code "54 193", with a single bisect separating the "54" and "193". The opposite side is marked with the company symbol.

4. CLINICAL PARTICULARS

4.1 Therapeutic indications

VIRAMUNE is indicated as part of combination therapy for the antiviral treatment of HIV-1 infected patients with advanced or progressive immunodeficiency (see section 4.4.).

Most of the experience with VIRAMUNE is in combination with nucleoside reverse transcriptase inhibitors (NRTIs). There is at present insufficient data on the efficacy of subsequent use of triple combination including protease inhibitors (PIs) after VIRAMUNE therapy (see section 5.1).

4.2 Posology and method of administration

Patients 16 years and older

The recommended dose of VIRAMUNE is one 200 mg tablet daily for the first 14 days (this lead-in period should be used because it has been found to lessen the frequency of rash), followed by one 200 mg tablet twice daily, in combination with at least two additional antiretroviral agents to which the patient has not been previously exposed. Resistant virus emerges rapidly and uniformly when VIRAMUNE is administered as monotherapy; therefore VIRAMUNE should always be administered in combination therapy. For concomitantly administered antiretroviral therapy, the recommended dosage and monitoring should be followed.

Paediatric (adolescent) patients

VIRAMUNE 200 mg tablets, following the dosing schedule described above, are suitable for larger children, particularly adolescents, below the age of 16 who weigh 50 kg or more. An oral suspension dosage form, which can be dosed according to body weight, is available for children in this age group weighing less than 50 kg (please refer to the Summary of Product Characteristics of VIRAMUNE oral suspension).

Dose management considerations

Clinical chemistry tests, which include liver function tests, should be performed prior to initiating VIRAMUNE therapy and at appropriate intervals during therapy.

For toxicities that require interruption of VIRAMUNE therapy, see section 4.4.

Patients experiencing rash during the 14-day lead-in period of 200 mg/day should not have their VIRAMUNE dose increased until the rash has resolved. The isolated rash should be closely monitored (please refer to section 4.4).

Patients who interrupt VIRAMUNE dosing for more than 7 days should restart the recommended lead-indosing, using one 200 mg tablet daily for the first 14 days followed by one 200 mg tablet twice daily.

VIRAMUNE should be administered by physicians who are experienced in the treatment of HIV infection.

4.3 Contraindications

Hypersensitivity to the active substance or to any of the excipients.

VIRAMUNE should not be readministered to patients who have required permanent discontinuation for severe rash, rash accompanied by constitutional symptoms, hypersensitivity reactions, or clinical hepatitis due to nevirapine.

VIRAMUNE should not be used in patients with severe hepatic impairment or pre-treatment ASAT or ALAT > 5 ULN until baseline ASAT/ALAT are stabilised < 5 ULN.

VIRAMUNE should not be readministered in patients who previously had ASAT or ALAT > 5 ULN during VIRAMUNE therapy and had recurrence of liver function abnormalities upon readministration of VIRAMUNE (see section 4.4).

Herbal preparations containing St John's Wort (*Hypericum perforatum*) must not be used while taking VIRAMUNE due to the risk of decreased plasma concentrations and reduced clinical effects of nevirapine (see section 4.5).

The available pharmacokinetic data suggest that the concomitant use of rifampicin and VIRAMUNE is not recommended (please also refer to section 4.5).

4.4 Special warnings and special precautions for use

On the basis of pharmacodynamic data VIRAMUNE should only be used with at least two other antiretroviral agents (see section 5.1).

The first 18 weeks of therapy with VIRAMUNE are a critical period which requires close monitoring of patients to disclose the potential appearance of severe and life-threatening skin reactions (including cases of Stevens-Johnson syndrome and toxic epidermal necrolysis) or serious hepatitis/hepatic failure. The greatest risk of hepatic events and skin reactions occurs in the first 6 weeks of therapy. However, the risk of any hepatic event continues past this period and monitoring should continue at frequent intervals. Female gender and higher CD4 counts at the initiation of therapy place patients at greater risk of hepatic adverse events. Unless the benefit outweighs the risk VIRAMUNE should not be initiated in adult females with CD4 cell counts greater than 250 cells/mm^3 or in adult males with CD4 cell counts greater than 400 cells/mm^3. This is based on the occurrence of serious and life threatening hepatotoxicity in controlled and uncontrolled studies.

In some cases, hepatic injury has progressed despite discontinuation of treatment. Patients developing signs or symptoms of hepatitis, severe skin reaction or hypersensitivity reactions must discontinue VIRAMUNE and seek medical evaluation immediately. Viramune should not be restarted following severe hepatic, skin or hypersensitivity reactions.

The dosage must be strictly adhered to, especially the 14-days lead-in period (see section 4.2).

Cutaneous reactions

Severe and life-threatening skin reactions, including fatal cases, have occurred in patients treated with VIRAMUNE mainly during the first 6 weeks of therapy. These have included cases of Stevens-Johnson syndrome, toxic epidermal necrolysis and hypersensitivity reactions characterised by rash, constitutional findings and visceral involvement. Patients should be intensively monitored during the first 18 weeks of treatment. Patients should be closely monitored if an isolated rash occurs. VIRAMUNE must be permanently discontinued in any patient experiencing severe rash or a rash accompanied by constitutional symptoms (such as fever, blistering, oral lesions, conjunctivitis, facial oedema, muscle or joint aches, or general malaise), including Stevens-Johnson syndrome, or toxic epidermal necrolysis. VIRAMUNE must be permanently discontinued in any patient experiencing hypersensitivity reaction (characterised by rash with constitutional symptoms, plus visceral involvement, such as hepatitis, eosinophilia, granulocytopenia, and renal dysfunction), see section 4.4.

VIRAMUNE administration above the recommended dose might increase the frequency and seriousness of skin reactions, such as Stevens-Johnson syndrome and toxic epidermal necrolysis.

Concomitant prednisone use (40 mg/day for the first 14 days of VIRAMUNE administration) has been shown not to decrease the incidence of VIRAMUNE-associated rash, and may be associated with an increase in incidence and severity of rash during the first 6 weeks of VIRAMUNE therapy.

Some risk factors for developing serious cutaneous reactions have been identified, they include failure to follow the initial dosing of 200 mg daily during the lead-in period and a long delay between the initial symptoms and medical consultation. Women appear to be at higher risk than men of developing rash, whether receiving VIRAMUNE or non-VIRAMUNE containing therapy.

Patients should be instructed that a major toxicity of VIRAMUNE is rash. They should be advised to promptly notify their physician of any rash and avoid delay between the initial symptoms and medical consultation. The majority of rashes associated with VIRAMUNE occur within the first 6 weeks of initiation of therapy. Therefore, patients should be monitored carefully for the appearance of rash during this period. Patients should be instructed that dose escalation is not to occur if any rash occurs during the two-week lead-in dosing period, until the rash resolves.

Any patient experiencing severe rash or a rash accompanied by constitutional symptoms such as fever, blistering, oral lesions, conjunctivitis, facial oedema, muscle or joint aches, or general malaise should discontinue medication and immediately seek medical evaluation. In these patients VIRAMUNE must not be restarted.

If patients present with a suspected VIRAMUNE-associated rash, liver function tests should be performed. Patients with moderate to severe elevations (ASAT or ALAT > 5 ULN) should be permanently discontinued from VIRAMUNE.

If a hypersensitivity reaction occurs, characterised by rash with constitutional symptoms such as fever, arthralgia, myalgia and lymphadenopathy, plus visceral involvement, such as hepatitis, eosinophilia, granulocytopenia, and renal dysfunction, VIRAMUNE should be permanently stopped and not be re-introduced.

Hepatic reactions

Severe and life-threatening hepatoxicity, including fatal fulminant hepatitis, has occurred in patients treated with VIRAMUNE. The first 18 weeks of treatment is a critical period which requires close monitoring. The risk of hepatic events is greatest in the first 6 weeks of therapy. However the risk continues past this period and monitoring should continue at frequent intervals throughout treatment.

Increased ASAT or ALAT levels ⩾ 2.5 ULN and/or co-infection with hepatitis B and/or C at the start of antiretroviral therapy is associated with greater risk of hepatic adverse reactions during antiretroviral therapy in general, including VIRAMUNE containing regimens.

Female gender and patients with higher CD4 counts are at increased risk of hepatic adverse events.

Women have a three fold higher risk than men for symptomatic, often rash-associated, hepatic events (5.8% versus 2.2%), and patients with higher CD4 counts at initiation of VIRAMUNE therapy are at higher risk for symptomatic hepatic events with VIRAMUNE. In a retrospective review, women with CD4 counts >250 cells/mm^3 had a 12 fold higher risk of symptomatic hepatic adverse events compared to women with CD4 counts <250 cells/mm^3 (11.0% versus 0.9%). An increased risk was observed in men with CD4 counts > 400 cells/mm^3 (6.3% versus 1,2 % for men with CD4 counts <400 cells/mm^3).

Patients should be informed that hepatic reactions are a major toxicity of VIRAMUNE requiring close monitoring during the first 18 weeks. They should be informed that occurrence of symptoms suggestive of hepatitis should lead them to discontinue VIRAMUNE and immediately seek medical evaluation, which should include liver function tests.

Liver monitoring

Abnormal liver function tests have been reported with VIRAMUNE, some in the first few weeks of therapy.

Asymptomatic elevations of liver enzymes are frequently described and are not necessarily a contraindication to use VIRAMUNE. Asymptomatic GGT elevations are not a contraindication to continue therapy.

Monitoring of hepatic tests should be done every two weeks during the first 2 months of treatment, at the 3rd month and then regularly thereafter. Liver test monitoring should be performed if the patient experiences signs or symptoms suggestive of hepatitis and/or hypersensitivity.

If ASAT or ALAT ⩾ 2.5 ULN before or during treatment, then liver tests should be monitored more frequently during regular clinic visits. VIRAMUNE should not be administered to patients with pre-treatment ASAT or ALAT > 5 ULN until baseline ASAT/ALAT are stabilised < 5 ULN.

Physicians and patients should be vigilant for prodromal signs or findings of hepatitis, such as anorexia, nausea, jaundice, bilirubinuria, acholic stools, hepatomegaly or liver tenderness. Patients should be instructed to seek medical attention promptly if these occur.

If ASAT or ALAT increase to > 5 ULN during treatment, VIRAMUNE should be immediately stopped. If ASAT and ALAT return to baseline values and if the patient had no clinical signs or symptoms of hepatitis, rash, constitutional symptoms or other findings suggestive of organ dysfunction, it may be possible to reintroduce VIRAMUNE, on a case by case basis, at the starting dosage regimen of 200 mg/day for 14 days followed by 400 mg/day. In these cases, more frequent liver monitoring is required. If liver function abnormalities recur, VIRAMUNE should be permanently discontinued.

If clinical hepatitis occurs, characterised by anorexia, nausea, vomiting, icterus AND laboratory findings (such as moderate or severe liver function test abnormalities (excluding GGT), VIRAMUNE must be permanently stopped. VIRAMUNE should not be readministered to patients who have required permanent discontinuation for clinical hepatitis due to nevirapine.

Liver disease

The safety and efficacy of VIRAMUNE has not been established in patients with significant underlying liver disorders. VIRAMUNE is contraindicated in patients with severe hepatic impairment (see section 4.3). Patients with chronic hepatitis B or C and treated with combination antiretroviral therapy are at an increased risk for severe and potentially fatal hepatic adverse events. In the case of concomitant antiviral therapy for hepatitis B or C, please refer also to the relevant product information for these medicinal products.

Patients with pre-existing liver dysfunction including chronic active hepatitis have an increased frequency of liver function abnormalities during combination antiretroviral therapy and should be monitored according to standard practice. If there is evidence of worsening liver disease in such patients, interruption or discontinuation of treatment must be considered.

Post-exposure-prophylaxis

Serious hepatotoxicity, including liver failure requiring transplantation, has been reported in HIV-uninfected individuals receiving multiple doses of VIRAMUNE in the setting of post-exposure-prophylaxis (PEP), an unapproved use. The use of VIRAMUNE has not been evaluated within a specific study on PEP, especially in term of treatment duration and therefore, is strongly discouraged.

Other warnings

Combination therapy with VIRAMUNE is not a curative treatment of patients infected with HIV-1; patients may continue to experience illnesses associated with advanced HIV-1 infection, including opportunistic infections.

The long-term effects of nevirapine are unknown at this time. Combination therapy with VIRAMUNE has not been shown to reduce the risk of transmission of HIV-1 to others through sexual contact or contaminated blood.

Combination antiretroviral therapy has been associated with the redistribution of body fat (lipodystrophy) in HIV infected patients. The long-term consequences of these events are currently unknown. Knowledge about the mechanism is incomplete. A connection between visceral lipomatosis and PIs and lipoatrophy and NRTIs has been hypothesised. A higher risk of lipodystrophy has been associated with individual factors such as older age, and with drug related factors such as longer duration of antiretroviral treatment and associated metabolic disturbances. Clinical examination should include evaluation for physical signs of fat redistribution. Consideration should be given to the measurement of fasting serum lipids and blood glucose. Lipid disorders should be managed as clinically appropriate (see section 4.8).

Nevirapine may interact with some medicinal products; therefore, patients should be advised to report to their doctor the use of any other medications.

Oral contraceptives and other hormonal methods of birth control should not be used as the sole method of contraception in women taking VIRAMUNE, since nevirapine might lower the plasma concentrations of these medications. For this reason, and to reduce the risk of HIV transmission, barrier contraception (e.g., condoms) is recommended. Additionally, when oral contraceptives are used for hormonal regulation during administration of VIRAMUNE the therapeutic effect should be monitored.

Pharmacokinetic results suggest caution should be exercised when VIRAMUNE is administered to patients with moderate hepatic dysfunction and should not be administered in patients with severe hepatic dysfunction. Overall, the results suggest that patients with mild to moderate hepatic dysfunction, defined as Child-Pugh Classification Score ⩽ 7, do not require an adjustment in VIRAMUNE dosing. In patients with renal dysfunction, who are undergoing dialysis, pharmacokinetic results suggest that supplementing VIRAMUNE therapy with an additional 200 mg dose of VIRAMUNE following each dialysis treatment would help offset the effects of dialysis on nevirapine clearance. Otherwise patients with CLcr ⩾ 20 ml/min do not require an adjustment in VIRAMUNE dosing (see section 5.2).

Immune reactivation syndrome

In HIV-infected patients with severe immune deficiency at the time of institution of combination antiretroviral therapy (CART), an inflammatory reaction to asymptomatic or residual opportunistic pathogens may arise and cause serious clinical conditions, or aggravation of symptoms. Typically, such reactions have been observed within the first few weeks or months of initiation of CART. Relevant examples are cytomegalovirus retinitis, generalised and/or focal mycobacterial infections, and Pneumocystis carinii pneumonia. Any inflammatory symptoms should be evaluated and treatment instituted when necessary.

4.5 Interaction with other medicinal products and other forms of Interaction

NRTIs: No dosage adjustments are required when VIRAMUNE is taken in combination with zidovudine, didanosine, or zalcitabine. When the zidovudine data were pooled from two studies (n = 33) in which HIV-1 infected patients received VIRAMUNE 400 mg/day either alone or in combination with 200-300 mg/day didanosine or 0.375 to 0.75 mg/day zalcitabine on a background of zidovudine therapy, nevirapine produced a non-significant decline of 13 % in zidovudine area under the curve (AUC) and a non-significant increase of 5.8 % in zidovudine C_{max}. In a subset of patients (n = 6) who were administered VIRAMUNE 400 mg/day and didanosine on a background of zidovudine therapy, nevirapine produced a significant decline of 32 % in zidovudine AUC and a non-significant decline of 27 % in zidovudine C_{max}. Paired data suggest that zidovudine had no effect on the pharmacokinetics of nevirapine. In one crossover study, nevirapine had no effect on the steady-state pharmacokinetics of either didanosine (n = 18) or zalcitabine (n = 6).

Results from a 36 day study in HIV infected patients (n = 25) administered VIRAMUNE, nelfinavir (750 mg t.i.d.) and stavudine (30-40 mg b.i.d.) showed no statistically significant changes in the AUC or C_{max} of stavudine. Furthermore, a population pharmacokinetic study of 90 patients assigned to receive lamivudine with VIRAMUNE or placebo revealed no changes to lamivudine apparent clearance and volume of distribution, suggesting no induction effect of nevirapine on lamivudine clearance.

Non-nucleoside reverse transcriptase inhibitors (NNRTIs): Results from a clinical trial (n=14) showed that steady-state pharmacokinetic parameters of nevirapine were not affected by co-administration of efavirenz. However, drug levels of efavirenz were significantly reduced in the presence of nevirapine. The AUC of efavirenz decreased by 22% and the C_{min} by 36%. When co-administered with nevirapine a dose increase of efavirenz to 800mg once daily may be warranted.

PIs: Nevirapine is a mild to moderate inducer of the hepatic enzyme CYP3A; therefore, it is possible that co-administration with PIs (also metabolised by CYP3A) may result in an alteration in the plasma concentration of either agent.

Results from a clinical trial (n = 31) with HIV infected patients administered VIRAMUNE and saquinavir (hard gelatin capsules; 600 mg t.i.d.) indicated that their co-administration leads to a mean reduction of 24 % (p = 0.041) in saquinavir AUC and no significant change in nevirapine plasma levels. The reduction in saquinavir levels due to this interaction may further reducethe marginal plasma levels of saquinavir which are achieved with the hard gelatin capsule formulation.

Another study (n=20) evaluated once daily dosing of saquinavir soft gel capsule (sgc) with a 100 mg dose of ritonavir. All patients concomitantly received VIRAMUNE. The study showed that the combination of saquinavir sgc and 100 mg of ritonavir had no measurable effect on the pharmacokinetic parameters of nevirapine, compared to historical controls. The effect of nevirapine on the pharmacokinetics of saquinavir sgc in the presence of 100 mg of ritonavir, was modest and clinically insignificant.

Results from a clinical trial (n = 25) with HIV infected patients administered VIRAMUNE and indinavir (800 mg q8h) indicated that their co-administration leads to a 28 % mean decrease (p < 0.01) in indinavir AUC and no significant change in nevirapine plasma levels. No definitive clinical conclusions have been reached regarding the potential impact of co-administration of nevirapine and indinavir. A dose increase of indinavir to 1000 mg q8h should be considered when indinavir is given with nevirapine 200 mg b.i.d.; however, there are no data currently available to establish that the short term or long term antiviral activity of indinavir 1000 mg q8h with nevirapine 200 mg b.i.d. will differ from that of indinavir 800 mg q8h with nevirapine 200 mg b.i.d.

Results from a clinical trial (n = 25) with HIV infected patients administered VIRAMUNE and ritonavir (600 mg b.i.d. [using a gradual dose escalation regimen]) indicated that their coadministration leads to no significant change in ritonavir or nevirapine plasma levels.

Results from a 36 day study in HIV infected patients (n = 25) administered VIRAMUNE, nelfinavir (750 mg t.i.d.) and stavudine (30-40 mg b.i.d.) showed no statistically significant changes in nelfinavir pharmacokinetic parameters after the addition of nevirapine (AUC + 4 %, C_{max} + 14 % and C_{min} - 2 %). Compared to historical controls nevirapine levels appeared to be unchanged.

There were no increased safety concerns noted with the coadministration of VIRAMUNE with any of these PIs when used in combination.

There was no apparent change in the pharmacokinetics of lopinavir when used concomitantly with VIRAMUNE in healthy volunteers. In single PI experienced patients, nevirapine, used in combination with lopinavir / ritonavir 400/100 mg (3 capsules) twice daily and NRTIs, provided very good virological response rates. Results from a pharmacokinetic study in paediatric patients revealed a decrease in lopinavir concentrations during nevirapine co-administration. The clinical significance of this interaction is unknown. However a dose increase of lopinavir / ritonavir to 533/133 mg (4 capsules or 6.5 ml) may be considered when used in combination with nevirapine in patients where reduced susceptibility to lopinavir / ritonavir is clinically suspected (by treatment history or laboratory evidence).

Ketoconazole: In one study, administration of nevirapine 200 mg b.i.d. with ketoconazole 400 mg q.d. resulted in a significant reduction (63 % median reduction in ketoconazole AUC and a 40 % median reduction in ketoconazole C_{max}). In the same study, ketoconazole administration resulted in a 15-28 % increase in the plasma levels of nevirapine compared to historical controls. Ketoconazole and VIRAMUNE should not be given concomitantly. The effects of nevirapine on itraconazole are not known.

Fluconazole: Co-administration of fluconazole and VIRAMUNE resulted in approximately 100% increase in nevirapine exposure compared with historical data where VIRAMUNE was administered alone. Because of the risk of increased exposure to nevirapine, caution should be exercised if the medicinal products are given concomitantly and patients should be monitored closely. There was no clinically relevant effect of nevirapine on fluconazole.

Oral Contraceptives: As oral contraceptives should not be used as the sole method of contraception in HIV infected patients, other means of contraception (such as barrier methods) are recommended in patients being treated with VIRAMUNE. Furthermore a pharmacokinetic interaction has been identified. Nevirapine 200 mg b.i.d. was co-administered with a single dose of an oral contraceptive containing ethinyl estradiol (EE) 0.035mg and norethindrone (NET) 1.0 mg. Compared to plasma concentrations observed prior to nevirapine administration, the median AUC for 17α-EE was significantly decreased by 29% after 28 days of nevirapine dosing. There was a significant reduction in EE mean resident time and half-life. There was a significant reduction (18%) in median AUC for NET, without changes in mean resident time or half-life. The magnitude of the effect suggests that the dose of the oral contraceptive should be adjusted to allow adequate treatment for indications other than contraception (e.g., endometriosis), if used with nevirapine.

Other medicinal products metabolised by CYP3A: Nevirapine is an inducer of CYP3A and potentially CYP2B6, with maximal induction occurring within 2-4 weeks of initiating multiple-dose therapy. Based on the known metabolism of methadone, nevirapine may decrease plasma concentrations of methadone by increasing its hepatic metabolism. Narcotic withdrawal syndrome has been reported in patients treated with VIRAMUNE and methadone concomitantly. Methadone-maintained patients beginning VIRAMUNE therapy should be monitored for evidence of withdrawal and methadone dose should be adjusted accordingly.

Other compounds that are substrates of *CYP3A and CYP2B6* may have decreased plasma concentrations when co-administered with VIRAMUNE. Therefore, careful monitoring of the therapeutic effectiveness of P450 metabolised medicinal products is recommended when taken in combination with VIRAMUNE.

CYP isoenzyme inhibitors: The results of a nevirapine-clarithromycin interaction study (n = 18) resulted in a significant reduction in clarithromycin AUC (30 %) and C_{max} (- 21 %) but a significant increase in the AUC (58 %) and C_{max} (62 %) of the active metabolite 14-OH clarithromycin. There was a significant increase in the nevirapine C_{min} (28 %) and a non-significant increase in nevirapine AUC (26 %) and C_{max} (24 %). These results would suggest that no dose adjustment is necessary for either clarithromycin and VIRAMUNE when the two medicinal products are co-administered. Close monitoring of hepatic abnormalities and activity against *Myobacterium avium*-intracellular complex (MAC) is nevertheless recommended.

Monitoring of steady-state nevirapine trough plasma concentrations in patients who received long-term VIRAMUNE treatment revealed that nevirapine trough concentrations were elevated in patients who received cimetidine (+ 7 %, n = 13).

CYP isoenzyme inducers: An open-label study (n = 14) to determine the effects of nevirapine on the steady state pharmacokinetics of rifampicin resulted in no significant change in rifampicin C_{max} and AUC. In contrast, rifampicin produced a significant lowering of nevirapine AUC (- 58 %), C_{max} (- 50 %) and C_{min} (- 68 %) compared to historical data.

The available pharmacokinetic data suggest that the concomitant use of rifampicin and VIRAMUNE is not recommended. Therefore, these medicinal products should not be used in combination. Physicians needing to treat patients co-infected with tuberculosis and using a VIRAMUNE containing regimen may consider use of rifabutin instead. Rifabutin and VIRAMUNE can be administered concurrently without dose adjustments (see below). Alternatively physicians may consider switching to a triple NRTI combination for a variable period of time, depending on the tuberculosis treatment regimen (see section 4.3).

In a pharmacokinetic study the concomitant administration of VIRAMUNE with rifabutin resulted in a non-significant 12 % (median) increase in the steady-state AUC, a non-significant 3% decrease in C_{minss} and a significant 20 % increase in the C_{maxss}. Non-significant changes were found on 25-O-desacetyl-rifabutin (rifabutin active metabolite) AUC, C_{minss} or C_{maxss}. A statistically significant increase in the apparent clearance of nevirapine (9 %) compared to historical pharmacokinetic data was reported. This study suggests that there is no clinically relevant interaction between nevirapine and rifabutin. Therefore, the two drugs can be administered concurrently without dose adjustments provided that a careful monitoring of the adverse reactions is performed.

Warfarin: The interaction between nevirapine and the antithrombotic agent warfarin is complex, with the potential for both increases and decreases in coagulation time when used concomitantly. The net effect of the interaction may change during the first weeks of co-administration or upon discontinuation of VIRAMUNE, and close monitoring of anticoagulation levels is therefore warranted.

Hypericum perforatum: Serum levels of nevirapine can be reduced by concomitant use of the herbal preparation St John's Wort (*Hypericum perforatum*). This is due to induction of drug metabolism enzymes and/or transport proteins by St John's Wort. Herbal preparations containing St John's Wort should therefore not be combined with VIRAMUNE. If patient is already taking St John's Wort check nevirapine and if possible viral levels and stop St John's Wort. Nevirapine levels may increase on stopping St John's Wort. The dose of VIRAMUNE may need adjusting. The inducing effect may persist for at least 2 weeks after cessation of treatment with St John's Wort.

Other information: Studies using human liver microsomes indicated that the formation of nevirapine hydroxylated metabolites was not affected by the presence of dapsone, rifabutin, rifampicin, and trimethoprim/sulfamethoxazole. Ketoconazole and erythromycin significantly inhibited the formation of nevirapine hydroxylated metabolites.

4.6 Pregnancy and lactation

No observable teratogenicity was detected in reproductive studies performed in pregnant rats and rabbits. There are no adequate and well-controlled studies in pregnant women. Therefore VIRAMUNE should only be used during pregnancy if the expected benefit justifies the possible risk to the child and caution should be exercised when prescribing VIRAMUNE to pregnant women.

Results from a pharmacokinetic study (ACTG 250) of 10 HIV-1 infected pregnant women who were administered a single oral dose of 100 or 200 mg VIRAMUNE at a median of 5.8 hours before delivery, have shown that nevirapine readily crosses the placenta and is found in breast milk.

It is recommended that HIV-infected mothers do not breast-feed their infants to avoid risking postnatal transmission of HIV and that mothers should discontinue nursing if they are receiving VIRAMUNE.

4.7 Effects on ability to drive and use machines

There are no specific studies on the ability to drive vehicles and use machinery.

4.8 Undesirable effects

The most frequently reported adverse events related to VIRAMUNE therapy, across all clinical trials, were rash, nausea, fatigue, fever, headache, vomiting, diarrhoea, abdominal pain and myalgia.

The postmarketing experience has shown that the most serious adverse reactions are Stevens-Johnson syndrome and toxic epidermal necrolysis and serious hepatitis/hepatic failure and hypersensitivity reactions, characterised by rash with constitutional symptoms such as fever, arthralgia, myalgia and lymphadenopathy, plus visceral involvement, such as hepatitis, eosinophilia, granulocytopenia, and renal dysfunction. The first 18 weeks of treatment is a critical period which requires close monitoring (see section 4.4).

The following adverse events which may be causally related to the administration of VIRAMUNE have been reported. The frequencies estimated are based on pooled clinical trial data for events considered related to VIRAMUNE treatment.

Frequency classes: very common (>1/10); common (>1/100, <1/10); uncommon (>1/1,000, <1/100); rare (>1/10,000, <1/1,000); very rare (<1/10,000)

Blood and lymphatic system disorders

rare: granulocytopenia, anaemia

Immune system disorders

common: allergic reactions

rare: hypersensitivity (syndrome), anaphylaxis

Nervous system disorders

common: headache

Gastrointestinal disorders

common: nausea

uncommon: vomiting, abdominal pain

rare: diarrhoea

Hepato-biliary disorders

common: hepatitis (1.2 %), liver function tests abnormal

uncommon: jaundice

rare: liver failure / fulminant hepatitis

Skin and subcutaneous tissue disorders

common: rash (9 %)

uncommon: Stevens Johnson syndrome (0.3 %), urticaria

rare: toxic epidermal necrolysis, angio-oedema

Musculoskeletal, connective tissue and bone disorders

uncommon: myalgia

rare: arthralgia

General disorders and administration site conditions

uncommon: fatigue, fever

Combination antiretroviral therapy has been associated with redistribution of body fat (lipodystrophy) in HIV infected patients including the loss of peripheral and facial subcutaneous fat, increased intra-abdominal and visceral fat, breast hypertrophy and dorsocervical fat accumulation (buffalo hump).

Combination antiretroviral therapy has been associated with metabolic abnormalities such as hypertriglyceridaemia, hypercholesterolaemia, insulin resistance, hyperglycaemia and hyperlactataemia (see section 4.4).

The following events have also been reported when VIRAMUNE has been used in combination with other antiretroviral agents: pancreatitis, peripheral neuropathy and thrombocytopaenia. These events are commonly associated with other antiretroviral agents and may be expected to occur when VIRAMUNE is used in combination with other agents; however it is unlikely that these events are due to VIRAMUNE treatment. Hepatic-renal failure syndromes have been rarely reported.

In HIV-infected patients with severe immune deficiency at the time of initiation of combination antiretroviral therapy (CART), an inflammatory reaction to asymptomatic or residual opportunistic infections may arise (see section 4.4).

Skin and subcutaneous tissues

The most common clinical toxicity of VIRAMUNE is rash, with VIRAMUNE attributable rash occurring in 9 % of patients in combination regimens in controlled studies. In these clinical trials 24 % of patients treated with a VIRAMUNE containing regimen experienced rash compared with 15 % of patients treated in control groups. Severe rash occurred in 1.7 % of VIRAMUNE-treated patients compared with 0.2 % of patients treated in the control groups.

Rashes are usually mild to moderate, maculopapular erythematous cutaneous eruptions, with or without pruritus, located on the trunk, face and extremities. Allergic reactions (anaphylaxis, angioedema and urticaria) have been reported. Rashes occur alone or in the context of hypersensitivity reactions, characterised by rash with constitutional symptoms such as fever, arthralgia, myalgia and lympadenopathy, plus visceral involvement, such as hepatitis, eosinophilia, granulocytopenia, and renal dysfunction.

Severe and life-threatening skin reactions have occurred in patients treated with VIRAMUNE, including Stevens-Johnson syndrome (SJS) and toxic epidermal necrolysis (TEN). Fatal cases of SJS, TEN and hypersensitivity reactions have been reported. The majority of severe rashes occurred within the first 6 weeks of treatment and some required hospitalisation, with one patient requiring surgical intervention.

Hepato-biliary

The most frequently observed laboratory test abnormalities are elevations in liver function tests (LFTs), including ALAT, ASAT, GGT, total bilirubin and alkaline phosphatase. Asymptomatic elevations of GGT levels are the most frequent. Cases of jaundice have been reported. Cases of hepatitis (severe and life-threatening hepatoxicity, including fatal fulminant hepatitis) have been reported in patients treated with VIRAMUNE. In a large clinical trial, the risk of a serious hepatic event among 1121 patients receiving VIRAMUNE for a median duration of greater than one year was 1.2 % (versus 0.6 % in placebo group). The best predictor of a serious hepatic event was elevated baseline liver function tests. The first 18 weeks of treatment is a critical period which requires close monitoring (see section 4.4).

Paediatric patients

Based on experience of 361 paediatric patients treated in clinical trials, the most frequently reported adverse events related to VIRAMUNE were similar to those observed in adults, with the exception of granulocytopaenia which was more commonly observed in children. In post-marketing surveillance anaemia has been more commonly observed in children. Isolated cases of Stevens-Johnson syndrome or Stevens-Johnson/toxic epidermal necrolysis transition syndrome have been reported in this population.

4.9 Overdose

There is no known antidote for VIRAMUNE overdosage. Cases of VIRAMUNE overdose at doses ranging from 800 to 6000 mg per day for up to 15 days have been reported. Patients have experienced oedema, erythema nodosum, fatigue, fever, headache, insomnia, nausea, pulmonary infiltrates, rash, vertigo, vomiting, increase in transaminases and weight decrease. All of these effects subsided following discontinuation of VIRAMUNE.

5. PHARMACOLOGICAL PROPERTIES

5.1 Pharmacodynamic properties

Pharmacotherapeutic group: antiviral agent, ATC code J05A G01.

Mechanism of action

Nevirapine is a NNRTI of HIV-1. Nevirapine binds directly to reverse transcriptase and blocks the RNA-dependent and DNA-dependent DNA polymerase activities by causing a disruption of the enzyme's catalytic site. The activity of nevirapine does not compete with template or nucleoside triphosphates. HIV-2 reverse transcriptase and eukaryotic DNA polymerases (such as human DNA polymerases α, β, γ, or δ) are not inhibited by nevirapine.

Resistance

HIV isolates with reduced susceptibility (100 to 250-fold) to nevirapine emerge *in vitro*. Phenotypic and genotypic changes occur in HIV isolates from patients treated with VIRAMUNE or VIRAMUNE + zidovudine over one to 12 weeks. By week 8 of VIRAMUNE monotherapy, 100 % of the patients tested had HIV isolates with a > 100-fold decrease in susceptibility to nevirapine, regardless of dose. VIRAMUNE + zidovudine combination therapy did not alter the emergence rate of nevirapine-resistant virus. Genotypic and phenotypic resistance was examined for patients receiving VIRAMUNE in triple and double therapy drug combination therapy, and in the non-VIRAMUNE comparative group from the INCAS study. Antiretroviral naive subjects with CD4 cells counts of 200-600/mm^3 were treated with either VIRAMUNE + zidovudine (n = 46), zidovudine + didanosine (n = 51) or VIRAMUNE + zidovudine + didanosine (n = 51) and followed for 52 weeks or longer on therapy. Virologic evaluations were performed at baseline, six months and 12 months. The phenotypic resistance test performed required a minimum of 1000 copies/ml HIV RNA in order to be able to amplify the virus. Of the three study groups, 16, 19 and 28 patients respectively had evaluable baseline isolates and subsequently remained in the study for at least 24 weeks. At baseline, there were five cases of phenotypic resistance to nevirapine; the IC_{50} values were 5 to 6.5-fold increased in three and >100 fold in two. At 24 weeks, all available isolates recoverable from patients receiving nevirapine were resistant to this agent, while 18/21 (86 %) patients carried such isolates at 30-60 weeks. In 16 subjects viral suppression was below the limits of detection (< 20 copies/ml = 14, < 400 copies/ml = 2). Assuming that suppression below < 20 copies/ml implies nevirapine susceptibility of the virus, 45 % (17/38) of patients had virus measured or imputed to be susceptible to nevirapine. All 11 subjects receiving VIRAMUNE + zidovudine who were tested for phenotypic resistance were resistant to nevirapine by six months. Over the entire period of observation, one case of didanosine resistance was seen. Zidovudine resistance emerged as more frequent after 30 - 60 weeks, especially in patients receiving double combination therapy. Based on the increase in IC_{50}, zidovudine resistance appeared lower in the VIRAMUNE + zidovudine + didanosine group than the other treatment groups.

With respect to nevirapine resistance, all isolates that were sequenced carried at least one mutation associated with resistance, the most common single changes being K103N and Y181C. Combinations of mutations were found in nine of the 12 patients observed. These data from INCAS illustrate that the use of highly active drug therapies is associated with a delay in the development of antiretroviral drug resistance.

The clinical relevance of phenotypic and genotypic changes associated with VIRAMUNE therapy has not been established.

In addition to the data presented above, there exists a risk of rapid emergence of resistance to NNRTIs in case of virological failure.

Cross-resistance

Rapid emergence of HIV strains which are cross-resistant to NNRTIs has been observed *in vitro*. Data on cross-resistance between the NNRTI nevirapine and NRTIs are very limited. In four patients, zidovudine-resistant isolates tested *in vitro* retained susceptibility to nevirapine and in six patients, nevirapine-resistant isolates were susceptible to zidovudine and didanosine. Cross-resistance between nevirapine and HIV PIs is unlikely because the enzyme targets involved are different.

Cross-resistance among the currently registered NNRTIs is broad. Some genotypic resistance data indicate that in most patients failing NNRTI, viral strains express cross-resistance to the other NNRTIs. The currently available data do not support sequential use of NNRTIs.

Pharmacodynamic effects

VIRAMUNE has been evaluated in both treatment naive and treatment experienced patients.

Results from a trial (ACTG 241) evaluated triple therapy with VIRAMUNE, zidovudine and didanosine compared to zidovudine + didanosine, in 398 HIV-1 infected patients (mean baseline 153 CD4+ cells/mm^3; plasma HIV1 RNA 4.59 log_{10} copies/ml), who had received at least 6 months of NRTI therapy prior to enrolment (median 115 weeks). These heavily experienced patients demonstrated a significant improvement of the triple therapy group over the double therapy group for one year in both viral RNA and CD4+ cell counts.

A durable response for at least one year was documented in a trial (INCAS) for the triple therapy arm with VIRAMUNE, zidovudine and didanosine compared to zidovudine + didanosine or VIRAMUNE + zidovudine in 151 HIV-1 infected, treatment naive patients with CD4+ cell counts of 200-600 cells/mm^3 (mean 376 cells/mm^3) and a mean baseline plasma HIV-1 RNA concentration of 4.41 log_{10} copies/ml (25,704 copies/ml). Treatment doses were VIRAMUNE, 200 mg daily for two weeks, followed by 200 mg twice daily, or placebo; zidovudine, 200 mg three times daily; didanosine, 125 or 200 mg twice daily (depending on the weight).

VIRAMUNE has also been studied in combination with other antiretroviral agents, e.g., zalcitabine, stavudine, lamivudine, indinavir, ritonavir, nelfinavir, saquinavir and lopinavir. No new and overt safety problems have been reported for these combinations.

Studies are on-going to evaluate the efficacy and safety of combination therapies with VIRAMUNE in patients failing PI therapy.

Perinatal transmission

Two studies evaluated the efficacy of VIRAMUNE to prevent vertical transmission of HIV-1 infection. Mothers received only study antiretroviral therapy during these trials.

In the HIVNET 012 study in Kampala (Uganda) mother-infant pairs were randomised to receive oral VIRAMUNE (mother: 200 mg at the onset of labour; infant: 2 mg/kg within 72 hours of birth), or an ultra-short oral zidovudine regimen (mother: 600 mg at the onset of labour and 300 mg every 3 hours until delivery; infant: 4 mg/kg twice daily for 7 days). The cumulative HIV-1 infant infection rate at 14-16 weeks was 13.1 % (n = 310) in the VIRAMUNE group, versus 25.1 % (n = 308 in the ultra-short zidovudine group (p = 0.00063).

In the SAINT study conducted in South Africa, mother-infant pairs were randomised to receive oral VIRAMUNE (mother: 200 mg during labor and 200 mg 24 to 48 hours postdelivery; infant: 6 mg 24 to 48 hours postdelivery); or a short oral zidovudine plus lamivudine regimen (mother: zidovudine 600 mg, then 300 mg every 3 hours during labour, followed by 300 mg b.i.d. for 7 days postdelivery plus lamivudine 150 mg b.i.d. during labour and for 7 days postdelivery; infant: zidovudine 12 mg b.i.d. plus lamivudine 6 mg b.i.d. for 7 days [if infant weight <2 kg, zidovudine 4 mg/kg b.i.d. plus lamivudine 2 mg/kg b.i.d. for 7 days]). There was no significant difference in HIV-1 transmission rates through 6 to 8 weeks between the VIRAMUNE group (5.7 %, n = 652) and the zidovudine plus lamivudine group (3.6 %, n = 649). There was greater risk of HIV-1 transmission to babies whose mothers received their VIRAMUNE or their zidovudine plus lamivudine doses less than 2 hours before delivery. In the SAINT study 68% of nevirapine-exposed mothers had resistant strains at approximately 4 weeks after delivery.

The clinical relevance of these data in European populations has not been established. Furthermore, in the case VIRAMUNE is used as single dose to prevent vertical transmission of HIV-1 infection, the risk of hepatotoxicity in mother and child cannot be excluded.

A blinded randomized clinical trial in women already taking antiretroviral therapy throughout pregnancy (PACTG 316) demonstrated no further reduction of vertical HIV-1 transmission when the mother and the child received a single VIRAMUNE dose during labour and after birth respectively. HIV-1 transmission rates were similarly low in both treatment groups (1.3% in the VIRAMUNE group, 1.4% in the placebo group). The vertical transmission decreased neither in women with HIV-1 RNA below the limit of quantification nor in women with HIV-1 RNA above the limit of quantification prior to partus. Of the 95 women who received intrapartum VIRAMUNE, 15% developed nevirapine resistance mutations at 6 weeks post partus.

5.2 Pharmacokinetic properties

Adults

Nevirapine is readily absorbed (> 90 %) after oral administration in healthy volunteers and in adults with HIV-1 infection. Absolute bioavailability in 12 healthy adults following single-dose administration was 93 ± 9 % (mean SD) for a 50 mg tablet and 91 ± 8 % for an oral solution. Peak plasma nevirapine concentrations of 2 ± 0.4 μg/ml (7.5 μM) were attained by 4 hours following a single 200 mg dose. Following multiple doses, nevirapine peak concentrations appear to increase linearly in the dose range of 200 to 400 mg/day. Data reported in the literature from 20 HIV infected patients suggest a steady state C_{max} of 5.74 μg/ml (5.00-7.44) and C_{min} of 3.73 μg/ml (3.20-5.08) with an AUC of 109.0 h-μg/ml (96.0-143.5) in patients taking 200 mg of nevirapine bid. Other published data support these conclusions. Long-term efficacy appears to be most likely in patients whose nevirapine trough levels exceed 3.5 μg/ml.

VIRAMUNE tablets and oral suspension have been shown to be comparably bioavailable and interchangeable at doses up to 200 mg.

The absorption of nevirapine is not affected by food, antacids or medicinal products which are formulated with an alkaline buffering agent (e.g., didanosine).

Nevirapine is lipophilic and is essentially nonionized at physiologic pH. Following intravenous administration to healthy adults, the volume of distribution (Vdss) of nevirapine was 1.21 ± 0.09 l/kg, suggesting that nevirapine is widely distributed in humans. Nevirapine readily crosses the placenta and is found in breast milk. Nevirapine is about 60 % bound to plasma proteins in the plasma concentration range of 1-10 μg/ml. Nevirapine concentrations in human cerebrospinal fluid (n = 6) were 45 % (± 5 %) of the concentrations in plasma; this ratio is approximately equal to the fraction not bound to plasma protein.

In vivo studies in humans and *in vitro* studies with human liver microsomes have shown that nevirapine is extensively biotransformed via cytochrome P450 (oxidative) metabolism to several hydroxylated metabolites. *In vitro* studies with human liver microsomes suggest that oxidative metabolism of nevirapine is mediated primarily by cytochrome P450 isozymes from the CYP3A family, although other isozymes may have a secondary role. In a mass balance/excretion study in eight healthy male volunteers dosed to steady state with nevirapine 200 mg given twice daily followed by a single 50 mg dose of 14C-nevirapine, approximately 91.4 ± 10.5 % of the radiolabelled dose was recovered, with urine (81.3 ± 11.1 %) representing the primary route of excretion compared to faeces (10.1 ± 1.5 %). Greater than 80 % of the radioactivity in urine was made up of glucuronide conjugates of hydroxylated metabolites. Thus cytochrome P450 metabolism, glucuronide conjugation, and urinary excretion of glucuronidated metabolites represent the primary route of nevirapine biotransformation and elimination in humans. Only a small fraction (< 5 %) of the radioactivity in urine (representing < 3 % of the total dose) was made up of parent compound; therefore, renal excretion plays a minor role in elimination of the parent compound.

Nevirapine has been shown to be an inducer of hepatic cytochrome P450 metabolic enzymes. The pharmacokinetics of autoinduction are characterised by an approximately 1.5 to 2 fold increase in the apparent oral clearance of nevirapine as treatment continues from a single dose to two-to-four weeks of dosing with 200-400 mg/day. Autoinduction also results in a corresponding decrease in the terminal phase half-life of nevirapine in plasma from approximately 45 hours (single dose) to approximately 25-30 hours following multiple dosing with 200-400 mg/day.

Renal dysfunction: The single-dose pharmacokinetics of nevirapine have been compared in 23 subjects with either mild (50 ⩽ CLcr < 80 ml/min), moderate (30 ⩽ CLcr < 50 ml/min) or severe renal dysfunction (CLcr < 30 ml/min), renal impairment or end-stage renal disease (ESRD) requiring dialysis, and 8 subjects with normal renal function (CLcr > 80 ml/min). Renal impairment (mild, moderate and severe) resulted in no significant change in the pharmacokinetics of nevirapine. However, subjects with ESRD requiring dialysis exhibited a 43.5 % reduction in nevirapine AUC over a one-week exposure period. There was also accumulation of nevirapine hydroxy-metabolites in plasma. The results suggest that supplementing VIRAMUNE therapy with an additional 200 mg dose of VIRAMUNE following each dialysis treatment would help offset the effects of dialysis on nevirapine clearance. Otherwise patients with CLcr ⩾ 20 ml/min do not require an adjustment in VIRAMUNE dosing.

Hepatic dysfunction: The single-dose pharmacokinetics of nevirapine have been compared in 10 subjects with hepatic dysfunction and 8 subjects with normal hepatic function. Overall, the results suggest that patients with mild to moderate hepatic dysfunction, defined as Child-Pugh Classification Score ⩽ 7, do not require an adjustment in VIRAMUNE dosing. However, the pharmacokinetics of nevirapine in one subject with a Child-Pugh score of 8 and moderate to severe ascites suggests that patients with worsening hepatic function may be at risk of accumulating nevirapine in the systemic circulation.

Although a slightly higher weight adjusted volume of distribution of nevirapine was found in female subjects compared to males, no significant gender differences in nevirapine plasma concentrations following single or multiple dose administrations were seen. Nevirapine pharmacokinetics in HIV-1 infected adults do not appear to change with age (range 19-68 years) or race (Black, Hispanic, or Caucasian). VIRAMUNE has not been specifically investigated in patients over the age of 65.

Paediatric patients

The pharmacokinetics of nevirapine have been studied in two open-label studies in children with HIV-1 infection. In one study, nine HIV infected children ranging in age from 9 months to 14 years were administered a single dose (7.5 mg, 30 mg, or 120 mg per m^2; n = 3 per dose) of VIRAMUNE oral suspension after an overnight fast. Nevirapine AUC and peak concentration increased in proportion with dose. Following absorption nevirapine mean plasma concentrations declined log linearly with time. Nevirapine terminal phase half-life following a single dose was 30.6 ± 10.2 hours.

In a second multiple dose study, VIRAMUNE oral suspension or tablets (240 to 400 mg/m^2/day) were administered as monotherapy or in combination with zidovudine or zidovudine and didanosine to 37 HIV-1 infected paediatric patients with the following demographics: male (54 %), racial minority groups (73 %), median age of 11 months (range: 2 months – 15 years). These patients received 120 mg/ m^2/day of nevirapine for approximately 4 weeks followed by 120 mg/ m^2/b.i.d. (patients > 9 years of age) or 200 mg/ m^2/b.i.d. (patients ⩽ 9 years of age). Nevirapine clearance adjusted for body weight reached maximum values by age 1 to 2 years and then decreased with increasing age. Nevirapine apparent clearance adjusted for body weight was approximately two-fold greater in children younger than 8 years compared to adults. Nevirapine half-life for the study group as a whole after dosing to steady state was 25.9 ± 9.6 hours. With long term drug administration, the mean values for nevirapine terminal half-life changed with age as follows: 2 months to 1 year (32 hours), 1 to 4 years (21 hours), 4 to 8 years (18 hours), greater than 8 years (28 hours).

5.3 Preclinical safety data

Preclinical data revealed no special hazard for humans other than those observed in clinical studies based on conventional studies of safety, pharmacology, repeated dose toxicity, and genotoxicity. In reproductive toxicology studies, evidence of impaired fertility was seen in rats. In carcinogenicity studies, nevirapine induces hepatic tumours in rats and mice. In rats these findings are most likely related to nevirapine being a strong inducer of liver enzymes, and not due to a genotoxic mode of action. The mechanism of tumours in mice is not yet clarified and therefore their relevance in humans remains to be determined.

6. PHARMACEUTICAL PARTICULARS

6.1 List of excipients

Microcrystalline cellulose, lactose monohydrate, povidone K26/28 or K/25, sodium starch glycolate, colloidal silicon dioxide and magnesium stearate.

6.2 Incompatibilities

Not applicable.

6.3 Shelf life

2 years

6.4 Special precautions for storage
No special precautions for storage.

6.5 Nature and contents of container
Polyvinyl chloride (PVC)/aluminium foil push-through blister units (blister card of 10 tablets, 6 blister cards per carton).

6.6 Instructions for use and handling
No special requirements.

7. MARKETING AUTHORISATION HOLDER
Boehringer Ingelheim International GmbH

Binger Strasse 173

55216 Ingelheim am Rhein, Germany

8. MARKETING AUTHORISATION NUMBER(S)
EU/1/97/055/001

9. DATE OF FIRST AUTHORISATION/RENEWAL OF THE AUTHORISATION
17th February 2003

10. DATE OF REVISION OF THE TEXT
April 2005
V1a/B/SPC/11

Virazole Aerosol

(Valeant Pharmaceuticals Ltd)

1. NAME OF THE MEDICINAL PRODUCT
Virazole (Ribavirin) Aerosol

2. QUALITATIVE AND QUANTITATIVE COMPOSITION
Ribavirin 6 g

International non-proprietary name (INN): Ribavirin

Chemical Name: 1-Beta-D-Ribofuranosyl-1H-1,2,4-triazole-3-carboxamide

3. PHARMACEUTICAL FORM
Powder for inhalation solution.

4. CLINICAL PARTICULARS
4.1 Therapeutic indications
Virazole is indicated in the treatment of infants and children with severe respiratory syncytial virus (RSV) bronchiolitis.

Important: Ribavirin aerosol is more effective when instituted within the first 3 days of the treatment of bronchiolitis. Treatment early in the course of the disease may be necessary to achieve efficacy.

Treatment with Virazole must be accompanied by, and does not replace, standard supportive respiratory and fluid management for infants and children with severe respiratory tract infection.

Nebulised bronchodilators, when clinically indicated, should be administered with the small particle aerosol generator (SPAG) generator or Aiolos nebuliser turned off.

4.2 Posology and method of administration
Ribavirin aerosol is only recommended for use in infants and children.

Aerosol administration or nebulisation should be carried out in a SPAG or Aiolos nebuliser. Before use read the relevant Operator's Manual for instructions.

Treatment is carried out for 12 to 18 hours per day for at least 3 and no more than 7 days and is part of a total treatment programme.

The daily dose is prepared by dissolving 6 g of ribavirin in a minimum of 75 ml Water for Injection BP. Shake well. Transfer dissolved drug and dilute to a total volume of 300 ml of Water for Injection BP to give a 20 mg/ml ribavirin solution.

In the SPAG unit and Aiolos nebuliser the average concentration for a 7 hour period is 190 μg/l of air.

Method of administration
Please see point 6.6 for instructions on preparation of the aerosol solution.

The aerosol is delivered to an infant oxygen hood from the SPAG aerosol generator or Aiolos nebuliser. Administration by face mask or oxygen tent may be necessary if a hood cannot be employed (see Operator's Manual). However, the volume of distribution and condensation area are larger in a tent and the efficacy of this method of administration has been evaluated only in a small number of patients.

4.3 Contraindications
Ribavirin is contra-indicated in females who are or may become pregnant and it should be noted that ribavirin can be detected in human blood even four weeks after oral administration has ceased.

4.4 Special warnings and special precautions for use
Precipitation of the drug in respiratory equipment and consequent accumulation of fluid in the tubing has caused difficulties for patients requiring assisted ventilation.

In infants requiring assisted ventilation, Virazole should only be used when there is constant monitoring of both patients and equipment.

Directions for use during assisted ventilation are given in the SPAG or Aiolos manual, which should be read carefully before such administration.

Occupational exposure
Nebulised Virazole may potentially escape into the hospital environment during therapy. However, ribavirin was not detected in the erythrocytes, plasma or urine of subjects exposed for a mean of 25 hours during 5 consecutive days. Reports of occupational asthma have been reported rarely although the causal link to ribavirin is unknown since respiratory viruses may induce reactive airways disease in addition to other symptoms including headache, fever, nasal congestion and wheezing. However, care should be exercised, particularly in healthcare workers with pre-existing reactive airways diseases.

Health care workers directly providing care to patients receiving aerosolised Virazole should be aware that ribavirin has been shown to be teratogenic in rabbits and rodents but not in baboons. However, no reports of teratogenicity in the offspring of mothers who were exposed to Virazole aerosol during pregnancy have been confirmed and the teratogenic risk of Virazole to humans is unknown. As a precaution, women who are pregnant or trying to become pregnant should avoid exposure to the Virazole aerosol.

It is good practice to avoid unnecessary occupational exposure to chemicals whenever possible. Several methods have been employed to lower environmental exposure during Virazole use. The most practical of these is to turn the SPAG or Aiolos Nebuliser off for 5 to 10 minutes prior to prolonged contact.

4.5 Interaction with other medicinal products and other forms of Interaction
None known.

4.6 Pregnancy and lactation
Ribavirin is contra-indicated in females who are or may become pregnant, and in nursing mothers. Ribavirin can be detected in human blood four weeks after administration has ceased. Although there are no pertinent human data, oral ribavirin has been found to be teratogenic in tested rodent species. Pregnant baboons given up to 120 mg/kg/day orally over a 4 week period and within 20 days of gestation failed to exhibit any teratogenic effects.

4.7 Effects on ability to drive and use machines
None known.

4.8 Undesirable effects
Side-effects: Several serious adverse events occurred in severely ill infants with life-threatening underlying disease, many of whom required assisted ventilation. These events included worsening of respiratory status, bacterial pneumonia and pneumothorax. The role of ribavirin aerosol in these events has not been determined.

Anaemia (often of a haemolytic variety) and reticulocytosis have been reported with oral and intravenous administration. Rarely, cases of non-specific anaemia and haemolysis have been reported spontaneously in association with the aerosol administration of Virazole.

4.9 Overdose
No overdoses have been reported.

5. PHARMACOLOGICAL PROPERTIES
5.1 Pharmacodynamic properties
Ribavirin has anti-viral inhibitory activity in vitro against respiratory syncytial virus, influenzae virus and herpes simplex virus. Ribavirin is also active against respiratory syncytial virus in experimentally infected cotton rats.

The inhibitory activity of ribavirin on RSV in cell cultures is selective. The mechanism of action is unknown, but there is evidence that ribavirin interferes with protein translation by mRNA of several other RNA viruses, possibly the result of interference with formation of the 5' cap structure of mRNA.

5.2 Pharmacokinetic properties
Assay for ribavirin in human materials is by a radioimmunoassay which detects ribavirin and at least one metabolite.

Ribavirin administered by aerosol is absorbed systemically. Four paediatric patients inhaling ribavirin aerosol administered by face mask for 2.5 hours each day had plasma concentrations ranging from 0.44 to 1.44 μM, with a mean concentration of 0.76 μM. The plasma half-life was reported to be 9.5 hours. Three paediatric patients inhaling ribavirin aerosol administered by face mask or mist tent for 20 hours each day for 5 days had plasma concentrations ranging from 1.5 to 14.3 μM, with a mean concentration of 6.8 μM.

It is likely that the concentration of ribavirin in respiratory tract secretions is much higher than plasma concentrations in view of the route of administration.

The bioavailability of ribavirin is unknown and may depend on the mode of aerosol delivery. After aerosol treatment, peak plasma concentrations are less than the concentration that reduced RSV plaque formation in tissue cultures by 85 to 98%. After aerosol treatment, respiratory tract secretions are likely to contain ribavirin in concentrations many fold higher than those required to reduce plaque formation. However, RSV is an intracellular virus and serum concentrations may better reflect intracellular concentrations in the respiratory tract than respiratory secretion concentrations.

5.3 Preclinical safety data
Pertinent information is included in the Pregnancy and Lactation section.

6. PHARMACEUTICAL PARTICULARS
6.1 List of excipients
Not applicable.

6.2 Incompatibilities
None known.

6.3 Shelf life
5 years. After reconstitution in Water for Injections, Virazole should be used within 24 hours.

6.4 Special precautions for storage
Store in a dry place. Store below 25°C.

6.5 Nature and contents of container
100 mlType 1 glass serum bottle with butyl rubber closure and aluminium seal with tear-off septum. Each bottle contains 6 g ribavirin as a lyophilised white cake. Virazole is packaged in cartons of three bottles.

6.6 Instructions for use and handling
By aseptic technique dissolve the powder in a minimum of 75 ml Water for Injections BP in the 100 ml vial. The solution should be adequately mixed to ensure complete dissolution. Shake well. It is not recommended that this solution is heated during dissolution. When using the SPAG generator, transfer the solution to the clean, sterilised 500 ml flask and dilute to a final volume of 300 ml with Water for Injections BP. When using the Aiolos nebuliser, transfer the solution into an infusion bag and dilute to a final volume of 300 ml with Water for Injections BP. The final concentration should be 20 mg/ml.

The Water for Injections BP used to make up the Virazole solution should not have any antimicrobial agent or any other substance added and all solutions should be inspected for particulate matter and discoloration prior to administration.

See guidelines for avoiding unwanted exposure to Virazole aerosol under 4.4. Special warnings and special precautions for use.

7. MARKETING AUTHORISATION HOLDER
Valeant Pharmaceuticals Ltd

Cedarwood

Chineham Business Park

Crockford Lane

Basingstoke

Hampshire RG24 8WD

8. MARKETING AUTHORISATION NUMBER(S)
PL 15142/0001 POM

9. DATE OF FIRST AUTHORISATION/RENEWAL OF THE AUTHORISATION
11 March 1996

10. DATE OF REVISION OF THE TEXT
January 2005

Viread 245 mg film-coated tablets

(Gilead Sciences International Limited)

1. NAME OF THE MEDICINAL PRODUCT
Viread 245 mg film-coated tablets ▼

2. QUALITATIVE AND QUANTITATIVE COMPOSITION
Each film-coated tablet contains 245 mg of tenofovir disoproxil (as fumarate), equivalent to 300 mg of tenofovir disoproxil fumarate, or 136 mg of tenofovir.

For excipients, see 6.1.

3. PHARMACEUTICAL FORM
Film-coated tablet.

Light blue, almond-shaped, film-coated tablets, debossed on one side with the markings "GILEAD" and "4331" and on the other side with the marking "300".

4. CLINICAL PARTICULARS
4.1 Therapeutic indications
Viread is indicated in combination with other antiretroviral medicinal products for the treatment of HIV 1 infected adults over 18 years of age.

The demonstration of benefit of Viread is based on results of one study in treatment naïve patients, including patients with a high viral load (> 100,000 copies/ml) and studies in which Viread was added to stable background therapy (mainly tritherapy) in antiretroviral pre-treated patients experiencing early virological failure (< 10,000 copies/ml, with the majority of patients having < 5,000 copies/ml).

The choice of Viread to treat antiretroviral experienced patients should be based on individual viral resistance testing and/or treatment history of patients.

4.2 Posology and method of administration
Therapy should be initiated by a physician experienced in the management of HIV infection.

In exceptional circumstances in patients having particular difficulty in swallowing, Viread can be administered following disintegration of the tablet in at least 100 ml of water, orange juice or grape juice.

Adults: The recommended dose is 245 mg (one tablet) once daily taken orally with food.

Children and adolescents: The safety and efficacy of Viread in patients under the age of 18 years have not been established (see 4.4). Viread must not be administered to children or adolescents until further data become available describing the safety and efficacy of tenofovir disoproxil fumarate in patients under the age of 18 years.

Elderly: No data are available on which to make a dose recommendation for patients over the age of 65 years (see 4.4).

Renal insufficiency: Tenofovir is eliminated by renal excretion and the exposure to tenofovir increases in patients with renal dysfunction (see 5.2). Dosing interval adjustment is required in all patients with creatinine clearance < 50 ml/min, as detailed below.

The proposed dose interval modifications are based on limited data and may not be optimal. The safety and efficacy of these dosing interval adjustment guidelines have not been clinically evaluated. Therefore, clinical response to treatment and renal function should be closely monitored in these patients (see 4.4).

(see Table 1)

No dosing recommendations could be drawn for non-haemodialysis patients with creatinine clearance < 10 ml/min.

Hepatic impairment: No dose adjustment is required in patients with hepatic impairment (see 4.4 and 5.2).

4.3 Contraindications

• Known hypersensitivity to tenofovir, tenofovir disoproxil fumarate, or to any of the excipients.

4.4 Special warnings and special precautions for use

Tenofovir disoproxil fumarate has not been studied in patients under the age of 18.

Tenofovir is principally eliminated via the kidney. Tenofovir exposure may be markedly increased in patients with moderate or severe renal impairment (creatinine clearance < 50 ml/min) receiving daily doses of tenofovir disoproxil 245 mg (as fumarate). Consequently, a dosing interval adjustment is required in all patients with creatinine clearance < 50 ml/min. Careful monitoring for signs of toxicity, such as deterioration of renal function, but also for changes in viral load is required in patients with pre-existing renal impairment once Viread has been started at prolonged dosing intervals. The safety and efficacy of Viread in patients with renal impairment have not been established (see 4.2 and 5.2).

Renal impairment, which may include hypophosphataemia, has been reported with the use of tenofovir disoproxil fumarate (see 4.8).

Monitoring of renal function (creatinine clearance and serum phosphate) is recommended before taking tenofovir disoproxil fumarate, every four weeks during the first year, and then every three months. In patients at risk for, or with a history of, renal dysfunction, and patients with renal insufficiency, consideration should be given to more frequent monitoring of renal function.

If serum phosphate is < 1.5 mg/dl (0.48 mmol/l) or creatinine clearance is decreased to < 50 ml/min, renal function should be re-evaluated within one week and the dose interval of Viread adjusted (see 4.2). Consideration should also be given to interrupting treatment with tenofovir disoproxil fumarate in patients with creatinine clearance decreased to < 50 ml/min or decreases in serum phosphate to < 1.0 mg/dl (0.32 mmol/l).

Tenofovir disoproxil fumarate has not been evaluated in patients receiving nephrotoxic medicinal products (e.g. aminoglycosides, amphotericin B, foscarnet, ganciclovir, pentamidine, vancomycin, cidofovir or interleukin 2). Use of tenofovir disoproxil fumarate should be avoided with concurrent or recent use of a nephrotoxic medicinal product. If concomitant use of tenofovir disoproxil fumarate and nephrotoxic agents is unavoidable, renal function should be monitored weekly.

Tenofovir disoproxil fumarate has not been clinically evaluated in patients receiving medicinal products which are secreted by the same renal transporter, human organic anion transporter 1 (hOAT1) (e.g. adefovir dipivoxil; cidofovir, a known nephrotoxic medicinal product). This renal transporter (hOAT1) may be responsible for tubular secretion and in part, renal elimination of tenofovir, adefovir and cidofovir. Consequently, the pharmacokinetics of these medicinal products might be modified if they are co administered. In healthy volunteers, a single dose of adefovir dipivoxil given with tenofovir disoproxil fumarate did not result in a relevant drug-drug interaction with regard to pharmacokinetics. However, the clinical safety including potential renal effects of the co-administration of adefovir dipivoxil and tenofovir disproxil fumarate is unknown. Unless clearly necessary, concomitant use of these medicinal products is not recommended, but if such use is unavoidable, renal function should be monitored weekly (see 4.5).

In a 144 week controlled clinical study that compared tenofovir disoproxil fumarate with stavudine in combination with lamivudine and efavirenz in antiretroviral naïve patients, small decreases in bone mineral density of the hip and spine were observed in both treatment groups. Decreases in bone mineral density of spine and changes in bone biomarkers from baseline were significantly greater in the tenofovir disoproxil fumarate treatment group at 144 weeks. Decreases in bone mineral density of hip were significantly greater in this group until 96 weeks. However, there was no increased risk of fractures or evidence for clinically relevant bone abnormalities over 144 weeks. If bone abnormalities are suspected then appropriate consultation should be obtained.

Tenofovir disoproxil fumarate should be avoided in antiretroviral experienced patients with strains harbouring the K65R mutation (see 5.1).

Tenofovir disoproxil fumarate has not been studied in patients over the age of 65. Elderly patients are more likely to have decreased renal function, therefore caution should be exercised when treating elderly patients with tenofovir disoproxil fumarate.

Liver disease: Tenofovir and tenofovir disoproxil fumarate are not metabolised by liver enzymes. A pharmacokinetic study has been performed in non-HIV infected patients with various degrees of hepatic impairment. No significant pharmacokinetic alteration has been observed in these patients (see 5.2).

The safety and efficacy data of tenofovir disoproxil fumarate are limited in patients with significant underlying liver disorders. Patients with chronic hepatitis B or C and treated with combination antiretroviral therapy are at an increased risk for severe and potentially fatal hepatic adverse events. In case of concomitant antiviral therapy for hepatitis B or C, please refer also to the relevant product information for these medicinal products.

Patients with pre-existing liver dysfunction including chronic active hepatitis have an increased frequency of liver function abnormalities during combination antiretroviral therapy and should be monitored according to standard practice. If there is evidence of worsening liver disease in such patients, interruption or discontinuation of treatment must be considered.

Lactic acidosis: Lactic acidosis, usually associated with hepatic steatosis, has been reported with the use of nucleoside analogues. The preclinical and clinical data suggest that the risk of occurrence of lactic acidosis, a class effect of nucleoside analogues, is low for tenofovir disoproxil fumarate. However, as tenofovir is structurally related to nucleoside analogues, this risk cannot be excluded. Early symptoms (symptomatic hyperlactatemia) include benign digestive symptoms (nausea, vomiting and abdominal pain), non specific malaise, loss of appetite, weight loss, respiratory symptoms (rapid and/or deep breathing) or neurological symptoms (including motor weakness). Lactic acidosis has a high mortality and may be associated with pancreatitis, liver failure or renal failure. Lactic acidosis generally occurred after a few or several months of treatment.

Treatment with nucleoside analogues should be discontinued in the setting of symptomatic hyperlactatemia and metabolic/lactic acidosis, progressive hepatomegaly, or rapidly elevating aminotransferase levels.

Caution should be exercised when administering nucleoside analogues to any patient (particularly obese women) with hepatomegaly, hepatitis or other known risk factors for liver disease and hepatic steatosis (including certain medicinal products and alcohol). Patients co infected with hepatitis C and treated with alpha interferon and ribavirin may constitute a special risk.

Patients at increased risk should be followed closely.

Combination antiretroviral therapy has been associated with the redistribution of body fat (lipodystrophy) in HIV patients. The long-term consequences of these events are currently unknown. Knowledge about the mechanism is incomplete. A connection between visceral lipomatosis and protease inhibitors and lipoatrophy and nucleoside reverse transcriptase inhibitors has been hypothesised. A higher risk of lipodystrophy has been associated with individual factors such as older age, and with drug related factors such as longer duration of antiretroviral treatment and associated metabolic disturbances. Clinical examination should include evaluation for physical signs of fat redistribution. Consideration should be given to the measurement of fasting serum lipids and blood glucose. Lipid disorders should be managed as clinically appropriate (see 4.8).

Tenofovir is structurally related to nucleoside analogues hence the risk of lipodystrophy cannot be excluded. However, 144 week clinical data from antiretroviral naïve patients indicate that the risk of lipodystrophy was lower with tenofovir disoproxil fumarate than with stavudine when administered with lamivudine and efavirenz.

Nucleoside and nucleotide analogues have been demonstrated *in vitro* and *in vivo* to cause a variable degree of mitochondrial damage. There have been reports of mitochondrial dysfunction in HIV negative infants exposed *in utero* and/or postnatally to nucleoside analogues. The main adverse events reported are haematological disorders (anaemia, neutropenia), metabolic disorders (hyperlactataemia, hyperlipasaemia). These events are often transitory. Some late-onset neurological disorders have been reported (hypertonia, convulsion, abnormal behaviour). Whether the neurological disorders are transient or permanent is currently unknown. Any child exposed *in utero* to nucleoside and nucleotide analogues, even HIV negative children, should have clinical and laboratory follow-up and should be fully investigated for possible mitochondrial dysfunction in case of relevant signs or symptoms. These findings do not affect current national recommendations to use antiretroviral therapy in pregnant women to prevent vertical transmission of HIV.

Immune Reactivation Syndrome: In HIV infected patients with severe immune deficiency at the time of institution of combination antiretroviral therapy (CART), an inflammatory reaction to asymptomatic or residual opportunistic pathogens may arise and cause serious clinical conditions, or aggravation of symptoms. Typically, such reactions have been observed within the first few weeks or months of initiation of CART. Relevant examples are cytomegalovirus retinitis, generalised and/or focal mycobacterium infections, and *Pneumocystis carinii* pneumonia. Any inflammatory symptoms should be evaluated and treatment instituted when necessary.

Co administration of tenofovir disoproxil fumarate and didanosine results in a 40 60% increase in systemic exposure to didanosine that may increase the risk for didanosine-related adverse events (see 4.5). Rare cases of pancreatitis and lactic acidosis, sometimes fatal, have been reported.

A reduced didanosine dose (250 mg) has been tested to avoid over exposure to didanosine in case of co administration with tenofovir disoproxil fumarate, but this has been associated with reports of high rate of virological failure and of emergence of resistance at early stage within several tested combinations. Co administration of tenofovir disoproxil fumarate and didanosine is therefore not recommended, especially in patients with high viral load and low CD4 cell count. If this combination is judged strictly necessary, patients should be carefully monitored for efficacy and didanosine related adverse events.

Triple nucleoside therapy: There have been reports of a high rate of virological failure and of emergence of resistance at early stage when tenofovir disoproxil fumarate was combined with lamivudine and abacavir as well as with lamivudine and didanosine as a once daily regimen.

Patients must be advised that antiretroviral therapies, including tenofovir disoproxil fumarate, have not been proven to prevent the risk of transmission of HIV to others through sexual contact or blood contamination. Appropriate precautions must continue to be used.

4.5 Interaction with other medicinal products and other forms of Interaction

Based on the results of *in vitro* experiments and the known elimination pathway of tenofovir, the potential for CYP450 mediated interactions involving tenofovir with other medicinal products is low.

Tenofovir is excreted renally, both by filtration and active secretion via the anionic transporter (hOAT1). Co-administration of tenofovir disoproxil fumarate with other medicinal products that are also actively secreted via the anionic transporter (e.g. cidofovir) may result in increased concentrations of tenofovir or of the co-administered medicinal product (see 4.4).

Concomitant antiretroviral medicinal products

Emtricitabine, lamivudine, indinavir and efavirenz: co administration with tenofovir disoproxil fumarate did not result in any interaction.

When tenofovir disoproxil fumarate was administered with lopinavir/ritonavir, no changes were observed in the pharmacokinetics of lopinavir and ritonavir. Tenofovir AUC was increased by approximately 30% when tenofovir disoproxil fumarate was administered with lopinavir/ritonavir.

Table 1

	Creatinine Clearance (ml/min)*		Haemodialysis Patients
	30-49	10-29	
Recommended 245 mg Dosing Interval	Every 48 hours	Every 72 to 96 hours	Every 7 days following completion of a haemodialysis session**

* Calculated using ideal (lean) body weight

**Generally, once weekly dosing assuming three haemodialysis sessions per week, each of approximately 4 hours duration or after 12 hours cumulative haemodialysis.

When didanosine gastro-resistant capsules were administered 2 hours prior to or concurrently with tenofovir disoproxil fumarate, the AUC for didanosine was on average increased by 48% and 60% respectively. The mean increase in the AUC of didanosine was 44% when the buffered tablets were administered 1 hour prior to tenofovir. In both cases the pharmacokinetic parameters for tenofovir administered with a light meal were unchanged. The co administration of tenofovir disoproxil fumarate and didanosine is not recommended (see 4.4).

When tenofovir disoproxil fumarate was administered with atazanavir, a decrease in concentrations of atazanavir was observed (decrease of 25% and 40% of AUC and C_{min} respectively compared to atazanavir 400 mg). When ritonavir was added to atazanavir, the negative impact of tenofovir on atazanavir C_{min} was significantly reduced, whereas the decrease of AUC was of the same magnitude (decrease of 25% and 26% of AUC and C_{min} respectively compared to atazanavir/ritonavir 300/100 mg). The co-administration of atazanavir with ritonavir in combination with tenofovir has been substantiated in a clinical study.

Other interactions

Co administration of tenofovir disoproxil fumarate, methadone, ribavirin, adefovir dipivoxil (see 4.4) or the hormonal contraceptive norgestimate/ethinyl oestradiol did not result in any pharmacokinetic interaction.

Tenofovir disoproxil fumarate must be taken with food, as food enhances the bioavailability of tenofovir (see 5.2).

4.6 Pregnancy and lactation

Pregnancy

No clinical data on exposed pregnancies are available for tenofovir disoproxil fumarate.

Animal studies do not indicate direct or indirect harmful effects of tenofovir disoproxil fumarate with respect to pregnancy, foetal development, parturition or postnatal development (see 5.3).

Tenofovir disoproxil fumarate should be used during pregnancy only if the potential benefit justifies the potential risk to the foetus.

However, given that the potential risks to developing human foetuses are unknown, the use of tenofovir disoproxil fumarate in women of childbearing potential must be accompanied by the use of effective contraception.

Lactation

In animal studies it has been shown that tenofovir is excreted into milk. It is not known whether tenofovir is excreted in human milk. Therefore, it is recommended that mothers being treated with tenofovir disoproxil fumarate do not breast-feed their infants.

As a general rule, it is recommended that HIV infected women do not breast-feed their infants in order to avoid transmission of HIV to the infant.

4.7 Effects on ability to drive and use machines

No studies on the effects on the ability to drive or use machines have been performed. However, patients should be informed that dizziness has been reported during treatment with tenofovir disoproxil fumarate.

4.8 Undesirable effects

Assessment of adverse reactions is based on post-marketing experience and experience in two studies in 653 treatment-experienced patients receiving treatment with tenofovir disoproxil fumarate (n = 443) or placebo (n = 210) in combination with other antiretroviral medicinal products for 24 weeks and also in a double blind comparative controlled study in which 600 treatment naïve patients received treatment with tenofovir disoproxil 245 mg (as fumarate) (n = 299) or stavudine (n = 301) in combination with lamivudine and efavirenz for 144 weeks.

Approximately one third of patients can be expected to experience adverse reactions following treatment with tenofovir disoproxil fumarate in combination with other antiretroviral agents. These reactions are usually mild to moderate gastrointestinal events.

The adverse reactions with suspected (at least possible) relationship to treatment are listed below by body system organ class and absolute frequency. Frequencies are defined as very common (≥ 1/10), common (≥ 1/100, < 1/10), uncommon (≥ 1/1000, < 1/100), rare (≥ 1/10,000, < 1/1000) or very rare (< 1/10,000) including isolated reports.

Metabolism and nutrition disorders:

Very common: hypophosphataemia

Rare: lactic acidosis

Nervous system disorders:

Very common: dizziness

Respiratory, thoracic and mediastinal disorders:

Very rare: dyspnoea

Gastrointestinal disorders:

Very common: diarrhoea, nausea, vomiting

Common: flatulence

Rare: pancreatitis

Hepatobiliary disorders:

Rare: increased transaminases

Very rare: hepatitis

Skin and subcutaneous tissue disorders:

Rare: rash

Renal and urinary disorders:

Rare: renal failure, acute renal failure, proximal tubulopathy (including Fanconi syndrome), increased creatinine

Very rare: acute tubular necrosis

General disorders and administration site conditions:

Very rare: asthenia

Approximately 1% of tenofovir disoproxil fumarate treated patients discontinued treatment due to the gastrointestinal events.

Combination antiretroviral therapy has been associated with metabolic abnormalities such as hypertriglyceridaemia, hypercholesterolaemia, insulin resistance, hyperglycaemia and hyperlactataemia (see 4.4).

Combination antiretroviral therapy has been associated with redistribution of body fat (lipodystrophy) in HIV patients including the loss of peripheral and facial subcutaneous fat, increased intra abdominal and visceral fat, breast hypertrophy and dorsocervical fat accumulation (buffalo hump).

In a 144 week controlled clinical study in antiretroviral naïve patients that compared tenofovir disoproxil fumarate with stavudine in combination with lamivudine and efavirenz, patients who received tenofovir disoproxil had a significantly lower incidence of lipodystrophy compared with patients who received stavudine. The tenofovir disoproxil fumarate arm also had significantly smaller mean increases in fasting triglycerides and total cholesterol than the comparator arm.

In HIV infected patients with severe immune deficiency at the time of initiation of combination antiretroviral therapy (CART), an inflammatory reaction to asymptomatic or residual opportunistic infections may arise (see section 4.4).

4.9 Overdose

If overdose occurs the patient must be monitored for evidence of toxicity (see 4.8 and 5.3), and standard supportive treatment applied as necessary.

Tenofovir can be removed by haemodialysis; the median haemodialysis clearance of tenofovir is 134 ml/min. The elimination of tenofovir by peritoneal dialysis has not been studied.

5. PHARMACOLOGICAL PROPERTIES

5.1 Pharmacodynamic properties

Pharmacotherapeutic group: Antiviral for systemic use, ATC code: J05AF07

Mechanism of action: Tenofovir disoproxil fumarate is the fumarate salt of the prodrug tenofovir disoproxil. Tenofovir disoproxil is absorbed and converted to the active substance tenofovir, which is a nucleoside monophosphate (nucleotide) analogue. Tenofovir is then converted to the active metabolite, tenofovir diphosphate, by constitutively expressed cellular enzymes through two phosphorylation reactions in both resting and activated T cells. Tenofovir diphosphate has an intracellular half-life of 10 hours in activated and 50 hours in resting peripheral blood mononuclear cells (PBMCs). Tenofovir diphosphate inhibits viral polymerases by direct binding competition with the natural deoxyribonucleotide substrate and, after incorporation into DNA, by DNA chain termination. Tenofovir diphosphate is a weak inhibitor of cellular polymerases α, β, and γ, with kinetic inhibition constants (K_i) that are > 200-fold higher against human DNA polymerase α (5.2 μmol/l) and > 3,000-fold higher against human DNA polymerase β and γ (81.7 and 59.5 μmol/l, respectively) than its K_i against HIV 1 reverse transcriptase (0.02 μmol/l). At concentrations of up to 300 μmol/l, tenofovir has also shown no effect on the synthesis of mitochondrial DNA or the production of lactic acid in *in vitro* assays.

Pharmacodynamic effects: Tenofovir has *in vitro* antiviral activity against retroviruses and hepadnaviruses.

The concentration of tenofovir required for 50% inhibition (IC_{50}) of the wild-type laboratory strain HIV 1_{IIIB} is 1 6 μmol/l in lymphoid cell lines and 1.1 μmol/l against primary HIV 1 subtype B isolates in PBMCs. Tenofovir is also active against HIV 1 subtypes A, C, D, E, F, G, and O and against HIV_{BaL} in primary monocyte/macrophage cells. Tenofovir shows activity *in vitro* against HIV 2, with an IC_{50} of 4.9 μmol/l in MT 4 cells and against hepatitis B virus, with an IC_{50} of 1.1 μmol/l in HepG2 2.2.15 cells.

The activity of tenofovir remains within twofold of wild-type IC_{50} against recombinant HIV 1 expressing didanosine resistance (L74V), zalcitabine resistance (T69D), and multinucleoside drug resistance (Q151M complex) mutations. The activity of tenofovir against HIV 1 strains with zidovudine-associated mutations appears to depend on the type and number of these resistance mutations. In the presence of mutation T215Y, a twofold increase of the IC_{50} was observed. In 10 samples which had multiple zidovudine-associated mutations (mean 3.4), a mean 3.7-fold increase of the IC_{50} was observed (range 0.8 to 8.4).

Multinucleoside resistant HIV 1 with T69S double insertions have reduced susceptibility to tenofovir (IC_{50} > 10-fold). Tenofovir shows full activity against non-nucleoside reverse transcriptase inhibitor resistant HIV 1 with K103N or Y181C mutations. Cross-resistance to protease inhibitor resistance mutations is not expected due to the different viral enzymes targeted.

Strains of HIV 1 with 3- to 4-fold reduced susceptibility to tenofovir and a K65R mutation in reverse transcriptase have been selected *in vitro*. The K65R mutation in reverse transcriptase can also be selected by zalcitabine, didanosine, and abacavir, and causes reduced susceptibility to zalcitabine, didanosine, abacavir, and lamivudine (14-, 4-, 3-, and 25-fold, respectively). Tenofovir disoproxil fumarate should be avoided in antiretroviral experienced patients with strains harbouring the K65R mutation (see also 4.4).

The clinical activity of tenofovir disoproxil fumarate has not been determined against hepatitis B virus (HBV) in humans. It is unknown whether treatment of patients co-infected with HIV 1 and HBV will result in the development of HBV resistance to tenofovir disoproxil fumarate or other medicinal products.

Clinical efficacy: The effects of tenofovir disoproxil fumarate in treatment experienced and treatment naïve HIV 1 infected adults have been demonstrated in trials of 48 weeks duration in treatment-experienced HIV 1 infected adults.

In study GS-99-907, 550 treatment-experienced patients were treated with placebo or tenofovir disoproxil 245 mg (as fumarate) for 24 weeks. The mean baseline CD4 cell count was 427 cells/mm^3, the mean baseline plasma HIV 1 RNA was 3.4 log_{10} copies/ml (78% of patients had a viral load of < 5,000 copies/ml) and the mean duration of prior HIV treatment was 5.4 years. Baseline genotypic analysis of HIV isolates from 253 patients revealed that 94% of patients had HIV 1 resistance mutations associated with nucleoside reverse transcriptase inhibitors, 58% had mutations associated with protease inhibitors and 48% had mutations associated with non-nucleoside reverse transcriptase inhibitors.

At week 24 the time-weighted average change from baseline in log_{10} plasma HIV 1 RNA levels ($DAVG_{24}$) was 0.03 log_{10} copies/ml and 0.61 log_{10} copies/ml for the placebo and tenofovir disoproxil 245 mg (as fumarate) recipients ($p < 0.0001$). Patients whose HIV expressed 3 or more thymidine analogue associated mutations (TAMs) that included either the M41L or L210W reverse transcriptase mutation showed reduced susceptibility to tenofovir disoproxil 245 mg (as fumarate) therapy. The virological response was substantially decreased in patients with viral strains of > 10-fold zidovudine phenotypic resistance. A statistically significant difference in favour of tenofovir disoproxil 245 mg (as fumarate) was seen in the time-weighted average change from baseline at week 24 ($DAVG_{24}$) for CD4 count (+13 cells/mm^3 for tenofovir disoproxil 245 mg (as fumarate) *versus* 11 cells/mm^3 for placebo, p value = 0.0008). The antiviral response to tenofovir disoproxil fumarate was durable through 48 weeks ($DAVG_{48}$ was 0.57 log_{10} copies/ml, proportion of patients with HIV 1 RNA below 400 or 50 copies/ml was 41% and 18% respectively). Eight (2%) tenofovir disoproxil 245 mg (as fumarate) treated patients developed the K65R mutation within the first 48 weeks.

The 144-week, double blind, active controlled phase of study GS 99 903 evaluated the efficacy and safety of tenofovir disoproxil 245 mg (as fumarate) *versus* stavudine when used in combination with lamivudine and efavirenz in HIV 1 infected patients naïve to antiretroviral therapy. The mean baseline CD4 cell count was 279 cells/mm^3, the mean baseline plasma HIV 1 RNA was 4.91 log_{10} copies/ml, 19% of patients had symptomatic HIV 1 infection and 18% had AIDS. Patients were stratified by baseline HIV 1 RNA and CD4 count. Forty three percent of patients had baseline viral loads > 100,000 copies/ml and 39% had CD4 cell counts < 200 cells/ml.

By intent to treat analysis (Missing data and switch in antiretroviral therapy (ART) considered as failure), the proportion of patients with HIV 1 RNA below 400 copies/ml and 50 copies/ml at 48 weeks of treatment was 80% and 76% respectively in the tenofovir disoproxil 245 mg (as fumarate) arm, compared to 84% and 80 % in the stavudine arm. At 144 weeks, the proportion of patients with HIV 1 RNA below 400 copies/ml and 50 copies/ml was 71% and 68% respectively in the tenofovir disoproxil 245 mg (as fumarate) arm, compared to 64% and 63% in the stavudine arm.

The average change from baseline for HIV 1 RNA and CD4 count at 48 weeks of treatment was similar in both treatment groups (3.09 and 3.09 log_{10} copies/ml; +169 and 167 cells/mm^3 in the tenofovir disoproxil 245 mg (as fumarate) and stavudine groups, respectively). At 144 weeks of treatment, the average change from baseline remained similar in both treatment groups (3.07 and 3.03 log_{10} copies/ml; +263 and +283 cells/mm^3 in the tenofovir disoproxil 245 mg (as fumarate) and stavudine groups, respectively). A consistent response to treatment with tenofovir disoproxil 245 mg (as fumarate) was seen regardless of baseline HIV 1 RNA and CD4 count.

The K65R mutation occurred in a slightly higher percentage of patients in the tenofovir disoproxil fumarate group than the active control group (2.7% *versu s* 0.7%). Efavirenz or lamivudine resistance either preceded or was coincident with the development of K65R in all cases. Eight patients had HIV that expressed K65R in the tenofovir disoproxil 245 mg (as fumarate) arm, 7 of these occurred during the first 48 weeks of treatment and the last one at week 96. No further K65R development was observed up to week 144.

From both the genotypic and phenotypic analyses there was no evidence for other pathways of resistance to tenofovir.

5.2 Pharmacokinetic properties

Tenofovir disoproxil fumarate is a water soluble ester prodrug which is rapidly converted *in vivo* to tenofovir and formaldehyde.

Tenofovir is converted intracellularly to tenofovir monophosphate and to the active component, tenofovir diphosphate.

Absorption

Following oral administration of tenofovir disoproxil fumarate to HIV infected patients, tenofovir disoproxil fumarate is rapidly absorbed and converted to tenofovir. Administration of multiple doses of tenofovir disoproxil fumarate with a meal to HIV infected patients resulted in mean (%CV) tenofovir C_{max}, $AUC_{0\infty}$, and C_{min} values of 326 (36.6%) ng/ml, 3,324 (41.2%) ng·hr/ml and 64.4 (39.4%) ng/ml, respectively. Maximum tenofovir concentrations are observed in serum within one hour of dosing in the fasted state and within two hours when taken with food. The oral bioavailability of tenofovir from tenofovir disoproxil fumarate in fasted patients was approximately 25%. Administration of tenofovir disoproxil fumarate with a high fat meal enhanced the oral bioavailability, with an increase in tenofovir AUC by approximately 40% and C_{max} by approximately 14%. Following the first dose of tenofovir disoproxil fumarate in fed patients, the median C_{max} in serum ranged from 213 to 375 ng/ml. However, administration of tenofovir disoproxil fumarate with a light meal did not have a significant effect on the pharmacokinetics of tenofovir.

Distribution

Following intravenous administration the steady-state volume of distribution of tenofovir was estimated to be approximately 800 ml/kg. After oral administration of tenofovir disoproxil fumarate, tenofovir is distributed to most tissues with the highest concentrations occurring in the kidney, liver and the intestinal contents (preclinical studies). *In vitro* protein binding of tenofovir to plasma or serum protein was less than 0.7 and 7.2%, respectively, over the tenofovir concentration range 0.01 to 25 μg/ml.

Biotransformation

In vitro studies have determined that neither tenofovir disoproxil fumarate nor tenofovir are substrates for the CYP450 enzymes. Moreover, at concentrations substantially higher (approximately 300-fold) than those observed *in vivo*, tenofovir did not inhibit *in vitro* drug metabolism mediated by any of the major human CYP450 isoforms involved in drug biotransformation (CYP3A4, CYP2D6, CYP2C9, CYP2E1, or CYP1A1/2). Tenofovir disoproxil fumarate at a concentration of 100 μmol/l had no effect on any of the CYP450 isoforms, except CYP1A1/2, where a small (6%) but statistically significant reduction in metabolism of CYP1A1/2 substrate was observed. Based on these data, it is unlikely that clinically significant interactions involving tenofovir disoproxil fumarate and medicinal products metabolised by CYP450 would occur.

Elimination

Tenofovir is primarily excreted by the kidney by both filtration and an active tubular transport system with approximately 70-80% of the dose excreted unchanged in urine following intravenous administration. Total clearance has been estimated to be approximately 230 ml/h/kg (approximately 300 ml/min). Renal clearance has been estimated to be approximately 160 ml/h/kg (approximately 210 ml/min), which is in excess of the glomerular filtration rate. This indicates that active tubular secretion is an important part of the elimination of tenofovir. Following oral administration the terminal half-life of tenofovir is approximately 12 to 18 hours.

Linearity/non-linearity

The pharmacokinetics of tenofovir were independent of tenofovir disoproxil fumarate dose over the dose range 75 to 600 mg and were not affected by repeated dosing at any dose level.

Age and gender

Limited data on the pharmacokinetics of tenofovir in women indicate no major gender effect.

Pharmacokinetic studies have not been performed in children and adolescents (under 18) or in the elderly (over 65).

Pharmacokinetics have not been specifically studied in different ethnic groups.

Renal impairment

Pharmacokinetic parameters of tenofovir were determined following administration of a single dose of tenofovir disoproxil 245 mg to 40 non HIV infected patients with varying degrees of renal impairment defined according to baseline creatinine clearance (CrCl) (normal renal function when CrCl > 80 ml/min; mild with CrCl = 50 79 ml/min; moderate with CrCl = 30 49 ml/min and severe with CrCl = 10 29 ml/min). Compared with patients with normal renal function, the mean (%CV) tenofovir exposure increased from 2,185 (12%) ng·h/ml in subjects with CrCl > 80 ml/min to respectively 3,064 (30%) ng·h/ml, 6,009 (42%) ng·h/ml and 15,985 (45%) ng·h/ml in patients with mild, moderate and severe renal impairment. The dosing recommendations in patients with renal impairment, with increased dosing interval, are expected to result in higher peak plasma concentrations and lower C_{min} levels in patients with renal impairment compared with patients with normal renal function. The clinical implications of this are unknown.

In patients with end-stage renal disease (ESRD) (CrCl < 10 ml/min) requiring haemodialysis, between dialysis tenofovir concentrations substantially increased over 48 hours achieving a mean C_{max} of 1,032 ng/ml and a mean AUC_{0-48h} of 42,857 ng·h/ml.

It is recommended that the dosing interval for tenofovir disoproxil 245 mg (as fumarate) is modified in patients with creatinine clearance < 50 ml/min or in patients who already have ESRD and require dialysis (see 4.2).

The pharmacokinetics of tenofovir in non-haemodialysis patients with creatinine clearance < 10 ml/min and in patients with ESRD managed by peritoneal or other forms of dialysis have not been studied.

Hepatic Impairment

A single 245 mg dose of tenofovir disoproxil was administered to non HIV infected patients with varying degrees of hepatic impairment defined according to Child Pugh Turcotte (CPT) classification. Tenofovir pharmacokinetics were not substantially altered in subjects with hepatic impairment suggesting that no dose adjustment is required in these subjects. The mean (%CV) tenofovir C_{max} and $AUC_{0\infty}$ values were 223 (34.8%) ng/ml and 2,050 (50.8%) ng·hr/ml, respectively, in normal subjects compared with 289 (46.0%) ng/ml and 2,310 (43.5%) ng·hr/ml in subjects with moderate hepatic impairment, and 305 (24.8%) ng/ml and 2,740 (44.0%) ng·hr/ml in subjects with severe hepatic impairment.

Intracellular pharmacokinetics

In non-proliferating human peripheral blood mononuclear cells (PBMCs) the half-life of tenofovir diphosphate was found to be approximately 50 hours, whereas the half-life in phytohaemagglutinin-stimulated PBMCs was found to be approximately 10 hours.

5.3 Preclinical safety data

Preclinical studies conducted in rats, dogs and monkeys revealed target organ effects in gastrointestinal tract, kidney, bone and a decrease in serum phosphate concentration. Bone toxicity was diagnosed as osteomalacia (monkeys) and reduced bone mineral density (rats and dogs). Findings in the rat and monkey studies indicated that there was a substance-related decrease in intestinal absorption of phosphate with potential secondary reduction in bone mineral density. However, no conclusion could be drawn on the mechanism(s) underlying these toxicities.

Reproductive studies were conducted in rats and rabbits. There were no effects on mating or fertility parameters or on any pregnancy or foetal parameter. There were no gross foetal alterations of soft or skeletal tissues. Tenofovir disoproxil fumarate reduced the viability index and weight of pups in peri-post natal toxicity studies.

Genotoxicity studies have shown that tenofovir disoproxil fumarate was negative in the *in vivo* mouse bone marrow micronucleus assay but was positive for inducing forward mutations in the *in vitro* L5178Y mouse lymphoma cell assay in the presence or absence of S9 metabolic activation. Tenofovir disoproxil fumarate was positive in the Ames test (strain TA 1535) in two out of three studies, once in the presence of S9 mix (6.2 to 6.8 fold-increase) and once without S9 mix. Tenofovir disoproxil fumarate was also weakly positive in an *in vivo / in vitro* unscheduled DNA synthesis test in primary rat hepatocytes.

Tenofovir disoproxil fumarate did not show any carcinogenic potential in a long-term oral carcinogenicity study in rats. A long term oral carcinogenicity study in mice showed a low incidence of duodenal tumours, considered likely related to high local concentrations of tenofovir disoproxil fumarate in the gastrointestinal tract at a dose of 600 mg/kg/day. While the mechanism of tumour formation is uncertain, the findings are unlikely to be of relevance to humans.

6. PHARMACEUTICAL PARTICULARS

6.1 List of excipients

Core:

Microcrystalline cellulose (E460)

Pregelatinised starch (gluten free)

Croscarmellose sodium

Lactose monohydrate

Magnesium stearate (E572)

Coating:

Lactose monohydrate

Hypromellose (E464)

Titanium dioxide (E171)

Glycerol triacetate (E1518)

Indigo carmine aluminium lake (E132)

6.2 Incompatibilities

Not applicable.

6.3 Shelf life

3 years

6.4 Special precautions for storage

This medicinal product does not require any special storage conditions.

6.5 Nature and contents of container

Viread is supplied in high density polyethylene (HDPE) bottles with a child-resistant closure containing 30 film-coated tablets with a silica gel desiccant.

6.6 Instructions for use and handling

No special requirements.

7. MARKETING AUTHORISATION HOLDER

Gilead Sciences International Limited

Cambridge

CB1 6GT

United Kingdom

8. MARKETING AUTHORISATION NUMBER(S)

EU/1/01/200/001

9. DATE OF FIRST AUTHORISATION/RENEWAL OF THE AUTHORISATION

5 February 2002

10. DATE OF REVISION OF THE TEXT

08/07/05

Virgan

(Chauvin Pharmaceuticals Ltd)

1. NAME OF THE MEDICINAL PRODUCT

VIRGAN eye gel.

2. QUALITATIVE AND QUANTITATIVE COMPOSITION

Active Ingredient.

Ganciclovir 0.15%

3. PHARMACEUTICAL FORM

Eye gel.

4. CLINICAL PARTICULARS

4.1 Therapeutic indications

Treatment of acute herpetic keratitis (dendritic and geographic ulcers).

4.2 Posology and method of administration

Instil one drop of gel in the inferior conjunctival sac of the eye to be treated, 5 times a day until complete corneal re-epithelialisation. Then 3 instillations a day for 7 days after healing. The treatment does not usually exceed 21 days.

Use in the elderly:

The dosage in the elderly is the same as in adults (see above). There is no need to adjust the dosage in the elderly as in clinical trials patients up to the age of 85 years have been treated and no specific health concerns were observed.

Use in children:

VIRGAN eye gel is not recommended for use in children.

Only limited clinical trial data are available. (7 children, range 2-14 years).

4.3 Contraindications

Hypersensitivity to ganciclovir or acyclovir or to any other ingredients of the product.

4.4 Special warnings and special precautions for use

The following special warnings and precautions for use should be borne in mind, although systemic effects after ocular instillation are very unlikely. In preclinical testing ganciclovir given systemically caused aspermatogenesis, mutagenicity, teratogenicity, carcinogenicity and suppression of female fertility. These effects in animal studies have been observed at plasma concentrations far exceeding those being seen in humans after therapeutic use of Virgan Eye Gel (see also 5.3). However, ganciclovir should be considered a potential carcinogen and teratogen in humans.

4.5 Interaction with other medicinal products and other forms of Interaction

In case of any additional local ocular treatment there should be an application interval of at least 5 minutes between the two medications. VIRGAN Eye Gel should be the last medication instilled.

Although the quantities of ganciclovir passing into the general circulation after ophthalmic use are small, the risk of drug interactions cannot be ruled out. Interactions with ganciclovir administered systemically have been observed.

Binding of ganciclovir to plasma proteins is only about 1-2% and drug interactions involving binding site displacement are not anticipated.

It is possible that drugs which inhibit replication of rapidly dividing cell populations such as bone marrow, spermatogonia and germinal layers of skin and gastrointestinal mucosa might have combined additive toxic effects when used concomitantly with, before, or after ganciclovir. Because of the possibility of additive toxicity with co-administration of drugs such as dapsone, pentamidine, flucystosine, vincristine, vinblastine, adriamycin, amphotericin B, trimethoprim/sulpha combinations or other nucleoside analogues, combination with ganciclovir therapy should be used only if the potential benefits outweigh the risks.

Since both zidovudine and ganciclovir can result in neutropenia, it is recommended that these two drugs should not be given concomitantly during induction treatment with ganciclovir. Maintenance ganciclovir treatment plus zidovudine at the recommended dose resulted in severe neutropenia in most patients studied to date.

Generalised seizures have been reported in patients taking ganciclovir and imipenem-cilastatin concomitantly.

It is also possible that probenecid, as well as other drugs which inhibit renal tubular secretion or resorption, may reduce renal clearance of ganciclovir and could increase the plasma half-life of ganciclovir.

4.6 Pregnancy and lactation
Teratogenicity has been observed in animal studies with systemic ganciclovir. There is no experience regarding the safety of VIRGAN eye gel in human pregnancy or lactation. Administration during pregnancy and lactation is therefore not recommended, except for compelling reasons.

4.7 Effects on ability to drive and use machines
Patients should refrain from driving a vehicle or operating machines on the occurrence of any visual disturbance or other visual symptomatology.

4.8 Undesirable effects
In some cases, adverse events which did not result in a treatment interruption were observed in relation to the use of VIRGAN eye gel; burning sensations or brief tingling sensations, superficial punctate keratitis, visual disturbance on application.

4.9 Overdose
There is practically no risk of adverse events due to accidental oral ingestion since a tube of 5g contains 7.5mg ganciclovir compared to the daily adult i.v dose of 500-1000mg.

In the unlikely event of overdose, dialysis and hydration may be of benefit in reducing drug plasma levels.

Toxic manifestations seen in animals given very high single intravenous doses of ganciclovir (500mg/kg) included emesis, hypersalivation, anorexia, bloody diarrhoea, inactivity, cytopenia, abnormal liver function tests and BUN, testicular atrophy and death.

5. PHARMACOLOGICAL PROPERTIES

5.1 Pharmacodynamic properties
VIRGAN® is a formulation of 0.15% ganciclovir in a transparent aqueous gel with a hydrophilic polymer base.

Ganciclovir, 9-(1,3-dihydroxy-2-propoxymethyl)guanine or DHPG, is a broad-spectrum virustatic agent which inhibits the replication of viruses, including viruses of the herpes group, both *in vivo* and *in vitro*: herpes simplex types 1 and 2 (HSV), cytomegalovirus (CMV), Epstein-Barr virus (EBV), herpes zoster (HZV).

The mean effective dose (ED50) *in vitro* of ganciclovir on ocular clinical isolates of the herpes simplex virus is on average 0.23μg/ml (0.06 - 0.50). Ganciclovir inhibits *in vitro* the replication of various adenovirus serotypes. The ED50 is 1.8 to 4.0μg/ml for Ad 8 and Ad 19, those most frequently seen in ophthalmology.

Herpetic viruses induce one or more cellular kinases in the host cells, which phosphorylise the ganciclovir into its triphosphate derivative. This phosphorylation is carried out mainly in infected cells, as the concentrations of ganciclovir-triphosphate in non-infected cells are 10 times lower.

Ganciclovir-triphosphate works as an antiviral agent by inhibiting the synthesis of viral DNA in two ways: competitive inhibition of viral DNA-polymerases and direct incorporation into viral DNA which has the effect of stopping its elongation.

5.2 Pharmacokinetic properties
Studies of ocular pharmacokinetics in rabbits have shown a rapid and relevant penetration of ganciclovir into the cornea and the anterior segment of the eye, allowing concentrations higher than the effective antiviral concentrations over several hours. In fact, after instillation of one drop of ganciclovir gel, the concentrations (Cmax) of ganciclovir measured in the cornea (17μg/g), the conjunctiva (160μg/g), the aqueous humour (1μg/g) and the iris/ciliary body (4μg/g), are higher than the inhibitory concentrations for herpes simplex viruses 1 and 2 (< 0.5μg/ml) over more than 4 hours.

The repeated instillation 4 times a day for 12 days in rabbits with herpetic keratitis does not result in an accumulation of ganciclovir in the plasma.

In man, after daily ocular instillations repeated 5 times a day for 11 to 15 days in the course of treatment of superficial herpetic keratitis, plasma levels determined by means of a precise analytical method (quantification limit: 0.005μg/ml) are very low: on average 0.013μg/ml (0 - 0.037) which is 640 times lower than levels following a one hour i.v infusion of 5mg/kg

(Cmax=8.0μg/ml). The oral bioavailability of ganciclovir is approximately 6% when taken with food. Ganciclovir has a half life of 2.9 hours, the systemic clearance is 3.64ml/min/kg and the major route of excretion of ganciclovir is via glomerular filtration of unchanged drug.

5.3 Preclinical safety data
Animal data indicate that a side-effect of systemic ganciclovir is inhibition of spermatogenesis which is reversible at lower doses and irreversible at higher doses. Animal data have also indicated that permanent suppression of fertility in women may occur.

Ganciclovir had no effect on developing mouse foetuses at daily intravenous doses of 36mg/kg, but caused maternal/foetal toxicity and embryo death at daily doses of 108mg/kg. In rabbits, ganciclovir had no effect on developing foetuses at daily intravenous doses of 6mg/kg, but caused foetal growth retardation, embryo death, teratogenicity and/or maternal toxicity at daily doses of 20 or 60mg/kg.

Ganciclovir did not cause point mutations in bacterial or yeast cells or dominant lethality in mice, but caused point mutations and chromosomal damage in mammalian cells *in vitro* and *in vivo*. Ganciclovir was positive in these tests at thousands of times the concentration in plasma of patients undergoing therapy with VIRGAN eye gel.

Ganciclovir was carcinogenic in the mouse after daily oral doses of 20 and 1000mg/kg/day. No carcinogenic effect occurred at the dose of 1mg/kg/day. Tumour incidence was slightly increased at plasma levels of ganciclovir approximately 50 times human levels following VIRGAN eye gel treatment.

6. PHARMACEUTICAL PARTICULARS

6.1 List of excipients
Benzalkonium chloride, Carbomer 974P, Sorbitol, Sodium hydroxide

Purified water

6.2 Incompatibilities
None known to date.

6.3 Shelf life
In the unopened container: 3 years.

In the opened container: 4 weeks.

6.4 Special precautions for storage
Do not store above 25°C.

6.5 Nature and contents of container
5g tube (polyethylene-aluminium) with dropper nozzle (polyethylene) and screw cap (polyethylene) fitted with a detachable plastic base. This base allows the tube to be placed vertically, with the dropper nozzle pointing downwards, thus avoiding an accumulation of air around the opening, which would inhibit the correct formation of drops.

6.6 Instructions for use and handling
The package remains sterile until the original closure is broken. Do not use VIRGAN eye gel for more than 28 days after first opening.

Administrative Data

7. MARKETING AUTHORISATION HOLDER
Chauvin Pharmaceuticals Ltd

106 London Road

Kingston-Upon-Thames

Surrey

KT2 6TN

United Kingdom

8. MARKETING AUTHORISATION NUMBER(S)
PL 00033/0158

9. DATE OF FIRST AUTHORISATION/RENEWAL OF THE AUTHORISATION
21 July 2000

10. DATE OF REVISION OF THE TEXT
February 2002

February 2003

[S1] Black triangle removed due to MHRA approval 10th May 2005

Viridal 10 Duo

(SCHWARZ PHARMA Limited)

1. NAME OF THE MEDICINAL PRODUCT
VIRIDAL 10 DUO

2. QUALITATIVE AND QUANTITATIVE COMPOSITION
1 double-chamber glass cartridge containing dry substance (47.8 mg) composed of alprostadil 10 micrograms (used as 1:1 clathrate complex with alfadex) and diluent (1 ml).

Diluent:

1 ml sterile sodium chloride solution 0.9% (w/v) PhEur.

3. PHARMACEUTICAL FORM
Double chamber glass cartridge containing lyophilised powder and diluent for reconstitution.

Administration devices

1 reusable injector (starter kit)

1 double-chamber cartridge with dry substance and 1 ml 0.9% sterile sodium chloride solution

1 injection needle 29 G × ½ (0.33 mm × 12.7 mm)

1 alcohol swab to be obtained for each injection.

Route of administration

For injection into the penile cavernous body.

4. CLINICAL PARTICULARS

4.1 Therapeutic indications
As an adjunct to the diagnostic evaluation of erectile dysfunction in adult males.

Treatment of erectile dysfunction in adult males.

4.2 Posology and method of administration
The drug solution should be prepared shortly before the injection.

Prior to injection the needle should be screwed onto the tip of the injector. After disinfecting the tip of the cartridge with one of the alcohol swabs, the cartridge should then be inserted into the injector. By screwing the thread part clockwise, the cartridge is fixed in the injector. Then, the dry substance, which is inside the front chamber of the cartridge, is reconstituted with 1 ml sterile sodium chloride solution 0.9% in the bottom chamber. While holding the device in a vertical position with the needle upwards, the thread part should be screwed slowly until it will not go any further. The solvent will by-pass the upper stopper into the front chamber and dissolve the dry substance within a few seconds. As soon as the dry substance is reconstituted, the larger external and the smaller inner protective cap have to be removed from the needle. The air should then be expelled out of the cartridge and the prescribed dose adjusted precisely.

Unused solution must be discarded immediately.

Viridal Duo is injected into either the right or the left cavernous body of the penile shaft. Once the needle is in the cavernous body, the injection should be done within 5 to 10 seconds and is very easy without much resistance if the needle is in the correct position.

The development of an erection will start approximately 5 – 15 minutes after the injection.

Dosage for injection in the clinic

Injections for diagnostic evaluation and dose titration must be performed by the attending physician. He will determine an individual dose suitable to produce an erectile response for diagnostic purposes.

The recommended starting dose is 2.5 mcg Viridal Duo in patients with primary psychogenic or neurogenic origin of erectile dysfunction. In all other patients with erectile dysfunction 5 mcg Viridal Duo should be used as a starting dose. Dose adjustments may be performed in increments of about 2.5 mcg to 5 mcg Viridal Duo. Most of the patients require between 10 and 20 mcg per injection. Some patients may need to be titrated to higher doses. Doses exceeding 20 mcg should be prescribed with particular care in patients with cardiovascular risk factors. The dose per injection should never exceed 40 mcg.

Dosage for self-injection therapy at home

Before starting treatment at home, each patient or the patient's partner has to be taught by a physician how to prepare the drug and perform the injection. In no cases should the injection therapy be started without precise instructions by the physician. The patient should only use his optimum individual dosage, which has been pre-determined by his physician using the above-mentioned procedure. This dose should allow the patient to have an erection at home, which should not last longer than one hour. If he experiences prolonged erections beyond 2 hours but less than 4 hours, the patient is recommended to contact his physician to re-establish the dose of the drug. Maximum injection frequency recommended is 2 or 3 times a week with an interval of at least 24 hours between the injections.

Follow-up

After the first injections and at regular intervals, e.g. every three months, the physician should re-evaluate the patient. Any local adverse reaction, e.g. haematoma, fibrosis or nodules should be noted and controlled. Following discussion with the patient, an adjustment of dosage may be necessary.

4.3 Contraindications
Hypersensitivity to alprostadil and/or alfadex (ingredients of Viridal Duo).

Patients with diseases causing priapism e.g. sickle-cell disease, leukaemia and multiple myeloma or patients with anatomical deformation of the penis as cavernosal fibrosis or Peyronie's disease. Patients with penis implants should not use Viridal Duo.

Viridal Duo should not be used in men for whom sexual activity is contraindicated.

4.4 Special warnings and special precautions for use
The physician should carefully select patients suitable for self-injection therapy.

Sexual stimulation and intercourse can lead to cardiac and/or pulmonary events in patients with coronary heart disease, congestive heart failure or pulmonary disease. Viridal Duo should be used with care in these patient groups and patients should be examined and cleared for stress resistance by a cardiologist before treatment.

Viridal Duo should be used with care in patients who have experienced transient ischaemic attacks.

Patients who experience a prolonged erection lasting longer than four hours should contact their physician immediately. Therefore it is recommended that the patient has an emergency telephone number of his attending physician or of a clinic experienced in therapy of erectile dysfunction. Prolonged erection may damage penile erectile tissue and lead to irreversible erectile dysfunction.

A benefit-risk evaluation is neccesary before using Viridal Duo in patients with pre-existing scarring, e.g. nodules of the cavernous body or pre-existing penile deviation or Peyronie's disease or clinically relevant phimosis, e.g. phimosis with risk of paraphimosis these patients should be treated with particular care, e.g. more frequent re-evaluation of the patient's condition.

Patients who have to be treated with alpha-adrenergic drugs due to prolonged erections (see: overdose) may in the case of concomitant therapy with monoamino-oxidase-inhibitors, develop a hypertensive crisis.

Other intracavernous drugs e.g. smooth muscle relaxing agents or alpha-adrenergic blocking agents may lead to prolonged erection and must not be used concomitantly. The effects of a combination therapy of alprostadil with oral, intraurethral or topical medicinal products for erectile dysfunction are currently unknown.

Patients with blood clotting disorders or patients on therapy influencing blood clotting parameters should be treated with special care, e.g. monitoring of the clotting parameters and advice to the patient to exercise sufficient manual pressure on the injection site. This is because of the increased risk of bleeding.

To prevent abuse, self-injection therapy with Viridal Duo should not be used by patients with drug addiction and/or disturbances of psychological or intellectual development.

In cases of excessive use, e.g. higher frequencies than recommended, an increased risk of penile scarring cannot be excluded.

Use of intracavernous alprostadil offers no protection from the transmission of sexually transmitted diseases. Individuals who use alprostadil should be counselled about the protective measures that are necessary to guard against the spread of sexually transmitted diseases, including the human immunodeficiency virus (HIV). In some patients, injection of Viridal Duo can induce a small amount of bleeding at the injection site. In patients infected with blood borne diseases, this could increase the transmission of such diseases to the partner. For this reason we recommend that a condom is used for intercourse after injecting Viridal Duo.

Viridal Duo is for intracavernous injection. Subcutaneous injection or injections at areas of the penis other than the cavernous body should be avoided.

The injection should be performed under hygienic conditions to avoid infections. In any condition that precludes safe self-injection like poor manual dexterity, poor visual acuity or morbid obesity, the partner should be trained in the injection technique and should perform the injection.

Up to now, there is no clinical experience in patients under 18 and over 75 years of age.

Viridal Duo does not interfere with ejaculation and fertility.

4.5 Interaction with other medicinal products and other forms of Interaction

Concomitant use of smooth muscle relaxing drugs like papaverine or other drugs inducing erection like alpha-adrenergic blocking agents may lead to prolonged erection and should not be used in parallel with Viridal Duo.

Risks exist when using alpha-adrenergic drugs to terminate prolonged erections in patients with cardiovascular disorders or receiving MAO inhibitors.

The effects of blood pressure lowering and vasodilating drugs may be increased.

4.6 Pregnancy and lactation

Not applicable.

Alprostadil did not cause any adverse effects on fertility or general reproductive performance in male and female rats treated with 40-200 mcg/kg/day. The high dose of 200 mcg/kg/day is about 300 times the maximum recommended human dose on a body weight basis (MHRD < 1 mcg/kg).

Alprostadil was not fetotoxic or teratogenic at doses up to 5000 mcg/kg/day (7500 times the MHRD) in rats, 200 mcg/kg/day (300 times the MHRD) in rabbits and doses up to 20 mcg/kg/day (30 times the MHRD) in guinea pigs or monkeys.

4.7 Effects on ability to drive and use machines

Viridal Duo may rarely induce hypotension with subsequent impairment of reactivity.

4.8 Undesirable effects

A burning sensation during injection is common (< 10 %) and generally subsides shortly afterwards. A sensation of tension in the penis and pain at the site of injection are common (< 10 %) and mostly of mild intensity. Spotlike haemorrhage/ spotlike bruises at the site of puncture occur uncommonly (< 1 %). Haemosiderin deposits, reddening and swellings at the site of injection are also uncommon (< 1 %). Other uncommon (< 1 %) reactions are swellings of the preputium or the glans, and headache.

Prolonged erections of more than 4 hours duration are uncommon (< 1 %) and are mainly seen during dose titration.

During long-term treatment, fibrotic alterations (e.g. fibrotic nodules, plaques at the site of injection or in the corpus cavernosum) may occur commonly (< 10 %) in follow up periods of up to 4 years. This may be associated with slight penile axis deviations in uncommon (< 1 %) cases. In rare cases (< 0.1%), fibrotic changes of the cavernous body may occur during treatment lasting up to 4 years.

Rare cases (< 0.1%) of circulatory effects such as short periods of hypotension and/or vertigo or dizziness have been observed after the intracavernous injection of Viridal Duo.

In rare cases (< 0.1%) allergic reactions ranging from cutaneous hypersensitivity such as rash, erythema, urticaria to anaphylactic/anaphylactoid reactions may occur.

4.9 Overdose

Symptoms

Full rigid erections lasting more than four hours.

If the patient experiences a prolonged erection, he is advised to contact his attending physician or a urologic clinic nearby immediately.

Treatment strategy

Treatment of prolonged erection should be done by a physician experienced in the field of erectile dysfunction. If prolonged erection occurs, the following is recommended:

If the erection has lasted less than six hours:

– observation of the erection because spontaneous flaccidity frequently occurs.

If the erection has lasted longer than six hours:

– cavernous body injection of alpha-adrenergic substances (e.g. phenylephrine or epinephrine (adrenaline)). Risks exist when using drugs in patients with cardiovascular disorders or receiving MAO inhibitors. All patients should be monitored for cardiovascular effects when these drugs are used to terminate prolonged erections.

or

– aspiration of blood from the cavernous body.

Accidental systemic injection of high doses

Single dose rising tolerance studies in healthy volunteers indicated that single intravenous doses of alprostadil from 1 to 120 mcg were well tolerated. Starting with a 40 mcg bolus intravenous dose, the frequency of drug-related adverse events increased in a dose-dependent manner, characterised mainly by facial flushing.

5. PHARMACOLOGICAL PROPERTIES

5.1 Pharmacodynamic properties

ATC Code: Other urologicals G04BX 05

Alprostadil [Prostaglandin E_1 (PGE_1)], the active ingredient of Viridal Duo, is an endogenous compound derived from the essential fatty acid dihomogammalinolenic acid. Alprostadil is a potent smooth muscle relaxant that produces vasodilation and occurs in high concentrations in the human seminal fluid. Pre-contracted isolated preparations of the human corpus cavernosum, corpus spongiosum and cavernous artery were relaxed by alprostadil, while other prostanoids were less effective. Alprostadil has been shown to bind to specific receptors in the cavernous tissue of human and non-human primates.

The binding of alprostadil to its receptors is accompanied by an increase in intracellular cAMP levels. Human cavernosal smooth muscle cells respond to alprostadil by releasing intracellular calcium. Since relaxation of smooth muscle is associated with a reduction of the cytoplasmic free calcium concentration, this effect may contribute to the relaxing activity of this prostanoid.

Intracavernous injection of alprostadil in healthy monkeys resulted in penile elongation and tumescence without rigidity. The cavernous arterial blood flow was increased for a mean duration of 20 min. In contrast, intracavernous application of alprostadil to rabbits and dogs caused no erectile response.

Systemic intravascular administration of alprostadil leads to a vasodilation and reduction of systemic peripheral vascular resistance. A decrease in blood pressure can be observed after administration of high doses. Alprostadil has also been shown in animal and *in vitro* tests to reduce platelet reactivity and neutrophil activation. Additional alprostadil activity has been reported: increase in fibrinolytic activity of fibroblasts, improvement of erythrocyte deformability and inhibition of erythrocyte aggregation; inhibition of the proliferative and mitotic activity of non-striated myocytes; inhibition of cholesterol synthesis and LDL-receptor activity; and an increase in the supply of oxygen and glucose to ischaemic tissue along with improved tissue utilisation of these substrates.

5.2 Pharmacokinetic properties

After reconstitution, alprostadil (PGE_1) dissociates from the α-cyclodextrin clathrate, and the two components have independent fates.

In symptomatic volunteers, systemic mean endogenous PGE_1 venous plasma concentrations measured before intracavernous injection are approximately 1pg/ml. After injection of 20 mcg of alprostadil, the PGE_1 venous plasma concentrations increase rapidly to concentrations of about 10-20 pg/ml. The PGE_1 plasma concentrations return to concentrations close to the baseline within a few minutes. Approximately 90% of PGE_1 found in plasma is protein-bound.

Metabolism

Enzymatic oxidation of the C15-hydroxy group and reduction of the C13,14 double bond produce the primary metabolites, 15-keto-PGE_1, PGE_0 (13,14-dihydro-PGE_1) and 15-keto-PGE_0. Only PGE_0 and 15-keto-PGE_0 have been detected in human plasma. Unlike the 15-keto metabolites, which are less pharmacologically active than the parent compound, PGE_0 has a potency similar to that of PGE_1 in most respects.

In symptomatic volunteers, the mean endogenous PGE_0 venous plasma concentrations measured before an intracavernous injection are approximately 1 pg/ml. After the injection of 20 mcg of alprostadil, the PGE_0 plasma concentrations increase to concentrations of about 5 pg/ml.

Excretion

After further degradation of the primary metabolites by beta and omega oxidation, the resulting, more polar metabolites are excreted primarily with the urine (88%) and the faeces (12%) and there is no evidence of tissue retention of PGE_1 or its metabolites.

5.3 Preclinical safety data

Studies on local tolerance following single and repeated intracavernous injections of alprostadil or alprostadil alfadex in rabbits and/or monkeys, in monkeys up to 6 months with daily injection revealed in general good local tolerance. Possible adverse effects like haematomas and inflammations are more likely related to the injection procedure.

Within the 6 months study in male monkeys, there were no adverse effects of alprostadil alfadex on male reproductive organs.

Mutagenicity studies with alprostadil alfadex revealed no risk of mutagenicity.

6. PHARMACEUTICAL PARTICULARS

6.1 List of excipients

Powder for injection:

Lactose monohydrates

Alfadex

Diluent:

Sodium chloride

Water for injection.

6.2 Incompatibilities

No incompatibilities have so far been demonstrated.

6.3 Shelf life

Shelf life for the product as packaged for sale: 4 years.

Shelf life after reconstitution: for immediate use only.

6.4 Special precautions for storage

Do not store above 25°C. Store in the original packaging.

6.5 Nature and contents of container

1. Cartons containing one colourless glass double-chamber cartridge, one injection needle 29 G × ½ (0.33 mm × 12.7 mm) and one reusable injector (starter kit).

2. Cartons containing two colourless glass double-chamber cartridges, two injection needles 29 G × ½ (0.33 mm × 12.7 mm) and one reusable injector (starter kit).

3. Cartons containing one, two or six colourless glass double-chamber cartridges and corresponding number of injection needles 29 G × ½ (0.33 mm × 12.7 mm) without reusable injector.

6.6 Instructions for use and handling

Fix the injection needle onto the front part of the injector.

Disinfect the tip of the cartridge with one of the alcohol swabs. Insert the cartridge into the re-usable injector and fix it by screwing the thread part. Dissolve the drug substance in the front chamber of the cartridge by completely screwing the thread-part into the injector thus moving both rubber stoppers to the top of the cartridge and allowing the solvent in to the bottom chamber to reach the dry substance via the bypass of the cartridge. Shake slightly until a clear solution is produced.

Expel the air and adjust the prescribed dosage precisely prior to intracavernous injection.

After preparation of the solution, the injection must be performed using aseptic procedures into either the left or right cavernous body of the penile shaft. Care should be taken not to inject into penile vessels or nerves on the upper side of the penis and into the urethra on the under side. The injection should be completed within 5 to 10 seconds and manual pressure should be applied to the injection site for 2 to 3 minutes.

Unused solution must be discarded immediately.

Advice

The content of the front chamber of the cartridge consists of a white, dry powder, which forms a compact layer, approximately 8 mm in height. The layer may show cracks and crumble slightly.

In case of damage to the cartridge, the usually dry content of the front chamber becomes moist and sticky and extensively loses volume. Viridal Duo must not be used in this case.

The bottom chamber contains the clear, colourless sodium chloride solvent solution.

The dry substance dissolves immediately after addition of the sodium chloride solution. Initially after reconstitution the solution may appear slightly opaque due to the presence of bubbles. This is of no relevance and disappears within a short time to give a clear solution.

7. MARKETING AUTHORISATION HOLDER
SCHWARZ PHARMA Limited

Schwarz House

East Street

Chesham

Bucks HP5 1DG

England

8. MARKETING AUTHORISATION NUMBER(S)
PL 04438/0049

9. DATE OF FIRST AUTHORISATION/RENEWAL OF THE AUTHORISATION
23 May 1997

10. DATE OF REVISION OF THE TEXT
January 2005

Viridal 20 Duo

(SCHWARZ PHARMA Limited)

1. NAME OF THE MEDICINAL PRODUCT
VIRIDAL 20 DUO

2. QUALITATIVE AND QUANTITATIVE COMPOSITION
1 double-chamber glass cartridge containing dry substance (48.2 mg) composed of alprostadil 20 micrograms (used as 1:1 clathrate complex with alfadex) and diluent (1 ml).

Diluent:

1 ml sterile sodium chloride solution 0.9% (w/v) Ph Eur.

3. PHARMACEUTICAL FORM
Double chamber glass cartridge containing lyophilised powder and diluent for reconstitution.

Administration devices

1 reusable injector (starter kit)

1 double-chamber cartridge with dry substance and 1 ml 0.9% sterile sodium chloride solution

1 injection needle 29 G × ½ (0.33 mm × 12.7 mm)

1 alcohol swab to be obtained for each injection

Route of administration

For injection into the penile cavernous body.

4. CLINICAL PARTICULARS

4.1 Therapeutic indications
As an adjunct to the diagnostic evaluation of erectile dysfunction in adult males.

Treatment of erectile dysfunction in adult males.

4.2 Posology and method of administration
The drug solution should be prepared shortly before the injection.

Prior to injection the needle should be screwed onto the tip of the injector. After disinfecting the tip of the cartridge with one of the alcohol swabs, the cartridge should then be inserted into the injector. By screwing the thread part clockwise, the cartridge is fixed in the injector. Then, the dry substance, which is inside the front chamber of the cartridge, is reconstituted with 1 ml sterile sodium chloride solution 0.9% in the bottom chamber. While holding the device in a vertical position with the needle upwards, the thread part should be screwed slowly until it will not go any further. The solvent will by-pass the upper stopper into the front chamber and dissolve the dry substance within a few seconds. As soon as the dry substance is reconstituted, the larger external and the smaller inner protective cap have to be removed from the needle. The air should then be expelled out of the cartridge and the prescribed dose adjusted precisely.

Unused solution must be discarded immediately.

Viridal Duo is injected into either the right or the left cavernous body of the penile shaft. Once the needle is in the cavernous body, the injection should be done within 5 to 10 seconds and is very easy without much resistance if the needle is in the correct position.

The development of an erection will start approximately 5 – 15 minutes after the injection.

Dosage for injection in the clinic

Injections for diagnostic evaluation and dose titration must be performed by the attending physician. He will determine an individual dose suitable to produce an erectile response for diagnostic purposes.

The recommended starting dose is 2.5 mcg Viridal Duo in patients with primary psychogenic or neurogenic origin of erectile dysfunction. In all other patients with erectile dysfunction 5 mcg Viridal Duo should be used as a starting dose. Dose adjustments may be performed in increments of about 2.5 mcg to 5 mcg Viridal Duo. Most of the patients require between 10 and 20 mcg per injection. Some patients may need to be titrated to higher doses. Doses exceeding 20 mcg should be prescribed with particular care in patients with cardiovascular risk factors. The dose per injection should never exceed 40 mcg.

Dosage for self-injection therapy at home
Before starting treatment at home, each patient or the patient's partner has to be taught by a physician how to prepare the drug and perform the injection. In no cases should the injection therapy be started without precise instructions by the physician. The patient should only use his optimum individual dosage which has been pre-determined by his physician using the above-mentioned procedure. This dose should allow the patient to have an erection at home which should not last longer than one hour. If he experiences prolonged erections beyond 2 hours but less than 4 hours, the patient is recommended to contact his physician to re-establish the dose of the drug. Maximum injection frequency recommended is 2 or 3 times a week with an interval of at least 24 hours between the injections.

Follow-up

After the first injections and at regular intervals, e.g. every three months, the physician should re-evaluate the patient. Any local adverse reaction, e.g. haematoma, fibrosis or nodules should be noted and controlled. Following discussion with the patient, an adjustment of dosage may be necessary.

4.3 Contraindications
Hypersensitivity to alprostadil and/or alfadex (ingredients of Viridal Duo).

Patients with diseases causing priapism e.g. sickle-cell disease, leukaemia and multiple myeloma or patients with anatomical deformation of the penis as cavernosal fibrosis or Peyronie's disease. Patients with penis implants should not use Viridal Duo.

Viridal Duo should not be used in men for whom sexual activity is contraindicated.

4.4 Special warnings and special precautions for use
The physician should carefully select patients suitable for self-injection therapy.

Sexual stimulation and intercourse can lead to cardiac and/or pulmonary events in patients with coronary heart disease, congestive heart failure or pulmonary disease. Viridal Duo should be used with care in these patient groups and patients should be examined and cleared for stress resistance by a cardiologist before treatment.

Viridal Duo should be used with care in patients who have experienced transient ischaemic attacks.

Patients who experience a prolonged erection lasting longer than four hours should contact their physician immediately. Therefore it is recommended that the patient has an emergency telephone number of his attending physician or of a clinic experienced in therapy of erectile dysfunction. Prolonged erection may damage penile erectile tissue and lead to irreversible erectile dysfunction.

A benefit-risk evaulation is neccesary before using Viridal Duo in patients with pre-existing scarring, e.g. nodules of the cavernous body or pre-existing penile deviation or Peyronie's disease or clinically relevant phimosis, e.g. phimosis with risk of paraphimosis these patients should be treated with particular care, e.g. more frequent re-evaluation of the patient's condition.

Patients who have to be treated with alpha-adrenergic drugs due to prolonged erections (see: overdose) may in the case of concomitant therapy with monoamino-oxidase-inhibitors, develop a hypertensive crisis.

Other intracavernous drugs e.g. smooth muscle relaxing agents or alpha-adrenergic blocking agents may lead to prolonged erection and must not be used concomitantly.

The effects of a combination therapy of alprostadil with oral, intraurethral or topical medicinal products for erectile dysfunction are currently unknown.

Patients with blood clotting disorders or patients on therapy influencing blood clotting parameters should be treated with special care, e.g. monitoring of the clotting parameters and advice to the patient to exercise sufficient manual pressure on the injection site. This is because of the increased risk of bleeding.

To prevent abuse, self-injection therapy with Viridal Duo should not be used by patients with drug addiction and/or disturbances of psychological or intellectual development.

In cases of excessive use, e.g. higher frequencies than recommended, an increased risk of penile scarring cannot be excluded.

Use of intracavernous alprostadil offers no protection from the transmission of sexually transmitted diseases. Individuals who use alprostadil should be counselled about the protective measures that are necessary to guard against the spread of sexually transmitted diseases, including the human immunodeficiency virus (HIV). In some patients, injection of Viridal Duo can induce a small amount of bleeding at the injection site. In patients infected with blood borne diseases, this could increase the transmission of such diseases to the partner. For this reason we recommend that a condom is used for intercourse after injecting Viridal Duo.

Viridal Duo is for intracavernous injection. Subcutaneous injection or injections at areas of the penis other than the cavernous body should be avoided.

The injection should be performed under hygienic conditions to avoid infections. In any condition that precludes safe self-injection like poor manual dexterity, poor visual acuity or morbid obesity, the partner should be trained in the injection technique and should perform the injection.

Up to now, there is no clinical experience in patients under 18 and over 75 years of age.

Viridal Duo does not interfere with ejaculation and fertility.

4.5 Interaction with other medicinal products and other forms of Interaction
Concomitant use of smooth muscle relaxing drugs like papaverine or other drugs inducing erection like alpha-adrenergic blocking agents may lead to prolonged erection and should not be used in parallel with Viridal Duo.

Risks exist when using alpha-adrenergic drugs to terminate prolonged erections in patients with cardiovascular disorders or receiving MAO inhibitors.

The effects of blood pressure lowering and vasodilating drugs may be increased.

4.6 Pregnancy and lactation
Not applicable.

Alprostadil did not cause any adverse effects on fertility or general reproductive performance in male and female rats treated with 40-200 mcg/kg/day. The high dose of 200 mcg/kg/day is about 300 times the maximum recommended human dose on a body weight basis (MHRD < 1 mcg/kg).

Alprostadil was not fetotoxic or teratogenic at doses up to 5000 mcg/kg/day (7500 times the MHRD) in rats, 200 mcg/kg/day (300 times the MHRD) in rabbits and doses up to 20 mcg/kg/day (30 times the MHRD) in guinea pigs or monkeys.

4.7 Effects on ability to drive and use machines
Viridal Duo may rarely induce hypotension with subsequent impairment of reactivity.

4.8 Undesirable effects
A burning sensation during injection is common (< 10 %) and generally subsides shortly afterwards. A sensation of tension in the penis and pain at the site of injection are common (< 10 %) and mostly of mild intensity. Spotlike haemorrhage/ spotlike bruises at the site of puncture occur uncommonly (< 1 %). Haemosiderin deposits, reddening and swellings at the site of injection are also uncommon (< 1 %). Other uncommon (< 1 %) reactions are swellings of the preputium or the glans, and headache.

Prolonged erections of more than 4 hours duration are uncommon (< 1 %) and are mainly seen during dose titration.

During long-term treatment, fibrotic alterations (e.g. fibrotic nodules, plaques at the site of injection or in the corpus cavernosum) may occur commonly (< 10 %) in follow up periods of up to 4 years. This may be associated with slight penile axis deviations in uncommon (< 1 %) cases. In rare cases (< 0.1%), fibrotic changes of the cavernous body may occur during treatment lasting up to 4 years,

Rare cases (< 0.1%) of circulatory effects such as short periods of hypotension and/or vertigo or dizziness have been observed after the intracavernous injection of Viridal Duo.

In rare cases (< 0.1%) allergic reactions ranging from cutaneous hypersensitivity such as rash, erythema, urticaria to anaphylactic/anaphylactoid reactions may occur.

4.9 Overdose
Symptoms
Full rigid erections lasting more than four hours.

If the patient experiences a prolonged erection, he is advised to contact his attending physician or a urologic clinic nearby immediately.

Treatment strategy
Treatment of prolonged erection should be done by a physician experienced in the field of erectile dysfunction. If prolonged erection occurs, the following is recommended:

If the erection has lasted less than six hours:

– observation of the erection because spontaneous flaccidity frequently occurs.

If the erection has lasted longer than six hours:

– cavernous body injection of alpha-adrenergic substances (e.g. phenylephrine or epinephrine (adrenaline)). Risks exist when using drugs in patients with cardiovascular disorders or receiving MAO inhibitors. All patients should be monitored for cardiovascular effects when these drugs are used to terminate prolonged erections.

or

– aspiration of blood from the cavernous body.

Accidental systemic injection of high doses

Single dose rising tolerance studies in healthy volunteers indicated that single intravenous doses of alprostadil from 1 to 120 mcg were well tolerated. Starting with a 40 mcg bolus intravenous dose, the frequency of drug-related adverse events increased in a dose-dependent manner, characterised mainly by facial flushing.

5. PHARMACOLOGICAL PROPERTIES

5.1 Pharmacodynamic properties
ATC Code: Other urologicals G04BX 05

Alprostadil [Prostaglandin E_1 (PGE_1)], the active ingredient of Viridal Duo, is an endogenous compound derived from the essential fatty acid dihomogammalinolenic acid. Alprostadil is a potent smooth muscle relaxant that produces vasodilation and occurs in high concentrations in the human seminal fluid. Pre-contracted isolated preparations of the human corpus cavernosum, corpus spongiosum and cavernous artery were relaxed by alprostadil, while other prostanoids were less effective.

Alprostadil has been shown to bind to specific receptors in the cavernous tissue of human and non-human primates.

The binding of alprostadil to its receptors is accompanied by an increase in intracellular cAMP levels. Human cavernosal smooth muscle cells respond to alprostadil by releasing intracellular calcium. Since relaxation of smooth muscle is associated with a reduction of the cytoplasmic free calcium concentration, this effect may contribute to the relaxing activity of this prostanoid.

Intracavernous injection of alprostadil in healthy monkeys resulted in penile elongation and tumescence without rigidity. The cavernous arterial blood flow was increased for a mean duration of 20 min. In contrast, intracavernous application of alprostadil to rabbits and dogs caused no erectile response.

Systemic intravascular administration of alprostadil leads to a vasodilation and reduction of systemic peripheral vascular resistance. A decrease in blood pressure can be observed after administration of high doses. Alprostadil has also been shown in animal and *in vitro* tests to reduce platelet reactivity and neutrophil activation. Additional alprostadil activity has been reported: increase in fibrinolytic activity of fibroblasts, improvement of erythrocyte deformability and inhibition of erythrocyte aggregation; inhibition of the proliferative and mitotic activity of non-striated myocytes; inhibition of cholesterol synthesis and LDL-receptor activity; and an increase in the supply of oxygen and glucose to ischaemic tissue along with improved tissue utilisation of these substrates.

5.2 Pharmacokinetic properties

After reconstitution, alprostadil (PGE_1) dissociates from the α-cyclodextrin clathrate, and the two components have independent fates.

In symptomatic volunteers, systemic mean endogenous PGE_1 venous plasma concentrations measured before intracavernous injection are approximately 1pg/ml. After injection of 20 mcg of alprostadil, the PGE_1 venous plasma concentrations increase rapidly to concentrations of about 10-20 pg/ml. The PGE_1 plasma concentrations return to concentrations close to the baseline within a few minutes. Approximately 90% of PGE_1 found in plasma is protein-bound.

Metabolism

Enzymatic oxidation of the C15-hydroxy group and reduction of the C13,14 double bond produce the primary metabolites, 15-keto- PGE_1, PGE (13,14-dihydro-PGE_1) and 15-keto-PGE_o. Only PGE_o and 15-keto-PGE_o have been detected in human plasma. Unlike the 15-keto metabolites, which are less pharmacologically active than the parent compound, PGE_o has a potency similar to that of PGE_1 in most respects.

In symptomatic volunteers, the mean endogenous PGE_o venous plasma concentrations measured before an intracavernous injection are approximately 1 pg/ml. After the injection of 20 mcg of alprostadil, the PGE_o plasma concentrations increase to concentrations of about 5 pg/ml.

Excretion

After further degradation of the primary metabolites by beta and omega oxidation, the resulting, more polar metabolites are excreted primarily with the urine (88%) and the faeces (12%) and there is no evidence of tissue retention of PGE_1 or its metabolites.

5.3 Preclinical safety data

Studies on local tolerance following single and repeated intracavernous injections of alprostadil or alprostadil alfadex in rabbits and/or monkeys, in monkeys up to 6 months with daily injection revealed in general good local tolerance. Possible adverse effects like haematomas and inflammations are more likely related to the injection procedure.

Within the 6 months study in male monkeys, there were no adverse effects of alprostadil alfadex on male reproductive organs.

Mutagenicity studies with alprostadil alfadex revealed no risk of mutagenicity.

6. PHARMACEUTICAL PARTICULARS

6.1 List of excipients

Powder for injection:

Lactose monohydrate

Alfadex

Diluent:

Sodium chloride

Water for injection.

6.2 Incompatibilities

No incompatibilities have so far been demonstrated.

6.3 Shelf life

Shelf life for the product as packaged for sale: 4 years.

Shelf life after reconstitution: for immediate use only.

6.4 Special precautions for storage

Do not store above 25°C. Store in the original packaging.

6.5 Nature and contents of container

1. Cartons containing one colourless glass double-chamber cartridge, one injection needle 29 G × ½ (0.33 mm × 12.7 mm) and one reusable injector (starter kit).

2. Cartons containing two colourless glass double-chamber cartridges, two injection needles 29 G × ½ (0.33 mm × 12.7 mm) and one reusable injector (starter kit).

3. Cartons containing one, two or six colourless glass double-chamber cartridges and corresponding number of injection needles 29 G × ½ (0.33 mm × 12.7 mm) without reusable injector.

6.6 Instructions for use and handling

Fix the injection needle onto the front part of the injector.

Disinfect the tip of the cartridge with one of the alcohol swabs. Insert the cartridge into the reusable injector and fix it by screwing the thread part. Dissolve the drug substance in the front chamber of the cartridge by completely screwing the thread-part into the injector thus moving both rubber stoppers to the top of the cartridge and allowing the solvent in to the bottom chamber to reach the dry substance via the bypass of the cartridge. Shake slightly until a clear solution is produced.

Expel the air and adjust the prescribed dosage precisely prior to intracavernous injection.

After preparation of the solution, the injection must be performed using aseptic procedures into either the left or right cavernous body of the penile shaft. Care should be taken not to inject into penile vessels or nerves on the upper side of the penis and into the urethra on the under side. The injection should be completed within 5 to 10 seconds and manual pressure should be applied to the injection site for 2 to 3 minutes.

Unused solution must be discarded immediately.

Advice

The content of the front chamber of the cartridge consists of a white, dry powder, which forms a compact layer, approximately 8 mm in height. The layer may show cracks and crumble slightly.

In case of damage to the cartridge, the usually dry content of the front chamber becomes moist and sticky and extensively loses volume. Viridal Duo must not be used in this case.

The bottom chamber contains the clear, colourless sodium chloride solvent solution.

The dry substance dissolves immediately after addition of the sodium chloride solution. Initially after reconstitution the solution may appear slightly opaque due to the presence of bubbles. This is of no relevance and disappears within a short time to give a clear solution.

7. MARKETING AUTHORISATION HOLDER

SCHWARZ PHARMA Limited

Schwarz House

East Street

Chesham

Bucks HP5 1DG

England

8. MARKETING AUTHORISATION NUMBER(S)

PL 04438/0050

9. DATE OF FIRST AUTHORISATION/RENEWAL OF THE AUTHORISATION

23 May 1997

10. DATE OF REVISION OF THE TEXT

January 2005

Viridal 40 Duo

(SCHWARZ PHARMA Limited)

1. NAME OF THE MEDICINAL PRODUCT

VIRIDAL 40 DUO

2. QUALITATIVE AND QUANTITATIVE COMPOSITION

1 double-chamber glass cartridge containing dry substance (48.8 mg) composed of alprostadil 40 micrograms (used as 1:1 clathrate complex with alfadex) and diluent (1 ml).

Diluent:

1 ml sterile sodium chloride solution 0.9% (w/v) Ph Eur

3. PHARMACEUTICAL FORM

Double chamber glass cartridge containing lyophilised powder and diluent for reconstitution.

Administration devices

1 reusable injector (starter kit)

1 double-chamber cartridge with dry substance and 1 ml 0.9% sterile sodium chloride solution

1 injection needle 29 G × ½ (0.33 mm × 12.7 mm)

1 alcohol swab to be obtained for each injection

Route of administration

For injection into the penile cavernous body.

4. CLINICAL PARTICULARS

4.1 Therapeutic indications

As an adjunct to the diagnostic evaluation of erectile dysfunction in adult males.

Treatment of erectile dysfunction in adult males.

4.2 Posology and method of administration

The drug solution should be prepared shortly before the injection.

Prior to injection the needle should be screwed onto the tip of the injector. After disinfecting the tip of the cartridge with one of the alcohol swabs, the cartridge should then be inserted into the injector. By screwing the thread part clockwise, the cartridge is fixed in the injector. Then, the dry substance, which is inside the front chamber of the cartridge, is reconstituted with 1 ml sterile sodium chloride solution 0.9% in the bottom chamber. While holding the device in a vertical position with the needle upwards, the thread part should be screwed slowly until it will not go any further. The solvent will by-pass the upper stopper into the front chamber and dissolve the dry substance within a few seconds. As soon as the dry substance is reconstituted, the larger external and the smaller inner protective cap have to be removed from the needle. The air should then be expelled out of the cartridge and the prescribed dose adjusted precisely.

Unused solution must be discarded immediately.

Viridal Duo is injected into either the right or the left cavernous body of the penile shaft. Once the needle is in the cavernous body, the injection should be done within 5 to 10 seconds and is very easy without much resistance if the needle is in the correct position.

The development of an erection will start approximately 5 – 15 minutes after the injection.

Dosage for injection in the clinic

Injections for diagnostic evaluation and dose titration must be performed by the attending physician. He will determine an individual dose suitable to produce an erectile response for diagnostic purposes.

The recommended starting dose is 2.5 mcg Viridal Duo in patients with primary psychogenic or neurogenic origin of erectile dysfunction. In all other patients with erectile dysfunction 5 mcg Viridal Duo should be used as a starting dose. Dose adjustments may be performed in increments of about 2.5 mcg to 5 mcg Viridal Duo. Most of the patients require between 10 and 20 mcg per injection. Some patients may need to be titrated to higher doses. Doses exceeding 20 mcg should be prescribed with particular care in patients with cardiovascular risk factors. The dose per injection should never exceed 40 mcg.

Dosage for self-injection therapy at home

Before starting treatment at home, each patient or the patient's partner has to be taught by a physician how to prepare the drug and perform the injection. In no cases should the injection therapy be started without precise instructions by the physician. The patient should only use his optimum individual dosage which has been pre-determined by his physician using the above-mentioned procedure. This dose should allow the patient to have an erection at home which should not last longer than one hour. If he experiences prolonged erections beyond 2 hours but less than 4 hours, the patient is recommended to contact his physician to re-establish the dose of the drug. Maximum injection frequency recommended is 2 or 3 times a week with an interval of at least 24 hours between the injections.

Follow-up

After the first injections and at regular intervals, e.g. every three months, the physician should re-evaluate the patient. Any local adverse reaction, e.g. haematoma, fibrosis or nodules should be noted and controlled. Following discussion with the patient, an adjustment of dosage may be necessary.

4.3 Contraindications

Hypersensitivity to alprostadil and/or alfadex (ingredients of Viridal Duo).

Patients with diseases causing priapism e.g. sickle-cell disease, leukaemia and multiple myeloma or patients with anatomical deformation of the penis as cavernosal fibrosis or Peyronie's disease. Patients with penis implants should not use Viridal Duo.

Viridal Duo should not be used in men for whom sexual activity is contraindicated.

4.4 Special warnings and special precautions for use

The physician should carefully select patients suitable for self-injection therapy.

Sexual stimulation and intercourse can lead to cardiac and/or pulmonary events in patients with coronary heart disease, congestive heart failure or pulmonary disease.

Viridal Duo should be used with care in these patient groups and patients should be examined and cleared for stress resistance by a cardiologist before treatment.

Viridal Duo should be used with care in patients who have experienced transient ischaemic attacks.

Patients who experience a prolonged erection lasting longer than four hours should contact their physician immediately. Therefore it is recommended that the patient has an emergency telephone number of his attending physician or of a clinic experienced in therapy of erectile dysfunction. Prolonged erection may damage penile erectile tissue and lead to irreversible erectile dysfunction.

A benefit-risk evaulation is neccesary before using Viridal Duo in patients with pre-existing scarring, e.g. nodules of the cavernous body or pre-existing penile deviation or Peyronie's disease or clinically relevant phimosis, e.g. phimosis with risk of paraphimosis these patients should be treated with particular care, e.g. more frequent re-evaluation of the patient's condition.

Patients who have to be treated with alpha-adrenergic drugs due to prolonged erections (see: overdose) may in the case of concomitant therapy with monoamino-oxidase-inhibitors, develop a hypertensive crisis.

Other intracavernous drugs e.g. smooth muscle relaxing agents or alpha-adrenergic blocking agents may lead to prolonged erection and must not be used concomitantly.

The effects of a combination therapy of alprostadil with oral, intraurethral or topical medicinal products for erectile dysfunction are currently unknown.

Patients with blood clotting disorders or patients on therapy influencing blood clotting parameters should be treated with special care, e.g. monitoring of the clotting parameters and advice to the patient to exercise sufficient manual pressure on the injection site. This is because of the increased risk of bleeding.

To prevent abuse, self-injection therapy with Viridal Duo should not be used by patients with drug addiction and/or disturbances of psychological or intellectual development.

In cases of excessive use, e.g. higher frequencies than recommended, an increased risk of penile scarring cannot be excluded.

Use of intracavernous alprostadil offers no protection from the transmission of sexually transmitted diseases. Individuals who use alprostadil should be counselled about the protective measures that are necessary to guard against the spread of sexually transmitted diseases, including the human immunodeficiency virus (HIV). In some patients, injection of Viridal Duo can induce a small amount of bleeding at the injection site. In patients infected with blood borne diseases, this could increase the transmission of such diseases to the partner. For this reason we recommend that a condom is used for intercourse after injecting Viridal Duo.

Viridal Duo is for intracavernous injection. Subcutaneous injection or injections at areas of the penis other than the cavernous body should be avoided.

The injection should be performed under hygienic conditions to avoid infections. In any condition that precludes safe self-injection like poor manual dexterity, poor visual acuity or morbid obesity, the partner should be trained in the injection technique and should perform the injection.

Up to now, there is no clinical experience in patients under 18 and over 75 years of age.

Viridal Duo does not interfere with ejaculation and fertility.

4.5 Interaction with other medicinal products and other forms of Interaction

Concomitant use of smooth muscle relaxing drugs like papaverine or other drugs inducing erection like alpha-adrenergic blocking agents may lead to prolonged erection and should not be used in parallel with Viridal Duo.

Risks exist when using alpha-adrenergic drugs to terminate prolonged erections in patients with cardiovascular disorders or receiving MAO inhibitors.

The effects of blood pressure lowering and vasodilating drugs may be increased.

4.6 Pregnancy and lactation

Not applicable.

Alprostadil did not cause any adverse effects on fertility or general reproductive performance in male and female rats treated with 40-200 mcg/kg/day. The high dose of 200 mcg/kg/day is about 300 times the maximum recommended human dose on a body weight basis (MHRD < 1 mcg/kg).

Alprostadil was not fetotoxic or teratogenic at doses up to 5000 mcg/kg/day (7500 times the MHRD) in rats, 200 mcg/kg/day (300 times the MHRD) in rabbits and doses up to 20 mcg/kg/day (30 times the MHRD) in guinea pigs or monkeys.

4.7 Effects on ability to drive and use machines

Viridal Duo may rarely induce hypotension with subsequent impairment of reactivity.

4.8 Undesirable effects

A burning sensation during injection is common (< 10 %) and generally subsides shortly afterwards. A sensation of tension in the penis and pain at the site of injection are common (< 10 %) and mostly of mild intensity. Spotlike haemorrhage/ spotlike bruises at the site of puncture occur uncommonly (< 1 %). Haemosiderin deposits, reddening and swellings at the site of injection are also uncommon (< 1 %). Other uncommon (< 1 %) reactions are swellings of the preputium or the glans, and headache.

Prolonged erections of more than 4 hours duration are uncommon (< 1 %) and are mainly seen during dose titration.

During long-term treatment, fibrotic alterations (e.g. fibrotic nodules, plaques at the site of injection or in the corpus cavernosum) may occur commonly (< 10 %) in follow up periods of up to 4 years. This may be associated with slight penile axis deviations in uncommon (< 1 %) cases. In rare cases (< 0.1%), fibrotic changes of the cavernous body may occur during treatment lasting up to 4 years.

Rare cases (< 0.1%) of circulatory effects such as short periods of hypotension and/or vertigo or dizziness have been observed after the intracavernous injection of Viridal Duo.

In rare cases (< 0.1%) allergic reactions ranging from cutaneous hypersensitivity such as rash, erythema, urticaria to anaphylactic/anaphylactoid reactions may occur.

4.9 Overdose

Symptoms

Full rigid erections lasting more than four hours.

If the patient experiences a prolonged erection, he is advised to contact his attending physician or a urologic clinic nearby immediately.

Treatment strategy

Treatment of prolonged erection should be done by a physician experienced in the field of erectile dysfunction. If prolonged erection occurs, the following is recommended:

If the erection has lasted less than six hours:

– observation of the erection because spontaneous flaccidity frequently occurs.

If the erection has lasted longer than six hours:

– cavernous body injection of alpha-adrenergic substances (e.g. phenylephrine or epinephrine (adrenaline)). Risks exist when using drugs in patients with cardiovascular disorders or receiving MAO inhibitors. All patients should be monitored for cardiovascular effects when these drugs are used to terminate prolonged erections.

or

– aspiration of blood from the cavernous body.

Accidental systemic injection of high doses

Single dose rising tolerance studies in healthy volunteers indicated that single intravenous doses of alprostadil from 1 to 120 mcg were well tolerated. Starting with a 40 mcg bolus intravenous dose, the frequency of drug-related adverse events increased in a dose-dependent manner, characterised mainly by facial flushing.

5. PHARMACOLOGICAL PROPERTIES

5.1 Pharmacodynamic properties

ATC Code: Other urologicals G04BX 05

Alprostadil [Prostaglandin E_1 (PGE_1)], the active ingredient of Viridal Duo, is an endogenous compound derived from the essential fatty acid dihomogammalinolenic acid. Alprostadil is a potent smooth muscle relaxant that produces vasodilation and occurs in high concentrations in the human seminal fluid. Pre-contracted isolated preparations of the human corpus cavernosum, corpus spongiosum and cavernous artery were relaxed by alprostadil, while other prostanoids were less effective. Alprostadil has been shown to bind to specific receptors in the cavernous tissue of human and non-human primates.

The binding of alprostadil to its receptors is accompanied by an increase in intracellular cAMP levels. Human cavernosal smooth muscle cells respond to alprostadil by releasing intracellular calcium. Since relaxation of smooth muscle is associated with a reduction of the cytoplasmic free calcium concentration, this effect may contribute to the relaxing activity of this prostanoid.

Intracavernous injection of alprostadil in healthy monkeys resulted in penile elongation and tumescence without rigidity. The cavernous arterial blood flow was increased for a mean duration of 20 min. In contrast, intracavernous application of alprostadil to rabbits and dogs caused no erectile response.

Systemic intravascular administration of alprostadil leads to a vasodilation and reduction of systemic peripheral vascular resistance. A decrease in blood pressure can be observed after administration of high doses. Alprostadil has also been shown in animal and *in vitro* tests to reduce platelet reactivity and neutrophil activation. Additional alprostadil activity has been reported: increase in fibrinolytic activity of fibroblasts, improvement of erythrocyte deformability and inhibition of erythrocyte aggregation; inhibition of the proliferative and mitotic activity of non-striated myocytes; inhibition of cholesterol synthesis and LDL-receptor activity; and an increase in the supply of oxygen and glucose to ischaemic tissue along with improved tissue utilisation of these substrates.

5.2 Pharmacokinetic properties

After reconstitution, alprostadil (PGE_1) dissociates from the α-cyclodextrin clathrate, and the two components have independent fates.

In symptomatic volunteers, systemic mean endogenous PGE_1 venous plasma concentrations measured before intracavernous injection are approximately 1 pg/ml. After injection of 20 mcg of alprostadil, the PGE_1 venous plasma concentrations increase rapidly to concentrations of about 10-20 pg/ml. The PGE_1 plasma concentrations return to concentrations close to the baseline within a few minutes. Approximately 90% of PGE_1 found in plasma is protein-bound.

Metabolism

Enzymatic oxidation of the C15-hydroxy group and reduction of the C13,14 double bond produce the primary metabolites, 15-keto-PGE_1, PGE (13,14-dihydro-PGE_1) and 15-keto-PGE_0. Only PGE_0 and 15-keto-PGE_0 have been detected in human plasma. Unlike the 15-keto metabolites, which are less pharmacologically active than the parent compound, PGE_0 has a potency similar to that of PGE_1 in most respects.

In symptomatic volunteers, the mean endogenous PGE_0 venous plasma concentrations measured before an intracavernous injection are approximately 1 pg/ml. After the injection of 20 mcg of alprostadil, the PGE_0 plasma concentrations increase to concentrations of about 5 pg/ml.

Excretion

After further degradation of the primary metabolites by beta and omega oxidation, the resulting, more polar metabolites are excreted primarily with the urine (88%) and the faeces (12%) and there is no evidence of tissue retention of PGE_1 or its metabolites.

5.3 Preclinical safety data

Studies on local tolerance following single and repeated intracavernous injections of alprostadil or alprostadil alfadex in rabbits and/or monkeys, in monkeys up to 6 months with daily injection revealed in general good local tolerance. Possible adverse effects like haematomas and inflammations are more likely related to the injection procedure.

Within the 6 months study in male monkeys, there were no adverse effects of alprostadil alfadex on male reproductive organs.

Mutagenicity studies with alprostadil alfadex revealed no risk of mutagenicity.

6. PHARMACEUTICAL PARTICULARS

6.1 List of excipients

Powder for injection:

Lactose monohydrate

Alfadex

Diluent:

Sodium chloride

Water for injection.

6.2 Incompatibilities

No incompatibilities have so far been demonstrated.

6.3 Shelf life

Shelf life for the product as packaged for sale: 4 years.

Shelf life after reconstitution: for immediate use only.

6.4 Special precautions for storage

Do not store above 25°C. Store in the original packaging.

6.5 Nature and contents of container

1. Cartons containing one colourless glass double-chamber cartridge, one injection needle 29 G × ½ (0.33 mm × 12.7 mm) and one reusable injector (starter kit).

2. Cartons containing two colourless glass double-chamber cartridges, two injection needles 29 G × ½ (0.33 mm × 12.7 mm) and one reusable injector (starter kit).

3. Cartons containing one, two or six colourless glass double-chamber cartridges and corresponding number of injection needles 29 G × ½ (0.33 mm × 12.7 mm) without reusable injector.

6.6 Instructions for use and handling

Fix the injection needle onto the front part of the injector.

Disinfect the tip of the cartridge with one of the alcohol swabs. Insert the cartridge into the reusable injector and fix it by screwing the thread part. Dissolve the drug substance in the front chamber of the cartridge by completely screwing the thread-part into the injector thus moving both rubber stoppers to the top of the cartridge and allowing the solvent in to the bottom chamber to reach the dry substance via the bypass of the cartridge. Shake slightly until a clear solution is produced.

Expel the air and adjust the prescribed dosage precisely prior to intracavernous injection.

After preparation of the solution, the injection must be performed using aseptic procedures into either the left or right cavernous body of the penile shaft. Care should be taken not to inject into penile vessels or nerves on the upper side of the penis and into the urethra on the under side. The injection should be completed within 5 to 10 seconds and manual pressure should be applied to the injection site for 2 to 3 minutes.

Unused solution must be discarded immediately.

Advice

The content of the front chamber of the cartridge consists of a white, dry powder, which forms a compact layer, approximately 8 mm in height. The layer may show cracks and crumble slightly.

In case of damage to the cartridge, the usually dry content of the front chamber becomes moist and sticky and extensively loses volume. Viridal Duo must not be used in this case.

The bottom chamber contains the clear, colourless sodium chloride solvent solution.

The dry substance dissolves immediately after addition of the sodium chloride solution. Initially after reconstitution the solution may appear slightly opaque due to the presence of bubbles. This is of no relevance and disappears within a short time to give a clear solution.

7. MARKETING AUTHORISATION HOLDER
SCHWARZ PHARMA Limited

Schwarz House

East Street

Chesham

Bucks HP5 1DG

England

8. MARKETING AUTHORISATION NUMBER(S)
PL 04438/0051

9. DATE OF FIRST AUTHORISATION/RENEWAL OF THE AUTHORISATION
7 October 1998

10. DATE OF REVISION OF THE TEXT
January 2005

VISCOTEARS Liquid Gel

(Novartis Pharmaceuticals UK Ltd)

1. NAME OF THE MEDICINAL PRODUCT
Viscotears® Liquid Gel.

2. QUALITATIVE AND QUANTITATIVE COMPOSITION
2.0mg/g Carbomer (polyacrylic acid).

3. PHARMACEUTICAL FORM
Eye drops.

4. CLINICAL PARTICULARS

4.1 Therapeutic indications
Substitute of tear fluid for management of dry eye conditions including keratoconjunctivitis sicca, and for unstable tear film.

4.2 Posology and method of administration
For ocular use.

Adults:

1 drop 3 - 4 times daily or as required, depending upon the severity of the disease

Elderly:

No dosage amendment is necessary in the elderly

Children:

No specific studies with Viscotears have been performed in children. Use in these patients, is therefore, at the responsibility of the physician.

4.3 Contraindications
Patients with known hypersensitivity to any of the ingredients.

4.4 Special warnings and special precautions for use
Contact lenses should not be worn during instillation of the drug. After instillation there should be an interval of at least 30 minutes before reinsertion.

4.5 Interaction with other medicinal products and other forms of Interaction
In case of any additional local ocular treatment (eg glaucoma therapy) there should be an application interval of at least 5 minutes between the two medications, Viscotears Liquid Gel always should be the last medication instilled.

4.6 Pregnancy and lactation
There is no experience regarding the safety of Viscotears Liquid Gel in human pregnancy or lactation. Administration during pregnancy and lactation is therefore not recommended, except for compelling reasons.

4.7 Effects on ability to drive and use machines
Viscotears Liquid Gel may temporarily influence the visual acuity. Patients with blurred vision driving a vehicle or operating machines should be alerted to the possibility of impaired reactions.

4.8 Undesirable effects
The following adverse events have been occasionally reported:

- mild, transient burning sensation
- sticky eyelid
- blurred vision after instillation of the gel

4.9 Overdose
Not applicable.

5. PHARMACOLOGICAL PROPERTIES

5.1 Pharmacodynamic properties
Viscotears Liquid Gel is a liquid gel containing Carbomer. After local instillation it spreads rapidly over the conjunctiva and cornea and forms a lubricating film with prolonged contact time.

The retention times of Viscotears Liquid Gel and a conventional tear substitute based on polyvinylalcohol were studied in 30 healthy volunteers with fluorescein staining. The retention time of Viscotears Liquid Gel was approximately 16 minutes compared with approximately 2 minutes for the conventional artificial tears eye drops.

Tear film stability was maintained for a period of up to 6 hours. Data of clinical studies on healthy volunteers, patients with dry eye and patients in intensive care or during operation suggest evidence that Viscotears Liquid Gel improves tear film stability and prolongs tear break-up time (BUT).

5.2 Pharmacokinetic properties
There are no controlled animal or human pharmacokinetic studies available. However, absorption or accumulation in eye tissues can presumably be excluded due to the high molecular weight of polyacrylic acid (4 mio D).

5.3 Preclinical safety data
The results of the preclinical tests do not add anything of further significance to the prescriber.

6. PHARMACEUTICAL PARTICULARS

6.1 List of excipients
Cetrimide, sodium hydroxide, sorbitol and water for injections.

6.2 Incompatibilities
None known.

6.3 Shelf life
Unopened: 36 months

Opened: 28 days

6.4 Special precautions for storage
Do not store above 25°C.

6.5 Nature and contents of container
Polyfoil (laminate) tube with cannula and closure containing 10g of liquid gel.

6.6 Instructions for use and handling

7. MARKETING AUTHORISATION HOLDER
Novartis Pharmaceuticals UK Limited

Frimley Business Park

Frimley

Camberley

Surrey GU16 7SR

8. MARKETING AUTHORISATION NUMBER(S)
PL 00101/0605

9. DATE OF FIRST AUTHORISATION/RENEWAL OF THE AUTHORISATION
07 December 2004

10. DATE OF REVISION OF THE TEXT
01 July 2002

LEGAL CATEGORY
P

VISCOTEARS Single Dose Unit 2.0mg/g Eye Gel

(Novartis Pharmaceuticals UK Ltd)

1. NAME OF THE MEDICINAL PRODUCT
Viscotears® Single Dose Unit 2.0mg/g Eye Gel

2. QUALITATIVE AND QUANTITATIVE COMPOSITION
2.0mg/g Carbomer

3. PHARMACEUTICAL FORM
Eye Gel

4. CLINICAL PARTICULARS

4.1 Therapeutic indications
Substitute tear fluid for the management of dry eye conditions including keratoconjunctivitis sicca, and for unstable tear film.

4.2 Posology and method of administration
For ocular use.

Adults:

1 drop 3 - 4 times daily or as required, depending upon the severity of the disease

Elderly:

No dosage amendment is necessary in the elderly

Children:

No specific studies with Viscotears have been performed in children. Use in these patients, is therefore, at the responsibility of the physician.

The exterior of the single-dose container is not sterile. To avoid contamination of the contents, do not touch the tip of the container to any surface.

Viscotears Single Dose Unit should be used immediately after opening and discarded after use.

4.3 Contraindications
Patients with known hypersensitivity to any of the ingredients.

4.4 Special warnings and special precautions for use
Although the product contains no preservative, contact lenses should not be worn during instillation of the drug due to the viscosity. After instillation there should be an interval of at least 30 minutes before reinsertion.

4.5 Interaction with other medicinal products and other forms of Interaction
In case of any additional local ocular treatment (eg glaucoma therapy) there should be an application interval of at least 5 minutes between the two medications, Viscotears Single Dose Unit always should be the last medication instilled.

4.6 Pregnancy and lactation
There is no experience regarding the safety of Viscotears Single Dose Unit in human pregnancy or lactation. Administration during pregnancy and lactation is therefore not recommended, except for compelling reasons.

4.7 Effects on ability to drive and use machines
Viscotears may temporarily influence the visual acuity. Patients with blurred vision driving a vehicle or operating machines should be alerted to the possibility of impaired reactions.

4.8 Undesirable effects
Adverse events with Viscotears Single Dose Unitare rare. However, based on experience with similar but preserved products, the following adverse events may be expected to occur with Viscotears Single Dose Unit:

- mild, transient burning sensation
- sticky eyelid
- blurred vision after instillation of the gel

4.9 Overdose
Not applicable.

5. PHARMACOLOGICAL PROPERTIES

5.1 Pharmacodynamic properties
Viscotears Single Dose Unit is a preservative-free liquid gel containing carbomer. After local instillation it spreads rapidly over the conjunctiva and cornea and forms a lubricating film with prolonged contact time.

The retention times of Viscotears Liquid Gel (a similar product containing a preservative) and a conventional tear substitute based on polyvinylalcohol were studied in 30 healthy volunteers with fluorescein staining. The retention time of Viscotears Liquid Gel was approximately 16 minutes compared with approximately 2 minutes for the conventional artificial tears eye drops. Tear film stability was maintained for a period of up to 6 hours. Data of clinical studies on healthy volunteers, patients with dry eye and patients in intensive care or during operation suggest evidence that Viscotears Liquid Gel improves tear film stability and prolongs tear break-up time (BUT).

5.2 Pharmacokinetic properties
There are no controlled animal or human pharmacokinetic studies available. However, absorption or accumulation in eye tissues can presumably be excluded due to the high molecular weight of polyacrylic acid (4 mio D).

5.3 Preclinical safety data
The results of the preclinical tests do not add anything of further significance to the prescriber.

6. PHARMACEUTICAL PARTICULARS

6.1 List of excipients
Sorbitol, sodium hydroxide and water for injections.

6.2 Incompatibilities
Not applicable.

6.3 Shelf life
2 years.

For single use only. Use immediately after first opening.

6.4 Special precautions for storage
Do not store above 25°C. Keep containers in outer carton.

6.5 Nature and contents of container
Transparent LDPE single-dose container containing 0.6ml of gel.

Available in packs of 5, 15, and 30 single dose units

6.6 Instructions for use and handling
Not applicable

7. MARKETING AUTHORISATION HOLDER
Novartis Pharmaceuticals UK Limited

Frimley Business Park

Frimley

Camberley

Surrey GU16 7SR

8. MARKETING AUTHORISATION NUMBER(S)
PL 00101/0652

9. DATE OF FIRST AUTHORISATION/RENEWAL OF THE AUTHORISATION
7 December 2004

10. DATE OF REVISION OF THE TEXT

7 April 2004.

LEGAL CATEGORY

P

Viskaldix Tablets

(Amdipharm)

1. NAME OF THE MEDICINAL PRODUCT

Viskaldix Tablets

2. QUALITATIVE AND QUANTITATIVE COMPOSITION

Each tablet contains 10 mg pindolol and 5 mg clopamide.

3. PHARMACEUTICAL FORM

Tablet.

4. CLINICAL PARTICULARS

4.1 Therapeutic indications

Mild to moderate hypertension.

4.2 Posology and method of administration

One tablet daily in the morning. If blood pressure is not satisfactorily lowered after 2 to 3 weeks then two tablets daily as a single dose in the morning. Maximum dose of three tablets daily, if required.

Children

There is no experience with Viskaldix in children.

Use in the elderly

There is no evidence that the dosage or tolerability of Viskaldix is directly affected by advanced age. However, because of the diuretic component, such patients should be carefully supervised as factors sometimes associated with aging, such as poor diet or impaired renal function may indirectly affect the dosage or tolerability.

Method of administration

Oral.

4.3 Contraindications

Untreated cardiac failure, sick sinus syndrome (including sino-atrial block), second and third degree heart block, Prinzmetal's angina, history of bronchospasm and bronchial asthma (a warning stating "do not take this medicine if you have a history of wheezing or asthma" will appear on the label), untreated phaeochromocytoma, metabolic acidosis, pronounced bradycardia, obstructive pulmonary disease, cor pulmonale, prolonged fasting hypokalaemia, refractory hypokalaemia, hyponatraemia, hypercalcaemia, Addison's disease, severe renal or hepatic impairment and symptomatic hyperuricaemia. Viskaldix should not be used with agents which inhibit calcium transport e.g. verapamil.

4.4 Special warnings and special precautions for use

Especially in patients with ischaemic heart disease, treatment should not be discontinued suddenly. The dosage should be gradually reduced, i.e. over 1-2 weeks, if necessary at the same time initiating replacement therapy, to prevent exacerbation of angina pectoris.

Patients with a poor cardiac reserve should be stabilised with digitalis before treatment with Viskaldix to prevent impairment of myocardial contractility.

As with all beta-blockers, Viskaldix should be used with caution in patients with a history of non-asthmatic chronic obstructive lung disease or recent myocardial infarction.

Patients with spontaneous hypoglycaemia or diabetes should be monitored closely as concomitant use of beta-blockers may intensify the blood sugar lowering effect of insulin and other antidiabetic drugs and also as thiazide diuretics can lower insulin tolerance. Use of beta-blockers may mask the symptoms of hypoglycaemia (tachycardia, tremor). Beta blockers may also mask the symptoms of thyrotoxicosis.

During treatment with Viskaldix, patients should not undergo anaesthesia with agents causing myocardial depression (e.g. halothane, cyclopropane, trichloroethylene, ether, chloroform). Viskaldix should be gradually withdrawn before elective surgery. In emergency surgery or cases where withdrawal of Viskaldix would cause deterioration in cardiac condition, atropine sulphate 1 to 2mg intravenously should be given to prevent severe bradycardia.

If a beta-blocker is indicated in a patient with phaeochromocytoma it must always be given in conjunction with an alpha-blocker. Pre-existing peripheral vascular disorders may be aggravated by beta-blockers. Patients with known psoriasis should take beta-blockers only after careful consideration.

Beta-blockers may increase both the sensitivity towards allergens and the seriousness of anaphylactic reactions.

There have been reports of skin rashes and/or dry eyes associated with the use of beta-adrenoceptor blocking drugs. The reported incidence is small and in most cases the symptoms have cleared when treatment was withdrawn. Discontinuance of the drug should be considered if any such reaction is not otherwise explicable. Cessation of therapy with a beta-blocker should be gradual.

In severe renal failure a further impairment of renal function following beta blockade has been reported in a few cases.

Potassium levels should be checked in patients with renal or hepatic failure and urate levels should be checked in patients with gout.

Dilutional hyponatraemia may occur in hot weather in oedematous patients on Viskaldix.

The appropriate therapy is water restriction rather than the administration of salt, except in rare instances when the hyponatraemia is life-threatening. In true salt depletion, appropriate replacement is the treatment of choice.

4.5 Interaction with other medicinal products and other forms of Interaction

Viskaldix should not be used during concomitant administration of lithium, or by patients with known hypersensitivity to sulphonamides.

Calcium-channel blocking agents: Viskaldix should not be used with calcium-channel blockers with negative inotropic effects e.g. verapamil and to a lesser extent diltiazem. The concomitant use of oral beta-blockers and calcium antagonists of the dihydropyridine type can be useful in hypertension or angina pectoris. However, because of their potential effect on the cardiac conduction system and contractility, the i.v. route must be avoided. The concomitant use with dihydropyridines e.g. nifedipine may increase the risk of hypotension. In patients with cardiac insufficiency, treatment with beta-blocking agents may lead to cardiac failure.

Use of digitalis glycosides in association with beta-blockers may increase atrio-ventricular conduction time.

Clonidine: when therapy is discontinued in patients receiving a beta-blocker and clonidine concurrently, the beta-blockers should be gradually discontinued several days before clonidine is discontinued, in order to reduce the potential risk of a clonidine withdrawal hypertensive crisis.

MAO inhibitors: concurrent use with beta-blockers is not recommended. Possibly significant hypertension may theoretically occur up to 14 days following discontinuation of the MAO inhibitor.

Caution should be exercised in the concurrent use of beta-blocking agents with class 1 antiarrhythmics (e.g. disopyramide, quinidine) and amiodarone.

Concomitant use of beta-blockers may intensify the blood sugar lowering effect of insulin and other antidiabetic drugs.

Cimetidine, hydralazine and alcohol may induce increased plasma level of beta-blockers.

Prostaglandin synthetase inhibiting drugs may decrease the hypotensive effects of beta-blockers

Sympathomimetics with beta-adrenergic stimulant activity and xanthines: concurrent use with beta-blockers may result in mutual inhibition of therapeutic effects; in addition, beta-blockers may decrease theophylline clearance.

Concomitant use of beta-blockers with tricyclic antidepressants, barbiturates and phenothiazines as well as other anti-hypertensive agents may increase the blood pressure lowering effect.

Reserpine: concurrent use may result in an additive and possibly excessive beta-adrenergic blockade.

4.6 Pregnancy and lactation

Viskaldix should not be given to pregnant or lactating women.

4.7 Effects on ability to drive and use machines

Because dizziness or fatigue may occur during initiation of treatment with antihypertensive drugs, patients driving vehicles or operating machinery should exercise caution until their individual reaction to treatment has been determined.

4.8 Undesirable effects

Side-effects associated with beta-blockade: bradycardia, a slowed av-conduction or increase of an existing av-block, hypotension, heart failure, cold and cyanotic extremities, Raynaud's phenomenon, paraesthesia of the extremities, increase of an existing intermittent claudication, fatigue, headaches, impaired vision, hallucinations, psychoses, confusion, impotence, dizziness, sleep disturbances, depression, nightmares. Gastro-intestinal problems, nausea, vomiting, diarrhoea. Bronchospasm in patients with bronchial asthma or a history of asthmatic complaints. Disorder of the skin, especially rash. Dry eyes. Beta-blockers may mask the symptoms of thyrotoxicosis or hypoglycaemia. An increase in ANA (anti-nuclear antibodies) has been seen; its clinical relevance is not clear.

Thiazide diuretics may cause postural hypotension and mild gastrointestinal effects; impotence (reversible on withdrawal of treatment); hypokalaemia, hypomagnesaemia, hyponatraemia, hypercalcaemia, hypochloraemic alkalosis, hyperuricaemia, gout, hyperglycaemia, and increases in plasma cholesterol. Less commonly rashes, photosensitivity; blood disorders (including neutropenia and thrombocytopenia), pancreatitis; intrahepatic cholestatis and hypersensitivity reactions (including pneumonitis, pulmonary oedema, severe skin reactions) have also been reported.

4.9 Overdose

Overdosage may cause alterations in heart rate, nausea, vomiting, orthostatic disturbances, collapse, hypokalaemia and its accompanying disorders. Treatment by elimination of any unabsorbed drug and general supportive measures.

Plasma electrolytes should be closely monitored. Marked bradycardia, as a result of overdosage (or idiosyncrasy) should be treated with atropine sulphate 1-2mg i.v.

If necessary isoprenaline hydrochloride can be administered by slow i.v. under constant supervision beginning with 25mcg (5mcg/min) until desired effect is achieved. A cardiac pacemaker may be required. Intravenous glucagon (5 to 10mg) has been reported to overcome some of the features of serious overdosage.

5. PHARMACOLOGICAL PROPERTIES

5.1 Pharmacodynamic properties

Viskaldix is a combination of pindolol and clopamide, both acting to lower blood pressure, although by two separate mechanisms.

Pindolol is a non-selective beta-adrenergic antagonist which blocks both B1 and B2 adrenoceptors for more than 24 hours following administration. It has negligible membrane stabilising activity. The intrinsic sympathomimetic activity (ISA) provides the heart with basal stimulation similar to that elicited by normal resting sympathetic activity. Thus, resting cardiac output and heart rate are not unduly depressed, subsequently reducing the risk of bradycardia.

Clopamide enhances the elimination of sodium and chloride by inhibiting their reabsorption in the renal tubules which, in turn, leads to increased water excretion. The mechanistic relationship to the diuretic action and reduced blood pressure is not fully understood, however the diuretic effect is proportional to the dosage. Diuresis is initiated after about 2 hours and can last for up to 24 hours with maximal effect after 3 to 6 hours.

This combination can produce a clear antihypertensive effect after a few days, but, in some cases, to achieve the full effect, two to three weeks treatment may be necessary.

5.2 Pharmacokinetic properties

The pharmacokinetics of the two active ingredients are very similar and are not influenced by their combination or by being taken with food. Both components are rapidly and almost completely absorbed. They show negligible hepatic first-pass metabolism. Thus, the bioavailability of both is at least 85%. The maximum plasma concentration of pindolol is reached within one hour after ingestion, and that of clopamide, one or two hours after ingestion. Plasma protein binding is 40% for pindolol, and 46% for clopamide. The volume of distribution is about 2L/Kg for pindolol, and 1.5L/Kg for clopamide. The total body clearance of pindolol is 400ml/min, that of clopamide is 165ml/min. The elimination half-life is 3-4 hours for pindolol, and 6 hours for clopamide. Approximately one third of the dose of both drugs is excreted unchanged in the urine. The excretion of clopamide occurs mainly via the kidneys, whereas pindolol shows a balanced excretion between the renal and hepatic routes.

5.3 Preclinical safety data

There are no pre-clinical data of relevance to the prescriber which are additional to that already included in other sections of the SmPC.

6. PHARMACEUTICAL PARTICULARS

6.1 List of excipients

Magnesium stearate, maize starch and lactose.

6.2 Incompatibilities

None.

6.3 Shelf life

5 years from date of manufacture.

6.4 Special precautions for storage

None.

6.5 Nature and contents of container

PVC/PVDC clear blister packs in a cardboard carton containing 28 tablets.

6.6 Instructions for use and handling

None.

7. MARKETING AUTHORISATION HOLDER

Amdipharm Plc
Regency House
Miles Gray Road
Basildon
Essex
SS14 3AF
United Kingdom

8. MARKETING AUTHORISATION NUMBER(S)

PL 20072/0023

9. DATE OF FIRST AUTHORISATION/RENEWAL OF THE AUTHORISATION

1 January 2005

10. DATE OF REVISION OF THE TEXT

Visken Tablets 15 mg

(Amdipharm)

1. NAME OF THE MEDICINAL PRODUCT
Visken Tablets 15 mg

2. QUALITATIVE AND QUANTITATIVE COMPOSITION
Each tablet contains 15 mg pindolol.

3. PHARMACEUTICAL FORM
Tablet.

4. CLINICAL PARTICULARS

4.1 Therapeutic indications
For the treatment of hypertension and the prophylaxis of angina pectoris.

4.2 Posology and method of administration
Adults
Hypertension: initially one 15 mg tablet daily, with breakfast, or 5 mg two or three times daily. Most patients respond to a once daily dose of from 15 to 30mg. If necessary, dosages may be increased at weekly intervals up to a maximum of 45 mg daily in single or divided doses. Patients not responding after 3-4 weeks at this dosage level rarely benefit from further elevation in dosage. Addition of Visken to existing diuretic therapy increases the hypotensive effect and combination with other antihypertensives enables reduction in dosage of these other agents.

Use in children
Experience with Visken in children is limited.

Use in the elderly
No data are available to show that elderly patients require different dosages or show different side-effects from younger patients.

Method of administration
Oral.

4.3 Contraindications
Untreated cardiac failure, cardiogenic shock, sick sinus syndrome, second and third degree heart block, Prinzmetals angina, history of bronchospasm and bronchial asthma (a warning stating "do not take this medicine if you have a history of wheezing or asthma" will appear on the label), untreated phaeochromocytoma, peripheral circulatory disease, pronounced bradycardia, obstructive pulmonary disease, history of cor pulmonale, metabolic acidosis, prolonged fasting, severe renal failure. Visken should not be taken in conjunction with agents which inhibit calcium transport e.g. verapamil.

4.4 Special warnings and special precautions for use
Patients with a poor cardiac reserve should be stabilised before treatment with Visken to prevent impairment of myocardial contractility.

As for other beta-blockers, and especially in patients with ischaemic heart disease, treatment should not be discontinued suddenly. The dosage should gradually be reduced, i.e. over 1-2 weeks, if necessary at the same time initiating replacement therapy, to prevent exacerbation of angina pectoris.

As with all beta-blockers, Visken should be used with caution in patients with a history of non-asthmatic chronic obstructive lung disease or recent myocardial infarction. Caution must be exercised when beta-blocking agents are administered to patients with spontaneous hypoglycaemia or diabetes under treatment with insulin or oral hypoglycaemic agents, since hypoglycaemia may occur during prolonged fasting and some of its symptoms (tachycardia, tremor) may be masked. Beta-blockers may also mask the symptoms of thyrotoxicosis.

During treatment with Visken, patients should not undergo anaesthesia with agents causing myocardial depression (e.g. halothane, cyclopropane, trichloroethylene, ether, chloroform). Visken should be gradually withdrawn before elective surgery. In emergency surgery or cases where withdrawal of Visken would cause deterioration in cardiac condition, atropine sulphate 1 to 2 mg intravenously should be given to prevent severe bradycardia.

If a beta-blocker is indicated in a patient with phaeochromocytoma it must always be given in conjunction with an alpha-blocker. Pre-existing peripheral vascular disorders may be aggravated by beta-blockers.

In severe renal failure a further impairment of renal function following beta blockade has been reported in a few cases.

There have been reports of skin rashes and/or dry eyes associated with the use of beta-adrenoceptor blocking drugs. The reported incidence is small and in most cases the symptoms have cleared when treatment is withdrawn. Discontinuance of the drug should be considered if any such reaction is not otherwise explicable.

Patients with known psoriasis should take beta-blockers only after careful consideration.

Beta-blockers may increase both the sensitivity towards allergens and the seriousness of anaphylactic reactions.

4.5 Interaction with other medicinal products and other forms of Interaction
Calcium-channel blocking agents: Visken should not be used with calcium-channel blockers with negative inotropic effects e.g. verapamil and to a lesser extent diltiazem. The concomitant use of oral beta-blockers and calcium antagonists of the dihydropyridine type can be useful in hypertension or angina pectoris. However, because of their potential effect on the cardiac conduction system and contractility, the i.v. route must be avoided. The concomitant use with dihydropyridines e.g. nifedipine may increase the risk of hypotension. In patients with cardiac insufficiency, treatment with beta-blocking agents may lead to cardiac failure.

Use of digitalis glycosides, in association with beta-adrenoceptor blocking drugs, may increase atrio-ventricular conduction time.

Clonidine: when therapy is discontinued in patients receiving a beta-blocker and clonidine concurrently, the beta-blockers should be gradually discontinued several days before clonidine is discontinued, in order to reduce the potential risk of a clonidine withdrawal hypertensive crisis.

MAO inhibitors: concurrent use with beta-blockers is not recommended. Possibly significant hypertension may theoretically occur up to 14 days following discontinuation of the MAO inhibitor.

Caution should be exercised in the concurrent use of beta-blocking agents with class 1 antiarrhythmics (e.g. disopyramide, quinidine) and amiodarone.

Concomitant use of beta-blockers may intensify the blood sugar lowering effect of insulin and other antidiabetic drugs. Use of beta-blockers may prevent appearance of the signs of hypocalcaemia (tachycardia).

Cimetidine, hydralazine and alcohol may induce increased plasma levels of hepatically metabolised beta-blockers.

Prostaglandin synthetase inhibiting drugs may decrease the hypotensive effects of beta-blockers.

Sympathomimetics with beta-adrenergic stimulant activity and xanthines: concurrent use with beta-blockers may result in mutual inhibition of therapeutic effects; in addition, beta-blockers may decrease theophylline clearance.

Concomitant use of beta-blockers with tricyclic antidepressants, barbiturates and phenothiazines as well as other anti-hypertensive agents may increase the blood pressure lowering effect.

Reserpine: concurrent use may result in an additive and possibly excessive beta-adrenergic blockade.

4.6 Pregnancy and lactation
Visken is contraindicated in pregnancy and passes in small quantities into breast milk. Breastfeeding is therefore not recommended following administration.

4.7 Effects on ability to drive and use machines
Because dizziness or fatigue may occur during initiation of treatment with beta-adrenoceptor blocking drugs, patients driving vehicles or operating machinery should exercise caution until their individual reaction to treatment has been determined.

4.8 Undesirable effects
Bradycardia, a slowed AV-conduction or increase of an existing AV-block, hypotension, heart failure, cold and cyanotic extremities, Raynaud's phenomenon, paraesthesia of the extremities, increase of an existing intermittent claudication. Fatigue, headaches, impaired vision, hallucinations, psychoses, confusion, impotence, dizziness, sleep disturbances, depression and nightmares. Gastrointestinal problems, nausea, vomiting, diarrhoea. Bronchospasm in patients with bronchial asthma or a history of asthmatic complaints. Disorder of the skin, especially rash and dry eyes. Beta-blockers may mask the symptoms of thyrotoxicosis or hypoglycaemia. An increase in ANA (antinuclear antibodies) has been seen, however, its clinical relevance is not clear.

4.9 Overdose
Treat by elimination of any unabsorbed drug and general supportive measures. Marked bradycardia as a result of overdosage or idiosyncrasy should be treated with atropine sulphate 1 or 2 mg intravenously. If necessary, isoprenaline hydrochloride can be administered by a slow intravenous injection, under constant supervision, beginning with 25 mcg (5 mcg/min) until the desired effect is achieved. A cardiac pacemaker may be required, i.v. glucagon (5-10 mg) has been reported to overcome some of the features of serious overdosage and may be useful.

5. PHARMACOLOGICAL PROPERTIES

5.1 Pharmacodynamic properties
Visken is a specific beta-adrenoceptor blocking agent with low cardiodepressant activity at therapeutic doses. Its beta-blocking activity prevents excessive sympathetic drive to the heart, resulting in a fall in heart rate and a decrease in cardiac work and myocardial oxygen consumption. Visken possesses some intrinsic sympathomimetic activity even at low dosage, which may prevent reduction of resting sympathetic tone to an undesirably low level and minimise myocardial depression.

5.2 Pharmacokinetic properties
The rapid, nearly complete absorption (>95%) and the negligible hepatic first-pass effect (13%) of Visken result in a high bioavailability (87%). Maximum plasma concentration is reached within one hour after oral administration. Visken has a plasma protein binding of 40%, a volume of distribution of 2-3 l/Kg and a total clearance of 500 ml/min. The elimination half-life of Visken is 3-4 hours. 30-40% is excreted unchanged in the urine, while 60-70% is excreted via kidney and liver as inactive metabolites. Visken crosses the placental barrier and passes in small quantities into breast milk.

5.3 Preclinical safety data
There are no pre-clinical data of relevance to the prescriber which are additional to that already included in other sections of the SmPC.

6. PHARMACEUTICAL PARTICULARS

6.1 List of excipients
Microcrystalline cellulose, starch, colloidal anhydrous silica, magnesium stearate.

6.2 Incompatibilities
None.

6.3 Shelf life
5 years from date of manufacture.

6.4 Special precautions for storage
None.

6.5 Nature and contents of container
PVC/PVDC clear blister packs in a cardboard carton containing 28 or 30 tablets.

6.6 Instructions for use and handling
None.

7. MARKETING AUTHORISATION HOLDER
Amdipharm Plc
Regency House
Miles Gray Road
Basildon
Essex
SS14 3AF
United Kingdom

8. MARKETING AUTHORISATION NUMBER(S)
PL 20072/0022

9. DATE OF FIRST AUTHORISATION/RENEWAL OF THE AUTHORISATION
1 January 2005

10. DATE OF REVISION OF THE TEXT

Visken Tablets 5 mg

(Amdipharm)

1. NAME OF THE MEDICINAL PRODUCT
Visken Tablets 5 mg

2. QUALITATIVE AND QUANTITATIVE COMPOSITION
Each tablet contains 5 mg pindolol.

3. PHARMACEUTICAL FORM
Tablet.

4. CLINICAL PARTICULARS

4.1 Therapeutic indications
Essential hypertension: For reduction in blood pressure in essential hypertension. Onset of action of Visken is usually rapid, most patients showing a response within the first one to two weeks of treatment. However, maximum response may take several weeks to develop.

Prophylactic treatment of angina pectoris: Prophylactic treatment with Visken reduces the frequency and severity of anginal attacks and increases work capacity.

4.2 Posology and method of administration
Adults
Hypertension: Initially one 5 mg tablet two or three times a day. According to the response of the patient the dose may be increased at weekly intervals to a maximum of 45 mg given in divided doses twice or three times daily.

Once daily dosage schedule: Further work shows that many patients respond to a once daily dosage regime. Initially 15 mg (3 tablets) should be taken once a day with breakfast and adjusted according to individual response up to a maximum of 45 mg (9 tablets). Most patients respond to a once daily dose of between 15-30 mg (3-6 tablets).

Angina pectoris: Usually 2.5 mg to 5 mg orally three times a day according to response.

Use in children
Experience with Visken in children is limited. Its use is therefore not recommended.

Use in the elderly
No evidence exists that elderly patients require different dosages or show different side-effects from younger patients.

Route of administration
Oral.

4.3 Contraindications
Untreated cardiac failure, cardiogenic shock, sick sinus syndrome, second and third degree heart block, Prinzmetals angina, history of bronchospasm and bronchial asthma (a warning stating "do not take this medicine if you have a history of wheezing or asthma" will appear on

the label), untreated phaeochromocytoma, peripheral circulatory disease, pronounced bradycardia, obstructive pulmonary disease, history of cor pulmonale, metabolic acidosis, prolonged fasting, severe renal failure. Visken should not be taken in conjunction with agents which inhibit calcium transport e.g. verapamil.

4.4 Special warnings and special precautions for use

Patients with a poor cardiac reserve should be stabilised with digitalis before treatment with Visken to prevent impairment of myocardial contractility.

As for other beta-blockers, and especially in patients with ischaemic heart disease, treatment should not be discontinued suddenly. The dosage should gradually be reduced, i.e. over 1-2 weeks, if necessary at the same time initiating replacement therapy, to prevent exacerbation of angina pectoris.

As with all beta-blockers, Visken should be used with caution in patients with a history of non-asthmatic chronic obstructive lung disease or recent myocardial infarction. Caution must be exercised when beta-blocking agents are administered to patients with spontaneous hypoglycaemia or diabetes under treatment with insulin or oral hypoglycaemic agents, since hypoglycaemia may occur during prolonged fasting and some of its symptoms (tachycardia, tremor) may be masked. Beta-blockers may also mask the symptoms of thyrotoxicosis.

During treatment with Visken, patients should not undergo anaesthesia with agents causing myocardial depression (e.g. halothane, cyclopropane, trichloroethylene, ether, chloroform). Visken should be gradually withdrawn before elective surgery. In emergency surgery or cases where withdrawal of Visken would cause deterioration in cardiac condition, atropine sulphate 1 to 2 mg intravenously should be given to prevent severe bradycardia.

If a beta-blocker is indicated in a patient with phaeochromocytoma it must always be given in conjunction with an alpha-blocker. Pre-existing peripheral vascular disorders may be aggravated by beta-blockers.

In severe renal failure a further impairment of renal function following beta blockade has been reported in a few cases.

There have been reports of skin rashes and/or dry eyes associated with the use of beta-adrenoceptor blocking drugs. The reported incidence is small and in most cases the symptoms have cleared when treatment is withdrawn. Discontinuance of the drug should be considered if any such reaction is not otherwise explicable.

Cessation of therapy with a beta-blocker should be gradual.

Patients with known psoriasis should take beta-blockers only after careful consideration.

Beta-blockers may increase both the sensitivity towards allergens and the seriousness of anaphylactic reactions.

4.5 Interaction with other medicinal products and other forms of Interaction

Calcium-channel blocking agents: Visken should not be used with calcium-channel blockers with negative inotropic effects e.g. verapamil and to a lesser extent diltiazem. The concomitant use of oral beta-blockers and calcium antagonists of the dihydropyridine type can be useful in hypertension or angina pectoris. However, because of their potential effect on the cardiac conduction system and contractility, the i.v. route must be avoided. The concomitant use with dihydropyridines e.g. nifedipine may increase the risk of hypotension. In patients with cardiac insufficiency, treatment with beta-blocking agents may lead to cardiac failure.

Use of digitalis glycosides, in association with beta-adrenoceptor blocking drugs, may increase atrio-ventricular conduction time.

Clonidine: when therapy is discontinued in patients receiving a beta-blocker and clonidine concurrently, the beta-blockers should be gradually discontinued several days before clonidine is discontinued, in order to reduce the potential risk of a clonidine withdrawal hypertensive crisis.

MAO inhibitors: concurrent use with beta-blockers is not recommended. Possibly significant hypertension may theoretically occur up to 14 days following discontinuation of the MAO inhibitor.

Caution should be exercised in the concurrent use of beta-blocking agents with class 1 antiarrhythmics (e.g. disopyramide, quinidine) and amiodarone.

Concomitant use of beta-blockers may intensify the blood sugar lowering effect of insulin and other antidiabetic drugs. Use of beta-blockers may prevent appearance of the signs of hypocalcaemia (tachycardia).

Cimetidine, hydralazine and alcohol may induce increased plasma levels of hepatically metabolised beta-blockers.

Prostaglandin synthetase inhibiting drugs may decrease the hypotensive effects of beta-blockers.

Sympathomimetics with beta-adrenergic stimulant activity and xanthines: concurrent use with beta-blockers may result in mutual inhibition of therapeutic effects; in addition, beta-blockers may decrease theophylline clearance.

Concomitant use of beta-blockers with tricyclic antidepressants, barbiturates and phenothiazines as well as other anti-hypertensive agents may increase the blood pressure lowering effect.

Reserpine: concurrent use may result in an additive and possibly excessive beta-adrenergic blockade.

4.6 Pregnancy and lactation

Visken is contraindicated in pregnancy and passes in small quantities into breast milk. Breastfeeding is therefore not recommended following administration.

4.7 Effects on ability to drive and use machines

Because dizziness or fatigue may occur during initiation of treatment with beta-adrenoceptor blocking drugs, patients driving vehicles or operating machinery should exercise caution until their individual reaction to treatment has been determined.

4.8 Undesirable effects

Bradycardia, a slowed AV-conduction or increase of an existing AV-block, hypotension, heart failure, cold and cyanotic extremities, Raynaud's phenomenon, paraesthesia of the extremities, increase of an existing intermittent claudication. Fatigue, headaches, impaired vision, hallucinations, psychoses, confusion, impotence, dizziness, sleep disturbances, depression, nightmares. Gastrointestinal disturbances (including diarrhoea, nausea and vomiting). Bronchospasm in patients with bronchial asthma or a history of asthmatic complaints. Disorder of the skin, especially rash. Dry eyes. Beta-blockers may mask the symptoms of thyrotoxicosis or hypoglycaemia. An increase in ANA (anti-nuclear antibodies) has been seen; its clinical relevance is not clear.

4.9 Overdose

Treat by elimination of any unabsorbed drug and general supportive measures. Marked bradycardia as a result of overdosage or idiosyncrasy should be treated with atropine sulphate 1 or 2 mg intravenously. If necessary, isoprenaline hydrochloride can be administered by a slow intravenous injection, under constant supervision, beginning with 25 mcg (5 mcg/min) until the desired effect is achieved. A cardiac pacemaker may be required, i.v. glucagon (5-10 mg) has been reported to overcome some of the features of serious overdosage and may be useful.

5. PHARMACOLOGICAL PROPERTIES

5.1 Pharmacodynamic properties

Visken is a potent beta-adrenoceptor antagonist (beta-blocker). It blocks both B- and B2-adrenoceptors for more than 24 hours after administration. It has negligible membrane-stabilising activity. As a beta-blocker, Visken protects the heart from beta-adrenoceptor stimulation by acetecholamines during physical exercise and mental stress, and also reduces the sympathetic drive to the heart at rest. Its intrinsic sympathomimetic activity (ISA), however, provides the heart with basal stimulation similar to that elicited by normal resting sympathetic activity, with the result that heart rate and contractility at rest and intracardiac conduction are not unduly depressed. The risk of bradycardia is therefore small and normal cardiac output is not reduced.

Visken is a beta-blocker with clinically relevant vasodilator activity. This results from the ISA exerted on B2-adrenoceptors in blood vessels. The high vascular resistance of established hypertension is lowered by Visken; tissue and organ perfusion is not impaired, and may even be improved.

In contrast to the potentially adverse changes in blood lipoprotein profiles seen during treatment with other beta-blockers (a decrease in the HDL/LDL ratio), the ratio of high density lipoproteins (HDL) to low density (for further information see product licence file).

5.2 Pharmacokinetic properties

The rapid, nearly complete absorption (>95%) and the negligible hepatic first-pass effect (13%) of Visken result in a high bioavailability (87%). Maximum plasma concentration is reached within one hour after oral administration. Visken has a plasma protein binding of 40%, a volume of distribution of 2-3 l/Kg and a total clearance of 500 ml/min. The elimination half-life of Visken is 3-4 hours. 30-40% is excreted unchanged in the urine, while 60-70% is excreted via kidney and liver as inactive metabolites. Visken crosses the placental barrier and passes in small quantities into breast milk.

Patients with impaired kidney or liver function may usually be treated with normal doses. Only in severe cases may a reduction of the daily dose be necessary.

5.3 Preclinical safety data

There are no pre-clinical data of relevance to the prescriber which are additional to that already included in other sections of the SmPC.

6. PHARMACEUTICAL PARTICULARS

6.1 List of excipients

Microcrystalline cellulose, starch, colloidal anhydrous silica, magnesium stearate.

6.2 Incompatibilities

None.

6.3 Shelf life

5 years.

6.4 Special precautions for storage

None.

6.5 Nature and contents of container

PVC/PVDC clear blister packs in a cardboard carton containing 56, 60 or 100 tablets.

6.6 Instructions for use and handling

None.

7. MARKETING AUTHORISATION HOLDER

Amdipharm Plc
Regency House
Miles Gray Road
Basildon
Essex
SS14 3AF
United Kingdom

8. MARKETING AUTHORISATION NUMBER(S)

PL 20072/0021

9. DATE OF FIRST AUTHORISATION/RENEWAL OF THE AUTHORISATION

1 January 2005

10. DATE OF REVISION OF THE TEXT

Vistide

(Pharmacia Limited)

1. NAME OF THE MEDICINAL PRODUCT

VISTIDE 75 mg/ml concentrate for solution for infusion

2. QUALITATIVE AND QUANTITATIVE COMPOSITION

Each vial contains cidofovir equivalent to 375 mg/5 ml (75 mg/ml) cidofovir anhydrous. The formulation is adjusted to pH 7.4.

For excipients, see 6.1.

3. PHARMACEUTICAL FORM

Concentrate for solution for infusion.

4. CLINICAL PARTICULARS

4.1 Therapeutic indications

VISTIDE is indicated for the treatment of CMV retinitis in patients with acquired immunodeficiency syndrome (AIDS) and without renal dysfunction. Until further experience is gained, VISTIDE should be used only when other agents are considered unsuitable.

4.2 Posology and method of administration

The therapy should be prescribed by a physician experienced in the management of HIV infection.

Before each administration of VISTIDE, serum creatinine and urine protein levels should be investigated.

The recommended dosage, frequency, or infusion rate must not be exceeded. VISTIDE must be diluted in 100 millilitres 0.9% (normal) saline prior to administration. To minimise potential nephrotoxicity, oral probenecid and intravenous saline prehydration must be administered with each VISTIDE infusion. Please see under section 4.4 Special warnings and special precautions for use for appropriate recommendations, and under section 6.6 for information on obtaining probenecid.

Dosage in adults

Induction treatment. The recommended dose of cidofovir is 5 mg/kg body weight (given as an intravenous infusion at a constant rate over 1 hour) administered once weekly for two consecutive weeks.

Maintenance treatment. Beginning two weeks after the completion of induction treatment, the recommended maintenance dose of cidofovir is 5 mg/kg body weight (given as an intravenous infusion at a constant rate over 1 hour) administered once every two weeks.

Suspension of maintenance treatment with cidofovir should be considered in accordance with local recommendations for the management of HIV-infected patients.

Dosage in elderly

The safety and efficacy of VISTIDE have not been established for the treatment of CMV disease in patients over 60 years of age. Since elderly individuals frequently have reduced glomerular function, particular attention should be paid to assessing renal function before and during administration of VISTIDE.

Dosage in children and neonates

The safety and efficacy of VISTIDE have not been established for the treatment of CMV disease in patients under 18 years of age. Therefore, VISTIDE is not recommended for use in children and neonates.

Dosage in renal insufficiency

Renal insufficiency is a contraindication for the use of VISTIDE (see section 4.3 Contraindications and section 4.4 Special warnings and special precautions for use, Prevention/reduction of nephrotoxicity).

Dosage in hepatic insufficiency

The safety and efficacy of VISTIDE have not been established in patients with hepatic disease.

4.3 Contraindications

Hypersensitivity to cidofovir or to any excipients.

VISTIDE is contraindicated in patients with renal impairment [serum creatinine > 133 μmol/l > 1.5 mg/dl) or creatinine clearance ⩽ 0.92 ml/s (⩽ 55 ml/min) or proteinuria ⩾ 100 mg/dl (⩾ 2+ proteinuria)]. Concomitant administration of VISTIDE and other potentially nephrotoxic agents is contraindicated (see section 4.4).

Direct intraocular injection of VISTIDE is contraindicated; direct injection may be associated with significant decreases in intraocular pressure and impairment of vision.

4.4 Special warnings and special precautions for use

VISTIDE is formulated for intravenous infusion only and should not be administered by intraocular injection. VISTIDE should be infused only into veins with adequate blood flow to permit rapid dilution and distribution. Therapy should be accompanied by administration of oral probenecid and adequate intravenous saline prehydration (see Prevention/reduction of nephrotoxicity, and under 6.6 for information on obtaining probenecid).

Prevention/reduction of nephrotoxicity

Treatment with VISTIDE should not be initiated in patients with serum creatinine > 133 μmol/l > 1.5 mg/dl), creatinine clearance ⩽ 0.92 ml/s (⩽ 55 ml/min), or ⩾ 2+ proteinuria (⩾ 100 mg/dl), as the optimum induction and maintenance doses for patients with moderate to severe renal impairment are not known.

To minimise the potential for nephrotoxicity, patients should receive a course of probenecid, administered orally with each cidofovir dose. All clinical trials relevant to clinical efficacy evaluation were performed using probenecid concomitantly with cidofovir. Two grams should be administered 3 hours prior to the cidofovir dose and one gram administered at 2 and again at 8 hours after completion of the 1 hour cidofovir infusion (for a total of 4 grams). In order to reduce the potential for nausea and/or vomiting associated with administration of probenecid, patients should be encouraged to eat food prior to each dose of probenecid. The use of an anti-emetic may be necessary.

In patients who develop allergic or hypersensitivity symptoms to probenecid (e.g., rash, fever, chills and anaphylaxis), prophylactic or therapeutic use of an appropriate antihistamine and/or paracetamol should be considered.

In patients unable to receive probenecid because of a clinically significant hypersensitivity to the drug or to other sulpha-containing medications, cidofovir administration should only be considered if the potential benefits of therapy outweigh the potential risks. Such use of cidofovir without concomitant probenecid has not been clinically investigated. A probenecid desensitisation program is not recommended for use.

In addition, to probenecid, patients must receive a total of one litre of 0.9% (normal) saline solution intravenously immediately prior to each infusion of cidofovir. Patients who can tolerate the additional fluid load may receive up to a total of 2 litres of 0.9% saline intravenously with each dose of cidofovir. The first litre of saline solution should be infused over a 1 hour period immediately before the cidofovir infusion, and the second litre, if given, infused over a 1-3 hour period beginning simultaneously with the cidofovir infusion or starting immediately after the infusion of cidofovir.

Renal function (serum creatinine and urine protein) must be monitored prior to each dose of cidofovir.

Interruption, and possibly discontinuation, is required for changes in renal function.

The safety of cidofovir has not been evaluated in patients receiving other known potentially nephrotoxic agents. It is recommended to discontinue potentially nephrotoxic agents at least 7 days before starting cidofovir.

Cidofovir therapy should be discontinued and intravenous hydration is advised if serum creatinine increases by ⩾ 44 μmol/l (⩾ 0.5 mg/dl), or if persistent proteinuria ⩾ 2+ develops. Proteinuria appears to be an early and sensitive indicator of cidofovir-induced nephrotoxicity. Patients receiving cidofovir must have their serum creatinine and urine protein levels determined on specimens obtained within 24 hours prior to the administration of each dose of cidofovir. In patients exhibiting ⩾ 2+ proteinuria, intravenous hydration should be performed and the test repeated. If following hydration, a ⩾ 2+ proteinuria is still observed, cidofovir therapy should be discontinued. Continued administration of cidofovir to patients with persistent ⩾ 2+ proteinuria following intravenous hydration may result in further evidence of proximal tubular injury, including glycosuria, decreases in serum phosphate, uric acid and bicarbonate, and elevations in serum creatinine.

During treatment, these parameters should be investigated prior to the administration of each infusion, and the treatment should be stopped in case of abnormality. In case of complete recovery, the reintroduction of cidofovir has not yet been evaluated. High flux haemodialysis has been shown to reduce the serum levels of cidofovir by approximately 75%. The fraction of the dose extracted during haemodialysis is 51.9 ± 11.0%.

Renal impairment

Dose-dependent nephrotoxicity is the major dose-limiting toxicity related to administration of cidofovir. Proteinuria, as measured by urinalysis in a clinical laboratory, may be an early indicator of nephrotoxicity. Patients receiving weekly intravenous cidofovir at a dose of 0.5 mg/kg or 1.0 mg/kg, without concomitant probenecid, with or without intravenous saline prehydration, did not show evidence of significant drug-related nephrotoxicity (as defined by serum creatinine ⩾ 177 μmol/l (⩾ 2.0 mg/dl), while patients treated at 3.0 mg/kg, 5.0 mg/kg or 10.0 mg/kg without concomitant probenecid developed evidence of proximal tubular cell injury, including glycosuria, and decreases in serum phosphate, uric acid and bicarbonate, and elevations in serum creatinine. The signs of nephrotoxicity were partially reversible in some patients.

Haematology

Reversible neutropenia has been observed in patients receiving cidofovir. This has not been associated with clinical sequelae and does not appear to be dose-dependent. Resolution has occurred in some cases while on continued cidofovir therapy and in others following discontinuation of the drug.

Laboratory tests

Renal function tests (routine urinalysis and serum creatinine) must be measured, and the results reviewed, prior to administration of each cidofovir dose. Neutrophil counts also should be monitored regularly.

Other

Cidofovir should be considered a potential carcinogen in humans (see section 5.3 Preclinical safety data).

Caution should be applied when considering cidofovir treatment of patients with diabetes mellitus due to the potential increased risk of developing ocular hypotony.

Male patients should be advised that cidofovir caused reduced testes weight and hypospermia in animals. Although not observed in clinical studies of cidofovir, such changes may occur in humans and cause infertility. Men should be advised to practice barrier contraceptive methods during and for 3 months after treatment with cidofovir.

White blood cell counts, including the differential neutrophil count, should also be performed prior to each dose of cidofovir.

Patients receiving cidofovir should be advised to have regular follow-up ophthalmologic examination.

4.5 Interaction with other medicinal products and other forms of Interaction

Probenecid is known to interact with the metabolism or renal tubular secretion of many drugs (e.g., paracetamol, acyclovir, angiotensin-converting enzyme inhibitors, aminosalicyclic acid, barbiturates, benzodiazepines, bumetanide, clofibrate, methotrexate, famotidine, furosemide, nonsteroidal anti-inflammatory agents, theophylline, and zidovudine).

Patients who are being treated with zidovudine should temporarily discontinue zidovudine administration or decrease their zidovudine dose by 50% on days when cidofovir is administered, because probenecid reduces the clearance of zidovudine.

Interactions of cidofovir, probenecid, and anti-HIV drugs, including anti-HIV protease inhibitors, have not been investigated in clinical trials.

4.6 Pregnancy and lactation

Cidofovir is embryotoxic in rats and rabbits at subtherapeutic dose levels. A significantly increased foetal incidence of external, soft tissue and skeletal anomalies occurred in rabbits at 1.0 mg/kg/day, which was also maternally toxic.

There are no studies of cidofovir in pregnant women. VISTIDE should not be used during pregnancy.

Women of childbearing potential should be advised to use effective contraception during and after treatment with cidofovir.

It is not known whether cidofovir is excreted in human milk. Because many substances are excreted in human milk, nursing mothers should be instructed to discontinue cidofovir or discontinue nursing if they continue to receive cidofovir. Passage of the placenta barrier of cidofovir-related compound was observed in pregnant rats. Excretion of cidofovir-related material into milk of lactating animals was not examined.

Refer to section 4.4 (Special warnings and special precautions for use) for further information

4.7 Effects on ability to drive and use machines

Adverse effects such as asthenia may occur during cidofovir therapy. The physician is advised to discuss this issue with the patient, and based upon the condition of the disease and the tolerance of medication, give his recommendation in the individual case.

4.8 Undesirable effects

The most commonly reported undesirable effect in controlled clinical trials was proteinuria occurring in 80% of patients. In addition, fever (43%), asthenia (32%), nausea with vomiting (26%), creatinine increase (24%), and rash (19%) were also very common. These incidence figures were calculated independent of relationship to study drugs (cidofovir or probenecid) or severity. Other adverse events occurring more commonly were:

Classification of expected frequencies:

Very common >10%), common (⩾1% and <10%), uncommon (⩾ 0.1% and <1%), rare (⩾ 0.01% and <0.1%) and very rare (<0.01%).

Blood disorders

Very common: Neutropenia.

Eye disorders

Common: Iritis/uveitis; decreased intraocular pressure (⩾ 50% decrease from pretreatment baseline).

Respiratory disorders

Common: Dyspnoea; pneumonia.

Gastrointestinal disorders

Very common: Nausea without vomiting.

Common: Nausea with vomiting.

Skin disorders

Very common: Alopecia.

Renal and urinary disorders

Very common: Proteinuria; creatinine increase.

General disorders

Very common: Asthenia; fever.

Common: Death; infection.

Very common undesirable effects in controlled clinical trials possibly or probably related to probenecid:

Gastrointestinal disorders: Nausea with and without vomiting.

Skin disorders: Rash.

General disorders: Fever.

Undesirable effects reported through the postmarketing spontaneous reporting system:

Eye disorders:

Uncommon: Uveitis/Iritis. Patients usually respond to treatment with topical corticosteroids with or without topical cycloplegic agents. Cidofovir should be discontinued if there is no response to treatment with a topical corticosteroid or the condition worsens, or if iritis/uveitis reoccurs after successful treatment.

Rare: Ocular hypotony.

Ear disorders

Very rare: Hearing disturbances.

Gastrointestinal disorders

Rare: Pancreatitis.

Renal and urinary disorders:

Uncommon: Renal failure. Reports of renal failure (plus events possibly caused by renal failure, e.g. creatinine increase, proteinuria, glycosuria) have been received and some of them were fatal. Cases of acute renal failure after only one or two doses of cidofovir have also been reported.

4.9 Overdose

Two cases of cidofovir overdose have been reported. In both cases, the overdose occurred during the first induction dose and no additional cidofovir therapy was administered. One patient received a single dose of 16.4 mg/kg and the other patient received a single dose of 17.3 mg/kg. Both patients were hospitalised and received prophylactic oral probenecid and vigorous hydration for 3 to 7 days. One of these patients experienced a minor transient change in renal function, while the other patient had no change in renal function.

5. PHARMACOLOGICAL PROPERTIES

5.1 Pharmacodynamic properties

Pharmacotherapeutic group: Antiviral for systemic use, ATC Code: J05

General

Cidofovir is a cytidine analogue with *in vitro* and *in vivo* activity against human cytomegalovirus (HCMV). HCMV strains resistant to ganciclovir may still be susceptible to cidofovir.

Mechanism of action

Cidofovir suppresses CMV replication by selective inhibition of viral DNA synthesis. Biochemical data support selective inhibition of HSV-1, HSV-2 and CMV DNA polymerases by cidofovir diphosphate, the active intracellular metabolite of cidofovir.

Cidofovir diphosphate inhibits these viral polymerases at concentrations that are 8- to 600-fold lower than those needed to inhibit human cellular DNA polymerases alpha, beta, and gamma. Incorporation of cidofovir into viral DNA results in reductions in the rate of viral DNA synthesis.

Cidofovir enters cells by fluid-phase endocytosis and is phosphorylated to cidofovir monophosphate and subsequently to cidofovir diphosphate. In addition, a cidofovir phosphate-choline adduct is formed. In contrast to ganciclovir, the metabolism of cidofovir is neither dependent on, nor facilitated by, viral infections. Prolonged antiviral effects of cidofovir are related to the half-lives of metabolites; cidofovir diphosphate persists inside cells with a half-life of 17-65 hours. Additionally, the phosphate-choline species has a half-life of 87 hours.

Antiviral activity

Cidofovir is active *in vitro* against CMV, a member of the herpesviridae family. Antiviral activity is seen at concentrations significantly below those which cause death in cell monolayers. The *in vitro* sensitivity to cidofovir is shown in the following table.

Cidofovir Inhibition of Virus Multiplication in Cell Culture

Virus	IC_{50} (μM)
wild-type CMV isolates	0.7 (± 0.6)
ganciclovir-resistant CMV isolates	7.5 (± 4.3)
foscarnet-resistant CMV isolates	0.59 (± 0.07)

In vivo activity against human CMV was confirmed with controlled clinical studies of cidofovir for the treatment of CMV retinitis in patients with AIDS, which demonstrated statistically significant delays in time to CMV retinitis progression for patients on cidofovir when compared to control patients. The median times to retinitis progression in the two studies relevant for efficacy assessment (studies GS-93-106 and GS-93-105, both conducted in patients previously untreated for CMV retinitis) were 120 days and not reached for the treatment arms vs. 22 days and 21 days for the untreated (deferred treatment) arms, respectively.

In study GS-93-107 conducted in patients who had relapsed after treatment with other agents, the median time to retinitis progression was 115 days.

Viral resistance

Following *in vitro* selection of ganciclovir-resistant human CMV isolates, cross-resistance between ganciclovir and cidofovir was seen with ganciclovir-selected mutations in the CMV DNA polymerase gene but not with mutations in the UL97 gene. No cross-resistance between foscarnet and cidofovir was seen with foscarnet-selected mutants. Cidofovir-selected mutants had a mutation in the DNA polymerase gene and were cross-resistant to ganciclovir, but susceptible to foscarnet.

5.2 Pharmacokinetic properties

The major route of elimination of cidofovir was by renal excretion of unchanged drug by a combination of glomerular filtration and tubular secretion. In patients with normal renal function, 80 to 100% of the intravenous dose was recovered in the urine over 24 hours as unchanged cidofovir. No metabolites of cidofovir have been detected in serum or urine of patients.

At the end of a one-hour infusion of cidofovir 5 mg/kg administered with concomitant oral probenecid, the mean (± SD) serum concentration of cidofovir was 19.6 (± 7.18) mcg/ml. The mean values of total serum clearance, volume of distribution at steady-state and terminal elimination half-life were 138 (± 36) ml/hr/kg, 388 (± 125) ml/kg and 2.2 (±0.5) hour, respectively.

Dose-independent kinetics were demonstrated with single doses of cidofovir given over the dose range 3 to 7.5 mg/kg.

In vitro protein binding

In vitro protein binding of cidofovir to plasma or serum protein was 10% or less over the cidofovir concentration range 0.25 to 25 mcg/ml.

5.3 Preclinical safety data

Preclinical animal studies demonstrated that nephrotoxicity was the major dose-limiting toxicity of cidofovir. Evidence for a nephroprotective effect for probenecid was shown in a 52-week study conducted in cynomolgus monkeys administered cidofovir 2.5 mg/kg once weekly intravenously with 1 g of probenecid given orally.

Carcinogenesis

In a 26-week intravenous toxicity study, a significant increase in incidence of mammary adenocarcinomas was seen in female rats and of Zymbal's gland carcinomas in male and female rats at subtherapeutic plasma levels of cidofovir. In a separate study, once weekly subcutaneous injections of cidofovir for 19 consecutive weeks resulted in mammary adenocarcinomas in female rats at doses as low as 0.6 mg/kg/week. In both studies, tumours were observed within 3 months of dosing. No tumours were observed in cynomolgus monkeys administered cidofovir intravenously once weekly for 52 weeks at doses up to 2.5 mg/kg/week.

Mutagenicity and reproductive toxicology

Studies have shown that cidofovir is clastogenic *in vitro* at 100 μg/ml and is embryotoxic in rats and rabbits.

No mutagenic response was elicited by cidofovir at dose levels up to 5 mg/plate, in the presence and absence of metabolic activation by rat liver S-9 fraction, in microbial assays involving *Salmonella typhimurium* for base pair substitutions or frameshift mutations (Ames) and *Escherichia coli* for reverse mutations.

An increase in formation of micronucleated polychromatic erythrocytes was observed *in vivo* in mice receiving a high, toxic intraperitoneal dose of cidofovir ($\geqslant$ 2000 mg/kg).

Cidofovir induced chromosomal aberrations in human peripheral blood lymphocytes *in vitro* without metabolic activation (S-9 fraction). At the 4 cidofovir levels (12.5 to 100 μg/ml) tested, the percentage of damaged metaphases and number of aberrations per cell increased in a concentration-dependent manner.

No adverse effects on fertility or general reproduction were seen following once weekly intravenous injections of cidofovir in male rats for 13 consecutive weeks at doses up to 15 mg/kg/week. Female rats dosed intravenously once weekly at 1.2 mg/kg/week or higher for up to 6 weeks prior to mating and for 2 weeks post mating had decreased litter sizes and live births per litter and increased early resorptions per litter. Peri- and post-natal development studies in which female rats received subcutaneous injections of cidofovir once daily at doses up to 1.0 mg/kg/day from day 7 of gestation through day 21 postpartum (approximately 5 weeks) resulted in no adverse effects on viability, growth, behaviour, sexual maturation or reproductive capacity in the offspring. Daily intravenous administration of cidofovir during the period of organogenesis led to reduced fetal body weights when administered to pregnant rats at 1.5 mg/kg/day and to pregnant rabbits at 1.0 mg/kg/day. The no-observable-effect dosages for embryotoxicity was 0.5 mg/kg/day in rats and 0.25 mg/kg/day in rabbits.

6. PHARMACEUTICAL PARTICULARS

6.1 List of excipients

Sodium Hydroxide

Hydrochloric Acid

Water for Injection

6.2 Incompatibilities

The chemical and physical stability of VISTIDE admixed with saline has been demonstrated in glass bottles, in infusion bags composed of either polyvinyl chloride (PVC) or ethylene/propylene copolymer, and in PVC based vented I.V. administration sets. Other types of I.V. set tubing and infusion bags have not been studied.

No data are available to support the addition of other medicinal products or supplements to the recommended admixture for intravenous infusion. Compatibility with Ringer's Solution, Lactated Ringer's Solution or bacteriostatic infusion fluids has not been evaluated.

6.3 Shelf life

3 years

6.4 Special precautions for storage

Do not store above 30°C. Do not refrigerate or freeze.

If not intended for use immediately after preparation, VISTIDE reconstituted solution for infusion may be stored temporarily for up to 24 hours in a refrigerator (2-8°C) when reconstitution is performed under aseptic conditions. Storage beyond 24 hours or freezing is not recommended. Refrigerated solutions should be allowed to warm to room temperature prior to use.

VISTIDE is supplied in single-use vials. Partially used vials should be discarded.

6.5 Nature and contents of container

Sterile VISTIDE solution is supplied in single use 5 ml clear glass vials with a 5 ml nominal fill volume. The container/closure components include: Type I clear borosilicate glass vials, Teflon faced grey butyl plug stoppers, and aluminium crimp seals with a flip off plastic tab. Each pack contains one 5 ml vial together with the package leaflet.

6.6 Instructions for use and handling

Method of preparation and administration

As with all parenteral products, VISTIDE vials should be visually inspected for particulate matter and discolouration prior to administration.

With a syringe, transfer under aseptic conditions the appropriate dose of VISTIDE from the vial to an infusion bag containing 100 ml 0.9% (normal) saline solution, and mix thoroughly. The entire volume should be infused intravenously into the patient at a constant rate over a period of 1 hour by use of a standard infusion pump. VISTIDE should be administered by health care professionals adequately experienced in the care of AIDS patients.

Handling and disposal

Adequate precautions including the use of appropriate safety equipment are recommended for the preparation, administration and disposal of VISTIDE. The preparation of VISTIDE reconstituted solution should be done in a laminar flow biological safety cabinet. Personnel preparing the reconstituted solution should wear surgical gloves, safety glasses and a closed front surgical-type gown with knit cuffs. If VISTIDE contacts the skin, wash membranes and flush thoroughly with water. Excess VISTIDE and all other materials used in the admixture preparation and administration should be placed in a leak-proof, puncture-proof container for disposal.

Obtaining probenecid

Probenecid is not supplied with VISTIDE and should be obtained via the Marketing Authorisation Holder of probenecid. However, in case of difficulty in obtaining probenecid the local representative of the Marketing Authorisation Holder of VISTIDE should be contacted for information (See also sections 4.2 and 4.4).

7. MARKETING AUTHORISATION HOLDER

Pfizer Enterprises SARL

51, Av JF Kennedy – Rond du Kirchberg

L - 1855 Luxembourg

G.D. Luxembourg

8. MARKETING AUTHORISATION NUMBER(S)

EU/1/97/037/001

9. DATE OF FIRST AUTHORISATION/RENEWAL OF THE AUTHORISATION

10 July 2002

10. DATE OF REVISION OF THE TEXT

September 2004

VISUDYNE

(Novartis Pharmaceuticals UK Ltd)

1. NAME OF THE MEDICINAL PRODUCT

Visudyne 15 mg, powder for solution for infusion

2. QUALITATIVE AND QUANTITATIVE COMPOSITION

Each vial contains 15 mg of verteporfin. For excipients see section 6.1.

3. PHARMACEUTICAL FORM

Powder for solution for infusion

4. CLINICAL PARTICULARS

4.1 Therapeutic indications

Visudyne is indicated for the treatment of patients with age-related macular degeneration with

- predominantly classic subfoveal choroidal neovascularisation,
- occult subfoveal choroidal neovascularisation with evidence of recent or ongoing disease progression (see section 5.1. Pharmacodynamic properties)

or

patients with subfoveal choroidal neovascularisation secondary to pathologic myopia.

4.2 Posology and method of administration

Visudyne should be used only by ophthalmologists experienced in the management of patients with age-related macular degeneration or with pathological myopia.

Visudyne therapy is a two-step process:

The first step is a 10-minute intravenous infusion of Visudyne at a dose of 6 mg/m^2 body surface area, diluted in 30 ml infusion solution (see 6.6 "Instruction for use/handling").

The second step is the light activation of Visudyne at 15 minutes after the start of the infusion. For this, a diode laser generating non-thermal red light (wavelength 689 nm ±3 nm) is used via a slit lamp mounted fibre optic device and a suitable contact lens. At the recommended light intensity of 600 mW/cm^2, it takes 83 seconds to deliver the required light dose of 50 J/cm^2.

The greatest linear dimension of the choroidal neovascular lesion is estimated using fluorescein angiography and fundus photography. Fundus cameras with a magnification within the range of 2.4 - 2.6X are recommended. The treatment spot should cover all neovasculature, blood and/or blocked fluorescence. To ensure treatment of poorly demarcated lesion borders, an additional margin of 500 μm should be added around the visible lesion. The nasal edge of the treatment spot must be at least 200 μm from the temporal edge of the optic disc. The maximum spot size used for the first treatment in the clinical studies was 6400 μm. For treatment of lesions that are larger than the maximum treatment spot size, apply the light to the greatest possible area of active lesion.

It is important to follow the above recommendations to achieve the optimal treatment effect.

Patients should be re-evaluated every 3 months. In the event of recurrent CNV leakage, Visudyne therapy may be given up to 4 times per year.

4.3 Contraindications

Visudyne is contra-indicated for patients with porphyria or a known hypersensitivity to verteporfin or to any of the excipients, and in patients with severe hepatic impairments.

4.4 Special warnings and special precautions for use

Patients who receive Visudyne will become photosensitive for 48 hours after the infusion. During that period, patients should avoid exposure of unprotected skin, eyes or other body organs to direct sunlight or bright indoor light such as tanning salons, bright halogen lighting, or high power lighting in surgery operating rooms or dentist offices. If patients have to go outdoors in daylight during the first 48 hours after treatment, they must protect their skin and eyes by wearing protective clothing and dark sunglasses. UV sunscreens are not effective in protecting against photosensitivity reactions.

Ambient indoor light is safe. Patients should not stay in the dark and should be encouraged to expose their skin to ambient indoor light, as it will help eliminate the drug quickly through the skin by a process called photobleaching.

Visudyne therapy should be considered carefully in patients with moderate hepatic impairment or biliary obstruction since no experience has been gained in these patients.

Patients who experience a severe decrease of vision (equivalent to 4 lines or more) within one week after treatment should not be re-treated, at least until their vision completely recovers to pre-treatment level and the potential benefits and risks of subsequent treatment are carefully considered by the treating physician.

Extravasation of Visudyne can cause severe pain, inflammation, swelling or discoloration at the injection site. The relief of pain may require analgesic treatment. If extravasation occurs, infusion should be stopped immediately. Protect the affected area thoroughly from bright direct light until swelling and discoloration have disappeared, and put cold compresses on the injection site. To avoid extravasation, a free-flowing IV line should be established before starting Visudyne infusion and the line should be monitored, the largest possible arm vein, preferably the antecubital, should be used for the infusion and small veins in the back of the hand should be avoided.

Chest pain, vaso-vagal reactions (procedure-related) and hypersensitivity reactions, which on rare occasions can be severe, have been reported. Both vaso-vagal and hypersensitivity reactions are associated with general symptoms such as syncope, sweating, dizziness, rash, dyspnoea, flushing, and changes in blood pressure and heart rate. Patients should be under close medical supervision during the Visudyne infusion.

There are no clinical data on the use of Visudyne in anaesthetised patients. In sedated or anaesthetised pigs, a Visudyne dose significantly higher than the recommended dose in patients given as a bolus injection caused severe haemodynamic effects including death, probably as a result of complement activation. Pre-dosing with diphenhydramine diminished these effects suggesting that histamine may play a role in this process. This effect was not observed in conscious nonsedated pigs, or in any other species including man. Verteporfin at more than 5 times the expected maximum plasma concentration in treated patients, caused a low level of complement activation in human blood *in vitro*. No clinically relevant complement activation was reported in clinical trials but anaphylactic reactions have been reported during post-marketing surveillance. Patients should be under close medical supervision during the Visudyne infusion and caution should be exercised when Visudyne treatment under general anaesthesia is considered.

There are no clinical data to support a concomitant treatment for the second eye. However, if the treatment of the second eye is deemed necessary, light should be applied to the second eye immediately after light application in the first eye but no later than 20 minutes from the start of the infusion.

No clinical experience is available in patients with unstable heart disease (class III or IV) and in patients with uncontrolled arterial hypertension.

4.5 Interaction with other medicinal products and other forms of Interaction

No specific drug-drug interaction studies have been conducted in humans.

It is possible that concomitant use of other photosensitising agents (e.g. tetracyclines, sulphonamides, phenothiazines, sulfonylurea, hypoglycemic agents, thiazide diuretics, and griseofulvin) could increase the potential for photosensitivity reactions.

4.6 Pregnancy and lactation

Visudyne has not been studied in pregnant women. In teratogenicity studies in rats, increasing incidences of anophthalmia/microphthalmia, wavy ribs and foetal alterations were observed at doses greater than approximately 70 times the exposure (based on AUC) of the recommended human dose. Therefore, Visudyne should be used in pregnant women only if the benefit justifies the potential risk to the foetus.

It is not known whether Visudyne is excreted in human milk, it should therefore not be administered to nursing mothers, or breast-feeding should be interrupted for 48 hours after administration.

4.7 Effects on ability to drive and use machines

Following Visudyne treatment, patients may develop transient visual disturbances such as abnormal vision, vision decrease, or visual field defects that may interfere with their ability to drive or use machines. Patients should not drive or use machines as long as these symptoms persist.

4.8 Undesirable effects

In clinical trials, the following adverse reactions were considered potentially related to Visudyne therapy.

Ocular side effects:

Common effects (1-10%): Abnormal vision such as blurry, hazy, fuzzy vision, or flashes of light, decreased vision, visual field defect such as grey or dark haloes, scotoma and black spots.

Severe vision decrease, equivalent of 4 lines or more, within seven days was reported in 2.1% of the verteporfin treated patients in the placebo-controlled ocular Phase III clinical studies and in less than 1% of patients in uncontrolled clinical studies. The event occurred mainly in patients with occult only (4.9%) or minimally classic CNV lesions in patients with AMD and was not reported for placebo-treated patients. A partial or complete recovery of vision to baseline values has been observed for most of these patients.

Uncommon effects (0.1-1%): Retinal detachment (non-rhegmatogenous), subretinal haemorrhage, vitreous haemorrhage.

Injection site side effects:

Common effects (1-10%): Pain, oedema, inflammation, extravasation.

Uncommon effects (0.1-1%): Haemorrhage, discoloration, and hypersensitivity.

Systemic side effects:

Common effects (1-10%): Infusion-related pain primarily presenting as back pain, but may also radiate to other areas such as the pelvis, shoulder girdle or rib cage, nausea, photosensitivity reaction, asthenia, pruritus, and hypercholesteraemia.

Photosensitivity reactions (in 2.2% of patients and $<1\%$ of Visudyne courses) occurred in the form of sunburn following exposure to sunlight usually within 24 hours from Visudyne treatment. Such reactions should be avoided by compliance with photosensitivity protection instructions under Section 4.4 "Warnings and precautions for use".

The higher incidence of back pain during infusion in the Visudyne group was not associated with any evidence of haemolysis or allergic reaction and usually resolved by the end of the infusion.

Uncommon effects (0.1-1%): Pain, hypertension, hypesthesia, fever.

Rare undesirable effects in clinical trials ($<0.1\%$) or spontaneously reported during post marketing surveillance included:

Ocular side effects: retinal or choroidal vessel nonperfusion;

Systemic side effects: chest pain, vaso-vagal reactions (procedure-related) and hypersensitivity reactions, which on rare occasions can be severe, have been reported. Both vaso-vagal and hypersensitivity reactions are associated with general symptoms such as syncope, sweating, dizziness, rash, dyspnoea, flushing, and changes in blood pressure and heart rate.

Most adverse reactions were mild to moderate and transient in nature. Undesirable effects reported in patients with pathologic myopia were similar to those reported in patients with AMD.

4.9 Overdose

No case of drug overdose has been reported. Overdose of drug and/or light in the treated eye may result in non-selective non-perfusion of normal retinal vessels with the possibility of severe vision decrease.

Overdose of the drug may result in the prolongation of the period during which the patient remains photosensitive. In such cases, the patient should prolong skin and eye protection from direct sunlight or bright indoor light for a period proportionate with the overdose given.

5. PHARMACOLOGICAL PROPERTIES

5.1 Pharmacodynamic properties

Pharmacotherapeutic group: Agents used in photodynamic therapy; ATC code L01 XD 02.

Verteporfin, also referred to as benzoporphyrin derivative monoacids (BPD-MA) consists of a 1:1 mixture of the equally active regioisomers BPD-MA_C and BPD-MA_D. It is used as a light-activated drug (photosensitiser).

By itself, the clinically recommended dose of verteporfin is not cytotoxic. It produces cytotoxic agents only when activated by light in the presence of oxygen. When energy absorbed by the porphyrin is transferred to oxygen, highly reactive short-lived singlet oxygen is generated. Singlet oxygen causes damage to biological structures within the diffusion range, leading to local vascular occlusion, cell damage and, under certain conditions, cell death.

The selectivity of PDT using verteporfin is based, in addition to the localised light exposure, on selective and rapid uptake and retention of verteporfin by rapidly proliferating cells including the endothelium of choroidal neovasculature.

Age-related Macular Degeneration with predominantly classic subfoveal lesions

Visudyne has been studied in two randomised, placebo-controlled, double-masked, multicentre studies (BPD OCR 002 A and B). A total of 609 patients were enrolled (402 Visudyne, 207 placebo).

The objective was to demonstrate the long-term efficacy and safety of Photodynamic Therapy (PDT) with verteporfin in limiting the decrease in visual acuity in patients with subfoveal choroidal neovascularisation (CNV) due to age–related macular degeneration (AMD).

The primary efficacy variable was responder rate, defined as the proportion of patients who lost less than 15 letters (equivalent to 3 lines) of visual acuity (measured with the ETDRS charts) at month 12 relative to baseline.

The following inclusion criteria were considered for the treatment: patients older than 50 years of age, presence of CNV secondary to AMD, presence of classic lesion components in the CNV (defined as a well-demarcated area of the fluorescence on angiography), CNV located subfoveally (involved the geometric centre of the foveal avascular zone), area of classic plus occult CNV $\geq 50\%$ of the total lesion surface, greatest linear dimension of the entire lesion ≤ 9 Macular Photocoagulation Study (MPS) disc area, and a best-corrected visual acuity between 34 and 73 letters (i.e. approximately 20/40 and 20/200) in the treated eye. Presence of occult CNV lesions (fluorescence not well demarcated on the angiogram) was allowed.

Results indicate that, at 12 months, Visudyne was statistically superior to placebo in terms of the proportion of patients responding to the treatment. The studies showed a difference of 15% between treatment groups (61% for Visudyne-treated patients compared to 46% placebo-treated patients, $p<0.001$, ITT analysis). This 15% difference between treatment groups was confirmed at 24 months (53% Visudyne versus 38% placebo, $p<0.001$).

The subgroup of patients with predominantly classic CNV lesions (N=243; Visudyne 159, placebo 84) were more likely to exhibit a larger treatment benefit). After 12 months, these patients showed a difference of 28% between treatment groups (67% for Visudyne patients compared to 39% for placebo patients, $p< 0.001$); the benefit was maintained at 24 months (59% versus 31%, $p<0.001$).

Age-related Macular Degeneration with occult with no classic lesions

Another randomised, placebo-controlled, double-masked, multicentre, 24-month study (BPD OCR 003 AMD) was conducted in patients with AMD characterised by occult with no classic subfoveal CNV with a visual acuity score of >50 letters (20/100), or classic-containing CNV with a visual acuity score >70 letters (20/40). Lesions with occult but no classic subfoveal CNV contained either blood or had shown disease progression within preceeding 3 months before randomisation. Disease progression was defined as a documented loss of 6 or more letters using the best corrected visual acuity assessment (ETDRS chart) or documented fluorescein angiographic evidence of a 10% or more increase in the lesion's greatest linear dimension. 339 patients (225 verteporfin, 114 placebo) were enrolled in this study. The efficacy parameter was the same as in BPD OCR 002 (see above).

At month 12, the study did not show any statistically significant results on the primary efficacy parameter (responder rate 49.3% versus 45.6%, $p=0.517$). At month 24, a statistically significant difference of 12.9% in favour of Visudyne compared to placebo was observed (46.2% versus 33.3%, $p=0.023$). A group of patients who had occult with no classic lesions (n=258), showed a statistically significant difference of 13.7% in favour of Visudyne compared to placebo (45.2% versus 31.5%, $p=0.032$)

Pathological Myopia

One multicentre, double-masked, placebo-controlled, randomised study (BPD OCR 003 PM) was conducted in patients with subfoveal choroidal neovascularisation caused by pathologic myopia. A total of 120 patients (81 Visudyne, 39 placebo) were enrolled in the study. The posology and retreatments were the same as in the AMD studies.

At month 12, there was a benefit of Visudyne for the primary efficacy endpoint (percentage of patients who lost less than 3 lines of visual acuity) – 86% for Visudyne versus 67% for placebo, $p=0.011$. The percentage of patients who lost less than 1.5 lines was 72% for Visudyne and 44% for placebo ($p=0.003$).

At Month 24, 79% Visudyne patients versus 72% placebo patients had lost less than 3 lines of visual acuity ($p=0.38$). The percentage of patients who lost less than 1.5 lines was 64% for Visudyne and 49% for placebo ($p=0.106$).

This indicates that clinical benefit may diminish over time.

5.2 Pharmacokinetic properties

Distribution

C_{max} after a 10-minute infusion of 6 and 12 mg/m^2 body surface area in the target population is approximately 1.5 and 3.5 μg/ml, respectively. These values are somewhat higher (26% for the proposed dose of 6 mg/m^2) than those observed in young healthy volunteers and may result in a higher exposure. The clinical relevance of this age-related difference is remote, as the risk/benefit assessment determined in the target population is favourable. A maximum 2-fold inter-individual variation in plasma concentrations at C_{max} (immediately after end of the infusion) and at the time of light administration was found for each Visudyne dose administered.

For both regioisomers, C_{max} and AUC values were proportional to dose. C_{max} values obtained at the end of infusion were higher for BPD-MA_D than for BPD-MA_C. The volume of distribution was 0.5 l/kg.

Protein-binding

In whole human blood, 90% of verteporfin is associated with plasma and 10% associated with blood cells, of which very little was membrane associated. In human plasma, 90% of verteporfin is associated with plasma lipoprotein fractions and approximately 6% are associated with albumin.

Metabolism

The ester group of verteporfin is hydrolysed via plasma and hepatic esterases, leading to the formation of benzoporphyrin derivative diacid (BPD-DA). BPD-DA is also a photosensitiser but its systemic exposure is low (5-10% of the verteporfin exposure suggesting that most of the drug is eliminated unchanged). *In vitro* studies did not show any significant involvement of oxidative metabolism by cytochrome P450 enzymes.

Elimination

Plasma elimination half-life mean values ranged from approximately 5-6 hours for verteporfin.

The mean area-under-the-curve (AUC) values for subjects with mild hepatic dysfunction were up to 1.4 times greater than those for subjects with normal hepatic function. This difference is not clinically relevant and does not require any dose adjustment to patients with mild hepatic impairment.

Combined excretion of verteporfin and BPD-DA in human urine was less than 1% suggesting a biliary excretion.

5.3 Preclinical safety data
In repeat-dose studies in rats and dogs (once per day without light for up to 4 weeks), mild extravascular haemolysis and haematopoietic responses were seen with exposure greater than approximately 70 times (rats) and 32 times (dogs) the exposure (based on AUC) of the recommended human dose.

Rapid administration of 2.0 mg/kg of verteporfin at a rate of 7 ml/minute to anaesthetised pigs resulted in haemodynamic effects and sometimes rapid death, occurring within 2 minutes of drug administration. Similar effects were observed in sedated pigs. Pre-dosing with diphenhydramine diminished these effects suggesting that histamine may play a role in this process. Non-anaesthetised non-sedated animals were not affected by these dosing parameters. No changes were recorded in either conscious and anaesthetised dogs receiving 20 mg/kg verteporfin at an infusion rate of 5 ml/minute. The effects may be resulting from complement activation. Verteporfin at more than 5 times the expected maximum plasma concentration in treated patients, caused a low level of complement activation in human blood *in vitro*.

Levels of ocular toxicity in normal rabbits and monkeys, particularly on the retina/choroid, correlated with drug dose, light dose, and time of light treatment. A retinal toxicity study in normal dogs with intravenous verteporfin and ambient light on the eye showed no treatment-related ocular toxicity.

In a teratology study rat foetuses of dams given greater than approximately 67 times the recommended human dose had increasing incidences of anophthalmia/microphthalmia, wavy ribs and foetal alterations. No teratogenicity was observed in foetuses from rabbits given 67 times the recommended human dose.

Verteporfin was not genotoxic in the absence or presence of light in the usual battery of genotoxic test.

Immunomodulatory effects have been observed in mice. Whole body light activation within 3 hours of verteporfin administration beneficially modified the course of several immunologically mediated pathologic conditions and diminished normal-skin immune responses without causing skin reactivity or generalised non-specific immune suppression.

6. PHARMACEUTICAL PARTICULARS
6.1 List of excipients
Lactose, egg phosphatidylglycerol, dimyristoyl phosphatidylcholine, ascorbyl palmitate, butylated hydroxytoluene

6.2 Incompatibilities
Visudyne precipitates in saline solutions. Do not use normal saline or other parenteral solutions. Do not mix Visudyne in the same solution with other drugs.

6.3 Shelf life
Shelf-life in the sealed vial: 3 years

Shelf-life after reconstitution and dilution: 4 hours

6.4 Special precautions for storage
Do not store above 25°C. Keep vial in the outer carton in order to protect from light.

After reconstitution and dilution protect from light until used, and use within a maximum of 4 hours.

6.5 Nature and contents of container
Glass vial, sealed with butyl stopper and aluminium cap.

6.6 Instructions for use and handling
Reconstitute Visudyne in 7.0 ml water for injection to produce 7.5 ml of a 2.0-mg/ml solution. For a dose of 6 mg/m^2 body surface (see 4.2 ''Posology and method of administration'') dilute the required amount of Visudyne solution in 5 % glucose for injection to a final volume of 30 ml. Do not use saline solution (see 6.2 ''Incompatibilities''). Use of a standard infusion line filter with hydrophylic membranes (such as polyethersulfon) of a pore size of not less than 1.2 μm is recommended.

If material is spilled, it should be contained and wiped up with a damp cloth. Eye and skin contact should be avoided. Use of rubber gloves and eye protection is recommended. All materials should be disposed of properly.

7. MARKETING AUTHORISATION HOLDER
Novartis Europharm Limited

Wimblehurst Road

Horsham

West Sussex, RH12 5AB

UNITED KINGDOM

8. MARKETING AUTHORISATION NUMBER(S)
EU/1/00/140/001

9. DATE OF FIRST AUTHORISATION/RENEWAL OF THE AUTHORISATION
27 July 2000

10. DATE OF REVISION OF THE TEXT
22/09/2003

Legal Category
POM

Vitamin E Suspension 100mg/ml

(Cambridge Laboratories)

1. NAME OF THE MEDICINAL PRODUCT
Vitamin E Suspension 100mg/ml

2. QUALITATIVE AND QUANTITATIVE COMPOSITION
Each 5ml of suspension contains 500mg of DL-alpha-tocopheryl acetate.

3. PHARMACEUTICAL FORM
Oral Suspension

4. CLINICAL PARTICULARS
4.1 Therapeutic indications
For the correction of Vitamin E deficiency occurring in malabsorption disorders ie. cystic fibrosis, chronic cholestasis and abetalipoproteinaemia.

4.2 Posology and method of administration
Route of administration: For oral use.

Adults (including the elderly)

For the treatment of malabsorption disorders the following doses should be administered:

Cystic fibrosis 100-200mg/day

Abetalipoproteinaemia 50-100mg/kg/day

Children

For the treatment of cystic fibrosis a dose of 50mg/day should be given to children less than 1 year and 100mg/day to children 1 year and over.

The adult dosage should be used for the treatment of abetalipoproteinaemia (50-100mg/kg/day).

Infants with vitamin E deficiency which is secondary to chronic cholestasis may be treated with doses of 150-200mg/kg/day.

4.3 Contraindications
Use in patients with a known hypersensitivity to Vitamin E.

4.4 Special warnings and special precautions for use
Vitamin E has been reported to increase the risk of thrombosis in patients predisposed to this condition, including patients taking oestrogens. This finding has not been confirmed but should be borne in mind when selecting patients for treatment, in particular women taking oral contraceptives containing oestrogens.

A higher incidence of necrotising enterocolitis has been noted in lower weight premature infants (less than 1.5kg) treated with vitamin E.

4.5 Interaction with other medicinal products and other forms of Interaction
Vitamin E may increase the risk of thrombosis in patients taking oestrogens (see 4.4 above).

4.6 Pregnancy and lactation
There is no evidence of the safety of high doses of vitamin E in pregnancy nor is there evidence from animal work that it is free from hazard, therefore do not use in pregnancy especially in the first trimester. No information is available on excretion in breast milk, therefore it is advisable not to use during lactation.

4.7 Effects on ability to drive and use machines
None known.

4.8 Undesirable effects
Diarrhoea and abdominal pain may occur with doses greater than 1g daily.

4.9 Overdose
Transient gastro-intestinal disturbances have been reported with doses greater than 1g daily and where necessary, general supportive measures should be employed.

5. PHARMACOLOGICAL PROPERTIES
5.1 Pharmacodynamic properties
The exact role of vitamin E in the animal organism has not yet been established. Vitamin E is known to exert an important physiological function as an antioxidant for fats, with a sparing action on vitamin A, carotenoids and on unsaturated fatty acids. Other work has demonstrated that vitamin E is connected with the maintenance of certain factors essential for the normal metabolic cycle.

5.2 Pharmacokinetic properties
Vitamin E is absorbed from the gastrointestinal tract. Most of the vitamin appears in the lymph and is then widely distributed to all tissues. Most of the dose is slowly excreted in the bile and the remainder is eliminated in the urine as glucuronides of tocopheronic acid or other metabolites.

5.3 Preclinical safety data
There are no pre-clinical data of relevance to the prescriber which are additional to that already included in other sections of the SPC.

6. PHARMACEUTICAL PARTICULARS
6.1 List of excipients
Castor oil polyethylene glycol ether

Benzoic acid

Sorbic acid

Glycerol

Syrup

Flavour raspberry

Purified Water

6.2 Incompatibilities
None.

6.3 Shelf life
Unopened: Two years.

After first opening: One month (The product will be stable after opening for the normal duration of treatment providing the cap is replaced after use and the recommended storage conditions on the label are observed).

6.4 Special precautions for storage
Store below 25°C.

6.5 Nature and contents of container
Amber glass bottles with aluminium screw caps or Vistop tamper-evident caps.

6.6 Instructions for use and handling
Vitamin E Suspension may be diluted with Syrup BP but should be used immediately and not stored.

7. MARKETING AUTHORISATION HOLDER
Cambridge Laboratories Limited

Deltic House

Kingfisher Way

Silverlink Business Park

Wallsend

Tyne & Wear

NE28 9NX

8. MARKETING AUTHORISATION NUMBER(S)
PL 12070/0010

9. DATE OF FIRST AUTHORISATION/RENEWAL OF THE AUTHORISATION
8 March 1993

10. DATE OF REVISION OF THE TEXT
March 2000

Vivaglobin 160mg/ml solution for injection (subcutaneous use)

(ZLB Behring UK Limited)

1. NAME OF THE MEDICINAL PRODUCT
Vivaglobin®, 160mg/ml solution for injection (subcutaneous use)

2. QUALITATIVE AND QUANTITATIVE COMPOSITION
1ml contains:

Human normal immunoglobulin (subcutaneous) 160mg*

*Corresponding to the total protein content of which at least 95% is IgG.

Distribution of IgG subclasses:

IgG_1	ca. 61 %
IgG_2	ca. 28 %
IgG_3	ca. 5 %
IgG_4	ca. 6 %
IgA	max. 1.7 mg/ml

For excipients, see 6.1.

3. PHARMACEUTICAL FORM
Solution for injection (subcutaneous use).

4. CLINICAL PARTICULARS
4.1 Therapeutic indications
Replacement therapy in adults and children in primary immunodeficiency (PID) syndromes such as:

– Congenital agammaglobulinaemia and hypogammaglobulinaemia

– Common variable immunodeficiency

– Severe combined immunodeficiency

– IgG subclass deficiencies with recurrent infections

Replacement therapy in myeloma or chronic lymphatic leukaemia with severe secondary hypogammaglobulinaemia and recurrent infections.

4.2 Posology and method of administration
Posology
The dosage may need to be individualized for each patient dependent on the pharmacokinetic and clinical response. The following dosage regimens are given as a guideline. The dosage regimen using the subcutaneous route should achieve a sustained plasma level of IgG.

A loading dose of at least 0.2 to 0.5 g/kg (1.3 to 3.1 ml/kg) bodyweight – divided over several days with a maximal daily dose of 0.1 to 0.15 g/kg bodyweight and as indicated by the treating physician - may be required. After steady state IgG levels have been attained, maintenance doses are administered at repeated intervals, ideally weekly, to reach a cumulative monthly dose of about 0.4 to 0.8 g/kg (2.5 to 5 ml/kg) bodyweight.

Trough levels of IgG should be measured in order to adjust the dose and dosage interval of Vivaglobin.

Method of administration

Vivaglobin should be administered via the subcutaneous route.

Subcutaneous infusion for home treatment should be initiated and monitored by a physician experienced in the treatment of immunodeficiency and in the guidance of patients for home treatment. The patient will be instructed in the use of a syringe driver, infusion techniques, the keeping of a treatment diary and measures to be taken in case of severe adverse events. The recommended infusion rate is 22 ml/hour. In a clinical study with 53 patients evaluated, during the training phase under supervision of a physician, the infusion rate was increased from initially 10 ml to 22 ml/hour.

Vivaglobin should preferentially be administered in the abdominal wall, thigh and/or buttocks. No more than 15ml should be injected into a single site. Doses over 15 ml should be divided and injected into 2 or more sites.

4.3 Contraindications
Hypersensitivity to any of the components of the product.

Vivaglobin must not be given intravascularly.

It must also not be administered intramuscularly in case of severe thrombocytopenia and in other disorders of haemostasis.

4.4 Special warnings and special precautions for use
Do not inject intravascularly! If Vivaglobin is accidentally administered into a blood vessel, patients could develop an anaphylactic shock.

The recommended infusion rate of Vivaglobin stated under "4.2 Method of administration" should be adhered to. Patients should be closely monitored and carefully observed for any adverse event throughout the infusion period.

Certain adverse reactions may occur more frequently in patients who receive human normal immunoglobulin for the first time or, in rare cases, when the product is switched or when treatment has been interrupted for more than eight weeks.

True hypersensitivity reactions are rare. They can occur in the very rare cases of IgA deficiency with anti-IgA antibodies and these patients should be treated with caution. Rarely, Vivaglobin can induce a fall in blood pressure with anaphylactic reaction, even in patients who had tolerated previous treatment with normal human immunoglobulin.

Potential complications can often be avoided by ensuring:

- that patients are not sensitive to human normal immunoglobulin, by first infusing the product slowly (see 4.2);
- that patients are carefully monitored for any symptoms throughout the infusion period. In particular, patients should be monitored during the first infusion and for the first hour thereafter, in order to detect potential adverse reactions in the following situations:
- patients naïve to human normal immunoglobulin,
- patients switched from an alternative product, or,
- when there has been a long interval since the previous infusion.

All other patients should be observed for at least 20 minutes after administration.

On suspicion of an allergic or anaphylactic reaction the administration has to be discontinued immediately. In case of shock, the current medical standards for shock treatment have to be applied.

Standard measures to prevent infections resulting from the use of medicinal products prepared from human blood or plasma include selection of donors, screening of individual donations and plasma pools for specific markers of infection, and the inclusion of effective manufacturing steps for the inactivation/removal of viruses. Despite this, when medicinal products prepared from human blood or plasma are administered, the possibility of transmitting infective agents cannot be totally excluded. This also applies to unknown or emerging viruses and other pathogens.

The measures are considered effective for enveloped viruses such as HIV, HBV and HCV, and for the non-enveloped viruses, HAV and parvovirus B19.

There is reassuring clinical experience regarding the lack of hepatitis A or parvovirus B19 transmission with immunoglobulins and it is also assumed that the antibody content makes an important contribution to the virus safety.

It is strongly recommended that every time that Vivaglobin is administered to a patient, the name and batch number of the product are recorded in order to maintain a link between the patient and the batch of the product.

4.5 Interaction with other medicinal products and other forms of Interaction
Live attenuated virus vaccines

Immunoglobulin administration may impair, for a period of at least 6 weeks and up to 3 months, the efficacy of live attenuated virus vaccines such as measles, rubella, mumps, and varicella vaccines. After administration of Vivaglobin, an interval of at least 3 months should elapse before vaccination with live attenuated virus vaccines.

In the case of measles, this impairment may persist for up to 1 year. Therefore, patients receiving measles vaccine should have their antibody status checked.

Interference with serological testing

It has to be considered that when serological test results are interpreted, the transitory rise of passively transferred antibodies after immunoglobulin injection may result in misleading positive test results.

Passive transmission of antibodies to erythrocyte antigens, e.g., A, B and D, may interfere with some serological tests for red cell allo-antibodies (e.g. Coombs test), reticulocyte count and haptoglobin.

4.6 Pregnancy and lactation
The safety of this medicinal product for use in human pregnancy has not been established in controlled clinical trials and therefore should only be given with caution to pregnant women or breast-feeding mothers. Clinical experience with immunoglobulins suggests that no harmful effects on the course of pregnancy, or on the foetus and the neonate are to be expected.

4.7 Effects on ability to drive and use machines
There are no indications that Vivaglobin may impair the ability to drive or use machines.

4.8 Undesirable effects
In a clinical study with s.c. administration in 60 subjects the following undesirable effects have been reported:

Very common injection site reactions of mostly mild severity (swelling, soreness, redness, induration, local heat, itching, bruising) at the beginning of the subcutaneous treatment and declining very rapidly within the first ten infusions, when subjects became used to this form of treatment. (In study patients who were treated with subcutaneous immunoglobulin for years before the trial, injection site reactions were not reported.)

In single cases:

– allergic reactions including fall in blood pressure

– generalized reactions such as chills, fever, headache, malaise, mild back pain, syncope, dizziness, rash, skin disorder, bronchospasm.

During post-marketing surveillance of product administered i.m. or s.c., the following undesirable effects have been reported in rare cases:

– allergic reactions including fall in blood pressure, dyspnoea, cutaneous reactions, in isolated cases reaching as far as anaphylactic shock, even when the patient has shown no hypersensitivity to previous administration.

– generalized reactions such as chills, fever, headache, malaise, nausea, vomiting, arthralgia and moderate back pain.

– cardiovascular reactions particularly if the product is inadvertently injected intravascularly.

– Local reactions at the infusion site: swelling, soreness, redness, induration, local heat, itching, bruising or rash.

For information on infectious disease risk see 4.4.

4.9 Overdose
Consequences of an overdose are not known.

5. PHARMACOLOGICAL PROPERTIES

5.1 Pharmacodynamic properties
Pharmacotherapeutic group: immune sera and immunoglobulins: immunoglobulins, normal human for extravascular administration, ATC code: J06B A01.

Human normal immunoglobulin contains mainly immunoglobulin G (IgG) having a broad spectrum of antibodies against various infectious agents.

Vivaglobin contains the immunoglobulin G antibodies present in the normal population. It is usually prepared from pooled plasma of at least 1,000 donors. It has a distribution of immunoglobulin G subclasses closely proportional to that in native human plasma. Adequate doses of this medicinal product may restore abnormally low immunoglobulin G levels to the normal range.

5.2 Pharmacokinetic properties
With subcutaneous administration of human normal immunoglobulin, peak levels are achieved in the recipient's circulation after a delay of approximately 2 days. Data from a clinical study (n=60) show that trough levels of approximately 8 to 9 g/l (n=53) in the plasma can be maintained by weekly doses between 0.05 and 0.15 g (0.3 to 0.9 ml/kg) Vivaglobin per kg bodyweight. This is commensurate to a monthly cumulative dosage of 0.2 to 0.6 g per kg bodyweight.

IgG and IgG-complexes are broken down in cells of the reticuloendothelial system.

5.3 Preclinical safety data
There are no preclinical data considered relevant to clinical safety beyond data included in other sections of the SPC.

6. PHARMACEUTICAL PARTICULARS

6.1 List of excipients
Glycine, sodium chloride, hydrochloric acid or sodium hydroxide (in small amounts for pH adjustment), water for injections.

6.2 Incompatibilities
In the absence of compatibility studies this medicinal product must not be mixed with other medicinal products.

6.3 Shelf life
3 years

Once an ampoule or injection vial has been opened its contents are to be used immediately.

6.4 Special precautions for storage
Store in a refrigerator (+2 to +8 °C) in the outer carton. Do not freeze!

6.5 Nature and contents of container
5ml of solution in an ampoule (Type I glass) – pack size 1 or 10

10 ml of solution in a vial (Type I glass) with a stopper (chlorobutyl) – pack of 1 or 10 or 20

6.6 Instructions for use and handling
Vivaglobin is a ready-for-use solution and should be administered at body temperature. Vivaglobin is a clear solution. The colour can vary from colourless to pale-yellow up to light brown during shelf-life. Do not use solutions that are cloudy or have deposits.

Any unused product or waste material should be disposed of in accordance with local requirements.

7. MARKETING AUTHORISATION HOLDER
ZLB Behring GmbH

Emil-von-Behring-Str. 76

D-35041 Marburg

Germany

8. MARKETING AUTHORISATION NUMBER(S)
PL 15036/0016

9. DATE OF FIRST AUTHORISATION/RENEWAL OF THE AUTHORISATION
21 February 2005

10. DATE OF REVISION OF THE TEXT
25 February 2005

Volmax Tablets 4mg, 8mg

(Allen & Hanburys)

1. NAME OF THE MEDICINAL PRODUCT
VOLMAX Tablets 4mg.

VOLMAX Tablets 8mg.

2. QUALITATIVE AND QUANTITATIVE COMPOSITION
Salbutamol Sulphate BP 4.82mg equivalent to Salbutamol 4mg per tablet.

Salbutamol Sulphate BP 9.64mg equivalent to Salbutamol 8mg per tablet.

3. PHARMACEUTICAL FORM
Controlled Release Tablets.

4. CLINICAL PARTICULARS

4.1 Therapeutic indications
Salbutamol is a selective Beta-2 adrenoceptor agonist.

Volmax Tablets are indicated for the treatment of asthma, bronchospasm and/or reversible airways obstruction.

Volmax Tablets are suitable oral therapy for children and adults who are unable to use an inhaler device. In these patients, the controlled-release formulation makes Volmax Tablets helpful in the management of nocturnal asthma.

4.2 Posology and method of administration
Volmax Tablets must be swallowed whole with a glass of water and not chewed or crushed.

Volmax Tablets sustain bronchodilation over a 12 hour period.

Adults

The recommended dose is one 8mg tablet twice daily. There is not need to adjust the dose in the elderly.

Children

In children aged 3 - 12 years, the recommended dose is one 4mg tablet twice daily.

For oral administration.

4.3 Contraindications
Although intravenous salbutamol and occasionally salbutamol tablets are used in the management of premature labour, uncomplicated by conditions such as placenta praevia, antepartum haemorrhage or toxaemia of pregnancy, salbutamol presentations should not be used for threatened abortion.

Volmax Tablets are contra-indicated in patients with a history of hypersensitivity to any of their components.

4.4 Special warnings and special precautions for use
Bronchodilators should not be the only or main treatment in patients with severe or unstable asthma. Severe asthma

requires regular medical assessment including lung function testing as patients are at risk of severe attacks and even death. Physicians should consider using oral corticosteroid therapy and/or the maximum recommended dose of inhaled corticosteroid in these patients.

Patients taking Volmax Tablets may also be receiving short-acting inhaled bronchodilators to relieve symptoms. Increasing use of bronchodilators, in particular short-acting inhaled Beta2-agonists to relieve symptoms, indicates deterioration of asthma control. If patients find that short acting relief bronchodilator treatment becomes less effective or they need more inhalations than usual, medical attention must be sought. Similarly, if patients find that treatment with Volmax becomes less effective, medical attention must be sought.

In these situations, patients should be reassessed and consideration given to the need for increased anti-inflammatory therapy (e.g. higher doses of inhaled corticosteroids or a course of oral corticosteroids). Severe exacerbations of asthma must be treated in the normal way.

Salbutamol and non-selective beta-blocking drugs, such as propranolol, should not usually be prescribed together.

Salbutamol should be administered cautiously to patients with thyrotoxicosis.

Potentially serious hypokalaemia may result from Beta-2 agonist therapy mainly from parenteral and nebulised administration. Particular caution is advised in acute severe asthma as this effect may be potentiated by concomitant treatment with xanthine derivatives, steroids, diuretics and hypoxia. It is recommended that serum potassium levels are monitored in such situations.

In common with other β-adrenoceptor agonists, salbutamol can induce reversible metabolic changes such as increased blood glucose levels. Diabetic patients may be unable to compensate for the increase in blood glucose and the development of ketoacidoses has been reported. Concurrent administration of corticosteroids can exaggerate this effect.

4.5 Interaction with other medicinal products and other forms of Interaction
None known.

4.6 Pregnancy and lactation
Administration of drugs during pregnancy should only be considered if the expected benefit to the mother is greater than any possible risk to the foetus.

As with the majority of drugs, there is little published evidence of the safety of salbutamol in the early stages of human pregnancy but in animal studies, there was evidence of some harmful effects on the foetus at very high dose levels.

As salbutamol is probably secreted in breast milk, its use in nursing mothers requires careful consideration. It is not known whether salbutamol has a harmful effect on the neonate and so its use should be restricted to situations where it is felt that the expected benefit to the mother is likely to outweigh any potential risk to the neonate.

4.7 Effects on ability to drive and use machines
None known.

4.8 Undesirable effects
Adverse events are listed below by system organ class and frequency. Frequencies are defined as: very common (⩾1/10), common (⩾1/100 and <1/10), uncommon (⩾1/1000 and <1/100), rare (⩾1/10,000 and <1/1000) and very rare (<1/10,000) including isolated reports. Very common and common events were generally determined from clinical trial data. Rare and very rare events were generally determined from spontaneous data.

Immune System Disorders

Very rare: Hypersensitivity reactions including angioedema, urticaria, bronchospasm, hypotension and collapse.

Metabolism and Nutrition Disorders

Rare: Hypokalaemia.

Potentially serious hypokalaemia may result from $beta_2$ agonist therapy.

Nervous System Disorders

Very common: Tremor

Common: Headache

Very rare: Hyperactivity.

Cardiac Disorders

Common: Tachycardia

Rare: Cardiac arrhythmias including atrial fibrillation, supraventricular tachycardia and extrasystoles.

Vascular Disorders

Rare: Peripheral vasodilatation

Musculoskeletal and Connective Tissue Disorders

Common: Muscle cramps.

Very rare: Feeling of muscle tension

4.9 Overdose
The preferred antidote for overdosage with salbutamol is a cardio-selective beta-blocking agent but beta-blocking drugs should be used with caution in patients with a history of bronchospasm.

Hypokalaemia may occur following overdose with salbutamol. Serum potassium levels should be monitored.

5. PHARMACOLOGICAL PROPERTIES

5.1 Pharmacodynamic properties
Salbutamol is a selective Beta-2 adrenoceptor agonist. At therapeutic doses, it acts on the Beta-2 adrenoceptors of bronchial muscle.

Volmax Tablets are a controlled release formulation of salbutamol.

5.2 Pharmacokinetic properties
Salbutamol administered intravenously has a half-life of 4 to 6 hours and is cleared partly renally and partly by metabolism to the inactive 4' - 0 - sulphate (phenolic sulphate) which is also excreted primarily in the urine. The faeces are a minor route of excretion, salbutamol is bound to plasma proteins to the extent of 10%.

After oral administration, salbutamol is absorbed from the gastrointestinal tract and undergoes considerable first-pass metabolism to the phenolic sulphate. Both unchanged drug and conjugate are excreted primarily in the urine. The bioavailability of orally administered salbutamol is about 50%.

Volmax Tablets are designed to deliver 90% of their salbutamol content in vitro over 9 hours. This corresponds to a release rate of 0.8mg/h for the 8mg tablet and 0.4mg/h for the 4mg tablet.

5.3 Preclinical safety data
There are no pre-clinical data of relevance to the prescriber which are additional to that already included in other sections of the SmPC.

6. PHARMACEUTICAL PARTICULARS

6.1 List of excipients
Tablet Core:

Sodium Chloride PhEur.

Povidone BP

Croscarmellose Sodium Type A USNF

Silica Gel USNF

Magnesium Stearate PhEur.

Industrial Methylated Spirit 99% HSE

or Ethanol IP

Purified Water PhEur.

Membrane:

Cellulose Acetate 398-10 USNF

Cellulose Acetate 320S USNF

Methylhydroxypropylcellulose PhEur.

Methylene Chloride USNF

Methyl Alcohol USNF

Colour:

Methylhydroxypropylcellulose PhEur.

Opaspray K-1-7000 HSE

Methylene Chloride USNF

Methyl Alcohol USNF

Printing Ink:

Opacode S-1-4362 HSE

6.2 Incompatibilities
None known.

6.3 Shelf life
36 months.

6.4 Special precautions for storage
Store at temperatures not exceeding 30° C.

6.5 Nature and contents of container
Double foil blister pack with a push through lid.

Pack size: 14 or 56 tablets.

6.6 Instructions for use and handling
No special instructions.

Administrative Data

7. MARKETING AUTHORISATION HOLDER
Glaxo Wellcome UK Ltd

Stockley Park West

Uxbridge

Middlesex UB11 1BT

8. MARKETING AUTHORISATION NUMBER(S)
VOLMAX Tablets 4mg PL10949/0089

VOLMAX Tablets 8mg PL10949/0090

9. DATE OF FIRST AUTHORISATION/RENEWAL OF THE AUTHORISATION
1 August 1994.

10. DATE OF REVISION OF THE TEXT
12 April 2005

11. Legal Status
POM

Voltarol 25mg, 50mg Rapid Tablets

(Novartis Pharmaceuticals UK Ltd)

1. NAME OF THE MEDICINAL PRODUCT
Voltarol® Rapid Tablets 25mg

Voltarol® Rapid Tablets 50mg

2. QUALITATIVE AND QUANTITATIVE COMPOSITION
Each tablet contains 25mg of diclofenac potassium

Chemical name: Potassium-[o-[(2,6-dichlorophenyl)-amino]-phenyl]-acetate

3. PHARMACEUTICAL FORM
Coated tablet

4. CLINICAL PARTICULARS

4.1 Therapeutic indications

- Rheumatoid arthritis
- Osteoarthrosis
- Low back pain
- Migraine attacks
- Acute musculo-skeletal disorders and trauma such as periarthritis (especially frozen shoulder), tendinitis, tenosynovitis, bursitis, sprains, strains and dislocations; relief of pain in fractures
- Ankylosing spondylitis
- Acute gout
- Control of pain and inflammation in orthopaedic, dental and other minor surgery
- Pyrophosphate arthropathy and associated disorders

4.2 Posology and method of administration
It is recommended that the tablets be taken with fluid.

Adults

The recommended daily dose is 100-150mg in two or three divided doses. For milder cases, 75-100 mg daily in two or three divided doses is usually sufficient.

In migraine an initial dose of 50 mg should be taken at the first signs of an impending attack. In cases where relief 2 hours after the first dose is not sufficient, a further dose of 50 mg may be taken. If needed, further doses of 50 mg may be taken at intervals of 4-6 hours, not exceeding a total dose of 200 mg per day.

Children

For children over 14 years of age, the recommended daily dose is 75-100 mg in two or three divided doses. Voltarol Rapid tablets are not recommended for children under 14 years of age.

The use of Voltarol Rapid (all forms) in migraine attacks has not been established in children.

Elderly

Although the pharmacokinetics of Voltarol Rapid are not impaired to any clinically relevant extent in elderly patients, non-steroidal anti-inflammatory drugs should be used with particular caution in older patients who generally are more prone to adverse reactions. In particular it is recommended that the lowest effective dosage be used in frail elderly patients or those with a low body weight (also see 'Precautions') and the patient should be monitored for GI bleeding for 4 weeks following initiation of NSAID therapy.

4.3 Contraindications

- Patients with a history of, or active or suspected, gastro-intestinal ulcers or bleeding.
- Previous sensitivity to diclofenac or to any of the excipients in Voltarol Rapid.
- Patients in whom attacks of asthma, urticaria or acute rhinitis are precipitated by aspirin or other non-steroidal anti-inflammatory agents.

4.4 Special warnings and special precautions for use

Warnings

Gastro-intestinal

Close medical surveillance is imperative in patients with symptoms indicative of gastro-intestinal disorders, with a history suggestive of gastro-intestinal ulceration, with ulcerative colitis, Crohn's disease, bleeding diathesis or haematological disorders.

Gastro-intestinal bleeding or ulceration/perforation, haematemesis and melaena have in general more serious consequences in the elderly. They can occur at any time during treatment with or without warning symptoms or a previous history. In the rare instances where gastro-intestinal bleeding or ulceration occurs in patients receiving Voltarol Rapid the drug should be withdrawn.

Hepatic

Close medical surveillance is imperative in patients suffering from severe impairment of hepatic function.

Hypersensitivity reactions

As with other non-steroidal anti-inflammatory drugs, allergic reactions, including anaphylactic/anaphylactoid reactions, can occur without earlier exposure to the drug.

Like other NSAIDs, Voltarol Rapid may mask the signs and symptoms of infection due to its pharmacodynamic properties.

Precautions

Renal, cardiac, hepatic, and elderly

Patients with renal, cardiac or hepatic impairment and the elderly should be kept under surveillance, since the use of NSAIDs may result in deterioration of renal function. The lowest effective dose should be used and renal function monitored.

The importance of prostaglandins in maintaining renal blood flow should be taken into account in patients with impaired cardiac or renal functions, those being treated with diuretics or recovering from major surgery. Effects on renal function are usually reversible on withdrawal of Voltarol Rapid.

Hepatic

If abnormal liver function tests persist or worsen, clinical signs or symptoms consistent with liver disease develop or if other manifestations occur (eosinophilia, rash), Voltarol Rapid should be discontinued. Hepatitis may occur without prodromal symptoms.

Use of Voltarol Rapid in patients with hepatic porphyria may trigger an attack.

Haematological

Voltarol Rapid may reversibly inhibit platelet aggregation (see "Interactions"). Patients with defects of haemostasis should be carefully monitored.

Long term treatment

All patients who are receiving long term treatment with non-steroidal, anti-inflammatory agents should be monitored as a precautionary measure eg renal function, hepatic function (elevation of liver enzymes may occur) and blood counts.

Like other drugs that inhibit prostaglandin synthetase activity, diclofenac sodium and other NSAIDs can precipitate bronchospasm if administered to patients suffering from, or with a previous history of, bronchial asthma.

Caution is required in patients with a history of heart failure or hypertension since oedema has been reported in association with NSAID administration.

4.5 Interaction with other medicinal products and other forms of Interaction

Lithium and digoxin

Voltarol Rapid may increase plasma concentrations of lithium and digoxin.

Anticoagulants

Although clinical investigations do not appear to indicate that Voltarol Rapid has an influence on the effect of anticoagulants, there are isolated reports of an increased risk of haemorrhage with the combined use of diclofenac and anticoagulant therapy. Therefore to be certain that no change in anticoagulant dosage is needed, close monitoring of such patients is required. As with other non-steroidal anti-inflammatory agents, diclofenac can reversibly inhibit platelet aggregation.

Antidiabetic agents

Clinical studies have shown that Voltarol Rapid can be given together with oral antidiabetic agents without influencing their clinical effect. However there have been isolated reports of hypoglycaemic and hyperglycaemic effects which have required adjustment to the dosage of hypoglycaemic agents.

Cyclosporin

Cases of nephrotoxicity have been reported in patients receiving concomitant cyclosporin and NSAIDs, including Voltarol Rapid. This might be mediated through combined renal anti-prostaglandin effects of both the NSAID and cyclosporin.

Methotrexate

Cases of serious toxicity have been reported when methotrexate and NSAIDs are given within 24 hours of each other. This interaction is mediated through accumulation of methotrexate resulting from impairment of renal excretion in the presence of the NSAID.

Quinolone Antibacterials

Convulsions may occur due to an interaction between quinolones and NSAIDs. This may occur in patients with or without a history of epilepsy or convulsions. Therefore, caution should be exercised when considering the use of a quinolone in patients already receiving an NSAID.

Other NSAIDs and corticosteroids

Co-administration of Voltarol Rapid with aspirin or corticosteroids may increase the risk of gastro-intestinal bleeding. Avoid concomitant use of two or more NSAIDs.

Diuretics

Like other NSAIDs, Voltarol Rapid may inhibit the activity of diuretics. Concomitant treatment with potassium sparing diuretics may be associated with increased serum potassium levels, which should therefore be monitored frequently.

Cardiac glycosides

Concomitant use of cardiac glycosides and NSAIDs in patients may exacerbate cardiac failure, reduce GFR and increase plasma glycoside levels.

Mifepristone

NSAIDs should not be used for 8-12 days after mifepristone administration as NSAIDs can reduce the effects of mifepristone.

Anti-hypertensives

Concomitant use of NSAIDs with antihypertensive drugs (i.e. beta-blockers, angiotensin converting enzyme (ACE) inhibitors, diuretics) may cause a decrease in their antihypertensive effect via inhibition of vasodilatory prostaglandin synthesis.

4.6 Pregnancy and lactation

Although animal studies have not demonstrated teratogenic effects, Voltarol Rapid should not be prescribed during pregnancy, unless there are compelling reasons for doing so. The lowest effective dosage should be used.

Congenital abnormalities have been reported in association with the administration of NSAIDs in man; however, these are low in frequency and do not appear to follow any discernible pattern.

In view of the known effects of NSAIDs on the foetal cardiovascular system (e.g. a premature closure of the ductus arteriosus) and in causing uterine intertia, use in late pregnancy should be avoided.

Following oral doses of 50 mg every 8 hours, traces of active substance have been detected in breast milk, but in quantities so small that no adverse effects on the breast-fed infant are to be expected.

4.7 Effects on ability to drive and use machines

Patients who experience dizziness or other central nervous disturbances while taking NSAIDs should refrain from driving or operating machinery.

4.8 Undesirable effects

If serious side-effects occur, Voltarol Rapid should be withdrawn.

Frequency estimate:

frequent: >10 %

occasional: >1 - 10 %

rare: >0.001 - 1 %

isolated cases: <0.001 %.

Gastro-intestinal tract:

Occasional: Epigastric pain, other gastro-intestinal disorders (e.g. nausea, vomiting, diarrhoea, abdominal cramps, dyspepsia, flatulence, anorexia).

Rare: Gastro-intestinal bleeding (haematemesis, melaena, bloody diarrhoea), gastro-intestinal ulcers with or without bleeding or perforation.

In isolated cases: Aphthous stomatitis, glossitis, oesophageal lesions, lower gut disorders (e.g. non-specific haemorrhagic colitis and exacerbations of ulcerative colitis or Crohn's proctocolitis, colonic damage and stricture formation), pancreatitis, constipation.

Central nervous system:

Occasional: Headache, dizziness, vertigo.

Rare: Drowsiness, tiredness.

In isolated cases: Disturbances of sensation, paraesthesia, memory disturbance, disorientation, insomnia, irritability, convulsions, depression, anxiety, nightmares, tremor, psychotic reactions, aseptic meningitis.

Special senses:

Isolated cases: Disturbances of vision (blurred vision, diplopia), impaired hearing, tinnitus, taste disturbances.

Skin:

Occasional: Rashes or skin eruptions.

Rare: Urticaria

In isolated cases: Bullous eruptions, eczema, erythema multiforme, Stevens- Johnson syndrome, Lyell's syndrome, (acute toxic epidermolysis), erythroderma (exfoliative dermatitis), loss of hair, photosensitivity reactions, purpura including allergic purpura.

Kidney:

Rare: Oedema

In isolated cases: Acute renal insufficiency, urinary abnormalities (e.g. haematuria, proteinuria), interstitial nephritis, nephrotic syndrome, papillary necrosis.

Liver:

Occasional: Elevation of serum amino-transferase enzymes (ALT, AST).

Rare: Liver function disorders including hepatitis with or without jaundice.

In isolated cases: Fulminant hepatitis.

Blood:

In isolated cases: Thrombocytopenia, leucopenia, agranulocytosis, haemolytic anaemia, aplastic anaemia.

Hypersensitivity:

Rare: Hypersensitivity reactions (e.g. bronchospasm, anaphylactic/ anaphylactoid systemic reactions including hypotension).

Isolated cases: Vasculitis, pneumonitis.

Cardiovascular system:

Isolated cases: Palpitations, chest pain, hypertension, congestive heart failure.

Other organ systems:

Isolated cases: Impotence.

4.9 Overdose

Management of acute poisoning with NSAIDs essentially consists of supportive and symptomatic measures. There is no typical clinical picture resulting from Voltarol Rapid overdosage.

The therapeutic measures to be taken are: absorption should be prevented as soon as possible after overdosage by means of gastric lavage and treatment with activated charcoal; supportive and symptomatic treatment should be given for complications such as hypotension, renal failure, convulsions, gastro-intestinal irritation, and respiratory depression; specific therapies such as forced diuresis, dialysis or haemoperfusion are unlikely to be helpful in eliminating NSAIDs due to their high rate of protein binding and extensive metabolism.

5. PHARMACOLOGICAL PROPERTIES

5.1 Pharmacodynamic properties

Pharmacotherapeutic group: Non-steroidal anti-inflammatory drug (NSAID).

Voltarol Rapid tablets contain the potassium salt of diclofenac, a non-steroidal compound with pronounced and clinically demonstrable analgesic, anti-inflammatory and anti-pyretic properties.

Diclofenac is a potent inhibitor of prostaglandin bio-synthesis and modulator of arachidonic acid release and uptake.

Voltarol Rapid tablets have a rapid onset of action and are, therefore, suitable for the treatment of acute episodes of pain and inflammation.

In migraine attacks Voltarol Rapid has been shown to be effective in relieving the headache and in improving the accompanying symptom of nausea.

Diclofenac *in vitro* does not suppress proteoglycan biosynthesis in cartilage at concentrations equivalent to the concentrations reached in human beings.

5.2 Pharmacokinetic properties

Absorption

Diclofenac is rapidly and completely absorbed from sugar-coated tablets. Food intake does not affect absorption.

Peak plasma concentration after one 50 mg sugar-coated tablet was 3.9 μmol/l after 20-60 minutes. The plasma concentrations show a linear relationship to the size of the dose.

Diclofenac undergoes first-pass metabolism and is extensively metabolised.

Distribution

Diclofenac is highly bound to plasma proteins (99.7%), chiefly albumin (99.4%)

Elimination

The total systemic clearance of diclofenac in plasma is 263 ± 56 ml/min (mean ± SD).

The terminal half-life in plasma is 1-2 hours.

Repeated oral administration of Voltarol Rapid for 8 days in daily doses of 50 mg t i d does not lead to accumulation of diclofenac in the plasma.

Approx. 60% of the dose administered is excreted in the urine in the form of metabolites, and less than 1% as unchanged substance. The remainder of the dose is eliminated as metabolites through the bile in the faeces.

Biotransformation

The biotransformation of diclofenac involves partly glucuronidation of the intact molecule but mainly single and multiple hydroxylation followed by glucuronidation.

Characteristics in patients

The age of the patient has no influence on the absorption, metabolism, or excretion of diclofenac.

In patients suffering from renal impairment, no accumulation of the unchanged active substance can be inferred from the single-dose kinetics when applying the usual dosage schedule. At a creatinine clearance of <10 ml/min the theoretical steady-state plasma levels of metabolites are about four times higher than in normal subjects. However, the metabolites are ultimately cleared through the bile.

In the presence of impaired hepatic function (chronic hepatitis, non-decompensated cirrhosis) the kinetics and metabolism are the same as for patients without liver disease.

5.3 Preclinical safety data

Relevant information on the safety of Voltarol Rapid is included in other sections of the Summary of Product Characteristics.

6. PHARMACEUTICAL PARTICULARS

6.1 List of excipients

Voltarol Rapid Tablets 25 mg

Silica aerogel

Calcium phosphate, tribasic

Magnesium stearate

Maize starch

Povidone (Polyvinylpyrrolidone K30 PH)

Sodium Starch Glycollate (Sodium carboxymethyl starch)

Microcrystalline cellulose

Iron oxide, red 17266 (E.172)

Macrogol 8000 (Polyethylene glycol 8000)

Sucrose, cryst

Talc PH

Titanium dioxide PH (E.171)

Each tablet contains 0.0748 mmol of Potassium.

Voltarol Rapid Tablets 50mg

Silica, colloidal anhydrous (Aerosil 200)

Calcium phosphate

Magnesium stearate

Maize starch

Povidone (Polyvinylpyrrolidone K30 PH)

Sodium Starch Glycollate (Sodium carboxymethyl starch)

Cellulose, Microcrystalline (Avicel PH 101)

Iron oxide, red 17266 (E.172)

Macrogol 8000 (Polyethylene glycol 8000)

Sucrose, cryst

Talc PH

Titanium dioxide PH (E.171)

Each tablet contains 0.1496 mmol of Potassium.

6.2 Incompatibilities
None.

6.3 Shelf life
60 months.

6.4 Special precautions for storage
Store in original packaging below 30°C and protect from moisture.

6.5 Nature and contents of container
PVC/PE/PVdC blister strips containing 28 tablets.

(PVC 190-275 micron, PE20-40 micron, PVdC 32-59 micron, aluminium foil 26-34 micron)

6.6 Instructions for use and handling
Medicines should be kept out of the reach of children.

7. MARKETING AUTHORISATION HOLDER
Name or style and permanent address or registered place of business of the holder of the marketing authorisation:

Novartis Pharmaceuticals UK Ltd

Trading as Geigy Pharmaceuticals

Frimley Business Park

Frimley

Camberley

Surrey, GU16 7SR

8. MARKETING AUTHORISATION NUMBER(S)
Voltarol Rapid Tablets 25 mg - PL 00101/0481

Voltarol Rapid Tablets 50mg - PL 00101/0482

9. DATE OF FIRST AUTHORISATION/RENEWAL OF THE AUTHORISATION
17 February 1998

10. DATE OF REVISION OF THE TEXT
30 September 2002

Legal Category
POM

Voltarol Ampoules

(Novartis Pharmaceuticals UK Ltd)

1. NAME OF THE MEDICINAL PRODUCT
Voltarol® Ampoules

2. QUALITATIVE AND QUANTITATIVE COMPOSITION
The active ingredient is sodium-[o-[(2,6-dichlorophenyl)-amino]-phenyl]-acetate) (diclofenac sodium).

Each 3ml ampoule contains 75mg diclofenac sodium Ph.Eur.

3. PHARMACEUTICAL FORM
Solution for injection in ampoules.

4. CLINICAL PARTICULARS

4.1 Therapeutic indications

Ampoules for im use

The ampoules are effective in acute forms of pain, including renal colic, exacerbations of osteo- and rheumatoid arthritis, acute back pain, acute gout, acute trauma and fractures, and post-operative pain.

Ampoules used in intravenous infusion

For treatment or prevention of post-operative pain in the hospital setting.

4.2 Posology and method of administration

Adults

Voltarol Ampoules (given i.m. or i.v.) should not be given for more than two days; if necessary, treatment can be continued with Voltarol Tablets or Suppositories.

Intramuscular injection

The following directions for intramuscular injection must be adhered to in order to avoid damage to a nerve or other tissue at the injection site.

One ampoule once (or in severe cases twice) daily intramuscularly by deep intragluteal injection into the upper outer quadrant. If two injections daily are required it is advised that the alternative buttock be used for the second injection. Alternatively, one ampoule of 75mg can be combined with other dosage forms of Voltarol (Tablets or Suppositories) up to the maximum daily dosage of 150mg.

Renal colic

One 75mg ampoule intramuscularly. A further ampoule may be administered after 30 minutes if necessary. The recommended maximum daily dose of Voltarol is 150mg.

Intravenous Infusion

Immediately before initiating an intravenous infusion, Voltarol must be diluted with 100-500ml of either sodium chloride solution (0.9%) or glucose solution (5%). Both solutions should be buffered with sodium bicarbonate solution (0.5ml 8.4% or 1ml 4.2%). Only clear solutions should be used.

Voltarol must not be given as an intravenous bolus injection.

Two alternative regimens are recommended:

For the *treatment* of moderate to severe post-operative pain, 75mg should be infused continuously over a period of 30 minutes to 2 hours. If necessary, treatment may be repeated after 4-6 hours, not exceeding 150mg within any period of 24 hours.

For the *prevention* of post-operative pain, a loading dose of 25mg-50mg should be infused after surgery over 15 minutes to 1 hour, followed by a continuous infusion of approx. 5mg per hour up to a maximum daily dosage of 150mg.

Children

Voltarol ampoules are not recommended for use in children.

Elderly

Although the pharmacokinetics of Voltarol are not impaired to any clinically relevant extent in elderly patients, non-steroidal anti-inflammatory drugs should be used with particular caution in such patients who generally are more prone to adverse reactions. In particular, it is recommended that the lowest effective dosage be used in frail elderly patients or those with a low body weight (see also "Precautions") and the patient should be monitored for GI bleeding for 4 weeks following initiation of NSAID therapy.

The recommended maximum daily dose of Voltarol is 150mg.

4.3 Contraindications

Patients with a history of or active or suspected gastro-intestinal ulcers or bleeding.

Patients who have previously shown hypersensitivity reactions (e.g. asthma, urticaria or acute rhinitis) to diclofenac sodium, aspirin or other non-steroidal anti-inflammatory drugs.

Hypersensitivity to the excipients sodium metabisulphite, benzyl alcohol, propylene glycol, mannitol.

Specifically for iv use

Concomitant NSAID or anticoagulant use (including low dose heparin).

History of haemorrhagic diathesis, a history of confirmed or suspected cerebrovascular bleeding.

Operations associated with a high risk of haemorrhage.

A history of asthma.

Moderate or severe renal impairment (serum creatinine >160mol/l). Hypovolaemia or dehydration from any cause.

4.4 Special warnings and special precautions for use

Warnings

Gastro-intestinal

Close medical surveillance is imperative in patients with symptoms indicative of gastro-intestinal disorders, with a history suggestive of gastro-intestinal ulceration, with ulcerative colitis or with Crohn's disease.

Gastro-intestinal bleeding or ulcerative/perforation, haematemesis and melaena have in general more serious consequences in the elderly. They can occur at any time during treatment, with or without warning symptoms or a previous history. In the rare instances where gastro-intestinal bleeding or ulceration occurs in patients receiving Voltarol, the drug should be withdrawn.

Hepatic

Close medical surveillance is also imperative in patients suffering from severe impairment of hepatic function.

Hypersensitivity reactions

As with other non-steroidal anti-inflammatory drugs, allergic reactions, including anaphylactic/anaphylactoid reactions, can also occur without earlier exposure to the drug.

Like other NSAIDs, Voltarol may mask the signs and symptoms of infection due to its pharmacodynamic properties.

Precautions

Renal

Patients with renal, cardiac or hepatic impairment and the elderly should be kept under surveillance, since the use of NSAIDS may result in deterioration of renal function. The lowest effective dose should be used and renal function monitored.

The importance of prostaglandins in maintaining renal blood flow should be taken into account in patients with impaired cardiac or renal function, those being treated with diuretics or recovering from major surgery. Effects on renal function are usually reversible on withdrawal of Voltarol.

Hepatic

If abnormal liver function tests persist or worsen, clinical signs or symptoms consistent with liver disease develop or if other manifestations occur (eosinophilia, rash), Voltarol should be discontinued. Hepatitis may occur without prodromal symptoms.

Use of Voltarol in patients with hepatic porphyria may trigger an attack.

Haematological

Voltarol may reversibly inhibit platelet aggregation (see anticoagulants in "Drug Interactions"). Patients with defects of haemostasis, bleeding diathesis or haematological abnormalities should be carefully monitored.

Long-term treatment

All patients who are receiving non-steroidal anti-inflammatory agents should be monitored as a precautionary measure e.g. renal function, hepatic function (elevation of liver enzymes may occur) and blood counts. This is particularly important in the elderly.

Like other drugs that inhibit prostaglandin synthetase activity, diclofenac sodium and other NSAIDs can precipitate bronchospasm if administered to patients suffering from, or with a previous history of, bronchial asthma.

Caution is required in patients with a history of heart failure or hypertension since oedema has been reported in association with NSAID administration.

4.5 Interaction with other medicinal products and other forms of Interaction

Lithium and digoxin

Voltarol may increase plasma concentrations of lithium and digoxin.

Anticoagulants

Although clinical investigations do not appear to indicate that Voltarol has an influence on the effect of anticoagulants, there are isolated reports of an increased risk of haemorrhage with the combined use of diclofenac and anticoagulant therapy. Therefore, to be certain that no change in anticoagulant dosage is required, close monitoring of such patients is required. As with other non-steroidal anti-inflammatory agents, diclofenac in a high dose can reversibly inhibit platelet aggregation.

Antidiabetic agents

Clinical studies have shown that Voltarol can be given together with oral antidiabetic agents without influencing their clinical effect. However, there have been isolated reports of hypoglycaemic and hyperglycaemic effects which have required adjustment to the dosage of hypoglycaemic agents.

Cyclosporin

Cases of nephrotoxicity have been reported in patients receiving concomitant cyclosporin and NSAIDS, including Voltarol. This might be mediated through combined renal antiprostaglandin effects of both the NSAID and cyclosporin.

Methotrexate

Cases of serious toxicity have been reported when methotrexate and NSAIDS are given within 24 hours of each other. This interaction is mediated through accumulation of methotrexate resulting from impairment of renal excretion in the presence of the NSAID.

Quinolone antimicrobials

Convulsions may occur due to an interaction between quinolones and NSAIDS. This may occur in patients with or without a previous history of epilepsy or convulsions. Therefore, caution should be exercised when considering the use of a quinolone in patients who are already receiving an NSAID.

Other NSAIDS and corticosteroids

Co-administration of Voltarol with aspirin or corticosteroids may increase the risk of gastro-intestinal bleeding. Avoid concomitant use of two or more NSAIDs.

Diuretics

Like other NSAIDS, Voltarol may inhibit the activity of diuretics. Concomitant treatment with potassium-sparing diuretics may be associated with increased serum potassium levels, which should therefore be monitored frequently.

Cardiac glycosides

Concomitant use of cardiac glycosides and NSAIDs in patients may exacerbate cardiac failure, reduce GFR and increase plasma glycoside levels.

Mifepristone

NSAIDs should not be used for 8-12 days after mifepristone administration as NSAIDs can reduce the effect of mifepristone.

Anti-hypertensives

Concomitant use of NSAIDs with antihypertensive drugs (i.e. beta-blockers, angiotensin converting enzyme (ACE) inhibitors, diuretics) may cause a decrease in their antihypertensive effect via inhibition of vasodilatory prostaglandin synthesis.

4.6 Pregnancy and lactation

Although animal studies have not demonstrated teratogenic effects, Voltarol should not be prescribed during pregnancy, unless there are compelling reasons for doing so. The lowest effective dosage should be used.

Congenital abnormalities have been reported in association with the administration of NSAIDs in man, however, these are low in frequency and do not appear to follow any discernible pattern.

In view of the known effects of NSAIDs on the foetal cardiovascular system (e.g. a premature closure of the ductus arteriosus) and in causing uterine inertia, use in late pregnancy should be avoided.

Following doses of 50mg enteric coated tablets every 8 hours, traces of active substance have been detected in breast milk, but in quantities so small that no adverse effects on the breast-fed infant are to be expected.

4.7 Effects on ability to drive and use machines

Patients who experience dizziness or other central nervous disturbances, while taking NSAIDS should refrain from driving or operating machinery.

4.8 Undesirable effects

If serious side-effects occur, Voltarol should be withdrawn.

Frequency estimate:

frequent: > 10 %

occasional: > 1 - 10 %

rare: > 0.001 - 1 %

isolated cases: < 0.001 %.

Gastro-intestinal tract

Occasional: Epigastric pain, other gastro-intestinal disorders (e.g. nausea, vomiting, diarrhoea, abdominal cramps, dyspepsia, flatulence, anorexia).

Rare: Gastro-intestinal bleeding (haematemesis, melaena, bloody diarrhoea), gastro-intestinal ulcers with or without bleeding or perforation.

In isolated cases: Aphthous stomatitis, glossitis, oesophageal lesions, lower gut disorders (e.g. non-specific haemorrhagic colitis and exacerbations of ulcerative colitis or Crohn's proctocolitis, colonic damage and stricture formation), pancreatitis, constipation.

Central Nervous System

Occasional: Headache, dizziness, or vertigo.

Rare: Drowsiness, tiredness.

In isolated cases: Disturbances of sensation, paraesthesia, memory disturbance, disorientation, insomnia, irritability, convulsions, depression, anxiety, nightmares, tremor, psychotic reactions, aseptic meningitis.

Special senses

Isolated cases: Disturbances of vision (blurred vision, diplopia), impaired hearing, tinnitus, taste disturbances.

Skin

Occasional: Rashes or skin eruptions.

Rare: Urticaria.

In isolated cases: Bullous eruptions, eczema, erythema multiforme, Stevens-Johnson syndrome, Lyell's syndrome, (acute toxic epidermolysis), erythroderma (exfoliative dermatitis), loss of hair, photosensitivity reactions, purpura including allergic purpura.

Kidney

Rare: Oedema

In isolated cases: Acute renal insufficiency, urinary abnormalities (e.g. haematuria, proteinuria), interstitial nephritis, nephrotic syndrome, papillary necrosis.

Liver

Occasional: Elevation of serum aminotransferase enzymes (ALT, AST).

Rare: Liver function disorders including hepatitis (in isolated cases fulminant) with or without jaundice.

Blood

In isolated cases: Thrombocytopenia, leucopenia, agranulocytosis, haemolytic anaemia, aplastic anaemia.

Hypersensitivity

Rare: Hypersensitivity reactions (e.g. bronchospasm, anaphylactic/anaphylactoid systemic reactions including hypotension).

Isolated cases: Vasculitis, pneumonitis.

Cardiovascular system

Isolated cases: Palpitations, chest pain, hypertension, congestive heart failure.

Other organ systems

Isolated cases: Impotence.

Reactions to the intramuscular injection

Occasional: Reactions such as local pain and induration.

Isolated cases: Abscesses and local necrosis at the intramuscular injection site.

4.9 Overdose

Management of acute poisoning with NSAIDS essentially consists of supportive and symptomatic measures. There is no typical clinical picture resulting from Voltarol overdosage.

Supportive and symptomatic treatment should be given for complications such as hypotension, renal failure, convulsions, gastro-intestinal irritation and respiratory depression.

Specific therapies such as forced diuresis, dialysis or haemoperfusion are probably of no help in eliminating NSAIDS due to their high rate of protein binding and extensive metabolism.

5. PHARMACOLOGICAL PROPERTIES

5.1 Pharmacodynamic properties

Pharmacotherapeutic group

Non-steroidal anti-inflammatory drugs (NSAIDs).

Mechanism of action

Voltarol is a non-steroidal agent with marked analgesic/anti-inflammatory properties. It is an inhibitor of prostaglandin synthetase, (cyclo-oxygenase). Diclofenac sodium *in vitro* does not suppress proteoglycan biosynthesis in cartilage at concentrations equivalent to the concentrations reached in human beings. When used concomitantly with opioids for the management of post-operative pain, Voltarol often reduces the need for opioids.

5.2 Pharmacokinetic properties

Absorption

After administration of 75mg diclofenac by intramuscular injection, absorption sets in immediately, and mean peak plasma concentrations of about 2.558 ± 0.968μg/ml (2.5μg/mL 8μmol/L) are reached after about 20 minutes. The amount absorbed is in linear proportion to the size of the dose.

Intravenous infusion

When 75mg diclofenac is administered as an intravenous infusion over 2 hours, mean peak plasma concentrations are about 1.875 ± 0.436μg/ml (1.9μg/mL 5.9μmol/L). Shorter infusions result in higher peak plasma concentrations, while longer infusions give plateau concentrations proportional to the infusion rate after 3 to 4 hours. This is in contrast to the rapid decline in plasma concentrations seen after peak levels have been achieved with oral, rectal or i.m. administration.

Bioavailability:

The area under the concentration curve (AUC) after intramuscular or intravenous administration is about twice as large as it is following oral or rectal administration as this route avoids "first-pass" metabolism.

Distribution

The active substance is 99.7% protein bound, mainly to albumin (99.4%).

Diclofenac enters the synovial fluid, where maximum concentrations are measured 2-4 hours after the peak plasma values have been attained. The apparent half-life for elimination from the synovial fluid is 3-6 hours. Two hours after reaching the peak plasma values, concentrations of the active substance are already higher in the synovial fluid than they are in the plasma and remain higher for up to 12 hours.

Metabolism

Biotransformation of diclofenac takes place partly by glucuronidation of the intact molecule, but mainly by single and multiple hydroxylation and methoxylation, resulting in several phenolic metabolites, most of which are converted to glucuronide conjugates. Two phenolic metabolites are biologically active, but to a much lesser extent than diclofenac.

Elimination

Total systemic clearance of diclofenac in plasma is 263 ± 56 mL/min (mean value ± SD). The terminal half-life in plasma is 1-2 hours. Four of the metabolites, including the two active ones, also have short plasma half-lives of 1-3 hours.

About 60% of the administered dose is excreted in the urine in the form of the glucuronide conjugate of the intact molecule and as metabolites, most of which are also converted to glucuronide conjugates. Less than 1% is excreted as unchanged substance. The rest of the dose is eliminated as metabolites through the bile in the faeces.

Characteristics in patients

Elderly

No relevant age-dependent differences in the drug's absorption, metabolism or excretion have been observed, other than the finding that in five elderly patients, a 15 minute i.v. infusion resulted in 50% higher plasma concentrations than expected with young healthy subjects.

Patients with renal impairment

In patients suffering from renal impairment, no accumulation of the unchanged active substance can be inferred from the single-dose kinetics when applying the usual dosage schedule. At a creatinine clearance of <10 mL/min, the calculated steady-state plasma levels of the hydroxy metabolites are about 4 times higher than in normal subjects. However, the metabolites are ultimately cleared through the bile.

Patients with hepatic disease

In patients with chronic hepatitis or non-decompensated cirrhosis, the kinetics and metabolism of diclofenac are the same as in patients without liver disease.

5.3 Preclinical safety data

None stated.

6. PHARMACEUTICAL PARTICULARS

6.1 List of excipients

Voltarol Ampoules also contain:

- Mannitol
- Sodium metabisulphite (E223)
- Benzyl alcohol
- Propylene glycol
- Sodium hydroxide
- Water.

6.2 Incompatibilities

The ampoules used i.m. or i.v. as an infusion should not be mixed with other injection solutions.

6.3 Shelf life

Two years.

6.4 Special precautions for storage

Protect from light and heat (store below 30 ° C).

Medicines should be kept out of the reach of children.

The infusion solution should not be used if crystals or precipitates are observed.

6.5 Nature and contents of container

The glass ampoules (Ph.Eur. Type I) contain colourless to faintly yellow liquid and come in packs of 10.

6.6 Instructions for use and handling

Intravenous infusions should be freshly made up and used immediately. Once prepared, the infusion should not be stored.

7. MARKETING AUTHORISATION HOLDER

Novartis Pharmaceuticals UK Ltd.,

Trading as Geigy Pharmaceuticals,

Frimley Business Park

Frimley

Camberley

Surrey

GU16 7SR.

8. MARKETING AUTHORISATION NUMBER(S)

PL 00101/0466

9. DATE OF FIRST AUTHORISATION/RENEWAL OF THE AUTHORISATION

11 July 1997

10. DATE OF REVISION OF THE TEXT

8 December 2000

LEGAL CATEGORY

POM

Voltarol Dispersible Tablets 50mg

(Novartis Pharmaceuticals UK Ltd)

1. NAME OF THE MEDICINAL PRODUCT

Voltarol® Dispersible Tablets 50mg

2. QUALITATIVE AND QUANTITATIVE COMPOSITION

The active ingredient is o-[(2,6-dichlorophenyl)amino]phenylacetic acid (diclofenac).

Each tablet contains 46.5mg of diclofenac free acid, which is equivalent to 50mg of diclofenac sodium.

3. PHARMACEUTICAL FORM

The tablets are pink, speckled with white, triangular shaped, uncoated, impressed GEIGY on one side with an embossed "V" on the other, with a blackcurrant odour.

4. CLINICAL PARTICULARS

4.1 Therapeutic indications

Adults and Elderly

The rapid onset of absorption of diclofenac from Voltarol Dispersible makes this preparation more suitable for short-term use in acute conditions for which treatment is required for no more than 3 months including: acute episodes of arthritic conditions, acute musculo-skeletal disorders and acute pain resulting from trauma.

There is no information on the use of Voltarol Dispersible for more than 3 months.

4.2 Posology and method of administration

Adults

100-150mg daily in two or three divided doses. The Voltarol Dispersible Tablet should be dropped into a glass of water, and the liquid stirred to aid dispersion, before swallowing.

The recommended maximum daily dose of Voltarol is 150mg.

Children

Not recommended.

Elderly

Although the pharmacokinetics of Voltarol are not impaired to any clinically relevant extent in elderly patients, non-steroidal anti-inflammatory drugs should be used with particular caution in such patients who generally are more prone to adverse reactions. In particular it is recommended that the lowest effective dosage be used in frail elderly patients or those with a low body weight (see also precautions) and the patient should be monitored for GI bleeding for 4 weeks following initiation of NSAID therapy.

4.3 Contraindications

Patients with a history of or active or suspected gastro-intestinal ulcers or bleeding.

Patients who have previously shown hypersensitivity reactions (e.g. asthma, urticaria or acute rhinitis) to diclofenac sodium, aspirin or other non-steroidal anti-inflammatory drugs.

4.4 Special warnings and special precautions for use

Warnings

Gastro-intestinal

Close medical surveillance is imperative in patients with symptoms indicative of gastro-intestinal disorders, with a history suggestive of gastro-intestinal ulceration, with ulcerative colitis, or with Crohn's disease.

Gastro-intestinal bleeding or ulcerative/perforation, haematemesis and melaena have, in general, more serious consequences in the elderly. They can occur at any time during treatment, with or without warning symptoms or a previous history. In the rare instances when gastro-intestinal bleeding or ulceration occurs in patients receiving Voltarol, the drug should be withdrawn.

In choosing to prescribe Voltarol Dispersible it should be remembered that any liquid NSAID preparation does not have the advantages of an enteric-coated tablet in relation to gastric tolerability. In clinical trials of three months duration, a slight increase in the frequency and reported severity of G.I. side-effects and higher rates of withdrawal because of these have been noted in patients receiving dispersible tablets compared with those receiving enteric-coated tablets.

An endoscopy study also revealed Voltarol Dispersible to have a slightly higher mucosal injury score than enteric-coated tablets, although no ulcers occurred with either treatment. These observations must be taken into account and weighed against the advantages of the dispersible formulation.

Hepatic

Close medical surveillance is also imperative in patients suffering from severe impairment of hepatic function.

Hypersensitivity reactions

As with other non-steroidal anti-inflammatory drugs, allergic reactions, including anaphylactic/anaphylactoid reactions, can also occur without earlier exposure to the drug.

Like other NSAIDs, Voltarol may mask the signs and symptoms of infection due to its pharmacodynamic properties.

Precautions

Renal

Patients with renal, cardiac or hepatic impairment and the elderly should be kept under surveillance, since the use of NSAIDS may result in deterioration of renal function. The lowest effective dose should be used and renal function monitored.

The importance of prostaglandins in maintaining renal blood flow should be taken into account in patients with impaired cardiac or renal function, those being treated with diuretics or recovering from major surgery. Effects on renal function are usually reversible on withdrawal of Voltarol.

Hepatic

If abnormal liver function tests persist or worsen, clinical signs or symptoms consistent with liver disease develop or if other manifestations occur (eosinophilia, rash), Voltarol should be discontinued. Hepatitis may occur without prodromal symptoms.

Use of Voltarol in patients with hepatic porphyria may trigger an attack.

Haematological

Voltarol may reversibly inhibit platelet aggregation (see anticoagulants in "Drug Interactions"). Patients with defects of haemostasis, bleeding diathesis or haematological abnormalities should be carefully monitored.

Long-term treatment

All patients who are receiving non-steroidal anti-inflammatory agents should be monitored as a precautionary measure e.g. renal function, hepatic function (elevation of liver enzymes may occur) and blood counts. This is particularly important in the elderly.

Like other drugs that inhibit prostaglandin synthetase activity, diclofenac sodium and other NSAIDs can precipitate bronchospasm if administered to patients suffering from, or with a previous history of, bronchial asthma.

Caution is required in patients with a history of heart failure or hypertension since oedema has been reported in association with NSAID administration.

4.5 Interaction with other medicinal products and other forms of Interaction

Lithium and digoxin

Voltarol may increase plasma concentrations of lithium and digoxin.

Anticoagulants

Although clinical investigations do not appear to indicate that Voltarol has an influence on the effect of anticoagulants, there are isolated reports of an increased risk of haemorrhage with the combined use of diclofenac and anticoagulant therapy. Therefore, to be certain that no change in anticoagulant dosage is required, close monitoring of such patients is required. As with other non-steroidal anti-inflammatory agents, diclofenac in high dose can reversibly inhibit platelet aggregation.

Antidiabetic agents

Clinical studies have shown that Voltarol can be given together with oral antidiabetic agents without influencing their clinical effect. However, there have been isolated reports of hypoglycaemic and hyperglycaemic effects which have required adjustment to the dosage of hypoglycaemic agents.

Cyclosporin

Cases of nephrotoxicity have been reported in patients receiving concomitant cyclosporin and NSAIDS, including Voltarol. This might be mediated through combined renal antiprostaglandin effects of both the NSAID and cyclosporin.

Methotrexate

Cases of serious toxicity have been reported when methotrexate and NSAIDS are given within 24 hours of each other. This interaction is mediated through accumulation of methotrexate resulting from impairment of renal excretion in the presence of the NSAID.

Quinolone antimicrobials

Convulsions may occur due to an interaction between quinolones and NSAIDS. This may occur in patients with or without a previous history of epilepsy or convulsions. Therefore, caution should be exercised when considering the use of a quinolone in patients who are already receiving an NSAID.

Other NSAIDs and corticosteroids

Co-administration of Voltarol with aspirin or corticosteroids may increase the risk of gastro-intestinal bleeding. Avoid concomitant use of two or more NSAIDs.

Diuretics

Like other NSAIDs, Voltarol may inhibit the activity of diuretics. Concomitant treatment with potassium-sparing diuretics may be associated with increased serum potassium levels, which should therefore be monitored frequently.

Cardiac glycosides

Concomitant use of cardiac glycosides and NSAIDs in patients may exacerbate cardiac failure, reduce GFR and increase plasma glycoside levels.

Mifepristone

NSAIDs should not be used for 8-12 days after mifepristone administration as NSAIDs can reduce the effect of mifepristone.

Anti-hypertensives

Concomitant use of NSAIDs with antihypertensive drugs (i.e. beta-blockers, angiotensin converting enzyme (ACE) inhibitors, diuretics) may cause a decrease in their antihypertensive effect via inhibition of vasodilatory prostaglandin synthesis.

4.6 Pregnancy and lactation

Although animal studies have not demonstrated teratogenic effects, Voltarol should not be prescribed during pregnancy, unless there are compelling reasons for doing so. The lowest effective dosage should be used.

Congenital abnormalities have been reported in association with the administration of NSAIDs in man, however, these are low in frequency and do not appear to follow any discernible pattern.

In view of the known effects of NSAIDs on the foetal cardiovascular system (e.g. a premature closure of the ductus arteriosus), use in late pregnancy should be avoided.

Following doses of 50mg enteric coated tablets every 8 hours, traces of active substance have been detected in breast milk, but in quantities so small that no adverse effects on the breast-fed infant are to be expected.

4.7 Effects on ability to drive and use machines

Patients who experience dizziness or other central nervous disturbances while taking NSAIDS should refrain from driving or operating machinery.

4.8 Undesirable effects

If serious side-effects occur, Voltarol should be withdrawn.

Frequency estimate:

frequent: $>$ 10 %

occasional: $>$ 1 - 10 %

rare: $>$ 0.001 - 1 %

isolated cases: $<$ 0.001 %.

Gastro-intestinal tract

Occasional: Epigastric pain, other gastro-intestinal disorders (e.g. nausea, vomiting, diarrhoea, abdominal cramps, dyspepsia, flatulence, anorexia).

Rare: Gastro-intestinal bleeding (haematemesis, melaena, bloody diarrhoea), gastro-intestinal ulcers with or without bleeding or perforation.

In isolated cases: Aphthous stomatitis, glossitis, oesophageal lesions, lower gut disorders (e.g. non-specific haemorrhagic colitis and exacerbations of ulcerative colitis or Crohn's proctocolitis, colonic damage and stricture formation), pancreatitis, constipation.

Central Nervous System

Occasional: Headache, dizziness or vertigo.

Rare: Drowsiness, tiredness.

In isolated cases: Disturbances of sensation, paraesthesia, memory disturbance, disorientation, insomnia, irritability, convulsions, depression, anxiety, nightmares, tremor, psychotic reactions, aseptic meningitis.

Special senses

Isolated cases: Disturbances of vision (blurred vision, diplopia), impaired hearing, tinnitus, taste disturbances.

Skin

Occasional: Rashes or skin eruptions.

Rare: Urticaria.

In isolated cases: Bullous eruptions, eczema, erythema multiforme, Stevens-Johnson syndrome, Lyell's syndrome, (acute toxic epidermolysis), erythroderma (exfoliative dermatitis), loss of hair, photosensitivity reactions, purpura including allergic purpura.

Kidney

Rare: Oedema.

In isolated cases: Acute renal insufficiency, urinary abnormalities (e.g. haematuria, proteinuria), interstitial nephritis, nephrotic syndrome, papillary necrosis.

Liver

Occasional: Elevation of serum aminotransferase enzymes (ALT, AST).

Rare: Liver function disorders including hepatitis (in isolated cases fulminant) with or without jaundice.

Blood

In isolated cases: Thrombocytopenia, leucopenia, agranulocytosis, haemolytic anaemia, aplastic anaemia.

Hypersensitivity

Rare: Hypersensitivity reactions (e.g. bronchospasm, anaphylactic/anaphylactoid systemic reactions including hypotension).

Isolated cases: Vasculitis, pneumonitis.

Cardiovascular system

Isolated cases: Palpitations, chest pain, hypertension, congestive heart failure.

Other organ systems

Isolated cases: Impotence.

4.9 Overdose

Management of acute poisoning with NSAIDS essentially consists of supportive and symptomatic measures. There is no typical clinical picture resulting from Voltarol overdosage.

The therapeutic measures to be taken are: Supportive and symptomatic treatment should be given for complications such as hypotension, renal failure, convulsions, gastro-intestinal irritation, and respiratory depression; special therapies such as forced diuresis, dialysis or haemoperfusion are probably of no help in eliminating NSAIDS due to their high rate of protein binding and extensive metabolism.

5. PHARMACOLOGICAL PROPERTIES

5.1 Pharmacodynamic properties

Pharmacotherapeutic group

Non-steroidal anti-inflammatory drugs (NSAIDs).

Mechanism of action

Voltarol is a non-steroidal agent with marked analgesic/anti-inflammatory properties. It is an inhibitor of prostaglandin synthetase, (cyclo-oxygenase).

Diclofenac sodium *in vitro* does not suppress proteoglycan biosynthesis in cartilage at concentrations equivalent to the concentrations reached in human beings.

5.2 Pharmacokinetic properties

Absorption

Absorption begins immediately upon administration. Mean peak plasma concentrations of diclofenac are reached at about 1 hour 0.9 ± 0.4μg/ml (1μg/mL 3μmol/L. Ingestion of dispersible tablets together with or immediately after a meal does not delay the onset of absorption but reduces the amount absorbed by on average of about 16% and the maximum concentrations by about 50%.

Bioavailability:

The bioavailability is 82% of that of enteric-coated tablets. Ingestion with food affects the bioavailability (see above).

Pharmacokinetic behaviour does not change on repeated administration. Accumulation does not occur, provided the recommended dosage intervals are observed.

Distribution

The active substance is 99.7% protein bound, mainly to albumin (99.4%).

Diclofenac enters the synovial fluid, where maximum concentrations are measured 2-4 hours after the peak plasma values have been attained. The apparent half-life for elimination from the synovial fluid is 3-6 hours. Two hours after reaching the peak plasma values, concentrations of the active substance are already higher in the synovial fluid than they are in the plasma and they remain higher for up to 12 hours.

Metabolism

Biotransformation of diclofenac takes place partly by glucuronidation of the intact molecule, but mainly by single and multiple hydroxylation and methoxylation, resulting in several phenolic metabolites, most of which are converted to glucuronide conjugates. Two phenolic metabolites are biologically active, but to a much lesser extent than diclofenac.

Elimination

The total systemic clearance of diclofenac in plasma is 263 ± 56 mL/min (mean value ± SD). The terminal half-life in plasma is 1-2 hours. Four of the metabolites, including the two active ones, also have short plasma half-lives of 1-3 hours.

About 60% of the administered dose is excreted in the urine in the form of the glucuronide conjugate of the intact molecule and as metabolites, most of which are also converted to glucuronide conjugates. Less than 1% is excreted as unchanged substance. The rest of the dose is eliminated as metabolites through the bile in the faeces.

Characteristics in patients

Elderly

No relevant age-dependent differences in the drug's absorption, metabolism, or excretion have been observed, other than the finding that in five elderly patients, a 15 minute i.v. infusion resulted in 50% higher plasma concentrations than expected with young healthy subjects.

Patients with renal impairment

In patients suffering from renal impairment, no accumulation of the unchanged active substance can be inferred from the single-dose kinetics when applying the usual dosage schedule. At a creatinine clearance of <10 mL/min, the calculated steady-state plasma levels of the hydroxy metabolites are about 4 times higher than in normal subjects. However, the metabolites are ultimately cleared through the bile.

Patients with hepatic disease

In patients with chronic hepatitis or non-decompensated cirrhosis, the kinetics and metabolism of diclofenac are the same as in patients without liver disease.

5.3 Preclinical safety data

None stated.

6. PHARMACEUTICAL PARTICULARS

6.1 List of excipients

The dispersible tablets also contain:

- Avicel PH 101
- Croscarmellose sodium type A
- Sodium starch glycollate
- Sodium saccharin
- Hydrogenated caster oil
- Purified talc special
- Aerosil 200 standard
- Blackcurrant and F.D. and C. red No. 3.

6.2 Incompatibilities

None known.

6.3 Shelf life

Five years.

6.4 Special precautions for storage

6.5 Nature and contents of container

Protect from heat (store below 30°C) and moisture.

Medicines should be kept out of the reach of children.

6.6 Instructions for use and handling

The dispersible tablets should be dissolved in water.

7. MARKETING AUTHORISATION HOLDER

Novartis Pharmaceuticals UK Ltd.

Trading as Geigy Pharmaceuticals,

Frimley Business Park

Frimley

Camberley

Surrey

GU16 7SR.

8. MARKETING AUTHORISATION NUMBER(S)

PL 00101/0467

9. DATE OF FIRST AUTHORISATION/RENEWAL OF THE AUTHORISATION

11 July 1997

10. DATE OF REVISION OF THE TEXT

8 December 2000

LEGAL CATEGORY

POM

Voltarol Emulgel

(Novartis Pharmaceuticals UK Ltd)

1. NAME OF THE MEDICINAL PRODUCT

Voltarol® Emulgel

2. QUALITATIVE AND QUANTITATIVE COMPOSITION

Diethylammonium-{-o-[2,6-dichlorophenyl)-amino]-phenyl}-acetate.

100g of Voltarol Emulgel contains 1.16g of the active substance diclofenac diethylammonium, which corresponds to 1g diclofenac sodium.

3. PHARMACEUTICAL FORM

Gel for topical administration.

4. CLINICAL PARTICULARS

4.1 Therapeutic indications

For the local symptomatic relief of pain and inflammation in:

- trauma of the tendons, ligaments, muscles and joints, e.g. due to sprains, strains and bruises

- localised forms of soft tissue rheumatism

It is recommended that treatment be reviewed after 14 days in these indications.

For the treatment of osteoarthritis of superficial joints such as the knee.

In the treatment of osteoarthritis, therapy should be reviewed after 4 weeks.

4.2 Posology and method of administration

Adults:

Voltarol Emulgel should be rubbed gently into the skin. Depending on the size of the affected site to be treated 2-4g (a circular shaped mass approximately 2.0-2.5cm in diameter) should be applied 3 - 4 times a daily. After application, the hands should be washed unless they are the site being treated.

Use in the elderly:

The usual adult dosage may be used.

Children:

Voltarol Emulgel is not recommended for use in children as dosage recommendations and indications for use in this group of patients have not been established.

Voltarol Emulgel is suitable for the transmission of ultrasound and may be used as a couplant in combination with ultrasound therapy. If large areas of the body are covered with gel, systemic absorption will be greater and the risk of side-effects increased, especially if the therapy is used frequently.

4.3 Contraindications

Patients with or without chronic asthma in whom attacks of asthma, urticaria or acute rhinitis are precipitated by aspirin or other non-steroidal anti-inflammatory agents. Hypersensitivity to diclofenac, acetylsalicylic acid or other non-steroidal anti-inflammatory drugs. Hypersensitivity to propylene glycol, isopropanol or other components of the gel base.

4.4 Special warnings and special precautions for use

4.4.1. Warnings

None stated.

4.4.2. Precautions

Concomitant use of oral NSAID's should be cautioned as the incidence of untoward effects, particularly systemic side effects, may increase. (See also 'Interactions')

Voltarol Emulgel should not be co-administered with other products containing diclofenac.

Voltarol Emulgel should be applied only to intact, non-diseased skin and not to skin wounds or open injuries. It should be not be used with occlusion. It should not be allowed to come into contact with the eyes or mucous membranes, and should never be taken by mouth.

Some possibility of gastro-intestinal bleeding in those with a significant history of this condition has been reported in isolated cases.

4.5 Interaction with other medicinal products and other forms of Interaction

Systemic absorption of Voltarol Emulgel is low and hence the risk of an interaction is small. There are no known interactions with Voltarol Emulgel but for a list of interactions known with oral diclofenac the data sheet for oral dosage forms should be consulted.

4.6 Pregnancy and lactation

Since no experience has been acquired with Voltarol Emulgel in pregnancy or lactation, it is not recommended for use in these circumstances.

During the last trimester of pregnancy the use of prostaglandin synthetase inhibitors may result in premature closure of the ductus arteriosus, or in uterine inertia.

Animal data has shown an increased incidence of dystonia and delayed parturition when drug administration is continued into late pregnancy.

4.7 Effects on ability to drive and use machines

None known.

4.8 Undesirable effects

Local reactions:

Voltarol Emulgel is usually well tolerated.

Occasional: allergic or non-allergic contact dermatitis (with symptoms and signs such as itching, reddening, oedema, papules, vesicles, bullae or scaling of skin).

Systemic reactions:

Isolated cases: generalised skin rash, hypersensitivity reactions (e.g. asthmatic attacks, angio-oedema), photosensitivity reactions.

Patients should be warned against excessive exposure to sunlight in order to reduce the incidence of photosensitivity.

General: Systemic absorption of Voltarol Emulgel is low compared with plasma levels obtained following administration of oral forms of Voltarol and the likelihood of systemic side-effects occurring with topical diclofenac is small compared with the frequency of side-effects associated with oral diclofenac. However, where Voltarol Emulgel is applied to a relatively large area of skin and over a prolonged period, the possibility of systemic side-effects cannot be completely excluded. If such usage is envisaged, the data sheet on Voltarol oral dosage forms should be consulted.

Asthma has been rarely reported in patients using topical NSAID preparations.

4.9 Overdose

Signs and symptoms

The low systemic absorption of Voltarol Emulgel renders overdosage extremely unlikely. In the event of accidental ingestion, resulting in significant systemic side-effects, general therapeutic measures normally adopted to treat poisoning with non-steroidal anti-inflammatory drugs should be used.

Treatment

Management of overdosage with NSAIDs essentially consists of supportive and symptomatic measures. There is no typical clinical picture resulting from Voltarol overdosage. Supportive and symptomatic treatment should be given for complications such as hypotension, renal failure, convulsions, gastro-intestinal irritation, and respiratory depression; specific therapies such as forced diuresis, dialysis or haemoperfusion are probably of no help in eliminating NSAIDs due to their high rate of protein binding and extensive metabolism.

5. PHARMACOLOGICAL PROPERTIES

5.1 Pharmacodynamic properties

Voltarol Emulgel is a non-steroidal anti-inflammatory (NSAID) and analgesic preparation designed for external application. Due to an aqueous-alcoholic base the gel exerts a soothing and cooling effect.

5.2 Pharmacokinetic properties

When Voltarol Emulgel is applied locally, the active substance is absorbed through the skin. In healthy volunteers approximately 6% of the dose applied is absorbed, as determined by urinary excretion of diclofenac and its hydroxylated metabolites. Findings in patients confirm that diclofenac penetrates inflamed areas following local application of Voltarol Emulgel.

After topical administration of Voltarol Emulgel to hand and knee joints diclofenac can be measured in plasma, synovial tissue and synovial fluid. Maximum plasma concentrations of diclofenac are about 100 times lower than after oral administration of Voltarol.

5.3 Preclinical safety data

None known.

6. PHARMACEUTICAL PARTICULARS

6.1 List of excipients

Diethylamine, carbomer, macrogol cetostearyl ether, cocyl caprylocaprate, isopropyl alcohol, liquid paraffin heavy, perfume creme 45, propylene glycol dist., and water.

6.2 Incompatibilities

None known.

6.3 Shelf life

Three years.

6.4 Special precautions for storage

Protect from heat (store below 30°C).

Voltarol Emulgel should be kept out of reach of children.

6.5 Nature and contents of container

Aluminium tubes with protective inner coating, available in packs of 20g and 100g

6.6 Instructions for use and handling

None

7. MARKETING AUTHORISATION HOLDER

Novartis Pharmaceuticals UK Ltd.

Trading as:

Geigy Pharmaceuticals

Frimley Business Park

Frimley

Surrey

GU16 7SR

8. MARKETING AUTHORISATION NUMBER(S)

PL 00101/0468

9. DATE OF FIRST AUTHORISATION/RENEWAL OF THE AUTHORISATION

11 July 1997

10. DATE OF REVISION OF THE TEXT

5 June 2001

Legal Category
POM

Voltarol Gel Patch

(Novartis Consumer Health)

1. NAME OF THE MEDICINAL PRODUCT
Voltarol Gel Patch 1%, medicated plaster

2. QUALITATIVE AND QUANTITATIVE COMPOSITION
Each 100 grams of gel contains diclofenac epolamine corresponding to 1 g of diclofenac sodium (1% w/w).

Each 10 cm × 14 cm plaster contains 14 g of gel.

For excipients, see 6.1.

3. PHARMACEUTICAL FORM
Medicated plaster.

White to pale yellow paste spread as a uniform layer onto unwoven cloth.

4. CLINICAL PARTICULARS
4.1 Therapeutic indications
Local symptomatic treatment of pain in epicondylitis and ankle sprain.

4.2 Posology and method of administration
Cutaneous use only

Posology

Adults

- Treatment of ankle sprains: 1 application a day

- Treatment of epicondylitis: 1 application morning and evening.

- Duration of administration

Voltarol Gel Patch is to be used for as short as possible depending on the indication:

- Treatment of ankle sprains: 3 days

- Treatment of epicondylitis: max. 14 days.

If there is no improvement, during the recommended duration of treatment, a doctor should be consulted.

Elderly

This medication should be used with caution in elderly patients who are more prone to adverse events. See also Section 4.4.

Children

Since no specific study has been performed, the use of Voltarol Gel Patch in children under 15 years old is not recommended.

Patients with hepatic or renal insufficiency

For the use of Voltarol Gel Patch in patients with hepatic or renal insufficiency see section

Method of administration

Cut the envelope containing the medicated plaster as indicated. Remove one medicated plaster, remove the plastic film used to protect the adhesive surface and apply it to painful joint or region. If necessary it can be held in place with an elastic net. Carefully reseal the envelope with the sliding closure.

The plaster should be used whole.

4.3 Contraindications
This medicinal product is contraindicated in the following cases:

- Hypersensitivity to diclofenac, acetylsalysilic acid or other non-steroidal anti-inflammatory drugs (NSAIDs) or any excipients of the finished medicinal product.

- damaged skin, whatever the lesion involved: exudative dermatitis, eczema, infected lesion, burn or wound.

- from the beginning of the 6th month of pregnancy (see 4.6 Pregnancy and lactation).

- Patients with active peptic ulceration.

4.4 Special warnings and special precautions for use
- The medicated plaster should not come into contact with or be applied to the mucosae or the eyes.

- Not for use with occlusive dressing.

- Discontinue the treatment immediately if a skin rash develops after applying the medicated plaster.

- Do not administer concurrently, by either the topical or the systemic route, any medicinal product containing diclofenac or other NSAIDs.

- Although systemic effects should be low, the plaster should be used with caution in patients with renal, cardiac or hepatic impairment, history of peptic ulceration or inflammatory bowel disease or bleeding diathesis. Non-steroidal anti-inflammatory drugs should be used with particular caution in elderly patients who are more prone to adverse events.

- This medicinal product containsmethylparahydroxybenzoate and propylparahydroxybenzoate. It may cause allergic reactions (possibly delayed). It also contains propylene glycol, which may cause skin irritation.

- Patients should be warned against exposure to direct and solarium sunlight in order to reduce the risk of photosensitivity.

- Bronchospasm may be precipitated in patients suffering from or with a previous history of bronchial asthma or allergenic disease or allergy to acetylsalicylic acid or other NSAID. The medicated plaster should be used with caution in patients with or without chronic asthma in whom attacks of asthma, urticaria or acute rhinitis are precipitated by aspirin or other non-steroidal anti-inflammatory agents (see 4.3 Contraindications).

4.5 Interaction with other medicinal products and other forms of Interaction
In view of the low rate of systemic transfer during normal use of the medicated plasters, the drug interactions reported for oral diclofenac are unlikely to be observed.

4.6 Pregnancy and lactation
By analogy with the other routes of administration

Pregnancy
There is insufficient experience for the use during pregnancy. Animal studies have shown reproductive toxicity (see section 5.3). The potential risk for humans is unknown. Therefore Voltarol Gel Patch should not be used during first and second trimester, and is contra-indicated from the beginning of the 6th month of pregnancy.

During the last trimester of pregnancy, the use of prostaglandine synthetase inhibitors may result in:

- Inhibition of uterine contractions, prolongation of pregnancy and delivery

- Pulmonary and cardiac toxicity in the foetus (pulmonary hypertension with preterm closing of the ductus arteriosus)

- Renal insufficiency in the foetus with oligohydramnios

- Increase possibility of bleeding in the mother and child and increased oedema formation in the mother.

Lactation
Experimental data regarding excretion of diclofenac epolamine in human or animal milk are not available therefore, Voltarol Gel Patch is not recommended in nursing mothers.

4.7 Effects on ability to drive and use machines
Patients who experienced dizziness or other central nervous disturbances while taking NSAID's should refrain from driving or operating machinery, but this would be very unlikely using topical preparations such as Voltarol Gel Patch.

4.8 Undesirable effects
Skin disorders are commonly reported.

Skin: pruritus, redness, erythema, rashes, application site reactions, allergic dermatitis.

1252 patients were treated with Voltarol Gel Patch and 734 with Placebo in clinical trials. The following adverse drug reactions were reported:

(see Table 1 above)

Table 1

System Organ Class	Very Common >1/10)	Common > 1/100, <1/10)	Uncommon > 1/1000, <1/100)	Rare >1/10'000, <1/1000)
Skin and subcutaneous tissue disorders		2.95%		
- Pruritus		2.3%		
- Redness			0.3%	
- Erythema				0.05%
- Dermatitis allergic			0.15%	
- Petechiae			0.1%	
- Dry skin				0.05%
General disorders and administration site conditions		1.05%		
- Application site rash			0.5%	
- Application site reaction			0.4%	
- Feeling hot			0.1%	
- Application site edema				0.05%

Undesirable effects may be reduced by using the minimum effective dose for the shortest possible duration.

In patients using topical NSAID preparations, in isolated cases, generalised skin rash, hypersensitivity reactions such as angioedema and reactions of anaphylactic type and photosensitivity reactions have been reported.

Systemic absorption of diclofenac is very low compared with plasma levels obtained following administration of oral forms of diclofenac and the likelihood of systemic side-effects reactions (like gastric and renal disorders) occurring with topical diclofenac is very small compared with the frequency of side-effects associated with oral diclofenac. However, where Voltarol Gel Patch is applied to a relatively large area of skin and over a prolonged period, the possibility of systemic side-effects cannot be excluded.

4.9 Overdose
Not applicable

5. PHARMACOLOGICAL PROPERTIES
5.1 Pharmacodynamic properties
Pharmacotherapeutic group: Antiinflammatory preparations, non-steroids for topical use.

ATC Code: M02AA15

Diclofenac hydroxyethylpyrrolidine or diclofenac epolamine is a water soluble salt of diclofenac.

Diclofenac is a nonsteroidal anti-inflammatory drug derived from phenylacetic acid which belongs to the aryl carboxylic acid group of compounds.

In the form of a medicated plaster, it has topical anti-inflammatory and analgesic activity.

5.2 Pharmacokinetic properties
Following cutaneous application of the medicated plaster, diclofenac epolamine is absorbed through the skin.

The absorption kinetics at steady state show a prolonged release of the active ingredient with a maximum diclofenac plasma level (Cmax) of 17.4 ±13.5 ng/ml, which is reached after about 5 hours (Tmax 5.4±3.7 hours).

Diclofenac is extensively bound to plasma protein (about 99 %).

Systemic transfer in healthy volunteers when using the medicated plaster, compared with oral forms of diclofenac, is of the order of 2%, as estimated from the urinary excretion of the drug and its metabolites and from a between study comparison.

5.3 Preclinical safety data
Preclinical data reveal no special hazard for humans, beyond the information included in other sections of the SPC. In the rat and rabbit, diclofenac epolamine and epolamine monosubstance have caused embryotoxicity and increased embryolethality after oral use.

6. PHARMACEUTICAL PARTICULARS
6.1 List of excipients
Gelatin, povidone (K90), liquid sorbitol (non crystallising), heavy kaolin, titanium dioxide (E171), propylene glycol, methyl parahydroxybenzoate, propyl parahydroxybenzoate, disodium edetate, tartaric acid, aluminium glycinate, carmellose sodium, sodium polyacrylate, 1,3-butylene glycol, polysorbate 80, Dalin PH perfume (propylene glycol, benzyl salicylate, phenylethyl alcohol, alpha amylcinnamic aldehyde, hydroxycitronellal, phenyethyl phenylacetate, cinnamyl acetate, benzyl acetate, terpineol, cinnamic alcohol, cyclamenaldehyde), purified water.

Unwoven polyester support.

6.2 Incompatibilities
Not applicable.

6.3 Shelf life
3 years.

After first opening the sealed envelope: 3 months.

6.4 Special precautions for storage
Do not store above 25°C.

6.5 Nature and contents of container

14 g of gel on a polyester fibre dressing measuring 10 cm × 14 cm with a removable polypropylene protective film, in a sealed envelope made of paper/PE/aluminium/ethylene and methacrylic acid copolymer. 10 medicated plasters per box, contained in one or two re-sealable envelopes.

6.6 Instructions for use and handling

Dispose of used plasters thoughtfully: After use the medicated plasters still contains substantial quantities of active ingredients. Remaining active ingredient of the plaster may pose a risk to the aquatic environment. Do not flush used plasters down the toilet. Place them in common waste disposal systems.

7. MARKETING AUTHORISATION HOLDER

Novartis Consumer Health,

Horsham,

RH12 5AB,

UK

8. MARKETING AUTHORISATION NUMBER(S)

PL 00030/0206

9. DATE OF FIRST AUTHORISATION/RENEWAL OF THE AUTHORISATION

March 2004

10. DATE OF REVISION OF THE TEXT

Scheduling status: POM.

VOLTAROL Ophtha

(Novartis Pharmaceuticals UK Ltd)

1. NAME OF THE MEDICINAL PRODUCT

Voltarol® Ophtha

2. QUALITATIVE AND QUANTITATIVE COMPOSITION

Eye drop solution containing 0.1% (w/v) diclofenac sodium in a preservative-free formulation.

3. PHARMACEUTICAL FORM

Eye drop solution presented in single dose units for administration by instillation in the conjunctival sac.

4. CLINICAL PARTICULARS

4.1 Therapeutic indications

i. Inhibition of peroperative miosis during cataract surgery (Voltarol Ophtha has no intrinsic mydriatic properties and does not replace standard mydriatic agents).

ii. Treatment of post-operative inflammation in cataract surgery.

iii. Control of ocular pain and discomfort associated with corneal epithelial defects after excimer PRK surgery or accidental trauma.

iv. Control of inflammation after Argon Laser Trabeculoplasty (ALT).

v. The relief of the ocular signs and symptoms of Seasonal Allergic Conjunctivitis (SAC).

vi. Treatment of inflammation and discomfort after strabismus surgery

vii. Treatment of ocular pain and discomfort after radial keratotomy

4.2 Posology and method of administration

Adults:

i. Prophylaxis of peroperative miosis: Apply 1 drop four times during the 2 hours before surgery

ii. Control of post-operative inflammation: Apply 1 drop 4 times daily for up to 28 days

iii. Control of Post PRK pain and discomfort: Apply 1 drop 2 times in the hour prior to surgery, one drop 2 times five minutes apart immediately after PRK surgery and then post-operatively 1 drop every 2-5 hours while awake for up to 24 hours.

iv. Control of ocular pain associated with corneal epithelial defects after accidental trauma: Apply one drop 4 times daily for up to 2 days

v. Control of post ALT inflammation: Apply one drop 4 times during the 2 hours before ALT, and then one drop 4 times daily for up to 7 days

vi. The relief of the ocular signs and symptoms of Seasonal Allergic Conjunctivitis: Apply one drop 4 times daily for as long as required

vii. Treatment of inflammation and discomfort after strabismus surgery – one drop 4 times daily in the 1st week, thrice daily in the 2nd week, twice daily in the 3rd week and as required in the 4th week.

viii. Treatment of ocular pain and discomfort after radial keratotomy – pre-operatively one drop before surgery, post-operatively one drop immediately after surgery, and then one drop 4 times daily for up to 2 days

NOTE: Each Voltarol Ophtha SDU is for single use only. Discard the single dose unit immediately after use. Do not save unused contents

4.3 Contraindications

Patients with known hypersensitivity to any of the ingredients.

Like other non-steroidal anti-inflammatory agents, Voltarol Ophtha is also contraindicated in patients in whom attacks of asthma, urticaria or acute rhinitis are precipitated by acetylsalicylic acid or by other drugs with prostaglandin synthetase inhibiting activity. Intraocular use during surgical procedure is also contraindicated.

4.4 Special warnings and special precautions for use

In the presence of infection, or if there is a risk of infection, appropriate therapy (e.g. antibiotics) should be given concurrently with Voltarol Ophtha.

Although there have been no reported adverse events, there is a theoretical possibility that patients receiving other medications which may prolong bleeding time, or with known haemostatic defects may experience exacerbation with Voltarol Ophtha.

4.5 Interaction with other medicinal products and other forms of Interaction

None reported to date. Clinical findings have shown that Voltarol Ophtha can if necessary be combined with steroid-containing eye drops. To prevent the active substances from being washed out when additional ophthalmic medication is used, an interval of at least 5 minutes between each application should be adhered to.

4.6 Pregnancy and lactation

There is no experience concerning the safety of Voltarol Ophtha in human pregnancy. Administration during pregnancy and lactation is therefore not recommended except for compelling reasons.

4.7 Effects on ability to drive and use machines

Patients with blurred vision should refrain from driving a vehicle or operating machines.

4.8 Undesirable effects

The following adverse events have been reported:

Frequent: a mild to moderate burning sensation

Rare: blurred vision immediately after instillation of the eye drops, hypersensitivity reactions with itching and reddening, photosensitivity, keratitis punctata, corneal epithelial discontinuity.

4.9 Overdose

There is practically no risk of adverse effects due to accidental oral ingestion, since the eye drop solution in a block of 10 units contains only 3mg of diclofenac sodium, corresponding to about 1.8% of the recommended maximum daily adult dose of Voltarol after oral administration. By way of comparison, the maximum oral daily dose for diclofenac sodium recommended in children is 2mg/kg body weight.

5. PHARMACOLOGICAL PROPERTIES

5.1 Pharmacodynamic properties

Voltarol Ophtha contains diclofenac sodium, a non-steroidal compound with pronounced anti-inflammatory and analgesic properties. Inhibition of prostaglandin biosynthesis, which has been demonstrated experimentally, is regarded as having an important bearing on its mechanism of action. Prostaglandins play a major role in the causation of inflammation and pain.

In clinical trials, Voltarol Ophtha has been found to:

i. inhibit miosis during cataract surgery

ii. reduce inflammation following surgical interventions

iii. reduce ocular pain and discomfort associated with corneal epithelial defects after excimer PRK surgery or accidental trauma.

iv. reduce the incidence of angiographic cystoid macular oedema after cataract surgery but clinical significance remains to be established.

v. reduce ocular inflammation and discomfort more effectively than topical steroids after strabismus surgery whilst avoiding steroidal adverse effects such as delayed conjunctival wound healing and raised intraocular pressure

vi. reduce ocular inflammation, pain and discomfort (photophobia, burning/stinging, foreign body sensation, deep headache-like ocular pain and itching) more effectively than placebo eye drops after corneal incisional surgery such as radial keratotomy.

The effective daily dose after ocular application of Voltarol Ophtha (approximately 0.25 - 0.5 mg diclofenac sodium) corresponds to less than 1% of the daily dose recommended for Voltarol in rheumatic indications.

5.2 Pharmacokinetic properties

In rabbits, peak concentrations of 14C-labelled diclofenac could be demonstrated in the cornea and conjunctiva 30 minutes after application. The highest amounts are found in these two tissues and in the choroid and retina. Elimination was fast and almost complete after 6 hours.

Penetration of diclofenac into the anterior chamber has been confirmed in humans. No measurable levels of diclofenac could be found in humans after ocular application of diclofenac sodium eye drops.

5.3 Preclinical safety data

The results of the preclinical tests do not add anything of further significance to the prescriber.

6. PHARMACEUTICAL PARTICULARS

6.1 List of excipients

Boric acid

Polyoxyl 35 castor oil

Tromethamine

Water for injections

6.2 Incompatibilities

None known to date

6.3 Shelf life

Unopened: 24 months

Blister opened: 28 days

Opened: Single Dose Unit

6.4 Special precautions for storage

Do not store above 25°C. Stable for 28 days after opening the blister.

6.5 Nature and contents of container

Sealed single dose units composed of low density polyethylene granulate. Each unit contains 0.3ml solution. Available in packs of 5 and 40.

6.6 Instructions for use and handling

7. MARKETING AUTHORISATION HOLDER

Novartis Pharmaceuticals UK Ltd

Frimley Business Park

Frimley

Surrey

GU16 7SR

8. MARKETING AUTHORISATION NUMBER(S)

PL 00101/0478

9. DATE OF FIRST AUTHORISATION/RENEWAL OF THE AUTHORISATION

11 July 1997

10. DATE OF REVISION OF THE TEXT

June 2001

Voltarol Ophtha Multidose 0.1% Eye Drops

(Novartis Pharmaceuticals UK Ltd)

1. NAME OF THE MEDICINAL PRODUCT

Voltarol® Ophtha Multidose 0.1% Eye Drops

2. QUALITATIVE AND QUANTITATIVE COMPOSITION

Contains diclofenac sodium 1mg/ml

3. PHARMACEUTICAL FORM

Eye drops solution

4. CLINICAL PARTICULARS

4.1 Therapeutic indications

i. Inhibition of peroperative miosis during cataract surgery (Voltarol Ophtha Multidose has no intrinsic mydriatic properties and does not replace standard mydriatic agents).

ii. Treatment of post-operative inflammation in cataract surgery.

iii. Control of ocular pain and discomfort associated with corneal epithelial defects after excimer PRK surgery or accidental trauma.

iv. Control of inflammation after Argon Laser Trabeculoplasty (ALT).

v. The relief of the ocular signs and symptoms of Seasonal Allergic Conjunctivitis (SAC).

vi. Treatment of inflammation and discomfort after strabismus surgery

vii. Treatment of ocular pain and discomfort after radial keratotomy

4.2 Posology and method of administration

Adults:

Prophylaxis of preoperative miosis.

Apply 1 drop four times during the 2 hours before surgery.

Control of post-operative inflammation.

Apply 1 drop 4 times daily for up to 28 days.

Control of Post-PRK pain and discomfort.

Apply 1 drop 2 times in the hour prior to surgery, 1 drop 2 times five minutes apart immediately after PRK surgery and then post-operatively 1 drop every 2-5 hours while awake for up to 24 hours.

Control of ocular pain associated with corneal epithelial defects after accidental trauma.

Apply 1 drop 4 times daily for up to 2 days

Control of post-ALT inflammation.

Apply one drop 4 times during the 2 hours before ALT, and then one drop 4 times daily for up to 7 days.

The relief of the ocular signs and symptoms of Seasonal Allergic Conjuctivitis.

Apply one drop 4 times daily for as long as required.

Treatment of inflammation and discomfort after strabismus surgery

One drop 4 times daily in the 1st week, thrice daily in the 2nd week, twice daily in the 3rd week and as required in the 4th week

Treatment of ocular pain and discomfort after radial keratotomy

Pre-operatively one drop before surgery, post-operatively one drop immediately after surgery, and then one drop 4 times daily for up to 2 days

Children:

No specific studies with Voltarol Ophtha Multidose have been performed in children.

4.3 Contraindications

Patients with known hypersensitivity to any of the ingredients.

Like other non-steroidal anti-inflammatory agents, Voltarol is also contraindicated in patients in whom attacks of asthma, urticaria or acute rhinitis are precipitated by acetylsalicylic acid or by other drugs with prostaglandin synthetase inhibiting activity. Intraocular use during surgical procedure is also contraindicated.

4.4 Special warnings and special precautions for use

This product contains benzalkonium chloride as a preservative, which may be deposited in soft contact lenses. Therefore this product should not be used while wearing soft contact lenses. The lenses must be removed before application of the drops and not reinserted earlier than 15 minutes after use.

In the presence of infection, or if there is a risk of infection, appropriate therapy (e.g. antibiotics) should be given concurrently with Voltarol Ophtha Multidose.

Although there have been no reported adverse events, there is a theoretical possibility that patients receiving other medications which may prolong bleeding time, or with known haemostatic defects may experience exacerbation with Voltarol Ophtha Multidose.

4.5 Interaction with other medicinal products and other forms of Interaction

None reported to date. Clinical studies using other formulations of Voltarol eye drops have shown that ocular diclofenac can, if necessary, be used in conjunction with steroid containing eye drops. An interval of at least five minutes between the application of the different medicinal products must be allowed.

4.6 Pregnancy and lactation

First and second trimester:

Animal studies to date have shown no risk to the foetus. No controlled studies in pregnant women are available.

Third trimester:

Voltarol Ophtha Multidose Eye Drops should not be used due to a possible risk of premature closure of the ductus arteriosus and possible inhibitions of contractions.

After oral administration of 50mg coated tablets (equivalent to 10 bottles of eye drops) only traces of diclofenac were detected in breast milk. The quantities were so small that no undesirable effects on the infant would be expected.

4.7 Effects on ability to drive and use machines

Patients with blurred vision should refrain from driving a vehicle or operating machines.

4.8 Undesirable effects

The following adverse events have been reported:

Frequent:

A mild to moderate burning sensation

Rare:

Blurred vision immediately after instillation of the eye drops, hypersensitivity reactions with itching and reddening, photosensitivity, keratitis punctata, corneal epithelial discontinuity.

4.9 Overdose

There is practically no risk of adverse effects due to accidental oral ingestion, since a 5ml bottle of the eye drops contains only 5mg of diclofenac sodium, corresponding to about 3% of the recommended maximum daily adult dose of Voltarol after oral administration. By way of comparison, the maximum oral daily dose for diclofenac sodium recommended in children is 2mg/kg body weight.

5. PHARMACOLOGICAL PROPERTIES

5.1 Pharmacodynamic properties

Voltarol Ophtha Multidose contains diclofenac sodium, a non-steroidal compound with pronounced anti-inflammatory and analgesic properties. Inhibition of prostaglandin biosynthesis, which has been demonstrated experimentally, is regarded as having an important bearing on its mechanism of action. Prostaglandins play a major role in the causation of inflammation and pain.

In clinical trials, Voltarol Ophtha has been found to:

i. inhibit miosis during cataract surgery

ii. reduce inflammation following surgical interventions

iii. reduce ocular pain and discomfort associated with corneal epithelial defects after excimer PRK surgery or accidental trauma.

iv. reduce the incidence of angiographic cystoid macular oedema after cataract surgery but clinical significance remains to be established.

v. reduce ocular inflammation and discomfort more effectively than topical steroids after strabismus surgery whilst avoiding steroidal adverse effects such as delayed conjunctival wound healing and raised intraocular pressure

vi. reduce ocular inflammation, pain and discomfort (photophobia, burning/stinging, foreign body sensation, deep headache-like ocular pain and itching) more effectively than placebo eye drops after corneal incisional surgery such as radial keratotomy.

The effective daily dose after ocular application of Voltarol Ophtha Multidose (approximately 0.25 - 0.5 mg diclofenac sodium) corresponds to less than 1% of the daily dose recommended for Voltarol in rheumatic indications.

Voltarol Ophtha Multidose Eye Drops contain a cyclodextrin, hydroxypropyl γ-cyclodextrin (HPγ-CD). Cyclodextrins (CDs) increase the aqueous solubility of some lipophilic water-insoluble drugs. It is believed that CDs act as true carriers by keeping hydrophobic drug molecules in solution and delivering them to the surface of biological membranes.

5.2 Pharmacokinetic properties

In rabbits, peak concentrations of ^{14}C-labelled diclofenac could be demonstrated in the cornea and conjunctiva 30 minutes after application. The highest amounts are found in these two tissues and in the choroid and retina. Elimination was fast and almost complete after 6 hours.

Penetration of diclofenac into the anterior chamber has been confirmed in humans. No measurable levels of diclofenac could be found in humans after ocular application of diclofenac sodium eye drops.

5.3 Preclinical safety data

Preclinical data reveal no special hazard for humans

6. PHARMACEUTICAL PARTICULARS

6.1 List of excipients

Benzalkonium chloride

Disodium edetate

Hydroxypropyl γ-cyclodextrin

Hydrochloric acid

Propylene glycol

Trometamol

Tyloxapol

Water for injections

6.2 Incompatibilities

None known

6.3 Shelf life

Unopened: 3 years

Opened: 4 weeks

6.4 Special precautions for storage

No special precautions for storage

6.5 Nature and contents of container

5ml white LDPE bottle with LDPE dropper and HDPE closure.

6.6 Instructions for use and handling

No special requirements

7. MARKETING AUTHORISATION HOLDER

Novartis Pharmaceuticals UK Limited

Frimley Business Park

Frimley

Surrey

GU16 7SR

8. MARKETING AUTHORISATION NUMBER(S)

PL 00101/0632

9. DATE OF FIRST AUTHORISATION/RENEWAL OF THE AUTHORISATION

22nd August 2002

10. DATE OF REVISION OF THE TEXT

LEGAL CATEGORY

POM

Voltarol SR and Retard Tablets

(Novartis Pharmaceuticals UK Ltd)

1. NAME OF THE MEDICINAL PRODUCT

Voltarol® 75mg SR and Retard tablets 100mg

2. QUALITATIVE AND QUANTITATIVE COMPOSITION

The active substance is sodium-[o-[(2,6-dichlorophenyl)-amino]-phenyl]-acetate (diclofenac sodium).

Each slow/sustained release tablet contains 75mg or 100mg diclofenac sodium Ph.Eur.

3. PHARMACEUTICAL FORM

Slow/sustained release, film-coated tablet.

4. CLINICAL PARTICULARS

4.1 Therapeutic indications

Adults and Elderly:

Relief of all grades of pain and inflammation in a wide range of conditions, including:

(i) arthritic conditions: rheumatoid arthritis, osteoarthritis, ankylosing spondylitis, acute gout,

(ii) acute musculo-skeletal disorders such as periarthritis (for example frozen shoulder), tendinitis, tenosynovitis, bursitis,

(iii) other painful conditions resulting from trauma, including fracture, low back pain, sprains, strains, dislocations, orthopaedic, dental and other minor surgery.

Children: Voltarol 75mg SR tablets and Retard tablets 100mg are not suitable for children.

4.2 Posology and method of administration

Adults:

One tablet once or twice daily, taken whole with liquid, preferably at meal times.

The recommended maximum daily dose of Voltarol is 150mg.

Children: Voltarol 75mg SR tablets and Retard tablets 100mg are not suitable for children.

Elderly: Although the pharmacokinetics of Voltarol are not impaired to any clinically relevant extent in elderly patients, non-steroidal anti-inflammatory drugs should be used with particular caution in such patients who generally are more prone to adverse reactions. In particular it is recommended that the lowest effective dosage be used in frail elderly patients or those with a low body weight (see also Precautions) and the patient should be monitored for GI bleeding for 4 weeks following initiation of NSAID therapy.

4.3 Contraindications

Patients with a history of, or active or suspected, gastro-intestinal ulcers or bleeding.

Patients who have previously shown hypersensitivity reactions (e.g. asthma, urticaria or acute rhinitis) to diclofenac sodium, aspirin or other non-steroidal anti-inflammatory drugs.

4.4 Special warnings and special precautions for use

Warnings:

Gastro-intestinal: Close medical surveillance is imperative in patients with symptoms indicative of gastro-intestinal disorders, with a history suggestive of gastric or intestinal ulceration, with ulcerative colitis, or with Crohn's disease. Gastro-intestinal bleeding or ulceration/perforation, haematemesis and melaena have in general more serious consequences in the elderly. They can occur at any time during treatment, with or without warning symptoms or a previous history. In the rare instances when gastro-intestinal bleeding or ulceration occur in patients receiving Voltarol, the drug should be withdrawn.

Hepatic: Close medical surveillance is also imperative in patients suffering from severe impairment of hepatic function.

Hypersensitivity reactions: As with other nonsteroidal anti-inflammatory drugs, allergic reactions, including anaphylactic/anaphylactoid reactions, can also occur without earlier exposure to the drug.

Like other NSAIDs, Voltarol may mask the signs and symptoms of infection due to its pharmacodynamic properties.

Precautions:

Renal: Patients with renal, cardiac or hepatic impairment and the elderly should be kept under surveillance, since the use of NSAIDS may result in deterioration of renal function. The lowest effective dose should be used and renal function monitored.

The importance of prostaglandins in maintaining renal blood flow should be taken into account in patients with impaired cardiac or renal function, those being treated with diuretics or recovering from major surgery. Effects on renal function are usually reversible on withdrawal of Voltarol.

Hepatic: If abnormal liver function tests persist or worsen, clinical signs or symptoms consistent with liver disease develop or if other manifestations occur (eosinophilia, rash), Voltarol should be discontinued. Hepatitis may occur without prodromal symptoms.

Use of Voltarol in patients with hepatic porphyria may trigger an attack.

Haematological: Voltarol may reversibly inhibit platelet aggregation (see anticoagulants in "Drug Interactions"). Patients with defects of haemostasis, bleeding diathesis or haematological abnormalities should be carefully monitored.

Long-term treatment: All patients who are receiving non-steroidal anti-inflammatory agents should be monitored as a precautionary measure e.g. renal function, hepatic function (elevation of liver enzymes may occur) and blood counts. This is particularly important in the elderly.

Like other drugs that inhibit prostaglandin synthetase activity, diclofenac sodium and other NSAIDs can precipitate bronchospasm if administered to patients suffering from, or with a previous history of, bronchial asthma.

Caution is required in patients with a history of heart failure or hypertension since oedema has been reported in association with NSAID administration.

4.5 Interaction with other medicinal products and other forms of Interaction

Lithium and digoxin: Voltarol may increase plasma concentrations of lithium and digoxin.

Anticoagulants: Although clinical investigations do not appear to indicate that Voltarol has an influence on the effect of anticoagulants, there are isolated reports of an increased risk of haemorrhage with the combined use of diclofenac and anticoagulant therapy. Therefore, to be certain that no change in anticoagulant dosage is required, close monitoring of such patients is required. As with other non-steroidal anti-inflammatory agents, diclofenac in high dose can reversibly inhibit platelet aggregation.

Antidiabetic agents: Clinical studies have shown that Voltarol can be given together with oral antidiabetic agents without influencing their clinical effect. However there have been isolated reports of hypoglycaemic and hyperglycaemic effects which have required adjustment to the dosage of hypoglycaemic agents.

Cyclosporin: Cases of nephrotoxicity have been reported in patients receiving concomitant cyclosporin and NSAIDS, including Voltarol. This might be mediated through combined renal antiprostaglandin effects of both the NSAID and cyclosporin.

Methotrexate: Cases of serious toxicity have been reported when methotrexate and NSAIDS are given within 24 hours of each other. This interaction is mediated through accumulation of methotrexate resulting from impairment of renal excretion in the presence of the NSAID.

Quinolone antimicrobials: Convulsions may occur due to an interaction between quinolones and NSAIDS. This may occur in patients with or without a previous history of epilepsy or convulsions. Therefore, caution should be exercised when considering the use of a quinolone in patients who are already receiving an NSAID.

Other NSAIDS and corticosteroids: Co-administration of Voltarol with aspirin or corticosteroids may increase the risk of gastro-intestinal bleeding. Avoid concomitant use of two or more NSAIDs.

Diuretics: Like other NSAIDS, Voltarol may inhibit the activity of diuretics. Concomitant treatment with potassium-sparing diuretics may be associated with increased serum potassium levels, which should therefore be monitored frequently.

Cardiac glycosides: Concomitant use of cardiac glycosides and NSAIDs in patients may exacerbate cardiac failure, reduce GFR and increase plasma glycoside levels.

Mifepristone: NSAIDs should not be used for 8-12 days after mifepristone administration as NSAIDs can reduce the effect of mifepristone.

Anti-hypertensives: Concomitant use of NSAIDs with anti-hypertensive drugs (i.e. beta-blockers, angiotensin converting enzyme (ACE) inhibitors, diuretics) may cause a decrease in their antihypertensive effect via inhibition of vasodilatory prostaglandin synthesis.

4.6 Pregnancy and lactation

Although animal studies have not demonstrated teratogenic effects, Voltarol should not be prescribed during pregnancy, unless there are compelling reasons for doing so. The lowest effective dosage should be used.

Congenital abnormalities have been reported in association with the administration of NSAIDs in man; however, these are low in frequency and do not appear to follow any discernible pattern.

In view of the known effects of NSAIDs on the foetal cardiovascular system (e.g. a premature closure of the ductus arteriosus) and in causing uterine inertia, use in late pregnancy should be avoided.

Following doses of 50mg enteric coated tablets every 8 hours, traces of active substance have been detected in breast milk, but in quantities so small that no adverse effects on the breast-fed infant are to be expected.

4.7 Effects on ability to drive and use machines

Patients who experience dizziness or other central nervous disturbances, while taking NSAIDS should refrain from driving or operating machinery.

4.8 Undesirable effects

If serious side effects occur, Voltarol should be withdrawn.

Frequency estimate: frequent: >10 %, occasional: >1 - 10 %, rare: >0.001 - 1 %, isolated cases: <0.001 %.

Gastro-intestinal tract

Occasional: Epigastric pain, other gastro-intestinal disorders (e.g. nausea, vomiting, diarrhoea, abdominal cramps, dyspepsia, flatulence, anorexia).

Rare: Gastro-intestinal bleeding (haematemesis, melaena, bloody diarrhoea), gastro-intestinal ulcers with or without bleeding or perforation.

In isolated cases: Aphthous stomatitis, glossitis, oesophageal lesions, lower gut disorders (e.g. non-specific haemorrhagic colitis and exacerbations of ulcerative colitis or Crohn's proctocolitis, colonic damage and stricture formation), pancreatitis, constipation.

Central Nervous System:

Occasional: Headache, dizziness, or vertigo.

Rare: Drowsiness, tiredness.

In isolated cases: Disturbances of sensation, paraesthesia, memory disturbance, disorientation, insomnia, irritability, convulsions, depression, anxiety, nightmares, tremor, psychotic reactions, aseptic meningitis.

Special senses:

Isolated cases: Disturbances of vision (blurred vision, diplopia), impaired hearing, tinnitus, taste disturbances.

Skin:

Occasional: Rashes or skin eruptions.

Rare: Urticaria.

In isolated cases: Bullous eruptions, eczema, erythema multiforme, Stevens-Johnson syndrome, Lyell's syndrome, (acute toxic epidermolysis), erythroderma (exfoliative dermatitis), loss of hair, photosensitivity reactions, purpura including allergic purpura.

Kidney:

Rare: Oedema

In isolated cases: Acute renal insufficiency, urinary abnormalities (e.g. haematuria, proteinuria), interstitial nephritis, nephrotic syndrome, papillary necrosis.

Liver:

Occasional: Elevation of serum aminotransferase enzymes (ALT, AST).

Rare: Liver function disorders including hepatitis (in isolated cases fulminant) with or without jaundice.

Blood:

In isolated cases: Thrombocytopenia, leucopenia, agranulocytosis, haemolytic anaemia, aplastic anaemia.

Hypersensitivity:

Rare: Hypersensitivity reactions (e.g. bronchospasm, anaphylactic/anaphylactoid systemic reactions including hypotension).

Isolated cases: Vasculitis, pneumonitis.

Cardiovascular system:

Isolated cases: Palpitations, chest pain, hypertension, congestive heart failure.

Other organ systems:

Isolated cases: Impotence.

4.9 Overdose

Management of acute poisoning with NSAIDS essentially consists of supportive and symptomatic measures. There is no typical clinical picture resulting from Voltarol overdosage.

The therapeutic measures to be taken are: Supportive and symptomatic treatment should be given for complications such as hypotension, renal failure, convulsions, gastro-intestinal irritation, and respiratory depression.

Special therapies such as forced diuresis, dialysis or haemoperfusion are probably of no help in eliminating NSAIDS due to the high rate of protein binding and extensive metabolism.

5. PHARMACOLOGICAL PROPERTIES

5.1 Pharmacodynamic properties

Pharmacotherapeutic group

Non-steroidal anti-inflammatory drugs (NSAIDs).

Mechanism of action

Voltarol is a non-steroidal agent with marked analgesic/anti- inflammatory properties. It is an inhibitor of prostaglandin synthetase, (cyclo-oxygenase).

Diclofenac sodium *in vitro* does not suppress proteoglycan biosynthesis in cartilage at concentrations equivalent to the concentrations reached in human beings.

5.2 Pharmacokinetic properties

Absorption

The same amount of active substance is released and absorbed from SR and Retard tablets as from enteric-coated tablets. Mean peak plasma concentrations of diclofenac are reached at 4 hours, 0.508 ± 0.185μg/ml (0.5μg/mL ≡ 1.6μmol/L) or 0.4 ± 0.184μg/ml (0.4μg/mL ≡ 1.25μmol/L) after Retard 100mg or 75mg SR, respectively. 75mg SR and Retard 100mg are modified release preparations and plasma concentrations of diclofenac of 13ng/mL (40μmol/L) can be recorded at 24 hours (Retard 100mg) and 16 hours (75mg SR) after administration. Absorption is unaffected by food.

Bioavailability:

The systemic availability of diclofenac from the SR formulations is on average 82% of that achieved with the same dose of enteric-coated tablets (possibly due to release rate dependent first-pass metabolism). As a result of the slower release of active substance, peak plasma concentrations are lower than for the equivalent enteric-coated tablets.

Pharmacokinetic behaviour does not change on repeated administration. Accumulation does not occur, provided the recommended dosage intervals are observed. Trough levels of diclofenac in the plasma after Retard 100mg daily or 75mg SR twice daily are around 22ng/ml or 25ng/ml (70nmol/l or 80nmol/l), respectively.

Distribution

The active substance is 99.7% protein bound, mainly to albumin (99.4%).

Diclofenac enters the synovial fluid, where maximum concentrations are measured 2-4 hours after the peak plasma values have been attained. The apparent half-life for elimination from the synovial fluid is 3-6 hours. Two hours after reaching the peak plasma values, concentrations of the active substance are already higher in the synovial fluid than they are in the plasma and remain higher for up to 12 hours.

Metabolism

Biotransformation of diclofenac takes place partly by glucuronidation of the intact molecule, but mainly by single and multiple hydroxylation and methoxylation, resulting in several phenolic metabolites, most of which are converted to glucuronide conjugates. Two phenolic metabolites are biologically active, but to a much lesser extent than diclofenac.

Elimination

The total systemic clearance of diclofenac in plasma is 263 ± 56 mL/min (mean value ± SD). The terminal half-life in plasma is 1-2 hours. Four of the metabolites, including the two active ones, also have short plasma half-lives of 1-3 hours.

About 60% of the administered dose is excreted in the urine in the form of the glucuronide conjugate of the intact molecule and as metabolites, most of which are also converted to glucuronide conjugates. Less than 1% is excreted as unchanged substance. The rest of the dose is eliminated as metabolites through the bile in the faeces.

Characteristics in patients

Elderly: No relevant age-dependent differences in the drug's absorption, metabolism, or excretion have been observed, other than the finding that in five elderly patients, a 15 minute iv infusion resulted in 50% higher plasma concentrations than expected with young healthy subjects.

Patients with renal impairment: In patients suffering from renal impairment, no accumulation of the unchanged active substance can be inferred from the single-dose kinetics when applying the usual dosage schedule. At a creatinine clearance of less than 10 mL/min, the calculated steady-state plasma levels of the hydroxy metabolites are about 4 times higher than in normal subjects. However, the metabolites are ultimately cleared through the bile.

Patients with hepatic disease: In patients with chronic hepatitis or non-decompensated cirrhosis, the kinetics and metabolism of diclofenac are the same as in patients without liver disease.

5.3 Preclinical safety data

None stated.

6. PHARMACEUTICAL PARTICULARS

6.1 List of excipients

The 75mg SR and Retard 100mg tablets also contain colloidal anhydrous silica, cetyl alcohol, sucrose (powder), povidone, magnesium stearate, hydroxypropyl methylcellulose, polysorbate 80, purified talc, titanium dioxide (E 171), red iron oxide (E.172) and purified water.

6.2 Incompatibilities

None known.

6.3 Shelf life

75mg SR tablets: Three years

Retard 100mg tablets: Five years.

6.4 Special precautions for storage

75mg SR tablets: Protect from moisture and heat (store below 30°C).

Retard 100mg tablets: There are no special precautions for storage.

Medicines should be kept out of the reach of children.

6.5 Nature and contents of container

75mg SR tablets are pale pink, triangular film-coated tablets embossed GEIGY on one face, V 75 SR on the other, and come in PVC/PVdC blister packs of 28, 56 and 70.

The Retard 100mg tablets are pale red, round, slightly convex, film coated tablets, impressed GEIGY on one side and VOLTAROL R on the other, and come in PVC/PVdC blister packs of 28 and 70.

6.6 Instructions for use and handling

The tablets should be swallowed whole with liquid, preferably with meals.

7. MARKETING AUTHORISATION HOLDER

Novartis Pharmaceuticals UK Ltd.

Trading as Geigy Pharmaceuticals,

Frimley Business Park

Frimley

Camberley

Surrey

GU16 7SR.

8. MARKETING AUTHORISATION NUMBER(S)

75mg SR tablets: PL 00101/0471

Retard 100mg tablets: PL 00101/0470

9. DATE OF FIRST AUTHORISATION/RENEWAL OF THE AUTHORISATION

11 July 1997

10. DATE OF REVISION OF THE TEXT

8 December 2000

LEGAL CATEGORY

POM

Voltarol Suppositories

(Novartis Pharmaceuticals UK Ltd)

1. NAME OF THE MEDICINAL PRODUCT

Voltarol® Suppositories 12.5mg, 25mg, 50mg and 100mg

2. QUALITATIVE AND QUANTITATIVE COMPOSITION

The active substance is sodium-[o-[(2,6-dichlorophenyl)-amino]-phenyl]-acetate (diclofenac sodium).

Each suppository contains 12.5mg, 25mg, 50mg and 100mg diclofenac sodium Ph.Eur.

3. PHARMACEUTICAL FORM

Suppositories.

4. CLINICAL PARTICULARS

4.1 Therapeutic indications

Adults and Elderly:

Relief of all grades of pain and inflammation in a wide range of conditions, including:

(i) arthritic conditions: rheumatoid arthritis, osteoarthritis, ankylosing spondylitis, acute gout,

(ii) acute musculo-skeletal disorders such as periarthritis (for example frozen shoulder), tendinitis, tenosynovitis, bursitis,

(iii) other painful conditions resulting from trauma, including fracture, low back pain, sprains, strains, dislocations, orthopaedic, dental and other minor surgery.

Children (aged 1-12 years):

Juvenile chronic arthritis (12.5mg and 25mg suppositories only).

Children (aged 6 years and above):

As monotherapy or as adjunct therapy with morphine or other opiates (due to its opiate-sparing effect) for the relief of acute post-operative pain. (12.5mg and 25mg suppositories only).

4.2 Posology and method of administration

Adults:

75-150mg daily, in divided doses (25mg, 50mg and 100mg).

The recommended maximum daily dose of Voltarol is 150mg. This may be administered using a combination of dosage forms, e.g. tablets and suppositories.

Children (aged 1-12 years):

1-3mg/kg per day in divided doses (12.5mg and 25mg suppositories only).

Children (aged 6-12 years)with acute post-operative pain:

1-2mg/kg per day in divided doses. Treatment of acute post-operative pain should be limited to 4 days treatment (12.5mg and 25mg suppositories only).

Elderly:

Although the pharmacokinetics of Voltarol are not impaired to any clinically relevant extent in elderly patients, non-steroidal anti-inflammatory drugs should be used with particular caution in such patients who generally are more prone to adverse reactions. In particular it is recommended that the lowest effective dosage be used in frail elderly patients or those with a low body weight (see also Precautions) and the patient should be monitored for GI bleeding for 4 weeks following initiation of NSAID therapy.

4.3 Contraindications

Patients with a history of, or active or suspected, gastro-intestinal ulcers or bleeding.

Patients who have previously shown hypersensitivity reactions (e.g. asthma, urticaria or acute rhinitis) to diclofenac sodium, aspirin or other non-steroidal anti-inflammatory drugs.

In ulcerative or acute inflammatory conditions of the anus, rectum (proctitis) and sigmoid colon.

4.4 Special warnings and special precautions for use

Warnings:

Gastro-intestinal:

Close medical surveillance is imperative in patients with symptoms indicative of gastro-intestinal disorders, with a history suggestive of gastric or intestinal ulceration, with ulcerative colitis, or with Crohn's disease.

Gastro-intestinal bleeding or ulceration/perforation, haematemesis and melaena have in general more serious consequences in the elderly. They can occur at any time during treatment, with or without warning symptoms or a previous history. They have in general more serious consequences in the elderly. In the rare instances when gastro-intestinal bleeding or ulceration occur in patients receiving Voltarol, the drug should be withdrawn.

Hepatic:

Close medical surveillance is also imperative in patients suffering from severe impairment of hepatic function.

Hypersensitivity reactions:

As with other nonsteroidal anti-inflammatory drugs, allergic reactions, including anaphylactic/anaphylactoid reactions, can also occur without earlier exposure to the drug.

Like other NSAIDs, Voltarol may mask the signs and symptoms of infection due to its pharmacodynamic properties.

Precautions:

Renal:

Patients with renal, cardiac or hepatic impairment and the elderly should be kept under surveillance, since the use of NSAIDS may result in deterioration of renal function. The lowest effective dose should be used and renal function monitored.

The importance of prostaglandins in maintaining renal blood flow should be taken into account in patients with impaired cardiac or renal function, those being treated with diuretics or recovering from major surgery. Effects on renal function are usually reversible on withdrawal of Voltarol.

Hepatic:

If abnormal liver function tests persist or worsen, clinical signs or symptoms consistent with liver disease develop or if other manifestations occur (eosinophilia, rash), Voltarol should be discontinued. Hepatitis may occur without prodromal symptoms.

Use of Voltarol in patients with hepatic porphyria may trigger an attack.

Haematological:

Voltarol may reversibly inhibit platelet aggregation (see anticoagulants in "Drug Interactions"). Patients with defects of haemostasis, bleeding diathesis or haematological abnormalities should be carefully monitored.

Long-term treatment:

All patients who are receiving non-steroidal anti-inflammatory agents should be monitored as a precautionary measure e.g. renal function, hepatic function (elevation of liver enzymes may occur) and blood counts. This is particularly important in the elderly.

Like other drugs that inhibit prostaglandin synthetase activity, diclofenac sodium and other NSAIDs can precipitate bronchospasm if administered to patients suffering from, or with a previous history of, bronchial asthma.

Caution is required in patients with a history of heart failure or hypertension since oedema has been reported in association with NSAID administration.

4.5 Interaction with other medicinal products and other forms of Interaction

Lithium and digoxin:

Voltarol may increase plasma concentrations of lithium and digoxin.

Anticoagulants:

Although clinical investigations do not appear to indicate that Voltarol has an influence on the effect of anticoagulants, there are isolated reports of an increased risk of haemorrhage with the combined use of diclofenac and anticoagulant therapy. Therefore, to be certain that no change in anticoagulant dosage is required, close monitoring of such patients is required. As with other non-steroidal anti-inflammatory agents, diclofenac in high dose can reversibly inhibit platelet aggregation.

Antidiabetic agents:

Clinical studies have shown that Voltarol can be given together with oral antidiabetic agents without influencing their clinical effect. However there have been isolated reports of hypoglycaemic and hyperglycaemic effects which have required adjustment to the dosage of hypoglycaemic agents.

Cyclosporin:

Cases of nephrotoxicity have been reported in patients receiving concomitant cyclosporin and NSAIDS, including Voltarol. This might be mediated through combined renal antiprostaglandin effects of both the NSAID and cyclosporin.

Methotrexate:

Cases of serious toxicity have been reported when methotrexate and NSAIDS are given within 24 hours of each other. This interaction is mediated through accumulation of methotrexate resulting from impairment of renal excretion in the presence of the NSAID.

Quinolone antimicrobials:

Convulsions may occur due to an interaction between quinolones and NSAIDS. This may occur in patients with or without a previous history of epilepsy or convulsions. Therefore, caution should be exercised when considering the use of a quinolone in patients who are already receiving an NSAID.

Other NSAIDS and corticosteroids:

Co-administration of Voltarol with aspirin or corticosteroids may increase the risk of gastro-intestinal bleeding. Avoid concomitant use of two or more NSAIDs.

Diuretics:

Like other NSAIDS, Voltarol may inhibit the activity of diuretics. Concomitant treatment with potassium-sparing diuretics may be associated with increased serum potassium levels, which should therefore be monitored frequently.

Cardiac glycosides:

Concomitant use of cardiac glycosides and NSAIDs in patients may exacerbate cardiac failure, reduce GFR and increase plasma glycoside levels.

Mifepristone:

NSAIDs should not be used for 8-12 days after mifepristone administration as NSAIDs can reduce the effect of mifepristone.

Anti-hypertensives:

Concomitant use of NSAIDs with antihypertensive drugs (i.e. beta-blockers, angiotensin converting enzyme (ACE) inhibitors, diuretics) may cause a decrease in their antihypertensive effect via inhibition of vasodilatory prostaglandin synthesis.

4.6 Pregnancy and lactation

Although animal studies have not demonstrated teratogenic effects, Voltarol should not be prescribed during pregnancy, unless there are compelling reasons for doing so. The lowest effective dosage should be used.

Congenital abnormalities have been reported in association with the administration of NSAIDs in man; however, these are low in frequency and do not appear to follow any discernible pattern.

In view of the known effects of NSAIDs on the foetal cardiovascular system (e.g. a premature closure of the ductus arteriosus) and in causing uterine inertia, use in late pregnancy should be avoided.

Following doses of 50mg enteric coated tablets every 8 hours, traces of active substance have been detected in breast milk, but in quantities so small that no adverse effects on the breast-fed infant are to be expected.

4.7 Effects on ability to drive and use machines

Patients who experience dizziness or other central nervous disturbances, while taking NSAIDS should refrain from driving or operating machinery.

4.8 Undesirable effects

If serious side-effects occur, Voltarol should be withdrawn.

Frequency estimate: frequent: >10 %, occasional: >1 - 10 %, rare: >0.001 - 1 %, isolated cases: <0.001 %.

Gastro-intestinal tract

Occasional: Epigastric pain, other gastro-intestinal disorders (e.g. nausea, vomiting, diarrhoea, abdominal cramps, dyspepsia, flatulence, anorexia).

Rare: Gastro-intestinal bleeding (haematemesis, melaena, bloody diarrhoea), gastro-intestinal ulcers with or without bleeding or perforation.

In isolated cases: Aphthous stomatitis, glossitis, oesophageal lesions, lower gut disorders (e.g. non-specific haemorrhagic colitis and exacerbations of ulcerative colitis or Crohn's proctocolitis, colonic damage and stricture formation), pancreatitis, constipation.

Suppositories only:

Occasional: Local reactions (e.g. itching, burning and increased bowel movement). In isolated cases: Exacerbation of haemorrhoids.

Central Nervous System:

Occasional: Headache, dizziness, or vertigo.

Rare: Drowsiness, tiredness.

In isolated cases: Disturbances of sensation, paraesthesia, memory disturbance, disorientation, insomnia, irritability, convulsions, depression, anxiety, nightmares, tremor, psychotic reactions, aseptic meningitis.

Special senses:

Isolated cases: Disturbances of vision (blurred vision, diplopia), impaired hearing, tinnitus, taste disturbances.

Skin:

Occasional: Rashes or skin eruptions.

Rare: Urticaria.

In isolated cases: Bullous eruptions, eczema, erythema multiforme, Stevens-Johnson syndrome, Lyell's syndrome, (acute toxic epidermolysis), erythroderma (exfoliative dermatitis), loss of hair, photosensitivity reactions, purpura including allergic purpura.

Kidney:

Rare: Oedema

In isolated cases: Acute renal insufficiency, urinary abnormalities (e.g. haematuria, proteinuria), interstitial nephritis, nephrotic syndrome, papillary necrosis.

Liver:

Occasional: Elevation of serum aminotransferase enzymes (ALT, AST).

Rare: Liver function disorders including hepatitis (in isolated cases fulminant) with or without jaundice.

Blood:

In isolated cases: Thrombocytopenia, leucopenia, agranulocytosis, haemolytic anaemia, aplastic anaemia.

Hypersensitivity:

Rare: Hypersensitivity reactions (e.g. bronchospasm, anaphylactic/anaphylactoid systemic reactions including hypotension).

Isolated cases: Vasculitis, pneumonitis.

Cardiovascular system:

Isolated cases: Palpitations, chest pain, hypertension, congestive heart failure.

Other organ systems:

Isolated cases: Impotence.

4.9 Overdose

Management of acute poisoning with NSAIDS essentially consists of supportive and symptomatic measures. There is no typical clinical picture resulting from Voltarol overdosage.

The therapeutic measures to be taken are: Supportive and symptomatic treatment should be given for complications such as hypotension, renal failure, convulsions, gastro-intestinal irritation, and respiratory depression.

Special therapies such as forced diuresis, dialysis or haemoperfusion are probably of no help in eliminating NSAIDS due to the high rate of protein binding and extensive metabolism.

5. PHARMACOLOGICAL PROPERTIES

5.1 Pharmacodynamic properties

Pharmacotherapeutic group

Non-steroidal anti-inflammatory drugs (NSAIDs).

Mechanism of action

Voltarol is a non-steroidal agent with marked analgesic/ anti- inflammatory properties. It is an inhibitor of prostaglandin synthetase, (cyclo-oxygenase).

Diclofenac sodium *in vitro* does not suppress proteoglycan biosynthesis in cartilage at concentrations equivalent to the concentrations reached in human beings.

5.2 Pharmacokinetic properties

Absorption

Absorption is rapid; although the rate of absorption is slower than from enteric-coated tablets administered orally. After the administration of 50mg suppositories, peak plasma concentrations are attained on average within 1 hour, but maximum concentrations per dose unit are about two thirds of those reached after administration of enteric-coated tablets (1.95 ± 0.8μg/ml (1.9μg/ml ≡ 5.9μmol/l)).

Bioavailability

As with oral preparations the AUC is approximately a half of the value obtained from a parenteral dose.

Pharmacokinetic behaviour does not change on repeated administration. Accumulation does not occur, provided the recommended dosage intervals are observed. The plasma concentrations attained in children given equivalent doses (mg/kg, b.w.) are similar to those obtained in adults.

Distribution

The active substance is 99.7% protein bound, mainly to albumin (99.4%).

Diclofenac enters the synovial fluid, where maximum concentrations are measured 2-4 hours after the peak plasma values have been attained. The apparent half-life for elimination from the synovial fluid is 3-6 hours. Two hours after reaching the peak plasma values, concentrations of the active substance are already higher in the synovial fluid than they are in the plasma and remain higher for up to 12 hours.

Metabolism

Biotransformation of diclofenac takes place partly by glucuronidation of the intact molecule, but mainly by single and multiple hydroxylation and methoxylation, resulting in several phenolic metabolites, most of which are converted to glucuronide conjugates. Two phenolic metabolites are biologically active, but to a much lesser extent than diclofenac.

Elimination

The total systemic clearance of diclofenac in plasma is 263 ± 56 mL/min (mean value ± SD). The terminal half-life in plasma is 1-2 hours. Four of the metabolites, including the two active ones, also have short plasma half-lives of 1-3 hours.

About 60% of the administered dose is excreted in the urine in the form of the glucuronide conjugate of the intact molecule and as metabolites, most of which are also converted to glucuronide conjugates. Less than 1% is excreted as unchanged substance. The rest of the dose is eliminated as metabolites through the bile in the faeces.

Characteristics in patients

No relevant age-dependent differences in the drug's absorption, metabolism, or excretion have been observed, other than the finding that in five elderly patients, a 15 minute iv infusion resulted in 50% higher plasma concentrations than expected with young healthy subjects.

Patients with renal impairment:

In patients suffering from renal impairment, no accumulation of the unchanged active substance can be inferred from the single-dose kinetics when applying the usual dosage schedule. At a creatinine clearance of less than 10 mL/min, the calculated steady-state plasma levels of the hydroxy metabolites are about 4 times higher than in normal subjects. However, the metabolites are ultimately cleared through the bile.

Patients with hepatic disease:

In patients with chronic hepatitis or non-decompensated cirrhosis, the kinetics and metabolism of diclofenac are the same as in patients without liver disease.

5.3 Preclinical safety data

None stated.

6. PHARMACEUTICAL PARTICULARS

6.1 List of excipients

Voltarol suppositories also contain suppository mass 5 (a waxy base composed of hard fat).

6.2 Incompatibilities

None known.

6.3 Shelf life

Three years.

6.4 Special precautions for storage

Protect from heat (store below 30 ° C).

Medicines should be kept out of the reach of children.

6.5 Nature and contents of container

The suppositories are white to yellowish, torpedo-shaped, with smooth surfaces and a slightly fatty odour, and are sealed in a composite foil made of polyvinylchloride (PVC) laminated with low-density polyethylene (LD-PE).

They come in packs of 10.

6.6 Instructions for use and handling

For rectal use only.

7. MARKETING AUTHORISATION HOLDER

Novartis Pharmaceuticals UK Ltd. Trading as Geigy Pharmaceuticals, Frimley Business Park Frimley Camberley Surrey GU16 7SR.

8. MARKETING AUTHORISATION NUMBER(S)

12.5mg: PL 00101/0472

25mg: PL 00101/0473

50mg: PL 00101/0474

100mg: PL 00101/0475

9. DATE OF FIRST AUTHORISATION/RENEWAL OF THE AUTHORISATION

11 July 1997

10. DATE OF REVISION OF THE TEXT

14 June 2005

Legal Category

POM

Voltarol Tablets

(Novartis Pharmaceuticals UK Ltd)

1. NAME OF THE MEDICINAL PRODUCT

Voltarol® Tablets 25mg and 50mg

2. QUALITATIVE AND QUANTITATIVE COMPOSITION

The active substance is sodium-[o-[(2,6-dichlorophenyl)-amino]-phenyl]-acetate (diclofenac sodium).

Each enteric coated tablet contains 25mg or 50mg diclofenac sodium Ph.Eur.

3. PHARMACEUTICAL FORM

Enteric coated tablet.

4. CLINICAL PARTICULARS

4.1 Therapeutic indications

Adults and Elderly:

Relief of all grades of pain and inflammation in a wide range of conditions, including:

(i) arthritic conditions: rheumatoid arthritis, osteoarthritis, ankylosing spondylitis, acute gout,

(ii) acute musculo-skeletal disorders such as periarthritis (for example frozen shoulder), tendinitis, tenosynovitis, bursitis,

(iii) other painful conditions resulting from trauma, including fracture, low back pain, sprains, strains, dislocations, orthopaedic, dental and other minor surgery.

Children (aged 1-12 years): Juvenile chronic arthritis (25mg tablet only).

4.2 Posology and method of administration

Adults:

75-150mg daily in two or three divided doses.

The recommended maximum daily dose of Voltarol is 150mg.

Children (aged 1-12 years): 1-3mg/kg per day in divided doses (25mg tablet only).

Elderly: Although the pharmacokinetics of Voltarol are not impaired to any clinically relevant extent in elderly patients, non-steroidal anti-inflammatory drugs should be used with particular caution in such patients who generally are more prone to adverse reactions. In particular it is recommended that the lowest effective dosage be used in frail elderly patients or those with a low body weight (see also Precautions) and the patient should be monitored for GI bleeding for 4 weeks following initiation of NSAID therapy.

4.3 Contraindications

Patients with a history of, or active or suspected, gastro-intestinal ulcers or bleeding

Patients who have previously shown hypersensitivity reactions (e.g. asthma, urticaria or acute rhinitis) to diclofenac sodium, aspirin or other non-steroidal anti-inflammatory drugs.

4.4 Special warnings and special precautions for use

Warnings:

Gastro-intestinal: ([a-z])lose medical surveillance is imperative in patients with symptoms indicative of gastro-intestinal disorders, with a history suggestive of gastric or intestinal ulceration, with ulcerative colitis, or with Crohn's disease.

Gastro-intestinal bleeding or ulceration/perforation, haematemesis and melaena have in general more serious consequences in the elderly. They can occur at any time during treatment, with or without warning symptoms or a previous history. In the rare instances when gastro-intestinal bleeding or ulceration occur in patients receiving Voltarol, the drug should be withdrawn.

Hepatic: Close medical surveillance is also imperative in patients suffering from severe impairment of hepatic function.

Hypersensitivity reactions: As with other nonsteroidal anti-inflammatory drugs, allergic reactions, including anaphylactic/anaphylactoid reactions, can also occur without earlier exposure to the drug.

Like other NSAIDs, Voltarol may mask the signs and symptoms of infection due to its pharmacodynamic properties.

Precautions:

Renal: Patients with renal, cardiac or hepatic impairment and the elderly should be kept under surveillance, since the use of NSAIDS may result in deterioration of renal function. The lowest effective dose should be used and renal function monitored.

The importance of prostaglandins in maintaining renal blood flow should be taken into account in patients with impaired cardiac or renal function, those being treated with diuretics or recovering from major surgery. Effects on renal function are usually reversible on withdrawal of Voltarol.

Hepatic: If abnormal liver function tests persist or worsen, clinical signs or symptoms consistent with liver disease develop or if other manifestations occur (eosinophilia, rash), Voltarol should be discontinued. Hepatitis may occur without prodromal symptoms.

Use of Voltarol in patients with hepatic porphyria may trigger an attack.

Haematological: Voltarol may reversibly inhibit platelet aggregation (see anticoagulants in "Drug Interactions"). Patients with defects of haemostasis, bleeding diathesis or haematological abnormalities should be carefully monitored.

Long-term treatment: All patients who are receiving non-steroidal anti-inflammatory agents should be monitored as a precautionary measure e.g. renal function, hepatic function (elevation of liver enzymes may occur) and blood counts. This is particularly important in the elderly.

Like other drugs that inhibit prostaglandin synthetase activity, diclofenac sodium and other NSAIDs can precipitate bronchospasm if administered to patients suffering from, or with a previous history of, bronchial asthma.

Caution is required in patients with a history of heart failure or hypertension since oedema has been reported in association with NSAID administration.

4.5 Interaction with other medicinal products and other forms of Interaction

Lithium and digoxin: Voltarol may increase plasma concentrations of lithium and digoxin.

Anticoagulants: Although clinical investigations do not appear to indicate that Voltarol has an influence on the effect of anticoagulants, there are isolated reports of an increased risk of haemorrhage with the combined use of diclofenac and anticoagulant therapy. Therefore, to be certain that no change in anticoagulant dosage is required, close monitoring of such patients is required. As with other non-steroidal anti-inflammatory agents, diclofenac in a high dose can reversibly inhibit platelet aggregation.

Antidiabetic agents: Clinical studies have shown that Voltarol can be given together with oral antidiabetic agents without influencing their clinical effect. However there have been isolated reports of hypoglycaemic and hyperglycaemic effects which have required adjustment to the dosage of hypoglycaemic agents.

Cyclosporin: Cases of nephrotoxicity have been reported in patients receiving concomitant cyclosporin and NSAIDS, including Voltarol. This might be mediated through combined renal antiprostaglandin effects of both the NSAID and cyclosporin.

Methotrexate: Cases of serious toxicity have been reported when methotrexate and NSAIDS are given within 24 hours of each other. This interaction is mediated through accumulation of methotrexate resulting from impairment of renal excretion in the presence of the NSAID.

Quinolone antimicrobials: Convulsions may occur due to an interaction between quinolones and NSAIDS. This may occur in patients with or without a previous history of epilepsy or convulsions. Therefore, caution should be exercised when considering the use of a quinolone in patients who are already receiving an NSAID.

Other NSAIDS and corticosteroids: Co-administration of Voltarol with aspirin or corticosteroids may increase the risk of gastro-intestinal bleeding. Avoid concomitant use of two or more NSAIDs.

Diuretics: Like other NSAIDS, Voltarol may inhibit the activity of diuretics. Concomitant treatment with potassium-sparing diuretics may be associated with increased serum potassium levels, which should therefore be monitored frequently.

Cardiac glycosides: Concomitant use of cardiac glycosides and NSAIDs in patients may exacerbate cardiac failure, reduce GFR and increase plasma glycoside levels.

Mifepristone: NSAIDs should not be used for 8-12 days after mifepristone administration as NSAIDs can reduce the effect of mifepristone.

Anti-hypertensives: Concomitant use of NSAIDs with antihypertensive drugs (i.e. beta-blockers, angiotensin converting enzyme (ACE) inhibitors, diuretics) may cause a decrease in their antihypertensive effect via inhibition of vasodilatory prostaglandin synthesis.

4.6 Pregnancy and lactation

Although animal studies have not demonstrated teratogenic effects, Voltarol should not be prescribed during pregnancy, unless there are compelling reasons for doing so. The lowest effective dosage should be used.

Congenital abnormalities have been reported in association with the administration of NSAIDs in man; however, these are low in frequency and do not appear to follow any discernible pattern.

In view of the known effects of NSAIDs on the foetal cardiovascular system (e.g. a premature closure of the ductus arteriosus) and in causing uterine inertia, use in late pregnancy should be avoided.

Following doses of 50mg enteric coated tablets every 8 hours, traces of active substance have been detected in breast milk, but in quantities so small that no adverse effects on the breast-fed infant are to be expected.

4.7 Effects on ability to drive and use machines

Patients who experience dizziness or other central nervous disturbances, while taking NSAIDS should refrain from driving or operating machinery.

4.8 Undesirable effects

If serious side-effects occur, Voltarol should be withdrawn.

Frequency estimate: frequent: >10 %, occasional: >1 - 10 %, rare: >0.001 - 1 %, isolated cases: <0.001 %.)

Gastro-intestinal tract

Occasional: Epigastric pain, other gastro-intestinal disorders (e.g. nausea, vomiting, diarrhoea, abdominal cramps, dyspepsia, flatulence, anorexia).

Rare: Gastro-intestinal bleeding (haematemesis, melaena, bloody diarrhoea), gastro-intestinal ulcers with or without bleeding or perforation.

In isolated cases: Aphthous stomatitis, glossitis, oesophageal lesions, lower gut disorders (e.g. non-specific haemorrhagic colitis and exacerbations of ulcerative colitis or Crohn's proctocolitis, colonic damage and stricture formation), pancreatitis, constipation.

Central Nervous System:

Occasional: Headache, dizziness, or vertigo.

Rare: Drowsiness, tiredness.

In isolated cases: Disturbances of sensation, paraesthesia, memory disturbance, disorientation, insomnia, irritability, convulsions, depression, anxiety, nightmares, tremor, psychotic reactions, aseptic meningitis.

Special senses:

Isolated cases: Disturbances of vision (blurred vision, diplopia), impaired hearing, tinnitus, taste disturbances.

Skin:

Occasional: Rashes or skin eruptions.

Rare: Urticaria.

In isolated cases: Bullous eruptions, eczema, erythema multiforme, Stevens-Johnson syndrome, Lyell's syndrome, (acute toxic epidermolysis), erythroderma (exfoliative dermatitis), loss of hair, photosensitivity reactions, purpura including allergic purpura.

Kidney:

Rare: Oedema

In isolated cases: Acute renal insufficiency, urinary abnormalities (e.g. haematuria, proteinuria), interstitial nephritis, nephrotic syndrome, papillary necrosis.

Liver:

Occasional: Elevation of serum aminotransferase enzymes (ALT, AST).

Rare: Liver function disorders including hepatitis (in isolated cases fulminant) with or without jaundice.

Blood:

In isolated cases: Thrombocytopenia, leucopenia, agranulocytosis, haemolytic anaemia, aplastic anaemia.

Hypersensitivity:

Rare: Hypersensitivity reactions (e.g. bronchospasm, anaphylactic/anaphylactoid systemic reactions including hypotension).

Isolated cases: Vasculitis, pneumonitis.

Cardiovascular system:

Isolated cases: Palpitations, chest pain, hypertension, congestive heart failure.

Other organ systems:

Isolated cases: Impotence.

4.9 Overdose

Management of acute poisoning with NSAIDS essentially consists of supportive and symptomatic measures. There is no typical clinical picture resulting from Voltarol overdosage.

The therapeutic measures to be taken are: Supportive and symptomatic treatment should be given for complications such as hypotension, renal failure, convulsions, gastro-intestinal irritation, and respiratory depression.

Special therapies such as forced diuresis, dialysis or haemoperfusion are probably of no help in eliminating NSAIDS due to the high rate of protein binding and extensive metabolism.

5. PHARMACOLOGICAL PROPERTIES

5.1 Pharmacodynamic properties

Pharmacotherapeutic group

Non-steroidal anti-inflammatory drugs (NSAIDs).

Mechanism of action

Voltarol is a non-steroidal agent with marked analgesic/anti- inflammatory properties. It is an inhibitor of prostaglandin synthetase, (cyclo-oxygenase).

Diclofenac sodium *in vitro* does not suppress proteoglycan biosynthesis in cartilage at concentrations equivalent to the concentrations reached in human beings.

5.2 Pharmacokinetic properties

Absorption

Absorption is complete but onset is delayed until passage through the stomach, which may be affected by food which delays stomach emptying. The mean peak plasma diclofenac concentration reached at about 2 hours (50mg dose produces 1.48 ± 0.65μg/ml (1.5μg/ml $\equiv$ 5μmol/l)).

Bioavailability

About half of the administered diclofenac is metabolised during its first passage through the liver ("first-pass" effect), the area under the concentrations curve (AUC) following oral administration is about half that following an equivalent parenteral dose.

Pharmacokinetic behaviour does not change on repeated administration. Accumulation does not occur, provided the recommended dosage intervals are observed. The plasma concentrations attained in children given equivalent doses (mg/kg, b.w.) are similar to those obtained in adults.

Distribution

The active substance is 99.7% protein bound, mainly to albumin (99.4%).

Diclofenac enters the synovial fluid, where maximum concentrations are measured 2-4 hours after the peak plasma values have been attained. The apparent half-life for elimination from the synovial fluid is 3-6 hours. Two hours after reaching the peak plasma values, concentrations of the active substance are already higher in the synovial fluid than they are in the plasma and remain higher for up to 12 hours.

Metabolism

Biotransformation of diclofenac takes place partly by glucuronidation of the intact molecule, but mainly by single and multiple hydroxylation and methoxylation, resulting in several phenolic metabolites, most of which are converted to glucuronide conjugates. Two phenolic metabolites are biologically active, but to a much lesser extent than diclofenac.

Elimination

The total systemic clearance of diclofenac in plasma is 263 ± 56 mL/min (mean value ± SD). The terminal half-life in plasma is 1-2 hours. Four of the metabolites, including the two active ones, also have short plasma half-lives of 1-3 hours.

About 60% of the administered dose is excreted in the urine in the form of the glucuronide conjugate of the intact molecule and as metabolites, most of which are also converted to glucuronide conjugates. Less than 1% is excreted as unchanged substance. The rest of the dose is eliminated as metabolites through the bile in the faeces.

Characteristics in patients

Elderly: No relevant age-dependent differences in the drug's absorption, metabolism, or excretion have been observed, other than the finding that in five elderly patients, a 15 minute iv infusion resulted in 50% higher plasma concentrations than expected with young healthy subjects.

Patients with renal impairment: In patients suffering from renal impairment, no accumulation of the unchanged active substance can be inferred from the single-dose kinetics when applying the usual dosage schedule. At a creatinine clearance of <10 mL/min, the calculated steady-state plasma levels of the hydroxy metabolites are about 4 times higher than in normal subjects. However, the metabolites are ultimately cleared through the bile.

Patients with hepatic disease: In patients with chronic hepatitis or non-decompensated cirrhosis, the kinetics and metabolism of diclofenac are the same as in patients without liver disease.

5.3 Preclinical safety data

None stated.

6. PHARMACEUTICAL PARTICULARS

6.1 List of excipients

The enteric-coated tablets also contain aerosil 200 standard, lactose, maize starch, sodium starch glycollate, povidone (K30), avicel PH 102, magnesium stearate, hydroxypropyl methylcellulose, cremophor RH40, yellow iron oxide (E.172), red iron oxide (E.172) *50mg tablet only,* purified talc special, titanium dioxide (E.171), eudragit L30D-55, polyethylene glycol 8000 flakes, silicone antifoam emulsion SE2, ammonia 25% and purified water.

6.2 Incompatibilities

None known.

6.3 Shelf life

5 years.

6.4 Special precautions for storage

Protect from moisture. Store below 30°C.

Medicines should be kept out of the reach of children.

6.5 Nature and contents of container

The 25mg tablets are yellow, round, biconvex, film coated tablets, impressed GEIGY on one face and VOLTAROL 25 on the other, and come in PVC/PVdC blister packs of 84.

The 50mg tablets are light brown, round, biconvex, film coated tablets, impressed GEIGY on one face and VOLTAROL 50 on the other, and come in PVC/PVdC blister packs of 14 and 84.

6.6 Instructions for use and handling

The enteric-coated tablets should be swallowed whole, preferably before meals.

7. MARKETING AUTHORISATION HOLDER

Novartis Pharmaceuticals UK Ltd.

Trading as Geigy Pharmaceuticals,

Frimley Business Park

Frimley

Camberley

Surrey, GU16 7SR.

8. MARKETING AUTHORISATION NUMBER(S)

25mg: PL 00101/0476

50mg: PL 00101/0477

9. DATE OF FIRST AUTHORISATION/RENEWAL OF THE AUTHORISATION

11 July 1997

10. DATE OF REVISION OF THE TEXT

8 December 2000

Legal Category:

POM

Warticon Cream

(Stiefel Laboratories (UK) Limited)

1. NAME OF THE MEDICINAL PRODUCT
Warticon 0.15% w/w Cream

2. QUALITATIVE AND QUANTITATIVE COMPOSITION
Podophyllotoxin 1.5 mg/g (0.15% w/w).

For excipients, see 6.1

3. PHARMACEUTICAL FORM
Topical cream

A homogenous white cream.

4. CLINICAL PARTICULARS
4.1 Therapeutic indications
Route of administration: Topical

For the topical treatment of condylomata acuminata affecting the penis and the external female genitalia.

4.2 Posology and method of administration
The affected area should be thoroughly washed with soap and water, and dried prior to application.

Using a fingertip, the cream is applied twice daily for 3 days using only enough cream to just cover each wart.

Residual warts should be treated with further courses of twice daily applications for three days at weekly intervals, if necessary for a total of 4 weeks of treatment.

Where lesions are greater than 4 cm^2, it is recommended that treatment takes place under the direct supervision of medical staff.

4.3 Contraindications
Known hypersensitivity to any of the ingredients

Open wounds eg. Following surgical procedures.

Use in children.

Hypersensitivity to podophyllotoxin.

Concomitant use with other podophyllotoxin containing preparations.

Pregnancy and lactation.

4.4 Special warnings and special precautions for use
Avoid contact with eyes. Should the cream accidentally come into the eye, the eye should be thoroughly rinsed with water.

The hands should be thoroughly washed after each application. Prolonged contact with healthy skin must be avoided since cream contains an active pharmaceutical substance which could be harmful on healthy skin.

4.5 Interaction with other medicinal products and other forms of Interaction
None presently known.

4.6 Pregnancy and lactation
The product is not for use in pregnancy or lactation.

Reproduction toxicity studies in animals have not given evidence of an increased incidence of foetal damage or other deleterious effects on the reproductive process. However, since podophyllotoxin is a mitosis inhibitor, Warticon Cream should not be used during pregnancy or lactation.

It is not known if the substance is excreted into breast milk.

Observations in man indicate that podophyllin, a crude mixture of lignans, can be harmful to pregnancy. Such observations have not been reported in patients treated with podophyllotoxin.

4.7 Effects on ability to drive and use machines
None presently known.

4.8 Undesirable effects
Local irritation may occur on the second or third day of application associated with the start of wart necrosis. In most cases the reactions are mild. Tenderness, itching, smarting, erythema, superficial epithelial ulceration and balanoposthitis have been reported. Local irritation decreases after treatment.

4.9 Overdose
There have been no reported overdosages with Warticon cream. However, excessive use of podophyllotoxin 0.5% solution has been reported as causing two cases of severe local reactions. In cases of excessive use of Warticon cream resulting in severe local reaction, the treatment should be stopped, the area washed and symptomatic treatment introduced.

No specific antidote is known. In the event of accidental ingestion, give emetic or stomach washout. Treatment should be symptomatic and in severe oral overdose ensure the airway is clear and give fluids. Check and correct electrolyte balance, monitor blood gases and liver function. Blood count should be monitored for at least 5 days.

5. PHARMACOLOGICAL PROPERTIES
5.1 Pharmacodynamic properties
Pharmaco-therapeutic group, D06BB antivirals

Podophyllotoxin is a metaphase inhibitor in dividing cells binding to at least one binding site on tubulin. Binding prevents tubulin polymerisation required for microtubule assembly. At higher concentrations, podophyllotoxin also inhibits nucleoside transport through the cell membrane.

The chemotherapeutic action of podophyllotoxin is assumed to be due to inhibition of growth and the ability to invade the tissue of the viral infected cells.

5.2 Pharmacokinetic properties
Systemic absorption of podophyllotoxin after topical application with a higher strength, 0.3% is low. Thus no study was performed on the present strength, 0.15%. The C_{max} (1.0 – 4.7 ng/ml) and T_{max} (0.5 – 36 hrs) are comparable for the 0.3% cream and 0.5% solution in both males and females.

5.3 Preclinical safety data
No relevant findings

6. PHARMACEUTICAL PARTICULARS
6.1 List of excipients
Purified Water

Methyl parahydroxybenzoate E218

Propyl parahydroxybenzoate E216

Sorbic acid

Phosphoric acid

Stearyl alcohol

Cetyl alcohol

Isopropyl myristate

Paraffin, liquid

Fractionated coconut oil

Butylhydroxyanisole (BHA) E320

Macrogol -7 stearyl ether

Macrogol – 10 stearyl ether

6.2 Incompatibilities
None known

6.3 Shelf life
3 years

6.4 Special precautions for storage
This medicinal product does not require any special storage precautions.

6.5 Nature and contents of container
A collapsible aluminium tube with imperforate nozzle membrane and internally coated with a protective lacquer. Tube cap of polyethylene with a spike on the upper end aimed to perforate the membrane when opening the tube for the first time. Size 5g.

6.6 Instructions for use and handling
No special requirements.

7. MARKETING AUTHORISATION HOLDER
Stiefel Laboratories (UK) Ltd.

Holtspur Lane,

Wooburn Green,

High Wycombe,

Bucks.

HP10 0AU

8. MARKETING AUTHORISATION NUMBER(S)
PL 00174/0210

9. DATE OF FIRST AUTHORISATION/RENEWAL OF THE AUTHORISATION
26 April 1999/18 January 2005

10. DATE OF REVISION OF THE TEXT
February 2005

Warticon Solution/Warticon FEM

(Stiefel Laboratories (UK) Limited)

1. NAME OF THE MEDICINAL PRODUCT
Warticon Solution/Warticon FEM

2. QUALITATIVE AND QUANTITATIVE COMPOSITION
Podophyllotoxin 5 mg/ml (0.5%w/v). The quality of podophyllotoxin fulfils in-house specification.

3. PHARMACEUTICAL FORM
Topical solution

4. CLINICAL PARTICULARS
4.1 Therapeutic indications
Warticon: For the topical treatment of condylomata penis.

Warticon Fem: For the treatment of condylomata acuminata affecting the external female genitalia.

4.2 Posology and method of administration
The affected area should be thoroughly washed with soap and water, and dried prior to application.

Warticon is applied twice daily for 3 days. If residual warts persist, this 3-day treatment may be repeated weekly, if necessary, for a total of 4 weeks of treatment.

Where lesions are greater than 4 cm^2, it is recommended that treatment takes place under the direct supervision of medical staff.

4.3 Contraindications
Open wounds following surgical procedures should not be treated with podophyllotoxin.

Hypersensitivity to podophyllotoxin is a contra-indication.

Use in children.

Concomitant use with other podophyllotoxin containing preparations.

Pregnancy and lactation.

4.4 Special warnings and special precautions for use
Avoid contact with eyes. Should the solution accidentally come into contact with the eye, the eye should be thoroughly rinsed with water.

The hands should be thoroughly washed after each application. Prolonged contact with healthy skin must be avoided since the solution contains an active pharmaceutical substance which could be harmful on healthy skin.

4.5 Interaction with other medicinal products and other forms of Interaction
None presently known.

4.6 Pregnancy and lactation
The product is not for use in pregnancy or lactation.

Reproduction toxicity studies in animals have not given evidence of an increased incidence of foetal damage or other deleterious effects on the reproductive process. However, since podophyllotoxin is a mitosis inhibitor, Warticon solution should not be used during pregnancy or lactation.

It is not known if the substance is excreted into breast milk.

Observations in man indicate that podophyllin, a crude mixture of lignans, can be harmful to pregnancy. Such observations have not been reported in patients treated with podophyllotoxin.

4.7 Effects on ability to drive and use machines
None presently known.

4.8 Undesirable effects
Local irritation may occur on the second or third day of application associated with the start of wart necrosis. In most cases the reactions are mild. Tenderness, itching, smarting, erythema, superficial epithelial ulceration and balanoposthitis have been reported. Local irritation decreases after treatment.

4.9 Overdose
There have been no reported overdosages with Warticon Solution. However, excessive use of podophyllotoxin 0.5% solution has been reported as causing two cases of severe local reactions. In cases of excessive use of Warticon Solution resulting in severe local reaction, the treatment should be stopped, the area washed and symptomatic treatment introduced.

No specific antidote is known. In the event of accidental ingestion, give emetic or stomach washout. Treatment should be symptomatic and in severe oral overdose ensure the airway is clear and give fluids. Check and correct electrolyte balance, monitor blood gases and liver function. Blood count should be monitored for at least 5 days.

5. PHARMACOLOGICAL PROPERTIES
5.1 Pharmacodynamic properties
Pharmaco-therapeutic group: D06B B Antivirals

Podophyllotoxin is a metaphase inhibitor in dividing cells binding to at least one binding site on tubulin. Binding prevents tubulin polymerisation required for microtubule assembly. At higher concentrations, podophyllotoxin also inhibits nucleoside transport through the cell membrane.

The chemotherapeutic action of podophyllotoxin is assumed to be due to inhibition of growth and the ability to invade the tissue of the viral infected cells.

5.2 Pharmacokinetic properties
Topical administration of a 0.5% solution of ethanolic podophyllotoxin in the majority of cases only requires volumes in the range of 0.1ml to 0.2ml. Studies monitoring serum drug level reveal that topical application of a twice daily dose of 100μl to the penile preputial cavity in 10 patients resulted in a maximum serum concentration of 0.25ng/ml.

5.3 Preclinical safety data
No relevant findings

6. PHARMACEUTICAL PARTICULARS

6.1 List of excipients

Phosphoric acid Ph Eur

Ethanol BP

Purified Water Ph Eur

Patent Blue V (E131)

6.2 Incompatibilities

None known

6.3 Shelf life

36 months

6.4 Special precautions for storage

Should be stored at below 25°C.

6.5 Nature and contents of container

An amber glass bottle with plastic child-proof cap. Each bottle contains 3ml of Warticon Solution. The outer carton also includes a tube containing plastic applicators. Each loop will carry approximately 5μl Warticon Solution.

Warticon Fem also contains a free-standing mirror to facilitate more accurate application.

6.6 Instructions for use and handling

The solution is applied by the plastic applicators provided.

7. MARKETING AUTHORISATION HOLDER

Stiefel Laboratories (UK) Ltd.

Holtspur Lane

Wooburn Green

High Wycombe

Bucks

HP10 0AU

8. MARKETING AUTHORISATION NUMBER(S)

PL 00174/0211

9. DATE OF FIRST AUTHORISATION/RENEWAL OF THE AUTHORISATION

08 October 2003

10. DATE OF REVISION OF THE TEXT

26 September 2005

Waxsol Ear Drops

(Norgine Limited)

1. NAME OF THE MEDICINAL PRODUCT

WAXSOL Ear Drops.

2. QUALITATIVE AND QUANTITATIVE COMPOSITION

WAXSOL Ear Drops contain the following active ingredient:

Docusate Sodium BP 0.5% w/v.

3. PHARMACEUTICAL FORM

Ear drops.

4. CLINICAL PARTICULARS

4.1 Therapeutic indications

WAXSOL Ear Drops are indicated as an aid in the removal of ear wax.

4.2 Posology and method of administration

Recommended dose and dosage schedules:

Adults (including the elderly): The application of ear drops sufficient to fill the affected ear on not more than two consecutive nights, prior to attending for syringing if this is necessary.

Children: As for adult dose.

4.3 Contraindications

Perforation of the ear drum or inflammation of the ear.

4.4 Special warnings and special precautions for use

If pain or inflammation is experienced, treatment should be discontinued.

4.5 Interaction with other medicinal products and other forms of Interaction

None known.

4.6 Pregnancy and lactation

There is no evidence to suggest that WAXSOL Ear Drops should not be used during pregnancy and lactation.

4.7 Effects on ability to drive and use machines

None known.

4.8 Undesirable effects

Rarely transient stinging or irritation may occur.

4.9 Overdose

None known.

5. PHARMACOLOGICAL PROPERTIES

5.1 Pharmacodynamic properties

The so-called "wax" which often obstructs the external auditory meatus of the ear contains less than 50% of fatty matter derived from secretions of the sebaceous ceruminous glands. The majority of the wax consists of desquamated epithelium, foreign matter and shed hairs. This non-fatty material forms a matrix holding together the granules of fatty matter to form the ceruminous mass.

The addition of oils or solvents binds the mass more firmly together, but aqueous solutions, if they are able to penetrate the matrix, cause a disintegration of the ceruminous mass.

WAXSOL Ear Drops, because of their low surface tension and miscibility, rapidly penetrate the dry matrix of the ceruminous mass, reducing the solid material to a semi-solid debris. This can be syringed away readily, or in less severe or chronic cases, is ejected by normal physiological processes.

5.2 Pharmacokinetic properties

Not applicable.

5.3 Preclinical safety data

None.

6. PHARMACEUTICAL PARTICULARS

6.1 List of excipients

Glycerin

Phenonip (solution of esters of 4-hydroxybenzoic acid in phenoxetol)

Water

6.2 Incompatibilities

None known.

6.3 Shelf life

3 years.

6.4 Special precautions for storage

Store below 25°C.

6.5 Nature and contents of container

Amber glass bottle with a dropper applicator, containing 10 or 11 ml of WAXSOL solution.

6.6 Instructions for use and handling

The dropper applicator must be filled before dripping WAXSOL Ear Drops into the affected ear.

7. MARKETING AUTHORISATION HOLDER

Norgine Limited

Chaplin House

Widewater Place

Moorhall Road

Harefield

UXBRIDGE

Middlesex, UB9 6NS

United Kingdom

8. MARKETING AUTHORISATION NUMBER(S)

PL 00322/5016R

9. DATE OF FIRST AUTHORISATION/RENEWAL OF THE AUTHORISATION

25 July 1985/28 October 2001

10. DATE OF REVISION OF THE TEXT

June 1998

Legal Category: **P**

Wellvone 750mg/5ml oral suspension

(GlaxoSmithKline UK)

1. NAME OF THE MEDICINAL PRODUCT

Wellvone 750mg/5ml oral suspension

2. QUALITATIVE AND QUANTITATIVE COMPOSITION

Atovaquone 150mg/ml

A unit dose of 5ml contains 750mg atovaquone.

For excipients, see section 6.1.

3. PHARMACEUTICAL FORM

Oral suspension.

4. CLINICAL PARTICULARS

4.1 Therapeutic indications

Wellvone Suspension is indicated for:

Acute treatment of mild to moderate *Pneumocystis carinii* pneumonia (PCP) (alveolar - arterial oxygen tension difference [(A-a)DO_2] $\leq$ 45 mmHg (6 kPa) and oxygen tension in arterial blood (PaO_2) $\geqslant$ 60 mmHg (8 kPa) breathing room air) in patients who are intolerant of co-trimoxazole therapy. (See Special Warnings and Precautions for Use).

4.2 Posology and method of administration

The importance of taking the full prescribed dose of Wellvone with food should be stressed to patients. The presence of food, particularly high fat food, increases bioavailability two to three fold.

Dosage in adults

Pneumocystis carinii pneumonia:

The recommended oral dose is 750 mg twice a day (1 × 5ml morning and evening) administered with food each day for 21 days.

Higher doses may be more effective in some patients (see section 5.2 Pharmacokinetic Properties).

Dosage in Children

Clinical efficacy has not been studied.

Dosage in the Elderly

There have been no studies of Wellvone in the elderly. (See Special Warnings and Precautions for Use).

Renal or hepatic impairment

Wellvone has not been specifically studied in patients with significant hepatic or renal impairment (see Pharmacokinetics in Adults). If it is necessary to treat such patients with Wellvone, caution is advised and administration should be closely monitored.

4.3 Contraindications

Wellvone Suspension is contra-indicated in individuals with known hypersensitivity to atovaquone or to any components of the formulation.

4.4 Special warnings and special precautions for use

Diarrhoea at the start of treatment has been shown to be associated with significantly lower atovaquone plasma levels. These in turn correlated with a higher incidence of therapy failures and a lower survival rate. Therefore, alternative therapies should be considered for such patients and for patients who have difficulty taking Wellvone with food.

The concomitant administration of atovaquone and rifampicin or rifabutin is not recommended (see Interaction with Other Medicaments section 4.5).

The efficacy of Wellvone has not been systematically evaluated i) in patients failing other PCP therapy, including co-trimoxazole, ii) for treatment of severe episodes of PCP [(A-a) $DO_2 > 45$ mmHg (6kPa)], iii) as a prophylactic agent for PCP, or iv) versus intravenous pentamidine for treatment of PCP.

No data are available in non-HIV immuno-compromised patients suffering with PCP.

As HIV infection is rarely observed in elderly patients, no clinical experience of atovaquone treatment has been gained. Therefore use in the elderly should be closely monitored.

Patients with pulmonary disease should be carefully evaluated for causes of disease other than PCP and treated with additional agents as appropriate. Wellvone is not expected to be effective therapy for other fungal, bacterial, mycobacterial or viral diseases.

4.5 Interaction with other medicinal products and other forms of Interaction

As experience is limited, care should be taken when combining other drugs with Wellvone.

Concomitant administration of rifampicin or rifabutin is known to reduce atovaquone levels by approximately 50% and 34%, respectively, and could result in sub therapeutic plasma concentrations in some patients (see Special Warnings and Precautions for Use).

Concomitant treatment with tetracycline or metoclopramide has been associated with significant decreases in plasma concentrations of atovaquone. Caution should be exercised in prescribing these drugs with Wellvone until the potential interaction has been further studied.

In clinical trials of Wellvone small decreases in plasma concentrations of atovaquone (mean < 3 μg/ml) were associated with concomitant administration of paracetamol, benzodiazepines, acyclovir, opiates, cephalosporins, anti-diarrhoeals and laxatives. The causal relationship between the change in plasma concentrations of atovaquone and the administration of the drugs mentioned above is unknown.

Clinical trials have evaluated the interaction of Wellvone Tablets with:

Zidovudine -Zidovudine does not appear to affect the pharmacokinetics of atovaquone. However, pharmacokinetic data have shown that atovaquone appears to decrease the rate of metabolism of zidovudine to its glucuronide metabolite (steady state AUC of zidovudine was increased by 33% and peak plasma concentration of the glucuronide was decreased by 19%). At zidovudine dosages of 500 or 600 mg/day it would seem unlikely that a three week, concomitant course of Wellvone for the treatment of acute PCP would result in an increased incidence of adverse reactions attributable to higher plasma concentrations of zidovudine.

Didanosine (ddI) - ddI does not affect the pharmacokinetics of atovaquone as determined in a prospective multi-dose drug interaction study of atovaquone and ddI. However, there was a 24% decrease in the AUC for ddI when co-administered with atovaquone which is unlikely to be of clinical significance.

Nevertheless, the modes of interaction being unknown, the effects of atovaquone administration on zidovudine and ddI may be greater with atovaquone suspension. The higher concentrations of atovaquone possible with the suspension might induce greater changes in the AUC values for zidovudine or ddI than those observed. Patients receiving atovaquone and zidovudine should be regularly monitored for zidovudine associated adverse effects.

Concomitant administration of Wellvone and indinavir results in a significant decrease in the C_{min} of indinavir (23% decrease; 90% CI 8-35%) and the AUC (9% decrease; 90% CI 1-18%). Caution should be exercised on the potential risk of failure of indinavir treatment if co-administered with atovaquone. No data are available regarding potential interactions of Wellvone and other protease inhibitor drugs.

In clinical trials of Wellvone the following medications were not associated with a change in steady state plasma concentrations of atovaquone: fluconazole, clotrimazole, ketoconazole, antacids, systemic corticosteroids, non-steroidal anti-inflammatory drugs, anti-emetics (excluding metoclopramide) and H_2-antagonists.

Atovaquone is highly bound to plasma proteins and caution should be used when administering Wellvone concurrently with other highly plasma protein bound drugs with narrow therapeutic indices. Atovaquone does not affect the pharmacokinetics, metabolism or extent of protein binding of phenytoin *in vivo*. *In vitro* there is no plasma protein binding interaction between atovaquone and quinine, phenytoin, warfarin, sulfamethoxazole, indometacin or diazepam.

4.6 Pregnancy and lactation

Thereis no information on the effects of atovaquone administration during human pregnancy. Atovaquone should not be used during pregnancy unless the benefit of treatment to the mother outweighs any possible risk to the developing foetus.

Insufficient data are available from animal experiments to assess the possible risk to reproductive potential or performance.

It is not known whether atovaquone is excreted in human milk, and therefore breast feeding is not recommended.

4.7 Effects on ability to drive and use machines

There have been no studies to investigate the effect of Wellvone on driving performance or the ability to operate machinery but a detrimental effect on such activities is not predicted from the pharmacology of the drug.

4.8 Undesirable effects

Patients participating in clinical trials with Wellvone have often had complications of advanced Human Immunodeficiency Virus (HIV) disease and therefore the causal relationship between the adverse experiences and atovaquone is difficult to evaluate.

Very common (greater than 1/10)

Gastrointestinal: nausea

Skin: rash

Common (greater than 1/100, less than 1/10)

Gastrointestinal: diarrhoea, vomiting

Neurology: headache, insomnia

Hepatobiliary tract & pancreas: elevated liver enzyme levels

Blood & lymphatic: anaemia, neutropenia

Endocrine & metabolic: hyponatraemia

Non-site specific: fever

Uncommon (greater than 1/1000, less than 1/100)

Hepatobiliary tract & pancreas: elevated amylase levels

4.9 Overdose

There is insufficient experience to predict the consequences or suggest specific management of atovaquone overdose. However, in the reported cases of overdosage, the observed effects were consistent with known undesirable effects of the drug. If overdosage occurs, the patient should be monitored and standard supportive treatment applied.

5. PHARMACOLOGICAL PROPERTIES

5.1 Pharmacodynamic properties

Pharmacotherapeutic group:Antiprotozoals,

ATC Code: P01A X06.

a. Mode of Action

Atovaquone belongs to a new therapeutic class with a novel mechanism of action. It is a selective and potent inhibitor of the eukaryotic mitochondrial electron transport chain in a number of parasitic protozoa. The site of action appears to be the cytochrome bc1 complex (complex III). The ultimate metabolic effect of such blockade is likely to be inhibition of nucleic acid and ATP synthesis.

b. Microbiology

Atovaquone has potent antiprotozoal activity, both *in vitro* and in animal models, particularly against the parasitic protozoan-like fungus *Pneumocystis carinii* (IC_{50} 0.1-1.0 μg/ml).

5.2 Pharmacokinetic properties

Atovaquone is a highly lipophilic compound with a low aqueous solubility. It is 99.9% bound to plasma proteins. The bioavailability of the drug demonstrates a relative decrease with single doses above 750 mg, and shows considerable inter-individual variability. Average absolute bioavailablility of a 750 mg single dose of atovaquone suspension administered with food to adult HIV positive males is 47% (compared to 23% for Wellvone tablets). Following the intravenous administration, the volume of distribution and clearance were calculated to be 0.62±0.19l/kg and 0.15±0.09ml/min/kg, respectively.

The bioavailability of atovaquone is greater when administered with food than in the fasting state. In healthy volunteers, a standardized breakfast (23 g fat; 610 kCal) increased bioavailability two to three-fold following a single 750 mg dose. The mean area under the atovaquone plasma concentration-time curve (AUC) was increased 2.5 fold and the mean C_{max} was increased 3.4 fold. The mean (±SD) AUC values for suspension were 324.3 (±115.0) μg/ml.h fasted and 800.6 (±319.8) μg/ml.h with food.

In a safety and pharmacokinetic study in patients with PCP, the following results were obtained:

Dose regimen	750 mg twice daily	1000 mg twice daily
Number of Patients	18	9
C avg, ss (range)	22 micrograms/ml (6-41)	25.7 micrograms/ml (15-36)
% of patients with C avg, ss >15 micrograms/ml	67%	100%

In a small safety and pharmacokinetic study of two higher dosing regimens [750 mg three times daily (n=8) and 1500 mg twice daily (n=8)] in HIV infected volunteers with severity criteria comparable to patients with PCP, similar Cavg were reached with the two doses [respectively for the 750mg tid and 1500 mg bid doses: 24.8 (7-40) and 23.4 micrograms/ml (7-35). Moreover, for both doses a Cavg, ss >15 μg/ml was reached in 87.5% of patients.

Average steady state concentrations above 15 micrograms/ml are predictive of a high (>90%) success rate.

In healthy volunteers and patients with AIDS, atovaquone has a half-life of 2 to 3 days.

In healthy volunteers there is no evidence that the drug is metabolised and there is negligible excretion of atovaquone in the urine, with parent drug being predominantly (>90%) excreted unchanged in faeces.

5.3 Preclinical safety data

a. Carcinogenicity

Oncogenicity studies in mice showed an increased incidence of hepatocellular adenomas and carcinomas without determination of the no observed adverse effect level. No such findings were observed in rats and mutagenicity tests were negative. These findings appear to be due to the inherent susceptibility of mice to atovaquone and are not predictive of a risk in the clinical situation.

b. Reproductive toxicity

In the dosage range of 600 to 1200 mg/kg studies in rabbits gave indications of maternal and embryotoxic effects.

6. PHARMACEUTICAL PARTICULARS

6.1 List of excipients

Benzyl alcohol

Xanthan Gum

Poloxamer 188

Saccharin Sodium

Purified water

Tutti Frutti Flavour (Firmenich 51.880/A) containing sweet orange oil, concentrated orange oil, propylene glycol, benzyl alcohol, vanillin, acetic aldehyde, amyl acetate and ethyl butyrate.

6.2 Incompatibilities

Not applicable

6.3 Shelf life

2 years

After first opening, the suspension may be stored for up to 21 days.

6.4 Special precautions for storage

Do not store above 25°C.

Do not freeze.

6.5 Nature and contents of container

A 240 ml high density polyethylene bottle with child resistant closure, containing 226 ml of atovaquone suspension.

A 5 ml measuring spoon (polypropylene) is included.

6.6 Instructions for use and handling

Do not dilute.

Administrative Data

7. MARKETING AUTHORISATION HOLDER

Glaxo Wellcome UK Ltd, trading as GlaxoSmithKline UK.

Stockley Park West,

Uxbridge,

Middlesex. UB11 1BT

8. MARKETING AUTHORISATION NUMBER(S)

PL 10949/0271

9. DATE OF FIRST AUTHORISATION/RENEWAL OF THE AUTHORISATION

21 August 1996

10. DATE OF REVISION OF THE TEXT

04 May 2004

11. Legal Status

POM

Xagrid 0.5mg hard capsule

(Shire Pharmaceuticals Limited)

1. NAME OF THE MEDICINAL PRODUCT

Xagrid ▼ 0.5mg hard capsule

2. QUALITATIVE AND QUANTITATIVE COMPOSITION

Each capsule contains 0.5 mg anagrelide (as 0.61 mg anagrelide hydrochloride)

For excipients, see 6.1.

3. PHARMACEUTICAL FORM

Capsule, hard

An opaque white hard capsule imprinted with S 063

4. CLINICAL PARTICULARS

4.1 Therapeutic indications

Xagrid is indicated for the reduction of elevated platelet counts in at risk essential thrombocythaemia patients who are intolerant to their current therapy or whose elevated platelet counts are not reduced to an acceptable level by their current therapy.

An at risk patient

An at risk essential thrombocythaemia patient is defined by one or more of the following features:

$>$60 years of age or

A platelet count $>$1000 $\times$ 10^9/l or

A history of thrombo-haemorrhagic events.

4.2 Posology and method of administration

Treatment with Xagrid capsules should be initiated by a clinician with experience in the management of essential thrombocythaemia (ET).

The recommended starting dosage of anagrelide is 1mg/day, which should be administered orally in two divided doses (0.5mg/dose).

The starting dose should be maintained for at least one week. After one week the dosage may be titrated, on an individual basis, to achieve the lowest effective dosage required to reduce and/or maintain a platelet count below 600 $\times$ 10^9/l and ideally at levels between 150 $\times$ 10^9/l and 400 $\times$ 10^9/l. The dosage increment must not exceed more than 0.5mg/day in any one-week and the recommended maximum single dose should not exceed 2.5mg (see section 4.9). During clinical development dosages of 10mg/day have been used.

The effects of treatment with anagrelide must be monitored on a regular basis (see section 4.4). If the starting dose is $>$1mg/day platelet counts should be performed every two days during the first week of treatment and at least weekly thereafter until a stable maintenance dose is reached. Typically, a fall in the platelet count will be observed within 14 to 21 days of starting treatment and in most patients an adequate therapeutic response will be observed and maintained at a dosage of 1 to 3mg/day (for further information on the clinical effects refer to section 5.1).

Elderly

No specific pharmacokinetic studies have been conducted in this patient population. However, during the clinical development approximately 50% of the patients treated with anagrelide were over 60 years of age and no age specific alterations in dosage were required in these patients. However, as expected, patients in this age group had twice the incidence of serious adverse events (mainly cardiac). Doses are titrated on an individual patient basis.

Renal impairment

Currently, there are no specific pharmacokinetic data for this patient population and the potential risk and benefits of anagrelide therapy in a patient with impairment of renal function should be assessed before treatment is commenced. Doses are titrated on an individual patient basis. Patients with mild to severe renal impairment have been treated with anagrelide at doses consistent with those used in patients without impairment (see section 4.3 and 4.4).

Hepatic impairment

Currently, there are no specific pharmacokinetic data for this patient population. However, hepatic metabolism represents the major route of drug clearance and liver function may therefore be expected to influence this process. Therefore it is recommended that patients with severe hepatic impairment are not treated with anagrelide. The potential risks and benefits of anagrelide therapy in a patient with mild or moderate impairment of hepatic function should be assessed before treatment is commenced (see section 4.3 and 4.4).

4.3 Contraindications

Hypersensitivity to anagrelide or to any of the excipients of the medicinal product.

Patients with severe hepatic impairment (Child-Pugh classification C).

Patients with severe renal impairment (creatinine clearance $<$30ml/min).

4.4 Special warnings and special precautions for use

Hepatic impairment: (see section 4.2 and 4.3) the potential risk and benefits of anagrelide therapy in a patient with mild or moderate impairment of hepatic function should be assessed before treatment is commenced. It is not recommended in patients with elevated transaminases $>$5 times the upper limit of normal).

Renal impairment: (see section 4.2 and 4.3) the potential risks and benefits of anagrelide therapy in a patient with impairment of renal function should be assessed before treatment is commenced.

General: therapy requires close clinical supervision of the patient which will include a full blood count (haemoglobin and white blood cells and platelet counts), and assessment of liver function (ALT and AST) and renal function (serum creatinine and urea) tests.

Platelets: the platelet count will increase within 4 days of stopping treatment with Xagrid capsules and will return to pre-treatment levels within 10 to 14 days.

Cardiovascular: Cases of cardiomegaly and congestive heart failure have been reported (see section 4.8). Anagrelide should be used with caution in patients of any age with known or suspected heart disease, and only if the potential benefits of therapy outweigh the potential risks. Anagrelide is an inhibitor of cyclic AMP phosphodiesterase III and because of its positive inotropic effects, a pre-treatment cardiovascular examination (including further investigation such as echocardiography, electrocardiogram) is recommended. Patients should be monitored during treatment for evidence of cardiovascular effects that may require further cardiovascular examination and investigation.

Paediatric patients: (see section 5.1) limited data are available on the use of anagrelide in the paediatric population and anagrelide should be used in this patient group with caution.

Clinically relevant interactions: anagrelide is an inhibitor of cyclic AMP phosphodiesterase III (PDE III). Concomitant use of anagrelide with other phosphodiesterase (PDEIII) inhibitors such as milrinone, amrinone, enoximone, olprinone and cilostazol is not recommended. The potential risks and benefits of the concomitant use of anagrelide with acetylsalicylic acid in patients with a platelet count greater than 1500 $\times$ 10^9/l and/or a history of haemorrhage should be assessed before treatment is commenced.

4.5 Interaction with other medicinal products and other forms of Interaction

Limited pharmacokinetic and/or pharmacodynamic studies investigating possible interactions between anagrelide and other medicinal products have been conducted.

Drug interactions: effects of other substances on anagrelide

Anagrelide is primarily metabolised by CYP1A2. It is known that CYP1A2 is inhibited by several medicinal products, including fluvoxamine and omeprazole, and such medicinal products could theoretically adversely influence the clearance of anagrelide.*In vivo* interaction studies in humans have demonstrated that digoxin and warfarin do not affect the pharmacokinetic properties of anagrelide.

Drug interactions: effects of anagrelide on other substances

Anagrelide demonstrates some limited inhibitory activity towards CYP1A2 which may present a theoretical potential for interaction with other co-administered medicinal products sharing that clearance mechanism e.g. theophylline. Anagrelide is an inhibitor of cyclic AMP phosphodiesterase III (PDE III). The effects of medicinal products with similar properties such as the inotropes milrinone, enoximone, amrinone, olprinone and cilostazol may be exacerbated by anagrelide. An *in vitro* study in human whole blood demonstrated that the anti-aggregatory effects of acetylsalicylic acid were additively, but not synergistically increased by the presence of anagrelide. *In vivo* interaction studies in humans have demonstrated that anagrelide does not affect the pharmacokinetic properties of digoxin or warfarin. At the doses recommended for use in the treatment of essential thrombocythaemia, anagrelide may theoretically potentiate the effects of other medicinal products that inhibit or modify platelet function e.g. acetylsalicylic acid. However, during clinical development, no such effects have been observed with acetylsalicylic acid. Anagrelide may cause intestinal disturbance in some patients and compromise the absorption of hormonal oral contraceptives. A preclinical *in vivo* pharmacokinetic interaction study in the dog investigating the potential effects of anagrelide and hydroxyurea when given in combination demonstrated no adverse effects on the kinetics of either medicinal product.

Food interactions:

Food delays the absorption of anagrelide but does not significantly alter systemic exposure. The effects of food on bioavailability are not considered clinically relevant to the use of anagrelide. Grapefruit juice has been shown to inhibit CYP1A2 and therefore could also reduce the clearance of anagrelide.

4.6 Pregnancy and lactation

Pregnancy:

There are no adequate data from the use of anagrelide in pregnant women.

Studies in animals have shown reproductive toxicity (see section 5.3). The potential risk for humans is unknown.

Use of Xagrid during pregnancy is not recommended. If Xagrid is used during pregnancy, or if the patient becomes pregnant while using the drug, they should be advised of the potential risk to the foetus.

Women of child-bearing potential should use adequate birth-control measures during treatment with anagrelide.

Lactation. It is not known whether anagrelide hydrochloride is excreted in milk. Since many medicinal products are excreted in human milk and because of the potential for adverse reactions in breast-feeding infants, mothers should discontinue breast-feeding when taking Xagrid.

4.7 Effects on ability to drive and use machines

No studies on the effects on the ability to drive and use machines have been performed. In clinical development, dizziness was commonly reported.

Patients are advised not to drive or operate machinery while taking Xagrid if dizziness is experienced.

4.8 Undesirable effects

The safety of anagrelide has been examined in 4 open label clinical studies. In 3 of the studies 942 patients who received anagrelide at a mean dose of approximately 2mg/day were assessed for safety. In these studies 22 patients received anagrelide for up to 4 years.

In the later study 3660 patients who received anagrelide at a mean dose of approximately 2mg/day were assessed for safety. In this study 34 patients received anagrelide for up to 5 years.

The most commonly reported drug related adverse reactions were headache occurring at approximately 14%, palpitations occurring at approximately 9%, fluid retention and nausea both occurring at approximately 6%, and diarrhoea occurring at 5%. These adverse drug reactions are expected based on the pharmacology of anagrelide (inhibition of phosphodiesterase III). Gradual dose titration may help diminish these effects (see section 4.2).

The following convention was used for frequency of adverse drug reactions: very common $>$1/10); common $>$1/100, $<$1/10); uncommon $>$1/1,000, $<$1/100); rare $>$1/10,000, $<$1/1,000).

Blood and lymphatic system disorders

Common: Anaemia

Uncommon: Thrombocytopaenia, pancytopaenia, ecchymosis, haemorrhage

Metabolism and nutrition disorders

Common: Fluid retention

Uncommon: Oedema, weight loss

Rare: Weight gain

Nervous system disorders

Very common: Headache

Common: Dizziness

Uncommon: Paraesthesia, insomnia, depression, confusion, hypoaesthesia, nervousness, dry mouth, amnesia

Rare: Somnolence, abnormal coordination, dysarthria

Special senses

Rare: Vision abnormal, tinnitus, diplopia

Cardiac disorders

Common: Palpitations, tachycardia

Uncommon: Congestive heart failure, hypertension, arrhythmia, atrial fibrillation, supraventricular tachycardia, ventricular tachycardia, syncope

Rare: Angina pectoris, myocardial infarction, cardiomegaly, pericardial effusion, vasodilatation, migraine, postural hypotension

Respiratory and thoracic disorders

Uncommon: Dyspnoea, epistaxis, pleural effusion, pneumonia

Rare: Pulmonary infiltrates

Gastrointestinal disorders

Common: Nausea, diarrhoea, abdominal pain, flatulence, vomiting

Uncommon: Dyspepsia, anorexia, pancreatitis, constipation, gastrointestinal haemorrhage, gastrointestinal disorder

Rare: Colitis, gastritis, gingival bleeding,

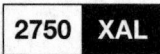

Skin and subcutaneous tissue

Common: Rash

Uncommon: Alopecia, skin discolouration, pruritus

Rare: Dry skin

Musculoskeletal and connective tissue disorders

Uncommon: Myalgia, arthralgia, back pain

Urogenital

Uncommon: Impotence

Rare: Nocturia, renal failure

Investigations

Rare: Blood creatinine increased

General disorders and administration site conditions

Common: Fatigue

Uncommon: Chest pain, weakness, chills, malaise, fever

Rare: Asthenia, pain, flu-like syndrome

4.9 Overdose

No case of overdose has been reported. A specific antidote for anagrelide has not been identified. In case of overdose, close clinical supervision of the patient is required; this includes monitoring of the platelet count for thrombocytopaenia, dosage should be decreased or stopped, as appropriate, until the platelet count returns to within the normal range.

Xagrid, at higher than recommended doses, has been shown to produce reductions in blood pressure with occasional instances of hypotension. A single 5mg dose of anagrelide can lead to a fall in blood pressure usually accompanied by dizziness.

5. PHARMACOLOGICAL PROPERTIES

5.1 Pharmacodynamic properties

Pharmacotherapeutic group:

Proposed ATC Code: L 01 X (Other Antineoplastic Agents)

The specific mechanism of action by which anagrelide reduces platelet count is not yet fully understood although it has been confirmed that anagrelide is platelet selective from *in vitro* and *in vivo* study information.

In vitro studies of human megakaryocytopoiesis established that anagrelide's inhibitory actions on platelet formation in man are mediated via retardation of maturation of megakaryocytes, and reducing their size and ploidy. Evidence of similar *in vivo* actions was observed in bone marrow biopsy samples from treated patients.

Anagrelide is an inhibitorof cyclic AMP phosphodiesterase III.

The safety and efficacy of anagrelide as a platelet lowering agent has been evaluated in four open-label, non-controlled clinical trials (study numbers 700-012, 700-014, 700-999 and 13970-301) including more than 4000 patients with myeloproliferative disorders (MPDs). In patients with essential thrombocythaemia complete response was defined as a decrease in platelet count to $\leqslant 600 \times 10^9/l$ or a $\geqslant 50\%$ reduction from baseline and maintenance of the reduction for at least 4 weeks. In studies 700-012, 700-014, 700-999 and study 13970-301 the time to complete response ranged from 4 to 12 weeks. Clinical benefit in terms of thrombohaemorrhagic events has not been convincingly demonstrated.

Children and adolescents: An open label clinical study with a 3 month treatment period did not raise any safety concerns for anagrelide in 17 children/adolescent patients with ET (age range 7-14 years) compared to 18 adult patients. Earlier during clinical development a limited number (12) of children (age range 5 - 17 years) with essential thrombocythaemia were treated with anagrelide.

5.2 Pharmacokinetic properties

Following oral administration of anagrelide in man, at least 70% is absorbed from the gastrointestinal tract. In fasted subjects, peak plasma levels occur about 1 hour after a 0.5mg dose; the plasma half-life is short, approximately 1.3 hours. Dose proportionality has been found in the dose range 0.5mg to 2mg.

Anagrelide is primarily metabolised by CYP1A2; less than 1% is recovered in the urine as anagrelide. Two major urinary metabolites, 2-amino-5, 6-dichloro-3, 4-dihydroquinazoline and N-(5,6-dichloro-3,4-dihydroquinazalin-2-yl)-2-oxoacetamide have been identified. The mean recovery of 2-amino-5, 6-dichloro-3, 4-dihydroquinazoline in urine is approximately 18-35% of the administered dose.

When a 0.5mg dose of anagrelide was taken following food, its bioavailability (based on AUC values) was modestly reduced by an average of 14% when compared with drug administered to the same subjects in the fasted state. The peak plasma levels were reduced by 45% and occurred approximately 3 hours after dosing. Excretion of the major urinary metabolite was decreased slightly. None of these changes induced by food were considered to be clinically significant.

As expected from its half-life, there is no evidence for anagrelide accumulation in the plasma. Additionally these results show no evidence of auto-induction of the anagrelide clearance.

Special populations

Children and adolescents

Pharmacokinetic data from fasting children and adolescents (age range 7 - 14 years) with essential thrombocythaemia indicate that dose and body weight normalised exposure, Cmax and AUC, of anagrelide were lower in children/adolescents compared to adults. There was also a trend to lower exposure to the active metabolite. These observations may be a reflection of more efficient metabolic clearance in younger subjects.

5.3 Preclinical safety data

Repeated dose toxicity.

Following repeated administration of anagrelide, at doses of 1mg/kg/day or higher, subendocardial haemorrhage and focal myocardial necrosis occurred in dogs. No cardiac toxicity occurred in rats or monkeys at doses up to 360 and 12 mg/kg/day, respectively.

Reproductive toxicology.

Maternally toxic doses of anagrelide (60 mg/kg/day and above) in rats and rabbits were associated with increased embryo resorption and foetal mortality.

Mutagenic and carcinogenic potential.

Studies on the genotoxic potential of anagrelide did not identify any mutagenic or clastogenic effects. Long-term carcinogenicity studies on anagrelide have not been conducted.

6. PHARMACEUTICAL PARTICULARS

6.1 List of excipients

Capsule contents

Povidone (E1201)

Anhydrous lactose

Lactose monohydrate

Microcrystalline cellulose (E460)

Crospovidone

Magnesium stearate

Capsule shell

Gelatin

Titanium dioxide (E171)

Printing ink

Shellac

Strong ammonium solution

Potassium hydroxide (E525)

Black iron oxide (E172)

6.2 Incompatibilities

Not applicable

6.3 Shelf life

3 years

6.4 Special precautions for storage

No special precautions for storage

6.5 Nature and contents of container

High-density polyethylene (HDPE) bottles containing desiccant with child-resistant closures containing 100 capsules

6.6 Instructions for use and handling

No special requirements

7. MARKETING AUTHORISATION HOLDER

Shire Pharmaceutical Contracts Ltd

Hampshire International Business Park

Chineham

Basingstoke

Hampshire RG24 8EP

United Kingdom

8. MARKETING AUTHORISATION NUMBER(S)

EU/1/04/295/001

9. DATE OF FIRST AUTHORISATION/RENEWAL OF THE AUTHORISATION

16/11/2004

10. DATE OF REVISION OF THE TEXT

12/09/2005

LEGAL STATUS

POM

Xalacom eye drops, solution

(Pharmacia Limited)

1. NAME OF THE MEDICINAL PRODUCT

Xalacom ▼ eye drops, solution.

2. QUALITATIVE AND QUANTITATIVE COMPOSITION

1ml solution contains latanoprost 50 micrograms and timolol maleate 6.8 mg equivalent to 5 mg timolol.

For excipients, see 6.1.

3. PHARMACEUTICAL FORM

Eye drops, solution

4. CLINICAL PARTICULARS

4.1 Therapeutic indications

Reduction of intraocular pressure (IOP) in patients with open angle glaucoma and ocular hypertension who are insufficiently responsive to topical beta-blockers.

4.2 Posology and method of administration

Recommended dosage for adults (including the elderly):

Recommended therapy is one eye drop in the affected eye(s) once daily in the morning.

If one dose is missed, treatment should continue with the next dose as planned. The dose should not exceed one drop in the affected eye(s) daily.

Administration:

If more than one topical ophthalmic drug is being used, the drugs should be administered at least five minutes apart.

Use in children and adolescents:

Safety and effectiveness in children and adolescents has not been established.

4.3 Contraindications

- Reactive airway disease including bronchial asthma or a history of bronchial asthma, severe chronic obstructive pulmonary disease.

- Sinus bradycardia, second or third degree atrioventricular block, overt cardiac failure, cardiogenic shock.

- Hypersensitivity to the active substances or to any of the excipients.

4.4 Special warnings and special precautions for use

Systemic effects

Like other topically applied ophthalmic agents, Xalacom may be absorbed systemically. Due to the beta-adrenergic component timolol, the same types of cardiovascular and pulmonary adverse reactions as seen with systemic beta-blockers may occur. Cardiac failure should be adequately controlled before beginning therapy with timolol. Patients with a history of severe cardiac disease should be watched for signs of cardiac failure and have their pulse rates checked. Respiratory reactions and cardiac reactions, including death due to bronchospasm in patients with asthma and, rarely, death in association with cardiac failures, have been reported following administration of timolol maleate. Beta-blockers should be administered with caution in patients subject to spontaneous hypoglycaemia or to diabetic patients (especially those with labile diabetes) as beta-blockers may mask the signs and symptoms of acute hypoglycaemia. Beta-blockers may also mask the signs of hyperthyroidism and cause worsening of Prinzmetal angina, severe peripheral and central circulatory disorders and hypotension.

Anaphylactic reactions

While taking beta-blockers, patients with a history of atopy or a history of severe anaphylactic reaction to a variety of allergens may be unresponsive to the usual doses of adrenaline used to treat anaphylactic reactions.

Concomitant therapy

Timolol may interact with other drugs, see 4.5 Interaction with other medicinal products and other forms of interaction.

The effect on intraocular pressure or the known effects of systemic beta-blockade may be potentiated when Xalacom is given to patients already receiving an oral beta-blocking agent. The use of two local beta-blockers or two local prostaglandins is not recommended.

Ocular effects

Latanoprost may gradually change the eye colour by increasing the amount of brown pigment in the iris. Similar to experience with latanoprost eye drops, increased iris pigmentation was seen in 16-20% of all patients treated with Xalacom for up to one year (based on photographs). This effect has predominantly been seen in patients with mixed coloured irides, i.e. green-brown, yellow-brown or blue/grey-brown, and is due to increased melanin content in the stromal melanocytes of the iris. Typically the brown pigmentation around the pupil spreads concentrically towards the periphery in affected eyes, but the entire iris or parts of it may become more brownish. In patients with homogeneously blue, grey, green or brown eyes, the change has only rarely been seen during two years of treatment in clinical trials with latanoprost. The change in iris colour occurs slowly and may not be noticeable for several months to years and it has not been associated with any symptom or pathological changes.

No further increase in brown iris pigment has been observed after discontinuation of treatment, but the resultant colour change may be permanent.

Neither naevi nor freckles of the iris have been affected by treatment.

Accumulation of pigment in the trabecular meshwork or elsewhere in the anterior chamber has not been observed but patients should be examined regularly and, depending on the clinical situation, treatment may be stopped if increased iris pigmentation ensues.

Before treatment is instituted patients should be informed of the possibility of a change in eye colour. Unilateral treatment can result in permanent heterochromia.

There is no documented experience with latanoprost in inflammatory, neovascular, chronic angle closure or congenital glaucoma, in open angle glaucoma of pseudophakic patients and in pigmentary glaucoma. Latanoprost has no or little effect on the pupil but there is no documented experience in acute attacks of closed angle glaucoma. It is recommended, therefore, that

Xalacom should be used with caution in these conditions until more experience is obtained.

Macular oedema, including cystoid macular oedema, has been reported during treatment with latanoprost. These reports have mainly occurred in aphakic patients, in pseudophakic patients with a torn posterior lens capsule, or in patients with known risk factors for macular oedema. Xalacom should be used with caution in these patients.

Choroidal detachment has been reported with administration of aqueous suppressant therapy (e.g. timolol, acetazolamide) after filtration procedures.

Use of contact lenses

Xalacom contains benzalkonium chloride, which may be absorbed by contact lenses. This may cause discoloration of soft contact lenses. Benzalkonium chloride may also cause eye irritation. The contact lenses should be removed before instillation of the eye drops and may be reinserted after 15 minutes.

4.5 Interaction with other medicinal products and other forms of Interaction

Specific medicinal product interaction studies have not been performed with Xalacom.

There is a potential for additive effects resulting in hypotension and/or marked bradycardia when eye drops with timolol are administered concomitantly with oral calcium channel blockers, guanethidine or beta-blocking agents, antiarrhythmics, digitalis glycosides or parasympathomimetics.

The hypertensive reaction to sudden withdrawal of clonidine can be potentiated when taking beta-blockers.

Beta-blockers may increase the hypoglycaemic effect of antidiabetic agents. Beta-blockers can mask the signs and symptoms of hypoglycaemia (see 4.4, Special warnings and special precautions for use).

4.6 Pregnancy and lactation

PREGNANCY

Latanoprost:

There are no adequate and well-controlled studies in pregnant women. Studies in animals have shown reproductive toxicity (see 5.3 Preclinical safety data). The potential risk for humans is unknown.

Timolol:

Well controlled epidemiological studies with systemic use of beta-blockers did not indicate malformative effects, but some pharmacological effects such as bradycardia have already been observed in foetuses or neonates.

Consequently Xalacom should not be used during pregnancy (see 5.3 Preclinical safety data).

LACTATION

Timolol is excreted into breast milk. Latanoprost and its metabolites may pass into breast milk. Xalacom should therefore not be used in women who are breast-feeding.

4.7 Effects on ability to drive and use machines

Instillation of eye drops may cause transient blurring of vision.

4.8 Undesirable effects

No adverse events specific for Xalacom have been observed in clinical studies. The adverse events have been limited to those earlier reported for latanoprost and timolol.

Based on evidence from consecutive photographs, increased iris pigmentation was seen in 16-20% of all patients treated with latanoprost/timolol in a fixed combination for up to one year. The most frequent findings of increased iris pigmentation were in patients with green-brown, yellow-brown and blue/grey-brown irides. In patients with homogeneously blue, grey, green or brown eyes, the change was only rarely seen. Darkening, thickening and lengthening of eyelashes were seen in 37% of patients.

Among other adverse reactions reported in clinical trials, the most frequent were:

Eye irritation, including stinging, burning and itching (12%), eye hyperaemia (7.4%), corneal disorders (3.0%), conjunctivitis (3.0%), blepharitis (2.5%), eye pain (2.3%), headache (2.3%) and skin rash (1.3%).

Additional adverse events that have been seen with one of the components and may potentially occur also with Xalacom:

Latanoprost:

Ocular: punctate epithelial erosions, periorbital oedema, corneal oedema and erosions, macular oedema (in aphakic, pseudophakic patients with torn posterior lens capsules or in patients with known risk factors for macular oedema), iritis/uveitis.

Cardiac disorders: Aggravation of angina in patients with pre-existing disease.

Respiratory: asthma, asthma exacerbation and dyspnoea.

Skin: darkening of the palpebral skin.

General disorders: Chest pain.

Timolol:

Special senses: signs and symptoms of ocular irritation including blepharitis, keratitis, decreased corneal sensitivity, and dry eyes, visual disturbances including refractive changes (due to withdrawal of miotic therapy in some cases), diplopia, ptosis, choroidal detachment (following filtration surgery), tinnitus

Cardiovascular: bradycardia, arrhythmia, hypotension, syncope, heart block, cerebrovascular accident, cerebral ischaemia, congestive heart failure, palpitation, cardiac arrest, oedema, claudication, Raynaud's phenomenon, cold hands and feet

Respiratory: bronchospasm (predominantly in patients with pre-existing bronchospastic disease), dyspnoea, cough

Body as a whole: headache, asthenia, fatigue, chest pain

Integumentary: alopecia, psoriasiform rash or exacerbation of psoriasis

Hypersensitivity: signs and symptoms of allergic reactions including angioedema, urticaria, localized and generalized rash

Nervous system/Psychiatric: dizziness, depression, insomnia, nightmares, memory loss, increase in signs and symptoms of myasthenia gravis, paresthaesia

Digestive: nausea, diarrhoea, dyspepsia, dry mouth

Urogenital: decreased libido, Peyronie's disease

Immunologic: systemic lupus erythematosus

4.9 Overdose

No data are available in humans with regard to overdose with Xalacom.

Symptoms of systemic timolol overdose are: bradycardia, hypotension, bronchospasm and cardiac arrest. If such symptoms occur the treatment should be symptomatic and supportive. Studies have shown that timolol does not dialyse readily.

Apart from ocular irritation and conjunctival hyperaemia no other ocular or systemic side effects are known if latanoprost is overdosed.

If latanoprost is accidentally ingested orally the following information may be useful: Treatment: Gastric lavage if needed. Symptomatic treatment. Latanoprost is extensively metabolised during the first pass through the liver. Intravenous infusion of 3 micrograms/kg in healthy volunteers induced no symptoms but a dose of 5.5-10 micrograms/kg caused nausea, abdominal pain, dizziness, fatigue, hot flushes and sweating. These events were mild to moderate in severity and resolved without treatment, within 4 hours after terminating the infusion.

5. PHARMACOLOGICAL PROPERTIES

5.1 Pharmacodynamic properties

Pharmacotherapeutic group:

Ophthalmological-betablocking agents - timolol, combinations

ATC code: S01ED51

Mechanism of action

Xalacom consists of two components: latanoprost and timolol maleate. These two components decrease elevated intraocular pressure (IOP) by different mechanisms of action and the combined effect results in additional IOP reduction compared to either compound administered alone.

Latanoprost, a prostaglandin F_{2alpha} analogue, is a selective prostanoid FP receptor agonist that reduces the IOP by increasing the outflow of aqueous humour. The main mechanism of action is increased uveoscleral outflow. Additionally, some increase in outflow facility (decrease in trabecular outflow resistance) has been reported in man. Latanoprost has no significant effect on the production of aqueous humour, the blood-aqueous barrier or the intraocular blood circulation. Chronic treatment with latanoprost in monkey eyes, which had undergone extracapsular lens extraction, did not affect the retinal blood vessels as determined by fluorescein angiography. Latanoprost has not induced fluorescein leakage in the posterior segment of pseudophakic human eyes during short-term treatment.

Timolol is a beta-1 and beta-2 (non-selective) adrenergic receptor blocking agent that has no significant intrinsic sympathomimetic, direct myocardial depressant or membrane-stabilising activity. Timolol lowers IOP by decreasing the formation of aqueous in the ciliary epithelium. The precise mechanism of action is not clearly established, but inhibition of the increased cyclic AMP synthesis caused by endogenous beta-adrenergic stimulation is probable. Timolol has not been found to significantly affect the permeability of the blood-aqueous barrier to plasma proteins. In rabbits, timolol was without effect on the regional ocular blood flow after chronic treatment.

Pharmacodynamic effects

Clinical effects

In dose finding studies, Xalacom produced significantly greater decreases in mean diurnal IOP compared to latanoprost and timolol administered once daily as monotherapy. In two well controlled, double masked six-month clinical studies the IOP reducing effect of Xalacom was compared with latanoprost and timolol monotherapy in patients with an IOP of at least 25 mm Hg or greater. Following a 2-4 week run-in with timolol (mean decrease in IOP from enrollment of 5 mm Hg), additional decreases in mean diurnal IOP of 3.1, 2.0 and 0.6 mm Hg were observed after 6 months of treatment for Xalacom, latanoprost and timolol (twice daily), respectively. The IOP lowering effect of Xalacom was maintained in 6 month open label extensions of these studies.

Onset of action of Xalacom is within one hour and maximal effect occurs within six to eight hours. Adequate IOP reducing effect has been shown to be present up to 24 hours post dosage after multiple treatments.

5.2 Pharmacokinetic properties

Latanoprost

Latanoprost is an isopropyl ester prodrug, which *per se* is inactive, but after hydrolysis by esterases in the cornea to the acid of latanoprost, becomes biologically active. The prodrug is well absorbed through the cornea and all drug that enters the aqueous humor is hydrolysed during the passage through the cornea. Studies in man indicate that the maximum concentration in the aqueous humour, approximately 15-30 ng/ml, is reached about 2 hours after topical administration of latanoprost alone. After topical application in monkeys latanoprost is distributed primarily in the anterior segment, the conjunctiva and the eyelids.

The acid of latanoprost has a plasma clearance of 0.40 l/h/kg and a small volume of distribution, 0.16 l/kg, resulting in a rapid half life in plasma, 17 minutes. After topical ocular administration the systemic bioavailability of the acid of latanoprost is 45%. The acid of latanoprost has a plasma protein binding of 87%.

There is practically no metabolism of the acid of latanoprost in the eye. The main metabolism occurs in the liver. The main metabolites, the 1,2-dinor and 1,2,3,4- tetranor metabolites, exert no or only weak biological activity in animal studies and are excreted primarily in the urine.

Timolol

The maximum concentration of timolol in the aqueous humor is reached about 1 hour after topical administration of eye drops. Part of the dose is absorbed systemically and a maximum plasma concentration of 1 ng/ml is reached 10-20 minutes after topical administration of one eye drop to each eye once daily (300 micrograms/day). The half life of timolol in plasma is about 6 hours. Timolol is extensively metabolised in the liver. The metabolites are excreted in the urine together with some unchanged timolol.

Xalacom

No pharmacokinetic interactions between latanoprost and timolol were observed although there was an approximate 2-fold increased concentration of the acid of latanoprost in aqueous humour 1-4 hours after administration of Xalacom compared to monotherapy.

5.3 Preclinical safety data

The ocular and systemic safety profile of the individual components is well established. No adverse ocular or systemic effects were seen in rabbits treated topically with the fixed combination or with concomitantly administered latanoprost and timolol ophthalmic solutions. Safety pharmacology, genotoxicity and carcinogenicity studies with each of the components revealed no special hazards for humans. Latanoprost did not affect corneal wound healing in the rabbit eye, whereas timolol inhibited the process in the rabbit and the monkey eye when administered more frequently than once a day.

For latanoprost, no effects on male and female fertility in rats and no teratogenic potential in rats and rabbits have been established. No embryotoxicity was observed in rats after intravenous doses of up to 250 micrograms/kg/day. Latanoprost, however, caused embryofetal toxicity, characterised by increased incidence of late resorption and abortion and by reduced foetal weight, in rabbits at intravenous doses of 5 micrograms/kg/day (approximately 100 times the clinical dose) and above. Timolol showed no effects on male and female fertility in rats or teratogenic potential in mice, rats and rabbits.

6. PHARMACEUTICAL PARTICULARS

6.1 List of excipients

Sodium chloride

Benzalkonium chloride

Sodium dihydrogen phosphate monohydrate

Disodium phosphate anhydrous

Hydrochloric acid solution (for adjustment to pH 6.0)

Sodium hydroxide solution (for adjustment to pH 6.0)

Water for injections

6.2 Incompatibilities

In vitro studies have shown that precipitation occurs when eye drops containing thiomersal are mixed with Xalatan. If such drugs are used concomitantly with Xalacom, the eye drops should be administered with an interval of at least five minutes.

6.3 Shelf life

2 years

After opening of container: 4 weeks

6.4 Special precautions for storage

Store at 2 °C - 8 °C.

Opened container: Do not store above 25 °C.

Keep the container in the outer carton.

6.5 Nature and contents of container

LDPE bottle (5 ml) and dropper applicator (dropper tip), HDPE screw cap, tamper evident LDPE overcap.

Each bottle contains 2.5 ml eye drop solution.

Pack sizes: 1 × 2.5 ml
3 × 2.5 ml
6 × 2.5 ml

Not all pack sizes may be marketed.

6.6 Instructions for use and handling
The tamper evident overcap should be removed before use.

Administrative Data

7. MARKETING AUTHORISATION HOLDER
Pharmacia Limited
Ramsgate RoadSandwich
Kent
CT 13 9NJ
United Kingdom

8. MARKETING AUTHORISATION NUMBER(S)
PL 00032/0288

9. DATE OF FIRST AUTHORISATION/RENEWAL OF THE AUTHORISATION
20 July 2001

10. DATE OF REVISION OF THE TEXT
4th May 2005
XM4_1

Xalatan 0.005% eye drops solution

(Pharmacia Limited)

1. NAME OF THE MEDICINAL PRODUCT
Xalatan® 0.005% eye drops solution.

2. QUALITATIVE AND QUANTITATIVE COMPOSITION
100 ml eye drops solution contains 0.005 g latanoprost.

One drop contains approximately 1.5 micrograms latanoprost.

For excipients, see 6.1.

3. PHARMACEUTICAL FORM
Eye drops, solution.

4. CLINICAL PARTICULARS

4.1 Therapeutic indications
Reduction of elevated intraocular pressure in patients with open angle glaucoma and ocular hypertension.

4.2 Posology and method of administration
Recommended dosage for adults (including the elderly):

Recommended therapy is one eye drop in the affected eye(s) once daily. Optimal effect is obtained if Xalatan is administered in the evening.

The dosage of Xalatan should not exceed once daily since it has been shown that more frequent administration decreases the intraocular pressure lowering effect.

If one dose is missed, treatment should continue with the next dose as normal.

As with any eye drops, to reduce possible systemic absorption, it is recommended that the lachrymal sac be compressed at the medial canthus (punctal occlusion) for one minute. This should be performed immediately following the instillation of each drop.

If more than one topical ophthalmic drug is being used, the drugs should be administered at least five minutes apart.

Children:

Safety and effectiveness in children has not been established. Therefore, Xalatan is not recommended for use in children.

4.3 Contraindications
Known hypersensitivity to any component in Xalatan.

Use of all contact lenses.

4.4 Special warnings and special precautions for use
Xalatan may gradually change eye colour by increasing the amount of brown pigment in the iris. Before treatment is instituted, patients should be informed of the possibility of a permanent change in eye colour. Unilateral treatment can result in permanent heterochromia.

This change in eye colour has predominantly been seen in patients with mixed coloured irides, i.e. blue-brown, grey-brown, yellow-brown and green-brown. The onset of the change is usually within the first 8 months of treatment, but may occur later in a small number of patients. The effect, based on evidence from consecutive photographs, has been seen in 30% of all patients during four years of treatment in clinical trials. The iris colour change is slight in the majority of cases and often not observed clinically. The incidence in patients with mixed colour irides ranged from 7 to 85%, with yellow-brown irides having the highest incidence. In patients with homogeneously blue eyes, no change has been observed and in patients with homogeneously grey, green or brown eyes, the change has only rarely been seen.

The colour change is due to increased melanin content in the stromal melanocytes of the iris and not to an increase in number of melanocytes. Typically, the brown pigmentation around the pupil spreads concentrically towards the periphery in affected eyes, but the entire iris or parts of it may become more brownish. No further increase in brown iris pigment has been observed after discontinuation of treatment. It has not been associated with any symptom or pathological changes in clinical trials to date.

Neither naevi nor freckles of the iris have been affected by treatment. Accumulation of pigment in the trabecular meshwork or elsewhere in the anterior chamber has not been observed in clinical trials. Based on 5 years clinical experience, increased iris pigmentation has not been shown to have any negative clinical sequelae and Xalatan can be continued if iris pigmentation ensues. However, patients should be monitored regularly and if the clinical situation warrants, Xalatan treatment may be discontinued.

There is limited experience of Xalatan in chronic angle closure glaucoma, open angle glaucoma of pseudophakic patients and in pigmentary glaucoma. There is no experience of Xalatan in inflammatory and neovascular glaucoma, inflammatory ocular conditions, or congenital glaucoma. Xalatan has no or little effect on the pupil, but there is no experience in acute attacks of closed angle glaucoma. Therefore, it is recommended that Xalatan should be used with caution in these conditions until more experience is obtained.

There are limited study data on the use of Xalatan during the peri-operative period of cataract surgery. Xalatan should be used with caution in these patients.

Caution is recommended when using Xalatan in aphakic patients, in pseudophakic patients with torn posterior lens capsule or anterior chamber lenses, or in patients with known risk factors for cystoid macular oedema, see also 4.8.

In patients with known predisposing risk factors for iritis/uveitis, Xalatan can be used with caution.

There is no experience in patients with severe or brittle asthma. Such patients should therefore be treated with caution until there is sufficient experience, see also 4.8.

Periorbital skin discolouration has been observed, the majority of reports being in Japanese patients. Experience to date shows that periorbital skin discolouration is not permanent and in some cases has reversed while continuing treatment with Xalatan.

4.5 Interaction with other medicinal products and other forms of Interaction
Definitive drug interaction data are not available.

4.6 Pregnancy and lactation
Pregnancy

The safety of this medicinal product for use in human pregnancy has not been established. It has potential hazardous pharmacological effects with respect to the course of pregnancy, to the unborn or the neonate. Therefore, Xalatan should not be used during pregnancy.

Lactation

Latanoprost and its metabolites may pass into breast milk and Xalatan should therefore not be used in nursing women or breast feeding should be stopped.

4.7 Effects on ability to drive and use machines
In common with other eye preparations, instillation of eye drops may cause transient blurring of vision.

4.8 Undesirable effects
Most undesirable effects observed relate to the ocular system.

Eye effects

Very common (> 1/10): Increased iris pigmentation; eye irritation (including slight foreign body sensation); eyelash changes (darkening, thickening, lengthening, increased number).

Common (> 1/100 and < 1/10): Mild to moderate conjunctival hyperaemia; transient punctate epithelial erosions, mostly without symptoms; blepharitis; eye pain.

Uncommon (> 1/1000 and < 1/100): Eyelid oedema.

Rare (< 1/1000): Iritis/uveitis; macular oedema; symptomatic corneal oedema and erosions; periorbital oedema; darkening of the palpebral skin; localised skin reaction on the eyelids; misdirected eyelashes sometimes resulting in eye irritation; increase in number, darkening, thickening and lengthening of vellus hair on the eyelid (vast majority of reports in Japanese population); extra row of cilia at the aperture of the meibomian glands (distichiasis).

Cardiac disorders

Very rare (<1/10,000): Aggravation of angina in patients with pre-existing disease.

Respiratory effects

Rare (< 1/1000): Asthma, asthma exacerbation and dyspnoea.

Skin effects

Uncommon (> 1/1000 and < 1/100): Skin rash.

General disorders

Very rare (< 1/10,000): Chest pain.

Xalatan may cause an increase in brown pigmentation of the iris, predominantly in patients with mixed coloured irides (i.e. blue-brown, grey-brown, yellow-brown, green-brown). This is due to increased melanin content in the stromal melanocytes of the iris. In some patients, the change in iris colour may be permanent, see also 4.4.

Macular oedema has been reported rarely during Xalatan treatment. These reports have mainly occurred in aphakic patients, in pseudophakic patients with torn posterior lens capsule or anterior chamber lenses, or in patients with known risk factors for cystoid macular oedema (such as diabetic retinopathy and retinal vein occlusion). An association between the use of Xalatan and unexplained macular oedema cannot be excluded, see also 4.4.

Rare cases of iritis/uveitis have been reported. The majority of patients in these cases had concomitant predisposing factors for developing iritis/uveitis.

Rare cases of asthma, asthma exacerbation and dyspnoea have been reported. There is limited experience from patients with asthma, but latanoprost has not been found to affect the pulmonary function when studied in small numbers of steroid and non-steroid treated patients suffering from moderate asthma. There is no experience in patients with severe or brittle asthma and such patients should therefore be treated with caution until there is sufficient experience.

4.9 Overdose
Apart from ocular irritation and conjunctival hyperaemia, no other ocular side effects are known if Xalatan is overdosed.

If Xalatan is accidentally ingested the following information may be useful: One bottle contains 125 micrograms latanoprost. More than 90% is metabolised during the first pass through the liver. Intravenous infusion of 3 micrograms/kg in healthy volunteers induced no symptoms, but a dose of 5.5-10 micrograms/kg caused nausea, abdominal pain, dizziness, fatigue, hot flushes and sweating. In monkeys, latanoprost has been infused intravenously in doses of up to 500 micrograms/kg without major effects on the cardiovascular system.

Intravenous administration of latanoprost in monkeys has been associated with transient bronchoconstriction. However, in patients with moderate bronchial asthma, bronchoconstriction was not induced by latanoprost when applied topically on the eyes in a dose of seven times the clinical dose of Xalatan.

If overdosage with Xalatan occurs, treatment should be symptomatic.

5. PHARMACOLOGICAL PROPERTIES

5.1 Pharmacodynamic properties
Pharmacotherapeutic group (ATC code): S 01 E E 01

The active substance latanoprost, a prostaglandin F2a analogue, is a selective prostanoid FP receptor agonist which reduces the intraocular pressure by increasing the outflow of aqueous humour. Reduction of the intraocular pressure in man starts about three to four hours after administration and maximum effect is reached after eight to twelve hours. Pressure reduction is maintained for at least 24 hours.

Studies in animals and man indicate that the main mechanism of action is increased uveoscleral outflow, although some increase in outflow facility (decrease in outflow resistance) has been reported in man.

Pivotal studies have demonstrated that Xalatan is effective as monotherapy. In addition, clinical trials investigating combination use have been performed. These include studies that show that latanoprost is effective in combination with beta-adrenergic antagonists (timolol). Short-term (1 or 2 weeks) studies suggest that the effect of latanoprost is additive in combination with adrenergic agonists (dipivalyl epinephrine), oral carbonic anhydrase inhibitors (acetazolamide) and at least partly additive with cholinergic agonists (pilocarpine).

Clinical trials have shown that latanoprost has no significant effect on the production of aqueous humour. Latanoprost has not been found to have any effect on the blood-aqueous barrier.

Latanoprost has no or negligible effects on the intraocular blood circulation when used at the clinical dose and studied in monkeys. However, mild to moderate conjunctival or episcleral hyperaemia may occur during topical treatment.

Chronic treatment with latanoprost in monkey eyes, which had undergone extracapsular lens extraction, did not affect the retinal blood vessels as determined by fluorescein angiography.

Latanoprost has not induced fluorescein leakage in the posterior segment of pseudophakic human eyes during short-term treatment.

Latanoprost in clinical doses has not been found to have any significant pharmacological effects on the cardiovascular or respiratory system.

5.2 Pharmacokinetic properties
Latanoprost (mw 432.58) is an isopropyl ester prodrug which per se is inactive, but after hydrolysis to the acid of latanoprost becomes biologically active.

The prodrug is well absorbed through the cornea and all drug that enters the aqueous humour is hydrolysed during the passage through the cornea.

Studies in man indicate that the peak concentration in the aqueous humour is reached about two hours after topical administration. After topical application in monkeys, latanoprost is distributed primarily in the anterior segment, the conjunctivae and the eyelids. Only minute quantities of the drug reach the posterior segment.

There is practically no metabolism of the acid of latanoprost in the eye. The main metabolism occurs in the liver. The half life in plasma is 17 minutes in man. The main metabolites, the 1,2-dinor and 1,2,3,4-tetranor metabolites, exert no or only weak biological activity in animal studies and are excreted primarily in the urine.

5.3 Preclinical safety data
The ocular as well as systemic toxicity of latanoprost has been investigated in several animal species. Generally, latanoprost is well tolerated with a safety margin between clinical ocular dose and systemic toxicity of at least 1000 times. High doses of latanoprost, approximately 100 times the clinical dose/kg body weight, administered intravenously to unanaesthetised monkeys have been shown to increase the respiration rate probably reflecting bronchoconstriction of short duration. In animal studies, latanoprost has not been found to have sensitising properties.

In the eye, no toxic effects have been detected with doses of up to 100 micrograms/eye/day in rabbits or monkeys (clinical dose is approximately 1.5 micrograms/eye/day). In monkeys, however, latanoprost has been shown to induce increased pigmentation of the iris.

The mechanism of increased pigmentation seems to be stimulation of melanin production in melanocytes of the iris with no proliferative changes observed. The change in iris colour may be permanent.

In chronic ocular toxicity studies, administration of latanoprost 6 micrograms/eye/day has also been shown to induce increased palpebral fissure. This effect is reversible and occurs at doses above the clinical dose level. The effect has not been seen in humans.

Latanoprost was found negative in reverse mutation tests in bacteria, gene mutation in mouse lymphoma and mouse micronucleus test. Chromosome aberrations were observed in vitro with human lymphocytes. Similar effects were observed with prostaglandin $F_{2\alpha}$, a naturally occurring prostaglandin, and indicates that this is a class effect.

Additional mutagenicity studies on in vitro/in vivo unscheduled DNA synthesis in rats were negative and indicate that latanoprost does not have mutagenic potency. Carcinogenicity studies in mice and rats were negative.

Latanoprost has not been found to have any effect on male or female fertility in animal studies. In the embryotoxicity study in rats, no embryotoxicity was observed at intravenous doses (5, 50 and 250 micrograms/kg/day) of latanoprost. However, latanoprost induced embryolethal effects in rabbits at doses of 5 micrograms/kg/day and above.

The dose of 5 micrograms/kg/day (approximately 100 times the clinical dose) caused significant embryofoetal toxicity characterised by increased incidence of late resorption and abortion and by reduced foetal weight.

No teratogenic potential has been detected.

6. PHARMACEUTICAL PARTICULARS

6.1 List of excipients
Sodium chloride

Benzalkonium chloride

Sodium dihydrogen phosphate monohydrate

Disodium phosphate anhydrous

Water for injections

6.2 Incompatibilities
In vitro studies have shown that precipitation occurs when eye drops containing thiomersal are mixed with Xalatan. If such drugs are used, the eye drops should be administered with an interval of at least five minutes.

6.3 Shelf life
Shelf life: 3 years

Shelf life after opening of container: 4 weeks

6.4 Special precautions for storage
Store at 2°C-8°C (in a refrigerator).

Keep the container in the outer carton in order to protect from light.

After first opening the container: do not store above 25°C and use within four weeks.

6.5 Nature and contents of container
Dropper container (5 ml) of polyethylene, screw cap, tamper evident overcap of polyethylene.

Each dropper container contains 2.5 ml eye drops solution corresponding to approximately 80 drops of solution.

Pack sizes: 1 × 2.5 ml, 3 × 2.5 ml, 6 × 2.5 ml.

Not all pack sizes may be marketed.

6.6 Instructions for use and handling
No special requirements.

7. MARKETING AUTHORISATION HOLDER
Pharmacia Limited

Ramsgate Road

Sandwich

Kent

CT13 9NJ

United Kingdom

8. MARKETING AUTHORISATION NUMBER(S)
PL 00032/0220

9. DATE OF FIRST AUTHORISATION/RENEWAL OF THE AUTHORISATION
16 December 1996/16 December 2001

10. DATE OF REVISION OF THE TEXT
4th May 2005

XN 5_1

Xanax Tablets 250 micrograms

(Pharmacia Limited)

1. NAME OF THE MEDICINAL PRODUCT
Xanax® Tablets 250 micrograms

2. QUALITATIVE AND QUANTITATIVE COMPOSITION
Alprazolam 250 micrograms

3. PHARMACEUTICAL FORM
White, oval, biconvex tablets containing 250 microgram (0.25 mg) alprazolam, scored on one side and marked "Upjohn 29" on the other.

4. CLINICAL PARTICULARS

4.1 Therapeutic indications
Xanax is indicated for the short-term treatment of moderate or severe anxiety states and anxiety associated with depression. It is only indicated when the disorder is severe, disabling or subjecting the individual to extreme distress.

Xanax should not be used to treat short-term mild anxiety, such as anxiety or tension associated with the stress of everyday life. As the efficacy of Xanax in depression and in phobic or obsessional states has yet to be established, specific treatment may have to be considered.

4.2 Posology and method of administration
Treatment should be as short as possible. It is recommended that the patient be reassessed at the end of no longer than 4 weeks' treatment and the need for continued treatment established, especially in case the patient is symptom free. The overall duration of treatment should not be more than 8-12 weeks, including a tapering off process.

In certain cases extension beyond the maximum treatment period may be necessary; if so, it should not take place without re-evaluation of the patient's status with special expertise. As with all benzodiazepines, physicians should be aware that long-term use might lead to dependence in certain patients.

The optimum dosage of Xanax should be based upon the severity of the symptoms and individual patient response. The lowest dose which can control symptoms should be used. Dosage should be reassessed at intervals of no more than 4 weeks. The usual dosage is stated below; in the few patients who require higher doses, the dosage should be increased cautiously to avoid adverse effects. When higher dosage is required, the evening dose should be increased before the daytime doses. In general, patients who have not previously received psychotropic medications will require lower doses than those so treated, or those with a history of chronic alcoholism.

Treatment should always be tapered off gradually. During discontinuation of alprazolam treatment, the dosage should be reduced slowly in keeping with good medical practice. It is suggested that the daily dosage of alprazolam be decreased by no more than 0.5 mg every three days. Some patients may require an even slower dosage reduction

There is a reduced clearance of the drug and, as with other benzodiazepines, an increased sensitivity to the drug in elderly patients.

Anxiety: 250 micrograms (0.25 mg) to 500 micrograms (0.5 mg) three times daily increasing if required to a total of 3 mg daily.

Geriatric patients or in the presence of debilitating disease: 250 micrograms (0.25 mg) two to three times daily to be gradually increased if needed and tolerated.

Children: Not recommended.

If side-effects occur, the dose should be lowered. It is advisable to review treatment regularly and to discontinue use as soon as possible. Should longer term treatment be necessary, then intermittent treatment may be considered to minimize the risk of dependence.

4.3 Contraindications
Myasthenia gravis

Hypersensitivity to benzodiazepines or any of the other constituents of the tablet

Severe respiratory insufficiency

Sleep apnoea syndrome

Severe hepatic insufficiency

4.4 Special warnings and special precautions for use

Tolerance
Some loss of efficacy to the hypnotic effects of benzodiazepines may develop after repeated use for a few weeks.

Dependence
Use of benzodiazepines may lead to the development of physical and psychic dependence upon these products. The risk of dependence increases with dose and duration of treatment; it is also greater in patients with a history of alcohol and drug abuse.

Once physical dependence has developed, abrupt termination of treatment will be accompanied by withdrawal symptoms. These may consist of headaches, muscle pain, extreme anxiety, tension, restlessness, confusion and irritability. In severe cases the following symptoms may occur: derealization, depersonalisation, hyperacusis, numbness and tingling of the extremities, hypersensitivity to light, noise and physical contact, hallucinations or epileptic seizures.

Rebound insomnia and anxiety: a transient syndrome whereby the symptoms that led to treatment with a benzodiazepine recur in an enhanced form, may occur on withdrawal of treatment. It may be accompanied by other reactions including mood changes, anxiety or sleep disturbances and restlessness. Since the risk of withdrawal phenomena/rebound phenomena is greater after abrupt discontinuation of treatment, it is recommended that the dosage be decreased gradually by no more than 0.5 mg every three days. Some patients may require an even slower dose reduction.

Duration of treatment
The duration of treatment should bed as short as possible (see posology) depending on the indication, but should not exceed eight to twelve weeks including tapering off process. Extension beyond these periods should not take place without re-evaluation of the situation.

It may be useful to inform the patient when treatment is started that it will be of limited duration and to explain precisely how the dosage will be progressively decreased. Moreover it is important that the patient should be aware of the possibility of rebound phenomena, thereby minimising anxiety over such symptoms should they occur while the medicinal product is being discontinued.

There are indications, that in the case of benzodiazepines with a short duration of action, withdrawal phenomena can become manifest within the dosage interval, especially when the dosage is high. When benzodiazepines with a long duration of action are being used it is important to warn against changing to a benzodiazepine with a short duration of action, as withdrawal symptoms may develop.

Amnesia
Benzodiazepines may induce anterograde amnesia. The condition occurs most often several hours after ingesting the product and therefore to reduce the risk patients should ensure that they will be able to have uninterrupted sleep of 7-8 ours (see also undesirable effects).

Psychiatric and 'paradoxical' reactions
Reactions like restlessness, agitation, irritability, aggressiveness, delusion, rages, nightmares, hallucinations, psychoses, inappropriate behaviour and other adverse behavioural effects are known to occur when using benzodiazepines. Should this occur, use of the drug should be discontinued.

They are more likely to occur in children and the elderly.

Specific patient groups
Benzodiazepines should not be given to children without careful assessment of the need to do so; the duration of treatment must be kept to a minimum. The elderly should be given a reduced dose (see posology). A lower dose is also recommended for patients with chronic respiratory insufficiency due to risk of respiratory depression.

Benzodiazepines are not indicated to treat patients with severe hepatic insufficiency as they may precipitate encephalopathy. Caution is recommended when treating patients with impaired renal or hepatic function.

Benzodiazepines are not recommended for the primary treatment of psychotic illness.

Benzodiazepines should not be used alone to treat depression of anxiety associated with depression (suicide may be precipitated in such patients). Administration to severely depressed or suicidal patients should be done with appropriate precautions and appropriate size of the prescription.

Benzodiazepines should be used with extreme caution in patients with a history of alcohol or drug abuse.

4.5 Interaction with other medicinal products and other forms of Interaction
§ Not recommended: Concomitant intake with alcohol

The sedative effects may be enhanced when the product is used in combination with alcohol. This affects the ability to drive or use machines.

§ Take into account: Combination with CNS depressants

Enhancement of the central depressive effect may occur in cases of concomitant use with antipsychotics (neuroleptics), hypnotics, anxiolytics/sedatives, antidepressant agents, narcotic analgesics, anti-epileptic drugs, anaesthetics and sedative antihistamines.

Pharmacokinetic interactions can occur when alprazolam is administered along with drugs that interfere with its metabolism. Compounds that inhibit certain hepatic enzymes (particularly cytochrome P450 3A4) may increase the concentration of alprazolam and enhance it's activity.

Data from clinical studies with alprazolam, in-vitro studies with alprazolam and clinical studies with drugs metabolised similarly to alprazolam provide evidence for varying degrees of interaction and possible interaction with alprazolam for a number of drugs. Based on the degree of interaction and the type of data available, the following recommendations are made:

§ The co-administration of alprazolam with ketoconazole, itraconazole, or other azole-type antifungals is not recommended.

§ Caution and consideration of dose reduction is recommended when alprazolam is co-administered with nefazodone, fluvoxamine and cimetidine.

§ Caution is recommended when alprazolam is co-administered with fluoxetine, propoxyphene, oral contraceptives, sertraline, diltiazem, or macrolide antibiotics such as erythromycin and troleandomycin.

§ Interactions involving HIV protease inhibitors (e.g. ritonavir) and alprazolam are complex and time dependent. Low doses of ritonavir resulted in a large impairment of alprazolam clearance, prolonged its elimination half-life and enhanced clinical effects, however, upon extended exposure to ritonavir, CYP3A induction offset this inhibition. This interaction will require a dose-adjustment or discontinuation of alprazolam.

4.6 Pregnancy and lactation

If the product is prescribed to a woman of childbearing potential, she should be warned to contact her physician regarding discontinuation of the product if she intends to become or suspects that she is pregnant. The data concerning teratogenicity and effects on postnatal development and behaviour following benzodiazepine treatment are inconsistent. There is evidence from some early studies with other members of the benzodiazepine class that in utero exposure may be associated with malformations. Later studies with the benzodiazepine class of drugs have provided no clear evidence of any type of defect.

If, for compelling medical reasons, the product is administered during the late phase of pregnancy, or during labour, effects on the neonate, such as hypothermia, hypotonia and moderate respiratory depression, can be expected, due to the pharmacological action of the compound.

Infants born to mothers who took benzodiazepines chronically during the latter stages of pregnancy may have developed physical dependence and may be at some risk of developing withdrawal symptoms in the postnatal period.

Since benzodiazepines are found in the breast milk, benzodiazepines should not be given to breast feeding mothers.

4.7 Effects on ability to drive and use machines

Sedation, amnesia, impaired concentration and impaired muscle function may adversely affect the ability to drive or use machines. If insufficient sleep occurs, the likelihood of impaired alertness may be increased (see also interactions).

These effects are potentiated by alcohol (see also interactions).

Patients should be cautioned about operating motor vehicles or engaging in other dangerous activities while taking Xanax.

4.8 Undesirable effects

Sedation/drowsiness, light-headedness, numbed emotions, reduced alertness, confusion, fatigue, headache, dizziness, muscle weakness, ataxia, double or blurred vision, insomnia, nervousness/anxiety, tremor, change in weight. These phenomena occur predominantly at the start of therapy and usually disappear with repeated administration. Other side effects like gastrointestinal disturbances, changes in libido or skin reactions have been reported occasionally.

In addition, the following adverse events have been reported in association with the use of alprazolam: dystonia, anorexia, slurred speech, jaundice, musculoskeletal weakness, sexual dysfunction/changes in libido, menstrual irregularities, incontinence, urinary retention, abnormal liver function and hyperprolactinaemia. Increased intraocular pressure have been rarely reported.

Withdrawal symptoms have occurred following rapid decrease or abrupt discontinuance of benzodiazepines including alprazolam. These can range from mild dysphoria and insomnia to a major syndrome, which may include abdominal and muscle cramps, vomiting, sweating, tremor and convulsions. In addition, withdrawal seizures have occurred upon rapid decrease or abrupt discontinuation of therapy with alprazolam.

Amnesia

Anterograde amnesia may occur at therapeutic dosages, the risk increasing at higher dosages. Amnesic effects may be associated with inappropriate behaviour (see warnings and precautions).

Depression

Pre-existing depression may be unmasked during benzodiazepam use.

Psychiatric and 'paradoxical' reactions

Reactions like restlessness, agitation, irritability, aggressiveness, delusion, rages, nightmares, hallucinations, psychoses, inappropriate behaviour and other adverse behavioural effects are known to occur when using benzodiazepines or benzodiazepine-like agents. They may be quite severe with this product. They are more likely to occur in children and the elderly.

In many of the spontaneous case reports of adverse behavioural effects, patients were receiving other CNS drugs concomitantly and/or were described as having underlying psychiatric conditions. Patients who have borderline personality disorder, a prior history of violent or aggressive behaviour, or alcohol or substance abuse may be at risk of such events. Instances of irritability, hostility and intrusive thoughts have been reported during discontinuance of alprazolam in patients with post-traumatic stress disorder.

Dependence

Use (even at therapeutic doses) may lead to the development of physical dependence: discontinuation of the therapy may result in withdrawal or rebound phenomena (see warnings and precautions). Psychic dependence may occur. Abuse of benzodiazepines have been reported.

4.9 Overdose

As with other benzodiazepines, overdose should not present a threat to life unless combined with other CNS depressants (including alcohol). In the management of overdose with any medicinal product, it should be borne in mind that multiple agents have been taken.

Following overdose with any medicinal product, vomiting may be induced (within 1 hour) if the patient is conscious or gastric lavage undertaken with the airway protected if the patient is unconscious. If there is no advantage in emptying the stomach, activated charcoal should be given to reduce absorption.

Special attention should be paid to respiratory and cardiovascular functions in intensive care.

Symptoms of overdose are extensions of its pharmacological activity and usually manifested by slurring of speech, motor incoordination and degrees of central nervous system depression ranging from drowsiness to coma. In mild cases, symptoms include drowsiness, mental confusion and lethargy, in more serious cases, symptoms may include ataxia, hypotonia, hypotension, respiratory depression, rarely coma and very rarely death.

Flumazenil may be useful as an antidote.

5. PHARMACOLOGICAL PROPERTIES

5.1 Pharmacodynamic properties

Alprazolam, like other benzodiazepines, has a high affinity for the benzodiazepine binding site in the brain. It facilitates the inhibitory neurotransmitter action of gamma-aminobutyric acid, which mediates both pre- and post synaptic inhibition in the central nervous system (CNS).

5.2 Pharmacokinetic properties

Alprazolam is readily absorbed. Following oral administration peak concentration in the plasma occurs after 1 - 2 hours.

The mean half-life is 12 - 15 hours. Repeated dosage may lead to accumulation and this should be borne in mind in elderly patients and those with impaired renal or hepatic function. Alprazolam and its metabolites are excreted primarily in the urine.

In vitro alprazolam is bound (80%) to human serum protein.

5.3 Preclinical safety data

None given

6. PHARMACEUTICAL PARTICULARS

6.1 List of excipients

Lactose monohydrate, microcrystalline cellulose, colloidal anhydrous silica, maize starch, magnesium stearate and docusate sodium with sodium benzoate.

6.2 Incompatibilities

None known.

6.3 Shelf life

5 years.

6.4 Special precautions for storage

Do not store above 25°C.

Blister pack: Keep container in the outer carton.

Bottle pack only: Store in the original container.

6.5 Nature and contents of container

Clear PVC/aluminium foil blister strips of 10 tablets, packed 6 strips to a box. Glass bottle with metal screw cap or HDPE bottle with LDPE tamper evident cap containing 100 or 1000 tablets.

6.6 Instructions for use and handling

Not applicable.

7. MARKETING AUTHORISATION HOLDER

Pharmacia Limited

Davy Avenue

Milton Keynes

MK5 8PH

United Kingdom

8. MARKETING AUTHORISATION NUMBER(S)

PL 0032/0092

9. DATE OF FIRST AUTHORISATION/RENEWAL OF THE AUTHORISATION

27 August 1982/23 January 2003

10. DATE OF REVISION OF THE TEXT

June 2003

Legal category: POM

Xanax Tablets 500 micrograms

(Pharmacia Limited)

1. NAME OF THE MEDICINAL PRODUCT

Xanax® Tablets 500 micrograms

2. QUALITATIVE AND QUANTITATIVE COMPOSITION

Alprazolam 500 micrograms

3. PHARMACEUTICAL FORM

Pink, oval, biconvex tablets containing 500 microgram (0.5 mg) alprazolam, scored on one side and marked "Upjohn 55" on the other.

4. CLINICAL PARTICULARS

4.1 Therapeutic indications

Xanax is indicated for the short-term treatment of moderate or severe anxiety states and anxiety associated with depression. It is only indicated when the disorder is severe, disabling or subjecting the individual to extreme distress.

Xanax should not be used to treat short-term mild anxiety, such as anxiety or tension associated with the stress of everyday life. As the efficacy of Xanax in depression and in phobic or obsessional states has yet to be established, specific treatment may have to be considered.

4.2 Posology and method of administration

Treatment should be as short as possible. It is recommended that the patient be reassessed at the end of no longer than 4 weeks' treatment and the need for continued treatment established, especially in case the patient is symptom free. The overall duration of treatment should not be more than 8-12 weeks, including a tapering off process.

In certain cases extension beyond the maximum treatment period may be necessary; if so, it should not take place without re-evaluation of the patient's status with special expertise. As with all benzodiazepines, physicians should be aware that long-term use might lead to dependence in certain patients.

The optimum dosage of Xanax should be based upon the severity of the symptoms and individual patient response. The lowest dose which can control symptoms should be used. Dosage should be reassessed at intervals of no more than 4 weeks. The usual dosage is stated below; in the few patients who require higher doses, the dosage should be increased cautiously to avoid adverse effects. When higher dosage is required, the evening dose should be increased before the daytime doses. In general, patients who have not previously received psychotropic medications will require lower doses than those so treated, or those with a history of chronic alcoholism.

Treatment should always be tapered off gradually. During discontinuation of alprazolam treatment, the dosage should be reduced slowly in keeping with good medical practice. It is suggested that the daily dosage of alprazolam be decreased by no more than 0.5 mg every three days. Some patients may require an even slower dosage reduction

There is a reduced clearance of the drug and, as with other benzodiazepines, an increased sensitivity to the drug in elderly patients.

Anxiety: 250 micrograms (0.25 mg) to 500 micrograms (0.5 mg) three times daily increasing if required to a total of 3 mg daily.

Geriatric patients or in the presence of debilitating disease: 250 micrograms (0.25 mg) two to three times daily to be gradually increased if needed and tolerated.

Children: Not recommended.

If side-effects occur, the dose should be lowered. It is advisable to review treatment regularly and to discontinue use as soon as possible. Should longer term treatment be necessary, then intermittent treatment may be considered to minimize the risk of dependence.

4.3 Contraindications

Myasthenia gravis

Hypersensitivity to benzodiazepines or any of the other constituents of the tablet

Severe respiratory insufficiency

Sleep apnoea syndrome

Severe hepatic insufficiency

4.4 Special warnings and special precautions for use

Tolerance

Some loss of efficacy to the hypnotic effects of benzodiazepines may develop after repeated use for a few weeks.

Dependence

Use of benzodiazepines may lead to the development of physical and psychic dependence upon these products. The risk of dependence increases with dose and duration of treatment; it is also greater in patients with a history of alcohol and drug abuse.

Once physical dependence has developed, abrupt termination of treatment will be accompanied by withdrawal symptoms. These may consist of headaches, muscle pain, extreme anxiety, tension, restlessness, confusion and irritability. In severe cases the following symptoms may occur: derealization, depersonalisation, hyperacusis, numbness and tingling of the extremities, hypersensitivity to light, noise and physical contact, hallucinations or epileptic seizures.

Rebound insomnia and anxiety: a transient syndrome whereby the symptoms that led to treatment with a benzodiazepine recur in an enhanced form, may occur on withdrawal of treatment. It may be accompanied by other reactions including mood changes, anxiety or sleep disturbances and restlessness. Since the risk of withdrawal phenomena/rebound phenomena is greater after abrupt discontinuation of treatment, it is recommended that the dosage be decreased gradually by no more than 0.5 mg every three days. Some patients may require an even slower dose reduction.

Duration of treatment

The duration of treatment should bed as short as possible (see posology) depending on the indication, but should not exceed eight to twelve weeks including tapering off process. Extension beyond these periods should not take place without re-evaluation of the situation.

It may be useful to inform the patient when treatment is started that it will be of limited duration and to explain precisely how the dosage will be progressively decreased. Moreover it is important that the patient should be aware of the possibility of rebound phenomena, thereby minimising anxiety over such symptoms should they occur while the medicinal product is being discontinued.

There are indications, that in the case of benzodiazepines with a short duration of action, withdrawal phenomena can become manifest within the dosage interval, especially when the dosage is high. When benzodiazepines with a long duration of action are being used it is important to warn against changing to a benzodiazepine with a short duration of action, as withdrawal symptoms may develop.

Amnesia

Benzodiazepines may induce anterograde amnesia. The condition occurs most often several hours after ingesting the product and therefore to reduce the risk patients should ensure that they will be able to have uninterrupted sleep of 7-8 ours (see also undesirable effects).

Psychiatric and 'paradoxical' reactions

Reactions like restlessness, agitation, irritability, aggressiveness, delusion, rages, nightmares, hallucinations, psychoses, inappropriate behaviour and other adverse behavioural effects are known to occur when using benzodiazepines. Should this occur, use of the drug should be discontinued.

They are more likely to occur in children and the elderly.

Specific patient groups

Benzodiazepines should not be given to children without careful assessment of the need to do so; the duration of treatment must be kept to a minimum. The elderly should be given a reduced dose (see posology). A lower dose is also recommended for patients with chronic respiratory insufficiency due to risk of respiratory depression.

Benzodiazepines are not indicated to treat patients with severe hepatic insufficiency as they may precipitate encephalopathy. Caution is recommended when treating patients with impaired renal or hepatic function.

Benzodiazepines are not recommended for the primary treatment of psychotic illness.

Benzodiazepines should not be used alone to treat depression of anxiety associated with depression (suicide may be precipitated in such patients). Administration to severely depressed or suicidal patients should be done with appropriate precautions and appropriate size of the prescription.

Benzodiazepines should be used with extreme caution in patients with a history of alcohol or drug abuse.

4.5 Interaction with other medicinal products and other forms of Interaction

§ Not recommended: Concomitant intake with alcohol

The sedative effects may be enhanced when the product is used in combination with alcohol. This affects the ability to drive or use machines.

§ Take into account: Combination with CNS depressants

Enhancement of the central depressive effect may occur in cases of concomitant use with antipsychotics (neuroleptics), hypnotics, anxiolytics/sedatives, antidepressant agents, narcotic analgesics, anti-epileptic drugs, anaesthetics and sedative antihistamines.

Pharmacokinetic interactions can occur when alprazolam is administered along with drugs that interfere with its metabolism. Compounds that inhibit certain hepatic enzymes (particularly cytochrome P450 3A4) may increase the concentration of alprazolam and enhance it's activity. Data from clinical studies with alprazolam, in-vitro studies with alprazolam and clinical studies with drugs metabolised similarly to alprazolam provide evidence for varying degrees of interaction and possible interaction with alprazolam for a number of drugs. Based on the degree of interaction and the type of data available, the following recommendations are made:

§ The co-administration of alprazolam with ketoconazole, itraconazole, or other azole-type antifungals is not recommended.

§ Caution and consideration of dose reduction is recommended when alprazolam is co-administered with nefazodone, fluvoxamine and cimetidine.

§ Caution is recommended when alprazolam is co-administered with fluoxetine, propoxyphene, oral contraceptives, sertraline, diltiazem, or macrolide antibiotics such as erythromycin and troleandomycin.

§ Interactions involving HIV protease inhibitors (e.g. ritonavir) and alprazolam are complex and time dependent. Low doses of ritonavir resulted in a large impairment of alprazolam clearance, prolonged its elimination half-life and enhanced clinical effects, however, upon extended exposure to ritonavir, CYP3A induction offset this inhibition. This interaction will require a dose-adjustment or discontinuation of alprazolam.

4.6 Pregnancy and lactation

If the product is prescribed to a woman of childbearing potential, she should be warned to contact her physician regarding discontinuance of the product if she intends to become or suspects that she is pregnant. The data concerning teratogenicity and effects on postnatal development and behaviour following benzodiazepine treatment are inconsistent. There is evidence from some early studies with other members of the benzodiazepine class that in utero exposure may be associated with malformations. Later studies with the benzodiazepine class of drugs have provided no clear evidence of any type of defect.

If, for compelling medical reasons, the product is administered during the late phase of pregnancy, or during labour, effects on the neonate, such as hypothermia, hypotonia and moderate respiratory depression, can be expected, due to the pharmacological action of the compound.

Infants born to mothers who took benzodiazepines chronically during the latter stages of pregnancy may have developed physical dependence and may be at some risk of developing withdrawal symptoms in the postnatal period.

Since benzodiazepines are found in the breast milk, benzodiazepines should not be given to breast feeding mothers.

4.7 Effects on ability to drive and use machines

Sedation, amnesia, impaired concentration and impaired muscle function may adversely affect the ability to drive or use machines. If insufficient sleep occurs, the likelihood of impaired alertness may be increased (see also interactions).

These effects are potentiated by alcohol (see also interactions).

Patients should be cautioned about operating motor vehicles or engaging in other dangerous activities while taking Xanax.

4.8 Undesirable effects

Sedation/drowsiness, light-headedness, numbed emotions, reduced alertness, confusion, fatigue, headache, dizziness, muscle weakness, ataxia, double or blurred vision, insomnia, nervousness/anxiety, tremor, change in weight. These phenomena occur predominantly at the start of therapy and usually disappear with repeated administration. Other side effects like gastrointestinal disturbances, changes in libido or skin reactions have been reported occasionally.

In addition, the following adverse events have been reported in association with the use of alprazolam: dystonia, anorexia, slurred speech, jaundice, musculoskeletal weakness, sexual dysfunction/changes in libido, menstrual irregularities, incontinence, urinary retention, abnormal liver function and hyperprolactinaemia. Increased intraocular pressure have been rarely reported.

Withdrawal symptoms have occurred following rapid decrease or abrupt discontinuance of benzodiazepines including alprazolam. These can range from mild dysphoria and insomnia to a major syndrome, which may include abdominal and muscle cramps, vomiting, sweating, tremor and convulsions. In addition, withdrawal seizures have occurred upon rapid decrease or abrupt discontinuation of therapy with alprazolam.

Amnesia

Anterograde amnesia may occur at therapeutic dosages, the risk increasing at higher dosages. Amnesic effects may be associated with inappropriate behaviour (see warnings and precautions).

Depression

Pre-existing depression may be unmasked during benzodiazepam use.

Psychiatric and 'paradoxical' reactions

Reactions like restlessness, agitation, irritability, aggressiveness, delusion, rages, nightmares, hallucinations, psychoses, inappropriate behaviour and other adverse behavioural effects are known to occur when using benzodiazepines or benzodiazepine-like agents. They may be quite severe with this product. They are more likely to occur in children and the elderly.

In many of the spontaneous case reports of adverse behavioural effects, patients were receiving other CNS drugs concomitantly and/or were described as having underlying psychiatric conditions. Patients who have borderline personality disorder, a prior history of violent or aggressive behaviour, or alcohol or substance abuse may be at risk of such events. Instances of irritability, hostility and intrusive thoughts have been reported during discontinuance of alprazolam in patients with post-traumatic stress disorder.

Dependence

Use (even at therapeutic doses) may lead to the development of physical dependence: discontinuation of the therapy may result in withdrawal or rebound phenomena (see warnings and precautions). Psychic dependence may occur. Abuse of benzodiazepines have been reported.

4.9 Overdose

As with other benzodiazepines, overdose should not present a threat to life unless combined with other CNS depressants (including alcohol). In the management of overdose with any medicinal product, it should be borne in mind that multiple agents have been taken.

Following overdose with any medicinal product, vomiting may be induced (within 1 hour) if the patient is conscious or gastric lavage undertaken with the airway protected if the patient is unconscious. If there is no advantage in emptying the stomach, activated charcoal should be given to reduce absorption.

Special attention should be paid to respiratory and cardiovascular functions in intensive care.

Symptoms of overdose are extensions of its pharmacological activity and usually manifested by slurring of speech, motor incoordination and degrees of central nervous system depression ranging from drowsiness to coma. In mild cases, symptoms include drowsiness, mental confusion and lethargy, in more serious cases, symptoms may include ataxia, hypotonia, hypotension, respiratory depression, rarely coma and very rarely death.

Flumazenil may be useful as an antidote.

5. PHARMACOLOGICAL PROPERTIES

5.1 Pharmacodynamic properties

Alprazolam, like other benzodiazepines, has a high affinity for the benzodiazepine binding site in the brain. It facilitates the inhibitory neurotransmitter action of gamma-aminobutyric acid, which mediates both pre- and post synaptic inhibition in the central nervous system (CNS).

5.2 Pharmacokinetic properties

Alprazolam is readily absorbed. Following oral administration peak concentration in the plasma occurs after 1 - 2 hours.

The mean half-life is 12 - 15 hours. Repeated dosage may lead to accumulation and this should be borne in mind in elderly patients and those with impaired renal or hepatic function. Alprazolam and its metabolites are excreted primarily in the urine.

In vitro alprazolam is bound (80%) to human serum protein.

5.3 Preclinical safety data

None given

6. PHARMACEUTICAL PARTICULARS

6.1 List of excipients

Lactose monohydrate, microcrystalline cellulose, colloidal anhydrous silica, maize starch, magnesium stearate and docusate sodium with sodium benzoate.

6.2 Incompatibilities

None known.

6.3 Shelf life

5 years.

6.4 Special precautions for storage

Do not store above 25°C.

Blister pack: Keep container in the outer carton.

Bottle pack only: Store in the original container.

6.5 Nature and contents of container

Clear PVC/aluminium foil blister strips of 10 tablets, packed 6 strips to a box. Glass bottle with metal screw cap or HDPE bottle with LDPE tamper evident cap containing 100 or 1000 tablets.

6.6 Instructions for use and handling

Not applicable.

7. MARKETING AUTHORISATION HOLDER

Pharmacia Limited

Davy Avenue

Milton Keynes

MK5 8PH

United Kingdom

8. MARKETING AUTHORISATION NUMBER(S)

PL 0032/0093

9. DATE OF FIRST AUTHORISATION/RENEWAL OF THE AUTHORISATION

27 August 1982/23 January 2003

10. DATE OF REVISION OF THE TEXT
June 2003

***Legal category:* POM**

Xatral

(sanofi-aventis)

1. NAME OF THE MEDICINAL PRODUCT
Xatral®

2. QUALITATIVE AND QUANTITATIVE COMPOSITION
Each tablet contains 2.5mg alfuzosin hydrochloride.

3. PHARMACEUTICAL FORM
White round, film coated tablet for oral administration marked Xatral 2.5 on one side.

4. CLINICAL PARTICULARS

4.1 Therapeutic indications
Treatment of the functional symptoms of benign prostatic hypertrophy.

4.2 Posology and method of administration
Xatral® tablets should be swallowed whole. The first dose should be given just before bedtime.

Adults

The usual dose is one tablet three times daily. The dose may be increased to a maximum of 4 tablets (10mg) per day depending on the clinical response.

Elderly and treated hypertensive patients

As a routine precaution when prescribing alfuzosin to elderly patients (aged over 65 years) and the treated hypertensive patient, the initial dose should be 1 tablet in the morning and 1 tablet in the evening.

Renal insufficiency

In patients with renal insufficiency, as a precaution, it is recommended that the dosing be started at Xatral® 2.5mg twice daily adjusted according to clinical response.

Hepatic insufficiency

In patients with mild to moderate hepatic insufficiency, it is recommended that therapy should commence with a single dose of Xatral® 2.5mg/day to be increased to Xatral® 2.5mg twice daily according to clinical response.

4.3 Contraindications
Hypersensitivity to the product. History of orthostatic hypotension. Combination with other α-blockers. Severe hepatic insufficiency.

4.4 Special warnings and special precautions for use
Warnings

In some subjects, in particular, patients receiving antihypertensive medications, postural hypotension with or without symptoms (dizziness, fatigue, sweating) may develop within a few hours following administration. In such cases, the patient should lie down until the symptoms have completely disappeared.

These effects are transient and do not usually prevent the continuation of treatment after adjustment of the dose. The patient should be warned of the possible occurrence of such events.

Precautions

Treatment should be initiated gradually in patients with hypersensitivity to α-1-blockers. Xatral® should be administered carefully to patients being treated with antihypertensives. Blood pressure should be monitored regularly, especially at the beginning of treatment.

In patients with coronary insufficiency specific anti-anginal therapy should be continued, but if the angina reappears or worsens Xatral® should be discontinued.

Patients with rare hereditary problems of galactose intolerance, the Lapp lactase deficiency or glucose-galactose malabsorption should not take this medicine.

4.5 Interaction with other medicinal products and other forms of Interaction
Combinations contraindicated:

- Alpha$_1$-receptor blockers (see 4.3 Contraindications)

Combinations to be taken into account:

- Antihypertensive drugs (see 4.4.2 Special precautions)

- Nitrates

The administration of general anaesthetics to patients receiving Xatral® could cause profound hypotension. It is recommended that Xatral® be withdrawn 24 hours before surgery.

Other forms of interaction

No pharmacodynamic or pharmacokinetic interaction has been observed in healthy volunteers between alfuzosin and the following drugs: warfarin, digoxin, hydrochlorothiazide and atenolol.

4.6 Pregnancy and lactation
Due to the type of indication this section is not applicable.

4.7 Effects on ability to drive and use machines
There are no data available on the effect on driving vehicles. Adverse reactions such as vertigo, dizziness and asthenia may occur. This has to be taken into account when driving vehicles and operating machinery.

4.8 Undesirable effects

- **CNS and psychiatric disorders**

Common: faintness/dizziness, vertigo, malaise, headache

Uncommon: drowsiness

- **Vision disorders**

Uncommon: vision abnormal

- **Cardiovascular disorders**

Common: hypotension (postural)

Uncommon: tachycardia, palpitations, syncope

Very rare: aggravation or recurrence of angina pectoris (see 4.4.)

- **Respiratory system disorders**

Uncommon: rhinitis

- **Gastro-intestinal disorders**

Common: nausea, abdominal pain, diarrhoea, dry mouth

- **Skin and appendages**

Uncommon: rash, pruritus

- **Body as a whole**

Common: asthenia

Uncommon: flushes, oedema, chest pain

Although only reported in isolated cases with alfuzosin, occurrence of priapism can not be excluded as it is generally accepted as being attributable to all other alpha adrenoreceptor blockers.

4.9 Overdose
In case of overdosage, the patient should be hospitalised, kept in the supine position, and conventional treatment of hypotension should take place.

Alfuzosin is not easily dialysable because of its high degree of protein binding.

5. PHARMACOLOGICAL PROPERTIES

5.1 Pharmacodynamic properties
Alfuzosin is an orally active quinazoline derivative. It is a selective, peripherally acting antagonist of post synaptic α_1-adrenoceptors.

In vitro pharmacological studies have documented the selectivity of alfuzosin for the alpha$_1$-adrenoreceptors located in the prostate, bladder base and prostatic urethra.

Clinical manifestations of Benign Prostatic Hypertrophy are associated with infra vesical obstruction which is triggered by both anatomical (static) and functional (dynamic) factors. The functional component of obstruction arises from the tension of prostatic smooth muscle which is mediated by α-adrenoceptors. Activation of α_1-adrenoceptors stimulates smooth muscle contraction, thereby increasing the tone of the prostate, prostatic capsule, prostatic urethra and bladder base, and, consequently, increasing the resistance to bladder outflow. This in turn leads to outflow obstruction and possible secondary bladder instability.

Alpha-blockade decreases infra vesical obstruction via a direct action on prostatic smooth muscle.

In vivo, animal studies have shown that alfuzosin decreases urethral pressure and therefore, resistance to urine flow during micturition. Moreover, alfuzosin inhibits the hypertonic response of the urethra more readily than that of vascular muscle and shows functional uroselectivity in conscious normotensive rats by decreasing urethral pressure at doses that do not affect blood pressure.

In man, alfuzosin improves voiding parameters by reducing urethral tone and bladder outlet resistance, and facilitates bladder emptying.

In placebo controlled studies in BPH patients, alfuzosin:

significantly increases peak flow rate (Qmax) in patients with Qmax $\leqslant$ 15ml/s by a mean of 30%. This improvement is observed from the first dose, significantly reduces the detrusor pressure and increases the volume producing a strong desire to void, significantly reduces the residual urine volume.

These favourable urodynamic effects lead to an improvement of lower urinary tract symptoms ie. Filling (irritative) as well as voiding (obstructive) symptoms.

Alfuzosin may cause moderate antihypertensive effects.

5.2 Pharmacokinetic properties
Xatral is well absorbed with a mean bioavailability of 64%, peak plasma levels are generally reached in 0.5-3 hours. Kinetics within the therapeutic range are linear. The kinetic profile is characterised by large interindividual fluctuations in plasma concentrations. The terminal half-life is 3-5 hours. Alfuzosin is 90% protein bound in plasma, 68.2% to human serum albumin and 52.5% to human serum alpha-glycoprotein. It is partially metabolised and excreted mainly in the bile and faeces.

None of the metabolites found in man has any pharmacodynamic activity. The pharmacokinetic profile is not affected by taking Xatral with food.

In subjects over 75 years, absorption is more rapid and peak plasma levels are higher. Bioavailability may be increased and in some patients the volume of distribution is reduced. The elimination half-life does not change.

The volume of distribution and clearance of alfuzosin are increased in renal insufficiency, with or without dialysis, owing to an increase in the free fraction. Chronic renal insufficiency even when severe (creatinine clearance between 15 and 40 mls/min) is not adversely affected by alfuzosin.

In patients with severe hepatic insufficiency, the elimination half-life is prolonged. A two-fold increase in Cmax values and a three-fold increase in the AUC is observed. Bioavailability is increased compared with healthy volunteers.

The pharmacokinetic profile of alfuzosin is not affected by chronic cardiac insufficiency.

5.3 Preclinical safety data
No data of therapeutic relevance.

6. PHARMACEUTICAL PARTICULARS

6.1 List of excipients
Tablet core: Microcrystalline cellulose, lactose, povidone, sodium starch glycollate, magnesium stearate, purified water.

Coating: Methylhydroxypropylcellulose, polyethylene glycol 400, titanium dioxide suspension (E171), purified water.

6.2 Incompatibilities
Not known.

6.3 Shelf life
3 years.

6.4 Special precautions for storage
Store in a dry place at or below 30°C.

6.5 Nature and contents of container
Boxes with 60 tablets in pvc/foil blister strips.

6.6 Instructions for use and handling
Please consult insert text before use.

Do not use after the stated expiry date on packaging and blisters.

Keep out of the reach of children.

7. MARKETING AUTHORISATION HOLDER
Sanofi-Synthelabo

PO Box 597

Guildford

Surrey

8. MARKETING AUTHORISATION NUMBER(S)
PL 11723/0329

9. DATE OF FIRST AUTHORISATION/RENEWAL OF THE AUTHORISATION
2 April 2002

10. DATE OF REVISION OF THE TEXT
April 2005

Legal category: POM

Xatral XL 10mg

(sanofi-aventis)

1. NAME OF THE MEDICINAL PRODUCT
Xatral® XL 10mg

2. QUALITATIVE AND QUANTITATIVE COMPOSITION
Each tablet contains 10mg alfuzosin hydrochloride.

3. PHARMACEUTICAL FORM
Prolonged release tablets.

4. CLINICAL PARTICULARS

4.1 Therapeutic indications
Treatment of the functional symptoms of benign prostatic hypertrophy (BPH).

For information on use in acute urinary retention (AUR) related to BPH see sections 4.2 and 5.1.

4.2 Posology and method of administration
Xatral® XL tablets should be swallowed whole.

BPH: The recommended dose is one 10mg tablet to be taken once daily after a meal.

AUR: In patients 65 years and older, one 10 mg tablet daily after a meal to be taken from the first day of catheterisation. The treatment should be administered for 3-4 days, 2-3 days during catheterisation and 1 day after its removal. In this indication no benefit has been established in patients under 65 years of age or if treatment is extended beyond 4 days.

4.3 Contraindications
Hypersensitivity to the product. History of orthostatic hypotension. Combination with other α-blockers. Hepatic insufficiency.

4.4 Special warnings and special precautions for use
Warnings

As with all alpha$_1$-blockers in some subjects, in particular patients receiving antihypertensive medications, postural hypotension with or without symptoms (dizziness, fatigue, sweating) may develop within a few hours following administration. In such cases, the patient should lie down until the symptoms have completely disappeared.

These effects are transient and do not usually prevent the continuation of treatment after adjustment of the dose. The patient should be warned of the possible occurrence of such events.

Precautions

Treatment should be initiated gradually in patients with hypersensitivity to α-1-blockers. Xatral® XL tablets 10mg should be administered carefully to patients being treated with antihypertensives. Blood pressure should be monitored regularly, especially at the beginning of treatment.

In patients with coronary insufficiency specific anti-anginal therapy should be continued, but if the angina reappears or worsens Xatral® XL tablets 10mg should be discontinued.

Experience in patients with severe renal impairment is limited and cautious use in these patients is recommended.

Patients should be warned that the tablet should be swallowed whole. Any other mode of administration, such as crunching, crushing, chewing, grinding or pounding to powder should be prohibited. These actions may lead to inappropriate release and absorption of the drug and therefore possible early adverse reactions.

4.5 Interaction with other medicinal products and other forms of Interaction

Combinations contra-indicated:

- Alpha$_1$-receptor blockers (see 4.3 Contra-indications).

Combinations to be taken into account:

- Antihypertensive drugs (see 4.4 Special Warnings and Precautions for Use).
- Nitrates

The administration of general anaesthetics to patients receiving Xatral® XL tablets 10mg could cause profound hypotension. It is recommended that the tablets be withdrawn 24 hours before surgery.

Other forms of interaction

No pharmacodynamic or pharmacokinetic interaction has been observed in healthy volunteers between alfuzosin and the following drugs: warfarin, digoxin, hydrochlorothiazide and atenolol.

4.6 Pregnancy and lactation

Due to the type of indication this section is not applicable.

4.7 Effects on ability to drive and use machines

There are no data available on the effect on driving vehicles. Adverse reactions such as vertigo, dizziness and asthenia may occur. This has to be taken into account when driving vehicles and operating machinery.

4.8 Undesirable effects

- **CNS and psychiatric disorders**

Common: faintness/dizziness, headache

Uncommon: vertigo, malaise, drowsiness

- **Cardiovascular disorders**

Uncommon: tachycardia, palpitations, hypotension (postural), syncope

Very rare: aggravation or recurrence of angina pectoris (see 4.4.)

- **Gastro-intestinal disorders**

Common: nausea, abdominal pain

Uncommon: diarrhoea, dry mouth

- **Skin and appendages**

Uncommon: rash, pruritus

- **Body as a whole**

Common: asthenia

Uncommon: flushes, oedema, chest pain

Although only reported in isolated cases with alfuzosin, occurrence of priapism can not be excluded as it is generally accepted as being attributable to all other alpha adrenoreceptor blockers.

4.9 Overdose

In case of overdosage, the patient should be hospitalized, kept in the supine position, and conventional treatment of hypotension should take place.

Alfuzosin is not dialysable because of its high degree of protein binding.

5. PHARMACOLOGICAL PROPERTIES

5.1 Pharmacodynamic properties

Alfuzosin is an orally active quinazoline derivative. It is a selective, peripherally acting antagonist of postsynaptic α_1-adrenoceptors.

In vitro pharmacological studies have documented the selectivity of alfuzosin for the alpha$_1$-adrenoreceptors located in the prostate, bladder base and prostatic urethra.

Clinical manifestations of Benign Prostatic Hypertrophy are associated with infra vesical obstruction which is triggered by both anatomical (static) and functional (dynamic) factors. The functional component of obstruction arises from the tension of prostatic smooth muscle which is mediated by α-adrenoceptors. Activation of α_1-adrenoceptors stimulates smooth muscle contraction, thereby increasing the tone of the prostate, prostatic capsule, prostatic urethra and bladder base, and, consequently, increasing the resistance to bladder outflow. This in turn leads to outflow obstruction and possible secondary bladder instability.

Alpha-blockade decreases infra vesical obstruction via a direct action on prostatic smooth muscle.

In vivo, animal studies have shown that alfuzosin decreases urethral pressure and therefore, resistance to urine flow during micturition. Moreover, alfuzosin inhibits the hypertonic response of the urethra more readily than that of vascular muscle and shows functional uroselectivity in conscious normotensive rats by decreasing urethral pressure at doses that do not affect blood pressure.

In man, alfuzosin improves voiding parameters by reducing urethral tone and bladder outlet resistance, and facilitates bladder emptying.

In placebo controlled studies in BPH patients, alfuzosin:

- significantly increases peak flow rate (Qmax) in patients with Qmax $\leqslant$ 15ml/s by a mean of 30%. This improvement is observed from the first dose,
- significantly reduces the detrusor pressure and increases the volume producing a strong desire to void,
- significantly reduces the residual urine volume.

These favourable urodynamic effects lead to an improvement of lower urinary tract symptoms ie. filling (irritative) as well as voiding (obstructive) symptoms.

Alfuzosin may cause moderate antihypertensive effects.

A lower frequency of acute urinary retention is observed in the alfuzosin treated patient than in the untreated patient.

AUR (related to BPH):

In the ALFAUR study, the effect of alfuzosin on the return of normal voiding was evaluated in 357 men over 50 years, presenting with a first episode of acute urinary retention (AUR), related to BPH. In this multicentre, randomised double blind parallel group study comparing alfuzosin 10mg/day and placebo, the evaluation of voiding was performed 24 hours after catheter removal, the morning after 2-3 days of treatment.

In men aged 65 years and over alfuzosin significantly increased the success rate of spontaneous voiding after catheter removal – see table. No benefit has been established in patients under 65 years of age or if treatment is extended beyond 4 days.

(see Table 1 below)

ALFAUR study: Percentage of patients (ITT population) successfully voiding post-catheter removal

5.2 Pharmacokinetic properties

Prolonged-release formulation:

The mean value of the relative bioavailability is 104.4 % versus the immediate release formulation (2.5 mg tid) in middle-aged healthy volunteers and the maximum plasma concentration is being achieved 9 hours after administration compared to 1 hour for the immediate release formulation.

The apparent elimination half-life is 9.1 hours.

Studies have shown that consistent pharmacokinetic profiles are obtained when the product is administered after a meal.

Under fed conditions, mean Cmax and Ctrough values are 13.6 (SD=5.6) and 3.2 (SD=1.6) ng/ml respectively. Mean AUC_{0-24} is 194 (SD=75) ng.h/ml. A plateau of concentration is observed from 3 to 14 hours with concentrations above 8.1 ng/ml (Cav) for 11 hours.

Compared to healthy middle aged volunteers, the pharmacokinetic parameters (Cmax and AUC) are not increased in elderly patients.

Compared to subjects with normal renal function, mean Cmax and AUC values are moderately increased in patients with renal impairment, without modification of the apparent elimination half-life. This change in the pharmacokinetic profile is not considered clinically relevant. Therefore, this does not necessitate a dosing adjustment.

The binding of alfuzosin to plasma proteins is about 90%.

Table 1

Age	Placebo N (%)	Alfuzosin N (%)	Relative difference vs placebo 95%CI	p value
65 years and above	30 (35.7%)	88 (56.1%)	1.57 (1.14-2.16)	0.003
Below 65 years	28 (75.7%)	58 (73.4%)	0.97 (0.77-1.22)	0.80
All patients (50 years and above)	58 (47.8%)	146 (61.9%)	1.29 (1.04-1.60)	0.012

Alfuzosin undergoes extensive metabolism by the liver, with only 11 % of the parent compound being excreted unchanged in the urine. The majority of the metabolites (which are inactive) are excreted in the faeces (75 to 91 %).

The pharmacokinetic profile of alfuzosin is not affected by chronic cardiac insufficiency.

5.3 Preclinical safety data

No data of therapeutic relevance.

6. PHARMACEUTICAL PARTICULARS

6.1 List of excipients

Ethylcellulose, hydrogenated castor oil, hypromellose, yellow ferric oxide, magnesium stearate, microcrystalline cellulose, povidone, silica colloidal hydrated, mannitol.

6.2 Incompatibilities

None known.

6.3 Shelf life

3 years.

6.4 Special precautions for storage

No special precautions for storage.

Store in the original container.

6.5 Nature and contents of container

Boxes with 10 and 30 tablets in pvc/foil blister strips.

6.6 Instructions for use and handling

Please consult patient leaflet before use.

Do not use after the stated expiry date on packaging and blisters.

Keep out of the reach of children.

Administrative Data

7. MARKETING AUTHORISATION HOLDER

Sanofi-Synthelabo

PO Box 597

Guildford,

Surrey

8. MARKETING AUTHORISATION NUMBER(S)

PL 11723/0370

9. DATE OF FIRST AUTHORISATION/RENEWAL OF THE AUTHORISATION

30 June 2000

10. DATE OF REVISION OF THE TEXT

April 2005

Legal category: POM

Xeloda

(Roche Products Limited)

1. NAME OF THE MEDICINAL PRODUCT

Xeloda ®▼150 mg and 500 mg film-coated tablets

2. QUALITATIVE AND QUANTITATIVE COMPOSITION

150 mg or 500 mg capecitabine

For excipients, see section 6.1.

3. PHARMACEUTICAL FORM

Film-coated tablet

4. CLINICAL PARTICULARS

4.1 Therapeutic indications

Xeloda is indicated for the adjuvant treatment of patients following surgery of stage III (Dukes' stage C) colon cancer (see section 5.1).

Xeloda is indicated for first line monotherapy of metastatic colorectal cancer (see section 5.1).

Xeloda in combination with docetaxel (see section 5.1) is indicated for the treatment of patients with locally advanced or metastatic breast cancer after failure of cytotoxic chemotherapy. Previous therapy should have included an anthracycline. Xeloda is also indicated as monotherapy for the treatment of patients with locally advanced or metastatic breast cancer after failure of taxanes and an anthracycline-containing chemotherapy regimen or for whom further anthracycline therapy is not indicated.

4.2 Posology and method of administration

Xeloda should only be prescribed by a qualified physician experienced in the utilisation of anti-neoplastic agents.

Recommended posology:

The recommended dose is 1250 mg/m^2 administered twice daily (morning and evening; equivalent to 2500 mg/m^2 total daily dose) for 14 days followed by a seven day rest period. Xeloda tablets should be swallowed with water within 30 minutes after a meal. Treatment should be discontinued if progressive disease or intolerable toxicity is observed. In combination with docetaxel, the recommended dose of Xeloda is 1250 mg/m^2 twice daily for 2 weeks followed by 1-week rest period, combined with docetaxel at 75 mg/m^2 as a 1 hour intravenous infusion every 3 weeks. Pre-medication with an oral corticosteroid such as dexamethasone according to the docetaxel summary of product characteristics should be started prior to docetaxel administration for patients receiving the Xeloda plus docetaxel combination.

Table 1 Xeloda dose calculation according to body surface area, standard starting dose

Dose level 1250 mg/m² (twice daily)		Number of tablets administered in the morning		Number of tablets administered in the evening	
Body Surface Area (m²)	Dose per administration (mg)	150 mg	500 mg	150 mg	500 mg
≤1.26	1500	-	3	-	3
1.27 - 1.38	1650	1	3	1	3
1.39 - 1.52	1800	2	3	2	3
1.53 - 1.66	2000	-	4	-	4
1.67 - 1.78	2150	1	4	1	4
1.79 - 1.92	2300	2	4	2	4
1.93 - 2.06	2500	-	5	-	5
2.07 - 2.18	2650	1	5	1	5
≥2.19	2800	2	5	2	5

Table 2 Calculated Xeloda dose, reduced to 75% of the standard starting dose

Dose level 950 mg/m² (twice daily)		Number of tablets administered in the morning		Number of tablets administered in the evening	
Body Surface Area (m²)	Dose per administration (mg)	150 mg	500 mg	150 mg	500 mg
≤1.26	1150	1	2	1	2
1.27 - 1.38	1300	2	2	2	2
1.39 - 1.52	1450	3	2	3	2
1.53 - 1.66	1500	-	3	-	3
1.67 - 1.78	1650	1	3	1	3
1.79 - 1.92	1800	2	3	2	3
1.93 - 2.06	1950	3	3	3	3
2.07 - 2.18	2000	-	4	-	4
≥2.19	2150	1	4	1	4

Table 3 Calculated Xeloda dose, reduced to 50% of the standard starting dose

Dose level 625 mg/m² (twice daily)		Number of tablets administered in the morning		Number of tablets administered in the evening	
Body Surface Area (m²)	Dose per administration (mg)	150 mg	500 mg	150 mg	500 mg
≤1.38	800	2	1	2	1
1.39 - 1.52	950	3	1	3	1
1.53 - 1.66	1000	-	2	-	2
1.67 - 1.78	1000	-	2	-	2
1.79 - 1.92	1150	1	2	1	2
1.93 - 2.06	1300	2	2	2	2
2.07 - 2.18	1300	2	2	2	2
≥2.19	1450	3	2	3	2

Table 1: Xeloda dose calculation according to body surface area, standard starting dose

(see Table 1 above)

Table 2: Calculated Xeloda dose, reduced to 75% of the standard starting dose

(see Table 2 above)

Table 3: Calculated Xeloda dose, reduced to 50% of the standard starting dose

(see Table 3 above)

Posology adjustments during treatment:

Toxicity due to Xeloda administration may be managed by symptomatic treatment and/or modification of the dose (treatment interruption or dose reduction). Once the dose has been reduced, it should not be increased at a later time. Patients taking Xeloda should be informed of the need to interrupt treatment immediately if moderate or worse toxicity occurs. Doses of Xeloda omitted for toxicity are not replaced or restored, instead the patient should resume the planned treatment cycle. The following are the recommended dose modifications for toxicity:

Table 4: Xeloda Monotherapy Dose Reduction Schedule

Toxicity NCIC grades*	During a course of therapy	Dose adjustment for next cycle (% of starting dose)
• *Grade 1*	Maintain dose level	Maintain dose level
• *Grade 2*		
-1st appearance	Interrupt until resolved to grade 0-1	100%
-2nd appearance	Interrupt until resolved to grade 0-1	75%
-3rd appearance	Interrupt until resolved to grade 0-1	50%
-4th appearance	Discontinue treatment permanently	
• *Grade 3*		
-1st appearance	Interrupt until resolved to grade 0-1	75%
-2nd appearance	Interrupt until resolved to grade 0-1	50%
-3rd appearance	Discontinue treatment permanently	
• *Grade 4*		
-1st appearance	Discontinue permanently *or* If physician deems it to be in the patient's best interest to continue, interrupt until resolved to grade 0-1	50%

*National Cancer Institute of Canada (NCIC) Common Toxicity Criteria (version 1) were used except for hand-foot syndrome.

The following are the recommended dose modifications for toxicity when Xeloda and docetaxel are used in combination:

Table 5: Xeloda (X) in Combination with Docetaxel (Taxotere®, T) Dose Reduction Schedule for Non-Haematological Toxicities (for dose modifications due to haematological toxicities, see section on haematological toxicity after the table)

	Recommended Dose Modifications	
	Xeloda dose changes within a treatment cycle	Dose adjustment on resumption of treatment
Toxicity grade[1]	Grade 1	
	100% of starting dose (no interruption)	X: 100% of starting dose T: 100% (75mg/m²)
Toxicity grade[1]	Grade 2	
1st appearance	Interrupt until resolved to grade 0-1	X: 100% of starting dose T: 100% (75mg/m²)
2nd appearance of same toxicity	Interrupt until resolved to (grade 0-1)	X:75% of starting dose T: Reduce to 55mg/m²
3rd appearance of same toxicity	Interrupt until resolved (grade 0-1)	X: 50% of starting dose T: Discontinue permanently
4th appearance of same toxicity	Discontinue permanently	
Toxicity grade[1]	Grade 3	
1st appearance	Interrupt until resolved (grade 0-1)	X: 75% of starting dose T: Reduce to 55mg/m²
2nd appearance	Interrupt until resolved (grade 0-1)	X: 50% of starting dose T: Discontinue permanently
3rd appearance	Discontinue permanently	
Toxicity grade[1]	Grade 4	
1st appearance	Discontinue permanently *or* (if physician deems it to be in the best interest of the patient) interrupt until resolved (grade 0-1)	X: Reduce to 50% T: Discontinue permanently
2nd appearance	Discontinue permanently	

1. National Cancer Institute of Canada Common Toxicity Criteria (NCIC CTC), version 1.0 revised December 1994.

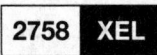

Specific dose adjustment in combination with docetaxel:

Xeloda and/or docetaxel dose modifications should be made according to the general dose modification scheme above, if nothing else is stated regarding specific dose adjustments. For those toxicities considered by the treating physician to be unlikely to become serious or life-threatening, e.g. alopecia, altered taste, nail changes, treatment can be continued at the same dose without reduction or interruption. At the beginning of a treatment cycle, if either a docetaxel or a Xeloda treatment delay is indicated, both docetaxel and Xeloda administration should be delayed until the requirements for restarting both drugs are met. For further information about docetaxel see also the summary of product characteristics for docetaxel (Taxotere®).

Haematology: Xeloda treatment may continue throughout a grade 3 neutropenic episode. However, the patient should be closely monitored and administration of Xeloda should be interrupted if any grade 2 clinical event (eg diarrhoea, stomatitis, fever) coincides with the grade 3 neutropenic episode. If grade 4 neutropenia occurs treatment with Xeloda should be interrupted until recovery to grade 0-1. Treatment should only be re-administered when the neutrophil count is $\geqslant 1.5 \times 10^9$/L (Grade 0 - 1).

Docetaxel dosage should be reduced from 75 mg/m^2 to 55 mg/m^2 in patients with neutropenia $<0.5 \times 10^9$/l (grade 4) for more than 1 week, or febrile (> 38°C) neutropenia. Docetaxel should be discontinued if grade 4 neutropenia or febrile neutropenia occurs at a dose of 55 mg/m^2 docetaxel. Patients with baseline neutrophil counts of $<1.5 \times 10^9$/l and/or thrombocyte counts of $<100 \times 10^9$/l should not be treated with the Xeloda/docetaxel combination.

Hypersensitivity: Patients who develop severe hypersensitivity reactions (hypotension with a decrease of $\geqslant$20 mm Hg, or bronchospasm, or generalised rash/erythema) should stop treatment immediately and be given appropriate therapy. These patients should not be rechallenged with the drug suspected to have caused hypersensitivity.

Peripheral neuropathy: For 1st appearance of grade 2 toxicity, reduce the docetaxel dose to 55 mg/m^2. If grade 3 toxicity appears, discontinue docetaxel treatment. In both instances follow the above dose modification scheme for Xeloda.

Fluid retention: Severe (grade 3 or 4) toxicity such as pleural effusion, pericardial effusion or ascites which is possibly related to docetaxel should be closely monitored. In case of appearance of such toxicity docetaxel treatment should be discontinued, Xeloda treatment may be continued without dose modification.

Hepatic impairment: Docetaxel should generally not be given to patients with serum bilirubin above the upper limit of normal. The following modifications should be applied to the docetaxel dose in the event of abnormal values for ASAT, ALAT, and/or alkaline phosphatase levels;

ASAT and/or ALAT values	Alkaline phosphatase values	Docetaxel Dose modification
$\leqslant 1.5 \times$ ULN	AND $\leqslant 5 \times$ ULN	no dose modification
$>1.5 \times$ ULN - $\leqslant 2.5 \times$ ULN	AND $\leqslant 2.5 \times$ ULN	no dose modification
$>2.5 \times$ ULN - $\leqslant 5 \times$ ULN	AND $\leqslant 2.5 \times$ ULN	reduce by 25% (not below 55 mg/m^2)
$>1.5 \times$ ULN - $\leqslant 5 \times$ ULN	AND $>2.5 \times$ ULN - $\leqslant 5 \times$ ULN	reduce by 25% (not below 55 mg/m^2)
$>5 \times$ ULN	OR $>5 \times$ ULN (unless bone metastasis are present in the absence of any liver disorder)	delay dose by a maximum of 2 weeks. If no recovery, discontinue docetaxel.

Once the docetaxel dose is reduced for a given cycle, no further dose reduction is recommended for subsequent cycles unless worsening of the parameters is observed. In case of recovery of liver function tests after previous reduction of the docetaxel dose, the docetaxel dose can be re-escalated to the previous dose level.

Diarrhoea: Follow the general dose modification scheme above (see also section 4.4).

Dehydration: Dehydration should be prevented or corrected at the onset. Patients with anorexia, asthenia, nausea, vomiting or diarrhoea may rapidly become dehydrated. If grade 2 (or higher) dehydration occurs, Xeloda treatment should be immediately interrupted and the dehydration corrected. Treatment should not be restarted until the patient is rehydrated and any precipitating causes have been corrected or controlled. Dose modifications applied should be those for the precipitating adverse event in accordance with the above guidelines.

Posology adjustments for special populations:

Hepatic impairment: Insufficient safety and efficacy data are available in patients with hepatic impairment to provide a dose adjustment recommendation. No information is available on hepatic impairment due to cirrhosis or hepatitis.

Renal impairment: Xeloda is contraindicated in patients with severe renal impairment (creatinine clearance below 30 ml/min [Cockroft and Gault] at baseline). The incidence of grade 3 or 4 adverse events in patients with moderate renal impairment (creatinine clearance 30-50 ml/min at baseline) is increased compared to the overall population. In patients with moderate renal impairment at baseline, a dose reduction to 75% of starting dose is recommended. In patients with mild renal impairment (creatinine clearance 51-80 ml/min at baseline) no adjustment of the starting dose is recommended. Careful monitoring and prompt treatment interruption is recommended if the patient develops a grade 2, 3 or 4 adverse event during treatment and subsequent dose adjustment as outlined in the table above. These dose adjustment recommendations for renal impairment apply both to monotherapy and combination use (see also section "Elderly" below).

Children (under 18 years): The safety and efficacy of Xeloda in children has not been studied.

Elderly: No adjustment of the starting dose is needed during Xeloda monotherapy. However, grade 3 or 4 treatment-related adverse events were more frequent in patients $\geqslant$60 years of age compared to younger patients. Careful monitoring of patients $\geqslant$60 years of age is advisable. In combination with docetaxel, an increased incidence of grade 3 or 4 treatment-related adverse events and treatment-related serious adverse events were observed in patients 60 years of age or more (see section 5.1). For patients 60 years of age or more treated with the combination of Xeloda plus docetaxel, a starting dose reduction of Xeloda to 75% (950 mg/m^2 twice daily) is recommended. If no toxicity is observed in patients $\geqslant$60 years of age treated with a reduced Xeloda starting dose in combination with docetaxel, the dose of Xeloda may be cautiously escalated to 1250 mg/m^2 twice daily.

4.3 Contraindications

History of severe and unexpected reactions to fluoropyrimidine therapy,

Known hypersensitivity to capecitabine, fluorouracil or any of the excipients,

In patients with known dihydropyrimidine dehydrogenase (DPD) deficiency,

During pregnancy and lactation,

In patients with severe leucopenia, neutropenia, or thrombocytopenia,

In patients with severe hepatic impairment,

In patients with severe renal impairment (creatinine clearance below 30 ml/min),

Treatment with sorivudine or its chemically related analogues, such as brivudine.

Contraindications for docetaxel also apply to the Xeloda plus docetaxel combination.

4.4 Special warnings and special precautions for use

Dose limiting toxicities include diarrhoea, abdominal pain, nausea, stomatitis and hand-foot syndrome (hand-foot skin reaction, palmar-plantar erythrodysesthesia). Most adverse events are reversible and do not require permanent discontinuation of therapy, although doses may need to be withheld or reduced.

Diarrhoea. Xeloda can induce the occurrence of diarrhoea, which has been observed in 50% of patients. Patients with severe diarrhoea should be carefully monitored and given fluid and electrolyte replacement if they become dehydrated. Standard antidiarrhoeal treatments (e.g. loperamide) may be used. NCIC CTC grade 2 diarrhoea is defined as an increase of 4 to 6 stools/day or nocturnal stools, grade 3 diarrhoea as an increase of 7 to 9 stools/day or incontinence and malabsorption. Grade 4 diarrhoea is an increase of $\geqslant$10 stools/day or grossly bloody diarrhoea or the need for parenteral support. If grade 2, 3 or 4 diarrhoea occurs, administration of Xeloda should be immediately interrupted until the diarrhoea resolves or decreases in intensity to grade 1. Following grade 3 or 4 diarrhoea, subsequent doses of Xeloda should be decreased or treatment discontinued permanently (grade 4).

Hand-foot syndrome (also known as hand-foot skin reaction or palmar-plantar erythrodysesthesia or chemotherapy induced acral erythema). Grade 1 hand- foot syndrome is defined as numbness, dysesthesia/paresthesia, tingling, painless swelling or erythema of the hands and/or feet and/or discomfort which does not disrupt the patient's normal activities.

Grade 2 hand- foot syndrome is painful erythema and swelling of the hands and/or feet and/or discomfort affecting the patient's activities of daily living.

Grade 3 hand- foot syndrome is moist desquamation, ulceration, blistering and severe pain of the hands and/or feet and/or severe discomfort that causes the patient to be unable to work or perform activities of daily living. If grade 2 or 3 hand- foot syndrome occurs, administration of Xeloda should be interrupted until the event resolves or decreases in intensity to grade 1. Following grade 3 hand- foot syndrome, subsequent doses of Xeloda should be decreased.

Cardiotoxicity. Cardiotoxicity has been associated with fluoropyrimidine therapy, including myocardial infarction, angina, dysrhythmias, cardiogenic shock, sudden death and electrocardiographic changes. These adverse events may be more common in patients with a prior history of coronary artery disease. Cardiac arrhythmias, angina pectoris, myocardial infarction, heart failure and cardiomyopathy have been reported in patients receiving Xeloda. Caution must be exercised in patients with history of significant cardiac disease, arrhythmias and angina pectoris (See section 4.8).

Hypo- or hypercalcaemia. Hypo- or hypercalcaemia has been reported during Xeloda treatment. Caution must be exercised in patients with pre-existing hypo- or hypercalcaemia (see section 4.8).

Central or peripheral nervous system disease. Caution must be exercised in patients with central or peripheral nervous system disease, e.g. brain metastasis or neuropathy (see section 4.8).

Diabetes mellitus or electrolyte disturbances. Caution must be exercised in patients with diabetes mellitus or electrolyte disturbances, as these may be aggravated during Xeloda treatment.

Coumarin-derivative anticoagulation. In a drug interaction study with single-dose warfarin administration, there was a significant increase in the mean AUC (+57%) of S-warfarin. These results suggest an interaction, probably due to an inhibition of the cytochrome P450 2C9 isoenzyme system by capecitabine. Patients receiving concomitant Xeloda and oral coumarin-derivative anticoagulant therapy should have their anticoagulant response (INR or prothrombin time) monitored closely and the anticoagulant dose adjusted accordingly (see section 4.5).

Hepatic impairment. In the absence of safety and efficacy data in patients with hepatic impairment, Xeloda use should be carefully monitored in patients with mild to moderate liver dysfunction, regardless of the presence or absence of liver metastasis. Administration of Xeloda should be interrupted if treatment-related elevations in bilirubin of $>3.0 \times$ ULN or treatment-related elevations in hepatic aminotransferases (ALT, AST) of $>2.5 \times$ ULN occur. Treatment with Xeloda monotherapy may be resumed when bilirubin decreases to $\leqslant 3.0 \times$ ULN or hepatic aminotransferases decrease to $\leqslant 2.5 \times$ ULN. For combination treatment with Xeloda and docetaxel, see also section 4.2.

Renal impairment. The incidence of grade 3 or 4 adverse events in patients with moderate renal impairment (creatinine clearance 30-50 ml/min) is increased compared to the overall population (see section 4.2 and 4.3).

4.5 Interaction with other medicinal products and other forms of Interaction

Interaction with other medicinal products:

Coumarin-derivative anticoagulants: Altered coagulation parameters and/or bleeding have been reported in patients taking Xeloda concomitantly with coumarin-derivative anticoagulants such as warfarin and phenprocoumon. These events occurred within several days and up to several months after initiating Xeloda therapy and, in a few cases, within one month after stopping Xeloda. In a clinical pharmacokinetic interaction study, after a single 20 mg dose of warfarin, Xeloda treatment increased the AUC of S-warfarin by 57% with a 91% increase in INR value. Since metabolism of R-warfarin was not affected, these results indicate that capecitabine down-regulates isozyme 2C9, but has no effect on isozymes 1A2 and 3A4. Patients taking coumarin-derivative anticoagulants concomitantly with Xeloda should be monitored regularly for alterations in their coagulation parameters (PT or INR) and the anti-coagulant dose adjusted accordingly.

Phenytoin: Increased phenytoin plasma concentrations resulting in symptoms of phenytoin intoxication in single cases have been reported during concomitant use of Xeloda with phenytoin. Patients taking phenytoin concomitantly with Xeloda should be regularly monitored for increased phenytoin plasma concentrations.

Folinic acid: A combination study with Xeloda and folinic acid indicated that folinic acid has no major effect on the pharmacokinetics of Xeloda and its metabolites. However, folinic acid has an effect on the pharmacodynamics of Xeloda: the maximum tolerated dose (MTD) of Xeloda alone using the intermittent regimen is 3000 mg/m^2 per day whereas it is only 2000 mg/ m^2 per day when Xeloda was combined with folinic acid (30 mg orally bid).

Sorivudine and analogues: A clinically significant drug-drug interaction between sorivudine and 5-FU, resulting from the inhibition of dihydropyrimidine dehydrogenase by sorivudine, has been described. This interaction, which leads to increased fluoropyrimidine toxicity, is potentially fatal. Therefore, Xeloda must not be administered with sorivudine or its chemically related analogues, such as brivudine (see section 4.3).

Antacid: The effect of an aluminum hydroxide and magnesium hydroxide-containing antacid on the pharmacokinetics of capecitabine was investigated. There was a small increase in plasma concentrations of capecitabine and one metabolite (5'-DFCR); there was no effect on the 3 major metabolites (5'-DFUR, 5-FU and FBAL).

Allopurinol: Interactions with allopurinol have been observed for 5-FU; with possible decreased efficacy of 5-FU. Concomitant use of allopurinol with Xeloda should be avoided.

Interaction with cytochrome P-450: For potential interactions with isozymes 1A2, 2C9 and 3A4, see interactions with coumarin-derivative anticoagulation.

Interferon alpha: The MTD of Xeloda was 2000 mg/m^2 per day when combined with interferon alpha-2a (3 MIU/m^2 per day) compared to 3000 mg/m^2 per day when Xeloda was used alone.

Radiotherapy: The MTD of Xeloda alone using the intermittent regimen is 3000 mg/m^2 per day, whereas, when combined with radiotherapy for rectal cancer, the MTD of Xeloda is 2000 mg/m^2 per day using either a continuous schedule or given daily Monday through Friday during a 6-week course of radiotherapy.

Food Interaction: In all clinical trials, patients were instructed to administer Xeloda within 30 minutes after a meal. Since current safety and efficacy data are based upon administration with food, it is recommended that Xeloda be administered with food. Administration with food decreases the rate of capecitabine absorption (see section 5.2).

4.6 Pregnancy and lactation

There are no studies in pregnant women using Xeloda; however, it should be assumed that Xeloda may cause foetal harm if administered to pregnant women. In reproductive toxicity studies in animals, Xeloda administration caused embryolethality and teratogenicity. These findings are expected effects of fluoropyrimidine derivatives. Xeloda is contraindicated during pregnancy. Women of childbearing potential should be advised to avoid becoming pregnant while receiving treatment with Xeloda. If the patient becomes pregnant while receiving Xeloda, the potential hazard to the foetus must be explained.

It is not known whether Xeloda is excreted in human breast milk. In lactating mice, considerable amounts of capecitabine and its metabolites were found in milk. Breast-feeding should be discontinued while receiving treatment with Xeloda.

4.7 Effects on ability to drive and use machines

Xeloda may cause dizziness, fatigue and nausea. These effects may impair the ability to drive and use machines.

4.8 Undesirable effects

The adverse reactions considered to be possibly, probably, or remotely related to the administration of Xeloda have been obtained from clinical studies conducted with Xeloda monotherapy (in adjuvant therapy of colon cancer, in metastatic colorectal cancer and metastatic breast cancer) and Xeloda in combination with docetaxel in metastatic breast cancer after failure of cytotoxic chemotherapy. The most commonly reported treatment-related adverse events were gastrointestinal disorders (especially diarrhoea, nausea, vomiting, abdominal pain, stomatitis), fatigue and hand-foot syndrome (palmar-plantar erythrodysesthesia).

Safety data of Xeloda monotherapy in adjuvant treatment for colon cancer (995 patients) and metastatic colorectal cancer (596 patients) were reported in three phase III trials (Table 6). The most frequently reported treatment-related adverse reactions in these trials were gastrointestinal disorders, especially diarrhoea, nausea, vomiting, stomatitis, and hand-foot syndrome (palmar-plantar erythrodysesthesia). The safety profile of Xeloda monotherapy for the breast cancer and colorectal cancer populations is comparable.

The following headings are used to rank the undesirable effects by frequency: Very common (>1/10), common (>1/100, < 1/10) and uncommon (>1/1,000, < 1/100).

Table 6: Summary of related adverse events reported in patients treated with Xeloda monotherapy in adjuvant treatment for colon cancer and metastatic colorectal cancer (total of 1591 patients)

(see Table 6 below)

Skin and subcutaneous tissue disorders (uncommon): Rash pruritic, skin discolouration, photosensitivity reaction, rash erythematous, dermatitis exfoliative, exanthema, onychorrhexis, hyperhidrosis, hypotrichosis, eczema, skin fissures, swelling face, onycholysis, palmar erythema, night sweats, skin ulcer, nail discolouration, nail ridging, rash generalised, rash maculo-papular, rash papular, penile ulceration, plantar erythema, skin lesion, actinic keratosis, localised exfoliation, nail dystrophy, pruritus generalised, rash vesicular, nail pigmentation, onychomadesis, urticaria, hyperkeratosis, purpura, rash scaly, skin inflammation.

Gastrointestinal disorders(uncommon): Oral pain, gastritis, dysphagia, dry lip, lip ulceration, abdominal pain lower, abdominal distension, oesophagitis, chapped lips, lip pain, rectal haemorrhage, abdominal discomfort, gastrooesophageal reflux disease, cheilitis, haemorrhoids, aphthous stomatitis, proctalgia, colitis, glossodynia, proctitis, salivary hypersecretion, frequent bowel movements, gingival pain, intestinal obstruction, pruritus ani, eructation, gastrointestinal haemorrhage, lip blister, small intestinal obstruction, aptyalism, enteritis, stomach discomfort, epigastric discomfort, abdominal tenderness, hypoaesthesia oral, rectal discharge, tongue ulceration, anal fissure, enterocolitis, haematochezia, melaena, ascites, bowel sounds abnormal, diarrhoea haemorrhagic, haematemesis.

General disorders and administration site conditions (uncommon): Chills, influenza like illness, non-cardiac chest pain, chest pain, pain, rigors, ill-defined disorder, thirst, chest discomfort, oedema, feeling cold, feeling hot, facial pain, pitting oedema, tenderness.

Metabolism and nutrition disorders (uncommon): Hypokalemia, cachexia, appetite disorder, diabetes mellitus inadequate control, hypertriglyceridaemia, malnutrition, diabetes mellitus, hypoalbuminaemia.

Nervous System Disorders (uncommon): Hypoaesthesia, paresthesia oral, ageusia, disturbance in attention, syncope, hyperaesthesia, burning sensation, balance disorder, somnolence, amnesia, memory impairment, dysaethesia, ataxia, parosmia, tremor, neuropathy peripheral, dizziness postural, aphasia, peripheral sensory neuropathy.

Eye disorders (uncommon): Eye pain, vision blurred, keratoconjunctivitis sicca, dry eye, eye pruritus, visual acuity reduced, eye discharge, eye redness, diplopia, conjunctival haemorrhage, eyelid pain.

Respiratory, thoracic and mediastinal disorders (uncommon): Pharyngolaryngeal pain, hiccups, dyspnoea exertional, rhinitis, nasal passage irritation, dry throat, nasal ulcer, pulmonary embolism, hoarseness, haemoptysis, productive cough, wheezing, asthma, nasal discomfort, postnasal drip, throat irritation, pneumothorax.

Muskuloskeletal and connective tissue disorders (uncommon): Myalgia, joint swelling, muscle cramp, bone pain, flank pain, facial pain, neck pain, musculoskeletal stiffness, muscular weakness.

Blood and lymphatic system disorders (uncommon): Febrile neutropenia, leucopenia, thrombocytopenia, granulocytopenia, haemolytic anaemia, pancytopenia.

Investigations (uncommon): Alanine aminotransferase increased, weight increased, hepatic enzyme increased, body temperature increased, aspartate aminotransferase increased, blood potassium decreased, haemoglobin decreased, liver function test abnormal, blood alkaline phosphatase increased, blood in stool, gamma-glutamyltransferase increased, international normalised ratio increased, blood creatinine increased.

Psychiatric disorders (uncommon): Anxiety, nervousness, confusional state, depressed mood, irritability, restlessness, mood altered, sleep disorder, anger, libido decreased, nightmare, panic attack.

Hepatobiliary disorders (uncommon): Hepatic steatosis, hepatomegaly, jaundice, hepatic pain.

Infections and infestations (uncommon): Oral candidiasis, urinary tract infection, upper respiratory tract infection, lower respiratory tract infection, localized infection, cystitis, pneumonia, pharyngitis, vaginal candidiasis, candidiasis, influenza, nail infection, bronchitis, gastroenteritis, sepsis, folliculitis, rhinitis, vaginitis, wound infection, fungal skin infection, paronychia, fungal infection, herpes virus infection, herpes zoster, infection, tooth abscess, cellulitis, onychomycosis, tonsillitis.

Vascular disorders (uncommon): Flushing, phlebitis, deep vein thrombosis, hypertension, hypotension, thrombophlebitis, hot flush, orthostatic hypotension, petechiae, thrombophlebitis superficial, peripheral coldness, phlebothrombosis, venous thrombosis limb.

Cardiac disorders (uncommon): Angina pectoris, palpitations, artrial fibrillation, arrhythmia, tachycardia, sinus tachycardia, angina unstable, myocardial ischaemia.

Injury, poisoning and procedural complications (uncommon): Blister, contusion, sunburn, overdose, stoma site reaction.

Reproductive system and breast disorders (uncommon): Balanitis, vaginal haemorrhage, vaginal burning sensation, genital erythema, genital pruritus male, phimosis.

Renal and urinary disorders (uncommon): Dysuria, pollakiuria, haematuria, chromaturia, urinary incontinence, hydronephrosis, nocturia.

Ear and labyrinth disorders (uncommon): Vertigo, ear pain.

Immune system disorders (uncommon): Hypersensitivity.

Neoplasm benign, malignant and unspecified (uncommon): Lipoma.

Table 7: Laboratory abnormalities reported in patients treated with Xeloda monotherapy in adjuvant treatment for colon cancer and metastatic colorectal cancer (total 1591 patients)

(see Table 7 on next page)

Xeloda and docetaxel in combination: The most frequent treatment-related undesirable effects (≥5%) reported in a phase III trial in breast cancer patients failing anthracycline treatment are presented in Table 8. Treatment-related undesirable effects reported in the comparator arm of this trial, using the standard dose of docetaxel, are also presented. Rare or uncommon undesirable effects, as described in the section on Xeloda monotherapy, can be expected for combination therapy as well. These are not listed in the following table.

Table 6 Summary of related adverse events reported in patients treated with Xeloda monotherapy in adjuvant treatment for colon cancer and metastatic colorectal cancer (total of 1591 patients)

Body System Adverse Event	Very Common	Common
Skin and subcutaneous tissue disorders	Palmar-plantar erythrodysesthesia syndrome (57%)	Rash (7%), alopecia (6%), erythema (6%), dry skin (5%), pruritus (2%), skin hyperpigmentation (2%), rash macular (1%); skin desquamation (1%), dermatitis (1%), pigmentation disorder (1%), nail disorder (1%)
Gastrointestinal disorders	Diarrhoea (47%), nausea (35%), stomatitis (23%), vomiting (18%), abdominal pain (11%)	Constipation (6%), upper abdominal pain (6%), dyspepsia (5%), flatulence (3%), dry mouth (3%), loose stools (2%),
General disorders and administration site conditions	Fatigue (16%), asthenia (10%)	Pyrexia (6%), lethargy (6%), oedema peripheral (3%), malaise (1%)
Metabolism and nutrition disorders	Anorexia (10%),	Dehydration (3%), decreased appetite (2%)
Nervous System Disorders	(none)	Dysgeusia (5%), dizziness (5%), headache (4%), paresthesia (3 %), lethargy (1%)
Eye disorders	(none)	Lacrimation increased (5%), conjunctivitis (4%), eye irritation (1%)
Hepatobiliary Disorders	(none)	Hyperbilirubinemia/blood bilirubin/blood bilirubin increased (3%)
Respiratory, thoracic and mediastinal disorders	(none)	Dyspnoea (3%), epistaxis (2%), cough (1%), rhinorrhea (1%)
Muskuloskeletal and connective tissue disorders	(none)	Pain in extremity (3%), back pain (2%), arthralgia (2%)
Investigations		Weight decreased (2%)
Blood and lymphatic system disorders	(none)	Neutropenia (2%), anaemia (2%)
Psychiatric disorders	(none)	Insomnia (2%), depression (1%)
Infections and infestations	(none)	Herpes simplex (1%), nasopharyngitis (1%)

Table 7 Laboratory abnormalities reported in patients treated with Xeloda monotherapy in adjuvant treatment for colon cancer and metastatic colorectal cancer (total 1591 patients)

	Patients with grade 1 to 4 abnormality (%)	Patients with grade 3/4 (%)	Patients with grade 4 (%)
Decreased haemoglobin	73.3	1.4	0.4
Decreased neutrophils/granulocytes	25.4	2.4	1.6
Decreased platelets	18.8	1.0	0.6
Decreased lymphocytes	83.5	21.9	4.0
Decreased sodium	26.0	0.6	0.1
Decreased potassium	24.3	0.6	0.1
Increased calcium	6.4	0.9	0.8
Decreased calcium	16.7	1.8	1.5
Increased bilirubin	49.4	21.06	2.6
Increased alkaline phosphatase	44.3	1.3	0.1
Increased ALAT (SGPT)	29.9	1.2	0.1
Increased ASAT (SGOT)	33.9	0.8	0.1

Table 8: Summary of adverse events reported in patient treated with Xeloda in combination with docetaxel for metastatic breast cancer after failure of cytotoxic chemotherapy

(see Table 8 on next page)

Table 9: Laboratory abnormalities: Xeloda in combination with docetaxel in metastatic breast cancer after failure of cytotoxic chemotherapy

Adverse Event	Xeloda 1250 mg/m^2/bid with Docetaxel 75 mg/m^2 / 3 weeks (n=251)	Docetaxel 100 mg/m^2 / 3 weeks (n=255)
Laboratory Abnormalities (according to NCIC/CTC)	**Grade 3 / 4 %**	**Grade 3 / 4 %**
Lymphopenia	89	84
Leucocytopenia	61	75
Neutropenia	63	72
Anaemia	10	6
Thrombocytopenia	3	3
Hyperbilirubinemia	9	3

Post-Marketing Experience

The following additional serious adverse events have been identified during post-marketing exposure:

- Very rare: lacrimal duct stenosis.

4.9 Overdose

The manifestations of acute overdose include nausea, vomiting, diarrhoea, mucositis, gastrointestinal irritation and bleeding, and bone marrow depression. Medical management of overdose should include customary therapeutic and supportive medical interventions aimed at correcting the presenting clinical manifestations and preventing their possible complications.

5. PHARMACOLOGICAL PROPERTIES

5.1 Pharmacodynamic properties

Pharmacotherapeutic group: Cytostatic (antimetabolite), ATC code: L01B C

Capecitabine is a non-cytotoxic fluoropyrimidine carbamate, which functions as an orally administered precursor of the cytotoxic moiety 5-fluorouracil (5-FU). Capecitabine is activated via several enzymatic steps (see section 5.2). The enzyme involved in the final conversion to 5-FU, thymidine phosphorylase (ThyPase), is found in tumour tissues, but also in normal tissues, albeit usually at lower levels. In human cancer xenograft models capecitabine demonstrated a synergistic effect in combination with docetaxel, which may be related to the upregulation of thymidine phosphorylase by docetaxel.

There is evidence that the metabolism of 5-FU in the anabolic pathway blocks the methylation reaction of deoxyuridylic acid to thymidylic acid, thereby interfering with the synthesis of deoxyribonucleic acid (DNA). The incorporation of 5-FU also leads to inhibition of RNA and protein synthesis. Since DNA and RNA are essential for cell division and growth, the effect of 5-FU may be to create a thymidine deficiency that provokes unbalanced growth and death of a cell. The effects of DNA and RNA deprivation are most marked on those cells which proliferate more rapidly and which metabolise 5-FU at a more rapid rate.

Adjuvant Therapy with Xeloda in colon cancer

Data from one multicentre, randomised, controlled phase 3 clinical trial in patients with stage III (Dukes' C) colon cancer supports the use of Xeloda for the adjuvant treatment of patients with colon cancer (XACT Study). In this trial, 1987 patients were randomised to treatment with Xeloda (1250 mg/m^2 twice daily for 2 weeks followed by a 1-week rest period and given as 3-week cycles for 24 weeks) or 5-FU and leucovorin (Mayo Clinic regimen: 20 mg/m^2 leucovorin IV followed by 425 mg/m^2 IV bolus 5-FU, on days 1 to 5, every 28 days for 24 weeks). Xeloda was at least equivalent to IV 5-FU/LV in disease-free survival in per protocol population (hazard ratio 0.89; 95% CI 0.76-1.04). In the all-randomised population, tests for difference of Xeloda vs 5-FU/LV in disease-free and overall survival showed hazard ratios of 0.87 (95% CI 0.75 – 1.00; p = 0.053) and 0.84 (95% CI 0.69 – 1.01; p = 0.071), respectively. Relapse-free survival, censoring patients at the time of last tumour assessment in case of death unrelated to disease progression or unrelated to treatment (for disease-free survival these death cases were considered as events), was statistically different in favour of Xeloda comparing to 5-FU/LV [HR 0.86 (95% CI 0.74 – 0.99; p = 0.041)]. The median follow up at the time of the analysis was 3.8 years.

Monotherapy with Xeloda in metastatic colorectal cancer

Data from two identically-designed, multicentre, randomised, controlled phase 3 clinical trials support the use of Xeloda for first line treatment of metastatic colorectal cancer. In these trials, 603 patients were randomised to treatment with Xeloda (1250 mg/m^2 twice daily for 2 weeks followed by a 1-week rest period and given as 3-week cycles). 604 patients were randomised to treatment with 5-FU and leucovorin (Mayo regimen: 20 mg/m^2 leucovorin IV followed by 425 mg/m^2 IV bolus 5-FU, on days 1 to 5, every 28 days). The overall objective response rates in the all-randomised population (investigator assessment) were 25.7% (Xeloda) vs. 16.7% (Mayo regimen); p <0.0002. The median time to progression was 140 days (Xeloda) vs. 144 days (Mayo regimen). Median survival was 392 days (Xeloda) vs. 391 days (Mayo regimen). Currently, no comparative data are available on Xeloda monotherapy in colorectal cancer in comparison with first line combination regimens.

Combination therapy with Xeloda and docetaxel in locally advanced or metastatic breast cancer

Data from one multicentre, randomised, controlled phase 3 clinical trial support the use of Xeloda in combination with docetaxel for treatment of patients with locally advanced or metastatic breast cancer after failure of cytotoxic chemotherapy, including an anthracycline. In this trial, 255 patients were randomised to treatment with Xeloda (1250 mg/m^2 twice daily for 2 weeks followed by 1-week rest period and docetaxel 75 mg/m^2 as a 1 hour intravenous infusion every 3 weeks). 256 patients were randomised to treatment with docetaxel alone (100 mg/ m^2 as a 1 hour intravenous infusion every 3 weeks). Survival was superior in the Xeloda + docetaxel combination arm (p=0.0126). Median survival was 442 days (Xeloda + docetaxel) vs. 352 days (docetaxel alone). The overall objective response rates in the all-randomised population (investigator assessment) were 41.6% (Xeloda + docetaxel) vs. 29.7% (docetaxel alone); p = 0.0058. Time to progressive disease was superior in the Xeloda + docetaxel combination arm (p<0.0001). The median time to progression was 186 days (Xeloda + docetaxel) vs. 128 days (docetaxel alone).

Monotherapy with Xeloda after failure of taxanes, anthracycline containing chemotherapy, and for whom anthracycline therapy is not indicated

Data from two multicentre phase 2 clinical trials support the use of Xeloda monotherapy for treatment of patients after failure of taxanes and an anthracycline-containing chemotherapy regimen or for whom further anthracycline therapy is not indicated. In these trials, a total of 236 patients were treated with Xeloda (1250 mg/m^2 twice daily for 2 weeks followed by 1-week rest period). The overall objective response rates (investigator assessment) were 20% (first trial) and 25% (second trial). The median time to progression was 93 and 98 days. Median survival was 384 and 373 days.

An analysis of safety data in patients treated with Xeloda monotherapy (colorectal cancer) with baseline renal impairment showed an increase in the incidence of treatment-related grade 3 and 4 adverse events compared to patients with normal renal function (36% in patients without renal impairment n=268, vs. 41% in mild n=257 and 54% in moderate n=59, respectively) (see section 5.2). Patients with moderately impaired renal function show an increased rate of dose reduction (44%) vs. 33% and 32% in patients with no or mild renal impairment and an increase in early withdrawals from treatment (21% withdrawals during the first two cycles) vs. 5% and 8% in patients with no or mild renal impairment.

An analysis of safety data in patients ⩾60 years of age treated with Xeloda monotherapy and an analysis of patients treated with Xeloda plus docetaxel combination therapy showed an increase in the incidence of treatment-related grade 3 and 4 adverse events and treatment-related serious adverse events compared to patients <60 years of age. Patients ⩾60 years of age treated with Xeloda plus docetaxel also had more early withdrawals from treatment due to adverse events compared to patients <60 years of age.

5.2 Pharmacokinetic properties

The pharmacokinetics of capecitabine have been evaluated over a dose range of 502-3514 mg/m^2/day. The parameters of capecitabine, 5'-deoxy-5-fluorocytidine (5'-DFCR) and 5'-deoxy-5-fluorouridine (5'-DFUR) measured on days 1 and 14 were similar. The AUC of 5-FU was 30%-35% higher on day 14. Capecitabine dose reduction decreases systemic exposure to 5-FU more than dose-proportionally, due to non-linear pharmacokinetics for the active metabolite.

Absorption: After oral administration, capecitabine is rapidly and extensively absorbed, followed by extensive conversion to the metabolites, 5'-DFCR and 5'-DFUR. Administration with food decreases the rate of capecitabine absorption, but only results in a minor effect on the AUC of 5'-DFUR, and on the AUC of the subsequent metabolite 5-FU. At the dose of 1250 mg/m^2 on day 14 with administration after food intake, the peak plasma concentrations (C_{max} in μg/ml) for capecitabine, 5'-DFCR, 5'-DFUR, 5-FU and FBAL were 4.67, 3.05, 12.1, 0.95 and 5.46 respectively. The time to peak plasma concentrations (T_{max} in hours) were 1.50, 2.00, 2.00, 2.00 and 3.34. The $AUC_{0-\infty}$ values in μg•h/ml were 7.75, 7.24, 24.6, 2.03 and 36.3.

Protein binding: *In vitro* human plasma studies have determined that capecitabine, 5'-DFCR, 5'-DFUR and 5-FU are 54%, 10%, 62% and 10% protein bound, mainly to albumin.

Metabolism: Capecitabine is first metabolised by hepatic carboxylesterase to 5'-DFCR, which is then converted to 5'-DFUR by cytidine deaminase, principally located in the liver and tumour tissues. Further catalytic activation of 5'-DFUR then occurs by thymidine phosphorylase (ThyPase). The enzymes involved in the catalytic activation are found in tumour tissues but also in normal tissues, albeit usually at lower levels. The sequential enzymatic biotransformation of capecitabine to 5-FU leads to higher concentrations within tumour tissues. In the case of colorectal tumours, 5-FU generation appears to be in large part localised in tumour stromal cells. Following oral administration of capecitabine to patients with colorectal cancer, the ratio of 5-FU concentration in colorectal tumours to adjacent tissues was 3.2 (ranged from 0.9 to 8.0). The ratio of 5-FU concentration in tumour to plasma was 21.4 (ranged from 3.9 to 59.9, n=8) whereas the ratio in healthy tissues to plasma was 8.9 (ranged from 3.0 to 25.8, n=8). Thymidine phosphorylase activity was measured and found to be 4 times greater in primary colorectal tumour than in adjacent normal tissue. According to immunohistochemical studies, thymidine phosphorylase appears to be in large part localised in tumour stromal cells.

5-FU is further catabolised by the enzyme dihydropyrimidine dehydrogenase (DPD) to the much less toxic dihydro-5-fluorouracil (FUH_2). Dihydropyrimidinase cleaves the pyrimidine ring to yield 5-fluoro-ureidopropionic acid (FUPA). Finally, β-ureido-propionase cleaves FUPA to α-fluoro-β-alanine (FBAL) which is cleared in the urine. Dihydropyrimidine dehydrogenase (DPD) activity is the rate limiting step. Deficiency of DPD may lead to increased toxicity of capecitabine (see section 4.3 and 4.4).

Elimination: The elimination half-life ($t_{1/2}$ in hours) of capecitabine, 5'-DFCR, 5'-DFUR, 5-FU and FBAL were 0.85, 1.11, 0.66, 0.76 and 3.23 respectively. Capecitabine and its metabolites are predominantly excreted in urine; 95.5% of

Table 8 Summary of adverse events reported in patient treated with Xeloda in combination with docetaxel for metastatic breast cancer after failure of cytotoxic chemotherapy

Adverse Event	Xeloda 1250 mg/m²/bid with Docetaxel 75 mg/m² / 3 weeks (n=251)		Docetaxel 100 mg/m² / 3 weeks (n=255)	
Body System/Adverse Event	**Total %**	**Grade 3 / 4 %**	**Total %**	**Grade 3 / 4 %**
Gastrointestinal				
Stomatitis	67	18	42	5
Diarrhoea	64	14	45	5
Nausea	43	6	35	2
Vomiting	33	4	22	1
Constipation	14	1	12	-
Abdominal pain	14	2	9	1
Dyspepsia	12	-	5	<1
Abdominal pain upper	9	-	6	1
Dry mouth	5	-	4	-
Skin and Subcutaneous				
Hand-foot syndrome	63	24	7	1
Alopecia	41	6	42	7
Nail disorder	14	2	15	-
Dermatitis	8	-	9	1
Rash erythematous	8	<1	4	-
Nail discolouration	6	-	4	<1
Onycholysis	5	1	5	1
General				
Asthenia	23	3	22	5
Pyrexia	21	1	29	<1
Fatigue	21	4	25	5
Weakness	13	1	9	2
Pain in limb	9	<1	8	<1
Lethargy	6	-	5	1
Pain	6	-	2	-
Blood & lymphatic system				
Neutropenic fever	16	16	21	21
Neurological				
Taste disturbance	15	<1	14	<1
Paresthesia	11	<1	15	1
Dizziness	9	-	6	<1
Headache	7	<1	8	1
Peripheral neuropathy	5	-	10	1
Metabolism				
Anorexia	12	1	10	1
Appetite decreased	10	-	4	-
Dehydration	8	2	5	1
Weight decreased	6	-	4	-
Eye				
Lacrimation increased	12	-	5	-
Musculoskeletal				
Myalgia	14	2	24	2
Arthralgia	11	1	18	2
Back pain	7	1	6	1
Cardiovascular				
Lower limb oedema	14	1	12	1
Respiratory				
Sore throat	11	2	7	<1
Dyspnoea	7	1	9	<1
Cough	6	<1	9	-
Epistaxis	5	<1	5	-
Infection				
Oral candidiasis	6	<1	7	<1

administered capecitabine dose is recovered in urine. Faecal excretion is minimal (2.6%). The major metabolite excreted in urine is FBAL, which represents 57% of the administered dose. About 3% of the administered dose is excreted in urine as unchanged drug.

Combination therapy: Phase I studies evaluating the effect of Xeloda on the pharmacokinetics of either docetaxel or paclitaxel and vice versa showed no effect by Xeloda on the pharmacokinetics of docetaxel or paclitaxel (C_{max} and AUC) and no effect by docetaxel or paclitaxel on the pharmacokinetics of 5'-DFUR.

Pharmacokinetics in special populations: A population pharmacokinetic analysis was carried out after Xeloda treatment of 505 patients with colorectal cancer dosed at 1250 mg/m² twice daily. Gender, presence or absence of liver metastasis at baseline, Karnofsky Performance Status, total bilirubin, serum albumin, ASAT and ALAT had no statistically significant effect on the pharmacokinetics of 5'-DFUR, 5-FU and FBAL.

Patients with hepatic impairment due to liver metastases: According to a pharmacokinetic study in cancer patients with mild to moderate liver impairment due to liver metastases, the bioavailability of capecitabine and exposure to 5-FU may increase compared to patients with no liver impairment. There are no pharmacokinetic data on patients with severe hepatic impairment.

Patients with renal impairment: Based on a pharmacokinetic study in cancer patients with mild to severe renal impairment, there is no evidence for an effect of creatinine clearance on the pharmacokinetics of intact drug and 5-FU. Creatinine clearance was found to influence the systemic exposure to 5'-DFUR (35% increase in AUC when creatinine clearance decreases by 50%) and to FBAL (114% increase in AUC when creatinine clearance decreases by 50%). FBAL is a metabolite without antiproliferative activity.

Elderly: Based on the population pharmacokinetic analysis, which included patients with a wide range of ages (27 to 86 years) and included 234 (46%) patients greater or equal to 65, age has no influence on the pharmacokinetics of 5'-DFUR and 5-FU. The AUC of FBAL increased with age (20% increase in age results in a 15% increase in the AUC of FBAL). This increase is likely due to a change in renal function.

Ethnic factors: Following oral administration of 825 mg/m² capecitabine twice daily for 14 days, Japanese patients (n=18) had about 36% lower C_{max} and 24% lower AUC for capecitabine than Caucasian patients (n=22). Japanese patients had also about 25% lower C_{max} and 34% lower AUC for FBAL than Caucasian patients. The clinical relevance of these differences is unknown. No significant differences occurred in the exposure to other metabolites (5'-DFCR, 5'-DFUR, and 5-FU).

5.3 Preclinical safety data

In repeat-dose toxicity studies, daily oral administration of capecitabine to cynomolgus monkeys and mice produced toxic effects on the gastrointestinal, lymphoid and haemopoietic systems, typical for fluoropyrimidines. These toxicities were reversible. Skin toxicity, characterised by degenerative/regressive changes, was observed with capecitabine. Capecitabine was devoid of hepatic and CNS toxicities. Cardiovascular toxicity (e.g. PR- and QT-interval prolongation) was detectable in cynomolgus monkeys after intravenous administration (100 mg/kg) but not after repeated oral dosing (1379 mg/m²/day).

A two-year mouse carcinogenicity study produced no evidence of carcinogenicity by capecitabine.

During standard fertility studies, impairment of fertility was observed in female mice receiving capecitabine; however, this effect was reversible after a drug-free period. In addition, during a 13-week study, atrophic and degenerative changes occurred in reproductive organs of male mice; however these effects were reversible after a drug-free period.

In embryotoxicity and teratogenicity studies in mice, dose-related increases in foetal resorption and teratogenicity were observed. In monkeys, abortion and embryolethality were observed at high doses, but there was no evidence of teratogenicity.

Capecitabine was not mutagenic *in vitro* to bacteria (Ames test) or mammalian cells (Chinese hamster V79/HPRT gene mutation assay). However, similar to other nucleoside analogues (ie, 5-FU), capecitabine was clastogenic in human lymphocytes (*in vitro*) and a positive trend occurred in mouse bone marrow micronucleus tests (*in vivo*).

6. PHARMACEUTICAL PARTICULARS

6.1 List of excipients

Tablet core: Anhydrous lactose, croscarmellose sodium, hypromellose, microcrystalline cellulose, magnesium stearate.

Tablet coating: Titanium dioxide (E171), yellow and red iron oxide (E172), talc.

6.2 Incompatibilities

Not applicable.

6.3 Shelf life

3 years.

6.4 Special precautions for storage

Do not store above 30°C.

6.5 Nature and contents of container

Nature: PVC/PE/PVDC blisters.

Content: 60 × 150 mg film-coated tablets (6 blisters of 10 tablets).

120 × 500 mg film-coated tablets (12 blisters of 10 tablets).

6.6 Instructions for use and handling

No special requirements.

7. MARKETING AUTHORISATION HOLDER

Roche Registration Limited
40 Broadwater Road
Welwyn Garden City
Hertfordshire, AL7 3AY
United Kingdom

8. MARKETING AUTHORISATION NUMBER(S)

EU/1/00/163/001 - 150 mg film-coated tablets
EU/1/00/163/002 - 500 mg film-coated tablets

9. DATE OF FIRST AUTHORISATION/RENEWAL OF THE AUTHORISATION

2 February 2001

10. DATE OF REVISION OF THE TEXT

30 March 2005

Xenazine 25

(Cambridge Laboratories)

1. NAME OF THE MEDICINAL PRODUCT

Xenazine(TM) 25

2. QUALITATIVE AND QUANTITATIVE COMPOSITION

Each tablet contains 25mg Tetrabenazine.

3. PHARMACEUTICAL FORM

Tablets.

4. CLINICAL PARTICULARS

4.1 Therapeutic indications

Movement disorders associated with organic central nervous system conditions, e.g. Huntington's chorea, hemiballismus and senile chorea.

Xenazine(TM) 25 is also indicated for the treatment of moderate to severe tardive dyskinesia, which is disabling and/or socially embarrassing. The condition

should be persistent despite withdrawal of antipsychotic therapy, or in cases where withdrawal of antipsychotic medication is not a realistic option; also where the condition persists despite reduction in dosage of antipsychotic medication or switching to atypical antipsychotic medication.

4.2 Posology and method of administration

The tablets are for oral administration.

Organic Central Nervous System Movement Disorders

Adults

Dosage and administration are variable and only a guide is given. An initial starting dose of 25mg three times a day is recommended. This can be increased by 25mg a day every three or four days until 200mg a day is being given or the limit of tolerance, as dictated by unwanted effects, is reached, whichever is the lower dose.

If there is no improvement at the maximum dose in seven days, it is unlikely that the compound will be of benefit to the patient, either by increasing the dose or by extending the duration of treatment.

Tardive Dyskinesia

Recommended starting dose of 12.5mg a day, subsequently titrated according to response. Medication should be discontinued if there is no clear benefit or if the side-effects cannot be tolerated

The elderly

No specific studies have been performed in the elderly, but Xenazine(TM) 25 has been administered to elderly patients in standard dosage without apparent ill effect.

Children

No specific dosage recommendations are made for the administration of Xenazine(TM) 25 to children, although it has been used without ill effect.

4.3 Contraindications

Xenazine(TM) 25 blocks the action of reserpine.

4.4 Special warnings and special precautions for use

Tardive Dyskinesia

The condition should be persistent despite withdrawal of antipsychotic therapy, or in cases where withdrawal of antipsychotic medication is not a realistic option; also where the condition persists despite reduction in dosage of antipsychotic medication or switching to atypical antipsychotic medication.

4.5 Interaction with other medicinal products and other forms of Interaction

Levodopa should be administered with caution in the presence of Xenazine(TM) 25.

4.6 Pregnancy and lactation

There is inadequate evidence of safety of the drug in human pregnancy and no evidence from animal work, but it has been in wide use for many years without apparent ill consequence. Tetrabenazine should be avoided in breast-feeding mothers.

4.7 Effects on ability to drive and use machines

Patients should be advised that Xenazine(TM) 25 may cause drowsiness and therefore may modify their performance at skilled tasks (driving ability, operation of machinery, etc.) to a varying degree, depending on dose and individual susceptibility.

4.8 Undesirable effects

Side-effects are usually mild with little hypotensive action and few digestive disorders. The main unwanted effect reported to date has been drowsiness, which occurs with higher doses. If depression occurs, it can be controlled by reducing the dose or by giving antidepressant drugs such as the monoamine oxidase inhibitors. However, Xenazine(TM) 25 should not be given immediately after a course of any of the monoamine oxidase inhibitors as such treatment may lead to a state of restlessness, disorientation and confusion. In man, a Parkinsonian-like syndrome has been reported on rare occasions, usually in doses above 200mg per day, but this disappears on reducing the dose.

Neuroleptic malignant syndrome (NMS) associated with the use of Tetrabenazine has been reported rarely. This may occur soon after initiation of therapy, following an increase in dosage or after prolonged treatment. The clinical features usually include hyperthermia, severe extra-pyramidal symptoms including muscular rigidity, autonomic dysfunction and altered levels of consciousness. Skeletal muscle damage may occur. If NMS is suspected Xenazine(TM) 25 should be withdrawn and appropriate supportive therapy instituted; treatment with Dantrolene and Bromocriptine may be effective.

4.9 Overdose

Signs and symptoms of overdosage may include drowsiness, sweating, hypotension and hypothermia. Treatment is symptomatic.

5. PHARMACOLOGICAL PROPERTIES

5.1 Pharmacodynamic properties

The central effects of Xenazine(TM) 25 closely resemble those of Reserpine, but it differs from the latter in having less peripheral activity and being much shorter acting.

5.2 Pharmacokinetic properties

Tetrabenazine has a low and erratic bioavailability. It appears to be extensively metabolised by first-pass metabolism. The major metabolite, hydroxytetrabenazine, is formed by reduction. Little unchanged Tetrabenazine can be detected in the urine. Since hydroxytetrabenazine is reported to be as active as Tetrabenazine in depleting brain amines, it is likely that this is the major therapeutic agent.

5.3 Preclinical safety data

It is known from animal experiments that Tetrabenazine intervenes in the metabolism of biogenic amines, such as serotonin and noradrenaline, and that this activity is mainly limited to the brain. It is thought that the effect of Tetrabenazine on brain amines explains its clinical effects in man.

6. PHARMACEUTICAL PARTICULARS

6.1 List of excipients

Starch BP

Lactose BP

Talc BP

Magnesium stearate BP

Iron oxide yellow E172

6.2 Incompatibilities

None known.

6.3 Shelf life

5 years.

6.4 Special precautions for storage

The recommended maximum storage temperature is 30°C.

6.5 Nature and contents of container

White HDPE bottle, pack size 112 tablets.

6.6 Instructions for use and handling

None.

7. MARKETING AUTHORISATION HOLDER

Lifehealth Limited

23 Winkfield Road

Windsor

BERKS

SL4 4BA

8. MARKETING AUTHORISATION NUMBER(S)

PL 14576/0005

9. DATE OF FIRST AUTHORISATION/RENEWAL OF THE AUTHORISATION

23 October 1995

10. DATE OF REVISION OF THE TEXT

July 2000

Xenical 120mg hard capsules

(Roche Products Limited)

1. NAME OF THE MEDICINAL PRODUCT

XENICAL® 120 mg hard capsules.

2. QUALITATIVE AND QUANTITATIVE COMPOSITION

Each hard capsule contains 120 mg orlistat.

For excipients, see 6.1.

3. PHARMACEUTICAL FORM

Capsule, hard.

The capsule has a turquoise cap and turquoise body bearing the imprint of "ROCHE XENICAL 120".

4. CLINICAL PARTICULARS

4.1 Therapeutic indications

XENICAL is indicated in conjunction with a mildly hypocaloric diet for the treatment of obese patients with a body mass index (BMI) greater or equal to 30 kg/m^2, or overweight patients (BMI $\geqslant$ 28 kg/m^2) with associated risk factors.

Treatment with orlistat should be discontinued after 12 weeks if patients have been unable to lose at least 5 % of the body weight as measured at the start of drug therapy.

4.2 Posology and method of administration

Adults

The recommended dose of orlistat is one 120 mg capsule taken with water immediately before, during or up to one hour after each main meal. If a meal is missed or contains no fat, the dose of orlistat should be omitted.

The patient should be on a nutritionally balanced, mildly hypocaloric diet that contains approximately 30 % of calories from fat. It is recommended that the diet should be rich in fruit and vegetables. The daily intake of fat, carbohydrate and protein should be distributed over three main meals.

Doses of orlistat above 120 mg three times daily have not been shown to provide additional benefit.

The effect of orlistat results in an increase in faecal fat as early as 24 to 48 hours after dosing. Upon discontinuation of therapy, faecal fat content usually returns to pre-treatment levels, within 48 to 72 hours.

Special populations

The effect of orlistat in patients with hepatic and/or renal impairment, children and elderly patients has not been studied. Orlistat is not intended to be used in children.

4.3 Contraindications

- Chronic malabsorption syndrome
- Cholestasis
- Breast-feeding
- Hypersensitivity to the active substance or to any of the excipients

4.4 Special warnings and special precautions for use

In clinical trials, the decrease in bodyweight with orlistat treatment was less in type II diabetic patients than in non-diabetic patients. Antidiabetic drug treatment may have to be closely monitored when taking orlistat.

Co-administration of orlistat with cyclosporine is not recommended (see section 4.5).

Patients should be advised to adhere to the dietary recommendations they are given (see section 4.2 Posology and method of administration). The possibility of experiencing gastrointestinal events (see section 4.8 Undesirable effects) may increase when orlistat is taken with a diet high in fat (e.g. in a 2000 kcal/day diet, > 30 % of calories from fat equates to > 67 g of fat). The daily intake of fat should be distributed over three main meals. If orlistat is taken with a meal very high in fat, the possibility of gastrointestinal adverse events may increase.

4.5 Interaction with other medicinal products and other forms of Interaction

Cyclosporine

A decrease in cyclosporine plasma levels has been observed in a drug-drug-interaction study and also reported in several cases, when orlistat was administered concomitantly. This can lead to a decrease of immunosuppressive efficacy. Therefore the combination is not recommended (see section 4.4). However, if such concomitant use is unavoidable, more frequent monitoring of cyclosporine blood levels should be performed both after addition of orlistat and upon discontinuation of orlistat in cyclosporine treated patients. Cyclosporine blood levels should be monitored until stabilised.

Acarbose

In the absence of pharmacokinetic interaction studies, the concomitant administration of orlistat with acarbose should be avoided.

Oral Anticoagulants

When warfarin or other anticoagulants are given in combination with orlistat, international normalised ratio (INR) values should be monitored.

Fat soluble vitamins

Treatment with orlistat may potentially impair the absorption of fat-soluble vitamins (A, D, E and K).

The vast majority of patients receiving up to four full years of treatment with orlistat in clinical studies had vitamin A, D, E and K and beta-carotene levels that stayed within normal range. In order to ensure adequate nutrition, patients on a weight control diet should be advised to have a diet rich in fruit and vegetables and use of a multivitamin supplement could be considered. If a multivitamin supplement is recommended, it should be taken at least two hours after the administration of orlistat or at bedtime.

Amiodarone

A small decrease in plasma levels of amiodarone, when given as a single dose, has been observed in a limited number of healthy volunteers who received orlistat concomitantly; in patients receiving amiodarone treatment, the clinical relevance of this effect remains unknown but may be of minor relevance. However, in patients receiving concomitant amiodarone treatment, reinforcement of clinical and ECG monitoring is warranted.

Lack of interactions

No interactions with amitriptyline, atorvastatin, biguanides, digoxin, fibrates, fluoxetine, losartan, phenytoin, oral contraceptives, phentermine, pravastatin, nifedipine Gastro-intestinal Therapeutic System (GITS), nifedipine slow release, sibutramine or alcohol have been observed. The absence of these interactions has been demonstrated in specific drug-drug-interaction studies.

4.6 Pregnancy and lactation

For orlistat no clinical data on exposed pregnancies are available.

Animal studies do not indicate direct or indirect harmful effects with respect to pregnancy, embryonal/foetal development, parturition or postnatal development (see 5.3, Preclinical safety data).

Caution should be exercised when prescribing to pregnant women.

As it is not known whether orlistat is secreted into human milk, orlistat is contra-indicated during breast-feeding.

4.7 Effects on ability to drive and use machines

XENICAL has no influence on the ability to drive and use machines.

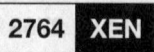

4.8 Undesirable effects

Adverse reactions to orlistat are largely gastrointestinal in nature. The incidence of adverse events decreased with prolonged use of orlistat.

The following table of undesirable effects (first year of treatment) is based on adverse events that occurred at a frequency of > 2 % and with an incidence ⩾ 1 % above placebo in clinical trials of 1 and 2 years duration:

(see Table 1 opposite)

In a 4 year clinical trial, the general pattern of adverse event distribution was similar to that reported for the 1 and 2 year studies with the total incidence of gastrointestinal related adverse events occurring in year 1 decreasing year on year over the four year period.

The following table of undesirable effects is based on post-marketing spontaneous reports:

• Immune System Disorders
Rare (0.01 - < 0.1%): Hypersensitivity (e.g. pruritus, rash, urticaria, angioedema, bronchospasm and anaphylaxis).
• Gastrointestinal disorders
Very rare (< 0.01%): Diverticulitis.
• Hepato-Biliary Disorders
Very rare (< 0.01%): Cholelithiasis. Hepatitis that may be serious.
• Skin and subcutaneous tissue disorders
Very rare (< 0.01%): Bullous eruptions.
• Investigations
Very rare (< 0.01%): Increase in liver transaminases and in alkaline phosphatase. Decreased prothrombin, increased INR and unbalanced anticoagulant treatment resulting in variations of haemostatic parameters have been reported in patients treated with anticoagulants in association with orlistat.

Table 1

System Organ Class	Adverse Event	Xenical	Placebo
• Infections and Infestations	*Very common (⩾ 10%):* Influenza	39.7%	36.2%
• Metabolism and Nutrition Disorders	*Very common (⩾ 10%):* Hypoglycaemia*	13.0%	10.0%
• Psychiatric Disorders	*Common (1 - < 10%):* Anxiety	4.7%	2.9%
• Nervous System Disorders	*Very common (⩾ 10%):* Headache	30.6%	27.6%
• Respiratory, Thoracic and Mediastinal Disorders	*Very common (⩾ 10%):* Upper respiratory infection	38.1%	32.8%
	Common (1 - < 10%): Lower respiratory infection	7.8%	6.6%
• Gastrointestinal Disorders	*Very common (⩾ 10%):*		
	Oily spotting from the rectum	26.6%	1.3%
	Abdominal pain/discomfort	25.5%	21.4%
	Flatus with discharge	23.9%	1.4%
	Faecal urgency	22.1%	6.7%
	Fatty/oily stool	20.0%	2.9%
	Flatulence	16.0%	13.1%
	Liquid stools	15.8%	11.4%
	Oily evacuation	11.9%	0.8%
	Increased defecation	10.8%	4.1%
	Common (1 - < 10%):		
	Soft stools	8.8%	6.8%
	Faecal incontinence	7.7%	0.9%
	Abdominal distension*	6.0%	4.0%
	Rectal pain/discomfort	5.2%	4.0%
	Tooth disorder	4.3%	3.1%
	Gingival disorder	4.1%	2.9%
• Renal and Urinary Disorders	*Common (1 - < 10%):* Urinary tract infection	7.5%	7.3%
• Reproductive System and Breast Disorders	*Common (1 - < 10%):* Menstrual irregularity	9.8%	7.4%
• General Disorders and Administration Site Conditions	*Common (1 - < 10%):* Fatigue	7.2%	6.4%

* only unique treatment adverse events that occurred at a frequency of > 2 % and with an incidence ⩾ 1 % above placebo in obese type 2 diabetic patients.

4.9 Overdose

Single doses of 800 mg orlistat and multiple doses of up to 400 mg three times daily for 15 days have been studied in normal weight and obese subjects without significant adverse findings. In addition, doses of 240 mg tid have been administered to obese patients for 6 months. The majority of orlistat overdose cases received during post-marketing reported either no adverse events or adverse events that are similar to those reported with recommended dose.

Should a significant overdose of orlistat occur, it is recommended that the patient be observed for 24 hours. Based on human and animal studies, any systemic effects attributable to the lipase-inhibiting properties of orlistat should be rapidly reversible.

5. PHARMACOLOGICAL PROPERTIES

5.1 Pharmacodynamic properties

Pharmaco-therapeutic group: Anti obesity agent, ATC code A08A B01.

Orlistat is a potent, specific and long-acting inhibitor of gastrointestinal lipases. It exerts its therapeutic activity in the lumen of the stomach and small intestine by forming a covalent bond with the active serine site of the gastric and pancreatic lipases. The inactivated enzyme is thus unavailable to hydrolyse dietary fat, in the form of triglycerides, into absorbable free fatty acids and monoglycerides.

In the 2-year studies and the 4-year study, a hypocaloric diet was used in association with treatment in both the orlistat and the placebo treated groups.

Pooled data from five 2 year studies with orlistat and a hypocaloric diet showed that 37 % of orlistat patients and 19 % of placebo patients demonstrated a loss of at least 5 % of their baseline body weight after 12 weeks of treatment. Of these, 49 % of orlistat treated patients and 40 % of placebo treated patients went on to lose ⩾10 % of their baseline body weight at one year. Conversely, of patients failing to demonstrate a loss of 5 % of their baseline body weight after 12 weeks of treatment, only 5 % of orlistat treated patients and 2 % of placebo treated patients went on to lose ⩾10 % of their baseline body weight at one year. Overall, after one year of treatment, the percentage of patients taking 120 mg orlistat who lost 10 % or more of their body weight was 20 % with orlistat 120 mg compared to 8 % of patients taking placebo. The mean difference in weight loss with the drug compared to placebo was 3.2 kg.

Data from the 4-year XENDOS clinical trial showed that 60 % of orlistat patients and 35 % of placebo patients demonstrated a loss of at least 5 % of their baseline body weight after 12 weeks of treatment. Of these, 62 % of orlistat treated patients and 52 % of placebo treated patients went on to lose ⩾10 % of their baseline body weight at one year. Conversely, of patients failing to demonstrate a loss of 5 % of their baseline body weight after 12 weeks of treatment, only 5 % of orlistat treated patients and 4 % of placebo treated patients went on to lose ⩾10 % of their baseline body weight at one year. After 1 year of treatment, 41 % of the orlistat treated patients versus 21 % of placebo treated patients lost ⩾10 % of body weight with a mean difference of 4.4 kg between the two groups. After 4 years of treatment 21 % of the orlistat treated patients compared to 10 % of the placebo treated patients had lost ⩾10 % of body weight, with a mean difference of 2.7 kg.

More patients on orlistat or placebo lost baseline body weight of at least 5 % at 12 weeks or 10 % at one year in the XENDOS study than in the five 2-year studies. The reason for this difference is that the five 2-year studies included a 4-week diet and placebo lead-in period during which patients lost on average 2.6 kg prior to commencing treatment.

Data from the 4-year clinical trial also suggested that weight loss achieved with orlistat delayed the development of type 2 diabetes during the study (cumulative diabetes cases incidences: 3.4 % in the orlistat group compared to 5.4 % in the placebo-treated group). The great majority of diabetes cases came from the subgroup of patients with impaired glucose tolerance at baseline, which represented 21 % of the randomised patients. It is not known whether these findings translate into long-term clinical benefits.

In obese type 2 diabetic patients insufficiently controlled by antidiabetic agents, data from four one-year clinical trials showed that the percentage of responders (⩾ 10 % of body weight loss) was 11.3 % with orlistat as compared to 4.5 % with placebo. In orlistat-treated patients, the mean difference from placebo in weight loss was 1.83 kg to 3.06 kg and the mean difference from placebo in HbA1c reduction was 0.18 % to 0.55 %. It has not been demonstrated that the effect on HbA1c is independent from weight reduction.

In a multi-centre (US, Canada), parallel-group, double-blind, placebo-controlled study, 539 obese adolescent patients were randomised to receive either 120 mg orlistat (n=357) or placebo (n=182) three times daily as an adjunct to a hypocaloric diet and exercise for 52 weeks. Both populations received multivitamin supplements. The primary endpoint was the change in body mass index (BMI) from baseline to the end of the study.

The results were significantly superior in the orlistat group (difference in BMI of 0.86 kg/m^2 in favour of orlistat). 9.5 % of the orlistat treated patients versus 3.3 % of the placebo treated patients lost ⩾ 10 % of body weight after 1 year with a mean difference of 2.6 kg between the two groups. The difference was driven by the outcome in the group of patients with ⩾ 5 % weight loss after 12 weeks of treatment with orlistat representing 19 % of the initial population. The side effects were generally similar to those observed in adults. However, there was an unexplained increase in the incidence of bone fractures (6 % versus 2.8 % in the orlistat and placebo groups, respectively).

5.2 Pharmacokinetic properties

Absorption:

Studies in normal weight and obese volunteers have shown that the extent of absorption of orlistat was minimal. Plasma concentrations of intact orlistat were non-measurable (< 5 ng/ml) eight hours following oral administration of orlistat.

In general, at therapeutic doses, detection of intact orlistat in plasma was sporadic and concentrations were extremely low (< 10 ng/ml or 0.02 μmol), with no evidence of accumulation, which is consistent with minimal absorption.

Distribution:

The volume of distribution cannot be determined because the drug is minimally absorbed and has no defined systemic pharmacokinetics. *In vitro* orlistat is > 99 % bound to plasma proteins (lipoproteins and albumin were the major binding proteins). Orlistat minimally partitions into erythrocytes.

Metabolism:

Based on animal data, it is likely that the metabolism of orlistat occurs mainly within the gastrointestinal wall. Based on a study in obese patients, of the minimal fraction of the dose that was absorbed systemically, two major metabolites, M1 (4-member lactone ring hydrolysed) and M3 (M1 with N-formyl leucine moiety cleaved), accounted for approximately 42 % of the total plasma concentration.

M1 and M3 have an open beta-lactone ring and extremely weak lipase inhibitory activity (1000- and 2500-fold less than orlistat respectively). In view of this low inhibitory activity and the low plasma levels at therapeutic doses (average of 26 ng/ml and 108 ng/ml respectively), these metabolites are considered to be pharmacologically inconsequential.

Elimination :

Studies in normal weight and obese subjects have shown that faecal excretion of the unabsorbed drug was the major route of elimination. Approximately 97 % of the administered dose was excreted in faeces and 83 % of that as unchanged orlistat.

The cumulative renal excretion of total orlistat-related materials was < 2 % of the given dose. The time to reach complete excretion (faecal plus urinary) was 3 to 5 days. The disposition of orlistat appeared to be similar between normal weight and obese volunteers. Orlistat, M1 and M3 are all subject to biliary excretion.

5.3 Preclinical safety data

Preclinical data reveal no special hazard for humans based on conventional studies of safety pharmacology, repeated dose toxicity, genotoxicity, carcinogenic potential, and toxicity to reproduction.

In animal reproductive studies, no teratogenic effect was observed. In the absence of a teratogenic effect in animals, no malformative effect is expected in man. To date, active substances responsible for malformations in man have been found teratogenic in animals when well-conducted studies were performed in two species.

6. PHARMACEUTICAL PARTICULARS

6.1 List of excipients

Capsule filling:

Microcrystalline cellulose (E 460),

sodium starch glycollate,

povidone (E 1201),

sodium lauryl sulphate and

talc.

Capsule shell:

Gelatine,

indigo carmine (E132),

titanium dioxide (E171) and

edible printing ink (black iron oxide, soya lecithin, polydimethylsiloxane, shellac).

6.2 Incompatibilities

Not applicable.

6.3 Shelf life

3 years.

6.4 Special precautions for storage

For blister strips: Do not store above 25°C. Store in original package in order to protect from moisture.

For glass bottles with desiccant: Do not store above 30°C. Keep the container tightly closed in order to protect from moisture.

6.5 Nature and contents of container

PVC/PE/PVDC blisters and glass bottles with desiccant containing 21, 42 and 84 hard capsules.

Not all pack sizes may be marketed.

6.6 Instructions for use and handling

No special requirements.

7. MARKETING AUTHORISATION HOLDER

Roche Registration Limited

40 Broadwater Road

Welwyn Garden City

Hertfordshire

AL7 3AY

United Kingdom.

8. MARKETING AUTHORISATION NUMBER(S)

EU/1/98/071/001-006

9. DATE OF FIRST AUTHORISATION/RENEWAL OF THE AUTHORISATION

29 July 1998 / 29 July 2003

10. DATE OF REVISION OF THE TEXT

June 2005

Xigris 20mg powder for solution for infusion, 5mg powder for solution for infusion

(Eli Lilly and Company Limited)

1. NAME OF THE MEDICINAL PRODUCT

Xigris*▼ 5mg powder for solution for infusion.

Xigris▼ 20mg powder for solution for infusion.

2. QUALITATIVE AND QUANTITATIVE COMPOSITION

Each vial contains: Drotrecogin alfa (activated): 2mg per ml after reconstitution.

Xigris 5mg: A vial contains 5mg of drotrecogin alfa (activated) to be reconstituted with 2.5ml of sterile water for injection.

Xigris 20mg: A vial contains 20mg of drotrecogin alfa (activated) to be reconstituted with 10ml of sterile water for injection.

Drotrecogin alfa (activated) is a recombinant version of the endogenous activated protein C and is produced by genetic engineering from an established human cell line.

For excipients, see section 6.1.

3. PHARMACEUTICAL FORM

Powder for solution for infusion.

4. CLINICAL PARTICULARS

4.1 Therapeutic indications

Xigris is indicated for the treatment of adult patients with severe sepsis with multiple organ failure when added to best standard care. The use of Xigris should be considered mainly in situations when therapy can be started within 24 hours after the onset of organ failure (for further information see section 5.1).

4.2 Posology and method of administration

Xigris should be used by experienced doctors in institutions skilled in the care of patients with severe sepsis.

Treatment should be started within 48 hours, and preferably within 24 hours, of onset of the first documented sepsis-induced organ dysfunction (see section 5.1).

The recommended dose of Xigris is 24µg/kg/hr given as a continuous intravenous infusion for a total duration of 96 hours. It is recommended that Xigris be infused with an infusion pump to accurately control the infusion rate. If the infusion is interrupted for any reason, Xigris should be restarted at the 24µg/kg/hr infusion rate and continued to complete the full recommended 96 hours of dosing administration. Dose escalation or bolus doses of Xigris are not necessary to account for the interruption in the infusion.

No dose adjustments are required in adult patients with severe sepsis with regard to age, gender, hepatic function (as measured by transaminase levels), or renal function. The pharmacokinetics of drotrecogin alfa (activated) have not been studied in patients with severe sepsis and pre-existing end-stage renal disease and chronic hepatic disease.

Paediatrics: Experience with Xigris in children and juveniles under the age of 18 is limited; the efficacy and safety of Xigris have not been established in this age group; therefore, no dosage recommendation can be made.

4.3 Contraindications

Because drotrecogin alfa (activated) may increase the risk of bleeding, Xigris is contra-indicated in the following situations:

- Active internal bleeding.
- Patients with intracranial pathology; neoplasm or evidence of cerebral herniation.
- Concurrent heparin therapy ⩾15 international units/kg/hr.
- Known bleeding diathesis except for acute coagulopathy related to sepsis.
- Chronic severe hepatic disease.
- Platelet count <30,000 × 10^6/l, even if the platelet count is increased after transfusions.
- Patients at increased risk for bleeding (for example):

a) Any major surgery, defined as surgery that requires general or spinal anaesthesia, performed within the 12-hour period immediately preceding drug infusion, or any postoperative patient who demonstrates evidence of active bleeding, or any patient with planned or anticipated surgery during the drug infusion period.

b) History of severe head trauma that required hospitalisation, intracranial or intraspinal surgery, or haemorrhagic stroke within the previous 3 months, or any history of intracerebral arteriovenous malformation, cerebral aneurysm, or central nervous system mass lesion; patients with an epidural catheter or who are anticipated to receive an epidural catheter during drug infusion.

c) History of congenital bleeding diatheses.

d) Gastro-intestinal bleeding within the last 6 weeks that has required medical intervention unless definitive surgery has been performed.

e) Trauma patients at increased risk of bleeding.

Xigris is also contra-indicated in patients with known hypersensitivity to drotrecogin alfa (activated), to any of the formulation excipients, or to bovine thrombin (a trace residue from the manufacturing process).

4.4 Special warnings and special precautions for use

Patients With Single Organ Dysfunction and Recent Surgery

Xigris is not approved for the treatment of patients with single organ dysfunction and should not be used in this particular subgroup of patients, especially if they had recent surgery (within 30 days). In each of two randomised, placebo-controlled trials, PROWESS and ADDRESS (see section 5.1), 28-day and in-hospital mortality were higher in patients treated with drotrecogin alfa (activated) compared to placebo for the subpopulation of patients with single organ dysfunction and recent surgery (n = 98 in PROWESS and n = 636 in ADDRESS).

Bleeding

Drotrecogin alfa (activated) increases the risk of bleeding. In the following conditions, the risks of the administration of Xigris should be weighed against the anticipated benefits:

- Recent administration (within 3 days) of thrombolytic therapy.
- Recent administration (within 7 days) of oral anticoagulants.
- Recent administration (within 7 days) of aspirin or other platelet inhibitors.
- Recent (within 3 months) ischaemic stroke.
- Any other condition in which the physician considers significant bleeding is likely.

For procedures with an inherent bleeding risk, discontinue Xigris for 2 hours prior to the start of the procedure. Xigris may be restarted 12 hours after major invasive procedures or surgery if adequate haemostasis has been achieved. Xigris may be restarted immediately after uncomplicated less invasive procedures if adequate haemostasis has been achieved.

As a component of routine care, measures of haemostasis (eg, activated partial thromboplastin time [APTT], prothrombin time [PT], and platelet count) should be obtained during the infusion of Xigris. If sequential tests of haemostasis indicate an uncontrolled or worsening coagulopathy that significantly increases the risk of bleeding, the benefits of continuing the infusion must be weighed against the potential increased risk of bleeding for that patient.

Laboratory Tests

Drotrecogin alfa (activated) has minimal effect on the PT. Prolongation of the APTT in patients with severe sepsis receiving Xigris may be due to the underlying coagulopathy, the pharmacodynamic effect of drotrecogin alfa (activated), and/or the effect of other concurrent medications. The pharmacodynamic effect of drotrecogin alfa (activated) on the APTT assay is dependent on the reagent and instrument used to perform the assay and the time that elapses between sample acquisition and assay performance. Drotrecogin alfa (activated) that is present in a blood or plasma sample drawn from a patient who is being infused with the drug will be gradually neutralised by endogenous plasma protease inhibitors present in the sample. Virtually no measurable activity of drotrecogin alfa (activated) is present 2 hours after obtaining the blood sample. Due to these biological and analytical variables, the APTT should not be used to assess the pharmacodynamic effect of drotrecogin alfa (activated). In addition, approximately 2 hours after terminating the infusion of the drug, there is virtually no measurable activity of drotrecogin alfa (activated) remaining in the circulation of the patient; blood samples drawn for APTT determination after this point are no longer affected by the drug. The interpretation of sequential determinations of the PT and/or APTT should take these variables into consideration.

Because drotrecogin alfa (activated) may affect the APTT assays, drotrecogin alfa (activated) present in plasma samples may interfere with one-stage coagulation assays based on the APTT (such as Factor VIII, IX, and XI assays). Drotrecogin alfa (activated) present in plasma samples does not interfere with one-stage factor assays based on the PT (such as Factor II, V, VII, and X assays).

If sequential measures of coagulopathy (including platelet count) indicate severe or worsening coagulopathy, the risk of continuing the infusion should be weighed against the expected benefit.

Immunogenicity

In patients with severe sepsis, the formation of anti-activated protein C antibodies was uncommon (<1%) after a single course of therapy. These antibodies were not capable of neutralising the effect of activated protein C on the APTT assay. However, the possibility of allergic reactions to constituents of the preparation cannot be completely excluded in certain predisposed patients. If allergic or anaphylactic reactions occur, treatment should be discontinued immediately and appropriate therapy initiated. Xigris has not been re-administered to patients with severe sepsis. If Xigris is re-administered to patients, caution should be employed. No anti-activated protein C antibody formation was detected in healthy subjects, even after repeat administration.

4.5 Interaction with other medicinal products and other forms of Interaction

Drug interactions with Xigris have not been studied in patients with sepsis.

Caution should be employed when Xigris is used with other drugs that affect haemostasis (see sections 4.3 and 4.4), including protein C, thrombolytics (eg, streptokinase, tPA, rPA, and urokinase), oral anticoagulants (eg, warfarin), hirudins, antithrombin, aspirin, and other anti-platelets agents, eg, non-steroidal anti-inflammatory drugs, ticlopidine and clopidogrel, glycoprotein IIb/IIIa antagonists (such as abciximab, eptifibatide, tirofiban), and prostacyclins, such as iloprost.

Heparin

Two-thirds of patients in the Phase 3 trial received prophylactic doses of unfractionated or low molecular weight heparin. There was no observed increase in the risk of bleeding events reported as serious adverse events in drotrecogin alfa (activated) patients receiving heparin. The effects of prophylactic low dose heparin and other coagulation-active medications on the efficacy of drotrecogin alfa (activated) have not been evaluated in a randomised controlled clinical trial.

4.6 Pregnancy and lactation

Animal studies with respect to effects on pregnancy, embryonal/foetal development, parturition, and postnatal development have not been conducted with Xigris. Therefore, the potential risk for humans is unknown. Xigris should not be used during pregnancy unless clearly necessary.

It is not known whether Xigris is excreted in human milk or if there is a potential effect on the nursed infant. Therefore, the patient should not breast-feed whilst treated with Xigris.

4.7 Effects on ability to drive and use machines

Not applicable.

4.8 Undesirable effects

Xigris increases the risk of bleeding.

The Phase 3, international, multi-centre, randomised, double-blind, placebo-controlled clinical trial (PROWESS) involved 850 drotrecogin alfa (activated)-treated and 840 placebo-treated patients. The percentage of patients experiencing at least one bleeding event in the two treatment groups was 24.9% and 17.7%, respectively. In both treatment groups, the majority of bleeding events were ecchymosis or gastro-intestinal tract bleeding. The difference in the incidence of serious bleeding events between the two treatment groups occurred primarily during study drug administration.

A total of 2,378 adult patients with severe sepsis received drotrecogin alfa (activated) in a Phase 3b, international, single-arm, open-label clinical trial (ENHANCE).

The incidence of serious bleeding events in the PROWESS and ENHANCE studies is provided below. In these studies, serious bleeding events included any intracranial haemorrhage, any life-threatening or fatal bleed, any bleeding event requiring the administration of ⩾3 units of packed red blood cells per day for 2 consecutive days, or any bleeding event assessed as serious by the investigator.

A Phase 3b, international, multi-centre, randomised, double-blind, placebo-controlled clinical trial (ADDRESS) of adult severe sepsis patients at low risk of death involved 1,317 drotrecogin alfa (activated)-treated and 1,293 placebo-treated patients. The percentage of patients experiencing at least one bleeding event in the two treatment groups was 10.9% and 6.4%, respectively ($P < 0.001$). Bleeding events included serious bleeding events, bleeding events assessed as possibly study drug related by the investigator, bleeding events associated with the need for a red blood cell transfusion, and bleeding events that led to permanent discontinuation of the study drug. In the ADDRESS trial, serious bleeding events included any fatal bleed, any life-threatening bleed, any CNS bleed, or any bleeding event assessed as serious by the investigator.

Serious Bleeding Events During the Infusion Period

The following table lists the percent of patients in PROWESS and ENHANCE experiencing serious bleeding events by site of haemorrhage during the study drug infusion period (defined as the duration of infusion plus the next full calendar day following the end of the infusion).

(see Table 1)

In ADDRESS, the percent of treated patients experiencing a serious bleeding event by site of haemorrhage was similar to that observed in PROWESS. The incidence of serious bleeding events during infusion (defined as study day 0 through study day 6) was 31 (2.4%) and 15 (1.2%) in drotrecogin alfa (activated)-treated and placebo-treated patients, respectively ($P = 0.02$). The incidence of CNS bleeds during infusion was 4 (0.3%) and 3 (0.2%) for drotrecogin alfa (activated)-treated and placebo-treated patients, respectively. Recent surgery (within 30 days prior to study entry) was associated with a numerically higher risk of serious bleeding during infusion in both the Xigris-treated and the placebo-treated patients (Xigris: 3.6% in patients with recent surgery versus 1.6% in patients without recent surgery; placebo: 1.6% versus 0.9%, respectively).

Serious Bleeding Events During the 28-Day Study Period

In PROWESS, the incidence of serious bleeding events during the 28-day study period was 3.5% and 2.0% in drotrecogin alfa (activated)-treated and placebo-treated patients, respectively. The incidence of CNS bleeds during the 28-day study period was 0.2% and 0.1% for drotrecogin alfa (activated)-treated and placebo-treated patients, respectively. The risk of CNS bleeding may increase with severe coagulopathy and severe thrombocytopenia (see sections 4.3 and 4.4).

In the open-label ENHANCE study, the incidence of serious bleeding events during the 28-day study period was 6.5%, and the incidence of CNS bleeds during the 28-day study period was 1.5%.

In the placebo-controlled ADDRESS study, the incidence of serious bleeding events during the 28-day study period was 51 (3.9%) and 28 (2.2%) in drotrecogin alfa (activated)-treated and placebo-treated patients, respectively ($P = 0.01$). The incidence of CNS bleeds during the 28-day study period was 6 (0.5%) and 5 (0.4%) for drotrecogin alfa (activated)-treated and placebo-treated patients, respectively.

In the Phase 1 studies, adverse events with a frequency of ⩾5% included headache (30.9%), ecchymosis (23.0%), and pain (5.8%).

Table 1

Site of Haemorrhage	Drotrecogin Alfa (Activated) [PROWESS] n = 850	Placebo [PROWESS] n = 840	Drotrecogin Alfa (Activated) [ENHANCE] n = 2,378
Gastro-intestinal	5 (0.6%)	4 (0.5%)	19 (0.8%)
Intra-abdominal	2 (0.2%)	3 (0.4%)	18 (0.8%)
Intra-thoracic	4 (0.5%)	0	11 (0.5%)
Retroperitoneal	3 (0.4%)	0	4 (0.2%)
Central nervous system (CNS)[1]	2 (0.2%)	0	15 (0.6%)
Genitourinary	2 (0.2%)	0	0
Skin/soft tissue	1 (0.1%)	0	16 (0.7%)
Nasopharyngeal	0	0	4 (0.2%)
Joint/bone	0	0	1 (0.04%)
Site unknown[2]	1 (0.1%)	1 (0.1%)	6 (0.3%)
Total	20 (2.4%)	8 (1.0%)	85[3] (3.6%)

[1]CNS bleeding is defined as any bleed in the central nervous system, including the following types of haemorrhage: petechial, parenchymal, subarachnoid, subdural, and stroke with haemorrhagic transformation.

[2]Patients requiring the administration of ⩾3 units of packed red blood cells per day for 2 consecutive days without an identified site of bleeding.

[3]In ENHANCE, six patients experienced multiple serious bleeding events during the study drug infusion period (94 events observed in 85 patients).

4.9 Overdose

In clinical trials, there has been one reported overdose of drotrecogin alfa (activated). This patient with severe sepsis received a dose of 181µg/kg/hr for 2 hours. There were no serious adverse events associated with the overdose.

Post-marketing experience: There have been reports of accidental overdosing. In the majority of cases, no reactions have been observed. For the other reports, the observed events were consistent with known undesirable effects of the drug (see section 4.8), effects of the drug on laboratory tests (see section 4.4), or consequences of the underlying condition of sepsis.

There is no known antidote for drotrecogin alfa (activated). In case of overdose, immediately stop the infusion (see section 5.2).

5. PHARMACOLOGICAL PROPERTIES

5.1 Pharmacodynamic properties

Pharmacotherapeutic group: Antithrombotic agents, enzymes. *ATC code:* B01AD10.

Mechanism of Action

Xigris is a recombinant version of the natural plasma-derived activated protein C, from which it differs only by unique oligosaccharides in the carbohydrate portion of the molecule. Activated protein C is a crucial coagulation regulator. It limits thrombin formation by inactivating Factors Va and VIIIa, thereby providing negative feedback regulation of coagulation. Excessive coagulation activation in the microcirculatory bed plays a significant part in the pathophysiology of severe sepsis. Furthermore, activated protein C is an important modulator of the systemic response to infection and has antithrombotic and profibrinolytic properties. Xigris has similar properties to those of endogenous human activated protein C.

Pharmacodynamic Effects

In placebo-controlled clinical trials in patients with severe sepsis, Xigris exerted an antithrombotic effect, by limiting thrombin generation, and improved sepsis-associated coagulopathy, as shown by a more rapid improvement in markers of coagulation and fibrinolysis. Xigris caused a more rapid decline in thrombotic markers, such as D-dimer, prothrombin F1.2, and thrombin-antithrombin levels, and a more rapid increase in protein C and antithrombin levels. Xigris also restored endogenous fibrinolytic potential, as evidenced by a more rapid trend toward normalisation in plasminogen levels and a more rapid decline in plasminogen activator inhibitor-1 levels. Additionally, patients with severe sepsis treated with Xigris had a more rapid decline in interleukin-6 levels, a global marker of inflammation, consistent with a reduction in the inflammatory response.

Clinical Efficacy

Xigris was studied in one Phase 3, international, multi-centre, randomised, double-blind, placebo-controlled trial (PROWESS) in 1,690 patients with severe sepsis. Severe sepsis is defined as sepsis associated with acute organ dysfunction. Patients meeting the clinical diagnosis of severe sepsis had: a) known or suspected infection; b) clinical evidence of systemic response to infection, including fever or hypothermia, leucopenia or leucocytosis, tachycardia and tachypnoea; and c) acute organ dysfunction. Organ dysfunction was defined as shock, hypotension or the need for vasopressor support despite adequate fluid resuscitation, relative hypoxemia (ratio of partial pressure of oxygen in arterial blood in mmHg to the percentage of oxygen in the inspired air expressed as a decimal [PaO_2/FiO_2 ratio] <250), oliguria despite adequate fluid resuscitation, marked reduction in blood platelet counts, and/or elevated lactic acid concentrations.

Exclusion criteria encompassed patients at high risk of bleeding (see sections 4.3 and 4.4), patients who were not expected to survive for 28 days due to a pre-existing, non-sepsis related medical condition, HIV positive patients whose most recent CD_4 count was ⩽50/mm^3, patients on chronic dialysis, and patients who had undergone bone marrow, lung, liver, pancreas, or small bowel transplantation, and patients with acute clinical pancreatitis without a proven source of infection.

In the PROWESS trial, treatment was initiated within 48 hours of onset of the first sepsis-induced organ dysfunction. The median duration of organ dysfunction prior to treatment was 18 hours. Patients were given a 96-hour constant rate infusion of Xigris at 24µg/kg/hr (n = 850) or placebo (n = 840). Xigris was added to best standard care. Best standard care includes adequate antibiotics, source control and supportive treatment (fluids, inotropes, vasopressors, and support of failing organs, as required).

Patients treated with Xigris experienced improved 28-day survival compared to those treated with placebo. At 28 days, the overall mortality rates were 24.7% for the Xigris-treated group and 30.8% for the placebo-treated group ($P = 0.005$).

Significant absolute death reduction was limited to the subgroup of patients with greater disease severity, ie, baseline APACHE II score ⩾25 or at least 2 acute organ dysfunctions at baseline. (The APACHE II score is designed to assess the risk of mortality based on Acute Physiology And Chronic Health Evaluation.) In the subgroup of patients with an APACHE II score ⩾25 at baseline, the mortality was 31% in the Xigris group (128 out of 414) and 44% in the placebo group (176 out of 403). No death reduction was observed in the subgroup of patients with lower disease severity. In the subgroup of patients with at least 2 acute organ dysfunctions at baseline, the mortality was 26.5% in the Xigris group (168 out of 634) and 33.9% in the placebo group (216 out of 637). No significant death reduction was observed in the subgroup of patients with less than 2 acute organ dysfunctions at baseline.

A consistent treatment effect on mortality with Xigris administration was observed across patient subgroups defined by age, gender, and infection type.

Heparin

Approximately ⅔ of the patients received prophylactic low dose heparin during the course of study. The mortality rate in patients receiving Xigris and concomitant prophylactic low dose heparin was 24.9% and the mortality rate in patients receiving placebo and concomitant prophylactic low dose heparin was 28.1% ($P = 0.20$). There is uncertainty if heparin could interfere with the activity of Xigris. The effect of low dose heparin on the efficacy of Xigris has not been evaluated in specific randomised controlled clinical trials.

PROWESS Follow-Up Study

Survival status was assessed in a follow-up study of PROWESS survivors. In-hospital and 3-month survival status was reported for 98% and 94% of the 1,690 PROWESS subjects, respectively. In the overall population, the in-hospital mortality was significantly lower in patients on Xigris than in patients on placebo (29.4% versus 34.6%; $P = 0.023$). Survival through 3 months was also better in the Xigris group compared to placebo (log rank $P = 0.048$). These data confirmed that the benefit of Xigris is limited to the more severely affected sepsis patients, such as patients with multiple organ failure and shock.

Further Clinical Experience

In a Phase 3b, international, single-arm, open-label clinical trial (ENHANCE), 2,378 adult patients with severe sepsis received drotrecogin alfa (activated). The entry criteria were similar to those employed in PROWESS. Patients received drotrecogin alfa (activated) within 48 hours of onset of the first sepsis-induced organ dysfunction. The median duration of organ dysfunction prior to treatment was 25 hours.

At 28 days, the mortality rate in the Phase 3b study was 25.3%. The mortality rate was lower for patients treated within 24 hours of organ dysfunction compared to those treated after 24 hours, even after adjustment for differences in disease severity.

A total of 2,640 adult patients with severe sepsis who were at low risk of death (eg, patients with APACHE II <25 or with only one sepsis-induced organ failure) were enrolled in a randomised, double-blind, placebo-controlled trial (ADDRESS). The trial was stopped after an interim analysis due to a low likelihood of demonstrating a significant difference in 28-day mortality by the end of the trial.

The ADDRESS trial did enrol 872 patients with multiple organ dysfunction. Compared to multiple organ dysfunction patients in PROWESS, those in ADDRESS had organ dysfunction for longer prior to receiving study drug (median 25 versus 18 hours), had lower APACHE II scores (median 20 versus 25), and were more likely to have two organ dysfunctions (76% versus 43%). At 28 days, the mortality rates for multiple organ dysfunction patients in ADDRESS were 20.7% versus 21.9% for drotrecogin alfa (activated)-treated and placebo-treated patients, respectively. In-hospital mortality rates were 23.1% and 25.3%, respectively. In the subgroup with two organ dysfunctions, the results were similar to those seen in the PROWESS trial.

In placebo-controlled clinical trials, the treatment effect was most evident at sites enrolling larger numbers of patients.

5.2 Pharmacokinetic properties

Drotrecogin alfa (activated) and endogenous human activated protein C are inactivated in plasma by endogenous protease inhibitors, but the mechanism by which they are cleared from plasma is unknown. Plasma concentrations of endogenous activated protein C in healthy subjects and patients with severe sepsis are usually below detection limits (<5ng/ml) and do not significantly influence the pharmacokinetic properties of drotrecogin alfa (activated).

In healthy subjects, greater than 90% of the steady-state condition is attained within 2 hours following the start of a constant-rate intravenous infusion of Xigris. Following the completion of an infusion, the decline in plasma drotrecogin alfa (activated) concentrations is biphasic and is comprised of a rapid initial phase ($t_{1/2\alpha}$ = 13 minutes) and a slower second phase ($t_{1/2\beta}$ = 1.6 hours). The short half-life of 13 minutes accounts for approximately 80% of the area under the plasma concentration curve and governs the initial rapid accrual of plasma drotrecogin alfa (activated) concentrations towards the steady-state. Plasma drotrecogin alfa (activated) steady-state concentrations are proportional to the infusion rate over a range of infusion rates from 12μg/kg/hr to 48μg/kg/hr. The mean steady-state plasma concentration of drotrecogin alfa (activated) in healthy subjects receiving 24μg/kg/hr is 72ng/ml.

In patients with severe sepsis, infusion of drotrecogin alfa (activated) from 12μg/kg/hr to 30μg/kg/hr rapidly produced steady-state plasma concentrations that were proportional to infusion rates. In the Phase 3 trial, the pharmacokinetics of drotrecogin alfa (activated) were evaluated in 342 patients with severe sepsis administered a 96-hour continuous infusion at 24μg/kg/hr. The pharmacokinetics of drotrecogin alfa (activated) were characterised by attainment of steady-state plasma concentration within 2 hours following the start of the infusion. In the majority of patients, measurements of activated protein C beyond 2 hours after termination of the infusion were below the quantifiable limit, suggesting rapid elimination of drotrecogin alfa (activated) from the systemic circulation. The plasma clearance of drotrecogin alfa (activated) is approximately 41.8 l/hr in sepsis patients as compared with 28.1 l/hr in healthy subjects.

In patients with severe sepsis, the plasma clearance of drotrecogin alfa (activated) was significantly decreased by renal impairment and hepatic dysfunction, but the magnitude of the differences in clearance (<30%) does not warrant any dosage adjustment.

5.3 Preclinical safety data

Changes observed in monkeys at, or in small excess of, the maximum human exposure during repeated dose studies were all related to the pharmacological effect of Xigris and include, beside the expected prolongation of APTT, decreases in haemoglobin, erythrocytes, and haematocrit, and increases in reticulocyte count and PT.

Drotrecogin alfa (activated) was not mutagenic in an *in vivo* micronucleus study in mice or in an *in vitro* chromosomal aberration study in human peripheral blood lymphocytes with or without rat liver metabolic activation.

Carcinogenicity studies and animal reproduction studies have not been conducted with Xigris. However, with respect to the latter, the potential risk for humans being unknown, Xigris should not be used during pregnancy unless clearly necessary (see section 4.6).

6. PHARMACEUTICAL PARTICULARS

6.1 List of excipients

Sucrose, sodium chloride, sodium citrate, citric acid, hydrochloric acid, and sodium hydroxide.

6.2 Incompatibilities

After reconstitution, Xigris should be compounded ONLY with 0.9% sodium chloride injection. The ONLY other solutions that can be administered through the same intravenous line are 0.9% sodium chloride injection, lactated Ringer's injection, dextrose, or dextrose and saline mixtures.

When administering drotrecogin alfa (activated) at low concentrations (less than approximately 200μg/ml), at low flow rates (less than approximately 5ml/hr), the infusion set must be primed for approximately 15 minutes at a flow rate of approximately 5ml/hr.

6.3 Shelf life

3 years.

After reconstitution, immediate use is recommended. However, the reconstituted solution in the vial may be held for up to 3 hours at room temperature (15 to 30°C). After preparation, the intravenous infusion solution can be used at room temperature (15 to 30°C) for a period up to 14 hours.

6.4 Special precautions for storage

Store at 2°C-8°C (in a refrigerator). Keep the vial in the outer carton in order to protect it from light.

6.5 Nature and contents of container

Xigris 5mg: 5mg of powder in vial (Type I glass) - pack of 1.

Xigris 20mg: 20mg of powder in vial (Type I glass) - pack of 1.

6.6 Instructions for use and handling

1. Use appropriate aseptic technique during the preparation of Xigris for intravenous administration.

2. Calculate the dose and the number of Xigris vials needed.

Xigris 5mg: Each Xigris vial contains 5mg of drotrecogin alfa (activated).

Xigris 20mg: Each Xigris vial contains 20mg of drotrecogin alfa (activated).

The vial contains an excess of drotrecogin alfa (activated) to facilitate delivery of the label amount.

3. *Xigris 5mg:* Prior to administration, 5mg vials of Xigris must be reconstituted with 2.5ml of sterile water for injection, resulting in a solution with a concentration of approximately 2mg/ml drotrecogin alfa (activated).

Xigris 20mg: Prior to administration, 20mg vials of Xigris must be reconstituted with 10ml of sterile water for injection, resulting in a solution with a concentration of approximately 2mg/ml drotrecogin alfa (activated).

Slowly add the sterile water for injection to the vial and avoid inverting or shaking the vial. Gently swirl each vial until the powder is completely dissolved.

4. The solution of reconstituted Xigris must be further diluted with sterile 0.9% sodium chloride injection. Slowly withdraw the appropriate amount of reconstituted drotrecogin alfa (activated) solution from the vial. Add the reconstituted drotrecogin alfa (activated) into a prepared infusion bag of sterile 0.9% sodium chloride injection. When adding the reconstituted drotrecogin alfa (activated) into the infusion bag, direct the stream to the side of the bag to minimise the agitation of the solution. Gently invert the infusion bag to obtain a homogeneous solution. Do not transport the infusion bag between locations using mechanical delivery systems.

5. After reconstitution, immediate use is recommended. However, the reconstituted solution in the vial may be held for up to 3 hours at room temperature (15 to 30°C). After preparation, the intravenous infusion solution can be used at room temperature (15 to 30°C) for a period up to 14 hours.

6. Parenteral drug products should be inspected visually for particulate matter and discolouration prior to administration.

7. **It is recommended that Xigris be infused with an infusion pump to accurately control the infusion rate.** The solution of reconstituted Xigris is typically diluted into an infusion bag containing sterile 0.9% sodium chloride injection to a final concentration of between 100μg/ml and 200μg/ml.

8. When administering drotrecogin alfa (activated) at low concentrations (less than approximately 200μg/ml), at low flow rates (less than approximately 5ml/hr), the infusion set must be primed for approximately 15 minutes at a flow rate of approximately 5ml/hr.

9. Xigris should be administered via a dedicated intravenous line or a dedicated lumen of a multi-lumen central venous catheter. The ONLY other solutions that can be administered through the same line are 0.9% sodium chloride injection, lactated Ringer's injection, dextrose, or dextrose and saline mixtures.

10. Avoid exposing drotrecogin alfa (activated) solutions to heat and/or direct sunlight. No incompatibilities have been observed between drotrecogin alfa (activated) and glass infusion bottles or infusion bags made of polyvinylchloride, polyethylene, polypropylene, or polyolefin. The use of other types of infusion sets could have a negative impact on the amount and potency of drotrecogin alfa (activated) administered.

11. Care should be taken to administer Xigris at the appropriate rate, calculated based on kg of bodyweight and infused for the correct duration. It is recommended that the bag be labelled accordingly.

7. MARKETING AUTHORISATION HOLDER

Eli Lilly Nederland BV, Grootslag 1-5, 3991 RA Houten, The Netherlands.

8. MARKETING AUTHORISATION NUMBER(S)

5mg vial: EU/1/02/225/001

20mg vial: EU/1/02/225/002

9. DATE OF FIRST AUTHORISATION/RENEWAL OF THE AUTHORISATION

Date of first authorisation: 22 August 2002

10. DATE OF REVISION OF THE TEXT

5 July 2005

LEGAL CATEGORY

POM

*XIGRIS (drotrecogin alfa [activated]) is a trademark of Eli Lilly and Company.

XIG5M

Xismox XL 60 Prolonged Release Tablets

(Genus Pharmaceuticals)

1. NAME OF THE MEDICINAL PRODUCT

Monosorb XL 60 Prolonged Release Tablets

and

Xismox® XL 60 Prolonged Release Tablets

(own-label name for distributor SCHEIN PHARMACEUTICAL UK LTD. trading as GENUS PHARMACEUTICALS)

2. QUALITATIVE AND QUANTITATIVE COMPOSITION

Isosorbide-5-mononitrate 60.0 mg

3. PHARMACEUTICAL FORM

Prolonged Release Tablets

Light yellow, biconvex, oval-shaped, prolonged release tablets, scored on both sides and marked "DX 31" on one side.

4. CLINICAL PARTICULARS

4.1 Therapeutic indications

Monosorb XL 60 is indicated for the prophylaxis of angina pectoris.

4.2 Posology and method of administration

Adults: The recommended dose of Monosorb XL 60 tablets is one Monosorb XL 60 tablet once daily to be taken in the morning. The dose may be increased to 120 mg (two tablets) daily, both to be taken once daily in the morning. The dose can be titrated, by initiating treatment with 30 mg (half tablet) for the first 2-4 days to minimize the possibility of headache.

Children: The safety and efficacy in children has not been established.

Elderly: No evidence of a need for routine dosage adjustment in the elderly has been found, but special care may be needed in those with increased susceptibility to hypotension or marked hepatic or renal insufficiency.

There is a risk of tolerance developing when nitrate therapy is given. For this reason it is important that Monosorb XL 60 tablets are taken once a day to achieve an interval with low nitrate concentration, thereby reducing the risk of tolerance development.

When necessary the product may be used in combination with beta-adrenoreceptor blockers and calcium antagonists. Dose adjustments of either class of agent may be necessary.

The tablets must not be chewed or crushed. They should be swallowed with half a glass of water.

4.3 Contraindications

Hypersensitivity to isosorbide mononitrate, or to any other ingredients in the tablets.

Sildenafil has been shown to potentiate the hypotensive effects of nitrates, and its co-administration with nitrates or nitric oxide donors is therefore contra-indicated.

Isosorbide mononitrate is contraindicated in constrictive pericarditis and pericardial tamponade.

4.4 Special warnings and special precautions for use

Use with extreme caution in hypotension with or without other signs of shock and in cases of cerebrovascular insufficiency.

Other special warnings and precautions with Isosorbide mononitrate:

Significant aortic or mitral valve stenosis.

Hypertrophic obstructive cardiomyopathy.

Anaemia. Hypoxaemia, Hypothyroidism.

Monosorb XL 60 is not indicated for relief of acute angina attacks.

4.5 Interaction with other medicinal products and other forms of Interaction

Isosorbide mononitrate may act as a physiological antagonist to noradrenaline, acetylcholine, histamine and many other agents. The effect of anti-hypertensive drugs may be enhanced. Alcohol may enhance the hypotensive effects of isosorbide mononitrate.

The hypotensive effects of nitrates are potentiated by concurrent administration of sildenafil.

4.6 Pregnancy and lactation

Monosorb XL 60 should not be used during pregnancy and lactation.

4.7 Effects on ability to drive and use machines

Patients experiencing headache or dizziness following initial treatment with

Monosorb XL 60 should become stabilised on treatment before driving or using machines.

4.8 Undesirable effects

Most of the adverse reactions are pharmacodynamically mediated and dose dependent. Headache may occur when treatment is initiated but usually disappears after continued treatment. Hypotension with symptoms such as dizziness and nausea has occasionally been reported. These symptoms generally disappear during long-term treatment.

Less common are vomiting and diarrhoea. Uncommon is fainting.

Skin rashes (dry rash, exfoliative dermatitis) and pruritus have been reported rarely with isosorbide mononitrate. Myalgia has been reported very rarely.

4.9 Overdose

Symptoms: Pulsing headache. More serious symptoms are excitation, flushing, cold perspiration, nausea, vomiting, vertigo, syncope, tachycardia and a fall in blood pressure. Very large doses may give rise to methaemoglobinaemia (Very rare).

Treatment: Induction of emesis, activated charcoal. In case of pronounced hypotension the patient should first be placed in the supine position with legs raised. If necessary, fluid should be administered intravenously.(In cases of cyanosis as a result of methaemoglobinaemia, methyl thionine (methylene blue) 1-2mg/Kg, slow intravenous delivery). Expert advice should be sought.

5. PHARMACOLOGICAL PROPERTIES

5.1 Pharmacodynamic properties

Isosorbide-5-mononitrate is an organic nitrate, the major active metabolite of isosorbide dinitrate and an active vasodilator in its own right. The mechanism of action of isosorbide-5-mononitrate, like other organic nitrates, is believed to involve peripheral vasodilation, both venous and arterial. Maximal venous dilatation is usually achieved with lower doses of the nitrate, while higher doses cause progressive dilatation of the arterial vasculature. Nitrates thus lead to pooling of blood in the veins and reduced left ventricular and diastolic pressure. As arterial vascular resistance is also decreased, arterial blood pressure is reduced. Isosorbide-5-mononitrate is an effective antianginal agent because it improves exertional angina by reducing myocardial oxygen demand, secondary to reduced preload and afterload. Organic nitrates release nitric oxide (NO), which induces protein phosphorylations, finally resulting in vascular smooth muscle relaxation.

In comparison to an immediate release product taken on a multiple dose basis, this prolonged release product has the advantage of both lowering the incidence of tolerance and increasing patient compliance.

5.2 Pharmacokinetic properties

Isosorbide-5-mononitrate is completely absorbed after oral administration. The absorption is not affected by simultaneous food intake. Contrary to many other nitrates, Isosorbide-5-mononitrate is not subject to first pass metabolism and its oral bioavailability is therefore close to 100%. This feature probably contributes to the relatively small intersubject variability in plasma levels that are achieved following ingestion of the drug. Peak plasma concentrations of isosorbide-5-mononitrate after oral ingestion of a prolonged release tablet usually occur within 3.1-4.5 hours. Isosorbide-5-mononitrate's volume of distribution is about 0.6 litres/kg, and its plasma protein binding is negligible (about 4%). Isosorbide-5-mononitrate is metabolised to form several inactive compounds. Elimination is primarily by denitration and conjugation in the liver. The metabolites are excreted mainly via the kidneys. About 2% of the dose is excreted intact via the kidneys. The half-life of isosorbide-5-mononitrate in the plasma of healthy volunteers as well as in most patients is about 6.5 hours after administration of prolonged release tablets. Neither renal nor hepatic disease influence the pharmacokinetic of isosorbide mononitrate. Monosorb XL 60 is a prolonged release formulation. The active substance is released independently of pH.

5.3 Preclinical safety data

Isosorbide-5-mononitrate is a well-established drug for which there is adequate published safety data.

6. PHARMACEUTICAL PARTICULARS

6.1 List of excipients

Hypromellose 2208, lactose, compressible Sugar (composed of sucrose and maltodextrin), magnesium stearate, colloidal anhydrous silica, iron oxide yellow.

6.2 Incompatibilities

None

6.3 Shelf life

3 years

6.4 Special precautions for storage

Do not store above 25°C.

6.5 Nature and contents of container

Blister pack PVDC- or ACLAR-coated-PVC/Aluminium 28 or 30 tablets

6.6 Instructions for use and handling

No specific requirements.

7. MARKETING AUTHORISATION HOLDER

Dexcel-Pharma Ltd.

1 Cottesbrooke Park

Heartlands Business Park

Daventry

Northamptonshire NN11 5YL

England

8. MARKETING AUTHORISATION NUMBER(S)

PL 14017/0020

9. DATE OF FIRST AUTHORISATION/RENEWAL OF THE AUTHORISATION

3 September 1997.

10. DATE OF REVISION OF THE TEXT

December 2002

Xylocaine 1% with Adrenaline (Epinephrine) 1:200,000.

(AstraZeneca UK Limited)

1. NAME OF THE MEDICINAL PRODUCT

Xylocaine 1% with Adrenaline (Epinephrine) 1:200,000.

2. QUALITATIVE AND QUANTITATIVE COMPOSITION

Each ml of solution for injection contains lidocaine hydrochloride monohydrate Ph. Eur., equivalent to 10 mg of lidocaine hydrochloride anhydrous (200 mg per 20 ml vial), 5 micrograms of adrenaline (epinephrine) as the acid tartrate (100 micrograms per 20 ml vial).

For excipients see 6.1

3. PHARMACEUTICAL FORM

Solution for injection

4. CLINICAL PARTICULARS

4.1 Therapeutic indications

Xylocaine with Adrenaline is indicated for the production of local anaesthesia by the following techniques:

- Local infiltration
- Minor and major nerve blocks
- Epidural block

4.2 Posology and method of administration

Adults and children above 12 years of age

The dosage is adjusted according to the response of the patient and the site of administration. The lowest concentration and smallest dose producing the required effect should be given. The maximum single dose of Xylocaine when given with adrenaline is 500 mg.

The dosages in the following table are recommended as a guide for the more commonly used techniques used in the average adult. The clinician's experience and knowledge of the patient's physical status are of importance in calculating the required dose. Elderly or debilitated patients require smaller doses, commensurate with age and physical status.

(see Table 1 on next page)

Unnecessarily high doses of local anaesthetics are to be avoided. In general, surgical anaesthesia (eg epidural administration) requires the use of higher concentrations and doses. When blocking smaller nerves, or when a less intense block is required, the use of a lower concentration is indicated. The volume of drug used will affect the extent and spread of anaesthesia.

Care should be taken to prevent acute toxic reactions by avoiding intravascular injection. Careful aspiration before and during the injection is recommended. When a large dose is to be injected, e.g. in epidural block, a test dose of 3-5 ml of lidocaine containing adrenaline is recommended. An accidental intravascular injection may be recognised by a temporary increase in heart rate. The main dose, should be injected slowly, at a rate of 100-200 mg/min, or in incremental doses, while keeping in constant verbal contact with the patient. If toxic symptoms occur, the injection should be stopped immediately.

Paediatric patients 1 to 12 years of age

In children, the dosage should be calculated on a weight basis up to 7 mg/kg. In children with a high body weight, a gradual reduction of the dosage is often necessary and should be based on the ideal body weight. Standard textbooks should be consulted for factors affecting specific block techniques and for individual patient requirements.

4.3 Contraindications

Known hypersensitivity to anaesthetics of the amide type or other components of the solution.

The use of a vasoconstrictor is contra-indicated for anaesthesia of fingers, toes, tip of nose, ears and penis.

4.4 Special warnings and special precautions for use

In common with other local anaesthetics, Xylocaine with Adrenaline should be used cautiously in patients with epilepsy, impaired cardiac conduction, impaired respiratory function and in patients with impaired hepatic function, if the dose or site of administration is likely to result in high blood levels. Patients with severe renal dysfunction, the elderly and patients in poor general condition also require special attention. Attempts should also be made to optimise the patient's condition before major blocks. Patients treated with anti-arrhythmic drugs class III (eg amiodarone) should be under close surveillance and ECG monitoring considered, since cardiac effects may be additive (see section 4.5 Interaction with other medicaments and other forms of interaction).

Xylocaine with Adrenaline should not be given intravenously.

Facilities for resuscitation should be available when local anaesthetics are administered.

The effect of local anaesthetics may be reduced if an injection is made into an inflamed or infected area.

Certain local anaesthetic procedures may be associated with serious adverse reactions, regardless of the local anaesthetic drug used, e.g.:

- Central nerve blocks may cause cardiovascular depression, especially in the presence of hypovolaemia, and therefore epidural anaesthesia should be used with caution in patients with impaired cardiovascular function.
- Retrobulbar injections may rarely reach the cranial subarachnoid space, causing serious / severe reactions, including cardiovascular collapse, apnoea, convulsions and temporary blindness.
- Retro- and peribulbar injections of local anaesthetics carry a low risk of persistent ocular muscle dysfunction. The primary causes include trauma and/or local toxic effects on muscles and/or nerves.

The severity of such tissue reactions is related to the degree of trauma, the concentration of the local anaesthetic and the duration of exposure of the tissue to the local anaesthetic. For this reason, as with all local anaesthetics, the lowest effective concentration and dose of local anaesthetic should be used. Vasoconstrictors may aggravate tissue reactions and should be used only when indicated.

- Injections in the head and neck regions may be made inadvertently into an artery, causing cerebral symptoms even at low doses.
- Paracervical block can sometimes cause fetal bradycardia/tachycardia, and careful monitoring of the foetal heart rate is necessary.

Epidural anaesthesia may lead to hypotension and bradycardia. This risk can be reduced by preloading the circulation with crystalloidal or colloidal solutions. Hypotension should be treated promptly with e.g. ephedrine 5-10 mg intravenously and repeated as necessary.

Solutions containing adrenaline should be used with caution in patients with hypertension, cardiac disease, cerebrovascular insufficiency hyperthyroidism, advanced diabetes and any other pathological condition that may be aggravated by the effects of adrenaline.

Table 1

Type of block	% Conc.	Each dose		Indication
		ml	mg	
Surgical Anaesthesia				
Lumbar epidural administration	2	15-25	300-500	Surgical operations
Thoracic epidural administration	2	10-15	150-225	Surgical operations
Caudal epidural block	1	20-30	200-300	Surgical operations and acute pain relief
	2	15-25	300-500	Surgical operations
Field Block (eg minor nerve blocks and infiltration)				
Infiltration	1	up to 40	up to 400	Surgical operations
Digital Block	1	1-5	10-50	Surgical operations
Intercostals (per nerve) (maximal number of nerves blocked at same time should be ⩽ 8)	1	2-5	20-50	Surgical operations Postoperative pain and fractured ribs
Retrobulbar	2	4	80	Ocular surgery
Peribulbar	1	10-15	100-150	Ocular surgery
Pudendal	1	10	100	Instrumental delivery
Major Nerve Block				
Paracervical (each side)	1	10	100	Surgical operations and dilatation of cervix Obstetric pain relief
Brachial plexus: Axillary	1	40-50	400-500	Surgical operations
Supraclavicular, intrascalene and subclavian perivascular	1	30-40	300-400	Surgical operations
Sciatic	2	15-20	300-400	Surgical operations
3 in 1	1	30-40	300-400	Surgical operations
(femoral, obturator and lateral cutaneous)				

Xylocaine with adrenaline contains sodium metabisulphite, which may cause allergic reactions including anaphylactic symptoms and life-threatening or less severe asthmatic episodes in certain susceptible people. The overall prevalence of sulphite sensitivity in the general population is unknown and probably low. Sulphite sensitivity is seen more frequently in asthmatic than non-asthmatic people.

4.5 Interaction with other medicinal products and other forms of Interaction

Lidocaine should be used with caution in patients receiving other local anaesthetics or agents structurally related to amide-type local anaesthetics eg, certain anti-arrhythmics, such as mexilitine, since the systemic toxic effects are additive. Specific interaction studies with lidocaine and anti-arrhythmic drugs class III (eg, amiodarone) have not been performed, but caution is advised (see also section 4.4 Special warnings and special precautions for use).

Solutions containing adrenaline should be used cautiously in patients taking tricyclic antidepressants, monoamine oxidase inhibitors or receiving potent general anaesthetic agents since severe, prolonged hypertension may be the result. In addition, the concurrent use of adrenaline-containing solutions and oxytocic drugs of the ergot type may cause severe, persistent hypertension and possibly cerebrovascular and cardiac accidents. Phenothiazines and butyrophenones may oppose the vasoconstrictor effects of adrenaline giving rise to hypotensive responses and tachycardia.

Solutions containing adrenaline should be used with caution in patients undergoing general anaesthesia with inhalation agents, such as halothane and enflurane, due to the risk of serious cardiac arrhythmias.

Non-cardioselective betablockers such as propranolol enhance the pressor effects of adrenaline, which may lead to severe hypertension and bradycardia.

4.6 Pregnancy and lactation

Pregnancy

Although there is no evidence from animal studies of harm to the foetus, as with all drugs, Xylocaine should not be given during early pregnancy unless the benefits are considered to outweigh the risks.

The addition of adrenaline may potentially decrease uterine blood flow and contractility, especially after inadvertent injection into maternal blood vessels.

Foetal adverse effects due to local anaesthetics, such as foetal bradycardia, seem to be most apparent in paracervical block anaesthesia. Such effects may be due to high concentrations of anaesthetic reaching the foetus.

Lactation

Lidocaine may enter the mother's milk, but in such small amounts that there is generally no risk of this affecting the neonate. It is not known whether adrenaline enters breast milk or not, but it is unlikely to affect the breast-fed child.

4.7 Effects on ability to drive and use machines

Besides the direct anaesthetic affect, local anaesthetics may have a very mild effect on mental function and co-ordination, even in the absence of overt CNS toxicity, and may temporarily impair locomotion and alertness.

4.8 Undesirable effects

In common with other local anaesthetics, adverse reactions to Xylocaine with Adrenaline are rare and are usually the result of excessively high blood concentrations due to inadvertent intravascular injection, excessive dosage, rapid absorption or occasionally to hypersensitivity, idiosyncrasy or diminished tolerance on the part of the patient. In such circumstances systemic effects occur involving the central nervous system and/or the cardiovascular system.

The following table gives a list of the frequencies of undesirable effects:

Common (>1/100 <1/10)	Vascular disorders: Hypotension Gastrointestinal disorders: Nausea Nervous system disorders: paraesthesia, dizziness Cardiac disorders: bradycardia
Uncommon (>1/1000 <1/100)	Nervous system disorders: Signs and symptoms of CNS toxicity (Convulsions, Numbness of tongue and Paraesthesia circumoral, Tinnitus, Tremor, Dysarthria, Hyperacusis, Visual disturbances, CNS depression)
Rare (<1/1000)	Cardiac disorders: Cardiac arrest, Cardiac arrhythmias Immune system disorders: Allergic reactions, Anaphylactic reaction Respiratory disorders: Respiratory depression Nervous system disorders: Neuropathy, peripheral nerve injury, Arachnoiditis Eye disorders: Diplopia

4.9 Overdose

Acute systemic toxicity

Central nervous system toxicity is a graded response with symptoms and signs of escalating severity. The first symptoms are circumoral paraesthesia, numbness of the tongue, light-headedness, hyperacusis and tinnitus. Visual disturbance and muscular tremors are more serious and precede the onset of generalized convulsions. These signs must not be mistaken for neurotic behaviour. Unconsciousness and grand mal convulsions may follow which may last from a few seconds to several minutes. Hypoxia and hypercarbia occur rapidly following convulsions due to the increased muscular activity, together with the interference with normal respiration and loss of the airway. In severe cases apnoea may occur. Acidosis increases the toxic effects of local anaesthetics.

Effects on the cardiovascular system may be seen in severe cases. Hypotension, bradycardia, arrhythmia and even cardiac arrest may occur as a result of high systemic concentrations.

Cardiovascular toxic effects are generally preceded by signs of toxicity in the central nervous system, unless the patient is receiving a general anaesthetic or is heavily sedated with drugs such as a benzodiazepine or barbiturate.

Recovery is due to redistribution of the local anaesthetic drug from the central nervous system and metabolism. Recovery may be rapid unless large amounts of the drug have been injected.

Treatment of acute toxicity

If signs of acute systemic toxicity appear, injection of the local anaesthetic should be immediately stopped.

Treatment will be required if convulsions occur. All drugs and equipment should be immediately available. The objectives of treatment are to maintain oxygenation, stop the convulsions and support the circulation. Oxygen must be given and ventilation assisted if necessary (mask and bag). An anticonvulsant should be given i.v. if the convulsions do not stop spontaneously in 15-20 sec. Thiopentone 1-3 mg/kg i.v. will abort the convulsions rapidly. Alternatively diazepam 0.1 mg/kg i.v. may be used, although its action is slower. Prolonged convulsions may jeopardise the patient's ventilation and oxygenation. If so, injection of a muscle relaxant (eg, suxamethonium 1 mg/kg) will facilitate ventilation, and oxygenation can be controlled. Early endotracheal intubation must be considered in such situations. If cardiovascular depression is evident (hypotension, bradycardia), ephedrine 5-10 mg i.v. should be given and repeated, if necessary, after 2-3 min.

Should circulatory arrest occur, immediate cardiopulmonary resuscitation should be instituted. Continual optimal oxygenation and ventilation and circulatory support as well as treatment of acidosis are of vital importance.

5. PHARMACOLOGICAL PROPERTIES

5.1 Pharmacodynamic properties

ATC code: N01B B52

Lidocaine is a local anaesthetic of the amide type. At high doses lidocaine has a quinidine like action on the myocardium i.e. cardiac depressant. All local anaesthetics stimulate the CNS and may produce anxiety, restlessness and tremors.

5.2 Pharmacokinetic properties

Lidocaine is readily absorbed from the gastro-intestinal tract, from mucous membranes and through damaged skin. It is rapidly absorbed from injection sites including muscle.

Elimination half-life is 2 hours.

Lidocaine undergoes first pass metabolism in the liver.

Less than 10% of a dose is excreted unchanged via the kidneys.

The speed of onset and duration of action of lidocaine are increased by the addition of a vasoconstrictor and absorption into the site of injection is reduced.

5.3 Preclinical safety data

Lidocaine and adrenaline are well-established active ingredients.

In animal studies, the signs and symptoms of toxicity noted after high doses of lidocaine are the results of the effects on the central nervous and cardiovascular systems. No drug related adverse effects were seen in the reproduction toxicity studies, neither did lidocaine show any mutagenic potential in either in vitro or in vivo mutagenicity tests. Cancer studies have not been performed with lidocaine, due to the area and duration of therapeutic use for this drug.

6. PHARMACEUTICAL PARTICULARS

6.1 List of excipients

Sodium chloride, sodium metabisulphite, methylparahydroxybenzoate, sodium hydroxide, hydrochloric acid and water for injections.

6.2 Incompatibilities

None

6.3 Shelf life

Two years.

Use within 3 days of first opening.

6.4 Special precautions for storage
Store between 2°C and 8°C.

6.5 Nature and contents of container
Multiple dose vials - 20 ml and 50 ml.

6.6 Instructions for use and handling
None

7. MARKETING AUTHORISATION HOLDER
AstraZeneca UK Ltd,
600 Capability Green,
Luton, LU1 3LU, UK.

8. MARKETING AUTHORISATION NUMBER(S)
PL 17901/0174

9. DATE OF FIRST AUTHORISATION/RENEWAL OF THE AUTHORISATION
21st May 2002

10. DATE OF REVISION OF THE TEXT
6th May 2005

Xylocaine 2% with Adrenaline (Epinephrine) 1:200,000.

(AstraZeneca UK Limited)

1. NAME OF THE MEDICINAL PRODUCT
Xylocaine 2% with Adrenaline (Epinephrine) 1:200,000.

2. QUALITATIVE AND QUANTITATIVE COMPOSITION
Each ml of solution for injection contains lidocaine hydrochloride monohydrate Ph. Eur., equivalent to 20 mg of lidocaine hydrochloride anhydrous (400 mg per 20 ml vial), 5 micrograms of adrenaline (epinephrine) as the acid tartrate (100 micrograms per 20 ml vial).

For excipients see 6.1

3. PHARMACEUTICAL FORM
Solution for injection

4. CLINICAL PARTICULARS

4.1 Therapeutic indications
Xylocaine with Adrenaline is indicated for the production of local anaesthesia by the following techniques:

- Local infiltration
- Minor and major nerve blocks
- Epidural block

4.2 Posology and method of administration
Adults and children above 12 years of age
The dosage is adjusted according to the response of the patient and the site of administration. The lowest concentration and smallest dose producing the required effect should be given. The maximum single dose of Xylocaine when given with adrenaline is 500 mg.

The dosages in the following table are recommended as a guide for the more commonly used techniques in the average adult. The clinician's experience and knowledge of the patient's physical status are of importance in calculating the required dose. Elderly or debilitated patients require smaller doses, commensurate with age and physical status.

(see Table 1)

Table 1

Type of block	% Conc.	Each dose ml	Each dose mg	Indication
Surgical Anaesthesia				
Lumbar epidural administration	2	15-25	300-500	Surgical operations
Thoracic epidural administration	2	10-15	150-225	Surgical operations
Caudal epidural block	1	20-30	200-300	Surgical operations and acute pain relief
	2	15-25	300-500	Surgical operations
Field Block (eg minor nerve blocks and infiltration)				
Infiltration	1	up to 40	up to 400	Surgical operations
Digital Block	1	1-5	10-50	Surgical operations
Intercostals (per nerve) (maximal number of nerves blocked at same time should be ⩽ 8)	1	2-5	20-50	Surgical operations Postoperative pain and fractured ribs
Retrobulbar	2	4	80	Ocular surgery
Peribulbar	1	10-15	100-150	Ocular surgery
Pudendal	1	10	100	Instrumental delivery
Major Nerve Block				
Paracervical (each side)	1	10	100	Surgical operations and dilatation of cervix Obstetric pain relief
Brachial plexus: Axillary	1	40-50	400-500	Surgical operations
Supraclavicular, intrascalene and subclavian perivascular	1	30-40	300-400	Surgical operations
Sciatic	2	15-20	300-400	Surgical operations
3 in 1 (femoral, obturator and lateral cutaneous)	1	30-40	300-400	Surgical operations

Unnecessarily high doses of local anaesthetics are to be avoided. In general, surgical anaesthesia (eg epidural administration) requires the use of higher concentrations and doses. When blocking smaller nerves, or when a less intense block is required, the use of a lower concentration is indicated. The volume of drug used will affect the extent and spread of anaesthesia.

Care should be taken to prevent acute toxic reactions by avoiding intravascular injection. Careful aspiration before and during the injection is recommended. When a large dose is to be injected, e.g. in epidural block, a test dose of 3-5 ml of lidocaine containing adrenaline is recommended. An accidental intravascular injection may be recognised by a temporary increase in heart rate. The main dose, should be injected slowly, at a rate of 100-200 mg/min, or in incremental doses, while keeping in constant verbal contact with the patient. If toxic symptoms occur, the injection should be stopped immediately.

Paediatric patients 1 to 12 years of age
In children, the dosage should be calculated on a weight basis up to 7 mg/kg. In children with a high body weight, a gradual reduction of the dosage is often necessary and should be based on the ideal body weight. Standard textbooks should be consulted for factors affecting specific block techniques and for individual patient requirements.

4.3 Contraindications
Known hypersensitivity to anaesthetics of the amide type or other components of the solution.

The use of a vasoconstrictor is contra-indicated for anaesthesia of fingers, toes, tip of nose, ears and penis.

4.4 Special warnings and special precautions for use
In common with other local anaesthetics, Xylocaine with Adrenaline should be used cautiously in patients with epilepsy, impaired cardiac conduction, impaired respiratory function and in patients with impaired hepatic function, if the dose or site of administration is likely to result in high blood levels. Patients with severe renal dysfunction, the elderly and patients in poor general condition also require special attention. Attempts should also be made to optimise the patient's condition before major blocks. Patients treated with anti-arrhythmic drugs class III (eg amiodarone) should be under close surveillance and ECG monitoring considered, since cardiac effects may be additive (see section 4.5 Interaction with other medicaments and other forms of interaction).

Xylocaine with Adrenaline should not be given intravenously.

Facilities for resuscitation should be available when local anaesthetics are administered.

The effect of local anaesthetics may be reduced if an injection is made into an inflamed or infected area.

Certain local anaesthetic procedures may be associated with serious adverse reactions, regardless of the local anaesthetic drug used, e.g.:

- Central nerve blocks may cause cardiovascular depression, especially in the presence of hypovolaemia, and therefore epidural anaesthesia should be used with caution in patients with impaired cardiovascular function.

- Retrobulbar injections may rarely reach the cranial subarachnoid space, causing serious / severe reactions, including cardiovascular collapse, apnoea, convulsions and temporary blindness.

- Retro- and peribulbar injections of local anaesthetics carry a low risk of persistent ocular muscle dysfunction. The primary causes include trauma and/or local toxic effects on muscles and/or nerves.

The severity of such tissue reactions is related to the degree of trauma, the concentration of the local anaesthetic and the duration of exposure of the tissue to the local anaesthetic. For this reason, as with all local anaesthetics, the lowest effective concentration and dose of local anaesthetic should be used. Vasoconstrictors may aggravate tissue reactions and should be used only when indicated.

- Injections in the head and neck regions may be made inadvertently into an artery, causing cerebral symptoms even at low doses.

- Paracervical block can sometimes cause fetal bradycardia/tachycardia, and careful monitoring of the foetal heart rate is necessary.

Epidural anaesthesia may lead to hypotension and bradycardia. This risk can be reduced by preloading the circulation with crystalloidal or colloidal solutions. Hypotension should be treated promptly with e.g. ephedrine 5-10 mg intravenously and repeated as necessary.

Solutions containing adrenaline should be used with caution in patients with hypertension, cardiac disease, cerebrovascular insufficiency hyperthyroidism, advanced diabetes and any other pathological condition that may be aggravated by the effects of adrenaline.

Xylocaine with adrenaline contains sodium metabisulphite, which may cause allergic reactions including anaphylactic symptoms and life-threatening or less severe asthmatic episodes in certain susceptible people. The overall prevalence of sulphite sensitivity in the general population is unknown and probably low. Sulphite sensitivity is seen more frequently in asthmatic than non-asthmatic people.

4.5 Interaction with other medicinal products and other forms of Interaction
Lidocaine should be used with caution in patients receiving other local anaesthetics or agents structurally related to amide-type local anaesthetics eg, certain anti-arrhythmics, such as mexilitine, since the systemic toxic effects are additive. Specific interaction studies with lidocaine and anti-arrhythmic drugs class III (eg, amiodarone) have not been performed, but caution is advised (see also section 4.4 Special warnings and special precautions for use).

Solutions containing adrenaline should be used cautiously in patients taking tricyclic antidepressants, monoamine oxidase inhibitors or receiving potent general anaesthetic agents since severe, prolonged hypertension may be the result. In addition, the concurrent use of adrenaline-containing solutions and oxytocic drugs of the ergot type may cause severe, persistent hypertension and possibly cerebrovascular and cardiac accidents. Phenothiazines and butyrophenones may oppose the vasoconstrictor effects of adrenaline giving rise to hypotensive responses and tachycardia.

Solutions containing adrenaline should be used with caution in patients undergoing general anaesthesia with inhalation agents, such as halothane and enflurane, due to the risk of serious cardiac arrhythmias.

Non-cardioselective betablockers such as propranolol enhance the pressor effects of adrenaline, which may lead to severe hypertension and bradycardia.

4.6 Pregnancy and lactation

Pregnancy

Although there is no evidence from animal studies of harm to the foetus, as with all drugs, Xylocaine should not be given during early pregnancy unless the benefits are considered to outweigh the risks.

The addition of adrenaline may potentially decrease uterine blood flow and contractility, especially after inadvertent injection into maternal blood vessels.

Foetal adverse effects due to local anaesthetics, such as foetal bradycardia, seem to be most apparent in paracervical block anaesthesia. Such effects may be due to high concentrations of anaesthetic reaching the foetus.

Lactation

Lidocaine may enter the mother's milk, but in such small amounts that there is generally no risk of this affecting the neonate. It is not known whether adrenaline enters breast milk or not, but it is unlikely to affect the breast-fed child.

4.7 Effects on ability to drive and use machines

Besides the direct anaesthetic affect, local anaesthetics may have a very mild effect on mental function and co-ordination, even in the absence of overt CNS toxicity, and may temporarily impair locomotion and alertness.

4.8 Undesirable effects

In common with other local anaesthetics, adverse reactions to Xylocaine with Adrenaline are rare and are usually the result of excessively high blood concentrations due to inadvertent intravascular injection, excessive dosage, rapid absorption or occasionally to hypersensitivity, idiosyncrasy or diminished tolerance on the part of the patient. In such circumstances systemic effects occur involving the central nervous system and/or the cardiovascular system.

The following table gives a list of the frequencies of undesirable effects:

Common (>1/100 <1/10)	Vascular disorders: Hypotension Gastrointestinal disorders: Nausea Nervous system disorders: paraesthesia, dizziness Cardiac disorders: bradycardia
Uncommon (>1/1000 <1/100)	Nervous system disorders: Signs and symptoms of CNS toxicity (Convulsions, Numbness of tongue and Paraesthesia circumoral, Tinnitus, Tremor, Dysarthria, Hyperacusis, Visual disturbances, CNS depression)
Rare (<1/1000)	Cardiac disorders: Cardiac arrest, Cardiac arrhythmias Immune system disorders: Allergic reactions, Anaphylactic reaction Respiratory disorders: Respiratory depression Nervous system disorders: Neuropathy, peripheral nerve injury, Arachnoiditis Eye disorders: Diplopia

4.9 Overdose

Acute systemic toxicity

Central nervous system toxicity is a graded response with symptoms and signs of escalating severity. The first symptoms are circumoral paraesthesia, numbness of the tongue, light-headedness, hyperacusis and tinnitus. Visual disturbance and muscular tremors are more serious and precede the onset of generalized convulsions. These signs must not be mistaken for neurotic behaviour. Unconsciousness and grand mal convulsions may follow which may last from a few seconds to several minutes. Hypoxia and hypercarbia occur rapidly following convulsions due to the increased muscular activity, together with the interference with normal respiration and loss of the airway. In severe cases apnoea may occur. Acidosis increases the toxic effects of local anaesthetics.

Effects on the cardiovascular system may be seen in severe cases. Hypotension, bradycardia, arrhythmia and even cardiac arrest may occur as a result of high systemic concentrations.

Cardiovascular toxic effects are generally preceded by signs of toxicity in the central nervous system, unless the patient is receiving a general anaesthetic or is heavily sedated with drugs such as a benzodiazepine or barbiturate.

Recovery is due to redistribution of the local anaesthetic drug from the central nervous system and metabolism. Recovery may be rapid unless large amounts of the drug have been injected.

Treatment of acute toxicity

If signs of acute systemic toxicity appear, injection of the local anaesthetic should be immediately stopped.

Treatment will be required if convulsions occur. All drugs and equipment should be immediately available. The objectives of treatment are to maintain oxygenation, stop the convulsions and support the circulation. Oxygen must be given and ventilation assisted if necessary (mask and bag). An anticonvulsant should be given i.v. if the convulsions do not stop spontaneously in 15-20 sec. Thiopentone 1-3 mg/kg i.v. will abort the convulsions rapidly. Alternatively diazepam 0.1 mg/kg i.v. may be used, although its action is slower. Prolonged convulsions may jeopardise the patient's ventilation and oxygenation. If so, injection of a muscle relaxant (eg, suxamethonium 1 mg/kg) will facilitate ventilation, and oxygenation can be controlled. Early endotracheal intubation must be considered in such situations. If cardiovascular depression is evident (hypotension, bradycardia), ephedrine 5-10 mg i.v. should be given and repeated, if necessary, after 2-3 min.

Should circulatory arrest occur, immediate cardiopulmonary resuscitation should be instituted. Continual optimal oxygenation and ventilation and circulatory support as well as treatment of acidosis are of vital importance.

5. PHARMACOLOGICAL PROPERTIES

5.1 Pharmacodynamic properties

ATC code: N01B B52

Lidocaine is a local anaesthetic of the amide type. At high doses lidocaine has a quinidine like action on the myocardium i.e. cardiac depressant. All local anaesthetics stimulate the CNS and may produce anxiety, restlessness and tremors.

5.2 Pharmacokinetic properties

Lidocaine is readily absorbed from the gastro-intestinal tract, from mucous membranes and through damaged skin. It is rapidly absorbed from injection sites including muscle.

Elimination half-life is 2 hours.

Lidocaine undergoes first pass metabolism in the liver.

Less than 10% of a dose is excreted unchanged via the kidneys.

The speed of onset and duration of action of lidocaine are increased by the addition of a vasoconstrictor and absorption into the site of injection is reduced.

5.3 Preclinical safety data

Lidocaine and adrenaline are well-established active ingredients.

In animal studies, the signs and symptoms of toxicity noted after high doses of lidocaine are the results of the effects on the central nervous and cardiovascular systems. No drug related adverse effects were seen in the reproduction toxicity studies, neither did lidocaine show any mutagenic potential in either *in vitro* or *in vivo* mutagenicity tests. Cancer studies have not been performed with lidocaine, due to the area and duration of therapeutic use for this drug.

6. PHARMACEUTICAL PARTICULARS

6.1 List of excipients

Sodium chloride, sodium metabisulphite, methylparahydroxybenzoate, sodium hydroxide, hydrochloric acid and water for injections.

6.2 Incompatibilities

None

6.3 Shelf life

Two years.

Use within 3 days of first opening.

6.4 Special precautions for storage

Store between 2°C and 8°C.

6.5 Nature and contents of container

Multiple dose vials - 20 ml and 50 ml.

6.6 Instructions for use and handling

None

7. MARKETING AUTHORISATION HOLDER

AstraZeneca UK Ltd,

600 Capability Green,

Luton, LU1 3LU, UK.

8. MARKETING AUTHORISATION NUMBER(S)

PL 17901/0175

9. DATE OF FIRST AUTHORISATION/RENEWAL OF THE AUTHORISATION

21st May 2002

10. DATE OF REVISION OF THE TEXT

6th May 2005

Xylocaine 4% Topical

(AstraZeneca UK Limited)

1. NAME OF THE MEDICINAL PRODUCT

Xylocaine 4% Topical

2. QUALITATIVE AND QUANTITATIVE COMPOSITION

Lidocaine Hydrochloride Ph. Eur. 42.8 mg/ml, corresponding to anhydrous lidocaine hydrochloride 40 mg/ml.

For excipients, see 6.1

3. PHARMACEUTICAL FORM

Solution for topical anaesthesia.

4. CLINICAL PARTICULARS

4.1 Therapeutic indications

Anaesthesia of mucous membranes of the oropharyngeal, tracheal and bronchial areas e.g. in bronchography, bronchoscopy, laryngoscopy, oesophagoscopy and endotracheal intubation.

Biopsy in the mouth and throat: Puncture of the maxillary sinus or polypectomy.

Tonsillectomy: Resection of nasal turbinates.

In dentistry: Surface anaesthesia may be achieved by instillation into a cavity or by spraying, e.g. using an atomiser or nebulizer. Xylocaine 4% Topical may also be applied from a swab.

4.2 Posology and method of administration

As with any local anaesthetic, reactions and complications are best averted by employing the minimal effective dosage. Debilitated or elderly patients and children should be given doses commensurate with their age and physical condition.

The degree of absorption from mucous membranes is variable but especially high from the bronchial tree. Application only to areas below the vocal cords may result in excessive plasma concentrations because of less transfer to the intestine and less first-pass loss. When inhaled from a nebulizer, the resulting plasma concentrations are lower than following spray applications.

The Xylocaine 4% Topical solution may be applied from a swab, which should be discarded after use. Surface anaesthesia may also be achieved by instillation into a cavity or on to a surface. When spraying, the solution should be transferred from the original container to an atomiser.

The recommended dosage for adults is 1-7.5 ml Xylocaine 4% Topical (= 40-300 mg lidocaine HCl). Doses exceeding 7.5 ml (= 300 mg lidocaine) may result in plasma levels associated with toxic manifestations. During prolonged procedures (>5 min) up to 400 mg lidocaine may be administered. In addition, when combined with other lidocaine products, the total dose should not exceed 400 mg. With applications mainly to the larynx, trachea and bronchi, the dose should not exceed 5 ml (200 mg lidocaine HCl). When inhaled from a nebulizer, 5-10 ml (200-400 mg lidocaine HCl) may be used.

In children, smaller amounts should be administered depending on their age and weight.

In children less than 12 years the dose should not exceed 3 mg/kg.

Biopsy: 3-4 ml may be sprayed on the area or the solution may be applied for a few minutes with a swab. Adrenaline may be added to this solution in order to produce vasoconstriction (add 1-2 drops, 0.05 ml, 1:1,000 solution to 5 ml Xylocaine 4% Topical).

Puncture of maxillary sinus or polypectomy: A swab soaked in the solution may be applied for two to three minutes. The addition of adrenaline is advised in these procedures, made up as indicated under 'Biopsy' above.

4.3 Contraindications

Known history of hypersensitivity to local anaesthetics of the amide type or other components of the solution.

4.4 Special warnings and special precautions for use

Absorption from wound surfaces and mucous membranes is relatively high, especially in the bronchial tree. Xylocaine 4% Topical should be used with caution in patients with traumatised mucosa and/or sepsis in the region of the proposed application.

If the dose or site of administration is likely to result in high blood levels, lidocaine, in common with other local anaesthetics, should be used with caution in patients with epilepsy, impaired cardiac conduction, bradycardia, impaired hepatic function, severe renal dysfunction and in severe shock. Lidocaine should also be used with caution in the elderly and patients in poor general health.

The oropharyngeal use of topical anaesthetic agents may interfere with swallowing and thus enhance the danger of aspiration. This is particularly important in children because of their frequency of eating. Numbness of the tongue or buccal mucosa may increase the danger of biting trauma.

Patients treated with anti-arrhythmic drugs Class III (e.g. amiodarone) should be kept under close surveillance and ECG monitoring considered, since cardiac effects may be additive.

4.5 Interaction with other medicinal products and other forms of Interaction

Lidocaine should be used with caution in patients receiving other local anaesthetics or agents structurally related to amide-type local anaesthetics, e.g. anti-arrhythmic drugs such as mexiletine, since the toxic effects are additive.

Specific interaction studies with lidocaine and anti-arrhythmic drugs class III (e.g. amiodarone) have not been performed, but caution is advised (see also section 4.4).

4.6 Pregnancy and lactation
There is no or inadequate evidence of safety of the drug in human pregnancy but it has been in wide use for many years without apparent ill consequence, animal studies have shown no hazard. If drug therapy is needed in pregnancy, this drug can be used if there is no safer alternative.

Lidocaine enters the mother's milk, but in such small quantities that there is generally no risk of affecting the child at therapeutic dose levels.

4.7 Effects on ability to drive and use machines
Depending on the dose, local anaesthetics may have a very mild effect on mental function and may temporarily impair locomotion and co-ordination.

4.8 Undesirable effects
In rare cases (<0.1%) amide-type local anaesthetic preparations have been associated with allergic reactions (in the most severe instances anaphylactic shock). Other constituents of the solution e.g. methyl parahydroxybenzoate, may also cause this type of reaction, which may be delayed.

Systemic adverse reactions are rare and may result from high plasma levels due to excessive dosage or rapid absorption or from hypersensitivity, idiosyncrasy or reduced tolerance on the part of the patient. Such reactions involve the central nervous system and/or the cardiovascular system.

CNS reactions are excitatory and/or depressant and may be characterised by nervousness, dizziness, convulsions, unconsciousness and possibly respiratory arrest. The excitatory reactions may be very brief or may not occur at all, in which case the first manifestations of toxicity may be drowsiness, merging into unconsciousness and respiratory arrest.

Cardiovascular reactions are depressant and may be characterised by hypotension, myocardial depression, bradycardia and possibly cardiac arrest.

4.9 Overdose
Acute systemic toxicity

Toxic reactions originate mainly in the central nervous system and the cardiovascular system.

Central nervous system toxicity is a graded response with symptoms and signs of escalating severity. The first symptoms are circumoral paraesthesia, numbness of the tongue, light-headedness, hyperacusis and tinnitus. Visual disturbance and muscular tremors are more serious and precede the onset of generalized convulsions. Unconsciousness and grand mal convulsions may follow, which may last from a few seconds to several minutes. Hypoxia and hypercarbia occur rapidly following convulsions due to the increased muscular activity, together with the interference with normal respiration. In severe cases apnoea may occur. Acidosis increases the toxic effects of local anaesthetics.

Cardiovascular effects are only seen in cases with high systemic concentrations. Severe hypotension, bradycardia, arrhythmia and cardiovascular collapse may be the result in such cases.

Cardiovascular toxic effects are generally preceded by signs of toxicity in the central nervous system, unless the patient is receiving a general anaesthetic or is heavily sedated with drugs such as a benzodiazepine or barbiturate.

Recovery is due to redistribution and metabolism of the local anaesthetic drug from the central nervous system. Recovery may be rapid unless large amounts of the drug have been administered.

Treatment of acute toxicity

The treatment of a patient with toxic manifestations consists of ensuring adequate ventilation and arresting convulsions. Ventilation should be maintained with oxygen by assisted or controlled respiration as required.

An anticonvulsant should be given i.v. if the convulsions do not stop spontaneously in 15-20 sec. Thiopentone sodium 1-3 mg/kg i.v. will abort the convulsions rapidly. Alternatively diazepam 0.1 mg/kg i.v. may be used, although its action is slower. Prolonged convulsions may jeopardise the patient's ventilation and oxygenation. If so, injection of a muscle relaxant (eg suxamethonium 1 mg/kg) will facilitate ventilation, and oxygenation can be controlled. Early endotracheal intubation must be considered in such situations.

If cardiovascular depression is evident (hypotension, bradycardia), ephedrine 5-10 mg i.v. should be given and repeated, if necessary, after 2-3 min.

Should circulatory arrest occur, immediate cardiopulmonary resuscitation should be instituted. Continual optimal oxygenation and ventilation and circulatory support as well as treatment of acidosis are of vital importance, since hypoxia and acidosis will increase the systemic toxicity of local anaesthetics.

Children should be given doses commensurate with their age and weight.

5. PHARMACOLOGICAL PROPERTIES

5.1 Pharmacodynamic properties
ATC code: N01B B02

Lidocaine stabilises the neuronal membrane and prevents the initiation of nerve impulses, thereby affecting local anaesthetic action.

When applied topically to accessible mucous membranes anaesthesia occurs within 1-5 minutes and persists for 15 - 30 minutes.

5.2 Pharmacokinetic properties
Lidocaine is absorbed systemically when applied to mucous membranes; absorption occurs most rapidly after intratracheal administration.

The drug is extensively metabolised in the liver, and metabolites and a small amount of unchanged drug are excreted by the kidneys.

5.3 Preclinical safety data
In animal studies, the toxicity noted after high doses of lidocaine consisted of effects on the central nervous and cardiovascular systems. No drug related adverse effects were seen in the reproduction toxicity studies; neither did lidocaine show any mutagenic potential in either *in vitro* or *in vivo* mutagenicity tests. Cancer studies have not been performed with lidocaine, due to the area and duration of therapeutic use for this drug.

6. PHARMACEUTICAL PARTICULARS

6.1 List of excipients
Methyl parahydroxybenzoate

Sodium hydroxide

Water for injections.

6.2 Incompatibilities
None stated.

6.3 Shelf life
3 years

6.4 Special precautions for storage
Do not store above 25°C. Avoid freezing.

6.5 Nature and contents of container
30ml brown soda glass bottles with pilfer-proof caps.

6.6 Instructions for use and handling
None stated.

7. MARKETING AUTHORISATION HOLDER
AstraZeneca UK Ltd.,

600 Capability Green,

Luton, LU1 3LU, UK.

8. MARKETING AUTHORISATION NUMBER(S)
PL 17901/0176

9. DATE OF FIRST AUTHORISATION/RENEWAL OF THE AUTHORISATION
7th May 2002

10. DATE OF REVISION OF THE TEXT
3rd May 2005

Xylocaine Spray

(AstraZeneca UK Limited)

1. NAME OF THE MEDICINAL PRODUCT
Xylocaine Spray

2. QUALITATIVE AND QUANTITATIVE COMPOSITION
Lidocaine Ph.Eur. 10 mg/dose.

For excipients see 6.1.

3. PHARMACEUTICAL FORM
Topical anaesthetic pump spray.

4. CLINICAL PARTICULARS

4.1 Therapeutic indications
For the prevention of pain associated with the following procedures:

- Otorhinolaryngology

- Puncture of the maxillary sinus and minor surgical procedures in the nasal cavity, pharynx and epipharynx.

- Paracentesis.

Obstetrics

During the final stages of delivery and before episiotomy and perineal suturing as supplementary pain control.

Introduction of instruments and catheters into the respiratory and digestive tract

Provides surface anaesthesia for the oropharyngeal and tracheal areas to reduce reflex activity, attenuate haemodynamic response and to facilitate insertion of the tube or the passage of instruments during endotracheal intubation, laryngoscopy, bronchoscopy and oesophagoscopy.

Dental practice

Before injections, dental impressions, X-ray photography, removal of calculus.

4.2 Posology and method of administration
As with any local anaesthetic, reactions and complications are best averted by employing the minimal effective dosage. Debilitated or elderly patients and children should be given doses commensurate with their age and physical condition.

Xylocaine spray should not be used on cuffs of endotracheal tubes (ETT) made of plastic (See also section 4.4).

Each activation of the metered dose valve delivers 10 mg lidocaine base. It is unnecessary to dry the site prior to application. No more than 20 spray applications should be used in any adult to produce the desired anaesthetic effect.

The number of sprays depend on the extent of the area to be anaesthetised.

- Dental practice

1-5 applications to the mucous membranes.

- Otorhinolaryngology

3 applications for puncture of the maxillary sinus.

- During delivery

Up to 20 applications (200 mg lidocaine base).

- Introduction of instruments and catheters into the respiratory and digestive tract

Up to 20 applications (200 mg lidocaine base) for procedures in pharynx, larynx, and trachea.

4.3 Contraindications
Known history of hypersensitivity to local anaesthetics of the amide type or to other components of the spray solution.

4.4 Special warnings and special precautions for use
Absorption from wound surfaces and mucous membranes is relatively high, especially in the bronchial tree. Xylocaine Spray should be used with caution in patients with traumatised mucosa and/or sepsis in the region of the proposed application.

If the dose or site of administration is likely to result in high blood levels, lidocaine, in common with other local anaesthetics, should be used with caution in patients with epilepsy, cardiovascular disease and heart failure, impaired cardiac conduction, bradycardia, severe renal dysfunction, impaired hepatic function and in severe shock. Lidocaine should also be used with caution in the elderly and patients in poor general health.

In paralysed patients under general anaesthesia, higher blood concentrations may occur than in spontaneously breathing patients. Unparalysed patients are more likely to swallow a large proportion of the dose which then undergoes considerable first-pass hepatic metabolism following absorption from the gut.

The oropharyngeal use of topical anaesthetic agents may interfere with swallowing and thus enhance the danger of aspiration. This is particularly important in children because of their frequency of eating. Numbness of the tongue or buccal mucosa may increase the danger of biting trauma.

Avoid contact with the eyes.

Patients treated with anti-arrhythmic drugs class III (e.g. amiodarone) should be under close surveillance and ECG monitoring considered, since cardiac effects may be additive.

Xylocaine spray should not be used on cuffs of endotracheal tubes (ETT) made of plastic. Lidocaine base in contact with both PVC and non-PVC cuffs of endotracheal tubes may cause damage of the cuff. This damage is described as pinholes, which may cause leakage that could lead to pressure loss in the cuff.

4.5 Interaction with other medicinal products and other forms of Interaction
Lidocaine should be used with caution in patients receiving other local anaesthetics or agents structurally related to amide-type local anaesthetics eg anti-arrhythmic drugs such as mexiletine, since the toxic effects are additive.

Specific interaction studies with lidocaine and anti-arrhythmic drugs class III (e.g. amiodarone) have not been performed, but caution is advised (see also section 4.4)

4.6 Pregnancy and lactation
There is no or inadequate evidence of safety of the drug in human pregnancy but it has been in wide use for many years without apparent ill consequence, animal studies have shown no hazard. If drug therapy is needed in pregnancy, this drug can be used if there is no safer alternative.

Lidocaine enters the mother's milk, but in such small quantities that there is generally no risk of the child being affected at therapeutic dose levels.

4.7 Effects on ability to drive and use machines
Depending on the dose, local anaesthetics may have a very mild effect on mental function and may temporarily impair locomotion and co-ordination.

4.8 Undesirable effects
In extremely rare cases amide type local anaesthetic preparations have been associated with allergic reactions (in the most severe instances anaphylactic shock).

Local irritation at the application site has been described. Following application to laryngeal mucosa before endotracheal intubation, reversible symptoms such as "sore throat", "hoarseness" and "loss of voice" have been reported. The use of Xylocaine pump spray provides surface anaesthesia during an endotracheal procedure but does not prevent post-intubation soreness.

Systemic adverse reactions are rare and may result from high plasma levels due to excessive dosage or rapid absorption (eg following application to areas below the vocal chords) or from hypersensitivity, idiosyncrasy or reduced tolerance on the part of the patient. Such reactions involve the central nervous system and/or the cardiovascular system.

CNS reactions are excitatory and/or depressant and may be characterised by nervousness, dizziness, convulsions, unconsciousness and possibly respiratory arrest. The excitatory reactions may be very brief or may not occur at all, in which case the first manifestations of toxicity may be drowsiness, merging into unconsciousness and respiratory arrest.

Cardiovascular reactions are depressant and may be characterised by hypotension, myocardial depression, bradycardia and possibly cardiac arrest.

4.9 Overdose

Acute systemic toxicity

Toxic reactions originate mainly in the central nervous and the cardiovascular systems.

Central nervous system toxicity is a graded response with symptoms and signs of escalating severity. The first symptoms are circumoral paraesthesia, numbness of the tongue, light-headedness, hyperacusis and tinnitus. Visual disturbance and muscular tremors are more serious and precede the onset of generalized convulsions. Unconsciousness and grand mal convulsions may follow, which may last from a few seconds to several minutes. Hypoxia and hypercarbia occur rapidly following convulsions due to the increased muscular activity, together with the interference with normal respiration. In severe cases apnoea may occur. Acidosis increases the toxic effects of local anaesthetics.

Cardiovascular effects are only seen in cases with high systemic concentrations. Severe hypotension, bradycardia, arrhythmia and cardiovascular collapse may be the result in such cases.

Cardiovascular toxic effects are generally preceded by signs of toxicity in the central nervous system, unless the patient is receiving a general anaesthetic or is heavily sedated with drugs such as a benzodiazepine or barbiturate.

Recovery is due to redistribution and metabolism of the local anaesthetic drug from the central nervous system. Recovery may be rapid unless large amounts of the drug have been administered.

Treatment of acute toxicity

The treatment of a patient with toxic manifestations consists of ensuring adequate ventilation and arresting convulsions. Ventilation should be maintained with oxygen by assisted or controlled respiration as required.

An anticonvulsant should be given i.v. if the convulsions do not stop spontaneously in 15-30 sec. Thiopentone sodium 1-3 mg/kg iv will abort the convulsions rapidly. Alternatively diazepam 0.1 mg/kg body-weight iv may be used, although its action will be slow. Prolonged convulsions may jeopardise the patient's ventilation and oxygenation. If so, injection of a muscle relaxant (e.g. succinylcholine 1 mg/kg body-weight) will facilitate ventilation, and oxygenation can be controlled. Early endotracheal intubation must be considered in such situations.

If cardiovascular depression is evident (hypotension, bradycardia), ephedrine 5-10 mg i.v. should be given and repeated, if necessary, after 2-3 min.

Should circulatory arrest occur, immediate cardiopulmonary resuscitation should be instituted. Optimal oxygenation and ventilation and circulatory support as well as treatment of acidosis are of vital importance, since hypoxia and acidosis will increase the systemic toxicity of local anaesthetics.

Children should be given doses commensurate with their age and weight.

5. PHARMACOLOGICAL PROPERTIES

5.1 Pharmacodynamic properties

ATC code: N01B B02

Lidocaine, like other local anaesthetics, causes a reversible blockade of impulse propagation along nerve fibres by preventing the inward movement of sodium ions through the nerve membrane. Local anaesthetics of the amide type are thought to act within the sodium channels of the nerve membrane.

Local anaesthetic drugs may also have similar effects on excitable membranes in the brain and myocardium. If excessive amounts of drug reach the systemic circulation rapidly, symptoms and signs of toxicity will appear, emanating from the central nervous and cardiovascular systems.

Central nervous system toxicity usually precedes the cardiovascular effects since it occurs at lower plasma concentrations. Direct effects of local anaesthetics on the heart include slow conduction, negative inotropism and eventually cardiac arrest.

5.2 Pharmacokinetic properties

Lidocaine is absorbed following topical administration to mucous membranes, its rate and extent of absorption being dependent upon the concentration and total dose administered, the specific site of application, and duration of exposure. In general, the rate of absorption of local anaesthetic agents following topical application is most rapid after intratracheal and bronchial administration. Lidocaine is also well-absorbed from the gastrointestinal tract, although little of the intact drug appears in the circulation because of biotransformation in the liver.

The plasma protein binding of lidocaine is dependent on the drug concentration, and the fraction bound decreases with increasing concentration. At concentrations of 1 to 4 μg of free base per ml, 60 to 80 percent of lidocaine is protein-bound. Binding is also dependent on the plasma concentration of the alpha-1-acid glycoprotein.

Lidocaine crosses the blood-brain and placental barriers, presumably by passive diffusion.

Lidocaine is metabolised rapidly by the liver, and metabolites and unchanged drug are excreted by the kidneys. Biotransformation includes oxidative N-dealkylation, ring hydroxylation, cleavage of the amide linkage and conjugation. N-dealkylation, a major pathway of biotransformation, yields the metabolites monoethylglycinexylidide and glycinexylidide. The pharmacological/toxicological actions of these metabolites are similar to, but less potent than, those of lidocaine. Approximately 90% of lidocaine administered is excreted in the form of various metabolites, and less than 10% is excreted unchanged. The primary metabolite in urine is a conjugate of 4-hydroxy-2,6-dimethylaniline.

The elimination half-life of lidocaine following an intravenous bolus injection is typically 1.5 to 2.0 hours. Because of the rapid rate at which lidocaine is metabolised, any condition that affects liver function may alter lidocaine kinetics. The half-life may be prolonged two-fold or more in patients with liver dysfunction. Renal dysfunction does not affect lidocaine kinetics but may increase the accumulation of metabolites.

Factors such as acidosis and the use of CNS stimulants and depressants affect the CNS levels of lidocaine required to produce overt systemic effects. Objective adverse manifestations become increasingly apparent with increasing venous plasma levels above 6.0 μg free base per ml.

5.3 Preclinical safety data

Lidocaine is a well established active ingredient.

6. PHARMACEUTICAL PARTICULARS

6.1 List of excipients

Ethanol, Macrogol 400, Essence of Banana, Menthol natural, Saccharin and Water purified.

6.2 Incompatibilities

None known.

6.3 Shelf life

3 years.

6.4 Special precautions for storage

Do not store above 25°C. During storage at temperatures below +8°C precipitation may occur. The precipitate dissolves on warming up to room temperature.

6.5 Nature and contents of container

50 ml spray bottles (approx. 500 spray doses) with a metering valve with applicator.

Each depression of the metered valve delivers 10 mg lidocaine base. The contents of the spray bottles are sufficient to provide approximately 500 sprays.

6.6 Instructions for use and handling

The spray nozzle is bent to ensure correct spray function. Do not try to alter the shape as this could affect its performance.

The nozzle must not be shortened, as it will affect the spray function.

To clean the nozzle, submerge in boiling water for 5 minutes.

7. MARKETING AUTHORISATION HOLDER

AstraZeneca UK Ltd.,

600 Capability Green,

Luton, LU1 3LU, UK.

8. MARKETING AUTHORISATION NUMBER(S)

PL 17901/0177

9. DATE OF FIRST AUTHORISATION/RENEWAL OF THE AUTHORISATION

7th May 2002

10. DATE OF REVISION OF THE TEXT

17th June 2004

Xyloproct Ointment

(AstraZeneca UK Limited)

1. NAME OF THE MEDICINAL PRODUCT

Xyloproct Ointment

2. QUALITATIVE AND QUANTITATIVE COMPOSITION

Composition for: 1g:

Lidocaine 50mg

Hydrocortisone Acetate micro Ph. Eur. 2.75mg

For excipients, see 6.1

3. PHARMACEUTICAL FORM

Rectal ointment.

White to slightly yellowish.

4. CLINICAL PARTICULARS

4.1 Therapeutic indications

For the relief of symptoms such as anal and peri-anal pruritus, pain and inflammation associated with haemorrhoids, anal fissure, fistulas and proctitis. Pruritus vulva.

4.2 Posology and method of administration

Route of administration: Topical.

To be applied several times daily according to the severity of the condition. For intrarectal use, apply the ointment with the special applicator. Cleanse the applicator thoroughly after use.

A daily dose of 6g ointment is well within safety limits. The duration of treatment may vary between ten days and three weeks. If the treatment is prolonged, a free interval can be recommended, especially if it is suspected that irritation due to lidocaine or hydrocortisone has occurred. If the local irritation disappears after the cessation of treatment, the possibility of sensitivity to lidocaine or hydrocortisone can be investigated, e.g. by a patch test.

Debilitated or elderly patients and children should be given doses commensurate with their age, weight and physical condition.

4.3 Contraindications

Known hypersensitivity to local anaesthetics of the amide type or any of the other ingredients. Use on atrophic skin. Xyloproct Ointment should not be used in patients with untreated infections of bacterial, viral, pathogenic fungal or parasitic origin.

4.4 Special warnings and special precautions for use

Xyloproct is intended for use for limited periods. Excessive dosage of lidocaine or short intervals between doses, may result in high plasma levels of lidocaine and serious adverse effects. Patients should be instructed to strictly adhere to recommended dosage.

Appropriate antibacterial, antiviral or antifungal therapy should be given with Xyloproct if infection is present at the site of application.

The possibility of malignancy should be excluded before use.

If irritation or rectal bleeding develops treatment should be discontinued.

When using the special applicator, care should be taken to avoid instillation of excessive amounts of Xyloproct Ointment into the rectum. This is of particular importance in infants and children.

Systemic absorption of lidocaine may occur from the rectum, and large doses may result in CNS side-effects. On rare occasions convulsions have occurred in children.

Prolonged and excessive use of hydrocortisone use may produce systemic corticosteroid effects or local effects such as skin atrophy. With the recommended dosage systemic effects of hydrocortisone are unlikely.

4.5 Interaction with other medicinal products and other forms of Interaction

Lidocaine should be used with caution in patients receiving antiarrhythmic drugs, since the toxic effects are additive.

4.6 Pregnancy and lactation

Do not use in pregnancy unless considered essential by the physician.

Lidocaine and hydrocortisone acetate are excreted into breast milk but in such small quantities that adverse effects on the child are unlikely at therapeutic doses.

4.7 Effects on ability to drive and use machines

Depending on the dose local anaesthetics may have a very mild effect on mental function and coordination even in the absence of overt CNS toxicity and may temporarily impair locomotion and alertness. With the recommended doses of Xyloproct adverse effects on the CNS are unlikely.

4.8 Undesirable effects

Contact sensitivity to lidocaine has been reported after perianal use. Contact sensitivity may also occur after the use of topical hydrocortisone. In extremely rare cases amide-type local anaesthetic preparations have been associated with allergic reactions (in the most severe instances anaphylactic shock).

4.9 Overdose

When using the special applicator care should be taken to avoid instillation of excessive amounts of Xyloproct Ointment into the rectum. This is of particular importance in infants and children.

Systemic absorption of lidocaine may occur from the rectum, and large doses may result in CNS side effects. On rare occasions convulsions have occurred in children.

5. PHARMACOLOGICAL PROPERTIES

5.1 Pharmacodynamic properties

ATC code: C05A A01

Lidocaine exerts a local anaesthetic effect by stabilising the neural membrane and preventing the initiation and conduction of nerve impulses.

Hydrocortisone acetate belongs to the mild group of corticosteroids and is effective because of its anti-inflammatory and anti-pruritic action.

5.2 Pharmacokinetic properties

The onset of action of lidocaine is 3 - 5 minutes on mucous membranes. Lidocaine can be absorbed following application to mucous membranes with metabolism taking place in the liver. Metabolites and unchanged drug are excreted in the urine.

Absorption of hydrocortisone may occur from normal intact skin and mucous membranes. Corticosteroids are metabolised mainly in the liver but also in the kidney, and are excreted in the urine.

5.3 Preclinical safety data

Lidocaine and hydrocortisone acetate are well established active ingredients.

6. PHARMACEUTICAL PARTICULARS

6.1 List of excipients

Zinc oxide

Aluminium acetate

Stearyl alcohol

Cetyl alcohol

Water purified

Macrogol (3350 and 400)

6.2 Incompatibilities

None known

6.3 Shelf life

The shelf-life of this product is 2 years when stored between 2°C and 8°C and 2 months when stored up to 25°C.

6.4 Special precautions for storage

Store at 2°C-8°C (in a refrigerator). The patient may store the product at temperatures up to 25°C for 2 months whilst in use. The remaining ointment should then be discarded.

6.5 Nature and contents of container

Aluminium tube 20g.

6.6 Instructions for use and handling

None

7. MARKETING AUTHORISATION HOLDER

AstraZeneca UK Ltd.,

600 Capability Green,

Luton,

LU1 3LU,

UK.

8. MARKETING AUTHORISATION NUMBER(S)

PL 17901/0179

9. DATE OF FIRST AUTHORISATION/RENEWAL OF THE AUTHORISATION

18th March 2002 / 17th September 2002

10. DATE OF REVISION OF THE TEXT

25th November 2003

Xyzal 5 mg film-coated Tablets

(UCB Pharma Limited)

1. NAME OF THE MEDICINAL PRODUCT

▼Xyzal 5 mg film-coated tablets.

2. QUALITATIVE AND QUANTITATIVE COMPOSITION

Each film-coated tablet contains 5 mg levocetirizine dihydrochloride.

For excipients, see 6.1.

3. PHARMACEUTICAL FORM

Film-coated tablet.

White to off-white, oval, film-coated tablet with a Y logo on one side.

4. CLINICAL PARTICULARS

4.1 Therapeutic indications

Symptomatic treatment of allergic rhinitis (including persistent allergic rhinitis) and chronic idiopathic urticaria.

4.2 Posology and method of administration

The film-coated tablet must be taken orally, swallowed whole with liquid and may be taken with or without food. It is recommended to take the daily dose in one single intake.

Adults and adolescents 12 years and above:

The daily recommended dose is 5 mg (1 film-coated tablet).

Elderly:

Adjustment of the dose is recommended in elderly patients with moderate to severe renal impairment (see Patients with renal impairment below).

Children aged 6 to 12 years:

The daily recommended dose is 5 mg (1 film-coated tablet).

For children aged less than 6 years no adjusted dosage is yet possible.

Patients with renal impairment:

The dosing intervals must be individualized according to renal function. Refer to the following table and adjust the dose as indicated. To use this dosing table, an estimate of the patient's creatinine clearance (CL_{cr}) in ml/min is needed. The CL_{cr} (ml/min) may be estimated from serum creatinine (mg/dl) determination using the following formula:

$$\frac{[140 - age(years)]\, x\, weight\ (kg)}{72\, x\, serum\, creatinine\ (mg/dl)}\ (x\, 0.85\ for\ women)$$

Dosing Adjustments for Patients with Impaired Renal Function:

Group	Creatinine clearance (ml/min)	Dosage and frequency
Normal	≥80	1 tablet once daily
Mild	50 – 79	1 tablet once daily
Moderate	30 – 49	1 tablet once every 2 days
Severe	< 30	1 tablet once every 3 days
End-stage renal disease - Patients undergoing dialysis	< 10-	Contra-indicated

Patients with hepatic impairment:

No dose adjustment is needed in patients with solely hepatic impairment. In patients with hepatic impairment and renal impairment, adjustment of the dose is recommended (see Patients with renal impairment above).

Duration of use:

The duration of use depends on the type, duration and course of the complaints. For hay fever 3-6 weeks, and in case of short-term pollen exposure as little as one week, is generally sufficient. Clinical experience with 5 mg levocetirizine as a film-coated tablet formulation is currently available for a 6-month treatment period. For chronic urticaria and chronic allergic rhinitis, up to one year's clinical experience is available for the racemate, and up to 18 months in patients with pruritus associated with atopic dermatitis.

4.3 Contraindications

History of hypersensitivity to levocetirizine or any of the other constituents of the formulation or to any piperazine derivatives.

Patients with severe renal impairment at less than 10 ml/min creatinine clearance.

4.4 Special warnings and special precautions for use

The use of Xyzal is not recommended in children aged less than 6 years since the currently available film-coated tablets do not yet allow dose adaptation.

Precaution is recommended with intake of alcohol (see Interactions).

Patients with rare hereditary problems of galactose intolerance, the Lapp lactase deficiency or glucose-galactose malabsorption should not take this medicine.

4.5 Interaction with other medicinal products and other forms of Interaction

No interaction studies have been performed with levocetirizine (including no studies with CYP3A4 inducers); studies with the racemate compound cetirizine demonstrated that there were no clinically relevant adverse interactions (with pseudoephedrine, cimetidine, ketoconazole, erythromycin, azithromycin, glipizide and diazepam). A small decrease in the clearance of cetirizine (16%) was observed in a multiple dose study with theophylline (400 mg once a day); while the disposition of theophylline was not altered by concomitant cetirizine administration.

The extent of absorption of levocetirizine is not reduced with food, although the rate of absorption is decreased.

In sensitive patients the simultaneous administration of cetirizine or levocetirizine and alcohol or other CNS depressants may have effects on the central nervous system, although it has been shown that the racemate cetirizine does not potentiate the effect of alcohol.

4.6 Pregnancy and lactation

For levocetirizine no clinical data on exposed pregnancies are available. Animal studies do not indicate direct or indirect harmful effects with respect to pregnancy, embyonal/fetal development, parturition or postnatal development. Caution should be exercised when prescribing to pregnant or lactating women.

4.7 Effects on ability to drive and use machines

Comparative clinical trials have revealed no evidence that levocetirizine at the recommended dose impairs mental alertness, reactivity or the ability to drive. Nevertheless, some patients could experience somnolence, fatigue and asthenia under therapy with Xyzal. Therefore, patients intending to drive, engage in potentially hazardous activities or operate machinery should take their response to the medicinal product into account.

4.8 Undesirable effects

In therapeutic studies in women and men aged 12 to 71 years, 15.1% of the patients in the levocetirizine 5 mg group had at least one adverse drug reaction compared to 11.3% in the placebo group. 91.6 % of these adverse drug reactions were mild to moderate.

In therapeutic trials, the drop out rate due to adverse events was 1.0% (9/935) with levocetirizine 5 mg and 1.8% (14/771) with placebo.

Clinical therapeutic trials with levocetirizine included 935 subjects exposed to the drug at the recommended dose of 5 mg daily. From this pooling, the following incidence of adverse drug reactions were reported at rates of 1 % or greater (common: >1/100, <1/10) under levocetirizine 5 mg or placebo:

Preferred Term (WHOART)	Placebo (n =771)	Levocetirizine 5 mg (n = 935)
Headache	25 (3.2 %)	24 (2.6 %)
Somnolence	11 (1.4 %)	49 (5.2 %)
Mouth dry	12 (1.6%)	24 (2.6%)
Fatigue	9 (1.2 %)	23 (2.5 %)

Further uncommon incidences of adverse reactions (uncommon >1/1000, <1/100) like asthenia or abdominal pain were observed.

The incidence of sedating adverse drug reactions such as somnolence, fatigue, and asthenia was altogether more common (8.1 %) under levocetirizine 5 mg than under placebo (3.1%).

In addition to the adverse reactions reported during clinical studies and listed above, very rare cases of the following adverse drug reactions have been reported in post-marketing experience.

Immune system disorders: hypersensitivity including anaphylaxis

Respiratory, thoracic, and mediastinal disorders: dyspnoea

Gastrointestinal disorders: nausea

Skin and subcutaneous tissue disorders: angioneurotic oedema, pruritus, rash, urticaria

Investigations: weight increased

4.9 Overdose

a) Symptoms

Symptoms of overdose may include drowsiness in adults and initially agitation and restlessness, followed by drowsiness in children.

b) Management of overdoses

There is no known specific antidote to levocetirizine.

Should overdose occur, symptomatic or supportive treatment is recommended. Gastric lavage should be considered following short-term ingestion. Levocetirizine is not effectively removed by haemodialysis.

5. PHARMACOLOGICAL PROPERTIES

5.1 Pharmacodynamic properties

Pharmacotherapeutic group: antihistamine for systemic use, piperazine derivative, ATC code: R06A E09.

Levocetirizine, the (R) enantiomer of cetirizine, is a potent and selective antagonist of peripheral H_1-receptors.

Binding studies revealed that levocetirizine has high affinity for human H_1-receptors (Ki = 3.2 nmol/l). Levocetirizine has an affinity 2-fold higher than that of cetirizine (Ki = 6.3 nmol/l). Levocetirizine dissociates from H_1-receptors with a half-life of 115 ± 38 min.

Pharmacodynamic studies in healthy volunteers demonstrate that, at half the dose, levocetirizine has comparable activity to cetirizine, both in the skin and in the nose.

In vitro studies (Boyden chambers and cell layers techniques) show that levocetirizine inhibits eotaxin-induced eosinophil transendothelial migration through both dermal and lung cells. A pharmacodynamic experimental study *in vivo* (skin chamber technique) showed three main inhibitory effects of levocetirizine 5 mg in the first 6 hours of pollen-induced reaction, compared with placebo in 14 adult patients: inhibition of VCAM-1 release, modulation of vascular permeability and a decrease in eosinophil recruitment.

The efficacy and safety of levocetirizine has been demonstrated in several double-blind, placebo controlled, clinical trials performed in patients suffering from seasonal allergic rhinitis or perennial allergic rhinitis.

A 6-month clinical study in 551 patients (including 276 levocetirizine-treated patients) suffering from persistent allergic rhinitis (symptoms present 4 days a week for at least 4 consecutive weeks) and sensitized to house dust mites and grass pollen demonstrated that levocetirizine 5 mg was clinically and statistically significantly more potent than placebo on the relief from the total symptom score of allergic rhinitis throughout the whole duration of the study, without any tachyphylaxis. During the whole duration of the study, levocetirizine significantly improved the quality of life of the patients.

Pharmacokinetic / pharmacodynamic relationship:

5 mg levocetirizine provide a similar pattern of inhibition of histamine-induced wheal and flare to 10 mg cetirizine. As for cetirizine, the action on histamine-induced skin reactions was out of phase with the plasma concentrations.

ECGs did not show relevant effects of levocetirizine on QT interval.

5.2 Pharmacokinetic properties

The pharmacokinetics of levocetirizine are linear with dose- and time-independent with low inter-subject variability. The pharmacokinetic profile is the same when given as the single enantiomer or when given as cetirizine. No chiral inversion occurs during the process of absorption and elimination.

Absorption:

Levocetirizine is rapidly and extensively absorbed following oral administration. Peak plasma concentrations are achieved 0.9 h after dosing. Steady state is achieved after two days. Peak concentrations are typically 270 ng/ml and 308 ng/ml following a single and a repeated 5 mg o.d. dose, respectively. The extent of absorption is dose-independent and is not altered by food, but the peak concentration is reduced and delayed.

Distribution:

No tissue distribution data are available in humans, neither concerning the passage of levocetirizine throughthe blood-brain-barrier. In rats and dogs, the highest tissue levels are found in liver and kidneys, the lowest in the CNS compartment.

Levocetirizine is 90% bound to plasma proteins. The distribution of levocetirizine is restrictive, as the volume of distribution is 0.4 l/kg.

Biotransformation:

The extent of metabolism of levocetirizine in humans is less than 14% of the dose and therefore differences resulting from genetic polymorphism or concomitant intake of enzyme inhibitors are expected to be negligible. Metabolic pathways include aromatic oxidation, N- and O- dealkylation and taurine conjugation. Dealkylation pathways are primarily mediated by CYP 3A4 while aromatic oxidation involved multiple and/or unidentified CYP isoforms. Levocetirizine had no effect on the activities of CYP isoenzymes 1A2, 2C9, 2C19, 2D6, 2E1 and 3A4 at concentrations well above peak concentrations achieved following a 5 mg oral dose.

Due to its low metabolism and absence of metabolic inhibition potential, the interaction of levocetirizine with other substances, or vice-versa, is unlikely.

Elimination:

The plasma half-life in adults is 7.9 ± 1.9 hours. The mean apparent total body clearance is 0.63 ml/min/kg. The major route of excretion of levocetirizine and metabolites is via urine, accounting for a mean of 85.4% of the dose. Excretion via feces accounts for only 12.9% of the dose. Levocetirizine is excreted both by glomerular filtration and active tubular secretion.

Renal impairment:

The apparent body clearance of levocetirizine is correlated to the creatinine clearance. It is therefore recommended to adjust the dosing intervals of levocetirizine, based on creatinine clearance in patients with moderate and severe renal impairment. In anuric end stage renal disease subjects, the total body clearance is decreased by approximately 80% when compared to normal subjects. The amount of levocetirizine removed during a standard 4-hour hemodialysis procedure was < 10%.

5.3 Preclinical safety data

Preclinical data reveal no special hazard for humans based on conventional studies of safety pharmacology, repeated dose toxicity, toxicity to reproduction, genotoxicity or carcinogenicity

6. PHARMACEUTICAL PARTICULARS

6.1 List of excipients

Core:

Microcrystalline cellulose

Lactose monohydrate

Colloidal anhydrous silica

Magnesium stearate

Coating:

Opadry® Y-1-7000 consisting of:

Hypromellose (E464)

Titanium dioxide (E 171)

Macrogol 400

6.2 Incompatibilities

Not applicable.

6.3 Shelf life

Three years.

6.4 Special precautions for storage

No special precaution for storage.

6.5 Nature and contents of container

Aluminium – OPA/aluminium/PVCblister

Pack sizes of 1, 2, 4, 5, 7, 10, 2 × 10, 10 × 10, 14, 15, 20, 21, 28, 30 40, 50, 60, 70, 90, 100.

Not all pack sizes may be marketed.

6.6 Instructions for use and handling

No special requirements.

7. MARKETING AUTHORISATION HOLDER

UCB Pharma Ltd

3 George Street

Watford

Hertfordshire, WD18 0UH

8. MARKETING AUTHORISATION NUMBER(S)

PL 08972/0036

9. DATE OF FIRST AUTHORISATION/RENEWAL OF THE AUTHORISATION

3 January 2001

10. DATE OF REVISION OF THE TEXT

13 April 2005

11. Legal category

POM

Yasmin film-coated tablets

(Schering Health Care Limited)

1. NAME OF THE MEDICINAL PRODUCT
Yasmin film-coated tablets

2. QUALITATIVE AND QUANTITATIVE COMPOSITION
Each tablet contains 3 mg drospirenone and 30 micrograms ethinylestradiol.

For excipients, see 6.1

3. PHARMACEUTICAL FORM
Film-coated tablet

Light yellow, round tablet with convex faces, one side embossed with the letters "DO" in a regular hexagon

4. CLINICAL PARTICULARS

4.1 Therapeutic indications
Oral contraception

4.2 Posology and method of administration

How to take Yasmin

The tablets must be taken every day at about the same time, if necessary with a little liquid, in the order shown on the blister pack. One tablet is to be taken daily for 21 consecutive days. Each subsequent pack is started after a 7-day tablet-free interval, during which time a withdrawal bleed usually occurs. This usually starts on day 2-3 after the last tablet and may not have finished before the next pack is started.

How to start Yasmin

• No preceding hormonal contraceptive use (in the past month)

Tablet-taking has to start on day 1 of the woman's natural cycle (i.e. the first day of her menstrual bleeding).

• Changing from another combined oral contraceptive (COC)

The woman should start with Yasmin on the day following the usual tablet-free or placebo tablet interval of her previous COC.

• Changing from a progestogen-only-method (minipill, injection, implant)

The woman may switch any day from the minipill (from an implant on the day of its removal, from an injectable when the next injection would be due).

• Following first-trimester abortion

The woman may start immediately. When doing so, she need not take additional contraceptive measures.

• Following delivery or second-trimester abortion

Women should be advised to start at day 21 to 28 after delivery or second-trimester abortion. When starting later, the woman should be advised to additionally use a barrier method for the first 7 days. However, if intercourse has already occurred, pregnancy should be excluded before the actual start of COC use or the woman has to wait for her first menstrual period.

For breastfeeding women see Section 4.6

Management of missed tablets

If the user is **less than 12 hours** late in taking any tablet, contraceptive protection is not reduced. The woman should take the tablet as soon as she remembers and should take further tablets at the usual time.

If she is **more than 12 hours** late in taking any tablet, contraceptive protection may be reduced. The management of missed tablets can be guided by the following two basic rules:

1. tablet-taking must never be discontinued for longer than 7 days

2. 7 days of uninterrupted tablet-taking are required to attain adequate suppression of the hypothalamic-pituitary-ovarian-axis.

Accordingly the following advice can be given in daily practice:

• Week 1

The user should take the last missed tablet as soon as she remembers, even if this means taking two tablets at the same time. She then continues to take tablets at her usual time. In addition, a barrier method such as a condom should be used for the next 7 days. If intercourse took place in the preceding 7 days, the possibility of a pregnancy should be considered. The more tablets are missed and the closer they are to the regular tablet-free interval, the higher the risk of a pregnancy.

• Week 2

The user should take the last missed tablet as soon as she remembers, even if this means taking two tablets at the same time. She then continues to take tablets at her usual time. Provided that the woman has taken her tablets correctly in the 7 days preceding the first missed tablet, there is no need to use extra contraceptive precautions. However, if she has missed more than 1 tablet, the woman should be advised to use extra precautions for 7 days.

• Week 3

The risk of reduced reliability is imminent because of the forthcoming 7 day tablet-free interval. However, by adjusting the tablet-intake schedule, reduced contraceptive protection can still be prevented. By adhering to either of the following two options, there is therefore no need to use extra contraceptive precautions, provided that in the 7 days preceding the first missed tablet the woman has taken all tablets correctly. If this is not the case, she should follow the first of these two options and use extra precautions for the next 7 days as well.

1. The user should take the last missed tablet as soon as she remembers, even if this means taking two tablets at the same time. She then continues to take tablets at her usual time. The next blister pack must be started as soon as the current blister pack is finished, i.e., no gap should be left between packs. The user is unlikely to have a withdrawal bleed until the end of the second pack, but she may experience spotting or breakthrough bleeding on tablet-taking days.

2. The woman may also be advised to discontinue tablet-taking from the current blister pack. She should then have a tablet-free interval of up to 7 days, including the days she missed tablets, and subsequently continue with the next blister pack.

If the woman missed tablets and subsequently has no withdrawal bleed in the first normal tablet-free interval, the possibility of a pregnancy should be considered.

Advice in case of vomiting or severe diarrhoea

If vomiting or severe diarrhoeaoccur within 3-4 hours after tablet-taking, absorption may not be complete. In such events, a new tablet should be taken as soon as possible. If more than 12 hours elapse, the advice concerning missed tablets, as given in Section 4.2 "Management of missed tablets", is applicable. If the woman does not want to change her normal tablet-taking schedule, she has to take the extra tablet(s) from another blister pack.

How to postpone a withdrawal bleed

To delay a period the woman should continue with another blister pack of Yasmin without a tablet-free interval. The extension can be carried on for as long as wished until the end of the second pack. During the extension the woman may experience breakthrough-bleeding or spotting. Regular intake of Yasmin is then resumed after the usual 7-day tablet-free interval.

To shift her periods to another day of the week than the woman is used to with her current scheme, she can be advised to shorten her forthcoming tablet-free interval by as many days as she likes. The shorter the interval, the higher the risk that she does not have a withdrawal bleed and will experience breakthrough-bleeding and spotting during the subsequent pack (just as when delaying a period).

4.3 Contraindications

Combined oral contraceptives (COCs) should not be used in the presence of any of the conditions listed below. Should any of the conditions appear for the first time during COC use, the product should be stopped immediately.

• Venous thrombosis presence or in history (deep venous thrombosis, pulmonary embolism).

• Arterial thrombosis presence or in history (e.g. cerebrovascular accident, myocardial infarction) or prodromal conditions (e.g. angina pectoris and transient ischaemic attack).

• The presence of a severe or multiple risk factor(s) for arterial thrombosis:

• diabetes mellitus with vascular symptoms

• severe hypertension

• severe dyslipoproteinaemia

• Hereditary or acquired predisposition for venous or arterial thrombosis, such as APC-resistance, antithrombin-III-deficiency, protein C deficiency, protein S deficiency, hyperhomocysteinaemia and antiphospholipid-antibodies (anticardiolipin-antibodies, lupus anticoagulant).

• Presence or history of severe hepatic disease as long as liver function values have not returned to normal.

• Severe renal insufficiency or acute renal failure.

• Presence or history of liver tumours (benign or malignant).

• Known or suspected malignant conditions of the genital organs or the breasts, if sex steroid-influenced.

• Undiagnosed vaginal bleeding.

• History of migraine with focal neurological symptoms.

• Hypersensitivity to the active substances or to any of the excipients of Yasmin film-coated tablets.

4.4 Special warnings and special precautions for use

Warnings

If any of the conditions/risk factors mentioned below is present, the benefits of COC use should be weighed against the possible risks for each individual woman and discussed with the woman before she decides to start using it. In the event of aggravation, exacerbation or first appearance of any of these conditions or risk factors, the woman should contact her physician. The physician should then decide on whether its use should be discontinued.

• Vascular Disorders

Epidemiological studies have shown that the incidence of VTE in users of oral contraceptives with low oestrogen content (<50 μg ethinylestradiol) (including Yasmin) ranges from about 20 to 40 cases per 100,000 women-years, but this risk estimate varies according to the progestogen. This compares with 5 to 10 cases per 100,000 women-years for non-users.

The use of any combined oral contraceptive carries an increased risk of venous thromboembolism (VTE) compared with no use. The excess risk of VTE is highest during the first year a woman ever uses a combined oral contraceptive. This increased risk is less than the risk of VTE associated with pregnancy, which is estimated as 60 cases per 100,000 pregnancies. VTE is fatal in 1-2% of cases.

Epidemiological studies have also associated the use of COCs with an increased risk for arterial (myocardial infarction, transient ischaemic attack) thromboembolism.

Extremely rarely, thrombosis has been reported to occur in other blood vessels, e.g. hepatic, mesenteric, renal or retinal veins and arteries, in contraceptive pill users. There is no consensus as to whether the occurrence of these events is associated with the use of hormonal contraceptives.

Symptoms of venous or arterial thrombosis can include:

• unusual unilateral leg pain and/ or swelling

• sudden severe pain in the chest, whether or not it radiates to the left arm

• sudden breathlessness

• sudden onset of coughing

• any unusual, severe, prolonged headache

• sudden partial or complete loss of vision

• diplopia

• slurred speech or aphasia

• vertigo

• collapse with or without focal seizure

• weakness or very marked numbness suddenly affecting one side or one part of the body

• motor disturbances

• 'acute' abdomen.

The risk for venous thromboembolic complications in COC users increases with:

- increasing age

- a positive family history (venous thromboembolism ever in a sibling or parent at a relatively early age). If a hereditary predisposition is suspected, the woman should be referred to a specialist for advice before deciding about any COC use

- prolonged immobilisation, major surgery, any surgery to the legs, or major trauma. In these situations it is advisable to discontinue the pill (in the case of elective surgery at least four weeks in advance) and not resume until two weeks after complete remobilisation. Antithrombotic treatment should be considered if the pills have not been discontinued in advance

- obesity (body mass index over 30 kg/m^2)

- there is no consensus about the possible role of varicose veins and superficial thrombophlebitis in the onset or progression of venous thrombosis.

The risk of arterial thrombo-embolic complications in COC users increases with:

- increasing age

- smoking (women over 35 years should be strongly advised not to smoke if they wish to use a COC)

- dyslipoproteinaemia

- hypertension

- valvular heart disease

- atrial fibrillation

The presence of one serious risk factor or multiple risk factors for venous or arterial disease, respectively, can also constitute a contra-indication. The possibility of anticoagulant therapy should also be taken into account. COC users should be specifically pointed out to contact their physician in case of possible symptoms of thrombosis. In case of suspected or confirmed thrombosis, COC use should be discontinued. Adequate alternative contraception should be initiated because of the teratogenicity of anticoagulant therapy (coumarins).

The increased risk of thromboembolism in the puerperium must be considered (for information on "Pregnancy and lactation" see Section 4.6).

Other medical conditions which have been associated with adverse vascular events include diabetes mellitus, systemic lupus erythematosus, haemolytic uraemic syndrome and chronic inflammatory bowel disease (Crohn's disease or ulcerative colitis).

An increase in frequency or severity of migraine during COC use (which may be prodromal of a cerebrovascular event) may be a reason for immediate discontinuation of the COC.

• Tumours

An increased risk of cervical cancer in long-term users of COCs has been reported in some epidemiological studies, but there continues to be controversy about the extent to which this finding is attributable to the confounding effects of sexual behaviour and other factors such as human papilloma virus (HPV).

A meta-analysis from 54 epidemiological studies reported that there is a slightly increased relative risk (RR = 1.24) of having breast cancer diagnosed in women who are currently using COCs. The excess risk gradually disappears during the course of the 10 years after cessation of COC use. Because breast cancer is rare in women under 40 years of age, the excess number of breast cancer diagnoses in current and recent COC users is small in relation to the overall risk of breast cancer. These studies do not provide evidence for causation. The observed pattern of increased risk may be due to an earlier diagnosis of breast cancer in COC users, the biological effects of COCs or a combination of both. The breast cancers diagnosed in ever-users tend to be less advanced clinically than the cancers diagnosed in never-users.

In rare cases, benign liver tumours, and even more rarely, malignant liver tumours have been reported in users of COCs. In isolated cases, these tumours have led to life-threatening intra-abdominal haemorrhages. A hepatic tumour should be considered in the differential diagnosis when severe upper abdominal pain, liver enlargement or signs of intra-abdominal haemorrhage occur in women taking COCs.

• Other conditions

Women using Yasmin and concomitant medications with the potential to increase serum potassium such as ACE-inhibitors, angiotensin-II-receptor-antagonists, aldosterone antagonists, potassium-sparing diuretics or NSAIDs used for long-term treatment should be tested for serum potassium during the first treatment cycle. See also section 4.5.

Potassium excretory capacity may be limited in patients with renal insufficiency.

Drospirenone intake did not show a significant effect on the serum potassium concentration in patients with mild or moderate renal impairment. However, if additionally concomitant potassium sparing drugs are taken, these patients should be monitored for hyperkalaemia.

Women with hypertriglyceridaemia, or a family history thereof, may be at an increased risk of pancreatitis when using COCs.

Although small increases in blood pressure have been reported in many women taking COCs, clinically relevant increases are rare. Only in these rare cases an immediate discontinuation of COC use is justified. A systematic relationship between COC use and clinical hypertension has not been established. If, during the use of a COC in pre-existing hypertension, constantly elevated blood pressure values or a significant increase in blood pressure do not respond adequately to antihypertensive treatment, the COC must be withdrawn. Where considered appropriate, COC use may be resumed if normotensive values can be achieved with antihypertensive therapy.

The following conditions have been reported to occur or deteriorate with both pregnancy and COC use, but the evidence of an association with COC use is inconclusive: jaundice and/or pruritus related to cholestasis; gallstones; porphyria; systemic lupus erythematosus; haemolytic uraemic syndrome; Sydenham's chorea; herpes gestationis; otosclerosis-related hearing loss.

Acute or chronic disturbances of liver function may necessitate the discontinuation of COC use until markers of liver function return to normal. Recurrence of cholestatic jaundice and/or cholestasis-related pruritus which previously occurred during pregnancy or during previous use of sex steroids necessitates the discontinuation of COCs.

Although COCs may have an effect on peripheral insulin resistance and glucose tolerance, there is no evidence for a need to alter the therapeutic regimen in diabetics using COCs. However, diabetic women should be carefully observed, particularly in the early stage of COC use.

Worsening of endogenous depression, of epilepsy, of Crohn's disease and of ulcerative colitis has been reported during COC use.

Chloasma may occasionally occur, especially in women with a history of chloasma gravidarum. Women with a tendency to chloasma should avoid exposure to the sun or ultraviolet radiation whilst taking COCs.

Medical examination/consultation

Prior to the initiation or reinstitution of Yasmin a complete medical history (including family history) should be taken and pregnancy must be ruled out. Blood pressure should be measured and a physical examination should be performed, guided by the contra-indications (section 4.3) and warnings (4.4). The woman should also be instructed to carefully read the user leaflet and to adhere to the advice given. The frequency and nature of examinations should be based on established practice guidelines and be adapted to the individual woman.

Women should be advised that oral contraceptives do not protect against HIV infections (AIDS) and other sexually transmissible diseases.

Reduced efficacy

The efficacy of COCs may be reduced in the event of missed tablets (Section 4.2), vomiting or severe diarrhoea(-Section 4.2) or concomitant medication (Section 4.5).

Reduced cycle control

With all COCs, irregular bleeding (spotting or breakthrough bleeding) may occur, especially during the first months of use. Therefore, the evaluation of any irregular bleeding is only meaningful after an adaptation interval of about three cycles.

If bleeding irregularities persist or occur after previously regular cycles, then non-hormonal causes should be considered and adequate diagnostic measures are indicated to exclude malignancy or pregnancy. These may include curettage.

In some women withdrawal bleeding may not occur during the tablet-free interval. If the COC has been taken according to the directions described in Section 4.2, it is unlikely that the woman is pregnant. However, if the COC has not been taken according to these directions prior to the first missed withdrawal bleed or if two withdrawal bleeds are missed, pregnancy must be ruled out before COC use is continued.

4.5 Interaction with other medicinal products and other forms of Interaction

Influence of other medication on Yasmin

Drug interactions which result in an increased clearance of sex hormones can lead to breakthrough bleeding and oral contraceptive failure. This has been established with hydantoins, barbiturates, primidone, carbamazepine and rifampicin; oxcarbazepine, topiramate, felbamate, ritonavir, griseofulvin and the herbal remedy St. John's Wort (hypericum perforatum) are also suspected. The mechanism of this interaction appears to be based on the hepatic enzyme-inducing properties of these drugs. Maximal enzyme induction is generally not seen for 2-3 weeks but may then be sustained for at least 4 weeks after the cessation of drug therapy.

Contraceptive failures have also been reported with antibiotics, such as ampicillin and tetracyclines. The mechanism of this effect has not been elucidated.

Women on short-term treatment (up to one week) with any of the above-mentioned classes of drugs or individual drugs should temporarily use a barrier method in addition to the COC, i.e. during the time of concomitant drug administration and for 7 days after their discontinuation.

For women on rifampicin a barrier method should be used in addition to the COC during the time of rifampicin administration and for 28 days after its discontinuation. If concomitant drug administration runs beyond the end of the tablets in the COC blister pack, the next COC pack should be started without the usual tablet-free interval.

In women on chronic treatment with hepatic enzyme-inducing drugs, experts have recommended to increase the contraceptive steroid dose. If a high contraceptive dosage is not desirable or appears to be unsatisfactory or unreliable, e.g. in the case of irregular bleeding, another, non-hormonal, method of contraception should be advised.

The main metabolites of drospirenone in human plasma are generated without involvement of the cytochrome P450 system. Inhibitors of this enzyme system are therefore unlikely to influence the metabolism of drospirenone.

• Influence of Yasmin on other medication

Based on in vitro inhibition studies and an in vivo interaction study in female volunteers using omeprazole as marker substrate, drospirenone shows little propensity to interact with the metabolism of other drugs.

• Other interactions

Women using Yasmin and concomitant medications with the potential to increase serum potassium such as ACE-inhibitors, angiotensin-II-receptor-antagonists, aldosterone antagonists, potassium-sparing diuretics or NSAIDs used for long-term treatment should be tested for serum potassium during the first treatment cycle. See also section 4.4.

• Laboratory tests

The use of contraceptive steroids may influence the results of certain laboratory tests, including biochemical parameters of liver, thyroid, adrenal and renal function, plasma levels of (carrier) proteins, e.g. corticosteroid-binding globulin and lipid/lipoprotein fractions, parameters of carbohydrate metabolism and parameters of coagulation and fibrinolysis. Changes generally remain within the normal laboratory range. Drospirenone causes an increase in plasma renin activity and plasma aldosterone induced by its mild antimineralocorticoid activity.

4.6 Pregnancy and lactation

Yasmin is not indicated during pregnancy.

If pregnancy occurs during medication with Yasmin, the preparation should be withdrawn immediately. However, extensive epidemiological studies have revealed neither an increased risk of birth defects in children born to women who used COCs prior to pregnancy, nor a teratogenic effect when COCs were taken inadvertently during pregnancy. No such studies have been carried out with Yasmin.

Animal studies have shown adverse effects during pregnancy and lactation (see Section 5.3). Based on these animal data, an adverse effect due to hormonal action of the active compounds cannot be excluded. However, general experience with COCs during pregnancy did not provide evidence for an actual adverse effect in humans.

The available data regarding the use of Yasmin during pregnancy are too limited to permit conclusions concerning negative effects of Yasmin on pregnancy, health of the foetus or neonate. Until now, no relevant epidemiological data are available.

Lactation may be influenced by COCs as they may reduce the quantity and change the composition of breast milk. Therefore, the use of COCs should generally not be recommended until the nursing mother has completely weaned her child. Small amounts of the contraceptive steroids and/or their metabolites may be excreted with the milk during COC use. These amounts may affect the child.

4.7 Effects on ability to drive and use machines

No effects on ability to drive and use machines have been observed.

4.8 Undesirable effects

For serious adverse effects in COC users see 4.4 Special warnings and special precautions for use.

The following adverse drug reactions have been reported during use of Yasmin:

(see Table 1 on next page)

The following serious adverse events have been reported in women using COCs, which are discussed in section 4.4 Special warnings and special precautions for use:

- Venous thromboembolic disorders;
- Arterial thromboembolic disorders;
- Hypertension;
- Liver tumours;
- Occurrence or deterioration of conditions for which association with COC use is not conclusive: Crohn's disease, ulcerative colitis, epilepsy, migraine, endometriosis, uterine myoma, porphyria, systemic lupus erythematosus, herpes gestationis, Sydenham's chorea, haemolytic uraemic syndrome, cholestatic jaundice;
- Chloasma.

The frequency of diagnosis of breast cancer is very slightly increased among OC users. As breast cancer is rare in women under 40 years of age the excess number is small in relation to the overall risk of breast cancer. Causation with COC use is unknown. For further information, see sections 4.3 Contraindications and 4.4 Special warnings and special precautions for use.

4.9 Overdose

There has not yet been any experience of overdose with Yasmin. On the basis of general experience with combined oral contraceptives, symptoms that may possibly occur in this case are:nausea, vomiting and, in young girls, slight vaginal bleeding. There are no antidotes and further treatment should be symptomatic.

5. PHARMACOLOGICAL PROPERTIES

5.1 Pharmacodynamic properties

Pharmacotherapeutic group (ATC): G03AA

The contraceptive effect of Yasmin is based on the interaction of various factors, the most important of which are seen as the inhibition of ovulation and the changes in the endometrium.

Yasmin is a combined oral contraceptive with ethinylestradiol and the progestogen drospirenone. In a therapeutic dosage, drospirenone also possesses antiandrogenic and mild antimineralocorticoid properties. It has no oestrogenic, glucocorticoid and antiglucocorticoid activity. This gives drospirenone a pharmacological profile closely resembling the natural hormone progesterone.

There are indications from clinical studies that the mild antimineralocorticoid properties of Yasmin result in a mild antimineralocorticoid effect.

With the use of the higher-dosed COCs (50 μg ethinylestradiol) the risk of endometrial and ovarian cancer is reduced. Whether this also applies to lower-dosed COCs remains to be confirmed.

5.2 Pharmacokinetic properties

• Drospirenone (3 mg)

Absorption

After repeated administration drospirenone is rapidly and completely absorbed. With a single administration, peak serum levels of approx. 35 ng/ml are reached 1-2 hours after ingestion. After repeated administration during a

Table 1 The following adverse drug reactions have been reported during use of Yasmin

Body System	Frequency of adverse reactions		
	Common	Uncommon	Rare
	≥1/100	< 1/100, ≥1/1000	< 1/1000
Immune system			asthma
Endocrine system	menstrual disorders, intermenstrual bleeding, breast pain		breast secretion
Nervous system	headache, depressive mood	changes in libido	
Ear and labyrinth			hypacusis
Vascular system	migraine	hypertension, hypotension	thromboembolism
Gastrointestinal system	nausea	vomiting	
Skin and subcutaneous system		acne, eczema, pruritus	
Reproductive system and breast	leucorrhoea, vaginal moniliasis,	vaginitis	
General		fluid retention, body weight changes	

treatment cycle, a maximum steady-state concentration of 60 ng/ml is reached after 7 to 14 days.

The absolute bioavailability of drospirenone is between 76 and 85 %. Concomitant ingestion of food has no influence on bioavailability.

Distribution

After oral administration, serum drospirenone levels decrease in two phases which are characterised by half-lives of 1.6 ± 0.7 h and 27.0 ± 7.5 h, respectively. Drospirenone is bound to serum albumin and does not bind to sex hormone binding globulin (SHBG) or corticoid binding globulin (CBG). Only 3 - 5 % of the total serum drug concentrations are present as free steroid. The ethinylestradiol-induced increase in SHBG does not influence the serum protein binding of drospirenone. The mean apparent volume of distribution of drospirenone is 3.7 ± 1.2 l/kg.

Metabolism

Drospirenone is extensively metabolised after oral administration. The major metabolites in the plasma are the acid form of drospirenone, generated by opening of the lactone ring, and the 4,5-dihydro-drospirenone-3-sulfate, both of which are formed without involvement of the P450 system. Drospirenone is metabolised to a minor extent by cytochrome P450 3A4 based on in vitro data.

Elimination

The metabolic clearance rate of drospirenone in serum is 1.5 ± 0.2 ml/min/kg. Drospirenone is excreted only in trace amounts in unchanged form. The metabolites of drospirenone are excreted with the faeces and urine at an excretion ratio of about 1.2 to 1.4. The half-life of metabolite excretion with the urine and faeces is about 40 h.

Steady-State Conditions

During a treatment cycle, maximum steady-state concentrations of drospirenone in serum of about 60 ng/ml are reached between day 7 and day 14 of treatment. Serum drospirenone levels accumulated by a factor of about 2 to 3 as a consequence of the ratio of terminal half-life and dosing interval. Further accumulation of drospirenone levels beyond treatment cycles was observed between cycles 1 and 6 but thereafter no further accumulation was observed.

• Ethinylestradiol (30 µg)

Absorption

Ethinylestradiol is rapidly and completely absorbed after ingestion. After administration of 30 µg, peak plasma concentrations of 100 pg/ml are reached 1-2 hours after ingestion. Ethinylestradiol undergoes an extensive first-pass effect, which displays great inter-individual variation. The absolute bioavailability is approx. 45 %.

Distribution

Ethinylestradiol has an apparent volume of distribution of 5 l/kg and binding to plasma proteins is approx. 98 %. Ethinylestradiol induces the hepatic synthesis of SHBG and CBG. During treatment with 30 µg ethinylestradiol the plasma concentration of SHBG increases from 70 to about 350 nmol/l.

Ethinylestradiol passes in small amounts into breast milk (0.02 % of the dose).

Metabolism

Ethinylestradiol is metabolised completely (metabolic plasma clearance 5 ml/min/kg).

Elimination

Ethinylestradiol is not excreted in unchanged form to any significant extent. The metabolites of ethinylestradiol are excreted at a urinary to biliary ratio of 4:6. The half-life of metabolite excretion is about 1 day. The elimination half-life is 20 hours.

Steady-state conditions

Steady-state conditions are reached during the second half of a treatment cycle and serum levels of ethinylestradiol accumulate by a factor of about 1.4 to 2.1.

5.3 Preclinical safety data

In laboratory animals, the effects of drospirenone and ethinylestradiol were confined to those associated with the recognised pharmacological action. In particular, reproduction toxicity studies revealed embryotoxic and foetotoxic effects in animals which are considered as species specific. At exposures to drospirenone exceeding those in users of Yasmin, effects on sexual differentiation were observed in rat foetuses but not in monkeys.

6. PHARMACEUTICAL PARTICULARS

6.1 List of excipients

Lactose monohydrate

Maize starch

Pregelatinised maize starch

Povidone K25

Magnesium stearate

Hypromellose

Macrogol 6000

Talc

Titanium dioxide (E 171)

Iron oxide pigment, yellow (E 172)

6.2 Incompatibilities

Not applicable.

6.3 Shelf life

3 years

6.4 Special precautions for storage

Do not store above 25 °C

Store in the original package

6.5 Nature and contents of container

PVC/Aluminium blister pack

Pack sizes:

21 tablets

3x21 tablets

6x21 tablets

13x21 tablets

Not all pack sizes listed are marketed in all EU countries.

6.6 Instructions for use and handling

No special requirements

7. MARKETING AUTHORISATION HOLDER

Schering Health Care Limited

The Brow

Burgess Hill

West Sussex RH15 9NE

8. MARKETING AUTHORISATION NUMBER(S)

PL/0053/0292

9. DATE OF FIRST AUTHORISATION/RENEWAL OF THE AUTHORISATION

23rd November 2000

10. DATE OF REVISION OF THE TEXT

30th July 2004

LEGAL CATEGORY

POM

Yentreve 20mg and 40mg hard gastro-resistant capsules

(Eli Lilly and Company Limited)

1. NAME OF THE MEDICINAL PRODUCT

Yentreve▼ 20mg and 40mg hard gastro-resistant capsules.

2. QUALITATIVE AND QUANTITATIVE COMPOSITION

The active ingredient in Yentreve is duloxetine.

Each 20mg capsule contains 20mg of duloxetine as duloxetine hydrochloride.

Each 40mg capsule contains 40mg of duloxetine as duloxetine hydrochloride.

For excipients, see section 6.1.

3. PHARMACEUTICAL FORM

Hard gastro-resistant capsule.

The 20mg capsule has an opaque blue body, imprinted with '20mg', and an opaque blue cap, imprinted with '9544'.

The 40mg capsule has an opaque orange body, imprinted with '40mg', and an opaque blue cap, imprinted with '9545'.

4. CLINICAL PARTICULARS

4.1 Therapeutic indications

Yentreve is indicated for women for the treatment of moderate to severe stress urinary incontinence (SUI), see section 5.1.

4.2 Posology and method of administration

The recommended dose of Yentreve is 40mg twice daily without regard to meals. After 2-4 weeks of treatment, patients should be re-assessed in order to evaluate the benefit and tolerability of the therapy. If a woman experiences troublesome adverse events beyond 4 weeks, the dose can be reduced to 20mg twice daily. However, limited data are available to support the efficacy of Yentreve 20mg twice daily. A 20mg capsule is also available.

The efficacy of Yentreve has not been evaluated for longer than 3 months in placebo-controlled studies. The benefit of treatment should be re-assessed at regular intervals.

Combining Yentreve with a pelvic floor muscle training (PFMT) programme may be more effective than either treatment alone. It is recommended that consideration be given to concomitant PFMT.

Hepatic insufficiency: Yentreve should not be used in women with liver disease resulting in hepatic impairment (see section 4.3).

Renal insufficiency: No dosage adjustment is necessary for patients with mild or moderate renal dysfunction (creatinine clearance 30 to 80ml/min).

Elderly: Caution should be exercised when treating the elderly.

Children and adolescents: The safety and efficacy of duloxetine in patients in these age groups have not been studied. Therefore, administration of Yentreve to children and adolescents is not recommended.

Discontinuation of treatment: When discontinuing Yentreve after more than 1 week of therapy, it is generally recommended that the dose be tapered (from 40mg twice daily to either 40mg once daily or 20mg twice daily) for 2 weeks before discontinuation in an effort to decrease the risk of possible discontinuation symptoms (see section 4.4).

4.3 Contraindications

Hypersensitivity to the active substance or to any of the excipients.

Liver disease resulting in hepatic impairment (see section 5.2).

Pregnancy and lactation (see section 4.6).

Yentreve should not be used in combination with non-selective, irreversible monoamine oxidase inhibitors (MAOIs), see section 4.5.

Yentreve should not be used in combination with CYP1A2 inhibitors, like fluvoxamine, ciprofloxacin, or enoxacine, since the combination results in elevated plasma concentrations of duloxetine (see section 4.5).

4.4 Special warnings and special precautions for use

Mania and seizures: Yentreve should be used with caution in patients with a history of mania or a diagnosis of bipolar disorder, and/or seizures.

Use with antidepressants: Caution should be exercised when using Yentreve in combination with antidepressants. In particular, the combination with selective reversible MAOIs is not recommended.

Mydriasis: Mydriasis has been reported in association with duloxetine, therefore, caution should be used when prescribing duloxetine in patients with increased intra-ocular pressure, or those at risk of acute narrow-angle glaucoma.

Renal impairment: Increased plasma concentrations of duloxetine occur in patients with severe renal impairment on haemodialysis (creatinine clearance <30ml/min). Patients with severe renal impairment are unlikely to be affected by SUI. See section 4.2 for information on patients with mild or moderate renal dysfunction.

Sucrose: Yentreve hard gastro-resistant capsules contain sucrose. Patients with rare hereditary problems of fructose intolerance, glucose-galactose malabsorption, or sucrose-isomaltase insufficiency should not take this medicine.

Haemorrhage: There have been reports of cutaneous bleeding abnormalities, such as ecchymoses and purpura, with selective serotonin reuptake inhibitors (SSRIs). Caution is advised in patients taking anticoagulants and/or medicinal products known to affect platelet function, and in patients with known bleeding tendencies.

Discontinuation of treatment: Some patients may experience symptoms on discontinuation of Yentreve, particularly if treatment is stopped abruptly (see section 4.2).

Hyponatraemia: Hyponatraemia has been reported rarely, predominantly in the elderly, when administering Yentreve and other drugs of the same pharmacodynamic class.

Suicidal ideation and behaviour: As with other drugs with similar pharmacological action (antidepressants), isolated cases of suicidal ideation and suicidal behaviours have been reported during duloxetine therapy or early after treatment discontinuation. Physicians should encourage patients to report any distressing thoughts or feelings at any time.

4.5 Interaction with other medicinal products and other forms of Interaction

Monoamine oxidase inhibitors (MAOIs): Due to the risk of serotonin syndrome, Yentreve should not be used in combination with non-selective, irreversible monoamine oxidase inhibitors (MAOIs), or within at least 14 days of discontinuing treatment with an MAOI. Based on the half-life of duloxetine, at least 5 days should be allowed after stopping Yentreve before starting an MAOI (see section 4.3).

Serotonin syndrome: In rare cases, serotonin syndrome has been reported in patients using SSRIs concomitantly with serotonergic medicinal products. Caution is advisable if Yentreve is used concomitantly with serotonergic antidepressants like SSRIs, tricyclics like clomipramine or amitriptyline, venlafaxine, or triptans, tramadol and tryptophan.

CNS drugs: Caution is advised when Yentreve is taken in combination with other centrally acting drugs or substances, including alcohol and sedative drugs (benzodiazepines, morphinomimetics, antipsychotics, phenobarbital, sedative antihistamines).

Effects of duloxetine on other drugs

Drugs metabolised by CYP1A2: In a clinical study, the pharmacokinetics of theophylline, a CYP1A2 substrate, were not significantly affected by co-administration with duloxetine (60mg twice daily). The study was performed in males and it cannot be excluded that females having a lower CYP1A2 activity and higher plasma concentrations of duloxetine may experience an interaction with a CYP1A2 substrate.

Drugs metabolised by CYP2D6: The co-administration of duloxetine (40mg twice daily) increases steady-state AUC of tolterodine (2mg twice daily) by 71% but does not affect the pharmacokinetics of its active 5-hydroxy metabolite, and no dosage adjustment is recommended. Caution is advised if duloxetine is co-administered with medicinal products that are predominantly metabolised by CYP2D6 if they have a narrow therapeutic index.

Oral contraceptives and other steroidal agents: Results of *in vitro* studies demonstrate that duloxetine does not induce the catalytic activity of CYP3A. Specific *in vivo* drug interaction studies have not been performed.

Effects of other drugs on duloxetine

Antacids and H_2 antagonists: Co-administration of Yentreve with aluminium- and magnesium-containing antacids or with famotidine had no significant effect on the rate or extent of duloxetine absorption after administration of a 40mg oral dose.

Inhibitors of CYP1A2: Because CYP1A2 is involved in duloxetine metabolism, concomitant use of Yentreve with potent inhibitors of CYP1A2 is likely to result in higher concentrations of duloxetine. Fluvoxamine (100mg once daily), a potent inhibitor of CYP1A2, decreased the apparent plasma clearance of duloxetine by about 77% and increased $AUC_{0\text{-}t}$ 6-fold. Therefore, Yentreve should not be administered in combination with potent inhibitors of CYP1A2 like fluvoxamine (see section 4.3).

4.6 Pregnancy and lactation

Pregnancy: There are no data on the use of duloxetine in pregnant women. Studies in animals have shown reproductive toxicity at systemic exposure levels (AUC) of duloxetine lower than the maximum clinical exposure (see section 5.3). The potential risk for humans is unknown. Withdrawal symptoms may occur in the neonate after maternal duloxetine use near term. Yentreve is contra-indicated during pregnancy (see section 4.3).

Breast-feeding: Duloxetine and/or its metabolites are excreted into the milk of lactating rats. Adverse behavioural effects were seen in offspring in a perinatal/postnatal toxicity study in rats (see section 5.3). Excretion of duloxetine and/or metabolites into human milk has not been studied. Yentreve is contra-indicated while breast-feeding (see section 4.3).

4.7 Effects on ability to drive and use machines

Although in controlled studies duloxetine has not been shown to impair psychomotor performance, cognitive function, or memory, it may be associated with sedation. Therefore, patients should be cautioned about their ability to drive a car or operate hazardous machinery.

4.8 Undesirable effects

The safety of Yentreve has been evaluated in four 12-week, placebo-controlled clinical trials in patients with SUI, including 958 duloxetine-treated and 955 placebo-treated patients. This represents 190 patient-years of exposure at 40mg twice daily.

The most commonly reported adverse events in patients treated with Yentreve were nausea, dry mouth, fatigue, insomnia, and constipation. Adverse events that occurred significantly more often in patients taking duloxetine than placebo and with a frequency of ≥2%, or were of potential clinical relevance, are displayed in Tables 1, 2, and 3.

The data analysis showed that the onset of the reported adverse events typically occurred in the first week of therapy. However, the majority of the most frequent adverse events were mild to moderate and resolved within 30 days of occurrence (eg, nausea).

Frequency estimate: Very common (≥10%), common (≥1% and <10%), and uncommon (≥0.1% and <1%).

Table 1

Very Common Undesirable Effects (≥10%)

(see Table 1)

Table 2

Common Undesirable Effects (≥1%, <10%)

(see Table 2)

Table 3

Uncommon Undesirable Effects (≥0.1%, <1%)

(see Table 3)

Dizziness (≥5%) was also reported as a common adverse event upon duloxetine discontinuation.

Duloxetine treatment, for up to 12 weeks in placebo-controlled clinical trials, was associated with small mean increases from baseline to endpoint in ALT, AST, and creatinine phosphokinase (CPK) (2.1 U/l, 1.3 U/l, and 5.8 U/l, respectively); infrequent, transient, abnormal values were observed more often for these analytes in duloxetine-treated patients compared with placebo-treated patients.

Electrocardiograms were obtained from 755 duloxetine-treated patients with SUI and 779 placebo-treated patients in 12-week clinical trials. The heart rate-corrected QT interval in duloxetine-treated patients did not differ from that seen in placebo-treated patients.

4.9 Overdose

There is limited clinical experience with duloxetine overdose in humans. In pre-marketing clinical trials, no cases of fatal overdose of duloxetine have been reported. Four non-fatal acute ingestions of duloxetine (300 to 1400mg), alone or in combination with other medicinal products, have been reported.

No specific antidote for duloxetine is known. A free airway should be established. Monitoring of cardiac and vital signs is recommended, along with appropriate symptomatic and supportive measures. Gastric lavage may be indicated if performed soon after ingestion or in symptomatic patients. Activated charcoal may be useful in limiting absorption. Duloxetine has a large volume of distribution and forced diuresis, haemoperfusion, and exchange perfusion are unlikely to be beneficial.

5. PHARMACOLOGICAL PROPERTIES

5.1 Pharmacodynamic properties

ATC code: Not yet assigned.

Duloxetine is a combined serotonin (5-HT) and norepinephrine (NE) reuptake inhibitor. It weakly inhibits dopamine reuptake with no significant affinity for histaminergic, dopaminergic, cholinergic, and adrenergic receptors.

In animal studies, increased levels of 5-HT and NE in the sacral spinal cord lead to increased urethral tone via enhanced pudendal nerve stimulation to the urethral striated sphincter muscle only during the storage phase of the micturition cycle. A similar mechanism in women is believed to result in stronger urethral closure during urine storage with physical stress that could explain the efficacy of duloxetine in the treatment of women with SUI.

The efficacy of duloxetine 40mg given twice daily in the treatment of SUI was established in four double-blind, placebo-controlled studies that randomised 1,913 women (22 to 83 years) with SUI; of these, 958 patients were randomised to duloxetine and 955 to placebo. The primary

Table 1 Very Common Undesirable Effects (≥10%)

System Organ Class	Adverse Event	Yentreve n = 958 (%)	Placebo n = 955 (%)
Psychiatric disorders	Insomnia	12.6	1.9
Gastro-intestinal disorders	Nausea Dry mouth Constipation	23.2 13.4 11.0	3.7 1.5 2.3
General disorders and administration site conditions	Fatigue	12.7	3.8

Table 2 Common Undesirable Effects (≥1%, <10%)

System Organ Class	Adverse Event	Yentreve n = 958 (%)	Placebo n = 955 (%)
Metabolism and nutrition disorders	Anorexia Appetite decreased Thirst	3.9 2.3 1.0	0.2 0.2 0.1
Psychiatric disorders	Sleep disorder Anxiety Libido decreased Anorgasmia	2.2 1.9 1.5 1.4	0.8 0.7 0.3 0.0
Nervous system disorders	Headache Dizziness (except vertigo) Somnolence Tremor Blurred vision Nervousness	9.7 9.5 6.8 2.7 1.3 1.1	6.6 2.6 0.1 0.0 0.1 0.0
Gastro-intestinal disorders	Diarrhoea Vomiting Dyspepsia	5.1 4.8 3.0	2.7 1.6 1.3
Skin and subcutaneous tissue disorders	Sweating increased	4.5	0.8
General disorders and administration site conditions	Lethargy Pruritus Weakness	2.6 1.4 1.3	0.3 0.3 0.3

Table 3 Uncommon Undesirable Effects (≥0.1%, <1%)

System Organ Class	Adverse Event	Yentreve n = 958 (%)	Placebo n = 955 (%)
Psychiatric disorders	Loss of libido	0.6	0.0

efficacy measures were incontinence episode frequency (IEF) from diaries and an incontinence specific quality of life questionnaire score (I-QOL).

Incontinence episode frequency: In all four studies the duloxetine-treated group had a 50% or greater median decrease in IEF compared with 33% in the placebo-treated group. Differences were observed at each visit after 4 weeks (duloxetine 54% and placebo 22%), 8 weeks (52% and 29%), and 12 weeks (52% and 33%) of medication.

In an additional study limited to patients with severe SUI, all responses with duloxetine were achieved within 2 weeks.

The efficacy of Yentreve has not been evaluated for longer than 3 months in placebo-controlled studies. The clinical benefit of Yentreve compared with placebo has not been demonstrated in women with mild SUI, defined in randomised trials as those with IEF <14 per week. In these women, Yentreve may provide no benefit beyond that afforded by more conservative behavioural interventions.

Quality of life: Incontinence quality of life (I-QOL) questionnaire scores were significantly improved in the duloxetine-treated patient group compared with the placebo-treated group (9.2 versus 5.9 score improvement, $P < .001$). Using a global improvement scale (PGI), significantly more women using duloxetine considered their symptoms of stress incontinence to be improved with treatment compared with women using placebo (64.6% versus 50.1%, $P < .001$).

Yentreve and prior continence surgery: There are limited data that suggest that the benefits of Yentreve are not diminished in women with stress urinary incontinence who have previously undergone continence surgery.

Yentreve and pelvic floor muscle training (PFMT): During a 12-week blinded, randomised, controlled study, Yentreve demonstrated greater reductions in IEF compared with either placebo treatment or with PFMT alone. Combined therapy (duloxetine + PFMT) showed greater improvement in both pad use and condition-specific quality of life measures than Yentreve alone or PFMT alone.

5.2 Pharmacokinetic properties

Duloxetine is administered as a single enantiomer. Duloxetine is extensively metabolised by oxidative enzymes (CYP1A2 and the polymorphic CYP2D6), followed by conjugation. The pharmacokinetics of duloxetine demonstrate large intersubject variability (generally 50-60%), partly due to gender, age, smoking status, and CYP2D6 metaboliser status.

Duloxetine is well absorbed after oral administration, with a C_{max} occurring 6 hours post dose. The absolute oral bioavailability of duloxetine ranged from 32% to 80% (mean of 50%; n = 8 subjects). Food delays the time to reach the peak concentration from 6 to 10 hours and it marginally decreases the extent of absorption (approximately 11%).

Duloxetine is approximately 96% bound to human plasma proteins. Duloxetine binds to both albumin and alpha$_1$ acid glycoprotein. Protein binding is not affected by renal or hepatic impairment.

Duloxetine is extensively metabolised and the metabolites are excreted principally in urine. Both CYP2D6 and CYP1A2 catalyse the formation of the two major metabolites, glucuronide conjugate of 4-hydroxy duloxetine and sulphate conjugate of 5-hydroxy,6-methoxy duloxetine. Based upon *in vitro* studies, the circulating metabolites of duloxetine are considered pharmacologically inactive. The pharmacokinetics of duloxetine in patients who are poor metabolisers with respect to CYP2D6 has not been specifically investigated. Limited data suggest that the plasma levels of duloxetine are higher in these patients.

The elimination half-life of duloxetine after an oral dose ranges from 8 to 17 hours (mean of 12 hours). After an intravenous dose, the plasma clearance of duloxetine ranges from 22 l/hr to 46 l/hr (mean of 36 l/hr). After an oral dose, the apparent plasma clearance of duloxetine ranges from 33 to 261 l/hr (mean 101 l/hr).

Special populations

Age: Pharmacokinetic differences have been identified between younger and elderly females ($\geqslant$65 years) (AUC increases by about 25% and half-life is about 25% longer in the elderly), although the magnitude of these changes is not sufficient to justify adjustments to the dose.

Renal impairment: End stage renal disease (ESRD) patients receiving dialysis had a 2-fold higher duloxetine C_{max} and AUC values compared to healthy subjects. Pharmacokinetic data on duloxetine is limited in patients with mild or moderate renal impairment.

Hepatic insufficiency: Moderate liver disease (Child Pugh Class B) affected the pharmacokinetics of duloxetine. Compared with healthy subjects, the apparent plasma clearance of duloxetine was 79% lower, the apparent terminal half-life was 2.3-times longer, and the AUC was 3.7-times higher in patients with moderate liver disease. The pharmacokinetics of duloxetine and its metabolites have not been studied in patients with mild or severe hepatic insufficiency.

5.3 Preclinical safety data

Duloxetine was not genotoxic in a standard battery of tests and was not carcinogenic in rats. Multinucleated cells were seen in the liver in the absence of other histopathological changes in the rat carcinogenicity study. The underlying mechanism and the clinical relevance are unknown.

Female mice receiving duloxetine for 2 years had an increased incidence of hepatocellular adenomas and carcinomas at the high dose only (144mg/kg/day), but these were considered to be secondary to hepatic microsomal enzyme induction. The relevance of this mouse data to humans is unknown. Female rats receiving duloxetine before and during mating and early pregnancy had a decrease in maternal food consumption and body weight, oestrous cycle disruption, decreased live birth indices and progeny survival, and progeny growth retardation at systemic exposure levels estimated to be at the most at maximum clinical exposure (AUC). In an embryotoxicity study in the rabbit, a higher incidence of cardiovascular and skeletal malformations was observed at systemic exposure levels below the maximum clinical exposure (AUC). No malformations were observed in another study testing a higher dose of a different salt of duloxetine. In a prenatal/postnatal toxicity study in the rat, duloxetine induced adverse behavioural effects in the offspring at systemic exposure levels below maximum clinical exposure (AUC).

6. PHARMACEUTICAL PARTICULARS

6.1 List of excipients

Capsule content:

Hypromellose

Hydroxypropyl methylcellulose acetate succinate

Sucrose

Sugar spheres

Talc

Titanium dioxide (E171)

Triethyl citrate

Capsule shell (20mg):

Gelatin, sodium lauryl sulfate, titanium dioxide (E171), indigo carmine (E132), edible black ink.

Capsule shell (40mg):

Gelatin, sodium lauryl sulfate, titanium dioxide (E171), indigo carmine (E132), red iron oxide (E172), yellow iron oxide (E172), edible black ink.

Edible ink: Black iron oxide-synthetic (E172), propylene glycol, shellac.

20 mg capsule shell cap colour:

Opaque blue

20 mg capsule shell body colour:

Opaque blue

40 mg capsule shell cap colour:

Opaque blue

40 mg capsule shell body colour:

Opaque orange

6.2 Incompatibilities

Not applicable.

6.3 Shelf life

2 years.

6.4 Special precautions for storage

Store in the original package. Do not store above 30°C.

6.5 Nature and contents of container

Polyvinylchloride (PVC), polyethylene (PE), and polychlorotrifluoroethylene (PCTFE) blister sealed with an aluminum foil.

20 mg capsules:

Packs of 56 capsules.

40 mg capsules:

Packs of 28, 56, 98, 140, and 196 (2 × 98) capsules.

Not all pack sizes may be marketed.

6.6 Instructions for use and handling

No special requirements.

7. MARKETING AUTHORISATION HOLDER

Eli Lilly Nederland BV, Grootslag 1-5, NL-3991 RA Houten, The Netherlands.

8. MARKETING AUTHORISATION NUMBER(S)

20mg, 56 capsules:	EU/1/04/280/001
40mg, 28 capsules:	EU/1/04/280/002
40mg, 56 capsules:	EU/1/04/280/003
40mg, 98 capsules:	EU/1/04/280/004
40mg, 140 capsules	EU/1/04/280/005
40mg, 98 × 2 capsules:	EU/1/04/280/006

9. DATE OF FIRST AUTHORISATION/RENEWAL OF THE AUTHORISATION

Date of first authorisation: 11 August 2004

10. DATE OF REVISION OF THE TEXT

-

LEGAL CATEGORY

POM

*YENTREVE (duloxetine) is a trademark of Eli Lilly and Company.

YEN1M

Zacin Cream 0.025%

(Zeneus Pharma Ltd)

1. NAME OF THE MEDICINAL PRODUCT
Zacin Cream 0.025%

2. QUALITATIVE AND QUANTITATIVE COMPOSITION
Capsaicin 0.025% w/w

3. PHARMACEUTICAL FORM
Cream for topical application

4. CLINICAL PARTICULARS

4.1 Therapeutic indications
For the symptomatic relief of pain associated with osteoarthritis.

4.2 Posology and method of administration
Adults and the elderly:

For topical administration to unbroken skin. Apply only a small amount of cream (pea size) to affected area 4 times daily. These applications should be evenly spaced throughout the waking hours and not more often than every 4 hours. The cream should be gently rubbed in, there should be no residue left on the surface. Hands should be washed immediately after application of Zacin unless hands and fingers are being treated. Zacin should not be applied near the eyes. Pain relief usually begins within the first week of treatment and increases with continuing regular application for the next two to eight weeks.

Not suitable for use in children.

4.3 Contraindications
Zacin cream is contra-indicated on broken or irritated skin.

Zacin Cream is contra-indicated in patients with known hypersensitivity to capsaicin or any of the excipients used in this product.

4.4 Special warnings and special precautions for use
Patients should avoid taking a hot bath or shower just before or after applying Zacin, as it can enhance the burning sensation.

Keep Zacin away from the eyes.

Medical advice should be sought if the condition worsens, or clears up then recurs.

Tight bandages should not be applied on top of Zacin cream.

4.5 Interaction with other medicinal products and other forms of Interaction
Not applicable.

4.6 Pregnancy and lactation
The safety of Zacin during pregnancy and lactation has not been established, in either humans or animals. However, in the small amounts absorbed transdermally from Zacin Cream, it is considered unlikely that capsaicin will cause any adverse effects in humans.

4.7 Effects on ability to drive and use machines
Not applicable.

4.8 Undesirable effects
Zacin may cause transient burning following application. This burning sensation generally disappears after several days of treatment, but may persist particularly when application schedules of less than 4 times daily are used. The burning can be enhanced if too much cream is used and if it is applied just before or after a bath or shower.

4.9 Overdose
Not applicable.

5. PHARMACOLOGICAL PROPERTIES

5.1 Pharmacodynamic properties
Although the precise mechanism of action of capsaicin is not fully understood, current evidence suggests that capsaicin exerts an analgesic effect by depleting and preventing reaccumulation of Substance P in peripheral sensory neurons. Substance P is thought to be the principal chemomediator of pain impulses from the periphery to the central nervous system.

5.2 Pharmacokinetic properties
Absorption after topical application is unknown. Average consumption of dietary spice from capsicum fruit has been estimated at 2.5g/person/day in India and 5.0g/person/day in Thailand. Capsaicin content in capsicum fruit is approximately 1% therefore dietary intake of capsaicin may range from 0.5-1mg/kg/day for a 50kg person. Application of two tubes of Zacin Cream 0.025% (90g) each week results in 3.21mg/day topical exposure. Assuming 100% absorption in a 50kg person, daily exposure would be 0.064mg/kg which is approximately one seventh to one eighth of the above mentioned dietary intake.

5.3 Preclinical safety data
The available animal toxicity data relating to capsicum, capsicum extracts and capsaicin do not suggest that, in usual doses, they pose any significant toxicity hazard to man. Thus, in both single and repeat dosing studies which have been reported, capsicum extracts and capsaicin are generally well-tolerated at many times even the highest estimated human intakes. The safety of Zacin for use in human pregnancy has not been established since no formal reproduction studies have been performed in either animals or man. However, there is no reason to suspect from human or animal studies currently available that any adverse effects in humans are likely.

Studies reported in the published literature which relate to potential genotoxic and carcinogenic action of capsaicin have produced inconclusive and conflicting data. However, it is unlikely that capsaicin, in the quantities absorbed transdermally from Zacin cream, will pose any significant hazard to humans.

6. PHARMACEUTICAL PARTICULARS

6.1 List of excipients
Purified Water

Sorbitol Solution

Isopropyl Myristate

Cetyl Alcohol

White Soft Paraffin

Glyceryl Stearate and Peg-100

Stearate (Arlacel 165)

Benzyl Alcohol

6.2 Incompatibilities
Not applicable.

6.3 Shelf life
3 years

6.4 Special precautions for storage
Store below 25°C.

Return any unused cream to your doctor or pharmacist.

6.5 Nature and contents of container
Aluminium tubes with epoxyphenolic lining and polypropylene spiked cap containing 45g of Zacin Cream 0.025%.

6.6 Instructions for use and handling
Not applicable.

7. MARKETING AUTHORISATION HOLDER
Elan Pharma International Ltd

W.I.L. House

Shannon Business Park

Shannon

Co. Clare

Ireland

8. MARKETING AUTHORISATION NUMBER(S)
PL 16804/0021

9. DATE OF FIRST AUTHORISATION/RENEWAL OF THE AUTHORISATION
19 February 2003

10. DATE OF REVISION OF THE TEXT
February 2005

11. Legal Category
POM

Zaditen Eye Drops

(Novartis Pharmaceuticals UK Ltd)

1. NAME OF THE MEDICINAL PRODUCT
ZADITEN® 0.25 mg/ml, eye drops, solution.

2. QUALITATIVE AND QUANTITATIVE COMPOSITION
One ml contains 0.345 mg ketotifen hydrogen fumarate corresponding to 0.25 mg ketotifen.

Each drop contains 8.5 microgram ketotifen hydrogen fumarate.

For excipients, see 6.1.

3. PHARMACEUTICAL FORM
Eye drops, solution.

Clear, colourless to faintly yellow solution

4. CLINICAL PARTICULARS

4.1 Therapeutic indications
Symptomatic treatment of seasonal allergic conjunctivitis

4.2 Posology and method of administration
Adults, elderly and children (age 3 and older): one drop of ZADITEN into the conjunctival sac twice a day.

The contents and dispenser remain sterile until the original closure is broken. To avoid contamination do not touch any surface with the dropper tip.

4.3 Contraindications
Hypersensitivity to ketotifen or to any of the excipients.

4.4 Special warnings and special precautions for use
The formulation of ZADITEN eye drops contains benzalkonium chloride as a preservative, which may be deposited in soft contact lenses; therefore ZADITEN eye drops should not be instilled while the patient is wearing these lenses. The lenses should be removed before application of the drops and not reinserted earlier than 15 minutes after use.

All eye drops preserved with benzalkonium chloride may possibly discolour soft contact lenses.

4.5 Interaction with other medicinal products and other forms of Interaction
If ZADITEN is used concomitantly with other eye medications there must be an interval of at least 5 minutes between the two medications.

The use of oral dosage forms of ketotifen may potentiate the effect of CNS depressants, antihistamines and alcohol. Although this has not been observed with ZADITEN eye drops, the possibility of such effects cannot be excluded.

4.6 Pregnancy and lactation
There are no adequate data from the use of ketotifen eye drops in pregnant women. Animal studies using maternally toxic oral doses showed increased pre- and postnatal mortality, but no teratogenicity. Systemic levels after ocular administration are much lower than after oral use. Caution should be exercised when prescribing to pregnant women.

Although animal data following oral administration show excretion into breast milk, topical administration to human is unlikely to produce detectable quantities in breast milk. ZADITEN eye drops can be used during lactation.

4.7 Effects on ability to drive and use machines
Any patient who experiences blurred vision or somnolence should not drive or operate machines.

4.8 Undesirable effects
At the recommended dose, the following undesirable effects have been reported:

Ocular side effects:

Between 1% and 2%: burning/stinging, punctate corneal epithelial erosion.

< 1%: blurring of vision upon drug instillation, dry eyes, eyelid disorder, conjunctivitis, eye pain, photophobia, subconjunctival haemorrhage.

Systemic side effects:

< 1%: headache, somnolence, skin rash, eczema, urticaria, dry mouth and allergic reaction.

4.9 Overdose
No case of overdose has been reported.

Oral ingestion of the contents of a 5 ml bottle would be equivalent to 1.25 mg of ketotifen which is 60% of a recommended oral daily dose for a 3 year old child. Clinical results have shown no serious signs or symptoms after oral ingestion of up to 20 mg of ketotifen.

5. PHARMACOLOGICAL PROPERTIES

5.1 Pharmacodynamic properties
Pharmacotherapeutic group: Ophthalmologicals, other anti-allergics

ATC code: S01GX08

Ketotifen is a histamine H_1-receptor antagonist. *In vivo* animal studies and *in vitro* studies suggest the additional activities of mast cell stabilisation and inhibition of infiltration, activation and degranulation of eosinophils.

5.2 Pharmacokinetic properties
In a pharmacokinetic study conducted in 18 healthy volunteers with ZADITEN eye drops, plasma levels of ketotifen after repeated ocular administration for 14 days were in most cases below the limit of quantitation (20 pg/ml).

After oral administration, ketotifen is eliminated biphasically with an initial half-life of 3 to 5 hours and a terminal half-life of 21 hours. About 1% of the substance is excreted unchanged in the urine within 48 hours and 60 to 70% as metabolites. The main metabolite is the practically inactive ketotifen-N-glucuronide.

5.3 Preclinical safety data
Preclinical data reveal no special hazard which is considered relevant in connection with use of ZADITEN eye drops in humans based on conventional studies of safety pharmacology, repeated dose toxicity, genotoxicity, carcinogenic potential and toxicity to reproduction.

6. PHARMACEUTICAL PARTICULARS

6.1 List of excipients
Benzalkonium chloride

Glycerol (E422)

Sodium hydroxide (E524)

Water for injections

6.2 Incompatibilities
Not applicable.

6.3 Shelf life
In unopened bottle: 2 years.

After opening: 4 weeks.

6.4 Special precautions for storage
Do not store above 25 °C.

6.5 Nature and contents of container
The container is a white-coloured LDPE bottle with a transparent LDPE dropper and a white HDPE screw cap with an integrated safety ring. One bottle contains 5 ml of the solution.

6.6 Instructions for use and handling
Any contents remaining 4 weeks after opening should be discarded.

7. MARKETING AUTHORISATION HOLDER
Novartis Pharmaceuticals UK Limited

Frimley Business Park

Frimley

Camberley

Surrey

GU16 7SR

United Kingdom

8. MARKETING AUTHORISATION NUMBER(S)
PL 00101/0614

9. DATE OF FIRST AUTHORISATION/RENEWAL OF THE AUTHORISATION
31 July 2001

10. DATE OF REVISION OF THE TEXT
18 December 2002

LEGAL CATEGORY
POM

Zaditen tablets 1mg and Zaditen Elixir 1mg/5ml

(Novartis Pharmaceuticals UK Ltd)

1. NAME OF THE MEDICINAL PRODUCT
Zaditen® Tablets 1mg

Zaditen® Elixir 1mg/5ml

2. QUALITATIVE AND QUANTITATIVE COMPOSITION
Tablets contain Ketotifen hydrogen fumarate 1.38mg (equivalent to 1mg ketotifen base).

Elixir contains Ketotifen hydrogen fumarate 1.38mg/5ml

3. PHARMACEUTICAL FORM
Tablets: White tablets, 7mm diameter, with breakline on one side and ZADITEN 1 on the other.

Elixir: Clear, colourless, strawberry flavoured elixir.

4. CLINICAL PARTICULARS

4.1 Therapeutic indications
Prophylactic treatment of bronchial asthma.

Symptomatic treatment of allergic conditions including rhinitis and conjunctivitis.

4.2 Posology and method of administration
Adults

1mg twice daily with food. If necessary the dose may be increased to 2mg twice daily.

Children

(From 2 years of age): 1mg twice daily with food.

Use in the elderly

No evidence exists that elderly patients require different dosages or show different side-effects from younger patients.

Patients known to be easily sedated should be given 0.5-1mg at night for the first few days.

4.3 Contraindications
Hypersensitivity to ketotifen or any of the excipients. A reversible fall in the thrombocyte count in patients receiving ZADITEN concomitantly with oral anti-diabetic agents has been observed in a few cases. This combination of drugs should therefore be avoided until this phenomenon has been satisfactorily explained.

4.4 Special warnings and special precautions for use
Post-marketing surveillance has shown exacerbation of asthma in approximately 2 per 1000 patients. Since some of these asthmatic attacks might have been related to stopping existing treatment it is important to continue such treatment for a minimum of 2 weeks after starting ZADITEN. This applies especially to systemic corticosteroids and ACTH because of the possible existence of adrenocortical insufficiency in steroid dependent patients: in such cases recovery of a normal pituitary-adrenal response to stress may take up to one year. If it is necessary to withdraw ZADITEN this should be done progressively over a period of 2 to 4 weeks. Symptoms of asthma may recur. If intercurrent infection occurs, ZADITEN treatment must be supplemented by specific antimicrobial therapy.

4.5 Interaction with other medicinal products and other forms of Interaction
ZADITEN may potentiate the effects of sedatives, hypnotics, antihistamines and alcohol. Patients should be warned not to take charge of vehicles or machinery until the effect of ZADITEN treatment on the individual is known.

4.6 Pregnancy and lactation
Although there is no evidence of any teratogenic effect, recommendation for ZADITEN in pregnancy cannot be given. Ketotifen is excreted in breast milk, therefore mothers receiving ZADITEN should not breast feed.

4.7 Effects on ability to drive and use machines
During the first few days of treatment with ZADITEN reactions may be impaired. Patients should be warned not to take charge of vehicles or machinery until the effect of ZADITEN treatment on the individual is known.

Elixir only: Patients should be advised to avoid alcoholic drinks.

4.8 Undesirable effects
Drowsiness and, in isolated cases, dry mouth and slight dizziness may occur at the beginning of treatment, but usually disappear spontaneously after a few days. Occasionally symptoms of CNS stimulation have been observed. Weight gain has been reported.

Cystitis has been rarely described in association with ZADITEN. Isolated cases of severe skin reactions (erythema multiforme, Stevens-Johnson syndrome) have been reported.

4.9 Overdose
The reported features of overdose include confusion, drowsiness, nystagmus, headache, disorientation, tachycardia, hypotension, reversible coma; especially in children, hyperexcitability or convulsions. Bradycardia and respiratory depression should be watched for. Elimination of the drug with gastric lavage or emesis is recommended. Otherwise, general supportive treatment is all that is required.

5. PHARMACOLOGICAL PROPERTIES

5.1 Pharmacodynamic properties
ZADITEN is a non-bronchodilator anti-asthmatic drug which inhibits the effect of certain endogenous substances known to be inflammatory mediators, and thereby exerts anti-allergic activity.

Laboratory experiments indicate that this anti-asthmatic activity may be due to the inhibition of release of allergic mediators such as histamine and leukotrienes and the inhibition of the development of airway hyperactivity associated with activation of platelets by PAF (platelet activating factor) or caused by neural activation following the use of sympathomimetic drugs or the exposure to allergen. In addition, ZADITEN exerts a non-competitive blocking effect on histamine (H1) receptors.

Experimental investigations in asthmatic subjects have shown that ZADITEN is as effective orally as a selective mast cell stabiliser administered by inhalation: antihistamines are ineffective in these tests. The effectiveness of ZADITEN in the prevention of bronchial asthma has been studied in long-term clinical trials. Asthma attacks were reduced in number, severity and duration and in some cases the patients were completely freed from attacks. Progressive reduction of corticosteroids and/or bronchodilators was also possible.

The prophylactic activity of ZADITEN may take several weeks to become fully established.

ZADITEN will not abort established attacks of asthma.

5.2 Pharmacokinetic properties
After oral administration the absorption of ZADITEN is nearly complete. Bioavailability amounts to approximately 50% due to a first pass effect of about 50% in the liver. Maximal plasma concentrations are reached within 2-4 hours. Protein binding is 75%. Ketotifen is eliminated biphasically with a short half-life of 3-5 hours and a longer one of 21 hours. In urine about 1% of the substance is excreted unchanged within 48 hours and 60-70% as metabolites. The main metabolite in the urine is the practically inactive ketotifen-N-glucuronide.

5.3 Preclinical safety data
Not stated.

6. PHARMACEUTICAL PARTICULARS

6.1 List of excipients
Tablets:

Magnesium stearate, pre-gel cornstarch, maize starch and lactose.

Elixir:

Strawberry flavour, propyl hydroxybenzoate, methyl hydroxybenzoate, citric acid anhydrous, disodium phosphate anhydrous, ethyl alcohol 96% w/w, maltitol liquid (grade 80/55) and purified water.

6.2 Incompatibilities
None known.

6.3 Shelf life
36 months

6.4 Special precautions for storage
Store below 25°C

6.5 Nature and contents of container
Tablets:

PVDC opaque blister pack (60 tablets).

Elixir:

Amber glass bottle with a child resistant, tamper evident closure, composed of a polypropylene or polyethylene outer, a polypropylene or polyethylene inner, with a wad faced with PP, PVDC or PET lining. Bottle size 300ml.

6.6 Instructions for use and handling
None

7. MARKETING AUTHORISATION HOLDER
Novartis Pharmaceuticals UK Limited

Trading as Sandoz Pharmaceuticals

Frimley Business Park

Frimley

Camberley

Surrey

GU16 7SR

8. MARKETING AUTHORISATION NUMBER(S)
Tablets: PL 0101/0125

Elixir: PL 0101/0137

9. DATE OF FIRST AUTHORISATION/RENEWAL OF THE AUTHORISATION
Tablets: 24 April 1980

Elixir: 18 April 1997

10. DATE OF REVISION OF THE TEXT
Tablets: 17 November 2000

Elixir: August 2000

LEGAL CATEGORY
POM

ZAMADOL 24hr 150 (200/300/400)mg TABLETS

(Viatris Pharmaceuticals Ltd)

1. NAME OF THE MEDICINAL PRODUCT
ZAMADOL 24hr 150 (200/300/400)mg TABLETS

2. QUALITATIVE AND QUANTITATIVE COMPOSITION
Each tablet contains 150 (200/300/400)mg of tramadol hydrochloride

For excipients, see 6.1

3. PHARMACEUTICAL FORM
Prolonged release tablet

White film coated tablets marked T 150 (200/300/400)

4. CLINICAL PARTICULARS

4.1 Therapeutic indications
Treatment of moderate to severe pain.

4.2 Posology and method of administration
ZAMADOL 24hr tablets should be taken at 24-hourly intervals and must be swallowed whole and not chewed.

As with all analgesic drugs, the dose of tramadol should be adjusted according to the severity of the pain and the clinical response of the individual patient. The correct dosage for any individual patient is that which controls the pain with no or tolerable side effects for a full 24 hours. Patients transferring from immediate release tramadol preparations should have their total daily dose calculated, and start on the nearest dose in the ZAMADOL 24hr range. It is recommended that patients are slowly titrated to higher doses to minimise transient side effects. The need for continued treatment should be assessed at regular intervals as withdrawal symptoms and dependence have been reported. (See Section 4.4 Special Warnings and Precautions for Use). A total daily dose of 400 mg should not be exceeded except in special clinical circumstances.

Adults and children over 12 years: The usual initial dose is one 150 mg tablet daily. If pain relief is not achieved, the dosage should be titrated upwards until pain relief is achieved.

Elderly patients: Dosing as for adults. The elimination half-life of tramadol may be prolonged in patients over 75 years. A starting dose of 150 mg daily is recommended. Dose titration upwards should be carefully monitored.

Patients with renal or hepatic insufficiency: The elimination half-life of tramadol may be prolonged in these patient populations. A starting dose of

150 mg daily is recommended. Dose titration upwards should be carefully monitored. Tramadol is not recommended for patients with severe renal impairment and/or severe hepatic impairment.

As tramadol is only removed very slowly by haemodialysis or by haemofiltration, post-dialysis administration to maintain analgesia is not usually necessary.

Children under 12 years: ZAMADOL 24hr has not been studied in children. Safety and efficacy of ZAMADOL 24hr have not been established and the product should not be used in children.

4.3 Contraindications

Hypersensitivity to tramadol or to any of the excipients; acute intoxication with alcohol, hypnotics, centrally acting analgesics, opioids or psychotropic drugs. Tramadol should not be administered to patients who are receiving monoamine oxidase inhibitors or within two weeks of their withdrawal.

Tramadol must not be used for narcotic withdrawal treatment.

4.4 Special warnings and special precautions for use

Warnings

At therapeutic doses withdrawal symptoms have been reported at a frequency of 1 in 8,000. Reports of dependence and abuse have been less frequent. Because of this potential the clinical need for continued analgesic treatment should be reviewed regularly.

In patients with a tendency to drug abuse or dependence, treatment should be for short periods and under strict medical supervision.

Tramadol is not suitable as a substitute in opioid-dependent patients. Although it is an opioid agonist, tramadol cannot suppress morphine withdrawal symptoms.

Precautions

Convulsions have been reported at therapeutic doses and the risk may be increased at doses exceeding the usual upper daily dose limit. Patients with a history of epilepsy or those susceptible to seizures should only be treated with tramadol if there are compelling reasons. The risk of convulsions may increase in patients taking tramadol and concomitant medication that can lower the seizure threshold. (See Section 4.5 Interactions with other Medicaments and other forms of Interaction).

Tramadol should be used with caution in patients with head injury, increased intracranial pressure, severe impairment of hepatic and renal function and in patients prone to convulsive disorders or in shock.

Care should be taken when treating patients with respiratory depression, or if concomitant CNS depressant drugs are being administered, as the possibility of respiratory depression cannot be excluded in these situations. At therapeutic doses respiratory depression has infrequently been reported.

4.5 Interaction with other medicinal products and other forms of Interaction

Concurrent administration of tramadol with other centrally acting drugs, including alcohol, may potentiate CNS depressant effects.

Simultaneous treatment with carbamazepine may shorten the analgesic effect as a result of a reduction in serum levels of tramadol and its active metabolite.

Co-administration with cimetidine is associated with a small prolongation of the half-life of tramadol, but this is not clinically relevant.

Tramadol can induce convulsions and increase the potential for selective serotonin re-uptake inhibitors (SSRIs), tricyclic anti-depressants (TCAs), anti-psychotics and other seizure threshold lowering drugs to cause convulsions (see Section 4.4 Special Warnings and Special Precautions for Use and 5.2 Pharmacokinetic Properties). Co-administration with SSRIs may lead to an increase of 5HT associated effects.

Co-administered ritonavir may increase serum concentration of tramadolresulting in tramadol toxicity.

Digoxin toxicity has occurred rarely during co-administration of digoxin and tramadol.

MAO inhibitors: A serotoninergic syndrome is likely to occur: diarrhoea, tachycardia, sweating, tremor, confusion, coma. In case of recent treatment with MAOIs, treatment with tramadol should not be started until 15 days after cessation of treatment with MAOIs.

Other morphine derivatives (including anti-tussives, substitution treatments), benzodiazepines, barbiturates: Increased risk of respiratory depression, that may be fatal in overdosage.

Mixed agonists/antagonists (eg buprenorphine, nalbuphine, pentazocine): The analgesic effect of tramadol which is a pure agonist may be reduced, and a withdrawal syndrome may occur.

There have been isolated reports of interaction with coumarin anticoagulants resulting in an increased INR and so care should be taken when commencing treatment with tramadol in patients on anticoagulants.

4.6 Pregnancy and lactation

There are no adequate data from the use of tramadol in pregnant women. Animal studies have shown reproductive toxicity, but not teratogenic effects (see section 5.3). Tramadol crosses the placental barrier and chronic use during pregnancy can cause withdrawal symptoms in the newborn baby. Therefore, it should not be used during pregnancy.

Tramadol administered before or during birth does not affect uterine contractility. In neonates it may induce changes in respiratory rate which are not usually clinically relevant.

During lactation very small amounts of tramadol and its metabolites (approximately 0.1% of an intravenous dose) are found in human breast milk. Therefore tramadol should not be administered during breast feeding.

4.7 Effects on ability to drive and use machines

Tramadol may cause drowsiness, blurred vision and dizziness which may be enhanced by alcohol or other CNS depressants. If affected, the patient should not drive or operate machinery.

4.8 Undesirable effects

Nervous system disorders	
Very Common (>10%)	Dizziness
Common (1 to 10%)	Muzziness
Uncommon (0.1 to 1%)	Headache
Rare (< 0.1%)	Paraesthesia, Blurred vision Hallucinations Nightmares Changes in mood (usually elation, occasionally dysphoria) Changes in activity (usually suppression, occasionally an increase) Changes in cognitive and sensorial capacity (e.g. decision behaviour, perception disorders) Epileptiform convulsions have occurred after administration of high doses of tramadol or after concomitant treatment with drugs which can lower the seizure threshold or themselves induce cerebral convulsions (eg anti-depressants or anti-psychotics)
Cardiovascular	
Uncommon (0.1 to 1%)	Palpitation Tachycardia Postural hypotension Cardiovascular collapse
Rare (< 0.1%)	Hypertension Bradycardia
Respiratory disorders	
Rare (< 0.1%)	Dyspnoea Worsening of asthma has been reported, though a causal relationship has not been established. Respiratory depression. If the recommended doses are considerably exceeded and other centrally depressant substances are administered concomitantly, respiratory depression may occur.
Gastro-intestinal disorders	
Very Common (> 10%)	Nausea
Common (1 to 10%)	Vomiting Dry mouth
Uncommon (0.1 to 1%)	Retching Constipation Gastrointestinal irritation
Rare (< 0.1%)	Anorexia Diarrhoea

Skin & appendages	
Common (1 to 10%)	sweating
Uncommon (0.1 to 1%)	pruritus, rash, urticaria
Urogenital	
Rare (<0.1%)	Micturition disorders (difficulty in passing urine and urinary retention)
Body as a whole	
Rare (<0.1%)	Muscle weakness Flushing Allergic reactions (eg dyspnoea, bronchospasm, wheezing, angioneurotic oedema) Anaphylaxis Dependence Withdrawal reactions, similar to those occurring during opiate withdrawal, may occur and include: agitation, anxiety, nervousness, insomnia, hyperkinesia, tremor and gastrointestinal symptoms. Increase in liver enzyme values have been reported in a temporal connection with the therapeutic use of tramadol

4.9 Overdose

Symptoms of overdosage are typical of other opioid analgesics, and include miosis, vomiting, cardiovascular collapse, sedation and coma, seizures and respiratory depression.

Supportive measures such as maintaining the patency of the airway and maintaining cardiovascular function should be instituted; naloxone should be used to reverse respiratory depression; fits can be controlled with diazepam.

Tramadol is minimally eliminated from the serum by haemodialysis or haemofiltration. Therefore treatment of acute intoxication with tramadol with haemodialysis or haemofiltration alone is not suitable for detoxification.

Emptying the gastric contents is useful to remove any unabsorbed drug, particularly when a modified release formulation has been taken.

5. PHARMACOLOGICAL PROPERTIES

5.1 Pharmacodynamic properties

Tramadol is a centrally acting analgesic (N02A X02). It is a non selective pure agonist at mu, delta and kappa opioid receptors with a higher affinity for the mu receptor. Other mechanisms that may contribute to its analgesic effect are inhibition of neuronal re-uptake of noradrenaline and 5HT.

5.2 Pharmacokinetic properties

Following oral administration of a single dose, tramadol is almost completely absorbed and the absolute bioavailability is approximately 70%. Tramadol is metabolised to O-desmethyltramadol, which has been shown to have analgesic activity in rodents. The elimination half life of tramadol is around 6 hours, although this is extended to around 16 hours following prolonged absorption from the ZAMADOL 24hr tablet.

Following administration of one ZAMADOL 24hr tablet 200 mg in the fasting state, a mean peak plasma concentration (Cmax) of 192 ng.ml-1 was attained. This was associated with a median t_{max} of 6 hours (range 4-8 hours). The availability of tramadol from the ZAMADOL 24hr tablet 200 mg was complete when compared with an immediate release tramadol solution 100 mg, after dose adjustment. In the presence of food, the availability and controlled release properties of ZAMADOL 24hr tablets were maintained, with no evidence of dose-dumping.

A single dose-proportionality study has confirmed a linear pharmacokinetic response (in relation to tramadol and O-desmethyltramadol) following administration of the 200 mg, 300 mg and 400 mg tablets. A steady state study has confirmed the dose adjusted bioequivalence of the 150 mg and 200 mg tablets administered once-daily. This study also confirmed that the ZAMADOL 24hr tablet 150 mg provided an equivalent peak concentration and extent of availability of tramadol to an immediate release capsule 50 mg administered 8-hourly. On this basis it is recommended that patients receiving immediate release tramadol should be transferred initially to the nearest daily dose of ZAMADOL 24hr tablets. It may be necessary to titrate the dose thereafter.

A further steady state study has demonstrated that immediate release tramadol tablets 50 mg, administered 6-hourly, provided plasma concentrations that were greater than would have been anticipated following administration of a single dose. This observation is consistent with a non-linear elimination of the drug substance. In contrast, the plasma concentrations from ZAMADOL 24hr tablet 200 mg administered once-daily were in line with single dose data, confirming that the controlled delivery of tramadol from ZAMADOL 24hr minimises the non-linearity associated with faster-releasing preparations. The more predictable plasma concentrations may lead to a more manageable dose titration process.

5.3 Preclinical safety data

Preclinical data reveal no special hazard for humans based on conventional studies of safety pharmacology, repeated dose toxicity, genotoxicity or carcinogenic potential.

Studies in rats and rabbits have revealed no teratogenic effects. However, embryotoxicity was shown in the form of delayed ossification. Fertility, reproductive performance and development of offspring were unaffected.

6. PHARMACEUTICAL PARTICULARS

6.1 List of excipients

Tablet core

Hydrogenated vegetable oil

Talc

Magnesium stearate

Film coat

Lactose Monohydrate

Hypromellose (E464)

Titanium dioxide (E171)

Macrogol 4000

6.2 Incompatibilities

None known.

6.3 Shelf life

3 years

6.4 Special precautions for storage

Do not store above 30C.

6.5 Nature and contents of container

1) PVC blisters with aluminium backing foil (containing 2, 7, 10, 14, 15, 20, 28, 30, 50,56, 60 or 100 tablets).

2) Polypropylene containers with polyethylene lids (containing 2, 7, 10, 14, 15, 20, 28, 30, 50,56, 60 or 100 tablets).

Not all pack sizes may be marketed

6.6 Instructions for use and handling

None.

Administrative Data

7. MARKETING AUTHORISATION HOLDER

Napp Pharmaceuticals Ltd

Cambridge Science Park

Milton Road

Cambridge CB4 0GW

UK

8. MARKETING AUTHORISATION NUMBER(S)

PL 16950/0084 (85/86/87)

9. DATE OF FIRST AUTHORISATION/RENEWAL OF THE AUTHORISATION

7 November 2001

10. DATE OF REVISION OF THE TEXT

December 2004

Zamadol Melt 50 mg Tablets

(Viatris Pharmaceuticals Ltd)

1. NAME OF THE MEDICINAL PRODUCT

Zamadol® Melt 50 mg Tablets

2. QUALITATIVE AND QUANTITATIVE COMPOSITION

Each tablet contains 50 mg of tramadol hydrochloride.

For excipients, see 6.1

3. PHARMACEUTICAL FORM

Orodispersible tablets and dispersible tablets.

Round, white, biconcave tablet, engraved 'T' on one side and '50' on the other side, with a characteristic mint flavour.

4. CLINICAL PARTICULARS

4.1 Therapeutic indications

Treatment of moderate to severe pain.

4.2 Posology and method of administration

As with all analgesic drugs, the dose of Zamadol Melt 50 mg Tablets should be adjusted according to the severity of the pain and the clinical response of the individual patient.

Adults and adolescents aged 12 years and over

For oral use:

Acute pain:

An initial dose is 50-100 mg depending on the intensity of pain. This can be followed by doses of 50 or 100 mg not more frequently than 4 hourly, and duration of therapy should be matched to clinical need. A total daily dose of 400 mg should not be exceeded except in special clinical circumstances.

Pain associated with chronic conditions:

Use an initial dose of 50 mg and then titrate dose according to pain severity. The initial dose may be followed if necessary by 50-100 mg every 4 to 6 hours. The recommended doses are intended as a guideline. Patients should always receive the lowest dose that provides effective pain control. A total daily dose of 400 mg should not be exceeded except in special clinical circumstances. The need for continued treatment should be assessed at regular intervals as withdrawal symptoms and dependence have been reported (see section 4.4 Special warnings and special precautions for use).

Elderly:

The usual dosagemay be used although it should be noted that in volunteers aged over 75 years the elimination half-life of tramadol was increased following oral administration. An adjustment of the dosage or increasing the dose interval should be considered.

Renal impairment/renal dialysis:

The elimination of tramadol may be prolonged. The usual initial dosage should be used. For patients with creatinine clearance < 30 ml/min, the dosage interval should be increased to 12 hours. Tramadol is not recommended for patients with severe renal impairment (creatinine clearance < 10 ml/min).

As tramadol is only removed very slowly by haemodialysis or haemofiltration, post-dialysis administration to maintain analgesia is not usually necessary.

Hepatic impairment:

The elimination of tramadol may be prolonged. The usual initial dosage should be used but in hepatic impairment the dosage interval should be increased to 12 hours and the dose reduced if necessary. Tramadol is not recommended for patients with severe hepatic impairment.

Children under 12 years:

Not recommended.

The tablet disperses rapidly in the mouth and is then swallowed. Alternatively, the tablet can be dispersed in half a glass of water, stirred and drunk immediately independently of meals.

4.3 Contraindications

Zamadol Melt 50 mg Tablets must not be administered to patients who have previously demonstrated hypersensitivity to the active substance or any of the excipients.

The product must not be administered to patients suffering from acute intoxication or overdose with alcohol, hypnotics, centrally acting analgesics, opioids or psychotropic drugs.

In common with other opioid analgesics it must not be administered to patients who are receiving monoamine oxidase inhibitors or within two weeks of their withdrawal. It must not be administered concomitantly with nalbuphine, buprenorphine or pentazocine (see 4.5, interactions with other medicinal products and other forms of interaction).

Contraindicated in patients suffering from uncontrolled epilepsy.

Tramadol must not be administered during breast-feeding if long term treatment is necessary.

Zamadol Melt 50 mg Tablets is not suitable for children under 12 years of age.

4.4 Special warnings and special precautions for use

Warnings:

At therapeutic doses, Zamadol Melt 50 mg Tablets has the potential to cause withdrawal symptoms. Rarely cases of dependence and abuse have been reported. However, Zamadol Melt should only be used for short periods and under strict medical supervision in patients with a tendency of drug abuse or dependence.

At therapeutic doses withdrawal symptoms have been reported at a reporting frequency of 1 in 8,000. Reports of dependence and abuse have been less frequent. Because of this potential the clinical need for continued analgesic treatment should be reviewed regularly. In patients with a tendency to drug abuse or dependence, treatment should be for short periods and under strict medical supervision.

Zamadol Melt is not suitable as a substitute in opioid-dependent patients. Although it is an opioid agonist, it cannot suppress morphine withdrawal symptoms.

Alcohol intake and concomitant use of carbamazepine are not recommended during treatment.

Precautions:

Zamadol Melt should be used with caution in patients with head injury, increased intracranial pressure, impairment of hepatic and renal function, decreased level of consciousness and in patients prone to convulsive disorders or in shock.

Convulsions have been reported at therapeutic doses and the risk may be increased at doses exceeding the usual upper daily dose limit. Patients with a history of epilepsy or those susceptible to seizures should only be treated with tramadol if there are compelling reasons. The risk of convulsions may increase in patients taking tramadol and concomitant medication that can lower the seizure threshold (see section 4.5 Interaction with other medicinal products and other forms of interaction).

At the recommended doses Zamadol Melt is unlikely to produce clinically relevant respiratory depression. However, care should be taken when treating patients with existing respiratory depression, or excessive bronchial secretion and in those patients taking concomitant CNS depressant drugs.

The ingredient aspartame contains a source of phenylalanine which may be harmful to people with phenylketonuria.

4.5 Interaction with other medicinal products and other forms of Interaction

Concomitant use of the following is contraindicated:

Patients treated with monoamine oxidase inhibitors within 14 days prior to the administration of the opioid pethidine have experienced life-threatening interactions affecting the central nervous system as well as the respiratory and circulatory centres (risk of serotonergic syndrome – see below). The possibility of similar interactions occurring between monoamine oxidase inhibitors (including the selective MAO A and B inhibitors and linezolid) and tramadol cannot be ruled out.

The combination of mixed agonists/ antagonists (e.g. buprenorphine, nalbuphine, pentazocine) and tramadol is not recommended because it is theoretically possible that the analgesic effect of a pure agonist is attenuated under these circumstances and that a withdrawal syndrome may occur.

Concomitant use of the following needs to be taken into consideration:

Isolated cases of serotonergic syndrome have been reported with the therapeutic use of tramadol in combination with other serotonergic agents such as selective serotonin re-uptake inhibitors (SSRIs). Signs of serotonergic syndrome may include: confusion, restlessness, agitation, fever, sweat, tachycardia, tremor, ataxia, hyper-reflexia, myoclonus, diarrhoea and possibly coma. Withdrawal of the serotonergic agent produces a rapid improvement.

Concomitant administration of Zamadol Melt with other centrally acting drugs(including other opioid derivatives, benzodiazepines, barbiturates, other anxiolytics, hypnotics, sedative anti-depressants, sedative anti-histamines, neuroleptics, centrally acting anti-hypotensive drugs, baclofen and alcohol) may potentiate CNS depressant effects including respiratory depression.

Simultaneous administration of carbamazepine markedly decreases serum concentrations of tramadol to an extent that a decrease in analgesic effectiveness and a shorter duration of action may occur.

Tramadol may increase the potential forselective serotonin reuptake inhibitors (SSRIs), tricyclic antidepressants (TCAs), anti-psychotics and other seizure threshold lowering drugs (e.g. bupropion and mefloquine) to cause convulsions (see sections 4.4 Special warnings and special precautions for use and 5.2 Pharmacokinetic properties).

There have been isolated reports of interaction with coumarin anticoagulants resulting in an increased international normalised ratio (INR) and so care should be taken when commencing treatment with tramadol in patients on anticoagulants.

4.6 Pregnancy and lactation

Pregnancy:

In humans, there are no sufficient data to assess malformative effect of tramadol when given during the first trimester of pregnancy. Animal studies have not shown any teratogenic effects, but at high doses, foetotoxicity due to maternotoxicity appeared (See 5.3 Preclinical data).

Tramadol crosses the placenta, therefore as with other opioid analgesics, chronic use of tramadol during the third trimester may induce a withdrawal syndrome in new-born. At the end of pregnancy, high dosages, even for short term treatment, may induce respiratory depression in new-born. There is inadequate evidence available on the safety of tramadol in human pregnancy, therefore Zamadol Melt should not be used in pregnant woman.

Lactation:

Tramadol and its metabolites are found in small amounts in human breast milk. An infant could ingest 0.1 % of the dose given to the mother. Zamadol Melt should not be administered during breast feeding.

4.7 Effects on ability to drive and use machines

Zamadol Melt may cause drowsiness and this effect may be potentiated by alcohol and other CNS depressants. Ambulant patients should be warned not to drive or operate machinery if affected.

4.8 Undesirable effects

The table below presents possible adverse drug reactions in system organ class order and sorted by frequency.

(see Table 1 on next page)

Psychic side-effects may occur following administration of tramadol which vary individually in intensity and nature (depending on personality and duration of medication). These include changes in mood (usually elation, occasionally dysphoria), changes in activity (usually suppression, occasionally increase) and changes in cognitive and sensorial capacity (e.g. decision behaviour, perception disorders), hallucinations, confusion, sleep disturbances and nightmares.

Prolonged administration of Zamadol Melt may lead to dependence (see section 4.4). Symptoms of withdrawal reactions, similar to those occurring during opiate withdrawal, may occur as follows: agitation, anxiety, nervousness, insomnia, hyperkinesia, tremor and gastrointestinal symptoms.

Epileptiform convulsions are rare and occur mainly after administration of high doses of tramadol or after concomitant treatment with drugs which can lower the seizure threshold or themselves induce cerebral convulsions (e.g. antidepressants or anti-psychotics, see section 4.5 "Interaction with other medicinal products and other forms of interaction".

Worsening of asthma has also been reported, though a causal relationship has not been established. Respiratory depression has been reported. If the recommended doses are considerably exceeded and other centrally depressant

Table 1

Organ System	Frequency	Adverse drug reaction
Immune system disorders	***Rare*** *(> 1/10.000, < 1/1.000)*	- allergic reactions (e.g. dyspnoea, bronchospasm, wheezing, angioneurotic oedema) and anaphylaxis.
Metabolism and Nutritional disorders	***Rare*** *(> 1/10.000, < 1/1.000)*	- changes in appetite.
Psychiatric disorders	***Rare*** *(> 1/10.000, < 1/1.000)*	The following may vary in nature and intensity depending on the individual (see below): - changes in mood (e.g. elation, dysphoria) - changes in activity (e.g. suppression, increase) - change in cognitive and sensorial capacity (e.g. decision behaviour, perception disorders) - hallucinations - confusion - sleep disturbances - nightmares - dependency (see below)
Nervous system disorders	***Very Common*** *(> 1/10)*	- dizziness
	Common *(> 1/100, < 1/10)*	- headache - drowsiness
	Rare *(> 1/10.000, < 1/1.000)*	- epileptiform convulsions (see below) - paraesthesia - tremor.
	Very rare (including isolated cases) *(< 1/10.000)*	- vertigo
Eye disorders	***Rare*** *(> 1/10.000, < 1/1.000*	- blurred vision
Cardiac disorders	***Uncommon*** *(> 1/1000, < 1/100)*	- cardiovascular regulation (e.g. palpitation, tachycardia, postural hypotension, cardiovascular collapse). These effects may occur especially on intravenous administration and in patients who are physically stressed.
	Rare *(> 1/10.000, < 1/1.000)*	- bradycardia, increase in blood pressure
Vascular disorders	***Very rare (including isolated cases)*** *(< 1/10.000)*	- flushing
Respiratory, thoracic and mediastinal disorders	***Very rare (including isolated cases)*** *(< 1/10.000)*	- worsening of asthma, respiratory depression (see below)
Gastrointestinal disorders	***Very Common*** *(> 1/10)*	- vomiting, nausea
	Common *(> 1/100, < 1/10)*	- constipation, dry mouth
	Uncommon *(> 1/1000, < 1/100)*	- retching, gastrointestinal irritation (a feeling of pressure in the stomach, bloating)
Hepato-biliary disorders	***Very rare (including isolated cases)*** *(< 1/10.000)*	- increase in liver enzyme values (a few isolated cases have been reported)
Skin and subcutaneous tissue disorders	***Common*** *(> 1/100 < 1/10)*	- sweating
	Uncommon *(> 1/1000, < 1/100)*	- dermal reactions (e.g. pruritus, rash, urticaria)
Musculoskeletal, connective tissue and bone disorders	***Rare*** *(> 1/10.000, < 1/1.000)*	- motorial weakness
Renal and urinary system disorders	***Rare*** *(> 1/10.000, < 1/1.000)*	- micturition disorders (difficulty in passing urine and urinary retention)
General disorders	***Common*** *(> 1/100, < 1/10)*	- fatigue

substances are administered concomitantly (see section 4.5 "Interaction with other medicinal products and other forms of interaction") respiratory depression may occur.

4.9 Overdose

Symptoms of overdose are typical of other opioid analgesics, and include miosis, vomiting, hypotension, cardiovascular collapse, sedation and coma, epileptic seizures and respiratory depression. Respiratory failure may also occur.

Supportive measures such as maintaining the patency of the airway and maintaining cardiovascular function should be instituted; naloxone should be used to reverse respiratory depression; fits can be controlled with diazepam. Naloxone administration may increase the risk of seizures. The use of benzodiazepines (intravenously) should be considered for patients with seizures.

Tramadol is minimally eliminated from the serum by haemodialysis or haemofiltration. Therefore treatment of acute intoxication with Zamadol Melt with haemodialysis or haemofiltration alone is not suitable for detoxification.

5. PHARMACOLOGICAL PROPERTIES

5.1 Pharmacodynamic properties

Analgesic, Other opioids, ATC code: N02AX02

Tramadol is a centrally acting analgesic. It is a non selective pure agonist at mu, delta and kappa opioid receptors with a higher affinity for the mu receptor. Other mechanisms which may contribute to its analgesic effect are inhibition of neuronal reuptake of noradrenaline and enhancement of serotonin release.

Tramadol has antitussive properties. Unlike morphine, tramadol does not depress breathing over a wide range of analgesic doses. The effects of tramadol on the cardiovascular system are comparatively small. The potency of tramadol is 1/10 to 1/6 that of morphine.

5.2 Pharmacokinetic properties

Absorption

After oral administration, tramadol is almost completely absorbed. Mean absolute bioavailability is approximately 70% following a single dose and increases to approximately 90% at steady state.

Following a single oral dose administration of tramadol 100 mg to young healthy volunteers, plasma concentrations were detectable within approximately 15-45 minutes with a mean C_{max} of 280 to 308 ng/ml and T_{max} of 1.6 to 2 hours.

In a specific study of comparing the Orodispersible tablets with Immediate Release capsules, the administration of a single dose of 50 mg Zamadol Melt in healthy volunteers produced a mean AUC 1102 ± 357 ng.h/ml, a mean Cmax 141 ± 39 ng/ml; and a mean T_{max} 1.5 hours. This demonstrated bioequivalence to 50 mg immediate release capsules (AUC 1008 ± 285 ng.h/ml; C_{max} 139 ± 37 ng/ml; T_{max} 1.5 hours).

Distribution

Plasma protein binding of tramadol is approximately 20%. It is independent of the plasma concentration of the drug within the therapeutic range.

Tramadol crosses the blood-brain barrier and the placental barrier. Tramadol and its metabolite O-desmethyltramadol are detectable in breast milk in very small amounts (0.1% and 0.02% of the administered doses, respectively).

Tramadol has a high tissue affinity, with an apparent volume of distribution of 3 to 4 l/kg.

Metabolism

Tramadol is metabolised by cytochrome P450 isoenzyme CYP2D6. It undergoes biotransformation to a number of metabolites mainly by means of N- and O-demethylation. O-desmethyl tramadol appears to be the most pharmacologically active metabolite, showing analgesic activity in rodents. It is 2 to 4 times more active than tramadol.

As humans excrete a higher percentage of unchanged tramadol than animals it is believed that the contribution made by this metabolite to analgesic activity is likely to be less in humans than animals. In humans the plasma concentration of this metabolite is about 25% that of unchanged tramadol.

The inhibition of one or both cytochrome P450 isoenzymes, CYP3A4 and CYP2D6 involved in the metabolism of tramadol, may affect the plasma concentration of tramadol or its active metabolite. The clinical consequences of any such interactions are not known.

Elimination

For tramadol, the terminal elimination half-life ($t_{½\beta}$) was 6.0 ± 1.5 hours in young volunteers. For O-desmethyltramadol, $t_{½\beta}$ (6 healthy volunteers) was 7.9 hours (range 5.4 – 9.6 hours).

When C^{14} labelled tramadol was administered to humans, approximately 90% was excreted via the kidneys with the remaining 10% appearing in the faeces.

Tramadol pharmacokinetics show little age dependence in volunteers up to the age of 75 years. In volunteers aged over 75 years, $t_{½\beta}$ was 7.0 ± 1.6 hours on oral administration.

Since tramadol is eliminated both metabolically and renally, the terminal half-life $t_{½\beta}$ may be prolonged in impaired hepatic or renal function. However, the increase in the $t_{½\beta}$ values is relatively low if at least one of these organs is functioning normally. In patients with liver cirrhosis $t_{½\beta}$ tramadol was a mean of 13.3 ± 4.9 hours; in patients with renal insufficiency (creatinine clearance ≤ 5 ml/min) it was 11.0 ± 3.2 hours.

PK/PD

Tramadol has a linear pharmacokinetic profile within the therapeutic dosage range.

The PK/PD relation is dose-dependent, but varies within a wide range. Generally, a serum concentration between 100 and 300 ng/ml is effective.

5.3 Preclinical safety data

In single and repeat-dose toxicity studies (rodents and dogs) exposure to tramadol 10 times that expected in man is required before toxicity (hepatotoxicity) is observed. Symptoms of toxicity are typical of opioids and include restlessness, ataxia, vomiting, tremor, dyspnoea and convulsions.

Exposure to tramadol (>that expected in man), in lifetime toxicity studies in rodents did not reveal any evidence of carcinogenic hazard, and a battery of *in-vitro* and *in-vivo* mutagenicity tests were negative.

No teratogenic effects have been observed in animal tests (rat and rabbit: the dosage of Tramadol given has been up to seven times higher than the dosage given to humans). Minimal embryo toxic effects (delayed ossification) were observed in the tests. No effect was observed on the fertility or the development of the offspring in the tests.

6. PHARMACEUTICAL PARTICULARS

6.1 List of excipients

ethylcellulose,

copovidone,

silicon dioxide,

mannitol (E421),

crospovidone,

aspartame (E951),

mint rootbeer flavouring,

magnesium stearate

6.2 Incompatibilities

Not applicable.

6.3 Shelf life

3 years.

6.4 Special precautions for storage

This medicinal product does not require any special storage precautions

6.5 Nature and contents of container

Tablets in blisters composed of two sheets:

- a complex of polyamide/ aluminium/poly(vinyl chloride)
- a sheet of aluminium.

Pack sizes: 10, 20, 28, 30, 40, 50, 56, 60 and 100 tablets.

'Not all pack sizes may be marketed.'

6.6 Instructions for use and handling

No special requirements.

7. MARKETING AUTHORISATION HOLDER

VIATRIS Pharmaceuticals Ltd
Beach Drive
Cambridge Research Park
Waterbeach
Cambridge, CB5 9PD
United Kingdom

8. MARKETING AUTHORISATION NUMBER(S)

UK: PL 19166/0036

9. DATE OF FIRST AUTHORISATION/RENEWAL OF THE AUTHORISATION

30 September 2003

10. DATE OF REVISION OF THE TEXT

8 July 2004

Zamadol SR Capsules 50mg, 100mg, 150mg, 200mg

(Viatris Pharmaceuticals Ltd)

1. NAME OF THE MEDICINAL PRODUCT

Zamadol® SR 50 mg Capsules
Zamadol® SR 100 mg Capsules
Zamadol® SR 150 mg Capsules
Zamadol® SR 200 mg Capsules

2. QUALITATIVE AND QUANTITATIVE COMPOSITION

One capsule contains 50 mg, 100 mg, 150 mg or 200 mg of tramadol hydrochloride

For excipients, see section 6.1

3. PHARMACEUTICAL FORM

Prolonged release capsule, hard.

The 50 mg capsules are darkgreen and marked T50SR.

The 100 mg capsules are white and marked T100SR.

The 150 mg capsules are dark green and marked T150SR.

The 200 mg capsules are yellow and marked T200SR.

4. CLINICAL PARTICULARS

4.1 Therapeutic indications

Treatment ofmoderate to severe pain.

4.2 Posology and method of administration

The capsules are intended for twice daily oral administration and can be taken independently of meal times, swallowed whole with water.

As with all analgesic drugs the dosing of Zamadol SR Capsules should be adjusted depending on the severity of the pain and the individual clinical response of the patient. The dose used should be the lowest dose that provides pain relief.

Adults:

The usual initial dose is 50-100 mg twice daily, morning and evening. This dose may be titrated up to 150-200 mg twice daily according to pain severity.

If long-term pain treatment with tramadol is necessary in view of the nature and severity of the illness, then careful and regular monitoring should be carried out (if necessary with breaks in treatment) to establish whether and to what extent further treatment is necessary.

A total oral daily dose of 400 mg should not be exceeded except in special clinical circumstances.

Elderly patients:

Dosing as for adults, however it should be noted that in patients over 75 years there tends to be an increase in absolute bioavailability of tramadol and a 17% increase in the terminal elimination half-life. An adjustment of the dosage or the dose interval may be required.

Patients with renal or hepatic insufficiency:

As the elimination of tramadol may be prolonged in patients with severe renal and/or hepatic impairment, the use of Zamadol SR Capsules is not recommended. In moderate cases an adjustment of the dosage interval may be required.

Patients who have difficulty in swallowing:

Zamadol SR Capsules can be opened, carefully, so that the pellets are deposited on a spoon. The spoon and pellets should be taken into the mouth, followed by a drink of water to rinse the mouth of all pellets. The pellets must not be chewed or crushed.

Children:

Over 12 years: Dosage as for adults.

Under 12 years: Zamadol SR Capsules have not been studied in children. Therefore, safety and efficacy have not been established and the product should not be used in children.

4.3 Contraindications

Zamadol SR Capsules should not be given to patients who have previously shown hypersensitivity to the active substance tramadol or to any of the excipients.

The product should not be administered to patients suffering from acute intoxication with hypnotics, centrally acting analgesics, opioids, psychotropic drugs or alcohol.

Tramadol should not be administered to patients who are receiving monoamine oxidase inhibitors or within 2 weeks of their withdrawal.

Contra-indicated in patients suffering from uncontrolled epilepsy.

Tramadol must not be used for narcotic withdrawal treatment.

4.4 Special warnings and special precautions for use

Warnings:

Tramadol has a low dependence potential. On long-term use tolerance, psychic and physical dependence may develop. In patients with a tendency to drug abuse or dependence, treatment should be for short periods under strict medical supervision. In rare cases at therapeutic doses, tramadol has the potential to cause withdrawal symptoms.

Zamadol SR Capsules are not a suitable substitute in opioid dependent patients. The product does not suppress morphine withdrawal symptoms although it is an opioid agonist.

Convulsions have been reported at therapeutic doses and the risk may be increased at doses exceeding the usual upper daily dose limit. Patients with a history of epilepsy or those susceptible to seizures should only be treated with tramadol if there are compelling reasons. The risk of convulsions may increase in patients taking tramadol and concomitant medication that can lower the seizure threshold (see section 4.5).

Precautions:

Zamadol SR Capsules should be used with prudence in patients who have shown previous hypersensitivity to opiates, and in patients with severe renal or hepatic impairment, head injury, decreased level of consciousness, increased intracranial pressure, or patients in shock or at risk of convulsions.

At recommended therapeutic doses Zamadol SR Capsules are unlikely to produce clinically relevant respiratory depression. Care should however be taken when administering Zamadol SR Capsules to patients with existing respiratory depression or excessive bronchial secretion and in those patients taking concomitant CNS depressant drugs.

4.5 Interaction with other medicinal products and other forms of Interaction

Patients treated with monoamine oxidase inhibitors within 14 days prior to the administration of the opioid pethidine have experienced life-threatening interactions affecting the central nervous system as well as the respiratory and circulatory centres. The possibility of similar interactions occurring between monoamine oxidase inhibitors and tramadol cannot be ruled out.

Tramadol may potentiate the CNS depressant effects of other centrally acting drugs (including alcohol) when administered concomitantly with such drugs.

Tramadol may increase the potential for selective serotonin re-uptake inhibitors (SSRIs), tricyclic antidepressants (TCAs), anti-psychotics and other seizure threshold lowering drugs to cause convulsions (See section 4.4).

Isolated cases of serotonergic syndrome have been reported with the therapeutic use of tramadol in combination with other serotonergic agents such as selective serotonin re-uptake inhibitors (SSRIs). Serotonergic syndrome can be manifested by symptoms such as confusion, restlessness, fever, sweat, ataxia, hyperreflexia, myoclonia and diarrhoea. Withdrawal of the serotonergic agent produces a rapid improvement.

Administration of Zamadol SR Capsules together with carbamazepine results in markedly decreased serum concentrations of tramadol which may reduce analgesic effectiveness and shorten the duration of action.

Caution should be exercised during concomitant treatment with tramadol and coumarin derivatives (e.g. warfarin) due to reports of increased INR and ecchymoses in some patients.

The combination of mixed agonists/antagonists (e.g. buprenorphine, nalbuphine, pentazocine) and tramadol is not recommended because it is theoretically possible that the analgesic effect of a pure agonist is attenuated under these circumstances.

There is no interaction with food.

4.6 Pregnancy and lactation

Pregnancy:

Zamadol SR Capsules should not be used during pregnancy as there is inadequate evidence available to assess the safety of tramadol in pregnant women. Tramadol - administered before or during birth - does not affect uterine contractility. In neonates it may induce changes in the respiratory rate which are usually not clinically relevant.

Lactation:

Zamadol SR Capsules should not be administered during breast feeding as tramadol and its metabolites have been detected in breast milk. 0.1% of the dose administered to the mother may be excreted in milk.

4.7 Effects on ability to drive and use machines

Zamadol SR Capsules may cause drowsiness and this effect may be potentiated by alcohol, anti-histamines and other CNS depressants. If patients are affected they should be warned not to drive or operate machinery.

4.8 Undesirable effects

The most commonly reported adverse drug reactions are nausea and dizziness, both occurring in more than 10% of patients.

Immune system disorders:

Rare >1/10,000, <1/1,000): Allergic reactions (e.g. dyspnoea, bronchospasm, wheezing, angioneurotic oedema) and anaphylaxis.

Metabolism and nutrition disorders:

Rare >1/10,000, <1/1,000): Changes in appetite.

Psychiatric disorders:

Rare >1/10,000, <1/1,000): psychic side-effects may occur following administration of tramadol which vary individually in intensity and nature (depending on personality and duration of medication). These include changes in mood (usually elation, occasionally dysphoria), changes in activity (usually suppression, occasionally increase) and changes in cognitive and sensorial capacity (e.g. decision behaviour, perception disorders), hallucinations, confusion, sleep disturbances and nightmares.

Prolonged administration of Zamadol SR Capsule may lead to dependence (see section 4.4). Symptoms of withdrawal reactions, similar to those occurring during opiate withdrawal, may occur as follows: agitation, anxiety, nervousness, insomnia, hyperkinesia, tremor and gastrointestinal symptoms.

Nervous system disorders:

Very common >1/10) dizziness.

Common >1/100, <1/10): headache, drowsiness.

Rare >1/10,000, ≤'1/1,000): epileptiform convulsions occurred mainly after administration of high doses of tramadol or after concomitant treatment with drugs which can lower the seizure threshold or themselves induce cerebral convulsions (e.g. antidepressants or anti-psychotics, see section 4.5 "Interaction with other medicinal products and other forms of interaction".

Paraesthesia and tremor.

Very rare (<1/10,000): vertigo

Eye disorders:

Rare >1/10,000, <1/1,000): blurred vision.

Cardiac disorders:

Uncommon >1/1,000, <1/100): effects on cardiovascular regulation (palpitation, tachycardia, postural hypotension or cardiovascular collapse). These adverse effects may occur especially on intravenous administration and in patients who are physically stressed.

Rare >1/10,000, <1/1,000): bradycardia, increase in blood pressure.

Vascular disorders:

Very rare (<1/10,000): flushing.

Respiratory disorders:

Worsening of asthma has also been reported, though a causal relationship has not been established.

Respiratory depression has been reported. If the recommended doses are considerably exceeded and other centrally depressant substances are administered concomitantly (see section 4.5 "Interaction with other medicinal products and other forms of interaction") respiratory depression may occur.

Gastrointestinal disorders:

Very common >1/10): vomiting, nausea.

Common >1/100, <1/10): constipation, dry mouth.

Uncommon >1/1,000, <1/100): retching, gastrointestinal irritation (a feeling of pressure in the stomach, bloating).

Hepato-biliary disorders:

In a few isolated cases an increase in liver enzyme values has been reported in a temporal connection with the therapeutic use of tramadol.

Skin and subcutaneous tissue disorders:

Common >1/100, <1/10): sweating.

Uncommon >1/1,000, <1/100): dermal reactions (e.g. pruritus, rash, urticaria).

Musculoskeletal, connective tissue and bone disorders:

Rare >1/10,000, <1/1,000): motorial weakness.

Renal and urinary system disorders:

Rare >1/10,000, <1/1,000): micturition disorders (difficulty in passing urine and urinary retention).

General disorders:

Common >1/100, <1/10): fatigue.

4.9 Overdose

Symptoms of tramadol overdose include vomiting, miosis, sedation, seizures, respiratory depression and hypotension, with circulatory failure and coma. Respiratory failure may also occur. Such symptoms are typical of opioid analgesics.

Treatment of overdose requires the maintenance of the airway and cardiovascular functions. Respiratory depression may be reversed using naloxone and fits controlled with diazepam. Naloxone administration may increase the risk of seizures.

The treatment of acute overdose of tramadol using haemodialysis or haemofiltration alone is not sufficient or suitable due to the slow elimination of tramadol from the serum by these routes.

5. PHARMACOLOGICAL PROPERTIES

5.1 Pharmacodynamic properties

Analgesic, ATC code: N02AX02

Tramadol is a centrally acting analgesic which possesses opioid agonist properties. Tramadol consists of two enantiomers, the (+)-isomer is predominantly active as an opioid with preferential activity for the μ-receptor. The (-)-isomer potentiates the analgesic effect of the (+)-isomer and is active as an inhibitor of noradrenaline and serotoninuptake thereby modifying the transmission of pain impulses.

Tramadol also has an antitussive action. At the recommended dosages, the effects of tramadol given orally on the respiratory and cardiovascular systems appear to be clinically insignificant. The potency of tramadol is reported to be 1/10 to 1/6 of morphine.

5.2 Pharmacokinetic properties

About 90% of tramadol released from Zamadol SR Capsules is absorbed after oral administration. The mean absolute bioavailability is approximately 70%, irrespective of concomitant intake of food.

The difference between absorbed and non-metabolised available tramadol is probably due to low first-pass effect. The first pass-effect after oral administration is a maximum of 30%.

Tramadol has a high tissue affinity with an apparent volume of distribution of 203 ± 40 litres after oral dosing in healthy volunteers. Protein binding is limited to 20%.

After single dose administration of Zamadol SR 50 mg Capsules the peak plasma concentration C_{max} 70 ± 16 ng/ml is reached after 5.3 h. After administration of Zamadol SR 100 mg Capsules C_{max} 137 ± 27 ng/ml is reached after 5.9 h. Following administration of Zamadol SR 200 mg Capsules C_{max} 294 ± 82 ng/ml is reached after 6.5 h. The reference product (Tramadol Immediate Release Capsules, given as a total dose of 200 mg tramadol hydrochloride) reached a peak concentration of C_{max} 640 ± 143 ng/ml after 2.0 hours.

The relative bioavailability for the slow release formulation after single dose administration is 89% and increases to 100% after multiple dose administration in comparison to the reference product.

Tramadol passes the blood-brain and placenta barriers. Very small amounts of the substance and its O-demethyl derivative are found in the breast-milk (0.1% and 0.02% respectively of the applied dose).

Elimination of half-life $t_{½,\beta}$ is approximately 6 h, irrespective of the mode of administration. In patients above 75 years of age it may be prolonged by a factor of 1.4.

In humans tramadol is mainly metabolised by means of N- and O-demethylation and conjugation of the O-demethylation products with glucuronic acid. Only O-desmethyltramadol is pharmacologically active. There are considerable interindividual quantitative differences between the other metabolites. So far, eleven metabolites have been found in the urine. Animal experiments have shown that O-desmethyltramadol is more potent than the parent substance by the factor 2-4. Its half life $t_{½,\beta}$ (6 healthy volunteers) is 7.9 h (range 5.4-9.6 h) and is approximately that of tramadol.

The inhibition of one or both cytochrome P450 isoenzymes, CYP3A4 and CYP2D6 involved in the metabolism of tramadol, may affect the plasma concentration of tramadol or its active metabolite. The clinical consequences of any such interactions are not known.

Tramadol and its metabolites are almost completely excreted via the kidneys. Cumulative urinary excretion is 90% of the total radioactivity of the administered dose. In cases of impaired hepatic and renal function the half-life may be slightly prolonged. In patients with cirrhosis of the liver, elimination half-lives of 13.3 ± 4.9 h (tramadol) and 18.5 ± 9.4 h (O-desmethyltramadol), in an extreme case 22.3 h and 36 h respectively have been determined. In patients with renal insufficiency (creatinine clearance < 5 ml/min) the values were 11 ± 3.2 h and 16.9 ± 3 h, in an extreme case 19.5 h and 43.2 h, respectively.

Tramadol has a linear pharmacokinetic profile within the therapeutic dosage range.

The relationship between serum concentrations and the analgesic effect is dose-dependent, but varies considerably in isolated cases. A serum concentration of 100 - 300 ng/ml is usually effective.

5.3 Preclinical safety data

Pre-clinical data reveal no special hazard for humans based on conventional studies of safety pharmacology, repeated dose toxicity, genotoxicity or carcinogenic potential. Studies of tramadol in rats and rabbits have revealed no teratogenic effects. However, embryo toxicity was shown in the form of delayed ossification. Fertility, reproductive performance and development of offspring were unaffected.

6. PHARMACEUTICAL PARTICULARS

6.1 List of excipients

Capsule Contents: Sugar spheres (sucrose and maize starch), colloidal anhydrous silica, ethylcellulose, shellac, talc.

Capsule Shell: Gelatin and Titanium Dioxide (E171).

The 50 mg and 150 mg capsules also contain Iron Oxide Yellow (E172) and Indigotin (E132).

The 200 mg capsules also contain Iron Oxide Yellow (E172).

Printing ink contains shellac, iron oxide black (E172), soya lecithin and antifoam DC 1510.

6.2 Incompatibilities

Not applicable.

6.3 Shelf life

3 years.

6.4 Special precautions for storage

Do not store above 25°C. Store in the original package.

6.5 Nature and contents of container

White opaque PVC/PVDC and aluminium foil blister strips. Each strip contains 10 capsules.

Each pack contains 10, 20, 30, 50, 60 or 100 capsules per pack.

Not all pack sizes may be marketed in all Member States.

6.6 Instructions for use and handling

No special requirements.

7. MARKETING AUTHORISATION HOLDER

VIATRIS Pharmaceuticals Ltd

Building 2000

Beach Drive

Cambridge Research Park

Waterbeach

Cambridge CB5 9PD

UK

8. MARKETING AUTHORISATION NUMBER(S)

PL 19166/0022

PL 19166/0023

PL 19166/0035

PL 19166/0025

9. DATE OF FIRST AUTHORISATION/RENEWAL OF THE AUTHORISATION

29 August 2002.

10. DATE OF REVISION OF THE TEXT

March 2003.

VIATRIS Pharmaceuticals Ltd

Zamadol is a registered trademark of VIATRIS

Zanaflex

(Zeneus Pharma Ltd)

1. NAME OF THE MEDICINAL PRODUCT

Zanaflex™

2. QUALITATIVE AND QUANTITATIVE COMPOSITION

Zanaflex tablets containing 4 mg of tizanidine as the hydrochloride.

For excipients, see 6.1.

3. PHARMACEUTICAL FORM

Tablet.

White to off-white, circular flat bevelled edge tablet. Cross scored on one side, 'A' and 594 on the other side.

4. CLINICAL PARTICULARS

4.1 Therapeutic indications

Treatment of spasticity associated with multiple sclerosis or with spinal cord injury or disease.

4.2 Posology and method of administration

For oral administration

The effect of Zanaflex on spasticity is maximal within 2-3 hours of dosing and it has a relatively short duration of action. The timing and frequency of dosing should therefore be tailored to the individual, and Zanaflex should be given in divided doses, up to 3-4 times daily, depending on the patient's needs. There is considerable variation in response between patients so careful titration is necessary. Care should be taken not to exceed the dose producing the desired therapeutic effect. It is usual to start with a single dose of 2 mg increasing by 2 mg increments at no less than half-weekly intervals.

The total daily dose should not exceed 36 mg, although it is usually not necessary to exceed 24 mg daily. Secondary pharmacological effects (see section 4.8 Undesirable Effects) may occur at therapeutic doses but these can be minimised by slow titration so that in the large majority of patients they are not a limiting factor.

Elderly

Experience in the elderly is limited and use of Zanaflex is not recommended unless the benefit of treatment clearly outweighs the risk. Pharmacokinetic data suggest that renal clearance in the elderly may be decreased by up to three fold.

Children

Experience with Zanaflex in patients under the age of 18 years is limited. Zanaflex is not recommended for use in children.

Patients with Renal impairment

In patients with renal insufficiency (creatinine clearance < 25mL/min) treatment should be started with 2 mg once daily with slow titration to achieve the effective dose. Dosage increases should be in increments of no more than 2 mg according to tolerability and effectiveness. It is advisable to slowly increase the once-daily dose before increasing the frequency of administration. Renal function should be monitored as appropriate in these patients.

Patients with Hepatic Impairment

Zanaflex is contraindicated in patients with significantly impaired hepatic function.

4.3 Contraindications

Hypersensitivity to tizanidine or any other component of the product.

The use of Zanaflex in patients with significantly impaired hepatic function is contraindicated, because tizanidine is extensively metabolised by the liver.

4.4 Special warnings and special precautions for use

Use in Renal Impairment

Patients with renal impairment may require lower doses and therefore caution should be exercised when using Zanaflex in these patients (see section 4.2 Posology and Method of Administration).

Liver Function

Hepatic dysfunction has been reported in association with Zanaflex. It is recommended that liver function tests should be monitored monthly for the first four months in all patients and in those who develop symptoms suggestive of liver dysfunction such as unexplained nausea, anorexia or tiredness. Treatment with Zanaflex should be discontinued if serum levels of SGPT and/or SGOT are persistently above three times the upper limit of normal range.

Zanaflex should be kept out of the reach of children.

4.5 Interaction with other medicinal products and other forms of Interaction

As Zanaflex may induce hypotension it may potentiate the effect of antihypertensive drugs, including diuretics, and caution should therefore be exercised in patients receiving blood pressure lowering drugs. Caution should also be exercised when Zanaflex is used concurrently with β-adrenoceptor blocking drugs or digoxin as the combination may potentiate hypotension or bradycardia.

Caution should be exercised when Zanaflex is prescribed with drugs known to increase the QT interval.

Pharmacokinetic data following single and multiple doses of Zanaflex suggested that clearance of Zanaflex was reduced by approximately 50% in women who were concurrently taking oral contraceptives. Although no specific pharmacokinetic study has been conducted to investigate a potential interaction between oral contraceptives and Zanaflex, the possibility of a clinical response and/or adverse effects occurring at lower doses of Zanaflex should be borne in mind when prescribing Zanaflex to a patient taking the contraceptive pill. Clinically significant drug-drug interactions have not been reported in clinical trials.

Alcohol or sedatives may enhance the sedative action of Zanaflex.

4.6 Pregnancy and lactation

Reproductive studies in rats and rabbits indicate that Zanaflex does not have embryotoxic or teratogenic potential but at maternally toxic doses of 10-100 mg/kg per day Zanaflex can retard foetal development due to its pharmacodynamic effects. Zanaflex and/or its metabolites have been found in the milk of rodents (see section 5.3 preclinical safety data). The safety of Zanaflex in pregnancy has not been established and its safety in breast-fed infants of mothers receiving Zanaflex is not known. Therefore Zanaflex should not be used in pregnant or nursing mothers unless the likely benefit clearly outweighs the risk.

4.7 Effects on ability to drive and use machines

Patients experiencing drowsiness should be advised against activities requiring a high degree of alertness, e.g. driving a vehicle or operating machinery.

4.8 Undesirable effects

The most frequently reported adverse events occurring in association with Zanaflex include drowsiness, fatigue, dizziness, dry mouth, nausea, gastrointestinal disturbances, and a reduction in blood pressure. With slow upward titration of the dose of Zanaflex these effects are usually not severe enough to require discontinuation of treatment. Insomnia, bradycardia and hallucinations have also been reported. The hallucinations are self-limiting, without evidence of psychosis, and have invariably occurred in patients concurrently taking potentially hallucinogenic drugs, e.g. anti-depressants. Increases in hepatic serum transaminases, which are reversible on stopping treatment, have occurred. Infrequent cases of acute hepatitis have been reported. Muscle weakness has been reported infrequently, although in controlled clinical trials it was clearly demonstrated that Zanaflex does not adversely affect muscle strength. Allergic reactions (e.g. pruritus and rash) have rarely been reported.

4.9 Overdose

Clinical experience is limited. In one adult case, who ingested 400mg Zanaflex, recovery was uneventful. This patient received mannitol and frusemide.

Symptoms: Nausea, vomiting, hypotension, dizziness, miosis, respiratory distress, coma, restlessness, somnolence.

Treatment: General supportive measures are indicated and an attempt should be made to remove uningested drug from the gastro-intestinal tract using gastric lavage or activated charcoal. The patient should be well hydrated.

5. PHARMACOLOGICAL PROPERTIES

5.1 Pharmacodynamic properties

Tizanidine is an α_2-adrenergic receptor agonist within the central nervous system at supra-spinal and spinal levels. This effect results in inhibition of spinal polysynaptic reflex activity. Tizanidine has no direct effect on skeletal muscle, the neuromuscular junction or on monosynaptic spinal reflexes.

In humans, tizanidine reduces pathologically increased muscle tone, including resistance to passive movements and alleviates painful spasms and clonus.

5.2 Pharmacokinetic properties

Tizanidine is rapidly absorbed, reaching peak plasma concentration in approximately 1 hour. Tizanidine is only about 30% bound to plasma proteins and, in animal studies, was found to readily cross the blood-brain barrier. Although tizanidine is well absorbed, first pass metabolism limits plasma availability to 34% of that of an intravenous dose. Tizanidine undergoes rapid and extensive metabolism in the liver and the pattern of biotransformation in animals and humans is qualitatively similar. The metabolites are primarily excreted via the renal route (approximately 70% of the administered dose) and appear to be inactive. Renal excretion of the parent compound is approximately 53% after a single 5 mg dose and 66% after dosing with 4 mg three times daily. The elimination half-life of tizanidine from plasma is 2-4 hours in patients.

Concomitant food intake has no influence on the pharmacokinetic profile of tizanidine tablets.

5.3 Preclinical safety data

Acute toxicity

Tizanidine possesses a low order of acute toxicity. Signs of overdosage were seen after single doses >40 mg/kg in animals and are related to the pharmacological action of the drug.

Repeat dose toxicity

The toxic effects of tizanidine are mainly related to its pharmacological action. At doses of 24 and 40 mg/kg per day in subchronic and chronic rodent studies, the α_2-agonist effects resulted in CNS stimulation, e.g. motor excitation, aggressiveness, tremor and convulsions.

Signs related to centrally mediated muscle relaxation, e.g. sedation and ataxia, were frequently observed at lower dose levels in subchronic and chronic oral studies with dogs. Such signs, related to the myotonolytic activity of the drug, were noted at 1 to 4 mg/kg per day in a 13 week dog study, and at 1.5 mg/kg per day in a 52-week dog study.

Prolongation of the QT interval and bradycardia were noted in chronic toxicity studies in dogs at doses of 1.0 mg/kg per day and above.

Slight increases in hepatic serum transaminases were observed in a number of toxicity studies at higher dose levels. They were not consistently associated with histopathological changes in the liver.

Mutagenicity

Various in vitro assays as well as in vivo assays produced no evidence of mutagenic potential of tizanidine.

Carcinogenicity

No evidence for carcinogenicity was demonstrated in two long-term dietary studies in mice (78 weeks) and rats (104 weeks), at dose levels up to 9 mg/kg per day in rats and up to 16 mg/kg per day in mice. At these dose levels, corresponding to the maximum tolerated dose, based on reductions in growth rate, no neoplastic or pre-neoplastic pathology, attributable to treatment, was observed.

Reproductive toxicity

No embryotoxicity or teratogenicity occurred in pregnant rats and rabbits at dose levels up to 30 mg/kg per day of tizanidine. However, doses of 10-100 mg/kg per day in rats were maternally toxic and resulted in developmental retardation of foetuses as seen by lower foetal body weights and retarded skeletal ossification.

In female rats, treated prior to mating through lactation or during late pregnancy until weaning of the young, a dose-dependent (10 and 30 mg/kg per day) prolongation of gestation time and dystocia occurred, resulting in an increased foetal mortality and delayed development. These effects were attributed to the pharmacological effect of tizanidine. No developmental effects occurred at 3mg/kg per day although sedation was induced in the treated dams.

Passage of tizanidine and/or its metabolites into milk of rodents is known to occur.

6. PHARMACEUTICAL PARTICULARS

6.1 List of excipients

silica, colloidal anhydrous

stearic acid

cellulose, microcrystalline

lactose, anhydrous.

6.2 Incompatibilities

None known.

6.3 Shelf life

5 years in both temperate and hot climates, and 5 years in tropical climate.

6.4 Special precautions for storage

No special precautions for storage.

6.5 Nature and contents of container

(PVC/PVDC/Al foil) blisters. Carton containing 4 blister strips of 30 tablets to givepack size of 120.

6.6 Instructions for use and handling

Not applicable.

7. MARKETING AUTHORISATION HOLDER

Elan Pharma International Ltd.

W.I.L House

Shannon Business Park

Shannon

Co. Clare

Ireland

Trading as:

Elan Pharma

Abel Smith House

Gunnels Wood Road

Stevenage

Hertfordshire

UK

SG1 2FG

8. MARKETING AUTHORISATION NUMBER(S)

PL 16804/0004

9. DATE OF FIRST AUTHORISATION/RENEWAL OF THE AUTHORISATION

March 2003

10. DATE OF REVISION OF THE TEXT

February 2003

Legal Category

POM

Zanaflex 2mg

(Zeneus Pharma Ltd)

1. NAME OF THE MEDICINAL PRODUCT

Zanaflex®

2. QUALITATIVE AND QUANTITATIVE COMPOSITION

Zanaflex tablets containing 2 mg of tizanidine as the hydrochloride.

For excipients, see 6.1

3. PHARMACEUTICAL FORM

Tablet

White to off-white, circular flat bevelled edge tablet. Scored on one side, 'A' and 592 on the other side.

4. CLINICAL PARTICULARS

4.1 Therapeutic indications

Treatment of spasticity associated with multiple sclerosis or with spinal cord injury or disease.

4.2 Posology and method of administration

For oral administration

The effect of Zanaflex on spasticity is maximal within 2-3 hours of dosing and it has a relatively short duration of action. The timing and frequency of dosing should therefore be tailored to the individual, and Zanaflex should be given in divided doses, up to 3-4 times daily, depending on the patient's needs. There is considerable variation in response between patients so careful titration is necessary. Care should be taken not to exceed the dose producing the desired therapeutic effect. It is usual to start with a single dose of 2 mg increasing by 2 mg increments at no less than half-weekly intervals.

The total daily dose should not exceed 36 mg, although it is usually not necessary to exceed 24 mg daily. Secondary pharmacological effects (see section 4.8 Undesirable Effects) may occur at therapeutic doses but these can be minimised by slow titration so that in the large majority of patients they are not a limiting factor.

Elderly

Experience in the elderly is limited and use of Zanaflex is not recommended unless the benefit of treatment clearly outweighs the risk. Pharmacokinetic data suggest that renal clearance in the elderly may be decreased by up to three fold.

Children

Experience with Zanaflex in patients under the age of 18 years is limited. Zanaflex is not recommended for use in children.

Patients with Renal impairment

In patients with renal insufficiency (creatinine clearance < 25mL/min) treatment should be started with 2 mg once daily with slow titration to achieve the effective dose. Dosage increases should be in increments of no more than 2 mg according to tolerability and effectiveness. It is advisable to slowly increase the once-daily dose before increasing the frequency of administration. Renal function should be monitored as appropriate in these patients.

Patients with Hepatic Impairment

Zanaflex is contraindicated in patients with significantly impaired hepatic function.

4.3 Contraindications

Hypersensitivity to tizanidine or any other component of the product.

The use of Zanaflex in patients with significantly impaired hepatic function is contraindicated, because tizanidine is extensively metabolised by the liver.

4.4 Special warnings and special precautions for use

Use in Renal Impairment

Patients with renal impairment may require lower doses and therefore caution should be exercised when using Zanaflex in these patients (see section 4.2 Posology and Method of Administration).

Liver Function

Hepatic dysfunction has been reported in association with Zanaflex. It is recommended that liver function tests should be monitored monthly for the first four months in all patients and in those who develop symptoms suggestive of liver dysfunction such as unexplained nausea, anorexia or tiredness. Treatment with Zanaflex should be discontinued if serum levels of SGPT and/or SGOT are persistently above three times the upper limit of normal range.

Zanaflex should be kept out of the reach of children.

4.5 Interaction with other medicinal products and other forms of Interaction

As Zanaflex may induce hypotension it may potentiate the effect of antihypertensive drugs, including diuretics, and caution should therefore be exercised in patients receiving blood pressure lowering drugs. Caution should also be exercised when Zanaflex is used concurrently with β-adrenoceptor blocking drugs or digoxin as the combination may potentiate hypotension or bradycardia.

Caution should be exercised when Zanaflex is prescribed with drugs known to increase the QT interval.

Pharmacokinetic data following single and multiple doses of Zanaflex suggested that clearance of Zanaflex was reduced by approximately 50% in women who were concurrently taking oral contraceptives. Although no specific pharmacokinetic study has been conducted to investigate a potential interaction between oral contraceptives and Zanaflex, the possibility of a clinical response and/or adverse effects occurring at lower doses of Zanaflex should be borne in mind when prescribing Zanaflex to a patient taking the contraceptive pill. Clinically significant drug-drug interactions have not been reported in clinical trials.

Alcohol or sedatives may enhance the sedative action of Zanaflex.

4.6 Pregnancy and lactation

Reproductive studies in rats and rabbits indicate that Zanaflex does not have embryotoxic or teratogenic potential but at maternally toxic doses of 10-100 mg/kg per day Zanaflex can retard foetal development due to its pharmacodynamic effects. Zanaflex and/or its metabolites have been found in the milk of rodents (see section 5.3 preclinical safety data). The safety of Zanaflex in pregnancy has not been established and its safety in breast-fed infants of mothers receiving Zanaflex is not known. Therefore Zanaflex should not be used in pregnant or nursing mothers unless the likely benefit clearly outweighs the risk.

4.7 Effects on ability to drive and use machines

Patients experiencing drowsiness should be advised against activities requiring a high degree of alertness, e.g. driving a vehicle or operating machinery.

4.8 Undesirable effects

The most frequently reported adverse events occurring in association with Zanaflex include drowsiness, fatigue, dizziness, dry mouth, nausea, gastrointestinal disturbances, and a reduction in blood pressure. With slow upward titration of the dose of Zanaflex these effects are usually not severe enough to require discontinuation of treatment. Insomnia, bradycardia and hallucinations have also been reported. The hallucinations are self-limiting, without evidence of psychosis, and have invariably occurred in patients concurrently taking potentially hallucinogenic drugs, e.g. anti-depressants. Increases in hepatic serum transaminases, which are reversible on stopping treatment, have occurred. Infrequent cases of acute hepatitis have been reported. Muscle weakness has been reported infrequently, although in controlled clinical trials it was clearly demonstrated that Zanaflex does not adversely affect muscle strength. Allergic reactions (e.g. pruritus and rash) have rarely been reported.

4.9 Overdose

Clinical experience is limited. In one adult case, who ingested 400mg Zanaflex, recovery was uneventful. This patient received mannitol and frusemide.

Symptoms: Nausea, vomiting, hypotension, dizziness, miosis, respiratory distress, coma, restlessness, somnolence.

Treatment: General supportive measures are indicated and an attempt should be made to remove uningested drug from the gastro-intestinal tract using gastric lavage or activated charcoal. The patient should be well hydrated.

5. PHARMACOLOGICAL PROPERTIES

5.1 Pharmacodynamic properties

Tizanidine is an α_2-adrenergic receptor agonist within the central nervous system at supra-spinal and spinal levels. This effect results in inhibition of spinal polysynaptic reflex activity. Tizanidine has no direct effect on skeletal muscle, the neuromuscular junction or on monosynaptic spinal reflexes.

In humans, tizanidine reduces pathologically increased muscle tone, including resistance to passive movements and alleviates painful spasms and clonus.

5.2 Pharmacokinetic properties

Tizanidine is rapidly absorbed, reaching peak plasma concentration in approximately 1 hour. Tizanidine is only about 30% bound to plasma proteins and, in animal studies, was found to readily cross the blood-brain barrier. Although tizanidine is well absorbed, first pass metabolism limits plasma availability to 34% of that of an intravenous dose. Tizanidine undergoes rapid and extensive metabolism in the liver and the pattern of biotransformation in animals and humans is qualitatively similar. The metabolites are primarily excreted via the renal route (approximately 70% of the administered dose) and appear to be inactive. Renal excretion of the parent compound is approximately 53% after a single 5 mg dose and 66% after dosing with 4 mg three times daily. The elimination half-life of tizanidine from plasma is 2-4 hours in patients.

Concomitant food intake has no influence on the pharmacokinetic profile of tizanidine tablets.

5.3 Preclinical safety data

Acute toxicity

Tizanidine possesses a low order of acute toxicity. Signs of overdosage were seen after single doses >40 mg/kg in animals and are related to the pharmacological action of the drug.

Repeat dose toxicity

The toxic effects of tizanidine are mainly related to its pharmacological action. At doses of 24 and 40 mg/kg per day in subchronic and chronic rodent studies, the α_2-agonist effects resulted in CNS stimulation, e.g. motor excitation, aggressiveness, tremor and convulsions.

Signs related to centrally mediated muscle relaxation, e.g. sedation and ataxia, were frequently observed at lower dose levels in subchronic and chronic oral studies with dogs. Such signs, related to the myotonolytic activity of the drug, were noted at 1 to 4 mg/kg per day in a 13 week dog study, and at 1.5 mg/kg per day in a 52-week dog study.

Prolongation of the QT interval and bradycardia were noted in chronic toxicity studies in dogs at doses of 1.0 mg/kg per day and above.

Slight increases in hepatic serum transaminases were observed in a number of toxicity studies at higher dose levels. They were not consistently associated with histopathological changes in the liver.

Mutagenicity

Various in vitro assays as well as in vivo assays produced no evidence of mutagenic potential of tizanidine.

Carcinogenicity

No evidence for carcinogenicity was demonstrated in two long-term dietary studies in mice (78 weeks) and rats (104 weeks), at dose levels up to 9 mg/kg per day in rats and up to 16 mg/kg per day in mice. At these dose levels, corresponding to the maximum tolerated dose, based on reductions in growth rate, no neoplastic or pre-neoplastic pathology, attributable to treatment, was observed.

Reproductive toxicity

No embryotoxicity or teratogenicity occurred in pregnant rats and rabbits at dose levels up to 30 mg/kg per day of tizanidine. However, doses of 10-100 mg/kg per day in rats were maternally toxic and resulted in developmental retardation of foetuses as seen by lower foetal body weights and retarded skeletal ossification.

In female rats, treated prior to mating through lactation or during late pregnancy until weaning of the young, a dose-dependent (10 and 30 mg/kg per day) prolongation of gestation time and dystocia occurred, resulting in an increased foetal mortality and delayed development. These effects were attributed to the pharmacological effect of tizanidine. No developmental effects occurred at 3mg/kg per day although sedation was induced in the treated dams.

Passage of tizanidine and/or its metabolites into milk of rodents is known to occur.

6. PHARMACEUTICAL PARTICULARS

6.1 List of excipients

silica, colloidal anhydrous

stearic acid

cellulose, microcrystalline

lactose, anhydrous.

6.2 Incompatibilities

None known.

6.3 Shelf life

5 years in both temperate and hot climates, and 5 years in tropical climate.

6.4 Special precautions for storage

No special precautions for storage

6.5 Nature and contents of container

PVC/PVDC/Al foil blisters. Carton containing 4 blister strips of 30 tablets to give pack size of 120.

6.6 Instructions for use and handling

Not applicable.

7. MARKETING AUTHORISATION HOLDER

Zeneus Pharma Limited

The Magdalen Centre

Oxford Science Park

Oxford

OX4 4GA

UK

8. MARKETING AUTHORISATION NUMBER(S)

PL 21799/0015

9. DATE OF FIRST AUTHORISATION/RENEWAL OF THE AUTHORISATION

15 September 2005

10. DATE OF REVISION OF THE TEXT

September 2005

11. LEGAL CATEGORY

POM

Zantac Effervescent Tablets 150mg

(GlaxoSmithKline UK)

1. NAME OF THE MEDICINAL PRODUCT

Zantac Effervescent Tablets 150 mg

2. QUALITATIVE AND QUANTITATIVE COMPOSITION

Each tablet contains ranitidine 150 mg (as the hydrochloride) and 14.3 mEq (328 mg) of sodium.

3. PHARMACEUTICAL FORM

Effervescent Tablet.

4. CLINICAL PARTICULARS

4.1 Therapeutic indications

Duodenal ulcer and benign gastric ulcer, including that associated with non-steroidal anti-inflammatory agents.

Prevention of non-steroidal anti-inflammatory drug (including aspirin) associated duodenal ulcers, especially in patients with a history of peptic ulcer disease.

Treatment of duodenal ulcers associated with *Helicobacter pylori* infection.

Post-operative ulcer.

Oesophageal reflux disease.

Symptom relief in gastro-oesophageal reflux disease.

Zollinger-Ellison Syndrome.

Chronic episodic dyspepsia, characterised by pain (epigastric or retrosternal) which is related to meals or disturbs sleep but not associated with the above conditions.

Prophylaxis of stress ulceration in seriously ill patients.

Prophylaxis of recurrent haemorrhage from peptic ulcer.

Prophylaxis of Mendelson's syndrome.

4.2 Posology and method of administration

Adults:

Duodenal ulcer and benign gastric ulcer:

Acute treatment:

The standard dosage regimen for duodenal or benign gastric ulcer is 150 mg twice daily or 300 mg nocte. In most cases of duodenal ulcer or benign gastric ulcer healing occurs within 4 weeks. Healing usually occurs after a further 4 weeks in those not fully healed after the initial 4 weeks.

Long-term management:

For the long-term management of duodenal or benign gastric ulcer the usual dosage regimen is 150 mg nocte.

In duodenal ulcer 300 mg twice daily for 4 weeks results in healing rates which are higher than those at 4 weeks with ranitidine 150 mg twice daily or 300 mg nocte. The increased dose has not been associated with an increased incidence of unwanted effects.

NSAID associated peptic ulceration:

Acute treatment:

In ulcers following non-steroidal anti-inflammatory drug therapy, or associated with continued non-steroidal anti-inflammatory drugs, 8-12 weeks treatment may be necessary with 150 mg twice daily or 300 mg nocte.

Prophylaxis:

For the prevention of non-steroidal anti-inflammatory drug associated duodenal ulcers ranitidine 150 mg twice daily may be given concomitantly with non-steroidal anti-inflammatory drug therapy.

For duodenal ulcers associated with *Helicobacter pylori* infection, ranitidine 300 mg at bedtime or 150 mg twice daily may be given with oral amoxycillin 750 mg three times daily and metronidazole 500 mg three times daily for two weeks. Therapy with ranitidine should continue for a further two weeks. This dose regimen significantly reduces the frequency of duodenal ulcer recurrence.

Postoperative ulcer:

The standard dosage regimen for postoperative ulcer is 150mg twice daily. Most cases heal within 4 weeks. Those not fully healed after the initial 4 weeks usually do so after a further 4 weeks.

Gastro-oesophageal reflux disease:

Symptom relief in gastro-oesophageal reflux disease.

In patients with gastro-oesophageal reflux disease, a dose regimen of 150 mg twice daily for 2 weeks is recommended and this can be repeated in patients in whom the initial symptomatic response is inadequate.

In the management of oesophageal reflux disease, the recommended course of treatment is either 150 mg twice daily or 300 mg at bedtime for up to 8 weeks or 12 weeks if necessary.

In patients with moderate to severe oesophagitis, the dosage of ranitidine may be increased to 150 mg 4 times daily for up to 12 weeks. The increased dose has not been associated with an increased incidence of unwanted effects.

Zollinger-Ellison syndrome:

The initial dosage regimen for Zollinger-Ellison syndrome is 150 mg three times daily, but this may be increased as necessary. Doses up to 6 grams per day have been well tolerated.

Chronic episodic dyspepsia:

The standard dosage regimen for patients with chronic episodic dyspepsia is 150 mg twice daily for up to 6 weeks. Anyone not responding or relapsing shortly afterwards should be investigated.

Prophylaxis of haemorrhage from stress ulceration in seriously ill patients or prophylaxis of recurrent haemorrhage in patients bleeding from peptic ulceration:

150 mg twice daily may be substituted for the injection once oral feeding commences.

Prophylaxis of Mendelson's syndrome:

150 mg 2 hours before anaesthesia, and preferably 150 mg the previous evening. Alternatively, the injection is also available. In obstetric patients in labour 150 mg every 6 hours, but if general anaesthesia is required it is recommended that a non-particulate antacid (e.g. sodium citrate) be given in addition.

Children:

The recommended oral dose for the treatment of peptic ulcer in children is 2 mg/kg to 4 mg/kg twice daily to a maximum of 300 mg ranitidine per day.

Renal Impairment:

Accumulation of ranitidine with resulting elevated plasma concentrations will occur in patients with severe renal impairment (creatinine clearance less than 50 ml/min). It is recommended that the daily dose of ranitidine in such patients should be 150 mg. In patients undergoing chronic ambulatory peritoneal dialysis or chronic haemodialysis, ranitidine (150 mg) should be taken immediately after dialysis.

For oral administration.

4.3 Contraindications

Ranitidine is contra-indicated in patients known to have hypersensitivity to any component of the preparation.

4.4 Special warnings and special precautions for use

Malignancy:

The possibility of malignancy should be excluded before commencement of therapy in patients with gastric ulcer (and if indications include dyspepsia; patients of middle age and over with new or recently changed dyspeptic symptoms) as treatment with ranitidine may mask symptoms of gastric carcinoma.

Renal Disease:

Ranitidine is excreted via the kidney and so plasma levels of the drug are increased in patients with severe renal impairment.

The dosage should be adjusted as detailed above under Dosage in Renal Impairment.

Regular supervision of patients who are taking non-steroidal anti-inflammatory drugs concomitantly with ranitidine is recommended, especially in the elderly and in those with a history of peptic ulcer.

Rare clinical reports suggest that ranitidine may precipitate acute porphyric attacks. Ranitidine should therefore be avoided in patients with a history of acute porphyria.

Zantac Effervescent Tablets contain sodium. Care should therefore be taken in treating patients in whom sodium restriction is indicated.

Zantac Effervescent Tablets contain aspartame. They should be used with caution in patients with phenylketonuria.

4.5 Interaction with other medicinal products and other forms of Interaction

Ranitidine, at blood levels produced by standard recommended doses, does not inhibit the hepatic cytochrome P450-linked mixed function oxygenase system. Accordingly, ranitidine in usual therapeutic doses does not potentiate the actions of drugs which are inactivated by this enzyme; these include diazepam, lignocaine, phenytoin, propranolol, theophylline and warfarin. There is no evidence of an interaction between ranitidine and amoxycillin or metronidazole.

4.6 Pregnancy and lactation

Ranitidine crosses the placenta and is excreted in human breast milk.

Like other drugs it should only be used during pregnancy and nursing if considered essential.

4.7 Effects on ability to drive and use machines

None reported.

4.8 Undesirable effects

The following convention has been utilised for the classification of undesirable effects: very common (>1/10), common (>1/100, <1/10), uncommon (>1/1000, <1/100), rare (>1/10,000, <1/1000), very rare (<1/10,000).

Adverse event frequencies have been estimated from spontaneous reports from post-marketing data.

Blood & Lymphatic System Disorders

Very Rare:

Blood count changes (leucopenia, thrombocytopenia). These are usually reversible. Agranulocytosis or pancytopenia, sometimes with marrow hypoplasia or marrow aplasia.

Immune System Disorders

Rare:

Hypersensitivity reactions (urticaria, angioneurotic oedema, ever, bronchospasm, hypotension and chest pain).

Very Rare:

Anaphylactic shock

These events have been reported after a single dose.

Psychiatric Disorders

Very Rare:

Reversible mental confusion, depression and hallucinations.

These have been reported predominantly in severely ill and elderly patients.

Nervous System Disorders

Very Rare:

Headache (sometimes severe), dizziness and reversible involuntary movement disorders.

Eye Disorders

Very Rare:

Reversible blurred vision.

There have been reports of blurred vision, which is suggestive of a change in accommodation.

Cardiac Disorders

Very Rare:

As with other H_2 receptor antagonists bradycardia and A-V Block.

Vascular Disorders

Very Rare:

Vasculitis.

Gastrointestinal Disorders

Very Rare:

Acute pancreatitis. Diarrhoea.

Hepatobiliary Disorders

Rare:

Transient and reversible changes in liver function tests.

Very Rare

Hepatitis (hepatocellular, hepatocanalicular or mixed) with or without jaundice, these were usually reversible.

Skin and Subcutaneous Tissue Disorders

Rare:

Skin Rash.

Very Rare:

Erythema multiforme, alopecia.

Musculoskeletal and Connective Tissue Disorders

Very Rare:

Musculoskeletal symptoms such as arthralgia and myalgia.

Renal and Urinary Disorders

Very rare:

Acute interstitial nephritis.

Reproductive System and Breast Disorders

Very Rare:

Reversible impotence. Breast symptoms in men.

4.9 Overdose

Ranitidine is very specific in action and accordingly no particular problems are expected following overdosage with the drug, clinicians should be aware of the sodium content (see Section 4.4 Special Warnings and Precautions for Use). Symptomatic and supportive therapy should be given as appropriate. If need be, the drug may be removed from the plasma by haemodialysis.

5. PHARMACOLOGICAL PROPERTIES

5.1 Pharmacodynamic properties

Ranitidine is a specific rapidly acting histamine H_2-antagonist. It inhibits basal and stimulated secretion of gastric acid, reducing both the volume and the acid and pepsin content of the secretion. Ranitidine has a relatively long duration of action and so a single 150 mg dose effectively suppresses gastric acid secretion for twelve hours.

5.2 Pharmacokinetic properties

The bioavailability of ranitidine is consistently about 50%. Absorption of ranitidine after oral administration is rapid and peak plasma concentrations are usually achieved 2-3 hours after administration. Absorption is not significantly impaired by food or antacids. Ranitidine is not extensively metabolised. Elimination of the drug is primarily by tubular secretion. The elimination half-life of ranitidine is 2-3 hours. In balance studies with 150 mg ^{3}H-ranitidine 60-70% of an oral dose was excreted in urine and 26% in faeces. Analysis of urine excreted in the first 24 hours after dosing showed that 35% of the oral dose was eliminated unchanged. About 6% of the dose is excreted as the N-Oxide, 2% as the S-Oxide, 2% as desmethyl ranitidine and 1-2% as the furoic acid analogue.

5.3 Preclinical safety data

No additional data of relevance.

6. PHARMACEUTICAL PARTICULARS

6.1 List of excipients

Monosodium Citrate Anhydrous

Sodium Bicarbonate

Aspartame

Povidone

Sodium Benzoate

Orange Flavour (IFF No. 6)

Grapefruit Flavour (IFF 18C 222)

Pharmaceutical Industrial Alcohol or Ethanol

6.2 Incompatibilities

None.

6.3 Shelf life

2 years.

6.4 Special precautions for storage

Store below 30°C in a dry place.

6.5 Nature and contents of container

Polypropylene tubes with polyethylene tamper evident cap, each tube contains 15 tablets packed in cartons of 15 or 60 tablets.

Aluminium foil strips of six tablets packed in cartons of 6 or 30 tablets.

6.6 Instructions for use and handling

Place the tablets in half a glass of water (minimum 75 ml) and allow to dissolve completely before swallowing.

Administrative Data

7. MARKETING AUTHORISATION HOLDER

Glaxo Wellcome UK Limited

trading as GlaxoSmithKline UK

Stockley Park West

Uxbridge

Middlesex

UB11 1BT

8. MARKETING AUTHORISATION NUMBER(S)

PL 10949/0137.

9. DATE OF FIRST AUTHORISATION/RENEWAL OF THE AUTHORISATION

28 April 2002

10. DATE OF REVISION OF THE TEXT

29 May 2004

11. Legal Status

POM

Zantac Effervescent Tablets 300mg

(GlaxoSmithKline UK)

1. NAME OF THE MEDICINAL PRODUCT

Zantac Effervescent Tablets 300 mg

2. QUALITATIVE AND QUANTITATIVE COMPOSITION

Each tablet contains ranitidine 300 mg (as the hydrochloride) and 20.8 mEq (479 mg) of sodium.

3. PHARMACEUTICAL FORM

Effervescent Tablet.

4. CLINICAL PARTICULARS

4.1 Therapeutic indications

- Duodenal ulcer and benign gastric ulcer, including that associated with non-steroidal anti-inflammatory agents.
- Treatment of duodenal ulcers associated with *Helicobacter pylori* infection.
- Post-operative ulcer.
- Oesophageal reflux disease.
- Zollinger-Ellison Syndrome.
- Chronic episodic dyspepsia, characterised by pain (epigastric or retrosternal) which is related to meals or disturbs sleep but not associated with the above conditions.
- Prophylaxis of stress ulceration in seriously ill patients.
- Prophylaxis of recurrent haemorrhage from peptic ulcer.
- Prophylaxis of Mendelson's syndrome.

4.2 Posology and method of administration

Adults:

Duodenal ulcer and benign gastric ulcer:

– Acute treatment:

The standard dosage regimen for duodenal or benign gastric ulcer is 150 mg twice daily or 300 mg nocte. In most cases of duodenal ulcer or benign gastric ulcer healing occurs within 4 weeks. Healing usually occurs after a further 4 weeks in those not fully healed after the initial 4 weeks.

– Long-term management:

For the long-term management of duodenal or benign gastric ulcer the usual dosage regimen is 150 mg nocte.

In duodenal ulcer 300 mg twice daily for 4 weeks results in healing rates which are higher than those at 4 weeks with ranitidine 150 mg twice daily or 300 mg nocte. The increased dose has not been associated with an increased incidence of unwanted effects.

NSAID associated peptic ulceration:

– Acute treatment:

In ulcers following non-steroidal anti-inflammatory drug therapy, or associated with continued non-steroidal anti-inflammatory drugs, 8-12 weeks treatment may be necessary with 150 mg twice daily or 300 mg nocte.

For duodenal ulcers associated with *Helicobacter pylori* infection, ranitidine 300 mg at bedtime or 150 mg twice daily may be given with oral amoxycillin 750mg three times daily and metronidazole 500 mg three times daily for two weeks. Therapy with ranitidine should continue for a further two weeks. This dose regimen significantly reduces the frequency of duodenal ulcer recurrence.

Postoperative ulcer:

The standard dosage regimen for postoperative ulcer is 150 mg twice daily. Most cases heal within 4 weeks. Those not fully healed after the initial 4 weeks usually do so after a further 4 weeks.

In the management of oesophageal reflux disease, the recommended course of treatment is either 150 mg twice daily or 300 mg at bedtime for up to 8 weeks or 12 weeks if necessary.

Zollinger-Ellison syndrome:

The initial dosage regimen for Zollinger-Ellison syndrome is 150 mg three times daily, but this may be increased as necessary. Doses up to 6 grams per day have been well tolerated.

Chronic episodic dyspepsia:

The standard dosage regimen for patients with chronic episodic dyspepsia is 150 mg twice daily for up to 6 weeks. Anyone not responding or relapsing shortly afterwards should be investigated.

Prophylaxis of haemorrhage from stress ulceration in seriously ill patients or prophylaxis of recurrent haemorrhage in patients bleeding from peptic ulceration:

150 mg twice daily may be substituted for the injection once oral feeding commences.

Prophylaxis of Mendelson's syndrome:

150 mg 2 hours before anaesthesia, and preferably 150 mg the previous evening. Alternatively, the injection is also available. In obstetric patients in labour 150 mg every 6 hours, but if general anaesthesia is required it is recommended that a non-particulate antacid (e.g. sodium citrate) be given in addition.

Children:

The recommended oral dose for the treatment of peptic ulcer in children is 2 mg/kg to 4 mg/kg twice daily to a maximum of 300 mg ranitidine per day.

Renal Impairment:

Accumulation of ranitidine with resulting elevated plasma concentrations will occur in patients with severe renal impairment (creatinine clearance less than 50 ml/min). It is recommended that the daily dose of ranitidine in such patients should be 150 mg. In patients undergoing chronic ambulatory peritoneal dialysis or chronic haemodialysis, ranitidine (150 mg) should be taken immediately after dialysis.

4.3 Contraindications

Ranitidine is contra-indicated in patients known to have hypersensitivity to any component of the preparation.

4.4 Special warnings and special precautions for use

Malignancy:

The possibility of malignancy should be excluded before commencement of therapy in patients with gastric ulcer (and if indications include dyspepsia; patients of middle age and over with new or recently changed dyspeptic symptoms) as treatment with ranitidine may mask symptoms of gastric carcinoma.

Renal Disease:

Ranitidine is excreted via the kidney and so plasma levels of the drug are increased in patients with severe renal impairment.

The dosage should be adjusted as detailed above under Dosage in Renal Impairment.

Regular supervision of patients who are taking non-steroidal anti-inflammatory drugs concomitantly with ranitidine is recommended, especially in the elderly and in those with a history of peptic ulcer.

Rare clinical reports suggest that ranitidine may precipitate acute porphyric attacks. Ranitidine should therefore be avoided in patients with a history of acute porphyria.

Zantac Effervescent Tablets contain sodium. Care should therefore be taken in treating patients in whom sodium restriction is indicated.

Zantac Effervescent Tablets contain aspartame. They should be used with caution in patients with phenylketonuria.

4.5 Interaction with other medicinal products and other forms of Interaction

Ranitidine, at blood levels produced by standard recommended doses, does not inhibit the hepatic cytochrome P450-linked mixed function oxygenase system. Accordingly, ranitidine in usual therapeutic doses does not potentiate the actions of drugs which are inactivated by this enzyme; these include diazepam, lignocaine, phenytoin, propranolol, theophylline and warfarin. There is no evidence of an interaction between ranitidine and amoxycillin or metronidazole.

4.6 Pregnancy and lactation

Ranitidine crosses the placenta and is excreted in human breast milk.

Like other drugs it should only be used during pregnancy and nursing if considered essential.

4.7 Effects on ability to drive and use machines

None reported.

4.8 Undesirable effects

The following convention has been utilised for the classification of undesirable effects: very common (>1/10), common (>1/100, <1/10), uncommon (>1/1000, <1/100), rare (>1/10,000, <1/1000), very rare (<1/10,000).

Adverse event frequencies have been estimated from spontaneous reports from post-marketing data.

Blood & Lymphatic System Disorders

Very Rare: Blood count changes (leucopenia, thrombocytopenia). These are usually reversible. Agranulocytosis or pancytopenia, sometimes with marrow hypoplasia or marrow aplasia.

Immune System Disorders

Rare: Hypersensitivity reactions (urticaria, angioneurotic oedema, fever, bronchospasm, hypotension and chest pain).

Very Rare: Anaphylactic shock

These events have been reported after a single dose.

Psychiatric Disorders

Very Rare: Reversible mental confusion, depression and hallucinations.

These have been reported predominantly in severely ill and elderly patients.

Nervous System Disorders

Very Rare: Headache (sometimes severe), dizziness and reversible involuntary movement disorders.

Eye Disorders

Very Rare: Reversible blurred vision.

There have been reports of blurred vision, which is suggestive of a change in accommodation.

Cardiac Disorders

Very Rare: As with other H_2 receptor antagonists bradycardia and A-V Block.

Vascular Disorders

Very Rare: Vasculitis.

Gastrointestinal Disorders

Very Rare: Acute pancreatitis. Diarrhoea.

Hepatobiliary Disorders

Rare: Transient and reversible changes in liver function tests.

Very Rare: Hepatitis (hepatocellular, hepatocanalicular or mixed) with or without jaundice, these were usually reversible.

Skin and Subcutaneous Tissue Disorders

Rare: Skin Rash.

Very Rare: Erythema multiforme, alopecia.

Musculoskeletal and Connective Tissue Disorders

Very Rare: Musculoskeletal symptoms such as arthralgia and myalgia.

Renal and Urinary Disorders

Very rare: Acute interstitial nephritis.

Reproductive System and Breast Disorders

Very Rare: Reversible impotence. Breast symptoms in men.

4.9 Overdose

Ranitidine is very specific in action and accordingly no particular problems are expected following overdosage with the drug, clinicians should be aware of the sodium content (see Precautions section). Symptomatic and supportive therapy should be given as appropriate. If need be, the drug may be removed from the plasma by haemodialysis.

5. PHARMACOLOGICAL PROPERTIES

5.1 Pharmacodynamic properties

Ranitidine is a specific rapidly acting histamine H_2-antagonist. It inhibits basal and stimulated secretion of gastric acid, reducing both the volume and the acid and pepsin content of the secretion. Ranitidine has a relatively long duration of action and so a single 150 mg dose effectively suppresses gastric acid secretion for twelve hours.

5.2 Pharmacokinetic properties

The bioavailability of ranitidine is consistently about 50%. Absorption of ranitidine after oral administration is rapid and peak plasma concentrations are usually achieved 2-3 hours after administration. Absorption is not significantly impaired by food or antacids. Ranitidine is not extensively metabolised. Elimination of the drug is primarily by tubular secretion. The elimination half-life of ranitidine is 2-3 hours. In balance studies with 150mg 3H-ranitidine 60-70% of an oral dose was excreted in urine and 26% in faeces. Analysis of urine excreted in the first 24 hours after dosing showed that 35% of the oral dose was eliminated unchanged. About 6% of the dose is excreted as the N-Oxide, 2% as the S-Oxide, 2% as desmethyl ranitidine and 1-2% as the furoic acid analogue.

5.3 Preclinical safety data

No additional data of relevance.

6. PHARMACEUTICAL PARTICULARS

6.1 List of excipients

Monosodium Citrate Anhydrous

Sodium Bicarbonate

Aspartame

Povidone

Sodium Benzoate

Orange Flavour (IFF No. 6)

Grapefruit Flavour (IFF 18C 222)

Pharmaceutical Industrial Alcohol or Ethanol

6.2 Incompatibilities

None.

6.3 Shelf life

2 years.

6.4 Special precautions for storage

Store below 30°C in a dry place.

6.5 Nature and contents of container

Polypropylene tubes with polyethylene tamper evident cap, each tube contains 15 tablets packed in cartons of 30 tablets.

Aluminium foil strips of six tablets packed in cartons of 30 tablets.

6.6 Instructions for use and handling

Place the tablets in half a glass of water (minimum 75 ml) and allow to dissolve completely before swallowing.

Administrative Data

7. MARKETING AUTHORISATION HOLDER

Glaxo Wellcome UK Limited

Stockley Park West

Uxbridge

Middlesex UB11 1BT

Trading as: GlaxoSmithKline UK

8. MARKETING AUTHORISATION NUMBER(S)

PL 10949/0138.

9. DATE OF FIRST AUTHORISATION/RENEWAL OF THE AUTHORISATION

26 January 2000

10. DATE OF REVISION OF THE TEXT

29 May 2004

11. Legal Status

POM

Zantac Injection 50mg/2ml

(GlaxoSmithKline UK)

1. NAME OF THE MEDICINAL PRODUCT

Zantac Injection 50 mg/2ml

2. QUALITATIVE AND QUANTITATIVE COMPOSITION

Ranitidine Hydrochloride HSE 56.0 mg/2ml equivalent to Ranitidine 50.0 mg/2ml.

3. PHARMACEUTICAL FORM

Injection (Aqueous solution)

4. CLINICAL PARTICULARS

4.1 Therapeutic indications

Zantac Injection is indicated for the treatment of duodenal ulcer, benign gastric ulcer, post - operative ulcer, reflux oesophagitis, Zollinger - Ellison Syndrome and the following conditions where reduction of gastric secretion and acid output is desirable:

The prophylaxis of gastrointestinal haemorrhage from stress ulceration in seriously ill patients, the prophylaxis of recurrent haemorrhage in patients with bleeding peptic ulcers and before general anaesthesia in patients considered to be at risk of acid aspiration (Mendelson's Syndrome), particularly obstetric patients during labour. For appropriate cases, Zantac tablets are also available.

4.2 Posology and method of administration

Adults (including elderly)

Zantac Injection may be given either as a slow (over a period of at least two minutes) intravenous injection of 50 mg, after dilution to a volume of 20 ml per 50 mg dose, which may be repeated every six to eight hours; or as an intermittent intravenous infusion at a rate of 25 mg per hour for two hours; the infusion may be repeated at six to eight hour intervals, or as an intramuscular injection of 50 mg (2ml) every six to eight hours.

In the prophylaxis of haemorrhage from stress ulceration in seriously ill patients or the prophylaxis of recurrent haemorrhage in patients bleeding from peptic ulceration, parenteral administration may be continued until oral feeding commences. Patients considered to be still at risk may then be treated with Zantac tablets 150 mg twice daily.

In the prophylaxis of upper gastro-intestinal haemorrhage from stress ulceration in seriously ill patients a priming dose of 50 mg as a slow intravenous injection followed by a continuous intravenous infusion of 0.125 - 0.250 mg/kg/hr may be preferred.

In patients considered to be at risk of developing acid aspiration syndrome, Zantac Injection 50 mg may be given intramuscularly or by slow intravenous injection 45 to 60 minutes before induction of general anaesthesia.

Children

The use of Zantac Injection in children has not been evaluated.

Route of Administration

Intravenous or intramuscular injection

4.3 Contraindications

Ranitidine is contraindicated for patients known to have hypersensitivity to any component of the preparation.

4.4 Special warnings and special precautions for use

Treatment with a histamine H_2-antagonist may mask the symptoms associated with carcinoma of the stomach and may therefore delay diagnosis of the condition. Accordingly, where gastric ulcer is suspected, the possibility of malignancy should be excluded before therapy with Zantac is instituted.

Ranitidine is excreted via the kidney and so plasma levels of the drug are increased in patients with renal impairment. Accordingly, it is recommended in such patients that Zantac be administered in doses of 25 mg.

Bradycardia in association with rapid administration of Zantac Injection has been reported rarely, usually in patients with factors predisposing to cardiac rhythm disturbances. Recommended rates of administration should not be exceeded.

It has been reported that the use of higher than recommended doses of intravenous H_2-antagonists has been associated with rises in liver enzymes when treatment has been extended beyond five days.

Although clinical reports of acute intermittent porphyria associated with ranitidine administration have been rare and inconclusive, ranitidine should be avoided in patients with a history of this condition.

4.5 Interaction with other medicinal products and other forms of Interaction

Ranitidine does not inhibit the hepatic cytochrome P450-linked mixed function oxygenase system. Accordingly, ranitidine does not potentiate the actions of drugs, which are inactivated by this enzyme; these include diazepam, lignocaine, phenytoin, propranolol, theophylline and warfarin.

4.6 Pregnancy and lactation

Zantac crosses the placenta but therapeutic doses administered to obstetric patients in labour or undergoing caesarean section have been without any adverse effect on labour, delivery or subsequent neonatal progress. Zantac is also excreted in human breast milk. Like other drugs, Zantac should only be used during pregnancy and nursing if considered essential.

4.7 Effects on ability to drive and use machines

None known.

4.8 Undesirable effects

The following convention has been utilised for the classification of undesirable effects: very common ($\geq$1/10), common ($\geq$1/100, <1/10), uncommon ($\geq$1/1000, <1/100), rare ($\geq$1/10,000, <1/1000), very rare (<1/10,000).

Adverse event frequencies have been estimated from spontaneous reports from post-marketing data.

Blood & Lymphatic System Disorders

Very Rare: Blood count changes (leucopenia, thrombocytopenia). These are usually reversible. Agranulocytosis or pancytopenia, sometimes with marrow hypoplasia or marrow aplasia.

Immune System Disorders

Rare: Hypersensitivity reactions (urticaria, angioneurotic oedema, fever, bronchospasm, hypotension and chest pain).

Very Rare: Anaphylactic shock

These events have been reported after a single dose.

Psychiatric Disorders

Very Rare: Reversible mental confusion, depression and hallucinations.

These have been reported predominantly in severely ill and elderly patients.

Nervous System Disorders

Very Rare: Headache (sometimes severe), dizziness and reversible involuntary movement disorders.

Eye Disorders

Very Rare: Reversible blurred vision.

There have been reports of blurred vision, which is suggestive of a change in accommodation.

Cardiac Disorders

Very Rare: As with other H_2 receptor antagonists bradycardia and A-V Block.

Vascular Disorders

Very Rare: Vasculitis.

Gastrointestinal Disorders

Very Rare: Acute pancreatitis. Diarrhoea.

Hepatobiliary Disorders

Rare: Transient and reversible changes in liver function tests.

Very Rare Hepatitis (hepatocellular, hepatocanalicular or mixed) with or without jaundice, these were usually reversible.

Skin and Subcutaneous Tissue Disorders

Rare: Skin Rash.

Very Rare: Erythema multiforme, alopecia.

Musculoskeletal and Connective Tissue Disorders

Very Rare: Musculoskeletal symptoms such as arthralgia and myalgia.

Renal and Urinary Disorders

Very rare: Acute interstitial nephritis.

Reproductive System and Breast Disorders

Very Rare: Reversible impotence. Breast symptoms in men.

4.9 Overdose

Zantac is very specific in action and accordingly, no particular problems are expected following overdosage with the drug. Symptomatic and supportive therapy should be given as appropriate. If need be, the drug may be removed from the plasma by haemodialysis.

5. PHARMACOLOGICAL PROPERTIES

5.1 Pharmacodynamic properties

Ranitidine is a specific, rapidly acting histamine H2-antagonist. It inhibits basal and stimulated secretion of gastric acid, reducing both the volume and the acid and pepsin content of the secretion.

5.2 Pharmacokinetic properties

Absorption of ranitidine after intramuscular injection is rapid and peak plasma concentrations are usually achieved within 15 minutes of administration. Ranitidine is not extensively metabolised. The elimination of the drug is primarily by tubular secretion. The elimination half-life of ranitidine is 2-3 hours. In balance, studies with 150mg 3H-ranitidine, 93% of an intravenous dose was excreted in urine and 5% in faeces. Analysis of urine excreted in the first 24 hours after dosing showed that 70% of the intravenous dose was eliminated unchanged. About 6% of the dose is excreted in the urine as the N-oxide, 2% as desmethyl ranitidine and 1-2% as the furoic acid analogue.

5.3 Preclinical safety data

There are no pre-clinical data of relevance to the prescriber which are additional to that already included in other sections of the SmPC.

6. PHARMACEUTICAL PARTICULARS

6.1 List of excipients

Sodium chloride	BP
Potassium Dihydrogen Orthophosphate	HSE
Disodium Hydrogen Orthophosphate	HSE
Water for Injection	BP

6.2 Incompatibilities

See 6.6 Instructions for Use/Handling.

6.3 Shelf life

36 months unopened.

6.4 Special precautions for storage

Store below 25°C, protect from light.

Zantac Injection should not be autoclaved.

6.5 Nature and contents of container

2 ml colourless Type I glass ampoules, Pack size: 5 ampoules.

6.6 Instructions for use and handling

Zantac Injection has been shown to be compatible with the following intravenous infusion fluids:-

0.9% Sodium Chloride BP

5% Dextrose BP

0.18% Sodium Chloride and 4% Dextrose BP

4.2% Sodium Bicarbonate BP

Hartmann's Solution.

All unused admixtures of Zantac Injection with infusion fluids should be discarded 24 hours after preparation.

Although compatibility studies have only been undertaken in polyvinyl chloride infusion bags (in glass for Sodium Bicarbonate BP) and a polyvinyl chloride administration set it is considered that adequate stability would be conferred by the use of a polyethylene infusion bag.

Administrative Data

7. MARKETING AUTHORISATION HOLDER

Glaxo Wellcome UK Ltd

T/A GlaxoSmithKline UK

Stockley Park West

Uxbridge

Middlesex, UB11 1BT

8. MARKETING AUTHORISATION NUMBER(S)

PL 10949/0109

9. DATE OF FIRST AUTHORISATION/RENEWAL OF THE AUTHORISATION

25 March 1998

10. DATE OF REVISION OF THE TEXT

29 May 2004

11. Legal Status

POM.

Zantac Syrup

(GlaxoSmithKline UK)

1. NAME OF THE MEDICINAL PRODUCT

Zantac Syrup

2. QUALITATIVE AND QUANTITATIVE COMPOSITION

Ranitidine Hydrochloride 168.0 mg (Equivalent to Ranitidine 150.0 mg)

3. PHARMACEUTICAL FORM

Syrup

4. CLINICAL PARTICULARS

4.1 Therapeutic indications

Zantac syrup is indicated for the treatment of duodenal ulcer and benign gastric ulcer, including that associated with non-steroidal anti-inflammatory agents. In addition, Zantac syrup is indicated for the prevention of NSAID associated duodenal ulcers. Zantac syrup is also indicated for the treatment of post-operative ulcer, Zollinger-Ellison Syndrome and oesophageal reflux disease including long term management of healed oesophagitis. Other patients with chronic episodic dyspepsia, characterised by pain (epigastric or retrosternal) which is related to meals or disturbs sleep but is not associated with the preceding conditions may benefit from ranitidine treatment. Zantac syrup is indicated for the following conditions where reduction of gastric secretion and acid output is desirable; the prophylaxis of gastro-intestinal haemorrhage from stress ulceration in seriously ill patients, the prophylaxis of recurrent haemorrhage in patients with bleeding peptic ulcers and before general anaesthesia in patients considered to be at risk of acid aspiration (Mendelson's Syndrome), particularly obstetric patients during labour. For appropriate cases Zantac injection is also available (see separate SPC).

4.2 Posology and method of administration

Route of administration: Oral

Adults (including the elderly):

The usual dosage is 150 mg twice daily, taken in the morning and evening. Alternatively, patients with duodenal ulceration, gastric ulceration or oesophageal reflux disease may be treated with a single bedtime dose of 300 mg. It is not necessary to time the dose in relation to meals. In most cases of duodenal ulcer, benign gastric ulcer and post operative ulcer, healing occurs in four weeks.

Healing usually occurs after a further 4 weeks of treatment in those patients whose ulcers have not fully healed after the initial course of therapy.

In ulcers following non-steroidal anti-inflammatory drug therapy or associated with continued non-steroidal anti-inflammatory drugs, 8 weeks treatment may be necessary.

For the prevention of non-steroidal anti-inflammatory drug associated duodenal ulcers ranitidine 150 mg twice daily may be given concomitantly with non-steroidal anti-inflammatory drug therapy.

In duodenal ulcer 300 mg twice daily for 4 weeks results in healing rates which are higher than those at 4 weeks with ranitidine 150 mg twice daily or 300 mg nocte. The increased dose has not been associated with an increased incidence of unwanted effects.

Maintenance treatment at a reduced dosage of 150 mg at bedtime is recommended for patients who have responded to short term therapy, particularly those with a history of recurrent ulcer.

In the management of oesophageal reflux disease, the recommended course of treatment is either 150 mg twice daily or 300 mg at bedtime for up to 8 weeks or if necessary 12 weeks.

In patients with moderate to severe oesophagitis, the dosage of ranitidine may be increased to 150 mg four times daily for up to twelve weeks. The increased dose has not been associated with an incidence of unwanted effects.

For the long-term management of oesophagitis the recommended adult oral dose is 150 mg twice daily. Long-term treatment is not indicated in the management of patients with unhealed oesophagitis with or without barrett's epithelium.

In patients with Zollinger-Ellison Syndrome, the starting dose is 150 mg three times daily and this may be increased as necessary. Patients with this syndrome have been given increasing doses up to 6 g per day and these doses have been well tolerated.

For patients with chronic episodic dyspepsia the recommended course of treatment is 150 mg twice daily for up to six weeks. Anyone not responding or relapsing shortly afterwards should be investigated.

In the prophylaxis of haemorrhage from stress ulceration in seriously ill patients or in the prophylaxis of recurrent haemorrhage in patients bleeding from peptic ulceration, treatment with Zantac tablets 150 mgs twice daily may be substituted for Zantac injection once oral feeding commences in patients considered to be still at risk from these conditions.

In patients thought to be at risk of acid aspiration syndrome an oral dose of 150 mg can be given 2 hours before induction of general anaesthesia, and preferably also 150 mg the previous evening.

In obstetric patients at commencement of labour, an oral dose of 150 mg may be given followed by 150 mg at six hourly intervals. It is recommended that since gastric emptying and drug absorption are delayed during labour, any patient requiring emergency general anaesthesia should be given, in addition, a non-particulate antacid (eg sodium citrate) prior to induction of anaesthesia. The usual precautions to avoid acid aspiration should also be taken.

Children:

The recommended oral dose for the treatment of peptic ulcer in children is 2 mg/kg to 4 mg/kg twice daily to a maximum of 300 mg ranitidine per day.

4.3 Contraindications

Ranitidine is contraindicated for patients known to have hypersensitivity to any component of the preparation.

4.4 Special warnings and special precautions for use

Treatment with a histamine H_2-antagonist may mask symptoms associated with carcinoma of the stomach and may therefore delay diagnosis of the condition. Accordingly, where gastric ulcer has been diagnosed or in patients of middle age and over with new or recently changed dyspeptic symptoms the possibility of malignancy should be excluded before therapy with Zantac is instituted.

Ranitidine is excreted via the kidney and so plasma levels of the drug are increased in patients with severe renal impairment. Accordingly, it is recommended that the therapeutic regimen for Zantac in such patients be 150 mg at night for 4 to 8 weeks. The same dose should be used for maintenance treatment should this be deemed necessary. If an ulcer has not healed after treatment, the standard dosage regimen of 150 mg twice daily should be instituted, followed, if need be, by maintenance treatment at 150 mg at night.

Regular supervision of patients who are taking non-steroidal anti-inflammatory drugs concomitantly with ranitidine is recommended, especially in the elderly. Current evidence shows that ranitidine protects against NSAID associated ulceration in the duodenum and not in the stomach.

Although clinical reports of acute intermittent porphyria associated with ranitidine administration have been rare and inconclusive, ranitidine should be avoided in patients with a history of this condition

Rates of healing of ulcers in clinical trial patients aged 65 and over have not been found to differ from those in younger patients. Additionally, there was no difference in the incidence of adverse effects.

4.5 Interaction with other medicinal products and other forms of Interaction

Ranitidine does not inhibit the hepatic cytochrome P450-linked mixed function oxygenase system. Accordingly, ranitidine does not potentiate the actions of drugs, which are inactivated by this enzyme; these include Diazepam, Lignocaine, Phenytoin, Propranolol, Theophylline and Warfarin.

4.6 Pregnancy and lactation

Zantac crosses the placenta but therapeutic doses administered to obstetric patients in labour or undergoing caesarean section have been without any adverse effect on labour, delivery or subsequent neonatal progress. Zantac is also excreted in human breast milk. Like other drugs, Zantac should only be used during pregnancy and nursing if considered essential.

4.7 Effects on ability to drive and use machines

Not applicable

4.8 Undesirable effects

The following convention has been utilised for the classification of undesirable effects: very common (>1/10), common (>1/100, <1/10), uncommon (>1/1000, <1/100), rare (>1/10,000, <1/1000), very rare (<1/10,000).

Adverse event frequencies have been estimated from spontaneous reports from post-marketing data.

Blood & Lymphatic System Disorders

Very Rare: Blood count changes (leucopenia, thrombocytopenia). These are usually reversible. Agranulocytosis or pancytopenia, sometimes with marrow hypoplasia or marrow aplasia.

Immune System Disorders

Rare: Hypersensitivity reactions (urticaria, angioneurotic oedema, fever, bronchospasm, hypotension and chest pain).

Very Rare: Anaphylactic shock

These events have been reported after a single dose.

Psychiatric Disorders

Very Rare: Reversible mental confusion, depression and hallucinations.

These have been reported predominantly in severely ill and elderly patients.

Nervous System Disorders

Very Rare: Headache (sometimes severe), dizziness and reversible involuntary movement disorders.

Eye Disorders

Very Rare: Reversible blurred vision.

There have been reports of blurred vision, which is suggestive of a change in accommodation.

Cardiac Disorders

Very Rare: As with other H_2 receptor antagonists bradycardia and A- V Block.

Vascular Disorders

Very Rare: Vasculitis.

Gastrointestinal Disorders

Very Rare: Acute pancreatitis. Diarrhoea.

Hepatobiliary Disorders

Rare: Transient and reversible changes in liver function tests.

Very Rare: Hepatitis (hepatocellular, hepatocanalicular or mixed) with or without jaundice, these were usually reversible.

Skin and Subcutaneous Tissue Disorders

Rare: Skin Rash.

Very Rare: Erythema multiforme, alopecia.

Musculoskeletal and Connective Tissue Disorders

Very Rare: Musculoskeletal symptoms such as arthralgia and myalgia.

Renal and Urinary Disorders

Very rare: Acute interstitial nephritis.

Reproductive System and Breast Disorders

Very Rare: Reversible impotence. Breast symptoms in men.

4.9 Overdose

Zantac is very specific in action and accordingly no particular problems are expected following overdosage with the drug. Symptomatic and supportive therapy should be given as appropriate. If need be, the drug may be removed from the plasma by haemodialysis.

5. PHARMACOLOGICAL PROPERTIES

5.1 Pharmacodynamic properties

Zantac is a specific, rapidly acting H_2-antagonist. It inhibits basal and stimulated secretion of gastric acid, reducing both the volume of the acid and pepsin content of the secretion. Zantac has a relatively long duration of action and a single 150 mg dose effectively suppresses gastric acid secretion for twelve hours.

5.2 Pharmacokinetic properties

The bioavailability of Ranitidine is consistently about 50 %. Absorption of ranitidine after oral administration is rapid and peak plasma concentrations are usually achieved 2-3 hours after administration. absorption is not significantly impaired by foods or antacids. Ranitidine is not extensively metabolised. Elimination of the drug is primarily by tubular secretion. The elimination half-life of ranitidine is 2-3 hours. In balance studies with 150 mg 3H-ranitidine 60-70% of an oral dose was excreted in urine and 26% in faeces. Analysis of urine excreted in the first 24 hours after dosing showed that 35% of the oral dose was eliminated unchanged. About 6% of the dose is excreted as the N-oxide, 2% as the S-oxide, 2% as desmethyl ranitidine and 1-2% as the furoic acid analogue.

5.3 Preclinical safety data

No clinically relevant findings were observed in preclinical studies.

6. PHARMACEUTICAL PARTICULARS

6.1 List of excipients

Hydroxypropyl methylcellulose USP

2906 or 2910

Ethanol (96%) BP

Propyl hydroxybenzoate BP

Butyl hydroxybenzoate BP

Potassium dihydrogen

Orthophosphate AR

Disodium hydrogen orthophosphat

Anhydrous AR

Sodium chloride BP

Saccharin sodium BP

Sorbitol solution 1973 BPC

Mint flavour IFF 17: 42: 3632

Purified water BP

6.2 Incompatibilities

Not applicable.

6.3 Shelf life

24 months

6.4 Special precautions for storage

Zantac syrup should be stored at a temperature not exceeding 25°C.

6.5 Nature and contents of container

Amber glass bottles with polypropylene child resistant caps, or plastic child resistant closures, or plastic child resistant tamper evident closures with either pet faced/al foil/epe wads, or pet faced/al foil/folding box board

Pack sizes: 300 ml, 2 × 150 ml

6.6 Instructions for use and handling

None

Administrative Data

7. MARKETING AUTHORISATION HOLDER

Glaxo Wellcome UK Ltd., trading as GlaxoSmithKline UK

Stockley Park West,

Uxbridge,

Middlesex, UB11 1BT

8. MARKETING AUTHORISATION NUMBER(S)

PL 10949/108

9. DATE OF FIRST AUTHORISATION/RENEWAL OF THE AUTHORISATION

17 April 2003

10. DATE OF REVISION OF THE TEXT

29 May 2004

11. Legal Status

POM

Zantac Tablets 150mg

(GlaxoSmithKline UK)

1. NAME OF THE MEDICINAL PRODUCT

Zantac Tablets 150 mg

2. QUALITATIVE AND QUANTITATIVE COMPOSITION

Each tablet contains ranitidine 150 mg (as the hydrochloride).

3. PHARMACEUTICAL FORM

Tablet.

4. CLINICAL PARTICULARS

4.1 Therapeutic indications

Duodenal ulcer and benign gastric ulcer, including that associated with non-steroidal anti-inflammatory agents.

Prevention of non-steroidal anti-inflammatory drug associated duodenal ulcers.

Treatment of duodenal ulcers associated with *Helicobacter pylori* infection.

Post-operative ulcer.

Oesophageal reflux disease including long term management of healed oesophagitis.

Symptomatic relief in gastro-oesophageal reflux disease.

Zollinger-Ellison Syndrome.

Chronic episodic dyspepsia, characterised by pain (epigastric or retrosternal) which is related to meals or disturbs sleep but not associated with the above conditions.

Prophylaxis of gastrointestinal haemorrhage from stress ulceration in seriously ill patients

Prophylaxis of recurrent haemorrhage with bleeding peptic ulcers.

Before general anaesthesia in patients at risk of acid aspiration (Mendelson's syndrome), particularly obstetric patients during labour.

For appropriate cases, Zantac injection is also available (see separate SPC).

4.2 Posology and method of administration

Adults:

Usual dosage is 150 mg twice daily, taken in the morning and evening.

Duodenal ulcer, gastric ulcer:

The standard dosage regimen is 150 mg twice daily or 300 mg at night. It is not necessary to time the dose in relation to meals.

In most cases of duodenal ulcer, benign gastric ulcer and post-operative ulcer, healing occurs within 4 weeks. Healing usually occurs after a further 4 weeks of treatment in those not fully healed after the initial course of therapy.

Ulcers following NSAID therapy or associated with continued NSAID's:

8 weeks treatment may be necessary

Prevention of NSAID associated duodenal ulcers:

150 mg twice daily may be given concomitantly with NSAID therapy.

In duodenal ulcer, 300 mg twice daily for 4 weeks results in healing rates which are higher than those at 4 weeks with ranitidine 150 mg twice daily or 300 mg at night. The increased dose has not been associated with an increased incidence of unwanted effects.

Duodenal ulcers associated with *Helicobacter pylori* infection:

For duodenal ulcers associated with *Helicobacter pylori* infection, ranitidine 300 mg at bedtime or 150 mg twice daily may be given with oral amoxycillin 750 mg three times daily and metronidazole 500 mg three times daily for two weeks. Therapy with ranitidine should continue for a further two weeks. This dose regimen significantly reduces the frequency of duodenal ulcer recurrence.

Maintenance treatment at a reduced dosage of 150 mg at bedtime is recommended for patients who have responded to short term therapy, particularly those with a history of recurrent ulcer.

Gastro-oesophageal reflux disease:

Symptom relief in gastro-oesophageal reflux disease. In patients with gastro-oesophageal reflux disease, a dose regimen of 150 mg twice daily for 2 weeks is recommended and this can be repeated in patients in whom the initial symptomatic response is inadequate

Oesophageal reflux disease:

In the management of oesophageal reflux disease, the recommended course of treatment is either 150 mg twice daily or 300 mg at bedtime for up to 8 weeks or 12 weeks if necessary.

In patients with moderate to severe oesophagitis, the dosage of ranitidine may be increased to 150 mg 4 times daily for up to 12 weeks. The increased dose has not been associated with an increased incidence of unwanted effects.

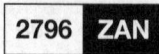

Healed oesophagitis:

For long term treatment, recommended adult dose is 150 mg twice daily. Long term treatment is not indicated in management of patients with unhealed oesophagitis with or without Barrett's epithelium.

Zollinger-Ellison syndrome:

The starting dose for Zollinger-Ellison syndrome is 150 mg three times daily, and this may be increased as necessary. Doses up to 6 grams per day have been well tolerated.

Chronic episodic dyspepsia:

The standard dosage regimen for patients with chronic episodic dyspepsia is 150 mg twice daily for up to 6 weeks. Anyone not responding or relapsing shortly afterwards should be investigated.

Prophylaxis of haemorrhage from stress ulceration in seriously ill patients or prophylaxis of recurrent haemorrhage in patients bleeding from peptic ulceration:

150 mg twice daily may be substituted for the injection once oral feeding commences.

Prophylaxis of acid aspiration (Mendelson's) syndrome:

150 mg oral dose can be given 2 hours before anaesthesia, and preferably also 150 mg the previous evening. Alternatively, the injection is also available. In obstetric patients in labour 150 mg every 6 hours, but if general anaesthesia is required it is recommended that a non-particulate antacid (e.g. sodium citrate) be given in addition. The usual precautions to avoid acid aspiration should also be taken.

Children:

The recommended oral dose for the treatment of peptic ulcer in children is 2 mg/kg to 4 mg/kg twice daily to a maximum of 300 mg ranitidine per day.

Renal Impairment:

Accumulation of ranitidine with resulting elevated plasma concentrations will occur in patients with severe renal impairment. Accordingly, it is recommended that the daily dose of ranitidine in such patients should be 150 mg at night for 4-8 weeks. The same dose should be used for maintenance treatment, if necessary. If an ulcer has not healed after treatment, 150 mg twice daily dosage should be instituted followed, if need be, by maintenance treatment of 150 mg at night.

4.3 Contraindications

Ranitidine is contra-indicated in patients known to have hypersensitivity to any component of the preparation.

4.4 Special warnings and special precautions for use

Malignancy:

The possibility of malignancy should be excluded before commencement of therapy in patients with gastric ulcer (and if indications include dyspepsia, patients of middle age and over with new or recently changed dyspeptic symptoms) as treatment with ranitidine may mask symptoms of gastric carcinoma.

Renal Disease:

Ranitidine is excreted via the kidney and so plasma levels of the drug are increased in patients with severe renal impairment.

The dosage should be adjusted as detailed above under Dosage in Renal Impairment.

Regular supervision of patients who are taking non-steroidal anti-inflammatory drugs concomitantly with ranitidine is recommended, especially in the elderly and in those with a history of peptic ulcer.

Rare clinical reports suggest that ranitidine may precipitate acute porphyric attacks. Ranitidine should therefore be avoided in patients with a history of acute porphyria.

Use in elderly patients:

Rates of healing of ulcers in clinical trial patients aged 65 and over have not been found to differ from those in younger patients. Additionally there was no difference in the incidence of adverse effects.

4.5 Interaction with other medicinal products and other forms of Interaction

Ranitidine does not inhibit the hepatic cytochrome P450-linked mixed function oxygenase system. Accordingly, ranitidine does not potentiate the actions of drugs which are inactivated by this enzyme; these include diazepam, lignocaine, phenytoin, propranolol, theophylline and warfarin. There is no evidence of an interaction between ranitidine and amoxycillin or metronidazole.

4.6 Pregnancy and lactation

Ranitidine crosses the placenta but therapeutic doses administered to obstetric patients in labour or undergoing caesarean section have been without any adverse effect on labour, delivery or subsequent neonatal progress. It is excreted in human breast milk.

Like other drugs it should only be used during pregnancy and nursing if considered essential.

4.7 Effects on ability to drive and use machines

Not applicable.

4.8 Undesirable effects

The following convention has been utilised for the classification of undesirable effects: very common ($>1/10$), common ($>1/100$, $<1/10$), uncommon ($>1/1000$, $<1/100$), rare ($>1/10,000$, $<1/1000$), very rare ($<1/10,000$).

Adverse event frequencies have been estimated from spontaneous reports from post-marketing data.

Blood & Lymphatic System Disorders

Very Rare:

Blood count changes (leucopenia, thrombocytopenia). These are usually reversible. Agranulocytosis or pancytopenia, sometimes with marrow hypoplasia or marrow aplasia.

Immune System Disorders

Rare:

Hypersensitivity reactions (urticaria, angioneurotic oedema, fever, bronchospasm, hypotension and chest pain).

Very Rare:

Anaphylactic shock

These events have been reported after a single dose.

Psychiatric Disorders

Very Rare:

Reversible mental confusion, depression and hallucinations.

These have been reported predominantly in severely ill and elderly patients.

Nervous System Disorders

Very Rare:

Headache (sometimes severe), dizziness and reversible involuntary movement disorders.

Eye Disorders

Very Rare:

Reversible blurred vision.

There have been reports of blurred vision, which is suggestive of a change in accommodation.

Cardiac Disorders

Very Rare:

As with other H_2 receptor antagonists bradycardia and A-V Block.

Vascular Disorders

Very Rare:

Vasculitis.

Gastrointestinal Disorders

Very Rare:

Acute pancreatitis. Diarrhoea.

Hepatobiliary Disorders

Rare:

Transient and reversible changes in liver function tests.

Very Rare:

Hepatitis (hepatocellular, hepatocanalicular or mixed) with or without jaundice, these were usually reversible.

Skin and Subcutaneous Tissue Disorders

Rare:

Skin Rash.

Very Rare:

Erythema multiforme, alopecia.

Musculoskeletal and Connective Tissue Disorders

Very Rare:

Musculoskeletal symptoms such as arthralgia and myalgia.

Renal and Urinary Disorders

Very rare:

Acute interstitial nephritis.

Reproductive System and Breast Disorders

Very Rare:

Reversible impotence. Breast symptoms in men.

4.9 Overdose

Ranitidine is very specific in action and accordingly no particular problems are expected following overdosage. Symptomatic and supportive therapy should be given as appropriate. If need be, the drug may be removed from the plasma by haemodialysis.

5. PHARMACOLOGICAL PROPERTIES

5.1 Pharmacodynamic properties

Ranitidine is a specific rapidly acting histamine H_2-antagonist. It inhibits basal and stimulated secretion of gastric acid, reducing both the volume and the acid and pepsin content of the secretion. Ranitidine has a relatively long duration of action and so a single 150 mg dose effectively suppresses gastric acid secretion for twelve hours.

5.2 Pharmacokinetic properties

Absorption of ranitidine after oral administration is rapid and peak plasma concentrations are usually achieved within two hours of administration. Absorption is not significantly impaired by food or antacids. The elimination half-life of ranitidine is approximately 2 hours. Ranitidine is excreted via the kidneys mainly as the free drug and in minor amounts as metabolites Its major metabolite is an N-oxide and there are smaller quantities of S-oxide and desmethyl ranitidine. The 24 hour urinary recovery of free ranitidine and its metabolites is about 40% with orally administered drug.

5.3 Preclinical safety data

No additional data of relevance.

6. PHARMACEUTICAL PARTICULARS

6.1 List of excipients

Tablet core:

Microcrystalline cellulose NF

Magnesium stearate EP

Methylhydroxypropyl cellulose (E464) EP

Film coat:

Titanium Dioxide E171 EP

Triacetin NF

6.2 Incompatibilities

None.

6.3 Shelf life

60 months.

6.4 Special precautions for storage

None necessary.

6.5 Nature and contents of container

Cartons of 30, 60 or 90 tablets, in aluminium foil strips or push through double foil blister packs.

6.6 Instructions for use and handling

No special instructions.

Administrative Data

7. MARKETING AUTHORISATION HOLDER

Glaxo Wellcome UK Limited

Trading as GlaxoSmithKline UK

Stockley Park West

Uxbridge

Middlesex

UB11 1BT

8. MARKETING AUTHORISATION NUMBER(S)

PL 10949/0042

9. DATE OF FIRST AUTHORISATION/RENEWAL OF THE AUTHORISATION

27 March 2002

10. DATE OF REVISION OF THE TEXT

29 May 2004

11. Legal Status

POM

Zantac Tablets 300mg

(GlaxoSmithKline UK)

1. NAME OF THE MEDICINAL PRODUCT

Zantac Tablets 300 mg

2. QUALITATIVE AND QUANTITATIVE COMPOSITION

Each tablet contains ranitidine 300 mg (as the hydrochloride).

3. PHARMACEUTICAL FORM

Tablet.

4. CLINICAL PARTICULARS

4.1 Therapeutic indications

Zantac Tablets are indicated for:

• treatment of duodenal ulcer and benign gastric ulcer, including that associated with non-steroidal anti-inflammatory agents.

- treatment of duodenal ulcers associated with *Helicobacter pylori* infection.
- treatment of post-operative ulcer
- Zollinger-Ellison syndrome
- oesophageal reflux disease
- chronic episodic dyspepsia, characterised by pain (epigastric or retrosternal) which is related to meals or disturbs sleep but is not associated with the preceding conditions may benefit from ranitidine treatment.

Zantac Tablets are indicated for the following conditions where reduction of gastric secretion and acid output is desirable:

- prophylaxis of gastrointestinal haemorrhage from stress ulceration in seriously ill patients
- prophylaxis of recurrent haemorrhage in patients with bleeding peptic ulcers
- before general anaesthesia in patients considered to be at risk of acid aspiration (Mendelson's syndrome), particularly obstetric patients during labour.

For appropriate cases Zantac Injection is also available (see separate SPC).

4.2 Posology and method of administration

Adults: The usual dosage is 150 mg twice daily, taken in the morning and evening. Alternatively, patients with duodenal ulceration, gastric ulceration or oesophageal reflux disease may be treated with a single bedtime dose of 300 mg. It is not necessary to time the dose in relation to meals. In most cases of duodenal ulcer, benign gastric ulcer and post operative ulcer, healing occurs in four weeks. Healing usually occurs after a further four weeks of treatment in those patients whose ulcers have not fully healed after the initial course of therapy.

In ulcers following non-steroidal anti-inflammatory drug therapy or associated with continued non-steroidal anti-inflammatory drugs, eight weeks treatment may be necessary.

In duodenal ulcer 300 mg twice daily for 4 weeks results in healing rates which are higher than those at 4 weeks with ranitidine 150 mg twice daily or 300 mg nocte. The increased dose has not been associated with an increased incidence of unwanted effects.

For duodenal ulcers associated with *Helicobacter pylori* infection Zantac 300 mg at bedtime or 150 mg twice daily may be given with oral amoxycillin 750 mg three times daily and metronidazole 500 mg three times daily for two weeks. Therapy with Zantac should continue for a further 2 weeks. This dose regimen significantly reduces the frequency of duodenal ulcer recurrence.

Maintenance treatment at a reduced dosage of 150 mg at bedtime is recommended for patients who have responded to short-term therapy, particularly those with a history of recurrent ulcer.

In the management of oesophageal reflux disease, the recommended course of treatment is either 150 mg twice daily or 300 mg at bedtime for up to 8 weeks or if necessary 12 weeks.

In patients with Zollinger-Ellison syndrome, the starting dose is 150 mg three times daily and this may be increased as necessary. Patients with this syndrome have been given increasing doses up to 6 g per day and these doses have been well tolerated.

For patients with chronic episodic dyspepsia the recommended course of treatment is 150 mg twice daily for up to six weeks. Anyone not responding or relapsing shortly afterwards should be investigated.

In the prophylaxis of haemorrhage from stress ulceration in seriously ill patients or the prophylaxis of recurrent haemorrhage in patients bleeding from peptic ulceration, treatment with Zantac Tablets 150 mg twice daily may be substituted for Zantac Injection (see separate SPC) once oral feeding commences in patients considered to be still at risk from these conditions.

In patients thought to be at risk of acid aspiration syndrome an oral dose of 150 mg can be given 2 hours before induction of general anaesthesia, and preferably also 150 mg the previous evening.

In obstetric patients at commencement of labour, an oral dose of 150 mg may be given followed by 150 mg at six hourly intervals. It is recommended that since gastric emptying and drug absorption are delayed during labour, any patient requiring emergency general anaesthesia should be given, in addition, a non-particulate antacid (e.g. sodium citrate) prior to induction of anaesthesia. The usual precautions to avoid acid aspiration should also be taken.

Children: The recommended oral dose for treatment of peptic ulcer in children is 2 mg/kg to 4 mg/kg twice daily to a maximum of 300 mg ranitidine per day.

Renal Impairment:

Accumulation of ranitidine with resulting elevated plasma concentrations will occur in patients with severe renal impairment. Accordingly, it is recommended that the daily dose of ranitidine in such patients should be 150 mg at night for 4-8 weeks. The same dose should be used for maintenance treatment, if necessary. If an ulcer has not healed after treatment, 150 mg twice daily dosage should be instituted followed, if need be, by maintenance treatment of 150 mg at night.

4.3 Contraindications

Ranitidine is contra-indicated in patients known to have hypersensitivity to any component of the preparation.

4.4 Special warnings and special precautions for use

Treatment with a histamine H2-antagonist may mask symptoms associated with carcinoma of the stomach and may therefore delay diagnosis of the condition. Accordingly, where gastric ulcer has been diagnosed or in patients of middle age and over with new or recently changed dyspeptic symptoms the possibility of malignancy should be excluded before therapy with Zantac Tablets is instituted.

Ranitidine is excreted via the kidney and so plasma levels of the drug are increased in patients with severe renal impairment. The dose should be adjusted as detailed above under Dosage in Renal Impairment.

Regular supervision of patients who are taking non-steroidal anti-inflammatory drugs concomitantly with ranitidine is recommended, especially in the elderly. Current evidence shows that ranitidine protects against NSAID associated ulceration in the duodenum and not in the stomach.

Although clinical reports of acute intermittent porphyria associated with ranitidine administration have been rare and inconclusive, ranitidine should be avoided in patients with a history of this condition.

Use in elderly patients:

Rates of healing of ulcers in clinical trial patients aged 65 and over have not been found to differ from those in younger patients. Additionally, there was no difference in the incidence of adverse effects.

4.5 Interaction with other medicinal products and other forms of Interaction

Ranitidine does not inhibit the hepatic cytochrome P450-linked mixed function oxygenase system. Accordingly, ranitidine does not potentiate the actions of drugs which are inactivated by this enzyme; these include diazepam, lignocaine, phenytoin, propranolol, theophylline and warfarin. There is no evidence of an interaction between ranitidine and amoxycillin or metronidazole.

4.6 Pregnancy and lactation

Zantac crosses the placenta but therapeutic doses administered to obstetric patients in labour or undergoing caesarean section have been without any adverse effect on labour, delivery or subsequent neonatal progress. Zantac is also excreted in human breast milk.

Like other drugs, Zantac should only be used during pregnancy and nursing if considered essential.

4.7 Effects on ability to drive and use machines

Not applicable.

4.8 Undesirable effects

The following convention has been utilised for the classification of undesirable effects: very common (>1/10), common (>1/100, <1/10), uncommon (>1/1000, <1/100), rare (>1/10,000, <1/1000), very rare (<1/10,000).

Adverse event frequencies have been estimated from spontaneous reports from post-marketing data.

Blood & Lymphatic System Disorders

Very Rare: Blood count changes (leucopenia, thrombocytopenia). These are usually reversible. Agranulocytosis or pancytopenia, sometimes with marrow hypoplasia or marrow aplasia.

Immune System Disorders

Rare: Hypersensitivity reactions (urticaria, angioneurotic oedema, fever, bronchospasm, hypotension and chest pain).

Very Rare: Anaphylactic shock

These events have been reported after a single dose.

Psychiatric Disorders

Very Rare: Reversible mental confusion, depression and hallucinations.

These have been reported predominantly in severely ill and elderly patients.

Nervous System Disorders

Very Rare: Headache (sometimes severe), dizziness and reversible involuntary movement disorders.

Eye Disorders

Very Rare: Reversible blurred vision.

There have been reports of blurred vision, which is suggestive of a change in accommodation.

Cardiac Disorders

Very Rare: As with other H_2 receptor antagonists bradycardia and A-V Block.

Vascular Disorders

Very Rare: Vasculitis.

Gastrointestinal Disorders

Very Rare: Acute pancreatitis. Diarrhoea.

Hepatobiliary Disorders

Rare: Transient and reversible changes in liver function tests.

Very Rare: Hepatitis (hepatocellular, hepatocanalicular or mixed) with or without jaundice, these were usually reversible.

Skin and Subcutaneous Tissue Disorders

Rare: Skin Rash.

Very Rare: Erythema multiforme, alopecia.

Musculoskeletal and Connective Tissue Disorders

Very Rare: Musculoskeletal symptoms such as arthralgia and myalgia.

Renal and Urinary Disorders

Very rare: Acute interstitial nephritis.

Reproductive System and Breast Disorders

Very Rare: Reversible impotence. Breast symptoms in men.

4.9 Overdose

Zantac is very specific in action and accordingly no particular problems are expected following overdosage. Symptomatic and supportive therapy should be given as appropriate. If need be, the drug may be removed from the plasma by haemodialysis.

5. PHARMACOLOGICAL PROPERTIES

5.1 Pharmacodynamic properties

Ranitidine is a specific rapidly acting histamine H_2-antagonist. It inhibits basal and stimulated secretion of gastric acid, reducing both the volume and the acid and pepsin content of the secretion. Ranitidine has a relatively long duration of action and so a single 150 mg dose effectively suppresses gastric acid secretion for twelve hours.

5.2 Pharmacokinetic properties

The bioavailability of ranitidine is consistently about 50%. Absorption of ranitidine after oral administration is rapid and peak plasma concentrations are usually achieved within 2-3 hours of administration. Absorption is not significantly impaired by food or antacids. Ranitidine is not extensively metabolised. Elimination of the drug is primarily by tubular secretion. The elimination half-life of ranitidine is 2-3 hours. In balanced studies with 150 mg 3H-Ranitidine 60-70% of an oral dose was excreted in urine and 25% in faeces. Analysis of urine excretion in the first 24 hours after dosing showed that 35% of the oral dose was eliminated unchanged. About 6% of the dose is excreted as the N-oxide, 2% as the S-oxide, 2% as desmethyl ranitidine and 1-2% as the furoic acid analogue.

5.3 Preclinical safety data

No additional data of relevance.

6. PHARMACEUTICAL PARTICULARS

6.1 List of excipients

Tablet core:

Microcrystalline cellulose

Croscarmellose sodium

Magnesium stearate

Film coat:

Methylhydroxypropyl cellulose (E464)

Titanium Dioxide (E171)

Triacetin

6.2 Incompatibilities

None.

6.3 Shelf life

3 years

6.4 Special precautions for storage

None necessary.

6.5 Nature and contents of container

Cartons of 30 tablets in aluminium foil strips or push through double foil blister packs.

6.6 Instructions for use and handling

No special instructions.

Administrative Data

7. MARKETING AUTHORISATION HOLDER

Glaxo Wellcome UK Limited

Trading as GlaxoSmithKline UK

Stockley Park West

Uxbridge

Middlesex

UB11 1BT

8. MARKETING AUTHORISATION NUMBER(S)

PL 10949/0043

9. DATE OF FIRST AUTHORISATION/RENEWAL OF THE AUTHORISATION

03 October 2000

10. DATE OF REVISION OF THE TEXT

29 May 2004

11. Legal Status

POM

Zarontin Syrup and Capsules

(Pfizer Limited)

1. NAME OF THE MEDICINAL PRODUCT
Zarontin Capsules 250 mg

Zarontin Syrup 250mg/ 5ml

2. QUALITATIVE AND QUANTITATIVE COMPOSITION
Each 250 mg capsule contains: Ethosuximide Ph Eur 250 mg.

Each 5 ml syrup contains: Ethosuximide 250 mg.

3. PHARMACEUTICAL FORM
Capsules: Clear pale yellow, dye-free, oblong soft gelatin capsules containing a clear, colourless solution.

Syrup: A clear, slightly yellowish to slightly pinkish, dye-free, raspberry flavoured syrup.

4. CLINICAL PARTICULARS

4.1 Therapeutic indications
Primarily useful in absence seizures. When generalised tonic clonic seizures (grand mal) and other forms of epilepsy co-exist with absence seizures, Zarontin may be administered in combination with other antiepileptic drugs.

4.2 Posology and method of administration
For oral use.

Adults (including the elderly) and children over six years
Capsules: Initially two capsules daily and adjusted thereafter to the patient's needs; daily dosage should be increased by small increments, for example, by one capsule every 4 to 7 days until control is achieved with minimal side effects. Although four to six capsules daily in divided doses often produces control of seizures, higher doses up to 8 capsules daily may occasionally be required.

Syrup: Initially two 5 ml spoonfuls daily and adjusted thereafter to the patient's needs; daily dosage should be increased by small increments, for example, by 5 ml every 4 to 7 days until control is achieved with minimal side effects. Although 20-30 ml daily in divided doses often produces control of seizures, higher doses up to 40 ml daily may occasionally be required.

Infants and children under six years
Zarontin Syrup is recommended for infants and children under six years.

The initial dose is 5 ml daily which is adjusted by small increments until control is achieved with minimal side effects. The optimal dose for most children is 20mg/kg/day. This dose has given average plasma levels within the accepted therapeutic range of 40 to 100mg/l.

4.3 Contraindications
Hypersensitivity to succinimides.

4.4 Special warnings and special precautions for use
Ethosuximide is capable of producing morphological and functional changes in the animal liver. In humans, abnormal liver and renal function studies have been reported. Zarontin should be used with caution in patients with impaired hepatic or renal function. Periodic urinalysis and liver function studies are advised for all patients receiving the drug.

If the patient has been receiving other antiepileptic medications the sudden withdrawal of these drugs may precipitate a series of attacks before Zarontin has been given in sufficient amounts to exercise control. This may be avoided by gradually replacing the antiepileptic medication previously used with Zarontin.

Sudden withdrawal of Zarontin should be avoided.

4.5 Interaction with other medicinal products and other forms of Interaction
Since ethosuximide may interact with concurrently administered antiepileptic drugs, periodic serum level determinations of these drugs may be necessary (e.g. ethosuximide may elevate phenytoin serum levels and valproic acid has been reported to both increase and decrease ethosuximide levels).

4.6 Pregnancy and lactation
There is some evidence that the succinimides may produce congenital abnormality in the offspring of a small number of epileptic patients and therefore they should only be used in pregnancy if in the judgement of the physician the potential benefits outweigh the risk.

The drug crosses the placental barrier and is also excreted in breast milk. Breast feeding is best avoided.

4.7 Effects on ability to drive and use machines
Ethosuximide may impair the mental and/or physical abilities required for the performance of potentially hazardous tasks such as driving or other such activities requiring alertness. Therefore, the patient should be cautioned accordingly.

4.8 Undesirable effects
Blood dyscrasias including some with fatal outcome have been reported to be associated with the use of ethosuximide. Should symptoms or signs of infection (e.g. sore throat, fever) develop, blood count determinations should be performed.

Ethosuximide when used alone in mixed types of epilepsy, may increase the frequency of generalised tonic-clonic (grand mal) seizures in some patients.

Other adverse reactions reported include: weight loss, diarrhoea, abdominal pain, gum hypertrophy, swelling of the tongue, hiccoughs, irritability, hyperactivity, lethargy, fatigue, sleep disturbances, night terrors, inability to concentrate, aggressiveness, paranoid psychosis, increased libido, myopia and vaginal bleeding.

Mild side effects, which are usually transient, may occur initially. These include apathy, drowsiness, depression, mild euphoria, extrapyramidal side effects, headache, ataxia, dizziness, anorexia, gastric upset, nausea and vomiting.

Psychotic states thought to be induced or exacerbated by anticonvulsant therapy have been reported.

Skin rashes have been seen in a few patients. Systemic lupus erythematosus has occasionally been associated with the use of ethosuximide. Additionally, lupus-like reactions have been reported in children given ethosuximide. They vary in severity from systemic immunological disorders, which include the nephrotic syndrome, to the asymptomatic presence of antinuclear antibodies. The nephrotic syndrome is rare and a complete recovery has usually been reported on drug withdrawal. Stevens-Johnson syndrome has also occurred during administration.

Cases of leucopenia, agranulocytosis, pancytopenia and aplastic anaemia have been reported. Monocytosis, leucocytosis and transitory mild eosinophilia have also been noted.

In most cases of leucopenia, the blood picture has been restored to normal on reduction of the dosage or discontinuation of the drug. Where leucopenia has occurred with other drugs, the polymorph count has in some cases increased steadily after starting treatment with ethosuximide and discontinuing the previous medication.

4.9 Overdose
Acute overdoses may produce nausea, vomiting and CNS depression including coma with respiratory depression. A relationship between ethosuximide toxicity and its plasma levels has not been established.

If less than 2g have been taken, fluids should be given by mouth. If a larger dose has been taken the stomach should be emptied, respiration maintained and any other symptoms treated accordingly. Activated charcoal and purgatives are known to be used in the treatment of overdosage. Haemodialysis may be useful. Forced diuresis and exchange transfusions are ineffective.

5. PHARMACOLOGICAL PROPERTIES

5.1 Pharmacodynamic properties
Ethosuximide is an anticonvulsant.

Ethosuximide suppresses the paroxysmal spike and wave pattern common to absence (petit mal) seizures. The frequency of epileptiform attacks is reduced, apparently by depression of the motor cortex and elevation of the threshold of the central nervous system to convulsive stimuli. Compared with other succinimide anticonvulsants, ethosuximide is more specific for pure absence seizures.

5.2 Pharmacokinetic properties
Ethosuximide is given by mouth. It is completely and rapidly absorbed from the gastrointestinal tract. Peak serum levels occur 1 to 7 hours after a single oral dose. Ethosuximide is not significantly bound to plasma proteins and therefore the drug is present in saliva and CSF in concentrations that approximate to that of the plasma. Therapeutic concentrations are in the range of 40 to 100 micrograms/ml. Ethosuximide is extensively metabolised to at least 3 plasma metabolites. Only between 12% and 20% of the drug is excreted unchanged in the urine. The elimination half life of ethosuximide is long, 40 to 60 hours in adults and 30 hours in children.

5.3 Preclinical safety data
The results of the preclinical tests do not add anything of further significance to the prescriber.

6. PHARMACEUTICAL PARTICULARS

6.1 List of excipients
Zarontin Capsules 250 mg contain the following excipients: Macrogol 400, gelatin, glycerol, purified water, triglycerides and soy lecithin.

Zarontin Syrup contains the following excipients: Sodium citrate, sodium benzoate, saccharin sodium, sucrose, glycerol, raspberry flavour, citric acid monohydrate and purified water.

6.2 Incompatibilities
None known.

6.3 Shelf life
3 years.

6.4 Special precautions for storage
Capsules: Do not store above 30°C. Keep the container tightly closed.

Syrup: Do not store above 25°C.

6.5 Nature and contents of container
Capsules: White high density polyethylene (HDPE) bottle fitted with a white low density polyethylene (LDPE) cap. Supplied in packs of 56 tablets.

Syrup: Amber round bottle with white aluminium. Each unit contains 200ml and is placed in folding carton.

6.6 Instructions for use and handling
No special instructions needed.

7. MARKETING AUTHORISATION HOLDER
Pfizer Limited

Ramsgate Road

Sandwich

Kent

CT13 9NJ

United Kingdom

8. MARKETING AUTHORISATION NUMBER(S)
Zarontin Capsules: PL 00057/0544

Zarontin Syrup: PA 00057/0545

9. DATE OF FIRST AUTHORISATION/RENEWAL OF THE AUTHORISATION
Capsules: 1 April 2003

Syrup: 1 March 2003

10. DATE OF REVISION OF THE TEXT
Capsules: June 2003

Syrup: October 2004

Ref: capsules: ZA2_0 UK

Syrup: ZA3_0 UK

Zavedos Capsules 10 mg

(Pharmacia Limited)

1. NAME OF THE MEDICINAL PRODUCT
Zavedos® Capsules 10 mg

2. QUALITATIVE AND QUANTITATIVE COMPOSITION
Idarubicin Hydrochloride 10.0 mg HSE

3. PHARMACEUTICAL FORM
Opaque red cap and white body, self-locking, hard gelatin capsule, size no. 4, containing an orange powder.

4. CLINICAL PARTICULARS

4.1 Therapeutic indications
Acute non-lymphocytic leukaemia (ANLL).

Whenever intravenous idarubicin cannot be employed e.g. for medical, psychological or social reasons, oral idarubicin can be used for remission induction in patients with previously untreated, relapsed or refractory acute non-lymphocytic leukaemia.

Zavedos may be used in combination chemotherapy regimens involving other cytotoxic agents.

As a single agent in the treatment of advanced breast cancer after failure of front line chemotherapy not including anthracyclines.

4.2 Posology and method of administration
Route of Administration: Oral

Dosage is usually calculated on the basis of body surface area.

In adult ANLL the recommended dose schedule suggested is 30 mg/m^2 orally given daily for 3 days as a single agent, or between 15 and 30 mg/m^2 orally daily for 3 days in combination with other anti-leukaemic agents.

In advanced breast cancer the recommended dose schedule as single agent is 45 mg/m^2 orally given either on a single day or divided over 3 consecutive days, to be repeated every 3 or 4 weeks based on the haematological recovery.

A maximum cumulative dose of 400 mg/m^2 is recommended.

These dosage schedules should, however, take into account the haematological status of the patient and the dosages of other cytotoxic drugs when used in combination.

In patients with hepatic impairment a dose reduction of Zavedos should be considered. (See special warnings.)

The capsules should be swallowed whole with some water and should not be sucked, bitten or chewed. Zavedos Capsules may also be taken with a light meal.

4.3 Contraindications
Zavedos should not be administered to individuals with hypersensitivity to idarubicin and/or other anthracyclines.

Zavedos therapy should not be started in patients with severe renal and liver impairment or patients with uncontrolled infections. See also "Use during pregnancy and lactation."

4.4 Special warnings and special precautions for use
Zavedos is intended for use under the direction of those experienced in antitumoral chemotherapy. The drug should not be given to patients with pre-existing bone marrow depression induced by previous drug therapy or radiotherapy unless the benefit warrants the risk. Pre-existing heart disease and previous therapy with anthracyclines, especially at high cumulative doses, or other potentially cardiotoxic agents are co-factors for increased risk of idarubicin-induced cardiac toxicity: the benefit to risk ratio of idarubicin therapy in such patients should be weighed before starting treatment with Zavedos. In absence of sufficient data, the use of oral idarubicin is

not recommended in patients with prior total body irradiation of bone marrow transplantation.

Like most other cytotoxic agents, idarubicin has mutagenic properties and is carcinogenic in rats.

Zavedos is a potent bone marrow suppressant. Myelosuppression, primarily of leukocytes, will therefore occur in all patients given a therapeutic dose of this agent and careful haematologic monitoring including granulocytes, red cells and platelets is required.

Facilities with laboratory and supportive resources adequate to monitor drug tolerability and protect and maintain a patient compromised by drug toxicity, should be available. It must be possible to treat rapidly and effectively a severe haemorrhagic condition and/or severe infection.

Myocardial toxicity as manifested by potentially fatal congestive heart failure (CHF), acute life-threatening arrhythmias or other cardiomyopathies may occur during therapy or several weeks after termination of therapy. Although a cumulative dose limit cannot yet be defined, available data on patients treated with Zavedos Capsules indicate that total cumulative doses up to at least 400 mg/m^2 have a low probability of cardiotoxicity. Should CHF occur, treatment with digitalis, diuretics, sodium restriction and bed rest is indicated. Cardiac function should be carefully monitored during treatment in order to minimise the risk of cardiac toxicity of the types described for other anthracycline compounds. The risk of such myocardial toxicity may be higher following concomitant or previous radiation to the mediastinal-pericardial area or treatment with other potentially cardiotoxic agents or in patients with a particular clinical situation due to their disease (anaemia, bone marrow depression, infections; leukaemic pericarditis and/or myocarditis). While there is no reliable method for predicting acute congestive heart failure, cardiomyopathy induced by anthracyclines is usually associated with persistent QRS voltage reduction, increase beyond normal limits of the systolic time interval (PEP/LVET) and a significant decrease of the left ventricular ejection fraction (LVEF) from pretreatment baseline values. An electrocardiogram or echocardiogram and a determination of left ventricular ejection fraction should be performed prior to starting therapy and during treatment with Zavedos. Early clinical diagnosis of drug-induced myocardial damage appears to be important for pharmacological treatment to be useful.

Occasional episodes of serious gastro-intestinal events (such as perforation or bleeding) have been observed in patients receiving oral idarubicin who had either acute leukaemia or a history of other pathologies/medications that might have led to G.I. complications. Therefore in the case of patients with active G.I. disease with increased risk of bleeding and/or perforation the physician must balance the benefit of Zavedos therapy against the risk.

Since hepatic function impairment can affect the disposition of idarubicin, liver function should be evaluated with conventional clinical laboratory tests (using serum bilirubin as indicator) prior to, and during, treatment. In a number of clinical trials, treatment was not given if bilirubin serum levels exceeded 2 mg/100 ml. With other anthracyclines a 50% dose reduction has been employed if bilirubin levels are in the range of 1.2-2.0 mg/100 ml in acute leukaemias. In some studies in breast cancer the oral idarubicin dose was reduced by 50% if bilirubin rose to 2-3 mg/100 ml during treatment or withdrawn with a bilirubin level > 3 mg/100 ml.

Therapy with Zavedos requires close observation of the patient and laboratory monitoring. Appropriate measures must be taken to control any systemic infection before beginning therapy. In acute leukaemia, patients over 55 years of age should be given vigorous supportive treatment during the aplastic period. Hyperuricaemia secondary to rapid lysis of leukaemic cells may be induced: blood uric acid levels should be monitored and appropriate therapy initiated if hyperuricaemia develops.

4.5 Interaction with other medicinal products and other forms of Interaction

Zavedos is a potent myelosuppressant and combination chemotherapy regimens which contain other agents having a similar action may be expected to lead to additive myelosuppressive effects.

An additive myelosuppressant effect is to be expected also with radiotherapy to metastases given concomitantly or within 2-3 weeks prior to treatment with Zavedos.

Food does not appear to reduce idarubicin absorption and Zavedos may therefore be given with a light meal.

4.6 Pregnancy and lactation

There is no information as to whether idarubicin may adversely affect human fertility, or cause teratogenesis. However, in rats (but not in rabbits) it is teratogenic and embryotoxic. Women of child bearing potential should be advised to avoid pregnancy. If Zavedos is to be used during pregnancy, or if the patient becomes pregnant during therapy, the patient should be informed of the potential hazard to the foetus. Mothers should be advised not to breast-feed whilst undergoing chemotherapy with this drug.

4.7 Effects on ability to drive and use machines

Special care should be taken if it is essential that patients drive or operate machinery while undergoing treatment especially if in a debilitated condition.

4.8 Undesirable effects

Severe myelosuppression and cardiac toxicity are the two major adverse effects. Other adverse reactions include: reversible alopecia in most patients treated at the dosage recommended in leukaemia and in about half of the patients treated at the doses recommended for breast cancer; acute nausea and vomiting; mucositis, usually involving the oral mucosa and appearing 3-10 days after starting treatment; oesophagitis; diarrhoea; fever and chills; skin rash; elevation of liver enzymes and bilirubin in about 10-20% of cases. Severe and sometimes fatal infections have been associated with idarubicin alone or in combination. Severe enterocolitis with perforation has been reported very rarely.

Idarubicin may impart a red colour to the urine for 1-2 days after administration and patients should be advised that this is no cause for alarm.

4.9 Overdose

Although the single-dose packaging is designed to minimise the risk of overdosage and no data on overdosage exists, should this occur, gastric lavage should be carried out as soon as possible. The patient should be observed for possible gastrointestinal haemorrhage and severe mucosal damage.

Very high doses of idarubicin may be expected to cause acute myocardial toxicity within 24 hours and severe myelosuppression within one or two weeks. Treatment should further aim to support the patient during this period and should utilise such measures as blood transfusions and reverse-barrier nursing. Delayed cardiac failure has been seen with the anthracyclines up to several months after an overdose. Patients should be observed carefully and if signs of cardiac failure arise, should be treated along conventional lines.

5. PHARMACOLOGICAL PROPERTIES

5.1 Pharmacodynamic properties

Idarubicin is an antimitotic and cytotoxic agent which intercalates with DNA and interacts with topoisomerase II and has an inhibitory effect on nucleic acid synthesis. The compound has a high lipophilicity which results in an increased rate of cellular uptake compared with doxorubicin and daunorubicin. Idarubicin has been shown to have a higher potency with respect to daunorubicin and to be an effective agent against murine leukaemia and lymphomas both by i.v. and oral routes. Studies *in-vitro* on human and murine anthracycline-resistant cells have shown a lower degree of cross-resistance for idarubicin compared with doxorubicin and daunorubicin. Cardiotoxicity studies in animals have indicated that idarubicin has a better therapeutic index than daunorubicin and doxorubicin. The main metabolite, idarubicinol, has shown *in-vitro* and *in-vivo* antitumoral activity in experimental models. In the rat, idarubicinol, administered at the same doses as the parent drug, is clearly less cardiotoxic than idarubicin.

5.2 Pharmacokinetic properties

After oral administration to patients with normal renal and hepatic function, idarubicin is rapidly absorbed, with a peak time of 2-4 H., is eliminated from systemic circulation with a terminal plasma T½ ranging between 10-35 H and is extensively metabolized to an active metabolite, idarubicinol, which is more slowly eliminated with a plasma T½ ranging between 33 and 60 H. The drug is mostly eliminated by biliary excretion, mainly in the form of idarubicinol, urinary excretion accounting for 1-2% of the dose as unchanged drug and for up to 4.6% as idarubicinol.

Average values of absolute bioavailability have been shown to range between 18 and 39% (individual values observed in the studies ranging between 3 and 77%), whereas the average values calculated on the data from the active metabolite, idarubicinol, are somewhat higher (29-58%; extremes 12-153%).

Studies of cellular (nucleated blood and bone marrow cells) drug concentrations in leukaemic patients have shown that uptake is rapid and almost parallels the appearance of the drug in plasma. Idarubicin and idarubicinol concentrations in nucleated blood and bone marrow cells are more than two hundred times the plasma concentrations. Idarubicin and idarubicinol disappearance rates in plasma and cells were almost comparable.

5.3 Preclinical safety data

No further preclinical safety data are available.

6. PHARMACEUTICAL PARTICULARS

6.1 List of excipients

Microcrystalline cellulose	Ph. Eur.
Glyceryl palmito-stearate	HSE
Capsule shell	
Red iron oxide (E172)	FP
Titanium dioxide (E171)	Ph Eur.
Gelatin	Ph Eur.
Sodium dodecyl sulphate	Ph. Eur.

6.2 Incompatibilities

Not known.

6.3 Shelf life

36 months.

6.4 Special precautions for storage

Store in a dry place.

6.5 Nature and contents of container

Type III amber glass bottles closed with an aluminium screw cap with a polyethylene gasket and a polyethylene cover cap. Aluminium/aluminium strips. Pack size: 1.

6.6 Instructions for use and handling

None stated.

7. MARKETING AUTHORISATION HOLDER

Pharmacia Limited
Davy Avenue
Milton Keynes
MK5 8PH
UK

8. MARKETING AUTHORISATION NUMBER(S)

PL 0032/0439

9. DATE OF FIRST AUTHORISATION/RENEWAL OF THE AUTHORISATION

25 March 2002

10. DATE OF REVISION OF THE TEXT

Legal Category

POM.

Zavedos Capsules 25 mg

(Pharmacia Limited)

1. NAME OF THE MEDICINAL PRODUCT

Zavedos® Capsules 25 mg

2. QUALITATIVE AND QUANTITATIVE COMPOSITION

Idarubicin Hydrochloride 25.0 mg HSE

3. PHARMACEUTICAL FORM

Opaque white cap and body, self-locking, hard gelatin capsule, size no. 2, containing an orange powder.

4. CLINICAL PARTICULARS

4.1 Therapeutic indications

Acute non-lymphocytic leukaemia (ANLL)

Whenever intravenous idarubicin cannot be employed e.g. for medical, psychological or social reasons, oral idarubicin can be used for remission induction in patients with previously untreated, relapsed or refractory acute non-lymphocytic leukaemia.

Zavedos may be used in combination chemotherapy regimens involving other cytotoxic agents.

As a single agent in the treatment of advanced breast cancer after failure of front line chemotherapy not including anthracyclines.

4.2 Posology and method of administration

Route of Administration: Oral

Dosage is usually calculated on the basis of body surface area.

In adult ANLL the recommended dose schedule suggested is 30 mg/m^2 orally given daily for 3 days as a single agent, or between 15 and 30 mg/m^2 orally daily for 3 days in combination with other anti-leukaemic agents.

In advanced breast cancer the recommended dose schedule as single agent is 45 mg/m^2 orally given either on a single day or divided over 3 consecutive days, to be repeated every 3 or 4 weeks based on the haematological recovery.

A maximum cumulative dose of 400 mg/m^2 is recommended.

These dosage schedules should, however, take into account the haematological status of the patient and the dosages of other cytotoxic drugs when used in combination. In patients with hepatic impairment a dose reduction of Zavedos should be considered. (See special warnings.)

The capsules should be swallowed whole with some water and should not be sucked, bitten or chewed. Zavedos capsules may also be taken with a light meal.

4.3 Contraindications

Zavedos should not be administered to individuals with hypersensitivity to idarubicin and/or other anthracyclines.

Zavedos therapy should not be started in patients with severe renal and liver impairment or patients with uncontrolled infections.

See also "Use during pregnancy and lactation."

4.4 Special warnings and special precautions for use

Zavedos is intended for use under the direction of those experienced in antitumoral chemotherapy. The drug should not be given to patients with pre-existing bone marrow depression induced by previous drug therapy or radiotherapy unless the benefit warrants the risk. Pre-existing heart disease and previous therapy with anthracyclines, especially at high cumulative doses, or other potentially cardiotoxic agents are co-factors for increased risk in idarubicin-induced cardiac toxicity: the benefit to risk ratio of idarubicin therapy in such patients should be weighed before starting treatment with Zavedos. In absence of sufficient data, the use of oral idarubicin is not recommended in patients with prior total body irradiation or bone marrow transplantation.

Like most other cytotoxic agents, idarubicin has mutagenic properties and is carcinogenic in rats.

Zavedos is a potent bone marrow suppressant. Myelosuppression, primarily of leukocytes, will therefore occur in all patients given a therapeutic dose of this agent and careful haematological monitoring including granulocytes, red cells and platelets is required.

Facilities with laboratory and supportive resources adequate to monitor drug tolerability and protect and maintain a patient compromised by drug toxicity, should be available. It must be possible to treat rapidly and effectively a severe haemorrhagic condition and/or severe infection.

Myocardial toxicity as manifested by potentially fatal congestive heart failure (CHF), acute life-threatening arrhythmias or other cardiomyopathies may occur during therapy or several weeks after termination of therapy. Although a cumulative dose limit cannot yet be defined, available data on patients treated with Zavedos Capsules indicate that total cumulative doses up to at least 400 mg/m^2 have a low probability of cardiotoxicity. Should CHF occur, treatment with digitalis, diuretics, sodium restriction and bed rest is indicated. Cardiac function should be carefully monitored during treatment in order to minimise the risk of cardiac toxicity of the types described for other anthracycline compounds. The risk of such myocardial toxicity may be higher following concomitant or previous radiation to the mediastinal-pericardial area or treatment with other potentially cardiotoxic agents or in patients with a particular clinical situation due to their disease (anaemia, bone marrow depression, infections; leukaemic pericarditis and/or myocarditis). While there is no reliable method for predicting acute congestive heart failure, cardiomyopathy induced by anthracyclines is usually associated with persistent QRS voltage reduction, increase beyond normal limits of the systolic time interval (PEP/LVET) and a significant decrease of the left ventricular ejection fraction (LVEF) from pretreatment baseline values. An electrocardiogram or echocardiogram and a determination of left ventricular ejection fraction should be performed prior to starting therapy and during treatment with Zavedos. Early clinical diagnosis of drug-induced myocardial damage appears to be important for pharmacological treatment to be useful.

Occasionally episodes of serious gastro-intestinal events (such as perforation or bleeding) have been observed in patients receiving oral idarubicin who had either acute leukaemia or a history of other pathologies/medications that might have led to G.I. complications. Therefore in the case of patients with active G.I. disease with increased risk of bleeding and/or perforation the physician must balance the benefit of Zavedos therapy against the risk.

Since hepatic function impairment can affect the disposition of idarubicin, liver function should be evaluated with conventional clinical laboratory tests (using serum bilirubin as indicator) prior to, and during, treatment. In a number of clinical trials, treatment was not given if bilirubin serum levels exceeded 2 mg/100 ml. With other antracyclines a 50% dose reduction has been employed if bilirubin levels are in the range of 1.2-2.0 mg/100 ml in acute leukaemias. In some studies in breast cancer the oral idarubicin dose was reduced by 50% if bilirubin rose to 2-3 mg/100 ml during treatment or withdrawn with a bilirubin level > 3 mg/100 ml.

Therapy with Zavedos requires a close observation of the patient and laboratory monitoring. Appropriate measures must be taken to control any systemic infection before beginning therapy. In acute leukaemia, patients over 55 years of age should be given vigorous supportive treatment during the aplastic period. Hyperuricaemia secondary to rapid lysis of leukaemic cells may be induced: blood uric acid levels should be monitored and appropriate therapy initiated if hyperuricaemia develops.

4.5 Interaction with other medicinal products and other forms of Interaction

Zavedos is a potent myelosuppressant and combination chemotherapy regimens which contain other agents having a similar action may be expected to lead to additive myelosuppressive effects.

An additive myelosuppressant effect is to be expected also with radiotherapy to metastases given concomitantly or within 2-3 weeks prior to treatment with Zavedos.

Food does not appear to reduce idarubicin absorption and Zavedos may therefore be given with a light meal.

4.6 Pregnancy and lactation

There is no information as to whether idarubicin may adversely affect human fertility, or cause teratogenesis. However, in rats (but not in rabbits) it is teratogenic and embryotoxic. Women of child bearing potential should be advised to avoid pregnancy. If Zavedos is to be used during pregnancy, or if the patient becomes pregnant during therapy, the patient should be informed of the potential hazard to the foetus. Mothers should be advised not to breast-feed whilst undergoing chemotherapy with this drug.

4.7 Effects on ability to drive and use machines

Special care should be taken if it is essential that patients drive or operate machinery while undergoing treatment especially if in a debilitated condition.

4.8 Undesirable effects

Severe myelosuppression and cardiac toxicity are the two major adverse effects. Other adverse reactions include: reversible alopecia in most patients; acute nausea and vomiting; mucositis, usually involving the oral mucosa and appearing 3-10 days after starting treatment; oesophagitis; diarrhoea; fever and chills; skin rash; elevation of liver enzymes and bilirubin in about 10-20% of cases. Severe and sometimes fatal infections have been associated with idarubicin alone or in combination. Severe enterocolitis with perforation has been reported very rarely.

Idarubicin may impart a red colour to the urine for 1-2 days after administration and patients should be advised that this is no cause for alarm.

4.9 Overdose

Although the single-dose packaging is designed to minimise the risk of overdosage and no data on overdosage exists, should this occur, gastric lavage should be carried out as soon as possible. The patient should be observed for possible gastrointestinal haemorrhage and severe mucosal damage.

Very high doses of idarubicin may be expected to cause acute myocardial toxicity within 24 hours and severe myelosuppression within one or two weeks. Treatment should further aim to support the patient during this period and should utilise such measures as blood transfusions and reverse-barrier nursing. Delayed cardiac failure has been seen with the anthracyclines up to several months after an overdose. Patients should be observed carefully and if signs of cardiac failure arise, should be treated along conventional lines.

5. PHARMACOLOGICAL PROPERTIES

5.1 Pharmacodynamic properties

Idarubicin is an antimitotic and cytotoxic agent which intercalates with DNA and interacts with topoisomerase II and has an inhibitory effect on nucleic acid synthesis. The compound has a high lipophilicity which results in an increased rate of cellular uptake compared with doxorubicin and daunorubicin. Idarubicin has been shown to have a higher potency with respect to daunorubicin and to be an effective agent against murine leukaemia and lymphomas both by i.v. and oral routes. Studies *in-vitro* on human and murine anthracycline-resistant cells have shown a lower degree of cross-resistance for idarubicin compared with doxorubicin and daunorubicin. Cardiotoxicity studies in animals have indicated that idarubicin has a better therapeutic index than daunorubicin and doxorubicin. The main metabolite, idarubicinol, has shown *in-vitro* and *in-vivo* antitumoral activity in experimental models. In the rat, idarubicinol, administered at the same doses as the parent drug, is clearly less cardiotoxic than idarubicin.

5.2 Pharmacokinetic properties

After oral administration to patients with normal renal and hepatic function, idarubicin is rapidly absorbed, with a peak time of 2-4 H., is eliminated from systemic circulation with a terminal plasma T½ ranging between 10-35 H and is extensively metabolized to an active metabolite, idarubicinol, which is more slowly eliminated with a plasma T½ ranging between 33 and 60 H. The drug is mostly eliminated by biliary excretion, mainly in the form of idarubicinol, urinary excretion accounting for 1-2% of the dose as unchanged drug and for up to 4.6% as idarubicinol.

Average values of absolute bioavailability have been shown to range between 18 and 39% (individual values observed in the studies ranged between 3 and 77%), whereas the average values calculated on the data from the active metabolite, idarubicinol, are somewhat higher (29-58%; extremes 12-153%).

Studies of cellular (nucleated blood and bone marrow cells) drug concentrations in leukaemic patients have shown that uptake is rapid and almost parallels the appearance of the drug in plasma. Idarubicin and idarubicinol concentrations in nucleated blood and bone marrow cells are more than two hundred times the plasma concentrations. Idarubicin and idarubicinol disappearance rates in plasma and cells were almost comparable.

5.3 Preclinical safety data

No further preclinical safety data are available.

6. PHARMACEUTICAL PARTICULARS

6.1 List of excipients

Microcrystalline cellulose	Ph. Eur.
Glyceryl palmito-stearate	HSE
Capsule shell	
Titanium dioxide (E171)	Ph. Eur.
Gelatin	Ph. Eur.
Sodium dodecyl sulphate	Ph. Eur.

6.2 Incompatibilities

Not known.

6.3 Shelf life

36 months.

6.4 Special precautions for storage

Store in a dry place.

6.5 Nature and contents of container

Type III amber glass bottles closed with an aluminium screw cap with a polyethylene gasket and a polyethylene cover cap. Aluminium/aluminium strips. Pack size: 1.

6.6 Instructions for use and handling

None stated.

7. MARKETING AUTHORISATION HOLDER

Pharmacia Limited
Davy Avenue
Milton Keynes
MK5 8PH
UK

8. MARKETING AUTHORISATION NUMBER(S)

PL 00032/0440

9. DATE OF FIRST AUTHORISATION/RENEWAL OF THE AUTHORISATION

10th May 2002

10. DATE OF REVISION OF THE TEXT

Legal Category

POM.

Zavedos Capsules 5 mg

(Pharmacia Limited)

1. NAME OF THE MEDICINAL PRODUCT

Zavedos® Capsules 5 mg

2. QUALITATIVE AND QUANTITATIVE COMPOSITION

Idarubicin Hydrochloride 5.0 mg HSE

3. PHARMACEUTICAL FORM

Opaque red cap and body, self-locking, hard gelatin capsules, size no. 4, containing an orange powder.

4. CLINICAL PARTICULARS

4.1 Therapeutic indications

Whenever intravenous idarubicin cannot be employed e.g. for medical, psychological or social reasons, oral idarubicin can be used for remission induction in patients with previously untreated, relapsed or refractory acute non-lymphocytic leukaemia.

Zavedos may be used in combination chemotherapy regimens involving other cytotoxic agents.

As a single agent in the treatment of advanced breast cancer after failure of front line chemotherapy not including anthracyclines.

4.2 Posology and method of administration

Route of Administration: Oral

Dosage is usually calculated on the basis of body surface area.

In adult ANLL the recommended dose schedule suggested is 30 mg/m^2 orally given daily for 3 days as a single agent, or between 15 and 30 mg/m^2 orally daily for 3 days in combination with other anti-leukaemic agents.

In advanced breast cancer the recommended dose schedule as single agent is 45 mg/m^2 orally given either on a single day or divided over 3 consecutive days, to be repeated every 3 or 4 weeks based on the haematological recovery.

A maximum cumulative dose of 400 mg/m^2 is recommended.

These dosage schedules should, however, take into account the haematological status of the patient and the dosages of other cytotoxic drugs when used in combination.

In patients with hepatic impairment a dose reduction of Zavedos should be considered. (See special warnings).

The capsules should be swallowed whole with some water and should not be sucked, bitten or chewed. Zavedos Capsules may also be taken with a light meal.

4.3 Contraindications

Zavedos should not be administered to individuals with hypersensitivity to idarubicin and/or other anthracyclines.

Zavedos therapy should not be started in patients with severe renal and liver impairment or patients with uncontrolled infections. See also "Use during pregnancy and lactation."

4.4 Special warnings and special precautions for use

Zavedos is intended for use under the direction of those experienced in antitumoral chemotherapy. The drug should not be given to patients with pre-existing bone marrow depression induced by previous drug therapy or radiotherapy unless the benefit warrants the risk. Pre-existing heart disease and previous therapy with anthracyclines, especially at high cumulative doses, or other potentially cardiotoxic agents are co-factors for increased risk of idarubicin-induced cardiac toxicity: the benefit to risk ratio of idarubicin therapy in such patients should be weighed before starting treatment with Zavedos. In absence of sufficient data, the use of oral idarubicin is not recommended in patients with prior total body irradiation or bone marrow transplantation.

Like most other cytotoxic agents, idarubicin has mutagenic properties and is carcinogenic in rats.

Zavedos is a potent bone marrow suppressant. Myelosuppression, primarily of leukocytes, will therefore occur in all patients given a therapeutic dose of this agent and careful haematologic monitoring including granulocytes, red cells and platelets is required.

Facilities with laboratory and supportive resources adequate to monitor drug tolerability and protect and maintain a patient compromised by drug toxicity, should be available. It must be possible to treat rapidly and effectively a severe haemorrhagic condition and/or severe infection.

Myocardial toxicity as manifested by potentially fatal congestive heart failure (CHF), acute life-threatening arrhythmias or other cardiomyopathies may occur during therapy or several weeks after termination of therapy. Although a cumulative dose limit cannot yet be defined, available data on patients treated with Zavedos Capsules indicate that total cumulative doses up to at least 400 mg/m^2 have a low probability of cardiotoxicity. Should CHF occur, treatment with digitalis, diuretics, sodium restriction and bed rest is indicated. Cardiac function should be carefully monitored during treatment in order to minimise the risk of cardiac toxicity of the types described for other anthracycline compounds. The risk of such myocardial toxicity may be higher following concomitant or previous radiation to the mediastinal-pericardial area or treatment with other potentially cardiotoxic agents or in patients with a particular clinical situation due to their disease (anaemia, bone marrow depression, infections; leukaemic pericarditis and/or myocarditis). While there is no reliable method for predicting acute congestive heart failure, cardiomyopathy induced by anthracyclines is usually associated with persistent QRS voltage reduction, increase beyond normal limits or the systolic time interval (PEP/LVET) and a significant decrease of the left ventricular ejection fraction (LVEF) from pretreatment baseline values. An electrocardiogram or echocardiogram and a determination of left ventricular ejection fraction should be performed prior to starting therapy and during treatment with Zavedos. Early clinical diagnosis of drug-induced myocardial damage appears to be important for pharmacological treatment to be useful.

Occasionally episodes of serious gastro-intestinal events (such as perforation or bleeding) have been observed in patients receiving oral idarubicin who had either acute leukaemia or a history of other pathologies/medications that might have led to G.I. complications. Therefore in the case of patients with active G.I. disease with increased risk of bleeding and/or perforation the physician must balance the benefit of Zavedos therapy against the risk.

Since hepatic function impairment can affect the disposition of idarubicin, liver function should be evaluated with conventional clinical laboratory tests (using serum bilirubin as indicator) prior to, and during, treatment. In a number of clinical trials, treatment was not given if bilirubin serum levels exceeded 2 mg/100 ml. With other anthracyclines a 50% dose reduction has been employed if bilirubin levels are in the range of 1.2-2.0 mg/100 ml in acute leukaemias. In some studies in breast cancer the oral idarubicin dose was reduced by 50% if bilirubin rose to 2-3 mg/100 ml during treatment or withdrawn with a bilirubin level > 3 mg/100 ml.

Therapy with Zavedos requires close observation of the patient and laboratory monitoring. Appropriate measures must be taken to control any systemic infection before beginning therapy. In acute leukaemia, patients over 55 years of age should be given vigorous supportive treatment during the aplastic period. Hyperuricaemia secondary to rapid lysis of leukaemic cells may be induced: blood uric acid levels should be monitored and appropriate therapy initiated if hyperuricaemia develops.

4.5 Interaction with other medicinal products and other forms of Interaction

Zavedos is a potent myelosuppressant and combination chemotherapy regimens which contain other agents having a similar action may be expected to lead to additive myelosuppressive effects.

An additive myelosuppressant effect is to be expected also with radiotherapy to metastases given concomitantly or within 2-3 weeks prior to the treatment with Zavedos.

Food does not appear to reduce idarubicin absorption and Zavedos may therefore be given with a light meal.

4.6 Pregnancy and lactation

There is no information as to whether idarubicin may adversely affect human fertility, or cause teratogenesis. However, in rats (but not in rabbits) it is teratogenic and embryotoxic. Women of child bearing potential should be advised to avoid pregnancy. If Zavedos is to be used during pregnancy, or if the patient becomes pregnant during therapy, the patient should be informed of the potential hazard to the foetus. Mothers should be advised not to breast-feed whilst undergoing chemotherapy with this drug.

4.7 Effects on ability to drive and use machines

Special care should be taken if it is essential that patients drive or operate machinery while undergoing treatment especially if in a debilitated condition.

4.8 Undesirable effects

Severe myelosuppression and cardiac toxicity are the two major adverse effects. Other adverse reactions include: reversible alopecia in most patients treated at the dosage recommended in leukaemia and in about half of the patients treated at the doses recommended for breast cancer; acute nausea and vomiting; mucositis, usually involving the oral mucosa and appearing 3-10 days after starting treatment; oesophagitis; diarrhoea; fever and chills; skin rash; elevation of liver enzymes and bilirubin in about 10-20% of cases. Severe and sometimes fatal infections have been associated with idarubicin alone or in combination. Severe enterocolitis with perforation has been reported very rarely.

Idarubicin may impart a red colour to the urine for 1-2 days after administration and patients should be advised that this is no cause for alarm.

4.9 Overdose

Although the single-dose packaging is designed to minimise the risk of overdosage and no data on overdosage exists, should this occur, gastric lavage should be carried out as soon as possible. The patient should be observed for possible gastrointestinal haemorrhage and severe mucosal damage.

Very high doses of idarubicin may be expected to cause acute myocardial toxicity within 24 hours and severe myelosuppression within one or two weeks. Treatment should further aim to support the patient during this period and should utilise such measures as blood transfusions and reverse-barrier nursing. Delayed cardiac failure has been seen with the anthracyclines up to several months after an overdose. Patients should be observed carefully and if signs of cardiac failure arise, should be treated along conventional lines.

5. PHARMACOLOGICAL PROPERTIES

5.1 Pharmacodynamic properties

Idarubicin is an antimitotic and cytotoxic agent which intercalates with DNA and interacts with topoisomerase II and has an inhibitory effect on nucleic acid synthesis. The compound has a high lipophilicity which results in an increased rate of cellular uptake compared with doxorubicin and daunorubicin. Idarubicin has been shown to have a higher potency with respect to daunorubicin and to be an effective agent against murine leukaemia and lymphomas both by i.v. and oral routes. Studies *in-vitro* on human and murine anthracycline-resistant cells have shown a lower degree of cross-resistance for idarubicin compared with doxorubicin and daunorubicin. Cardiotoxicity studies in animals have indicated that idarubicin has a better therapeutic index than daunorubicin and doxorubicin. The main metabolite, idarubicinol, has shown *in-vitro* and *in-vivo* antitumoral activity in experimental models. In the rat, idarubicinol, administered at the same doses as the parent drug, is clearly less cardiotoxic than idarubicin.

5.2 Pharmacokinetic properties

After oral administration to patients with normal renal and hepatic function, idarubicin is rapidly absorbed, with a peak time of 2-4 H., is eliminated from systemic circulation with a terminal plasma T½ ranging between 10-35 H and is extensively metabolized to an active metabolite, idarubicinol, which is more slowly eliminated with a plasma T½ ranging between 33 and 60 H. The drug is mostly eliminated by biliary excretion, mainly in the form of idarubicinol, urinary excretion accounting for 1-2% of the dose as unchanged drug and for up to 4.6% as idarubicinol.

Average values of absolute bioavailability have been shown to range between 18 and 39% (individual values observed in the studies ranging between 3 and 77%), whereas the average values calculated on the data from the active metabolite, idarubicinol, are somewhat higher (29-58%; extremes 12-153%).

Studies of cellular (nucleated blood and bone marrow cells) drug concentrations in leukaemic patients have shown that uptake is rapid and almost parallels the appearance of the drug in plasma. Idarubicin and idarubicinol concentrations in nucleated blood and bone marrow cells are more than two hundred times the plasma concentrations. Idarubicin and idarubicinol disappearance rates in plasma and cells were almost comparable.

5.3 Preclinical safety data

No further preclinical safety data are available.

6. PHARMACEUTICAL PARTICULARS

6.1 List of excipients

Microcrystalline cellulose	Ph. Eur.
Glyceryl palmito-stearate	HSE
Capsule shell	
Red iron oxide (E172)	FP
Titanium dioxide (E171)	Ph. Eur.
Gelatin	Ph. Eur.
Sodium dodecyl sulphate	Ph. Eur.

6.2 Incompatibilities

Not known.

6.3 Shelf life

36 months.

6.4 Special precautions for storage

Store in a dry place.

6.5 Nature and contents of container

Type III amber glass bottles closed with an aluminium screw cap with a polyethylene gasket and a polyethylene cover cap. Aluminium/aluminium strips. Pack size: 1.

6.6 Instructions for use and handling

None stated.

7. MARKETING AUTHORISATION HOLDER

Pharmacia Limited
Davy Avenue
Milton Keynes
MK5 8PH
UK

8. MARKETING AUTHORISATION NUMBER(S)

PL 00032/0441

9. DATE OF FIRST AUTHORISATION/RENEWAL OF THE AUTHORISATION

10th May 2002

10. DATE OF REVISION OF THE TEXT

Legal Category

POM.

Zavedos Injection 5mg/10mg

(Pharmacia Limited)

1. NAME OF THE MEDICINAL PRODUCT

Zavedos Injection

2. QUALITATIVE AND QUANTITATIVE COMPOSITION

Each vial contains:

Idarubicin HCl 5 mg or10mg

3. PHARMACEUTICAL FORM

Powder for Solution for Injection

Sterile, pyrogen-free, orange-red, freeze-dried powder in vial containing:

5mg injection: 5mg of idarubicin hydrochloride, with 50mg of lactose monohydrate.

10mg injection: 10mg of idarubicin hydrochloride, with 100mg of lactose monohydrate.

4. CLINICAL PARTICULARS

4.1 Therapeutic indications

For the treatment of acute non-lymphoblastic leukaemia (ANLL) in adults, for remission induction in untreated patients or for remission induction in relapsed or refractory patients.

In the treatment of relapsed acute lymphoblastic leukaemia (ALL) as second line treatment in adults and children.

Zavedos may be used in combination chemotherapy regimens involving other cytotoxic agents.

4.2 Posology and method of administration

Dosage is calculated on the basis of body surface area.

Warning: Not for intrathecal use.

For reconstitution the contents of the:

5 mg vial should be dissolved in 5 ml of water for injections (Ph. Eur).

10 mg vial should be dissolved in 10 ml of water for injections (Ph. Eur).

Zavedos must be administered only by the intravenous route and the reconstituted solution should be given via the tubing of a freely running intravenous infusion of 0.9% sodium chloride injection taking 5 to 10 minutes over the injection. This technique minimises the risk of thrombosis or perivenous extravasation which can lead to severe cellulitis and necrosis. Venous sclerosis may result from injection into small veins or repeated injections into the same vein.

Acute non-lymphoblastic leukaemia (ANLL)

- Adults

- 12 mg/m^2/day i.v. daily for 3 days in combination with cytarabine.

or

- 8 mg/m^2/day i.v. daily for 5 days with/without combination.

Acute lymphoblastic leukaemia (ALL)

Adults

As single agent in ALL the suggested dose in adults is 12 mg/m^2 i.v. daily for 3 days.

Children

10 mg/m^2 i.v. daily for 3 days, as a single agent.

All of these dosage schedules should, however, take into account the haematological status of the patient and the dosages of other cytotoxic drugs when used in combination.

4.3 Contraindications

Zavedos therapy should not be started in patients with severe renal and liver impairment or patients with uncontrolled infections.

4.4 Special warnings and special precautions for use
Not for intrathecal use.

Zavedos is intended for use under the direction of those experienced in leukaemia chemotherapy. The drug should not be given to patients with pre existing bone-marrow suppression induced by previous drug therapy or radiotherapy unless the benefit warrants the risk. Pre-existing heart disease and previous therapy with anthracyclines at high cumulative doses or other potentially cardiotoxic agents are co-factors for increased risk of idarubicin-induced cardiac toxicity and the benefit to risk ratio of idarubicin therapy in such patients should be weighed before starting treatment with Zavedos. Like most other cytotoxic agents, idarubicin has mutagenic properties and it is carcinogenic in rats.

Zavedos is a potent bone marrow suppressant. Myelosuppression, primarily of leukocytes, will therefore occur in all patients given a therapeutic dose of this agent and careful haematological monitoring including granulocytes, red cells and platelets is required.

Facilities with laboratory and supportive resources adequate to monitor drug tolerability and protect and maintain a patient compromised by drug toxicity should be available. It must be possible to treat rapidly and completely a severe haemorrhagic condition and/or severe infection.

Myocardial toxicity as manifested by potentially fatal congestive heart failure, acute life-threatening arrhythmias or other cardiomyopathies may occur during therapy or several weeks after termination of therapy. Treatment with digitalis, diuretics, sodium restriction and bed-rest is indicated. Cardiac function should be carefully monitored during treatment in order to minimise the risk of cardiac toxicity of the type described for other anthracycline compounds. The risk of such myocardial toxicity may be higher following concomitant or previous radiation to the mediastinal-pericardial area or treatment with other potentially cardiotoxic agents or in patients with a particular clinical situation due to their disease (anaemia, bone marrow depression, infection, leukaemic pericarditis and/or myocarditis).

On the basis of the recommended dosage schedules the total cumulative dose administered over two courses can be expected to reach 60 - 80 mg/m^2. Although a cumulative dose limit cannot yet be defined, a specific cardiological evaluation in cancer patients showed no significant modifications of cardiac function in patients treated with Zavedos at a mean cumulative dose of 93 mg/m^2.

Whilst there is no reliable method for predicting acute congestive heart failure, cardiomyopathy induced by anthracyclines is usually associated with persistent QRS voltage reduction, increased beyond normal limits of the systolic time interval (PEP/LVET) and decrease of the left ventricular ejection fraction (LVET) from pre-treatment baseline values.

An electrocardiogram or echocardiogram and a determination of left ventricular ejection fraction should be performed prior to starting therapy and during treatment with Zavedos. Early clinical diagnosis of drug-induced myocardial damage appears to be important for pharmacological treatment to be useful.

Since hepatic and/or renal function impairment can affect the disposition of idarubicin, liver and kidney function should be evaluated with conventional clinical laboratory tests (using serum bilirubin and serum creatinine as indicators) prior to, and during treatment. In a number of Phase III clinical trials, treatment was not given if bilirubin and/or creatinine serum levels exceeded 2 mg%. With other anthracyclines a 50% dose reduction is generally employed if bilirubin and creatinine levels are in the range 1.2 - 2.0 mg%.

Therapy with Zavedos requires close observation of the patient and laboratory monitoring. Patients aged over 55 years should be given vigorous supportive treatment during the aplastic period. Hyperuricaemia secondary to rapid lysis of leukaemic cells may be induced: blood uric acid levels should be monitored and appropriate therapy initiated if hyperuricaemia develops. Appropriate measures must be taken to control any systemic infection before beginning therapy.

Extravasation of Zavedos at the site of i.v. injection can cause severe local tissue necrosis. The risk of thrombophlebitis at the injection site may be minimised by following the recommended procedure of administration. A stinging or burning sensation at the site of administration signifies a small degree of extravasation and the infusion should be stopped and restarted in another vein.

4.5 Interaction with other medicinal products and other forms of Interaction

Zavedos is a potent myelosuppressant and combination chemotherapy regimens which contain other agents having a similar action may be expected to lead to additive myelosuppressive effects. Prolonged contact with any solution of an alkaline pH should be avoided as it will result in degradation of the drug. Zavedos should not be mixed with heparin as a precipitate may form and it is not recommended that it be mixed with other drugs.

4.6 Pregnancy and lactation

There is no information as to whether idarubicin may adversely affect human fertility, or cause teratogenesis. However, in rats (but not rabbits) it is teratogenic and embryotoxic. Women of child bearing potential should be advised to avoid pregnancy. If Zavedos is to be used during pregnancy or if the patient becomes pregnant during therapy, the patient should be informed of the potential hazard to the foetus. Mothers should be advised not to breast-feed whilst undergoing chemotherapy with this drug.

4.7 Effects on ability to drive and use machines

None stated.

4.8 Undesirable effects

Severe myelosuppression and cardiac toxicity are the two major adverse effects. Other adverse reactions include: reversible alopecia in most patients; acute nausea and vomiting; mucositis, usually involving the oral mucosa and appearing 3 - 10 days after starting treatment; oesophagitis and diarrhoea; fever, chills, skin rash; elevation of liver enzymes and bilirubin in about 20 - 30% of cases. Severe and sometimes fatal infections have been associated with idarubicin alone or in combination with cytarabine.

Idarubicin may impart a red colour to the urine for 1 - 2 days after administration and patients should be advised that this is no cause for alarm.

4.9 Overdose

Very high doses of Zavedos may be expected to cause acute myocardial toxicity within 24 hours and severe myelosuppression within one to two weeks. Treatment should aim to support the patient during this period and should utilise such measures as blood transfusion and reverse-barrier nursing. Delayed cardiac failure has been seen with the anthracyclines up to several months after the overdose. Patients should be observed carefully and if signs of cardiac failure arise, should be treated along conventional lines.

5. PHARMACOLOGICAL PROPERTIES

5.1 Pharmacodynamic properties

Idarubicin is a DNA intercalating anthracycline which interacts with the enzyme topoisomerase II and has an inhibitory effect on nucleic acid synthesis.

The modification of position 4 of the anthracycline structure gives the compound a high lipophilicity which results in an increased rate of cellular uptake compared with doxorubicin and daunorubicin.

Idarubicin has been shown to have a higher potency with respect to daunorubicin and to be an effective agent against murine leukaemia and lymphomas both by i.v. and oral routes. Studies *in-vitro* on human and murine anthracycline-resistant cells have shown a lower degree of cross-resistance for idarubicin compared with doxorubicin and daunorubicin. Cardiotoxicity studies in animals have indicated that idarubicin has a better therapeutic index than daunorubicin and doxorubicin. The main metabolite, idarubicinol, has shown, *in-vitro* and *in-vivo*, antitumoural activity in experimental models. In the rat, idarubicinol administered at the same doses as the parent drug, is clearly less cardiotoxic than idarubicin.

5.2 Pharmacokinetic properties

After i.v. administration to patients with normal renal and hepatic function, idarubicin is eliminated from systemic circulation (terminal plasma $T_{1/2}$ ranging between 11 - 25 hours) and is extensively metabolised to an active metabolite, idarubicinol, which is slowly eliminated with a plasma $T_{1/2}$ ranging between 41 - 69 hours). The drug is eliminated by biliary and renal excretion, mostly in the form or idarubicinol.

Studies of cellular (nucleated blood and bone marrow cells) in leukaemic patients have shown that peak cellular idarubicin concentrations are reached a few minutes after injection. Idarubicin and idarubicinol concentrations in nucleated blood and bone marrow cells are more than a hundred times the plasma concentrations. Idarubicin disappearance rates in plasma and cells were comparable, with a terminal half-life of about 15 hours. The terminal half-life of idarubicinol in cells was about 72 hours.

5.3 Preclinical safety data

Idarubicin has mutagenic properties and it is carcinogenic in rats.

Reproduction studies in animals have shown that idarubicin is embryotoxic and teratogenic in rats but not rabbits.

6. PHARMACEUTICAL PARTICULARS

6.1 List of excipients

Lactose monohydrate Ph. Eur.

6.2 Incompatibilities

None known.

6.3 Shelf life

The shelf-life expiry date for this product shall not exceed three years from the date of its manufacture.

6.4 Special precautions for storage

Unreconstituted solution: None

Reconstituted solution: The reconstituted solution is chemically stable when stored for at least 48 hours at 2-8°C and 24 hours at room temperature (20°C - 25°C); however, it is recommended that, in line with good pharmaceutical practice, the solution should not normally be stored for longer than 24 hours at 2-8°C.

The product does not contain any antibacterial preservative. Therefore of aseptic preparation cannot be ensured, the product must be prepared immediately before use and any unused portion discarded.

6.5 Nature and contents of container

Colourless glass vial, type I, with chlorobutyl rubber bung and aluminium seal with insert yellow polypropylene disk.

6.6 Instructions for use and handling

The following protective recommendations are given due to the toxic nature of this substance:

- Pregnant staff should be excluded from working with this drug
- Personnel handling idarubicin should wear protective clothing: goggles, gowns and disposable gloves and masks
- All items used for administration or cleaning, including gloves, should be placed in high risk, waste disposal bags for high temperature incineration.

5mg Injection: Reconstitute with 5ml of Water for Injections

10mg Injection: Reconstitute with 10ml of Water for Injections to produce a 1mg/ml solution for injection (i.v.). See section 6.4 also.

Spillage or leakage should be treated with dilute sodium hypochlorite (1% available chlorine) solution, preferably by soaking, and then with water.

All cleaning materials should be disposed of as indicated previously. Accidental contact with the skin and eyes should be treated immediately by copious lavage with water, or sodium bicarbonate solution, medical attention should be sought.

Discard any unused solution.

7. MARKETING AUTHORISATION HOLDER

Pharmacia Limited
Davy Avenue
Milton Keynes
MK5 8PH

8. MARKETING AUTHORISATION NUMBER(S)

5mg Injection: PL 00032/0438
10mg Injection: PL 00032/0349

9. DATE OF FIRST AUTHORISATION/RENEWAL OF THE AUTHORISATION

5mg Injection: 23 May 2002
10mg Injection: 10th May 2002
20mg Injection: 25 March 2002

10. DATE OF REVISION OF THE TEXT

September 2004

ZD_2_0

Zavesca

(Actelion Pharmaceuticals UK)

1. NAME OF THE MEDICINAL PRODUCT

Zavesca ▼ 100 mg hard capsules.

2. QUALITATIVE AND QUANTITATIVE COMPOSITION

Each capsule contains 100 mg miglustat.

For excipients, see section 6.1.

3. PHARMACEUTICAL FORM

Capsule, hard.

White capsules with "OGT 918" printed in black on the cap and "100" printed in black on the body.

4. CLINICAL PARTICULARS

4.1 Therapeutic indications

Zavesca is indicated for the oral treatment of mild to moderate type 1 Gaucher disease. Zavesca may be used only in the treatment of patients for whom enzyme replacement therapy is unsuitable (see sections 4.4 and 5.1).

4.2 Posology and method of administration

Therapy should be directed by physicians who are knowledgeable in the management of Gaucher disease.

Adults

The recommended starting dose for the treatment of patients with type 1 Gaucher disease is 100 mg three times a day.

Dose reduction to 100 mg once or twice a day may be necessary in some patients because of diarrhoea.

Zavesca can be taken with or without food.

Children, Adolescents and the Elderly

There is no experience with the use of Zavesca in patients under the age of 18 and over the age of 70. The use in children and adolescents is not recommended.

Renal Impairment

Pharmacokinetic data indicate increased systemic exposure to miglustat in patients with renal impairment. In patients with an adjusted creatinine clearance of 50-70 ml/min/1.73 m^2, administration should commence at a dose of 100 mg twice daily. In patients with an adjusted creatinine clearance of 30-50 ml/min/1.73 m^2, administration should commence at a dose of one 100 mg capsule per day. Use in patients with severe renal impairment (creatinine clearance <30 ml/min/1.73 m^2) is not recommended (see section 4.4 and 5.2).

Hepatic Impairment

Zavesca has not been evaluated in patients with hepatic impairment.

4.3 Contraindications

Hypersensitivity to the active substance or to any of the excipients.

4.4 Special warnings and special precautions for use

Although no direct comparisons with Enzyme Replacement Therapy (ERT) have been performed in treatment naïve patients, it appears that it would take longer to achieve an effect with Zavesca and there is no evidence of an efficacy or safety advantage over ERT. ERT is the standard of care for patients who require treatment for type 1 Gaucher disease (see section 5.1). The efficacy and safety of Zavesca has not been evaluated in patients with severe Gaucher disease, defined as a haemoglobin concentration below 9 g/dl or a platelet count below 50 × 10^9/l or active bone disease.

Approximately 30% of patients have reported tremor or exacerbation of existing tremor on treatment. These tremors were described as an exaggerated physiological tremor of the hands. Tremor usually began within the first month and in many cases resolved between 1 to 3 months during treatment. Dose reduction may ameliorate the tremor usually within days but discontinuation with treatment may sometimes be required.

Regular monitoring of vitamin B_{12} level is recommended because of the high prevalence of vitamin B_{12} deficiency in patients with type 1 Gaucher disease.

Cases of peripheral neuropathy have been reported in patients treated with Zavesca with or without concurrent conditions such as vitamin B_{12}deficiency and monoclonal gammopathy. All patients should undergo baseline and repeat neurological evaluation. Patients who develop symptoms such as numbness and tingling should have a careful re-assessment of risk-benefit and may require cessation of treatment.

Isolated cases of cognitive dysfunction have been reported during clinical trials of Zavesca in type 1 Gaucher disease. Baseline and periodic assessment of cognitive functions is recommended in all patients on Zavesca treatment.

Male patients should maintain reliable contraceptive methods whilst taking Zavesca. Studies in the rat have shown that miglustat adversely affects spermatogenesis, sperm parameters and reduces fertility (see section 5.3). Until further information is available, it is advised that before seeking to conceive, male patients should cease Zavesca and maintain reliable contraceptive methods for 3 months thereafter.

Due to limited experience, Zavesca should be used with caution in patients with renal or hepatic impairment. There is a close relationship between renal function and clearance of miglustat. Exposure of miglustat is markedly increased in patients with severe renal impairment (see section 5.2). At present, there is insufficient clinical experience in these patients to provide dosing recommendations. Use in patients with severe renal impairment (creatinine clearance < 30 ml/min/1.73 m^2) is not recommended.

4.5 Interaction with other medicinal products and other forms of Interaction

Limited data suggest that co-administration of Zavesca and Cerezyme mayresult in decreased exposure to miglustat (approximately a 22% reduction in C_{max} and a 14% reduction in AUC was observed in a small parallel-group study). This study also indicates that Zavesca has no or limited effect on the pharmacokinetics of Cerezyme.

4.6 Pregnancy and lactation

There are no adequate data from the use of miglustat in pregnant women. Studies in animals have shown effects on reproductive toxicity, including dystocia (see section 5.3).

The potential risk for humans is unknown. Miglustat crosses the placenta. Zavesca should not be used during pregnancy. Contraceptive measures should be used by women of childbearing potential.

It is not known if miglustat is secreted in breast milk. Zavesca should not be used during breast-feeding.

4.7 Effects on ability to drive and use machines

No studies on the effects on the ability to drive or to use machines have been performed. However, dizziness has been reported as a very common adverse event and patients suffering from dizziness should not drive or operate machinery.

4.8 Undesirable effects

Adverse events reported in clinical trials with Zavesca in 82 patients are listed in the table below by body system and frequency (very common: >1/10, common >1/100, <1/10). Most events were of mild to moderate severity.

Metabolism and Nutrition Disorders	
Very Common	Weight loss
Common	Decreased appetite, weight increase

Nervous System Disorders	
Very Common	Tremor, dizziness, headache, leg cramps
Common	Paraesthesia, peripheral neuropathy, cognitive dysfunction

Eye Disorders	
Very Common	Visual disturbance

Gastrointestinal Disorders	
Very Common	Diarrhoea, flatulence, abdominal pain, nausea, constipation, vomiting
Common	Dyspepsia, distension

Weight loss has been observed in approximately 60% of patients. The nadir was at 12 months with a mean weight loss of 6-7% of body weight and a subsequent tendency for an increase in weight towards the baseline value.

Gastrointestinal events have been observed in more than 80% of patients either at the outset of treatment, or intermittently during treatment. The majority of cases are mild and are expected to resolve spontaneously or after dose reduction. The mechanism is probably inhibition of disaccharidases in the gastrointestinal tract. The diarrhoea responds to loperamide.

4.9 Overdose

No acute symptoms of overdose have been identified. Zavesca has been administered at doses of up to 3000 mg/day for up to six months in HIV positive patients during clinical trials. Adverse events observed included granulocytopenia, dizziness and paraesthesia. Leukopenia and neutropenia have also been observed in a similar group of patients receiving 800 mg/day or higher dose.

5. PHARMACOLOGICAL PROPERTIES

5.1 Pharmacodynamic properties

Pharmacotherapeutic group: Other alimentary tract and metabolism products.

ATC Code: A16AX06

Gaucher disease is an inherited metabolic disorder caused by a failure to degrade glucosylceramide resulting in lysosomal storage of this material and widespread pathology. Miglustat is an inhibitor of the enzyme glucosylceramide synthase, the enzyme responsible for the first step in the synthesis of most glycolipids. *In vitro* and *in vivo* studies have shown that miglustat can reduce the synthesis of glucosylceramide. This inhibitory action forms the rationale for substrate reduction therapy in Gaucher disease.

The pivotal trial of Zavesca was conducted in patients unable or unwilling to receive ERT. Reasons for not receiving ERT included the burden of intravenous infusions and difficulties in venous access. Twenty-eight patients with mild to moderate type 1 Gaucher disease were enrolled in this 12 month non-comparative study and twenty-two patients completed the study. At 12 months, there was a mean reduction in liver organ volume of 12.1% and a mean reduction in spleen volume of 19.0%. A mean increase in haemoglobin concentration of 0.26 g/dl as well as a mean platelet count increase of 8.29 × 10^9/l were observed. Eighteen patients then continued to receive Zavesca in an optional extended treatment protocol. Clinical benefit has been assessed at 24 and 36 months in 13 patients. After 3 years of continuous Zavesca treatment, mean reductions in liver and spleen organ volume were 17.5% and 29.6%, respectively. There was a mean increase of 22.2 × 10^9/l in platelet count and a mean increase of 0.95 g/dl in haemoglobin concentration.

A second open controlled study randomised 36 patients who had received a minimum of two years treatment with ERT into three treatment groups: continuation with Cerezyme, Cerezyme in combination with Zavesca, or switch to Zavesca. This study was conducted over a six-month period. In patients who were switched to Zavesca, there were small reductions in liver and spleen organ volume. However, there were reductions in platelet count and increases in chitotriosidase activity in some patients, indicating that Zavesca monotherapy may not be sufficient to maintain the same control of disease activity in all patients.

A total daily dose of 300 mg Zavesca administered in three divided doses was used in the above two studies. An additional monotherapy study was performed in 18 patients at a total daily dose of 150 mg and results indicate reduced efficacy compared to a total daily dose of 300 mg.

5.2 Pharmacokinetic properties

Pharmacokinetic parameters of miglustat were assessed in a small number of patients with type 1 Gaucher disease.

The kinetics of miglustat appear to be dose linearand time independent.

Miglustat is rapidly absorbed. Maximum plasma concentrations are reached about 2 h after dose. Absolute bioavailability has not been determined. Concomitant administration of food decreases the rate of absorption (C_{max} was decreased by 36% and t_{max} delayed 2 hours) but has no statistically significant effect on the extent of absorption of miglustat (AUC decreased by 14%).

The apparent volume of distribution is 83 l. Miglustat does not bind to plasma proteins. Information from a study using a prodrug of miglustat indicates that the major route of excretion is renal. Apparent oral clearance (CL/F) is 230 ± 39 ml/min. The average half-life is 6-7 hours.

Limited data in patients with Fabry disease and impaired renal function showed thatCL/F decreases with decreasing renal function. While the numbers of subjects with mild and moderate renal impairment were very small, the data suggest an approximate decrease in CL/F of 40% and 60%, respectively, in mild and moderate renal impairment (see section 4.2). Data in severe renal impairment are limited to two patients with creatinine clearance in the range 18-29 ml/min and cannot be extrapolated below this range. These data suggest a decrease in CL/F by at least 70% in patients with severe renal impairment.

Over the range of data available, no significant relationships or trends were noted between miglustat pharmacokinetic parameters and demographic variables (age, BMI, gender or race).

There are no pharmacokinetic data available in patients with liver impairment, in children or adolescents(<18 years) or in elderly (>70 years).

5.3 Preclinical safety data

The main effects common to all species were weight loss and diarrhoea, and, at higher doses, damage to the gastrointestinal mucosa (erosions and ulceration). Further, effects seen in animals at doses that result in exposure levels moderately higher than the clinical exposure level were: changes in lymphoid organs in all species tested, transaminase changes, vacuolation of thyroid and pancreas, cataracts, nephropathy and myocardial changes in rats. These findings were considered to be secondary to debilitation.

Repeated dose toxicity studies in rats showed effects on the seminiferous epithelium of the testes. Other studies revealed changes in sperm parameters (motility and morphology) consistent with an observed reduction in fertility. These effects occurred at exposure levels similar to those in patients but showed reversibility. Miglustat affected embryo/foetal survival in rats and rabbits; dystocia was reported; postimplantation losses were increased and an increased incidence of vascular anomalies occurred in rabbits. These effects may be partly related to maternal toxicity.

Changes in lactation were observed in female rats in a 1-year study. The mechanism for this effect is unknown.

Miglustat did not show any potential for mutagenic or clastogenic effects in the standard battery of genotoxicity tests. Long term studies on the carcinogenic potential have not been conducted.

6. PHARMACEUTICAL PARTICULARS

6.1 List of excipients

Capsule contents: sodium starch glycollate, povidone (K30), magnesium stearate.

Capsule shell: gelatin, water, titanium dioxide (E171).

Printing ink: comprising black iron oxide (E172), shellac, soya lecithin and antifoam.

6.2 Incompatibilities

Not applicable.

6.3 Shelf life

3 years

6.4 Special precautions for storage

Do not store above 30°C.

6.5 Nature and contents of container

ACLAR/ALU blister strips supplied as a box of 4 blister strips each blister strip containing 21 capsules providing a total of 84 capsules.

6.6 Instructions for use and handling

No special requirements.

7. MARKETING AUTHORISATION HOLDER

Actelion Registration Ltd

BSI Building 13th Floor

389 Chiswick High Road

London W4 4AL

United Kingdom

8. MARKETING AUTHORISATION NUMBER(S)
EU/1/02/238/001

9. DATE OF FIRST AUTHORISATION/RENEWAL OF THE AUTHORISATION
20 November 2002

10. DATE OF REVISION OF THE TEXT
17 March 2005

Zeffix 100 mg film-coated tablets

(GlaxoSmithKline UK)

1. NAME OF THE MEDICINAL PRODUCT
Zeffix 100 mg film-coated tablets

2. QUALITATIVE AND QUANTITATIVE COMPOSITION
Zeffix film-coated tablets contain 100 mg lamivudine

For excipients see section 6.1.

3. PHARMACEUTICAL FORM
Film-coated tablet

The tablets are butterscotch coloured, film-coated, capsule shaped, biconvex and engraved "GX CG5" on one face.

4. CLINICAL PARTICULARS

4.1 Therapeutic indications

Zeffix is indicated for the treatment of chronic hepatitis B in adults with:

§ compensated liver disease with evidence of active viral replication, persistently elevated serum alanine aminotransferase (ALT) levels and histological evidence of active liver inflammation and / or fibrosis.

§ decompensated liver disease.

4.2 Posology and method of administration

Therapy with Zeffix should be initiated by a physician experienced in the management of chronic hepatitis B.

The recommended dosage of Zeffix is 100 mg once daily. Zeffix can be taken with or without food.

Duration of treatment:

• In patients with HBeAg positive chronic hepatitis B (CHB) treatment should be administered until HBeAg seroconversion (HBeAg and HBV DNA loss with HBeAb detection) on two consecutive serum samples at least 3 months apart or until HBsAg seroconversion. This recommendation is based on limited data (see section 5.1).

• In patients with HBeAg negative CHB (pre-core mutant), the optimal duration of treatment is unknown. Treatment discontinuation may be considered following HBsAg seroconversion.

• In patients with either HBeAg positive or HBeAg negative CHB, the development of YMDD variant HBV may result in a diminished therapeutic response to lamivudine, indicated by a rise in HBV DNA and ALT from previous on-treatment levels. In patients with extended-duration YMDD variant HBV, a switch to or addition of an alternative agent should be considered (see section 5.1).

• In patients with decompensated liver disease and liver transplant recipients, treatment cessation is not recommended. If there is a loss of efficacy attributable to the emergence of YMDD variant HBV in these patients, additional or alternative therapies should be considered (see section 5.1).

If Zeffix is discontinued, patients should be periodically monitored for evidence of recurrent hepatitis (see section 4.4).

Renal impairment:

Lamivudine serum concentrations (AUC) are increased in patients with moderate to severe renal impairment due to decreased renal clearance. The dosage should therefore be reduced for patients with a creatinine clearance of < 50 ml/minute. When doses below 100 mg are required Zeffix oral solution should be used (see Table 1 below).

Table 1: Dosage of Zeffix in patients with decreased renal clearance.

Creatinine clearance ml/min	First Dose of Zeffix oral solution *	Maintenance Dose Once daily
30 to < 50	20 ml (100 mg)	10 ml (50 mg)
15 to < 30	20 ml (100 mg)	5 ml (25 mg)
5 to < 15	7 ml (35 mg)	3 ml (15 mg)
< 5	7 ml (35 mg)	2 ml (10 mg)

* Zeffix oral solution containing 5 mg/ml lamivudine.

Data available in patients undergoing intermittent haemodialysis (for less than or equal to 4 hrs dialysis 2-3 times weekly), indicate that following the initial dosage reduction of lamivudine to correct for the patient's creatinine clearance, no further dosage adjustments are required while undergoing dialysis.

Hepatic impairment:

Data obtained in patients with hepatic impairment, including those with end-stage liver disease awaiting transplant, show that lamivudine pharmacokinetics are not significantly affected by hepatic dysfunction. Based on these data, no dose adjustment is necessary in patients with hepatic impairment unless accompanied by renal impairment.

4.3 Contraindications

Zeffix is contraindicated in patients with known hypersensitivity to lamivudine or to any ingredient of the preparation.

4.4 Special warnings and special precautions for use

Lamivudine has been administered to children (2 years and above) and adolescents with compensated chronic hepatitis B. However, due to limitations of the data, the administration of lamivudine to this patient population is not currently recommended (see section 5.1).

The efficacy of lamivudine in patients co-infected with Delta hepatitis or hepatitis C has not been established.

Data are limited on the use of lamivudine in HBeAg negative (pre-core mutant) patients and in those receiving concurrent immunosuppressive regimes, including cancer chemotherapy.

During treatment with Zeffix patients should be monitored regularly. Serum ALT levels should be monitored at 3 month intervals and HBV DNA and HBeAg should be assessed every 6 months.

HBV viral subpopulations with reduced susceptibility to lamivudine (YMDD variant HBV) have been identified with extended therapy. In some patients the development of YMDD variant HBV can lead to exacerbation of hepatitis, primarily detected by serum ALT elevations and re-emergence of HBV DNA. In patients who have YMDD variant HBV and worsening liver disease (increasing ALT with or without decompensated cirrhosis) or recurrent hepatitis B after liver transplantation, a switch to or addition of an alternative agent should be considered.

If Zeffix is discontinued or there is a loss of efficacy due to the development of YMDD variant HBV (see section 4.2), some patients may experience clinical or laboratory evidence of recurrent hepatitis. If Zeffix is discontinued, patients should be periodically monitored both clinically and by assessment of serum liver function tests (ALT and bilirubin levels), for at least four months, and then as clinically indicated. Exacerbation of hepatitis has primarily been detected by serum ALT elevations, in addition to the re-emergence of HBV DNA. See Table 3 in Section 5.1 Clinical experience for more information regarding frequency of post treatment ALT elevations. Most events have been self-limited, however some fatalities have been observed.

For patients who develop evidence of recurrent hepatitis post-treatment, there are insufficient data on the benefits of re-initiation of lamivudine treatment.

Transplantation recipients and patients with advanced liver disease are at greater risk from active viral replication. Due to the marginal liver function in these patients, hepatitis reactivation at discontinuation of lamivudine or loss of efficacy during treatment may induce severe and even fatal decompensation. These patients should be monitored for clinical, virological and serological parameters associated with hepatitis B, liver and renal function, and antiviral response during treatment (at least every month), and, if treatment is discontinued for any reason, for at least 6 months after treatment. Laboratory parameters to be monitored should include (as a minimum) serum ALT, bilirubin, albumin, blood urea nitrogen, creatinine, and virological status: HBV antigen/antibody, and serum HBV DNA concentrations when possible. Patients experiencing signs of hepatic insufficiency during or post-treatment should be monitored more frequently as appropriate.

For the treatment of patients who are co-infected with HIV and are currently receiving or plan to receive treatment with lamivudine or the combination lamivudine-zidovudine, the dose of lamivudine prescribed for HIV infection (usually 150 mg/twice daily in combination with other antiretrovirals) should be maintained. For HIV co-infected patients not requiring anti-retroviral therapy, there is a risk of HIV mutation when using lamivudine alone for treating chronic hepatitis B.

There is no information available on maternal-foetal transmission of hepatitis B virus in pregnant women receiving treatment with lamivudine. The standard recommended procedures for hepatitis B virus immunisation in infants should be followed.

Patients should be advised that therapy with lamivudine has not been proven to reduce the risk of transmission of hepatitis B virus to others and therefore, appropriate precautions should still be taken.

4.5 Interaction with other medicinal products and other forms of Interaction

The likelihood of metabolic interactions is low due to limited metabolism and plasma protein binding and almost complete renal elimination of unchanged substance.

Lamivudine is predominantly eliminated by active organic cationic secretion. The possibility of interactions with other medicinal products administered concurrently should be considered, particularly when their main route of elimination is active renal secretion via the organic cationic transport system e.g. trimethoprim. Other medicinal products (e.g. ranitidine, cimetidine) are eliminated only in part by this mechanism and were shown not to interact with lamivudine.

Substances shown to be predominately excreted either via the active organic anionic pathway, or by glomerular filtration are unlikely to yield clinically significant interactions with lamivudine.

Administration of trimethoprim/sulphamethoxazole 160 mg/800 mg increased lamivudine exposure by about 40 %. Lamivudine had no effect on the pharmacokinetics of trimethoprim or sulphamethoxazole. However, unless the patient has renal impairment, no dosage adjustment of lamivudine is necessary.

A modest increase in C_{max} (28 %) was observed for zidovudine when administered with lamivudine, however overall exposure (AUC) was not significantly altered. Zidovudine had no effect on the pharmacokinetics of lamivudine (see section 5.2).

Lamivudine has no pharmacokinetic interaction with alpha-interferon when the two medicinal products are concurrently administered. There were no observed clinically significant adverse interactions in patients taking lamivudine concurrently with commonly used immunosuppressant medicinal products (e.g. cyclosporin A). However, formal interaction studies have not been performed.

Lamivudine may inhibit the intracellular phosphorylation of zalcitabine when the two medicinal products are used concurrently. Zeffix is therefore not recommended to be used in combination with zalcitabine.

4.6 Pregnancy and lactation

Pregnancy:

The safety of lamivudine in human pregnancy has not been established. Studies in animals have shown reproductive toxicity (see section 5.3). Consistent with passive transmission of the substance across the placenta, lamivudine concentrations in infant serum at birth were similar to those in maternal and cord serum at delivery.

Although animal reproductive studies are not always predictive of the human response, administration is not recommended during the first three months of pregnancy (see section 4.4).

Lactation:

Following oral administration, lamivudine was excreted in breast milk at similar concentrations to those found in serum. It is therefore recommended that mothers taking lamivudine do not breast feed their infants.

4.7 Effects on ability to drive and use machines

No studies on the effects on the ability to drive and use machines have been performed.

4.8 Undesirable effects

In clinical studies of patients with chronic hepatitis B, lamivudine was well tolerated. The incidence of adverse events and laboratory abnormalities (with the exception of elevations of ALT and CPK, see below) were similar between placebo and lamivudine treated patients). The most common adverse events reported were malaise and fatigue, respiratory tract infections, throat and tonsil discomfort, headache, abdominal discomfort and pain, nausea, vomiting and diarrhoea.

Adverse reactions are listed below by system organ class and frequency. Frequency categories are only assigned to those adverse reactions considered to be at least possibly causally related to lamivudine. Frequencies are defined as: very common (⩾ 1/10), common (⩾ 1/100, < 1/10), uncommon (⩾ 1/1000, < 1/100), rare (⩾ 1/10,000, < 1/1000) and very rare (< 1/10,000).

The frequency categories assigned to the adverse reactions below are estimates: for most events, suitable data for calculating incidence are not available. Very common and common adverse drug reaction frequency categories were determined from clinical trial data and the background incidence in placebo groups was not taken into account. Adverse drug reactions identified through post-marketing surveillance were categorised as rare or very rare.

Clinical trial data:

Hepatobiliary disorders:

Very common: ALT elevations (see section 4.4).

Musculoskeletal and connective tissue disorders:

Common: Elevations of CPK

Post-marketing experience:

In addition to adverse events reported from clinical trials, the following events have been identified during post-approval use of Zeffix.

Blood and lymphatic system disorders:

Very rare: Thrombocytopenia.

Musculoskeletal and connective tissue disorders:

Very rare: Muscle disorders, including myalgia and cramps.

In patients with HIV infection, cases of pancreatitis and peripheral neuropathy (or paresthesia) have been reported. In patients with chronic hepatitis B there was no observed difference in incidence of these events between placebo and lamivudine treated patients.

Cases of lactic acidosis, sometimes fatal, usually associated with severe hepatomegaly and hepatic steatosis, have been reported with the use of combination nucleoside analogue therapy in patients with HIV. There have been rare reports of lactic acidosis in patients receiving lamivudine for hepatitis B.

4.9 Overdose

Administration of lamivudine at very high dose levels in acute animal studies did not result in any organ toxicity. Limited data are available on the consequences of ingestion of acute overdoses in humans. No fatalities occurred, and the patients recovered. No specific signs or symptoms have been identified following such overdose.

If overdose occurs the patient should be monitored and standard supportive treatment applied as required. Since lamivudine is dialysable, continuous haemodialysis could be used in the treatment of overdose, although this has not been studied.

5. PHARMACOLOGICAL PROPERTIES

5.1 Pharmacodynamic properties

Pharmacotherapeutic group - nucleoside analogue, ATC Code: J05A F05.

Lamivudine is an antiviral agent which is active against hepatitis B virus in all cell lines tested and in experimentally infected animals.

Lamivudine is metabolised by both infected and uninfected cells to the triphosphate (TP) derivative which is the active form of the parent compound. The intracellular half life of the triphosphate in hepatocytes is 17-19 hours *in vitro*. Lamivudine-TP acts as a substrate for the HBV viral polymerase.

The formation of further viral DNA is blocked by incorporation of lamivudine-TP into the chain and subsequent chain termination.

Lamivudine-TP does not interfere with normal cellular deoxynucleotide metabolism. It is also only a weak inhibitor of mammalian DNA polymerases alpha and beta. Furthermore, lamivudine-TP has little effect on mammalian cell DNA content.

In assays relating to potential substance effects on mitochondrial structure and DNA content and function, lamivudine lacked appreciable toxic effects. It has a very low potential to decrease mitochondrial DNA content, is not permanently incorporated into mitochondrial DNA, and does not act as an inhibitor of mitochondrial DNA polymerase gamma.

Clinical experience

Experience in patients with HBeAg positive CHB and compensated liver disease: in controlled studies, 1 year of lamivudine therapy significantly suppressed HBV DNA replication [34-57 % of patients were below the assay detection limits (Abbott Genostics solution hybridization assay, LLOD < 1.6pg/ml)], normalised ALT level (40-72 % of patients), induced HBeAg seroconversion (HBeAg loss and HBeAb detection with HBV DNA loss [by conventional assay], 16-18 % of patients), improved histology (38-52 % of patients had a ⩾ 2 point decrease in the Knodell Histologic Activity Index [HAI]) and reduced progression of fibrosis (in 3-17 % of patients) and progression to cirrhosis.

Continued lamivudine treatment for an additional 2 years in patients who had failed to achieve HBeAg seroconversion in the initial 1 year controlled studies resulted in further improvement in bridging fibrosis. In patients with YMDD variant HBV, 41/82 (50 %) patients had improvement in liver inflammation and 40/56 (71 %) patients without YMDD variant HBV had improvement. Improvement in bridging fibrosis occurred in 19/30 (63 %) patients without YMDD variant and 22/44 (50 %) patients with the variant. Five percent (3/56) of patients without the YMDD variant and 13 % (11/82) of patients with YMDD variant showed worsening in liver inflammation compared to pre-treatment. Progression to cirrhosis occurred in 4/68 (6 %) patients with the YMDD variant, whereas no patients without the variant progressed to cirrhosis.

In an extended treatment study in Asian patients (NUCB3018) the HBeAg seroconversion rate and ALT normalisation rate at the end of the 5 year treatment period was 48 % (28/58) and 47 % (15/32), respectively. HBeAg seroconversion was increased in patients with elevated ALT levels; 77 % (20/26) of patients with pre-treatment ALT> 2 × ULN seroconverted. At the end of 5 years, all patients had HBV DNA levels that were undetectable or lower than pre-treatment levels.

Further results from the trial by YMDD variant status are summarised in Table 2.

Table 2: Efficacy results 5 years by YMDD status (Asian Study) NUCB3018

(see Table 2 below)

Comparative data according to YMDD status were also available for histological assessment but only up to three years. In patients with YMDD variant HBV, 18/39 (46 %) had improvements in necroinflammatory activity and 9/39 (23 %) had worsening. In patients without the variant, 20/27 (74 %) had improvements in necroinflammatory activity and 2/27 (7 %) had worsening.

Following HBeAg seroconversion, serologic response and clinical remission are generally durable after stopping lamivudine. However, relapses have been identified in patients although they obtained HBeAg seroconversion. Therefore, following HBeAg seroconversion, patients should be periodically monitored to determine that serologic and clinical responses are being maintained. In patients who do not maintain a sustained serological response, consideration should be given to retreatment with either lamivudine or an alternative antiviral agent for resumption of clinical control of HBV.

In patients followed for up to 16 weeks after discontinuation of treatment at one year, post-treatment ALT elevations were observed more frequently in patients who had received lamivudine than in patients who had received placebo. A comparison of post-treatment ALT elevations between weeks 52 and 68 in patients who discontinued lamivudine at week 52 and patients in the same studies who received placebo throughout the treatment course is shown in Table 3. The proportion of patients who had post-treatment ALT elevations in association with an increase in bilirubin levels was low and similar in patients receiving either lamivudine or placebo.

Table 3: Post-treatment ALT Elevations in 2 Placebo-Controlled Studies in Adults

	Patients with ALT Elevation/ Patients with Observations*	
Abnormal Value	Lamivudine	Placebo
ALT ⩾ 2 × baseline value	37/137 (27 %)	22/116 (19 %)
ALT ⩾ 3 × baseline value†	29/137 (21 %)	9/116 (8 %)
ALT ⩾ 2 × baseline value and absolute ALT> 500 IU/l	21/137 (15 %)	8/116 (7 %)
ALT ⩾2 × baseline value; and bilirubin >2 × ULN and ⩾2 × baseline value	1/137 (0.7 %)	1/116 (0.9 %)

*Each patient may be represented in one or more category.

†Comparable to a Grade 3 toxicity in accordance with modified WHO criteria.

ULN = Upper limit of normal.

Experience in patients with HBeAg negative CHB: initial data indicate the efficacy of lamivudine in patients with HBeAg negative CHB is similar to patients with HBeAg positive CHB, with 71 % of patients having HBV DNA suppressed below the detection limit of the assay, 67 % ALT normalisation and 38 % with improvement in HAI after one year of treatment. When lamivudine was discontinued, the majority of patients (70 %) had a return of viral replication. Data is available from an extended treatment study in HBeAg negative patients (NUCAB3017) treated with lamivudine. After two years of treatment in this study, ALT normalisation and undetectable HBV DNA occurred in 30/69 (43 %) and 32/68 (47 %) patients respectively and improvement in necroinflammatory score in 18/49 (37 %) patients. In patients without YMDD variant HBV, 14/22 (64 %) showed improvement in necroinflammatory score and 1/22 (5 %) patients worsened compared to pre-treatment. In patients with the variant, 4/26 (15 %) patients showed improvement in necroinflammatory score and 8/26 (31 %) patients worsened compared to pre-treatment. No patients in either group progressed to cirrhosis.

Frequency of emergence of YMDD variant HBV and impact on the treatment response: lamivudine monotherapy results in the selection of YMDD variant HBV in approximately 24 % of patients following one year of therapy, increasing to 67 % following 4 years of therapy. Development of YMDD variant HBV is associated with reduced treatment response in some patients, as evidenced by increased HBV DNA levels and ALT elevations from previous on-therapy levels, progression of signs and symptoms of hepatitis disease and/or worsening of hepatic necroinflammatory findings. The optimal therapeutic management of patients with YMDD variant HBV has not yet been established (see section 4.4).

In a double-blind study in CHB patients with YMDD variant HBV and compensated liver disease (NUC20904), with a reduced virological and biochemical response to lamivudine (n=95), the addition of adefovir dipivoxil 10 mg once daily to ongoing lamivudine 100mg for 52 weeks resulted in a median decrease in HBV DNA of 4.6 $\log_{10}$ copies/ml compared to a median increase of 0.3 $\log_{10}$ copies/ml in those patients receiving lamivudine monotherapy. Normalisation of ALT levels occurred in 31 % (14/45) of patients receiving combined therapy versus 6 % (3/47) receiving lamivudine alone.

Forty patients (HBeAg negative or HBeAg positive) with either decompensated liver disease or recurrent HBV following liver transplantation and YMDD variant were also enrolled into an open label arm of the study. Addition of 10 mg adefovir dipivoxil once daily to ongoing lamivudine 100mg for 52 weeks resulted in a median decrease in HBV

Table 2 Efficacy results 5 years by YMDD status (Asian Study) NUCB3018

	Subjects, % (no.)			
YMDD variant HBV status	YMDD[1]		Non-YMDD[1]	
HBeAg seroconversion				
All patients	38	(15/40)	72	(13/18)
- Baseline ALT ⩽ 1 × ULN[2]	9	(1/11)	33	(2/6)
- Baseline ALT> 2 × ULN	60	(9/15)	100	(11/11)
Undetectable HBV DNA				
- Baseline [3]	5	(2/40)	6	(1/18)
- Week 260 [4]				
negative	8	(2/25)	0	
positive < baseline	92	(23/25)	100	(4/4)
positive > baseline	0		0	
ALT normalisation				
- Baseline				
normal	28	(11/40)	33	(6/18)
above normal	73	(29/40)	67	(12/18)
- Week 260				
normal	46	(13/28)	50	(2/4)
above normal <baseline	21	(6/28)	0	
above normal >baseline	32	(9/28)	50	(2/4)

1 Patients designated as YMDD variant were those with ⩾5% YMDD variant HBV at any annual time-point during the 5-year period. Patients categorised as non-YMDD variant were those with > 95% wild-type HBV at all annual time-points during the 5-year study period

2 Upper limit of normal

3 Abbott Genostics solution hybridisation assay (LLOD < 1.6 pg/ml

4 Chiron Quantiplex assay (LLOD 0.7 Meq/ml)

DNA of 4.6 log_{10} copies/ml. Improvement in liver function was also seen after one year of therapy

Experience in patients with decompensated liver disease: placebo controlled studies have been regarded as inappropriate in patients with decompensated liver disease, and have not been undertaken. In non-controlled studies, where lamivudine was administered prior to and during transplantation, effective HBV DNA suppression and ALT normalisation was demonstrated. When lamivudine therapy was continued post transplantation there was reduced graft re-infection by HBV, increased HBsAg loss and on one-year survival rate of 76 – 100 %.

As anticipated due to the concomitant immunosuppression, the rate of emergence of YMDD variant HBV after 52 weeks treatment was higher (36 % - 64 %) in the liver transplant population than in the immunocompetent CHB patients (14 % - 32 %).

Experience in CHB patients with advanced fibrosis or cirrhosis: in a placebo-controlled study in 651 patients with clinically compensated chronic hepatitis B and histologically confirmed fibrosis or cirrhosis, lamivudine treatment (median duration 32 months) significantly reduced the rate of overall disease progression (34/436, 7.8 % for lamivudine versus 38/215, 17.7 % for placebo, p=0.001), demonstrated by a significant reduction in the proportion of patients having increased Child-Pugh scores (15/436, 3.4 % versus 19/215, 8.8 %, p=0.023) or developing hepatocellular carcinoma (17/436, 3.9 % versus 16/215, 7.4 %, p=0.047). The rate of overall disease progression in the lamivudine group was higher for subjects with detectable YMDD variant HBV DNA (23/209, 11 %) compared to those without detectable YMDD variant HBV (11/221, 5 %). However, disease progression in YMDD subjects in the lamivudine group was lower than the disease progression in the placebo group (23/209, 11 % versus 38/214, 18 % respectively). Confirmed HBeAg seroconversion occurred in 47 % (118/252) of subjects treated with lamivudine and 93 % (320/345) of subjects receiving lamivudine became HBV DNA negative (VERSANT [version 1], bDNA assay, LLOD < 0.7 MEq/ml) during the study.

Experience in children and adolescents: lamivudine has been administered to children and adolescents with compensated CHB in a placebo controlled study of 286 patients aged 2 to 17 years. This population primarily consisted of children with minimal hepatitis B. A dose of 3 mg/kg once daily (up to a maximum of 100 mg daily) was used in children aged 2 to 11 years and a dose of 100 mg once daily in adolescents aged 12 years and above. This dose needs to be further substantiated. The difference in the HBeAg seroconversion rates (HBeAg and HBV DNA loss with HBeAb detection) between placebo and lamivudine was not statistically significant in this population (rates after one year were 13 % (12/95) for placebo versus 22 % (42/191) for lamivudine; p=0.057). The incidence of YMDD variant HBV was similar to that observed in adults, ranging from 19 % at week 52 up to 45 % in patients treated continuously for 24 months.

5.2 Pharmacokinetic properties

Absorption: Lamivudine is well absorbed from the gastrointestinal tract, and the bioavailability of oral lamivudine in adults is normally between 80 and 85 %. Following oral administration, the mean time (t_{max}) to maximal serum concentrations (C_{max}) is about an hour. At therapeutic dose levels i.e.

100 mg once daily, C_{max} is in the order of 1.1-1.5 μg/ml and trough levels were 0.015-0.020 μg/ml.

Co-administration of lamivudine with food resulted in a delay of t_{max} and a lower C_{max} (decreased by up to 47 %). However, the extent (based on the AUC) of lamivudine absorbed was not influenced, therefore lamivudine can be administered with or without food.

Distribution: From intravenous studies the mean volume of distribution is 1.3 l/kg. Lamivudine exhibits linear pharmacokinetics over the therapeutic dose range and displays low plasma protein binding to albumin.

Limited data shows lamivudine penetrates the central nervous system and reaches the cerebro-spinal fluid (CSF). The mean lamivudine CSF/serum concentration ratio 2-4 hours after oral administration was approximately 0.12.

Metabolism: Lamivudine is predominately cleared by renal excretion of unchanged substance. The likelihood of metabolic substance interactions with lamivudine is low due to the small (5-10 %) extent of hepatic metabolism and the low plasma protein binding.

Elimination: The mean systemic clearance of lamivudine is approximately 0.3 l/h/kg. The observed half-life of elimination is 5 to 7 hours. The majority of lamivudine is excreted unchanged in the urine via glomerular filtration and active secretion (organic cationic transport system). Renal clearance accounts for about 70 % of lamivudine elimination.

Special populations:

Studies in patients with renal impairment show lamivudine elimination is affected by renal dysfunction. Dose reduction in patients with a creatinine clearance of < 50 ml/min is necessary (see section 4.2).

The pharmacokinetics of lamivudine are unaffected by hepatic impairment. Limited data in patients undergoing liver transplantation, show that impairment of hepatic function does not impact significantly on the pharmacokinetics of lamivudine unless accompanied by renal dysfunction.

In elderly patients the pharmacokinetic profile of lamivudine suggests that normal ageing with accompanying renal decline has no clinically significant effect on lamivudine exposure, except in patients with creatinine clearance of < 50 ml/min (see section 4.2).

5.3 Preclinical safety data

Administration of lamivudine in animal toxicity studies at high doses was not associated with any major organ toxicity. At the highest dosage levels, minor effects on indicators of liver and kidney function were seen together with occasional reduction in liver weights. Reduction of erythrocytes and neutrophil counts were identified as the effects most likely to be of clinical relevance. These events were seen infrequently in clinical studies.

Lamivudine was not mutagenic in bacterial tests but, like many nucleoside analogues showed activity in an *in vitro* cytogenetic assay and the mouse lymphoma assay. Lamivudine was not genotoxic *in vivo* at doses that gave plasma concentrations around 60-70 times higher than the anticipated clinical plasma levels. As the *in vitro* mutagenic activity of lamivudine could not be confirmed by *in vivo* tests, it is concluded that lamivudine should not represent a genotoxic hazard to patients undergoing treatment.

Reproductive studies in animals have not shown evidence of teratogenicity and showed no effect on male or female fertility. Lamivudine induces early embryolethality when administered to pregnant rabbits at exposure levels comparable to those achieved in man, but not in the rat even at very high systemic exposures.

The results of long term carcinogenicity studies with lamivudine in rats and mice did not shown any carcinogenic potential.

6. PHARMACEUTICAL PARTICULARS

6.1 List of excipients

Tablet core: Tablet film coat:

Microcrystalline Cellulose Hypromellose

Sodium Starch Glycollate Titanium Dioxide

Magnesium Stearate Macrogol 400

Polysorbate 80

Synthetic yellow and red iron oxides

6.2 Incompatibilities

Not applicable

6.3 Shelf life

Three years

6.4 Special precautions for storage

Do not store above 30°C.

6.5 Nature and contents of container

Boxes containing 28 or 84 film-coated tablets in double foil blisters, laminated with polyvinyl chloride.

6.6 Instructions for use and handling

No special requirements

Administrative Data

7. MARKETING AUTHORISATION HOLDER

Glaxo Group Ltd
Greenford Road
Greenford
Middlesex UB6 0NN
United Kingdom

8. MARKETING AUTHORISATION NUMBER(S)

EU/1/99/114/001
EU/1/99/114/002

9. DATE OF FIRST AUTHORISATION/RENEWAL OF THE AUTHORISATION

Date of first authorisation: 29 July 1999

Date of renewal of authorisation: 20 September 2004

10. DATE OF REVISION OF THE TEXT

26 April 2005

Zeffix 5 mg/ml oral solution

(GlaxoSmithKline UK)

1. NAME OF THE MEDICINAL PRODUCT

Zeffix 5 mg/ml oral solution

2. QUALITATIVE AND QUANTITATIVE COMPOSITION

Zeffix oral solution contains 5 mg/ml lamivudine

For excipients see section 6.1.

3. PHARMACEUTICAL FORM

Oral solution

The solution is clear, colourless to pale yellow in colour.

4. CLINICAL PARTICULARS

4.1 Therapeutic indications

Zeffix is indicated for the treatment of chronic hepatitis B in adults with:

§ compensated liver disease with evidence of active viral replication, persistently elevated serum alanine aminotransferase (ALT) levels and histological evidence of active liver inflammation and / or fibrosis.

§ decompensated liver disease.

4.2 Posology and method of administration

Therapy with Zeffix should be initiated by a physician experienced in the management of chronic hepatitis B.

The recommended dosage of Zeffix is 100 mg once daily. Zeffix can be taken with or without food.

Duration of treatment:

- In patients with HBeAg positive chronic hepatitis B (CHB) treatment should be administered until HBeAg seroconversion (HBeAg and HBV DNA loss with HBeAb detection) on two consecutive serum samples at least 3 months apart or until HBsAg seroconversion. This recommendation is based on limited data (see section 5.1).
- In patients with HBeAg negative CHB (pre-core mutant), the optimal duration of treatment is unknown. Treatment discontinuation may be considered following HBsAg seroconversion.
- In patients with either HBeAg positive or HBeAg negative CHB the development of YMDD variant HBV may result in a diminished therapeutic response to lamivudine, indicated by a rise in HBV DNA and ALT from previous on-treatment levels. In patients with extended-duration YMDD variant HBV, a switch to or addition of an alternative agent should be considered (see section 5.1).
- In patients with decompensated liver disease and liver transplant recipients, treatment cessation is not recommended. If there is a loss of efficacy attributable to the emergence of YMDD variant HBV in these patients, additional or alternative therapies should be considered (see section 5.1).

If Zeffix is discontinued, patients should be periodically monitored for evidence of recurrent hepatitis (see section 4.4).

Renal impairment:

Lamivudine serum concentrations (AUC) are increased in patients with moderate to severe renal impairment due to decreased renal clearance. The dosage should therefore be reduced for patients with a creatinine clearance of < 50 ml/minute. When doses below 100 mg are required Zeffix oral solution should be used (see Table 1 below).

Table 1: Dosage of Zeffix in patients with decreased renal clearance.

Creatinine clearance ml/min	First Dose of Zeffix oral solution	Maintenance Dose Once daily
30 to < 50	20 ml (100 mg)	10 ml (50 mg)
15 to < 30	20 ml (100 mg)	5 ml (25 mg)
5 to < 15	7 ml (35 mg)	3 ml (15 mg)
< 5	7 ml (35 mg)	2 ml (10 mg)

Data available in patients undergoing intermittent haemodialysis (for less than or equal to 4 hrs dialysis 2-3 times weekly), indicate that following the initial dosage reduction of lamivudine to correct for the patient's creatinine clearance, no further dosage adjustments are required while undergoing dialysis.

Hepatic impairment:

Data obtained in patients with hepatic impairment, including those with end-stage liver disease awaiting transplant, show that lamivudine pharmacokinetics are not significantly affected by hepatic dysfunction. Based on these data, no dose adjustment is necessary in patients with hepatic impairment unless accompanied by renal impairment.

4.3 Contraindications

Zeffix is contraindicated in patients with known hypersensitivity to lamivudine or to any ingredient of the preparation.

4.4 Special warnings and special precautions for use

Lamivudine has been administered to children (2 years and above) and adolescents with compensated chronic hepatitis B. However, due to limitations of the data, the administration of lamivudine to this patient population is not currently recommended (see section 5.1).

The efficacy of lamivudine in patients co-infected with Delta hepatitis or hepatitis C has not been established.

Data are limited on the use of lamivudine in HBeAg negative (pre-core mutant) patients and in those receiving concurrent immunosuppressive regimes, including cancer chemotherapy.

During treatment with Zeffix patients should be monitored regularly. Serum ALT levels should be monitored at 3 month intervals and HBV DNA and HBeAg should be assessed every 6 months.

HBV viral subpopulations with reduced susceptibility to lamivudine (YMDD variant HBV) have been identified with extended therapy. In some patients the development of YMDD variant HBV can lead to exacerbation of hepatitis, primarily detected by serum ALT elevations and re-emergence of HBV DNA. In patients who have YMDD variant HBV and worsening liver disease (increasing ALT with or without decompensated cirrhosis) or recurrent hepatitis B after liver transplantation, a switch to or addition of an alternative agent should be considered.

If Zeffix is discontinued or there is a loss of efficacy due to the development of YMDD variant HBV (see section 4.2), some patients may experience clinical or laboratory evidence of recurrent hepatitis. If Zeffix is discontinued, patients should be periodically monitored both clinically and by assessment of serum liver function tests (ALT and bilirubin levels), for at least four months, and then as clinically indicated. Exacerbation of hepatitis has primarily been detected by serum ALT elevations, in addition to the re-emergence of HBV DNA. See Table 3 in Section 5.1 Clinical experience for more information regarding frequency of post treatment ALT elevations. Most events have been self-limited, however some fatalities have been observed.

For patients who develop evidence of recurrent hepatitis post-treatment, there are insufficient data on the benefits of re-initiation of lamivudine treatment.

Transplantation recipients and patients with advanced liver disease are at greater risk from active viral replication. Due to the marginal liver function in these patients, hepatitis reactivation at discontinuation of lamivudine or loss of efficacy during treatment may induce severe and even fatal decompensation. These patients should be monitored for clinical, virological and serological parameters associated with hepatitis B, liver and renal function, and antiviral response during treatment (at least every month), and, if treatment is discontinued for any reason, for at least 6 months after treatment. Laboratory parameters to be monitored should include (as a minimum) serum ALT, bilirubin, albumin, blood urea nitrogen, creatinine, and virological status: HBV antigen/antibody, and serum HBV DNA concentrations when possible. Patients experiencing signs of hepatic insufficiency during or post-treatment should be monitored more frequently as appropriate.

For the treatment of patients who are co-infected with HIV and are currently receiving or plan to receive treatment with lamivudine or the combination lamivudine-zidovudine, the dose of lamivudine prescribed for HIV infection (usually 150 mg/twice daily in combination with other antiretrovirals) should be maintained. For HIV co-infected patients not requiring anti-retroviral therapy, there is a risk of HIV mutation when using lamivudine alone for treating chronic hepatitis B.

There is no information available on maternal-foetal transmission of hepatitis B virus in pregnant women receiving treatment with lamivudine. The standard recommended procedures for hepatitis B virus immunisation in infants should be followed.

Patients should be advised that therapy with lamivudine has not been proven to reduce the risk of transmission of hepatitis B virus to others and therefore, appropriate precautions should still be taken.

Patients with rare hereditary problems of fructose intolerance, glucose-galactose malabsorption or sucrase-isomaltase insufficiency should not take this medicine.

Diabetic patients should be advised that each dose of oral solution (100 mg = 20 ml) contains 4 g of sucrose.

The oral solution contains propyl and methyl parahydroxybenzoate. These products may cause an allergic reaction in some individuals. This reaction may be delayed.

4.5 Interaction with other medicinal products and other forms of Interaction

The likelihood of metabolic interactions is low due to limited metabolism and plasma protein binding and almost complete renal elimination of unchanged substance.

Lamivudine is predominantly eliminated by active organic cationic secretion. The possibility of interactions with other medicinal products administered concurrently should be considered, particularly when their main route of elimination is active renal secretion via the organic cationic transport system e.g. trimethoprim. Other medicinal products (e.g. ranitidine, cimetidine) are eliminated only in part by this mechanism and were shown not to interact with lamivudine.

Substances shown to be predominately excreted either via the active organic anionic pathway, or by glomerular filtration are unlikely to yield clinically significant interactions with lamivudine.

Administration of trimethoprim/sulphamethoxazole 160 mg/800 mg increased lamivudine exposure by about 40 %. Lamivudine had no effect on the pharmacokinetics of trimethoprim or sulphamethoxazole. However, unless the patient has renal impairment, no dosage adjustment of lamivudine is necessary.

A modest increase in C_{max} (28 %) was observed for zidovudine when administered with lamivudine, however overall exposure (AUC) was not significantly altered. Zidovudine had no effect on the pharmacokinetics of lamivudine (see section 5.2).

Lamivudine has no pharmacokinetic interaction with alpha-interferon when the two medicinal products are concurrently administered. There were no observed clinically significant adverse interactions in patients taking lamivudine concurrently with commonly used immunosuppressant medicinal products (e.g. cyclosporin A). However, formal interaction studies have not been performed.

Lamivudine may inhibit the intracellular phosphorylation of zalcitabine when the two medicinal products are used concurrently. Zeffix is therefore not recommended to be used in combination with zalcitabine.

4.6 Pregnancy and lactation

Pregnancy:

The safety of lamivudine in human pregnancy has not been established. Studies in animals have shown reproductive toxicity (see section 5.3). Consistent with passive transmission of the substance across the placenta, lamivudine concentrations in infant serum at birth were similar to those in maternal and cord serum at delivery.

Although animal reproductive studies are not always predictive of the human response, administration is not recommended during the first three months of pregnancy (see section 4.4).

Lactation:

Following oral administration, lamivudine was excreted in breast milk at similar concentrations to those found in serum. It is therefore recommended that mothers taking lamivudine do not breast feed their infants.

4.7 Effects on ability to drive and use machines

No studies on the effects on the ability to drive and use machines have been performed.

4.8 Undesirable effects

In clinical studies of patients with chronic hepatitis B, lamivudine was well tolerated. The incidence of adverse events and laboratory abnormalities (with the exception of elevations of ALT and CPK, see below) were similar between placebo and lamivudine treated patients). The most common adverse events reported were malaise and fatigue, respiratory tract infections, throat and tonsil discomfort, headache, abdominal discomfort and pain, nausea, vomiting and diarrhoea.

Adverse reactions are listed below by system organ class and frequency. Frequency categories are only assigned to those adverse reactions considered to be at least possibly causally related to lamivudine. Frequencies are defined as: very common ($\geq$ 1/10), common ($\geq$ 1/100, $<$ 1/10), uncommon ($\geq$ 1/1000, $<$ 1/100), rare ($\geq$ 1/10,000, $<$ 1/1000) and very rare ($<$ 1/10,000).

The frequency categories assigned to the adverse reactions below are estimates: for most events, suitable data for calculating incidence are not available. Very common and common adverse drug reaction frequency categories were determined from clinical trial data and the background incidence in placebo groups was not taken into account. Adverse drug reactions identified through post-marketing surveillance were categorised as rare or very rare.

Clinical trial data:

Hepatobiliary disorders:

Very common: ALT elevations (see section 4.4).

Musculoskeletal and connective tissue disorders:

Common: Elevations of CPK

Post-marketing experience:

In addition to adverse events reported from clinical trials, the following events have been identified during post-approval use of Zeffix.

Blood and lymphatic system disorders:

Very rare: Thrombocytopenia.

Musculoskeletal and connective tissue disorders:

Very rare: Muscle disorders, including myalgia and cramps.

In patients with HIV infection, cases of pancreatitis and peripheral neuropathy (or paresthesia) have been reported. In patients with chronic hepatitis B there was no observed difference in incidence of these events between placebo and lamivudine treated patients.

Cases of lactic acidosis, sometimes fatal, usually associated with severe hepatomegaly and hepatic steatosis, have been reported with the use of combination nucleoside analogue therapy in patients with HIV. There have been rare reports of lactic acidosis in patients receiving lamivudine for hepatitis B.

4.9 Overdose

Administration of lamivudine at very high dose levels in acute animal studies did not result in any organ toxicity. Limited data are available on the consequences of ingestion of acute overdoses in humans. No fatalities occurred, and the patients recovered. No specific signs or symptoms have been identified following such overdose.

If overdose occurs the patient should be monitored, and standard supportive treatment applied as required. Since lamivudine is dialysable, continuous haemodialysis could be used in the treatment of overdose, although this has not been studied.

5. PHARMACOLOGICAL PROPERTIES

5.1 Pharmacodynamic properties

Pharmacotherapeutic group - nucleoside analogue, ATC Code: J05A F05.

Lamivudine is an antiviral agent which is active against hepatitis B virus in all cell lines tested and in experimentally infected animals.

Lamivudine is metabolised by both infected and uninfected cells to the triphosphate (TP) derivative which is the active form of the parent compound. The intracellular half life of the triphosphate in hepatocytes is 17-19 hours *in vitro*. Lamivudine-TP acts as a substrate for the HBV viral polymerase.

The formation of further viral DNA is blocked by incorporation of lamivudine-TP into the chain and subsequent chain termination.

Lamivudine-TP does not interfere with normal cellular deoxynucleotide metabolism. It is also only a weak inhibitor of mammalian DNA polymerases alpha and beta. Furthermore, lamivudine-TP has little effect on mammalian cell DNA content.

In assays relating to potential substance effects on mitochondrial structure and DNA content and function, lamivudine lacked appreciable toxic effects. It has a very low potential to decrease mitochondrial DNA content, is not permanently incorporated into mitochondrial DNA, and does not act as an inhibitor of mitochondrial DNA polymerase gamma.

Clinical experience

Experience in patients with HBeAg positive CHB and compensated liver disease: in controlled studies, 1 year of lamivudine therapy significantly suppressed HBV DNA replication (34-57 % of patients were below the assay detection limits (Abbott Genostics solution hybridization assay, LLOD $<$ 1.6pg/ml)], normalised ALT level (40-72 % of patients), induced HBeAg seroconversion (HBeAg loss and HBeAb detection with HBV DNA loss [by conventional assay], 16-18 % of patients), improved histology (38-52 % of patients had a $\geq$ 2 point decrease in the Knodell Histologic Activity Index [HAI]) and reduced progression of fibrosis (in 3-17 % of patients) and progression to cirrhosis.

Continued lamivudine treatment for an additional 2 years in patients who had failed to achieve HBeAg seroconversion in the initial 1 year controlled studies resulted in further improvement in bridging fibrosis. In patients with YMDD variant HBV, 41/82 (50 %) patients had improvement in liver inflammation and 40/56 (71 %) patients without YMDD variant HBV had improvement. Improvement in bridging fibrosis occurred in 19/30 (63 %) patients without YMDD variant and 22/44 (50 %) patients with the variant. Five percent (3/56) of patients without the YMDD variant and 13 % (11/82) of patients with YMDD variant showed worsening in liver inflammation compared to pre-treatment. Progression to cirrhosis occurred in 4/68 (6 %) patients with the YMDD variant, whereas no patients without the variant progressed to cirrhosis.

In an extended treatment study in Asian patients (NUCB3018) the HBeAg seroconversion rate and ALT normalisation rate at the end of the 5 year treatment period was 48 % (28/58) and 47 % (15/32), respectively. HBeAg seroconversion was increased in patients with elevated ALT levels; 77 % (20/26) of patients with pre-treatment ALT$>$ 2 $\times$ ULN seroconverted. At the end of 5 years, all patients had HBV DNA levels that were undetectable or lower than pre-treatment levels.

Further results from the trial by YMDD variant status are summarised in Table 2.

Table 2: Efficacy results 5 years by YMDD status (Asian Study) NUCB3018

(see Table 2 on next page)

Comparative data according to YMDD status were also available for histological assessment but only up to three years. In patients with YMDD variant HBV, 18/39 (46 %) had improvements in necroinflammatory activity and 9/39 (23 %) had worsening. In patients without the variant, 20/27 (74 %) had improvements in necroinflammatory activity and 2/27 (7 %) had worsening.

Following HBeAg seroconversion, serologic response and clinical remission are generally durable after stopping lamivudine. However, relapses have been identified in patients although they obtained HBeAg seroconversion. Therefore, following HBeAg seroconversion, patients should be periodically monitored to determine that serologic and clinical responses are being maintained. In patients who do not maintain a sustained serological response, consideration should be given to retreatment with either lamivudine or an alternative antiviral agent for resumption of clinical control of HBV.

In patients followed for up to 16 weeks after discontinuation of treatment at one year, post-treatment ALT elevations were observed more frequently in patients who had received lamivudine than in patients who had received placebo. A comparison of post-treatment ALT elevations between weeks 52 and 68 in patients who discontinued lamivudine at week 52 and patients in the same studies who received placebo throughout the treatment course is shown in Table 3. The proportion of patients who had post-treatment ALT elevations in association with an increase in bilirubin levels was low and similar in patients receiving either lamivudine or placebo.

Table 2 Efficacy results 5 years by YMDD status (Asian Study) NUCB3018

	Subjects, % (no.)			
YMDD variant HBV status	YMDD[1]		Non-YMDD[1]	
HBeAg seroconversion				
All patients	38	(15/40)	72	(13/18)
- Baseline ALT ≤ 1 × ULN[2]	9	(1/11)	33	(2/6)
- Baseline ALT> 2 × ULN	60	(9/15)	100	(11/11)
Undetectable HBV DNA				
- Baseline [3]	5	(2/40)	6	(1/18)
- Week 260 [4]				
negative	8	(2/25)	0	
positive < baseline	92	(23/25)	100	(4/4)
positive > baseline	0		0	
ALT normalisation				
- Baseline				
normal	28	(11/40)	33	(6/18)
above normal	73	(29/40)	67	(12/18)
- Week 260				
normal	46	(13/28)	50	(2/4)
above normal <baseline	21	(6/28)	0	
above normal >baseline	32	(9/28)	50	(2/4)

1 Patients designated as YMDD variant were those with ≥5% YMDD variant HBV at any annual time-point during the 5-year period. Patients categorised as non-YMDD variant were those with > 95% wild-type HBV at all annual time-points during the 5-year study period

2 Upper limit of normal

3 Abbott Genostics solution hybridisation assay (LLOD < 1.6 pg/ml

4 Chiron Quantiplex assay (LLOD 0.7 Meq/ml)

Table 3: Post-treatment ALT Elevations in 2 Placebo-Controlled Studies in Adults

	Patients with ALT Elevation/ Patients with Observations*	
Abnormal Value	Lamivudine	Placebo
ALT ≥ 2 × baseline value	37/137 (27 %)	22/116 (19 %)
ALT ≥ 3 × baseline value[†]	29/137 (21 %)	9/116 (8 %)
ALT ≥ 2 × baseline value and absolute ALT> 500 IU/l	21/137 (15 %)	8/116 (7 %)
ALT ≥ 2 × baseline value; and bilirubin > 2 × ULN and ≥ 2 × baseline value	1/137 (0.7 %)	1/116 (0.9 %)

*Each patient may be represented in one or more category.

[†]Comparable to a Grade 3 toxicity in accordance with modified WHO criteria.

ULN = Upper limit of normal.

Experience in patients with HBeAg negative CHB: initial data indicate the efficacy of lamivudine in patients with HBeAg negative CHB is similar to patients with HBeAg positive CHB, with 71 % of patients having HBV DNA suppressed below the detection limit of the assay, 67 % ALT normalisation and 38 % with improvement in HAI after one year of treatment. When lamivudine was discontinued, the majority of patients (70 %) had a return of viral replication. Data is available from an extended treatment study in HBeAg negative patients (NUCAB3017) treated with lamivudine. After two years of treatment in this study, ALT normalisation and undetectable HBV DNA occurred in 30/69 (43 %) and 32/68 (47 %) patients respectively and improvement in necroinflammatory score in 18/49 (37 %) patients. In patients without YMDD variant HBV, 14/22 (64 %) showed improvement in necroinflammatory score and 1/22 (5 %) patients worsened compared to pre-treatment. In patients with the variant, 4/26 (15%) patients showed improvement in necroinflammatory score and 8/26 (31 %) patients worsened compared to pre-treatment. No patients in either group progressed to cirrhosis.

Frequency of emergence of YMDD variant HBV and impact on the treatment response: lamivudine monotherapy results in the selection of YMDD variant HBV in approximately 24 % of patients following one year of therapy, increasing to 67 % following 4 years of therapy. Development of YMDD variant HBV is associated with reduced treatment response in some patients, as evidenced by increased HBV DNA levels and ALT elevations from previous on-therapy levels, progression of signs and symptoms of hepatitis disease and/or worsening of hepatic necroinflammatory findings. The optimal therapeutic management of patients with YMDD variant HBV has not yet been established (see section 4.4).

In a double-blind study in CHB patients with YMDD variant HBV and compensated liver disease (NUC20904), with a reduced virological and biochemical response to lamivudine (n=95), the addition of adefovir dipivoxil 10 mg once daily to ongoing lamivudine 100mg for 52 weeks resulted in a median decrease in HBV DNA of 4.6 $\log_{10}$ copies/ml compared to a median increase of 0.3 $\log_{10}$ copies/ml in those patients receiving lamivudine monotherapy. Normalisation of ALT levels occurred in 31 % (14/45) of patients receiving combined therapy versus 6 % (3/47) receiving lamivudine alone.

Forty patients (HBeAg negative or HBeAg positive) with either decompensated liver disease or recurrent HBV following liver transplantation and YMDD variant were also enrolled into an open label arm of the study. Addition of 10 mg adefovir dipivoxil once daily to ongoing lamivudine 100mg for 52 weeks resulted in a median decrease in HBV DNA of 4.6 $\log_{10}$ copies/ml. Improvement in liver function was also seen after one year of therapy.

Experience in patients with decompensated liver disease: placebo controlled studies have been regarded as inappropriate in patients with decompensated liver disease, and have not been undertaken. In non-controlled studies, where lamivudine was administered prior to and during transplantation, effective HBV DNA suppression and ALT normalisation was demonstrated. When lamivudine therapy was continued post transplantation there was reduced graft re-infection by HBV, increased HBsAg loss and on one-year survival rate of 76 – 100 %.

As anticipated due to the concomitant immunosuppression, the rate of emergence of YMDD variant HBV after 52 weeks treatment was higher (36 % - 64 %) in the liver transplant population than in the immunocompetent CHB patients (14 % - 32 %).

Experience in CHB patients with advanced fibrosis or cirrhosis: in a placebo-controlled study in 651 patients with clinically compensated chronic hepatitis B and histologically confirmed fibrosis or cirrhosis, lamivudine treatment (median duration 32 months) significantly reduced the rate of overall disease progression (34/436, 7.8 % for lamivudine versus 38/215, 17.7 % for placebo, p=0.001), demonstrated by a significant reduction in the proportion of patients having increased Child-Pugh scores (15/436, 3.4 % versus 19/215, 8.8 %, p=0.023) or developing hepatocellular carcinoma (17/436, 3.9 % versus 16/215, 7.4 %, p=0.047). The rate of overall disease progression in the lamivudine group was higher for subjects with detectable YMDD variant HBV DNA (23/209, 11 %) compared to those without detectable YMDD variant HBV (11/221, 5 %). However, disease progression in YMDD subjects in the lamivudine group was lower than the disease progression in the placebo group (23/209, 11 % versus 38/214, 18 % respectively). Confirmed HBeAg seroconversion occurred in 47 % (118/252) of subjects treated with lamivudine and 93 % (320/345) of subjects receiving lamivudine became HBV DNA negative (VERSANT [version 1], bDNA assay, LLOD < 0.7 MEq/ml) during the study.

Experience in children and adolescents: lamivudine has been administered to children and adolescents with compensated CHB in a placebo controlled study of 286 patients aged 2 to 17 years. This population primarily consisted of children with minimal hepatitis B. A dose of 3 mg/kg once daily (up to a maximum of 100 mg daily) was used in children aged 2 to 11 years and a dose of 100 mg once daily in adolescents aged 12 years and above. This dose needs to be further substantiated. The difference in the HBeAg seroconversion rates (HBeAg and HBV DNA loss with HBeAb detection) between placebo and lamivudine was not statistically significant in this population (rates after one year were 13 % (12/95) for placebo versus 22 % (42/191) for lamivudine; p=0.057). The incidence of YMDD variant HBV was similar to that observed in adults, ranging from 19 % at week 52 up to 45 % in patients treated continuously for 24 months.

5.2 Pharmacokinetic properties

Absorption: Lamivudine is well absorbed from the gastrointestinal tract, and the bioavailability of oral lamivudine in adults is normally between 80 and 85 %. Following oral administration, the mean time (t_{max}) to maximal serum concentrations (C_{max}) is about an hour. At therapeutic dose levels i.e.

100 mg once daily, C_{max} is in the order of 1.1-1.5 μg/ml and trough levels were 0.015-0.020 μg/ml.

Co-administration of lamivudine with food resulted in a delay of t_{max} and a lower C_{max} (decreased by up to 47 %). However, the extent (based on the AUC) of lamivudine absorbed was not influenced, therefore lamivudine can be administered with or without food.

Distribution: From intravenous studies the mean volume of distribution is 1.3 l/kg. Lamivudine exhibits linear pharmacokinetics over the therapeutic dose range and displays low plasma protein binding to albumin.

Limited data shows lamivudine penetrates the central nervous system and reaches the cerebro-spinal fluid (CSF). The mean lamivudine CSF/serum concentration ratio 2-4 hours after oral administration was approximately 0.12.

Metabolism: Lamivudine is predominately cleared by renal excretion of unchanged substance. The likelihood of metabolic substance interactions with lamivudine is low due to the small (5-10 %) extent of hepatic metabolism and the low plasma protein binding.

Elimination: The mean systemic clearance of lamivudine is approximately 0.3 l/h/kg. The observed half-life of elimination is 5 to 7 hours. The majority of lamivudine is excreted unchanged in the urine via glomerular filtration and active secretion (organic cationic transport system). Renal clearance accounts for about 70 % of lamivudine elimination.

Special populations:

Studies in patients with renal impairment show lamivudine elimination is affected by renal dysfunction. Dose reduction in patients with a creatinine clearance of < 50 ml/min is necessary (see section 4.2).

The pharmacokinetics of lamivudine are unaffected by hepatic impairment. Limited data in patients undergoing liver transplantation, show that impairment of hepatic function does not impact significantly on the pharmacokinetics of lamivudine unless accompanied by renal dysfunction.

In elderly patients the pharmacokinetic profile of lamivudine suggests that normal ageing with accompanying renal decline has no clinically significant effect on lamivudine exposure, except in patients with creatinine clearance of < 50 ml/min (see section 4.2).

5.3 Preclinical safety data

Administration of lamivudine in animal toxicity studies at high doses was not associated with any major organ toxicity. At the highest dosage levels, minor effects on indicators of liver and kidney function were seen together with occasional reduction in liver weights. Reduction of erythrocytes and neutrophil counts were identified as the effects most likely to be of clinical relevance. These events were seen infrequently in clinical studies.

Lamivudine was not mutagenic in bacterial tests but, like many nucleoside analogues showed activity in an *in vitro* cytogenetic assay and the mouse lymphoma assay. Lamivudine was not genotoxic *in vivo* at doses that gave plasma concentrations around 60-70 times higher than the anticipated clinical plasma levels. As the *in vitro* mutagenic activity of lamivudine could not be confirmed by *in vivo* tests, it is concluded that lamivudine should not represent a genotoxic hazard to patients undergoing treatment.

Reproductive studies in animals have not shown evidence of teratogenicity and showed no effect on male or female fertility. Lamivudine induces early embryolethality when administered to pregnant rabbits at exposure levels comparable to those achieved in man, but not in the rat even at very high systemic exposures.

The results of long term carcinogenicity studies with lamivudine in rats and mice did not shown any carcinogenic potential.

6. PHARMACEUTICAL PARTICULARS

6.1 List of excipients

Sucrose (20 % w/v)

Methyl Parahydroxybenzoate (E218)

Propyl Parahydroxybenzoate (E216)

Citric Acid (anhydrous)

Propylene Glycol

Sodium Citrate

Artificial strawberry flavour

Artificial banana flavour

Purified water

6.2 Incompatibilities

Not applicable

6.3 Shelf life

Two years

After first opening the container: 1 month

6.4 Special precautions for storage

Do not store above 25 °C.

6.5 Nature and contents of container

Cartons containing 240 ml lamivudine oral solution 5 mg/ml in an opaque, white, high-density polyethylene (HDPE) Bottle with a polypropylene child resistant closure. The pack includes a clear polypropylene oral dosing syringe and a polyethylene syringe-adapter.

6.6 Instructions for use and handling

No special requirements

An oral dosing syringe is provided for accurate measurement of the prescribed dose of oral solution. Instructions for use are included in the pack.

Administrative Data

7. MARKETING AUTHORISATION HOLDER

Glaxo Group Ltd

Greenford Road

Greenford

Middlesex UB6 0NN

United Kingdom

8. MARKETING AUTHORISATION NUMBER(S)

EU/1/99/114/003

9. DATE OF FIRST AUTHORISATION/RENEWAL OF THE AUTHORISATION

Date of first authorisation: 29 July 1999

Date of renewal of authorisation: 20 September 2004

10. DATE OF REVISION OF THE TEXT

26 April 2005

Zelapar

(Zeneus Pharma Ltd)

1. NAME OF THE MEDICINAL PRODUCT

Zelapar 1.25 mg Oral Lyophilisate.

2. QUALITATIVE AND QUANTITATIVE COMPOSITION

Each Zelapar Oral Lyophilisate contains 1.25 mg of selegiline hydrochloride, equivalent to 1.05 mg selegiline free base. For excipients, see section 6.1.

3. PHARMACEUTICAL FORM

Oral lyophilisate.

A pale yellow round tablet with the letter A on one side.

4. CLINICAL PARTICULARS

4.1 Therapeutic indications

Adjunctive therapy in combination with levodopa (with a peripheral decarboxylase inhibitor) in the treatment of Parkinson's disease. Zelapar in combination with maximal levodopa therapy is indicated particularly in patients who experience fluctuations in their condition such as 'end-dose' type fluctuations, 'on-off' symptoms or other dyskinesias.

Zelaparmay be used alone in early Parkinson's disease for symptomatic relief and/or to delay the need for levodopa.

4.2 Posology and method of administration

When prescribed as monotherapy for the first time in the early stage of Parkinson's disease or as an adjuvant to levodopa, the dose of Zelaparis one 1.25 mg unit placed on the tongue in the morning, at least five minutes before breakfast and allowed to dissolve. The unit will dissolve rapidly (in less than 10 seconds) in the mouth. The patient should not eat, drink, rinse or wash-out out their mouth for five minutes after taking their medicine to enable selegiline to be absorbed pre-gastrically.

When Zelaparadjunctive therapy is prescribed a reduction (10 to 30%) in the dose of levodopa is usually required. Reduction of the levodopa dose should be gradual in steps of 10% every 3 to 4 days.

No dosage adjustment is required for patients with renal or hepatic impairment.

Do not push the Zelapar tablet through the foil blister. Peel back the foil and carefully remove the unit.

Unused tablets must be disposed of after three months of a sachet opening.

4.3 Contraindications

Zelapar is contra-indicated in patients with known hypersensitivity (including severe dizziness or hypotension) to conventional selegiline tablets or liquid or any of the excipients used in this product.

Zelapar is contra-indicated in patients receiving treatment with serotonin-agonists (e.g. sumatriptan, naratriptan, zolmitriptan and rizatriptan).

Zelapar is contra-indicated in patients with phenylketonuria due to the content of aspartame, a source of phenylalanine.

Selegiline is also contra-indicated for concomitant use with pethidine and other opioids.

Selegiline should not be used in patients with other extrapyramidal disorders not related to dopamine deficiency.

Selegiline should not be used in patients with active duodenal or gastric ulcer.

Selegiline should not be used in patients who are being treated with antidepressant drugs, including MAO inhibitors and selective serotonin reuptake inhibitors (e.g citalopram, escitalopram, fluoxetine, fluvoxamine, paroxetine, sertraline and venlafaxine. See section 4.5 interactions).

Selegiline should also not be used with other drugs which are also monoamine oxidase inhibitors, e.g. linezolid.

Selegiline in combination with levodopa is contra-indicated in severe cardiovascular disease, arterial hypertension, hyperthyroidism, phaeochromocytoma, narrow-angle glaucoma, prostatic adenoma with appearance of residual urine, tachycardia, arrhythmias, severe angina pectoris, psychoses, advanced dementia and thyrotoxicosis.

4.4 Special warnings and special precautions for use

One unit of Zelapar contains 1.25 mg selegiline. It is recommended that patients be warned that the correct dose of Zelapar is one oral lyophilisate.

Special care should be taken when administering selegiline to patients who have labile hypertension, cardiac arrhythmias, severe angina pectoris, psychosis or a history of peptic ulceration.

Although serious hepatic toxicity has not been observed, caution is recommended in patients with a history of hepatic dysfunction. Transient or continuing abnormalities with a tendency for elevated plasma concentrations of liver enzymes have been described during long-term therapy with conventional tablets of selegiline.

The selectivity for MAO-B following administration of conventional selegiline tablets may be diminished with doses above 10 mg/day. A non-selective dose of Zelapar above 10 mg/day has not been determined. The precise dose at which selegiline becomes a non-selective inhibitor of all MAO has not been determined, but with doses higher than 10 mg/day there is a theoretical risk of hypertension after ingestion of tyramine-rich food.

Concomitant treatment with medicines which inhibit MAO-A, (or non-selective MAO inhibitors) can cause hypotensive reactions. Hypotension, sometimes sudden in onset, has been reported with conventional selegiline.

Since selegiline potentiates the effects of levodopa, the adverse effects of levodopa may be increased. When selegiline is added to the maximum tolerated dose of levodopa, involuntary movements and agitation may occur. Levodopa should be reduced by about 10 to 30% when selegiline is added to the treatment (see section 4.2 Posology and Method of Administration). When an optimum dose of levodopa is reached, adverse effects from the combination are less than those observed with levodopa on its own.

Although conventional tablets of selegiline, at doses of 5 to 10 mg/day, have been in widespread use for many years, the full spectrum of possible responses to Zelapar may not have been observed to date. Therefore patients should be observed closely for atypical responses.

Mouth ulcers may occur during treatment with Zelapar 1.25 mg oral lyophilisate.

4.5 Interaction with other medicinal products and other forms of Interaction

Selegiline should not be administered with any type of antidepressant.

When selegiline is used at its recommended dose, it selectively inhibits MAO-B. The combined use of the SSRI, fluoxetine and Zelapar, should only be used under clinical supervision. Use of Zelapar beyond the recommended dose could lead to non-selectivity and serious adverse effects.

Serious reactions with signs and symptoms that may include diaphoresis, flushing, ataxia, tremor, hyperthermia, hyper/hypotension, seizures, palpitation, dizziness and mental changes that include agitation, confusion and hallucinations progressing to delirium and coma have been reported in some patients receiving a combination of selegiline and fluoxetine. Similar experience has been reported in patients receiving selegiline and two other serotonin reuptake inhibitors, sertraline and paroxetine. There is a potential risk of interaction with fluvoxamine and venlafaxine.

Death has been reported to occur following the initiation of therapy with non-selective MAO inhibitors shortly after discontinuation of fluoxetine. Fluoxetine and its active metabolite have long half-lives; therefore MAO inhibitor therapy should not be started until at least 5 weeks after discontinuation of fluoxetine. Selegiline should not be started until 2 weeks after stopping sertraline. For all other serotonin reuptake inhibitors, a time interval of 1 week is recommended between discontinuation of the serotonin reuptake inhibitor and initiation of selegiline. In general, selegiline should not be introduced after a drug that is known to interact with selegiline, until after 5 half lives of that drug have elapsed.

At least 14 days should lapse between the discontinuation of selegiline and initiation of treatment with any drug known to interact with selegiline.

A time interval of 24 hours is recommended between the discontinuation of selegiline and initiation of serotonin agonists.

Patients being treated with selegiline currently or within the past 2 weeks should receive dopamine only after careful risk-benefit assessment, as this combination enhances the risk of hypertensive reactions.

Selegiline should not be given in conjunction with non-specific MAO inhibitors, e.g. linezolid.

Severe CNS toxicity has been reported in patients with the combination of tricyclic antidepressants and selegiline. In one patient receiving amitriptyline and selegiline this included hyperpyrexia and death, and another patient receiving protriptyline and selegiline experienced tremor, agitation, and restlessness followed by unresponsiveness and death two weeks after selegiline was added.

Other adverse reactions occasionally reported in patients receiving a combination of selegiline with various tricyclic antidepressants include hyper/hypotension, dizziness, diaphoresis, tremor, seizures and changes in behavioural and mental status.

Concomitant use of sympathomimetics, nasal decongestants, hypertensive agents, anti-hypertensives, psychostimulants, central suppressant drugs (sedatives, hypnotics) and alcohol should be avoided.

The combination of selegiline and oral contraceptives or drugs for hormone replacement therapy, should be avoided, as this combination may multiply the bioavailability of selegiline.

Foodstuffs containing tyramine have not been found to cause hypertensive reactions during therapy with conventional selegiline tablets at dosages recommended for the treatment of Parkinson's disease. As the selectivity of action of Zelapar for MAO-B is identical to that of conventional tablets of selegiline given in the same dosage (10 mg), no adverse interactions with foodstuffs containing tyramine are anticipated with Zelapar.

Concomitant administration of amantadine and anticholinergic drugs can lead to an increased occurrence of side-effects.

In view of the high degree of binding to plasma proteins by selegiline particular attention must be given to patients who are being treated with medicines with a narrow therapeutic margin such as digitalis and/or anticoagulants.

Four patients receiving altretamine and a monamine oxidase inhibitor experienced symptomatic hypotension after four to seven days of concomitant therapy.

Interactions between non-selective MAO-inhibitors and pethidine as well as selegiline and pethidine have been described. The mechanism of this interaction is not fully understood and therefore, use of pethidine concomitantly with selegiline should be avoided (see contra-indications).

4.6 Pregnancy and lactation

Selegiline is indicated for the treatment of Parkinson's disease which, in most cases, is a disease occurring after childbearing age. As no work has been done to assess the effects of selegiline on pregnancy and lactation, it should not be used in such cases.

Selegiline should not be used by mothers when breastfeeding as information is lacking concerning whether selegiline passes into breast milk.

4.7 Effects on ability to drive and use machines

Even when used correctly, this medicine can affect reaction capacity to the extent that driving or operating machinery is affected and therefore patients should avoid these activities.

4.8 Undesirable effects

In clinical trials, Zelaparwas associated with the following adverse reactions in 5% or more of patients: back pain, dizziness, tremor, sore throat. Adverse reactions occurring with Zelapar at a frequency of less than 5% include stomatitis, mouth ulceration, impaired balance, muscle cramps, joint pain, falling, insomnia, abnormal dreams, hallucinations, nasal congestion, constipation, diarrhoea and pharyngitis.

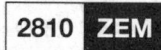

In the first 5 years of post-marketing, no adverse reactions have been reported with Zelapar at a frequency greater than 0.1%. The following adverse reactions were reported at the frequencies given: nausea (0.1%), confusional state (0.08%), dizziness (0.08%), hallucinations NOS (0.06%) and vertigo (0.06%).

Serious adverse reactions with selegiline in monotherapy have been reported as follows: depression, chest pain, myopathy, hypotension and diarrhoea. Other reported adverse reactions included dry mouth, insomnia, tiredness, headache, nausea, dizziness and vertigo. Transient increases in liver enzyme values have also been observed.

As selegiline potentiates the effect of levodopa, the side-effects of levodopa may be emphasised unless the dosage of levodopa is reduced. The most common undesirable effect reported for conventional tablets is dyskinesia (e.g. hyperkinesia - 10 to 15% of patients). Commonly reported undesirable effects for selegiline > 1%): dizziness, orthostatic hypotension, problems in sleeping, dry mouth, nausea, transient transaminase increase (ALAT), confusion, hallucinations and psychoses. Other side-effects reported for selegiline include loss of appetite and other gastrointestinal disorders, headache, agitation, anxiety, irritability, micturition disorders, dyspnoea, palpitations, arrhythmias, angina pectoris, tiredness, depression, loss of balance, hypertension, syncope, excessive perspiration, ankle oedema, hair loss, blurred vision, skin eruptions, leucocytopenia and thrombocytopenia. Once the optimum levodopa dose level has been established, the side-effects produced by this combination will usually be less than those caused by the levodopa therapy on its own.

4.9 Overdose

Zelapar is rapidly metabolised and the metabolites rapidly excreted. In cases of suspected overdosage the patient should be kept under observation for 24 to 48 hours.

No specific information is available about clinically significant overdoses with Zelapar. However, experience gained in use of conventional tablets of selegiline reveals that some individuals exposed to doses of 60 mg/day suffered severe hypotension and psychomotor agitation.

Since the selective inhibition of MAO-B by selegiline hydrochloride is achieved only at doses in the range recommended for the treatment of Parkinson's disease, overdoses are likely to cause significant inhibition of both MAO-A and MAO-B. Consequently, the signs and symptoms of overdose may resemble those observed with non-selective MAOIs (e.g. tranylcypromine, isocarboxazide and phenelzine) and are dizziness, ataxia, irritability, pyrexia, tremor, convulsions, hypomania, psychosis, convulsions, euphoria, respiratory depression, hypotension, hypertension (sometimes with sub-arachnoid haemorrhage), coma and extra-pyramidal symptoms.

5. PHARMACOLOGICAL PROPERTIES

5.1 Pharmacodynamic properties

ATC Code: N04B D01

Zelaparselectively inhibits MAO-B. It prevents dopamine and β-phenylethylamine breakdown in the brain. Selegiline can be used as monotherapy and permits the initiation of treatment with levodopa to be significantly postponed. It potentiates and prolongs the effect of concomitantly administered levodopa. Since it does not interfere with the breakdown of 5-hydroxytryptamine (serotonin) or noradrenaline, it does not cause any hypertensive crises or changes in the plasma or urinary metabolites of these monoamines. Although dietary restrictions are not necessary during Zelapar treatment, the inhibition of MAO-B in blood platelets can lead to a slight potentiation of the circulatory effects of any tyramine not broken down by gastrointestinal MAO-A during absorption. This effect is no greater with Zelapar than with conventional selegiline in equal doses.

The magnitude of increase in the urinary excretion of β-phenylethylamine over 24 hours is simply related to the area under the selegiline plasma concentration-time curve after any selegiline product. Urinary β-phenylethylamine increase reflects the degree of inhibition of MAO-B. Zelapar gives rise to a similar increase in β-phenylethylamine as 10 mg conventional selegiline tablets.

Combined with levodopa therapy selegiline reduces, in particular, fluctuation in the condition of patients who suffer from parkinsonism, e.g. on-off symptoms or end-of-dose akinesia.

In a clinical trial where patients were switched from 10 mg conventional selegiline tablets to 1.25 mg Zelapar oral lyophilisate, control of motor symptoms was maintained.

Zelapar may be useful in those patients with Parkinson's disease who experience difficulties in swallowing.

5.2 Pharmacokinetic properties

Zelapar dissolves completely within 10 seconds of placing on the tongue and, in contrast to conventional tablets, selegiline is absorbed primarily pregastrically.

The plasma concentrations of selegiline following single doses of Zelapar 1.25 mg are of the same order as those obtained with conventional 10 mg tablets of selegiline, but are much less variable. The range of AUCs for plasma selegiline is 0.22 to 2.82 ng.h/ml for Zelapar 1.25 mg and 0.05 to 23.64 ng.h/ml for conventional 10 mg tablets. The Cmax ranges are 0.32 to 4.58 ng/ml and 0.07 to 16.0 ng/ml respectively.

After Zelapar 1.25 mg, plasma concentrations of selegiline metabolites, *N*-desmethylselegiline, *l*-methamphetamine and *l*-amphetamine, were reduced by between 88% and 92% in comparison with the concentrations reached after conventional selegiline tablets 10 mg.

Ninety-four per cent of plasma selegiline is reversibly bound to plasma protein. Selegiline is mainly eliminated by metabolism. It is excreted mainly in the urine as metabolites (mainly *l*-methamphetamine) and the remainder in the faeces.

5.3 Preclinical safety data

Selegiline has not been sufficiently tested for reproductive toxicity. Studies with selegiline revealed no evidence of mutagenic or carcinogenic effects. The only safety concerns for human use derived from animal studies were effects associated with an exaggerated pharmacological action.

6. PHARMACEUTICAL PARTICULARS

6.1 List of excipients

Gelatin

Mannitol

Glycine

Aspartame

Citric Acid anhydrous

Grapefruit flavour

Yellow Colouring (yellow iron oxide [E172], hypromellose [E464]).

6.2 Incompatibilities

Not applicable.

6.3 Shelf life

Sealed sachets - 3 years.

Opened sachets - 3 months.

6.4 Special precautions for storage

Do not store above 25°C.

6.5 Nature and contents of container

PVC/PE/PVdC blister packs sealed with aluminium foil enclosed in a paper/PE/aluminium foil/PE sachet. Each pack contains 10, 30, 60 or 100 oral lyophilisates. Not all pack sizes may be marketed.

6.6 Instructions for use and handling

No special requirements.

7. MARKETING AUTHORISATION HOLDER

Elan Pharma International Limited

WIL House

Shannon Business Park

Shannon

County Clare

Ireland

8. MARKETING AUTHORISATION NUMBER(S)

PL 16804/0001

9. DATE OF FIRST AUTHORISATION/RENEWAL OF THE AUTHORISATION

18 September 1998

10. DATE OF REVISION OF THE TEXT

July 2005

11. Legal Category

POM

Zemplar 5 microgram/ml Solution for Injection

(Abbott Laboratories Limited)

1. NAME OF THE MEDICINAL PRODUCT

Zemplar▼ 5 microgram/ml Solution for Injection

2. QUALITATIVE AND QUANTITATIVE COMPOSITION

Each 1ml of Zemplar solution for injection contains 5 micrograms of paricalcitol.

Each 1ml ampoule contains 5 micrograms of paricalcitol.

Each 2 ml ampoule contains 10 micrograms of paricalcitol.

For excipients, see section 6.1.

3. PHARMACEUTICAL FORM

Solution for Injection

A sterile, clear and colourless aqueous solution

4. CLINICAL PARTICULARS

4.1 Therapeutic indications

Paricalcitol is indicated for the prevention and treatment of secondary hyperparathyroidism associated with chronic renal failure.

4.2 Posology and method of administration

The usual route of administration of Zemplar solution for injection is via a central line during haemodialysis. For patients without a haemodialysis access, Zemplar Injection should be given by slow intravenous injection, for not less than 30 seconds, to minimise pain on administration.

Adults

1) Initial Dose should be calculated based on baseline PTH levels:

An intact PTH (iPTH) assay has been used as the measurement of biologically active PTH in patients with CRF.

The initial dose of paricalcitol is based on the following formula:

$$\text{Initial dose (micrograms)} = \frac{\text{baseline iPTH level in pg/ ml}}{80}$$

and administered as an intravenous (IV) bolus dose no more frequently then every other day at any time during dialysis.

The maximum dose safely administered in clinical studies was as high as 40 μg.

2) Titration Dose:

The currently accepted target range for PTH levels in end-stage renal failure subjects undergoing dialysis is no more than 1.5 to 3 times the non-uremic upper limit of normal (150-300 pg/ml for iPTH). Close monitoring and individual dose titration are necessary to reach appropriate physiological endpoints. During any dose adjustment period, serum calcium (corrected for hypoalbuminaemia) and phosphate levels should be monitored more frequently. If an elevated corrected calcium (Ca) level (>11.2 mg/dl) or persistently elevated phosphate (P) levels (>6.5 mg/dl) are noted, the drug dosage should be adjusted until these parameters are normalised. If hypercalcaemia or a persistently elevated corrected Ca × P product greater than 65 is noted, the drug dosage should be reduced or interrupted until these parameters are normalised. Then, paricalcitol administration should be reinitiated at a lower dose. Doses may need to be decreased as the PTH levels decrease in response to therapy. Thus, incremental dosing must be individualised.

If a satisfactory response is not observed, the dose may be increased by 2-4 microgram at 2- to 4-week intervals. If at any time iPTH levels decrease to less than 150 pg/ml, the drug dosage should be decreased.

The following table is a suggested approach for dose titration:

Suggested Dosing Guidelines

PTH Level	Paricalcitol Dose
the same or increasing	Increase by 2-4 μg
decreasing by < 30%	Increase by 2-4 μg
decreasing by > 30%, < 60%	Maintain
decreasing by > 60%	Decrease by 2-4 μg
one and one-half to three times upper limit of normal	Maintain

Once dosage has been established, serum calcium and phosphate should be measured at least monthly. Serum iPTH measurements are recommended every three months. During dose adjustment with paricalcitol, laboratory tests may be required more frequently.

During treatment with paricalcitol patients should take adequate amounts of calcium either nutritionally or by supplements in line with the RDA.

Hepatic insufficiency

Unbound concentrations of paricalcitol in patients with mild to moderate hepatic impairment are similar to healthy subjects and dose adjustment is not necessary in this patient population. There is no experience in patients with severe hepatic impairment.

Pediatric Use

Safety and efficacy of paricalcitol in paediatric patients have not been established.

Geriatric Use

There is a limited amount of experience with patients 65 years of age or over receiving paricalcitol in the phase III studies. In these studies, no overall differences in efficacy or safety were observed between patients 65 years or older and younger patients.

4.3 Contraindications

Paricalcitol should not be given to patients with evidence of Vitamin D toxicity, hypercalcemia, or hypersensitivity to any ingredient in this product.

4.4 Special warnings and special precautions for use

Acute overdose of paricalcitol may cause hypercalcemia, and require emergency attention. During dose adjustment, serum calcium and phosphate levels should be monitored closely (e.g., twice weekly). If clinically significant hypercalcemia (>11.2 mg/dl)develops, the dose should be reduced or interrupted. Chronic administration of paricalcitol may place patients at risk of hypercalcemia, elevated Ca × P product, and metastatic calcification. Signs and symptoms of vitamin D intoxication associated with hypercalcaemia include:

Early: Weakness, headache, somnolence, nausea, vomiting, dry mouth, constipation, muscle pain, bone pain and metallic taste.

Late: Anorexia, weight loss, conjunctivitis (calcific), pancreatitis, photophobia, rhinorrhoea, pruritus, hyperthermia, decreased libido, elevated BUN, hypercholesterolaemia, elevated AST and ALT, ectopic calcification, hypertension, cardiac arrhythmias, somnolence, death, and rarely, overt psychosis.

Treatment of patients with clinically significant hypercalcaemia consists of immediate dose reduction or interruption of paricalcitol therapy and includes a low calcium diet, withdrawal of calcium supplements, patient mobilisation, attention to fluid and electrolyte imbalances, assessment of electrocardiographic abnormalities (critical in patients receiving digitalis), and haemodialysis or peritoneal dialysis against a calcium-free dialysate, as warranted. Serum calcium levels should be monitored frequently until normocalcaemia ensues.

Adynamic bone lesions (low-turnover bone disease) may develop if PTH levels are suppressed to abnormal levels.

Zemplar contains 30% v/v of propyleneglycol as an excipient. Isolated cases of Central Nervous System depression, haemolysis and lactic acidosis have been reported as toxic effect associated with propyleneglycol administration at high doses. Although they are not expected to be found with Zemplar administration as propyleneglycol is eliminated during the dialysis process, the risk of toxic effect in overdosing situations has to be taken into account.

This product contains 20% v/v of ethanol. Dosing is variable dependent on the severity of disease and response to treatment, however each dose may contain up to 1.3g of ethanol based on the maximum dose seen in clinical trials. Ethanol may be harmful for those suffering from liver disease, alcoholism, epilepsy, brain injury or disease as well as for pregnant women and children, and may modify or increase the effect of other medicines.

4.5 Interaction with other medicinal products and other forms of Interaction

Specific interaction studies were not performed. Digitalis toxicity is potentiated by hypercalcaemia of any cause, so caution should be applied when digitalis compounds are prescribed concomitantly with paricalcitol.

Phosphate or vitamin D-related compounds should not be taken concomitantly with paricalcitol, due to an increased risk of hypercalcaemia and CaxP product elevation.

Aluminium-containing preparations (e.g., antacids, phosphate-binders) should not be administered chronically with Vitamin D preparations, as increased blood levels of aluminium and aluminium bone toxicity may occur.

High doses of calcium-containing preparations or thiazide diuretics may increase the risk of hypercalcaemia.

Magnesium-containing preparations (e.g. antacids) should not be taken concomitantly with vitamin D preparations, because hypermagnesemia may occur.

4.6 Pregnancy and lactation

There is no adequate data on the use of paricalcitol in pregnant women. Animal studies have shown reproductive toxicity (see section 5.3). Potential risk in human use is not known and it can be used during pregnancy only if the potential benefit outweighs the potential risk for the foetus.

Lactation: It is not known whether paricalcitol is excreted in human milk. Because many drugs are excreted in human milk, caution should be exercised when paricalcitol is administered to a nursing woman.

4.7 Effects on ability to drive and use machines

No studies on the effects on the ability to drive a car and use machines have been performed.

Zemplar solution for injection contains 20 % v/v ethanol.

4.8 Undesirable effects

The safety of Zemplar has been investigated in 600 patients in Phase II/III/IV clinical trials.

The most common adverse events (>1%) associated with Zemplar therapy were hypercalcaemia, hyperphosphataemia,, parathyroid disorder, pruritus, and taste perversion occurring in 4.7 %, 1.7 %, 1.2%, 1.1% and 1.1% of patients, respectively. Hypercalcaemia and hyperphosphataemia were mainly dependent on the level of PTH oversuppression and can be minimised by proper dose titration. No adverse events with possible or probable or definite relationship to Zemplar have been reported in >2% of patients.

Uncommon adverse reactions (>0.1 and < 1 % of patients) listed below by body system:

Haematological and Lymphatic System: anaemia, leucopoenia, lymphadenopathy, and increased bleeding time.

Metabolic and Nutritional Disorders: oedema,, peripheral oedema, increased AST, and weight loss.

Nervous System: abnormal gait, agitation, confusion, delirium, depersonalisation, dizziness, hypesthesia, insomnia, myoclonus, nervousness, paraesthesia and stupor.

Special Senses: conjunctivitis, ear disorder, and glaucoma.

Cardiovascular System: arrhythmia, atrial flutter, cerebral ischaemia, cerebrovascular accident, cardiac arrest, hypotension, hypertension, and syncope.

Respiratory System: asthma, increased cough, dyspnoea, epistaxis, pulmonary oedema, pharyngitis, and pneumonia.

Gastrointestinal System: anorexia, colitis, constipation, diarrhoea, dry mouth, dyspepsia, dysphagia, gastrointestinal disorder, gastritis, nausea, rectal haemorrhage, thirst, and vomiting.

Skin and Appendages: alopecia, hirsutism, rash, sweating, and vesiculobullous rash.

Musculoskeletal System: arthralgia, myalgia, joint disorder, and twitching.

Urogenital System: breast carcinoma, breast pain, impotence, and vaginitis.

Others: allergic reaction, back pain, chest pain, fever, flu syndrome, infection, injection site pain, malaise, pain, and sepsis.

4.9 Overdose

Overdosage of paricalcitol may lead to hypercalcemia (see Warnings and precautions).

Paricalcitol is not significantly removed by dialysis.

The content of propylene glycol as excipient is eliminated by dialysis.

5. PHARMACOLOGICAL PROPERTIES

5.1 Pharmacodynamic properties

Pharmaco-therapeutic group: ATC code: A11CC

Mechanism of action:

Paricalcitol is a synthetic vitamin D analog. Vitamin D and paricalcitol have been shown to reduce parathyroid hormone (PTH) levels.

5.2 Pharmacokinetic properties

Distribution

The pharmacokinetics of paricalcitol have been studied in patients with chronic renal failure (CRF) requiring haemodialysis. Paricalcitol is administered as an intravenous bolus injection. Within two hours after administering doses ranging from 0.04 to 0.24 microgram/kg, concentrations of paricalcitol decreased rapidly; thereafter, concentrations of paricalcitol declined log-linearly with a mean half-life of about 15 hours. No accumulation of paricalcitol was observed with multiple dosing.

Elimination

In healthy subjects, a study was conducted with a single 0.16 microgram/kg intravenous bolus dose of ^{3}H-paricalcitol (n=4), plasma radioactivity was attributed to parent drug. Paricalcitol was eliminated primarily by hepatobiliary excretion, as 74% of the radioactive dose was recovered in faeces and only 16% was found in urine.

Metabolism

Several unknown metabolites were detected in both the urine and faeces, with no detectable paricalcitol in the urine. These metabolites have not been characterised and have not been identified. Together, these metabolites contributed 51% of the urinary radioactivity and 59% of the faecal radioactivity. *In vitro* plasma protein binding of paricalcitol was extensive (>99.9%) and nonsaturable over the concentration range of 1 to 100 ng/mL.

Paricalcitol Pharmacokinetic Characteristics in CRF Patients (0.24 μ g/kg dose)

Parameter	N	Values (Mean ± SD)
C_{max} (5 minutes after bolus)	6	1850± 664 (pg/mL)
$AUC_{0-¥}$	5	27382 ± 8230 (pg •hr/mL)
CL	5	0.72 ± 0.24 (L/hr)
V_{ss}	5	6 ± 2 (L)

Special Populations

Gender, Race and Age: No age or gender related pharmacokinetic differences have been observed in adult patients studied. Pharmacokinetic differences due to race have not been identified.

Hepatic insufficiency: Unbound concentrations of paricalcitol in patients with mild to moderate hapatic inpairment is similar to healthy subjects and dose adjustement is not necessary in this patient population. There is no experience in patients with severe hepatic impairment.

5.3 Preclinical safety data

The effects seen in repeat-dose toxicity studies in rodents and dogs fell into two general categories: those related and those unrelated to paricalcitol's calcaemic activity.

Effects not clearly related to hypercalcaemia included decreased white blood cell counts and thymic atrophy in dogs, and altered APTT values (increased in dogs, decreased in rats). Except for reductions in WBCs, similar effects were seen in rats and dogs treated with calcitriol. Such WBC changes were not observed in clinical trials of paricalcitol.

Paricalcitol did not affect fertility in rats and there was no evidence of teratogenic activity in rats or rabbits. Paricalcitol was shown to affect foetal viability, as well as to promote a significant increase of peri-natal and post-natal mortality of newborn rats, when administered at maternally toxic doses.

Increases in benign and malignant phaeochromocytomas (adrenal tumours) were observed in a carcinogenicity study conducted in rats. Rats are unusually prone to developing these tumours following chronic exposures to agents that increase calcium absorption. Therefore increased incidences of these tumours with paricalcitol is expected to have limited relevance in humans.

Limitations of the animal models (animals without renal insufficiency) precluded the administration of high doses of paricalcitol in studies on repeated dose toxicity, reproductive toxicity and carcinogenicity. Doses administered and/or systemic exposures to paricalcitol were slightly higher than therapeutic doses/systemic exposures.

Paricalcitol did not exhibit genotoxic potential in a set of *in-vitro* and *in-vivo* genotoxicity assays.

6. PHARMACEUTICAL PARTICULARS

6.1 List of excipients

Solution for injection contains:

Ethanol (20 % v/v),

Propylene glycol,

Purified water.

6.2 Incompatibilities

Propylene glycol interacts with heparin and neutralises its effect. Zemplar contains propylene glycol as an excipient and its administration with heparin must be avoided.

Not to be mixed with other medicinal products.

6.3 Shelf life

24 months.

6.4 Special precautions for storage

Do not store above 30°C.

6.5 Nature and contents of container

Zemplar Injection 5 microgram/ ml is presented in single dose Type I glass ampoule.

- 5 ampoules containing 1 ml each
- 5 ampoules containing 2 ml each

6.6 Instructions for use and handling

Parenteral drug products should be inspected visually for particulate matter and discoloration prior to administration whenever solution and container permit.

Discard unused portion.

7. MARKETING AUTHORISATION HOLDER

Abbott Laboratories Limited

Queenborough

Kent

ME11 5EL

8. MARKETING AUTHORISATION NUMBER(S)

PL 00037/0403

9. DATE OF FIRST AUTHORISATION/RENEWAL OF THE AUTHORISATION

21/07/2003

10. DATE OF REVISION OF THE TEXT

APRIL 2005

Zenapax

(Roche Products Limited)

1. NAME OF THE MEDICINAL PRODUCT

Zenapax▼, 5 mg/ml concentrate for solution for infusion.

2. QUALITATIVE AND QUANTITATIVE COMPOSITION

Daclizumab*................................. 5 mg per 1 ml infusion.

One vial of 5 ml contains 25 mg of daclizumab* (5 mg/ml).

* Recombinant humanised IgG1 anti-Tac antibody produced in a murine NSO myeloma cell line using a glutamine synthetase (GS) expression system (NS_GSO) by recombinant DNA technology.

For excipients, see section 6.1.

3. PHARMACEUTICAL FORM

Concentrate for solution for infusion.

4. CLINICAL PARTICULARS

4.1 Therapeutic indications

Zenapax is indicated for the prophylaxis of acute organ rejection in *de novo* allogenic renal transplantation and is to be used concomitantly with an immunosuppressive regimen, including ciclosporin and corticosteroids in patients who are not highly immunised.

4.2 Posology and method of administration

Zenapax should be prescribed only by physicians who are experienced in the use of immunosuppressive therapy following organ transplantation.

The recommended dose for Zenapax in adult and paediatric patients is 1 mg/kg. The volume of Zenapax containing the appropriate dose is added to 50 ml of sterile 0.9% saline solution and is administered intravenously over a 15 minute period. It may be given via a peripheral or central vein.

Zenapax should initially be given within 24 hours before transplantation. The next and each subsequent dose should be given at intervals of fourteen days, for a total of five doses.

Elderly

Experience with Zenapax in elderly patients (older than 65 years) is limited because of the small number of older patients who undergo renal transplantation, but there is no evidence that elderly patients require a different dosage from younger patients.

Patients with severe renal impairment

No dosage adjustment is necessary for patients with severe renal impairment.

Patients with severe hepatic impairment

No data are available for patients with severe hepatic impairment.

4.3 Contraindications

Zenapax is contraindicated in patients with known hypersensitivity to daclizumab or to any excipients of this product (see section 6.1 ''List of Excipients'').

Zenapax is contraindicated during pregnancy and lactation.

4.4 Special warnings and special precautions for use

There is no experience of the use of Zenapax in patients who are highly immunised.

Anaphylactic reactions following the administration of proteins can occur. Severe, acute (onset within 24 hours) hypersensitivity reactions on both initial and subsequent exposure to Zenapax have been reported rarely. The clinical manifestations of these reactions include hypotension, tachycardia, hypoxia, dyspnoea, wheezing, laryngeal oedema, pulmonary oedema, flushing, diaphoresis, temperature increase, rash and pruritus. Medications for the treatment of severe hypersensitivity reactions should therefore be available for immediate use.

Patients on immunosuppressive therapy following transplantation are at increased risk for developing lymphoproliferative disorders (LPDs) and opportunistic infections. While Zenapax is an immunosuppressive drug, to date no increase in LPDs or opportunistic infections have been observed in patients treated with Zenapax.

In transplant recipients there is no experience of exposure to second or subsequent treatment courses using Zenapax.

In a single randomised controlled clinical trial in cardiac transplant recipients which compared Zenapax to placebo, each used in combination with mycophenolate mofetil (CellCept 1.5 g bid), ciclosporin, and corticosteroids, there were more infection related deaths among patients who received Zenapax. At 1 year post-transplant 14 to 216 patients (6.5%) who received Zenapax and 4 of 207 (1.9%) patients who received placebo died of an infection, a difference of 4.6% (95% CI: 0.3%, 8.8%). Of these 14 Zenapax patients, 4 died more than 90 days after receiving their last dose of Zenapax, making it unlikely that Zenapax had a role in the infection related death. Overall, use of polyclonal antilymphocyte antibody therapy (OKT3, ATG, ATGAM) was similar in patients who received Zenapax and in patients who received placebo, 18.5% and 17.9%, respectively. However, of the 40 patients who received both Zenapax and antilymphocyte therapy, 8 (20.0%) died whereas of the 37 patients who received both placebo and antilymphocyte therapy, 2 (5.4%) died. Concomitant use of Zenapax with another antilymphocyte antibody therapy in the context of intensive immunosuppression with ciclosporin, mycophenolate mofetil and corticosteroids may be a factor leading to fatal infection.

4.5 Interaction with other medicinal products and other forms of Interaction

Because Zenapax is an immunoglobulin, no metabolic drug-drug interactions are to be expected.

The following transplant medications have been administered in clinical trials with Zenapax without any interactions: ciclosporin, mycophenolate mofetil, gancyclovir, acyclovir, tacrolimus, azathioprine, antithymocyte immune globulin, muromonab-CD3 (OKT3), and corticosteroids.

4.6 Pregnancy and lactation

Zenapax is contraindicated during pregnancy and lactation. Because of its immunosuppressive potential it has potentially hazardous effects with respect to the course of gestation and the suckling infant exposed to daclizumab in breast milk.

Women of childbearing potential must use an effective contraceptive method during Zenapax therapy and continue its use for an additional 4 months following the last dose of Zenapax.

4.7 Effects on ability to drive and use machines

There is no evidence to indicate that Zenapax will impair ability to drive or use machinery.

4.8 Undesirable effects

The safety profile of Zenapax was studied in comparison to placebo in patients who concomitantly received immunosuppressive regimens containing ciclosporin and corticosteroids alone, with the addition of azathioprine or with the addition of mycophenolate mofetil. The incidence and types of adverse events were similar in both placebo-treated and Zenapax-treated patients. Adverse events were reported by 95% of placebo and 96% of daclizumab treated patients. Serious adverse events were reported by 44.4% of the patients in the placebo-treated group and 39.9% of the patients in the Zenapax-treated group.

Humanised Anti-Tac (Ro 24-7375)

Prevention of Renal Allograft Rejection

Protocol O14392, O14393, O14874, and O15301 Pooled

Table 1: Percentage (Number) of Patients with Adverse Events during the First 3 Months Post-transplant **(only Adverse Events occurring with a frequency of ⩾ 5% of patients in either group are listed)**

Body System and Adverse Event	Placebo (N = 293)	HAT* (N = 336)
Gastro-Intestinal System Disorders	**68**	**67**
Constipation	38	35
Nausea	26	27
Diarrhoea	16	15
Vomiting	14	15
Abdominal pain	13	10
Pyrosis	10	8
Dyspepsia	5	7
Abdominal distention	4	6
Epigastric pain not food-related	4	5
Metabolic and Nutritional Disorders	**50**	**45**
Oedema extremities	30	28
Oedema	18	16
Fluid overload	6	3
Central & periph. Nervous syst. disorders	**41**	**46**
Tremor	16	19
Headache	15	16
Dizziness	7	5
Urinary Systems Disorders	**45**	**39**
Oliguria	11	10
Dysuria	12	6
Renal tubular necrosis	7	7
Renal damage	8	5
Body As a Whole – General Disorders	**40**	**37**
Pain post traumatic	20	21
Chest pain	9	9
Fever	10	5
Pain	8	7
Shivering	5	3
Autonomic Nervous System Disorder	**36**	**38**
Hypertension	21	25
Hypotension	10	9
Aggravated hypertension	7	7
Respiratory System Disorders	**37**	**35**
Dyspnoea	15	12
Pulmonary oedema	4	6
Coughing	5	5
Skin and appendages disorders	**28**	**32**
Impaired wound healing without infection	10	12
Acne	7	9
Pruritus	6	4
Psychiatric disorders	**29**	**25**
Insomnia	14	13
Fatigue	10	7
Anxiety	6	2
Musculo-skeletal systems disorders	**26**	**26**
Musculoskeletal pain	12	13
Back pain	8	7
Heart rate and rhythm	**12**	**11**
Tachycardia	7	7
Vascular extracardiac	**10**	**12**
Thrombosis	4	5
Platelet, Bleeding and clotting disorders	**11**	**8**
Bleeding	11	7
Haemic and lymphatic	**8**	**8**
Lymphocele	7	7
Application Site Disorders	**5**	**5**
Application site reaction	5	5

**HAT = humanised anti-Tac*

Other less frequently (⩾ 2% and <5%) occurring adverse events were observed for a number of body systems and included flatulence, gastritis, haemorrhoids, diabetes mellitus, dehydration, hydronephrosis, urinary tract bleeding, urinary tract disorder, renal insufficiency, generalised weakness, urinary retention, leg cramps, prickly sensation, atelectasis, congestion, pharyngitis, rhinitis, hypoxia, rales, abnormal breath sounds, pleural effusion, hirsutism, rash, night sweats, increased sweating, depression, arthralgia, myalgia and blurred vision.

Incidence of malignancies: Three years after treatment, the incidence of malignancies was 7.8% in the placebo group compared with 6.4% in the Zenapax group. Addition of Zenapax did not increase the number of post-transplant lymphomas, which occurred with a frequency of 1.5% in the placebo-treated group and 0.7% in the Zenapax-treated group.

Hyperglycaemia: No differences in abnormal haematologic or chemical laboratory test results were seen between placebo-treated and Zenapax-treated groups with the exception of fasting blood glucose. Fasting blood glucose was measured in a small number of placebo- and Zenapax-treated patients. A total of 16% (10 of 64 patients) of placebo-treated and 32% (28 of 88 patients) of Zenapax-treated patients had high fasting blood glucose values. Most of these high values occurred either on the first day post-transplant when patients received high doses of corticosteroids or in patients with diabetes.

Deaths occurring during the first 6 months post-transplant were reported in 3.4% of the placebo- and in 0.6% of the Zenapax-treated groups. The twelve months mortality was 4.4% in the placebo- and 1.5% in the Zenapax-treated groups.

Infectious episodes, including viral infections, fungal infections, bacteraemia and septicaemia, and pneumonia, were reported in 72% of the placebo-treated patients and in 68% of Zenapax-treated patients. The type of infections reported was similar in both the Zenapax- and the placebo-treated groups. Cytomegalovirus infection was reported in 16% of the patients in the placebo group and in 13% of the patients in the Zenapax group.

In rare cases severe hypersensitivity reactions following administration of Zenapax have been reported (see section 4.4 Special warnings and special precautions for use).

Paediatric patients: The safety profile for the use of Zenapax in paediatric patients was shown to be comparable to that in adult patients. However, the following adverse events occurred more frequently in paediatric patients: diarrhoea (41%), post-operative pain (38%), fever (33%), vomiting (33%), hypertension (28%), pruritus (21%) and infections of the upper respiratory tract (20%) and urinary tract (18%).

4.9 Overdose

A maximum tolerated dose has not been determined in patients and could not be achieved in animals that received Zenapax. A dose of 1.5 mg/kg has been administered to bone marrow transplant recipients without any associated adverse events. In a single dose toxicity study a dose of 125 mg/kg was administered intravenously to mice and showed no evidence of toxicity.

5. PHARMACOLOGICAL PROPERTIES

Pharmacotherapeutic group: selective immunosuppressive agents.

ATC code: L04A A08.

5.1 Pharmacodynamic properties

Clinical pharmacology

Zenapax contains daclizumab, a recombinant, humanised IgG1 anti-Tac antibody, and functions as an interleukin 2 (IL-2) receptor antagonist. Daclizumab binds with high specificity to the alpha or Tac subunit of the high affinity IL-2 receptor complex (expressed on activated T cells), and inhibits IL-2 binding and biological activity. Administration of Zenapax inhibits IL-2-mediated activation of lymphocytes, a critical pathway in the cellular immune response involved in allograft rejection. Daclizumab saturates the Tac receptor for approximately 90 days at the recommended dosage regimen for the majority of patients. Antibodies to daclizumab developed in approximately 9% of Zenapax-treated patients in clinical studies but did not appear to affect efficacy, safety, serum daclizumab levels, or any other clinically relevant parameter examined.

No gross changes to circulating lymphocyte numbers or cell phenotypes were observed by fluorescence-activated cell sorter (FACS) analysis other than the expected transient decrease in Tac+ cells.

Combination Therapy in Renal Allograft Recipients

In the Phase III trials, Zenapax was added to a standard immunosuppressive regimen of ciclosporin (5 mg/kg), steroids (prednisone or methylprednisolone), with or without the addition of azathioprine (4 mg/kg).

Both trials showed a statistically significant superiority to placebo in reducing the rate of acute renal allograft rejection to six months post-transplant as confirmed by biopsy. From pooled data the difference in biopsy-proven acute rejection remained statistically different at one-year post-transplant (43% as compared with 28%). Three year graft survival rates were significantly higher among those patients who did not experience acute rejection within the first year posttransplant (n=345) compared with those who experienced acute rejection during the first year (n=190) regardless of treatment. The three year graft survival was not significantly different between placebo and daclizumab in the triple immunosuppressant trial (83% Vs. 84%) or the double immunosuppressant trial (78% Vs 82%). The three year patient survival rate was significantly different between placebo and daclizumab in the double immunosuppressant trial (88% Vs. 96%; p = 0.017), but not in the triple immunosuppressant trial (94% Vs. 92%).

Renal function evaluated by serum creatinine and GFR was similar in both groups at three years post-transplant.

The beneficial effect of Zenapax prophylaxis upon the incidence of acute rejection after renal transplantation was not associated with adverse clinical sequelae, including the development of Post-Transplant Lymphoproliferative Disease (PTLD), at 3 years post-transplant.

5.2 Pharmacokinetic properties

In clinical trials involving renal allograft patients treated with 1 mg/kg of Zenapax every 14 days for a total of 5 doses, average peak serum concentrations (mean ± standard deviation) rose between the first dose (21 ± 14μg/ml) and fifth doses (32 ± 22μg/ml). The mean ± standard deviation trough serum concentration prior to fifth dose was 7.6 ± 4.0μg/ml. Serum levels of 0.5 to 0.9μg/ml are needed to saturate the IL-2 receptor and levels of 5 - 10μg/ml are needed to inhibit IL-2 mediated biologic activity. The recommended regimen of daclizumab will maintain serum concentrations sufficient to saturate IL-2R alpha receptors on activated T lymphocytes for more than 90 days post-transplantation in the majority of patients. This first three months, is the most critical period post-transplantation.

The estimated terminal elimination half-life of daclizumab ranged from 270 to 919 hours (average 480 hours) in renal allograft patients and is equivalent to that reported for human IgG which ranged from 432 to 552 hours (average 480 hours). This is attributable to the humanisation of the protein.

Population pharmacokinetic analysis showed that the systemic clearance of daclizumab was influenced by total body weight, age, gender, proteinuria, and race. The identified body weight influence on systemic clearance supports the dosing of Zenapax on a mg/kg basis and maintains drug exposure within 30% of the reference exposure for patient groups with wide range of demographic characteristics. No dosage adjustments based on other identified covariates (gender, proteinuria, race and age) are required for renal allograft patients.

Paediatric patients: Pharmacokinetic and pharmacodynamic properties were evaluated in 61 paediatric patients treated with 1 mg/kg I.V. dose of Zenapax every 14 days for a total of 5 doses. Peak serum concentrations (peak ± SD) rose between the first dose (16 ± 12μg/ml) and the fifth dose (21 ± 14μg/ml). The mean trough serum concentration before the fifth dose was 5.0 ± 2.7μg/ml. The Tac subunit of the IL-2 receptor was saturated immediately after the first dose of 1.0 mg/kg of daclizumab and remained saturated for at least the first three months post-transplant. Saturation of the Tac subunit of the IL-2 receptor was similar to that observed in adult patients receiving the same dose regimen.

There is no pharmacokinetic interaction between Zenapax and mycophenolic acid, the active metabolite of mycophenolate mofetil (CellCept).

5.3 Preclinical safety data

Daclizumab was well tolerated after single bolus intravenous or subcutaneous doses ranging from 50 to 125 mg/kg in mice, rats, and rabbits and after 28 days administration of 15 mg/kg to monkeys. One of 18 monkeys had an anaphylactic reaction to daclizumab. Appreciable daclizumab serum levels were maintained except in 2 out of 18 monkeys that developed anti-daclizumab antibodies. There was no cross reactivity *in vitro* between daclizumab and human cryosections (28 organs) at concentrations up to 56 mg/ml, demonstrating the absence of non specific binding. Daclizumab was not genotoxic in standard tests.

6. PHARMACEUTICAL PARTICULARS

6.1 List of excipients

Polysorbate 80

Sodium chloride

Sodium dihydrogen phosphate anhydrous

Disodium phosphate anhydrous

Hydrochloric acid, concentrated

Sodium hydroxide

Water for injections

6.2 Incompatibilities

No incompatibility between Zenapax and polyvinyl chloride bags or infusion sets has been observed.

6.3 Shelf life

2 years.

After dilution an immediate use is recommended. Chemical and physical in-use stability has been demonstrated for 24 hours at 2-8°C or for 4 hours at 25°C. From a microbiological point of view, however, the diluted product should be used immediately. The product is not intended to be stored after dilution unless the dilution has taken place under controlled and validated aseptic conditions. If not used immediately, in use storage times and conditions prior to use are the responsibility of the user.

6.4 Special precautions for storage

– Store in a refrigerator (2-8°C).

– Do not freeze.

– Store in the original package in order to protect from light.

6.5 Nature and contents of container

5 ml in a vial (Type I glass). Pack sizes of 1 or 3.

Not all pack sizes may be marketed.

6.6 Instructions for use and handling

Zenapax is NOT for direct injection. It should be diluted in 50 ml of sterile 0.9% sodium chloride solution before intravenous administration to the patients. For mixing the solution, do not shake, gently invert the bag in order to avoid foaming. Care must be taken to assure sterility of prepared solution, since the drug product does not contain any antimicrobial preservative or bacteriostatic agents. Zenapax is a colourless solution provided as a single use vial. Any unused product or waste material should be disposed of in accordance with local requirements. Parenteral drug products should be inspected visually for particulate matter and discoloration before administration. Once the infusion is prepared it should be administered intravenously immediately. If diluted aseptically it may be stored for 24 hours when refrigerated between 2 - 8°C or for 4 hours at 25°C.

Other drug/substances should not be added or infused simultaneously through the same intravenous line.

7. MARKETING AUTHORISATION HOLDER

Roche Registration Limited, 40 Broadwater Road, Welwyn Garden City, Hertfordshire AL7 3AY, UK.

8. MARKETING AUTHORISATION NUMBER(S)

EU/1/99/098/001 (single vial pack)

EU/1/99/098/002 (3 vial pack)

9. DATE OF FIRST AUTHORISATION/RENEWAL OF THE AUTHORISATION

26 February 1999

10. DATE OF REVISION OF THE TEXT

April 2004

In Ireland further information is available on request from Roche Products (Ireland) Limited, 3004 Lake Drive, City West, Naas Road, Dublin 24, Ireland.

Zenapax is a registered trade mark

P983018/504

Zerit 15 mg, 20 mg, 30 mg and 40 mg Hard Capsules

(Bristol-Myers Squibb Pharmaceuticals Ltd)

1. NAME OF THE MEDICINAL PRODUCT

Zerit 15® mg hard capsules

Zerit 20® mg hard capsules

Zerit 30® mg hard capsules

Zerit 40® mg hard capsules

2. QUALITATIVE AND QUANTITATIVE COMPOSITION

Each hard capsule contains 15 mg, 20 mg, 30 mg, or 40 mg of stavudine.

For excipients, see section 6.1.

3. PHARMACEUTICAL FORM

15mg Capsules: The hard capsules are red and yellow, opaque and imprinted with "BMS" over a BMS code "1964" on one side and "15" on the other side.

20mg Capsules: The hard capsules are brown, opaque and imprinted with "BMS" over a BMS code "1965" on one side and "20" on the other side.

30mg Capsules: The hard capsules are light and dark orange, opaque and imprinted with "BMS" over a BMS code "1966" on one side and "30" on the other side.

40mg Capsules: The hard capsules are dark orange, opaque and imprinted with "BMS" over a BMS code "1967" on one side and "40" on the other side.

4. CLINICAL PARTICULARS

4.1 Therapeutic indications

Zerit is indicated in combination with other antiretroviral medicinal products for the treatment of HIV infected patients.

4.2 Posology and method of administration

Oral use.

The therapy should be initiated by a doctor experienced in the management of HIV infection.

Adults: the recommended dosage is:

Patient weight	Zerit dosage
< 60 kg ≥ 60 kg	30 mg twice daily (every 12 hours) 40 mg twice daily

Adolescents, children and infants over the age of 3 months: the recommended dosage is:

Patient weight	Zerit dosage
< 30 kg ≥ 30 kg	1 mg/kg twice daily (every 12 hours) adult dosing

For optimal absorption, Zerit should be taken on an empty stomach (i.e. at least 1 hour prior to meals) but, if this is not possible, it may be taken with a light meal. Zerit may also be administered by carefully opening the hard capsule and mixing the contents with food.

Infants under the age of 3 months: please refer to the Summary of Product Characteristics of the powder formulation.

Elderly: Zerit has not been specifically investigated in patients over the age of 65.

Dose adjustments

Peripheral neuropathy: if symptoms of peripheral neuropathy develop (usually characterised by persistent numbness, tingling, or pain in the feet and/or hands) (see section 4.4), switching the patient to an alternate treatment regimen should be considered. In the rare cases when this is inappropriate, treatment with Zerit may be continued at 50% of the previous dosage while the symptoms of peripheral neuropathy are under close monitoring.

Hepatic impairment: no initial dosage adjustment is necessary.

Renal impairment: the following dosages are recommended:

	Zerit dosage (according to creatinine clearance)	
Patient weight	26-50 ml/min	≤ 25 ml/min (including dialysis dependence*)

< 60 kg	15 mg twice daily	15 mg every 24 hours
⩾ 60 kg	20 mg twice daily	20 mg every 24 hours

* Patients on haemodialysis should take Zerit after the completion of haemodialysis, and at the same time on non-dialysis days.

Since urinary excretion is also a major route of elimination of stavudine in paediatric patients, the clearance of stavudine may be altered in paediatric patients with renal impairment. Although there are insufficient data to recommend a specific dosage adjustment of Zerit in this patient population, a reduction in the dose and/or an increase in the interval between doses proportional to the reduction for adults should be considered.

4.3 Contraindications

Hypersensitivity to stavudine or to any of the excipients (see section 6.1).

4.4 Special warnings and special precautions for use

Peripheral neuropathy: patients with a history of peripheral neuropathy are at increased risk for development of neuropathy. If Zerit must be administered in this setting, careful clinical monitoring is essential. Symptoms of peripheral neuropathy are characterised by persistent numbness, tingling, or pain in the feet and/or hands.

Pancreatitis: patients with a history of pancreatitis had an incidence of approximately 5% on Zerit, as compared to approximately 2% in patients without such a history. Patients with a high risk of pancreatitis or those receiving products known to be associated with pancreatitis should be closely followed for symptoms of this condition.

Lactic acidosis:
lactic acidosis, usually associated with hepatomegaly and hepatic steatosis has been reported with the use of nucleoside reverse transcriptase inhibitors (NRTIs). Early symptoms (symptomatic hyperlactatemia) include benign digestive symptoms (nausea, vomiting and abdominal pain), non-specific malaise, loss of appetite, weight loss, respiratory symptoms (rapid and/or deep breathing) or neurological symptoms (including motor weakness). Lactic acidosis has a high mortality and may be associated with pancreatitis, liver failure, renal failure, or motor paralysis.
Lactic acidosis generally occurred after a few or several months of treatment.
Treatment with NRTIs should be discontinued if there is symptomatic hyperlactatemia and metabolic/lactic acidosis, progressive hepatomegaly, or rapidly elevating aminotransferase levels. Caution should be exercised when administering NRTIs to any patient (particularly obese women) with hepatomegaly, hepatitis or other known risk factors for liver disease and hepatic steatosis (including certain medicinal products and alcohol).
Patients co-infected with hepatitis C and treated with alpha interferon and ribavirin may constitute a special risk.
Patients at increased risk should be followed closely (see also section 4.6).

Liver disease: hepatitis or liver failure, which was fatal in some cases, has been reported. The safety and efficacy of Zerit has not been established in patients with significant underlying liver disorders. Patients with chronic hepatitis B or C and treated with combination antiretroviral therapy are at an increased risk of severe and potentially fatal hepatic adverse events. In case of concomitant antiviral therapy for hepatitis B or C, please refer also to the relevant product information for these medicinal products.

Patients with pre-existing liver dysfunction including chronic active hepatitis have an increased frequency of liver function abnormalities during combination antiretroviral therapy and should be monitored according to standard practice. If there is evidence of worsening liver disease in such patients, interruption or discontinuation of treatment must be considered.

In the event of rapidly elevating transaminase levels (ALT/AST, > 5 times upper limit of normal, ULN), discontinuation of Zerit and any potentially hepatotoxic medicinal products should be considered.

Immune reactivation syndrome: in HIV-infected patients with severe immune deficiency at the time of institution of combination antiretroviral therapy (CART), an inflammatory reaction to asymptomatic or residual opportunistic pathogens may arise and cause serious clinical conditions, or aggravation of symptoms. Typically, such reactions have been observed within the first few weeks or months of initiation of CART. Relevant examples are cytomegalovirus retinitis, generalised and/or focal mycobacterial infections, and Pneumocystis carinii pneumonia. Any inflammatory symptoms should be evaluated and treatment instituted when necessary.

Lipodystrophy and metabolic abnormalities: combination antiretroviral therapy has been associated with the redistribution of body fat (lipodystrophy) in HIV patients. The long-term consequences of these events are currently unknown. Knowledge about the mechanism is incomplete. A connection between visceral lipomatosis and Protease Inhibitors and lipoatrophy and NRTIs has been hypothesised. A higher risk of lipodystrophy has been associated with individual factors such as older age, and with drug related factors such as longer duration of antiretroviral treatment and associated metabolic disturbances. Clinical examination should include evaluation for physical signs of fat redistribution. Consideration should be given to the measurement of fasting serum lipids and blood glucose. Lipid disorders should be managed as clinically appropriate (see section 4.8).

Elderly: Zerit has not been specifically investigated in patients over the age of 65.

Infants under the age of 3 months: safety data is available from clinical trials up to 6 weeks of treatment in 179 newborns and infants < 3 months of age (see section 4.8).

Special consideration should be given to the antiretroviral treatment history and the resistance profile of the HIV strain of the mother.

Mitochondrial dysfunction: nucleoside and nucleotide analogues have been demonstrated *in vitro* and *in vivo* to cause a variable degree of mitochondrial damage. There have been reports of mitochondrial dysfunction in HIV-negative infants exposed *in utero* and/or post-natally to nucleoside analogues (see also section 4.8). The main adverse events reported are haematological disorders (anaemia, neutropenia), metabolic disorders (hyperlactatemia, hyperlipasemia). These events are often transitory. Some late-onset neurological disorders have been reported (hypertonia, convulsion, abnormal behaviour). Whether the neurological disorders are transient or permanent is currently unknown. Any child exposed *in utero* to nucleoside and nucleotide analogues, even HIV-negative children, should have clinical and laboratory follow-up and should be fully investigated for possible mitochondrial dysfunction in case of relevant signs or symptoms. These findings do not affect current national recommendations to use antiretroviral therapy in pregnant women to prevent vertical transmission of HIV.

Not recommended combinations: pancreatitis (fatal and nonfatal) and peripheral neuropathy (severe in some cases) have been reported in HIV infected patients receiving stavudine in association with hydroxyurea and didanosine. Hepatotoxicity and hepatic failure resulting in death were reported during postmarketing surveillance in HIV infected patients treated with antiretroviral agents and hydroxyurea; fatal hepatic events were reported most often in patients treated with stavudine, hydroxyurea and didanosine. Hence, hydroxyurea should not be used in the treatment of HIV infection.

Lactose intolerance: the hard capsules contain lactose (120 mg). Patients with rare hereditary problems of galactose intolerance, the Lapp lactase deficiency or glucose-galactose malabsorption, should not take this medicine.

4.5 Interaction with other medicinal products and other forms of Interaction

Since stavudine is actively secreted by the renal tubules, interactions with other actively secreted medicinal products are possible, e.g. with trimethoprim. No clinically relevant pharmacokinetic interaction has, however, been seen with lamivudine.

Zidovudine and stavudine are phosphorylated by the cellular enzyme (thymidine kinase), which preferentially phosphorylates zidovudine, thereby decreasing the phosphorylation of stavudine to its active triphosphate form. Zidovudine is therefore not recommended to be used in combination with stavudine.

In vitro studies indicate that the activation of stavudine is inhibited by doxorubicin and ribavirin but not by other medicinal products used in HIV infection which are similarly phosphorylated, e.g. didanosine, zalcitabine, ganciclovir and foscarnet. Stavudine's influence on the phosphorylation kinetics of nucleoside analogues other than zidovudine has not been investigated.

Clinically significant interactions of stavudine or stavudine plus didanosine with nelfinavir have not been observed.

Stavudine does not inhibit the major cytochrome P450 isoforms CYP1A2, CYP2C9, CYP2C19, CYP2D6, and CYP3A4; therefore, it is unlikely that clinically significant drug interactions will occur with drugs metabolised through these pathways.

Because stavudine is not protein-bound, it is not expected to affect the pharmacokinetics of protein-bound drugs.

There have been no formal interaction studies with other medicinal products.

4.6 Pregnancy and lactation

Clinical experience in pregnant women is limited, but congenital anomalies and abortions have been reported.

In study AI455-094, performed in South-Africa, 362 mother-infant pairs were included in a prevention of mother-to-child-transmission study. Treatment naive pregnant women were enrolled into the study at gestation week 34-36 and given antiretroviral treatment until delivery. Antiretroviral prophylaxis, the same medications as given to the mother, was given to the new-born infant within 36 hours of delivery and continued for 6 weeks. In the stavudine containing arms, the neonates were treated for 6 weeks with stavudine 1 mg/kg BID. The follow-up time was up to 24 weeks of age.

The mother-infant pairs were randomised to receive either stavudine (N= 91), didanosine (N= 94), stavudine + didanosine (N= 88) or zidovudine (N= 89).

95% Confidence intervals for the mother-to-child-transmission rates were 5.4-19.3% (stavudine), 5.2-18.7% (didanosine); 1.3-11.2% (stavudine + didanosine); and 1.9-12.6% for zidovudine.

Preliminary safety data from this study (see also section 4.8), showed an increased infant mortality in the stavudine + didanosine (10%) treatment group compared to the stavudine (2%), didanosine (3%) or zidovudine (6%) groups, with a higher incidence of stillbirths in the stavudine + didanosine group. Data on lactic acid in serum were not collected in this study.

However, lactic acidosis (see section 4.4), sometimes fatal, has been reported in pregnant women who received the combination of didanosine and stavudine with or without other anti-retroviral treatment. Embryo-foetal toxicities were seen only at high exposure levels in animals. Preclinical studies showed placental transfer of stavudine (see section 5.3). Until additional data become available, Zerit should be given during pregnancy only after special consideration; there is insufficient information to recommend Zerit for prevention of mother-to-child transmission of HIV. Furthermore, the combination of stavudine and didanosine should be used with caution during pregnancy and is recommended only if the potential benefit clearly outweighs the potential risk.

It is recommended that HIV infected women should not breast-feed under any circumstances in order to avoid transmission of HIV.

The data available on stavudine excretion into human breast milk are insufficient to assess the risk to the infant. Studies in lactating rats showed that stavudine is excreted in breast milk. Therefore, mothers should be instructed to discontinue breast-feeding prior to receiving Zerit.

4.7 Effects on ability to drive and use machines

Based on the pharmacodynamic properties of stavudine it is unlikely that Zerit affects the ability to drive or operate machinery.

4.8 Undesirable effects

Adults: extensive safety experience is available for Zerit immediate-release formulations used as monotherapy and in combination regimens. Many of the serious undesirable effects with stavudine were consistent with the course of HIV infection or with the side effects of concomitant therapies.

The safety of Zerit prolonged-release hard capsules has been compared to Zerit immediate-release formulations, each in combination with efavirenz and lamivudine, in two randomised double-blind clinical trials. The safety profile of the prolonged-release capsule was not substantially different from that of the immediate-release form.

Peripheral neuropathy: in two clinical trials comparing Zerit immediate-release with Zerit prolonged-release, the frequency of peripheral neurologic symptoms was 19% (6% for moderate to severe) for Zerit immediate-release, with a rate of discontinuation due to neuropathy of 2%. Dose-related peripheral neuropathy requiring dose modification occurred in monotherapy trials with Zerit immediate-release (see sections 4.2 and 4.4). The patients usually experienced resolution of symptoms after dose reduction or interruption.

Pancreatitis: pancreatitis, occasionally fatal, has been reported in up to 2-3% of patients enrolled in monotherapy clinical studies(see section 4.4). Pancreatitis was reported in < 1% of patients for Zerit in studies comparing Zerit prolonged-release capsule with Zerit immediate-release.

Lactic acidosis: cases of lactic acidosis, sometimes fatal, usually associated with severe hepatomegaly and hepatic steatosis, have been reported with the use of nucleoside analogues (see section 4.4).

Hepatitis or liver failure, which was fatal in some cases, has been reported with the use of stavudine and with other nucleoside analogues (see section 4.4).

Immune reactivation syndrome: in HIV-infected patients with severe immune deficiency at the time of initiation of combination antiretroviral therapy (CART), an inflammatory reaction to asymptomatic or residual opportunistic infections may arise (see section 4.4).

Lipodystrophy and metabolic abnormalities: combination antiretroviral therapy has been associated with redistribution of body fat (lipodystrophy) in HIV patients including the loss of peripheral and facial subcutaneous fat, increased intra-abdominal and visceral fat, breast hypertrophy and dorsocervical fat accumulation (buffalo hump).

Combination antiretroviral therapy has been associated with metabolic abnormalities such as hypertriglyceridaemia, hypercholesterolaemia, insulin resistance, hyperglycaemia and hyperlactataemia (see section 4.4).

The frequency of adverse reactions listed below is defined using the following convention:

very common (⩾ 1/10); common (⩾ 1/100, < 1/10); uncommon (⩾ 1/1,000, < 1/100); rare (⩾ 1/10,000, < 1/1,000); very rare (< 1/10,000).

Undesirable effects (moderate to severe) were reported from 467 patients treated with Zerit immediate-release in combination with lamivudine and efavirenz in two randomised clinical trials and an ongoing long-term follow-up study (total follow-up: median 56 weeks ranging up to 119 weeks). The following undesirable effects considered possibly related to study regimen based on investigators' attribution, have been identified:

Endocrine disorders:	uncommon: gynaecomastia
Gastrointestinal disorders:	common: diarrhoea, nausea, abdominal pain, dyspepsia uncommon: pancreatitis, vomiting
General disorders and administration site conditions:	common: fatigue uncommon: asthenia
Hepato-biliary disorders:	uncommon: hepatitis or jaundice
Metabolism and nutrition disorders:	common: lipodystrophy uncommon: lactic acidosis (in some cases involving motor weakness), anorexia
Musculoskeletal, connective tissue and bone disorders:	uncommon: arthralgia, myalgia
Nervous system disorders:	common: peripheral neurologic symptoms including peripheral neuropathy, paresthesia, and peripheral neuritis; dizziness; abnormal dreams; headache, insomnia; abnormal thinking; somnolence
Psychiatric disorders:	common: depression uncommon: anxiety, emotional lability
Skin and subcutaneous disorders:	common: rash, pruritus uncommon: urticaria

Discontinuation due to undesirable events was 7% for the patients treated with Zerit immediate-release.

Laboratory abnormalities reported in these two trials and an ongoing follow-up study included elevations of ALT (> 5 × ULN) in 3%, of AST (> 5 × ULN) in 3%, of lipase (≥ 2.1 ULN) in 3% of the patients in the Zerit group. Neutropenia (< 750 cells/mm^3) was reported in 5%, thrombocytopenia (platelets < 50,000/mm^3) in 2%, and low haemoglobin (< 8 g/dl) in < 1% of patients receiving Zerit.

Macrocytosis was not evaluated in these trials, but was found to be associated with Zerit immediate-release in an earlier trial (MCV > 112 fl occurred in 30% of patients treated with Zerit immediate-release).

Adolescents, children and infants: undesirable effects and serious laboratory abnormalities reported to occur in paediatric patients ranging in age from birth through adolescence who received stavudine in clinical studies were generally similar in type and frequency to those seen in adults. However, clinically significant peripheral neuropathy is less frequent. These studies include ACTG 240, where 105 paediatric patients ages 3 month to 6 years received Zerit 2 mg/kg/day for a median of 6.4 months; a controlled clinical trial where 185 newborns received Zerit 2 mg/kg/day either alone or in combination with didanosine from birth through 6 weeks of age; and a clinical trial where 8 newborns received Zerit 2 mg/kg/day in combination with didanosine and nelfinavir from birth through 4 weeks of age.

In study AI455-094 (see also section 4.6), the safety follow-up period was restricted to only six months, which may be insufficient to capture long-term data on neurological adverse events and mitochondrial toxicity. Relevant grade 3-4 laboratory abnormalities in the 91 stavudine treated infants were low neutrophils in 7%, low hemoglobin in 1%, ALT increase in 1% and no lipase abnormality. Data on lactic acid in serum were not collected. No notable differences in the frequency of adverse drug reactions were seen between treatment groups. There was, however, an increased infant mortality in the stavudine + didanosine (10%) treatment group compared to the stavudine (2%), didanosine (3%) or zidovudine (6%) groups, with a higher incidence of stillbirths in the stavudine + didanosine group.

Postmarketing

The following events have been reported spontaneously during postmarketing experience (the calculation for the frequency is based on a rough estimate of patient exposure):

Blood and lymphatic system disorders:	very rare: thrombocytopenia
Metabolic and nutrition disorders:	common: asymptomatic hyperlactatemia, rare: lactic acidosis
Hepato-biliary disorders:	very rare: hepatic steatosis, hepatitis and liver failure
Nervous system disorders:	very rare: motor weakness (most often reported in the setting of symptomatic hyperlactatemia or lactic acidosis syndrome)

Mitochondrial dysfunction: review of the postmarketing safety database shows that adverse events indicative of mitochondrial dysfunction have been reported in the neonate and infant population exposed to one or more nucleoside analogues (see also section 4.4). The HIV status for the newborns and infants ≤ 3 months of age was negative, for older infants it tended to be positive. The profile of the adverse events for newborns and infants ≤ 3 months of age showed increases in lactic acid levels, neutropenia, anaemia, thrombocytopenia, hepatic transaminase increases and increased lipids, including hypertriglyceridaemia. The number of reports in older infants was too small to identify a pattern.

4.9 Overdose

Experience in adults treated with up to 12 times the recommended daily dosage revealed no acute toxicity. Complications of chronic overdosage could include peripheral neuropathy and hepatic dysfunction. The mean haemodialysis clearance of stavudine is 120 ml/min. The contribution of this to the total elimination in an overdose situation is unknown. It is not known whether stavudine is removed by peritoneal dialysis.

5. PHARMACOLOGICAL PROPERTIES

5.1 Pharmacodynamic properties

Pharmacotherapeutic group: Nucleoside reverse transcriptase inhibitor

ATC code: J05AF04.

Stavudine, a thymidine analog, is an antiviral agent with *in vitro* activity against HIV in human cells. It is phosphorylated by cellular kinases to stavudine triphosphate which inhibits HIV reverse transcriptase by competing with the natural substrate, thymidine triphosphate. It also inhibits viral DNA synthesis by causing DNA chain termination due to a lack of the 3'-hydroxyl group necessary for DNA elongation. Cellular DNA polymerase γ is also sensitive to inhibition by stavudine triphosphate, while cellular polymerases α and β are inhibited at concentrations 4,000-fold and 40-fold higher, respectively, than that needed to inhibit HIV reverse transcriptase.

Stavudine treatment can select for and/or maintain mutations associated with zidovudine resistance. Isolates containing these mutations remain sensitive to stavudine. The clinical relevance of these findings is unknown.

The activity of stavudine is affected by multi-drug resistance associated mutations such as Q151 M. A more than 10-fold reduced sensitivity to stavudine has been reported for some strains with reduced sensitivity to zidovudine and lamivudine. No mutations associated with high degree resistance specifically to stavudine have been revealed *in vivo*.

Clinical efficacy

Zerit immediate-release has been studied in combination with other antiretroviral agents, e.g. didanosine, lamivudine, ritonavir, indinavir, saquinavir, efavirenz, and nelfinavir.

Two double-blind triple-therapy studies have demonstrated similar antiviral efficacy and tolerability with Zerit prolonged-release capsule compared to Zerit immediate-release, each given in combination of lamivudine and efavirenz.

Study AI455-099 was a 48-week, randomised, double-blind study comparing Zerit prolonged-release capsule (100 mg once daily) with Zerit (40 mg twice daily), each in combination with lamivudine (150 mg twice daily) plus efavirenz (600 mg once daily), in 783 treatment-naive patients, with a median CD4 cell count of 277 cells/mm^3 (range 61 to 1,215 cells/mm^3) and a median plasma HIV-1 RNA of 4.80 $\log_{10}$ copies/ml (range 2.6 to 5.9 $\log_{10}$ copies/ml) at baseline. Patients were primarily males (69%) and non-white (58%) with a median age of 33 years (range 18 to 69 years).

Study AI455-096 was a 48-week, randomised, double-blind study comparing Zerit prolonged-release capsule (100 mg once daily) with Zerit (40 mg twice daily), each in combination with lamivudine (150 mg twice daily) plus efavirenz (600 mg once daily), in 150 treatment-naive patients, with a median CD4 cell count of 285 cells/mm^3 (range 63 to 962 cells/mm^3) and a median plasma HIV-1 RNA of 4.65 $\log_{10}$ copies/ml (range 2.3 to 5.9 $\log_{10}$ copies/ml) at baseline. Patients were primarily males (75%) and white (70%) with a median age of 34 years (range 20 to 69 years).

The results of AI455-099 and AI455-096 are presented in the table below:

(see Table 1 below)

In adolescents, children and infants, use of stavudine is supported by evidence from adequate and well-controlled studies in adults with additional pharmacokinetic and safety data in paediatric patients (see also sections 4.8 and 5.2).

5.2 Pharmacokinetic properties

Adults

Absorption: the absolute bioavailability is 86±18%. After multiple oral administration of 0.5-0.67 mg/kg doses, a Cmax value of 810±175 ng/ml was obtained. Cmax and AUC increased proportionally with dose in the dose ranges, intravenous 0.0625-0.75 mg/kg, and oral 0.033-4.0 mg/kg.

In eight patients receiving 40 mg twice daily in the fasted state, steady-state AUC_{0-12h} was 1284±227 ng>/>h/ml (18%) (mean ± SD [% CV]), Cmax was 536±146 ng/ml (27%), and C_{min} was 9±8 ng/ml (89%). A study in asymptomatic patients demonstrated that systemic exposure is similar while Cmax is lower and T_{max} is prolonged when stavudine is administered with a standardised, high-fat meal compared with fasting conditions. The clinical significance of this is unknown.

Distribution: the apparent volume of distribution at steady state is 46±21 l. It was not possible to detect stavudine in cerebrospinal fluid until at least 2 hours after oral administration. Four hours after administration, the CSF/plasma ratio was 0.39±0.06. No significant accumulation of stavudine is observed with repeated administration every 6, 8, or 12 hours.

Binding of stavudine to serum proteins was negligible over the concentration range of 0.01 to 11.4 μg/ml. Stavudine distributes equally between red blood cells and plasma.

Metabolism: The metabolism of stavudine has not been elucidated in humans. Studies in monkeys indicate that approximately 50% is excreted unchanged in the urine, most of the remainder is hydrolysed to thymine and sugar.

Elimination: the terminal elimination half-life is 1.3±0.2 hours after a single dose, and 1.4±0.2 hours after multiple doses, and is independent of dose. *In vitro*, stavudine triphosphate has an intracellular half-life of 3.5 hours in CEM T-cells (a human T-lymphoblastoid cell line) and peripheral blood mononuclear cells, supporting twice daily dosing.

Total clearance of stavudine is 594±164 ml/min, and renal clearance is 237±98 ml/min, indicating active tubular

Table 1

Study	Percent of patients with HIV RNA < 400 copies/ml Treatment response (%)[a]	Percent of patients with HIV RNA < 50 copies/ml Treatment response (%)[a]	HIV RNA Mean Change from Baseline ($\log_{10}$ copies/ml)	CD4 Mean change from Baseline (cells/mm^3)
AI455-099 (48 weeks)				
Zerit prolonged-release capsule + lamivudine + efavirenz (n = 392)	78	54	-2.86	+202
Zerit immediate-release + lamivudine + efavirenz (n = 391)	73	55	-2.83	+182
AI455-096 (48 weeks)				
Zerit prolonged-release capsule + lamivudine + efavirenz (n = 74)	70	41	-2.74	+232
Zerit immediate-release + lamivudine + efavirenz (n = 76)	66	38	-2.64	+195

[a] Percent of patients who have HIV RNA < 400 c/ml or < 50 c/ml and do not meet any criteria for treatment failure including the occurrence of a new AIDS-defining diagnosis.

secretion in addition to glomerular filtration. After intravenous administration, 42±7% of dose is excreted unchanged in the urine. The corresponding values after oral single and multiple dose administration are 34±5% and 40±12%, respectively. The remaining 60% of the drug is presumably eliminated by endogenous pathways. The half-life of stavudine is approximately 2 hours.

The pharmacokinetics of stavudine was independent of time, since the ratio between $AUC_{(ss)}$ at steady state and the $AUC_{(0-t)}$ after the first dose was approximately 1. Intra- and interindividual variation in pharmacokinetic characteristics of stavudine is low, approximately 15% and 25%, respectively, after oral administration.

Special Populations

Adolescents, children and infants: total exposure to stavudine was comparable between adolescents, children and infants ≥ 14 days receiving the 2 mg/kg/day dose and adults receiving 1 mg/kg/day. Apparent oral clearance was approximately 14 ml/min/kg for infants ages 5 weeks to 15 years, 12 ml/min/kg for infants ages 14 to 28 days, and 5 ml/min/kg for infants on the day of birth. Two to three hours post-dose, CSF/plasma ratios of stavudine ranged from 16% to 125% (mean of 59%±35%).

Renal impairment: the clearance of stavudine decreases as creatinine clearance decreases; therefore, it is recommended that the dosage of Zerit be adjusted in patients with reduced renal function (see section 4.2).

Hepatic impairment: stavudine pharmacokinetics in patients with hepatic impairment were similar to those in patients with normal hepatic function.

5.3 Preclinical safety data

Animal data showed embryo-foetal toxicity at very high exposure levels. An *ex vivo* study using a term human placenta model demonstrated that stavudine reaches the foetal circulation by simple diffusion. A rat study also showed placental transfer of stavudine, with the foetal tissue concentration approximately 50% of the maternal plasma concentration.

Stavudine was genotoxic in *in vitro* tests in human lymphocytes possessing triphosphorylating activity (in which no no-effect level was established), in mouse fibroblasts, and in an *in vivo* test for chromosomal aberrations. Similar effects have been observed with other nucleoside analogues.

Stavudine was carcinogenic in mice (liver tumours) and rats (liver tumours: cholangiocellular, hepatocellular, mixed hepatocholangiocellular, and/or vascular; and urinary bladder carcinomas) at very high exposure levels. No carcinogenicity was noted at doses of 400 mg/kg/day in mice and 600 mg/kg/day in rats, corresponding to exposures ~ 39 and 168 times the expected human exposure, respectively, suggesting an insignificant carcinogenic potential of stavudine in clinical therapy.

6. PHARMACEUTICAL PARTICULARS

6.1 List of excipients

Capsule contents:

Lactose

Magnesium stearate

Microcrystalline cellulose

Sodium starch glycolate

Capsule shell:

Gelatin

Iron oxide colorant (E172)

Silicon dioxide

Sodium laurilsulphate

Titanium dioxide (E171)

The capsule shells are marked using edible black printing ink containing:

Shellac

Propylene Glycol

Purified Water

Potassium Hydroxide

Iron Oxide (E172)

6.2 Incompatibilities

Not applicable.

6.3 Shelf life

2 years.

6.4 Special precautions for storage

Do not store above 30°C.

Store in the original carton.

6.5 Nature and contents of container

Aclar/aluminum blisters with 14 hard capsules per card and 4 cards (56 hard capsules) per carton.

6.6 Instructions for use and handling

No special requirements.

7. MARKETING AUTHORISATION HOLDER

BRISTOL-MYERS SQUIBB PHARMA EEIG

Uxbridge Business Park

Sanderson Road

Uxbridge UB8 1DH

United Kingdom

8. MARKETING AUTHORISATION NUMBER(S)

Capsules 15mg	Blister pack of 56	EU/1/96/009/002
Capsules 20mg	Blister pack of 56	EU/1/96/009/004
Capsules 30mg	Blister pack of 56	EU/1/96/009/006
Capsules 40mg	Blister pack of 56	EU/1/96/009/008

9. DATE OF FIRST AUTHORISATION/RENEWAL OF THE AUTHORISATION

Date of first authorisation: 08 May 1996

Date of last renewal: 08 June 2001

10. DATE OF REVISION OF THE TEXT

August 2005

Zerit 200 mg Powder for Oral Solution

(Bristol-Myers Squibb Pharmaceuticals Ltd)

1. NAME OF THE MEDICINAL PRODUCT

Zerit 200 mg powder for oral solution

2. QUALITATIVE AND QUANTITATIVE COMPOSITION

Stavudine 200 mg.

The reconstituted solution contains 1 mg of stavudine per ml.

For excipients, see section 6.1.

3. PHARMACEUTICAL FORM

Powder for oral solution.

4. CLINICAL PARTICULARS

4.1 Therapeutic indications

Zerit is indicated in combination with other antiretroviral medicinal products for the treatment of HIV infected patients.

4.2 Posology and method of administration

Oral use.

The therapy should be initiated by a doctor experienced in the management of HIV infection.

Adults: the recommended dosage is:

Patient weight	Zerit dosage
< 60 kg ≥ 60 kg	30 mg twice daily (every 12 hours) 40 mg twice daily (every 12 hours)

Adolescents, children and infants: the recommended dosage is:

Patient age and/or weight	Zerit dosage
From birth* to 13 days old	0.5 mg/kg twice daily (every 12 hours)
At least 14 days old and < 30 kg	1 mg/kg twice daily (every 12 hours)
≥ 30 kg	adult dosing

*The reduced posology in neonates from 0 to 13 days is based on average study data and may not correspond to invidual variation in kidney maturation. Dosing recommendations are not available for neonates with a gestational age < 37 weeks.

For optimal absorption, Zerit should be taken on an empty stomach (i.e. at least 1 hour prior to meals) but, if this is not possible, it may be taken with a light meal.

Elderly: Zerit has not been specifically investigated in patients over the age of 65.

Dose adjustments

Peripheral neuropathy: if symptoms of peripheral neuropathy develop (usually characterised by persistent numbness, tingling, or pain in the feet and/or hands) (see section 4.4), switching the patient to an alternate treatment regimen should be considered. In the rare cases when this is inappropriate, treatment with Zerit may be continued at 50% of the previous dosage while the symptoms of peripheral neuropathy are under close monitoring.

Hepatic impairment: no initial dosage adjustment is necessary.

Renal impairment: the following dosages are recommended:

	Zerit dosage (according to creatinine clearance)	
Patient weight	26-50 ml/min	≤ 25 ml/min (including dialysis dependence*)
< 60 kg	15 mg twice daily	15 mg every 24 hours
≥ 60 kg	20 mg twice daily	20 mg every 24 hours

* Patients on haemodialysis should take Zerit after the completion of haemodialysis, and at the same time on non-dialysis days.

Since urinary excretion is also a major route of elimination of stavudine in paediatric patients, the clearance of stavudine may be altered in paediatric patients with renal impairment. Although there are insufficient data to recommend a specific dosage adjustment of Zerit in this patient population, a reduction in the dose and/or an increase in the interval between doses proportional to the reduction for adults should be considered.

4.3 Contraindications

Hypersensitivity to stavudine or to any of the excipients (see section 6.1).

4.4 Special warnings and special precautions for use

Peripheral neuropathy: patients with a history of peripheral neuropathy are at increased risk for development of neuropathy. If Zerit must be administered in this setting, careful monitoring is essential. Symptoms of peripheral neuropathy are characterised by persistent numbness, tingling, or pain in the feet and/or hands.

Pancreatitis: patients with a history of pancreatitis had an incidence of approximately 5% on Zerit, as compared to approximately 2% in patients without such a history. Patients with a high risk of pancreatitis or those receiving products known to be associated with pancreatitis should be closely followed for symptoms of this condition.

Lactic acidosis:

lactic acidosis, usually associated with hepatomegaly and hepatic steatosis has been reported with the use of nucleoside reverse transcriptase inhibitors (NRTIs). Early symptoms (symptomatic hyperlactatemia) include benign digestive symptoms (nausea, vomiting and abdominal pain), non-specific malaise, loss of appetite, weight loss, respiratory symptoms (rapid and/or deep breathing) or neurological symptoms (including motor weakness). Lactic acidosis has a high mortality and may be associated with pancreatitis, liver failure, renal failure, or motor paralysis.

Lactic acidosis generally occurred after a few or several months of treatment.

Treatment with NRTIs should be discontinued if there is symptomatic hyperlactatemia and metabolic/lactic acidosis, progressive hepatomegaly, or rapidly elevating aminotransferase levels. Caution should be exercised when administering NRTIs to any patient (particularly obese women) with hepatomegaly, hepatitis or other known risk factors for liver disease and hepatic steatosis (including certain medicinal products and alcohol).

Patients co-infected with hepatitis C and treated with alpha interferon and ribavirin may constitute a special risk.

Patients at increased risk should be followed closely (see also section 4.6).

Liver disease: hepatitis or liver failure, which was fatal in some cases, has been reported. The safety and efficacy of Zerit has not been established in patients with significant underlying liver disorders. Patients with chronic hepatitis B or C and treated with combination antiretroviral therapy are at an increased risk of severe and potentially fatal hepatic adverse events. In case of concomitant antiviral therapy for hepatitis B or C, please refer also to the relevant product information for these medicinal products.

Patients with pre-existing liver dysfunction including chronic active hepatitis have an increased frequency of liver function abnormalities during combination antiretroviral therapy and should be monitored according to standard practice. If there is evidence of worsening liver disease in such patients, interruption or discontinuation of treatment must be considered.

In the event of rapidly elevating transaminase levels (ALT/AST, > 5 times upper limit of normal, ULN), discontinuation of Zerit and any potentially hepatotoxic medicinal products should be considered.

Immune reactivation syndrome: in HIV-infected patients with severe immune deficiency at the time of institution of combination antiretroviral therapy (CART), an inflammatory reaction to asymptomatic or residual opportunistic pathogens may arise and cause serious clinical conditions, or aggravation of symptoms. Typically, such reactions have been observed within the first few weeks or months of initiation of CART. Relevant examples are cytomegalovirus retinitis, generalised and/or focal mycobacterial infections, and Pneumocystis carinii pneumonia. Any inflammatory symptoms should be evaluated and treatment instituted when necessary.

Lipodystrophy and metabolic abnormalities: combination antiretroviral therapy has been associated with the redistribution of body fat (lipodystrophy) in HIV patients. The long-term consequences of these events are currently unknown. Knowledge about the mechanism is incomplete. A connection between visceral lipomatosis and Protease Inhibitors and lipoatrophy and NRTIs has been hypothesised. A higher risk of lipodystrophy has been associated with individual factors such as older age, and with drug related factors such as longer duration of antiretroviral treatment and associated metabolic disturbances. Clinical examination should include evaluation for physical signs of fat redistribution. Consideration should be given to the measurement of fasting serum lipids and blood glucose.

Lipid disorders should be managed as clinically appropriate (see section 4.8).

Elderly: Zerit has not been specifically investigated in patients over the age of 65.

Diabetic patients: the constituted powder for oral solution contains 50 mg sucrose per ml of constituted solution.

Infants under the age of 3 months: safety data is available from clinical trials up to 6 weeks of treatment in 179 newborns and infants < 3 months of age (see section 4.6).

Special consideration should be given to the antiretroviral treatment history and the resistance profile of the HIV strain of the mother.

Mitochondrial dysfunction: nucleoside and nucleotide analogues have been demonstrated *in vitro* and *in vivo* to cause a variable degree of mitochondrial damage. There have been reports of mitochondrial dysfunction in HIV-negative infants exposed *in utero* and/or post-natally to nucleoside analogues (see also section 4.8). The main adverse events reported are haematological disorders (anaemia, neutropenia), metabolic disorders (hyperlactatemia, hyperlipasemia). These events are often transitory. Some late-onset neurological disorders have been reported (hypertonia, convulsion, abnormal behaviour). Whether the neurological disorders are transient or permanent is currently unknown. Any child exposed *in utero* to nucleoside and nucleotide analogues, even HIV-negative children, should have clinical and laboratory follow-up and should be fully investigated for possible mitochondrial dysfunction in case of relevant signs or symptoms. These findings do not affect current national recommendations to use antiretroviral therapy in pregnant women to prevent vertical transmission of HIV.

Not recommended combinations: pancreatitis (fatal and nonfatal) and peripheral neuropathy (severe in some cases) have been reported in HIV infected patients receiving stavudine in association with hydroxyurea and didanosine. Hepatotoxicity and hepatic failure resulting in death were reported during postmarketing surveillance in HIV infected patients treated with antiretroviral agents and hydroxyurea; fatal hepatic events were reported most often in patients treated with stavudine, hydroxyurea and didanosine. Hence, hydroxyurea should not be used in the treatment of HIV infection.

4.5 Interaction with other medicinal products and other forms of Interaction

Since stavudine is actively secreted by the renal tubules, interactions with other actively secreted medicinal products are possible, e.g. with trimethoprim. No clinically relevant pharmacokinetic interaction has, however, been seen with lamivudine.

Zidovudine and stavudine are phosphorylated by the cellular enzyme (thymidine kinase), which preferentially phosphorylates zidovudine, thereby decreasing the phosphorylation of stavudine to its active triphosphate form. Zidovudine is therefore not recommended to be used in combination with stavudine.

In vitro studies indicate that the activation of stavudine is inhibited by doxorubicin and ribavirin but not by other medicinal products used in HIV infection which are similarly phosphorylated, e.g. didanosine, zalcitabine, ganciclovir and foscarnet. Stavudine's influence on the phosphorylation kinetics of nucleoside analogues other than zidovudine has not been investigated.

Clinically significant interactions of stavudine or stavudine plus didanosine with nelfinavir have not been observed.

Stavudine does not inhibit the major cytochrome P450 isoforms CYP1A2, CYP2C9, CYP2C19, CYP2D6, and CYP3A4; therefore, it is unlikely that clinically significant drug interactions will occur with drugs metabolised through these pathways.

Because stavudine is not protein-bound, it is not expected to affect the pharmacokinetics of protein-bound drugs.

There have been no formal interaction studies with other medicinal products.

4.6 Pregnancy and lactation

Clinical experience in pregnant women is limited, but congenital anomalies and abortions have been reported with the use of nucleoside analogues.

In study AI455-094, performed in South-Africa, 362 mother-infant pairs were included in a prevention of mother-to-child-transmission study. Treatment naive pregnant women were enrolled into the study at gestation week 34-36 and given antiretroviral treatment until delivery. Antiretroviral prophylaxis, the same medications as given to the mother, was given to the new-born infant within 36 hours of delivery and continued for 6 weeks. In the stavudine containing arms, the neonates were treated for 6 weeks with stavudine 1 mg/kg BID. The follow-up time was up to 24 weeks of age.

The mother-infant pairs were randomised to receive either stavudine (N= 91), didanosine (N= 94), stavudine + didanosine (N= 88) or zidovudine (N= 89).

95% Confidence intervals for the mother-to-child-transmission rates were 5.4-19.3% (stavudine), 5.2-18.7% (didanosine); 1.3-11.2% (stavudine + didanosine); and 1.9-12.6% for zidovudine.

Preliminary safety data from this study (see also section 4.8), showed an increased infant mortality in the stavudine + didanosine (10%) treatment group compared to the stavudine (2%), didanosine (3%) or zidovudine (6%) groups, with a higher incidence of stillbirths in the stavudine + didanosine group. Data on lactic acid in serum were not collected in this study.

However, lactic acidosis (see section 4.4), sometimes fatal, has been reported in pregnant women who received the combination of didanosine and stavudine with or without other anti-retroviral treatment. Embryo-foetal toxicities were seen only at high exposure levels in animals. Preclinical studies showed placental transfer of stavudine (see section 5.3). Until additional data become available, Zerit should be given during pregnancy only after special consideration; there is insufficient information to recommend Zerit for prevention of mother-to-child transmission of HIV. Furthermore, the combination of stavudine and didanosine should be used with caution during pregnancy and is recommended only if the potential benefit clearly outweighs the potential risk.

It is recommended that HIV infected women should not breast-feed under any circumstances in order to avoid transmission of HIV.

The data available on stavudine excretion into human breast milk are insufficient to assess the risk to the infant. Studies in lactating rats showed that stavudine is excreted in breast milk. Therefore, mothers should be instructed to discontinue breast-feeding prior to receiving Zerit.

4.7 Effects on ability to drive and use machines

Based on the pharmacodynamic properties of stavudine it is unlikely that Zerit affects the ability to drive or operate machinery.

4.8 Undesirable effects

Adults: extensive safety experience is available for Zerit immediate-release formulations used as monotherapy and in combination regimens. Many of the serious undesirable effects with stavudine were consistent with the course of HIV infection or with the side effects of concomitant therapies.

The safety of Zeritprolonged-release hard capsules has been compared to Zerit immediate-release formulations, each in combination with efavirenz and lamivudine, in two randomised double-blind clinical trials. The safety profile of the prolonged-release capsule was not substantially different from that of the immediate-release form.

Peripheral neuropathy: in two clinical trials comparing 200 immediate-release with Zerit prolonged-release, the frequency of peripheral neurologic symptoms was 19% (6% for moderate to severe) for Zerit immediate-release, with a rate of discontinuation due to neuropathy of 2%. Dose-related peripheral neuropathy requiring dose modification occurred in monotherapy trials with Zerit immediate-release (see sections 4.2 and 4.4). The patients usually experienced resolution of symptoms after dose reduction or interruption.

Pancreatitis: pancreatitis, occasionally fatal, has been reported in up to 2-3% of patients enrolled in monotherapy clinical studies(see section 4.4). Pancreatitis was reported in < 1% of patients for Zerit in studies comparing Zerit prolonged-release capsule with Zerit immediate-release.

Lactic Acidosis: cases of lactic acidosis, sometimes fatal, usually associated with severe hepatomegaly and hepatic steatosis, have been reported with the use of nucleoside analogues (see section 4.4).

Hepatitis or liver failure, which was fatal in some cases, has been reported with the use of stavudine and with other nucleoside analogues (see section 4.4).

Immune reactivation syndrome: in HIV-infected patients with severe immune deficiency at the time of initiation of combination antiretroviral therapy (CART), an inflammatory reaction to asymptomatic or residual opportunistic infections may arise (see section 4.4).

Lipodystrophy and metabolic abnormalities: combination antiretroviral therapy has been associated with redistribution of body fat (lipodystrophy) in HIV patients including the loss of peripheral and facial subcutaneous fat, increased intra-abdominal and visceral fat, breast hypertrophy and dorsocervical fat accumulation (buffalo hump).

Combination antiretroviral therapy has been associated with metabolic abnormalities such as hypertriglyceridaemia, hypercholesterolaemia, insulin resistance, hyperglycaemia and hyperlactataemia (see section 4.4).

The frequency of adverse reactions listed below is defined using the following convention:

very common (⩾ 1/10); common (⩾ 1/100, < 1/10); uncommon (⩾ 1/1,000, < 1/100); rare (⩾ 1/10,000, < 1/1,000); very rare (< 1/10,000).

Undesirable effects (moderate to severe) were reported from 467 patients treated with Zerit immediate-release in combination with lamivudine and efavirenz in two randomised clinical trials and an ongoing long-term follow-up study (total follow-up: median 56 weeks ranging up to 119 weeks). The following undesirable effects considered possibly related to study regimen based on investigators' attribution, have been identified:

Endocrine disorders:	uncommon: gynaecomastia
Gastrointestinal disorders:	common: diarrhoea, nausea, abdominal pain, dyspepsia uncommon: pancreatitis, vomiting
General disorders and administration site conditions:	common: fatigue uncommon: asthenia
Hepato-biliary disorders:	uncommon: hepatitis or jaundice
Metabolism and nutrition disorders:	common: lipodystrophy uncommon: lactic acidosis (in some cases involving motor weakness), anorexia
Musculoskeletal, connective tissue and bone disorders:	uncommon: arthralgia, myalgia
Nervous system disorders:	common: peripheral neurologic symptoms including peripheral neuropathy, paresthesia, and peripheral neuritis; dizziness; abnormal dreams; headache, insomnia; abnormal thinking; somnolence
Psychiatric disorders:	common: depression uncommon: anxiety, emotional lability
Skin and subcutaneous disorders:	common: rash, pruritus uncommon: urticaria

Discontinuation due to undesirable events was 7% for the patients treated with Zerit immediate-release.

Laboratory abnormalities reported in these two trials and an ongoing follow-up study included elevations of ALT (> 5 × ULN) in 3%, of AST (> 5 × ULN) in 3%, of lipase (⩾ 2.1 ULN) in 3% of the patients in the Zerit group. Neutropenia (< 750 cells/mm^3) was reported in 5%, thrombocytopenia (platelets < 50,000/mm^3) in 2%, and low haemoglobin (< 8 g/dl) in < 1% of patients receiving Zerit.

Macrocytosis was not evaluated in these trials, but was found to be associated with Zerit immediate-release in an earlier trial (MCV > 112 fl occurred in 30% of patients treated with Zerit immediate-release).

Adolescents, children and infants: undesirable effects and serious laboratory abnormalities reported to occur in paediatric patients ranging in age from birth through adolescence who received stavudine in clinical studies were generally similar in type and frequency to those seen in adults. However, clinically significant peripheral neuropathy is less frequent. These studies include ACTG 240, where 105 paediatric patients ages 3 months to 6 years received Zerit 2 mg/kg/day for a median of 6.4 months; a controlled clinical trial where 185 newborns received Zerit 2 mg/kg/day either alone or in combination with didanosine from birth through 6 weeks of age; and a clinical trial where 8 newborns received Zerit 2 mg/kg/day in combination with didanosine and nelfinavir from birth through 4 weeks of age.

In study AI455-094 (see also section 4.6), the safety follow-up period was restricted to only six months, which may be insufficient to capture long-term data on neurological adverse events and mitochondrial toxicity. Relevant grade 3-4 laboratory abnormalities in the 91 stavudine treated infants were low neutrophils in 7%, low hemoglobin in 1%, ALT increase in 1% and no lipase abnormality. Data on lactic acid in serum were not collected. No notable differences in the frequency of adverse drug reactions were seen between treatment groups. There was, however, an increased infant mortality in the stavudine + didanosine (10%) treatment group compared to the stavudine (2%), didanosine (3%) or zidovudine (6%) groups, with a higher incidence of stillbirths in the stavudine + didanosine group.

Postmarketing

The following events have been reported spontaneously during postmarketing experience (the calculation for the frequency is based on a rough estimate of patient exposure):

Blood and lymphatic system disorders:	very rare: thrombocytopenia
Metabolic and nutrition disorders:	common: asymptomatic hyperlactatemia, rare: lactic acidosis
Hepato-biliary disorders:	very rare: hepatic steatosis, hepatitis and liver failure
Nervous system disorders:	very rare: motor weakness (most often reported in the setting of symptomatic hyperlactatemia or lactic acidosis syndrome)

Mitochondrial dysfunction: review of the postmarketing safety database shows that adverse events indicative of mitochondrial dysfunction have been reported in the neonate and infant population exposed to one or more nucleoside analogues (see also section 4.4). The HIV status for the newborns and infants ⩽ 3 months of age was negative, for older infants it tended to be positive. The profile of the adverse events for newborns and infants ⩽ 3 months of age showed increases in lactic acid levels, neutropenia, anaemia, thrombocytopenia, hepatic transaminase increases and increased lipids, including hypertriglyceridaemia. The number of reports in older infants was too small to identify a pattern.

4.9 Overdose

Experience in adults treated with up to 12 times the recommended daily dosage revealed no acute toxicity. Complications of chronic overdosage could include peripheral neuropathy and hepatic dysfunction. The mean haemodialysis clearance of stavudine is 120 ml/min. The contribution of this to the total elimination in an overdose situation is unknown. It is not known whether stavudine is removed by peritoneal dialysis.

5. PHARMACOLOGICAL PROPERTIES

5.1 Pharmacodynamic properties

Pharmacotherapeutic group: Nucleoside reverse transcriptase inhibitor

ATC code: J05AF04.

Stavudine, a thymidine analogue, is an antiviral agent with *in vitro* activity against HIV in human cells. It is phosphorylated by cellular kinases to stavudine triphosphate which inhibits HIV reverse transcriptase by competing with the natural substrate, thymidine triphosphate. It also inhibits viral DNA synthesis by causing DNA chain termination due to a lack of the 3'-hydroxyl group necessary for DNA elongation. Cellular DNA polymerase γ is also sensitive to inhibition by stavudine triphosphate, while cellular polymerases α and β are inhibited at concentrations 4,000-fold and 40-fold higher, respectively, than that needed to inhibit HIV reverse transcriptase.

Stavudine treatment can select for and/or maintain mutations associated with zidovudine resistance. Isolates containing these mutations remain sensitive to stavudine. The clinical relevance of these findings is unknown.

The activity of stavudine is affected by multi-drug resistance associated mutations such as Q151 M. A more than 10-fold reduced sensitivity to stavudine has been reported for some strains with reduced sensitivity to zidovudine and lamivudine. No mutations associated with high degree resistance specifically to stavudine have been revealed *in vivo*.

Clinical efficacy

Zerit immediate-release has been studied in combination with other antiretroviral agents, e.g. didanosine, lamivudine, ritonavir, indinavir, saquinavir, efavirenz, and nelfinavir.

Two double-blind triple-therapy studies have demonstrated similar antiviral efficacy and tolerability of Zerit prolonged-release capsule compared to Zerit immediate-release, each given in combination of lamivudine and efavirenz.

Study AI455-099 was a 48-week, randomised, double-blind study comparing Zerit prolonged-release capsule (100 mg once daily) with Zerit (40 mg twice daily), each in combination with lamivudine (150 mg twice daily) plus efavirenz (600 mg once daily), in 783 treatment-naive patients, with a median CD4 cell count of 277 cells/mm^3 (range 61 to 1,215 cells/mm^3) and a median plasma HIV-1 RNA of 4.80 $\log_{10}$ copies/ml (range 2.6 to 5.9 $\log_{10}$ copies/ml) at baseline. Patients were primarily males (69%) and non-white (58%) with a median age of 33 years (range 18 to 69 years).

Study AI455-096 was a 48-week, randomised, double-blind study comparing Zerit prolonged-release capsule (100 mg once daily) with Zerit (40 mg twice daily), each in combination with lamivudine (150 mg twice daily) plus efavirenz (600 mg once daily), in 150 treatment-naive patients, with a median CD4 cell count of 285 cells/mm^3 (range 63 to 962 cells/mm^3) and a median plasma HIV-1 RNA of 4.65 $\log_{10}$ copies/ml (range 2.3 to 5.9 $\log_{10}$ copies/ml) at baseline. Patients were primarily males (75%) and white (70%) with a median age of 34 years (range 20 to 69 years).

The results of AI455-099 and AI455-096 are presented in the table below:

(see Table 1 below)

In adolescents, children and infants, use of stavudine is supported by evidence from adequate and well-controlled studies in adults with additional pharmacokinetic and safety data in paediatric patients (see also sections 4.8 and 5.2).

5.2 Pharmacokinetic properties

Adults

Absorption: the absolute bioavailability is 86±18%. After multiple oral administration of 0.5-0.67 mg/kg doses, a Cmax value of 810±175 ng/ml was obtained. Cmax and AUC increased proportionally with dose in the dose ranges, intravenous 0.0625-0.75 mg/kg, and oral 0.033-4.0 mg/kg.

In eight patients receiving 40 mg twice daily in the fasted state, steady-state AUC_{0-12h} was 1284±227 ng>/>h/ml (18%) (mean ± SD [% CV]), Cmaxwas 536±146 ng/ml (27%), and C_{min} was 9±8 ng/ml (89%). A study in asymptomatic patients demonstrated that systemic exposure is similar while Cmax is lower and T_{max} is prolonged when stavudine is administered with a standardised, high-fat meal compared with fasting conditions. The clinical significance of this is unknown.

Distribution: the apparent volume of distribution at steady state is 46±21 l. It was not possible to detect stavudine in cerebrospinal fluid until at least 2 hours after oral administration. Four hours after administration, the CSF/plasma ratio was 0.39±0.06. No significant accumulation of stavudine is observed with repeated administration every 6, 8, or 12 hours.

Binding of stavudine to serum proteins was negligible over the concentration range of 0.01 to 11.4 μg/ml. Stavudine distributes equally between red blood cells and plasma.

Metabolism: The metabolism of stavudine has not been elucidated in humans. Studies in monkeys indicate that approximately 50% is excreted unchanged in the urine, most of the remainder is hydrolysed to thymine and sugar.

Elimination: the terminal elimination half-life is 1.3±0.2 hours after a single dose, and 1.4±0.2 hours after multiple doses, and is independent of dose. *In vitro*, stavudine triphosphate has an intracellular half-life of 3.5 hours in CEM T-cells (a human T-lymphoblastoid cell line) and peripheral blood mononuclear cells, supporting twice daily dosing.

Total clearance of stavudine is 594±164 ml/min, and renal clearance is 237±98 ml/min, indicating active tubular secretion in addition to glomerular filtration. After intravenous administration, 42±7% of dose is excreted unchanged in the urine. The corresponding values after oral single and multiple dose administration are 34±5% and 40±12%, respectively. The remaining 60% of the drug is presumably eliminated by endogenous pathways. The half-life of stavudine is approximately 2 hours.

The pharmacokinetics of stavudine was independent of time, since the ratio between $AUC_{(ss)}$ at steady state and the $AUC_{(0-t)}$ after the first dose was approximately 1. Intra- and interindividual variation in pharmacokinetic characteristics of stavudine is low, approximately 15% and 25%, respectively, after oral administration.

Special Populations

Adolescents, children and infants: total exposure to stavudine was comparable between adolescents, children and infants ⩾ 14 days receiving the 2 mg/kg/day dose and adults receiving 1 mg/kg/day. Apparent oral clearance was approximately 14 ml/min/kg for infants ages 5 weeks to 15 years, 12 ml/min/kg for infants ages 14 to 28 days, and 5 ml/min/kg for infants on the day of birth. Two to three hours post-dose, CSF/plasma ratios of stavudine ranged from 16% to 125% (mean of 59%±35%).

Renal impairment: the clearance of stavudine decreases as creatinine clearance decreases; therefore, it is recommended that the dosage of Zerit be adjusted in patients with reduced renal function (see section 4.2).

Hepatic impairment: stavudine pharmacokinetics in patients with hepatic impairment were similar to those in patients with normal hepatic function.

5.3 Preclinical safety data

Animal data showed embryo-foetal toxicity at very high exposure levels. An *ex vivo* study using a term human placenta model demonstrated that stavudine reaches the foetal circulation by simple diffusion. A rat study also showed placental transfer of stavudine, with the foetal tissue concentration approximately 50% of the maternal plasma concentration.

Stavudine was genotoxic in *in vitro* tests in human lymphocytes possessing triphosphorylating activity (in which no no-effect level was established), in mouse fibroblasts, and in an *in vivo* test for chromosomal aberrations. Similar effects have been observed with other nucleoside analogues.

Stavudine was carcinogenic in mice (liver tumours) and rats (liver tumours: cholangiocellular, hepatocellular, mixed hepatocholangiocellular, and/or vascular; and urinary bladder carcinomas) at very high exposure levels. No carcinogenicity was noted at doses of 400 mg/kg/day in mice and 600 mg/kg/day in rats, corresponding to exposures ~ 39 and 168 times the expected human exposure, respectively, suggesting an insignificant carcinogenic potential of stavudine in clinical therapy.

6. PHARMACEUTICAL PARTICULARS

6.1 List of excipients

Cherry flavour

Methylparaben

Propylparaben

Silicon dioxide

Simethicone

Sodium carmellose

Sorbic acid

Stearate emulsifiers

Sucrose

6.2 Incompatibilities

Not applicable.

6.3 Shelf life

2 years.

6.4 Special precautions for storage

Keep the bottle tightly closed.

After reconstitution, store the solution in tightly closed bottles at 2°C-8°C.

6.5 Nature and contents of container

HDPE bottle with child resistant screw cap, fill mark (200 ml of solution after constitution) and measuring cup.

6.6 Instructions for use and handling

Constitute with water to a 200 ml deliverable volume solution (stavudine concentration of 1 mg/ml):

Add 202 ml of water to the original bottle (when the patient makes up the solution, they should be instructed to fill to the mark). Replace the cap.

Shake the bottle well until the powder dissolves completely. The solution may remain slightly hazy.

Dispense the solution with the measuring cup provided, or for doses less than 10 ml, dispense with a syringe. The patient should be instructed to shake the bottle well prior to measuring each dose.

7. MARKETING AUTHORISATION HOLDER

BRISTOL-MYERS SQUIBB PHARMA EEIG

Uxbridge Business Park

Sanderson Road

Uxbridge UB8 1DH

United Kingdom

8. MARKETING AUTHORISATION NUMBER(S)

EU/1/96/009/009

Table 1

Study	Percent of patients with HIV RNA < 400 copies/ml Treatment response (%)[a]	Percent of patients with HIV RNA < 50 copies/ml Treatment response (%)[a]	HIV RNA Mean Change from Baseline ($\log_{10}$ copies/ml)	CD4 Mean change from Baseline (cells/mm^3)
AI455-099 (48 weeks)				
Zerit prolonged-release capsule + lamivudine + efavirenz (n = 392)	78	54	-2.86	+202
Zerit immediate-release + lamivudine + efavirenz (n = 391)	73	55	-2.83	+182
AI455-096 (48 weeks)				
Zerit prolonged-release capsule + lamivudine + efavirenz (n = 74)	70	41	-2.74	+232
Zerit immediate-release + lamivudine + efavirenz (n = 76)	66	38	-2.64	+195

[a]Percent of patients who have HIV RNA < 400 c/ml or < 50 c/ml and do not meet any criteria for treatment failure including the occurrence of a new AIDS-defining diagnosis.

9. DATE OF FIRST AUTHORISATION/RENEWAL OF THE AUTHORISATION

Date of first authorisation: 08 May 1996

Date of last renewal: 08 June 2001

10. DATE OF REVISION OF THE TEXT

August 2005

Zestoretic 10

(AstraZeneca UK Limited)

1. NAME OF THE MEDICINAL PRODUCT

'Zestoretic' 10.

2. QUALITATIVE AND QUANTITATIVE COMPOSITION

Each tablet contains lisinopril dihydrate (equivalent to 10 mg anhydrous lisinopril) and hydrochlorothiazide Ph. Eur. 12.5 mg.

3. PHARMACEUTICAL FORM

Tablet.

4. CLINICAL PARTICULARS

4.1 Therapeutic indications

'Zestoretic' 10 is indicated in the management of mild to moderate hypertension in patients who have been stabilised on the individual components given in the same proportions.

4.2 Posology and method of administration

The usual dosage is one tablet, administered once daily. As with all other medication taken once daily, 'Zestoretic' 10 should be taken at approximately the same time each day.

In general, if the desired therapeutic effect cannot be achieved in a period of 2 to 4 weeks at this dose level, the dose can be increased to two tablets administered once daily.

No adjustment of dosage is required in the elderly.

Safety and effectiveness in children have not been established.

Dosage in Renal Insufficiency

Thiazides may not be appropriate diuretics for use in patients with renal impairment and are ineffective at creatinine clearance values of 30 ml/min or below (i.e. moderate or severe renal insufficiency).

'Zestoretic' 10 is not to be used as initial therapy in any patient with renal insufficiency.

In patients with creatinine clearance of >30 and <80 ml/min, 'Zestoretic' 10 may be used, but only after titration of the individual components.

Prior Diuretic Therapy

Symptomatic hypotension may occur following the initial dose of 'Zestoretic' 10; this is more likely in patients who are volume and/or salt depleted as a result of prior diuretic therapy. The diuretic therapy should be discontinued for 2-3 days prior to initiation of therapy with 'Zestoretic' 10. If this is not possible, treatment should be started with lisinopril alone, in a 2.5 mg dose.

4.3 Contraindications

'Zestoretic' 10 is contraindicated in pregnancy and treatment should be stopped if pregnancy is suspected (see also Section 4.6).

'Zestoretic' 10 is contraindicated in patients with anuria.

'Zestoretic' 10 is contraindicated in patients who are hypersensitive to any component of this product and in patients with a history of angioneurotic oedema relating to previous treatment with an angiotensin-converting enzyme inhibitor and in patients with hereditary or idiopathic angioedema.

'Zestoretic' 10 is contraindicated in patients who are hypersensitive to other sulphonamide-derived drugs.

4.4 Special warnings and special precautions for use

Hypotension and Electrolyte/Fluid Imbalance

As with all antihypertensive therapy, symptomatic hypotension may occur in some patients. This was rarely seen in uncomplicated hypertensive patients but is more likely in the presence of fluid or electrolyte imbalance, eg. volume depletion, hyponatraemia, hypochloraemic alkalosis, hypomagnesaemia or hypokalaemia which may occur from prior diuretic therapy, dietary salt restriction, dialysis, or during intercurrent diarrhoea or vomiting. Periodic determination of serum electrolytes should be performed at appropriate intervals in such patients.

In patients at increased risk of symptomatic hypotension, initiation of therapy and dose adjustment should be monitored under close medical supervision.

Particular consideration should be given when therapy is administered to patients with ischaemic heart or cerebrovascular disease because an excessive fall in blood pressure could result in a myocardial infarction or cerebrovascular accident.

If hypotension occurs, the patient should be placed in the supine position and, if necessary, should receive an intravenous infusion of normal saline. A transient hypotensive response is not a contraindication to further doses. Following restoration of effective blood volume and pressure, reinstitution of therapy at reduced dosage may be possible; or either of the components may be used appropriately alone.

As with other vasodilators, 'Zestoretic' 10 should be given with caution to patients with aortic stenosis or hypertrophic cardiomyopathy.

Renal Function Impairment

Thiazides may not be appropriate diuretics for use in patients with renal impairment and are ineffective at creatinine clearance values of 30ml/min or below (i.e. moderate or severe renal insufficiency).

'Zestoretic' 10 should not be administered to patients with renal insufficiency (creatinine clearance ⩽80 ml/min) until titration of the individual components has shown the need for the doses present in the combination tablet.

In some patients with bilateral renal artery stenosis or stenosis of the artery to a solitary kidney, who have been treated with angiotensin converting enzyme inhibitors, increases in blood urea and serum creatinine, usually reversible upon discontinuation of therapy have been seen. This is especially likely in patients with renal insufficiency. If renovascular hypertension is also present there is an increased risk of severe hypotension and renal insufficiency. In these patients, treatment should be started under close medical supervision with low doses and careful dose titration. Since treatment with diuretics may be a contributory factor to the above, renal function should be monitored during the first few weeks of 'Zestoretic' 10 therapy.

Some hypertensive patients with no apparent pre-existing renal disease have developed usually minor and transient increases in blood urea and serum creatinine when lisinopril has been given concomitantly with a diuretic. If this occurs during therapy with 'Zestoretic' 10, the combination should be discontinued. Reinstitution of therapy at reduced dosage may be possible; or either of the components may be used appropriately alone.

Hepatic Disease

Thiazides should be used with caution in patients with impaired hepatic function or progressive liver disease, since minor alterations of fluid and electrolyte balance may precipitate hepatic coma.

Surgery/Anaesthesia

In patients undergoing major surgery or during anaesthesia with agents that produce hypotension, lisinopril may block angiotensin II formation secondary to compensatory renin release. If hypotension occurs and is considered to be due to this mechanism, it can be corrected by volume expansion.

Metabolic and Endocrine Effects

Thiazide therapy may impair glucose tolerance. Dosage adjustment of antidiabetic agents, including insulin, may be required.

Thiazides may decrease urinary calcium excretion and may cause intermittent and slight elevation of serum calcium. Marked hypercalcaemia may be evidence of hidden hyperparathyroidism. Thiazides should be discontinued before carrying out tests for parathyroid function.

Increases in cholesterol and triglyceride levels may be associated with thiazide diuretic therapy.

Thiazide therapy may precipitate hyperuricaemia and/or gout in certain patients. However, lisinopril may increase urinary uric acid and thus may attenuate the hyperuricaemic effect of hydrochlorothiazide.

Hypersensitivity/Angioneurotic Oedema

Angioneurotic oedema of the face, extremities, lips, tongue, glottis and/or larynx has been reported rarely in patients treated with angiotensin converting enzyme inhibitors, including lisinopril. In such cases, 'Zestoretic' 10 should be discontinued promptly and appropriate monitoring should be instituted to ensure complete resolution of symptoms prior to dismissing the patient. In those instances where swelling has been confined to the face and lips, the condition generally resolved without treatment, although antihistamines have been useful in relieving symptoms.

Angioneurotic oedema associated with laryngeal oedema may be fatal. Where there is involvement of the tongue, glottis or larynx, likely to cause airway obstruction, appropriate emergency therapy should be administered promptly. This may include administration of adrenaline and/or the maintenance of a patent airway. The patient should be under close medical supervision until complete and sustained resolution of symptoms has occurred. Angioedema may also affect the intestines and present with acute abdominal pain, nausea, vomiting and diarrhoea.

Angiotensin converting enzyme inhibitors cause a higher rate of angioedema in black patients than in non-black patients.

Patients with a history of angioedema unrelated to ACE inhibitor therapy may be at increased risk of angioedema while receiving an ACE inhibitor. (See also Section 4.3).

In patients receiving thiazides, sensitivity reactions may occur with or without a history of allergy or bronchial asthma. Exacerbation or activation of systemic lupus erythematosus has been reported with the use of thiazides.

Race

Angiotensin converting enzyme inhibitors cause a higher rate of angioedema in black patients than in non-black patients.

Desensitisation

Patients receiving ACE inhibitors during desensitisation treatment (eg. hymenoptera venom) have sustained anaphylactoid reactions. In the same patients, these reactions have been avoided when ACE inhibitors were temporarily withheld but they reappeared upon inadvertent rechallenge.

Haemodialysis Membranes

See Section 4.5

Cough

Cough has been reported with the use of ACE inhibitors. Characteristically, the cough is non-productive, persistent and resolves after discontinuation of therapy. ACE inhibitor-induced cough should be considered as part of the differential diagnosis of cough.

Paediatric Use

Safety and effectiveness in children have not been established.

Use in the Elderly

In clinical studies the efficacy and tolerability of lisinopril and hydrochlorothiazide, administered concomitantly, were similar in both elderly and younger hypertensive patients.

4.5 Interaction with other medicinal products and other forms of Interaction

Prior Diuretic Therapy

Symptomatic hypotension may occur following the initial dose of 'Zestoretic' 10; this is more likely in patients who are volume and/or salt depleted as a result of prior diuretic therapy. The diuretic therapy should be discontinued for 2-3 days prior to initiation of therapy with 'Zestoretic' 10. If this is not possible, treatment should be started with lisinopril alone, in a 2.5 mg dose.

Haemodialysis Membranes

The use of 'Zestoretic' 10 is not indicated in patients requiring dialysis for renal failure. A high incidence of anaphylactoid reactions have been reported in patients dialysed with high-flux membranes (eg. AN 69) and treated concomitantly with an ACE inhibitor. This combination should therefore be avoided.

Serum Potassium

The potassium losing effect of thiazide diuretics is usually attenuated by the potassium conserving effect of lisinopril. The use of potassium supplements, potassium-sparing agents or potassium-containing salt substitutes, particularly in patients with impaired renal function, may lead to a significant increase in serum potassium. If concomitant use of 'Zestoretic' 10 and any of these agents is deemed appropriate, they should be used with caution and with frequent monitoring of serum potassium.

Lithium

Lithium generally should not be given with diuretics or ACE inhibitors. Diuretic agents and ACE inhibitors reduce the renal clearance of lithium and add a high risk of lithium toxicity. Refer to the prescribing information for lithium preparations before use of such preparations.

Other Agents

Indomethacin may diminish the antihypertensive effect of concomitantly-administered 'Zestoretic' 10. In some patients with compromised renal function who are being treated with non-steroidal anti-inflammatory drugs (NSAIDs), the co-administration of lisinopril may result in a further deterioration of renal function.

The antihypertensive effect of 'Zestoretic' 10 may be potentiated when given concomitantly with other agents likely to cause postural hypotension.

Thiazides may increase the responsiveness to tubocurarine.

4.6 Pregnancy and lactation

'Zestoretic' 10 is contraindicated in pregnancy and treatment should be stopped if pregnancy is suspected.

ACE inhibitors can cause foetal and neonatal morbidity and mortality when administered to pregnant women during the second and third trimesters. Use of ACE inhibitors during this period has been associated with foetal and neonatal injury including hypotension, renal failure, hyperkalaemia and/or skull hypoplasia in the newborn. Maternal oligohydramnios, presumably representing decreased foetal renal function, has occurred and may result in limb contractures, craniofacial deformations and hypoplastic lung development.

These adverse effects to the embryo and foetus do not appear to have resulted from intrauterine ACE inhibitor exposure limited to the first trimester.

Infants whose mothers have taken lisinopril should be closely observed for hypotension, oliguria and hyperkalaemia. Lisinopril, which crosses the placenta, has been removed from the neonatal circulation by peritoneal dialysis with some clinical benefit, and theoretically may be removed by exchange transfusion. There is no experience with the removal of hydrochlorothiazide, which also crosses the placenta, from the neonatal circulation.

Nursing Mothers

It is not known whether lisinopril is secreted in human milk; however, thiazides do appear in human milk. Because of the potential for serious reactions in breast-fed infants, a decision should be made whether to discontinue breast feeding or to discontinue 'Zestoretic' 10, taking into account the importance of the drug to the mother.

4.7 Effects on ability to drive and use machines

None known.

4.8 Undesirable effects

Side Effects with the Combination

'Zestoretic' 10 is usually well tolerated. In clinical studies, side effects have usually been mild and transient, and in most instances have not required interruption of therapy. The side effects that have been observed have been limited to those reported previously with lisinopril or hydrochlorothiazide.

One of the most common clinical side effects was dizziness, which generally responded to dosage reduction and seldom required discontinuation of therapy.

Other side effects were headache, dry cough, fatigue and hypotension including orthostatic hypotension.

Less common were diarrhoea, nausea, vomiting, dry mouth, rash, gout, palpitations, chest discomfort, muscle cramps and weakness, paraesthesia, asthenia and impotence.

Pancreatitis has been reported rarely with lisinopril and with hydrochlorothiazide and, therefore, is a potential side effect of 'Zestoretic' 10.

Hypersensitivity/Angioneurotic Oedema

Angioneurotic oedema of the face, extremities, lips, tongue, glottis and/or larynx has been reported rarely (see Section 4.4). In very rare cases, intestinal angioedema has been reported.

A symptom complex has been reported which may include one or more of the following: fever, vasculitis, myalgia, arthralgia/arthritis, a positive ANA, elevated ESR, eosinophilia and leucocytosis, rash, photosensitivity, or other dermatological manifestations.

Laboratory Test Findings

Laboratory side effects have rarely been of clinical importance. Occasional hyperglycaemia, hyperuricaemia and hyper- or hypokalaemia have been noted. Usually minor and transient increases in blood urea nitrogen and serum creatinine have been seen in patients without evidence of pre-existing renal impairment. If such increases persist, they are usually reversible upon discontinuation of 'Zestoretic' 10. Bone marrow depression, manifest as anaemia and/or thrombocytopenia and/or leucopenia has been reported. Agranulocytosis has been rarely reported. Small decreases in haemoglobin and haematocrit have been reported frequently in hypertensive patients treated with 'Zestoretic' 10 but were rarely of clinical importance unless another cause of anaemia co-existed. Rarely, elevations of liver enzymes and/or serum bilirubin have occurred, but a causal relationship to 'Zestoretic' 10 has not been established.

Other Side Effects Reported with the Individual Components Alone

These may be potential side effects with 'Zestoretic' 10 and include:

Hydrochlorothiazide: anorexia, gastric irritation, constipation, jaundice (intrahepatic cholestatic jaundice), pancreatitis, sialoadenitis, vertigo, xanthopsia, leucopenia, agranulocytosis, thrombocytopenia, aplastic anaemia, haemolytic anaemia, purpura, photosensitivity, urticaria, necrotizing angiitis (vasculitis) (cutaneous vasculitis), fever, respiratory distress including pneumonitis and pulmonary oedema, anaphylactic reactions, hyperglycaemia, glycosuria, hyperuricaemia, electrolyte imbalance including hyponatraemia, muscle spasm, restlessness, transient blurred vision, renal failure, renal dysfunction and interstitial nephritis.

Lisinopril: myocardial infarction or cerebrovascular accident possibly secondary to excessive hypotension in high risk patients, tachycardia, abdominal pain and indigestion, mood alterations, mental confusion, vertigo have occurred; as with other angiotensin converting enzyme inhibitors, taste disturbance and sleep disturbance have been reported; bronchospasm, rhinitis, sinusitis, alopecia, urticaria, diaphoresis, pruritus, psoriasis and severe skin disorders, (including pemphigus, toxic epidermal necrolysis, Stevens-Johnson Syndrome and erythema multiforme), have been reported; hyponatraemia, uraemia, oliguria/anuria, renal dysfunction, acute renal failure, hepatitis (hepatocellular or cholestatic), jaundice and haemolytic anaemia.

4.9 Overdose

No specific information is available on the treatment of overdosage with 'Zestoretic' 10. Treatment is symptomatic and supportive. Therapy with 'Zestoretic' 10 should be discontinued and the patient should be kept under very close supervision. Therapeutic measures depend on the nature and severity of the symptoms. Measures to prevent absorption and methods to speed elimination should be employed.

Lisinopril: The most likely features of overdosage would be hypotension, electrolyte disturbance and renal failure. If severe hypotension occurs, the patient should be placed in the shock position and an intravenous infusion of normal saline should be given rapidly. Treatment with angiotensin II (if available) may be considered. Angiotensin converting enzyme inhibitors may be removed from the general circulation by haemodialysis. The use of high-flux polyacrylonitrile dialysis membranes should be avoided. Serum electrolytes and creatinine should be monitored frequently.

Hydrochlorothiazide: The most common signs and symptoms observed are those caused by electrolyte depletion (hypokalaemia, hypochloraemia, hyponatraemia) and dehydration resulting from excessive diuresis. If digitalis has also been administered hypokalaemia may accentuate cardiac arrhythmias.

5. PHARMACOLOGICAL PROPERTIES

5.1 Pharmacodynamic properties

'Zestoretic' 10 is a fixed dose combination product containing lisinopril, an inhibitor of angiotensin converting enzyme (ACE) and hydrochlorothiazide, a thiazide diuretic. Both components have complementary modes of action and exert an additive antihypertensive effect.

Lisinopril is a peptidyl dipeptidase inhibitor. It inhibits the angiotensin converting enzyme (ACE) that catalyses the conversion of angiotensin I to the vasoconstrictor peptide, angiotensin II. Angiotensin II also stimulates aldosterone secretion by the adrenal cortex. Inhibition of ACE results in decreased concentrations of angiotensin II which results in decreased vasopressor activity and reduced aldosterone secretion. The latter decrease may result in an increase in serum potassium concentration. While the mechanism through which lisinopril lowers blood pressure is believed to be primarily suppression of the renin-angiotensin-aldosterone system, lisinopril is antihypertensive even in patients with low-renin hypertension. ACE is identical to kininase II, an enzyme that degrades bradykinin. Whether increased levels of bradykinin, a potent vasodilatory peptide, play a role in the therapeutic effects of lisinopril remains to be elucidated.

Hydrochlorothiazide is a diuretic and an antihypertensive agent. It affects the distal renal tubular mechanism of electrolyte reabsorption and increases excretion of sodium and chloride in approximately equivalent amounts. Natriuresis may be accompanied by some loss of potassium and bicarbonate. The mechanism of the antihypertensive effect of the thiazides is unknown. Thiazides do not usually affect normal blood pressure.

When combined with other antihypertensive agents, additive falls in blood pressure may occur.

5.2 Pharmacokinetic properties

Concomitant administration of lisinopril and hydrochlorothiazide has little or no effect on the bioavailability of either drug. The combination tablet is bioequivalent to concomitant administration of the separate entities.

Lisinopril

Following oral administration of lisinopril, peak serum concentrations occur within about 7 hours. On multiple dosing lisinopril has an effective half life of accumulation of 12.6 hours. Declining serum concentrations exhibit a prolonged terminal phase which does not contribute to drug accumulation. This terminal phase probably represents saturable binding to ACE and is not proportional to dose. Lisinopril does not appear to bind to other serum proteins.

Impaired renal function decreases elimination of lisinopril, which is excreted via the kidneys, but this decrease becomes clinically important only when the glomerular filtration rate is below 30 ml/min. Older patients have higher blood levels and higher values for the area under the plasma concentration time curve than younger patients. Lisinopril can be removed by dialysis.

Based on urinary recovery, the mean extent of absorption of lisinopril is approximately 25%, with interpatient variability (6-60%) at all doses tested (5-80 mg).

Lisinopril does not undergo metabolism and absorbed drug is excreted unchanged entirely in the urine. Lisinopril absorption is not affected by the presence of food in the gastrointestinal tract.

Studies in rats indicate that lisinopril crosses the blood-brain barrier poorly.

Hydrochlorothiazide

When plasma levels have been followed for at least 24 hours, the plasma half-life has been observed to vary between 5.6 and 14.8 hours. At least 61% of the dose is eliminated unchanged within 24 hours. After oral hydrochlorothiazide, diuresis begins within 2 hours, peaks in about 4 hours and lasts 6 to 12 hours. Hydrochlorothiazide crosses the placental but not the blood-brain barrier.

5.3 Preclinical safety data

Lisinopril and hydrochlorthiazide are both drugs on which extensive clinical experience has been obtained, both separately and in combination. All relevant information for the prescriber is provided elsewhere in the Summary of Product Characteristics.

6. PHARMACEUTICAL PARTICULARS

6.1 List of excipients

Calcium Hydrogen Phosphate Dihydrate Ph. Eur.

Iron Oxide E172.

Magnesium Stearate Ph. Eur.

Maize Starch Ph. Eur.

Mannitol Ph. Eur.

Pregelatinised Starch Ph. Eur.

6.2 Incompatibilities

None known, but see Section 4.5.

6.3 Shelf life

2.5 years stored in the sales package.

6.4 Special precautions for storage

Store below 30°C and protect from light. If blister packs are removed from the carton, they should be protected from light.

6.5 Nature and contents of container

Blister packs of 28 tablets

6.6 Instructions for use and handling

Not applicable.

7. MARKETING AUTHORISATION HOLDER

AstraZeneca UK Limited,
600 Capability Green,
Luton, LU1 3LU, UK.

8. MARKETING AUTHORISATION NUMBER(S)

PL 17901/0058

9. DATE OF FIRST AUTHORISATION/RENEWAL OF THE AUTHORISATION

8 June 2000

10. DATE OF REVISION OF THE TEXT

4th March 2004

Zestoretic 20

(AstraZeneca UK Limited)

1. NAME OF THE MEDICINAL PRODUCT

'Zestoretic' 20.

2. QUALITATIVE AND QUANTITATIVE COMPOSITION

Each tablet contains lisinopril dihydrate (equivalent to 20 mg anhydrous lisinopril) and hydrochlorothiazide Ph. Eur. 12.5 mg.

3. PHARMACEUTICAL FORM

Tablet.

4. CLINICAL PARTICULARS

4.1 Therapeutic indications

'Zestoretic' 20 is indicated in the management of mild to moderate hypertension in patients who have been stabilised on the individual components given in the same proportions.

4.2 Posology and method of administration

The usual dosage is one tablet, administered once daily. As with all other medication taken once daily, 'Zestoretic' 20 should be taken at approximately the same time each day.

In general, if the desired therapeutic effect cannot be achieved in a period of 2 to 4 weeks at this dose level, the dose can be increased to two tablets administered once daily.

Use in the elderly

In clinical studies the efficacy and tolerability of lisinopril and hydrochlorothiazide, administered concomitantly, were similar in both elderly and younger hypertensive patients.

Lisinopril was equally effective in elderly (65 years or older) and non-elderly hypertensive patients. In elderly hypertensive patients, monotherapy with lisinopril was as effective in reducing diastolic blood pressure as monotherapy with either hydrochlorothiazide or atenolol in clinical studies, age did not affect the tolerability of lisinopril.

Safety and effectiveness in children have not been established.

Dosage in Renal Insufficiency

Thiazides may not be appropriate diuretics for use in patients with renal impairment and are ineffective at creatinine clearance values of 30 ml/min or below (i.e. moderate or severe renal insufficiency).

'Zestoretic' 20 is not to be used as initial therapy in any patient with renal insufficiency.

In patients with creatinine clearance of >30 and <80 ml/min, 'Zestoretic' 20 may be used, but only after titration of the individual components.

Prior Diuretic Therapy

Symptomatic hypotension may occur following the initial dose of 'Zestoretic' 20; this is more likely in patients who are volume and/or salt depleted as a result of prior diuretic therapy. The diuretic therapy should be discontinued for 2-3 days prior to initiation of therapy with 'Zestoretic' 20. If this is not possible, treatment should be started with lisinopril alone, in a 2.5 mg dose.

4.3 Contraindications

'Zestoretic' 20 is contraindicated in pregnancy and treatment should be stopped if pregnancy is suspected (see also Section 4.6).

'Zestoretic' 20 is contraindicated in patients with anuria.

'Zestoretic' 20 is contraindicated in patients who are hypersensitive to any component of this product and in patients with a history of angioneurotic oedema relating to previous treatment with an angiotensin-converting enzyme inhibitor and in patients with hereditary or idiopathic angioedema.

'Zestoretic' 20 is contraindicated in patients who are hypersensitive to other sulphonamide-derived drugs.

4.4 Special warnings and special precautions for use

Hypotension and Electrolyte/Fluid Imbalance

As with all antihypertensive therapy, symptomatic hypotension may occur in some patients. This was rarely seen in uncomplicated hypertensive patients but is more likely in the presence of fluid or electrolyte imbalance, eg. volume depletion, hyponatraemia, hypochloraemic alkalosis, hypomagnesaemia or hypokalaemia which may occur from prior diuretic therapy, dietary salt restriction, dialysis, or during intercurrent diarrhoea or vomiting. Periodic determination of serum electrolytes should be performed at appropriate intervals in such patients.

In patients at increased risk of symptomatic hypotension, initiation of therapy and dose adjustment should be monitored under close medical supervision.

Particular consideration should be given when therapy is administered to patients with ischaemic heart or cerebrovascular disease because an excessive fall in blood pressure could result in a myocardial infarction or cerebrovascular accident.

If hypotension occurs, the patient should be placed in the supine position and, if necessary, should receive an intravenous infusion of normal saline. A transient hypotensive response is not a contraindication to further doses. Following restoration of effective blood volume and pressure, reinstitution of therapy at reduced dosage may be possible; or either of the components may be used appropriately alone.

As with other vasodilators, 'Zestoretic' 20 should be given with caution to patients with aortic stenosis or hypertrophic cardiomyopathy.

Renal Function Impairment

Thiazides may not be appropriate diuretics for use in patients with renal impairment and are ineffective at creatinine clearance values of 30ml/min or below (i.e. moderate or severe renal insufficiency).

'Zestoretic' 20 should not be administered to patients with renal insufficiency (creatinine clearance ⩽80 ml/min) until titration of the individual components has shown the need for the doses present in the combination tablet.

In some patients with bilateral renal artery stenosis or stenosis of the artery to a solitary kidney, who have been treated with angiotensin enzyme inhibitors, increases in blood urea and serum creatinine, usually reversible upon discontinuation of therapy, have been seen. This is especially likely in patients with renal insufficiency. If renovascular hypertension is also present there is an increased risk of severe hypotension and renal insufficiency. In these patients, treatment should be started under close medical supervision with low doses and careful dose titration. Since treatment with diuretics may be a contributory factor to the above, renal function should be monitored during the first few weeks of 'Zestoretic' 20 therapy.

Some hypertensive patients with no apparent pre-existing renal disease have developed usually minor and transient increases in blood urea and serum creatinine when lisinopril has been given concomitantly with a diuretic. If this occurs during therapy with 'Zestoretic' 20, the combination should be discontinued. Reinstitution of therapy at reduced dosage may be possible; or either of the components may be used appropriately alone.

Hepatic Disease

Thiazides should be used with caution in patients with impaired hepatic function or progressive liver disease, since minor alterations of fluid and electrolyte balance may precipitate hepatic coma.

Surgery/Anaesthesia

In patients undergoing major surgery or during anaesthesia with agents that produce hypotension, lisinopril may block angiotensin II formation secondary to compensatory renin release. If hypotension occurs and is considered to be due to this mechanism, it can be corrected by volume expansion.

Metabolic and Endocrine Effects

Thiazide therapy may impair glucose tolerance. Dosage adjustment of antidiabetic agents, including insulin, may be required.

Thiazides may decrease urinary calcium excretion and may cause intermittent and slight elevation of serum calcium. Marked hypercalcaemia may be evidence of hidden hyperparathyroidism. Thiazides should be discontinued before carrying out tests for parathyroid function.

Increases in cholesterol and triglyceride levels may be associated with thiazide diuretic therapy.

Thiazide therapy may precipitate hyperuricaemia and/or gout in certain patients. However, lisinopril may increase urinary uric acid and thus may attenuate the hyperuricaemic effect of hydrochlorothiazide.

Hypersensitivity/Angioneurotic Oedema

Angioneurotic oedema of the face, extremities, lips, tongue, glottis and/or larynx has been reported rarely in patients treated with angiotensin converting enzyme inhibitors, including lisinopril. In such cases, 'Zestoretic' 20 should be discontinued promptly and appropriate monitoring should be instituted to ensure complete resolution of symptoms prior to dismissing the patient. In those instances where swelling has been confined to the face and lips, the condition generally resolved without treatment, although antihistamines have been useful in relieving symptoms.

Angioneurotic oedema associated with laryngeal oedema may be fatal. Where there is involvement of the tongue, glottis or larynx, likely to cause airway obstruction, appropriate emergency therapy should be administered promptly. This may include administration of adrenaline and/or the maintenance of a patent airway. The patient should be under close medical supervision until complete and sustained resolution of symptoms has occurred.

Angioedema may also affect the intestines and present with acute abdominal pain, nausea, vomiting and diarrhoea.

Angiotensin converting enzyme inhibitors cause a higher rate of angioedema in black patients than in non-black patients.

Patients with a history of angioedema unrelated to ACE inhibitor therapy may be at increased risk of angioedema while receiving an ACE inhibitor. (See also Section 4.3).

In patients receiving thiazides, sensitivity reactions may occur with or without a history of allergy or bronchial asthma. Exacerbation or activation of systemic lupus erythematosus has been reported with the use of thiazides.

Race

Angiotensin converting enzyme inhibitors cause a higher rate of angioedema in black patients than in non-black patients.

Desensitisation

Patients receiving ACE inhibitors during desensitisation treatment (e.g. hymenoptera venom) have sustained anaphylactoid reactions. In the same patients, these reactions have been avoided when ACE inhibitors were temporarily withheld but they reappeared upon inadvertent rechallenge.

Haemodialysis Membranes

(See Section 4.5).

Cough

Cough has been reported with the use of ACE inhibitors. Characteristically, the cough is non-productive, persistent and resolves after discontinuation of therapy. ACE inhibitor-induced cough should be considered as part of the differential diagnosis of cough.

Paediatric Use

Safety and effectiveness in children have not been established.

Use in the Elderly

In clinical studies the efficacy and tolerability of lisinopril and hydrochlorothiazide, administered concomitantly, were similar in both elderly and younger hypertensive patients.

4.5 Interaction with other medicinal products and other forms of Interaction

Prior Diuretic Therapy

Symptomatic hypotension may occur following the initial dose of 'Zestoretic' 20; this is more likely in patients who are volume and/or salt depleted as a result of prior diuretic therapy. The diuretic therapy should be discontinued for 2-3 days prior to initiation of therapy with 'Zestoretic' 20. If this is not possible, treatment should be started with lisinopril alone, in a 2.5 mg dose.

Haemodialysis Membranes

The use of 'Zestoretic' 20 is not indicated in patients requiring dialysis for renal failure. A high incidence of anaphylactoid reactions have been reported in patients dialysed with high-flux membranes (e.g. AN 69) and treated concomitantly with an ACE inhibitor. This combination should therefore be avoided.

Serum Potassium

The potassium losing effect of thiazide diuretics is usually attenuated by the potassium conserving effect of lisinopril. The use of potassium supplements, potassium-sparing agents or potassium-containing salt substitutes, particularly in patients with impaired renal function, may lead to a significant increase in serum potassium. If concomitant use of 'Zestoretic' 20 and any of these agents is deemed appropriate, they should be used with caution and with frequent monitoring of serum potassium.

Lithium

Lithium generally should not be given with diuretics or ACE inhibitors. Diuretic agents and ACE inhibitors reduce the renal clearance of lithium and add a high risk of lithium toxicity. Refer to the prescribing information for lithium preparations before use of such preparations.

Other Agents

Indomethacin may diminish the antihypertensive effect of concomitantly administered 'Zestoretic' 20. In some patients with compromised renal function who are being treated with non-steroidal anti-inflammatory drugs (NSAIDs), the co-administration of lisinopril may result in a further deterioration of renal function.

The antihypertensive effect of 'Zestoretic' 20 may be potentiated when given concomitantly with other agents likely to cause postural hypotension.

Thiazides may increase the responsiveness to tubocurarine.

4.6 Pregnancy and lactation

'Zestoretic' 20 is contraindicated in pregnancy and treatment should be stopped if pregnancy is suspected.

ACE inhibitors can cause foetal and neonatal morbidity and mortality when administered to pregnant women during the second and third trimesters. Use of ACE inhibitors during this period has been associated with foetal and neonatal injury including hypotension, renal failure, hyperkalaemia and/or skull hypoplasia in the newborn. Maternal oligohydramnios, presumably representing decreased foetal renal function, has occurred and may result in limb contractures, craniofacial deformations and hypoplastic lung development.

These adverse effects to the embryo and foetus do not appear to have resulted from intrauterine ACE inhibitor exposure limited to the first trimester.

Infants whose mothers have taken lisinopril should be closely observed for hypotension, oliguria and hyperkalaemia. Lisinopril, which crosses the placenta, has been removed from the neonatal circulation by peritoneal dialysis with some clinical benefit, and theoretically may be removed by exchange transfusion. There is no experience with the removal of hydrochlorothiazide, which also crosses the placenta, from the neonatal circulation.

Nursing Mothers

It is not known whether lisinopril is secreted in human milk; however, thiazides do appear in human milk. Because of the potential for serious reactions in breast-fed infants, a decision should be made whether to discontinue breast feeding or to discontinue 'Zestoretic' 20, taking into account the importance of the drug to the mother.

4.7 Effects on ability to drive and use machines

None known.

4.8 Undesirable effects

Side Effects with the Combination

'Zestoretic' 20 is usually well tolerated. In clinical studies, side effects have usually been mild and transient, and in most instances have not required interruption of therapy. The side effects that have been observed have been limited to those reported previously with lisinopril or hydrochlorothiazide.

One of the most common clinical side effects was dizziness, which generally responded to dosage reduction and seldom required discontinuation of therapy.

Other side effects were headache, dry cough, fatigue and hypotension including orthostatic hypotension.

Less common were diarrhoea, nausea, vomiting, dry mouth, rash, gout, palpitations, chest discomfort, muscle cramps and weakness, paraesthesia, asthenia and impotence.

Pancreatitis has been reported rarely with lisinopril and with hydrochlorothiazide and, therefore, is a potential side effect of 'Zestoretic' 20.

Hypersensitivity/Angioneurotic Oedema

Angioneurotic oedema of the face, extremities, lips, tongue, glottis and/or larynx has been reported rarely (see Section 4.4). In very rare cases, intestinal angioedema has been reported.

A symptom complex has been reported which may include one or more of the following: fever, vasculitis, myalgia, arthralgia/arthritis, a positive ANA, elevated ESR, eosinophilia and leucocytosis, rash, photosensitivity, or other dermatological manifestations.

Laboratory Test Findings

Laboratory side effects have rarely been of clinical importance. Occasional hyperglycaemia, hyperuricaemia and hyper- or hypokalaemia have been noted. Usually minor and transient increases in blood urea nitrogen and serum creatinine have been seen in patients without evidence of pre-existing renal impairment. If such increases persist, they are usually reversible upon discontinuation of 'Zestoretic' 20. Bone marrow depression, manifest as anaemia and/or thrombocytopenia and/or leucopenia has been reported. Agranulocytosis has been rarely reported. Small decreases in haemoglobin and haematocrit have been reported frequently in hypertensive patients treated with 'Zestoretic' 20 but were rarely of clinical importance unless another cause of anaemia co-existed. Rarely, elevations of liver enzymes and/or serum bilirubin have occurred, but a causal relationship to 'Zestoretic' 20 has not been established.

Other Side Effects Reported with the Individual Components Alone

These may be potential side effects with 'Zestoretic' 20 and include:

Hydrochlorothiazide: anorexia, gastric irritation, constipation, jaundice (intrahepatic cholestatic jaundice), pancreatitis, sialoadenitis, vertigo, xanthopsia, leucopenia, agranulocytosis, thrombocytopenia, aplastic anaemia, haemolytic anaemia, purpura, photosensitivity, urticaria, necrotizing angiitis (vasculitis) (cutaneous vasculitis), fever, respiratory distress including pneumonitis and pulmonary oedema, anaphylactic reactions, hyperglycaemia, glycosuria, hyperuricaemia, electrolyte imbalance including hyponatraemia, muscle spasm, restlessness, transient blurred vision, renal failure, renal dysfunction and interstitial nephritis.

Lisinopril: myocardial infarction or cerebrovascular accident possibly secondary to excessive hypotension in high risk patients, tachycardia, abdominal pain and indigestion, mood alterations, mental confusion, vertigo have occurred; as with other angiotensin converting enzyme inhibitors, taste disturbance and sleep disturbance have been reported; bronchospasm, rhinitis, sinusitis, alopecia, urticaria, diaphoresis, pruritus, psoriasis and severe skin disorders, (including pemphigus, toxic epidermal necrolysis, Stevens-Johnson Syndrome and erythema multiforme), have been reported; hyponatraemia, uraemia, oliguria/anuria, renal dysfunction, acute renal failure, hepatitis (hepatocellular or cholestatic), jaundice and haemolytic anaemia.

4.9 Overdose

No specific information is available on the treatment of overdosage with 'Zestoretic' 20. Treatment is symptomatic and supportive. Therapy with 'Zestoretic' 20 should be discontinued and the patient should be kept under very close supervision. Therapeutic measures depend on the nature and severity of the symptoms. Measures to prevent absorption and methods to speed elimination should be employed.

Lisinopril: The most likely features of overdosage would be hypotension, electrolyte disturbance and renal failure. If severe hypotension occurs, the patient should be placed in the shock position and an intravenous infusion of normal saline should be given rapidly. Treatment with angiotensin II (if available) may be considered. Angiotensin converting enzyme inhibitors may be removed from the general circulation by haemodialysis. The use of high-flux polyacrylonitrile dialysis membranes should be avoided. Serum electrolytes and creatinine should be monitored frequently.

Hydrochlorothiazide: The most common signs and symptoms observed are those caused by electrolyte depletion (hypokalaemia, hypochloraemia, hyponatraemia) and dehydration resulting from excessive diuresis. If digitalis has also been administered hypokalaemia may accentuate cardiac arrhythmias.

5. PHARMACOLOGICAL PROPERTIES

5.1 Pharmacodynamic properties

'Zestoretic' 20 is a fixed dose combination product containing lisinopril, an inhibitor of angiotensin converting enzyme (ACE) and hydrochlorothiazide, a thiazide diuretic. Both components have complementary modes of action and exert an additive antihypertensive effect.

Lisinopril is a peptidyl dipeptidase inhibitor. It inhibits the angiotensin converting enzyme (ACE) that catalyses the conversion of angiotensin I to the vasoconstrictor peptide, angiotensin II. Angiotensin II also stimulates aldosterone secretion by the adrenal cortex. Inhibition of ACE results in decreased concentrations of angiotensin II which results in decreased vasopressor activity and reduced aldosterone secretion. The latter decrease may result in an increase in serum potassium concentration.

While the mechanism through which lisinopril lowers blood pressure is believed to be primarily suppression of the renin-angiotensin-aldosterone system, lisinopril is antihypertensive even in patients with low-renin hypertension. ACE is identical to kininase II, an enzyme that degrades bradykinin. Whether increased levels of bradykinin, a potent vasodilatory peptide, play a role in the therapeutic effects of lisinopril remains to be elucidated.

Hydrochlorothiazide is a diuretic and an antihypertensive agent. It affects the distal renal tubular mechanism of electrolyte reabsorption and increases excretion of sodium and chloride in approximately equivalent amounts. Natriuresis may be accompanied by some loss of potassium and bicarbonate. The mechanism of the antihypertensive effect of the thiazides is unknown. Thiazides do not usually affect normal blood pressure.

When combined with other antihypertensive agents, additive falls in blood pressure may occur.

5.2 Pharmacokinetic properties

Concomitant administration of lisinopril and hydrochlorothiazide has little or no effect on the bioavailability of either drug. The combination tablet is bioequivalent to concomitant administration of the separate entities.

Lisinopril:

Following oral administration of lisinopril, peak serum concentrations occur within about 7 hours. On multiple dosing lisinopril has an effective half life of accumulation of 12.6 hours. Declining serum concentrations exhibit a prolonged terminal phase which does not contribute to drug accumulation. This terminal phase probably represents saturable binding to ACE and is not proportional to dose. Lisinopril does not appear to bind to other serum proteins.

Impaired renal function decreases elimination of lisinopril, which is excreted via the kidneys, but this decrease becomes clinically important only when the glomerular filtration rate is below 30 ml/min. Older patients have higher blood levels and higher values for the area under the plasma concentration time curve than younger patients. Lisinopril can be removed by dialysis.

Based on urinary recovery, the mean extent of absorption of lisinopril is approximately 25%, with interpatient variability (6-60%) at all doses tested (5-80 mg).

Lisinopril does not undergo metabolism and absorbed drug is excreted unchanged entirely in the urine. Lisinopril absorption is not affected by the presence of food in the gastrointestinal tract.

Studies in rats indicate that lisinopril crosses the blood-brain barrier poorly.

Hydrochlorothiazide:

When plasma levels have been followed for at least 24 hours, the plasma half-life has been observed to vary between 5.6 and 14.8 hours. At least 61% of the dose is eliminated unchanged within 24 hours. After oral hydrochlorothiazide, diuresis begins within 2 hours, peaks in about 4 hours and lasts 6 to 12 hours. Hydrochlorothiazide crosses the placental but not the blood-brain barrier.

5.3 Preclinical safety data

Lisinopril and hydrochlorthiazide are both drugs on which extensive clinical experience has been obtained, both separately and in combination. All relevant information for the prescriber is provided elsewhere in the Summary of Product Characteristics.

6. PHARMACEUTICAL PARTICULARS

6.1 List of excipients

Calcium Hydrogen Phosphate Dihydrate Ph. Eur.

Magnesium Stearate Ph. Eur

Maize Starch Ph. Eur.

Mannitol Ph. Eur.

Pregelatinised Maize Starch Ph. Eur.

6.2 Incompatibilities

None known, but see Section 4.5.

6.3 Shelf life

2.5 years stored in the sales package.

6.4 Special precautions for storage

Store below 30°C and protect from light.

6.5 Nature and contents of container

Blister packs of 28 tablets

6.6 Instructions for use and handling

Not applicable.

7. MARKETING AUTHORISATION HOLDER

AstraZeneca UK Limited,

600 Capability Green,

Luton, LU1 3LU, UK.

8. MARKETING AUTHORISATION NUMBER(S)

PL 17901/0059

9. DATE OF FIRST AUTHORISATION/RENEWAL OF THE AUTHORISATION

8 June 2000

10. DATE OF REVISION OF THE TEXT

4th March 2004

Zestril 2.5mg, 5mg, 10mg, 20mg and 30mg tablets.

(AstraZeneca UK Limited)

1. NAME OF THE MEDICINAL PRODUCT

Zestril 2.5mg, 5mg, 10mg, 20mg and 30mg tablets.

2. QUALITATIVE AND QUANTITATIVE COMPOSITION

Each tablet contains lisinopril dihydrate equivalent to 2.5mg, 5mg, 10mg, 20mg or 30mg anhydrous lisinopril.

For excipients, see 6.1 List of excipients.

3. PHARMACEUTICAL FORM

2.5 mg tablets are white, round and biconvex. They have a diameter of 6 mm.

5 mg tablets are pink, round and biconvex. They have a diameter of 6 mm.

10 mg tablets are pink, round and biconvex. They have a diameter of 8 mm.

20 mg tablets are pink, round and biconvex. They have a diameter of 8 mm.

30 mg tablets are pink, round and biconvex. They have a diameter of 9 mm.

All tablets are marked on one side with a number denoting the tablet strength.

4. CLINICAL PARTICULARS

4.1 Therapeutic indications

Hypertension

Treatment of hypertension.

Heart failure

Treatment of symptomatic heart failure.

Acute myocardial infarction

Short-term (6 weeks) treatment of haemodynamically stable patients within 24 hours of an acute myocardial infarction.

Renal complications of diabetes mellitus

Treatment of renal disease in hypertensive patients with Type 2 diabetes mellitus and incipient nephropathy (see section 5.1).

4.2 Posology and method of administration

Zestril should be administered orally in a single daily dose. As with all other medication taken once daily, Zestril should be taken at approximately the same time each day. The absorption of Zestril tablets is not affected by food.

The dose should be individualised according to patient profile and blood pressure response (see section 4.4).

Hypertension

Zestril may be used as monotherapy or in combination with other classes of antihypertensive therapy.

Starting dose

In patients with hypertension the usual recommended starting dose is 10 mg. Patients with a strongly activated renin-angiotensin-aldosterone system (in particular, renovascular hypertension, salt and /or volume depletion, cardiac decompensation, or severe hypertension) may experience an excessive blood pressure fall following the initial dose. A starting dose of 2.5-5 mg is recommended in such patients and the initiation of treatment should take place under medical supervision. A lower starting dose is required in the presence of renal impairment (see Table 1 below).

Maintenance dose

The usual effective maintenance dosage is 20 mg administered in a single daily dose. In general if the desired therapeutic effect cannot be achieved in a period of 2 to 4 weeks on a certain dose level, the dose can be further increased. The maximum dose used in long-term, controlled clinical trials was 80 mg/day.

Diuretic-treated tatients

Symptomatic hypotension may occur following initiation of therapy with Zestril. This is more likely in patients who are being treated currently with diuretics. Caution is recommended therefore, since these patients may be volume and/or salt depleted. If possible, the diuretic should be discontinued 2 to 3 days before beginning therapy with Zestril. In hypertensive patients in whom the diuretic cannot be discontinued, therapy with Zestril should be initiated with a 5 mg dose. Renal function and serum potassium should be monitored. The subsequent dosage of Zestril should be adjusted according to blood pressure response. If required, diuretic therapy may be resumed (see section 4.4 and section 4.5).

Dosage adjustment In renal impairment

Dosage in patients with renal impairment should be based on creatinine clearance as outlined in Table 1 below.

Table 1 Dosage adjustment in renal impairment.

Creatinine Clearance (ml/min)	Starting Dose (mg/day)
Less than 10 ml/min (including patients on dialysis)	2.5 mg*
10-30 ml/min	2.5-5 mg
31-80 ml/min	5-10 mg

* Dosage and/or frequency of administration should be adjusted depending on the blood pressure response.

The dosage may be titrated upward until blood pressure is controlled or to a maximum of 40 mg daily.

Heart failure

In patients with symptomatic heart failure, Zestril should be used as adjunctive therapy to diuretics and, where appropriate, digitalis or beta-blockers. Zestril may be initiated at a starting dose of 2.5 mg once a day, which should be administered under medical supervision to determine the initial effect on the blood pressure. The dose of Zestril should be increased:

- By increments of no greater than 10 mg
- At intervals of no less than 2 weeks
- To the highest dose tolerated by the patient up to a maximum of 35 mg once daily

Dose adjustment should be based on the clinical response of individual patients.

Patients at high risk of symptomatic hypotension e.g. patients with salt depletion with or without hyponatraemia, patients with hypovolaemia or patients who have been receiving vigorous diuretic therapy should have these conditions corrected, if possible, prior to therapy with Zestril. Renal function and serum potassium should be monitored (see section 4.4).

Acute myocardial infarction

Patients should receive, as appropriate, the standard recommended treatments such as thrombolytics, aspirin, and beta-blockers. Intravenous or transdermal glyceryl trinitrate may be used together with Zestril.

Starting dose (first 3 days after infarction)

Treatment with Zestril may be started within 24 hours of the onset of symptoms. Treatment should not be started if systolic blood pressure is lower than 100 mm Hg. The first dose of Zestril is 5 mg given orally, followed by 5 mg after 24 hours, 10 mg after 48 hours and then 10 mg once daily. Patients with a low systolic blood pressure (120 mm Hg or less) when treatment is started or during the first 3 days after the infarction should be given a lower dose - 2.5 mg orally (see section 4.4).

In cases of renal impairment (creatinine clearance < 80 ml/min), the initial Zestril dosage should be adjusted according to the patient's creatinine clearance (see Table 1).

Maintenance dose

The maintenance dose is 10 mg once daily. If hypotension occurs (systolic blood pressure less than or equal to 100 mm Hg) a daily maintenance dose of 5 mg may be given with temporary reductions to 2.5 mg if needed. If prolonged hypotension occurs (systolic blood pressure less than 90 mm Hg for more than 1 hour) Zestril should be withdrawn.

Treatment should continue for 6 weeks and then the patient should be re-evaluated. Patients who develop symptoms of heart failure should continue with Zestril (see section 4.2)

Renal complications of diabetes mellitus

In hypertensive patients with type 2 diabetes mellitus and incipient nephropathy, the dose is 10 mg Zestril once daily which can be increased to 20 mg once daily, if necessary, to achieve a sitting diastolic blood pressure below 90 mm Hg.

In cases of renal impairment (creatinine clearance < 80 ml/min), the initial Zestril dosage should be adjusted according to the patient's creatinine clearance (see Table 1).

Paediatric use

Efficacy and safety of use in children has not been fully established. Therefore, use in children is not recommended.

Use in the elderly

In clinical studies, there was no age-related change in the efficacy or safety profile of the drug. When advanced age is associated with decrease in renal function, however, the guidelines set out in Table 1 should be used to determine the starting dose of Zestril. Thereafter, the dosage should be adjusted according to the blood pressure response.

Use in kidney transplant patients

There is no experience regarding the administration of Zestril in patients with recent kidney transplantation. Treatment with Zestril is therefore not recommended.

4.3 Contraindications

- Hypersensitivity to Zestril, to any of the excipients or any other angiotensin converting enzyme (ACE) inhibitor.
- History of angioedema associated with previous ACE inhibitor therapy
- Hereditary or idiopathic angioedema.
- Second or third trimesters of pregnancy (see section 4.6).

4.4 Special warnings and special precautions for use

Symptomatic hypotension

Symptomatic hypotension is seen rarely in uncomplicated hypertensive patients. In hypertensive patients receiving Zestril, hypotension is more likely to occur if the patient has been volume-depleted e.g. by diuretic therapy, dietary salt restriction, dialysis, diarrhoea or vomiting, or has severe renin-dependent hypertension (see section 4.5 and section 4.8). In patients with heart failure, with or without associated renal insufficiency, symptomatic hypotension has been observed. This is most likely to occur in those patients with more severe degrees of heart failure, as reflected by the use of high doses of loop diuretics, hyponatraemia or functional renal impairment. In patients at increased risk of symptomatic hypotension, initiation of therapy and dose adjustment should be closely monitored. Similar considerations apply to patients with ischaemic heart or cerebrovascular disease in whom an excessive fall in blood pressure could result in a myocardial infarction or cerebrovascular accident.

If hypotension occurs, the patient should be placed in the supine position and, if necessary, should receive an intravenous infusion of normal saline. A transient hypotensive response is not a contraindication to further doses, which can be given usually without difficulty once the blood pressure has increased after volume expansion.

In some patients with heart failure who have normal or low blood pressure, additional lowering of systemic blood pressure may occur with Zestril. This effect is anticipated and is not usually a reason to discontinue treatment. If hypotension becomes symptomatic, a reduction of dose or discontinuation of Zestril may be necessary.

Hypotension in acute myocardial infarction

Treatment with Zestril must not be initiated in acute myocardial infarction patients who are at risk of further serious haemodynamic deterioration after treatment with a vasodilator. These are patients with systolic blood pressure of 100 mm Hg or lower or those in cardiogenic shock. During the first 3 days following the infarction, the dose should be reduced if the systolic blood pressure is 120 mm Hg or lower. Maintenance doses should be reduced to 5 mg or temporarily to 2.5 mg if systolic blood pressure is 100 mm Hg or lower. If hypotension persists (systolic blood pressure less than 90 mm Hg for more than 1 hour) then Zestril should be withdrawn.

Aortic and mitral valve stenosis/hypertrophic cardiomyopathy

As with other ACE inhibitors, Zestril should be given with caution to patients with mitral valve stenosis and obstruction in the outflow of the left ventricle such as aortic stenosis or hypertrophic cardiomyopathy.

Renal function impairment

In cases of renal impairment (creatinine clearance < 80 ml/min), the initial Zestril dosage should be adjusted according to the patient's creatinine clearance (see Table 1 in section 4.2) and then as a function of the patient's response to treatment. Routine monitoring of potassium and creatinine is part of normal medical practice for these patients.

In patients with heart failure, hypotension following the initiation of therapy with ACE inhibitors may lead to some further impairment in renal function. Acute renal failure, usually reversible, has been reported in this situation.

In some patients with bilateral renal artery stenosis or with a stenosis of the artery to a solitary kidney, who have been treated with angiotensin converting enzyme inhibitors, increases in blood urea and serum creatinine, usually reversible upon discontinuation of therapy, have been seen. This is especially likely in patients with renal insufficiency. If renovascular hypertension is also present there is an increased risk of severe hypotension and renal insufficiency. In these patients, treatment should be started under close medical supervision with low doses and careful dose titration. Since treatment with diuretics may be a contributory factor to the above, they should be discontinued and renal function should be monitored during the first weeks of Zestril therapy.

Some hypertensive patients with no apparent pre-existing renal vascular disease have developed increases in blood urea and serum creatinine, usually minor and transient, especially when Zestril has been given concomitantly with a diuretic. This is more likely to occur in patients with pre-existing renal impairment. Dosage reduction and/or discontinuation of the diuretic and/or Zestril may be required.

In acute myocardial infarction, treatment with Zestril should not be initiated in patients with evidence of renal dysfunction, defined as serum creatinine concentration exceeding 177 micromol/l and/or proteinuria exceeding 500 mg/24 h. If renal dysfunction develops during treatment with Zestril (serum creatinine concentration exceeding 265 micromol/l or a doubling from the pre-treatment value) then the physician should consider withdrawal of Zestril.

Hypersensitivity/Angioedema

Angioedema of the face, extremities, lips, tongue, glottis and/or larynx has been reported rarely in patients treated with angiotensin converting enzyme inhibitors, including Zestril. This may occur at any time during therapy. In such cases, Zestril should be discontinued promptly and appropriate treatment and monitoring should be instituted to ensure complete resolution of symptoms prior to dismissing the patients. Even in those instances where swelling of only the tongue is involved, without respiratory distress, patients may require prolonged observation since treatment with antihistamines and corticosteroids may not be sufficient.

Very rarely, fatalities have been reported due to angioedema associated with laryngeal oedema or tongue oedema. Patients with involvement of the tongue, glottis or larynx, are likely to experience airway obstruction, especially those with a history of airway surgery. In such cases emergency therapy should be administered promptly. This may include the administration of adrenaline and/or the maintenance of a patent airway. The patient should be under close medical supervision until complete and sustained resolution of symptoms has occurred.

Angiotensin converting enzyme inhibitors cause a higher rate of angioedema in black patients than in non-black patients.

Patients with a history of angioedema unrelated to ACE inhibitor therapy may be at increased risk of angioedema while receiving an ACE inhibitor (see section 4.3).

Anaphylactoid reactions in haemodialysis patients

Anaphylactoid reactions have been reported in patients dialysed with high flux membranes (e.g. AN 69) and treated concomitantly with an ACE inhibitor. In these patients consideration should be given to using a different type of dialysis membrane or different class of antihypertensive agent.

Anaphylactoid reactions during low-density lipoproteins (LDL) apheresis

Rarely, patients receiving ACE inhibitors during low-density lipoproteins (LDL) apheresis with dextran sulphate have experienced life-threatening anaphylactoid reactions. These reactions were avoided by temporarily withholding ACE inhibitor therapy prior to each apheresis.

Desensitisation

Patients receiving ACE inhibitors during desensitisation treatment (e.g. hymenoptera venom) have sustained anaphylactoid reactions. In the same patients, these reactions have been avoided when ACE inhibitors were temporarily withheld but they have reappeared upon inadvertent re-administration of the medicinal product.

Hepatic failure

Very rarely, ACE inhibitors have been associated with a syndrome that starts with cholestatic jaundice and progresses to fulminant necrosis and (sometimes) death. The mechanism of this syndrome is not understood. Patients receiving Zestril who develop jaundice or marked elevations of hepatic enzymes should discontinue Zestril and receive appropriate medical follow-up.

Neutropenia/Agranulocytosis

Neutropenia/agranulocytosis, thrombocytopenia and anaemia have been reported in patients receiving ACE inhibitors. In patients with normal renal function and no other complicating factors, neutropenia occurs rarely. Neutropenia and agranulocytosis are reversible after discontinuation of the ACE inhibitor. Zestril should be used with extreme caution in patients with collagen vascular disease, immunosuppressant therapy, treatment with allopurinol or procainamide, or a combination of these complicating factors, especially if there is pre-existing impaired renal function. Some of these patients developed serious infections, which in a few instances did not respond to intensive antibiotic therapy. If Zestril is used in such patients, periodic monitoring of white blood cell counts is advised and patients should be instructed to report any sign of infection.

Race

Angiotensin converting enzyme inhibitors cause a higher rate of angioedema in black patients than in non-black patients.

As with other ACE inhibitors, Zestril may be less effective in lowering blood pressure in black patients than in non-blacks, possibly because of a higher prevalence of low-renin states in the black hypertensive population.

Cough

Cough has been reported with the use of ACE inhibitors. Characteristically, the cough is non-productive, persistent and resolves after discontinuation of therapy. ACE inhibitor-induced cough should be considered as part of the differential diagnosis of cough.

Surgery/Anaesthesia

In patients undergoing major surgery or during anaesthesia with agents that produce hypotension, Zestril may block angiotensin II formation secondary to compensatory renin release. If hypotension occurs and is considered to be due to this mechanism, it can be corrected by volume expansion.

Hyperkalaemia

Elevations in serum potassium have been observed in some patients treated with ACE inhibitors, including Zestril. Patients at risk for the development of hyperkalaemia include those with renal insufficiency, diabetes mellitus, or those using concomitant potassium-sparing diuretics, potassium supplements or potassium-containing salt substitutes, or those patients taking other drugs associated with increases in serum potassium (e.g. heparin). If concomitant use of the above-mentioned agents is deemed appropriate, regular monitoring of serum potassium is recommended (see section 4.5).

Diabetic patients

In diabetic patients treated with oral antidiabetic agents or insulin, glycaemic control should be closely monitored during the first month of treatment with an ACE inhibitor (see 4.5 Interaction with other medicinal products and other forms of interaction).

Lithium

The combination of lithium and Zestril is generally not recommended (see section 4.5).

Pregnancy and lactation

Lisinopril should not be used during the first trimester of pregnancy. Zestril is contraindicated in the second and third trimesters of pregnancy (see section 4.3). When pregnancy is detected, lisinopril treatment should discontinue as soon as possible (see section 4.6).

Use of lisinopril is not recommended during breast-feeding.

4.5 Interaction with other medicinal products and other forms of Interaction

Diuretics

When a diuretic is added to the therapy of a patient receiving Zestril the antihypertensive effect is usually additive.

Patients already on diuretics and especially those in whom diuretic therapy was recently instituted, may occasionally experience an excessive reduction of blood pressure when Zestril is added. The possibility of symptomatic hypotension with Zestril can be minimised by discontinuing the diuretic prior to initiation of treatment with Zestril (see section 4.4 and section 4.2).

Potassium supplements, potassium-sparing diuretics or potassium-containing salt substitutes

Although in clinical trials, serum potassium usually remained within normal limits, hyperkalaemia did occur in some patients. Risk factors for the development of hyperkalaemia include renal insufficiency, diabetes mellitus, and concomitant use of potassium-sparing diuretics (e.g. spironolactone, triamterene or amiloride), potassium supplements or potassium-containing salt substitutes. The use of potassium supplements, potassium-sparing diuretics or potassium-containing salt substitutes, particularly in patients with impaired renal function, may lead to a significant increase in serum potassium.

If Zestril is given with a potassium-losing diuretic, diuretic-induced hypokalaemia may be ameliorated.

Lithium

Reversible increases in serum lithium concentrations and toxicity have been reported during concomitant administration of lithium with ACE inhibitors. Concomitant use of thiazide diuretics may increase the risk of lithium toxicity and enhance the already increased lithium toxicity with ACE inhibitors. Use of Zestril with lithium is not recommended, but if the combination proves necessary, careful monitoring of serum lithium levels should be performed (see section 4.4).

Non steroidal anti-inflammatory drugs (NSAIDs) including acetylsalicylic acid ⩾ 3g/day

Chronic administration of NSAIDs may reduce the antihypertensive effect of an ACE inhibitor. NSAIDs and ACE inhibitors exert an additive effect on the increase in serum potassium and may result in a deterioration of renal function. These effects are usually reversible. Rarely, acute renal failure may occur, especially in patients with compromised renal function such as the elderly or dehydrated.

Other antihypertensive agents

Concomitant use of these agents may increase the hypotensive effects of Zestril. Concomitant use with glyceryl trinitrate and other nitrates, or other vasodilators, may further reduce blood pressure.

Tricyclic antidepressants/Antipsychotics /Anaesthetics

Concomitant use of certain anaesthetic medicinal products, tricyclic antidepressants and antipsychotics with ACE inhibitors may result in further reduction of blood pressure (see section 4.4).

Sympathomimetics

Sympathomimetics may reduce the antihypertensive effects of ACE inhibitors.

Antidiabetics

Epidemiological studies have suggested that concomitant administration of ACE inhibitors and antidiabetic medicines (insulins, oral hypoglycaemic agents) may cause an increased blood glucose lowering effect with risk of hypoglycaemia. This phenomenon appeared to be more likely to occur during the first weeks of combined treatment and in patients with renal impairment.

Acetylsalicylic acid, thrombolytics, beta-blockers, nitrates

Zestril may be used concomitantly with acetylsalicylic acid (at cardiologic doses), thrombolytics, beta-blockers and/or nitrates.

4.6 Pregnancy and lactation

Pregnancy

Zestril should not be used during the first trimester of pregnancy. When pregnancy is planned or confirmed the switch to an alternative treatment should be initiated as soon as possible. Controlled studies with ACE inhibitors have not been done in humans, but a limited number of cases with first trimester toxicity exposure have not appeared to manifest malformations consistent with human foetotoxicity as described below.

Zestril is contraindicated during the second and third trimester of pregnancy.

Prolonged ACE inhibitor exposure during the second and third trimesters is known to induce human foetotoxicity (decreased renal function, oligohydramnios, skull ossification retardation) and neonatal toxicity (renal failure, hypotension, hyperkalaemia (see also section 5.3).

Should exposure to Zestril have occurred from the second trimester of pregnancy, an ultrasound check of renal function and the skull is recommended.

Infants whose mothers have taken Zestril should be closely observed for hypotension, oliguria and hyperkalaemia. Zestril, which crosses the placenta, has been removed from the neonatal circulation by peritoneal dialysis with some clinical benefit, and theoretically may be removed by exchange transfusion.

Lactation

It is not known whether Zestril is excreted into human breast milk. Lisinopril is excreted into the milk of lactating rats. The use of Zestril is not recommended in women who are breast-feeding.

4.7 Effects on ability to drive and use machines

When driving vehicles or operating machines it should be taken into account that occasionally dizziness or tiredness may occur.

4.8 Undesirable effects

The following undesirable effects have been observed and reported during treatment with Zestril and other ACE inhibitors with the following frequencies: Very common (⩾10%), common (⩾1%, <10%), uncommon (⩾0.1, <1%), rare (⩾0.01, <0.1%), very rare (<0.01%) including isolated reports.

Blood and the lymphatic system disorders:

rare: decreases in haemoglobin, decreases in haematocrit.

very rare: bone marrow depression, anaemia, thrombocytopenia, leucopenia, neutropenia, agranulocytosis (see section 4.4), haemolytic anaemia, lymphadenopathy, autoimmune disease.

Metabolism and nutrition disorders:

very rare: hypoglycaemia.

Nervous system and psychiatric disorders:

common: dizziness, headache

uncommon: mood alterations, paraesthesia, vertigo, taste disturbance, sleep disturbances.

rare: mental confusion.

Cardiac and vascular disorders:

common: orthostatic effects (including hypotension)

uncommon: myocardial infarction or cerebrovascular accident, possibly secondary to excessive hypotension in high risk patients (see section 4.4), palpitations, tachycardia. Raynaud's phenomenon.

Respiratory, thoracic and mediastinal disorders:

common: cough

uncommon: rhinitis

very rare: bronchospasm, sinusitis. Allergic alveolitis/eosinophilic pneumonia.

Gastrointestinal disorders:

common: diarrhoea, vomiting

uncommon: nausea, abdominal pain and indigestion

rare: dry mouth

very rare: pancreatitis, intestinal angioedema, hepatitis - either hepatocellular or cholestatic, jaundice and hepatic failure (see section 4.4).

Skin and subcutaneous tissue disorders:

uncommon: rash, pruritus

rare: hypersensitivity/angioneurotic oedema: angioneurotic oedema of the face, extremities, lips, tongue, glottis, and/or larynx (see section 4.4), urticaria, alopecia, psoriasis.

very rare: diaphoresis, pemphigus, toxic epidermal necrolysis, Stevens-Johnson Syndrome, erythema multiforme.

A symptom complex has been reported which may include one or more of the following: fever, vasculitis, myalgia, arthralgia/arthritis, a positive antinuclear antibodies (ANA), elevated red blood cell sedimentation rate (ESR), eosinophilia and leucocytosis, rash, photosensitivity or other dermatological manifestations may occur.

Renal and urinary disorders:

common: renal dysfunction

rare: uraemia, acute renal failure

very rare: oliguria/anuria.

Reproductive system and breast disorders:

uncommon: impotence

rare: gynaecomastia.

General disorders and administration site conditions:

uncommon: fatigue, asthenia.

Investigations:

uncommon: increases in blood urea, increases in serum creatinine, increases in liver enzymes, hyperkalaemia.

rare: increases in serum bilirubin, hyponatraemia.

4.9 Overdose

Limited data are available for overdose in humans. Symptoms associated with overdosage of ACE inhibitors may include hypotension, circulatory shock, electrolyte disturbances, renal failure, hyperventilation, tachycardia, palpitations, bradycardia, dizziness, anxiety and cough.

The recommended treatment of overdose is intravenous infusion of normal saline solution. If hypotension occurs, the patient should be placed in the shock position. If available, treatment with angiotensin II infusion and/or intravenous catecholamines may also be considered. If ingestion is recent, take measures aimed at eliminating Zestril (e.g. emesis, gastric lavage, administration of absorbents and sodium sulphate). Zestril may be removed from the general circulation by haemodialysis (see 4.4 special warning and precautions for use). Pacemaker therapy is indicated for therapy-resistant bradycardia. Vital signs, serum electrolytes and creatinine concentrations should be monitored frequently.

5. PHARMACOLOGICAL PROPERTIES

5.1 Pharmacodynamic properties

Pharmacotherapeutic group: Angiotensin converting enzyme inhibitors, ATC code: C09A A03.

Zestril is a peptidyl dipeptidase inhibitor. It inhibits the angiotensin converting enzyme (ACE) that catalyses the conversion of angiotensin I to the vasoconstrictor peptide, angiotensin II. Angiotensin II also stimulates aldosterone secretion by the adrenal cortex. Inhibition of ACE results in decreased concentrations of angiotensin II which results in decreased vasopressor activity and reduced aldosterone secretion. The latter decrease may result in an increase in serum potassium concentration.

Whilst the mechanism through which lisinopril lowers blood pressure is believed to be primarily suppression of the renin-angiotensin-aldosterone system, lisinopril is antihypertensive even in patients with low renin hypertension. ACE is identical to kininase II, an enzyme that degrades bradykinin. Whether increased levels of bradykinin, a potent vasodilatory peptide, play a role in the therapeutic effects of lisinopril remains to be elucidated.

The effect of Zestril on mortality and morbidity in heart failure has been studied by comparing a high dose (32.5 mg or 35 mg once daily) with a low dose (2.5 mg or 5 mg once daily). In a study of 3164 patients, with a median follow up period of 46 months for surviving patients, high dose Zestril produced a 12% risk reduction in the combined endpoint of all-cause mortality and all-cause hospitalisation (p = 0.002) and an 8% risk reduction in all-cause mortality and cardiovascular hospitalisation (p = 0.036) compared with low dose. Risk reductions for all-cause mortality (8%; p = 0.128) and cardiovascular mortality (10%; p = 0.073) were observed. In a post-hoc analysis, the number of hospitalisations for heart failure was reduced by 24% (p=0.002) in patients treated with high-dose Zestril compared with low dose. Symptomatic benefits were similar in patients treated with high and low doses of Zestril.

The results of the study showed that the overall adverse event profiles for patients treated with high or low dose Zestril were similar in both nature and number. Predictable events resulting from ACE inhibition, such as hypotension or altered renal function, were manageable and rarely led to treatment withdrawal. Cough was less frequent in patients treated with high dose Zestril compared with low dose.

In the GISSI-3 trial, which used a 2x2 factorial design to compare the effects of Zestril and glyceryl trinitrate given alone or in combination for 6 weeks versus control in 19,394, patients who were administered the treatment within 24 hours of an acute myocardial infarction, Zestril produced a statistically significant risk reduction in mortality of 11% versus control (2p=0.03). The risk reduction with glyceryl trinitrate was not significant but the combination of Zestril and glyceryl trinitrate produced a significant risk reduction in mortality of 17% versus control (2p=0.02). In the sub-groups of elderly (age > 70 years) and females, pre-defined as patients at high risk of mortality, significant benefit was observed for a combined endpoint of mortality and cardiac function. The combined endpoint for all patients, as well as the high-risk sub-groups, at 6 months also showed significant benefit for those treated with Zestril or Zestril plus glyceryl trinitrate for 6 weeks, indicating a prevention effect for Zestril. As would be expected from any vasodilator treatment, increased incidences of hypotension and renal dysfunction were associated with Zestril treatment but these were not associated with a proportional increase in mortality.

In a double-blind, randomised, multicentre trial which compared Zestril with a calcium channel blocker in 335 hypertensive Type 2 diabetes mellitus subjects with incipient nephropathy characterised by microalbuminuria, Zestril 10 mg to 20 mg administered once daily for 12 months, reduced systolic/diastolic blood pressure by 13/10 mmHg and urinary albumin excretion rate by 40%. When compared with the calcium channel blocker, which produced a similar reduction in blood pressure, those treated with Zestril showed a significantly greater reduction in urinary albumin excretion rate, providing evidence that the ACE inhibitory action of Zestril reduced microalbuminuria by a direct mechanism on renal tissues in addition to its blood pressure lowering effect.

Lisinopril treatment does not affect glycaemic control as shown by a lack of significant effect on levels of glycated haemoglobin (HbA_{1c}).

5.2 Pharmacokinetic properties

Lisinopril is an orally active non-sulphydryl-containing ACE inhibitor.

Absorption

Following oral administration of lisinopril, peak serum concentrations occur within about 7 hours, although there was a trend to a small delay in time taken to reach peak serum concentrations in acute myocardial infarction patients. Based on urinary recovery, the mean extent of absorption of lisinopril is approximately 25% with interpatient variability of 6-60% over the dose range studied (5-80 mg). The absolute bioavailability is reduced approximately 16% in patients with heart failure. Lisinopril absorption is not affected by the presence of food.

Distribution

Lisinopril does not appear to be bound to serum proteins other than to circulating angiotensin converting enzyme (ACE). Studies in rats indicate that lisinopril crosses the blood-brain barrier poorly.

Elimination

Lisinopril does not undergo metabolism and is excreted entirely unchanged into the urine on multiple dosing lisinopril has an effective half-life of accumulation of 12.6 hours. The clearance of lisinopril in healthy subjects is approximately 50 ml/min. Declining serum concentrations exhibit a prolonged terminal phase, which does not contribute to drug accumulation. This terminal phase probably represents saturable binding to ACE and is not proportional to dose.

Hepatic impairment

Impairment of hepatic function in cirrhotic patients resulted in a decrease in lisinopril absorption (about 30% as determined by urinary recovery) but an increase in exposure (approximately 50%) compared to healthy subjects due to decreased clearance.

Renal impairment

Impaired renal function decreases elimination of lisinopril, which is excreted via the kidneys, but this decrease becomes clinically important only when the glomerular filtration rate is below 30 ml/min. In mild to moderate renal impairment (creatinine clearance 30-80 ml/min) mean AUC was increased by 13% only, while a 4.5- fold increase in mean AUC was observed in severe renal impairment (creatinine clearance 5-30 ml/min).

Lisinopril can be removed by dialysis. During 4 hours of haemodialysis, plasma lisinopril concentrations decreased on average by 60%, with a dialysis clearance between 40 and 55 ml/min.

Heart failure

Patients with heart failure have a greater exposure of lisinopril when compared to healthy subjects (an increase in AUC on average of 125%), but based on the urinary recovery of lisinopril, there is reduced absorption of approximately 16% compared to healthy subjects.

Elderly

Older patients have higher blood levels and higher values for the area under the plasma concentration time curve (increased approximately 60%) compared with younger subjects.

5.3 Preclinical safety data

Preclinical data reveal no special hazard for humans based on conventional studies of general pharmacology, repeated dose toxicity, genotoxicity, and carcinogenic potential. Angiotensin converting enzyme inhibitors, as a class, have been shown to induce adverse effects on the late foetal development, resulting in foetal death and congenital effects, in particular affecting the skull. Foetotoxicity, intrauterine growth retardation and patent ductus arteriosus have also been reported. These developmental anomalies are thought to be partly due to a direct action of ACE inhibitors on the foetal renin-angiotensin system and partly due to ischaemia resulting from maternal hypotension and decreases in foetal-placental blood flow and oxygen/nutrients delivery to the foetus.

6. PHARMACEUTICAL PARTICULARS

6.1 List of excipients

Mannitol

Calcium Hydrogen Phosphate dihydrate

Red Iron Oxide, in all except the 2.5 mg (E172)

Maize Starch

Pregelatinised Starch

Magnesium Stearate.

6.2 Incompatibilities

None known.

6.3 Shelf life

2.5mg: 24 months

5mg, 10mg, 20mg and 30mg: 48 months.

6.4 Special precautions for storage

Store below 30 Degrees C.

6.5 Nature and contents of container

2.5mg, 5mg, 10mg and 20mg: Blister of packs of 28 or 84 tablets.

30mg: PVC/Aluminium foil blister packs of 28 tablets.

Not all pack sizes may be marketed.

6.6 Instructions for use and handling

No special instructions.

7. MARKETING AUTHORISATION HOLDER

AstraZeneca UK Limited,

600 Capability Green,

Luton, LU1 3LU, UK.

8. MARKETING AUTHORISATION NUMBER(S)

2.5mg: PL 17901/0060

5mg: PL 17901/0061

10mg: PL 17901/0062

20mg: PL 17901/0063

30mg: PL 17901/0072

9. DATE OF FIRST AUTHORISATION/RENEWAL OF THE AUTHORISATION

8 June 2000.

10. DATE OF REVISION OF THE TEXT

18 March 2004.

Zevalin 1.6 mg/ml, Kit for radiopharmaceutical preparation for infusion

(Schering Health Care Limited)

1. NAME OF THE MEDICINAL PRODUCT

▼Zevalin 1.6 mg/ml, Kit for radiopharmaceutical preparation for infusion

2. QUALITATIVE AND QUANTITATIVE COMPOSITION

Ibritumomab tiuxetan* 1.6 mg per ml

One vial contains 3.2 mg of ibritumomab tiuxetan

*produced by a genetically engineered Chinese Hamster Ovary (CHO) cell line conjugated to the chelating agent MX-DTPA

Zevalin is supplied as a kit for the preparation of yttrium-90 radiolabelled ibritumomab tiuxetan.

The final formulation after radiolabelling contains 2.08 mg ibritumomab tiuxetan in a total volume of 10 ml.

For excipients, see 6.1.

3. PHARMACEUTICAL FORM

Kit for radiopharmaceutical preparation for infusion

4. CLINICAL PARTICULARS

4.1 Therapeutic indications

The [^{90}Y]-radiolabelled Zevalin is indicated for the treatment of adult patients with rituximab relapsed or refractory CD20+ follicular B-cell non-Hodgkin's lymphoma (NHL).

4.2 Posology and method of administration

[^{90}Y]-radiolabelled Zevalin should only be handled and administered by qualified personnel with appropriate authorisation for the use and manipulation of radionuclides within a designated clinical setting. Its preparation, use, transfer, storage and disposal are subject to the regulations and/or appropriate authorisation. Infusions should be administered under the close supervision of an experienced physician with full resuscitation facilities immediately available (for radiopharmaceutical precautions see also sections 4.4 and 6.6).

Zevalin should be used following pre-treatment with rituximab.

Refer to the product information of rituximab for detailed guidance on its use.

The prepared infusion solution must be given as a slow intravenous administration over 10 minutes. Do not use as an intravenous bolus.

The [^{90}Y]-radiolabelled Zevalin solution must be prepared according to section 6.6: "Instructions for use/handling".

Before administration to the patient, the percent radio-incorporation of the prepared [^{90}Y]-radiolabelled Zevalin must be checked according to the procedure outlined in section 6.6.

If the average radiochemical purity is less than 95%, the preparation should not be administered.

The recommended radioactivity is:

- for patients with 150,000 platelets per mm^3 and more: 15 MBq [^{90}Y]-radiolabelled Zevalin per kg body weight up to a maximum of 1200 MBq.

- for patients with less than 150,000 but more than 100,000 platelets per mm^3: 11 MBq [^{90}Y]-radiolabelled Zevalin per kg body weight up to a maximum of 1200 MBq.

[^{90}Y]-radiolabelled Zevalin may be infused directly by stopping the flow from an infusion bag and administering it directly into the line. A 0.2 or 0.22 micron low protein binding filter must be on line between the patient and the infusion port. Flush the line with at least 10 ml of sodium chloride 9 mg/ml (0.9%) solution after the infusion of [^{90}Y]-radiolabelled Zevalin.

Treatment consists of two intravenous administrations of rituximab and one administration of [^{90}Y]-radiolabelled Zevalin in the following order:

Day 1: an intravenous infusion of rituximab.

Rituximab infusion dose schedule: 250 mg/m^2 of rituximab.

Day 7, 8, or 9: an intravenous infusion of rituximab shortly before the administration of [^{90}Y]-radiolabelled Zevalin.

Rituximab infusion dose schedule: 250 mg/m^2 of rituximab.

[^{90}Y]-radiolabelled Zevalin infusion: 10 minute intravenous infusion of [^{90}Y]-radiolabelled Zevalin is given up to a maximum dose of 1200 MBq. If the average radiochemical purity is less then 95%, the preparation should not be administered.

Repeated use

Data on the re-treatment of patients with [^{90}Y]-radiolabelled Zevalin are not available.

4.3 Contraindications

Hypersensitivity to ibritumomab tiuxetan, to yttrium chloride, to other murine proteins or to any of the excipients.

Pregnancy and lactation.

4.4 Special warnings and special precautions for use

Radiopharmaceutical agents should only be used by qualified personnel with the appropriate government authorisation for the use and manipulation of radionuclides. This radiopharmaceutical may be received, used and administered only by authorised persons in designated settings. Its receipt, storage, use, transfer, and disposal are subject to the regulations and/or appropriate licences of the local competent official organisations. Radiopharmaceuticals should be prepared by the user in a manner which satisfies both radiation safety and pharmaceutical quality requirements. Appropriate aseptic precautions should be taken, complying with the requirements of Good Manufacturing Practice for pharmaceuticals.

[^{90}Y]-radiolabelled Zevalin should not be administered to patients who are likely to develop life-threatening haematological toxicity signs.

Zevalin should not be administered in the patients mentioned below as safety and efficacy has not been established:

- patients in whom more than 25% of the bone marrow has been infiltrated by lymphoma cells

- patients who have received prior external beam radiation involving more than 25% of active bone marrow

- patients with platelet counts $<100{,}000/mm^3$ or neutrophil counts $<1{,}500/mm^3$

- patients who have received prior bone marrow transplant or stem cell support

- children and adolescents under 18 years of age.

Special caution is required with respect to bone marrow depletion.

Patients who had received murine-derived proteins before Zevalin treatment, should be tested for human anti-mouse antibodies (HAMA). Patients who have developed HAMA may have allergic or hypersensitivity reactions when treated with Zevalin or other murine-derived proteins.

Severe infusion reactions may occur during or following rituximab infusion, which may be associated with chest pain, cardiogenic shock, myocardial infarction, pulmonary edema, ventricular fibrillation, apnea, bronchospasm, dyspnea, hypoxia, angioneurotic edema, flushing, hypotension, ARDS, and lung infiltration. Infusion–related reactions due to Zevalin are less common and less severe.

Anaphylactic and other hypersensitivity reactions have been reported in less than 1 % of patients following the intravenous administration of proteins to patients. Medicinal products for the treatment of hypersensitivity reactions, e.g. adrenaline, antihistamines and corticosteroids, should be available for immediate use in the event of an allergic reaction during administration of Zevalin.

After use of Zevalin, patients should generally be tested for HAMA before any further treatment with mouse derived proteins.

Long-term animal studies on the effect on fertility and reproductive function have not been performed. Due to the nature of the compound, females of child-bearing potential, as well as males, should use effective contraceptive measures during treatment with Zevalin and for 12 months afterwards.

The safety of immunisation with any vaccine, particularly live viral vaccines, following therapy with Zevalin has not been studied. The ability to generate a primary or anamnestic humoral response to any vaccine has also not been studied.

4.5 Interaction with other medicinal products and other forms of Interaction

There are no known interactions with other medicinal products. Formal drug interaction studies have not been carried out.

4.6 Pregnancy and lactation

Animal reproduction studies were not conducted with ibritumomab tiuxetan. Since IgG is known to pass the placenta and because of the concomitant use of radiation, Zevalin must not be used during pregnancy. Pregnancy must be excluded before the start of treatment in women. Females of childbearing potential as well as males should use effective contraceptive methods during treatment with Zevalin and for 12 months afterwards. When it is necessary to administer Zevalin to women of childbearing potential, information should always be sought about pregnancy. Any woman who has missed a period should be assumed to be pregnant until proven otherwise and alternative therapies which do not involve ionising radiation should be then considered.

It is not known whether ibritumomab tiuxetan is excreted in human milk. Because human IgG is excreted in human milk and because the potential for absorption and immunosuppression in the infant is unknown, women must discontinue breast-feeding.

4.7 Effects on ability to drive and use machines

Zevalin could affect the ability to drive and to use machines, as dizziness has been reported as a common side effect.

4.8 Undesirable effects

The radiation dose resulting from therapeutic exposure may result in secondary malignancies and in development of hereditary defects. It is necessary to ensure that the risks of the radiation are less than from the disease itself.

The majority of patients may be expected to experience adverse reactions.

The frequencies of the adverse reactions reported below (very common ⩾1/10, common ⩾1/100, <1/10, uncommon ⩾ 1/1,000, <1/100, rare: ⩾ 1/10,000, <1/1,000; very rare: <1/10,000) are based on clinical trial data.

Anaphylactic reactions and hypersensitivity

Anaphylactic and other hypersensitivity reactions have been reported in less than 1 % of patients following the intravenous administration of proteins to patients. Medicinal products for the treatment of hypersensitivity reactions, e.g. adrenaline, antihistamines and corticosteroids, should be available for immediate use in the event of an allergic reaction during administration of Zevalin.

Haematological adverse reactions

Haematological toxicity has been very commonly observed in clinical trials, and is dose-limiting. Median time to blood platelet and granulocyte nadirs were around 60 days after start of treatment. Grade 3 or 4 thrombocytopenia was reported with median times to recovery of 13 and 21 days and grade 3 or 4 neutropenia with median times to recovery of 8 and 14 days.

Infections

During the first 13 weeks after treatment with Zevalin, patients very commonly developed infections. Grade 3 and grade 4 infections were reported commonly. During follow-up, infections occurred commonly. Of these, grade 3 was common, grade 4 uncommon.

Secondary malignancies

Myelodysplasia / acute myeloid leukaemia (AML) has been reported in five out of 211 patients assigned to treatment with Zevalin. The risk of developing secondary myelodysplasia or leukaemia following therapy with alkylating agents is well known. Since all of these patients were pre-treated with alkylating agents, available results provide insufficient data on whether Zevalin contributes to an increased risk of myelodysplasia, or on the extent of risk.

Incidence of adverse reactions by body system

The table below reports adverse events by body system:

In total, infections of any cause occurred very commonly but are listed in the table under the specifically reported term.

(see Table 1 below)

Disease progression is the natural evolution of the underlying disease.

4.9 Overdose

Overdose as high as 19.2 MBq/kg of [^{90}Y]-radiolabelled Zevalin occurred in clinical trials. Expected haematological toxicity was observed, comprising Grade 3 or 4. Patients recovered from these toxicity signs, and overdoses were not associated with serious or fatal outcome.

There is no known specific antidote for [^{90}Y]-radiolabelled Zevalin overdosage. Treatment consists of discontinuation of Zevalin and supportive therapy, which may include growth factors. If available, autologous stem cell support should be administered to manage haematological toxicity.

For accidental administration of the pure radiopharmaceutical precursor product yttrium-90, refer to the product information of yttrium-90.

5. PHARMACOLOGICAL PROPERTIES

5.1 Pharmacodynamic properties

Pharmacotherapeutic group: monoclonal antibodies, ATC code: L01XC

Table 1

System organ class	Adverse Reactions			
	Very common (⩾1/10)	Common (⩾ 1/100, < 1/10)	Uncommon (⩾ 1/1,000, < 1/100)	Rare (⩾ 1/10,000, < 1/1,000)
Blood and lymphatic system disorders	Anemia, leukocytopenia, neutropenia, thrombocytopenia	Febrile neutropenia, lymphocytopenia, pancytopenia		
Cardiac disorders			Tachycardia	
Gastrointestinal disorders	Nausea	Abdominal pain, constipation, diarrhoea, dyspepsia, throat irritation, vomiting		
General disorders and administration site conditions	Asthenia, pyrexia, rigors	Flu syndrome, hemorrhage while thrombocytopenic, malaise, pain, peripheral edema		
Immune system disorders		Hypersensitivity		
Infections and infestations		Infection, Oral moniliasis, Pneumonia, Sepsis, Urinary tract infection		
Metabolism and nutrition disorders		Anorexia		
Musculoskeletal, connective tissue and bone disorders		Arthralgia, back pain, myalgia, neck pain		
Neoplasms (benign and malignant)		Tumour pain	Myelodysplastic syndrome	Acute myeloid leukemia, meningioma
Nervous system disorders		Dizziness (except vertigo), headache, insomnia		
Psychiatric disorders		Anxiety		
Respiratory, thoracic, and mediastinal disorders		Cough, rhinitis		
Skin and subcutaneous tissue disorders		Pruritus, rash, sweating increased		
Vascular disorders				Intracranial hemorrhage while thrombocytopenic

Ibritumomab tiuxetan is a recombinant murine IgG_1 kappa monoclonal antibody specific for the B-cell antigen CD20. Ibritumomab tiuxetan targets the antigen CD20 which is located on the surface of malignant and normal B-lymphocytes. During B-cell maturation, CD20 is first expressed in the midstage of B-lymphoblast (pre-B-cell), and is lost during the final stage of B-cell maturation to plasma cells. It is not shed from the cell surface and does not internalise on antibody binding. The conjugated antibody has an apparent affinity constant for the CD20 antigen of approximately 17 nM. The binding pattern is very restricted, with no cross-reactivity to other leukocytes or to other types of human tissue.

[^{90}Y]-radiolabelled Zevalin binds specifically to B-cells, including CD20-expressing malignant cells. The isotope yttrium-90 is a pure β-emitter and has a mean path length of about 5 mm. This results in the ability to kill both targeted and neighbouring cells.

Rituximab pre-treatment is necessary to clear circulating B-cells, enabling Zevalin to deliver radiation more specifically to the lymphomas. Rituximab is administered in a reduced dose when compared with the approved monotherapy.

Treatment with [^{90}Y]-radiolabelled Zevalin also leads to depletion of normal CD20+ B-cells. Pharmacodynamic analysis demonstrated that this was a temporary effect; recovery of normal B-cells began within 6 months and median counts of B-cells were within normal range within 9 months after treatment.

The safety and efficacy of the Zevalin therapeutic regimen were evaluated in two multi-center trials enrolling a total of 197 subjects. The Zevalin therapeutic regimen was administered in two steps (see 4.2). The efficacy and toxicity of a variation of the Zevalin therapeutic regimen employing a reduced activity of [^{90}Y]-Zevalin was further defined in a third study enrolling a total of 30 patients who had mild thrombocytopenia (platelet count 100,000 to 149,000 cells/mm^3).

Study 1 was a single arm study of 54 patients with relapsed follicular lymphoma refractory to rituximab treatment. Patients were considered refractory if their last prior treatment with rituximab did not result in a complete or partial response, or if time to disease progression (TTP) was <6 months. The primary efficacy endpoint of the study was the overall response rate (ORR) using the International Workshop Response Criteria (IWRC). Secondary efficacy endpoints included time to disease progression (TTP) and duration of response (DR). In a secondary analysis comparing objective response to the Zevalin therapeutic regimen with that observed with the most recent treatment with rituximab, the median duration of response following the Zevalin therapeutic regimen was 6 vs. 4 months. Table 2 summarizes efficacy data from this study.

Study 2 was a randomized, controlled, multicenter study comparing the Zevalin therapeutic regimen to treatment with rituximab. The trial was conducted in 143 patients with relapsed or refractory low-grade or follicular non-Hodgkin's lymphoma (NHL), or transformed B-cell NHL. A total of 73 patients received the Zevalin therapeutic regimen, and 70 patients received rituximab given as an intravenous infusion at 375 mg/m^2 weekly times 4 doses. The primary efficacy endpoint of the study was to determine the ORR using the IWRC (see Table 2). The ORR was significantly higher (80% vs. 56%, $p = 0.002$) for patients treated with the Zevalin therapeutic regimen. The secondary endpoints, duration of response and time to progression, were not significantly different between the two treatment arms.

(see Table 2 on next page in right hand column)

5.2 Pharmacokinetic properties

In patients given IV infusions of 250 mg/m^2 rituximab followed by intravenous injections of 15 MBq/kg of [^{90}Y]-radiolabelled Zevalin, the median serum effective half-life of [^{90}Y]-radiolabelled Zevalin was 28 h.

As yttrium-90 forms a stable complex with ibritumomab tiuxetan, the biodistribution of the radiolabel follows the biodistribution of the antibody. Irradiation by the emitted beta particles from yttrium-90 occurs in a radius of 5 mm around the isotope.

5.3 Preclinical safety data

The human radiation dose estimates derived from biodistribution studies in mice with [^{90}Y]- or [^{111}In]-radiolabelled ibritumomab tiuxetan predicted acceptable radiation to normal human tissue with limited levels of skeleton and bone marrow radiation. The linker chelate tiuxetan forms a stable complex with the radioisotopes yttrium-90 and indium-111 and only negligible degradation due to radiolysis is expected.

The single and repeated dose toxicity studies of the non-radioactive compound in cynomolgus monkeys did not indicate any other risk than the expected B-cell depletion arising from the use of ibritumomab tiuxetan alone or in combination with rituximab.

Studies on reproductive and developmental toxicity as well as on the mutagenic and carcinogenic potential have not been performed (see sections 4.4 and 4.6).

Studies on the mutagenic and carcinogenic potential of Zevalin have not been performed. Due to the exposure to ionising radiation derived from the radiolabel, a risk of mutagenic and carcinogenic effects has to be taken into account.

5.4 Radiation dosimetry

Yttrium-90 decays by the emission of high-energy beta particles, with a physical half-life of 64.1 hours (2.67 days). The product of radioactive decay is stable zirconium-90. The path length of beta emission (χ_{90}) by yttrium-90 in tissue is 5 mm.

Analyses of estimated radiation absorbed dose were carried out using quantitative imaging with the gamma-emitter [^{111}In]-radiolabelled Zevalin, blood sampling, and the MIRDOSE3 software program. The imaging dose of [^{111}In]-radiolabelled Zevalin was always given immediately following an infusion with rituximab at 250 mg/m^2 to deplete peripheral CD20+ cells and to optimise bio-distribution. Following administration of [^{111}In]-radiolabelled Zevalin, whole body scans were performed at up to eight time-points, acquiring both anterior and posterior images. Blood samples, used to calculate residence times for red marrow, were drawn up to eight time-points.

Based upon dosimetry studies with [^{111}In]-radiolabelled Zevalin, performed with 179 patients treated in four clinical studies; the estimated radiation dosimetry for individual organs following administration of [^{90}Y]-radiolabelled Zevalin at activities of 15 MBq/kg and 11 MBq/kg was calculated according to Medical Internal Radiation Dosimetry (MIRD) (Table 3). The estimated radiation-absorbed doses to normal organs were substantially below recognised upper safety limits. Individual patient dosimetry results were not predictive for [^{90}Y]-radiolabelled Zevalin toxicity.

Table 3.
Estimated Radiation Absorbed Doses From [^{90}Y]-Zevalin

Organ	[^{90}Y]-Zevalin mGy/MBq	
	Median	Range
Spleen[1]	9.4	1.8 - 14.4
Testes[1]	9.1	5.4 - 11.4
Liver[1]	4.8	2.3 - 8.1
Lower Large Intestinal Wall[1]	4.8	3.1 – 8.2
Upper Large Intestinal Wall[1]	3.6	2.0 – 6.7
Heart Wall[1]	2.8	1.5 - 3.2
Lungs[1]	2.0	1.2 - 3.4
Small Intestine[1]	1.4	0.8 – 2.1
Red Marrow[2]	1.3	0.7 - 1.8
Urinary Bladder Wall[3]	0.9	0.7 - 2.1
Bone Surfaces [2]	0.9	0.5 - 1.2
Ovaries[3]	0.4	0.3 - 0.5
Uterus[3]	0.4	0.3 - 0.5
Adrenals[3]	0.3	0.0 - 0.5
Brain[3]	0.3	0.0 - 0.5
Breasts[3]	0.3	0.0 - 0.5
Gallbladder Wall[3]	0.3	0.0 - 0.5
Muscle[3]	0.3	0.0 - 0.5
Pancreas[3]	0.3	0.0 - 0.5
Skin[3]	0.3	0.0 - 0.5
Stomach[3]	0.3	0.0 - 0.5
Thymus[3]	0.3	0.0 - 0.5
Thyroid[3]	0.3	0.0 - 0.5
Kidneys[1]	0.1	0.0 - 0.2
Total Body[3]	0.5	0.2 - 0.7

1 Organ region of interest
2 Sacrum region of interest
3 Whole body region of interest

6. PHARMACEUTICAL PARTICULARS

6.1 List of excipients

Ibritumomab tiuxetan vial:

Sodium chloride

Water for injections

Table 2 Summary of Efficacy Data[1]

	Study 1	Study 2	
	Zevalin therapeutic regimen	Zevalin therapeutic regimen	Rituximab
	N = 54	N = 73	N = 70
Overall Response Rate (%)	74	80	56
Complete Response Rate (%)	15	30	16
CRu Rate[2](%)	0	4	4
Median DR[3,4] (Months) [Range[5]]	6.4 [0.5-24.9+]	13.9 [1.0-30.1+]	11.8 [1.2-24.5]
Median TTP[3,6] (Months) [Range[5]]	6.8 [1.1-25.9+]	11.2 [0.8-31.5+]	10.1 [0.7-26.1]

[1] IWRC: International Workshop response criteria
[2] CRu: Unconfirmed complete response
[3] Estimated with observed range.
[4] Duration of response: interval from the onset of response to disease progression.
[5]"+" indicates an ongoing response.
[6] Time to Disease Progression: interval from the first infusion to disease progression.

Study 3 was a single arm study of 30 patients with relapsed or refractory low-grade, follicular, or transformed B-cell NHL who had mild thrombocytopenia (platelet count 100,000 to 149,000 cells/mm^3). Excluded from the study were patients with ≥25% lymphoma marrow involvement and/or impaired bone marrow reserve. Patients were considered to have impaired bone marrow reserve if they had any of the following: prior myeloablative therapy with stem cell support; prior external beam radiation to > 25% of active marrow; a platelet count < 100,000 cells/mm^3; or neutrophil count < 1,500 cells/mm^3. In this study, a modification of the Zevalin therapeutic regimen with a lower [^{90}Y]-Zevalin activity per body weight (11 MBq/kg) was used. Objective, durable clinical responses were observed [67% ORR (95% CI: 48-85%), 11.8 months median DR (range: 4-17 months)] and resulted in a greater incidence of haematologic toxicity (see 4.8) than in Studies 1 and 2.

Sodium acetate vial:
Sodium acetate
Water for injections

Formulation buffer vial:
Human albumin solution
Sodium chloride
Disodium phosphate dodecahydrate
Sodium hydroxide
Potassium dihydrogen phosphate
Potassium chloride
Pentetic acid
Hydrochloric acid, diluted
Water for injections

6.2 Incompatibilities

This medicinal product must not be mixed with other medicinal products

6.3 Shelf life

3 years

After radiolabelling, an immediate use is recommended. Chemical and physical in-use stability has been demonstrated for 8 hours at 2°C - 8°C and protected from light.

6.4 Special precautions for storage

Store at 2°C - 8°C (in a refrigerator).

Do not freeze.

Store in the original package in order to protect from light.

After radiolabelling: Store at 2°C - 8°C (in a refrigerator) and protect from light.

Storage should be in accordance with national regulations for radioactive materials.

6.5 Nature and contents of container

2 ml of solution of ibritumomab tiuxetan in a vial (type I glass) with a rubber stopper (teflon-lined bromobutyl)

2 ml of solution of sodium acetate solution in a vial (type I glass) with a rubber stopper (teflon-lined bromobutyl)

10 ml of formulation buffer in a vial (type I glass) with a rubber stopper (teflon-lined bromobutyl)

10 ml empty reaction vial (type I glass) with a rubber stopper (teflon-lined bromobutyl)

Pack size of 1 kit

6.6 Instructions for use and handling

Read complete directions thoroughly before starting the preparation procedure.

Proper aseptic technique and precautions for handling radioactive materials should be employed. Waterproof gloves should be utilised in the preparation and during the determination of radiochemical purity of [^{90}Y]-radiolabelled Zevalin.

No incompatibilities have been observed between Zevalin and infusion sets.

The administration of radiopharmaceuticals creates risks for other persons from external radiation or contamination from spills of urine, vomiting, etc. Radiation protection precaution in accordance with local regulations must therefore be taken.

Any unused product or waste material should be disposed of in accordance with local requirements. Contaminated materials must be disposed of as radioactive waste by the authorised route.

Characteristics of yttrium-90

- The following minimum yttrium-90 characteristics are recommended:

Radioactivity concentration at time of use	1.67 to 3.34 GBq/ml
Total extractable activity to deliver at time of use	≥ 1.48 GBq corresponding to 0.44 ml to 0.89 ml of yttrium-90 solution
HCl concentration	0.035-0.045 M
Chloride identification	Positive
Yttrium identification	Positive
Radiochemical purity of the yttrium-90 chloride solution	≥ 95% of free ionic yttrium-90
Bacterial endotoxins	≤150 EU/ml
Sterility	No growth
Radionuclidic purity strontium-90 content	≤ 0.74 MBq strontium-90 / 37 GBq yttrium-90
Metal impurities	
Total metals*	≤50 ppm
Individual metals*	≤ 10 ppm each

* Metals to be included need to be based on the specific manufacturing process. Control of these metals can be achieved either through process validation or release test.

- Additional testing that might be required for suitability assessment:

Process-specific impurities:

Total organic carbon (e.g. organic chelators)	Below limit of quantitation*
Process residuals (e.g. ammonia, nitrate)	Below limit of quantitation*
Total Alpha impurities	Below limit of quantitation*

Total other Beta impurities (non-strontium-90)	Below limit of quantitation*
Total Gamma impurities	Below limit of quantitation*

* Needs to be included as release test or controlled through process validation if above limit of quantitation

Directions for radio-labelling of Zevalin with yttrium-90:

Sterile, pyrogen-free yttrium-90 chloride of the above specified quality must be used for the preparation of [^{90}Y]-radiolabelled Zevalin.

Before radiolabelling, bring refrigerated Zevalin cold kit to room temperature 25°C.

Clean the rubber stopper of all cold kit vials and the yttrium-90 chloride vial with a suitable alcohol swab and allow to air dry.

Place cold kit reaction vial in a suitable dispensing shield (plastic enclosed in lead).

Step 1: Transfer sodium acetate solution to the reaction vial

Using a 1-ml sterile syringe, transfer sodium acetate solution to reaction vial. The volume of sodium acetate solution added is equivalent to 1.2 times the volume of yttrium-90 chloride to be transferred in step 2.

Step 2: Transfer yttrium-90 chloride to the reaction vial

Aseptically transfer 1500 MBq of yttrium-90 chloride with a 1 ml sterile syringe to the reaction vial containing the sodium acetate solution transferred in step 1. Mix completely by coating the entire inner surface of the reaction vial. Mix by inversion, rolling the container, avoid foaming or agitating the solution.

Step 3: Transfer ibritumomab tiuxetan solution to the reaction vial

Using a 2-3 ml sterile syringe, transfer 1.3 ml ibritumomab tiuxetan solution to the reaction vial. Mix completely by coating the entire inner surface of the reaction vial. Mix by inversion, rolling the container, avoid foaming or agitating the solution.

Incubate the yttrium-90 chloride/acetate/ibritumomab tiuxetan solution at room temperature for five minutes. Labelling time longer than six minutes or shorter than four minutes will result in inadequate radioincorporation.

Step 4: Add the formulation buffer to the reaction vial

Using a 10-ml syringe with a large bore needle (18-20 G), draw formulation buffer that will result in a combined total volume of 10 ml.

After the five-minute incubation period, add the formulation buffer to the reaction vial terminating incubation. Immediately prior to this addition withdraw an equal volume of air from the reaction vial in order to normalise pressure. Gently add the formulation buffer down the side of the reaction vial. Do not foam, shake, or agitate the mixture.

Step 5: Assay the [^{90}Y]-radiolabelled Zevalin solution for its specific radioactivity

Radiochemical purity of the radiolabelled preparation applies as long as more than 95% of yttrium-90 is incorporated into the monoclonal antibody.

Before administration to the patient, the percent radioincorporation of the prepared [^{90}Y]-radiolabelled Zevalin must be checked according to the procedure outlined below.

Caution: Patient dose not to exceed 1200 MBq.

Instructions for determining the percent radioincorporation.

The radioincorporation assay for radiochemical purity, is performed by Instant Thin Layer Chromatography (ITLC) and should be carried out according to the following procedure.

Required materials not supplied in the Zevalin kit:

- Developing chamber for chromatography

- Mobile phase: sodium chloride 9 mg/ml (0.9%) solution, bacteriostatic-free

- ITLC strips (e.g. ITLC silica gel (SG) plates Art. No. 61885, Gelman Sciences, Ann Arbor, Michigan, USA or equivalent; dimensions: 0.5 cm × 6 cm, origin: 1.4 cm, cut line: 3.5 cm, solvent front: 5.4 cm)

- Scintillation vials

- Liquid scintillation cocktail (e.g. Ultima Gold, catalog No. 6013329, Packard Instruments, USA or equivalent)

Assay procedure:

1.) Add approximately 0.8 ml 0.9% sodium chloride solution to developing chamber assuring the liquid will not touch the 1.4 cm origin mark on the ITCL strip.

2.) Using a 1 ml insulin syringe with a 25- to 26-G needle, place a hanging drop (7-10 μl) of [^{90}Y]-radiolabelled Zevalin onto the ITLC strip at its origin. Spot one strip at a time and run three ITLC strips. It may be necessary to perform a dilution (1:100) before application of the [^{90}Y]-radiolabelled Zevalin to the ITLC strips.

3.) Place ITLC strip in the developing chamber and allow the solvent front to migrate past the 5.4 cm mark.

4.) Remove ITLC strip and cut in half at the 3.5 cm cut line. Place each half into separate scintillation vials to which 5 ml LSC cocktail should be added (e.g. Ultima Gold, catalog No. 6013329, Packard Instruments, USA or equivalent). Count each vial in a beta counter or in an appropriate counter for one minute (CPM), record net counts, corrected for background.

5.) Calculate the average Radiochemical Purity (RCP) as follows:

6.) $$\text{Average \% RCP} = \frac{\text{net CPM bottom half}}{\text{net CPM top half + net CPM bottom half}} \times 100$$

7.) If the average radiochemical purity is less than 95%, the preparation should not be administered.

7. MARKETING AUTHORISATION HOLDER
Schering AG

13342 Berlin

Germany

8. MARKETING AUTHORISATION NUMBER(S)
EU/1/03/264/001

9. DATE OF FIRST AUTHORISATION/RENEWAL OF THE AUTHORISATION
January 2004

10. DATE OF REVISION OF THE TEXT
July 2005

LEGAL CATEGORY
POM

Ziagen 20 mg/ml Oral Solution

(GlaxoSmithKline UK)

1. NAME OF THE MEDICINAL PRODUCT
Ziagen 20 mg/ml oral solution

2. QUALITATIVE AND QUANTITATIVE COMPOSITION
Oral solution containing 20 mg/ml of abacavir as abacavir sulfate.

For excipients see section 6.1.

3. PHARMACEUTICAL FORM
Oral solution

The oral solution is clear to slightly opalescent yellowish, aqueous solution with strawberry and banana flavouring.

4. CLINICAL PARTICULARS

4.1 Therapeutic indications
Ziagen is indicated in antiretroviral combination therapy for the treatment of Human Immunodeficiency Virus (HIV) infection.

The demonstration of the benefit of Ziagen is mainly based on results of studies performed in treatment-naïve adult patients on combination therapy with a twice daily regimen (see section 5.1).

4.2 Posology and method of administration
Ziagen should be prescribed by physicians experienced in the management of HIV infection.

Adults and adolescents over 12 years: the recommended dose of Ziagen is 600 mg daily (30 ml). This may be administered as either 300 mg (15 ml) twice daily or 600 mg (30 ml) once daily (see sections 4.4 and 5.1).

Patients changing to the once daily regimen should take 300 mg (15 ml) twice a day and switch to 600 mg (30 ml) once a day the following morning. Where an evening once daily regimen is preferred, 300 mg (15 ml) of Ziagen should be taken on the first morning only, followed by 600 mg (30 ml) in the evening. When changing back to a twice daily regimen, patients should complete the day's treatment and start 300 mg (15 ml) twice a day the following morning.

Children from three months to 12 years: the recommended dose is 8 mg/kg twice daily up to a maximum of 600 mg (30 ml) daily.

Children less than three months: the data available on the use of Ziagen in this age group are very limited (see section 5.2).

Ziagen can be taken with or without food.

Ziagen is also available as a tablet formulation.

Renal impairment: no dosage adjustment of Ziagen is necessary in patients with renal dysfunction. However, Ziagen should be avoided in patients with end-stage renal disease (see section 5.2).

Hepatic impairment: abacavir is primarily metabolised by the liver. No dose recommendation can be made in patients with mild hepatic impairment. No data are available in patients with moderate hepatic impairment, therefore the use of abacavir is not recommended unless judged necessary. In patients with mild and moderate hepatic impairment close monitoring is required, and if feasible, monitoring of abacavir plasma levels is recommended (see section 5.2). Abacavir is contraindicated in patients with severe hepatic impairment (see section 4.3 and 4.4).

Elderly: no pharmacokinetic data is currently available in patients over 65 years of age.

4.3 Contraindications

Ziagen is contraindicated in patients with known hypersensitivity to abacavir or to any of the excipients of Ziagen oral solution. See BOXED INFORMATION ON HYPERSENSITIVITY REACTIONS in sections 4.4. and 4.8.

Ziagen is contraindicated in patients with severe hepatic impairment.

4.4 Special warnings and special precautions for use *(see Table 1 on next page)*
Lactic acidosis: lactic acidosis, usually associated with hepatomegaly and hepatic steatosis, has been reported with the use of nucleoside analogues. Early symptoms (symptomatic hyperlactatemia) include benign digestive symptoms (nausea, vomiting and abdominal pain), non-specific malaise, loss of appetite, weight loss, respiratory symptoms (rapid and/or deep breathing) or neurological symptoms (including motor weakness).

Lactic acidosis has a high mortality and may be associated with pancreatitis, liver failure, or renal failure.

Lactic acidosis generally occurred after a few or several months of treatment.

Treatment with nucleoside analogues should be discontinued in the setting of symptomatic hyperlactatemia and metabolic/lactic acidosis, progressive hepatomegaly, or rapidly elevating aminotransferase levels.

Caution should be exercised when administering nucleoside analogues to any patient (particularly obese women) with hepatomegaly, hepatitis or other known risk factors for liver disease and hepatic steatosis (including certain medicinal products and alcohol). Patients co-infected with hepatitis C and treated with alpha interferon and ribavirin may constitute a special risk.

Patients at increased risk should be followed closely.

Mitochondrial dysfunction: nucleoside and nucleotide analogues have been demonstrated *in vitro* and *in vivo* to cause a variable degree of mitochondrial damage. There have been reports of mitochondrial dysfunction in HIV-negative infants exposed *in utero* and/or post-natally to nucleoside analogues. The main adverse events reported are haematological disorders (anaemia, neutropenia), metabolic disorders (hyperlactatemia, hyperlipasemia). These events are often transitory. Some late-onset neurological disorders have been reported (hypertonia, convulsion, abnormal behaviour). Whether the neurological disorders are transient or permanent is currently unknown. Any child exposed *in utero* to nucleoside and nucleotide analogues, even HIV-negative children, should have clinical and laboratory follow-up and should be fully investigated for possible mitochondrial dysfunction in case of relevant signs or symptoms. These findings do not affect current national recommendations to use antiretroviral therapy in pregnant women to prevent vertical transmission of HIV.

Lipodystrophy: combination antiretroviral therapy has been associated with the redistribution of body fat (lipodystrophy) in HIV patients. The long-term consequences of these events are currently unknown. Knowledge about the mechanism is incomplete. A connection between visceral lipomatosis and protease inhibitors (PIs) and lipoatrophy and nucleoside reverse transcriptase inhibitors (NRTIs) has been hypothesised. A higher risk of lipodystrophy has been associated with individual factors such as older age, and with drug related factors such as longer duration of antiretroviral treatment and associated metabolic disturbances. Clinical examination should include evaluation for physical signs of fat redistribution. Consideration should be given to the measurement of fasting serum lipids and blood glucose. Lipid disorders should be managed as clinically appropriate (see section 4.8).

Pancreatitis: pancreatitis has been reported, but a causal relationship to Ziagen treatment is uncertain.

Triple nucleoside therapy: in patients with high viral load >100,000 copies/ml) the choice of a triple combination with abacavir, lamivudine and zidovudine needs special consideration (see section 5.1).

There have been reports of a high rate of virological failure and of emergence of resistance at an early stage when abacavir was combined with tenofovir disoproxil fumarate and lamivudine as a once daily regimen.

Once daily administration (abacavir 600 mg): the benefit of abacavir as a once daily regimen is mainly based on a study performed in combination with efavirenz and lamivudine, in antiretroviral-naïve adult patients (see section 5.1).

Liver disease: the safety and efficacy of Ziagen has not been established in patients with significant underlying liver disorders. Ziagen is contraindicated in patients with severe hepatic impairment (see section 4.3). Patients with chronic hepatitis B or C and treated with combination antiretroviral therapy are at an increased risk of severe and potentially fatal hepatic adverse events. In case of concomitant antiviral therapy for hepatitis B or C, please refer also to the relevant product information for these medicinal products.

Patients with pre-existing liver dysfunction, including chronic active hepatitis, have an increased frequency of

Table 1

Hypersensitivity Reaction
(see also section 4.8):

In clinical studies approximately 5% of subjects receiving abacavir develop a hypersensitivity reaction; some of these cases were life-threatening and resulted in a fatal outcome despite taking precautions.

• **Description**
Hypersensitivity reactions are characterised by the appearance of symptoms indicating multi-organ system involvement. Almost all hypersensitivity reactions will have fever and/or rash as part of the syndrome.

Other signs and symptoms may include respiratory signs and symptoms such as dyspnoea, sore throat, cough and abnormal chest x-ray findings (predominantly infiltrates, which can be localised), gastrointestinal symptoms, such as nausea, vomiting, diarrhoea, or abdominal pain, **and may lead to misdiagnosis of hypersensitivity as respiratory disease (pneumonia, bronchitis, pharyngitis), or gastroenteritis.**

Other frequently observed signs or symptoms of the hypersensitivity reaction may include lethargy or malaise and musculoskeletal symptoms (myalgia, rarely myolysis, arthralgia).

The symptoms related to this hypersensitivity reaction worsen with continued therapy and can be life-threatening. These symptoms usually resolve upon discontinuation of Ziagen.

• **Management**
Hypersensitivity reaction symptoms usually appear within the first six weeks of initiation of treatment with abacavir, although these reactions **may occur at any time during therapy.**

Patients should be monitored closely, especially during the first two months of treatment with Ziagen, with consultation every two weeks.

Patients who are diagnosed with a hypersensitivity reaction whilst on therapy **MUST discontinue Ziagen immediately.**

Ziagen, or any other medicinal product containing abacavir (i.e. Kivexa, Trizivir), MUST NEVER be restarted in patients who have stopped therapy due to a hypersensitivity reaction.

Restarting abacavir following a hypersensitivity reaction results in a prompt return of symptoms within hours. This recurrence is usually more severe than on initial presentation, and may include life-threatening hypotension and death.

To avoid a delay in diagnosis and minimise the risk of a life-threatening hypersensitivity reaction, Ziagen must be permanently discontinued if hypersensitivity cannot be ruled out, even when other diagnoses are possible (respiratory diseases, flu-like illness, gastroenteritis or reactions to other medications).

Special care is needed for those patients simultaneously starting treatment with Ziagen and other medicinal products known to induce skin toxicity (such as non-nucleoside reverse transcriptase inhibitors - NNRTIs). This is because it is currently difficult to differentiate between rashes induced by these products and abacavir related hypersensitivity reactions.

• **Management after an interruption of Ziagen therapy**
If therapy with Ziagen has been discontinued for any reason and restarting therapy is under consideration, the reason for discontinuation must be established to assess whether the patient had any symptoms of a hypersensitivity reaction. **If a hypersensitivity reaction cannot be ruled out, Ziagen or any other medicinal product containing abacavir (i.e. Kivexa, Trizivir) must not be restarted.**

Hypersensitivity reactions with rapid onset, including life-threatening reactions have occurred after restarting Ziagen in patients who had only one of the key symptoms of hypersensitivity (skin rash, fever, gastrointestinal, respiratory or constitutional symptoms such as lethargy and malaise) prior to stopping Ziagen. The most common isolated symptom of a hypersensitivity reaction was a skin rash. Moreover, on very rare occasions hypersensitivity reactions have been reported in patients who have restarted therapy, and who had no preceding symptoms of a hypersensitivity reaction.

In both cases, if a decision is made to restart Ziagen this must be done in a setting where medical assistance is readily available.

• **Essential patient information**
Prescribers must ensure that patients are fully informed regarding the following information on the hypersensitivity reaction:

- patients must be made aware of the possibility of a hypersensitivity reaction to abacavir that may result in a life-threatening reaction or death.

- patients developing signs or symptoms possibly linked with a hypersensitivity reaction **MUST CONTACT their doctor IMMEDIATELY.**

- patients who are hypersensitive to abacavir should be reminded that they must never take Ziagen or any other medicinal product containing abacavir (i.e. Kivexa, Trizivir)

- in order to avoid restarting Ziagen, patients who have experienced a hypersensitivity reaction should be asked to return the remaining Ziagen tablets or oral solution to the pharmacy.

- patients who have stopped Ziagen for any reason, and particularly due to possible adverse reactions or illness, must be advised to contact their doctor before restarting.

- patients should be advised of the importance of taking Ziagen regularly.

- each patient should be reminded to read the Package Leaflet included in the Ziagen pack. They should be reminded of the importance of removing the Alert Card included in the pack, and keeping it with them at all times.

liver function abnormalities during combination antiretroviral therapy, and should be monitored according to standard practice. If there is evidence of worsening liver disease in such patients, interruption or discontinuation of treatment must be considered.

A pharmacokinetic study has been performed in patients with mild hepatic impairment. However, a definitive recommendation on dose reduction is not possible due to substantial variability of drug exposure in this patient population (see section 5.2). The clinical safety data available with abacavir in hepatically impaired patients is very limited. Due to the potential increases in exposure (AUC) in some patients, close monitoring is required. No data are available in patients with moderate or severe hepatic impairment. Plasma concentrations of abacavir are expected to substantially increase in these patients. Therefore, the use of abacavir in patients with moderate hepatic impairment is not recommended unless judged necessary and requires close monitoring of these patients. For patients with severe hepatic impairment, Ziagen is contraindicated (see section 4.3).

Renal disease: Ziagen should not be administered to patients with end-stage renal disease (see section 5.2).

Excipients: Ziagen oral solution contains 340 mg/ml of sorbitol. When taken according to the dosage recommendations each 15 ml dose contains approximately 5 g of sorbitol. Patients with rare hereditary problems of fructose intolerance should not take this medicine. Sorbitol can have a mild laxative effect. The calorific value of sorbitol is 2.6 kcal/g.

Immune Reactivation Syndrome: In HIV-infected patients with severe immune deficiency at the time of institution of combination antiretroviral therapy (CART), an inflammatory reaction to asymptomatic or residual opportunistic pathogens may arise and cause serious clinical conditions, or aggravation of symptoms. Typically, such reactions have been observed within the first few weeks or months of initiation of CART. Relevant examples are cytomegalovirus retinitis, generalised and/or focal mycobacterium infections, and Pneumocystis carinii pneumonia. Any inflammatory symptoms should be evaluated and treatment instituted when necessary.

Opportunistic infections: patients receiving Ziagen or any other antiretroviral therapy may still develop opportunistic infections and other complications of HIV infection. Therefore patients should remain under close clinical observation by physicians experienced in the treatment of these associated HIV diseases.

Transmission: patients should be advised that current antiretroviral therapy, including Ziagen, have not been proven to prevent the risk of transmission of HIV to others through sexual contact or blood contamination. Appropriate precautions should continue to be taken.

4.5 Interaction with other medicinal products and other forms of Interaction
Based on the results of *in vitro* experiments and the known major metabolic pathways of abacavir, the potential for P450 mediated interactions with other medicinal products involving abacavir is low. P450 does not play a major role in the metabolism of abacavir, and abacavir does not inhibit metabolism mediated by CYP 3A4. Abacavir has also been shown *in vitro* not to inhibit CYP 3A4, CYP2C9 or CYP2D6 enzymes at clinically relevant concentrations. Induction of hepatic metabolism has not been observed in clinical studies. Therefore, there is little potential for interactions with antiretroviral PIs and other medicinal products metabolised by major P450 enzymes. Clinical studies have shown that there are no clinically significant interactions between abacavir, zidovudine, and lamivudine.

Potent enzymatic inducers such as rifampicin, phenobarbital and phenytoin may via their action on UDP-glucuronyltransferases slightly decrease the plasma concentrations of abacavir.

Ethanol: the metabolism of abacavir is altered by concomitant ethanol resulting in an increase in AUC of abacavir of about 41%. These findings are not considered clinically significant. Abacavir has no effect on the metabolism of ethanol.

Methadone: in a pharmacokinetic study, coadministration of 600 mg abacavir twice daily with methadone showed a 35% reduction in abacavir C_{max} and a one hour delay in t_{max} but the AUC was unchanged. The changes in abacavir pharmacokinetics are not considered clinically relevant. In this study abacavir increased the mean methadone systemic clearance by 22%. The induction of drug metabolising enzymes cannot therefore be excluded. Patients being treated with methadone and abacavir should be monitored for evidence of withdrawal symptoms indicating under dosing, as occasionally methadone re-titration may be required.

Retinoids: retinoid compounds are eliminated via alcohol dehydrogenase. Interaction with abacavir is possible but has not been studied.

4.6 Pregnancy and lactation
Pregnancy: Ziagen is not recommended during pregnancy. The safe use of abacavir in human pregnancy has not been established. Placental transfer of abacavir and/or its related metabolites has been shown to occur in animals. Toxicity to the developing embryo and foetus occurred in rats, but not in rabbits (see section 5.3). The teratogenic potential of abacavir could not be established from studies in animals.

Lactation: abacavir and its metabolites are secreted into the milk of lactating rats. It is expected that these will also be secreted into human milk, although this has not been confirmed. There are no data available on the safety of abacavir when administered to babies less than three months old. It is therefore recommended that mothers do not breast-feed their babies while receiving treatment with abacavir. Additionally, it is recommended that HIV infected women do not breast-feed their infants under any circumstances in order to avoid transmission of HIV.

4.7 Effects on ability to drive and use machines
No studies on the effects on ability to drive and use machines have been performed.

4.8 Undesirable effects
(see Table 2 on next page)
For many of the other adverse events reported, it is unclear whether they are related to Ziagen, to the wide range of medicinal products used in the management of HIV infection or as a result of the disease process.

Many of those listed below occur commonly (nausea, vomiting, diarrhoea, fever, lethargy, rash) in patients with abacavir hypersensitivity. Therefore, patients with any of these symptoms should be carefully evaluated for the presence of this hypersensitivity reaction. If Ziagen has been discontinued in patients due to experiencing any one

Table 2

Hypersensitivity
(see also section 4.4):

In clinical studies, approximately 5% of subjects receiving abacavir developed a hypersensitivity reaction. In clinical studies with abacavir 600 mg once daily the reported rate of hypersensitivity remained within the range recorded for abacavir 300 mg twice daily.

Some of these hypersensitivity reactions were life-threatening and resulted in fatal outcome despite taking precautions. This reaction is characterised by the appearance of symptoms indicating multi-organ/body-system involvement.

Almost all patients developing hypersensitivity reactions will have fever and/or rash (usually maculopapular or urticarial) as part of the syndrome, however reactions have occurred without rash or fever.

The signs and symptoms of this hypersensitivity reaction are listed below. These have been identified either from clinical studies or post marketing surveillance. Those reported **in at least 10% of patients** with a hypersensitivity reaction are in bold text.

Skin	**Rash** (usually maculopapular or urticarial)
Gastrointestinal tract	**Nausea, vomiting, diarrhoea, abdominal pain**, mouth ulceration
Respiratory tract	**Dyspnoea, cough**, sore throat, adult respiratory distress syndrome, respiratory failure
Miscellaneous	**Fever, lethargy, malaise**, oedema, lymphadenopathy, hypotension, conjunctivitis, anaphylaxis
Neurological/Psychiatry	**Headache**, paraesthesia
Haematological	Lymphopenia
Liver/pancreas	**Elevated liver function tests,** hepatitis, hepatic failure
Musculoskeletal	**Myalgia**, rarely myolysis, arthralgia, elevated creatine phosphokinase
Urology	Elevated creatinine, renal failure

Rash (81% vs 67% respectively) and gastrointestinal manifestations (70% vs 54% respectively) were more frequently reported in children compared to adults.

Some patients with hypersensitivity reactions were initially thought to have gastroenteritis, respiratory disease (pneumonia, bronchitis, pharyngitis) or a flu-like illness. This delay in diagnosis of hypersensitivity has resulted in Ziagen being continued or re-introduced, leading to more severe hypersensitivity reactions or death. Therefore, the diagnosis of hypersensitivity reaction should be carefully considered for patients presenting with symptoms of these diseases.

Symptoms usually appeared within the first six weeks (median time to onset 11 days) of initiation of treatment with abacavir, although these reactions may occur at any time during therapy. Close medical supervision is necessary during the first two months, with consultations every two weeks.

Risk factors that may predict the occurrence or severity of hypersensitivity to abacavir have not been identified. However, it is likely that intermittent therapy may increase the risk of developing sensitisation and therefore occurrence of clinically significant hypersensitivity reactions. Consequently, patients should be advised of the importance of taking Ziagen regularly.

Restarting Ziagen following a hypersensitivity reaction results in a prompt return of symptoms within hours. This recurrence of the hypersensitivity reaction was usually more severe than on initial presentation, and may include life-threatening hypotension and death. **Patients who develop this hypersensitivity reaction must discontinue Ziagen and must never be rechallenged with Ziagen, or any other medicinal product containing abacavir (i.e. Kivexa, Trizivir).**

To avoid a delay in diagnosis and minimise the risk of a life-threatening hypersensitivity reaction, Ziagen must be permanently discontinued if hypersensitivity cannot be ruled out, even when other diagnoses are possible (respiratory diseases, flu-like illness, gastroenteritis or reactions to other medications).

Hypersensitivity reactions with rapid onset, including life-threatening reactions have occurred after restarting Ziagen in patients who had only one of the key symptoms of hypersensitivity (skin rash, fever, gastrointestinal, respiratory or constitutional symptoms such as lethargy and malaise) prior to stopping Ziagen. The most common isolated symptom of a hypersensitivity reaction was a skin rash. Moreover, on very rare occasions hypersensitivity reactions have been reported in patients who have restarted therapy and who had no preceding symptoms of a hypersensitivity reaction.

In both cases, if a decision is made to restart Ziagen this must be done in a setting where medical assistance is readily available.

Each patient must be warned about this hypersensitivity reaction to abacavir.

of these symptoms and a decision is made to restart a medicinal product containing abacavir, this must be done in a setting where medical assistance is readily available (see section 4.4.). Very rarely cases of erythema multiforme, Stevens Johnson syndrome or toxic epidermal necrolysis have been reported where abacavir hypersensitivity could not be ruled out. In such cases medicinal products containing abacavir should be permanently discontinued.

Many of the adverse reactions have not been treatment limiting. The following convention has been used for their classification: very common >1/10), common >1/100, <1/10), uncommon >1/1,000, <1/100), rare >1/10,000, <1/1,000) very rare (<1/10,000).

Metabolism and nutrition disorders

Common: anorexia

Nervous system disorders

Common: headache

Gastrointestinal disorders

Common: nausea, vomiting, diarrhoea

Rare: pancreatitis

Skin and subcutaneous tissue disorders

Common: rash (without systemic symptoms)

Very rare: erythema multiforme, Stevens-Johnson syndrome and toxic epidermal necrolysis

General disorders and administration site conditions

Common: fever, lethargy, fatigue

Cases of lactic acidosis, sometimes fatal, usually associated with severe hepatomegaly and hepatic steatosis, have been reported with the use of nucleoside analogues(see section 4.4).

Combination antiretroviral therapy has been associated with redistribution of body fat (lipodystrophy) in HIV patients including the loss of peripheral and facial subcutaneous fat, increased intra-abdominal and visceral fat, breast hypertrophy and dorsocervical fat accumulation (buffalo hump).

Combination antiretroviral therapy has been associated with metabolic abnormalities such as hypertriglyceridaemia, hypercholesterolaemia, insulin resistance, hyperglycaemia and hyperlactataemia (see section 4.4).

In HIV-infected patients with severe immune deficiency at the time of initiation of combination antiretroviral therapy (CART) an inflammatory reaction to asymptomatic or residual opportunistic infections may arise (see section 4.4).

Laboratory abnormalities

In controlled clinical studies laboratory abnormalities related to Ziagen treatment were uncommon, with no differences in incidence observed between Ziagen treated patients and the control arms.

4.9 Overdose

Single doses up to 1200 mg and daily doses up to 1800 mg of Ziagen have been administered to patients in clinical studies. No unexpected adverse reactions were reported. The effects of higher doses are not known. If overdose occurs the patient should be monitored for evidence of toxicity (see section 4.8), and standard supportive treatment applied as necessary. It is not known whether abacavir can be removed by peritoneal dialysis or haemodialysis.

5. PHARMACOLOGICAL PROPERTIES

5.1 Pharmacodynamic properties

Pharmacotherapeutic group: nucleoside reverse transcriptase inhibitors, ATC Code: J05A F06

Abacavir is a NRTI. It is a potent selective inhibitor of HIV-1 and HIV-2, including HIV-1 isolates with reduced susceptibility to zidovudine, lamivudine, zalcitabine, didanosine or nevirapine. Abacavir is metabolised intracellularly to the active moiety, carbovir 5'- triphosphate (TP). *In vitro* studies have demonstrated that its mechanism of action in relation to HIV is inhibition of the HIV reverse transcriptase enzyme, an event which results in chain termination and interruption of the viral replication cycle. Abacavir shows synergy *in vitro* in combination with nevirapine and zidovudine. It has been shown to be additive in combination with didanosine, zalcitabine, lamivudine and stavudine.

Abacavir-resistant isolates of HIV-1 have been selected *in vitro* and are associated with specific genotypic changes in the reverse transcriptase (RT) codon region (codons M184V, K65R, L74V and Y115F). Viral resistance to abacavir develops relatively slowly *in vitro* and *in vivo*, requiring multiple mutations to reach an eight-fold increase in IC_{50} over wild-type virus, which may be a clinically relevant level. Isolates resistant to abacavir may also show reduced sensitivity to lamivudine, zalcitabine and/or didanosine, but remain sensitive to zidovudine and stavudine.

Cross-resistance between abacavir and PIs or NNRTIs is unlikely. Reduced susceptibility to abacavir has been demonstrated in clinical isolates of patients with uncontrolled viral replication, who have been pretreated with and are resistant to other nucleoside inhibitors. Clinical isolates with three or more mutations associated with NRTIs are unlikely to be susceptible to abacavir.

Clinical Experience

The demonstration of the benefit of Ziagen is mainly based on results of studies performed in adult treatment-naïve patients using a regimen of Ziagen 300 mg twice daily in combination with zidovudine and lamivudine.

Twice daily (300 mg) administration:

• *Therapy naïve adults*

In adults treated with abacavir in combination with lamivudine and zidovudine the proportion of patients with undetectable viral load (<400 copies/ml) was approximately 70% (intention to treat analysis at 48 weeks) with corresponding rise in CD4 cells.

One randomised, double blind, placebo controlled clinical study in adults has compared the combination of abacavir, lamivudine and zidovudine to the combination of indinavir, lamivudine and zidovudine. Due to the high proportion of premature discontinuation (42% of patients discontinued randomised treatment by week 48), no definitive conclusion can be drawn regarding the equivalence between the treatment regimens at week 48. Although a similar antiviral effect was observed between the abacavir and indinavir containing regimens in terms of proportion of patients with undetectable viral load (≤400 copies/ml; intention to treat analysis (ITT), 47% versus 49%; as treated analysis (AT), 86% versus 94% for abacavir and indinavir combinations respectively), results favoured the indinavir combination, particularly in the subset of patients with high viral load >100,000 copies/ml at baseline; ITT, 46% versus 55%; AT, 84% versus 93% for abacavir and indinavir respectively).

In a multicentre, double-blind, controlled study (CNA30024), 654 HIV-infected, antiretroviral therapy-naïve patients were randomised to receive either abacavir 300 mg twice daily or zidovudine 300 mg twice daily, both in combination with lamivudine 150 mg twice daily and efavirenz 600 mg once daily. The duration of double-blind treatment was at least 48 weeks. In the intent-to-treat (ITT) population, 70% of patients in the abacavir group, compared to 69% of patients in the zidovudine group, achieved a virologic response of plasma HIV-1 RNA ≤50 copies/ml by Week 48 (point estimate for treatment difference: 0.8, 95% CI -6.3, 7.9). In the as treated (AT) analysis the difference between both treatment arms was more noticeable (88% of patients in the abacavir group, compared to 95% of patients in the zidovudine group (point estimate for treatment difference: -6.8, 95% CI -11.8; -1.7). However, both analyses were compatible with a conclusion of non-inferiority between both treatment arms.

• *Therapy naïve children*

In a study comparing the unblinded NRTI combinations (with or without blinded nelfinavir) in children, a greater proportion treated with abacavir and lamivudine (71%) or abacavir and zidovudine (60%) had HIV-1 RNA $\leqslant$400 copies/ml at 48 weeks, compared with those treated with lamivudine and zidovudine (47%)[p=0.09, intention to treat analysis]. Similarly, greater proportions of children treated with the abacavir containing combinations had HIV-1 RNA $\leqslant$50 copies/ml at 48 weeks (53%, 42% and 28% respectively, p=0.07).

• *Therapy experienced patients*

In adults moderately exposed to antiretroviral therapy the addition of abacavir to combination antiretroviral therapy provided modest benefits in reducing viral load (median change 0.44 $\log_{10}$ copies/ml at 16 weeks).

In heavily NRTI pretreated patients the efficacy of abacavir is very low. The degree of benefit as part of a new combination regimen will depend on the nature and duration of prior therapy which may have selected for HIV-1 variants with cross-resistance to abacavir.

Once daily (600 mg) administration:

• *Therapy naïve adults*

The once daily regimen of abacavir is supported by a 48 weeks multi-centre, double-blind, controlled study (CNA30021) of 770 HIV-infected, therapy-naïve adults. These were primarily asymptomatic HIV infected patients (CDC stage A). They were randomised to receive either abacavir 600 mg once daily or 300 mg twice daily, in combination with efavirenz and lamivudine given once daily. Similar clinical success (point estimate for treatment difference -1.7, 95% CI -8.4, 4.9) was observed for both regimens. From these results, it can be concluded with 95% confidence that the true difference is no greater than 8.4% in favour of the twice daily regimen. This potential difference is sufficiently small to draw an overall conclusion of non-inferiority of abacavir once daily over abacavir twice daily.

There was a low, similar overall incidence of virologic failure (viral load $>$50 copies/ml) in both the once and twice daily treatment groups (10% and 8% respectively). In the small sample size for genotypic analysis, there was a trend toward a higher rate of NRTI-associated mutations in the once daily versus the twice daily abacavir regimens. No firm conclusion could be drawn due to the limited data derived from this study. Long term data with abacavir used as a once daily regimen (beyond 48 weeks) are currently limited.

• *Therapy experienced patients*

In study CAL30001, 182 treatment-experienced patients with virologic failure were randomised to receive either the fixed-dose combination of abacavir/lamivudine (FDC) once daily or abacavir 300 mg twice daily plus lamivudine 300 mg once daily, both in combination with tenofovir and a PI or an NNRTI for 48 weeks. Preliminary data at 24 weeks indicate that the FDC group was non-inferior to the abacavir twice daily group, based on similar reductions in HIV-1 RNA as measured by average area under the curve minus baseline (AAUCMB, -1.6 versus -1.87 respectively, 95% CI -0.06, 0.37). Proportions with HIV-1 RNA $<$ 50 copies/ml (56% versus 47%) and $<$ 400 copies/ml (65% versus 63%) were also similar in each group. However, as there were only moderately experienced patients included in this study with an imbalance in baseline viral load and treatment discontinuations between the arms, these results should be interpreted with caution.

In study ESS30008, 260 patients with virologic suppression on a first line therapy regimen containing abacavir 300 mg plus lamivudine 150 mg, both given twice daily and a PI or NNRTI, were randomised to continue this regimen or switch to abacavir/lamivudine FDC plus a PI or NNRTI for 48 weeks. Preliminary data at 24 weeks indicate that the FDC group was associated with a similar virologic outcome (non-inferior) compared to the abacavir plus lamivudine group, based on proportions of subjects with HIV-1 RNA $<$ 50 copies/ml (91% and 86% respectively, 95% CI -11.1, 1.9).

Additional information:

The safety and efficacy of Ziagen in a number of different multidrug combination regimens is still not completely assessed (particularly in combination with NNRTIs).

Abacavir penetrates the cerebrospinal fluid (CSF) (see section 5.2), and has been shown to reduce HIV-1 RNA levels in the CSF. However, no effects on neuropsychological performance were seen when it was administered to patients with AIDS dementia complex.

5.2 Pharmacokinetic properties

Absorption: abacavir is rapidly and well absorbed following oral administration. The absolute bioavailability of oral abacavir in adults is about 83%. Following oral administration, the mean time (t_{max}) to maximal serum concentrations of abacavir is about 1.5 hours for the tablet formulation and about 1.0 hour for the solution formulation.

There are no differences observed between the AUC for the tablet or solution. At therapeutic dosages a dosage of 300 mg twice daily, the mean (CV) steady state C_{max} and C_{min} of abacavir are approximately 3.00 μg/ml (30%) and 0.01 μg/ml (99%), respectively. The mean (CV) AUC over a dosing interval of 12 hours was 6.02 μg.h/ml (29%), equivalent to a daily AUC of approximately 12.0 μg.h/ml. The C_{max} value for the oral solution is slightly higher than the tablet. After a 600 mg abacavir tablet dose, the mean (CV) abacavir C_{max} was approximately 4.26 μg/ml (28%) and the mean AUC was 11.95 μg.h/ml (21%).

Food delayed absorption and decreased C_{max} but did not affect overall plasma concentrations (AUC). Therefore Ziagen can be taken with or without food.

Distribution: following intravenous administration, the apparent volume of distribution was about 0.8 l/kg, indicating that abacavir penetrates freely into body tissues.

Studies in HIV infected patients have shown good penetration of abacavir into the cerebrospinal fluid (CSF), with a CSF to plasma AUC ratio of between 30 to 44%. The observed values of the peak concentrations are 9 fold greater than the IC_{50} of abacavir of 0.08 μg/ml or 0.26 μM when abacavir is given at 600 mg twice daily.

Plasma protein binding studies *in vitro* indicate that abacavir binds only low to moderately (~49%) to human plasma proteins at therapeutic concentrations. This indicates a low likelihood for interactions with other medicinal products through plasma protein binding displacement.

Metabolism: abacavir is primarily metabolised by the liver with approximately 2% of the administered dose being renally excreted, as unchanged compound. The primary pathways of metabolism in man are by alcohol dehydrogenase and by glucuronidation to produce the 5'-carboxylic acid and 5'-glucuronide which account for about 66% of the administered dose. The metabolites are excreted in the urine.

Elimination: the mean half-life of abacavir is about 1.5 hours. Following multiple oral doses of abacavir 300 mg twice a day there is no significant accumulation of abacavir. Elimination of abacavir is via hepatic metabolism with subsequent excretion of metabolites primarily in the urine. The metabolites and unchanged abacavir account for about 83% of the administered abacavir dose in the urine. The remainder is eliminated in the faeces.

Intracellular pharmacokinetics

In a study of 20 HIV-infected patients receiving abacavir 300 mg twice daily, with only one 300 mg dose taken prior to the 24 hour sampling period, the geometric mean terminal carbovir-TP intracellular half-life at steady-state was 20.6 hours, compared to the geometric mean abacavir plasma half-life in this study of 2.6 hours. Similar intracellular kinetics are expected from abacavir 600 mg once daily. These data support the use of abacavir 600 mg once daily for the treatment of HIV infected patients. Additionally, the efficacy of abacavir given once daily has been demonstrated in a pivotal clinical study (CNA30021- See section 5.1 Clinical experience).

Special populations

Hepatically impaired: abacavir is metabolised primarily by the liver. The pharmacokinetics of abacavir have been studied in patients with mild hepatic impairment (Child-Pugh score 5-6) receiving a single 600 mg dose. The results showed that there was a mean increase of 1.89 fold [1.32; 2.70] in the abacavir AUC, and 1.58 [1.22; 2.04] fold in the elimination half-life. No recommendation on dosage reduction is possible in patients with mild hepatic impairment due to the substantial variability of abacavir exposure.

Renally impaired: abacavir is primarily metabolised by the liver with approximately 2% of abacavir excreted unchanged in the urine. The pharmacokinetics of abacavir in patients with end-stage renal disease is similar to patients with normal renal function. Therefore no dosage reduction is required in patients with renal impairment. Based on limited experience Ziagen should be avoided in patients with end-stage renal disease.

Children: according to clinical trials performed in children abacavir is rapidly and well absorbed from an oral solution administered to children. The overall pharmacokinetic parameters in children are comparable to adults, with greater variability in plasma concentrations. The recommended dose for children from three months to 12 years is 8 mg/kg twice daily. This will provide slightly higher mean plasma concentrations in children, ensuring that the majority will achieve therapeutic concentrations equivalent to 300 mg twice daily in adults.

There are insufficient safety data to recommend the use of Ziagen in infants less than three months old. The limited data available indicate that a dose of 2 mg/kg in neonates less than 30 days old provides similar or greater AUCs, compared to the 8 mg/kg dose administered to older children.

Elderly: the pharmacokinetics of abacavir have not been studied in patients over 65 years of age.

5.3 Preclinical safety data

Abacavir was not mutagenic in bacterial tests but showed activity *in vitro* in the human lymphocyte chromosome aberration assay, the mouse lymphoma assay, and the *in vivo* micronucleus test. This is consistent with the known activity of other nucleoside analogues. These results indicate that abacavir has a weak potential to cause chromosomal damage both *in vitro* and *in vivo* at high test concentrations.

Carcinogenicity studies with orally administered abacavir in mice and rats showed an increase in the incidence of malignant and non-malignant tumours. Malignant tumours occurred in the preputial gland of males and the clitoral gland of females of both species, and in rats in the thyroid gland of males and the liver, urinary bladder, lymph nodes and the subcutis of females.

The majority of these tumours occurred at the highest abacavir dose of 330 mg/kg/day in mice and 600 mg/kg/day in rats. The exception was the preputial gland tumour which occurred at a dose of 110 mg/kg in mice. The systemic exposure at the no effect level in mice and rats was equivalent to 3 and 7 times the human systemic exposure during therapy. While the carcinogenic potential in humans is unknown, these data suggest that a carcinogenic risk to humans is outweighed by the potential clinical benefit.

In pre-clinical toxicology studies, abacavir treatment was shown to increase liver weights in rats and monkeys. The clinical relevance of this is unknown. There is no evidence from clinical studies that abacavir is hepatotoxic. Additionally, autoinduction of abacavir metabolism or induction of the metabolism of other medicinal products hepatically metabolised has not been observed in man.

Mild myocardial degeneration in the heart of mice and rats was observed following administration of abacavir for two years. The systemic exposures were equivalent to 7 to 24 times the expected systemic exposure in humans. The clinical relevance of this finding has not been determined.

In reproductive toxicity studies, embryo and foetal toxicity have been observed in rats but not in rabbits. These findings included decreased foetal body weight, foetal oedema, and an increase in skeletal variations/malformations, early intra-uterine deaths and still births. No conclusion can be drawn with regard to the teratogenic potential of abacavir because of this embryo-foetal toxicity.

A fertility study in the rat has shown that abacavir had no effect on male or female fertility.

6. PHARMACEUTICAL PARTICULARS

6.1 List of excipients

Sorbitol 70% (E420), saccharin sodium, sodium citrate, citric acid anhydrous, methyl parahydroxybenzoate (E218), propyl parahydroxybenzoate (E216), propylene glycol (E1520), maltodextrin, lactic acid, glyceryl triacetate, natural and artificial strawberry and banana flavours, purified water, and sodium hydroxide and/or hydrochloric acid for pH adjustment.

6.2 Incompatibilities

Not applicable

6.3 Shelf life

2 years

After first opening the container: 2 months

6.4 Special precautions for storage

Do not store above 30°C

6.5 Nature and contents of container

Ziagen oral solution is supplied in high density polyethylene bottles with child-resistant closures, containing 240 ml of oral solution. A 10 ml polypropylene oral dosing syringe and a polyethylene adapter are also included in the pack.

6.6 Instructions for use and handling

A plastic adapter and oral dosing syringe are provided for accurate measurement of the prescribed dose of oral solution. The adapter is placed in the neck of the bottle and the syringe attached to this. The bottle is inverted and the correct volume withdrawn. Instructions for use are included in the package leaflet.

Adminstrative Data

7. MARKETING AUTHORISATION HOLDER

Glaxo Group Ltd

Greenford

Middlesex UB6 0NN

United Kingdom

8. MARKETING AUTHORISATION NUMBER(S)

EU/1/99/112/002

9. DATE OF FIRST AUTHORISATION/RENEWAL OF THE AUTHORISATION

Date of first authorisation: 8 July 1999

Date of renewal: 18 August 2004

10. DATE OF REVISION OF THE TEXT

17 December 2004

Ziagen 300 mg Film Coated Tablets

(GlaxoSmithKline UK)

1. NAME OF THE MEDICINAL PRODUCT

Ziagen 300 mg film-coated tablets

2. QUALITATIVE AND QUANTITATIVE COMPOSITION

Each film-coated tablet contains 300 mg of abacavir as abacavir sulfate.

For excipients see section 6.1.

3. PHARMACEUTICAL FORM

Film-coated tablet

The biconvex, capsule shaped tablets are yellow and engraved with GX 623 on one side.

4. CLINICAL PARTICULARS

4.1 Therapeutic indications

Ziagen is indicated in antiretroviral combination therapy for the treatment of Human Immunodeficiency Virus (HIV) infection.

The demonstration of the benefit of Ziagen is mainly based on results of studies performed with a twice daily regimen, in treatment-naïve adult patients on combination therapy (see section 5.1).

4.2 Posology and method of administration

Ziagen should be prescribed by physicians experienced in the management of HIV infection.

Adults and adolescents over 12 years: the recommended dose of Ziagen is 600 mg daily. This may be administered as either 300 mg (one tablet) twice daily or 600 mg (two tablets) once daily (see sections 4.4 and 5.1).

Patients changing to the once daily regimen should take 300 mg twice a day and switch to 600 mg once a day the following morning. Where an evening once daily regimen is preferred, 300 mg of Ziagen should be taken on the first morning only, followed by 600 mg in the evening. When changing back to a twice daily regimen, patients should complete the day's treatment and start 300 mg twice a day the following morning.

Children from three months to 12 years: the recommended dose is 8 mg/kg twice daily up to a maximum of 600 mg daily.

Children less than three months: the data available on the use of Ziagen in this age group are very limited (see section 5.2).

Ziagen can be taken with or without food.

Ziagen is available as an oral solution for use in children and for those patients for whom the tablets are inappropriate.

Renal impairment: no dosage adjustment of Ziagen is necessary in patients with renal dysfunction. However, Ziagen should be avoided in patients with end-stage renal disease (see section 5.2).

Hepatic impairment: abacavir is primarily metabolised by the liver. No dose recommendation can be made in patients with mild hepatic impairment. No data are available in patients with moderate hepatic impairment, therefore the use of abacavir is not recommended unless judged necessary. In patients with mild and moderate hepatic impairment close monitoring is required, and if feasible, monitoring of abacavir plasma levels is recommended (see section 5.2). Abacavir is contraindicated in patients with severe hepatic impairment (see section 4.3 and 4.4).

Elderly: no pharmacokinetic data is currently available in patients over 65 years of age.

4.3 Contraindications

Ziagen is contraindicated in patients with known hypersensitivity to abacavir or to any of the excipients of Ziagen tablets. See BOXED INFORMATION ON HYPERSENSITIVITY REACTIONS in sections 4.4. and 4.8.

Ziagen is contraindicated in patients with severe hepatic impairment.

4.4 Special warnings and special precautions for use *(see Table 1)*

Lactic acidosis: lactic acidosis, usually associated with hepatomegaly and hepatic steatosis, has been reported with the use of nucleoside analogues. Early symptoms (symptomatic hyperlactatemia) include benign digestive symptoms (nausea, vomiting and abdominal pain), non-specific malaise, loss of appetite, weight loss, respiratory symptoms (rapid and/or deep breathing) or neurological symptoms (including motor weakness).

Lactic acidosis has a high mortality and may be associated with pancreatitis, liver failure, or renal failure.

Lactic acidosis generally occurred after a few or several months of treatment.

Treatment with nucleoside analogues should be discontinued in the setting of symptomatic hyperlactatemia and metabolic/lactic acidosis, progressive hepatomegaly, or rapidly elevating aminotransferase levels.

Caution should be exercised when administering nucleoside analogues to any patient (particularly obese women) with hepatomegaly, hepatitis or other known risk factors for liver disease and hepatic steatosis (including certain medicinal products and alcohol). Patients co-infected with hepatitis C and treated with alpha interferon and ribavirin may constitute a special risk.

Patients at increased risk should be followed closely.

Mitochondrial dysfunction: nucleoside and nucleotide analogues have been demonstrated *in vitro* and *in vivo* to cause a variable degree of mitochondrial damage. There have been reports of mitochondrial dysfunction in HIV-negative infants exposed *in utero* and/or post-natally to nucleoside analogues. The main adverse events reported are haematological disorders (anaemia, neutropenia), metabolic disorders (hyperlactatemia, hyperlipasemia). These events are often transitory. Some late-onset neurological disorders have been reported (hypertonia, convulsion, abnormal behaviour). Whether the neurological disorders are transient or permanent is currently unknown. Any child exposed *in utero* to nucleoside and nucleotide analogues, even HIV-negative children, should have clinical and laboratory follow-up and should be fully investigated for possible mitochondrial dysfunction in case of relevant signs or symptoms. These findings do not affect current national recommendations to use antiretroviral therapy in pregnant women to prevent vertical transmission of HIV.

Lipodystrophy: combination antiretroviral therapy has been associated with the redistribution of body fat (lipodystrophy) in HIV patients. The long-term consequences of these events are currently unknown. Knowledge about the mechanism is incomplete. A connection between visceral lipomatosis and protease inhibitors (PIs) and lipoatrophy and nucleoside reverse transcriptase inhibitors (NRTIs) has been hypothesised. A higher risk of lipodystrophy has been associated with individual factors such as older age, and with drug related factors such as longer duration of antiretroviral treatment and associated metabolic disturbances. Clinical examination should include evaluation for physical signs of fat redistribution. Consideration should be given to the measurement of fasting serum lipids and blood glucose. Lipid disorders should be managed as clinically appropriate (see section 4.8).

Pancreatitis: pancreatitis has been reported, but a causal relationship to Ziagen treatment is uncertain.

Triple nucleoside therapy: in patients with high viral load >100,000 copies/ml) the choice of a triple combination with abacavir, lamivudine and zidovudine needs special consideration (see section 5.1).

Table 1

Hypersensitivity Reaction
(see also section 4.8):

In clinical studies approximately 5% of subjects receiving abacavir develop a hypersensitivity reaction; some of these cases were life-threatening and resulted in a fatal outcome despite taking precautions.

• **Description**

Hypersensitivity reactions are characterised by the appearance of symptoms indicating multi-organ system involvement. Almost all hypersensitivity reactions will have fever and/or rash as part of the syndrome.

Other signs and symptoms may include respiratory signs and symptoms such as dyspnoea, sore throat, cough and abnormal chest x-ray findings (predominantly infiltrates, which can be localised), gastrointestinal symptoms, such as nausea, vomiting, diarrhoea, or abdominal pain, **and may lead to misdiagnosis of hypersensitivity as respiratory disease (pneumonia, bronchitis, pharyngitis), or gastroenteritis.**

Other frequently observed signs or symptoms of the hypersensitivity reaction may include lethargy or malaise and musculoskeletal symptoms (myalgia, rarely myolysis, arthralgia).

The symptoms related to this hypersensitivity reaction worsen with continued therapy and can be life-threatening. These symptoms usually resolve upon discontinuation of Ziagen.

• **Management**

Hypersensitivity reaction symptoms usually appear within the first six weeks of initiation of treatment with abacavir, although these reactions **may occur at any time during therapy.**

Patients should be monitored closely, especially during the first two months of treatment with Ziagen, with consultation every two weeks.

Patients who are diagnosed with a hypersensitivity reaction whilst on therapy **MUST discontinue Ziagen immediately.**

Ziagen, or any other medicinal product containing abacavir (i.e. Kivexa, Trizivir), MUST NEVER be restarted in patients who have stopped therapy due to a hypersensitivity reaction.

Restarting abacavir following a hypersensitivity reaction results in a prompt return of symptoms within hours. This recurrence is usually more severe than on initial presentation, and may include life-threatening hypotension and death.

To avoid a delay in diagnosis and minimise the risk of a life-threatening hypersensitivity reaction, Ziagen must be permanently discontinued if hypersensitivity cannot be ruled out, even when other diagnoses are possible (respiratory diseases, flu-like illness, gastroenteritis or reactions to other medications).

Special care is needed for those patients simultaneously starting treatment with Ziagen and other medicinal products known to induce skin toxicity (such as non-nucleoside reverse transcriptase inhibitors - NNRTIs). This is because it is currently difficult to differentiate between rashes induced by these products and abacavir related hypersensitivity reactions.

• **Management after an interruption of Ziagen therapy**

If therapy with Ziagen has been discontinued for any reason and restarting therapy is under consideration, the reason for discontinuation must be established to assess whether the patient had any symptoms of a hypersensitivity reaction. **If a hypersensitivity reaction cannot be ruled out, Ziagen or any other medicinal product containing abacavir (i.e. Kivexa, Trizivir) must not be restarted.**

Hypersensitivity reactions with rapid onset, including life-threatening reactions have occurred after restarting Ziagen in patients who had only one of the key symptoms of hypersensitivity (skin rash, fever, gastrointestinal, respiratory or constitutional symptoms such as lethargy and malaise) prior to stopping Ziagen. The most common isolated symptom of a hypersensitivity reaction was a skin rash. Moreover, on very rare occasions hypersensitivity reactions have been reported in patients who have restarted therapy, and who had no preceding symptoms of a hypersensitivity reaction. In both cases, if a decision is made to restart Ziagen this must be done in a setting where medical assistance is readily available.

• **Essential patient information**

***Prescribers* must ensure that patients are fully informed regarding the following information on the hypersensitivity reaction:**

- patients must be made aware of the possibility of a hypersensitivity reaction to abacavir that may result in a life-threatening reaction or death.

- patients developing signs or symptoms possibly linked with a hypersensitivity reaction **MUST CONTACT their doctor IMMEDIATELY.**

- patients who are hypersensitive to abacavir should be reminded that they must never take Ziagen or any other medicinal product containing abacavir (i.e. Kivexa, Trizivir)

- in order to avoid restarting Ziagen, patients who have experienced a hypersensitivity reaction should be asked to return the remaining Ziagen tablets or oral solution to the pharmacy.

- patients who have stopped Ziagen for any reason, and particularly due to possible adverse reactions or illness, must be advised to contact their doctor before restarting.

- patients should be advised of the importance of taking Ziagen regularly.

- each patient should be reminded to read the Package Leaflet included in the Ziagen pack. They should be reminded of the importance of removing the Alert Card included in the pack, and keeping it with them at all times.

There have been reports of a high rate of virological failure and of emergence of resistance at an early stage when abacavir was combined with tenofovir disoproxil fumarate and lamivudine as a once daily regimen.

Once daily administration (abacavir 600 mg): the benefit of abacavir as a once daily regimen is mainly based on a study performed in combination with efavirenz and lamivudine, in antiretroviral-naïve adult patients (see section 5.1).

Liver disease: the safety and efficacy of Ziagen has not been established in patients with significant underlying liver disorders. Ziagen is contraindicated in patients with severe hepatic impairment (see section 4.3). Patients with chronic hepatitis B or C and treated with combination antiretroviral therapy are at an increased risk of severe and potentially fatal hepatic adverse events. In case of concomitant antiviral therapy for hepatitis B or C, please refer also to the relevant product information for these medicinal products.

Patients with pre-existing liver dysfunction, including chronic active hepatitis, have an increased frequency of liver function abnormalities during combination antiretroviral therapy, and should be monitored according to standard practice. If there is evidence of worsening liver disease in such patients, interruption or discontinuation of treatment must be considered.

A pharmacokinetic study has been performed in patients with mild hepatic impairment. However, a definitive recommendation on dose reduction is not possible due to substantial variability of drug exposure in this patient population (see section 5.2). The clinical safety data available with abacavir in hepatically impaired patients is very limited. Due to the potential increases in exposure (AUC) in some patients, close monitoring is required. No data are available in patients with moderate or severe hepatic impairment. Plasma concentrations of abacavir are expected to substantially increase in these patients. Therefore, the use of abacavir in patients with moderate hepatic impairment is not recommended unless judged necessary and requires close monitoring of these patients. For patients with severe hepatic impairment, Ziagen is contraindicated (see section 4.3).

Renal disease: Ziagen should not be administered to patients with end-stage renal disease (see section 5.2).

Immune Reactivation Syndrome: In HIV-infected patients with severe immune deficiency at the time of institution of combination antiretroviral therapy (CART), an inflammatory reaction to asymptomatic or residual opportunistic pathogens may arise and cause serious clinical conditions, or aggravation of symptoms. Typically, such reactions have been observed within the first few weeks or months of initiation of CART. Relevant examples are cytomegalovirus retinitis, generalised and/or focal mycobacterium infections, and Pneumocystis carinii pneumonia. Any inflammatory symptoms should be evaluated and treatment instituted when necessary.

Opportunistic infections: patients receiving Ziagen or any other antiretroviral therapy may still develop opportunistic infections and other complications of HIV infection. Therefore patients should remain under close clinical observation by physicians experienced in the treatment of these associated HIV diseases.

Transmission: patients should be advised that current antiretroviral therapy, including Ziagen, have not been proven to prevent the risk of transmission of HIV to others through sexual contact or blood contamination. Appropriate precautions should continue to be taken.

Table 2

Hypersensitivity (see also section 4.4):	
In clinical studies, approximately 5% of subjects receiving abacavir developed a hypersensitivity reaction. In clinical studies with abacavir 600 mg once daily the reported rate of hypersensitivity remained within the range recorded for abacavir 300 mg twice daily.	
Some of these hypersensitivity reactions were life-threatening and resulted in fatal outcome despite taking precautions. This reaction is characterised by the appearance of symptoms indicating multi-organ/body-system involvement.	
Almost all patients developing hypersensitivity reactions will have fever and/or rash (usually maculopapular or urticarial) as part of the syndrome, however reactions have occurred without rash or fever.	
The signs and symptoms of this hypersensitivity reaction are listed below. These have been identified either from clinical studies or post marketing surveillance. Those reported **in at least 10% of patients** with a hypersensitivity reaction are in bold text.	
Skin	**Rash** (usually maculopapular or urticarial)
Gastrointestinal tract	**Nausea, vomiting, diarrhoea, abdominal pain**, mouth ulceration
Respiratory tract	**Dyspnoea, cough**, sore throat, adult respiratory distress syndrome, respiratory failure
Miscellaneous	**Fever, lethargy, malaise**, oedema, lymphadenopathy, hypotension, conjunctivitis, anaphylaxis
Neurological/Psychiatry	**Headache**, paraesthesia
Haematological	Lymphopenia
Liver/pancreas	**Elevated liver function tests,** hepatitis, hepatic failure
Musculoskeletal	**Myalgia**, rarely myolysis, arthralgia, elevated creatine phosphokinase
Urology	Elevated creatinine, renal failure
Rash (81% vs 67% respectively) and gastrointestinal manifestations (70% vs 54% respectively) were more frequently reported in children compared to adults.	
Some patients with hypersensitivity reactions were initially thought to have gastroenteritis, respiratory disease (pneumonia, bronchitis, pharyngitis) or a flu-like illness. This delay in diagnosis of hypersensitivity has resulted in Ziagen being continued or re-introduced, leading to more severe hypersensitivity reactions or death. Therefore, the diagnosis of hypersensitivity reaction should be carefully considered for patients presenting with symptoms of these diseases.	
Symptoms usually appeared within the first six weeks (median time to onset 11 days) of initiation of treatment with abacavir, although these reactions may occur at any time during therapy. Close medical supervision is necessary during the first two months, with consultations every two weeks.	
Risk factors that may predict the occurrence or severity of hypersensitivity to abacavir have not been identified. However, it is likely that intermittent therapy may increase the risk of developing sensitisation and therefore occurrence of clinically significant hypersensitivity reactions. Consequently, patients should be advised of the importance of taking Ziagen regularly.	
Restarting Ziagen following a hypersensitivity reaction results in a prompt return of symptoms within hours. This recurrence of the hypersensitivity reaction was usually more severe than on initial presentation, and may include life-threatening hypotension and death. **Patients who develop this hypersensitivity reaction must discontinue Ziagen and must never be rechallenged with Ziagen, or any other medicinal product containing abacavir (i.e. Kivexa, Trizivir).**	
To avoid a delay in diagnosis and minimise the risk of a life-threatening hypersensitivity reaction, Ziagen must be permanently discontinued if hypersensitivity cannot be ruled out, even when other diagnoses are possible (respiratory diseases, flu-like illness, gastroenteritis or reactions to other medications).	
Hypersensitivity reactions with rapid onset, including life-threatening reactions have occurred after restarting Ziagen in patients who had only one of the key symptoms of hypersensitivity (skin rash, fever, gastrointestinal, respiratory or constitutional symptoms such as lethargy and malaise) prior to stopping Ziagen. The most common isolated symptom of a hypersensitivity reaction was a skin rash. Moreover, on very rare occasions hypersensitivity reactions have been reported in patients who have restarted therapy and who had no preceding symptoms of a hypersensitivity reaction.	
In both cases, if a decision is made to restart Ziagen this must be done in a setting where medical assistance is readily available.	
Each patient must be warned about this hypersensitivity reaction to abacavir.	

4.5 Interaction with other medicinal products and other forms of Interaction

Based on the results of *in vitro* experiments and the known major metabolic pathways of abacavir, the potential for P450 mediated interactions with other medicinal products involving abacavir is low. P450 does not play a major role in the metabolism of abacavir, and abacavir does not inhibit metabolism mediated by CYP 3A4. Abacavir has also been shown *in vitro* not to inhibit CYP 3A4, CYP2C9 or CYP2D6 enzymes at clinically relevant concentrations. Induction of hepatic metabolism has not been observed in clinical studies. Therefore, there is little potential for interactions with antiretroviral PIs and other medicinal products metabolised by major P450 enzymes. Clinical studies have shown that there are no clinically significant interactions between abacavir, zidovudine, and lamivudine.

Potent enzymatic inducers such as rifampicin, phenobarbital and phenytoin may via their action on UDP-glucuronyltransferases slightly decrease the plasma concentrations of abacavir.

Ethanol: the metabolism of abacavir is altered by concomitant ethanol resulting in an increase in AUC of abacavir of about 41%. These findings are not considered clinically significant. Abacavir has no effect on the metabolism of ethanol.

Methadone: in a pharmacokinetic study, coadministration of 600 mg abacavir twice daily with methadone showed a 35% reduction in abacavir C_{max} and a one hour delay in t_{max} but the AUC was unchanged. The changes in abacavir pharmacokinetics are not considered clinically relevant. In this study abacavir increased the mean methadone systemic clearance by 22%. The induction of drug metabolising enzymes cannot therefore be excluded. Patients being treated with methadone and abacavir should be monitored for evidence of withdrawal symptoms indicating under dosing, as occasionally methadone re-titration may be required.

Retinoids: retinoid compounds are eliminated via alcohol dehydrogenase. Interaction with abacavir is possible but has not been studied.

4.6 Pregnancy and lactation

Pregnancy: Ziagen is not recommended during pregnancy. The safe use of abacavir in human pregnancy has not been established. Placental transfer of abacavir and/or its related metabolites has been shown to occur in animals. Toxicity to the developing embryo and foetus occurred in rats, but not in rabbits (see section 5.3). The teratogenic potential of abacavir could not be established from studies in animals.

Lactation: abacavir and its metabolites are secreted into the milk of lactating rats. It is expected that these will also be secreted into human milk, although this has not been confirmed. There are no data available on the safety of abacavir when administered to babies less than three months old. It is therefore recommended that mothers do not breast-feed their babies while receiving treatment with abacavir. Additionally, it is recommended that HIV infected women do not breast-feed their infants under any circumstances in order to avoid transmission of HIV.

4.7 Effects on ability to drive and use machines

No studies on the effects on ability to drive and use machines have been performed.

4.8 Undesirable effects

(see Table 2 above)

For many of the other adverse events reported, it is unclear whether they are related to Ziagen, to the wide range of medicinal products used in the management of HIV infection or as a result of the disease process.

Many of those listed below occur commonly (nausea, vomiting, diarrhoea, fever, lethargy, rash) in patients with abacavir hypersensitivity. Therefore, patients with any of these symptoms should be carefully evaluated for the presence of this hypersensitivity reaction. If Ziagen has been discontinued in patients due to experiencing any one of these symptoms and a decision is made to restart a medicinal product containing abacavir, this must be done in a setting where medical assistance is readily available (see section 4.4.). Very rarely cases of erythema multiforme, Stevens Johnson syndrome or toxic epidermal necrolysis have been reported where abacavir hypersensitivity could not be ruled out. In such cases medicinal products containing abacavir should be permanently discontinued.

Many of the adverse reactions have not been treatment limiting. The following convention has been used for their classification: very common >1/10), common >1/100, <1/10), uncommon >1/1,000, <1/100), rare >1/10,000, <1/1,000) very rare (<1/10,000).

Metabolism and nutrition disorders

Common: anorexia

Nervous system disorders

Common: headache

Gastrointestinal disorders

Common: nausea, vomiting, diarrhoea

Rare: pancreatitis

Skin and subcutaneous tissue disorders

Common: rash (without systemic symptoms)

Veryrare: erythema multiforme, Stevens-Johnson syndrome and toxic epidermal necrolysis

General disorders and administration site conditions

Common: fever, lethargy, fatigue

Cases of lactic acidosis, sometimes fatal, usually associated with severe hepatomegaly and hepatic steatosis, have been reported with the use of nucleoside analogues (see section 4.4).

Combination antiretroviral therapy has been associated with redistribution of body fat (lipodystrophy) in HIV patients including the loss of peripheral and facial subcutaneous fat, increased intra-abdominal and visceral fat, breast hypertrophy and dorsocervical fat accumulation (buffalo hump).

Combination antiretroviral therapy has been associated with metabolic abnormalities such as hypertriglyceridaemia, hypercholesterolaemia, insulin resistance, hyperglycaemia and hyperlactataemia (see section 4.4).

In HIV-infected patients with severe immune deficiency at the time of initiation of combination antiretroviral therapy (CART) an inflammatory reaction to asymptomatic or residual opportunistic infections may arise (see section 4.4).

Laboratory abnormalities

In controlled clinical studies laboratory abnormalities related to Ziagen treatment were uncommon, with no differences in incidence observed between Ziagen treated patients and the control arms.

4.9 Overdose

Single doses up to 1200 mg and daily doses up to 1800 mg of Ziagen have been administered to patients in clinical studies. No unexpected adverse reactions were reported. The effects of higher doses are not known. If overdose occurs the patient should be monitored for evidence of toxicity (see section 4.8), and standard supportive treatment applied as necessary. It is not known whether abacavir can be removed by peritoneal dialysis or haemodialysis.

5. PHARMACOLOGICAL PROPERTIES

5.1 Pharmacodynamic properties

Pharmacotherapeutic group: nucleoside reverse transcriptase inhibitors, ATC Code: J05A F06

Abacavir is a NRTI. It is a potent selective inhibitor of HIV-1 and HIV-2, including HIV-1 isolates with reduced susceptibility to zidovudine, lamivudine, zalcitabine, didanosine or nevirapine. Abacavir is metabolised intracellularly to the active moiety, carbovir 5'- triphosphate (TP). *In vitro* studies have demonstrated that its mechanism of action in relation to HIV is inhibition of the HIV reverse transcriptase enzyme, an event which results in chain termination and interruption of the viral replication cycle. Abacavir shows synergy *in vitro* in combination with nevirapine and zidovudine. It has been shown to be additive in combination with didanosine, zalcitabine, lamivudine and stavudine.

Abacavir-resistant isolates of HIV-1 have been selected *in vitro* and are associated with specific genotypic changes in the reverse transcriptase (RT) codon region (codons M184V, K65R, L74V and Y115F). Viral resistance to abacavir develops relatively slowly *in vitro* and *in vivo*, requiring multiple mutations to reach an eight-fold increase in IC_{50} over wild-type virus, which may be a clinically relevant level. Isolates resistant to abacavir may also show reduced sensitivity to lamivudine, zalcitabine and/or didanosine, but remain sensitive to zidovudine and stavudine.

Cross-resistance between abacavir and PIs or NNRTIs is unlikely. Reduced susceptibility to abacavir has been demonstrated in clinical isolates of patients with uncontrolled viral replication, who have been pretreated with and are resistant to other nucleoside inhibitors. Clinical isolates with three or more mutations associated with NRTIs are unlikely to be susceptible to abacavir.

Clinical Experience

The demonstration of the benefit of Ziagen is mainly based on results of studies performed in adult treatment-naïve patients using a regimen of Ziagen 300 mg twice daily in combination with zidovudine and lamivudine.

Twice daily (300 mg) administration:

• *Therapy naïve adults*

In adults treated with abacavir in combination with lamivudine and zidovudine the proportion of patients with undetectable viral load (<400 copies/ml) was approximately 70% (intention to treat analysis at 48 weeks) with corresponding rise in CD4 cells.

One randomised, double blind, placebo controlled clinical study in adults has compared the combination of abacavir, lamivudine and zidovudine to the combination of indinavir, lamivudine and zidovudine. Due to the high proportion of premature discontinuation (42% of patients discontinued randomised treatment by week 48), no definitive conclusion can be drawn regarding the equivalence between the treatment regimens at week 48. Although a similar antiviral effect was observed between the abacavir and indinavir containing regimens in terms of proportion of patients with undetectable viral load (⩽400 copies/ml; intention to treat analysis (ITT), 47% versus 49%; as treated analysis (AT), 86% versus 94% for abacavir and indinavir combinations respectively), results favoured the indinavir combination, particularly in the subset of patients with high viral load >100,000 copies/ml at baseline; ITT, 46% versus 55%; AT, 84% versus 93% for abacavir and indinavir respectively).

In a multicentre, double-blind, controlled study (CNA30024), 654 HIV-infected, antiretroviral therapy-naïve patients were randomised to receive either abacavir 300 mg twice daily or zidovudine 300 mg twice daily, both in combination with lamivudine 150 mg twice daily and efavirenz 600 mg once daily. The duration of double-blind treatment was at least 48 weeks. In the intent-to-treat (ITT) population, 70% of patients in the abacavir group, compared to 69% of patients in the zidovudine group, achieved a virologic response of plasma HIV-1 RNA ⩽50 copies/ml by Week 48 (point estimate for treatment difference: 0.8, 95% CI -6.3, 7.9). In the as treated (AT) analysis the difference between both treatment arms was more noticeable (88% of patients in the abacavir group, compared to 95% of patients in the zidovudine group (point estimate for treatment difference: -6.8, 95% CI -11.8; -1.7). However, both analyses were compatible with a conclusion of non-inferiority between both treatment arms.

• *Therapy naïve children*

In a study comparing the unblinded NRTI combinations (with or without blinded nelfinavir) in children, a greater proportion treated with abacavir and lamivudine (71%) or abacavir and zidovudine (60%) had HIV-1 RNA ⩽400 copies/ml at 48 weeks, compared with those treated with lamivudine and zidovudine (47%)[p=0.09, intention to treat analysis]. Similarly, greater proportions of children treated with the abacavir containing combinations had HIV-1 RNA ⩽50 copies/ml at 48 weeks (53%, 42% and 28% respectively, p=0.07).

• *Therapy experienced patients*

In adults moderately exposed to antiretroviral therapy the addition of abacavir to combination antiretroviral therapy provided modest benefits in reducing viral load (median change 0.44 $\log_{10}$ copies/ml at 16 weeks).

In heavily NRTI pretreated patients the efficacy of abacavir is very low. The degree of benefit as part of a new combination regimen will depend on the nature and duration of prior therapy which may have selected for HIV-1 variants with cross-resistance to abacavir.

Once daily (600 mg) administration:

• *Therapy naïve adults*

The once daily regimen of abacavir is supported by a 48 weeks multi-centre, double-blind, controlled study (CNA30021) of 770 HIV-infected, therapy-naïve adults. These were primarily asymptomatic HIV infected patients (CDC stage A). They were randomised to receive either abacavir 600 mg once daily or 300 mg twice daily, in combination with efavirenz and lamivudine given once daily. Similar clinical success (point estimate for treatment difference -1.7, 95% CI -8.4, 4.9) was observed for both regimens. From these results, it can be concluded with 95% confidence that the true difference is no greater than 8.4% in favour of the twice daily regimen. This potential difference is sufficiently small to draw an overall conclusion of non-inferiority of abacavir once daily over abacavir twice daily.

There was a low, similar overall incidence of virologic failure (viral load >50 copies/ml) in both the once and twice daily treatment groups (10% and 8% respectively). In the small sample size for genotypic analysis, there was a trend toward a higher rate of NRTI-associated mutations in the once daily versus the twice daily abacavir regimens. No firm conclusion could be drawn due to the limited data derived from this study. Long term data with abacavir used as a once daily regimen (beyond 48 weeks) are currently limited.

• *Therapy experienced patients*

In study CAL30001, 182 treatment-experienced patients with virologic failure were randomised to receive either the fixed-dose combination of abacavir/lamivudine (FDC) once daily or abacavir 300 mg twice daily plus lamivudine 300 mg once daily, both in combination with tenofovir and a PI or an NNRTI for 48 weeks. Preliminary data at 24 weeks indicate that the FDC group was non-inferior to the abacavir twice daily group, based on similar reductions in HIV-1 RNA as measured by average area under the curve minus baseline (AAUCMB, -1.6 versus -1.87 respectively, 95% CI -0.06, 0.37). Proportions with HIV-1 RNA < 50 copies/ml (56% versus 47%) and < 400 copies/ml (65% versus 63%) were also similar in each group. However, as there were only moderately experienced patients included in this study with an imbalance in baseline viral load and treatment discontinuations between the arms, these results should be interpreted with caution.

In study ESS30008, 260 patients with virologic suppression on a first line therapy regimen containing abacavir 300 mg plus lamivudine 150 mg, both given twice daily and a PI or NNRTI, were randomised to continue this regimen or switch to abacavir/lamivudine FDC plus a PI or NNRTI for 48 weeks. Preliminary data at 24 weeks indicate that the FDC group was associated with a similar virologic outcome (non-inferior) compared to the abacavir plus lamivudine group, based on proportions of subjects with HIV-1 RNA < 50 copies/ml (91% and 86% respectively, 95% CI -11.1, 1.9).

Additional information:

The safety and efficacy of Ziagen in a number of different multidrug combination regimens is still not completely assessed (particularly in combination with NNRTIs).

Abacavir penetrates the cerebrospinal fluid (CSF) (see section 5.2), and has been shown to reduce HIV-1 RNA levels in the CSF. However, no effects on neuropsychological performance were seen when it was administered to patients with AIDS dementia complex.

5.2 Pharmacokinetic properties

Absorption: abacavir is rapidly and well absorbed following oral administration. The absolute bioavailability of oral abacavir in adults is about 83%. Following oral administration, the mean time (t_{max}) to maximal serum concentrations of abacavir is about 1.5 hours for the tablet formulation and about 1.0 hour for the solution formulation.

At therapeutic dosages a dosage of 300 mg twice daily, the mean (CV) steady state C_{max} and C_{min} of abacavir are approximately 3.00 μg/ml (30%) and 0.01 μg/ml (99%), respectively. The mean (CV) AUC over a dosing interval of 12 hours was 6.02 μg.h/ml (29%), equivalent to a daily AUC of approximately 12.0 μg.h/ml. The C_{max} value for the oral solution is slightly higher than the tablet. After a 600 mg abacavir tablet dose, the mean (CV) abacavir C_{max} was approximately 4.26 μg/ml (28%) and the mean AUC was 11.95 μg.h/ml (21%).

Food delayed absorption and decreased C_{max} but did not affect overall plasma concentrations (AUC). Therefore Ziagen can be taken with or without food.

Distribution: following intravenous administration, the apparent volume of distribution was about 0.8 l/kg, indicating that abacavir penetrates freely into body tissues.

Studies in HIV infected patients have shown good penetration of abacavir into the cerebrospinal fluid (CSF), with a CSF to plasma AUC ratio of between 30 to 44%. The observed values of the peak concentrations are 9 fold greater than the IC_{50} of abacavir of 0.08 μg/ml or 0.26 μM when abacavir is given at 600 mg twice daily.

Plasma protein binding studies *in vitro* indicate that abacavir binds only low to moderately (~49%) to human plasma proteins at therapeutic concentrations. This indicates a low likelihood for interactions with other medicinal products through plasma protein binding displacement.

Metabolism: abacavir is primarily metabolised by the liver with approximately 2% of the administered dose being renally excreted, as unchanged compound. The primary pathways of metabolism in man are by alcohol dehydrogenase and by glucuronidation to produce the 5'-carboxylic acid and 5'-glucuronide which account for about 66% of the administered dose. The metabolites are excreted in the urine.

Elimination: the mean half-life of abacavir is about 1.5 hours. Following multiple oral doses of abacavir 300 mg twice a day there is no significant accumulation of abacavir. Elimination of abacavir is via hepatic metabolism with subsequent excretion of metabolites primarily in the urine. The metabolites and unchanged abacavir account for about 83% of the administered abacavir dose in the urine. The remainder is eliminated in the faeces.

Intracellular pharmacokinetics

In a study of 20 HIV-infected patients receiving abacavir 300 mg twice daily, with only one 300 mg dose taken prior to the 24 hour sampling period, the geometric mean terminal carbovir-TP intracellular half-life at steady-state was 20.6 hours, compared to the geometric mean abacavir plasma half-life in this study of 2.6 hours. Similar intracellular kinetics are expected from abacavir 600 mg once daily. These data support the use of abacavir 600 mg once daily for the treatment of HIV infected patients. Additionally, the efficacy of abacavir given once daily has been demonstrated in a pivotal clinical study (CNA30021- See section 5.1 Clinical experience).

Special populations

Hepatically impaired: abacavir is metabolised primarily by the liver. The pharmacokinetics of abacavir have been studied in patients with mild hepatic impairment

(Child-Pugh score 5-6) receiving a single 600 mg dose. The results showed that there was a mean increase of 1.89 fold [1.32; 2.70] in the abacavir AUC, and 1.58 [1.22; 2.04] fold in the elimination half-life. No recommendation on dosage reduction is possible in patients with mild hepatic impairment due to the substantial variability of abacavir exposure.

Renally impaired: abacavir is primarily metabolised by the liver with approximately 2% of abacavir excreted unchanged in the urine. The pharmacokinetics of abacavir in patients with end-stage renal disease is similar to patients with normal renal function. Therefore no dosage reduction is required in patients with renal impairment. Based on limited experience Ziagen should be avoided in patients with end-stage renal disease.

Children: according to clinical trials performed in children abacavir is rapidly and well absorbed from an oral solution administered to children. The overall pharmacokinetic parameters in children are comparable to adults, with greater variability in plasma concentrations. The recommended dose for children from three months to 12 years is 8 mg/kg twice daily. This will provide slightly higher mean plasma concentrations in children, ensuring that the majority will achieve therapeutic concentrations equivalent to 300 mg twice daily in adults.

There are insufficient safety data to recommend the use of Ziagen in infants less than three months old. The limited data available indicate that a dose of 2 mg/kg in neonates less than 30 days old provides similar or greater AUCs, compared to the 8 mg/kg dose administered to older children.

Elderly: the pharmacokinetics of abacavir have not been studied in patients over 65 years of age.

5.3 Preclinical safety data

Abacavir was not mutagenic in bacterial tests but showed activity *in vitro* in the human lymphocyte chromosome aberration assay, the mouse lymphoma assay, and the *in vivo* micronucleus test. This is consistent with the known activity of other nucleoside analogues. These results indicate that abacavir has a weak potential to cause chromosomal damage both *in vitro* and *in vivo* at high test concentrations.

Carcinogenicity studies with orally administered abacavir in mice and rats showed an increase in the incidence of malignant and non-malignant tumours. Malignant tumours occurred in the preputial gland of males and the clitoral gland of females of both species, and in rats in the thyroid gland of males and the liver, urinary bladder, lymph nodes and the subcutis of females.

The majority of these tumours occurred at the highest abacavir dose of 330 mg/kg/day in mice and 600 mg/kg/day in rats. The exception was the preputial gland tumour which occurred at a dose of 110 mg/kg in mice. The systemic exposure at the no effect level in mice and rats was equivalent to 3 and 7 times the human systemic exposure during therapy. While the carcinogenic potential in humans is unknown, these data suggest that a carcinogenic risk to humans is outweighed by the potential clinical benefit.

In pre-clinical toxicology studies, abacavir treatment was shown to increase liver weights in rats and monkeys. The clinical relevance of this is unknown. There is no evidence from clinical studies that abacavir is hepatotoxic. Additionally, autoinduction of abacavir metabolism or induction of the metabolism of other medicinal products hepatically metabolised has not been observed in man.

Mild myocardial degeneration in the heart of mice and rats was observed following administration of abacavir for two years. The systemic exposures were equivalent to 7 to 24 times the expected systemic exposure in humans. The clinical relevance of this finding has not been determined.

In reproductive toxicity studies, embryo and foetal toxicity have been observed in rats but not in rabbits. These findings included decreased foetal body weight, foetal oedema, and an increase in skeletal variations/malformations, early intra-uterine deaths and still births. No conclusion can be drawn with regard to the teratogenic potential of abacavir because of this embryo-foetal toxicity.

A fertility study in the rat has shown that abacavir had no effect on male or female fertility.

6. PHARMACEUTICAL PARTICULARS

6.1 List of excipients

Core: microcrystalline cellulose, sodium starch glycollate, magnesium stearate, colloidal anhydrous silica.

Coating: triacetin, methylhydroxypropylcellulose, titanium dioxide, polysorbate 80, iron oxide yellow.

6.2 Incompatibilities

Not applicable

6.3 Shelf life

3 years

6.4 Special precautions for storage

Do not store above 30°C

6.5 Nature and contents of container

Ziagen tablets are available in polyvinyl chloride/foil blister packs containing 60 tablets.

6.6 Instructions for use and handling

No special requirements

Administrative Data

7. MARKETING AUTHORISATION HOLDER

Glaxo Group Ltd

Greenford

Middlesex UB6 0NN

United Kingdom

8. MARKETING AUTHORISATION NUMBER(S)

EU/1/99/112/001

9. DATE OF FIRST AUTHORISATION/RENEWAL OF THE AUTHORISATION

Date of first authorisation: 8 July 1999

Date of renewal: 18 August 2004

10. DATE OF REVISION OF THE TEXT

17 December 2004

Zibor 2,500 and 3,500 IU anti-Xa/0.2 ml; Zibor 25,000 IU anti-Xa/ml

(Amdipharm)

1. NAME OF THE MEDICINAL PRODUCT

Zibor® 2,500 IU anti-Xa/0.2 ml solution for injection in pre-filled syringes. ▼

Zibor® 3,500 IU anti-Xa/0.2 ml solution for injection in pre-filled syringes. ▼

Zibor® 25,000 IU anti-Xa/ml solution for injection in pre-filled syringes. ▼

2. QUALITATIVE AND QUANTITATIVE COMPOSITION

Zibor 2,500 IU:

Bemiparin sodium (INN): 2,500 IU (anti-Factor Xa*) per 0.2 ml pre-filled syringe (equivalent to 12500 IU (anti-Factor Xa*) per millilitre solution for injection).

Zibor 3,500 IU:

Bemiparin sodium (INN): 3,500 IU (anti-Factor Xa*) per 0.2 ml pre-filled syringe (equivalent to 17500 IU (anti-Factor Xa*) per millilitre solution for injection).

Zibor 25,000 IU/ml:

Bemiparin sodium (INN): 25,000 IU (anti-Factor Xa*) per ml solution for injection, equivalent to:

5,000 IU (anti-Factor Xa) per 0.2 ml pre-filled syringe

7,500 IU (anti-Factor Xa) per 0.3 ml pre-filled syringe

10,000 IU (anti-Factor Xa) per 0.4 ml pre-filled syringe

*Potency is described in International anti-Factor Xa activity units (IU) of the 1st International Low Molecular Weight Heparin Reference Standard.

For excipients, see 6.1.

3. PHARMACEUTICAL FORM

Solution for injection in pre-filled syringe.

Colourless (or slightly yellowish for Zibor 25,000 IU/ml), clear solution free of visible particles.

4. CLINICAL PARTICULARS

4.1 Therapeutic indications

Zibor 2,500 IU: Prevention of thromboembolic disease in patients undergoing general surgery. Prevention of clotting in the extracorporeal circuit during haemodialysis.

Zibor 3,500 IU: Prevention of thromboembolic disease in patients undergoing orthopaedic surgery. Prevention of clotting in the extracorporeal circuit during haemodialysis.

Zibor 25,000 IU/ml: The treatment of established deep vein thrombosis, with or without pulmonary embolism, during the acute phase.

4.2 Posology and method of administration

WARNING: The different low molecular weight heparins are not necessarily equivalent. Therefore compliance with the dosage regimen and the specific method of use for each of these medicinal products is required.

Adults:

Prevention

General surgery with moderate risk of venous thromboembolism:

On the day of the surgical procedure, Zibor 2,500 IU anti-Xa is to be administered by subcutaneous (sc) route, 2 hours before or 6 hours after surgery. On subsequent days, Zibor 2,500 IU anti-Xa sc is to be administered every 24 hours.

Orthopaedic surgery with high risk of venous thromboembolism:

On the day of the surgical procedure, Zibor 3,500 IU anti-Xa is to be administered by subcutaneous (sc) route, 2 hours before or 6 hours after surgery. On subsequent days, Zibor 3,500 IU anti-Xa sc is to be administered every 24 hours.

Prophylactic treatment must be followed in accordance with the physician's opinion during the period of risk or until the patient is mobilised. As a general rule, it is considered necessary to maintain prophylactic treatment for at least 7 – 10 days after the surgical procedure and until the risk of thromboembolic disease has decreased.

Prevention of clotting in the extracorporeal circuit during haemodialysis:

For patients undergoing repeated haemodialysis of no longer than 4 hours in duration and with no risk of bleeding, the prevention of clotting in the extracorporeal circuit during haemodialysis is obtained by injecting a single dose in the form of bolus into the arterial line at the beginning of the dialysis session. For patients weighing less than 60kg, the dose will be 2,500 IU, whereas for patients weighing more than 60kg, the dose will be 3,500 IU.

Treatment

Treatment of deep vein thrombosis

Zibor 25,000 IU anti-Factor Xa/ml solution for injection should be administered by the subcutaneous route at a dose of 115 IU anti-Xa/kg weight, once daily. The recommended duration of treatment is 7 ± 2 days. The daily dose generally corresponds - depending on the body weight range - to the following doses and volumes of the product in pre-filled syringes: < 50 kg, 0.2 ml (5,000 IU anti-Xa); 50-70 kg, 0.3 ml (7,500 IU anti-Xa), > 70 kg, 0.4 ml (10,000 IU anti-Xa). In patients weighing more than 100 kg body-weight, the dose should be calculated on the basis of 115 IU anti-Xa/kg/day, where the concentration of anti-Xa is 25,000 IU/ml.

In the absence of any contra-indication, oral anticoagulation should be commenced 3-5 days after beginning Zibor 25,000 IU/ml first administration, and the dose adjusted so as to keep the International Normalized Ratio (INR) value between 2-3 times the control value.

Bemiparin administration can be stopped as soon as the said INR value is achieved. Oral anticoagulation should be continued for at least 3 months.

Children: The safety and efficacy of the use of bemiparin in children has not been established, therefore the usage in children is not recommended.

Elderly: No dose adjustment required.

Renal and hepatic impairment: There are insufficient data to recommend a dose adjustment of bemiparin in this group of patients.

Method of administration. Subcutaneous injection technique:

The pre-filled syringes are ready for immediate use and must not be purged before the subcutaneous injection. When Zibor is administered subcutaneously, the injection should be given in the subcutaneous cell tissue of the anterolateral or posterolateral abdominal waist, alternately on the left and right sides. The needle should be fully inserted, perpendicularly and not tangentially, into the thick part of a skin fold held between the thumb and the forefinger; the skin fold should be held throughout the whole injection. Do not rub the injection site.

4.3 Contraindications

Hypersensitivity to bemiparin sodium, heparin or substances derived from pigs.

History of confirmed or suspected immunologically mediated heparin induced thrombocytopenia (HIT) (see 4.4: *Special warnings and precautions for use*).

Active haemorrhage or increased risk of bleeding due to impairment of haemostasis.

Severe impairment of liver and pancreas function.

Injuries to and operations on the central nervous system, eyes and ears within the last 2 months.

Disseminated Intravascular Coagulation (DIC) attributable to heparin-induced thrombocytopenia.

Acute bacterial endocarditis and endocarditis lenta.

Organic lesion with high risk of bleeding (e.g. active peptic ulcer, haemorrhagic stroke, cerebral aneurysm or cerebral neoplasms).

In patients receiving heparin for treatment rather than for prophylaxis, locoregional anaesthesia in elective surgical procedures is contra-indicated.

4.4 Special warnings and special precautions for use

Do not administer by the intramuscular route.

Due to risk of haematoma during bemiparin administration the intramuscular injection of other agents should be avoided.

Caution should be exercised in patients with liver or renal failure, uncontrolled arterial hypertension, history of gastro-duodenal ulcer disease, thrombocytopenia, nephrolithiasis and/or urethrolithiasis, choroid and retinal vascular disease, or any other organic lesion with an increased risk of bleeding complications, or in patients undergoing spinal or epidural anaesthesia and /or lumbar puncture.

Bemiparin, like other LMWHs, can suppress adrenal secretion of aldosterone leading to hyperkalaemia, particularly in patients such as those with diabetes mellitus, chronic renal failure, pre-existing metabolic acidosis, a raised plasma potassium or taking potassium sparing drugs. The risk of hyperkalaemia appears to increase with the duration of therapy but is usually reversible. Serum electrolytes should be measured in patients at risk before starting bemiparin therapy and monitored regularly thereafter particularly if treatment is prolonged beyond about 7 days.

Occasionally a mild transient thrombocytopenia (type I) at the beginning of therapy with heparin with platelet counts between 100,000/mm^3 and 150,000/mm^3 due to temporary platelet activation has been observed (see 4.8: *Undesirable effects*). As a rule, no complications occur, therefore treatment can be continued.

In rare cases antibody-mediated severe thrombocytopenia (type II) with platelet counts clearly below 100,000/mm^3 has been observed (see 4.8: *Undesirable effects*). This effect usually occurs within 5 to 21 days after the beginning of treatment; in patients with a history of heparin-induced thrombocytopenia this may occur sooner.

Platelet counts are recommended before administration of bemiparin, on the first day of therapy and then regularly 3 to 4 days and at the end of therapy with bemiparin. In practice, treatment must be discontinued immediately and an alternative therapy initiated if a significantly reduced platelet count is observed (30 to 50%) associated with positive or unknown results of in-vitro tests for antiplatelet antibody in the presence of bemiparin or other LMWHs and/or heparins.

As with other heparins, cases of cutaneous necrosis, sometimes preceded by purpura or painful erythematous blotches have been reported with bemiparin (see 4.8: *Undesirable effects*). In such cases, treatment should be discontinued immediately.

In patients undergoing epidural or spinal anaesthesia or lumbar puncture, the prophylactic use of heparin may very rarely be associated with epidural or spinal haematoma, resulting in prolonged or permanent paralysis (see 4.8: *Undesirable effects*). The risk is increased by the use of an epidural or spinal catheter for anaesthesia, by the concomitant use of drugs affecting haemostasis such as non-steroidal anti-inflammatory drugs (NSAIDs), platelet inhibitors or anticoagulants (see 4.5: *Interaction with other medicinal products and other forms of interaction*), and by traumatic or repeated puncture.

When reaching a decision as to the interval between the last heparin administration at prophylactic doses and the placement or removal of an epidural or spinal catheter, the product characteristics and the patient profile should be taken into account. The subsequent dose of bemiparin should not take place until at least four hours after removal of the catheter. The subsequent dose should be delayed until the surgical procedure is completed.

Should a physician decide to administer anticoagulation treatment in the context of epidural or spinal anaesthesia, extreme vigilance and frequent monitoring must be exercised to detect any signs and symptoms of neurological impairment, such as back pain, sensory and motor deficits (numbness and weakness in lower limbs) and bowel or bladder dysfunction. Nurses should be trained to detect such signs and symptoms. Patients should be instructed to inform a nurse or a clinician immediately if they experience any of these symptoms.

If signs or symptoms of epidural or spinal haematoma are suspected, urgent diagnosis and treatment including medullary/spinal cord decompression should be initiated.

4.5 Interaction with other medicinal products and other forms of Interaction

Bemiparin interactions with other medicinal products have not been investigated and the information given on this section is derived from data available from other LMWH.

The concomitant administration of bemiparin and the following medicinal products is not advisable:

Vitamin K antagonists and other anticoagulants, acetyl salicylic acid and other salicylates and NSAIDs, ticlopidine, clopidogrel and other platelet inhibitors, systemic glucocorticoids and dextran.

All these drugs increase the pharmacological effect of bemiparin by interfering with its action on coagulation and/or platelet function and increasing the risk of bleeding.

If the combination cannot be avoided, it should be used with careful clinical and laboratory monitoring.

Medicinal products that increase the serum potassium concentration should only be taken concomitantly under especially careful medical supervision.

Interaction of heparin with intravenous nitroglycerine (which can result in a decrease in efficacy) cannot be ruled out for bemiparin.

4.6 Pregnancy and lactation

Pregnancy: No reproductive toxicity studies have been performed with bemiparin. Animal studies have not shown any evidence of teratogenic effects with the use of LMWHs (see 5.3: *Preclinical safety data*).

There are no data to evaluate the possible teratogenic or foetotoxic effect of bemiparin in pregnant women, so that the potential risk for humans is unknown. Therefore Zibor is not recommended for use in pregnancy unless clearly necessary.

It is unknown whether bemiparin crosses placental barrier.

Lactation: Insufficient information is available as to whether bemiparin passes into breast milk. Therefore, where it is necessary for lactating mothers to receive Zibor, they should be advised to avoid breast-feeding.

4.7 Effects on ability to drive and use machines

Bemiparin has no influence on the ability to drive and use precision or dangerous machinery.

4.8 Undesirable effects

The most commonly reported adverse reaction is haematoma and/or ecchymosis at the injection site, occurring in approximately 15% of patients receiving Zibor.

Osteoporosis has been associated with long-term heparin treatment.

The frequency of adverse events (AEs) reported with bemiparin are similar to those reported with other LMWHs and is as follows:

Very common (≥1/10):	Ecchymosis at injection site.
Common (≥1/100, <1/10):	Haematoma and pain at injection site. Bleeding complications (skin, mucous membranes, wounds, gastro-intestinal tract, urogenital tract). Mild and transient elevations of transaminases (ASAT, ALAT) and gamma-GT levels.
Uncommon (≥1/1000, <1/100):	Cutaneous allergic reactions (urticaria, pruritus). Mild and transient thrombocytopenia (type I) (see 4.4: *Special warnings and precautions for use*).
Rare (<1/1000):	Anaphylactic reactions (nausea, vomiting, fever, dyspnoea, bronchospasm, glottis oedema, hypotension, urticaria, pruritus). Severe thrombocytopenia (type II) (see 4.4: *Special warnings and precautions for use*). Cutaneous necrosis at the injection site (see 4.4: *Special warnings and precautions for use*). Epidural and spinal haematoma following epidural or spinal anaesthesia and lumbar puncture. These haematomas have caused various degrees of neurological impairment, including prolonged or permanent paralysis (see 4.4: *Special warnings and precautions for use*).

4.9 Overdose

Bleeding is the main symptom of overdose. Bemiparin should be discontinued depending on the severity of the haemorrhage and the risk of thrombosis.

Minor haemorrhages rarely need specific treatment. In case of major haemorrhages, administration of protamine sulphate may be needed.

The neutralisation of bemiparin with protamine sulphate has been studied *in-vitro* and *in-vivo*, with the aim of observing the reduction of anti-Xa activity and the effect on the APTT.

Protamine sulphate exerts a partial decrease on anti-Xa activity for 2 hours after its intravenous administration, at a dose of 1.4mg of protamine sulphate each 100 IU anti-Xa administered.

5. PHARMACOLOGICAL PROPERTIES

5.1 Pharmacodynamic properties

Pharmacotherapeutic group: antithrombotic agent, heparin group. ATC code B01AB.

Bemiparin sodium is a LMWH obtained by depolymerization of heparin sodium from porcine intestinal mucosa. Its mean molecular weight (MW) is approximately 3,600 daltons.

The percentage of chains with MW lower than 2,000 daltons is less than 35%. The percentage of chains with MW from 2,000 to 6,000 daltons ranges between 50-75%. The percentage of chains with MW higher than 6,000 daltons is less than 15%.

The anti-Xa activity ranges between 80 and 120 anti-Xa IU per mg and the anti-IIa activity ranges between 5 and 20 anti-IIa IU per mg, calculated in relation to dry matter. The anti-Xa/anti-IIa ratio is approximately 8.

In animal experiment models, bemiparin has shown antithrombotic activity and moderate haemorrhagic effect.

In humans, bemiparin has confirmed its antithrombotic activity and, at the recommended doses, it does not significantly prolong global clotting tests.

5.2 Pharmacokinetic properties

The pharmacokinetic properties of bemiparin have been determined by measuring the plasma anti-Xa activity using the amydolitic method; it is based on reference to the W.H.O. First International Low Molecular Weight Heparin Reference Standard (National Institute for Biological Standards and Control, NIBSC).

The absorption and elimination processes follow a linear kinetic of the 1st order.

Absorption: Bemiparin sodium is rapidly absorbed following subcutaneous injection and the bioavailability is estimated to be 96%. The maximum plasma anti-Xa effect at prophylactic doses of 2,500 IU and 3,500 IU occurs 2 to 3 hours after subcutaneous injection of bemiparin, reaching peak activities in the order of 0.34 ± 0.08 and 0.45 ± 0.07 IU anti-Xa/ml, respectively. Anti-IIa activity was not detected at these doses. The maximum plasma anti-Xa effect at treatment doses of 5,000 IU, 7,500 IU, 10,000 IU and 12,500 IU occurs 3 to 4 hours after subcutaneous injection of bemiparin, reaching peak activities in the order of 0.54 ± 0.06, 1.22 ± 0.27, 1.42 ± 0.19 and 2.03 ± 0.25 IU anti-Xa/ml, respectively. Anti-IIa activity of 0.01 IU/ ml was detected at doses of 7,500 IU, 10,000 IU and 12,500 IU.

Elimination: Bemiparin administered in the dose range of 2,500 IU to 12,500 IU has an approximate half-life of between 5 and 6 hours, and should therefore be administered once daily.

There are currently no data available with regards to plasma protein binding, metabolism and excretion of bemiparin in humans.

5.3 Preclinical safety data

Preclinical data for bemiparin reveal no special hazard for humans based on conventional studies of safety pharmacology, single and repeated dose toxicity and genotoxicity.

Acute and repeated dose toxicity studies following subcutaneous administration of bemiparin in animals have revealed alterations consisting essentially in haemorrhagic lesions at the injection sites, which were reversible and directly dose-dependent. The alterations recorded could be considered as relating to their pharmacological effects rather than to a strictly toxic action, although pharmacokinetic data were not obtained for these animal species.

No reproductive toxicity or carcinogenicity studies have been performed with bemiparin. Previously published studies of reproductive toxicity performed with other LMWHs in pregnant rats and rabbits, did not indicate any direct or indirect damaging effect that provided experimental evidence of impairment of fertility, embryo-foetal toxicity or impairment of peri and post-natal development.

6. PHARMACEUTICAL PARTICULARS

6.1 List of excipients

Water for injections

6.2 Incompatibilities

Zibor should not be mixed with any other injections or infusions.

6.3 Shelf life

2 years.

After first opening, Zibor should be used immediately.

6.4 Special precautions for storage

Zibor 2,500 IU and 3,500 IU:

Do not store above 30°C. Do not freeze.

Zibor 25,000 IU/ml:

Do not store above 25°C. Do not freeze.

6.5 Nature and contents of container

Zibor 2,500 IU and 3,500 IU:

0.2 ml solution in pre-filled syringe (Type I glass) with a rubber plunger rod (polypropylene), rubber plunger stopper (chlorobutyl) and injection needle (stainless steel). Packs of 2 and 10 syringes.

Zibor 25,000 IU/ml:

0.2 ml, 0.3 ml and 0.4 ml of solution in pre-filled syringe (Type I glass) with a rubber plunger rod (polypropylene), rubber plunger stopper (chlorobutyl) and injection needle (stainless steel). Packs of 2 and 10 syringes.

6.6 Instructions for use and handling

Single-dose container. Discard any unused content. Do not use if the protective package is opened or damaged. Only clear and colourless (or slightly yellowish for Zibor 25,000 IU) solutions, free of visible particles, should be used. Any unused product and injection needles should be disposed of in accordance with local requirements.

Administrative Data

7. MARKETING AUTHORISATION HOLDER

Laboratorios Pan Química-Farmacéutica, S.A.

Rufino González, 50

28037 Madrid

Spain

8. MARKETING AUTHORISATION NUMBER(S)

Zibor 2,500 IU anti-Xa: PL 19119/0001

Zibor 3,500 IU anti-Xa: PL 19119/0002

Zibor 25,000 IU anti-Xa/ml: PL 19119/0003

9. DATE OF FIRST AUTHORISATION/RENEWAL OF THE AUTHORISATION

Zibor 2,500 and 3,500 IU:

18 March 2002

Zibor 25,000 IU/ml:

24 July 2003

10. DATE OF REVISION OF THE TEXT

July 2003

Zidoval

(3M Health Care Limited)

1. NAME OF THE MEDICINAL PRODUCT

Zidoval[TM]7.5 mg/g vaginal gel

2. QUALITATIVE AND QUANTITATIVE COMPOSITION

Metronidazole 0.75% w/w, 7.5 mg/g

For excipients, see 6.1.

3. PHARMACEUTICAL FORM

Vaginal gel

A colourless to straw coloured gel

4. CLINICAL PARTICULARS

4.1 Therapeutic indications

Zidoval vaginal gel is indicated for the treatment of bacterial vaginosis.

4.2 Posology and method of administration

For vaginal administration.

Adults

One application of Zidoval vaginal gel (5g) inserted into the vagina once daily, at bedtime, for 5 consecutive days.

Directions for use: Pierce sealed end of tube and screw open end of applicator tightly onto tube of gel. Squeeze tube, filling the applicator with gel. Remove applicator from tube and gently insert applicator into vagina as far as it will comfortably go. Push the plunger to release the gel. Dispose of applicator as instructed.

Elderly

Bacterial vaginosis is not commonly seen in the elderly population and consequently clinical assessment in this age group has not been carried out.

Children

Notrecommended for use in children and adolescents under 18 years since safety and efficacyhave not been established.

4.3 Contraindications

Zidoval vaginal gel is contraindicated in patients with a prior history of hypersensitivity to metronidazole, other nitroimidazoles, parabens or any other ingredient of the gel.

4.4 Special warnings and special precautions for use

Use during menses is not recommended.

Known or previously unrecognised candidiasis may present more prominent symptoms during therapy with Zidoval vaginal gel and may require treatment with a candicidal agent.

Metronidazole is a nitroimidazole and should be used with care in patients with evidence of a history of blood dyscrasias.

As with all vaginal infections, sexual intercourse during the infection and during treatment with Zidoval vaginal gel is not recommended.

4.5 Interaction with other medicinal products and other forms of Interaction

Oral metronidazole has been associated with a disulfiram-like reaction in combination with alcohol. Acute psychotic reactions and confusion have occurred during concomitant use of disulfiram with oral metronidazole. At the low serum concentrations which result from the use of Zidoval vaginal gel, the possibility of similar reactions is unlikely although cannot be excluded.

Oral metronidazole has been shown to increase the plasma concentrations of warfarin, lithium, cyclosporin and 5-fluorouracil. Similar effects after vaginal administration of metronidazole are not expected due to the low plasma concentrations but cannot be completely ruled out.

Metronidazole may interfere with certain types of determination of serum chemistry values, such as aspartate aminotransferase (AST, SGOT), alanine aminotransferase (ALT, SGPT), lactic dehydrogenase (LDH), triglycerides and hexokinase glucose. Values of zero may be observed.

4.6 Pregnancy and lactation

Pregnancy

Data on a large number (several hundred) of exposed pregnancies indicate no adverse effects of metronidazole on the foetus/newborn child. There have been no formal studies with Zidoval vaginal gel in pregnant women. Caution should, therefore, be exercised when prescribing to pregnant women.

Lactation

The ratio of serum concentrations of Zidoval vaginal gel/oral metronidazole is approximately 0.02. Metronidazole is excreted in milk at concentrations similar to those in maternal serum and the ratio of serum concentrations ofmetronidazole in the breastfed infant/mother is approximately 0.15. Caution should be exercised when prescribing to lactating women.

4.7 Effects on ability to drive and use machines

None.

4.8 Undesirable effects

In controlled clinical trials involving 759 patients, the most commonly reported ADRs were urogenital (26%) and gastrointestinal (14%).

Common >1/100, <1/10)	Neurological: Headache, dizziness. GI: GI discomfort/abdominal cramps, nausea and/or vomiting, unpleasant taste/unusual feeling on tongue, decreased appetite. Urogenital: Vaginal candidiasis, vaginal itching/irritation/burning/numbness, pelvic discomfort, vaginal discharge.
Uncommon >1/1000, <1/100)	Psychiatric: Depression, fatigue, irritability, trouble sleeping. Neurological: Unusual sensation in extremities. GI: Diarrhoea, constipation, stomach gurgling/bloating/gas, thirsty/dry mouth, metallic taste. Skin: Itching. Urinary: Urinary tract infection symptoms, darkened urine. Urogenital: Vulvar swelling, menstrual discomfort/irregularities, vaginal spotting/bleeding, medication leakage. General: Cramping.

4.9 Overdose

There is no human experience of overdosage with Zidoval vaginal gel. There is no specific treatment. Metronidazole is readily removed from the plasma by haemodialysis.

5. PHARMACOLOGICAL PROPERTIES

5.1 Pharmacodynamic properties

ATC classification: G01 AF01

Metronidazole is a synthetic antibacterial agent which also possesses amoebicidal activity. Zidoval vaginal gel has been shown *in vivo* to be active against the vaginal pathogens Gardnerella vaginalis and bacteroides species.

Significant increases in lactobacilli are observed in bacterial vaginosis patients following therapy with Zidoval.

5.2 Pharmacokinetic properties

Bioavailability studies on the administration of a single 5 gram dose of Zidoval vaginal gel into the vagina of 12 normal subjects showed a mean C_{max} serum concentration of 237 nanogram/ml or about 2% of the mean maximum serum concentration of a 500 mg tablet taken orally (mean C_{max} = 12,785 ng/ml). Under normal usage, the formulation therefore affords minimal serum concentrations of metronidazole.

Metronidazole has a large apparent volume of distribution and has the ability to penetrate the blood brain barrier and blood cerebro-spinal fluid barrier at concentrations similar to serum concentrations.

Metronidazole is metabolised in the liver by side chain oxidation and glucuronide formation and a large portion of the absorbed dose is excreted as metabolites. Both unchanged drug and metabolites are excreted mainly in the urine.

5.3 Preclinical safety data

At highdoses metronidazolehas been found to be mutagenic in bacteria but not in mammalian cells *in vitro* or *in vivo*. A carcinogenic potential has been demonstrated in mouse and rat but not in hamster. In epidemiological studies, no evidence of increased risk of cancer as a consequence of exposure to metronidazole has been observed.

6. PHARMACEUTICAL PARTICULARS

6.1 List of excipients

Carbomer (Carbopol) 974P, disodium edetate, methyl parahydroxybenzoate, propyl parahydroxybenzoate, propylene glycol, sodium hydroxide, purified water.

6.2 Incompatibilities

None known

6.3 Shelf life

3years

6.4 Special precautions for storage

Do not store above 25 °C.

6.5 Nature and contents of container

Aluminium tubes lined with an epoxy phenolic resinwith polyethylene screw caps containing 40 g product. The product is packaged with 5 disposable vaginal applicators, each to deliver 5 g of gel.

6.6 Instructions for use and handling

Not applicable.

7. MARKETING AUTHORISATION HOLDER

3M Health Care Limited

3M House

Morley Street

Loughborough

Leics

LE111EP

8. MARKETING AUTHORISATION NUMBER(S)

00068/0169

9. DATE OF FIRST AUTHORISATION/RENEWAL OF THE AUTHORISATION

31 January 1997 / 27 July 2000.

10. DATE OF REVISION OF THE TEXT

July 2000

Zimbacol XL tablets

(Link Pharmaceuticals Ltd)

1. NAME OF THE MEDICINAL PRODUCT

Zimbacol® XL

2. QUALITATIVE AND QUANTITATIVE COMPOSITION

Each tablet contains 400mg bezafibrate

3. PHARMACEUTICAL FORM

Modified release tablets

4. CLINICAL PARTICULARS

4.1 Therapeutic indications

Zimbacol XL is indicated for use in hyperlipidaemia of Type IIa, IIb, III, IV and V under the Frederikson Classification.

Bezafibrate should be administered only to patients with a fully defined and diagnosed lipid abnormality where changes in diet or lifestyle (for example greater physical activity and weight reduction) cannot control the condition and in whom the long term risks associated with the condition warrant treatment. The rationale for use of bezafibrate is to control abnormal increases in serum lipid and lipoprotein levels or prevent long term adverse effects that have been shown by many epidemiological studies to be positively and strongly correlated with such hyperlipidaemias.

4.2 Posology and method of administration

Adults

Zimbacol XL should be taken orally. The dosage is one 400mg tablet daily. Tablets should be swallowed whole with a little fluid after a meal, either morning or night.

The response to therapy is normally rapid, but a gradual improvement may occur over several weeks. Treatment should be stopped if an adequate response has not been achieved within 3 to 4 months.

Elderly

There are no specific dosage requirements for elderly patients.

Children

There is currently insufficient information available to recommend an appropriate dosage in children.

4.3 Contraindications

Bezafibrate is contraindicated in patients with severe hepatic disease (other than fatty infiltration of the liver associated with raised triglyceride values), gall bladder disease with or without cholelithiasis, nephrotic syndrome and severe renal disorders (serum creatinine greater than 135 μmoles/l or creatinine clearance less than 60ml/min). Bezafibrate is contraindicated in patients hypersensitive to bezafibrate.

4.4 Special warnings and special precautions for use

Zimbacol XL is contraindicated in patients with renal impairment (serum creatinine greater than 135 μmoles/l or creatinine clearance less than 60ml/min). Such patients may be treated with conventional bezafibrate tablets (200mg bezafibrate) using a reduced daily dosage.

4.5 Interaction with other medicinal products and other forms of Interaction

Care is required in administering bezafibrate to patients receiving coumarin-type anti-coagulant therapy. The dose of anti-coagulant should be reduced initially by 50% and adjusted according to prothrombin time.

As bezafibrate can improve glucose utilisation, the action of anti-diabetic medication might be potentiated. Although hypoglycaemia has not been observed, caution must be taken and monitoring of glycaemic status may be warranted.

Bezafibrate should not be administered with MAO-inhibitors with hepatoxic potential.

HMG CoA reductase inhibitors taken in combination with fibrates may increase the risk of myopathy and should therefore be used with caution. Patients predisposed to myopathy (impaired renal function, severe infection, trauma, surgery, disturbances of hormone or electrolyte balance) should not be given this combination therapy.

If combined therapy with an ion-exchange resin is necessary, to avoid impairment of bezafibrate absorption, there should be an interval of two hours between intake of the resin and Zimbacol XL.

Oestrogens may lead to a rise in lipid levels and therefore the necessity for treatment with Zimbacol XL in patients receiving oestrogens or oestrogen containing preparations should be considered on an individual basis.

4.6 Pregnancy and lactation

Bezafibrate has not been shown to have any adverse effects on the foetus during animal studies, however, it is recommended that bezafibrate should not be administered to women either when they are pregnant or breast-feeding.

4.7 Effects on ability to drive and use machines
None stated.

4.8 Undesirable effects
The most frequent adverse effects during treatment with bezafibrate are gastrointestinal in nature, such as nausea, loss of appetite, vomiting, diarrhoea, dyspepsia, flatulence and abdominal discomfort. These symptoms are generally transient and resolve without drug withdrawal or dosage adjustment. Other less frequently occurring adverse effects include weight gain, headache, dizziness, fatigue or drowsiness, skin rashes, pruritus, alopecia, impotence, anaemia and leucopenia. Rarely, muscle cramps and weakness may occur, accompanied by increases in creatinine phosphokinase concentrations and serum myoglobin. These adverse effects are generally rapidly resolved following withdrawal of therapy.

Serum creatinine has been observed to increase in patients with normal renal function. For patients with renal dysfunction care should be taken as failure to follow dosage guidelines could result in rhabdomyolysis.

There have been isolated reports of cholecystitis, gallstones and sometimes pancreatitis in patients receiving fibrates. However, there is no evidence that the administration of bezafibrate is associated with these problems.

4.9 Overdose
In cases of acute overdosage, treatment, where necessary, should be symptomatic. There is no evidence of serious clinical or biochemical effects following bezafibrate overdosage.

5. PHARMACOLOGICAL PROPERTIES
5.1 Pharmacodynamic properties
Bezafibrate is a fibric acid derivative with hypolipidaemic activity. It has the isobutyric group in common with clofibrate, but it is 10 times more potent than clofibrate at reducing serum cholesterol and triglycerides. Bezafibrate has four separate metabolic effects: a limitation of substrate availability for triglyceride synthesis in the liver; promotion of the action of lipoprotein lipase; modulation of low density lipoprotein (LDL) receptor/ligand interaction; and stimulation of reverse cholesterol transport.

5.2 Pharmacokinetic properties
Bezafibrate is rapidly and almost completely absorbed from the gastrointestinal tract and there is no presystemic metabolism. Maximum plasma concentrations occur at approximately 4 hours after administration of Zimbacol XL (average plasma half-life 3.4 hours). The protein-binding of bezafibrate in serum is approximately 95%. Elimination is mainly in urine (>90%) either as polar metabolites or unchanged bezafibrate. A small percentage of the dose is excreted in the faeces. Elimination may be increased in forced diuresis.

5.3 Preclinical safety data
Chronic administration of a high dose of bezafibrate to rats was associated with hepatic tumour formation in females. However, the dosage was in the order of 30 to 40 times the human dosage and no similar effect was observed at lower dose levels correlating more closely to the lipid lowering dose in humans.

6. PHARMACEUTICAL PARTICULARS
6.1 List of excipients
Zimbacol XL contains the following excipients: Maize starch, sodium starch glycollate, lactose, poly(ethyl acrylate-methyl methacrylate), magnesium stearate, polysorbate 80, hypromellose, talc, calcium carbonate, povidone, arabic gum, titanium dioxide (E171), glucose, sucrose, purified water, Macrogol 6000 EP

6.2 Incompatibilities
None stated.

6.3 Shelf life
36 months.

6.4 Special precautions for storage
Do not store above 25°C.

6.5 Nature and contents of container
Zimbacol XL is available in rigid PVC film/ Aluminium foil blister strips packed in outer cardboard cartons.

6.6 Instructions for use and handling
None stated.

7. MARKETING AUTHORISATION HOLDER
Link Pharmaceuticals Limited, Bishops Weald House, Albion Way, Horsham, West Sussex, RH12 1AH

8. MARKETING AUTHORISATION NUMBER(S)
PL 12406/0010

9. DATE OF FIRST AUTHORISATION/RENEWAL OF THE AUTHORISATION
16 May 2000

10. DATE OF REVISION OF THE TEXT

11. Legal Category
POM

® Zimbacol is a registered trade mark

Zimovane

(sanofi-aventis)

1. NAME OF THE MEDICINAL PRODUCT
Zimovane
Zimovane LS

2. QUALITATIVE AND QUANTITATIVE COMPOSITION
Zopiclone 7.5 mg or 3.75mg.

3. PHARMACEUTICAL FORM
Zopiclone is intended to be administered by the oral route in the form of white, elliptical film-coated tablets with a score-line on one side (Zimovane) or white, round, biconvex, film-coated tablets (Zimovane LS).

4. CLINICAL PARTICULARS
4.1 Therapeutic indications
Short term treatment of insomnia, including difficulties in falling asleep, nocturnal awakening and early awakening, transient, situational or chronic insomnia, and insomnia secondary to psychiatric disturbances, in situations where the insomnia is debilitating or is causing severe distress for the patient. Long term continuous use is not recommended. A course of treatment should employ the lowest effective dose.

4.2 Posology and method of administration
Adults: The recommended dose is one Zimovane tablet (7.5mg zopiclone) by the oral route shortly before retiring.

Elderly: A lower dose of 3.75mg zopiclone should be employed to start treatment in the elderly. Depending on effectiveness and acceptability, the dosage subsequently may be increased if clinically necessary.

Patients with hepatic insufficiency: As elimination of zopiclone may be reduced in patients with hepatic dysfunction, a lower dose of 3.75mg zopiclone nightly is recommended. The standard dose of 7.5mg zopiclone may be used with caution in some cases, depending on effectiveness and acceptability.

Renal insufficiency: Accumulation of zopiclone or its metabolites has not been seen during treatment of insomnia in patients with renal insufficiency. However, it is recommended that patients with impaired renal function should start treatment with 3.75mg.

Treatment duration
Transient insomnia 2 - 5 days. Short term insomnia 2 - 3 weeks. A single course of treatment should not continue for longer than 4 weeks including any tapering off.

Route of administration
Oral. Each tablet should be swallowed whole without sucking, chewing or breaking.

4.3 Contraindications
Zimovane is contraindicated in patients with myasthenia gravis, respiratory failure, severe sleep apnoea syndrome, severe hepatic insufficiency and those people with a hypersensitivity to zopiclone. As with all hypnotics Zimovane should not be used in children.

4.4 Special warnings and special precautions for use
Use in hepatic insufficiency: A reduced dosage is recommended, see Posology.

Use in renal insufficiency: A reduced dosage is recommended, see Posology.

Risk of dependence: Clinical experience to date with Zimovane suggests that the risk of dependence is minimal when the duration of treatment is limited to not more than 4 weeks.

Use of benzodiazepines and benzodiazepine-like agents (even at therapeutic doses) may lead to the development of physical and psychological dependence upon these products. The risk of dependence increases with dose and duration of treatment; it is also greater in patients with a history of alcohol and or drug abuse, or those who have marked personality disorders. The decision to use a hypnotic in such patients should be taken only with this clearly in mind. If physical dependence has developed, abrupt termination of treatment will be accompanied by withdrawal symptoms (see warnings and precautions). These may consist of headaches, muscle pain, extreme anxiety, tension, restlessness, confusion and irritability. In severe cases the following symptoms may occur: derealisation, depersonalisation, hyperacusis, numbness and tingling of the extremities, hypersensitivity to light, noise and physical contact, hallucinations or epileptic seizures. Rare cases of abuse have been reported.

Withdrawal: The termination of treatment with Zimovane is unlikely to be associated with withdrawal effects when duration of treatment is limited to 4 weeks. Patients may benefit from tapering of the dose before discontinuation. (See also section 4.8. Undesirable Effects).

Depression: Zopiclone does not constitute a treatment for depression. Any underlying cause of the insomnia should also be addressed before symptomatic treatment to avoid under treating potentially serious effects of depression.

Tolerance: Some loss of efficacy to the hypnotic effect of benzodiazepines and benzodiazepine-like agents may develop after repeated use for a few weeks. However, with Zimovane there is an absence of any marked tolerance during treatment periods of up to 4 weeks.

Rebound insomnia is a transient syndrome where the symptoms which led to treatment with a benzodiazepine or benzodiazepine-like agent recur in an enhanced form on discontinuation of therapy. It may be accompanied by other reactions including mood changes, anxiety and restlessness. Since the risk of withdrawal/rebound phenomena may be increased after prolonged treatment, or abrupt discontinuation of therapy, decreasing the dosage in a stepwise fashion may be helpful.

A course of treatment should employ the lowest effective dose for the minimum length of time necessary for effective treatment. See Posology for guidance on possible treatment regimen. A course of treatment should not continue for longer than 4 weeks including any tapering off. (See also section 4.8 Undesirable Effects).

Amnesia: Amnesia is rare, but anterograde amnesia may occur, especially when sleep is interrupted or when retiring to bed is delayed after taking the tablet. Therefore, patients should ensure that they take the tablet when certain of retiring for the night and they are able to have a full night's sleep.

Driving: It has been reported that the risk that zopiclone adversely affects driving ability is increased by the concomitant intake of alcohol. Therefore, it is recommended not to drive while taking zopiclone and alcohol concomitantly.

4.5 Interaction with other medicinal products and other forms of Interaction
The sedative effect of zopiclone may be enhanced when used in combination with alcohol, concomitant use is therefore not recommended. In particular this could affect the patient's ability to drive or use machines.

In combination with CNS depressants an enhancement of the central depressive effect may occur. The therapeutic benefit of co-adminstration with antipsychotics (neuroleptics), hypnotics, anxiolytics/sedatives, antidepressant agents, narcotic analgesics, anti-epileptic drugs, anaesthetics and sedative antihistamines should therefore be carefully weighed. Concomitant use of benzodiazepines or benzodiazepine-like agents with narcotic analgesics may enhance their euphoric effect and could lead to an increase in psychic dependence. Compounds which inhibit certain hepatic enzymes (particularly cytochrome P450) may enhance the activity of benzodiazepines and benzodiazepine-like agents.

The effect of erythromycin on the pharmacokinetics of zopiclone has been studied in 10 healthy subjects. The AUC of zopiclone is increased by 80% in presence of erythromycin which indicates that erythromycin can inhibit the metabolism of drugs metabolised by CYP 3A4. As a consequence, the hypnotic effect of zopiclone may be enhanced.

Since zopiclone is metabolised by the cytochrome P450 (CYP) 3A4 isoenzyme (see section 5.2 Pharmacokinetic properties), plasma levels of zopiclone may be increased when co-adminstered with CYP3A4 inhibitors such as erythromycin, clarithromycin, ketoconazole, itraconazole and ritonavir. A dose reduction for zopiclone may be required when it is co-adminstered with CYP3A4 inhibitors.

Conversely, plasma levels of zopiclone may be decreased when co-administered with CYP3A4 inducers such as rifampicin, carbamazepine, phenobarbital, phenytoin and St. John's wort. A dose increase for zopiclone may be required when it is co-adminstered with CYP3A4 inducers.

4.6 Pregnancy and lactation
Use during pregnancy: Experience of use of zopiclone during pregnancy in humans is limited although there have been no adverse findings in animals. Use in pregnancy is therefore not recommended. If the product is prescribed to a woman of child bearing potential, she should be advised to contact her physician about stopping the product if she intends to become pregnant, or suspects that she is pregnant.

Moreover, if zopiclone is used during the last three months of pregnancy or during labour, due to the pharmacological action of the product, effects on the neonate, such as hypothermia, hypnotic and respiratory depression can be expected.

Infants born to mothers who took benzodiazepines or benzodiazepine-like agents chronically during the latter stages of pregnancy may have developed physical dependence and may be at some risk of developing withdrawal symptoms in the postnatal period.

Use during lactation: Zopiclone is excreted in breast milk and use in nursing mothers must be avoided.

4.7 Effects on ability to drive and use machines
Although residual effects are rare and generally of minor significance, patients should be advised not to drive or operate machinery the day after treatment until it is established that their performance is unimpaired. The risk is increased by concomitant intake of alcohol (see section 4.4 Special Warnings and Precautions for Use).

4.8 Undesirable effects
A mild bitter or metallic after-taste is the most frequently reported adverse effect. Less commonly, mild gastrointestinal disturbances, including nausea and vomiting, dizziness, headache, drowsiness and dry mouth have occurred.

Psychological and behavioural disturbances, such as irritability, aggressiveness, confusion, depressed mood, anterograde amnesia, hallucinations and nightmares have been reported. Rarely these reactions may be severe and may be more likely to occur in the elderly. Rarely allergic and allied manifestations such as urticaria or rashes have been observed and, more rarely, light headedness and incoordination. Angiodema and/or anaphylactic reactions have been reported very rarely.

Withdrawal syndrome has been reported upon discontinuation of zopiclone. (See section 4.4. Special Warnings and Precautions for Use). Withdrawal symptoms vary and may include rebound insomnia, anxiety, tremor, sweating, agitation, confusion, headache, palpitations, tachycardia, delirium, nightmares, hallucinations, panic attacks, muscle aches/cramps, gastrointestinal disturbances and irritability. In very rare cases, seizures may occur.

Mild to moderate increases in serum transaminases and/or alkaline phosphatase have been reported very rarely.

4.9 Overdose

Overdose is usually manifested by varying degrees of central nervous system depression ranging from drowsiness to coma according to the quantity ingested. In mild cases, symptoms include drowsiness, confusion, and lethargy; in more serious cases, symptoms may include ataxia, hypotonia, hypotension, respiratory depression and coma. Other risk factors, such as combining zopiclone with other CNS depressants (including alcohol), the presence of concomitant illness and the debilitated state of the patient, may contribute to the severity of the symptoms and very rarely can result in fatal outcome.

Symptomatic and supportive treatment in an adequate clinical environment is recommended. Attention should be paid to respiratory and cardiovascular functions. Gastric lavage is only useful when performed soon after ingestion. Haemodialysis is of no value due to the large volume of distribution of zopiclone. Flumazenil may be a useful antidote.

5. PHARMACOLOGICAL PROPERTIES

5.1 Pharmacodynamic properties

Zopiclone is an hypnotic agent, and a member of the cyclopyrrolone group of compounds. It rapidly initiates and sustains sleep without reduction of total REM sleep and with preservation of slow wave sleep. Negligible residual effects are seen the following morning. Its pharmacological properties include hypnotic, sedative, anxiolytic, anticonvulsant and muscle-relaxant actions. These are related to its high affinity and specific agonist action at central receptors belonging to the 'GABA' macromolecular receptor complex modulating the opening of the chloride ion channel. However, it has been shown that zopiclone and other cyclopyrrolones act on a different site to those of benzodiazepines including different conformational changes in the receptor complex.

5.2 Pharmacokinetic properties

Absorption: Zopiclone is absorbed rapidly. Peak concentrations are reached within 1.5 - 2 hours and they are approximately 30 ng/ml and 60 ng/ml after administration of 3.75mg and 7.5mg respectively. Absorption is not modified by gender, food or repetition of doses.

Distribution: The product is rapidly distributed from the vascular compartment. Plasma protein binding is weak (approximately 45%) and non saturable. There is very little risk of drug interactions due to protein binding. The volume of distribution is 91.8 - 104.6 litres.

At doses between 3.75 - 15mg, plasma clearance does not depend on dose. The elimination half life is approximately 5 hours. After repeated administration, there is no accumulation, and inter-individual variations appear to be very small.

Metabolism: Zopiclone is exensively metabolised in humans to two major metabolites, N-oxide zopiclone (pharmacologically active in animals) and N-desmethyl zopiclone (pharmacologically inactive in animals). An *in-vitro* study indicates that cytochrome P450 (CYP) 3A4 is the major isoenzyme involved in the metabolism of zopiclone to both metabolites, and that CYP2C8 is also involved with N-desmethyl zopiclone formation. Their apparent half-lives (evaluated from the urinary data) are approximately 4.5 hours and 1.5 hours respectively. No significant accumulation is seen on repeated dosing (15mg) for 14 days. In animals, no enzyme induction has been observed even at high doses.

Excretion: The low renal clearance value of unchanged zopiclone (mean 8.4ml/min) compared with the plasma clearance (232ml/min) indicates that zopiclone clearance is mainly metabolic. The product is eliminated by the urinary route (approximately 80%) in the form of free metabolites (n-oxide and n-desmethyl derivatives) and in the faeces (approximately 16%).

Special patient groups: In elderly patients, notwithstanding a slight decrease in hepatic metabolism and lengthening of elimination half-life to approximately 7 hours, various studies have shown no plasma accumulation of drug substance on repeated dosing. In renal insufficiency, no accumulation of zopiclone or of its metabolites has been detected after prolonged administration. Zopiclone crosses dialysis membranes. In cirrhotic patients, the plasma clearance of zopiclone is clearly reduced by the slowing of the desmethylation process: dosage will therefore have to be modified in these patients.

5.3 Preclinical safety data

There are no preclinical data of relevance to the prescriber which are additional to that already included in other sections of the SPC.

6. PHARMACEUTICAL PARTICULARS

6.1 List of excipients

Zimovane: Lactose, calcium hydrogen phosphate, wheat-starch, sodium starch glycollate, magnesium stearate, hydroxypropyl methylcellulose, titanium dioxide, absolute ethanol and purified water.

Zimovane LS: Lactose, calcium hydrogen phosphate, wheat starch, macrogol 6000, sodium starch glycollate, magnesium stearate, hydroxypropyl methylcellulose, titanium dioxide and purified water.

6.2 Incompatibilities

None stated.

6.3 Shelf life

Clear PVC/aluminium foil blister 24 months.

6.4 Special precautions for storage

Store in a dry place below 30°C. Protect from light.

6.5 Nature and contents of container

Zimovane are provided in clear PVC/aluminium foil blisters containing 28 tablets.

6.6 Instructions for use and handling

No special instructions.

7. MARKETING AUTHORISATION HOLDER

Rhône-Poulenc Rorer
RPR House
50 Kings Hill Avenue
Kings Hill
West Malling
Kent ME19 4AH

8. MARKETING AUTHORISATION NUMBER(S)

Zimovane: PL 00012/0259

Zimovane LS: PL 00012/0260

9. DATE OF FIRST AUTHORISATION/RENEWAL OF THE AUTHORISATION

18 March 2005

10. DATE OF REVISION OF THE TEXT

July 2005

Legal category: POM

Zinacef

(GlaxoSmithKline UK)

1. NAME OF THE MEDICINAL PRODUCT

Zinacef®

Cefuroxime (as sodium) INN for Injection or Infusion.

2. QUALITATIVE AND QUANTITATIVE COMPOSITION

Vials contain either 250mg, 750mg or 1.5g cefuroxime (as sodium).

3. PHARMACEUTICAL FORM

Cefuroxime is a white to cream powder to which appropriate amounts of water are added to prepare an off-white suspension for intramuscular use or a yellowish solution for intravenous administration.

4. CLINICAL PARTICULARS

4.1 Therapeutic indications

Zinacef is a bactericidal cephalosporin antibiotic which is resistant to most beta-lactamases and is active against a wide range of Gram-positive and Gram-negative organisms. It is indicated for the treatment of infections before the infecting organism has been identified or when caused by sensitive bacteria. In addition, it is an effective prophylactic against post-operative infection in a variety of operations. Usually Zinacef will be effective alone, but when appropriate it may be used in combination with an aminoglycoside antibiotic, or in conjunction with metronidazole, orally or by suppository or injection, (see Pharmaceutical precautions).

In situations where mixed aerobic and anaerobic infections are encountered or suspected (e.g. peritonitis, aspiration pneumonia, abscesses in the lung, pelvis and brain), or are likely to occur (e.g. in association with colorectal or gynaecological surgery) it is appropriate to administer Zinacef in combination with metronidazole.

Most of these infections will respond to an i.v. regimen of Zinacef (750mg) plus metronidazole injection (500mg/100ml) administered eight-hourly. In more severe or well established mixed infections, an i.v. regimen of Zinacef (1.5g) plus metronidazole injection (500mg/100ml) eight-hourly may be indicated. For the prophylaxis of infection in surgery (e.g. colorectal and gynaecological) a single dose of 1.5g Zinacef plus metronidazole injection (500mg/100ml) is appropriate.

Alternatively this may be followed by two 750mg doses of Zinacef plus metronidazole.

Indications include:

Respiratory tract infections for example, acute and chronic bronchitis, infected bronchiectasis, bacterial pneumonia, lung abscess and post operative chest infections.

Ear, nose and throat infections for example, sinusitis, tonsillitis and pharyngitis.

Urinary tract infections for example acute and chronic pyelonephritis, cystitis and asymptomatic bacteriuria.

Soft-tissue infections for example cellulitis, erysipelas, peritonitis and wound infections.

Bone and joint infections for example, osteomyelitis and septic arthritis.

Obstetric and gynaecological infections pelvic inflammatory diseases.

Gonorrhoea particularly when penicillin is unsuitable.

Other infections including septicaemia and meningitis.

Prophylaxis against infection in abdominal, pelvic, orthopaedic, cardiac, pulmonary, oesophageal and vascular surgery where there is increased risk from infection.

Cefuroxime is also available as the axetil ester (Zinnat) for oral administration.

This permits the use of sequential therapy with the same antibiotic, when a change from parenteral to oral therapy is clinically indicated. Where appropriate Zinacef is effective when used prior to oral therapy with Zinnat (cefuroxime axetil) in the treatment of pneumonia and acute exacerbations of chronic bronchitis.

4.2 Posology and method of administration

Intramuscular

Add 1ml water for injections to 250mg Zinacef or 3ml water for injections to 750mg Zinacef. Shake gently to produce an opaque suspension.

Intravenous

Dissolve Zinacef in water for injections using at least 2ml for 250mg, at least 6ml for 750mg or 15ml for 1.5g. For short intravenous infusion (e.g. up to 30 minutes), 1.5g may be dissolved in 50ml water for injections. These solutions may be given directly into the vein or introduced into the tubing of the giving set if the patient is receiving parenteral fluids.

General Recommendations

Adults: Many infections will respond to 750mg t.i.d. by im or iv injection. For more severe infections, this dose should be increased to 1.5g t.i.d. iv. The frequency of im or iv injection can be increased to six-hourly if necessary, giving total doses of 3g to 6g daily.

Where clinically indicated adults with pneumonia and acute exacerbations of chronic bronchitis have been shown to respond to 750mg or 1.5g bd, followed by oral therapy with Zinnat (see Sequential therapy).

Infants and Children: Doses of 30 to 100mg/kg/day given as three or four divided doses. A dose of 60mg/kg/day will be appropriate for most infections.

Neonates: Doses of 30 to 100mg/kg/day given as two or three divided doses. In the first weeks of life the serum half-life of cefuroxime can be three to five times that in adults.

Elderly: See dosage in adults.

Other Recommendations

Gonorrhoea: 1.5g should be given as a single dose. This may be given as 2 × 750mg injections into different sites eg each buttock.

Meningitis: Zinacef is suitable for sole therapy of bacterial meningitis due to sensitive strains. The following dosages are recommended.

Infants and Children: 200 to 240mg/kg/day iv in three or four divided doses. This dosage may be reduced to 100mg/kg/day iv after three days or when clinical improvement occurs.

Neonates: The initial dosage should be 100mg/kg/day iv. A reduction to 50mg/kg/day iv may be made when clinically indicated.

Adults: 3g iv every eight hours. Data are not yet sufficient to recommend a dose for intrathecal administration.

Prophylaxis: The usual dose is 1.5g iv with induction of anaethesia for abdominal, pelvic and orthopaedic operations, but may be supplemented with two 750mg im doses eight and sixteen hours later. In cardiac pulmonary oesophageal and vascular operations, the usual dose is 1.5g iv with induction of anaesthesia continuing with 750mg im t.d.s. for a further 24 to 48 hours.

In total joint replacement, 1.5g cefuroxime powder may be mixed dry with each pack of methyl methacrylate cement polymer before adding the liquid monomer.

Sequential therapy:

Pneumonia:

1.5g bd (iv or im) for 48-72 hours, followed by 500mg bd Zinnat (cefuroxime axetil) oral therapy for 7 days.

Acute exacerbations of chronic bronchitis:

750mg bd (iv or im) for 48-72 hours, followed by 500mg bd Zinnat (cefuroxime axetil) oral therapy for 5-7 days.

Duration of both parenteral and oral therapy is determined by the severity of the infection and the clinical status of the patient.

Dosage in impaired renal function

Cefuroxime is excreted by the kidneys. Therefore, as with all such antibiotics, in patients with markedly impaired renal function it is recommended that the dosage of Zinacef should be reduced to compensate for its slower excretion. However, it is not necessary to reduce the dose until the creatinine clearance falls below 20ml/min. In adults with marked impairment (creatinine clearance 10-20ml/min) 750mg bd is recommended and with severe impairment (creatinine clearance <10ml/min) 750mg once daily is adequate. For patients on haemodialysis a further 750mg dose should be given at the end of each dialysis. When continuous peritoneal dialysis is being used, a suitable dosage is usually 750mg twice daily.

For patients in renal failure on continuous arteriovenous haemodialysis or high-flux haemofiltration in intensive therapy units a suitable dosage is 750mg twice daily. For low-flux haemofiltration follow the dosage recommended under impaired renal function.

Cefuroxime is also available as the axetil ester (Zinnat) for oral administration. This permits parenteral therapy with cefuroxime to be followed by oral therapy in situations where a change from parenteral to oral is clinically indicated.

4.3 Contraindications

Hypersensitivity to cephalosporin antibiotics

4.4 Special warnings and special precautions for use

Special care is indicated in patients who have experienced an allergic reaction to penicillins or beta-lactams.

There may be some variation on the results of biochemical tests of renal function, but these do not appear to be of clinical importance. As a precaution, renal function should be monitored if this is already impaired.

Delayed sterilisation of the CSF in patients with Haemophilus influenzae meningitis may result in an adverse outcome such as deafness and /or neurological sequelae. Persistence of positive CSF cultures of H. influenzae at 18-36 hours has been noted in some patients treated with cefuroxime sodium injection and, as with other therapeutic regimens used in the treatment of meningitis, hearing loss has been reported in some children.

With a sequential therapy regime the timing of change to oral therapy is determined by severity of the infection, clinical status of the patient and susceptibility of the pathogens involved. The change to oral therapy should only be made once there is a clear clinical improvement. If there has been no clinical improvement after 72 hours of parenteral treatment, then the patient's treatment should be reviewed. Please refer to the relevant prescribing information for cefuroxime axetil before initiating sequential therapy.

4.5 Interaction with other medicinal products and other forms of Interaction

Cephalosporin antibiotics at high dosage should be given with caution to patients receiving concurrent treatment with potent diuretics such as frusemide and aminoglycosides, as these combinations are suspected of adversely affecting renal function. Clinical experience with Zinacef has shown that this is not likely to be a problem at the recommended dose levels.

Zinacef does not interfere in enzyme-based tests for glycosuria. Slight interference with copper reduction methods (Benedict's, Fehling's, Clinitest) may be observed. However, this should not lead to false-positive results, as may be experienced with some other cephalosporins.

It is recommended that either the glucose oxidase or hexokinase methods are used to determine blood/plasma glucose levels in patients receiving Zinacef. This antibiotic does not interfere in the alkaline picrate assay for creatinine.

4.6 Pregnancy and lactation

There is no experimental evidence of embryopathic or teratogenic effects attributable to Zinacef but, as with all drugs, it should be administered with caution during the early months of pregnancy.

Cefuroxime is excreted in human milk, and consequently caution should be exercised when Zinacef is administered to a nursing mother.

4.7 Effects on ability to drive and use machines

None reported.

4.8 Undesirable effects

Adverse reactions to Zinacef have occurred relatively infrequently and have been generally mild and transient in nature.

There have been rare reports of hypersensitivity reactions including skin rashes, urticaria, pruritus, interstitial nephritis, drug fever and very rarely anaphylaxis.

As with other cephalosporins, there have been rare reports of erythema multiforme, Stevens-Johnson syndrome and toxic epidermal necrolysis (exanthematic necrolysis).

As with other antibiotics, prolonged use may result in the overgrowth of non-susceptible organisms, eg. candida. Gastrointestinal disturbance, including, very rarely, symptoms of pseudomembranous colitis may occur during or after treatment. The principal changes in haematological parameters seen in some patients have been of decreased haemoglobin concentration and of eosinophilia, leukopenia and neutropenia.

Cephalosporins as a class tend to be absorbed onto the surface of red cell membranes and react with antibodies directed against the drug to produce a positive Coombs test (which can interfere with cross-matching of blood) and very rarely haemolytic anaemia.

Although there are sometimes transient rises in serum liver enzymes or serum bilirubin, particularly in patients with pre-existing liver disease, there is no evidence of hepatic involvement.

Transient pain may be experienced at the site of intramuscular injection. This is more likely to occur with higher doses. However, it is unlikely to be a cause for discontinuation of treatment. Occasionally, thrombophlebitis may follow intravenous injection.

As with other cephalosporins, there have been very rare reports of thrombocytopenia.

4.9 Overdose

Overdosage of cephalosporins can cause cerebral irritation leading to convulsions. Serum levels of cefuroxime can be reduced by haemodialysis or peritoneal dialysis.

5. PHARMACOLOGICAL PROPERTIES

5.1 Pharmacodynamic properties

Cefuroxime is a bactericidal cephalosporin antibiotic which is resistant to most beta-lactamases and is active against a wide range of Gram-positive and Gram-negative organisms.

It is highly active against *Staphylococcus aureus*, including strains which are resistant to penicillin (but not the rare methicillin-resistant strains), *Staph. epidermidis, Haemophilus influenzae*, Klebsiella spp., Enterobacter spp., *Streptococcus pyogenes, Escherichia coli, Str. mitis (viridans group)*, Clostridium spp., *Proteus mirabilis*, Pr. rettgeri, *Salmonella typhi, S. typhimurium* and other Salmonella spp., Shigella spp., Neisseria spp. (including beta-lactamase producing strains of *N. gonorrhoea*) and *Bordetella pertussis*. It is also moderately active against strains of *Pr. vulgaris, Morganella morganii* (formerly *Proteus morganii*) and *Bacteroides fragilis*.

The following organisms are not susceptible to cefuroxime: *Clostridium difficile*, Pseudomonas spp., Campylobacter spp., *Acinetobacter calcoaceticus*, Legionella spp. and methicillin-resistant strains of *Staph. aureus* and *Staph. epidermidis*.

Some strains of the following genera have also been found not to be susceptible to Zinacef:

Strep. faecalis, Morganella morganii, Proteus vulgaris, Enterobacter spp., Citrobacter spp., Serratia spp. and *Bacteroides fragilis*.

In vitro the activities of Zinacef and aminoglycoside antibiotics in combination have been shown to be at least additive with occasional evidence of synergy.

5.2 Pharmacokinetic properties

Peak levels of cefuroxime are achieved within 30 to 45 minutes after intramuscular administration. The serum half-life after either intramuscular or intravenous injection is approximately 70 minutes. Concurrent administration of probenecid prolongs the excretion of the antibiotic and produces an elevated peak serum level. There is almost complete recovery of unchanged cefuroxime in the urine within 24 hours of administration, the major part being eliminated in the first six hours. Approximately 50% is excreted through the renal tubules and approximately 50% by glomerular filtration. Concentrations of cefuroxime in excess of the minimum inhibitory levels for common pathogens can be achieved in bone, synovial fluid and aqueous humor. Cefuroxime passes the blood-brain barrier when the meninges are inflamed.

5.3 Preclinical safety data

None stated

6. PHARMACEUTICAL PARTICULARS

6.1 List of excipients

None.

6.2 Incompatibilities

Cefuroxime is compatible with most commonly used intravenous fluids and electrolyte solutions.

The pH of 2.74% w/v sodium bicarbonate injection BP considerably affects the colour of solutions and therefore this solution is not recommended for the dilution of Zinacef. However, if required, for patients receiving sodium bicarbonate injection by infusion the Zinacef may be introduced into the tube of the giving set.

Zinacef should not be mixed in the syringe with aminoglycoside antibiotics.

6.3 Shelf life

Two years when stored below 25°C and protected from light.

6.4 Special precautions for storage

Store below 25°C and protect from light.

After constitution, Zinacef should be stored at 2 - 8°C for no longer than 24 hours.

6.5 Nature and contents of container

1) Moulded glass (type 1 or III) vials with bromobutyl or fluoro-resin laminated butyl rubber plug, overseal and flip-off cap containing either 250mg, 750mg or 1.5g Zinacef.

2) A bulk pack of 100 vials.

3) Monovial containing either 750mg or 1.5g Zinacef with transfer needle.

*Only the 1.5g injection pack is marketed (the infusion pack is not)

6.6 Instructions for use and handling

None.

Administrative Data

7. MARKETING AUTHORISATION HOLDER

Glaxo Operations UK Limited, Greenford, Middlesex UB6 0HE

Trading as

GlaxoSmithKline UK, Stockley Park West, Uxbridge, Middlesex UB11 1BT

8. MARKETING AUTHORISATION NUMBER(S)

PL 00004/0263.

9. DATE OF FIRST AUTHORISATION/RENEWAL OF THE AUTHORISATION

28 April 2002

10. DATE OF REVISION OF THE TEXT

3 January 2003

11. Legal Status

POM

Zincaband

(Medlock Medical Ltd)

1. NAME OF THE MEDICINAL PRODUCT

Zincaband.

2. QUALITATIVE AND QUANTITATIVE COMPOSITION

Zinc Oxide BP 15% w/w.

3. PHARMACEUTICAL FORM

Open-wove bleached cotton bandage impregnated with a paste formulation.

4. CLINICAL PARTICULARS

4.1 Therapeutic indications

For use in the treatment of leg ulcers. Where venous insufficiency exists, the paste bandage should be adjunct to graduated pressure bandaging. For use in the treatment of chronic eczema/dermatitis, where occlusion is indicated, including lichenification.

4.2 Posology and method of administration

For topical administration only. The product is a medicated paste bandage. Frequency of dressing changes is at the discretion of the responsible physician (Differentiation between patients of differing age groups is less important when considering the 'dosage' regime than the apparent healing rate of the wound/condition).

4.3 Contraindications

Hypersensitivity to an ingredient of the paste and acute eczematous lesions.

4.4 Special warnings and special precautions for use

Avoid use on grossly macerated skin. The skin of leg ulcer patients is easily sensitised to topical medicaments including preservatives. Sensitisation should be suspected in patients, particularly where there is deterioration of the ulcer or surrounding skin. Such patients should be referred for specialist diagnosis including patch testing. One of the functions of occlusive bandages is to increase absorption. Care should therefore be taken if it is decided to apply topical steroid preparations under these bandages as their absorption may be significantly increased.

4.5 Interaction with other medicinal products and other forms of Interaction

None known.

4.6 Pregnancy and lactation

No special precautions required.

4.7 Effects on ability to drive and use machines

Not applicable.

4.8 Undesirable effects

Not applicable.

4.9 Overdose

None known.

5. PHARMACOLOGICAL PROPERTIES

5.1 Pharmacodynamic properties

The product is a paste bandage with the active constituent presented in glycerine, modified starch and castor oil paste, spread onto a cotton bandage. Zinc oxide, as a zinc salt, has astringent properties and is well established in use. Much of the therapeutic action of paste bandages is attributable to the bandaging technique, the physical support and protection provided, and to the maintenance of moist wound healing conditions.

5.2 Pharmacokinetic properties

The pharmacokinetics are those relevant to topical application of the substances through whole or broken skin. Contemporary literature describes the biochemical properties but, with the exception of zinc salts, does not directly relate these properties to the disease states being treated.

5.3 Preclinical safety data
None known.

6. PHARMACEUTICAL PARTICULARS

6.1 List of excipients
Glycerine; castor oil; modified starch; citric acid; propyl hydroxybenzoate; purified water; open wove cotton bandage.

6.2 Incompatibilities
None known.

6.3 Shelf life
30 months unopened.

6.4 Special precautions for storage
Store in a dry place not exceeding 25°C.

6.5 Nature and contents of container
Individually wrapped in waxed paper or polythene film, within a sealed polythene bag, or foil/nylon/polythene laminate bag, and cardboard carton. 12 cartons per corrugated cardboard carton.

6.6 Instructions for use and handling
None stated.

7. MARKETING AUTHORISATION HOLDER
Seton Healthcare Group plc, Tubiton House, Oldham, OL1 3HS.

8. MARKETING AUTHORISATION NUMBER(S)
PL 0223/5000R.

9. DATE OF FIRST AUTHORISATION/RENEWAL OF THE AUTHORISATION
11th October 1989 / 10th January 2002.

10. DATE OF REVISION OF THE TEXT
June 2003.

Zineryt

(Astellas Pharma Limited)

1. NAME OF THE MEDICINAL PRODUCT
Zineryt.

2. QUALITATIVE AND QUANTITATIVE COMPOSITION
Erythromycin 40 mg and zinc acetate 12 mg per ml on constitution.

3. PHARMACEUTICAL FORM
Dry powder bottle and solvent bottle to be admixed on dispensing.

4. CLINICAL PARTICULARS

4.1 Therapeutic indications
Topical treatment of acne vulgaris.

4.2 Posology and method of administration
For children, adults, and the elderly. Apply twice daily over the whole of the affected area for a period of 10 to 12 weeks.

4.3 Contraindications
Zineryt is contraindicated in patients who are hypersensitive to erythromycin or other macrolide antibiotics, or to zinc, di-isopropyl sebacate or ethanol.

4.4 Special warnings and special precautions for use
Cross resistance may occur with other antibiotics of the macrolide group and also with lincomycin and clindamycin. Contact with the eyes or the mucous membranes of the nose and mouth should be avoided.

4.5 Interaction with other medicinal products and other forms of Interaction
None known.

4.6 Pregnancy and lactation
There is no contraindication to the use of Zineryt in pregnancy or lactation.

4.7 Effects on ability to drive and use machines
None.

4.8 Undesirable effects
Occasionally a burning sensation or a slight redness of the skin may be observed; this is due to the alcohol base of Zineryt and is transient and of minor clinical significance.

4.9 Overdose
It is not expected that overdosage would occur in normal use. Patients showing idiosyncratic hypersensitivity should wash the treated area with copious water and simple soap.

5. PHARMACOLOGICAL PROPERTIES

5.1 Pharmacodynamic properties
Erythromycin is known to be efficacious, at 4%, in the topical treatment of acne vulgaris. Zinc, topically, is established as an aid to wound healing. The zinc acetate is solubilised by complexing with the erythromycin, and delivery of the complex is enhanced by the chosen vehicle.

5.2 Pharmacokinetic properties
The complex does not survive in the skin, and erythromycin and zinc penetrate independently. The erythromycin penetrates, and is partially systemically absorbed (0 - 10% in vitro, 40 - 50% in animal studies); that portion absorbed is excreted in 24 - 72 hours. The zinc is not absorbed systemically.

5.3 Preclinical safety data
No relevant pre-clinical safety data has been generated.

6. PHARMACEUTICAL PARTICULARS

6.1 List of excipients
Di-isopropyl sebacate, ethanol.

6.2 Incompatibilities
None known.

6.3 Shelf life
2 years; 5 weeks after constitution.

6.4 Special precautions for storage
Do not store above 25°C.

6.5 Nature and contents of container
Screw-capped HDPE bottles; an applicator assembly is fitted when dispensed. When constituted packs are of 30 ml and 90 ml.

6.6 Instructions for use and handling
None

Administrative Data

7. MARKETING AUTHORISATION HOLDER
Yamanouchi Pharma Ltd
Yamanouchi House
Pyrford Road
West Byfleet
Surrey KT14 6RA

8. MARKETING AUTHORISATION NUMBER(S)
Product licence 0166/0109.

9. DATE OF FIRST AUTHORISATION/RENEWAL OF THE AUTHORISATION
First authorisation granted 7 March 1990/ 29 March 2001

10. DATE OF REVISION OF THE TEXT
Date of Partial revision = 14th August 2003.

11. Legal category
POM

Zinnat Suspension

(GlaxoSmithKline UK)

1. NAME OF THE MEDICINAL PRODUCT
Zinnat Suspension 125mg/5ml

2. QUALITATIVE AND QUANTITATIVE COMPOSITION
Cefuroxime 125mg/5ml (as 150 mg cefuroxime axetil)

3. PHARMACEUTICAL FORM
Granules for constitution with water to form a suspension for oral administration.

4. CLINICAL PARTICULARS

4.1 Therapeutic indications
Cefuroxime axetil is an oral prodrug of the bactericidal cephalosporin antibiotic cefuroxime, which is resistant to most β-lactamases and is active against a wide range of Gram-positive and Gram-negative organisms.

It is indicated for the treatment of infections caused by sensitive bacteria.

Indications include: Lower respiratory tract infections for example, acute bronchitis, acute exacerbations of chronic bronchitis and pneumonia.

Upper respiratory tract infections for example, ear, nose, throat infections, such as otitis media, sinusitis, tonsillitis and pharyngitis.

Genito-urinary tract infections for example, pyelonephritis, cystitis and urethritis.

Skin and soft tissue infections for example, furunculosis, pyoderma and impetigo.

Gonorrhoea acute uncomplicated gonococcal urethritis, and cervicitis.

Treatment of early Lyme disease and subsequent prevention of late Lyme disease in adults and children over 12 years old.

Cefuroxime is also available as the sodium salt (Zinacef) for parenteral administration. This permits the use of sequential therapy with the same antibiotic, when a change from parenteral to oral therapy is clinically indicated.

Where appropriate Zinnat is effective when used following initial parenteral Zinacef (cefuroxime sodium) in the treatment of pneumonia and acute exacerbations of chronic bronchitis.

4.2 Posology and method of administration
Adults: Most infections will respond to 250mg b.d. In mild to moderate lower respiratory tract infections e.g. bronchitis 250mg b.d. should be given. For more severe lower respiratory tract infections, or if pneumonia is suspected then 500mg b.d. should be given. For urinary tract infections a dose of 125mg b.d. is usually adequate; in pyelonephritis the recommended dose is 250mg b.d. A single dose of one gram is recommended for the treatment of uncomplicated gonorrhoea.

Lyme disease in adults and children over the age of 12 years: the recommended dose is 500mg b.d. for 20 days.

Sequential therapy:

Pneumonia:

1.5g Zinacef bd (iv or im) for 48-72 hours, followed by 500mg bd Zinnat (cefuroxime axetil) oral therapy for 7 days.

Acute exacerbations of chronic bronchitis:

750mg Zinacef bd (iv or im) for 48-72 hours, followed by 500mg Zinnat (cefuroxime axetil) oral therapy for 5-7 days.

Duration of both parenteral and oral therapy is determined by the severity of the infection and the clinical status of the patient.

Children: The usual dose is 125mg b.d. (1 × 125mg tablet or 5ml of suspension or 1 × 125mg sachet), or 10mg/kg b.d. to a maximum of 250mg daily. For otitis media, in children less than 2 years of age the usual dosage is 125mg b.d. (1 × 125mg tablet or 5ml of suspension or 1 × 125mg sachet), or 10mg/kg b.d. to a maximum of 250mg daily and in children over 2 years of age, 250mg b.d. (1 × 250mg tablet or 10ml of suspension or 2 × 125mg sachets), or 15mg/kg b.d. to a maximum of 500mg daily. There is no experience in children under 3 months of age.

Zinnat Tablets should not be crushed, therefore in younger children the suspension is more appropriate.

Elderly and Patients with Renal Impairment: No special precautions are necessary in patients with renal impairment or on renal dialysis or in the elderly at dosages up to the normal maximum of 1g per day.

The usual course of therapy is seven days.

Zinnat should be taken after food for optimum absorption.

4.3 Contraindications
Hypersensitivity to cephalosporin antibiotics.

4.4 Special warnings and special precautions for use
Special care is indicated in patients who have experienced an allergic reaction to penicillins or other beta-lactams.

As with other antibiotics, prolonged use of cefuroxime axetil may result in the overgrowth of non-susceptible organisms (e.g. Candida, Enterococci, *Clostridium difficile*), which may require interruption of treatment. Pseudomembranous colitis has been reported with the use of broad-spectrum antibiotics, therefore, it is important to consider its diagnosis in patients who develop serious diarrhoea during or after antibiotic use.

The Jarisch-Herxheimer reaction has been seen following Zinnat treatment of Lyme disease. It results from the bactericidal activity of Zinnat on the causative organism of Lyme disease, the spirochaete *Borrelia burgdorferi*. Patients should be reassured that this is a common and usually self-limited consequence of antibiotic treatment of Lyme disease.

With a sequential therapy regime the timing of change to oral therapy is determined by severity of the infection, clinical status of the patient and susceptibility of the pathogens involved. The change to oral therapy should only be made once there is a clear clinical improvement. If there has been no clinical improvement after 72 hours of parenteral treatment, then the patient's treatment should be reviewed. Please refer to the relevant prescribing information for cefuroxime sodium before initiating sequential therapy.

Zinnat suspension contain aspartame, which is a source of phenylalanine and so should be used with caution in patients with phenylketonuria.

4.5 Interaction with other medicinal products and other forms of Interaction
It is recommended that either the glucose oxidase or hexokinase methods are used to determine blood/plasma glucose levels in patients receiving cefuroxime axetil. This antibiotic does not interfere in the alkaline picrate assay for creatinine.

4.6 Pregnancy and lactation
There is no experimental evidence of embryopathic or teratogenic effects attributable to cefuroxime axetil but, as with all drugs, it should be administered with caution during early months of pregnancy. Cefuroxime is excreted in human milk, and consequently caution should be exercised when cefuroxime axetil is administered to a nursing mother.

4.7 Effects on ability to drive and use machines
Not applicable.

4.8 Undesirable effects
Adverse reactions to cefuroxime axetil have been generally mild and transient in nature.

As with other cephalosporins, there have been rare reports of interstitial nephritis, erythema multiforme, Stevens-Johnson syndrome, toxic epidermal necrolysis (exanthematic necrolysis) and hypersensitivity reactions including skin rashes, urticaria, pruritus, drug fever, serum sickness, and very rarely anaphylaxis.

Gastrointestinal disturbances including diarrhoea and nausea and vomiting have been reported. Diarrhoea, although uncommon, is more likely to be associated with higher doses.

As with other broad-spectrum antibiotics, there have been occasional reports of pseudomembranous colitis.

Headache has also been reported.

There have been rare reports of thrombocytopenia and leucopenia (sometimes profound).

Eosinophilia and transient increases of hepatic enzyme levels [ALT (SGPT), AST (SGOT) and LDH] have been noted during Zinnat therapy.

Cephalosporins as a class tend to be absorbed on to the surface of red cell membranes and react with antibodies directed against the drug to produce a positive Coombs test (which can interfere with cross-matching of blood) and very rarely haemolytic anaemia.

4.9 Overdose
Overdosage of cephalosporins can cause cerebral irritancy leading to convulsions.

Serum levels of cefuroxime can be reduced by haemodialysis or peritoneal dialysis.

5. PHARMACOLOGICAL PROPERTIES

5.1 Pharmacodynamic properties
Cefuroxime axetil is an oral prodrug of the bactericidal cephalosporin antibiotic cefuroxime, which is resistant to most beta-lactamases and is active against a wide range of gram-positive and gram-negative organisms.

Microbiology:

Cefuroxime axetil owes its *in vivo* bactericidal activity to the parent compound, cefuroxime. Cefuroxime is a well-characterized and effective antibacterial agent which has broad-spectrum bactericidal activity against a wide range of common pathogens, including beta-lactamase-producing strains. Cefuroxime has good stability to bacterial beta-lactamase and consequently, is active against many ampicillin-resistant and amoxycillin-resistant strains. The bactericidal action of cefuroxime results from inhibition of cell-wall synthesis by binding to essential target proteins.

Cefuroxime is usually active against the following organisms *in vitro*:

Aerobes, Gram-negative: *Haemophilus influenzae* (including ampicillin-resistant strains); *Haemophilus parainfluenzae; Moraxella catarrhalis; Escherichia coli;* Klebsiella species; *Proteus mirabilis; Proteus inconstans;* Providencia species; *Proteus rettgeri* and *Neisseria gonorrhoea* (including penicillinase and non-penicillinase-producing strains).

Some strains of *Morganella morganii,* Enterobacter species and Citrobacter species have been shown by *in vitro* tests to be resistant to cefuroxime and other beta-lactam antibiotics.

Aerobes, Gram-positive: *Staphylococcus aureus* (including penicillinase-producing strains but excluding methicillin-resistant strains); *Staphylococcus epidermidis,* (including penicillinase producing strains but excluding methicillin-resistant strains); *Streptococcus pyogenes (*and betahaemolytic streptococci), *Streptococcus pneumoniae*; Streptococcus Group B (*Streptococcus agalactiae)* and Propionibacterium species.

Certain strains of enterococci, eg. *Streptococcus faecalis,* are resistant.

Anaerobes, Gram-positive and Gram-negative cocci (including Peptococcus and Peptostreptococcus species); Gram-positive bacilli (including Clostridium species) and Gram-negative bacilli (including Bacteroides and Fusobacterium species). Most strains of *Bacteroides fragilis* are resistant.

Other organisms, *Borrelia burgdorferi*.

Pseudomonas species, Campylobacter species, *Acinetobacter calcoaceticus*, *Listeria monocytogenes,* Legionella species and most strains of Serratia and *Proteus vulgaris* and *Clostridium difficile* are resistant to many cephalosporins including cefuroxime.

5.2 Pharmacokinetic properties
After oral administration, cefuroxime axetil is absorbed from the gastrointestinal tract and rapidly hydrolysed in the intestinal mucosa and blood to release cefuroxime into the circulation. Optimum absorption occurs when it is administered after a meal. Peak serum cefuroxime levels occur approximately two to three hours after oral dosing. The serum half life is about 1.2 hours. Approximately 50% of serum cefuroxime is protein bound. Cefuroxime is not metabolised and is excreted by glomerular filtration and tubular secretion.

Concurrent administration of probenecid increases the area under the mean serum concentration time curve by 50%. Serum levels of cefuroxime are reduced by dialysis.

5.3 Preclinical safety data
No additional data of relevance.

6. PHARMACEUTICAL PARTICULARS

6.1 List of excipients
Aspartame
Xanthan gum
Acesulfame potassium
Povidone K30
Stearic Acid
Sucrose
Tutti Frutti Flavour
Purified Water

6.2 Incompatibilities
None.

6.3 Shelf life
The shelf life of unconstituted Zinnat Suspension from date of manufacture is 24 months stored below 30°C. The reconstituted suspension when refrigerated between 2 and 8°C can be kept for up to 10 days.

6.4 Special precautions for storage
Zinnat Suspension granules should be stored below 30°C.

Bottles: Store the reconstituted suspension must be refrigerated between 2 and 8 °C.

Sachets: Reconstituted suspension should be taken immediately.

6.5 Nature and contents of container
Zinnat Suspension 125mg/5ml, granules for oral suspension are supplied in multidose bottles* of 50, 70, 100, 140 and 200ml and in 125 and 250mg sachets (heat-sealed laminate of paper/polyethylene/foil/ethylene-methacrylic acid ionomer).

125mg sachets are packed as either 1 duplex sachet in a carton or 7 duplex sachets in a carton (i.e. 2 or 14 doses).

250mg sachets are packed as 7 duplex sachets in a carton (i.e. 14 doses).

*Ph Eur Type III amber glass multiple unit bottles with a closure containing a heat-sealed induction membrane and a re-seal liner.

6.6 Instructions for use and handling
Directions for reconstituting suspension in bottles: Shake the bottle to loosen dry granules, add water as directed on the label and replace cap. INVERT bottle and shake granules down into water using a rocking action. Continue to shake the bottle until the suspension is well dispersed.

If desired the dose of the reconstituted suspension may be added to cold children's drinks such as fruit drinks or cold milk immediately prior to administration.

Directions for reconstituting suspension from sachets: Empty granules from sachet into a glass, add 10ml water, or 10ml cold children's drinks such as fruit drinks or milk, stir well and drink straight away.

The reconstituted suspension when refrigerated between 2 and 8 °C.can be kept for up to 10 days. The reconstituted suspension (from sachets) and the further diluted suspension from multidose bottles in cold children's drinks should be taken immediately.

The reconstituted suspension retains potency for up to 10 days when stored in a refrigerator between 2 and 8 °C.

Zinnat granules should not be reconstituted in hot drinks. The reconstituted suspension should not be mixed with hot drinks.

Administrative Data

7. MARKETING AUTHORISATION HOLDER
Glaxo Wellcome UK Limited
t/a Glaxo Laboratories
Stockley Park West
Uxbridge
Middlesex UB11 1BT

8. MARKETING AUTHORISATION NUMBER(S)
PL10949/0094

9. DATE OF FIRST AUTHORISATION/RENEWAL OF THE AUTHORISATION
1 July 1993

10. DATE OF REVISION OF THE TEXT
13 June 2003

11. Legal Status
POM

Zinnat Tablets 125mg

(GlaxoSmithKline UK)

1. NAME OF THE MEDICINAL PRODUCT
Zinnat Tablets 125mg

2. QUALITATIVE AND QUANTITATIVE COMPOSITION
Each tablet contains 125mg cefuroxime (as cefuroxime axetil).

3. PHARMACEUTICAL FORM
White, film-coated, capsule-shaped tablet plain on one side and engraved with 'GXES5' on the other.

4. CLINICAL PARTICULARS

4.1 Therapeutic indications
Cefuroxime axetil is indicated for the treatment of infections caused by sensitive bacteria.

Lower respiratory tract infections for example, acute bronchitis, acute exacerbations of chronic bronchitis, and pneumonia.

Upper respiratory tract infections for example, ear, nose, throat infections, such as otitis media, sinusitis, tonsillitis and pharyngitis.

Genito-urinary tract infections for example, pyelonephritis, cystitis and urethritis.

Skin and soft tissue infections for example, furunculosis, pyoderma and impetigo.

Treatment of early Lyme disease and subsequent prevention of late Lyme disease in adults and children over 12 years old.

Gonorrhoea acute uncomplicated gonococcal urethritis, and cervicitis.

Cefuroxime is also available as the sodium salt (Zinacef) for parenteral administration. This permits the use of sequential therapy with the same antibiotic, when a change from parenteral to oral therapy is clinically indicated.

Where appropriate Zinnat is effective when used following initial parenteral Zinacef (cefuroxime sodium) in the treatment of pneumonia and acute exacerbations of chronic bronchitis.

4.2 Posology and method of administration
Route of administration: oral

Dosage in adults

Most infections will respond to 250mg bd. In mild to moderate lower respiratory tract infections e.g. bronchitis 250mg bd should be given. For more severe lower respiratory tract infections, or if pneumonia is suspected then 500mg bd should be given. For urinary tract infections a dose of 125mg bd is usually adequate; in pyelonephritis the recommended dose is 250mg bd. A single dose of one gram is recommended for the treatment of uncomplicated gonorrhoea. Lyme disease in adults and children over the age of 12 years: the recommended dose is 500mg bd for 20 days.

Sequential therapy:

Pneumonia:

1.5g Zinacef bd (iv or im) for 48-72 hours, followed by 500mg bd Zinnat (cefuroxime axetil) oral therapy for 7 days.

Acute exacerbations of chronic bronchitis:

750mg Zinacef bd (iv or im) for 48-72 hours, followed by 500mg bd Zinnat (cefuroxime axetil) oral therapy for 5-7 days.

Duration of both parenteral and oral therapy is determined by the severity of the infection and the clinical status of the patient.

Dosage in children

The usual dose is 125mg bd or 10mg/kg bd to a maximum of 250mg daily. For otitis media, in children less than 2 years of age the usual dosage is 125mg bd or 10mg/kg bd to a maximum of 250mg daily and in children over 2 years of age, 250mg bd or 15mg/kg bd to a maximum of 500mg daily. There is no experience in children under 3 months of age.

Zinnat Tablets should not be crushed, therefore in younger children the suspension is more appropriate.

Elderly and patients with renal impairment

No special precautions are necessary in patients with renal impairment or on renal dialysis or in the elderly at dosages up to the normal maximum of 1g per day.

The usual course of therapy is seven days.

Zinnat should be taken after food for optimum absorption.

4.3 Contraindications
Hypersensitivity to cephalosporin antibiotics.

4.4 Special warnings and special precautions for use
Special care is indicated in patients who have experienced an allergic reaction to penicillins or other beta-lactams.

As with other antibiotics, prolonged use of cefuroxime axetil may result in the overgrowth of non-susceptible organisms (e.g. Candida, Enterococci, *Clostridium difficile*), which may require interruption of treatment. Pseudomembranous colitis has been reported with the use of broad-spectrum antibiotics, therefore, it is important to consider its diagnosis in patients who develop serious diarrhoea during or after antibiotic use.

It is recommended that either the glucose oxidase or hexokinase methods are used to determine blood/plasma glucose levels in patients receiving cefuroxime axetil. This antibiotic does not interfere in the alkaline picrate assay for creatinine.

The Jarisch-Herxheimer reaction has been seen following Zinnat treatment of Lyme disease. It results from the bactericidal activity of Zinnat on the causative organism of Lyme disease, the spirochaete Borrelia burgdorferi. Patients should be reassured that this is common and usually self-limited consequence of antibiotic treatment of Lyme disease.

With a sequential therapy regime the timing of change to oral therapy is determined by severity of the infection, clinical status of the patient and susceptibility of the pathogens involved. The change to oral therapy should only be made once there is a clear clinical improvement. If there has been no clinical improvement after 72 hours of parenteral treatment, then the patient's treatment should be reviewed. Please refer to the relevant prescribing information for cefuroxime sodium before initiating sequential therapy.

4.5 Interaction with other medicinal products and other forms of Interaction

Concurrent administration of probenecid increases the area under the mean serum concentration time curve by 50%. Serum levels of cefuroxime are reduced by dialysis.

A positive Coomb's test has been reported during treatment with cephalosporins. This phenomenon can interfere with cross matching of blood.

4.6 Pregnancy and lactation

There is no experimental evidence of embryopathic or teratogenic effects attributable to cefuroxime axetil but, as with all drugs, it should be administered with caution during early months of pregnancy. Cefuroxime is excreted in human milk, and consequently caution should be exercised when cefuroxime axetil is administered to a nursing mother.

4.7 Effects on ability to drive and use machines

None reported

4.8 Undesirable effects

Adverse reactions to cefuroxime axetil have been generally mild and transient in nature.

As with other cephalosporins, there have been rare reports of interstitial nephritis, erythema multiforme, Stevens-Johnson syndrome, toxic epidermal necrolysis (exanthematic necrolysis) and hypersensitivity reactions including skin rashes, urticaria, pruritus, drug fever, serum sickness, and very rarely anaphylaxis.

Gastrointestinal disturbances including diarrhoea and nausea and vomiting have been reported. Diarrhoea, although uncommon, is more likely to be associated with higher doses.

As with other broad-spectrum antibiotics, there have been occasional reports of pseudomembranous colitis.

Headache has also been reported.

There have been rare reports of thrombocytopenia and leucopenia (sometimes profound).

Eosinophilia and transient increases of hepatic enzyme levels [ALT (SGPT), AST (SGOT) and LDH] have been noted during Zinnat therapy. As with other cephalosporins, jaundice has been reported very rarely.

Cephalosporins as a class tend to be absorbed onto the surface of red cell membranes and react with antibodies directed against the drug to produce a positive Coombs test (which can interfere with cross-matching of blood) and very rarely haemolytic anaemia.

4.9 Overdose

Overdosage of cephalosporins can cause cerebral irritancy leading to convulsions.

Serum levels of cefuroxime can be reduced by haemodialysis or peritoneal dialysis.

5. PHARMACOLOGICAL PROPERTIES

5.1 Pharmacodynamic properties

Cefuroxime axetil is an oral prodrug of the bactericidal cephalosporin antibiotic cefuroxime, which is resistant to most beta-lactamases and is active against a wide range of gram-positive and gram-negative organisms.

Microbiology

Cefuroxime axetil owes its *in vivo* bactericidal activity to the parent compound, cefuroxime. Cefuroxime is a well-characterized and effective antibacterial agent which has broad-spectrum bactericidal activity against a wide range of common pathogens, including beta-lactamase-producing strains.

Cefuroxime has good stability to bacterial beta-lactamase and consequently, is active against many ampicillin-resistant and amoxycillin-resistant strains. The bactericidal action of cefuroxime results from inhibition of cell-wall synthesis by binding to essential target proteins.

Cefuroxime is usually active against the following organisms *in vitro*:

Aerobes, Gram-negative: *Haemophilus influenzae* (including ampicillin-resistant strains); *Haemophilus parainfluenzae; Moraxella catarrhalis; Escherichia coli;* Klebsiella species; *Proteus mirabilis; Proteus inconstans;* Providencia species; *Proteus rettgeri* and *Neisseria gonorrhoea* (including penicillinase and non-penicillinase-producing strains).

Some strains of *Morganella morganii,* Enterobacter species and Citrobacter species have been shown by *in vitro* tests to be resistant to cefuroxime and other beta-lactam antibiotics.

Aerobes, Gram-positive: *Staphylococcus aureus* (including penicillinase-producing strains but excluding methicillin-resistant strains); *Staphylococcus epidermis,* (including penicillinase - producing strains but excluding methicillin-resistant strains); *Streptococcus pyogenes* (and other betahaemolytic streptococci); *Streptococcus pneumonia* Streptococcus Group B (*Streptococcus agalactiae*) and Propionibacterium species. Certain strains of enterococci, eg. *Streptococcusfaecalis,* are resistant.

Anaerobes, Gram-positive and Gram-negative cocci (including Peptococcus and Peptostreptococcus species); Gram-positive bacilli (including Clostridium species) and Gram-negative bacilli (including Bacteroides and Fusobacterium species). Most strains of Bacteroides fragilis are resistant.

Other organisms, *Borrelia burgdorferi.*

Pseudomonas species, Campylobacter species, Acinetobacter calcoaceticus, Listeria monocytogenes, Legionella species and most strains of Serratia and Proteus vulgaris and Clostridium difficile are resistant to many cephalosporins including cefuroxime.

5.2 Pharmacokinetic properties

After oral administration, cefuroxime axetil is absorbed from the gastro-intestinal tract and rapidly hydrolysed in the intestinal mucosa and blood to release cefuroxime into the circulation. Optimum absorption occurs when it is administered after a meal. Peak serum cefuroxime levels occur approximately two to three hours after oral dosing. The serum half life is about 1.2 hours. Approximately 50% of serum cefuroxime is protein bound. Cefuroxime is not metabolised and is excreted by glomerular filtration and tubular secretion. Concurrent administration of probenecid increases the area under the mean serum concentration time curve by 50%.

5.3 Preclinical safety data

No additional data of relevance.

6. PHARMACEUTICAL PARTICULARS

6.1 List of excipients

Microcrystalline cellulose EP

Croscarmellose sodium, Type A USNF

Sodium lauryl sulphate EP

Hydrogenated vegetable oil USNF

Colloidal silicon dioxide USNF

Methylhydroxypropyl cellulose EP

Propylene glycol EP

Methyl parahydroxybenzoate EP

Propyl parahydroxybenzoate EP

Opaspray white M-1-7120

6.2 Incompatibilities

A positive Coombs' test has been reported during treatment with cephalosporins - this phenomenon can interfere with cross-matching of blood.

6.3 Shelf life

36 months in aluminium foil strips or blister packs.

24 months in HDPE bottles (not marketed in the UK)

6.4 Special precautions for storage

Cefuroxime axetil tablets in foil strips or blisters should be stored below 30°C.

Cefuroxime axetil tablets in HDPE bottles should be stored below 25°C (not marketed in the UK)

6.5 Nature and contents of container

Aluminium foil blister pack with an aluminium lid.

Pack size: 2, 4, 14 and 50

(2 and 4 not marketed in the UK)

Aluminium foil strips coated with surlyn polymer.

Pack size: 14 and 50

(not marketed in the UK)

White opaque, high density polyethylene bottles fitted with a clic-loc child resistant closure containing a pulp board wad to which is wax-bonded a 'lectraseal' membrane.

Pack size: 14 and 60

(not marketed in the UK)

6.6 Instructions for use and handling

None stated.

Administrative Data

7. MARKETING AUTHORISATION HOLDER

Glaxo Wellcome UK Limited trading as GlaxoSmithKline UK

Stockley Park West

Uxbridge

Middlesex

UB11 1BT

8. MARKETING AUTHORISATION NUMBER(S)

PL 10949/0095

9. DATE OF FIRST AUTHORISATION/RENEWAL OF THE AUTHORISATION

15 October 1998

10. DATE OF REVISION OF THE TEXT

29 January 2003

11. Legal Status

POM

Zinnat Tablets 250mg

(GlaxoSmithKline UK)

1. NAME OF THE MEDICINAL PRODUCT

Zinnat Tablets 250mg

2. QUALITATIVE AND QUANTITATIVE COMPOSITION

Each tablet contains 250mg cefuroxime (as cefuroxime axetil).

3. PHARMACEUTICAL FORM

White, film-coated, capsule-shaped tablet plain on one side and engraved with 'GXES7' on the other.

4. CLINICAL PARTICULARS

4.1 Therapeutic indications

Cefuroxime axetil is indicated for the treatment of infections caused by sensitive bacteria.

Lower respiratory tract infections for example, acute bronchitis, acute exacerbations of chronic bronchitis, and pneumonia.

Upper respiratory tract infections for example, ear, nose, throat infections, such as otitis media, sinusitis, tonsillitis and pharyngitis.

Genito-urinary tract infections for example, pyelonephritis, cystitis and urethritis.

Skin and soft tissue infections for example, furunculosis, pyoderma and impetigo.

Treatment of early Lyme disease and subsequent prevention of late Lyme disease in adults and children over 12 years old.

Gonorrhoea acute uncomplicated gonococcal urethritis, and cervicitis.

Cefuroxime is also available as the sodium salt (Zinacef) for parenteral administration. This permits the use of sequential therapy with the same antibiotic, when a change from parenteral to oral therapy is clinically indicated.

Where appropriate Zinnat is effective when used following initial parenteral Zinacef (cefuroxime sodium) in the treatment of pneumonia and acute exacerbations of chronic bronchitis.

4.2 Posology and method of administration

Route of administration: oral

Dosage in adults

Most infections will respond to 250mg bd. In mild to moderate lower respiratory tract infections e.g. bronchitis 250mg bd should be given. For more severe lower respiratory tract infections, or if pneumonia is suspected then 500mg bd should be given. For urinary tract infections a dose of 125mg bd is usually adequate; in pyelonephritis the recommended dose is 250mg bd. A single dose of one gram is recommended for the treatment of uncomplicated gonorrhoea. Lyme disease in adults and children over the age of 12 years: the recommended dose is 500mg bd for 20 days.

Sequential therapy:

Pneumonia:

1.5g Zinacef bd (iv or im) for 48-72 hours, followed by 500mg bd Zinnat (cefuroxime axetil) oral therapy for 7 days.

Acute exacerbations of chronic bronchitis:

750mg Zinacef bd (iv or im) for 48-72 hours, followed by 500mg bd Zinnat (cefuroxime axetil) oral therapy for 5-7 days.

Duration of both parenteral and oral therapy is determined by the severity of the infection and the clinical status of the patient.

Dosage in children

The usual dose is 125mg bd or 10mg/kg bd to a maximum of 250mg daily. For otitis media, in children less than 2 years of age the usual dosage is 125mg bd or 10mg/kg bd to a maximum of 250mg daily and in children over 2 years of age, 250mg bd or 15mg/kg bd to a maximum of 500mg daily. There is no experience in children under 3 months of age.

Zinnat Tablets should not be crushed, therefore in younger children the suspension is more appropriate.

Elderly and patients with renal impairment

No special precautions are necessary in patients with renal impairment or on renal dialysis or in the elderly at dosages up to the normal maximum of 1g per day.

The usual course of therapy is seven days.

Zinnat should be taken after food for optimum absorption.

4.3 Contraindications

Hypersensitivity to cephalosporin antibiotics.

4.4 Special warnings and special precautions for use

Special care is indicated in patients who have experienced an allergic reaction to penicillins or other beta-lactams.

As with other antibiotics, prolonged use of cefuroxime axetil may result in the overgrowth of non-susceptible organisms (e.g. Candida, Enterococci, *Clostridium difficile*), which may require interruption of treatment. Pseudomembranous colitis has been reported with the use of broad-spectrum antibiotics, therefore, it is important to consider its diagnosis in patients who develop serious diarrhoea during or after antibiotic use.

It is recommended that either the glucose oxidase or hexokinase methods are used to determine blood/plasma glucose levels in patients receiving cefuroxime axetil. This antibiotic does not interfere in the alkaline picrate assay for creatinine.

The Jarisch-Herxheimer reaction has been seen following Zinnat treatment of Lyme disease. It results from the bactericidal activity of Zinnat on the causative organism of Lyme disease, the spirochaete Borrelia burgdorferi. Patients should be reassured that this is common and usually self-limited consequence of antibiotic treatment of Lyme disease.

With a sequential therapy regime the timing of change to oral therapy is determined by severity of the infection, clinical status of the patient and susceptibility of the pathogens involved. The change to oral therapy should only be made once there is a clear clinical improvement. If there has been no clinical improvement after 72 hours of parenteral treatment, then the patient's treatment should be reviewed. Please refer to the relevant prescribing information for cefuroxime sodium before initiating sequential therapy.

4.5 Interaction with other medicinal products and other forms of Interaction

Concurrent administration of probenecid increases the area under the mean serum concentration time curve by 50%. Serum levels of cefuroxime are reduced by dialysis.

A positive Coomb's test has been reported during treatment with cephalosporins. This phenomenon can interfere with cross matching of blood.

4.6 Pregnancy and lactation

There is no experimental evidence of embryopathic or teratogenic effects attributable to cefuroxime axetil but, as with all drugs, it should be administered with caution during early months of pregnancy. Cefuroxime is excreted in human milk, and consequently caution should be exercised when cefuroxime axetil is administered to a nursing mother.

4.7 Effects on ability to drive and use machines

None reported.

4.8 Undesirable effects

Adverse reactions to cefuroxime axetil have been generally mild and transient in nature.

As with other cephalosporins, there have been rare reports of interstitial nephritis, erythema multiforme, Stevens-Johnson syndrome, toxic epidermal necrolysis (exanthematic necrolysis) and hypersensitivity reactions including skin rashes, urticaria, pruritus, drug fever, serum sickness, and very rarely anaphylaxis.

Gastrointestinal disturbances including diarrhoea and nausea and vomiting have been reported. Diarrhoea, although uncommon, is more likely to be associated with higher doses.

As with other broad-spectrum antibiotics, there have been occasional reports of pseudomembranous colitis.

Headache has also been reported.

There have been rare reports of thrombocytopenia and leucopenia (sometimes profound).

Eosinophilia and transient increases of hepatic enzyme levels [ALT (SGPT), AST (SGOT) and LDH] have been noted during Zinnat therapy. As with other cephalosporins, jaundice has been reported very rarely.

Cephalosporins as a class tend to be absorbed onto the surface of red cell membranes and react with antibodies directed against the drug to produce a positive Coombs test (which can interfere with cross-matching of blood) and very rarely haemolytic anaemia.

4.9 Overdose

Overdosage of cephalosporins can cause cerebral irritancy leading to convulsions.

Serum levels of cefuroxime can be reduced by haemodialysis or peritoneal dialysis.

5. PHARMACOLOGICAL PROPERTIES

5.1 Pharmacodynamic properties

Cefuroxime axetil is an oral prodrug of the bactericidal cephalosporin antibiotic cefuroxime, which is resistant to most beta-lactamases and is active against a wide range of gram-positive and gram-negative organisms.

Microbiology

Cefuroxime axetil owes its *in vivo* bactericidal activity to the parent compound, cefuroxime. Cefuroxime is a well-characterized and effective antibacterial agent which has broad-spectrum bactericidal activity against a wide range of common pathogens, including beta-lactamase-producing strains.

Cefuroxime has good stability to bacterial beta-lactamase and consequently, is active against many ampicillin-resistant and amoxycillin-resistant strains. The bactericidal action of cefuroxime results from inhibition of cell-wall synthesis by binding to essential target proteins.

Cefuroxime is usually active against the following organisms *in vitro*:

Aerobes, Gram-negative: *Haemophilus influenzae* (including ampicillin-resistant strains); *Haemophilus parainfluenzae; Moraxella catarrhalis; Escherichia coli;* Klebsiella species; *Proteus mirabilis; Proteus inconstans;* Providencia species; *Proteus rettgeri* and *Neisseria gonorrhoea* (including penicillinase and non-penicillinase-producing strains).

Some strains of *Morganella morganii,* Enterobacter species and Citrobacter species have been shown by *in vitro* tests to be resistant to cefuroxime and other beta-lactam antibiotics.

Aerobes, Gram-positive: *Staphylococcus aureus* (including penicillinase-producing strains but excluding methicillin-resistant strains); *Staphylococcus epidermis,* (including penicillinase-producing strains but excluding methicillin-resistant strains); *Streptococcus pyogenes (*and other betahaemolytic streptococci); *Streptococcus pneumonia* Streptococcus Group B (*Streptococcus agalactiae)* and Propionibacterium species. Certain strains of enterococci, eg. *Streptococcusfaecalis,* are resistant.

Anaerobes, Gram-positive and Gram-negative cocci (including Peptococcus and Peptostreptococcus species); Gram-positive bacilli (including Clostridium species) and Gram-negative bacilli (including Bacteroides and Fusobacterium species). Most strains of Bacteroides fragilis are resistant.

Other organisms, *Borrelia burgdorferi.*

Pseudomonas species, *Campylobacter* species, *Acinetobacter calcoaceticus, Listeria monocytogenes, Legionella species* and most strains of Serratia and *Proteus vulgaris* and *Clostridium difficile* are resistant to many cephalosporins including cefuroxime.

5.2 Pharmacokinetic properties

After oral administration, cefuroxime axetil is absorbed from the gastro-intestinal tract and rapidly hydrolysed in the intestinal mucosa and blood to release cefuroxime into the circulation. Optimum absorption occurs when it is administered after a meal. Peak serum cefuroxime levels occur approximately two to three hours after oral dosing. The serum half life is about 1.2 hours. Approximately 50% of serum cefuroxime is protein bound. Cefuroxime is not metabolised and is excreted by glomerular filtration and tubular secretion. Concurrent administration of probenecid increases the area under the mean serum concentration time curve by 50%.

5.3 Preclinical safety data

No additional data of relevance.

6. PHARMACEUTICAL PARTICULARS

6.1 List of excipients

Microcrystalline cellulose EP

Croscarmellose sodium, Type A USNF

Sodium lauryl sulphate EP

Hydrogenated vegetable oil USNF

Colloidal silicon dioxide USNF

Methylhydroxypropyl cellulose EP

Propylene glycol EP

Methyl parahydroxybenzoate EP

Propyl parahydroxybenzoate EP

Opaspray white M-1-7120

6.2 Incompatibilities

A positive Coombs' test has been reported during treatment with cephalosporins - this phenomenon can interfere with cross-matching of blood.

6.3 Shelf life

36 months in aluminium foil strips or blister packs.

24 months in HDPE bottles (not marketed in the UK)

6.4 Special precautions for storage

Cefuroxime axetil tablets in foil strips or blisters should be stored below 30°C.

Cefuroxime axetil tablets in HDPE bottles should be stored below 25°C (not marketed in the UK)

6.5 Nature and contents of container

Aluminium foil blister pack with an aluminium lid.

Pack size: 2, 4, 14 and 50

(2 and 4 not marketed in the UK)

Aluminium foil strips coated with surlyn polymer.

Pack size: 14 and 50

(not marketed in the UK)

White opaque, high density polyethylene bottles fitted with a clic-loc child resistant closure containing a pulp board wad to which is wax-bonded a 'lectraseal' membrane.

Pack size: 14 and 60

(not marketed in the UK)

6.6 Instructions for use and handling

None stated

Administrative Data

7. MARKETING AUTHORISATION HOLDER

Glaxo Wellcome UK Limited trading as GlaxoSmithKline UK

Stockley Park West

Uxbridge

Middlesex

UB11 1BT

8. MARKETING AUTHORISATION NUMBER(S)

PL10949/0096

9. DATE OF FIRST AUTHORISATION/RENEWAL OF THE AUTHORISATION

15 October 1998

10. DATE OF REVISION OF THE TEXT

29 January 2003

11. Legal Status

POM

Zirtek Allergy Solution

(UCB Pharma Limited)

1. NAME OF THE MEDICINAL PRODUCT

Zirtek Allergy Solution 1mg/ml.

2. QUALITATIVE AND QUANTITATIVE COMPOSITION

Cetirizine hydrochloride 1 mg / ml

3. PHARMACEUTICAL FORM

Solution for oral administration.

4. CLINICAL PARTICULARS

4.1 Therapeutic indications

Cetirizine is indicated for the symptomatic treatment of seasonal allergic rhinitis, perennial rhinitis and chronic idiopathic urticaria in adults and children aged six years and over, and additionally for the symptomatic treatment of seasonal allergic rhinitis in children between two to five years of age.

4.2 Posology and method of administration

Adults and children 6 years and above: 10mg daily.

Adults and children aged 12 years and above: 10ml once daily.

Children aged between 6 to 11 years: Either 5ml twice daily or 10ml once daily.

Children aged between 2-5 years: 5mg daily.

Either 5ml once daily or 2.5ml twice daily.

At present there is insufficient clinical data to recommend the use of cetirizine in children under 2 years of age.

There is no data to suggest that the dose should be reduced in elderly patients.

In patients with renal insufficiency the dosage should be reduced to half the normal recommended daily dose.

4.3 Contraindications

A history of hypersensitivity to any of the constituents of the formulation.

4.4 Special warnings and special precautions for use

Do not exceed the recommended dose.

In patients with renal insufficiency the dosage should be reduced to half the usual recommended dose.

For patients whose symptoms persist, it is advised to consult a doctor or pharmacist.

4.5 Interaction with other medicinal products and other forms of Interaction

To date there are no known interactions with other drugs. Studies with diazepam and cimetidine have revealed no evidence of interactions. As with other antihistamines it is advisable to avoid excessive alcohol consumption.

4.6 Pregnancy and lactation

No adverse effects have been reported from animal studies. There has been little or no use of cetirizine during pregnancy. As with other drugs the use of cetirizine in pregnancy should be avoided.

Cetirizine is contraindicated in lactating women as it is excreted in breast milk.

4.7 Effects on ability to drive and use machines

Studies in healthy volunteers at 20 and 25 mg/day have not revealed effects on alertness or reaction time; however patients are advised not to exceed the recommended dose if driving or operating machinery.

4.8 Undesirable effects

In objective tests of psychomotor function the incidence of sedation with cetirizine was similar to that of placebo. There have been occasional reports of mild and transient side effects such as drowsiness, headache, dizziness, agitation, dry mouth and gastro-intestinal discomfort. If desired the dose might be taken as 5mg in the morning and 5 mg in the evening. Convulsions have very rarely been reported.

4.9 Overdose

Drowsiness can be a symptom of overdosage. In children agitation can occur. In the case of massive overdosage gastric lavage should be performed together with the usual supportive measures. To date there is no specific antidote.

5. PHARMACOLOGICAL PROPERTIES

5.1 Pharmacodynamic properties

Cetirizine is a potent antihistamine with a low potential for drowsiness at pharmacologically active doses and which has additional anti-allergic properties. It is a selective H_1-antagonist with negligible effects on other receptors and so is virtually free from anti-cholinergic and anti-serotonin effects. Cetirizine inhibits the histamine-mediated "early" phase of the allergic reaction and also reduces the migration of inflammatory cells and the release of certain mediators associated with the "late" allergic response.

5.2 Pharmacokinetic properties

Peak blood levels in the order of 0.3 micrograms / ml are attained between 30 and 60 minutes following the administration of a 10 mg oral dose of cetirizine.

The terminal half-life is approximately ten hours in adults and six hours in children aged between 6 to 12 years. This is consistent with the urinary excretion half-life of the drug.

The cumulative urinary excretion represents about two thirds of the dose given for both adults and children.

The apparent plasma clearance in children is higher than that measured in adults. A high proportion of cetirizine is bound to human plasma proteins.

5.3 Preclinical safety data
None Stated.

6. PHARMACEUTICAL PARTICULARS

6.1 List of excipients
Sorbitol solution
Glycerol
Propylene glycol
Saccharin sodium
Methyl parahydroxybenzoate
Propyl parahydroxybenzoate
Banana flavouring
Sodium acetate
Acetic acid
Purified water

6.2 Incompatibilities
None

6.3 Shelf life
3 years.

6.4 Special precautions for storage
Store below 30°C.

6.5 Nature and contents of container
75 ml, 100 ml or 200 ml in a type III amber glass bottle.

6.6 Instructions for use and handling
No special requirements

7. MARKETING AUTHORISATION HOLDER
UCB Pharma Limited
3 George Street
Watford
Herts WD18 0UH.

8. MARKETING AUTHORISATION NUMBER(S)
PL 08972/0033.

9. DATE OF FIRST AUTHORISATION/RENEWAL OF THE AUTHORISATION
5 May 2000 / 31 October 2001.

10. DATE OF REVISION OF THE TEXT
January 2003.

Zirtek Allergy Tablets

(UCB Pharma Limited)

1. NAME OF THE MEDICINAL PRODUCT
Zirtek Allergy/ Zirtek Allergy Relief

2. QUALITATIVE AND QUANTITATIVE COMPOSITION
Cetirizine hydrochloride: 10 mg per tablet.

3. PHARMACEUTICAL FORM
Film-coated tablet.

4. CLINICAL PARTICULARS

4.1 Therapeutic indications
Cetirizine is indicated for the symptomatic treatment of perennial rhinitis, seasonal allergic rhinitis and chronic idiopathic urticaria.

4.2 Posology and method of administration
P Pack

Adults and children aged 6 years and over: 10 mg daily.

Adults 10 mg once daily

Children between 6 to 12 years of age: either 5 mg twice daily or 10 mg once daily.

GSL Pack

Adults and Children aged 12 years and over: 10 mg once daily

All Packs

At present there are insufficient clinical data to recommend use of cetirizine in children under the age of 6.

For the time being, there is no data to suggest that the dose needs to be reduced in elderly patients.

In patients with renal insufficiency the dosage should be reduced to half the usual recommended daily dose.

4.3 Contraindications
A history of hypersensitivity to any of the constituents of the formulation.

4.4 Special warnings and special precautions for use
Do not exceed the stated dose. If symptoms persist consult your doctor.

4.5 Interaction with other medicinal products and other forms of Interaction
To date, there are no known interactions with other drugs. Studies with diazepam and cimetidine have revealed no evidence of interactions. As with other antihistamines it is advisable to avoid excessive alcohol consumption.

4.6 Pregnancy and lactation
No adverse effects have been reported from animal studies. There has been little or no clinical experience of cetirizine in pregnancy. As with other drugs, the use of cetirizine in pregnancy should be avoided.

Cetirizine is contraindicated in lactating women since it is excreted in breast milk.

4.7 Effects on ability to drive and use machines
Antihistamines can cause drowsiness in some patients. Although this has not been reported with cetirizine at the recommended dose please be cautious whilst driving or operating machinery.

4.8 Undesirable effects
In objective tests of psychomotor function the incidence of sedation with cetirizine was similar to that of placebo. There have been occasional reports of mild and transient side effects such as headache, dizziness, drowsiness, agitation, dry mouth, and gastrointestinal discomfort. If affected the dose may be taken as 5 mg in the morning and 5 mg in the evening. Convulsions have very rarely been reported.

4.9 Overdose
Drowsiness can be a symptom of overdosage. In children agitation can occur. In the case of massive overdosage lavage should be performed together with the usual supportive measures. To date there is no specific antidote.

5. PHARMACOLOGICAL PROPERTIES

5.1 Pharmacodynamic properties
Cetirizine is a potent antihistamine with a low potential for drowsiness at normal therapeutic doses which has additional anti-allergic properties. It is a selective H_1 antagonist with negligible effects on other receptors and so is virtually free from anti-cholinergic and anti-serotonin effects. Cetirizine inhibits the histamine-mediated early phase of the allergic reaction and also reduces the migration of certain inflammatory cells and the release of certain mediators associated with the late allergic response.

5.2 Pharmacokinetic properties
Peak blood levels of the order of 0.3 micrograms/ml are reached between 30 and 60 minutes after the oral administration of a 10 mg dose of cetirizine. The terminal half-life is approximately ten hours in adults and six hours in children aged 6 - 12 years.

This is consistent with the urinary excretion half-life of the drug. The cumulative urinary excretion represents about two thirds of the administered dose for both adults and children.

The apparent plasma clearance in children is higher than that measured in adults. A high proportion of cetirizine is bound to human plasma proteins.

5.3 Preclinical safety data
None stated

6. PHARMACEUTICAL PARTICULARS

6.1 List of excipients
Tablet core:
Microcrystalline cellulose
Lactose
Colloidal anhydrous silica
Magnesium stearate
Film coating:
Opadry Y-1-7000
- Hydroxypropylmethylcellulose (E464)
- Titanium dioxide (E 171)
- Polyethlene glycol

6.2 Incompatibilities
None.

6.3 Shelf life
60 months

6.4 Special precautions for storage
No special precautions for storage.

6.5 Nature and contents of container
Aluminium / PVC blister packs:

P packs containing 7, 14, 21, 28, 30 or 60 tablets.

GSL packs containing 4, 5, or 7 tablets

6.6 Instructions for use and handling
No special requirements

7. MARKETING AUTHORISATION HOLDER
UCB Pharma Limited,
3 George Street,
Watford,
Hertfordshire WD18 0UH.

8. MARKETING AUTHORISATION NUMBER(S)
PL 08972/0032

9. DATE OF FIRST AUTHORISATION/RENEWAL OF THE AUTHORISATION
5 May 2000 / 31 October 2001

10. DATE OF REVISION OF THE TEXT
February 2003.

Zispin SolTab 15 mg

(Organon Laboratories Limited)

1. NAME OF THE MEDICINAL PRODUCT
Zispin SolTab 15 mg orodispersible tablet

2. QUALITATIVE AND QUANTITATIVE COMPOSITION
Each tablet contains 15 mg of mirtazapine.

3. PHARMACEUTICAL FORM
Orodispersible tablet

The tablets are round, white, standard bevelled-edge tablets marked with the code TZ/1 on one side.

4. CLINICAL PARTICULARS

4.1 Therapeutic indications
Treatment of depressive illness.

4.2 Posology and method of administration
(see Table 1 on next page)

<u>**Major Depressive Episode**</u>

Treatment should begin with 15mg daily. As with all anti-depressant medicinal products, dosage should be reviewed and adjusted if necessary within 2 to 4 weeks of initiation of therapy and thereafter as judged clinically appropriate. Although there may be an increased potential for undesirable effects at higher doses, if after some weeks on the recommended dose insufficient response is seen some patients may benefit from having their dose increased gradually up to a maximum of 45mg a day (see section 5.1). Dosage adjustments should be made carefully on an individual patient basis, to maintain the patients at the lowest effective dose. If there is no response within 2-4 weeks at 45mg/day, then treatment should be stopped. Patients with depression should be treated for a sufficient period of at least 6 months to ensure that they are free from symptoms. After this, treatment can be gradually discontinued.

Elderly: The recommended dose is the same as that for adults. In elderly patients an increase in dosing should be done under close supervision to elicit a satisfactory and safe response.

Children: Since safety and efficacy of Zispin has not been established in children, it is not recommended to treat children with Zispin. Two randomised placebo-controlled trials failed to demonstrate efficacy for Zispin in the treatment of children and adolescents with major depressive disorder. Safety and efficacy of Zispin in paediatric depression can not be extrapolated from adult data.

The clearance of mirtazapine may be decreased in patients with renal or hepatic insufficiency. This should be taken into account when prescribing Zispin to this category of patients.

Mirtazapine has a half-life of 20-40 hours and therefore Zispin is suitable for once-a-day administration. It should be taken preferably as a single night-time dose before going to bed. Zispin may also be given in sub-doses equally divided over the day (once in the morning and once at night-time).

Treatment should preferably be continued until the patient has been completely symptom-free for 4-6 months. After this, treatment can be gradually discontinued. Treatment with an adequate dose should result in a positive response within 2-4 weeks. With an insufficient response, the dose can be increased up to the maximum dose. If there is no response within a further 2-4 weeks, then treatment should be stopped.

<u>**Withdrawal symptoms seen on discontinuation of Mirtazapine**</u>

Abrupt discontinuation should be avoided (see section 4.4 Special Warnings and Special Precautions for Use and section 4.8 Undesirable Effects). If intolerable symptoms occur following a decrease in the dose or upon discontinuation of treatment, then resuming the previously prescribed dose may be considered. Subsequently, the physician may continue decreasing the dose, but at a more gradual rate.

4.3 Contraindications
Hypersensitivity to mirtazapine or any of the other ingredients of Zispin.

4.4 Special warnings and special precautions for use
Reversible white blood cell disorders including agranulocytosis, leukopenia and granulocytopenia have been reported as a rare occurrence with Zispin. This mostly appears after 4-6 weeks of treatment and is in general reversible after termination of treatment With respect to agranulocytosis the physician should be alert to symptoms such as fever, sore throat, stomatitis or other signs of infection; when such symptoms occur, treatment should be stopped and blood counts taken. Patients should also be advised of the importance of these symptoms.

Careful dosing as well as regular and close monitoring is necessary in patients with:

- epilepsy and organic brain syndrome. As with other antidepressants, mirtazapine should be introduced cautiously in patients who have a history of seizures. Treatment should be discontinued in any patient who develops seizures, or where there is an increase in seizure frequency. Antidepressants should be avoided in patients with

Table 1

In order to prevent crushing the tablet, do not push against the tablet pocket. *(Figure A).*

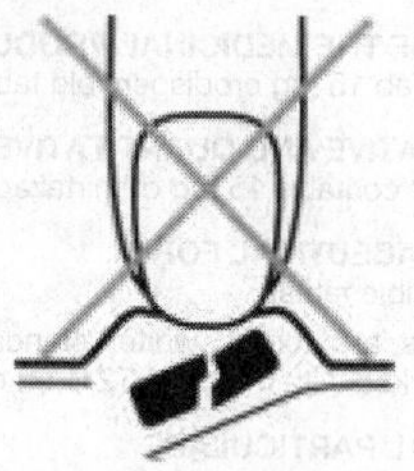

Figure A

Each strip contains six tablet pockets, which are separated by perforations. Tear off one tablet pocket along the dotted lines. *(Figure 1)*

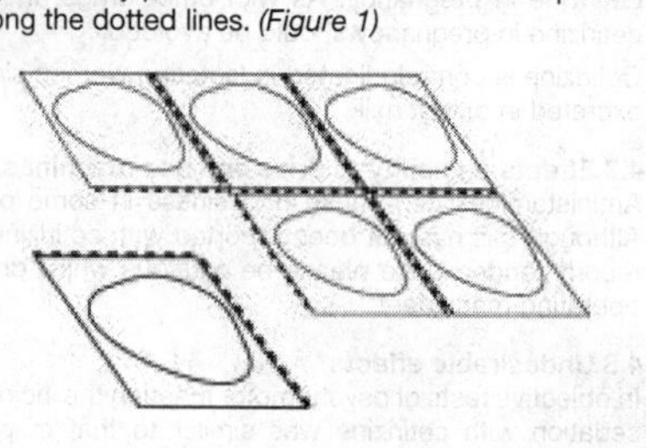

Figure 1

Carefully peel off the lidding foil, starting in the corner indicated by the arrow. *(Figures 2 and 3)*

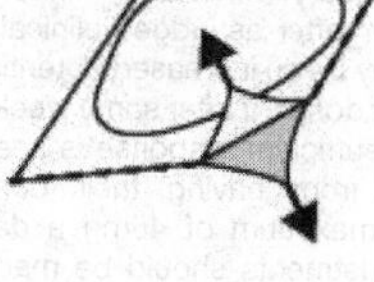

Figure 2

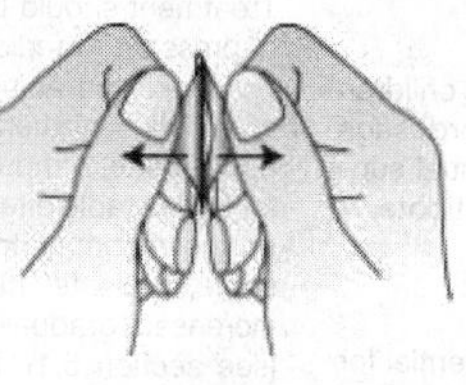

Figure 3

The tablet should be taken out of the strip with dry hands and should be placed on the tongue. *(Figure 4)*

The tablet will rapidly disintegrate and can be swallowed with or without water.

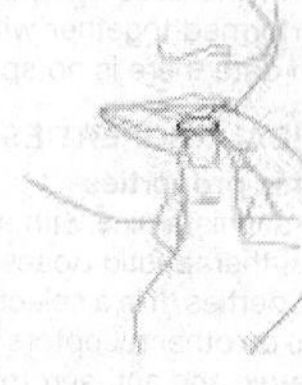

Figure 4

unstable seizure disorders/epilepsy and patients with controlled epilepsy should be carefully monitoredFrom clinical experience it appears that insults occur rarely in patients treated with Zispin

- hepatic or renal insufficiency

- cardiac diseases like conduction disturbances, angina pectoris and recent myocardial infarct, where normal precautions should be taken and concomitant medicines carefully administered

- low blood pressure.

- diabetes mellitus. In patients with diabetes, antidepressants may alter glycaemic control. Insulin and/or oral hypoglycaemic dosage may need to be adjusted and close monitoring is recommended.

As with other antidepressants care should be taken in patients with:

- micturition disturbances like prostate hypertrophy (although problems are not to be expected because Zispin possesses only very weak anticholinergic activity)

- acute narrow-angle glaucoma and increased intra-ocular pressure (also here little chance of problems with Zispin because of its very weak anticholinergic activity)

Treatment should be discontinued if jaundice occurs.

Moreover, as with other antidepressants, the following should be taken into account:

- worsening of psychotic symptoms can occur when antidepressants are administered to patients with schizophrenia or other psychotic disturbances; paranoid thoughts can be intensified

- when the depressive phase of manic-depressive psychosis is being treated, it can transform into the manic phase

- as improvement may not occur during the first few weeks of treatment, in common with all antidepressants, patients should be closely monitored during this period. The possibility of suicide is inherent in depression, and may persist until significant remission occurs. It is general clinical experience with all therapies for depression, that the risk of suicide may increase in the early stages of recovery.

- elderly patients are often more sensitive, especially with regard to the side-effects of antidepressants. During clinical research with Zispin, side-effects have not been reported more often in elderly patients than in other age groups; however, experience until now is limited.

- Zispin SolTab contains aspartame a source of phenylalanine. Each tablet with 15 mg mirtazapine corresponds to 2.6 mg phenylalanine, respectively. May be harmful for patients with phenylketonuria.

- Suicide/suicidal thoughts

- Depression is associated with an increased risk of suicidal thoughts, self harm and suicide (suicide-related events). This risk persists until significant remission occurs. As improvement may not occur during the first few weeks or more of treatment, patients should be closely monitored until such improvement occurs. It is general clinical experience that the risk of self harm is highest shortly after presentation and the risk of suicide may increase again in the early stages of recovery. Furthermore, there is evidence that in a small group of people, antidepressants may increase the risk of suicidal thoughts and self-harm.

- Other psychiatric conditions for which mirtazapine is prescribed can also be associated with an increased risk of suicide-related events. In addition, these conditions may be co-morbid with major depressive disorder. The same precautions observed when treating patients with major depressive disorder should therefore be observed when treating patients with other psychiatric disorders.

- Patients with a history of suicide-related events, those exhibiting a significant degree of suicidal ideation prior to commencement of treatment, and young adults, are at a greater risk of suicidal thoughts or suicide attempts, and should receive careful monitoring during treatment.

- Patients, (and caregivers of patients) should be alerted about the need to monitor for the emergence of suicidal thoughts and to seek medical advice immediately if these symptoms present

Psychomotor restlessness

The use of mirtazapine has been associated with the development of psychomotor restlessness, which clinically may be very similar to akathisia, characterised by a subjectively unpleasant or distressing restlessness and need to move often accompanied by an inability to sit or stand still. This is most likely to occur within the first few weeks of treatment. In patients who develop these symptoms, increasing the dose may be detrimental and it may be necessary to review the use of mirtazapine.

Withdrawal symptoms seen on discontinuation of mirtazapine treatment

Withdrawal symptoms when treatment is discontinued are common, particularly if discontinuation is abrupt (see section 4.8 Undesirable effects). In clinical trials adverse events seen on treatment discontinuation occurred in approximately 15% of patients treated with mirtazapine. The risk of withdrawal symptoms may be dependent on several factors including the duration and dose of therapy and the rate of dose reduction.

Dizziness, agitation, anxiety, headache and nausea and/or vomiting are the most commonly reported reactions. Generally these symptoms are mild to moderate, however, in some patients they may be severe in intensity. They usually occur within the first few days of discontinuing treatment, but there have been very rare reports of such symptoms in patients who have inadvertently missed a dose. Generally these symptoms are self-limiting and usually resolve within 2 weeks, though in some individuals they may be prolonged (2-3 months or more). It is therefore advised that mirtazapine should be gradually tapered when discontinuing treatment over a period of several weeks, according to the patient's needs (see "Withdrawal Symptoms Seen on Discontinuation of Mirtazapine", Section 4.2 Posology and Method of Administration).

4.5 Interaction with other medicinal products and other forms of Interaction

- Mirtazapine may potentiate the central nervous dampening action of alcohol; patients should therefore be advised to avoid alcohol during treatment with Zispin.

- Zispin should not be administered concomitantly with MAO inhibitors or within two weeks of cessation of therapy with these agents.

- Mirtazapine may potentiate the sedative effects of benzodiazepines; caution should be taken when these drugs are prescribed together with Zispin.

- In vitro data suggest that mirtazapine is a very weak competitive inhibitor of the cytochrome P450 enzymes CYP1A2, CYP2D6 and CYP3A.

- Caution is needed when strong CYP3A4 inhibitors, such as the HIV protease inhibitors, azole antifungals, erythromycin and nefazodone are co-administered with mirtazapine.

· Co-administration of the potent inhibitor of CYP3A4, ketoconazole increased the peak plasma levels and AUC by approximately 30 and 45% respectively.

· Carbamazepine, an inducer of CYP3A4, increased mirtazapine clearance about twofold, resulting in a decrease in plasma levels of 45-60%. Phenytoin increased the clearance of mirtazapine in a similar fashion. When carbamazepine or another inducer of drug metabolism (such as rifampicin) is added to mirtazapine therapy, the mirtazapine dose may have to be increased. If treatment with an inducer is stopped, mirtazapine dosing may have to be decreased.

· Bioavailability of mirtazapine increased by more than 50% when co-administered with cimetidine. The mirtazapine dose may have to be decreased when concomitant treatment with cimetidine is started or increased when cimetidine treatment is ended.

· Mirtazapine caused a small but clinically insignificant increase in INR in subjects treated with warfarin.

Absence of interactions

· In *in vivo* interaction studies, mirtazapine did not influence the pharmacokinetics of risperidone or paroxetine (CYP2D6 substrate), carbamazepine (CYP3A4 substrate), amitriptyline and cimetidine.

· No relevant clinical effects or changes in pharmacokinetics have been observed in man with concurrent administration of mirtazapine and lithium.

· A number of clinical interaction studies, and a study of mirtazapine treatment following mirtazapine treatment failure have been performed with mirtazapine and SSRIs. Until now no clinical interactions, pharmacodynamic or pharmacokinetic, have been encountered.

4.6 Pregnancy and lactation

The safety of Zispin in human pregnancy has not been established.

Reproduction studies in pregnant rats and rabbits at doses up to 100 mg/kg and 40 mg/kg (approx. 3 and 5 times respectively the maximum recommended human dose on the basis of exposure) have revealed no evidence of teratogenic effects. There was, however, in rats an increase in post-implantation loss; there was also an increase in pup deaths during the first three days of lactation (cause of death unknown) and a decrease in pup birth weights. These findings are common with CNS-active drugs at high dose levels in animals.

As the relevance of these findings to humans is not certain the use of Zispin during pregnancy is not recommended. Women of child-bearing potential should employ an adequate method of contraception if taking Zispin.

Although animal experiments show that mirtazapine is excreted only in very small amounts in the milk, the use of Zispin in nursing mothers is not recommended since no human data in breast milk are available.

4.7 Effects on ability to drive and use machines

In some patients, particularly the elderly, Zispin may have transient sedative properties and may initially impair alertness and concentration. Patients treated with Zispin should therefore be cautioned about their ability to drive a car or operate hazardous machinery.

4.8 Undesirable effects

Depressed patients display a number of symptoms that are associated with the illness itself. It is therefore sometimes difficult to ascertain which symptoms are a result of the illness itself and which are a result of treatment with Zispin.

The following adverse effects have been reported:

(see Table 2 on next page)

Withdrawal symptoms seen on discontinuation of Mirtazapine treatment

Discontinuation of mirtazapine (particularly when abrupt) commonly leads to withdrawal symptoms. Dizziness, agitation, anxiety, headache and nausea and/or vomiting are the most commonly reported reactions. Generally these events are mild to moderate and are self-limiting, however, in some patients they may be severe and/or prolonged. It is therefore advised that when mirtazapine treatment is no longer required, gradual discontinuation by dose tapering should be carried out (see section 4.2 Posology and Method of Administration and section 4.4 Special Warnings and Special Precautions for use).

4.9 Overdose

Present experience concerning overdose with Zispin alone indicates that symptoms are usually mild.

Depression of the central nervous system with disorientation and prolonged sedation have been reported, together with tachycardia and mild hyper- or hypotension.

Cases of overdose should be treated by gastric lavage with appropriate symptomatic and supportive therapy for vital functions.

Table 2

	Rare >1/10,000)	Uncommon >1/1000)	Common >1/100)
Blood and the lymphatic system disorders	Reversible agranulocytosis has been reported as a rare occurrence with Zispin. (see also section 4.4 'Special warnings and special precautions for use')		
Metabolism and nutrition disorders			Increase in appetite and weight gain
Psychiatric disorders	Nightmares/vivid dreams Psychomotor restlessness* (see section 4.4 Special Warnings and Special Precautions for Use)		
Nervous system disorders	Mania, convulsions (insults), tremor, myoclonus. There have been rare reports of agitation and hallucinations although these symptoms may be related to underlying disease. Paraesthesia	Dizziness, Headache	
Cardiac disorders	(Orthostatic) hypotension.		
Hepato-biliary disorders		Increases in liver enzyme levels	
Skin and subcutaneous tissue disorders	Rash		
Musculoskeletal, connective tissue and bone disorders	Restless legs, Arthralgia/ myalgia		
General disorders			Generalised or local oedema. Drowsiness/ sedation/ fatigue, generally occurring during the first few weeks of treatment. (N.B. dose reduction generally does not lead to less sedation but can jeopardise antidepressant efficacy)

* including akathisia

5. PHARMACOLOGICAL PROPERTIES

Zispin (mirtazapine) is an antidepressant, which can be given as treatment for episodes of major depression. The presence of symptoms such as anhedonia, psychomotor inhibition, sleep disturbances (early wakening) and weight loss, increase the chance of a positive response. Other symptoms are: loss of interest, suicidal thoughts and changes in mood (better in the evening than in the morning). Zispin begins to exert its effect in general after 1-2 weeks of treatment.

5.1 Pharmacodynamic properties

Pharmacotherapeutic group: Antidepressant

(ATC code: NO6AX11)

Mirtazapine is a centrally active presynaptic α_2-antagonist, which increases central noradrenergic and serotonergic neurotransmission. The enhancement of serotonergic neurotransmission is specifically mediated via 5-HT_1 receptors, because 5-HT_2 and 5-HT_3 receptors are blocked by mirtazapine. Both enantiomers of mirtazapine are presumed to contribute to the antidepressant activity, the S(+) enantiomer by blocking α_2 and 5-HT_2 receptors and the R(-) enantiomer by blocking 5-HT_3 receptors.

The histamine H_1-antagonistic activity of mirtazapine is responsible for its sedative properties. Mirtazapine is generally well tolerated. It has practically no anticholinergic activity and, at therapeutic doses, has practically no effect on the cardiovascular system.

__Dose response__

No formal clinical trials were conducted investigating the dose response of mirtazapine. However, it is clinical experience that up-titrating the dose might be beneficial for some patients.

5.2 Pharmacokinetic properties

After oral administration of Zispin tablets, the active constituent mirtazapine is rapidly and well absorbed (bioavailability 50%), reaching peak plasma levels after about 2 hours. Binding of mirtazapine to plasma proteins is approx. 85%. The mean half-life of elimination is 20-40 hours; longer half-lives, up to 65 hours, have occasionally been recorded and shorter half-lives have been seen in young men. The half-life of elimination is sufficient to justify once-a-day dosing. Steady state is reached after 3-4 days, after which there is no further accumulation. Mirtazapine displays linear pharmacokinetics within the recommended dose range. Food intake has no influence on the pharmacokinetics of mirtazapine. Mirtazapine is extensively metabolised and eliminated via the urine and faeces within a few days. Major pathways of biotransformation are demethylation and oxidation, followed by conjugation. In vitro data from human liver microsomes indicate that cytochrome P450 enzymes CYP2D6 and CYP1A2 are involved in the formation of the 8-hydroxy metabolite of mirtazapine, whereas CYP3A4 is considered to be responsible for the formation of the N-demethyl and N-oxide metabolites. The demethyl metabolite is pharmacologically active and appears to have the same pharmacokinetic profile as the parent compound. There are no differences in the pharmacokinetic parameters of racemic mirtazapine or its demethyl metabolite in extensive and poor metabolisers. Plasma metabolite profiles for the individual enantiomers are qualitatively similar in extensive and poor metabolisers.

The clearance of mirtazapine may be decreased as a result of renal or hepatic insufficiency.

5.3 Preclinical safety data

No special particulars.

6. PHARMACEUTICAL PARTICULARS

6.1 List of excipients

Sugar spheres, hydroxypropyl methylcellulose, polyvinylpyrrolidone (povidone), magnesium stearate, aminoalkyl methacrylate copolymer E aspartame (contains 2.6 mg phenylalanine), citric acid, crospovidone, mannitol, microcrystalline cellulose, natural and artificial orange flavour and sodium bicarbonate.

6.2 Incompatibilities

Not known.

6.3 Shelf life

The shelf life for Zispin SolTab is 3 years. Zispin SolTab should not be used after the expiry date indicated on the package.

6.4 Special precautions for storage

Do not store above 30°C. Store in the original pack.

6.5 Nature and contents of container

Zispin SolTab tablets are packed in a child-resistant, peel-to-open, rigid strip, formed from a laminate of aluminium foil and plastic films sealed to a paper-based laminate of aluminium foil coated with a heat seal lacquer. Tablet pockets in the strip are separated by perforations.

The following packages are available:

- Peel-to-open strips with 6 tablets each, available in packs of 6, 30 and 90 tablets.

6.6 Instructions for use and handling

See 4.2

7. MARKETING AUTHORISATION HOLDER

Organon Laboratories Ltd, Science Park, Milton Road, Cambridge, CB4 0FL, UK.

8. MARKETING AUTHORISATION NUMBER(S)

PL 00065/0180

9. DATE OF FIRST AUTHORISATION/RENEWAL OF THE AUTHORISATION

15th July 2003

10. DATE OF REVISION OF THE TEXT

December 2004

Ref: US Zisp 15mg SOLTAB v8.0

Zispin SolTab 30 mg

(Organon Laboratories Limited)

1. NAME OF THE MEDICINAL PRODUCT

Zispin SolTab 30 mg orodispersible tablet.

2. QUALITATIVE AND QUANTITATIVE COMPOSITION

Each tablet contains 30 mg of mirtazapine.

3. PHARMACEUTICAL FORM

Orodispersible tablet

The tablets are round, white, standard bevelled-edge tablets marked with the code TZ/2 on one side.

4. CLINICAL PARTICULARS

4.1 Therapeutic indications

Treatment of depressive illness.

4.2 Posology and method of administration

(see Table 1 on next page)

__**Major Depressive Episode**__

Treatment should begin with 15mg daily. As with all antidepressant medicinal products, dosage should be reviewed and adjusted if necessary within 2 to 4 weeks of initiation of therapy and thereafter as judged clinically appropriate. Although there may be an increased potential for undesirable effects at higher doses, if after some weeks on the recommended dose insufficient response is seen some patients may benefit from having their dose increased gradually up to a maximum of 45mg a day (see section 5.1). Dosage adjustments should be made carefully on an individual patient basis, to maintain the patients at the lowest effective dose. If there is no response within 2-4 weeks at 45mg/day, then treatment should be stopped. Patients with depression should be treated for a sufficient period of at least 6 months to ensure that they are free from symptoms. After this, treatment can be gradually discontinued.

Elderly: The recommended dose is the same as that for adults. In elderly patients an increase in dosing should be done under close supervision to elicit a satisfactory and safe response.

Children: Since safety and efficacy of Zispin has not been established in children, it is not recommended to treat children with Zispin. Two randomised placebo-controlled trials failed to demonstrate efficacy for Zispin in the treatment of children and adolescents with major depressive disorder. Safety and efficacy of Zispin in paediatric depression can not be extrapolated from adult data.

The clearance of mirtazapine may be decreased in patients with renal or hepatic insufficiency. This should be taken into account when prescribing Zispin to this category of patients.

Mirtazapine has a half-life of 20-40 hours and therefore Zispin is suitable for once-a-day administration. It should be taken preferably as a single night-time dose before going to bed. Zispin may also be given in sub-doses equally divided over the day (once in the morning and once at night-time).

Treatment should preferably be continued until the patient has been completely symptom-free for 4-6 months. After this, treatment can be gradually discontinued. Treatment with an adequate dose should result in a positive response within 2-4 weeks. With an insufficient response, the dose can be increased up to the maximum dose. If there is no response within a further 2-4 weeks, then treatment should be stopped.

__**Withdrawal symptoms seen on discontinuation of Mirtazapine**__

Abrupt discontinuation should be avoided (see section 4.4 Special Warnings and Special Precautions for Use and section 4.8 Undesirable Effects). If intolerable symptoms occur following a decrease in the dose or upon discontinuation of treatment, then resuming the previously prescribed dose may be considered. Subsequently, the physician may continue decreasing the dose, but at a more gradual rate.

4.3 Contraindications

Hypersensitivity to mirtazapine or any of the other ingredients of Zispin.

4.4 Special warnings and special precautions for use

Reversible white blood cell disorders including agranulocytosis, leukopenia and granulocytopenia have been reported as a rare occurence with Zispin. This mostly appears after 4-6 weeks of treatment and is in general reversible after termination of treatment. With respect to agranulocytosis the physician should be alert to symptoms such as fever, sore throat, stomatitis or other signs of infection; when such symptoms occur, treatment should be stopped and blood counts taken. Patients should also be advised of the importance of these symptoms.

Careful dosing as well as regular and close monitoring is necessary in patients with:

- epilepsy and organic brain syndrome. As with other antidepressants, mirtazapine should be introduced cautiously in patients who have a history of seizures.

Table 1

In order to prevent crushing the tablet, do not push against the tablet pocket. *(Figure A)*.

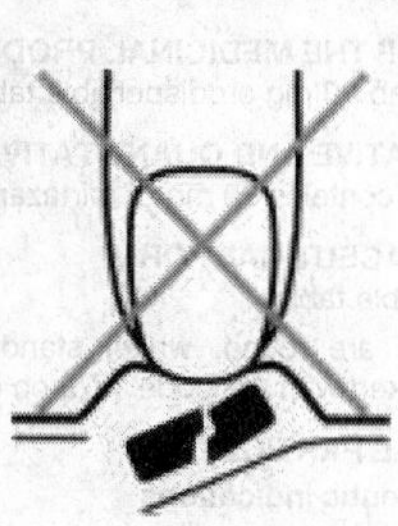

Figure A

Each strip contains six tablet pockets, which are separated by perforations. Tear off one tablet pocket along the dotted lines. *(Figure 1)*

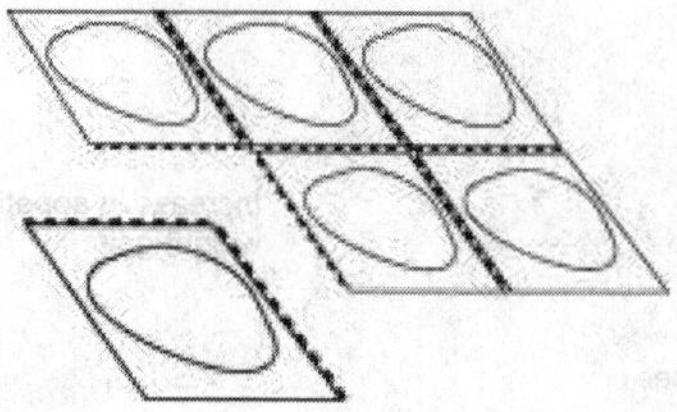

Figure 1

Carefully peel off the lidding foil, starting in the corner indicated by the arrow. *(Figures 2 and 3)*

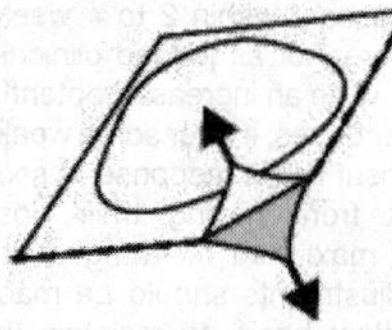

Figure 2

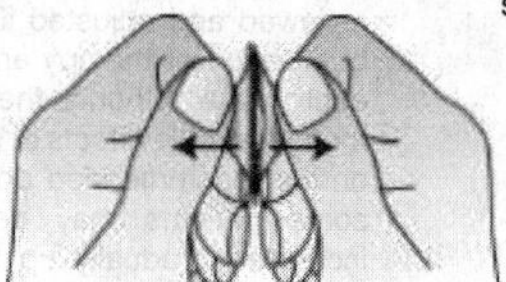

Figure 3

The tablet should be taken out of the strip with dry hands and should be placed on the tongue. *(Figure 4)* The tablet will rapidly disintegrate and can be swallowed with or without water.

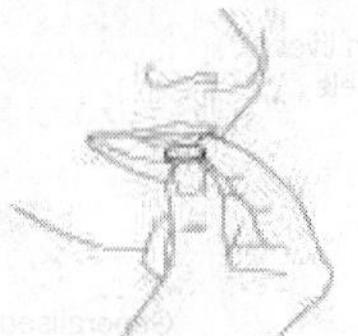

Figure 4

Treatment should be discontinued in any patient who develops seizures, or where there is an increase in seizure frequency. Antidepressants should be avoided in patients with unstable seizure disorders/epilepsy and patients with controlled epilepsy should be carefully monitored. From clinical experience it appears that insults occur rarely in patients treated with Zispin

- hepatic or renal insufficiency

- cardiac diseases like conduction disturbances, angina pectoris and recent myocardial infarct, where normal precautions should be taken and concomitant medicines carefully administered

- low blood pressure.

- diabetes mellitus. In patients with diabetes, antidepressants may alter glycaemic control. Insulin and/or oral hypoglycaemic dosage may need to be adjusted and close monitoring is recommended.

As with other antidepressants care should be taken in patients with:

- micturition disturbances like prostate hypertrophy (although problems are not to be expected because Zispin possesses only very weak anticholinergic activity)

- acute narrow-angle glaucoma and increased intra-ocular pressure (also here little chance of problems with Zispin because of its very weak anticholinergic activity)

Treatment should be discontinued if jaundice occurs.

Moreover, as with other antidepressants, the following should be taken into account:

- worsening of psychotic symptoms can occur when antidepressants are administered to patients with schizophrenia or other psychotic disturbances; paranoid thoughts can be intensified

- when the depressive phase of manic-depressive psychosis is being treated, it can transform into the manic phase

- as improvement may not occur during the first few weeks of treatment, in common with all antidepressants, patients should be closely monitored during this period. The possibility of suicide is inherent in depression, and may persist until significant remission occurs. It is general clinical experience with all therapies for depression, that the risk of suicide may increase in the early stages of recovery

- elderly patients are often more sensitive, especially with regard to the side-effects of antidepressants. During clinical research with Zispin, side-effects have not been reported more often in elderly patients than in other age groups; however, experience until now is limited

- Zispin SolTab contains aspartame a source of phenylalanine. Each tablet with 30 mg mirtazapine corresponds to 5.2 mg phenylalanine, respectively. May be harmful for patients with phenylketonuria.

<u>**Suicide/suicidal thoughts**</u>

- Depression is associated with an increased risk of suicidal thoughts, self harm and suicide (suicide-related events). This risk persists until significant remission occurs. As improvement may not occur during the first few weeks or more of treatment, patients should be closely monitored until such improvement occurs. It is general clinical experience that the risk of self harm is highest shortly after presentation and the risk of suicide may increase again in the early stages of recovery. Furthermore, there is evidence that in a small group of people, antidepressants may increase the risk of suicidal thoughts and self-harm.

- Other psychiatric conditions for which mirtazapine is prescribed can also be associated with an increased risk of suicide-related events. In addition, these conditions may be co-morbid with major depressive disorder. The same precautions observed when treating patients with major depressive disorder should therefore be observed when treating patients with other psychiatric disorders.

- Patients with a history of suicide-related events, those exhibiting a significant degree of suicidal ideation prior to commencement of treatment, and young adults, are at a greater risk of suicidal thoughts or suicide attempts, and should receive careful monitoring during treatment.

- Patients, (and caregivers of patients) should be alerted about the need to monitor for the emergence of suicidal thoughts and to seek medical advice immediately if these symptoms present

<u>Psychomotor restlessness</u>

The use of mirtazapine has been associated with the development of psychomotor restlessness, which clinically may be very similar to akathisia, characterised by a subjectively unpleasant or distressing restlessness and need to move often accompanied by an inability to sit or stand still. This is most likely to occur within the first few weeks of treatment. In patients who develop these symptoms, increasing the dose may be detrimental and it may be necessary to review the use of mirtazapine.

<u>**Withdrawal symptoms seen on discontinuation of mirtazapine treatment**</u>

Withdrawal symptoms when treatment is discontinued are common, particularly if discontinuation is abrupt (see section 4.8 Undesirable effects). In clinical trials adverse events seen on treatment discontinuation occurred in approximately 15% of patients treated with mirtazapine. The risk of withdrawal symptoms may be dependent on several factors including the duration and dose of therapy and the rate of dose reduction.

Dizziness, agitation, anxiety, headache and nausea and/or vomiting are the most commonly reported reactions. Generally these symptoms are mild to moderate, however, in some patients they may be severe in intensity. They usually occur within the first few days of discontinuing treatment, but there have been very rare reports of such symptoms in patients who have inadvertently missed a dose. Generally these symptoms are self-limiting and usually resolve within 2 weeks, though in some individuals they may be prolonged (2-3 months or more). It is therefore advised that mirtazapine should be gradually tapered when discontinuing treatment over a period of several weeks, according to the patient's needs (see "Withdrawal Symptoms Seen on Discontinuation of Mirtazapine", Section 4.2 Posology and Method of Administration).

4.5 Interaction with other medicinal products and other forms of Interaction

- Mirtazapine may potentiate the central nervous dampening action of alcohol; patients should therefore be advised to avoid alcohol during treatment with Zispin.

- Zispin should not be administered concomitantly with MAO inhibitors or within two weeks of cessation of therapy with these agents.

- Mirtazapine may potentiate the sedative effects of benzodiazepines; caution should be taken when these drugs are prescribed together with Zispin.

- In vitro data suggest that mirtazapine is a very weak competitive inhibitor of the cytochrome P450 enzymes CYP1A2, CYP2D6 and CYP3A.

- Caution is needed when strong CYP3A4 inhibitors, such as the HIV protease inhibitors, azole antifungals, erythromycin and nefazodone are co-administered with mirtazapine.

- Co-administration of the potent inhibitor of CYP3A4, ketoconazole increased the peak plasma levels and AUC by approximately 30 and 45% respectively.

- Carbamazepine, an inducer of CYP3A4, increased mirtazapine clearance about twofold, resulting in a decrease in plasma levels of 45-60%. Phenytoin increased the clearance of mirtazapine in a similar fashion. When carbamazepine or another inducer of drug metabolism (such as rifampicin) is added to mirtazapine therapy, the mirtazapine dose may have to be increased. If treatment with an inducer is stopped, mirtazapine dosing may have to be decreased.

- Bioavailability of mirtazapine increased by more than 50% when co-administered with cimetidine. The mirtazapine dose may have to be decreased when concomitant treatment with cimetidine is started or increased when cimetidine treatment is ended.

- Mirtazapine caused a small but clinically insignificant increase in INR in subjects treated with warfarin.

<u>*Absence of interactions*</u>

- In *in vivo* interaction studies, mirtazapine did not influence the pharmacokinetics of risperidone or paroxetine (CYP2D6 substrate), carbamazepine (CYP3A4 substrate), amitriptyline and cimetidine.

- No relevant clinical effects or changes in pharmacokinetics have been observed in man with concurrent administration of mirtazapine and lithium.

- A number of clinical interaction studies, and a study of mirtazapine treatment following mirtazapine treatment failure have been performed with mirtazapine and SSRIs. Until now no clinical interactions, pharmacodynamic or pharmacokinetic, have been encountered.

4.6 Pregnancy and lactation

The safety of Zispin in human pregnancy has not been established.

Reproduction studies in pregnant rats and rabbits at doses up to 100 mg/kg and 40 mg/kg (approx. 3 and 5 times respectively the maximum recommended human dose on the basis of exposure) have revealed no evidence of teratogenic effects. There was, however, in rats an increase in post-implantation loss; there was also an increase in pup deaths during the first three days of lactation (cause of death unknown) and a decrease in pup birth weights. These findings are common with CNS-active drugs at high dose levels in animals.

As the relevance of these findings to humans is not certain the use of Zispin during pregnancy is not recommended. Women of child-bearing potential should employ an adequate method of contraception if taking Zispin.

Although animal experiments show that mirtazapine is excreted only in very small amounts in the milk, the use of Zispin in nursing mothers is not recommended since no human data in breast milk are available.

4.7 Effects on ability to drive and use machines

In some patients, particularly the elderly, Zispin may have transient sedative properties and may initially impair alertness and concentration. Patients treated with Zispin should therefore be cautioned about their ability to drive a car or operate hazardous machinery.

4.8 Undesirable effects

Depressed patients display a number of symptoms that are associated with the illness itself. It is therefore sometimes difficult to ascertain which symptoms are a result of the illness itself and which are a result of treatment with Zispin.

The following adverse effects have been reported:

(see Table 2 on next page)

<u>**Withdrawal symptoms seen on discontinuation of Mirtazapine treatment**</u>

Discontinuation of mirtazapine (particularly when abrupt) commonly leads to withdrawal symptoms. Dizziness, agitation, anxiety, headache and nausea and/or vomiting are the most commonly reported reactions. Generally these events are mild to moderate and are self-limiting, however, in some patients they may be severe and/or prolonged. It is therefore advised that when mirtazapine treatment is no longer required, gradual discontinuation by dose tapering should be carried out (see section 4.2 Posology and Method of Administration and section 4.4 Special Warnings and Special Precautions for use).

4.9 Overdose

Present experience concerning overdose with Zispin alone indicates that symptoms are usually mild.

Table 2

	Rare (> 1/10,000)	Uncommon (> 1/1000)	Common (> 1/100)
Blood and the lymphatic system disorders	Reversible agranulocytosis has been reported as a rare occurrence with Zispin. (see also section 4.4 'Special warnings and special precautions for use')		
Metabolism and nutrition disorders			Increase in appetite and weight gain
Psychiatric disorders	Nightmares/vivid dreams Psychomotor restlessness* (see section 4.4 Special Warnings and Special Precautions for Use)		
Nervous system disorders	Mania, convulsions (insults), tremor, myoclonus. There have been rare reports of agitation and hallucinations although these symptoms may be related to underlying disease. Paraesthesia	Dizziness, Headache	
Cardiac disorders	(Orthostatic) hypotension.		
Hepato-biliary disorders		Increases in liver enzyme levels	
Skin and subcutaneous tissue disorders	Rash		
Musculoskeletal, connective tissue and bone disorders	Restless legs, Arthralgia/ myalgia		
General disorders			Generalised or local oedema. Drowsiness/ sedation/ fatigue, generally occurring during the first few weeks of treatment. (N.B. dose reduction generally does not lead to less sedation but can jeopardise antidepressant efficacy)

* Including akathisia

Depression of the central nervous system with disorientation and prolonged sedation have been reported, together with tachycardia and mild hyper- or hypotension.

Cases of overdose should be treated by gastric lavage with appropriate symptomatic and supportive therapy for vital functions.

5. PHARMACOLOGICAL PROPERTIES

Zispin (mirtazapine) is an antidepressant, which can be given as treatment for episodes of major depression. The presence of symptoms such as anhedonia, psychomotor inhibition, sleep disturbances (early wakening) and weight loss, increase the chance of a positive response. Other symptoms are: loss of interest, suicidal thoughts and changes in mood (better in the evening than in the morning). Zispin begins to exert its effect in general after 1-2 weeks of treatment.

5.1 Pharmacodynamic properties

Pharmacotherapeutic group: Antidepressant

(ATC code: NO6AX11)

Mirtazapine is a centrally active presynaptic α2-antagonist, which increases central noradrenergic and serotonergic neurotransmission. The enhancement of serotonergic neurotransmission is specifically mediated via 5-HT1 receptors, because 5-HT2 and 5-HT3 receptors are blocked by mirtazapine. Both enantiomers of mirtazapine are presumed to contribute to the antidepressant activity, the S(+) enantiomer by blocking α2 and 5-HT2 receptors and the R(-) enantiomer by blocking 5-HT3 receptors.

The histamine H1-antagonistic activity of mirtazapine is responsible for its sedative properties. Mirtazapine is generally well tolerated. It has practically no anticholinergic activity and, at therapeutic doses, has practically no effect on the cardiovascular system.

Dose response

No formal clinical trials were conducted investigating the dose response of mirtazapine. However, it is clinical experience that up-titrating the dose might be beneficial for some patients.

5.2 Pharmacokinetic properties

After oral administration of Zispin tablets, the active constituent mirtazapine is rapidly and well absorbed (bioavailability 50%), reaching peak plasma levels after about 2 hours. Binding of mirtazapine to plasma proteins is approx. 85%. The mean half-life of elimination is 20-40 hours; longer half-lives, up to 65 hours, have occasionally been recorded and shorter half-lives have been seen in young men. The half-life of elimination is sufficient to justify once-a-day dosing. Steady state is reached after 3-4 days, after which there is no further accumulation. Mirtazapine displays linear pharmacokinetics within the recommended dose range. Food intake has no influence on the pharmacokinetics of mirtazapine. Mirtazapine is extensively metabolised and eliminated via the urine and faeces within a few days. Major pathways of biotransformation are demethylation and oxidation, followed by conjugation. In vitro data from human liver microsomes indicate that cytochrome P450 enzymes CYP2D6 and CYP1A2 are involved in the formation of the 8-hydroxy metabolite of mirtazapine, whereas CYP3A4 is considered to be responsible for the formation of the N-demethyl and N-oxide metabolites. The demethyl metabolite is pharmacologically active and appears to have the same pharmacokinetic profile as the parent compound. There are no differences in the pharmacokinetic parameters of racemic mirtazapine or its demethyl metabolite in extensive and poor metabolisers. Plasma metabolite profiles for the individual enantiomers are qualitatively similar in extensive and poor metabolisers.

The clearance of mirtazapine may be decreased as a result of renal or hepatic insufficiency.

5.3 Preclinical safety data

No special particulars.

6. PHARMACEUTICAL PARTICULARS

6.1 List of excipients

Sugar spheres, hydroxypropyl methylcellulose, polyvinylpyrrolidone (povidone), magnesium stearate, aminoalkyl methacrylate copolymer E, aspartame (contains 5.2 mg phenylalanine), citric acid, crospovidone, mannitol, microcrystalline cellulose, natural and artificial orange flavour and sodium bicarbonate.

6.2 Incompatibilities

Not known.

6.3 Shelf life

The shelf life for Zispin SolTab is 3 years. Zispin SolTab should not be used after the expiry date indicated on the package.

6.4 Special precautions for storage

Do not store above 30°C. Store in the original pack.

6.5 Nature and contents of container

Zispin SolTab tablets are packed in a child-resistant, peel-to-open, rigid strip, formed from a laminate of aluminium foil and plastic films sealed to a paper-based laminate of aluminium foil coated with a heat seal lacquer. Tablet pockets in the strip are separated by perforations.

The following packages are available:

- Peel-to-open strips with 6 tablets each, available in packs of 30 and 90 tablets.

6.6 Instructions for use and handling

See 4.2

7. MARKETING AUTHORISATION HOLDER

Organon Laboratories Ltd, Science Park, Milton Road, Cambridge, CB4 0FL, UK.

8. MARKETING AUTHORISATION NUMBER(S)

PL 00065/0181

9. DATE OF FIRST AUTHORISATION/RENEWAL OF THE AUTHORISATION

15th July 2003

10. DATE OF REVISION OF THE TEXT

December 2004

Ref: US Zisp 30mg SOLTAB v7.0

Zispin SolTab 45 mg

(Organon Laboratories Limited)

1. NAME OF THE MEDICINAL PRODUCT

Zispin SolTab 45 mg orodispersible tablet

2. QUALITATIVE AND QUANTITATIVE COMPOSITION

Each tablet contains 45 mg of mirtazapine.

3. PHARMACEUTICAL FORM

Orodispersible tablet

The tablets are round, white, standard bevelled-edge tablets marked with the code TZ/4on one side.

4. CLINICAL PARTICULARS

4.1 Therapeutic indications

Treatment of depressive illness.

4.2 Posology and method of administration

(see Table 1 on next page)

Major Depressive Episode

Treatment should begin with 15mg daily. As with all antidepressant medicinal products, dosage should be reviewed and adjusted if necessary within 2 to 4 weeks of initiation of therapy and thereafter as judged clinically appropriate. Although there may be an increased potential for undesirable effects at higher doses, if after some weeks on the recommended dose insufficient response is seen some patients may benefit from having their dose increased gradually up to a maximum of 45mg a day (see section 5.1). Dosage adjustments should be made carefully on an individual patient basis, to maintain the patients at the lowest effective dose. If there is no response within 2-4 weeks at 45mg/day, then treatment should be stopped. Patients with depression should be treated for a sufficient period of at least 6 months to ensure that they are free from symptoms. After this, treatment can be gradually discontinued.

Elderly: The recommended dose is the same as that for adults. In elderly patients an increase in dosing should be done under close supervision to elicit a satisfactory and safe response.

Children: Since safety and efficacy of Zispin has not been established in children, it is not recommended to treat children with Zispin. Two randomised placebo- controlled trials failed to demonstrate efficacy for Zispin in the treatment of children and adolescents with major depressive disorder. Safety and efficacy of Zispin in paediatric depression can not be extrapolated from adult data.

The clearance of mirtazapine may be decreased in patients with renal or hepatic insufficiency. This should be taken into account when prescribing Zispin to this category of patients.

Mirtazapine has a half-life of 20-40 hours and therefore Zispin is suitable for once-a-day administration. It should be taken preferably as a single night-time dose before going to bed. Zispin may also be given in sub-doses equally divided over the day (once in the morning and once at night-time).

Treatment should preferably be continued until the patient has been completely symptom-free for 4-6 months. After this, treatment can be gradually discontinued. Treatment with an adequate dose should result in a positive response within 2-4 weeks. With an insufficient response, the dose can be increased up to the maximum dose. If there is no response within a further 2-4 weeks, then treatment should be stopped.

Withdrawal symptoms seen on discontinuation of Mirtazapine

Abrupt discontinuation should be avoided (see section 4.4 Special Warnings and Special Precautions for Use and section 4.8 Undesirable Effects). If intolerable symptoms occur following a decrease in the dose or upon

Table 1

In order to prevent crushing the tablet, do not push against the tablet pocket. *(Figure A)*.

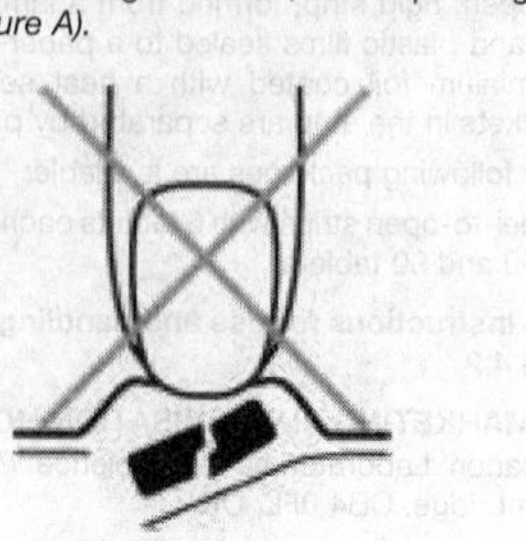

Figure A

Each strip contains six tablet pockets, which are separated by perforations. Tear off one tablet pocket along the dotted lines. *(Figure 1)*

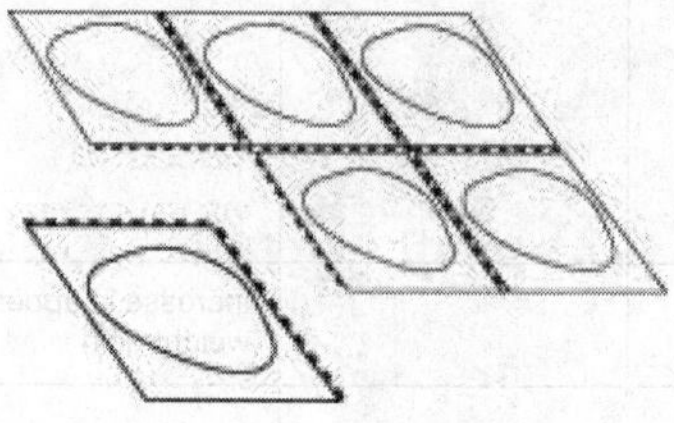

Figure 1

Carefully peel off the lidding foil, starting in the corner indicated by the arrow. *(Figures 2 and 3)*

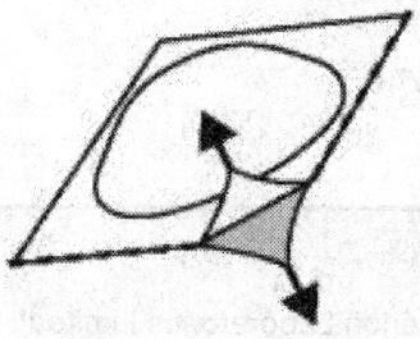

Figure 2

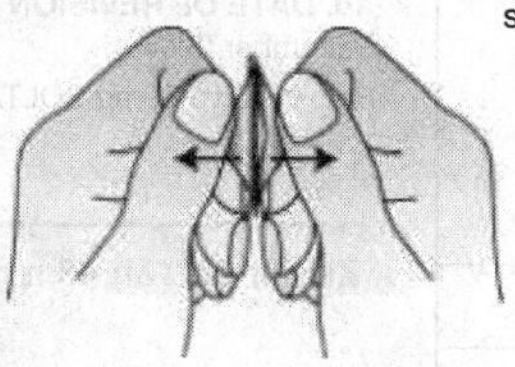

Figure 3

The tablet should be taken out of the strip with dry hands and should be placed on the tongue. *(Figure 4)* The tablet will rapidly disintegrate and can be swallowed with or without water.

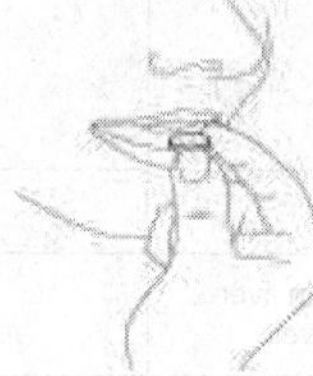

Figure 4

discontinuation of treatment, then resuming the previously prescribed dose may be considered. Subsequently, the physician may continue decreasing the dose, but at a more gradual rate.

4.3 Contraindications

Hypersensitivity to mirtazapine or any of the other ingredients of Zispin.

4.4 Special warnings and special precautions for use

Reversible white blood cell disorders including agranulocytosis, leukopenia and granulocytopenia have been reported as a rare occurence with Zispin. This mostly appears after 4-6 weeks of treatment and is in general reversible after termination of treatment. With respect to agranulocytosis the physician should be alert to symptoms such as fever, sore throat, stomatitis or other signs of infection; when such symptoms occur, treatment should be stopped and blood counts taken. Patients should also be advised of the importance of these symptoms.

Careful dosing as well as regular and close monitoring is necessary in patients with:

- epilepsy and organic brain syndrome. As with other antidepressants, mirtazapine should be introduced cautiously in patients who have a history of seizures. Treatment should be discontinued in any patient who develops seizures, or where there is an increase in seizure frequency. Antidepressants should be avoided in patients with unstable seizure disorders/epilepsy and patients with controlled epilepsy should be carefully monitored. From clinical experience it appears that insults occur rarely in patients treated with Zispin

- hepatic or renal insufficiency

- cardiac diseases like conduction disturbances, angina pectoris and recent myocardial infarct, where normal precautions should be taken and concomitant medicines carefully administered

- low blood pressure.

- diabetes mellitus. In patients with diabetes, antidepressants may alter glycaemic control. Insulin and/or oral hypoglycaemic dosage may need to be adjusted and close monitoring is recommended.

As with other antidepressants care should be taken in patients with:

- micturition disturbances like prostate hypertrophy (although problems are not to be expected because Zispin possesses only very weak anticholinergic activity)

- acute narrow-angle glaucoma and increased intra-ocular pressure (also here little chance of problems with Zispin because of its very weak anticholinergic activity)

Treatment should be discontinued if jaundice occurs.

Moreover, as with other antidepressants, the following should be taken into account:

- worsening of psychotic symptoms can occur when antidepressants are administered to patients with schizophrenia or other psychotic disturbances; paranoid thoughts can be intensified

- when the depressive phase of manic-depressive psychosis is being treated, it can transform into the manic phase

- as improvement may not occur during the first few weeks of treatment, in common with all antidepressants, patients should be closely monitored during this period. The possibility of suicide is inherent in depression, and may persist until significant remission occurs. It is general clinical experience with all therapies for depression, that the risk of suicide may increase in the early stages of recovery

- elderly patients are often more sensitive, especially with regard to the side-effects of antidepressants. During clinical research with Zispin, side-effects have not been reported more often in elderly patients than in other age groups; however, experience until now is limited

- Zispin SolTab contains aspartame a source of phenylalanine. Each tablet with 45 mg mirtazapine corresponds to 7.8 mg phenylalanine, respectively. May be harmful for patients with phenylketonuria.

-Suicide/suicidal thoughts

- Depression is associated with an increased risk of suicidal thoughts, self harm and suicide (suicide-related events). This risk persists until significant remission occurs. As improvement may not occur during the first few weeks or more of treatment, patients should be closely monitored until such improvement occurs. It is general clinical experience that the risk of self harm is highest shortly after presentation and the risk of suicide may increase again in the early stages of recovery. Furthermore, there is evidence that in a small group of people, antidepressants may increase the risk of suicidal thoughts and self-harm.

- Other psychiatric conditions for which mirtazapine is prescribed can also be associated with an increased risk of suicide-related events. In addition, these conditions may be co-morbid with major depressive disorder. The same precautions observed when treating patients with major depressive disorder should therefore be observed when treating patients with other psychiatric disorders.

- Patients with a history of suicide-related events, those exhibiting a significant degree of suicidal ideation prior to commencement of treatment, and young adults, are at a greater risk of suicidal thoughts or suicide attempts, and should receive careful monitoring during treatment.

- Patients, (and caregivers of patients) should be alerted about the need to monitor for the emergence of suicidal thoughts and to seek medical advice immediately if these symptoms present

Psychomotor restlessness

The use of mirtazapine has been associated with the development of psychomotor restlessness, which clinically may be very similar to akathisia, characterised by a subjectively unpleasant or distressing restlessness and need to move often accompanied by an inability to sit or stand still. This is most likely to occur within the first few weeks of treatment. In patients who develop these symptoms, increasing the dose may be detrimental and it may be necessary to review the use of mirtazapine.

Withdrawal symptoms seen on discontinuation of mirtazapine treatment

Withdrawal symptoms when treatment is discontinued are common, particularly if discontinuation is abrupt (see section 4.8 Undesirable effects). In clinical trials adverse events seen on treatment discontinuation occurred in approximately 15% of patients treated with mirtazapine. The risk of withdrawal symptoms may be dependent on several factors including the duration and dose of therapy and the rate of dose reduction.

Dizziness, agitation, anxiety, headache and nausea and/or vomiting are the most commonly reported reactions. Generally these symptoms are mild to moderate, however, in some patients they may be severe in intensity. They usually occur within the first few days of discontinuing treatment, but there have been very rare reports of such symptoms in patients who have inadvertently missed a dose. Generally these symptoms are self-limiting and usually resolve within 2 weeks, though in some individuals they may be prolonged (2-3 months or more). It is therefore advised that mirtazapine should be gradually tapered when discontinuing treatment over a period of several weeks, according to the patient's needs (see "Withdrawal Symptoms Seen on Discontinuation of Mirtazapine", Section 4.2 Posology and Method of Administration).

4.5 Interaction with other medicinal products and other forms of Interaction

- Mirtazapine may potentiate the central nervous dampening action of alcohol; patients should therefore be advised to avoid alcohol during treatment with Zispin.

- Zispin should not be administered concomitantly with MAO inhibitors or within two weeks of cessation of therapy with these agents.

- Mirtazapine may potentiate the sedative effects of benzodiazepines; caution should be taken when these drugs are prescribed together with Zispin.

- In vitro data suggest that mirtazapine is a very weak competitive inhibitor of the cytochrome P450 enzymes CYP1A2, CYP2D6 and CYP3A.

- Caution is needed when strong CYP3A4 inhibitors, such as the HIV protease inhibitors, azole antifungals, erythromycin and nefazodone are co-administered with mirtazapine.

- Co-administration of the potent inhibitor of CYP3A4, ketoconazole increased the peak plasma levels and AUC by approximately 30 and 45% respectively.

- Carbamazepine, an inducer of CYP3A4, increased mirtazapine clearance about twofold, resulting in a decrease in plasma levels of 45-60%. Phenytoin increased the clearance of mirtazapine in a similar fashion. When carbamazepine or another inducer of drug metabolism (such as rifampicin) is added to mirtazapine therapy, the mirtazapine dose may have to be increased. If treatment with an inducer is stopped, mirtazapine dosing may have to be decreased.

- Bioavailability of mirtazapine increased by more than 50% when co-administered with cimetidine. The mirtazapine dose may have to be decreased when concomitant treatment with cimetidine is started or increased when cimetidine treatment is ended.

- Mirtazapine caused a small but clinically insignificant increase in INR in subjects treated with warfarin.

-Absence of interactions

- In *in vivo* interaction studies, mirtazapine did not influence the pharmacokinetics of risperidone or paroxetine (CYP2D6 substrate), carbamazepine (CYP3A4 substrate), amitriptyline and cimetidine.

- No relevant clinical effects or changes in pharmacokinetics have been observed in man with concurrent administration of mirtazapine and lithium.

- A number of clinical interaction studies, and a study of mirtazapine treatment following mirtazapine treatment failure have been performed with mirtazapine and SSRIs. Until now no clinical interactions, pharmacodynamic or pharmacokinetic, have been encountered.

4.6 Pregnancy and lactation

The safety of Zispin in human pregnancy has not been established.

Reproduction studies in pregnant rats and rabbits at doses up to 100 mg/kg and 40 mg/kg (approx. 3 and 5 times respectively the maximum recommended human dose on the basis of exposure) have revealed no evidence of teratogenic effects. There was, however, in rats an increase in post-implantation loss; there was also an increase in pup deaths during the first three days of lactation (cause of death unknown) and a decrease in pup birth weights. These findings are common with CNS-active drugs at high dose levels in animals.

As the relevance of these findings to humans is not certain the use of Zispin during pregnancy is not recommended. Women of child-bearing potential should employ an adequate method of contraception if taking Zispin.

Although animal experiments show that mirtazapine is excreted only in very small amounts in the milk, the use of Zispin in nursing mothers is not recommended since no human data in breast milk are available.

4.7 Effects on ability to drive and use machines

In some patients, particularly the elderly, Zispin may have transient sedative properties and may initially impair alertness and concentration. Patients treated with Zispin should therefore be cautioned about their ability to drive a car or operate hazardous machinery.

4.8 Undesirable effects

Depressed patients display a number of symptoms that are associated with the illness itself. It is therefore sometimes difficult to ascertain which symptoms are a result of the illness itself and which are a result of treatment with Zispin.

The following adverse effects have been reported:

(see Table 2 below)

Withdrawal symptoms seen on discontinuation of Mirtazapine treatment

Discontinuation of mirtazapine (particularly when abrupt) commonly leads to withdrawal symptoms. Dizziness, agitation, anxiety, headache and nausea and/or vomiting are the most commonly reported reactions. Generally these events are mild to moderate and are self-limiting, however, in some patients they may be severe and/or prolonged. It is therefore advised that when mirtazapine treatment is no longer required, gradual discontinuation by dose tapering should be carried out (see section 4.2 Posology and Method of Administration and section 4.4 Special Warnings and Special Precautions for use).

4.9 Overdose

Present experience concerning overdose with Zispin alone indicates that symptoms are usually mild.

Depression of the central nervous system with disorientation and prolonged sedation have been reported, together with tachycardia and mild hyper- or hypotension.

Cases of overdose should be treated by gastric lavage with appropriate symptomatic and supportive therapy for vital functions.

5. PHARMACOLOGICAL PROPERTIES

Zispin (mirtazapine) is an antidepressant, which can be given as treatment for episodes of major depression. The presence of symptoms such as anhedonia, psychomotor inhibition, sleep disturbances (early wakening) and weight loss, increase the chance of a positive response. Other symptoms are: loss of interest, suicidal thoughts and changes in mood (better in the evening than in the morning). Zispin begins to exert its effect in general after 1-2 weeks of treatment.

5.1 Pharmacodynamic properties

Pharmacotherapeutic group: Antidepressant

(ATC code: NO6AX11)

Mirtazapine is a centrally active presynaptic α_2-antagonist, which increases central noradrenergic and serotonergic neurotransmission. The enhancement of serotonergic neurotransmission is specifically mediated via 5-HT_1 receptors, because 5-HT_2 and

5-HT_3 receptors are blocked by mirtazapine. Both enantiomers of mirtazapine are presumed to contribute to the antidepressant activity, the S(+) enantiomer by blocking α_2 and 5-HT_2 receptors and the R(-) enantiomer by blocking 5-HT_3 receptors.

The histamine H_1-antagonistic activity of mirtazapine is responsible for its sedative properties. Mirtazapine is generally well tolerated. It has practically no anticholinergic activity and, at therapeutic doses, has practically no effect on the cardiovascular system.

Dose response

No formal clinical trials were conducted investigating the dose response of mirtazapine. However, it is clinical experience that up-titrating the dose might be beneficial for some patients.

5.2 Pharmacokinetic properties

After oral administration of Zispin tablets, the active constituent mirtazapine is rapidly and well absorbed (bioavailability 50%), reaching peak plasma levels after about 2 hours. Binding of mirtazapine to plasma proteins is approx. 85%. The mean half-life of elimination is 20-40 hours; longer half-lives, up to 65 hours, have occasionally been recorded and shorter half-lives have been seen in young men. The half-life of elimination is sufficient to justify once-a-day dosing. Steady state is reached after 3-4 days, after which there is no further accumulation. Mirtazapine displays linear pharmacokinetics within the recommended dose range. Food intake has no influence on the pharmacokinetics of mirtazapine. Mirtazapine is extensively metabolised and eliminated via the urine and faeces within a few days. Major pathways of biotransformation are demethylation and oxidation, followed by conjugation. In vitro data from human liver microsomes indicate that cytochrome P450 enzymes CYP2D6 and CYP1A2 are involved in the formation of the 8-hydroxy metabolite of mirtazapine, whereas CYP3A4 is considered to be responsible for the formation of the N-demethyl and N-oxide metabolites. The demethyl metabolite is pharmacologically active and appears to have the same pharmacokinetic profile as the parent compound. There are no differences in the pharmacokinetic parameters of racemic mirtazapine or its demethyl metabolite in extensive and poor metabolisers. Plasma metabolite profiles for the individual enantiomers are qualitatively similar in extensive and poor metabolisers.

The clearance of mirtazapine may be decreased as a result of renal or hepatic insufficiency.

5.3 Preclinical safety data

No special particulars.

6. PHARMACEUTICAL PARTICULARS

6.1 List of excipients

Sugar spheres, hydroxypropyl methylcellulose, polyvinylpyrrolidone (povidone), magnesium stearate, aminoalkyl methacrylate copolymer E, aspartame (contains 7.8 mg phenylalanine), citric acid, crospovidone, mannitol, microcrystalline cellulose, natural and artificial orange flavour and sodium bicarbonate.

6.2 Incompatibilities

Not known.

6.3 Shelf life

The shelf life for Zispin SolTab is 3 years. Zispin SolTab should not be used after the expiry date indicated on the package.

6.4 Special precautions for storage

Do not store above 30°C. Store in the original pack.

6.5 Nature and contents of container

Zispin SolTab tablets are packed in a child-resistant, peel-to-open, rigid strip, formed from a laminate of aluminium foil and plastic films sealed to a paper-based laminate of aluminium foil coated with a heat seal lacquer. Tablet pockets in the strip are separated by perforations.

The following packages are available:

- Peel-to-open strips with 6 tablets each, available in packs of 30 and 90 tablets.

6.6 Instructions for use and handling

See 4.2

7. MARKETING AUTHORISATION HOLDER

Organon Laboratories Ltd, Science Park, Milton Road, Cambridge, CB4 0FL, UK.

8. MARKETING AUTHORISATION NUMBER(S)

PL 00065/0182

9. DATE OF FIRST AUTHORISATION/RENEWAL OF THE AUTHORISATION

15th July 2003

10. DATE OF REVISION OF THE TEXT

December 2004

Ref: US Zisp 45mg SOLTAB v7.0

Table 2

	Rare >1/10,000)	Uncommon>1/1000)	Common >1/100)
Blood and the lymphatic system disorders	Reversible agranulocytosis has been reported as a rare occurrence with Zispin. (see also section 4.4 'Special warnings and special precautions for use')		
Metabolism and nutrition disorders			Increase in appetite and weight gain
Psychiatric disorders	Nightmares/vivid dreams Psychomotor restlessness* (see section 4.4 Special Warnings and Special Precautions for Use)		
Nervous system disorders	Mania, convulsions (insults), tremor, myoclonus. There have been rare reports of agitation and hallucinations although these symptoms may be related to underlying disease. Paraesthesia	Dizziness, Headache	
Cardiac disorders	(Orthostatic) hypotension.		
Hepato-biliary disorders		Increases in liver enzyme levels	
Skin and subcutaneous tissue disorders	Rash		
Musculoskeletal, connective tissue and bone disorders	Restless legs, Arthralgia/ myalgia		
General disorders			Generalised or local oedema. Drowsiness/ sedation/ fatigue, generally occurring during the first few weeks of treatment. (N.B. dose reduction generally does not lead to less sedation but can jeopardise antidepressant efficacy)

* Including akathisia

Zithromax Capsules, Suspension

(Pfizer Limited)

1. NAME OF THE MEDICINAL PRODUCT

ZITHROMAX(TM) CAPSULES ZITHROMAX(TM) SUSPENSION

2. QUALITATIVE AND QUANTITATIVE COMPOSITION

Active ingredient: azithromycin.

Zithromax Capsules contain azithromycin dihydrate equivalent to 250mg azithromycin.

Zithromax Powder for Oral Suspension is a dry blend of azithromycin dihydrate containing the equivalent of 200mg azithromycin per 5ml on reconstitution with water.

3. PHARMACEUTICAL FORM

Zithromax Capsules are white, hard gelatin capsules marked Pfizer and ZTM 250.

Zithromax Powder for Oral Suspension is a dry powder which reconstitutes with water to give a cherry/banana flavoured suspension with a slight vanilla odour.

4. CLINICAL PARTICULARS

4.1 Therapeutic indications

Zithromax is indicated for infections caused by susceptible organisms; in lower respiratory tract infections including bronchitis and pneumonia, skin and soft tissue infections, otitis media and in upper respiratory tract infections including sinusitis and pharyngitis/tonsillitis.

In sexually transmitted diseases in men and women, Zithromax is indicated in the treatment of uncomplicated genital infections due to *Chlamydia trachomatis*.

4.2 Posology and method of administration

Zithromax should be given as a single daily dose. In common with many other antibiotics Zithromax Capsules should be taken at least 1 hour before or 2 hours after food.

Zithromax Suspension can be taken with food.

Adults: For the treatment of sexually transmitted diseases caused by *Chlamydia trachomatis*, the dose is 1g given as a single dose.

For all other indications, the dose is 1.5g, which should be given as 500mg daily for 3 days.

In the elderly: The same dose range as in younger patients may be used in the elderly.

In children: Zithromax Suspension should be used for children under 45kg. There is no information on children under 6 months of age. The dose in children is 10mg/kg as a single daily dose for 3 days:

Up to 15kg: Measure the dose as closely as possible using the 10ml oral dosing

(less than syringe provided. The syringe is graduated in 0.25ml divisions,

3 years) providing 10mg of azithromycin in every graduation.

For children weighing more than 15kg, Zithromax Suspension should be administered using the spoon provided according to the following guidance:

15-25 kg: 5ml (200mg) given as 1 × 5ml spoonful, once daily for 3 days.

(3-7 years)

26-35 kg: 7.5ml (300mg) given as 1 × 7.5ml spoonful, once daily for 3 days.

(8-11 years)

36-45 kg: 10ml (400mg) given as 1 × 10ml spoonful, once daily for 3 days.

(12-14 years)

Over 45 kg: Dose as per adults.

See Nature and contents of container, section 6.5, for appropriate pack size to use depending on age/body weight of child.

The specially supplied measure should be used to administer Zithromax suspension to children.

In patients with renal impairment: No dose adjustment is necessary in patients with mild to moderate (GFR 10 - 80 ml/min) or severe (GFR < 10 ml/min) renal impairment (see section 4.4 - **Special Warnings and Precautions for Use**).

In patients with hepatic impairment: See Special warnings and special precautions for use, section 4.4.

Zithromax Capsules and Zithromax Suspension are for oral administration only.

4.3 Contraindications

Zithromax is contra-indicated in patients with a known hypersensitivity to azithromycin or any of the macrolide antibiotics.

Because of the theoretical possibility of ergotism, Zithromax and ergot derivatives should not be coadministered.

4.4 Special warnings and special precautions for use

As with erythromycin and other macrolides, rare serious allergic reactions including angioneurotic oedema and anaphylaxis (rarely fatal), have been reported. Some of these reactions with Zithromax have resulted in recurrent symptoms and required a longer period of observation and treatment.

Prolonged cardiac repolarisation and QT interval, imparting a risk of developing cardiac arrhythmia and torsades de pointes, have been seen in treatment with other macrolides. A similar effect with azithromycin cannot be completely ruled out in patients at increased risk for prolonged cardiac repolarisation (see section 4.8 Undesirable Effects).

As with any antibiotic preparation, observation for signs of superinfection with non-susceptible organisms, including fungi is recommended.

Use in renal impairment: In patients with severe renal impairment (GFR <10 ml/min) a 33% increase in systemic exposure to azithromycin was observed (see section 5.2 - **Pharmacokinetic Properties**).

Use in hepatic impairment: As the liver is the principal route of excretion of azithromycin, it should not be used in patients with hepatic disease.

4.5 Interaction with other medicinal products and other forms of Interaction

Antacids: In patients receiving Zithromax and antacids, Zithromax should be taken at least 1 hour before or 2 hours after the antacid.

Carbamazepine: In a pharmacokinetic interaction study in healthy volunteers, no significant effect was observed on the plasma levels of carbamazepine or its active metabolite.

Cimetidine: A single dose of cimetidine administered 2 hours before Zithromax had no effect on the pharmacokinetics of azithromycin.

Cyclosporin: In a pharmacokinetic study with healthy volunteers that were administered a 500 mg/day oral dose of azithromycin for 3 days and were then administered a single 10 mg/kg oral dose of cyclosporin, the resulting cyclosporin C_{max} and AUC_{0-5} were found to be significantly elevated (by 24% and 21% respectively), however no significant changes were seen in $AUC_{0-\infty}$. Consequently, caution should be exercised before considering coadministration of these two drugs. If coadministration is necessary, cyclosporin levels should be monitored and the dose adjusted accordingly.

Digoxin: Some of the macrolide antibiotics have been reported to impair the metabolism of digoxin (in the gut) in some patients. Therefore, in patients receiving concomitant Zithromax and digoxin the possibility of raised digoxin levels should be borne in mind, and digoxin levels monitored.

Ergot derivatives: Because of the theoretical possibility of ergotism, Zithromax and ergot derivatives should not be coadministered.

Methylprednisolone: In a pharmacokinetic interaction study in healthy volunteers, Zithromax had no significant effect on the pharmacokinetics of methylprednisolone.

Terfenadine: Because of the occurrence of serious dysrhythmias secondary to prolongation of the QTc interval in patients receiving other anti-infectives in conjunction with terfenadine, pharmacokinetic interaction studies have been performed. These studies have reported no evidence of an interaction between azithromycin and terfenadine. There have been rare cases reported where the possibility of such an interaction could not be entirely excluded; however there was no specific evidence that such an interaction had occurred. As with other macrolides, Zithromax should be administered with caution in combination with terfenadine.

Theophylline: Theophylline levels may be increased in patients taking Zithromax.

Coumarin-Type Oral Anticoagulants: In a pharmacodynamic interaction study, Zithromax did not alter the anticoagulant effect of a single 15mg dose of warfarin administered to healthy volunteers. There have been reports received in the post-marketing period of potentiated anticoagulation subsequent to coadministration of azithromycin and coumarin-type oral anticoagulants. Although a causal relationship has not been established, consideration should be given to the frequency of monitoring prothrombin time when azithromycin is used in patients receiving coumarin-type oral anticoagulants.

Zidovudine: Single 1000mg doses and multiple 1200mg or 600mg doses of azithromycin did not affect the plasma pharmacokinetics or urinary excretion of zidovudine or its glucuronide metabolite. However, administration of azithromycin increased the concentrations of phosphorylated zidovudine, the clinically active metabolite, in peripheral blood mononuclear cells. The clinical significance of this finding is unclear, but it may be of benefit to patients.

Didanosine: Coadministration of daily doses of 1200mg azithromycin with didanosine in 6 subjects did not appear to affect the pharmacokinetics of didanosine as compared with placebo.

Rifabutin: Coadministration of azithromycin and rifabutin did not affect the serum concentrations of either drug.

Neutropenia was observed in subjects receiving concomitant treatment of azithromycin and rifabutin. Although neutropenia has been associated with the use of rifabutin, a causal relationship to combination with azithromycin has not been established (see section 4.8. Undesirable effects).

4.6 Pregnancy and lactation

Use in pregnancy: Animal reproduction studies have demonstrated that azithromycin crosses the placenta, but have revealed no evidence of harm to the foetus. There are no adequate and well controlled studies in pregnant women. Since animal studies are not always predictive of human response, Zithromax should be used during pregnancy only if adequate alternatives are not available.

Use in lactation: No data on secretion of azithromycin in breast milk are available, so that Zithromax should only be used in lactating women where adequate alternatives are not available.

4.7 Effects on ability to drive and use machines

There is no evidence to suggest that Zithromax may have an effect on a patient's ability to drive or operate machinery.

4.8 Undesirable effects

Zithromax is well tolerated with a low incidence of side effects.

Infections and Infestations: Moniliasis and vaginitis

Blood and Lymphatic System Disorders: Thrombocytopenia. Transient mild reductions in neutrophil counts have occasionally been observed in clinical trials.

Immune system disorders: Anaphylaxis (rarely fatal) (see Special Warnings and Special Precautions for Use, Section 4.4)

Metabolism and nutrition disorders: Anorexia

Psychiatric Disorders: Aggressive reaction, nervousness, agitation and anxiety.

Nervous System Disorders: Dizziness, convulsions (as seen with other macrolides), headache, somnolence, parasthesia, hyperactivity and syncope.

There have been rare reports of taste perversion.

Ear and Labyrinth Disorders: Vertigo, hearing impairment has been reported with macrolide antibiotics. There have been reports of hearing impairment, including hearing loss, deafness and/or tinnitus in some patients receiving azithromycin. Many of these have been associated with prolonged use of high doses in investigational studies. In those cases where follow-up information were available the majority of these events was reversible.

Cardiac Disorders: Palpitations and arrythmias including ventricular tachycardia (as seen with macrolides) have been reported. There have been rare reports of QT prolongation and torsades de pointes (see section 4.4 Special Warnings and Special Precautions for Use).

Vascular Disorders: Hypotension

Gastrointestinal Disorders: Nausea, vomiting/diarrhoea (rarely resulting in dehydration), loose stools, dyspepsia, abdominal discomfort (pain/cramps), constipation, flatulence, pseudomembranous colitis, pancreatitis and rare reports of tongue discoloration.

Hepatobiliary Disorders: Abnormal liver function including hepatitis and cholestatic jaundice have been reported, as well as rare cases of hepatic necrosis and hepatic failure, which have rarely resulted in death.

Skin and Subcutaneous Tissue Disorders: Allergic reactions including, pruritus, rash, photosensitivity, oedema, urticaria and angioedema (see Special Warnings and Special Precautions for Use, Section 4.4).

Rarely, serious skin reactions including erythema multiforme, Stevens Johnson Syndrome and toxic epidermal necrolysis have occurred.

Musculoskeletal and Connective Tissue Disorders: Arthralgia

Renal and Urinary Disorders: Interstitial nephritis and acute renal failure.

General Disorders and Administration Site Conditions: Asthenia, fatigue and malaise have been reported.

4.9 Overdose

Adverse events experienced in higher than recommended doses were similar to those seen at normal doses. In the event of overdosage, general symptomatic and supportive measures are indicated as required.

5. PHARMACOLOGICAL PROPERTIES

5.1 Pharmacodynamic properties

Zithromax is an azalide, derived from the macrolide class of antibiotics. The mode of action of azithromycin is inhibition of protein synthesis in bacteria by binding to the 50s ribosomal subunit and preventing translocation of peptides.

Azithromycin demonstrates activity *in vitro* against a wide variety of Gram-positive and Gram-negative bacteria including: *Staphylococcus aureus, Streptococcus pneumoniae, Streptococcus pyogenes* (Group A) and other Streptococcal species; *Haemophilus influenzae* and *parainfluenzae*; *Branhamella catarrhalis*; anaerobes including *Bacteroides fragilis; Escherichia coli; Bordetella pertussis; Bordetella parapertussis; Borrelia burgdorferi; Haemophilus ducreyi; Neisseria gonorrhoeae* and *Chlamydia trachomatis*. Azithromycin also demonstrates *in vitro* activity against *Legionella pneumophila, Mycoplasma pneumoniae* and *hominis*, Campylobacter sp., *Toxoplasma gondii* and *Treponema pallidum*.

5.2 Pharmacokinetic properties

Following oral administration in humans, azithromycin is widely distributed throughout the body; bioavailability is approximately 37%. The time taken to peak plasma levels is 2-3 hours. The plasma terminal elimination half-life closely reflects the tissue depletion half-life of 2 to 4 days.

Kinetic studies have shown markedly higher azithromycin levels in tissue than in plasma (up to 50 times the maximum observed concentration in plasma) indicating that the drug is heavily tissue bound. Concentrations in target tissues such as lung, tonsil, and prostate exceed the MIC90 for likely pathogens after a single dose of 500 mg.

Following a single dose of azithromycin 1 gram orally, the pharmacokinetics in subjects with mild to moderate renal impairment (GFR 10 - 80 ml/min) were not affected. Statistically significant differences in AUC_{0-120} (8.8 μg*hr/ml vs. 11.7 μg*hr/ml), C_{max} (1.0 μg/ml vs. 1.6 μg/ml) and CLr (2.3 ml/min/kg vs. 0.2 ml/min/kg) were observed between the group with normal renal function and the group with severe renal impairment (GFR < 10 ml/min).

6. PHARMACEUTICAL PARTICULARS

6.1 List of excipients

Zithromax Capsules contain: Lactose, magnesium stearate, maize starch, and sodium lauryl sulphate. The capsule shells contain: Gelatin, iron oxide-black (E172), shellac, sulphur dioxide and titanium dioxide.

Zithromax Powder for Oral Suspension contains: Hydroxypropylcellulose, sodium phosphate tribasic anhydrous, sucrose, xanthan gum. Flavours: artificial banana, artificial cherry, artificial creme de vanilla.

6.2 Incompatibilities

None known

6.3 Shelf life

Zithromax Capsules 60 months.

Powder for Oral Suspension 3 years.

Once reconstituted with water, Zithromax Suspension has a shelf-life of 5 days.

6.4 Special precautions for storage

No special storage conditions required.

6.5 Nature and contents of container

Zithromax Capsules are available as:

Packs of 4 capsules. Aluminium/PVC blister strips, 4 capsules per strip, 1 strip in a carton box.

Pack of 6 capsules. Aluminium/PVC blister strips, 6 capsules per strip, 1 strip in a carton box.

Zithromax Powder for Oral Suspension is available as:

600mg (15ml) Pack: (Recommended for use in children up to 7 years (25kg)).

Packs of powder equivalent to 600mg azithromycin in a polypropylene container with child resistant screw cap (with or without a tamper evident seal), in a carton box. Pack contains a double-ended multi-dosing spoon and 10ml oral dosing syringe with detachable adaptor. A sticker for the syringe is appended to the bottle label. Reconstitute with 9ml of water to give 15ml suspension.

900mg (22.5ml) Pack: (Recommended for use in children aged from 8-11 years (26-35kg)). Packs of powder equivalent to 900mg azithromycin in a polypropylene container with child resistant screw cap (with or without a tamper evident seal), in a carton box. Pack contains a double-ended multi-dosing spoon. Reconstitute with 12ml of water to give 22.5ml suspension.

1200mg (30ml) Pack:(Recommended for use in children aged from 12-14 years (36-45kg)). Packs of powder equivalent to 1200mg azithromycin in a polypropylene container with child resistant screw cap (with or without a tamper evident seal), in a carton box. Pack contains a double-ended multi-dosing spoon. Reconstitute with 15ml of water to give 30ml suspension.

Multi-dosing spoon delivers doses as follows:

Small end to graduation 2.5ml (100mg)

brimful 5ml (200mg)

Large end to graduation 7.5ml (300mg)

brimful 10ml (400mg)

Each pack contains a Patient information/instruction leaflet.

6.6 Instructions for use and handling
When dispensing the 15ml pack, advice should be given as to whether the dose should be measured using the oral dosing syringe or the spoon provided and on correct usage.

If the dose is to be given using the oral dosing syringe, before dispensing, the syringe adaptor should be detached from the syringe and inserted into the bottle neck and the cap replaced.

The sticker provided should be used to mark the syringe at the appropriate level once the correct daily dosage has been calculated.

When dispensing 22.5ml and 30ml packs, advice should be given as to the correct usage of the multi-dosing spoon.

Zithromax Capsules should be swallowed whole.

7. MARKETING AUTHORISATION HOLDER
Pfizer Limited
Ramsgate Road
Sandwich
Kent CT13 9NJ
United Kingdom

8. MARKETING AUTHORISATION NUMBER(S)
Zithromax Capsules 250mg PL0057/0335

Zithromax Powder for Oral Suspension 200mg/5ml PL0057/0336

9. DATE OF FIRST AUTHORISATION/RENEWAL OF THE AUTHORISATION
Zithromax Capsules 250mg: 4 April 1996

Zithromax Powder for Oral Suspension 200mg/5ml: 4 April 1996

10. DATE OF REVISION OF THE TEXT
July 2004

11. LEGAL CATEGORY
POM

ZX_10.0

Zocor

(Merck Sharp & Dohme Limited)

1. NAME OF THE MEDICINAL PRODUCT
Zocor 10 mg, film-coated tablets.

Zocor 20 mg, film-coated tablets.

Zocor 40 mg, film-coated tablets.

Zocor 80 mg, film-coated tablets.

2. QUALITATIVE AND QUANTITATIVE COMPOSITION
Each tablet contains 10 mg of simvastatin.

Each tablet contains 20 mg of simvastatin.

Each tablet contains 40 mg of simvastatin.

Each tablet contains 80 mg of simvastatin.

For excipients, see section 6.1.

3. PHARMACEUTICAL FORM
Film-coated tablet.

The peach-coloured, oval-shaped tablets marked 'Zocor 10' contain 10 mg simvastatin. The tan-coloured, oval-shaped tablets marked 'Zocor 20' contain 20 mg simvastatin. The brick-red coloured, oval-shaped tablets marked 'MSD 749' contain 40 mg simvastatin. The brick-red coloured, capsule-shaped tablets marked '543' on one side and '80' on the other contain 80 mg simvastatin.

4. CLINICAL PARTICULARS
4.1 Therapeutic indications
Hypercholesterolaemia

Treatment of primary hypercholesterolaemia or mixed dyslipidaemia, as an adjunct to diet, when response to diet and other non-pharmacological treatments (e.g. exercise, weight reduction) is inadequate.

Treatment of homozygous familial hypercholesterolaemia as an adjunct to diet and other lipid-lowering treatments (e.g. LDL apheresis) or if such treatments are not appropriate.

Cardiovascular prevention

Reduction of cardiovascular mortality and morbidity in patients with manifest atherosclerotic cardiovascular disease or diabetes mellitus, with either normal or increased cholesterol levels, as an adjunct to correction of other risk factors and other cardioprotective therapy (see section 5.1).

4.2 Posology and method of administration
The dosage range is 5-80 mg/day given orally as a single dose in the evening. Adjustments of dosage, if required, should be made at intervals of not less than 4 weeks, to a maximum of 80 mg/day given as a single dose in the evening. The 80-mg dose is only recommended in patients with severe hypercholesterolaemia and high risk for cardiovascular complications.

Hypercholesterolaemia

The patient should be placed on a standard cholesterol-lowering diet, and should continue on this diet during treatment with 'Zocor'. The usual starting dose is 10-20 mg/day given as a single dose in the evening. Patients who require a large reduction in LDL-C (more than 45 %) may be started at 20-40 mg/day given as a single dose in the evening. Adjustments of dosage, if required, should be made as specified above.

Homozygous familial hypercholesterolaemia

Based on the results of a controlled clinical study, the recommended dosage is 'Zocor' 40 mg/day in the evening or 80 mg/day in 3 divided doses of 20 mg, 20 mg, and an evening dose of 40 mg. 'Zocor' should be used as an adjunct to other lipid-lowering treatments (e.g., LDL apheresis) in these patients or if such treatments are unavailable.

Cardiovascular prevention

The usual dose of 'Zocor' is 20 to 40 mg/day given as a single dose in the evening in patients at high risk of coronary heart disease (CHD, with or without hyperlipidaemia). Drug therapy can be initiated simultaneously with diet and exercise. Adjustments of dosage, if required, should be made as specified above.

Concomitant therapy

'Zocor' is effective alone or in combination with bile acid sequestrants. Dosing should occur either > 2 hours before or > 4 hours after administration of a bile acid sequestrant.

In patients taking cyclosporine, gemfibrozil, other fibrates (except fenofibrate) or lipid-lowering doses (⩾ 1 g/day) of niacin concomitantly with 'Zocor', the dose of 'Zocor' should not exceed 10 mg/day. In patients taking amiodarone orverapamil concomitantly with 'Zocor', the dose of 'Zocor' should not exceed 20 mg/day. (See sections 4.4 and 4.5.)

Dosage in renal insufficiency

No modification of dosage should be necessary in patients with moderate renal insufficiency.

In patients with severe renal insufficiency (creatinine clearance < 30 ml/min), dosages above 10 mg/day should be carefully considered and, if deemed necessary, implemented cautiously.

Use in the elderly

No dosage adjustment is necessary.

Use in children and adolescents

Efficacy and safety of use in children have not been established. Therefore 'Zocor' is not recommended for paediatric use.

4.3 Contraindications

- Hypersensitivity to simvastatin or to any of the excipients
- Active liver disease or unexplained persistent elevations of serum transaminases
- Pregnancy and lactation (see section 4.6)
- Concomitant administration of potent CYP3A4 inhibitors (e.g. itraconazole, ketoconazole, HIV protease inhibitors, erythromycin, clarithromycin, telithromycin and nefazodone) (see section 4.5).

4.4 Special warnings and special precautions for use
Myopathy/Rhabdomyolysis

Simvastatin, like other inhibitors of HMG-CoA reductase, occasionally causes myopathy manifested as muscle pain, tenderness or weakness with creatine kinase (CK) above ten times the upper limit of normal (ULN). Myopathy sometimes takes the form of rhabdomyolysis with or without acute renal failure secondary to myoglobinuria, and very rare fatalities have occurred. The risk of myopathy is increased by high levels of HMG-CoA reductase inhibitory activity in plasma.

The risk of myopathy/rhabdomyolysis is dose related. The incidence in clinical trials, in which patients were carefully monitored and some interacting medicinal products were excluded, has been approximately 0.03 % at 20 mg, 0.08 % at 40 mg and 0.4 % at 80 mg.

Creatine Kinase measurement

Creatine Kinase (CK) should not be measured following strenuous exercise or in the presence of any plausible alternative cause of CK increase as this makes value interpretation difficult. If CK levels are significantly elevated at baseline (> 5 × ULN), levels should be re-measured within 5 to 7 days later to confirm the results.

Before the treatment

All patients starting therapy with simvastatin, or whose dose of simvastatin is being increased, should be advised of the risk of myopathy and told to report promptly any unexplained muscle pain, tenderness or weakness.

Caution should be exercised in patients with pre-disposing factors for rhabdomyolysis. In order to establish a reference baseline value, a CK level should be measured before starting a treatment in the following situations:

- Elderly (age > 70 years)
- Renal impairment
- Uncontrolled hypothyroidism
- Personal or familial history of hereditary muscular disorders
- Previous history of muscular toxicity with a statin or fibrate
- Alcohol abuse.

In such situations, the risk of treatment should be considered in relation to possible benefit, and clinical monitoring is recommended. If a patient has previously experienced a muscle disorder on a fibrate or a statin, treatment with a different member of the class should only be initiated with caution. If CK levels are significantly elevated at baseline (> 5 × ULN), treatment should not be started.

Whilst on treatment

If muscle pain, weakness or cramps occur whilst a patient is receiving treatment with a statin, their CK levels should be measured. If these levels are found, in the absence of strenuous exercise, to be significantly elevated (> 5 × ULN), treatment should be stopped. If muscular symptoms are severe and cause daily discomfort, even if CK levels are < 5 × ULN, treatment discontinuation may be considered. If myopathy is suspected for any other reason, treatment should be discontinued.

If symptoms resolve and CK levels return to normal, then re-introduction of the statin or introduction of an alternative statin may be considered at the lowest dose and with close monitoring.

Therapy with simvastatin should be temporarily stopped a few days prior to elective major surgery and when any major medical or surgical condition supervenes.

Measures to reduce the risk of myopathy caused by medicinal product interactions (see also section 4.5)

The risk of myopathy and rhabdomyolysis is significantly increased by concomitant use of simvastatin with potent inhibitors of CYP3A4 (such as itraconazole, ketoconazole, erythromycin, clarithromycin, telithromycin, HIV protease inhibitors, nefazodone), as well as gemfibrozil and cyclosporine (see section 4.2)

The risk of myopathy and rhabdomyolysis is also increased by concomitant use of other fibrates, lipid-lowering doses (⩾ 1 g/day) of niacin or by concomitant use of amiodarone or verapamil with higher doses of simvastatin (see sections 4.2 and 4.5). There is also a slight increase in risk when diltiazem is used with simvastatin 80 mg.

Consequently, regarding CYP3A4 inhibitors, the use of simvastatin concomitantly with itraconazole, ketoconazole, HIV protease inhibitors, erythromycin, clarithromycin, telithromycin and nefazodone is contraindicated (see sections 4.3 and 4.5). If treatment with itraconazole, ketoconazole, erythromycin, clarithromycin or telithromycin is unavoidable, therapy with simvastatin must be suspended during the course of treatment. Moreover, caution should be exercised when combining simvastatin with certain other less potent CYP3A4 inhibitors: cyclosporine, verapamil, diltiazem (see sections 4.2 and 4.5). Concomitant intake of grapefruit juice and simvastatin should be avoided.

The dose of simvastatin should not exceed 10 mg daily in patients receiving concomitant medication with cyclosporine, gemfibrozil, or lipid-lowering doses (⩾ 1 g/day) of niacin. The combined use of simvastatin with gemfibrozil should be avoided, unless the benefits are likely to outweigh the increased risks of this drug combination. The benefits of the combined use of simvastatin 10 mg daily with other fibrates (except fenofibrate), niacin or cyclosporine should be carefully weighed against the potential risks of these combinations. (See sections 4.2 and 4.5.)

Caution should be used when prescribing fenofibrate with simvastatin, as either agent can cause myopathy when given alone.

The combined use of simvastatin at doses higher than 20 mg daily with amiodarone or verapamil should be avoided unless the clinical benefit is likely to outweigh the increased risk of myopathy (see sections 4.2 and 4.5).

Hepatic effects

In clinical studies, persistent increases (to > 3 × ULN) in serum transaminases have occurred in a few adult patients who received simvastatin. When simvastatin was interrupted or discontinued in these patients, the transaminase levels usually fell slowly to pre-treatment levels.

It is recommended that liver function tests be performed before treatment begins and thereafter when clinically indicated. Patients titrated to the 80-mg dose should receive an additional test prior to titration, 3 months after titration to the 80-mg dose, and periodically thereafter (e.g., semi-annually) for the first year of treatment. Special attention should be paid to patients who develop elevated serum transaminase levels, and in these patients, measurements should be repeated promptly and then performed more frequently. If the transaminase levels show evidence of progression, particularly if they rise to 3 × ULN and are persistent, simvastatin should be discontinued.

The product should be used with caution in patients who consume substantial quantities of alcohol.

As with other lipid-lowering agents, moderate (< 3 × ULN) elevations of serum transaminases have been reported following therapy with simvastatin. These changes appeared soon after initiation of therapy with simvastatin, were often transient, were not accompanied by any symptoms and interruption of treatment was not required.

4.5 Interaction with other medicinal products and other forms of Interaction

Pharmacodynamic interactions

Interactions with lipid-lowering medicinal products that can cause myopathy when given alone

The risk of myopathy, including rhabdomyolysis, is increased during concomitant administration with fibrates and niacin (nicotinic acid) (⩾ 1 g/day). Additionally, there is a pharmacokinetic interaction with gemfibrozil resulting in increased simvastatin plasma levels (see below *Pharmacokinetic interactions* and sections 4.2 and 4.4). When simvastatin and fenofibrate are given concomitantly, there is no evidence that the risk of myopathy exceeds the sum of the individual risks of each agent. Adequate pharmacovigilance and pharmacokinetic data are not available for other fibrates.

Pharmacokinetic interactions

Effects of other medicinal products on simvastatin

Interactions involving CYP3A4

Simvastatin is a substrate of cytochrome P450 3A4. Potent inhibitors of cytochrome P450 3A4 increase the risk of myopathy and rhabdomyolysis by increasing the concentration of HMG-CoA reductase inhibitory activity in plasma during simvastatin therapy. Such inhibitors include itraconazole, ketoconazole, erythromycin, clarithromycin, telithromycin, HIV protease inhibitors, and nefazodone. Concomitant administration of itraconazole resulted in a more than 10-fold increase in exposure to simvastatin acid (the active beta-hydroxyacid metabolite). Telithromycin caused an 11-fold increase in exposure to simvastatin acid.

Therefore, combination with itraconazole, ketoconazole, HIV protease inhibitors, erythromycin, clarithromycin, telithromycin and nefazodone is contraindicated. If treatment with itraconazole, ketoconazole, erythromycin, clarithromycin or telithromycin is unavoidable, therapy with simvastatin must be suspended during the course of treatment. Caution should be exercised when combining simvastatin with certain other less potent CYP3A4 inhibitors: cyclosporine, verapamil, diltiazem (see sections 4.2 and 4.4).

Cyclosporine

The risk of myopathy/rhabdomyolysis is increased by concomitant administration of cyclosporine particularly with higher doses of simvastatin (see sections 4.2 and 4.4). Therefore, the dose of simvastatin should not exceed 10 mg daily in patients receiving concomitant medication with cyclosporine. Although the mechanism is not fully understood, cyclosporine increases the AUC of simvastatin acid presumably due, in part, to inhibition of CYP3A4.

Gemfibrozil

Gemfibrozil increases the AUC of simvastatin acid by 1.9-fold, possibly due to inhibition of the glucuronidation pathway (see sections 4.2 and 4.4).

Amiodarone and verapamil

The risk of myopathy and rhabdomyolysis is increased by concomitant administration of amiodarone or verapamil with higher doses of simvastatin (see section 4.4). In an ongoing clinical trial, myopathy has been reported in 6 % of patients receiving simvastatin 80 mg and amiodarone.

An analysis of the available clinical trials showed an approximately 1 % incidence of myopathy in patients receiving simvastatin 40 mg or 80 mg and verapamil. In a pharmacokinetic study, concomitant administration with verapamil resulted in a 2.3-fold increase in exposure of simvastatin acid, presumably due, in part, to inhibition of CYP3A4. Therefore, the dose of simvastatin should not exceed 20 mg daily in patients receiving concomitant medication with amiodarone or verapamil, unless the clinical benefit is likely to outweigh the increased risk of myopathy and rhabdomyolysis.

Diltiazem

An analysis of the available clinical trials showed a 1 % incidence of myopathy in patients receiving simvastatin 80 mg and diltiazem. The risk of myopathy in patients taking simvastatin 40 mg was not increased by concomitant diltiazem(see section 4.4). In a pharmacokinetic study, concomitant administration of diltiazem caused a 2.7-fold increase in exposure of simvastatin acid, presumably due to inhibition of CYP3A4. Therefore, the dose of simvastatin should not exceed 40 mg daily in patients receiving concomitant medication with diltiazem, unless the clinical benefit is likely to outweigh the increased risk of myopathy and rhabdomyolysis.

Grapefruit juice

Grapefruit juice inhibits cytochrome P450 3A4. Concomitant intake of large quantities (over 1 litre daily) of grapefruit juice and simvastatin resulted in a 7-fold increase in exposure to simvastatin acid. Intake of 240 ml of grapefruit juice in the morning and simvastatin in the evening also resulted in a 1.9-fold increase. Intake of grapefruit juice during treatment with simvastatin should therefore be avoided.

Oral anticoagulants

In two clinical studies, one in normal volunteers and the other in hypercholesterolaemic patients, simvastatin 20-40 mg/day modestly potentiated the effect of coumarin anticoagulants: the prothrombin time, reported as International Normalized Ratio (INR), increased from a baseline of 1.7 to 1.8 and from 2.6 to 3.4 in the volunteer and patient studies, respectively. Very rare cases of elevated INR have been reported. In patients taking coumarin anticoagulants, prothrombin time should be determined before starting simvastatin and frequently enough during early therapy to ensure that no significant alteration of prothrombin time occurs. Once a stable prothrombin time has been documented, prothrombin times can be monitored at the intervals usually recommended for patients on coumarin anticoagulants. If the dose of simvastatin is changed or discontinued, the same procedure should be repeated. Simvastatin therapy has not been associated with bleeding or with changes in prothrombin time in patients not taking anticoagulants.

Effects of simvastatin on the pharmacokinetics of other medicinal products

Simvastatin does not have an inhibitory effect on cytochrome P450 3A4. Therefore, simvastatin is not expected to affect plasma concentrations of substances metabolised via cytochrome P450 3A4.

4.6 Pregnancy and lactation

Pregnancy

'Zocor' is contraindicated during pregnancy (see section 4.3).

Safety in pregnant women has not been established. No controlled clinical trials with simvastatin have been conducted in pregnant women. Rare reports of congenital anomalies following intrauterine exposure to HMG-CoA reductase inhibitors have been received. However, in an analysis of approximately 200 prospectively followed pregnancies exposed during the first trimester to 'Zocor' or another closely related HMG-CoA reductase inhibitor, the incidence of congenital anomalies was comparable to that seen in the general population. This number of pregnancies was statistically sufficient to exclude a 2.5-fold or greater increase in congenital anomalies over the background incidence.

Although there is no evidence that the incidence of congenital anomalies in offspring of patients taking 'Zocor' or another closely related HMG-CoA reductase inhibitor differs from that observed in the general population, maternal treatment with 'Zocor' may reduce the foetal levels of mevalonate which is a precursor of cholesterol biosynthesis. Atherosclerosis is a chronic process, and ordinarily discontinuation of lipid-lowering medicinal products during pregnancy should have little impact on the long-term risk associated with primary hypercholesterolaemia. For these reasons, 'Zocor' should not be used in women who are pregnant, trying to become pregnant or suspect they are pregnant. Treatment with 'Zocor' should be suspended for the duration of pregnancy or until it has been determined that the woman is not pregnant. (See section 4.3.)

Lactation

It is not known whether simvastatin or its metabolites are excreted in human milk. Because many medicinal products are excreted in human milk and because of the potential for serious adverse reactions, women taking 'Zocor' should not breast-feed their infants (see section 4.3).

4.7 Effects on ability to drive and use machines

'Zocor' has no or negligible influence on the ability to drive and use machines. However, when driving vehicles or operating machines, it should be taken into account that dizziness has been reported rarely in post-marketing experiences.

4.8 Undesirable effects

The frequencies of the following adverse events, which have been reported during clinical studies and/or post-marketing use, are categorized based on an assessment of their incidence rates in large, long-term, placebo-controlled, clinical trials including HPS and 4S with 20,536 and 4,444 patients, respectively (see section 5.1). For HPS, only serious adverse events were recorded as well as myalgia, increases in serum transaminases and CK. For 4S, all the adverse events listed below were recorded. If the incidence rates on simvastatin were less than or similar to that of placebo in these trials, and there were similar reasonably causally related spontaneous report events, these adverse events are categorized as "rare".

In HPS (see section 5.1) involving 20,536 patients treated with 40 mg/day of 'Zocor' (n = 10,269) or placebo (n = 10,267), the safety profiles were comparable between patients treated with 'Zocor' 40 mg and patients treated with placebo over the mean 5 years of the study. Discontinuation rates due to side effects were comparable (4.8 % in patients treated with 'Zocor' 40 mg compared with 5.1 % in patients treated with placebo). The incidence of myopathy was < 0.1 % in patients treated with 'Zocor' 40 mg. Elevated transaminases (> 3 × ULN confirmed by repeat test) occurred in 0.21 % (n = 21) of patients treated with 'Zocor' 40 mg compared with 0.09 % (n = 9) of patients treated with placebo.

The frequencies of adverse events are ranked according to the following: Very common > 1/10), Common (⩾ 1/100, < 1/10), Uncommon (⩾ 1/1000, < 1/100), Rare (⩾ 1/10,000, < 1/1000), Very Rare (< 1/10,000) including isolated reports.

Blood and lymphatic system disorders:

Rare: anaemia

Nervous system disorders:

Rare: headache, paresthesia, dizziness, peripheral neuropathy

Gastrointestinal disorders:

Rare: constipation, abdominal pain, flatulence, dyspepsia, diarrhoea, nausea, vomiting, pancreatitis

Hepato-biliary disorders:

Rare: hepatitis/jaundice

Skin and subcutaneous tissue disorders:

Rare: rash, pruritus, alopecia

Musculoskeletal, connective tissue and bone disorders:

Rare: myopathy, rhabdomyolysis (see section 4.4), myalgia, muscle cramps

General disorders and administration site conditions:

Rare: asthenia

An apparent hypersensitivity syndrome has been reported rarely which has included some of the following features: angioedema, lupus-like syndrome, polymyalgia rheumatica, dermatomyositis, vasculitis, thrombocytopenia, eosinophilia, ESR increased, arthritis and arthralgia, urticaria, photosensitivity, fever, flushing, dyspnoea and malaise.

Investigations:

Rare: increases in serum transaminases (alanine aminotransferase, aspartate aminotransferase, γ-glutamyl transpeptidase) (see section 4.4 *Hepatic effects*), elevated alkaline phosphatase; increase in serum CK levels (see section 4.4).

4.9 Overdose

To date, a few cases of overdosage have been reported; the maximum dose taken was 3.6 g. All patients recovered without sequelae. There is no specific treatment in the event of overdose. In this case, symptomatic and supportive measures should be adopted.

5. PHARMACOLOGICAL PROPERTIES

5.1 Pharmacodynamic properties

Pharmacotherapeutic group: HMG-CoA reductase inhibitor

ATC-Code: C10A A01

After oral ingestion, simvastatin, which is an inactive lactone, is hydrolyzed in the liver to the corresponding active beta-hydroxyacid form which has a potent activity in inhibiting HMG-CoA reductase (3 hydroxy – 3 methylglutaryl CoA reductase). This enzyme catalyses the conversion of HMG-CoA to mevalonate, an early and rate-limiting step in the biosynthesis of cholesterol.

'Zocor' has been shown to reduce both normal and elevated LDL-C concentrations. LDL is formed from very-low-density protein (VLDL) and is catabolised predominantly by the high affinity LDL receptor. The mechanism of the LDL-lowering effect of 'Zocor' may involve both reduction of VLDL-cholesterol (VLDL-C) concentration and induction of the LDL receptor, leading to reduced production and increased catabolism of LDL-C. Apolipoprotein B also falls substantially during treatment with 'Zocor'. In addition, 'Zocor' moderately increases HDL-C and reduces plasma TG. As a result of these changes the ratios of total- to HDL-C and LDL- to HDL-C are reduced.

High Risk of Coronary Heart Disease (CHD) or Existing Coronary Heart Disease

In the Heart Protection Study (HPS), the effects of therapy with 'Zocor' were assessed in 20,536 patients (age 40-80 years), with or without hyperlipidaemia, and with coronary heart disease, other occlusive arterial disease or diabetes mellitus. In this study, 10,269 patients were treated with 'Zocor' 40 mg/day and 10,267 patients were treated with placebo for a mean duration of 5 years. At baseline, 6,793 patients (33 %) had LDL-C levels below 116 mg/dL; 5,063 patients (25 %) had levels between 116 mg/dL and 135 mg/dL; and 8,680 patients (42 %) had levels greater than 135 mg/dL.

Treatment with 'Zocor' 40 mg/day compared with placebo significantly reduced the risk of all cause mortality (1328 [12.9 %] for simvastatin-treated patients versus 1507 [14.7 %] for patients given placebo; p = 0.0003), due to an 18 % reduction in coronary death rate (587 [5.7 %] versus 707 [6.9 %]; p = 0.0005; absolute risk reduction of 1.2 %). The reduction in non-vascular deaths did not reach statistical significance. 'Zocor' also decreased the risk of major coronary events (a composite endpoint comprised of non-fatal MI or CHD death) by 27 % (p < 0.0001). 'Zocor' reduced the need for undergoing coronary revascularization procedures (including coronary artery bypass grafting or percutaneous transluminal coronary angioplasty) and peripheral and other non-coronary revascularization procedures by 30 % (p < 0.0001) and 16 % (p = 0.006), respectively. 'Zocor' reduced the risk of stroke by 25 % (p < 0.0001), attributable to a 30 % reduction in ischemic stroke (p < 0.0001). In addition, within the subgroup of patients with diabetes, 'Zocor' reduced the risk of developing macrovascular complications, including peripheral revascularization procedures (surgery or angioplasty), lower limb amputations, or leg ulcers by 21 % (p = 0.0293). The proportional reduction in event rate was similar in each subgroup of patients studied, including those without coronary disease but who had cerebrovascular or peripheral artery disease, men and women, those aged either under or over 70 years at entry into the study, presence or absence of hypertension, and notably those with LDL cholesterol below 3.0 mmol/l at inclusion.

In the Scandinavian Simvastatin Survival Study (4S), the effect of therapy with 'Zocor' on total mortality was assessed in 4,444 patients with CHD and baseline total cholesterol 212-309 mg/dL (5.5-8.0 mmol/L). In this multicenter, randomised, double-blind, placebo-controlled study, patients with angina or a previous myocardial infarction (MI) were treated with diet, standard care, and either 'Zocor' 20-40 mg/day (n = 2,221) or placebo (n = 2,223) for a median duration of 5.4 years. 'Zocor' reduced the risk of death by 30 % (absolute risk reduction of 3.3 %). The risk of CHD death was reduced by 42 % (absolute risk reduction of 3.5 %). 'Zocor' also decreased the risk of having major coronary events (CHD death plus hospital-verified and silent nonfatal MI) by 34 %. Furthermore, 'Zocor' significantly reduced the risk of fatal plus nonfatal cerebrovascular events (stroke and transient ischemic attacks) by 28 %. There was no statistically significant difference between groups in non-cardiovascular mortality.

Primary Hypercholesterolaemia and Combined Hyperlipidaemia

In studies comparing the efficacy and safety of simvastatin 10, 20, 40 and 80 mg daily in patients with hypercholesterolemia, the mean reductions of LDL-C were 30, 38, 41 and 47 %, respectively. In studies of patients with combined (mixed) hyperlipidaemia on simvastatin 40 mg and 80 mg, the median reductions in triglycerides were 28 and 33 % (placebo: 2 %), respectively, and mean increases in HDL-C were 13 and 16 % (placebo: 3 %), respectively.

5.2 Pharmacokinetic properties

Simvastatin is an inactive lactone which is readily hydrolyzed *in vivo* to the corresponding beta-hydroxyacid, a potent inhibitor of HMG-CoA reductase. Hydrolysis takes place mainly in the liver; the rate of hydrolysis in human plasma is very slow.

Absorption

In man simvastatin is well absorbed and undergoes extensive hepatic first-pass extraction. The extraction in the liver is dependent on the hepatic blood flow. The liver is the primary site of action of the active form. The availability of the beta-hydroxyacid to the systemic circulation following an oral dose of simvastatin was found to be less than 5 % of the dose. Maximum plasma concentration of active inhibitors is reached approximately 1-2 hours after administration of simvastatin. Concomitant food intake does not affect the absorption.

The pharmacokinetics of single and multiple doses of simvastatin showed that no accumulation of medicinal product occurred after multiple dosing.

Distribution

The protein binding of simvastatin and its active metabolite is > 95 %.

Elimination

Simvastatin is a substrate of CYP3A4 (see sections 4.3 and 4.5). The major metabolites of simvastatin present in human plasma are the beta-hydroxyacid and four additional active metabolites. Following an oral dose of radioactive simvastatin to man, 13 % of the radioactivity was excreted in the urine and 60 % in the faeces within 96 hours. The amount recovered in the faeces represents absorbed medicinal product equivalents excreted in bile as well as unabsorbed medicinal product. Following an intravenous injection of the beta-hydroxyacid metabolite, its half-life averaged 1.9 hours. An average of only 0.3 % of the IV dose was excreted in urine as inhibitors.

5.3 Preclinical safety data

Based on conventional animal studies regarding pharmacodynamics, repeated dose toxicity, genotoxicity and carcinogenicity, there are no other risks for the patient than may be expected on account of the pharmacological mechanism. At maximally tolerated doses in both the rat and the rabbit, simvastatin produced no foetal malformations, and had no effects on fertility, reproductive function or neonatal development.

6. PHARMACEUTICAL PARTICULARS

6.1 List of excipients

Each simvastatin tablet strength contains the following excipients:

Ascorbic acid E300, butylated hydroxyanisole E320, citric acid monohydrate E330, lactose, magnesium stearate E572, hydroxypropylcellulose E463, microcrystalline cellulose E460, pregelatinised maize starch (pregelatinised starch), talc E553 (b) titanium dioxide E171, hydroxypropylmethylcellulose E464 (hypromellose). In addition 'Zocor' 10 mg, 20 mg, 40 mg and 80 mg tablets also contain red iron oxide E172 and 'Zocor' 10 mg and 20 mg tablets also contain yellow iron oxide E172.

6.2 Incompatibilities

None.

6.3 Shelf life

24 months.

6.4 Special precautions for storage

Do not store above 30°C.

6.5 Nature and contents of container

Blister packs of trilaminate foil composed of polyvinyl chloride/polyethylene/polyvinylidene chloride (PVC/PE/PVDC) lidded with aluminium foil containing 28 tablets, 4 tablets or 1 tablet.

White high density polyethylene or polypropylene bottles or amber glass bottles containing 50 tablets.

Not all pack sizes may be marketed.

6.6 Instructions for use and handling

No special requirements.

7. MARKETING AUTHORISATION HOLDER

Merck Sharp & Dohme Limited, Hertford Road, Hoddesdon, Hertfordshire EN11 9BU, UK.

8. MARKETING AUTHORISATION NUMBER(S)

10 mg Tablet: PL0025/0241

20 mg Tablet: PL0025/0242

40 mg Tablet: PL0025/0243

80 mg Tablet: PL0025/0366.

9. DATE OF FIRST AUTHORISATION/RENEWAL OF THE AUTHORISATION

10 mg, 20 mg, 40 mg: Licence first granted April 1989. Last renewed November 2001.

80 mg: Licence first granted March 2000.

10. DATE OF REVISION OF THE TEXT

July 2004.

LEGAL CATEGORY

POM

® denotes registered trademark of Merck & Co., Inc., Whitehouse Station, NJ, USA.

SPC.ZCR.04.UK.1096

Zofran Injection, Flexi-Amp Injection

(GlaxoSmithKline UK)

1. NAME OF THE MEDICINAL PRODUCT

Zofran Injection 2mg/ml. Zofran Flexi-amp Injection 2mg/ml.

2. QUALITATIVE AND QUANTITATIVE COMPOSITION

Zofran Injection 2mg/ml: 2ml glass ampoules each containing 4mg ondansetron (as hydrochloride dihydrate) in aqueous solution for intramuscular or intravenous administration. 4ml glass ampoules each containing 8mg ondansetron (as hydrochloride dihydrate) in aqueous solution for intravenous or intramuscular administration.

Zofran Flexi-amp injection 2mg/ml: 2ml plastic ampoules each containing 4 mg ondansetron (as hydrochloride dihydrate) in aqueous solution for intramuscular or intravenous administration. 4ml plastic ampoules each containing 8 mg ondansetron (as hydrochloride dihydrate) in aqueous solution for intravenous or intramuscular administration.

3. PHARMACEUTICAL FORM

Injection (aqueous solution).

4. CLINICAL PARTICULARS

4.1 Therapeutic indications

Zofran is indicated for the management of nausea and vomiting induced by cytotoxic chemotherapy and radiotherapy, and for the prevention and treatment of post-operative nausea and vomiting (PONV).

4.2 Posology and method of administration
Chemotherapy and radiotherapy:

Adults: The emetogenic potential of cancer treatment varies according to the doses and combinations of chemotherapy and radiotherapy regimens used. The route of administration and dose of Zofran should be flexible in the range of 8-32mg a day and selected as shown below.

Emetogenic chemotherapy and radiotherapy: Zofran can be given either by rectal, oral (tablets or syrup), intravenous or intramuscular administration.

For most patients receiving emetogenic chemotherapy or radiotherapy, Zofran 8mg should be administered as a slow intravenous or intramuscular injection immediately before treatment, followed by 8mg orally twelve hourly.

To protect against delayed or prolonged emesis after the first 24 hours, oral or rectal treatment with Zofran should be continued for up to 5 days after a course of treatment.

Highly emetogenic chemotherapy: For patients receiving highly emetogenic chemotherapy, e.g. high-dose cisplatin, Zofran can be given either by rectal, intravenous or intramuscular administration. Zofran has been shown to be equally effective in the following dose schedules over the first 24 hours of chemotherapy:

A single dose of 8mg by slow intravenous or intramuscular injection immediately before chemotherapy.

A dose of 8mg by slow intravenous or intramuscular injection immediately before chemotherapy, followed by two further intravenous or intramuscular doses of 8mg two to four hours apart, or by a constant infusion of 1mg/hour for up to 24 hours.

A single dose of 32mg diluted in 50-100ml of saline or other compatible infusion fluid *(see Pharmaceutical Precautions)* and infused over not less than 15 minutes immediately before chemotherapy.

The selection of dose regimen should be determined by the severity of the emetogenic challenge.

The efficacy of Zofran in highly emetogenic chemotherapy may be enhanced by the addition of a single intravenous dose of dexamethasone sodium phosphate, 20mg administered prior to chemotherapy.

To protect against delayed or prolonged emesis after the first 24 hours, oral or rectal treatment with Zofran should be continued for up to 5 days after a course of treatment.

Children: Zofran may be administered as a single intravenous dose of $5mg/m^2$ immediately before chemotherapy, followed by 4mg orally twelve hours later. 4mg orally twice daily should be continued for up to 5 days after a course of treatment.

Elderly: Zofran is well tolerated by patients over 65 years and no alteration of dosage, dosing frequency or route of administration are required.

Patients with Renal Impairment:

No alteration of daily dosage or frequency of dosing, or route of administration are required.

Patients with hepatic Impairment:

Clearance of Zofran is significantly reduced and serum half-life significantly prolonged in subjects with moderate or severe impairment of hepatic function. In such patients a total daily dose of 8mg should not be exceeded.

Post-operative nausea and vomiting (PONV):

Adults: For the prevention of PONV Zofran can be administered orally or by intravenous or intramuscular injection.

Zofran may be administered as a single dose of 4mg given by intramuscular or slow intravenous injection at induction of anaesthesia.

For treatment of established PONV a single dose of 4mg given by intramuscular or slow intravenous injection is recommended.

Children (aged 2 years and over): For prevention of PONV in paediatric patients having surgery performed under general anaesthesia, ondansetron may be administered by slow intravenous injection at a dose of 0.1mg/kg up to a maximum of 4mg either prior to, at or after induction of anaesthesia.

For treatment of established PONV in paediatric patients, ondansetron may be administered by slow intravenous injection at a dose of 0.1mg/kg up to a maximum of 4mg.

There is limited data on the use of Zofran in the prevention and treatment of PONV in children under 2 years of age.

Elderly: There is limited experience in the use of Zofran in the prevention and treatment of PONV in the elderly, however Zofran is well tolerated in patients over 65 years receiving chemotherapy.

Patients with renal impairment: No alteration of daily dosage or frequency of dosing, or route of administration are required.

Patients with hepatic impairment: Clearance of Zofran is significantly reduced and serum half life significantly prolonged in subjects with moderate or severe impairment of hepatic function. In such patients a total daily dose of 8mg should not be exceeded.

Patients with poor sparteine/debrisoquine metabolism: The elimination half-life of ondansetron is not altered in subjects classified as poor metabolisers of sparteine and debrisoquine. Consequently in such patients repeat dosing will give drug exposure levels no different from those of the general population. No alteration of daily dosage or frequency of dosing are required.

4.3 Contraindications

Hypersensitivity to any component of the preparation.

4.4 Special warnings and special precautions for use

Hypersensitivity reactions have been reported in patients who have exhibited hypersensitivity to other selective $5HT_3$ receptor antagonists.

As ondansetron is known to increase large bowel transit time, patients with signs of subacute intestinal obstruction should be monitored following administration

4.5 Interaction with other medicinal products and other forms of Interaction

There is no evidence that ondansetron either induces or inhibits the metabolism of other drugs commonly co-administered with it. Specific studies have shown that there are no pharmacokinetic interactions when ondansetron is administered with alcohol, temazepan, furosemide, tramadol or propofol.

Ondansetron is metabolised by multiple hepatic cytochrome P-450 enzymes: CYP3A4, CYP2D6 and CYP1A2. Due to the multiplicity of metabolic enzymes capable of metabolising ondansetron, enzyme inhibition or reduced activity of one enzyme (e.g. CYP2D6 genetic deficiency) is normally compensated by other enzymes and should result in little or no significant change in overall ondansetron clearance or dose requirement.

Phenytoin, Carbamazepine and Rifampicin: In patients treated with potent inducers of CYP3A4 (i.e. phenytoin, carbamazepine, and rifampicin), the oral clearance of ondansetron was increased and ondansetron blood concentrations were decreased.

Tramadol: Data from small studies indicate that ondansetron may reduce the analgesic effect of tramadol.

4.6 Pregnancy and lactation
The safety of ondansetron for use in human pregnancy has not been established. Evaluation of experimental animal studies does not indicate direct or indirect harmful effects with respect to the development of the embryo, or foetus, the course of gestation and peri- and post-natal development. However as animal studies are not always predictive of human response the use of ondansetron in pregnancy is not recommended.

Tests have shown that ondansetron passes into the milk of lactating animals. It is therefore recommended that mothers receiving Zofran should not breast-feed their babies.

4.7 Effects on ability to drive and use machines
In psychomotor testing ondansetron does not impair performance nor cause sedation.

4.8 Undesirable effects
Ondansetron is known to increase large bowel transit time and may cause constipation in some patients. The following side effects can occur: headache, a sensation of flushing or warmth, hiccups and occasional asymptomatic increases in liver functiontests. There have been rare reports of immediate hypersensitivity reactions sometimes severe including anaphylaxis. Rare cases of transient visual disturbances (e.g. blurred vision) and dizziness have been reported during rapid intravenous administration of ondansetron. There have been rare reports suggestive of involuntary movement disorders such as extrapyramidal reactions e.g. oculogyric crisis/dystonic reactions without definitive evidence of persistent clinical sequelae and seizures have been rarely observed although no known pharmacological mechanism can account for ondansetron causing these effects. Chest pain with or without ST segment depression, cardiac arrhythmias, hypotension and bradycardia have been rarely reported.

Occasionally, hypersensitivity reactions around the injection site (e.g. rash, urticaria, itching) may occur, sometimes extending along the drug administration vein.

4.9 Overdose
Little is known at present about overdosage with ondansetron, however, a limited number of patients received overdoses. Manifestations that have been reported include visual disturbances, severe constipation, hypotension and a vasovagal episode with transient second degree AV block. In all instances, the events resolved completely. There is no specific antidote for ondansetron, therefore in all cases of suspected overdose, symptomatic and supportive therapy should be given as appropriate.

5. PHARMACOLOGICAL PROPERTIES

5.1 Pharmacodynamic properties
Ondansetron is a potent, highly selective 5HT3 receptor-antagonist. Its precise mode of action in the control of nausea and vomiting is not known. Chemotherapeutic agents and radiotherapy may cause release of 5HT in the small intestine initiating a vomiting reflex by activating vagal afferents via 5HT3 receptors. Ondansetron blocks the initiation of this reflex. Activation of vagal afferents may also cause a release of 5HT in the area postrema, located on the floor of the fourth ventricle, and this may also promote emesis through a central mechanism. Thus, the effect of ondansetron in the management of the nausea and vomiting induced by cytotoxic chemotherapy and radiotherapy is probably due to antagonism of 5HT3 receptors on neurons located both in the peripheral and central nervous system. The mechanisms of action in post-operative nausea and vomiting are not known but there may be common pathways with cytotoxic induced nausea and vomiting.

Ondansetron does not alter plasma prolactin concentrations.

The role of ondansetron in opiate-induced emesis is not yet established.

5.2 Pharmacokinetic properties
Following oral administration, ondansetron is passively and completely absorbed from the gastrointestinal tract and undergoes first pass metabolism. Peak plasma concentrations of about 30ng/ml are attained approximately 1.5 hours after an 8mg dose. For doses above 8mg the increase in ondansetron systemic exposure with dose is greater than proportional; this may reflect some reduction in first pass metabolism at higher oral doses. Bioavailability, following oral administration, is slightly enhanced by the presence of food but unaffected by antacids. Studies in healthy elderly volunteers have shown slight, but clinically insignificant, age-related increases in both oral bioavailability (65%) and half-life (5 hours) of ondansetron. Gender differences were shown in the disposition of ondansetron, with females having a greater rate and extent of absorption following an oral dose and reduced systemic clearance and volume of distribution (adjusted for weight).

The disposition of ondansetron following oral, intramuscular(IM) and intravenous(IV) dosing is similar with a terminal half life of about 3 hours and steady state volume of distribution of about 140L. Equivalent systemic exposure is achieved after IM and IV administration of ondansetron.

A 4mg intravenous infusion of ondansetron given over 5 minutes results in peak plasma concentrations of about 65ng/ml. Following intramuscular administration of ondansetron, peak plasma concentrations of about 25ng/ml are attained within 10 minutes of injection.

Following administration of ondansetron suppository, plasma ondansetron concentrations become detectable between 15 and 60 minutes after dosing. Concentrations rise in an essentially linear fashion, until peak concentrations of 20-30 ng/ml are attained, typically 6 hours after dosing. Plasma concentrations then fall, but at a slower rate than observed following oral dosing due to continued absorption of ondansetron. The absolute bioavailability of ondansetron from the suppository is approximately 60% and is not affected by gender. The half life of the elimination phase following suppository administration is determined by the rate of ondansetron absorption, not systemic clearance and is approximately 6 hours. Females show a small, clinically insignificant, increase in half-life in comparison with males.

Ondansetron is not highly protein bound (70-76%). Ondansetron is cleared from the systemic circulation predominantly by hepatic metabolism through multiple enzymatic pathways. Less than 5% of the absorbed dose is excreted unchanged in the urine. The absence of the enzyme CYP2D6 (the debrisoquine polymorphism) has no effect on ondansetron's pharmacokinetics. The pharmacokinetic properties of ondansetron are unchanged on repeat dosing.

In a study of 21 paediatric patients aged between 3 and 12 years undergoing elective surgery with general anaesthesia, the absolute values for both the clearance and volume of distribution of ondansetron following a single intravenous dose of 2mg (3-7 years old) or 4mg (8-12 years old) were reduced. The magnitude of the change was age-related, with clearance falling from about 300mL/min at 12 years of age to 100mL/min at 3 years. Volume of distribution fell from about 75L at 12 years to 17L at 3 years. Use of weight-based dosing (0.1mg/kg up to 4mg maximum) compensates for these changes and is effective in normalising systemic exposure in paediatric patients.

In patients with renal impairment (creatinine clearance 15-60 ml/min), both systemic clearance and volume of distribution are reduced following IV administration of ondansetron, resulting in a slight, but clinically insignificant, increase in elimination half-life (5.4h). A study in patients with severe renal impairment who required regular haemodialysis (studied between dialyses) showed ondansetron's pharmacokinetics to be essentially unchanged following IV administration.

Specific studies in the elderly or patients with renal impairment have been limited to IV and oral administration. However, it is anticipated that the half-life of ondansetron after rectal administration in these populations will be similar to that seen in healthy volunteers, since the rate of elimination of ondansetron following rectal administration is not determined by systemic clearance.

Following oral, intravenous or intramuscular dosing in patients with severe hepatic impairment, ondansetron's systemic clearance is markedly reduced with prolonged elimination half-lives (15-32 h) and an oral bioavailability approaching 100% due to reduced pre-systemic metabolism. The pharmacokinetics of ondansetron following administration as a suppository have not been evaluated in patients with hepatic impairment.

5.3 Preclinical safety data
No additional data of relevance.

6. PHARMACEUTICAL PARTICULARS

6.1 List of excipients
Citric acid monohydrate, sodium citrate, sodium chloride, Water for Injections.

6.2 Incompatibilities
Zofran injection should not be administered in the same syringe or infusion as any other medication.

6.3 Shelf life
36 months (unopened). 24 hours (dilutions stored 2 - 8°C).

6.4 Special precautions for storage
Protect from light. Store below 30°C.

Dilutions of Zofran injection in compatible intravenous infusion fluids are stable under normal room lighting conditions or daylight for at least 24 hours, thus no protection from light is necessary while infusion takes place.

6.5 Nature and contents of container
Zofran Injection: Type I clear glass snap-ring ampoules.

Zofran Flexi-amp injection: Polypropylene blow-fill-sealed ampoules with a twist-off top and overwrapped in a double foil blister.

5 ampoules are packed in a carton.

6.6 Instructions for use and handling
Zofran Injection and Zofran Flexi-amp injection should not be autoclaved.

Compatibility with intravenous fluids

Zofran injection should only be admixed with those infusion solutions which are recommended:

Sodium Chloride Intravenous Infusion BP 0.9%w/v

Glucose Intravenous Infusion BP 5%w/v

Mannitol Intravenous Infusion BP 10%w/v

Ringers Intravenous Infusion

Potassium Chloride 0.3%w/v and Sodium Chloride 0.9%w/v Intravenous Infusion BP

Potassium Chloride 0.3%w/v and Glucose 5%w/v Intravenous Infusion BP

In keeping with good pharmaceutical practice dilutions of Zofran injection in intravenous fluids should be prepared at the time of infusion or stored at 2-8°C for no more than 24 hours before the start of administration.

Compatibility studies have been undertaken in polyvinyl chloride infusion bags and polyvinyl chloride administration sets. It is considered that adequate stability would also be conferred by the use of polyethylene infusion bags or Type 1 glass bottles. Dilutions of Zofran in sodium chloride 0.9%w/v or in glucose 5%w/v have been demonstrated to be stable in polypropylene syringes. It is considered that Zofran injection diluted with other compatible infusion fluids would be stable in polypropylene syringes.

Compatibility with other drugs: Zofran may be administered by intravenous infusion at 1mg/hour, e.g. from an infusion bag or syringe pump. The following drugs may be administered via the Y-site of the Zofran giving set for ondansetron concentrations of 16 to 160 micrograms/ml (e.g. 8 mg/500 ml and 8 mg/50 ml respectively);

Cisplatin: Concentrations up to 0.48 mg/ml (e.g. 240 mg in 500 ml) administered over one to eight hours.

5 -Fluorouracil:

Concentrations up to 0.8 mg/ml (e.g. 2.4g in 3 litres or 400mg in 500ml) administered at a rate of at least 20 ml per hour (500 ml per 24 hours). Higher concentrations of 5-fluorouracil may cause precipitation of ondansetron. The 5-fluorouracil infusion may contain up to 0.045%w/v magnesium chloride in addition to other excipients shown to be compatible.

Carboplatin: Concentrations in the range 0.18 mg/ml to 9.9 mg/ml (e.g. 90 mg in 500 ml to 990 mg in 100 ml), administered over ten minutes to one hour.

Etoposide: Concentrations in the range 0.14 mg/ml to 0.25 mg/ml (e.g. 72 mg in 500 ml to 250 mg in 1 litre), administered over thirty minutes to one hour.

Ceftazidime: Doses in the range 250 mg to 2000 mg reconstituted with Water for Injections BP as recommended by the manufacturer (e.g. 2.5 ml for 250 mg and 10 ml for 2g ceftazidime) and given as an intravenous bolus injection over approximately five minutes.

Cyclophosphamide: Doses in the range 100 mg to 1g, reconstituted with Water for Injections BP, 5 ml per 100 mg cyclophosphamide, as recommended by the manufacturer and given as an intravenous bolus injection over approximately five minutes.

Doxorubicin: Doses in the range 10-100mg reconstituted with Water for Injections BP, 5 ml per 10 mg doxorubicin, as recommended by the manufacturer and given as an intravenous bolus injection over approximately 5 minutes.

Dexamethasone: Dexamethasone sodium phosphate 20mg may be administered as a slow intravenous injection over 2-5 minutes via the Y-site of an infusion set delivering 8 or 32mg of ondansetron diluted in 50-100ml of a compatible infusion fluid over approximately 15 minutes. Compatibility between dexamethasone sodium phosphate and ondansetron has been demonstrated supporting administration of these drugs through the same giving set resulting in concentrations in line of 32 microgram - 2.5mg/ml for dexamethasone sodium phosphate and 8 microgram - 1mg/ml for ondansetron.

Administrative Data

7. MARKETING AUTHORISATION HOLDER
Glaxo Operations UK Limited,

Greenford Road,

Greenford,

Middlesex, UB6 0HE

Trading as

GlaxoSmithKline UK

Stockley Park West

Uxbridge

Middlesex UB11 1BT

8. MARKETING AUTHORISATION NUMBER(S)
PL00004/0375

9. DATE OF FIRST AUTHORISATION/RENEWAL OF THE AUTHORISATION
23rd October 2001

10. DATE OF REVISION OF THE TEXT
28 September 2004

11. Legal Status
POM

Zofran Melt 8mg, 4mg

(GlaxoSmithKline UK)

1. NAME OF THE MEDICINAL PRODUCT
Zofran Melt 8mg

Zofran Melt 4mg

2. QUALITATIVE AND QUANTITATIVE COMPOSITION

White, round, plano-convex, freeze dried, fast dispersing oral dosage form.

Each Melt contains ondansetron 4mg or 8mg.

3. PHARMACEUTICAL FORM

Oral lyophilisate.

4. CLINICAL PARTICULARS

4.1 Therapeutic indications

The management of nausea and vomiting induced by cytotoxic chemotherapy and radiotherapy, and for the prevention of post-operative nausea and vomiting in adults.

4.2 Posology and method of administration

Place the Melt on top of the tongue, where it will disperse within seconds, then swallow

Chemotherapy and radiotherapy induced nausea and vomiting

Adults:

The emetogenic potential of cancer treatment varies according to the doses and combinations of chemotherapy and radiotherapy regimens used. The route of administration and dose of Zofran should be flexible and selected as shown below.

Emetogenic chemotherapy and radiotherapy: Zofran can be given either by rectal, oral (as Melt, tablets or syrup) intravenous or intramuscular administration.

For oral administration: 8mg 1-2 hours before treatment, followed by 8mg 12 hours later.

To protect against delayed or prolonged emesis after the first 24 hours, oral or rectal treatment with Zofran should be continued for up to 5 days after a course of treatment.

The recommended dose for oral administration is 8mg twice daily.

Highly emetogenic chemotherapy (e.g. high dose cisplatin): Zofran can be given either by rectal, intravenous or intramuscular administration.

To protect against delayed or prolonged emesis after the first 24 hours, oral or rectal treatment with Zofran should be continued for up to 5 days after a course of treatment.

The recommended dose for oral administration is 8mg twice daily.

Children:

Zofran may be administered as a single intravenous dose of 5mg/m2 immediately before chemotherapy, followed by 4mg orally twelve hours later. 4mg orally twice daily should be continued for up to 5 days after a course of treatment.

Elderly:

Zofran is well tolerated by patients over 65 years and no alteration of dosage, dosing frequency or route of administration are required.

POST OPERATIVE NAUSEA AND VOMITING (PONV)

Adults:

For the prevention of PONV: Zofran may be administered either orally (as Melt, tablets or syrup) or by intravenous or intramuscular injection.

For oral administration: 16mg one hour prior to anaesthesia. Alternatively, 8mg one hour prior to anaesthesia followed by two further doses of 8mg at eight hourly intervals.

For the treatment of established PONV: Intravenous or intramuscular administration is recommended.

Children (aged 2 years and over):

For the prevention and treatment of PONV: Slow intravenous injection is recommended.

Elderly:

There is limited experience in the use of Zofran in the prevention and treatment of PONV in the elderly, however Zofran is well tolerated in patients over 65 years receiving chemotherapy.

For both indications

Patients with renal impairment:

No special requirements.

Patients with hepatic impairment:

Clearance of Zofran is significantly reduced and serum half life significantly prolonged in subjects with moderate or severe impairment of hepatic function. In such patients a total daily dose of 8mg should not be exceeded.

Patients with poor sparteine/debrisoquine metabolism:

The elimination half-life of ondansetron is not altered in subjects classified as poor metabolisers of sparteine and debrisoquine. Consequently in such patients repeat dosing will give drug exposure levels no different from those of the general population. No alteration of daily dosage or frequency of dosing are required.

4.3 Contraindications

Hypersensitivity to any component of the preparation.

4.4 Special warnings and special precautions for use

Hypersensitivity reactions have been reported in patients who have exhibited hypersensitivity to other selective 5HT3 receptor antagonists.

Patients with signs of subacute intestinal obstruction should be monitored following administration.

Caution in patients with phenylketonuria.

4.5 Interaction with other medicinal products and other forms of Interaction

There is no evidence that ondansetron either induces or inhibits the metabolism of other drugs commonly co-administered with it. Specific studies have shown that there are no pharamcokinetic interactions when ondansetron is administered with alcohol, temazepam, furosemide, tramadol or propofol.

Ondansetron is metabolised by multiple hepatic cytochrome P-450 enzymes: CYP3A4, CYP2D6 and CYP1A2. Due to the multiplicity of metabolic enzymes capable of metabolising ondansetron, enzyme inhibition or reduced activity of one enzyme (e.g. CYP2D6 genetic deficiency) is normally compensated by other enzymes and should result in little or no significant change in overall ondansetron clearance or dose requirement.

Phenytoin, Carbamazepine and Rifampicin: In patients treated with potent inducers of CYP3A4 (i.e. phenytoin, carbamazepine, and rifampicin), the oral clearance of ondansetron was increased and ondansetron blood concentrations were decreased.

Tramadol: Data from small studies indicate that ondansetron may reduce the analgesic effect of tramadol.

4.6 Pregnancy and lactation

The safety of ondansetron for use in human pregnancy has not been established. Evaluation of experimental animal studies does not indicate direct or indirect harmful effects with respect to the development of the embryo, or the foetus, the course of gestation and peri- and post-natal development. However, as animal studies are not always predictive of human response the use of ondansetron in pregnancy is not recommended.

Tests have shown that ondansetron passes into the milk of lactating animals. It is therefore recommended that mothers receiving Zofran should not breast-feed their babies.

4.7 Effects on ability to drive and use machines

None reported

4.8 Undesirable effects

There have been rare reports of immediate hypersensitivity reactions, sometimes severe, including anaphylaxis.

Chest pain with or without ST segment depression, cardiac arrhythmias, hypotension and bradycardia have been rarely reported.

There have been rare reports suggestive of involuntary movement disorders such as extrapyramidal reactions e.g. oculogyric crisis/dystonic reactions, without definitive evidence of persistent clinical sequelae, and seizures have been rarely observed, although no known pharmacological mechanism can account for ondansetron causing these effects.

Ondansetron is known to increase large bowel transit time and may cause constipation in some patients.

The following side effects can occur: headache, a sensation of flushing or warmth, hiccups and occasional transient, asymptomatic increases in liver function tests.

4.9 Overdose

Little is known at present about overdosage with ondansetron, however, a limited number of patients received overdoses. Manifestations that have been reported include visual disturbances, severe constipation, hypotension and a vasovagal episode with transient second degree AV block. In all instances, the events resolved completely. There is no specific antidote for ondansetron, therefore in all cases of suspected overdose, symptomatic and supportive therapy should be given as appropriate.

5. PHARMACOLOGICAL PROPERTIES

5.1 Pharmacodynamic properties

Ondansetron is a potent, highly selective 5HT3 receptor-antagonist. Its precise mode of action in the control of nausea and vomiting is not known. Chemotherapeutic agents and radiotherapy may cause release of 5HT in the small intestine initiating a vomiting reflex by activating vagal afferents via 5HT3 receptors. Ondansetron blocks the initiation of this reflex. Activation of vagal afferents may also cause a release of 5HT in the area postrema, located on the floor of the fourth ventricle, and this may also promote emesis through a central mechanism. Thus, the effect of ondansetron in the management of the nausea and vomiting induced by cytotoxic chemotherapy and radiotherapy is probably due to antagonism of 5HT3 receptors on neurons located both in the peripheral and central nervous system. The mechanisms of action in post-operative nausea and vomiting are not known but there may be common pathways with cytotoxic induced nausea and vomiting.

Ondansetron does not alter plasma prolactin concentrations.

The role of ondansetron in opiate-induced emesis is not yet established.

5.2 Pharmacokinetic properties

Following oral administration of ondansetron, absorption is rapid with maximum peak plasma concentrations of about 30ng/ml being attained and achieved in approximately 1.5 hours after an 8mg dose. The syrup and tablet formulations are bioequivalent and have an absolute oral bioavailability of 60%. The disposition of ondansetron following oral, intravenous and intramuscular dosing is similar with a terminal elimination half-life of approximately 3 hours and a steady-state volume of distribution of about 140L. Ondansetron is not highly protein bound (70-76%) and is cleared from the systemic circulation predominantly by hepatic metabolism through multiple enzymatic pathways. Less than 5% of the absorbed dose is excreted unchanged in the urine. The absence of the enzyme CYP2D6 (the debrisoquine polymorphism) has no effect on the pharmacokinetics of ondansetron. The pharmacokinetic properties of ondansetron are unchanged on repeat dosing.

Studies in healthy elderly volunteers have shown a slight but clinically insignificant, age-related increases in both oral bioavailability (65%) and half-life (5h) of ondansetron. Gender differences were shown in the disposition of ondansetron, with females having a greater rate and extent of absorption following an oral dose and reduced systemic clearance and volume of distribution (adjusted for weight).

In a study of 21 paediatric patients aged between 3 and 12 years undergoing elective surgery with general anaesthesia, the absolute values for both the clearance and volume of distribution of ondansetron following a single intravenous dose of 2mg (3-7 years old) or 4mg (8-12 years old) were reduced. The magnitude of the change was age-related, with clearance falling from about 300ml/min at 12 years of age to 100ml/min at 3 years. Volume of distribution fell from about 75L at 12 years to 17L at 3 years. Use of weight-based dosing (0.1mg/kg up to 4mg maximum) compensates for these changes and is effective in normalising systemic exposure in paediatric patients.

In patients with renal impairment (creatinine clearance >15 ml/min), systemic clearance and volume of distribution are reduced, resulting in a slight, but clinically insignificant increase in elimination half-life (5.4h). A study in patients with severe renal impairment who required regular haemodialysis (studied between dialyses) showed ondansetron's pharmacokinetics to be essentially unchanged.

In patients with severe hepatic impairment, systemic clearance is markedly reduced with prolonged elimination half-lives (15-32h) and an oral bioavailability approaching 100% because of reduced pre-systemic metabolism.

5.3 Preclinical safety data

No additional data of relevance.

6. PHARMACEUTICAL PARTICULARS

6.1 List of excipients

Gelatin

Mannitol

Aspartame

Sodium methyl hydroxybenzoate

Sodium propyl hydroxybenzoate

Strawberry flavour

6.2 Incompatibilities

None reported.

6.3 Shelf life

3 years.

6.4 Special precautions for storage

Store below 30°C.

6.5 Nature and contents of container

Double aluminium foil blister strip containing 10 tablets

6.6 Instructions for use and handling

Do not attempt to push Zofran Melt through the lidding foil.

Peel back the lidding foil of one blister and gently remove the Zofran Melt.

Place the Melt on top of the tongue, where it will disperse within seconds then swallow.

Administrative Data

7. MARKETING AUTHORISATION HOLDER

Glaxo Wellcome UK Limited trading as GlaxoSmithKline UK

Stockley Park West

Uxbridge

Middlesex, UB11 1BT

8. MARKETING AUTHORISATION NUMBER(S)

PL10949/0264 - Zofran Melt 8 mg

PL 10949/0263 - Zofran Melt 4 mg

9. DATE OF FIRST AUTHORISATION/RENEWAL OF THE AUTHORISATION

3rd April 1998

10. DATE OF REVISION OF THE TEXT

30 November 2004

11. Legal Status

POM

Zofran Suppositories 16mg

(GlaxoSmithKline UK)

1. NAME OF THE MEDICINAL PRODUCT

Zofran Suppositories 16mg

2. QUALITATIVE AND QUANTITATIVE COMPOSITION
White torpedo shaped suppositories containing 16mg of ondansetron.

3. PHARMACEUTICAL FORM
Suppositories.

4. CLINICAL PARTICULARS

4.1 Therapeutic indications
The management of nausea and vomiting induced by cytotoxic chemotherapy and radiotherapy.

4.2 Posology and method of administration
Adults (including the elderly):

The emetogenic potential of cancer treatment varies according to the doses and combinations of chemotherapy and radiotherapy regimens used. The route of administration and dose of Zofran should be flexible and selected as shown below.

Emetogenic chemotherapy and radiotherapy: Zofran can be given either by rectal, oral (tablets or syrup), intravenous or intramuscular administration.

For rectal administration: One suppository (16mg ondansetron) 1-2 hours before treatment.

To protect against delayed or prolonged emesis after the first 24 hours, oral or rectal treatment with Zofran should be continued for up to 5 days after a course of treatment. The recommended dose for rectal administration is one suppository daily.

Highly emetogenic chemotherapy (e.g. high dose cisplatin): Zofran can be given either by rectal, intravenous or intramuscular administration.

For rectal administration: One suppository (16mg ondansetron) 1-2 hours before treatment.

The efficacy of Zofran in highly emetogenic chemotherapy may be enhanced by the addition of a single intravenous dose of dexamethasone sodium phosphate 20mg, administered prior to chemotherapy.

To protect against delayed or prolonged emesis after the first 24 hours, oral or rectal treatment with Zofran should be continued for up to 5 days after a course of treatment. The recommended dose for rectal administration is one suppository daily.

Children:

The use of Zofran Suppositories in children is not recommended.

Zofran may be administered as a single intravenous dose of $5mg/m^2$ immediately before chemotherapy, followed by 4mg orally twelve hours later. 4mg orally twice daily should be continued for up to 5 days after a course of treatment.

Patients with renal impairment:

No special requirements.

Patients with hepatic impairment:

Clearance of Zofran is significantly reduced and serum half-life significantly prolonged in subjects with moderate or severe impairment of hepatic function. In such patients a total daily dose of 8mg should not be exceeded and therefore intravenous or oral administration is recommended.

Patients with poor sparteine/debrisoqine metabolism:

The elimination half-life of ondansetron is not altered in subjects classified as poor metabolisers of sparteine and debrisoquine. Consequently in such patients repeat dosing will give drug exposure levels no different from those of the general population. No alteration of daily dosage or frequency of dosing are required.

4.3 Contraindications
Hypersensitivity to any ingredient.

4.4 Special warnings and special precautions for use
Hypersensitivity reactions have been reported in patients who have exhibited hypersensitivity to other selective $5HT_3$ receptor antagonists.

As ondansetron is known to increase large bowel transit time, patients with signs of subacute intestinal obstruction should be monitored following administration.

4.5 Interaction with other medicinal products and other forms of Interaction
There is no evidence that ondansetron either induces or inhibits the metabolism of other drugs commonly co-administered with it. Specific studies have shown that there are no pharamcokinetic interactions when ondansetron is administered with alcohol, temazepam, furosemide, tramadol or propofol.

Ondansetron is metabolised by multiple hepatic cytochrome P-450 enzymes: CYP3A4, CYP2D6 and CYP1A2. Due to the multiplicity of metabolic enzymes capable of metabolising ondansetron, enzyme inhibition or reduced activity of one enzyme (e.g. CYP2D6 genetic deficiency) is normally compensated by other enzymes and should result in little or no significant change in overall ondansetron clearance or dose requirement.

Phenytoin, Carbamazepine and Rifampicin: In patients treated with potent inducers of CYP3A4 (i.e. phenytoin, carbamazepine, and rifampicin), the oral clearance of ondansetron was increased and ondansetron blood concentrations were decreased.

Tramadol: Data from small studies indicate that ondansetron may reduce the analgesic effect of tramadol.

4.6 Pregnancy and lactation
The safety of ondansetron for use in human pregnancy has not been established. Evaluation of experimental animal studies does not indicate direct or indirect harmful effects with respect to the development of the embryo, or foetus, the course of gestation and peri- and post-natal development. However as animal studies are not always predictive of human response the use of ondansetron in pregnancy is not recommended.

Tests have shown that ondansetron passes into the milk of lactating animals. It is therefore recommended that mothers receiving Zofran should not breast-feed their babies.

4.7 Effects on ability to drive and use machines
None reported.

4.8 Undesirable effects
There have been rare reports of immediate hypersensitivity reactions, sometimes severe, including anaphylaxis.

Chest pain with or without ST segment depression, cardiac arrhythmias, hypotension and bradycardia have been rarely reported.

There have been rare reports suggestive of extrapyramidal reactions such as oculogyric crisis/dystonic reactions without definitive evidence of persistent clinical sequelae, and seizures have been rarely observed, although no known pharmacological mechanism can account for ondansetron causing these effects.

Ondansetron is known to increase large bowel transit time and may cause constipation in some patients.

The following side effects can occur: headache, a sensation of flushing or warmth, hiccups and occasional asymptomatic increases in liver function tests.

There have been rare reports of a local anal/rectal burning sensation following insertion of a suppository.

4.9 Overdose
Little is known at present about overdosage with ondansetron, however, a limited number of patients received overdoses. Manifestations that have been reported include visual disturbances, severe constipation, hypotension and a vasovagal episode with transient second degree AV block. In all instances, the events resolved completely. There is no specific antidote for ondansetron, therefore in all cases of suspected overdose, symptomatic and supportive therapy should be given as appropriate.

5. PHARMACOLOGICAL PROPERTIES

5.1 Pharmacodynamic properties
Ondansetron is a potent, highly selective $5HT_3$ receptor-antagonist. The precise mode of action in the control of nausea and vomiting is not known. Chemotherapeutic agents and radiotherapy may cause release of 5HT in the small intestine initiating a vomiting reflex by activating vagal afferents via $5HT_3$ receptors. Ondansetron blocks the initiation of this reflex. Activation of vagal afferents may also cause a release of 5HT in the area postrema, located on the floor of the fourth ventricle, and this may also promote emesis through a central mechanism. Thus, the effect of ondansetron in the management of the nausea and vomiting induced by cytotoxic chemotherapy and radiotherapy is probably due to antagonism of $5HT_3$ receptors on neurons located both in the peripheral and central nervous system. The mechanisms of action in post-operative nausea and vomiting are not known but there may be common pathways with cytotoxic induced nausea and vomiting.

Ondansetron does not alter plasma prolactin concentrations.

The role of ondansetron in opiate-induced emesis is not yet established.

5.2 Pharmacokinetic properties
Following oral administration, ondansetron is passively and completely absorbed from the gastrointestinal tract and undergoes first pass metabolism. Peak plasma concentrations of about 30ng/ml are attained approximately 1.5 hours after an 8mg dose. For doses above 8mg the increase in ondansetron systemic exposure with dose is greater than proportional; this may reflect some reduction in first pass metabolism at higher oral doses. Bioavailability, following oral administration, is slightly enhanced by the presence of food but unaffected by antacids. Studies in healthy elderly volunteers have shown slight, but clinically insignificant, age-related increases in both oral bioavailability (65%) and half-life (5 hours) of ondansetron. Gender differences were shown in the disposition of ondansetron, with females having a greater rate and extent of absorption following an oral dose and reduced systemic clearance and volume of distribution (adjusted for weight).

The disposition of ondansetron following oral, intramuscular(IM) and intravenous(IV) dosing is similar with a terminal half life of about 3 hours and steady state volume of distribution of about 140L. Equivalent systemic exposure is achieved after IM and IV administration of ondansetron.

A 4mg intravenous infusion of ondansetron given over 5 minutes results in peak plasma concentrations of about 65ng/ml. Following intramuscular administration of ondansetron, peak plasma concentrations of about 25ng/ml are attained within 10 minutes of injection.

Following administration of ondansetron suppository, plasma ondansetron concentrations become detectable between 15 and 60 minutes after dosing. Concentrations rise in an essentially linear fashion, until peak concentrations of 20-30 ng/ml are attained, typically 6 hours after dosing. Plasma concentrations then fall, but at a slower rate than observed following oral dosing due to continued absorption of ondansetron. The absolute bioavailability of ondansetron from the suppository is approximately 60% and is not affected by gender. The half life of the elimination phase following suppository administration is determined by the rate of ondansetron absorption, not systemic clearance and is approximately 6 hours. Females show a small, clinically insignificant, increase in half-life in comparison with males.

Ondansetron is not highly protein bound (70-76%). Ondansetron is cleared from the systemic circulation predominantly by hepatic metabolism through multiple enzymatic pathways. Less than 5% of the absorbed dose is excreted unchanged in the urine. The absence of the enzyme CYP2D6 (the debrisoquine polymorphism) has no effect on ondansetron's pharmacokinetics. The pharmacokinetic properties of ondansetron are unchanged on repeat dosing.

In a study of 21 paediatric patients aged between 3 and 12 years undergoing elective surgery with general anaesthesia, the absolute values for both the clearance and volume of distribution of ondansetron following a single intravenous dose of 2mg (3-7 years old) or 4mg (8-12 years old) were reduced. The magnitude of the change was age-related, with clearance falling from about 300mL/min at 12 years of age to 100mL/min at 3 years. Volume of distribution fell from about 75L at 12 years to 17L at 3 years. Use of weight-based dosing (0.1mg/kg up to 4mg maximum) compensates for these changes and is effective in normalising systemic exposure in paediatric patients.

In patients with renal impairment (creatinine clearance 15-60 ml/min), both systemic clearance and volume of distribution are reduced following IV administration of ondansetron, resulting in a slight, but clinically insignificant, increase in elimination half-life (5.4h). A study in patients with severe renal impairment who required regular haemodialysis (studied between dialyses) showed ondansetron's pharmacokinetics to be essentially unchanged following IV administration.

Specific studies in the elderly or patients with renal impairment have been limited to IV and oral administration. However, it is anticipated that the half-life of ondansetron after rectal administration in these populations will be similar to that seen in healthy volunteers, since the rate of elimination of ondansetron following rectal administration is not determined by systemic clearance.

Following oral, intravenous or intramuscular dosing in patients with severe hepatic impairment, ondansetron's systemic clearance is markedly reduced with prolonged elimination half-lives (15-32 h) and an oral bioavailability approaching 100% due to reduced pre-systemic metabolism. The pharmacokinetics of ondansetron following administration as a suppository have not been evaluated in patients with hepatic impairment.

5.3 Preclinical safety data
No additional data of relevance.

6. PHARMACEUTICAL PARTICULARS

6.1 List of excipients
Witepsol S58.

6.2 Incompatibilities
None reported.

6.3 Shelf life
3 years.

6.4 Special precautions for storage
Store below 30°C.

6.5 Nature and contents of container
Each suppository is in an individually sealed cavity enclosed in a perforated cardboard mount and packed into a carton.

6.6 Instructions for use and handling
Insert into the rectum.

For detailed instructions see the patient information leaflet included in every pack.

Administrative Data

7. MARKETING AUTHORISATION HOLDER
Glaxo Wellcome UK Limited trading as GlaxoSmithKline UK

Stockley Park West

Uxbridge

Middlesex, UB11 1BT

8. MARKETING AUTHORISATION NUMBER(S)
PL10949/0247

9. DATE OF FIRST AUTHORISATION/RENEWAL OF THE AUTHORISATION
15th January 2002

10. DATE OF REVISION OF THE TEXT
30 November 2004

11. Legal Status
POM

Zofran Syrup

(GlaxoSmithKline UK)

1. NAME OF THE MEDICINAL PRODUCT
Zofran® Syrup

2. QUALITATIVE AND QUANTITATIVE COMPOSITION
Sugar-free strawberry flavoured liquid.

Each 5ml contains 4mg of ondansetron as the hydrochloride dihydrate.

3. PHARMACEUTICAL FORM
Oral solution.

4. CLINICAL PARTICULARS

4.1 Therapeutic indications
The management of nausea and vomiting induced by cytotoxic chemotherapy and radiotherapy, and for the prevention of post-operative nausea and vomiting in adults.

4.2 Posology and method of administration
Chemotherapy and radiotherapy induced nausea and vomiting

Adults (including the elderly):

The emetogenic potential of cancer treatment varies according to the doses and combinations of chemotherapy and radiotherapy regimens used. The route of administration and dose of Zofran should be flexible and selected as shown below.

Emetogenic chemotherapy and radiotherapy: Zofran can be given either by rectal, oral (tablets or syrup), intravenous or intramuscular administration.

For oral administration: 8mg 1-2 hours before treatment, followed by 8mg 12 hours later.

To protect against delayed or prolonged emesis after the first 24 hours, oral or rectal treatment with Zofran should be continued for up to 5 days after a course of treatment.

The recommended dose for oral administration is 8mg twice daily.

Highly emetogenic chemotherapy (e.g. high dose cisplatin): Zofran can be given either by rectal, intravenous or intramuscular administration.

To protect against delayed or prolonged emesis after the first 24 hours, oral or rectal treatment with Zofran should be continued for up to 5 days after a course of treatment.

The recommended dose for oral administration is 8mg twice daily.

Children:

Zofran may be administered as a single intravenous dose of 5mg/m^2 immediately before chemotherapy, followed by 4mg orally twelve hours later. 4mg orally twice daily should be continued for up to 5 days after a course of treatment.

Post operative nausea and vomiting (ponv).

Adults:

For the prevention of PONV: Zofran can be administered orally or by intravenous or intramuscular injection.

For oral administration: 16mg one hour prior to anaesthesia. Alternatively, 8mg one hour prior to anaesthesia followed by two further doses of 8mg at eight hourly intervals.

For the treatment of established PONV: Intravenous or intramuscular administration is recommended.

Children (aged 2 years and over):

For the prevention and treatment of PONV: Slow intravenous injection is recommended.

Elderly:

There is limited experience in the use of Zofran in the prevention and treatment of PONV in the elderly, however Zofran is well tolerated in patients over 65 years receiving chemotherapy.

For both indications

Patients with renal impairment:

No special requirements.

Patients with hepatic impairment:

Clearance of Zofran is significantly reduced and serum half life significantly prolonged in subjects with moderate or severe impairment of hepatic function. In such patients a total daily dose of 8mg should not be exceeded.

Patients with poor sparteine/debrisoquine metabolism:

The elimination half-life of ondansetron is not altered in subjects classified as poor metabolisers of sparteine and debrisoquine. Consequently in such patients repeat dosing will give drug exposure levels no different from those of the general population. No alteration of daily dosage or frequency of dosing are required.

4.3 Contraindications
Hypersensitivity to any ingredient.

4.4 Special warnings and special precautions for use
Hypersensitivity reactions have been reported in patients who have exhibited hypersensitivity to other selective $5HT_3$ receptor antagonists.

As ondansetron is known to increase large bowel transit time, patients with signs of subacute intestinal obstruction should be monitored following administration.

4.5 Interaction with other medicinal products and other forms of Interaction
There is no evidence that ondansetron either induces or inhibits the metabolism of other drugs commonly co-administered with it. Specific studies have shown that there are no pharamcokinetic interactions when ondansetron is administered with alcohol, temazepam, furosemide, tramadol or propofol.

Ondansetron is metabolised by multiple hepatic cytochrome P-450 enzymes: CYP3A4, CYP2D6 and CYP1A2. Due to the multiplicity of metabolic enzymes capable of metabolising ondansetron, enzyme inhibition or reduced activity of one enzyme (e.g. CYP2D6 genetic deficiency) is normally compensated by other enzymes and should result in little or no significant change in overall ondansetron clearance or dose requirement.

Phenytoin, Carbamazepine and Rifampicin: In patients treated with potent inducers of CYP3A4 (i.e. phenytoin, carbamazepine, and rifampicin), the oral clearance of ondansetron was increased and ondansetron blood concentrations were decreased.

Tramadol: Data from small studies indicate that ondansetron may reduce the analgesic effect of tramadol.

4.6 Pregnancy and lactation
The safety of ondansetron for use in human pregnancy has not been established. Evaluation of experimental animal studies does not indicate direct or indirect harmful effects with respect to the development of the embryo, or foetus, the course of gestation and peri- and post-natal development. However as animal studies are not always predictive of human response the use of ondansetron in pregnancy is not recommended.

Tests have shown that ondansetron passes into the milk of lactating animals. It is therefore recommended that mothers receiving Zofran should not breast-feed their babies.

4.7 Effects on ability to drive and use machines
None reported

4.8 Undesirable effects
There have been rare reports of immediate hypersensitivity reactions, sometimes severe, including anaphylaxis.

Chest pain with or without ST segment depression, cardiac arrhythmias, hypotension and bradycardia have been rarely reported.

There have been rare reports suggestive of involuntary movement disorders such as extrapyramidal reactions e.g. oculogyric crisis/dystonic reactions without definitive evidence of persistent clinical sequelae and seizures have been rarely observed, although no known pharmacological mechanism can account for ondansetron causing these effects.

Ondansetron is known to increase large bowel transit time and may cause constipation in some patients.

The following side effects can occur: headache, a sensation of flushing or warmth, hiccups and occasional asymptomatic increases in liver function tests.

4.9 Overdose
Little is known at present about overdosage with ondansetron, however, a limited number of patients received overdoses. Manifestations that have been reported include visual disturbances, severe constipation, hypotension and a vasovagal episode with transient second degree AV block. In all instances, the events resolved completely. There is no specific antidote for ondansetron, therefore in all cases of suspected overdose, symptomatic and supportive therapy should be given as appropriate.

5. PHARMACOLOGICAL PROPERTIES

5.1 Pharmacodynamic properties
Ondansetron is a potent, highly selective 5HT3 receptor-antagonist. Its precise mode of action in the control of nausea and vomiting is not known. Chemotherapeutic agents and radiotherapy may cause release of 5HT in the small intestine initiating a vomiting reflex by activating vagal afferents via 5HT3 receptors. Ondansetron blocks the initiation of this reflex. Activation of vagal afferents may also cause a release of 5HT in the area postrema, located on the floor of the fourth ventricle, and this may also promote emesis through a central mechanism. Thus, the effect of ondansetron in the management of the nausea and vomiting induced by cytotoxic chemotherapy and radiotherapy is probably due to antagonism of 5HT3 receptors on neurons located both in the peripheral and central nervous system. The mechanisms of action in post-operative nausea and vomiting are not known but there may be common pathways with cytotoxic induced nausea and vomiting.

Ondansetron does not alter plasma prolactin concentrations.

The role of ondansetron in opiate-induced emesis is not yet established.

5.2 Pharmacokinetic properties
Following oral administration, ondansetron is passively and completely absorbed from the gastrointestinal tract and undergoes first pass metabolism. Peak plasma concentrations of about 30ng/ml are attained approximately 1.5 hours after an 8mg dose. For doses above 8mg the increase in ondansetron systemic exposure with dose is greater than proportional; this may reflect some reduction in first pass metabolism at higher oral doses. Bioavailability, following oral administration, is slightly enhanced by the presence of food but unaffected by antacids. Studies in healthy elderly volunteers have shown slight, but clinically insignificant, age-related increases in both oral bioavailability (65%) and half-life (5 hours) of ondansetron. Gender differences were shown in the disposition of ondansetron, with females having a greater rate and extent of absorption following an oral dose and reduced systemic clearance and volume of distribution (adjusted for weight).

The disposition of ondansetron following oral, intramuscular(IM) and intravenous(IV) dosing is similar with a terminal half life of about 3 hours and steady state volume of distribution of about 140L. Equivalent systemic exposure is achieved after IM and IV administration of ondansetron.

A 4mg intravenous infusion of ondansetron given over 5 minutes results in peak plasma concentrations of about 65ng/ml. Following intramuscular administration of ondansetron, peak plasma concentrations of about 25ng/ml are attained within 10 minutes of injection.

Following administration of ondansetron suppository, plasma ondansetron concentrations become detectable between 15 and 60 minutes after dosing. Concentrations rise in an essentially linear fashion, until peak concentrations of 20-30 ng/ml are attained, typically 6 hours after dosing. Plasma concentrations then fall, but at a slower rate than observed following oral dosing due to continued absorption of ondansetron. The absolute bioavailability of ondansetron from the suppository is approximately 60% and is not affected by gender. The half life of the elimination phase following suppository administration is determined by the rate of ondansetron absorption, not systemic clearance and is approximately 6 hours. Females show a small, clinically insignificant, increase in half-life in comparison with males.

Ondansetron is not highly protein bound (70-76%). Ondansetron is cleared from the systemic circulation predominantly by hepatic metabolism through multiple enzymatic pathways. Less than 5% of the absorbed dose is excreted unchanged in the urine. The absence of the enzyme CYP2D6 (the debrisoquine polymorphism) has no effect on ondansetron's pharmacokinetics. The pharmacokinetic properties of ondansetron are unchanged on repeat dosing.

In a study of 21 paediatric patients aged between 3 and 12 years undergoing elective surgery with general anaesthesia, the absolute values for both the clearance and volume of distribution of ondansetron following a single intravenous dose of 2mg (3-7 years old) or 4mg (8-12 years old) were reduced. The magnitude of the change was age-related, with clearance falling from about 300mL/min at 12 years of age to 100mL/min at 3 years. Volume of distribution fell from about 75L at 12 years to 17L at 3 years. Use of weight-based dosing (0.1mg/kg up to 4mg maximum) compensates for these changes and is effective in normalising systemic exposure in paediatric patients.

In patients with renal impairment (creatinine clearance 15-60 ml/min), both systemic clearance and volume of distribution are reduced following IV administration of ondansetron, resulting in a slight, but clinically insignificant, increase in elimination half-life (5.4h). A study in patients with severe renal impairment who required regular haemodialysis (studied between dialyses) showed ondansetron's pharmacokinetics to be essentially unchanged following IV administration.

Specific studies in the elderly or patients with renal impairment have been limited to IV and oral administration. However, it is anticipated that the half-life of ondansetron after rectal administration in these populations will be similar to that seen in healthy volunteers, since the rate of elimination of ondansetron following rectal administration is not determined by systemic clearance.

Following oral, intravenous or intramuscular dosing in patients with severe hepatic impairment, ondansetron's systemic clearance is markedly reduced with prolonged elimination half-lives (15-32 h) and an oral bioavailability approaching 100% due to reduced pre-systemic metabolism. The pharmacokinetics of ondansetron following administration as a suppository have not been evaluated in patients with hepatic impairment.

5.3 Preclinical safety data
No additional data of relevance.

6. PHARMACEUTICAL PARTICULARS

6.1 List of excipients
Citric acid

Sodium citrate dihydrate

Sodium benzoate

Sorbitol solution

Strawberry flavour

Purified water

6.2 Incompatibilities
None reported.

6.3 Shelf life
3 years.

6.4 Special precautions for storage
Store upright below 30°C. Do not refrigerate.

6.5 Nature and contents of container
60ml amber glass bottle with a child resistant cap containing 50ml of Zofran Syrup.

6.6 Instructions for use and handling
For oral administration. For detailed information see the patient information leaflet included in every pack.

Administrative Data

7. MARKETING AUTHORISATION HOLDER
Glaxo Wellcome UK Limited trading as GlaxoSmithKline UK
Stockley Park West
Uxbridge
Middlesex, UB11 1BT

8. MARKETING AUTHORISATION NUMBER(S)
PL 10949/0246

9. DATE OF FIRST AUTHORISATION/RENEWAL OF THE AUTHORISATION
17th August 2001

10. DATE OF REVISION OF THE TEXT
30 November 2004

11. Legal Status
POM

Zofran Tablets 4mg, 8mg

(GlaxoSmithKline UK)

1. NAME OF THE MEDICINAL PRODUCT
Zofran Tablets 4mg

Zofran Tablets 8mg

2. QUALITATIVE AND QUANTITATIVE COMPOSITION
Each Zofran Tablet 4mg is a yellow, oval, film coated tablet engraved "GLAXO" on one face and "4" on the other. Each tablet contains ondansetron 4mg (as hydrochloride dihydrate).

Each Zofran Tablet 8mg is a yellow, oval, film coated tablet engraved "GLAXO" on one face and "8" on the other. Each tablet contains ondansetron 8mg (as hydrochloride dihydrate).

3. PHARMACEUTICAL FORM
Film coated tablet.

4. CLINICAL PARTICULARS

4.1 Therapeutic indications
Zofran is indicated for the management of nausea and vomiting induced by cytotoxic chemotherapy and radiotherapy, and for the prevention and treatment of post-operative nausea and vomiting.

4.2 Posology and method of administration
Chemotherapy and radiotherapy induced nausea and vomiting

Adults:

The emetogenic potential of cancer treatment varies according to the doses and combinations of chemotherapy and radiotherapy regimens used. The route of administration and dose of Zofran should be flexible in the range of 8-32mg a day and selected as shown below.

Emetogenic Chemotherapy and Radiotherapy: Zofran can be given either by rectal, oral (tablets or syrup), intravenous or intramuscular administration.

For oral administration: 8mg 1-2 hours before treatment, followed by 8mg 12 hours later.

To protect against delayed or prolonged emesis after the first 24 hours, oral or rectal treatment with Zofran should be continued for up to 5 days after a course of treatment.

The recommended dose for oral administration is 8mg twice daily.

Highly Emetogenic Chemotherapy: For patients receiving highly emetogenic chemotherapy, eg. high-dose cisplatin, Zofran can be given either by rectal, intravenous or intramuscular administration.

To protect against delayed or prolonged emesis after the first 24 hours, oral or rectal treatment with Zofran should be continued for up to 5 days after a course of treatment.

The recommended dose for oral administration is 8mg twice daily.

Children:

Zofran may be administered as a single intravenous dose of 5mg/m^2 immediately before chemotherapy, followed by 4mg orally twelve hours later. 4mg orally twice daily should be continued for up to 5 days after a course of treatment.

Elderly:

Zofran is well tolerated by patients over 65 years and no alteration of dosage, dosing frequency or route of administration are required.

Patients with Renal Impairment:

No alteration of daily dosage or frequency of dosing, or route of administration are required.

Patients with hepatic Impairment:

Clearance of Zofran is significantly reduced and serum half-life significantly prolonged in subjects with moderate or severe impairment of hepatic function. In such patients a total daily dose of 8mg should not be exceeded.

Post operative nausea and vomiting:

Adults:

For the prevention of PONV: Zofran can be administered orally or by intravenous or intramuscular injection.

For oral administration: 16mg one hour prior to anaesthesia. Alternatively, 8mg one hour prior to anaesthesia followed by two further doses of 8mg at eight hourly intervals.

For the treatment of established PONV: Intravenous or intramuscular administration is recommended.

Children (aged 2 years and over):

For the prevention and treatment of PONV: Slow intravenous injection is recommended.

Elderly:

There is limited experience in the use of Zofran in the prevention and treatment of post-operative nausea and vomiting in the elderly, however Zofran is well tolerated in patients over 65 years receiving chemotherapy.

Patients with renal impairment:

No alteration of daily dosage or frequency of dosing, or route of administration are required.

Patients with hepatic impairment:

Clearance of Zofran is significantly reduced and serum half life significantly prolonged in subjects with moderate or severe impairment of hepatic function. In such patients a total daily dose of 8mg should not be exceeded.

Patients with poor sparteine/debrisoquine metabolism:

The elimination half-life of ondansetron is not altered in subjects classified as poor metabolisers of sparteine and debrisoquine. Consequently in such patients repeat dosing will give drug exposure levels no different from those of the general population. No alteration of daily dosage or frequency of dosing are required.

4.3 Contraindications
Hypersensitivity to any component of the preparation.

4.4 Special warnings and special precautions for use
Hypersensitivity reactions have been reported in patients who have exhibited hypersensitivity to other selective $5HT_3$ receptor antagonists.

As ondansetron is known to increase large bowel transit time, patients with signs of subacute intestinal obstruction should be monitored following administration.

4.5 Interaction with other medicinal products and other forms of Interaction
There is no evidence that ondansetron either induces or inhibits the metabolism of other drugs commonly coadministered with it. Specific studies have shown that there are no pharamcokinetic interactions when ondansetron is administered with alcohol, temazepam, furosemide, tramadol or propofol.

Ondansetron is metabolised by multiple hepatic cytochrome P-450 enzymes: CYP3A4, CYP2D6 and CYP1A2. Due to the multiplicity of metabolic enzymes capable of metabolising ondansetron, enzyme inhibition or reduced activity of one enzyme (e.g. CYP2D6 genetic deficiency) is normally compensated by other enzymes and should result in little or no significant change in overall ondansetron clearance or dose requirement.

Phenytoin, Carbamazepine and Rifampicin: In patients treated with potent inducers of CYP3A4 (i.e. phenytoin, carbamazepine, and rifampicin), the oral clearance of ondansetron was increased and ondansetron blood concentrations were decreased.

Tramadol: Data from small studies indicate that ondansetron may reduce the analgesic effect of tramadol.

4.6 Pregnancy and lactation
The safety of ondansetron for use in human pregnancy has not been established. Evaluation of experimental animal studies does not indicate direct or indirect harmful effects with respect to the development of the embryo, or foetus, the course of gestation and peri- and post-natal development. However as animal studies are not always predictive of human response the use of ondansetron in pregnancy is not recommended.

Tests have shown that ondansetron passes into the milk of lactating animals. It is therefore recommended that mothers receiving Zofran should not breast-feed their babies.

4.7 Effects on ability to drive and use machines
In psychomotor testing ondansetron does not impair performance nor cause sedation.

4.8 Undesirable effects
Ondansetron is known to increase large bowel transit time and may cause constipation in some patients. The following side effects can occur: headache, a sensation of flushing or warmth, hiccups and occasional asymptomatic increases in liver function tests. There have been rare reports of immediate hypersensitivity reactions sometimes severe including anaphylaxis. Rare cases of transient visual disturbances (e.g: blurred vision) and dizziness have been reported during rapid intravenous administration of ondansetron. There have been rare reports suggestive of extrapyramidal reactions such as oculogyric crisis/dystonic reactions without definitive evidence of persistent clinical sequelae, and seizures have been rarely observed although no known pharmacological mechanism can account for ondansetron causing these effects. Chest pain with or without ST segment depression, cardiac arrhythmias, hypotension and bradycardia have been rarely reported.

4.9 Overdose
Little is known at present about overdosage with ondansetron, however, a limited number of patients received overdoses. Manifestations that have been reported include visual disturbances, severe constipation, hypotension and a vasovagal episode with transient second degree AV block. In all instances, the events resolved completely. There is no specific antidote for ondansetron, therefore in all cases of suspected overdose, symptomatic and supportive therapy should be given as appropriate.

5. PHARMACOLOGICAL PROPERTIES

5.1 Pharmacodynamic properties
Ondansetron is a potent, highly selective 5HT3 receptor-antagonist. Its precise mode of action in the control of nausea and vomiting is not known. Chemotherapeutic agents and radiotherapy may cause release of 5HT in the small intestine initiating a vomiting reflex by activating vagal afferents via 5HT3 receptors. Ondansetron blocks the initiation of this reflex. Activation of vagal afferents may also cause a release of 5HT in the area postrema, located on the floor of the fourth ventricle, and this may also promote emesis through a central mechanism. Thus, the effect of ondansetron in the management of the nausea and vomiting induced by cytotoxic chemotherapy and radiotherapy is probably due to antagonism of 5HT3 receptors on neurons located both in the peripheral and central nervous system. The mechanisms of action in post-operative nausea and vomiting are not known but there may be common pathways with cytotoxic induced nausea and vomiting.

Ondansetron does not alter plasma prolactin concentrations.

5.2 Pharmacokinetic properties
Following oral administration, ondansetron is passively and completely absorbed from the gastrointestinal tract and undergoes first pass metabolism. Peak plasma concentrations of about 30ng/ml are attained approximately 1.5 hours after an 8mg dose. For doses above 8mg the increase in ondansetron systemic exposure with dose is greater than proportional; this may reflect some reduction in first pass metabolism at higher oral doses. Bioavailability, following oral administration, is slightly enhanced by the presence of food but unaffected by antacids. Studies in healthy elderly volunteers have shown slight, but clinically insignificant, age-related increases in both oral bioavailability (65%) and half-life (5 hours) of ondansetron. Gender differences were shown in the disposition of ondansetron, with females having a greater rate and extent of absorption following an oral dose and reduced systemic clearance and volume of distribution (adjusted for weight).

The disposition of ondansetron following oral, intramuscular(IM) and intravenous(IV) dosing is similar with a terminal half life of about 3 hours and steady state volume of distribution of about 140L. Equivalent systemic exposure is achieved after IM and IV administration of ondansetron.

A 4mg intravenous infusion of ondansetron given over 5 minutes results in peak plasma concentrations of about 65ng/ml. Following intramuscular administration of ondansetron, peak plasma concentrations of about 25ng/ml are attained within 10 minutes of injection.

Following administration of ondansetron suppository, plasma ondansetron concentrations become detectable between 15 and 60 minutes after dosing. Concentrations rise in an essentially linear fashion, until peak concentrations of 20-30 ng/ml are attained, typically 6 hours after dosing. Plasma concentrations then fall, but at a slower rate than observed following oral dosing due to continued absorption of ondansetron. The absolute bioavailability of ondansetron from the suppository is approximately 60% and is not affected by gender. The half life of the elimination phase following suppository administration is determined by the rate of ondansetron absorption, not systemic clearance and is approximately 6 hours. Females show a small, clinically insignificant, increase in half-life in comparison with males.

Ondansetron is not highly protein bound (70-76%). Ondansetron is cleared from the systemic circulation predominantly by hepatic metabolism through multiple enzymatic pathways. Less than 5% of the absorbed dose is excreted unchanged in the urine. The absence of the enzyme CYP2D6 (the debrisoquine polymorphism) has no effect on ondansetron's pharmacokinetics. The pharmacokinetic properties of ondansetron are unchanged on repeat dosing.

In a study of 21 paediatric patients aged between 3 and 12 years undergoing elective surgery with general anaesthesia, the absolute values for both the clearance and volume of distribution of ondansetron following a single intravenous dose of 2mg (3-7 years old) or 4mg (8-12 years old) were reduced. The magnitude of the change was age-related, with clearance falling from about 300mL/min at 12 years of age to 100mL/min at 3 years. Volume of distribution fell from about 75L at 12 years to 17L at 3 years.

Use of weight-based dosing (0.1mg/kg up to 4mg maximum) compensates for these changes and is effective in normalising systemic exposure in paediatric patients.

In patients with renal impairment (creatinine clearance 15-60 ml/min), both systemic clearance and volume of distribution are reduced following IV administration of ondansetron, resulting in a slight, but clinically insignificant, increase in elimination half-life (5.4h). A study in patients with severe renal impairment who required regular haemodialysis (studied between dialyses) showed ondansetron's pharmacokinetics to be essentially unchanged following IV administration.

Specific studies in the elderly or patients with renal impairment have been limited to IV and oral administration. However, it is anticipated that the half-life of ondansetron after rectal administration in these populations will be similar to that seen in healthy volunteers, since the rate of elimination of ondansetron following rectal administration is not determined by systemic clearance.

Following oral, intravenous or intramuscular dosing in patients with severe hepatic impairment, ondansetron's systemic clearance is markedly reduced with prolonged elimination half-lives (15-32 h) and an oral bioavailability approaching 100% due to reduced pre-systemic metabolism. The pharmacokinetics of ondansetron following administration as a suppository have not been evaluated in patients with hepatic impairment.

5.3 Preclinical safety data
No additional data of relevance.

6. PHARMACEUTICAL PARTICULARS

6.1 List of excipients
Lactose, microcrystalline cellulose, pregelatinised maize starch, magnesium stearate, methylhydroxypropylcellulose, titanium dioxide (E171), iron oxide (E172).

6.2 Incompatibilities
None reported.

6.3 Shelf life
36 months

6.4 Special precautions for storage
Store below 30°C.

6.5 Nature and contents of container
Zofran Tablets 4mg: Blister packs of 10 or 30 tablets comprising aluminium/PVC blister film and aluminium foil lidding. Securitainer packs of 30 or 100 tablets.

Marketed Pack size: 30 Tablets (blister pack)

Zofran tablets 8mg: Blister packs of 10, 15, or 30 tablets comprising aluminium/PVC blister film and aluminium foil lidding. Securitainer packs of 30 or 100 tablets.

Marketed Pack Size: 10 Tablets (blister pack)

6.6 Instructions for use and handling
None stated.

Administrative Data

7. MARKETING AUTHORISATION HOLDER
Glaxo Wellcome UK Limited

Trading as GlaxoSmithKline UK

Stockley Park West

Uxbridge

Middlesex UB11 1BT

8. MARKETING AUTHORISATION NUMBER(S)
Zofran Tablets 4mg: PL10949/0110

Zofran Tablets 8mg: PL 10949/0111

9. DATE OF FIRST AUTHORISATION/RENEWAL OF THE AUTHORISATION
9th January 2002

10. DATE OF REVISION OF THE TEXT
30 November 2004

11. Legal Status
POM

Zofran Tablets and Flexi-Amp Injection

(GlaxoSmithKline UK)

1. NAME OF THE MEDICINAL PRODUCT
Zofran Flexi-amp® Injection 2mg/ml.

Zofran Tablets 4mg

Zofran Tablets 8mg

2. QUALITATIVE AND QUANTITATIVE COMPOSITION
Zofran Flexi-amp injection 2mg/ml: 2ml plastic ampoules each containing 4 mg ondansetron (as hydrochloride dihydrate) in aqueous solution for intramuscular or intravenous administration. 4ml plastic ampoules each containing 8 mg ondansetron (as hydrochloride dihydrate) in aqueous solution for intravenous or intramuscular administration.

Each Zofran Tablet 4mg is a yellow, oval, film coated tablet engraved "GLAXO" on one face and "4" on the other. Each tablet contains ondansetron 4mg (as hydrochloride dihydrate).

Each Zofran Tablet 8mg is a yellow, oval, film coated tablet engraved "GLAXO" on one face and "8" on the other. Each tablet contains ondansetron 8mg (as hydrochloride dihydrate).

3. PHARMACEUTICAL FORM
Injection (aqueous solution).

Film coated tablet.

4. CLINICAL PARTICULARS

4.1 Therapeutic indications
Zofran is indicated for the management of nausea and vomiting induced by cytotoxic chemotherapy and radiotherapy, and for the prevention and treatment of post-operative nausea and vomiting (PONV).

4.2 Posology and method of administration

CHEMOTHERAPY AND RADIOTHERAPY INDUCED NAUSEA AND VOMITING:

Adults:

The emetogenic potential of cancer treatment varies according to the doses and combinations of chemotherapy and radiotherapy regimens used. The route of administration and dose of Zofran should be flexible in the range of 8-32mg a day and selected as shown below.

Emetogenic chemotherapy and radiotherapy:

Zofran can be given either by rectal, oral (tablets or syrup), intravenous or intramuscular administration.

For most patients receiving emetogenic chemotherapy or radiotherapy, Zofran 8mg should be administered as a slow intravenous or intramuscular injection immediately before treatment, or orally 1 – 2 hours before treatment, followed by 8mg orally twelve hourly.

To protect against delayed or prolonged emesis after the first 24 hours, oral or rectal treatment with Zofran should be continued for up to 5 days after a course of treatment.

The recommended dose for oral administration is 8mg twice daily.

Highly emetogenic chemotherapy:

For patients receiving highly emetogenic chemotherapy, e.g. high-dose cisplatin, Zofran can be given either by rectal, intravenous or intramuscular administration. Zofran has been shown to be equally effective in the following dose schedules over the first 24 hours of chemotherapy:

A single dose of 8mg by slow intravenous or intramuscular injection immediately before chemotherapy.

A dose of 8mg by slow intravenous or intramuscular injection immediately before chemotherapy, followed by two further intravenous or intramuscular doses of 8mg two to four hours apart, or by a constant infusion of 1mg/hour for up to 24 hours.

A single dose of 32mg diluted in 50-100ml of saline or other compatible infusion fluid *(see Pharmaceutical Precautions)* and infused over not less than 15 minutes immediately before chemotherapy.

The selection of dose regimen should be determined by the severity of the emetogenic challenge.

The efficacy of Zofran in highly emetogenic chemotherapy may be enhanced by the addition of a single intravenous dose of dexamethasone sodium phosphate, 20mg administered prior to chemotherapy.

To protect against delayed or prolonged emesis after the first 24 hours, oral or rectal treatment with Zofran should be continued for up to 5 days after a course of treatment.

The recommended dose for oral administration is 8mg twice daily.

Children:

Zofran may be administered as a single intravenous dose of 5mg/m^2 immediately before chemotherapy, followed by 4mg orally twelve hours later. 4mg orally twice daily should be continued for up to 5 days after a course of treatment.

Elderly:

Zofran is well tolerated by patients over 65 years and no alteration of dosage, dosing frequency or route of administration are required.

Patients with renal impairment:

No alteration of daily dosage or frequency of dosing, or route of administration are required.

Patients with hepatic impairment:

Clearance of Zofran is significantly reduced and serum half-life significantly prolonged in subjects with moderate or severe impairment of hepatic function. In such patients a total daily dose of 8mg should not be exceeded.

POST OPERATIVE NAUSEA AND VOMITING (PONV):

Adults:

For the prevention of PONV: Zofran can be administered orally or by intravenous or intramuscular injection.

Zofran may be administered as a single dose of 4mg given by intramuscular or slow intravenous injection at induction of anaesthesia.

For oral administration: 16mg one hour prior to anaesthesia. Alternatively, 8mg one hour prior to anaesthesia followed by two further doses of 8mg at eight hourly intervals.

For treatment of established PONV: a single dose of 4mg given by intramuscular or slow intravenous injection is recommended.

Children (aged 2 years and over):

For prevention of PONV in paediatric patients having surgery performed under general anaesthesia, ondansetron may be administered by slow intravenous injection at a dose of 0.1mg/kg up to a maximum of 4mg either prior to, at or after induction of anaesthesia.

For treatment of established PONV in paediatric patients, ondansetron may be administered by slow intravenous injection at a dose of 0.1mg/kg up to a maximum of 4mg.

There is limited data on the use of Zofran in the prevention and treatment of PONV in children under 2 years of age.

Elderly:

There is limited experience in the use of Zofran in the prevention and treatment of PONV in the elderly, however Zofran is well tolerated in patients over 65 years receiving chemotherapy.

Patients with renal impairment:

No alteration of daily dosage or frequency of dosing, or route of administration are required.

Patients with hepatic impairment:

Clearance of Zofran is significantly reduced and serum half life significantly prolonged in subjects with moderate or severe impairment of hepatic function. In such patients a total daily dose of 8mg should not be exceeded.

Patients with poor sparteine/debrisoquine metabolism:

The elimination half-life of ondansetron is not altered in subjects classified as poor metabolisers of sparteine and debrisoquine. Consequently in such patients repeat dosing will give drug exposure levels no different from those of the general population. No alteration of daily dosage or frequency of dosing are required.

4.3 Contraindications
Hypersensitivity to any component of the preparation.

4.4 Special warnings and special precautions for use
Hypersensitivity reactions have been reported in patients who have exhibited hypersensitivity to other selective 5HT3 receptor antagonists.

As ondansetron is known to increase large bowel transit time, patients with signs of subacute intestinal obstruction should be monitored following administration

4.5 Interaction with other medicinal products and other forms of Interaction
There is no evidence that ondansetron either induces or inhibits the metabolism of other drugs commonly co-administered with it. Specific studies have shown that there are no pharamcokinetic interactions when ondansetron is administered with alcohol, temazepam, furosemide, tramadol or propofol.

Ondansetron is metabolised by multiple hepatic cytochrome P-450 enzymes: CYP3A4, CYP2D6 and CYP1A2. Due to the multiplicity of metabolic enzymes capable of metabolising ondansetron, enzyme inhibition or reduced activity of one enzyme (e.g. CYP2D6 genetic deficiency) is normally compensated by other enzymes and should result in little or no significant change in overall ondansetron clearance or dose requirement.

Phenytoin, Carbamazepine and Rifampicin: In patients treated with potent inducers of CYP3A4 (i.e. phenytoin, carbamazepine, and rifampicin), the oral clearance of ondansetron was increased and ondansetron blood concentrations were decreased.

Tramadol: Data from small studies indicate that ondansetron may reduce the analgesic effect of tramadol.

4.6 Pregnancy and lactation
The safety of ondansetron for use in human pregnancy has not been established. Evaluation of experimental animal studies does not indicate direct or indirect harmful effects with respect to the development of the embryo, or foetus, the course of gestation and peri- and post-natal development. However as animal studies are not always predictive of human response the use of ondansetron in pregnancy is not recommended.

Tests have shown that ondansetron passes into the milk of lactating animals. It is therefore recommended that mothers receiving Zofran should not breast-feed their babies.

4.7 Effects on ability to drive and use machines
In psychomotor testing ondansetron does not impair performance nor cause sedation.

4.8 Undesirable effects
Ondansetron is known to increase large bowel transit time and may cause constipation in some patients. The following side effects can occur: headache, a sensation of flushing or warmth, hiccups and occasional asymptomatic increases in liver functiontests. There have been rare reports of immediate hypersensitivity reactions sometimes severe including anaphylaxis. Rare cases of transient visual disturbances (e.g. blurred vision) and dizziness have been reported during rapid intravenous administration of ondansetron. There have been rare reports suggestive of involuntary movement disorders such as extrapyramidal reactions e.g. oculogyric crisis/dystonic reactions without definitive evidence of persistent clinical sequelae and seizures have been rarely observed although no known pharmacological mechanism can account for ondansetron

causing these effects. Chest pain with or without ST segment depression, cardiac arrhythmias, hypotension and bradycardia have been rarely reported.

Occasionally, hypersensitivity reactions around the injection site (e.g. rash, urticaria, itching) may occur, sometimes extending along the drug administration vein.

4.9 Overdose

Little is known at present about overdosage with ondansetron, however, a limited number of patients received overdoses. Manifestations that have been reported include visual disturbances, severe constipation, hypotension and a vasovagal episode with transient second degree AV block. In all instances, the events resolved completely. There is no specific antidote for ondansetron, therefore in all cases of suspected overdose, symptomatic and supportive therapy should be given as appropriate.

5. PHARMACOLOGICAL PROPERTIES

5.1 Pharmacodynamic properties

Ondansetron is a potent, highly selective 5HT3 receptor-antagonist. Its precise mode of action in the control of nausea and vomiting is not known. Chemotherapeutic agents and radiotherapy may cause release of 5HT in the small intestine initiating a vomiting reflex by activating vagal afferents via 5HT3 receptors. Ondansetron blocks the initiation of this reflex. Activation of vagal afferents may also cause a release of 5HT in the area postrema, located on the floor of the fourth ventricle, and this may also promote emesis through a central mechanism. Thus, the effect of ondansetron in the management of the nausea and vomiting induced by cytotoxic chemotherapy and radiotherapy is probably due to antagonism of 5HT3 receptors on neurons located both in the peripheral and central nervous system. The mechanisms of action in post-operative nausea and vomiting are not known but there may be common pathways with cytotoxic induced nausea and vomiting.

Ondansetron does not alter plasma prolactin concentrations.

The role of ondansetron in opiate-induced emesis is not yet established.

5.2 Pharmacokinetic properties

Following oral administration, ondansetron is passively and completely absorbed from the gastrointestinal tract and undergoes first pass metabolism. Peak plasma concentrations of about 30ng/ml are attained approximately 1.5 hours after an 8mg dose. For doses above 8mg the increase in ondansetron systemic exposure with dose is greater than proportional; this may reflect some reduction in first pass metabolism at higher oral doses. Bioavailability, following oral administration, is slightly enhanced by the presence of food but unaffected by antacids. Studies in healthy elderly volunteers have shown slight, but clinically insignificant, age-related increases in both oral bioavailability (65%) and half-life (5 hours) of ondansetron. Gender differences were shown in the disposition of ondansetron, with females having a greater rate and extent of absorption following an oral dose and reduced systemic clearance and volume of distribution (adjusted for weight).

The disposition of ondansetron following oral, intramuscular(IM) and intravenous(IV) dosing is similar with a terminal half life of about 3 hours and steady state volume of distribution of about 140L. Equivalent systemic exposure is achieved after IM and IV administration of ondansetron.

A 4mg intravenous infusion of ondansetron given over 5 minutes results in peak plasma concentrations of about 65ng/ml. Following intramuscular administration of ondansetron, peak plasma concentrations of about 25ng/ml are attained within 10 minutes of injection.

Following administration of ondansetron suppository, plasma ondansetron concentrations become detectable between 15 and 60 minutes after dosing. Concentrations rise in an essentially linear fashion, until peak concentrations of 20-30 ng/ml are attained, typically 6 hours after dosing. Plasma concentrations then fall, but at a slower rate than observed following oral dosing due to continued absorption of ondansetron. The absolute bioavailability of ondansetron from the suppository is approximately 60% and is not affected by gender. The half life of the elimination phase following suppository administration is determined by the rate of ondansetron absorption, not systemic clearance and is approximately 6 hours. Females show a small, clinically insignificant, increase in half-life in comparison with males.

Ondansetron is not highly protein bound (70-76%). Ondansetron is cleared from the systemic circulation predominantly by hepatic metabolism through multiple enzymatic pathways. Less than 5% of the absorbed dose is excreted unchanged in the urine. The absence of the enzyme CYP2D6 (the debrisoquine polymorphism) has no effect on ondansetron's pharmacokinetics. The pharmacokinetic properties of ondansetron are unchanged on repeat dosing.

In a study of 21 paediatric patients aged between 3 and 12 years undergoing elective surgery with general anaesthesia, the absolute values for both the clearance and volume of distribution of ondansetron following a single intravenous dose of 2mg (3-7 years old) or 4mg (8-12 years old) were reduced. The magnitude of the change was age-related, with clearance falling from about 300mL/min at 12 years of age to 100mL/min at 3 years. Volume of distribution fell from about 75L at 12 years to 17L at 3 years. Use of weight-based dosing (0.1mg/kg up to 4mg maximum) compensates for these changes and is effective in normalising systemic exposure in paediatric patients.

In patients with renal impairment (creatinine clearance 15-60 ml/min), both systemic clearance and volume of distribution are reduced following IV administration of ondansetron, resulting in a slight, but clinically insignificant, increase in elimination half-life (5.4h). A study in patients with severe renal impairment who required regular haemodialysis (studied between dialyses) showed ondansetron's pharmacokinetics to be essentially unchanged following IV administration.

Specific studies in the elderly or patients with renal impairment have been limited to IV and oral administration. However, it is anticipated that the half-life of ondansetron after rectal administration in these populations will be similar to that seen in healthy volunteers, since the rate of elimination of ondansetron following rectal administration is not determined by systemic clearance.

Following oral, intravenous or intramuscular dosing in patients with severe hepatic impairment, ondansetron's systemic clearance is markedly reduced with prolonged elimination half-lives (15-32 h) and an oral bioavailability approaching 100% due to reduced pre-systemic metabolism. The pharmacokinetics of ondansetron following administration as a suppository have not been evaluated in patients with hepatic impairment.

5.3 Preclinical safety data

No additional data of relevance.

6. PHARMACEUTICAL PARTICULARS

6.1 List of excipients

Injection

Citric acid monohydrate, sodium citrate, sodium chloride, Water for Injections.

Tablets

Lactose, microcrystalline cellulose, pregelatinised maize starch, magnesium stearate, methylhydroxypropylcellulose, titanium dioxide (E171), iron oxide (E172).

6.2 Incompatibilities

Injection

Zofran injection should not be administered in the same syringe or Infusion as any other medication.

Tablets

None reported.

6.3 Shelf life

Injection 36 months (unopened).

24 hours (dilutions stored 2 - 8°C).

Tablets 36 months

6.4 Special precautions for storage

Injection Protect from light. Store below 30°C.

Dilutions of Zofran injection in compatible intravenous infusion fluids are stable under normal room lighting conditions or daylight for at least 24 hours, thus no protection from light is necessary while infusion takes place.

Tablets Store below 30°C.

6.5 Nature and contents of container

Zofran Flexi-amp injection: Polypropylene blow-fill-sealed ampoules with a twist-off top and overwrapped in a double foil blister.

5 ampoules are packed in a carton.

4mg Tablets: Blister packs of 30 tablets comprising aluminium/PVC blister film and aluminium foil lidding.

8mg Tablets: Blister packs of 10 tablets comprising aluminium/PVC blister film and aluminium foil lidding.

6.6 Instructions for use and handling

Zofran Flexi-amp injection should not be autoclaved.

Tablets None stated.

Compatibility with intravenous fluids

Zofran injection should only be admixed with those infusion solutions which are recommended:

Sodium Chloride Intravenous Infusion BP 0.9%w/v

Glucose Intravenous Infusion BP 5%w/v

Mannitol Intravenous Infusion BP 10%w/v

Ringers Intravenous Infusion

Potassium Chloride 0.3%w/v and Sodium Chloride 0.9%w/v Intravenous Infusion BP

Potassium Chloride 0.3%w/v and Glucose 5%w/v Intravenous Infusion BP

In keeping with good pharmaceutical practice dilutions of Zofran injection in intravenous fluids should be prepared at the time of infusion or stored at 2-8°C for no more than 24 hours before the start of administration.

Compatibility studies have been undertaken in polyvinyl chloride infusion bags and polyvinyl chloride administration sets. It is considered that adequate stability would also be conferred by the use of polyethylene infusion bags or Type 1 glass bottles. Dilutions of Zofran in sodium chloride 0.9%w/v or in glucose 5%w/v have been demonstrated to be stable in polypropylene syringes. It is considered that Zofran injection diluted with other compatible infusion fluids would be stable in polypropylene syringes.

Compatibility with other drugs

Zofran may be administered by intravenous infusion at 1mg/hour, e.g. from an infusion bag or syringe pump. The following drugs may be administered via the Y-site of the Zofran giving set for ondansetron concentrations of 16 to 160 micrograms/ml (e.g. 8 mg/500 ml and 8 mg/50 ml respectively);

Cisplatin: Concentrations up to 0.48 mg/ml (e.g. 240 mg in 500 ml) administered over one to eight hours.

5 -Fluorouracil:

Concentrations up to 0.8 mg/ml (e.g. 2.4g in 3 litres or 400mg in 500ml) administered at a rate of at least 20 ml per hour (500 ml per 24 hours). Higher concentrations of 5-fluorouracil may cause precipitation of ondansetron. The 5-fluorouracil infusion may contain up to 0.045%w/v magnesium chloride in addition to other excipients shown to be compatible.

Carboplatin: Concentrations in the range 0.18 mg/ml to 9.9 mg/ml (e.g. 90 mg in 500 ml to 990 mg in 100 ml), administered over ten minutes to one hour.

Etoposide: Concentrations in the range 0.14 mg/ml to 0.25 mg/ml (e.g. 72 mg in 500 ml to 250 mg in 1 litre), administered over thirty minutes to one hour.

Ceftazidime: Doses in the range 250 mg to 2000 mg reconstituted with Water for Injections BP as recommended by the manufacturer (e.g. 2.5 ml for 250 mg and 10 ml for 2g ceftazidime) and given as an intravenous bolus injection over approximately five minutes.

Cyclophosphamide: Doses in the range 100 mg to 1g, reconstituted with Water for Injections BP, 5 ml per 100 mg cyclophosphamide, as recommended by the manufacturer and given as an intravenous bolus injection over approximately five minutes.

Doxorubicin: Doses in the range 10-100mg reconstituted with Water for Injections BP, 5 ml per 10 mg doxorubicin, as recommended by the manufacturer and given as an intravenous bolus injection over approximately 5 minutes.

Dexamethasone: Dexamethasone sodium phosphate 20mg may be administered as a slow intravenous injection over 2-5 minutes via the Y-site of an infusion set delivering 8 or 32mg of ondansetron diluted in 50-100ml of a compatible infusion fluid over approximately 15 minutes. Compatibility between dexamethasone sodium phosphate and ondansetron has been demonstrated supporting administration of these drugs through the same giving set resulting in concentrations in line of 32 microgram - 2.5mg/ml for dexamethasone sodium phosphate and 8 microgram - 1mg/ml for ondansetron.

Administrative Data

7. MARKETING AUTHORISATION HOLDER

Zofran Flexi-amp Injection 2mg/ml

Glaxo Operations UK Limited, Greenford, Middlesex, UB6 0HE

Zofran Tablets 4mg and 8mg

Glaxo Wellcome UK Limited, Stockley park, Middlesex, UB11 1BT

Trading as GlaxoSmithKline UK, Stockley Park West, Uxbridge, Middlesex, UB11 1BT

8. MARKETING AUTHORISATION NUMBER(S)

Zofran Flexi-amp Injection 2mg/ml 00004/0375

Zofran Tablets 4mg 10949/0110

Zofran Tablets 8mg 10949/0111

9. DATE OF FIRST AUTHORISATION/RENEWAL OF THE AUTHORISATION

Zofran Flexi-amp Injection 2mg/ml 23rd October 2001

Zofran Tablets 4mg 9th January 2002

Zofran Tablets 8mg 9th January 2002

10. DATE OF REVISION OF THE TEXT

30 November 2004 (Tablets)

28 September 2004 (Injection)

11. Legal Status

POM

Zoladex

(AstraZeneca UK Limited)

1. NAME OF THE MEDICINAL PRODUCT

Zoladex®

2. QUALITATIVE AND QUANTITATIVE COMPOSITION

Goserelin Acetate

(equivalent to 3.6mg goserelin)

3. PHARMACEUTICAL FORM

Implant, in pre-filled syringe.

4. CLINICAL PARTICULARS

4.1 Therapeutic indications

(i) Prostate Cancer: Zoladex is indicated in the management of prostate cancer suitable for hormonal manipulation.

(ii) Advanced breast cancer in pre- and peri-menopausal women suitable for hormonal manipulation.

(iii) Zoladex 3.6mg is indicated as an alternative to chemotherapy in the standard of care for pre-/ peri-menopausal women with oestrogen receptor (ER) positive early breast cancer.

(iv) Endometriosis: In the management of endometriosis, Zoladex alleviates symptoms, including pain, and reduces the size and number of endometrial lesions.

(v) Endometrial thinning: Zoladex is indicated for the pre-thinning of the uterine endometrium prior to endometrial ablation or resection.

(vi) Uterine fibroids: In conjunction with iron therapy in the haematological improvement of anaemic patients with fibroids prior to surgery.

(vii) Assisted reproduction: Pituitary downregulation in preparation for superovulation.

4.2 Posology and method of administration

Adults

One 3.6mg depot of Zoladex injected subcutaneously into the anterior abdominal wall, every 28 days. No dosage adjustment is necessary for patients with renal or hepatic impairment or in the elderly.

Endometriosis should be treated for a period of six months only, since at present there are no clinical data for longer treatment periods. Repeat courses should not be given due to concern about loss of bone mineral density. In patients receiving Zoladex for the treatment of endometriosis, the addition of hormone replacement therapy (a daily oestrogenic agent and a progestogenic agent) has been shown to reduce bone mineral density loss and vasomotor symptoms.

For use in endometrial thinning, four or eight weeks treatment. The second depot may be required for the patient with a large uterus or to allow flexible surgical timing.

For women who are anaemic as a result of uterine fibroids, Zoladex 3.6mg depot with supplementary iron may be administered for up to three months before surgery.

Assisted reproduction: Zoladex 3.6 mg is administered to downregulate the pituitary gland, as defined by serum oestradiol levels similar to those observed in the early follicular phase (approximately 150 pmol/l). This will usually take between 7 and 21 days.

When downregulation is achieved, superovulation (controlled ovarian stimulation) with gonadotrophin is commenced. The downregulation achieved with a depot agonist is more consistent suggesting that, in some cases, there may be an increased requirement for gonadotrophin. At the appropriate stage of follicular development, gonadotrophin is stopped and human chorionic gonadotrophin (hCG) is administered to induce ovulation. Treatment monitoring, oocyte retrieval and fertilisation techniques are performed according to the normal practice of the individual clinic.

Children

Zoladex is not indicated for use in children.

For correct administration of 'Zoladex', see instructions on the instruction card.

4.3 Contraindications

Zoladex should not be given to patients with a known hypersensitivity to Zoladex or to other LHRH analogues. Zoladex should not be used in pregnancy (see section 4.6).

4.4 Special warnings and special precautions for use

Zoladex is not indicated for use in children, as safety and efficacy have not been established in this group of patients.

Males

The use of Zoladex in men at particular risk of developing ureteric obstruction or spinal cord compression should be considered carefully and the patients monitored closely during the first month of therapy. Consideration should be given to the initial use of an anti-androgen (eg. cyproterone acetate 300mg daily for three days before and three weeks after commencement of Zoladex) at the start of LHRH analogue therapy since this has been reported to prevent the possible sequelae of the initial rise in serum testosterone. If spinal cord compression or renal impairment due to ureteric obstruction are present or develop, specific standard treatment of these complications should be instituted.

Females

The use of LHRH agonists in women may cause a loss of bone mineral density.

Following two years treatment for early breast cancer, the average loss of bone mineral density was 6.2% and 11.5% at the femoral neck and lumbar spine respectively. This loss has been shown to be partially reversible at the one year off treatment follow-up with recovery to 3.4% and 6.4% relative to baseline at the femoral neck and lumbar spine respectively although this recovery is based on very limited data.

In patients receiving Zoladex for the treatment of endometriosis, the addition of hormone replacement therapy (a daily oestrogenic agent and a progestogenic agent) has been shown to reduce bone mineral density loss and vasomotor symptoms.

Zoladex should be used with caution in women with known metabolic bone disease.

Zoladex may cause an increase in uterine cervical resistance, which may result in difficulty in dilating the cervix.

Currently, there are no clinical data on the effect of treating benign gynaecological conditions with Zoladex for periods in excess of six months.

Zoladex should only be administered as part of a regimen for assisted reproduction under the supervision of a specialist experienced in the area.

As with other LHRH agonists, there have been reports of ovarian hyperstimulation syndrome (OHSS), associated with the use of Zoladex 3.6 mg in combination with gonadotrophin. It has been suggested that the downregulation achieved with a depot agonist may lead, in some cases, to an increased requirement for gonadotrophin. The stimulation cycle should be monitored carefully to identify patients at risk of developing OHSS because its severity and incidence may be dependent on the dose regimen of gonadotrophin. Human chorionic gonadotrophin (hCG) should be withheld, if appropriate.

It is recommended that Zoladex is used with caution in assisted reproduction regimens in patients with polycystic ovarian syndrome as follicle recruitment may be increased.

4.5 Interaction with other medicinal products and other forms of Interaction

None Known.

4.6 Pregnancy and lactation

Pregnancy: Although reproductive toxicity in animals gave no evidence of teratogenic potential, Zoladex should not be used in pregnancy as there is a theoretical risk of abortion or foetal abnormality if LHRH agonists are used during pregnancy. Potentially fertile women should be examined carefully before treatment to exclude pregnancy. Non hormonal methods of contraception should be employed during therapy and in the case of endometriosis should be continued until menses are resumed.

Pregnancy should be excluded before Zoladex is used for assisted reproduction. The clinical data from use in this setting are limited but the available evidence suggests there is no causal association between Zoladex and any subsequent abnormalities of oocyte development or pregnancy and outcome.

Lactation: The use of Zoladex during breast feeding is not recommended.

4.7 Effects on ability to drive and use machines

There is no evidence that Zoladex results in impairment of these activities.

4.8 Undesirable effects

General

Rare incidences of hypersensitivity reactions, which may include some manifestations of anaphylaxis, have been reported.

Arthralgia has been reported. Non-specific paraesthesias have been reported. Skin rashes have been reported which are generally mild, often regressing without discontinuation of therapy.

Changes in blood pressure, manifest as hypotension or hypertension, have been occasionally observed in patients administered Zoladex. The changes are usually transient, resolving either during continued therapy or after cessation of therapy with Zoladex. Rarely, such changes have been sufficient to require medical intervention including withdrawal of treatment from Zoladex.

As with other agents in this class, very rare cases of pituitary apoplexy have been reported following initial administration.

Occasional local reactions include mild bruising at the subcutaneous injection site.

Males

Pharmacological effects in men include hot flushes and sweating and a decrease in libido, seldom requiring withdrawal of therapy. Breast swelling and tenderness have been noted infrequently. Initially, prostate cancer patients may experience a temporary increase in bone pain, which can be managed symptomatically. Isolated cases of ureteric obstruction and spinal cord compression have been recorded.

The use of LHRH agonists in men may cause a loss of bone mineral density.

Females

Pharmacological effects in women include hot flushes and sweating, and loss in libido, seldom requiring withdrawal of therapy. Headaches, mood changes including depression, vaginal dryness and change in breast size have been noted. During early treatment with Zoladex some women may experience vaginal bleeding of variable duration and intensity. If vaginal bleeding occurs it is usually in the first month after starting treatment. Such bleeding probably represents oestrogen withdrawal bleeding and is expected to stop spontaneously.

Initially breast cancer patients may experience a temporary increase in signs and symptoms, which can be managed symptomatically. In women with fibroids, degeneration of fibroids may occur.

Rarely, breast cancer patients with metastases have developed hypercalcaemia on initiation of therapy.

Rarely, some women may enter the menopause during treatment with LHRH analogues and not resume menses on cessation of therapy. This may simply be a physiological change.

In Assisted Reproduction: As with other LHRH agonists, there have been reports of ovarian hyperstimulation syndrome (OHSS), associated with the use of Zoladex 3.6 mg in combination with gonadotrophin. It has been suggested that the downregulation achieved with a depot agonist may lead, in some cases, to an increased requirement for gonadotrophin. The stimulation cycle should be monitored carefully to identify patients at risk of developing OHSS because its severity and incidence may be dependent on the dose regimen of gonadotrophin. Human chorionic gonadotrophin (hCG) should be withheld, if appropriate.

Follicular and luteal ovarian cysts have been reported to occur following LHRH therapy. Most cysts are asymptomatic, non functional, varying in size and resolve spontaneously.

4.9 Overdose

There is limited experience of overdosage in humans. In cases where Zoladex has unintentionally been re-administered early or given at a higher dose, no clinically relevant adverse effects have been seen. Animal tests suggest that no effect other than the intended therapeutic effects on sex hormone concentrations and on the reproductive tract will be evident with higher doses of Zoladex. If overdosage occurs, this should be managed symptomatically.

5. PHARMACOLOGICAL PROPERTIES

5.1 Pharmacodynamic properties

Zoladex (D-Ser(Bu^t)^6 Azgly^{10} LHRH) is a synthetic analogue of naturally occurring LHRH. On chronic administration Zoladex results in inhibition of pituitary LH secretion leading to a fall in serum testosterone concentrations in males and serum oestradiol concentrations in females. This effect is reversible on discontinuation of therapy. Initially, Zoladex, like other LHRH agonists, may transiently increase serum testosterone concentration in men and serum oestradiol concentration in women.

In men by around 21 days after the first depot injection testosterone concentrations have fallen to within the castrate range and remain suppressed with continuous treatment every 28 days. This inhibition leads to prostate tumour regression and symptomatic improvement in the majority of patients.

In women serum oestradiol concentrations are suppressed by around 21 days after the first depot injection and, with continuous treatment every 28 days, remain suppressed at levels comparable with those observed in postmenopausal women. This suppression is associated with a response in hormone dependent advanced breast cancer, uterine fibroids, endometriosis and suppression of follicular development within the ovary. It will produce endometrial thinning and will result in amenorrhoea in the majority of patients.

During treatment with LHRH analogues patients may enter the menopause. Rarely some women do not resume menses on cessation of therapy.

Zoladex in combination with iron has been shown to induce amenorrhoea and improve haemoglobin concentrations and related haematological parameters in women with fibroids who are anaemic. The combination produced a mean haemoglobin concentration 1g/dl above that achieved by iron therapy alone.

5.2 Pharmacokinetic properties

The bioavailability of Zoladex is almost complete. Administration of a depot every four weeks ensures that effective concentrations are maintained with no tissue accumulations. Zoladex is poorly protein bound and has a serum elimination half-life of two to four hours in subjects with normal renal function. The half-life is increased in patients with impaired renal function. For the compound given monthly in a depot formulation, this change will have minimal effect. Hence, no change in dosing is necessary in these patients. There is no significant change in pharmacokinetics in patients with hepatic failure.

5.3 Preclinical safety data

Following long-term repeated dosing with Zoladex, an increased incidence of benign pituitary tumours has been observed in male rats. Whilst this finding is similar to that previously noted in this species following surgical castration, any relevance to man has not been established.

In mice, long term repeated dosing with multiples of the human dose produced histological changes in some regions of the digestive system manifested by pancreatic islet cell hyperplasia and a benign proliferative condition in the pyloric region of the stomach, also reported as a spontaneous lesion in this species. The clinical relevance of these findings is unknown.

6. PHARMACEUTICAL PARTICULARS

6.1 List of excipients

Lactide/glycolide co-polymer.

6.2 Incompatibilities

None known.

6.3 Shelf life

36 months.

6.4 Special precautions for storage

Do not store above 25°C.

6.5 Nature and contents of container

Single dose Safe System® syringe applicator with a protective sleeve.

6.6 Instructions for use and handling
Use as directed by the prescriber. Use only if pouch is undamaged. Use immediately after opening pouch. Dispose of the syringe in an approved sharps collector.

7. MARKETING AUTHORISATION HOLDER
AstraZeneca UK Limited,

600 Capability Green,

Luton, LU1 3LU, UK.

8. MARKETING AUTHORISATION NUMBER(S)
PL 17901/0064

9. DATE OF FIRST AUTHORISATION/RENEWAL OF THE AUTHORISATION
1st May 2001 (formerly 13.05.1993)

10. DATE OF REVISION OF THE TEXT
12th November 2003

Zoladex LA 10.8mg

(AstraZeneca UK Limited)

1. NAME OF THE MEDICINAL PRODUCT
'Zoladex' LA 10.8mg.

2. QUALITATIVE AND QUANTITATIVE COMPOSITION
Each depot contains goserelin acetate equivalent to 10.8 mg goserelin.

3. PHARMACEUTICAL FORM
Implant, in pre-filled syringe.

4. CLINICAL PARTICULARS

4.1 Therapeutic indications
'Zoladex' LA is indicated for prostate cancer suitable for hormonal manipulation.

4.2 Posology and method of administration
Adult males (including the elderly) - one depot of 'Zoladex' LA injected subcutaneously into the anterior abdominal wall every 12 weeks.

Children - 'Zoladex' LA is not indicated for use in children.

Renal Impairment - no dosage adjustment is necessary for patients with renal impairment.

Hepatic Impairment - no dosage adjustment for patients with hepatic impairment.

For correct administration of 'Zoladex', see instructions on the instruction card.

4.3 Contraindications
'Zoladex' LA should not be given to patients with a known hypersensitivity to 'Zoladex' or to other LHRH analogues.

4.4 Special warnings and special precautions for use
'Zoladex' LA is not indicated for use in females, since there is insufficient evidence of reliable suppression of serum oestradiol. For female patients requiring treatment with goserelin, refer to the prescribing information for 'Zoladex' 3.6 mg.

'Zoladex' LA is not indicated for use in children, as safety and efficacy have not been established in this group of patients.

The use of 'Zoladex' LA in patients at particular risk of developing ureteric obstruction or spinal cord compression should be considered carefully and the patients monitored closely during the first month of therapy. Consideration should be given to the initial use of an antiandrogen (eg. cyproterone acetate 300mg daily for three days before and three weeks after commencement of 'Zoladex') at the start of LHRH analogue therapy since this has been reported to prevent the possible sequelae of the initial rise in serum testosterone.

If spinal cord compression or renal impairment due to ureteric obstruction are present or develop, specific standard treatment of these complications should be instituted.

4.5 Interaction with other medicinal products and other forms of Interaction
None known.

4.6 Pregnancy and lactation
'Zoladex' LA is not indicated for use in females.

4.7 Effects on ability to drive and use machines
There is no evidence that 'Zoladex' LA results in impairment of ability to drive or operate machinery.

4.8 Undesirable effects
Rare incidences of hypersensitivity reactions, which may include some manifestations of anaphylaxis, have been reported.

Arthralgia has been reported. Non-specific paraesthesias have been reported. Skin rashes have also been reported which are generally mild, often regressing without discontinuation of therapy.

Pharmacological effects in men include hot flushes and sweating and a decrease in libido, seldom requiring withdrawal of therapy. Breast swelling and tenderness have been noted infrequently. Initially, prostate cancer patients may experience a temporary increase in bone pain, which can be managed symptomatically. Isolated cases of spinal cord compression have been recorded.

The use of LHRH agonists in men may cause a loss of bone mineral density.

Changes in blood pressure, manifest as hypotension or hypertension, have been occasionally observed in patients administered 'Zoladex'. The changes are usually transient, resolving either during continued therapy or after cessation of therapy with 'Zoladex'. Rarely, such changes have been sufficient to require medical intervention including withdrawal of treatment from 'Zoladex'.

As with other agents in this class, very rare cases of pituitary apoplexy have been reported following initial administration of 'Zoladex' 3.6 mg.

Following the administration of 'Zoladex' 3.6mg isolated cases of ureteric obstruction have been recorded.

4.9 Overdose
There is limited experience of overdosage in humans. In cases where 'Zoladex' has unintentionally been readministered early or given at a higher dose, no clinically relevant adverse effects have been seen. Animal tests suggest that no effect other than the intended therapeutic effects on sex hormone concentrations and on the reproductive tract will be evident with higher doses of 'Zoladex' LA. If overdosage occurs, this should be managed symptomatically.

5. PHARMACOLOGICAL PROPERTIES

5.1 Pharmacodynamic properties
'Zoladex' (D-Ser(Bu^t)^{6}Azgly^{10} LHRH) is a synthetic analogue of naturally occurring luteinising-hormone releasing hormone (LHRH). On chronic administration 'Zoladex' LA results in inhibition of pituitary luteinising hormone secretion leading to a fall in serum testosterone concentrations in males. Initially, 'Zoladex' LA like other LHRH agonists transiently increases serum testosterone concentrations.

In men by around 21 days after the first depot injection, testosterone concentrations have fallen to within the castrate range and remain suppressed with continuous treatment every 12 weeks.

5.2 Pharmacokinetic properties
Administration of 'Zoladex' LA every 12 weeks ensures that exposure to goserelin is maintained with no clinically significant accumulation. 'Zoladex' is poorly protein bound and has a serum elimination half-life of two to four hours in subjects with normal renal function. The half-life is increased in patients with impaired renal function. For the compound given in a 10.8 mg depot formulation every 12 weeks this change will not lead to any accumulation. Hence, no change in dosing is necessary in these patients. There is no significant change in pharmacokinetics in patients with hepatic failure.

5.3 Preclinical safety data
Following long-term repeated dosing with 'Zoladex', an increased incidence of benign pituitary tumours has been observed in male rats. Whilst this finding is similar to that previously noted in this species following surgical castration, any relevance to humans has not been established.

In mice, long term repeated dosing with multiples of the human dose produced histological changes in some regions of the digestive system. This is manifested by pancreatic islet cell hyperplasia and a benign proliferative condition in the pyloric region of the stomach, also reported as a spontaneous lesion in this species. The clinical relevance of these findings is unknown.

6. PHARMACEUTICAL PARTICULARS

6.1 List of excipients
A blend of high and low molecular weight lactide/glycolide copolymers.

6.2 Incompatibilities
None known.

6.3 Shelf life
36 months.

6.4 Special precautions for storage
Do not store above 25°C.

6.5 Nature and contents of container
'Zoladex' LA is supplied as a single dose SafeSystem™ syringe applicator with a protective sleeve in a sealed pouch which contains a desiccant.

6.6 Instructions for use and handling
Use as directed by the prescriber. Use only if pouch is undamaged. Use immediately after opening pouch. Dispose of the syringe in an approved sharps collector.

7. MARKETING AUTHORISATION HOLDER
AstraZeneca UK Limited,

600 Capability Green,

Luton, LU1 3LU, UK.

8. MARKETING AUTHORISATION NUMBER(S)
PL 17901/0065

9. DATE OF FIRST AUTHORISATION/RENEWAL OF THE AUTHORISATION
1st May 2001

10. DATE OF REVISION OF THE TEXT
12th November 2003

Zolvera 40mg/5ml Oral Solution

(Rosemont Pharmaceuticals Limited)

1. NAME OF THE MEDICINAL PRODUCT
ZOLVERA 40mg/5ml Oral Solution

2. QUALITATIVE AND QUANTITATIVE COMPOSITION
Verapamil Hydrochloride 40mg/5ml

For excipients see Section 6.1

3. PHARMACEUTICAL FORM
Oral Solution

4. CLINICAL PARTICULARS

4.1 Therapeutic indications
1. Treatment of mild to moderate hypertension.

2. Treatment and prophylaxis of chronic stable angina, vasospastic angina and unstable angina.

3. Treatment and prophylaxis of paroxysmal supraventricular tachycardia and the reduction of ventricular rate in atrial flutter/fibrillation. Verapamil should not be used when atrial flutter/fibrillation complicates Wolff-Parkinson-White syndrome (see Precautions).

4.2 Posology and method of administration
Adults:

Hypertension: Initially 120mg b.d. increasing to 160mg b.d. when necessary. In some cases, dosages of up to 480mg daily, in divided doses, have been used. A further reduction in blood pressure may be obtained by combining verapamil with other antihypertensive agents, in particular diuretics. For concomitant administration with beta-blockers see Precautions.

Angina: 120mg t.d.s. is recommended. 80mg t.d.s. can be completely satisfactory in some patients with angina of effort. Less than 120mg t.d.s is not likely to be effective in variant angina.

Supraventricular tachycardias: 40-120mg, t.d.s. according to the severity of the condition.

Children:

Up to 2 years: 20mg, 2-3 times a day.

2 years and above: 40-120mg, 2-3 times a day, according to age and effectiveness.

Elderly:

The adult dose is recommended unless liver or renal function is impaired (see Precautions).

4.3 Contraindications
Hypersensitivity to verapamil or any of the ingredients

Cardiogenic shock

Acute myocardial infarction complicated by bradycardia, hypotension or left ventricular failure

Second or third degree atrioventricular block

Sino-atrial block

Sick sinus syndrome

Uncompensated heart failure

Bradycardia of less than 50 beats/minute

Hypotension of less than 90mmHg systolic

Concomitant ingestion of grapefruit juice.

4.4 Special warnings and special precautions for use
Since verapamil is extensively metabolised in the liver, careful dose titration of verapamil is required in patients with liver disease. The disposition of verapamil in patients with renal impairment has not been fully established and therefore careful patient monitoring is recommended. Verapamil is not removed during dialysis.

Verapamil may affect impulse conduction and therefore verapamil solution should be used with caution in patients with first degree AV block. Patients with atrial flutter/fibrillation in association with an accessory pathway (e.g. WPW syndrome) may develop increased conduction across the anomalous pathway and ventricular tachycardia may be precipitated.

Verapamil may affect left ventricular contractility; this effect is small and normally not important but cardiac failure may be precipitated or aggravated.

In patients with incipient cardiac failure, therefore, verapamil should be given only after such cardiac failure has been controlled with appropriate therapy, e.g. digitalis.

When treating hypertension with verapamil, monitoring of the patient's blood pressure at regular intervals is required.

This preparation contains benzoic acid which can irritate skin, eyes and mucous membranes. It may also increase the risk of jaundice in newborn babies.

It also contains liquid maltitol which may cause diarrhoea.

4.5 Interaction with other medicinal products and other forms of Interaction
Interactions between verapamil and the following medications have been reported:

Digoxin: Verapamil has been shown to increase the serum concentration of digoxin and caution should be exercised with regard to digitalis toxicity. The digitalis level should be determined and the glycoside dose reduced, if required.

Beta-blockers, anti-arrhythmic agents or inhaled anaesthetics: The combination with verapamil may lead to additive cardiovascular effects (e.g. AV block, bradycardia, hypotension, heart failure). Intravenous beta-blockers should not be given to patients under treatment with verapamil.

Carbamazepine, ciclosporin and theophylline: Use of verapamil has resulted in increased serum levels of these medications, which could lead to increased side effects.

Rifampicin, phenytoin and phenobarbital: Serum levels of verapamil are reduced.

Lithium: Serum levels of lithium may be reduced (pharmacokinetic effect); there may be increased sensitivity to lithium causing enhanced neurotoxicity (pharmacodynamic effect).

Cimetidine: Increase in verapamil serum level is possible.

Neuromuscular blocking agents employed in anaesthesia: The effects may be potentiated.

The effects of verapamil may be additive to other hypotensive agents.

Grapefruit Juice: An increase in verapamil levels has been reported.

4.6 Pregnancy and lactation

Although animal studies have not shown any teratogenic effects, verapamil should not be given during the first trimester of pregnancy unless, in the clinician's judgement, it is essential for the welfare of the patient.

Verapamil is excreted into the breast milk in small amounts and is unlikely to be harmful. However, rare hypersensitivity reactions have been reported with verapamil and, therefore, it should only be used during lactation if, in the clinician's judgement, it is essential for the welfare of the patient.

4.7 Effects on ability to drive and use machines

Depending on individual susceptibility, the patient's ability to drive a vehicle or operate machinery may be impaired. This is particularly true in the initial stages of treatment, or when changing over from another medication. Like many other common medicines, verapamil has been shown to increase the blood levels of alcohol and slow its elimination. Therefore, the effects of alcohol may be exaggerated.

4.8 Undesirable effects

Verapamil is generally well tolerated. Side effects are usually mild and transient and discontinuation of therapy is rarely necessary.

Endocrine: On very rare occasions, gynaecomastia has been observed in elderly male patients under long-term verapamil treatment, which was fully reversible in all cases when the drug was discontinued.

Rises in prolactin levels have been reported.

Cardiac: Particularly when given in high doses or in the presence of previous myocardial damage, some cardiovascular effects of verapamil may occasionally be greater than therapeutically desired: bradycardic arrhythmias, such as sinus bradycardia, sinus arrest with asystole, second and third degree AV block, bradyarrhythmia in atrial fibrillation, hypotension, development or aggravation of heart failure.

Hepato-biliary: A reversible impairment of liver function, characterised by an increase in transaminase and/or alkaline phosphatase may occur on very rare occasions during verapamil treatment and is most probably a hypersensitivity reaction.

General: Constipation may occur. Flushing is observed occasionally and headaches, nausea, vomiting, dizziness, fatigue and ankle oedema have been reported rarely.

Allergic reactions (e.g. erythema, pruritus, urticaria, Quincke's oedema, Stevens-Johnson syndrome) are very rarely seen.

Gingival hyperplasia may very rarely occur when the drug is administered over prolonged periods, and is fully reversible when the drug is discontinued. Erythromelalgia and paraesthesia may occur. In very rare cases, there may be myalgia and arthralgia.

4.9 Overdose

The course of symptoms in verapamil intoxication depends on the amount taken, the point in time at which detoxification measures are taken and myocardial contractility (age-related). The main symptoms are as follows: blood pressure fall (at times to values not detectable), shock symptoms, loss of consciousness, first and second degree AV block (frequently as Wenckebach's phenomenon with or without escape rhythms), total AV block with total AV dissociation, escape rhythm, asystole, sinus bradycardia, sinus arrest. The therapeutic measures to be taken depend on the point in time at which verapamil was taken and the type and severity of intoxication symptoms. Gastric lavage, taking the usual precautionary measures may be appropriate. The usual intensive resuscitation measures, such as extrathoracic heart massage, respiration, defibrillation and/or pacemaker therapy. Specific measures to be taken: Elimination of cardiodepressive effects, hypotension or bradycardia. The specific antidote is calcium, e.g. 10-20ml of a 10% calcium gluconate solution administered intravenously (2.25 - 4.5mmol), repeated if necessary or given as a continuous drip infusion (e.g. 5mmol/hour). The following measures may also be necessary: In case of second and third degree AV block, sinus bradycardia, asystole: atropine, isoprenaline, orciprenaline or pacemaker therapy. In case of hypotension after appropriate positioning of the patient: dopamine, dobutamine, noradrenaline. If there are signs of continuing myocardial failure: dopamine, dobutamine, cardiac glycosides or if necessary, repeated calcium gluconate injections.

5. PHARMACOLOGICAL PROPERTIES

5.1 Pharmacodynamic properties

Verapamil is a calcium antagonist which blocks the inward movement of calcium ions in cardiac muscle cells, in smooth muscle cells of the coronary and systemic arteries and in the cells of the intracardiac conduction system. Verapamil lowers peripheral vascular resistance with no reflex tachycardia. Its efficacy in reducing both raised systolic and diastolic blood pressure is thought to be due to this mode of action. The decrease in systemic and coronary vascular resistance and the sparing effect on intracellular oxygen consumption appear to explain the anti-anginal properties of the drug. Because of its effect on the movement of calcium in the intracardiac conduction system, verapamil reduces automaticity, decreases conduction velocity and increases the refractory period.

5.2 Pharmacokinetic properties

Over 90% of verapamil is absorbed following administration with peak plasma concentrations occurring between 1 and 2 hours and does not appear to be affected markedly by food.

Verapamil is subject to pre-systemic hepatic metabolism with up to 80% of the dose eliminated this way. Because of rapid biotransformation of verapamil during its first pass through the portal circulation, absolute bioavailability ranges from 20-35%. Verapamil is widely distributed throughout the body with a distribution half-life of 15-30 mins. Verapamil is 90% bound to plasma proteins, mainly to albumin and α1 glycoprotein. The half life of verapamil after a single oral dose is between 2 and 7h. However, after repeated administration it increases to 4.5 to 12h resulting in accumulation of the drug.

5.3 Preclinical safety data

Verapamil is a drug on which extensive clinical experience has been obtained. Relevant information for the prescriber is provided elsewhere in the Summary of Product Characteristics.

6. PHARMACEUTICAL PARTICULARS

6.1 List of excipients

Propylene glycol, benzoic acid, liquid maltitol, dill water concentrate, liquorice flavour, citric acid monohydrate, sodium citrate and purified water.

6.2 Incompatibilities

Not applicable.

6.3 Shelf life

36 months

3 months once open

6.4 Special precautions for storage

Do not store above 25°C.

6.5 Nature and contents of container

Bottle: Amber (Type III) glass

Closures: a) Aluminium, EPE wadded, roll-on pilfer proof screw cap.

b) HDPE, EPE wadded, tamper evident screw cap.

c) HDPE, EPE wadded, tamper evident, child resistant closure.

Pack Size: 150ml

6.6 Instructions for use and handling

Not applicable.

Administrative Data

7. MARKETING AUTHORISATION HOLDER

Rosemont Pharmaceuticals Ltd, Rosemont House, Yorkdale Industrial Park, Braithwaite Street, Leeds, LS11 9XE, UK.

8. MARKETING AUTHORISATION NUMBER(S)

PL 00427/0130

9. DATE OF FIRST AUTHORISATION/RENEWAL OF THE AUTHORISATION

23 May 2001

10. DATE OF REVISION OF THE TEXT

May 2005

Zomacton 4mg Injection

(Ferring Pharmaceuticals Ltd)

1. NAME OF THE MEDICINAL PRODUCT

ZOMACTON® 4mg Injection.

2. QUALITATIVE AND QUANTITATIVE COMPOSITION

Somatropin* 4mg

(1.3mg/ml or 3.3mg/ml after reconstitution)

* Produced by genetic engineering from *E. coli*

For excipients, see 6.1.

3. PHARMACEUTICAL FORM

Powder and solvent for solution for injection.

ZOMACTON is a white to off-white lyophilised powder which after reconstitution with benzyl alcohol preserved saline solvent forms a clear and colourless solution for injection.

4. CLINICAL PARTICULARS

4.1 Therapeutic indications

ZOMACTON is indicated for the long-term treatment of children who have growth failure due to inadequate secretion of growth hormone and for the long-term treatment of growth retardation due to Turner's Syndrome confirmed by chromosome analysis.

4.2 Posology and method of administration

The dosage and schedule of administration of ZOMACTON should be individualised for each patient.

The duration of treatment, usually a period of several years, will depend on maximum achievable therapeutic benefit.

The subcutaneous administration of growth hormone may lead to loss or increase of adipose tissue at the injection site. Therefore, injection sites should be alternated.

Growth Hormone Deficiency

Generally a dose of 0.17 - 0.23mg/kg bodyweight (approximating to 4.9mg/m^2 – 6.9mg/m^2 body surface area) per week divided into 6 - 7 s.c. injections is recommended (corresponding to a daily injection of 0.02 – 0.03mg/kg bodyweight or 0.7 - 1.0mg/m^2 body surface area). The total weekly dose of 0.27mg/kg bodyweight or 8mg/m^2 body surface area should not be exceeded (corresponding to daily injections of up to about 0.04mg/kg).

Turner's Syndrome

Generally a dose of 0.33mg/kg bodyweight (approximating to 9.86mg/m^2 body surface area) per week divided into 6 - 7 s.c. injections is recommended (corresponding to a daily injection of 0.05mg/kg bodyweight or 1.40-1.63mg/m^2 body surface area).

4.3 Contraindications

ZOMACTON should not be used in children with closed epiphyses.

Patients with evidence of progression of an underlying intra-cranial lesion or other active neoplasms should not receive ZOMACTON, since the possibility of a tumor growth promoting effect cannot be excluded. Prior to the initiation of therapy with ZOMACTON, neoplasms must be inactive and anti-tumor therapy completed.

Pregnancy and lactation (see section 4.6).

Hypersensitivity to somatropin or to any of the excipients.

Patients with a known sensitivity to benzyl alcohol, neonates and children under the age of 3 years in whom the administration of benzyl alcohol has been associated with toxicity, should not receive ZOMACTON 4mg as the solvent contains benzyl alcohol

Patients with acute critical illness suffering complications following open-heart surgery, abdominal surgery, multiple accidental trauma, acute respiratory failure, or similar conditions should not be treated with ZOMACTON (see section 4.4).

4.4 Special warnings and special precautions for use

ZOMACTON therapy should be used only under the supervision of a qualified physician experienced in the management of patients with growth hormone deficiency.

Patients should be observed for evidence of glucose intolerance because growth hormone may induce a state of insulin resistance. ZOMACTON should be used with caution in patients with diabetes mellitus or with a family history predisposing for the disease. Strict monitoring of urine and blood glucose is necessary in these patients. In children with diabetes, the dose of insulin may need to be increased to maintain glucose control during ZOMACTON therapy.

In patients with growth hormone deficiency secondary to an intra-cranial lesion, frequent monitoring for progression or recurrence of the underlying disease process is advised. Discontinue ZOMACTON therapy if progression or recurrence of the lesion occurs.

In patients with previous malignant diseases special attention should be given to signs and symptoms of relapse.

Rare cases of benign intra-cranial hypertension have been reported. In the event of severe or recurring headache, visual problems, and nausea/vomiting, a funduscopy for papilla edema is recommended. If papilla edema is confirmed, diagnosis of benign intra-cranial hypertension should be considered and if appropriate, growth hormone treatment should be discontinued (see also section 4.8).

Hypothyroidism may develop during treatment with growth hormone. Inadequate treatment of hypothyroidism may prevent optimal response to ZOMACTON. Therefore, patients should have periodic thyroid function tests and be treated with thyroid hormone when indicated.

Leukaemia has been reported in a small number of growth hormone deficient patients treated with Somatropin as well as in untreated patients. Based on clinical experience of more than 10 years, the incidence of leukaemia in GH-treated patients without risk factors is not greater than that in the general population.

Slipped capital femoral epiphysis may occur more frequently in patients with endocrine disorders. A patient treated with ZOMACTON who develops a limp or complains of hip or knee pain should be evaluated by a physician.

The effects of treatment with growth hormone on recovery were studied in two placebo controlled trials involving 522 critically ill adult patients suffering complications following open heart surgery, abdominal surgery, multiple accidental trauma, or acute respiratory failure.

Mortality was higher (42% vs. 19%) among patients treated with growth hormones (doses 5.3 to 8mg/day) compared to those receiving placebo. Based on this information, such patients should not be treated with growth hormones. As there is no information available on the safety of growth hormone substitution therapy in acutely critically ill patients, the benefits of continued treatment in this situation should be weighed against the potential risks involved.

In all patients developing other or similar acute critical illness, the possible benefit of treatment with growth hormone must be weighed against the possible risk involved.

4.5 Interaction with other medicinal products and other forms of Interaction

Glucocorticoid therapy may inhibit the growth promoting effect of ZOMACTON. Patients with coexisting ACTH deficiency should have their glucocorticoid replacement dose carefully adjusted to avoid impairment of the growth promoting effect of ZOMACTON.

High doses of androgens, oestrogens, or anabolic steroids can accelerate bone maturation and may, therefore, diminish gain in final height.

Because somatropin can induce a state of insulin resistance, insulin dose may have to be adjusted in diabetic patients receiving concomitant ZOMACTON.

Data from an interaction study performed in growth hormone deficient adults suggests that somatropin administration may increase the clearance of compounds known to be metabolised by cytochrome P450 isoenzymes. The clearance of compounds metabolised by cytochrome P450 3A4 (e.g. sex steroids, corticosteroids, anticonvulsants and cyclosporin) may be especially increased resulting in lower plasma levels of these compounds. The clinical significance of this is unknown.

4.6 Pregnancy and lactation

ZOMACTON should not be used during pregnancy or lactation:

There is no evidence from either human or animal studies of the safety of growth hormone treatment during pregnancy. Also, no information is available as to whether peptide hormones pass into breast milk.

4.7 Effects on ability to drive and use machines

No effects on the ability to drive and use machines have been observed.

4.8 Undesirable effects

Common (> 1/100, < 1/10):	Local injection site reaction, formation of antibodies, hypoglycemia.
Rare (> 1/10000, < 1/1000):	Peripheral oedema, pain and itchy rash at injection site, diabetes mellitus Type II, myalgia, transient headache, intracranial hypertension.
Very rare (< 1/10000):	Leukaemia.

The subcutaneous administration of growth hormone may lead to loss or increase of adipose tissue at the injection site. On rare occasions patients have developed pain and an itchy rash at the site of injection.

Somatropin has given rise to the formation of antibodies in approximately 1% of patients. The binding capacity of these antibodies has been low and no clinical changes have been associated with their formation.

Rare cases of benign intra-cranial hypertension have been reported with somatropin (see section 4.4).

Very rare cases of leukaemia have been reported in growth hormone deficient children treated with somatropin, but the incidence appears to be similar to that in children without growth hormone deficiency.

4.9 Overdose

The recommended dose of ZOMACTON should not be exceeded.

Although there have been no reports of overdose with ZOMACTON, acute overdose may result in an initial hypoglycaemia followed by a subsequent hyperglycaemia.

The effects of long-term, repeated use of ZOMACTON in doses exceeding those recommended, are unknown. However, it is possible that such use might produce signs and symptoms consistent with the known effects of excess human growth hormone (e.g. acromegaly).

5. PHARMACOLOGICAL PROPERTIES

5.1 Pharmacodynamic properties

Identical to pituitary-derived human growth hormone (pit-hGH) in amino acid sequence, chain length (191 amino acids) and pharmacokinetic profile. ZOMACTON can be expected to produce the same pharmacological effects as the endogenous hormone.

Skeletal system:

Growth hormone produces a generally proportional growth of the skeletal bone in man. Increased linear growth in children with confirmed deficiency in pit-hGH has been demonstrated after exogenous administration of ZOMACTON. The measurable increase in height after administration of ZOMACTON results from an effect on the epiphyseal plates of long bones. In children who lack adequate amounts of pit-hGH, ZOMACTON produces increased growth rates and increased IGF-1 (Insulin-like Growth Factor/Somatomedin-C) concentrations that are similar to those seen after therapy with pit-hGH. Elevations in mean serum alkaline phosphatase concentrations are also involved.

Other organs and tissues:

An increase in size, proportional to total increase in body weight, occurs in other tissues in response to growth hormone, as well.

Changes include: increased growth of connective tissues, skin and appendages; enlargement of skeletal muscle with increase in number and size of cells; growth of the thymus; liver enlargement with increased cellular proliferation; and a slight enlargement of the gonads, adrenals, and thyroid. Disproportionate growth of the skin and flat bones, and accelerated sexual maturation have not been reported in association with the growth hormone replacement therapy.

Protein, carbohydrate and lipid metabolism:

Growth hormone exerts a nitrogen-retaining effect and increases the transport of amino acids into tissue. Both processes augment the synthesis of protein. Carbohydrate use and lipogenesis are depressed by growth hormone. With large doses or in the absence of insulin, growth hormone acts as a diabetogenic agent, producing effects seen typically during fasting (i.e. intolerance to carbohydrate, inhibition of lipogenesis, mobilisation of fat and ketosis).

Mineral metabolism:

Conservation of sodium, potassium, and phosphorous occurs after treatment with growth hormone. Increased calcium loss by the kidney is offset by increased absorption in the gut. Serum calcium concentrations are not significantly altered in patients treated with ZOMACTON or with pit-hGH. Increased serum concentrations of inorganic phosphates have been shown to occur both after ZOMACTON and pit-hGH. Accumulation of these minerals signals an increased demand during tissue synthesis.

5.2 Pharmacokinetic properties

Eight healthy subjects received 0.1mg somatropin/kg body weight. Peak plasma levels of about 64ng/ml were found 6 hours after administration.

5.3 Preclinical safety data

Single dose toxicity:

Single dose toxicity studies were performed in rats (intramuscular application of 10mg/kg), dogs and monkeys (intramuscular dose of 5mg/kg, corresponding to the 50 - 100 fold of the human therapeutic dose). There was no evidence of drug-related toxicity in any of these species.

Repeated dose toxicity:

No relevant toxicological signs were observed in a rat study in which doses of 1.10mg/kg/day for 30 days and 0.37mg/kg/day for 90 days were administered to the animals.

Reproduction toxicology, mutagenic and carcinogenic potential:

Genetically engineered somatropin is identical to endogenous human pituitary growth hormone. It has the same biological properties and it is usually administered in physiological doses. Therefore, it was not deemed necessary to perform the full range of such toxicological studies. Untoward effects on reproduction organs, on pregnancy and lactation are unlikely and also no carcinogenic potential has to be expected. A mutagenicity study showed the absence of mutagenic potential.

6. PHARMACEUTICAL PARTICULARS

6.1 List of excipients

Powder:

Mannitol

Solvent:

Sodium chloride

Benzyl alcohol

Water for injections

6.2 Incompatibilities

In the absence of compatibility studies, this medicinal product must not be mixed with other medicinal products.

6.3 Shelf life

2 years

After reconstitution, chemical and physical stability has been demonstrated during 14 days at + 2°C to + 8°C

6.4 Special precautions for storage

Store at + 2°C to + 8°C (in a refrigerator); keep in the outer carton in order to protect from light.

After reconstitution, store at + 2°C to + 8°C (in a refrigerator). Store vials in an upright position.

6.5 Nature and contents of container

ZOMACTON is supplied in various packs subject to national approvals:

a) Powder in a borosilicate vial (type I glass) with a red halobutyl rubber stopper, a seal and a "flip-off" top + 3.5ml solvent in borosilicate ampoule (type I glass).

Pack: 1

6.6 Instructions for use and handling

Reconstitution:

ZOMACTON should be reconstituted only with the solvent provided.

ZOMACTON powder is reconstituted by introducing the benzyl alcohol preserved isotonic saline solvent into the vial.

Two concentrations can be prepared: 3.3mg/ml for use with the ZOMAJET 2 Vision or conventional syringes and 1.3mg/ml for conventional syringes only.

The solution for injection 3.3mg/ml is prepared by reconstituting the ZOMACTON powder with 1.3ml benzyl alcohol preserved saline solvent using a graduated disposable syringe.

The solution for injection 1.3mg/ml is prepared by reconstituting ZOMACTON powder with 3.2ml of benzyl alcohol preserved saline solvent using a disposable syringe.

To prevent foaming of the solution, the stream of solvent should be aimed against the side of the vial. The vial must then be swirled with a gentle rotary motion until the contents are completely dissolved and a clear, colorless solution is produced. Since ZOMACTON is a protein, shaking or vigorous mixing is not recommended. If after mixing, the solution is cloudy or contains particulate matter, the contents must be discarded. In the case of cloudiness after refrigeration, the product should be allowed to warm to room temperature. If cloudiness persists or coloration appears, discard the vial and its contents.

Administrative Data

The required ZOMACTON dose is administered by using the ZOMAJET 2 Vision, a needle free device or alternatively a conventional syringe.

Specific instructions for use of the ZOMAJET 2 Vision are given in a brochure supplied with the device.

7. MARKETING AUTHORISATION HOLDER

Ferring Pharmaceuticals Limited

The Courtyard

Waterside Drive

Langley

SL3 6EZ

8. MARKETING AUTHORISATION NUMBER(S)

PL 03194/0052

9. DATE OF FIRST AUTHORISATION/RENEWAL OF THE AUTHORISATION

17th March 1995/27th August 2001

10. DATE OF REVISION OF THE TEXT

November 2002

11. Legal Category

POM

Zometa 4mg/5ml Concentrate for Solution for Infusion

(Novartis Pharmaceuticals UK Ltd)

1. NAME OF THE MEDICINAL PRODUCT

▼Zometa® 4 mg/5 ml concentrate for solution for infusion

2. QUALITATIVE AND QUANTITATIVE COMPOSITION

One vial with 5 ml concentrate contains 4 mg zoledronic acid (anhydrous).

One ml concentrate contains zoledronic acid (as monohydrate) corresponding to 0.8 mg zoledronic acid (anhydrous).

For excipients, see 6.1.

3. PHARMACEUTICAL FORM

Concentrate for solution for infusion

4. CLINICAL PARTICULARS

4.1 Therapeutic indications

Prevention of skeletal related events (pathological fractures, spinal compression, radiation or surgery to bone, or tumour-induced hypercalcaemia) in patients with advanced malignancies involving bone.

Treatment of tumour-induced hypercalcaemia (TIH).

4.2 Posology and method of administration

Zometa must only be used by clinicians experienced in the administration of intravenous bisphosphonates.

<u>**Prevention of skeletal related events in patients with advanced malignancies involving bone**</u>

<u>Adults and elderly</u>

The recommended dose in the prevention of skeletal related events in patients with advanced malignancies involving bone is 4 mg zoledronic acid. The concentrate must be further diluted with 100 ml sterile 0.9 % w/v sodium chloride or 5 % w/v glucose solution and given in no less than a 15-minute intravenous infusion every 3 to 4 weeks.

Patients should also be administered an oral calcium supplement of 500 mg and 400 IU vitamin D daily.

Treatment of TIH

Adults and elderly

The recommended dose in hypercalcaemia (albumin-corrected serum calcium ⩾ 12.0 mg/dl or 3.0 mmol/l) is 4 mg zoledronic acid. The concentrate must be further diluted with 100 ml sterile 0.9 % w/v sodium chloride or 5 % w/v glucose solution and given as a single intravenous infusion in no less than 15 minutes. Patients must be maintained well hydrated prior to and following administration of Zometa.

Renal impairment

TIH:

Zometa treatment in TIH patients who also have severe renal impairment should be considered only after evaluating the risks and benefits of treatment. In the clinical studies, patients with serum creatinine > 400 μmol/l or > 4.5 mg/dl were excluded. No dose adjustment is necessary in TIH patients with serum creatinine < 400 μmol/l or < 4.5 mg/dl (see section 4.4, "Special warnings and special precautions for use").

Prevention of skeletal related events in patients with advanced malignancies involving bone:

When initiating treatment with Zometa in patients with multiple myeloma or metastatic bone lesions from solid tumours, serum creatinine and creatinine clearance (CrCl) should be determined. CrCl is calculated from serum creatinine using the Cockcroft-Gault formula. Zometa is not recommended for patients presenting with severe renal impairment prior to initiation of therapy, which is defined for this population as CrCl < 30 ml/min. In clinical trials with Zometa, patients with serum creatinine > 265 μmol/l or > 3.0 mg/dl were excluded.

In patients with bone metastases presenting with mild to moderate renal impairment prior to initiation of therapy, which is defined for this population as CrCl 30–60 ml/min, the following Zometa dose is recommended (see also section 4.4, "Special warnings and special precautions for use"):

Baseline Creatinine Clearance (ml/min)	Zometa Recommended Dose*
> 60	4.0 mg
50 – 60	3.5 mg*
40 – 49	3.3 mg*
30 - 39	3.0 mg*

*Doses have been calculated assuming target AUC of 0.66 (mg•hr/l) (CrCl=75 ml/min). The reduced doses for patients with renal impairment are expected to achieve the same AUC as that seen in patients with creatinine clearance of 75 ml/min.

Following initiation of therapy, serum creatinine should be measured prior to each dose of Zometa and treatment should be withheld if renal function has deteriorated. In the clinical trials, renal deterioration was defined as follows:

- For patients with normal baseline serum creatinine (< 1.4 mg/dl or < 124 μmol/l), an increase of 0.5 mg/dl or 44 μmol/l;

- For patients with an abnormal baseline creatinine (> 1.4 mg/dl or > 124 μmol/l), an increase of 1.0 mg/dl or 88 μmol/l.

In the clinical studies, Zometa treatment was resumed only when the creatinine level returned to within 10 % of the baseline value (see section 4.4, "Special warnings and special precautions for use"). Zometa treatment should be resumed at the same dose as that prior to treatment interruption.

Instructions for preparing reduced doses of Zometa

Withdraw an appropriate volume of the concentrate needed, as follows:4.4 ml for 3.5 mg dose 4.1 ml for 3.3 mg dose 3.8 ml for 3.0 mg dose

The withdrawn amount of concentrate must be further diluted in 100 ml of sterile 0.9 % w/v sodium chloride solution or 5 % w/v glucose solution. The dose must be given as a single intravenous infusion over no less than 15 minutes.

The use of Zometa in paediatric patients has not been studied. Zometa should not be used in that patient population until further data becomes available.

4.3 Contraindications

Zometa concentrate is contraindicated in pregnancy, breast-feeding women, in patients with clinically significant hypersensitivity to zoledronic acid, other bisphosphonates or any of the excipients in the formulation of Zometa.

4.4 Special warnings and special precautions for use

Patients must be assessed prior to administration of Zometa to ensure that they are adequately hydrated.

Standard hypercalcaemia-related metabolic parameters, such as serum levels of calcium, phosphate and magnesium, should be carefully monitored after initiating Zometa therapy. If hypocalcaemia, hypophosphataemia, or hypomagnesaemia occurs, short-term supplemental therapy may be necessary.

Untreated hypercalcaemia patients generally have some degree of renal function impairment, therefore careful renal function monitoring should be considered.

Patients with TIH with evidence of deterioration in renal function should be appropriately evaluated with consideration given as to whether the potential benefit of treatment with Zometa outweighs the possible risk.

The decision to treat patients with bone metastases for the prevention of skeletal related events should consider that the onset of treatment effect is 2-3 months.

As with other bisphosphonates, Zometa has been associated with reports of renal dysfunction. Factors that may increase the potential for deterioration in renal function include dehydration, pre-existing renal impairment, multiple cycles of Zometa and other bisphosphonates as well as use of other nephrotoxic drugs. While the risk is reduced with a dose of Zometa 4 mg administered over 15 minutes, deterioration in renal function may still occur. Increases in serum creatinine also occur in some patients with chronic administration of Zometa at recommended doses for prevention of skeletal related events, although less frequently.

Patients should have their serum creatinine levels assessed prior to each dose of Zometa. Upon initiation of treatment in patients with bone metastases with mild to moderate renal impairment, lower doses of Zometa are recommended. In patients who show evidence of renal deterioration during treatment, Zometa should be withheld. Zometa should only be resumed when serum creatinine returns to within 10% of baseline (see section 4.2, "Posology and method of administration").

In view of the potential impact of bisphosphonates, including Zometa, on renal function, the lack of clinical safety data in patients with severe renal impairment (in clinical trials defined as serum creatinine ⩾ 400 μmol/l or ⩾ 4.5 mg/dl for patients with TIH and ⩾ 265 μmol/l or ⩾ 3.0 mg/dl for patients with cancer and bone metastases, respectively) at baseline and only limited pharmacokinetic data in patients with severe renal impairment at baseline (creatinine clearance < 30 ml/min), the use of Zometa is not recommended in patients with severe renal impairment.

As only limited clinical data are available in patients with severe hepatic insufficiency, no specific recommendations can be given for this patient population.

Overhydration should be avoided in patients at risk of cardiac failure.

The safety and efficacy of Zometa in paediatric patients have not been established.

Osteonecrosis of the jaw has been reported in patients with cancer receiving treatment regimens including bisphosphonates. Many of these patients were also receiving chemotherapy and corticosteroids. The majority of reported cases have been associated with dental procedures such as tooth extraction. Many had signs of local infection including osteomyelitis.

A dental examination with appropriate preventive dentistry should be considered prior to treatment with bisphosphonates in patients with concomitant risk factors (e.g. cancer, chemotherapy, corticosteroids, poor oral hygiene).

While on treatment, these patients should avoid invasive dental procedures if possible. For patients who develop osteonecrosis of the jaw while on bisphosphonate therapy, dental surgery may exacerbate the condition. For patients requiring dental procedures, there are no data available to suggest whether discontinuation of bisphosphonate treatment reduces the risk of osteonecrosis of the jaw. Clinical judgement of the treating physician should guide the management plan of each patient based on individual benefit/risk assessment.

4.5 Interaction with other medicinal products and other forms of Interaction

In clinical studies, Zometa has been administered concomitantly with commonly used anticancer agents, diuretics, antibiotics and analgesics without clinically apparent interactions occurring. Zoledronic acid shows no appreciable binding to plasma proteins and does not inhibit human P450 enzymes *in vitro* (see section 5.2, "Pharmacokinetic properties"), but no formal clinical interaction studies have been performed. Caution is advised when bisphosphonates are administered with aminoglycosides, since both agents may have an additive effect, resulting in a lower serum calcium level for longer periods than required. Caution is indicated when Zometa is used with other potentially nephrotoxic drugs. Attention should also be paid to the possibility of hypomagnesaemia developing during treatment.

In multiple myeloma patients, the risk of renal dysfunction may be increased when intravenous bisphosphonates are used in combination with thalidomide.

4.6 Pregnancy and lactation

There are no adequate data on the use of zoledronic acid in pregnant women. Animal reproduction studies with zoledronic acid have shown reproductive toxicity (see section 5.3, "Preclinical safety data"). Dystocia was observed at the lowest dose (0.01 mg/kg bodyweight) tested in the rat. The potential risk for humans is unknown. Zometa should not be used during pregnancy.

It is not known whether zoledronic acid is excreted into human milk. Zometa should not be used by breast-feeding women (see section 4.3, "Contraindications").

4.7 Effects on ability to drive and use machines

No studies on the effects on the ability to drive and use machines have been performed.

4.8 Undesirable effects

Frequencies of adverse reactions for Zometa 4 mg are mainly based on data collection from chronic treatment. Adverse reactions to Zometa are similar to those reported for other bisphosphonates and can be expected to occur in approximately one third of patients. Intravenous administration has been most commonly associated with a flu-like syndrome in about 9 % of patients, including bone pain (9.1 %), fever (7.2 %), fatigue (4.1 %) and rigors (2.9 %). Occasionally cases of arthralgia and myalgia in approximately 3 % have been reported. No information is available on the reversibility of these adverse effects.

Frequently, the reduction in renal calcium excretion is accompanied by a fall in serum phosphate levels (in approximately 20 % of patients), which is asymptomatic not requiring treatment. The serum calcium may fall to asymptomatic hypocalcaemic levels in approximately 3 % of patients.

Gastrointestinal reactions, such as nausea (5.8 %) and vomiting (2.6 %) have been reported following intravenous infusion of Zometa. Occasionally local reactions at the infusion site such as redness or swelling and/or pain were also observed in less than 1 % of the patients.

Anorexia was reported in 1.5 % of patients treated with Zometa 4 mg.

Few cases of rash or pruritus have been observed (below 1 %).

As with other bisphosphonates, cases of conjunctivitis in approximately 1 % have been reported.

There have been some reports of impaired renal function (2.3 %), although the aetiology appears to be multifactorial in many cases.

Based on pooled analysis of placebo-controlled studies, severe anaemia (Hb < 8.0 g/dl) was reported in 5.2 % of patients receiving Zometa 4 mg versus 4.2 % on placebo.

The following adverse drug reactions, listed in Table 1, have been accumulated from clinical studies following predominantly chronic treatment with zoledronic acid:

Table 1

Adverse reactions are ranked under headings of frequency, the most frequent first, using the following convention: Very common (⩾ 1/10), common (⩾ 1/100, < 1/10), uncommon (⩾ 1/1,000, < 1/100), rare (⩾ 1/10,000, < 1/1,000), very rare (< 1/10,000), including isolated reports.

Blood and lymphatic system disorders		
	Common:	Anaemia
	Uncommon:	Thrombocytopenia, leukopenia
	Rare:	Pancytopenia
Nervous system disorders		
	Common:	Headache
	Uncommon:	Dizziness, paraesthesia, taste disturbance, hypoaesthesia, hyperaesthesia, tremor
Psychiatric disorders		
	Uncommon:	Anxiety, sleep disturbance
	Rare:	Confusion
Eye disorders		
	Common:	Conjunctivitis
	Uncommon:	Blurred vision
	Very rare:	Uveitis, episcleritis
Gastrointestinal disorders		
	Common:	Nausea, vomiting, anorexia
	Uncommon:	Diarrhoea, constipation, abdominal pain, dyspepsia, stomatitis, dry mouth

Respiratory, thoracic and mediastinal disorders		
	Uncommon:	Dyspnoea, cough
Skin and subcutaneous tissue disorders		
	Uncommon:	Pruritus, rash (including erythematous and macular rash), increased sweating
Musculoskeletal, connective tissue and bone disorders		
	Common:	Bone pain, myalgia, arthralgia, generalised pain
	Uncommon:	Muscle cramps
Cardiovascular disorders		
	Uncommon:	Hypertension
	Rare:	Bradycardia
Renal and urinary disorders		
	Common:	Renal impairment
	Uncommon:	Acute renal failure, haematuria, proteinuria
Immune system disorders		
	Uncommon:	Hypersensitivity reaction
	Rare:	Angioneurotic oedema
General disorders and administration site conditions		
	Common:	Fever, flu-like syndrome (including fatigue, rigors, malaise and flushing)
	Uncommon:	Asthenia, peripheral oedema, injection site reactions (including pain, irritation, swelling, induration), chest pain, weight increase
Laboratory abnormalities		
	Very common:	Hypophosphataemia
	Common:	Blood creatinine and blood urea increased, hypocalcaemia
	Uncommon:	Hypomagnesaemia, hypokalaemia
	Rare:	Hyperkalaemia, hypernatraemia

Postmarketing: Rare cases of osteonecrosis (primarily of the jaws) have been reported in patients treated with bisphosphonates. Many had signs of local infection including osteomyelitis. The majority of the reports refer to cancer patients following tooth extractions or other dental surgeries. Osteonecrosis of the jaws has multiple well documented risk factors including a diagnosis of cancer, concomitant therapies (e.g. chemotherapy, radiotherapy, corticosteroids) and co-morbid conditions (e.g. anaemia, coagulopathies, infection, pre-existing oral disease). Although causality cannot be determined, it is prudent to avoid dental surgery as recovery may be prolonged (see section 4.4, "Special warnings and special precautions for use").

4.9 Overdose

There is no experience of acute intoxication with Zometa. Patients who have received doses higher than those recommended should be carefully monitored. In the event of clinically significant hypocalcaemia, reversal may be achieved with an infusion of calcium gluconate.

5. PHARMACOLOGICAL PROPERTIES

5.1 Pharmacodynamic properties

Pharmacotherapeutic group: Bisphosphonate

ATC code: M05 BA 08

Zoledronic acid belongs to the class of bisphosphonates and acts primarily on bone. It is an inhibitor of osteoclastic bone resorption.

The selective action of bisphosphonates on bone is based on their high affinity for mineralised bone, but the precise molecular mechanism leading to the inhibition of osteoclastic activity is still unclear. In long-term animal studies, zoledronic acid inhibits bone resorption without adversely affecting the formation, mineralisation or mechanical properties of bone.

In addition to being a potent inhibitor of bone resorption, zoledronic acid also possesses several anti-tumour properties that could contribute to its overall efficacy in the treatment of metastatic bone disease. The following properties have been demonstrated in preclinical studies:

In vivo: Inhibition of osteoclastic bone resorption, which alters the bone marrow microenvironment, making it less conducive to tumour cell growth, anti-angiogenic activity and anti-pain activity.

In vitro: Inhibition of osteoblast proliferation, direct cytostatic and pro-apoptotic activity on tumour cells, synergistic cytostatic effect with other anti-cancer drugs, anti-adhesion/invasion activity.

Clinical trial results in the prevention of skeletal related events in patients with advanced malignancies involving bone

The first randomised, double-blind, placebo-controlled study compared Zometa to placebo for the prevention of skeletal related events (SREs) in prostate cancer patients. Zometa 4 mg significantly reduced the proportion of patients experiencing at least one skeletal related event (SRE), delayed the median time to first SRE by > 5 months, and reduced the annual incidence of events per patient - skeletal morbidity rate. Multiple event analysis showed a 36 % risk reduction in developing SREs in the Zometa group compared with placebo. Patients receiving Zometa reported less increase in pain than those receiving placebo, and the difference reached significance at months 3, 9, 21 and 24. Fewer Zometa patients suffered pathological fractures. The treatment effects were less pronounced in patients with blastic lesions. Efficacy results are provided in Table 2.

In a second study including solid tumours other than breast or prostate cancer, Zometa 4 mg significantly reduced the proportion of patients with an SRE, delayed the median time to first SRE by > 2 months, and reduced the skeletal morbidity rate. Multiple event analysis showed 30.7 % risk reduction in developing SREs in the Zometa group compared with placebo. Efficacy results are provided in Table 3.

(see Table 2)

(see Table 3 on next page)

In a third phase III randomised, double-blind trial, 4 mg Zometa or 90 mg pamidronate every 3 to 4 weeks were compared in patients with multiple myeloma or breast cancer with at least one bone lesion. The results demonstrated that Zometa 4 mg showed comparable efficacy to 90 mg pamidronate in the prevention of SREs. The multiple event analysis revealed a significant risk reduction of 16 % in patients treated with Zometa 4 mg in comparison with patients receiving pamidronate. Efficacy results are provided in Table 4.

(see Table 4 on next page)

Clinical trial results in the treatment of TIH

Clinical studies in tumour-induced hypercalcaemia (TIH) demonstrated that the effect of zoledronic acid is characterised by decreases in serum calcium and urinary calcium excretion. In Phase I dose finding studies in patients with mild to moderate tumour-induced hypercalcaemia (TIH), effective doses tested were in the range of approximately 1.2-2.5 mg.

To assess the effects of Zometa versus pamidronate 90 mg, the results of two pivotal multicentre studies in patients with TIH were combined in a pre-planned analysis. There was faster normalisation of corrected serum calcium at day 4 for Zometa 8 mg and at day 7 for Zometa 4 mg and 8 mg. The following response rates were observed:

Table 5: Proportion of complete responders by day in the combined TIH studies

(see Table 5 on next page)

Median time to normocalcaemia was 4 days. Median time to relapse (re-increase of albumin-corrected serum calcium ⩾ 2.9 mmol/l) was 30 to 40 days for patients treated with Zometa versus 17 days for those treated with pamidronate 90 mg (p-values: 0.001 for 4 mg and 0.007 for 8 mg). There were no statistically significant differences between the two Zometa doses.

In clinical trials 69 patients who relapsed or were refractory to initial treatment (Zometa 4 mg, 8 mg or pamidronate 90 mg) were retreated with Zometa 8 mg. The response rate in these patients was about 52%. Since those patients were retreated with the 8 mg dose only, there are no data available allowing comparison with the 4 mg dose.

In clinical trials performed in patients with tumour-induced hypercalcaemia (TIH), the overall safety profile amongst all three treatment groups (zoledronic acid 4 and 8 mg and pamidronate 90 mg) was similar in types and severity.

5.2 Pharmacokinetic properties

Single and multiple 5- and 15-minute infusions of 2, 4, 8 and 16 mg zoledronic acid in 64 patients with bone metastases yielded the following pharmacokinetic data, which were found to be dose independent.

After initiating the infusion of zoledronic acid, the plasma concentrations of drug rapidly increased, achieving their peak at the end of the infusion period, followed by a rapid decline to < 10 % of peak after 4 hours and < 1 % of peak after 24 hours, with a subsequent prolonged period of very low concentrations not exceeding 0.1 % of peak prior to the second infusion of drug on day 28.

Intravenously administered zoledronic acid is eliminated by a triphasic process: rapid biphasic disappearance from the systemic circulation, with half-lives of $t_{½\alpha}$ 0.24 and $t_{½\beta}$ 1.87 hours, followed by a long elimination phase with a terminal elimination half-life of $t_{½\gamma}$ 146 hours. There was no accumulation of drug in plasma after multiple doses of the drug given every 28 days. Zoledronic acid is not metabolised and is excreted unchanged via the kidney. Over the first 24 hours, 39 ± 16 % of the administered dose is recovered in the urine, while the remainder is principally bound to bone tissue. From the bone tissue it is released very slowly back into the systemic circulation and eliminated via the kidney. The total body clearance is 5.04 ± 2.5 l/h, independent of dose, and unaffected by gender, age, race, and body weight. Increasing the infusion time from 5 to 15 minutes caused a 30 % decrease in zoledronic acid concentration at the end of the infusion, but had no effect on the area under the plasma concentration versus time curve.

The interpatient variability in pharmacokinetic parameters for zoledronic acid was high, as seen with other bisphosphonates.

Table 2 Efficacy results (prostate cancer patients receiving hormonal therapy)

	Any SRE (+TIH)		Fractures*		Radiation therapy to bone	
	Zometa 4 mg	Placebo	Zometa 4 mg	Placebo	Zometa 4 mg	Placebo
N	214	208	214	208	214	208
Proportion of patients with SREs (%)	38	49	17	25	26	33
p-value	0.028		0.052		0.119	
Median time to SRE (days)	488	321	NR	NR	NR	640
p-value	0.009		0.020		0.055	
Skeletal morbidity rate	0.77	1.47	0.20	0.45	0.42	0.89
p-value	0.005		0.023		0.060	
Risk reduction of suffering from multiple events** (%)	36	-	NA	NA	NA	NA
p-value	0.002		NA		NA	

* Includes vertebral and non-vertebral fractures

** Accounts for all skeletal events, the total number as well as time to each event during the trial

NR Not Reached

NA Not Applicable

Carcinogenicity studies in rats and mice were conducted at the highest feasible doses and gave no suggestion of tumorogenicity.

Reproductive studies in male and female rats, at dose levels limited by toxicity, revealed no effect on fertility.

6. PHARMACEUTICAL PARTICULARS

6.1 List of excipients

Each Zomig Nasal Spray vial contains the following excipients:

Citric acid

Disodium phosphate

Purified Water

6.2 Incompatibilities

None known.

6.3 Shelf life

30 months.

6.4 Special precautions for storage

Do not store above 25°C.

6.5 Nature and contents of container

Ph Eur Type I glass vials which are closed with chlorobutyl rubber stoppers. The vials are assembled into a unit dose nasal spray device, comprising of a vial holder, an actuation device and a protection cover.

Packs containing 1, 2, or 6 single use devices.

6.6 Instructions for use and handling

The protection cover must not be removed until immediately before use. For instructions for use see the patient information leaflet.

7. MARKETING AUTHORISATION HOLDER

AstraZeneca UK Limited

600 Capability Green

Luton

LU1 3LU

UK

8. MARKETING AUTHORISATION NUMBER(S)

PL 17901/0095

9. DATE OF FIRST AUTHORISATION/RENEWAL OF THE AUTHORISATION

19th September 2002

10. DATE OF REVISION OF THE TEXT

19th May 2005

Zomig Rapimelt 2.5mg

(AstraZeneca UK Limited)

1. NAME OF THE MEDICINAL PRODUCT

'Zomig Rapimelt'

2. QUALITATIVE AND QUANTITATIVE COMPOSITION

Oro-dispersible tablets containing 2.5 mg of zolmitriptan.

For excipients, see Section 6.1.

3. PHARMACEUTICAL FORM

Oro-dispersible tablets.

4. CLINICAL PARTICULARS

4.1 Therapeutic indications

'Zomig Rapimelt' is indicated for the acute treatment of migraine with or without aura.

4.2 Posology and method of administration

The recommended dose of 'Zomig Rapimelt' to treat a migraine attack is 2.5mg. 'Zomig Rapimelt' rapidly dissolves when placed on the tongue and is swallowed with the patient's saliva. A drink of water is not required when taking 'Zomig Rapimelt'. 'Zomig Rapimelt' can be taken when water is not available thus allowing early administration of treatment for a migraine attack. This formulation may also be beneficial for patients who suffer from nausea and are unable to drink during a migraine attack, or for patients who do not like swallowing conventional tablet.

If symptoms persist or return within 24 hours, a second dose of zolmitriptan has been shown to be effective. If a second dose is required, it should not be taken within 2 hours of the initial dose.

If a patient does not achieve satisfactory relief with 2.5 mg doses, subsequent attacks can be treated with 5 mg doses of 'Zomig Rapimelt'. In those patients who respond, significant efficacy is apparent within 1 hour of dosing with zolmitriptan.

Zolmitriptan is equally effective whenever the tablets are taken during a migraine attack; although it is advisable that 'Zomig Rapimelt' is taken as early as possible after the onset of migraine headache.

In the event of recurrent attacks, it is recommended that the total intake of 'Zomig Rapimelt' in a 24 hour period should not exceed 10 mg.

'Zomig Rapimelt' is not indicated for prophylaxis of migraine.

Use in Children

Safety and efficacy of 'Zomig Rapimelt' in paediatric patients have not been established.

Use in Patients Aged Over 65 years

Safety and efficacy of 'Zomig Rapimelt' in individuals aged over 65 years have not been established.

Patients with Hepatic Impairment

Metabolism is reduced in patients with hepatic impairment (See Section 5.2 Pharmacokinetic properties). Therefore for patients with moderate or severe hepatic impairment a maximum dose of 5 mg in 24 hours is recommended.

Patients with Renal Impairment

No dosage adjustment required (see Section 5.2 Pharmacokinetic Properties).

4.3 Contraindications

'Zomig Rapimelt' is contraindicated in patients with:

- Known hypersensitivity to any component of the product.
- Uncontrolled hypertension.
- Ischaemic heart disease.
- Coronary vasospasm/Prinzmetal's angina.
- A history of cerebrovascular accident (CVA) or transient ischaemic attack (TIA)
- Concomitant administration of Zomig with ergotamine or ergotamine derivatives or other 5-HT$_1$ receptor agonists.

4.4 Special warnings and special precautions for use

'Zomig Rapimelt' should only be used where a clear diagnosis of migraine has been established. Care should be taken to exclude other potentially serious neurological conditions. There are no data on the use of 'Zomig Rapimelt' in hemiplegic or basilar migraine. Migraineurs may be at risk of certain cerebrovascular events. Cerebral haemorrhage, subarachnoid haemorrhage, stroke, and other cerebrovascular events have been reported in patients treated with 5HT$_{1B/1D}$ agonists.

'Zomig Rapimelt' should not be given to patients with symptomatic Wolff-Parkinson-White syndrome or arrhythmias associated with other cardiac accessory conduction pathways.

In very rare cases, as with other 5HT$_{1B/1D}$ agonists, coronary vasospasm, angina pectoris and myocardial infarction have been reported. In patients with risk factors for ischaemic heart disease, cardiovascular evaluation prior to commencement of treatment with this class of compounds, including 'Zomig Rapimelt', is recommended (see Section 4.3 Contraindications). These evaluations, however, may not identify every patient who has cardiac disease, and in very rare cases, serious cardiac events have occurred in patients without underlying cardiovascular disease.

As with other 5HT$_{1B/1D}$ agonists, atypical sensations over the precordium (see Section 4.8 Undesirable Effects) have been reported after the administration of zolmitriptan. If chest pain or symptoms consistent with ischaemic heart disease occur, no further doses of zolmitriptan should be taken until after appropriate medical evaluation has been carried out.

As with other 5HT$_{1B/1D}$ agonists transient increases in systemic blood pressure have been reported in patients with and without a history of hypertension; very rarely these increases in blood pressure have been associated with significant clinical events.

As with other 5HT$_{1B/1D}$ agonists, there have been rare reports of anaphylaxis/anaphylactoid reactions in patients receiving Zomig.

Patients with phenylketonuria should be informed that 'Zomig Rapimelt' contains phenylalanine (a component of aspartame). Each 2.5 mg orally dispersible tablet contains 2.81 mg of phenylalanine.

Excessive use of an acute anti-migraine medicinal product may lead to an increased frequency of headache, potentially requiring withdrawal of treatment.

4.5 Interaction with other medicinal products and other forms of Interaction

There is no evidence that concomitant use of migraine prophylactic medications has any effect on the efficacy or unwanted effects of zolmitriptan (for example beta blockers, oral dihydroergotamine, pizotifen).

The pharmacokinetics and tolerability of 'Zomig', when administered as the conventional tablet, were unaffected by acute symptomatic treatments such as paracetamol, metoclopramide and ergotamine. Concomitant administration of other 5HT$_{1B/1D}$ agonists within 12 hours of 'Zomig Rapimelt' treatment should be avoided.

Data from healthy subjects suggest there are no pharmacokinetic or clinically significant interactions between Zomig and ergotamine, however, the increased risk of coronary vasospasm is a theoretical possibility. Therefore, it is advised to wait at least 24 hours following the use of ergotamine containing preparations before administering Zomig. Conversely it is advised to wait at least six hours following use of Zomig before administering any ergotamine preparation (see Section 4.3 Contraindications).

Following administration of moclobemide, a specific MAO-A inhibitor, there was a small increase (26%) in AUC for zolmitriptan and a 3-fold increase in AUC of the active metabolite. Therefore, a maximum intake of 5 mg 'Zomig Rapimelt' in 24 hours is recommended in patients taking an MAO-A inhibitor.

Following the administration of cimetidine, a general P450 inhibitor, the half life of zolmitriptan was increased by 44% and the AUC increased by 48%. In addition the half life and AUC of the active N-desmethylated metabolite (183C91) were doubled. A maximum dose of 5 mg 'Zomig Rapimelt' in 24 hours is recommended in patients taking cimetidine. Based on the overall interaction profile, an interaction with inhibitors of the cytochrome P450 isoenzyme CYP1A2 cannot be excluded. Therefore, the same dosage reduction is recommended with compounds of this type, such as fluvoxamine and the quinolone antibiotics (eg ciprofloxacin).

Fluoxetine does not affect the pharmacokinetic parameters of zolmitriptan. Therapeutic doses of the specific serotonin reuptake inhibitors, fluoxetine, sertraline, paroxetine and citalopram do not inhibit CYP1A2.

As with other 5HT$_{1b/1d}$ agonists, there is the potential for dynamic interactions with the herbal remedy St John's wort (Hypericum perforatum) which may result in an increase in undesirable effects.

4.6 Pregnancy and lactation

Pregnancy

'Zomig Rapimelt' should be used in pregnancy only if the benefits to the mother justify potential risk to the foetus. There are no studies in pregnant women, but there is no evidence of teratogenicity in animal studies. (See Section 5.3 Preclinical Safety Data).

Lactation

Studies have shown that zolmitriptan passes into the milk of lactating animals. No data exist for passage of zolmitriptan into human breast milk. Therefore, caution should be exercised when administering 'Zomig Rapimelt' to women who are breast-feeding.

4.7 Effects on ability to drive and use machines

There was no significant impairment of performance of psychomotor tests with doses up to 20 mg zolmitriptan. Use is unlikely to result in an impairment of the ability of patients to drive or operate machinery. However it should be taken into account that somnolence may occur.

4.8 Undesirable effects

Zomig is well tolerated. Adverse reactions are typically mild/moderate, transient, not serious and resolve spontaneously without additional treatment.

Possible adverse reactions tend to occur within 4 hours of dosing and are no more frequent following repeated dosing.

The incidences of ADRs associated with ZOMIG therapy are tabulated below according to the format recommended by the Council for International Organizations of Medical Sciences (CIOMS III Working Group; 1995).

Frequency	System organ class	Event
Common (⩾1% - <10%)	Gastrointestinal Disorders	Dry mouth Nausea
	Musculoskeletal and Connective Tissue Disorders	Muscle weakness Myalgia
	Nervous System Disorders	Abnormalities or disturbances of sensation Asthenia Dizziness Dysaesthesia Heaviness, tightness, pain or pressure in throat, neck, limbs or chest Paraesthesia Somnolence Warm sensation
Rare (⩾0.01% - <0.1%)	Cardiac Disorders	Palpitations Tachycardia
	Immune System Disorders	Anaphylaxis/ Anaphylactoid Reactions[1] Hypersensitivity reactions[1]
	Nervous System Disorders	Headache[2]
	Skin and Subcutaneous Tissue disorders	Angioedema[1] Urticaria[1]
Very rare (<0.01%)	Cardiac Disorders	Angina pectoris[3] Coronary Vasospasm[3] Myocardial Infarction[3]

	Gastrointestinal Disorders	Abdominal pain[4] Bloody diarrhoea[4] Gastrointestinal infarction or necrosis[4] Gastrointestinal ischaemic events[4] Ischaemic colitis[4] Splenic Infarction
	Renal and Urinary Disorders	Polyuria Urinary frequency Urinary Urgency
	Vascular Disorders	Transient increases in systemic blood pressure very rarely associated with significant clinical events[5]

[1]As with other 5HT $_{1B/1D}$ agonists, there have been rare reports of hypersensitivity reactions, including anaphylaxis/anaphylactoid reactions, urticaria and angioedema.

[2]As with other acute migraine treatments, including 5HT $_{1B/1D}$ agonists, there have been rare reports of headache.

[3]In very rare cases, as with other 5HT $_{1B/1D}$ agonists, angina pectoris, myocardial infarction have been reported.

[4]As with other 5HT $_{1B/1D}$ agonists very rare reports of gastrointestinal ischaemic events including ischaemic colitis, gastrointestinal infarction or necrosis, which may present as bloody diarrhoea or abdominal pain, have been received.

[5]As with other 5HT $_{1B/1D}$ agonists, transient increases in systemic blood pressure, very rarely associated with significant clinical events, have been reported.

4.9 Overdose

Volunteers receiving single oral doses of 50 mg commonly experienced sedation. The elimination half-life of zolmitriptan is 2.5 to 3 hours, (see Section 5.2 Pharmacokinetic Properties) and therefore monitoring of patients after overdose with 'Zomig Rapimelt' should continue for at least 15 hours or while symptoms or signs persist.

There is no specific antidote to zolmitriptan. In cases of severe intoxication, intensive care procedures are recommended, including establishing and maintaining a patent airway, ensuring adequate oxygenation and ventilation, and monitoring and support of the cardiovascular system.

It is unknown what effect haemodialysis or peritoneal dialysis has on the serum concentrations of zolmitriptan.

5. PHARMACOLOGICAL PROPERTIES

5.1 Pharmacodynamic properties

In pre-clinical studies, zolmitriptan has been demonstrated to be a selective agonist for the vascular human recombinant $5HT_{1B}$ and $5HT_{1D}$ receptor subtypes. Zolmitriptan is a high affinity $5HT_{1B/1D}$ receptor agonist with modest affinity for $5HT_{1A}$ receptors. Zolmitriptan has no significant affinity (as measured by radioligand binding assays) or pharmacological activity at $5HT_2$-, $5HT_3$-, $5HT_4$-, alpha$_1$-, alpha$_2$-, or beta$_1$-, adrenergic; H_1-, H_2-, histaminic; muscarinic; dopaminergic$_1$, or dopaminergic$_2$ receptors. The $5HT_{1D}$ receptor is predominately located presynaptically at both the peripheral and central synapses of the trigeminal nerve and preclinical studies have shown that zolmitriptan is able to act at both these sites.

5.2 Pharmacokinetic properties

Following oral administration of 'Zomig' conventional tablets zolmitriptan is rapidly and well absorbed (at least 64%) in man. The mean absolute bioavailability of the parent compound is approximately 40%. There is an active metabolite (183C91, the N-desmethyl metabolite) which is also a 5HT $_{1B/1D}$ agonist and is 2 to 6 times as potent, in animal models, as zolmitriptan.

In healthy subjects, when given as a single dose, zolmitriptan and its active metabolite 183C91, display dose-proportional AUC and C_{max} over the dose range 2.5 to 50 mg. Absorption is rapid with 75% of C_{max} achieved within 1 hour and plasma concentrations are sustained subsequently for 4 to 6 hours. Zolmitriptan absorption is unaffected by the presence of food. There is no evidence of accumulation on multiple dosing of zolmitriptan.

Zolmitriptan is eliminated largely by hepatic biotransformation followed by urinary excretion of the metabolites. There are three major metabolites: the indole acetic acid, (the major metabolite in plasma and urine), the N-oxide and N-desmethyl analogues. The N-desmethylated metabolite (183C91) is active whilst the others are not. Plasma concentrations of 183C91 are approximately half those of the parent drug, hence it would therefore be expected to contribute to the therapeutic action of 'Zomig Rapimelt'. Over 60% of a single oral dose is excreted in the urine (mainly as the indole acetic acid metabolite) and about 30% in faeces, mainly as unchanged parent compound.

A study to evaluate the effect of liver disease on the pharmacokinetics of zolmitriptan showed that the AUC and C_{max} were increased by 94% and 50% respectively in patients with moderate liver disease and by 226% and 47% in patients with severe liver disease compared with healthy volunteers. Exposure to the metabolites, including the active metabolite, was decreased. For the 183C91 metabolite, AUC and C_{max} were reduced by 33% and 44% in patients with moderate liver disease and by 82% and 90% in patients with severe liver disease.

The plasma half-life ($t_{½}$) of zolmitriptan was 4.7 hours in healthy volunteers, 7.3 hours in patients with moderate liver disease and 12 hours in those with severe liver disease. The corresponding $t_{½}$ values for the 183C91 metabolite were 5.7 hours, 7.5 hours and 7.8 hours respectively.

Following intravenous administration, the mean total plasma clearance is approximately 10 ml/min/kg, of which one third is renal clearance. Renal clearance is greater than glomerular filtration rate suggesting renal tubular secretion. The volume of distribution following intravenous administration is 2.4 L/kg. Plasma protein binding is low (approximately 25%). The mean elimination half-life of zolmitriptan is 2.5 to 3 hours. The half-lives of its metabolites are similar, suggesting their elimination is formation-rate limited.

Renal clearance of zolmitriptan and all its metabolites is reduced (7 to 8 fold) in patients with moderate to severe renal impairment compared to healthy subjects, although the AUC of the parent compound and the active metabolite were only slightly higher (16 and 35% respectively) with a 1 hour increase in half-life to 3 to 3.5 hours. These parameters are within the ranges seen in healthy volunteers.

In a small group of healthy individuals there was no pharmacokinetic interaction with ergotamine. Concomitant administration of zolmitriptan with ergotamine/caffeine was well tolerated and did not result in any increase in adverse events or blood pressure changes as compared with zolmitriptan alone.

Following the administration of rifampicin, no clinically relevant differences in the pharmacokinetics of zolmitriptan or its active metabolite were observed.

Selegiline, an MAO-B inhibitor, and fluoxetine (a selective serotonin reuptake inhibitor; SSRI) had no effect on the pharmacokinetic parameters of zolmitriptan.

The pharmacokinetics of zolmitriptan in healthy elderly subjects were similar to those in healthy young volunteers.

'Zomig Rapimelt' was demonstrated to be bioequivalent with the conventional tablet in terms of AUC and C_{max} for zolmitriptan and its active metabolite 183C91. Clinical pharmacology data show that the t_{max} for zolmitriptan can be later for the orally dispersible tablet (range 0.6 to 5h, median 3h) compared to the conventional tablet (range 0.5 to 3h, median 1.5h). The t_{max} for the active metabolite was similar for both formulations (median 3h).

5.3 Preclinical safety data

An oral teratology study of zolmitriptan has been conducted. At the maximum tolerated doses, 1200 mg/kg/day (AUC 605 μg/ml.h: approx. 3700 × AUC of the human maximum recommended daily intake of 15 mg) and 30 mg/kg/day (AUC 4.9 μg/ml.h: approx. 30 × AUC of the human maximum recommended daily intake of 15 mg) in rats and rabbits, respectively, no signs of teratogenicity were apparent.

Five genotoxicity tests have been performed. It was concluded that 'Zomig Rapimelt' is not likely to pose any genetic risk in humans.

Carcinogenicity studies in rats and mice were conducted at the highest feasible doses and gave no suggestion of tumorogenicity.

Reproductive studies in male and female rats, at dose levels limited by toxicity, revealed no effect on fertility.

6. PHARMACEUTICAL PARTICULARS

6.1 List of excipients

Each 'Zomig Rapimelt' orodispersible tablet contains the following excipients:

Aspartame

Citric Acid Anhydrous

Silica Colloidal Anhydrous

Crospovidone

Magnesium Stearate

Mannitol

Microcrystalline Cellulose

Orange Flavour SN027512

Sodium Hydrogen Carbonate

6.2 Incompatibilities

None known.

6.3 Shelf life

3 years.

6.4 Special precautions for storage

Do not store above 30°C.

6.5 Nature and contents of container

PVC aluminium/aluminium blister pack of 2 tablets (sample pack)* or 6 tablets (3 strips of 2 tablets) with a plastic reusable wallet.

6.6 Instructions for use and handling

The blister pack should be peeled open as shown on the foil (tablets should not be pushed through the foil). The 'Zomig Rapimelt' tablet should be placed on the tongue, where it will dissolve and be swallowed with the saliva.

7. MARKETING AUTHORISATION HOLDER

AstraZeneca UK Ltd

600 Capability Green

Luton LU1 3LU

United Kingdom

8. MARKETING AUTHORISATION NUMBER(S)

PL 17901/0076

9. DATE OF FIRST AUTHORISATION/RENEWAL OF THE AUTHORISATION

20 June 2001

10. DATE OF REVISION OF THE TEXT

1st February 2005

'Zomig Rapimelt' is a trademark property of the AstraZeneca Group of Companies.

Zomig Rapimelt 5 mg Orodispersible Tablets

(AstraZeneca UK Limited)

1. NAME OF THE MEDICINAL PRODUCT

'Zomig Rapimelt'5 mg Orodispersible Tablets

2. QUALITATIVE AND QUANTITATIVE COMPOSITION

Orodispersible tablets containing 5 mg of zolmitriptan.

For excipients, see Section 6.1.

3. PHARMACEUTICAL FORM

Orodispersible tablet.

4. CLINICAL PARTICULARS

4.1 Therapeutic indications

'Zomig Rapimelt' is indicated for the acute treatment of migraine with or without aura.

4.2 Posology and method of administration

The recommended dose of 'Zomig Rapimelt' to treat a migraine attack is 2.5 mg. 'Zomig Rapimelt' rapidly dissolves when placed on the tongue and is swallowed with the patient's saliva. A drink of water is not required when taking 'Zomig Rapimelt'. 'Zomig Rapimelt' can be taken when water is not available thus allowing early administration of treatment for a migraine attack. This formulation may also be beneficial for patients who suffer from nausea and are unable to drink during a migraine attack, or for patients who do not like swallowing conventional tablets.

If symptoms persist or return within 24 hours, a second dose of zolmitriptan has been shown to be effective. If a second dose is required, it should not be taken within 2 hours of the initial dose.

If a patient does not achieve satisfactory relief with 2.5 mg doses, subsequent attacks can be treated with 5 mg doses of 'Zomig Rapimelt'. In those patients who respond, significant efficacy is apparent within 1 hour of dosing with zolmitriptan.

Zolmitriptan is equally effective whenever the tablets are taken during a migraine attack; although it is advisable that 'Zomig Rapimelt' is taken as early as possible after the onset of migraine headache.

In the event of recurrent attacks, it is recommended that the total intake of 'Zomig Rapimelt' in a 24 hour period should not exceed 10 mg.

'Zomig Rapimelt' is not indicated for prophylaxis of migraine.

Use in Children

Safety and efficacy of 'Zomig Rapimelt' in paediatric patients have not been established.

Use in Patients Aged Over 65 years

Safety and efficacy of 'Zomig Rapimelt' in individuals aged over 65 years have not been established. Patients with Hepatic Impairment Metabolism is reduced in patients with hepatic impairment (See Section 5.2 Pharmacokinetic properties). Therefore for patients with moderate or severe hepatic impairment a maximum dose of 5 mg in 24 hours is recommended. Patients with Renal Impairment

No dosage adjustment required (see Section 5.2 Pharmacokinetic Properties).

4.3 Contraindications

'Zomig Rapimelt' is contraindicated in patients with:

- Known hypersensitivity to any component of the product.
- Uncontrolled hypertension.
- Ischaemic heart disease.
- Coronary vasospasm/Prinzmetal's angina.
- A history of cerebrovascular accident (CVA) or transient ischaemic attack (TIA).
- Concomitant administration of Zomig with ergotamine or ergotamine derivatives or other $5\text{-}HT_1$ receptor agonists.

4.4 Special warnings and special precautions for use

'Zomig Rapimelt' should only be used where a clear diagnosis of migraine has been established. Care should be taken to exclude other potentially serious neurological conditions. There are no data on the use of 'Zomig Rapimelt' in hemiplegic or basilar migraine. Migraneurs may be at risk of certain cerebrovascular events. Cerebral haemorrhage, subarachnoid haemorrhage, stroke, and other cerebrovascular events have been reported in patients treated with $5HT_{1B/1D}$ agonists.

'Zomig Rapimelt' should not be given to patients with symptomatic Wolff-Parkinson-White syndrome or arrhythmias associated with other cardiac accessory conduction pathways.

In very rare cases, as with other $5HT_{1B/1D}$ agonists, coronary vasospasm, angina pectoris and myocardial infarction have been reported. In patients with risk factors for ischaemic heart disease, cardiovascular evaluation prior to commencement of treatment with this class of compounds, including 'Zomig Rapimelt', is recommended (see Section 4.3 Contraindications). These evaluations, however, may not identify every patient who has cardiac disease, and in very rare cases, serious cardiac events have occurred in patients without underlying cardiovascular disease.

As with other $5HT_{1B/1D}$ agonists, atypical sensations over the precordium (see Section 4.8 Undesirable Effects) have been reported after the administration of zolmitriptan. If chest pain or symptoms consistent with ischaemic heart disease occur, no further doses of zolmitriptan should be taken until after appropriate medical evaluation has been carried out.

As with other $5HT_{1B/1D}$ agonists transient increases in systemic blood pressure have been reported in patients with and without a history of hypertension; very rarely these increases in blood pressure have been associated with significant clinical events.

As with other $5HT_{1B/1D}$ agonists, there have been rare reports of anaphylaxis/anaphylactoid reactions in patients receiving Zomig.

Patients with phenylketonuria should be informed that 'Zomig Rapimelt' contains phenylalanine (a component of aspartame). Each 5 mg orally dispersible tablet contains 5.62 mg of phenylalanine.

Excessive use of an acute anti-migraine medicinal product may lead to an increased frequency of headache, potentially requiring withdrawal of treatment.

4.5 Interaction with other medicinal products and other forms of Interaction

There is no evidence that concomitant use of migraine prophylactic medications has any effect on the efficacy or unwanted effects of zolmitriptan (for example beta blockers, oral dihydroergotamine, pizotifen).

The pharmacokinetics and tolerability of 'Zomig', when administered as the conventional tablet, were unaffected by acute symptomatic treatments such as paracetamol, metoclopramide and ergotamine. Concomitant administration of other $5HT_{1B/1D}$ agonists within 12 hours of 'Zomig Rapimelt' treatment should be avoided.

Data from healthy subjects suggest there are no pharmacokinetic or clinically significant interactions between Zomig and ergotamine, however, the increased risk of coronary vasospasm is a theoretical possibility. Therefore, it is advised to wait at least 24 hours following the use of ergotamine containing preparations before administering Zomig. Conversely it is advised to wait at least six hours following use of Zomig before administering any ergotamine preparation (see Section 4.3 Contraindications).

Following administration of moclobemide, a specific MAO-A inhibitor, there was a small increase (26%) in AUC for zolmitriptan and a 3-fold increase in AUC of the active metabolite. Therefore, a maximum intake of 5 mg 'Zomig Rapimelt' in 24 hours is recommended in patients taking an MAO-A inhibitor.

Following the administration of cimetidine, a general P450 inhibitor, the half life of zolmitriptan was increased by 44% and the AUC increased by 48%. In addition the half life and AUC of the active N-desmethylated metabolite (183C91) were doubled. A maximum dose of 5 mg 'Zomig Rapimelt' in 24 hours is recommended in patients taking cimetidine. Based on the overall interaction profile, an interaction with inhibitors of the cytochrome P450 isoenzyme CYP1A2 cannot be excluded. Therefore, the same dosage reduction is recommended with compounds of this type, such as fluvoxamine and the quinolone antibiotics (e.g. ciprofloxacin).

Fluoxetine does not affect the pharmacokinetic parameters of zolmitriptan. Therapeutic doses of the specific serotonin reuptake inhibitors, fluoxetine, sertraline, paroxetine and citalopram do not inhibit CYP1A2.

As with other $5HT_{1b/1d}$ agonists, there is the potential for dynamic interactions with the herbal remedy St John's wort (Hypericum perforatum) which may result in an increase in undesirable effects.

4.6 Pregnancy and lactation

Pregnancy

'Zomig Rapimelt' should be used in pregnancy only if the benefits to the mother justify potential risk to the foetus. There are no studies in pregnant women, but there is no evidence of teratogenicity in animal studies. (See Section 5.3 Preclinical Safety Data).

Lactation

Studies have shown that zolmitriptan passes into the milk of lactating animals. No data exist for passage of zolmitriptan into human breast milk. Therefore, caution should be exercised when administering 'Zomig Rapimelt' to women who are breast-feeding.

4.7 Effects on ability to drive and use machines

There was no significant impairment of performance of psychomotor tests with doses up to 20 mg zolmitriptan. Use is unlikely to result in an impairment of the ability of patients to drive or operate machinery. However it should be taken into account that somnolence may occur.

4.8 Undesirable effects

Zomig is well tolerated. Adverse reactions are typically mild/moderate, transient, not serious and resolve spontaneously without additional treatment.

Possible adverse reactions tend to occur within 4 hours of dosing and are no more frequent following repeated dosing.

The incidences of ADRs associated with ZOMIG therapy are tabulated below according to the format recommended by the Council for International Organizations of Medical Sciences (CIOMS III Working Group; 1995).

Frequency	System organ class	Event
Common (≥1% - <10%)	Gastrointestinal Disorders	Dry mouth Nausea
	Musculoskeletal and Connective Tissue Disorders	Muscle weakness Myalgia
	Nervous System Disorders	Abnormalities or disturbances of sensation Asthenia Dizziness Dysaesthesia Heaviness, tightness, pain or pressure in throat, neck, limbs or chest Paraesthesia Somnolence Warm sensation
Rare (≥0.01% - <0.1%)	Cardiac Disorders	Palpitations Tachycardia
	Immune System Disorders	Anaphylaxis/Anaphylactoid Reactions[1] Hypersensitivity reactions[1]
	Nervous System Disorders	Headache[2]
	Skin and Subcutaneous Tissue disorders	Angioedema[1] Urticaria[1]
Very rare (<0.01%)	Cardiac Disorders	Angina pectoris[3] Coronary Vasospasm[3] Myocardial Infarction[3]
	Gastrointestinal Disorders	Abdominal pain[4] Bloody diarrhoea[4] Gastrointestinal infarction or necrosis[4] Gastrointestinal ischaemic events[4] Ischaemic colitis[4] Splenic Infarction
	Renal and Urinary Disorders	Polyuria Urinary frequency Urinary Urgency
	Vascular Disorders	Transient increases in systemic blood pressure very rarely associated with significant clinical events[5]

[1]As with other $5HT_{1B/1D}$ agonists, there have been rare reports of hypersensitivity reactions, including anaphylaxis/anaphylactoid reactions, urticaria and angioedema.

[2]As with other acute migraine treatments, including $5HT_{1B/1D}$ agonists, there have been rare reports of headache.

[3]In very rare cases, as with other $5HT_{1B/1D}$ agonists, angina pectoris, myocardial infarction have been reported.

[4]As with other $5HT_{1B/1D}$ agonists very rare reports of gastrointestinal ischaemic events including ischaemic colitis, gastrointestinal infarction or necrosis, which may present as bloody diarrhoea or abdominal pain, have been received.

[5]As with other $5HT_{1B/1D}$ agonists, transient increases in systemic blood pressure, very rarely associated with significant clinical events, have been reported.

4.9 Overdose

Volunteers receiving single oral doses of 50 mg commonly experienced sedation.

The elimination half-life of zolmitriptan is 2.5 to 3 hours, (see Section 5.2 Pharmacokinetic Properties) and therefore monitoring of patients after overdose with 'Zomig Rapimelt' should continue for at least 15 hours or while symptoms or signs persist.

There is no specific antidote to zolmitriptan. In cases of severe intoxication, intensive care procedures are recommended, including establishing and maintaining a patent airway, ensuring adequate oxygenation and ventilation, and monitoring and support of the cardiovascular system.

It is unknown what effect haemodialysis or peritoneal dialysis has on the serum concentrations of zolmitriptan.

5. PHARMACOLOGICAL PROPERTIES

Pharmacotherapeutic group: Selective serotonin ($5HT_1$) agonists

Therapeutic classification: N02CC03

5.1 Pharmacodynamic properties

In pre-clinical studies, zolmitriptan has been demonstrated to be a selective agonist for the vascular human recombinant $5HT_{1B}$ and $5HT_{1D}$ receptor subtypes. Zolmitriptan is a high affinity $5HT_{1B/1D}$ receptor agonist with modest affinity for $5HT_{1A}$ receptors. Zolmitriptan has no significant affinity (as measured by radioligand binding assays) or pharmacological activity at $5HT_2$-, $5HT_3$-, $5HT_4$-, alpha$_1$-, alpha$_2$-, or beta$_1$-, adrenergic; H_1-, H_2-, histaminic; muscarinic; dopaminergic$_1$, or dopaminergic$_2$ receptors. The $5HT_{1D}$ receptor is predominately located presynaptically at both the peripheral and central synapses of the trigeminal nerve and preclinical studies have shown that zolmitriptan is able to act at both these sites.

5.2 Pharmacokinetic properties

Following oral administration of 'Zomig' conventional tablets zolmitriptan is rapidly and well absorbed (at least 64%) in man. The mean absolute bioavailability of the parent compound is approximately 40%. There is an active metabolite (183C91, the N-desmethyl metabolite) which is also a $5HT_{1B/1D}$ agonist and is 2 to 6 times as potent, in animal models, as zolmitriptan.

In healthy subjects, when given as a single dose, zolmitriptan and its active metabolite 183C91, display dose-proportional AUC and C_{max} over the dose range 2.5 to 50 mg. Absorption is rapid with 75% of C_{max} achieved within 1 hour and plasma concentrations are sustained subsequently for 4 to 6 hours. Zolmitriptan absorption is unaffected by the presence of food. There is no evidence of accumulation on multiple dosing of zolmitriptan.

Zolmitriptan is eliminated largely by hepatic biotransformation followed by urinary excretion of the metabolites. There are three major metabolites: the indole acetic acid, (the major metabolite in plasma and urine), the N-oxide and N-desmethyl analogues. The N-desmethylated metabolite (183C91) is active whilst the others are not. Plasma concentrations of 183C91 are approximately half those of the parent drug, hence it would therefore be expected to contribute to the therapeutic action of 'Zomig Rapimelt'. Over 60% of a single oral dose is excreted in the urine (mainly as the indole acetic acid metabolite) and about 30% in faeces, mainly as unchanged parent compound.

A study to evaluate the effect of liver disease on the pharmacokinetics of zolmitriptan showed that the AUC and C_{max} were increased by 94% and 50% respectively in patients with moderate liver disease and by 226% and 47% in patients with severe liver disease compared with healthy volunteers. Exposure to the metabolites, including the active metabolite, was decreased. For the 183C91 metabolite, AUC and C_{max} were reduced by 33% and 44% in patients with moderate liver disease and by 82% and 90% in patients with severe liver disease.

The plasma half-life ($t_{½}$) of zolmitriptan was 4.7 hours in healthy volunteers, 7.3 hours in patients with moderate liver disease and 12 hours in those with severe liver disease. The corresponding $t_{½}$ values for the 183C91 metabolite were 5.7 hours, 7.5 hours and 7.8 hours respectively.

Following intravenous administration, the mean total plasma clearance is approximately 10 ml/min/kg, of which one third is renal clearance. Renal clearance is greater than glomerular filtration rate suggesting renal tubular secretion. The volume of distribution following intravenous administration is 2.4 L/kg. Plasma protein binding is low (approximately 25%). The mean elimination half-life of zolmitriptan is 2.5 to 3 hours. The half-lives of its metabolites are similar, suggesting their elimination is formation-rate limited.

Renal clearance of zolmitriptan and all its metabolites is reduced (7 to 8 fold) in patients with moderate to severe renal impairment compared to healthy subjects, although the AUC of the parent compound and the active metabolite were only slightly higher (16 and 35% respectively) with a 1 hour increase in half-life to 3 to 3.5 hours. These parameters are within the ranges seen in healthy volunteers.

In a small group of healthy individuals there was no pharmacokinetic interaction with ergotamine. Concomitant administration of zolmitriptan with ergotamine/caffeine was well tolerated and did not result in any increase in adverse events or blood pressure changes as compared with zolmitriptan alone.

Following the administration of rifampicin, no clinically relevant differences in the pharmacokinetics of zolmitriptan or its active metabolite were observed.

Selegiline, an MAO-B inhibitor, and fluoxetine (a selective serotonin reuptake inhibitor; SSRI) had no effect on the pharmacokinetic parameters of zolmitriptan.

The pharmacokinetics of zolmitriptan in healthy elderly subjects were similar to those in healthy young volunteers.

'Zomig Rapimelt' was demonstrated to be bioequivalent with the conventional tablet in terms of AUC and C_{max} for zolmitriptan and its active metabolite 183C91. Clinical pharmacology data show that the t_{max} for zolmitriptan can be later for the orally dispersible tablet (range 0.6 to 5h, median 3h) compared to the conventional tablet (range 0.5 to 3h, median 1.5h). The t_{max} for the active metabolite was similar for both formulations (median 3h).

5.3 Preclinical safety data

An oral teratology study of zolmitriptan has been conducted. At the maximum tolerated doses, 1200 mg/kg/day (AUC 605 μg/ml.h: approx. 3700 × AUC of the human maximum recommended daily intake of 15 mg) and 30 mg/kg/day (AUC 4.9 μg/ml.h: approx. 30 × AUC of the human maximum recommended daily intake of 15 mg) in rats and rabbits, respectively, no signs of teratogenicity were apparent.

Five genotoxicity tests have been performed. It was concluded that 'Zomig Rapimelt' is not likely to pose any genetic risk in humans.

Carcinogenicity studies in rats and mice were conducted at the highest feasible doses and gave no suggestion of tumorogenicity.

Reproductive studies in male and female rats, at dose levels limited by toxicity, revealed no effect on fertility.

6. PHARMACEUTICAL PARTICULARS

6.1 List of excipients

Each 'Zomig Rapimelt' orodispersible tablet contains the following excipients:

Aspartame

Citric Acid Anhydrous

Silica Colloidal Anhydrous

Crospovidone

Magnesium Stearate

Mannitol

Microcrystalline Cellulose

Orange Flavour SN027512

Sodium Hydrogen Carbonate

6.2 Incompatibilities

None known

6.3 Shelf life

2 years

6.4 Special precautions for storage

Do not store above 30°C.

6.5 Nature and contents of container

PVC aluminium/aluminium blister pack of 6 tablets (1 strip of 6 tablets) with a plastic re-usable wallet.

6.6 Instructions for use and handling

The blister pack should be peeled open as shown on the foil (tablets should not be pushed through the foil). The 'Zomig Rapimelt' tablet should be placed on the tongue, where it will dissolve and be swallowed with the saliva.

7. MARKETING AUTHORISATION HOLDER

AstraZeneca UK Ltd

600 Capability Green

Luton LU1 3LU

United Kingdom

8. MARKETING AUTHORISATION NUMBER(S)

PL 17901/0230

9. DATE OF FIRST AUTHORISATION/RENEWAL OF THE AUTHORISATION

21st September 2004

10. DATE OF REVISION OF THE TEXT

21st September 2004

'Zomig Rapimelt' is a trademark property of the AstraZeneca Group of Companies.

Zomorph capsules

(Link Pharmaceuticals Ltd)

1. NAME OF THE MEDICINAL PRODUCT

Zomorph® capsules 10mg, 30mg, 60mg, 100mg and 200mg

2. QUALITATIVE AND QUANTITATIVE COMPOSITION

Morphine sulphate BP 10mg

Morphine sulphate BP 30mg

Morphine sulphate BP 60mg

Morphine sulphate BP 100mg

Morphine sulphate BP 200mg

3. PHARMACEUTICAL FORM

Sustained-release capsules.

4. CLINICAL PARTICULARS

4.1 Therapeutic indications

Severe chronic pain and/or pain resistant to other analgesics, in particular pain associated with cancer.

4.2 Posology and method of administration

Route of administration: oral.

As directed by a medical practitioner.

Recommended dosage

Adults: Recommended dosage is one capsule twice daily, at 12-hourly intervals.

Elderly: As with all narcotics, a reduction in dosage may be advisable in the elderly, as appropriate.

Children: Not recommended.

The capsules should not be chewed and should normally be swallowed whole.

The dosage varies according to the severity of pain and the previous analgesic treatments received by the patient.

If the pain persists, or if the patient develops tolerance to morphine, the dosage may be increased by prescribing the 10mg, 30mg, 60mg, 100mg and 200mg capsules either alone or in various combinations to obtain the desired relief.

Patients previously treated with immediate-release oral morphine should receive the same total daily dose of sustained-release capsules, but in two divided doses at 12-hourly intervals.

Patients previously treated with parenteral morphine should be given a sufficiently increased dosage to compensate for any reduction of the analgesic effect associated with oral administration. The dosage should be adjusted to meet the individual requirements of each patient.

For patients who cannot swallow the capsules, their contents can be administered directly in semi-solid food (e.g. puree, jam or yoghurt) or via gastric or gastrostomy tubes of a diameter of more than 16 F.G. with an open distal end or lateral pores. It is sufficient to rinse the tube with 30ml to 50ml of water.

4.3 Contraindications

Respiratory impairment, acute abdominal syndrome of unknown origin, severely impaired liver function, cranial trauma and raised intracranial pressure, convulsive state, acute alcoholic intoxication and delirium tremens, children, risk of paralytic ileus, known hypersensitivity to any of the ingredients contained in Zomorph capsules, concurrent treatment with MAO (MAO = monoamine oxidase) inhibitors or within two weeks of their use.

4.4 Special warnings and special precautions for use

Caution should be exercised in:

- elderly subjects.
- patients with impaired hepatic and/or renal functions. The dose of Zomorph capsules should be reduced, or its use should be avoided in cases of hepatic or renal failure.
- patients with hypothyroidism or hypoadrenalism.
- patients in a state of shock or with asthma.
- patients suffering from the following conditions: hypotension, convulsive disorders, dependence (severe withdrawal symptoms if withdrawn abruptly) and prostatic hypertrophy.

Urinary retention may occur in patients with urethral disease or prostatic hypertrophy.

4.5 Interaction with other medicinal products and other forms of Interaction

As serious and sometimes fatal reactions have occurred following administration of pethidine to patients receiving monoamine oxidase inhibitors (MAOI's), pethidine and related drugs are contraindicated in patients taking MAOI's or within 14 days of stopping such treatment: morphine and other opioid analgesics should be given with extreme caution.

The depressant effects of opioid analgesics are enhanced by depressants of the central nervous system such as alcohol, anaesthetics, antipsychotics, anxiolytics, hypnotics and sedatives, tricyclic antidepressants and phenothiazines.

Cyclizine may counteract the haemodynamic benefits of opioids.

Opioid analgesics with some antagonist activity such as buprenorphine, butorphanol, nalbuphine or pentazocine may precipitate opioid withdrawal symptoms in patients who have recently used pure agonists such as morphine. The actions of opioids may in turn affect the activities of other compounds, for instance their gastro-intestinal effects may delay absorption as with mexiletine or may be counteractive as with metoclopramide, domperidone and possibly cisapride.

Plasma concentrations of morphine are possibly increased by ritonavir.

4.6 Pregnancy and lactation

Since this product rapidly crosses the placental barrier, it should not be used during the second stage of labour or in premature delivery because of the risk of secondary respiratory depression in the new-born infant. If the mother is addicted a withdrawal syndrome is observed in the new-born infant characterised by: convulsions, irritability, vomiting and increased mortality. As with all drugs, it is not advisable to administer morphine during pregnancy.

4.7 Effects on ability to drive and use machines

Because of the decrease in vigilance induced by this drug, attention is drawn to the possible dangers incurred by drivers of vehicles or machine operators.

4.8 Undesirable effects

The most common side effects at usual doses are nausea, constipation, confusion and occasionally vomiting.

Other possible effects include: urticaria, pruritus, rashes, decreased libido or potency, mood changes, drowsiness, dry mouth, sweating, headache, facial flushing, vertigo, bradycardia, tachycardia, palpitations, postural hypotension, dysphoria, hypotension, hypothermia, miosis, dysuria, sedation or excitation (particularly in elderly subjects in whom delirium and hallucinations may occur), increased intracranial pressure which may aggravate existing cerebral disorders, increased pressure in the main bile duct and urinary retention in cases of prostatic adenoma or urethral stenosis. Mild respiratory depression occurs even at therapeutic doses and in the event of overdosage it may be severe, serious or even fatal. Physical and psychic dependence may appear after administration of therapeutic doses for periods of 1 to 2 weeks. Some cases of dependence have been observed after only 2 to 3 days.

Withdrawal syndrome: this may occur a few hours after withdrawal of a prolonged treatment, and is maximal between the 36th and 72nd hours.

4.9 Overdose

Symptoms include respiratory depression, extreme miosis, hypotension, hypothermia and coma. Treatment is by intravenous injection of naloxone 0.4mg, repeated every 2 to 3 minutes if necessary, or by an infusion of 2mg in 500ml of normal saline or 5% dextrose (0.004mg/ml).

In subjects dependent on morphine-like drugs, withdrawal symptoms may occur following injection of a high dose of naloxone. It should therefore be injected in gradually increasing doses to such subjects.

5. PHARMACOLOGICAL PROPERTIES

5.1 Pharmacodynamic properties

Morphine is an opioid analgesic. It acts mainly on the central nervous system and smooth muscle.

Morphine exerts an analgesic action, and affects psychomotor behaviour: depending on the dose administered, it induces sedation (>1cg) or, in some cases, excitation (<1cg). At high doses, greater than those required to produce analgesia, it induces somnolence and sleep.

5.2 Pharmacokinetic properties

Absorption

This is a sustained-release form, which makes possible twice-daily oral administration. Morphine is immediately absorbed from the digestive tract following oral administration. The maximum serum concentrations of morphine are obtained in 2 to 4 hours.

Distribution

The percentage of binding to plasma proteins after absorption is low (about 34%). There is no clearly defined correlation between the plasma concentration of morphine and the analgesic effect.

Metabolism

A considerable quantity of morphine is metabolised by the liver to glucuronides, which undergo enterohepatic recirculation.

Excretion

The product is eliminated essentially in the urine, by glomerular filtration, mainly as glucuronides. A small amount (less than 10%) is eliminated in the faeces.

5.3 Preclinical safety data

There are no pre-clinical safety data of relevance to the prescriber which are additional to those already included in other sections of the Summary of Product Characteristics.

6. PHARMACEUTICAL PARTICULARS

6.1 List of excipients

Sucrose, maize starch, polyethylene glycol 4000, ethyl cellulose, cetyl alcohol, sodium lauryl sulphate, dibutyl sebacate, talc, gelatin, iron oxide ink (E172), titanium dioxide (E171)[1].

The 10mg capsules also contain quinoline yellow (E104), the 30mg capsules erythrosine (E127), and the 60mg capsules sunset yellow (E110).

[1] The 200mg capsules do not contain titanium dioxide (E171).

6.2 Incompatibilities

Not applicable.

6.3 Shelf life

36 months.

6.4 Special precautions for storage

Store below 25°C in a dry place protected from heat.

6.5 Nature and contents of container

Blister packs (aluminium/PVC).

Boxes of 60 capsules.

6.6 Instructions for use and handling
Not applicable.

7. MARKETING AUTHORISATION HOLDER
Laboratoires Ethypharm, 17 - 21 rue Saint Matthieu, 78550 Houdan, France

Distributed in the UK by

Link Pharmaceuticals Limited, Bishops Weald House, Albion Way, Horsham, West Sussex, RH12 1AH

8. MARKETING AUTHORISATION NUMBER(S)
Zomorph 10mg, 30mg, 60mg, 100mg PL 06934/0006/0007/0008/0009

Zomorph 200mg PL 06934/0016

9. DATE OF FIRST AUTHORISATION/RENEWAL OF THE AUTHORISATION
Zomorph 10mg, 30mg, 60mg, 100mg May 1995 / July 2000

Zomorph 200mg August 1995 / July 2000

10. DATE OF REVISION OF THE TEXT
July 2000

® Zomorph is a registered trade mark

Zonegran capsules

(Eisai Ltd)

1. NAME OF THE MEDICINAL PRODUCT
25 mg: Zonegran ▼ 25 mg hard capsules.
50 mg: Zonegran ▼ 50 mg hard capsules.
100 mg: Zonegran ▼ 100 mg hard capsules.

2. QUALITATIVE AND QUANTITATIVE COMPOSITION
25 mg: Each Zonegran hard capsule contains 25 mg of zonisamide.

50 mg: Each Zonegran hard capsule contains 50 mg of zonisamide.

100 mg: Each Zonegran hard capsule contains 100 mg of zonisamide.

For excipients, see Section 6.1.

3. PHARMACEUTICAL FORM
Hard capsule.

25 mg: A white opaque body and a white opaque cap printed with a logo and "ZONEGRAN 25" in black.

50 mg: A white opaque body and a grey opaque cap printed with a logo and "ZONEGRAN 50" in black.

100 mg: A white opaque body and a red opaque cap printed with a logo and "ZONEGRAN 100" in black

4. CLINICAL PARTICULARS
4.1 Therapeutic indications
Zonegran is indicated as adjunctive therapy in the treatment of adult patients with partial seizures, with or without secondary generalisation.

4.2 Posology and method of administration
Zonegran hard capsules are for oral use.

Adults
Zonegran must be added to existing therapy and the dose should be titrated on the basis of clinical effect. Doses of 300 mg to 500 mg per day have been shown to be effective, though some patients, especially those not taking CYP3A4-inducing agents, may respond to lower doses.

The recommended initial daily dose is 50 mg in two divided doses. After one week the dose may be increased to 100 mg daily and thereafter the dose may be increased at one weekly intervals, in increments of up to 100 mg.

Use of two weekly intervals should be considered for patients with renal or hepatic impairment and patients not receiving CYP3A4-inducing agents (see Section 4.5).

Zonegran can be administered once or twice daily after the titration phase.

Elderly
Caution should be exercised at initiation of treatment in elderly patients as there is limited information on the use of Zonegran in these patients. Prescribers should also take account of the safety profile of Zonegran (see Section 4.8).

Children and adolescents
The safety and effectiveness in children and adolescents under 18 years have not been established. Therefore use in these patients is not recommended.

Patients with renal impairment
Caution must be exercised in treating patients with renal impairment, as there is limited information on use in such patients and a slower titration of Zonegran might be required. Since zonisamide and its metabolites are excreted renally, it should be discontinued in patients who develop acute renal failure or where a clinically significant sustained increase in serum creatinine is observed.

In subjects with renal impairment, renal clearance of single doses of zonisamide was positively correlated with creatinine clearance. The plasma AUC of zonisamide was increased by 35% in subjects with creatinine clearance < 20 ml/min.

Patients with hepatic impairment
Use in patients with hepatic impairment has not been studied. Therefore use in patients with severe hepatic impairment is not recommended. Caution must be exercised in treating patients with mild to moderate hepatic impairment, and a slower titration of Zonegran may be required.

Effect of food
Zonegran may be taken with or without food (see Section 5.2).

Withdrawal of Zonegran
When Zonegran treatment is to be discontinued, it should be withdrawn gradually. In clinical studies, dose reductions of 100 mg at weekly intervals have been used with concurrent adjustment of other anti-epileptic drug doses.

4.3 Contraindications
Hypersensitivity to zonisamide, to any of the excipients or to sulphonamides.

4.4 Special warnings and special precautions for use
In accordance with current clinical practice, discontinuation of Zonegran in patients with epilepsy must be accomplished by gradual dose reduction, to reduce the possibility of seizures on withdrawal. There are insufficient data for the withdrawal of concomitant anti-epileptic medications once seizure control with Zonegran has been achieved in the add-on situation, in order to reach monotherapy with Zonegran. Therefore withdrawal of concomitant anti-epileptic agents must be undertaken with caution.

Zonegran is a benzisoxazole derivative, which contains a sulphonamide group. Serious immune based adverse reactions that have been associated with medicinal products containing a sulphonamide group include rash, allergic reaction and major haematological disturbances including aplastic anaemia.

Serious rashes have occurred in association with Zonegran therapy, including isolated cases of Stevens-Johnson syndrome.

Consideration must be given to discontinuing Zonegran in patients who develop an otherwise unexplained rash. All patients who develop a rash while taking Zonegran must be closely supervised, with additional levels of caution applied to those patients receiving concomitant anti-epileptic agents that may independently induce skin rashes.

Isolated cases of agranulocytosis, thrombocytopenia, leukopenia, aplastic anaemia, pancytopenia and leucocytosis have been reported. There is inadequate information to assess the relationship, if any, between dose and duration of treatment and these events.

Kidney stones have occurred in patients treated with Zonegran. Zonegran should be used with caution in patients who have risk factors for nephrolithiasis, including prior stone formation, a family history of nephrolithiasis and hypercalcuria. Such patients may be at increased risk for renal stone formation and associated signs and symptoms such as renal colic, renal pain or flank pain. In addition, patients taking other medications associated with nephrolithiasis may be at increased risk. Increasing fluid intake and urine output may help reduce the risk of stone formation, particularly in those with predisposing risk factors.

Zonegran should be used with caution in patients being treated concomitantly with carbonic anhydrase inhibitors such as topiramate, as there are insufficient data to rule out a pharmacodynamic interaction (see Section 4.5).

Cases of decreased sweating and elevated body temperature have been reported mainly in paediatric patients. Heat stroke requiring hospital treatment was diagnosed in some cases. Most reports occurred during periods of warm weather. Patients or their carers must be warned to take care to maintain hydration and avoid exposure to excessive temperatures. Caution should be used when Zonegran is prescribed with other medicinal products that predispose patients to heat related disorders; these include carbonic anhydrase inhibitors and medicinal products with anticholinergic activity.

In patients taking Zonegran who develop the clinical signs and symptoms of pancreatitis, it is recommended that pancreatic lipase and amylase levels are monitored. If pancreatitis is evident, in the absence of another obvious cause, it is recommended that discontinuation of Zonegran be considered and appropriate treatment initiated.

In patients taking Zonegran, in whom severe muscle pain and/or weakness develop either in the presence or absence of a fever, it is recommended that markers of muscle damage be assessed, including serum creatine phosphokinase and aldolase levels. If elevated, in the absence of another obvious cause such as trauma or grand mal seizures, it is recommended that Zonegran discontinuation be considered and appropriate treatment initiated.

Women of child-bearing potential must use adequate contraception during treatment with Zonegran and for one month after discontinuation (see section 4.6). Physicians treating patients with Zonegran should try to ensure that appropriate contraception is used, and should use clinical judgement when assessing whether OCs (oral contraceptive), or the doses of the OC components, are adequate based on the individual patient's clinical situation.

Zonegran 100 mg hard capsules contain a yellow colour called sunset yellow FCF (E110), which may cause allergic reactions.

There is limited data from clinical studies in patients with a body weight of less than 40 kg. Therefore these patients should be treated with caution.

Zonegran may cause weight loss. A dietary supplement or increased food intake may be considered if the patient is losing weight or is underweight whilst on this medication. If substantial undesirable weight loss occurs, discontinuation of Zonegran should be considered.

4.5 Interaction with other medicinal products and other forms of Interaction
Effect of Zonegran on cytochrome P450 enzymes.

In vitro studies using human liver microsomes show no or little (< 25%) inhibition of cytochrome P450 isozymes 1A2, 2A6, 2C9, 2C19, 2D6, 2E1 or 3A4 at zonisamide levels approximately two-fold or greater than clinically relevant unbound serum concentrations. Therefore Zonegran is not expected to affect the pharmacokinetics of other medicinal products via cytochrome P450-mediated mechanisms, as demonstrated for carbamazepine, phenytoin, ethinylestradiol and desipramine *in vivo*.

Potential for Zonegran to affect other medicinal products

Anti-epileptic drugs
In epileptic patients, steady-state dosing with Zonegran resulted in no clinically relevant pharmacokinetic effects on carbamazepine, lamotrigine, phenytoin, or sodium valproate.

Oral contraceptives
In clinical studies in healthy subjects, steady-state dosing with Zonegran did not affect serum concentrations of ethinylestradiol or norethisterone in a combined oral contraceptive.

Carbonic anhydrase inhibitors

There are insufficient data to rule out possible pharmacodynamic interactions with carbonic anhydrase inhibitors such as topiramate.

Potential medicinal product interactions affecting Zonegran

In clinical studies co-administration of lamotrigine had no apparent effect on zonisamide pharmacokinetics. The combination of Zonegran with other medicinal products that may lead to urolithiasis may enhance the risk of developing kidney stones; therefore the concomitant administration of such medicinal products should be avoided.

Zonisamide is metabolised partly by CYP3A4 (reductive cleavage), and also by N-acetyl-transferases and conjugation with glucuronic acid; therefore, substances that can induce or inhibit these enzymes may affect the pharmacokinetics of zonisamide:

- Enzyme Induction: Exposure to zonisamide is lower in epileptic patients receiving CYP3A4-inducing agents such as phenytoin, carbamazepine, and phenobarbitone. These effects are unlikely to be of clinical significance when Zonegran is added to existing therapy; however, changes in zonisamide concentrations may occur if concomitant CYP3A4-inducing anti-epileptic or other medicinal products are withdrawn, dose adjusted or introduced, and an adjustment of the Zonegran dose may be required. Rifampicin is a potent CYP3A4 inducer. If co-administration is necessary, the patient should be closely monitored and the dose of Zonegran and other CYP3A4 substrates adjusted as needed.

- CYP3A4 Inhibition: Based upon clinical data, known specific and non-specific CYP3A4 inhibitors appear to have no clinically relevant effect on zonisamide pharmacokinetic exposure parameters. Steady-state dosing of either ketoconazole (400 mg/day) or cimetidine (1200 mg/day) had no clinically relevant effects on the single-dose pharmacokinetics of zonisamide given to healthy subjects. Therefore, modification of Zonegran dosing should not be necessary when co-administered with known CYP3A4 inhibitors.

4.6 Pregnancy and lactation
Zonegran must not be used during pregnancy unless clearly necessary and only if the potential benefit is considered to justify the risk to the foetus. The need for anti-epileptic treatment should be reviewed in patients planning to become pregnant. If Zonegran is prescribed, careful monitoring is recommended.

Specialist advice should be given to women who are likely to become pregnant in order to consider the optimal treatment during pregnancy. Women of child-bearing potential should be counselled to use contraception during treatment with Zonegran, and for one month after discontinuation.

There are no adequate data from the use of Zonegran in pregnant women. Studies in animals have shown reproductive toxicity (see Section 5.3).

No sudden discontinuation of anti-epileptic therapy should be undertaken as this may lead to breakthrough seizures which could have serious consequences for both mother and child.

Zonisamide is excreted in human milk; the concentration in breast milk is similar to maternal plasma. A decision must be made whether to discontinue breast-feeding or to discontinue/abstain from Zonegran therapy. Due to the long retention time of zonisamide in the body, breast-feeding must not be resumed until one month after Zonegran therapy is completed.

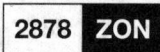

4.7 Effects on ability to drive and use machines

Some patients may experience drowsiness or difficulty with concentration, particularly early in treatment or after a dose increase. Patients must be advised to exercise caution during activities requiring a high degree of alertness, e.g., driving or operating machinery.

4.8 Undesirable effects

Zonegran has been administered to over 1,200 patients in clinical studies, more than 400 of whom received Zonegran for at least 1 year. In addition there has been extensive post-marketing experience with zonisamide in Japan since 1989 and in the USA since 2000.

The most common adverse reactions in controlled adjunctive-therapy studies were somnolence, dizziness and anorexia. Adverse reactions associated with Zonegran obtained from clinical studies and post-marketing surveillance are tabulated below. The frequencies are arranged according to the following scheme:

very common	> 1/10
common	> 1/100 < 1/10
uncommon	> 1/1,000 < 1/100
rare	> 1/10,000 < 1/1,000
very rare	< 1/10,000 including isolated reports

(see Table 1)

Table 1

System Organ Class (MedDRA terminology)	Very Common	Common	Uncommon	Very Rare
Infections and infestation			Pneumonia Urinary tract infection	
Blood and lymphatic system disorders				Agranulocytosis Aplastic anaemia Leucocytosis Leucopoenia Lymphadenopathy Pancytopenia, Thrombocytopenia
Immune system disorders		Hypersensitivity		
Metabolism and nutrition disorders	Anorexia		Hypokalaemia	Metabolic acidosis
Psychiatric Disorders	Agitation Irritability Confusional state Depression		Psychotic disorder	Hallucination Insomnia Suicidal ideation
Nervous system disorders	Ataxia Dizziness Memory impairment Somnolence	Disturbance in attention Speech disorder	Convulsion	Amnesia Coma Grand mal seizure Myasthenic syndrome Neuroleptic malignant syndrome
Eye disorders	Diplopia			
Respiratory, thoracic and mediastinal disorders				Dyspnoea Pneumonia aspiration Respiratory disorder
Gastrointestinal disorders		Abnormal pain Diarrhoea Nausea	Vomiting	Pancreatitis
Hepatobiliary disorders			Cholecystitis Cholelithiasis	Hepatocellular damage
Skin and subcutaneous tissue disorders		Rash		Anhidrosis Erythema multiforme Pruritis Stevens-Johnson syndrome
Musculoskeletal and connective tissue disorders				Rhabdomyolysis
Renal and urinary disorders			Calculus urinary Nephrolithiasis	Hydronephrosis Renal insufficiency Urine abnormality
General disorders and administration site conditions		Pyrexia		
Investigations		Weight decreased		Blood creatine phosphokinase increased Blood urea increased Liver function tests abnormal
Injury, poisoning and procedural complications				Heat stroke

In addition there have been isolated cases of Sudden Unexplained Death in Epilepsy Patients (SUDEP) receiving Zonegran.

4.9 Overdose

There have been cases of accidental and intentional overdose in adult and paediatric patients. In some cases, the overdoses were asymptomatic, particularly where emesis or lavage was prompt. In other cases, the overdose was followed by symptoms such as somnolence, nausea, gastritis, nystagmus, myoclonus, coma, bradycardia, reduced renal function, hypotension and respiratory depression. A very high plasma concentration of 100.1 μg/ml zonisamide was recorded approximately 31 hours after a patient took an overdose of Zonegran and clonazepam; the patient became comatose and had respiratory depression, but recovered consciousness five days later and had no sequelae.

Treatment

No specific antidotes for Zonegran overdose are available. Following a suspected recent overdose, emptying the stomach by gastric lavage or by induction of emesis may be indicated with the usual precautions to protect the airway. General supportive care is indicated, including frequent monitoring of vital signs and close observation. Zonisamide has a long elimination half-life so its effects may be persistent. Although not formally studied for the treatment of overdose, haemodialysis reduced plasma concentrations of zonisamide in a patient with reduced renal function, and may be considered as treatment of overdose if clinically indicated.

5. PHARMACOLOGICAL PROPERTIES

Zonisamide is benzisoxazole derivative. It is an anti-epileptic medicine with weak carbonic anhydrase activity *in-vitro*. It is chemically unrelated to other anti-epileptic agents.

5.1 Pharmacodynamic properties

Pharmacotherapeutic group:Anti-epileptics, ATC code: N03A X15

Efficacy has been demonstrated with Zonegran in 4 double-blind, placebo-controlled studies of periods of up to 24 weeks with either once or twice daily dosing. These studies show that the median reduction in partial seizure frequency is related to Zonegran dose with sustained efficacy at doses of 300-500 mg per day.

The anticonvulsant activity of zonisamide has been evaluated in a variety of models, in several species with induced or innate seizures, and zonisamide appears to act as a broad-spectrum anti-epileptic in these models. Zonisamide prevents maximal electroshock seizures and restricts seizure spread, including the propagation of seizures from cortex to sub-cortical structures and suppresses epileptogenic focus activity. Unlike phenytoin and carbamazepine however, zonisamide acts preferentially on seizures originating in the cortex.

The mechanism of action of zonisamide is not fully elucidated, but it appears to act on voltage-sensitive sodium and calcium channels, thereby disrupting synchronised neuronal firing, reducing the spread of seizure discharges and disrupting subsequent epileptic activity. Zonisamide also has a modulatory effect on GABA-mediated neuronal inhibition.

5.2 Pharmacokinetic properties

Absorption

Zonisamide is almost completely absorbed after oral administration, generally reaching peak serum or plasma concentrations within 2 to 5 hours of dosing. The first-pass metabolism is believed to be negligible. Absolute bioavailability is estimated to be approximately 100%. Oral bioavailability is not affected by food, although peak plasma and serum concentrations may be delayed.

Zonisamide AUC and C_{max} values increased almost linearly after single dose over the dose range of 100-800 mg and after multiple doses over the dose range of 100-400 mg once daily. The increase at steady state was slightly more than expected on the basis of dose, probably due to the saturable binding of zonisamide to erythrocytes. Steady state was achieved within 13 days. Slightly greater than expected accumulation occurs relative to single dosing.

Distribution

Zonisamide is 40 - 50 % bound to human plasma proteins, with *in vitro* studies showing that this is unaffected by the presence of various anti-epileptic medicinal products (i.e., phenytoin, phenobarbitone, carbamazepine, and sodium valproate). The apparent volume of distribution is about 1.1 – 1.7 l/kg in adults indicating that zonisamide is extensively distributed to tissues. Erythrocyte/plasma ratios are about 15 at low concentrations and about 3 at higher concentrations.

Metabolism

Zonisamide is metabolised primarily through reductive cleavage of the benzisoxazole ring of the parent drug by CYP3A4 to form 2-sulphamoylacetylphenol (SMAP) and also by N-acetylation. Parent drug and SMAP can additionally be glucuronidated. The metabolites, which could not be detected in plasma, are devoid of anticonvulsant activity. There is no evidence that zonisamide induces its own metabolism.

Elimination

Apparent clearance of zonisamide at steady-state after oral administration is about 0.70 l/h and the terminal elimination half-life is about 60 hours in the absence of CYP3A4 inducers. The elimination half-life was independent of dose and not affected by repeat administration. Fluctuation in serum or plasma concentrations over a dosing interval is low (< 30 %). The main route of excretion of zonisamide metabolites and unchanged drug is via the urine. Renal clearance of unchanged zonisamide is relatively low (approximately 3.5 ml/min); about 15 - 30 % of the dose is eliminated unchanged.

Special patient groups

In subjects with renal impairment, renal clearance of single doses of zonisamide was positively correlated with creatinine clearance. The plasma AUC of zonisamide was increased by 35% in subjects with creatinine clearance <20 ml/min (see also section 4.2.).

Patients with an impaired liver function: The pharmacokinetics of zonisamide in patients with impaired liver function have not been adequately studied.

Elderly: No clinically significant differences were observed in the pharmacokinetics between young (aged 21-40 years) and elderly (65-75 years).

Adolescents (12-18 years): Limited data indicate that pharmacokinetics in adolescents dosed to steady state at 1, 7 or 12 mg/kg daily, in divided doses, are similar to those observed in adults, after adjustment for bodyweight.

Other characteristics

No clear Zonegran dose-concentration-response relationship has been defined. When comparing the same dose level, subjects of higher total body weight appear to have lower steady-state serum concentrations, but this effect appears to be relatively modest. Age (⩾ 12 years) and gender, after adjustment for body weight effects, have no apparent effect on zonisamide exposure in epileptic patients during steady-state dosing.

5.3 Preclinical safety data

Findings not observed in clinical studies, but seen in the dog at exposure levels similar to clinical use, were liver changes (enlargement, dark-brown discolouration, mild hepatocyte enlargement with concentric lamellar bodies in the cytoplasm and cytoplasmic vacuolation) associated with increased metabolism.

Zonisamide was not genotoxic and has no carcinogenic potential.

Zonisamide caused developmental abnormalities in mice, rats, and dogs, and was embryolethal in monkeys, when administered during the period of organogenesis at zonisamide dosage and maternal plasma levels similar to or lower than therapeutic levels in humans.

6. PHARMACEUTICAL PARTICULARS

6.1 List of excipients

Capsule contents:

Microcrystalline cellulose

Hydrogenated vegetable oil

Sodium laurilsulfate.

The capsule shells contain:

Gelatin

Titanium dioxide (E171)

Shellac

Propylene glycol

Potassium hydroxide

Black iron oxide (E172)

Additionally the 100 mg capsule shells contain:

Allura red AC (E129)

Sunset yellow FCF (E110)

6.2 Incompatibilities

Not applicable.

6.3 Shelf life

2 years.

6.4 Special precautions for storage

Do not store above 30°C.

6.5 Nature and contents of container

25 mg: PVC/PCTFE/aluminium blisters, packs of 14, 28 and 56 hard capsules.

50 mg: PVC/PCTFE/aluminium blisters, packs of 14, 28 and 56 hard capsules.

100 mg: PVC/PCTFE/aluminium blisters, packs of 28, 56, 98 and 196 hard capsules.

Not all pack sizes may be marketed.

6.6 Instructions for use and handling

No special requirements.

7. MARKETING AUTHORISATION HOLDER

Eisai Limited

3 Shortlands

London

W6 8EE

United Kingdom

8. MARKETING AUTHORISATION NUMBER(S)

25 mg 14 capsules: EU/1/04/307/001

25 mg 28 capsules: EU/1/04/307/005

25 mg 56 capsules: EU/1/04/307/002

50 mg 14 capsules: EU/1/04/307/010

50 mg 28 capsules: EU/1/04/307/009

50 mg 56 capsules: EU/1/04/307/003

100 mg 28 capsules: EU/1/04/307/006

100 mg 56 capsules: EU/1/04/307/004

100 mg 98 capsules: EU/1/04/307/007

100 mg 196 capsules: EU/1/04/307/008

9. DATE OF FIRST AUTHORISATION/RENEWAL OF THE AUTHORISATION

10 March 2005

10. DATE OF REVISION OF THE TEXT

26 April 2005

11. LEGAL CATEGORY

POM - Medicinal product subject to medical prescription

Zorac 0.05% Gel

(Allergan Ltd)

1. NAME OF THE MEDICINAL PRODUCT

ZORAC 0.05%, gel

2. QUALITATIVE AND QUANTITATIVE COMPOSITION

100 g gel contains: tazarotene 0.05 g

For excipients, see 6.1.

3. PHARMACEUTICAL FORM

Gel.

Zorac is a colourless to light yellow, translucent to homogeneous cloudy, gel.

4. CLINICAL PARTICULARS

4.1 Therapeutic indications

For the topical treatment of mild to moderate plaque psoriasis involving up to 10% body surface area.

4.2 Posology and method of administration

Zorac gel is available in two concentrations.

To initiate a treatment with Zorac, it is advisable to start with Zorac 0.05 % in order to evaluate the skin response and tolerance before progressing to Zorac 0.1 % if necessary.

Treatment with the lower concentration gel is associated with a somewhat lower incidence of local adverse events (see section 4.8 and 5).

Treatment with the higher concentration gel gives a faster and numerically higher response rate.

The physician should choose the concentration to be used based on clinical circumstances and the principle of using the least concentration of drug to achieve the desired effect.

Individual variations with respect to efficacy and tolerability are possible. It is thus advisable for patients to consult their physician on a weekly basis when initiating therapy.

A thin film of the gel should be applied once daily in the evening; care should be taken to apply it only to areas of affected skin, avoiding application to healthy skin or in skin folds. Treatment is limited to 10% body surface area (approximately equivalent to the total skin area of one arm).

If the patient experiences more drying or irritation, an effective greasy emollient (without pharmaceutically active ingredients) can be applied to the areas of the skin to be treated to improve tolerability. Healthy skin around the psoriatic plaques can be covered by using zinc paste, for example, to prevent irritation.

Usually, the treatment period is up to 12 weeks. Clinical experience, particularly on tolerability, is available on periods of use of up to 12 months.

4.3 Contraindications

Hypersensitivity to any ingredient of the medication(s)

Pregnancy or in women planning a pregnancy

Breast-feeding mothers

Since there is, as yet, no clinical experience, Zorac should not be used in the treatment of psoriasis pustulosa and psoriasis exfoliativa, and the gel should not be applied to intertriginous areas, to the face or to hair-covered scalp.

4.4 Special warnings and special precautions for use

Care should be taken to ensure that Zorac is applied only to psoriatic lesions, as application to normal, eczematous or inflamed skin or skin affected by other pathologies may cause irritation. Patients should be advised to wash their hands after application of the gel to avoid accidental transfer to the eyes.

If psoriatic areas on the skin of the hands are being treated, particular care should be taken to ensure that no gel is transferred to facial skin or the eyes.

If skin irritation develops, treatment with Zorac should be interrupted.

The safety of use on more than 10% of the body surface area has not been established. There is limited experience of application to up to 20% of the body surface area.

Patients should be advised to avoid excessive exposure to UV light (including sunlight, use of a solarium, PUVA or UVB therapy) during treatment with Zorac (see section 5.3).

No therapeutic studies using Zorac under occlusion or concomitantly with other antipsoriatic agents (including tar shampoos) have been carried out. To minimise interference with absorption and to avoid unnecessary spreading of the medication, topical application of emollients and cosmetics should not be applied within 1 hour of applying Zorac.

The safety and efficacy of Zorac have not been established in patients under the age of 18 years.

This medicinal product contains butylhydroxyanisole and butylhydroxytoluene and therefore may cause local skin reactions (e.g. contact dermatitis) or irritation to the eyes and mucous membranes.

4.5 Interaction with other medicinal products and other forms of Interaction

Concomitant use of pharmaceutical and cosmetic preparations which cause irritation or have a strong drying effect should be avoided.

4.6 Pregnancy and lactation

Pregnancy

Although in animals no malformations were observed after dermal application, skeletal alterations were seen in the foetuses, which may be attributable to systemic retinoid effects. Teratogenic effects were observed after oral administration.

In view of these findings Zorac gel must not be used by pregnant women or women planning a pregnancy.

Women of childbearing potential should be informed of the potential risk and adopt adequate birth control measures when Zorac is used.

Lactation

Although no data are available on the excretion of tazarotene in human milk, animal data indicate that excretion into milk is possible. For that reason Zorac gel should not be used during breast feeding.

4.7 Effects on ability to drive and use machines

None known.

4.8 Undesirable effects

The most frequently reported adverse reactions in controlled clinical trials of Zorac in the treatment of psoriasis were pruritus (incidence 20-25%), burning, erythema, and irritation (10-20%), desquamation, non-specific rash, irritant contact dermatitis, skin pain, and a worsening of psoriasis (5-10 %).

More rarely observed were stinging and inflamed and dry skin (1-3 %).

The incidence of adverse reactions appears to be concentration-related and dependent on duration of use. The higher concentration gel (0.1%) may cause up to 5% more cases of severe skin irritation than the lower concentration gel (0.05%), especially during the first 4 weeks of use.

4.9 Overdose

Excessive dermal use of Zorac may result in marked redness, peeling, or local discomfort.

Inadvertent ingestion of Zorac is a theoretical possibility. In such a case, the signs and symptoms associated with hypervitaminosis A (severe headache, nausea, vomiting, drowsiness, irritability, and pruritus) may occur. However, it is likely that these symptoms would prove to be reversible.

5. PHARMACOLOGICAL PROPERTIES

Both gels have demonstrated therapeutic effects as early as 1 week after commencement of a course of treatment. A good clinical response was seen in up to 65% of the patients after 12 weeks of treatment.

The therapeutic effect of the higher concentration gel is more rapidly apparent and the efficacy more marked.

In various studies in which patients were also evaluated for 12 weeks following cessation of therapy, it was found that patients continued to show a certain clinical benefit, however, no difference between the higher and lower concentrations with regard to this effect was observed.

5.1 Pharmacodynamic properties

Topical antipsoriatic agent; ATC-code: D05AX05

Tazarotene, a member of the acetylenic class of retinoids, is a prodrug which is converted to its active free form, tazarotenic acid, by de-esterification in the skin area.

Tazarotenic acid is the only known metabolite of tazarotene to have retinoid activity.

The active metabolite specifically regulates gene expression, thus modulating cell proliferation, hyperplasia, and differentiation in a wide range of tissues, as has been demonstrated in *in vitro* and *in vivo* trials.

The exact mechanism of action of tazarotene in psoriasis is, as yet, unknown.

Improvement in psoriatic patients occurs in association with restoration of normal cutaneous morphology, and reduction of the inflammatory markers ICAM-1 and HLA-DR, and of markers of epidermal hyperplasia and abnormal differentiation, such as elevated keratinocyte transglutaminase, involucrin, and keratin 16.

5.2 Pharmacokinetic properties

A) *General characteristics*

Absorption

Results of a pharmacokinetic study of single topical application of 0.1% ^{14}C-tazarotene gel show that approximately

5% is absorbed when applied to normal skin under occlusion.

After a single topical application of tazarotene gel to 20% body surface area for 10 hours in healthy volunteers, tazarotene was not detectable in the plasma. Maximum plasma levels for the active metabolite tazarotenic acid of 0.3 ± 0.2 ng/ml (for the 0.05% strength) and 0.5 ± 0.3 ng/ml (0.1% gel) were measured after approximately 15 hours. The AUC was 40% higher for the 0.1% gel compared with the 0.05% gel. Thus, the two strengths of the gel are not strictly dose proportional with respect to systemic absorption.

Repeated topical application of the 0.1% gel over 7 days led to maximum plasma levels for tazarotenic acid of 0.7 ± 0.6 ng/ml after 9 hours.

Biotransformation

After dermal application, tazarotene undergoes esterase hydrolysis to form its free acid, tazarotenic acid, and oxidative metabolism to form inactive sulphoxide and sulphone derivatives.

Elimination

Secondary metabolites of tazarotenic acid (the sulphoxide, the sulphone and an oxygenated derivative of tazarotenic acid) have been detected in human urine and faeces. The elimination half-life of tazarotenic acid after dermal application of tazarotene is approximately 18 hours in normal and psoriatic subjects.

After intravenous administration, the half-life of tazarotene was approximately 6 hours and that of tazarotenic acid 14 hours.

B) *Characteristics after use in patients*

After single topical application of 0.1% ^{14}C-tazarotene gel for 10 hours to psoriatic lesions (without occlusion), 4.5% of the dose was recovered in the stratum corneum and 2.4% in the epidermal/dermal layers. Less than 1% of the dose was absorbed systemically. More than 75% of drug elimination was completed within 72 hours.

In a small five patient study, repeated topical application of tazarotene 0.1% gel over 13 days results in a mean peak plasma level of tazarotenic acid of 12 ± 8 ng/ml. These patients had psoriatic lesions on 8-18% of body surface area. In a larger 24 psoriatic patient study, tazarotene 0.05% and 0.1% gels were applied for 3 months and yielded a Cmax of 0.45 ± 0.78 ng/ml and 0.83 ± 1.22 ng/ml, respectively.

In a 1 year clinical study with 0.05% and 0.1% tazarotene gel, tazarotene was detected in 3 out of 112 patients at plasma concentrations below 1 ng/ml, while its active metabolite tazarotenic acid was found in 31 patients. Only four patients had plasma concentrations of tazarotenic acid greater than or equal to 1 ng/ml (maximum 2.8 ng/ml).

5.3 Preclinical safety data

Subacute/Chronic toxicity

The safety of daily dermal application of tazarotene gel was tested in mouse, rat and mini-pig over periods of up to one year. The main observation was reversible skin irritation. In the case of the mini-pig, an incomplete healing of the dermal irritation was observed after an 8 week recovery period. The rat appears to be the most sensitive species to tazarotene, as is the case with other retinoids. Here, dermal application induced severe skin reactions and clinically significant retinoid-like systemic effects. No adverse systemic effects were observed in the other species.

After oral administration of 0.025 mg/kg/day for 1 year in the cynomolgus monkey, no toxic effects were observed. At higher doses, typical symptoms of retinoid toxicity were seen.

Reproductive toxicity

Safety of use during pregnancy has not been established. Teratogenic and embryotoxic effects were observed after oral administration in the rat and rabbit. In dermal application studies during foetal development, skeletal alterations and decreased pup weight at birth and at the end of the lactation period were observed.

Animal tests suggest that tazarotene or its active metabolite is excreted in breast milk and passes the placenta barrier.

No effects on fertility are reported after topical application in the male and female rat.

Mutagenicity/Carcinogenicity

No evidence of a mutagenic potential of tazarotene has been reported in *in vitro* and *in vivo* trials.

In long term investigations of the effects of dermal and oral administration in animals, no carcinogenic effects were observed.

There was an increased incidence of photocarcinogenic effects in the hairless mouse when exposed to UV light after topical application of tazarotene.

Local tolerability

Tazarotene gel has a considerable irritative potential on skin in all animal species investigated.

Instillation of tazarotene gel in the eye of the rabbit resulted in irritation with marked hyperaemia of the conjunctiva, but there was no corneal damage.

6. PHARMACEUTICAL PARTICULARS

6.1 List of excipients

Benzyl alcohol,

Macrogol 400,

Hexylene glycol,

Carbomer 974P,

Trometamol,

Poloxamer 407,

Polysorbate 40,

Ascorbic acid,

Butylhydroxyanisole (E320),

Butylhydroxytoluene (E321),

Disodium edetate,

Purified water.

6.2 Incompatibilities

Tazarotene is susceptible to oxidising agents and may undergo ester hydrolysis when in contact with bases.

6.3 Shelf life

3 years.

After first opening of the container: 6 months.

6.4 Special precautions for storage

Do not store above 30°C.

6.5 Nature and contents of container

Aluminium tube, internally lacquered, epoxyphenolic, with white polypropylene cap.

Pack sizes: 10 g, 15 g, 30 g, 50 g, 60 g, and 100 g gel.

6.6 Instructions for use and handling

No special requirements.

7. MARKETING AUTHORISATION HOLDER

Allergan Pharmaceuticals Ireland

Castlebar Road

Westport

County Mayo

Ireland

8. MARKETING AUTHORISATION NUMBER(S)

PL 05179/0003

9. DATE OF FIRST AUTHORISATION/RENEWAL OF THE AUTHORISATION

20th January 2003

10. DATE OF REVISION OF THE TEXT

Zorac 0.1% Gel

(Allergan Ltd)

1. NAME OF THE MEDICINAL PRODUCT

ZORAC 0.1%, gel

2. QUALITATIVE AND QUANTITATIVE COMPOSITION

100 g gel contains: tazarotene 0.1 g

For excipients, see 6.1.

3. PHARMACEUTICAL FORM

Gel.

Zorac is a colourless to light yellow, translucent to homogeneous cloudy, gel.

4. CLINICAL PARTICULARS

4.1 Therapeutic indications

For the topical treatment of mild to moderate plaque psoriasis involving up to 10% body surface area.

4.2 Posology and method of administration

Zorac gel is available in two concentrations.

To initiate a treatment with Zorac, it is advisable to start with Zorac 0.05 % in order to evaluate the skin response and tolerance before progressing to Zorac 0.1 % if necessary.

Treatment with the lower concentration gel is associated with a somewhat lower incidence of local adverse events (see section 4.8 and 5).

Treatment with the higher concentration gel gives a faster and numerically higher response rate.

The physician should choose the concentration to be used based on clinical circumstances and the principle of using the least concentration of drug to achieve the desired effect.

Individual variations with respect to efficacy and tolerability are possible. It is thus advisable for patients to consult their physician on a weekly basis when initiating therapy.

A thin film of the gel should be applied once daily in the evening; care should be taken to apply it only to areas of affected skin, avoiding application to healthy skin or in skin folds. Treatment is limited to 10% body surface area (approximately equivalent to the total skin area of one arm).

If the patient experiences more drying or irritation, an effective greasy emollient (without pharmaceutically active ingredients) can be applied to the areas of the skin to be treated to improve tolerability. Healthy skin around the psoriatic plaques can be covered by using zinc paste, for example, to prevent irritation.

Usually, the treatment period is up to 12 weeks. Clinical experience, particularly on tolerability, is available on periods of use of up to 12 months.

4.3 Contraindications

Hypersensitivity to any ingredient of the medication(s)

Pregnancy or in women planning a pregnancy

Breast-feeding mothers

Since there is, as yet, no clinical experience, Zorac should not be used in the treatment of psoriasis pustulosa and psoriasis exfoliativa, and the gel should not be applied to intertriginous areas, to the face or to hair-covered scalp.

4.4 Special warnings and special precautions for use

Care should be taken to ensure that Zorac is applied only to psoriatic lesions, as application to normal, eczematous or inflamed skin or skin affected by other pathologies may cause irritation. Patients should be advised to wash their hands after application of the gel to avoid accidental transfer to the eyes. If psoriatic areas on the skin of the hands are being treated, particular care should be taken to ensure that no gel is transferred to facial skin or the eyes.

If skin irritation develops, treatment with Zorac should be interrupted.

The safety of use on more than 10% of the body surface area has not been established. There is limited experience of application to up to 20% of the body surface area.

Patients should be advised to avoid excessive exposure to UV light (including sunlight, use of a solarium, PUVA or UVB therapy) during treatment with Zorac (see section 5.3).

No therapeutic studies using Zorac under occlusion or concomitantly with other antipsoriatic agents (including tar shampoos) have been carried out. To minimise interference with absorption and to avoid unnecessary spreading of the medication, topical application of emollients and cosmetics should not be applied within 1 hour of applying Zorac.

The safety and efficacy of Zorac have not been established in patients under the age of 18 years.

This medicinal product contains butylhydroxyanisole and butylhydroxytoluene and therefore may cause local skin reactions (e.g. contact dermatitis) or irritation to the eyes and mucous membranes.

4.5 Interaction with other medicinal products and other forms of Interaction

Concomitant use of pharmaceutical and cosmetic preparations which cause irritation or have a strong drying effect should be avoided.

4.6 Pregnancy and lactation

Pregnancy

Although in animals no malformations were observed after dermal application, skeletal alterations were seen in the foetuses, which may be attributable to systemic retinoid effects. Teratogenic effects were observed after oral administration.

In view of these findings Zorac gel must not be used by pregnant women or women planning a pregnancy.

Women of childbearing potential should be informed of the potential risk and adopt adequate birth control measures when Zorac is used.

Lactation

Although no data are available on the excretion of tazarotene in human milk, animal data indicate that excretion into milk is possible. For that reason Zorac gel should not be used during breast feeding.

4.7 Effects on ability to drive and use machines

None known.

4.8 Undesirable effects

The most frequently reported adverse reactions in controlled clinical trials of Zorac in the treatment of psoriasis were pruritus (incidence 20-25%), burning, erythema, and irritation (10-20%), desquamation, non-specific rash, irritant contact dermatitis, skin pain, and a worsening of psoriasis (5-10 %).

More rarely observed were stinging and inflamed and dry skin (1-3 %).

The incidence of adverse reactions appears to be concentration-related and dependent on duration of use. The higher concentration gel (0.1%) may cause up to 5% more cases of severe skin irritation than the lower concentration gel (0.05%), especially during the first 4 weeks of use.

4.9 Overdose

Excessive dermal use of Zorac may result in marked redness, peeling, or local discomfort.

Inadvertent ingestion of Zorac is a theoretical possibility. In such a case, the signs and symptoms associated with hypervitaminosis A (severe headache, nausea, vomiting, drowsiness, irritability, and pruritus) may occur. However, it is likely that these symptoms would prove to be reversible.

5. PHARMACOLOGICAL PROPERTIES

Both gels have demonstrated therapeutic effects as early as 1 week after commencement of a course of treatment. A good clinical response was seen in up to 65% of the patients after 12 weeks of treatment.

The therapeutic effect of the higher concentration gel is more rapidly apparent and the efficacy more marked.

In various studies in which patients were also evaluated for 12 weeks following cessation of therapy, it was found that patients continued to show a certain clinical benefit, however, no difference between the higher and lower concentrations with regard to this effect was observed.

5.1 Pharmacodynamic properties

Topical antipsoriatic agent; ATC-code: D05AX05.

Tazarotene, a member of the acetylenic class of retinoids, is a prodrug which is converted to its active free form, tazarotenic acid, by de-esterification in the skin area.

Tazarotenic acid is the only known metabolite of tazarotene to have retinoid activity.

The active metabolite specifically regulates gene expression, thus modulating cell proliferation, hyperplasia, and differentiation in a wide range of tissues, as has been demonstrated in *in vitro* and *in vivo* trials.

The exact mechanism of action of tazarotene in psoriasis, is, as yet, unknown.

Improvement in psoriatic patients occurs in association with restoration of normal cutaneous morphology, and reduction of the inflammatory markers ICAM-1 and HLA-DR, and of markers of epidermal hyperplasia and abnormal differentiation, such as elevated keratinocyte transglutaminase, involucrin, and keratin 16.

5.2 Pharmacokinetic properties

A) *General characteristics*

Absorption

Results of a pharmacokinetic study of single topical application of 0.1% ^{14}C-tazarotene gel show that approximately 5% is absorbed when applied to normal skin under occlusion.

After a single topical application of tazarotene gel to 20% body surface area for 10 hours in healthy volunteers, tazarotene was not detectable in the plasma. Maximum plasma levels for the active metabolite tazarotenic acid of 0.3 ± 0.2 ng/ml (for the 0.05% strength) and 0.5 ± 0.3 ng/ml (0.1% gel) were measured after approximately 15 hours. The AUC was 40% higher for the 0.1% gel compared with the 0.05% gel. Thus, the two strengths of the gel are not strictly dose proportional with respect to systemic absorption.

Repeated topical application of the 0.1% gel over 7 days led to maximum plasma levels for tazarotenic acid of 0.7 ± 0.6 ng/ml after 9 hours.

Biotransformation

After dermal application, tazarotene undergoes esterase hydrolysis to form its free acid, tazarotenic acid, and oxidative metabolism to form inactive sulphoxide and sulphone derivatives.

Elimination

Secondary metabolites of tazarotenic acid (the sulphoxide, the sulphone and an oxygenated derivative of tazarotenic acid) have been detected in human urine and faeces. The elimination half-life of tazarotenic acid after dermal application of tazarotene is approximately 18 hours in normal and psoriatic subjects.

After intravenous administration, the half-life of tazarotene was approximately 6 hours and that of tazarotenic acid 14 hours.

B) *Characteristics after use in patients*

After single topical application of 0.1% ^{14}C-tazarotene gel for 10 hours to psoriatic lesions (without occlusion), 4.5% of the dose was recovered in the stratum corneum and 2.4% in the epidermal/dermal layers. Less than 1% of the dose was absorbed systemically. More than 75% of drug elimination was completed within 72 hours.

In a small five patient study, repeated topical application of tazarotene 0.1% gel over 13 days results in a mean peak plasma level of tazarotenic acid of 12 ± 8 ng/ml.

These patients had psoriatic lesions on 8-18% of body surface area. In a larger 24 psoriatic patient study, tazarotene 0.05% and 0.1% gels were applied for 3 months and yielded a Cmax of 0.45 ± 0.78 ng/ml and 0.83 ± 1.22 ng/ml, respectively.

In a 1 year clinical study with 0.05% and 0.1% tazarotene gel, tazarotene was detected in 3 out of 112 patients at plasma concentrations below 1 ng/ml, while its active metabolite tazarotenic acid was found in 31 patients. Only four patients had plasma concentrations of tazarotenic acid greater than or equal to 1 ng/ml (maximum 2.8 ng/ml).

5.3 Preclinical safety data

Subacute/Chronic toxicity

The safety of daily dermal application of tazarotene gel was tested in mouse, rat and mini-pig over periods of up to one year. The main observation was reversible skin irritation. In the case of the mini-pig, an incomplete healing of the dermal irritation was observed after an 8 week recovery period. The rat appears to be the most sensitive species to tazarotene, as is the case with other retinoids. Here, dermal application induced severe skin reactions and clinically significant retinoid-like systemic effects. No adverse systemic effects were observed in the other species.

After oral administration of 0.025 mg/kg/day for 1 year in the cynomolgus monkey, no toxic effects were observed.

At higher doses, typical symptoms of retinoid toxicity were seen.

Reproductive toxicity

Safety of use during pregnancy has not been established. Teratogenic and embryotoxic effects were observed after oral administration in the rat and rabbit. In dermal application studies during foetal development, skeletal alterations and decreased pup weight at birth and at the end of the lactation period were observed.

Animal tests suggest that tazarotene or its active metabolite is excreted in breast milk and passes the placenta barrier.

No effects on fertility are reported after topical application in the male and female rat.

Mutagenicity/Carcinogenicity

No evidence of a mutagenic potential of tazarotene has been reported in in vitro and in vivo trials.

In long term investigations of the effects of dermal and oral administration in animals, no carcinogenic effects were observed.

There was an increased incidence of photocarcinogenic effects in the hairless mouse when exposed to UV light after topical application of tazarotene.

Local tolerability

Tazarotene gel has a considerable irritative potential on skin in all animal species investigated.

Instillation of tazarotene gel in the eye of the rabbit resulted in irritation with marked hyperaemia of the conjunctiva, but there was no corneal damage.

6. PHARMACEUTICAL PARTICULARS

6.1 List of excipients

Benzyl alcohol,

Macrogol 400,

Hexylene glycol,

Carbomer 974P,

Trometamol,

Poloxamer 407,

Polysorbate 40,

Ascorbic acid,

Butylhydroxyanisole (E320),

Butylhydroxytoluene (E321),

Disodium edetate,

Purified water.

6.2 Incompatibilities

Tazarotene is susceptible to oxidising agents and may undergo ester hydrolysis when in contact with bases.

6.3 Shelf life

3 years.

After first opening of the container: 6 months.

6.4 Special precautions for storage

Do not store above 30°C.

6.5 Nature and contents of container

Aluminium tube, internally lacquered, epoxyphenolic, with white polypropylene cap.

Pack sizes: 10 g, 15 g, 30 g, 50 g, 60 g, and 100 g gel.

6.6 Instructions for use and handling

No special requirements.

7. MARKETING AUTHORISATION HOLDER

Allergan Pharmaceuticals Ireland

Castlebar Road

Westport

County Mayo

Ireland

8. MARKETING AUTHORISATION NUMBER(S)

PL 05179/0002

9. DATE OF FIRST AUTHORISATION/RENEWAL OF THE AUTHORISATION

20th January 2003

10. DATE OF REVISION OF THE TEXT

Zoton Capsules

(Wyeth Pharmaceuticals)

1. NAME OF THE MEDICINAL PRODUCT

Zoton Capsules 15 mg.

Zoton Capsules 30 mg.

2. QUALITATIVE AND QUANTITATIVE COMPOSITION

Capsules containing 15 mg or 30 mg of lansoprazole (INN).

3. PHARMACEUTICAL FORM

Zoton Capsules 15 mg: Opaque, yellow capsules for oral administration. Each capsule contains white to off-white enteric-coated granules.

Zoton Capsules 30 mg: Two tone lilac/purple capsules for oral administration. Each capsule contains white to off-white enteric-coated granules.

4. CLINICAL PARTICULARS

4.1 Therapeutic indications

Uses

Zoton is effective in the treatment of acid-related disorders of the upper gastro-intestinal tract, with the benefit of rapid symptom relief. Zoton is also effective in combination with antibiotics in the eradication of *Helicobacter pylori* (*H. pylori*).

Indications

Healing and long term management of Gastro Oesophageal Reflux Disease (GORD).

Healing and maintenance therapy for patients with duodenal ulcer.

Relief of reflux-like symptoms (eg. heartburn) and/or ulcer-like symptoms (eg. upper epigastric pain) associated with acid-related dyspepsia.

Healing of benign gastric ulcer.

Treatment and prophylaxis of NSAID-associated benign gastric ulcers, duodenal ulcers and relief of symptoms in patients requiring continued NSAID treatment.

Long term management of pathological hypersecretory conditions including Zollinger-Ellison syndrome.

Zoton is also effective in patients with benign peptic lesions, including reflux oesophagitis, unresponsive to H_2 receptor antagonists.

Eradication of H. pylori from the upper gastrointestinal tract when used in combination with appropriate antibiotics in patients with ulcer-like dyspepsia leading to the prevention of symptom recurrence.

Eradication of *H. pylori* from the upper gastrointestinal tract when used in combination with appropriate antibiotics in patients with gastritis or duodenal ulcer leading to the healing and prevention of relapse of the ulcer.

4.2 Posology and method of administration

Dosage:

Gastro Oesophageal Reflux Disease: Zoton 30mg once daily for 4 weeks. The majority of patients will be healed after the first course. For those patients not fully healed at this time, a further 4 weeks treatment at the same dosage should be given.

For long term management, a maintenance dose of Zoton 15mg or 30mg once daily can be used dependent upon patient response.

Duodenal ulcer: Zoton 30mg once daily for 4 weeks.

For prevention of relapse, the recommended maintenance dose is Zoton 15mg once daily.

Acid-related dyspepsia: Intermittent courses, as required, of Zoton 15mg or 30mg once daily for 2-4 weeks depending on the severity and persistence of symptoms. Patients who do not respond after 4 weeks, or who relapse shortly afterwards, should be investigated.

Benign gastric ulcer: Zoton 30mg once daily for 8 weeks.

Treatment of NSAID-associated benign gastric and duodenal ulcers and relief of symptoms: Zoton 15mg or 30mg once daily for 4 or 8 weeks. Most patients will be healed after 4 weeks; for those patients not fully healed, a further 4 weeks treatment can be given.

For patients at particular risk or with ulcers that may be difficult to heal, the higher dose and/or the longer treatment duration should be used.

Prophylaxis of NSAID-associated benign gastric ulcers, duodenal ulcers and symptoms: Zoton 15mg or 30mg once daily.

Hypersecretory conditions: The initial dose should be Zoton 60mg once daily. The dosage should then be adjusted individually. Treatment should be continued for as long as clinically indicated.

For patients who require 120mg or more per day, the dose should be divided and administered twice daily.

Eradication of *H. pylori*: The following combinations have been shown to be effective when given for 7 days:

Zoton 30mg twice daily plus clarithromycin 250-500mg twice daily and amoxycillin 1g twice daily or

Zoton 30mg twice daily plus clarithromycin 250-500mg twice daily and metronidazole 400mg twice daily or

Zoton 30mg twice daily plus amoxycillin 1g twice daily and metronidazole 400mg twice daily.

The best eradication results are obtained when clarithromycin is combined with either amoxycillin or metronidazole. When used in combination with the recommended antibiotics, Zoton is associated with *H. pylori*-eradication rates of up to 90%.

Eradication of *H. pylori* with any one of the above regimens has been shown to result in the healing of duodenal ulcers, without the need for continued anti-ulcer drug therapy. The risk of reinfection is low and relapse following successful eradication is, therefore, unlikely.

For the optimal prevention of symptom recurrence in patients with ulcer-like dyspepsia, eradication of H. pylori should be followed by continued lansoprazole treatment (see acid-related dyspepsia).

To achieve the optimal acid inhibitory effect, and hence most rapid healing and symptom relief, Zoton 'once daily' should be administered in the morning before food. Zoton 'twice daily' should be administered once in the morning before food, and once in the evening.

The capsules should be swallowed whole. Do not crush or chew.

Elderly: Dose adjustment is not required in the elderly. The normal daily dosage should be given.

Children: There is no experience with Zoton in children.

Impaired Hepatic and Renal Function:

Lansoprazole is metabolised substantially by the liver. Clinical trials in patients with liver disease indicate that metabolism of lansoprazole is prolonged when daily doses of 30mg are administered to patients with severe hepatic impairment. It is therefore recommended that the daily dose for patients with severe liver disease is individually adjusted to 15mg or 30mg. These patients should be kept under regular supervision and a daily dosage of 30mg should not be exceeded.

There is no need to alter the dosage in patients with mild to moderate impairment of hepatic function or impaired renal function.

4.3 Contraindications

The use of Zoton is contra-indicated in patients with a history of hypersensitivity to any of the ingredients of Zoton capsules.

4.4 Special warnings and special precautions for use

In common with other anti-ulcer therapies, the possibility of malignancy should be excluded when gastric ulcer is suspected, as symptoms may be alleviated and diagnosis delayed. Similarly, the possibility of serious underlying disease such as malignancy should be excluded before treatment for dyspepsia commences, particularly in patients of middle age or older who have new or recently changed dyspeptic symptoms.

Before using Zoton with antibiotics to eradicate *H. pylori*, prescribers should refer to the full prescribing information of the respective antibiotics for guidance.

Zoton should be used with caution in patients with severe hepatic dysfunction. These patients should be kept under regular supervision and a daily dosage of 30mg should not be exceeded (See Section 4.2 Posology and Method of Administration).

Decreased gastric acidity due to any means, including proton pump inhibitors, increases gastric counts of bacteria normally present in the gastrointestinal tract. Treatment with acid-reducing drugs may lead to a slightly increased risk of gastrointestinal infections such as *Salmonella* and *Campylobacter*.

4.5 Interaction with other medicinal products and other forms of Interaction

Lansoprazole is hepatically metabolised and studies indicate that it is a weak inducer of Cytochrome P450. There is the possibility of interaction with drugs which are metabolised by the liver. Caution should be exercised when oral contraceptives and preparations such as phenytoin, carbamazepine, theophylline, or warfarin are taken concomitantly with the administration of Zoton.

No clinically significant effects on NSAIDs or diazepam have been found.

Antacids and sucralfate may reduce the bioavailability of lansoprazole and should, therefore, not be taken within an hour of Zoton.

4.6 Pregnancy and lactation

There is insufficient experience to recommend the use of Zoton in pregnancy. Animal studies do not reveal any teratogenic effect. Reproduction studies indicate slightly reduced litter survival and weights in rats and rabbits given very high doses of lansoprazole. The use of Zoton in pregnancy should be avoided.

Animal studies indicate that lansoprazole is secreted in breast milk. There is no information on the secretion of lansoprazole into breast milk in humans. The use of Zoton during breast feeding should be avoided unless considered essential.

4.7 Effects on ability to drive and use machines

Zoton is not known to affect ability to drive or operate machines.

4.8 Undesirable effects

Zoton is well-tolerated, with adverse events generally being mild and transient.

The most commonly reported adverse events are headache, dizziness, fatigue and malaise.

Gastrointestinal effects include diarrhoea, constipation, abdominal pain, nausea, vomiting, flatulence and dry or sore mouth or throat.

As with other PPIs, very rarely, cases of colitis have been reported. In severe and/or protracted cases of diarrhoea, discontinuation of therapy should be considered. In the majority of cases symptoms resolve on discontinuation of therapy.

Alterations in liver function test values and, rarely, jaundice or hepatitis, have been reported.

Dermatological reactions include skin rashes, urticaria and pruritus. These generally resolve on discontinuation of drug therapy. Serious dermatological reactions are rare but there have been occasional reports of Stevens-Johnson Syndrome, toxic epidermal necrolysis and erythematous or bullous rashes including erythema multiforme. Cases of hair thinning and photosensitivity have also been reported.

Other hypersensitivity reactions include angioedema, wheezing, and very rarely, anaphylaxis. Cases of interstitial nephritis have been reported which have sometimes resulted in renal failure.

Haematological effects (thrombocytopenia, agranulocytosis, eosinophilia, leucopenia and pancytopenia) have occurred rarely. Bruising, purpura and petechiae have also been reported.

Other reactions include arthralgia, myalgia, depression, peripheral oedema and, rarely, paraesthesia, blurred vision, taste disturbances, vertigo, confusion and hallucinations.

Gynaecomastia and impotence have been reported rarely.

4.9 Overdose

There is no information on the effect of overdosage. However, Zoton has been given at doses up to 120mg/day without significant adverse effects. Symptomatic and supportive therapy should be given as appropriate.

5. PHARMACOLOGICAL PROPERTIES

5.1 Pharmacodynamic properties

Lansoprazole is a member of a class of drugs called proton pump inhibitors. Its mode of action is to inhibit specifically the H^+ / K^+ ATPase (proton pump) of the parietal cell in the stomach, the terminal step in acid production, thus reducing gastric acidity, a key requirement for healing of acid-related disorders such as gastric ulcer, duodenal ulcer and reflux oesophagitis. It is believed that the parent drug is biotransformed into its active form(s) in the acidic environment of the parietal cell, whereupon it reacts with the sulphydryl group of the H^+ / K^+ ATPase causing inhibition. This inhibition is reversible *in vitro* by intrinsic and extrinsic reducing agents. Lansoprazole's mode of action differs significantly from the H_2 antagonists which inhibit one of the three pathways involved in stimulation of acid production. A single dose of 30mg inhibits pentagastrin-stimulated acid secretion by approximately 80%, indicating effective acid inhibition from the first day of dosing.

Lansoprazole has a prolonged pharmacological action providing effective acid suppression over 24 hours, thereby promoting rapid healing and symptom relief.

By reducing gastric acidity, Zoton creates an environment in which appropriate antibiotics can be effective against *H. pylori. In vitro* studies have shown that lansoprazole has a direct antimicrobial effect on *H. pylori.*

5.2 Pharmacokinetic properties

Lansoprazole exhibits high (80-90%) bioavailability with a single dose. As a result, effective acid inhibition is achieved rapidly. Peak plasma levels occurred within 1.5 to 2.0 hours. The plasma elimination half-life ranges from 1 to 2 hours following single or multiple doses in healthy subjects. There is no evidence of accumulation following multiple doses in healthy subjects. The plasma protein binding is 97%.

Following absorption, lansoprazole is extensively metabolised and is excreted by both the renal and biliary route. A study with ^{14}C-labelled lansoprazole indicated that up to 50% of the dose was excreted in the urine. Lansoprazole is metabolised substantially by the liver.

5.3 Preclinical safety data

Gastric tumours have been observed in life-long studies in rats.

An increased incidence of spontaneous retinal atrophy has been observed in life-long studies in rats. These lesions which are common to albino laboratory rats have not been observed in monkeys or dogs or life-long studies in mice. They are considered to be rat specific. No such treatment related changes have been observed in patients treated continuously for long periods.

6. PHARMACEUTICAL PARTICULARS

6.1 List of excipients

Gastro-resistant Granules: Magnesium Carbonate, Sugar Spheres, Sucrose, Maize Starch, Low Substituted Hydroxypropyl Cellulose, Hydroxypropylcellulose, Methacrylic Acid – Ethyl Acrylate Copolymer (1:1) Dispersion 30 per cent, Talc, Macrogol 8000, Titanium Dioxide, Polysorbate 80, Colloidal Anhydrous Silica, Purified Water. **Capsule Shells:** Gelatin, Opacode Black 1007, Titanium Dioxide (E171), Erythrosine (E127, 30mg capsules only), Indigo Carmine (E132, 30mg capsules only), Iron Oxide Yellow (E172, 15mg capsules only).

6.2 Incompatibilities

None known.

6.3 Shelf life

Zoton Capsules may be stored in bottles or blister packs for up to 3 years.

The bottles incorporate an aluminium membrane seal. The capsules should retain potency and physical properties for three months after opening. Discard any remaining capsules after this period.

Capsules may be dispensed into a tightly closed container.

6.4 Special precautions for storage

Do not store above 25°C. Store in the original package.

6.5 Nature and contents of container

Zoton Capsules 15 mg: Blister packs of 28, 56 or 84 (maintenance pack) capsules.

Zoton Capsules 30 mg: Blister packs of 2, 7, 14, 28, 42 or 56 capsules.

White plastic bottles of 50 capsules.

6.6 Instructions for use and handling

Not applicable.

7. MARKETING AUTHORISATION HOLDER

John Wyeth & Brother Limited

Trading as Wyeth Pharmaceuticals

Huntercombe Lane South

Taplow

Maidenhead

Berkshire SL6 0PH

UK

8. MARKETING AUTHORISATION NUMBER(S)

Zoton Capsules 15 mg: PL 00011/0288

Zoton Capsules 30 mg: PL 00011/0287

9. DATE OF FIRST AUTHORISATION/RENEWAL OF THE AUTHORISATION

Zoton Capsules 15 mg: 26 January 2004

Zoton Capsules 30 mg: 26 January 2004

10. DATE OF REVISION OF THE TEXT

31 July 2005

Zoton FasTab

(Wyeth Pharmaceuticals)

1. NAME OF THE MEDICINAL PRODUCT

Zoton FasTab* 15 mg

Zoton FasTab* 30 mg

Lansoprazole oro-dispersible tablets 15mg and 30mg

2. QUALITATIVE AND QUANTITATIVE COMPOSITION

Oro-dispersible tablet containing 15 mg or 30 mg of lansoprazole.

For excipients, see 6.1.

3. PHARMACEUTICAL FORM

Oro-dispersible tablet.

Zoton FasTab 15mg and 30mg are white to yellowish white, circular flat bevelled-edge oro-dispersible tablets speckled with orange to dark brown gastro-resistant microgranules.

4. CLINICAL PARTICULARS

4.1 Therapeutic indications

Uses

Zoton is effective in the treatment of acid-related disorders of the upper gastro-intestinal tract, with the benefit of rapid symptom relief. Zoton is also effective in combination with antibiotics in the eradication of *Helicobacter pylori* (*H. pylori*).

Indications

Healing and long term management of Gastro Oesophageal Reflux Disease (GORD).

Healing and maintenance therapy for patients with duodenal ulcer.

Relief of reflux-like symptoms (eg. heartburn) and/or ulcer-like symptoms (eg. upper epigastric pain) associated with acid-related dyspepsia.

Healing of benign gastric ulcer.

Treatment and prophylaxis of NSAID-associated benign gastric ulcers, duodenal ulcers and relief of symptoms in patients requiring continued NSAID treatment.

Long term management of pathological hypersecretory conditions including Zollinger-Ellison syndrome.

Zoton is also effective in patients with benign peptic lesions, including reflux oesophagitis, unresponsive to H_2-receptor antagonists.

Eradication of *H. pylori* from the upper gastrointestinal tract when used in combination with appropriate antibiotics in patients with ulcer-like dyspepsia leading to the prevention of symptom recurrence.

Eradication of *H. pylori* from the upper gastrointestinal tract when used in combination with appropriate antibiotics in patients with gastritis or duodenal ulcer leading to the healing and prevention of relapse of the ulcer.

4.2 Posology and method of administration

For oral administration. Zoton FasTab is strawberry flavoured and should be placed on the tongue and gently sucked. The tablet rapidly disperses in the mouth, releasing the gastro-resistant microgranules which are swallowed with the patient's saliva. Alternatively, the tablet can be swallowed whole with a drink of water.

The tablets should not be crushed or chewed.

To achieve the optimal acid inhibitory effect, and hence most rapid healing and symptom relief, Zoton 'once daily' should be administered in the morning before food. Zoton 'twice daily' should be administered once in the morning before food, and once in the evening.

Dosage:

Gastro Oesophageal Reflux Disease: Zoton 30mg once daily for 4 weeks. The majority of patients will be healed after the first course. For those patients not fully healed at this time, a further 4 weeks treatment at the same dosage should be given.

For long term management, a maintenance dose of Zoton 15mg or 30mg once daily can be used dependent upon patient response.

Duodenal ulcer: Zoton 30mg once daily for 4 weeks.

For prevention of relapse, the recommended maintenance dose is Zoton 15mg once daily.

Acid-related dyspepsia: Intermittent courses, as required, of Zoton 15mg or 30mg once daily for 2-4 weeks depending on the severity and persistence of symptoms. Patients who do not respond after 4 weeks, or who relapse shortly afterwards, should be investigated.

Benign gastric ulcer: Zoton 30mg once daily for 8 weeks.

Treatment of NSAID-associated benign gastric and duodenal ulcers and relief of symptoms: Zoton 15mg or 30mg once daily for 4 or 8 weeks. Most patients will be healed after 4 weeks; for those patients not fully healed, a further 4 weeks treatment can be given.

For patients at particular risk or with ulcers that may be difficult to heal, the higher dose and/or the longer treatment duration should be used.

Prophylaxis of NSAID-associated benign gastric ulcers, duodenal ulcers and symptoms: Zoton 15mg or 30mg once daily.

Hypersecretory conditions: The initial dose should be Zoton 60mg once daily. The dosage should then be adjusted individually. Treatment should be continued for as long as clinically indicated.

For patients who require 120mg or more per day, the dose should be divided and administered twice daily.

Eradication of *H. pylori*: The following combinations have been shown to be effective when given for 7 days:

Zoton 30mg twice daily plus clarithromycin 250-500mg twice daily and amoxycillin 1g twice daily or

Zoton 30mg twice daily plus clarithromycin 250-500mg twice daily and metronidazole 400mg twice daily or

Zoton 30mg twice daily plus amoxycillin 1g twice daily and metronidazole 400mg twice daily.

The best eradication results are obtained when clarithromycin is combined with either amoxycillin or metronidazole. When used in combination with the recommended antibiotics, Zoton is associated with *H. pylori*-eradication rates of up to 90%.

Eradication of *H. pylori* with any one of the above regimens has been shown to result in the healing of duodenal ulcers, without the need for continued anti-ulcer drug therapy. The risk of reinfection is low and relapse following successful eradication is, therefore, unlikely.

For the optimal prevention of symptom recurrence in patients with ulcer-like dyspepsia, eradication of *H. pylori* should be followed by continued lansoprazole treatment (see acid-related dyspepsia).

Elderly: Dose adjustment is not required in the elderly. The normal daily dosage should be given.

Children: There is no experience with Zoton in children.

Impaired Hepatic and Renal Function:

Lansoprazole is metabolised substantially by the liver. Clinical trials in patients with liver disease indicate that metabolism of lansoprazole is prolonged when daily doses of 30mg areadministered to patients with severe hepatic impairment. It is therefore recommended that the daily dose for patients with severe liver disease is individually adjusted to 15mg or 30mg. These patients should be kept under regular supervision and a daily dose of 30mg should not be exceeded.

There is no need to alter the dosage in patients with mild to moderate impairment of hepaticfunction or impaired renal function.

4.3 Contraindications

The use of Zoton FasTab is contra-indicated in patients with a history of hypersensitivity to any of the ingredients of Zoton FasTab.

4.4 Special warnings and special precautions for use

In common with other anti-ulcer therapies, the possibility of malignancy should be excluded when gastric ulcer is suspected, as symptoms may be alleviated and diagnosis delayed. Similarly, the possibility of serious underlying disease such as malignancy should be excluded before treatment for dyspepsia commences, particularly in patients of middle age or older who have new or recently changed dyspeptic symptoms.

Before using Zoton with antibiotics to eradicate *H. pylori*, prescribers should refer to the full prescribing information of the respective antibiotics for guidance.

Zoton should be used with caution in patients with severe hepatic dysfunction. These patients should be kept under regular supervision, and a daily dosage of 30mg should not be exceeded (See Section 4.2 Posology and Method of Administration).

Decreased gastric acidity due to any means, including proton pump inhibitors, increases gastric counts of bacteria normally present in the gastrointestinal tract. Treatment with acid-reducing drugs may lead to a slightly increased risk of gastrointestinal infections such as *Salmonella* and *Campylobacter*.

4.5 Interaction with other medicinal products and other forms of Interaction

Lansoprazole is hepatically metabolised and studies indicate that it is a weak inducer of Cytochrome P450. There is the possibility of interaction with drugs which are metabolised by the liver. Caution should be exercised when oral contraceptives and preparations such as phenytoin, carbamazepine, theophylline, or warfarin are taken concomitantly with the administration of Zoton.

No clinically significant effects on NSAIDs or diazepam have been found.

Antacids and sucralfate may reduce the bioavailability of lansoprazole and should, therefore, not be taken within an hour of Zoton.

4.6 Pregnancy and lactation

There is insufficient experience to recommend the use of Zoton in pregnancy. Animal studies do not reveal any teratogenic effect. Reproduction studies indicate slightly reduced litter survival and weights in rats and rabbits given very high doses of lansoprazole. The use of Zoton in pregnancy should be avoided.

Animal studies indicate that lansoprazole is secreted in breast milk. There is no information on the secretion of lansoprazole into breast milk in humans. The use of Zoton during breast feeding should be avoided unless considered essential.

4.7 Effects on ability to drive and use machines

Zoton is not known to affect ability to drive or operate machines.

4.8 Undesirable effects

Zoton is well-tolerated, with adverse events generally being mild and transient.

The most commonly reported adverse events are headache, dizziness, fatigue and malaise.

Gastrointestinal effects include diarrhoea, constipation, abdominal pain, nausea, vomiting, flatulence and dry or sore mouth or throat.

As with other PPIs, very rarely, cases of colitis have been reported. In severe and/or protracted cases of diarrhoea, discontinuation of therapy should be considered. In the majority of cases symptoms resolve on discontinuation of therapy.

Alterations in liver function test values and, rarely, jaundice or hepatitis, have been reported.

Dermatological reactions include skin rashes, urticaria and pruritus. These generally resolve on discontinuation of drug therapy. Serious dermatological reactions are rare but there have been occasional reports of Stevens-Johnson syndrome, toxic epidermal necrolysis and erythematous or bullous rashes including erythema multiforme. Cases of hair thinning and photosensitivity have also been reported.

Other hypersensitivity reactions include angioedema, wheezing, and very rarely, anaphylaxis. Cases of interstitial nephritis have been reported which have sometimes resulted in renal failure.

Haematological effects (thrombocytopenia, agranulocytosis, eosinophilia, leucopenia and pancytopenia) have occurred rarely. Bruising, purpura and petechiae have also been reported.

Other reactions include arthralgia, myalgia, depression, peripheral oedema and, rarely, paraesthesia, blurred vision, taste disturbances, vertigo, confusion and hallucinations.

Gynaecomastia and impotence have been reported rarely.

4.9 Overdose

There is no information on the effect of overdosage. However, Zoton has been given at doses up to 120mg/day without significant adverse effects. Symptomatic and supportive therapy should be given as appropriate.

5. PHARMACOLOGICAL PROPERTIES

5.1 Pharmacodynamic properties

Lansoprazole is a member of a class of drugs called proton pump inhibitors. Its mode of action is to inhibit specifically the H^+ / K^+ ATPase (proton pump) of the parietal cell in the stomach, the terminal step in acid production, thus reducing gastric acidity, a key requirement for healing of acid-related disorders such as gastric ulcer, duodenal ulcer and reflux oesophagitis. It is believed that the parent drug is biotransformed into its active form(s) in the acidic environment of the parietal cell, whereupon it reacts with the sulphydryl group of the H^+ / K^+ ATPase causing inhibition. This inhibition is reversible *in vitro* by intrinsic and extrinsic reducing agents. Lansoprazole's mode of action differs significantly from the H_2-antagonists which inhibit one of the three pathways involved in stimulation of acid production. A single dose of 30mg inhibits pentagastrin-stimulated acid secretion by approximately 80%, indicating effective acid inhibition from the first day of dosing.

Lansoprazole has a prolonged pharmacological action providing effective acid suppression over 24 hours, thereby promoting rapid healing and symptom relief.

By reducing gastric acidity, Zoton creates an environment in which appropriate antibiotics can be effective against *H. pylori*. *In vitro* studies have shown that lansoprazole has a direct antimicrobial effect on *H. pylori*.

5.2 Pharmacokinetic properties

Lansoprazole exhibits high (80-90%) bioavailability with a single dose. As a result, effective acid inhibition is achieved rapidly. Peak plasma levels occurred within 1.5 to 2.0 hours. The plasma elimination half-life ranges from 1 to 2 hours following single or multiple doses in healthy subjects. There is no evidence of accumulation following multiple doses in healthy subjects. The plasma protein binding is 97%.

Following absorption, lansoprazole is extensively metabolised and is excreted by both the renal and biliary route. A study with ^{14}C-labelled lansoprazole indicated that up to 50% of the dose was excreted in the urine. Lansoprazole is metabolised substantially by the liver.

5.3 Preclinical safety data

Gastric tumours have been observed in life-long studies in rats.

An increased incidence of spontaneous retinal atrophy has been observed in life-long studies in rats. These lesions which are common to albino laboratory rats have not been observed in monkeys or dogs or life-long studies in mice. They are considered to be rat specific. No such treatment related changes have been observed in patients treated continuously for long periods.

6. PHARMACEUTICAL PARTICULARS

6.1 List of excipients

Gastro-resistant microgranules: Lactose monohydrate, microcrystalline cellulose, heavy magnesium carbonate, low-substituted hydroxypropylcellulose, hydroxypropyl cellulose, hypromellose, titanium dioxide, talc, mannitol, methacrylic acid – ethyl acrylate copolymer (1:1) 30 per cent, polyacrylate dispersion 30 per cent, macrogol 8000, citric acid anhydrous, glyceryl monostearate, polysorbate 80, mannitol, iron oxide yellow (E172) and iron oxide red (E172).

Other excipients: Mannitol, microcrystalline cellulose, low-substituted hydroxypropylcellulose, citric acid anhydrous, crospovidone, magnesium stearate, strawberry flavour and aspartame.

6.2 Incompatibilities

None known.

6.3 Shelf life

3 years.

6.4 Special precautions for storage

Do not store above 25°C. Store in the original package.

6.5 Nature and contents of container

Zoton FasTab 15mg: Aluminium blister packs of 28 or 56 Tablets.

Zoton FasTab 30mg: Aluminium blister packs of 2, 7, 14 or 28 Tablets.

6.6 Instructions for use and handling

Not applicable.

7. MARKETING AUTHORISATION HOLDER

John Wyeth & Brother Limited

Trading as Wyeth Pharmaceuticals

Huntercombe Lane South

Taplow

Maidenhead

Berkshire SL6 0PH

UK

8. MARKETING AUTHORISATION NUMBER(S)

Zoton FasTab 15mg: PL 00011/0290

Zoton FasTab 30mg: PL 00011/0289

9. DATE OF FIRST AUTHORISATION/RENEWAL OF THE AUTHORISATION

Zoton FasTab 15mg: 26 January 2004

Zoton FasTab 30mg: 26 January 2004

10. DATE OF REVISION OF THE TEXT

31 July 2005

* Zoton and Zoton FasTab are trade marks of and under Licence Agreement from Takeda Chemical Industries Ltd., Japan.

Zoton Suspension

(Wyeth Pharmaceuticals)

1. NAME OF THE MEDICINAL PRODUCT

Zoton Suspension 30mg

2. QUALITATIVE AND QUANTITATIVE COMPOSITION

Each single dose sachet contains 30 mg of lansoprazole (INN).

3. PHARMACEUTICAL FORM

Gastro-resistant granules for oral suspension.

When reconstituted in water the granules give a pink suspension with a strawberry flavour.

4. CLINICAL PARTICULARS

4.1 Therapeutic indications

Uses:

Zoton is effective in the treatment of acid-related disorders of the upper gastro-intestinal tract, with the benefit of rapid symptom relief. Zoton is also effective in combination with antibiotics in the eradication of *Helicobacter pylori* (*H. pylori*).

Zoton Suspension may be particularly useful for patients who have difficulty swallowing, such as the elderly or patients with oesophageal strictures or dysphagia caused by severe oesophagitis.

Indications:

Healing and long term management of Gastro Oesophageal Reflux Disease (GORD).

Healing and maintenance therapy for patients with duodenal ulcer.

Relief of reflux-like symptoms (eg. heartburn) and/or ulcer-like symptoms (eg. upper epigastric pain) associated with acid-related dyspepsia.

Healing of benign gastric ulcer.

Treatment and prophylaxis of NSAID-associated benign gastric ulcers, duodenal ulcers and relief of symptoms in patients requiring continued NSAID treatment.

Long term management of pathological hypersecretory conditions including Zollinger-Ellison syndrome.

Zoton is also effective in patients with benign peptic lesions, including reflux oesophagitis, unresponsive to H_2 receptor antagonists.

Eradication of *H. pylori* from the upper gastrointestinal tract when used in combination with appropriate antibiotics in patients with ulcer-like dyspepsia leading to the prevention of symptom recurrence.

Eradication of *H. pylori* from the upper gastrointestinal tract when used in combination with appropriate antibiotics in patients with gastritis or duodenal ulcer leading to the healing and prevention of relapse of the ulcer.

4.2 Posology and method of administration

The contents of one sachet should be reconstituted by stirring into 30ml (2 tablespoons) of tap water, and swallowed immediately.

Dosage:

For patients requiring 30mg lansoprazole daily, Zoton Capsules 30mg or Zoton Suspension may be used.

For patients requiring 15mg lansoprazole daily, Zoton Capsules 15mg should be used.

Gastro Oesophageal Reflux Disease: Zoton 30mg once daily for 4 weeks. The majority of patients will be healed after the first course. For those patients not fully healed at this time, a further 4 weeks treatment at the same dosage should be given.

For long term management, a maintenance dose of Zoton 15mg or 30mg once daily can be used, dependent upon patient response.

Duodenal ulcer: Zoton 30mg once daily for 4 weeks.

For prevention of relapse, the recommended maintenance dose is Zoton Capsules 15mg once daily.

Acid-related dyspepsia: Intermittent courses, as required, of Zoton 15mg or 30mg once daily for 2-4 weeks depending on the severity and persistence of symptoms. Patients who do not respond after 4 weeks, or who relapse shortly afterwards, should be investigated.

Benign gastric ulcer: Zoton 30mg once daily for 8 weeks.

Treatment of NSAID-associated benign gastric and duodenal ulcers and relief of symptoms: Zoton 15mg or 30mg once daily for 4 or 8 weeks. Most patients will be healed after 4 weeks; for those patients not fully healed, a further 4 weeks treatment can be given.

For patients at particular risk or with ulcers that may be difficult to heal, the higher dose and/or the longer treatment duration should be used.

Prophylaxis of NSAID-associated benign gastric ulcers, duodenal ulcers and symptoms: Zoton 15mg or 30mg once daily.

Hypersecretory conditions: The initial dose should be Zoton 60mg once daily. The dosage should then be adjusted individually. Treatment should be continued for as long as clinically indicated.

For patients who require 120mg or more per day, the dose should be divided and administered twice daily.

Eradication of *H. pylori*: The following combinations have been shown to be effective when given for 7 days:

Zoton 30mg twice daily plus clarithromycin 250-500mg twice daily and amoxycillin 1g twice daily or

Zoton 30mg twice daily plus clarithromycin 250-500mg twice daily and metronidazole 400mg twice daily or

Zoton 30mg twice daily plus amoxycillin 1g twice daily and metronidazole 400mg twice daily.

The best eradication results are obtained when clarithromycin is combined with either amoxycillin or metronidazole. When used in combination with the recommended antibiotics, Zoton is associated with *H. pylori*-eradication rates of up to 90%.

Eradication of *H. pylori* with any one of the above regimens has been shown to result in the healing of duodenal ulcers, without the need for continued anti-ulcer drug therapy. The risk of reinfection is low and relapse following successful eradication is, therefore, unlikely.

For the optimal prevention of symptom recurrence in patients with ulcer-like dyspepsia, eradication of H. pylori should be followed by continued lansoprazole treatment (see acid-related dyspepsia).

Zoton should be taken once daily, except when used to eradicate *H. pylori*. To achieve the optimal acid inhibitory effect, and hence most rapid healing and symptom relief, Zoton should be administered in the morning before food.

Elderly: Dose adjustment is not required in the elderly. The normal daily dosage should be given.

Children: There is no experience with Zoton in children.

Impaired Hepatic and Renal Function:

Lansoprazole is metabolised substantially by the liver. Clinical trials in patients with liver disease indicate that metabolism of lansoprazole is prolonged when daily doses of 30mg are administered to patients with severe hepatic impairment. It is therefore recommended that the daily dose for patients with severe liver disease is individually adjusted to 15mg or 30mg. These patients should be kept under regular supervision and a daily dosage of 30mg should not be exceeded.

There is no need to alter the dosage in patients with mild to moderate impairment of hepatic function or impaired renal function.

4.3 Contraindications

The use of Zoton is contra-indicated in patients with a history of hypersensitivity to any of the ingredients of Zoton Suspension.

4.4 Special warnings and special precautions for use

In common with other anti-ulcer therapies, the possibility of malignancy should be excluded when gastric ulcer is suspected, as symptoms may be alleviated and diagnosis delayed. Similarly, the possibility of serious underlying disease such as malignancy should be excluded before treatment for dyspepsia commences, particularly in patients of middle age or older who have new or recently changed dyspeptic symptoms.

Before using Zoton with antibiotics to eradicate *H. pylori*, prescribers should refer to the full prescribing information of the respective antibiotics for guidance.

Zoton should be used with caution in patients with severe hepatic dysfunction. These patients should be kept under regular supervision and a daily dosage of 30mg should not be exceeded (see Section 4.2 Posology and Method of Administration).

Decreased gastric acidity due to any means, including proton pump inhibitors, increases gastric counts of bacteria normally present in the gastrointestinal tract. Treatment with acid-reducing drugs may lead to a slightly increased risk of gastrointestinal infections such as *Salmonella* and *Campylobacter*.

4.5 Interaction with other medicinal products and other forms of Interaction

Lansoprazole is hepatically metabolised and studies indicate that it is a weak inducer of Cytochrome P450. There is the possibility of interaction with drugs which are metabolised by the liver. Caution should be exercised when oral contraceptives and preparations such as phenytoin, carbamazepine, theophylline, or warfarin are taken concomitantly with the administration of Zoton.

No clinically significant effects on NSAIDs or diazepam have been found.

Antacids and sucralfate may reduce the bioavailability of lansoprazole and should, therefore, not be taken within an hour of Zoton.

4.6 Pregnancy and lactation

There is insufficient experience to recommend the use of Zoton in pregnancy. Animal studies do not reveal any teratogenic effect. Reproduction studies indicate slightly reduced litter survival and weights in rats and rabbits given very high doses of lansoprazole.

The use of Zoton in pregnancy should be avoided.

Animal studies indicate that lansoprazole is secreted in breast milk. There is no information on the secretion of lansoprazole into breast milk in humans.

The use of Zoton during breast feeding should be avoided unless considered essential.

4.7 Effects on ability to drive and use machines

Zoton is not known to affect ability to drive or operate machines.

4.8 Undesirable effects

Zoton is well-tolerated, with adverse events generally being mild and transient.

The most commonly reported adverse events are headache, dizziness, fatigue and malaise.

Gastrointestinal effects include diarrhoea, constipation, abdominal pain, nausea, vomiting, flatulence and dry or sore mouth or throat.

As with other PPIs, very rarely, cases of colitis have been reported. In severe and/or protracted cases of diarrhoea, discontinuation of therapy should be considered. In the majority of cases symptoms resolve on discontinuation of therapy.

Alterations in liver function test values and, rarely, jaundice or hepatitis, have been reported.

Dermatological reactions include skin rashes, urticaria and pruritus. These generally resolve on discontinuation of drug therapy. Serious dermatological reactions are rare but there have been occasional reports of Stevens-Johnson Syndrome, toxic epidermal necrolysis and erythematous or bullous rashes including erythema multiforme. Cases of hair thinning and photosensitivity have also been reported.

Other hypersensitivity reactions include angioedema, wheezing, and very rarely, anaphylaxis. Cases of interstitial nephritis have been reported which have sometimes resulted in renal failure.

Haematological effects (thrombocytopenia, agranulocytosis, eosinophilia, leucopenia and pancytopenia) have occurred rarely. Bruising, purpura and petechiae have also been reported.

Other reactions include arthralgia, myalgia, depression, peripheral oedema and, rarely, paraesthesia, blurred vision, taste disturbances, vertigo, confusion and hallucinations.

Gynaecomastia and impotence have been reported rarely.

4.9 Overdose

There is no information on the effect of overdosage. However, Zoton has been given at doses up to 120mg/day without significant adverse effects. Symptomatic and supportive therapy should be given as appropriate.

5. PHARMACOLOGICAL PROPERTIES

5.1 Pharmacodynamic properties

Lansoprazole is a member of a class of drugs called proton pump inhibitors. Its mode of action is to inhibit specifically the H^+ / K^+ ATPase (proton pump) of the parietal cell in the stomach, the terminal step in acid production, thus reducing gastric acidity, a key requirement for healing of acid-related disorders such as gastric ulcer, duodenal ulcer and reflux oesophagitis.

It is believed that the parent drug is biotransformed into its active form(s) in the acidic environment of the parietal cell, whereupon it reacts with the sulphydryl group of the H^+ / K^+ ATPase causing inhibition. This inhibition is reversible *in-vitro* by intrinsic and extrinsic reducing agents. Lansoprazole's mode of action differs significantly from the H_2 antagonists which inhibit one of the three pathways involved in stimulation of acid production. A single dose of 30mg inhibits pentagastrin-stimulated acid secretion by approximately 80%, indicating effective acid inhibition from the first day of dosing.

Lansoprazole has a prolonged pharmacological action providing effective acid suppression over 24 hours, thereby promoting rapid healing and symptom relief.

By reducing gastric acidity, Zoton creates an environment in which appropriate antibiotics can be effective against *H. pylori*. *In-vitro* studies have shown that lansoprazole has a direct antimicrobial effect on *H. pylori*.

5.2 Pharmacokinetic properties

One sachet of Zoton Suspension 30mg is bioequivalent to one Zoton Capsule 30mg.

Lansoprazole exhibits high (80-90%) bioavailability with a single dose. As a result, effective acid inhibition is achieved rapidly. Peak plasma levels occurred within 1.5 to 2.0 hours. The plasma elimination half-life ranges from 1 to 2 hours following single or multiple doses in healthy subjects. There is no evidence of accumulation following multiple doses in healthy subjects. The plasma protein binding is 97%.

Following absorption, lansoprazole is extensively metabolised and is excreted by both the renal and biliary route. A study with ^{14}C-labelled lansoprazole indicated that up to 50% of the dose was excreted in the urine. Lansoprazole is metabolised substantially by the liver.

5.3 Preclinical safety data

Gastric tumours have been observed in life-long studies in rats.

An increased incidence of spontaneous retinal atrophy has been observed in life-long studies in rats. These lesions which are common to albino laboratory rats have not been observed in monkeys or dogs or life-long studies in mice. They are considered to be rat specific. No such treatment related changes have been observed in patients treated continuously for long periods.

6. PHARMACEUTICAL PARTICULARS

6.1 List of excipients

Gastro-resistant Granules:

Magnesium Carbonate, Sugar Spheres, Sucrose, Maize Starch, Low Substituted Hydroxypropyl Cellulose, Hydroxypropylcellulose, Methacrylic Acid – Ethyl Acrylate Copolymer (1:1) Dispersion 30 per cent, Talc, Macrogol 8000, Titanium Dioxide, Polysorbate 80, Colloidal Anhydrous Silica, Purified Water.

Suspending Granules:

Sucrose, Mannitol, Docusate Sodium, Crospovidone, Xanthan Gum, Strawberry flavour (J2161), Citric Acid, Red Iron Oxide (E172), Colloidal Anhydrous Silica, Magnesium Stearate, Ethanol.

6.2 Incompatibilities
None known.

6.3 Shelf life
3 years.

Once opened Zoton Suspension should be suspended in water and consumed immediately.

6.4 Special precautions for storage
Zoton Suspension sachets should be stored at room temperature (below 25°C) in a dry place.

6.5 Nature and contents of container
Sachets consisting of paper, polythene, aluminium foil and ionomer laminate.

2, 14 or 28 sachets / carton

6.6 Instructions for use and handling
Patients Instructions:

Directions for constituting suspension from sachets:

1. Add two tablespoons (30ml) of water to a glass
2. Empty the granules from a sachet into the glass
3. Stir well and drink immediately

7. MARKETING AUTHORISATION HOLDER
John Wyeth & Brother Limited

t/a Wyeth Pharmaceuticals

Huntercombe Lane South

Taplow

Maidenhead

Berkshire SL6 0PH

8. MARKETING AUTHORISATION NUMBER(S)
PL 00011/0291

9. DATE OF FIRST AUTHORISATION/RENEWAL OF THE AUTHORISATION
28 July 1998.

10. DATE OF REVISION OF THE TEXT
31 July 2005

Zovirax 200mg Tablets

(GlaxoSmithKline UK)

1. NAME OF THE MEDICINAL PRODUCT
Zovirax Tablets 200 mg.

2. QUALITATIVE AND QUANTITATIVE COMPOSITION
Aciclovir BP 200 mg

3. PHARMACEUTICAL FORM
Dispersible film-coated tablet.

4. CLINICAL PARTICULARS
4.1 Therapeutic indications
Zovirax Tablets are indicated for the treatment of herpes simplex virus infections of the skin and mucous membranes including initial and recurrent genital herpes.

Zovirax Tablets are indicated for the suppression (prevention of recurrences) of recurrent herpes simplex infections in immunocompetent patients.

Zovirax Tablets are indicated for the prophylaxis of herpes simplex infections in immunocompromised patients.

Zovirax Tablets are indicated for the treatment of varicella (chickenpox) and herpes zoster (shingles) infections.

Route of administration: Oral.

4.2 Posology and method of administration
Zovirax tablets may be dispersed in a minimum of 50 ml of water or swallowed whole with a little water. Ensure that patients on high doses of aciclovir are adequately hydrated.

Dosage in adults

Treatment of herpes simplex infections: 200 mg Zovirax should be taken five times daily at approximately four hourly intervals omitting the night time dose. Treatment should continue for 5 days, but in severe initial infections this may have to be extended.

In severely immunocompromised patients (e.g. after marrow transplant) or in patients with impaired absorption from the gut the dose can be doubled to 400 mg Zovirax or alternatively intravenous dosing could be considered.

Dosing should begin as early as possible after the start of an infection; for recurrent episodes this should preferably be during the prodromal period or when lesions first appear.

Suppression of herpes simplex infections in immunocompetent patients: 200 mg Zovirax should be taken four times daily at approximately six-hourly intervals.

Many patients may be conveniently managed on a regimen of 400 mg Zovirax twice daily at approximately twelve-hourly intervals.

Dosage titration down to 200 mg Zovirax taken thrice daily at approximately eight-hourly intervals or even twice daily at approximately twelve-hourly intervals may prove effective.

Some patients may experience break-through infection on total daily doses of 800 mg Zovirax.

Therapy should be interrupted periodically at intervals of six to twelve months, in order to observe possible changes in the natural history of the disease.

Prophylaxis of herpes simplex infections in immunocompromised patients: 200 mg Zovirax should be taken four times daily at approximately six-hourly intervals.

In severely immunocompromised patients (e.g. after marrow transplant) or in patients with impaired absorption from the gut, the dose can be doubled to 400 mg Zovirax, or alternatively, intravenous dosing could be considered.

The duration of prophylactic administration is determined by the duration of the period at risk.

Treatment of varicella and herpes zoster infections: 800 mg Zovirax should be taken five times daily at approximately four-hourly intervals, omitting the night time dose. Treatment should continue for seven days.

In severely immunocompromised patients (e.g. after marrow transplant) or in patients with impaired absorption from the gut, consideration should be given to intravenous dosing.

Dosing should begin as early as possible after the start of an infection: Treatment of herpes zoster yields better results if initiated as soon as possible after the onset of the rash. Treatment of chickenpox in immunocompetent patients should begin within 24 hours after onset of the rash.

Dosage in children

Treatment of herpes simplex infections, and prophylaxis of herpes simplex infections in the immunocompromised: Children aged two years and over should be given adult dosages and children below the age of two years should be given half the adult dose.

Treatment of varicella infection

6 years and over:	800 mg Zovirax four times daily.
2 - 5 years:	400mg Zovirax four times daily.
Under 2 years:	200mg Zovirax four times daily.

Treatment should continue for five days.

Dosing may be more accurately calculated as 20 mg/kg bodyweight (not to exceed 800 mg) Zovirax four times daily.

No specific data are available on the suppression of herpes simplex infections or the treatment of herpes zoster infections in immunocompetent children.

Dosage in the elderly: In the elderly, total aciclovir body clearance declines along with creatinine clearance. Adequate hydration of elderly patients taking high oral doses of Zovirax should be maintained. Special attention should be given to dosage reduction in elderly patients with impaired renal function.

Dosage in renal impairment: In the management of herpes simplex infections in patients with impaired renal function, the recommended oral doses will not lead to accumulation of aciclovir above levels that have been established by intravenous infusion. However for patients with severe renal impairment (creatinine clearance less than 10 ml/minute) an adjustment of dosage to 200 mg aciclovir twice daily at approximately twelve-hourly intervals is recommended.

In the treatment of herpes zoster infections it is recommended to adjust the dosage to 800 mg aciclovir twice daily at approximately twelve - hourly intervals for patients with severe renal impairment (creatinine clearance less than 10 ml/minute), and to 800 mg aciclovir three times daily at intervals of approximately eight hours for patients with moderate renal impairment (creatinine clearance in the range 10 – 25 ml/minute).

4.3 Contraindications
Zovirax tablets are contra-indicated in patients known to be hypersensitive to aciclovir or valaciclovir.

4.4 Special warnings and special precautions for use
Hydration status: Care should be taken to maintain adequate hydration in patients receiving higher dose oral regimens e.g. for the treatment of herpes zoster infection (4g daily), in order to avoid the risk of possible renal toxicity.

The results of a wide range of mutagenicity tests *in vitro* and *in vivo* indicate that aciclovir is unlikely to pose a genetic risk to man. Aciclovir was not found to be carcinogenic in long term studies in the rat and the mouse. Largely reversible adverse effects on spermatogenesis in association with overall toxicity in rats and dogs have been reported only at doses of aciclovir greatly in excess of those employed therapeutically. Two generation studies in mice did not reveal any effect of aciclovir on fertility. There is no experience of the effect of Zovirax double strength suspension on human female fertility. Zovirax double strength suspension has been shown to have no definite effect upon sperm count, morphology or motility in man.

The data currently available from clinical studies is not sufficient to conclude that treatment with Zovirax reduces the incidence of chickenpox-associated complications in immunocompetent patients.

4.5 Interaction with other medicinal products and other forms of Interaction
No clinically significant interactions have been identified.

Aciclovir is eliminated primarily unchanged in the urine via active renal tubular secretion. Any drugs administered concurrently that compete with this mechanism may increase aciclovir plasma concentrations. Probenecid and cimetidine increase the AUC of aciclovir by this mechanism, and reduce aciclovir renal clearance. Similarly increases in plasma AUCs of aciclovir and of the inactive metabolite of mycophenolate mofetil, an immunosuppresant agent used in transplant patients have been shown when the drugs are coadministered. However no dosage adjustment is necessary because of the wide therapeutic index of aciclovir.

4.6 Pregnancy and lactation
A post-marketing aciclovir pregnancy registry has documented pregnancy outcomes in women exposed to any formulation of Zovirax. The birth defects described amongst Zovirax exposed subjects have not shown any uniqueness or consistent pattern to suggest a common cause.

Caution should however be exercised by balancing the potential benefits of treatment against any possible hazard.

Following oral administration of 200 mg Zovirax five times a day, aciclovir has been detected in breast milk at concentrations ranging from 0.6 to 4.1 times the corresponding plasma levels. These levels would potentially expose nursing infants to aciclovir dosages of up to 0.3 mg/kg/day. Caution is therefore advised if aciclovir is to be administered to a nursing woman.

Systemic administration of aciclovir in internationally accepted standard tests did not produce embryotoxic or teratogenic effects in rats, rabbits or mice.

In a non-standard test in rats, foetal abnormalities were observed, but only following such high subcutaneous doses that maternal toxicity was produced. The clinical relevance of these findings is uncertain.

4.7 Effects on ability to drive and use machines
None known.

4.8 Undesirable effects
Gastrointestinal: nausea, vomiting, diarrhoea and abdominal pains have been reported.

Haematological: very rarely, anaemia, leukopenia and thrombocytopenia.

Hypersensitivity and skin: rashes including photosensitivity, urticaria, pruritis and rarely dyspnoea, angioedema and anaphylaxis.

Kidney: rare reports of increases in blood urea and creatinine. Acute renal failure has been reported on vary rare occasions.

Liver: rare reports of reversible rises in bilirubin and liver related enzymes. Hepatitis and jaundice have been reported on vary rare occasions.

Neurological: headaches. Occasionally, reversible neurological reactions, notably dizziness, confusional states, hallucinations, somnolence, convulsions and coma have been reported, usually in patients with renal impairment in whom the dosage was in excess of that recommended or with other predisposing factors.

Other: fatigue. Occasional reports of accelerated diffuse hair loss. As this type of hair loss has been associated with a wide variety of disease processes and medicines, the relationship of the event to aciclovir therapy is uncertain.

4.9 Overdose
Symptoms and signs:- Aciclovir is only partly absorbed in the gastrointestinal tract. Patients have ingested overdoses of up to 20g aciclovir on a single occasion, usually without toxic effects. Accidental, repeated overdoses of oral aciclovir over several days have been associated with gastrointestinal effects (such as nausea and vomiting) and neurological effects (headache and confusion).

Overdosage of intravenous aciclovir has resulted in elevations of serum creatinine, blood urea nitrogen and subsequent renal failure. Neurological effects including confusion, hallucinations, agitation, seizures and coma have been described in association with intravenous overdosage.

Management:- Patients should be observed closely for signs of toxicity. Haemodialysis significantly enhances the removal of aciclovir from the blood and may, therefore, be considered a management option in the event of symptomatic overdose.

5. PHARMACOLOGICAL PROPERTIES
5.1 Pharmacodynamic properties
Aciclovir is a synthetic purine nucleoside analogue with *in vitro* and *in vivo* inhibitory activity against human herpes viruses, including herpes simplex virus (HSV) types I and II and varicella zoster virus (VZV).

The inhibitory activity of aciclovir for HSV I, HSV II and VZV is highly selective. The enzyme thymidine kinase (TK) of normal, uninfected cells does not use aciclovir effectively as a substrate, hence toxicity of mammalian host cells is low; however, TK encoded by HSV and VZV converts aciclovir to aciclovir monophosphate, a nucleoside analogue which is further converted to the diphosphate and finally to the triphosphate by cellular enzymes. Aciclovir triphosphate interferes with the viral DNA polymerase and inhibits viral DNA replication with resultant chain termination following its incorporation into the viral DNA.

Prolonged or repeated courses of aciclovir in severely immune-compromised individuals may result in the selection of virus strains with reduced sensitivity, which may not respond to continued aciclovir treatment. Most of the clinical isolates with reduced sensitivity have been relatively deficient in viral TK, however, strains with altered viral TK or viral DNA polymerase have also been reported. *In vitro* exposure of HSV isolates to aciclovir can also lead to the emergence of less sensitive strains. The relationship between the *in vitro* determined sensitivity of HSV isolates and clinical response to aciclovir therapy is not clear.

5.2 Pharmacokinetic properties
Aciclovir is only partially absorbed from the gut. Mean steady state peak plasma concentrations (C^{ss}max) following doses of 200 mg administered four-hourly were 3.1 microMol (0.7 micrograms/ml) and equivalent trough plasma levels (C^{ss}min) were 1.8 microMol (0.4 micrograms/ml). Corresponding C^{ss}max levels following doses of 400 mg and 800 mg administered four-hourly were 5.3 microMol (1.2 micrograms/ml) and 8 microMol (1.8 micrograms/ml) respectively and equivalent C^{ss}min levels were 2.7 microMol (0.6 micrograms/ml) and 4 microMol (0.9 micrograms/ml).

In adults the terminal plasma half-life of aciclovir after administrations of intravenous aciclovir is about 2.9 hours. Most of the drug is excreted unchanged by the kidney. Renal clearance of aciclovir is substantially greater than creatinine clearance, indicating that tubular secretion, in addition to glomerular filtration contributes to the renal elimination of the drug. 9-carboxymethoxymethylguanine is the only significant metabolite of aciclovir, and accounts for approximately 10 - 15% of the administered dose recovered from the urine. When aciclovir is given one hour after 1 gram of probenecid the terminal half-life and the area under the plasma concentration time curve is extended by 18% and 40% respectively.

In adults, mean steady state peak plasma concentrations (C^{ss}max) following a one hour infusion of 2.5 mg/kg, 5 mg/kg and 10 mg/kg were 22.7 microMol (5.1 micrograms/ml), 43.6 microMol (9.8 micrograms/ml) and 92 microMol (20.7 micrograms/ml), respectively. The corresponding trough levels (C^{ss}min) 7 hours later were 2.2 microMol (0.5 micrograms/ml), 3.1 microMol (0.7 micrograms/ml), and 10.2 microMol (2.3 micrograms/ml), respectively.

In children over 1 year of age similar peak (C^{ss}max) and trough (C^{ss}min) levels were observed when a dose of 250 mg/m^2 was substituted for 5 mg/kg and a dose of 500 mg/m^2 was substituted for 10 mg/kg. In neonates and young infants (0 to 3 months of age) treated with doses of 10 mg/kg administered by infusion over a one-hour period every 8 hours the C^{ss}max was found to be 61.2 microMol (13.8 micrograms/ml) and C^{ss}min to be 10.1 microMol (2.3 micrograms/ml). The terminal plasma half-life in these patients was 3.8 hours. In the elderly, total body clearance falls with increasing age associated with decreases in creatinine clearance although there is little change in the terminal plasma half-life.

In patients with chronic renal failure the mean terminal half-life was found to be 19.5 hours. The mean aciclovir half-life during haemodialysis was 5.7 hours. Plasma aciclovir levels dropped approximately 60% during dialysis.

Cerebrospinal fluid levels are approximately 50% of corresponding plasma levels. Plasma protein binding is relatively low (9 to 33%) and drug interactions involving binding site displacement are not anticipated.

5.3 Preclinical safety data
There are no preclinical data of relevance to the prescriber which are additional to those already included in other sections of the SPC.

6. PHARMACEUTICAL PARTICULARS
6.1 List of excipients
Core:
Microcrystalline cellulose
Aluminium magnesium silicate
Sodium starch glycollate
Povidone K30
Magnesium stearate
Purified water
Industrial methylated spirit
Or
Ethanol
Or
Absolute alcohol
Film coat*:
Colour concentrate Y-1-7000, White
Purified water
Coating concentrate contains:
Hypromellose
Polyethylene glycol 400
Titanium dioxide
Polish:
Polyethylene glycol 8000
Purified water

6.2 Incompatibilities
None known.

6.3 Shelf life
36 months.

6.4 Special precautions for storage
Store below 30°C.

Keep dry.

Protect from light.

6.5 Nature and contents of container
Amber glass bottles with polyethylene snap fitting caps.

PVC/PVDC/Aluminium foil blister packs.

Pack size: 25 tablets.

6.6 Instructions for use and handling
No special instructions

Administrative Data
7. MARKETING AUTHORISATION HOLDER
The Wellcome Foundation Limited
Glaxo Wellcome House
Berkeley Avenue
Greenford
Middlesex
UB6 0NN
Trading as
GlaxoSmithKline UK
Stockley Park West
Uxbridge
Middlesex UB11 1BT

8. MARKETING AUTHORISATION NUMBER(S)
PL 00003/0344

9. DATE OF FIRST AUTHORISATION/RENEWAL OF THE AUTHORISATION
13 September 2001

10. DATE OF REVISION OF THE TEXT
02 July 2003

11. Legal Status
POM

Zovirax 400mg Tablets

(GlaxoSmithKline UK)

1. NAME OF THE MEDICINAL PRODUCT
Zovirax Tablets 400 mg

2. QUALITATIVE AND QUANTITATIVE COMPOSITION
Aciclovir BP 400 mg

3. PHARMACEUTICAL FORM
Dispersible film-coated tablet.

4. CLINICAL PARTICULARS
4.1 Therapeutic indications
Zovirax dispersible tablets are indicated for the treatment of herpes simplex virus infections of the skin and mucous membranes including initial and recurrent genital herpes.

Zovirax dispersible tablets are indicated for the suppression (prevention of recurrences) of recurrent herpes simplex infections in immunocompetent patients.

Zovirax dispersible tablets are indicated for the prophylaxis of herpes simplex infections in immunocompromised patients.

Zovirax dispersible tablets are indicated for the treatment of varicella (chickenpox) and herpes zoster (shingles) infections.

4.2 Posology and method of administration
Route of administration: Oral

Zovirax dispersible tablets my be dispersed in a minimum of 50 ml of water or swallowed whole with a little water. Ensure that patients on high doses of aciclovir are adequately hydrated.

Dosage in adults

Treatment of herpes simplex infections: 200 mg Zovirax should be taken five times daily at approximately four hourly intervals omitting the night time dose. Treatment should continue for 5 days, but in severe initial infections this may have to be extended.

In severe immunocompromised patients (e.g. after marrow transplant) or in patients with impaired absorption from the gut the dose can be doubled to 400 mg Zovirax or alternatively intravenous dosing could be considered.

Dosing should begin as early as possible after the start of an infection: for recurrent episodes this should preferably be during the prodromal period or when lesions first appear.

Suppression of herpes infections in immunocompetent patients: 200 mg Zovirax should be taken four times daily at approximately six-hourly intervals.

Many patients may be conveniently managed on a regimen of 400 mg Zovirax twice daily at approximately twelve-hourly intervals.

Dosage titration down to 200 mg Zovirax taken thrice daily at approximately eight-hourly intervals or even twice daily at approximately twelve-hourly intervals may prove, effective.

Some patients may experience break-through infection on total daily doses of 800 mg Zovirax.

Therapy should be interrupted periodically at intervals of six to twelve months, in order to observe possible chances in the natural history of the disease.

Prophylaxis of herpes simplex infections in immunocompromised patients: 200 mg Zovirax should be taken four times daily at approximately six-hourly intervals.

In severely immunocompromised patients (e.g. after marrow transplant) or in patients with impaired absorption from the gut, the dose can be doubled to 400 mg Zovirax or alternatively, intravenous dosing could be considered.

The duration of prophylactic administration is determined by the duration of the period at risk.

Treatment of varicella and herpes zoster infections 800 mg Zovirax should be taken five times daily at approximately four-hourly intervals, omitting the night time dose. Treatment should continue for seven days.

In severely, immunocompromised patients (e.g. after marrow transplant) or in patients with impaired absorption from the gut, consideration should be given to intravenous dosing.

Dosing should begin as early as possible after the start of an infection: Treatment of herpes zoster yields better results if initiated as soon as possible after the onset of the rash. Treatment of chickenpox in immunocompetent patients should begin within 24 hours after onset of the rash.

Dosage in children

Treatment of herpes simplex infections and prophylaxis of herpes simplex infections in the immunocompromised: Children aged two years and over should be given adult dosages and children below the age of two years should be given half the adult dose.

Treatment of varicella infection

6 years and over; 800 mg Zovirax four times daily

2-5 years; 400 mg Zovirax four times daily

Under 2 years; 200 mg Zovirax four times daily

Treatment should continue for five days.

No specific data are available on the suppression of herpes simplex infections or the treatment of herpes zoster infections in immunocompetent children.

Dosage in renal impairment: In the management of herpes simplex infections in patients with impaired renal function, the recommended oral doses will not lead to accumulation of aciclovir above levels that have been established by intravenous infusion. However for patients with severe renal impairment (creatinine clearance less than 10ml/minute) an adjustment of dosage to 200 mg aciclovir twice daily at approximately twelve-hourly intervals is recommended.

In the treatment of herpes zoster infections it is recommended to adjust the dosage to 800 mg aciclovir twice daily at approximately twelve hourly intervals for patients with severe renal impairment (creatinine clearance less than 10ml/minute), and to 800 mg aciclovir three times daily at intervals of approximately eight hours for patients with moderate renal impairment (creatinine clearance in the range 10-25ml/minute).

4.3 Contraindications
Aciclovir tablets are contra-indicated in patients known to be hypersensitive to aciclovir or valaciclovir.

4.4 Special warnings and special precautions for use
Hydration status: Care should be taken to maintain adequate hydration in patients receiving higher dose oral regimens e.g. for the treatment of herpes zoster infection (4g daily), in order to avoid the risk of possible renal toxicity.

The results of a wide range of mutagenicity tests in vitro and in vivo indicate that aciclovir is unlikely to pose a genetic risk to man. Aciclovir was not found to be carcinogenic in long term studies in the rat and the mouse. Largely reversible adverse effects on spermatogenesis in association with overall toxicity in rats and dogs have been reported only at doses of aciclovir greatly in excess of those employed therapeutically. Two generation studies in mice did not reveal any effect of aciclovir on fertility. There is no experience of the effect of Zovirax double strength suspension on human female fertility. Zovirax double strength suspension has been shown to have no definite effect upon sperm count, morphology or motility in man.

The data currently available from clinical studies is not sufficient to conclude that treatment with Zovirax reduces the incidence of chickenpox-associated complications in immunocompetent patients.

4.5 Interaction with other medicinal products and other forms of Interaction
No clinically significant interactions have been identified.

Aciclovir is eliminated primarily unchanged in the urine via active renal tubular secretion. Any drugs administered concurrently that compete with this mechanism may increase aciclovir plasma concentrations. Probenecid and cimetidine increase the AUC of aciclovir by this mechanism, and reduce aciclovir renal clearance. Similarly increases in plasma AUCs of aciclovir and of the inactive metabolite of mycophenolate mofetil, an immunosuppresant agent used in transplant patients have been shown when the drugs are coadministered. However no dosage adjustment is necessary because of the wide therapeutic index of aciclovir.

4.6 Pregnancy and lactation

A post-marketing aciclovir pregnancy registry has documented pregnancy outcomes in women exposed to any formulation of Zovirax. The birth defects described amongst Zovirax exposed subjects have not shown any uniqueness or consistent pattern to suggest a common cause.

Caution should however be exercised by balancing the potential benefits of treatment against any possible hazard.

Following oral administration of 200 mg Zovirax five times a day, aciclovir has been detected in breast milk at concentrations ranging from 0.6 to 4.1 times the corresponding plasma levels. These levels would potentially expose nursing infants to aciclovir dosages of up to 0.3 mg/kg/day. Caution is therefore advised if Zovirax is to be administered to a nursing woman.

Systemic administration of aciclovir in internationally accepted standard tests did not produce embryotoxic or teratogenic effects in rats, rabbits or mice.

In a non-standard test in rats, foetal abnormalities were observed. But only following such high subcutaneous doses that maternal toxicity was produced. The clinical relevance of these findings is uncertain.

4.7 Effects on ability to drive and use machines

None known.

4.8 Undesirable effects

Gastrointestinal: nausea, vomiting, diarrhoea and abdominal pains have been reported.

Haematological: very rarely, anaemia, leukopenia and thrombocytopenia.

Hypersensitivity and skin: rashes including photosensitivity, urticaria, pruritis and rarely dyspnoea, angioedema and anaphylaxis.

Kidney: rare reports of increases in blood urea and creatinine. Acute renal failure has been reported on very rare occasions.

Liver: rare reports of reversible rises in bilirubin and liver related enzymes. Hepatitis and jaundice have been reported on very rare occasions.

Neurological: headaches. Occasionally, reversible neurological reactions, notably dizziness, confusional states, hallucinations, somnolence, convulsions and coma have been reported, usually in patients with renal impairment in whom the dosage was in excess of that recommended or with other predisposing factors.

Other: fatigue. Occasional reports of accelerated diffuse hair loss. As this type of hair loss has been associated with a wide variety of disease processes and medicines, the relationship of the event to aciclovir therapy is uncertain.

4.9 Overdose

Symptoms & signs:- Aciclovir is only partly absorbed in the gastrointestinal tract. Patients have ingested overdoses of up to 20g aciclovir on a single occasion, usually without toxic effects. Accidental, repeated overdoses of oral aciclovir over several days have been associated with gastrointestinal effects (such as nausea and vomiting) and neurological effects (headache and confusion).

Overdosage of intravenous aciclovir has resulted in elevations of serum creatinine, blood urea nitrogen and subsequent renal failure. Neurological effects including confusion, hallucinations, agitation, seizures and coma have been described in association with intravenous overdosage.

Management: patients should be observed closely for signs of toxicity. Haemodialysis significantly enhances the removal of aciclovir from the blood and may, therefore, be considered a management option in the event of symptomatic overdose.

5. PHARMACOLOGICAL PROPERTIES

5.1 Pharmacodynamic properties

Aciclovir is a synthetic purine nucleoside analogue with in vitro and in vivo inhibitory activity against human herpes viruses, including herpes simplex virus (HSV) types I and II and varicella zoster virus (VZV). The inhibitory activity of aciclovir for HSV I, HSV II and VZV is highly selective. The enzyme thymidine kinase (TK) of normal uninfected cells does not use aciclovir effectively as a substrate, hence toxicity of mammalian host cells is low. However, TK encoded by HSV and VZV converts aciclovir to aciclovir monophosphate, a nucleoside, analogue which is further converted to the diphosphate and finally to the triphosphate by cellular enzymes. Aciclovir triphosphate interferes with the viral DNA polymerase and inhibits viral DNS replication with resultant chain termination following its incorporation into the viral DNA.

Prolonged or repeated courses of aciclovir is severely immune-compromised individuals may result in the selective of virus strains with reduced sensitivity, which may not respond to continued aciclovir treatment. Most of the clinical isolates with reduced sensitivity have been relatively deficient in viral TK. However, strains with altered viral TK or DNA polymerase have also been reported. In vitro exposure of HSV isolates to aciclovir can also lead to the emergence of less sensitive strains. The relationship between the in vitro determined sensitivity of HSV isolate and clinical response to aciclovir therapy is not clear.

5.2 Pharmacokinetic properties

Aciclovir is only partially absorbed from the gut. Mean steady state peak plasma concentration (C^{ss}Max) following doses of 200 mg administered four-hourly were 3.1 micromol (0.7 micrograms/ml) and equivalent trough plasma levels (C^{ss}Min) were 1.8 micromol (0.4 micrograms/ml). Corresponding C^{ss}Max levels following doses of 400 mg and 800 mg administered four-hourly were 5.3 micromol (1.2 micrograms/ml) and 8 micromol (1.8 micrograms/ml) respectively and equivalent C^{ss}Min levels were 2.7 micromol (0.6 micrograms/ml) and 4 microMol (0.9 micrograms/ml).

In adults the terminal plasma half life after administration of intravenous aciclovir is about 2.9 hours. Most of the drug is excreted unchanged by the kidney. Renal clearance of aciclovir is substantially greater than creatinine clearance, indicating that tubular secretion in addition to glomerular filtration contributes to the renal elimination of the drug. 9-carboxymethoxymethyl-guanine is the only significant metabolite of aciclovir and accounts for approximately 10-15% of the administered dose recovered from the urine. When aciclovir is given one hour after 1 gram of probenecid the terminal half life and the area under the plasma concentration time curve is extended by 18% and 40% respectively.

In adults, mean steady state peak plasma concentrations (C^{ss}max) following a one hour infusion of 2.5mg/kg, 5mg/kg and 10mg/kg were 22.7 microMol (5.1 micrograms/ml), 43.6 microMol (9.8 micrograms/ml) and 92 microMol (20.7 micrograms/ml), respectively. The corresponding trough levels (C^{ss}min) 7 hours later were 2.2 microMol (0.5 micrograms/ml), 3.1 microMol (0.7 micrograms/ml), and 10.2 microMol (2.3 micrograms/ml), respectively.

In children over 1 year of age similar mean peak (C^{ss}max) and trough (C^{ss}min) levels were observed when a dose of 250 mg/m^2 was substituted for 5 mg/kg and a dose of 500 mg/m^2 was substituted for 5 mg/kg and a dose of 500 mg/m^2 was substituted for 10 mg/kg. In neonates and young infants (0-3 months of age) treated with doses of 10mg/kg administered by infusion over a one-hour period every 8 hours the C^{ss}max was found to be 61.2 microMol (13.8 micrograms/ml) and C^{ss}min to be 10.1 microMol (2.3 micrograms/ml). The terminal plasma half life in these patients was 3.8 hours. In the elderly total body clearance falls with increasing age associated with decreases in creatinine clearance although there is little changes in the terminal plasma half life.

In patients with chronic renal failure the mean terminal half life was found to be 19.5 hours. The mean aciclovir half life during haemodialysis was 5.7 hours. Plasma aciclovir levels dropped approximately 60% during dialysis.

Cerebrospinal fluid levels are approximately 50% of corresponding plasma levels. Plasma protein binding is relatively low (9 to 33%) and drug interactions involving binding site displacement are not anticipated.

5.3 Preclinical safety data

There are no preclinical data of relevance to the prescriber which are additional to that in other sections of this SPC.

6. PHARMACEUTICAL PARTICULARS

6.1 List of excipients

Core:

Microcrystalline cellulose

Aluminium magnesium silicate

Sodium starch glycollate

Povidone, K30

Magnesium stearate

Iron oxide, red E172

Industrial methylated spirit

Purified water

*Ethanol (96 per cent) or Absolute alcohol may be used as an alternative to industrial methylated spirit

Film coat:

Colour concentrate Y-1-7000, White*

Purified water

Methylated spirit

*The coating concentrate contains:

Hypromellose

Titanium dioxide

Polyethylene glycol 400

Polish:

Polyethylene glycol 8000

Purified water

6.2 Incompatibilities

None known.

6.3 Shelf life

36 months.

6.4 Special precautions for storage

Store below 30°C

Keep dry

Protect from light

6.5 Nature and contents of container

Amber glass bottles with polyethylene snap fitting caps.

PVC/PVDC/Aluminium foil blister packs.

Pack size: 56 tablets

6.6 Instructions for use and handling

Not applicable.

Administrative Data

7. MARKETING AUTHORISATION HOLDER

The Wellcome Foundation Limited

Glaxo Wellcome House

Berkeley Avenue

Greenford

Middlesex

UB6 ONN

Trading as:

GlaxoSmithKline UK

Stockley Park West

Uxbridge

Middlesex UB11 1BT

8. MARKETING AUTHORISATION NUMBER(S)

PL 00003/0345

9. DATE OF FIRST AUTHORISATION/RENEWAL OF THE AUTHORISATION

4 June 2003.

10. DATE OF REVISION OF THE TEXT

May 2003

11. Legal Status

POM

Zovirax 800mg Tablets

(GlaxoSmithKline UK)

1. NAME OF THE MEDICINAL PRODUCT

Zovirax Tablets BP 800mg

2. QUALITATIVE AND QUANTITATIVE COMPOSITION

Aciclovir 800mg BP

3. PHARMACEUTICAL FORM

Dispersible film coated tablet

4. CLINICAL PARTICULARS

4.1 Therapeutic indications

Zovirax tablets 800 mg are indicated for the treatment of varicella (chickenpox) and herpes zoster (shingles) infections.

4.2 Posology and method of administration

Dosage in adults:

Treatment of varicella and herpes zoster infections: 800 mg Zovirax should be taken five times daily at approximately four-hourly intervals, omitting the night time dose. Treatment should continue for seven days.

In severely immunocompromised patients (e.g. after marrow transplant) or in patients with impaired absorption from the gut, consideration should be given to intravenous dosing.

Dosing should begin as early as possible after the start of an infection: Treatment of herpes zoster yields better results if initiated as soon as possible after the onset of the rash. Treatment of chickenpox in immunocompetent patients should begin within 24 hours after the onset of the rash.

Dosage in children:

Treatment of varicella infections:

6 years and over: 800 mg Zovirax four times daily.

Treatment should continue for five days.

No specific data are available on the treatment of herpes zoster infections in immunocompetent children.

Dosage in the elderly:

In the elderly, total Aciclovir body clearance declines along with creatinine clearance. Adequate hydration of elderly patients taking high oral doses of Zovirax should be maintained. Special attention should be given to dosage reduction in elderly patients with impaired renal function.

Dosage in renal impairment:

In the treatment of herpes zoster infections it is recommended to adjust the dosage to 800 mg Aciclovir twice daily at approximately twelve-hourly intervals for patients with severe renal impairment (creatinine clearance less than 10 ml/minute) and to 800 mg Aciclovir three times daily at intervals of approximately eight hours for patients with moderate renal impairment (creatinine clearance in the range of 10-25 ml/minute).

Administration

Zovirax tablets are for oral administration and may be dispersed in a minimum of 50 ml of water or swallowed whole with a little water. Ensure that patients on high doses of aciclovir are adequately hydrated.

4.3 Contraindications

Zovirax tablets are contra-indicated in patients known to be hypersensitive to aciclovir or valaciclovir.

4.4 Special warnings and special precautions for use

Hydration status: Care should be taken to maintain adequate hydration in patients receiving high doses of aciclovir.

The results of a wide range of mutagenicity tests *in vitro* and *in vivo* indicate that Aciclovir is unlikely to pose a genetic risk to man. Aciclovir was not found to be carcinogenic in long term studies in the rat and the mouse. Largely reversible adverse effects on spermatogenesis in association with overall toxicity in rats and dogs have been reported only at doses of Aciclovir greatly in excess of those employed therapeutically. Two generation studies in mice did not reveal any effect of Aciclovir on fertility. There is no experience of the effect of Zovirax double strength suspension on human female fertility. Zovirax double strength suspension has been shown to have no definite effect upon sperm count, morphology or motility in man.

The data currently available from clinical studies is not sufficient to conclude that treatment with Zovirax reduces the incidence of chickenpox-associated complications in immunocompetent patients.

4.5 Interaction with other medicinal products and other forms of Interaction

No clinically significant interactions have been identified.

Aciclovir is eliminated primarily unchanged in the urine via active renal tubular secretion. Any drugs administered concurrently that compete with this mechanism may increase aciclovir plasma concentrations. Probenecid and cimetidine increase the AUC of aciclovir by this mechanism, and reduce aciclovir renal clearance. Similarly increases in plasma AUCs of aciclovir and of the inactive metabolite of mycophenolate mofetil, an immunosuppresant agent used in transplant patients have been shown when the drugs are coadministered. However no dosage adjustment is necessary because of the wide therapeutic index of aciclovir.

4.6 Pregnancy and lactation

A post-marketing aciclovir pregnancy registry has documented pregnancy outcomes in women exposed to any formulation of Zovirax. The birth defects described amongst Zovirax exposed subjects have not shown any uniqueness or consistent pattern to suggest a common cause.

Caution should however be exercised by balancing the potential benefits of treatment against any possible hazard.

Following oral administration of 200 mg Zovirax five times a day, Aciclovir has been detected in breast milk at concentrations ranging from 0.6 to 4.1 times the corresponding plasma levels. These levels would potentially expose nursing infants to Aciclovir dosages of up to 0.3 mg/kg/day. Caution is therefore advised if Zovirax is to be administered to a nursing woman.

Systemic administration of Aciclovir in internationally accepted standard tests did not produce embryotoxic or teratogenic effects in rats, rabbits or mice.

In a non-standard test in rats, foetal abnormalities were observed, but only following such high subcutaneous doses that maternal toxicity was produced. The clinical relevance of these findings is uncertain.

4.7 Effects on ability to drive and use machines

None known.

4.8 Undesirable effects

Gastrointestinal: nausea, vomiting, diarrhoea and abdominal pains have been reported.

Haematological: very rarely, anaemia, leukopenia and thrombocytopenia.

Hypersensitivity and skin: rashes including photosensitivity, urticaria, pruritis and rarely dyspnoea, angioedema and anaphylaxis.

Kidney: rare reports of increases in blood urea and creatinine. Acute renal failure has been reported on vary rare occasions.

Liver: rare reports of reversible rises in bilirubin and liver related enzymes. Hepatitis and jaundice have been reported on vary rare occasions.

Neurological: headaches. Occasionally, reversible neurological reactions, notably dizziness, confusional states, hallucinations, somnolence, convulsions and coma have been reported, usually in patients with renal impairment in whom the dosage was in excess of that recommended or with other predisposing factors.

Other: fatigue. Occasional reports of accelerated diffuse hair loss. As this type of hair loss has been associated with a wide variety of disease processes and medicines, the relationship of the event to aciclovir therapy is uncertain.

4.9 Overdose

Aciclovir is only partly absorbed in the gastrointestinal tract.

Patients have ingested overdoses of up to 20g aciclovir on a single occasion, usually without toxic effects. Accidental, repeated overdoses of oral aciclovir over several days have been associated with gastrointestinal effects (such as nausea and vomiting) and neurological effects (headache and confusion).

Overdosage of intravenous aciclovir has resulted in elevations of serum creatinine, blood urea nitrogen and subsequent renal failure. Neurological effects including confusion, hallucinations, agitation, seizures and coma have been described in association with intravenous overdosage.

Management: patients should be observed closely for signs of toxicity. Haemodialysis significantly enhances the removal of aciclovir from the blood and may, therefore, be considered a management option in the event of symptomatic overdose.

5. PHARMACOLOGICAL PROPERTIES

5.1 Pharmacodynamic properties

Aciclovir is a synthetic purine nucleoside analogue with *in vitro* and *in vivo* inhibitory activity against human herpes viruses, including herpes simplex virus (HSV) types I and II and varicella zoster virus (VZV). The inhibitory activity of Aciclovir for HSV I and HSV II and VZV is highly selective. The enzyme thymidine kinase (TK) of normal, uninfected cells does not use Aciclovir effectively as a substrate, hence toxicity to mammalian host cells is low; however, TK encoded by HSV and VZV converts Aciclovir to Aciclovir monophosphate, a nucleoside analogue which is further converted to the diphosphate and finally to the triphosphate by cellular enzymes. Aciclovir triphosphate interferes with the viral DNA polymerase and inhibits viral DNA replication with resultant chain termination following its incorporation into the viral DNA.

Prolonged or repeated courses of Aciclovir in severely immuno-compromised individuals may result in the selection of virus strains with reduced sensitivity, which may not respond to continued Aciclovir treatment. Most of the clinical isolates with reduced sensitivity have been relatively deficient in viral TK, however, strains with altered viral TK or viral DNA polymerase have also been reported. *In vitro* exposure of HSV isolates to Aciclovir can also lead to the emergence of less sensitive strains. The relationship between the *in vitro*-determined sensitivity of HSV isolates and clinical response to Aciclovir therapy is not clear.

5.2 Pharmacokinetic properties

Aciclovir is only partially absorbed from the gut. Mean study state peak plasma concentrations ($C^{ss}max$) following doses of 800 mg Aciclovir administered four-hourly were 8 microMol (1.8 micrograms/ml) and equivalent trough plasma levels were 4 microMol (0.9 micrograms/ml).

In adults the terminal plasma half-life after administration of intravenous Aciclovir is about 2.9 hours. Most of the drug is excreted unchanged by the kidney. Renal clearance of Aciclovir is substantially greater than creatinine clearance, indicating that tubular secretion, in addition to glomerular filtration, contributes to the renal elimination of the drug. 9-carboxymethoxymethylguanine is the only significant metabolite of Aciclovir, and accounts for 10-15% of the dose excreted in the urine. When Aciclovir is given one hour after 1 gram of probenecid the terminal half-life and the area under the plasma concentration time curve is extended by 18% and 40% respectively.

In adults, mean steady state peak plasma concentrations ($C^{ss}max$) following a one hour infusion of 2.5 mg/kg, 5 mg/kg and 10 mg/kg were 22.7 microMol (5.1 micrograms/ml), 43.6 microMol (9.8 micrograms/ml) and 92 microMol (20.7 micrograms/ml), respectively. The corresponding trough levels ($C^{ss}min$) 7 hours later were 2.2 microMol (0.5 micrograms/ml), 3.1 microMol (0.7 micrograms/ml) and 10.2 microMol (2.3 micrograms/ml), respectively. In children over 1 year of age similar mean peak ($C^{ss}max$) and trough ($C^{ss}min$) levels were observed when a dose of 250 mg/m^2 was substituted for 5 mg/kg and a dose of 500 mg/m^2 was substituted for 10 mg/kg. In neonates and young infants (0 to 3 months of age) treated with doses of 10 mg/kg administered by infusion over a one-hour period every 8 hours the $C^{ss}max$ was found to be 61.2 microMol (13.8 micrograms/ml) and $C^{ss}min$ to be 10.1 microMol (2.3 micrograms/ml). The terminal plasma half-life in these patients was 3.8 hours. In the elderly, total body clearance falls with increasing age associated with decreases in creatinine clearance although there is little change in the terminal plasma half-life.

In patients with chronic renal failure the mean terminal half-life was found to be 19.5 hours. The mean Aciclovir half-life during haemodialysis was 5.7 hours. Plasma Aciclovir levels dropped approximately 60% during dialysis.

Cerebrospinal fluid levels are approximately 50% of corresponding plasma levels. Plasma protein binding is relatively low (9 to 33%) and drug interactions involving binding site displacement are not anticipated.

5.3 Preclinical safety data

There are no preclinical data of relevance to the prescriber which are additional to that in other sections of this SPC.

6. PHARMACEUTICAL PARTICULARS

6.1 List of excipients

Microcrystalline Cellulose Ph Eur

Aluminium Magnesium Silicate BP

Sodium Starch Glycollate BP

Povidone (K30) Ph Eur

Magnesium Stearate Ph Eur

Filmcoat

Hypromellose HSE

Titanium Dioxide HSE

Polyethylene glycol 400 HSE

Polish

Polyethylene Glycol 8000 NF

6.2 Incompatibilities

None known

6.3 Shelf life

36 months

6.4 Special precautions for storage

Store below 30°C

Keep dry

Protect from light

6.5 Nature and contents of container

PVC/Aluminium foil blisterpack (5 tablets per blister strip)

Pack size: 35 tablets (marketed).

Polypropylene container with polyethylene snap-on lid.

Pack size: 35 and 800 tablets (non-marketed)

PVC/Aluminium foil blister sample pack.

Pack size: 5 and 2 tablets(non-marketed).

Polyethylene bag in a rigid polypropylene container with a polypropylene lid.

Pack size: 8000 tablets (non-marketed).

6.6 Instructions for use and handling

No special instructions for use.

Administrative Data

7. MARKETING AUTHORISATION HOLDER

The Wellcome Foundation Ltd

Glaxo Wellcome House

Berkeley Avenue

Greenford

Middlesex UB6 ONN

Trading as

GlaxoSmithKline UK

Stockley Park West

Uxbridge

Middlesex UB11 1BT

8. MARKETING AUTHORISATION NUMBER(S)

PL 00003/0299

9. DATE OF FIRST AUTHORISATION/RENEWAL OF THE AUTHORISATION

16 April 1997

10. DATE OF REVISION OF THE TEXT

2 April 2003

11. Legal Status

POM

Zovirax Cream

(GlaxoSmithKline UK)

1. NAME OF THE MEDICINAL PRODUCT

Zovirax Cream

2. QUALITATIVE AND QUANTITATIVE COMPOSITION

Aciclovir BP 5.0% w/w

3. PHARMACEUTICAL FORM

Topical Cream

4. CLINICAL PARTICULARS

4.1 Therapeutic indications

Zovirax Cream is indicated for the treatment of Herpes Simplex virus infections of the skin including initial and recurrent genital herpes and herpes labialis.

Route of administration: topical.

Do not use in eyes.

4.2 Posology and method of administration

Adults and Children: Zovirax Cream should be applied five times daily at approximately four hourly intervals, omitting the night time application. Treatment should be continued for 5 days. If, after 5 days, healing is not complete then treatment may be continued for up to an additional 5 days. Zovirax Cream should be applied to the lesion or impending lesion as early as possible after the start of an infection. It is particularly important to start treatment of recurrent episodes during the prodromal period or when lesions first appear.

Use in the elderly: No special comment

4.3 Contraindications

Zovirax Cream is contraindicated in patients known to be hypersensitive to aciclovir or propylene glycol.

4.4 Special warnings and special precautions for use

Zovirax Cream is not recommended for application to mucous membranes such as in the mouth, eye or vagina, as it may be irritant.

Particular care should be taken to avoid accidental introduction into the eye.

In severely immunocompromised patients (eg AIDS patients or bone marrow transplant recipients) oral Zovirax dosing should be considered. Such patients should be encouraged to consult a physician concerning the treatment of any infection.

Largely reversible adverse effects on spermatogenesis in association with overall toxicity in rats and dogs have been reported only at doses of aciclovir greatly in excess of those employed therapeutically. There has been no experience of the effect of Zovirax cream on human fertility. Two generation studies in mice did not reveal any effect of (orally administered) aciclovir on fertility. Zovirax Tablets have been shown to have no definite effect upon sperm count, morphology or motility in man.

The results of a wide range of mutagenicity tests *in vitro* and *in vivo* indicate that aciclovir does not pose a genetic risk to man.

Aciclovir was not found to be carcinogenic in long term studies in the rat and the mouse.

Zovirax Cream contains a specially formulated base and should not be diluted or used as a base for the incorporation of other medicaments.

4.5 Interaction with other medicinal products and other forms of Interaction

Probenecid increases the mean half-life and area under the plasma concentration curve of systemically administered aciclovir. However, this is likely to be of little relevance to the topical application of aciclovir.

4.6 Pregnancy and lactation

Systemic administration of aciclovir in internationally accepted standard tests did not produce embryotoxic or teratogenic effects in rats, rabbits or mice.

In a non-standard test in rats, foetal abnormalities were observed, but only following such high subcutaneous doses that maternal toxicity was produced. The clinical relevance of these findings is uncertain.

A post-marketing aciclovir pregnancy registry has documented pregnancy outcomes in women exposed to any formulation of Zovirax. The birth defects described amongst Zovirax exposed subjects have not shown any uniqueness or consistent pattern to suggest a common cause.

The use of Zovirax Cream should be considered only when the potential benefits outweigh the possibility of unknown risks.

Limited human data show that the drug does pass into breast milk following systemic administration.

4.7 Effects on ability to drive and use machines

Not applicable

4.8 Undesirable effects

Transient burning or stinging following application of Zovirax Cream may occur in some patients. Mild drying or flaking of the skin has occurred in about 5% of patients. Erythema and itching have been reported in a small proportion of patients.

Contact dermatitis has been reported rarely following application. Where sensitivity tests have been conducted the reactive substances have most often been shown to be components of the cream base rather than aciclovir

There have been very rare reports of immediate hypersensitivity reactions including angioedema with topical aciclovir.

4.9 Overdose

No untoward effects would be expected if the entire contents of a Zovirax Cream 10 g tube containing 500 mg of aciclovir were ingested orally. Oral doses of 800 mg five times daily (4 g per day), have been administered for seven days without adverse effects. Single intravenous doses of up to 80 mg/kg have been inadvertently administered without adverse effects. Aciclovir is dialysable.

5. PHARMACOLOGICAL PROPERTIES

5.1 Pharmacodynamic properties

Aciclovir is an antiviral agent which is highly active *in vitro* against herpes simplex virus (HSV) types I and II and varicella zoster virus. Toxicity to mammalian host cells is low.

Aciclovir is phosphorylated after entry into herpes infected cells to the active compound aciclovir triphosphate. The first step in this process is dependent on the presence of the HSV-coded thymidine kinase. Aciclovir triphosphate acts as an inhibitor of, and substrate for, the herpes-specified DNA polymerase, preventing further viral DNA synthesis without affecting normal cellular processes

5.2 Pharmacokinetic properties

From studies with intravenous aciclovir, the terminal plasma half-life has been determined as about 2.9 hours. Most of the drug is excreted unchanged by the kidney. Renal clearance of aciclovir is substantially greater than creatinine clearance, indicating that tubular secretion in addition to glomerular filtration contributes to the renal elimination of the drug. 9-carboxymethoxymethlguanine is the only significant metabolite of aciclovir, and accounts for 10-15% of the dose excreted in the urine. In patients with chronic renal failure, the mean terminal half-life was found to be 19.5 hours.

5.3 Preclinical safety data

There are no preclinical data of relevance to the prescriber which are additional to that in other sections of this SPC.

6. PHARMACEUTICAL PARTICULARS

6.1 List of excipients

Poloxamer 407	NF
Cetostearyl alcohol	Ph Eur
Sodium lauryl sulphate	Ph Eur
White soft paraffin	BP
Liquid paraffin	Ph Eur
Propylene glycol	Ph Eur
Purified water	Ph Eur

6.2 Incompatibilities

None known.

6.3 Shelf life

3 years

6.4 Special precautions for storage

Store below 25°C. Do not refrigerate.

6.5 Nature and contents of container

Collapsible aluminium tubes with plastic screw caps

Pack size: 2g or 10g tubes

6.6 Instructions for use and handling

No special instructions.

7. MARKETING AUTHORISATION HOLDER

The Wellcome Foundation
Glaxo Wellcome House
Berkeley Avenue
Greenford
Middlesex UB6 0NN
Trading as
GlaxoSmithKline UK
Stockley Park West
Uxbridge
Middlesex UB11 1BT

8. MARKETING AUTHORISATION NUMBER(S)

PL 00003/0180

9. DATE OF FIRST AUTHORISATION/RENEWAL OF THE AUTHORISATION

28 October 1999/ 28 October 2004

10. DATE OF REVISION OF THE TEXT

13 April 2005

11. LEGAL STATUS

POM

Zovirax Double-Strength Suspension

(GlaxoSmithKline UK)

1. NAME OF THE MEDICINAL PRODUCT

Zovirax Double Strength Suspension

2. QUALITATIVE AND QUANTITATIVE COMPOSITION

Aciclovir BP 400mg/5ml

3. PHARMACEUTICAL FORM

Suspension

4. CLINICAL PARTICULARS

4.1 Therapeutic indications

Zovirax Double Strength Suspension is indicated for the treatment of herpes simplex virus infections of the skin and mucous membranes including initial and recurrent genital herpes.

Zovirax Double Strength Suspension is indicated for the suppression (prevention of recurrences) of recurrent herpes simplex infections in immunocompetent patients.

Zovirax Double Strength Suspension is indicated for the prophylaxis of herpes simplex infections in immunocompromised patients.

Zovirax Double Strength Suspension is indicated for the treatment of varicella (chickenpox) and herpes zoster (shingles) infections.

Route of Administration: Oral

4.2 Posology and method of administration

Dosage in Adults

Treatment of herpes simplex infections: 200mg Zovirax should be taken five times daily at approximately four hourly intervals omitting the night time dose. Treatment should continue for 5 days, but in severe initial infections this may have to be extended.

In severely immunocompromised patients (eg after marrow transplant) or in patients with impaired absorption from the gut the dose can be doubled to 400mg Zovirax or alternatively intravenous dosing could be considered.

Dosing should begin as early as possible after the start of an infection; for recurrent episodes this should preferably be during the prodromal period or when lesions first appear.

Suppression of herpes simplex infections in immunocompetent patients:

200mg Zovirax should be taken four times daily at approximately six-hourly intervals.

Many patients may be conveniently managed on a regimen of 400mg Zovirax twice daily at approximately twelve-hourly intervals.

Dosage titration down to 200mg Zovirax taken thrice daily at approximately eight-hourly intervals or even twice daily at approximately twelve-hourly intervals, may prove effective.

Some patients may experience break-through infection on total daily doses of 800mg Zovirax.

Therapy should be interrupted periodically at intervals of six to twelve months, in order to observe possible changes in the natural history of the disease.

Prophylaxis of herpes simplex infections in immunocompromised patients:

200mg Zovirax should be taken four times daily at approximately six hourly intervals.

In severely immunocompromised patients (eg after marrow transplant) or in patients with impaired absorption from the gut, the dose can be doubled to 400mg Zovirax or, alternatively, intravenous dosing could be considered.

The duration of prophylactic administration is determined by the duration of the period at risk.

Treatment of varicella and herpes zoster infections: 800mg Zovirax should be taken five times daily at approximately four-hourly intervals, omitting the night time dose. Treatment should continue for seven days.

In severely immunocompromised patients (eg after marrow transplant) or in patients with impaired absorption from the gut, consideration should be given to intravenous dosing.

Dosing should begin as early as possible after the start of an infection: treatment of herpes zoster yields better results if initiated as soon as possible after the onset of the rash. Treatment of chickenpox in immunocompetent patients should begin within 24 hours after onset of the rash.

Dosage in Children

Treatment of herpes simplex infections, and prophylaxis of herpes simplex infections in the immunocompromised: Children aged two years and over should be given adult dosages and children below the age of two years should be given *half* the adult dose.

Treatment of varicella infections:

6 years and over:

800mg Zovirax four times daily.

2 - 6 years:

400mg Zovirax four times daily.

Under 2 years: 200mg Zovirax four times daily.

Treatment should continue for five days.

Dosing may be more accurately calculated as 20mg/kg body weight (not to exceed 800mg) Zovirax four times daily.

No specific data are available on the *suppression* of *herpes simplex* infections or the treatment of herpes *zoster* infections in immunocompetent children.

Zovirax Double Strength Suspension may be diluted with an equal volume of either Syrup BP or Sorbitol Solution (70%) (non-crystallising) BP. The diluted product is stable for 4 weeks at 25°C but it is recommended that all dilutions are freshly prepared.

Dosage in the Elderly

In the elderly, total aciclovir body clearance declines along with creatinine clearance. Adequate hydration of elderly patients taking high oral doses of Zovirax should be maintained. Special attention should be given to dosage reduction in elderly patients with impaired renal function.

Dosage in Renal Impairment

In the management of herpes simplex infections in patients with impaired renal function, the recommended oral doses will not lead to accumulation of aciclovir above levels that have been established by intravenous infusion. However, for patients with severe renal impairment (creatinine clearance less than 10ml/minute) an adjustment of dosage to 200mg aciclovir twice daily at approximately twelve-hourly intervals is recommended.

In the treatment of herpes zoster infections it is recommended to adjust the dosage to 800mg aciclovir twice daily at approximately twelve-hourly intervals for patients with severe renal impairment (creatinine clearance less than 10ml/minute), and to 800mg aciclovir three times daily at intervals of approximately eight hours for patients with moderate renal impairment (creatinine clearance in the range 10 to 25ml/minute).

4.3 Contraindications
Zovirax Double Strength Suspension is contra-indicated in patients known to be hypersensitive to aciclovir or valaciclovir.

4.4 Special warnings and special precautions for use
Hydration status: Care should be taken to maintain adequate hydration in patients receiving high oral dose regimens e.g. for the treatment of herpes zoster infection (4g daily), in order to avoid the risk of possible renal toxicity.

The data currently available from clinical studies is not sufficient to conclude that treatment with Zovirax reduces the incidence of chickenpox-associated complications in immunocompetent patients.

4.5 Interaction with other medicinal products and other forms of Interaction
No clinically significant interactions have been identified.

Aciclovir is eliminated primarily unchanged in the urine via active renal tubular secretion. Any drugs administered concurrently that compete with this mechanism may increase aciclovir plasma concentrations. Probenecid and cimetidine increase the AUC of aciclovir by this mechanism, and reduce aciclovir renal clearance. Similarly increases in plasma AUCs of aciclovir and of the inactive metabolite of mycophenolate mofetil, an immunosuppressant agent used in transplant patients have been shown when the drugs are coadministered. However no dosage adjustment is necessary because of the wide therapeutic index of aciclovir.

4.6 Pregnancy and lactation
A post-marketing aciclovir pregnancy registry has documented pregnancy outcomes in women exposed to any formulation of Zovirax. The birth defects described amongst Zovirax exposed subjects have not shown any uniqueness or consistent pattern to suggest a common cause. Findings from reproduction toxicology studies are included in section 5.3.

Caution should however be exercised by balancing the potential benefits of treatment against any possible hazard.

Following oral administration of 200mg Zovirax five times a day, aciclovir has been detected in breast milk at concentrations ranging from 0.6 to 4.1 times the corresponding plasma levels. These levels would potentially expose nursing infants to aciclovir dosages of up to 0.3mg/kg/day. Caution is therefore advised if Zovirax is to be administered to a nursing woman.

4.7 Effects on ability to drive and use machines
No studies on the effects on the ability to drive and use machines have been performed.

4.8 Undesirable effects
Gastrointestinal: Nausea, vomiting, diarrhoea and abdominal pains have been reported.

Haematological: Very rarely, anaemia, leukopenia and thrombocytopenia.

Hypersensitivity and Skin: Rashes including photosensitivity, urticaria, pruritis and rarely dyspnoea, angioedema and anaphylaxis.

Kidney: Rare reports of increases in blood urea and creatinine. Acute renal failure has been reported on very rare occasions.

Liver: Rare reports of reversible rises in bilirubin and liver related enzymes. Hepatitis and jaundice have been reported on very rare occasions.

Neurological: Headaches. Occasionally, reversible neurological reactions, notably dizziness, confusional states, hallucinations, somnolence, convulsions and coma have been reported, usually in patients with renal impairment in whom the dosage was in excess of that recommended or with other predisposing factors.

Other: Fatigue. Occasional reports of accelerated diffuse hair loss. As this type of hair loss has been associated with a wide variety of disease processes and medicines, the relationship of the event to aciclovir therapy is uncertain.

4.9 Overdose
Symptoms & signs:- Aciclovir is only partly absorbed in the gastrointestinal tract. Patients have ingested overdoses of up to 20g aciclovir on a single occasion, usually without toxic effects. Accidental, repeated overdoses of oral aciclovir over several days have been associated with gastrointestinal effects (such as nausea and vomiting) and neurological effects (headache and confusion).

Overdosage of intravenous aciclovir has resulted in elevations of serum creatinine, blood urea nitrogen and subsequent renal failure. Neurological effects including confusion, hallucinations, agitation, seizures and coma have been described in association with intravenous overdosage.

Management:- Patients should be observed closely for signs of toxicity. Haemodialysis significantly enhances the removal of aciclovir from the blood and may, therefore, be considered a management option in the event of symptomatic overdose.

5. PHARMACOLOGICAL PROPERTIES

5.1 Pharmacodynamic properties
Aciclovir is a synthetic purine nucleoside analogue with *in vitro* and *in vivo* inhibitory activity against human herpes viruses, including herpes simplex virus (HSV) types I and II and varicella zoster virus (VSV).

The inhibitory activity of aciclovir for HSV I, HSV II, and VZV is highly selective. The enzyme thymidine kinase (TK) of normal, uninfected cells does not use aciclovir effectively as a substrate, hence toxicity to mammalian host cells is low; however, TK encoded by HSV and VZV converts aciclovir to aciclovir monophosphate, a nucleoside analogue which is further converted to the diphosphate and finally to the triphosphate by cellular enzymes. Aciclovir triphosphate interferes with the viral DNA polymerase and inhibits viral DNA replication with the resultant chain termination following its incorporation into the viral DNA.

Prolonged or repeated courses of aciclovir in severely immunocompromised individuals may result in the selection of virus strains with reduced sensitivity, which may not respond to continued aciclovir treatment. Most of the clinical isolates with reduced sensitivity have been relatively deficient in viral TK, however, strains with altered viral TK or viral DNA polymerase have also been reported. *In vitro* exposure of HSV isolates to aciclovir can also lead to the emergence of less sensitive strains. The relationship between the *in vitro* determined sensitivity of HSV isolates and clinical response to aciclovir therapy is not clear.

5.2 Pharmacokinetic properties
Aciclovir is only partially absorbed from the gut. Mean steady state peak plasma concentrations ($C^{SS}max$) following doses of 200mg aciclovir administered four-hourly were 3.1 microMol (0.7 microgram/ml) and the equivalent trough plasma levels ($C^{SS}min$) were 1.8 microMol (0.4 microgram/ml). Corresponding steady-state plasma concentrations following doses of 400mg and 800mg aciclovir administered four-hourly were 5.3 microMol (1.2 microgram/ml) and 8 microMol (1.8 microgram/ml) respectively, and equivalent trough plasma levels were 2.7 microMol (0.6 microgram/ml) and 4 microMol (0.9 microgram/ml).

In adults the terminal plasma half-life after administration of intravenous aciclovir is about 2.9 hours. Most of the drug is excreted unchanged by the kidney. Renal clearance of aciclovir is substantially greater than creatinine clearance, indicating that tubular secretion, in addition to glomerular filtration, contributes to the renal elimination of the drug.

9-carboxymethoxymethylguanine is the only significant metabolite of aciclovir, and accounts for 10-15% of the dose excreted in the urine. When aciclovir is given one hour after 1 gram of probenecid the terminal half-life and the area under the plasma concentration time curve is extended by 18% and 40% respectively.

In adults, mean steady state peak plasma concentrations ($C^{SS}max$) following a one hour infusion of 2.5mg/kg, 5mg/kg and 10mg/kg were 22.7 microMol (5.1 microgram/ml), 43.6 microMol (9.8 microgram/ml) and 92 microMol (20.7 microgram/ml), respectively. The corresponding trough levels ($C^{SS}min$) 7 hours later were 2.2 microMol (0.5 microgram/ml), 3.1 microMol (0.7 microgram/ml) and 10.2 microMol (2.3 microgram/ml), respectively.

In children over 1 year of age similar mean peak ($C^{SS}max$) and trough ($C^{SS}min$) levels were observed when a dose of 250mg/m^2 was substituted for 5mg/kg and a dose of 500mg/m^2 was substituted for 10mg/kg. In neonates (0 to 3 months of age) treated with doses of 10mg/kg administered by infusion over a one-hour period every 8 hours the $C^{SS}max$ was found to be 61.2 microMol (13.8 microgram/ml) and $C^{SS}min$ to be 10.1 microMol (2.3 microgram/ml). The terminal plasma half-life in these patients was 3.8 hours.

In the elderly total body clearance falls with increasing age associated with decreases in creatinine clearance although there is little change in the terminal plasma half-life.

In patients with chronic renal failure the mean terminal half-life was found to be 19.5 hours. The mean aciclovir half-life during haemodialysis was 5.7 hours. Plasma aciclovir levels dropped approximately 60% during dialysis.

Cerebrospinal fluid levels are approximately 50% of corresponding plasma levels. Plasma protein binding is relatively low (9 to 33%) and drug interactions involving binding site displacement are not anticipated.

5.3 Preclinical safety data
Mutagenicity:- The results of a wide range of mutagenicity tests *in vitro* and *in vivo* indicate that aciclovir is unlikely to pose a genetic risk to man.

Carcinogenicity:- Aciclovir was not found to be carcinogenic in long term studies in the rat and the mouse.

Teratogenicity:- Systemic administration of aciclovir in internationally accepted standard tests did not produce embryotoxic or teratogenic effects in rats, rabbits or mice.

In a non-standard test in rats, foetal abnormalities were observed, but only following such high subcutaneous doses that maternal toxicity was produced. The clinical relevance of these findings is uncertain.

Fertility:- Largely reversible adverse effects on spermatogenesis in association with overall toxicity in rats and dogs have been reported only at doses of aciclovir greatly in excess of those employed therapeutically. Two generation studies in mice did not reveal any effect of aciclovir on fertility. There is no information on the effect of Zovirax Double Strength Suspension on human female fertility. In patients with normal sperm count, chronically administered oral aciclovir has been shown to have no clinically significant effect on sperm count, motility or morphology.

6. PHARMACEUTICAL PARTICULARS

6.1 List of excipients
Sorbitol Solution, 70%, non-crystallising EP

Glycerol EP

Dispersible cellulose BP

Methyl parahydroxybenzoate EP

Propyl parahydroxybenzoate EP

Flavour, orange, 52.570/T HSE

Purified water EP

6.2 Incompatibilities
None Known.

6.3 Shelf life
3 years.

6.4 Special precautions for storage
Store below 30°C

6.5 Nature and contents of container
Amber glass bottles fitted with white, child resistant caps with an EPE/Saranex liner or metal roll-on closures lined with PVDC-faced wads.

Pack sizes: 50ml[1], 100ml, 175ml[2], 350ml[3]

The 100ml pack contains a double-ended measuring spoon.

6.6 Instructions for use and handling
No special instructions.

Administrative Data

7. MARKETING AUTHORISATION HOLDER
The Wellcome Foundation Ltd

Glaxo Wellcome House

Berkeley Avenue

Greenford

Middlesex

UB6 ONN

Trading as

GlaxoSmithKline UK

Stockley Park West

Uxbridge

Middlesex UB11 1BT

8. MARKETING AUTHORISATION NUMBER(S)
PL 00003/0264

9. DATE OF FIRST AUTHORISATION/RENEWAL OF THE AUTHORISATION
26 April 2001

10. DATE OF REVISION OF THE TEXT
29 November 2004

11. Legal Status
POM

[1] Non-marketed pack size

[2] Non-marketed pack size

[3] Non-marketed pack size

Zovirax Eye Ointment

(GlaxoSmithKline UK)

1. NAME OF THE MEDICINAL PRODUCT
Zovirax Eye Ointment

2. QUALITATIVE AND QUANTITATIVE COMPOSITION
Aciclovir 3.0% W/W

3. PHARMACEUTICAL FORM
Ophthalmic Ointment

4. CLINICAL PARTICULARS

4.1 Therapeutic indications
Treatment of herpes simplex keratitis.

4.2 Posology and method of administration
Topical administration to the eye.

Adults: 1cm ribbon of ointment should be placed inside the lower conjunctival sac five times a day at approximately four hourly intervals, omitting the night time application. Treatment should continue for at least 3 days after healing is complete.

Children: As for adults

Use in the elderly: As for adults.

4.3 Contraindications
Zovirax eye ointment is contra-indicated in patients with a known hypersensitivity to aciclovir.

4.4 Special warnings and special precautions for use
None

4.5 Interaction with other medicinal products and other forms of Interaction
Probenecid increases the aciclovir mean half-life and area under the plasma concentration curve of systematically administered aciclovir. Other drugs affecting renal

physiology could potentially influence the pharmacokinetics of aciclovir. However, clinical experience has not identified other drug interactions with aciclovir.

4.6 Pregnancy and lactation

Systemic administration of aciclovir in internationally accepted standard tests did not produce embryotoxic or teratogenic effects in rats, rabbits or mice.

In a non-standard test in rats, foetal abnormalities were observed, but only following such high subcutaneous doses that maternal toxicity was produced. The clinical relevance of these findings is uncertain.

A post-marketing aciclovir pregnancy registry has documented pregnancy outcomes in women exposed to any formulation of Zovirax. The birth defects described amongst Zovirax exposed subjects have not shown any uniqueness or consistent pattern to suggest a common cause.

The use of Zovirax Eye Ointment should be considered only when the potential benefits outweigh the possibility of unknown risks.

There is no information on the effect of Zovirax Eye Ointment on human female fertility. Two-generation studies in mice did not reveal any effect of (orally administered) aciclovir on fertility.

Limited human data show that the drug does pass into breast milk.

4.7 Effects on ability to drive and use machines

Not applicable

4.8 Undesirable effects

FOR OPHTHALMIC USE ONLY

Transient mild stinging immediately following application may occur in a small proportion of patients. Superficial punctate keratopathy has been reported but has not resulted in patients being withdrawn from therapy, and healing has occurred without apparent sequelae. Local irritation and inflammation such as blepharitis and conjunctivitis have also been reported.

The results of a wide range of mutagenicity tests *in vitro* and *in vivo* indicate that aciclovir does not pose a genetic risk to man. Aciclovir was not found to be carcinogenic in long-term studies in the rat and the mouse. Largely reversible adverse effects on spermatogenesis in association with overall toxicity in rats and dogs have been reported only at doses of aciclovir greatly in excess of those employed therapeutically. Zovirax Tablets have been shown to have no definite effect upon sperm count, morphology or motility in man.

There have been very rare reports of immediate hypersensitivity reactions including angioedema with topical aciclovir.

4.9 Overdose

No untoward effects would be expected if the entire contents of the tube containing 135 mg of aciclovir were ingested orally. Oral doses of 800 mg five times daily (4 g per day) have been administered for seven days without adverse effects.

Single intravenous doses of up to 80 mg/kg have been inadvertently administered without adverse effects. Aciclovir is dialysable by haemodialysis.

5. PHARMACOLOGICAL PROPERTIES

5.1 Pharmacodynamic properties

Aciclovir is an antiviral agent which is highly active *in vitro* against herpes simplex (HSV) types I and II, but its toxicity to mammalian cells is low.

Aciclovir is phosphorylated to the active compound aciclovir triphosphate after entry into a herpes infected cell. The first step in this process requires the presence of the HSV coded thymidine kinase. Aciclovir triphosphate acts as an inhibitor of, and substrate for, herpes specified DNA polymerase, preventing further viral DNA synthesis without affecting normal cellular processes

5.2 Pharmacokinetic properties

Aciclovir is rapidly absorbed from the ophthalmic ointment through the corneal epithelium and superficial ocular tissues, achieving antiviral concentrations in the aqueous humor. It has not been possible by existing methods to detect aciclovir in the blood after topical application to the eye. However, trace quantities are detectable in the urine. These levels are not therapeutically significant.

5.3 Preclinical safety data

There are no preclinical data of relevance to the prescriber which are additional to that in other sections of the SmPC.

6. PHARMACEUTICAL PARTICULARS

6.1 List of excipients

White petrolatum USP

6.2 Incompatibilities

None known

6.3 Shelf life

5 years

6.4 Special precautions for storage

Store below 25°C

6.5 Nature and contents of container

Laminate ophthalmic ointment tubes closed with high-density polyethylene screw caps or tamper evident screw caps.

Pack size: 4.5G

6.6 Instructions for use and handling

No special instructions

Administrative Data

7. MARKETING AUTHORISATION HOLDER

The Wellcome Foundation Ltd

Glaxo Wellcome House

Berkeley Avenue

Greenford

Middlesex

UB6 ONN

Trading as

GlaxoSmithKline UK

Stockley Park West

Uxbridge

Middlesex UB11 1BT

8. MARKETING AUTHORISATION NUMBER(S)

PL 00003/0150

9. DATE OF FIRST AUTHORISATION/RENEWAL OF THE AUTHORISATION

16 October 1996

10. DATE OF REVISION OF THE TEXT

2 April 2003

11. Legal Status

POM

Zovirax IV 250mg, 500mg

(GlaxoSmithKline UK)

1. NAME OF THE MEDICINAL PRODUCT

Zovirax IV 250mg

Zovirax IV 500mg

2. QUALITATIVE AND QUANTITATIVE COMPOSITION

250mg Aciclovir OR

500mg Aciclovir in each vial

3. PHARMACEUTICAL FORM

Intravenous injection

4. CLINICAL PARTICULARS

4.1 Therapeutic indications

Zovirax I.V. is indicated for the treatment of *Herpes simplex* infections in immunocompromised patients and severe initial genital herpes in the non-immunocompromised.

Zovirax I.V. is indicated for the prophylaxis of *Herpes simplex* infections inimmunocompromised patients.

Zovirax I.V. is indicated for the treatment of *Varicella zoster* infections.

Zovirax I.V. is indicated for the treatment of herpes encephalitis.

Zovirax I.V. is indicated for the treatment of *Herpes simplex* infections in the neonate and infant up to 3 months of age.

4.2 Posology and method of administration

Route of administration:

Slow intravenous infusion

A course of treatment with Zovirax I.V. usually lasts 5 days, but this may be adjusted according to the patient's condition and response to therapy. Treatment for herpes encephalitis and neonatal *Herpes simplex* infections usually lasts 10 days.

The duration of prophylactic administration of Zovirax I.V. is determined by the duration of the period at risk.

Dosage in adults:

Patients with *Herpes simplex* (except herpes encephalitis) or *Varicella zoster* infections should be given Zovirax I.V. in doses of 5 mg/kg bodyweight every 8 hours.

Immunocompromised patients with *Varicella zoster* infections or patients with herpes encephalitis should be given Zovirax I.V. in doses of 10 mg/kg bodyweight every 8 hours provided renal function is not impaired (see *Dosage in renal impairment*).

Dosage in children:

The dose of Zovirax I.V. for children aged between 3 months and 12 years is calculated on the basis of body surface area.

Children with *Herpes simplex* (except herpes encephalitis) or *Varicella zoster* infections should be given Zovirax I.V. in doses of 250 mg per square metre of body surface area every 8 hours.

In immunocompromised children with *Varicella zoster* infections or children with herpes encephalitis, Zovirax I.V. should be given in doses of 500 mg per square metre body surface area every 8 hours if renal function is not impaired.

Children with impaired renal function require an appropriately modified dose, according to the degree of impairment.

The dosage of Zovirax I.V. in neonates and infants up to 3 months of age is calculated on the basis of bodyweight.

Neonates and infants up to 3 months of age with *Herpes simplex* infections should be given Zovirax I.V. in doses of 10 mg/kg bodyweight every 8 hours. Treatment for neonatal herpes simplex infections usually lasts 10 days.

Dosage in the elderly:

In the elderly, total aciclovir body clearance declines in parallel with creatinine clearance. Special attention should be given to dosage reduction in elderly patients with impaired creatinine clearance.

Caution is advised when administering Zovirax I.V. to patients with impaired renal function. The following adjustments in dosage are suggested:

Creatinine Clearance

Dosage 25 to 50 ml/min

The dose recommended above (5 or 10 mg/kg bodyweight) should be given every 12 hours.

10 to 25 ml/min

The dose recommended above (5 or 10 mg/kg bodyweight) should be given every 24 hours.

0(anuric) to 10 ml/min

In patients receiving continuous ambulatory peritoneal dialysis (CAPD) the dose recommended above (5 or 10 mg/kg bodyweight) should be halved and administered every 24 hours. In patients receiving haemodialysis the dose recommended above (5 or 10 mg/kg bodyweight) should be halved and administered every 24 hours and after dialysis.

4.3 Contraindications

Zovirax IV is contraindicated in patients known to be previously hypersensitive to aciclovir or valaciclovir.

4.4 Special warnings and special precautions for use

The dose of Zovirax I.V. must be adjusted in patients with impaired renal function in order to avoid accumulation of aciclovir in the body (see *Dosage in renal impairment*).

In patients receiving Zovirax I.V. at higher doses (e.g. for herpes encephalitis), specific care regarding renal function should be taken, particularly when patients are dehydrated or have any renal impairment.

Reconstituted Zovirax I.V. has a pH of approximately 11.0 and should not be administered by mouth.

Zovirax I.V. contains no antimicrobial preservative. Reconstitution and dilution should therefore be carried out under full aseptic conditions immediately before use and any unused solution discarded. The reconstituted or diluted solutions should not be refrigerated.

Other warnings and precautions

The labels shall contain the following statements:

For intravenous infusion only

Keep out of reach of children

Store below 25°C

Prepare immediately for use

Discard unused solution

4.5 Interaction with other medicinal products and other forms of Interaction

No clinically significant interactions have been identified.

Aciclovir is eliminated primarily unchanged in the urine via active renal tubular secretion. Any drugs administered concurrently that compete with this mechanism may increase aciclovir plasma concentrations. Probenecid and cimetidine increase the AUC of aciclovir by this mechanism, and reduce aciclovir renal clearance. However no dosage adjustment is necessary because of the wide therapeutic index of aciclovir.

In patients receiving intravenous Zovirax, caution is required during concurrent administration with drugs which compete with aciclovir for elimination, because of the potential for increased plasma levels of one or both drugs or their metabolites. Increases in plasma AUCs of aciclovir and of the inactive metabolite of mycophenolate mofetil, an immunosuppressant agent used in transplant patients, have been shown when the drugs are coadministered.

Care is also required (with monitoring for changes in renal function) if administering intravenous Zovirax with drugs which affect other aspects of renal physiology (e.g. ciclosporin, tacrolimus).

4.6 Pregnancy and lactation

A post-marketing aciclovir pregnancy registry has documented pregnancy outcomes in women exposed to any formulation of Zovirax. The birth defects described amongst Zovirax exposed subjects have not shown any uniqueness or consistent pattern to suggest a common cause.

Caution should however be exercised by balancing the potential benefits of treatment against any possible hazard. Findings from reproduction toxicology studies are included in Section 5.3.

Following oral administration of 200 mg five times a day, aciclovir has been detected in human breast milk at concentrations ranging from 0.6 to 4.1 times the corresponding plasma levels. These levels would potentially expose nursing infants to aciclovir dosages of up to 0.3 mg/kg bodyweight/day. Caution is therefore advised if Zovirax is to be administered to a nursing woman.

4.7 Effects on ability to drive and use machines
No studies on the effects on the ability to drive and use machines have been performed.

4.8 Undesirable effects
Gastrointestinal: Nausea and vomiting have been reported.

Haematological: Decreases in haematological indices (anaemia, thrombocytopenia, leucopenia).

Hypersensitivity and Skin: Rashes including photosensitivity, urticaria, pruritus, fevers and rarely dyspnoea, angioedema and anaphylaxis.

Severe local inflammatory reactions sometimes leading to breakdown of the skin have occurred when Zovirax I.V. has been inadvertently infused into extravascular tissues.

Kidney: Rapid increases in blood urea and creatinine levels may occasionally occur in patients given Zovirax I.V. This is believed to be related to peak plasma levels and the state of hydration of the patient. To avoid this effect the drug should not be given as an intravenous bolus injection but by slow infusion over a one hour period.

Adequate hydration of the patient should be maintained. Renal impairment developing during treatment with Zovirax I.V. usually responds rapidly to rehydration of the patient and/or dosage reduction or withdrawal of the drug. Progression to acute renal failure, however, can occur in exceptional cases.

Liver: Reversible increases in bilirubin and liver-related enzymes. Hepatitis and jaundice have been reported on very rare occasions.

Neurological: Reversible neurological reactions such as confusion, hallucinations, agitation, tremors, somnolence, psychosis, convulsions and coma have been associated with Zovirax I.V. therapy, usually in medically complicated cases.

4.9 Overdose
Overdosage of intravenenous aciclovir has resulted in elevations of serum creatinine, blood urea nitrogen and subsequent renal failure. Neurological effects including confusion, hallucinations, agitation, seizures and coma have been described in association with overdosage. Haemodialysis significantly enhances the removal of aciclovir from the blood and may, therefore, be considered an option in the management of overdose of this drug.

5. PHARMACOLOGICAL PROPERTIES
5.1 Pharmacodynamic properties
Aciclovir is a synthetic purine nucleoside analogue with *in vitro* and *in vivo* inhibitory activity against human herpes viruses, including *Herpes simplex* virus types 1 and 2 and *Varicella zoster* virus (VZV), Epstein Barr virus (EBV) and Cytomegalovirus (CMV). In cell culture aciclovir has the greatest antiviral activity against HSV-1, followed (in decreasing order of potency) by HSV-2, VZV, EBV, and CMV.

The inhibitory activity of aciclovir for HSV-1, HSV-2, VZV and EBV is highly selective. The enzyme thymidine kinase (TK) of normal, uninfected cells does not use aciclovir effectively as a substrate, hence toxicity to mammalian host cells is low; however, TK encoded by HSV, VZV and EBV converts aciclovir to aciclovir monophosphate, a nucleoside analogue, which is further converted to the diphosphate and finally to the triphosphate by cellular enzymes. Aciclovir triphosphate interferes with the viral DNA polymerase and inhibits viral DNA replication with resultant chain termination following its incorporation into the viral DNA.

5.2 Pharmacokinetic properties
In adults, the terminal plasma half-life of aciclovir after administration of Zovirax I.V. is about 2.9 hours. Most of the drug is excreted unchanged by the kidney. Renal clearance of aciclovir is substantially greater than creatinine clearance, indicating that tubular secretion, in addition to glomerular filtration, contributes to the renal elimination of the drug. 9-carboxymethoxymethylguanine is the only significant metabolite of aciclovir and accounts for 10 to 15% of the dose excreted in the urine.

When aciclovir is given one hour after 1 gram of probenecid the terminal half-life and the area under the plasma concentration time curve, are extended by 18% and 40% respectively.

In adults, mean steady state peak plasma concentrations (C^{ss}max) following a one-hour infusion of 2.5 mg/kg, 5 mg/kg, and 10 mg/kg were 22.7 micromolar (5.1 microgram/ml), 43.6 micromolar (9.8 microgram/ml), and 92 micromolar (20.7 microgram/ml) respectively. The corresponding trough levels (C^{ss}min) 7 hours later were 2.2 micromolar (0.5 microgram/ml), 3.1 micromolar (0.7 microgram/ml) and 10.2 micromolar (2.3 microgram/ml) respectively. In children over 1 year of age similar mean peak (C^{ss}max) and trough (C^{ss}min) levels were observed when a dose of 250 mg/m^2 was substituted for 5 mg/kg and a dose of 500 mg/m^2 was substituted for 10 mg/kg. In neonates (0 to 3 months of age) treated with doses of 10 mg/kg administered by infusion over a one-hour period every 8 hours the C^{ss}max was found to be 61.2 micromolar (13.8 microgram/ml) and the C^{ss}min.to be 10.1 micromolar (2.3 microgram/ml).

The terminal plasma half-life in these patients was 3.8 hours. In the elderly, total body clearance falls with increasing age and is associated with decreases in creatinine clearance although there is little change in the terminal plasma half-life.

In patients with chronic renal failure the mean terminal half-life was found to be 19.5 hours. The mean aciclovir half-life during haemodialysis was 5.7 hours. Plasma aciclovir levels dropped approximately 60% during dialysis.

Cerebrospinal fluid levels are approximately 50% of corresponding plasma levels.

Plasma protein binding is relatively low (9 to 33%) and drug interactions involving binding site displacement are not anticipated.

5.3 Preclinical safety data
Mutagenicity:- The results of a wide range of mutagenicity tests *in vitro* and *in vivo* indicate that aciclovir is unlikely to pose a genetic risk to man.

Carcinogenicity:- Aciclovir was not found to be carcinogenic in long-term studies in the rat and the mouse.

Teratogenicity:- Systemic administration of aciclovir in internationally accepted standard tests did not produce embryotoxic or teratogenic effects in rabbits, rats or mice

In a non-standard test in rats, foetal abnormalities were observed but only following such high subcutaneous doses that maternal toxicity was produced. The clinical relevance of these findings is uncertain.

Fertility:- Largely reversible adverse effects on spermatogenesis in association with overall toxicity in rats and dogs have been reported only at doses of aciclovir greatly in excess of those employed therapeutically. Two-generation studies in mice did not reveal any effect of (orally administered) aciclovir on fertility.

There is no information on the effect of Zovirax I.V. on human female fertility. In patients with normal sperm count, chronically administered oral aciclovir has been shown to have no clinically significant effect on sperm count, motility or morphology.

6. PHARMACEUTICAL PARTICULARS
6.1 List of excipients
Sodium hydroxide (used to adjust pH)

6.2 Incompatibilities
None known

6.3 Shelf life
60 months

6.4 Special precautions for storage
Store below 25°C

6.5 Nature and contents of container
Neutral glass vials closed with butyl rubber closures secured by aluminium collars.

17ml-nominal capacity of vial containing 250mg aciclovir.

20ml-nominal capacity of vial containing 500mg aciclovir.

6.6 Instructions for use and handling
Reconstitution:

Zovirax I.V. should be reconstituted using the following volumes of either Water for Injections BP or Sodium Chloride Intravenous Injection BP (0.9% w/v) to provide a solution containing 25 mg aciclovir per ml:

Formulation	Volume of fluid for reconstitution
250 mg vial	10 ml
500 mg vial	20 ml

From the calculated dose, determine the appropriate number and strength of vials to be used. To reconstitute each vial add the recommended volume of infusion fluid and shake gently until the contents of the vial have dissolved completely.

Administration:

The required dose of Zovirax I.V. should be administered by slow intravenous infusion over a one-hour period.

After reconstitution Zovirax I.V. may be administered by a controlled-rate infusion pump.

Alternatively, the reconstituted solution may be further diluted to give an Aciclovir concentration of not greater than 5 mg/ml (0.5% w/v) for administration by infusion:

Add the required volume of reconstituted solution to the chosen infusion solution, as recommended below, and shake well to ensure adequate mixing occurs.

For children and neonates, where it is advisable to keep the volume of infusion fluid to a minimum, it is recommended that dilution is on the basis of 4 ml reconstituted solution (100 mg Aciclovir) added to 20 ml of infusion fluid.

For adults, it is recommended that infusion bags containing 100 ml of infusion fluid are used, even when this would give an aciclovir concentration substantially below 0.5% w/v. Thus one 100 ml infusion bag may be used for any dose between 250 mg and 500 mg aciclovir (10 and 20 ml of reconstituted solution) but a second bag must be used for doses between 500 and 1000 mg.

When diluted in accordance with the recommended schedules, Zovirax I.V. is known to be compatible with the following infusion fluids and stable for up to 12 hours at room temperature (15C to 25C):

Sodium Chloride Intravenous Infusion BP (0.45% and 0.9% w/v);

Sodium Chloride (0.18% w/v) and Glucose (4% w/v) Intravenous Infusion BP;

Sodium Chloride (0.45% w/v) and Glucose (2.5% w/v) Intravenous Infusion BP;

Compound Sodium Lactate Intravenous Infusion BP (Hartmann's Solution).

Zovirax I.V. when diluted in accordance with the above schedule will give an aciclovir concentration not greater than 0.5% w/v.

Since no antimicrobial preservative is included, reconstitution and dilution must be carried out under full aseptic conditions, immediately before use, and any unused solution discarded.

Should any visible turbidity or crystallisation appear in the solution before or during infusion, the preparation should be discarded.

Administrative Data
7. MARKETING AUTHORISATION HOLDER
The Wellcome Foundation Ltd

Glaxo Wellcome House

Berkeley Avenue

Greenford

Middlesex

UB6 ONN

Trading as

GlaxoSmithKline UK

Stockley Park West

Uxbridge

Middlesex UB11 1BT

8. MARKETING AUTHORISATION NUMBER(S)
PL 00003/0159

9. DATE OF FIRST AUTHORISATION/RENEWAL OF THE AUTHORISATION
9 June 1997

10. DATE OF REVISION OF THE TEXT
7 December 2004

11. Legal Status
POM

Zovirax Suspension

(GlaxoSmithKline UK)

1. NAME OF THE MEDICINAL PRODUCT
Zovirax Suspension

2. QUALITATIVE AND QUANTITATIVE COMPOSITION
Aciclovir 200mg/5ml

3. PHARMACEUTICAL FORM
Suspension

4. CLINICAL PARTICULARS
4.1 Therapeutic indications
Zovirax Suspension is indicated for the treatment of herpes simplex virus infections of the skin and mucous membranes including initial and recurrent genital herpes.

Zovirax Suspension is indicated for the suppression (prevention of recurrences) of recurrent herpes simplex infections in immunocompetent patients.

Zovirax Suspension is indicated for the prophylaxis of herpes simplex infections in immunocompromised patients.

Zovirax Suspension is indicated for the treatment of varicella (chickenpox) and herpes zoster (shingles) infections.

4.2 Posology and method of administration
Dosage in Adults

Treatment of herpes simplex infections: 200mg Zovirax should be taken five times daily at approximately four hourly intervals omitting the night time dose. Treatment should continue for 5 days, but in severe initial infections this may have to be extended.

In severely immunocompromised patients (e.g. after marrow transplant) or in patients with impaired absorption from the gut the dose can be doubled to 400mg Zovirax or alternatively intravenous dosing could be considered.

Dosing should begin as early as possible after the start of an infection; for recurrent episodes this should preferably be during the prodromal period or when lesions first appear.

Suppression of herpes simplex infections in immunocompetent patients:

200mg Zovirax should be taken four times daily at approximately six-hourly intervals.

Many patients may be conveniently managed on a regimen of 400mg Zovirax twice daily at approximately twelve-hourly intervals.

Dosage titration down to 200mg Zovirax taken thrice daily at approximately eight-hourly intervals or even twice daily at approximately twelve-hourly intervals, may prove effective.

Some patients may experience break-through infection on total daily doses of 800mg Zovirax.

Therapy should be interrupted periodically at intervals of six to twelve months, in order to observe possible changes in the natural history of the disease.

Prophylaxis of herpes simplex infections in immunocompromised patients:

200mg Zovirax should be taken four times daily at approximately six hourly intervals.

In severely immunocompromised patients (e.g. after marrow transplant) or in patients with impaired absorption from the gut, the dose can be doubled to 400mg Zovirax or, alternatively, intravenous dosing could be considered.

The duration of prophylactic administration is determined by the duration of the period at risk.

Treatment of varicella and herpes zoster infections: 800mg Zovirax should be taken five times daily at approximately four-hourly intervals, omitting the night time dose. Treatment should continue for seven days.

In severely immunocompromised patients (e.g. after marrow transplant) or in patients with impaired absorption from the gut, consideration should be given to intravenous dosing.

Dosing should begin as early as possible after the start of an infection: treatment of herpes zoster yields better results if initiated as soon as possible after the onset of the rash. Treatment of chickenpox in immunocompetent patients should begin within 24 hours after onset of the rash.

Dosage in Children

Treatment of herpes simplex infections, and prophylaxis of herpes simplex infections in the immunocompromised: Children aged two years and over should be given adult dosages and children below the age of two years should be given halfthe adult dose.

Treatment of varicella infections:

6 years and over:

800mg Zovirax four times daily.

2 to 5 years:

400mg Zovirax four times daily.

Under 2 years: 200mg Zovirax four times daily.

Treatment should continue for five days.

Dosing may be more accurately calculated as 20mg/kg body weight (not to exceed 800mg) Zovirax four times daily.

No specific data are available on the *suppression* of *herpes simplex* infections or the treatment of herpes *zoster* infections in immunocompetent children.

Zovirax Suspension may be diluted with an equal volume of either Syrup BP or Sorbitol Solution (70%) (non-crystallising) BP. The diluted product is stable for 4 weeks at $25^{\circ}C$ but it is recommended that all dilutions are freshly prepared.

Dosage in the Elderly

In the elderly, total aciclovir body clearance declines along with creatinine clearance. Adequate hydration of elderly patients taking high oral doses of Zovirax should be maintained. Special attention should be given to dosage reduction in elderly patients with impaired renal function.

Dosage in Renal Impairment

In the management of herpes simplex infections in patients with impaired renal function, the recommended oral doses will not lead to accumulation of aciclovir above levels that have been established by intravenous infusion. However, for patients with severe renal impairment (creatinine clearance less than 10ml/minute) an adjustment of dosage to 200mg aciclovir twice daily at approximately twelve-hourly intervals is recommended.

In the treatment of herpes zoster infections it is recommended to adjust the dosage to 800mg aciclovir twice daily at approximately twelve-hourly intervals for patients with severe renal impairment (creatinine clearance less than 10ml/minute), and to 800mg aciclovir three times daily at intervals of approximately eight hours for patients with moderate renal impairment (creatinine clearance in the range 10 to 25ml/minute).

4.3 Contraindications

Zovirax Suspension is contra-indicated in patients known to be hypersensitive to aciclovir or valaciclovir.

4.4 Special warnings and special precautions for use

Hydration status: Care should be taken to maintain adequate hydration in patients receiving high oral dose regimens e.g. for the treatment of herpes zoster infection (4g daily), in order to avoid the risk of possible renal toxicity.

The data currently available from clinical studies is not sufficient to conclude that treatment with Zovirax reduces the incidence of chickenpox-associated complications in immunocompetent patients.

4.5 Interaction with other medicinal products and other forms of Interaction

No clinically significant interactions have been identified.

Aciclovir is eliminated primarily unchanged in the urine via active renal tubular secretion. Any drugs administered concurrently that compete with this mechanism may increase aciclovir plasma concentrations. Probenecid and cimetidine increase the AUC of aciclovir by this mechanism, and reduce aciclovir renal clearance. Similarly increases in plasma AUCs of aciclovir and of the inactive metabolite of mycophenolate mofetil, an immunosuppressant agent used in transplant patients have been shown when the drugs are coadministered. However no dosage adjustment is necessary because of the wide therapeutic index of aciclovir.

4.6 Pregnancy and lactation

A post-marketing aciclovir pregnancy registry has documented pregnancy outcomes in women exposed to any formulation of Zovirax. The birth defects described amongst Zovirax exposed subjects have not shown any uniqueness or consistent pattern to suggest a common cause.

Caution should however be exercised by balancing the potential benefits of treatment against any possible hazard. Findings from reproduction toxicology studies are included in Section 5.3.

Following oral administration of 200mg Zovirax five times a day, aciclovir has been detected in breast milk at concentrations ranging from 0.6 to 4.1 times the corresponding plasma levels. These levels would potentially expose nursing infants to aciclovir dosages of up to 0.3mg/kg/day. Caution is therefore advised if Zovirax is to be administered to a nursing woman.

4.7 Effects on ability to drive and use machines

No studies on the effects on the ability to drive and use machines have been performed.

4.8 Undesirable effects

Gastrointestinal: Nausea, vomiting, diarrhoea and abdominal pains have been reported.

Haematological: Very rarely, anaemia, leukopenia and thrombocytopenia.

Hypersensitivity and Skin: Rashes including photosensitivity, urticaria, pruritis and rarely dyspnoea, angioedema and anaphylaxis.

Kidney: Rare reports of increases in blood urea and creatinine. Acute renal failure has been reported on very rare occasions.

Liver: Rare reports of reversible rises in bilirubin and liver related enzymes. Hepatitis and jaundice have been reported on very rare occasions.

Neurological: Headaches. Occasionally, reversible neurological reactions, notably dizziness, confusional states, hallucinations, somnolence, convulsions and coma have been reported, usually in patients with renal impairment in whom the dosage was in excess of that recommended or with other predisposing factors.

Other: Fatigue. Occasional reports of accelerated diffuse hair loss. As this type of hair loss has been associated with a wide variety of disease processes and medicines, the relationship of the event to aciclovir therapy is uncertain.

4.9 Overdose

Symptoms & signs:- Aciclovir is only partly absorbed in the gastrointestinal tract. Patients have ingested overdoses of up to 20g aciclovir on a single occasion, usually without toxic effects. Accidental, repeated overdoses of oral aciclovir over several days have been associated with gastrointestinal effects (such as nausea and vomiting) and neurological effects (headache and confusion).

Overdosage of intravenous aciclovir has resulted in elevations of serum creatinine, blood urea nitrogen and subsequent renal failure. Neurological effects including confusion, hallucinations, agitation, seizures and coma have been described in association with intravenous overdosage.

Management:- Patients should be observed closely for signs of toxicity. Haemodialysis significantly enhances the removal of aciclovir from the blood and may, therefore, be considered a management option in the event of symptomatic overdose.

5. PHARMACOLOGICAL PROPERTIES

5.1 Pharmacodynamic properties

Aciclovir is a synthetic purine nucleoside analogue with *in vitro* and *in vivo* inhibitory activity against human herpes viruses, including herpes simplex virus (HSV) types I and II and varicella zoster virus (VSV).

The inhibitory activity of aciclovir for HSV I, HSV II, and VZV is highly selective. The enzyme thymidine kinase (TK) of normal, uninfected cells does not use aciclovir effectively as a substrate, hence toxicity to mammalian host cells is low; however, TK encoded by HSV and VZV converts aciclovir to aciclovir monophosphate, a nucleoside analogue which is further converted to the diphosphate and finally to the triphosphate by cellular enzymes. Aciclovir triphosphate interferes with the viral DNA polymerase and inhibits viral DNA replication with the resultant chain termination following its incorporation into the viral DNA.

Prolonged or repeated courses of aciclovir in severely immunocompromised individuals may result in the selection of virus strains with reduced sensitivity, which may not respond to continued aciclovir treatment. Most of the clinical isolates with reduced sensitivity have been relatively deficient in viral TK, however, strains with altered viral TK or viral DNA polymerase have also been reported. *In vitro* exposure of HSV isolates to aciclovir can also lead to the emergence of less sensitive strains. The relationship between the *in vitro* determined sensitivity of HSV isolates and clinical response to aciclovir therapy is not clear.

5.2 Pharmacokinetic properties

Aciclovir is only partially absorbed from the gut. Mean steady state peak plasma concentrations ($C^{SS}max$) following doses of 200mg aciclovir administered four-hourly were 3.1 microMol (0.7 microgram/ml) and the equivalent trough plasma levels ($C^{SS}min$) were 1.8 microMol (0.4 microgram/ml). Corresponding steady-state plasma concentrations following doses of 400mg and 800mg aciclovir administered four-hourly were 5.3 microMol (1.2 microgram/ml) and 8 microMol (1.8 microgram/ml) respectively, and equivalent trough plasma levels were 2.7 microMol (0.6 microgram/ml) and 4 microMol (0.9 microgram/ml).

In adults the terminal plasma half-life after administration of intravenous aciclovir is about 2.9 hours. Most of the drug is excreted unchanged by the kidney. Renal clearance of aciclovir is substantially greater than creatinine clearance, indicating that tubular secretion, in addition to glomerular filtration, contributes to the renal elimination of the drug.

9-carboxymethoxymethylguanine is the only significant metabolite of aciclovir, and accounts for 10-15% of the dose excreted in the urine. When aciclovir is given one hour after 1 gram of probenecid the terminal half-life and the area under the plasma concentration time curve is extended by 18% and 40% respectively.

In adults, mean steady state peak plasma concentrations ($C^{SS}max$) following a one hour infusion of 2.5mg/kg, 5mg/kg and 10mg/kg were 22.7 microMol (5.1 microgram/ml), 43.6 microMol (9.8 microgram/ml) and 92 microMol (20.7 microgram/ml), respectively. The corresponding trough levels ($C^{SS}min$) 7 hours later were 2.2 microMol (0.5 microgram/ml), 3.1 microMol (0.7 microgram/ml) and 10.2 microMol (2.3 microgram/ml), respectively.

In children over 1 year of age similar mean peak ($C^{SS}max$) and trough ($C^{SS}min$) levels were observed when a dose of $250mg/m^2$ was substituted for 5mg/kg and a dose of $500mg/m^2$ was substituted for 10mg/kg. In neonates (0 to 3 months of age) treated with doses of 10mg/kg administered by infusion over a one-hour period every 8 hours the $C^{SS}max$ was found to be 61.2 microMol (13.8 microgram/ml) and $C^{SS}min$ to be 10.1 microMol (2.3 microgram/ml). The terminal plasma half-life in these patients was 3.8 hours.

In the elderly total body clearance falls with increasing age associated with decreases in creatinine clearance although there is little change in the terminal plasma half-life.

In patients with chronic renal failure the mean terminal half-life was found to be 19.5 hours. The mean aciclovir half-life during haemodialysis was 5.7 hours. Plasma aciclovir levels dropped approximately 60% during dialysis.

Cerebrospinal fluid levels are approximately 50% of corresponding plasma levels. Plasma protein binding is relatively low (9 to 33%) and drug interactions involving binding site displacement are not anticipated.

5.3 Preclinical safety data

Mutagenicity:- The results of a wide range of mutagenicity tests *in vitro* and *in vivo* indicate that aciclovir is unlikely to pose a genetic risk to man.

Carcinogenicity:- Aciclovir was not found to be carcinogenic in long term studies in the rat and the mouse.

Teratogenicity:-Systemic administration of aciclovir in internationally accepted standard tests did not produce embryotoxic or teratogenic effects in rats, rabbits or mice.

In a non-standard test in rats, foetal abnormalities were observed, but only following such high subcutaneous doses that maternal toxicity was produced. The clinical relevance of these findings is uncertain.

Fertility:- Largely reversible adverse effects on spermatogenesis in association with overall toxicity in rats and dogs have been reported only at doses of aciclovir greatly in excess of those employed therapeutically. Two generation studies in mice did not reveal any effect of aciclovir on fertility.

There is no information on the effect of Zovirax Suspension on human female fertility. In patients with normal sperm count, chronically administered oral aciclovir has been shown to have no clinically significant effect on sperm count, motility or morphology.

6. PHARMACEUTICAL PARTICULARS

6.1 List of excipients

Sorbitol Solution, 70%, non-crystallising

Glycerol

Dispersible cellulose

Methyl parahydroxybenzoate

Propyl parahydroxybenzoate

Flavour, banana 5708023

Vanillin

Purified water

6.2 Incompatibilities

None Known.

6.3 Shelf life

3 years.

6.4 Special precautions for storage

Store below 25°C

6.5 Nature and contents of container

Neutral amber glass bottles sealed with white, child resistant caps with an EPE/Saranex liner, polyolefin screw caps or metal roll-on closures fitted with sealing wads of agglomerate cork faced with saran-coated paper or saran-coated expanded polyethylene wads.

This container and these closures are applicable to both pack sizes 25ml and 125ml.

The 25ml pack is a starter pack.

The 125ml pack contains a double-ended measuring spoon.

6.6 Instructions for use and handling

No special instructions.

Administrative Data

7. MARKETING AUTHORISATION HOLDER

The Wellcome Foundation Ltd

Glaxo Wellcome House

Berkeley Avenue

Greenford

Middlesex

UB6 ONN

Trading as

GlaxoSmithKline UK

Stockley Park West

Uxbridge

Middlesex UB11 1BT

8. MARKETING AUTHORISATION NUMBER(S)

PL 00003/0202

9. DATE OF FIRST AUTHORISATION/RENEWAL OF THE AUTHORISATION

30 April 2001

10. DATE OF REVISION OF THE TEXT

29 November 2004

11. Legal Status

POM

Zumenon 1mg

(Solvay Healthcare Limited)

1. NAME OF THE MEDICINAL PRODUCT

Zumenon® 1 mg

2. QUALITATIVE AND QUANTITATIVE COMPOSITION

This product contains 1 mg estradiol hemihydrate Ph.Eur. equivalent to 1 mg estradiol per tablet.

3. PHARMACEUTICAL FORM

White, round, biconvex, film-coated tablets imprinted 'S' on one side and '379' on the other.

4. CLINICAL PARTICULARS

4.1 Therapeutic indications

For the treatment of symptoms of oestrogen deficiency as a result of natural menopause or oophorectomy, e.g. hot flushes, nocturnal perspiration and atrophic changes in the genito-urinary tract.

In women with a uterus, a progestogen should be added to Zumenon for 10-14 days each month.

4.2 Posology and method of administration

One tablet daily without interruption. If clinical response is inadequate, dosage may be increased to two tablets daily, but should be reduced to one tablet daily as soon as practicable.

Treatment of hysterectomized women and postmenopausal women may be started on any convenient day. If the patient is menstruating, treatment is started on day 5 of bleeding.

4.3 Contraindications

Known, suspected or past history of carcinoma of the breast, endometrial carcinoma or other hormone dependent neoplasia.

Acute or chronic liver disease or history of liver disease where the liver function tests have failed to return to normal.

Active deep venous thrombosis, thromboembolic disorders, or a history of confirmed venous thromboembolism.

Cerebral vascular accident.

Abnormal genital bleeding of unknown aetiology.

Known or suspected pregnancy.

4.4 Special warnings and special precautions for use

Assessment of each woman prior to taking hormone replacement therapy (and at regular intervals thereafter) should include a personal and family medical history. Physical examination should be guided by this and by the contra-indications (section 4.3) and warnings (section 4.4) for this product. During assessment of each individual woman clinical examination of the breasts and pelvic examination should be performed where clinically indicated rather than as a routine procedure. Women should be encouraged to participate in the national breast cancer screening programme (mammography) and the national cervical cancer screening programme (cervical cytology) as appropriate for their age). Breast awareness should also be encouraged and women advised to report any changes in their breasts to their doctor or nurse.

A reanalysis of original data from 51 epidemiological studies reported a small or moderate increase in the probability of having breast cancer *diagnosed* in women currently or recently using HRT. The findings may be due to biological effects of HRT, earlier diagnosis, or a combination of both. The relative risk increased with duration of treatment (by 2.3% per year of use) and returned to normal in the course of five years cessation of HRT use. This is comparable to the increase in relative risk when natural menopause is delayed in the absence of HRT. Breast cancers diagnosed in current or recent users of HRT are more likely to be localised to the breast than those found in non-users. HRT use may not be associated with increased mortality from breast cancer.

Between the ages of 50 and 70, about 45 women in every 1000 not using HRT will have breast cancer diagnosed. It is estimated that among those who use HRT for 5 years starting at 50, 2 extra cases of breast cancer will be detected by age 70 in every 1000 women. For those who use HRT for 10 years there will be 6 extra cases of breast cancer, and for 15 years use, 12 extra cases of breast cancer in every 1000 women during the 20 year period until age 70.

It is important that the increased risk of being diagnosed with breast cancer is discussed with the patient and weighed against the known benefits of HRT.

Patients with an intact uterus should not be treated with unopposed oestrogen. There is an increased risk of endometrial hyperplasia or carcinoma associated with unopposed oestrogen. However, the appropriate addition of a progestogen to an oestrogen regimen lowers this risk.

Breakthrough bleeding may occasionally occur and can be the result of poor compliance or concurrent antibiotic use. It may however indicate endometrial pathology and therefore any doubt as to the cause of breakthrough bleeding is an indication for endometrial evaluation including endometrial biopsy.

Patients with or developing epilepsy, migraine, diabetes mellitus, cardiac failure, multiple sclerosis, hypertension, porphyria, haemoglobinopathies or otosclerosis should be carefully observed during treatment, as oestrogens may worsen these conditions. In patients with a past history of liver disease it is advisable to check liver functions on a regular basis.

Special care should be taken in patients with uterine leiomyomata and patients with (a history of) endometriosis as oestrogens may influence these conditions.

The indications for immediate withdrawal of therapy are:

- deep venous thrombosis
- thromboembolic disorders
- the appearance of jaundice
- the emergence of migraine - type headache
- sudden visual disturbances
- significant increase in blood pressure
- pregnancy

Epidemiological studies have suggested that hormone replacement therapy (HRT) is associated with an increased relative risk of developing venous thromboembolism (VTE) i.e. deep vein thrombosis or pulmonary embolism. The studies find a 2-3 fold increase for users compared with non-users which for healthy women amounts to a low risk of one extra case of VTE each year for every 5000 patients taking HRT.

Generally recognised risk factors for VTE include a personal or family history and severe obesity (Body Mass Index $>30\ kg/m^2$). In women with these factors the benefits of treatment with HRT need to be carefully weighed against risks.

The risk of VTE may be temporarily increased with prolonged immobilisation, major trauma or major surgery. In women on HRT scrupulous attention should be given to prophylactic measures to prevent VTE following surgery. Where prolonged immobilisation is liable to follow elective surgery, particularly abdominal or orthopaedic surgery to the lower limbs, consideration should be given to temporarily stopping HRT 4 weeks earlier, if this is possible.

If venous thromboembolism develops after initiating therapy the drug should be discontinued.

4.5 Interaction with other medicinal products and other forms of Interaction

Oestrogens interact with liver enzyme inducing drugs with increased metabolism of oestrogens, which may reduce the oestrogen effect. Interactions are documented for the following liver enzyme inducing drugs: barbiturates, phenytoin, rifampicin, carbamazepine.

4.6 Pregnancy and lactation

Known, or suspected pregnancy is a contra-indication to Zumenon therapy.

Lactation: this product is not indicated during this period.

4.7 Effects on ability to drive and use machines

No effects known.

4.8 Undesirable effects

During the first few months of treatment with Zumenon, breast tenderness may occur. Nausea, headache and oedema occur rarely. Symptoms are normally transient. Furthermore, skin reactions have been reported.

4.9 Overdose

There have been no reports of ill-effects from overdosing. If overdosage is discovered within two or three hours and is so large that treatment seems desirable, gastric lavage can safely be used. There is no specific antidote and further treatment should be symptomatic.

5. PHARMACOLOGICAL PROPERTIES

5.1 Pharmacodynamic properties

Estradiol is chemically and biologically identical to the endogenous human estradiol and is, therefore, classified as a human estrogen. Estradiol is the primary estrogen and the most active of the ovarian hormones. The endogenous estrogens are involved in certain functions of the uterus and accessory organs, including the proliferation of the endometrium and the cyclic changes in the cervix and vagina.

Estrogens are known to play an important role for bone and fat metabolism. Furthermore, estrogens also affect the autonomic nervous system and may have indirect positive psychotropic actions.

5.2 Pharmacokinetic properties

Following oral administration, micronised estradiol is readily absorbed, but extensively metabolised. The major unconjugated and conjugated metabolites are estrone and estrone sulphate. These metabolites can contribute to the estrogen activity, either directly or after conversion to estradiol. Estrone sulphate may undergo enterohepatic circulation. In urine, the major compounds are the glucuronides of estrone and estradiol.

Estrogens are secreted in the milk of nursing mothers.

5.3 Preclinical safety data

Supraphysiologically high doses (prolonged overdoses) of estradiol have been associated with the induction of tumours in estrogen-dependent target organs for all rodent species tested. Pronounced species differences in toxicology, pharmacology and pharmacodynamics exist.

6. PHARMACEUTICAL PARTICULARS

6.1 List of excipients

Lactose, methylhydroxypropyl cellulose, maize starch, colloidal anhydrous silica, magnesium stearate, polyethylene glycol 400, E171.

6.2 Incompatibilities

Not applicable

6.3 Shelf life

3 years.

6.4 Special precautions for storage

Do not store above 30°C.

6.5 Nature and contents of container

The tablets are packed in blister strips of 28. The blister strips are made of PVC film with covering Aluminium foil. Each carton contains 84 tablets.

6.6 Instructions for use and handling

Not applicable.

7. MARKETING AUTHORISATION HOLDER

Solvay Healthcare Limited

Mansbridge Road

West End

Southampton

SO18 3JD

8. MARKETING AUTHORISATION NUMBER(S)

PL 00512/0141

9. DATE OF FIRST AUTHORISATION/RENEWAL OF THE AUTHORISATION

16 August 2001

10. DATE OF REVISION OF THE TEXT

May 2001

Legal category

POM

Zumenon 2mg

(Solvay Healthcare Limited)

1. NAME OF THE MEDICINAL PRODUCT
Zumenon® 2 mg

2. QUALITATIVE AND QUANTITATIVE COMPOSITION
This product contains 2 mg estradiol hemihydrate Ph.Eur. equivalent to 2 mg estradiol per tablet.

3. PHARMACEUTICAL FORM
Brick-red, round, biconvex, film-coated tablets imprinted '$' on one side and '379' on the other.

4. CLINICAL PARTICULARS

4.1 Therapeutic indications
Hormone replacement therapy (HRT) for estrogen deficiency symptoms in peri and postmenopausal women.

Second line therapy for prevention of osteoporosis in postmenopausal women at high risk of future fractures who are intolerant of, or contraindicated for, other medicinal products approved for the prevention of osteoporosis.

The experience in treating women older than 65 years is limited.

4.2 Posology and method of administration
Adults (including the elderly):

Climacteric Symptoms
Therapy should be initiated with Zumenon 1 mg. The dosage may be increased if required by using Zumenon 2 mg. For maintenance therapy the lowest effective dose should be used.

One tablet daily without interruption. If clinical response is inadequate, dosage may be increased to two tablets daily, but should be reduced to one tablet daily as soon as practicable.

Prevention of Osteoporosis
One 2 mg tablet daily without interruption. Treatment should start as soon as possible after the onset of menopause and certainly within 2 or 3 years. Protection appears to be effective for as long as treatment continues, however data beyond 10 years are limited. A careful reappraisal of the risk benefit ratio should be undertaken before treating for longer than 5-10 years. For long term use see also Special Warnings and Precautions for Use.

Treatment of hysterectomised women and post-menopausal women may be started on any convenient day. If the patient is menstruating, treatment is started on day 5 of bleeding.

Breakthrough bleeding may occasionally occur in the first few weeks after initiating treatment and will usually settle.

Children

Zumenon is not indicated in children.

4.3 Contraindications
1. Known, suspected or past history of carcinoma of the breast, endometrial carcinoma or other hormone dependent neoplasia.
2. Acute or chronic liver disease or history of liver disease where the liver function tests have failed to return to normal.
3. Active deep venous thrombosis, thromboembolic disorders, or a history of confirmed venous thromboembolism.
4. Cerebral vascular accident.
5. Abnormal genital bleeding of unknown aetiology.
6. Rotor syndrome or Dubin-Johnson syndrome.
7. Severe cardiac or renal disease.
8. Known or suspected pregnancy.

4.4 Special warnings and special precautions for use
Assessment of each woman prior to taking hormone replacement therapy (and at regular intervals thereafter) should include a personal and family medical history. Physical examination should be guided by this and by the contraindications (section 4.3) and warnings (section 4.4) for this product. During assessment of each individual woman clinical examination of the breasts and pelvic examination should be performed where clinically indicated rather than as a routine procedure. Women should be encouraged to participate in the national breast cancer screening programme (mammography) and the national cervical cancer screening programme (cervical cytology) as appropriate for their age). Breast awareness should also be encouraged and women advised to report any changes in their breasts to their doctor or nurse.

A reanalysis of original data from 51 epidemiological studies reported a small or moderate increase in the probability of having breast cancer *diagnosed* in women currently or recently using HRT. The findings may be due to biological effects of HRT, earlier diagnosis, or a combination of both. The relative risk increased with duration of treatment (by 2.3% per year of use) and returned to normal in the course of five years cessation of HRT use. This is comparable to the increase in relative risk when natural menopause is delayed in the absence of HRT. Breast cancers diagnosed in current or recent users of HRT are more likely to be localised to the breast than those found in non-users. HRT use may not be associated with increased mortality from breast cancer.

Between the ages of 50 and 70, about 45 women in every 1000 not using HRT will have breast cancer diagnosed. It is estimated that among those who use HRT for 5 years starting at 50, 2 extra cases of breast cancer will be detected by age 70 in every 1000 women. For those who use HRT for 10 years there will be 6 extra cases of breast cancer, and for 15 years use, 12 extra cases of breast cancer in every 1000 women during the 20 year period until age 70.

It is important that the increased risk of being diagnosed with breast cancer is discussed with the patient and weighed against the known benefits of HRT.

Patients with an intact uterus should not be treated with unopposed oestrogen. There is an increased risk of endometrial hyperplasia or carcinoma associated with unopposed oestrogen. However, the appropriate addition of a progestogen to an oestrogen regimen lowers this risk.

Breakthrough bleeding may occasionally occur and can be the result of poor compliance or concurrent antibiotic use. It may however indicate endometrial pathology and therefore any doubt as to the cause of breakthrough bleeding is an indication for endometrial evaluation including endometrial biopsy.

Certain diseases may be made worse by hormone replacement therapy and patients with these conditions should be closely monitored. These include otosclerosis, multiple sclerosis, systemic lupus erythematosus, porphyria, melanoma, epilepsy, migraine, asthma, haemoglobinopathies, diabetes mellitus. In patients with a past history of liver disease it is advisable to check liver functions on a regular basis. In addition, pre-existing fibroids may increase in size during oestrogen therapy and symptoms associated with endometriosis may be exacerbated.

Epidemiological studies have suggested that hormone replacement therapy (HRT) is associated with an increased relative risk of developing venous thromboembolism (VTE) i.e. deep vein thrombosis or pulmonary embolism. The studies find a 2-3 fold increase for users compared with non-users which for healthy women amounts to a low risk of one extra case of VTE each year for every 5000 patients taking HRT.

Generally recognised risk factors for VTE include a personal or family history and severe obesity (Body Mass Index >30 kg/m^2). In women with these factors the benefits of treatment with HRT need to be carefully weighed against risks.

The risk of VTE may be temporarily increased with prolonged immobilisation, major trauma or major surgery. In women on HRT scrupulous attention should be given to prophylactic measures to prevent VTE following surgery. Where prolonged immobilisation is liable to follow elective surgery, particularly abdominal or orthopaedic surgery to the lower limbs, consideration should be given to temporarily stopping HRT 4 weeks earlier, if this is possible.

If venous thromboembolism develops after initiating therapy the drug should be discontinued.

As oestrogens may cause fluid retention, patients with cardiac or renal dysfunction should be carefully observed.

Zumenon is not an oral contraceptive. Women of childbearing potential should be advised to use non-hormonal contraceptive methods.

Most studies indicate that oestrogen replacement therapy has little effect on blood pressure and some indicate that oestrogen use may be associated with a small decrease. In addition, most studies on combined therapy indicate that the addition of progestogen also has little effect on blood pressure. Rarely, idiosyncratic hypertension may occur.

When oestrogens are administered to hypertensive women, supervision is necessary and blood pressure should be monitored at regular intervals.

It has been reported that there is an increase in the risk of surgically confirmed gall bladder disease in women receiving post-menopausal oestrogens.

4.5 Interaction with other medicinal products and other forms of Interaction
Oestrogens interact with liver enzyme inducing drugs with increased metabolism of oestrogens, which may reduce the oestrogen effect. Interactions are documented for the following liver enzyme inducing drugs: barbiturates, phenytoin, rifampicin, carbamazepine.

Changes in oestrogen serum concentrations may affect the results of certain endocrine or liver function tests.

4.6 Pregnancy and lactation
Known, or suspected pregnancy is a contra-indication to Zumenon therapy.

Lactation: this product is not indicated during this period.

4.7 Effects on ability to drive and use machines
No effects known.

4.8 Undesirable effects
The following side effects have been reported with oestrogen/progestogen therapy:

1. Genito-urinary system - Breakthrough bleeding, spotting, change in menstrual flow, dysmenorrhoea, premenstrual-like syndrome, amenorrhoea, increase in size of uterine fibromyomata, vaginal candidiasis, change in cervical erosion and in degree of cervical secretion, cystitis-like syndrome.
2. Breasts - Tenderness, enlargement, secretion.
3. Gastrointestinal - Nausea, vomiting, abdominal cramps, bloating, cholestatic jaundice.
4. Skin - Chloasma or melasma which may persist when drug is discontinued, erythema multiforme, erythema nodosum, haemorrhagic eruption.
5. Eyes - Steepening of corneal curvature, intolerance to contact lenses.
6. CNS - Headaches, migraine, dizziness, mental depression, chorea.
7. Miscellaneous - Increase or decrease in weight, reduced carbohydrate tolerance, aggravation of porphyria, oedema, changes in libido, leg cramps.

4.9 Overdose
There have been no reports of ill-effects following overdose. Overdose of oestrogen may cause nausea, and withdrawal bleeding may occur in females.

If overdosage is discovered within two or three hours and is so large that treatment seems desirable, gastric lavage can safely be used. There is no specific antidote and further treatment should be symptomatic.

5. PHARMACOLOGICAL PROPERTIES

5.1 Pharmacodynamic properties
Estradiol is chemically and biologically identical to the endogenous human estradiol and is, therefore, classified as a human oestrogen. Estradiol is the primary oestrogen and the most active of the ovarian hormones. The endogenous oestrogens are involved in certain functions of the uterus and accessory organs, including the proliferation of the endometrium and the cyclic changes in the cervix and vagina.

Oestrogens are known to play an important role for bone and fat metabolism. Furthermore, oestrogens also affect the autonomic nervous system and may have indirect positive psychotropic actions.

5.2 Pharmacokinetic properties
Following oral administration, micronised estradiol is readily absorbed, but extensively metabolised. The major unconjugated and conjugated metabolites are estrone and estrone sulphate. These metabolites can contribute to the oestrogen activity, either directly or after conversion to estradiol. Estrone sulphate may undergo enterohepatic circulation. In urine, the major compounds are the glucuronides of estrone and estradiol.

Oestrogens are secreted in the milk of nursing mothers.

5.3 Preclinical safety data
Supraphysiologically high doses (prolonged overdoses) of estradiol have been associated with the induction of tumours in oestrogen-dependent target organs for all rodent species tested. Pronounced species differences in toxicology, pharmacology and pharmacodynamics exist.

6. PHARMACEUTICAL PARTICULARS

6.1 List of excipients
Lactose, methylhydroxypropyl cellulose, maize starch, colloidal anhydrous silica, magnesium stearate, polyethylene glycol 400, titanium dioxide (E171), black, red and yellow iron oxides (E172).

6.2 Incompatibilities
Not applicable.

6.3 Shelf life
3 years.

6.4 Special precautions for storage
Do not store below 30°C.

Keep container in outer carton.

6.5 Nature and contents of container
The tablets are packed in blister strips of 28. The blister strips are made of PVC film with covering Aluminium foil. Each carton contains 84 tablets.

6.6 Instructions for use and handling
Not applicable

7. MARKETING AUTHORISATION HOLDER
Solvay Healthcare Ltd

Mansbridge Road

West End

Southampton

SO18 3JD

8. MARKETING AUTHORISATION NUMBER(S)
PL 00512/0100

9. DATE OF FIRST AUTHORISATION/RENEWAL OF THE AUTHORISATION
14 May 1997

10. DATE OF REVISION OF THE TEXT
December 2003

Zyban

(GlaxoSmithKline UK)

1. NAME OF THE MEDICINAL PRODUCT

Zyban ▼150 mg prolonged release film-coated tablets.

2. QUALITATIVE AND QUANTITATIVE COMPOSITION

Each tablet contains bupropion hydrochloride 150 mg.

For excipients, see 6.1.

3. PHARMACEUTICAL FORM

Prolonged release film-coated tablet.

White, film-coated, biconvex, round tablet printed on one side with GX CH7 and plain on the other side.

4. CLINICAL PARTICULARS

4.1 Therapeutic indications

Zyban tablets are indicated as an aid to smoking cessation in combination with motivational support in nicotine-dependent patients.

4.2 Posology and method of administration

Zyban should be used in accordance with smoking cessation guidelines.

Prescribers should assess the patient's motivation to quit. Smoking cessation therapies are more likely to succeed in those patients whom are motivated to quit and have motivational support.

Zyban tablets should be swallowed whole and not crushed or chewed.

Patients should be treated for 7-9 weeks.

Although discontinuation reactions are not expected with Zyban, a tapering-off period may be considered.

If at seven weeks no effect is seen, treatment should be discontinued.

Use in Adults

It is recommended that treatment is started while the patient is still smoking and a "target stop date" set within the first two weeks of treatment with Zyban, preferably in the second week.

The initial dose is 150mg to be taken daily for six days, increasing on day seven to 150mg twice daily.

There should be an interval of at least 8 hours between successive doses.

The maximum single dose must not exceed 150mg and the maximum total daily dose must not exceed 300mg.

Insomnia is a very common adverse event which can be reduced by avoiding bedtime doses of Zyban (provided there is at least 8 hours between doses).

Use in Children and Adolescents

Use in patients under 18 years of age is not recommended as the safety and efficacy of Zyban tablets have not been evaluated in these patients.

Use in Elderly Patients

Zyban should be used with caution in elderly patients. Greater sensitivity in some elderly individuals cannot be ruled out. The recommended dose in the elderly is 150mg once a day.

Use in Patients with Hepatic Insufficiency

Zyban should be used with caution in patients with hepatic impairment. Because of increased variability in the pharmacokinetics in patients with mild to moderate impairment the recommended dose in these patients is 150mg once a day.

Use in Patients with Renal Insufficiency

Zyban should be used with caution in patients with renal insufficiency. The recommended dose in these patients is 150mg once a day.

4.3 Contraindications

Zyban is contraindicated in patients with hypersensitivity to bupropion or any of the excipients.

Zyban is contraindicated in patients with a current seizure disorder or any history of seizures.

Zyban is contraindicated in patients with a known central nervous system (CNS) tumour.

Zyban is contraindicated in patients who, at any time during treatment, are undergoing abrupt withdrawal from alcohol or any medicinal product known to be associated with risk of seizures on withdrawal (in particular benzodiazepines and benzodiazepine-like agents).

Zyban is contraindicated in patients with a current or previous diagnosis of bulimia or anorexia nervosa.

Zyban is contraindicated for use in patients with severe hepatic cirrhosis.

Concomitant use of Zyban and monoamine oxidase inhibitors (MAOIs) is contraindicated. At least 14 days should elapse between discontinuation of irreversible MAOIs and initiation of treatment with Zyban. For reversible MAOIs, a 24 hour period is sufficient.

Zyban is contraindicated in patients with a history of bipolar disorder as it may precipitate a manic episode during the depressed phase of their illness.

Zyban should not be administered to patients being treated with any other medicinal product containing bupropion as the incidence of seizures is dose dependent.

4.4 Special warnings and special precautions for use

<u>Seizures</u>

The recommended dose of Zyban must not be exceeded, since bupropion is associated with a dose-related risk of seizure. At doses up to the maximum recommended daily dose (300mg of Zyban daily), the incidence of seizures is approximately 0.1% (1/1,000).

There is an increased risk of seizures occurring with the use of Zyban in the presence of predisposing risk factors which lower the seizure threshold. Zyban must not be used in patients with predisposing risk factors unless there is a compelling clinical justification for which the potential medical benefit of smoking cessation outweighs the potential increased risk of seizure. In these patients, a maximum dose of 150mg daily should be considered for the duration of treatment.

All patients should be assessed for predisposing risk factors, which include:

- concomitant administration of other medicinal products-known to lower the seizure threshold (e.g., antipsychotics, antidepressants, antimalarials, tramadol, theophylline, systemic steroids, quinolones and sedating antihistamines). For patients prescribed such medicinal products whilst taking Zyban, a maximum dose of150mg daily for the remainder of their treatment should be considered.
- alcohol abuse (see also 4.3 Contraindications)
- history of head trauma
- diabetes treated with hypoglycaemics or insulin
- use of stimulants or anorectic products.

Zyban should be discontinued and not recommenced in patients who experience a seizure while on treatment.

<u>Interactions (see 4.5 Interaction with other medicinal products and other forms of interaction)</u>

Due to pharmacokinetic interactions plasma levels of bupropion or its metabolites may be altered, which may increase the potential for undesirable effects (e.g. dry mouth, insomnia, seizures). Therefore care should be taken when bupropion is given concomitantly with medicinal products which can induce or inhibit the metabolism of bupropion.

Bupropion inhibits metabolism by cytochrome P450 2D6. Caution is advised when medicinal products metabolised by this enzyme are administered concomitantly.

<u>Neuropsychiatry</u>

Zyban is a centrally-acting noradrenaline (norepinephrine)/ dopamine reuptake inhibitor and as such the pharmacology resembles that of some antidepressants. Neuropsychiatric reactions have been reported (see 4.8 Undesirable Effects). In particular, psychotic and manic symptomatology have been reported mainly in patients with a known history of psychiatric illness.

Depressed mood may be a symptom of nicotine withdrawal. Depression, rarely including suicidal ideation, has been reported in patients undergoing a smoking cessation attempt. These symptoms have also been reported during Zyban treatment, and generally occurred early during the treatment course. Clinicians should be aware of the possible emergence of significant depressive symptomatology in patients undergoing a smoking cessation attempt, and should advise patients accordingly.

Data in animals suggest a potential for drug abuse. However, studies on abuse liability in humans and extensive clinical experience show that bupropion has low abuse potential.

<u>Hypersensitivity</u>

Zyban should be discontinued if patients experience hypersensitivity reactions during treatment. Clinicians should be aware that symptoms may progress or recur following the discontinuation of Zyban and should ensure symptomatic treatment is administered for an adequate length of time (at least one week). Symptoms typically include skin rash, pruritus, urticaria or chest pain but more severe reactions may include angioedema, dyspnoea/ bronchospasm, anaphylactic shock, erythema multiforme or Stevens-Johnson Syndrome. Arthralgia, myalgia and fever have also been reported in association with rash and other symptoms suggestive of delayed hypersensitivity. These symptoms may resemble serum sickness (See 4.8 Undesirable Effects). In most patients symptoms improved after stopping bupropion and initiating treatment with antihistamine or corticosteroids, and resolved over time.

<u>Hypertension</u>

In clinical practice, hypertension, which in some cases may be severe (see 4.8 Undesirable Effects) and require acute treatment, has been reported in patients receiving bupropion alone and in combination with nicotine replacement therapy. This has been observed in patients with and without pre-existing hypertension. A baseline blood pressure should be obtained at the start of treatment with subsequent monitoring, especially in patients with pre-existing hypertension. Consideration should be given to discontinuation of Zyban if a clinically significant increase in blood pressure is observed.

Limited clinical trial data suggest that higher smoking cessation rates may be achieved by the combination use of Zyban together with Nicotine Transdermal System (NTS). However, a higher rate of treatment-emergent hypertension was noted in the combination therapy group. If combination therapy with a NTS is used, caution must be exercised and weekly monitoring of blood pressure is recommended. Prior to initiation of combination therapy prescribers should consult the prescribing information of the relevant NTS.

<u>Specific patient groups</u>

Elderly – Clinical experience with bupropion has not identified any differences in tolerability between elderly and other adult patients. However, greater sensitivity of some elderly individuals cannot be ruled out. Elderly patients are more likely to have decreased renal function, hence 150 mg once a day is the recommended dose in these patients.

Hepatically-impaired - Bupropion is extensively metabolised in the liver to active metabolites, which are further metabolised. No statistically significant differences in the pharmacokinetics of bupropion were observed in patients with mild to moderate hepatic cirrhosis compared with healthy volunteers, but bupropion plasma levels showed a higher variability between individual patients. Therefore Zyban should be used with caution in patients with mild to moderate hepatic impairment and 150 mg once a day is the recommended dose in these patients.

All patients with hepatic impairment should be closely monitored for possible undesirable effects (e.g., insomnia, dry mouth) that could indicate high drug or metabolite levels.

Renally-impaired - Patients with impaired renal function were not studied. Bupropion is mainly excreted into urine as its metabolites. Therefore 150 mg once a day is the recommended dose in patients with renal impairment, as bupropion and its metabolites may accumulate in such patients to a greater extent than usual. The patient should be closely monitored for possible undesirable effects that could indicate high drug or metabolite levels.

4.5 Interaction with other medicinal products and other forms of Interaction

In patients receiving medicinal products known to lower the seizure threshold, Zyban must only be used if there is a compelling clinical justification for which the potential medical benefit of smoking cessation outweighs the increased risk of seizure (see 4.4 Special Warnings and Precautions for use).

<u>The effect of bupropion on other medicinal products:</u>

Although not metabolised by the CYP2D6 isoenzyme, bupropion and its main metabolite, hydroxybupropion, inhibit the CYP2D6 pathway. Co-administration of bupropion hydrochloride and desipramine to healthy volunteers known to be extensive metabolisers of the CYP2D6 isoenzyme resulted in large (2- to 5-fold) increases in the C_{max} and AUC of desipramine. Inhibition of CYP2D6 was present for at least 7 days after the last dose of bupropion hydrochloride.

Although not formally studied, concomitant therapy with medicinal products with narrow therapeutic indices that are predominantly metabolised by CYP2D6 should be initiated at the lower end of the dose range of the concomitant medicinal product. Such medicinal products include certain antidepressants (e.g. desipramine, imipramine, paroxetine), antipsychotics (e.g. risperidone, thioridazine), beta-blockers (e.g. metoprolol), and Type 1C antiarrhythmics (e.g. propafanone, flecainide). If Zyban is added to the treatment regimen of a patient already receiving such a medicinal product, the need to decrease the dose of the original medicinal product should be considered. In these cases the expected benefit of treatment with Zyban should be carefully considered compared with the potential risks.

<u>The effect of other medicinal products on bupropion:</u>

In vitro findings indicate that bupropion is metabolised to its major active metabolite hydroxybupropion primarily by the cytochrome P450 CYP2B6 (see 5.2 Pharmacokinetic Properties). Care should therefore be exercised when Zyban is co-administered with medicinal products that may affect the CYP2B6 isoenzyme (e.g.: orphenadrine, cyclophosphamide, ifosfamide).

Since bupropion is extensively metabolised, caution is advised when bupropion is co-administered with medicinal products known to induce metabolism (e.g. carbamazepine, phenytoin) or inhibit metabolism (e.g. valproate), as these may affect its clinical efficacy and safety.

Nicotine, administered transdermally by patches, did not affect the pharmacokinetics of bupropion and its metabolites.

<u>Other interactions:</u>

Smoking is associated with an increase in CYP1A2 activity. After cessation of smoking, reduced clearance of medicinal products metabolised by this enzyme, with subsequent increases in plasma levels, may occur. This may be particularly important for those medicinal products primarily metabolised by CYP1A2 with narrow therapeutic windows (e.g. theophylline, tacrine and clozapine). The clinical consequences of smoking cessation on other medicinal products that are partially metabolised by CYP1A2 (e.g., imipramine, olanzapine, clomipramine, and fluvoxamine) are unknown. In addition, limited data indicate that the metabolism of flecainide or pentazocine may also be induced by smoking.

Administration of Zyban to patients receiving either levodopa or amantadine concurrently should be undertaken with caution. Limited clinical data suggest a higher incidence of undesirable effects (e.g. nausea, vomiting, and neuropsychiatric events – see 4.8 Undesirable Effects) in patients receiving bupropion concurrently with either levodopa or amantadine.

Although clinical data do not identify a pharmacokinetic interaction between bupropion and alcohol, there have been rare reports of adverse neuropsychiatric events or reduced alcohol tolerance in patients drinking alcohol during Zyban treatment. The consumption of alcohol during Zyban treatment should be minimised or avoided.

Since monoamine oxidase A and B inhibitors also enhance the catecholaminergic pathways, by a different mechanism from bupropion, concomitant use of Zyban and monoamine oxidase inhibitors (MAOIs) is contraindicated (see 4.3 Contra-indications) as there is an increased possibility of adverse reactions from their co-administration. At least 14 days should elapse between discontinuation of irreversible MAOIs and initiation of treatment with Zyban. For reversible MAOIs, a 24 hour period is sufficient.

4.6 Pregnancy and lactation

The safety of Zyban for use in human pregnancy has not been established.

Evaluation of experimental animal studies does not indicate direct or indirect harmful effects with respect to the development of the embryo or foetus, the course of gestation and peri-natal or post-natal development. Exposure in animals was, however, similar to the systemic exposure achieved in humans at the maximum recommended dose. The potential risk in humans is unknown.

Pregnant women should be encouraged to quit smoking without the use of pharmacotherapy. Zyban should not be used in pregnancy.

As bupropion and its metabolites are excreted in human breast milk mothers should be advised not to breast feed while taking Zyban.

4.7 Effects on ability to drive and use machines

As with other CNS acting drugs bupropion may affect ability to perform tasks that require judgement or motor and cognitive skills. Zyban has also been reported to cause dizziness and lightheadedness. Patients should therefore exercise caution before driving or use of machinery until they are reasonably certain Zyban does not adversely affect their performance.

4.8 Undesirable effects

The list below provides information on the undesirable effects identified from clinical experience, categorised by incidence and body system. It is important to note that smoking cessation is often associated with nicotine withdrawal symptoms (e.g. agitation, insomnia, tremor, sweating), some of which are also recognised as adverse events associated with Zyban.

Undesirable effects are ranked under headings of frequency using the following convention; very common (>1/10); common (>1/100, <1/10); uncommon (>1/1,000, <1/100); rare (>1/10000, <1/1,000).

Cardiovascular	Uncommon	Tachycardia, increased blood pressure (sometimes severe), flushing
	Rare	Vasodilation, postural hypotension, syncope, palpitations
CNS	Very common	Insomnia (see 4.2 Posology and Method of Administration)
	Common	Tremor, concentration disturbance, headache, dizziness, depression (see 4.4 Special Warnings and Precautions for Use), agitation, anxiety
	Uncommon	Confusion
	Rare	Seizures (see below), irritability, hostility, hallucinations, depersonalisation, dystonia, ataxia, Parkinsonism, twitching, incoordination, abnormal dreams including nightmares, memory impairment, paraesthesia
Endocrine and metabolic	Uncommon	Anorexia.
	Rare	Blood glucose disturbances
Gastrointestinal	Common	Dry mouth, gastrointestinal disturbance including nausea and vomiting, abdominal pain, constipation
General (body)	Common	Fever
	Uncommon	Chest pain, asthenia
Genitourinary	Rare	Urinary frequency and/or retention
Hepatobiliary	Rare	Elevated liver enzymes, jaundice, hepatitis
Skin / Hypersensitivity:	Common	Rash, pruritus, sweating. Hypersensitivity reactions such as urticaria.
	Rare	More severe hypersensitivity reactions including angioedema, dyspnoea/ bronchospasm and anaphylactic shock. Arthralgia, myalgia and fever have also been reported in association with rash and other symptoms suggestive of delayed hypersensitivity. These symptoms may resemble serum sickness. Erythema multiforme and Stevens Johnson syndrome have also been reported. Exacerbation of psoriasis
Special senses	Common	Taste disorders
	Uncommon	Tinnitus, visual disturbance

The incidence of seizures is approximately 0.1% (1/1,000). The most common type of seizures is generalised tonic-clonic seizures, a seizure type which can result in some cases in post-ictal confusion or memory impairment. (See 4.4 Special Warnings And Precautions for Use).

4.9 Overdose

Acute ingestion of doses in excess of 10 times the maximum therapeutic dose has been reported. In addition to those events reported as Undesirable Effects, overdose has resulted in symptoms including drowsiness, loss of consciousnessand/or ECG changes such as conduction disturbances, arrhythmias and tachycardia. Experimental and clinical data do not rule out potential for QT prolongation and widening of the QRS at supra-therapeutic levels. Although most patients recovered without sequelae, deaths associated with overdoses of bupropion have been reported rarely in patients ingesting massive doses of the drug.

Treatment: In the event of overdose, hospitalisation is advised. ECG and vital signs should be monitored.

Ensure an adequate airway, oxygenation and ventilation. Gastric lavage may be indicated if performed soon after ingestion. The use of activated charcoal is also recommended. No specific antidote for bupropion is known.

5. PHARMACOLOGICAL PROPERTIES

5.1 Pharmacodynamic properties

Pharmacotherapeutic group: drugs used in nicotine dependence, ATC code: N07B A02.

Bupropion is a selective inhibitor of the neuronal re-uptake of catecholamines (noradrenaline (norepinephrine) and dopamine) with minimal effect on the re-uptake of indolamines (serotonin) and does not inhibit either monoamine oxidase. The mechanism by which bupropion enhances the ability of patients to abstain from smoking is unknown. However, it is presumed that this action is mediated by noradrenergic and/or dopaminergic mechanisms.

5.2 Pharmacokinetic properties

Absorption

After oral administration of 150 mg bupropion hydrochloride as a prolonged release tablet to healthy volunteers, maximum plasma concentrations (C_{max}) of approximately 100 nanograms per ml are observed after about 2.5 to 3 hours. The AUC and C_{max} values of bupropion and its active metabolites hydroxybupropion and threohydrobupropion increase dose proportionally over a dose range of 50-200 mg following single dosing and over a dose range of 300-450 mg/day following chronic dosing. The C_{max} and AUC values of hydroxybupropion are approximately 3 and 14 times higher, respectively, than bupropion C_{max} and AUC values. The C_{max} of threohydrobupropion is comparable with the C_{max} of bupropion, while the AUC of threohydrobupropion is approximately 5 times higher than that of bupropion. Peak plasma levels of hydroxybupropion and threohydrobupropion are reached after about 6 hours following administration of a single dose of bupropion. Plasma levels of erythrohydrobupropion (an isomer of threohydrobupropion, which is also active) are not quantifiable after single dosing with bupropion.

After chronic dosing with bupropion 150 mg bid, the C_{max} of bupropion is similar to values reported after single dosing. For hydroxybupropion and threohydrobupropion, the C_{max} values are higher (about 4 and 7 times respectively) at steady-state than after a single dosing. Plasma levels of erythrohydrobupropion are comparable to steady-state plasma levels of bupropion. Steady-state of bupropion and its metabolites is reached within 5-8 days. The absolute bioavailability of bupropion is not known; excretion data in urine, however, show that at least 87% of the dose of bupropion is absorbed. The absorption of bupropion is not significantly influenced when taken concurrently with food.

Distribution

Bupropion is widely distributed with an apparent volume of distribution of approximately 2000 L.

Bupropion, hydroxybupropion and threohydrobupropion bind moderately to plasma proteins (84%, 77% and 42%, respectively).

Bupropion and its active metabolites are excreted in human breast milk. Animal studies show that bupropion and its active metabolites pass the blood-brain barrier and the placenta.

Metabolism

Bupropion is extensively metabolised in humans. Three pharmacologically active metabolites have been identified in plasma: hydroxybupropion and the amino-alcohol isomers, threohydrobupropion and erythrohydrobupropion. These may have clinical importance, as their plasma concentrations are as high or higher than those of bupropion. The active metabolites are further metabolised to inactive metabolites (some of which have not been fully characterised but may include conjugates) and excreted in the urine.

In vitro studies indicate that bupropion is metabolised to its major active metabolite hydroxybupropion primarily by the CYP2B6, while CYP1A2, 2A6, 2C9, 3A4 and 2E1 are less involved. In contrast, formation of threohydrobupropion involves carbonyl reduction but does not involve cytochrome P450 isoenzymes. (See 4.5 Interaction with Other Medicinal Products and Other Forms of Interaction)

The inhibition potential of threohydrobupropion and erythrohydrobupropion towards cytochrome P450 has not been studied.

Bupropion and hydroxybupropion are both inhibitors of the CYP2D6 isoenzyme with K_i values of 21 and 13.3μM, respectively (See 4.5 Interaction with Other Medicinal Products and Other Forms of Interaction).

Following oral administration of a single 150-mg dose of bupropion, there was no difference in C_{max}, half-life, T_{max}, AUC, or clearance of bupropion or its major metabolites between smokers and non-smokers.

Bupropion has been shown to induce its own metabolism in animals following sub-chronic administration. In humans, there is no evidence of enzyme induction of bupropion or hydroxybupropion in volunteers or patients receiving recommended doses of bupropion hydrochloride for 10 to 45 days.

Elimination

Following oral administration of 200mg of ^{14}C-bupropion in humans, 87% and 10% of the radioactive dose were recovered in the urine and faeces, respectively. The fraction of the dose of bupropion excreted unchanged was only 0.5%, a finding consistent with the extensive metabolism of bupropion. Less than 10% of this ^{14}C dose was accounted for in the urine as active metabolites.

The mean apparent clearance following oral administration of bupropion hydrochloride is approximately 200 L/hr and the mean elimination half-life of bupropion is approximately 20 hours.

The elimination half-life of hydroxybupropion is approximately 20 hours. The elimination half-lives for threohydrobupropion and erythrohydrobupropion are longer (37 and 33 hours, respectively).

Special Patient Groups:

Patients with renal impairment

The effect of renal disease on the pharmacokinetics of bupropion has not been studied. The elimination of the major metabolites of bupropion may be affected by reduced renal function. (See 4.4 Special Warnings and Precautions for Use).

Patients with hepatic impairment

The pharmacokinetics of bupropion and its active metabolites were not statistically significantly different in patients with mild to moderate cirrhosis when compared to healthy volunteers, although more variability was observed between individual patients. (see 4.4 Special Warnings And Precautions for Use) For patients with severe hepatic cirrhosis, the bupropion Cmax and AUC were substantially increased (mean difference approximately 70% and 3-fold, respectively) and more variable when compared to the values in healthy volunteers; the mean half-life was also longer (by approximately 40%). For hydroxybupropion, the mean Cmax was lower (by approximately 70%), the mean AUC tended to be higher (by approximately 30%), the median Tmax was later (by approximately 20 hrs), and the mean half-lives were longer (by approximately 4-fold) than in healthy volunteers. For threohydrobupropion and erythrohydrobupropion, the mean Cmax tended to be lower (by approximately 30%), the mean AUC tended to be higher (by approximately 50%), the median Tmax was later (by approximately 20 hrs), and the mean half-life was longer (by approximately 2-fold) than in healthy volunteers. (see 4.3 Contraindications)

Elderly patients

Pharmacokinetic studies in the elderly have shown variable results. A single dose study showed that the pharmacokinetics of bupropion and its metabolites in the elderly do not differ from those in the younger adults. Another pharmacokinetic study, single and multiple dose, has suggested that accumulation of bupropion and its metabolites may occur to a greater extent in the elderly. Clinical experience has not identified differences in tolerability between elderly and younger patients, but greater sensitivity in older patients cannot be ruled out. (see 4.4 Special Warnings And Precautions for Use)

5.3 Preclinical safety data

In animal experiments bupropion doses several times higher than therapeutic doses in humans caused, amongst others, the following dose-related symptoms: ataxia and convulsions in rats, general weakness, trembling and emesis in dogs and increased lethality in both species. Due to enzyme induction in animals but not in humans, systemic exposures in animals were similar to the systemic exposures seen in humans at the maximum recommended dose.

Liver changes are seen in animal studies but these reflect the action of a hepatic enzyme inducer. At recommended doses in humans, bupropion does not induce its own metabolism. This suggests that the hepatic findings in laboratory animals have only limited importance in the evaluation and risk assessment of bupropion.

Genotoxicity data indicate that bupropion is a weak bacterial mutagen, but not a mammalian mutagen, and therefore is of no concern as a human genotoxic agent. Mouse and rat studies confirm the absence of carcinogenicity in these species.

6. PHARMACEUTICAL PARTICULARS

6.1 List of excipients

Tablet core

Microcrystalline cellulose

Hypromellose

Cysteine hydrochloride monohydrate

Magnesium stearate

Film coat

Hypromellose

Macrogol 400

Titanium dioxide (E171)

Carnauba wax

Printing ink

Iron oxide black (E172)

Hypromellose

6.2 Incompatibilities

Not applicable

6.3 Shelf life

2 years.

6.4 Special precautions for storage

Do not store above 25°C. Store in the original package.

6.5 Nature and contents of container

Cartons containing cold form foil / foil blister packs (PA-Alu-PVC / Alu).

30, 40, 50, 60 or 100 tablets are supplied in each pack. Each blister strip contains 10 tablets. Not all pack sizes may be marketed.

6.6 Instructions for use and handling

No special requirements.

Administrative Details

7. MARKETING AUTHORISATION HOLDER

Glaxo Wellcome UK Limited

trading as

GlaxoSmithKline UK

Stockley Park West

Uxbridge

Middlesex UB11 1BT

UK

8. MARKETING AUTHORISATION NUMBER(S)

PL 10949/0340

9. DATE OF FIRST AUTHORISATION/RENEWAL OF THE AUTHORISATION

7 June 2000 / 1 December 2004

10. DATE OF REVISION OF THE TEXT

20 July 2005

Issue number: 8

Zyloric Tablets 100mg, 300mg

(GlaxoSmithKline UK)

1. NAME OF THE MEDICINAL PRODUCT

Zyloric 100 mg Tablets

Zyloric 300 mg Tablets

2. QUALITATIVE AND QUANTITATIVE COMPOSITION

Allopurinol 100 mg (Zyloric Tablets)

Allopurinol 300 mg (Zyloric-300 Tablets)

3. PHARMACEUTICAL FORM

Tablet

4. CLINICAL PARTICULARS

4.1 Therapeutic indications

Zyloric is indicated for reducing urate/uric acid formation in conditions where urate/uric acid deposition has already occurred (e.g. gouty arthritis, skin tophi, nephrolithiasis) or is a predictable clinical risk (e.g. treatment of malignancy potentially leading to acute uric acid nephropathy). The main clinical conditions where urate/uric acid deposition may occur are: idiopathic gout; uric acid lithiasis; acute uric acid nephropathy; neoplastic disease and myeloproliferative disease with high cell turnover rates, in which high urate levels occur either spontaneously, or after cytotoxic therapy; certain enzyme disorders which lead to overproduction of urate, for example: hypoxanthine-guanine phosphoribosyltransferase, including Lesch-Nyhan syndrome; glucose-6-phosphatase including glycogen storage disease; phosphoribosylpyrophosphate synthetase, phosphoribosylpyrophosphate amidotransferase; adenine phosphoribosyltransferase. Zyloric is indicated for management of 2,8-dihydroxyadenine (2,8-DHA) renal stones related to deficient activity of adenine phosphoribosyltransferase.

Zyloric is indicated for the management of recurrent mixed calcium oxalate renal stones in the presence of hyperuricosuria, when fluid, dietary and similar measures have failed.

4.2 Posology and method of administration

Dosage in Adults: Zyloric should be introduced at low dosage e.g. 100mg/day to reduce the risk of adverse reactions and increased only if the serum urate response is unsatisfactory. Extra caution should be exercised if renal function is poor (*see Dosage in renal impairment*). The following dosage schedules are suggested:

100 to 200 mg daily in mild conditions,

300 to 600 mg daily in moderately severe conditions,

700 to 900 mg daily in severe conditions.

If dosage on a mg/kg bodyweight basis is required, 2 to 10 mg/kg bodyweight/day should be used.

Dosage in children: Children under 15 years: 10 to 20 mg/kg bodyweight/day up to a maximum of 400 mg daily. Use in children is rarely indicated, except in malignant conditions (especially leukaemia) and certain enzyme disorders such as Lesch-Nyhan syndrome.

Dosage in the elderly: In the absence of specific data, the lowest dosage which produces satisfactory urate reduction should be used. Particular attention should be paid to advice in *Dosage in renal impairment* and *Precautions and Warnings*.

Dosage in renal impairment: Since allopurinol and its metabolites are excreted by the kidney, impaired renal function may lead to retention of the drug and/or its metabolites with consequent prolongation of plasma half-lives. In severe renal insufficiency, it may be advisable to use less than 100 mg per day or to use single doses of 100mg at longer intervals than one day.

If facilities are available to monitor plasma oxipurinol concentrations, the dose should be adjusted to maintain plasma oxipurinol levels below 100 micromol/litre (15.2 mg/litre).

Allopurinol and its metabolites are removed by renal dialysis. If dialysis is required two to three times a week consideration should be given to an alternative dosage schedule of 300-400 mg Zyloric immediately after each dialysis with none in the interim.

Dosage in hepatic impairment: Reduced doses should be used in patients with hepatic impairment. Periodic liver function tests are recommended during the early stages of therapy.

Treatment of high urate turnover conditions, e.g. neoplasia, Lesch-Nyhan syndrome: It is advisable to correct existing hyperuricaemia and/or hyperuricosuria with Zyloric before starting cytotoxic therapy. It is important to ensure adequate hydration to maintain optimum diuresis and to attempt alkalinisation of urine to increase solubility of urinary urate/uric acid. Dosage of Zyloric should be at the lower end of the recommended dosage schedule.

If urate nephropathy or other pathology has compromised renal function, the advice given in *Dosage in renal impairment* should be followed.

These steps may reduce the risk of xanthine and/or oxipurinol deposition complicating the clinical situation. See also *Drug Interactions And Adverse Reactions.*

Monitoring Advice: The dosage should be adjusted by monitoring serum urate concentrations and urinary urate/uric acid levels at appropriate intervals.

Instructions for Use: Zyloric may be taken orally once a day after a meal. It is well tolerated, especially after food. Should the daily dosage exceed 300 mg and gastrointestinal intolerance be manifested, a divided doses regimen may be appropriate.

4.3 Contraindications

Zyloric should not be administered to individuals known to be hypersensitive to allopurinol or to any of the components of the formulation.

4.4 Special warnings and special precautions for use

Zyloric should be withdrawn *immediately* when a skin rash or other evidence of sensitivity occurs. Reduced doses should be used in patients with hepatic or renal impairment. Patients under treatment for hypertension or cardiac insufficiency, for example with diuretics or ACE inhibitors, may have some concomitant impairment of renal function and allopurinol should be used with care in this group.

Asymptomatic hyperuricaemia per se is generally not considered an indication for use of Zyloric. Fluid and dietary modification with management of the underlying cause may correct the condition.

Acute gouty attacks: Allopurinol treatment should not be started until an acute attack of gout has completely subsided, as further attacks may be precipitated.

In the early stages of treatment with Zyloric, as with uricosuric agents, an acute attack of gouty arthritis may be precipitated. Therefore it is advisable to give prophylaxis with a suitable anti-inflammatory agent or colchicine for at least one month. The literature should be consulted for details of appropriate dosage and precautions and warnings.

If acute attacks develop in patients receiving allopurinol, treatment should continue at the same dosage while the acute attack is treated with a suitable anti-inflammatory agent.

Xanthine deposition: In conditions where the rate of urate formation is greatly increased (e.g. malignant disease and its treatment, Lesch-Nyhan syndrome) the absolute concentration of xanthine in urine could, in rare cases, rise sufficiently to allow deposition in the urinary tract. This risk may be minimised by adequate hydration to achieve optimal urine dilution.

Impaction of uric acid renal stones: Adequate therapy with Zyloric will lead to dissolution of large uric acid renal pelvic stones, with the remote possibility of impaction in the ureter.

4.5 Interaction with other medicinal products and other forms of Interaction

6 -mercaptopurine and azathioprine:

Azathioprine is metabolised to 6-mercaptopurine which is inactivated by the action of xanthine oxidase. When 6-mercaptopurine or azathioprine is given concurrently with Zyloric, only one-quarter of the usual dose of 6-mercaptopurine or azathioprine should be given because inhibition of xanthine oxidase will prolong their activity.

Vidarabine (Adenine Arabinoside): Evidence suggests that the plasma half-life of vidarabine is increased in the presence of allopurinol. When the two products are used concomitantly extra vigilance is necessary, to recognise enhanced toxic effects.

Salicylates and uricosuric agents: oxipurinol, the major metabolite of allopurinol and itself therapeutically active, is excreted by the kidney in a similar way to urate. Hence, drugs with uricosuric activity such as probenecid or large doses of salicylate may accelerate the excretion of oxipurinol. This may decrease the therapeutic activity of Zyloric, but the significance needs to be assessed in each case.

Chlorpropamide: If Zyloric is given concomitantly with chlorpropamide when renal function is poor, there may be an increased risk of prolonged hypoglycaemic activity because allopurinol and chlorpropamide may compete for excretion in the renal tubule.

Coumarin anticoagulants

There have been rare reports of increased effect of warfarin and other coumarin anticoagulants when co-administered with allopurinol, therefore, all patients receiving anticoagulants must be carefully monitored.

Phenytoin: Allopurinol may inhibit hepatic oxidation of phenytoin but the clinical significance has not been demonstrated.

Theophylline: Inhibition of the metabolism of theophylline has been reported. The mechanism of the interaction may be explained by xanthine oxidase being involved in the biotransformation of theophylline in man. Theophylline levels should be monitored in patients starting or increasing allopurinol therapy.

Ampicillin/Amoxicillin: An increase in frequency of skin rash has been reported among patients receiving ampicillin or amoxicillin concurrently with allopurinol compared to patients who are not receiving both drugs. The cause of the reported association has not been established. However, it is recommended that in patients receiving allopurinol an alternative to ampicillin or amoxicillin is used where available.

Cyclophosphamide, doxorubicin, bleomycin, procarbazine, mechloroethamine: Enhanced bone marrow suppression by cyclophosphamide and other cytotoxic agents has been reported among patients with neoplastic disease (other than leukaemia), in the presence of allopurinol. However, in a well-controlled study of patients treated with cyclophosphamide, doxorubicin, bleomycin, procarbazine and/or mechloroethamine (chlormethine hydrochloride) allopurinol did not appear to increase the toxic reaction of these cytotoxic agents.

Ciclosporin: Reports suggest that the plasma concentration of ciclosporin may be increased during concomitant treatment with allopurinol. The possibility of enhanced ciclosporin toxicity should be considered if the drugs are co-administered.

4.6 Pregnancy and lactation

There is inadequate evidence of safety of Zyloric in human pregnancy, although it has been in wide use for many years without apparent ill consequence.

Use in pregnancy only when there is no safer alternative and when the disease itself carries risk for the mother or unborn child.

Reports indicate that allopurinol and oxipurinol are excreted in human breast milk. Concentrations of 1.4mg/litre allopurinol and 53.7 mg/litre oxipurinol have been demonstrated in breast milk from woman taking Zyloric 300 mg/day. However, there are no data concerning the effects of allopurinol or its metabolites on the breast-fed baby.

4.7 Effects on ability to drive and use machines

Since adverse reactions such as somnolence, vertigo and ataxia have been reported in patients receiving allopurinol, patients should exercise caution before driving, using machinery or participating in dangerous activities until they are reasonably certain that allopurinol does not adversely affect performance.

4.8 Undesirable effects

Adverse reactions in association with Zyloric are rare in the overall treated population and mostly of a minor nature. The incidence is higher in the presence of renal and/or hepatic disorder.

Skin and hypersensitivity reactions: These are the most common reactions and may occur at any time during treatment. They may be pruritic, maculopapular, sometimes scaly, sometimes purpuric and rarely exfoliative. Fixed drug eruptions occur very rarely. Zyloric should be withdrawn *immediately* should such reactions occur. After recovery from mild reactions, Zyloric may, if desired, be re-introduced at a small dose (e.g. 50mg/day) and gradually increased. If the rash recurs, Zyloric should be *permanently* withdrawn as more severe hypersensitivity reactions may occur.

Skin reactions associated with exfoliation, fever, lymphadenopathy, arthralgia and/or eosinophilia including Stevens-Johnson Syndrome and Toxic Epidermal Necrolysis occur rarely. Associated vasculitis and tissue response may be manifested in various ways including hepatitis, renal impairment and very rarely, seizures. If such reactions do occur, it may be at any time during treatment, Zyloric should be withdrawn *immediately and permanently.*

Corticosteroids may be beneficial in overcoming hypersensitivity skin reactions. When generalised hypersensitivity reactions have occurred, renal and/or hepatic disorder has usually been present particularly when the outcome has been fatal.

Very rarely acute anaphylactic shock has been reported.

Angioimmunoblastic lymphadenopathy: Angioimmunoblastic lymphadenopathy has been described rarely following biopsy of a generalised lymphadenopathy. It appears to be reversible on withdrawal of Zyloric.

Hepatic functions: Rare reports of hepatic dysfunction ranging from asymptomatic rises in liver function tests to hepatitis (including hepatic necrosis and granulomatous hepatitis) have been reported without overt evidence of more generalised hypersensitivity.

Gastrointestinal disorder: In early clinical studies, nausea and vomiting were reported. Further reports suggest that this reaction is not a significant problem and can be avoided by taking Zyloric after meals. Recurrent haematemesis has been reported as an extremely rare event, as has steatorrhoea.

Blood and lymphatic system: Occasional reports have been received of thrombocytopenia, agranulocytosis and aplastic anaemia, particularly in individuals with impaired renal and/or hepatic function, reinforcing the need for particular care in this group of patients.

Miscellaneous: the following complaints have been reported occasionally; fever, general malaise, asthenia, headache, vertigo, ataxia, somnolence, coma depression, paralysis, paraesthesiae, neuropathy, visual disorder, cataract, macular changes, taste perversion, stomatitis, changed bowel habit, infertility, impotence, diabetes mellitus, hyperlipaemia, furunculosis, alopecia, discoloured hair, angina, hypertension, bradycardia, oedema, uraemia, haematuria, angioedema, gynacomastia.

4.9 Overdose

Ingestion of up to 22.5 g allopurinol without adverse effect has been reported. Symptoms and signs including nausea, vomiting, diarrhoea and dizziness have been reported in a patient who ingested 20 g allopurinol. Recovery followed general supportive measures. Massive absorption of Zyloric may lead to considerable inhibition of xanthine oxidase activity, which should have no untoward effects unless affecting concomitant medication, especially with 6-mercaptopurine and/or azathioprine. Adequate hydration to maintain optimum diuresis facilitates excretion of allopurinol and its metabolites. If considered necessary haemodialysis may be used.

5. PHARMACOLOGICAL PROPERTIES

5.1 Pharmacodynamic properties

Allopurinol is a xanthine-oxidase inhibitor. Allopurinol and its main metabolite oxipurinol lower the level of uric acid in plasma and urine by inhibition of xanthine oxidase, the enzyme catalyzing the oxidation of hypoxanthine to xanthine and xanthine to uric acid. In addition to the inhibition of purine catabolism in some but not all hyperuricaemic patients, de novo purine biosynthesis is depressed via feedback inhibition of hypoxanthine-guanine phosphoribosyltransferase. Other metabolites of allopurinol include allopurinol-riboside and oxipurinol-7 riboside.

5.2 Pharmacokinetic properties

Allopurinol is active when given orally and is rapidly absorbed from the upper gastrointestinal tract. Studies have detected allopurinol in the blood 30-60 minutes after dosing. Estimates of bioavailability vary from 67% to 90%. Peak plasma levels of allopurinol generally occur approximately 1.5 hours after oral administration of Zyloric, but fall rapidly and are barely detectable after 6 hours. Peak levels of oxipurinol generally occur after 3-5 hours after oral administration of Zyloric and are much more sustained.

Allopurinol is negligibly bound by plasma proteins and therefore variations in protein binding are not thought to significantly alter clearance. The apparent volume of distribution of allopurinol is approximately 1.6 litre/kg which suggests relatively extensive uptake by tissues. Tissue concentrations of allopurinol have not been reported in humans, but it is likely that allopurinol and oxipurinol will be present in the highest concentrations in the liver and intestinal mucosa where xanthine oxidase activity is high.

Approximately 20% of the ingested allopurinol is excreted in the faeces. Elimination of allopurinol is mainly by metabolic conversion to oxipurinol by xanthine oxidase and aldehyde oxidase, with less than 10% of the unchanged drug excreted in the urine. Allopurinol has a plasma half-life of about 1 to 2 hours.

Oxipurinol is a less potent inhibitor of xanthine oxidase than allopurinol, but the plasma half-life of oxipurinol is far more prolonged. Estimates range from 13 to 30 hours in man. Therefore effective inhibition of xanthine oxidase is maintained over a 24 hour period with a single daily dose of Zyloric. Patients with normal renal function will gradually accumulate oxipurinol until a steady-state plasma oxipurinol concentration is reached. Such patients, taking 300 mg of allopurinol per day will generally have plasma oxipurinol concentrations of 5-10 mg/litre.

Oxipurinol is eliminated unchanged in the urine but has a long elimination half-life because it undergoes tubular reabsorption. Reported values for the elimination half-life range from 13.6 hours to 29 hours. The large discrepancies in these values may be accounted for by variations in study design and/or creatinine clearance in the patients.

Pharmacokinetics in patients with renal impairment.

Allopurinol and oxipurinol clearance is greatly reduced in patients with poor renal function resulting in higher plasma levels in chronic therapy. Patients with renal impairment, where creatinine clearance values were between 10 and 20ml/min, showed plasma oxipurinol concentrations of approximately 30mg/litre after prolonged treatment with 300 mg allopurinol per day. This is approximately the concentration which would be achieved by doses of 600 mg/day in those with normal renal function. A reduction in the dose of Zyloric is therefore required in patients with renal impairment.

Pharmacokinetics in elderly patients.

The kinetics of the drug are not likely to be altered other than due to deterioration in renal function (see Pharmacokinetics in patients with renal impairment).

5.3 Preclinical safety data

A. Mutagenicity

Cytogenetic studies show that allopurinol does not induce chromosome aberrations in human blood cells *in vitro* at concentrations up to 100 micrograms/ml and *in vivo* at doses up to 600 mg/day for mean period of 40 months.

Allopurinol does not produce nitraso compounds *in vitro* or affect lymphocyte transformation *in vitro.*

Evidence from biochemical and other cytological investigations strongly suggests that allopurinol has no deleterious effects on DNA at any stage of the cell cycle and is not mutagenic.

B. Carcinogenicity

No evidence of carcinogenicity has been found in mice and rats treated with allopurinol for up to 2 years.

C. Teratogenicity

One study in mice receiving intraperitoneal doses of 50 or 100 mg/kg on days 10 or 13 of gestation resulted in foetal abnormalities, however in a similar study in rats at 120 mg/kg on day 12 of gestation no abnormalities were observed. Extensive studies of high oral doses of allopurinol in mice up to 100 mg/kg/day, rats up to 200 mg/kg/day and rabbits up to 150 mg/kg/day during days 8 to 16 of gestation produced no teratogenic effects.

An *in vitro* study using foetal mouse salivary glands in culture to detect embryotoxicity indicated that allopurinol would not be expected to cause embryotoxicity without also causing maternal toxicity.

6. PHARMACEUTICAL PARTICULARS

6.1 List of excipients

Lactose

Maize Starch

Povidone

Magnesium Stearate

Purified Water

6.2 Incompatibilities

None known.

6.3 Shelf life

5 years.

6.4 Special precautions for storage

Do not store above 25°C. Store in the original package

6.5 Nature and contents of container

Zyloric 100mg Tablets

PVC/aluminium foil blister pack

Zyloric-300 Tablets

PVC/aluminium foil blister pack

6.6 Instructions for use and handling

No special instructions.

Administrative Data

7. MARKETING AUTHORISATION HOLDER

The Wellcome Foundation Ltd

Glaxo Wellcome House

Berkeley Avenue

Greenford

Middlesex

Trading as GlaxoSmithKline UK

Stockley Park West

Uxbridge

Middlesex

UB11 1BT

8. MARKETING AUTHORISATION NUMBER(S)

PL 0003/5207R – Zyloric 100mg Tablets

PL 0003/0092 - Zyloric-300 Tablets

9. DATE OF FIRST AUTHORISATION/RENEWAL OF THE AUTHORISATION

Zyloric 100mg TabletsZyloric-300 Tablets

MAA: 20.03.80 14.07.80

Renewal: 06.06.90 18.02.91

Renewal: 14.11.95 25.11.98

10. DATE OF REVISION OF THE TEXT

11 August 2004

11. Legal Status

POM

Zyprexa 2.5mg, 5mg, 7.5mg, 10mg, and 15mg coated tablets. Zyprexa Velotab 5mg, 10mg, and 15mg orodispersible tablets

(Eli Lilly and Company Limited)

1. NAME OF THE MEDICINAL PRODUCT

Zyprexa* 2.5mg, 5mg, 7.5mg, 10mg, and 15mg coated tablets.

Zyprexa Velotab* 5mg, 10mg, and 15mg orodispersible tablets.

2. QUALITATIVE AND QUANTITATIVE COMPOSITION

Each coated tablet contains 2.5mg olanzapine.

Each coated tablet contains 5mg olanzapine.

Each coated tablet contains 7.5mg olanzapine.

Each coated tablet contains 10mg olanzapine.

Each coated tablet contains 15mg olanzapine.

Each orodispersible tablet contains 5mg olanzapine.

Each orodispersible tablet contains 10mg olanzapine.

Each orodispersible tablet contains 15mg olanzapine.

For excipients, see section 6.1.

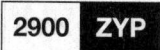

3. PHARMACEUTICAL FORM

Coated tablets

Zyprexa 2.5mg tablets are round, white, coated tablets imprinted with 'LILLY' and a numeric identicode '4112'.

Zyprexa 5mg tablets are round, white, coated tablets imprinted with 'LILLY' and a numeric identicode '4115'.

Zyprexa 7.5mg tablets are round, white, coated tablets imprinted with 'LILLY' and a numeric identicode '4116'.

Zyprexa 10mg tablets are round, white, coated tablets imprinted with 'LILLY' and a numeric identicode '4117'.

Zyprexa 15mg tablets are elliptical, blue, coated tablets debossed with 'LILLY' and a numeric identicode '4415'.

Orodispersible tablet

Zyprexa Velotab 5mg, 10mg, and 15mg orodispersible tablet is a yellow, round, freeze-dried, rapid-dispersing preparation to be placed in the mouth or alternatively to be dispersed in water or other suitable beverage for administration.

4. CLINICAL PARTICULARS

4.1 Therapeutic indications

Olanzapine is indicated for the treatment of schizophrenia.

Olanzapine is effective in maintaining the clinical improvement during continuation therapy in patients who have shown an initial treatment response.

Olanzapine is indicated for the treatment of moderate to severe manic episode.

In patients whose manic episode has responded to olanzapine treatment, olanzapine is indicated for the prevention of recurrence in patients with bipolar disorder (see section 5.1).

4.1.1 Further information on clinical trials

In a multinational, double-blind, comparative study of schizophrenia, schizoaffective and related disorders, which included 1,481 patients with varying degrees of associated depressive symptoms (baseline mean of 16.6 on the Montgomery-Asberg Depression Rating Scale), a prospective secondary analysis of baseline to endpoint mood score change demonstrated a statistically significant improvement (P = 0.001) favouring olanzapine (-6.0) versus haloperidol (-3.1).

4.2 Posology and method of administration

Schizophrenia: The recommended starting dose for olanzapine is 10mg/day.

Manic episode: The starting dose is 15mg as a single daily dose in monotherapy or 10mg daily in combination therapy (see section 5.1).

Preventing recurrence in bipolar disorder: The recommended starting dose is 10mg/day. For patients who have been receiving olanzapine for treatment of manic episode, continue therapy for preventing recurrence at the same dose. If a new manic, mixed, or depressive episode occurs, olanzapine treatment should be continued (with dose optimisation as needed), with supplementary therapy to treat mood symptoms, as clinically indicated.

During treatment for schizophrenia, manic episode, and recurrence prevention in bipolar disorder, daily dosage may subsequently be adjusted on the basis of individual clinical status within the range 5-20mg/day. An increase to a dose greater than the recommended starting dose is advised only after appropriate clinical reassessment and should generally occur at intervals of not less than 24 hours. Olanzapine can be given without regard for meals, as absorption is not affected by food. Gradual tapering of the dose should be considered when discontinuing olanzapine.

Zyprexa Velotab orodispersible tablet should be placed in the mouth, where it will rapidly disperse in saliva, so it can be easily swallowed. Removal of the intact orodispersible tablet from the mouth is difficult. Since the orodispersible tablet is fragile, it should be taken immediately on opening the blister. Alternatively, it may be dispersed in a full glass of water or other suitable beverage (orange juice, apple juice, milk, or coffee) immediately before administration.

Olanzapine orodispersible tablet is bioequivalent to olanzapine coated tablets, with a similar rate and extent of absorption. It has the same dosage and frequency of administration as olanzapine coated tablets. Olanzapine orodispersible tablets may be used as an alternative to olanzapine coated tablets.

Children and adolescents: Olanzapine has not been studied in subjects under 18 years of age.

Elderly patients: A lower starting dose (5mg/day) is not routinely indicated but should be considered for those 65 and over when clinical factors warrant (see also section 4.4).

Patients with renal and/or hepatic impairment: A lower starting dose (5mg) should be considered for such patients. In cases of moderate hepatic insufficiency (cirrhosis, Child-Pugh class A or B), the starting dose should be 5mg and only increased with caution.

Gender: The starting dose and dose range need not be routinely altered for female patients relative to male patients.

Smokers: The starting dose and dose range need not be routinely altered for non-smokers relative to smokers.

When more than one factor is present which might result in slower metabolism (female gender, geriatric age, non-smoking status), consideration should be given to decreasing the starting dose. Dose escalation, when indicated, should be conservative in such patients.

In cases where dose increments of 2.5mg are considered necessary, Zyprexa coated tablets should be used.

(See also section 4.5 and section 5.2.)

4.3 Contraindications

Hypersensitivity to olanzapine or to any of the excipients. Patients with known risk for narrow-angle glaucoma.

4.4 Special warnings and special precautions for use

Hyperglycaemia and/or development or exacerbation of diabetes, occasionally associated with ketoacidosis or coma, has been reported very rarely, including some fatal cases. In some cases, a prior increase in body weight has been reported, which may be a predisposing factor. Appropriate clinical monitoring is advisable, particularly in diabetic patients and in patients with risk factors for the development of diabetes mellitus.

Acute symptoms, such as sweating, insomnia, tremor, anxiety, nausea, or vomiting, have been reported very rarely (<0.01%) when olanzapine is stopped abruptly. Gradual dose reduction should be considered when discontinuing olanzapine.

Concomitant illnesses: While olanzapine demonstrated anticholinergic activity *in vitro*, experience during the clinical trials revealed a low incidence of related events. However, as clinical experience with olanzapine in patients with concomitant illness is limited, caution is advised when prescribing for patients with prostatic hypertrophy, or paralytic ileus and related conditions.

The use of olanzapine in the treatment of dopamine agonist associated psychosis in patients with Parkinson's disease is not recommended. In clinical trials, worsening of Parkinsonian symptomatology and hallucinations were reported very commonly and more frequently than with placebo (see also section 4.8), and olanzapine was not more effective than placebo in the treatment of psychotic symptoms. In these trials, patients were initially required to be stable on the lowest effective dose of anti-Parkinsonian medications (dopamine agonist) and to remain on the same anti-Parkinsonian medications and dosages throughout the study. Olanzapine was started at 2.5mg/day and titrated to a maximum of 15mg/day based on investigator judgement.

Olanzapine is not approved for the treatment of dementia-related psychosis and/or behavioural disturbances, and is not recommended for use in this particular group of patients because of an increase in mortality and the risk of cerebrovascular accident. In placebo-controlled clinical trials (6-12 weeks duration) of elderly patients (mean age 78 years) with dementia-related psychosis and/or disturbed behaviours, there was a 2-fold increase in the incidence of death in olanzapine-treated patients compared to patients treated with placebo (3.5% versus 1.5%, respectively). The higher incidence of death was not associated with olanzapine dose (mean daily dose 4.4mg) or duration of treatment. Risk factors that may predispose this patient population to increased mortality include age >65 years, dysphagia, sedation, malnutrition and dehydration, pulmonary conditions (eg, pneumonia, with or without aspiration), or concomitant use of benzodiazepines. However, the incidence of death was higher in olanzapine-treated than in placebo-treated patients, independent of these risk factors.

In the same clinical trials, cerebrovascular adverse events (CVAE, eg, stroke, transient ischaemic attack), including fatalities, were reported. There was a 3-fold increase in CVAE in patients treated with olanzapine compared to patients treated with placebo (1.3% versus 0.4%, respectively). All olanzapine- and placebo-treated patients who experienced a cerebrovascular event had pre-existing risk factors. Age >75 years and vascular/mixed type dementia were identified as risk factors for CVAE in association with olanzapine treatment. The efficacy of olanzapine was not established in these trials.

During antipsychotic treatment, improvement in the patient's clinical condition may take several days to some weeks. Patients should be closely monitored during this period.

Phenylalanine: Zyprexa Velotab orodispersible tablet contains aspartame, which is a source of phenylalanine.

Mannitol: Zyprexa Velotab orodispersible tablet contains mannitol.

Sodium methyl parahydroxybenzoate and sodium propyl parahydroxybenzoate: Olanzapine orodispersible tablet contains sodium methyl parahydroxybenzoate and sodium propyl parahydroxybenzoate. These preservatives are known to cause urticaria. Generally, delayed type reactions, such as contact dermatitis, may occur, but rarely immediate reactions with bronchospasm may occur.

Lactose: Zyprexa tablets contain lactose.

Transient, asymptomatic elevations of hepatic transaminases, ALT, AST have been seen commonly, especially in early treatment. Caution should be exercised in patients with elevated ALT and/or AST, in patients with signs and symptoms of hepatic impairment, in patients with pre-existing conditions associated with limited hepatic functional reserve, and in patients who are being treated with potentially hepatotoxic medicines. In the event of elevated ALT and/or AST during treatment, follow-up should be organised and dose reduction should be considered. In cases where hepatitis has been diagnosed, olanzapine treatment should be discontinued.

As with other neuroleptic medicines, caution should be exercised in patients with low leucocyte and/or neutrophil counts for any reason, in patients receiving medicines known to cause neutropenia, in patients with a history of drug-induced bone marrow depression/toxicity, in patients with bone marrow depression caused by concomitant illness, radiation therapy or chemotherapy, and in patients with hypereosinophilic conditions or with myeloproliferative disease. Neutropenia has been reported commonly when olanzapine and valproate are used concomitantly (see section 4.8).

There are limited data on co-medication with lithium and valproate (see section 5.1). There are no clinical data available on olanzapine and carbamazepine co-therapy; however, a pharmacokinetic study has been conducted (see section 4.5).

Neuroleptic malignant syndrome (NMS): NMS is a potentially life-threatening condition associated with antipsychotic medication. Rare cases reported as NMS have also been received in association with olanzapine. Clinical manifestations of NMS are hyperpyrexia, muscle rigidity, altered mental status, and evidence of autonomic instability (irregular pulse or blood pressure, tachycardia, diaphoresis, and cardiac dysrhythmia). Additional signs may include elevated creatinine phosphokinase, myoglobinuria (rhabdomyolysis), and acute renal failure. If a patient develops signs and symptoms indicative of NMS, or presents with unexplained high fever without additional clinical manifestations of NMS, all antipsychotic medicines, including olanzapine, must be discontinued.

Olanzapine should be used cautiously in patients who have a history of seizures or are subject to factors which may lower the seizure threshold. Seizures have been reported to occur rarely in patients when treated with olanzapine. In most of these cases, a history of seizures or risk factors for seizures were reported.

Tardive dyskinesia: In comparator studies of one year or less duration, olanzapine was associated with a statistically significant lower incidence of treatment emergent dyskinesia. However, the risk of tardive dyskinesia increases with long-term exposure, and therefore if signs or symptoms of tardive dyskinesia appear in a patient on olanzapine, a dose reduction or discontinuation should be considered. These symptoms can temporally deteriorate or even arise after discontinuation of treatment.

Given the primary CNS effects of olanzapine, caution should be used when it is taken in combination with other centrally acting medicines and alcohol. As it exhibits *in vitro* dopamine antagonism, olanzapine may antagonise the effects of direct and indirect dopamine agonists.

Postural hypotension was infrequently observed in the elderly in olanzapine clinical trials. As with other antipsychotics, it is recommended that blood pressure is measured periodically in patients over 65 years.

In clinical trials, olanzapine was not associated with a persistent increase in absolute QT intervals. Only 8 of 1,685 subjects had increased QT corrected (QTc) interval on multiple occasions. However, as with other antipsychotics, caution should be exercised when olanzapine is prescribed with medicines known to increase QTc interval, especially in the elderly, in patients with congenital long QT syndrome, congestive heart failure, heart hypertrophy, hypokalaemia, or hypomagnesaemia.

Temporal association of olanzapine treatment and venous thromboembolism has very rarely (<0.01%) been reported. A causal relationship between the occurrence of venous thromboembolism and treatment with olanzapine has not been established. However, since patients with schizophrenia often present with acquired risk factors for venous thromboembolism, all possible risk factors of VTE, eg, immobilisation of patients, should be identified and preventive measures undertaken.

4.5 Interaction with other medicinal products and other forms of Interaction

Caution should be exercised in patients who receive medicinal products that can cause central nervous system depression.

Potential interactions affecting olanzapine

Since olanzapine is metabolised by CYP1A2, substances that can specifically induce or inhibit this isoenzyme may affect the pharmacokinetics of olanzapine.

Induction of CYP1A2: The metabolism of olanzapine may be induced by smoking and carbamazepine, which may lead to reduced olanzapine concentrations. Only slight to moderate increase in olanzapine clearance has been observed. The clinical consequences are likely to be limited, but clinical monitoring is recommended and an increase of olanzapine dose may be considered if necessary (see section 4.2).

Inhibition of CYP1A2: Fluvoxamine, a specific CYP1A2 inhibitor, has been shown to significantly inhibit the metabolism of olanzapine. The mean increase in olanzapine C_{max} following fluvoxamine was 54% in female non-smokers and 77% in male smokers. The mean increase in olanzapine AUC was 52% and 108%, respectively. A lower starting dose of olanzapine should be considered in patients who are using fluvoxamine or any other CYP1A2 inhibitors, such as ciprofloxacin. A decrease in the dose of olanzapine should be considered if treatment with an inhibitor of CYP1A2 is initiated.

Decreased bioavailability: Activated charcoal reduces the bioavailability of oral olanzapine by 50 to 60% and should be taken at least 2 hours before or after olanzapine.

Fluoxetine (a CYP2D6 inhibitor), single doses of antacid (aluminium, magnesium) or cimetidine have not been found to significantly affect the pharmacokinetics of olanzapine.

Potential for olanzapine to affect other medicinal products

Olanzapine may antagonise the effects of direct and indirect dopamine agonists.

Olanzapine does not inhibit the main CYP450 isoenzymes *in vitro* (eg, 1A2, 2D6, 2C9, 2C19, 3A4). Thus, no particular interaction is expected, as verified through *in vivo* studies, where no inhibition of metabolism of the following active substances was found: tricyclic antidepressant (representing mostly CYP2D6 pathway), warfarin (CYP2C9), theophylline (CYP1A2), or diazepam (CYP3A4 and 2C19).

Olanzapine showed no interaction when co-administered with lithium or biperiden.

Therapeutic monitoring of valproate plasma levels did not indicate that valproate dosage adjustment is required after the introduction of concomitant olanzapine.

4.6 Pregnancy and lactation

Pregnancy: There are no adequate and well-controlled studies in pregnant women. Patients should be advised to notify their physician if they become pregnant or intend to become pregnant during treatment with olanzapine. Nevertheless, because human experience is limited, olanzapine should be used in pregnancy only if the potential benefit justifies the potential risk to the foetus.

Spontaneous reports have been very rarely received on tremor, hypertonia, lethargy, and sleepiness, in infants born to mothers who had used olanzapine during the 3rd trimester.

Lactation: In a study in lactating, healthy women, olanzapine was excreted in breast milk. Mean infant exposure (mg/kg) at steady-state was estimated to be 1.8% of the maternal olanzapine dose (mg/kg). Patients should be advised not to breast-feed an infant if they are taking olanzapine.

4.7 Effects on ability to drive and use machines

Because olanzapine may cause somnolence and dizziness, patients should be cautioned about operating machinery, including motor vehicles.

4.8 Undesirable effects

Very common (>10%) undesirable effects associated with the use of olanzapine in clinical trials were somnolence and weight gain.

In clinical trials in elderly patients with dementia, olanzapine treatment was associated with a higher incidence of death and cerebrovascular adverse events compared to placebo (see also section 4.4). Very common (>10%) undesirable effects associated with the use of olanzapine in this patient group were abnormal gait and falls. Pneumonia, increased body temperature, lethargy, erythema, visual hallucinations, and urinary incontinence were observed commonly (1-10%).

In clinical trials in patients with drug-induced (dopamine agonist) psychosis associated with Parkinson's disease, worsening of Parkinsonian symptomatology and hallucinations were reported very commonly and more frequently than with placebo.

In one clinical trial in patients with bipolar mania, valproate combination therapy with olanzapine resulted in an incidence of neutropenia of 4.1%; a potential contributing factor could be high plasma valproate levels. Olanzapine administered with lithium or valproate resulted in increased levels (>10%) of tremor, dry mouth, increased appetite, and weight gain. Speech disorder was also reported commonly (1% to 10%). During treatment with olanzapine in combination with lithium or divalproex, an increase of ⩾7% from baseline body weight occurred in 17.4% of patients during acute treatment (up to 6 weeks). Long-term olanzapine treatment (up to 12 months) for recurrence prevention in patients with bipolar disorder was associated with an increase of ⩾7% from baseline body weight in 39.9% of patients.

The following table of undesirable effects is based on adverse event reporting and laboratory investigations from clinical trials.

Blood and lymphatic system disorders
Common (1-10%): Eosinophilia.

Metabolism and nutrition disorders
Very common (>10%): Weight gain.
Common (1-10%): Increased appetite. Elevated glucose levels (see note 1 below). Elevated triglyceride levels.

Nervous system disorders
Very common (>10%): Somnolence.
Common (1-10%): Dizziness, akathisia, parkinsonism, dyskinesia (see also note 2 below).

Cardiac disorders
Uncommon (0.1-1%): Bradycardia, with or without hypotension or syncope.

Vascular disorders
Common (1-10%): Orthostatic hypotension.

Gastro-intestinal disorders
Common (1-10%): Mild, transient anticholinergic effects, including constipation and dry mouth.

Hepato-biliary disorders
Common (1-10%): Transient, asymptomatic elevations of hepatic transaminases (ALT, AST), especially in early treatment (see also section 4.4).

Skin and subcutaneous tissue disorders
Uncommon (0.1-1%): Photosensitivity reaction.

General disorders and administration site conditions
Common (1-10%): Asthenia, oedema.

Investigations
Very common (>10%): Elevated plasma prolactin levels, but associated clinical manifestations (eg, gynaecomastia, galactorrhoea, and breast enlargement) were rare. In most patients, levels returned to normal ranges without cessation of treatment.
Uncommon (0.1-1%): High creatine phosphokinase.

[1] In clinical trials with olanzapine in over 5,000 patients with baseline non-fasting glucose levels ⩽7.8mmol/l, the incidence of non-fasting plasma glucose levels ⩾11mmol/l (suggestive of diabetes) was 1.0%, compared to 0.9% with placebo. The incidence of non-fasting plasma glucose levels ⩾8.9mmol/l but <11mmol/l (suggestive of hyperglycaemia) was 2.0%, compared to 1.6% with placebo. Hyperglycaemia is also reported as a very rare (<0.01%) spontaneous event.

[2] In clinical trials, the incidence of parkinsonism and dystonia in olanzapine-treated patients was numerically higher, but not statistically significantly different from placebo. Olanzapine-treated patients had a lower incidence of parkinsonism, akathisia, and dystonia compared with titrated doses of haloperidol. In the absence of detailed information on the pre-existing history of individual acute and tardive extrapyramidal movement disorders, it can not be concluded at present that olanzapine produces less tardive dyskinesia and/or other tardive extrapyramidal syndromes.

The following table of undesirable effects is based on post-marketing spontaneous reports.

Blood and lymphatic system disorders
Rare (0.01-0.1%): Leucopenia.
Very rare (<0.01%): Thrombocytopenia. Neutropenia.

Immune system disorders
Very rare (<0.01%): Allergic reaction (eg, anaphylactoid reaction, angioedema, pruritus, or urticaria).

Metabolism and nutrition disorders
Very rare (<0.01%): Hyperglycaemia and/or development or exacerbation of diabetes, occasionally associated with ketoacidosis or coma, has been spontaneously reported very rarely, including some fatal cases (see also note 1 above and section 4.4). Hypertriglyceridaemia, hypothermia.

Nervous system disorders
Rare (0.01-0.1%): Seizures have been reported to occur rarely in patients treated with olanzapine. In most of these cases, a history of seizures or risk factors for seizures were reported.
Very rare (<0.01%): Cases reported as neuroleptic malignant syndrome (NMS) have been received in association with olanzapine (see also section 4.4). Parkinsonism, dystonia, and tardive dyskinesia have been reported very rarely with olanzapine.
Acute symptoms, such as sweating, insomnia, tremor, anxiety, nausea, or vomiting, have been reported very rarely when olanzapine is stopped abruptly.

Vascular disorders
Very rare (<0.01%): Thromboembolism (including pulmonary embolism and deep vein thrombosis).

Gastro-intestinal disorders
Very rare (<0.01%): Pancreatitis.

Hepato-biliary disorders
Very rare (<0.01%): Hepatitis.

Musculoskeletal and connective tissue and bone disorders
Very rare (<0.01%): Rhabdomyolysis.

Skin and subcutaneous tissue disorders
Rare (0.01-0.1%): Rash.

Renal and urinary disorders
Very rare (< 0.01%): Urinary hesitation.

Reproductive system and breast disorders
Very rare (<0.01%): Priapism.

4.9 Overdose

Signs and symptoms

Very common symptoms in overdose (>10% incidence) include tachycardia, agitation/aggressiveness, dysarthria, various extrapyramidal symptoms, and reduced level of consciousness ranging from sedation to coma.

Other medically significant sequelae of overdose include delirium, convulsion, coma, possible neuroleptic malignant syndrome, respiratory depression, aspiration, hypertension or hypotension, cardiac arrhythmias (<2% of overdose cases), and cardiopulmonary arrest. Fatal outcomes have been reported for acute overdoses as low as 450mg, but survival has also been reported following acute overdose of 1,500mg.

Management of overdose

There is no specific antidote for olanzapine. Induction of emesis is not recommended. Standard procedures for management of overdose may be indicated (ie, gastric lavage, administration of activated charcoal). The concomitant administration of activated charcoal was shown to reduce the oral bioavailability of olanzapine by 50 to 60%.

Symptomatic treatment and monitoring of vital organ function should be instituted according to clinical presentation, including treatment of hypotension and circulatory collapse and support of respiratory function. Do not use epinephrine, dopamine, or other sympathomimetic agents with beta-agonist activity, since beta stimulation may worsen hypotension. Cardiovascular monitoring is necessary to detect possible arrhythmias. Close medical supervision and monitoring should continue until the patient recovers.

5. PHARMACOLOGICAL PROPERTIES

5.1 Pharmacodynamic properties

Pharmacotherapeutic group: Antipsychotic. *ATC code:* N05A H03.

Olanzapine is an antipsychotic, antimanic, and mood stabilising agent that demonstrates a broad pharmacologic profile across a number of receptor systems.

In preclinical studies, olanzapine exhibited a range of receptor affinities (Ki; <100nM) for serotonin $5HT_{2A/2C}$, $5HT_3$, $5HT_6$; dopamine D_1, D_2, D_3, D_4, D_5; cholinergic muscarinic receptors m_1-m_5; alpha$_1$ adrenergic; and histamine H_1 receptors. Animal behavioural studies with olanzapine indicated 5HT, dopamine, and cholinergic antagonism, consistent with the receptor-binding profile. Olanzapine demonstrated a greater *in vitro* affinity for serotonin $5HT_2$ than dopamine D_2 receptors and greater $5HT_2$ than D_2 activity in *in vivo* models. Electrophysiological studies demonstrated that olanzapine selectively reduced the firing of mesolimbic (A10) dopaminergic neurons, while having little effect on the striatal (A9) pathways involved in motor function. Olanzapine reduced a conditioned avoidance response, a test indicative of antipsychotic activity, at doses below those producing catalepsy, an effect indicative of motor side-effects. Unlike some other antipsychotic agents, olanzapine increases responding in an 'anxiolytic' test.

In a single oral dose (10mg) Positron Emission Tomography (PET) study in healthy volunteers, olanzapine produced a higher $5HT_{2A}$ than dopamine D_2 receptor occupancy. In addition, a Single Photon Emission Computed Tomography (SPECT) imaging study in schizophrenic patients revealed that olanzapine-responsive patients had lower striatal D_2 occupancy than some other antipsychotic- and risperidone-responsive patients, while being comparable to clozapine-responsive patients.

In two of two placebo- and two of three comparator-controlled trials with over 2,900 schizophrenic patients presenting with both positive and negative symptoms, olanzapine was associated with statistically significantly greater improvements in negative as well as positive symptoms.

In patients with a manic or mixed episode of bipolar disorder, olanzapine demonstrated superior efficacy to placebo and valproate semisodium (divalproex) in reduction of manic symptoms over 3 weeks. Olanzapine also demonstrated comparable efficacy results to haloperidol in terms of the proportion of patients in symptomatic remission from mania and depression at 6 and 12 weeks. In a co-therapy study of patients treated with lithium or valproate for a minimum of 2 weeks, the addition of olanzapine 10mg (co-therapy with lithium or valproate) resulted in a greater reduction in symptoms of mania than lithium or valproate monotherapy after 6 weeks.

In a 12-month recurrence prevention study in manic episode patients who achieved remission on olanzapine and were then randomised to olanzapine or placebo, olanzapine demonstrated statistically significant superiority over placebo on the primary endpoint of bipolar recurrence. Olanzapine also showed a statistically significant advantage over placebo in terms of preventing either recurrence into mania or recurrence into depression.

In a second 12-month recurrence prevention study in manic episode patients who achieved remission with a combination of olanzapine and lithium and were then randomised to olanzapine or lithium alone, olanzapine was statistically non-inferior to lithium on the primary endpoint of bipolar recurrence (olanzapine 30.0%, lithium 38.3%; $P = 0.055$).

In an 18-month co-therapy study in manic or mixed episode patients stabilised with olanzapine plus a mood stabiliser (lithium or valproate), long-term olanzapine co-therapy with lithium or valproate was not statistically significantly superior to lithium or valproate alone in delaying bipolar recurrence, defined according to syndromic (diagnostic) criteria.

5.2 Pharmacokinetic properties

Olanzapine orodispersible tablet is bioequivalent to olanzapine coated tablets, with a similar rate and extent of absorption. Olanzapine orodispersible tablets may be used as an alternative to olanzapine coated tablets.

Olanzapine is well absorbed after oral administration, reaching peak plasma concentrations within 5 to 8 hours. The absorption is not affected by food. Absolute oral bioavailability relative to intravenous administration has not been determined.

Olanzapine is metabolised in the liver by conjugative and oxidative pathways. The major circulating metabolite is the 10-N-glucuronide, which does not pass the blood brain barrier. Cytochromes P450-CYP1A2 and P450-CYP2D6 contribute to the formation of the N-desmethyl and 2-hydroxymethyl metabolites; both exhibited significantly less *in vivo* pharmacological activity than olanzapine in animal studies. The predominant pharmacologic activity is from the parent, olanzapine. After oral administration, the mean terminal elimination half-life of olanzapine in healthy subjects varied on the basis of age and gender.

In healthy elderly (65 and over) versus non-elderly subjects, the mean elimination half-life was prolonged (51.8 versus 33.8 hours) and the clearance was reduced (17.5 versus 18.2 l/hr). The pharmacokinetic variability observed in the elderly is within the range for the non-elderly. In 44 patients with schizophrenia >65 years of age, dosing from 5 to 20mg/day was not associated with any distinguishing profile of adverse events.

In female versus male subjects, the mean elimination half-life was somewhat prolonged (36.7 versus 32.3 hours) and the clearance was reduced (18.9 versus 27.3 l/hr). However, olanzapine (5-20mg) demonstrated a comparable safety profile in female (n = 467) as in male patients (n = 869).

In renally impaired patients (creatinine clearance <10ml/min) versus healthy subjects, there was no significant difference in mean elimination half-life (37.7 versus 32.4 hours) or clearance (21.2 versus 25.0 l/hr). A mass balance study showed that approximately 57% of radiolabelled olanzapine appeared in urine, principally as metabolites.

In smoking subjects with mild hepatic dysfunction, mean elimination half-life (39.3 hours) was prolonged and clearance (18.0 l/hr) was reduced analogous to non-smoking healthy subjects (48.8 hours and 14.1 l/hr, respectively).

In non-smoking versus smoking subjects (males and females), the mean elimination half-life was prolonged (38.6 versus 30.4 hours) and the clearance was reduced (18.6 versus 27.7 l/hr).

The plasma clearance of olanzapine is lower in elderly versus young subjects, in females versus males, and in non-smokers versus smokers. However, the magnitude of the impact of age, gender, or smoking on olanzapine clearance and half-life is small in comparison to the overall variability between individuals.

In a study of Caucasians, Japanese, and Chinese subjects, there were no differences in the pharmacokinetic parameters among the three populations.

The plasma protein binding of olanzapine was about 93% over the concentration range of about 7 to about 1,000ng/ml. Olanzapine is bound predominantly to albumin and alpha$_1$-acid-glycoprotein.

5.3 Preclinical safety data

Acute (single-dose) toxicity

Signs of oral toxicity in rodents were characteristic of potent neuroleptic compounds: hypoactivity, coma, tremors, clonic convulsions, salivation, and depressed weight gain. The median lethal doses were approximately 210mg/kg (mice) and 175mg/kg (rats). Dogs tolerated single oral doses up to 100mg/kg without mortality. Clinical signs included sedation, ataxia, tremors, increased heart rate, laboured respiration, miosis, and anorexia. In monkeys, single oral doses up to 100mg/kg resulted in prostration and, at higher doses, semi-consciousness.

Repeated-dose toxicity

In studies up to 3 months duration in mice and up to 1 year in rats and dogs, the predominant effects were CNS depression, anticholinergic effects, and peripheral haematological disorders. Tolerance developed to the CNS depression. Growth parameters were decreased at high doses. Reversible effects consistent with elevated prolactin in rats included decreased weights of ovaries and uterus and morphologic changes in vaginal epithelium and in mammary gland.

Haematologic toxicity: Effects on haematology parameters were found in each species, including dose-related reductions in circulating leucocytes in mice and non-specific reductions of circulating leucocytes in rats; however, no evidence of bone marrow cytotoxicity was found. Reversible neutropenia, thrombocytopenia, or anaemia developed in a few dogs treated with 8 or 10mg/kg/day (total olanzapine exposure [area under the curve - AUC] is 12- to 15-fold greater than that of a man given a 12mg dose). In cytopenic dogs, there were no adverse effects on progenitor and proliferating cells in the bone marrow.

Reproductive toxicity

Olanzapine had no teratogenic effects. Sedation affected mating performance of male rats. Oestrous cycles were affected at doses of 1.1mg/kg (3-times the maximum human dose) and reproduction parameters were influenced in rats given 3mg/kg (9-times the maximum human dose). In the offspring of rats given olanzapine, delays in foetal development and transient decreases in offspring activity levels were seen.

Mutagenicity

Olanzapine was not mutagenic or clastogenic in a full range of standard tests, which included bacterial mutation tests and *in vitro* and *in vivo* mammalian tests.

Carcinogenicity

Based on the results of studies in mice and rats, it was concluded that olanzapine is not carcinogenic.

6. PHARMACEUTICAL PARTICULARS

6.1 List of excipients

Zyprexa tablet

Tablet core

Lactose monohydrate

Hydroxypropylcellulose

Crospovidone

Microcrystalline cellulose

Magnesium stearate

Tablet coat

2.5 mg, 5mg, 7.5mg, and 10mg tablets:

Hypromellose

Colour mixture white (hypromellose, titanium dioxide [E171], macrogol, polysorbate 80)

Carnauba wax

Edible blue ink (shellac, macrogol, indigo carmine [E132])

15 mg tablets:

Hypromellose

Colour mixture light blue (titanium dioxide [E171], lactose monohydrate, hypromellose, triacetin, indigo carmine [E132])

Carnauba wax

Zyprexa Velotab

Gelatin

Mannitol (E421)

Aspartame (E951)

Sodium methyl parahydroxybenzoate (E219)

Sodium propyl parahydroxybenzoate (E217)

6.2 Incompatibilities

Not applicable.

6.3 Shelf life

Zyprexa tablets: Three years (5mg, 7.5mg, 10mg, and 15mg).

Zyprexa tablets: Two years (2.5mg).

Zyprexa Velotabs: Two years.

6.4 Special precautions for storage

Zyprexa tablets: Store in the original package.

Zyprexa Velotabs: Store in the original package in order to protect from light and moisture.

6.5 Nature and contents of container

Aluminium blister strips.

Zyprexa 2.5mg tablets are available in cold-formed aluminium blister strips in cartons of 28 tablets per carton.

Zyprexa 5mg tablets are available in cold-formed aluminium blister strips in cartons of 28 tablets per carton.

Zyprexa 7.5mg tablets are available in cold-formed aluminium blister strips in cartons of 56 tablets per carton.

Zyprexa 10mg tablets are available in cold-formed aluminium blister strips in cartons of 28 or 56 tablets per carton.

Zyprexa 15mg tablets are available in cold-formed aluminium blister strips in cartons of 28 tablets per carton.

Zyprexa Velotab 5mg, 10mg, and 15mg is supplied in aluminium blister strips in cartons of 28 or 56 orodispersible tablets per carton.

Not all packs may be marketed in every country.

6.6 Instructions for use and handling

No special requirements.

7. MARKETING AUTHORISATION HOLDER

Eli Lilly Nederland BV, Grootslag 1-5, NL-3991 RA Houten, The Netherlands.

8. MARKETING AUTHORISATION NUMBER(S)

EU/1/96/022/002:	Zyprexa 2.5mg coated tablets - 28 tablets per box
EU/1/96/022/004:	Zyprexa 5mg coated tablets - 28 tablets per box
EU/1/96/022/006:	Zyprexa 7.5mg coated tablets - 56 tablets per box
EU/1/96/022/009:	Zyprexa 10mg coated tablets - 28 tablets per box
EU/1/96/022/010:	Zyprexa 10mg coated tablets - 56 tablets per box
EU/1/96/022/012:	Zyprexa 15mg coated tablets - 28 tablets per box
EU/1/99/125/001:	5mg × 28 Velotabs
EU/1/99/125/005:	5mg × 56 Velotabs
EU/1/99/125/002:	10mg × 28 Velotabs
EU/1/99/125/006:	10mg × 56 Velotabs
EU/1/99/125/003:	15mg × 28 Velotabs
EU/1/99/125/007:	15mg × 56 Velotabs

9. DATE OF FIRST AUTHORISATION/RENEWAL OF THE AUTHORISATION

2.5mg, 5mg, 7.5mg, 10mg, and 15mg Zyprexa tablets:

Date of first authorisation: 27 September 1996

Date of last renewal of the authorisation: 20 November 2001

Zyprexa Velotabs:

Date of first authorisation: 3 February 2000

Date of last renewal of the authorisation: 5 November 2004

10. DATE OF REVISION OF THE TEXT

February 2005

LEGAL CATEGORY

POM

*ZYPREXA (olanzapine) and VELOTAB are trademarks of Eli Lilly and Company.

ZY29M

Zyprexa Powder for Solution for Injection

(Eli Lilly and Company Limited)

1. NAME OF THE MEDICINAL PRODUCT

Zyprexa*▼ 10mg Powder for Solution for Injection.

2. QUALITATIVE AND QUANTITATIVE COMPOSITION

Each vial contains 10mg olanzapine. It provides a solution containing 5mg/ml olanzapine when reconstituted as recommended.

For excipients, see section 6.1.

3. PHARMACEUTICAL FORM

Powder for Solution for Injection.

Yellow lyophilised powder in a clear glass vial.

4. CLINICAL PARTICULARS

4.1 Therapeutic indications

Zyprexa Powder for Solution for Injection is indicated for the rapid control of agitation and disturbed behaviours in patients with schizophrenia or manic episode, when oral therapy is not appropriate. Treatment with Zyprexa Powder for Solution for Injection should be discontinued, and the use of oral olanzapine should be initiated, as soon as clinically appropriate.

4.2 Posology and method of administration

For intramuscular use. Do not administer intravenously or subcutaneously. Zyprexa Powder for Solution for Injection is intended for short-term use only, for up to a maximum of three consecutive days.

The maximum daily dose of olanzapine (including all formulations of olanzapine) is 20mg.

The recommended initial dose for olanzapine injection is 10mg, administered as a single intramuscular injection. A lower dose (5mg or 7.5mg) may be given, on the basis of individual clinical status, which should also include consideration of medications already administered either for maintenance or acute treatment (see section 4.4). A second injection, 5-10mg, may be administered 2 hours after the first injection, on the basis of individual clinical status.

Not more than three injections should be given in any 24-hour period and the maximum daily dose of olanzapine of 20mg (including all formulations) should not be exceeded.

Zyprexa Powder for Solution for Injection should be reconstituted in accordance with the recommendation in section 6.6.

For further information on continued treatment with oral olanzapine (5 to 20mg daily), see the Summary of Product Characteristics for Zyprexa coated tablets or Zyprexa Velotab orodispersible tablets.

Children and adolescents: Zyprexa has not been studied in subjects under 18 years of age. It should not be used in this population until relevant clinical data are available.

Elderly patients: The recommended starting dose in elderly patients (>60 years) is 2.5-5mg. Depending on the patient's clinical status (see section 4.4), a second injection, 2.5-5mg, may be administered 2 hours after the first injection. Not more than 3 injections should be given in any

24-hour period and the maximum daily dose of 20mg (including all formulations) of olanzapine should not be exceeded.

Patients with renal and/or hepatic impairment: A lower starting dose (5mg) should be considered for such patients. In cases of moderate hepatic insufficiency (cirrhosis, Child-Pugh class A or B), the starting dose should be 5mg and only increased with caution.

Gender: The dose and dose range need not be routinely altered for female patients relative to male patients.

Smokers: The dose and dose range need not be routinely altered for non-smokers relative to smokers.

When more than one factor is present which might result in slower metabolism (female gender, geriatric age, non-smoking status), consideration should be given to decreasing the dose. Additional injections, when indicated, should be conservative in such patients.

(See also section 4.5 and section 5.2.)

4.3 Contraindications

Hypersensitivity to olanzapine or to any of the excipients. Patients with known risk of narrow-angle glaucoma.

4.4 Special warnings and special precautions for use

The efficacy of IM olanzapine has not been established in patients with agitation and disturbed behaviours related to conditions other than schizophrenia or manic episode.

IM olanzapine should not be administered to patients with unstable medical conditions, such as acute myocardial infarction, unstable angina pectoris, severe hypotension and/or bradycardia, sick sinus syndrome, or following heart surgery. If the patient's medical history with regard to these unstable medical conditions cannot be determined, the risks and benefits of IM olanzapine should be considered in relation to other alternative treatments.

Simultaneous injection of intramuscular olanzapine and parenteral benzodiazepine is not recommended (see also section 4.5 and section 6.2). If the patient is considered to need parenteral benzodiazepine treatment, this should not be given until at least one hour after IM olanzapine administration. If the patient has received parenteral benzodiazepine, IM olanzapine administration should only be considered after careful evaluation of clinical status, and the patient should be closely monitored for excessive sedation and cardiorespiratory depression.

It is extremely important that patients receiving intramuscular olanzapine should be closely observed for hypotension, including postural hypotension, bradyarrhythmia, and/or hypoventilation, particularly for the first 4 hours following injection, and close observation should be continued after this period if clinically indicated. Blood pressure, pulse, respiratory rate, and level of consciousness should be observed regularly and remedial treatment provided if required. Patients should remain recumbent if dizzy or drowsy after injection until examination indicates that they are not experiencing hypotension, including postural hypotension, bradyarrhythmia, and/or hypoventilation.

Special caution is necessary in patients who have received treatment with other medicinal products having haemodynamic properties similar to those of intramuscular olanzapine, including other antipsychotics (oral and/or intramuscular) and benzodiazepines (see also section 4.5). Temporal association of treatment with IM olanzapine with hypotension, bradycardia, respiratory depression, and death has been very rarely (<0.01%) reported, particularly in patients who have received benzodiazepines and/or other antipsychotics (see section 4.8).

The safety and efficacy of IM olanzapine has not been evaluated in patients with alcohol or drug intoxication (either with prescribed or illicit drugs) (see also section 4.5).

Hyperglycaemia and/or development or exacerbation of diabetes, occasionally associated with ketoacidosis or coma, has been reported very rarely, including some fatal cases. In some cases, a prior increase in body weight has been reported, which may be a predisposing factor. Appropriate clinical monitoring is advisable, particularly in diabetic patients and in patients with risk factors for the development of diabetes mellitus.

Acute symptoms, such as sweating, insomnia, tremor, anxiety, nausea, or vomiting, have been reported very rarely (<0.01%) when olanzapine is stopped abruptly. Gradual dose reduction should be considered when discontinuing olanzapine.

While olanzapine demonstrated anticholinergic activity *in vitro*, experience during oral clinical trials revealed a low incidence of related events. However, as clinical experience with olanzapine in patients with concomitant illness is limited, caution is advised when prescribing for patients with prostatic hypertrophy, or paralytic ileus and related conditions.

The use of olanzapine in the treatment of dopamine agonist associated psychosis in patients with Parkinson's disease is not recommended. In clinical trials, worsening of Parkinsonian symptomatology and hallucinations were reported very commonly and more frequently than with placebo (see also section 4.8), and olanzapine was not more effective than placebo in the treatment of psychotic symptoms. In these trials, patients were initially required to be stable on the lowest effective dose of anti-Parkinsonian medications (dopamine agonist) and to remain on the same anti-Parkinsonian medications and dosages throughout the study. Olanzapine was started at 2.5mg/day and titrated to a maximum of 15mg/day based on investigator judgement.

Olanzapine is not approved for the treatment of dementia-related psychosis and/or behavioural disturbances, and is not recommended for use in this particular group of patients because of an increase in mortality and the risk of cerebrovascular accident. In placebo-controlled clinical trials (6-12 weeks duration) of elderly patients (mean age 78 years) with dementia-related psychosis and/or disturbed behaviours, there was a 2-fold increase in the incidence of death in olanzapine-treated patients compared to patients treated with placebo (3.5% versus 1.5%, respectively). The higher incidence of death was not associated with olanzapine dose (mean daily dose 4.4mg) or duration of treatment. Risk factors that may predispose this patient population to increased mortality include age >65 years, dysphagia, sedation, malnutrition and dehydration, pulmonary conditions (eg, pneumonia, with or without aspiration), or concomitant use of benzodiazepines. However, the incidence of death was higher in olanzapine-treated than in placebo-treated patients, independent of these risk factors.

In the same clinical trials, cerebrovascular adverse events (CVAE, eg, stroke, transient ischaemic attack), including fatalities, were reported. There was a 3-fold increase in CVAE in patients treated with olanzapine compared to patients treated with placebo (1.3% versus 0.4%, respectively). All olanzapine- and placebo-treated patients who experienced a cerebrovascular event had pre-existing risk factors. Age >75 years and vascular/mixed type dementia were identified as risk factors for CVAE in association with olanzapine treatment. The efficacy of olanzapine was not established in these trials.

Transient, asymptomatic elevations of hepatic transaminases, ALT, AST have been seen commonly, especially in early treatment. Caution should be exercised in patients with elevated ALT and/or AST, in patients with signs and symptoms of hepatic impairment, in patients with pre-existing conditions associated with limited hepatic functional reserve, and in patients who are being treated with potentially hepatotoxic medicines. In the event of elevated ALT and/or AST during treatment, follow-up should be organised and dose reduction should be considered. In cases where hepatitis has been diagnosed, olanzapine treatment should be discontinued.

As with other antipsychotic medicines, caution should be exercised in patients with low leucocyte and/or neutrophil counts for any reason, in patients receiving medicines known to cause neutropenia, in patients with a history of drug-induced bone marrow depression/toxicity, in patients with bone marrow depression caused by concomitant illness, radiation therapy or chemotherapy, and in patients with hypereosinophilic conditions or with myeloproliferative disease. Neutropenia has been reported commonly when olanzapine and valproate are used concomitantly (see section 4.8).

There are limited data on co-medication with lithium and valproate (see section 5.1). There are no clinical data available on olanzapine and carbamazepine co-therapy; however, a pharmacokinetic study has been conducted (see section 4.5).

Neuroleptic malignant syndrome (NMS): NMS is a potentially life-threatening condition associated with antipsychotic medication. Rare cases reported as NMS have also been received in association with olanzapine. Clinical manifestations of NMS are hyperpyrexia, muscle rigidity, altered mental status, and evidence of autonomic instability (irregular pulse or blood pressure, tachycardia, diaphoresis, and cardiac dysrhythmia). Additional signs may include elevated creatinine phosphokinase, myoglobinuria (rhabdomyolysis), and acute renal failure. If a patient develops signs and symptoms indicative of NMS, or presents with unexplained high fever without additional clinical manifestations of NMS, all antipsychotic medicines, including olanzapine, must be discontinued.

Olanzapine should be used cautiously in patients who have a history of seizures or are subject to factors which may lower the seizure threshold. Seizures have been reported to occur rarely in patients when treated with olanzapine. In most of these cases, a history of seizures or risk factors for seizures were reported.

Tardive dyskinesia: In comparator oral studies of one year or less duration, olanzapine was associated with a statistically significant lower incidence of treatment emergent dyskinesia. However, the risk of tardive dyskinesia increases with long-term exposure, and therefore, if signs or symptoms of tardive dyskinesia appear in a patient on olanzapine, a dose reduction or discontinuation should be considered. These symptoms can temporally deteriorate or even arise after discontinuation of treatment.

Given the primary CNS effects of olanzapine, caution should be used when it is taken in combination with other centrally acting medicines and alcohol. As it exhibits *in vitro* dopamine antagonism, olanzapine may antagonise the effects of direct and indirect dopamine agonists.

Postural hypotension was infrequently observed in the elderly in oral olanzapine clinical trials. As with other antipsychotics, it is recommended that blood pressure is measured periodically in patients over 65 years.

In clinical trials with Zyprexa Powder for Solution for Injection, olanzapine was not associated with a persistent increase in absolute QT or in QTc intervals. In clinical trials with oral administration, olanzapine was not associated with a persistent increase in absolute QT intervals. Only 8 of 1,685 subjects had increased QTc interval on multiple occasions. However, as with other antipsychotics, caution should be exercised when olanzapine is prescribed with medicines known to increase QTc interval, especially in the elderly, in patients with congenital long QT syndrome, congestive heart failure, heart hypertrophy, hypokalaemia, or hypomagnesaemia.

Temporal association of olanzapine treatment and venous thromboembolism has very rarely (<0.01%) been reported. A causal relationship between the occurrence of venous thromboembolism and treatment with olanzapine has not been established. However, since patients with schizophrenia often present with acquired risk factors for venous thromboembolism, all possible risk factors of VTE, eg, immobilisation of patients, should be identified and preventive measures undertaken.

4.5 Interaction with other medicinal products and other forms of Interaction

IM olanzapine has not been studied in patients with alcohol or drug intoxication (see also section 4.4).

Caution should be exercised in patients who receive medicinal products that can induce hypotension, bradycardia, respiratory or central nervous system depression (see also section 4.4).

Potential for interaction, following intramuscular injection

In a single dose intramuscular study of olanzapine 5mg, administered 1 hour before intramuscular lorazepam 2mg (metabolised by glucuronidation), the pharmacokinetics of both medicines were unchanged. However, the combination added to the somnolence observed with either medicine alone. Concomitant injection of olanzapine and parenteral benzodiazepine is not recommended (see section 4.4 and section 6.2).

Potential interactions affecting olanzapine

Since olanzapine is metabolised by CYP1A2, substances that can specifically induce or inhibit this isoenzyme may affect the pharmacokinetics of olanzapine.

Induction of CYP1A2: The metabolism of olanzapine may be induced by smoking and carbamazepine, which may lead to reduced olanzapine concentrations. Only slight to moderate increase in olanzapine clearance has been observed. The clinical consequences are likely to be limited, but clinical monitoring is recommended and an increase of olanzapine dose may be considered if necessary (see section 4.2).

Inhibition of CYP1A2: Fluvoxamine, a specific CYP1A2 inhibitor, has been shown to significantly inhibit the metabolism of olanzapine. The mean increase in olanzapine C_{max} following fluvoxamine was 54% in female non-smokers and 77% in male smokers. The mean increase in olanzapine AUC was 52% and 108%, respectively. A lower starting dose of olanzapine should be considered in patients who are using fluvoxamine or any other CYP1A2 inhibitors, such as ciprofloxacin. A decrease in the dose of olanzapine should be considered if treatment with an inhibitor of CYP1A2 is initiated.

Decreased bioavailability: Activated charcoal reduces the bioavailability of oral olanzapine by 50 to 60% and should be taken at least 2 hours before or after olanzapine.

Fluoxetine (a CYP2D6 inhibitor), single doses of antacid (aluminium, magnesium) or cimetidine have not been found to significantly affect the pharmacokinetics of olanzapine.

Potential for olanzapine to affect other medicinal products

Olanzapine may antagonise the effects of direct and indirect dopamine agonists (see section 6.2).

Olanzapine does not inhibit the main CYP450 isoenzymes *in vitro* (eg, 1A2, 2D6, 2C9, 2C19, 3A4). Thus, no particular interaction is expected, as verified through *in vivo* studies, where no inhibition of metabolism of the following active substances was found: tricyclic antidepressant (representing mostly CYP2D6 pathway), warfarin (CYP2C9), theophylline (CYP1A2), or diazepam (CYP3A4 and 2C19).

Olanzapine showed no interaction when co-administered with lithium or biperiden.

Therapeutic monitoring of valproate plasma levels did not indicate that valproate dosage adjustment is required after the introduction of concomitant olanzapine.

4.6 Pregnancy and lactation

Pregnancy: There are no adequate and well-controlled studies in pregnant women. Patients should be advised to notify their physician if they become pregnant or intend to become pregnant during treatment with olanzapine. Nevertheless, because human experience is limited, olanzapine should be used in pregnancy only if the potential benefit justifies the potential risk to the foetus.

Spontaneous reports have been very rarely received on tremor, hypertonia, lethargy, and sleepiness, in infants born to mothers who had used olanzapine during the 3rd trimester.

Lactation: In a study in lactating, healthy women, olanzapine was excreted in breast milk. Mean infant exposure (mg/kg) at steady-state was estimated to be 1.8% of the maternal olanzapine dose (mg/kg). Patients should be advised not to breast-feed an infant if they are taking olanzapine.

4.7 Effects on ability to drive and use machines

Because olanzapine may cause somnolence and dizziness, patients should be cautioned about operating machinery, including motor vehicles.

4.8 Undesirable effects

A common (1-10%) undesirable effect associated with the use of intramuscular olanzapine in clinical trials was somnolence.

In post-marketing reports, temporal association of treatment with IM olanzapine with cases of respiratory depression, hypotension or bradycardia, and death have been very rarely reported, mostly in patients who concomitantly received benzodiazepines, and/or other antipsychotic drugs or who were treated in excess of olanzapine recommended daily doses (see section 4.4 and section 4.5).

The following table is based on the undesirable effects and laboratory investigations from clinical trials with Zyprexa Powder for Solution for Injection rather than oral olanzapine.

Cardiac disorders *Common (1-10%):* Bradycardia, with or without hypotension or syncope, tachycardia. *Uncommon (0.1-1%):* Sinus pause.
Vascular disorders *Common (1-10%):* Postural hypotension, hypotension.
Respiratory disorders *Uncommon (0.1-1%):* Hypoventilation.
General disorders and administration site conditions *Common (1-10%):* Injection site discomfort.

The undesirable effects listed below have been observed following administration of oral olanzapine, but may also occur following administration of Zyprexa Powder for Solution for Injection.

Very common (>10%) undesirable effects associated with the use of oral olanzapine in clinical trials were somnolence and weight gain.

In clinical trials in elderly patients with dementia, olanzapine treatment was associated with a higher incidence of death and cerebrovascular adverse events compared to placebo (see also section 4.4). Very common (>10%) undesirable effects associated with the use of olanzapine in this patient group were abnormal gait and falls. Pneumonia, increased body temperature, lethargy, erythema, visual hallucinations, and urinary incontinence were observed commonly (1-10%).

In clinical trials in patients with drug-induced (dopamine agonist) psychosis associated with Parkinson's disease, worsening of Parkinsonian symptomatology and hallucinations were reported very commonly and more frequently than with placebo.

In one clinical trial in patients with bipolar mania, valproate combination therapy with olanzapine resulted in an incidence of neutropenia of 4.1%; a potential contributing factor could be high plasma valproate levels. Olanzapine administered with lithium or valproate resulted in increased levels (>10%) of tremor, dry mouth, increased appetite, and weight gain. Speech disorder was also reported commonly (1% to 10%). During treatment with olanzapine in combination with lithium or divalproex, an increase of ⩾7% from baseline body weight occurred in 17.4% of patients during acute treatment (up to 6 weeks). Long-term olanzapine treatment (up to 12 months) for recurrence prevention in patients with bipolar disorder was associated with an increase of ⩾7% from baseline body weight in 39.9% of patients.

The following table of undesirable effects is based on adverse event reporting and laboratory investigations from clinical trials with oral olanzapine.

Blood and lymphatic system disorders *Common (1-10%):* Eosinophilia.
Metabolism and nutrition disorders *Very common (>10%):* Weight gain. *Common (1-10%):* Increased appetite. Elevated glucose levels (see note 1 below). Elevated triglyceride levels.
Nervous system disorders *Very common (>10%):* Somnolence. *Common (1-10%):* Dizziness, akathisia, parkinsonism, dyskinesia (see also note 2 below).
Cardiac disorders *Uncommon (0.1-1%):* Bradycardia, with or without hypotension or syncope.
Vascular disorders *Common (1-10%):* Orthostatic hypotension.
Gastro-intestinal disorders *Common (1-10%):* Mild, transient anticholinergic effects, including constipation and dry mouth.
Hepato-biliary disorders *Common (1-10%):* Transient, asymptomatic elevations of hepatic transaminases (ALT, AST), especially in early treatment (see also section 4.4).
Skin and subcutaneous tissue disorders *Uncommon (0.1-1%):* Photosensitivity reaction.
General disorders and administration site conditions *Common (1-10%):* Asthenia, oedema.
Investigations *Very common (>10%):* Elevated plasma prolactin levels, but associated clinical manifestations (eg, gynaecomastia, galactorrhoea, and breast enlargement) were rare. In most patients, levels returned to normal ranges without cessation of treatment. *Uncommon (0.1-1%):* High creatine phosphokinase.

[1]In clinical trials with olanzapine in over 5,000 patients with baseline non-fasting glucose levels ⩽7.8mmol/l, the incidence of non-fasting plasma glucose levels ⩾11mmol/l (suggestive of diabetes) was 1.0%, compared to 0.9% with placebo. The incidence of non-fasting plasma glucose levels ⩾8.9mmol/l but <11mmol/l (suggestive of hyperglycaemia) was 2.0%, compared to 1.6% with placebo. Hyperglycaemia is also reported as a very rare (<0.01%) spontaneous event.

[2]In clinical trials, the incidence of parkinsonism and dystonia in olanzapine-treated patients was numerically higher, but not statistically significantly different from placebo. Olanzapine-treated patients had a lower incidence of parkinsonism, akathisia, and dystonia compared with titrated doses of haloperidol. In the absence of detailed information on the pre-existing history of individual acute and tardive extrapyramidal movement disorders, it can not be concluded at present that olanzapine produces less tardive dyskinesia and/or other tardive extrapyramidal syndromes.

The following table of undesirable effects is based on post-marketing spontaneous reports with oral olanzapine.

Blood and lymphatic system disorders *Rare (0.01-0.1%):* Leucopenia. *Very rare (<0.01%):* Thrombocytopenia. Neutropenia.
Immune system disorders *Very rare (<0.01%):* Allergic reaction (eg, anaphylactoid reaction, angioedema, pruritus, or urticaria).
Metabolism and nutrition disorders *Very rare (<0.01%):* Hyperglycaemia and/or development or exacerbation of diabetes, occasionally associated with ketoacidosis or coma, has been spontaneously reported very rarely, including some fatal cases (see also note 1 above and section 4.4). Hypertriglyceridaemia, hypothermia.
Nervous system disorders *Rare (0.01-0.1%):* Seizures have been reported to occur rarely in patients treated with olanzapine. In most of these cases, a history of seizures or risk factors for seizures were reported. *Very rare (<0.01%):* Cases reported as neuroleptic malignant syndrome (NMS) have been received in association with olanzapine (see also section 4.4). Parkinsonism, dystonia, and tardive dyskinesia have been reported very rarely with olanzapine. Acute symptoms, such as sweating, insomnia, tremor, anxiety, nausea, or vomiting, have been reported very rarely when olanzapine is stopped abruptly.
Vascular disorders *Very rare (<0.01%):* Thromboembolism (including pulmonary embolism and deep vein thrombosis).
Gastro-intestinal disorders *Very rare (<0.01%):* Pancreatitis.
Hepato-biliary disorders *Very rare (<0.01%):* Hepatitis.
Musculoskeletal and connective tissue and bone disorders *Very rare (<0.01%):* Rhabdomyolysis.
Skin and subcutaneous tissue disorders *Rare (0.01-0.1%):* Rash.
Renal and urinary disorders *Very rare (<0.01%):* Urinary hesitation.
Reproductive system and breast disorders *Very rare (<0.01%):* Priapism.

4.9 Overdose

Signs and symptoms

Very common symptoms in overdose (>10% incidence) include tachycardia, agitation/aggressiveness, dysarthria, various extrapyramidal symptoms, and reduced level of consciousness, ranging from sedation to coma.

Other medically significant sequelae of overdose include delirium, convulsion, coma, possible neuroleptic malignant syndrome, respiratory depression, aspiration, hypertension or hypotension, cardiac arrhythmias (<2% of overdose cases), and cardiopulmonary arrest. Fatal outcomes have been reported for acute overdoses as low as 450mg, but survival has also been reported following acute overdose of 1,500mg.

Management of overdose

There is no specific antidote for olanzapine. Induction of emesis is not recommended. Standard procedures for management of overdose may be indicated (ie, gastric lavage, administration of activated charcoal). The concomitant administration of activated charcoal was shown to reduce the oral bioavailability of olanzapine by 50 to 60%.

Symptomatic treatment and monitoring of vital organ function should be instituted according to clinical presentation, including treatment of hypotension and circulatory collapse, and support of respiratory function. Do not use epinephrine, dopamine, or other sympathomimetic agents with beta-agonist activity, since beta stimulation may worsen hypotension. Cardiovascular monitoring is necessary to detect possible arrhythmias. Close medical supervision and monitoring should continue until the patient recovers.

5. PHARMACOLOGICAL PROPERTIES

5.1 Pharmacodynamic properties

Pharmacotherapeutic group: Antipsychotic. *ATC code*: N05A H03.

Olanzapine is an antipsychotic, antimanic, and mood stabilising agent that demonstrates a broad pharmacologic profile across a number of receptor systems.

In preclinical studies, olanzapine exhibited a range of receptor affinities (Ki; <100nM) for serotonin 5-$HT_{2A/2C}$, 5-HT_3, 5-HT_6; dopamine D_1, D_2, D_3, D_4, D_5; cholinergic muscarinic receptors m_1-m_5; alpha$_1$-adrenergic; and histamine H_1 receptors. Animal behavioural studies with olanzapine indicated 5HT, dopamine, and cholinergic antagonism, consistent with the receptor-binding profile. Olanzapine demonstrated a greater *in vitro* affinity for serotonin 5-HT_2 than dopamine D_2 receptors and greater 5-HT_2 than D_2 activity in *in vivo* models. Electrophysiological studies demonstrated that olanzapine selectively reduced the firing of mesolimbic (A10) dopaminergic neurons, while having little effect on the striatal (A9) pathways involved in motor function. Olanzapine reduced a conditioned avoidance response, a test indicative of antipsychotic activity, at doses below those producing catalepsy, an effect indicative of motor side-effects. Unlike some other antipsychotic agents, olanzapine increases responding in an 'anxiolytic' test.

In a single oral dose (10mg) Positron Emission Tomography (PET) study in healthy volunteers, olanzapine produced a higher 5-HT_{2A} than dopamine D_2 receptor occupancy. In addition, a SPECT imaging study in schizophrenic patients revealed that olanzapine-responsive patients had lower striatal D_2 occupancy than some other antipsychotic- and risperidone-responsive patients, while being comparable to clozapine-responsive patients.

In two of two placebo- and two of three comparator-controlled trials with oral olanzapine, in over 2,900 schizophrenic patients presenting with both positive and negative symptoms, olanzapine was associated with statistically significantly greater improvements in negative as well as positive symptoms.

In patients with manic or mixed episode of bipolar disorder, oral olanzapine demonstrated superior efficacy to placebo and valproate semisodium (divalproex) in reduction of manic symptoms over 3 weeks. Oral olanzapine also demonstrated comparable efficacy results to haloperidol in terms of the proportion of patients in symptomatic remission from mania and depression at 6 and 12 weeks. In a co-therapy study of patients treated with lithium or valproate for a minimum of 2 weeks, the addition of oral olanzapine 10mg (co-therapy with lithium or valproate) resulted in a greater reduction in symptoms of mania than lithium or valproate monotherapy after 6 weeks.

In a 12-month recurrence prevention study in manic episode patients who achieved remission on olanzapine and were then randomised to olanzapine or placebo, olanzapine demonstrated statistically significant superiority over placebo on the primary endpoint of bipolar recurrence. Olanzapine also showed a statistically significant advantage over placebo in terms of preventing either recurrence into mania or recurrence into depression.

In a second 12-month recurrence prevention study in manic episode patients who achieved remission with a combination of olanzapine and lithium and were then randomised to olanzapine or lithium alone, olanzapine was statistically non-inferior to lithium on the primary endpoint of bipolar recurrence (olanzapine 30.0%, lithium 38.3%; $P = 0.055$).

In an 18-month co-therapy study in manic or mixed episode patients stabilised with olanzapine plus a mood stabiliser (lithium or valproate), long-term olanzapine co-therapy with lithium or valproate was not statistically significantly superior to lithium or valproate alone in delaying bipolar recurrence, defined according to syndromic (diagnostic) criteria.

5.2 Pharmacokinetic properties
In a pharmacokinetic study in healthy volunteers, a dose of 5mg of Zyprexa Powder for Solution for Injection produced a maximum plasma concentration (C_{max}) approximately 5-times higher than that seen with the same dose of olanzapine administered orally. The C_{max} occurs earlier after intramuscular compared to oral use (15 to 45 minutes versus 5 to 8 hours). As with oral use, C_{max} and area under the curve after intramuscular use are directly proportional to the dose administered. For the same dose of olanzapine administered intramuscularly and orally, the associated area under the curve, half-life, clearance, and volume of distribution are similar. The metabolic profiles following intramuscular and oral use are similar.

In non-smoking versus smoking subjects (males and females) administered olanzapine intramuscularly, the mean elimination half-life was prolonged (38.6 versus 30.4 hours) and the clearance was reduced (18.6 versus 27.7 l/hr).

Additional pharmacokinetic data following administration of oral olanzapine are described below.

Olanzapine is metabolised in the liver by conjugative and oxidative pathways. The major circulating metabolite is the 10-N-glucuronide, which does not pass the blood brain barrier. Cytochromes P450-CYP1A2 and P450-CYP2D6 contribute to the formation of the N-desmethyl and 2-hydroxymethyl metabolites; both exhibited significantly less *in vivo* pharmacological activity than olanzapine in animal studies. The predominant pharmacologic activity is from the parent, olanzapine. After oral administration, the mean terminal elimination half-life of olanzapine in healthy subjects varied on the basis of age and gender.

In healthy elderly (65 and over) versus non-elderly subjects administered oral olanzapine, the mean elimination half-life was prolonged (51.8 versus 33.8 hours) and the clearance was reduced (17.5 versus 18.2 l/hr). The pharmacokinetic variability observed in the elderly is within the range for the non-elderly. In 44 patients with schizophrenia >65 years of age, dosing from 5 to 20mg/day was not associated with any distinguishing profile of adverse events.

In female versus male subjects administered oral olanzapine, the mean elimination half-life was somewhat prolonged (36.7 versus 32.3 hours) and the clearance was reduced (18.9 versus 27.3 l/hr). However, olanzapine (5-20mg) demonstrated a comparable safety profile in female (n = 467) as in male patients (n = 869).

In renally impaired patients (creatinine clearance <10ml/min) versus healthy subjects administered oral olanzapine, there was no significant difference in mean elimination half-life (37.7 versus 32.4 hours) or clearance (21.2 versus 25.0 l/hr). A mass balance study showed that approximately 57% of radiolabelled olanzapine appeared in urine, principally as metabolites.

In smoking subjects with mild hepatic dysfunction administered olanzapine orally, mean elimination half-life (39.3 hours) was prolonged and clearance (18.0 l/hr) was reduced analogous to non-smoking healthy subjects (48.8 hours and 14.1 l/hr, respectively).

The plasma clearance of olanzapine is lower in elderly versus young subjects, in females versus males, and in non-smokers versus smokers. However, the magnitude of the impact of age, gender, or smoking on olanzapine clearance and half-life is small in comparison to the overall variability between individuals.

In a study of Caucasians, Japanese, and Chinese subjects, there were no differences in the pharmacokinetic parameters among the three populations.

The plasma protein binding of olanzapine was about 93% over the concentration range of about 7 to about 1,000ng/ml. Olanzapine is bound predominantly to albumin and alpha$_1$-acid-glycoprotein.

5.3 Preclinical safety data
Acute (single-dose) toxicity
Signs of oral toxicity in rodents were characteristic of potent antipsychotic compounds: hypoactivity, coma, tremors, clonic convulsions, salivation, and depressed weight gain. The median lethal doses were approximately 210mg/kg (mice) and 175mg/kg (rats). Dogs tolerated single oral doses up to 100mg/kg without mortality. Clinical signs included sedation, ataxia, tremors, increased heart rate, laboured respiration, miosis, and anorexia. In monkeys, single oral doses up to 100mg/kg resulted in prostration and, at higher doses, semi-consciousness.

Repeated-dose toxicity
In studies up to 3 months duration in mice and up to 1 year in rats and dogs, the predominant effects were CNS depression, anticholinergic effects, and peripheral haematological disorders. Tolerance developed to the CNS depression. Growth parameters were decreased at high doses. Reversible effects consistent with elevated prolactin in rats included decreased weights of ovaries and uterus, and morphologic changes in vaginal epithelium and in mammary gland.

Haematologic toxicity: Effects on haematology parameters were found in each species, including dose-related reductions in circulating leucocytes in mice and non-specific reductions of circulating leucocytes in rats; however, no evidence of bone marrow cytotoxicity was found. Reversible neutropenia, thrombocytopenia, or anaemia developed in a few dogs treated with 8 or 10mg/kg/day (total olanzapine exposure [AUC] is 12- to 15-fold greater than that of a man given a 12mg dose). In cytopenic dogs, there were no undesirable effects on progenitor and proliferating cells in the bone marrow.

Reproductive toxicity
Olanzapine had no teratogenic effects. Sedation affected mating performance of male rats. Oestrous cycles were affected at doses of 1.1mg/kg (3-times the maximum human dose) and reproduction parameters were influenced in rats given 3mg/kg (9-times the maximum human dose). In the offspring of rats given olanzapine, delays in foetal development and transient decreases in offspring activity levels were seen.

Mutagenicity
Olanzapine was not mutagenic or clastogenic in a full range of standard tests, which included bacterial mutation tests and *in vitro* and oral *in vivo* mammalian tests.

Carcinogenicity
Based on the results of oral studies in mice and rats, it was concluded that olanzapine is not carcinogenic.

6. PHARMACEUTICAL PARTICULARS
6.1 List of excipients
Lactose monohydrate

Tartaric acid (E334)

Hydrochloric acid. This may have been added to adjust pH.

Sodium hydroxide. This may have been added to adjust pH.

6.2 Incompatibilities
Reconstitute Zyprexa Powder for Solution for Injection only with water for injections (see section 6.6).

Zyprexa Powder for Solution for Injection must not be combined in the syringe with any commercially available drugs. See examples of incompatibilities below.

Olanzapine for injection should not be combined in a syringe with diazepam injection because precipitation occurs when these products are mixed.

Lorazepam injection should not be used to reconstitute olanzapine for injection as this combination results in a delayed reconstitution time.

Olanzapine for injection should not be combined in a syringe with haloperidol injection because the resulting low pH has been shown to degrade olanzapine over time.

6.3 Shelf life
Vial: 2 years.

Solution (after reconstitution): 1 hour.

6.4 Special precautions for storage
Do not store above 25°C. Protect from light. Do not freeze the solution following reconstitution of the vial.

6.5 Nature and contents of container
Zyprexa 10mg Powder for Solution for Injection: Type I glass vial.

One carton contains 1 vial.

Not all packs may be marketed in every country.

6.6 Instructions for use and handling
Reconstitute Zyprexa only with water for injections, using standard aseptic techniques for reconstitution of parenteral products. No other solutions should be used for reconstitution (see section 6.2).

1. Withdraw 2.1ml of water for injection into a sterile syringe. Inject into a vial of Zyprexa.

2. Rotate the vial until the contents have completely dissolved, giving a yellow coloured solution. The vial contains 11.0mg olanzapine as a solution of 5mg/ml (1mg olanzapine is retained in the vial and syringe, thus allowing delivery of 10mg olanzapine).

3. The following table provides injection volumes for delivering various doses of olanzapine:

Dose (mg)	Volume of Injection (ml)
10	2.0
7.5	1.5
5	1.0

4. Administer the solution intramuscularly. Do not administer intravenously or subcutaneously.

5. Discard the syringe and any unused solution in accordance with appropriate clinical procedures.

6. Use the solution immediately within 1 hour of reconstitution. Do not store above 25°C. Do not freeze.

Parenteral medicines should be inspected visually for particulate matter prior to administration.

7. MARKETING AUTHORISATION HOLDER
Eli Lilly Nederland BV, Grootslag 1-5, NL-3991 RA, Houten, The Netherlands.

8. MARKETING AUTHORISATION NUMBER(S)
EU/1/96/022/016

9. DATE OF FIRST AUTHORISATION/RENEWAL OF THE AUTHORISATION

Date of first authorisation:	27 September 1996
Date of last renewal of authorisation:	20 November 2001

10. DATE OF REVISION OF THE TEXT
February 2005

LEGAL CATEGORY
POM

*ZYPREXA (olanzapine) and VELOTAB are trademarks of Eli Lilly and Company.

ZY30M

Zyvox 600 mg Film-Coated Tablets, 100 mg/5 ml Granules for Oral Suspension, 2 mg/ml Solution for Infusion

(Pharmacia Limited)

1. NAME OF THE MEDICINAL PRODUCT
Zyvox ▼600 mg Film-Coated Tablets

Zyvox ▼ 100 mg/5 ml Granules for Oral Suspension

Zyvox ▼ 2 mg/ml Solution for Infusion

2. QUALITATIVE AND QUANTITATIVE COMPOSITION
Zyvox 600 mg Film-Coated Tablets

Each tablet contains 600 mg linezolid.

Zyvox 100 mg/5 ml Granules for Oral Suspension

Following reconstitution with 123 ml water, each 5 ml contains 100 mg linezolid.

Zyvox 2 mg/ml Solution for Infusion

1 ml contains 2 mg linezolid. 300 ml infusion bags contain 600 mg linezolid.

For excipients, see section 6.1.

3. PHARMACEUTICAL FORM
Zyvox 600 mg Film-Coated Tablets

Film-coated tablet.

White, ovaloid tablet with "ZYVOX 600 mg" printed on one side.

Zyvox 100 mg/5 ml Granules for Oral Suspension

Granules for oral suspension.

White to light-yellow, orange flavoured granules.

Zyvox 2 mg/ml Solution for Infusion

Solution for infusion.

Isotonic, clear, colourless to yellow solution.

4. CLINICAL PARTICULARS
4.1 Therapeutic indications
Zyvox is indicated for the treatment of the following infections when known or suspected to be caused by susceptible Gram positive bacteria. In determining whether Zyvox is an appropriate treatment, the results of microbiological tests or information on the prevalence of resistance to antibacterial agents among Gram positive bacteria should be taken into consideration. (See section 5.1 for the appropriate organisms).

- Nosocomial pneumonia
- Community acquired pneumonia
- Complicated skin and soft tissue infections (see section 4.4)

Linezolid should only be initiated in a hospital environment and after consultation with a relevant specialist.

Combination therapy will be necessary if a concomitant Gram negative pathogen is documented or suspected. (See section 5.1).

Consideration should be given to official guidance on the appropriate use of antibacterial agents.

4.2 Posology and method of administration
Zyvox solution for infusion, film-coated tablets or oral suspension may be used as initial therapy. Patients who commence treatment on the parenteral formulation may be switched to either oral presentation when clinically indicated. In such circumstances, no dose adjustment is required as linezolid has an oral bioavailability of approximately 100%.

Recommended dosage and duration of treatment for adults: The duration of treatment is dependent on the pathogen, the site of infection and its severity, and on the patient's clinical response.

The following recommendations for duration of therapy reflect those used in the clinical trials. Shorter treatment regimens may be suitable for some types of infection but have not been evaluated in clinical trials.

To date, the maximum treatment duration has been 28 days (see section 4.4).

No increase in the recommended dosage or duration of treatment is required for infections associated with concurrent bacteraemia.

The dose recommendation for the solution for infusion and the tablets/granules for oral suspension are identical and are as follows:

Infections	Dosage	Duration of treatment
Nosocomial pneumonia	600 mg twice daily	10-14 Consecutive days
Community acquired pneumonia	600 mg twice daily	10-14 Consecutive days
Complicated skin and soft tissue infections	600 mg twice daily	10-14 Consecutive days

Children: There are insufficient data on the safety and efficacy of linezolid in children and adolescents (< 18 years old) to establish dosage recommendations (see section 5.2). Therefore, until further data are available, use of linezolid in this age group is not recommended.

Elderly patients: No dose adjustment is required.

Patients with renal insufficiency: No dose adjustment is required (see sections 4.4 and 5.2).

Patients with severe renal insufficiency (i.e. CL_{CR} < 30 ml/min): No dose adjustment is required. Due to the unknown clinical significance of higher exposure (up to 10 fold) to the two primary metabolites of linezolid in patients with severe renal insufficiency, linezolid should be used with special caution in these patients and only when the anticipated benefit is considered to outweigh the theoretical risk.

As approximately 30% of a linezolid dose is removed during 3 hours of haemodialysis, linezolid should be given after dialysis in patients receiving such treatment. The primary metabolites of linezolid are removed to some extent by haemodialysis, but the concentrations of these metabolites are still very considerably higher following dialysis than those observed in patients with normal renal function or mild to moderate renal insufficiency.

Therefore, linezolid should be used with special caution in patients with severe renal insufficiency who are undergoing dialysis and only when the anticipated benefit is considered to outweigh the theoretical risk.

To date, there is no experience of linezolid administration to patients undergoing continuous ambulatory peritoneal dialysis (CAPD) or alternative treatments for renal failure (other than haemodialysis).

Patients with hepatic insufficiency: No dose adjustment is required. However, there are limited clinical data and it is recommended that linezolid should be used in such patients only when the anticipated benefit is considered to outweigh the theoretical risk (see sections 4.4 and 5.2).

Method of administration: The recommended linezolid dosage should be administered intravenously or orally twice daily.

Zyvox 600 mg Film-Coated Tablets

Route of administration: Oral use.

The film-coated tablets may be taken with or without food.

Zyvox 100 mg/5 ml Granules for Oral Suspension

Route of administration: Oral use.

The oral suspension may be taken with or without food.

A 600 mg dose is provided by 30 ml of reconstituted suspension (i.e. six 5 ml spoonfuls).

Zyvox 2 mg/ml Solution for Infusion

Route of administration: Intravenous use.

The solution for infusion should be administered over a period of 30 to 120 minutes.

4.3 Contraindications

Patients hypersensitive to linezolid or any of the excipients (see section 6.1).

Linezolid should not be used in patients taking any medicinal product which inhibits monoamine oxidases A or B (e.g. phenelzine, isocarboxazid, selegiline, moclobemide) or within two weeks of taking any such medicinal product.

Unless there are facilities available for close observation and monitoring of blood pressure, linezolid should not be administered to patients with the following underlying clinical conditions or on the following types of concomitant medications:

- Patients with uncontrolled hypertension, phaeochromocytoma, carcinoid, thyrotoxicosis, bipolar depression, schizoaffective disorder, acute confusional states.

- Patients taking any of the following medications: serotonin re-uptake inhibitors, tricyclic antidepressants, serotonin 5-HT_1 receptor agonists (triptans), directly and indirectly acting sympathomimetic agents (including the adrenergic bronchodilators, pseudoephedrine and phenylpropanolamine), vasopressive agents (e.g. epinephrine, norepinephrine), dopaminergic agents (e.g. dopamine, dobutamine), pethidine or buspirone.

Animal data suggest that linezolid and its metabolites may pass into breast milk and, accordingly, breastfeeding should be discontinued prior to and throughout administration (see section 4.6).

4.4 Special warnings and special precautions for use

Linezolid is a reversible, non-selective inhibitor of monoamine oxidase (MAOI); however, at the doses used for antibacterial therapy, it does not exert an anti-depressive effect. There are very limited data from drug interaction studies and on the safety of linezolid when administered to patients with underlying conditions and/or on concomitant medications which might put them at risk from MAO inhibition. Therefore, linezolid is not recommended for use in these circumstances unless close observation and monitoring of the recipient is possible (see sections 4.3 and 4.5).

Patients should be advised against consuming large amounts of tyramine rich foods (see section 4.5).

Zyvox 100 mg/5 ml Granules for Oral Suspension

The reconstituted oral suspension contains a source of phenylalanine (aspartame) equivalent to 20 mg/5 ml. Therefore, this formulation may be harmful for people with phenylketonuria. For patients with phenylketonuria, Zyvox solution for infusion or tablets are recommended.

The suspension also contains sucrose, mannitol and sodium equivalent to 1.7 mg/ml.

Therefore, it should not be administered to patients with rare hereditary problems of fructose intolerance, glucose-galactose malabsorption or sucrase-isomaltase insufficiency. Due to its mannitol content, the oral suspension may have a mild laxative effect. The product contains 8.5 mg sodium per 5 ml dose. The sodium content should be taken into account in patients on a controlled sodium diet.

Zyvox 2 mg/ml Solution for Infusion

Each ml of the solution contains 45.7 mg (i.e. 13.7 g/300 ml) glucose. This should be taken into account in patients with diabetes mellitus or other conditions associated with glucose intolerance. Each ml of solution also contains 0.38 mg (114 mg/300 ml) sodium.

Myelosuppression (including anaemia, leucopenia, pancytopenia and thrombocytopenia) has been reported in patients receiving linezolid. In cases where the outcome is known, when linezolid was discontinued, the affected haematologic parameters have risen toward pretreatment levels. The risk of these effects appears to be related to the duration of treatment. Thrombocytopenia may occur more commonly in patients with severe renal insufficiency, whether or not on dialysis. Therefore, close monitoring of blood counts is recommended in patients who: have pre-existing anaemia, granulocytopenia or thrombocytopenia; are receiving concomitant medications that may decrease haemoglobin levels, depress blood counts or adversely affect platelet count or function; have severe renal insufficiency; receive more than 10-14 days of therapy. Linezolid should be administered to such patients only when close monitoring of haemoglobin levels, blood counts and platelet counts is possible.

If significant myelosuppression occurs during linezolid therapy, treatment should be stopped unless it is considered absolutely necessary to continue therapy, in which case intensive monitoring of blood counts and appropriate management strategies should be implemented.

In addition, it is recommended that complete blood counts (including haemoglobin levels, platelets, and total and differentiated leucocyte counts) should be monitored weekly in patients who receive linezolid regardless of baseline blood count.

Controlled clinical trials did not include patients with diabetic foot lesions, decubitus or ischaemic lesions, severe burns or gangrene. Therefore, experience in the use of linezolid in the treatment of these conditions is limited.

Linezolid should be used with special caution in patients with severe renal insufficiency and only when the anticipated benefit is considered to outweigh the theoretical risk (see sections 4.2 and 5.2).

It is recommended that linezolid should be given to patients with severe hepatic insufficiency only when the perceived benefit outweighs the theoretical risk (see sections 4.2 and 5.2).

Pseudomembranous colitis has been reported with nearly all antibacterial agents, including linezolid. Therefore, it is important to consider this diagnosis in patients who present with diarrhoea subsequent to the administration of any antibacterial agent. In cases of suspected or verified antibiotic-associated colitis, discontinuation of linezolid may be warranted. Appropriate management measures should be instituted.

The effects of linezolid therapy on normal flora have not been evaluated in clinical trials.

The use of antibiotics may occasionally result in an overgrowth of non-susceptible organisms. For example, approximately 3% of patients receiving the recommended linezolid doses experienced drug-related candidiasis during clinical trials. Should superinfection occur during therapy, appropriate measures should be taken.

The safety and effectiveness of linezolid when administered for periods longer than 28 days have not been established.

Linezolid reversibly decreased fertility and induced abnormal sperm morphology in adult male rats at exposure levels approximately equal to those expected in humans; possible effects of linezolid on the human male reproductive system are not known (see section 5.3).

4.5 Interaction with other medicinal products and other forms of Interaction

Linezolid is a reversible, non-selective inhibitor of monoamine oxidase (MAOI). There are very limited data from drug interaction studies and on the safety of linezolid when administered to patients on concomitant medications that might put them at risk from MAO inhibition. Therefore, linezolid is not recommended for use in these circumstances unless close observation and monitoring of the recipient is possible (see section 4.3).

In normotensive healthy volunteers, linezolid enhanced the increases in blood pressure caused by pseudoephedrine and phenylpropanolamine hydrochloride. Co-administration of linezolid with either pseudoephedrine or phenylpropanolamine resulted in mean increases in systolic blood pressure of the order of 30-40 mmHg, compared with 11-15 mmHg increases with linezolid alone, 14-18 mmHg with either pseudoephedrine or phenylpropanolamine alone and 8-11 mmHg with placebo. Similar studies in hypertensive subjects have not been conducted. It is recommended that doses of drugs with a vasopressive action, including dopaminergic agents, should be carefully titrated to achieve the desired response when co-administered with linezolid.

The potential drug-drug interaction with dextromethorphan was studied in healthy volunteers. Subjects were administered dextromethorphan (two 20 mg doses given 4 hours apart) with or without linezolid. No serotonin syndrome effects (confusion, delirium, restlessness, tremors, blushing, diaphoresis, hyperpyrexia) have been observed in normal subjects receiving linezolid and dextromethorphan.

Post marketing experience: there has been one report of a patient experiencing serotonin syndrome-like effects while taking linezolid and dextromethorphan which resolved on discontinuation of both medications.

During clinical use of linezolid with serotonin re-uptake inhibitors, cases of serotonin syndrome have been very rarely reported (see sections 4.3 and 4.8).

No significant pressor response was observed in subjects receiving both linezolid and less than 100 mg tyramine. This suggests that it is only necessary to avoid ingesting excessive amounts of food and beverages with a high tyramine content (e.g. mature cheese, yeast extracts, undistilled alcoholic beverages and fermented soya bean products such as soy sauce).

Linezolid is not detectably metabolised by the cytochrome P450 (CYP) enzyme system and it does not inhibit any of the clinically significant human CYP isoforms (1A2, 2C9, 2C19, 2D6, 2E1, 3A4). Similarly, linezolid does not induce P450 isoenzymes in rats. Therefore, no CYP450-induced drug interactions are expected with linezolid.

When warfarin was added to linezolid therapy at steady-state, there was a 10% reduction in mean maximum INR on co-administration with a 5% reduction in AUC INR. There are insufficient data from patients who have received warfarin and linezolid to assess the clinical significance, if any, of these findings.

4.6 Pregnancy and lactation

There are no adequate data from the use of linezolid in pregnant women. Studies in animals have shown reproductive toxicity (see section 5.3). A potential risk for humans exists.

Linezolid should not be used during pregnancy unless clearly necessary i.e. only if the potential benefit outweighs the theoretical risk.

Animal data suggest that linezolid and its metabolites may pass into breast milk and, accordingly, breastfeeding should be discontinued prior to and throughout administration.

4.7 Effects on ability to drive and use machines

Patients should be warned about the potential for dizziness whilst receiving linezolid and should be advised not to drive or operate machinery if dizziness occurs.

4.8 Undesirable effects

The information provided is based on data generated from clinical studies in which more than 2,000 adult patients received the recommended linezolid doses for up to 28 days.

Approximately 22% of patients experienced adverse reactions; those most commonly reported were headache (2.1%), diarrhoea (4.2%), nausea (3.3%) and candidiasis (particularly oral [0.8%] and vaginal [1.1%] candidiasis, see table below).

The most commonly reported drug-related adverse events which led to discontinuation of treatment were headache, diarrhoea, nausea and vomiting. About 3% of patients discontinued treatment because they experienced a drug-related adverse event.

(see Table 1 on next page)

The following adverse reactions to linezolid were considered to be serious in isolated cases: localised abdominal

Table 1

Adverse drug reactions occurring at frequencies > 0.1%		
General body	Common	Headache; candidiasis (particularly oral and vaginal candidiasis) or fungal infection.
	Uncommon	Localised or general abdominal pain; chills; fatigue; fever; injection site pain; phlebitis / thrombophlebitis; localised pain.
Blood and the lymphatic system disorders	Uncommon	(Frequency as reported by clinician): Eosinophilia, leucopenia, neutropenia, thrombocytopenia.
Metabolism and nutrition disorders	Common	Abnormal liver function tests.
Nervous system disorders	Uncommon:	Dizziness, hypoaesthesia, insomnia, paraesthesia
Special senses	Common:	Taste perversion (metallic taste).
	Uncommon:	Blurred vision, tinnitus.
Cardiovascular disorders	Uncommon:	Hypertension
Gastrointestinal disorders	Common:	Diarrhoea, nausea, vomiting.
	Uncommon:	Constipation; dry mouth; dyspepsia; gastritis; glossitis; increased thirst; loose stools; pancreatitis; stomatitis; tongue discolouration or disorder.
Skin disorders	Uncommon:	Dermatitis, diaphoresis, pruritus, rash, urticaria.
Urogenital disorders	Uncommon:	Vulvovaginal disorder, polyuria, vaginitis.
Laboratory abnormalities (according to definitions applied during clinical trials) occurring at frequencies > 0.1%		
Chemistry	Common:	Increased AST, ALT, LDH, alkaline phosphatase, BUN, creatine kinase, lipase, amylase or non fasting glucose. Decreased total protein, albumin, sodium or calcium. Increased or decreased potassium or bicarbonate.
	Uncommon:	Increased total bilirubin, creatinine, sodium or calcium. Decreased non fasting glucose. Increased or decreased chloride.
Haematology	Common:	Increased neutrophils or eosinophils. Decreased haemoglobin, haematocrit or red blood cell count. Increased or decreased platelet or white blood cell counts.
	Uncommon:	Increased reticulocyte count. Decreased neutrophils.
Common	> 1/100 and < 1/10 or > 1% and < 10%	
Uncommon	> 1/1,000 and < 1/100 or > 0.1% and < 1%	

pain, transient ischaemic attacks, hypertension, pancreatitis and renal failure.

During clinical trials, a single case of arrhythmia (tachycardia) was reported as drug related. Seizures were reported in 10 patients of which none was considered to be drug related.

Post marketing experience: There have been reports of anaemia, leucopenia, neutropenia, thrombocytopenia, pancytopenia and myelosuppression (see section 4.4). Neuropathy (peripheral, optic) has been rarely reported in patients treated with linezolid; these reports have primarily been in patients treated for longer than the maximum recommended duration of 28 days. Cases of serotonin syndrome have been very rarely reported (see sections 4.3 and 4.5). Very rare reports of bullous skin disorders such as those described as Stevens-Johnson syndrome have been received.

4.9 Overdose

No specific antidote is known.

No cases of overdose have been reported. However, the following information may prove useful:

Supportive care is advised together with maintenance of glomerular filtration. Approximately 30% of a linezolid dose is removed during 3 hours of haemodialysis, but no data are available for the removal of linezolid by peritoneal dialysis or haemoperfusion. The two primary metabolites of linezolid are also removed to some extent by haemodialysis.

Signs of toxicity in rats following doses of 3000 mg/kg/day linezolid were decreased activity and ataxia whilst dogs treated with 2000 mg/kg/day experienced vomiting and tremors.

5. PHARMACOLOGICAL PROPERTIES

5.1 Pharmacodynamic properties

Pharmacotherapeutic group: Other antibacterials.

ATC code: J 01 X X 08

General Properties

Linezolid is a synthetic, antibacterial agent that belongs to a new class of antimicrobials, the oxazolidinones. It has in vitro activity against aerobic Gram positive bacteria, some Gram negative bacteria and anaerobic micro-organisms. Linezolid selectively inhibits bacterial protein synthesis via a unique mechanism of action. Specifically, it binds to a site on the bacterial ribosome (23S of the 50S subunit) and prevents the formation of a functional 70S initiation complex which is an essential component of the translation process.

The in vitro postantibiotic effect (PAE) of linezolid for *Staphylococcus aureus* was approximately 2 hours. When measured in animal models, the in vivo PAE was 3.6 and 3.9 hours for *Staphylococcus aureus* and *Streptococcus pneumoniae*, respectively. In animal studies, the key pharmacodynamic parameter for efficacy was the time for which the linezolid plasma level exceeded the minimum inhibitory concentration (MIC) for the infecting organism.

Breakpoints

◆ The general MIC breakpoint to identify organisms susceptible to linezolid is ⩽ 2 mg/l.

◆ There are limited data to suggest that staphylococcal and enterococcal species for which the MIC linezolid is 4 mg/l may be successfully treated.

◆ All organisms for which the MIC of linezolid is ⩾ 8 mg/l (i.e.> 4 mg/l) linezolid should be considered resistant.

Susceptibility

The prevalence of resistance may vary geographically and with time for selected species and local information on resistance is desirable, particularly when treating severe infections. Only micro-organisms relevant to the given clinical indications are presented here.

Category
Susceptible organisms
Gram positive aerobes:
Enterococcus faecalis
*Enterococcus faecium**
*Staphylococcus aureus**
Coagulase negative staphylococci
*Streptococcus agalactiae**
Streptococcus pneumoniae*
*Streptococcus pyogenes**
Group C streptococci
Group G streptococci
Gram positive anaerobes:
Clostridium perfringens
Peptostreptococcus anaerobius
Peptostreptococcus species
Resistant organisms
Haemophilus influenzae
Moraxella catarrhalis
Neisseria species
Enterobacteriaceae
Pseudomonas species

*Clinical efficacy has been demonstrated for susceptible isolates in approved clinical indications.

Whereas linezolid shows some in vitro activity against *Legionella, Chlamydia pneumoniae* and *Mycoplasma pneumoniae*, there are insufficient data to demonstrate clinical efficacy.

Resistance

Cross resistance

Linezolid's mechanism of action differs from those of other antibiotic classes. In vitro studies with clinical isolates (including methicillin-resistant staphylococci, vancomycin-resistant enterococci, and penicillin- and erythromycin-resistant streptococci) indicate that linezolid is usually active against organisms which are resistant to one or more other classes of antimicrobial agents.

Resistant mutant frequency

Resistant mutant frequency to linezolid occurs in vitro at a frequency of 1×10^{-9} to 1×10^{-11} and is associated with point mutations in the 23S rRNA. Linezolid-resistant organisms were recovered from six patients infected with *E. faecium* (four patients received 200 mg Q12h and two patients received 600 mg Q12h) in clinical trials and in eight patients with *E. faecium* and in one patient with *E. faecalis* treated in the expanded access programme. All patients had prosthetic devices that were not removed or abscesses that were not drained.

5.2 Pharmacokinetic properties

Zyvox primarily contains (s)-linezolid which is biologically active and is metabolised to form inactive derivatives.

Absorption

Linezolid is rapidly and extensively absorbed following oral dosing. Maximum plasma concentrations are reached within 2 hours of dosing. Absolute oral bioavailability of linezolid (oral and intravenous dosing in a crossover study) is complete (approximately 100%). Absorption is not significantly affected by food and absorption from the oral suspension is similar to that achieved with the film-coated tablets.

Plasma linezolid Cmax and Cmin (mean and [SD]) at steady-state following twice daily intravenous dosing of 600 mg have been determined to be 15.1 [2.5] mg/l and 3.68 [2.68] mg/l, respectively.

In another study following oral dosing of 600 mg twice daily to steady-state, Cmax and Cmin were determined to be 21.2 [5.8] mg/l and 6.15 [2.94] mg/l, respectively. Steady-state conditions are achieved by the second day of dosing.

Distribution

Volume of distribution at steady-state averages at about 40-50 litres in healthy adults and approximates to total body water. Plasma protein binding is about 31% and is not concentration dependent.

Linezolid concentrations have been determined in various fluids from a limited number of subjects in volunteer studies following multiple dosing. The ratio of linezolid in saliva and sweat relative to plasma was 1.2:1.0 and 0.55:1.0, respectively. The ratio for epithelial lining fluid and alveolar cells of the lung was 4.5:1.0 and 0.15:1.0, when measured at steady-state Cmax, respectively. In a small study of subjects with ventricular-peritoneal shunts and essentially non-inflamed meninges, the ratio of linezolid in cerebrospinal fluid to plasma at Cmax was 0.7:1.0 after multiple linezolid dosing.

Metabolism

Linezolid is primarily metabolised by oxidation of the morpholine ring resulting mainly in the formation of two inactive open-ring carboxylic acid derivatives; the aminoethoxyacetic acid metabolite (PNU-142300) and the hydroxyethyl glycine metabolite (PNU-142586). The hydroxyethyl glycine metabolite (PNU-142586) is the predominant human metabolite and is believed to be formed by a non-enzymatic process. The aminoethoxyacetic acid metabolite

(PNU-142300) is less abundant. Other minor, inactive metabolites have been characterised.

Elimination

In patients with normal renal function or mild to moderate renal insufficiency, linezolid is primarily excreted under steady-state conditions in the urine as PNU-142586 (40%), parent drug (30%) and PNU-142300 (10%). Virtually no parent drug is found in the faeces whilst approximately 6% and 3% of each dose appears as PNU-142586 and PNU-142300, respectively. The elimination half-life of linezolid averages at about 5-7 hours.

Non-renal clearance accounts for approximately 65% of the total clearance of linezolid. A small degree of non-linearity in clearance is observed with increasing doses of linezolid. This appears to be due to lower renal and non-renal clearance at higher linezolid concentrations. However, the difference in clearance is small and is not reflected in the apparent elimination half-life.

Special Populations

Patients with renal insufficiency: After single doses of 600 mg, there was a 7-8 fold increase in exposure to the two primary metabolites of linezolid in the plasma of patients with severe renal insufficiency (i.e. creatinine clearance < 30 ml/min). However, there was no increase in AUC of parent drug. Although there is some removal of the major metabolites of linezolid by haemodialysis, metabolite plasma levels after single 600 mg doses were still considerably higher following dialysis than those observed in patients with normal renal function or mild to moderate renal insufficiency.

In 24 patients with severe renal insufficiency, 21 of whom were on regular haemodialysis, peak plasma concentrations of the two major metabolites after several days dosing were about 10 fold those seen in patients with normal renal function. Peak plasma levels of linezolid were not affected.

The clinical significance of these observations has not been established as limited safety data are currently available (see sections 4.2 and 4.4).

Patients with hepatic insufficiency: Limited data indicate that the pharmacokinetics of linezolid, PNU-142300 and PNU-142586 are not altered in patients with mild to moderate hepatic insufficiency (i.e. Child-Pugh class A or B). The pharmacokinetics of linezolid in patients with severe hepatic insufficiency (i.e. Child-Pugh class C) have not been evaluated. However, as linezolid is metabolised by a non-enzymatic process, impairment of hepatic function would not be expected to significantly alter its metabolism (see sections 4.2 and 4.4).

Children and adolescents (< 18 years old): There are insufficient data on the safety and efficacy of linezolid in children and adolescents (< 18 years old) and therefore, use of linezolid in this age group is not recommended.(see section 4.2). Further studies are needed to establish safe and effective dosage recommendations. Pharmacokinetic studies indicate that after single and multiple doses in children (1 week to 12 years), linezolid clearance (based on kg body weight) was greater in paediatric patients than in adults, but decreased with increasing age.

In children 1 week to 12 years old, administration of 10 mg/kg every 8 hours daily gave exposure approximating to that achieved with 600 mg twice daily in adults.

In neonates up to 1 week of age, the systemic clearance of linezolid (based on kg body weight) increases rapidly in the first week of life. Therefore, neonates given 10 mg/kg every 8 hours daily will have the greatest systemic exposure on the first day after delivery. However, excessive accumulation is not expected with this dosage regimen during the first week of life as clearance increases rapidly over that period.

In adolescents (12 to 17 years old), linezolid pharmacokinetics were similar to that in adults following a 600mg dose. Therefore, adolescents administered 600 mg every 12 hours daily will have similar exposure to that observed in adults receiving the same dosage.

Elderly patients: The pharmacokinetics of linezolid are not significantly altered in elderly patients aged 65 and over.

Female patients: Females have a slightly lower volume of distribution than males and the mean clearance is reduced by approximately 20% when corrected for body weight. Plasma concentrations are higher in females and this can partly be attributed to body weight differences. However, because the mean half life of linezolid is not significantly different in males and females, plasma concentrations in females are not expected to substantially rise above those known to be well tolerated and, therefore, dose adjustments are not required.

5.3 Preclinical safety data

Linezolid decreased fertility and reproductive performance of male rats at exposure levels approximately equal to those expected in humans. In sexually mature animals these effects were reversible. However, these effects did not reverse in juvenile animals treated with linezolid for nearly the entire period of sexual maturation. Abnormal sperm morphology in testis of adult male rats, and epithelial cell hypertrophy and hyperplasia in the epididymis were noted. Linezolid appeared to affect the maturation of rat spermatozoa. Supplementation of testosterone had no effect on linezolid-mediated fertility effects. Epididymal hypertrophy was not observed in dogs treated for 1 month, although changes in the weights of prostate, testes and epididymis were apparent.

Reproductive toxicity studies in mice and rats showed no evidence of a teratogenic effect at exposure levels 4 times or equivalent, respectively, to those expected in humans. The same linezolid concentrations caused maternal toxicity in mice and were related to increased embryo death including total litter loss, decreased fetal body weight and an exacerbation of the normal genetic predisposition to sternal variations in the strain of mice. In rats, slight maternal toxicity was noted at exposures lower than expected clinical exposures. Mild fetal toxicity, manifested as decreased fetal body weights, reduced ossification of sternebrae, reduced pup survival and mild maturational delays were noted. When mated, these same pups showed evidence of a reversible dose-related increase in pre-implantation loss with a corresponding decrease in fertility.

Linezolid and its metabolites are excreted into the milk of lactating rats and the concentrations observed were higher than those in maternal plasma.

Linezolid produced reversible myelosupression in rats and dogs.

Preclinical data, based on conventional studies of repeated-dose toxicity and genotoxicity, revealed no special hazard for humans beyond those addressed in other sections of this Summary of Product Characteristics. Carcinogenicity / oncogenicity studies have not been conducted in view of the short duration of dosing and lack of genotoxicity in the standard battery of studies.

6. PHARMACEUTICAL PARTICULARS

6.1 List of excipients

Zyvox 600 mg Film-Coated Tablets

Tablet core:

Microcrystalline cellulose (E460)

Maize starch

Sodium starch glycollate type A

Hydroxypropylcellulose (E463)

Magnesium stearate (E572)

Film coat:

Hypromellose (E464)

Titanium dioxide (E171)

Macrogol 400

Carnauba wax (E903)

Red ink

Red iron oxide (E172)

Zyvox 100 mg/5 ml Granules for Oral Suspension

Sucrose

Mannitol (E421)

Microcrystalline cellulose (E460)

Carboxymethylcellulose sodium (E466)

Aspartame (E951)

Anhydrous colloidal silica (E551)

Sodium citrate (E331)

Xanthan gum (E415)

Sodium benzoate (E211)

Citric acid anhydrous (E330)

Sodium chloride

Sweetners (fructose, maltodextrin, monoammonium glycyrrhizinate, sorbitol)

Orange, Orange Cream, Peppermint, Vanilla flavourings (acetoin, alpha tocopherols acetaldehyde, anisic aldehyde, beta-caryophyllene, n-butyric acid, butyl butyryl lactate, decalactone delta, dimethyl benzyl carb acetate, ethyl alcohol, ethyl butyrate, ethyl maltol, ethyl vanillin, furaneol, grapefruit terpenes, heliotropin, maltodextrin, modified food starch, monomethyl succinate, orange aldehyde, orange oil FLA CP, orange oil Valencia 2X, orange oil 5X Valencia, orange essence oil, orange juice carbonyls, orange terpenes, peppermint essential oil, propylene glycol, tangerine oil, vanilla extract, vanillin, water)

Zyvox 2 mg/ml Solution for Infusion

Glucose monohydrate

Sodium citrate (E331)

Citric acid anhydrous (E330)

Hydrochloric acid (E507)

Sodium hydroxide (E524)

Water for injections

6.2 Incompatibilities

Zyvox 600 mg Film-Coated Tablets and Zyvox 100 mg/5 ml Granules for Oral Suspension

Not applicable.

Zyvox 2 mg/ml Solution for Infusion

Additives should not be introduced into this solution. If linezolid is to be given concomitantly with other drugs, each drug should be given separately in accordance with its own directions for use. Similarly, if the same intravenous line is to be used for sequential infusion of several drugs, the line should be flushed prior to and following linezolid administration with a compatible infusion solution (see section 6.6).

Zyvox solution for infusion is known to be physically incompatible with the following compounds: amphotericin B, chlorpromazine hydrochloride, diazepam, pentamidine isethionate, erythromycin lactobionate, phenytoin sodium and sulphamethoxazole / trimethoprim. Additionally, it is chemically incompatible with ceftriaxone sodium.

6.3 Shelf life

Zyvox 600 mg Film-Coated Tablets

2 years.

Zyvox 100 mg/5 ml Granules for Oral Suspension

Before reconstitution:	2 years.
After reconstitution:	3 weeks.

Zyvox 2 mg/ml Solution for Infusion

Before opening: 3 years.

After opening: From a microbiological point of view, unless the method of opening precludes the risk of microbial contamination, the product should be used immediately. If not used immediately, in-use storage times and conditions are the responsibility of the user.

6.4 Special precautions for storage

Zyvox 600 mg Film-Coated Tablets

No special precautions for storage.

Zyvox 100 mg/5 ml Granules for Oral Suspension

Before reconstitution:	Keep the container tightly closed.
After reconstitution:	Keep the container in the outer carton.

Zyvox 2 mg/ml Solution for Infusion

Store in the original package (overwrap and carton) until ready to use.

6.5 Nature and contents of container

Zyvox 600 mg Film-Coated Tablets

White, HDPE bottle with a polypropylene screw cap containing either 10*, 14*, 20*, 24, 30, 50 or 60 tablets.

White, HDPE bottle with a polypropylene screw cap containing 100 tablets (for hospital use only).

Note:

*The above bottles may also be supplied in "hospital packs" of 5 or 10.

Polyvinylchloride (PVC)/foil blisters of 10 tablets packaged in a box. Each box contains either 10*, 20*, 30, 50 or 60 tablets.

Polyvinylchloride (PVC)/foil blisters of 10 tablets packaged in a box. Each box contains 100 tablets (for hospital use only).

Note:

*The above boxes may also be supplied in "hospital packs" of 5 or 10.

Not all package sizes may be marketed.

Zyvox 100 mg/5 ml Granules for Oral Suspension

Amber, Type III glass bottles with a nominal volume of 240 ml containing 66 g granules for oral suspension. Each bottle has a polypropylene, child resistant screw cap and is packaged in a box with a 2.5 ml/5 ml measuring spoon.

Note:

The above bottles may also be supplied in "hospital packs" of 5 or 10.

Not all package sizes may be marketed.

Zyvox 2 mg/ml Solution for Infusion

Single use, ready-to-use, latex-free, multilayered (inner layer: ethylene propylene copolymer and styrene/ethylene butylene/styrene copolymer; middle layer: styrene/ethylene butylene/styrene copolymer; outer layer: copolyester) film infusion bags sealed inside a foil laminate overwrap. The bag holds 300 ml solution and is packaged in a box. Each box contains 1*, 2**, 5, 10, 20 or 25 infusion bags.

Note:

The above boxes may also be supplied in "hospital" packs of:

*5, 10 or 20

**3, 6 or 10

Not all package sizes may be marketed.

6.6 Instructions for use and handling

Zyvox 600 mg Film-Coated Tablets

No special requirements.

Zyvox 100 mg/5 ml Granules for Oral Suspension

Loosen the granules and reconstitute using 123 ml water in two approximately equal aliquots to produce 150 ml oral suspension. The suspension should be vigorously shaken between each addition of water.

Before use, gently invert the bottle a few times. Do not shake.

Zyvox 2 mg/ml Solution for Infusion

For single use only. Remove overwrap only when ready to use, then check for minute leaks by squeezing the bag firmly. If the bag leaks, do not use as sterility may be impaired. The solution should be visually inspected prior to use and only clear solutions, without particles should be used. Do not use these bags in series connections. Any unused solution must be discarded. Do not reconnect partially used bags.

Zyvox solution for infusion is compatible with the following solutions: 5% glucose intravenous infusion, 0.9% sodium chloride intravenous infusion, Ringer-lactate solution for injection (Hartmann's solution for injection).

7. MARKETING AUTHORISATION HOLDER

Pharmacia Limited
Ramsgate Road
Sandwich
Kent
CT13 9NJ

8. MARKETING AUTHORISATION NUMBER(S)

Zyvox 600 mg Film-Coated Tablets - PL 00032/0261

Zyvox 100 mg/5 ml Granules for Oral Suspension - PL 00032/0259

Zyvox 2 mg/ml Solution for Infusion - PL 00032/0262

9. DATE OF FIRST AUTHORISATION/RENEWAL OF THE AUTHORISATION

5 January 2001/4 January 2006

10. DATE OF REVISION OF THE TEXT

24 November 2004

CODE OF PRACTICE for the PHARMACEUTICAL INDUSTRY

INTRODUCTION

Promoting Appropriate Use of Medicines

The pharmaceutical industry in the United Kingdom is committed to benefiting patients by operating in a professional, ethical and transparent manner to ensure the appropriate use of medicines and support the provision of high quality healthcare. This commitment applies to all with whom the industry interacts. To demonstrate this commitment The Association of the British Pharmaceutical Industry (ABPI), which represents the UK industry, decided that certain activities should be covered in detail and thus agreed the ABPI Code of Practice for the Pharmaceutical Industry. The Code covers the promotion of medicines for prescribing to both health professionals and appropriate administrative staff. In addition it sets standards for the provision of information about prescription only medicines to the public and patients, including patient organisations.

In addition to the Code there is extensive UK and European law relating to the promotion of medicines. The Code reflects and extends beyond the relevant UK law.

The aim of the Code is to ensure that the promotion of medicines to health professionals and to administrative staff is carried out within a robust framework to support high quality patient care. As well as covering printed materials, it controls samples, meetings, promotional aids and the provision of medical and educational goods and services. The Code also sets standards relating to the provision of information to patients and the public as well as relationships with patient groups. The industry considers that provided the requirements of the Code are met, working with patients and patient organisations can bring significant public health benefits. These requirements also apply to working with all user groups, such as disability associations, relative and carer associations and consumer associations.

In summary, companies must ensure that their materials are appropriate, factual, fair and capable of substantiation and that all other activities are appropriate and reasonable.

Ensuring High Standards

The detailed provisions in the Code are to ensure that pharmaceutical companies operate in a responsible, ethical and professional manner. Whilst the industry has a legitimate right to promote medicines to health professionals, the Code recognises and seeks to achieve a balance between the needs of patients, health professionals and the public, bearing in mind the political and social environment within which the industry operates and the statutory controls governing medicines. The availability of accurate up-to-date information is vital to the appropriate use of medicines. Pharmaceutical companies must ensure that enquiries about their medicines are answered appropriately in a timely manner.

Strong support is given to the Code by the industry with all companies devoting considerable resources to ensure that their activities comply with it. Any complaint made against a company under the Code is regarded as a serious matter both by that company and by the industry as a whole. Sanctions are applied against a company ruled in breach of the Code.

Companies must ensure that all relevant personnel are appropriately trained in the requirements of the Code and must have robust operating procedures under which all materials and activities covered by the Code are reviewed to ensure compliance both with the Code and with the appropriate legal requirements.

The Code incorporates the principles set out in:

- the International Federation of Pharmaceutical Manufacturers and Associations' (IFPMA) Code of Pharmaceutical Marketing Practices
- The European Federation of Pharmaceutical Industries and Associations' (EFPIA) Code of Practice on the Promotion of Medicines
- Directive 2001/83/EC on the community code relating to medicinal products for human use, as amended by Directive 2004/27/EC
- The World Health Organisation's Ethical criteria for medicinal drug promotion.

The Code covers the industry's activities only. However those interacting with industry as individuals or organisations also have a responsibility to ensure that their interactions comply with relevant legal requirements and are asked to follow the Code where relevant and not make requests that are not in accordance with the Code. Most of those interacting with the industry, other than patients, are covered by a selection of professional codes and guidance. For example, the General Medical Council guidance 'Duties of a Doctor', the Royal Pharmaceutical Society of Great Britain Code of Ethics and Standards and the Nursing & Midwifery Council Code of Professional Conduct: standards for conduct, performance and ethics. Patient organisations are likely to be covered by Charity Commission rules as well as their own codes. The pharmaceutical industry is encouraged to take into account all relevant codes and guidance as well as the ABPI Code.

Transparency

The industry recognises that transparency is an important means of maintaining confidence. The operation of the Code, including the complaints procedure, is a demonstration of the industry's commitment to transparency as are the requirement to declare pharmaceutical company involvement in activities and materials and the publication of detailed reports of cases considered under the Code. Although not a requirement of this Code, the industry's global agreement to disclose certain clinical trial data is another example of the industry's commitment to transparency. Further information can be found in the Joint Position on the Disclosure of Clinical Trial Information via Clinical Trial Registries and Databases 2005.

Sanctions

In each case where a breach of the Code is ruled, the company concerned must give an undertaking that the practice in question has ceased forthwith and that all possible steps have been taken to avoid a similar breach in the future. An undertaking must be accompanied by details of the action taken to implement the ruling. At the conclusion of a case a detailed case report is published.

Additional sanctions are imposed in serious cases. These can include:

- the audit of a company's procedures to comply with the Code, followed by the possibility of a requirement for the pre-vetting of future material
- recovery of material from those to whom it has been given
- the issue of a corrective statement
- a public reprimand
- advertising in the medical and pharmaceutical press of brief details of cases in which companies were ruled in breach of Clause 2 of the Code, were required to issue a corrective statement or were the subject of a public reprimand
- suspension or expulsion from the ABPI.

Monitoring of Activities and Guidance

The Prescription Medicines Code of Practice Authority (PMCPA) arranges for advertising and meetings to be regularly monitored. The PMCPA also provides informal guidance about the Code and its operation.

Promoting Health

The commitment of Britain's pharmaceutical industry to providing high quality effective medicines brings major benefits to both the nation's health and economy.

The National Health Service spends more than £9.4 billion a year on medicines, representing less than 11 per cent of its total expenditure. Medicine exports are worth over £12.3 billion a year – the UK's third largest foreign exchange earner in manufactured goods. Nearly a quarter of the world's top 100 medicines were discovered in Britain.

Investment into researching and developing new products in the UK is now running at around £3.2 billion a year and each new medicine takes an average of ten to twelve years to develop before it is authorized for use, with no guarantee of commercial success.

The Association of the British Pharmaceutical Industry and its Code of Practice

The Association of the British Pharmaceutical Industry (ABPI) is the trade association representing manufacturers of prescription medicines. It was formed in 1930 and now represents about seventy-five companies which supply more than 80% per cent of the medicines used by the National Health Service.

The Code has been regularly revised since its inception in 1958 and is drawn up in consultation with the British Medical Association, the Royal Pharmaceutical Society of Great Britain and the Medicines and Healthcare products Regulatory Agency of the Department of Health. This edition of the Code was drawn up following consultation with many stakeholders, including patient organisations. Any individual who wished to comment was invited to do so via the ABPI website.

It is a condition of membership of the ABPI to abide by the Code in both the spirit and the letter. Companies which are not members of the ABPI may give their formal agreement to abide by the Code and accept the jurisdiction of the Prescription Medicines Code of Practice Authority and about sixty have done so. The current list can be found on the PMCPA website www.pmcpa.org.uk. Thus the Code is accepted by virtually all pharmaceutical companies operating in the UK.

Administering the Code of Practice

The Code is administered by the Prescription Medicines Code of Practice Authority which is responsible for the provision of advice, guidance and training on the Code as well as for the complaints procedure. The PMCPA operates independently of the ABPI itself. The relationship between the PMCPA and the ABPI is set out in a protocol of agreement. Financial information about the PMCPA is published in its Annual Report.

PMCPA publications can all be found on the website or are supplied on request.

Complaints which are made under the Code are considered by the Code of Practice Panel and, where required, by the Code of Practice Appeal Board. Reports on completed cases are published by the PMCPA. The PMCPA publishes a list of ongoing cases on its website.

How to Complain

Complaints should be submitted to the Director of the Prescription Medicines Code of Practice Authority, 12 Whitehall, London SW1A 2DY, telephone 020-7930 9677, facsimile 020-7930 4554, email complaints@pmcpa.org.uk.

PROVISIONS OF THE CODE OF PRACTICE

Clause 1 Scope of the Code and Definition of Certain Terms

1.1 This Code applies to the promotion of medicines to members of the United Kingdom health professions and to appropriate administrative staff.

The Code also applies to a number of areas which are non-promotional, including information made available to the general public about prescription only medicines.

It does not apply to the promotion of over-the-counter medicines to members of the health professions when the object of that promotion is to encourage their purchase by members of the public.

Clause 1.1 Scope of the Code

For the purposes of the application of the Code, the United Kingdom includes the Channel Islands and the Isle of Man.

The Code applies to the promotion of medicines to members of the health professions and to appropriate administrative staff as specified in Clause 1.1. This includes promotion at meetings for UK residents held outside the UK. It also applies to promotion to UK health professionals and administrative staff at international meetings held outside the UK, except that the promotional material distributed at such meetings will need to comply with local requirements.

Some of the requirements of the Code are not necessarily related to promotion. Examples include declaration of sponsorship in Clause 9.10, certain aspects of the provision of medicines and samples in Clause 17 and the provision of information to the public in Clause 20.

The Code does not apply to the promotion of over-the-counter medicines to members of the health professions when the object of that promotion is to encourage their purchase by members of the public as specified in Clause 1.1. Thus, for example, an advertisement to doctors for an over-the-counter medicine does not come within the scope of the Code if its purpose is to encourage doctors to recommend the purchase of the medicine by patients. Where the advertisement is designed to encourage doctors to prescribe the medicine, then it comes within the scope of the Code.

Advertisements for over-the-counter medicines to pharmacists are outside the scope of the Code. Advertisements to pharmacists for other medicines come within the scope of the Code.

Clause 1.1 Journals with an International Distribution

The Code applies to the advertising of medicines in professional journals which are produced in the UK and/or intended for a UK audience.

International journals which are produced in English in the UK are subject to the Code even if only a small proportion of their circulation is to a UK audience. It is helpful in these circumstances to indicate that the information in the advertisement is consistent with the UK marketing authorization.

It should be noted that the Medicines and Healthcare products Regulatory Agency's guidance 'Advertising and Promotion of Medicines in the UK', The Blue Guide, differs from the above by stating 'Advertising material in professional journals intended primarily for circulation in the UK whether or not in the English language must comply with UK legislation and with the UK marketing authorization for the product'.

Where a journal is produced in the UK but intended for distribution solely to overseas countries local requirements and/or the requirements of the International Federation of Pharmaceutical Manufacturers and Associations' (IFPMA) Code of Pharmaceutical Marketing Practices should be borne in mind.

Clause 1.1 Advertising to the Public and Advertising Over-the-Counter Medicines to Health Professionals and the Retail Trade

The promotion of medicines to the public for self medication is covered by the Code of Standards of Advertising Practice for Over-the-Counter Medicines of the Proprietary Association of Great Britain (PAGB). The PAGB also has a Code of Practice for Advertising Over-the-Counter Medicines to Health Professionals and the Retail Trade.

Clause 1.1 Promotion to Administrative Staff

The provisions of the Code apply in their entirety to the promotion of medicines to appropriate administrative staff except where the text indicates otherwise. For example, the prescribing information required under Clause 4 must be included in promotional material provided to administrative staff but it is not permissible to provide samples of medicines to them as this is proscribed by Clause 17.1.

Particular attention is drawn to the provisions of Clause 12.1 and the supplementary information to that clause, which concern the appropriateness of promotional material to those to whom it is addressed.

1.2 The term 'promotion' means any activity under-taken by a pharmaceutical company or with its authority which promotes the prescription, supply, sale or administration of its medicines.

It includes:

- journal and direct mail advertising
- the activities of representatives including detail aids and other printed material used by representatives
- the supply of samples
- the provision of inducements to prescribe, supply, administer, recommend, buy or sell medicines by the gift, offer or promise of any benefit or bonus, whether in money or in kind
- the provision of hospitality for promotional purposes
- the sponsorship of promotional meetings
- the sponsorship of scientific meetings including payment of travelling and accommodation expenses in connection therewith
- all other sales promotion in whatever form, such as participation in exhibitions, the use of audio-cassettes, films, records, tapes, video recordings, radio, television, the Internet, electronic media, interactive data systems and the like.

It does not include:

- replies made in response to individual enquiries from members of the health professions or appropriate administrative staff or in response to specific communications from them whether of enquiry or comment, including letters published in professional journals, but only if they relate solely to the subject matter of the letter or enquiry, are accurate and do not mislead and are not promotional in nature
- factual, accurate, informative announcements and reference material concerning licensed medicines and relating, for example, to pack changes, adverse-reaction warnings, trade catalogues and price lists, provided they include no product claims
- information supplied by pharmaceutical companies to national public organizations, such as the National Institute for Health and Clinical Excellence (NICE), the All Wales Medicines Strategy Group (AWMSG) and the Scottish Medicines Consortium (SMC) is exempt from the Code provided the information is factual, accurate and not misleading
- measures or trade practices relating to prices, margins or discounts which were in regular use by a significant proportion of the pharmaceutical industry on 1 January 1993
- summaries of product characteristics
- European public assessment reports
- UK public assessment reports
- the labelling on medicines and accompanying package leaflets insofar as they are not promotional for the medicines concerned; the contents of labels and package leaflets are covered by regulations
- information relating to human health or diseases provided there is no reference, either direct or indirect, to specific medicines.

Clause 1.2 Replies Intended for Use in Response to Individual Enquiries

The exemption for replies made in response to individual enquiries from members of the health professions or appropriate administrative staff relates to unsolicited enquiries only. An unsolicited enquiry is one without any prompting from the company. In answering an unsolicited enquiry a company can offer to provide further information. If the enquirer subsequently requests additional information this can be provided and would be exempt from the Code provided the additional information met the requirements of the exemption. A solicited enquiry would be one where a company invites a person to make a request. For example, material offering further information to readers would be soliciting a request for that information. Placing documents on exhibition stands amounts to an invitation to take them. Neither can take the benefit of this exemption.

Replies intended for use in response to enquiries which are received on a regular basis may be drafted in advance provided that they are used only when they directly and solely relate to the particular enquiry. Documents must not have the appearance of promotional material.

1.3 The term 'medicine' means any branded or unbranded medicine intended for use in humans which requires a marketing authorization.

1.4 The term 'health professional' includes members of the medical, dental, pharmacy and nursing professions and any other persons who in the course of their professional activities may prescribe, supply or administer a medicine.

1.5 The term 'over-the-counter medicine' means those medicines or particular packs of medicines which are primarily advertised to the general public for use in self medication.

1.6 The term 'representative' means a representative calling on members of the health professions and administrative staff in relation to the promotion of medicines.

Clause 1.6 Representatives

'Medical representatives' and 'generic sales representatives' are distinguished in Clause 16.4 relating to examinations for representatives.

1.7 Pharmaceutical companies must comply with all applicable codes, laws and regulations to which they are subject.

Clause 1.7 Applicability of Codes

Pharmaceutical companies must ensure that they comply with all applicable codes, laws and regulations to which they are subject. This is particularly relevant when activities/materials involve more than one country or when a pharmaceutical company based in one country is involved in activities in another country.

Activities carried out and materials used by a pharmaceutical company located in a European country must comply with the national code of that European country as well as the national code of the country in which the activities take place or the materials are used. Activities carried out and materials used in a European country by a pharmaceutical company located in a country other than a European country must comply with the EFPIA Code as well as the national code of the country in which the activities are carried out and materials are used.

For example a company located in the UK carrying out an activity outside the UK but within Europe, such as in France, must comply with the UK Code and the French Code regardless of whether or not UK health professionals or appropriate administrative staff are involved. Conversely a company located in France carrying out an activity in the UK must comply with the ABPI Code regardless of whether or not UK health professionals or appropriate administrative staff are involved. Details of the various codes can be found at www.efpia.org or www.ifpma.org.

By 'company' is meant any legal entity that organizes or sponsors promotion which takes place within Europe, whether such entity be a parent company (eg the headquarters, principal office, or controlling company of a commercial enterprise), subsidiary company or any other form of enterprise or organization.

In the event of a conflict of requirements the more restrictive requirements would apply.

All international events, that is to say events that take place outside the responsible pharmaceutical company's home country, must be notified in advance to any relevant local subsidiary or local advice taken.

1.8 Each company must appoint a senior employee to be responsible for ensuring that the company meets the requirements of the Code.

Clause 1.8 Responsible Person

There is an assumption that the responsible person is the managing director or chief executive or equivalent unless other formal arrangements have been made within the company.

Clause 2 Discredit to, and Reduction of Confidence in, the Industry

Activities or materials associated with promotion must never be such as to bring discredit upon, or reduce confidence in, the pharmaceutical industry.

Clause 2 Discredit to, and Reduction of Confidence in, the Industry

A ruling of a breach of this clause is a sign of particular censure and is reserved for such circumstances.

Examples of activities that are likely to be in breach of Clause 2 include prejudicing patient safety and/or public health, excessive hospitality, inducements to prescribe, inadequate action leading to a breach of undertaking, promotion prior to the grant of a marketing authorization, conduct of company employees/agents that falls short of competent care and multiple/cumulative breaches of a similar and serious nature in the same therapeutic area within a short period of time.

Clause 3 Marketing Authorization

Clause 3 Marketing Authorization

The legitimate exchange of medical and scientific information during the development of a medicine is not prohibited provided that any such information or activity does not constitute promotion which is prohibited under this or any other clause.

Clause 3 Promotion at International Meetings

The promotion of medicines at international meetings held in the UK may on occasion pose certain problems with regard to medicines or indications for medicines which do not have a marketing authorization in the UK although they are so authorized in another major industrialised country.

The display and provision of promotional material for such medicines is permitted at international meetings in the UK provided that the following conditions are met:

- *the meeting must be a truly international meeting of high scientific standing with a significant proportion of attendees from outside the UK*
- *the medicine or indication must be relevant and proportional to the purpose of the meeting*
- *promotional material for a medicine or indication that does not have a UK marketing authorization must be clearly and prominently labelled to that effect*
- *in relation to an unlicensed indication, UK approved prescribing information must be readily available for a medicine authorized in the UK even though it will not refer to the unlicensed indication*
- *the name must be given of at least one major industrialised country (such as EU member states, EFTA countries, Australia, Canada, Israel, Japan, New Zealand, South Africa and the United States of America) in which the medicine or indication is authorized and it must be stated that registration conditions differ from country to country*
- *the material is certified in accordance with Clause 14 except that the signatories need certify only that in their belief the material is a fair and truthful presentation of the facts about the medicine.*

3.1 A medicine must not be promoted prior to the grant of the marketing authorization which permits its sale or supply.

Clause 3.1 Advance Notification of New Products or Product Changes

Health authorities and health boards and their equivalents, trust hospitals and primary care trusts and groups need to estimate their likely budgets two to three years in advance in order to meet Treasury requirements and there is a need for them to receive advance information about the introduction of new medicines, or changes to existing medicines, which may significantly affect their level of expenditure during future years.

At the time this information is required, the medicines concerned (or the changes to them) will not be the subject of marketing authorizations (though applications will often have been made) and it would thus be contrary to the Code for them to be promoted. Information may, however, be provided on the following basis:

i) *the information must relate to:*

   (a) *a product which contains a new active substance, or*

   (b) *a product which contains an active substance prepared in a new way, such as by the use of biotechnology, or*

   (c) *a product which is to have a significant addition to the existing range of authorized indications, or*

   (d) *a product which has a novel and innovative means of administration*

ii) *information should be directed to those responsible for making policy decisions on budgets rather than those expected to prescribe*

iii) *whether or not a new medicine or a change to an existing medicine is the subject of a marketing* authorization in the UK must be made clear in advance information

v) the likely cost and budgetary implications must be indicated and must be such that they will make significant differences to the likely expenditure of health authorities and trust hospitals and the like

vi) only factual information must be provided which should be limited to that sufficient to provide an adequate but succinct account of the product's properties; other products should only be mentioned to put the new product into context in the therapeutic area concerned

vii) the information may be attractively presented and printed but should not be in the style of promotional material – product specific logos should be avoided but company logos may be used; the brand name of the product may be included in moderation but it should not be stylized or used to excess

viii) the information provided should not include mock up drafts of either summaries of product characteristics or patient information leaflets

viii) if requested, further information may be supplied or a presentation made.

3.2 The promotion of a medicine must be in accordance with the terms of its marketing authorization and must not be inconsistent with the particulars listed in its summary of product characteristics.

Clause 3.2 Unauthorized Indications

The promotion of indications not covered by the marketing authorization for a medicine is prohibited by this clause.

Clause 4 Prescribing Information and Other Obligatory Information

4.1 The prescribing information listed in Clause 4.2 must be provided in a clear and legible manner in all promotional material for a medicine except for abbreviated advertisements (see Clause 5) and for promotional aids which meet the requirements of Clause 18.3.

The prescribing information must be positioned for ease of reference and must not be presented in a manner such that the reader has to turn the material round in order to read it, for example by providing it diagonally or around the page borders.

The prescribing information must form part of the promotional material and must not be separate from it.

Clause 4.1 Prescribing Information and Summaries of Product Characteristics

Each promotional item for a medicine must be able to stand alone. For example, when a 'Dear Doctor' letter on a medicine is sent in the same envelope as a brochure about the same medicine, each item has to include the prescribing information. It does not suffice to have the prescribing information on only one of the items. The inclusion of a summary of product characteristics moreover does not suffice to conform with the provisions of this clause.

The prescribing information must be consistent with the summary of product characteristics for the medicine.

Clause 4.1 Legibility of Prescribing Information

The prescribing information is the essential information which must be provided in promotional material. It follows therefore that the information must be given in a clear and legible manner which assists readability.

Legibility is not simply a question of type size. The following recommendations will help to achieve clarity:

- *type size should be such that a lower case letter 'x' is no less than 1 mm in height*
- *lines should be no more than 100 characters in length, including spaces*
- *sufficient space should be allowed between lines to facilitate easy reading*
- *a clear style of type should be used*
- *there should be adequate contrast between the colour of the text and the background*
- *dark print on a light background is preferable*
- *emboldening headings and starting each section on a new line aids legibility.*

Clauses 4.1 and 4.9 Date of Prescribing Information and Material

All prescribing information must include the date that the prescribing information was drawn up or last revised.

In addition, promotional material (other than journal advertising) must include the date that the material as a whole, ie the copy plus the prescribing information, was drawn up or last revised.

Clause 4.1 Electronic Journals

The first part of an advertisement in an electronic journal, such as the banner, is often the only part of the advertisement that is seen by readers. It must therefore include a clear, prominent statement as to where the prescribing information can be found. This should be in the form of a direct link. The first part is often linked to other parts and in such circumstances the linked parts will be considered as one advertisement.

If the first part mentions the product name then this is the most prominent display of the brand name and the non-proprietary name of the medicine or a list of the active ingredients using approved names where such exist must appear immediately adjacent to the most prominent display of the brand name. The size must be such that the information is easily readable. If the product is one that is required to show an inverted black triangle on its promotional material then the black triangle symbol should also appear adjacent to the product name. That is not, however, a requirement of the Code (see supplementary information to Clause 4.3). The requirement of Clause 10 that promotional material and activities should not be disguised should also be borne in mind.

Clause 4.1 Advertisements for Devices

Where an advertisement relates to the merits of a device used for administering medicines, such as an inhaler, which is supplied containing a variety of medicines, the prescribing information for one only need be given if the advertisement makes no reference to any particular medicine.

Full prescribing information must, however, be included in relation to each particular medicine which is referred to.

Clause 4.1 Prescribing Information at Exhibitions

The prescribing information for medicines promoted on posters and exhibition panels at meetings must either be provided on the posters or panels themselves or must be available at the company stand. If the prescribing information is made available at the company stand, this should be referred to on the posters or panels.

4.2 The prescribing information consists of the following:

- the name of the medicine (which may be either a brand name or a non-proprietary name)
- a quantitative list of the active ingredients, using approved names where such exist, or other non-proprietary names; alternatively, the non-proprietary name of the product if it is the subject of an accepted monograph
- at least one authorized indication for use consistent with the summary of product characteristics
- a succinct statement of the information in the summary of product characteristics relating to the dosage and method of use relevant to the indications quoted in the advertisement and, where not otherwise obvious, the route of administration
- a succinct statement of common side-effects likely to be encountered in clinical practice, serious side-effects and precautions and contra-indications relevant to the indications in the advertisement, giving, in an abbreviated form, the substance of the relevant information in the summary of product characteristics, together with a statement that prescribers should consult the summary of product characteristics in relation to other side-effects
- any warning issued by the Medicines Commission, the Commission on Human Medicines, the Committee on Safety of Medicines or the licensing authority, which is required to be included in advertisements
- the cost (excluding VAT) of either a specified package of the medicine to which the advertisement relates, or a specified quantity or recommended daily dose, calculated by reference to any specified package of the product, except in the case of advertisements in journals printed in the UK which have more than 15 per cent of their circulation outside the UK and audio-visual advertisements and prescribing information provided in association with them
- the legal classification of the product
- the number of the relevant marketing authorization and the name and address of the holder of the authorization or the name and address of the part of the business responsible for its sale or supply
- the date the prescribing information was drawn up or last revised.

The information specified above in relation to dosage, method of use, side-effects, precautions and contra-indications and any warning which is required to be included in advertisements, must be placed in such a position in the advertisement that its relationship to the claims and indications for the product can be appreciated by the reader.

4.3 In addition, the non-proprietary name of the medicine or a list of the active ingredients using approved names where such exist must appear immediately adjacent to the most prominent display of the brand name in bold type of a size such that a lower case 'x' is no less than 2mm in height or in type of such a size that the non-proprietary name or list of active ingredients occupies a total area no less than that taken up by the brand name.

Clause 4.3 Non-Proprietary Name

'Immediately adjacent to . . . ' means immediately before, immediately after, immediately above or immediately below.

It should be noted that in a promotional letter the most prominent display of the brand name will usually be that in the letter itself, rather than that in prescribing information provided on the reverse of the letter.

Clause 4.3 Black Triangle Symbol

Certain medicines are required to show an inverted black triangle on their promotional material, other than promotional aids, to denote that special reporting is required in relation to adverse reactions. This is not a Code of Practice or a statutory requirement.

The agreement between the Committee on Safety of Medicines and the ABPI on the use of the black triangle is that:

The symbol should always be black and its size should normally be not less than 5mm per side but with a smaller size of 3mm per side for A5 size advertisements and a larger size of 7.5mm per side for A3 size advertisements:

- *the symbol should appear once and be located adjacent to the most prominent display of the name of the product*
- *no written explanation of the symbol is necessary.*

4.4 In the case of audio-visual material such as films, video recordings and suchlike and in the case of inter-active data systems, the prescribing information may be provided either:

- by way of a document which is made available to all persons to whom the material is shown or sent, or
- by inclusion on the audio-visual recording or in the interactive data system itself.

When the prescribing information is included in an interactive data system instructions for accessing it must be clearly displayed.

Clause 4.4 Prescribing Information on Audio-Visual Material

Where prescribing information is shown in the audio-visual material as part of the recording, it must be of sufficient clarity and duration so that it is easily readable. The prescribing information must be an integral part of the advertisement and must appear with it. It is not acceptable for the advertisement and the prescribing information to be separated by any other material.

4.5 In the case of audio material, ie. material which consists of sound only, the prescribing information must be provided by way of a document which is made available to all persons to whom the material is played or sent.

4.6 In the case of promotional material included on the Internet, there must be a clear, prominent statement as to where the prescribing information can be found.

In the case of an advertisement included in an independently produced electronic journal on the Internet, there must be a clear and prominent statement in the form of a direct link between the first page of the advertisement and the prescribing information.

The non-proprietary name of the medicine or the list of active ingredients, as required by Clause 4.3, must appear immediately adjacent to the brand name at its first appearance in a size such that the information is readily readable.

4.7 In the case of a journal advertisement where the prescribing information appears overleaf, at either the beginning or the end of the advertisement, a reference to where it can be found must appear on the outer edge of the other page of the advertisement in a type size such that a lower case 'x' is no less than 2mm in height.

4.8 In the case of printed promotional material consisting of more than four pages, a clear reference must be given to where the prescribing information can be found.

4.9 Promotional material other than advertisements appearing in professional publications must include the date on which the promotional material was drawn up or last revised.

Clause 4.9 Date Drawn Up or Last Revised

This is in addition to the requirement in Clause 4.2 that the date of the prescribing information be included.

Clause 4.9 Dates on Loose Inserts

A loose insert is not regarded for this purpose as appearing in the professional publication with which it is sent and must therefore bear the date on which it was drawn up or last revised.

4.10 All promotional material, other than promotional aids, must include prominent information about adverse event reporting mechanisms.

Clause 4.10 Adverse Event Reporting

The requirements of this clause can be met by the inclusion of the statement 'Information about adverse event reporting can be found at www.yellowcard.gov.uk' or similar and 'Adverse events should also be reported to [the relevant pharmaceutical company]'. A telephone number for the relevant department of the company may be included. Text is more likely to be deemed to be prominent if it is presented in a larger type size than that used for the prescribing information.

Clause 5 Abbreviated Advertisements

5.1 Abbreviated advertisements are advertisements which are exempt from the requirement to include prescribing information for the advertised medicine, provided that they meet with the requirements of this clause.

5.2 Abbreviated advertisements may only appear in professional publications i.e. publications sent or delivered wholly or mainly to members of the health professions and/or appropriate administrative staff. A loose insert in such a publication cannot be an abbreviated advertisement.

Abbreviated advertisements are not permitted in audio-visual material or in interactive data systems or on the Internet, including journals on the Internet.

Clause 5.2 Abbreviated Advertisements – Professional Publications

Abbreviated advertisements are largely restricted to journals and other such professional publications sent or delivered wholly or mainly to members of the health professions etc. A promotional mailing or representative leavepiece cannot be an abbreviated advertisement and an abbreviated advertisement cannot appear as part of another promotional item, such as in a brochure consisting of a full advertisement for another of the company's medicines.

Diaries and desk pads bearing a number of advertisements are considered to be professional publications and may include abbreviated advertisements for medicines. Similarly, video programmes and suchlike sent to doctors etc may be considered professional publications and an abbreviated advertisement may be affixed to the side of the video cassette or included on the box containing the video. The prescribing information must, however, be made available for any advertisement for a medicine appearing on audio-visual material or in an interactive data system or on the Internet, including journals on the Internet. Such advertisements cannot be deemed abbreviated advertisements.

5.3 Abbreviated advertisements must be no larger than 420 square centimetres in size.

5.4 Abbreviated advertisements must provide the following information in a clear and legible manner:

- the name of the medicine (which may be either a brand name or a non-proprietary name)
- the non-proprietary name of the medicine or a list of the active ingredients using approved names where such exist
- at least one indication for use consistent with the summary of product characteristics
- a statement that prescribers are recommended to consult the summary of product characteristics before prescribing, particularly in relation to side-effects, precautions and contra-indications
- the legal classification of the product
- any warning issued by the Medicines Commission, the Commission on Human Medicines, the Committee on Safety of Medicines or the licensing authority which is required to be included in advertisements
- the name and address of the holder of the marketing authorization or the name and address of the part of the business responsible for its sale or supply
- a statement that further information is available on request to the holder of the marketing authorization or that it may be found in the summary of product characteristics.

Clauses 5.4, 5.5, 5.6 and 5.7 Abbreviated Advertisements – Permitted Information

The contents of abbreviated advertisements are restricted as set out in Clauses 5.4, 5.5, 5.6 and 5.7 and the following information should not therefore be included in abbreviated advertisements:

- *marketing authorization numbers*
- *references*
- *dosage particulars*
- *details of pack sizes*
- *cost.*

There may be exceptions to the above if the information provided, for example the cost of the medicine or the frequency of its dosage or its availability as a patient pack, is given as the reason why the medicine is recommended for the indication or indications referred to in the advertisement.

Artwork used in abbreviated advertisements must not convey any information about a medicine which is additional to that permitted under Clauses 5.4, 5.5, 5.6 and 5.7.

Telephone numbers may be included in abbreviated advertisements.

5.5 In addition, the non-proprietary name of the medicine or a list of the active ingredients using approved names where such exist must appear immediately adjacent to the most prominent display of the brand name in bold type of a size such that a lower case 'x' is no less than 2mm in height or in type of such a size that the non-proprietary name or list of active ingredients occupies a total area no less than that taken up by the brand name.

Clause 5.5 Non-Proprietary Name

'Immediately adjacent to . . . ' means immediately before, immediately after, immediately above or immediately below.

Clause 5.5 Black Triangle Symbol

Certain medicines are required to show an inverted black triangle on their promotional material, other than promotional aids, to denote that special reporting is required in relation to adverse reactions. This is not a Code of Practice or a statutory requirement.

The agreement between the Committee on Safety of Medicines and the ABPI on the use of the black triangle is that:

The symbol should always be black and its size should normally be not less than 5mm per side but with a smaller size of 3mm per side for A5 size advertisements and a larger size of 7.5mm per side for A3 size advertisements:

- *the symbol should appear once and be located adjacent to the most prominent display of the name of the product*
- *no written explanation of the symbol is necessary.*

5.6 In addition, abbreviated advertisements must include prominent information about adverse event reporting mechanisms.

Clause 5.6 Adverse Event Reporting

The requirements of this clause can be met by the inclusion of the statement 'Information about adverse event reporting can be found at www.yellowcard.gov.uk' or similar and 'Adverse events should also be reported to [the relevant pharmaceutical company]'.

5.7 Abbreviated advertisements may in addition con-tain a concise statement consistent with the summary of product characteristics, giving the reason why the medicine is recommended for the indication or indications given.

Clause 6 Journal Advertising

Clause 6 Journal Advertisements

See Clause 4 and in particular Clause 4.7 regarding the requirements for prescribing information in journal advertisements.

A two page journal advertisement is one where the pages follow on without interruption by intervening editorial text or other copy. Thus, for example, promotional material on two successive right hand pages cannot be a single advertisement. Each such page would need to be treated as a separate advertisement for the purposes of prescribing information.

Similarly, if promotional material appears on the outer edges of the left and right hand pages of a double page spread, and the promotional material is separated by intervening editorial matter, then again each page would need to be treated as a separate advertisement.

6.1 Where the pages of a two page advertisement are not facing, neither must be false or misleading when read in isolation.

6.2 No advertisement taking the form of a loose insert in a journal may consist of more than a single sheet of a size no larger than the page size of the journal itself, printed on one or both sides.

Clause 6.2 Advertising on the Outside of Journals

Advertising such as cards stapled to a journal and 'wrap-arounds' must not have a greater surface area than that outlined for loose inserts under Clause 6.2.

6.3 No issue of a journal may bear advertising for a particular product on more than two pages.

Clause 6.3 Limitation on Number of Pages of Advertising

Advertisements taking the form of inserts, whether loose or bound in, count towards the two pages allowed by Clause 6.3. A loose insert printed on both sides counts as two pages.

A summary of product characteristics is permitted as an insert in addition to the two pages of advertising which is allowed.

Inserts and supplements which are not advertisements as such, though they may be regarded as promotional material, for example reports of conference proceedings, are not subject to the restrictions of Clauses 6.2 and 6.3.

Clause 7 Information, Claims and Comparisons

Clause 7 General

The application of this clause is not limited to information or claims of a medical or scientific nature. It includes, inter alia, information or claims relating to pricing and market share. Thus, for example, any claim relating to the market share of a product must be substantiated without delay upon request as required under Clause 7.5.

It should be borne in mind that claims in promotional material must be capable of standing alone as regards accuracy etc. In general claims should not be qualified by the use of footnotes and the like.

7.1 Upon reasonable request, a company must promptly provide members of the health professions and appropriate administrative staff with accurate and relevant information about the medicines which the company markets.

7.2 Information, claims and comparisons must be accurate, balanced, fair, objective and unambiguous and must be based on an up-to-date evaluation of all the evidence and reflect that evidence clearly. They must not mislead either directly or by implication, by distortion, exaggeration or undue emphasis.

Material must be sufficiently complete to enable the recipient to form their own opinion of the therapeutic value of the medicine.

Clause 7.2 Misleading Information, Claims and Comparisons

The following are areas where particular care should be taken by companies:

- ***claims for superior potency in relation to weight*** *are generally meaningless and best avoided unless they can be linked with some practical advantage, for example, reduction in side-effects or cost of effective dosage*
- ***the use of data derived from in-vitro studies, studies in healthy volunteers and in animals.*** *Care must be taken with the use of such data so as not to mislead as to its significance. The extrapolation of such data to the clinical situation should only be made where there is data to show that it is of direct relevance and significance*
- ***economic evaluation of medicines.*** *The economic evaluation of medicines is a relatively new science. Care must be taken that any claim involving the economic evaluation of a medicine is borne out by the data available and does not exaggerate its significance*

To be acceptable as the basis of promotional claims, the assumptions made in an economic evaluation must be clinically appropriate and consistent with the marketing authorization

Attention is drawn to guidance on good practice in the conduct of economic evaluations of medicines which has been given by the Department of Health and the ABPI and which is available upon request from the Prescription Medicines Code of Practice Authority

- ***emerging clinical or scientific opinion.*** *Where a clinical or scientific issue exists which has not been resolved in favour of one generally accepted viewpoint, particular care must be taken to ensure that the issue is treated in a balanced manner in promotional material*
- ***hanging comparisons*** *whereby a medicine is described as being better or stronger or suchlike without stating that with which the medicine is compared must not be made*
- ***price comparisons.*** *Price comparisons, as with any comparison, must be accurate, fair and must not mislead. Valid comparisons can only be made where like is compared with like. It follows therefore that a price comparison should be made on the basis of the equivalent dosage requirement for the same indications. For example, to compare the cost per ml for topical preparations is likely to mislead unless it can be shown that their usage rates are similar or, where this is not possible, for the comparison to be qualified in such a way as to indicate that usage rates may vary*
- ***statistical information.*** *Care must be taken to ensure that there is a sound statistical basis for all information, claims and comparisons in promotional material. Differences which do not reach statistical significance must not be presented in such a way as to mislead.*

Instances have occurred where claims have been based on published papers in which the arithmetic and/or statistical methodology was incorrect. Accordingly, before statistical information is included in promotional material it must have been subjected to statistical appraisal.

7.3 A comparison is only permitted in promotional material if:

- it is not misleading
- medicines or services for the same needs or intended for the same purpose are compared
- one or more material, relevant, substantiable and representative features are compared
- no confusion is created between the medicine advertised and that of a competitor or between the advertiser's trade marks, trade names, other distinguishing marks and those of a competitor
- the trade marks, trade names, other distinguishing marks, medicines, services, activities or circumstances of a competitor are not discredited or denigrated
- no unfair advantage is taken of the reputation of a trade mark, trade name or other distinguishing marks of a competitor
- medicines or services are not presented as imitations or replicas of goods or services bearing a competitor's trade mark or trade name.

Clause 7.3 Comparisons

The Code does not preclude the use of other companies' brand names when making comparisons.

7.4 Any information, claim or comparison must be capable of substantiation.

7.5 Substantiation for any information, claim or comparison must be provided as soon as possible, and certainly within ten working days, at the request of members of the health professions or appropriate administrative staff. It need not be provided, however, in relation to the validity of indications approved in the marketing authorization.

Clause 7.5 Data from Clinical Trials

Companies must provide substantiation following a request for it, as set out in Clause 7.5. In addition, when data from clinical trials is used companies must ensure that where necessary that data has been registered in accordance with the Joint Position on the Disclosure of Clinical Trial Information via Clinical Trial Registries and Databases 2005.

7.6 When promotional material refers to published studies, clear references must be given.

Clause 7.6 References

Clause 7.6 applies to references to published material, including the use of quotations, tables, graphs and other illustrative matters.

7.7 When promotional material refers to data on file, the relevant part of this data must be provided without delay at the request of members of the health professions or appropriate administrative staff.

7.8 All artwork including illustrations, graphs and tables must conform to the letter and spirit of the Code and, when taken from published studies, a reference must be given. Graphs and tables must be presented in such a way as to give a clear, fair, balanced view of the matters with which they deal, and must not be included unless they are relevant to the claims or comparisons being made.

Clause 7.8 Artwork, Illustrations, Graphs and Tables

Care must be taken to ensure that artwork does not mislead as to the nature of a medicine or any claim or comparison and that it does not detract from any warnings or contraindications. For example, anatomical drawings used to show results from a study must not exaggerate those results and depictions of children should not be used in relation to products not authorized for use in children in any way which might encourage such use.

Particular care should be taken with graphs and tables to ensure that they do not mislead, for example by their incompleteness or by the use of suppressed zeros or unusual scales. Differences which do not reach statistical significance must not be presented in such a way as to mislead.

Graphs and tables must be adequately labelled so that the information presented can be readily understood. When taken from published studies, the source of the artwork must be given (see also Clause 7.6). If a graph, table or suchlike is taken from a published study it must be faithfully reproduced except where modification is needed in order to comply with the Code. In such circumstances it must be clearly stated that the material has been modified. Any such adaptation must not distort or mislead as to the significance of that graph, table etc. Care should be taken not to mislead when expressing data as percentages; patient numbers should be included wherever possible. It should also be noted that if a table, graph etc in a paper is unacceptable in terms of the requirements of the Code, because, for example, it gives a visually misleading impression as to the data shown, then it must not be used or reproduced in promotional material.

7.9 Information and claims about side-effects must reflect available evidence or be capable of substantiation by clinical experience. It must not be stated that a product has no side-effects, toxic hazards or risks of addiction or dependency. The word 'safe' must not be used without qualification.

Clause 7.9 Use of the Word 'Safe'

The restrictions on the word 'safe' apply equally to grammatical derivatives of the word such as 'safety'. For example, 'demonstrated safety' or 'proven safety' are prohibited under this clause.

7.10 Promotion must encourage the rational use of a medicine by presenting it objectively and without exaggerating its properties. Exaggerated or all-embracing claims must not be made and superlatives must not be used except for those limited circumstances where they relate to a clear fact about a medicine. Claims should not imply that a medicine or an active ingredient has some special merit, quality or property unless this can be substantiated.

Clause 7.10 Benefit/Risk Profile

The benefit/risk profile of a medicine must be presented in promotional campaigns in such a way as to comply with the Code. Particular attention should be paid to Clauses 7.2, 7.9 and 7.10.

Clause 7.10 Superlatives

Superlatives are those grammatical expressions which denote the highest quality or degree, such as best, strongest, widest etc. A claim that a product was 'the best' treatment for a particular condition, for example, could not be substantiated as there are too many variables to enable such a sweeping claim to be proven. The use of a superlative is acceptable only if it can be substantiated as a simple statement of fact which can be very clearly demonstrated, such as that a particular medicine is the most widely prescribed in the UK for a certain condition, if this is not presented in a way which misleads as to its significance.

Clause 7.10 Use of the Words 'The' and 'Unique'

In certain circumstances the use of the word 'the' can imply a special merit, quality or property for a medicine which is unacceptable under this clause if it cannot be substantiated. For example, a claim that a product is 'The analgesic' implies that it is in effect the best, and might not be acceptable under this clause.

Similarly, great care needs to be taken with the use of the word 'unique'. Although in some circumstances the word unique may be used to describe some clearly defined special feature of a medicine, in many instances it may simply imply a general superiority. In such instances it is not possible to substantiate the claim as the claim itself is so ill defined.

7.11 The word 'new' must not be used to describe any product or presentation which has been generally available, or any therapeutic indication which has been generally promoted, for more than twelve months in the UK.

Clause 8 Disparaging References

8.1 The medicines, products and activities of other pharmaceutical companies must not be disparaged.

Clause 8.1 Disparaging References

Much pharmaceutical advertising contains comparisons with other products and, by the nature of advertising, such comparisons are usually made to show an advantage of the advertised product over its comparator. Provided that such critical references to another company's products are accurate, balanced, fair etc, and can be substantiated, they are acceptable under the Code.

Unjustified knocking copy in which the products or activities of a competitor are unfairly denigrated is prohibited under this clause.

Attention is drawn to the requirements for comparisons set out in Clauses 7.2 to 7.5.

8.2 The health professions and the clinical and scientific opinions of health professionals must not be disparaged.

Clause 9 High Standards, Format, Suitability and Causing Offence, Sponsorship

9.1 High standards must be maintained at all times.

9.2 All material and activities must recognise the special nature of medicines and the professional standing of the audience to which they are directed and must not be likely to cause offence.

Clauses 9.1 and 9.2 Suitability and Taste

The special nature of medicines and the professional audience to which the material is directed require that the standards set for the promotion of medicines are higher than those which might be acceptable for general commodity advertising.

It follows therefore that certain types, styles and methods of promotion, even where they might be acceptable for the promotion of products other than medicines, are unacceptable. These include:

- *the display of naked or partially naked people for the purpose of attracting attention to the material or the use of sexual imagery for that purpose*
- *'teaser' advertising whereby promotional material is intended to 'tease' the recipient by eliciting an interest in something which will be following or will be available at a later date without providing any actual information about it*
- *the provision of rubber stamps to doctors for use as aids to prescription writing*
- *the provision of private prescription forms preprinted with the name of a medicine.*

9.3 The name or photograph of a member of a health profession must not be used in any way that is contrary to the conventions of that profession.

9.4 Promotional material must not imitate the devices, copy, slogans or general layout adopted by other companies in a way that is likely to mislead or confuse.

9.5 Promotional material must not include any reference to the Medicines Commission, the Commission on Human Medicines, the Committee on Safety of Medicines, the Medicines and Healthcare products Regulatory Agency, the Medicines Control Agency or the licensing authority, unless this is specifically required by the licensing authority.

9.6 Reproductions of official documents must not be used for promotional purposes unless permission has been given in writing by the appropriate body.

9.7 Extremes of format, size or cost of promotional material must be avoided.

Clause 9.7 Extremes of Format, Size or Cost

Particular care needs to be taken in this regard in the first six months following the launch of a medicine to avoid criticism of the industry.

9.8 Postcards, other exposed mailings, envelopes or wrappers must not carry matter which might be regarded as advertising to the general public, contrary to Clause 20.1.

Clause 9.8 Reply Paid Cards

Reply paid cards which are intended to be returned to companies through the post and which relate to a prescription only medicine should not bear both the name of the medicine and information as to its usage but may bear one or the other.

9.9 The telephone, text messages, email, telemessages, facsimile, automated calling systems and other electronic data communications must not be used for promotional purposes, except with the prior permission of the recipient.

9.10 Material relating to medicines and their uses, whether promotional in nature or not, which is sponsored by a pharmaceutical company must clearly indicate that it has been sponsored by that company.

The only exception to this is market research material which need not reveal the name of the company involved but must state that it is sponsored by a pharmaceutical company.

Clause 9.10 Declaration of Sponsorship

The declaration of sponsorship must be sufficiently prominent to ensure that readers of sponsored material are aware of it at the outset.

Clause 9.10 Market Research

Where market research is carried out by an agency on behalf of a pharmaceutical company, the agency must reveal the name of its client to the Prescription Medicines Code of Practice Authority when the Authority requests it to do so. When commissioning market research, a company must take steps to ensure that its identity would be so made known to the Authority should a request for that information be made.

Clause 10 Disguised Promotion

10.1 Promotional material and activities must not be disguised.

Clause 10.1 Disguised Promotional Material

Promotional material sent in the guise of personal communications, for example by using envelopes or postcards addressed in real or facsimile handwriting is inappropriate. Envelopes must not be used for the dispatch of promotional material if they bear words implying that the contents are non-promotional, for example that the contents provide information relating to safety.

When a company pays for, or otherwise secures or arranges the publication of promotional material in journals, such material must not resemble independent editorial matter. Care must be taken with company sponsored reports of meetings and the like to ensure that they are not disguised promotion. Sponsorship must be declared in accordance with Clause 9.10.

10.2 Market research activities, post-marketing surveillance studies, clinical assessments and the like must not be disguised promotion. Post-marketing surveillance studies, clinical assessments and the like must be conducted with a primarily scientific or educational purpose.

Clause 10.2 Guidelines for Company Sponsored Safety Assessment of Marketed Medicines

Attention is drawn to the Guidelines for Company Sponsored Safety Assessment of Marketed Medicines (SAMM) which have been produced jointly by the ABPI, the British Medical Association, the Committee on Safety of Medicines, the Medicines and Healthcare products Regulatory Agency and the Royal College of General Practitioners. These state that SAMM studies should not be undertaken for the purposes of promotion.

Clause 10.2 Market Research

Market research is the collection and analysis of information and must be unbiased and non-promotional. The use to which the statistics or information is put may be promotional. The two phases must be kept distinct.

Attention is drawn to guidelines – The Legal and Ethical Framework for Healthcare Market Research – produced by the British Healthcare Business Intelligence Association in consultation with the ABPI.

Market research material should be examined to ensure that it does not contravene the Code.

Where market research is carried out by an agency on behalf of a pharmaceutical company, the agency must reveal the name of its client to the Prescription Medicines Code of Practice Authority when the Authority requests it to do so. When commissioning market research, a company must take steps to ensure that its identity would be so made known to the Authority should a request for that information be made.

Clause 11 Provision of Reprints and the Use of Quotations

11.1 Reprints of articles in journals must not be provided unsolicited unless the articles have been refereed.

Clause 11.1 Provision of Reprints

The provision of an unsolicited reprint of an article about a medicine constitutes promotion of that medicine and all relevant requirements of the Code must therefore be observed. Particular attention must be paid to the requirements of Clause 3.

When providing an unsolicited reprint of an article about a medicine, it should be accompanied by prescribing information.

11.2 Quotations from medical and scientific literature or from personal communications must be faithfully reproduced (except where adaptation or modification is required in order to comply with the Code) and must accurately reflect the meaning of the author. The precise source of the quotation must be identified.

Clause 11.2 Quotations

Any quotation chosen by a company for use in promotional material must comply with the requirements of the Code itself. For example, to quote from a paper which stated that a certain medicine was 'safe and effective' would not be acceptable even if it was an accurate reflection of the meaning of the author of the paper, as it is prohibited under Clause 7.9 of the Code to state without qualification in promotional material that a medicine is safe.

Quotations can only be adapted or modified in order to comply with the Code. In such circumstances it must be clearly stated that the quotation has been amended.

Care should be taken in quoting from any study or the like to ensure that it does not mislead as to its overall significance. (See Clause 7.2 which prohibits misleading information, claims etc in promotional material). Attention is drawn to the provisions of Clause 7.6 which requires that when promotional material refers to published studies clear references must be given to where they can be found.

11.3 Quotations relating to medicines taken from public broadcasts, for example on radio and television, and from private occasions, such as medical conferences or symposia, must not be used without the formal permission of the speaker.

11.4 The utmost care must be taken to avoid ascribing claims or views to authors when these no longer represent the current views of the authors concerned.

Clause 11.4 Current Views of Authors

If there is any doubt as to the current view of an author, companies should check with the author prior to its use in promotional material.

Clause 12 Distribution of Promotional Material

12.1 Promotional material should only be sent or distributed to those categories of persons whose need for, or interest in, the particular information can reasonably be assumed.

Clause 12.1 Distribution of Promotional Material

Promotional material should be tailored to the audience to whom it is directed. For example, promotional material devised for general practitioners might not be appropriate for hospital doctors and, similarly, material devised for clinicians might not be appropriate for use with National Health Service administrative staff.

12.2 Restraint must be exercised on the frequency of distribution and on the volume of promotional material distributed.

Clause 12.2 Frequency of Mailings

The style of mailings is relevant to their acceptability to doctors and criticism of their frequency is most likely to arise where their informational content is limited or where they appear to be elaborate and expensive.

In the first six months following the launch of a new medicine, a health professional may be sent an initial mailing giving detailed information about its use, including, for example, the summary of product characteristics, the public assessment report, the package leaflet and the product monograph, and no more than three other mailings about the medicine.

No more than eight mailings for a particular medicine may be sent to a health professional in a year.

Mailings concerned solely with safety issues can be sent in addition to the above.

12.3 Mailing lists must be kept up-to-date. Requests to be removed from promotional mailing lists must be complied with promptly and no name may be restored except at the addressee's request or with their permission.

Clause 13 Scientific Service Responsible for Information

Companies must have a scientific service to compile and collate all information, whether received from medical representatives or from any other source, about the medicines which they market.

Clause 14 Certification

14.1 Promotional material must not be issued unless its final form, to which no subsequent amendments will be made, has been certified by two persons on behalf of the company in the manner provided for by this clause. One of the two persons must be a registered medical practitioner or, in the case of a product for dental use only, a registered medical practitioner or a dentist.

A practising UK registered pharmacist working under the direction of a registered medical practitioner may certify certain promotional material instead of a registered medical practitioner. The promotional material that can be so certified is promotional material for products or indications that have been on the market in the UK for more than one year and which is not part of a new and novel promotional campaign. All other material, including that referred to in Clause 14.3 below, must be certified by a registered medical practitioner or, in the case of a product for dental use only, a registered medical practitioner or a dentist.

The second person certifying on behalf of the company must be an appropriately qualified person or senior official of the company or an appropriately qualified person whose services are retained for that purpose.

Clause 14.1 Certification

An acceptable way to comply with Clause 14.1 is for the final proof to be certified but this is not obligatory provided that that which is certified is in its final form to which no subsequent amendments will be made. Companies may use validated electronic signatures for certifying material. Written copies of certificates and material etc must be preserved in order to comply with Clause 14.6.

All promotional material must be certified in this way including audio and audio-visual material, promotional material on databases, interactive data systems and the Internet, promotional aids and representatives' technical briefing materials.

Account should be taken of the fact that a non-promotional item can be used for a promotional purpose and therefore come within the scope of the Code.

In certifying audio and audio-visual material and promotional material on databases, interactive systems and the Internet, companies must ensure that a written transcript of the material is certified including reproductions of any graphs, tables and the like that appear in it. In the event of a complaint, a copy of the written material will be requested. Alternatively companies may certify material on interactive systems by means of producing an electronic copy, for example on a CD Rom or data stick, if the electronic copy is write protected and unable to be changed.

The guidelines on company procedures relating to the Code which are on page 47 give further information on certification.

See also the supplementary information to Clause 3 on promotion at international conferences regarding the certification of such material.

Clause 14.1 Suitable Qualifications for Signatories

In deciding whether a person can be a nominated signatory, account should be taken of product knowledge, relevant experience both within and outwith the industry, length of service and seniority. In addition signatories must have an up to date, detailed knowledge of the Code. Pharmacists certifying certain promotional material instead of registered medical practitioners must have not less than one year's experience of working with the product concerned.

Clause 14.1 Joint Ventures and Co-Promotion

In a joint venture in which a third party provides a service on behalf of a number of pharmaceutical companies, the pharmaceutical companies involved are responsible for any activity carried out by that third party on their behalf.

It follows therefore that the pharmaceutical companies involved should be aware of all aspects of the service carried out on their behalf and take this into account when certifying the material or activity involved. Similarly if two or more pharmaceutical companies organise a joint meeting each company should ensure that the arrangements for the meeting are acceptable.

Under co-promotion arrangements whereby companies jointly promote the same medicine and the promotional material bears both company names, each company should certify the promotional material involved as they will be held jointly responsible for it under the Code.

14.2 All meetings which involve travel outside the UK must be certified in advance in a manner similar to that provided for by Clause 14.1.

Clause 14.2 Meetings involving Travel outside the UK

When certifying meetings which involve travel outside the UK, the signatories should ensure that all the arrangements are examined, including the programme, the venue, the reasons for using that venue, the intended audience, the anticipated cost and the nature of the hospitality and the like.

14.3 The following must be certified in advance in a manner similar to that provided for by Clause 14.1:

- educational material for the public or patients issued by companies which relates to diseases or medicines but is not intended as promotion for those medicines, including material relating to working with patient organisations as described in Clause 20.3 and its supplementary information
- non promotional material for patients or health professionals relating to the provision of medical and educational goods and services, including relevant internal company instructions, as described in Clause 18.4 and paragraph 8 of its supplementary information.

Clause 14.3 Examination of Other Material

Other material issued by companies which relates to medicines but which is not intended as promotional material for those medicines per se, such as corporate advertising, press releases, market research material, financial information to inform shareholders, the Stock Exchange and the like, and written responses from medical information departments or similar to unsolicited enquiries from the public etc, should be examined to ensure that it does not contravene the Code or the relevant statutory requirements.

14.4 The names of those nominated, together with their qualifications, shall be notified in advance to the Product Information and Advertising Unit of the Post Licensing Division of the Medicines and Healthcare products Regulatory Agency and to the Prescription Medicines Code of Practice Authority. The names and qualifications of designated alternative signatories must also be given. Changes in the names of nominees must be promptly notified.

14.5 The certificate for promotional material must certify that the signatories have examined the final form of the material and that in their belief it is in accordance with the requirements of the relevant advertising regulations and this Code, is not inconsistent with the marketing authorization and the summary of product characteristics and is a fair and truthful presentation of the facts about the medicine.

The certificates for the following must certify that the signatories have examined the final form of the material and that in their belief it complies with the Code:

- educational material for the public or patients issued by companies which relates to diseases or medicines but is not intended as promotion for those medicines including material relating to working with patient organisations as described in Clause 20.3 and its supplementary information
- non promotional material for patients or health professionals relating to the provision of medical and educational goods and services, including relevant internal company instructions, as described in Clause 18.4 and paragraph 8 of its supplementary information.

Material which is still in use must be recertified at intervals of no more than two years to ensure that it continues to conform with the relevant advertising regulations and the Code.

The certificate for meetings involving travel outside the UK must certify that the signatories have examined all the proposed arrangements for the meeting and that in their belief the arrangements are in accordance with the relevant advertising regulations and the Code.

14.6 Companies shall preserve all certificates. In relation to certificates for promotional material, the material in the form certified and information indicating the persons to whom it was addressed, the method of dissemination and the date of first dissemination must also be preserved. In relation to certificates for meetings involving travel outside the UK, details of the programme, the venue, the reasons for using the venue, the audience, the anticipated and actual costs and the nature of the hospitality and the like must also be preserved.

Companies shall preserve certificates and the relevant accompanying information for not less than three years after the final use of the promotional material or the date of the meeting and produce them on request from the Medicines and Healthcare products Regulatory Agency or the Prescription Medicines Code of Practice Authority.

Clause 14.6 Retention of Documentation

Companies should note that the Medicines and Healthcare products Regulatory Agency is entitled to request particulars of an advertisement, including particulars as to the content and form of the advertisement, the method of dissemination and the date of first dissemination, and such a request is not subject to any time limit. This does not apply to the certificates themselves in respect of which the three year limit in Clause 14.6 is applicable.

Clause 15 Representatives

Clause 15 Representatives

All provisions in the Code relating to the need for accuracy, balance, fairness, good taste etc apply equally to oral representations as well as to printed material. Representatives must not make claims or comparisons which are in any way inaccurate, misleading, disparaging, in poor taste etc, or which are outside the terms of the marketing authorization for the medicine or are inconsistent with the summary of product characteristics. Indications for which the medicine does not have a marketing authorization must not be promoted.

Attention is drawn to the provisions of Clause 9.9 which prohibit the use of the telephone, text messages, email, telemessages and facsimile etc for promotional purposes, except with the prior permission of the recipient.

Clause 15 Contract Representatives

Companies employing or using contract representatives are responsible for their conduct and must ensure that they comply with the provisions of this and all other relevant clauses in the Code, and in particular the training requirements under Clauses 15.1, 16.1, 16.3 and 16.4.

15.1 Representatives must be given adequate training and have sufficient scientific knowledge to enable them to provide full and accurate information about the medicines which they promote.

15.2 Representatives must at all times maintain a high standard of ethical conduct in the discharge of their duties and must comply with all relevant requirements of the Code.

15.3 Representatives must not employ any inducement or subterfuge to gain an interview. No fee should be paid or offered for the grant of an interview.

Clause 15.3 Hospitality and Payments for Meetings

Attention is drawn to the requirements of Clauses 18 and 19 which prohibit the provision of any financial inducement for the purposes of sales promotion and require that any hospitality provided is secondary to the purpose of a meeting, is not out of proportion to the occasion and does not extend beyond members of the health professions or appropriate administrative staff.

Meetings organised for groups of doctors, other health professionals and/or appropriate administrative staff which are wholly or mainly of a social or sporting nature are unacceptable.

Representatives organising meetings are permitted to provide appropriate hospitality and/or to meet any reasonable, actual costs which may have been incurred. For example, if the refreshments have been organised and paid for by a medical practice the cost may be reimbursed as long as it is reasonable in relation to what was provided and the refreshments themselves were appropriate for the occasion.

Donations in lieu of hospitality are unacceptable as they are inducements for the purpose of holding a meeting. If hospitality is not required at a meeting there is no obligation or right to provide some benefit of an equivalent value.

Clause 15.3 Donations to Charities

Donations to charities in return for representatives gaining interviews are prohibited under Clause 15.3.

Clause 15.3 Items Delivered by Representatives

Reply paid cards which refer to representatives delivering items which have been offered to health professionals or appropriate administrative staff should explain that there is no obligation to grant the representative an interview when the item is delivered. This is to avoid the impression that there is such an obligation, which would be contrary to Clause 15.3 which prohibits the use of any inducement to gain an interview.

Clause 15.3 General Medical Council

The General Medical Council is the regulatory body for the medical profession and is responsible for giving guidance on standards of professional conduct and on medical ethics. In its guidance, the Council advises doctors that 'You must act in your patients' best interests when making referrals and providing or arranging treatment or care. So you must not ask for or accept any inducement, gift or hospitality which may affect or be seen to affect your judgement'.

15.4 Representatives must ensure that the frequency, timing and duration of calls on health professionals, administrative staff in hospitals and health authorities and the like, together with the manner in which they are made, do not cause inconvenience. The wishes of individuals on whom representatives wish to call and the arrangements in force at any particular establishment, must be observed.

Clause 15.4 Frequency and Manner of Calls on Doctors and Other Prescribers

The number of calls made on a doctor or other prescriber and the intervals between successive visits are relevant to the determination of frequency.

Companies should arrange that intervals between visits do not cause inconvenience. The number of calls made on a doctor or other prescriber by a representative each year should not normally exceed three on average. This does not include the following which may be additional to those three visits:

- *attendance at group meetings, including audio-visual presentations and the like*
- *a visit which is requested by a doctor or other prescriber or a call which is made in order to respond to a specific enquiry*
- *a visit to follow up a report of an adverse reaction.*

Representatives must always endeavour to treat prescribers' time with respect and give them no cause to believe that their time might have been wasted. If for any unavoidable reasons, an appointment cannot be kept, the longest possible notice must be given.

15.5 In an interview, or when seeking an appointment for one, representatives must at the outset take reasonable steps to ensure that they do not mislead as to their identity or that of the company they represent.

15.6 Representatives must transmit forthwith to the scientific service referred to in Clause 13 any information which they receive in relation to the use of the medicines which they promote, particularly reports of side-effects.

15.7 Representatives must be paid a fixed basic salary and any addition proportional to sales of medicines must not constitute an undue proportion of their remuneration.

15.8 Representatives must provide, or have available to provide if requested, a copy of the summary of product characteristics for each medicine which they are to promote.

Clause 15.8 Provision of Summary of Product Characteristics

If discussion on a medicine is initiated by the person or persons on whom a representative calls, the representative is not obliged to have available the information on that medicine referred to in this clause.

15.9 Companies must prepare detailed briefing material for medical representatives on the technical aspects of each medicine which they will promote. A copy of such material must be made available to the Medicines and Healthcare products Regulatory Agency and the Prescription Medicines Code of Practice Authority on request. Briefing material must comply with the relevant requirements of the Code and, in particular, is subject to the certification requirements of Clause 14.

Briefing material must not advocate, either directly or indirectly, any course of action which would be likely to lead to a breach of the Code.

Clause 15.9 Briefing Material

The detailed briefing material referred to in this clause consists of both the training material used to instruct medical representatives about a medicine and the instructions given to them as to how the product should be promoted.

15.10 Companies are responsible for the activities of their representatives if these are within the scope of their employment even if they are acting contrary to the instructions which they have been given.

Clause 16 Training

16.1 All relevant personnel including representatives and members of staff (including persons retained by way of contract with third parties) concerned in any way with the preparation or approval of promotional material or of information to be provided to members of the UK health professions and to appropriate administrative staff or of information to be provided to the public and recognised patient organisations must be fully conversant with the requirements of the Code and the relevant laws and regulations.

Clause 16.1 Training

Extensive in house training on the Code is carried out by companies and by the Prescription Medicines Code of Practice Authority.

In addition, the Authority runs seminars on the Code which are open to all companies and personnel from advertising agencies, public relations agencies and the like which act for the pharmaceutical industry. Details of these seminars can be obtained from the Authority.

16.2 All personnel (including persons retained by way of contract with third parties) must be fully conversant with pharmacovigilance requirements relevant to their work and this must be documented.

16.3 Representatives must pass the appropriate ABPI representatives examination, as specified in Clause 16.4. They must be entered for the appropriate examination within their first year of such employment. Prior to passing the appropriate examination, they may be engaged in such employment for no more than two years, whether continuous or otherwise.

Clause 16.3 Time Allowed to Pass Examination

Prior to passing the appropriate ABPI examination, representatives may be engaged in such employment for no more than two years, whether continuous or otherwise and irrespective of whether with one company or with more than one company. A representative cannot, for example, do eighteen months with one company and eighteen months with another and so on, thus avoiding the examination.

In the event of extenuating circumstances, such as prolonged illness or no or inadequate opportunity to take the examination, the Director of the Prescription Medicines Code of Practice Authority may agree to the continued employment of a person as a representative past the end of the two year period, subject to the representative passing the examination within a reasonable time.

Service as a representative prior to 1 January 2006 by persons who were exempt from taking the appropriate examination by virtue of Clause 16.4 of the 2003 edition of the Code does not count towards the two year limit on employment as a representative prior to passing the appropriate examination. In order to comply with Clause 16.3 such persons must be entered for the appropriate examination before 1 January 2007 and must pass it before 1 January 2008.

16.4 The Medical Representatives Examination is appropriate for, and must be taken by, representatives whose duties comprise or include one or both of:

- calling upon doctors and/or dentists and/or other prescribers
- the promotion of medicines on the basis, inter alia, of their particular therapeutic properties.

The Generic Sales Representatives Examination is appropriate for, and must be taken by, representatives who promote medicines primarily on the basis of price, quality and availability.

Clause 16.4 Medical Representatives and Generic Sales Representatives

The ABPI examinations for medical representatives and generic sales representatives are based on a syllabus published by the ABPI which covers, as appropriate, subjects such as body systems, disease processes and pharmacology, the classification of medicines and pharmaceutical technology. Information on the National Health Service and pharmaceutical industry forms an additional core part of the syllabus. The syllabus is complementary to, and may be incorporated within, the company's induction training which is provided to representatives as a pre-requisite to carrying out their function.

16.5 Persons who have passed the Medical Representatives Examination whose duties change so as to become those specified in Clause 16.4 as being appropriate to the Generic Sales Representatives Examination are exempt from the need to take that examination.

Persons who have passed the Generic Sales Representatives Examination whose duties change so as to become those specified in Clause 16.4 as being appropriate to the Medical Representatives Examination must pass that examination within two years of their change of duties.

16.6 Details of the numbers of medical and generic sales representatives who have passed the respective examinations above, together with the examination status of others, must be provided to the Prescription Medicines Code of Practice Authority on request.

Clause 17 Provision of Medicines and Samples

Clause 17 Definition of Sample

A sample is a small supply of a medicine provided to health professionals so that they may familiarise themselves with it and acquire experience in dealing with it. A sample of a medicine may be provided only to a health professional qualified to prescribe that particular medicine.

A small sample which is provided only for identification or similar purposes and which is not intended to be used in treatment may be provided to any health professional but is otherwise subject to the requirements of Clause 17.

Titration packs, free goods and bonus stock provided to pharmacists and others are not samples. Neither are starter packs classified as samples. This is because they are not for the purposes described above.

Starter packs are small packs designed to provide sufficient medicine for a primary care prescriber to initiate treatment in such circumstances as a call out in the night or in other instances where there might be some undesirable or unavoidable delay in having a prescription dispensed. It follows from this that the types of medicines for which starter packs are appropriate are limited to those where immediate commencement of treatment is necessary or desirable, such as analgesics and antibiotics. Starter packs are not samples and should not be labelled as such. The quantity of medicine in a starter pack should be modest, only being sufficient to tide a patient over until their prescription can be dispensed.

Titration packs are packs containing various strengths of a medicine for the purpose of establishing a patient on an effective dose.

17.1 Samples of a product may be provided only to a health professional qualified to prescribe that product. They must not be provided to administrative staff.

17.2 No more than ten samples of a particular medicine may be provided to an individual health professional during the course of a year.

17.3 Samples may only be supplied in response to written requests which have been signed and dated.

Clause 17.3 Sample Requests

This clause does not preclude the provision of a preprinted sample request form bearing the name of the product for signing and dating by the applicant.

All signed and dated written requests for samples should be retained for not less than one year.

17.4 A sample of a medicine must be no larger than the smallest presentation of the medicine on the market in the UK.

17.5 Each sample must be marked 'free medical sample – not for resale' or words to that effect and must be accompanied by a copy of the summary of product characteristics.

17.6 The provision of samples is not permitted for any medicine which contains a substance listed in any of Schedules I, II or IV to the Narcotic Drugs Convention (where the medicine is not a preparation listed in Schedule III to that Convention) or a substance listed in any of Schedules I to IV of the Psychotropic Substances Convention (where the medicine is not a preparation which may be exempted from measures of control in accordance with Paragraphs 2 and 3 of Article 3 of that Convention).

17.7 Samples distributed by representatives must be handed direct to the health professionals requesting them or persons authorized to receive them on their behalf.

17.8 The provision of medicines and samples in hospitals must comply with individual hospital requirements.

17.9 Companies must have adequate systems of control and accountability for samples which they distribute and for all medicines handled by representatives.

Clause 17.9 Control and Accountability

Companies should ensure that their systems of control and accountability relating to medicines held by representatives cover such matters as the security of delivery to them, the security of medicines held by them, the audit of stocks held by them, including expiry dates, and the return to the companies of medicines no longer to be held by representatives.

17.10 Medicines which are sent by post must be packed so as to be reasonably secure against being opened by young children. No unsolicited medicine must be sent through the post.

17.11 Medicines may not be sold or supplied to members of the general public for promotional purposes.

Clause 18 Gifts, Inducements, Promotional Aids and the Provision of Medical and Educational Goods and Services

18.1 No gift, benefit in kind or pecuniary advantage shall be offered or given to members of the health professions or to administrative staff as an inducement to prescribe, supply, administer, recommend, buy or sell any medicine, subject to the provisions of Clause 18.2.

Clause 18.1 General Medical Council

The General Medical Council is the regulatory body for the medical profession and is responsible for giving guidance on standards of professional conduct and on medical ethics. In its guidance, the Council advises doctors that 'You must act in your patients' best interests when making referrals and providing or arranging treatment or care. So you must not ask for or accept any inducement, gift or hospitality which may affect or be seen to affect your judgement'.

Clause 18.1 Terms of Trade

Measures or trade practices relating to prices, margins and discounts which were in regular use by a significant proportion of the pharmaceutical industry on 1 January 1993 are outside the scope of the Code (see Clause 1.2) and are excluded from the provisions of this clause. Other trade practices are subject to the Code. The terms 'prices', 'margins' and 'discounts' are primarily financial terms.

Schemes which enable health professionals to obtain personal benefits, for example gift vouchers for high street stores, in relation to the purchase of medicines are unacceptable even if they are presented as alternatives to financial discounts.

The Royal Pharmaceutical Society of Great Britain has issued guidance in relation to the acceptance of gifts and inducements to prescribe or supply. The Society states that pharmacists accepting items such as gift vouchers, bonus points, discount holidays, sports equipment etc would be in breach of UK law and advises pharmacists not to participate in such offers.

Clause 18.1 Package Deals

Clause 18.1 does not prevent the offer of package deals whereby the purchaser of particular medicines receives with them other associated benefits, such as apparatus for administration, provided that the transaction as a whole is fair and reasonable and the associated benefits are relevant to the medicines involved.

Clause 18.1 Donations to Charities

Donations to charities made by companies in return for health professionals' attendance at company stands at meetings are not unacceptable under this clause provided that the level of donation for each individual is modest, the money is for a reputable charity and any action required of the health professional is not inappropriate. Any donation to a charity must not constitute a payment that would otherwise be unacceptable under the Code. For example, it would not be acceptable for a representative to pay into a practice equipment fund set up as a charity as this would be a financial inducement prohibited under Clause 18.1. Donations to charities in return for representatives gaining interviews are also prohibited under Clause 15.3 of the Code.

Any offer by a company of a donation to a charity which is conditional upon some action by a health professional must not place undue pressure on the health professional to fulfil that condition. At all times the provisions of Clauses 2 and 9.1 must be kept in mind.

18.2 Promotional aids, whether related to a particular product or of general utility, may be distributed to members of the health professions and to appropriate administrative staff, provided that the promotional aids are inexpensive and relevant to the practice of their profession or employment.

Clause 18.2 Gifts

Items provided on long term or permanent loan to a doctor or other prescriber or a practice are regarded as gifts and are subject to the requirements of this clause.

Promotional aids must be inexpensive and relevant to the recipients' work and are more likely to be acceptable if they benefit patient care. An 'inexpensive' promotional aid means one which has cost the donor company no more than £6, excluding VAT. The perceived value to the recipient must be similar.

Items for the personal benefit of health professionals or appropriate administrative staff must not be offered or provided.

Items of general utility which are acceptable promotional aids for health professionals as being inexpensive and of relevance to their work include stationery items, such as computer accessories for business use, pens, pads, diaries and calendars and clinical items, such as nail brushes, surgical gloves, tongue depressors, tissues and peak flow meters. It is permissible to give a coffee mug.

Items which are for use in the home or car are unacceptable. Examples of unacceptable items include table mats, coasters, clocks, desk thermometers, fire extinguishers, rugs, thermos flasks, coffee pots, tea pots, lamps, travel adaptors, toolboxes, umbrellas, neck cushions, plant seeds, road atlases and compact discs of music.

Names of medicines should not be used on promotional aids when it would be inappropriate to do so, for example when it might mislead as to the nature of the item.

Certain independently produced medical/educational publications such as textbooks have been held to be acceptable gifts under Clause 18.2. The content of publications used in this way has to be considered carefully and must comply with the Code as regards any references to the donor's or competitors' products. It might be possible to give certain medical/educational publications in accordance with Clause 18.4 – Provision of Medical and Educational Goods and Services.

Clause 18.2 Competitions and Quizzes

The use of competitions, quizzes and suchlike, and the giving of prizes, are unacceptable methods of promotion.

Clause 18.2 Gifts To or for Use by Patients

Some items distributed as promotional aids are intended for use by patients and these are not generally unacceptable provided that they meet the requirements of Clause 18.2; for example, puzzles and toys for a young child to play with during a visit to the doctor.

Other items which may be made available to patients, for example by completing a request card enclosed with a medicine, should meet the relevant principles set out in Clause 18.2, that is they should be inexpensive and related to either the condition under treatment or general health. Care must be taken that any such activity meets all the requirements of the Code and in particular Clause 20.

No gift or promotional aid for use by patients must be given for the purpose of encouraging patients to request a particular medicine.

18.3 The prescribing information for a medicine as required under Clause 4 does not have to be included on a promotional aid if the promotional aid includes no more than the following about the medicine:

- the brand name or the non-proprietary name of the medicine
- an indication that the name of the medicine is a trade mark
- the name of the company responsible for marketing the product.

Clause 18.3 Promotional Aids – Name of the Medicine

A promotional aid may bear the names of more than one medicine.

Clause 18.3 Prescribing Information on Note Pads and Calendars

If a promotional aid consists of a note pad or calendar in which the individual pages bear advertising material, there is no need for the individual pages to comply with Clause 4 provided that the information required by that clause is given elsewhere; for example, on the cover.

18.4 Medical and educational goods and services which enhance patient care, or benefit the NHS and maintain patient care, can be provided subject to the provisions of Clause 18.1. Medical and educational goods and services must not bear the name of any medicine.

Clause 18.4 Provision of Medical and Educational Goods and Services

Clauses 18.1 and 18.4 do not prevent the provision of medical and educational goods and services. In order to comply with the Code such goods and services must be in the interests of patients or benefit the NHS whilst maintaining patient care.

Medical and educational goods and services may bear a corporate name. The involvement of a pharmaceutical company in such activities must be made clear to relevant health professionals and/or administrative staff receiving the service. In addition the involvement of a pharmaceutical company in therapy review services should be made clea[r] to patients. However, if there are no materials for patient[s] this would be a matter for the relevant health professional. [If] there are materials for patients the requirements fo[r] declaration of sponsorship set out in Clause 9.10 woul[d] apply.

The following guidance is intended to assist companies i[n] relation to medical and educational goods and services.

1 (i) The role of medical/generic representatives in relatio[n] to the provision of goods and services supplied i[n] accordance with Clauses 18.1 and 18.4 needs to be i[n] accordance with the principles set out below. In thi[s] context companies should consider using staff othe[r] than medical/generic representatives.

(ii) If medical/generic representatives provide, deliver o[r] demonstrate medical and educational goods an[d] services then this must not be linked in any way t[o] the promotion of products.

In order to comply with this stipulation the represen[-]tative must not carry out both activities at the sam[e] visit. Representatives may introduce a service b[y] means of a brief description and/or delivering materi[-]als but may not instigate a detailed discussion abou[t] the service at the same time as a call at which pro[-]ducts are promoted.

(iii) The acceptability of the role of medical/generic repre[-]sentatives will depend on the nature of the goods an[d] services provided and the method of provision.

(iv) The nature of the service provider, the person asso[-]ciated with the provision of medical and educationa[l] goods and services, is important ie is the servic[e] provider a medical/generic representative or is th[e] service provider some other appropriately qualifie[d] person, such as a sponsored registered nurse? If th[e] goods and services require patient contact, for exam[-]ple either directly or by identification of patients fro[m] patient records and the like, then medical/generi[c] representatives must not be involved. Only an appro[-]priately qualified person, for example a sponsore[d] registered nurse, not employed as a medical/generi[c] representative, may undertake activities relating t[o] patient contact and/or patient identification. Medi[-]cal/generic representatives could provide adminis[-]trative support in relation to the provision of [a] screening service, but must not be present durin[g] the actual screening and must not discuss or hel[p] interpret individual clinical findings.

(v) Neither the company nor its medical/generic repre[-]sentatives may be given access to data/records tha[t] could identify, or could be linked to, particula[r] patients.

(vi) Sponsored health professionals should not b[e] involved in the promotion of specific products[.] Registered nurses, midwives and health visitor[s] are required to comply with the Nursing & Midwifer[y] Council Code of professional conduct. That Cod[e] requires, inter alia, that registration status is n[o]t used in the promotion of commercial products o[r] services.

2 The remuneration of those not employed as medica[l/] generic representatives but who are sponsored o[r] employed as service providers in relation to the prov[i]sion of medical and educational goods and service[s] must not be linked to sales in any particular territory o[r] place or to sales of a specific product or products and, i[n] particular, may not include a bonus scheme linked t[o] such sales. Bonus schemes linked to a company's over[-]all national performance, or to the level of service pro[-]vided, may be acceptable.

3 Companies must ensure that patient confidentiality [is] maintained at all times and that data protection legisla[-]tion is complied with.

4 Service providers must operate to detailed writte[n] instructions provided by the company. These shoul[d] be similar to the briefing material for representatives a[s] referred to in Clause 15.9. The written instruction[s] should set out the role of the service provider an[d] should cover patient confidentiality issues. Instruction[s] on how the recipients are to be informed etc should b[e] included. The written instructions must not advocat[e] either directly or indirectly, any course of action whic[h] would be likely to lead to a breach of the Code.

5 Service providers must abide by the principle set out i[n] Clause 15.5 that in an interview, or when seeking a[n] appointment, reasonable steps must be taken to ensur[e] that they do not mislead as to their identity or that of th[e] company they represent.

6 A recipient of a service must be provided with a writte[n] protocol to avoid misunderstandings as to what th[e] recipient has agreed. The identity of the sponsorin[g] pharmaceutical company must be given. For exampl[e] a general practitioner allowing a sponsored registere[d] nurse access to patient records should be informed i[n] writing of any data to be extracted and the use to whic[h] those data will be put.

7 Any printed material designed for use in relation to th[e] provision of medical and educational goods and se[r]vices must be non-promotional. It is not acceptabl[e] for such materials to promote the prescription, suppl[y,] sale or administration of the sponsoring company'[s] medicines: Nor is it acceptable for materials to criticise competitor products as this might be seen as promotional. All printed materials must identify the sponsoring pharmaceutical company.

8 *Material relating to the provision of medical and educational goods and services, such as internal instructions, external instructions, the written protocol for recipients and other printed material, including material relating to therapy reviews, etc, must be certified by the Code of Practice signatories within companies to ensure that the requirements of the Code are met as required by Clause 14.3.*

A copy of the materials must be made available to the Prescription Medicines Code of Practice Authority on request.

9 *Companies are recommended to inform relevant parties such as NHS trusts, health authorities, health boards and primary care organisations of their activities where appropriate. This is particularly recommended where companies are proposing to provide medical and educational goods and services which would have budgetary implications for the parties involved. For example the provision of a screening service for a limited period might mean that funds would have to be found in the future when company sponsorship stopped. Another example might be the provision of diagnostic or laboratory services and the like, which the NHS trust, health authority, health board or primary care organisation would normally be expected to provide.*

Clause 18.4 Switch and Therapy Review Programmes

Clauses 18.1 and 18.4 prohibit switch services paid for or facilitated directly or indirectly by a pharmaceutical company whereby a patient's medicine is simply changed to another. For example it would be unacceptable if patients on medicine A were changed to medicine B, without any clinical assessment, at the expense of a pharmaceutical company promoting either or both medicines. It would be acceptable for a company to promote a simple switch from one product to another but not to assist a health professional in implementing that switch even if assistance was by means of a third party such as a sponsored nurse or similar. Such arrangements are seen as companies in effect paying for prescriptions and are unacceptable.

A therapeutic review is different to a switch service. A therapeutic review which aims to ensure that patients receive optimal treatment following a clinical assessment is a legitimate activity for a pharmaceutical company to support and/or assist. The result of such clinical assessments might require, among other things, possible changes of treatment including changes of dose or medicine or cessation of treatment. A genuine therapeutic review should include a comprehensive range of relevant treatment choices, including non-medicinal choices, for the health professional and should not be limited to the medicines of the sponsoring pharmaceutical company. The arrangements for therapeutic review must enhance patient care, or benefit the NHS and maintain patient care, and must otherwise be in accordance with Clause 18.4 and the supplementary information on the provision of medical and educational goods and services. The decision to change or commence treatment must be made for each individual patient by the prescriber and every decision to change an individual patient's treatment must be documented with evidence that it was made on rational grounds.

Clause 19 Meetings and Hospitality

19.1 Companies must not provide hospitality to members of the health professions and appropriate administrative staff except in association with scientific meetings, promotional meetings, scientific congresses and other such meetings. Meetings must be held in appropriate venues conducive to the main purpose of the event. Hospitality must be strictly limited to the main purpose of the event and must be secondary to the purpose of the meeting ie subsistence only. The level of subsistence offered must be appropriate and not out of proportion to the occasion. The costs involved must not exceed that level which the recipients would normally adopt when paying for themselves. It must not extend beyond members of the health professions or appropriate administrative staff.

Clause 19.1 Meetings and Hospitality

The provision of hospitality is limited to refreshments/subsistence (meals and drinks), accommodation, genuine registration fees and the payment of reasonable travel costs which a company may provide to sponsor a delegate to attend a meeting. The payment of travel expenses and the like for persons accompanying the delegate is not permitted. Funding must not be offered or provided to compensate merely for the time spent by health professionals in attending meetings. The payment of reasonable honoraria and reimbursement of out of pocket expenses, including travel, for speakers, advisory board members and the providers of other professional services, is permissible. The arrangements for meetings must comply with Clause 19.1 with regard to hospitality and venues.

Companies should only offer or provide economy air travel to delegates sponsored to attend meetings. Delegates may of course organise and pay at their own expense the genuine difference between economy travel and business class or first class.

Pharmaceutical companies may appropriately sponsor a wide range of meetings. These range from small lunchtime audio-visual presentations in a group practice, hospital meetings and meetings at postgraduate education centres, launch meetings for new products, management training courses, meetings of clinical trialists, patient support group meetings, satellite symposia through to large international meetings organised by independent bodies with sponsorship from pharmaceutical companies.

With any meeting, certain basic principles apply:

- *the meeting must have a clear educational content*
- *the venue must be appropriate and conducive to the main purpose of the meeting; lavish or deluxe venues must not be used and companies should avoid using venues that are renowned for their entertainment facilities*
- *the subsistence associated with the meeting must be secondary to the nature of the meeting, must be appropriate and not out of proportion to the occasion and*
- *any hospitality provided must not extend to a spouse or other such person unless that person is a member of the health professions or appropriate administrative staff and qualifies as a proper delegate or participant at the meeting in their own right*
- *spouses and other accompanying persons, unless qualified as above, may not attend the actual meeting and may not receive any associated hospitality at the company's expense; the entire costs which their presence involves are the responsibility of those they accompany.*

Administrative staff may be invited to meetings where appropriate. For example, receptionists might be invited to a meeting in a general practice when the subject matter related to practice administration.

A useful criterion in determining whether the arrangements for any meeting are acceptable is to apply the question 'would you and your company be willing to have these arrangements generally known?' The impression that is created by the arrangements for any meeting must always be kept in mind.

Meetings organised for groups of doctors, other health professionals and/or for administrative staff which are wholly or mainly of a social or sporting nature are unacceptable.

Meetings organised by pharmaceutical companies which involve UK health professionals at venues outside the UK are not necessarily unacceptable. There have, however, to be valid and cogent reasons for holding meetings at such venues. These are that most of the invitees are from outside the UK and, given their countries of origin, it makes greater logistical sense to hold the meeting outside the UK or, given the location of the relevant resource or expertise that is the object or subject matter of the meeting, it makes greater logistical sense to hold the meeting outside the UK. As with meetings held in the UK, in determining whether such a meeting is acceptable or not, consideration must also be given to the educational programme, overall cost, facilities offered by the venue, nature of the audience, subsistence provided and the like. As with any meeting it should be the programme that attracts delegates and not the associated hospitality or venue.

The requirements of the Code do not apply to the provision of hospitality other than to those referred to in Clause 19.1 and in the supplementary information to Clauses 20.2 and 20.3.

Clause 19.1 Certification of Meetings

Pharmaceutical companies must ensure that all meetings which are planned are checked to see that they comply with the Code. Companies must have a written document that sets out their policies on meetings and hospitality and the associated allowable expenditure. In addition, meetings which involve travel outside the UK must be formally certified as set out in Clause 14.2 of the Code.

Clause 19.1 General Medical Council

The General Medical Council is the regulatory body for the medical profession and is responsible for giving guidance on standards of professional conduct and on medical ethics. In its guidance, the Council advises doctors that 'You must act in your patients' best interests when making referrals and providing or arranging treatment or care. So you must not ask for or accept any inducement, gift or hospitality which may affect or be seen to affect your judgement'.

Clause 19.1 Continuing Professional Development (CPD) Meetings and Courses

The provisions of this and all other relevant clauses in the Code apply equally to meetings and courses organised or sponsored by pharmaceutical companies which are continuing professional development (CPD) approved, such as postgraduate education allowance (PGEA) approved meetings and courses. The fact that a meeting or course has CPD approval does not mean that the arrangements are automatically acceptable under the Code. The relevant provisions of the Code and, in particular, those relating to hospitality, must be observed.

19.2 Payments may not be made to doctors or groups of doctors or to other prescribers, either directly or indirectly, for rental for rooms to be used for meetings.

Clause 19.2 Payment of Room Rental

This provision does not preclude the payment of room rental to postgraduate medical centres and the like.

Payment of room rental to doctors or groups of doctors or to other prescribers is not permissible even if such payment is made to equipment funds or patients' comforts funds and the like or to charities or companies.

19.3 When meetings are sponsored by pharmaceutical companies, that fact must be disclosed in all of the papers relating to the meetings and in any published proceedings. The declaration of sponsorship must be sufficiently prominent to ensure that readers are aware of it at the outset.

Clause 19.3 Sponsorship and Reports of Meetings

Attention is drawn to Clause 9.10 which requires that all material relating to medicines and their uses, whether promotional or not, which is sponsored by a pharmaceutical company must clearly indicate that it has been sponsored by that company.

It should be noted that where companies are involved in the sponsorship and/or distribution of reports on meetings or symposia etc, these reports may constitute promotional material and thus be fully subject to the requirements of the Code.

Clause 20 Relations with the General Public and the Media

20.1 Prescription only medicines must not be advertised to the general public. This prohibition does not apply to vaccination campaigns carried out by companies and approved by the health ministers.

Clause 20.1 Advertising of Medicines to the General Public

The advertising of prescription only medicines to the public is also prohibited by the Advertising Regulations.

The promotion of medicines to the public for self medication purposes is covered by the Code of Standards of Advertising Practice for Over-the-Counter Medicines of the Proprietary Association of Great Britain (PAGB).

Methods of sale of medicines through pharmacies are also covered by the Code of Ethics and Standards of the Royal Pharmaceutical Society of Great Britain.

20.2 Information about prescription only medicines which is made available to the public either directly or indirectly must be factual and presented in a balanced way. It must not raise unfounded hopes of successful treatment or be misleading with respect to the safety of the product.

Statements must not be made for the purpose of encouraging members of the public to ask their health professional to prescribe a specific prescription only medicine.

Clause 20.2 Information to the Public

This clause allows for the provision of non-promotional information about prescription only medicines to the public either in response to a direct enquiry from an individual, including enquiries from journalists, or by dissemination of such information via press conferences, press announcements, television and radio reports, public relations activities and the like. It also includes information provided by means of posters distributed for display in surgery waiting rooms etc and reference information made available by companies on their websites or otherwise as a resource for members of the public.

Any information so provided must observe the principles set out in this clause; that is, it should be factual, balanced and must not be made for the purpose of encouraging members of the public to ask their doctors or other prescribers to prescribe a specific prescription only medicine. It must not constitute the advertising of prescription only medicines to the public prohibited under Clause 20.1. The provisions of Clause 20.4 must be observed if an enquiry is from an individual member of the public.

Information to the public falls into one of three categories depending on its purpose, how it is supplied and how the public is made aware of the information.

Proactive information is supplied to the public without a direct request. This includes booklets on diseases and/or medicines supplied directly or via a health professional, press releases, briefings, conferences, mailings to patient organisations and disease awareness advertising.

Reference information is intended to provide a comprehensive up-to-date resource that companies should make available on their websites or by way of a link from their website or by some other means. The primary purpose of reference information is to be a library resource for members of the public giving information relating to prescription only medicines which have marketing authorizations. Pharmaceutical companies are not obliged to provide reference information but it is considered good practice to provide as a minimum the regulatory information comprising the summary of product characteristics (SPC), the package information leaflet (PIL) and the public assessment report (PAR) (UK or European) where such a document exists. Reference information may also include the registration studies used for marketing authorization applications and variations and any other studies published or not including those referred to in the SPC, PIL, EPAR or UKPAR or available on clinical trial databases. Reference information may also include material supplied for health technology assessments to bodies such as the National Institute for Health and Clinical Excellence (NICE), the All Wales Medicines Strategy Group (AWMSG) and the Scottish Medicines Consortium (SMC).

Reference information may also include medicine guides where available, studies (published or not), information about diseases and information about specific medicines etc.

Where companies decide to make reference information available this must represent fairly the current body of evidence relating to a medicine and its benefit/risk profile.

Reactive information is supplied to the public in response to a direct request and must be limited to that information necessary to respond to the request.

It is good practice to include the summary of product characteristics with a press release or press pack relating to a medicine. Companies should also consider including references to other credible sources of information about a condition or a medicine.

Particular care must be taken in responding to approaches from the media to ensure that the provisions of this clause are upheld.

In the event of a complaint which relates to the provisions of this clause, companies will be asked to provide copies of any information supplied, including copies of any relevant press releases and the like. This information will be assessed to determine whether it fulfils the requirements of this clause.

Public assessment reports (European or UK), summaries of product characteristics and package leaflets may be provided to members of the public on request.

Companies may provide members of the health professions with leaflets concerning a medicine with a view to their provision to patients to whom the medicine has already been prescribed, provided that such a leaflet is factual and non-promotional in nature.

A company may conduct a disease awareness or public health campaign provided that the purpose is to encourage members of the public to seek treatment for their symptoms while in no way promoting the use of a specific medicine. The use of brand or non-proprietary names and/or restricting the range of treatments described in the campaign might be likely to lead to the use of a specific medicine. Particular care must be taken where the company's product, even though not named, is the only medicine relevant to the disease or symptoms in question.

Attention is drawn to the Disease Awareness Campaigns Guidelines produced by the Medicines and Healthcare products Regulatory Agency.

The requirements of Clause 7 relating to information (Clauses 7.2, 7.4, 7.5, 7.8, 7.9, 7.10 and 7.11) also apply to information to the public.

Meetings organised for or attended by members of the public, journalists and patient organisations must comply with Clause 19.

Items for patients or for use by patients are covered in the supplementary information to Clause 18.2.

Clause 20.2 Financial Information

Information made available in order to inform shareholders, the Stock Exchange and the like by way of annual reports and announcements etc. may relate to both existing medicines and those not yet marketed. Such information must be factual and presented in a balanced way. Business press releases should identify the business importance of the information.

Clause 20.2 Information to Current or Prospective Employees

Information about pharmaceutical companies provided to current or prospective employees may relate to both existing medicines and those not yet marketed. Such information must be factual and presented in a balanced way.

Clause 20.2 Approval of Information

Information on medicines made available under this clause other than responses from medical information departments or similar to unsolicited enquiries from the public must be certified in advance as required by Clause 14.3.

Clause 20.2 Health Technology Assessments

Companies may supply information to relevant patient organisations, the public or patients in relation to forthcoming health technology assessments by public national organisations such as NICE, AWMSG or SMG, provided the information is accurate, not misleading, not promotional in nature and otherwise complies with Clause 20.2.

20.3 Pharmaceutical companies can work with patient organisations but when doing so must ensure that the involvement of the company is made clear and that all of the arrangements comply with the Code. This includes the need to declare sponsorship (Clause 9.10) and the prohibition on advertising prescription only medicines to the public (Clause 20.1). The requirements of Clause 19, which covers meetings for health professionals and appropriate administrative staff, also apply to pharmaceutical companies supporting patient organisation meetings.

Clause 20.3 Relationships with Patient Organisations

Pharmaceutical companies can interact with patient organisations or any user organisation such as disability organisations, carer or relative organisations and consumer organisations to support their work, including assistance in the provision of appropriate information to the public, patients and carers. Any involvement a pharmaceutical company has with a patient organisation must be declared and transparent. Companies must make public by means of information on their websites or in their annual report a list of all patient organisations to which they provide financial support. This might include sponsoring materials and meetings. Matters to be borne in mind include arrangements for meetings (Clause 19), the need to declare sponsorship (Clause 9.10) and the prohibition on advertising prescription only medicines to the general public (Clause 20.1).

Companies working with patient organisations must have in place a written agreement setting out exactly what has been agreed, including funding, in relation to every significant activity or ongoing relationship. The written agreement should set out the activities agreed and the level of funding and refer to the approval process for each party. Attention is drawn to the certification requirements set out in Clause 14.3.

There are other codes and guidelines which cover patient groups, including the Long Term Medical Conditions Alliance guidelines and Charity Commission requirements etc.

Pharmaceutical companies should take into account the purpose of materials and/or activities. The purpose of information supplied to a patient organisation must be made clear. For example, there is a difference between providing information to be supplied to the members of a patient organisation and providing background information to enable a patient organisation to respond to a health technology assessment or similar.

20.4 Requests from individual members of the public for advice on personal medical matters must be refused and the enquirer recommended to consult his or her own doctor or other prescriber or other health professional.

Clause 20.4 Requests for Information or Advice on Personal Medical Matters

This clause prohibits the provision of advice on personal medical matters to individual members of the public requesting it. The intention behind this prohibition is to ensure that companies do not intervene in the patient/ doctor or patient/prescriber relationship by offering advice or information which properly should be in the domain of the doctor or other prescriber.

Pharmaceutical companies can provide information appropriate to support the use of medicines and enhance patient welfare. Emergency advice, for example action needed in the event of an overdose, can be provided. Other information may also be given, including information on medicines prescribed for the enquirer, provided that it complies with the requirements of Clauses 20.1 and 20.2 and does not impinge on the principle behind this clause. For example, answering requests from members of the public as to whether a particular medicine contains sucrose or some other inactive ingredient, or whether there would be problems associated with drinking alcohol whilst taking the medicine or whether the medicine should be taken before or after a meal, is acceptable. Particular care needs to be taken with regard to enquiries relating to side-effects, the indications for a medicine and suchlike.

All requests from members of the public must be handled with great care and a company should refer the enquirer to other sources where appropriate. These might include health professionals, NHS Direct and patient organisations, etc.

A request from a patient for information may in some instances best be handled by passing the information to the patient's doctor or other prescriber for discussion with them rather than providing the information direct to the patient concerned. This should not be done without the patient's consent.

20.5 The introduction of a new medicine must not be made known to the public until reasonable steps have been taken to inform the medical and pharmaceutical professions of its availability.

20.6 Companies are responsible for information about their products which is issued by their public relations agencies.

Clause 21 The Internet

21.1 Access to promotional material directed to a UK audience provided on the Internet in relation to prescription only medicines should generally be limited to health professionals and appropriate administrative staff.

Clause 21.1 Access

Promotional material should ideally be access restricted. If, however, access restriction is not applied, a pharmaceutical company website or a company sponsored website must provide information for the public as well as promotion to health professionals with the sections for each target audience clearly separated and the intended audience identified. This is to avoid the public needing to access material for health professionals unless they choose to. The MHRA Blue Guide states that the public should not be encouraged to access material which is not intended for them.

21.2 Information or promotional material about medicines covered by Clause 21.1 above which is placed on the Internet outside the UK will be regarded as coming within the scope of the Code if it was placed there by a UK company or an affiliate of a UK company or at the instigation or with the authority of such a company and it makes specific reference to the availability or use of the medicine in the UK.

21.3 Information about medicines covered by Clauses 21.1 and 21.2 above which is provided on the Internet and which can be accessed by members of the public must comply with Clause 20.2 of the Code.

21.4 Notwithstanding the provisions of Clauses 21.1 and 21.3 above, a medicine covered by Clause 21.1 may be advertised in a relevant independently produced electronic journal intended for health professionals or appropriate administrative staff which can be accessed by members of the public.

Clause 21.4 Advertisements in Electronic Journals

It should be noted that the MHRA Blue Guide states that each page of an advertisement for a prescription only medicine should be clearly labelled as intended for health professionals.

21.5 Public assessment reports (European or UK), summaries of product characteristics, package leaflets and reference material for prescription only medicines may be included on the Internet and be accessible by members of the public provided that they are not presented in such a way as to be promotional in nature.

Clause 21.5 MHRA Guidance

The MHRA Blue Guide states that the public should not need to access non-UK websites or non-UK parts of websites to obtain basic information about a company's products, such as patient information leaflets, summaries of product characteristics, public assessment reports and other non promotional material. It is good practice for each page of a company website to include a statement identifying the intended audience.

Clause 21.5 Information on Clinical Trials

Information on clinical trials as agreed in the Joint Position on the Disclosure of Clinical Trial Information via Clinical Trial Registries and Databases 2005 may be available at a UK or a non UK website.

21.6 It should be made clear when a user is leaving any of the company's sites, or sites sponsored by the company, or is being directed to a site which is not that of the company.

Clause 21.6 Sites Linked via Company Sites

Sites linked via company sites are not necessarily covered by the Code.

Clause 22 Compliance with Undertakings

When an undertaking has been given in relation to a ruling under the Code, the company concerned must ensure that it complies with that undertaking.

PRESCRIPTION MEDICINES CODE OF PRACTICE AUTHORITY: Constitution and Procedure

Operative on 1 January 2006 except for paragraphs 5, 6, 7, 8, 10, 11, 12, 13, 16.3 and 21 which are operative in respect of complaints received on and after 1 January 2006.

INTRODUCTION

The Code of Practice for the Pharmaceutical Industry is administered by the Prescription Medicines Code of Practice Authority. The Authority is responsible for the provision of advice, guidance and training on the Code of Practice as well as for the complaints procedure. It is also responsible for arranging for conciliation between companies when requested to do so and for scrutinising advertising and meetings on a regular basis. Complaints made under the Code about promotional material or the promotional activities of companies are considered by the Code of Practice Panel and, where required, by the Code of Practice Appeal Board. Reports on cases are published by the Authority and are available on request and on the Authority's website www.pmcpa.org.uk.

The names of individuals complaining from outside the pharmaceutical industry are kept confidential. In exceptional cases it may be necessary for a company to know the identity of the complainant so that the matter can be properly investigated. Even in these instances, the name of the complainant is only disclosed with the complainant's permission.

Complaints about the promotion of medicines should be submitted to the Director of the Prescription Medicines Code of Practice Authority, 12 Whitehall,

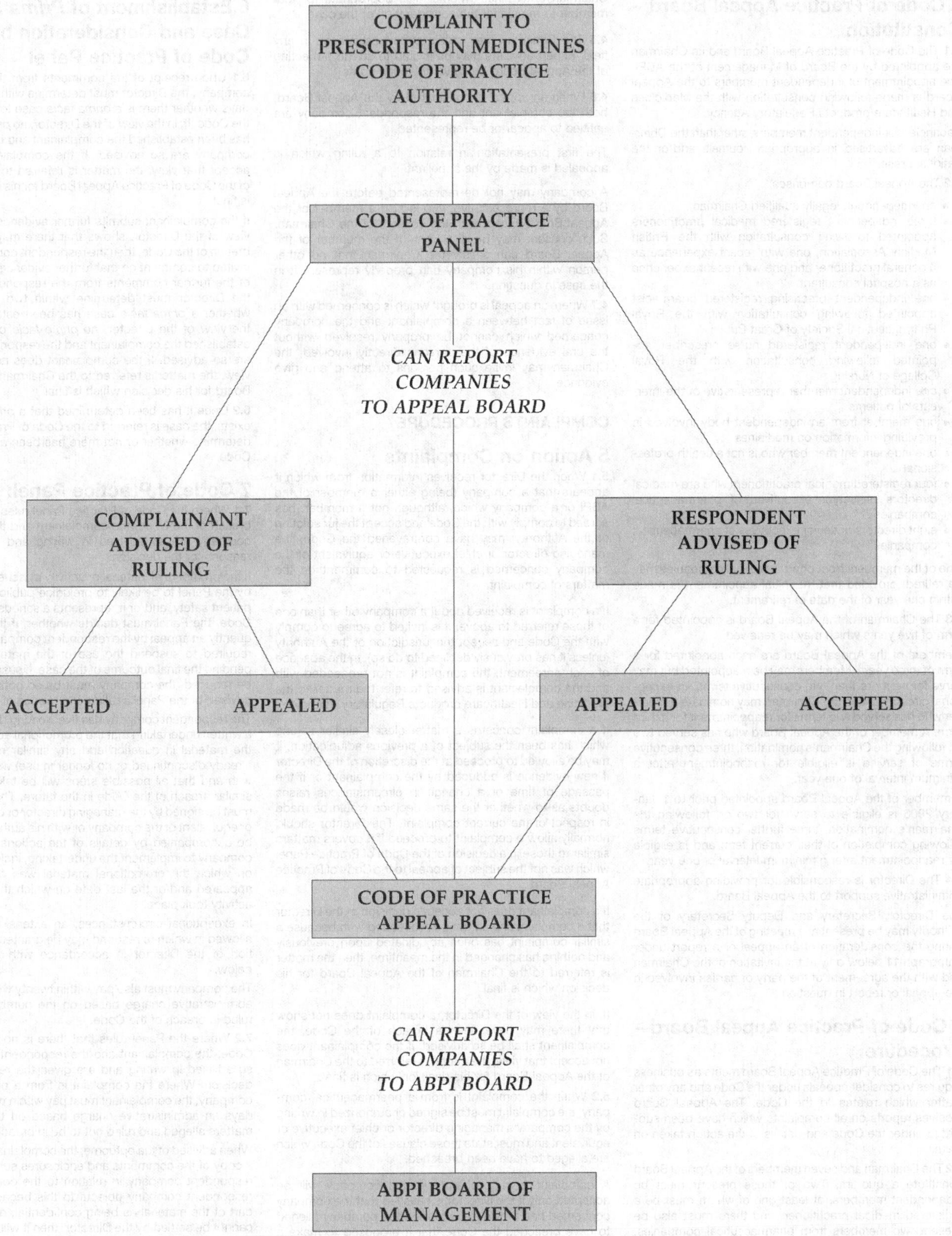

London SW1A 2DY, telephone 020-7930 9677, facsimile 020-7930 4554, email complaints@pmcpa.org.uk.

STRUCTURE AND RESPONSIBILITIES

1 Prescription Medicines Code of Practice Authority

1.1 The Prescription Medicines Code of Practice Authority is responsible for the administration of the Code of Practice for the Pharmaceutical Industry including the provision of advice, guidance and training on the Code. It is also responsible for arranging for conciliation between companies when requested to do so and for scrutinising advertising and meetings on a regular basis.

1.2 The Authority also administers the complaints procedure by which complaints made under the Code are considered by the Code of Practice Panel and, where required, by the Code of Practice Appeal Board.

1.3 The Authority is appointed by and reports to the Board of Management of The Association of the British Pharmaceutical Industry (ABPI) and consists of the Director, Secretary and Deputy Secretary.

The Director reports to the Appeal Board for guidance on the interpretation of the Code and the operation of the complaints procedure and to the President of the ABPI for administrative purposes.

In the absence of the Director, the Secretary is authorised to act on his behalf.

1.4 The Director has the authority to request copies of any relevant material from a pharmaceutical company, including copies of the certificates authorizing any such material and copies of relevant briefing material for representatives.

1.5 The Authority may consult the Appeal Board upon any matter concerning the Code or its administration.

2 Code of Practice Panel – Constitution and Procedure

2.1 The Code of Practice Panel consists of the members of the Prescription Medicines Code of Practice Authority and meets as business requires to consider complaints made under the Code.

2.2 Two members of the Authority form a quorum for a meeting of the Panel. Decisions are made by majority voting. The Director or, in his absence, the Secretary, acts as Chairman of the Panel and has both an original and a casting vote.

2.3 The Director may obtain expert assistance in any field. Expert advisers who are consulted may be invited to attend a meeting of the Panel but have no voting rights.

3 Code of Practice Appeal Board – Constitution

3.1 The Code of Practice Appeal Board and its Chairman are appointed by the Board of Management of the ABPI. The appointment of independent members to the Appeal Board is made following consultation with the Medicines and Healthcare products Regulatory Agency.

Vacancies for independent members other than the Chairman are advertised in appropriate journals and/or the national press.

3.2 The Appeal Board comprises:

- an independent, legally qualified Chairman
- three independent registered medical practitioners appointed following consultation with the British Medical Association, one with recent experience as a general practitioner and one with recent experience as a hospital consultant
- one independent practising registered pharmacist appointed following consultation with the Royal Pharmaceutical Society of Great Britain
- one independent registered nurse prescriber appointed following consultation with the Royal College of Nursing
- one independent member representative of the interests of patients
- one member from an independent body involved in providing information on medicines
- one independent member who is not a health professional
- four registered medical practitioners who are medical directors or senior executives of pharmaceutical companies
- eight directors or senior executives of pharmaceutical companies.

One of the members from pharmaceutical companies may be retired, provided that the initial appointment is made within one year of the date of retirement.

3.3 The Chairman of the Appeal Board is appointed for a term of five years which may be renewed.

Members of the Appeal Board are each appointed for a term of three years. Members may be reappointed but may serve for no more than two consecutive terms. In exceptional circumstances the Chairman may nominate a member who has served two terms for reappointment for a third term. A member of the Appeal Board who has served two or, following the Chairman's nomination, three consecutive terms of service is eligible for reappointment after a minimum interval of one year.

A member of the Appeal Board appointed prior to 1 January 2006 is eligible to serve for two or, following the Chairman's nomination, three further consecutive terms following completion of their current term and is eligible for reappointment after a minimum interval of one year.

3.4 The Director is responsible for providing appropriate administrative support to the Appeal Board.

The Director, Secretary and Deputy Secretary of the Authority may be present at a meeting of the Appeal Board during the consideration of an appeal or a report under Paragraph 11 below only at the invitation of the Chairman and with the agreement of the party or parties involved in the appeal or report in question.

4 Code of Practice Appeal Board – Procedure

4.1 The Code of Practice Appeal Board meets as business requires to consider appeals under the Code and any other matter which relates to the Code. The Appeal Board receives reports on all complaints which have been submitted under the Code and details of the action taken on them.

4.2 The Chairman and seven members of the Appeal Board constitute a quorum. Two of those present must be independent members, at least one of whom must be a registered medical practitioner, and there must also be present two members from pharmaceutical companies, at least one of whom must be a registered medical practitioner.

In the event that a quorum cannot be attained for the consideration of a case because of the number of members barred under Paragraph 4.4 below, or for any other reason, the Chairman may co-opt appropriate persons who are former members of the Appeal Board, or who are on a list of persons approved for co-option to the Appeal Board, so as to enable a quorum to be achieved. The list of persons approved for co-option is drawn up following procedures similar to those for appointing members of the Appeal Board.

4.3 Decisions are made by majority voting. The Chairman has both an original and a casting vote.

4.4 If a member of the Appeal Board is concerned in a case either as complainant or respondent, that member does not receive copies of the papers circulated in connection with the case and is required to withdraw from the Appeal Board during its consideration.

Members of the Appeal Board are also required to declare any other interest in a case prior to its consideration. The Chairman determines whether it is appropriate for that member to remain for the consideration of the case.

4.5 The Chairman may obtain expert assistance in any field. Expert advisers may be invited to attend a meeting of the Appeal Board but have no voting rights.

4.6 When an appeal is considered by the Appeal Board, both the complainant and the respondent company are entitled to appear or be represented.

The first presentation in relation to a ruling which is appealed is made by the appellant.

A company may not be represented before the Appeal Board by a representative who is also a member of the Appeal Board except with the consent of the Chairman. Such consent may be given only if the member of the Appeal Board can satisfy the Chairman that no other person within his company can properly represent it in the case in question.

4.7 Where an appeal is brought which is concerned with an issue of fact between a complainant and the company concerned which cannot be properly resolved without the oral evidence of the persons directly involved, the Chairman may invite such persons to attend and give evidence.

COMPLAINTS PROCEDURE

5 Action on Complaints

5.1 When the Director receives information from which it appears that a company (being either a member of the ABPI or a company which, although not a member, has agreed to comply with the Code and accept the jurisdiction of the Authority) may have contravened the Code, the managing director or chief executive or equivalent of the company concerned is requested to comment on the matters of complaint.

If a complaint is received about a company other than one of those referred to above, it is invited to agree to comply with the Code and accept the jurisdiction of the Authority (unless it has previously declined to do so). In the absence of such agreement, the complaint is not proceeded with and the complainant is advised to refer the matter to the Medicine and Healthcare products Regulatory Agency.

If a complaint concerns a matter closely similar to one which has been the subject of a previous adjudication, it may be allowed to proceed at the discretion of the Director if new evidence is adduced by the complainant or if the passage of time or a change in circumstances raises doubts as to whether the same decision would be made in respect of the current complaint. The Director should normally allow a complaint to proceed if it covers matters similar to those in a decision of the Code of Practice Panel which was not the subject of appeal to the Code of Practice Appeal Board.

If a complainant does not accept a decision of the Director that a complaint should not be proceeded with because a similar complaint has been adjudicated upon previously and nothing has changed in the meantime, then the matter is referred to the Chairman of the Appeal Board for his decision which is final.

If, in the view of the Director, a complaint does not show that there may have been a breach of the Code, the complainant shall be so advised. If the complainant does not accept that view, the matter is referred to the Chairman of the Appeal Board for his decision which is final.

5.2 When the complaint is from a pharmaceutical company, the complaint must be signed or authorized in writing by the company's managing director or chief executive or equivalent and must state those clauses of the Code which are alleged to have been breached.

A complaint from a pharmaceutical company will be accepted only if the Director is satisfied that the company concerned has previously informed the company alleged to have breached the Code that it proposed to make a formal complaint and offered inter-company dialogue at a senior level in an attempt to resolve the matter, but that this offer was refused or dialogue proved unsuccessful. A formal statement detailing the actions taken must be provided.

Attention is drawn to the availability of conciliation prior to making a complaint as referred to in Paragraph 19.2 below. Information about conciliation is available from the Authority.

5.3 Upon receipt of a complaint, the company concerned has ten working days in which to submit its comments in writing.

5.4 When a company advises the Authority that it may have breached the Code, the Director shall treat the matter as a complaint if it relates to a potentially serious breach of the Code or if the company fails to take appropriate action to address the matter. The company's comments are invited and the Director must then determine within two working days whether a prima facie case has been established. If a prima facie case is established the procedures under Paragraph 6.2 below onwards shall be followed.

6 Establishment of *Prima Facie* Case and Consideration by the Code of Practice Panel

6.1 Upon receipt of the comments from the respondent company, the Director must determine within two working days whether there is a *prima facie* case to answer under the Code. If, in the view of the Director, no *prima facie* case has been established the complainant and the respondent company are so advised. If the complainant does not accept that view, the matter is referred to the Chairman of the Code of Practice Appeal Board for his decision which is final.

If the complainant submits further evidence which, in the view of the Director, shows that there may have been a breach of the Code, then the respondent company shall be invited to comment on that further evidence. Upon receipt of the further comments from the respondent company, the Director must determine within two working days whether a *prima facie* case has been established. If, in the view of the Director, no *prima facie* case has been established the complainant and the respondent company are so advised. If the complainant does not accept that view, the matter is referred to the Chairman of the Appeal Board for his decision which is final.

6.2 Once it has been determined that a *prima facie* case exists, the case is referred to the Code of Practice Panel to determine whether or not there has been a breach of the Code.

7 Code of Practice Panel: Rulings

7.1 Where the Code of Practice Panel rules that there is a breach of the Code, the complainant and the respondent company are so advised in writing and are given the reasons for the decision.

If the promotional material or activity at issue is considered by the Panel to be likely to prejudice public health and/or patient safety, and/or it represents a serious breach of the Code, the Panel must decide whether, if there is subsequently an appeal by the respondent company, it would be required to suspend the use of the material or activity pending the final outcome of the case. If suspension would be required, the company must be so notified when it is advised of the Panel's ruling of a breach of the Code.

The respondent company has five working days to provide a written undertaking that the promotional activity or use of the material in question and any similar material (if not already discontinued or no longer in use) will cease forthwith and that all possible steps will be taken to avoid a similar breach of the Code in the future. This undertaking must be signed by the managing director or chief executive or equivalent of the company or with his authority and must be accompanied by details of the actions taken by the company to implement the undertaking, including the date on which the promotional material was finally used or appeared and/or the last date on which the promotional activity took place.

In exceptional circumstances, an extension in the time allowed in which to respond may be granted at the discretion of the Director in accordance with Paragraph 14 below.

The company must also pay within twenty working days an administrative charge based on the number of matters ruled in breach of the Code.

7.2 Where the Panel rules that there is no breach of the Code, the complainant and the respondent company are so advised in writing and are given the reasons for the decision. Where the complaint is from a pharmaceutical company, the complainant must pay within twenty working days an administrative charge based on the number of matters alleged and ruled not to be in breach of the Code.

When advised of the outcome, the complainant will be sent a copy of the comments and enclosures submitted by the respondent company in relation to the complaint. If the respondent company objects to this because it regards part of the material as being confidential, and the matter cannot be settled by the Director, then it will be referred to the Chairman of the Code of Practice Appeal Board for his decision which is final.

7.3 The complainant or the respondent company may appeal against a ruling of the Panel to the Appeal Board. Appeals must be accompanied by reasons as to why the Panel's ruling is not accepted. These reasons will be circulated to the Appeal Board.

An appeal by the complainant must be lodged within ten working days of notification of the ruling of the Panel.

Where the respondent company appeals, it must give notice of appeal within five working days of notification of the ruling of the Panel and must lodge the appeal within ten working days of notification of the ruling of the Panel.

If the Panel has so required in accordance with Paragraph 7.1 above, where the respondent company gives notice of appeal it must, within five working days of notification of the Panel's ruling, suspend the use of the promotional material or activity at issue, pending the final outcome of the case, and must notify the Authority that such action has been taken.

If the respondent company accepts one or more of the Panel's rulings of breaches of the Code, but appeals one or nore other such rulings, then within five working days of otification of the Panel's rulings it must provide the underaking required by Paragraph 7.1 above in respect of the uling or rulings which it is not appealing.

n exceptional circumstances, an extension in the time llowed in which to respond may be granted at the discreion of the Director in accordance with Paragraph 14 elow.

.4 Where an appeal is lodged by the complainant, the espondent company has five working days to comment on he reasons given by the complainant for the appeal and hese comments will be circulated to the Appeal Board.

he complainant has five working days to comment on the espondent company's comments upon the reasons given y the complainant for the appeal and these comments will e circulated to the respondent company and the Appeal Board.

n the event that the respondent company objects to ertain of its comments being made available to the comlainant on the grounds of confidentiality, and the matter annot be settled by the Director, then it will be referred to he Chairman of the Appeal Board who will decide whether hose particular comments can be included in the evidence which goes before the Appeal Board. The Chairman's decision is final.

.5 Where an appeal is lodged by the respondent company, the complainant has five working days to comment on the reasons given by the respondent company for the appeal and these comments will be circulated to the espondent company and the Appeal Board.

n the event that the respondent company objects to certain details of its appeal being made available to the complainant on the grounds of confidentiality, and the matter cannot be settled by the Director, then it will be eferred to the Chairman of the Appeal Board who will decide whether those particular details can be included n the evidence which goes before the Appeal Board. The Chairman's decision is final.

Where an appeal is lodged by the respondent company, he complainant is sent a copy of the initial comments and enclosures submitted by the respondent company in relaion to the complaint. If the respondent company objects to his because it regards part of the material as being confidential, and the matter cannot be settled by the Director, hen it will be referred to the Chairman of the Appeal Board or his decision which is final.

8 Code of Practice Panel: Reports to the Code of Practice Appeal Board

8.1 Failure to comply with the procedures set out in Paragraphs 5, 6 and 7 above shall be reported to the Code of Practice Appeal Board.

8.2 The Code of Practice Panel may also report to the Appeal Board any company whose conduct in relation to the Code, or in relation to a particular case before it, or because it repeatedly breaches the Code such that it raises concerns about the company's procedures, warrants consideration by the Appeal Board. Such a report to the Appeal Board may be made notwithstanding the fact that a company has provided an undertaking requested by the Panel.

9 Action on Complaints about Safety from the Medicines and Healthcare products Regulatory Agency

9.1 In the event of the Medicines and Healthcare products Regulatory Agency making a complaint which relates to the safety or proper use of a medicine, and requesting that an advertisement be withdrawn, the respondent company has five working days to respond with its comments.

9.2 If the Code of Practice Panel upholds the complaint, the company is required to suspend the advertisement or practice forthwith pending the final outcome of the case.

10 Code of Practice Appeal Board: Rulings

10.1 Where the Code of Practice Appeal Board rules that there is no breach of the Code, the complainant and the respondent company are so advised in writing and are given the reasons for the decision.

Where a complainant pharmaceutical company appeals and the Appeal Board upholds the ruling that there is no breach of the Code, the complainant pharmaceutical company must pay within twenty working days an administrative charge based on the number of matters taken to appeal on which no breach is ruled.

Where a respondent company appeals and the Appeal Board rules that there is no breach of the Code, the complainant pharmaceutical company must pay within twenty working days an administrative charge based on the number of matters taken to appeal on which no breach is ruled.

10.2 Where the Appeal Board rules that there is a breach of the Code, the respondent company is so advised in writing and is given the reasons for the decision. The respondent company then has five working days to provide a written undertaking providing the information specified in Paragraph 7.1 above.

The company must also pay within twenty working days an administrative charge based on the number of matters ruled in breach of the Code.

10.3 Where the Appeal Board rules that there is a breach of the Code, the company may be required by the Appeal Board to take steps to recover items given in connection with the promotion of a medicine or non promotional items provided to members of the public and the like. Details of the action taken must be provided in writing to the Appeal Board.

10.4 Where the Appeal Board rules that there is a breach of the Code, the Appeal Board may require an audit of the company's procedures in relation to the Code to be carried out by the Prescription Medicines Code of Practice Authority and, following that audit, decide whether to impose requirements on the company concerned to improve its procedures in relation to the Code. These could include a further audit and/or a requirement that promotional material be submitted to the Authority for pre-vetting for a specified period. The Authority must arrange for material submitted for pre-vetting to be examined for compliance with the Code but the Authority cannot approve such material.

The Appeal Board may also require an audit if a company repeatedly breaches the Code.

10.5 Where the Appeal Board rules that there is a breach of the Code, the Appeal Board may reprimand the company and publish details of that reprimand.

10.6 Where the Appeal Board rules that there is a breach of the Code, the Appeal Board may require the company to issue a corrective statement. Details of the proposed content and mode and timing of dissemination of the corrective statement must be provided to the Appeal Board for approval prior to use.

11 Reports to the Code of Practice Appeal Board

11.1 Where the Panel reports a company to the Code of Practice Appeal Board under the provisions of Paragraphs 8.1 and 8.2 above, or where the Panel reports the failure of a company to comply with the procedures set out in Paragraph 9 above, or where the Authority reports the failure of a company to comply with the procedures set out in Paragraph 10 above, the procedures set out below shall apply. These procedures also apply if the Appeal Board, having received a report on a case completed at the Panel level, in accordance with Paragraph 4.1 above, considers that additional sanctions may be appropriate.

11.2 The company concerned is provided with a copy of the report prior to its consideration and is entitled to have a representative or representatives appear before the Appeal Board to state the company's case.

A company may not be represented before the Appeal Board by a representative who is also a member of the Appeal Board except with the consent of the Chairman. Such consent may be given only if the member of the Appeal Board can satisfy the Chairman that no other person within his company can properly represent it in the matter in question.

11.3 The Appeal Board may decide:

- to reprimand the company and publish details of that reprimand
- to require an audit of the company's procedures in relation to the Code to be carried out by the Prescription Medicines Code of Practice Authority and, following that audit, decide whether to impose requirements on the company concerned to improve its procedures in relation to the Code; these could include a further audit and/or a requirement that promotional material be submitted to the Authority for pre-vetting for a specified period; the Authority must arrange for material submitted for pre-vetting to be examined for compliance with the Code but the Authority cannot approve such material
- to require the company to issue a corrective statement; details of the proposed content and mode and timing of dissemination of the corrective statement must be provided to the Appeal Board for approval prior to use
- to take steps to recover items given in connection with the promotion of a medicine; details of the action taken must be provided in writing to the Appeal Board.

11.4 Where a company not in membership of the ABPI fails to comply with the procedures set out in Paragraphs 5, 6, 7, 9 or 10 above and indicates that it no longer wishes to accept the jurisdiction of the Authority, the Appeal Board may decide that the company should be removed from the list of non member companies which have agreed to abide by the Code and the Medicines and Healthcare products Regulatory Agency advised that responsibility for that company under the Code can no longer continue to be accepted.

The Board of Management of the ABPI must be advised that such action has been taken.

12 Code of Practice Appeal Board: Reports to the ABPI Board of Management

12.1 Where the Code of Practice Appeal Board considers that the conduct of a company in relation to the Code or a particular case before it warrants such action, it may report the company to the Board of Management of the ABPI for it to consider whether further sanctions should be applied against that company. Such a report may be made notwithstanding the fact that the company has provided an undertaking requested by either the Code of Practice Panel or the Appeal Board.

12.2 Where such a report is made to the Board of Management, the Board of Management may decide:

- to reprimand the company and publish details of that reprimand
- to require an audit of the company's procedures in relation to the Code to be carried out by the Prescription Medicines Code of Practice Authority and, following that audit, decide whether to impose requirements on the company concerned to improve its procedures in relation to the Code; these could include a further audit and/or a requirement that promotional material be submitted to the Authority for pre-vetting for a specified period; the Authority must arrange for material submitted for pre-vetting to be examined for compliance with the Code but the Authority cannot approve such material
- to require the company to issue a corrective statement; details of the proposed content and mode and timing of dissemination of the corrective statement must be provided to the Appeal Board for approval prior to use
- to suspend or expel the company from the ABPI or
- in the case of companies not in membership of the ABPI, to remove the company from the list of non member companies which have agreed to abide by the Code and to advise the Medicines and Healthcare products Regulatory Agency that responsibility for that company under the Code can no longer continue to be accepted.

12.3 If a member of the Board of Management is concerned in a case which has led to the report, as either complainant or respondent, that member does not receive a copy of the report and is required to withdraw from the Board of Management during its consideration.

Members of the Board of Management are also required to declare any other interest in a report prior to its consideration. The President (or Chairman in the absence of the President) determines whether it is appropriate for that member to remain for the consideration of the report.

12.4 Where a report is made to the Board of Management under Paragraph 12.1 above, the company concerned is provided with a copy of the report prior to its consideration and is entitled to have a representative or representatives appear before the Board of Management to state the company's case.

13 Case Reports

13.1 At the conclusion of any case under the Code, the complainant is advised of the outcome and a report is published summarising the details of the case.

13.2 The respondent company and the medicine concerned are named in the report.

In a case where the complaint was initiated by a company or by an organisation or official body, that company or organisation or official body is named in the report. The information given must not, however, be such as to identify any individual person.

Where expert assistance has been obtained by either the Code of Practice Panel or the Code of Practice Appeal Board, the report will include the name and qualifications of the expert concerned.

Where a company has been required to issue a corrective statement, the report will reproduce its text and provide details of how the corrective statement was disseminated.

13.3 A copy of the report on a case is made available to both the complainant and the respondent company prior to publication. Any amendments to the report suggested by these parties are considered by the Director, consulting with the other party where appropriate. If either party does not accept the Director's decision as to whether or not a report should be amended, the matter is referred to the Chairman of the Appeal Board for his decision which is final.

13.4 Copies of all case reports are submitted to the Appeal Board prior to publication. Copies of the reports are sent to the ABPI Board of Management for information following publication.

13.5 Full case reports in printed form are published by the Authority on a quarterly basis.

Copies of the reports are sent to the Medicines and Healthcare products Regulatory Agency, the Office of Fair

Trading, the British Medical Association, the Royal Pharmaceutical Society of Great Britain, the Royal College of Nursing and the Editors of the BMJ, The Pharmaceutical Journal and the Nursing Standard. Copies are also available to anyone on request.

13.6 In addition to the printed reports, full case reports appear on the Authority's website. The website also carries brief details of all complaints in which a prima facie case has been established and which are currently under consideration but not yet resolved and the texts and modes of dissemination of any corrective statements that companies have been required to issue during the previous twelve months.

Access to the Authority's website is unrestricted.

13.7 Following publication of the relevant case reports, the Authority advertises in the medical and pharmaceutical press brief details of cases in which companies were ruled in breach of Clause 2 of the Code, were required to issue a corrective statement or were the subject of a public reprimand. Such advertisements also appear on the Authority's website.

GENERAL PROVISIONS

14 Time Periods for Responding to Matters under the Code

The number of working days within which companies or complainants must respond to enquiries etc, from the Prescription Medicines Code of Practice Authority, as referred to in the above procedures, are counted from the date of receipt of the notification in question.

An extension in time to respond to such notifications may be granted at the discretion of the Director.

15 Withdrawal of Complaints and Notices of Appeal

15.1 A complaint may be withdrawn by a complainant with the consent of the respondent company up until such time as the respondent company's comments on the complaint have been received by the Prescription Medicines Code of Practice Authority, but not thereafter.

15.2 Notice of appeal may be withdrawn by a complainant with the consent of the respondent company up until such time as the respondent company's comments on the reasons for the appeal have been received by the Authority, but not thereafter.

15.3 Notice of appeal may be withdrawn by a respondent company at any time but if notice is given after the papers relating to its appeal have been circulated to the Code of Practice Appeal Board, then the higher administrative charge will be payable.

16 Code of Practice Levy and Charges

16.1 An annual Code of Practice levy is paid by members of the ABPI. The levy together with the administrative charges referred to in Paragraphs 7 and 10 above and the charges for audits carried out in accordance with Paragraphs 10.4, 11.3 and 12.2 above are determined by the Board of Management of the ABPI subject to approval at a General Meeting of the ABPI by a simple majority of those present and voting.

16.2 Administrative charges are payable only by pharmaceutical companies and companies are liable for such charges whether they are members of the ABPI or not.

There are two levels of administrative charge.

The lower level is payable by a company which accepts either a ruling of the Code of Practice Panel that it was in breach of the Code or a rejection by the Panel of its allegation against another company. The lower level is also payable by a complainant company if a ruling of the Panel that there was a breach of the Code is subsequently overturned by the Code of Practice Appeal Board and by a respondent company if a ruling of the Panel that there was no breach of the Code is subsequently overturned by the Appeal Board.

The higher level is paid by a company which unsuccessfully appeals a decision of the Panel.

16.3 Where two or more companies are ruled in breach of the Code in relation to a matter involving co-promotion, each company shall be separately liable to pay any administrative charge which is payable.

16.4 The number of administrative charges which apply in a case is determined by the Director. If a company does not agree with the Director's decision, the matter is referred to the Chairman of the Appeal Board for his decision which is final.

16.5 Failure to pay any of the charges provided for by this paragraph must be reported by the Director to the Appeal Board or the Board of Management of the ABPI as appropriate.

17 Possible Breaches identified by the Code of Practice Panel or Code of Practice Appeal Board

Where the Code of Practice Panel or Code of Practice Appeal Board identifies a possible breach of the Code which has not been addressed by the complainant in a case, the Director shall treat the matter as a complaint. The company's comments are invited and the Director must then determine within two working days whether a prima facie case has been established. If a prima facie case is established the procedures under Paragraph 6.2 above onwards shall be followed.

18 Scrutiny

18.1 Samples of advertisements, detail aids, leavepieces, other promotional items and meetings are scrutinised by the Prescription Medicines Code of Practice Authority on a continuing basis in relation to the requirements of the Code.

To facilitate such scrutiny, the Director has the authority to request relevant material from pharmaceutical companies, including copies of the certificates authorizing such material, and companies must respond to such requests within ten working days.

18.2 Where a prima facie breach of the Code is identified under this procedure, the company concerned is requested to comment in writing within ten working days of receipt of the notification.

18.3 If the company accepts that there is a breach of the Code, the company is requested to provide an undertaking providing the information specified in Paragraph 7.1 above. No administrative charge shall be payable in these circumstances and there shall be no case report on the matter in question.

18.4 If the company does not accept that there is a breach of the Code and, having considered the company's comments, the Director decides that there is no prima facie case to answer under the Code, then the procedure is brought to a close. There shall be no case report on the matter in question.

18.5 If the company does not accept that there is a breach of the Code but, having considered the company's comments, the Director considers that a prima facie case has been established, the procedures under Paragraph 6.2 above onwards shall be followed.

19 Provision of Advice and Assistance with Conciliation

19.1 The Prescription Medicines Code of Practice Authority is willing and able to provide informal guidance and advice in relation to the requirements of the Code and, where appropriate, may seek the views of the Code of Practice Appeal Board.

19.2 Companies wishing to seek the assistance of a conciliator with the view to reaching agreement on inter-company differences about promotion may contact the Director for advice and assistance.

20 Amendments to the Code of Practice and Constitution and Procedure

20.1 The Code of Practice for the Pharmaceutical Industry and this Constitution and Procedure may be amended by a simple majority of those present and voting at a General Meeting of the ABPI.

20.2 The views of the Prescription Medicines Code of Practice Authority and the Code of Practice Appeal Board must be sought on any proposal to amend the Code or this Constitution and Procedure. The views of the Medicines and Healthcare products Regulatory Agency, the British Medical Association, the Royal Pharmaceutical Society of Great Britain and the Royal College of Nursing must also be invited.

20.3 The Prescription Medicines Code of Practice Authority and the Code of Practice Appeal Board may, in the light of their experience, make recommendations for amendment of the Code and this Constitution and Procedure.

21 Annual Report

An annual report of the Prescription Medicines Code of Practice Authority is published each year with the approval of the Code of Practice Appeal Board. This report includes details of the work of the Authority, the Code of Practice Panel and the Appeal Board during the year and provides a list of all companies ruled in breach of the Code during the year which specifically identifies those ruled to have breached Clause 2.

INDEX

Key
numbers refer to clauses in the Code
si refers to supplementary information to a clause in the Code
¶ followed by number refers to a paragraph in the Constitution and Procedure

DIRECTORY of PARTICIPANTS

This directory is included in the Compendium so that doctors and other healthcare professionals may obtain additional nformation about products from the participating pharmaceutical companies.

M HEALTH CARE LIMITED
M House
orley Street
oughborough
eics LE11 1EP
el: +44 (0)1509 611 611
ax: +44 (0)1509 237 288
ledical Information fax: +44 (0)1509 613 415
mail: innovation.uk@mmm.com
Vebsite: http://www.3m.com/uk

. MENARINI PHARMA U.K. S.R.L.
lenarini House
lercury Park
Vycombe Lane
Vooburn Green
uckinghamshire HP10 0HH
el: +44 (0)1628 856 400
ax: +44 (0)1628 856 402
Careline: +44 (0)1793 710 700
mail: Medinfo@menarini.com

ABBOTT LABORATORIES LIMITED
bbott House
orden Road
laidenhead
erkshire SL6 4XE
el: +44 (0)1628 773 355
ax: +44 (0)1628 644 185
Vebsite: http://www.abbottuk.com

ACTELION PHARMACEUTICALS UK
SI Building 13th Floor
89 Chiswick High Road
hiswick
ondon W4 4AL
el: +44 (0)208 987 3333
ax: +44 (0)208 987 3322
ledical Information only: +44 (0)845 075 0555
Vebsite: http://www.actelion.com

ALLEN & HANBURYS
Stockley Park West
Jxbridge
liddlesex UB11 1BT
el: +44 (0)800 221 441
ax: +44 (0)208 990 4321
mail: customercontactuk@gsk.com

ALLERGAN LTD
Coronation Road
ligh Wycombe
ucks HP12 3SH
el: +44 (0)1494 444 722
ax: +44 (0)1494 427 057
ledical Information only: +44 (0)1494 427 026
ledical Information fax: +44 (0)1494 427 057
mail: UK_MedInfo@Allergan.com
Vebsite: http://www.allergan.co.uk

ALLIANCE PHARMACEUTICALS
vonbridge House
ath Road
hippenham
Viltshire SN15 2BB
el: +44 (0)1249 466 966
ax: +44 (0)1249 466 977
mail: info@alliancepharma.co.uk
Vebsite: http://www.alliancepharma.co.uk

ALPHARMA LIMITED
Vhiddon Valley
arnstaple
lorth Devon EX32 8NS
el: +44 (0)1271 311 200
ax: +44 (0)1271 346 106
ledical Information only: +44 (0)1271 311 257
ledical Information fax: +44 (0)1271 311 329
mail: med.info@alpharma.co.uk
Vebsite: http://www.alpharma.co.uk

ALTANA PHARMA LIMITED
Three Globeside Business Park
Fieldhouse Lane
Marlow
Buckinghamshire SL7 1HZ
Tel: +44 (0)1628 646 400
Fax: +44 (0)1628 646 401
Medical Information only: +44 (0)1628 646 463
Medical Information fax: +44 (0)1628 646 534
email: medinfo@altanapharma.co.uk

AMDIPHARM
Regency House
Miles Gray Road
Basildon
Essex SS14 3AF
Tel: +44 (0)870 777 7675
Fax: +44 (0)870 777 7875
email: medinfo@amdipharm.com

ASTELLAS PHARMA LIMITED
Lovett House
Lovett Road
Staines
Middlesex TW18 3AZ
Tel: +44 (0)1784 419 615
Fax: +44 (0)1784 419 583

ASTRAZENECA UK LIMITED
Horizon Place
600 Capability Green
Luton
Bedfordshire LU1 3LU
Tel: +44 (0)1582 836 000
Fax: +44 (0)1582 838 000
Medical Information only: +44 (0)1582 836 836
Medical Information fax: +44 (0)1582 838 003
Careline: +44 (0)1582 837 837
email: medical.informationgb@astrazeneca.com

BAYER PLC
Bayer House
Strawberry Hill
Newbury
Berkshire RG14 1JA
Tel: +44 (0)1635 563 000
Fax: +44 (0)1635 563 393
Website: http://www.bayer.co.uk

BEACON PHARMACEUTICALS
85 High Street
Tunbridge Wells TN1 1YG
Tel: +44 (0)1892 600 930
Fax: +44 (0)1892 600 937
email: info@beaconpharma.co.uk
Website: http://www.beaconpharma.co.uk

BIOGEN IDEC LTD
5 Roxborough Way
Foundation Park
Maidenhead
Berks SL6 3UD
Tel: +44 (0)1628 501 000
Fax: +44 (0)1628 501 010
Medical Information only: +44 (0)8000 286 639

BOEHRINGER INGELHEIM LIMITED
Ellesfield Avenue
Bracknell
Berkshire RG12 8YS
Tel: +44 (0)1344 424 600
Fax: +44 (0)1344 741 298
Medical Information only: +44 (0)1344 741 286
email: medinfo@bra.boehringer-ingelheim.com
Website: http://www.boehringer-ingelheim.co.uk

BOEHRINGER INGELHEIM LIMITED SELF-MEDICATION DIVISION
Ellesfield Avenue
Bracknell
Berkshire RG12 8YS
Tel: +44 (0)1344 424 600
Fax: +44 (0)1344 741 399
Medical Information only: +44 (0)1344 741 286
Medical Information fax: +44 (0)1344 741 298
Careline: +44 (0)1344 741 186
email: medinfo@bra.boehringer-ingelheim.com
Website: http://www.boehringer-ingelheim.co.uk

BRISTOL-MYERS PHARMACEUTICALS
Bristol-Myers Squibb House
Uxbridge Business Park
Sanderson Road
Uxbridge
Middlesex UB8 1DH
Tel: +44 (0)1895 523 000
Fax: +44 (0)1895 523 010
Medical Information only: +44 (0)1895 523 740
Medical Information fax: +44 (0)1895 523 677
email: medical.information@bms.com

BRISTOL-MYERS SQUIBB PHARMACEUTICALS LTD
Bristol-Myers Squibb House
Uxbridge Business Park
Sanderson Road
Uxbridge
Middlesex UB8 1DH
Tel: +44 (0)1895 523 000
Fax: +44 (0)1895 523 010
Medical Information only: +44 (0)1895 523 740
Medical Information fax: +44 (0)1895 523 677
email: medical.information@bms.com

BRITANNIA PHARMACEUTICALS LIMITED
41-51 Brighton Road
Redhill
Surrey RH1 6YS
Tel: +44 (0)1737 773 741
Fax: +44 (0)1737 762 672
email: medicalservices@forumgroup.co.uk
Website: http://www.britannia-pharm.co.uk

CAMBRIDGE LABORATORIES
Deltic House
Kingfisher Way
Silverlink Business Park
Wallsend
Tyne & Wear NE28 9NX
Tel: +44 (0)191 296 9369
Fax: +44 (0)191 296 9368
Medical Information only: +44 (0)191 296 9339
Careline: +44 (0)191 296 9300
email: medicines.information@camb-labs.com

CELLTECH MANUFACTURING SERVICES LIMITED
Vale of Bardsley
Ashton-under-Lyne
Lancashire OL7 9RR
Tel: +44 (0)161 342 6000
Fax: +44 (0)161 342 6018
Medical Information only: +44 (0)1753 447 690
Medical Information fax: +44 (0)1753 447 647
Careline: +44 (0)800 953 0183
email: medicalinformationuk@ucb-group.com

CELLTECH PHARMACEUTICALS LIMITED
208 Bath Road
Slough
Berkshire SL1 3WE
Tel: +44 (0)1753 534 655
Fax: +44 (0)1753 536 632
Medical Information only: +44 (0)1753 447 690
Medical Information fax: +44 (0)1753 447 647
Careline: +44 (0)800 953 0183
email: medicalinformationuk@ucb-group.com

CEPHALON UK LIMITED
20 Alan Turing Road
Surrey Research Park
Guildford
Surrey GU2 7EH
Tel: +44 (0)1483 453 360
Fax: +44 (0)1483 453 324
Medical Information only: +44 (0)800 783 4869
email: ukmedinfo@cephalon.com

CHAUVIN PHARMACEUTICALS LTD
106 London Road
Kingston-upon-Thames
Surrey KT2 6TN
Tel: +44 (0)208 781 5500
Fax: +44 (0)208 781 5547
Medical Information only: +44 (0)1277 243 442
Medical Information fax: +44 (0)1277 243 441
Careline: +44 (0)208 781 2800

CHEMIDEX PHARMA LTD
Chemidex House
Egham Business Village
Crabtree Road
Egham
Surrey TW20 8RB
Tel: +44 (0)1784 477 167
Fax: +44 (0)1784 471 776
email: info@chemidex.co.uk
Website: http://www.chemidex.co.uk

CHIRON CORPORATION LIMTED
Symphony House
7 Cowley Business Park
High Street
Cowley
Uxbridge UB8 2AD
Tel: +44 (0)208 580 4000
Fax: +44 (0)208 580 4001
Medical Information only: +44 (0)208 580 4053
Medical Information fax: +44 (0)208 580 4095
Careline: +44 (0)208 580 4040
email: Medicalinfo-europe@chiron.com
Website: http://www.chiron.com

CHUGAI PHARMA UK LIMITED
Mulliner House
Flanders Road
Turnham Green
London W4 1NN
Tel: +44 (0)208 987 5600
Fax: +44 (0)208 987 5660

DERMAL LABORATORIES LIMITED
Tatmore Place
Gosmore
Hitchin
Herts SG4 7QR
Tel: +44 (0)1462 458 866
Fax: +44 (0)1462 420 565
Website: http://www.dermal.co.uk

DR FALK PHARMA UK LIMITED
Unit K, Bourne End Business Park
Cores End Road
Bourne End
Buckinghamshire SL8 5AS
Tel: +44 (0)1628 536 600
Fax: +44 (0)1628 536 601
Medical Information only: +44 (0)1628 536 616
Medical Information fax: +44 (0)1628 536 601
Careline: +44 (0)1628 536 600

E. C. DE WITT & COMPANY LIMITED
Tudor Road
Manor Park
Runcorn
Cheshire WA7 1SZ
Tel: +44 (0)1928 579 029
Fax: +44 (0)1928 579 712
email: meddep@ecdewitt.com
Website: http://www.ecdewitt.co.uk

E. R. SQUIBB & SONS LIMITED
Uxbridge Business Park
Sanderson Road
Uxbridge
Middlesex UB8 1DH
Tel: +44 (0)1895 523 000
Fax: +44 (0)1895 523 010
Medical Information only: +44 (0)1895 523 740
Medical Information fax: +44 (0)1895 523 677
email: medical.information@bms.com

EISAI LTD
Hammersmith International Centre
3 Shortlands
London W6 8EE
Tel: +44 (0)208 600 1400
Fax: +44 (0)208 600 1486
email: Lmedinfo@eisai.net

ELI LILLY AND COMPANY LIMITED
Lilly House
Priestley Road
Basingstoke
Hampshire RG24 9NL
Tel: +44 (0)1256 315 000
Fax: +44 (0)1256 775 858
Medical Information fax: +44 (0)1256 775 569
Careline: +44 (0)1256 315 999
Website: http://www.lilly.co.uk

EXELGYN LABORATOIRES
6 Rue Christophe Colomb
75008 Paris
France
Tel: +44 (0)1491 642 137
Fax: +44 (0)1491 642 137
Medical Information only: +44 (0)800 7316 120 Freephone
Medical Information fax: +44 (0)800 7316 120
email: exelgyn.uk@btinternet.com

FERRING PHARMACEUTICALS LTD
The Courtyard
Waterside Drive
Langley
Berkshire SL3 6EZ
Tel: +44 (0)1753 214 800
Fax: +44 (0)1753 214 802
Medical Information only: +44 (0)1753 214 845
Medical Information fax: +44 (0)1753 214 801
email: medical@ferring.com
Website: http://www.ferring.co.uk

FLYNN PHARMA LTD
Alton House
4 Herbert Street
Dublin 2
Republic of Ireland
Tel: +353 1 209 0241
Fax: +353 1 288 3310
Medical Information only: +44 (0)1462 458 974
Medical Information fax: + (0)1462 450 755
Careline: +44 (0)1773 510 123

FOREST LABORATORIES UK LIMITED
Bourne Road
Bexley
Kent DA5 1NX
Tel: +44 (0)1322 550 550
Fax: +44 (0)1322 555 469
email: medinfo@forest-labs.co.uk
Website: http://www.forestlabs.com

FOURNIER PHARMACEUTICALS LIMITED
19 – 20 Progress Business Centre
Whittle Parkway
Slough
Berkshire SL1 6DQ
Tel: +44 (0)1753 740 400
Fax: +44 (0)1753 740 444

FUJISAWA LTD
Now use Astellas Pharma Limited contact details

GALDERMA (U.K.) LTD
Galderma House
Church Lane
Kings Langley
Hertfordshire WD4 8JP
Tel: +44 (0)1923 291 033
Fax: +44 (0)1923 291 060

GALEN LIMITED
Seagoe Industrial Estate
Craigavon
Co Armagh
Ireland BT63 5UA
Tel: +44 (0)28 3833 4974
Fax: +44 (0)28 3835 0206
email: customer.services@galen.co.uk
Website: http://www.galen.co.uk

GENUS PHARMACEUTICALS
Benham Valence
Newbury
Berkshire RG20 8LU
Tel: +44 (0)1635 568 400
Fax: +44 (0)1635 568 401
Medical Information only: +44 (0)1793 710 700
Medical Information fax: +44 (0)1793 710 387
Careline: +44 (0)1635 568 445
email: genus@medinformation.co.uk

GILEAD SCIENCES INTERNATIONAL LIMITED
Granta Park
Abington
Cambridge CB1 6GT
Tel: +44 (0)1223 897 300
Fax: +44 (0)1223 897 282
Medical Information only: +44 (0)1223 897 555
Medical Information fax: +44 (0)1223 897 281
Careline: +44 (0)1223 897 355
email: ukmedinfo@gilead.com

GLAXOSMITHKLINE UK
Stockley Park West
Uxbridge
Middlesex UB11 1BT
Tel: +44 (0)800 221 441
Fax: +44 (0)208 990 4321
email: customercontactuk@gsk.com

GLENWOOD LABORATORIES LTD
Jenkins Dale
Chatham
Kent ME4 5RD
Tel: +44 (0)1634 830 535
Fax: +44 (0)1634 831 345

HK PHARMA LIMITED
PO Box 105
HITCHIN
Herts SG5 2GG
Tel: +44 (0)1462 433 993
Fax: +44 (0)1462 450 755

INTERNATIONAL MEDICATION SYSTEMS (UK) LTD
208 Bath Road
Slough
Berkshire SL1 3WE
Tel: +44 (0)1753 534 655
Fax: +44 (0)1753 536 632
Medical Information only: +44 (0)1753 447 690
Medical Information fax: +44 (0)1753 447 647
Careline: +44 (0)800 953 0183
email: medicalinformationuk@ucb-group.com
Website: http://www.celltechgroup.com

INTRAPHARM LABORATORIES LTD
60 Boughton Lane
Maidstone
Kent ME15 9QS
Tel: +44 (0)1622 749 222
Medical Information fax: +44 (0)1622 743 816
email: sales@intrapharmlabs.com

IPSEN LTD
190 Bath Road
Slough
Berkshire SL1 3XE
Tel: +44 (0)1753 627 700
Fax: +44 (0)1753 627 701
email: medical.information.uk@ipsen.com

JANSSEN-CILAG LTD
Saunderton
High Wycombe
Bucks HP14 4HJ
Tel: +44 (0)1494 567 567
Fax: +44 (0)1494 567 568
Medical Information only: +44 (0)800 731 8450
Careline: +44 (0)800 731 5550
email: medinfo@janssen-cilag.co.uk

KING PHARMACEUTICALS LTD
Donegal Street
Ballybofey
County Donegal
Tel: +353 1 209 0246
Fax: +353 1 209 0246
Medical Information only: +44 (0)1462 434 366
Medical Information fax: +44 (0)1462 450 755

KYOWA HAKKO UK LTD
258 Bath Road
Slough
Berkshire SL1 4DX
Tel: +44 (0)1753 566 020
Fax: +44 (0)1753 566 030
Medical Information fax: +44 (0)1753 566 030
email: medinfo@kyowa-uk.co.uk

LABORATOIRE HRA PHARMA
15, rue Beranger
75003 Paris
France
Tel: +33 1 40 33 11 30
Fax: +33 1 40 33 12 31
email: product-support@hra-pharma.com
Website: http://www.hra-pharma.com

LABORATORIES FOR APPLIED BIOLOGY LIMITED
91 Amhurst Park
London N16 5DR
Tel: +44 (0)208 800 2252
Fax: +44 (0)208 809 6884
email: enquiries@cerumol.co.uk

LEO LABORATORIES LIMITED
Longwick Road
Princes Risborough
Bucks HP27 9RR
Tel: +44 (0)1844 347 333
Fax: +44 (0)1844 342 278
email: medical-info.uk@leo-pharma.com

LINK PHARMACEUTICALS LTD
Bishops Weald House
Albion Way
Horsham
West Sussex RH12 1AH
Tel: +44 (0)1403 272 451
Fax: +44 (0)1403 272 455
email: medical.information@linkpharm.co.uk
Website: http://www.linkpharm.co.uk

LUNDBECK LIMITED
Lundbeck House
Caldecotte Lake Business Park
Caldecotte
Milton Keynes MK7 8LF
Tel: +44 (0)1908 649 966
Fax: +44 (0)1908 647 888
Careline: +44 (0)1908 638 935
email: ukmedicalinformation@lundbeck.com
Website: http://www.lundbeck.co.uk

MASTA LTD
Moorfield Road
Yeadon
Leeds LS19 7BN
Tel: +44 (0)113 2387 500
Fax: +44 (0)113 2387 501
Medical Information only: +44 (0)113 2387 500 (option 3)
Careline: +44 (0)113 2387 500 (option 1)
email: medical@masta.org
Website: http://www.masta.org

MEDA PHARMACEUTICALS
Regus House
Herald Way
Pegasus Business Park
Castle Donington
Derbyshire DE74 2TZ
Tel: +44 (0)1332 638 033
Fax: +44 (0)1332 638 192
Medical Information only: +44 (0)1748 828 810
Medical Information fax: +44 (0)1748 828 801
email: meda@professionalinformation.co.uk

MEDAC GMBH
Fehlandtstrasse 3
20354 Hamburg
Germany
Tel: +44 (0)141 332 8464
Fax: +44 (0)141 332 8619
email: info@medac-uk.co.uk

MEDLOCK MEDICAL LTD
Tubiton House
Medlock Street
Oldham
Greater Manchester OL1 3HS
Tel: +44 (0)161 621 2100
Fax: +44 (0)161 621 0932
Medical Information only: +44 (0)161 621 2121
Medical Information fax: +44 (0)161 621 2126
Careline: +44 (0)161 621 2020
email: medical.information@medlockmedical.com
Website: http://www.medlockmedical.com

MERCK PHARMACEUTICALS
Harrier House
High Street
West Drayton
Middlesex UB7 7QG
Tel: +44 (0)1895 452 200
Fax: +44 (0)1895 420 605
Medical Information only: +44 (0)1895 452 307
Medical Information fax: +44 (0)1895 452 286
email: medinfo@merckpharma.co.uk
Website: http://www.merckpharma.co.uk

MERCK SHARP & DOHME LIMITED
Hertford Road
Hoddesdon
Hertfordshire EN11 9BU
Tel: +44 (0)1992 467 272
Fax: +44 (0)1992 451 066

MSD-SP LTD
Hertford Road
Hoddesdon
Hertfordshire EN11 9BU
Tel: +44 (0)1992 467 272
Fax: +44 (0)1992 451 066
Medical Information fax: +44 (0)1707 363 763

NAPP PHARMACEUTICALS LIMITED
Cambridge Science Park
Milton Road
Cambridge
Cambridgeshire CB4 0GW
Tel: +44 (0)1223 424 444
Fax: +44 (0)1223 424 441
Medical Information fax: +44 (0)1223 424 912
Website: http://www.napp.co.uk

NORGINE LIMITED
Chaplin House
Widewater Place
Moorhall Road
Harefield
Middlesex UB9 6NS
Tel: +44 (0)1895 826 600
Fax: +44 (0)1895 825 865
email: medinfo@norgine.com

NOVARTIS CONSUMER HEALTH
Wimblehurst Road
Horsham
West Sussex RH32 5AB
Tel: +44 (0)1403 210 211
Fax: +44 (0)1403 323 939
Medical Information only: +44 (0)1403 323 046
Careline: +44 (0)1403 218 211
email: medical.affairs.uk@novartis.com

NOVARTIS PHARMACEUTICALS UK LTD
Frimley Business Park
Frimley
Camberley
Surrey GU16 7SR
Tel: +44 (0)1276 692 255
Fax: +44 (0)1276 698 449
Medical Information only: +44 (0)1276 698 370
Careline: +44 (0)845 741 9442
email: medicalinfo.phgbfr@pharma.novartis.com

NOVO NORDISK LIMITED
Broadfield Park
Brighton Road
Crawley
West Sussex RH11 9RT
Tel: +44 (0)1293 613 555
Fax: +44 (0)1293 613 535
Medical Information only: +44 (0)845 600 5055
Medical Information fax: +44 (0)1293 613 211
Careline: +44 (0)845 600 5055
email: ukmedicalinfo@novonordisk.com

ORGANON LABORATORIES LIMITED
Cambridge Science Park
Milton Road
Cambridge
Cambridgeshire CB4 0FL
Tel: +44 (0)1223 432 700
Fax: +44 (0)1223 424 368
Medical Information only: +44 (0)1223 432 756
Medical Information fax: +44 (0)1223 432 733
email: medrequest@organon.co.uk
Website: http://www.organon.co.uk

ORION PHARMA (UK) LIMITED
Leat House
Overbridge Square
Hambridge Lane
Newbury
Berkshire RG14 5UX
Tel: +44 (0)1635 520 300
Fax: +44 (0)1635 349 94
email: medicalinformation@orionpharma.com

OTSUKA PHARMACEUTICALS (UK) LTD
BSi Tower
389 Chiswich High Road
Chiswick
London W4 4AJ
Tel: +44 (0)208 742 4300
Fax: +44 (0)208 994 8548
email: medinfo@otsuka-europe.com
Website: http://www.otsuka-europe.com

PAINES & BYRNE LIMITED
Lovett House
Lovett Road
Staines
Middlesex TW18 3AZ
Tel: +44 (0)1784 419 615
Fax: +44 (0)1784 419 583

PARKE DAVIS
Ramsgate Road
Sandwich
Kent CT13 9NJ
Tel: +44 (0)1304 616161
Fax: +44 (0)1304 656 221
Medical Information only: +44 (0)1737 331 111

PFIZER CONSUMER HEALTHCARE
Walton Oaks
Dorking Road
Walton-on-the-Hill
Surrey KT20 7NS
Tel: +44 (0)1304 616 161
Fax: +44 (0)1304 656 221
Careline: +44 (0)1737 331 186
email: medinfo.ch@pfizer.com

PFIZER LIMITED
Ramsgate Road
Sandwich
Kent CT13 9NJ
Tel: +44 (0)1304 616 161
Fax: +44 (0)1304 656 221
Medical Information only: +44 (0)1737 331 111

PHARMACIA LIMITED
Ramsgate Road
Sandwich
Kent CT13 9NJ
Tel: +44 (0)1304 616 161
Fax: +44 (0)1304 656 221
Medical Information only: +44 (0)1737 331 111

PHARMACIA LTD - (CONSUMER PRODUCTS)
Pfizer Limited
Walton Oaks
Dorking Road
Walton-on-the-Hill
Surrey KT20 7NT
Tel: +44 (0)1304 616 161
Fax: +44 (0)1304 656 221
Careline: +44 (0)1737 331 186
email: medinfo.ch@pfizer.com

PIERRE FABRE LIMITED
Hyde Abbey House
23 Hyde Street
Winchester
Hampshire SO23 7DR
Tel: +44 (0)1962 856 956
Fax: +44 (0)1962 844 014
Medical Information only: +44 (0)1962 874 435
Medical Information fax: +44 (0)1962 874 413
Careline: +44 (0)1962 874 402
email: medicalinformation@pierre-fabre.co.uk

PLIVA PHARMA LTD
Vision House
Bedford Road
Petersfield
Hampshire GU32 3QB
Tel: +44 (0)1730 710 900
Fax: +44 (0)1730 710 901
Medical Information only: +44 (0)1730 710 944
Careline: +44 (0)1730 710 910
email: medinfo@pliva-pharma.co.uk

PROCTER & GAMBLE PHARMACEUTICALS UK LIMITED
Rusham Park Technical Centre
Whitehall Lane
Egham
Surrey TW20 9NW
Tel: +44 (0)1784 474 900
Fax: +44 (0)1784 474 705

PROFILE PHARMA LIMITED
Heath Place
Bognor Regis
West Sussex PO22 9SL
Tel: +44 (0)870 770 2025
Fax: +44 (0)870 770 2224
email: info@profilepharma.com
Website: http://www.profilepharma.com

PROVALIS HEALTHCARE
Newtech Square
Deeside Industrial Park
Deeside
Flintshire CH5 2NT
Tel: +44 (0)1244 288 888
Fax: +44 (0)1244 280 342
Medical Information only: +44 (0)1244 833 518

RECKITT BENCKISER HEALTHCARE (UK) LTD
Dansom Lane
Hull HU7 8DS
Tel: +44 (0)1482 326 151
Fax: +44 (0)1482 582 532
Medical Information only: +44 (0)1482 582 070
Medical Information fax: +44 (0)1482 582 526
Careline: +44 (0)500 455 456
email: MIU@reckittbenckiser.com
Website: http://www.reckittbenckiser.com

ROCHE PRODUCTS LIMITED
Hexagon Place
6 Falcon Way
Shire Park
Welwyn Garden City
Hertfordshire AL7 1TW
Tel: +44 (0)1707 366 000
Fax: +44 (0)1707 338 297
Medical Information only: +44 (0)800 328 1629
Medical Information fax: +44 (0)1707 384 555
Careline: +44 (0)800 731 5711
email: medinfo.uk@roche.com
Website: http://www.rocheuk.com

ROSEMONT PHARMACEUTICALS LIMITED
Rosemont House
Yorkdale Industrial Park
Braithwaite Street
Leeds
Yorkshire LS11 9XE
Tel: +44 (0)113 244 1400
Fax: +44 (0)113 246 0738
Careline: +44 (0)800 919 312
Website: http://www.rosemontpharma.com

SANKYO PHARMA UK LIMITED
Sankyo House
Repton Place
White Lion Road
Little Chalfont
Amersham
Bucks HP7 9LP
Tel: +44 (0)1494 766 866
Medical Information only: +44 (0)1494 766 866
Medical Information fax: +44 (0)1494 766 557
Careline: +44 (0)800 0687 616
email: medinfo@sankyo.co.uk

SANOFI-AVENTIS
1 Onslow Street
Guildford
Surrey GU1 4YS
Tel: +44 (0)1483 505 515
Fax: +44 (0)1483 535 432
email: uk-medicalinformation@sanofi-aventis.com

SANOFI-AVENTIS BRISTOL MYERS SQUIBB

One Onslow Street Guildford Surrey GU1 4YS	Bristol Myers Squibb House Uxbridge Business Park, Sanderson Road, Uxbridge, Middlesex UB8 1DH
Tel: +44 (0)1483 505 515 - Plavix Fax: +44 (0)1483 535 432 email: uk-medicalinformation@sanofi-aventis.com	Tel: +44 (0)800 731 1736 - Aprovel & Co-Aprovel Fax: +44 (0)1895 52 3677 email: medical.information@bms.com

SANOFI PASTEUR MSD
Mallards Reach
Bridge Avenue
Maidenhead
Berkshire SL6 1QP
Tel: +44 (0)1628 785 291
Fax: +44 (0)1628 671 722
Careline: +44 (0)1628 773 737

SCHERING HEALTH CARE LIMITED
The Brow
Burgess Hill
West Sussex RH15 9NE
Tel: +44 (0)1444 232 323
Fax: +44 (0)1444 246 613
Medical Information fax: +44 (0)1444 465 878
Careline: +44 (0)845 609 6767
email: customer.care@schering.co.uk
Website: http://www.schering.co.uk

SCHERING-PLOUGH LTD
Schering-Plough House
Shire Park
Welwyn Garden City
Herts AL7 1TW
Tel: +44 (0)1707 363 636
Medical Information fax: +44 (0)1707 363 763
email: medical.info@spcorp.com

SCHWARZ PHARMA LIMITED
Schwarz House
East Street
Chesham
Bucks HP5 1DG
Tel: +44 (0)1494 797 500
Fax: +44 (0)1494 773 934

SERONO LTD
Bedfont Cross
Stanwell Road
Feltham
Middlesex TW14 8NX
Tel: +44 (0)208 818 7200
Fax: +44 (0)208 818 7222
Medical Information only: +44 (0)208 818 7373

SERVIER LABORATORIES LIMITED
Gallions
Wexham Springs
Framewood Road
Wexham
Slough
Berkshire SL3 6RJ
Tel: +44 (0)1753 662 744
Fax: +44 (0)1753 663 456

SHIRE PHARMACEUTICALS LIMITED
Hampshire International Business Park
Chineham
Basingstoke
Hampshire RG24 8EP
Tel: +44 (0)1256 894 000
Medical Information only: +44 (0)1256 894 894
Medical Information fax: +44 (0)1256 894 714
Careline: +44 (0)1256 894 107
email: medinfo@uk.shire.com
Website: http://www.shire.com

SOLVAY HEALTHCARE LIMITED
Mansbridge Road
West End
Southampton SO18 3JD
Tel: +44 (0)2380 467 000
Fax: +44 (0)2380 465 350
Medical Information fax: +44 (0)2380 465 350
Careline: +44 (0)1753 650 099
email: medinfo.shl@solvay.com

SOVEREIGN MEDICAL
Sovereign House
Miles Gray Road
Basildon
Essex SS14 3FR
Tel: +44 (0)1268 535 200
Fax: +44 (0)1268 535 299
Medical Information only: +44 (0)1268 823 049
Medical Information fax: +44(0)1268 535 287
email: medinfo@amdipharm.com

SSL INTERNATIONAL PLC
Venus
1 Old Park Lane
Trafford Park
Urmston
Manchester M41 7HA
UK
Tel: +44 (0)8701 222 690
Fax: +44 (0)8701 222 696
Medical Information only: +44 (0)161 638 2027
Medical Information fax: +44 (0)161 615 8819
Careline: +44 (0)161 638 2399
email: medical.information@ssl-international.com
Website: http://www.ssl-international.com

STD PHARMACEUTICAL PRODUCTS LTD
Plough Lane
Hereford
Herefordshire HR4 0EL
Tel: +44 (0)1432 373 555
Fax: +44 (0)1432 373 556
Website: http://www.stdpharm.co.uk

STIEFEL LABORATORIES (UK) LIMITED
Holtspur Lane
Wooburn Green
High Wycombe
Buckinghamshire HP10 0AU
Tel: +44 (0)1628 524 966
Fax: +44 (0)1628 810 021

STRAKAN PHARMACEUTICALS LTD
Buckholm Mill
Buckholm Mill Brae
Galashiels TD1 2HB
Tel: +44 (0)1896 668 060
Fax: +44 (0)1896 668 061
email: medinfo@strakan.com
Website: http://www.Strakan.com

TAKEDA UK LTD
Takeda House
Mercury Park
Wycombe Lane
Wooburn Green
High Wycombe
Buckinghamshire HP10 0HH
Tel: +44 (0)1628 537 900
Fax: +44 (0)1628 526 617
Medical Information only: +44 (0)1628 537 900
Medical Information fax: +44 (0)1628 526 617
Website: http://www.Takeda.co.uk

UCB PHARMA LIMITED
208 Bath Road
Slough
Berkshire SL1 3WE
Tel: +44 (0)1753 534 655
Fax: +44 (0)1753 536 632
Medical Information only: +44 (0)1923 475 503
Careline: +44 (0)1923 471 010
email: medicalinformationuk@ucb-group.com

VALEANT PHARMACEUTICALS LTD
Cedarwood
Chineham Business Park
Crockford Lane
Basingstoke
Hampshire RG24 8WD
Tel: +44 (0)1256 707 744
Fax: +44 (0)1256 707 334
Medical Information only: +44 (0)1256 374 646
email: ukmedical@valeant.com
Website: http://www.valeant.com

VIATRIS PHARMACEUTICALS LTD
Building 2000
Beach Drive
Cambridge Research Park
Waterbeach
Cambridge CB5 9PD
Tel: +44 (0)1223 205 999
Fax: +44 (0)1223 205 998
Medical Information only: +44 (0)1223 205 991
email: lorraine.stephens@viatrisuk.co.uk

WOCKHARDT UK LTD
Ash Road North
Wrexham Industrial Estate
Wrexham LL13 9UF
Tel: +44 (0)1978 661 261
Fax: +44 (0)1978 660 130

WYETH CONSUMER HEALTHCARE
Huntercombe Lane South
Taplow
Maidenhead
Berks SL6 0PH
Tel: +44 (0)1628 669 011
Fax: +44 (0)1628 669 846
Medical Information only: +44 (0)845 111 0151 (Care Line)
Medical Information fax: +44 (0)1628 414 870
email: carelineUK@wyeth.com
Website: http://www.wyethconsumerhealthcare.co.uk

WYETH PHARMACEUTICALS
Huntercombe Lane South
Taplow
Maidenhead
Berks SL6 0PH
Tel: +44 (0)1628 604 377
Fax: +44 (0)1628 666 368
Medical Information only: +44 (0)1628 415 330
email: ukmedinfo@wyeth.com

YAMANOUCHI PHARMA LTD
Now use Astellas Pharma Limited contact details

ZENEUS PHARMA LTD
Abel Smith House
Gunnels Wood Road
Stevenage
Hertfordshire SG1 2BT
Tel: +44 (0)1438 731 731
Fax: +44 (0)1438 765 008
Medical Information only: +44 (0)1438 765 100
Medical Information fax: +44 (0)1438 765 008
Website: http://www.zeneuspharma.com

ZLB BEHRING UK LIMITED
Hayworth House,
Market Place
Haywards Heath
West Sussex RH16 1DB
Tel: +44 (0)1444 447 400
Fax: +44 (0)1444 447 401
Medical Information only: +44 (0)1444 447 405
Careline: +44 (0)1444 447 402
email: medinfo@zlbbehring.com

INDEX by COMPANY

Astellas Pharma Limited

AstraZeneca UK Limited

Bayer plc

Beacon Pharmaceuticals

Biogen Idec Ltd

Boehringer Ingelheim Limited

Glenwood Laboratories Ltd

HK Pharma Limited

International Medication Systems (UK) Ltd

Intrapharm Laboratories Ltd

Ipsen Ltd

Janssen-Cilag Ltd

Norgine Limited

Novartis Consumer Health

Novartis Pharmaceuticals UK Ltd

Novo Nordisk Limited

Organon Laboratories Limited

Orion Pharma (UK) Limited

Otsuka Pharmaceuticals (UK) Ltd

Paines & Byrne Limited

Parke Davis

Pfizer Consumer Healthcare

Pfizer Limited

Pharmacia Limited

Pharmacia Ltd - (Consumer Products)

Pierre Fabre Limited

Pliva Pharma Ltd

Procter & Gamble Pharmaceuticals UK Limited

Profile Pharma Limited

Provalis Healthcare

Reckitt Benckiser Healthcare (UK) Ltd

Roche Products Limited

Rosemont Pharmaceuticals Limited

Sankyo Pharma UK Limited

Sanofi Pasteur MSD

Sanofi Pharma Bristol-Myers Squibb SNC

sanofi-aventis

Schering Health Care Limited

Schering-Plough Ltd

SCHWARZ PHARMA Limited

Serono Ltd

Servier Laboratories Limited

Shire Pharmaceuticals Limited

Solvay Healthcare Limited

Sovereign Medical

SSL International plc

STD Pharmaceutical Products Ltd

Stiefel Laboratories (UK) Limited

Strakan Pharmaceuticals Ltd

Takeda UK Ltd

UCB Pharma Limited

Valeant Pharmaceuticals Ltd

Viatris Pharmaceuticals Ltd

Wockhardt UK Ltd

Wyeth Consumer Healthcare

Wyeth Pharmaceuticals

Zeneus Pharma Ltd

ZLB Behring UK Limited

INDEX by PRODUCT

Proprietary names are in ordinary type, generic names in *italics*. It should be noted that although different products may contain the same active ingredients this does not imply that they are equivalent in regard to bio-availability or therapeutic activity.

UK REGIONAL MEDICINES INFORMATION UNITS

The Medicines Information (MI) service in the United Kingdom is provided on a national basis by specialist pharmacists, the majority of whom are based within hospital trusts located across the UK. Their work is supported by regional MI centres which provide additional resources and support to local centres.

For details of your nearest regional centre, please see below:

England

East Anglia

East Anglian Medicines Information Service
Ipswich Hospital NHS Trust
Heath Road
Ipswich
Suffolk
IP4 5PD

Tel:	01473 704 430
	01473 704 431
Fax:	01473 704 433
eMail:	mike.brandon@dial.pipex.com

London – Northwick Park

Medicines Information
Pharmacy Department
Northwick Park Hospital
Watford Road
Harrow
Middlesex
HA1 3UJ

Tel:	0208 869 3973
	0208 869 2763
Fax:	0208 869 2764
eMail:	med.info@nwlh.nhs.uk

London and South East

Pharmacy Department
Guy's Hospital
St Thomas' Street
London
SE1 9RT

Tel:	0207 378 0023
	0207 188 3849/0207 188 3855
Fax:	0207 188 3857
eMail:	medicines.information@gstt.nhs.uk

North West

North West Medicines Information Centre
Pharmacy Practice Unit
70 Pembroke Place
Liverpool
L69 3GF

Tel:	0151 794 8117
Fax:	0151 794 8118
eMail:	druginfo@liv.ac.uk

Northern & Yorkshire (Leeds)
Pharmacy Department
Leeds General Infirmary
Great George Street
Leeds
LS1 3EX

Tel:	0113 392 5076
	0113 392 3547
Fax:	0113 244 5849
eMail:	medicines.information@leedsth.nhs.uk

Northern & Yorkshire (Newcastle)
Wolfson Unit
Regional Drug & Therapeutics Centre
24 Claremont Place
Newcastle upon Tyne
NE2 4HH

Tel:	0191 232 1525
Fax:	0191 260 6192
eMail:	nydrtc.di@ncl.ac.uk

South West
South West Medicines Information & Training
Bristol Royal Infirmary
Marlborough Street
Bristol
BS2 8HW

Tel:	0117 928 2867
Fax:	0117 928 3818
eMail:	swmi@ubht.swest.nhs.uk

Trent
Trent Medicines Information Service
Leicester Royal Infirmary
Leicester
LE1 5WW

Tel:	0116 255 5779
	0116 258 6491
Fax:	0116 258 5680
eMail:	medicines.info@uhl-tr.nhs.uk

Wessex
Wessex Drug & Medicines Information Centre
Mailpoint 31
Southampton General Hospital
Tremona Road
Southampton
SO16 6YD

Tel:	023 8079 6908
	023 8079 6909
Fax:	023 8079 4467
eMail:	medicinesinformation@suht.swest.nhs.uk

West Midlands
West Midlands Medicines Information Service
Good Hope Hospital NHS Trust
Sutton Coldfield
B75 7RR

Tel:	0121 311 1974
	0121 378 2211 Ext: 2296/2297
Fax:	0121 378 1594
eMail:	druginfo@goodhope.nhs.uk

Northern Ireland

Belfast

Regional Medicines & Poisons Information Service
The Royal Hospitals
Grosvenor Road
Belfast
BT12 6BA

Tel:	028 90 632 032
	028 90 633 847
Fax:	028 90 248 030
eMail:	eilish.smith@royalhospitals.n-i.nhs.uk

Scotland

Aberdeen

Aberdeen Royal Infirmary
Pharmacy Department
Foresterhill Site
Aberdeen
AB25 2ZN

Tel:	01224 552 316
Fax:	01224 553 371
eMail:	druginfo@arh.grampian.scot.nhs.uk

Dundee

Ninewells Hospital & Medical School
Pharmacy Department
Dundee
DD1 9SY

Tel:	01382 632 351
Fax:	01382 632 599
eMail:	medinfo@tuth.scot.nhs.uk

Edinburgh

Royal Infirmary of Edinburgh
NHS Lothian – University Hospitals Division
51 Little France Crescent
Old Dalkeith Road
Edinburgh
EH16 4SA

Tel:	0131 242 2920
	0131 536 1000 Ext: 22920
Fax:	0131 242 2925

Glasgow

Glasgow Royal Infirmary
Pharmacy Department
84 Castle Street
Glasgow
G4 0SF

Tel:	0141 211 4407
Fax:	0141 552 8170
eMail:	med.info@northglasgow.scot.nhs.uk

Wales

Cardiff

Welsh Medicines Information Centre
University Hospital of Wales
Heath Park
Cardiff
CF14 4XW

Tel:	02920 742 979
	02920 743 877
Fax:	02920 743 879
eMail:	fiona.woods@cardiffandvale.wales.nhs.uk

In Confidence

COMMITTEE ON SAFETY OF MEDICINES

MHRA
Medicines and Healthcare products Regulatory Agency
Safeguarding public health

SUSPECTED ADVERSE DRUG REACTIONS

If you are suspicious that an adverse reaction may be related to a drug or combination of drugs please complete this Yellow Card.

For reporting advice please see over. Do not be put off reporting because some details are not known.

PATIENT DETAILS Patient Initials: ________ Sex: M / F Weight if known (kg): ________

Age (at time of reaction): ________ Identification (Your Practice / Hospital Ref.)*: ________

SUSPECTED DRUG(S)

Give brand name of drug and batch number if known	Route	Dosage	Date started	Date stopped	Prescribed for

SUSPECTED REACTION(S)

Please describe the reaction(s) and any treatment given:

Outcome
Recovered ☐
Recovering ☐
Continuing ☐
Other ☐

Date reaction(s) started: ________ Date reaction (s) stopped: ________

Do you consider the reaction to be serious? Yes / No

If *yes*, please indicate why the reaction is considered to be serious (please tick all that apply):

Patient died due to reaction ☐ Involved or prolonged inpatient hospitalisation ☐

Life threatening ☐ Involved persistent or significant disability or incapacity ☐

Congenital abnormality ☐ Medically significant; please give details: ________

* This is to enable you to identify the patient in any future correspondence concerning this report

Please attach additional pages if necessary

In Confidence

COMMITTEE ON SAFETY OF MEDICINES

MHRA
Medicines and Healthcare products Regulatory Agency
Safeguarding public health

SUSPECTED ADVERSE DRUG REACTIONS

If you are suspicious that an adverse reaction may be related to a drug or combination of drugs please complete this Yellow Card.

For reporting advice please see over. Do not be put off reporting because some details are not known.

PATIENT DETAILS Patient Initials: ________ Sex: M / F Weight if known (kg): ________

Age (at time of reaction): ________ Identification (Your Practice / Hospital Ref.)*: ________

SUSPECTED DRUG(S)

Give brand name of drug and batch number if known | Route | Dosage | Date started | Date stopped | Prescribed for

SUSPECTED REACTION(S)

Please describe the reaction(s) and any treatment given:

Outcome
Recovered ☐
Recovering ☐
Continuing ☐
Other ☐

Date reaction(s) started: ________ Date reaction (s) stopped: ________

Do you consider the reaction to be serious? Yes / No

If yes, please indicate why the reaction is considered to be serious (please tick all that apply):

Patient died due to reaction ☐ Involved or prolonged inpatient hospitalisation ☐

Life threatening ☐ Involved persistent or significant disability or incapacity ☐

Congenital abnormality ☐ Medically significant; please give details: ________

* This is to enable you to identify the patient in any future correspondence concerning this report

Please attach additional pages if necessary

OTHER DRUGS (including self-medication & herbal remedies)

Did the patient take any other drugs in the last 3 months prior to the reaction? Yes / No

If *yes*, please give the following information if known:

Drug (Brand, if known)	Route	Dosage	Date started	Date stopped	Prescribed for

Additional relevant information e.g. medical history, test results, known allergies, rechallenge (if performed), suspected drug interactions. For congenital abnormalities please state all other drugs taken during pregnancy and the date of the last menstrual period.

REPORTER DETAILS

Name and Professional Address:

Post code: Tel No:

Speciality:

Signature: Date:

CLINICIAN (if not the reporter)

Name and Professional Address:

Post code:

Tel No: Speciality:

If you would like information about other adverse reactions associated with the suspected drug, please tick this box ☐

Send to **MHRA (medicines) , CSM FREEPOST, London, SW8 5BR** or if you are in one of the following NHS regions:

to **CSM Mersey, FREEPOST, Liverpool, L3 3AB**

or **CSM Wales, FREEPOST, Cardiff, CF4 1ZZ**

or **CSM Northern and Yorkshire, FREEPOST, Newcastle upon Tyne, NE1 1BR**

or **CSM West Midlands, FREEPOST, Birmingham, B18 7BR**

CSM Scotland, 51 Little France Crescent, Old Dalkeith Road, Edinburgh, EH16 4SA

OTHER DRUGS (including self-medication & herbal remedies)

Did the patient take any other drugs in the last 3 months prior to the reaction? Yes / No

If *yes*, please give the following information if known:

Drug (Brand, if known)	Route	Dosage	Date started	Date stopped	Prescribed for

Additional relevant information e.g. medical history, test results, known allergies, rechallenge (if performed), suspected drug interactions. For congenital abnormalities please state all other drugs taken during pregnancy and the date of the last menstrual period.

REPORTER DETAILS

Name and Professional Address:

Post code: Tel No:

Speciality:

Signature: Date:

CLINICIAN (if not the reporter)

Name and Professional Address:

Post code:

Tel No: Speciality:

If you would like information about other adverse reactions associated with the suspected drug, please tick this box ☐

Send to **MHRA (medicines) , CSM FREEPOST, London, SW8 5BR** or if you are in one of the following NHS regions:

to **CSM Mersey, FREEPOST, Liverpool, L3 3AB**

or **CSM Wales, FREEPOST, Cardiff, CF4 1ZZ**

or **CSM Northern and Yorkshire, FREEPOST, Newcastle upon Tyne, NE1 1BR**

or **CSM West Midlands, FREEPOST, Birmingham, B18 7BR**

CSM Scotland, 51 Little France Crescent, Old Dalkeith Road, Edinburgh, EH16 4SA

In Confidence

COMMITTEE ON SAFETY OF MEDICINES

MHRA
Medicines and Healthcare products Regulatory Agency
Safeguarding public health

SUSPECTED ADVERSE DRUG REACTIONS

If you are suspicious that an adverse reaction may be related to a drug or combination of drugs please complete this Yellow Card.

For reporting advice please see over. Do not be put off reporting because some details are not known.

PATIENT DETAILS Patient Initials: ________ Sex: M / F Weight if known (kg): ________

Age (at time of reaction): ________ Identification (Your Practice / Hospital Ref.)*: ________

SUSPECTED DRUG(S)

Give brand name of drug and batch number if known	Route	Dosage	Date started	Date stopped	Prescribed for

SUSPECTED REACTION(S)

Please describe the reaction(s) and any treatment given:

Outcome

Recovered ☐
Recovering ☐
Continuing ☐
Other ☐

Date reaction(s) started: ________ Date reaction (s) stopped: ________

Do you consider the reaction to be serious? Yes / No

If *yes*, please indicate why the reaction is considered to be serious (please tick all that apply):

Patient died due to reaction ☐ Involved or prolonged inpatient hospitalisation ☐

Life threatening ☐ Involved persistent or significant disability or incapacity ☐

Congenital abnormality ☐ Medically significant; please give details: ________

* This is to enable you to identify the patient in any future correspondence concerning this report

Please attach additional pages if necessary

In Confidence

COMMITTEE ON SAFETY OF MEDICINES

MHRA
Medicines and Healthcare products Regulatory Agency
Safeguarding public health

SUSPECTED ADVERSE DRUG REACTIONS

If you are suspicious that an adverse reaction may be related to a drug or combination of drugs please complete this Yellow Card.

For reporting advice please see over. Do not be put off reporting because some details are not known.

PATIENT DETAILS Patient Initials: ________ Sex: M / F Weight if known (kg): ________

Age (at time of reaction): ________ Identification (Your Practice / Hospital Ref.)*: ________

SUSPECTED DRUG(S)

Give brand name of drug and batch number if known	Route	Dosage	Date started	Date stopped	Prescribed for

SUSPECTED REACTION(S)

Please describe the reaction(s) and any treatment given:

Outcome

Recovered ☐
Recovering ☐
Continuing ☐
Other ☐

Date reaction(s) started: ________ Date reaction (s) stopped: ________

Do you consider the reaction to be serious? Yes / No

If *yes*, please indicate why the reaction is considered to be serious (please tick all that apply):

Patient died due to reaction ☐ Involved or prolonged inpatient hospitalisation ☐

Life threatening ☐ Involved persistent or significant disability or incapacity ☐

Congenital abnormality ☐ Medically significant; please give details: ________

* This is to enable you to identify the patient in any future correspondence concerning this report

Please attach additional pages if necessary

OTHER DRUGS (including self-medication & herbal remedies)

Did the patient take any other drugs in the last 3 months prior to the reaction? Yes / No

If *yes*, please give the following information if known:

Drug (Brand, if known)	Route	Dosage	Date started	Date stopped	Prescribed for

Additional relevant information e.g. medical history, test results, known allergies, rechallenge (if performed), suspected drug interactions. For congenital abnormalities please state all other drugs taken during pregnancy and the date of the last menstrual period.

REPORTER DETAILS

Name and Professional Address: ______________________

Post code: ____________ Tel No: ____________

Speciality: ______________________

Signature: ____________ Date: ____________

CLINICIAN (if not the reporter)

Name and Professional Address: ______________________

Post code: ____________

Tel No: ____________ Speciality: ____________

If you would like information about other adverse reactions associated with the suspected drug, please tick this box ☐

Send to **MHRA (medicines)**, **CSM FREEPOST, London, SW8 5BR** or if you are in one of the following NHS regions:

to **CSM Mersey, FREEPOST, Liverpool, L3 3AB**

or **CSM Northern and Yorkshire, FREEPOST, Newcastle upon Tyne, NE1 1BR**

CSM Scotland, 51 Little France Crescent, Old Dalkeith Road, Edinburgh, EH16 4SA

or **CSM Wales, FREEPOST, Cardiff, CF4 1ZZ**

or **CSM West Midlands, FREEPOST, Birmingham, B18 7BR**

OTHER DRUGS (including self-medication & herbal remedies)

Did the patient take any other drugs in the last 3 months prior to the reaction? Yes / No

If *yes*, please give the following information if known:

Drug (Brand, if known)	Route	Dosage	Date started	Date stopped	Prescribed for

Additional relevant information e.g. medical history, test results, known allergies, rechallenge (if performed), suspected drug interactions. For congenital abnormalities please state all other drugs taken during pregnancy and the date of the last menstrual period.

REPORTER DETAILS

Name and Professional Address: ______________________

Post code: ____________ Tel No: ____________

Speciality: ______________________

Signature: ____________ Date: ____________

CLINICIAN (if not the reporter)

Name and Professional Address: ______________________

Post code: ____________

Tel No: ____________ Speciality: ____________

If you would like information about other adverse reactions associated with the suspected drug, please tick this box ☐

Send to **MHRA (medicines)**, **CSM FREEPOST, London, SW8 5BR** or if you are in one of the following NHS regions:

to **CSM Mersey, FREEPOST, Liverpool, L3 3AB**

or **CSM Northern and Yorkshire, FREEPOST, Newcastle upon Tyne, NE1 1BR**

CSM Scotland, 51 Little France Crescent, Old Dalkeith Road, Edinburgh, EH16 4SA

or **CSM Wales, FREEPOST, Cardiff, CF4 1ZZ**

or **CSM West Midlands, FREEPOST, Birmingham, B18 7BR**

In Confidence

COMMITTEE ON SAFETY OF MEDICINES

MHRA
Medicines and Healthcare products Regulatory Agency
Safeguarding public health

SUSPECTED ADVERSE DRUG REACTIONS

If you are suspicious that an adverse reaction may be related to a drug or combination of drugs please complete this Yellow Card.

For reporting advice please see over. Do not be put off reporting because some details are not known.

PATIENT DETAILS Patient Initials: ________ Sex: M / F Weight if known (kg): ________

Age (at time of reaction): ________ Identification (Your Practice / Hospital Ref.)*: ________

SUSPECTED DRUG(S)

Give brand name of drug and batch number if known	Route	Dosage	Date started	Date stopped	Prescribed for

SUSPECTED REACTION(S)

Please describe the reaction(s) and any treatment given:

Outcome

Recovered ☐
Recovering ☐
Continuing ☐
Other ☐

Date reaction(s) started: ________ Date reaction (s) stopped: ________

Do you consider the reaction to be serious? Yes / No

If *yes*, please indicate why the reaction is considered to be serious (please tick all that apply):

Patient died due to reaction ☐
Life threatening ☐
Congenital abnormality ☐
Involved or prolonged inpatient hospitalisation ☐
Involved persistent or significant disability or incapacity ☐
Medically significant; please give details: ________

* This is to enable you to identify the patient in any future correspondence concerning this report

Please attach additional pages if necessary

In Confidence

COMMITTEE ON SAFETY OF MEDICINES

MHRA
Medicines and Healthcare products Regulatory Agency
Safeguarding public health

SUSPECTED ADVERSE DRUG REACTIONS

If you are suspicious that an adverse reaction may be related to a drug or combination of drugs please complete this Yellow Card.

For reporting advice please see over. Do not be put off reporting because some details are not known.

PATIENT DETAILS Patient Initials: ________ Sex: M / F Weight if known (kg): ________

Age (at time of reaction): ________ Identification (Your Practice / Hospital Ref.)*: ________

SUSPECTED DRUG(S)

Give brand name of drug and batch number if known | Route | Dosage | Date started | Date stopped | Prescribed for

SUSPECTED REACTION(S)

Please describe the reaction(s) and any treatment given:

Outcome

Recovered ☐
Recovering ☐
Continuing ☐
Other ☐

Date reaction(s) started: ________ Date reaction (s) stopped: ________

Do you consider the reaction to be serious? Yes / No

If yes, please indicate why the reaction is considered to be serious (please tick all that apply):

Patient died due to reaction ☐
Life threatening ☐
Congenital abnormality ☐
Involved or prolonged inpatient hospitalisation ☐
Involved persistent or significant disability or incapacity ☐
Medically significant; please give details: ________

* This is to enable you to identify the patient in any future correspondence concerning this report

Please attach additional pages if necessary

OTHER DRUGS (including self-medication & herbal remedies)

Did the patient take any other drugs in the last 3 months prior to the reaction? Yes / No

If *yes*, please give the following information if known:

Drug (Brand, if known)	Route	Dosage	Date started	Date stopped	Prescribed for

Additional relevant information e.g. medical history, test results, known allergies, rechallenge (if performed), suspected drug interactions. For congenital abnormalities please state all other drugs taken during pregnancy and the date of the last menstrual period.

REPORTER DETAILS

Name and Professional Address:

Post code: Tel No:

Speciality:

Signature: Date:

CLINICIAN (if not the reporter)

Name and Professional Address:

Post code:

Tel No: Speciality:

If you would like information about other adverse reactions associated with the suspected drug, please tick this box ☐

Send to **MHRA (medicines), CSM FREEPOST, London, SW8 5BR** or if you are in one of the following NHS regions:

to **CSM Mersey, FREEPOST, Liverpool, L3 3AB**

or **CSM Northern and Yorkshire, FREEPOST, Newcastle upon Tyne, NE1 1BR**

CSM Scotland, 51 Little France Crescent, Old Dalkeith Road, Edinburgh, EH16 4SA

or **CSM Wales, FREEPOST, Cardiff, CF4 1ZZ**

or **CSM West Midlands, FREEPOST, Birmingham, B18 7BR**

OTHER DRUGS (including self-medication & herbal remedies)

Did the patient take any other drugs in the last 3 months prior to the reaction? Yes / No

If *yes*, please give the following information if known:

Drug (Brand, if known)	Route	Dosage	Date started	Date stopped	Prescribed for

Additional relevant information e.g. medical history, test results, known allergies, rechallenge (if performed), suspected drug interactions. For congenital abnormalities please state all other drugs taken during pregnancy and the date of the last menstrual period.

REPORTER DETAILS

Name and Professional Address:

Post code: Tel No:

Speciality:

Signature: Date:

CLINICIAN (if not the reporter)

Name and Professional Address:

Post code:

Tel No: Speciality:

If you would like information about other adverse reactions associated with the suspected drug, please tick this box ☐

Send to **MHRA (medicines), CSM FREEPOST, London, SW8 5BR** or if you are in one of the following NHS regions:

to **CSM Mersey, FREEPOST, Liverpool, L3 3AB**

or **CSM Northern and Yorkshire, FREEPOST, Newcastle upon Tyne, NE1 1BR**

CSM Scotland, 51 Little France Crescent, Old Dalkeith Road, Edinburgh, EH16 4SA

or **CSM Wales, FREEPOST, Cardiff, CF4 1ZZ**

or **CSM West Midlands, FREEPOST, Birmingham, B18 7BR**

In Confidence

COMMITTEE ON SAFETY OF MEDICINES

MHRA
Medicines and Healthcare products Regulatory Agency
Safeguarding public health

SUSPECTED ADVERSE DRUG REACTIONS

If you are suspicious that an adverse reaction may be related to a drug or combination of drugs please complete this Yellow Card.

For reporting advice please see over. Do not be put off reporting because some details are not known.

PATIENT DETAILS Patient Initials: ____________ Sex: M / F Weight if known (kg): ____________

Age (at time of reaction): ____________ Identification (Your Practice / Hospital Ref.)*: ____________

SUSPECTED DRUG(S)

Give brand name of drug and batch number if known	Route	Dosage	Date started	Date stopped	Prescribed for

SUSPECTED REACTION(S)

Please describe the reaction(s) and any treatment given:

Outcome

Recovered ☐
Recovering ☐
Continuing ☐
Other ☐

Date reaction(s) started: ____________ Date reaction (s) stopped: ____________

Do you consider the reaction to be serious? Yes / No

If *yes*, please indicate why the reaction is considered to be serious (please tick all that apply):

Patient died due to reaction ☐ Involved or prolonged inpatient hospitalisation ☐

Life threatening ☐ Involved persistent or significant disability or incapacity ☐

Congenital abnormality ☐ Medically significant; please give details: ____________

* This is to enable you to identify the patient in any future correspondence concerning this report

Please attach additional pages if necessary

In Confidence

COMMITTEE ON SAFETY OF MEDICINES

MHRA
Medicines and Healthcare products Regulatory Agency
Safeguarding public health

SUSPECTED ADVERSE DRUG REACTIONS

If you are suspicious that an adverse reaction may be related to a drug or combination of drugs please complete this Yellow Card.

For reporting advice please see over. Do not be put off reporting because some details are not known.

PATIENT DETAILS Patient Initials: ____________ Sex: M / F Weight if known (kg): ____________

Age (at time of reaction): ____________ Identification (Your Practice / Hospital Ref.)*: ____________

SUSPECTED DRUG(S)

Give brand name of drug and batch number if known	Route	Dosage	Date started	Date stopped	Prescribed for

SUSPECTED REACTION(S)

Please describe the reaction(s) and any treatment given:

Outcome

Recovered ☐
Recovering ☐
Continuing ☐
Other ☐

Date reaction(s) started: ____________ Date reaction (s) stopped: ____________

Do you consider the reaction to be serious? Yes / No

If *yes*, please indicate why the reaction is considered to be serious (please tick all that apply):

Patient died due to reaction ☐ Involved or prolonged inpatient hospitalisation ☐

Life threatening ☐ Involved persistent or significant disability or incapacity ☐

Congenital abnormality ☐ Medically significant; please give details: ____________

* This is to enable you to identify the patient in any future correspondence concerning this report

Please attach additional pages if necessary

OTHER DRUGS (including self-medication & herbal remedies)

Did the patient take any other drugs in the last 3 months prior to the reaction? Yes / No

If *yes*, please give the following information if known:

Drug (Brand, if known)	Route	Dosage	Date started	Date stopped	Prescribed for

Additional relevant information e.g. medical history, test results, known allergies, rechallenge (if performed), suspected drug interactions. For congenital abnormalities please state all other drugs taken during pregnancy and the date of the last menstrual period.

REPORTER DETAILS

Name and Professional Address: ______

Post code: ______ Tel No: ______

Speciality: ______

Signature: ______ Date: ______

CLINICIAN (if not the reporter)

Name and Professional Address: ______

Post code: ______

Tel No: ______ Speciality: ______

If you would like information about other adverse reactions associated with the suspected drug, please tick this box ☐

Send to **MHRA (medicines) , CSM FREEPOST, London, SW8 5BR** or if you are in one of the following NHS regions:

to **CSM Mersey, FREEPOST, Liverpool, L3 3AB**

or **CSM Northern and Yorkshire, FREEPOST, Newcastle upon Tyne, NE1 1BR**

CSM Scotland, 51 Little France Crescent, Old Dalkeith Road, Edinburgh, EH16 4SA

or **CSM Wales, FREEPOST, Cardiff, CF4 1ZZ**

or **CSM West Midlands, FREEPOST, Birmingham, B18 7BR**

OTHER DRUGS (including self-medication & herbal remedies)

Did the patient take any other drugs in the last 3 months prior to the reaction? Yes / No

If *yes*, please give the following information if known:

Drug (Brand, if known)	Route	Dosage	Date started	Date stopped	Prescribed for

Additional relevant information e.g. medical history, test results, known allergies, rechallenge (if performed), suspected drug interactions. For congenital abnormalities please state all other drugs taken during pregnancy and the date of the last menstrual period.

REPORTER DETAILS

Name and Professional Address: ______

Post code: ______ Tel No: ______

Speciality: ______

Signature: ______ Date: ______

CLINICIAN (if not the reporter)

Name and Professional Address: ______

Post code: ______

Tel No: ______ Speciality: ______

If you would like information about other adverse reactions associated with the suspected drug, please tick this box ☐

Send to **MHRA (medicines) , CSM FREEPOST, London, SW8 5BR** or if you are in one of the following NHS regions:

to **CSM Mersey, FREEPOST, Liverpool, L3 3AB**

or **CSM Northern and Yorkshire, FREEPOST, Newcastle upon Tyne, NE1 1BR**

CSM Scotland, 51 Little France Crescent, Old Dalkeith Road, Edinburgh, EH16 4SA

or **CSM Wales, FREEPOST, Cardiff, CF4 1ZZ**

or **CSM West Midlands, FREEPOST, Birmingham, B18 7BR**